Laboratory	Conventional Units	Conversion Factor	SI Units
CD8 lymphocyte count	18–39% of total lymphocytes		
Cerebrospinal fluid (CSF)			
Pressure	75–175 mm H_2O		
Glucose	40–70 mg/dL	0.0555	2.2–3.9 mmol/L
Protein	15–45 mg/dL	0.01	0.15–0.45 g/L
WBC	Less than 10/mm^3		
Ceruloplasmin	18–45 mg/dL	10	180–450 mg/L
		0.063	1.1–2.8 μmol/L
Chloride	97–110 mEq/L	1	97–110 mmol/L
Cholesterol			
Desirable	Less than 200 mg/dL	0.0259	Less than 5.18 mmol/L
Borderline high	200–239 mg/dL	0.0259	5.18–6.19 mmol/L
High	Greater than or equal to 240 mg/dL	0.0259	Greater than or equal to 6.2 mmol/L
Chorionic gonadotropin (β-hCG)	Less than 5 milliunits/mL	1	Less than 5 units/L
Clozapine	Minimum trough 300–350 ng/mL or mcg/L	3.06	918–1071 nmol/L
CO_2 content	22–30 mEq/L	1	22–30 mmol/L
Complement component 3 (C3)	70–160 mg/dL	0.01	0.7–1.6 g/L
Complement component 4 (C4)	20–40 mg/dL	0.01	0.2–0.4 g/L
Copper	70–150 mcg/dL	0.157	11–24 μmol/L
Cortisol (fasting, morning)	5–25 mcg/dL	27.6	138–690 nmol/L
Cortisol (free, urinary)	10–100 mcg/day	2.76	28–276 nmol/day
Creatine kinase			
Male	30–200 IU/L	0.01667	0.50–3.33 μkat/L
Female	20–170 IU/L	0.01667	0.33–2.83 μkat/L
MB fraction	0–7 IU/L	0.01667	0.0–0.12 μkat/L
Creatinine clearance (CrCl) (urine)	85–135 mL/minute/1.73 m^2	0.00963	0.82–1.3 mL/s/m^2
Creatinine			
Male 4–20 years	0.2–1.0 mg/dL	88.4	18–88 μmol/L
Female 4–20 years	0.2–1.0 mg/dL	88.4	18–88 μmol/L
Male (adults)	0.7–1.3 mg/dL	88.4	62–115 μmol/L
Female (adults)	0.6–1.1 mg/dL	88.4	53–97 μmol/L
Cyclosporin			
Renal transplant	100–300 ng/mL or mcg/L	0.832	83–250 nmol/L
Cardiac, liver, or pancreatic transplant	200–350 ng/mL or mcg/L	0.832	166–291 nmol/L
Cryptococcal antigen	Negative		
D-dimers	Less than 250 ng/mL	1	Less than 250 mcg/L
Desipramine	75–300 ng/mL or mcg/L	3.75	281–1125 mmol/L
Dexamethasone suppression test (DST) (overnight)	8:00 am cortisol less than 5 mcg/dL	0.0276	Less than 0.14 μmol/L
DHEAS			
Male	170–670 mcg/dL	0.0271	4.6–18.2 μmol/L
Female			
Premenopausal	50–540 mcg/dL	0.0271	1.4–14.7 μmol/L
Postmenopausal	30–260 mcg/dL	0.0271	0.8–7.1 μmol/L
Digoxin, therapeutic	0.5–1.0 ng/mL or mcg/L	1.28	0.6–1.3 nmol/L
Erythrocyte count (blood) See under Red blood cell count			
Erythrocyte sedimentation rate (ESR)			
Westergren			
Male	0–20 mm/hour		
Female	0–30 mm/hour		
Wintrobe			
Male	0–9 mm/hour		
Female	0–15 mm/hour		
Erythropoietin	2–25 mIU/mL	1	2–25 IU/L
Estradiol			
Male	10–36 pg/mL	3.67	37–132 pmol/L
Female	34–170 pg/mL	3.67	125–624 pmol/L
Ethanol, legal intoxication	Greater than or equal to 50–100 mg/dL	0.217	10.9–21.7 mmol/L
	Greater than or equal to 0.05–0.1%	217	
Ethosuccimide, therapeutic	40–100 mg/L or mcg/mL	7.08	283–708 μmol/L
Factor VIII or factor IX			
Severe hemophilia	Less than 1 IU/dL	0.01	Less than 0.01 units/mL
Moderate hemophilia	1–5 IU/dL	0.01	0.01–0.05 units/mL
Mild hemophilia	Greater than 5 IU/dL	0.01	Greater than 0.05 units/mL
Usual adult levels	60–140 IU/dL	0.01	0.60–1.40 units/mL
Ferritin			
Male	20–250 ng/mL	1	20–250 mcg/L
Female	10–150 ng/mL	1	10–150 mcg/L
Fibrin degradation products (FDP)	2–10 mg/L		
Fibrinogen	200–400 mg/dL	0.01	2.0–4.0 g/L
Folate (plasma)	3.1–12.4 ng/mL	2.266	7.0–28.1 nmol/L
Folic acid (RBC)	125–600 ng/mL	2.266	283–1360 nmol/L
Follicle-stimulating hormone (FSH)			
Male	1–7 mIU/mL	1	1–7 IU/L
Female			
Follicular phase	1–9 mIU/mL	1	1–9 IU/L
Midcycle	6–26 mIU/mL	1	6–26 IU/L
Luteal phase	1–9 mIU/mL	1	1–9 IU/L
Postmenopausal	30–118 mIU/mL	1	30–118 IU/L
Free thyroxine index (FT_4I)	6.5–12.5		
Gamma glutamyl transferase (GGT)	0–30 IU/L	0.01667	0–0.5 μkat/L
Gastrin (fasting)	0–130 pg/mL	1	0–130 ng/L
Gentamicin, therapeutic	4–10 mg/L peak	2.09	8.4–21 μmol/L peak
	Less than or equal to 2 mg/L trough		Less than or equal to 4.2 μmol/L trough
Globulin	2.3–3.5 g/dL	10	23–35 g/L
Glucose (fasting, plasma)	65–109 mg/dL	0.0555	3.6–6.00 mmol/L
Glucose, two hour postprandial blood (PPBG)	Less than 140 mg/dL	0.0555	Less than 7.8 mmol/L
Granulocyte count	1.8–6.6 × 10^3/μL	10^6	1.8–6.6 × 10^9/L
Growth hormone (fasting)			
Male	Less than 5 ng/mL	1	Less than 5 mcg/L
Female	Less than 10 ng/mL	1	Less than 10 mcg/L

(continued on back inside cover)

Pharmacotherapy

A Pathophysiologic Approach

Seventh Edition

NOTICE

Pharmacotherapy

A Pathophysiologic Approach

Seventh Edition

Joseph T. DiPiro, PharmD, FCCP
Executive Dean and Professor, South Carolina
College of Pharmacy, University of South Carolina, Columbia, South Carolina
and Medical University of South Carolina, Charleston, South Carolina

Robert L. Talbert, PharmD, FCCP, BCPS, CLS
SmithKline Professor, College of Pharmacy, University of Texas at Austin,
Professor, Department of Medicine, University of Texas Health
Science Center at San Antonio, San Antonio, Texas

Gary C. Yee, PharmD, FCCP, BCOP
Professor, Department of Pharmacy Practice,
College of Pharmacy, University of Nebraska Medical Center,
Omaha, Nebraska

Gary R. Matzke, PharmD, FCP, FCCP
Professor of Pharmacy and Pharmaceutics and Associate
Dean for Clinical Research and Public Policy, School of Pharmacy,
Professor of Internal Medicine, Nephrology Division, School of Medicine,
Virginia Commonwealth University, Richmond, Virginia

Barbara G. Wells, PharmD, FASHP, FCCP, BCPP
Dean and Professor, Executive Director of the Research Institute
of Pharmaceutical Sciences, School of Pharmacy,
The University of Mississippi, Oxford, Mississippi

L. Michael Posey, BSPharm
Editorial Director, Periodicals Department, American Pharmacists Association,
Washington, D.C.

McGraw Hill Medical

New York Chicago San Francisco Lisbon London Madrid Mexico City
Milan New Delhi San Juan Seoul Singapore Sydney Toronto

The McGraw·Hill Companies

Pharmacotherapy: A Pathophysiologic Approach, Seventh Edition

1 2 3 4 5 6 7 8 9 0 CTP/CTP 0 9 8

ISBN 978-0-07-147899-1
MHID 0-07-147899-X

Please tell the authors and publisher what you think of this book by sending your comments to *pharmacotherapy@mcgraw-hill.com*. Please put the author and title of the book in subject line.

This book was set in Minion by Silverchair Science + Communications.
The editors were Michael Weitz and Kim J. Davis.
The production supervisor was Catherine H. Saggese.
Project management was provided by Sylvia Rebert of Progressive Publishing Alternatives.
The text designer was Alan Barnett.
The cover designer was Aimee Davis.
Kay Cole prepared the index.
China Translation and Printing Services was printer and binder.

This book is printed on acid-free paper.

Library of Congress Cataloging-in-Publication Data
Pharmacotherapy : a pathophysiologic approach / editors, Joseph T. DiPiro ... [et al.]. -- 7th ed.
p. ; cm.
Includes bibliographical references and index.
ISBN 978-0-07-147899-1 (hardcover : alk. paper) 1. Chemotherapy. 2. Physiology, Pathological. I. DiPiro, Joseph T.
[DNLM: 1. Drug Therapy. WB 330 P5357 2008]
RM263.P56 2008
615.5'8--dc22

2007039929

Illustration of the death of a tumor after effective anti-angiogenic therapy, static "time lapse" rendering. The treatment causes new tumor vasculature (angiogenesis) to collapse and retreat. The tumor is shown changing from robust (upper left corner) to anoxic and dying (lower right corner). Tumor necrosis occurs from the inside out.

DEDICATION

To our patients, who have challenged and inspired us
and given meaning to all our endeavors.

To practitioners, who continue to improve patient health outcomes
and thereby serve as role models for their colleagues and students
while clinging tenaciously to the highest standards of practice.

To our mentors, whose vision provided educational and training
programs that encouraged our professional growth and challenged us
to be innovators in our patient care, research, and education.

To our faculty colleagues for their efforts and support for our mission
to provide a comprehensive and challenging educational
foundation for the pharmacists of the future.

And finally to our families for the time that they have sacrificed
so that this seventh edition would become a reality.

IN MEMORIAM

Mario M. Zeolla (1974–2007) earned his Bachelor of Science and Doctor of Pharmacy degrees from the Albany College of Pharmacy, completed a Community Pharmacy Residency at the University of Maryland School of Pharmacy, and was a Board Certified Pharmacotherapy Specialist. In his brief but productive career as a pharmacy practitioner and educator at the Albany College of Pharmacy, Dr. Zeolla quickly rose to the rank of Associate Professor in the Department of Pharmacy Practice. In addition, he was the Patient Care Pharmacist at Eckerd (and later Brooks) Pharmacy in Loudonville, New York, where he developed innovative community-based clinical pharmacy services. He was an author in previous editions of *Pharmacotherapy: A Pathophysiologic Approach* and published several scholarly papers related to community pharmacy practice and dietary supplements/herbal therapies. Dr. Zeolla was considered one of the brightest stars on the Albany College of Pharmacy faculty and a passionate advocate for pharmacy. He was a popular teacher, trusted advisor, and beloved peer.

CONTENTS

🖱 The complete chapter, learning objectives, and other resources can be found at **www.pharmacotherapyonline.com**.

ⓦ The complete chapter, learning objectives, and other resources can be found at **www.pharmacotherapyonline.com**.

SECTION 6
Neurologic Disorders
Section Editor: Barbara G. Wells

SECTION 7
Psychiatric Disorders
Section Editor: Barbara G. Wells

SECTION 8
Endocrinologic Disorders
Section Editor: Robert L. Talbert

The complete chapter, learning objectives, and other resources can be found at **www.pharmacotherapyonline.com**.

SECTION 9

Gynecologic Disorders

Section Editor: Barbara G. Wells

SECTION 10

Urologic Disorders

Section Editor: L. Michael Posey

SECTION 11

Immunologic Disorders

Section Editor: Gary C. Yee

SECTION 12

Rheumatologic Disorders

Section Editor: L. Michael Posey

SECTION 13

Ophthalmic and Otolaryngologic Disorders

Section Editor: L. Michael Posey

SECTION 14

Dermatologic Disorders

Section Editor: L. Michael Posey

SECTION 15

Hematologic Disorders

Section Editor: Gary C. Yee

SECTION 18

Nutrition Disorders

Section Editor: Gary R. Matzke

The complete chapter, learning objectives, and other resources can be found at **www.pharmacotherapyonline.com**.

CONTRIBUTORS

Val R. Adams, PharmD, FCCP, BCOP
Associate Professor, University of Kentucky, College of Pharmacy, Lexington, Kentucky
Chapter 135

Jeffrey R. Aeschlimann, PharmD
University of Connecticut, School of Pharmacy, Storrs, Connecticut
Chapter 108

Rondall E. Allen, PharmD
Clinical Assistant Professor and Assistant Dean for Program Assessment, Xavier University of Louisiana College of Pharmacy, New Orleans, Louisana
Chapter 40

J. V. Anandan, PharmD
Adjunct Associate Professor, Eugene Applebaum College of Pharmacy and Health Sciences, Wayne State University; Pharmacy Specialist, Center for Drug Use Analysis and Information, Department of Pharmacy Services, Henry Ford Hospital, Detroit, Michigan
Chapter 119

Peter L. Anderson, PharmD
Assistant Professor, School of Pharmacy, University of Colorado, Denver, Colorado
Chapter 129

Shawn Anderson, PharmD
Postdoctoral Fellow, Colleges of Pharmacy and Medicine, Departments of Pharmacy Practice and Family Medicine, University of Florida, Gainesville, Florida
Chapter 79

Tami R. Argo, PharmD, MS, BCPP
Clinical Assistant Professor, Department of Pharmacy Practice, College of Pharmacy, University of Texas at Austin, Austin, Texas
Chapter 70

Edward P. Armstrong, PharmD
Professor, Department of Pharmacy Practice and Science, College of Pharmacy, University of Arizona, Tucson, Arizona
Chapter 122

Jacquelyn L. Bainbridge, PharmD
Associate Professor, Department of Clinical Pharmacy and Department of Neurology, University of Colorado at Denver and The Health Sciences Center, Denver, Colorado
Chapter 57

Jeffrey F. Barletta, PharmD, FCCM
Clinical Specialist-Critical Care, Department of Pharmacy, Spectrum Health, Adjunct Assistant Professor, College of Pharmacy, Ferris State University, Grand Rapids, Michigan
Chapter 14

Kimberly A. Bauer, MD
Clinical Research Fellow, Department of Dermatology, Feinberg School of Medicine, Northwestern University, Chicago, Illinois
Chapters 100 and 101

Larry A. Bauer, PharmD, FCP, FCCP
Professor, Departments of Pharmacy and Laboratory Medicine, University of Washington, Seattle, Washington
Chapter 5

Jerry L. Bauman, PharmD, FACC, FCCP
Professor and Dean, College of Pharmacy; Professor, Department of Medicine, College of Medicine, University of Illinois, Chicago, Illinois
Chapter 19

Terry J. Baumann, PharmD, BCPS
Clinical Manager, Munson Medical Center, Traverse City, Michigan; Adjunct Assistant Professor of Pharmacy, Ferris State University, College of Pharmacy, Big Rapids, Michigan
Chapter 62

Rosemary R. Berardi, PharmD, FCCP, FASHP, FAPhA
Professor of Pharmacy, College of Pharmacy, University of Michigan; Clinical Pharmacist, Gastrointestinal/Liver Diseases, Department of Pharmacy, University of Michigan Health System, Ann Arbor, Michigan
Chapters 35 and 41

Charles J. Billington, MD
Professor, Department of Medicine, University of Minnesota, Minneapolis VA Medical Center, Minneapolis, Minnesota
Chapter 148

Lisa A. Boothby, PharmD, BCPS
Coordinator, Drug Information Services, Columbus Regional Healthcare System; Affiliate Clinical Associate Professor, Auburn University Harrison School of Pharmacy, Columbus, Georgia
Chapters 68 and 69

Bradley A. Boucher, PharmD, FCCP, FCCM
Professor, Department of Clinical Pharmacy, College of Pharmacy, University of Tennessee, Memphis, Tennessee
Chapter 60

Sharya V. Bourdet, PharmD, BCPS

Critical Care Pharmacist, Veterans Affairs Medical Center, San Francisco, Health Sciences Assistant Clinical Professor, School of Pharmacy, University of California, San Francisco, San Francisco, California

Chapter 29

Denise Boudreau, RPh, PhD

Scientific Investigator, Group Health Center for Health Studies, Seattle, Washington

Chapter 9

Rebecca Boudreaux, PharmD

Clinical Instructor, College of Pharmacy, University of Texas at Austin; Department of Medicine, University of Texas Health Science Center at San Antonio, San Antonio, Texas

Chapter 30

Nancy Brahm, PharmD, MS, BCPP

Clinical Associate Professor, Department of Pharmacy, Clinical and Administrative Sciences, University of Oklahoma College of Pharmacy, Tulsa, Oklahoma

Chapter 76

Donald F. Brophy, PharmD, MSc, FCCP, BCPS

Associate Professor of Pharmacy and Internal Medicine, Virginia Commonwealth University Medical College of Virginia Campus, School of Pharmacy, Richmond, Virginia

Chapter 54

Jason E. Brouillard, PharmD

Adjunct Clinical Instructor, Department of Pharmacotherapy, College of Pharmacy, Washington State University; Critical Care Pharmacist, Department of Pharmacy, Sacred Heart Medical Center, Spokane, Washington

Chapter 11

Robert C. Brown, MD

Adjunct Clinical Associate Professor, University of Oklahoma College of Pharmacy, Department of Pharmacy, Clinical and Administrative Sciences, Oklahoma City, Oklahoma

Chapter 76

Thomas E. R. Brown, PharmD

Associate Professor, Leslie Dan Faculty of Pharmacy, University of Toronto, and Clinical Coordinator, Women's Health Sunnybrook Health Sciences Centre, Toronto, Ontario

Chapter 124

Edward M. Buchanan, MD

Department of Family Medicine, Thomas Jefferson University, Philadelphia, Pennsylvania

Chapter 83

Peter F. Buckley, MD

Professor and Chairman, Department of Psychiatry, Associate Dean of Leadership Development, Medical College of Georgia, Augusta, Georgia

Chapter 70

David S. Burgess, PharmD, FCCP

Clinical Professor of Pharmacy and Medicine, Center for Advancement of Research and Education in Infectious Diseases, University of Texas at Austin College of Pharmacy and Pharmacotherapy Education and Research Center, University of Texas Health Science Center, San Antonio, Texas

Chapter 109

Julianna A. Burzynski, PharmD, BCPS, BCOP

Pharmacy Specialist-Hematology/Oncology, Mayo Clinic, Rochester, Minnesota

Chapter 140

Lucinda M. Buys, PharmD

Associate Professor , Clinical and Administrative Pharmacy Division, University of Iowa, College of Pharmacy and the Siouxland Medical Education Foundation, Sioux City, Iowa

Chapter 95

Karim Anton Calis, PharmD, MPH, FASHP, FCCP

Director, Drug Information Service and Clinical Specialist, Endocrinology and Women's Health, Mark O. Hatfield Clinical Research Center, National Institutes of Health, Bethesda, Maryland; Professor of Pharmacy, School of Pharmacy, Virginia Commonwealth University, Richmond, Virginia; Clinical Professor, Department of Pharmacy Practice and Science, School of Pharmacy, University of Maryland, Baltimore, Maryland; Clinical Professor, Department of Pharmacy Practice, School of Pharmacy, Shenandoah University, Winchester, Virginia

Chapters 80 and 85

Kimberly A. Cappuzzo, PharmD, MS, CGP

Assistant Professor of Pharmacy, School of Pharmacy, Virginia Commonwealth University; Clinical Pharmacist/Geriatric Pharmacotherapy Specialist, Virginia Commonwealth University Medical Center, Richmond, Virginia

Chapter 90

Peggy L. Carver, PharmD, FCCP

Associate Professor of Pharmacy, College of Pharmacy, and Clinical Pharmacist, University of Michigan Health System, Ann Arbor, Michigan

Chapter 125

Larisa H. Cavallari, PharmD, BCPS

Assistant Professor, Department of Pharmacy Practice, University of Illinois College of Pharmacy, Chicago, Illinois

Chapters 6 and 16

Jose E. Cavazos, MD, PhD

Director of Research and Education, South Texas Comprehensive Epilepsy Center, University of Texas Health Science Center, San Antonio, Texas

Chapter 58

C. Y. Jennifer Chan, PharmD

Clinical Assistant Professor of Pharmacy, University of Texas in Austin, College of Pharmacy, Clinical Associate Professor of Pediatrics, University of Texas Health Science Center in San Antonio; Clinical Manager, Pediatric Pharmacy Services, Methodist Children's Hospital, San Antonio, Texas

Chapter 106

Nina H. Cheigh, PharmD

Clinical Associate Professor, University of Illinois College of Pharmacy, Rye, New York

Chapters 99 and 102

Jack J. Chen, PharmD, BCPS, CGP

Loma Linda University, School of Medicine, Department of Neurology and School of Pharmacy, Department of Pharmacotherapy, Outcomes and Research, Loma Linda, California

Chapter 61

Katherine Hammond Chessman, PharmD, FCCP, BCPS, BCNSP

Associate Professor, Department of Pharmacy and Clinical Sciences, South Carolina College of Pharmacy, MUSC Campus; Clinical Pharmacy Specialist, Pediatrics/Pediatric Surgery, Department of Pharmacy Services, Medical University of South Carolina Children's Hospital, Charleston, South Carolina

Chapters 143 and 146

Robert Chilton, DO, FACC, FAHA

Professor, Department of Medicine, University of Texas Health Science Center, San Antonio, Texas

Chapter 13

Thomas W. F. Chin, PharmD, BSc, FCSHP

Clinical Pharmacy Specialist/Leader-Antimicrobials and Infectious Diseases, St. Michael's Hospital; Assistant Professor, Leslie Dan Faculty of Pharmacy, University of Toronto, Toronto, Ontario, Canada

Chapter 124

Elaine Chiquette, PharmD, BCPS

Senior Medical Science Division, Medical Affairs, Amylin Pharmaceuticals, Inc., San Antonio, Texas

Chapter 3

Marie A. Chisholm-Burns, PharmD, MPH, FCCP, FASHP

Professor and Head, Department of Pharmacy Practice and Science, University of Arizona College of Pharmacy, Tuscon, Arizona

Chapter 33

Peter A. Chyka, PharmD, FAACT, DABAT

Professor, Department of Clinical Pharmacy and Associate Dean, Knoxville Campus, College of Pharmacy, University of Tennessee, Knoxville, Tennessee

Chapter 10

Elizabeth C. Clark, MD, MPH

University of Medicine and Denistry of New Jersey, Robert Wood Johnson Medical School, Department of Family Medicine, Somerset, New Jersey

Chapter 96

Stephen Joel Coons, PhD

Professor, Department of Pharmacy Practice and Service, College of Pharmacy, University of Arizona, Tuscon, Arizona

Chapter 2

John R. Corboy, MD

Professor, Department of Neurology, University of Colorado School of Medicine; Denver Veteran's Affairs Medical Center, Denver, Colorado

Chapter 57

Lindsay J. Corporon, PharmD, BCDP

Assistant Professor of Pharmacy and Therapeutics, University of Pittsburgh, School of Pharmacy; Clinical Specialist in Oncology, Magee Women's Hospital, Pittsburgh, Pennsylvania

Chapter 141

Lisa T. Costanigro, Pharm D

Infectious Diseases Pharmacy Resident; Deaconess Medical Center, Washington State University College of Pharmacy, Spokane, Washington

Chapter 11

Elizabeth A. Coyle, PharmD, BCPS

Clinical Associate Professor, University of Houston College of Pharmacy, Houston, Texas

Chapter 120

James D. Coyle, PharmD

Assistant Professor of Clinical Pharmacy, College of Pharmacy, Ohio State University, Columbus, Ohio

Chapter 52

Michael Craig, MD

Assistant Professor, Department of Medicine, Section of Hematology/Oncology, West Virginia University, Morgantown, West Virginia

Chapter 103

Catherine M. Crill, PharmD, BCPS, BCNSP

Associate Professor, Department of Clinical Pharmacy; Assistant Professor, Department of Pediatrics, University of Tennessee Health Science Center, Memphis, Tennessee

Chapter 144

M. Lynn Crismon, PharmD, FCCP, BCPP

Dean, James T. Doluisio Chair and Behrens Professor, College of Pharmacy, University of Texas at Austin, Austin, Texas

Chapter 70

Michael A. Crouch, PharmD, BCPS

Professor and Chair, Department of Pharmacy Practice, South University, Savannah, Georgia

Chapter 115

William E. Dager, PharmD, FCSHP

Pharmacist Specialist, UC Davis Medical Center, Clinical Professor of Medicine, UC Davis School of Medicine, Sacramento, California; Clinical Professor of Pharmacy, UC San Francisco School of Pharmacy, San Francisco, California

Chapter 45

Joseph F. Dasta, MSc, FCCM, FCCP

Professor Emeritus, Ohio State University, College of Pharmacy, Columbus, Ohio; Adjunct Professor, University of Texas, Austin, Texas

Chapter 25

Lisa E. Davis, PharmD, FCCP, BCPS, BCOP

Associate Professor and Vice Chair of Research, Philadelphia College of Pharmacy, University of the Sciences in Philadelphia, Philadelphia, Pennsylvania

Chapter 133

Susan R. Davis, MD, PhD, FRAPC

Chair of Women's Health, Department of Medicine, Monash University, Clayton, Victoria, Australia

Chapter 85

Larry H. Danziger, PharmD

Professor of Pharmacy, Department of Pharmacy Practice, Interim Vice Chancellor for Research, University of Illinois, Chicago, Illinois

Chapter 114

Simon de Denus, MSc, BPharm
Assistant Professor, Faculty of Pharmacy, University of Montreal, Montreal Heart Institute, Montreal, Quebec, Canada
Chapter 18

Jeffrey C. Delafuente, MS, FCCP, FASCP
Associate Dean for Professional Education; Professor of Pharmacy and Director of Geriatric Programs, School of Pharmacy, Virginia Commonwealth University, Richmond, Virginia
Chapter 90

Mark DeLegge, MD
Professor and Director, Digestive Disease Center, School of Medicine, Medical University of South Carolina, Charleston, South Carolina
Chapter 147

Paulina Deming, PharmD
Assistant Professor, College of Pharmacy and Department of Internal Medicine, University of New Mexico, Albuquerque, New Mexico
Chapter 42

Marcel Devetten, MD
Associate Professor of Medicine and Director of Hematopoietic Cell Transplant Program, University of Nebraska Medical Center, Omaha, Nebraska
Chapter 138

John W. Devlin, PharmD, FCCP, FCCM, BCPS
Associate Professor, Department of Pharmacy Practice, School of Pharmacy, Northeastern University; Adjunct Associate Professor, School of Medicine, Tufts University, Boston, Massachusetts
Chapters 55 and 127

Vanessa A. Diaz, MD, MS
Assistant Professor, Department of Family Medicine, Medical University of South Carolina, Charleston, South Carolina
Chapter 82

Lori M. Dickerson, PharmD, FCCP, BCPS
Associate Professor and Associate Residency Program Director, Department of Family Medicine, Medical University of South Carolina, Charleston, South Carolina
Chapter 82

Cecily V. DiPiro, PharmD
Consultant Pharmacist, Mt. Pleasant, South Carolina
Chapter 37

Joseph T. DiPiro, PharmD, FCCP
Executive Dean and Professor, South Carolina College of Pharmacy, Medical University of South Carolina, Charleston, South Carolina; University of South Carolina, Columbia, South Carolina
Chapters 36, 91, 118, and 123

Paul L. Doering, MS
Distinguished Service Professor of Pharmacy Practice, College of Pharmacy, University of Florida, Gainesville, Florida
Chapters 68 and 69

Julie Ann Dopheide, PharmD, BCPP
Associate Professor of Clinical Pharmacy, Psychiatry and the Behavioral Sciences, University of Southern California Schools of Pharmacy and Medicine, Los Angeles, California
Chapter 65

John M. Dopp, PharmD
Assistant Professor, Pharmacy Practice Division, School of Pharmacy, University of Wisconsin-Madison, Madison, Wisconsin
Chapter 75

Thomas C. Dowling, PharmD, PhD
Associate Professor, Director, Renal Clinical Pharmacology Lab, School of Pharmacy, University of Maryland, Baltimore, Maryland
Chapter 44

Shannon J. Drayton, PharmD
Assistant Professor, Department of Pharmacy and Clinical Sciences, South Carolina College of Pharmacy, Medical University of South Carolina Campus, Charleston, South Carolina
Chapter 72

Deepak P. Edward, MD, FACS
Chair and Program Director; Professor/NEOUCOM, Department of Ephthalmology, Summa Health System, Akron, Ohio
Chapter 97

Mary Elizabeth Elliott, PharmD, PhD
Associate Professor and Vice-Chair, Pharmacy Practice Division, School of Pharmacy, University of Wisconsin-Madison, Madison, Wisconson, Clinical Pharmacist, Osteoporosis Clinic, VA Medical Center, Madison, Wisconsin
Chapter 95

Michael E. Ernst, PharmD, BCPS
Associate Professor (Clinical), Division of Clinical and Administrative Pharmacy, College of Pharmacy; Department of Family Medicine, Carver College of Medicine, University of Iowa, Iowa City, Iowa
Chapter 96

Brian L. Erstad, PharmD
Professor, Department of Pharmacy Practice and Science, College of Pharmacy, University of Arizona, Tucson, Arizona
Chapter 26

Janet L. Espirito, PharmD, BCOP
Clinical Pharmacy Specialist-Breast Oncology, Division of Pharmacy, University of Texas M.D. Anderson Cancer Center, Houston, Texas
Chapter 131

Francisco J. Esteva, MD, PhD
Associate Professor of Medicine, Departments of Breast Medical Oncology and Molecular and Cellular Oncology, University of Texas, M.D. Anderson Cancer Center, Houston, Texas
Chapter 131

Susan C. Fagan, PharmD, BCPS
Professor, Clinical and Administrative Pharmacy, College of Pharmacy, University of Georgia and Adjunct Professor of Neurology, Medical College of Georgia, Augusta, Georgia
Chapters 22 and 56

Chris Fausel, PharmD, BCPS, BCOP

Clinical Pharmacist, Hematology/Oncology/BMT, Indiana University Cancer Center, Indianapolis, Indiana

Chapter 130

Richard G. Fiscella, BS Pharm, MPH

Clinical Professor, Department of Pharmacy Practice, Adjunct Assistant Professor, Department of Ophthalmology, University of Illinois, Chicago, Illinois

Chapter 97

Douglas N. Fish, PharmD

Professor, Department of Clinical Pharmacy, School of Pharmacy; Clinical Associate Professor, Division of Respiratory and Critical Care Medicine, School of Medicine, University of Colorado, Denver, Colorado

Chapters 114 and 126

Courtney V. Fletcher, PharmD

Dean and Professor, College of Pharmacy, University of Nebraska Medical Center, Omaha, Nebraska

Chapter 129

Edward F. Foote, PharmD, FCCP, BCPS

Professor and Chair, Pharmacy Practice Department, Nesbitt College of Pharmacy and Nursing, Wilkes-Barre University, Wilkes-Barre, Pennsylvania

Chapter 48

Sarah Forgie, MD, FRCP(C)

Assistant Professor, Pediatrics, Division of Infectious Diseases, University of Alberta; Associate Director, Infection Control, Stollery Children's Hospital, Edmonton, Alberta, Canada

Chapter 112

Nora Franceschini, MD, MPH

Department of Epidemiology, School of Public Health, University of North Carolina at Chapel Hill, Chapel Hill, North Carolina

Chapter 46

Allan D. Friedman, MD, MPH

Professor and Chair, Division of General Pediatrics, Virginia Commonwealth University, Richmond, Virginia

Chapter 122

Deborah A. Frieze, PharmD, BCOP

Clinical Pharmacist, Hematology/Oncology; Clinical Instructor, Seattle Cancer Care Alliance; University of Washington Medical Center, Seattle, Washington

Chapter 132

Reginald F. Frye, PharmD, PhD

Associate Professor, Departments of Pharmacy Practice and Pharmaceutics, College of Pharmacy, University of Florida, Gainesville, Florida

Chapter 51

Todd W. B. Gehr, MD

Professor and Chairman, Division of Nephrology, Department of Internal Medicine, Virginia Commonwealth University, Richmond, Virginia

Chapter 54

Mark L. Glover, PharmD, BS Pharm

Associate Professor and Director, West Palm Beach Program, Department of Pharmacy Practice, College of Pharmacy, Nova Southeastern University, Palm Beach Gardens, Florida

Chapter 111

Shelly L. Gray, PharmD, MS

Professor, School of Pharmacy, University of Washington, Seattle, Washington

Chapter 8

Jessica S. Gruber, PhD, MPH

Washington State University, College of Pharmacy, Deaconess Medical Center, Spokane, Washington

Chapter 11

David R. P. Guay, Pharm D

Professor, Department of Experimental and Clinical Pharmacology, College of Pharmacy, University of Minnesota; Department of Geriatrics, Health Partners, Inc., Minneapolis, Minnesota

Chapters 8 and 88

John G. Gums, PharmD

Professor of Pharmacy and Medicine, Departments of Pharmacy Practice and Family Medicine, Director of Clinical Research in Family Medicine, University of Florida, Gainesville, Florida

Chapter 79

Stuart T. Haines, PharmD, BCPS

Professor and Vice Chair, University of Maryland School of Pharmacy; Clinical Specialist, University of Maryland Medical System, Baltimore, Maryland

Chapter 21

Emily R. Hajjar, PharmD

Assistant Professor, Jefferson School of Pharmacy, Thomas Jefferson University, Philadelphia, Pennsylvania

Chapter 8

Philip D. Hall, PharmD, FCCP, BCPS, BCOP

Associate Dean and Associate Professor, South Carolina College of Pharmacy, Medical University of South Carolina Campus, Hollings Cancer Center, Charleston, South Carolina

Chapter 89

Steven M. Handler, MP, MS, CMD

Assistant Professor, Department of Medicine, Division of Geriatic Medicine and Department of Biomedical Informatics, University of Pittsburgh, Pittsburgh, Pennsylvania

Chapter 8

Joseph T. Hanlon, PharmD, MS, BCPS

Professor, Division of Geriatrics and Gerontology, Department of Medicine, School of Medicine; Department of Pharmacy and Therapeutics, School of Pharmacy, University of Pittsburgh; Research Health Scientist, Center for Health Equity Research and Promotion, Geriatric Research Education (CHERP) and Clinical Center (GRECC), Pittsburgh, Pennsylvania

Chapter 8

Michelle Harkins, MD

Associate Professor, Department of Internal Medicine, Pulmonary and Critical Care, University of New Mexico Health Sciences Center, Albuquerque, New Mexico

Chapter 31

David W. Hawkins, PharmD
Professor and Dean, California Northstate College of Pharmacy, Sacramento, California
Chapter 96

Peggy E. Hayes, PharmD
President, Hayes CNS Services, LLC, San Diego, California
Chapter 71

Mary S. Hayney, PharmD, FCCP, BCPS
Associate Professor of Pharmacy (CHS) University of Wisconsin-Madison, School of Pharmacy, Madison, Wisconsin
Chapter 128

Thomas K. Hazlet, PharmD, DrPH
Pharmaceutical Outcomes Research and Policy Program University of Washington School of Pharmacy, Seattle, Washington
Chapter 9

Brian A. Hemstreet, PharmD, BCPS
Assistant Professor, University of Colorado at Denver and Health Sciences Center School of Pharmacy, Department of Clinical Pharmacy, Denver, Colorado
Chapter 36

Elizabeth D. Hermsen, PharmD, MBA, BCPS
Antimicrobial Specialist and Research Associate, Nebraska Medical Center; Adjunct Assistant Professor, University of Nebraska Medical Center, College of Pharmacy and Medicine, Omaha, Nebraska
Chapters 110 and 113

David C. Hess, MD
Professor and Chair, Department of Neurology, Medical College of Georgia, Augusta, Georgia
Chapter 22

Angela Massey Hill, PharmD, BCPP
Professor, Division Director of Pharmacy Practice, Florida A&M University College of Pharmacy, Tallahassee, Florida
Chapter 67

Jonathan Himmelfarb, MD
Director, Division of Nephrology and Transplantation; Associate Chair for Research, Department of Medicine; Director of Clinical and Translational Research, Maine Medical Center, Portland, Maine
Chapter 49

Brian M. Hodges, PharmD, BCPS, BCNSP
Assistant Professor, Department of Clinical Pharmacy, School of Pharmacy, West Virginia University, Morgantown, West Virginia
Chapter 147

Barbara J. Hoeben, PharmD, MSPharm, BCPS
Clinical Pharmacy Flight Commander, 59 MDW, Wilford Hall Medical Center, Lackland Airforce Base; Clinical Assistant Professor, Department of General Medicine, University of Texas Health Science Center, San Antonio, Texas
Chapter 24

Collin A. Hovinga, PharmD
Assistant Professor, Pharmacy and Pediatrics, University of Tennessee Health Science Center, Memphis, Tennessee
Chapter 59

Thomas R. Howdieshell, MD, FACS, FCCP
Professor of Surgery, Section of Trauma/Surgical Critical Care, Department of Surgery, University of New Mexico Health Sciences Center, Albuquerque, New Mexico
Chapter 118

Joanna Q. Hudson, PharmD, BCPS, FASN
Associate Professor, Departments of Clinical Pharmacy and Medicine (Nephrology), Schools of Pharmacy and Medicine, University of Tennessee; Clinical Pharmacist, Methodist University Hospital, Memphis, Tennessee
Chapter 47

Beata A. Ineck, PharmD, BCPS, CDE
Inpatient Clinical Staff Pharmacist, St. Luke's Meridian Medical Center, Meridian, Idaho
Chapter 104

William L. Isley, MD
Consultant, Mayo Clinic; Associate Professor of Medicine, Mayo Clinic College of Medicine, Rochester, Minnesota (Deceased)
Chapter 77

Mark W. Jackson, MD
Gastroenterologist, Fort Sanders Regional Medical Center and Baptist Hospital of East Tennessee, Knoxville, Tennesseee
Chapter 33

Thomas E. Johns, PharmD, BCPS
Assistant Director, Clinical Pharmacy Services, Shands at the University of Florida, Gainesville, Florida
Chapter 107

Heather J. Johnson, PharmD, BCPS, FASN
Assistant Professor, School of Pharmacy, University of Pittsburgh; Clinical Pharmacist, University of Pittsburgh Medical Center, Pittsburgh, Pennsylvania
Chapter 92

Melanie S. Joy, PharmD
Associate Professor, Division of Nephrology and Hypertension, UNC Kidney Center, School of Medicine, Division of Pharmacotherapy and Experimental Therapeutics, School of Pharmacy, University of North Carolina at Chapel Hill, Chapel Hill, North Carolina
Chapters 46 and 52

Rose Jung, PharmD, BCPS
Prestige Associate Professor, Department of Pharmacy Practice, University of Toledo, College of Pharmacy, Toledo, Ohio
Chapter 117

Thomas N. Kakuda, PharmD
Director, Human Pharmacokinetics, Tibotec, Inc., Yardley, Pennsylvania
Chapter 129

Sophia N. Kalantaridou, MD, PhD
Associate Professor of Obstetrics and Gynecology, Division of Reproductive Endocrinology, University of Ioannina Medical School, Ioannina, Greece
Chapter 85

Judith C. Kando, PharmD, BCPP
Senior Scientific Affairs Liaison, Ortho-McNeil Janssen Scientific Affairs, LLC, Tewksbury, Massachusetts
Chapter 71

S. Lena Kang-Birken, PharmD, FCCP

Associate Professor, Department of Pharmacy Practice, Thomas J. Long School of Pharmacy and Health Sciences, University of the Pacific, Stockton, California

Chapter 123

Salmaan Kanji, PharmD, MSc

Clinical Pharmacy Specialist, Ottawa Health Research Institute, Ottawa, Ontario, Canada

Chapter 127

H. William Kelly, PharmD

Professor Emeritus, Department of Pediatrics, School of Medicine, University of New Mexico Health Sciences Center, Albuquerque, New Mexico

Chapter 28

W. Klugh Kennedy, PharmD, BCPP

Clinical Associate Professor , University of Georgia College of Pharmacy; Associate Professor, Mercer University School of Medicine, Savannah, Georgia

Chapter 69

Yasmin Khaliq, PharmD

Ottawa Hospital, Ottawa, Ontario, Canada

Chapter 112

William R. Kirchain, PharmD

Wilbur and Mildred Robichaux Endowed Professor of Pharmacy, Xavier University, College of Pharmacy, New Orleans, Louisana

Chapter 40

Cynthia K. Kirkwood, PharmD, BCPP

Associate Professor of Pharmacy, Vice Chair for Education, Department of Pharmacy, School of Pharmacy, Virginia Commonwealth University, Richmond, Virginia

Chapters 73 and 74

Leroy C. Knodel, PharmD

Associate Professor, Department of Surgery, University of Texas Health Science Center, San Antonio, Texas; Clinical Associate Professor, College of Pharmacy, University of Texas, Austin, Texas

Chapter 121

Jill M. Kolesar, PharmD, FCCP, BCPS

Associate Professor, School of Pharmacy, University of Wisconsin, Madison, Wisconsin

Chapter 134

Connie R. Kraus, PharmD, BCPS

Clinical Professor, School of Pharmacy, University of Wisconsin-Madison, Madison, Wisconsin

Chapter 81

Abhijit Kshirsagar, MD, MPH

Assistant Professor of Medicine, Division of Nephrology and Hypertension, UNC Kidney Center, School of Medicine, University of North Carolina at Chapel Hill, Chapel Hill, North Carolina

Chapter 46

Vanessa J. Kumpf, PharmD, BCNSP

Clinical Specialist, Nutrition Support, Vanderbilt University Medical Center, Nashville, Tennessee

Chapters 143 and 146

Thomas Lackner, PharmD

Professor, Department of Experimental and Clinical Pharmacy, College of Pharmacy, University of Minnesota, Minneapolis, Minnesota

Chapter 88

Y. W. Francis Lam, PharmD, FCCP

Associate Professor of Pharmacology and Medicine, Clinical Associate Professor of Pharmacy, Departments of Pharmacology and Medicine, University of Texas Health Science Center, San Antonio, Texas

Chapters 6 and 43

Alan H. Lau, PharmD

Professor, Department of Pharmacy Practice, College of Pharmacy, University of Illinois, Chicago, Illinois

Chapter 50

Helen L. Leather, BPharm

Clinical Pharmacy Specialist BMT/Leukemia, Shands at the University of Florida, Department of Pharmacy, Gainesville, Florida

Chapter 137

Mary Lee, PharmD, BCPS, FCCP

Professor of Pharmacy Practice, Chicago College of Pharmacy; Vice President and Chief Academic Officer, Pharmacy and Health Science Education, Midwestern University, Downers Grove, Illinois

Chapters 86 and 87

Timonthy S. Lesar, PharmD

Director of Pharmacy, Patient Care Service Director, Department of Pharmacy, Albany Medical Center, Albany, New York

Chapter 97

Stephanie M. Levine, MD

Professor of Medicine, Division of Pulmonary and Critical Care Medicine, University of Texas Health Science Center, San Antonio, Texas

Chapter 27

Amy Loyd, DO, CPT, MC

Resident, Army Medical Corps, Brooke Army Medical Center, San Antonio, Texas

Chapters 100 and 101

William L. Lyons, MD

Assistant Professor, Section of Geriatrics and Gerontology, University of Nebraska Medical Center, Omaha, Nebraska

Chapter 104

George E. MacKinnon, III, PhD, RPh, FASHP

Vice President of Academic Affairs, American Association of Colleges of Pharmacy, Alexandria, Virginia

Chapter 4

Neil J. MacKinnon, PhD, RPh, FCSHP

Associate Director for Research and Associate Professor, Dalhousie University College of Pharmacy, Halifax, Nova Scotia, Canada

Chapter 4

Robert MacLaren, PharmD, BSc

Associate Professor, Department of Clinical Pharmacy, University of Colorado, Denver, School of Pharmacy, Aurora, Colorado

Chapter 25

Eric J. MacLaughlin, PharmD, BS Pharm
Associate Professor, Texas Tech University Health Sciences Center, School of Pharmacy, Amarillo, Texas
Chapter 15

Eugene H. Makela, PharmD, BCPP
Associate Professor, Schools of Pharmacy and Medicine, West Virginia University, Morgantown, West Virginia
Chapter 74

Michael Malkin, MD
Director, Juvenile Court Mental Health Services, Los Angeles County Department of Mental Health; Assistant Professor, UCLA Department of Psychiatry, Los Angeles, California
Chapter 65

Harold J. Manley, PharmD, FASN, FCCP, BCPS
Director of Clinical Pharmacy, Village Health Disease Management, Glenmont, New York
Chapter 48

Patricia A. Marken, PharmD, FCCP, BCPP
Professor and Chair of Pharmacy Practice, School of Pharmacy; Professor of Psychiatry, School of Medicine, University of Missouri, Kansas City, Missouri
Chapter 64

Patricia L. Marshik, PharmD
Associate Professor, University of New Mexico Health Sciences Center, College of Pharmacy, Albuquerque, New Mexico
Chapter 31

Steven Martin, PharmD, BCPS, FCCP, FCCM
Professor and Chairman, Department of Pharmacy Practice, University of Toledo, College of Pharmacy, Toledo, Ohio
Chapter 117

Barbara J. Mason, PharmD, FASHP
Professor and Vice Chair, Idaho State University College of Pharmacy; Ambulatory Core Clinical Pharmacist, Boise VA Medical Center, Boise, Idaho
Chapter 104

Todd W. Mattox, PharmD, BCNSP
Coordinator, Nutrition Support Team, H. Lee Moffitt Cancer Center and Research Institute, Tampa, Florida
Chapter 145

Gary R. Matzke, PharmD, FCP, FCCP
Professor of Pharmacy and Pharmaceutics and Associate Dean for Clinical Research and Public Policy, School of Pharmacy, Professor of Internal Medicine, Nephrology Division, School of Medicine, Virginia Commonwealth University, Richmond, Virginia
Chapters 51 and 55

J. Russell May, PharmD, FASHP
Clinical Professor, Department of Clinical and Administrative Pharmacy, University of Georgia College of Pharmacy; Clinical Pharmacy Specialist, Medical College of Georgia, Augusta, Georgia
Chapter 98

Jeannine S. McCune, PharmD, BCPS, BCOP
Associate Professor, University of Washington, School of Pharmacy; Affiliate Investigator, Fred Hutchinson Cancer Research Center, Seattle, Washington
Chapter 132

Timothy R. McGuire, PharmD, FCCP, BCOP
Associate Professor, College of Pharmacy, University of Nebraska Medical Center, Omaha, Nebraska
Chapters 138 and 139

Jerry R. McKee, PharmD, MS, BCPP
Clinical Assistant Professor, Department of Pharmacotherapy, University of North Carolina School of Pharmacy, Chapel Hill, North Carolina; Pharmacy Director-Broughton Hospital, Morganton, North Carolina
Chapter 76

Trevor McKibbin, PharmD, BCPS, MSc
Assistant Professor, Department of Clinical Pharmacy, College of Pharmacy, University of Tennessee Health Science Center, Memphis, Tennessee
Chapter 140

Patrick J. Medina, PharmD, BCOP
Associate Professor, University of Oklahoma College of Pharmacy, Oklahoma City, Oklahoma
Chapters 130 and 133

Sarah T. Melton, PharmD, BCPP, CGP
Adjunct Associate Professor of Pharmacy Practice, University of Appalachia College of Pharmacy; Clinical Pharmacist, Lebanon, Virginia
Chapter 73

Giuseppe Micali, MD
Professor and Chairman, Dermatology Clinic, University of Catania, Catania, Italy
Chapters 100 and 101

Laura Boehnke Michaud, PharmD, BCOP, FASHP
Manager, Clinical Pharmacy and Clinical Pharmacy Specialist–Breast Oncology, University of Texas M. D. Anderson Cancer Center, Houston, Texas
Chapter 131

Gary Milavetz, PharmD, RPh, BS, FCCP
Associate Professor of Pharmacy, Division of Clinical and Administrative Pharmacy, College of Pharmacy, University of Iowa, Iowa City, Iowa
Chapter 32

Deborah S. Minor, PharmD
Associate Professor, Department of Medicine, School of Medicine, University of Mississippi Medical Center, Jackson, Mississippi
Chapter 63

Isaac F. Mitropoulos, PharmD
Research Fellow, Experimental and Clinical Pharmacology, College of Pharmacy, University of Minnesota, Minneapolis, Minnesota
Chapter 110

Patricia A. Montgomery, PharmD
Clinical Pharmacy Specialist, Mercy General Hospital, Sacramento, California
Chapter 41

Reginald H. Moore, MD
Clinical Associate Professor, Department of Pediatrics, University of Texas Health Science Center, San Antonio, Texas
Chapter 106

Stuart Munro, MD

Chair, Department of Psychiatry, School of Medicine, University of Missouri-Kansas City, Kansas City, Missouri

Chapter 64

Maria Letizia Musumeci, MD, PhD

Assistant, Dermatology Clinic, University of Catania, Catania, Italy

Chapter 101

Milap C. Nahata, PharmD, MS, FCCP

Professor of Pharmacy, Pediatrics and Internal Medicine; Division Chair, Pharmacy Practice and Administration, Ohio State University, College of Pharmacy, Associate Director, Department of Pharmacy, Ohio State University Medical Center, Columbus, Ohio

Chapter 7

Jean M. Nappi, PharmD, FCCP, BCPS

Professor of Pharmacy and Clinical Sciences, South Carolina College of Pharmacy-MUSC Campus; Professor of Medicine, Medical University of South Carolina, Charleston, South Carolina

Chapter 20

Merlin V. Nelson, MD, PharmD

Neurologist, Affiliated Community Medical Centers, Willmar, Minnesota

Chapter 61

Fenwick T. Nichols, III, MD

Professor, Department of Neurology, Medical College of Georgia, Augusta, Georgia

Chapter 56

Thomas D. Nolin, PharmD, PhD

Clinical Pharmacologist, Department of Pharmacy Services, Division of Nephrology and Transplantation, Department of Medicine, Maine Medical Center, Portland, Maine

Chapter 49

Edith A. Nutescu, PharmD, FCCP

Clinical Associate Professor, Director, Antithrombosis Center, University of Chicago College of Pharmacy and Medical Center, Chicago, Illinois

Chapter 21

Mary Beth O'Connell, PharmD, BCPS

Department of Pharmacy Practice, Wayne State University, Detroit, Michigan

Chapter 93

Keith M. Olsen, PharmD, FCCP, FCCM

Professor and Chair, Department of Pharmacy Practice, College of Pharmacy, University of Nebraska Medical Center, Omaha, Nebraska

Chapter 33

Rebecca L. Owens, PharmD

Clinical Instructor, College of Pharmacy, University of Texas, Austin, Texas; Department of Medicine, University of Texas Health Science Center at San Antonio, San Antonio, Texas

Chapter 30

Robert L. Page, II, PharmD, CGP, BCPS

Associate Professor of Clinical Pharmacy and Physical Medicine; Clinical Specialist, Division of Cardiology, UHCSC, Schools of Pharmacy and Medicine, Denver, Colorado

Chapter 20

Amy Barton Pai, PharmD, BCPS, FASN

Associate Professor of Pharmacy, College of Pharmacy; School of Medicine, University of New Mexico, Albuquerque, New Mexico

Chapter 53

Paul M. Palevsky, MD

Chief Renal Section, VA Pittsburgh Healthcare System; Professor of Medicine, Renal-Electrolyte Division, School of Medicine, University of Pittsburgh, Pittsburgh, Pennsylvania

Chapter 55

Robert B. Parker, PharmD, FCCP

Professor, University of Tennessee College of Pharmacy, Memphis, Tennessee

Chapter 16

Charles A. Peloquin, PharmD

Director, Infectious Disease Pharmacokinetics Laboratory, National Jewish Medical and Research Center, Denver, Colorado

Chapter 116

Susan L. Pendland, PharmD, MS

Adjunct Associate Professor, Department of Pharmacy Practice, College of Pharmacy, University of Illinois at Chicago, Chicago, Illinois; Clinical Staff Pharmacist, Saint Joseph Berea Hospital, Berea, Kentucky

Chapter 114

Janelle B. Perkins, Pharm D

Assistant Professor, Department of Interdisciplinary Oncology, Blood and Marrow Transplant Program, Moffitt Cancer Center, Tampa, Florida

Chapter 142

Jay I. Peters, MD

Professor of Medicine, Pulmonary/Critical Care Division, University of Texas Health Science Center, San Antonio, Texas

Chapter 27

William P. Petros, PharmD, FCCP

Mylan Chair of Pharmacology, Professor of Pharmacy and Medicine, West Virginia University Health Sciences Center; Associate Director of Anti-Cancer Drug Development, Mary Babb Randolph Cancer Center, Morgantown, West Virginia

Chapter 103

Stephanie J. Phelps, PharmD, BCPS

Professor, Department of Clinical Pharmacy, University of Tennessee, Memphis, Tennessee

Chapter 59

Bradley G. Phillips, PharmD, BCPS, FCCP

Milliken-Reeve Professor and Head, Department of Clinical and Administrative Pharmacy, College of Pharmacy, University of Georgia, Athens, Georgia

Chapter 75

Amy M. Pick, PharmD, BCOP

Assistant Professor of Pharmacy Practice, Creighton University School of Pharmacy and Health Professions; Clinical Pharmacist, Nebraska Methodist Hospital, Omaha, Nebraska

Chapter 138

Denise L. Walbrandt Pigarelli, PharmD, BC-ADM
Clinical Associate Professor, University of Wisconsin-Madison, School of Pharmacy, Madison, Wisconsin
Chapter 81

Betsy Bickert Poon, PharmD
Oncology/Stem Cell Transplant Clinical Pharmacist, Children's Hospital of Philadelphia, Philadelphia, Pennsylvania
Chapters 105 and 137

L. Michael Posey, BSPharm
Editorial Director, Periodicals Department, American Pharmacists Association, Washington, D.C.
Chapter 3

Beth E. Potter, MD
Associate Professor, Department of Family Medicine, School of Medicine and Public Health, University of Wisconsin-Madison, Madison, Wisconsin
Chapter 81

Randall A. Prince, PharmD
Professor, University of Houston, College of Pharmacy, Houston, Texas
Chapter 120

Hengameh H. Raissy, PharmD
University of New Mexico, School of Medicine, Albuquerque, New Mexico
Chapter 31

Charles A. Reasner, II, MD
Professor, Department of Endocrinology, Metabolism, and Diabetes, University of Texas Health Science Center: Medical Director, Texas Diabetes Institute, San Antonio, Texas
Chapter 77

Michael D. Reed, PharmD, FCCP, FCP
Director, Division of Clinical Pharmacology and Toxicology, Department of Pediatrics, Children's Hospital Medical Center, Akron, Ohio
Chapter 111

Pamela D. Reiter, PharmD
Clinical Pharmacy Specialist, Pediatric ICU and Trauma, The Children's Hospital of Denver; Clinical Associate Professor, University of Colorado of Denver Health Sciences Center, School of Pharmacy, Denver, Colorado
Chapter 145

Jo E. Rodgers, PharmD, BCPS (AQ Cardiology)
Clinical Assistant Professor, Department of Pharmacotherapy and Experimental Therapeutics, School of Pharmacy, University of North Carolina at Chapel Hill, Chapel Hill, North Carolina
Chapter 16

Susan J. Rogers, PharmD, BCPS
Assistant Clinical Professor, University of Texas at Austin; Clinical Pharmacy Specialist Neurology, South Texas Healthcare System, Audie L. Murphy Memorial Veterans Hospital, San Antonio, Texas
Chapter 58

Mark Rohrscheib, MD
Assistant Professor, Department of Internal Medicine, Division of Nephrology, University of New Mexico Health Sciences Center, Albuquerque, New Mexico
Chapter 53

John C. Rotschafer, PharmD, FCCP
Professor, Department of Experimental and Clinical Pharmacy, College of Pharmacy, University of Minnesota, Minneapolis, Minnesota
Chapter 110

Eric S. Rovner, MD
Associate Professor of Urology, Department of Urology, Medical University of South Carolina, Charleston, South Carolina
Chapter 88

Maria I. Rudis, PharmD, FCCM
Assistant Professor of Clinical Pharmacy, School of Pharmacy; Assistant Professor of Clinical Emergency Medicine, Keck School of Medicine, University of Southern California, Los Angeles, California
Chapter 25

Mark E. Rupp, MD
Professor, Department of Internal Medicine, University of Nebraska Medical Center; Medical Director, Department of Healthcare Epidemiology, Nebraska Medical Center, Omaha, Nebraska
Chapter 113

Michael J. Rybak, PharmD, MPH
Professor of Pharmacy and Medicine, Associate Dean for Research, Director, Anti-Infective Research Laboratory, Eugene Applebaum College of Pharmacy and Health Sciences, Wayne State University, Detroit, Michigan
Chapter 108

Gordon Sacks, PharmD
Clinical Professor and Chair, Pharmacy Practice Division, School of Pharmacy, University of Wisconsin-Madison, Madison, Wisconsin
Chapter 144

Lisa Sanchez, PharmD
PE Applications, Highlands Ranch, Colorado
Chapter 1

Cynthia A. Sanoski, PharmD, BS
Associate Professor of Clinical Pharmacy, Department of Pharmacy Practice and Pharmacy Administration, Philadelphia College of Pharmacy, University of the Sciences, Philadelphia, Pennsylvania
Chapter 19

Joseph J. Saseen, PharmD, FCCP, BCPS
Associate Professor, University of Colorado-Denver, Department of Clinical Pharmacy, School of Pharmacy; Department of Family Medicine, School of Medicine, Aurora, Colorado
Chapter 15

Robert R. Schade, MD, FACP, AGAF, FACG, FASGE
Professor of Medicine, Chief, Division of Gastroenterology/Hepatology, Medical College of Georgia, Division of Gastroenterology/Hepatology, Augusta, Georgia
Chapter 34

Jeremy A. Schafer, PharmD

Manager of Formulary Development, Prime Therapeutics, Eagan, Minnesota

Chapter 110

Mark E. Schneiderhan, PharmD, BCPP

Clinical Assistant Professor, Department of Pharmacy Practice, Clinical Pharmacist, Department of Psychiatry, University of Illinois, College of Pharmacy, Chicago, Illinois

Chapter 64

Marieke Dekker Schoen, PharmD, BCPS

Clinical Associate Professor, Department of Pharmacy and Department of Medicine, University of Illinois, Chicago, Illinois

Chapter 19

Kristine S. Schonder, PharmD

Assistant Professor, Pharmacy and Therapeutics Department, School of Pharmacy, University of Pittsburgh; Clinical Pharmacist, Thomas E. Starzl Transplantation Institute, University of Pittsburgh Medical Center, Pittsburgh, Pennsylvania

Chapter 92

Arthur A. Schuna, MS

Clinical Coordinator, William S. Middleton VA Medical Center, Clinical Professor, University of Wisconsin-Madison, School of Pharmacy, Madison, Wisconsin

Chapter 94

Richard B. Schwartz, MD

Associate Professor, Department of Emergency Medicine, Medical College of Georgia, Augusta, Georgia

Chapter 12

Rowena N. Schwartz, PharmD, BCOP

Director of Weinberg and Oncology Pharmacy, Johns Hopkins Hospital, Baltimore, Maryland

Chapter 141

Laura Scuderi, MD

Assistant, Dermatology Clinic, University of Catania, Catania, Italy

Chapter 100

Julie M. Sease, PharmD, BCPS

Clinical Assistant Professor, Department of Clinical Pharmacy and Outcome Sciences, South Carolina, College of Pharmacy, University of South Carolina, Columbia, South Carolina

Chapter 39

Amy Heck Sheehan, PharmD

Associate Professor of Pharmacy Practice, Purdue University School of Pharmacy and Pharmaceutical Sciences, Indianapolis, Indiana

Chapter 80

Greene Shepherd, PharmD

Clinical Associate Professor, College of Pharmacy, University of Georgia, Augusta, Georgia

Chapter 12

Steven I. Sherman, MD

Chair and Professor, Department of Endocrine Neoplasia and Hormonal Disorders, University of Texas M.D. Anderson Cancer Center; Adjunct Associate Professor, Baylor College of Medicine, Houston, Texas

Chapter 78

Sarah P. Shrader, PharmD, BCPS

Assistant Professor, Department of Pharmacy and Clinical Sciences, South Carolina College of Pharmacy-MUSC Campus, Charleston, South Carolina

Chapter 82

Patricia W. Slattum, PharmD, PhD

Associate Professor, Geriatric Pharmacotherapy Program, Department of Pharmacy, School of Pharmacy, Virginia Commonwealth University, Richmond, Virginia

Chapter 67

Judith A. Smith, PharmD, FCCP, BCOP

Assistant Professor, Department of Gynecologic Oncology, University of Texas MD Anderson Cancer Center, Houston, Texas

Chapter 136

Philip H. Smith, MD

Section of Allergy and Immunology, Rheumatology, Department of Internal Medicine, Medical College of Georgia, Augusta, Georgia

Chapter 98

Christine A. Sorkness, PharmD

Professor, Department of Pharmacy Practice, School of Pharmacy; Professor, Department of Medicine, Division of Allergy, Pulmonary and Critical Care Medicine, School of Medicine and Public Health, University of Wisconsin-Madison, Madison, Wisconsin

Chapter 28

Anne P. Spencer, PharmD

Associate Professor, Department of Clinical Pharmacy and Outcome Sciences, South Carolina College of Pharmacy, Medical University of South Carolina, Charleston, South Carolina

Chapter 45

Sarah A. Spinler, PharmD, BCPS (AQ Cardiology)

Professor, College of Pharmacy, University of the Sciences, Philadelphia, Pennsylvania

Chapter 18

William J. Spruill, PharmD, FCCP, FASHP

Professor, University of Georgia, College of Pharmacy, Athens, Georgia

Chapter 38

John V. St. Peter, BCPS

Adjunct Associate Professor of Pharmacy, College of Pharmacy, University of Minnesota, Minneapolis, Minnesota; Clinical and Outcomes Manager, Takeda Pharmaceuticals North America, Deerfield, Illinois

Chapter 48

Catherine I. Starner, PharmD, BCPS, CGP

Senior Clinical Pharmacist, Prime Theapeutics; Clinical Assistant Professor, University of Minnesota, College of Pharmacy, Eagan, Minnesota

Chapter 8

Andy Stergachis, PhD, RPh

Professor of Epidemiology and Global Health, Adjunct Professor of Pharmacy, University of Washington, Seattle, Washington

Chapter 9

Steven C. Stoner, PharmD, BCPP
UMKC School of Pharmacy, Division of Pharmacy Practice, Clinical Associate Professor, Kansas City, Missouri
Chapter 66

James J. Stragand, MD, PhD, FACG, FACP
Attendant Gastroenterologist, St. Charles Medical Center, Bend, Oregon
Chapter 39

Jennifer Strickland, PharmD, BCPS
Pain and Palliative Care Specialists, Lakeland Regional Medical Center, Lakeland, Florida
Chapter 62

Deborah A. Sturpe, PharmD, BCPS
Assistant Professor, Department of Pharmacy Practice and Science, University of Maryland, School of Pharmacy, Baltimore, Maryland
Chapter 84

Weijing Sun, MD
Associate Professor of Medicine, University of Pennsylvania, Abramson Cancer Center, Philadelphia, Pennsylvania
Chapter 133

Russell H. Swerdlow, MD
Professor of Neurology, Molecular and Integrative Physiology, University of Kansas School of Medicine, Kansas City, Kansas
Chapter 67

David M. Swope, MD
Associate Professor of Neurology, Loma Linda University, Loma Linda, California
Chapter 61

Carol Taketomo, PharmD
Pharmacy Manager, Children's Hospital of Los Angeles, Adjunct Assistant Professor of Pharmacy Practice, University of Southern California School of Pharmacy, Los Angeles, California
Chapter 7

Robert L. Talbert, PharmD, FCCP, BCPS, CLS
SmithKline Professor, College of Pharmacy, University of Texas at Austin; Professor, Department of Medicine, University of Texas Health Science Center at San Antonio, San Antonio, Texas
Chapters 13, 17, 23, 24, 30, and 78

Colleen M. Terriff, PharmD
Assistant Professor, Pharmacy Department, College of Pharmacy, Washington State University; Clinical Pharmacist, Deaconess Medical Center, Spokane, Washington
Chapter 11

Jane Tran Tesoro, PharmD, BCPP
Clinical Pharmacist, Juvenile Court Mental Health Services, Los Angeles, California
Chapter 65

Christian J. Teter, PharmD, BCPP
Assistant Professor, School of Pharmacy, Northwestern University, Boston, Massachusetts; Clinical Research Pharmacist, Alcohol and Drug Abuse Treatment Program, McLean Hospital, Belmont, Massachusetts
Chapter 71

Edward G. Timm, PharmD, MS
Senior Clinical Pharmacy Specialist, Critical Care and Adjunct Assistant Professor, Albany Medical Center Hospital and Albany College of Pharmacy, Albany, New York
Chapter 39

Shelly D. Timmons, MD, PhD, FACS
Semmes-Murphey Clinic, Assistant Professor and Chief of Neurotrauma Division, University of Tennessee Health Science Center, Memphis, Tennessee
Chapter 60

Curtis L. Triplitt, PharmD, CDE
Texas Diabetes Institute; Assistant Professor, Department of Medicine, Division of Diabetes, University of Texas Health Science Center, San Antonio, Texas
Chapter 77

Elena M. Umland, PharmD
Associate Dean for Academic Affairs, Jefferson School of Pharmacy, Thomas Jefferson University, Philadelphia, Pennsylvania
Chapter 83

Angie Veverka, PharmD
Assistant Professor of Pharmacy, Wingate University School of Pharmacy, Wingate, North Carolina
Chapter 115

Sheryl F. Vondracek, PharmD, FCCP, BCPS
Associate Professor, Department of Clinical Pharmacy, University of Colorado-Denver; School of Pharmacy, Aurora, Colorado
Chapter 93

William E. Wade, PharmD, FASHP, FCCP
Professor, College of Pharmacy, University of Georgia, Athens, Georgia
Chapter 38

Nicole A. Weimert, PharmD, BCPS
Clinical Specialist, Solid Organ Transplantation, Department of Pharmacy Services; Assistant Clinical Professor, South Carolina College of Pharmacy, Medical University of South Carolina Campus, Charleston, South Carolina
Chapter 89

Benjamin L. Weinstein, MD
Assistant Professor, Department of Psychiatry, Medical University of South Carolina, Charleston, South Carolina
Chapter 72

Lara C. Weinstein, MD
Assistant Professor, Department of Family and Community Medicine, Thomas Jefferson University, Philadelphia, Pennsylvania
Chapter 83

Lynda S. Welage, PharmD, FCCP
Professor of Pharmacy, College of Pharmacy and Associate Dean for Academic Affairs, University of Michigan; Clinical Pharmacist, Critical Care, Department of Pharmacy, University of Michigan Health-System, Ann Arbor, Michigan
Chapter 35

Barbara G. Wells, PharmD, FASHP, FCCP, BCPP
Dean and Professor, Executive Director of the Research Institute of Pharmaceutical Sciences, School of Pharmacy, University of Mississippi, Oxford, Mississippi
Chapters 71 and 74

Lee E. West, BS
Clinical Pharmacist, Northwestern Memorial Hospital, Chicago, Illinois
Chapters 100 and 101

Dennis P. West, PhD, FCCP, CIP
Vincent W. Foglia Family Research Professor of Dermatology; Director, Dermatology Program, Chair for Administrative Review, IRB, Office for the Protection of Research Subjects, Feinberg School of Medicine, Chicago, Illinois
Chapters 100 and 101

James W. Wheless, MD
Professor and Chief of Pediatric Neurology, LeBonheur Chair in Pediatric Neurology, University of Tennessee Health Science Center; Director, Neuroscience Institute and LeBonheur Comprehensive Epilepsy Program, LeBonheur Children's Medical Center, Memphis, Tennessee
Chapter 59

Dale H. Whitby, PharmD, BCPS
Pediatric Editor, Clinical Pharmacology, Gold Standard, Inc., Tampa, Florida
Chapter 107

Dennis M. Williams, PharmD, BCPS
Associate Professor, Division of Pharmacotherapy and Experiemental Therapeutics, School of Pharmacy, University of North Carolina, Chapel Hill, North Carolina
Chapter 29

Dianne B. Williams, PharmD, BCPS
Drug Information and Formulary Coordinator, MCG Health, Inc.; Associate Clinical Professor, University of Georgia College of Pharmacy, Augusta, Georgia
Chapter 34

Jeffrey L. Wilt, MD, FACP, FCCP
Program Director, Critical Care Fellowship, Michigan State University, Kalamazoo Center for Medical Studies; Associate Professor, College of Human Medicine, Michigan State University, Kalamazoo, Michigan
Chapter 14

Char Witmer, MD
Assistant Professor, Department of Pediatrics, Division of Hematology, Philadelphia, Pennsylvania
Chapter 105

Daniel M. Witt, PharmD, FCCP, BCPS, CACP
Manager, Clinical Pharmacy Services, Kaiser Permanente Colorado, Aurora, Colorado
Chapter 21

Marion R. Wofford, MD, MPH
Associate Professor, Department of Medicine, School of Medicine, University of Mississippi Medical Center, Jackson, Mississippi
Chapter 63

Judith K. Wolf, MD
Associate Professor, Department of Gynecologic Oncology, University of Texas MD Anderson Cancer Center, Houston, Texas
Chapter 136

Jean Wyman, PhD, RN
Professor and Cora, Meldi Siehl Chair in Nursing Research; Clinical Director, Minnesota Continence Associates, University of Minnesota School of Nursing, Minneapolis, Minnesota
Chapter 88

Jack A. Yanovski, MD, PhD
Head, Unit on Growth and Obesity, Program on Developmental Endocrinology and Genetics, National Institute of Child Health and Human Development, National Institutes of Health, Bethesda, Maryland
Chapter 80

Gary C. Yee, PharmD, FCCP, BCOP
Professor, Department of Pharmacy Practice, College of Pharmacy, University of Nebraska Medical Center, Omaha, Nebraska
Chapters 135 and 142

George Zhanel, PharmD, PhD
Professor, Department of Medical Microbiology; Faculty of Medicine, University of Manitoba; Coordinator, Antimicrobial Resistance Program, Departments of Clinical Microbiology and Medicine, Health Sciences Center of Clinical Microbiology and Medicine, Health Sciences Centre, Winnipeg, Manitoba, Canada
Chapter 112

FOREWORD

It's a safe assumption that you didn't purchase this seventh edition of *Pharmacotherapy: A Pathophysiologic Approach* for its foreword. It's probable that most of you will never read these musings. The value of this text lies in its succeeding pages, in the collective knowledge and wisdom conveyed by its authors, and in its ability to help you provide better care for your patients.

It's also a safe assumption that many—perhaps most—readers had not yet begun their careers in pharmacy when the first edition of *Pharmacotherapy: A Pathophysiologic Approach* was published in 1988. This seventh edition will mark the text's 20th anniversary. Noting this milestone, it's appropriate to reflect on a few "then and now" comparisons.

Knowing the time required to conceive and create a new publication of the scope and depth of *Pharmacotherapy: A Pathophysiologic Approach*, I imagine that work began on its first edition sometime around 1985. In February of that year, about 150 pharmacy practitioners and educators gathered in Hilton Head, South Carolina for an Invitational Conference on Directions for Clinical Pharmacy Practice. Organized by the American Society of Hospital (now Health-System) Pharmacists (ASHP), the conference objectives included an evaluation of the status of clinical pharmacy practice and education, and identification of practical ways for advancing clinical practice.[1] Today, most readers of *Pharmacotherapy: A Pathophysiologic Approach* would probably concisely describe their professional mission as "ensuring optimal medication therapy outcomes for patients," or something to that effect. But in 1985, pharmacy's perception of its professional mission could probably best be described by the concept of "drug use control" as articulated by Don Brodie: assuring "optimal safety in the distribution and use of medications."[2] Our emphasis had been focused more on the distribution of medicines and was only just beginning to emphasize how those medicines were used. The Hilton Head Conference, as it came to be known, helped to catalyze a change in how organized pharmacy and individual pharmacists viewed their professional mission—their societal purpose. As noted by Max Ray, who was key in organizing the conference as a member of the ASHP staff at the time, the conference represented ". . . a commitment to the establishment of pharmacy as a true clinical profession." Subsequently, a more specific definition of clinical pharmacy would emerge, the practice philosophy embodied by pharmaceutical care, and today, the set of pharmacist services referred to as medication therapy management.

In 1985, 361 pharmacists graduated from ASHP accredited residency programs. By 2006, that number had increased to nearly 1500 per year. In 1985, 33 schools of pharmacy awarded the Doctor of Pharmacy (PharmD) degree to 812 graduates (most as post-baccalaureate degrees). Responding to evolving trends and future needs within the profession, the Accreditation Council for Pharmacy Education (ACPE) began to implement new accreditation standards and guidelines in 2000. The PharmD degree is now pharmacy's entry-level degree. Accordingly, the number of PharmD graduates has increased more than ten-fold (9040 in 2006). In 1988, Pharmacotherapy and Nutritional Support were formally recognized as specialty areas of pharmacy practice by the Board of Pharmaceutical Specialties. Psychiatric Pharmacy and Oncology Pharmacy followed in 1992 and 1996, respectively. By 2007, more than 5200 pharmacy specialists had become board certified in one or more of these clinical specialties. Research in a variety of care settings has demonstrated the beneficial impact of pharmacists' services on the clinical, humanistic, and economic outcomes of medication use.[3,4] Research conducted by pharmacists contributes important new knowledge to rational pharmacotherapy. We've made real progress. But is it good enough? Our focus has shifted from predominantly emphasizing the control of drug distribution to assuring that our patients receive the optimal benefits and outcomes from their use of medicines. Or has it?

In 1985, spending for prescription drugs in the United States was just over $22 billion. By 2005, that figure had increased to just over $200 billion (i.e., almost ten-fold in 20 years!), and is predicted to rise to almost $500 billion in 2016.[5] A hefty sum indeed, but not the complete picture. Consider that in addition to these costs for the medications themselves, an additional $177 billion is estimated to be spent annually because of treatment failure or drug-related morbidity and mortality among ambulatory patients alone.[6] Add to this the human and financial costs associated with medication errors, drug-related problems among nursing home residents, and adverse drug events among hospitalized patients, and the real cost is truly staggering.[7,8] It is not hyperbole to say that we are in the midst of a public health crisis.

In 2004, the Joint Commission of Pharmacy Practitioners (JCPP) and the eleven national pharmacy organizations that comprise its membership endorsed a future vision of pharmacy practice:

> *Pharmacists will be the health care professionals responsible for providing patient care that ensures optimal medication therapy outcomes.*

The JCPP vision statement goes on to describe pharmacy practice and how pharmacy will benefit patients and society in 2015.[9] It is my hope that all readers of *Pharmacotherapy: A Pathophysiologic Approach* would adopt this statement not just as a lofty vision for the future of our profession but as their own professional mission—the reason we exist today!

But consider, by "optimal" do we mean "as good as can be expected under the circumstances" the way many dictionaries would define the word? Or do we mean "best possible"? If we're satisfied with the former definition, then let's declare victory and break out the champagne. However, I hope you agree that we could do better for our patients. This public health crisis demands rapid and significant transformation of our medication use system and more effective deployment of resources within that system. One such resource is the nation's pharmacists. As significant as our accomplishments of the past 20 years may appear to be, we cannot rely on a similar, largely evolutionary process as we address this crisis of medication use over the next decade or two. On the whole, today's generation of pharmacists is better educated and trained as clinicians than any other in our history. But as important as that foundation is, it will not suffice alone.

Our pharmacy practices—from the corner drug store in rural America to the most specialized tertiary care center—must adopt a philosophy of practice that emphasizes the pharmacist's patient care responsibilities. The use of support personnel and technology must be optimized so pharmacists can devote the majority of their effort to these patient care responsibilities. Management must adopt different benchmarks for assessing pharmacist productivity. No longer should the key measurement be the number of prescriptions filled. Our metrics must focus instead on patient outcomes that are affected by pharmacists' medication therapy management and other patient care responsibilities (e.g., wellness, disease prevention).

Of course, this practice model must be economically viable. Currently, payment for pharmacy services is largely based on payment for the drug product and the act of dispensing it. Concerted efforts are underway to change the payment policies of both private and government payers and develop the infrastructure needed to enable a different paradigm. However, we cannot wait until all of the payment ducks have been put in a row to broadly implement the philosophy and model of practice alluded to above. We should not expect private and government health plans to cover pharmacists' medication therapy management and other patient care services if their customers (i.e., our patients) aren't demanding that they do so. In turn, we should not expect our customers (e.g., patients, other health professionals) to demand something they have not personally experienced and come to value. It is our responsibility to create that demand through every encounter with a patient, caregiver, family member, or other health professional.

It must begin with us. With our professional knowledge, skills, and attitudes. With a commitment to care for, and about, patients. With a commitment to drive change in a system that needs a lot of change. Our patients need and deserve nothing less than our true best.

Robert M. Elenbaas, PharmD, FCCP

Kansas City, Missouri

Executive Director, American College of Clinical Pharmacy (1986–2003)

Director, ACCP Research Institute (2004–2006)

References

1. Directions for clinical practice in pharmacy. Proceedings of an invitational conference conducted by the ASHP Research and Education Foundation and the American Society of Hospital Pharmacists. February 10–13, 1985. Am J Health Syst Pharm 1985;42:1287–1292.
2. Brodie DC. Drug use control: Keystone to pharmaceutical service. Drug Intell Clin Pharm 1967;1:63–65
3. Schumock GT, Butler MG, Meek PD, et al. Evidence of the economic benefit of clinical pharmacy services: 1996–2000. Pharmacotherapy 2003;23:113–132.
4 Schumock GT, Meek PD, Ploetz PA, Vermeulen LC. Economic evaluations of clinical pharmacy services—1988–1995. Pharmacotherapy 1996;16:1188–1208.
5. Kaiser Family Foundation. Prescription drug trends. May 2007. Available from kff.org/rxdrugs/upload/3057_06.pdf. Accessed October 23, 2007.
6. Ernst FR, Grizzle AJ. Drug-related morbidity and mortality: Updating the cost-of-illness model. J Am Pharm Assoc 2001;41:192–199.
7. Lazarou J, Pomeranz BH, Corey PN. Incidence of adverse drug reactions in hospitalized patients. A meta-analysis of prospective studies. JAMA 1998;279:1200–1205.
8. Gurwitz JH. Improving the quality of medication use in elderly patients. A not-so-simple prescription. Arch Intern Med 2002;162: 1670–1672.
9. JCPP future vision of pharmacy practice. Available from aacp.org/Docs/MainNavigation/Resources/6725_JCPPFutureVisionofPharmacyPracticeFINAL.pdf. Accessed October 23, 2007.

FOREWORD TO THE FIRST EDITION

Evidence of the maturity of a profession is not unlike that characterizing the maturity of an individual; a child's utterances and behavior typically reveal an unrealized potential for attainment, eventually, of those attributes characteristic of an appropriately confident, independently competent, socially responsible, sensitive, and productive member of society.

Within a period of perhaps 15 or 20 years, we have witnessed a profound maturation within the profession of pharmacy. The utterances of the profession, as projected in its literature, have evolved from mostly self-centered and self-serving issues of trade protection to a composite of expressed professional interests that prominently include responsible explorations of scientific/technological questions and ethical issues that promote the best interests of the clientele served by the profession. With the publication of *Pharmacotherapy: A Pathophysiologic Approach*, pharmacy's utterances bespeak a matured practitioner who is able to call upon unique knowledge and skills so as to function as an appropriately confident, independently competent pharmacotherapeutics expert.

In 1987, the Board of Pharmaceutical Specialties (BPS), in denying the petition filed by the American College of Clinical Pharmacy (ACCP) to recognize "clinical pharmacy" as a specialty, conceded nonetheless that the petitioning party had documented in its petition a specialist who does in fact exist within the practice of pharmacy and whose expertise clearly can be extricated from the performance characteristics of those in general practice. A refiled petition from ACCP requests recognition of "pharmacotherapy" as a Specialty Area of Pharmacy Practice. While the BPS had issued no decision when this book went to press, it is difficult to comprehend the basis for a rejection of the second petition.

Within this book one will find the scientific foundation for the essential knowledge required of one who may aspire to specialty practice as a pharmacotherapist. As is the case with any such publication, its usefulness to the practitioner or the future practitioner is limited to providing such a foundation. To be socially and professionally responsible in practice, the pharmacotherapist's foundation must be continually supplemented and complemented by the flow of information appearing in the primary literature. Of course this is not unique to the general or specialty practice of pharmacy; it is essential to the fulfillment of obligations to clients in any occupation operating under the code of professional ethics.

Because of the growing complexity of pharmacotherapeutic agents, their dosing regimens, and techniques for delivery, pharmacy is obligated to produce, recognize, and remunerate specialty practitioners who can fulfill the profession's responsibilities to society for service expertise where the competence required in a particular case exceeds that of the general practitioner. It simply is a component of our covenant with society and is as important as any other facet of that relationship existing between a profession and those it serves.

The recognition by BPS of pharmacotherapy as an area of specialty practice in pharmacy will serve as an important statement by the profession that we have matured sufficiently to be competent and willing to take unprecedented responsibilities in the collaborative, pharmacotherapeutic management of patient-specific problems. It commits pharmacy to an intention that will not be uniformly or rapidly accepted within the established healthcare community. Nonetheless, this formal action places us on the road to an avowed goal, and acceptance will be gained as the pharmacotherapists proliferate and establish their importance in the provision of optimal, cost-effective drug therapy.

Suspecting that other professions in other times must have faced similar quests for recognition of their unique knowledge and skills I once searched the literature for an example that might parallel pharmacy's modern-day aspirations. Writing in the *Philadelphia Medical Journal*, May 27, 1899, D. H. Galloway, MD, reflected on the need for specialty training and practice in a field of medicine lacking such expertise at that time. In an article entitled "The Anesthetizer as a Specialty," Galloway commented:

> *The anesthetizer will have to make his own place in medicine: the profession will not make a place for him, and not until he has demonstrated the value of his services will it concede him the position which the importance of his duties entitles him to occupy. He will be obliged to define his own rights, duties and privileges, and he must not expect that his own estimate of the importance of his position will be conceded without opposition. There are many surgeons who are unwilling to share either the credit or the emoluments of their work with anyone, and their opposition will be overcome only when they are shown that the importance of their work will not be lessened, but enhanced, by the increased safety and dispatch with which operations may be done. . . .*

It has been my experience that, given the opportunity for one-on-one, collaborative practice with physicians and other health professionals, pharmacy practitioners who have been educated and trained to perform at the level of pharmacotherapeutics specialists almost invariably have convinced the former that "the importance of their work will not be lessened, but enhanced, by the increased safety and dispatch with which" individualized problems of drug therapy could be managed in collaboration with clinical pharmacy practitioners.

It is fortuitous—the coinciding of the release of *Pharmacotherapy: A Pathophysiologic Approach* with ACCP's petitioning of BPS for recognition of the pharmacotherapy specialist. The utterances of a maturing profession as revealed in the contents of this book, and the intraprofessional recognition and acceptance of a higher level of responsibility in the safe, effective, and economical use of drugs and drug products, bode well for the future of the profession and for the improvement of patient care with drugs.

Charles A. Walton, PhD
San Antonio, Texas

PREFACE

Pharmacists and other healthcare professionals who evaluate, design, and recommend pharmacotherapy for the management of their patients face many new and exciting challenges as the twenty-first century matures. With this seventh edition of *Pharmacotherapy: A Pathophysiologic Approach*, we recognize just how complicated our tasks as editors have become. Balancing the need for accurate, thorough, and unbiased information about the treatment of diseases against the publishing realities of deadlines, page counts, and book length, we strive to adhere to our founding precepts:

- Advance the quality of patient care through evidence-based medication therapy management based on sound pharmacotherapeutic principles.
- Enhance the health of our communities by incorporating contemporary health promotion and disease-prevention strategies in our practice environments.
- Motivate young practitioners to enhance the breadth, depth, and quality of care they provide to their patients.
- Challenge pharmacists and other primary-care providers to learn new concepts and refine their understanding of the pathophysiology tenets that undergird the development of individualized therapeutic regimens.
- Present the pharmacy and health care communities with innovative patient assessment, triage, and pharmacotherapy management skills.

While our emphasis in past editions has been to incorporate diseases that were previously untreatable with pharmacologic agents, this seventh edition is focused on application of evidence-based pharmacotherapy. Most of the disease-oriented chapters have incorporated evidence-based treatment guidelines that include, when available, rating indicators for the key therapeutic approaches. Also, as in recent editions:

- Key concepts are listed at the beginning of each chapter and are identified in the text with numbered icons so that the reader can easily jump to the material of interest.
- The most common signs and symptoms of diseases are presented in highlighted Clinical Presentation boxes in disease-specific chapters.
- Clinical controversies in treatment or patient management are highlighted to assure that the reader is aware of these issues and discuss how practitioners are responding to them.
- Each chapter has about 100 of the most important and current references relevant to each disease, with most published since 2000.
- For easy reference, abbreviations and acronyms and their meanings are presented at the end of each chapter.
- A glossary of the medical terms used throughout the text is presented at the end of the book.
- Finally, the diagnostic flow diagrams, treatment algorithms, dosing guideline recommendations, and monitoring approaches that were present in the sixth edition have been refined.

This edition includes eight new chapters. The new Influenza chapter addresses changing presentation of this group of infections and focuses on public health and management of the individual. We have incorporated the influence of the emerging pharmacogenetic knowledge on drug metabolism into an integrated authoritative chapter entitled: Drug Therapy Individualization for Patients with Hepatic Disease or Altered Drug-Metabolizing Status. In the respiratory section of this edition, Primary Pulmonary Hypertension replaces Adult Respiratory Distress Syndrome. Other new chapters include Developmental Disabilities and two oncology chapters, Multiple Myeloma and Myelodysplastic Syndromes.

To make room for these new chapters and stay with a single volume of *Pharmacotherapy*, 11 chapters of this edition are being published in our Pharmacotherapy Online Learning Center, accessible at www.pharmacotherapyonline.com or http://highered.mcgraw-hill.com/sites/0071416137/information_center_view0/. The chapters chosen for Web publication include those of specialized application that may be predominantly used by practitioners rather than serving as core elements of the pharmacotherapy sequences at colleges of pharmacy. In addition, seven introductory chapters provide students and practitioners with an overview of topics typically covered in other courses. Two of the new chapters in this edition are online chapters that focus on the healthcare community's need for accurate, definitive, and concise information regarding emergency preparedness: Identification and Management of Biological Exposures, and Identification and Clinical Management of Chemical and Radiological Exposures. These 11 online chapters are accessible to anyone via the Online Learning Center; users need not have purchased the print text to read this material. Thus, the online chapters are actually more available than are the chapters published in print for this edition.

While preparing for this edition, we sought the advice of users and colleagues to guide modifications. During editing, we reviewed each passage of text—and the references cited—for continued relevance and accuracy. We made deletions, asked authors to summarize concepts more succinctly or use tables to present details more concisely, included new medications as they entered the U.S. market or emerged in other countries, and updated references. This process continued as the book entered production, and even during the review of final proofs, we continued to make changes to ensure that this book is as current and complete as is possible.

As the world increasingly relies on electronic means of communication, we are committed to keeping *Pharmacotherapy* and its companion works, *Pharmacotherapy Casebook: A Patient-Focused Approach* and *Pharmacotherapy Handbook* integral components of clinicians' toolboxes. Two other new works have been created in parallel with the preparation of this edition, *Pharmacotherapy Principles and Practice* and *Pharmacotherapy: A Primary Care Approach*. These texts are intended to meet the needs of additional audiences, including nurse practitioner and physician assistant programs and practicing primary care physicians, nurse practitioners, and physician assistants. The Online Learning Center continues to provide unique features designed to benefit students, practitioners, and faculty around the world. The site includes learning objectives and self-assessment questions for each chapter, and the full text of this book is now available on the publisher's Access Pharmacy site (www.accesspharmacy.com).

In closing, we acknowledge the many hours that *Pharmacotherapy*'s 200 authors contributed to this labor of love. Without their devotion to the cause of improved pharmacotherapy and dedication in maintaining the accuracy, clarity, and relevance of their chapters, this text would unquestionably not be possible. In addition, we thank Michael Weitz, Kim Davis, and James Shanahan and their colleagues at McGraw-Hill for their consistent support of the *Pharmacotherapy* family of resources, insights into trends in publishing and higher education, and the critical attention to detail so necessary in pharmacotherapy.

The Editors
March 2008

SECTION 1
FOUNDATION ISSUES

CHAPTER 1

Pharmacoeconomics: Principles, Methods, and Applications

LISA A. SANCHEZ

KEY CONCEPTS

1. Pharmacoeconomics identifies, measures, and compares the costs and consequences of drug therapy to healthcare systems and society.
2. The perspective of a pharmacoeconomic evaluation is paramount because the study results will be highly dependent on the perspective selected.
3. Healthcare costs can be categorized as direct medical, direct nonmedical, indirect nonmedical, intangible, opportunity, and incremental costs.
4. Economic, humanistic, and clinical outcomes should be considered and valued using pharmacoeconomic methods, to inform local decision making whenever possible.
5. To compare various healthcare choices, economic valuation methods are used, including cost-minimization, cost-benefit, cost-effectiveness, and cost-utility analyses. These methods all provide the means to compare competing treatment options and are similar in the way they measure costs (dollar units). They differ, however, in their measurement of outcomes and expression of results.
6. In today's healthcare settings, pharmacoeconomic methods can be applied for effective formulary management, individual patient treatment, medication policy determination, and resource allocation.
7. When evaluating published pharmacoeconomic studies, the following factors should be considered: study objective, study perspective, pharmacoeconomic method, study design, choice of interventions, costs and consequences, discounting, study results, sensitivity analysis, study conclusions, and sponsorship.
8. Use of economic models and conducting pharmacoeconomic analyses on a local level both can be useful and relevant sources of pharmacoeconomic data when rigorous methods are employed, as outlined in this chapter.

WWW

The complete chapter, learning objectives, and other resources can be found at **www.pharmacotherapyonline.com.**

Today's cost-sensitive healthcare environment has created a competitive and challenging workplace for clinicians. Competition for diminishing resources has necessitated that the appraisal of healthcare goods and services extends beyond evaluations of safety and efficacy and considers the economic impact of these goods and services on the cost of healthcare. A challenge for healthcare professionals is to provide quality patient care while assuring an efficient use of resources.

Defining the *value* of medicine is a common thread that unites today's healthcare practitioners. With serious concerns about rising medication costs and consistent pressure to decrease pharmacy expenditures and budgets, clinicians/prescribers, pharmacists, and other healthcare professionals must answer the question, "What is the value of the pharmaceutical goods and services I provide?" *Pharmacoeconomics*, or the discipline of placing a value on drug therapy,[1] has evolved to answer this question.

Challenged to provide high-quality patient care in the least expensive way, clinicians have developed strategies aimed at containing costs. However, most of these strategies focus solely on determining the least expensive alternative rather than the alternative that represents the best value for the money. The "cheapest" alternative—with respect to drug acquisition cost—is not always the best value for patients, departments, institutions, and healthcare systems.

Quality patient care must not be compromised while attempting to contain costs. The products and services delivered by today's health professionals should demonstrate *pharmacoeconomic value*, that is, a balance of economic, humanistic, *and* clinical outcomes. Pharmacoeconomics can provide the systematic means for this quantification. This chapter discusses the principles and methods of pharmacoeconomics and how they can be applied to clinical pharmacy practice and thereby how they can assist in the valuation of pharmacotherapy and other modalities of treatment in clinical practice.

CHAPTER 2 Health Outcomes and Quality of Life

STEPHEN JOEL COONS

KEY CONCEPTS

❶ The evaluation of healthcare is increasingly focused on the assessment of the *outcomes* of medical interventions.

❷ An essential patient-reported outcome is self-assessed function and well-being, or health-related quality of life (HRQOL).

❸ In certain chronic conditions, HRQOL may be the most important health outcome to consider in assessing treatment.

❹ Information about the impact of pharmacotherapy on HRQOL can provide additional data for making decisions regarding medication use.

❺ HRQOL instruments can be categorized as generic/general or targeted/specific.

❻ In HRQOL research, the quality of the data collection tool is the major determinant of the overall quality of the results.

Although it has not involved the comprehensive reform that may be necessary,[1] the medical care marketplace in the United States continues to experience change in both the financing and delivery of care.[2] This change is evidenced by a variety of developments, including an increase in investor-owned organizations, heightened competition, numerous mergers and acquisitions, increasingly sophisticated clinical and administrative information systems, and new financing and organizational structures. In this dynamic and increasingly competitive environment, there is a concern that healthcare quality is being compromised in the push to contain costs. ❶ As a consequence, there has been a growing movement to focus the evaluation of healthcare on the assessment of the end results, or *outcomes,* associated with medical care delivery systems as well as specific medical interventions. The primary objective of this effort is to maximize the net health benefit derived from the use of finite healthcare resources.[3] However, there is a serious lack of critical information as to what value is received for the tremendous amount of resources expended on medical care.[4] This lack of critical information as to the outcomes produced is an obstacle to optimal healthcare decision making at all levels.

The complete chapter, learning objectives, and other resources can be found at **www.pharmacotherapyonline.com.**

HEALTH OUTCOMES

Although the implicit objective of medical care is to improve health outcomes, until relatively recently, little attention was paid to the explicit measurement of them. An outcome is one of the three components of the conceptual framework articulated by Donabedian for assessing and ensuring the quality of healthcare: *structure, process,* and *outcome.*[5] For far too long, the approach to evaluating healthcare had emphasized the structure and processes involved in medical care delivery rather than the outcomes. However, healthcare regulators, payers, providers, manufacturers, and patients are placing increasing emphasis on the outcomes that medical care products and services produce.[6] As stated by Ellwood, outcomes research is "designed to help patients, payers, and providers make rational medical care choices based on better insight into the effect of these choices on the patient's life."[7]

TYPES OF OUTCOMES

The types of outcomes that result from medical care interventions can be described in a number of ways. One classic list, called the *five D's*—death, disease, disability, discomfort, and dissatisfaction—captures a limited range of outcomes for use in assessing the quality of medical care.[7] The *five D's* do not reflect any positive health outcomes and, as a result, have little value in contemporary outcomes research.

A more comprehensive conceptual framework, the ECHO model, places outcomes into three categories: *e*conomic, *c*linical, and *h*umanistic *o*utcomes.[8] As described by Kozma et al.,[8] *economic outcomes* are the direct, indirect, and intangible costs compared with the consequences of a medical intervention. *Clinical outcomes* are the medical events that occur as a result of the condition and/or its treatment. ❷ *Humanistic outcomes,* which now are more commonly called *patient-reported outcomes,*[9] are the consequences of the disease and/or its treatment as perceived and reported by the patient.

Patient-reported outcomes (PROs) refer to a number of important outcomes, including self-assessed health status, symptom experience, treatment satisfaction, and functioning and perceived well-being. PROs are increasingly being used to complement safety data, survival rates, and traditional indicators of clinical efficacy in therapeutic intervention trials.[10]

CHAPTER 3

Evidence-Based Medicine

ELAINE CHIQUETTE AND L. MICHAEL POSEY

KEY CONCEPTS

1. The best current evidence integrated into clinical expertise ensures optimal care for patients.
2. The four steps in the process of applying evidence-based medicine (EBM) in practice are (a) formulate a clear question from a patient's problem, (b) identify relevant information, (c) critically appraise available evidence, and (d) implement the findings in clinical practice.
3. The decision as to whether to implement the results of a specific study, conclusions of a review article, or another piece of evidence in clinical practice depends on the quality (i.e., internal validity) of the evidence, its clinical importance, whether benefits outweigh risks and costs, and its relevance in the clinical setting and patient's circumstances.
4. EBM strategies can be applied to help in keeping current.
5. EBM is realistic.

In the information age, clinicians are presented with a daunting number of diseases and possible treatments to consider as they care for patients each day. As knowledge increases and as the technology for accessing information becomes widely available, healthcare professionals are expected to stay current in their fields of expertise and to remain competent throughout their careers. In addition, the number of information sources for the typical practitioner has ballooned, and clinicians must sort out information from many sources: college courses and continuing education (including seminars and journals), pharmaceutical representatives, and colleagues, as well as guidelines from committees of healthcare facilities, governmental agencies, and expert committees and organizations.

❶ How does the healthcare professional find valid information from such a cacophony? Increasingly, clinicians are turning to the principles of evidence-based medicine (EBM) to identify the best course of action for each patient. EBM strategies help healthcare professionals to ferret out these gold nuggets, enabling them to integrate the best current evidence into their pharmacotherapeutic decision making. These strategies can help physicians, pharmacists, and other healthcare professionals to distinguish reliably beneficial pharmacotherapies from those that are ineffective or harmful. Also, EBM approaches can be applied to keep up-to-date and to make an overwhelming task seem more manageable.

This chapter describes the principles of EBM, offers guidance for finding EBM sources on the World Wide Web, provides a model for applying EBM in patient care, and explains how EBM strategies can help a practitioner stay current.

WHAT IS EVIDENCE-BASED MEDICINE?

EBM is an approach to medical practice that uses the results of patient care research and other available objective evidence as a component of clinical decision making. Similarly, evidence-based pharmacotherapy, defined by Etminan et al.,[1] is an approach to decision making whereby clinicians appraise the scientific evidence and its strength in support of their therapeutic decisions.

Although few would argue against the necessity for basing clinical decisions on the best possible evidence available, considerable controversy actually surrounds the practice of EBM. Critics note that not all questions relevant to the care of a patient are of a scientific nature and that EBM favors a "cookbook" approach. In fact, EBM integrates knowledge from research with other factors affecting clinical decision making. EBM does not replace clinical judgment. Rather, it informs clinical judgment with the current best evidence. The expertise and experience of the clinician who understands the disease are crucial in determining whether the external evidence applies to the patient and whether it should be integrated in the therapeutic plan. Also, nonmedical factors affect decision making, such as the patient's preferences and readiness and the healthcare delivery system's characteristics.

Other critics state that EBM considers randomized controlled trials (RCTs) as the only evidence to be used in clinical decision making. Actually, EBM seeks the best existing evidence, from basic science to clinical research, with which to inform clinical decision. For example, a decision about the accuracy of a diagnostic test is best informed by evidence from a cross-sectional study, not a RCT. A cohort study, not a RCT, best answers a question about prognosis. However, in selecting a treatment, the RCT is the best study design to provide the most accurate estimate of treatment efficacy and safety.

WWW

The complete chapter, learning objectives, and other resources can be found at **www.pharmacotherapyonline.com.**

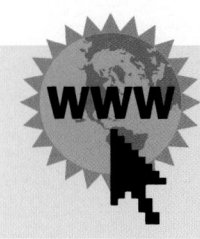

CHAPTER 4

Documentation of Pharmacy Services

GEORGE E. MACKINNON III AND NEIL J. MACKINNON

KEY CONCEPTS

1. Documentation of pharmacists' interventions, their actions, and the impact on patient outcomes is central to the process of pharmaceutical care.
2. Unless pharmacists in all practice settings document their activities and communicate with other health professionals, they may not be considered an essential and integral part of the healthcare team.
3. Manual systems of documentation for pharmacists have been described in detail, but increasingly electronic systems are used to facilitate integration with other clinicians, payer records, and healthcare systems.
4. Integrated electronic information systems can facilitate provision of seamless care as patients move among ambulatory, acute, and long-term care settings.
5. Medication reconciliation, a process of ensuring documentation of the patient's correct medication profile, has become a central part of patient safety activities in recent years.
6. Systems of pharmacy documentation are becoming increasingly important models in the United States as the Medicare Part D Prescription Drug Plan and accompanying Medication Therapy Management Services are implemented and revised.
7. Electronic medical records and prescribing systems have several advantages over manual systems that will facilitate access by community pharmacists and their participation as fully participating and acknowledged members of the healthcare team.

As the opportunities to become more patient-focused increase and market pressures exert increased accountability for pharmacists' actions, the importance of documenting pharmacists' professional activities related to patient care will become paramount in the years to come. Processes to document the clinical activities and therapeutic interventions of pharmacists have been described extensively in the pharmacy literature, yet universal adoption of documentation throughout pharmacy practice remains inconsistent, incomplete, and misunderstood.

(1) Documentation is central to the provision of patient-centered care/pharmaceutical care.[1] Pharmaceutical care is provided through a "system" in which feedback loops are established for monitoring purposes. This has advantages compared with the traditional medication-use process because the system enhances communication among members of the healthcare team and the patient. Pharmaceutical care requires responsibility by the provider to identify drug/medication-related problems (DRPs), provide a therapeutic monitoring plan, and ensure that patients receive the most appropriate medicines and ultimately achieve their desired level of health-related quality of life (HRQOL).

To provide pharmaceutical care, the pharmacist, patient, and other providers enter a covenantal relationship that is considered to be mutually beneficial to all parties. The patient grants the pharmacist the opportunity to provide care, and the pharmacist, in turn, must accept this and the responsibility it entails. Documentation enables the pharmaceutical care model of pharmacy practice to be maximized and communicated to vested parties. Communication among sites of patient care must be accurate and timely to facilitate pharmaceutical care. As discussed by Hepler and Stand,[1] documentation supports care that is coordinated, efficient, and cooperative.

Conversely, failure to document activities and patient outcomes can directly affect patients' quality of care. There are several reasons for failure to document in the medication-use system, and they are related to the process of documentation, the specific data collected on a consistent basis, how documentation is shared (e.g., other pharmacists, healthcare providers, patients, insurers), and methods by which the data are shared.

The contributions of Denise Sprague to the content of this chapter are acknowledged.

WWW

The complete chapter, learning objectives, and other resources can be found at **www.pharmacotherapyonline.com.**

CHAPTER 5

Clinical Pharmacokinetics and Pharmacodynamics

LARRY A. BAUER

KEY CONCEPTS

1. Clinical pharmacokinetics is the discipline that describes the absorption, distribution, metabolism, and elimination of drugs in patients requiring drug therapy.

2. Clearance is the most important pharmacokinetic parameter because it determines the steady-state concentration for a given dosage rate. Physiologically, clearance is determined by blood flow to the organ that metabolizes or eliminates the drug and the efficiency of the organ in extracting the drug from the bloodstream.

3. The volume of distribution is a proportionality constant that relates the amount of drug in the body to the serum concentration. The volume of distribution is used to calculate the loading dose of a drug that will immediately achieve a desired steady-state concentration. The value of the volume of distribution is determined by the physiologic volume of blood and tissues and how the drug binds in blood and tissues.

4. Half-life is the time required for serum concentrations to decrease by one-half after absorption and distribution are complete. Half-life is important because it determines the time required to reach steady state and the dosage interval. Half-life is a dependent kinetic variable because its value depends on the values of clearance and volume of distribution.

5. The fraction of drug absorbed into the systemic circulation after extravascular administration is defined as its bioavailability.

6. Most drugs follow linear pharmacokinetics, whereby steady-state serum drug concentrations change proportionally with long-term daily dosing.

7. Some drugs do not follow the rules of linear pharmacokinetics. Instead of steady-state drug concentration changing proportionally with dose, serum concentration changes more or less than expected. These drugs follow nonlinear pharmacokinetics.

8. Pharmacokinetic models are useful to describe data sets, to predict serum concentrations after several doses or different routes of administration, and to calculate pharmacokinetic constants such as clearance, volume of distribution, and half-life. The simplest case uses a single compartment to represent the entire body.

Learning objectives, review questions, and other resources can be found at **www.pharmacotherapyonline.com.**

9. Factors to be taken into consideration when deciding on the best drug dose for a patient include age, gender, weight, ethnic background, other concurrent disease states, and other drug therapy.

10. Cytochrome P450 is a generic name for the group of enzymes that are responsible for most drug metabolism oxidation reactions. Several P450 isozymes have been identified, including CYP1A2, CYP2C9, CYP2C19, CYP2D6, CYP2E1, and CYP3A4.

11. The importance of transport proteins in drug bioavailability and elimination is now better understood. The principal transport protein involved in the movement of drugs across biologic membranes is P-glycoprotein. P-glycoprotein is present in many organs, including the gastrointestinal tract, liver, and kidney.

12. When deciding on initial doses for drugs that are renally eliminated, the patient's renal function should be assessed. A common, useful way to do this is to measure the patient's serum creatinine concentration and convert this value into an estimated creatinine clearance ($CL_{cr\ est}$). For drugs that are eliminated primarily by the kidney (≥60% of the administered dose), some agents will need minor dosage adjustments for $CL_{cr\ est}$ between 30 and 60 mL/min, moderate dosage adjustments for $CL_{cr\ est}$ between 15 and 30 mL/min, and major dosage adjustments for $CL_{cr\ est}$ less than 15 mL/min. Supplemental doses of some medications also may be needed for patients receiving hemodialysis if the drug is removed by the artificial kidney or for patients receiving hemoperfusion if the drug is removed by the hemofilter.

13. When deciding on initial doses for drugs that are hepatically eliminated, the patient's liver function should be assessed. The Child-Pugh score can be used as an indicator of a patient's ability to metabolize drugs that are eliminated by the liver. In the absence of specific pharmacokinetic dosing guidelines for a medication, a Child-Pugh score equal to 8 or 9 is grounds for a moderate decrease (~25%) in initial daily drug dose for agents that are metabolized primarily hepatically (≥60%), and a score of 10 or greater indicates that a significant decrease in initial daily dose (~50%) is required for drugs that are metabolized mostly hepatically.

14. For drugs that exhibit linear pharmacokinetics, steady-state drug concentration (C_{ss}) changes proportionally with dose (D). To adjust a patient's drug therapy, a reasonable starting dose is administered for an estimated three to five half-lives. A serum concentration is obtained, assuming that it will reflect C_{ss}. Independent of the route of administration, the new dose (D_{new}) needed to attain the desired C_{ss} ($C_{ss,new}$) is calculated: $D_{new} = D_{old}(C_{ss,new}/C_{ss,old})$, where D_{old} and $C_{ss,old}$ are the old dose and old C_{ss}, respectively.

⓯ If it is necessary to determine the pharmacokinetic constants for a patient to individualize the patient's dose, a small pharmacokinetic evaluation is conducted in the individual. Additionally, Bayesian computer programs that aid in the individualization of therapy are available for many different drugs.

⓰ Pharmacodynamics is the study of the relationship between the concentration of a drug and the response obtained in a patient. If pharmacologic effect is plotted versus concentration for most drugs, a hyperbola results with an asymptote equal to maximum attainable effect.

Pharmacokinetic concepts have been used successfully by pharmacists to individualize patient drug therapy for about a quarter of a century. Pharmacokinetic consultant services and individual clinicians routinely provide patient-specific drug-dosing recommendations that increase the efficacy and decrease the toxicity of many medications. Laboratories routinely measure patient serum or plasma samples for many drugs, including antibiotics (e.g., aminoglycosides and vancomycin), theophylline, antiepileptics (e.g., phenytoin, carbamazepine, valproic acid, phenobarbital, and ethosuximide), methotrexate, lithium, antiarrhythmics (e.g., lidocaine, procainamide, quinidine, and digoxin), and immunosuppressants (e.g., cyclosporine and tacrolimus). Combined with a knowledge of the disease states and conditions that influence the disposition of a particular drug, kinetic concepts can be used to modify doses to produce serum drug concentrations that result in desirable pharmacologic effects without unwanted side effects. This narrow range of concentrations within which the pharmacologic response is produced and adverse effects prevented in most patients is defined as the *therapeutic range* of the drug. Table 5–1 lists the therapeutic ranges for commonly used medications.

Although most individuals experience favorable effects with serum drug concentrations in the therapeutic range, the effects of a given serum concentration can vary widely among individuals. Clinicians should never assume that a serum concentration within the therapeutic range will be safe and effective for every patient. The response to the drug, such as number of seizures a patient experiences while taking an antiepileptic agent, always should be assessed when serum concentrations are measured.

TABLE 5-1 Selected Therapeutic Ranges

Drug	Therapeutic Range
Digoxin	0.5–2 ng/mL
Lidocaine	1.5–5 mcg/mL
Procainamide/N-acetylprocainamide	10–30 mcg/mL (total)
Quinidine	2–5 mcg/mL
Amikacin[a]	20–30 mcg/mL (peak) <5 mcg/mL (trough)
Gentamicin, tobramycin, netilmicin[a]	5–10 mcg/mL (peak) <2 mcg/mL (trough)
Vancomycin	20–40 mcg/mL (peak) 5–10 mcg/mL (trough)
Chloramphenicol	10–20 mcg/mL
Lithium	0.6–1.4 mEq/L
Carbamazepine	4–12 mcg/mL
Ethosuximide	40–100 mcg/mL
Phenobarbital	15–40 mcg/mL
Phenytoin	10–20 mcg/mL
Primidone	5–12 mcg/mL
Valproic acid	50–100 mcg/mL
Theophylline	10–20 mcg/mL
Cyclosporine	150–400 ng/mL (blood)

[a]Using a multiple-dose-per-day dosage schedule.

TABLE 5-2 Pharmacokinetic Abbreviations

Abbreviation	Definition
CL	Clearance
k_0	Intravenous infusion rate
C_{SS}	Steady-state concentration
D	Dose
τ	Dosage interval
F	Fraction of drug absorbed into the systemic circulation
Q	Blood flow
E	Extraction ratio
f_b	Fraction of drug in the blood that is unbound
CL_{int}	Intrinsic clearance
$C_{ss,u}$	Steady-state concentration of unbound drug
V_D	Volume of distribution
LD	Loading dose
MD	Maintenance dose
$t_{1/2}$	Half-life
k	Elimination rate constant
k_a	Absorption rate constant
α	Distribution rate constant
β	Terminal rate constant
t′	Postinfusion time
T	Duration of infusion
AUC	Area under serum- or blood-concentration-versus-time curve
V_{max}	Maximum rate of drug metabolism
K_m	Serum concentration at which the rate of metabolism equals $V_{max}/2$
C_{max}	Maximum serum or blood concentration
C_{min}	Minimum serum or blood concentration
DR	Dosage rate
P-gp	P-glycoprotein

Throughout this chapter, abbreviations for various pharmacokinetic parameters are used frequently. Table 5–2 lists commonly used abbreviations.

CLINICAL PHARMACOKINETIC CONCEPTS

❶ Clinical pharmacokinetics is the discipline that describes the absorption, distribution, metabolism, and elimination of drugs in patients requiring drug therapy. When a drug is administered extravascularly to patients, it must be absorbed across biologic membranes to reach the systemic circulation. If the drug is given orally, the drug molecules must pass through the gastrointestinal tract wall into capillaries. For transdermal patches, the drug must penetrate the skin to enter the vascular system. In general, the pharmacologic effect of the drug is delayed when it is given extravascularly because time is required for the drug to be absorbed into the vascular system.

The vascular system generally provides the "transportation" for the drug molecule to its site of activity. After the drug reaches the systemic circulation, it can leave the vasculature and penetrate the various tissues or remain in the blood. If the drug remains in the blood, it may bind to endogenous proteins such as albumin or α_1-acid glycoprotein. This binding usually is reversible, and an equilibrium is created between protein-bound drug and unbound drug. Unbound drug in the blood provides the driving force for distribution of the agent to body tissues. If unbound drug leaves the bloodstream and distributes to tissue, it may become tissue-bound, it may remain unbound in the tissue, or if the tissue can metabolize or eliminate the drug, it may be rendered inactive and/or eliminated from the body. If the drug becomes tissue-bound, it may bind to the receptor that causes its pharmacologic or toxic effect or to a nonspecific binding site that causes no effect. Again, tissue binding is usually reversible so that the tissue-bound drug is in equilibrium with unbound drug in the tissue.

Certain organs—such as the liver, gastrointestinal tract wall, and lung—possess enzymes that metabolize drugs. The resulting metabolite may be inactive or have a pharmacologic effect of its own. The blood also contains esterases, which cleave ester bonds in drug molecules and generally render them inactive.

Drug metabolism usually occurs in the liver through one or both of two types of reactions. Phase I reactions generally make the drug molecule more polar and water soluble so that it is prone to elimination by the kidney. Phase I modifications include oxidation, hydrolysis, and reduction. Phase II reactions involve conjugation to form glucuronides, acetates, or sulfates. These reactions generally inactivate the pharmacologic activity of the drug and may make it more prone to elimination by the kidney.

Other organs have the ability to eliminate drugs or metabolites from the body. The kidney can excrete drugs by glomerular filtration or by such active processes as proximal tubular secretion. Drugs also can be eliminated via bile produced by the liver or air expired by the lungs.

LINEAR PHARMACOKINETICS

(6) Most drugs follow linear pharmacokinetics: Serum drug concentrations change proportionally with long-term daily dosing. For example, if a drug dose were doubled from 300 to 600 mg/day, the patient's serum drug concentration would double.

When a drug is given by continuous intravenous infusion, serum concentrations increase until an equilibrium is established between the drug dosage rate and the rate of drug elimination. At that point, the rate of drug administration equals the rate of drug elimination, and the serum concentrations remain constant (Fig. 5–1). For example, if a patient were receiving a continuous intravenous infusion of theophylline at 40 mg/h, the theophylline serum concentration would increase until the patient's body was eliminating theophylline at 40 mg/h. When serum drug concentrations reach a constant value, steady state is achieved.

If the drug is given at intermittent dosage intervals, such as 250 mg every 6 hours, steady state is achieved when the serum-concentration-versus-time curves for each dosage interval are superimposable. The amount of drug eliminated during the dosage interval equals the dose.

BIOAVAILABILITY AND BIOEQUIVALENCE

When drugs are administered extravascularly, drug molecules must be released from the dosage form (dissolution) and pass through several biologic barriers before reaching the vascular system (5) (absorption). The fraction of drug absorbed into the systemic circulation (F) after extravascular administration is defined as its *bioavailability* and can be calculated after single intravenous and extravascular doses as[1]

$$F = \frac{D_{iv}(AUC_{0-\infty})}{D(AUC_{iv,0-\infty})}$$

where D and D_{iv} are the extravascular and intravenous doses, respectively, and $AUC_{iv,0\text{-}\infty}$ and $AUC_{0\text{-}\infty}$ are the intravenous and extravascular areas under the serum- or blood-concentration-versus-time curves, respectively, from time zero to infinity. The AUC represents the body's total exposure to the drug and is a function of the fraction of the drug dose that enters the systemic circulation via the administered route and clearance (Fig. 5–2). When F is less than 1 for a drug administered extravascularly, either the dosage form did not release all the drug contained in it, or some of the drug was eliminated or destroyed (by stomach acid or other means) before it reached the systemic circulation.

When the extravascular dose is administered orally, part of the dose may be metabolized by enzymes or removed by transport proteins contained in the gastrointestinal tract wall or liver before it reaches the systemic circulation.[2,3] This occurs commonly when drugs have a high liver extraction ratio or are subject to gastrointestinal tract wall metabolism because, after oral administration, the drug must pass through the gastrointestinal tract wall and into the portal circulation of the liver. Transport proteins are also present in the gastrointestinal tract wall that can actively pump drug molecules that already have been absorbed back into the lumen of the gastrointestinal tract. P-glycoprotein (P-gp) is the primary transport protein that interferes with drug absorption by this mechanism. For example, if an orally administered drug is 100% absorbed from the gastrointestinal tract but has a hepatic extraction ratio of 0.75, only 25% of the original dose enters the systemic circulation. This first-pass effect through the liver and/or gastrointestinal tract wall is avoided when the drug is given by other routes of administration. The computation of F does not separate loss of oral drug metabolized by the first-pass effect and drug not absorbed by the gastrointestinal tract. Special techniques are needed to determine the fraction of drug absorbed orally for drugs with high liver extraction ratios or substantial gut wall metabolism.

Two different dosage forms of the same drug are considered to be bioequivalent when the $AUC_{0\text{-}\infty}$, maximum serum or blood concen-

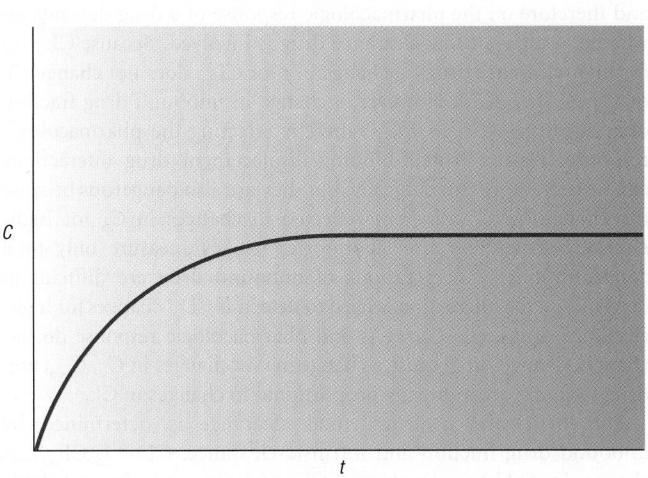

FIGURE 5-1. Normal serum concentration-time curve following a continuous intravenous infusion.

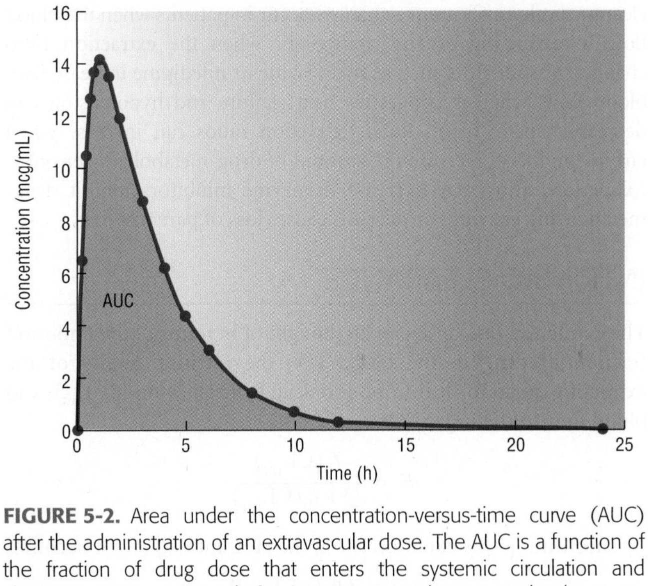

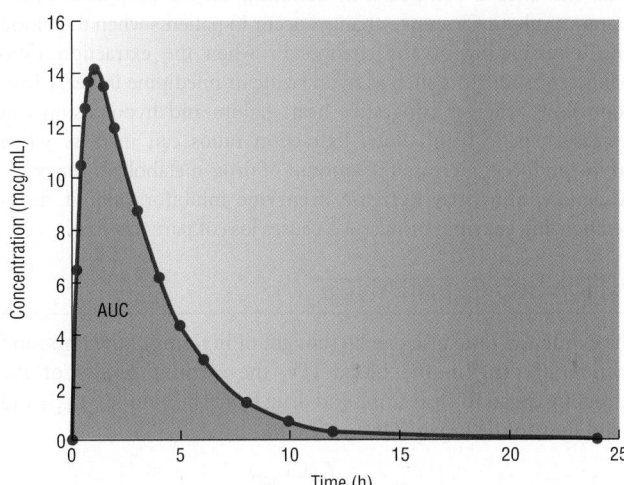

FIGURE 5-2. Area under the concentration-versus-time curve (AUC) after the administration of an extravascular dose. The AUC is a function of the fraction of drug dose that enters the systemic circulation and clearance. AUCs measured after intravenous and extravascular doses can be used to determine bioavailability for the extravascular dose.

trations (C_{max}), and the times that C_{max} occurs (t_{max}) are neither clinically nor statistically different. When this occurs, the serum-concentration-versus-time curves for the two dosage forms should be superimposable and identical. Bioequivalence studies have become very important as expensive drugs become available in less costly generic form. Most bioequivalence studies involve 18 to 25 healthy adults who are given the brand-name product and the generic product in a randomized, crossover study design.

CLEARANCE

❷ Clearance (CL) is the most important pharmacokinetic parameter because it determines the steady-state concentration for a given dosage rate. When a drug is given at a continuous intravenous infusion rate equal to k_0, the steady-state concentration (C_{ss}) is determined by the quotient of k_0 and CL ($C_{ss} = k_0/CL$). If the drug is administered as individual doses (D) at a given dosage interval (τ), the average steady-state concentration (C_{ss}) over the dosage interval is given by the equation[4]

$$C_{ss} = \frac{F(D/\tau)}{\mathrm{CL}}$$

where F is the fraction of dose absorbed into the systemic vascular system. The average steady-state concentration over the dosage interval is the steady-state concentration that would have occurred had the same dose been given as a continuous intravenous infusion (e.g., 300 mg every 6 hours would produce an average C_{ss} equivalent to the actual C_{ss} produced by a continuous infusion administered at a rate of 50 mg/h).

Physiologically, clearance is determined by (a) blood flow (Q) to the organ that metabolizes (liver) or eliminates (kidney) the drug and (b) the efficiency of the organ in extracting the drug from the bloodstream.[5] Efficiency is measured using an extraction ratio *(E)*, calculated by subtracting the concentration in the blood leaving the extracting organ (C_{out}) from the concentration in the blood entering the organ (C_{in}) and then dividing the result by C_{in}:

$$E = \frac{C_{in} - C_{out}}{C_{in}}$$

Clearance for that organ is calculated by taking the product of Q and E (CL = QE). For example, if liver blood flow equals 1.5 L/min and the drug's extraction ratio is 0.33, hepatic clearance equals 0.5 L/min. Total clearance is computed by summing all the individual organ clearance values. Clearance changes occur in patients when the blood flow to extracting organs changes or when the extraction ratio changes. Vasodilators such as hydralazine or nifedipine increase liver blood flow, whereas congestive heart failure and hypotension can decrease hepatic blood flow. Extraction ratios can increase when enzyme inducers increase the amount of drug-metabolizing enzyme. Extraction ratios may decrease if enzyme inhibitors inhibit drug-metabolizing enzymes or necrosis causes loss of parenchyma.

INTRINSIC CLEARANCE

The extraction ratio also can be thought of in terms of the unbound fraction of drug in the blood (f_b), the intrinsic ability of the extracting organ to clear unbound drug from the blood (CL_{int}), and blood flow to the organ (Q)[6,7]:

$$E = \frac{f_b(CL_{int})}{Q + f_b(CL_{int})}$$

By substituting this equation for E, the clearance equation becomes

$$CL = \frac{Q[f_b(CL_{int})]}{Q + f_b(CL_{int})}$$

Clearance changes will occur when blood flow to the clearing organ changes (in conditions where blood flow is reduced, e.g., shock, congestive heart failure, or where blood flow is increased, e.g., administration of medications such as vasodilators, resolution of shock or congestive heart failure), binding in the blood changes (e.g., if the concentration of binding proteins is low or highly protein-bound drugs are displaced), or intrinsic clearance of unbound drug changes (e.g., when metabolizing enzymes are induced or inhibited by other drug therapy or functional organ tissue is destroyed by disease processes).

If CL_{int} is large (enzymes have a high capacity to metabolize the drug), the product of f_b and CL_{int} is much larger than Q. When $f_b(CL_{int})$ is much greater than Q, the sum of Q and $f_b(CL_{int})$ in the denominator of the clearance equation almost equals $f_b(CL_{int})$:

$$f_b(CL_{int}) \approx Q + f_b(CL_{int})$$

Substituting this expression in the denominator of the clearance equation and canceling common terms leads to the following expression for drugs with a large CL_{int}: CL ≈ Q. In this case, clearance of the drug is equal to blood flow to the organ; such drugs are called *high-clearance drugs* and have large extraction ratios. Propranolol, verapamil, morphine, and lidocaine are examples of high-clearance drugs. High-clearance drugs such as these typically exhibit high first-pass effects when administered orally.

If CL_{int} is small (enzymes have a limited capacity to metabolize the drug), Q is much larger than the product of f_b and CL_{int}. When Q is much greater than $f_b(CL_{int})$, the sum of Q and $f_b(CL_{int})$ in the denominator of the clearance equation becomes almost equal to Q: $Q \approx Q + f_b(CL_{int})$. Substituting this expression in the denominator of the clearance equation and canceling common terms leads to the following expression for drugs with a small CL_{int}: $CL \approx f_b(CL_{int})$. In this case, clearance of the drug is equal to the product of the fraction unbound in the blood and the intrinsic ability of the organ to clear unbound drug from the blood; such drugs are known as *low-clearance drugs* and have small extraction ratios. Warfarin, theophylline, diazepam, and phenobarbital are examples of low-clearance drugs.

As mentioned previously, the concentration of unbound drug in the blood is probably more important pharmacologically than the total (bound plus unbound) concentration. The unbound drug in the blood is in equilibrium with the unbound drug in the tissues and reflects the concentration of drug at its site of action. Therefore, the pharmacologic effect of a drug is thought to be a function of the concentration of unbound drug in the blood. The unbound steady-state concentration ($C_{ss,u}$) can be calculated by multiplying C_{ss} and f_b: $C_{ss,u} = C_{ss}f_b$. The effect that changes in Q, f_b, and CL_{int} have on $C_{ss,u}$ and therefore on the pharmacologic response of a drug depends on whether a high- or low-clearance drug is involved. Because CL = Q for high-clearance drugs, a change in f_b or CL_{int} does not change CL or C_{ss} ($C_{ss} = k_0/CL$). However, a change in unbound drug fraction does alter $C_{ss,u}$ ($C_{ss,u} = f_bC_{ss}$), thereby affecting the pharmacologic response. Plasma-protein-binding displacement drug interactions can be very important clinically, but they are also dangerous because the changes in $C_{ss,u}$ are not reflected in changes in C_{ss} for high-clearance drugs. Because laboratories usually measure only total concentrations (concentrations of unbound drug are difficult to determine), the interaction is hard to detect. If CL_{int} changes for high-clearance drugs, CL, C_{ss}, $C_{ss,u}$, and pharmacologic response do not change. Changes in Q cause a change in CL; changes in C_{ss}, $C_{ss,u}$, and drug response are indirectly proportional to changes in CL.

For low-clearance drugs, total clearance is determined by unbound drug fraction and intrinsic clearance: $CL = f_b(CL_{int})$. A change in Q does not change CL, C_{ss}, $C_{ss,u}$, or pharmacologic response. However, a change in f_b or CL_{int} does alter CL and C_{ss} ($C_{ss} = k_0/CL$). Changes in CL_{int} will cause a proportional change in CL.

Changes in C_{ss}, $C_{ss,u}$, and drug response are indirectly proportional to changes in CL. Altering f_b for low-clearance drugs produces interesting results. A change in f_b alters CL and C_{ss} ($C_{ss} = k_0/CL$). Because CL and C_{ss} change in opposite directions with changes in f_b, $C_{ss,u}$ ($C_{ss,u} = f_b C_{ss}$) and pharmacologic response do not change with alterations in the fraction of unbound drug in the blood. For example, a low-clearance drug is administered to a patient until steady-state is achieved:

$$CL = f_b(CL_{int})$$

$$C_{ss} = \frac{k_0}{CL}$$

Suppose that another drug is administered to the patient that displaces the first drug from plasma-protein-binding sites and doubles f_b (f_b now equals $2f_b$). CL doubles because of the protein-binding displacement [$2CL = 2f_b(CL_{int})$], and C_{ss} decreases by one-half because of the change in clearance [$^1/_2\,(C_{ss}) = k_0/(2Cl)$]. $C_{ss,u}$ does not change because even though f_b is doubled, C_{ss} decreased by one-half ($C_{ss,u} = f_b C_{ss}$). The potential for error in this situation is that clinicians may increase the dose of a low-clearance drug after a protein-binding displacement interaction because C_{ss} decreased. Because $C_{ss,u}$ and the pharmacologic effect do not change, the dose should remain unaltered. Plasma protein binding decreases occur commonly in patients taking phenytoin. Low albumin concentrations (as in trauma or pregnant patients), high concentrations of endogenous plasma protein-binding displacers (as with high concentrations of bilirubin), or plasma protein-binding drug interactions (as with concomitant therapy with valproic acid) can result in subtherapeutic total phenytoin concentrations. Despite this fact, unbound phenytoin concentrations usually are within the therapeutic range, and often the patient is responding appropriately to treatment. Thus, in these situations, unbound rather than total phenytoin serum concentrations should be monitored and used to guide future therapeutic decisions.

CLEARANCES FOR DIFFERENT ROUTES OF ELIMINATION AND METABOLIC PATHWAYS

Clearances for individual organs can be computed if the excretion the organ produces can be obtained. For example, renal clearance can be calculated if urine is collected during a pharmacokinetic experiment. The patient empties his or her bladder immediately before the dose is given. Subsequent urine production is collected until the last serum concentration (C_{last}) is obtained. Renal clearance (CL_R) is computed by dividing the amount of drug excreted in the urine by $AUC_{0-t,last}$. Biliary and other clearance values are computed in a similar fashion.

Clearances also can be calculated for each metabolite that is formed from the parent drug. This computation is particularly useful in drug-interaction studies to determine which metabolic pathway is stimulated or inhibited. In the following metabolic scheme, the parent drug (D) is metabolized into two different metabolites (M_1, M_2) that subsequently are eliminated by the kidney (M_{1R}, M_{2R}):

$$D \xrightarrow{CL_{FM1}} M_1 \xrightarrow{\text{kidney}} M_1$$

$$D \xrightarrow{CL_{FM2}} M_2 \xrightarrow[\text{kidney}]{} M_{2R}$$

To compute the formation clearance of M_1 and M_2 (CL_{FM1}, CL_{FM2}), urine would be collected for five or more half-lives after a single dose or during a dosage interval at steady state. The amount of metabolite eliminated in the urine is then determined. The fraction of the dose (in moles, because the molecular weights of the parent drug and metabolites are not equal) eliminated by each metabolic pathway ($f_{M1} = M_{1R}/D$ and $f_{M2} = M_{2R}/D$) can then be computed. Formation clearance for each pathway can be calculated using the following equations: $CL_{FM1} = f_{M1}CL_M$ and $CL_{FM2} = f_{M2}CL_M$, where CL_M is the metabolic clearance for the parent drug.

VOLUME OF DISTRIBUTION

❸ The volume of distribution (V_D) is a proportionality constant that relates the amount of drug in the body to the serum concentration (amount in body = CV_D). V_D is used to calculate the loading dose (LD) of a drug that will immediately achieve a desired C_{ss} (LD = $C_{ss}V_D$). However, in practice, the patient's own V_D is not known at the time the loading dose is administered. In this case, an average V_D is assumed and used to calculate a loading dose. Because the patient's V_D is almost always different from the average V_D for the drug, a loading dose does not attain the calculated C_{ss}, but it hopefully achieves a therapeutic concentration. As usual, steady-state conditions are achieved in three to five half-lives for the drug.

The numeric value for the volume of distribution is determined by the physiologic volume of blood and tissues and how the drug binds in blood and tissues[8]:

$$V_D = V_b + (f_b/f_t)V_t$$

where V_b and V_t are the volumes of blood and tissues, respectively, and f_b and f_t are the fractions of unbound drug in blood and tissues, respectively.

HALF-LIFE

❹ Half-life ($t_{1/2}$) is the time required for serum concentrations to decrease by one-half after absorption and distribution are complete. It takes the same amount of time for serum concentrations to drop from 200 to 100 mg/L as it does for concentrations to decline from 2 to 1 mg/L (Fig. 5–3).

Half-life is important because it determines the time required to reach steady state and the dosage interval. It takes approximately three to five half-lives to reach steady-state concentrations during continuous dosing. In three half-lives, serum concentrations are at approximately 90% of their ultimate steady-state values. Because most serum drug assays have approximately a 10% error, it is difficult to differentiate concentrations that are within 10% of each

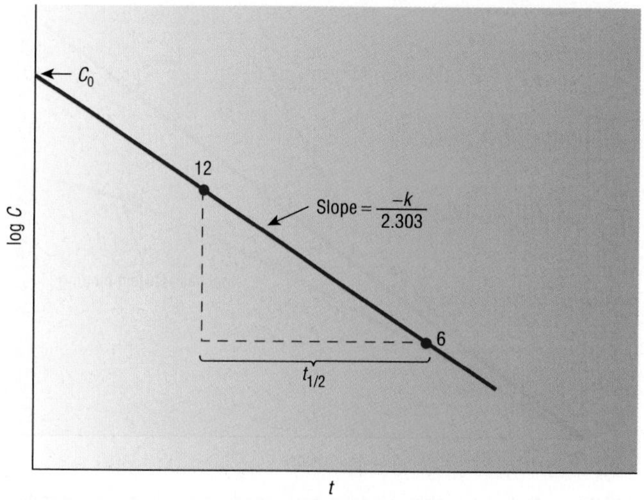

FIGURE 5-3. Calculation of the half-life of a drug following intravenous bolus dosing.

other. For this reason, many clinicians consider concentrations obtained after three half-lives to be C_{ss}.

Half-life is also used to determine the dosage interval for a drug. For instance, it may be desirable to maintain maximum steady-state concentrations at 20 mg/L and minimum steady-state concentrations at 10 mg/L. In this case, it would be necessary to administer the drug every half-life because the minimum desirable concentration is one-half the maximum desirable concentration.

Half-life is a dependent kinetic variable because its value depends on the values of CL and V_D.[8] The equation that describes the relationship among the three variables is $t_{1/2} = 0.693V_D/\text{CL}$. Changes in $t_{1/2}$ can result from a change in either V_D or CL; a change in $t_{1/2}$ does not necessarily indicate that CL has changed. Half-life can change solely because of changes in V_D. The elimination rate constant (k) is related to the half-life by the following equation: $k = 0.693/t_{1/2}$. Both the half-life and elimination rate constant describe how quickly serum concentrations decrease in the serum or blood.

NONLINEAR PHARMACOKINETICS

Michaelis-Menten Kinetics

7 Some drugs do not follow the rules of linear pharmacokinetics. Instead of C_{ss} and AUC increasing proportionally with dose, serum concentrations change more or less than expected (Fig. 5–4). One explanation for the greater-than-expected increase in C_{ss} and AUC after an increase in dose is that the enzymes responsible for the metabolism or elimination of the drug may start to become saturated. When this occurs, the maximum rate of metabolism (V_{max}) for the drug is approached. This is called *Michaelis-Menten kinetics.* The serum concentration at which the rate of metabolism equals $V_{max}/2$ is K_m. Practically speaking, K_m is the serum concentration at which nonproportional changes in C_{ss} and AUC start to occur when dose is increased. The Michaelis-Menten constants (V_{max} and K_m) determine the dosage rate (DR) needed to maintain a given C_{ss}: DR $= V_{max}C_{ss}/(K_m + C_{ss})$. Most drugs eliminated by the liver are metabolized by enzymes but still appear to follow linear kinetics. The reason for this disparity is that the therapeutic range for most drugs is well below the K_m of the enzyme system that metabolizes the agent. The therapeutic range is higher than K_m for some commonly used drugs. The average K_m for phenytoin is about 4 mg/L. The therapeutic range for phenytoin is usually 10 to 20 mg/L. Most patients experience Michaelis-Menten kinetics while taking phenytoin.

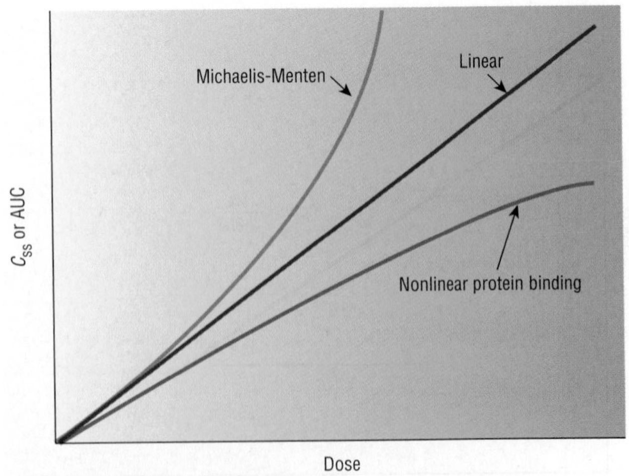

FIGURE 5-4. Relationship of dose and steady-state drug concentration (C_{ss}) or area under the concentration-versus-time curve (AUC) under linear and nonlinear conditions.

Nonlinear Protein Binding

Another type of nonlinear kinetics can occur if C_{ss} and AUC increase less than expected after an increase in dose of a low-clearance drug. This usually indicates that plasma protein-binding sites are starting to become saturated so that f_b increases with increases in dose (see Fig. 5–4). For a low-clearance drug, CL depends on the values of f_b and CL_{int} ($\text{CL} = f_b\text{CL}_{int}$). When a dosage increase takes place, f_b increases because nearly all plasma-protein-binding sites are occupied and no binding sites are available. If f_b increases, CL increases and C_{ss} increases less than expected with the dosage change ($C_{ss} = k_0/\text{CL}$). However, $C_{ss,u}$ increases proportionally with dose because $C_{ss,u}$ depends on CL_{int} for low-clearance drugs ($C_{ss,u} = k_0/\text{CL}_{int}$). Valproic acid[9] and disopyramide[10] both follow saturable protein-binding pharmacokinetics.

PHARMACOKINETIC MODELS AND EQUATIONS

8 Pharmacokinetic models are useful to describe data sets, to predict serum concentrations after several doses or different routes of administration, and to calculate pharmacokinetic constants such as CL, V_D, and $t_{1/2}$.[11] Compartmental models depict the body as one or more discrete compartments to which drug is distributed and/or from which drug is eliminated. The shape of the serum-concentration-versus-time curve determines the number of compartments in the pharmacokinetic model and the equation used in computations (Fig. 5–5). First-order rate constants, known as *microconstants,* describe the rate of transfer from one compartment to another. Each compartment also has its own V_D. For clinical dosage adjustment purposes using drug concentrations, a one-compartment model is the most commonly used pharmacokinetic model.

One-Compartment Model

The simplest case uses a single compartment to represent the entire body (see Fig. 5–5). Drug enters the compartment by continuous intravenous infusion (k_0), absorption from an extravascular site with an absorption rate constant of k_a, or intravenous bolus (D). After an intravenous bolus, serum concentrations decline in a straight line when plotted on semilogarithmic coordinates (see Fig. 5–3). The slope of the line is $-k/2.303$; $t_{1/2}$ can be computed by determining the time required for concentrations to decrease by one-half ($t_{1/2} = 0.693/k$). The equation that describes the data is $C = (D/V_D)e^{-kt}$. V_D is calculated by dividing the intravenous dose by the y intercept (the concentration at time zero, C_0) of the graph. CL is computed by taking the product of k and V_D. Once V_D and k are known, concentrations at any time after the dose can be computed [$C = (D/V_D)e^{-kt}$].

When an extravascular dose is given, one-compartment-model serum concentrations rise during absorption, reach C_{max}, and then

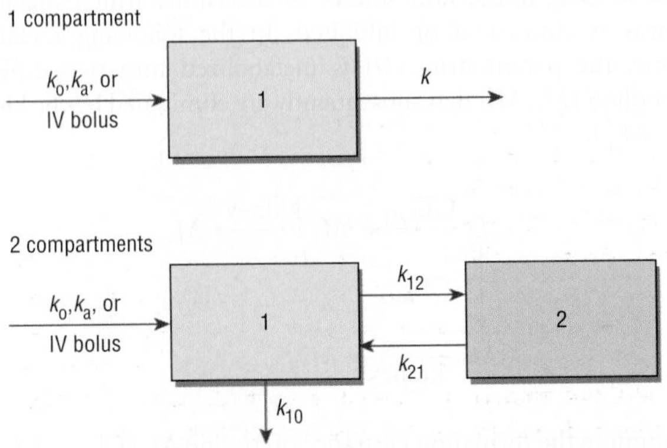

FIGURE 5-5. Visual representations of one- and two-compartment drug-distribution models.

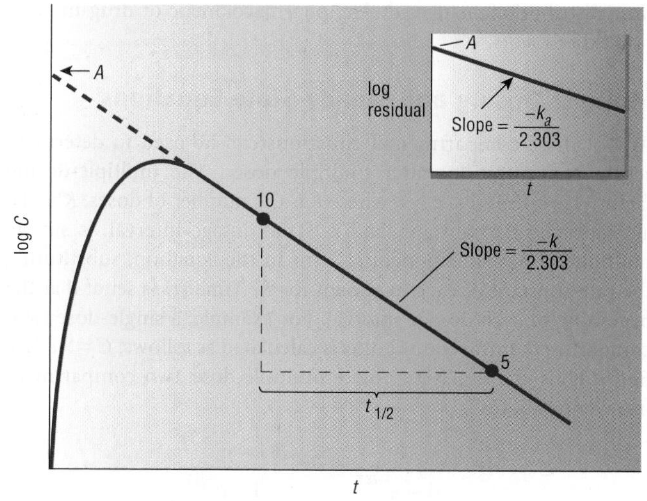

FIGURE 5-6. Calculation of the half-life of a drug following oral, intramuscular, or other extravascular dosing route.

decrease in a straight line with a slope equal to $-k/2.303$. The equation that describes the data is $C = \{(FDk_a)/[V_D(k_a - k)]\}(e^{-kt} - e^{-k_at})$, where F is the fraction of the dose absorbed into the systemic circulation. The absorption rate constant (k_a) is obtained using the method of residuals.

The method of residuals is used to obtain the individual rate constants (Fig. 5–6). A is determined by extrapolating the terminal slope to the y axis; k_a can be obtained by calculating the slope or $t_{1/2}$ and using the formulas given for the intravenous bolus case. At each time point in the absorption portion of the curve, the concentration value from the extrapolated line is noted and called the *extrapolated concentration.* For each point, the actual concentration is subtracted from the extrapolated concentration to compute the *residual concentration.* When the residual concentrations are plotted on semilogarithmic coordinates, a line with y intercept equal to A and slope equal to $-k_a/2.303$ is obtained. When these values are calculated, they can be placed into the equation ($C = Ae^{-kt} - Ae^{-k_at}$, where $A = FDk_a/[V_D(k_a - k)]$) and used to compute the serum concentration at any time after the extravascular dose. The intercepts and rate constants also can be used to compute CL and V_D: $CL = FD/(A/k - A/k_a)$ and $V_D = CL/k$, where F is the fraction of the dose absorbed into the systemic circulation.

During a continuous intravenous infusion, the serum concentrations in a one-compartment model change according to the following function: $C = (k_0/CL)(1 - e^{-kt})$. If the infusion has been running for more than three to five half-lives, the patient will be at steady state, and CL can be calculated ($CL = k_0/C_{ss}$). When the infusion is discontinued, serum concentrations appear to decline in a straight line when plotted on semilogarithmic paper with a slope of $-k/2.303$. V_D is computed by dividing CL by k (Fig. 5–7).

Multicompartment Model

After an intravenous bolus dose, serum concentrations often decline in two or more phases. During the early phases, drug leaves the bloodstream by two mechanisms: (a) distribution into tissues and (b) metabolism and/or elimination. Because the drug is leaving the bloodstream through these two mechanisms, serum concentrations decline rapidly. After tissues and blood are in equilibrium, only metabolism and/or elimination remove drug from the blood. During this terminal phase, serum concentrations decline more slowly. The half-life is measured during the terminal phase by determining the time required for concentrations to decline by one-half.

After an intravenous bolus dose, serum concentrations decrease as if the drug were being injected into a central compartment that not

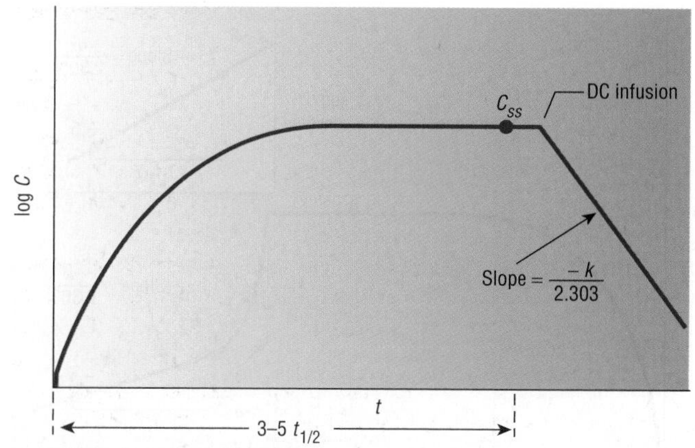

FIGURE 5-7. Achievement of steady-state serum concentrations after three to five half-lives of a drug. Note the elimination phase after discontinuance of the infusion.

only metabolizes and eliminates drug but also distributes drug to one or more other compartments. Of these multicompartment models, the two-compartment model is encountered most commonly (see Fig. 5–5). After an intravenous bolus injection, serum concentrations decrease in two distinct phases described by the equation:

$$C = \frac{D(\alpha - k_{21})}{V_{D_1}(\alpha - \beta)}e^{-\alpha t} + \frac{D(k_{21} - \beta)}{V_{D_1}(\alpha - \beta)}e^{-\beta t}$$

or $C = Ae^{-\alpha t} + Be^{-\beta t}$, where k_{21} is the first-order rate constant that reflects the transfer of drug from compartment 2 to compartment 1, V_{D1} is the V_D of compartment 1, $A = D(\alpha - k_{21})/[V_{D1}(\alpha - \beta)]$ and $B = D(k_{21} - \beta)/[V_{D1}(\alpha - \beta)]$. The rate constants α and β found in the exponents of the equations describe the distribution and elimination of the drug, respectively (Fig. 5–8). A and B are the y intercepts of the lines that describe drug distribution and elimination, respectively, on the log concentration-versus-time plot.

The residual line is calculated as before using the method of residuals. The terminal line is extrapolated to the y axis, and extrapolated concentrations are determined for each time point. Because actual concentrations are greater in this case, residual concentrations are calculated by subtracting the extrapolated concentrations from the actual concentrations. When plotted on semilogarithmic paper, the residual line has a y intercept equal to A. The slope of the residual line is used to compute α (slope $= -\alpha/2.303$). With the rate constants (α and β) and the intercepts (A and B), concentrations can be calculated for any time after the intravenous

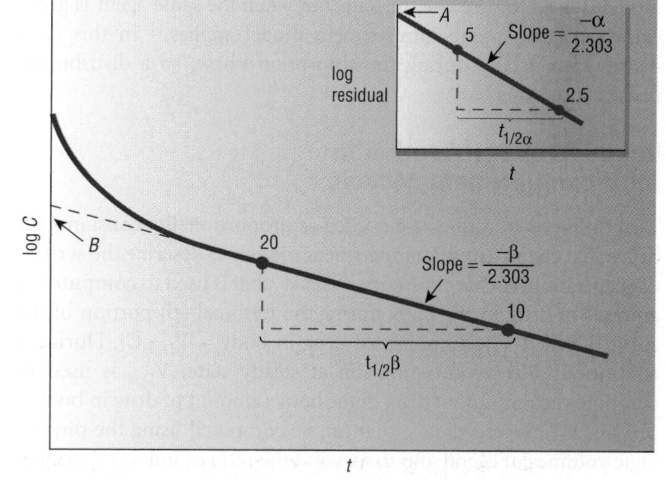

FIGURE 5-8. Calculation of α and β half-lives following intravenous dosing.

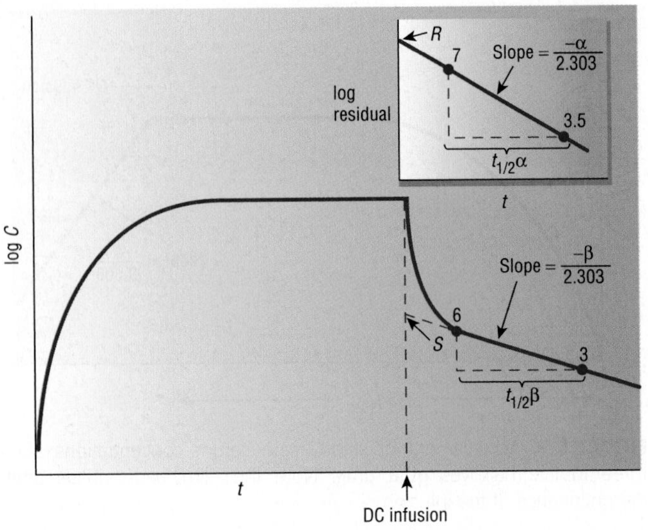

FIGURE 5-9. Calculation of α and β half-lives following a steady-state infusion.

bolus dose ($C = Ae^{-\alpha t} + Be^{-\beta t}$), or pharmacokinetic constants can be computed: $CL = D/[(A/\alpha) + (B/\beta)]$, $V_{D,\beta} = CL/\beta$, $V_{D,ss} = \{D[(A/\alpha^2) + (B/\beta^2)]\}/[(A/\alpha) + (B/\beta)]^2$.

If serum concentrations of a drug given as a continuous intravenous infusion decline in a biphasic manner after the infusion is discontinued, a two-compartment model describes the data set (Fig. 5–9).[12,13] In this instance, the postinfusion concentrations decrease according to the equation $C = Re^{-\alpha t'} + Se^{-\beta t'}$, where t' is the postinfusion time ($t' = 0$ when infusion is discontinued) and R, S, α, and β are determined from the postinfusion concentrations using the method of residuals with the y axis set at $t' = 0$. R and S are used to compute A and B. A and B are the y intercepts that would have occurred had the total dose given during the infusion ($D = k_0T$) been administered as an intravenous bolus dose.

$$A = \frac{RD\alpha}{k_0(1 - e^{-\alpha T})}$$

$$B = \frac{SD\beta}{k_0(1 - e^{-\beta T})}$$

where T is the duration of infusion. Once A, B, α, and β are known, the equations for an intravenous bolus are used to compute the pharmacokinetic constants. Often, when a drug is given as an intravenous bolus or continuous intravenous infusion, a two-compartment model is used to describe the data, but when the same agent is given extravascularly, a one-compartment model applies.[14] In this case, distribution occurs during the absorption phase, so a distribution phase is not observed.

Volumes of Distribution in Multicompartment Models

Two different V_D values are needed as proportionality constants for drugs that require multicompartment models to describe the serum-concentration-versus-time curve. The V_D that is used to compute the amount of drug in the body during the terminal (β) portion of the curve is called $V_{D,\beta}$ (amount of drug in body = $V_{D,\beta}$ C). During a continuous intravenous infusion at steady state, $V_{D,ss}$ is used to compute the amount of drug in the body (amount of drug in body = $V_{D,ss}C$). $V_{D,ss}$ is also the V_D that can be computed using the physiologic volumes of blood and tissues and the ratio of unbound drug in blood to that in tissues [$V_{D,ss} = V_b + (f_b/f_t)V_t$]. Because the value of $V_{D,\beta}$ changes when CL changes, $V_{D,ss}$ should be used to indicate if drug distribution changes during pharmacokinetic or drug-interaction experiments.

Multiple Dosing and Steady-State Equations

Any of these compartmental equations can be used to determine serum concentrations after multiple doses. The multiple-dosing factor $(1 - e^{-nK\tau})/(1 - e^{-K\tau})$, where n is the number of doses, K is the appropriate rate constant, and τ is the dosage interval, is simply multiplied by each exponential term in the equation, substituting the rate constant of each exponent for K. Time (t) is set at 0 at the beginning of each dosage interval. For example, a single-dose two-compartment intravenous bolus is calculated as follows: $C = Ae^{-\alpha t} + Be^{-\beta t}$. Thus the equation for a multiple-dose two-compartment intravenous bolus is

$$C = Ae^{-\alpha t}\frac{1 - e^{-n\alpha\tau}}{1 - e^{-\alpha\tau}} + Be^{-\beta t}\frac{1 - e^{-n\beta\tau}}{1 - e^{-\beta\tau}}$$

A single-dose one-compartment intravenous bolus is calculated as $C = (D/V_D)e^{-kt}$. For a multiple-dose one-compartment intravenous bolus, the concentration is $C = (D/V_D)e^{-kt}[(1 - e^{nk\tau})/(1 - e^{-k\tau})]$.

At steady state, the number of doses becomes large, $e^{-nK\tau}$ approaches zero, and the multiple-dosing factor equals $1/(1 - e^{-K\tau})$. Therefore, the steady-state versions of the equations are simpler than their multiple-dose counterparts:

$$C = \frac{Ae^{-\alpha t}}{1 - e^{-\alpha\tau}} + \frac{Be^{-\beta t}}{1 - e^{-\beta\tau}}$$

and

$$C = \frac{(D/V_D)e^{-kt}}{1 - e^{-k\tau}}$$

for a steady-state two-compartment intravenous bolus and a steady-state one-compartment intravenous bolus, respectively.

USE OF PHARMACOKINETIC CONCEPTS FOR INDIVIDUALIZATION OF DRUG THERAPY

9 Many factors must be taken into consideration when deciding on the best drug dose for a patient. For example, the age of the patient is important because the dose (in milligrams per kilogram) for pediatric patients may be higher and for geriatric patients may be lower than the typically prescribed dose for young adults. Gender also can be a factor because males and females metabolize and eliminate some drugs differently. Patients who are significantly obese or cachectic also may require different drug doses because of clearance and volume of distribution changes. Other drug therapy that could cause drug interactions needs to be considered. Disease states and conditions may alter the drug-dosage regimen for a patient. Three disease states that deserve special mention are congestive heart failure, renal disease, and hepatic disease. Renal and hepatic diseases cause loss of organ function and decreased drug elimination and metabolism. Congestive heart failure causes decreased blood flow to organs that clear the drug from the body.

Many drug compounds are racemic mixtures of stereoisomers. In most cases, one of the isomers is more pharmacologically active than the other isomer, and each isomer may exhibit different pharmacokinetic properties. Warfarin, propranolol, verapamil, and ibuprofen are all racemic mixtures of stereoisomers. Some drug interactions inhibit or increase the elimination of only one stereoisomer. The importance of the drug interaction depends on which isomer is affected. Other drugs, such as dextromethorphan, levofloxacin, and diltiazem, are composed of just one stereoisomer.

10 Genetics also plays a role in drug metabolism. *Cytochrome P450* is a generic term for the group of enzymes that are responsible for most drug metabolism oxidation reactions. Several cytochrome P450 (CYP) isozymes have been identified that are responsible for the metabolism of many important drugs (Table 5–3). CYP2C19 is responsible for aromatic hydroxylation of (S)-mephenytoin, and CYP2D6 oxidizes debrisoquine.[15] These subsets of the cytochrome P450 enzyme family are also responsible for the metabolism of several other drugs (CYP2D6: many tricyclic antidepressants, codeine, (S)-metoprolol; CYP2C19: most proton pump inhibitors, sertraline, voriconazole). CYP2C9, CYP2C19, and CYP2D6 isozymes appear to be under genetic control. As a consequence, there are "poor metabolizers" who have a defective mutant gene for the isozyme, cannot manufacture a fully functional isozyme, and therefore cannot metabolize the drug substrate very well. "Extensive metabolizers" have the standard gene for the isozyme and metabolize the drugs normally. Poor metabolizers usually are a minority of the general population. They may achieve toxic concentrations of drug when usual doses are prescribed for them or, if the active drug moiety is a metabolite, may fail to have any pharmacologic effect from the drug. The ethnic background of the patient can affect the likelihood that the patient will be a poor metabolizer.[15] For example, the incidence of poor metabolizers for CYP2D6 is approximately 5% to 10% for whites and approximately 0% to 1% for Asians, whereas for CYP2C19, poor metabolizers make up approximately 3% to 6% of the white population and approximately 20% of the Asian population. Approximately 7% of the white population are poor metabolizers for CYP2C9 substrates.

TABLE 5-3 Cytochrome P450 (CYP) Enzyme Family and Selected Substrates

CYP1A2	CYP2E1
Acetaminophen	Enflurane
Caffeine	Ethanol
Ondansetron	Halothane
Tacrine	Isoflurane
Theophylline	CYP3A4
R-Warfarin	Alfentanil
Zileuton	Alprazolam
CYP2C9	Astemizole
Candesartan	Carbamazepine
Diclofenac	Cyclosporine
Ibuprofen	Diltiazem
Losartan	Erythromycin
Naproxen	Felodipine
Phenytoin	Itraconazole
Tolbutamide	Ketoconazole
Valsartan	Lidocaine
S-Warfarin	Lovastatin
CYP2C19	Midazolam
Diazepam	Nifedipine
Lansoprazole	Quinidine
(S)-Mephenytoin	Simvastatin
Nelfinavir	Tacrolimus
Omeprazole	Verapamil
Pantoprazole	Ziprasidone
Voriconazole	
CYP2D6	
Carvedilol	
Codeine	
Debrisoquine	
Dextromethorphan	
Encainide	
Fluoxetine	
Haloperidol	
(S)-Metoprolol	
Paroxetine	
Propafenone	
Risperidone	
Thioridazine	
Venlafaxine	

Other cytochrome P450 isozymes have been isolated.[15] CYP1A2 is the enzyme that is responsible for the demethylation of caffeine and theophylline; CYP2C9 metabolizes phenytoin, tolbutamide, losartan, and ibuprofen; some antiretroviral protease inhibitors, cyclosporine, nifedipine, lovastatin, simvastatin, and atorvastatin are metabolized by CYP3A4; and ethanol is a substrate for CYP2E1. It is important to recognize that a drug may be metabolized by more than one cytochrome P450 isozyme. Although most tricyclic antidepressants are hydroxylated by CYP2D6, *N*-demethylation probably is mediated by a combination of CYP2C19, CYP1A2, and CYP3A4. Acetaminophen appears to be metabolized by both CYP1A2 and CYP2E1. The 4-hydroxy metabolite of propranolol is produced by CYP2D6, but side-chain oxidation of propranolol is probably a product of CYP2C19. The CYP3A enzyme family comprises approximately 90% of the drug-metabolizing enzyme present in the intestinal wall but only approximately 30% of the drug-metabolizing enzyme found in the liver. The remainder of hepatic drug-metabolizing enzyme is approximately 20% for the CYP2C family, approximately 13% for CYP1A2, approximately 7% for CYP2E1, and approximately 2% for CYP2D6.

Understanding which cytochrome P450 isozyme is responsible for the metabolism of a drug is extraordinarily useful in predicting and understanding drug interactions. Some drug-metabolism inhibitors and inducers are highly selective for certain cytochrome P450 isozymes.[15] Quinidine is an extremely potent inhibitor of the CYP2D6 enzyme system[15]; a single 50-mg dose of quinidine can change a rapid metabolizer of debrisoquine into a poor metabolizer. Ciprofloxacin and zileuton inhibit, whereas tobacco or marijuana smoke induce, CYP1A2. Some drugs that are enzyme inhibitors are also substrates for that same enzyme system and appear to cause drug interactions by being a competitive inhibitor. For example, erythromycin is both a substrate for and an inhibitor of CYP3A4. Obviously, if one knows that a new drug is metabolized by a given cytochrome P450 enzyme system, it is logical to assume that the new drug will exhibit drug interactions with the known inducers and inhibitors of that cytochrome P450 isozyme.

⓫ The importance of transport proteins in drug bioavailability and elimination is now better understood. A principal transport protein involved in the movement of drugs across biologic membranes is P-gp. P-gp is present in many organs, including the gastrointestinal tract, liver, and kidney. If a drug is a substrate for P-gp, its oral absorption may be decreased when P-gp transports drug molecules that have been absorbed back into the gastrointestinal tract lumen. In the liver, some drugs are transported by P-gp from the blood into the bile, where the drug is eliminated by biliary secretion. Similarly, some drugs eliminated by the kidney are transported from the blood into the urine by P-gp. Digoxin is a substrate of P-gp. Other possible mechanisms for drug interactions are when two drugs that are substrates for P-gp compete for transport by the protein and when a drug is an inhibitor or inducer of P-gp. Drug interactions involving inhibition of P-gp decrease drug transportation in these organs and potentially can increase gastrointestinal absorption of orally administered drug, decrease biliary secretion of the drug, or decrease renal elimination of drug molecules. The drug interaction between amiodarone and digoxin probably involves all three of these mechanisms, and this explains why digoxin concentrations increase so dramatically in patients receiving amiodarone. Many drugs that are metabolized by CYP3A4 are also substrates for P-gp, and some of the drug interactions attributed to inhibition of CYP3A4 may be a result of decreased drug transportation by P-gp. Drug interactions involving induction of P-gp have the opposite effect in these organs and may decrease gastrointestinal absorption of orally administered drug, increase biliary secretion of the drug, or increase renal elimination of drug molecules.

SELECTION OF INITIAL DRUG DOSES

⓬ When deciding on initial doses for drugs that are eliminated renally, the patient's renal function should be assessed. A common, useful way to do this is to measure the patient's serum creatinine concentration and convert this value into an $CL_{cr\ est}$. Serum creatinine values alone should not be used to assess renal function because they do not include the effects of age, body weight, or gender. The Cockcroft-Gault equation[16] is probably the most widely used method to estimate creatinine clearance (in milliliters per minute) in adults (age 18 years or older) who are within approximately 30% of their ideal body weight and have stable renal function:

$$\text{Male: } CL_{cr\ est} = \frac{(140 - \text{age})BW}{S_{cr} \times 72}$$

$$\text{Female: } CL_{cr\ est} = \frac{0.85(140 - \text{age})BW}{S_{cr} \times 72}$$

where BW is body weight (in kilograms), age is the patient's age (in years), 0.85 is a correction factor to account for lower muscle mass in females, and S_{cr} is serum creatinine (in milligrams per deciliter). For children, the following estimation equations are available according to the age of the child[17]: age 0 to 1 years: $CL_{cr\ est}$ (in mL/min/1.73 m^2) = $(0.45 \times Lt)/S_{cr}$; age 1 to 20 years: $CL_{cr\ est}$ (in mL/min/1.73 m^2) = $(0.55 \times Lt)/S_{cr}$, where Lt is patient length in centimeters. Other methods to determine $CL_{cr\ est}$ for obese adults[18] and patients with rapidly changing renal function[19] are available. Creatinine is a by-product of muscle breakdown in the body, so none of these estimation methods work well in patients with muscle disease, such as multiple sclerosis, or diseases that alter muscle mass, such as cachexia, malnutrition, cancer, or spinal cord injury. Nomograms that adjust initial doses according to a patient's renal function are available for several drugs, including digoxin,[20] vancomycin,[21] and the aminoglycoside antibiotics.[22]

For drugs that are eliminated primarily by the kidney (≥60% of the administered dose), some agents will need minor dosage adjustments for $CL_{cr\ est}$ between 30 and 60 mL/min, moderate dosage adjustments for $CL_{cr\ est}$ between 15 and 30 mL/min, and major dosage adjustments for $CL_{cr\ est}$ less than 15 mL/min. Specific recommendations for dosage adjustments of other drugs for patients with renal disease are available.[23,24] Supplemental doses of some medications also may be needed for patients receiving hemodialysis if the drug is removed by the artificial kidney or for patients receiving hemoperfusion if the drug is removed by the hemofilter.[24]

⓭ A similar assessment of liver function should be made for drugs that are metabolized hepatically. Unfortunately, there is no single test that can estimate liver drug-metabolism capacity accurately, and those that are used do not always prove accurate. High aminotransferase (aspartate aminotransferase [AST] and alanine aminotransferase [ALT]) and alkaline phosphatase concentrations usually indicate acute hepatic cellular damage and do not establish poor liver drug metabolism reliably. Abnormal values for three tests that usually indicate that drugs will be metabolized poorly by the liver are high serum bilirubin concentration, low serum albumin concentration, and a prolonged prothrombin time. Bilirubin is metabolized by the liver, and albumin and clotting factors are manufactured by the liver, so aberrant values for all three of these tests are a more reliable indicator of abnormal liver drug metabolism. The Child-Pugh score,[25] a widely used clinical classification for liver disease that incorporates clinical signs and symptoms (ascites and hepatic encephalopathy) in addition to these three laboratory tests, can be used as an indicator of a patient's ability to metabolize drugs that are eliminated by the liver. A score in excess of 10 suggests very poor liver function. As a general rule, patients with cirrhosis have the most severe decreases in liver drug metabolism. Patients with acute or chronic hepatitis often retain relatively normal or slightly decreased hepatic drug-metabolism capacity. In the absence of specific pharmacokinetic dosing guidelines for a medication, a Child-Pugh score equal to 8 to 9 is grounds for a moderate decrease (approximately 25%) in initial daily drug dose for agents that are metabolized primarily (≥60%) hepatically, and a score of 10 or greater indicates that a significant decrease in initial daily dose (approximately 50%) is required for drugs that are metabolized mostly by the liver. As in any patient with or without liver dysfunction, initial doses are meant as starting points for dosage titration based on patient response and avoidance of adverse effects.

Because there are no good markers of liver function, clinicians have come to rely on pharmacokinetic parameters derived in various patient populations to compute initial doses of drugs that are eliminated hepatically. Table 5–4 contains average pharmacokinetic parameters for theophylline in several disease states. Initial doses of many liver-metabolized drugs are computed by determining which disease states and/or conditions the patient has that are known to alter the kinetics of the drug and by using these average pharmacokinetic constants to calculate doses. The patient is then monitored for therapeutic and adverse effects, and drug serum concentrations are obtained to ensure that concentrations are appropriate and to adjust doses, if necessary. The following computations illustrate the estimated intravenous loading dose and the intravenous continuous infusion necessary to achieve a theophylline concentration of 10 mg/L for a 55-year-old, 70-kg male with liver cirrhosis (mean kinetic parameters obtained from Table 5–4):

$$V_D = (0.5 \text{ L/kg})(70 \text{ kg}) = 35 \text{ L}$$

$$LD = C_{ss} V_D = (10 \text{ mg/L})(35 \text{ L})$$

$$= 350 \text{ mg theophylline infused over 20 to 30 min}$$

$$CL(\text{in L/h}) = \frac{(0.35 \text{ mL/min/kg})(70 \text{ kg})(60 \text{ min/h})}{1000 \text{ mL}/L}$$

$$= 1.5 \text{ L/h}$$

$$k_0 = C_{ss}CL = (10 \text{ mg/L})(1.5 \text{ L/h})$$

$$= 15 \text{ mg/h of theophylline to begin after loading dose is given}$$

If theophylline is to be given as the aminophylline salt form, each dose would need to be changed to reflect the fact that aminophylline contains only 85% theophylline (LD = 350 mg of theophylline/0.85 = 410 mg of aminophylline infused over 20 to 30 minutes, k_0 = 15 mg/h of theophylline/0.85 = 18 mg/h of aminophylline to begin after loading dose is given).

Heart failure is often overlooked as a disease state that can alter drug disposition. Severe heart failure decreases cardiac output and therefore reduces liver blood flow. Theophylline,[26] lidocaine,[27] and

TABLE 5-4 Theophylline Pharmacokinetic Parameters for Selected Disease States/Conditions

Disease State/Condition	Mean Clearance (mL/min/kg)	Mean Dose (mg/kg/h)
Children age 1–9 y	1.4	0.8
Children age 9–12 y or adult smokers	1.25	0.7
Adolescents age 12–16 y or elderly smokers (>65 y)	0.9	0.5
Adult nonsmokers	0.7	0.4
Elderly nonsmokers (age >65 y)	0.5	0.3
Decompensated congestive heart failure, cor pulmonale, cirrhosis	0.35	0.2

Mean volume of distribution = 0.5 L/kg.
Adapted from reference 49.

drugs with high extraction ratios are compounds whose clearance declines with decreased liver blood flow. Initial dosages of these drugs should be reduced in patients with moderate to severe heart failure (New York Heart Association class III or IV) by 25% to 50% until steady-state concentrations and response can be determined.

USE OF STEADY-STATE DRUG CONCENTRATIONS

Serum drug concentrations are readily available to clinicians to use as guides for the individualization of drug therapy. The therapeutic ranges for several drugs have been identified, and it is likely that new drugs also will be monitored using serum concentrations. Although several individualization methods have been advocated for specific ⓮ drugs, one simple, reliable method is used commonly. For drugs that exhibit linear pharmacokinetics, C_{ss} changes proportionally with dose. To adjust a patient's drug therapy, a reasonable starting dose is administered for an estimated three to five half-lives. A serum concentration is obtained, assuming that it will reflect C_{ss}. Independent of the route of administration, the new dose (D_{new}) needed to attain the desired C_{ss} ($C_{ss,new}$) is calculated: $D_{new} = D_{old}(C_{ss,new}/C_{ss,old})$, where D_{old} and $C_{ss,old}$ are the old dose and old C_{ss}, respectively. To use this method, $C_{ss,old}$ must reflect steady-state conditions. Often patients are noncompliant with regard to their drug dosage and therefore are not at steady state. This occurs not only in outpatients but also in hospital inpatients. Inpatients can spit out oral doses or alter the infusion rates on intravenous pump rates after the nurse leaves the hospital room. Doses also can be missed if the patient is absent from his or her room at the time medications are to be administered. If $C_{ss,old}$ is much larger or smaller than expected for the D_{old} the patient is taking, one should suspect noncompliance and repeat the serum concentration determination after another three to five half-lives or change the patient's dose cautiously and monitor for signs of toxicity or lack of effect.

MEASUREMENT OF PHARMACOKINETIC PARAMETERS IN PATIENTS

⓯ If it is necessary to determine the kinetic constants for a patient to individualize his or her dose, a small kinetic evaluation is conducted in the individual. In these cases, the number of serum concentrations obtained from the patient is held to the minimum needed to calculate accurate pharmacokinetic parameters and doses. The reason for using fewer serum drug concentration determinations is to be as cost-effective as possible because these laboratory tests generally cost $20 to $50 each.

Although many drugs follow two-compartment-model pharmacokinetics (especially after intravenous administration), a one-compartment model is used to compute kinetic parameters in patients because too many serum concentration determinations would be needed to determine accurately both the distribution and elimination phases found in the two-compartment model. Because of this, serum concentrations usually are not measured in patients during the distribution phase. Another important reason serum concentrations are not measured during the distribution phase for therapeutic drug-monitoring purposes in patients is that drug in the blood and drug in the tissues are not in equilibrium during this time so that serum concentrations do not reflect tissue concentrations. When drug serum concentrations are obtained in patients for the purpose of assessing efficacy or toxicity, it is important that they be measured in the postdistribution phase when drug in the blood is in equilibrium with drug at the site of action.

In the case where the patient has received enough doses to be at steady state, pharmacokinetic parameters can be computed using a predose minimum concentration and a postdose maximum concentration. Under steady-state conditions, serum concentrations after each dose are identical, so the predose minimum concentration is the same before each dose (Fig. 5–10). This situation allows the predose concentration to be used to compute both the patient's $t_{1/2}$ and V. If the drug was given extravascularly or has a significant distribution phase, the postdose concentration should be determined after absorption or distribution is finished. To ensure that steady-state conditions have been achieved, the patient needs to receive the drug on schedule for at least three to five estimated half-lives. To make sure that this is the case, inpatients should have their medication administration records checked, and the patient's nurse should be consulted regarding missed or late doses. Outpatients should be interviewed about compliance with the prescribed dosage regimen. When compliance with the dosage regimen has been verified, steady-state conditions reasonably can be assumed.

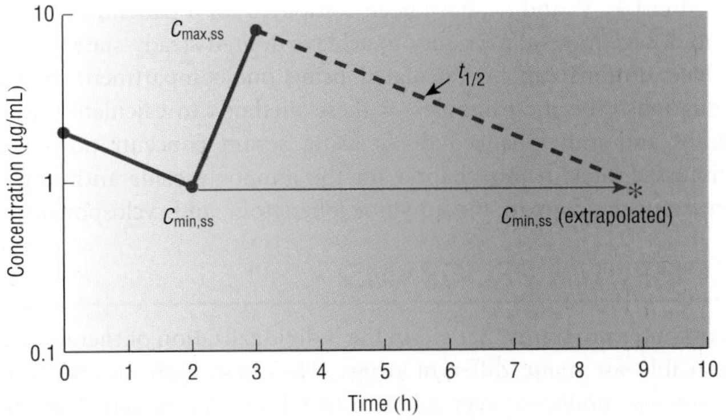

FIGURE 5-10. When a patient has received enough doses to be at steady state, steady-state maximum ($C_{max,ss}$) and minimum ($C_{min,ss}$) concentrations can be used to compute clearance, volume of distribution, and half-life. At steady state, consecutive $C_{min,ss}$ values are equal, so the predose value can be extrapolated to the time before the next dose and be used to calculate half-life *(dashed line)*.

If the patient is not at steady state, an additional postdose serum concentration determination should be done to compute the patient's pharmacokinetic parameters. Ideally, the third concentration (C_3) should be acquired approximately one estimated half-life after the postdose maximum concentration. Determining serum concentrations too close together will hamper the drug assay's ability to measure differences between them, and getting the third sample too late could result in a concentration too low for the assay to detect. In this situation, the predose minimum and postdose maximum concentrations are used to compute V, and both postdose concentrations are used to calculate $t_{1/2}$ (Fig. 5–11).

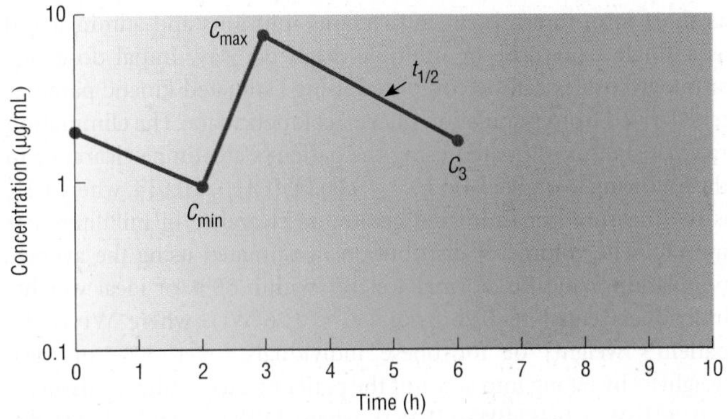

FIGURE 5-11. If a patient has not received enough doses to be at steady state, or doses have been given on an irregular schedule, the minimum concentration (C_{min}), maximum concentration (C_{max}), and an additional postdose concentration (C_3) can be used to compute clearance, volume of distribution, and half-life.

After CL, V, and $t_{1/2}$ have been computed for a patient, the dose and dosage interval necessary to achieve desired steady-state serum concentrations can be calculated using one-compartment-model equations. Specific examples of these methods to calculate initial doses and individualized doses using serum concentrations are discussed later in this chapter for the aminoglycoside antibiotics, vancomycin, digoxin, theophylline, phenytoin, and cyclosporine.

COMPUTER PROGRAMS

Computer programs that aid in the individualization of therapy are available for many different drugs. The most sophisticated programs use nonlinear regression to fit CL and V_D to actual serum concentrations obtained in a patient.[28] After drug doses and serum concentrations are entered into the computer, nonlinear least-squares regression programs adjust CL and V_D until the sum of the squared error between actual (C_{act}) and computer-estimated concentrations (C_{est}) is at a minimum [$\Sigma (C_{est} - C_{act})^2$]. Once estimates of CL and V_D are available, doses are calculated easily.

Many programs also take into account what the CL and V_D should be on the basis of disease states and conditions present in the patient.[29] Incorporation of expected population-based parameters allows the computer to use a limited number of serum concentrations (one or two) to provide estimates of CL and V_D. This type of computer program is called *Bayesian* because it incorporates portions of Bayes' theorem during the fitting routine.[30] Bayesian pharmacokinetic dosing programs are used widely to adjust the dose of a variety of drugs. In the case of renally eliminated drugs (e.g., aminoglycosides, vancomycin, and digoxin), population estimates for kinetic parameters are generated by entering the patient's age, weight, height, gender, and serum creatinine concentration into the computer program. For hepatically eliminated drugs (e.g., theophylline and phenytoin), population estimates for kinetic parameters are computed using the patient's age, weight, and gender, as well as other factors that might change hepatic clearance, such as the presence or absence of disease states (e.g., cirrhosis or congestive heart failure) or other drug therapy that might cause a drug interaction. The Bayesian estimates of the pharmacokinetic parameters are then modified using nonlinear least-squares regression fits of serum concentrations to result in individualized parameters for the patient. The individualized parameters are used to compute doses for the patient that will result in desired steady-state concentrations of the drug.

Aminoglycosides

Although aminoglycoside pharmacokinetics follow multicompartment models,[31] a one-compartment model appears sufficient to individualize doses in patients.[32] Aminoglycosides usually are given as short-term intermittent intravenous infusions and administered as a single daily dose or multiple doses per day. Initial doses for aminoglycosides can be computed using estimated kinetic parameters derived from population pharmacokinetic data. The elimination rate constant is estimated using the patient's creatinine clearance in the following formula: k (in h^{-1}) = $0.00293(CL_{cr}) + 0.014$, where CL_{cr} is the measured or estimated creatinine clearance in milliliters per minute. The volume of distribution is estimated using the average population value for normal-weight (within 30% of ideal weight) individuals equal to 0.26 L/kg [$V = 0.26(\text{Wt})$, where Wt is the patient's weight] or for obese individuals (over 30% of ideal weight)[33] by taking into account the patient's excess adipose tissue: $V = 0.26[\text{IBW} + 0.4(\text{TBW} - \text{IBW})]$, where TBW is total body weight, IBW is ideal body weight [IBW_{males} (in kilograms) = 50 + 2.3(Ht – 60) or $\text{IBW}_{females}$ (in kilograms) = 45 + 2.3(Ht – 60), and Ht is the patient's height in inches]. Additional volume of distribution population estimates are available for other disease states and conditions such as cystic fibrosis,[34] ascites,[35] and neonates.[36]

Appropriate $C_{max,ss}$ and $C_{min,ss}$ values are selected for the patient based on the site and severity of the infection and the sensitivity of the known or suspected pathogen, as well as avoidance of adverse effects. For example, $C_{max,ss}$ values of 8 to 10 mg/L generally are selected for gram-negative pneumonia patients, whereas $C_{min,ss}$ values of less than 2 mg/L usually are chosen to avoid aminoglycoside-induced nephrotoxicity when tobramycin and gentamicin are prescribed using conventional multiple-daily-dosing regimens. Once appropriate steady-state serum concentrations are selected, the dosage interval required to achieve those concentrations is calculated, and τ is rounded to a clinically acceptable value (e.g., 8, 12, 18, 24, 36, or 48 hours): $\tau = [(\ln C_{max,ss} - \ln C_{min,ss})/k] + T$. Finally, a dose is computed for the patient using the one-compartment-model intermittent intravenous infusion equation at steady state, and the dose is rounded off to the nearest 5 to 10 mg:

$$D = TkV_D C_{max,ss} \frac{1 - e^{-k\tau}}{1 - e^{-kT}}$$

The Hull and Sarrubi aminoglycoside dosage nomogram (Table 5–5) is based on this dosage-calculation method and includes precalculated doses and dosage intervals for a variety of creatinine clearance

TABLE 5-5 Aminoglycoside Dosage Chart

1. Compute patient's creatinine clearance (CL_{cr}) using Cockcroft-Gault method: $CL_{cr} = [(140 - \text{age})\text{BW}]/(S_{cr} \times 72)$. Multiply by 0.85 for females.
2. Use patient's weight if within 30% of IBW; otherwise use adjusted dosing weight = IBW + [0.40(TBW – IBW)].
3. Select loading dose in mg/kg to provide peak serum concentrations in range listed below for the desired aminoglycoside antibiotic:

Aminoglycoside	Usual Loading Doses	Expected Peak Serum Concentrations
Tobramycin Gentamicin Netilmicin	1.5 to 2.0 mg/kg	4 to 10 mcg/mL
Amikacin Kanamycin	5.0 to 7.5 mg/kg	15 to 30 mcg/mL

4. Select maintenance dose (as percentage of loading dose) to continue peak serum concentrations indicated above according to desired dosage interval and the patient's creatinine clearance. To maintain usual peak to trough ratio, use dosage intervals in unshaded areas below.

Percentage of Loading Dose Required for Dosage Interval Selected

CL_{cr} (mL/min)	Estimated Half-Life (h)	8 h (%)	12 h (%)	24 h (%)
>90	2–3	90	–	–
90	3.1	84	–	–
80	3.4	80	91	–
70	3.9	76	88	–
60	4.5	71	84	–
50	5.3	65	79	–
40	6.5	57	72	92
30	8.4	48	63	86
25	9.9	43	57	81
20	11.9	37	50	75
17	13.6	33	46	70
15	15.1	31	42	67
12	17.9	27	37	61
10[a]	20.4	24	34	56
7[a]	25.9	19	28	47
5[a]	31.5	16	23	41
2[a]	46.8	11	16	30
0[a]	69.3	8	11	21

BW, body weight; CL_{cr}, creatine clearance; IBW, ideal body weight; S_{cr}, serum creatinine; TBW, total body weight.

[a]Note: Dosing for patients with $CL_{cr} \leq 10$ mL/min should be assisted by measuring serum concentrations.

Adapted from reference 22.

values.[22] The nomogram assumes that $V_D = 0.26$ L/kg and should not be used to compute doses for disease states with altered V_D.

For extended-interval therapy, $C_{max,ss}$ values of 20 to 30 mg/L and $C_{min,ss}$ values less than 1 mg/L generally are accepted as appropriate for gram-negative pneumonia patients. A minimum 24-hour dosage interval is chosen for this dosing technique, and the dosing interval is increased in 12- to 24-hour increments for patients with renal dysfunction.

An example of this initial dosage scheme for a typical case is provided to illustrate the use of the various equations. Mr. JJ is a 65-year-old, 80-kg, 6-ft-tall man with the diagnosis of gram-negative pneumonia. His serum creatinine concentration is 2.1 mg/dL and is stable. Compute a conventional gentamicin dosage regimen (infused over 1 hour) that would provide approximate peak and trough concentrations of $C_{max,ss} = 8$ mg/L and $C_{min,ss} = 1.5$ mg/L, respectively. The patient is within 30% of his ideal body weight [$IBW_{male} = 50 + 2.3(72 \text{ in} - 60) = 78$ kg] and has stable renal function, so the Cockcroft-Gault creatinine clearance estimation equation can be used: $CL_{cr\,est} = [(140 - 65\text{ y})80\text{ kg}]/[72(2.1\text{ mg/dL})] = 40$ mL/min. The patient's weight and estimated creatinine clearance are used to compute his V and k, respectively: $V = 0.26$ L/kg(80 kg) = 20.8 L; $k = 0.00293(40\text{ mL/min}) + 0.014 = 0.131\text{ h}^{-1}$ or $t_{1/2} = 0.693/0.131\text{ h}^{-1}) = 5.3$ h. The dosage interval and dose for the desired serum concentrations would then be calculated: $\tau = [(\ln 8\text{ mg/L} - \ln 1.5\text{ mg/L})/0.131\text{ h}^{-1}] + 1\text{ h} = 13.7$ h rounded to 12 h; $D = (1\text{ h})(0.131\text{ h}^{-1})(20.8\text{ L})(8\text{ mg/L})[1 - e^{-(0.131h-1(12h)}/1 - e^{-(0.131h-1(1h)}] = 140$ mg. Thus the prescribed dose would be gentamicin 140 mg every 12 hours administered as a 1-hour infusion. If a loading dose were deemed necessary, it would be given as the first dose [LD = (20.8 L)(8 mg/L) = 166 mg rounded to 170 mg infused over 1 hour], and the first maintenance dose would be administered 12 hours (e.g., one dosage interval) later. Using the Hull and Sarrubi nomogram for the same patient, the loading dose is 160 mg (gentamicin loading dose for serious gram-negative infection is 2 mg/kg: 2 mg/kg × 80 kg = 160 mg), and the maintenance dose is 115 mg every 12 hours (for a 12-hour dosage interval and $CL_{cr\,est} = 40$ mL/min, maintenance dose is 72% of the loading dose: 0.72 × 160 mg = 115 mg).

CLINICAL CONTROVERSY

Some clinicians use conventional dosing or extended-interval dosing exclusively for patients requiring aminoglycosides, whereas others use a mix of both approaches according to the perceived benefit to the patient. Definitive, authoritative recommendations to guide the choice of one method of aminoglycoside dosing over the other are not available.

If appropriate aminoglycoside serum concentrations are available, kinetic parameters can be calculated at any point in therapy. When the patient is not at steady state, serum aminoglycoside concentrations are obtained before a dose (C_{min}), after a dose administered as an intravenous infusion of about 1 hour or as a 30-minute infusion followed by a 30-minute waiting period to allow for drug distribution (C_{max}), and at one additional postdose time (C_3) approximately one estimated half-life after C_{max}. The $t_{1/2}$ and k values are computed using C_{max} and C_3: $k = (\ln C_{max} - \ln C_3)/\Delta t$ and $t_{1/2} = 0.693/k$, where Δt is the time that expired between the times C_{max} and C_3 were obtained. If the patient is at steady state, serum aminoglycoside concentrations are obtained before a dose ($C_{min,ss}$) and after a dose administered as an intravenous infusion of about 1 hour or as a 30-minute infusion followed by a 30-minute waiting period to allow for drug distribution ($C_{max,ss}$). The $t_{1/2}$ and k values are computed using $C_{max,ss}$ and $C_{min,ss}$: $k = (\ln C_{max,ss} - \ln C_{min,ss})/(\tau - T)$ and $t_{1/2} = 0.693/k$, where τ is the dosage interval and T is the dose infusion time or dose infusion time plus waiting time.

Assuming a one-compartment model, the following equation is used to compute V_D[32]:

$$V_D = \frac{(D/T)(1 - e^{-kT})}{k(C_{max} - C_{min}e^{-kT})}$$

where D is dose and T is duration of infusion. Once these are known, the dose and dosage interval (τ) can be calculated for any desired maximum C_{ss} ($C_{max,ss}$) and minimum C_{ss} ($C_{min,ss}$):

$$\tau = \frac{\ln C_{max,ss} - \ln C_{min,ss}}{k} + T$$

$$D = TkV_D C_{max,ss}\frac{1 - e^{-k\tau}}{1 - e^{-kT}}$$

The dose and dosage interval should be rounded to provide clinically accepted values (every 8, 12, 18, 24, 36, and 48 hours for dosage interval, nearest 5 to 10 mg for conventional dosing or every 24, 36, and 48 hours for dosage interval, nearest 10 to 25 mg for extended interval dosing). This method also has been used to individualize intravenous theophylline dosage regimens.[37]

To provide an example of this technique, the problem given previously will be extended to include steady-state concentrations. Mr. JJ was prescribed gentamicin 140 mg every 12 hours (infused over 1 hour) for the treatment of gram-negative pneumonia. Steady-state trough ($C_{min,ss}$) and peak ($C_{max,ss}$) values were obtained before and after the fourth dose was given (more than three to five estimated half-lives), respectively, and equaled $C_{min,ss} = 2.8$ mg/L and $C_{max,ss} = 8.5$ mg/L. Clinically, the patient was improving with decreased white blood cell counts and body temperatures and a resolving chest radiograph. However, the serum creatinine value had increased to 2.5 mg/dL. Because of this, a new dosage regimen with a similar peak (to maintain high intrapulmonary levels) but lower trough (to decrease the risk of drug-induced nephrotoxicity) concentrations was suggested. The patient's elimination rate constant and half-life can be computed using the following formulas: $k = (\ln 8.5\text{ mg/L} - \ln 2.8\text{ mg/L})/(12\text{ h} - 1\text{ h}) = 0.101\text{ h}^{-1}$ and $t_{1/2} = 0.693/0.101\text{ h}^{-1} = 6.9$ h. The patient's volume of distribution can be calculated using the following equation:

$$V = \frac{(140\text{ mg}/1\text{ h})\left[1 - e^{-(0.101h^{-1})(1h)}\right]}{(0.101\text{ h}^{-1})\left\{8.5\text{ mg/L} - \left[(2.8\text{ mg/L})e^{-(0.101h^{-1})(1h)}\right]\right\}} = 22.3\text{L}$$

Thus the patient's volume of distribution was larger and half-life was longer than originally estimated, and this led to higher serum concentrations than anticipated. To achieve the desired serum concentrations ($C_{min,ss} = 1.5$ mg/L and $C_{max,ss} = 8$ mg/L), the patient's actual kinetic parameters are used to compute a new dose and dosage interval: $\tau = [(\ln 8\text{ mg/L} - \ln 1.5\text{ mg/L})/0.101\text{ h}^{-1}] + 1\text{ h} = 17.6$ h, rounded to 18 h and

$$D = (1\text{h})(0.101\text{h}^{-1})(22.3\text{L})(8\text{ mg/L})\frac{\left(1 - e^{-(0.101\text{h}^{-1})(18\text{h})}\right)}{\left(1 - e^{-(0.101\text{h}^{-1})(1\text{h})}\right)}$$

$$= 157\text{ mg, round to 160 mg}$$

Thus the new dose would be gentamicin 160 mg every 18 hours and infused over 1 hour; the first dose of the new dosage regimen would be given 18 hours (e.g., the new dosage interval) after the last dose of the old dosage regimen.

Because aminoglycoside antibiotics exhibit concentration-dependent bacterial killing and the postantibiotic effect is longer with higher concentrations, investigators studied the possibility of giving a higher dose of aminoglycoside using an extended-dosage interval (24 hours or longer, depending on renal function). Generally, these studies have shown comparable microbiologic and clinical cure rates for many infections and about the same rate of nephrotoxicity (approximately 5% to 10%) as with conventional dosing. Ototoxicity has not been monitored using audiometry in most of these investigations, but loss of hearing in the conversational range, as well as signs and symptoms of vestibular toxicity, usually has been assessed and found to be similar to that with aminoglycoside therapy dosed conventionally. Based on these data, clinicians are using extended-interval dosing in selected patients. For *Pseudomonas aeruginosa* infections where the organism has an expected minimum inhibitory concentration (MIC) ≈ 2 mg/L, peak concentrations between 20 and 30 mg/L and trough concentrations of less than 1 mg/L for gentamicin or tobramycin have been suggested.[38]

At the present time, there is no consensus on how to approach concentration monitoring using this mode of administration. Some clinicians obtain steady-state peak and trough concentrations and use the kinetic equations given earlier to adjust the dose and dosage interval in order to attain appropriate target levels. Other clinicians measure only trough concentrations, trusting that the large doses administered to patients achieve adequate peak concentrations.

Also, a nomogram that adjusts extended-interval doses based on a single postdose concentration to achieve these steady-state concentration goals has been proposed (Fig. 5–12). The dose is 7 mg/kg of gentamicin or tobramycin. The initial dosage interval is set according to the patient's creatinine clearance (see Fig. 5–12). The Hartford nomogram includes a method to adjust doses based on serum concentrations. This portion of the nomogram contains average serum concentration time lines for gentamicin or tobramycin in patients with creatinine clearances of 60, 40, and 20 mL/min. A serum concentration is measured 6 to 14 hours after the first dose is given, and this concentration/time point is plotted on the graph (see Fig. 5–12). The modified dosage interval is indicated by which zone the serum concentration/time point falls in. Because cystic fibrosis patients have a different volume of distribution (0.35 L/kg) than assumed by this dosing technique and extended-interval dosing has not been tested adequately in patients with endocarditis, the Hartford nomogram should not be used in these situations.

To illustrate how the nomogram is used, the same patient example used previously will be repeated for this dosage approach. Mr. JJ is an 80-kg man with a $CL_{cr\ est}$ of 40 mL/min. Using the Hartford nomogram, the patient would receive gentamicin 560 mg every 36 hours (7 mg/kg × 80 kg = 560 mg; the initial dosage interval for $CL_{cr\ est}$ = 40 mL/min is 36 hours). Ten hours after the first dose was given, the serum gentamicin concentration is 8.2 mg/L. According to the graph contained in the nomogram, the dosage interval should be changed to 48 hours. The new dose is 560 mg every 48 hours.

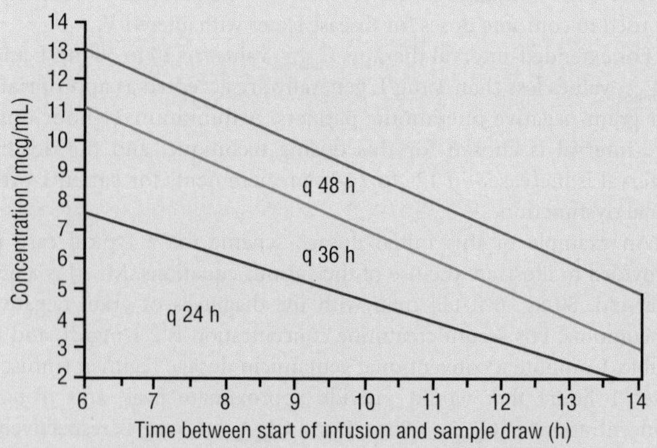

1. Administer 7 mg/kg gentamicin with initial dosage interval:

Estimated CL_{cr} (mL/min)	Initial dosage interval
≥60 mL/min	q 24 h
40–59 mL/min	q 36 h
20–39 mL/min	q 48 h
<20 mL/min	Monitor serial concentrations and administer next dose when <1 mcg/mL.

2. Obtain timed serum concentration 6 to 14 hours after dose (ideally first dose).
3. Alter dosage interval to that indicated by the nomogram zone (above q 48 h zone, monitor serial concentrations and administer next dose when <1 mcg/mL)

FIGURE 5-12. Hartford nomogram for extended-interval aminoglycosides. *(Adapted with permission from reference 38.)*

CLINICAL CONTROVERSY

"Trough only" measurement of steady-state vancomycin concentrations is a mainstream method to monitor therapy. The exact range for this value is uncertain. Some clinicians recommend 5 to 10 mcg/mL, whereas others suggest 5 to 15 mcg/mL. For some sites of infection with specific organisms (such as hospital-acquired pneumonia caused by multidrug-resistant organisms) guidelines suggest vancomycin trough concentrations as high as 15 to 20 mcg/mL may be necessary. Some clinicians continue to measure both steady-state peak and trough vancomycin concentrations.

Vancomycin

Vancomycin requires multicompartment models to completely describe its serum-concentration-versus-time curves. However, if peak serum concentrations are obtained after the distribution phase is completed (usually 30 minutes to 1 hour after a 1-hour intravenous infusion), a one-compartment model can be used for patient dosage calculations. Also, because vancomycin has a relatively long half-life compared with the infusion time, only a small amount of drug is eliminated during infusion, and it is usually unnecessary to use more complex intravenous infusion equations. Thus simple intravenous bolus equations can be used to calculate vancomycin doses for most patients. Although a recent review paper[39] questioned the clinical usefulness of measuring vancomycin concentrations on a routine basis, research articles[40,41] have shown potential benefits in obtaining vancomycin concentrations in selected patient populations. Some clinicians advocate monitoring only steady-state trough concentrations of vancomycin.[42] The decision to conduct vancomycin concentration monitoring should be made on a patient-by-patient basis.

Initial doses of vancomycin can be computed for adult patients using estimated kinetic parameters derived from population pharmacokinetic data. Clearance is estimated using the patient's creatinine clearance in the following equation[41]: CL (in mL/min/kg) = 0.695(CL_{cr} in mL/min/kg) + 0.05. The volume of distribution is computed assuming the standard value of 0.7 L/kg: $V_D = 0.7(\text{Wt})$, where Wt is the patient's weight. In the case of obese patients, actual or total body weight is used in the calculation of clearance, but ideal body weight is used to compute volume of distribution.[44] The elimination rate constant is calculated using clearance and volume of distribution estimates, correcting for possible differences in units for these parameters: $k = CL/V_D$. A nomogram that uses this type of approach for vancomycin therapy is available to determine initial doses rapidly for patients (Table 5–6).[45]

TABLE 5-6 Vancomycin Dosage Chart

1. Compute patient's creatinine clearance (CL_{cr}) using Cockcroft-Gault method: $CL_{cr} = [(140 - age)BW]/(S_{cr} \times 72)$. Multiply by 0.85 for females.
2. Use patient's total body weight to compute doses.
3. Dosage chart designed to achieve peak serum concentrations of 30 μg/mL and trough concentrations of 7.5 μg/mL.
4. Compute loading dose of 25 mg/kg.
5. Compute maintenance dose of 19 mg/kg given at the dosage interval listed in the following chart for the patient's CL_{cr}:

CL_{cr} (mL/min)	Dosage Interval (Days)
≥120	0.5
100	0.6
80	0.75
60	1.0
40	1.5
30	2.0
20	2.5
10	4.0
5	6.0
0	12.0

Adapted from reference 45.

Steady-state peak and trough concentrations are chosen for the patient based on the site and severity of the infection, as well as the known or suspected pathogen and avoidance of potential side effects. $C_{max,ss}$ values of between 20 and 40 mg/L and $C_{min,ss}$ values of between 5 and 15 mg/L typically are used for patients with moderate to severe methicillin-resistant *Staphylococcus aureus, Staphylococcus epidermidis,* or penicillin-resistant enterococcal infections. After appropriate steady-state concentrations are chosen, the dosage interval required to attain those concentrations is computed, and τ is rounded to a clinically acceptable value (12, 18, 24, 36, 48, or 72 hours): $\tau = (\ln C_{max,ss} - \ln C_{min,ss})/k$. Finally, the maintenance dose is computed for the patient using a one-compartment-model intravenous bolus equation at steady state, and the dose is rounded off to the nearest 100 to 250 mg:

$$D = C_{max,ss}\, V_D\, (1 - e^{-k\tau})$$

If desired, a loading dose can be computed using the following equation:

$$LD = V_D\, C_{max,ss}$$

The following case will illustrate the use of this dosage methodology. Ms. HJ is a 65-year-old, 68-kg, 5-ft 4-in tall patient who has developed a surgical wound infection with *S. aureus* the suspected pathogen. Her serum creatinine concentration is 1.8 mg/dL and stable. Compute a vancomycin dosage regimen that would provide approximate peak (obtained 1 hour after a 1-hour infusion) and trough concentrations of 30 and 7 mg/L, respectively. The patient is within 30% of her ideal body weight [$IBW_{female} = 45 + 2.3(64 \text{ in} - 60) = 54$ kg] and has stable renal function, so the Cockcroft-Gault creatinine clearance estimation formula can be used: $CL_{cr\ est} = 0.85[(140 - 65\ y)68\ kg]/[72(1.8\ mg/dL)] = 33$ mL/min. The patient's weight and estimated creatinine clearance are used to calculate her estimated CL, V_D, and k, respectively: CL = 0.695 (33 mL/min/68 kg) + 0.05 = 0.387 mL/min/kg; V_D = 0.7 L/kg(68 kg) = 48 L; and k = [(0.387 mL/min/kg)(68 kg)(60 min/h)]/[(48 L)(1,000 mL/L)] = 0.033 h^{-1} or $t_{1/2}$ = 0.693/0.033 h^{-1} = 21 h. The dosage interval, maintenance dose, and loading dose for the desired serum concentrations then can be computed: τ = (ln 30 mg/L – ln 7 mg/L)/0.033 h^{-1} = 44 h, rounded to 48 h; D = (30 mg/L) (48 L)(1 – $e^{-(0.033h\text{-}1)(48h)}$) = 1,145 mg, rounded to 1,200 mg; LD = (48 L)(30 mg/L) = 1,440 mg, rounded to 1,450 mg. Therefore, the prescribed doses would be vancomycin 1,200 mg every 48 hours administered as a 1-hour infusion. If a loading dose was used, it would be given as the first dose, and the first maintenance dose would be administered 48 hours (one dosage interval) later. Using the Matzke nomogram for the same patient, the loading dose would be 1,700 mg (vancomycin loading dose is 25 mg/kg: 25 mg/kg × 68 kg = 1,700 mg), followed by a maintenance dose of 1,300 mg every 48 hours (for $CL_{cr\ est}$ = 30 mL/min, maintenance dose is 19 mg/kg every 2 days: 19 mg/kg × 68 kg = 1,292 mg, rounded to 1,300 mg).

If appropriate vancomycin serum concentrations are available, kinetic parameters can be computed at any point in therapy. When the patient is not at steady state, serum vancomycin concentrations are obtained before a dose (C_{min}), after a dose administered as an intravenous infusion of 1 hour followed by a 30-minute to 1-hour waiting period to allow for drug distribution (C_{max}), and at one additional postdose time (C_3) approximately one estimated half-life after C_{max}. The $t_{1/2}$ and k values are computed using C_{max} and C_3: $k = (\ln C_{max} - \ln C_3)/\Delta t$ and $t_{1/2} = 0.693/k$, where Δt is the time that expired between the times C_{max} and C_3 were obtained. If the patient is at steady state, serum vancomycin concentrations are obtained before a dose ($C_{min,ss}$) and after a dose administered as an intravenous infusion of about 1 hour followed by a 30-minute to 1-hour waiting period to allow for drug distribution ($C_{max,ss}$). The $t_{1/2}$ and k values are computed using $C_{max,ss}$ and $C_{min,ss}$: $k = (\ln C_{max,ss} - \ln C_{min,ss})/(\tau - T_{max})$ and $t_{1/2} = 0.693/k$, where τ is the dosage interval and T_{max} is the dose infusion time plus waiting time.

Assuming a one-compartment model, the following equation is used to compute V_D:

$$V_D = \frac{D}{C_{max} - C_{min}}$$

where D is dose. Once these are known, the dose and dosage interval (τ) can be calculated for any desired maximum C_{ss} ($C_{max,ss}$) and minimum C_{ss} ($C_{min,ss}$):

$$\tau = \frac{\ln C_{max,ss} - \ln C_{min,ss}}{k}$$

$$D = C_{max,ss} V_D (1 - e^{-k\tau})$$

The dose and dosage interval should be rounded to provide clinically accepted values (every 12, 18, 24, 36, 48, or 72 hours for dosage interval, nearest 100 to 250 mg for dose).

To provide an example for this dosage-calculation method, the preceding problem will be extended to include steady-state concentrations. Ms. HJ was prescribed vancomycin 1,200 mg every 48 hours (infused over 1 hour) for the treatment of a surgical wound infection. Steady-state trough ($C_{min,ss}$) and peak ($C_{max,ss}$) values ($C_{max,ss}$ obtained 1 hour after the end of the infusion) were obtained before and after the third dose was given (more than three to five estimated half-lives), respectively, and equaled $C_{min,ss}$ = 2.5 mg/L and $C_{max,ss}$ = 22.4 mg/L. Clinically, the patient had improved somewhat, but her white blood cell count was still elevated, and the patient was still febrile. Because of this, a modified dosage regimen with a $C_{max,ss}$ = 30 mg/L and $C_{min,ss}$ = 7 mg/L was suggested to maintain trough concentrations three to five times above the MIC for the suspected pathogen. The patient's actual elimination rate constant and half-life can be calculated using the following formulas: k = (ln 22.4 mg/L – ln 2.5 mg/L)/(48 h – 2 h) = 0.048 h^{-1} and $t_{1/2}$ = 0.693/0.048 h^{-1} = 14.4 h. The patient's volume of distribution can be calculated using the following equation:

$$V_D = \frac{1{,}200\text{mg}}{22.4\text{ mg/L} - 2.5\text{ mg/L}} = 60\text{ L}$$

Thus the patient's volume of distribution was larger and half-life shorter than originally estimated, and this led to lower serum concentrations than anticipated. To achieve the desired serum concentrations ($C_{max,ss}$ = 30 mg/L and $C_{min,ss}$ = 7 mg/L), the patient's actual kinetic parameters are used to calculate a new dose and dosage interval:

$$\tau = \frac{\ln 30\ \text{mg/L} - \ln 7\ \text{mg/L}}{0.048\text{h}^{-1}}$$

$$= 30\ \text{h, rounded to 36 h}$$

$$D = (30\ \text{mg/L})(60\text{L})\left(1 - e^{-(0.048\text{h}^{-1})(36\text{h})}\right)$$

$$= 1{,}480\ \text{mg, rounded to 1,500 mg}$$

The new dose would be vancomycin 1,500 mg every 36 hours (infused over 1 hour); the first dose of the new dosage regimen would be given 36 hours (the new dosage interval) after the last dose of the old dosage regimen.

Many clinicians measure only steady-state vancomycin trough concentrations in patients. The justification for this approach is that because vancomycin exhibits time-dependent bacterial killing, the minimum concentration is the most important with regard to therapeutic outcome. Vancomycin pharmacokinetics also support this approach because the volume of distribution is relatively stable and is not changed by many disease states or conditions. Because of this important point, it is difficult to attain peak steady-state concentrations in the toxic range when the steady-state vancomycin trough is in the therapeutic range if typical doses are used (15 mg/kg or ≈1,000 mg for average-weight individuals). Also, toxic peak concentrations (generally greater than 80 to 100 mg/L) are quite a bit higher than therapeutic peak concentrations, which adds a safety margin between effective concentrations and those yielding adverse drug effects.

Coupled with trough-only vancomycin concentration monitoring is a widening of the therapeutic steady-state trough concentration range from 5 to 15 mg/L. The justification for increasing the top of the range from 10 to 15 mg/L comes from limited retrospective[41] and prospective[42] studies, and until more clinical evidence is available, should be reserved for severely ill patients, infections caused by bacteria with higher MICs, and patients who are not responding to trough concentrations within the usual 5- to 10-mg/L range. Trough concentrations in the range of 15 to 20 mg/L should only be used for specific clinical situations, such as hospital-acquired pneumonia caused by multidrug-resistant organisms.[56]

When trough-only monitoring of vancomycin concentrations is chosen by a clinician, a simple variant of linear pharmacokinetics can be used to adjust the dose (D) and dosage interval (τ): $(D_{new}/\tau_{new}) = (D_{old}/\tau_{old})(C_{ss,new}/C_{ss,old})$, where *new* and *old* indicate the new target trough concentration and the old measured trough concentration, respectively. In practice, the dose (typically 1,000 mg) is held constant and only the dosage interval is changed. This equation is an approximation of the actual new steady-state trough concentration that will be attained in the patient because, mathematically, $C_{ss,new}$ is an exponential function of τ.

An example of this approach is given in the following case. Mr. MK (72 years old, 72-kg weight, 5 ft 9 in tall) was prescribed vancomycin 1,000 mg every 12 hours (infused over 1 hour) for the treatment of an *S. epidermidis* central venous catheter infection. A steady-state trough ($C_{min,ss}$) value was obtained before the fifth dose was given (more than three to five estimated half-lives), and $C_{min,ss}$ equaled 19 mg/L. Clinically, the patient was improving, but the trough concentration was judged to be too high. Because of this, a modified dosage regimen with a $C_{min,ss}$ = 10 mg/L was suggested to maintain trough concentrations three to five times above the MIC for the suspected pathogen: (D_{new}/τ_{new}) = (1,000 mg/12 h)(10 mg/L/19 mg/L) = 44 mg/h. Because the patient is near his ideal weight, the same dose of 1,000 mg can be used (D_{new}), and the new dosage interval (τ_{new}) can be computed: τ = 1,000 mg/44 mg/h = 23 h, rounded to 24 h. The new prescribed dose for the patient would be 1,000 mg every 24 hours.

Digoxin

Digoxin pharmacokinetics are best described by a two-compartment model. However, because digoxin has a long half-life compared with its dosage interval and a very long distribution phase, simple pharmacokinetic equations can be used to individualize dosing when postdistribution serum concentrations are used. Digoxin can be given as an intravenous injection and orally as elixir (F = 0.8), tablets (F = 0.7), or capsules (F = 0.9). When given orally, the appropriate bioavailability fraction must be used to compute the correct dose. Initial doses of digoxin can be computed using population pharmacokinetic data obtained from published studies. Digoxin clearance is estimated using the patient's creatinine clearance in the following formula[20]: CL (in milliliters per minute) = 1.303(CL_{cr} in milliliters per minute) + CL_m, where CL_m is metabolic clearance and equals 40 mL/min for patients with no or mild heart failure or 20 mL/min for patients with moderate to severe heart failure. The volume of distribution decreases with declining renal function and is estimated using the following equation[20]: V_D (in liters) = 226 + [298(CL_{cr} in milliliters per minute)]/(29.1 + CL_{cr} in milliliters per minute). The elimination rate constant can be computed by taking the product of CL and V_D: $k = CL/V_D$. For obese individuals, digoxin dosing should be based on ideal body weight.[46]

Appropriate C_{ss} values are chosen for the patient based on the disease state being treated, the goal of therapy, and avoidance of adverse effects. The inotropic effects of digoxin occur at lower concentrations than do the chronotropic effects. Therefore, initial serum concentrations of digoxin for the treatment of heart failure generally are 1 ng/mL or less and for the treatment of atrial fibrillation are 1 to 1.5 ng/mL. Once the appropriate C_{ss} is selected, a dose is computed for the patient: $D/\tau = (C_{ss}CL)/F$.

An example of this initial dosage scheme is provided in the following case. Mr. PO is a 72-year-old, 83-kg, 5-ft 11-in tall man admitted to the hospital for the treatment of community-acquired pneumonia. While in the hospital, Mr. PO develops atrial fibrillation, and the decision is made to treat him with digoxin to provide ventricular rate control. His serum creatinine concentration is 2.5 mg/dL and stable. Calculate an intravenous loading dose and oral maintenance dose that will achieve a C_{ss} of 1.5 ng/mL. The Cockcroft-Gault equation can be used to estimate the patient's creatinine clearance because his serum creatinine concentration is stable and he is within 30% of his ideal weight [IBW_{male} = 50 + 2.3(71 in – 60) = 75 kg]: CL_{cr} = [(140 – 72 y)83 kg]/[72(2.5 mg/dL)] = 31 mL/min. Using the estimated CL_{cr}, both CL and V_D can be computed:

$$CL = 1.303(31\ \text{mL/min}) + 40 = 80\ \text{mL/min}$$

$$V_D = 226 + \frac{298(31\ \text{mL/min})}{29.1 + 31\ \text{mL/min}} = 380\ \text{L}$$

The maintenance dose will be given as digoxin tablets, so F = 0.7 in the dosing equation: D/τ = [(1.5 mcg/L)(80 mL/min)(60 min/h)(24 h/day)]/[0.7(1,000 mL/L)] = 247 mcg/day, rounded to 250 mcg/day. The loading dose will be given intravenously as a digoxin injection: LD = (1.5 mcg/L)(380 L) = 570 mcg, rounded to 500 mcg. The loading dose would be given 50% now (250 mcg), 25% (125 mcg) in 4 to 6 hours after monitoring the patient's heart rate and blood pressure and assessing the patient for digoxin adverse effects, and the final 25% (125 mcg) 4 to 6 hours later after monitoring the same clinical parameters. The first maintenance dose would be given one dosage interval (in this case 24 hours) after the first part of the loading dose was given.

Adjustment of digoxin doses using steady-state concentrations is accomplished using linear pharmacokinetics and dosage ratios: $D_{new} = D_{old}(C_{ss,new}/C_{ss,old})$. For example, Mr. PO's atrial fibrillation responded to digoxin therapy, and he was discharged after resolution of his pneumonia. A month later he was followed up in the clinic with moderate nausea, possibly a result of digoxin toxicity. His heart rate was 51 beats per minute. A steady-state digoxin concentration was determined and reported by the clinical laboratory as 2.2 mcg/L. Compute a new dose for the patient to achieve a C_{ss} of 1.5 mcg/L. The digoxin C_{ss} and old dose would be used to calculate a new dose using the linear pharmacokinetic equation: D_{new} = 250 mcg/day[(1.5 mcg/L)/(2.2 mcg/L)] = 170 mcg/day. This approximate average daily dose could be achieved by having the patient alternate take two 125-mcg tablets (250 mcg) and one 125-mcg tablet daily, giving an average dose equal to 187.5 mcg/day [(250 mcg + 125 mcg)/2 = 187.5 mcg/day].

Theophylline

Theophylline disposition is described most accurately by nonlinear kinetics.[47,48] However, at the usual doses, theophylline acts as if it obeys linear kinetics in most patients. Initial theophylline doses are computed by taking a detailed medical history of the patient and noting disease states and conditions that are known to change theophylline disposition. Age, smoking of tobacco-containing products, heart failure, and liver disease are among the important factors that alter theophylline kinetic parameters and dosage requirements. Once the patient has been assessed, average theophylline kinetic parameters obtained from the literature for patients similar to the one being currently treated are used to compute either oral or intravenous doses. Dosage guidelines that take into account most common disease states and conditions that change theophylline kinetic parameters are available (see Table 5–4).[49] Once theophylline is administered, the patient is monitored for the therapeutic effect and potential adverse effects. Theophylline concentrations then are used to individualize the theophylline dose that the patient receives. An example of this approach was given previously for a patient in the section on drug dosing in patients with liver disease.

Continuous intravenous infusions of theophylline (or its salt, aminophylline) can be individualized rapidly by determining the patient's CL before steady state occurs.[50] Assuming that the patient receives theophylline only by continuous intravenous infusion (previous doses of sustained-release oral theophylline are completely absorbed), two serum theophylline concentration determinations are done 4 hours or more apart. The infusion rate (k_0) cannot be changed between the times the samples are drawn. With one-compartment model equations, the first (C_1) and second (C_2) theophylline concentrations are used to calculate theophylline CL:

$$CL = \frac{2k_0}{C_1 + C_2} + \frac{2V_D(C_1 - C_2)}{(C_1 + C_2)(t_2 - t_1)}$$

V_D is assumed to be 0.5 L/kg, and t_1 and t_2 are the times at which C_1 and C_2, respectively, are obtained. Once CL is known, k_0 can be computed easily for any desired C_{ss} ($C_{ss} = k_0/CL$). This method probably can be applied to other drugs that are administered as continuous intravenous infusions, such as intravenous antiarrhythmics, when rapid individualization of drug dosage is desirable.

An example of this approach can be obtained by continuing the theophylline patient case from the section on drug dosing in liver disease. In this example, a 55-year-old, 70-kg man with liver cirrhosis was prescribed a loading dose of theophylline 350 mg intravenously over 20 to 30 minutes, followed by a maintenance dose of 15 mg/h of theophylline as a continuous infusion. The infusion began at 9 AM, blood samples were obtained at 10 AM and 4 PM, and the clinical laboratory reported the theophylline serum concentrations as 10.9 and 12.3 mg/L, respectively. The patient's theophylline clearance and revised continuous infusion to maintain a C_{ss} of 15 mg/L can be computed as follows (patient's V_D estimated at 0.5 L/kg):

$$CL = \frac{2(15\text{ mg/h})}{10.9\text{ mg/L} + 12.3\text{ mg/L}} + \frac{2(0.5\text{ L/kg} \times 70\text{ kg})(10.9\text{ mg/L} - 12.3\text{ mg/L})}{(10.9\text{ mg/L} + 12.3\text{ mg/L})(16 - 10\text{ h})} = 0.59\text{ L/h}$$

$$k_0 = C_{ss}CL = (15\text{ mg/L})(0.59\text{ L/h}) = 9\text{ mg/h theophylline}$$

If theophylline is to be given as the aminophylline salt form, the doses would need to be changed to reflect the fact that aminophylline contains only 85% theophylline (k_0 = 9 mg/h theophylline/0.85 = 11 mg/h aminophylline).

If continuous intravenous infusions or oral dosage regimens are given long enough for steady state to occur (three to five estimated half-lives based on previous studies conducted in similar patients), linear pharmacokinetics can be used to adjust doses for either route of administration: $D_{new} = D_{old}\,(C_{ss,new}/C_{ss,old})$. For example, a patient receiving 200 mg of sustained-release oral theophylline every 12 hours with a theophylline steady-state serum concentration of 9.5 mcg/mL can have the dose required to achieve a new steady-state concentration equal to 15 mcg/mL computed by applying linear pharmacokinetics: D_{new} = 200 mg[(15 mcg/mL)/(9.5 mcg/mL)] = 316 mg, rounded to 300 mg. Thus the new theophylline dose would be 300 mg every 12 hours.

Phenytoin

Phenytoin doses are very difficult to individualize because the drug follows Michaelis-Menten kinetics, and there is a large amount of interpatient variability in V_{max} and K_m. Initial maintenance doses of phenytoin in adults usually range between 4 and 7 mg/kg per day, yielding starting doses of 300 to 400 mg/day in most individuals. If needed, loading doses of phenytoin or fosphenytoin (a prodrug of phenytoin used intravenously) can be administered in adults at a dose of 15 mg/kg, which is approximately 1,000 mg in many individuals. Loading doses of phenytoin can be given orally but need to be administered in divided doses separated by several hours in order to avoid decreased bioavailability and gastrointestinal intolerance (400 mg, 300 mg, and then 300 mg with each dose separated by 4 to 6 hours). Since phenytoin is metabolized hepatically, decreased doses may be needed in patients with liver disease. Because phenytoin follows dose-dependent pharmacokinetics, the half-life of phenytoin increases for a patient as the maintenance dose increases. Therefore, the time to steady-state phenytoin concentrations increases with dose. On average, at a phenytoin dose of 300 mg/day, it takes approximately 5 to 7 days to achieve steady state; at a dose of 400 mg/day, it takes approximately 10 to 14 days to achieve steady state; and at a dose of 500 mg/day, it takes approximately 21 to 28 days to achieve steady state. It should be noted that the injectable and capsule dosage forms of phenytoin are phenytoin sodium, and the labeled dosage amounts contain 92% of active phenytoin (300-mg phenytoin sodium capsules contain 276 mg [300 mg × 0.92 = 276 mg] of active phenytoin). Unbound phenytoin concentrations are useful in patients with hypoalbuminemia (e.g., liver disease, nephrotic syndrome, pregnancy, cystic fibrosis, burns, trauma, and malnourishment, as well as in the elderly), in patients in whom displacement with endogenous compounds is possible (e.g., hyperbilirubinemia, liver disease, or end-stage renal disease), and in patients receiving other drugs that may displace phenytoin from plasma protein-binding sights (e.g., valproic acid, aspirin therapy of more than 2 g/day, warfarin, and nonsteroidal antiinflammatory drugs with high albumin binding).[57]

After steady state has occurred, phenytoin serum concentrations can be obtained as an aid to dosage adjustment. A simple, easy way to approximate new serum concentrations after a dosage adjustment with phenytoin is to temporarily assume linear pharmacokinetics and then add 15% to 33% for a dosage increase or subtract

15% to 33% for a dosage decrease to account for Michaelis-Menten kinetics. To avoid large disproportionate changes in phenytoin concentrations when using this empirical method, dosage adjustments should be limited to 50 to 100 mg/day. This technique is only intended to provide a rough approximation of the resulting phenytoin steady-state concentration after an appropriate dosage adjustment has been made.

For example, Ms. PP is a 35-year-old, 65-kg patient with grand mal seizures who is receiving phenytoin capsules 300 mg orally at bedtime. A steady-state concentration of 9.2 mcg/mL is measured. It is observed that her seizure frequency decreased by only approximately 15% and that she has had no adverse effects as a consequence of phenytoin treatment. Because of this, her phenytoin dose is increased to 400 mg orally at bedtime. The expected phenytoin steady-state concentration would be estimated using linear pharmacokinetics [$C_{new} = (D_{new}/D_{old})C_{old}$ = (400 mg/300 mg)/(9.2 mcg/mL) = 12.3 mcg/mL] and then increased by 15% to 33% to account for nonlinear kinetics [C_{new} = 1.15(12.3 mcg/mL) = 14.1 mcg/mL or C_{new} = 1.33 (12.3 mcg/mL) = 16.4 mcg/mL]. Thus the patient would be expected to have a steady-state phenytoin concentration of approximately 14 to 16 mcg/mL as a consequence of the dosage increase. An alternative approach would be to use a graphic Bayesian method that allows an estimate of V_{max} and K_m from one steady-state phenytoin concentration and the prediction of new steady-state concentrations when doses are changed.[51]

Other methods used to individualize phenytoin doses involve rearrangements of the Michaelis-Menten equation [DR = $V_{max}C_{ss}/(K_m + C_{ss})$, in which DR is the dosage rate at steady state] so that two or more doses and C_{ss} values can be used to obtain graphic solutions for V_{max} and K_m. One rearrangement[52] is DR = $-K_m$(DR/C_{ss}) + V_{max}. When DR is plotted on the *y* axis and DR/C_{ss} is plotted on the *x* axis of Cartesian graph paper, a straight line with a *y* intercept of V_{max} and slope equal to $-K_m$ is found (Fig. 5–13). To use this method, patients are prescribed an initial phenytoin dose, and C_{ss} is obtained. The phenytoin dose is then changed, and a second C_{ss} from the new dose is obtained. Each dose is divided by its respective C_{ss} to derive DR/C_{ss} values. The DR/C_{ss} and C_{ss} values are plotted on the graph to calculate V_{max} (*y* intercept) and K_m (minus slope). The steady-state Michaelis-Menten equation can be used to compute C_{ss} for a given DR or a DR for any C_{ss}.

Cyclosporine

Because of the large amount of variability in cyclosporine pharmacokinetics, even when concurrent disease states and conditions are identified, many clinicians believe that the use of standardized initial cyclosporine doses for various situations is warranted. Indeed, most transplant centers use doses that are determined employing a locally derived cyclosporine dosage protocol. The original computations of these doses were based on the pharmacokinetic dosing methods described in preceding sections and subsequently modified based on clinical experience. In general, the expected cyclosporine steady-state concentration used to compute these doses depends on the type of transplanted tissue and the posttransplantation time line. Generally speaking, initial oral doses of 8 to 18 mg/kg per day or intravenous doses of 3 to 6 mg/kg per day (one-third the oral dose to account for approximately 30% oral bioavailability) are used and vary greatly from institution to institution. For obese individuals (more than 30% over ideal body weight), ideal body weight should be used to compute initial doses.

It is likely that doses computed using patient population characteristics will not always produce cyclosporine concentrations that are expected or desirable. Additionally, there is a very high amount of interday variation in cyclosporine concentrations. Because of pharmacokinetic variability, the narrow therapeutic index of cyclosporine, and the severity of cyclosporine adverse side effects, measurement of cyclosporine concentrations is mandatory for patients to ensure that therapeutic, nontoxic levels are present. When cyclosporine concentrations are measured in patients and a dosage change is necessary, clinicians should seek to use the simplest, most straightforward method available to determine a dose that will provide safe and effective treatment. In most cases, a simple dosage ratio can be used to change cyclosporine doses using steady-state concentrations and assuming that the drug follows linear pharmacokinetics:

$$D_{new} = D_{old}\frac{C_{ss,new}}{C_{ss,old}}$$

For example, LK is a 50-year-old, 75-kg, 5-ft 11-in male renal transplant recipient who is receiving oral cyclosporine 400 mg every 12 hours. The current steady-state blood cyclosporine concentration is 375 ng/mL. To compute a cyclosporine dose that will provide a steady-state concentration of 200 ng/mL, linear pharmacokinetic equations can be used. The new dose to attain the desired concentration should be proportional to the old dose that produced the measured concentration (total daily dose = 400 mg/dose × 2 doses/day = 800 mg/day):

$$D_{new} = D_{old}\frac{C_{ss,new}}{C_{ss,old}} = 800 \text{ mg/day}\frac{200 \text{ ng/mL}}{375 \text{ ng/mL}}$$
$$= 427 \text{ mg/day, round to } 400 \text{ mg/day}$$

The new suggested dose would be 400 mg/day or 200 mg every 12 hours of cyclosporine capsules to be started at the next scheduled dosing time.

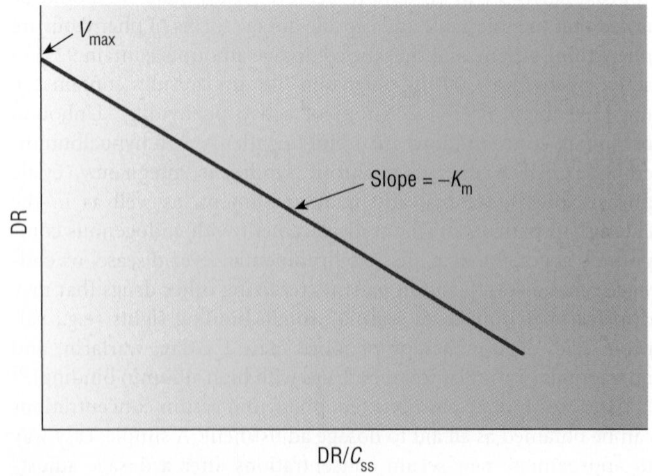

FIGURE 5-13. Relationship between dosage rate (DR) and steady-state serum concentrations (C_{ss}).

CLINICAL PHARMACODYNAMICS

⓰ Pharmacodynamics is the study of the relationship between the concentration of a drug and the response obtained in a patient. Originally, investigators examined the dose–response relationship of drugs in humans but found that the same dose of a drug usually resulted in different concentrations in individuals because of pharmacokinetic differences in clearance and volume of distribution. Examples of quantifiable pharmacodynamic measurements include changes in blood pressure during antihypertensive drug therapy, decreases in heart rate during *β*-blocker treatment, and alterations in prothrombin time or international normalized ratio during warfarin therapy.

For drugs that exhibit a direct and reversible effect, the following diagram describes what occurs at the level of the drug receptor:

Drug + receptor ↔ drug – receptor complex ↔ response

According to this scheme, there is a drug receptor located within the target organ or tissue. When a drug molecule "finds" the receptor, it forms a complex that causes the pharmacologic response to occur. The drug and receptor are in dynamic equilibrium with the drug-receptor complex.

THE E_{MAX} AND SIGMOID E_{MAX} MODELS

The mathematical model that comes from the classic drug receptor theory shown previously is known as the E_{max} model:

$$E = \frac{E_{max} \times C}{EC_{50} + C}$$

where E is the pharmacologic effect elicited by the drug, E_{max} is the maximum effect the drug can cause, EC_{50} is the concentration causing one-half the maximum drug effect ($E_{max}/2$), and C is the concentration of drug at the receptor site. EC_{50} can be used as a measure of drug potency (a lower EC_{50} indicating a more potent drug), whereas E_{max} reflects the intrinsic efficacy of the drug (a higher E_{max} indicating greater efficacy). If pharmacologic effect is plotted versus concentration in the E_{max} equation, a hyperbola results with an asymptote equal to E_{max} (Fig. 5–14). At a concentration of zero, no measurable effect is present.

When dealing with human studies in which a drug is administered to a patient and pharmacologic effect is measured, it is very difficult to determine the concentration of drug at the receptor site. Because of this, serum concentrations (total or unbound) usually are used as the concentration parameter in the E_{max} equation. Therefore, the values of E_{max} and EC_{50} are much different than if the drug were added to an isolated tissue contained in a laboratory beaker.

The result is that a much more empirical approach is used to describe the relationship between concentration and effect in clinical pharmacology studies. After a pharmacodynamic experiment has been conducted, concentration–effect plots are generated. The shape of the concentration–effect curve is used to determine which pharmacodynamic model will be used to describe the data. Because of this, the pharmacodynamic models used in a clinical pharmacology study are deterministic in the same way that the shape of the serum-concentration-versus-time curve determines which pharmacokinetic model is used in clinical pharmacokinetic studies.

Sometimes a hyperbolic function does not describe the concentration–effect relationship at lower concentrations adequately. When this is the case, the sigmoid E_{max} equation may be superior to the E_{max} model:

$$E = \frac{E_{max} \times C^n}{EC_{50}^n + C^n}$$

where n is an exponent that changes the shape of the concentration–effect curve. When $n > 1$, the concentration–effect curve is S- or sigmoid-shaped at lower serum concentrations. When $n < 1$, the concentration–effect curve has a steeper slope at lower concentrations (Fig. 5–15).

With both the E_{max} and sigmoid E_{max} models, the largest changes in drug effect occur at the lower end of the concentration scale. Small changes in low serum concentrations cause large changes in effect. As serum concentrations become larger, further increases in serum concentration result in smaller changes in effect. Using the E_{max} model as an example and setting E_{max} = 100 units and EC_{50} = 20 mg/L, doubling the serum concentration from 5 to 10 mg/L increases the effect from 20 to 33 units (a 67% increase), whereas doubling the serum concentration from 40 to 80 mg/L only increases the effect from 67 to 80 units (a 19% increase). This is an important concept for clinicians to remember when doses are being titrated in patients.

LINEAR MODELS

When serum concentrations obtained during a pharmacodynamic experiment are between 20% and 80% of E_{max}, the concentration–effect curve may appear to be linear (Fig. 5–16). This occurs often because lower drug concentrations may not be detectable with the analytic technique used to assay serum samples, and higher drug concentrations may be avoided to prevent toxic side effects. The equation used is that of a simple line: $E = S \times C + I$, where E is the drug effect, C is the drug concentration, S is the slope of the line, and I is the y intercept. In this situation, the value of S can be used as a measure of drug potency (the larger the value of S, the more potent the drug). The linear model can be derived from the E_{max} model. When EC_{50} is much greater than C, $E = (E_{max}/EC_{50})C = S \times C$, where $S = E_{max}/EC_{50}$.

The linear model allows a nonzero value for effect when the concentration equals zero. This may be a baseline value for the effect that is present without the drug, the result of measurement error when determining effect, or model misspecification. Also, this model does not allow the prediction of a maximum response.

Some investigators have used a log-linear model in pharmacodynamic experiments: $E = S \times (\log C) + I$, where the symbols have the

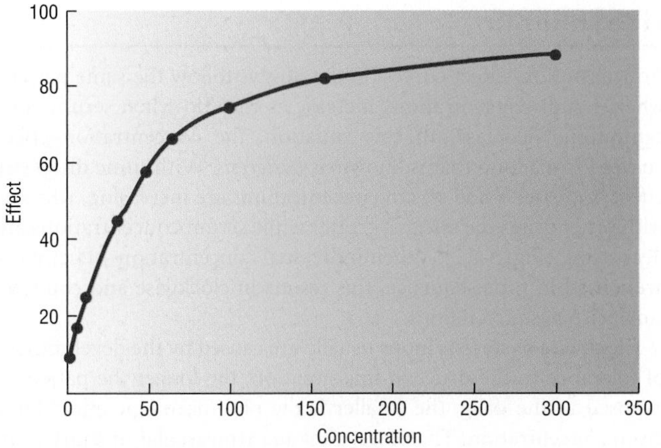

FIGURE 5-14. The E_{max} model [$E = (E_{max} \times C)/(EC_{50} + C)$] has the shape of a hyperbola with an asymptote equal to E_{max}. EC_{50} is the concentration where effect = $E_{max}/2$.

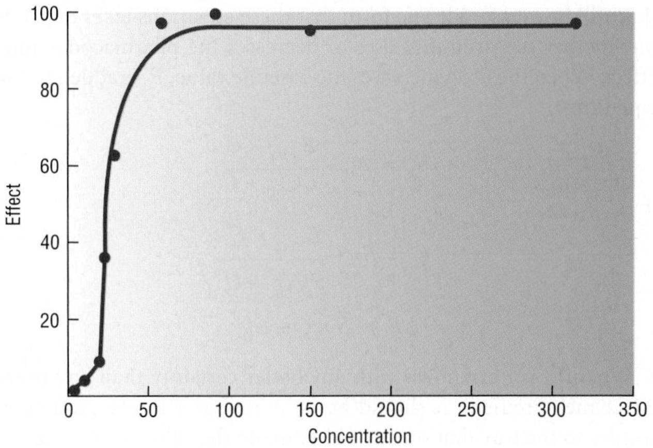

FIGURE 5-15. The sigmoid E_{max} model [$E = (E_{max} \times C^n)/(EC^n_{50} + C^n)$] has an S-shaped curve at lower concentrations. In this example, E_{max} and EC_{50} have the same values as in Fig. 5–14.

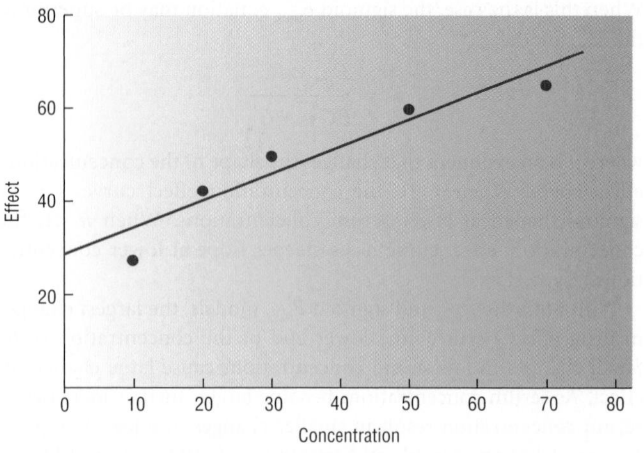

FIGURE 5-16. The linear model ($E = S \times C + I$) is often used as a pharmacodynamic model when the measured pharmacologic effect is 20% to 80% of E_{max}. In this situation, the determination of E_{max} and EC_{50} is not possible. To illustrate this, effect measurements from Fig. 5–14 between 20% and 80% of E_{max} are graphed using the linear pharmacodynamic model.

same meaning as in the linear model. The advantages of this model are that the concentration scale is compressed on concentration–effect plots for experiments where wide concentration ranges were used, and the concentration values are transformed so that linear regression can be used to compute model parameters. The disadvantages are that the model cannot predict a maximum effect or an effect when the concentration equals zero. With the increased availability of nonlinear regression programs that can compute the parameters of nonlinear functions such as the E_{max} model easily, use of the log-linear model has been discouraged.[53]

BASELINE EFFECTS

At times, the effect measured during a pharmacodynamic study has a value before the drug is administered to the patient. In these cases, the drug changes the patient's baseline value. Examples of these types of measurements are heart rate and blood pressure. In addition, a given drug may increase or decrease the baseline value. Two basic techniques are used to incorporate baseline values into pharmacodynamic data. One way incorporates the baseline value into the pharmacodynamic model; the other way transforms the effect data to take baseline values into account.

Incorporation of the baseline value into the pharmacodynamic model involves the addition of a new term to the previous equations. E_0 is the symbol used to denote the baseline value of the effect that will be measured. The form that these equations takes depends on whether the drug increases or decreases the pharmacodynamic effect. When the drug increases the baseline value, E_0 is added to the equations:

$$E = E_0 + \frac{E_{max} \times C}{EC_{50} + C}$$

$$E = E_0 + \frac{E_{max} \times C^n}{EC_{50}^n + C^n}$$

$$E = S \times C + E_0$$

When E_0 is not known with any better certainty than any other effect measurement, it should be estimated as a model parameter similar to the way that one would estimate the values of E_{max}, EC_{50}, S, or n.[54,55] If the baseline effect is well known and has only a small amount of measurement error, it can be subtracted from the effect determined in the patient during the experiment and not estimated as a model parameter. This approach can lead to better estimates of the remaining model parameters.[55] Using the linear model as an example, the equation used would be $E - E_0 = S \times C$.

If the drug decreases the baseline value, the drug effect is subtracted from E_0 in the pharmacodynamic models:

$$E = E_0 - \frac{E_{max} \times C}{IC_{50} + C}$$

$$E = E_0 - \frac{E_{max} \times C^n}{IC_{50}^n + C^n}$$

$$E = E_0 - S \times C$$

where E_{max} represents the maximum reduction in effect caused by the drug, and IC_{50} is the concentration that produces a 50% inhibition of E_{max}. These forms of the equations have been called the *inhibitory* E_{max} and *inhibitory sigmoidal* E_{max} *equations*, respectively. In this arrangement of the pharmacodynamic model, E_0 is a model parameter and can be estimated. If the baseline effect is well known and has little measurement error, the effect in the presence of the drug can be subtracted from the baseline effect and not estimated as a model parameter. Using the inhibitory E_{max} model as an example, the formula would be $E_0 - E = (E_{max} \times C)/(IC_{50} + C)$.

When using the inhibitory E_{max} model, a special situation occurs if the baseline effect can be obliterated completely by the drug (e.g., decreased premature ventricular contractions during antiarrhythmic therapy). In this situation, $E_{max} = E_0$, and the equation simplifies to a rearrangement known as the *fractional* E_{max} *equation:*

$$E = E_0\left(1 - \frac{C}{IC_{50} + C}\right)$$

This form of the model relates drug concentration to the fraction of the maximum effect.

An alternative approach to the pharmacodynamic modeling of drugs that alter baseline effects is to transform the effect data so that they represent a percentage increase or decrease from the baseline value.[55] For drugs that increase the effect, the following transformation equation would be used: percent effect$_t$ = [(treatment$_t$ – baseline)/baseline] × 100. For drugs that decrease the effect, the following formula would be applied to the data: percent inhibition$_t$ = [(baseline – treatment$_t$)/baseline] × 100. The subscript indicates the treatment, effect, or inhibition that occurred at time t during the experiment. If the study included a placebo control phase, baseline measurements made at the same time as treatment measurements (i.e., heart rate determined 2 hours after placebo and 2 hours after drug treatment) could be used in the appropriate transformation equation.[55] The appropriate model (excluding E_0) then would be used.

HYSTERESIS

Concentration–effect curves do not always follow the same pattern when serum concentrations increase as they do when serum concentrations decrease. In this situation, the concentration–effect curves form a loop that is known as *hysteresis*. With some drugs the effect is greater when serum concentrations are increasing, whereas with other drugs the effect is greater while serum concentrations are decreasing (Fig. 5–17). When individual concentration–effect pairs are joined in time sequence, this results in clockwise and counterclockwise hysteresis loops.

Clockwise hysteresis loops usually are caused by the development of tolerance to the drug. In this situation, the longer the patient is exposed to the drug, the smaller is the pharmacologic effect for a given concentration. Therefore, after an extravascular or short-term infusion dose of the drug, the effect is smaller when serum concentrations are decreasing compared with the time when serum concentrations are increasing during the infusion or absorption phase.

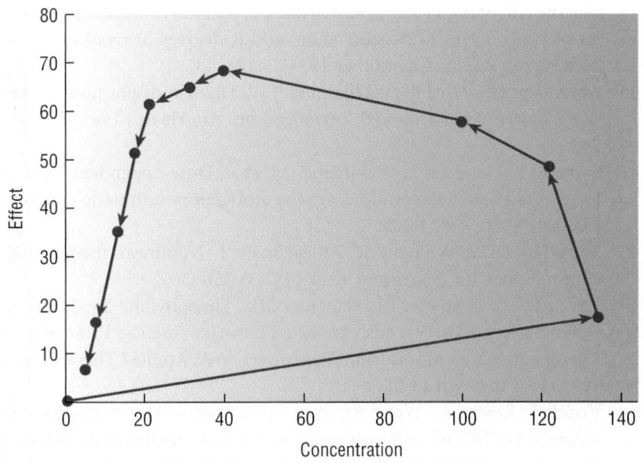

FIGURE 5-17. Hysteresis occurs when effect measurements are different at the same concentration. This is commonly seen after short-term intravenous infusions or extravascular doses where concentrations increase and subsequently decrease. Counterclockwise hysteresis loops are found when concentration–effect points are joined as time increases *(shown by arrows)* and effect is larger at the same concentration but at a later time. Clockwise hysteresis loops are similar, but the concentration–effect points are joined in clockwise order and the effect is smaller at a later time.

Accumulation of a drug metabolite that acts as an antagonist also can cause clockwise hysteresis.

Counterclockwise hysteresis loops can be caused by the accumulation of an active metabolite, sensitization to the drug, or delay in time in equilibration between serum concentration and concentration of drug at the site of action. Combined pharmacokinetic-pharmacodynamic models have been devised that allow equilibration lag times to be taken into account.

CONCLUSIONS

The availability of inexpensive, rapidly achievable serum drug concentrations has changed the way clinicians monitor drug therapy in patients. The therapeutic range for many drugs is known, and it is likely that more drugs will be monitored using serum concentrations in the future. Clinicians need to remember that the therapeutic range is merely an average guideline and to take into account interindividual pharmacodynamic variability when treating patients. Individual patients may respond to smaller concentrations or require concentrations that are much greater to obtain a therapeutic effect. Conversely, patients may show toxic effects at concentrations within or below the therapeutic range. Serum concentrations should never replace clinical judgment.

Three kinetic constants determine the dosage requirements of patients. Clearance determines the maintenance dose ($MD = CLC_{ss}$), volume of distribution determines the loading dose ($LD = V_DC_{ss}$), and half-life determines the time to steady state and the dosage interval. Several methods are available to compute these parameters.

Methods available to individualize drug therapy range from clinical pharmacokinetic techniques using simple mathematical relationships that hold for all drugs that obey linear pharmacokinetics to very complex computer programs that are specific to one drug.

REFERENCES

1. Koup JR, Gibaldi M. Some comments on the evaluation of bioavailability data. Drug Intell Clin Pharm 1980;14:327–330.
2. Gibaldi M, Boyes RN, Feldman S. Influence of first pass effect on availability of drugs on oral administration. J Pharm Sci 1971;60:1338–1340.
3. Wu C-Y, Benet LZ, Hebert MF, et al. Differentiation of absorption and first-pass gut and hepatic metabolism in humans: Studies with cyclosporine. Clin Pharmacol Ther 1995;58:492–497.
4. Wagner JG, Northam JI, Alway CD, et al. Blood levels of drug at the equilibrium state after multiple dosing. Nature 1965;207:1301–1302.
5. Rowland M, Benet LZ, Graham GG. Clearance concepts in pharmacokinetics. J Pharmacokinet Biopharm 1973;1:123–136.
6. Wilkinson GR, Shand DG. A physiological approach to hepatic drug clearance. Clin Pharmacol Ther 1975;18:377–390.
7. Nies AS, Shand DG, Wilkinson GR. Altered hepatic blood flow and drug disposition. Clin Pharmacokinet 1976;1:135–155.
8. Gibaldi M, Koup JR. Pharmacokinetic concepts: Drug binding, apparent volume of distribution and clearance. Eur J Clin Pharmacol 1981;20:299–305.
9. Bowdle TA, Patel IH, Levy RH, et al. Valproic acid dosage and plasma protein binding and clearance. Clin Pharmacol Ther 1980;28:486–492.
10. Lima JJ, Boudonlas H, Blanford M. Concentration-dependence of disopyramide binding to plasma protein and its influence on kinetics and dynamics. J Pharmacol Exp Ther 1981;219:741–747.
11. Gibaldi M, Perrier D. Pharmacokinetics, 2d ed. New York: Marcel Dekker, 1980.
12. Gibaldi M. Estimation of the pharmacokinetic parameters of the two-compartment open model from post-infusion plasma concentration data. J Pharm Sci 1969;58:1133–1135.
13. Loo JCK, Riegelman S. Assessment of pharmacokinetic constants from postinfusion blood curves obtained after IV infusion. J Pharm Sci 1970;59:53–55.
14. Wagner JG. Model-independent linear pharmacokinetics. Drug Intell Clin Pharm 1976;10:179–180.
15. Hansten PD, Horn JR. The Top 100 Drug Interactions: A Guide to Patient Management, 2007 ed. Freeland, WA: H&H Publications, 2007.
16. Cockcroft DW, Gault MH. Prediction of creatinine clearance from serum creatinine. Nephron 1976;16:31–41.
17. Traub SL, Johnson CE. Comparison of methods of estimating creatinine clearance in children. Am J Hosp Pharm 1980;37:195–201.
18. Salazar DE, Corcoran GB. Predicting creatinine clearance and renal drug clearance in obese patients from estimated fat-free body mass. Am J Med 1988;84:1053–1060.
19. Jelliffe RW, Jelliffe SM. A computer program for estimation of creatinine clearance from unstable serum creatinine levels, age, sex, and weight. Math Biosci 1972;14:17–24.
20. Koup JR, Jusko WJ, Elwood CM, Kohli RK. Digoxin pharmacokinetics: Role of renal failure in dosage regimen design. Clin Pharmacol Ther 1975;18:9–21.
21. Matzke GR, McGory RW, Halstenson CE, Keane WF. Pharmacokinetics of vancomycin in patients with various degrees of renal function. Antimicrob Agents Chemother 1984;25:433–437.
22. Sarubbi FA, Hull JH. Amikacin serum concentrations: Predictions of levels and dosage guidelines. Ann Intern Med 1978;89:612–618.
23. Sivan SK, Bennett WM. Drug dosing guidelines in patients with renal failure. West J Med 1992;156:633–638.
24. Brier ME, Aronoff GR. Drug Prescribing in Renal Failure, 5th ed. Philadelphia: American College of Physicians, 2007.
25. Pugh RNH, Murray-Lyon IM, Dawson JL, et al. Transection of the oesophagus for bleeding oesophageal varices. Br J Surg 1973;60:646–649.
26. Jusko WJ, Gardner MJ, Mangione A, et al. Factors affecting theophylline clearances: Age, tobacco, marijuana, cirrhosis, congestive heart failure, obesity, oral contraceptives, benzodiazepines, barbiturates, and ethanol. J Pharm Sci 1979;68:1358–1366.
27. Thomson PD, Melmon KL, Richardson JA, et al. Lidocaine pharmacokinetics in advanced heart failure, liver disease, and renal failure in humans. Ann Intern Med 1973;78:499–508.
28. Koup JR, Killen T, Bauer LA. Multiple-dose nonlinear regression analysis program: Aminoglycoside dose prediction. Clin Pharmacokinet 1983;8:456–462.
29. Sheiner LB, Beal S, Rosenberg B, et al. Forecasting individual pharmacokinetics. Clin Pharmacol Ther 1979;26:294–305.
30. Sheiner LB, Beal SL. Bayesian individualization of pharmacokinetics: Simple implementation and comparison with non-Bayesian methods. J Pharm Sci 1982;71:1344–1348.

31. Schentag JJ, Jusko WJ. Renal clearance and tissue accumulation of gentamicin. Clin Pharmacol Ther 1977;22:364–370.
32. Sawchuk RJ, Zaske DE, Cipolle RJ, et al. Kinetic model for gentamicin dosing with the use of individual patient parameters. Clin Pharmacol Ther 1977;21:362–369.
33. Bauer LA, Edwards WAD, Dellinger EP, Simonowitz DA. Influence of weight on aminoglycoside pharmacokinetics in normal weight and morbidly obese patients. Eur J Clin Pharmacol 1983;24:643–647.
34. Bauer LA, Piecoro JJ, Wilson HD, Blouin RA. Gentamicin and tobramycin pharmacokinetics in patients with cystic fibrosis. Clin Pharm 1983;2:262–264.
35. Sampliner R, Perrier D, Powell R, Finley P. Influence of ascites on tobramycin pharmacokinetics. J Clin Pharmacol 1984;24:43–46.
36. Zank KE, Miwa L, Cohen JL, et al. Effect of body weight on gentamicin pharmacokinetics in neonates. Clin Pharm 1984;3:170–173.
37. Pancorbo S, Sawchuk RJ, Dashe C, et al. Use of a pharmacokinetic model for individual intravenous doses of aminophylline. Eur J Clin Pharmacol 1979;16:251–254.
38. Nicolau DP, Freeman CD, Belliveau PP, et al. Experience with a once-daily aminoglycoside program administered to 2184 adult patients. Antimicrob Agents Chemother 1995;39:650–655.
39. Cantu TG, Yamanaka-Yuen NA, Lietman PS. Serum vancomycin concentrations: Reappraisal of their clinical value. Clin Infect Dis 1994;18:533–543.
40. Welty TE, Copa AK. Impact of vancomycin therapeutic drug monitoring on patient care. Ann Pharmacother 1994;28:1335–1339.
41. Zimmermann AE, Katona BG, Plaisance KI. Association of vancomycin serum concentrations with outcomes in patients with gram-positive bacteremia. Pharmacotherapy 1995;15:85–91.
42. Karam CM, McKinnon PS, Neuhauser MM, Rybak MJ. Outcome assessment of minimizing vancomycin monitoring and dosage adjustments. Pharmacotherapy 1999;19:257–266.
43. Moellering RC Jr, Krogstad DJ, Greenblatt DJ. Vancomycin therapy in patients with impaired renal function: A nomogram for dosage. Ann Intern Med 1981;94:343–346.
44. Blouin RA, Bauer LA, Miller DD, et al. Vancomycin pharmacokinetics in normal and morbidly obese subjects. Antimicrob Agents Chemother 1982;21:575–580.
45. Matzke GR, McGory RW, Halstenson CE, Keane WF. Pharmacokinetics of vancomycin in patients with various degrees of renal function. Antimicrob Agents Chemother 1984;25:433–437.
46. Abernethy DR, Greenblatt DJ, Smith TW. Digoxin disposition in obesity: Clinical pharmacokinetic investigations. Am Heart J 1981;102:740–744.
47. Sarrazin E, Hendeles L, Weinberger M, et al. Dose-dependent kinetics for theophylline: Observations among ambulatory asthmatic children. J Pediatr 1980;97:825–828.
48. Tang-Liu DDS, Williams RL, Riegelman S. Nonlinear theophylline elimination. Clin Pharmacol Ther 1982;31:358–369.
49. Edwards DJ, Zarowitz BJ, Slaughter RL. Theophylline In: Evans E, Schentag JJ, Jusko WJ, eds. Applied Pharmacokinetics: Principles of Therapeutic Drug Monitoring. Vancouver, WA: Applied Therapeutics, 1992, 13-1 through 13-38.
50. Vozeh S, Kewitz G, Wenk M, et al. Rapid prediction of steady-state serum theophylline concentrations in patients treated with intravenous aminophylline. Eur J Clin Pharmacol 1980;18:473–477.
51. Vozeh S, Muir KT, Sheiner LB, Follath F. Predicting individual phenytoin dosage. J Pharmacokinet Biopharm 1991;9:131–146.
52. Ludden TM, Allen JP, Valutsky WA, et al. Individualization of phenytoin dosage regimens. Clin Pharmacol Ther 1977;21:287–293.
53. Holford NHG, Sheiner LB. Understanding the dose-effect relationship: Clinical application of pharmacokinetic-pharmacodynamic models. Clin Pharmacokinet 1981;6:429–453.
54. Schwinghammer TL, Kroboth PD. Basic concepts in pharmacodynamic modeling. J Clin Pharmacol 1988;28:388–394.
55. Sheiner LB, Stanski DR, Vozeh S, et al. Simultaneous modeling of pharmacokinetics and pharmacodynamics: Application to *d*-tubocurarine. Clin Pharmacol Ther 1979;25:358.
56. Niederman MS, Craven DE. Guidelines for the management of adults with hospital-acquired, ventilator-associated, and healthcare-associated pneumonia. Am J Respir Crit Care Med 2005;171(4):388–416.
57. Bauer LA. Use of mixed-effect modeling to determine the influence of albumin, bilirubin, valproic acid, warfarin, and aspirin on phenytoin unbound fraction and pharmacokinetics. J Am Pharm Assoc 2004;44:236–237.

CHAPTER 6

Pharmacogenetics

LARISA H. CAVALLARI AND Y.W. FRANCIS LAM

KEY CONCEPTS

1. Genetic variations contribute to interpatient differences in drug response.
2. Genetic variations occur for drug metabolism, drug transporter, and drug target proteins as well as for disease-associated genes.
3. Genetic polymorphisms may be linked to drug efficacy and toxicity.
4. Pharmacogenetics is the study of the impact of genetic polymorphisms on drug response.
5. The goals of pharmacogenetics are to optimize drug efficacy and limit drug toxicity based on an individual's DNA.
6. Single nucleotide polymorphisms are the most common variations in the human genome.
7. Gene therapy aims to cure disease caused by genetic defects by changing gene expression.
8. Inadequate gene delivery and expression and serious adverse effects are obstacles to successful gene therapy.

Individuals vary greatly in their response to drug therapy, and predicting how effective or safe a medication will be for a particular patient often is difficult. For example, when treating a patient with hypertension, several agents or a combination of agents may be attempted before adequate blood pressure control with acceptable tolerability is achieved. A number of nongenetic factors influence drug response, including pharmacokinetics, age, and concomitant drug use. However, considering these factors alone often is insufficient for predicting the likelihood of drug efficacy or safety for a given patient. For instance, identical antihypertensive therapy in two patients with similar demographic characteristics, medical histories, and concomitant drug therapy may produce inadequate blood pressure reduction in one patient and symptomatic hypotension in the other.

❶ ❷ The observed interpatient variability in drug response may result largely from genetically determined differences in drug metabolism, drug distribution, and drug target proteins. The influence of heredity on drug response was demonstrated as early as 1956 with the discovery that an inherited deficiency of glucose-6-phosphate dehydrogenase was responsible for hemolytic reactions to the antimalarial drug primaquine.[1] Variations in genes encoding cytochrome P450 (CYP450) and other drug-metabolizing enzymes now are well-recognized causes of interindividual differences in plasma concentrations of certain drugs. These variations may have serious implications for drugs with a narrow therapeutic index, such as warfarin, phenytoin, and mercaptopurine.[2–4] More recent interest focuses on associations between drug response and variations in genes for drug transporters such as P-glycoprotein and drug targets such as receptors, enzymes, and proteins involved in intracellular signal transduction. Genetic variations of drug-metabolizing enzymes and drug transporter proteins may influence pharmacokinetic drug properties, thus altering drug disposition. Drug target genes may alter pharmacodynamic mechanisms by affecting sensitivity to a drug at its target site. Finally, genes associated with disease severity have been correlated with drug efficacy despite having no direct effect on pharmacokinetic or pharmacodynamic mechanisms.

Learning objectives, review questions, and other resources can be found at **www.pharmacotherapyonline.com.**

PHARMACOGENETICS: A DEFINITION

❸ ❹ Pharmacogenetics involves the search for genetic variations that lead to interindividual differences in drug response. The term *pharmacogenetics* often is used interchangeably with the term *pharmacogenomics*. However, *pharmacogenetics* generally refers to monogenetic variants that affect drug response, whereas *pharmacogenomics* refers to the entire spectrum of genes that interact to determine drug efficacy and safety. For example, a pharmacogenetic study would examine the influence of the β_1-adrenergic receptor gene on blood pressure response to carvedilol. A pharmacogenomic study might examine the interaction between CYP2D6 and β_1-, β_2-, and α_1-adrenergic receptor genes on carvedilol effects. To date, most studies of gene–drug responses are pharmacogenetic in nature. However, given that multiple proteins are involved in determining the ultimate response to most drugs, many investigators are taking a more pharmacogenomic approach to elucidating genetic contributions to drug response. For simplicity, this chapter treats pharmacogenetics and pharmacogenomics as synonymous.

❺ The goals of pharmacogenetics are to optimize drug therapy and limit drug toxicity based on an individual's genetic profile. Thus, pharmacogenetics aims to use genetic information to choose a drug, drug dose, and treatment duration that will have the greatest likelihood of achieving therapeutic outcomes with the least potential for harm in a given patient. The results of pharmacogenetic research ultimately will provide opportunities for clinicians to use genetic tests to predict individual responses to drug treatments, specifically to select medications for patients based on DNA profiles and to develop novel strategies for disease treatment and prevention based on an understanding of genetic control of cellular functions.

Although there has been considerable interest in genetic influences of drug response in recent years, pharmacogenetics is not a new area. In 1957, shortly after the discovery of a genetic predisposition toward primaquine-induced toxicity, Arno Motulsky pro-

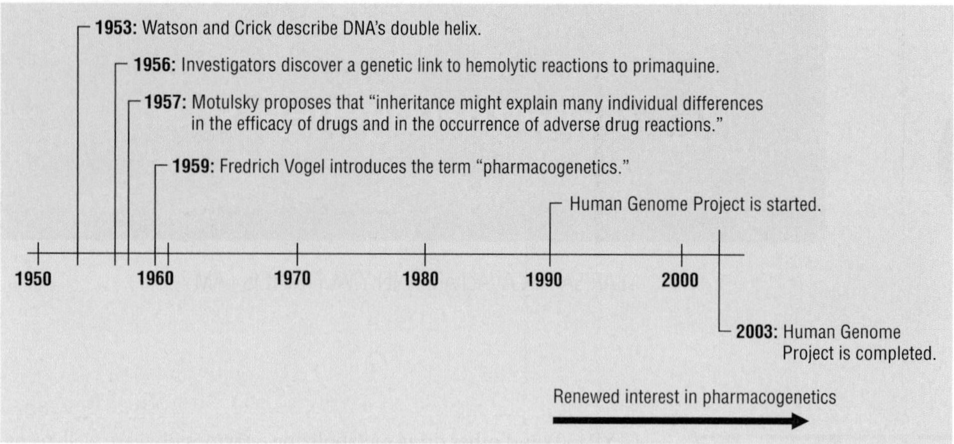

FIGURE 6-1. Time line of genomic discoveries.

posed that inheritance might underlie much of the disparity in drug response among individuals (Fig. 6–1).[5] Two years later, Fredrich Vogel introduced the term *pharmacogenetics*.[6] With the advent of the Human Genome Project in 1990 came a resurgence of interest in determining genetic contributions to drug response.

HUMAN GENOME PROJECT

In 1988, Congress commissioned the Department of Energy and the National Institutes of Health to plan and implement the Human Genome Project. The goal of the Human Genome Project was to determine the entire sequence of the human genome by 2005. Mapping of the human genome, which officially began in 1990, has led to a better understanding of genetic contributions to disease susceptibility. To encourage research and ultimately maximize the societal benefits of the Human Genome Project, sequence data from the Human Genome Project have been deposited into a freely accessible database run by the National Center for Biotechnology Information (*www.ncbi.nlm.nih.gov*). As a consequence of these shared data, research efforts in the 1990s accelerated the discovery of genetic variations affecting treatment response and the development of new treatments and preventive strategies for human disease.

Largely because of advances in biotechnology, the initial working draft of the human genome sequence was completed in 2000, well ahead of schedule.[7] In April 2003, 50 years after James Watson and Francis Crick described the double-helix structure of DNA and more than 2 years ahead of schedule, researchers announced the completion of the Human Genome Project.[8] The final version contains 99% of the gene-containing sequence, with 99.9% accuracy.

Following completion of the Human Genome Project, the National Human Genome Research Institute announced its vision for the future of genomic research with the goal of improving human health and well-being.[9] One of the challenges set forth to meet this goal is to develop genome-based approaches to predict drug response. This challenge involves the accurate, unbiased determination of genetic variants linked to drug response, advanced technology to efficiently determine genotype, and appropriate integration of genetic testing into the therapeutic decision process. The National Human Genome Research Institute also challenges investigators to develop new, gene-based approaches to disease management, which will require a thorough understanding of genetic determinants of disease susceptibility and progression.

GENETIC CONCEPTS

The human genome contains approximately three billion nucleotide bases, which code for approximately 20,000 to 25,000 protein-coding genes. Two purine nucleotide bases, adenine (A) and guanine (G), and two pyrimidine nucleotide bases, cytosine (C) and thymidine (T), are present in DNA. Purines and pyrimidines always pair together as A-T and C-G in the two strands that make up the DNA structure. Most nucleotide base pairs are identical from person to person, with only 0.1% contributing to individual differences.

According to the central dogma, when one strand of DNA is transcribed into RNA and translated to make proteins, three consecutive nucleotides form a *codon*. Each codon specifies an amino acid or amino acid chain termination. For example, the nucleotide sequence, or codon, GGA specifies the amino acid glycine. The genetic code has substantial redundancy, in that two or more codons code for the same amino acid. For example, GGC, GGG, and GGT also code for glycine. Amino acids are the basic constituents of proteins, which mediate all cellular functions. Only 20 different amino acids, in various arrangements, form the basic units of all the proteins in the human body.

A *gene* is a series of codons that specifies a particular protein. Genes contain several regions: *exons* that encode for the final protein, *introns* that consist of intervening noncoding regions, and *regulatory regions* that control gene transcription. In most cases, an individual carries two alleles, one from each parent, at each gene locus. An *allele* is defined as the sequence of nucleic acid bases at a given gene chromosomal locus. Two identical alleles make up a *homozygous* genotype. Two different alleles make up a *heterozygous* genotype. The *phenotype* refers to the outward expression of the genotype.

TYPES OF GENETIC VARIATIONS

Genetic variations occur as either rare defects or polymorphisms. *Polymorphisms* are defined as variations that occur at a frequency of at least 1% in the human population. For example, the genes encoding the CYP450 enzymes CYP2A6, CYP2C9, CYP2C19, CYP2D6, and CYP3A4 are polymorphic, with functional mutations of >1% occurring in different ethnic groups. In contrast, rare mutations occur in <1% of the population and cause inherited diseases such as cystic fibrosis, hemophilia, and Huntington's disease. Common diseases, such as essential hypertension and diabetes mellitus, are polygenic in that multiple genetic polymorphisms likely interact with environmental factors to contribute to the disease susceptibility.

❻ Single nucleotide polymorphisms (SNPs; pronounced "snips") are the most common genetic variations in human DNA, occurring approximately once in every 100 to 300 base pairs. To date more than four million SNPs have been mapped in the human genome. SNPs occur when one nucleotide base pair replaces another (Fig. 6–2). Thus, SNPs are single-base differences that exist between individuals. Nucleotide substitution results in two possible alleles. One allele, typically either the most commonly occurring

A. "Wild-type" allele

Codon	13	14	15	16	17	18	19
Nucleotide	...GCA	CCC	AAT	<u>A</u>GA	AGC	CAT	GCG ...
Amino acid	Ala	Pro	Asn	**Arg**	Ser	His	Ala

B. "Variant" allele

Codon	13	14	15	16	17	18	19
Nucleotide	...GCA	CCC	AAT	<u>G</u>GA	AGC	CAT	GCG ...
Amino acid	Ala	Pro	Asn	**Gly**	Ser	His	Ala

FIGURE 6-2. Nucleotide sequence of the β_2-adrenergic receptor gene from codons 13 through 19. *A.* Nucleotide sequence of the wild-type allele with adenine (A) at nucleotide position 46 *(underlined)* located in codon 16 of the β_2-adrenergic receptor gene. The AGA codon designates the amino acid arginine (Arg), with an average frequency of 39% in the human population. *B.* Nucleotide sequence of the variant allele with guanine (G) at nucleotide position 46 *(underlined)*, located in codon 16. The GGA codon designates the amino acid glycine (Gly), which occurs at an average frequency of 61%. Although the Arg16 polymorphism occurs less commonly than the Gly16 polymorphism, it is referred to as the wild type because it was identified first.

allele or the allele originally sequenced, is considered the *wild type;* the alternative allele is considered the *variant allele.*

A SNP may change the codon resulting in amino acid substitution, which may or may not alter the amount or function of the encoded protein. For example, in Fig. 6–2, guanine (G) is substituted for adenine (A) at nucleotide 46 in the β_2-adrenergic receptor gene. This results in the substitution of glycine for arginine at amino acid position (codon) 16 and alterations in receptor downregulation upon prolonged exposure to β_2-receptor agonists.[10] SNPs such as this that result in amino acid substitution are referred to as *nonsynonymous.* SNPs that do not result in amino acid substitution are called *synonymous.* Referring to a previous example of redundancy in the genetic code, replacement of adenine (A) with cytosine (C) in the codon AGA is an example of a synonymous SNP because the resulting amino acid still is glycine. Synonymous SNPs usually are abbreviated based on the nucleotides involved and the nucleotide base position. For example, A1166C or A1166→C indicates that cytosine is substituted for adenine at nucleotide position 1166 of a given gene region. Nonsynonymous SNPs usually are designated by the amino acids and codon involved. For example, Arg16Gly or Arg16→Gly indicates that glycine is substituted for arginine at codon 16. If a SNP changes the amount or function of a protein that contributes to drug response, it may alter a patient's sensitivity to a drug or predispose the patient to adverse reactions to drug therapy.

Other examples of genetic variants include the following:

- *Insertion–deletion polymorphisms,* in which a nucleotide or nucleotide sequence either is added to or deleted from a DNA sequence
- *Tandem repeats,* in which a nucleotide sequence repeats in tandem (e.g., if "AG" is the nucleotide repeat unit, "AGAGAGAGAG" is a five-tandem repeat)
- *Frameshift mutation,* in which there is an insertion/deletion polymorphism and the number of nucleotides added or lost is not a multiple of three, resulting in disruption of the gene's reading frame
- *Defective splicing,* in which an internal polypeptide segment is abnormally removed, and the ends of the remaining polypeptide chain are joined
- *Aberrant splice site,* in which processing of the protein occurs at an alternate site
- *Premature stop codon polymorphisms,* in which there is premature termination of the polypeptide chain by a stop codon (specific sequence of three nucleotides that do not code for an amino acid but rather specify polypeptide chain termination)

SNPs may occur in exon, intron, or regulatory regions of a gene. Those occurring in exon regions may alter the function of a protein, whereas those in regulatory regions may alter the amount of protein that is produced. Variations in the intron region often are silent unless they affect intron splicing. Multiple SNPs may be in *linkage disequilibrium* with each other, meaning that two or more SNPs are inherited together more frequently than expected based on chance alone. For example, if two SNPs, A46T and G72C, are possible in a given gene and if a T at position 46 always occurs with a C at position 72, the two SNPs are said to be in *complete linkage disequilibrium.* A set of SNPs that are inherited together is called a *haplotype.* For more detailed information about genetic concepts, refer to the recommended genetics textbook.[11]

Most common diseases are polygenic in nature. For example, genes for numerous proteins involved in the renin–angiotensin system, sympathetic nervous system, and renal sodium transport have been associated with the risk for essential hypertension.[12] Environmental factors are well-known risk factors for diseases such as hypertension and often interact with genetic factors to influence disease susceptibility and progression. Given the complex pathophysiology of most common diseases, genes linked to disease susceptibility are not discussed in this chapter. Rather, this chapter focuses on genetic variations linked to responses to pharmacologic agents.

POLYMORPHISMS IN GENES FOR DRUG-METABOLIZING ENZYMES

❸ Polymorphisms in the drug-metabolizing enzymes represent the first recognized and the most documented examples of genetic variants with consequences in drug response and toxicity. The major phase I enzymes are the CYP450 superfamily of isoenzymes. *N*-acetyltransferase, uridine diphosphate glucuronosyltransferase (UGT), and glutathione *S*-transferase are examples of phase II metabolizing enzymes that exhibit genetic polymorphisms. Thiopurine *S*-methyltransferase (TPMT) and dihydropyrimidine dehydrogenase (DPD) are examples of nucleotide base-metabolizing enzymes. Table 6–1 lists selected examples of polymorphic metabolizing enzymes, corresponding drug substrates, and consequences of altered enzyme function as a result of gene variation.

CYTOCHROME P450 ENZYMES

Currently, 57 different CYP450 isoenzymes have been documented to be present in humans, with 42 involved in the metabolism of exogenous xenobiotics and endogenous substances such as steroids and prostaglandins.[12] Fifteen of these isoenzymes are known to be involved in the metabolism of drugs, but significant interindividual variabilities in enzyme activity exist as a result of induction, inhibition, and genetic inheritance. Functional genetic polymorphism has been discovered for CYP2A6, CYP2C9, CYP2C19, CYP2D6,[13] and, more recently, CYP3A4/5.[14,15] A polymorphism in the regulatory region of the gene encoding for CYP1A2 has been identified,[16] but its functional importance remains to be determined.

CYP2D6

Polymorphisms in the *CYP2D6* gene are the best characterized of the CYP450 variants. At least 48 gene variants and 53 alleles in the

TABLE 6-1 Selected Examples of Genetic Polymorphisms in Drug-Metabolizing Enzymes and Response to Drug Therapy

Genetic Variants/Genes	Drug	Drug Effect Associated with Polymorphism
*CYP2D6*4, CYP2D6*5*	Perhexiline	Neuropathy[18]
	Codeine	Significant reduction in analgesic effect[22,23]
	Tramadol	
*CYP2D6*2 (n > l)*	Tricyclic antidepressants (e.g., desipramine, nortriptyline)	Inadequate antidepressant response[30,31]
*CYP2D6*10*	Antipsychotics (e.g., haloperidol)	Elevated plasma concentrations and exaggerated responses[34]
*CYP2CP*2, CYP2C9*3*	Warfarin	Hemorrhage[2]
CYP2C9, CYP2C19	Phenytoin	Phenytoin toxicity[3]
CYP2C19	Omeprazole	Improved cure rates for *Helicobacter pylori*[42]
Glutathione-*S*-transferase	Primaquine	Hemolytic reactions[1]
Thiopurine methyltransferase	Mercaptopurine	Bone marrow depression[4]
N-Acetyltransferase slow acetylator	Isoniazid	More prone to peripheral neuropathy[105]
	Procainamide	More prone to development of systemic lupus erthematosus-like syndrome[106,107]
	Hydralazine	
	Sulfonamides	Increased hematologic and gastrointestinal adverse reactions[108]
Uridine diphosphate glucuronosyltransferase	Irinotecan	Increased severity of diarrhea and neutropenia in carrier of $(TA)^{7}TAA$ allele[62]

CYP2D6 gene have been identified.[17] Nevertheless, the CYP2D6 extensive-metabolizer (EM) and poor-metabolizer (PM) phenotypes (outward expression of genotypes) can be predicted with up to 99% confidence with six genotypic variants. *CYP2D6*1* is considered the wild-type variant and exhibits normal enzyme activity. *CYP2D6*2* has the same activity as *CYP2D6*1* but is capable of duplication or amplification. Both variants are present in EMs. The *CYP2D6*4* (defective splicing) and *CYP2D6*5* (gene deletion) variants are predominantly found in white PMs (5% to 10% of the Caucasian population)[17] and result in an inactive enzyme and an absence of enzyme, respectively. The predominant variants in people of Asian and African heritage are *CYP2D6*10* (Pro34Ser) and *CYP2D6*17* (Arg296Cys), respectively. Both result in a single amino acid substitution and consequent reduction in enzyme activity.

Poor CYP2D6 metabolizers carry two defective alleles, such as *CYP2D6*3, CYP2D6*4* (more common), *CYP2D6*5*, and *CYP2D6*6*, resulting in a total absence of active enzyme and an impaired ability to metabolize CYP2D6-dependent substrates. Examples of CYP2D6 substrates include neuroleptic medications, antidepressants such as tricyclic antidepressants and mianserin, antiarrhythmic drugs such as propafenone, and β-adrenergic antagonists such as metoprolol (see Table 6–1). Depending on the importance of the affected CYP2D6 pathway to overall drug metabolism and the drug's therapeutic index, clinically significant side effects may occur in PMs as a result of elevated parent drug concentrations. For example, compared with EMs, PMs develop neuropathy after treatment with the antianginal agent perhexiline[18] and have experienced more adverse effects with propafenone[19] and neuroleptic agents such as perphenazine.[20,21]

The therapeutic implication of CYP2D6 polymorphism is different if the substrate in question is a prodrug. In this case, PMs would not be able to convert the drug into the therapeutically active metabolite. Two examples of prodrugs dependent on CYP2D6-mediated conversion to active forms are codeine and tramadol. Codeine and tramadol are converted by CYP2D6 to morphine and *O*-desmethyltramadol, respectively; thus, poor CYP2D6 metabolizers experience little or no analgesic relief after taking these drugs.[22,23] Another example is CYP2D6-catalyzed conversion of tamoxifen to the more potent antiestrogen metabolite 4-hydroxytamoxifen.[24]

Although PMs are at a disadvantage from the standpoint of drug toxicity for most CYP2D6 substrates and lack of efficacy for CYP2D6 prodrugs, data suggest that they may be "protected" from abusing opiates such as codeine, oxycodone, and hydrocodone. This idea is primarily based on the observation that no PMs were found among opiate-dependent subjects, which likely reflects their inability to convert these drugs of abuse into their respective "pharmacologically active" moieties.[25] Given the reduced potential for opiate abuse among CYP2D6 PMs, investigators have used daily doses of fluoxetine 20 mg, a CYP2D6 inhibitor, as adjunctive therapy in the management of opiate abuse to "metabolically convert" drug abusers who are EMs to PMs.[26]

The potential and magnitude of drug interactions involving competitive inhibition of CYP2D6 are much greater in EMs versus PMs, who have either deficient or absent enzyme activity.[27,28] For example, Hamelin et al.[29] showed that hemodynamic responses to metoprolol (a CYP2D6 substrate) were pronounced and prolonged during concomitant diphenhydramine administration in EMs but not in PMs. Thus, potent CYP2D6 inhibitors may reduce the metabolic capacity of EMs significantly so that EMs appear phenotypically as PMs.

Patients who are EMs have a wide range of CYP2D6 activity, with ultrarapid metabolizers (UMs) on one end of the spectrum and subjects with diminished activity on the other end. Both have clinical implications in terms of dosage adjustment for CYP2D6 substrates. UMs carry a duplicated or amplified mutant allele, resulting in two or multiple copies of the functional *CYP2D6*1* or *CYP2D6*2* allele, and therefore show very high CYP2D6 activity. Nontherapeutic plasma concentrations of nortriptyline, a CYP2D6 substrate, were observed in a UM given normal doses of the drug.[30] The CYP2D6 enzyme converts nortriptyline to 10-hydroxynortriptyline, and one study demonstrated a directly proportional relationship between the number of functional *CYP2D6* genes and the concentration of 10-hydroxynortriptyline after nortriptyline administration.[31] A patient with three copies of *CYP2D6*2* required nortriptyline doses threefold to fivefold higher than normally recommended to achieve therapeutic plasma concentrations (50 to 150 mcg/mL).[30,32] In the same report, another patient with duplicated *CYP2D6*2* required twice the usual recommended daily dose (300 mg versus 25 to 150 mg) to achieve adequate therapeutic response.[32] On the other hand, UMs administered the usual therapeutic dose of codeine might exhibit symptoms of narcotic overdose associated with high morphine concentration. The UM genotype also has been reported to affect the potential for drug interaction with paroxetine, a CYP2D6 substrate as well as a potent CYP2D6 inhibitor.[33]

The high prevalence of *CYP2D6*10* (associated with lower enzyme activity) in the Asian population provides a biologic and molecular explanation for the higher drug concentrations and/or lower dosage requirements of neuroleptic medications and mianserin in people of Asian heritage.[34,35] The widespread presence of the *CYP2D6*17* variant among people of African heritage suggests that native African populations metabolize CYP2D6 substrates at a slower rate than do other ethnic or racial groups.[36,37] However, no current genotype- and phenotype-based data document the need for prescribing lower doses of psychotropics and other CYP2D6 substrates in native African populations.

In addition to the therapeutic implications of genetic polymorphisms, one study showed that the CYP2D6 polymorphism has an economic impact.[38] The annual cost of treating UMs and PMs (carriers of two nonfunctional CYP2D6 alleles) was $4,000 to $6,000 higher than the cost of treating EMs or intermediate metabolizers (carriers of one nonfunctional allele and one allele associated with diminished activity). The cost of genotyping can be considerably less than that incurred in a patient with a serious adverse drug reaction. Brockmoller et al.[39] suggested how CYP2D6 genotyping can be used to achieve higher therapeutic success with the CYP2D6 substrate haloperidol. Along these lines, the Food and Drug Administration (FDA) approved the AmpliChip CYP450 Test (Roche Diagnostics) for analyzing 27 CYP2D6 alleles in addition to the *CYP2C19*1*, **2*, and **3* alleles (discussed below) to assist clinicians in individualizing therapy with drugs metabolized through the CYP2D6 and CYP2C19 pathways.

CYP2C19

The principal defective alleles for the CYP2C19 genetic polymorphism are *CYP2C19*2* (aberrant splice site) and *CYP2C19*3* (premature stop codon), which result in inactive CYP2C19 enzymes and the PM phenotype. Clinical implication of the CYP2C19 polymorphism has not been examined as extensively as that of the CYP2D6 polymorphism. However, PMs for the CYP2C19 polymorphism showed a more than 12-fold increase in the area under the curve (AUC) of the CYP2C19 substrate omeprazole compared with EMs.[40] In a separate study, the steady-state AUC of omeprazole and other CYP2C19 substrate proton pump inhibitors was five-fold higher in PMs versus EMs.[41]

The presence of a defective CYP2C19 allele has been associated with improved *Helicobacter pylori* cure rates after dual (omeprazole and amoxicillin)[42] or triple therapy (omeprazole, amoxicillin, and clarithromycin) with omeprazole[43] as well as with lansoprazole.[44] This difference likely reflects the higher achievable intragastric pH in the PM group.[45] The cure rate achieved with dual therapy was 100% in PMs compared with 60% and 29% in heterozygous and homozygous EMs, respectively.[42] In two studies, EMs had *H. pylori* eradication rates of 41% with dual therapy and 74% to 83% with triple therapy.[43,44] In contrast, both dual- and triple-therapy regimens produced 100% cure rates in all 15 PMs included in the same studies. Interestingly, EMs who did not respond to initial triple therapy (lansoprazole, clarithromycin, and amoxicillin) and were retreated with high-dose lansoprazole (30 mg four times daily) and amoxicillin achieved 97% *H. pylori* eradication.[46]

Similar to the CYP2D6 polymorphism, people of Asian heritage also metabolize most CYP2C19 substrates at a slower rate than do white people.[47] This reflects the higher prevalence of both PMs (13% to 20% versus 2% to 6% in white people) and heterozygotes for the defective *CYP2C19* allele in Asians.[48] This genotypic difference may explain the practice of prescribing lower diazepam dosages for patients of Chinese heritage.[49]

CYP2C9

Warfarin, phenytoin, and tolbutamide are examples of drugs with a narrow therapeutic index that are metabolized by CYP2C9. Warfarin is a racemic mixture, and the *S*-isomer, which possesses about three times the anticoagulant effects of the *R*-isomer, is metabolized by CYP2C9. *CYP2C9*2* and *CYP2C9*3* are the two most common CYP2C9 variants. Both exhibit single amino acid substitutions at positions critical for enzyme activity.[50] This could have clinically important consequences in warfarin-treated patients. For example, a 90% reduction in *S*-warfarin clearance was reported in *CYP2C9*3* homozygotes compared with subjects homozygous for the wild-type allele.[51] In another study, an overrepresentation of *CYP2C9* variant alleles was observed in 81% of patients requiring low-dose warfarin therapy (≤1.5 mg/day).[2] The low-dose group was reported to have more difficulty with warfarin induction, requiring longer hospital stays to stabilize the warfarin regimen and experiencing a higher incidence of bleeding complications. In addition, a profound therapeutic response to usual doses of warfarin was observed in a patient homozygous for the *CYP2C9*3* allele, necessitating dose reduction to 0.5 mg/day.[52]

CYP2A6

A polymorphism has been characterized for CYP2A6, with identification of several variants—*CYP2A6*1* (wild type), *CYP2A6*2* (single amino acid substitution), *CYP2A6*3* (gene conversion)—and three gene-deletion alleles—*CYP2A6*4A*, *CYP2A6*4B*, and *CYP2A6*4D*.[53] Deletion of the *CYP2A6* gene is very common in Asian patients,[53,54] which likely accounts for the dramatic difference in the frequency of PMs in Asian (20%) versus European and white populations (≤1%). Nicotine is metabolized by CYP2A6, and the clinical relevance of the CYP2A6 polymorphism lies in management of tobacco abuse.[55] Investigators reported that nonsmokers were more likely to carry the defective *CYP2A6* allele than were smokers. Smokers who had the defective *CYP2A6* allele smoked fewer cigarettes and were more likely to quit.[55] The inability to metabolize nicotine, secondary to the presence of a defective *CYP2A6* allele, likely leads to enhanced nicotine tolerance and increased adverse effects from nicotine. Based on these observations, CYP2A6 inhibition may have a role in the management of tobacco dependency.[56]

CYP3A4/5

Within the CYP3A subfamily, at least three isoenzymes, namely, CYP3A4, CYP3A5, and CYP3A7, have been characterized. Despite as much as 40-fold interindividual variability in its expression, functional CYP3A4 is expressed in most adults, with intestinal expression playing a significant role in the first-pass metabolism of numerous drugs. CYP3A4 variants with amino acid substitutions in exons 7 and 12 have been associated with altered catalytic activity for the CYP3A4 substrate nifedipine.[14] The clinical importance of this finding needs further elucidation and confirmation.

CYP3A5 is reported to be polymorphic in 60% of African Americans and 33% of white people. In contrast to individuals with the *CYP3A5*1* allele, subjects with variant alleles such as *CYP3A5*3* (aberrant splice site) in intron 3 have no functional CYP3A5 enzyme.[15] With overlapping substrate specificities, whether there are clinically used drugs that are substrates for CYP3A5 but not CYP3A4 and vice versa is unknown. Although variability exists between dose-adjusted concentration and CYP3A5 genotypes, studies have shown a correlation between pharmacokinetics of tacrolimus and *CYP3A5* genetic constitution.[57,58]

PHASE II AND NUCLEOTIDE-BASE METABOLIZING ENZYMES

The clinical relevance of genetic polymorphisms in TPMT, DPD, and UGT enzymes has been demonstrated in the treatment of cancer.[4,59,60] The *TPMT* gene has three mutant alleles: *TPMT*3A* (the most common), *TPMT*2*, and *TPMT*3C*. Patients who are homozygous or heterozygous for the *TPMT* mutant alleles are at higher risk for developing serious anemias during mercaptopurine treatment.[4] DPD mediates the metabolism of 5-fluorouracil, and patients with a defective allele of the *DPD* gene cannot metabolize 5-fluorouracil and thus may experience enhanced drug-related neurotoxicity.[59] The camptothecin derivative irinotecan (CPT-11) is activated by carboxylesterase to SN-38, which is a potent topoisomerase I inhibitor. SN-38 is inactivated by glucuronidation via the polymorphic UGT1A1 enzyme, which may play a role in CPT-11–related toxicity. A polymorphism in the promoter region of the *UGT1A1* gene results in the *(TA)⁷TAA* allele, which possesses lower enzyme activity than the wild-type *(TA)⁶TAA* allele. A patient homozygous for the *(TA)⁷TAA* allele had impaired SN-38 glucuronidation.[60] Abnormally high SN-38 concentrations have been associated with neutropenia and severe diarrhea.[61] Diarrhea likely results from increased SN-38 excretion into the gut lumen, predisposing patients with the *(TA)⁷TAA* allele to developing diarrhea with usual CPT-11 doses. This observation was confirmed in a prospective clinical trial that demonstrated more severe diarrhea and neutropenia in irinotecan-treated patients who are homozygous or heterozygous carriers of the *(TA)⁷TAA* allele.[62] The FDA approved the Invader UGT1A1 Molecular Assay (Third Wave Technologies) to genotype for *UGT1A1* alleles and revised the labeling for irinotecan to recommend therapy adjustment for individuals who are homozygous for the *(TA)⁷TAA* allele.

POLYMORPHISMS IN DRUG TRANSPORTER GENES

Certain membrane-spanning proteins facilitate drug transport across the gastrointestinal tract, drug excretion into the bile and urine, and drug distribution across the blood–brain barrier. Genetic variations for drug transport proteins may affect the distribution of drugs that are substrates for these proteins and alter drug concentrations at their therapeutic sites of action. P-glycoprotein is one of the most recognized of the drug transport proteins that exhibit genetic polymorphism. P-glycoprotein is an energy-dependent transmembrane efflux pump encoded by the *ABCB1* gene (also known as the multidrug resistance-1 [MDR1] gene), which is a member of the ATP-binding cassette (ABC) transporter superfamily. P-glycoprotein was first recognized for its ability to actively export anticancer agents from cancer cells and promote multidrug resistance to cancer chemotherapy. P-glycoprotein later was discovered to be widely distributed on normal cell types, including intestinal enterocytes, hepatocytes, renal proximal tubule cells, and endothelial cells lining the blood–brain barrier. At these locations, P-glycoprotein serves a protective role by transporting toxic substances or metabolites out of cells. P-glycoprotein affects the distribution of some nonchemotherapeutic agents, including digoxin, the immunosuppressants cyclosporine and tacrolimus, and antiretroviral protease inhibitors (Fig. 6–3). Increased intestinal expression of P-glycoprotein can limit the absorption of P-glycoprotein substrates, thus reducing their bioavailability and preventing attainment of therapeutic plasma concentrations. Conversely, decreased P-glycoprotein expression may result in supratherapeutic plasma concentrations of relevant drugs and drug toxicity.

CLINICAL CONTROVERSY

Much of the data on individual variations in the *ABCB1* gene and response to P-glycoprotein substrates are inconsistent, even conflicting, and require clarification. The combination of multiple variations in the *ABCB1* gene eventually may prove to be a stronger predictor of drug response than any individual variation.

A number of polymorphisms have been identified in the promoter and exon regions of the *ABCB1* gene. Common SNPs occur in exons 12 (C1236T), 21 (G2677T), and 26 (C3435T). The exon 21 and 26 SNPs have been associated with intestinal *ABCB1* expression, P-glycoprotein activity, and digoxin plasma concentrations in healthy volunteers.[63] These data imply that the *ABCB1* genotype is useful in predicting digoxin concentrations in patients with atrial arrhythmias or heart failure and in appropriate selection of initial digoxin doses.

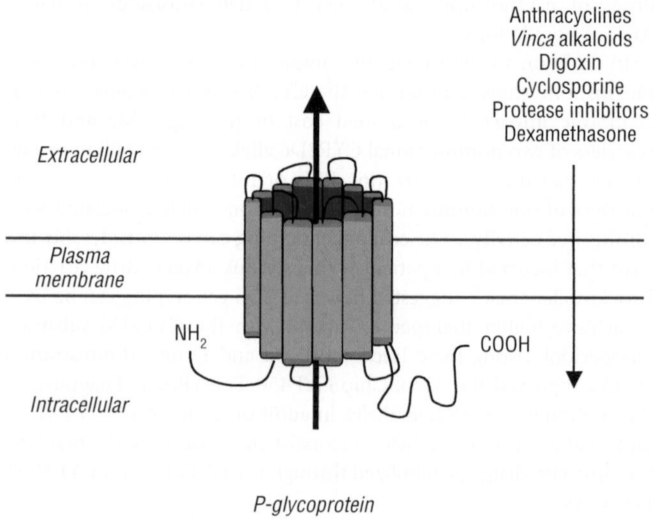

FIGURE 6-3. Active transport of drugs out of the cell by P-glycoprotein.

The *ABCB1* exon 26 polymorphism also has been associated with plasma concentrations and clinical effects of protease inhibitors in patients infected with the human immunodeficiency virus (HIV).[64] Specifically, following 6 months of therapy with efavirenz or nelfinavir, a greater rise in CD4 cell counts was observed in individuals with the exon 26 TT genotype compared with CC homozygotes. This finding suggests a role for *ABCB1* genotyping in predicting hematologic responses to protease inhibitors and individualizing antiretroviral drug therapy for HIV-infected patients.

Other examples of polymorphic drug transporter proteins include the dipeptide transporter, organic anion and cation transporters, and L-amino acid transporter. Their effects on drug distribution are the focus of ongoing research.

POLYMORPHISMS IN DRUG TARGET GENES

❺ Genetic polymorphisms occur commonly for drug target proteins, including receptors, enzymes, ion channels, and intracellular signaling proteins. Drug target genes may work in concert with genes that affect pharmacokinetic properties to contribute to overall drug response. Table 6–2 provides examples of drug target genes linked to drug response in clinical studies. The following section highlights some of the receptor, enzyme, ion channel, and cell-signaling protein genes that influence the efficacy and safety of various pharmacologic agents.

RECEPTOR GENOTYPES AND DRUG RESPONSE

The β_1- and β_2-adrenergic receptor genes have been the focus of much research into genetic determinants of responses to β-adrenergic receptor agonists and antagonists. β_1-Receptors are located in the heart and kidney, where they are involved in the regulation of heart rate, cardiac contractility, and blood pressure. Two common nonsynonymous SNPs in the β_1-receptor gene are located at codons 49 (Ser→Gly) and 389 (Arg→Gly), and there is evidence of their involvement in blood pressure control.[10] Investigators have examined the influence of the β_1-receptor gene on blood pressure response to β_1-receptor blockade with metoprolol. Hypertensive patients who were homozygous for both the Ser49 and Arg389 alleles

TABLE 6-2 Genetic Polymorphisms in Drug Targets and Response to Drug Therapy

Gene	Drug/Drug Class	Drug Effect Associated with Polymorphism
α-Adducin	Hydrochlorothiazide	Blood pressure reduction[78]
ACE	ACE inhibitors	Blood pressure reduction, regression of left ventricular hypertrophy, renoprotective effects[77,78]
Epithelial sodium channel	Amiloride	Blood pressure reduction[83]
Angiotensinogen	ACE inhibitors	Blood pressure reduction[78]
β_1-Adrenergic receptor	β-Blockers	Blood pressure lowering[65]
β_2-Adrenergic receptor	β_2-Agonists	Bronchodilation[68]
Cyclooxygenase-1	Aspirin	Antiplatelet effects[109]
Dopamine D_3 receptor	Levodopa, neuroleptics	Tardive dyskinesia[84]
3-Hydroxy-3-methylglutaryl-coenzyme A reductase	Statins	Magnitude of cholesterol lowering[110]
Inhibitory GTP-binding protein β_3-subunit	Antidepressants	Antidepressant response[80]
5-Lipoxygenase	Leukotriene modifier	Change in FEV_1[111]
Combination of H_2, 5-HT_{2A}, 5-HT_{2C}, 5-HT transporter	Clozapine	Response in schizophrenia[70]
Serotonin transporter	Selective serotonin reuptake inhibitors	Antidepressant response[80]
Stimulatory GTP-binding protein α-subunit	β-Blockers	Blood pressure lowering[78]
Vitamin K epoxide reductase complex subunit-1	Warfarin	Dose requirements[73]

ACE, angiotensin-converting enzyme; H, histamine; FEV_1, forced expiratory volume in the first second of expiration; 5-HT, serotonin.

had greater reductions in diastolic blood pressure with metoprolol monotherapy compared with carriers of the Gly49 and/or Gly389 alleles.[65] These data suggest that β_1-receptor genotype may be an important determinant of blood pressure response to β-blockers in the management of hypertension. Given that a significant percentage of hypertensive patients fail to derive adequate blood pressure reduction with β-blocker monotherapy,[66] the ability to predict the likelihood of response based on genotype would have important clinical implications. Specifically, β-blockers could be started in patients expected to respond well to this drug class based on their β_1-receptor genotype, whereas other classes of antihypertensive agents could be used in patients expected to respond poorly to β-blockers.

β_2-Receptors are located on bronchial smooth muscle cells, where they mediate bronchodilation upon exposure to the β_2-receptor agonists. Inhaled β_2-agonists are the most effective agents for acute reversal of bronchospasm; however, the magnitude of their effects varies substantially among asthmatic patients.[67] More than 11 SNPs have been identified in the β_2-receptor gene, three of which occur frequently and result in amino acid changes. Two common nonsynonymous SNPs are found in the gene's coding block region, at codons 16 and 27, and a third occurs upstream from the coding block in the gene's promoter region.

A number of studies have examined the association between the codon 16 or 27 polymorphisms and bronchodilatory response to β_2-receptor agonists in asthma; however, the results of these studies have been largely inconsistent.[68] More recently, investigators found that the combination of SNPs in the gene's coding block and promoter region was a better determinant of β_2-agonist response than any individual SNP.[69] These data suggest that an individual SNP in the β_2-receptor gene is an insufficient predictor of β_2-agonist effects and that multiple receptor gene variations more accurately correlate with bronchodilatory response to β_2-agonists.

Clozapine is an example of a drug for which evidence indicates that multiple receptor genes interact to influence the drug's effects. Clozapine is an atypical antipsychotic used for the treatment of schizophrenia. Because of its potential to produce agranulocytosis in 0.5% to 2% of treated patients, clozapine is reserved for schizophrenic patients who are unresponsive to other drug therapies. However, only 30% to 60% of patients with refractory schizophrenia respond to clozapine.[70] Clozapine's effects are believed to be mediated through dopaminergic, serotoninergic, adrenergic, and histaminergic receptors in the central nervous system. Although several studies have demonstrated relationships between single genetic variants for these receptor subtypes and clozapine response, the data are inconsistent.[71] In a more recent study, a combination of six polymorphisms in the histamine and serotonin 2A and 2C receptor genes and the serotonin transporter gene were 77% predictive of antipsychotic response to clozapine.[70] These findings imply that, similar to other drug target gene–drug response relationships, a combination of polymorphisms, rather than any single polymorphism, provides more accurate prediction of clozapine response.

ENZYME GENES AND DRUG RESPONSE

Vitamin K epoxide reductase (VKOR) is an example of an enzyme with genetic contributions to drug response. Warfarin exerts its anticoagulant effects by inhibiting VKOR, thus preventing carboxylation of clotting factors II, VII, IX, and X. The vitamin K epoxide reductase complex subunit-1 gene (*VKORC1*) encodes for VKOR. Mutations in the *VKORC1* coding region cause rare cases of warfarin resistance. Carriers of these mutations either require exceptionally high warfarin doses (>100 mg/wk) to achieve effective anticoagulation or fail to respond to any dose of warfarin.[72]

Aside from rare cases of warfarin resistance, among patients there is substantial variability with regard to the dose of warfarin necessary to produce optimal anticoagulation, defined as an international normalized ratio of 2.0 to 3.0 for most indications. Common SNPs in the *VKORC1* promoter and intron regions have been identified and found to contribute to the interpatient variability in warfarin dose requirements.[73] These SNPs are in linkage disequilibrium (i.e., inherited together) and form several haplotypes. *VKORC1* haplotype, together with *CYP2C9* genotype, explains approximately 30% to 40% of the interpatient variability in warfarin dose requirements.[74] Much of the remainder of the variability is believed to be due to differences in demographic characteristics and dietary habits. Warfarin dosing algorithms that incorporate both genetic and nongenetic (e.g., age, body size) factors have been developed, and their accuracy in prospectively predicting warfarin dose is being tested.[75,76] In the future, it may be possible to use these algorithms to accurately predict warfarin dose requirements for a given patient, thus reducing the patient's risk for thrombosis and bleeding associated with subtherapeutic or supratherapeutic anticoagulation, respectively.

The angiotensin-converting enzyme (ACE) gene is probably the most widely studied of the enzyme genes. An insertion/deletion (I/D) polymorphism in intron 16 of the *ACE* gene results in the presence or absence of a 287-base-pair fragment. This polymorphism has been linked consistently to plasma concentrations of ACE, the enzyme responsible for conversion of angiotensin I to the

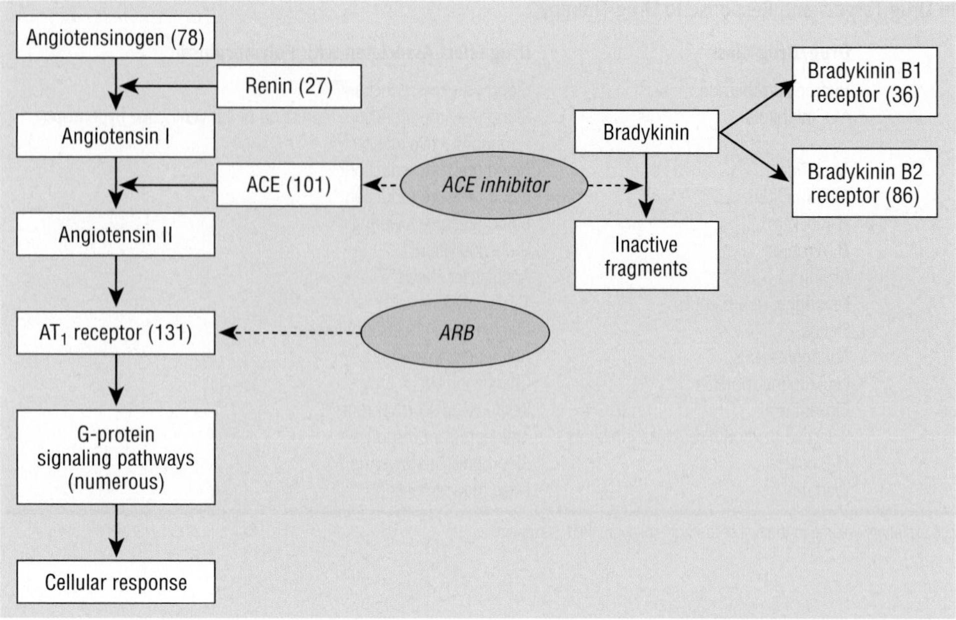

FIGURE 6-4. Single nucleotide polymorphisms (SNPs) identified for renin–angiotensin system genes. The number of polymorphisms identified for each protein is shown in parentheses after the protein name *(http://snp.cshl.org)*. (ACE, angiotensin-converting enzyme; ARB, angiotensin receptor blocker.)

potent vasoconstrictor angiotensin II.[77] Given its association with ACE concentrations, a number of investigators have examined whether the I/D polymorphism contributes to the interpatient variability in ACE inhibitor response. However, much of the data with the I/D polymorphism and blood pressure response to ACE inhibitors are inconsistent and even conflicting, with some studies demonstrating greater response with the DD genotype but others showing greater response with the II genotype.[78] In the largest pharmacogenetic study (including nearly 38,000 patients) to date, no association has been found between the ACE I/D genotype and either blood pressure response or cardiovascular or renal outcome with antihypertensive therapy.[79]

The negative findings with regard to the *ACE* gene and ACE inhibitor response are not surprising given that numerous proteins are involved in the complex signaling pathway of the renin–angiotensin system (Fig. 6–4). Multiple genetic polymorphisms have been identified for many of these proteins. Thus, one explanation for the lack of an association between the *ACE* gene and ACE inhibitor response is that a single polymorphism contributes little to the overall response to an ACE inhibitor. Rather, response to ACE inhibition may be best determined by a combination of multiple polymorphisms occurring in multiple genes involved in the renin–angiotensin pathway. Indeed, other renin–angiotensin system genes, including the gene for angiotensinogen and aldosterone synthase, have been correlated with antihypertensive responses to ACE inhibitors and angiotensin receptor blockers,[78] suggesting that genes for ACE, angiotensinogen, aldosterone synthase, and probably other renin–angiotensin system proteins interact to influence ACE inhibitor response. Thus, before genotype can be used as a predictor of response to renin–angiotensin antagonists, the combination of genetic variants in the renin–angiotensin system that best determines drug response first must be elucidated.

There is evidence of racial differences in response to ACE inhibitors as well as many other pharmacologic agents. Specifically, African Americans in general are believed to have diminished antihypertensive responses to ACE inhibitors compared with white people.[66] The frequencies of many SNPs in the renin–angiotensin system vary between African American and white populations and may contribute to the observed racial differences in ACE inhibitor response. Indeed, most racial differences in drug response probably can be attributed to racial differences in genotype frequencies, although this is yet to be determined.

GENES FOR INTRACELLULAR SIGNALING PROTEINS, ION CHANNELS, AND DRUG RESPONSE

Cellular responses to many drugs are mediated through GTP-binding proteins, also called *G proteins*. The β_1-adrenergic receptor is an example of a G-protein–coupled receptor in which a stimulatory G (G_s) protein couples the receptor to intracellular signaling mechanisms to elicit a cellular response (Fig. 6–5). Receptor-coupled G_s proteins contain α-, β-, and γ-subunits that mediate the activation of adenylyl cyclase and the generation of cyclic AMP following receptor stimulation. A SNP in the α-subunit of G_s protein has been linked to the blood pressure response to β-blockers.[78] Whether the G_s protein α-subunit gene interacts with the β_1-adrenergic receptor gene or other intracellular signaling-protein genes to determine β-blocker response remains to be determined.

Disturbances in G-protein–mediated signal transduction have been implicated in the response to antidepressant drugs.[80] A common SNP (C825T) occurs in the gene for the inhibitory G (G_i) protein β_3-subunit and has been associated with enhanced intracellular signal transduction.[81] The TT genotype has been correlated with greater improvement in depression symptoms among patients treated with either a tricyclic antidepressant or serotonin reuptake

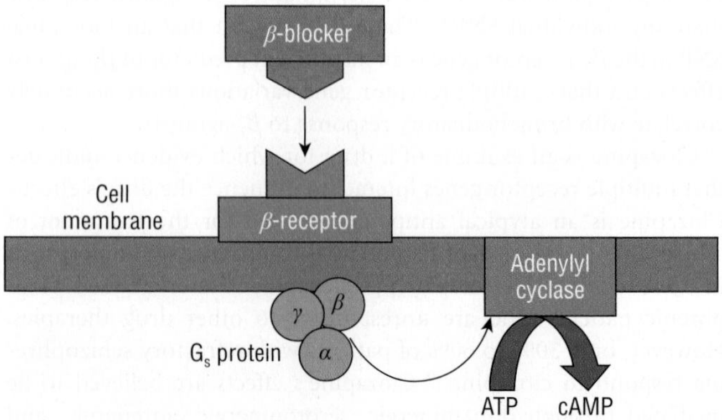

FIGURE 6-5. β_1-receptor coupled to intracellular signaling mechanisms by a stimulatory G (G_s) protein.

inhibitor,[80] implying that the G_i protein β_3-subunit gene may have a role in therapeutic decisions for depression management.

The epithelial sodium channel (ENaC) is an example of an ion channel with genetic contributions to drug response. The ENaC is located in the distal renal tubule and collecting duct of the nephron, where it serves as the final site for sodium reabsorption. The channel is composed of α-, β-, and γ-subunits. Mutations in the β- or γ-subunit cause excessive sodium reabsorption and an inherited form of hypertension called Liddle syndrome. The more common variant Thr594Met occurs exclusively in blacks and is associated with high blood pressure in this population.[82] Amiloride blocks the ENaC but is a relatively weak diuretic with minimal effects on blood pressure when used as monotherapy in most hypertensive individuals. However, evidence indicates that amiloride monotherapy is as effective as combination therapy with more potent agents in blacks carrying the Thr594Met variant.[83] These data suggest that genotyping for the Thr594Met polymorphism may be appropriate for black patients whose blood pressure is resistant to traditional antihypertensive drugs, in whom treatment with amiloride could be instituted if the polymorphism is present.

The examples of drug target genes given thus far relate to drug efficacy. There are also examples of drug target genes linked to drug toxicity. One example is the Ser9Gly polymorphism of the dopamine D_3 receptor gene, which has been associated with neuroleptic-induced tardive dyskinesia.[84] Tardive dyskinesia is a debilitating adverse effect that occurs in up 30% of patients treated with typical antipsychotics. Genetic influences of adverse effects that occur less frequently, such as ACE inhibitor–induced angioedema, are more difficult to delineate because of the large sample size needed to establish a definite genetic cause. Investigators for many multicenter clinical drug trials now are asking participants to provide consent for the collection of genetic material so that genetic contributions to rare but serious adverse drug effects can be elucidated in future studies.

DISEASE-ASSOCIATED GENES

Numerous genes have been correlated with disease outcomes, and many of these have been found subsequently to influence response to pharmacologic disease management. These gene–drug response associations often occur despite the lack of a direct effect on pharmacokinetic or pharmacodynamic drug properties. Examples of disease-associated genes are given in the following.

FACTOR V AND PROTHROMBIN GENES AND ORAL CONTRACEPTION

Use of oral contraceptives is associated with an increased risk for developing thromboembolic disorders, including deep-vein thrombosis, pulmonary embolism, and thrombotic stroke. Variations in the genes for the coagulation factors prothrombin and factor V Leiden also have been identified as risk factors for thromboembolic disorders.[85] In case-control studies, the presence of a factor V Leiden or prothrombin gene variation markedly increased the risk for deep-vein thrombosis and cerebral vein thrombosis among oral contraceptive users.[85] These data suggest that women who are known to carry a prothrombin or factor V Leiden mutation should use alternative birth control measures.

CONGENITAL LONG QT SYNDROME AND DRUG-INDUCED TORSADES DE POINTES

Drug-induced QT-interval prolongation may precipitate the serious, potentially life-threatening arrhythmia called *torsades de pointes*. It is well recognized that many antiarrhythmic drugs can cause QT-interval prolongation and torsade de pointes. In addition, numerous noncardiovascular agents can induce torsade de pointes, and many have been withdrawn from the market as a result. Such drugs include the antihistamines terfenadine and astemizole, the fluoroquinolone antibiotic grepafloxacin, and the motility agent cisapride. Given the serious and unpredictable nature of torsade de pointes, there has been great interest in identifying genetic markers that predispose individuals to its occurrence.

Abnormalities in ion flux across the cardiac cell membrane resulting in an excess of intracellular positive ions and delayed ventricular repolarization are characteristic of long QT syndromes. Mutations in genes for the pore-forming channel proteins that affect potassium and sodium transport across the cardiac cell membrane underlie congenital long QT syndromes.[86] There is evidence that these mutations also may increase the risk for drug-induced torsade de pointes.[86] The ability to screen for mutations associated with drug-induced torsade de pointes would be of clinical significance, so that individuals with a genetic predisposition for this life-threatening arrhythmia could be spared exposure to potentially causative agents and treated with alternative therapies.

CORONARY DISEASE PROGRESSION GENE AND RESPONSE TO STATIN THERAPY

Several large clinical trials in patients with coronary heart disease, including the Scandinavian Simvastatin Survival Study (4S), have demonstrated significant reductions in coronary events and mortality with β-hydroxy-β-methylglutaryl-coenzyme A (HMG-CoA) reductase inhibitors, or statins.[87] The gene for apolipoprotein E has been correlated with hepatic cholesterol uptake and the risk for coronary heart disease.[88] Its contribution to coronary heart disease progression and statin response was examined in the 4S population.[89] Investigators found that the variant $\varepsilon 4$ allele was associated with increased risk for all-cause mortality among placebo-treated study participants. However, no such association was observed in the simvastatin group, suggesting that simvastatin abolished the excess mortality risk associated with the $\varepsilon 4$ allele.

Several other genes have been associated with responses to statins in coronary heart disease. These include the genes for the cholesteryl ester transfer protein, which is involved in the metabolism of high-density lipoprotein cholesterol; β-fibrinogen, which influences plasma fibrinogen concentrations; and stromelysin-1, which is involved in remodeling of the extracellular matrix of atherosclerotic plaques.[88] In each case, the gene linked to worse disease progression or clinical outcomes also was associated with the greatest response to statin therapy. These data imply that genotype is useful in identifying which coronary heart disease patients are at increased risk for coronary events and death, in whom treatment with a statin would be of particular benefit.

NOVEL SITES FOR DRUG DEVELOPMENT

The discovery of genes that confer disease has led to an improved understanding of the molecular mechanisms involved in disease pathophysiology. Once associations between genes and diseases are discovered, scientists can elucidate the functions of the encoded proteins and more clearly define the consequences of genetic mutations. Insight into the genetic control of cellular functions may reveal new strategies for disease treatment and prevention.

For example, overexpression of the human epidermal growth factor receptor-2 (HER2) secondary to HER2 gene amplification occurs in 20% to 30% of metastatic breast cancers and is associated with decreased survival.[90] The discovery of HER2 overexpression and its effects on cancer prognosis led to the development of trastuzumab, a recombinant monoclonal antibody that targets and blocks HER2. The addition of trastuzumab to cancer chemotherapy significantly slows the progression of cancer and improves tumor response rates in women with HER2-positive tumors.[90] Testing for HER2 overexpression is necessary to determine which patients may benefit from trastuzumab. The FDA has approved several tests that detect HER2 overexpression either directly by measuring the amount of protein or indirectly by measuring gene amplification.

The discovery that the apolipoprotein E gene is strongly linked to Alzheimer's disease[91] and that the α-synuclein gene is associated with Parkinson's disease[92] raises the possibility of examining these genes as targets for drug therapy for psychiatric and neurologic diseases.

GENE THERAPY

❼ Gene therapy has emerged as a possible approach to treating and curing disease by altering gene expression. Initially, the focus of gene therapy was treatment of inherited disorders such as cystic fibrosis, sickle cell anemia, hemophilia, and adenosine deaminase deficiency. Gene therapy trials later were expanded to include patients with acquired diseases such as cancer and heart disease. The goal of gene therapy for inherited diseases is to correct genetic defects permanently and thereby restore normal cellular function. Gene therapy for acquired diseases aims to cure disease by targeting pathogenic processes.

Most gene therapy techniques for inherited diseases attempt to replace defective genes with normally functioning ones. Exogenous genes, called *transgenes,* can be transferred into either somatic (body) or germ-line (egg or sperm) cells of the recipient. In somatic cell gene transfer, genetic changes do not affect future generations. In contrast, germ-line cell transfer, which currently is prohibited by the FDA, results in the passage of genetic alterations to offspring.

The first clinical gene therapy trial for treatment of adenosine deaminase deficiency began in 1990.[93] B and T lymphocytes fail to develop in this autosomal recessive disease, resulting in a severe combined immunodeficiency syndrome (SCID) made famous by the "bubble boys" whose lives were confined to tents in an effort to keep them in a germ-free environment. Only two patients were included in this trial, and although both boys continued to demonstrate clinical improvement 10 years later, gene therapy did not cure the disease, as investigators had hoped.

Since then, the FDA has approved more than 700 clinical gene therapy trials (*www.clinicaltrials.gov*). Most of these trials involve cancer patients; however, a number of studies also target inherited disorders. The results of gene therapy trials to date have been disappointing, with reports of serious toxicities and few therapeutic successes.

OBSTACLES TO SUCCESS

Reasons for limited success with gene therapy include inefficient gene delivery to target cells, inadequate gene expression, and unacceptable adverse effects.[93]

Sufficient amounts of the transgene must be inserted into a sufficient number of recipient cells to produce a therapeutic response. In addition, the transgene must be inserted into the correct chromosomal position of the correct cell nucleus so as not to disrupt normal gene function and expression. Incorrect chromosomal insertion of the transgene is a problem referred to as *insertional mutagenesis.* Once the therapeutic gene is integrated correctly into host DNA, it must be expressed at adequate levels and at appropriate times to restore normal cell function. Finally, the gene delivery system and delivery technique should lack any potential to cause unwanted effects in the transgene recipient.

RETROVIRAL GENE DELIVERY

❽ Because of their efficiency in integrating into human DNA, viruses are the most common vectors used to deliver therapeutic genes to recipient cell targets. Disease-causing genes are replaced with the desired therapeutic genes; the viral genes that control delivery mechanisms are retained.

The first viral vectors introduced were retroviruses, which are RNA viruses that integrate into the host cell genome and replicate during cell division. Thus, retroviral gene transfer is capable of permanently altering gene expression. Retroviruses can be used to deliver genes through either direct infusion into target organs or ex vivo manipulation of harvested cells followed by reinfusion into the recipient. The disadvantages of retroviral vectors are the limited size of the gene they can carry, relatively low efficiency, and risk of insertional mutagenesis. In fact, the FDA temporarily halted retroviral gene delivery into hematopoietic tissue in early 2003 after leukemia developed as a result of insertional mutagenesis in two of 11 SCID-affected children treated with retroviral gene therapy.[94] A third child later developed cancer.

Since research with retroviral gene therapy has resumed, some success with this mode of gene delivery has been reported in the area of oncology. In 2003, the FDA granted orphan drug status for a retroviral gene therapy that targets the cyclin G1 gene in the treatment of pancreatic cancer. Retroviruses also have been used in the development of recombinant cancer vaccines designed to stimulate the immune system to recognize and destroy cancer cells. One such vaccine was associated with regression of metastatic lesions in two of 15 patients with advanced melanoma.[95]

ADENOVIRAL GENE DELIVERY

Unlike retroviruses, adenoviruses do not integrate into the host genome and thus do not replicate. As a result, genes delivered by adenoviruses are active only temporarily. Adenoviral-mediated gene therapy is used commonly in cancer patients because permanent gene expression is unnecessary in this patient population.

Tumor cells have been infused with adenoviral vectors carrying the herpes simplex virus-1 thymidine kinase gene and then exposed to ganciclovir as a mode of cancer chemotherapy.[96] Thymidine kinase converts ganciclovir to its active, cytotoxic form, which is incorporated in the DNA of tumor cells, leading to their death. Adenoviruses can be grown in high titers and do not carry the risk of insertional mutagenesis. The major disadvantage of adenoviruses is their immunogenic potential, which has resulted in one death and prompted federal oversight of gene therapy trials.[97]

OTHER MEANS OF GENE DELIVERY

Adeno-associated viruses are human DNA-containing viruses that do not appear to trigger immune responses upon injection. Similar to retroviruses, adeno-associated viruses are incapable of carrying a large amount of genetic material, and their use entails the risk of insertional mutagenesis. Investigators have reported some success in treating hemophilia B using intramuscular injections of an adeno-associated virus vector that expresses the human coagulation factor IX gene.[98]

Scientists are experimenting with nonviral delivery methods such as the use of direct DNA injection, liposomes, and electroporation. Some success with intramyocardial transfection of plasmid DNA encoding for vascular endothelial growth factor into patients with severe, intractable angina has been reported.[99] Initially, the procedure improved myocardial perfusion and angina in this patient population, with few major adverse events. One year later, patients continued to report some improvement in anginal symptoms.[100]

Scientists have enjoyed few successes with gene therapy for inherited diseases. Improvements in gene delivery techniques and a better understanding of molecular processes controlling gene expression are necessary before gene therapy can correct genetic defects successfully and thus cure associated diseases without inducing adverse effects. Because of limited success with traditional approaches to gene therapy, scientists are exploring other strategies, such as repairing or regulating ("turning off") defective genes rather than replacing them.[101] Scientists have reported more success with gene therapy for acquired diseases, such as cancer, and a number of phase II and III clinical trials in this area are underway. While gene therapy research is evolving, much progress is needed before effective and safe therapies are available.

ETHICAL CONSIDERATIONS

PHARMACOGENETICS

Traditionally, *genetic testing* refers to screening human genetic material to identify genotypes associated with disease susceptibility or carrier status for inherited diseases, such as Huntington's disease, Alzheimer's disease, and breast cancer. This kind of testing can have profound legal, ethical, and social implications. For example, knowledge that a patient is at risk for developing a genetic disorder could result in discrimination by employers or insurance companies. In addition, this information likely would cause emotional distress for the individual at risk and his or her family members.

Within the context of pharmacogenetics, however, testing involves searching for genetic variations linked to drug efficacy or toxicity rather than to disease susceptibility. In many instances, this form of testing will carry little risk for ethical, legal, and social concerns. For example, knowledge that a person has a genotype associated with poor blood pressure response to a β-blocker is of little consequence because a number of alternative therapies are available. However, more serious implications may arise if a person is predicted to respond poorly to a drug based on genotype, and treatment options are limited. Thus, ethical considerations associated with pharmacogenetic testing may need to be addressed before testing is widely accepted by the public.

GENE THERAPY

Many of the ethical concerns with gene therapy center on transgenic manipulation of somatic versus germ-line cells. Somatic gene therapy only affects the recipient, that is, genetic alterations introduced by gene therapy are not passed on to future generations. In contrast, with manipulation of germ-line cells, alterations are passed on to children of the treated patient. Some argue that this is unethical because it violates the rights of future generations. Thus, it appears that most gene therapy in the foreseeable future will focus on somatic gene transfer.

ROLE OF PHARMACISTS

Although pharmacogenetics provides opportunities to improve drug therapy outcomes, it likely will increase the complexity of drug prescribing. In addition to considering factors such as age, concomitant drug therapy, and renal and hepatic function, prescribers will have to interpret the results of genetic analyses when making drug therapy decisions. The FDA has already incorporated genetic information into the package insert for a number of drugs, including irinotecan, azathioprine, mercaptopurine, fluoxetine, and celecoxib.

Further complicating the drug-prescribing process are many medications whose effects are not determined by single polymorphisms in single genes. Rather, pharmacologic effects for most medications likely are determined by the interaction of polymorphisms in multiple genes that encode proteins involved in the various pathways of drug metabolism, distribution, and effects. For example, the immunosuppressants cyclosporine and tacrolimus are believed to be substrates for both P-glycoprotein and the CYP450, CYP3A4, and possibly CPY3A5 enzymes.[112] Thus, it is possible that genes for both MDR1 and CYP450 enzymes interact to influence cyclosporine and tacrolimus distribution and plasma concentrations.

Pharmacists are broadly trained in a number of medication-related areas, including pharmacology, pharmacokinetics, and pharmacodynamics. This training places pharmacists in a unique position to deal with the complexities of the drug-decision process in the age of pharmacogenetics. Pharmacists will be in key positions to interpret the results of genetic tests, determine the ultimate effects of multiple genetic variations on drug response, and choose the most appropriate drug for a given patient based on the individual's DNA. Thus, it will be essential for pharmacists to stay abreast of significant discoveries in genotype–drug response relationships and understand how best to incorporate this genomic information into pharmacotherapeutic decisions.

Recognizing the challenges in healthcare delivery with advancing genetic discoveries, the National Coalition for Health Professional Education in Genetics established core competencies related to genetics for healthcare professionals that are available through the coalition's website (*www.nchpeg.org*). The objective of these competencies is to encourage clinicians to incorporate genetics knowledge, skills, and attitudes into their clinical practices. Subsequently, the American Association of Colleges of Pharmacy developed recommendations to guide academic institutions on how to instill these competencies in future pharmacists so that pharmacists will be prepared to provide appropriate pharmacotherapy in the age of genomics.[102]

APPLICATION OF PHARMACOGENETIC DATA TO DISEASE MANAGEMENT

Pharmacogenetics has the potential to greatly improve the pharmacologic management of disease. Clinicians may be able to predict the likelihood that an individual will respond to a particular medication based on the patient's genotype. Medications may be avoided or prescribed in lower doses with careful monitoring in patients genetically predisposed to the drugs' adverse effects. This would be of particular benefit for drugs with a narrow therapeutic index. For example, warfarin may be initiated at lower doses, with closer monitoring in patients with a *VKORC1* haplotype associated with increased warfarin sensitivity or a *CYP2C9* allele associated with reduced warfarin metabolism.

With pharmacogenetics, it may be possible to eliminate the trial-and-error approach to drug prescribing for many diseases. Instead, clinicians may be able to use genetic information to match the right drug to the right patient at the right dose while minimizing adverse effects. For example, the current approach to hypertension management involves the trial of various antihypertensives until blood pressure goals are achieved with acceptable drug tolerability. Commonly, the initial agent fails to lower blood pressure to goal or produces intolerable adverse effects (Fig. 6–6). Trials of additional or alternative antihypertensive medications must be undertaken until treatment is deemed successful. In the interim, the patient remains hypertensive and at risk for hypertension-related target-organ damage. With pharmacogenetics, clinicians may choose the antihypertensive drug expected to provide the greatest response with the best tolerability for a particular patient based on his or her DNA.

New drugs may be developed based on knowledge about genetic control of cellular functions. For example, the discovery that chronic myeloid leukemia was caused by chromosome translocation and consequent production of an enzyme capable of producing life-threatening lymphocyte levels led to accelerated FDA approval of Gleevec (also known as STI-571), an inhibitor of the transloca-

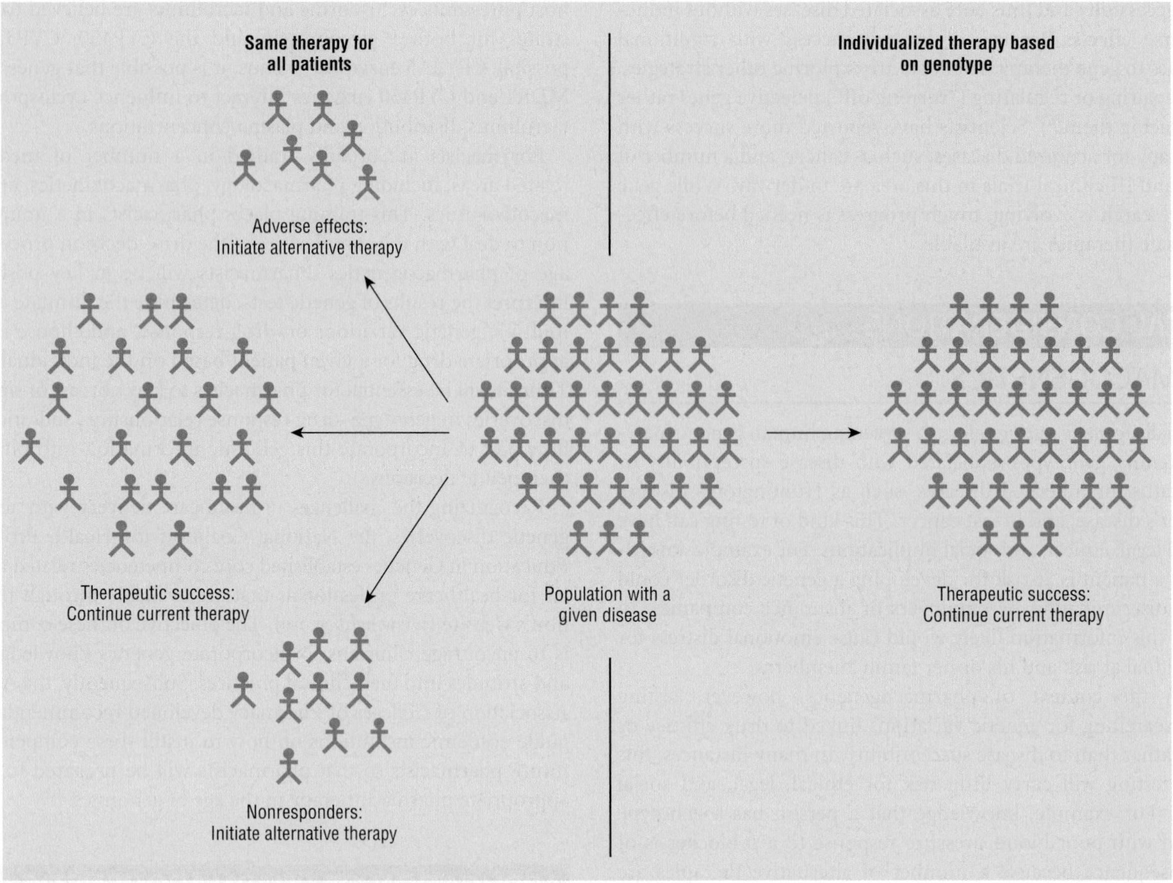

FIGURE 6-6. Current and future approaches to pharmacologic management of disease.

tion-created enzyme, for treatment of chronic myeloid leukemia.[103] In addition, future drug development may focus on treating specific genetic subgroups instead of broadly treating all individuals with a particular disease. Along these lines, the FDA is encouraging pharmaceutical companies to submit pharmacogenetic data during the drug development process.[104] Ultimately, pharmacogenetics may improve the quality and reduce the overall costs of healthcare by decreasing the number of treatment failures and the number of adverse drug reactions and leading to the discovery of new genetic targets and therapeutic interventions for disease management.

CLINICAL CONTROVERSY

For many drugs, such as warfarin, variations in genes affecting both pharmacokinetic and pharmacodynamic drug properties may interact to determine the ultimate effects of drug therapy. Thus, the challenge for researchers will be to identify the combination of gene variations that best predicts response for these drugs.

ABBREVIATIONS

A: adenine

ACE: angiotensin-converting enzyme

AUC: area under the curve

C: cytosine

CYP450: cytochrome P450

DPD: dihydropyrimidine dehydrogenase

EM: extensive metabolizer

FDA: Food and Drug Administration

G: guanine

HIV: human immunodeficiency virus

I/D: insertion/deletion

MDR1: multidrug resistance-1

PM: poor metabolizer

SCID: severe combined immunodeficiency syndrome

SNPs: single nucleotide polymorphisms

T: thymidine

TPMT: thiopurine *S*-methyltransferase

UGT: uridine diphosphate glucuronosyltransferase

UM: ultrarapid metabolizer

REFERENCES

1. Alving AS, Carson PE, Flanagan CL, Ickes CE. Enzymatic deficiency in primaquine-sensitive erythrocytes. Science 1956;124:484–485.
2. Aithal GP, Day CP, Kesteven PJ, Daly AK. Association of polymorphisms in the cytochrome P450 CYP2C9 with warfarin dose requirement and risk of bleeding complications. Lancet 1999;353:717–719.
3. Mamiya K, Ieiri I, Shimamoto J, et al. The effects of genetic polymorphisms of CYP2C9 and CYP2C19 on phenytoin metabolism in Japanese adult patients with epilepsy: Studies in stereoselective hydroxylation and population pharmacokinetics. Epilepsia 1998;39:1317–1323.
4. Relling MV, Hancock ML, Rivera GK, et al. Mercaptopurine therapy intolerance and heterozygosity at the thiopurine S-methyltransferase gene locus. J Natl Cancer Inst 1999;91:2001–2008.
5. Motulsky AG. Drug reactions, enzymes and biochemical genetics. JAMA 1957;165:835–837.

6. Vogel F. Moderne Probleme der Humangenetick. Ergebn Inn Med Kinderheilk 1959;12:52–125.
7. Lander ES, Linton LM, Birren B, et al. Initial sequencing and analysis of the human genome. Nature 2001;409:860–921.
8. Human Genome Program. Genomics and Its Impact On Medicine and Society: A 2003 Primer. Washington, DC: U.S. Department of Energy, 2003.
9. Collins FS, Green ED, Guttmacher AE, Guyer MS. A vision for the future of genomics research. Nature 2003;422:835–847.
10. Johnson JA, Terra SG. Beta-adrenergic receptor polymorphisms: Cardiovascular disease associations and pharmacogenetics. Pharm Res 2002;19:1779–1787.
11. Strachan T, Read AP. Human Molecular Genetics, 3rd ed. New York: Garland Science, 2004.
12. Ferrari P, Bianchi G. Genetic mapping and tailored antihypertensive therapy. Cardiovasc Drugs Ther 2000;14:387–395.
13. Evans WE, Relling MV. Pharmacogenomics: Translating functional genomics into rational therapeutics. Science 1999;286:487–491.
14. Sata F, Sapone A, Elizondo G, et al. CYP3A4 allelic variants with amino acid substitutions in exons 7 and 12: Evidence for an allelic variant with altered catalytic activity. Clin Pharmacol Ther 2000;67:48–56.
15. Kuehl P, Zhang J, Lin Y, et al. Sequence diversity in CYP3A promoters and characterization of the genetic basis of polymorphic CYP3A5 expression. Nat Genet 2001;27:383–391.
16. Sachse C, Brockmoller J, Bauer S, Roots I. Functional significance of a CA polymorphism in intron 1 of the cytochrome P450 CYP1A2 gene tested with caffeine. Br J Clin Pharmacol 1999;47:445–449.
17. Marez D, Legrand M, Sabbagh N, et al. Polymorphism of the cytochrome P450 CYP2D6 gene in a European population: Characterization of 48 mutations and 53 alleles, their frequencies and evolution. Pharmacogenetics 1997;7:193–202.
18. Shah RR, Oates NS, Idle JR, et al. Impaired oxidation of debrisoquine in patients with perhexiline neuropathy. Br Med J (Clin Res Ed) 1982;284:295–299.
19. Lee JT, Kroemer HK, Silberstein DJ, et al. The role of genetically determined polymorphic drug metabolism in the beta-blockade produced by propafenone. N Engl J Med 1990;322:1764–1768.
20. Dahl-Puustinen ML, Liden A, Alm C, Nordin C, Bertilsson L. Disposition of perphenazine is related to polymorphic debrisoquin hydroxylation in human beings. Clin Pharmacol Ther 1989;46:78–81.
21. Spina E, Ancione M, Di Rosa AE, Meduri M, Caputi AP. Polymorphic debrisoquine oxidation and acute neuroleptic-induced adverse effects. Eur J Clin Pharmacol 1992;42:347–348.
22. Poulsen L, Arendt-Nielsen L, Brosen K, Sindrup SH. The hypoalgesic effect of tramadol in relation to CYP2D6. Clin Pharmacol Ther 1996;60:636–644.
23. Sindrup SH, Brosen K, Bjerring P, et al. Codeine increases pain thresholds to copper vapor laser stimuli in extensive but not poor metabolizers of sparteine. Clin Pharmacol Ther 1990;48:686–693.
24. Dehal SS, Kupfer D. CYP2D6 catalyzes tamoxifen 4-hydroxylation in human liver. Cancer Res 1997;57:3402–3406.
25. Tyndale RF, Droll KP, Sellers EM. Genetically deficient CYP2D6 metabolism provides protection against oral opiate dependence. Pharmacogenetics 1997;7:375–379.
26. Romach MK, Otton SV, Somer G, Tyndale RF, Sellers EM. Cytochrome P450 2D6 and treatment of codeine dependence. J Clin Psychopharmacol 2000;20:43–45.
27. Alfaro CL, Lam YW, Simpson J, Ereshefsky L. CYP2D6 status of extensive metabolizers after multiple-dose fluoxetine, fluvoxamine, paroxetine, or sertraline. J Clin Psychopharmacol 1999;19:155–163.
28. Alfaro CL, Lam YW, Simpson J, Ereshefsky L. CYP2D6 inhibition by fluoxetine, paroxetine, sertraline, and venlafaxine in a crossover study: Intraindividual variability and plasma concentration correlations. J Clin Pharmacol 2000;40:58–66.
29. Hamelin BA, Bouayad A, Methot J, et al. Significant interaction between the nonprescription antihistamine diphenhydramine and the CYP2D6 substrate metoprolol in healthy men with high or low CYP2D6 activity. Clin Pharmacol Ther 2000;67:466–477.
30. Bertilsson L, Aberg-Wistedt A, Gustafsson LL, Nordin C. Extremely rapid hydroxylation of debrisoquine: A case report with implication for treatment with nortriptyline and other tricyclic antidepressants. Ther Drug Monit 1985;7:478–480.
31. Dalen P, Dahl ML, Ruiz ML, Nordin J, Bertilsson L. 10-Hydroxylation of nortriptyline in white persons with 0, 1, 2, 3, and 13 functional CYP2D6 genes. Clin Pharmacol Ther 1998;63:444–452.
32. Bertilsson L, Dahl ML, Sjoqvist F, et al. Molecular basis for rational megaprescribing in ultrarapid hydroxylators of debrisoquine. Lancet 1993;341:63.
33. Lam YW, Gaedigk A, Ereshefsky L, Alfaro CL, Simpson J. CYP2D6 inhibition by selective serotonin reuptake inhibitors: Analysis of achievable steady-state plasma concentrations and the effect of ultrarapid metabolism at CYP2D6. Pharmacotherapy 2002;22:1001–1006.
34. Lin KM, Finder E. Neuroleptic dosage for Asians. Am J Psychiatry 1983;140:490–491.
35. Mihara K, Otani K, Tybring G, Dahl ML, Bertilsson L, Kaneko S. The CYP2D6 genotype and plasma concentrations of mianserin enantiomers in relation to therapeutic response to mianserin in depressed Japanese patients. J Clin Psychopharmacol 1997;17:467–471.
36. Masimirembwa C, Persson I, Bertilsson L, Hasler J, Ingelman-Sundberg M. A novel mutant variant of the CYP2D6 gene (CYP2D6*17) common in a black African population: Association with diminished debrisoquine hydroxylase activity. Br J Clin Pharmacol 1996;42:713–719.
37. Droll K, Bruce-Mensah K, Otton SV, Gaedigk A, Sellers EM, Tyndale RF. Comparison of three CYP2D6 probe substrates and genotype in Ghanaians, Chinese and Caucasians. Pharmacogenetics 1998;8:325–333.
38. Chou WH, Yan FX, de Leon J, et al. Extension of a pilot study: Impact from the cytochrome P450 2D6 polymorphism on outcome and costs associated with severe mental illness. J Clin Psychopharmacol 2000;20:246–251.
39. Brockmoller J, Kirchheiner J, Schmider J, et al. The impact of the CYP2D6 polymorphism on haloperidol pharmacokinetics and on the outcome of haloperidol treatment. Clin Pharmacol Ther 2002;72:438–452.
40. Andersson T, Regardh CG, Lou YC, Zhang Y, Dahl ML, Bertilsson L. Polymorphic hydroxylation of S-mephenytoin and omeprazole metabolism in Caucasian and Chinese subjects. Pharmacogenetics 1992;2:25–31.
41. Andersson T, Holmberg J, Rohss K, Walan A. Pharmacokinetics and effect on caffeine metabolism of the proton pump inhibitors, omeprazole, lansoprazole, and pantoprazole. Br J Clin Pharmacol 1998;45:369–375.
42. Furuta T, Ohashi K, Kamata T, et al. Effect of genetic differences in omeprazole metabolism on cure rates for *Helicobacter pylori* infection and peptic ulcer. Ann Intern Med 1998;129:1027–1030.
43. Tanigawara Y, Aoyama N, Kita T, et al. CYP2C19 genotype-related efficacy of omeprazole for the treatment of infection caused by *Helicobacter pylori*. Clin Pharmacol Ther 1999;66:528–534.
44. Kawabata H, Habu Y, Tomioka H, et al. Effect of different proton pump inhibitors, differences in CYP2C19 genotype and antibiotic resistance on the eradication rate of *Helicobacter pylori* infection by a 1-week regimen of proton pump inhibitor, amoxicillin and clarithromycin. Aliment Pharmacol Ther 2003;17:259–264.
45. Furuta T, Ohashi K, Kosuge K, et al. CYP2C19 genotype status and effect of omeprazole on intragastric pH in humans. Clin Pharmacol Ther 1999;65:552–561.
46. Furuta T, Shirai N, Takashima M, et al. Effect of genotypic differences in CYP2C19 on cure rates for *Helicobacter pylori* infection by triple therapy with a proton pump inhibitor, amoxicillin, and clarithromycin. Clin Pharmacol Ther 2001;69:158–168.
47. Ghoneim MM, Korttila K, Chiang CK, et al. Diazepam effects and kinetics in Caucasians and Orientals. Clin Pharmacol Ther 1981;29:749–756.
48. Kalow W. Interethnic variation of drug metabolism. Trends Pharmacol Sci 1991;12:102–107.
49. Kumana CR, Lauder IJ, Chan M, Ko W, Lin HJ. Differences in diazepam pharmacokinetics in Chinese and white Caucasians—Relation to body lipid stores. Eur J Clin Pharmacol 1987;32:211–215.
50. Stubbins MJ, Harries LW, Smith G, Tarbit MH, Wolf CR. Genetic analysis of the human cytochrome P450 CYP2C9 locus. Pharmacogenetics 1996;6:429–439.
51. Takahashi H, Kashima T, Nomoto S, et al. Comparisons between in-vitro and in-vivo metabolism of (S)-warfarin: Catalytic activities of cDNA-expressed CYP2C9, its Leu359 variant and their mixture versus unbound clearance in patients with the corresponding CYP2C9 genotypes. Pharmacogenetics 1998;8:365–373.
52. Steward DJ, Haining RL, Henne KR, et al. Genetic association between sensitivity to warfarin and expression of CYP2C9*3. Pharmacogenetics 1997;7:361–367.

53. Nunoya K, Yokoi T, Kimura K, et al. A new deleted allele in the human cytochrome P450 2A6 (CYP2A6) gene found in individuals showing poor metabolic capacity to coumarin and (+)-cis-3,5-dimethyl-2-(3-pyridyl)thiazolidin-4-one hydrochloride (SM-12502). Pharmacogenetics 1998;8:239–249.
54. Nunoya KI, Yokoi T, Kimura K, et al. A new CYP2A6 gene deletion responsible for the in vivo polymorphic metabolism of (+)-cis-3,5-dimethyl-2-(3-pyridyl)thiazolidin-4-one hydrochloride in humans. J Pharmacol Exp Ther 1999;289:437–442.
55. Pianezza ML, Sellers EM, Tyndale RF. Nicotine metabolism defect reduces smoking. Nature 1998;393:750.
56. Sellers EM, Tyndale RF. Mimicking gene defects to treat drug dependence. Ann N Y Acad Sci 2000;909:233–246.
57. Hesselink DA, van Schaik RH, van der Heiden IP, et al. Genetic polymorphisms of the CYP3A4, CYP3A5, and MDR-1 genes and pharmacokinetics of the calcineurin inhibitors cyclosporine and tacrolimus. Clin Pharmacol Ther 2003;74:245–254.
58. Zheng H, Zeevi A, Schuetz E, et al. Tacrolimus dosing in adult lung transplant patients is related to cytochrome P4503A5 gene polymorphism. J Clin Pharmacol 2004;44:135–140.
59. Lu Z, Zhang R, Carpenter JT, Diasio RB. Decreased dihydropyrimidine dehydrogenase activity in a population of patients with breast cancer: Implication for 5-fluorouracil-based chemotherapy. Clin Cancer Res 1998;4:325–329.
60. Ando Y, Saka H, Asai G, Sugiura S, Shimokata K, Kamataki T. UGT1A1 genotypes and glucuronidation of SN-38, the active metabolite of irinotecan. Ann Oncol 1998;9:845–847.
61. Wasserman E, Myara A, Lokiec F, et al. Severe CPT-11 toxicity in patients with Gilbert's syndrome: Two case reports. Ann Oncol 1997;8:1049–1051.
62. Iyer L, Das S, Janisch L, et al. UGT1A1*28 polymorphism as a determinant of irinotecan disposition and toxicity. Pharmacogenomics J 2002;2:43–47.
63. Johne A, Kopke K, Gerloff T, et al. Modulation of steady-state kinetics of digoxin by haplotypes of the P-glycoprotein MDR1 gene. Clin Pharmacol Ther 2002;72:584–594.
64. Fellay J, Marzolini C, Meaden ER, et al. Response to antiretroviral treatment in HIV-1–infected individuals with allelic variants of the multidrug resistance transporter 1: A pharmacogenetics study. Lancet 2002;359:30–36.
65. Johnson JA, Zineh I, Puckett BJ, McGorray SP, Yarandi HN, Pauly DF. Beta 1-adrenergic receptor polymorphisms and antihypertensive response to metoprolol. Clin Pharmacol Ther 2003;74:44–52.
66. Materson BJ, Reda DJ, Cushman WC. Department of Veterans Affairs single-drug therapy of hypertension study. Revised figures and new data. Department of Veterans Affairs Cooperative Study Group on Antihypertensive Agents. Am J Hypertens 1995;8:189–192.
67. Drazen JM, Israel E, Boushey HA, et al. Comparison of regularly scheduled with as-needed use of albuterol in mild asthma. Asthma Clinical Research Network. N Engl J Med 1996;335:841–847.
68. Litonjua AA. The significance of β2-adrenergic receptor polymorphisms in asthma. Curr Opin Pulm Med 2006;12:12–17.
69. Drysdale CM, McGraw DW, Stack CB, et al. Complex promoter and coding region β2-adrenergic receptor haplotypes alter receptor expression and predict in vivo responsiveness. Proc Natl Acad Sci USA 2000;97:10483–10488.
70. Arranz MJ, Munro J, Birkett J, et al. Pharmacogenetic prediction of clozapine response. Lancet 2000;355:1615–1616.
71. Masellis M, Basile VS, Ozdemir V, Meltzer HY, Macciardi FM, Kennedy JL. Pharmacogenetics of antipsychotic treatment: Lessons learned from clozapine. Biol Psychiatry 2000;47:252–266.
72. Rost S, Fregin A, Ivaskevicius V, et al. Mutations in VKORC1 cause warfarin resistance and multiple coagulation factor deficiency type 2. Nature 2004;427:537–541.
73. Rieder MJ, Reiner AP, Gage BF, et al. Effect of VKORC1 haplotypes on transcriptional regulation and warfarin dose. N Engl J Med 2005;352:2285–2293.
74. Carlquist JF, Horne BD, Muhlestein JB, et al. Genotypes of the cytochrome p450 isoform, CYP2C9, and the vitamin K epoxide reductase complex subunit 1 conjointly determine stable warfarin dose: A prospective study. J Thromb Thrombolysis 2006;22:191–197.
75. Sconce EA, Khan TI, Wynne HA, et al. The impact of CYP2C9 and VKORC1 genetic polymorphism and patient characteristics upon warfarin dose requirements: Proposal for a new dosing regimen. Blood 2005;106:2329–2333.
76. Voora D, Eby C, Linder MW, et al. Prospective dosing of warfarin based on cytochrome P-450 2C9 genotype. Thromb Haemost 2005;93:700–705.
77. Scharplatz M, Puhan MA, Steurer J, Bachmann LM. What is the impact of the ACE gene insertion/deletion (I/D) polymorphism on the clinical effectiveness and adverse events of ACE inhibitors? Protocol of a systematic review. BMC Med Genet 2004;5:23.
78. Arnett DK, Claas SA, Glasser SP. Pharmacogenetics of antihypertensive treatment. Vasc Pharmacol 2006;44:107–118.
79. Arnett DK, Davis BR, Ford CE, et al. Pharmacogenetic association of the angiotensin-converting enzyme insertion/deletion polymorphism on blood pressure and cardiovascular risk in relation to antihypertensive treatment: The Genetics of Hypertension-Associated Treatment (GenHAT) study. Circulation 2005;111:3374–3383.
80. Serretti A, Benedetti F, Zanardi R, Smeraldi E. The influence of Serotonin Transporter Promoter Polymorphism (SERTPR) and other polymorphisms of the serotonin pathway on the efficacy of antidepressant treatments. Prog Neuropsychopharmacol Biol Psychiatry 2005;29:1074–1084.
81. Siffert W, Rosskopf D, Moritz A, et al. Enhanced G protein activation in immortalized lymphoblasts from patients with essential hypertension. J Clin Invest 1995;96:759–766.
82. Su YR, Menon AG. Epithelial sodium channels and hypertension. Drug Metab Dispos 2001;29:553–556.
83. Baker EH, Duggal A, Dong Y, et al. Amiloride, a specific drug for hypertension in black people with T594M variant? Hypertension 2002;40:13–17.
84. de Leon J, Susce MT, Pan RM, Koch WH, Wedlund PJ. Polymorphic variations in GSTM1, GSTT1, PgP, CYP2D6, CYP3A5, and dopamine D2 and D3 receptors and their association with tardive dyskinesia in severe mental illness. J Clin Psychopharmacol 2005;25:448–456.
85. Martinelli I, Battaglioli T, Mannucci PM. Pharmacogenetic aspects of the use of oral contraceptives and the risk of thrombosis. Pharmacogenetics 2003;13:589–594.
86. Roepke TK, Abbott GW. Pharmacogenetics and cardiac ion channels. Vasc Pharmacol 2006;44:90–106.
87. Executive Summary of The Third Report of The National Cholesterol Education Program (NCEP) Expert Panel on Detection, Evaluation, and Treatment of High Blood Cholesterol in Adults (Adult Treatment Panel III). JAMA 2001;285:2486–2497.
88. Maitland-van der Zee AH, Klungel OH, Stricker BH, et al. Genetic polymorphisms: Importance for response to HMG-CoA reductase inhibitors. Atherosclerosis 2002;163:213–222.
89. Gerdes LU, Gerdes C, Kervinen K, et al. The apolipoprotein ε4 allele determines prognosis and the effect on prognosis of simvastatin in survivors of myocardial infarction: A substudy of the Scandinavian simvastatin survival study. Circulation 2000;101:1366–1371.
90. Harries M, Smith I. The development and clinical use of trastuzumab (Herceptin). Endocr Relat Cancer 2002;9:75–85.
91. Brickell KL, Steinbart EJ, Rumbaugh M, et al. Early-onset Alzheimer's disease in families with late-onset Alzheimer's disease: A potential important subtype of familial Alzheimer's disease. Arch Neurol 2006;63:1307–1311.
92. Mizuno Y, Hattori N, Yoshino H, et al. Progress in familial Parkinson's disease. J Neural Transm Suppl 2006:191–204.
93. Fibison WJ. Gene therapy. Nurs Clin North Am 2000;35:757–772.
94. Marshall E. Gene therapy. Second child in French trial is found to have leukemia. Science 2003;299:320.
95. Morgan RA, Dudley ME, Wunderlich JR, et al. Cancer regression in patients after transfer of genetically engineered lymphocytes. Science 2006;314:126–129.
96. Morris JC, Ramsey WJ, Wildner O, Muslow HA, Aguilar-Cordova E, Blaese RM. A phase I study of intralesional administration of an adenovirus vector expressing the HSV-1 thymidine kinase gene (AdV.RSV-TK) in combination with escalating doses of ganciclovir in patients with cutaneous metastatic malignant melanoma. Hum Gene Ther 2000;11:487–503.
97. Marshall E. Gene therapy death prompts review of adenovirus vector. Science 1999;286:2244–2245.
98. Jiang H, Pierce GF, Ozelo MC, et al. Evidence of multiyear factor IX expression by AAV-mediated gene transfer to skeletal muscle in an individual with severe hemophilia B. Mol Ther 2006;14:452–455.
99. Symes JF, Losordo DW, Vale PR, et al. Gene therapy with vascular endothelial growth factor for inoperable coronary artery disease. Ann Thorac Surg 1999;68:830–836.

100. Fortuin FD, Vale P, Losordo DW, et al. One-year follow-up of direct myocardial gene transfer of vascular endothelial growth factor-2 using naked plasmid deoxyribonucleic acid by way of thoracotomy in no-option patients. Am J Cardiol 2003;92:436–439.
101. Sullenger BA. Targeted genetic repair: An emerging approach to genetic therapy. J Clin Invest 2003;112:310–311.
102. Johnson JA, Bootman JL, Evans WE, et al. Pharmacogenomics: A scientific revolution in pharmaceutical sciences and pharmacy practice. Report of the 2001–2002 Academic Affairs Committee. Am J Pharm Educ 2002;66:12S–15S.
103. Johnson JR, Bross P, Cohen M, et al. Approval summary: Imatinib mesylate capsules for treatment of adult patients with newly diagnosed Philadelphia chromosome-positive chronic myelogenous leukemia in chronic phase. Clin Cancer Res 2003;9:1972–1979.
104. Ratner M. FDA pharmacogenomics guidance sends clear message to industry. Nat Rev Drug Discov 2005;4:359.
105. Devadatta S, Gangadharam PRJ, Andrews RH. Peripheral neuritis due to isoniazid. Bull World Health Organ 1960;23:587–598.
106. Henningsen NC, Cederberg A, Hanson A, Johansson BW. Effects of long-term treatment with procaine amide. A prospective study with special regard to ANF and SLE in fast and slow acetylators. Acta Med Scand 1975;198:475–482.
107. Strandberg I, Boman G, Hassler L, Sjoqvist F. Acetylator phenotype in patients with hydralazine-induced lupoid syndrome. Acta Med Scand 1976;200:367–371.
108. Pullar T, Hunter JA, Capell HA. Effect of acetylator phenotype on efficacy and toxicity of sulfphasalazine in rheumatoid arthritis. Ann Rheum Dis 1985;44:831–837.
109. Maree AO, Curtin RJ, Chubb A, et al. Cyclooxygenase-1 haplotype modulates platelet response to aspirin. J Thromb Haemost 2005;3:2340–2345.
110. Chasman DI, Posada D, Subrahmanyan L, Cook NR, Stanton VP Jr, Ridker PM. Pharmacogenetic study of statin therapy and cholesterol reduction. JAMA 2004;291:2821–2827.
111. Drazen JM, Yandava CN, Dube L, et al. Pharmacogenetic association between ALOX5 promoter genotype and the response to anti-asthma treatment. Nat Genet 1999;22:168–170.
112. Hesselink DA, van Schaik RH, van der Heiden IP, et al. Genetic polymorphisms of the CYP3A4, CYP3A5, and MDR-1 genes and pharmacokinetics of the calcineurin inhibitors cyclosporin and tacrolimus. Clin Pharmacol Ther 2003;74:245–254.

CHAPTER 7

Pediatrics

MILAP C. NAHATA AND CAROL TAKETOMO

KEY CONCEPTS

1. Children are not just "little adults," and lack of data on important pharmacokinetic and pharmacodynamic differences has led to several disastrous situations in pediatric care.
2. Variations in absorption of medications from the gastrointestinal tract, intramuscular injection sites, and skin are important in pediatric patients, especially in premature and other newborn infants.
3. The rate and extent of organ function development and the distribution, metabolism, and elimination of drugs differ not only between pediatric versus adult patients but also among pediatric age groups.
4. The effectiveness and safety of drugs may vary among various age groups and from one drug to another in pediatric versus adult patients.
5. Concomitant diseases may influence dosage requirements to achieve a targeted effect for a specific disease in children.
6. The myth that neonates and young infants do not experience pain has led to inadequate pain management in this pediatric population.
7. Special methods of drug administration are needed for infants and young children.
8. Many medicines needed for pediatric patients are not available in appropriate dosage forms; thus, the dosage forms of drugs marketed for adults may require modification for use in infants and children, necessitating assurance of potency and safety of drug use.
9. The pediatric medication-use process is complex and error-prone because of the multiple steps required in calculating, verifying, preparing, and administering doses.

Remarkable progress has been made in the clinical management of disease in pediatric patients. This chapter highlights important principles of pediatric pharmacotherapy that must be considered when the diseases discussed in other chapters of this book occur in pediatric patients, defined as those younger than 18 years. Newborn infants born before 37 weeks of gestational age are termed *premature;* those between 1 day and 1 month of age are *neonates;* 1 month to 1 year are *infants;* 1 to 11 years are *children;* and 12 to 16 years are *adolescents.* This chapter covers notable examples of problems in pediatrics, pharmacokinetic differences in pediatric patients, drug efficacy and toxicity in this patient group, and various factors affecting pediatric pharmacotherapy. Specific examples of problems and special considerations in pediatric patients are cited to enhance understanding.

1 Infant mortality has declined from 200 per 1,000 births in the 19th century to 75 per 1,000 births in 1925 to 6.79 per 1,000 births in 2004.[1] This success has resulted largely from improvements in identification, prevention, and treatment of diseases once common during delivery and the period of infancy. Although most marketed drugs are used in pediatric patients, only one fourth of the drugs approved by the Food and Drug Administration (FDA) have indications specific for use in the pediatric population. Data on the pharmacokinetics, pharmacodynamics, efficacy, and safety of drugs in infants and children are scarce. Lack of this type of information led to disasters such as gray baby syndrome from chloramphenicol, phocomelia from thalidomide, and kernicterus from sulfonamide therapy. Gray baby syndrome was first reported in two neonates who died after excessive doses of chloramphenicol (100–300 mg/kg/day); the serum concentrations of chloramphenicol immediately before death were 75 and 100 mcg/mL. Patients with gray baby syndrome usually have abdominal distension, vomiting, diarrhea, a characteristic gray color, respiratory distress, hypotension, and progressive shock.

Thalidomide is well known for its teratogenic effects. Clearly implicated as the cause of multiple congenital fetal abnormalities (particularly limb deformities), thalidomide also can cause polyneuritis, nerve damage, and mental retardation. Isotretinoin (Accutane) is another teratogen. Because it is used to treat severe acne vulgaris, which is common in teenage patients who may be sexually active but not willing to acknowledge that activity to healthcare professionals, isotretinoin has presented a difficult problem in patient education since its marketing in the 1980s.

Kernicterus was reported in neonates receiving sulfonamides, which displaced bilirubin from protein-binding sites in the blood to cause a hyperbilirubinemia. This results in deposition of bilirubin in the brain and induces encephalopathy in infants.

Another area of concern in pediatrics is identifying an optimal dosage. Dosage regimens cannot be based simply on body weight or surface area of a pediatric patient extrapolated from adult data. Bioavailability, pharmacokinetics, pharmacodynamics, efficacy, and adverse-effect information can differ markedly between pediatric and adult patients, as well as among pediatric patients, because of differences in age, organ function, and disease state. Significant progress has been made in the area of pediatric pharmacokinetics during the last 2 decades, but few such studies have correlated pharmacokinetics with the outcomes of efficacy, adverse effects, or quality of life.

Several additional factors should be considered in optimizing pediatric drug therapy. Many drugs prescribed widely for infants and children are not available in suitable dosage forms. For example, extemporaneous liquid dosage forms of amiodarone, captopril, omeprazole, and spironolactone are prepared for infants and children who cannot swallow tablets or capsules, and injectable dosage forms of aminophylline, methylprednisolone, morphine, and phenobarbital are diluted to accurately measure small doses for infants. Alteration (dilution or reformulation) of dosage forms intended for adult patients raises questions about the bioavailability, stability, and compatibility of these drugs. Because of low fluid volume requirements and limited access to intravenous sites, special methods must be used for delivery of intravenous drugs to infants and children. As simple as it may seem, administration of oral drugs to young patients continues to be a difficult task for nurses and parents. Similarly, ensuring adherence to pharmacotherapy in pediatric patients poses a special challenge.

Finally, the need for additional pharmacologic or therapeutic research brings up the issue of ethical justification for conducting research. Investigators proposing studies and institutional review committees approving human studies must assess the risk-to-benefit ratio of each study to be fair to children who are not in a position to accept or reject the opportunity to participate in the research project.

Enormous progress in pharmacokinetics has been made in pediatric patients. Two factors have contributed to this progress: (a) the availability of sensitive and specific analytic methods to measure drugs and their metabolites in small volumes of biologic fluids and (b) awareness of the importance of clinical pharmacokinetics in optimization of drug therapy. Absorption, distribution, metabolism, and elimination of many drugs are different in premature infants, full-term infants, and older children, and this topic is discussed in detail in the next few sections.

ABSORPTION

GASTROINTESTINAL TRACT

❷ Two factors affecting the absorption of drugs from the gastrointestinal tract are pH-dependent passive diffusion and gastric emptying time. Both processes are strikingly different in premature infants compared with older children and adults. In a full-term infant, gastric pH ranges from 6 to 8 at birth but declines to 1 to 3 within 24 hours.[2] In contrast, gastric pH remains elevated in premature infants because of immature acid secretion.[3]

In premature infants, higher serum concentrations of acid-labile drugs, such as penicillin,[4] ampicillin,[5] and nafcillin,[6] and lower serum concentrations of a weak acid such as phenobarbital[7] can be explained by higher gastric pH. Because of a lack of extensive data comparing serum concentration–time profiles after oral versus intravenous drug administration, differences in the bioavailability of drugs in premature infants are poorly understood. Although little is known about the influence of developmental changes with age on drug absorption in pediatric patients, a few studies with drugs (e.g., digoxin and phenobarbital) and nutrients (e.g., arabinose and xylose) have suggested that the processes of both passive and active transport may be fully developed by approximately 4 months of age.[8] Little is known about the development and expression of the efflux transporter P-glycoprotein and the intestinal drug-metabolizing enzymes and their impact on drug absorption and bioavailability in infants and children.

Studies have shown that gastric emptying is slow in a premature infant.[9] Thus, drugs with limited absorption in adults may be absorbed efficiently in a premature infant because of prolonged contact time with gastrointestinal mucosa.

INTRAMUSCULAR SITES

Drug absorption from an intramuscular site may be altered in premature infants. Differences in relative muscle mass, poor perfusion to various muscles, peripheral vasomotor instability, and insufficient muscular contractions in premature infants compared with older children and adults can influence drug absorption from the intramuscular site. The net effect of these factors on drug absorption is impossible to predict; phenobarbital has been reported to be absorbed rapidly,[10] whereas diazepam absorption may be delayed.[11] Thus, intramuscular dosing is used rarely in neonates except in emergencies or when an intravenous site is inaccessible.

SKIN

Percutaneous absorption may be increased substantially in newborns because of an underdeveloped epidermal barrier (stratum corneum) and increased skin hydration. Furthermore, because the ratio of total body surface area to total body weight is highest in the youngest group, the relative systemic exposure of topically applied drugs, including corticosteroids, may be higher in infants and young children than in adults. The increased exposure can produce toxic effects after topical use of hexachlorophene soaps and powders,[12] salicylic acid ointment, and rubbing alcohol.[13] Interestingly, a study has shown that a therapeutic serum concentration of theophylline can be achieved for control of apnea in premature infants less than 30 weeks' gestation after topical application of gel containing a standard dose of theophylline.[14] Use of this route of administration may minimize the unpredictability of oral and intramuscular absorption and the complications of intravenous drug administration for certain drugs. A transdermal patch formulation of methylphenidate has been approved for use in children 6 to 12 years of age for treatment of attention-deficit/hyperactivity disorder (ADHD). The patch can be applied once daily and can remain on during normal activities such as bathing, swimming, and exercising.

DISTRIBUTION

❸ Drug distribution is determined by the physicochemical properties of the drug itself (pK_a, molecular weight, partition coefficient) and the physiologic factors specific to the patient. Although the physicochemical properties of the drug are constant, the physiologic functions often vary in different patient populations. Some important patient-specific factors include extracellular and total body water, protein binding by the drug in plasma, and presence of pathologic conditions modifying physiologic function. Total body water, as a percentage of total body weight, has been estimated to be 94% in fetuses, 85% in premature infants, 78% in full-term infants, and 60% in adults.[14] Extracellular fluid volume also is markedly different in premature infants compared with older children and adults; the extracellular fluid volume may account for 50% of body weight in premature infants, 35% in 4- to 6-month-old infants, 25% in children 1 year old, and 19% in adults.[15] This conforms to the observed gentamicin distribution volumes of 0.48 L/kg in neonates and 0.20 L/kg in adults.[16] Studies have shown that the distribution volume of tobramycin is largest in the most premature infants and decreases with increases in gestational age and birth weight of the infant.[17]

Binding of drugs to plasma proteins is decreased in newborn infants because of decreased plasma protein concentration, lower binding capacity of protein, decreased affinity of proteins for drug binding, and competition for certain binding sites by endogenous compounds such as bilirubin. The plasma protein binding of many drugs, including phenobarbital, salicylates, and phenytoin, is significantly less in the neonate than in the adult.[18] The decrease in plasma protein binding of drugs can increase their apparent volumes of distribution. Therefore, premature infants require a larger loading dose than do older children and adults to achieve a therapeutic serum concentration of drugs such as phenobarbital[19] and phenytoin.[20]

The consequences of increased concentrations of free or unbound drug in the serum and tissues must be considered. Pharmacologic and toxic effects are related directly to the concentration of free drug in the body. Increases in free drug concentrations may result directly from decreases in plasma protein binding or indirectly from, for example, drug displacement from binding sites. The increased mortality from the development of kernicterus secondary to displacement of bilirubin by sulfisoxazole in neonates is well documented.[21] However, because drug bound to plasma proteins cannot be eliminated by the kidney, an increase in free drug concentration also may increase its clearance.[22]

The amount of body fat is substantially lower in neonates than in adults, which may affect drug therapy. Certain highly lipid-soluble drugs are distributed less widely in infants than in adults. The apparent volume of distribution of diazepam has ranged from 1.4 to 1.8 L/kg in neonates and from 2.2 to 2.6 L/kg in adults.[23] In recent years, the numbers of mothers breast-feeding their infants has climbed. Thus, certain drugs distributed in breast milk may pose problems for the infants. The American Academy of Pediatrics recommends that bromocriptine, cyclophosphamide, cyclosporine, doxorubicin, ergotamine, lithium, methotrexate, phenindione, and all drugs of abuse (e.g., amphetamine, cocaine, heroin, marijuana, and phencyclidine [PCP]) not be used during breast-feeding. Use of nuclear medicines should be stopped temporarily during breast-feeding.[24] Note that these recommendations are based on limited data; other drugs taken over a prolonged period by the mother also may be toxic to the infant. For example, acebutolol, aspirin, atenolol, clemastine, phenobarbital, primidone, sulfasalazine, and 5-aminosalicylic acid have been associated with adverse effects in some nursing infants.[24,25] Unless the benefits outweigh the risks, the mother should avoid using any drug during pregnancy and while breast-feeding.

METABOLISM

Drug metabolism is substantially slower in infants than in older children and adults. There are important differences in the maturation of various pathways of metabolism within a premature infant. For example, the sulfation pathway is well developed but the glucuronidation pathway is undeveloped in infants.[26] Although acetaminophen metabolism by glucuronidation is impaired in infants compared with adults, it is partly compensated for by the sulfation pathway. The cause of the tragic chloramphenicol-induced gray baby syndrome in newborn infants is decreased metabolism of chloramphenicol by glucuronyltransferases to the inactive glucuronide metabolite.[27] This metabolic pathway appears to be age related[28] and may take several months to 1 year to develop fully, as evidenced by the increase in clearance with age up to 1 year.[29]

Interestingly, higher serum concentrations of morphine are required to achieve efficacy in premature infants than in adults, in part because infants are not able to metabolize morphine adequately to its 6-glucuronide metabolite (20 times more active than morphine).[30] This is balanced to some degree by the fact that the clearance of morphine quadruples between 27 and 40 weeks of postconceptional age.

Metabolism of drugs such as theophylline, phenobarbital, and phenytoin by oxidation also is impaired in newborn infants. However, the rate of metabolism is more rapid with phenobarbital and phenytoin than with theophylline, perhaps because of the involvement of different cytochrome P450 isozymes. Total clearance of phenytoin by CYP2C9 and, to a lesser extent, by CYP2C19 surpasses adult values by 2 weeks of age, whereas theophylline clearance is not fully developed for several months.[18] Two additional observations about theophylline metabolism by CYP1A2 in pediatric patients should be noted. First, in premature infants receiving theophylline for treatment of apnea, a significant amount of its active metabolite caffeine may be present, unlike the case in older children and adults.[18] Second, theophylline clearance in children 1 to 9 years of age exceeds the values in infants as well as adults. Thus, a child with asthma often requires markedly higher doses on a weight basis of theophylline compared with an adult.[31] Because of decreased metabolism, doses of drugs such as theophylline, phenobarbital, phenytoin, and diazepam should be decreased in premature infants.

The clearance of unbound *S*-warfarin, a substrate of CYP2C9, was substantially greater in prepubertal children than among pubertal children and adults even after adjustment for total body weight.[32] Finally, clearance of caffeine, metabolized by demethylation, declines to adult values when girls reach Tanner stage II (early puberty) and boys reach Tanner stages IV and V (late puberty).[33] The knowledge of pharmacogenetics and pharmacogenomics now is being applied to patient care in some instances. 6-Mercaptopurine (6-MP), a drug commonly used in pediatric leukemias, undergoes catabolism that is facilitated by thiopurine methyltransferase (TPMT). The inherited deficiency (an autosomal recessive trait), which occurs in 6% to 11% of patients, is primarily explained by three polymorphisms in the *TPMT* gene (*2, *3A, and *3C). Children homozygous for one of the variant alleles require 6-MP dose reduction of approximately 90%, and heterozygotic children need a dose reduction of approximately 50% to achieve survival rates observed in patients receiving full doses in the absence of TPMT deficiency. Thus, *TPMT* screening is recommended to identify patients with genotypes associated with TPMT deficiency who may benefit from dose reductions to prevent toxicity.[34]

ELIMINATION

Drugs and their metabolites are often eliminated by the kidney. The glomerular filtration rate (GFR) may be as low as 0.6 to 0.8 mL/min per 1.73 m^2 in preterm infants and approximately 2 to 4 mL/min per 1.73 m^2 in term infants. The processes of glomerular filtration, tubular secretion, and tubular reabsorption determine the efficiency of renal excretion. These processes may not develop fully for several weeks to 1 year after birth.

Studies in infants have shown that tobramycin clearance during the first postnatal week may increase with an increase in gestational age.[17] In infants up to 1 month after birth, postnatal age also was correlated directly with aminoglycoside clearance.[29] Thus, premature infants require a lower daily dose of drugs eliminated by the kidney during the first week of life; the dosage requirement then increases with age.

Because of immature renal elimination, chloramphenicol succinate can accumulate in premature infants. Although chloramphenicol succinate is inactive, this accumulation may be the reason for an increased bioavailability of chloramphenicol in premature infants compared with older children.[28] These data indicate that dose-related toxicity may result from an underdeveloped glucuronidation pathway as well as increased bioavailability of chloramphenicol in premature infants.

DRUG EFFICACY AND TOXICITY

❹ Besides the pharmacokinetic differences previously identified between pediatric and older patients, factors related to drug efficacy and toxicity also should be considered in planning pediatric pharmacotherapy. Unique pathophysiologic changes occur in pediatric patients with some disease states.

Examples of pathophysiologic and pharmacodynamic differences are numerous. Clinical presentation of chronic asthma differs in children and adults.[35] Children present almost exclusively with a reversible extrinsic type of asthma, whereas adults have nonspecific, nonatopic bronchial irritability.[35] This explains the value of adjunctive hyposensitization therapy in the management of pediatric patients with extrinsic asthma.[36,37]

The maintenance dose of digoxin is substantially higher in infants than in adults. This is explained by a lower binding affinity of receptors in the myocardium for digoxin and increased digoxin-binding sites on neonatal erythrocytes compared with adult erythrocytes.[38] Insulin requirement is highest during adolescence because of the individual's rapid growth. Growth hormone therapy has allowed children with growth hormone deficiency to attain greater adult height. However, a study has shown that in "normal" short children (without growth hormone deficiency), early and rapid pubertal progression by growth hormone therapy may lead to a shorter final adult height than may have been attained naturally.[39] This finding emphasizes the need for identifying specific indications for the effective and safe use of drugs in pediatric patients.

Certain adverse effects of drugs are most common in the newborn period, whereas other toxic effects may continue to be important for many years of childhood. Promethazine now is contraindicated for use in children younger than 2 years because of the risk of severe respiratory depression. Chloramphenicol toxicity is increased in newborns because of immature metabolism and enhanced bioavailability. Similarly, propylene glycol, which is added to many injectable drugs, including phenytoin, phenobarbital, digoxin, diazepam, vitamin D, and hydralazine, to increase their stability, can cause hyperosmolality in infants.[40] Benzyl alcohol was a popular preservative used in intravascular flush solutions until a syndrome of metabolic acidosis, seizures, neurologic deterioration, gasping respirations, hepatic and renal abnormalities, cardiovascular collapse, and death was described in premature infants. A decline in both mortality and the incidence of major intraventricular hemorrhage was documented after use of solutions containing benzyl alcohol was stopped in low-birth-weight infants.[41]

Tetracyclines are contraindicated for use in pregnant women, nursing mothers, and children younger than 8 years because these drugs can cause dental staining and defects in enamelization of deciduous and permanent teeth, as well as a decrease in bone growth.[42] However, the Centers for Disease Control and Prevention has recommended the use of doxycycline for initial prophylaxis following suspected bioterrorism related exposure to *Bacillus anthracis* (anthrax); the potential benefits outweigh potential risks among infants and children.

CLINICAL CONTROVERSY

Are fluoroquinolones safe in pediatric patients younger than 1 year? Antibiotics of the fluoroquinolone class (e.g., ciprofloxacin) are generally not recommended for pediatric patients or pregnant women because of an association between these drugs and the development of permanent lesions of the cartilage of weight-bearing joints and other signs of arthropathy in immature animals of various species.[43] However, there are exceptions. The manufacturer states that ciprofloxacin can be used in pediatric patients **only** for inhalation anthrax (postexposure) or for treatment of complicated urinary tract infections and pyelonephritis caused by susceptible ***Escherichia coli***. The American Academy of Pediatrics and Infectious Disease Society of America suggest that their use may be justified for certain other conditions (e.g., endocarditis and multidrug-resistant gram-negative infections). Reversible arthralgia, sometimes accompanied by synovial effusion, was associated with ciprofloxacin therapy in 1.8% of pediatric patients with cystic fibrosis.[44] Although these drugs are used to treat certain infections in pediatric populations, additional safety data are needed before these drugs can be prescribed routinely, especially in infants.

CLINICAL CONTROVERSY

Are antidepressants safe and effective in children and adolescents? Because of observations of increased suicidality among adolescents (and adults, for that matter), experts are questioning whether these medications merely bring out an increased suicide risk that the patient has suppressed or has been too depressed to act on, or these medications actually increase the risk per se through some pharmacologic effect. Some selective serotonin reuptake inhibitors (SSRIs)—fluoxetine, sertraline, and fluvoxamine—are approved for use in pediatric patients in the United States. The British regulatory agency banned the use of another SSRI, paroxetine, in 2003 after analysis of the data indicated the occurrence of suicidal thoughts or episodes of self-harm at a rate 1.5 to 3.2 times higher than that with placebo. Subsequently, the FDA added a black-box warning about the use of and need for monitoring SSRI therapy in pediatric patients, and FDA action has continued in this arena.

Some drugs may be less toxic in pediatric patients than in adults. Aminoglycosides appear to be less toxic in infants than in adults. In adults, aminoglycoside toxicity is related to both peripheral compartment accumulation and the individual patient's inherent sensitivity to these tissue concentrations.[45] Although neonatal peripheral tissue compartments for gentamicin have been reported to closely resemble those of adults with similar renal function,[16] gentamicin rarely is nephrotoxic in infants. This dissimilarity in the incidence of nephrotoxicity implies that newborn infants have less inherent tissue sensitivity for toxicity than do adults.

The differences in efficacy, toxicity, and protein binding of drugs in pediatric versus adult patients raise an important question about the acceptable therapeutic range in children. Therapeutic ranges for drugs are first established in adults and often are applied directly to pediatric patients, but specific studies should be conducted in pediatric patients to define optimal therapeutic ranges of drugs.

FACTORS AFFECTING PEDIATRIC THERAPY

DISEASES

❺ Because most drugs are either metabolized by the liver or eliminated by the kidney, hepatic and renal diseases are expected to decrease the dosage requirements in patients. Nevertheless, not all diseases require lower doses of drugs. For instance, patients with cystic fibrosis require larger doses of certain drugs to achieve therapeutic concentrations.[46]

Hepatic Disease

Because the liver is the main organ for drug metabolism, drug clearance usually is decreased in patients with hepatic disease. However, most studies on the influence of hepatic disease on dosage requirements have been performed in adults, and these data may not be extrapolated uniformly to pediatric patients.

Drug metabolism by the liver depends on complex interactions among hepatic blood flow, ability of the liver to extract the drug from the blood, drug binding in the blood, and both type and severity of hepatic disease. Routine hepatic function tests, such as determinations of serum aspartate aminotransferase, serum alanine aminotransferase, alkaline phosphatase, and bilirubin levels, have not correlated consistently with drug pharmacokinetics. Furthermore, because of different pathologic changes in various types of hepatic diseases, patients with acute viral hepatitis may have different abilities to metabolize drugs than patients with alcoholic cirrhosis.[47]

On the basis of hepatic extraction characteristics, drugs can be divided into two categories. The first category consists of drugs with a high hepatic extraction ratio (>0.7; such drugs include morphine, meperidine, lidocaine, and propranolol). Clearance of these drugs is affected by hepatic blood flow. A decreased hepatic blood flow in the presence of disease states such as cirrhosis and congestive heart failure is expected to decrease the clearance of drugs with high extraction ratios. The second category consists of drugs with a low extraction ratio (<0.2) and a low affinity for plasma proteins. Metabolism of these drugs (e.g., theophylline, chloramphenicol, and acetaminophen) is influenced mainly by hepatocellular function and not as much by changes in hepatic blood flow or plasma protein binding. One report suggested that theophylline clearance may decrease by 45% in a child with acute viral hepatitis.[48] Because of a lack of specific data on dosage adjustment in hepatic disease, drug therapy should be monitored closely in pediatric patients to avoid potential toxicity from excessive doses, particularly for drugs with narrow therapeutic indices.

Renal Disease

Renal failure decreases the dosage requirement of drugs eliminated by the kidney. Once again, because of limited studies, dosage adjustments in pediatric patients are based largely on data obtained in adults. For many important drugs, such as aminoglycoside antibiotics, renal clearance or rate of elimination is directly proportional to the GFR, as measured by endogenous renal creatinine clearance.

In clinical practice, GFR can be estimated from prediction equations such as the Schwartz formula, which takes into account serum creatinine concentration and the patient's height, gender, and age. The advantage of estimating GFR using the Schwartz equation is rapid determination and the avoidance of a cumbersome 24-hour urine collection.[49,50] The following formula is used to estimate GFR:

$$\text{GFR} = K \times L / S_{Cr} \qquad (7\text{–}1)$$

where GFR is expressed in milliliters per minute per 1.73 m^2, K = age-specific constant of proportionality (see below), L = child's length in centimeters, and S_{Cr} = serum creatinine concentration in milligrams per deciliter.

Age	K
<1 year of age, low-birth-weight infant	0.33
<1 year of age, full-term infant	0.45
2- to 12-year-old child	0.55
13- to 21-year-old female	0.55
13- to 21-year-old male	0.70

Studies comparing the Schwartz-predicted GFR versus measured GFR noted that the Schwartz formula overestimated GFR in patients with decreasing GFR. The formula may not provide an accurate estimation of GFR in patients with rapidly changing serum creatinine concentrations, as seen in the critical care setting, in infants younger than 1 week, and in patients with obesity, malnutrition, or muscle wasting. Factors that interfere with serum creatinine measurement also may cause errors in estimation of GFR.

Serum drug concentrations should be monitored for drugs with narrow therapeutic indices and eliminated largely by the kidney (e.g., aminoglycosides and vancomycin) to optimize therapy in pediatric patients with renal dysfunction. For drugs with wide therapeutic ranges (e.g., penicillins and cephalosporins), dosage adjustment may be necessary only in patients with moderate-to-severe renal failure.

Cystic Fibrosis

Drug therapy in pediatric patients with cystic fibrosis has been reviewed.[51] For unknown reasons, these patients require increased doses of certain drugs. Studies have reported higher clearance of drugs such as gentamicin, tobramycin, netilmicin, amikacin, dicloxacillin, cloxacillin, azlocillin, piperacillin, and theophylline in patients with cystic fibrosis compared with patients without the disease. The apparent volume of distribution of certain drugs also may be altered in cystic fibrosis.[51] Severity of the illness may influence the change in dosage requirements, but this is not certain. Chapter 32 reviews these changes in detail.

Other Diseases

Although specific dosage guidelines are not available, pediatric patients with gastrointestinal disease (e.g., celiac disease, gastroenteritis, and severe malabsorption) may require dosage adjustments.[46] Hypoxemia also has been shown to decrease the elimination of amikacin in low-birth-weight infants.[52] Critically ill adult and pediatric patients with severe head trauma require higher than normal doses of phenytoin in part because of increased intrinsic clearance.[53]

ISSUES IN PEDIATRIC DRUG THERAPY

PAIN MANAGEMENT

❻ For many years, the term *pain* could not be found in the index of any major pediatric medicine or pediatric surgical textbooks.[54] The prevailing wisdom was that neonates did not experience pain because of their inadequately developed neuroendocrine systems and nerve pathways. During the last years of the 20th century, however, many research and clinical studies have been performed in the areas of pain management and assessment of neonates, infants, children, and adolescents. Today, results of these discoveries have been incorporated into clinical practice, making effective pain therapy a standard of care and pain assessment the fifth vital sign in modern pediatric practice.[55]

The basic mechanisms of pain perception in infants and children are similar to those of adults, except that pain impulse transmission in neonates occurs primarily along slow-conducting, nonmyelinated C fibers rather than along myelinated Aδ fibers. In addition, pain signal transmission in the spinal cord is less precise, and descending inhibitory neurotransmitters are lacking. As a result, neonates and young infants may perceive pain more intensely and be more sensitive to pain than are older children or adults.[56,57] It is now known that previous pain experience leads to long-term consequences such as alterations in response to a subsequent painful event.[58] Taddio et al.[59,60] reported that boys circumcised with the topical anesthetic eutectic mixture of local anesthetics (EMLA) had a lower pain response to subsequent immunizations than those who were circumcised without topical anesthesia. An inadequately treated initial painful procedure may decrease the effect of adequate analgesia in subsequent procedures as a result of altered pain response patterns.

Children consistently report that needles and shots are what they fear most. However, with the current immunization schedule that recommends 14 to 33 injections before adolescence, interventions to decrease injection pain need to be performed (Table 7–1).

Pharmacologic pain management for medical conditions and surgical and postoperative events has progressed considerably over the past decade with the use of continuous opioid infusions, epidural anesthesia, peripheral nerve blockade, local anesthetics, nonsteroidal antiinflammatory drugs, different routes for traditional agents (i.e., transmucosal and transdermal), and nonopioid adjuvant drugs (Table 7–2). New pain management techniques, education, research, and increasing awareness of pain management options have helped to improve the quality of life in children.

TABLE 7-1 Techniques for Minimizing Pain Caused by Injection

Pharmacologic methods	
EMLA[61] (eutectic mixture of lidocaine and prilocaine)	*Advantages:* Penetrates the skin to provide anesthesia to a depth of 5 mm; effective in decreasing the pain of IM and subcutaneous injections, venipuncture, IV cannulation, lumbar puncture, circumcision, skin-graft harvesting, and laser dermal therapy; safe and effective in newborns >37 weeks' gestation.
	Disadvantages: Requires 1 hour before onset of adequate anesthesia, has a vasoconstrictive effect that may make starting IV catheters difficult, may induce methemoglobinemia.
Numby Stuff (lidocaine iontophoresis)[62]	*Advantages:* Provides dermal anesthesia to a depth of 10 mm within 10–20 min; effective in decreasing the pain of IM injection, IV cannulation, venipuncture, lumbar puncture, skin biopsy, and bone marrow aspiration.
	Disadvantage: Tingling, itching, or burning sensation from the electric current used to transport drug to the tissues.
Vapocoolant sprays (ethyl chloride or dichlorodifluoromethane)[63]	*Advantages:* Vapocoolant is sprayed directly onto the skin or applied to a cotton ball that is held on the area to be anesthetized; provides local anesthesia within 15 seconds; effective in reducing injection pain in children 4–6 years of age.
	Disadvantages: Brief duration of action, so procedure should be completed in 1 or 2 min; may not be effective in reducing injection pain in infants aged 2–6 months.
Local anesthetic (lidocaine)[64]	*Advantage:* Reduces the pain of subsequent needle insertion.
	Disadvantage: Local anesthetic injection itself is associated with pain and burning sensation.
Pacifier with sucrose[65,66]	*For preterm neonates:* 0.1–0.4 mL of a 12%–24% sucrose solution (place on pacifier or the tongue 2 min before procedure). *For term neonates:* 1–2 mL of a 12%–24% sucrose solution (place on pacifier or the tongue 2 min before procedure).
	Advantage: Noninvasive method to reduce pain associated with needle insertion in infants.
	Disadvantage: Sucrose solution's effect in reducing pain gradually decreases over time.
Other techniques	
Site selection[67]	*For children older than 18 months:* Use of the deltoid muscle for IM injections is associated with less pain than injections administered in the thigh. *For children older than 3 years:* Use of the ventrogluteal area for injection is associated with less pain than the anterior thigh or dorsogluteal area.
Z-tract technique	Z-tract intramuscular injection technique is less painful (pull skin taut at the injection site, give injection, then release the skin); use a higher-gauge needle when the injectable solution is not viscous.
Behavioral	Use of distraction methods (e.g., blowing bubbles, providing music by headphones, relaxation, imagery, self-hypnosis, or having parents present for the procedure) can be helpful.

TABLE 7-2 Opioid Administration for Acute and Severe Pain

Intermittent IV or PO bolus administration (not as needed)	Weak opioids (e.g., codeine, hydrocodone, oxycodone) often are combined with acetaminophen or a nonsteroidal antiinflammatory agent (NSAID) for moderate pain. With dose escalation of combination oral products, be aware that the dose does not exceed recommended daily amounts for acetaminophen or ibuprofen. IV administration of codeine has been associated with allergic reactions related to histamine release. Parenteral administration of codeine is not recommended. Intermittent opioid administration is associated with wide fluctuation between peak and trough levels, so the patient may alternate between peak blood levels associated with untoward effects and trough levels associated with inadequate pain relief when being treated for severe pain.
	Oxycodone and morphine are available in a sustained-release formulation for use with chronic pain (not acute pain). Tablet must be swallowed whole and cannot be administered to patients through gastric tubes.
Intravenous continuous infusion[68,69]	Loading dose is administered to achieve rapidly a therapeutic blood level and pain relief (i.e., morphine loading dose of 0.05–0.15 mg/kg in children; 0.1 mg/kg infused over 90 min in neonates). Loading dose is followed by a maintenance continuous infusion. Doses that are considered safe in children can cause respiratory depression and seizures in neonates because of decreased clearance, immature blood–brain barrier at birth that is more permeable to morphine, and an increased unbound fraction of morphine that increases CNS effects of the drug.
Patient-controlled analgesia (PCA)[70]	Gives patient some control over his/her pain therapy. PCA allows the patient to self-administer small opioid doses. The PCA-Plus (Abbott, Chicago, IL) pump allows the patient to receive a continuous infusion together with a set number of self-administered doses per hour. PCA helps to eliminate wide peak and trough fluctuations so that levels remain in a therapeutic range. Children as young as 6 or 7 years of age can master the use of PCA.
Epidural and intrathecal analgesia[71]	Effective in the management of severe postoperative, chronic, or cancer pain. Spinal opioids can be administered by a single bolus injection into the epidural or subarachnoid space or by continuous infusion via an indwelling catheter. Dosage requirement by these routes is significantly less than with IV administration (epidural opioid doses: 10-fold lower than IV doses; intrathecal opioid doses: 100-fold lower than IV doses). Morphine, hydromorphone, fentanyl, and sufentanil are effective when administered intrathecally. Bupivacaine is the most commonly used local anesthetic in continuous epidural infusions. Fentanyl, morphine, or hydromorphone usually is combined with bupivacaine for epidural infusions.
Transmucosal administration	Fentanyl lozenge is absorbed transmucosally. It is useful for providing analgesia during painful procedures. Advantages include rapid onset of action (within 15 min), short duration of action (60–90 min), and painless administration because no injection is needed. A common side effect is vomiting and mild-to-moderate oxygen desaturation. Doses of 10–15 mcg/kg provide blood levels equivalent to 3–5 mcg/kg IV.

DRUG ADMINISTRATION

7 Drugs often are given by the intravenous route to seriously ill patients. Syringe pumps are widely used for administration of intravenous drugs. Important steps in successfully administering intravenous drugs include selecting the drug, calculating the dose, preparing the infusion, programming the infusion pump, and delivering the infusion. Use of "smart" pumps is preferred because they can recognize syringes and have drug libraries and dose limits as safety features. The pumps should be accurate; precise; easy to use; accept syringes and administration sets from various manufacturers; offer extensive delivery mode combinations including milliliters per hour, body weight, mass, volume over time, custom dilution and intermittent, loading dose, bolus dose, standby, volume limit; wide-ranging flow rates and rate to keep vein open; and adequate internal battery capacity.

No single infusion system is ideal for delivery of all drugs in all institutions for all patients. Each facility must be cognizant of problems of drug delivery and develop specific guidelines for intravenous infusions. At our institution, specific guidelines are provided for administration of each drug. These guidelines take into account various infusion rates and provide consistency of delivery with each dose. As long as the time for actual delivery is known, times to obtain blood samples for measurement of drug concentration can be adjusted accordingly to generate meaningful data.

ALTERATION OF DOSAGE FORMS

❽ Many drugs used in pediatric patients are not available in suitable dosage forms. This necessitates dilution of high concentrations of drugs intended for adult patients. Examples of these drugs include atropine, carbamazepine, diazepam, digoxin, epinephrine, hydralazine, insulin, morphine, phenobarbital, and phenytoin. Volumes ranging from 0.01 to 0.1 mL must be measured to dispense these drugs for use in infants. This obviously can be associated with large errors in measurements, and such errors have caused intoxication with digoxin[72] and morphine[73] in infants. One solution to this problem is to dilute these concentrated products, but such alterations can influence the stability or compatibility of these drugs. Because of limited data, pharmacists justifiably may be reluctant to alter dosage forms of certain drugs.

Selection of the appropriate vehicle to dilute the adult dosage forms for use in pediatric patients can be difficult. Phenobarbital sodium contains propylene glycol in the original product to improve drug stability. Because propylene glycol can cause hyperosmolality in infants,[40] further addition of this vehicle may not be wise. Because of limited access to intravenous sites in pediatric patients, drugs must be administered through the same site; however, data on drug compatibilities often are missing. Newborn infants often require aminoglycosides for presumed or proven sepsis and calcium gluconate for correction of hypocalcemia. Tobramycin and calcium gluconate have been found to be compatible, at least during a 1-hour administration at the same site.[73]

Administration of oral drugs continues to challenge parents and nurses. Alteration of these drugs by crushing or mixing, refusal of patients to accept the medication, and loss of drug during administration are some factors that can affect pediatric therapy. A common practice is to mix medications in applesauce, syrup, ice cream, or other vehicles just before administration to make the drugs palatable.

A number of extemporaneous formulations for oral, intravenous, and rectal administration are included in a compilation of products for use in pediatric patients.[74] However, a specific reference on the stability of many drug formulations is lacking and emphasizes the need for continued research in this area.

Drug administration into the middle ear, nose, or eye of a child requires special attention. Certain drugs (e.g., sodium valproate and morphine) can be administered rectally to infants who have limited access for intravenous drug administration or if oral drug administration cannot be accomplished.

Transdermal drug delivery can be used in pediatric patients (a) to avoid problems of drug absorption from the oral route and complications from the intravenous route and (b) to maximize duration of effect and minimize adverse effects of drugs. As discussed earlier in this chapter, methylphenidate (Daytrana) now is available as a transdermal patch for children with ADHD. Unfortunately, the commercially available transdermal dosage forms (e.g., clonidine and scopolamine) are not intended for pediatric patients; these would deliver doses much higher than needed for infants and children.

MEDICATION ADHERENCE

The issue of medication adherence is more complex in pediatric patients than in adults. Caregivers of young patients must appreciate the importance of understanding and following the prescribing information.

In one study, medication adherence was considered to be a problem in nearly 60% of adolescents (age 12 to 15 years) with asthma. Approximately 40% of patients had severe denial regarding their asthma and its severity. Nearly 80% of patients had preventable asthma exacerbations.[75]

Among the factors that can negatively affect adherence are poor communication between the physician and patient or parent; insufficient prescribing information; lack of understanding about the severity of illness by the patient or parent; lack of interest (e.g., among adolescents); fear of side effects; failure of the patient or parent to remember to administer the drugs; inconvenient dosage forms or dosing schedules involving administration of three or more doses daily; and unpalatability of drug products.[76] Studies in pediatric volunteers have compared the palatability of antibiotics,[77] and the data may have important implications for adherence in children.

DOSE REQUIREMENTS

Medication doses often are based on the body weight of neonates, infants, and children, for example, milligrams per kilogram of body weight per day to be given in one or more portions daily. However, certain drugs, including antineoplastic agents, may be given based on body surface area, for example, milligrams per square meter in one or more doses daily. In either case, the total amount of weight- or surface area-based individual or daily dose in a pediatric patient, especially an adolescent, should not exceed the amount of drug indicated in an adult patient.

An additional challenge in managing pediatric drug therapy is understanding the effects of obesity on a population that relies on weight-based dosing. According to the Centers for Disease Control and Prevention, the prevalence of overweight and obese children in the United States nearly doubled from 15% during 1976 to 1980 to more than 30% during 1999 to 2002.[78] Using ideal body weight versus total body weight to calculate a weight-based dose or to determine body surface area can result in a large variance in obese patients. Additional pharmacokinetic studies are needed to study the effects of obesity on drug distribution, protein binding, and clearance and to identify whether dosing should be adjusted according to total body weight or ideal body weight to achieve consistent drug exposure for individual drugs.[79,80] Generally, the highest drug dose recommended for a child is the maximum dose approved for adults. However, determining the highest dose of certain drugs for use in children without a known maximum dose for adults (e.g., intravenous immunoglobulin, infliximab, rituximab, and liposomal amphotericin B [AmBisome]) can be difficult.

DRUG INTERACTIONS

Drug interaction studies in pediatric age groups generally are lacking. The data often are extrapolated from studies in adult populations. Special attention should be given to adolescents, who may concurrently use alcohol, recreational/illicit drugs, or other prescription or nonprescription medications without the knowledge of the primary healthcare provider, who must attempt to determine their use to avoid drug interactions.

COMPLEMENTARY AND ALTERNATIVE THERAPY

In a study of patients between 3 weeks and 18 years (mean 5.3 years) of age, 45% of caregivers were giving a product to the children; 27% had given three or more products in the past year. The most commonly used products were aloe plant/juice (44% of those reporting use of herbal therapies), echinacea (33%), and sweet oil (25%). The most dangerous combination was ephedra (which was withdrawn from the U.S. market in 2004) with albuterol given to adolescents with asthma. Most caregivers did not recognize potential adverse effects or drug interactions associated with herbs. Friends or relatives were the main source of information for 80% of caregivers.[81]

Little is known about the efficacy of herbal products in infants, children, and adolescents. Healthcare professionals must ask caregivers specifically about the use of complementary and alternative treatments to minimize the adverse effects and costs associated with ineffective therapies.

MEDICATION SAFETY

9 The Institute of Medicine reported that between 44,000 and 98,000 Americans each year die as a result of medical errors in hospitals.[82] According to this report, the vast majority of medical errors that cause harm to patients are preventable. Healthcare professionals have a responsibility for creating a safe medication environment and reducing risk to a vulnerable pediatric population.

Pediatric medication errors commonly occur at the medication-ordering step because of the multiple calculations required for weight-based dosing and the adjustments needed for providing therapy to the developing pediatric patient.[83–85] The United States Pharmacopeia (USP) Center for the Advancement of Patient Safety states that risk to patients when performing repeated calculations involving multiple steps can be minimized using computer-based algorithms.[86] Since the medication-preparation step is also a high-hazard point owing to the need for dilution or manipulation of commercially available products only available in adult doses, the USP recommends that compounded pediatric medications be prepared and labeled in the pharmacy and verified by a pharmacist. Among drug administration–related errors, wrong dose, wrong technique, and wrong drug are the three most common errors and may be related to an inability to access pediatric drug information. In 2001, the Agency for Healthcare Research and Quality (AHRQ) published an evidence-based assessment of patient safety practices that prevent or reduce medication errors.[87] Risk-reduction strategies include placing a clinical pharmacist on pediatric wards in hospitals, simplifying the medication-use system, ordering standardized concentrations and doses, implementing computerized physician order-entry systems with dose range checking, dispensing pharmacy-prepared/ready-to-administer doses, standardizing infusion equipment, using smart infusion pumps, using bar-coded medications and bar-coding systems that check the medication at the point of care, and implementing computerized adverse event detection systems.[85,87–89] Identifying and understanding the high-hazard areas or points of failure in the medication-use process will help in designing strategies that prevent problems before they arise.

CONCLUSIONS

Although tremendous progress has been made in the area of pediatric pharmacotherapy, many questions remain unanswered. The pharmacokinetics of many important drugs have been elucidated, but their pharmacodynamics have not been explored fully. Similarly, the effect of disease states and patient characteristics, such as genetic status, have not been studied for most drugs. The effect of these factors on the development of cytochrome P450 isozymes (e.g., CYP3A4, CYP2D6, CYP1A2, CYP2C9, and CYP2C19), other enzymes, and P-glycoprotein needs to be studied (see Chaps. 5 and 6). Similarly, comparative efficacy and safety data for many therapies are unavailable. Studies on the influence of drug therapy on clinical and economic outcomes and on quality of life in pediatric patients are needed.

The development of new drugs has contributed to improved patient care. The new FDA regulations (Best Pharmaceuticals for Children Act of 2002) can require the industry to conduct studies and seek labeling of important drugs for use in pediatric patients. As an incentive, a 6-month patent extension and waiver of supplemental new drug application fee are offered to the industry. This should encourage the industry to develop and market more drugs for the pediatric population. However, greater emphasis also should be placed on disease prevention. Millions of children die because of preventable diseases, particularly in developing countries of the world. Administration of vaccines and control of diarrhea alone could save millions of these lives annually. However, the developed countries face different problems. The infant mortality rate in the United States is nearly twice as high among blacks as whites. Improved prenatal care, educational programs, and avoidance of alcohol, smoking, and drugs of abuse during pregnancy may decrease mortality as well as morbidity from illnesses, including acquired immunodeficiency syndrome.

Finally, efforts should be made to offer evidence-based pharmacotherapy. This often is difficult in pediatric populations when the drugs must be used outside the guidelines and indications approved by the FDA. Institutions should develop guidelines for the use of drugs in specific diseases and for the use of high-cost drugs such as colony-stimulating factors, monoclonal antibodies, dornase-alfa, epoetin-alfa, immunoglobulins, surfactants, and growth hormones.

Although much needs to be learned about the optimization of therapy, it is encouraging to witness the continued growth of knowledge in this area that has improved the quality of life and survival from pharmacotherapy in pediatric patients.

ABBREVIATIONS

FDA: Food and Drug Administration

GFR: glomerular filtration rate

SSRI: selective serotonin reuptake inhibitor

USP: United States Pharmacopeia

REFERENCES

1. Miniño AM, Heron M, Murphy SL, Kochanet KD. Deaths: Final Data for 2004. National Center for Health Statistics. 2006, *http://www.cdc.gov/nchs/products/pubs/pubd/hestats/finaldeaths04/finaldeaths04.htm*.
2. Avery GB, Randolph JG, Weaver T. Gastric acidity in the first day of life. Pediatrics 1966;37:1005–1007.
3. Agunod M, Yamaguchi N, Lopex R, et al. Correlative study of hydrochloric acid, pepsin, and intrinsic factor secretion in newborns and infants. Am J Dig Dis 1969;14:400–414.
4. Huang NN, High RN. Comparison of serum levels following the administration of oral and parenteral preparations of penicillin to infants and children of various age groups. J Pediatr 1953;42:657–668.
5. Silverio J, Poole JW. Serum concentrations of ampicillin in newborn infants after oral administration. Pediatrics 1973;51:578–580.
6. O'Connor WJ, Warren GH, Edrada LS, et al. Serum concentrations of sodium nafcillin in infants during the perinatal period. Antimicrob Agents Chemother 1965;5:220–222.
7. Jalling B. Plasma concentrations of phenobarbital in the treatment of seizures in newborns. Acta Paediatr Scand 1975;64:514–524.
8. Kearns GL, Abdel-Rahman SM, Alander SW, et al. Drug therapy: Developmental pharmacology—Drug disposition, action, and therapy in infants and children. N Engl J Med 2003;349:1157–1167.
9. Signer E, Fridrich R. Gastric emptying in newborns and young infants. Acta Paediatr Scand 1975;64:525–530.

10. Boreus IO. Plasma concentrations of phenobarbital in mother and child after combined prenatal and postnatal administration for prophylaxis of hyperbilirubinemia. J Pediatr 1978;93:695.
11. Morselli PL. Serum levels and pharmacokinetics of anticonvulsants in the management of seizure disorders. In: Merkin B, ed. Clinical Pharmacology. Chicago: Mosby Year Book, 1978:89.
12. Tyrala FF, Hillman LS, Hillman RE, et al. Clinical pharmacology of hexa-chlorophene in newborn infants. J Pediatr 1977;91:481–486.
13. McFadden S, Haddow JE. Coma produced by topical application of isopropanol. Pediatrics 1969;43:622–623.
14. Evans NJ, Rutter N, Hadgraft J, et al. Percutaneous administration of theophylline in preterm infant. J Pediatr 1985;107:307–311.
15. Friis-Hansen B. Body water compartments in children: Changes during growth and related changes in body composition. Pediatrics 1961;28:169–181.
16. Haughey DB, Hilligoss DM, Grassi A, et al. Two-compartment gentamicin pharmacokinetics in premature neonates: A comparison to adults with decreased glomerular filtration rates. J Pediatr 1980;96:325–330.
17. Nahata MC, Powell DA, Durrell DE, et al. Effect of gestational age and birth weight on tobramycin kinetics in newborn infants. J Antimicrob Chemother 1984;14:59–65.
18. Roberts RJ. Pharmacologic principles in therapeutics in infants. In: Drug Therapy in Infants: Pharmacologic Principles and Clinical Experience. Philadelphia: WB Saunders, 1984:3–12.
19. Pitlick W, Painter M, Pippenger C. Phenobarbital pharmacokinetics in neonates. Clin Pharmacol Ther 1978;23:346–350.
20. Painter MJ, Pippenger C, MacDonald H, et al. Phenobarbital and diphenylhydantoin levels in neonates with seizures. J Pediatr 1978;92:315–319.
21. Silverman WA, Anderson DH, Blanc WA, et al. A difference in mortality rate and incidence of kernicterus among premature infants allotted to two prophylactic antibacterial regimens. Pediatrics 1956;18:614–624.
22. Odell GB. The dissociation of bilirubin from albumin and its clinical implications. J Pediatr 1959;55:268–279.
23. Morselli PL. Clinical pharmacokinetics in neonates. Clin Pharmacokinet 1976;1:81–98.
24. Committee on Drugs, American Academy of Pediatrics. The transfer of drugs and other chemicals into human milk. Pediatrics 1994;93:137–150.
25. Anderson PO. Drugs and breast milk. J Pediatr 1995;95:957.
26. Rane A. Basic principles of drug disposition and action in infants and children. In: Yaffe JF, ed. Pediatric Pharmacology: Therapeutic Principles in Practice. New York: Grune & Stratton, 1980:7–28.
27. Weiss CF, Glazko AJ, Weston JK. Chloramphenicol in the newborn infant: A physiologic explanation of its toxicity when given in excessive doses. N Engl J Med 1960;262:787–794.
28. Nahata MC, Powell DA. Comparative bioavailability and pharmacokinetics of chloramphenicol after intravenous chloramphenicol succinate in premature infants and older patients. Dev Pharmacol Ther 1983;6:23–32.
29. Kuhn R, Nahata MC, Powell DA, et al. Netilmicin pharmacokinetics in newborn infants. Eur J Clin Pharmacol 1986;29:635–637.
30. Cha PCW, Duffy BJ, Walker JS. Pharmacokinetic-pharmacodynamic relationships of morphine in neonates. Clin Pharmacol Ther 1992;51:334–342.
31. Edwards DJ, Zarowitz BJ, Slaughter RL. Theophylline. In: Evans WE, Schentag JJ, Jusko WJ, eds. Applied Pharmacokinetics, 3rd ed. Vancouver, WA: Applied Therapeutics, 1992:1–47.
32. Takahashi H, Ishikawa S, Nomoto S, et al. Developmental changes in pharmacokinetics and pharmacodynamics of warfarin enantiomers in Japanese children. Clin Pharmacol Ther 2000;68:541–555.
33. Lambert GH, Schoeller DA, Kotake AN, et al. The effect of age, gender, and sexual maturation on the caffeine breath test. Dev Pharmacol Ther 1986;9:375–388.
34. McLeod HL, Krynetski ER, Relling MV, Evans WE. Genetic polymorphism of thiopurine methyltransferase and its clinical relevance for childhood acute lymphoblastic leukemia. Leukemia 2000;14:567–572.
35. Leffert FL. The management of chronic asthma. J Pediatr 1980;97:875–885.
36. Johnston DE. Immunotherapy in children: Past, present, and future, part I. Ann Allergy 1981;46:1–7.
37. Johnston DE. Immunotherapy in children: Past, present, and future, part II. Ann Allergy 1981;46:59–66.
38. Kearin M, Kelly JG, O'Malley K. Digoxin "receptors" in neonates: An explanation of less sensitivity to digoxin than in adults. Clin Pharmacol Ther 1980;28:346–349.
39. Kawai M, Momoi T, Yorifuji, T, et al. Unfavorable effects of growth hormone therapy on the final height of boys with short stature not caused by growth hormone deficiency. J Pediatr 1997;130:205–209.
40. Glasgow AM, Boeckx RL, Miller MK, et al. Hyperosmolality in small infants due to propylene glycol. Pediatrics 1983;72:353–355.
41. Hiller JL, Benda GI, Rahatzad M, et al. Benzyl alcohol toxicity: Impact of mortality and intraventricular hemorrhage among very low birth weight infants. Pediatrics 1986;77:500–506.
42. Grossman ER, Walchek A, Freedman H. Tetracyclines and permanent teeth: The relation between dose and tooth color. Pediatrics 1971;47:567–570.
43. Walker RC, Wright AJ. The quinolones. Mayo Clin Proc 1987;62:1007–1012.
44. Chysky V, Kapla M, Hullman R, et al. Safety of ciprofloxacin in children: Worldwide clinical experience based on compassionate usage. Infection 1991;19:289–296.
45. Schentag JJ, Plaut ME, Cerra FB, et al. Aminoglycoside nephrotoxicity in critically ill surgical patients. J Surg Res 1979;26:270–279.
46. Kauffman RE, Habersange R. Modification of dosage regimens in disease states of childhood. In: Mirking BL, ed. Clinical Pharmacology and Therapeutics: A Pediatric Perspective. Chicago: Mosby Year Book, 1978:73–88.
47. Roberts RJ. Special considerations in drug therapy in infants. In: Drug Therapy in Infants: Pharmacologic Principles and Clinical Experience. Philadelphia: WB Saunders, 1984:25–35.
48. Feinstein RA, Miles MV. The effect of acute viral hepatitis on theophylline clearance. Clin Pediatr 1985;24:357–358.
49. Hogg RJ, Furth S, Lemley KV, et al. National Kidney Foundation's kidney disease outcomes quality initiative clinical practice guidelines for chronic kidney disease in children and adolescents: Evaluation, classification, and stratification. Pediatrics 2003;111:1416–1421.
50. Schwartz Gj, Brion LP, Spitzer A. The use of plasma creatinine concentration for estimating glomerular filtration rate in infants, children and adolescents. Pediatr Clin North Am 1987;34:571–590.
51. Wallace CS, Hall M, Kuhn RJ. Pharmacologic management of cystic fibrosis. Clin Pharm 1993;12:657–674.
52. Myers MG, Roberts JF, Mirhig NJ. Effect of gestational age, birth weight, and hypoxemia on the pharmacokinetics of amikacin in serum of infants. Antimicrob Agents Chemother 1977;11:1027.
53. Bahal-O'Mara N, Jones R, Nahata MC, et al. Pharmacokinetics of phenytoin in children with acute neurotrauma. Crit Care Med 1995;23:1418–1424.
54. Rana SR. Pain: A subject ignored [letter]. Pediatrics 1987;79:309.
55. Franch LS, Greenberg CS, Stevens B. Pain assessment in infants and children. Pediatr Clin North Am 2000;47:487–512.
56. Anand KJS. Consensus statement for the prevention and management of pain in the newborn. Arch Pediatr Adolesc Med 2001;155:173–180.
57. American Academy of Pediatrics at Canadian Paediatric Society. Prevention and management of pain and stress in the neonate. Pediatrics 2000;105:454–461.
58. Fitzgerald M, Anand KJS. Development neuroanatomy and neurophysiology of pain. In: Schechter NL, Berde CB, Yaster M, eds. Pain in Infants, Children and Adolescents. Baltimore: Williams & Wilkins, 1993:11–31.
59. Taddio A, Katz J, Ilersich Al, et al. Effect of neonatal circumcision on pain response during subsequent routine vaccination. Lancet 1997;349:559–603.
60. Taddio A, Ohlsson A, Einarson T, et al. A systematic review of lidocaine-prilocaine cream for neonatal circumcision pain. N Engl J Med 1997;336:1197–1201.
61. Uhari M. Eutectic mixture of lidocaine and prilocaine for alleviating vaccination pain in infants. Pediatrics 1993;92:719–721.
62. Zempsky, WT, Anand KS, Sullivan KM, et al. Lidocaine iontophoresis for topical anesthesia before intravenous line placement in children. J Pediatr 1998;132:1061–1063.
63. Reis EC, Holobukov R. Vapocoolant spray is equally effective as EMLA cream in reducing immunization pain in school aged children. Pediatrics 1997;100:5.
64. Bartfield JM, Connis P, Barbera J, et al. Buffered versus plain lidocaine as a local anesthetic for simple laceration repair. Ann Emerg Med 1990;19:1387–1390.

65. Annand KHS; International Evidenced Based Group for Neonatal Pain. Consensus statement for the prevention and management of pain in the newborn. Arch Pediatr Adolesc Med 2001;155:173–180.
66. Schechter NL, Berde CB, Yaster M, et al. Pain in Infants, Children, and Adolescents. Baltimore: Lippincott Williams & Wilkins, 2003.
67. Keen MF. Comparison of intramuscular injection techniques to reduce site discomfort and lesions. Nurs Res 1986;35:207–210.
68. Golianu B, Krane EJ, Galloway KS, et al. Pediatric acute pain management. Pediatr Clin North Am 2000;47:559–587.
69. Chay PCW, Duffy BJ, Walker JS. Pharmacokinetic–pharmacodynamic relationship of morphine in neonates. Clin Pharmacol Ther 1992;51:334–342.
70. Berde CB, Lehn BM, Yee JD, et al. Patient-controlled analgesia in children and adolescents: A randomized, prospective comparison with intramuscular administration of morphine for postoperative analgesia. J Pediatr 1991;118:460–466.
71. Nichols DG, Yaster M, Lynn AM, et al. Disposition and respiratory effects of intrathecal morphine in children. Anesthesiology 1993;79:733–738.
72. Berman W. Whitman V, Marks KH, et al. Inadvertent overadministration of digoxin to low birth weight infants. J Pediatr 1978;92:1024.
73. Zenk KE, Anderson S. Improving the accuracy of minivolume injections. Infusion 1982;Jan–Feb:7–11.
74. Nahata MC, Pai V, Hipple TF. Pediatric Drug Formulations, 5th ed. Cincinnati, OH: Harvey Whitney Books, 2003:1–307.
75. Martin AJ, Campbell DA, Gluyas PA, et al. Characteristics of near-fatal asthma in childhood. Pediatr Pulmonol 1995;20:1–8.
76. Boreus LO. Drug compliance. In: Yaffe SJ, ed. Principles of Pediatric Pharmacology. New York: Churchill-Livingstone, 1982:176–192.
77. Matsui D, Barron A, Rieder MJ. Assessment of the palatability of antistaphylococcal antibiotics in pediatric volunteers. Ann Pharmacother 1996;30:586–588.
78. Hedley AA, Ogden CL, Johnson CL, et al. Prevalence of overweight and obesity among US children, adolescents and adults, 1999–2002. JAMA 2004;291:2847–2850.
79. Cheymol G. Effects of obesity on pharmacokinetics: Implications for drug therapy. Clin Pharmacokinetics 2000;39:215–231.
80. Vance-Bryan K, Guay DR, Gilliland SS, et al. Effect of obesity on vancomycin pharmacokinetic parameters as determined by using a Bayesian forecasting technique. Antimicrob Agents Chemother 1993;37:436–440.
81. Lanski SL, Greenwald M, Perkins A, et al. Herbal therapy use in a pediatric emergency department population: Expect the unexpected. Pediatrics 2003;111:981–985.
82. Institute of Medicine, Committee on Quality of Health Care in American. To Err is Human: Building a Safer Health System. Washington, DC: National Academy Press, 2000.
83. Raju TN, Kecskes S, Thornton JP, et al. Medication errors in neonatal and paediatric intensive-care units. Lancet 1989;2:374–376.
84. Folli HL, Poole RL, Benitz WE, et al. Medication error prevention by clinical pharmacists in two children's hospitals. Pediatrics 1987;79:718–722.
85. Kaushal R, Bates DW, Landrigan C, et al. Medication errors and adverse drug events in pediatric inpatients. JAMA 2001;285:2114–2120.
86. USP Center for the Advancement of Patient Safety. USP issues recommendations for preventing medication errors in children. January 21, 2003.
87. American Academy of Pediatrics Committee on Drugs and Committee on Hospital Care. Prevention of medication errors in pediatric inpatient setting. Pediatrics 2003;112:431–436.
88. Agency for Healthcare Research and Quality. Making Health Care Safer: A Critical Analysis of Patient Safety Practices. AHRQ Publication No. 01-E058. Washington, DC: Agency for Healthcare Research and Quality, 2001.
89. Larsen GY, Parker HB, Cash J, et al. Standard drug concentrations and smart-pump technology reduce continuous-medication-infusion errors in pediatric patients. Pediatrics 2005;116:21–25.

CHAPTER 8

Geriatrics

CATHERINE I. STARNER, SHELLY L. GRAY, DAVID R.P. GUAY, EMILY R. HAJJAR, STEVEN M. HANDLER, AND JOSEPH T. HANLON

KEY CONCEPTS

1. The population of persons aged 65 years and older is increasing.
2. Age-related changes in physiology can affect the pharmacokinetics and pharmacodynamics of numerous drugs.
3. Improving and maintaining functional status is a cornerstone of care for older adults.
4. Drug-related problems in older adults are common and cause considerable morbidity.
5. Pharmacists can play a major role in optimizing drug therapy and preventing drug-related problems in older adults.

Pharmacotherapy for older adults can cure or palliate disease as well as enhance health-related quality of life (HRQOL). HRQOL considerations for older adults include focusing on improvements in physical functioning (e.g., activities of daily living), psychological functioning (e.g., cognition, depression), social functioning (e.g., social activities, support systems), and overall health (e.g., general health perception).[1] Despite the benefits of pharmacotherapy, HRQOL can be compromised by drug-related problems. The prevention of drug-related adverse consequences in older adults requires that health professionals become knowledgeable about a number of age-specific issues. To address these knowledge needs, this chapter discusses the epidemiology of aging; physiologic changes associated with aging, with emphasis on those changes that can affect the pharmacokinetics and pharmacodynamics of drugs; clinical conditions commonly seen in older adult patients; epidemiology of drug-related problems in older adults; and an approach to reducing drug-related problems through the provision of comprehensive geriatric assessment.

EPIDEMIOLOGY OF AGING

❶ The older American population is highly diverse and heterogeneous with respect to health status. The demographics and health characteristics of persons aged 65 to 74 years are different from those of persons 85 years of age and older, as are those of persons who are institutionalized compared with those living in the community. It is teasing apart the various threads of wellness and illness, independence and dependence, and function and dysfunction that make the available demographic and health status data relevant for clinical practice. Understanding this diversity and growth of the older population will allow society to plan for the training, research, and resources needed for future clinical practice and adequate healthcare.

In 2000, persons aged 65 and older accounted for 12.4% (35 million) of the total U.S. population.[2] Among those older than 65 years, women outnumbered men and accounted for 58.8% of this segment of the population. The gender gap widens with increasing age, with women accounting for 71.1% of the cohort aged 85 years and older and 80% of centenarians.[2]

In 2011, the first baby boomers will turn 65 years old; this will mark a rapid increase in the older population in the years between 2010 and 2030. By 2030, the older population is projected to double in size relative to the year 2000, with one in five (20%) Americans older than 65 years. This 20% projection for persons aged 65 years and older will remain relatively stable through 2050. However, the proportion of the oldest old (>85 years) will continue to grow. In 2000, the oldest old represented 12.1% of the older population but are projected to double by 2050. The increase in the number of older persons is due not just to the higher post–World War II birth rate but also to the declining mortality rate and the overall better health among older adults.[2] The decline in early death and the better health of older adults arise for a variety of reasons: (a) public health measures affecting all age groups (e.g., immunizations, prenatal care), (b) advances in medical technology, (c) promotion of a healthy lifestyle, and (d) improvements in living conditions.[3] More relevant to providers of care to older Americans is life expectancy at age 65 years. In 2000, white women 65 years of age can expect an average additional 19.2 years of life; black women, 17.4 years; white men, 16.3 years; and black men, 14.5 years.[2] For a person who survived to age 85 years in 2000, another 5.6 years of life can be expected for men and 6.7 years for women. Given this increase in life expectancy, the increase in the number of centenarians from 37,000 in 1990 to 50,000 in 2000 is not surprising.[2]

Along with changes in the life expectancy of future older adults, the older population will become more diverse in racial/ethnic composition. In 2000, an estimated 84% of persons aged 65 years and older were non-Hispanic white, 8% were black, 5% were Hispanic, and 2.3% were Asian. By 2050, the percent of non-Hispanic white older adults is projected to decline to 61%, whereas Hispanics will account for 18% and Asians 8% of the older population.[2]

Most older persons are self-sufficient and live in the community. However, as they age in the community, the likelihood of living alone increases, more so for women than for men. Only 4.5% of older persons reside in a long-term care facility, a decrease since 1990 (5.1%). This decline may be due to the improved health of older adults or the use of alternative long-term care services (e.g., assisted-living facilities, in-home healthcare). Nursing homes resi-

Learning objectives, review questions, and other resources can be found at **www.pharmacotherapyonline.com.**

dents are predominately 85 years and older (45%), followed by persons 75 to 84 years (33.5%), 65 to 74 years (12.2%), and younger than 65 years (9.5%).[2] Oldest old women (>85 years) compose 42% of nursing home residents.

Physical activity has many positive health benefits in adults, including disease reduction (e.g., cardiovascular disease), weight maintenance, and reduction in physical disability. Only 22% of older adults engage in regular leisure-time physical activity, and this percentage decreases with increasing age.[4] It is no surprise that obesity is a growing problem in both men (33%) and women (36%) aged 65 to 74 years. The prevalence of obesity decreases to approximately one in four for those older than 75 years.[4]

An important goal in the care of older adults is allowing them to maintain independence and avoid the need for institutionalization for as long as possible. Functional loss or disability often is a final common pathway of many clinical problems in older persons, especially among those older than 75 years. In 2000, 28.6% of older adults reported a physical disability (e.g., difficulty walking, climbing stairs, reaching, lifting, carrying), and 9.5% reported disability with self-care or *basic* activities of daily living (ADLs; e.g., dressing, bathing, transferring, feeding, toileting).[5] Disability increases with increasing age and is higher in institutionalized older persons, among whom approximately 80% have some problems with mobility and 65% have difficulty with bowel control.[6] Segments of the population that are especially vulnerable to disability include women, minorities, and those in lower socioeconomic classes. Disability rates have declined significantly during the last 2 decades.[2] The decline in late-life disability was greatest for limitations in *instrumental* ADLs (e.g., housekeeping chores, shopping, going outside, medication management) and physical disability. Conflicting evidence exists for basic ADL disability, the most severe type of disability that often leads to institutionalization. Multiple factors likely are responsible for the decline in disability prevalence, including improved medical treatment, change in health behaviors (e.g., reduced smoking), and widespread use of assistive devices.[2]

Chronic diseases or impairments, such as heart disease, stroke, and diabetes, are major causes of disability in older adults. An estimated 80% of older adults have at least one chronic health condition, and more than half have at least two concomitant conditions. Many chronic conditions can be prevented or improved with behavioral modification, such as diet and physical activity. The prevalence of select common conditions in 2003 to 2004 included hypertension (52%), arthritis (50%), heart disease (32%), any cancer (21%), diabetes (17%), stroke (9%), and asthma (9%). Sensory impairments are common in older adults and pose challenges for maintaining functional independence and interactions with healthcare providers. In 2004, 40% of older adults reported some trouble hearing, and 17% reported difficulties with vision. Furthermore, 13% of older adults have moderate or severe memory impairment, which is a major risk factor for nursing home admission. The prevalence of memory impairment increases dramatically (to 32%) for the oldest old.[4]

Chronic diseases are the primary cause of death in older adults. The leading causes of death among older adults have changed little over the last 20 years. Fig. 8–1 illustrates the leading casues of death from 2004.[4] Some important trends have emerged over the past 2 decades. First, the death rates for heart disease and stroke have decreased. This trend is secondary to the gains made in the prevention and treatment of these diseases. Second, death secondary to Alzheimer's disease has increased rapidly in recent years. The increased rate is due in part to improvements in the diagnosis and awareness of Alzheimer's disease in the medical community.[4]

Older adults are devoted consumers of medical and prescription drug resources. With older persons accounting for 36% of all hospital stays and 49% of all days of care in hospitals, elders consume almost one third of total U.S. healthcare expenditures.[7] By 2030, healthcare spending by the U.S. population is projected to increase by 25% simply because of aging demographics.[7] Although older persons compose 12.4% of the U.S. population, they account for 34% of all prescription drug expenditures.[8] Overall in 2002, prescription drug spending was estimated to be between $91 and $117 billion.[9] National estimates in 2002 indicated that individuals older than 65 years filled nearly 32 prescriptions per year and that their average annual expenditure for prescription drugs was $1,740.[4] In 2003, approximately one fourth (27%) of older adults had no prescription drug coverage, with the poor disproportionately affected (34%).[10] The Medicare Prescription Drug, Improvement and Modernization Act (MMA) began offering coverage to the 43 million Medicare beneficiaries as of January 1, 2006, and this has improved prescription drug coverage for older adults. However, as

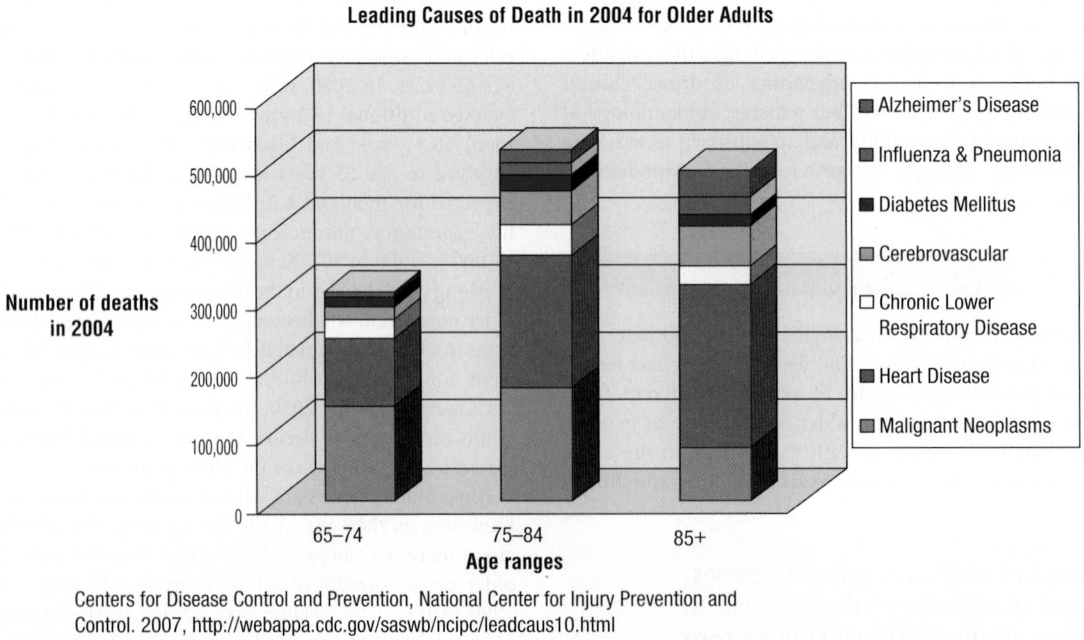

FIGURE 8-1. Leading causes of death in 2004, by age group. *(Data from Centers for Disease Control and Prevention, National Center for Injury Prevention and Control. 2007, http://webappa.cdc.gov/sasweb/ncipc/leadcaus10.htm.)*

of June 2006, five million beneficiaries still did not have coverage under MMA or other sources of credible coverage.[9]

HUMAN AGING AND CHANGES IN DRUG PHARMACOKINETICS AND PHARMACODYNAMICS

❷ There is a progressive functional decline in many organ systems with advancing age. Table 8–1 reviews some common physiologic changes associated with aging, with an emphasis on those changes that can affect pharmacotherapy. For more detailed information, readers are referred to excellent reviews.[11,12]

Age-associated physiologic changes may cause reductions in functional reserve capacity (i.e., ability to respond to physiologic challenges or stresses) and the ability to preserve homeostasis, thus making elders susceptible to decompensation in stressful situations.[11–13] To deal with physiologic challenges or stresses, older individuals may require up to 95% of their remaining reserve capacity.[11,12] The cardiovascular, musculoskeletal, and central nervous systems appear to be most affected.[12] Examples of homeostatic mechanisms that may become impaired include postural or gait stability, orthostatic blood pressure responses, thermoregulation, cognitive reserve, and bowel and bladder function. An event resulting in functional impairment may involve an insult for which the body cannot compensate, and relatively small stresses may result in major morbidity and mortality.[11–13]

TABLE 8-1 Physiologic Changes with Aging

Organ System	Manifestation
Body composition	↓ Total body water
	↓ Lean body mass
	↑ Body fat
	↔ or ↓ Serum albumin
	↑ α_1-Acid glycoprotein (↔ or ↑ by several disease states)
Cardiovascular	↓ Myocardial sensitivity to β-adrenergic stimulation
	↓ Baroreceptor activity
	↓ Cardiac output
	↑ Total peripheral resistance
Central nervous system	↓ Weight and volume of the brain
	Alterations in several aspects of cognition
Endocrine	Thyroid gland atrophies with age
	Increased incidence of diabetes mellitus, thyroid disease
	Menopause
Gastrointestinal	↑ Gastric pH
	↓ Gastrointestinal blood flow
	Delayed gastric emptying
	Slowed intestinal transit
Genitourinary	Atrophy of the vagina due to decreased estrogen
	Prostatic hypertrophy due to androgenic hormonal changes
	Age-related changes may predispose to incontinence
Immune	↓ Cell-mediated immunity
Liver	↓ Hepatic size
	↓ Hepatic blood flow
Oral	Altered dentition
	↓ Ability to taste sweetness, sourness, bitterness
Pulmonary	↓ Respiratory muscle strength
	↓ Chest wall compliance
	↓ Total alveolar surface
	↓ Vital capacity
	↓ Maximal breathing capacity
Renal	↓ Glomerular filtration rate
	↓ Renal blood flow
	↑ Filtration fraction
	↓ Tubular secretory function
	↓ Renal mass
Sensory	↓ Accommodation of the lens of the eye, causing farsightedness
	Presbycusis (loss of auditory acuity)
	↓ Conduction velocity
Skeletal	Loss of skeletal bone mass (osteopenia)
Skin/hair	Skin dryness, wrinkling, changes in pigmentation, epithelial thinning, loss of dermal thickness
	↓ Number of hair follicles
	↓ Number of melanocytes in hair bulbs

From Kane et al.[11] and Masoro.[12]

A number of age-related physiologic changes occur that could affect drug pharmacokinetics and pharmacodynamics (see Table 8–1). Unfortunately, data on the pharmacokinetics and pharmacodynamics of individual drugs commonly used in older adults are limited. This information gap may improve with implementation of Food and Drug Administration guidelines calling for pharmacokinetic studies by pharmaceutical companies for new molecular entities likely to be used in older adults.[14]

ALTERED PHARMACOKINETICS

Table 8–2 and the following discussion summarize what is known about the effect of aging on each of the four major facets of pharmacokinetics.[13,15] Of interest, when multivariate population pharmacokinetic analyses are conducted, age by itself seldom is a significant predictor of individual pharmacokinetic parameters (e.g., clearance). Aging-associated changes in drug absorption, distribution, metabolism, and elimination are more important predictors of altered pharmacokinetics than is aging, per se.

Absorption

Most drugs are taken orally; thus, a number of age-related changes in gastrointestinal physiology could affect the absorption of medications. Fortunately, most drugs are absorbed via passive diffusion, and age-related physiologic changes appear to have little influence on drug bioavailability.[16] A few drugs require active transport for absorption, so their bioavailability may be reduced (e.g., calcium in the setting of hypochlorhydria). However, there is evidence for a decreased first-pass effect on hepatic and/or gut wall metabolism that results in increased bioavailability and higher plasma concentrations of drugs such as propranolol and morphine.[16] Increased drug bioavailability also may be seen with the concurrent ingestion of grapefruit juice. Constituents of this product inhibit cytochrome P450 (CYP450) isoenzyme CYP3A4, thus decreasing first-pass metabolism and resulting in exaggerated pharmacologic effects.[17]

TABLE 8-2 Age-Related Changes in Drug Pharmacokinetics

Pharmacokinetic Phase	Pharmacokinetic Parameters
Gastrointestinal absorption	Unchanged passive diffusion and no change in bioavailability for most drugs
	↓ Active transport and ↓ bioavailability for some drugs
	↓ First-pass extraction and ↑ bioavailability for some drugs
Distribution	↓ Volume of distribution and ↑ plasma concentration of water-soluble drugs
	↑ Volume of distribution and ↑ terminal disposition half-life ($t_{1/2}$) for fat-soluble drugs
	↑ or ↓ Free fraction of highly plasma protein-bound drugs
Hepatic metabolism	↓ Clearance and ↑ $t_{1/2}$ for some oxidatively metabolized drugs
	↓ Clearance and ↑ $t_{1/2}$ for drugs with high hepatic extraction ratios
Renal excretion	↓ Clearance and ↑ $t_{1/2}$ for renally eliminated drugs and active metabolites

From Cusack[13] and Chapron.[15]

Distribution

The distribution of medications in the body depends on factors such as blood flow, plasma protein binding, and body composition, each of which may be altered with age. For example, the volume of distribution of water-soluble drugs is decreased, whereas lipophilic drugs exhibit an increased volume of distribution.[13,15] Changes in the volume of distribution can have a direct impact on the amount of medication that must be given as a loading dose.

P-glycoprotein, a member of the multidrug resistance (MDR)-associated protein family of efflux transporters, influences the transport of drugs across the blood–brain barrier. Studies using verapamil labeled with carbon-11 (a positron emitter) and positron emission tomography have demonstrated decreased P-glycoprotein activity in the blood–brain barrier with aging. As a result of this, the brain of aged individuals may be exposed to higher than normal levels of drugs and toxins.[18]

The two major plasma proteins to which medications can bind are albumin and α_1-acid glycoprotein, and concentrations of these proteins may change with concurrent pathologies seen with increasing age.[19] For acidic drugs such as naproxen, phenytoin, tolbutamide, and warfarin, decreased serum albumin may lead to an increase in free fraction. An increase in α_1-acid glycoprotein induced by burns, cancer, inflammatory disease, or trauma may lead to a decreased free fraction of basic drugs such as lidocaine, propranolol, quinidine, and imipramine. In the absence of compromise in excretory pathways, these potential changes are unlikely to have any deleterious clinical effect. However, they may be important to consider when interpreting serum concentrations of these drugs because usually only total drug concentrations (sum of free and protein-bound drug) are reported.

Metabolism

The liver is the major organ responsible for drug metabolism, including phase I (oxidative) and phase II (conjugative) reactions.[20] The most remarkable characteristic of hepatic function in older adults is the increase in interindividual variability compared with other age groups, a feature that may obscure true age-related changes.[20] Data suggest that age-related declines in phase I metabolism more likely are the result of reduced hepatic volume than reduced hepatic enzymatic activity.[21] Decreased phase I metabolism (e.g., hydroxylation, dealkylation) producing decreased drug clearance and increased terminal disposition half-life ($t_{1/2}$) has been reported in elders for medications such as diazepam, piroxicam, theophylline, and quinidine. Phase II metabolism (e.g., glucuronidation, acetylation) of medications such as lorazepam and oxazepam appears to be relatively unaffected by advancing age. Hepatic enzyme induction (e.g., by rifampin, phenytoin) or inhibition (e.g., by fluoroquinolone and macrolide antimicrobials, cimetidine) does not appear to be affected by the aging process.[20,22]

Age-related decreases in hepatic blood flow can decrease significantly the metabolism of drugs with high hepatic extraction ratios, such as imipramine, lidocaine, morphine, and propranolol.[20] The effect of aging on polymorphic drug metabolism has not been well studied. Advancing age has been reported both to have no significant effect and to reduce significantly the activity of the CYP450 isoenzyme CYP3A4.[23,24] Other available data suggest that advancing age has no significant effect on drug acetylation or on CYP450 isoenzyme CYP2D6 or CYP2C9 isoenzyme-mediated metabolism.[25–28] A single-point blood sampling method for evaluating CYP450 isoenzyme CYP3A4 activity in older adults has been described.[29] A number of potential confounding factors, including race, sex, frailty, smoking, diet, and drug–drug interactions, may significantly affect hepatic metabolism in older adults.[20]

Elimination

Renal excretion is the primary route of elimination for many drugs. Although age-related reductions in glomerular filtration are well documented, as many as one third of "normal" older adult subjects may have no reduction as measured by creatinine clearance.[13,15] Moreover, emerging information suggests that renal tubular secretion may not decline in proportion to other renal processes.[30] The estimation of creatinine clearance, although not entirely accurate in individual patients, can serve as a useful screening approximation. Cockcroft and Gault[31] created one of the most commonly used equations for adults with stable renal function whose actual weight is within 30% of ideal body weight:

$$\text{Creatinine clearance} = \frac{(140 - \text{Age})\ (\text{Actual body weight})}{72\ (\text{Serum creatinine concentration})}$$

where age is given in years, actual body weight in kilograms, and serum creatinine concentration in milligrams per deciliter. For women, multiply this result by 0.85. The Modified Diet in Renal Disease[32] equation has become more widely used for estimation of glomerular filtration rate. However, dosing guidelines for medications that primarily are renally cleared still are based on estimated creatinine clearance determined using the Cockcroft and Gault equation. In the future, use of another protein, cystatin C, a low-molecular-mass protein that is produced by all nucleated cells, is freely filtered at the glomerulus, and is not secreted by the renal tubules, may prove to be superior to use of creatinine. This could be the case especially with coexisting conditions such as cachexia, sedentary lifestyle, malnutrition, and hepatic disease, because creatinine clearance is a poor predictor of glomerular filtration in the presence of these conditions.[33]

Medications whose excretion is primarily renal and for which there is evidence of age-related reduction in renal and total body clearance include (but are not limited to) amantadine, aminoglycosides, atenolol, captopril, cimetidine, digoxin, lithium, and vancomycin. Some hepatically metabolized medications can yield active, primarily renally excreted metabolites, such as *N*-acetylprocainamide, normeperidine, and morphine-6-glucuronide, which can accumulate with advancing age because of reduced renal function.

CLINICAL CONTROVERSY

When using the Cockcroft and Gault equation to estimate creatinine clearance in older adults, some clinicians round the value up to 1 if the patient's serum creatinine concentration is less than 1. Rounding the serum creatinine concentration may provide an underestimation of creatinine clearance and result in improper dose adjustment of renally eliminated medications. It is important to realize that the equation is merely an estimate, and attempts should be made to determine creatinine clearance accurately when use of certain medications (e.g., metformin) is being contemplated.

ALTERED PHARMACODYNAMICS

There is some evidence of altered drug response or "sensitivity" in older adults. Four possible mechanisms have been suggested: (a) changes in receptor numbers, (b) changes in receptor affinity, (c) postreceptor alterations, and (d) age-related impairment of homeostatic mechanisms.[13,34] For example, muscarinic, parathyroid hormone, β-adrenergic, α_1-adrenergic, and μ-opioid receptors exhibit reduced density with increasing age.[13,34] Evidence from epidemiologic and experimental studies suggests that, independent of pharmacokinetic alterations, older adults are more sensitive to the central nervous system effects of benzodiazepines.[13,34] Older adults exhibit a greater analgesic responsiveness to opioids compared with their younger counterparts, even when pharmacokinetic parameters are similar in the two groups.[13,34] In addition, older adults demonstrate an enhanced responsiveness to anticoagulants such as warfarin and heparin as well as to thrombolytic therapy but not to the direct thrombin inhibitor ximelagatran.[13,34,35] In contrast, older adults exhibit decreased responsiveness to certain drugs (e.g., β-agonists/antagonists).[13,34] Reflex tachycardia, seen commonly with vasodilator therapy, often is blunted in older adults, perhaps because of dampened baroreceptor function. For some drugs (e.g., calcium channel blockers), both enhanced responsiveness (as demonstrated by greater reduction in blood pressure) and decreased responsiveness (as demonstrated by reduced atrioventricular nodal blockade) can occur simultaneously in older adults.[13,34]

CLINICAL GERIATRICS

❸ Maintenance of independence and prevention of disability are primary goals in the clinical care of persons 65 years of age and older. To achieve these goals, it is necessary that all healthcare professionals understand the concept of functional status. Functional status is a proxy measure of a patient's ability to live independently and can be determined in part by inquiring about an older person's ability to perform specific tasks. As mentioned previously, the two types of functional measurements are basic ADLs and the more complex instrumental ADLs.[36,37] However, to fully assess functional status, the patient's psychological state, financial resources, physical function, and social circumstances also must be considered.[1]

One of the challenges of maintaining and improving functional status in geriatric individuals is recognizing and managing conditions frequently seen in older adults. Problems found more commonly in older persons sometimes are referred to as the "*I*'s of geriatrics" (Table 8–3).[11] These problems are often due to underlying disease processes that may or may not be diagnosed. Examples of diseases and syndromes that can present as common problems in older adults include Parkinson's disease, falls, hip fractures, benign prostatic hypertrophy, dementia, glaucoma, postherpetic neuralgia, and tuberculosis.

Another factor contributing to the challenge of clinical geriatrics is that approximately 50% of older patients present with atypical symptoms or complaints, so use of the classic medical model for diagnosis is difficult. For example, cardiac ischemia in an older person may present as syncope or weakness rather than the typical presentation of chest pain. Confusion may be the presenting symptom of an acute abdominal process rather than the expected severe pain, rigid abdominal muscles, and leukocytosis. Serious adverse consequences may result if a diagnosis is delayed or missed because of these atypical presentations. Such unusual presentations may be due to age-related physiologic changes, the presence of multiple comorbid illnesses or compromised function, and the presence of psychological stressors.[38] Table 8–4 lists other examples of medical illnesses that often present atypically in older adults.[38–40] For very frail older adults, delirium, falls, and nonspecific functional decline (e.g., failure to thrive) frequently are presenting problems.[38–40]

Multiple coexisting chronic illnesses are another common threat to independence that distinguishes older adults from younger patients. Older patients usually have multiple comorbidities, such as osteoarthritis, heart disease, and diabetes. Although multiple comorbidities can have a substantial impact on a patient's functional status, the mere existence of multiple diseases alone does not determine functional impairment.

TABLE 8-3 The *I*'s of Geriatrics: Common Problems in Older Adults

Immobility	Instability
Isolation	Intellectual impairment
Incontinence	Impotence
Infection	Immunodeficiency
Inanition (malnutrition)	Insomnia
Impaction	Iatrogenesis
Impaired senses	

From Kane et al.[11]

TABLE 8-4 Atypical Disease Presentation in Older Adults

Disease	Presentation
Acute myocardial infarction	Only ~50% present with chest pain. In general, older adults present with weakness, confusion, syncope, and abdominal pain; however, electrocardiographic findings are similar to those in younger patients.
Congestive heart failure	Instead of dyspnea, the older patient may present with hypoxic symptoms, lethargy, restlessness, and confusion.
Gastrointestinal bleed	Although the mortality rate is ~10%, presenting symptoms are nonspecific, ranging from altered mental status to syncope with hemodynamic collapse. Abdominal pain often is absent.
Upper respiratory infection	Older patients typically present with lethargy, confusion, anorexia, and decompensation of a preexisting medical condition. Fever, chills, and a productive cough may or may not be present.
Urinary tract infection	Dysuria, fever, and flank pain may be absent. More commonly, older adults present with incontinence, confusion, abdominal pain, nausea/vomiting, and azotemia.

From Fried et al.,[38] Jarrett et al.,[39] and Merck Manual of Geriatrics, 3rd ed, Whitehouse Station, NJ.[40]

DRUG-RELATED PROBLEMS IN OLDER ADULTS

❹ Although medications used by older adults can lead to improvement in HRQOL, negative outcomes due to drug-related problems are considerable.[41–43] Three important and potentially preventable negative outcomes due to drug-related problems that can occur in older adults are adverse drug withdrawal events (ADWEs), which are clinically significant sets of symptoms or signs caused by the removal of a drug; therapeutic failure (inadequate or inappropriate drug therapy and not related to the natural progression of disease); and adverse drug reactions (ADRs), defined as reactions that are noxious and unintended and occur at dosages normally used in humans for prophylaxis, diagnosis, or therapy.[41–43]

Data on the prevalence of ADWEs and therapeutic failures in older adults are limited. Graves et al.[44] reported ADWEs in 38 of 124 male outpatients who had discontinued taking 238 medications. Kaiser et al.[45] reported that 11% of hospital admissions in a group of older frail men were related to therapeutic failure. ADRs occur commonly in older adults, with reported rates ranging from 2.5% to 50.6% depending on the study population and methodology used.[41] In a large study of more than 30,000 Medicare outpatients, Gurwitz et al.[46] reported that 5% experienced an ADR in a 1-year period, with more serious reactions more likely to be preventable. In contrast, Hanlon et al.[47] reported that 33% of frail male outpatients had one or more ADRs in a 1-year period. A review suggests that ADRs are the most common type of medication-related problem in elderly nursing home patients.[42]

ADRs and other drug-related problems (e.g., ADWEs, therapeutic failure) are major threats to the HRQOL of outpatient elders and account for billions of healthcare dollars per year.[48] In the nursing home setting alone, a cost-of-illness study estimated that drug-related problems (including ADRs and therapeutic failure) cost $4 billion per year.[49]

RISK FACTORS

Overuse

Polypharmacy can be defined as either the concomitant use of multiple drugs or the administration of more medications than are indicated clinically.[50] Polypharmacy is common and increasing among older adults. Community-based surveys reveal that older adults take an average of two to nine prescription and nonprescription medications each day.[50–52] A study of community-dwelling older adults in Finland reported an increase in polypharmacy, with the largest growth among patients older than 85 years.[53] Increased use of dietary supplements, such as herbal products, vitamins, and minerals, may add to the increase in polypharmacy. In a nationwide survey, Kaufman et al.[54] found that 59% of women and 46% of men older than 65 years used a vitamin or mineral supplement and that 14% of these women and 11% of these men used an herbal product. Outside of the community, a nursing facility survey found that institutionalized older persons took an average of 6.69 routine medications and 27.1% took nine or more medications on a regular basis.[55] Drug-use studies that defined polypharmacy as use of one or more unnecessary medications showed that polypharmacy occurs in 55% to 59% of older outpatients.[56,57] A study of frail veterans at hospital discharge reported that 44% of patients were taking one or more unnecessary medications, with 25% of patients starting the medication(s) during hospitalization.[58] Multiple medication use has been strongly associated with ADRs.[41] Polypharmacy also is problematic for older adults because it may increase the risk of geriatric syndromes (e.g., falls, cognitive impairment), diminished functional status, and healthcare costs.[50,59,60]

Inappropriate Prescribing

Inappropriate prescribing can be defined as prescribing medications outside the bounds of accepted medical standards.[61] This phenomenon occurs commonly in older outpatients, as exemplified by one study in which 92% of patients were taking at least one medication with one or more inappropriate ratings based on clinical review applying explicit criteria.[62] Studies using explicit drug-use review criteria have found that between 15% and 21% of community-dwelling older adults take one or more medications that have a dose, duration, duplication, or drug-interaction problem.[63,64]

Alternatively, inappropriate prescribing can be defined as prescribing drugs whose use should be avoided because their risk outweighs their potential benefit.[65] A European study found that 20% of older home-care patients used at least one inappropriate medicine as defined by explicit criteria.[66] A study of inappropriate drug use in U.S. long-term care facilities found that 25% of residents took one or more inappropriate medications as defined by explicit criteria.[67]

CLINICAL CONTROVERSY

At present, the best way to measure inappropriate prescribing is not clear. The association between explicit criteria developed by Beers et al. (known commonly as the Beers' criteria)[65] for inappropriate prescribing or other measures of inappropriate prescribing and health outcomes has been mixed.[68] We recommend further studies of the predictive validity of evidence-based standards for measuring inappropriate prescribing of medications in older adults.

Underuse

An important and increasingly recognized problem in elders is *underuse,* defined as the omission of drug therapy that is indicated for treatment or prevention of a disease or condition.[61] A study of community-dwelling elders found that 50% of 372 vulnerable adults were not prescribed an indicated medication. The most common problems were the lack of a gastroprotective agent for high-risk nonsteroidal antiinflammatory drug users, no angiotensin-converting enzyme inhibitor for patients with diabetes and proteinuria, and no calcium and/or vitamin D for those with osteoporosis.[69] A study of older adults in assisted-living facilities revealed that 62% of residents with a diagnosis of heart failure did not take an angiotensin-converting enzyme inhibitor, and 61% of those with osteoporosis did not take calcium supplements.[70]

Underuse may have an important relationship with negative health outcomes in older adults, including functional disability, death, and health services use.[61] Underuse of medication in general because of limiting access of Medicaid patients to medications more than doubled the risk of admission to a nursing home.[71] Tamblyn et al.[72] studied the effects of a deductible and a 25% coinsurance fee for medications taken by elders in Canada. This reform led to a decrease in the number of essential medications (e.g., furosemide, anticoagulants, angiotensin-converting enzyme inhibitors) used by older patients and increased costs owing to adverse events and emergency department visits.

Medication Nonadherence

The World Health Organization (WHO) defines *medication adherence* as "the extent to which a person's behavior—taking medication…corresponds with agreed recommendations from a healthcare provider."[73] Given that definition, nonadherence could be defined as not filling the prescription, stopping use of the medication before the entire supply is consumed, or taking more or less of the medication than stated by the label. The prevalence rate of medication nonadherence in older adults ranges from 40% to 80% (mean approximately 50%).[74,75] Older and younger patients have similar adherence when the number of drugs taken is similar.[76] In fact, some evidence indicates that adherence may be better in older adults for some conditions.[74,77,78] According to the AARP (formerly the American Association for Retired Persons) and a study in the Medicare population, cost is a common reason why older adults do not fill their prescriptions.[79,80] Older patients also may not adhere to their regimens because of possible adverse effects, an inability to read product labels, or a lack of full understanding of information about the prescribed medication.[79,81]

Limited retrospective data suggest that nonadherence is associated with increased health services use and ADRs. In a 2001 study, nonadherence was the possible cause of more than 10% of older adult hospital admissions.[82] A study by Col et al. [83] evaluated 315 consecutive older patients admitted to a hospital and determined that 11.4% of admissions resulted from nonadherence. Gurwitz et al.[46] found that 21% of preventable ADRs in elderly outpatients were due to errors in patient adherence. On the positive side, a study found that increased medication adherence was associated with fewer hospitalizations and decreased cost in patients with certain chronic medical conditions (e.g., diabetes, hypertension).[84]

PROVISION OF COMPREHENSIVE GERIATRIC ASSESSMENT

❺ Given that drug-related problems are common, costly, and clinically important, how can they be prevented/managed? A solution may lie in comprehensive geriatric assessment. The term *comprehensive geriatric assessment* has been applied to geriatric evaluation and management (GEM), in which GEM clinicians (which often include pharmacists) manage the patient. Comprehensive geriatric assessment has become a cornerstone in the care of older adults. A comprehensive review has summarized its effectiveness in improving suboptimal prescribing and reducing ADRs.[61]

Pharmacists can independently play a significant role in optimizing pharmacotherapy for older adults. The results from 13 randomized controlled studies show that clinical pharmacy interventions can reduce drug-related problems and improve health outcomes in older adults.[85] Subsequent published studies also have demonstrated the value of pharmacists in improving drug therapy for elders.[61,86,87]

The following subsections provide an approach to how pharmacists in any practice setting (especially those providing medication therapy management services under the new Medicare Part D program) can optimize medication use through the provision of comprehensive geriatric assessment.

HISTORY TAKING

Several difficulties may occur while taking medication histories from older adults. They include (a) communication problems (impaired hearing and vision), (b) underreporting (e.g., health beliefs, cognitive impairment), (c) reporting of vague or nonspecific symptoms (altered presentation), (d) coexistence of multiple diseases and/or use of multiple medications, (e) reliance on a caregiver for the history, and (f) lack of medical records to confirm findings. Despite these potential difficulties, health professionals should find value in collecting this vital medication history information.

The importance of inquiring about use of nonprescription medications and dietary supplements in older adults cannot be overstressed. A national survey reported that half of community-dwelling older adults take one or more vitamins or minerals and another 12% take one or more herbal/botanical agents.[54]

Asking older adults and their caregivers about methods they use to keep track of medicines is important. This will allow design of solutions to any problems detected and prevent repeating of ineffective, previously used methods.

Patients and caregivers should be asked about risk factors for prescribing problems (e.g., utilizing multiple physicians and pharmacies) and adherence problems (e.g., impaired hearing, vision, and/or cognition; inability to open safety caps, pay for medicines, or swallow medications).[88] The drug history should end with an inquiry about any past allergies to medications and whether patients currently or in the recent past experienced any adverse effects, unwanted reactions, or other problems with their medications.[89]

ASSESSING AND MONITORING DRUG THERAPY

The first step in the assessment is to determine whether drug-related problems are causing any of the patient's symptoms/problems. In particular, consider whether any current medications are causing any geriatric syndrome (e.g., falls, urinary incontinence, cognitive impairment). Table 8–5 lists medications for which there is evidence that use increases the risk of cognitive impairment.[90] The next step is to match the medical problem list with the drug list. If a drug does not have a match with the problem list, the drug may not be needed. Conversively, if the patient has a chronic condition and is not taking a medication, consider whether the patient would benefit from an essential evidence-based drug to treat the condition. Next, examine laboratory test results and vital signs that can be used to monitor the efficacy and toxicity of each medication. Table 8–6 lists laboratory monitoring recommendations for medications used in long-term care facilities.[91] Finally, assess the appropriateness of the remaining medications. A variety of approaches can be used.[61] One standardized measure with demonstrated reliability and validity is the Medication Appropriateness Index (MAI).[68,92] The MAI consists of 10 questions that should be asked about each medication (Table 8–7). Some other factors to consider during drug regimen review include medication storage problems and drug interactions with food and/or laboratory test results.

TABLE 8-5 Drugs/Drug Classes Associated with Altered Cognition and/or Cognitive Disorders

Antiarrhythmic agents (e.g., disopyramide)
Antiemetic/antivertigo agents (e.g., meclizine)
Antihistamines (e.g., diphenhydramine, hydroxyzine)
Antiparkinsonian agents (e.g., benztropine, trihexyphenidyl)
Antipsychotic agents (e.g., thioridazine)
Antispasmodic agents (e.g., belladonna, flavoxate)
Benzodiazepines
Central nervous system drugs, especially when several agents are used concomitantly (as in polypharmacy)
Digoxin
Histamine H_2 receptor antagonists
Nonsteroidal antiinflammatory drugs
Opioid agonists (especially meperidine, pentazocine)
Skeletal muscle relaxants (e.g., cyclobenzaprine)
Tricyclic antidepressants (e.g., amitriptyline)

Data from Kotylar M, Gray SL, Lindblad CI, Hanlon JT. Psychiatric Manifestations of Medications in the Elderly. In Malletta G, Agronin M (editors). Principles and Practice of Geriatric Psychiatry, 1st ed. Philadelphia, PA: Lippincott Williams and Wilkins 2005;605–615.

TABLE 8-6 Centers for Medicare and Medicaid Services Guidelines for Monitoring Medication Use

Drug	Monitoring
Acetaminophen (>4 g/day)	Hepatic function tests
Aminoglycosides	Serum creatinine, drug levels
Hypoglycemic agents	Blood sugar levels
Antiepileptic agents (older)	Drug levels
Angiotensin-converting enzyme inhibitors	Potassium levels
Antipsychotic agents	Extrapyramidal adverse effects
Appetite stimulants	Weight, appetite
Digoxin	Serum creatinine, drug levels
Diuretic	Potassium levels
Erythropoiesis stimulants	Blood pressure, iron and ferritin levels, complete blood count
Fibrates	Hepatic function test, complete blood count
Iron	Iron and ferritin levels, complete blood count
Lithium	Drug levels
Niacin	Blood sugar levels, hepatic function tests
Statins	Hepatic function tests
Theophylline	Drug levels
Thyroid replacement	Thyroid function tests
Warfarin	Prothrombin time/international normalized ratio

From reference 91.

CLINICAL CONTROVERSY

An increasing number of clinical trials are enrolling older adult patients. For example, we now have evidence supporting the cardiac benefits of pravastatin in older adults.[93] Clinicians must weigh the risks and benefits of adding drug therapy to a patient's drug regimen because increasing the number of drugs may decrease adherence and lead to an increased risk for ADRs. Furthermore, a clinician must decide whether adding drug therapy in patients who may not live long enough to benefit from the medication is ethical.

DOCUMENTING PROBLEMS AND FORMULATING A THERAPEUTIC PLAN

The clinician must document the problems that have been detected, develop a therapeutic plan to resolve them, and establish reasonable

TABLE 8-7 Medication Appropriateness Index

Questions to Ask About Each Individual Medication

1. Is there an indication for the medication?
2. Is the medication effective for the condition?
3. Is the dosage correct?
4. Are the directions correct?
5. Are the directions practical?
6. Are there clinically significant drug–drug interactions?
7. Are there clinically significant drug–disease/condition interactions?
8. Is there unnecessary duplication with other medication(s)?
9. Is the duration of therapy acceptable?
10. Is this medication the least expensive alternative compared with others of equal utility?

Reprinted and adapted from J Clin Epidemiol, Vol. 45, Hanlon JT, Schmader KE, Samsa GP, et al. A method for assessing drug therapy appropriateness, Pages 1045–1051, Copyright 1992, with permission from Elsevier.

therapeutic end points. Remember that what may be a reasonable end point for a 40-year-old patient may not be as reasonable for an 80-year-old patient when comorbidities, functional status, and life expectancy are taken into consideration.

CONSULTING THE PHYSICIAN REGARDING PROBLEMS AND CONCERNS

In most cases, the pharmacist or other healthcare professional should contact a patient's physician regarding problems and concerns that have been detected and documented. In discussing the patient in this context, the importance of optimizing the prescribing for the older adult patient before implementing strategies to enhance his or her adherence cannot be overstressed. Otherwise, adherence intervention, if effective, may result in patient harm. Similarly, in institutional settings, strategies to reduce medication errors may not improve patient outcomes if prescribing is not improved beforehand.

COUNSELING AND ADHERENCE AIDS

Before dispensing medication, consider some general factors that may enhance adherence by older adults, such as modifying medication schedules to fit patients' lifestyles, prescribing generic agents to reduce costs, and using easy-to-open bottles, easy-to-swallow dosage forms, and larger type on direction and auxiliary labels.[94] The WHO suggests clinicians consider five dimensions when assessing medication adherence: social/economic factors (e.g., cultural beliefs), provider–patient/healthcare system factors (e.g., provider–patient relationship), condition-related factors (e.g., chronic conditions), therapy-related factors (e.g., regimen complexity), and patient-related factors (e.g., visual or hearing impairment).[73] Finally, when dispensing medications (particularly new medications or previously used medications that have changed in appearance or directions for use), provide both written and oral drug information to the patient and caregiver.

To improve the likelihood of adherence, the healthcare professional should recruit active patient and caregiver involvement, stress the importance of adherence, and consider the use of adherence-enhancing aids (e.g., special packaging, a medication record, a drug calendar, medication boxes, magnification for insulin syringes, dose-measuring devices, and spacers for metered-dose inhalers).[95,96] In institutional settings, discussion of special considerations (e.g., medications that can be crushed and given via feeding tube) with healthcare professionals responsible for medication administration is prudent.

DOCUMENTING INTERVENTIONS AND MONITORING PATIENT PROGRESS

All interventions must be documented, and the steps just outlined must be repeated over time with older adult patients. During followup contacts, minimum inquiry should include asking patients whether they have any questions or concerns regarding medicines and determining whether the therapeutic end points previously established have been achieved. To assess potential ADRs, ask patients whether they currently or recently have experienced any side effects, unwanted reactions, or other problems with their medications.

TARGETING HIGH-RISK OLDER ADULTS

In busy practices, the approach outlined may not be feasible for every patient. Therefore, practitioners may consider targeting these activities to patients at high risk for developing drug-related problems. Geriatric experts have identified risk factors for preventable ADRs in older adult nursing home patients.[97] These include the following medication-related factors: (a) polypharmacy (i.e., use of seven or more medications or more than three cardiac medications), and (b) taking specific high-risk drugs (e.g., anticoagulant, antidepressant, antiinfective, antipsychotic, anticonvulsant, opioid analgesic, sedative/hypnotic, skeletal muscle relaxant). Another study of geriatric experts identified 21 risk factors for ADRs in ambulatory older adults.[98] Other unique risk factors include (a) medication-related issues (i.e., with anticholinergics, benzodiazepines, chlorpropamide, corticosteroids, nonsteroidal antiinflammatory drugs), (b) certain patient characteristics (e.g., multiple comorbidities, multiple prescribers, age 85 years and older, dementia, regular use of alcohol, decreased renal function), (c) use of drugs with narrow therapeutic ranges (e.g., lithium, theophylline), (d) history of an ADR, and (e) recent hospitalization.

CONCLUSIONS

The number of people older than 65 years is growing in the United States and around the world, and individuals older than 85 years are the fastest growing segment of the U.S. population. A number of physiologic changes associated with age, especially hepatic metabolism and renal excretion, affect the pharmacokinetics and pharmacodynamics of drugs. Improving and maintaining the patient's functional status and managing the patient's comorbidities are hallmarks of clinical geriatrics. Certain medical conditions are restricted to older adults, and drug-related problems represent a major concern for this group. Innovative approaches, such as the provision of comprehensive geriatric assessment by pharmacists and other healthcare professionals, are needed to decrease the occurrence of these drug-related problems.

ABBREVIATIONS

ADL: activity of daily living

ADR: adverse drug reaction

ADWE: adverse drug withdrawal event

CYP450: cytochrome P450

GEM: geriatric evaluation and management

HRQOL: health-related quality of life

MAI: Medication Appropriateness Index

MMA: Medicare Prescription Drug, Improvement and Modernization Act

WHO: World Health Organization

REFERENCES

1. Rubenstein LZ, Rubenstein LV. Multidimensional geriatric assessment. In: Tallis R, Fillit H, eds. Brocklehurst's Textbook of Geriatric Medicine, 6th ed. London: Churchill-Livingstone, 2003:291–299.
2. He W, Sengupta M, Velkoff VA, DeBarros KA. U.S. Census Bureau, Current Population Reports. P23-P209, 65+ in the United States: 2005. Washington, DC: U.S. Government Printing Office, 2005.
3. Olshansky SJ. The demography of aging. In: Cassel CK, Leipzig RM, Cohen HJ, Larson EB, Meier DE, eds. Geriatric Medicine: An Evidence-based Approach, 4th ed. New York: Springer-Verlag, 2003:37–44.
4. Centers for Disease Control and Prevention. National Center for Injury Prevention and Control. 2007. Accessed at *http://webappa.cdc.gov/sasweb/ncipc/leadcaus10.html*, October 19, 2007.
5. Waldrop J, Stern SM. Disability Status, 2000. Census 2000 Brief. March Report Number C2KBR-17. Washington, DC: U.S. Department of Commerce, Economics and Statistics Administration, U.S. Census Bureau, 2003.
6. National Center for Health Statistics. Health, United States, 2000. Hyattsville, MD: U.S. Department of Health and Human Services, 2000.
7. National Center for Chronic Disease Prevention and Health Promotion. Healthy Aging: Preventing Disease and Improving Quality of Life

Among Older Americans: At-a-Glance 2000. Atlanta, GA: Centers for Disease Control and Prevention, 2000.
8. Stuart B, Shea D, Briesacher B. Dynamics in drug coverage of Medicare beneficiaries: Finders, losers, switchers. Health Affairs 2001;20:86–99.
9. Henry J. Kaiser Foundation: Prescription Drug Trends, Fact Sheet. 2007, *http://www.kff.org/rxdrugs/upload/3057–05.pdf.*
10. Safran DG, Neuman P, Schoen C, et al. Rogers Prescription drug coverage and seniors: Findings from a 2003 national survey. Health Aff (Millwood). 2005;Jan–Jun;Suppl Web Exclusives:W5-152–W5-166.
11. Kane RL, Ouslander JG, Abrass IB. Clinical implications of the aging process. In: Essentials of Clinical Geriatrics, 5th ed. New York: McGraw-Hill, 2004:3–15.
12. Masoro EJ. Physiology of aging. In: Tallis R, Fillit H, eds. Brocklehurst's Textbook of Geriatric Medicine, 6th ed. London, Churchill-Livingstone, 2003:291–299.
13. Cusack BJ. Pharmacokinetics in older persons. Am J Geriatr Pharm 2004;2:274–302.
14. U.S. Food and Drug Administration. Guideline for industry: Studies in support of special populations. Geriatrics, ICH-E7. 1994, *http://www.fda.gov/cder/guidance/iche7.pdf.*
15. Chapron DJ. Drug disposition and response. In: Delafuente JC, Stewart RB, eds. Therapeutics in the Elderly, 3rd ed. Cincinnati, OH: Harvey Whitney, 2000:257–288.
16. Iber FL, Murphy PA, Connor ES. Age-related changes in the gastrointestinal system: Effects on drug therapy. Drugs Aging 1994;5:34–48.
17. Dresser GK, Bailey DG, Carruthers SG. Grapefruit juice–felodipine interaction in the elderly. Clin Pharmacol Ther 2000;68:28–34.
18. Toornvliet R, vanBerckel BNM, Luurtsema G, et al. Effect of age on functional P-glycoprotein in the blood-brain barrier measured by use of (R)-[^{11}C]verapamil and positron emission tomography. Clin Pharmacol Ther 2006;79:540–548.
19. Grandison MK, Boudinot FD. Age-related changes in protein binding of drugs: Implications for therapy. Clin Pharmacokinet 2000;38:271–290.
20. Herrlinger C, Klotz U. Drug metabolism and drug interactions in the elderly. Best Pract Res Clin Gastroenterol 2001;15:897–918.
21. Sotaniemi EA, Arranto AJ, Pelkonen O, Pasanen M. Age and cytochrome P450–linked drug metabolism in humans. Clin Pharmacol Ther 1997;61:331–339.
22. Dilger K, Hofmann U, Klotz U. Enzyme induction in the elderly: Effect of rifampin on the pharmacokinetics and pharmacodynamics of propafenone. Clin Pharmacol Ther 2000;67:512–520.
23. Schwartz JB. Race not age affects erythromycin breath test results in older hypertensive men. J Clin Pharmacol 2001;41:324–329.
24. Krecic-Shepard ME, Barnas CR, Slimko J, Schwartz JB. Faster clearance of sustained release verapamil in men versus women: Continuing observations on sex-specific differences after oral administration of verapamil. Clin Pharmacol Ther 2000;68:286–292.
25. Korrapati MR, Sorkin JD, Andres R, et al. Acetylator phenotype in relation to age and gender in the Baltimore Longitudinal Study of Aging. J Clin Pharmacol 1997;37:83–91.
26. Agundez JA, Rodriguez I, Olivera M, et al. C4P2D6 NAT2 and C4P2E1 genetic polymorphisms in nonagenarians. Age Ageing 1997;26:147–151.
27. Taioli E, Mari D, Franceschi C, et al. Polymorphisms of drug-metabolizing enzymes in healthy nonagenarians and centenarians: Difference at GSTT1 locus. Biochem Biophys Res Commun 2001;280:1389–1392.
28. Brenner SS, Herrlinger C, Dilger K, et al. Influence of age and cytochrome P450 2C9 genotype on the steady-state disposition of diclofenac and celecoxib. Clin Pharmacokinet 2003;42:283–292.
29. Krupka E, Venisse N, Lafay C, et al. Probe of CYP3A by a single-point blood measurement after oral administration of midazolam in healthy elderly volunteers. Eur J Clin Pharmacol 2006;62:653–659.
30. Ujhelyi MR, Bottorff MB, Schur M, et al. Aging effects on the organic base transporter and stereoselective renal clearance. Clin Pharmacol Ther 1997;62:117–128.
31. Cockcroft DW, Gault MH. Prediction of creatinine clearance from serum creatinine. Nephron 1976;16:31–41.
32. Levey AS, Bosch JP, Lewis JB, et al. A more accurate method to estimate glomerular filtration rate from serum creatinine: A new prediction equation. Modification of Diet in Renal Disease Study Group. Ann Intern Med 1999;130:461–470.
33. Hermida J, Tutor JC. Serum cystatin C for the prediction of glomerular filtration rate with regard to the dose adjustment of amikacin, gentamicin, tobramycin, and vancomycin. Ther Drug Monit 2006;28:326–331.
34. Guay D, Artz MB, Hanlon JT, Schmader KE. The pharmacology of aging. In: Tallis R, Fillit H, eds. Brocklehurst's Textbook of Geriatric Medicine, 6th ed. London: Churchill-Livingstone, 2003:155–161.
35. Wernevik LC, Nystrom P, Andersson M, et al. Comparable pharmacokinetics and pharmacodynamics of melagatran in Japanese and Caucasian volunteers after oral administration of the direct thrombin inhibitor ximelagatran. Clin Pharmacokinet 2006;45:85–94.
36. Katz S, Akpom CA. A measure of primary sociobiologic functions. Int J Health Serv 1976;6:493–507.
37. Fillenbaum GG. Screening the elderly: A brief instrumental ADL measure. J Am Geriatr Soc 1985;33:698–706.
38. Fried LP, Storer DJ, King DE, et al. Diagnosis of illness presentation in the elderly. J Am Geriatr Soc 1991;39:117–123.
39. Jarrett PG, Rockwood K, Carver D, et al. Illness presentation in elderly patients. Arch Intern Med 1995;155:1060–1064.
40. Beers MH, Berkow R, eds. History and physical examination. In: Merck Manual of Geriatrics, 3rd ed. Whitehouse Station, NJ: Merck, 2000:24–40.
41. Hanlon JT, Schmader K, Gray SL. Adverse drug reactions. In: Delafuente JC, Stewart RB, eds. Therapeutics in the Elderly, 3rd ed. Cincinnati, OH: Harvey Whitney, 2000:289–314.
42. Handler SM, Wright RM, Ruby CM, Hanlon JT. Epidemiology of medication-related adverse events in nursing homes. Am J Geriatr Pharmacother 2006;4:264–272.
43. Institute of Medicine. Committee on Identifying and Preventing Medication Errors: Preventing Medication Errors: Quality Chasm Series. Washington, DC: National Academy Press, 2006.
44. Graves T, Hanlon JT, Schmader KE, et al. Adverse events after discontinuing medications in elderly outpatients. Arch Intern Med 1997;157:2205–2210.
45. Kaiser RM, Schmader KE, Pieper CF, Lindblad CI, Ruby CM, Hanlon JT. Therapeutic failure-related hospitalisations in the frail elderly. Drugs Aging 2006;23:579–586.
46. Gurwitz JH, Field TS, Harrold LR, et al. Incidence and preventability of adverse drug events among older persons in the ambulatory setting. JAMA 2003;289:1107–1116.
47. Hanlon JT, Pieper CF, Hajjar ER, et al. Incidence and predictors of all and preventable adverse drug reactions in frail elderly post hospital stay. J Gerontol Med Sci 2006;61A:511–515.
48. Ernst FR, Grizzle AJ. Drug-related morbidity and mortality: Updating the cost-of-illness model. J Am Pharm Assoc 2001;41:192–199.
49. Bootman JL, Harrison DL, Cox E. The health care cost of drug-related morbidity and mortality in nursing facilities. Arch Intern Med 1997;157:2089–2096.
50. Stewart RB, Cooper JW. Polypharmacy in the aged: Practical solutions. Drugs Aging 1994;4:449–461.
51. Hanlon JT, Fillenbaum GG, Burchett B, et al. Drug-use patterns among black and nonblack community dwelling elderly. Ann Pharmacother 1992;26:679–685.
52. Roth MT, Ivet JL. Self-reported medication use in community-residing older adults: A pilot study. Am J Geriatr Pharmacother 2005;3:196–204.
53. Linjakumpu T, Hartikainen S, Klaukka T, Veijola J. Use of medications and polypharmacy are increasing among the elderly. J Clin Epidemiol 2002;55:809–817.
54. Kaufman DW, Kelly JP, Rosenberg L, et al. Recent Patterns of Medication Use in the Ambulatory Adult Population of the United States: The Slone Survey. JAMA 2002;287:337–344.
55. Tobias DE, Sey M. General and psychotherapeutic medication use in 328 nursing facilities: A year 2000 national survey. Consult Pharm 2001;16:54–64.
56. Schmader K, Hanlon JT, Weinberger M, et al. Appropriateness of medication prescribing in ambulatory elderly patients. J Am Geriatr Soc 1994;42:1241–1247.
57. Lipton HL, Bird JA. The impact of clinical pharmacists' consultations on geriatric patients' compliance and medical care use: A randomized, controlled trial. Gerontologist 1994;34:307–315.
58. Hajjar EH, Hanlon JT, Sloane RJ, et al. Unnecessary drug use in frail older people at hospital discharge. J Am Geriatr Soc 2005;53:1518–1523.

59. Montamat SC, Cusack B. Overcoming problems with polypharmacy and drug misuse in the elderly. Clin Geriatr Med 1992;8:143–158.
60. Hanlon JT, Schmader KE, Ruby CM, Weinberger M. Suboptimal prescribing in older inpatients and outpatients. J Am Geriatr Soc 2001;49:200–209.
61. Spinewine A, Schmader KE, Barber N, et al. Appropriate prescribing in elderly people: How well can it be measured and optimised? Lancet 2007;370:173–184.
62. Hanlon JT, Artz MB, Pieper CF, et al. Inappropriate medication use among frail elderly inpatients. Ann Pharmacother 2004;38:9–14.
63. Hanlon JT, Schmader KE, Boult C, et al. Use of inappropriate prescription drugs by older people. J Am Geriatr Soc 2002;50:26–34.
64. Lindblad CI, Hanlon JT, Gross CR, et al. Clinically important drug-disease interactions and their prevalence in older adults. Clin Ther 2006;28:1133–1143.
65. Fick DM, Cooper JW, Wade WE, et al. Updating the Beers criteria for potentially inappropriate medication use in older adults: Results of a US consensus panel of experts. Arch Intern Med 2003;163:2716–2724.
66. Fialova D, Topinkova E, Gambassi G, et al. Potentially inappropriate medication use among elderly home care patients in Europe. JAMA 2005;293:1348–1358.
67. Briesacher B, Limcangco R, Simoni-Wastila L, et al. Evaluation of nationally mandated drug use reviews to improve patient safety in nursing homes: A natural experiment. J Am Geriatr Soc 2005;53:991–996.
68. Spinewine A, Dumont C, Mallet L, Swine C. Medication Appropriateness Index: Reliability and recommendations for future use. J Am Geriatr Soc 2006;54:720–722.
69. Higashi T, Shekelle PG, Solomon DH, et al. The quality of pharmacologic care for vulnerable older patients. Ann Intern Med 2004;140:714–720.
70. Sloane PD, Gruber-Baldini Al, Zimmerman S, et al. Medication undertreatment in assisted living settings. Arch Intern Med 2004;164;2031–2037.
71. Soumerai SB, Ross-Degnan D, Avorn J, et al. Effects of Medicaid drug-payment limits on admission to hospitals and nursing homes. N Engl J Med 1991;325:1072–1077.
72. Tamblyn R, Laprise R, Hanley JA, et al. Adverse events associated with prescription drug cost-sharing among poor and elderly persons. JAMA 2001;285:421–429.
73. World Health Organization. Adherence to long-term therapies: Evidence for action. 2003, *http://www.who.int/topics/patient_adherence/en/*.
74. Hughes CM. Medication non-adherence in the elderly: How big is the problem? Drugs Aging 2004;21:793–811.
75. American Society on Aging and American Society of Consultant Pharmacists Foundation 2006. Medication adherence—Where are we today? 2007, *http://www.adultmeducation.com.*
76. German PS, Klein LE, McPhee SJ, et al. Knowledge of and compliance with drug regimens in the elderly. J Am Geriatr Soc 1982;30:568–571.
77. Park DC, Hertzog C, Leventhal H, et al. Medication adherence in rheumatoid arthritis patients: Older is wiser. J Am Geriatr Soc 1999;47:172–183.
78. Buist DSM, LaCroix AZ, Black DM, et al. Inclusion of older women in randomized clinical trials: Factors associated with taking study medication in the Fracture Intervention Trial. J Am Geriatr Soc 2000;48:1126–1131.
79. AARP. Prescription drug use among midlife and older Americans. Washington, DC: AARP, December 2004.
80. Soumerai SB, Pierre-Jacques M, Zhang F, et al. Cost-related medication nonadherence among elderly and disabled medicare beneficiaries: A national survey 1 year before the medicare drug benefit. Arch Intern Med 2007;166:1829–1835.
81. Moisan J, Gaudet M, Gregoire JP, et al. Non-compliance with drug treatment and reading difficulties with regard to prescription labeling among seniors. Gerontology 2002;48:44–51.
82. Vermiere E, Hearnshaw H, Van Royen P, et al. Patient adherence to treatment: Three decades of research: A comprehensive review. J Clin Pharm Ther 2001;26:331–342.
83. Col N, Fanale JE, Kronholm P. The role of medication noncompliance and adverse drug reactions in hospitalizations in the elderly. Arch Intern Med 1990;150:841–845.
84. Sokol MC, McGuigan KA, Verbrugge, Epstein RS. Impact of medication adherence on hospitalization and health care cost. Med Care 2005;43:521–530.
85. Hanlon JT, Lindblad CI, Gray SL. Evidence that clinical pharmacy services can have a positive impact on drug-related problems and health outcomes in community based older adults. Am J Geriatr Pharmacother 2003;1:38–43.
86. Zermansky AG, Alldred DP, Petty DR, et al. Clinical medication review by a pharmacist of elderly people living in care homes—Randomised controlled trial. Age Ageing 2006;35:586–591.
87. Lee JK, Grace KA, Taylor AJ. Effect of a pharmacy care program on medication adherence and persistence, blood pressure, and low-density lipoprotein cholesterol. A randomized controlled trial. JAMA 2006;296:2563–2571.
88. Orwig D, Brandt N, Gruber-Baldini AL. Medication management assessment for older adults in the community. Gerontologist 2006;46:661–668.
89. Chrischilles E, Rubenstein L, Van Gilder R, et al. Risk factors for adverse drug events in older adults with mobility limitations in the community setting. J Am Geriatric Soc 2007;55:29–34.
90. Kotylar M, Gray SL, Lindblad CI, Hanlon JT. Psychiatric manifestations of medications in the elderly. In: Malletta G, Agronin M, eds. Principles and Practice of Geriatric Psychiatry. Philadelphia: Lippincott Williams & Wilkins 2005:605–615.
91. Center for Medicaid and Medicare Services Unnecessary Medication Use (Tag F329) 2007, *http://www.cms.hhs.gov/transmittals/downloads/R22SOMA.pdf.*
92. Hanlon JT, Schmader KE, Samsa GP, et al. A method for assessing drug therapy appropriateness. J Clin Epidemiol 1992;45:1045–1051.
93. Shepherd J, Blauw GJ, Murphy MB, et al. PROspective Study of Pravastatin in the Elderly at Risk. Pravastatin in elderly individuals at risk of vascular disease (PROSPER): A randomized, controlled trial. Lancet 2002;360:1623–1630.
94. Ryan AA. Medication compliance and older people: A review of the literature. Int J Nurs Stud 1999;36:153–162.
95. van Eijken M, Tsang S, Wensing M, et al. Interventions to improve medication compliance in older patients living in the community: A systematic review of the literature. Drugs Aging 2003;20:229–240.
96. Cramer JA. Enhancing patient compliance in the elderly: Role of packaging aids and monitoring. Drugs Aging 1998;12:7–15.
97. Lapane, KL. Hughes, CM. Identifying nursing home residents at high risk for preventable adverse drug events: Modifying a tool for use in the Fleetwood Phase III study. Consult Pharm 2004;19:533–537.
98. Hajjar E, Artz MB, Lindblad CI, et al. Risk factors and prevalence for adverse drug reactions in an ambulatory elderly population. J Am Geriatr Soc 2004;52:S30–S31.

CHAPTER 9 Pharmacoepidemiology

ANDY STERGACHIS, THOMAS K. HAZLET, AND DENISE BOUDREAU

KEY CONCEPTS

1. Risks and benefits are commonly identified only after a drug is used widely by the general population.
2. Observational study designs are essential for the study of risks and benefits associated with marketed drugs.
3. Not all associations represent a cause-and-effect relationship.
4. Regulatory agencies are under pressure to identify and respond to postapproval drug safety issues.

(1) The practice of pharmacotherapy presents numerous challenges to clinicians as they apply knowledge of the benefits and risks of pharmaceuticals to individual and population-based patient care. A great deal of our understanding about the efficacy and short-term safety of drugs arises from well-controlled studies conducted during the drug development and approval process. However, many additional risks and, increasingly, additional benefits are only identified after the drug is used widely by the general population. Our gaps in knowledge of risks and benefits at the time a drug is marketed is a result of numerous characteristics of preapproval studies, including limited sample size, relatively short study followup, restricted characteristics of persons studied, and differences in research settings from real-life conditions once a drug is marketed. Benefits and risks learned following a drug's approval may range from relatively minor to clinically important effects that seriously alter an individual drug's risk-to-benefit profile. The association between certain appetite-suppressant drugs and primary pulmonary hypertension and valvular heart disease, and between some cyclooxygenase-2 inhibitors and cardiovascular events, are two examples where serious adverse effects were discovered only after these drugs had come into widespread use.[1–4] These examples highlight the inherent limitations of the drug development process, the limitations of the regulatory framework for contemporary medical products (drugs, biologics, and medical devices), and the need to study populations receiving medications obtained through usual clinical practice. The liver toxicity seen with troglitazone and more recently, rosiglitazone, is another example of the valuable contribution of close monitoring to drug safety. The first thiazolidinedione introduced for treatment of type 2 diabetes mellitus in 1997, troglitazone was withdrawn from the market based on reports of serious hepatocellular injury. In mid-2007, heart attacks and related deaths were observed in pooled clinical trials data for some patients receiving rosiglitazone, another thiazolidinedione subsequently approved for diabetes.[5] Medical products must also be monitored closely following their introduction into the marketplace, and this information has value when applied to clinical practice. This chapter describes the role of pharmacoepidemiology in drug development and therapeutics and characterizes the primary methods and contemporary issues in this field.

WWW
The complete chapter, learning objectives, and other resources can be found at **www.pharmacotherapyonline.com.**

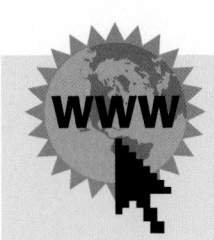

CHAPTER 10 Clinical Toxicology

PETER A. CHYKA

KEY CONCEPTS

1. Poisoning can result from exposure to excessive doses of any chemical, with medicines being responsible for most childhood and adult poisonings.
2. The total number and rate of poisonings have been increasing, but preventive measures, such as child-resistant containers, have reduced mortality in young children.
3. Immediate first aid may reduce the development of serious poisoning, and consultation with a poison control center may indicate the need for further therapy.
4. The use of ipecac syrup, gastric lavage, and cathartics has fallen out of favor as routine therapies, whereas activated charcoal and whole-bowel irrigation still are useful for gastric decontamination of appropriate patients.
5. Antidotes can prevent or reduce the toxicity of certain poisons, but symptomatic and supportive care is essential for all patients.
6. Acute acetaminophen poisoning produces severe liver injury and occasionally kidney failure. A determination of serum acetaminophen concentration may indicate whether there is risk of hepatotoxicity and the need for acetylcysteine therapy.
7. Anticholinesterase insecticides may produce life-threatening respiratory distress and paralysis by all routes of exposure and can be treated with symptomatic care, atropine, and pralidoxime.
8. An overdose of calcium channel antagonists will produce severe hypotension and bradycardia and can be treated with supportive care, calcium, glucagon, and insulin with supplemental dextrose.
9. Poisoning with iron-containing drugs produces vomiting, gross gastrointestinal bleeding, shock, metabolic acidosis, and coma and can be treated with supportive care and deferoxamine.
10. Overdoses of tricyclic antidepressants can cause arrhythmias, such as prolonged QRS intervals and ventricular dysrhythmias, coma, respiratory depression, and seizures and are treated with symptomatic care and intravenous sodium bicarbonate.

Poisoning is an adverse effect from a chemical that has been taken in excessive amounts. The body is able to tolerate and, in some cases, detoxify a certain dose of a chemical; however, once a critical threshold is exceeded, toxicity results. Poisoning can produce minor local effects that can be treated readily in the outpatient setting or systemic life-threatening effects that require intensive medical intervention. This spectrum of toxicity is typical for many chemicals with which humans come in contact. Virtually any chemical can become a poison when taken in sufficient quantity, but the potency of some compounds leads to serious toxicity with small quantities (Table 10–1).[1] Poisoning by chemicals includes exposure to drugs, industrial chemicals, household products, plants, venomous animals, and agrochemicals. This chapter describes some examples of this spectrum of toxicity, outlines means to recognize poisoning risk, and presents principles of treatment.

Learning objectives, review questions, and other resources can be found at **www.pharmacotherapyonline.com.**

EPIDEMIOLOGY

Each year poisonings account for approximately 30,000 deaths and at least 1.4 million emergency department visits in the United States.[2,3] Adults, 20 to 59 years of age are at greatest risk for a poisoning death, and males have a twofold higher incidence of death than do females. One fifth of all adult poisoning deaths are due to suicide. Poisoning deaths in adults are most commonly caused by motor vehicle exhaust (carbon monoxide), opioids, antidepressants, benzodiazepines, sedatives, alcohol, and cocaine.[3,4] Approximately 0.2% of poisoning deaths involve children younger than 5 years. The number and rates of poisoning deaths from all circumstances have been increasing steadily, with a 50% increase from 1999 to 2004.[3] Age-adjusted annual rates for unintentional poisoning deaths increased from 4.4 per 100,000 population in 1999 to 7.1 in 2004 (63% increase).[5] This increase in mortality is attributed to poisonings from drugs (primarily prescription opioids; secondarily cocaine and prescription psychotherapeutic drugs, e.g., sedatives), which increased by 68% compared to an increase of 1% from other substances.[5]

1 Several databases in the United States provide different levels of insight into and documentation of the poisoning problem (Table 10–2). Poisonings documented by U.S. poison centers are compiled in the annual report of the American Association of Poison Control Centers' National Poison Data System (AAPCC-NPDS).[6] Although it represents the largest database on poisoning, it

TABLE 10-1 Serious Toxicity in a Child Associated with Ingestion of One Mouthful or One Dosage Unit

Acids[a]	Cocaine
Anticholinesterase insecticides[a]	Colchicine
Caustics or alkalis[a]	Cyanide[a]
Cationic detergents[a]	Hydrocarbons[a]
Chloroquine	Methanol[a]
Clonidine	Phencyclidine or LSD

[a]Concentrated or undiluted form.

TABLE 10-2 Comparison of Various Poisoning Databases

Database (Abbreviation)	Characteristics
Death certificates from state health departments compiled by the National Center for Health Statistics (NCHS) *www.cdc.gov/ncipc/wisqars*	Compiles all death certificates whether the cause of death was by disease or external forces. Data typically verified by laboratory and clinical observations.
National Electronic Injury Surveillance System of U.S. Consumer Product Safety Commission (NEISS) *www.cdc.gov/ncipc/wisqars*	Surveys electronically all injuries, including poisonings, treated daily at a sample of approximately 100 emergency departments. Used to identify product-related injuries.
Drug Abuse Warning Network (DAWN) of the Federal Substance Abuse and Mental Health Services Administration *www.dawninfo.samhsa.gov* (SAMHSA)	Identifies substance abuse–related episodes and deaths as reported to approximately 420 hospitals and 120 medical examiners.
The American Association of Poison Control Centers'-National Poison Data System (AAPCC-NPDS) *www.aapcc.org*	Represents largest database of poisonings with high representation of children based on voluntary reporting to poison control centers.

is not complete because it relies on individuals voluntarily contacting a poison control center. The AAPCC-NPDS dataset captures approximately 5% of the annual number of deaths from poisoning tabulated in death certificates.[4] Despite this shortcoming, AAPCC-NPDS provides valuable insight into the characteristics and frequency of poisonings. In the 2005 AAPCC-NPDS summary, 2,424,180 poisoning exposures were reported by 61 participating poison centers that served a population of 296 million people.[6] Children younger than 6 years accounted for 51% of cases. The home was the site of exposure in 93% of the cases, and a single substance was involved in 91% of cases. An acute exposure accounted for 92% of cases, 84% of which were unintentional or accidental exposures. Only 13% were intentional. Fatalities accounted for 1,261 (0.05%) cases, of which 2% were children younger than 6 years. The distribution of substances most frequently involved in pediatric and adult exposures differed; however, medicines were the most frequently involved (51%) substances (Table 10–3). Seventy-four percent of the poison exposures were treated at the scene, typically a home. In summary, children account for most of the reported poisonings with morbidity, but adults account for a greater proportion of mortality from poisoning.

ECONOMIC IMPACT OF POISONING

Poisoning accounted for a total lifetime cost of $12.6 billion annually in 2003 dollars.[7] Estimates of the lifetime cost of injury include related health care costs and lost lifetime earnings of the victim; however, they do not include the costs of suffering, reduced productivity of caregivers, or legal costs. The definition of poisoning for this economic estimate excluded poisoning from alcohol and illicit drugs.

TABLE 10-3 Poison Exposure by Age Group and Fatal Outcome, Ranked in Decreasing Order

Pediatric	Adult	Fatal Outcome
Medicines	Medicines	Medicines
Cosmetics and personal care items	Cleaning substances	Alcohols
Cleaning substances	Bites or envenomations	Gases and fumes
Foreign bodies	Alcohols	Chemicals
Plants	Pesticides	Cleaning substances
Pesticides	Cosmetics and personal care items	Pesticides
Arts and crafts or office supplies	Food products or food poisoning	Automotive products

From Lai et al.[6]

TABLE 10-4 Examples of Products Requiring Child-Resistant Closures

Acetaminophen	Kerosene
Aspirin	Methanol
Diphenhydramine	Oral prescription drugs[a]
Ethylene glycol	Permanent hair wave neutralizers containing sodium bromate
Glue removers containing acetonitrile	Sodium hydroxide
Ibuprofen	Sulfuric acid
Iron pharmaceuticals	Turpentine

[a]With certain exceptions such as nitroglycerin and oral contraceptives.

POISON PREVENTION STRATEGIES

❷ The number of poisoning deaths in children has declined dramatically over the past three decades, due, in part, to the implementation of several poison prevention approaches.[7,8] These include the Poison Prevention Packaging Act (PPPA) of 1970, the evolution of regional poison control centers, the application of prompt first aid measures, improvements in overall critical care, development of less toxic product formulations, better clarity in the packaging and labeling of products, and public education on the risks and prevention of poisoning.[9] Although all these factors play a role in minimizing poisoning dangers, particularly in children, the PPPA has perhaps had the most significant influence.[8] The intent of the PPPA was to develop packaging that is difficult for children younger than 5 years to open or to obtain harmful amounts within a reasonable period of time. However, the packaging was not to be difficult for normal adults to use properly. Safety packaging is required for a number of products and product categories (Table 10–4). Child-resistant containers are not totally childproof and may be opened by children, which can result in poisoning. Despite the success of child-resistant containers, many adults disable the hardware or simply use no safety cap, thus placing children at risk.[10] Fatigue of the packaging materials can occur, which underscores the need for new prescription ware for refills, as required in the PPPA.[11]

Poison prevention requires constant vigilance because of new generations of families in which parents and grandparents must be educated on poisoning risks and prevention strategies. New products and changes in product formulations present different poisoning dangers and must be studied to provide optimal management. Strategies to prevent poisonings should consider the various psychosocial circumstances of poisoning (Table 10–5), prioritize risk groups and behaviors, and customize an intervention for specific situations.[12,13]

TABLE 10-5 Psychosocial Characteristics of Poisoning Patients

Children	Young Adults	Elderly
Act purposefully or are poisoned by caretaker or sibling	Intentional abuse or suicidal intent is possible	Suicidal intent or unintentional misuse
Act with developmentally appropriate curiosity	Disregard or cannot read directions	Confuse product identity and directions for use
Attracted by product appearance	Do not recognize poisoning risk	Do not recognize poisoning risk
Ingest substances that adults find unpleasant	Reluctant to seek assistance until ill	Comorbid conditions complicate toxicity
React to stressful and disrupted household	Exaggerate or misrepresent situation	Unable or unwilling to describe situation
Imitate adult behaviors (e.g., taking medicine)	Peer pressure to experiment with drugs	Multiple drugs may lead to adverse reactions

TABLE 10-6 Considerations in Evaluating the Results of Some Common Immunoassays Used for Urine Drug Screening

Drug	Detection after Stopping Use	Comments
Amphetamines	2–5 days	Many sympathomimetic amines, such as pseudoephedrine, ephedra, phenylephrine, fenfluramine, and phentermine, may cause positive results.
	Up to 2 weeks with prolonged or heavy use	Other drugs, such as selegiline, chlorpromazine, trazodone, bupropion, and amantadine, may cause false-positive results depending on the assay.
Benzodiazepines	Up to 2 weeks Up to 6 weeks with chronic use of some drugs	Ability to detect benzodiazepines varies by drug.
Cannabinoid metabolite (marijuana)	7–10 days Up to 1–2 months with prolonged or heavy use	Extent and duration of use will affect detection time. Drugs such as ibuprofen and naproxen may cause false-positive results depending on the assay.
Cocaine metabolite (benzoylecgonine)	12–72 hours Up to 1–3 weeks with prolonged or heavy use	Cocaine is metabolized rapidly, and specific metabolites are typically the substance detected. False-positive results from "caine" anesthetics and other drugs are unlikely.
Opioids	2–3 days Up to 6 days with sustained-release formulations Up to 1 week with prolonged or heavy use	Because the assay was made to detect morphine, detection of other opioids, such as codeine, oxycodone, hydrocodone, and other semisynthetic opioids, may be limited. Some synthetic opioids, such as fentanyl and meperidine, may not be detected. Drugs such as rifampin and some fluoroquinolones may cause false-positive results depending on the assay.
Phencyclidine	2–10 days 1 month or more with prolonged or heavy use	Drugs such as ketamine, dextromethorphan, diphenhydramine, and sertraline may cause false-positive results depending upon the assay.

RECOGNITION AND ASSESSMENT

The clinician's initial responsibility is to determine whether a poisoning has occurred or a potential for development of a poisoning exists. Some patients provide a clear account of an exposure that occurred with a known quantity of a specific agent. Other patients appear with an unexplained illness characterized by nonspecific signs and symptoms and no immediate history of ingestion. Exposure to folk remedies, dietary supplements, and environmental toxins also should be considered. Patients with suicide gestures can deliberately give an unclear history, and poisoning should be suspected routinely. Poisoning and drug overdoses should be suspected in any patient with a sudden, unexplained illness or with a puzzling combination of signs and symptoms, particularly in high-risk age groups. Nearly any symptom can be seen with poisoning, but some signs and symptoms are suggestive of a particular toxin exposure.[14] Compounds that produce characteristic clinical pictures (toxidromes), such as or–ganophosphate poisoning with pinpoint pupils, rales, bradycardia, central nervous system depression, sweating, excessive salivation, and diarrhea, are most readily recognizable.[15] The recognition of chemicals responsible for acute mass emergencies resulting from industrial disasters, hazardous materials accidents, or acts of terrorism may be aided by evaluating characteristic signs and symptoms.[16] Assessment of the patient may be aided by consultation with a poison control center. The center can provide information on product composition, typical symptoms, range of toxicity, laboratory analysis, treatment options, and bibliographic references. Furthermore, the center will have specially trained physicians, pharmacists, nurses, and toxicologists on staff or available for consultation to assist with difficult cases. Consultation with a poison control center also may identify changes in recommended therapy. A nationwide toll-free poison center access number (1-800-222-1222) routes callers to the local poison control center.

When the circumstances of a poison exposure indicate that it is minimally toxic, many poisonings can be managed successfully at the scene of the poisoning.[6,17] Poison control centers typically monitor the victim by telephone during the first 2 to 6 hours of the exposure to assess the patient's status and outcome of first aid.

Once a poisoning is suspected and confirmation of the diagnosis is needed for medical or legal purposes, appropriate biologic material should be sent to the laboratory for analysis. Gastric contents may contain the greatest concentration of drug, but they are difficult to analyze. Blood or urine can be tested by qualitative screening in order to detect a drug's presence.[18,19] The results of a qualitative drug screen can be misleading because of interfering or low-level substances (Table 10–6); it rarely guides emergency therapy and thus has questionable value for nonspecific, general screening purposes.[18,19] Consultation with the laboratory technician and review of the assay package insert will help to determine the sensitivity and specificity of the assay. Quantitative determination of serum concentrations may be important for the assessment of some poisonings, such as those containing acetaminophen, ethanol, methanol, iron, theophylline, and digoxin.[20]

PHARMACOKINETICS OF OVERDOSE

The pharmacokinetic characteristics of drugs taken in overdose may differ from those observed following therapeutic doses (Table 10–7).[21,22] These differences are the result of dose-dependent changes in absorption, distribution, metabolism, or elimination;

TABLE 10-7 Examples of the Influence of Drug Overdosage on Pharmacokinetic and Pharmacodynamic Characteristics

Effect of Overdosage[a]	Examples
Slowed absorption due to formation of poorly soluble concretions in the gastrointestinal tract	Aspirin, lithium, phenytoin, sustained-release theophylline
Slowed absorption due to slowed gastrointestinal motility	Benztropine, nortriptyline
Slowed absorption due to toxin-induced hypoperfusion	Procainamide
Decreased serum protein binding	Lidocaine, salicylates, valproic acid
Increased volume of distribution associated with toxin-induced acidemia	Salicylates
Slowed elimination due to saturation of biotransformation pathways	Ethanol, phenytoin, salicylates, theophylline
Slowed elimination due to toxin-induced hypothermia (<35°C)	Ethanol, propranolol
Prolonged toxicity due to formation of longer-acting metabolites	Carbamazepine, dapsone, glutethimide, meperidine

[a]Compared to characteristics following therapeutic doses or resolution of toxicity.

pharmacologic effects of the drug; or pathophysiologic consequences of the overdose. Dose-dependent changes may decrease the rate and extent of absorption, whereas the bioavailability of the agent may be increased due to saturation of first-pass metabolism. The distribution of a compound may be altered due to saturation of protein-binding sites. Metabolism and elimination of a compound may be retarded due to saturation of biotransformation pathways leading to nonlinear elimination kinetics. Delayed gastric emptying by anticholinergic drugs or as the result of general central nervous system depression caused by many drugs may alter the rate and extent of absorption. Patients with a drug overdose may inherently exhibit prolonged gastric emptying and gastric hypomotility.[23] The formation of concretions or bezoars of solid dosage forms may delay the onset, prolong the duration, or complicate the therapy for an acute overdose.[24] A combination of pharmacokinetic and pharmacodynamic factors may lead to delayed onset of toxicity of several toxins, such as thyroid hormones, oral anticoagulants, acetaminophen, and drugs in sustained-release dosage forms.[25] Drug-induced hypoperfusion may affect drug distribution and result in reduced hepatic or renal clearance. Changes in blood pH may alter the distribution of weak acids and bases. Drug-induced renal or hepatic injury also can decrease clearance significantly. Implications of these changes for poisoning management include delayed achievement of peak concentrations with a corresponding longer period of opportunity to remove the drug from the gastrointestinal tract. The expected duration of effects may be much greater than that observed with therapeutic doses because of continued absorption and impaired clearance. The application of pharmacokinetic variables, such as percentage protein binding and volume of distribution, from therapeutic doses may not be appropriate in poisoning cases.[21] Data on toxicokinetics often are difficult to interpret and compare because the doses and times of ingestion are uncertain, the duration of sampling is inadequate, active metabolites may not be measured, protein binding typically is not assessed, and the severity of toxicity may vary dramatically.

TREATMENT

Clinical Toxicology

GENERAL APPROACHES TO TREATMENT OF THE POISONED PATIENT

■ PREHOSPITAL CARE

First Aid

❸ The presence of adequate airway, breathing, and circulation should be assessed, and cardiopulmonary resuscitation should be started if needed. The most important step in preventing a minor exposure from progressing to a serious intoxication is early decontamination of the poison. Basic poisoning first aid and decontamination measures (Table 10–8) should be instituted immediately at the scene of the poisoning. If there is any question about the potential severity of the poison exposure, a poison control center should be consulted immediately (1-800-222-1222). While awaiting transport, placing the patient on the left side may afford easier clearance of the airway if emesis occurs and may slow absorption of drug from the gastrointestinal tract.[26]

TABLE 10-8 First Aid for Poison Exposures

Inhaled poison
Immediately get the person to fresh air. Avoid breathing fumes. Open doors and windows. If victim is not breathing, start artificial respiration.
Poison on the skin
Remove contaminated clothing and flood skin with water for 10 minutes. Wash gently with soap and water and rinse. Avoid further contamination of victim or first aid providers.
Poison in the eye
Flood the eye with lukewarm or cool water poured from a glass 2 or 3 inches from the eye. Repeat for 10–15 continuous minutes. Keep eye open, but do not force the eyelid open.
Swallowed poison
Unless the patient is unconscious, having convulsions, or cannot swallow, give 2–4 ounces of water immediately and then seek further help.

Ipecac Syrup

❹ Ipecac syrup, a nonprescription drug, has been used in the United States for the past 50 years as a means to induce vomiting for treatment of ingested poisons. Despite its widespread use, concerns about its effectiveness and safety have been raised recently. An expert panel of North American and European toxicologists concluded that its routine use in the emergency department should be abandoned.[27] In 2003 the American Academy of Pediatrics issued a policy statement indicating that ipecac syrup was no longer to be used routinely to treat poisonings at home and that parents should discard any ipecac.[28] The key reason for the policy change was that research failed to show benefits in children who were treated with ipecac syrup. It likely will take several years for these recommendations to be adopted fully by parents and healthcare professionals, and rare exceptions may arise. In the 2005 AAPCC-NPDS report, 0.1% of 2.4 million cases received ipecac syrup, with or without poison center direction.[6]

There are several contraindications to the use of ipecac syrup or any form of induced emesis, such as gagging.[27] If the patient is without a gag reflex; is lethargic, comatose, or convulsing; or is expected to become unresponsive within the next 30 minutes, emesis should not be induced. If a fruitful emesis has occurred spontaneously shortly after ingestion, further emesis may not be necessary. Ingestions of caustics, corrosives, ammonia, and bleach are definite contraindications to induced emesis. Ingestion of aliphatic hydrocarbons (e.g., gasoline, kerosene, and charcoal lighter fluid) typically does not require emesis. When the agent is definitely known to be nontoxic, induction of emesis is purposeless and potentially dangerous. The rapid onset of coma or seizures or the potential to exaggerate the toxic effects of the poison may preclude the induction of emesis. Some examples include poisonings with diphenoxylate, propoxyphene, clonidine, tricyclic antidepressants, hypoglycemic agents, nicotine, strychnine, β-blocking agents, and calcium channel blockers. Debilitated, pregnant, and elderly patients may be further compromised by induction of emesis.

■ HOSPITAL TREATMENT

General Care

Supportive and symptomatic care is the mainstay of treatment of a poisoned patient. In the search for specific antidotes and methods to increase excretion of the drug, attention to vital signs and organ functions should not be neglected. Establishment of adequate oxygenation and maintenance of adequate circulation are the highest priorities. Other components of the acute supportive care plan include the management of seizures, arrhythmias, hypotension, acid–base balance, fluid status, electrolyte balance, and hypoglycemia. Placement of intravenous and urinary catheters is typical to ensure delivery of fluids and drugs when necessary and to monitor urine production, respectively.

Gastric Lavage

Gastric lavage involves the placement of an orogastric tube and washing out of the gastric contents through repetitive instillation and withdrawal of fluid. Gastric lavage may be considered only if a potentially toxic agent has been ingested within the past hour for most patients. If the patient is comatose or lacks a gag reflex, gastric lavage should be performed only after intubation with a cuffed or well-fitting endotracheal tube. The largest orogastric tube that can be passed (external diameter at least 12 mm in adults and 8 mm in children) should be used to ensure adequate evacuation, especially of undissolved tablets. Lavage should be performed with warm (37°C to 38°C) normal saline or tap water until the gastric return is clear; this usually requires 2 to 4 L or more of fluid. Relative contraindications for gastric lavage include ingestion of a corrosive or hydrocarbon agent. Complications of gastric lavage include aspiration pneumonitis, laryngospasm, mechanical injury to the esophagus and stomach, hypothermia, and fluid and electrolyte imbalance.[29] Use of gastric lavage has declined in recent years as evidenced by the finding that only 2.2% of 553,292 cases treated at a healthcare facility received gastric lavage.[6]

Single-Dose Activated Charcoal

Reduction of toxin absorption can be achieved by administration of activated charcoal. It is a highly purified, adsorbent form of carbon that prevents gastrointestinal absorption of a drug by chemically binding (adsorbing) the drug to the charcoal surface. There are no toxin-related contraindications to its use, but it is generally ineffective for iron, lead, lithium, simple alcohols, and corrosives. It is not indicated for aliphatic hydrocarbons because of the increased risk for emesis and pulmonary aspiration. Activated charcoal is most effective when given within the first few hours after ingestion, ideally within the first hour.[30] The recommended dose of activated charcoal for a child (1 to 12 years old) is 25 to 50 g; for an adolescent or adult the recommended dose is 25 to 100 g. Children younger than 1 year can receive 1 g/kg.[9] Activated charcoal is mixed with water to make a slurry, shaken vigorously, and administered orally or via a nasogastric tube. Activated charcoal is contraindicated when the gastrointestinal tract is not intact. Activated charcoal is relatively nontoxic, but two identified risks are (a) emesis following administration and (b) pulmonary aspiration of charcoal and gastric contents leading to pneumonitis in patients with an unprotected airway or absent gag reflex.[30] Some activated charcoal products contain sorbitol, a cathartic that may be associated with an increased incidence of emesis following use.[31] Single-dose activated charcoal use has remained relatively steady during the past decade, with 4.9% of 2.4 million cases having received it according to the 2005 AAPCC-NPDS report.[6]

Cathartics

Cathartics, such as magnesium citrate and sorbitol, were thought to decrease the rate of absorption by increasing gastrointestinal elimination of the poison and the poison-activated charcoal complex, but their value is unproven. Poisoned patients do not routinely require a cathartic, and it is rarely, if ever, given without concurrent activated charcoal administration.[32] If used, a cathartic should be administered only once and only if bowel sounds are present. Infants, the elderly, and patients with renal failure should be given saline cathartics cautiously, if at all.[9,32]

CLINICAL CONTROVERSY

Activated charcoal has been promoted for use at home as a replacement for ipecac syrup, but some have contended that little evidence indicates activated charcoal can be used safely and properly in this setting.

Whole-Bowel Irrigation

Polyethylene glycol electrolyte solutions, such as GoLYTELY and Colyte, are used routinely as whole-bowel irrigants prior to colonoscopy and bowel surgery.[33] These solutions also can be used to decontaminate the gastrointestinal tract of ingested toxins.[9,14,34] Large volumes of these osmotically balanced solutions are administered continuously through a nasogastric or duodenal tube for 4 to 12 hours or more. They quickly cause gastrointestinal evacuation and are continued until the rectal discharge is relatively clear. This procedure may be indicated for certain patients in whom the ingestion occurred several hours prior to hospitalization and the drug still is suspected to be in the gastrointestinal tract, such as drug smugglers who swallow condoms filled with cocaine.[35] In addition, patients who have ingested delayed-release or enteric-coated drug formulations or have ingested substances such as iron that are not well adsorbed by activated charcoal may benefit from whole-bowel irrigation.[34] It should not be used in patients with a bowel perforation or obstruction, gastrointestinal hemorrhage, ileus, or intractable emesis. Emesis, abdominal cramps, and intestinal bloating have been reported with whole-bowel irrigation.[34] During 2005, whole-bowel irrigation was used in 0.5% of 553,292 cases managed at a healthcare facility.[6]

CLINICAL CONTROVERSY

Some clinicians believe that whole-bowel irrigation should be used more routinely as a rapid means to evacuate the gastrointestinal tract. Others recognize that it does have a quick onset but point out that little proof indicates whole-bowel irrigation makes a difference in patient outcome.

Perspectives on Gastric Decontamination

Although there are a variety of options for gastric decontamination, two clinical toxicology groups (the American Academy of Clinical Toxicology and the European Association of Poison Centers and Clinical Toxicologists) have concluded that no means of gastric decontamination should be used routinely for a poisoned patient without careful consideration.[27,29,30,32,34] They indicate that therapy is most effective within the first hour and that effectiveness beyond this time cannot be supported or refuted with the available data. A clinical policy statement by the American College of Emergency Physicians concludes that although no definitive recommendation can be made on the use of ipecac syrup, gastric lavage, cathartics, or whole-bowel irrigation, activated charcoal is advocated for most patients when appropriate.[36] The clinical policy also states that ipecac syrup is rarely of value in the emergency department and that the use of whole-bowel irrigation following ingestion of substances not well adsorbed by activated charcoal is not supported by evidence. The efficacy of activated charcoal has been demonstrated for many compounds,[30] but a randomized, controlled clinical trial of poisoned patients indicated that charcoal therapy did not reduce length of hospital stay or positively influence patient outcomes.[37] Although gastric lavage can reduce drug absorption if performed within 1 hour of ingestion, its use is not recommended routinely.[29,36,38] In recent years, the use of ipecac syrup has declined markedly in part because of its apparent lower efficacy compared with activated charcoal in minimizing drug absorption.[6,27,30] The American Academy of Pediatrics has recommended that ipecac syrup no longer be used for treatment of poisonings at home and has called for its removal from the home.[28] Recently, activated charcoal has been promoted for treatment of poisonings at home, but issues of safety, patient compliance, and effectiveness have not been proven in the home setting.[28,39] Poison control centers may be a source of guidance on the contemporary application of gastric decontamination techniques for a specific patient.

Enhanced Elimination Numerous methods have been used to increase the rate of excretion of poisons from the body. Of these, only diuresis, multiple-dose activated charcoal, and hemodialysis have demonstrated usefulness. These approaches should be considered only if the risks of the procedure are significantly outweighed by the expected benefits or if the recovery of the patient is seriously in doubt and the method has been shown to be helpful.

Diuresis Diuresis can be used for poisons excreted predominantly by the renal route; however, most drugs and poisons are metabolized, and only a good urine flow (e.g., 2 to 3 mL/kg/h) needs to be maintained for most patients. Fluid and electrolyte balance should be monitored closely. Ionized diuresis by altering urinary pH may increase excretion of certain chemicals that are weak acids or bases by trapping ionized drug in the renal tubule and minimizing reabsorption.[14] Alkalinization of the urine to achieve a urine pH of 7.5 or greater for poisoning by weak acids such as salicylates or phenobarbital can be achieved by intravenous administration of sodium bicarbonate 1 to 2 mEq/kg over a 1- to 2-hour period. Complications of urinary alkalinization include alkalosis, fluid and electrolyte disturbances, and inability to achieve target urinary pH values.[40] Acid diuresis may enhance the excretion of weak bases, such as amphetamines, but it is rarely, if ever, used because it risks worsening rhabdomyolysis commonly associated with amphetamine overdose.[14] Generally, diuresis or ionized diuresis is rarely indicated for poisoned patients because it is inefficient relative to other methods of enhancing elimination, it is associated with a risk of unacceptable adverse effects, and renal elimination of most drugs is not enhanced dramatically.

Multiple-Dose Activated Charcoal Multiple doses of activated charcoal can augment the body's clearance of certain drugs by enhanced passage from the bloodstream into the gastrointestinal tract and subsequent adsorption. This process, termed *charcoal intestinal dialysis* or *charcoal-enhanced intestinal exsorption,* describes the attraction of drug molecules across the capillary bed of the intestine by activated charcoal in the intestinal lumen and subsequent adsorption of the drug to the charcoal.[41] Furthermore, it may interrupt the enterohepatic recirculation of certain drugs.[14,41] Once the drug is adsorbed to the charcoal, it is eliminated with the charcoal in the stool. Systemic clearance of several drugs has been shown to be enhanced up to severalfold.[41,42] An international toxicology group's position statement on multiple-dose activated charcoal concluded that it should be considered only if a patient has ingested a life-threatening amount of carbamazepine, dapsone, phenobarbital, quinine, or theophylline.[42] Although a prospective, randomized study of the effects of multiple-dose activated charcoal on phenobarbital-overdosed patients demonstrated increased drug elimination, no demonstrable effect on patient outcome was observed.[43]

This approach provides a rapid onset of action that is limited by blood flow and a maximal "ceiling effect" related to the dose of charcoal present in the intestine. The response to multiple-dose activated charcoal is greatest for drugs with the following characteristics: good affinity for adsorption by activated charcoal, low intrinsic clearance, sufficient residence time in the body (long serum half-life), long distributive phase, and nonrestrictive protein binding. A small volume of distribution is desirable, but it has a marginal influence as an isolated characteristic,[44] particularly if multiple-dose activated charcoal is instituted during the toxin's distributive phase. A typical dosage schedule is 15 to 25 g of activated charcoal every 2 to 6 hours until serious symptoms abate or the serum concentration of the toxin is below the toxic range. This procedure has been used in premature and full-term infants in doses of 1 g/kg every 1 to 4 hours. Serious complications, such as pulmonary aspiration, occur in <1% of patients.[45] The risks of aspiration pneumonitis in obtunded or uncooperative patients and of intestinal obstruction in patients prone to ileus following a period of bowel ischemia (e.g., after cardiopulmonary arrest in the elderly) may be higher.[46] Contraindications are the same as those for single-dose charcoal.

Hemodialysis Hemodialysis may be necessary for certain severe cases of poisoning. Dialysis should be considered when the duration of symptoms is expected to be prolonged, normal pathways of excretion are compromised, clinical deterioration is present, the drug is dialyzable, and appropriate personnel and equipment are available. Drugs that are hemodialyzable usually have a low molecular weight, are not highly or tightly protein bound, and are not highly distributed to tissues. The principles of hemodialysis for acutely ill individuals are described in Chap. 48. Hemodialysis and charcoal hemoperfusion are efficient methods of dialysis, but both pose serious risks related to anticoagulation, blood transfusions, loss of blood elements, fluid and electrolyte disturbances, and infection.[47] Hemodialysis may be lifesaving for methanol and ethylene glycol poisoning and effective for other poisons, such as lithium, salicylates, ethanol, and theophylline.[14,36] Charcoal hemoperfusion was popular in the 1970s and 1980s as a means to remove toxins, but this approach has fallen out of favor because of poor clinical results, inappropriate use for drugs with large volumes of distribution, and limited availability of charcoal hemoperfusion columns.[48] Continuous hemofiltration transports drugs across a semipermeable membrane by convection in response to hydrostatic pressure gradients.[14,47] Limited experience is reported with the use of hemofiltration for poisonings, but it may be attractive for the hemodynamically unstable patient who cannot tolerate hemodialysis.

Antidotes

❺ The search for and use of an antidote should never replace good supportive care.[36] Specific systemic antidotes are available for many common poisonings (Table 10–9). [49,50] Inadequate availability of antidotes at acute care hospitals has been noted throughout the United States and can complicate the care of a poisoned patient. An evidenced-based consensus of experts has recommended minimum stocking requirements for 16 antidotes for acute care hospitals.[51] These recommendations may provide guidance to pharmacy and therapeutics committees in establishing a hospital's antidote needs. Drugs used conventionally for nonpoisoning situations may act as antidotes to reverse acute toxicity, such as glucagon for β-adrenergic blocker or calcium channel antagonist overdose and octreotide for sulfonylurea-induced hypoglycemia.[52] As our understanding of drug toxicity increases, antidotes may have applications beyond contemporary indications, such as for acetylcysteine, which has shown promise for treating approximately 25 different poisonings and adverse drug reactions.[53] The use of toxin-specific antibodies (e.g., fragment antigen binding [Fab] antibody fragments for digoxin[54] or crotalid snake venom[55]) has offered a new approach to treatment of poisoning victims.

Assessing the Effectiveness of Therapies

Our knowledge of poisoning treatment is derived from case reports, clinical studies, human volunteer studies, animal investigations, and in vitro tests. Each of these approaches has limited applicability to the care of humans who have been poisoned. Case reports often are difficult to assess because they are uncontrolled, the histories are uncertain, and multiple therapies frequently are used. However, they can be useful to describe unique or new toxicities or characterize adverse effects associated with a therapy. Although clinical studies may describe tens to hundreds of patients, they can exhibit

TABLE 10-9 Systemic Antidotes Available in the United States

Toxic Agent	Antidote
Acetaminophen	Acetylcysteine
Anticholinesterase insecticides	Atropine
Anticoagulants	Phytonadione
Benzodiazepines	Flumazenil
Botulism	Botulism antitoxin
Carbon monoxide	Oxygen
Cyanide	Cyanide antidote kit (amyl nitrite, sodium nitrate, and sodium thiosulfate)
Cyanide	Hydroxocobalamin
Digoxin	Digoxin immune Fab
Ethylene glycol, methanol	Ethanol
Ethylene glycol, methanol	Fomepizole
Heavy metals (arsenic, inorganic mercury, lead, gold)	Dimercaprol
Heavy metals (copper, lead)	Penicillamine
Iron	Deferoxamine
Isoniazid	Pyridoxine
Lead	Calcium EDTA
Lead	Succimer
Methemoglobinemia	Methylene blue
Opioids	Nalmefene
Opioids	Naloxone
Organophosphate insecticides	Pralidoxime
Radioactive americium, curium, plutonium	Diethylenetriamene pentaacetate
Radioactive iodine	Potassium iodide
Snake, coral	*Micrurus fulvius* antivenin
Snakes (rattlesnakes, cotton-mouth, copperhead)	*Crotalidae* polyvalent antivenin
	Crotalidae polyvalent immune Fab
Spider, black widow	*Lactrodectus mactans* antivenin
Thallium	Prussian blue

serious shortcomings, such as weak randomization procedures, no laboratory confirmation or correlation with history, insufficient number of severe cases, no control group, and no quantitative measure of outcome. Extrapolation of data from human volunteer studies to patients who overdose is difficult because of potential or unknown variations in pharmacokinetics (e.g., differing dissolution, gastric emptying, and absorption rates) seen with toxic as opposed to therapeutic doses,[21,22] differences in time to institute therapy in the emergency setting, and differences in absorption in fasted human volunteers compared with the full stomach of some patients who overdose. However, these studies provide the most controlled and objective measures of the efficacy of a treatment. Experiences from animal studies cannot be applied directly to humans because of interspecies differences in toxicity and metabolism. In vitro tests serve to screen the efficacy of some approaches, such as activated charcoal adsorption, but they do not mimic physiologic conditions sufficiently to allow direct clinical application of the findings. Despite their limitations, these data compose the basis for the therapy of poisoned patients and are tempered with the consideration of nonpoisoning-related factors such as a particular patient's underlying medical condition, age, and need for concurrent supportive measures.

CLINICAL SPECTRUM OF POISONING

Poisoning and drug overdose with acetaminophen, anticholinesterase insecticides, calcium channel blockers, iron, and tricyclic antidepressants are the focus of the remainder of this chapter because they represent commonly encountered poisonings for which pharmacotherapy is indicated. These agents also were chosen because they represent common examples with different mechanisms of toxicity, and they illustrate the application of general treatment approaches as well as some agent-specific interventions.

ACETAMINOPHEN

Clinical Presentation

❻ Acute acetaminophen poisoning characteristically results in hepatotoxicity[56,57] and is the leading cause of acute liver failure in the United States.[58] Clinical presentation (see below) is dependent on the time since ingestion, presence of risk factors, and the ingestion of other drugs. During the first 12 to 24 hours after ingestion, nausea, vomiting, anorexia, and diaphoresis may be observed; however, many patients are asymptomatic. During the next 1 to 3 days, which is a latent phase of lessened symptoms, patients often have an asymptomatic rise in liver enzymes and bilirubin. Signs and symptoms of hepatic injury become manifest 3 to 5 days after ingestion and include right upper quadrant abdominal tenderness, jaundice, hypoglycemia, and encephalopathy. Prolongation of the prothrombin time worsens as hepatic necrosis progresses and may lead to disseminated intravascular coagulopathy. Patients with hepatic damage may develop hepatic coma and hepatorenal syndrome, and death can occur.[56,57,59] Even in patients with severe hepatotoxicity, usually no residual functional or histologic abnormalities of the liver are noted within 1 to 6 months of the incident.[57]

CLINICAL PRESENTATION OF ACUTE ACETAMINOPHEN POISONING

General

- No or mild nonspecific symptoms within 6 hours of ingestion

Symptoms

- Nausea, vomiting, and abdominal discomfort within 1 to 12 hours after ingestion
- Right upper abdominal quadrant tenderness typically within 1 to 2 days

Signs

- Typically no signs present within first day
- Jaundice, scleral icterus, bleeding within 3 to 10 days
- Oliguria occasionally within 2 to 7 days
- With severe poisoning, hepatic encephalopathy (delirium, depressed reflexes, coma) within 5 to 10 days

Laboratory Tests

- Toxic serum acetaminophen concentration no earlier than 4 hours after ingestion by comparison with nomogram
- Elevated aspartate aminotransferase (AST), alanine aminotransferase (ALT), serum bilirubin, and international normalization ratio (INR); hypoglycemia within 1 to 3 days
- Elevated serum creatinine and blood urea nitrogen (BUN) within 2 to 7 days

Mechanism of Toxicity

Acetaminophen is metabolized in the liver primarily to glucuronide or sulfate conjugates, which are excreted into the urine with small amounts (<5%) of unchanged drug. Approximately 5% of a therapeutic dose is metabolized by the cytochrome P450 mixed-function oxygenase system, primarily CYP2E1, to a reactive metabolite, *N*-acetyl-*p*-benzoquinoneimine (NAPQI). This metabolite normally is conjugated with glutathione, a sulfhydryl-containing compound, in the hepatocyte and excreted in the urine as a mercapturate conjugate (Fig. 10–1).[59]

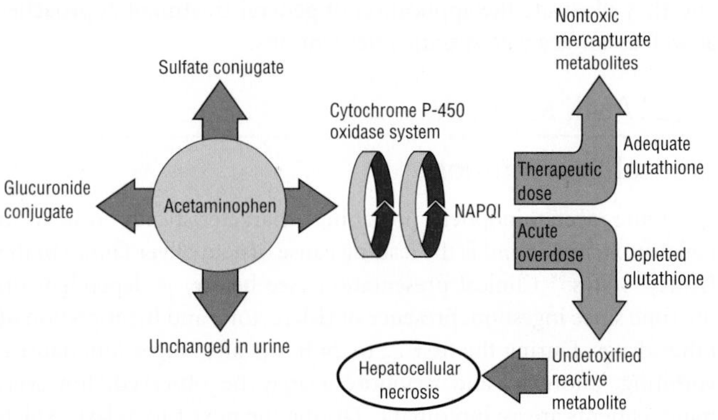

FIGURE 10-1. Pathway of acetaminophen metabolism and basis for hepatotoxicity. (NAPQI, *N*-acetyl-*p*-benzoquinoneimine, a reactive acetaminophen metabolite.)

In an acute overdose situation, sulfate stores are depleted, shifting more drug through the cytochrome system, thereby depleting the available glutathione used to detoxify the reactive metabolite. The reactive metabolite NAPQI then reacts with other hepatocellular sulfhydryl compounds such as those in the cytosol, cell wall, and endoplasmic reticulum. This results in centrilobular hepatic necrosis.[59] Several other mechanisms, such as cytokine release and oxidative stress, also may be initiated by the initial cellular injury.[59]

In many cases of severe hepatotoxicity, renal injury also is present and may range from oliguria to acute renal failure. The etiology of the renal injury may be a direct effect of the toxic metabolite of acetaminophen, NAPQI, generated by renal cytochrome oxidase, or a consequence of hepatic injury resulting in hepatorenal syndrome.[60]

Causative Agents

Acetaminophen, also known as paracetamol, is available widely without prescription as an analgesic and antipyretic. It is available in various oral dosage forms, including extended-release preparations. Acetaminophen may be combined with other drugs, such as antihistamines or opioid analgesics, and marketed in cough and cold preparations, menstrual remedies, and allergy products.

Incidence

Acetaminophen is one of the drugs most commonly ingested by small children and is used commonly in suicide attempts by adolescents and adults. The 2005 AAPCC-NPDS report documented 67,393 nonfatal exposures and 138 deaths from acetaminophen, with 49% of the exposures in children younger than 6 years.[6]

Age-based differences in the metabolism of acetaminophen appear to be responsible for major differences in the incidence of serious toxicity. Despite the common ingestion of acetaminophen by young children, few develop hepatotoxicity from acute overdosage.[6] In children younger than 9 to 12 years, acetaminophen undergoes more sulfation and less glucuronidation. The reduced fraction available for metabolism by the cytochrome system may explain the rare development of serious toxicity in young children who take large overdoses. Earlier treatment intervention and spontaneous emesis also may reduce the risk of toxicity in children.

Risk Assessment

There is a risk of developing hepatotoxicity when patients 6 years or older acutely ingest at least 10 g or 200 mg/kg, whichever is less, of acetaminophen or when children younger than 6 years acutely ingest 200 mg/kg or more.[61] Patients have survived much larger doses, particularly with early treatment. Initial symptoms, if present, do not predict how serious the toxicity eventually may become.

Chronic exposure to drugs that induce the cytochrome oxidase system—specifically isoenzyme CYP2E1, which is responsible for most of the formation of NAPQI—may increase the risk of acetaminophen hepatotoxicity. Poorer outcomes have been noted in patients who chronically ingest alcohol and those receiving anticonvulsants, both known to induce CYP2E1.[57,62] Patients with chronic alcoholism have a 3.5 greater odds of mortality with acute acetaminophen poisoning.[63] Concurrent acute ingestion of alcohol and acetaminophen may decrease the risk of acetaminophen-induced hepatotoxicity by ethanol acting as a competitive substrate for CYP2E1, thus reducing NAPQI formation.[64] Ethanol coingestion is not advocated as a preventive measure, and it is difficult to account for its specific impact on care.

Repeated ingestion of supratherapeutic doses of acetaminophen (defined for patients <6 years: ≥200 mg/kg over 8 to 24 hours, ≥150 mg/kg/day for 2 days, ≥100 mg/kg/day for 3 days or longer; for patients ≥6 years: ≥10 g or 200 mg/kg (whichever is less) over a single 24-hour period, ≥6 g or 150 mg/kg (whichever is less) per 24-hour period for ≥48 hours) has been associated with hepatotoxicity.[57,61] Patients who are fasting or have ingested alcohol in the preceding 5 days appear to be at greater risk.[65] Young children who receive repetitive supratherapeutic doses of acetaminophen have a higher risk of developing hepatotoxicity, particularly when they have been acutely fasting as the result of a febrile illness or gastroenteritis.[61,66] Patients with suspected risk factors, such as alcoholism, isoniazid therapy, or prolonged fasting, should be referred for medical evaluation if there is evidence that the ingestion exceeded 4 g/day or 100 mg/kg/day, whichever is less.[61]

The risk of developing hepatotoxicity may be predicted from a nomogram (Fig. 10–2) based on the acetaminophen serum concentration and time after ingestion.[56] The treatment line of the nomogram (150 mcg/mL at 4 hours), which allows a margin of error in laboratory analysis and time of ingestion, should be used to make treatment decisions. The other lines on the nomogram indicate differing levels of risk for hepatotoxicity based on a multicenter study of 11,195 patients.[56]

If the plasma concentration plotted on the nomogram falls above the nomogram treatment line, indicating that hepatic damage is possible, a full course of treatment with acetylcysteine is indicated. When the results of the acetaminophen determination will be available later than 8 hours after the ingestion, acetylcysteine therapy should be initiated based on the history and later discontinued if the results indicate nontoxic concentrations. The nomogram has not been evaluated and thus is not useful for assessing chronic exposure to acetaminophen. Some have advocated that patients with chronic alcoholism should be treated with acetylcysteine regardless of the risk estimation.[63]

Management of Toxicity

Therapy of an acute acetaminophen overdose depends on the amount ingested, time after ingestion, and serum concentration of acetaminophen. When excessive amounts are ingested, the history is unclear, or an intentional ingestion is suspected, the patient should be evaluated at an emergency department and acetaminophen serum concentrations obtained.[61] No prehospital care generally is indicated, and ipecac syrup typically is not recommended.[61] If the patient presents to the emergency department within 4 hours of the ingestion or ingestion of other drugs is suspected, one dose of activated charcoal can be administered.

Acetylcysteine (also known as *N*-acetylcysteine), a sulfhydryl-containing compound, replenishes the hepatic stores of glutathione by serving as a glutathione surrogate that combines directly with reactive metabolites or by serving as a source of sulfate, thus preventing hepatic damage.[67] It should be started within 10 hours of the ingestion to be most effective.[56] Initiation of therapy 24 to 36 hours after the ingestion may be of value in some patients, particu-

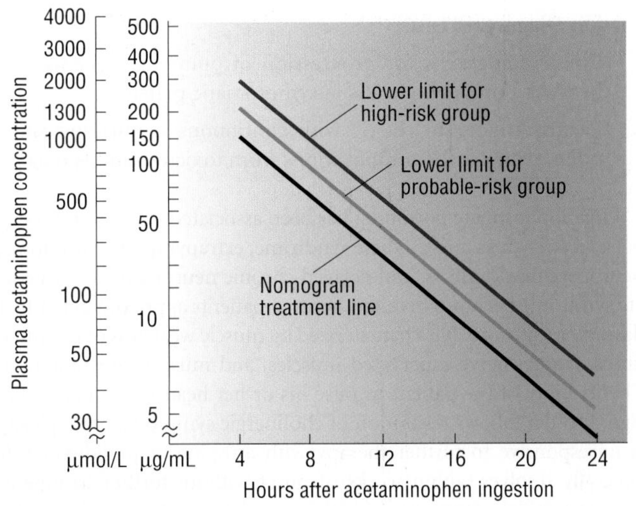

FIGURE 10-2. Nomogram for assessing hepatotoxic risk following acute ingestion of acetaminophen. *(Adapted from reference 56.)*

larly those with measurable serum acetaminophen concentrations.[67,68] Patients with fulminant hepatic failure may benefit through other mechanisms by the administration or initiation of acetylcysteine several days after ingestion.[67]

CLINICAL CONTROVERSY

The routine administration of acetylcysteine more than 24 hours after acetaminophen overdose has been proposed. Case reports and animal studies indicate that it is relatively safe and that its use may minimize hepatotoxicity. Although accepted criteria for its use are lacking, it may be considered for patients with fulminant hepatoxicity, when acetaminophen is still measurable in the serum, or when the ingestion was not recognized within 24 hours and liver toxicity is apparent.

Therapy should be initiated with acetylcysteine within 10 hours of ingestion when indicated. The oral liquid was the only approved form of acetylcysteine in the United States until 2004, when the Food and Drug Administration (FDA) approved an intravenous formulation.[69] The dosage regimen for the intravenous form is based on one used in Europe for two decades, and outcomes similar to the 72-hour oral regimen have been reported.[53,70] A systematic review of the literature indicated that acetylcysteine is superior to supportive care, but there is no clear evidence of which regimen is better.[71] Although there are several notable differences (Table 10–10),[53,56,69,70] a clear preference for the oral or intravenous form of acetylcysteine likely will not evolve until further experience with IV formulation accumulates. When acetaminophen plasma concentrations are below the nomogram treatment line, there is little risk of toxicity, protective therapy with acetylcysteine is not necessary, and medical therapy likely is unnecessary.[56] The acetaminophen blood sample should be drawn no sooner than 4 hours after the ingestion to ensure that peak acetaminophen concentrations have been reached. If a concentration is obtained less than 4 hours after ingestion, it is uninterpretable, and a second determination should be done at least 4 hours after ingestion. Serial determinations of a serum concentration, 4 to 6 hours apart, typically are unnecessary unless there is some evidence of slowed gastrointestinal motility as the result of the ingestion of certain drugs (e.g., opioids, antihistamines, or anticholinergics) or unless an extended-release product is involved. Therapy with acetylcysteine is continued if any concentration is above the treatment line of the nomogram, and provisional therapy is discontinued when both concentrations are below the treatment line.

TABLE 10-10 Comparison of Intravenous and Oral Regimens for Acetylcysteine in the Treatment of Acute Acetaminophen Poisoning

Characteristic	Intravenous	Oral
Regimen	150 mg/kg in 200 mL D_5W infused over 1 hour, then 50 mg/kg in 500 mL D_5W over 4 hours, followed by 100 mg/kg in 1,000 mL D_5W over 16 hours[a]	140 mg/kg, followed 4 hours later by 70 mg/kg every 4 hours for 17 doses diluted to 5% with juice or soft drinks
Total dose (mg/kg)	300	1,330
Duration (h)	21	72
Adverse effects	Anaphylactoid reactions (rash, hypotension, wheezing, dyspnea); acute flushing and erythema in first hour of the infusion that typically resolves spontaneously	Nausea, vomiting
Ancillary therapy, if needed	Antihistamines and epinephrine for severe anaphylactic reactions	Antiemetics, e.g., metoclopramide, ondansetron, or droperidol
Trade name	Acetadote	Mucomyst
Available strength	20%	10%, 20%

[a]For patients <40 kg and those requiring fluid restriction, the total volume for dilution should be reduced as directed in the package insert.
D_5W, 5% dextrose in water for injection.

Although young children have an inherently lower risk of acetaminophen-induced hepatotoxicity, these patients should be managed in the same manner as adults. When acetaminophen plasma concentrations predict that toxicity is probable, young children should receive acetylcysteine in the dosing regimen described previously.[66] If fulminant hepatic failure develops, the approaches described in Chap. 39 should be considered. In unresponsive patients, liver transplantation is a lifesaving option.[57]

Monitoring and Prevention

Baseline liver function tests (AST, ALT, bilirubin, prothrombin time), serum creatinine determination, and urinalysis should be obtained on admission and repeated at 24-hour intervals until at least 96 hours have elapsed for patients at risk. Most patients with liver injury develop elevated transaminase concentrations within 24 hours of ingestion. AST or ALT concentrations >1,000 international units per liter commonly are associated with other signs of liver dysfunction and have been used as the threshold concentration in outcome studies to define severe liver toxicity.[56] The extent of transaminase elevation is not correlated directly with the severity of hepatic injury, with nonfatal cases demonstrating peak concentrations as high as 30,000 international units per liter between 48 and 72 hours after ingestion.[57]

Prevention of acetaminophen poisoning is based on recognition of the maximum daily therapeutic doses, observance of general poison prevention practices, and early intervention in cases of suspected overdose. The frequent involvement of acetaminophen in poisonings and overdoses, whether or not declared by the patient, has led to the routine determination of acetaminophen concentrations in patients admitted to emergency departments for any overdose.[18]

ANTICHOLINESTERASE INSECTICIDES

Clinical Presentation

❼ The clinical manifestations of anticholinesterase insecticide poisoning include any or all of the following: pinpoint pupils, excessive

TABLE 10-11 Effects of Acetylcholinesterase Inhibition at Muscarinic, Nicotinic, and CNS Receptors

Muscarinic receptors	Nicotinic–sympathetic neurons
Diarrhea	Increased blood pressure
Urination	Sweating and piloerection
Miosis[a]	Mydriasis[a]
Bronchorrhea	Hyperglycemia
Bradycardia[a]	Tachycardia[a]
Emesis	Priapism
Lacrimation	**Nicotinic–neuromuscular neurons**
Salivation	Muscular weakness
CNS receptors (mixed type)	Cramps
Coma	Fasciculations
Seizures	Muscular paralysis

[a]Generally muscarinic effects predominate, but nicotinic effects can be observed.

lacrimation, excessive salivation, bronchorrhea, bronchospasm and expiratory wheezes, hyperperistalsis producing abdominal cramps and diarrhea, bradycardia, excessive sweating, fasciculations and weakness of skeletal muscles, paralysis of skeletal muscles (particularly those involved with respiration), convulsions, and coma.[72] Symptoms of anticholinesterase poisoning and their response to antidotal therapy depend on the action of excessive acetylcholinesterase at different receptor types (Table 10–11).

The time of onset and severity of symptoms depend on the route of exposure, potency of the agent, and total dose received (see presentation box below). Toxic signs and symptoms develop most rapidly after inhalation or intravenous injection and slowest after skin contact. Anticholinesterase insecticides are absorbed through the skin, lungs, conjunctivae, and gastrointestinal tract. Severe symptoms can occur from absorption by any route. Most patients are symptomatic within 6 hours, and death may occur within 24 hours without treatment. Death typically is caused by respiratory failure resulting from the combination of pulmonary and cardiovascular effects (Fig. 10–3).[72] Poisoning may be complicated by aspiration pneumonia, urinary tract infections, and sepsis.[73]

CLINICAL PRESENTATION OF ANTICHOLINESTERASE INSECTICIDE POISONING

General

- Mild symptoms may resolve spontaneously; life-threatening toxicity may develop with 1 to 6 hours of exposure

Symptoms

- Diarrhea, diaphoresis, excessive urination, miosis, blurred vision, pulmonary congestion, dyspnea, vomiting, lacrimation, salivation, and shortness of breath within 1 hour
- Headache, confusion, coma, and seizures possible within 1 to 6 hours

Signs

- Increased bronchial secretions, tachypnea, rales, and cyanosis within 1 to 6 hours
- Muscle weakness, fasciculations, and respiratory paralysis within 1 to 6 hours
- Bradycardia, atrial fibrillation, atrioventricular block, and hypotension within 1 to 6 hours

Laboratory Tests

- Markedly depressed serum pseudocholinesterase activity below normal range
- Altered arterial blood gases (acidosis), serum electrolytes, BUN, and serum creatinine in response to respiratory distress and shock within 1 to 6 hours

Other Diagnostic Tests

- Chest radiographs for progression of pulmonary edema or hydrocarbon pneumonitis in symptomatic patients
- Electrocardiogram (ECG) with continuous monitoring and pulse oximetry for complications from toxicity and hypoxia

Organophosphate poisoning has been associated with several residual effects, such as intermediate syndrome, extrapyramidal symptoms, neuropsychiatric effects, and delayed chronic neuropathy. Intermediate syndrome becomes manifest in some patients approximately 1 to 3 days after exposure. It is characterized by muscle weakness of proximal limbs, cranial nerve innervated muscles, and muscles of respiration. The inability of the patient to raise his or her head is often an initial sign. It often follows resolution of cholinergic symptoms but typically is unresponsive to further therapy with atropine or pralidoxime. It generally resolves within weeks of onset without further treatment. Extrapyramidal symptoms, which may develop 1 to 7 days after exposure, usually resolve spontaneously within a few days of onset. Neuropsychiatric effects, such as confusion, lethargy, memory impairment, headache, and depression, typically begin weeks to months after exposure and may last for years. The etiology is unclear. Delayed chronic neuropathy often presents as cramping muscle pain in the legs (upper extremities are sometimes involved), followed by rapidly progressive weakness and paralysis. Paresthesia and pain may be present. The onset often is delayed by 1 to 5 weeks after recovery from the acute poisoning exposure. It is unresponsive to further atropine or pralidoxime therapy. Improvement may be delayed for months to years, and in some cases the patient develops permanent disability. It is not associated with all organophosphates.[72,74]

Mechanism of Toxicity

Anticholinesterase insecticides phosphorylate the active site of cholinesterase in all parts of the body.[72,75] Inhibition of this enzyme leads to accumulation of acetylcholine at affected receptors and results in widespread toxicity. Acetylcholine is the neurohormone responsible for physiologic transmission of nerve impulses from preganglionic and postganglionic neurons of the cholinergic (parasympathetic) nervous system, preganglionic adrenergic (sympathetic) neurons, neuromuscular junction in skeletal muscles, and multiple nerve endings in the central nervous system (Fig. 10–4).

Causative Agents

Anticholinesterase insecticides include organophosphate and carbamate insecticides. These insecticides are currently in widespread use throughout the world for eradication of insects in dwellings and crops. Carbamates typically are less potent and inactivate cholinesterase in a more reversible fashion through carbamylation compared with organophosphates.[72] The prototype anticholinesterase agent is the organophosphate, which is the focus of this discussion. A large number of organophosphates are used as pesticides (e.g., dichlorphos disulfoton, malathion, mevinphos, phosmet), and several were specifically developed for use as potent chemical warfare agents (see Chap. 12).[72,73,76,77] The chemical warfare agents act like organophosphate insecticides, but they are highly potent, are quickly absorbed, and can be deadly to humans within minutes (see Chap. 12).[77,78] An anticholinesterase insecticide typically is stored in a garage, chemical storage area, or living area. Anticholinesterase agents also can be found in occupational (e.g., pest exterminators) or agricultural (e.g., crop dusters or farm workers) settings. These agents also have been used as a means for suicide or homicide.

Incidence

Anticholinesterase insecticides are among the most poisonous substances commonly used for pest control and are a frequent source of

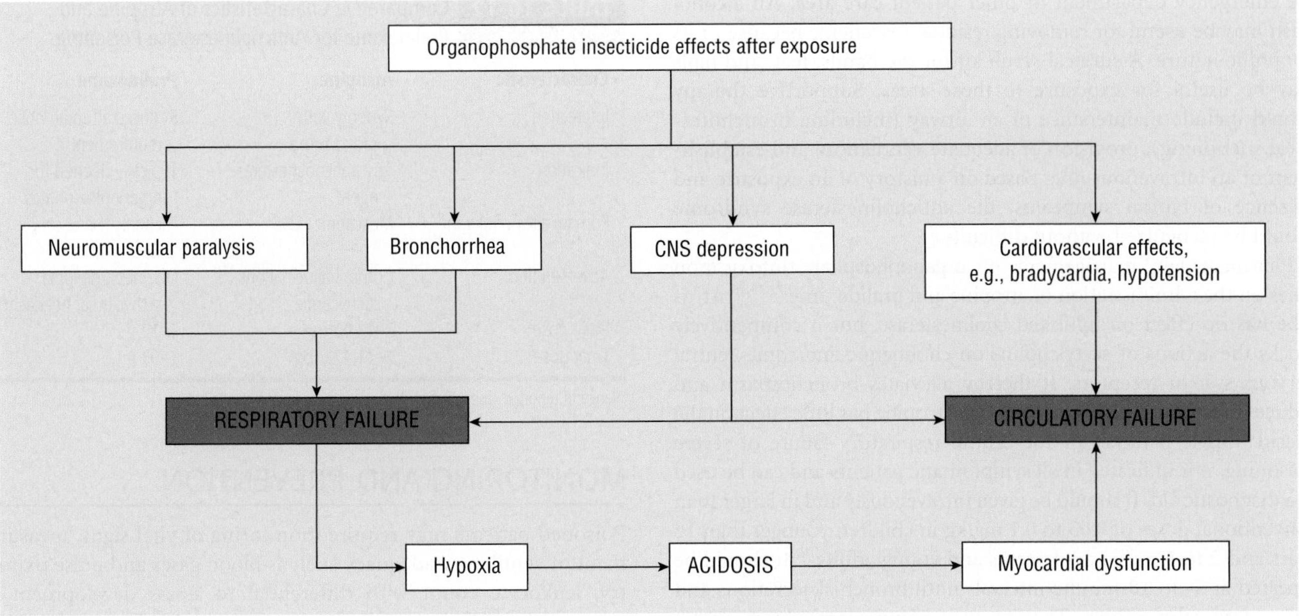

FIGURE 10-3. Pathogenesis of life-threatening effects of organophosphate poisoning. (CNS, central nervous system.)

serious poisoning in children and adults in rural and urban settings. The 2005 AAPCC-NPDS report documented 9,942 nonfatal exposures and 12 deaths from anticholinesterase insecticides alone or in combination with other pesticides, with 29% of exposures in children younger than 6 years.[6]

Risk Assessment

The triad of miosis, bronchial secretions, and muscle fasciculations should suggest the possibility of anticholinesterase insecticide poisoning and warrants a therapeutic trial of the antidote atropine. In cases of low-level exposure, failure to develop signs within 6 hours indicates a low likelihood of subsequent toxicity.[72] Ruling out other chemical exposures may be guided initially by symptoms at presentation.[16]

Although the lethal dose for parathion is approximately 4 mg/kg, as little as 10 to 20 mg can be lethal to an adult and 2 mg (0.1 mg/kg) to a child. Small children may be more susceptible to toxicity because less pesticide is required per body weight to produce toxicity.[72,76] Estimation of an exact dose is impossible in most cases of acute poisoning; thus, tabulated "toxic" doses generally are not helpful in assessing risk of toxicity. Generally, ingestion of a small mouthful (~5 mL) of the concentrated forms of an organophosphate intended to be diluted for commercial or agricultural use will produce serious, life-threatening toxicity, whereas a mouthful of an already diluted household product, such as an aerosol insecticide for household use, typically does not produce serious toxic effects.[76]

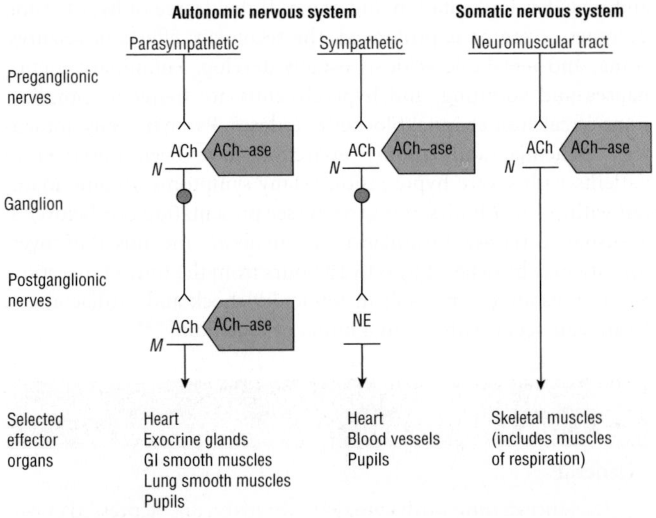

FIGURE 10-4. Organization of neurotransmitters of the peripheral nervous system and site of acetylcholinesterase action. (ACh, acetylcholine; ACh-ase, acetylcholinesterase; M, muscarinic receptor; N, nicotinic receptor; NE, norepinephrine.)

Measurement of acetylcholinesterase activity at the neuronal synapse is not feasible clinically. Cholinesterase activity can be measured in the blood as the pseudocholinesterase (butylcholinesterase) activity of the plasma and acetylcholinesterase activity in the erythrocyte. Both cholinesterases will be depressed with anticholinesterase insecticide poisoning.[72,79] Severity can be estimated roughly by the extent of depressed activity in relation to the low end of normal values. Because there are several methods to measure and report cholinesterase activity, each particular laboratory's normal range must be considered. Clinical toxicity usually is seen only after a 50% reduction in enzyme activity, and severe toxicity typically is observed at levels 20% or less of the normal range.[75,76,79] The intrinsic activity of acetylcholinesterase may be depressed in some individuals, but the absence of any manifestations in most people does not permit recognition of the relative deficiency in the general population. Therapy should not be delayed pending laboratory confirmation when insecticide poisoning is clinically suspected.

Management of Toxicity

People handling the patient should wear gloves and aprons to protect themselves against contaminated clothing, skin, or gastric fluid of the patient.[72,76] Because many insecticides are dissolved in a hydrocarbon vehicle, there is an additional risk of pulmonary aspiration of the hydrocarbon leading to pneumonitis. The risks and benefits of gastric decontamination (e.g., gastric lavage, activated charcoal) should be considered carefully and should involve consultation with a poison control center or clinical toxicologist. Symptomatic cases of anticholinesterase insecticide exposure typically are referred to an emergency department for evaluation and treatment.

If the poison has been ingested within the hour, gastric lavage should be considered and followed by the administration of activated charcoal. For the patient with skin contamination, contaminated clothing should be removed and the patient washed with copious amounts of soap and water before he or she is admitted to the emergency department or other patient care area. An alcohol wash may be useful for removing residual insecticide because of its lipophilic nature. A surgical scrub kit for the hands, feet, and nails may be useful for exposure to those areas. Supportive therapy should include maintenance of an airway (including bronchotracheal suctioning), provision of adequate ventilation, and establishment of an intravenous line. Based on a history of an exposure and presence of typical symptoms, the anticholinesterase syndrome should be recognized without difficulty.

Pharmacologic management of organophosphate intoxication relies on the administration of atropine and pralidoxime.[72,75,76] Atropine has no effect on inhibited cholinesterase, but it competitively blocks the actions of acetylcholine on cholinergic and some central nervous system receptors. It thereby alleviates bronchospasm and reduces bronchial secretions. Although atropine has little effect on the flaccid muscle paralysis or the central respiratory failure of severe poisoning, it is indicated in all symptomatic patients and can be used as a diagnostic aid. It should be given intravenously and in larger than conventional doses of 0.05 to 0.1 mg/kg in children younger than 12 years and 2 to 5 mg in adolescents and young adults.[76] It should be repeated at 5- to 10-minute intervals until bronchial secretions and pulmonary rales resolve. Therapy may require large doses over a period of several days until all absorbed organophosphate is metabolized, and acetylcholinesterase activity is restored.

Restoration of enzyme activity is necessary for severe poisoning, characterized by a reduction of cholinesterase activity to <20% of normal, profound weakness, and respiratory distress. Pralidoxime (Protopam), also called 2-PAM or 2-pyridine aldoxime methiodide, breaks the covalent bond between the cholinesterase and organophosphate and regenerates enzyme activity. Organophosphate-cholinesterase binding is reversible initially, but it gradually becomes irreversible. Therefore, therapy with pralidoxime should be initiated as soon as possible, preferably within 36 to 72 hours of exposure.[76] The drug should be given at a dose of 25 to 50 mg/kg up to 1 g intravenously over 5 to 20 minutes. If muscle weakness persists or recurs, the dose can be repeated after 1 hour and again if needed. A continuous infusion of pralidoxime has been shown to be effective in adults when administered at 2 to 4 mg/kg/h preceded by a loading dose of 4 to 5 mg/kg[80] and in children at 10 to 20 mg/kg/h with a loading dose of 15 to 50 mg/kg.[81] Both atropine and pralidoxime should be given together because they have complementary actions (Table 10–12). Systematic reviews of the literature indicate that the effectiveness of pralidoxime and similar oxime compounds in the treatment of organophosphate poisoning is inconclusive because of problems with study design.[82,83] Carbamate insecticide poisonings typically do not require the administration of pralidoxime.

CLINICAL CONTROVERSY

Some references indicate that pralidoxime should be avoided in the treatment of carbamate (another type of anticholinesterase insecticide) poisoning because of reports of worsened toxicity in animals. Pralidoxime may be considered when exposure to carbamates is not known but an anticholinesterase is suspected based on symptoms or when respiratory paralysis due to nicotinic effects is not managed sufficiently by mechanical ventilation.

One of the pitfalls of therapy is the delay in administering sufficient doses of atropine or pralidoxime.[72,76] The adverse effects of atropine and pralidoxime, predictable extensions of their anticholinergic actions, are minimally important compared with the life-threatening effects of severe anticholinesterase poisoning and can be minimized easily by decreasing the dose.

TABLE 10-12 Comparative Characteristics of Atropine and Pralidoxime for Anticholinesterase Poisoning

Characteristic	Atropine	Pralidoxime
Interaction	Synergy with pralidoxime	Reduces atropine dose requirement
Indication	Any anticholinesterase agent	Typically needed for organophosphates
Primary sites of action	Muscarinic, CNS	Nicotinic > muscarinic > CNS
Adverse effects	Coma, hallucinations, tachycardia	Dizziness, diplopia, tachycardia, headache
Daily dose[a]	2–1,600 mg	1–12 g
Total dose[a]	2–11,422 mg	1–92 g

[a]Range of reported cases; higher doses may be required in rare cases.

MONITORING AND PREVENTION

Poisoned patients may require monitoring of vital signs, measurement of ventilatory adequacy such as blood gases and pulse oximetry, leukocyte count with differential to assess development of pneumonia, and chest radiographs to assess the degree of pulmonary edema or development of hydrocarbon pneumonitis. Workers involved in the formulation and application of pesticides should be monitored by periodic measurement of cholinesterase activity in their bloodstream. Untreated, anticholinesterase-depressed acetylcholinesterase activity returns to normal values in approximately 120 days. Long-term followup for severe cases of poisoning may be necessary to detect the presence of delayed or persistent neuropsychiatric effects.

Many anticholinesterase insecticide poisonings are unintentional as a result of misuse, improper storage, failure to follow instructions for mixing or application, or inability to read directions for use. Training and vigilant adherence to directions may minimize some poisonings. Storing pesticides in original or labeled containers can minimize the risk of unintentional ingestion. Keeping pesticides out of children's reach may decrease the risk of childhood poisoning.[84]

CALCIUM CHANNEL BLOCKERS

Clinical Presentation

8 Overdosage with calcium channel blockers typically results in bradycardia and hypotension (Fig. 10–5). Many patients become lethargic and may develop agitation and coma. If the degree of hypotension becomes severe or is prolonged, the secondary effects of seizures, coma, and metabolic acidosis usually develop. Pulmonary edema, nausea and vomiting, and hyperglycemia are frequent complications of calcium channel blocker overdoses. Paralytic ileus, mesenteric ischemia, and colonic infarction have been observed in patients with severe hypotension. Many symptoms become manifest within 1 to 2 hours of ingestion (see presentation box below). If a sustained-release formulation is involved, the onset of overt toxicity may be delayed by 6 to 18 hours from the time of ingestion. Severe poisoning can result in refractory shock and cardiac arrest. Death can occur within 3 to 4 hours of ingestion.[85–88]

CLINICAL PRESENTATION OF CALCIUM CHANNEL BLOCKER POISONING

General

- Life-threatening cardiac toxicity (bradycardia, depressed contractility, dysrhythmias) within 1 to 3 hours of ingestion, delayed by 12 to 18 hours if a sustained-release product is involved

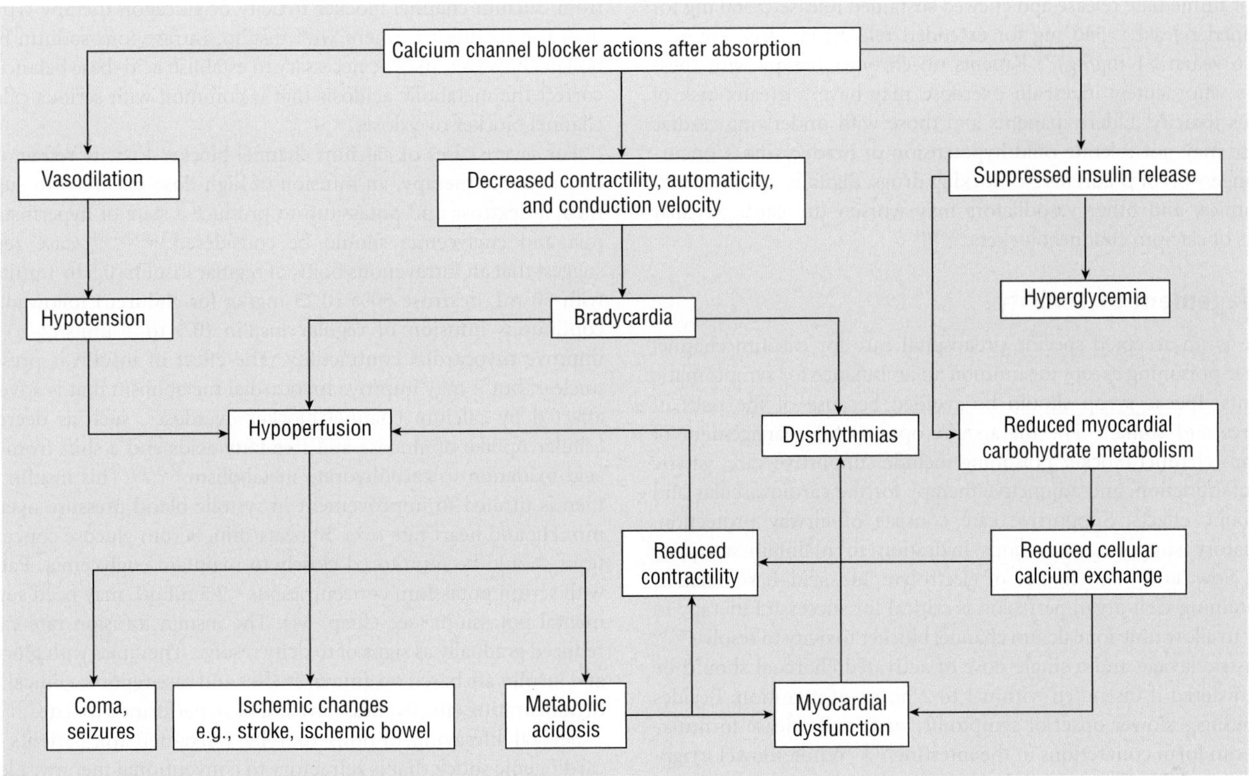

FIGURE 10-5. Pathophysiologic changes associated with calcium channel blocker poisoning.

Symptoms

- Nausea and vomiting within 1 hour
- Dizziness, lethargy, coma, and seizures within 1 to 3 hours

Signs

- Hypotension and bradycardia within 1 to 6 hours
- Unresponsiveness and depressed reflexes within 1 to 6 hours
- Atrioventricular block, intraventricular conduction defects, and ventricular dysrhythmias on ECG

Laboratory Tests

- Hyperglycemia typically resolves spontaneously if it occurs
- Altered arterial blood gases (metabolic acidosis), serum electrolytes, BUN, and serum creatinine in response to shock within 1 to 6 hours

Other Diagnostic Tests

- ECG with continuous monitoring and pulse oximetry to monitor for toxicity and shock
- Monitor for complications of pulmonary aspiration such as hypoxia and pneumonia by physical findings and chest radiographs

Mechanism of Toxicity

Most toxic effects of calcium channel blockers are produced by three basic actions on the cardiovascular system: vasodilation through relaxation of smooth muscles, decreased contractility by action on cardiac tissue, and decreased automaticity and conduction velocity through slow recovery of calcium channels. Calcium channel blockers interfere with calcium entry by inhibiting one or more of the several types of calcium channels and binding at one or more cellular binding sites. Selectivity of these actions varies with the calcium channel blocker and provides some therapeutic distinctions, but these differences are less clear with overdosage.[88] Calcium channel blockers also inhibit insulin secretion, which results in hyperglycemia and changes in fatty acid oxidation in the myocardium that alter myocardial calcium flow and reduce contractility.[89] Current experiences suggest that the signs and symptoms of calcium channel blocker toxicity are similar among the drugs in this class.

Causative Agents

Approximately 10 calcium channel antagonists are marketed in the United States for treatment of hypertension, certain dysrhythmias, and some forms of angina. The calcium channel blockers are classified by their chemical structure as phenylalkylamines (e.g., verapamil), benzothiapines (e.g., diltiazem), and dihydropyridines (e.g., amlodipine, felodipine, nicardipine, and nifedipine). Several of these agents, namely, diltiazem, nicardipine, nifedipine, and verapamil, are formulated as sustained-release oral dosage forms or have a slow onset of action and longer half-life (e.g., amlodipine[90]), allowing once-daily administration.

Incidence

In 2005, the AAPCC-NPDS report documented 10,500 toxic exposures to a calcium channel blocker in 9,650 individuals; 384 patients exhibited and survived major toxic effects, and 75 died.[6] Poison control center reports have shown a steady increase in the number of cases of morbidity and mortality following calcium channel blocker overdosage.

Risk Assessment

Ingestion of doses near or in excess of 1 g of diltiazem, nifedipine, or verapamil may result in life-threatening symptoms or death in an adult.[85] Ingestion of an amount that exceeds the usual maximum single therapeutic dose or a dose equal to or greater than the lowest reported toxic dose (whichever is less) warrants referral to a poison control center and/or an emergency department. The threshold doses of several agents and dosage forms vary (e.g., diltiazem: adults, >120 mg for immediate release and chewed sustained release, >360 mg for sustained release, >540 mg for extended release; children younger than 6 years: >1 mg/kg).[91] Patients on chronic therapy with these agents who acutely ingest an overdose may have a greater risk of serious toxicity. Elderly patients and those with underlying cardiac disease may not tolerate mild hypotension or bradycardia. Concurrent ingestion of β-adrenergic blocking drugs, digitalis, class I antiarrhythmics, and other vasodilators may worsen the cardiovascular effects of calcium channel blockers.[86,88,91]

Management of Toxicity

There is no accepted specific prehospital care for calcium channel blocker poisoning except to summon an ambulance for symptomatic patients. Ipecac syrup should be avoided because of the risks of seizures and coma.[91] The therapeutic options for management of calcium channel blocker poisoning include supportive care, gastric decontamination, and adjunctive therapy for the cardiovascular and metabolic effects. Supportive care consists of airway protection, ventilatory support, intravenous hydration to maintain adequate urine flow, and maintenance of electrolyte and acid–base balance. Maintaining vital organ perfusion is critical for successful therapy in order to allow time for calcium channel blocker toxicity to resolve.[87,88]

Gastric lavage and a single dose of activated charcoal should be administered if instituted within 1 to 2 hours of ingestion. Besides exhibiting a slower onset of symptoms, sustained-release formulations can form concretions in the intestine.[87,88] Whole-bowel irrigation with polyethylene glycol electrolyte solution may accelerate rectal elimination of the sustained-release tablets and should be considered routinely for ingestion of sustained-release calcium channel blocker formulations.[34,92]

Adjunctive therapy is focused on treating hypotension, bradycardia, and resulting shock. Hypotension is treated primarily by correction of coexisting dysrhythmias (e.g., bradycardia, heart block) and implementation of conventional measures to treat decreased blood pressure. Infusion of normal saline and placement of the patient in the Trendelenburg position are initial therapies. Further fluid therapy should be guided by central venous pressure monitoring. Dopamine and epinephrine in conventional doses for cardiogenic shock should be considered next. If hypotension persists, dysrhythmias are present, or other signs of serious toxicity are present, calcium should be administered intravenously.[85,88]

A calcium chloride bolus test dose (10 to 20 mg/kg up to 1 to 3 g) is the preferred therapy for patients with serious toxicity. In adults, calcium chloride 10% can be diluted in 100 mL normal saline and infused over 5 minutes through a central venous line. If a positive cardiovascular response is achieved with this test dose, a continuous infusion of calcium chloride (20 to 50 mg/kg/h) should be started. Calcium gluconate is less desirable to use because it contains less elemental calcium per milligram of final dosage form. Intravenous calcium salts can produce vomiting and tissue necrosis on extravasation.[52,88] Atropine also may be considered for treatment of bradycardia, but it is seldom sufficient as a sole therapy.[87]

If the bradycardia and hypotension are refractory to the foregoing therapy, a bolus infusion of glucagon (0.05 to 0.20 mg/kg, initial adult dose is 3 to 5 mg over 1 to 2 minutes) should be considered. Benefit typically is observed within 5 minutes of administration and can be sustained with a continuous intravenous infusion (0.05 to 0.1 mg/kg/h) titrated to clinical response.[93] Glucagon possesses chronotropic and inotropic effects in part by stimulating adenyl cyclase and increasing cyclic adenosine monophosphate, which may promote intracellular entry of calcium through calcium channels. It thereby may improve hypotension and bradycardia.[52] Vomiting is not uncommon with these large doses of glucagon, and the airway should be protected to prevent pulmonary aspiration. Hyperglycemia may occur or be exacerbated in those patients receiving glucagon therapy. Hyperglycemia from calcium channel blocker toxicity or glucagon therapy typically does not require treatment with insulin. Intravenous sodium bicarbonate, however, may be necessary to establish acid–base balance and correct the metabolic acidosis that is common with serious calcium channel blocker overdoses.

For severe cases of calcium channel blocker toxicity refractory to conventional therapy, an infusion of high-dose insulin with supplemental dextrose and potassium to produce a state of hyperinsulinemia and euglycemia should be considered.[52,85,87–89] Case reports suggest that an intravenous bolus of regular insulin (0.5 to 1 units/kg) with 50 mL dextrose 50% (0.25 mg/kg for children) followed by a continuous infusion of regular insulin (0.5 to 1 units/kg/h) may improve myocardial contractility. The effect of insulin is presently unclear, but it may improve myocardial metabolism that is adversely affected by calcium channel blocker overdoses, such as decreased cellular uptake of glucose and free fatty acids and a shift from fatty acid oxidation to carbohydrate metabolism.[85,87,89] This insulin regimen is titrated to improvement in systolic blood pressure over 100 mm Hg and heart rate over 50 beats/min. Serum glucose concentrations should be monitored closely to maintain euglycemia. Patients with serum potassium concentrations <2.5 mEq/L may need supplemental potassium (see Chap. 54). The insulin infusion rate can be reduced gradually as signs of toxicity resolve. Therapies with glucagon and insulin are based on animal studies and case reports; clinical trials demonstrating effectiveness have not been performed to date.[52,85,87–89]

Several lifesaving options may be warranted for patients with cardiogenic shock that is refractory to conventional therapy. Electrical cardiac pacing may restore an acceptable heart rate in patients with severe bradycardia.[88] Intraaortic balloon counterpulsation or cardiopulmonary bypass may improve shock in patients unresponsive to other therapies.[52,88,94,95]

Measures to enhance elimination from the bloodstream by hemodialysis or multiple-dose activated charcoal have not been shown to be effective and are not indicated for calcium channel blocker poisoning.[42,86,88,96]

CLINICAL CONTROVERSY

Some clinicians believe that hyperinsulinemia/euglycemia or glucagon therapy for calcium channel blocker poisoning should be used early in the course of therapy. Others reserve it for life-threatening symptoms not responsive to other therapy. More safety and effectiveness data are needed to define the place of these two agents in therapy.

Monitoring and Prevention

Regular monitoring of vital signs and ECG is essential in suspected calcium channel blocker poisoning. Determinations of serum electrolytes, serum glucose, arterial blood gases, urine output, and renal function are indicated to assess and monitor symptomatic patients. If serious toxicity is likely to develop, overt symptoms will manifest within 6 hours of ingestion.[91] For ingestions of sustained-release products in toxic doses, observation for 24 hours in a critical care unit may be prudent because the onset of symptoms may be slow and delayed up to 12 to 18 hours after ingestion.[85,91,92,96,97] Serum concentrations of these agents in overdose patients do not correlate well with the ingested dose, degree of toxicity, or outcome.

Poisonings resulting from these agents are likely to increase as their therapeutic indications and use increase. These poisonings may be the result of an intentional suicide or unintentional ingestion by young children. Prevention of calcium channel blocker poisonings in children rests with the education of patients receiving these agents, particularly of grandparents and those who have children visit their homes infrequently, of their dangers on overdosage. Safe storage and use of child-resistant closures may reduce the opportunities for unintentional poisonings by children.[86]

IRON

Clinical Presentation

❾ In the first few hours after ingestion of toxic amounts of iron, symptoms of gastrointestinal irritation (e.g., nausea, vomiting, and diarrhea) are common (see presentation box below). In certain severe cases, acidosis and shock can become manifest within 6 hours of ingestion. Some have observed a quiescent phase between 6 and 48 hours after ingestion when symptoms improve or abate, but this phenomenon is poorly characterized.[98] Continued gastrointestinal symptoms, poor perfusion, and oliguria should suggest the development of severe toxicity, with other effects still to become manifest. Generally, within 24 to 36 hours of the ingestion, central nervous system involvement with coma and seizures; hepatic injury characterized by jaundice, increased prothrombin time, increased bilirubin, and hypoglycemia; cardiovascular shock; and acidosis also develop.[98,99] Adult respiratory distress syndrome (ARDS) may develop in patients with severe cardiovascular shock and further compromise recovery.[100] Coagulopathy with decreased thrombin formation is one of the early direct effects of excessive iron concentrations, and later disturbances of coagulation (after 24 to 48 hours of ingestion) are a consequence of hepatotoxicity.[101] Mucosal injury, an iron-rich circulation, or deferoxamine therapy may promote septicemia with *Yersinia enterocolitica* during iron overdose; other bacteria or viruses also may cause septicemia.[98] Two to four weeks after the exposure, a few rare patients experience persistent vomiting from gastric outlet obstruction as the result of pyloric and duodenal stenosis from the earlier gastric mucosal necrosis. Autopsy findings in children indicate prominent iron deposition in intestinal mucosa and periportal necrosis of the liver that correlate with the primary symptoms of serious iron poisoning.[102]

CLINICAL PRESENTATION OF ACUTE IRON POISONING

General

- Gastrointestinal symptoms shortly after ingestion with possible rapid progression to shock and coma

Symptoms

- Vomiting, abdominal pain, and diarrhea within 1 to 6 hours
- Lethargy, coma, seizures, bloody vomiting, bloody diarrhea, and shock within 6 to 24 hours

Signs

- Hypotension and tachycardia within 6 to 24 hours
- Liver dysfunction and failure possible in 2 to 5 days

Laboratory Tests

- Toxic serum iron concentrations >500 mcg/dL
- Altered arterial blood gases and serum electrolytes associated with a high anion gap metabolic acidosis within 3 to 24 hours
- Elevated BUN, serum creatinine, AST, ALT, and INR within 1 to 2 days

Other Diagnostic Tests

- Guaiac test of stools for the presence of blood
- Abdominal radiograph to detect solid iron tablets in gastrointestinal tract

Mechanism of Toxicity

The toxicity of acute iron poisoning includes local effects on the gastrointestinal mucosa and systemic effects induced by excessive iron in the body.[98,100] Iron is irritating to the gastric and duodenal mucosa, which may result in hemorrhage and occasional perforations. Once absorbed, iron is taken up by tissues, particularly the liver, and acts as a mitochondrial poison. It occasionally causes hepatic injury. Iron may inhibit aerobic glycolysis and perturb the electron transport system. Further, iron may shunt electrons away from the electron transport system, thereby reducing the efficiency of oxidative phosphorylation. These biochemical factors, along with the cardiovascular effects of iron, lead to metabolic acidosis. The pathogenesis of shock is not well understood but may include the development of hypovolemia and lactic acidosis, release of endogenous vasodilators, and the direct vasodepressant effects of iron and ferritin on the circulation (Fig. 10–6).

Causative Agents

Iron poisoning results from the ingestion and absorption of excessive amounts of iron from iron tablets, multiple vitamins with iron, and prenatal vitamins. Different iron salts and formulations contain varying amounts of elemental iron (see Chap. 104). Generally, children's chewable vitamins are less likely to produce systemic iron poisoning in part because of their lower iron content.[103]

Incidence

Acute iron poisoning can produce death in children and adults.[102,103] The 2005 AAPCC-NPDS report documented 3,635 nonfatal and 4 fatal cases, respectively, of iron poisoning, with 54% of the exposures in children younger than 6 years. Multiple vitamins with iron were involved in 24,599 cases, with 84% of ingestions occurring in those younger than 6 years. No deaths were associated with these products.[6]

Risk Assessment

A patient who exhibits lethargy, paleness, persistent or bloody emesis, or diarrhea should be immediately referred to an emergency department.[103] Ingestion of 10 to 20 mg/kg elemental iron usually elicits mild gastrointestinal symptoms. Ingestion of 20 to 40 mg/kg is not likely to produce systemic toxicity, and typically these patients can be conservatively managed at home. Ingestions of 40 mg/kg or more of elemental iron are often associated with serious toxicity and require immediate medical attention.[103] Psychiatric as well as medical intervention is indicated for adults and adolescents who intentionally ingest iron as a suicide gesture.[98,100,103]

An abdominal radiograph may help to confirm the ingestion of iron tablets and indicate the need for aggressive gastrointestinal evacuation with whole-bowel irrigation. An abdominal radiograph is most useful within 2 hours of ingestion. The visualization of radiopaque iron tablets is confounded by the presence of other hard-coated tablets and some extended-release tablets that also are radiopaque. Furthermore, the radiopacity of iron tablets diminishes as the tablets disintegrate, and chewable and liquid formulations typically are not radiopaque.[104]

Iron poisoning causes vomiting and diarrhea, but these symptoms are poor indicators of later serious toxicity. The presence of a combination of findings such as coma, radiopacities, leukocytosis, and increased anion gap, however, is associated with dangerously high serum concentrations >500 mcg/dL. The presence of single signs and symptoms, such as vomiting, leukocytosis, or hyperglycemia, is not a reliable indicator of the severity of iron poisoning in adults or children.[105,106]

Once iron is absorbed, it is eliminated only as the result of blood loss or sloughing of the intestinal and epidermal cells. Thus, iron kinetics essentially represent a closed system with multiple compartments. The serum iron concentration represents a small fraction of the total-body content of iron and is at its greatest concentration in

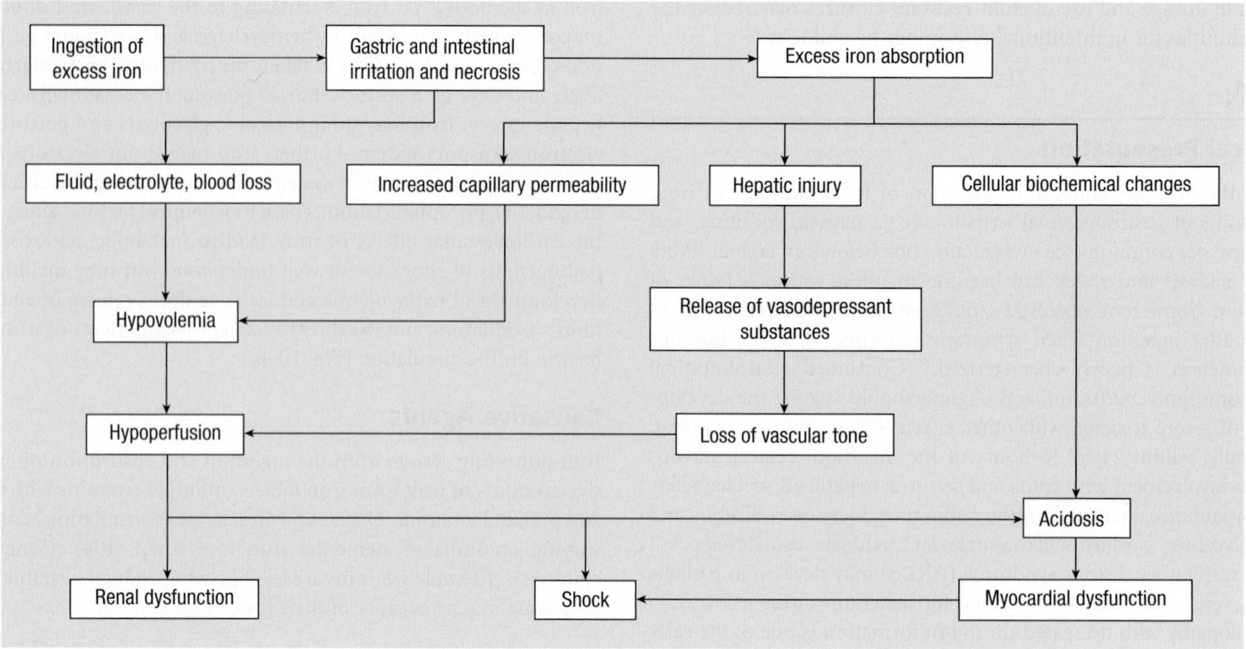

FIGURE 10-6. Pathophysiology of acute iron poisoning.

the postabsorptive and distributive phases, typically 2 to 10 hours after ingestion.[107] Serum iron concentrations >500 mcg/dL have been associated with severe toxicity, whereas concentrations <350 mcg/dL typically are not associated with severe toxicity; however, exceptions have been reported for both thresholds.[107] Serious toxicity is best determined by assessing the development of gross gastrointestinal bleeding, metabolic acidosis, shock, and coma regardless of the serum iron concentration.[100] The serum iron concentration serves as a guide for further assessment and treatment options. The ratio of the serum iron concentration to the total iron-binding capacity previously has been advocated to assess acute iron poisoning, but it is no longer used. This procedure is unreliable, insensitive, and has little relationship to toxicity.[106]

Management of Toxicity

Many patients vomit spontaneously, and ipecac syrup should be avoided.[103] At the emergency department, gastric lavage with normal saline can be considered. Lavage with normal saline may remove iron tablet fragments and dissolved iron, but because the lumen of the tube is often smaller than some whole tablets, effective removal is unlikely.[98] Activated charcoal administration is not warranted routinely because it adsorbs iron poorly. If abdominal radiographs reveal a large number of iron tablets, whole-bowel irrigation with polyethylene glycol electrolyte solution typically is necessary.[34] Although removal by gastrostomy has been used in a few cases,[100] early and aggressive decontamination and evacuation of the gastrointestinal tract usually will be adequate to minimize iron absorption and thereby reduce the risk of systemic toxicity.

Patients with systemic symptoms (e.g., shock, coma, or gross gastrointestinal bleeding or metabolic acidosis) should receive deferoxamine as soon as possible. If the serum iron concentration is >500 mcg/dL, deferoxamine is also indicated because serious systemic toxicity is likely.[98,100] Its use is less clear in patients with serum iron concentrations in the range from 350 to 500 mcg/dL because many of these patients do not develop systemic symptoms.[107]

Deferoxamine is a highly selective chelator of iron that theoretically binds ferric (Fe^{3+}) iron in a 1:1 molar ratio (100 mg deferoxamine to 8.5 mg ferric iron) that is more stable than the binding of iron to transferrin. Deferoxamine removes excess iron from the circulation and some iron from transferrin by chelating ferric complexes in equilibrium with transferrin. The resulting iron–deferoxamine complex, ferrioxamine, is then excreted in the urine. Its action on intracellular iron is unclear, but it may have a protective intracellular effect or may chelate extramitochondrial iron.[100] The parenteral administration of deferoxamine produces an orange–red-colored urine within 3 to 6 hours because of the presence of ferrioxamine in the urine.[98] For mild-to-moderate cases of iron poisoning, where its use is unclear, the presence of discolored urine indicates the persistent presence of chelatable iron and the need to continue deferoxamine. The reliance on discolored urine as a therapeutic end point has been challenged because it is not sensitive and is difficult to detect.[108]

An initial intravenous infusion of 15 mg/kg/h generally is indicated, although some have used up to 30 mg/kg/h for life-threatening cases. In these situations, the dose must be titrated carefully to minimize deferoxamine-induced hypotension.[98,100,109] The rapid intravenous infusion of deferoxamine (>15 mg/kg/h) has been associated with tachycardia, hypotension, shock, generalized erythema, and urticaria.[98,110] Anaphylaxis has been reported rarely. The use of deferoxamine for more than 24 hours at doses used for treatment of acute poisoning has been associated with exacerbation or development of ARDS.[110–112] Although the manufacturer states that the total dose in 24 hours should not exceed 6 g, the basis for this recommendation is unclear, and daily doses as high as 37.1 g have been administered without incident.[109,111] Good hydration and urine output may moderate some of the secondary physiologic effects of iron toxicity and ensure urinary elimination of ferrioxamine. In the patient who develops renal failure, hemodialysis or hemofiltration does not remove excess iron but will remove ferrioxamine.[98]

CLINICAL CONTROVERSY

There is little evidence on how much deferoxamine should be given for iron poisoning or for how long it should be administered. The dosage regimen should balance the benefits of increased iron removal in patients with exceedingly high serum iron concentrations versus the risk of developing ARDS when therapy lasts for more than 1 to 3 days.

The desired end point for deferoxamine therapy is not clear. Some have suggested that deferoxamine therapy should cease when the serum iron concentration falls below 150 mcg/dL.[100] The decline of serum iron concentrations, however, may not account for the potential cellular action of deferoxamine irrespective of its effect on iron elimination. The cessation of orange–red urine production that is indicative of ferrioxamine excretion is not reliable because many individuals cannot distinguish its presence in the urine.[108] Considering these shortcomings, deferoxamine therapy should be continued for 12 hours after the patient is asymptomatic and the urine returns to normal color or until the serum iron concentration falls below 350 mcg/dL and approaches 150 mcg/dL.

Other Therapies

Lavage solutions of phosphate or deferoxamine have been proposed previously as a means to render iron insoluble, but they were found ineffective and dangerous.[95] Oral iron chelating agents, such as deferiprone and deferasirox, are available for the management of chronic iron overload states such as sickle cell anemia, but their role in the treatment of acute iron poisoning remains to be determined.[113,114]

Monitoring and Prevention

Once a poisoning has occurred, acid–base balance (anion gap and arterial blood gases), fluid and electrolyte balance, and perfusion should be monitored. Other indicators of organ toxicity, such as ALT, AST, bilirubin, prothrombin time, serum glucose and creatinine concentrations, as well as markers of physiologic stress or infection such as leukocytosis, also should be monitored.

Iron poisoning often is not recognized as a potentially serious problem by parents or victims until symptoms develop; thus, valuable time to institute treatment is lost. Parents should be made aware of the potential risks and asked to observe basic poison prevention measures. Some hard-coated iron tablets resemble candy-coated chocolates and are confused easily by children. Based on these considerations and the frequency of this poisoning, iron tablets are packaged in child-resistant containers.

TRICYCLIC ANTIDEPRESSANTS

Clinical Presentation

⑩ Patients may deteriorate rapidly and progress from no symptoms to life-threatening cardiotoxicity or seizures within 1 hour.[115,116] Major symptoms of tricyclic antidepressant overdose typically are manifest within 6 hours of ingestion.[115] The principal effects of tricyclic antidepressant poisoning involve the cardiovascular system and the central nervous system and can result in arrhythmias, hypotension, coma, and seizures (see presentation box below).

CLINICAL PRESENTATION OF TRICYCLIC ANTIDEPRESSANT POISONING

General

- Sedating and cardiovascular effects observed within 1 hour of ingestion, quickly leading to life-threatening symptoms; death is possible within 1 to 2 hours

Symptoms

- Lethargy, coma, and seizures occur within 1 to 6 hours
- Dry mouth, mydriasis, urinary retention, and hypoactive bowel sounds, develop within 1 to 6 hours

Signs

- Tachycardia within 1 to 3 hours
- Mild hypertension early will change to severe hypotension and shock within 1 to 6 hours
- Unresponsiveness and depressed reflexes within 1 to 3 hours
- Depressed respiratory rate and depth depending on the degree of coma
- Common arrhythmias, such as prolonged QRS and QT intervals to ventricular dysrhythmias, within 1 to 6 hours

Laboratory Tests

- Altered arterial blood gases associated with metabolic acidosis from hypoxia and seizures
- Altered serum electrolytes, BUN, and serum creatinine in response to seizures and shock within 3 to 12 hours

Other Diagnostic Tests

- ECG with continuous monitoring and pulse oximetry to monitor for toxicity and shock
- Monitor for complications of pulmonary aspiration, such as hypoxia and pneumonia, by physical findings and chest radiograph

Prolongation of the QRS complex on ECG indicating nonspecific intraventricular conduction delay or bundle-branch block is the most distinctive feature of tricyclic antidepressant overdose.[116] Sinus tachycardia with rates typically <160 beats/min is common and does not cause serious hemodynamic changes in most patients. Ventricular tachycardia is a common ventricular arrhythmia, but it may be difficult to distinguish from sinus tachycardia in the presence of QRS complex prolongation and the apparent absence of P waves. It often occurs in patients with marked QRS complex prolongation or hypotension and may be precipitated by seizures.[116,117] High rates of mortality are associated with ventricular tachycardia; ventricular fibrillation is the terminal rhythm. Torsade de pointes is observed infrequently with tricyclic antidepressant poisoning. With massive tricyclic antidepressant overdose, slow ventricular rhythms may be observed. Hypotension is a significant factor in most cases of tricyclic antidepressant poisoning. Refractory hypotension leading to death is due to vasodilation and impaired cardiac contractility.[116] Other factors, such as extreme heart rates, intravascular volume depletion, hypoxia, hyperthermia, seizures, and acidosis, may contribute to refractory hypotension.

Coma usually is present in patients with tricyclic antidepressant poisoning and may or may not be associated with QRS complex prolongation. In severe cases, coma is sufficient to depress respirations. Delirium, manifest as agitation or disorientation, may occur early in the course of severe poisoning or with poisoning of moderate severity. Seizures often occur within 2 hours of ingestion and usually are generalized, single, and brief. Seizures may result in acidosis, hyperthermia, or rhabdomyolysis, and 10% to 20% of patients may abruptly develop cardiovascular deterioration.[116] Myoclonus also may be observed with tricyclic antidepressant overdose.

Hyperthermia often results from seizure and myoclonic activity in the presence of decreased sweating and is associated with a high incidence of neurologic sequelae and mortality. Anticholinergic symptoms, such as urinary retention, ileus, and dry mucous membranes, often are observed with tricyclic antidepressant overdose.[115,116] Pupil size is variable. Tricyclic antidepressant overdose can be staged based on the patient's symptoms and recovery time. In stage 1, patients are responsive to pain, have sinus tachycardia, and recover within 24 hours. In stage 2, seizures, coma, and cardiac conduction problems are evident; respiratory support typically is needed. Patients recover within 24 to 48 hours of ingestion. Stage 3 is characterized by the features of stage 2 with the addition of respiratory arrest, hypotension, ventricular dysrhythmias, and asystole, which may occur within 1 to 24 hours of ingestion. Typically symptoms appear within 2 hours, and more serious effects usually are not seen until 6 hours postingestion; rarely rapid clinical deterioration is observed within 1 to 2 hours.[118]

Amoxapine, bupropion, and maprotiline are atypical antidepressants associated with a higher incidence of seizures on overdose; amoxapine produces minimal cardiotoxicity,[116,119] but venlafaxine has been associated with greater mortality.[120] The selective serotonin reuptake inhibitors (SSRIs) generally produce a common toxicity profile on overdose despite their structural and pharmacologic distinctions.[121] The SSRIs inhibit presynaptic neuronal uptake of serotonin, resulting in increased synaptic serotonin levels. When ingested in excess, SSRIs rarely cause death and typically produce nausea, vomiting, diarrhea, tremor, and decreased level of consciousness.[121] Tachycardia and seizures are infrequent.[116,119,122]

Serotonin syndrome is a condition in which associated drugs (e.g., meperidine, nonselective monoamine oxidase inhibitors, dextromethorphan, linezolid, tricyclic antidepressants, SSRIs) acutely increase serotonin levels and develops within minutes to hours (typically within 6 hours) after starting a medication, increasing the dose of a medication, or overdosing. It is characterized by a collection of neurobehavioral (e.g., confusion, agitation, coma, seizures), autonomic (e.g., hyperthermia, diaphoresis, tachycardia, hypertension), and neuromuscular (e.g., myoclonus, rigidity, tremor, ataxia, shivering, nystagmus) signs and symptoms.[123] Most cases are mild and resolve spontaneously within 24 to 72 hours. Cardiac arrest, coma, and multiorgan system failure have been reported as consequences of serotonin syndrome.[123] Recognition of the syndrome is based on a high index of suspicion and identification of risk factors.

Mechanism of Toxicity

Many of the toxic effects of tricyclic antidepressants are associated with an exaggeration of their pharmacologic action. The tricyclic antidepressants, such as type Ia antiarrhythmic drugs, inhibit the fast sodium channel so that phase 0 depolarization of the myocardium is slowed.[116] This action leads to QRS complex prolongation, atrioventricular block, ventricular tachycardia, and decreased myocardial contractility. Tricyclic antidepressants also block vascular α-adrenergic receptors, resulting in vasodilation, which contributes to hypotension. Sinus tachycardia is related to the inhibition of norepinephrine reuptake and anticholinergic effects. Other anticholinergic effects include urinary retention, ileus, dry mucous membranes, and impaired sweating. Inhibition of norepinephrine reuptake also may account for the early, transient, and self-limiting elevation of blood pressure observed in some patients. The central nervous system toxicity of tricyclic antidepressants is not well understood.

Causative Agents

Tricyclic antidepressants and SSRIs are used to treat a variety of behavioral conditions (see Chaps. 71–73). The tricyclic antidepressants include drugs such as amitriptyline, desipramine, doxepin, imipramine, and nortriptyline. Atypical agents include amoxapine, bupropion, maprotiline, nefazodone, trazodone, and venlafaxine. The SSRIs include fluoxetine, paroxetine, and sertraline. The tricyclic antidepressants are generally highly protein bound, exhibit a large volume of distribution, and possess elimination half-lives of 8 to 24 hours or more. Virtually none of the drug is eliminated unchanged in the urine. Metabolism of the parent drug produces active metabolites in most cases (e.g., amitriptyline to nortriptyline) that may contribute to toxicity after the first 12 to 24 hours.[116] Genetic polymorphism at CYP2D6 may lead to slower recovery in patients who are slow hydroxylators.[124]

Incidence

Tricyclic antidepressant poisoning is a common cause of death from drug overdose.[116,117] The 2005 AAPCC-NPDS report documented 11,198 patients with exposures to tricyclic antidepressants; 63% of these cases were considered to be intentional overdoses. A total of 1,256 people experienced a major effect, and 101 people died.[6] The SSRIs accounted for 48,161 nonfatal exposures and 118 deaths.

Risk Assessment

Referral to an emergency department is warranted for ingestions >5 mg/kg of amitriptyline, clomipramine, doxepin, and imipramine; >2.5 mg/kg of desipramine, nortriptyline, and trimipramine; and >1 mg/kg of protriptyline.[118] Patients who exhibit weakness, drowsiness, dizziness, tremulousness, and palpitations after an ingestion of a tricyclic antidepressant and patients suspected of a suicide gesture or those who are suspected victims of malicious poisoning should be promptly referred to an emergency department.[118] A QRS complex >160 milliseconds or progressive prolongation of the QRS complex is an indicator of toxicity such as seizures or ventricular arrhythmias and often precedes the onset of serious symptoms.[115,117,125] The QRS complex duration should not be used as the sole indicator of risk for tricyclic antidepressant poisoning.[125] Although urine drug analyses routinely screen for tricyclic antidepressants, the qualitative result can only suggest or confirm a potential risk for the development of toxicity.

Patients with coexisting cardiovascular and pulmonary conditions (e.g., ARDS, pulmonary infection, pulmonary aspiration) may be more susceptible to the toxic effects or complications of tricyclic antidepressant poisoning.[118] Tricyclic antidepressants interact with other central nervous system depressant drugs, which together may lead to increased central nervous system and respiratory depression.

Consult a poison control center for current recommendations for doses of SSRIs that would warrant referral to an emergency department.[126] The risk of serotonin syndrome may be increased shortly after dosage increases of SSRIs or when drug interactions increase serotonin activity.[123] Concomitant or proximal use of SSRIs, tricyclic antidepressants, or nonselective monoamine oxidase inhibitors may cause serotonin syndrome. Furthermore, the addition of certain drugs, such as tryptophan, dextromethorphan, cocaine, or sympathomimetics, to SSRI therapy may increase the risk of developing serotonin syndrome.[123]

Management of Toxicity

Once the ingestion of an overdose of tricyclic antidepressant is suspected or for any intentional ingestions, medical evaluation and treatment should be sought promptly. If the patient is symptomatic, it may be prudent to call for an ambulance because of the rapid progression of some cases. At the emergency department, the patient should be monitored carefully, have vital signs assessed regularly, and have an intravenous line started. Supportive and symptomatic care includes oxygen, intravenous fluids, and other treatments as indicated. Prompt administration of activated charcoal may decrease the absorption of any remaining tricyclic antidepressant. It also may be useful beyond the first hour of ingestion because of decreased gastrointestinal motility from the anticholinergic action of tricyclic antidepressants. Gastric lavage may be considered if the time of the ingestion is unknown or if ingestion occurred within the past 1 to 2 hours. Some practitioners avoid gastric lavage altogether.[116] Ipecac syrup should be avoided in patients who ingest tricyclic antidepressants because the rapid onset of toxicity limits its usefulness. Multiple-dose activated charcoal has been shown to increase the elimination of some tricyclic antidepressants in human volunteers[42] and has been used in poisoned patients.[115,116] It may be most useful during the first 12 hours of ingestion while the drug is distributing to tissue compartments. Because the tricyclic antidepressants possess a large volume of distribution, little of the drug is present in the bloodstream; thus hemodialysis is not useful for the extracorporeal removal of tricyclic antidepressants.

Intravenous sodium bicarbonate is part of the first-line treatment of QRS complex prolongation, ventricular arrhythmias, and hypotension caused by tricyclic antidepressant overdose.[52,116,127] Typically 1 to 2 mEq/kg sodium bicarbonate (1 mEq/mL) is administered as a bolus infusion (usually a 50-mEq ampule in an adult) and repeated as necessary to achieve an arterial blood pH of 7.50 to 7.55 or abatement of toxicity.[115,116] A therapeutic effect usually is observed within minutes. Excessive use of sodium bicarbonate may produce dangerous alkalemia, which by itself is associated with ventricular arrhythmias.[116] The mechanism of action of sodium bicarbonate is unclear. Although some practitioners have proposed that sodium bicarbonate increases protein binding of tricyclic antidepressants, this theory has been discounted. Sodium may play an important role by stabilizing tricyclic antidepressant–induced changes to the sodium gradient of the myocardium.[116,128] Regardless of its action, it is effective and generally safe. Hyperventilation to produce a mild state of respiratory alkalosis has been used to treat some dysrhythmias, but it is used less widely than sodium bicarbonate.[115,116]

CLINICAL CONTROVERSY

Because intravenous sodium bicarbonate is used as therapy for certain arrhythmias and hypotension caused by tricyclic antidepressant poisoning, some practitioners have advocated its prophylactic use. Little evidence indicates which patients would benefit from prophylactic use. The risks of potentially producing alkalosis in a patient who is not seriously toxic should be considered.

Treatment of the complications of tricyclic antidepressant poisoning is outlined in Table 10–13 and includes pharmacologic and nonpharmacologic approaches.[115,116] Several agents generally should be avoided in the treatment of tricyclic antidepressant poisoning. Other drugs that inhibit the fast sodium channel, such as procainamide and quinidine, are contraindicated. Phenytoin has limited usefulness in treating tricyclic antidepressant seizures and has questionable efficacy in managing cardiotoxicity.[115] Physostigmine was used in the past as a treatment of tricyclic antidepressant cardiotoxicity and seizures because it antagonizes anticholinergic actions. However, physostigmine has been associated with bradycardia and asystole[116,129] and has been avoided in the contemporary treatment of tricyclic antidepressant cardiovascular or central nervous system toxicity. Flumazenil is used to antagonize the effects of benzodiazepines, but its use in the presence of a tricyclic antidepressant has been associated with the development of seizures and should be avoided.[130]

Treatment of an overdose of the atypical antidepressants and SSRIs is directed primarily toward decontamination of the gastrointestinal tract with activated charcoal, symptomatic treatment, and general supportive care. Management of the serotonin syndrome involves discontinuation of the serotoninergic agent and supportive therapy. Benzodiazepines, propranolol, and cyproheptadine, a serotonin antagonist, have been used successfully.[123]

Monitoring and Prevention

Measurement of vital signs, electrolytes, and BUN and a urinalysis are indicated for initial assessment. Patients should be monitored continuously by ECG, and a 12-lead ECG should be obtained if QRS complex prolongation is noted. If patients start to show signs of

TABLE 10-13 Treatment Options for Acute Tricyclic Antidepressant Toxicity

Toxicity	Treatment
Cardiovascular	
QRS prolongation, if progressive or >0.16 s	Intravenous sodium bicarbonate to a blood pH of 7.5 even in the absence of acidosis; generally avoid other antiarrhythmic drugs
Hypotension	Intravascular fluids; intravenous sodium bicarbonate; consider norepinephrine or dopamine
Ventricular tachycardia	Intravenous sodium bicarbonate; lidocaine, overdrive pacing
Ventricular bradycardia	Epinephrine drip; cardiac pacemaker
Atrioventricular block type II, second or third degree	Cardiac pacemaker
Cardiac arrest	Advanced cardiac life support, prolonged resuscitation may be needed
Neurologic	
Seizures, agitation	Benzodiazepines; neuromuscular blockade may be needed if hyperthermia or acidosis is present
Coma	Endotracheal intubation; mechanical ventilation if needed
Homeostatic	
Hyperthermia	Treat seizures and agitation; consider cooling blanket, ice water lavage, and cool water mist of body
Acidosis	Intravenous sodium bicarbonate

cardiotoxicity, arterial blood gases should be determined. Patients who show no signs of toxicity during 6 hours of observation and have received activated charcoal promptly require no further medical monitoring. Psychiatric evaluation is indicated for adolescents and adults. When signs of tricyclic antidepressant toxicity are present in a patient, cardiac monitoring generally is recommended for at least 24 hours after the patient is without findings.[116]

Prevention of tricyclic antidepressant poisoning poses unique challenges. Many of the dosage forms are small in size, and adults and children can consume large numbers easily. In the course of treating depression, several antidepressant agents may be tried to achieve results. By not discarding unused medicines, a storehouse of potentially deadly drugs may be available for children to discover or for the despondent patient to use to attempt suicide. Although patients take tricyclic antidepressants for therapeutic relief of depression, they are also a group likely to contemplate suicide with tricyclic antidepressants. Strategies that would limit the amount of tricyclic antidepressant prescribed at one time also potentially would impair adherence to a dosage regimen and thereby compromise the therapeutic potential of these agents.[116,127] Patients with a history of suicidal gestures may be candidates for the atypical antidepressants or SSRIs, which possess less cardiotoxicity. General poison prevention measures may limit childhood poisonings, and monitoring depressed patients for suicidal ideation may identify patients at risk.[131]

ABBREVIATIONS

AAPCC-NPDS: American Association of Poison Control Centers' National Poison Data System

ALT: alanine aminotransferase

ARDS: adult respiratory distress syndrome

AST: aspartate aminotransferase

BUN: blood urea nitrogen

ECG: electrocardiogram

INR: international normalized ratio

NAPQI: *N*-acetyl-*p*-benzoquinoneimine

PPPA: Poison Prevention Packaging Act (of 1970)

REFERENCES

1. Bar-Oz B, Levichek A, Koren G. Medications that can be fatal for a toddler with one tablet or teaspoonful: A 2004 update. Pediatr Drugs 2004;6:123–126.
2. Substance Abuse and Mental Health Services Administration, Office of Applied Studies. Drug Abuse Warning Network, 2005: National Estimates of Drug-Related Emergency Department Visits. DAWN Series D-29, DHHS Publication No. (SMA) 07–4256, Rockville, MD, 2007. *http://dawninfo.samhsa.gov/files/DAWN-ED-2005-Web.pdf.*
3. Centers for Disease Control and Prevention. Web-based Injury Statistics Query and Reporting System (WISQARS) (online). Washington, National Center for Injury Prevention and Control, Centers for Disease Control and Prevention, *www.cdc.gov/ncipc/wisqars.*
4. Hoppe-Roberts JH, Lloyd LM, Chyka PA. Poisoning mortality in the United States: Comparison of national mortality statistics and poison control center reports. Ann Emerg Med 2000;35:440–448.
5. Centers for Disease Control and Prevention. Unintentional poisoning deaths—United States, 1999–2004. MMWR Morb Mortal Wkly Rep 2007;56:93–96.
6. Lai MW, Klein-Schwartz W, Rodgers GC, et al. 2005 Annual Report of the American Association of Poison Control Centers" National Poisoning and Exposure Database. Clin Toxicol (Phila) 2006;44:803–932. *http://www.aapcc.org/annual.htm.*
7. Institute of Medicine. Forging a Poison Prevention and Control System. Committee on Poison Prevention and Control. Board on Health Promotion and Disease Prevention. Washington, DC: National Academy Press, 2004.
8. Rodgers GB. The safety effects of child-resistant packaging for oral prescription drugs: Two decades of experience. JAMA 1996;275:1661–1665.
9. Shannon M. Ingestion of toxic substances by children. N Engl J Med 2000;342:186–191.
10. King WD, Palmisano PA. Ingestion of prescription drugs by children: An epidemiologic study. South Med J 1989;82:1468–1478.
11. Poison Prevention Packaging: A Textbook for Pharmacists and Physicians. Publication number 384. Washington, DC: US Consumer Product Safety Commission, 2005. *http://www.cpsc.gov/cpscpub/pubs/384.pdf.*
12. Buckley NA, Whyte IM, Dawson AH, et al. Correlations between prescriptions and drugs taken in self-poisoning. Med J Aust 1995;162:194–197.
13. Haselberger MB, Kroner BA. Drug poisoning in older patients: Preventative and management strategies. Drugs Aging 1995;7:292–297.
14. Mokhlesi B, Leiken JB, Mirray P, Corbridge TC. Adult toxicology in critical care: I. General approach to the intoxicated patient. Chest 2003;123:577–592.
15. Liang HK. Clinical evaluation of the poisoned patient and toxic syndromes. Clin Chem 1996;42:1350–1355.
16. Kales SN, Christiani DC. Acute chemical emergencies. N Engl J Med 2004;350:800–808.
17. Kearney TE, Van Bebber SL, Hiatt PH, Olson KR. Protocols for pediatric poisonings from nontoxic substances: Are they valid? Pediatr Emerg Care 2006;22:215–221.
18. Chyka PA. Substance abuse and toxicological tests. In: Lee M, ed. Basic Skills in Interpreting Laboratory Data, 3rd ed. Bethesda, MD: American Society of Health System Pharmacists, 2004:61–86.
19. Tests for drugs of abuse. Med Lett Drug Ther 2002;44:71–73.
20. Wu AB, McKay C, Broussard LA, et al. National Academy of Clinical Biochemistry Laboratory Medicine Practice Guidelines: Recommendations for the use of laboratory tests to support poisoned patients who present to the emergency department. Clin Chem 2003;49:357–379.
21. Rosenberg J, Benowitz NL, Pond S. Pharmacokinetics of drug overdose. Clin Pharmacokinet 1981;6:161–192.
22. Young-Jin S, Shannon M. Pharmacokinetics of drugs in overdose. Clin Pharmacokinet 1992;23:93–105.
23. Adams BK, Mann MD, Aboo A, et al. Prolonged gastric emptying half-time and gastric hypomotility after drug overdose. Am J Emerg Med 2004;22:548–554.
24. Taylor JR, Streetman DS, Castle SS. Medication bezoars: A literature review and report of a case. Ann Pharmacother 1998;32:940–946.
25. Bosse GM, Matyunas NJ. Delayed toxidromes. J Emerg Med 1999;17:679–690.
26. Vance MV, Selden BS, Clark RF. Optimal patient position for transport and initial management of toxic ingestions. Ann Emerg Med 1992;21:243–246.
27. Krenzelok EP, McGuigan M, Lheur P. American Academy of Clinical Toxicology, European Association of Poison Centres and Clinical Toxicologists. Position statement: Ipecac syrup. J Toxicol Clin Toxicol 1997;35:699–709.
28. Committee on Injury, Violence, and Poison Prevention. American Academy of Pediatrics policy statement: Poison treatment in the home. Pediatrics 2003:112:1180–1181.
29. Vale JA. American Academy of Clinical Toxicology, European Association of Poison Centres and Clinical Toxicologists. Position statement: Gastric lavage. J Toxicol Clin Toxicol 1997;35:711–719.
30. Chyka PA, Seger D, Krenzelok EP, Vale JA; American Academy of Clinical Toxicology; European Association of Poisons Centres and Clinical Toxicologists. Position paper: Single-dose activated charcoal. Clin Toxicol (Phila) 2005;43:61–87.
31. McFarland AK III, Chyka PA. Selection of activated charcoal products for the treatment of poisonings. Ann Pharmacother 1993;27:358–361.
32. Barceloux D, McGuigan M, Hartigan-Go K. American Academy of Clinical Toxicology, European Association of Poisons Centres and Clinical Toxicologists. Position statement: Cathartics. J Toxicol Clin Toxicol 1997;35:743–752.
33. Oral electrolyte solutions for colonic lavage before colonoscopy or barium enema. Med Lett Drugs Ther 1985;27:39–40.
34. Tenenbein M. American Academy of Clinical Toxicology, European Association of Poison Centres and Clinical Toxicologists. Position statement: Whole bowel irrigation. Clin Toxicol 2004;42:843–854.
35. Traub SJ, Hoffman RS, Nelson LS. Body packing: The internal concealment of illicit drugs. N Engl J Med 2003;349:2519–2526.
36. American College of Emergency Physicians. Clinical policy for the initial approach to patients presenting with acute toxic ingestion or dermal or inhalation exposure. Ann Emerg Med 1999;33:735–761.
37. Cooper GM, Le Couteur DG, Richardson D, Buckley NA. A randomized clinical trial of activated charcoal for the routine management of oral drug overdose. QJM 2005;98:655–660.
38. Bond GR. The role of activated charcoal and gastric emptying in gastrointestinal decontamination: A state-of-the-art review. Ann Emerg Med 2002:39:273–286.
39. McGuigan MA. Activated charcoal in the home. Clin Pediatr Emerg Med 2000;1:191–194.
40. Elenbaas RM. Critical review of forced alkaline diuresis in acute salicylism. Crit Care Q 1982;4:89–95.
41. Chyka PA. Multiple-dose activated charcoal and enhancement of systemic drug clearance: Summary of studies in animals and humans. J Toxicol Clin Toxicol 1995;33:399–405.
42. American Academy of Clinical Toxicology, European Association of Poison Centres and Clinical Toxicologists. Position statement and practice guidelines on the use of multidose activated charcoal in the treatment of acute poisoning. J Toxicol Clin Toxicol 1999;37:731–751.
43. Pond SM, Olson KR, Osterloh JD, et al. Randomized study of the treatment of phenobarbital overdose with repeated doses of activated charcoal. JAMA 1984;251:3104–3108.
44. Chyka PA, Holley JE, Mandrell TM, Sugathan P. Correlation of drug pharmacokinetics and effectiveness of multiple-dose activated charcoal therapy. Ann Emerg Med 1995;25:356–362.
45. Dorrington CL, Johnson DW, Brant R, et al. The frequency of complications associated with the use of multiple-dose activated charcoal. Ann Emerg Med 2003;42:370–377.
46. Tomaszewski C. Activated charcoal: Treatment or toxin? (editorial). Clin Toxicol 1999;37:17–18.
47. Zimmerman JL. Poisonings and overdoses in the intensive care unit: General and specific management issues. Crit Care Med 2003;31:2794–2801.
48. Shalkham AS, Kirrane BM, Hoffman RS, et al. The availability and use of charcoal hemoperfusion in the treatment of poisoned patients. Am J Kidney Dis 2006;48:239–241.

49. Calello DP, Osterhoudt KC, Henretig FM. New and novel antidotes in pediatrics. Pediatr Emerg Care 2006;22:523–530.
50. Trujillo MH, Guerrero J, Fragachan C, Fernandez MA. Pharmacologic antidotes in critical care medicine: A practical guide for drug administration. Crit Care Med 1998;26:377–391.
51. Dart RC, Goldfrank L, Chyka PA, et al. Combined evidence-based literature analysis and consensus guidelines for stocking of emergency antidotes in the United States. Ann Emerg Med 2000;36:126–132.
52. Albertson TE, Dawson A, de Latorre F, et al. Tox-ACLS: Toxicologic-oriented advanced cardiac life support. Ann Emerg Med 2001;37:S78–S90.
53. Chyka PA, Butler AY, Holliman BJ, Herman MI. Utility of *N*-acetylcysteine in treating poisonings and adverse drug reactions. Drug Saf 2000;22:123–148.
54. Antman EM, Wenger TL, Butler VP, et al. Treatment of 150 cases of life-threatening digitalis intoxication with digoxin-specific Fab antibody fragments. Circulation 1990;81:1744–1752.
55. Dart RC, Seifert SA, Boyer LV, et al. A randomized multicenter trial of Crotalidae polyvalent immune Fab (ovine) antivenom for the treatment for crotaline snakebite in the United States. Arch Intern Med 2001;161:2030–2036.
56. Smilkstein MJ, Knapp GL, Kulig KW, Rumack BH. Efficacy of oral *N*-acetylcysteine in the treatment of acetaminophen overdose: Analysis of the national multicenter study (1976–1985). N Engl J Med 1988;319:1557–1562.
57. Makin AJ, Wendon J, Williams R. A 7-year experience of severe acetaminophen-induced hepatotoxicity (1987–1993). Gastroenterology 1995;109:1907–1916.
58. Larson AM, Polson J, Fontana RJ, et al. Acetaminophen-induced acute liver failure: Results of a United States multicenter, prospective study. Hepatology 2005;42:1364–1372.
59. James LP, Mayeux PR, Hinson JA. Acetaminophen-induced hepatotoxicity. Drug Metab Dispos 2003;31:1499–1506.
60. Blantz RC. Acetaminophen: Acute and chronic effects on renal function. Am J Kidney Dis 1996;28(Suppl 1):S3–S6.
61. Dart RC, Erdman AR, Olson KR, et al. Acetaminophen poisoning: An evidence-based consensus guideline for out-of-hospital management. Clin Toxicol (Phila) 2006;44:1–18.
62. Bray GP, Harrison PM, O'Grady JG, et al. Long-term anticonvulsant therapy worsens outcome in paracetamol-induced fulminant hepatic failure. Hum Exp Toxicol 1992;11:265–270.
63. Schmidt LE, Dalhoff K, Poulsen HE. Acute versus chronic alcohol consumption in acetaminophen-induced hepatoxicity. Hepatology 2002;35:876–882.
64. Lee WM. Drug-induced hepatotoxicity. N Engl J Med 2003;349:474–485.
65. Draganov P, Durrence H, Cox C, Reuben A. Alcohol-acetaminophen syndrome: Even moderate social drinkers are at risk. Postgrad Med 2000;107:189–195.
66. Kearns GL, Leeder JS, Wasserman GS. Acetaminophen intoxication during treatment: What you don't know can hurt you. Clin Pediatr 2000;39:133–144.
67. Jones AL. Mechanism of action and value of *N*-acetylcysteine in the treatment of early and late acetaminophen poisoning: A critical review. J Toxicol Clin Toxicol 1998;36:277–285.
68. Tucker JR. Late-presenting acute acetaminophen toxicity and the role of *N*-acetylcysteine. Pediatr Emerg Care 1998;14:424–426.
69. Acetadote (acetylcysteine) Injection, manufacturer's package insert. Nashville, TN: Cumberland Pharmaceuticals, 2006.
70. Kanter MZ. Comparison of oral and i.v. acetylcysteine in the treatment of acetaminophen poisoning. Am J Health Syst Pharm 2006;63:1821–1827.
71. Brok J, Buckley N, Gluud C. Interventions for paracetamol (acetaminophen) overdose. Cochrane Database Syst Rev 2006;(2):CD003328.
72. Reigart JR, Roberts JR. Recognition and Management of Pesticide Poisonings, 5th ed. Washington, DC: US Environmental Protection Agency, 1999. *http://www.epa.gov/oppfead1/safety/healthcare/handbook/handbook.pdf.*
73. Sungar M, Guven M. Intensive care management of organophosphate insecticide poisoning. Crit Care 2001;5:211–215.
74. Abou-Donia MB. Organophosphorus ester-induced chronic neurotoxicity. Arch Environ Health 2003;58:484–497.
75. Kwong TC. Organophosphate pesticides: Biochemistry and clinical toxicology. Ther Drug Monit 2002;24:144–149.
76. Klasco RK, ed. Organophosphates Management. Poisindex System. Greenwood Village, CO: Thomson Micromedex.
77. Okumura T, Takasu N, Ishimatsu S, et al. Report on 640 victims of the Tokyo subway sarin attack. Ann Emerg Med 1996;28:129–135.
78. Evison D, Hinsley D, Rice P. Chemical weapons. Br Med J 2002;324:332–335.
79. Aygun D, Doganay Z, Altintop L, et al. Serum acetylcholinesterase and prognosis of acute organophosphate poisoning. J Toxicol Clin Toxicol 2002;40:903–910.
80. Medicis JJ, Stork CM, Howland MA, et al. Pharmacokinetics following a loading dose plus a continuous infusion of pralidoxime compared with the traditional short infusion regimen in human volunteers. J Toxicol Clin Toxicol 1996;34:289–295.
81. Farrar HC, Wells TG, Kearns GL. Use of continuous infusion of pralidoxime for treatment of organophosphate poisoning in children. J Pediatr 1990;116:658–661.
82. Buckley NA, Eddleston M, Szinicz L. Oximes for acute organophosphate pesticide poisoning. Cochrane Database Syst Rev 2005;(1):CD005085.
83. Peter JV, Moran JL, Graham P. Oxime therapy and outcomes in human organophosphate poisoning: An evaluation using meta-analytic techniques. Crit Care Med 2006;34:502–510.
84. Pesticides: Health and Safety. Washington, DC: US Environmental Protection Agency. *http://www.epa.gov/pesticides/health.*
85. Salhanick SD, Shannon MW. Management of calcium channel antagonist overdose. Drug Saf 2003;26:65–79.
86. Pearigen PD, Benowitz NL. Poisoning due to calcium antagonists: Experience with verapamil, diltiazem, and nifedipine. Drug Saf 1991;6:408–430.
87. DeWitt CR, Waksman JC. Pharmacology, pathophysiology and management of calcium channel blocker and beta-blocker toxicity. Toxicol Rev 2004;23:223–238.
88. Harris NS. Case records of the Massachusetts General Hospital. Case 24–2006. A 40-year-old woman with hypotension after an overdose of amlodipine. N Engl J Med 2006;355:602–611.
89. Shepherd G. Treatment of poisoning caused by beta-adrenergic and calcium-channel blockers. Am J Health Syst Pharm 2006;63:1828–1835.
90. Adams BD, Browne WT. Amlodipine overdose causes prolonged calcium channel blocker toxicity. Am J Emerg Med 1998;16:527–528.
91. Olson KR, Erdman AR, Woolf AD, et al. Calcium channel blocker ingestion: An evidence-based consensus guideline for out-of-hospital management. Clin Toxicol (Phila) 2005;43:797–821.
92. Buckley N, Dawson AH, Howarth D, Whyte IM. Slow-release verapamil poisoning: Use of polyethylene glycol whole-bowel lavage and high-dose calcium. Med J Aust 1993;158:202–204.
93. Papadopoulos J, O'Neil MG. Utilization of a glucagon infusion in the management of a massive nifedipine overdose. J Emerg Med 2000;18:453–455.
94. Holzer M, Sterz F, Schoerkhuber W, et al. Successful resuscitation of a verapamil-intoxicated patient with percutaneous cardiopulmonary bypass. Crit Care Med 1999;27:2818–2823.
95. Durward A, Guerguerian AM, Lefebvre M, Shemie SD. Massive diltiazem overdose treated with extracorporeal membrane oxygenation. Pediatr Crit Care Med 2003;4:372–376.
96. Luomanmaki K, Tiula E, Kivisto KT, Neuvonen PJ. Pharmacokinetics of diltiazem in massive overdose. Ther Drug Monit 1997;19:240–242.
97. Morimoto S, Sasaki S, Kiyama M, et al. Sustained-release diltiazem overdose. J Hum Hypertens 1999;13:643–644.
98. Fine JS. Iron poisoning. Curr Probl Pediatr 2000;30:71–90.
99. Robertson A, Tenenbein M. Hepatotoxicity in acute iron poisoning. Hum Exp Toxicol 2005;24:559–562.
100. Chyka PA, Banner W Jr. Hematopoietic agents. In: Dart RC, ed. Medical Toxicology, 3rd ed. Philadelphia: Lippincott Williams & Wilkins, 2004:605–614.
101. Tenenbein M, Israels SJ. Early coagulopathy in severe iron poisoning. J Pediatr 1988;113:695–697.
102. Pestaner JP, Ishak KG, Mullick FG, Centeno JA. Ferrous sulfate toxicity: A review of autopsy findings. Biol Trace Element Res 1999;69:191–198.
103. Manoguerra AS, Erdman AR, Booze LL, et al. Iron ingestion: An evidence-based consensus guideline for out-of-hospital management. Clin Toxicol (Phila) 2005;43:553–570.

104. Everson GW, Oukjhane K, Young LW, et al. Effectiveness of abdominal radiographs in visualizing chewable iron supplements following overdose. Am J Emerg Med 1989;7:459–463.
105. Palatnick W, Tenenbein M. Leukocytosis, hyperglycemia, vomiting, and positive x-rays are not indicators of severity of iron overdose in adults. Am J Emerg Med 1996;14:454–455.
106. Chyka PA, Butler AY. Assessment of acute iron poisoning by laboratory and clinical observations. Am J Emerg Med 1993;11:99–103.
107. Chyka PA, Butler AY, Holley JE. Serum iron concentrations and symptoms of acute iron poisoning in children. Pharmacother 1996;16:1053–1058.
108. Eisen TF, Lacouture PG, Woolf A. Visual detection of ferrioxamine color changes in urine. Vet Hum Toxicol 1988;30:369–370.
109. Peck M, Rogers J, Riverbach J. Use of high doses of deferoxamine (Desferal) in an adult patient with acute iron overdosage. J Toxicol Clin Toxicol 1982;19:865–869.
110. Howland MA. Risks of parenteral deferoxamine for acute iron poisoning. J Toxicol Clin Toxicol 1996;34:491–497.
111. Shannon M. Desferrioxamine in acute iron poisoning [letter]. Lancet 1992;339:1601.
112. Tenenbein M, Kowalski S, Sienko A, et al. Pulmonary toxic effects of continuous desferrioxamine administration in acute iron poisoning. Lancet 1992;339:699–701.
113. VanOrden HE, Hagemann TM. Deferasirox—An oral agent for chronic iron overload. Ann Pharmacother 2006;40:1110–1117.
114. Berkovitch M, Livne A, Lushkov G, et al. The efficacy of oral deferiprone in acute iron poisoning. Am J Emerg Med 2000;18:36–40.
115. Kerr GW, McGuffie AC, Wilkie S. Tricyclic antidepressant overdose: A review. Emerg Med J 2001:18:236–241.
116. Pentel PR, Keyler DE, Haddad LM. Tricyclic antidepressants and selective serotonin reuptake inhibitors. In: Haddad LM, Shannon MW, Winchester JI, eds. Clinical Management of Poisoning and Drug Overdose, 3rd ed. Philadelphia: WB Saunders, 1998:437–451.
117. James LP, Kearns GL. Cyclic antidepressant toxicity in children and adolescents. J Clin Pharmacol 1995;35:343–350.
118. Woolf AD, Erdman AR, Nelson LS, et al. Tricyclic antidepressant poisoning: An evidence-based consensus guideline for out-of-hospital management. Clin Toxicol (Phila) 2007;45:203–233.
119. Henry JA. Epidemiology and relative toxicity of antidepressant drugs in overdose. Drug Saf 1997;16:374–390.
120. Buckley NA, McManus PR. Fatal toxicity of serotoninergic and other antidepressant drugs: Analysis of United Kingdom mortality data. Br Med J 2002;325:1332–1333.
121. Barbey JT, Roose SP. SSRI safety and overdose. J Clin Psychiatry 1998;59(Suppl 15):42–48.
122. Borys DJ, Setzer SC, Ling LJ, et al. Acute fluoxetine overdose: A report of 234 cases. Am J Emerg Med 1992;10:115–120.
123. Boyer EW, Shannon M. The serotonin syndrome. N Engl J Med 2005; 352:1112–1120.
124. Spina E, Henthorn TK, Eleborg L, et al. Desmethylimipramine overdose: Nonlinear kinetics in a slow hydroxylator. Ther Drug Monit 1985;7:239–241.
125. Buckley NA, Chevalier S, Leditschke A, et al. The limited utility of electrocardiography variables used to predict arrhythmia in psychotropic drug overdose. Crit Care 2003;7:R102–R107. *http://ccforum.com/content/7/5/R101*.
126. Nelson LS, Erdman AR., Booze LL, et al. Selective serotonin reuptake inhibitor poisoning: An evidence-based consensus guideline for out-of-hospital management. Clin Toxicol (Phila) 2007;45:315–332.
127. Smilkstein MJ. Reviewing cyclic antidepressant cardiotoxicity: Wheat and chaff. J Emerg Med 1990;8:645–648.
128. McCabe JL, Cobaugh DJ, Mengazzi JJ, Fata J. Experimental tricyclic antidepressant toxicity: A randomized, controlled comparison of hypertonic saline solution, sodium bicarbonate, and hyperventilation. Ann Emerg Med 1998;32:329–333.
129. Suchard JR. Assessing physostigmine's contraindication in cyclic antidepressant ingestions. J Emerg Med 2003;25:185–191.
130. Weinbroum AA, Flaishon R, Sorkine P. A risk-benefit assessment of flumazenil in the management of benzodiazepine overdose. Drug Saf 1997;17:181–196.
131. Friedman RA, Leon AC. Expanding the Black Box—depression, antidepressants, and the risk of suicide. N Engl J Med 2007;356:2343–2346.

CHAPTER 11 Emergency Preparedness: Identification and Management of Biological Exposures

COLLEEN M. TERRIFF, JASON E. BROUILLARD, LISA T. COSTANIGRO, AND JESSICA S. GRUBER

KEY CONCEPTS

1. Bioterrorism agents are organisms or toxins that can cause disease and death in humans, animals, or plants and elicit terror.
2. Category A bioterrorism agents include anthrax (*Bacillus anthracis*), tularemia (*Francisella tularensis*), smallpox (*variola major*), plague (*Yersinia pestis*), botulinum toxin (*Clostridium botulinum*), and viral hemorrhagic fevers.
3. Many bioterrorism agents cause symptoms similar to other more common infectious diseases, like seasonal influenza, and may be difficult to differentiate without confirmatory laboratory testing.
4. Anthrax is a highly virulent, lethal infection; human-to-human transmission, however, has not been documented.
5. Individuals with signs and symptoms of botulism should be administered a test dose prior to receiving equine antitoxin therapy.
6. Prompt initiation of appropriate empiric therapy, after cultures are obtained, is vital to decreasing the mortality rate associated with plague.
7. Emergency preparedness for those at risk and response efforts for those exposed to smallpox involves mass vaccination campaigns.
8. Viral hemorrhagic fever, caused by one of a variety of viruses, can manifest as a febrile illness with a large range of sequela, including bleeding complications.

The fall of 2001 forever changed how many people through out the world felt about flying, airport security, and even opening their mail. Terrorism, especially bioterrorism, became a common term used by the media, military analysts, both governments and public health officials, and the public at large. Anxiety caused by the 2001 intentional anthrax release through the United States mail system, and the ensuing exposures and deaths, was further escalated by numerous false alarms surrounding the delivery of parcels containing unidentified white powder.[1] Recent devastating natural disasters, such as tsunamis and hurricanes, have reawakened our appreciation of the power and destruction associated with natural disasters. Isolated reports during the past decade have heightened concern about a global outbreak of severe acute respiratory syndrome (SARS) or avian influenza and as a result many levels of the community, including schools, businesses, health systems, first responders, and governments, have begun to address the need for planning for public health emergencies. Stockpiling of antibiotics for bioterrorism attacks and antivirals for pandemic influenza is becoming a crucial public health issue. Healthcare providers need to play an active role in awareness and preparedness for biological threats released by terrorists or nature, and the decision-making process regarding postexposure prophylaxis (PEP), mass vaccination, and treatment of biologic exposures to help protect the public.

(1) Bioterrorism agents—organisms or toxins that can cause disease and death in humans, animals or plants for the purpose of eliciting terror—have been used against civilians and military personnel for centuries. Thousands of years ago crude, but effective methods were used for bioterrorism. Filth, human cadavers, and animal carcasses were flung over city walls, poisons were dropped in drinking wells, and contaminated clothing and blankets were offered as gifts to cause disease and, ultimately, death to enemies. More recently, sophisticated methods have been utilized, such as aerosolized technology for spraying plague and an umbrella-looking device used to shoot ricin toxin pellets for a targeted assassination.[2,3] Over the past 80 years a variety of methods to weaponize biologic agents—enhance the shelf-life or dissemination properties (i.e., aerosolize) and/or fill munitions—have been researched.[3] Approximately 12 countries throughout the world are believed to have active biological weapons programs, ranging from conducting research on the virulence of selected agents to actually weaponizing them.[4]

This chapter describes the natural history, symptomatology, diagnostic procedures, pharmacologic and nonpharmacologic treatment of biological agents of highest concern that could be used in a bioterrorism attack, such as anthrax, botulinum toxin, plague, smallpox, tularemia, viral hemorrhagic fevers and select Category B and C agents. The potential consequences of infectious disease outbreaks surrounding natural disasters, which rival bioterrorist events in their devastating potential, are also discussed. An evidence-based approach evaluating the various treatment options, including those for special populations, is presented, when the relevant data is available. Finally, information about the roles of healthcare providers in emergency preparedness and response is shared.

The complete chapter, learning objectives, and other resources can be found at **www.pharmacotherapyonline.com.**

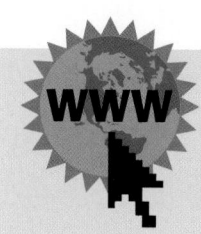

CHAPTER 12 Emergency Preparedness: Identification and Management of Chemical and Radiological Exposures

GREENE SHEPHERD AND RICHARD B. SCHWARTZ

KEY CONCEPTS

1. In mass casualty events with chemical or radiologic exposure, the majority of victims can be managed with decontamination, observation and supportive care. Antidotal therapies should be reserved for more critically injured victims.
2. Nerve agent poisoning is similar to organophosphate insecticide poisoning with atropine and pralidoxime being the primary antidotes.
3. Cyanide gas exposure can be rapidly fatal but most victims that are conscious upon arrival to the hospital will not require antidote therapy.
4. Respiratory problems caused by pulmonary agents with low water solubility may take several hours to develop thus requiring extended observation.
5. Vesicant chemical weapons are less lethal than other chemical weapons but cause significant morbidity leaving many survivors that need extensive care.
6. Therapeutic agents are available that can block the uptake or enhance the elimination of radioactive contamination.
7. Clinicians, especially pharmacists need to be prepared to take an active role in the design and operationalization of disaster plans for their workplace and community. Pharmacists may participate on established disaster response teams that may be deployed to assist in the care of individuals outside of their local area.

Life-threatening hazardous material exposures may happen anywhere and at any time. The exposure may be due to an unintentional release or at the other extreme be the result of an intentional and catastrophic act of terrorism.[1–6] A hazardous material is defined as any substance that poses a substantial risk to the health or safety of individuals, or the environment when improperly handled, stored, transported, or disposed.[1] The specific risks are dependent on the quantity and concentration of the substance exposure and the physical, chemical, or infectious characteristics of the material. Many of these substances have the potential to be used as weapons. Small quantities of hazardous materials are used in many commercial products, such as pesticides. Larger and more concentrated quantities are found at industrial sites and in their waste byproducts. Injuries from hazardous materials are relatively common as evidenced by the tens of thousands of hazardous material incidents recorded by the U.S. Environmental Protection Agency during the last decade. The majority of these incidents occur during transport rather than at the site of manufacture or use and represent a complex and significant danger for emergency healthcare workers.[1] At the other extreme, a hazardous material exposure may be the result of an intentional and catastrophic act of terrorism. Historically, acts of chemical or radiologic terrorism have been rare but have had very high visibility and marked psychological impact. Terrorism represents a profound threat to many countries around the world. Terrorists, whether representing foreign governments, organized religious sects, or individuals, have the capacity to endanger our communities with hazardous materials. Even a single patient contaminated with a hazardous material has the potential to overwhelm an unprepared healthcare facility.

The complete chapter, learning objectives, and other resources can be found at www.pharmacotherapyonline.com.

(1) A common thread in all disasters is that community healthcare systems are severely strained by limited communication, lack of personnel with disaster training or experience, lack of plans for facility surge capacity and limited availability of medical supplies. If chemical or radiologic contamination occurs the system is strained even further because of a lack of decontamination training and equipment at hospitals. Preplanning and early detection systems need to be in place to facilitate early recognition of the event and the substances involved if the community has any likelihood of being able to mount an effective response to a chemical or radiologic disaster. In all disasters, the normal flow of care is disrupted and the influx of victims becomes the major focus of the healthcare community. Preplanning for acute care needs for large numbers of patients, may include devising a method for expanding bed and surgical capacity as well as preparing specialized antidotes. Even if only minor injuries result from the event a significant portion of the affected population will need access to critical every day medications, such as insulin and personal needs, such as food and shelter.

This chapter discusses the major groups of hazardous materials that have been used as weapons. Chemical and radiologic events that have occurred in recent years are reviewed to provide an understanding of the scope, size, and complexity of such events. The clinical presentation, mechanisms of toxicity, and relevant diagnostic approaches are discussed for each type of agent. The community and individual preventative measures that can be taken to minimize the risks associated with the major types of chemical and radiologic threats are reviewed and the nonpharmacologic and pharmacologic treatment options are critically evaluated. Because controlled clinical trial data is lacking in this area the majority of treatment recommendations in this chapter are based on animal studies, anecdotal experience, and expert opinion. Finally, the ways in which clinicians can actively participate in disaster planning and response at the local, state and national level are presented.

SECTION 2
CARDIOVASCULAR DISORDERS

CHAPTER 13

Cardiovascular Testing

ROBERT CHILTON AND ROBERT L. TALBERT

KEY CONCEPTS

1. A careful patient history and physical examination are extremely important in diagnosing cardiovascular disease and should be done prior to any test.
2. Heart sounds and heart murmurs are important in identifying heart valve abnormalities and other structural cardiac defects.
3. Elevated jugular venous pressure is an important sign of heart failure and may be used to assess severity and response to therapy.
4. Electrocardiography is useful for determining rhythm disturbances (tachy- or bradyarrhythmias) and changes in ventricular and atrial size.
5. Exercise stress testing provides important information concerning the likelihood and severity of coronary artery disease; changes in the electrocardiogram, blood pressure, and heart rate are used to assess the response to exercise.
6. Cardiac catheterization and angiography are used to assess coronary anatomy and ventricular performance.
7. Echocardiography is used to assess valve structure and function as well as ventricular wall motion; transesophogeal echocardiography is more sensitive for detecting thrombus and vegetations than transthoracic echocardiography.
8. Radionuclides such as technetium-99m and thallium-201 are used to assess wall motion and myocardial viability in patients with coronary artery disease and heart failure.
9. Pharmacologic stress testing is used when patients cannot perform physical exercise to assess the likelihood of coronary artery disease.

Learning objectives, review questions, and other resources can be found at **www.pharmacotherapyonline.com.**

Every 36 seconds 1 person dies from cardiovascular disease and each day about 2,500 people die in the United States. Cardiovascular disease exceeds the next four leading causes of death combined (cancer, lung disease, accidents, and diabetes).[1] Another important factor in cardiovascular disease is that greater than 60% of unexpected cardiac deaths occur *without* prior history of heart disease and 70% of patients having a myocardial infarction have coronary artery blockages of about 40% to 60% (Fig. 13–1).

Cardiovascular disease affects 71,300,000 Americans, with one-third being older than age 65 years based on the National Health and Nutrition Examination Survey.[2] The current increase in patients older than age 65 years with cardiovascular disease will undoubtedly generate a large financial burden on the economy and families. Adding to the increasing burden of cardiovascular disease is information from Centers for Disease Control and Prevention revealing a marked increase in the number of patients with obesity; additionally, the projected 2050 growth rate in both obesity and diabetes is staggering. In 1997, the percentage of patient with obesity was approximately 19.5% of the U.S. population, and in 2004 it was found to have increased by 25% (24.3%). Along with this increase in obesity there was a 30% increase in diabetes from 5.3% to 6.9% over this same period of time.[3] The rise of obesity and diabetes will undoubtedly lead to increases in heart disease prevalence.

Another area of concern in cardiovascular disease is illustrated by the Framingham Heart Study, which has followed patients for more than 40 years and found that the average annual rate of first major cardiovascular events increase significantly with age. Patients ages 35 to 44 years were found to have 7 major cardiovascular events per 1,000 men and to increase to 68 per 1,000 men by age 85 years, a 9-fold increase.[4]

In summary, one of the most important pieces of information that patients need to know is that lifestyle changes, that is, healthy-smart eating with reasonable caloric intake and frequent exercise, are major keys to a productive healthy life. The importance of lifestyle in saving lives is well illustrated from a recent study by Chiuve et al., which studied 42,847 men in the Health Professionals Follow-up Study (cohort) who were 40 to 75 years of age and free of disease in 1986.[5] The healthy lifestyle was defined as no smoking, body mass index <25 kg/m^2, moderate to vigorous activity >30 min/day, moderate alcohol consumption (5 to 30 g/day), and a healthy diet score. Tracking nonfatal myocardial infarctions and fatal coronary heart disease using a multivariate-adjusted Cox proportional hazards model, men complying with these five lifestyle factors had a

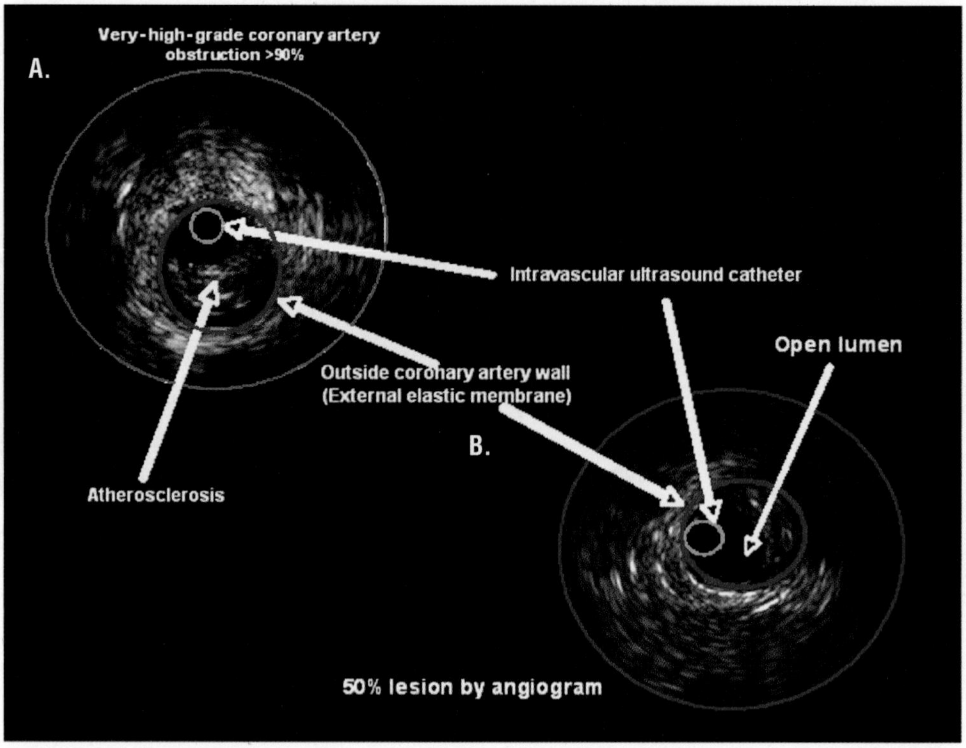

FIGURE 13-1. Intravascular ultrasound (IVUS) of a coronary artery. *A.* High-grade obstruction which on angiogram was thought to be only approximately 50% stenotic. *B.* Another coronary artery segment with 50% stenosis but more prone to rupture.

lower risk of coronary heart disease (relative risk: 0.13; 95% confidence interval [CI]: 0.09 to 0.19) compared with men who were at low risk with no lifestyle factors. Using population-attributable risk calculations (proportion of cases within the population that could have been avoided had all the men adhered to the low-risk lifestyle) adherence to five lifestyle changes could prevent 62% of men from having a coronary event. If patients were taking medication for hypertension or hypercholesterolemia they still would have a 57% reduction ([95% confidence interval (CI) 0.07 to 0.43]).

THE HISTORY

A comprehensive history is the cornerstone of a cardiovascular workup. The value of the history depends on the clinician's ability to elicit relevant information. Family history is very important because of the genetic links involved in many cardiovascular diseases from early myocardial infarction, strokes, diabetes, valvular heart disease, hypertension and familial hypercholesterolemia. The elements of a comprehensive history include the chief complaint, present problems, past medical history, review of systems, and social history.

The chief complaint needs to be narrowed down and focused if possible. Usually the chief complaint/main concern is a short brief statement as to the reason why the patient seeks medical care (get to the point). The duration of the chief complaint is important, along with any prior history of the same problem, the severity of the problem, and whether there are any limitations on the patient's daily activities. Other areas that need to be addressed are character, any types of motion or other things that increase or decrease the discomfort, any association with additional signs or symptoms, and whether the discomfort is increasing in frequency or duration. All these and many other matters need to be considered as the clinician does the intake interview with a new patient.

CARDIOVASCULAR HISTORY

❶ Ischemic heart disease is the most common cardiovascular disease seen in clinical practice. A focus on chest pain history is very important. The clinical syndrome of angina is frequently described by patients as a discomfort from chest ache, pain, or pressure, to dull pain in the jaw, back, shoulder, or either arm. Many research studies have found that family/work stress or exertion brings on increased symptoms of angina and rest or nitroglycerin frequently relieves it.[6] Another important consideration when one considers angina is that in addition to epicardial large-vessel coronary artery disease (CAD), angina can develop in patients with valvular heart disease, obstructive cardiomyopathies, and hypertension. Symptoms of angina can occur in patients with noncardiac conditions such as gastrointestinal (esophageal), chest wall, or pulmonary disease (see Chap. 17). Angina does not necessarily relate to the severity or extent of CAD obstruction. Angina that is increasing in severity, longer in duration or occurring at rest is consistent with unstable angina and should be evaluated immediately.[7]

Initial evaluation of chest pain requires a good history and physical examination.[8,9] The quality of chest pain, its location and duration, and factors that provoke or relieve the chest pain are important elements. Rarely do patients with ischemic heart disease describe their pain as sharp or stabbing. Commonly, patients state they do not have chest pain but a heaviness or pressure in the chest. Ischemic chest pain typically lasts only a few minutes and is generally brought on by exertion or emotional stress, and is commonly relieved by rest or nitroglycerin. Based on the history, classify the patient's symptoms. Three characteristics to consider are (a) whether the substernal chest discomfort has a classic quality and duration that is (b) provoked by exertion or emotional stress and (c) relieved by rest or nitroglycerin. If all three of these conditions are met, then the patient has classical angina; if only two of these conditions exist, the pain is considered to be atypical or probably angina; and if none are met, it is considered to be noncardiac chest pain. It is equally important that the patient inform the healthcare professional that the discomfort the patient is experiencing, which could be atypical, is the patient's "angina equivalent." Important information when taking a history of patients with angina is being aware of the grading of angina pectoris by the Canadian Cardiovascular Society (see Chap. 17).

It is important in an ischemic chest to differentiate angina from acute coronary syndrome. Acute coronary syndrome is more frequent, dramatic, and severe (see Chap. 18).

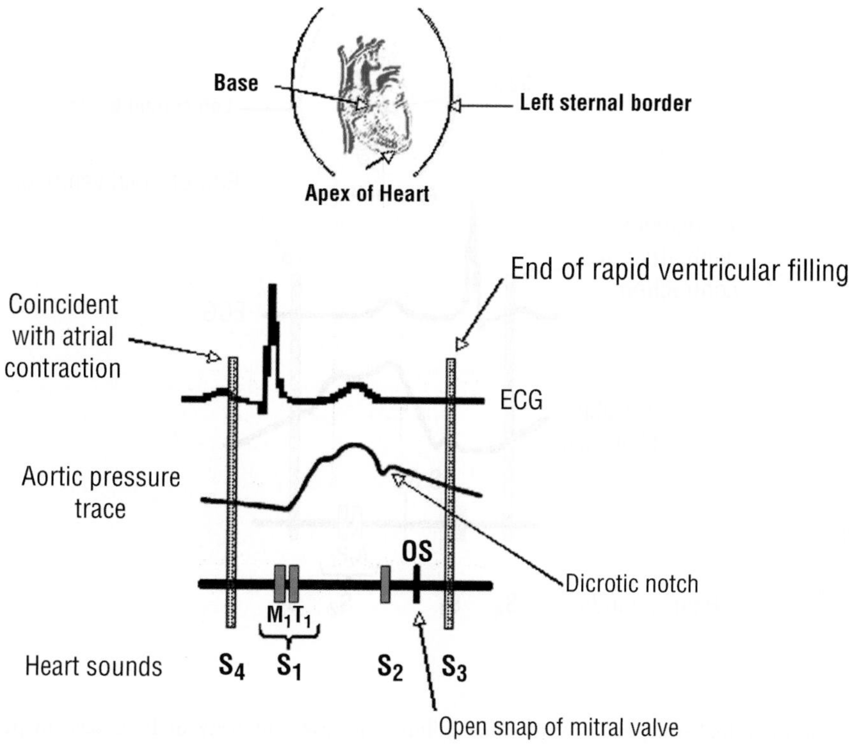

FIGURE 13-2. Correlation of the electrocardiogram (ECG) with an aortic pressure tracing and heart sounds. Normal heart sounds are S_1 and S_2; S_3 and S_4 are abnormal, as is an opening snap (OS), which is heard with mitral stenosis. S_1 may be split in some conditions (M_1, mitral; T_1, tricuspid.)

PHYSICAL EXAMINATION

The cardiovascular physical examination is divided into four categories:

1. Global examination of the patient for signs of cardiovascular disease (CVD) and a review of all body systems.
2. Observation and assessment of physical findings (e.g., jugular venous pressure).
3. Measurement of parameters of CVD function (pulse, blood pressure).
4. Auscultation, percussion, and palpation of the chest and related cardiac structures.

The initial part of the physical examination consists of inspection of the precordium for normal patterns of rise and fall and any abnormal markings or shape. The chest is then palpated for normal pulses, thrills (humming vibrations like the throat of a purring cat), and heaves (lifting of the chest wall). Thrills may indicate murmurs, and heaves may indicate enlargement of one of the heart chambers or an abnormal vessel such as an aneurysm. The apical pulse (also known as the *point of maximum impulse*) is helpful to estimate heart size and rotation. This is usually located in the fifth intercostal space in the midsternal line and radiates in an arc of 1 to 2 cm. Heightened intensity and/or displacement laterally suggests left or right ventricle enlargement, and reduced intensity may be a sign of fluid overload or pericardial effusion. Factors such as obesity, large breasts, muscularity, and pulmonary disease can interfere with determination of the apical pulse. The carotid pulse is examined for its intensity and, concurrently with the apical pulse, for concordance within the cardiac cycle. Decreased carotid pulsations may be a result of reduced stroke volume or atherosclerotic narrowing of the carotid artery.

Important physical correlations need to be carefully noted, as shown in Figs. 13–2 and 13–3. These critical associations are basic facts needed to understanding the physical examination of the human heart.

HEART SOUNDS

❷ Auscultation with a stethoscope is used to characterize heart sounds. Auscultation is conducted in a systematic manner to ensure that all sites where normal and abnormal sounds are heard are reviewed. Respiratory pattern, various maneuvers such as handgrip and the Valsalva maneuver, sitting versus standing, and pharmacologic agents (e.g., amyl nitrate) also may be used in the evaluation of heart sounds to accentuate or diminish the intensity of these sounds. Auscultation is an acquired art and requires considerable practice to become competent.

The normal heart sounds include S_1 (first heart sound—closure of the mitral and tricuspid valves) and S_2 (second heart sound—aortic and pulmonic valves). Normally the second heart sound becomes split during inspiration because of delayed closure of the pulmonic valve (prolongation of right ventricle systole secondary to an increase in venous return) or because of an inspiratory decrease in impedance of the pulmonary bed.

Other sounds, such as S_3 (third heart sound) and S_4 (fourth heart sound) and murmurs, are not considered normal but provide important diagnostic information. Initially, the patient is examined lying partially on the left side to accentuate left-sided S_3 and S_4 and mitral murmurs, with the bell on the point of maximum impulse. To identify S_1 and S_2, the patient can be examined lying or sitting. The other areas that are auscultated are the apex or base of the heart (mitral sounds), the lower left sternal border (tricuspid sounds), the second left interspace (pulmonic sounds), and the second right interspace (aortic sounds). At each of these locations, S_1 and S_2 should be heard (Fig. 13–4).

Heart sounds are characterized by location, pitch, intensity, duration, and timing within the cardiac cycle. High-pitched sounds such as S_1 and S_2, murmurs of aortic and mitral regurgitation, and pericardial friction rubs are best heard with the diaphragm. The bell is preferred for low-pitched sounds such as S_3 and S_4. S_1 is heard as a click at the end of diastole and usually is synchronous with the apical pulse. The intensity of S_1 can be increased if systole begins

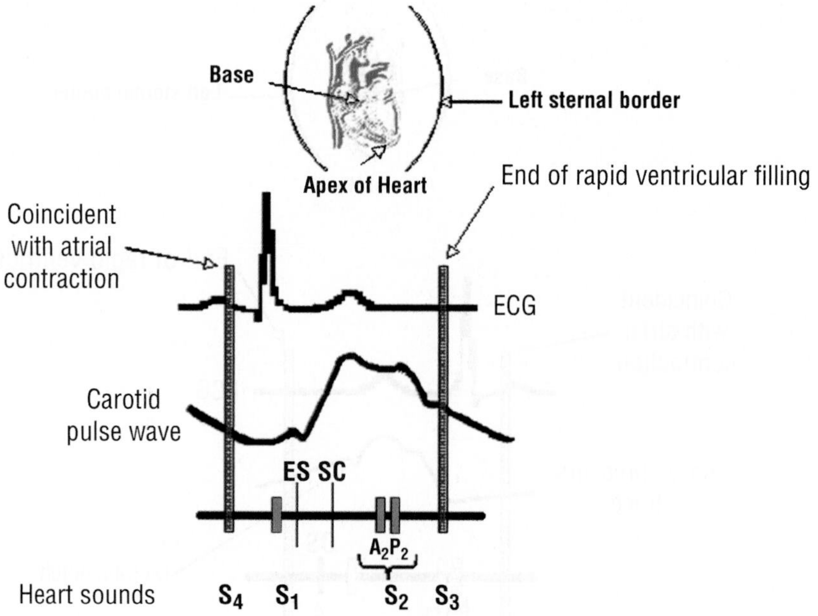

FIGURE 13-3. Correlation of the electrocardiogram (ECG) with a carotid pulse pressure tracing and heart sounds. A split S_2 is heard in some conditions (A_2, aortic; P_2, pulmonic).

prior to the mitral valve closing, which may occur in high-output states (e.g., exercise, tachycardia, anemia, or hyperthyroidism) and mitral valve stenosis. S_1 intensity is decreased in first-degree heart block, mitral regurgitation, states of reduced myocardial contractility (such as heart failure or coronary artery disease), obesity (difficult to hear), and systemic or pulmonary hypertension. S_2 is heard at the end of systole and is best heard at the tricuspid and mitral areas. Most of the sound arises from aortic valve closure. Heart sounds may be "spilt" if the two valves do not close synchronously. Physiologic splitting of S_1 or S_2 is accentuated by inspiration and may disappear with expiration. Splitting of S_2 creates a pulmonic (P_2) and aortic (A_2) sound. S_2 frequently is heard as a split sound and is most predominant at the height of inspiration. Although S_1 also may be split, this is often difficult to hear.

Pathologic splitting of S_2 during expiration is described as *wide splitting, fixed splitting,* and *paradoxical splitting* and may be indicative of both stenosis and regurgitation. With right-sided heart failure, right bundle-branch block, pulmonic stenosis, or atrial septal defects, S_2 may be split owing to delayed closure of the pulmonic valve. Fixed splitting of S_2 is associated with large atrial septal defects and right ventricular failure. Increased intensity of P_2 is seen in pulmonary hypertension and dilated pulmonary arteries and with atrial septal defects. Decreased or absent P_2 occurs with aging and in pulmonic stenosis. Extra heart sounds in systole include early systolic ejection sounds and clicks and midsystolic clicks. Early ejection sounds such as aortic or pulmonic ejection sounds often are associated with valvular disease. Midsystolic to late systolic clicks usually are a result of mitral valve prolapse. Mitral valve prolapse is best heard at or medial to the apex, but also may be heard at the left lower sternal border.

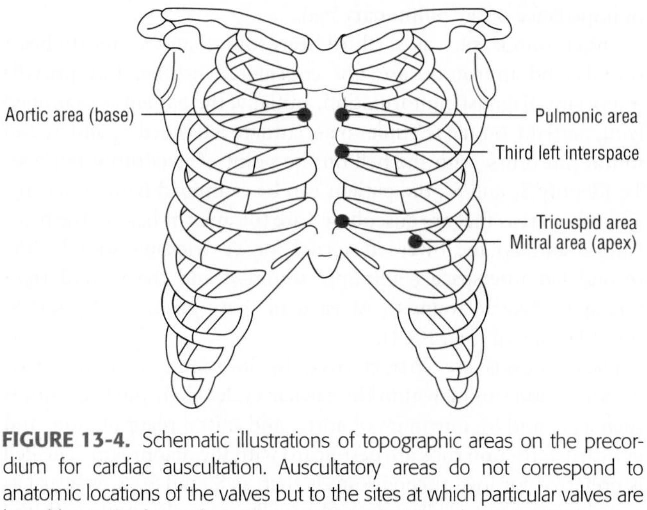

FIGURE 13-4. Schematic illustrations of topographic areas on the precordium for cardiac auscultation. Auscultatory areas do not correspond to anatomic locations of the valves but to the sites at which particular valves are heard best. *(Redrawn from Kinney MR, Packa DR, eds. Andreoli's Comprehensive Cardiac Care, 8th ed. St. Louis: Mosby, 1996, with permission.)*

The S_3 heart sound, or ventricular gallop, is an abnormal low-pitched sound usually heard at the apex of the heart. It is thought to be caused by rapid filling and stretching of the left ventricle when the left ventricle is somewhat noncompliant. This heart sound is characteristic of volume overloading, such as in congestive heart failure (especially left-sided heart failure), tricuspid or mitral valve insufficiency, and atrial and/or ventricular septal defects. A physiologic S_3 is heard commonly in children and may persist into young adulthood. Localization of S_3 is helpful for determining heart rotation within the chest cavity.

The S_4 diastolic sound is a dull, low-pitched postsystolic atrial gallop (rapid blood flow) usually caused by reduced ventricular compliance. It is best heard at the apex in the left lateral position. Like S_3, it occurs with reduced ventricular compliance and is present in conditions such as aortic stenosis, hypertension, hypertrophic cardiomyopathies, and coronary artery disease. It is less specific for congestive heart failure than S_3.

The frequency range of S_3 and S_4 is below 100 Hz and requires the bell of the stethoscope to be used most of the time. This should be lightly touched to the skin to obtain the best results.

HEART MURMURS

Murmurs are auditory vibrations heard on auscultation, and they occur because of turbulent blood flow within the heart chambers or through the valves.[10] They are classified by timing and duration within the cardiac cycle (systolic, diastolic, and continuous), location, intensity, shape (configuration or pattern), pitch (frequency), quality, and radiation (Table 13–1). It is important to first note where it is heard best and where it radiates for example from apex to left axilla. Using S_1 and S_2 as a marker for timing, ask yourself this

TABLE 13-1 Characteristics of Heart Sounds

Type of Murmur	Examples	Location	Pitch	Radiation	Quality
Midsystolic	Aortic stenosis	2nd RICS	Medium	Neck, left sternal border	Harsh
	Pulmonic stenosis	2nd and 3rd LICS	Medium	Left shoulder and neck	Harsh
	Hypertrophic cardiomyopathy	3rd and 4th LICS	Medium	Left sternal border to apex	Harsh
Pansystolic	Mitral regurgitation	Apex	Medium to high	Left axilla	Blowing
	Tricuspid regurgitation	Lower left sternal border	Medium	Right sternum, xiphoid	Blowing
	Ventricular septal defect	3rd, 4th, and 5th LICS	High		Often harsh
Diastolic	Aortic regurgitation	2nd to 4th LICS	High	Apex	Blowing
	Mitral stenosis	Apex	Low	Little or none	

LICS, left intercostal space; RICS, right intercostal space.

question: Does the murmur occur in systole or diastole? Next carefully listen to see if the murmur completely fills that phase of the systolic cycle (i.e., holosystolic), or if it has discrete start and end points. Murmurs that occur after second heart sound are considered diastolic murmurs and most commonly relate to mitral stenosis or aortic insufficiency; however there are many other possibilities. Regurgitant murmurs for example, mitral valve insufficiency, usually fill the entire phase, while ejection murmurs, like aortic stenosis, usually have discrete beginning and end points within systole (between S_1 and S_2). Next the shape and quality of the murmur should be described along with descriptive terms about the murmur, that is, blowing, harsh, rumbling, machinery, musical, and others.

Some murmurs are considered innocent or physiologic and result from rapid, turbulent flow of blood into the left ventricle during atrial systole and through the aorta during ventricular systole. Fever, anxiety, anemia, hyperthyroidism, and pregnancy exacerbate physiologic murmurs, and these murmurs need to be distinguished from those suggestive of valvular abnormalities. Another important consideration is the grading of heart murmurs. The intensity or loudness of a murmur is graded using a scale of I to VI. Below are the different grades.

- I — Lowest intensity; difficult to hear even by expert listeners
- II — Low intensity, but usually audible by all listeners
- III — Medium intensity; easy to hear even by inexperienced listeners but without a palpable thrill
- IV — Medium intensity with a palpable thrill
- V — Loud intensity with a palpable thrill; audible even with the stethoscope placed on the chest with the edge of the diaphragm
- VI — Loudest intensity with a palpable thrill; audible even with the stethoscope raised above the chest

Multiple factors determine the grade, which includes the amount of blood ejected across a valve, severity of the lesion, and chest anatomy.

Systolic murmurs begin with or after S_1 and end at or before S_2, depending on the origin of the murmur. They are classified based on time of onset and termination within systole: midsystolic, holosystolic (pansystolic), early, or late. Some examples of pathologic midsystolic murmurs are pulmonic stenosis, aortic stenosis, and hypertrophic cardiomyopathy. Midsystolic murmurs may include obstruction to ventricular outflow (a common example is aortic stenosis; Fig. 13–5), dilation of the aortic root or pulmonary trunk, an increased flow in the great arteries, anatomic changes in the semilunar valves, and some forms of regurgitation. Holosystolic murmurs occur when blood flows from a chamber of higher pressure to one of lower pressure, such as with mitral or tricuspid regurgitation and ventricular septal defects. Early systolic murmurs can be decrescendo and may be associated with ventricular septal defects, mitral regurgitation, or tricuspid regurgitation. A late systolic murmur preceded by one or more midsystolic to late systolic clicks is the hallmark of mitral valve

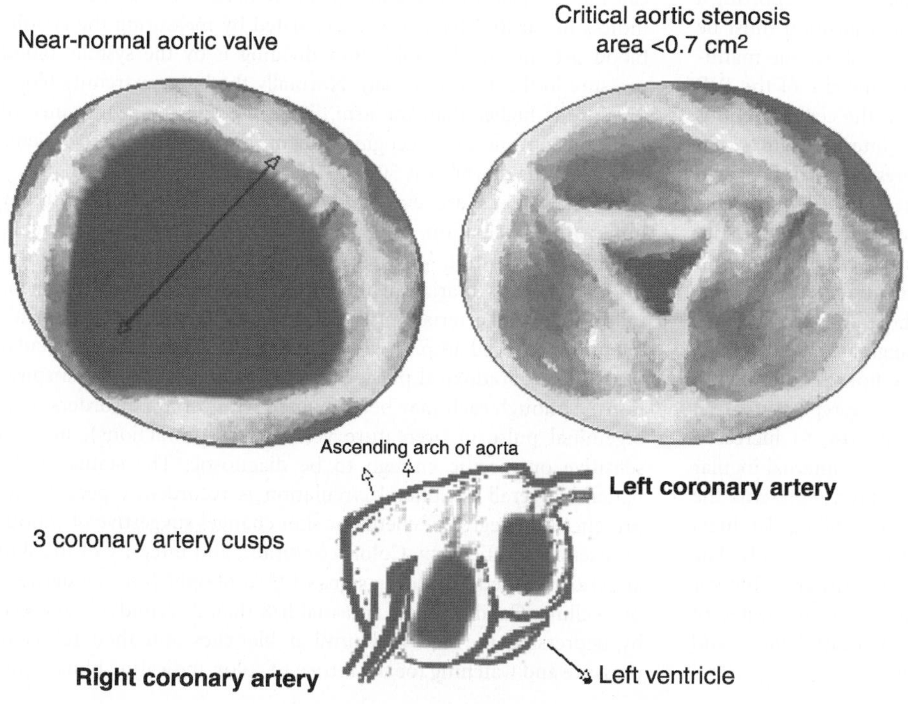

FIGURE 13-5. Aortic valve anatomy. A near-normal aortic valve is shown on the left and critical stenosis is shown on the right. The relationship of the aortic valve to coronary artery anatomy is shown below.

prolapse, which classically moves during changes in ventricular volume. Atherosclerotic obstruction of the carotid, subclavicular, or iliofemoral artery can give rise to a crescendo–decrescendo extracardiac systolic arterial murmur.

Early diastolic murmurs that are heard more commonly are mitral stenosis and aortic regurgitation. Aortic regurgitation begins with A_2 and generally is decrescendo, reflecting the progressive decline in volume and rate of regurgitant flow during diastole. Aortic regurgitation is best heard by having the patient lean forward while holding his or her breath and listening with the diaphragm along the mid left sternal border. Pulmonary hypertension (Graham Steell murmur: an early diastolic murmur caused by pulmonary insufficiency secondary to pulmonary hypertension) also may cause an early diastolic murmur. Middiastolic murmurs occur across the atrioventricular valves (mitral or tricuspid) during rapid filling and are consistent with mitral stenosis or mitral stenosis along with a ventricular septal defect or tricuspid regurgitation with an atrial septal defect. The Austin Flint murmur is a consequence of blood jets from the aortic regurgitation hitting the anterior leaflet of the mitral valve, leading to a middiastolic, low-pitched rumbling best heard at the cardiac apex that results in early mitral valve closure because of simultaneous rapid left ventricular filling (volume overload) from aortic regurgitation. Continuous murmurs begin in systole and continue without interruption into all or part of diastole. Such murmurs are mainly a result of aortopulmonary connections (e.g., patent ductus arteriosus), arteriovenous connections (e.g., arteriovenous fistula, coronary artery fistula), and disturbances of flow patterns in arteries or veins.

Anatomic correlation of murmurs may require cardiac catheterization or echocardiography with Doppler, where direct visualization of the blood flow abnormality and calculation of flow and chamber pressures can be obtained. In special cases the use of positron emission tomography (PET) and magnetic resonance imaging (MRI) are also possible options to evaluate flow patterns and gradients of murmurs across heart valves.

JUGULAR VENOUS PRESSURE

❸ The jugular venous pressure (JVP) is used as an indirect measure of right atrial pressure.[10] The JVP is measured in centimeters from the sternal angle and is best visualized with the patient's head rotated to the left. The JVP is described for its quality and character, effects of respiration, and patient position-induced changes. When reporting a JVP, both the extent of elevation and the patient position must be reported. The JVP can be reported as centimeters above the manubrium, or this value plus 5 to 7 cm to indicate the rise of the JVP above the right ventricle. For persons in whom the central venous pressure is normal, JVP is observed in the right internal jugular vein with the patient supine at 30° or less. In the presence of an elevated central venous pressure, the JVP is measured at 60 to 90°. In patients with poor myocardial function, the accuracy of the JVP as a measure of central venous pressure is reduced, and central venous pressure is best measured directly by means of a Swan-Ganz catheter.

The normal JVP is a *v* wave 1 to 2 cm above the sternal ridge. Elevation in JVP more than halfway to the jaw angle are elevated. Both the degree of elevation of the JVP and its wave flow in conjunction with the heartbeat are noted. The first wave, or *a* wave, represents atrial contraction and occurs just prior to S_1, giving rise to increased pressure. It is seen as an undulating pulsation in the internal jugular vein. The second and much larger wave, the *v* wave, represents the increased venous pressure that occurs during venous filling. To interpret the JVP accurately, the carotid pulse is palpated concurrently. The *a* wave occurs just before the pulse and the *v* wave just after. Jugular venous pressure is often elevated in heart failure, and the degree of elevation can be used to assess the severity of heart failure, and diminution of JVP can be used to assess therapy.

PERIPHERAL CIRCULATION AND ARTERIAL PULSES

In recent years the recognition of peripheral arterial disease (PAD) has become very important because of the marked number of patients with asymptomatic disease. PAD affects about 8 million Americans and is associated with significant morbidity and mortality.[11,12] PAD affects 12% to 20% of Americans age 65 years and older. Despite its prevalence and cardiovascular risk implications, only 25% of PAD patients are undergoing treatment.[13] Approximately 40% do not complain of leg pain and only approximately 10% of persons with PAD have the classic symptoms of intermittent claudication (see Chap. 24).

It includes a variety of arterial syndromes (noncoronary artery) that are caused by pathobiologic changes of the arteries that supply the brain, visceral organs, and the limbs. Terminology is also important in discussing this area of arterial disease. Peripheral arterial disease includes an assorted group of disorders that lead to progressive stenosis or occlusion, or aneurysmal dilation, of the aorta and its noncoronary branch arteries, including the carotid, upper extremity, visceral, and lower extremity arterial branches. PAD is the preferred clinical term that should be used to denote stenotic, occlusive, and aneurysmal diseases of the aorta and its branch arteries, exclusive of the coronary arteries. Peripheral vascular disease includes pathophysiologic syndromes that affect the arterial, venous, and lymphatic circulations.

Current American College of Cardiologists/American Heart Association (ACC/AHA) guidelines[11] for the management of peripheral artery disease recommend a vascular history and physical examination (class I) for patients who are at risk for lower extremity PAD, age less than 50 years with diabetes and one other atherosclerosis risk factor (smoking, dyslipidemia, hypertension, or hyperhomocysteinemia), age 50 to 69 years and a history of smoking or diabetes, age 70 years and older, ischemic leg symptoms with exertion (intermittent claudication) or ischemic rest pain, abnormal lower extremity pulse examination, or known atherosclerotic coronary, carotid, or renal artery disease. They also recommend that patients older than 50 years of age should be asked if they have a family history of a first-degree relative with an abdominal aortic aneurysm.

One of the most important tests that can be easily done in patients suspected of PAD is to do an ankle–brachial index. An ankle–brachial index of <0.90 is 90% sensitive and 95% specific for PAD. Severe PAD causing rest pain or ulceration generally occurs with ankle–brachial indices of <0.40. This is easily calculated by measuring the systolic blood pressure in the ankle and dividing it by the systolic blood pressure in the arm (brachial). Normally the lower extremity blood pressure is higher than the arm. To appreciate the significance of PAD, one only needs to recognize that over a 5-year period in patients with PAD the mortality is 30%.[14]

Arterial pulses are evaluated and characterized bilaterally by observation, palpation, and auscultation for presence, character, pattern, and rhythm. Various arterial pulse patterns are described: pulsus alternans (variation in amplitude beat to beat), bisferiens pulse (increased arterial pulse with a double systolic peak), bigeminal pulse (reduced amplitude associated with premature ventricular beats), and paradoxical pulse (decrease in amplitude with inspiration). Although each may be associated with certain disorders (e.g., bigeminal pulse in premature ventricular contractions), none is sensitive or specific enough to be diagnostic. The status of the patient's overall peripheral circulation is recorded, especially the presence and degree of edema or skin changes suggestive of venous or arterial insufficiency. Color, condition, and integrity of the skin are also recorded, including signs of thrombophlebitis, tenderness, or swelling. Capillary refill (normal less than 2 seconds) is assessed by depressing the nail bed until it blanches and then releasing pressure and watching for the return of color, indicating blood flow.

HEART RATE

Heart rate is described by both rate and rhythm. The arterial pulse usually is taken at the radius, but carotid or other arterial pulses may be used. In healthy individuals, the heart rate is usually assessed by counting the pulse for 15 seconds and multiplying by 4. In patients with irregular rhythms, the pulse should be taken over an extended period, approximately 1 to 2 minutes, to try to determine the patient's average pulse and rhythm.

Arterial pulses are an accurate measure of the ventricular rate in healthy persons with good ventricular function. In patients with a rapid ventricular rate—because of supraventricular tachyarrhythmias such as atrial flutter or fibrillation or rapid ventricular rates (e.g., ventricular tachycardia or premature ventricular beats)—extremity pulses (e.g., radial pulse) may be considerably slower than the true ventricular rate. A more accurate ventricular rate is determined by listening to the ventricles with the stethoscope (usually at the apex) or counting from an electrocardiogram (ECG). In patients with atrial fibrillation and a fast ventricular rate, a pulse deficit (measure of the difference in true ventricular rate and peripheral pulse rate) may exist. This may be as much as 10 to 20 beats per minute. Consequently, the location of the pulse (radial or apical) should be recorded. The pulse deficit will be reduced as the ventricular rate is controlled with drug therapy or normal sinus rhythm is restored.

PRACTICE GUIDELINES FOR DIAGNOSTIC AND PROGNOSTIC TESTING IN CARDIOVASCULAR DISEASE TESTING

The American Heart Association (AHA) and American College of Cardiology (ACC) task force on practice guidelines publishes guidelines as to the recommended uses for many diagnostic testing methods. Such guidelines were first developed in the 1980s and are updated as more information is available. These are evidence-based recommendations that rank the indications and uses of tests into three primary classes. Class I indications are those where there is evidence or agreement that the specific procedure is useful and effective. Class II indications are those situations where there is divergence of opinion as to the usefulness of the method. Class III indications are those where there is evidence or agreement that a diagnostic test is not useful. Each class (usually class II) may be broken down into two or three subcategories. Class IIa indications are those where there is evidence or opinion in favor of the test, whereas class IIb indications are those where there is less evidence favoring the test. With each class of recommendation for a specific clinical scenario, the guidelines indicate the level of evidence for the recommendation. Level A evidence is given if the recommendation is based on the availability of multiple randomized clinical trials. Level B evidence is given if only a single randomized trial or multiple nonrandomized trials exist. Level C evidence is given if the recommendation is afforded based on expert opinion only.

Each guideline provides a preamble to indicate how it was constructed and the peer review process. These documents provide the clinician with an extensive database on the testing methodologies and are endorsed by both organizations as acceptable standards of practice.

TESTING MODALITIES

CHEST RADIOGRAPHY

The chest radiograph provides supplemental information to the physical examination and is usually the first diagnostic test in a cardiac workup. It does not provide details of internal cardiac structures but gives global information about position and size of the heart and chambers and surrounding anatomy. The standard chest radiographs for evaluation of lungs and heart are standing posteroanterior and lateral views taken at maximal inspiration. Portable chest radiographs usually are less satisfactory because of penetration difficulties, patient rotation, and poor inspiratory effort.

Initial assessment of the chest radiograph evaluates the quality of the film for patient rotation, inspiratory effort, and penetration. Rotation is assessed by evaluating symmetry of the clavicles and central placement of the carina. Inspiratory effect is considered adequate if the diaphragms are pulled below the ninth rib. Lack of inspiratory effort and obesity lead to a poor-quality chest radiograph, which makes it more difficult to assess the presence of pleural effusions and fluid in the costophrenic angles. Where possible, comparison with previous or baseline films is done to determine the quality of film and comparison of structures.

The posteroanterior view chest radiograph outlines the superior vena cava, right atrium on the right and left sides, aortic knob, main pulmonary artery, left atrial appendage (especially if enlarged), and left ventricle. In the lateral view, the chest radiograph visualizes the right ventricle, inferior vena cava, and left ventricle. These structures are visualized as shadows of differing density rather than discrete structures.

The chest radiograph is approached from two perspectives: (a) observation and (b) clinical correlation. Observation notes gross anatomic features such as size and placement of the cardiac silhouette, definition of the cardiac border, chamber enlargement, pulmonary vasculature, air–fluid levels, and diaphragm. Cardiac enlargement is determined by the cardiothoracic ratio, which is the maximal transverse diameter of the heart divided by the maximal transverse diameter of the thorax of a posteroanterior view. Normal averages 0.45, but it may be up to 0.55 in subjects with large stroke volumes (e.g., highly trained athletes). Heart conditions, such as heart failure and hypertension, may enlarge the heart and so the cardiothoracic ratio. Individual chamber enlargement can be seen on the chest radiograph. Right ventricle enlargement is best seen on the lateral film, where the heart appears to occupy the retrosternal space. Left atrial enlargement is suspected if there is elevation of the left bronchus or an increase in the atrial appendage bulge. Left ventricular enlargement is the most common feature identified on chest radiograph and is seen as an elongation and downward displacement of the apex of the heart. Sometimes a characteristic "boot" or "water bottle" outline is seen with left ventricular enlargement, as in heart failure.

The pulmonary vessels are examined for plumpness and definition of vessel walls. Decreased pulmonary flow (e.g., tetralogy of Fallot) causes central and peripheral vessels to be decreased in size. Increased pulmonary flow is associated with high-output states such as hyperthyroidism and atrial septal defects. This may lead to enlargement and tortuosity of the central and peripheral vessels. Pulmonary arterial hypertension (increased pulmonary resistance) is identified by enlargement of the central vessels and diminished peripheral vessels. Pulmonary venous hypertension usually is caused by mitral stenosis or left ventricular failure. This is characterized by larger-than-normal vessels in the upper lung zones owing to recruitment of upper vessels from blood diverted from the lower constricted vessels (cephalization of flow).

Heart failure causes Kerley B lines (edema of interlobular septa), which appear as thin, horizontal reticular lines in the costophrenic angles. At higher pressures, alveolar edema and pleural effusions appear in the pleural space or as blunting of the costophrenic angles. Pericardial effusions also may appear as a large heart, but because it usually occurs rapidly, there is no evidence of pulmonary venous congestion.

ELECTROCARDIOGRAM

❹ Measurement of electrical activity in the heart, now known as the ECG, was introduced about 75 years ago by Willem Einthoven. The

TABLE 13-2 Drugs That May Affect the Electrocardiogram

Digoxin	Pentamidine
Antiarrhythmics–classes I–IV	Lithium
Tricyclic antidepressants	Catecholamines (e.g., dopamine, albuterol)
H_1 antagonists	Diuretics (electrolyte abnormalities)
Methylxanthines	
Doxorubicin	

ECG is simple to perform and is the most frequently used, least invasive, and cheapest cardiovascular test.[15,16] It remains the procedure of first choice for evaluation of chest pain, dizziness, or syncope. In its simplest interpretation, the ECG characterizes rhythms and conduction abnormalities. However, the ECG also provides, by inference, information about the anatomy and structures of the heart, pathophysiologic changes, and hemodynamics of the CVD system.[17] ECG abnormalities are often the earliest sign of adverse drug effects, ischemia, and electrolyte abnormalities.

Although few ECG recordings are highly specific or sensitive to a disease state, correlation of findings with clinical and pathologic states affords the ECG significant diagnostic and prognostic capabilities. Sensitivity and specificity of ECG changes depend primarily on the clinical setting, recording technique, and skill of interpreters. Sensitivity and specificity of findings are increased by interpretation in conjunction with patient information such as age, gender, medical history, and medications. Additionally, prior and/or serial ECGs should be obtained for comparison prior to identifying new findings on a current ECG as diagnostic. This is particularly important in patients with significant cardiac disease or on medications that alter the ECG (Table 13–2). The ECG is sensitive in detecting rhythm abnormalities, but it does not record the actual activity of the conduction tissue.[18,19]

The ECG can be used to evaluate ischemia following angioplasty or other surgical interventions and to monitor responses to antiarrhythmic agents or in patients receiving drugs with potential cardiac effects.

Electrocardiography is based on the measurement of change in summated three-dimensional electrical vectors or forces that result from depolarization and repolarization of cells in the conduction system and heart muscle. The standard external 12-lead ECG uses two sets of leads: limb and chest (Fig. 13–6). The six limb leads look at the heart in a single frontal plane. Limb lead nomenclature is as follows: lead I, right arm/left arm; lead II, right arm/left leg; lead III, left arm/left leg. Altering resistances create the augmented limb leads, which are called aVR, aVL, and aVF. Unipolar chest leads are positioned across the chest and labeled V_1 to V_6. V_1 is positioned slightly to the right of the midline, and V_6 is positioned in the left midaxillary line (Fig. 13–7). Leads aVR and V_1 are considered right-sided leads, so they appear inverted, and leads aVL, I, II, V_5 and V_6 are left-sided leads, so they appear upright on the ECG. Leads II, III, and aVF are inferior leads. Leads V_1 to V_4 are anterior wall leads. Single-lead ECGs or ECG monitors frequently use lead II.

Recording of the ECG has several standard features. The paper is divided into squares of 1 mm; each 10 mm (10 small boxes) is equivalent to 1 mV. Paper speed is 25 mm per second. Each small box on the tracing paper equals 0.04 second (40 milliseconds), and each big box is 0.2 second. If there is one QRS complex per six big boxes (6 × 0.20 second), the patient has a heart rate of 50 beats per minute, whereas one QRS per big box indicates a heart rate of 300 beats per minute.

The ECG pattern is named alphabetically and is read from left to right, beginning with the P wave. Electrical activation (depolarization) of the right and then the left atrium as a result of discharge from the sinoatrial nodes causes an upward or positive deflection in lead II called the *P wave.* The normal duration of the P wave is up to 0.12 second, and it has an amplitude of 0.25 mV (i.e., 2.5 small boxes). The *PR segment* is created by passage of the impulse through the atrioventricular node and the bundle of His and its branches, and it has a duration of 0.12 to 0.21 second. The *QRS complex* primarily traces the electrical depolarization of the ventricles. Initially, there is a negative deflection, the *Q wave,* followed by a positive deflection, the *R wave,* and finally a negative deflection, the *S wave.* Q-wave duration is normally 0.4 second or less, and the amplitude is 25% or less of the overall height of the QRS complex. Normal duration of the QRS complex is 0.12 second. The QRS complex is positive in left-sided leads and negative in right-sided leads because the left ventricle is much thicker than the right, and the forces going left during depolarization dominate.

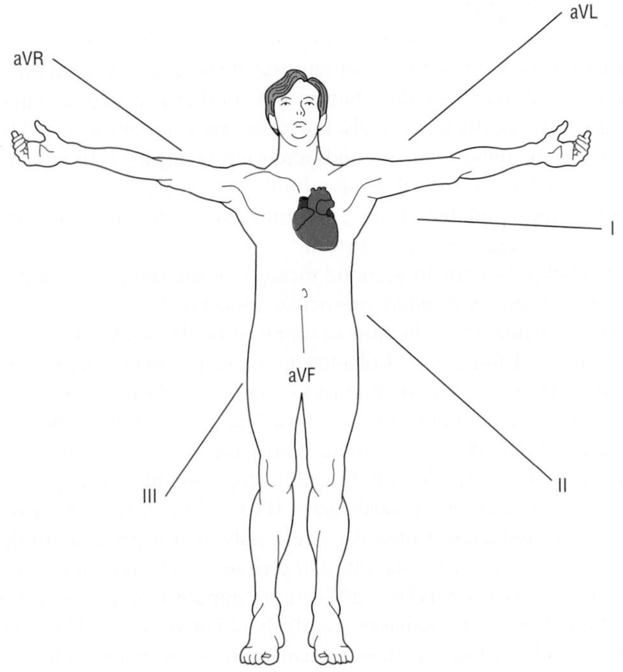

FIGURE 13-6. The torso with the six limb leads in a single frontal plane.

Following the QRS complex is a plateau phase called the *ST segment,* which extends from the end of the QRS complex (called the *J point*) to the beginning of the T wave. The ST segment is evaluated from its position relevant to the baseline, configuration, and leads where changes occur. The ST segment is normally on or slightly above the baseline. Configuration changes, convexity upward or downward, identify the presence of myocardial ischemia. Lead localization of ST-segment changes indicates the area of ischemia. The *QT interval* is measured from the start of the QRS complex to the end of the T wave. This varies with heart rate and is corrected (QTc) for heart rates greater than 60 beats per minute. The normal QTc is less than 0.42 second in men and 0.43 second in women.

Repolarization of the ventricle leads to the *T wave.* The T wave usually goes in the same direction as the QRS complex. The normal axis of the ECG is 30° (above the horizontal) to +110° (away from the horizontal) (see Fig. 13–7). The six frontal plane (A) and the six horizontal plane (B) leads provide a three-dimensional representation of cardiac electrical activity.

The ECG is evaluated in a systematic manner to avoid omission of important characteristics. All ECGs are interpreted for the following elements: rate, general rhythm, intervals, voltage, axis, waveforms, abnormal features (e.g., Q waves), and technical aspects such as adequacy of lead placement and calibration.[20] The number of P waves and QRS complexes (*RR interval*) is also used to determine rate. QRS complexes may be more useful if heart block exists. The rhythm from the ECG is identified by the following features:

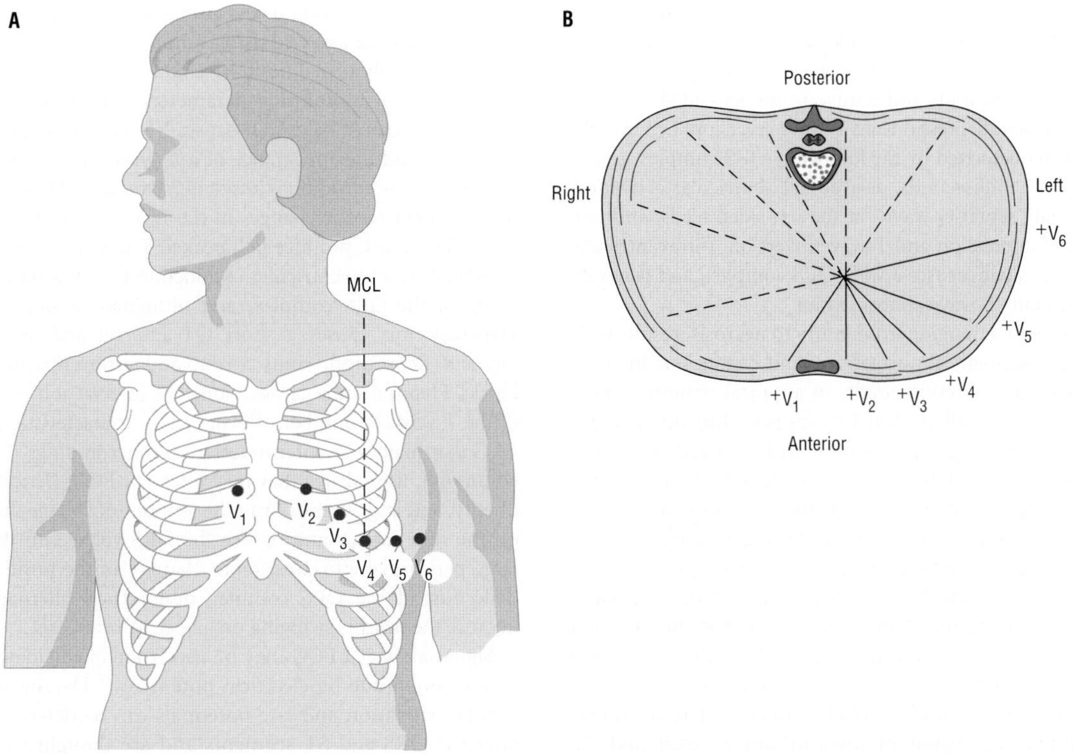

FIGURE 13-7. *A.* Electrode positions of the precordial leads. (MCL, midclavicular line; V_1, fourth intercostal space at the right sternal border; V_2, fourth intercostal space at the left sternal border; V_3, halfway between V_2 and V_4; V_4, fifth intercostal space at the midclavicular line; V_5, anterior axillary line directly lateral to V_4; V_6, anterior axillary space directly lateral V_5.) *B.* The precordial reference figure. Leads V_1 and V_2 are called right-sided precordial leads; leads V_3 and V_4, midprecordial leads; and leads V_5 and V_6, left-sided precordial leads. *(Redrawn from Kinney MR, Packa DR, eds. Andreoli's Comprehensive Cardiac Care, 8th ed. St. Louis: Mosby, 1996, with permission.)*

1. The rate of the QRS (>100/min is tachycardia and <60/min is bradycardia).
2. The regularity of the QRS. (The presence or absence of the QRS complex with each P wave helps to identify if the rhythm is atrial or ventricular in origin and if each atrial beat [P wave] is being conducted to the ventricles. The regularity of the QRS identifies conditions such as atrial fibrillation and extra beats.)
3. Configuration of the QRS—wide or narrow—indicating if it is generated from electrical activity that arose in the atria or ventricles.

Always reported are the RR, PR, QRS, and QT intervals and the duration, magnitude, and configuration of the P waves, QRS complexes, ST segments, T waves, and U waves.[21] Computer interpretation of the ECG provides a standardized reading and records and calculates basic rhythm patterns, heart rate, and intervals but does not interpret arrhythmias. Independent review of the ECG is necessary for accurate translation of findings. In epidemiologic studies, the ECG is used to assess physical fitness, document the prevalence of ischemic heart disease (IHD), and identify subclinical heart disease. The sensitivity and specificity of ECG changes are highly dependent on the pretest probability of heart disease. As the pretest probability of heart disease increases, the sensitivity and specificity of ECG findings increase. The use and value of the ECG as a screening tool are controversial. It is only used where the diagnosis of heart disease would preclude active employment, such as in airline pilots. The ECG frequently is used in conjunction with other diagnostic tests to provide additional data, to monitor the patient, and to identify if abnormalities detected during tests correlate with ECG changes.[20–22]

Gating, or linkage of and simultaneous recording of an ECG and other diagnostic tests, such as echocardiography and computed tomography (CT) scans, allow for correlation of images with the cardiac cycle. Gating is either prospective, where a certain portion of the cardiac cycle is predetermined as the time during which the images are obtained, or retrospective, where the ECG and image are recorded simultaneously but independently and later matched for concurrent events. This allows multiple cardiac cycles to be overlaid, thus increasing the sensitivity to detect abnormalities.

Anomalies on the ECG include abnormal intervals, altered waveform configurations, and rate variability. Other findings give evidence for various forms of heart block, ischemia, infarction, atrial and ventricular enlargement and hypertrophy, atrial and ventricular rhythm disorders, pericarditis, metabolic abnormalities, drug-induced changes, and pacemaker-related changes. ECG patterns found on consecutive leads can help to identify where a particular conduction defect or impulse generation is occurring or anatomic problem is located. For example, ST-segment elevation in V_2 to V_6 is indicative of anterior wall myocardial infarction from occlusion of the left anterior descending coronary artery. Single-lead abnormalities most frequently are attributed to poor lead placement, position of the patient, or recording artifacts.[22]

Examples of some common findings will be discussed briefly. Short PR intervals are associated with the Wolff-Parkinson-White and Lown-Ganong-Levine syndromes and reflect the presence of accessory pathways. Long PR intervals are measures of heart block. The presence of a Q wave is a marker for loss of electrically functioning myocardium and suggests a prior myocardial infarction. It also may be present in congenital heart disorders, hypertrophic cardiomyopathy, left ventricular hypertrophy, conduction defects such as Wolff-Parkinson-White syndrome, and intraventricular conduction defects. U waves are relatively nonspecific, the most common cause being hypertension. Bundle-branch blocks are frequent findings and indicate conduction defects in one of the bundles of His. Their presence confounds the interpretation of important ECG findings such as ischemia. Right bundle-branch block is associated with an R wave and the following abnormalities: QRS complex greater than or equal to 12 milliseconds, delayed right ventricular forces resulting in terminal R waves in the right-sided leads and S wave in the left-sided lead, and right-sided ST-segment depression and T-wave inversion. Left bundle-branch block is characterized by the following: QRS complex greater than or equal to 12 milliseconds, delayed left ventricular activation, loss of the normal "septal Q wave" in the left-sided leads, and left-sided ST-segment depression and T-wave inversion. Intraventricular conduction delay usually causes a wide QRS complex, and generally there are ST-segment–T-wave abnormalities.

Myocardial ischemia, ranging from injury to necrosis, results in T-wave changes, ST-segment abnormalities, and changes in the QRS complex. Myocardial infarction results in a typical pattern of ECG changes that begins with tall, peaked T waves persisting up to several hours, followed by ST-segment elevation with a coved (convexity upward) configuration, and inverted T waves. Development of a new Q wave has a high specificity but low sensitivity for acute myocardial ischemia. Q waves that are 4 milliseconds or longer in duration and 25% or greater of the overall QRS height are considered diagnostic and occur within minutes to hours of occlusion. Although Q waves usually evolve within hours of infarction, they may not become evident for several days. The finding of new and significant Q waves on an ECG is indicative of a previous infarction. Q waves persist indefinitely in 80% to 90% of myocardial infarctions. The location of Q waves identifies the region of myocardium affected and the coronary artery blocked (e.g., inferior infarction will result in Q waves in II, III, and aVF associated with blockage in the right coronary artery). Non–Q-wave (subendocardial) myocardial infarction implies that the Q wave does not meet the diagnostic criteria for Q-wave infarction. ST-segment depression may be present.

ST-segment changes are very common and always should be compared with a previous ECG. ST-segment elevation may be seen in persons with no known coronary disease but is usually indicative of hyperacute ischemia. ST-segment depression is never considered a normal finding. ST-segment scooping (convexity downward) may be normal, but coving (convexity upward) is abnormal. Depression of the ST segment that does not return quickly to normal and changes in multiple leads suggests clinically significant heart disease. Diffuse ST-segment elevation in all leads except V_1 and aVR suggests the diagnosis of pericarditis. Exertion in normal individuals may cause J-point depression with a rapid rise of the ST segment, and this may be confused with ST-segment depression because of the configuration. Poor R-wave progression (usually increase in size moving from V_1 to V_6) suggests anterior myocardial infarction, but smaller R waves also can occur in diseases such as chronic obstructive pulmonary disease. T-wave changes are the most frequent and most sensitive abnormality on the ECG but are also the least specific and frequently are found in persons with no heart disease.

Left atrial enlargement is characterized by a P wave that is ≥12 mV in lead II, or the negative component of the biphasic P wave is 4 mV in duration and 0.1 mV in depth in lead V_1. In right atrial enlargement, the P wave in lead II can exceed 0.25 mV and usually has a vertical axis. Ventricular hypertrophy results in increased deflection of the QRS complex because of the increased muscle mass. Left ventricular hypertrophy (LVH) is diagnosed from the ECG using several different sets of criteria; none are considered highly sensitive or specific. LVH often is indicative of hypertension and resulting ventricular enlargement and strain. Commonly used voltage criteria indicating LVH are summation of the S wave in V_1 and the R wave in V_5 or the S wave in V_2 and the R wave in V_6 that exceeds 3.5 mV (35 small boxes) or the R wave in lead aVL that exceeds 1.1 mV (11 small boxes). Right ventricular hypertrophy is characterized by an R wave in V_1 that is equal to or greater than the S wave in that lead. In persons who are obese, increased voltage may not be apparent, making voltage criteria a less useful tool to identify hypertrophy. LVH also may be assessed using echocardiography.

Electrolyte abnormalities have characteristic signs on the ECG and can be used as monitoring parameters. Hypokalemia may increase ventricular ectopic beats and causes ST-segment depression, T-wave flattening, and the appearance of a U wave (usually when the serum potassium concentration is less than 3.0 mEq/L). Hyperkalemia results in very characteristic changes in the ECG. Potassium concentrations above 6.0 mEq/L produce tall, peaked T waves. As the concentration rises further, intraventricular conduction becomes blocked, with widening of the QRS complex, and ultimately, a sine wave develops. Hypercalcemia causes a short QT interval and, occasionally, ST-segment depression, sinus arrest, and atrioventricular conduction blocks. Hypocalcemia causes a long QT interval and some broadening of the T wave. A number of drugs cause characteristic changes in the ECG that may mask interpretation of other findings. Table 13–2 lists commonly used drugs that may alter the ECG. Pericardial effusion, obesity, and large breasts limit the amount of voltage that is measured on the skin surface and reduce the QRS voltage. In the presence of large pericardial effusions, rapid changes in the positive to negative deflection of the QRS complex or electrical alternans may occur because the heart is swinging on a beat-to-beat basis.

Signal-averaged ECG may be used to help elucidate the presence of low-amplitude bioelectrical potentials.[23] Derangements of ventricular activation and late potentials can be detected on the ECG after the QRS and ST segments and are thought to be associated with increased risk of ventricular arrhythmias. Traditional ECGs are unable to detect these potentials because they are "lost" in the noise of the ECG recording. Signal-averaged ECG improves the signal-to-noise ratio, enabling the low-amplitude potentials to be interpreted. Signal-averaged ECG can be used to identify patients at risk for developing sustained ventricular tachycardia after myocardial infarction. Patients with IHD and unexplained syncope who are at risk for sustained ventricular tachycardia also may be candidates for signal-averaged ECG. Other potential uses of signal-averaged ECG include patients with nonischemic cardiomyopathy with sustained ventricular tachycardia, detection of acute rejection of heart transplant, and assessment of the proarrhythmia potential of antiarrhythmic drug therapy.

AMBULATORY ELECTROCARDIOGRAM MONITORING

Ambulatory ECG monitoring (AECG), or Holter monitoring, named for its inventor, is an aid to detect, document, characterize, and evaluate arrhythmias and other ECG abnormalities over extended periods of time.[24,25] AECG provides information regarding random abnormal cardiac electrical activity during daily activity and helps relate altered electrical activity to precipitating factors and patient symptomatology. algorithms. AECG also helps in the discovery and investigation of arrhythmias and ST-segment deviation along with more sophisticated analyses of R-R intervals, QRS-T morphology including late potentials, Q-T dispersion, and T-wave alternans. Additionally, some findings on AECG have been used to determine prognostic implications. Different types of recording systems are discussed later in this chapter in the Echocardiogram section: one version is noninvasive, which can be patient activated and varies in duration of recording from hours to days, and the other version is invasive, which can be implanted like a pacemaker and removed later and can record for years. Most of the current new recording systems are digital (recommended guidelines by AHA/ACC) and have a diagnostic frequency response range for more accurate investigation of ST-segment deviations.

Although controversial, AECG is used as a diagnostic and screening tool for asymptomatic ischemia. It is difficult to interpret changes in the ST segment recorded during AECG owing to amplitude, and definitions of significant changes recorded with AECG are still in evolution. As a prognostic tool, it is used primarily to evaluate patients with known CVD who have symptoms that may be associated with an arrhythmia. It is also used in clinical trials to evaluate the efficacy of drug therapy.[26]

Guidelines as to the recommended uses of AECG are available from AHA/ACC. The major class I indications for AECG include diagnosis in patients with symptoms suggestive of arrhythmias, prognostic delineation in patients with cardiac disease considered at risk for arrhythmia-related events, and measurement of efficacy of interventions in patients with known and characterized arrhythmias. Examples of indications and clinical rhythm disturbances are listed in Tables 13–3, 13–4, and 13–5.

A major limitation of AECG is the amount of data collected with ECG abnormalities that are of unknown clinical significance. High day-to-day variability of frequency and type of arrhythmias means that repeat AECG may demonstrate as much as a 90% difference in the number of premature ventricular contractions. Little correlation of arrhythmia suppression and clinical outcomes is available. No AECG study has shown a mortality advantage when used in conjunction with antiarrhythmic drugs or devices. Following an intervention (drugs or device), at least a 63% to 95% reduction in arrhythmia frequency is required for AECG to be considered a valuable arrhythmia detection and evaluation tool. Compared with electrophysiology testing in the Electrophysiologic Study Versus Electrocardiographic Monitoring (ESVEM) study, AECG was equivalent but not superior to electrophysiology testing in the ability to select initial drug therapy.[22] The Asymptomatic Cardiac Ischemia Pilot (ACIP) study found that 75% of patients with asymptomatic evidence of ischemia on AECG had multivessel coronary artery disease on angiography.[26]

During AECG, the patient wears a portable ECG recorder that weighs about 8 to 16 oz. The recorder uses two to four chest leads (V_5 and V_3 most commonly). Additional leads do not improve the sensitivity of AECG significantly. If ST-segment changes are known to occur in certain leads, these can be used during AECG. Most AECG recordings are for 24 to 48 hours, but they can extend to weeks or months where the frequency of events related to ECG abnormalities is low. Implantable devices are used when long periods of monitoring are necessary. Currently used equipment is able to detect and analyze arrhythmias, ST-segment deviations, QRS complexes, RR intervals, and late potentials.

Three types of monitors are available: (a) continuous monitors, which record an ECG strip over the duration of the test, (b) event or intermittent recorders, which continuously monitor the ECG but only record preprogrammed abnormal ECG events or are patient-activated based on occurrence of symptoms, and (c) real-time analytical recorders, which record throughout the monitoring period and analyze each beat as it occurs. Monitors digitize, encode, and store the information in a solid-state memory or on magnetic tape. Event monitors are preprogrammed to record parameters such as the number of premature ventricular contractions and heart rate. During monitoring, the patient maintains a diary, in which the occurrence, duration, and severity of symptoms (e.g., light-headedness, chest pain) are recorded, plus any specific activities undertaken, development of symptoms with the activity, and any interventions such as the taking of medication. A clocking device in the recorder allows later correlation of the patient's diary with the recorded ECG.

Evaluation and analysis of the ECG record are complex. Computer-assisted interpretation is used to scan the ECG and identify irregular rhythms, rates, and specific preprogrammed changes. The main advantage of computer analysis is to reduce interpretation of artifact recordings. Each beat recorded during AECG is evaluated for its arrhythmia potential and classified as normal or abnormal. The morphology of each QRS-T section is examined for ischemia potential, although, as indicated previously, baseline ST-segment abnormalities and adjustments in amplitude of the recording may preclude interpretation of these segments. The ACC/AHA guidelines provide detail as to the suitability of using ST segments for analysis of ischemia.[27] Various drugs, such as digoxin and the tricyclic antidepressants that cause baseline ECG abnormalities, may preclude patients from being evaluated with AECG.

Sections identified by the computer as abnormal or those correlating with patient symptoms are then evaluated and characterized

TABLE 13-3 Indications for Ambulatory Electrocardiogram Monitoring to Assess Symptoms Possibly Related to Rhythm Disturbances

Class I
Patients with unexplained syncope, near syncope, or episodic dizziness in whom the cause is not obvious
Patients with unexplained recurrent palpitation
Class IIb
Patients with episodic shortness of breath, chest pain, or fatigue that is not otherwise explained
Patients with neurologic events when transient atrial fibrillation or flutter is suspected
Patients with symptoms such as syncope, near syncope, episodic dizziness, or palpitation in whom a probable cause other than an arrhythmia has been identified but in whom symptoms persist despite treatment of this other cause
Class III
Patients with symptoms such as syncope, near syncope, episodic dizziness, or palpitation in whom other causes have been identified by history, physical examination, or laboratory tests
Patients with cerebrovascular accidents, without other evidence of arrhythmia

TABLE 13-4 Indications for Ambulatory Electrocardiogram Arrhythmia Detection to Assess Risk for Future Cardiac Events in Patients without Symptoms from Arrhythmia

Class I
None
Class IIb
1. Post-myocardial infarction patients with left ventricular dysfunction (ejection fraction <40%)
2. Patients with congestive heart failure
3. Patients with idiopathic hypertrophic cardiomyopathy
Class III
1. Patients who have sustained myocardial contusion
2. Systemic hypertensive patients with left ventricular hypertrophy
3. Post-myocardial infarction patients with normal left ventricular function
4. Preoperative arrhythmia evaluation of patients for noncardiac surgery
5. Patients with sleep apnea
6. Patients with valvular heart disease

Adapted from AHA/ACC guidelines.

TABLE 13-5 Indication for Ambulatory Electrocardiogram Monitoring for Ischemia

Class I
None
Class IIa
1. Patients with suspected variant angina
Class IIb
1. Evaluation of patients with chest pain who cannot exercise
2. Preoperative evaluation for vascular surgery of patients who cannot exercise
3. Patients with known coronary artery disease and atypical chest pain syndrome
Class III
1. Initial evaluation of patients with chest pain who are able to exercise
2. Routine screening of asymptomatic subjects

Adapted from AHA/ACC guidelines.

TABLE 13-6 Confounding Factors in Ambulatory Electrocardiogram Monitoring

Patient Factors	Equipment Factors
Electrolyte abnormalities	Battery failure
Hyperventilation	Loose lead
Lead interference by patient	Mechanical failure of recorder
Medications	Motor failure
Physiologic variations in waveforms	Overrecording
Medications	Computer inability to detect arrhythmia
Patient activities (e.g., sudden exercise)	
Presence of atrial fibrillation	

further (e.g., potentially pathologic rhythms) by technical personnel and physicians. Confounding factors when using AECG can arise from the patient and the device (Table 13–6). AECG is evolving rapidly, primarily related to improved technology with respect to data interpretation, signal quality, and improved understanding of the implications of ECG changes.

EXERCISE STRESS TESTING

5 Exercise stress (tolerance) testing (ETT) is a noninvasive test used to evaluate clinical and cardiovascular responses to exercise.[27–29] ETT is used frequently as an initial test, in conjunction with physical examination and patient symptoms, to aid in the selection of additional testing modalities. It is a simple test that can be conducted in a physician's office and is about 20 times less expensive than an angiogram and almost three times less expensive than stress echocardiography. Almost two-thirds of ETTs billed to Medicare in 1996 were conducted in physicians' offices, and one-third was conducted by noncardiologists.[27]

Central facts to remember about ETT is that its value to diagnose CAD is largely dependent on the risk of the population studied. For example, it is not very helpful in identifying CAD if one does ETT on patients who are young and without risk factors because their risk is extremely low; but if one tests a population of people that has multiple risk factors and is older, it is more useful (Table 13–7). Even though one uses these considerations, randomized trial data on the clinical value of screening exercise testing are absent and it is not known whether a strategy of routine screening exercise testing in selected subjects reduces the risk for premature mortality or major cardiac morbidity. A recent report from the U.S. Preventive Services Task Force[26] recommended against the use of exercise testing as a screening tool, in a large part because most studies were completed in asymptomatic patients, and because of the well-established Bayesian argument.

One of most important parts of exercising testing is functional capacity, even though it is rarely measured directly. Functional capacity can be obtained by directly measuring the oxygen consumption but this is not routinely available because of complexity and cost of equipment. If one uses functional capacity to exercise capacity, prediction of cardiovascular risk can be assessed.[30] It is also essential to evaluate the inability of the heart rate to increase appropriately during exercise (chronotropic incompetence) testing. Peak heart rate, age related predicted maximum heart rate have important prognostic importance. Heart rate during exercise is an expression of decreased parasympathetic tone and increased sympathetic tone. In disease states affecting electrical conduction or possibly heart failure this becomes important. The second important area is heart rate recovery after exercise testing. Normal individuals and especially athletes have a rapid fall in heart rate during the first 30 seconds after exercise vs a patient with heart disease who has slow fall in heart rate. This heart rate response is markedly influenced by parasympathetic tone.

The ETT provides diagnostic information in patients with known or suspected IHD and prognostic information in patients after myocardial infarction or revascularization. However, there are no data that support its use as a screening tool for CAD or for detection of early CAD in asymptomatic subjects.

The principle behind ETT is to increase myocardial oxygen demand above myocardial oxygen supply and coronary reserve, thereby provoking ischemia (inadequate myocardial perfusion), using exercise as a stressor. Ischemia is detected by patient symptoms, ECG changes, and/or hemodynamic changes. The type of ECG changes, leads affected, and patient performance are used as an index of severity and location of disease. ETT is a very practical test in that it can assess patients' functional capacity.[30]

Some examples of classes I, II, and III indications from the ACC/AHA guidelines for ETT are presented here.[31] The major class I indications are evaluation of males older than age 40 years who have symptoms suggestive of CAD and risk factors for CAD or atypical symptoms suggestive of CAD. Another class I indication is to help assess prognosis and functional capacity in patients with confirmed CAD.[32] Frequently, the ETT is performed following an acute myocardial infarction for this purpose (Table 13–8). Class II indications

TABLE 13-7 Comparing Pretest Likelihoods of Coronary Artery Disease in Low-Risk Symptomatic Patients with High-Risk Symptomatic Patients—Duke Database

Age (Years)	Nonanginal Chest Pain		Atypical Angina		Typical Angina	
	Men	*Women*	*Men*	*Women*	*Men*	*Women*
35	3–35	1–19	8–59	2–39	30–88	10–78
45	9–47	2–22	21–70	5–43	51–92	20–79
55	23–59	4–25	45–79	10–47	80–95	38–82
65	49–69	9–29	71–86	20–51	93–97	56–84

Each value represents the percent with significant coronary artery disease (CAD). The first is the percentage for a low-risk, mid-decade patient without diabetes, smoking, or hyperlipidemia. The second is that of the same age patient with diabetes, smoking, and hyperlipidemia. Both high- and low-risk patients have normal resting electrocardiograms. If ST-T–wave changes or Q waves had been present, the likelihood of CAD would be higher in each entry of the table.

TABLE 13-8 Exercise Stress Testing after Myocardial Infarction

Class I

1. Before discharge for prognostic assessment, activity prescription, evaluation of medical therapy (submaximal at about 4 to 76 days).
2. Early after discharge for prognostic assessment, activity prescription, evaluation of medical therapy, and cardiac rehabilitation if the predischarge exercise test was not done (symptom limited; about 14–21 days).
3. Late after discharge for prognostic assessment, activity prescription, evaluation of medical therapy, and cardiac rehabilitation if the early exercise test was submaximal (symptom limited; about 3 to 6 weeks).

Class IIa

After discharge for activity counseling and/or exercise training as part of cardiac rehabilitation in patients who have undergone coronary revascularization.

Class IIb

Periodic monitoring in patients who continue to participate in exercise training or cardiac rehabilitation.

Class III

1. Severe comorbidity likely to limit life expectancy and/or candidacy for revascularization.
2. At any time to evaluate patients with acute myocardial infarction who have uncompensated congestive heart failure, cardiac arrhythmia, or noncardiac conditions that severely limit their ability to exercise. (*Level of Evidence: C*)
3. Before discharge to evaluate patients who have already been selected for, or have undergone, cardiac catheterization. Although a stress test may be useful before or after catheterization to evaluate or identify ischemia in the distribution of a coronary lesion of borderline severity, stress imaging tests are recommended. (*Level of Evidence: C*)

Adapted from AHA/ACC guidelines.

TABLE 13-9 2002 Exercise Testing Guideline Recommendations

Class I

1. Patients undergoing initial evaluation with suspected or known CAD, including those with complete right bundle-branch block or less than 1 mm of resting ST depression.
2. Patients with suspected or known CAD, previously evaluated, now presenting with significant change in clinical status.
3. Low-risk unstable angina patients 8 to 12 hours after presentation who have been free of active ischemic or heart failure symptoms.
4. Intermediate-risk unstable angina patients 2 to 3 days after presentation who have been free of active ischemic or heart failure symptoms.

Class IIa

1. Intermediate-risk unstable angina patients who have initial cardiac markers that are normal, a repeat ECG without significant change, and cardiac markers 6 to 12 hours after the onset of symptoms that are normal and no other evidence of ischemia during observation. (*Level of Evidence: B*)

Class IIb

1. Patients with the following resting ECG abnormalities:
   Preexcitation (Wolff-Parkinson-White) syndrome.
   Electronically paced ventricular rhythm.
   1 mm or more of resting ST depression.
   Complete left bundle-branch block or any interventricular conduction defect with a QRS duration greater than 120 ms.
2. Patients with a stable clinical course who undergo periodic monitoring to guide treatment.

Class III

1. Patients with severe comorbidity likely to limit life expectancy and/or candidacy for revascularization.
2. High-risk unstable angina patients.

CAD, coronary artery disease; ECG, electrocardiogram.
Adapted from AHA/ACC guidelines.

are patients with variant angina or women with a history of typical or atypical chest pain (Table 13–9). Examples of class III indications are patients with simple premature ventricular contractions on a resting ECG with no other signs or symptoms of CAD. Additionally, ETT is used to assess symptoms such as chest pain or breathlessness. ETT should be used only if the results are able to alter patient management or to assess patient function.

Guidelines for conducting and interpreting the tests and details of testing equipment and environment are outlined in the 2002 ACC/AHA guidelines on ETT standards.[33] ETT is conducted on a treadmill or bicycle ergometer or by means of a handgrip. These dynamic methods are used to assess exercise tolerance because they induce both a volume and pressure load on the heart. Both modalities also allow the degree of stress to be delivered in a graded and calibrated manner. Treadmill walking is preferred over the ergometer because it involves more muscle mass and the maximal oxygen consumption (VO_2max) achieved with cycle ergometer is 10% to 15% lower than with the treadmill.

Many protocols have been designed and validated for use with ETT, but the two used most commonly are the Bruce and Naughton protocols. Protocols help to decrease inter- and intrapatient variability and allow for standardization in the interpretation of the tests. Protocols may be customized for individual patients to ensure an exercise time of 6 to 12 minutes and a heart rate of 85% to 90% of maximum predicted (adjusted for age and gender). Protocols detail gradient, speed, and rates of change of these parameters during the test.

In preparation for ETT, patients fast prior to the test for a minimum of 3 hours, may not exercise 12 hours prior to the test, and must dress suitably for exercise. Baseline evaluation consists of history and physical examination, blood pressure, heart rate, and ECG. The test begins with a 1-minute warmup period to orient the patient to the equipment. Each stage of the test is maintained for at least 3 minutes. Continuous blood pressure, heart rate, and ECG recordings are obtained, with definitive readings 2 minutes into each stage. Patients are questioned 2 to 3 minutes into each stage of the test about symptoms such as headache, dizziness, and chest pain. Clinical symptoms assessed include color of skin, level of perspiration, and evidence of peripheral cyanosis and light-headedness. Patients are encouraged to exercise as vigorously as they can to ensure an optimal test result. Onset, nature, and duration of all changes in symptoms, hemodynamics, and ECG are noted. Following the test there is a cool-down period during which the patient is seated or lying and is observed for changes as described earlier.

ETT requires considerable effort, with many patients requiring encouragement to perform to the best of their ability. Some patients use the test as a personal challenge and perform better on repeated attempts. This is referred to as a *training effect* and may be a confounding factor in using ETT to assess the effect of drug therapy or after interventions for IHD in clinical trials.

Interpretation of the test requires correlation of clinical, ECG, and other parameters measured during the test with the patient's history (e.g., age, gender, concurrent risk factors, and medical history) and concomitant therapy. Results of ETT can be used as a guide to future patient management, including suitability for interventional cardiology and selection of pharmacotherapy. A positive test is defined as 1 mm of horizontal or downsloping depression or elevation of the ST segment for 60 to 80 milliseconds after the QRS complex. For patients with baseline ST-segment depression, combinations of abnormal responses (e.g., 2 mm of ST-segment depression with hemodynamic abnormalities) would be necessary to call a test positive. ST-segment depression of 2 mm or more, especially in conjunction with heart rates of less than 120 beats per minute, low levels of stress, or depression persisting for up to 6 minutes after the cessation of the test, is associated with a poor prognosis. Depression of the ST segment in multiple leads is also significant. Other ECG changes include development of U waves and increased complexity and/or frequency of premature ventricular contractions or beats, especially if associated with bigeminy or periods of ventricular tachycardia.

Although ECG changes and heart rate responses are used as objective end points of ETT, patient and clinical end points are actually preferred. The use of the 85% to 90% maximally predicted heart rate is highly variable among patients and often is not achieved because of concomitant drug therapy and different levels of fitness. Symptom-limited or patient-directed tests are continued to the predetermined end point(s) unless the patient tires or certain characteristics are noted. Clinical symptoms, exhaustion, chest pain, and changes in blood pressure, heart rate, and the ECG (rhythm, configuration, and rate) are used as end points for such *open-ended tests*. Also, patient performance, measured as exercise duration, time until symptoms, stress at which symptoms occur, and hemodynamic parameters, is a better indicator of an adequate test than is heart rate response. *Close-ended testing* is the use of fixed end points such as time on the treadmill or maximal heart rate.

The product of blood pressure and heart rate (*double product*) is a measure of myocardial oxygen demand. In patients with stable angina, the double product is reproducible on repeat ETTs; consequently, it is used as an objective parameter to follow an individual patient's disease. Inappropriate or inadequate responses in blood pressure and/or heart rate to exercise suggest heart disease. A reduction in heart rate or a flat response (failure to increase heart rate above 120 beats per minute) with increasing levels of stress has a poor prognosis. Likewise, failure to increase the systolic blood pressure or the finding of a sustained decrease of more than 10 mm Hg is also associated with a worse prognosis. Such responses indicate that the heart has an inadequate reserve to respond to stress. Patients who are unable to progress beyond stage II of the Bruce protocol have a poor prognosis and more severe IHD. Other rating scales (e.g., Borg, which measures perceived exertion) may be

TABLE 13-10 MET Relationship to Activity and Function

METS	Level of Activity	ET Result
1	Resting	<6 METS
2	Level walking at 2 miles/h	Symptom-limited lifestyle
4	Level walking at 4 miles/h	Sedentary lifestyle tolerated
13	Cycling 9–10 miles/h	Little or no activity-limited lifestyle
20	Shoveling heavy snow	No limitations on lifestyle

ET, exercise testing; METS, metabolic equivalents of task.

used in conjunction with the objective results from the ETT to classify patients into high- and low-risk groups. Silent ischemia may confound the interpretation of ETT because blood pressure and ECG changes may occur in the absence of symptoms.

To provide standardized comparability between tests and patients, metabolic equivalents (METS) are used as a measure of VO_2max. A MET is a measure of resting oxygen uptake. Activity energy demands then can be calculated in terms of METS. For example, 4 METS is equivalent to walking at 4 miles per hour. The number of METS a patient can undertake without symptoms of ischemia correlates with prognosis and helps to guide appropriate management strategies. Table 13–10 has examples of METS and activity correlations. Exercise capacities of less than 5 METS are associated with a poor prognosis; those greater than 13 METS have a good prognosis despite the presence of disease.

Meta-analysis of more than 24,000 patients in 147 studies showed a mean sensitivity of 68% and specificity of 77% for ETT as a diagnostic test. The specificity of ETT to detect the presence of CAD, compared with angiography, is 84%. Sensitivity ranges from 40% to 90%, depending on the number of vessels affected, with a mean of 66%.

As a prognostic test, ETT is very popular after myocardial infarction and can be conducted within 3 days of an acute event. It can be used to determine functional capacity, assess the degree of rehabilitation, and identify patients at risk for further cardiovascular events. Immediately after myocardial infarction, a modified protocol is used; the test is terminated when a heart rate of 70% to 75% of age- and gender-predicted maximum is reached (e.g., 140 beats per minute for those younger than age 40 years and 130 beats per minute for those older than age 40 years) or a METS level of 5 for patients older than age 40 years or of 7 for those younger than age 40 years. Tests usually are done prior to discharge or within 6 weeks of infarction. In the periinfarction period, mortality and reinfarction rates caused by ETT are 0.02% and 0.09%, respectively. Patients may be stratified into low-, intermediate-, and high-risk categories, depending on the evidence for ischemia and the level of exercise tolerance.[33]

TABLE 13-11 Exercise Testing before and after Revascularization

Class I
1. Demonstration of ischemia before revascularization.
2. Evaluation of patients with recurrent symptoms that suggest ischemia after revascularization.

Class IIa
After discharge for activity counseling and/or exercise training as part of cardiac rehabilitation in patients who have undergone coronary revascularization.

Class IIb
1. Detection of restenosis in selected, high-risk asymptomatic patients within the first 12 months after percutaneous coronary intervention.
2. Periodic monitoring of selected, high-risk asymptomatic patients for restenosis, graft occlusion, incomplete coronary revascularization, or disease progression.

Class III
1. Localization of ischemia for determining the site of intervention.
2. Routine, periodic monitoring of asymptomatic patients after percutaneous coronary intervention or coronary artery bypass grafting without specific indications.

Adapted from AHA/ACC guidelines.

TABLE 13-12 Contraindications to Exercise Testing

Absolute
- Acute myocardial infarction (within 2 days)
- High-risk unstable angina
- Uncontrolled cardiac arrhythmias causing symptoms or hemodynamic compromise
- Symptomatic severe aortic stenosis
- Uncontrolled symptomatic heart failure
- Acute pulmonary embolus or pulmonary infarction
- Acute myocarditis or pericarditis
- Acute aortic dissection

Relative
- Left main coronary stenosis
- Moderate stenotic valvular heart disease
- Electrolyte abnormalities
- Severe arterial hypertension
- Tachyarrhythmias or bradyarrhythmias
- Hypertrophic cardiomyopathy and other forms of outflow tract obstruction
- Mental or physical impairment leading to inability to exercise adequately
- High-degree atrioventricular block

Adapted from AHA/ACC guidelines.

ETT is relatively safe, with an estimated risk of acute myocardial infarction or death of 10 per 10,000 tests overall. Most adverse effects are cardiac in nature, including arrhythmias (primarily bradyarrhythmias), sudden death, hypotension, and myocardial infarction. Patients in whom ETT is contraindicated are those who are unable or who should not exercise because of physiologic or psychological limitations and indications for termination (Tables 13–11, 13–12, and 13–13). Unstable angina is usually a contraindication to ETT because of the instability of the patient's disease state and because patients cannot exercise to a satisfactory level for the test to be considered adequate. However, once such a patient is stable, ETT is excellent for prognostic evaluation. In patients with untreated life-threatening arrhythmias or congestive heart failure, ETT is also contraindicated. Patients with comorbid diseases such as chronic obstructive pulmonary disease or peripheral vascular disease may be limited in their exercise capacity, whereas lower-limb amputees are unable to perform the standard treadmill test. For patients with disabilities or other medical conditions that limit their exercise capacity independent of heart disease, pharmacologic stress testing with dipyridamole, adenosine, or dobutamine is an alternative (see Pharmacologic Stress Testing below).

Drug therapy rarely is discontinued for the test primarily because few data exist to support better test results off drug therapy. Patients on β-blockers or calcium channel blockers may not achieve maximal heart rates, but ETT helps to demonstrate patients' exercise capacity on drug therapy. Nitrates do not alter exercise capacity directly and theoretically may improve patient response because they relieve or prevent symptoms of ischemia. Digoxin interferes with interpretation of ST-segment changes, and patients rarely achieve ST-segment changes greater than 1 mm even in the face of significant ischemia.

TABLE 13-13 Indications for Terminating Exercise Testing

Absolute indications
- Drop in systolic blood pressure of >10 mm Hg from baseline blood pressure despite an increase in workload, when accompanied by other evidence of ischemia
- Moderate to severe angina
- Increasing nervous system symptoms (e.g., ataxia, dizziness, or near syncope)
- Signs of poor perfusion (cyanosis or pallor)
- Technical difficulties in monitoring electrocardiogram or systolic blood pressure
- Subject's desire to stop
- Sustained ventricular tachycardia
- ST elevation (>1.0 mm) in leads without diagnostic Q-waves (other than V1 or aVR)

Adapted from AHA/ACC guidelines.

Because of its long half-life, digoxin does not need to be discontinued prior to the test (see Table 13–2).

ECHOCARDIOGRAM

❼ The echocardiogram (ECHO) is the use of ultrasound to visualize anatomic structures, such as the valves, within the heart and to describe wall motion.[34,35] Clinically, the ECHO is the most frequently used noninvasive cardiovascular test, aside from the ECG. It competes well with invasive techniques, such as cardiac catheterization with angiography, for the evaluation of ischemia and valvular abnormalities. ECHO is relatively cheap to perform and can be done at the bedside, in the operating room, or in the physician's office. The major disadvantages of the ECHO relate to technical limitations of operator-dependent images and competition from other noninvasive technologies such as MRI and CT scanning that provide similar information with superior tissue-type resolution. The ECHO is often used as an initial evaluative tool following auscultation detection of an abnormality, thus providing a baseline visual characterization. Serial determinations in a given patient, especially following a change in clinical condition or a procedure, allow evaluation of progression of disease over time.

The ECHO remains the procedure of choice in the diagnosis and evaluation of a number of conditions such as valvular dysfunction (aortic and mitral stenosis and regurgitation and endocarditis), wall motion abnormalities associated with ischemia, and congenital abnormalities, such as ventricular or atrial septal defects. Images obtained from ECHO are used to estimate chamber wall thickness and left ventricle ejection fraction, assess ventricular function, and detect abnormalities of the pericardium such as effusions or thickening.

Echocardiography is based on the principle of differential acoustic impedance (or tissue density) and the laws of reflection and refraction. Sound waves directed across tissues from a transducer will reflect back sound waves of different frequencies. The ability of the ultrasonic beam to penetrate chest wall structures is inversely proportional to the frequency of the signal. With transthoracic echocardiography, frequencies of 2.0 to 5.0 MHz are commonly used in adults, and frequencies of 3.5 to 10.0 MHz are used in children. Serial determinations in a given patient using the same conditions and ECHO images (windows) provide the best form of internal control to allow comparisons of test results. In clinical trials, echocardiograms are read and interpreted independently by two or three clinicians to provide a means of control.

Two primary approaches to ECHO are used in clinical practice. Transthoracic echocardiography (TTE) is conducted with the transducer on the chest wall, whereas transesophageal echocardiography (TEE) is conducted with the transducer in the esophagus. In TTE, several modes of operation are possible, the most common being M-mode (motion) and two-dimensional (2D) imaging. Both M-mode and 2D echocardiography provide visualization of heart structures and can indicate numerous structural abnormalities such as aneurysms, wall thickness abnormalities, chamber collapse (e.g., tamponade), and valvular stenosis. TEE is used primarily for assessment of valvular anatomy and function or to image intracardiac masses such as tumors or thrombi and valvular vegetations.[36]

In M-mode echocardiography, the transducer is placed at a single site on the chest (usually along the sternal border), and the ultrasound is directed posteriorly. M-mode echocardiography records only static objects in one plane, producing a single picture of a small region of the heart, or an "ice pick view." Results depend on the exact placement of the transducer with respect to the underlying structures. Conventional M-mode echocardiography provides visualization of the right ventricle, left ventricle, and posterior left ventricular wall and pericardium. If the transducer is swept in an arc from the apex to the base of the heart, virtually the whole heart can

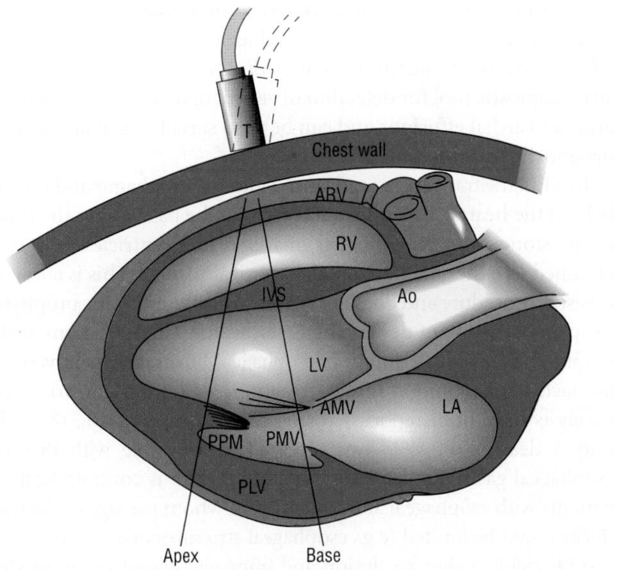

FIGURE 13-8. Schematic of two-dimensional echocardiography to illustrate location of cardiac structures as "seen" by the transducer. The transducer is swept in an arc so that several pictures of the heart are obtained to generate the final electrocardiogram. (Ao, aorta; AMV, anterior mitral valve; ARV, anterior right ventricle; IVS, interventricular septum; LA, left atrium; LV, left ventricle; PLV, posterior left ventricle; PMV, posterior mitral valve; PPM, posterior papillary muscle; RV, right ventricle.) *(Redrawn from Coryu BC, et al. Application of electrocardiography in acute myocardial infarction. Cardiovasc Clin 1995;2:113, with permission.)*

be visualized, including the valves and left atrium. Images are displayed as "windows."

Two-dimensional echocardiography employs multiple windows of the heart, and each view provides a wedge-shaped image. Windows most commonly used include parasternal long- and short-axis and apical two- and four-chamber views (Fig. 13–8). These views are processed onto a videotape to produce a motion picture of the heart. Two-dimensional echocardiography renders increased accuracy in calculating ventricular volumes, wall thickness, and degree of valvular stenosis compared with M-mode echocardiography. Patient-specific calculated parameters such as ejection fraction and wall thickness are compared with standardized values (population-based) or with previously obtained values from the patient. Although ejection fraction is still commonly obtained with echocardiography, it is a derived number, so it is considered subjective. Other tests to determine ejection fraction provide different numbers and highlight the difficulty of comparing results between tests. Ejection fraction from echocardiography is also limited by the diminished views of total ventricular volume able to be visualized, especially in persons with distorted ventricles. Despite these limitations, echocardiography remains the most common modality for ejection fraction determination.

The ECHO can be used for diagnosis and prognosis and as a serial evaluation tool to assess acute and chronic ischemic heart disease and regional left ventricular function. Areas of ischemic myocardium are seen on the ECHO as aberrations in wall motion. Wall motion abnormalities are seen as altered thicknesses of various segments of the heart. Wall motion abnormalities are graded using descriptive terms such as *akinetic, hypokinetic, dyskinetic,* and *hyperkinetic.* It is possible to visualize the complete ventricle (in segments), allowing both global and regional left ventricular function to be assessed. Studies show that the locations of segmental ventricular wall motion abnormalities correspond with areas of CAD. Echocardiography can be linked with the various stress tests (ETT, dipyridamole or dobutamine) to assess stress-induced structural or functional abnormalities (e.g., changes in wall motion). As a serial monitoring test, echocardiography is comparable with angiography as a prognostic tool and can be used as a treatment planning tool. After myocardial infarction, echocardiography is a useful noninvasive diagnostic tool for detection of ventricular aneurysms, thrombi, and pericardial effusions and can be used serially for diagnostic and prognostic information.

In TEE, the transducer is advanced into the esophagus and rests just behind the heart.[37] The transducer also can be passed into the fundus of the stomach to obtain better images of the ventricles. Images are obtained in either the horizontal or vertical plane.[38] This is a low-risk invasive procedure and does not require routine antibiotic prophylaxis for patients at risk of developing endocarditis. Complications such as esophageal tears or perforation, esophageal burns, transient ventricular tachycardia, minor throat irritation, and transient vocal cord paralysis have been reported rarely. In one series of 10,218 studies, only 1 death (0.0098%) was reported, comparable with that with esophageal gastroduodenoscopy (0.004%). TEE is contraindicated in patients with esophageal abnormalities, in whom passage of the transducer might be limited (e.g., esophageal strictures or varices).

TEE yields higher resolution and improved visualization of structures, especially pulmonary veins and valves, compared with TTE. Interference of ribs, lungs, and subcutaneous tissues is reduced, enabling TEE to be more useful in patients in whom TTE is limited because of pulmonary disease, mechanical ventilation, or obesity. A high-frequency transducer (5 MHz for adults) is used, thus producing better image resolution. TEE is used for the same indications as TTE. Visualization of the heart valves—in particular, the mitral valve—is superior, allowing more accurate evaluation of both native and prosthetic valves. Clinical studies show that it is possible to visualize valvular vegetations as small as 5 mm with TEE. The ACC/AHA guidelines recommend TEE if the TTE is equivocal and the patient has staphylococcal bacteremia. In a study comparing vegetation visualization, TEE detected vegetations in 90% of patients, compared to TTE detecting vegetations in 58%. It also can help to define complications of endocarditis such as thrombosis or valve leakage. In aortic dissection, TEE is able to identify the initial flap and origin of dissection and has an overall sensitivity and specificity of 97% and 100%, respectively. CT remains the diagnostic method of choice for aortic dissection, but TEE offers a sensitive and fast test that can be conducted in the emergency room.

Other uses of TEE include identification of cardiac thrombus, especially thrombi in the left atrium, and assessment of atrial dilation. After transient ischemic attacks or cerebrovascular accidents, TEE may enable identification of the site of cardiac emboli by providing excellent images of likely sources, namely, ventricular or atrial thrombus, valvular vegetation, cardiac shunts, cardiac tumors, or atrial and ventricular septal defects. In a study of almost 1,500 patients with cerebral ischemia or nonvalvular atrial fibrillation, atrial thrombi were seen in 183 patients when evaluated by TEE versus only in 2 patients when evaluated by TTE. TEE can be used for intraoperative cardiac imaging to ascertain development of ischemia.

Another advance with echocardiography has been the addition of Doppler and color-flow Doppler technology. The Doppler principle involves reflecting sound off a moving object—in the case of echocardiography, the red blood cell. As the red cell moves in relation to the transducer, a frequency shift occurs in the reflected wave. Assessment with Doppler echocardiography combines structural images and hemodynamic monitoring. Thus it is possible to evaluate the impact of structural disease on cardiac function and quantify the associated hemodynamics. Color enhancement allows flow direction to be visualized; different colors are used for antegrade and retrograde flow. These improve resolution of structures, identify patterns of blood flow, and allow calculation of flow gradients.

Doppler echocardiography is used primarily in conjunction with traditional echocardiography for analysis of valvular function or blood flow patterns. It allows measurement of transvalvular pressure gradients, valve area, and pressure changes on either side of the valve. Doppler echocardiography is either continuous or pulsed; the former is used to assess pressure changes, whereas the latter is used to localize points of origin and creation of turbulent and high blood flow. Color Doppler is used to visualize blood flow (e.g., regurgitation). Turbulence associated with valvular and wall motion abnormalities can be visualized and quantified clearly. In aortic regurgitation, Doppler echocardiography is one of the best noninvasive technique to assess the pressure and severity of regurgitation. Color-flow mapping allows tracing of the jet direction and an indication of its volume, point of wall contact, and width. Because Doppler echocardiography distinguishes different types of turbulence, it can simultaneously identify more than one type of valvular abnormality (e.g., aortic regurgitation and mitral stenosis) and the source of concomitant heart murmur.

The ACC/AHA 2003 task force has published clinical guidelines for application of echocardiography. In recent years, the use of intraoperative TEE has significantly increased and standard for valvular heart surgery and other types of cardiovascular surgery (Table 13–14).

NUCLEAR CARDIOLOGY[39,40]

Nuclear cardiology continues to be a major advance as a noninvasive testing method. Radionuclides with short half-lives, which can be

TABLE 13-14 Recommendations for Intraoperative Echocardiography

Class I

1. Evaluation of acute, persistent, and life-threatening hemodynamic disturbances in which ventricular function and its determinants are uncertain and have not responded to treatment.
2. Surgical repair of valvular lesions, hypertrophic obstructive cardiomyopathy, and aortic dissection with possible aortic valve involvement.
3. Evaluation of complex valve replacements requiring homografts or coronary reimplantation, such as the Ross prodecure.
4. Surgical repair of most congenital heart lesions that require cardiopulmonary bypass.
5. Surgical intervention for endocarditis when preoperative testing was inadequate or extension to perivalvular tissue is suspected.
6. Placement of intracardiac devices and monitoring of their position during port-access and other cardiac surgical interventions.
7. Evaluation of pericardial window procedures in patients with posterior or loculated pericardial effusions.

Class IIa

1. Surgical procedures in patients at increased risk of myocardial ischemia, myocardial infarction, or hemodynamic disturbances.
2. Evaluation of valve replacement, aortic atheromatous disease, the Maze procedure, cardiac aneurysm repair, removal of cardiac tumors, intracardiac thrombectomy, and pulmonary embolectomy.
3. Detection of air emboli during cardiotomy, heart transplant operations, and upright neurosurgical procedures.

Class IIb

1. Evaluation of suspected cardiac trauma, repair of acute thoracic aortic dissection without valvular involvement, and anastomotic sites during heart and/or lung transplantation.
2. Evaluation of regional myocardial function during and after off-pump coronary artery bypass graft procedures.
3. Evaluation of pericardiectomy, pericardial effusions, and pericardial surgery.
4. Evaluation of myocardial perfusion, coronary anatomy, or graft patency.
5. Dobutamine stress testing to detect inducible demand ischemia or to predict functional changes after myocardial revascularization.
6. Assessment of residual duct flow after interruption of patent ductus arteriosus.

Class III

1. Surgical repair of uncomplicated secundum atrial septal defect.

Cheitlin MD, Armstrong WF, Aurigemma GP, et al. ACC/AHA/ASE 2003 guideline update for the clinical application of echocardiography–summary article. J Am Coll Cardiol 2003;42(5):954-970. Full text at http://content.onlinejacc.org/.[41]

used either alone or combined with other substances to form agents with particular properties, such as technetium-99m pyrophosphate, have expanded the role for nuclear imaging in cardiology.

Nuclear imaging techniques have demonstrated equal sensitivity and specificity to many of the invasive "gold standard" testing modalities. The major limitations of nuclear cardiology are the availability of suitable radionuclides and correlation of nuclear images with cardiovascular function.

Despite the availability of new radionuclides, technetium-99m (^{99m}Tc) and thallium-201 (^{201}Tl) remain the two most commonly used radionuclides. ^{99m}Tc is ideal for clinical imaging because it has a half-life of about 6 hours, a single 140-keV photon peak suitable for available imaging systems, primarily gamma ray emission, and the ability to be combined with multiple pharmaceuticals. It is generated in-house by a benchtop generator that reduces transportation costs and provides immediate availability. The short half-life means high doses and repeat injections can be given to evaluate efficacy of interventional therapy over a relatively short period of time. ^{201}Tl has a much longer half-life of 73 hours, which prevents the use of multiple doses close together but does mean that delayed imaging is possible following administration of the agent. Uptake into cells depends on blood flow. The energy from ^{201}Tl is x-ray, with an energy level of 69 to 83 keV. Production of ^{201}Tl requires a cyclotron. Images are obtained with a conventional gamma camera.

Technetium Scanning

Technetium scanning is used for the evaluation of blood pool and myocardial perfusion and as an infarct-avid agent to identify damaged myocardium. Analysis of the blood pool, as in multigated angiography, uses technetium either alone or as a red blood cell complex. The former obtains images following a bolus of technetium and traces its passage from the venous system through the heart to the aorta and is known as *first-pass angiography.* Equilibrium tests where technetium is bound to red blood cells provide an imaging time of several hours, which allows serial images to be obtained. These tests are used to determine right and left ventricular ejection fractions, detect cardiac shunts, estimate ventricular volumes, and view wall motion.[42]

Infarct-avid radionuclides such as technetium-pyrophosphate (^{99m}Tc-PYP) are used to describe the presence and extent of damaged myocardium after myocardial infarction, in suspected myocardial contusion, and following chest wall injuries. Imaging with ^{99m}Tc-PYP is applicable when myocardial infarction is suspected clinically, but patient history, ECG changes, and laboratory evidence are not definitive. Uptake of ^{99m}Tc-PYP into infarcted tissue depends on regional blood flow, myocardial calcium concentration, the degree of irreversible myocardial injury, and time after infarction. ^{99m}Tc-PYP attaches to calcium deposited in the infarcted area, so the approach is known as *hot-spot scanning.* False hot spots may occur where there is necrotic myocardial tissue, as in myocarditis, myocardial abscesses, old infarctions, and myocardial trauma. Additionally, uptake has been seen during unstable angina and ventricular dyskinesia and at sites of ventricular aneurysms, suggesting that these are associated with transient low blood flow. In infarcted tissue, ^{99m}Tc-PYP levels can be as high as 18 to 20 times that of normal myocardium, which gives rise to very distinct borders between the infarcted and normal myocardium. Uptake of ^{99m}Tc-PYP into necrotic myocardium is delayed and not measurable until after about 4 hours of coronary occlusion. Scans prior to this time are usually negative and become positive about 12 hours after occlusion. Peak intensity of ^{99m}Tc-PYP is reached at 48 hours. Washout occurs over 5 to 7 days, so ^{99m}Tc-PYP is a useful late marker of infarction, especially in patients who present late or with a silent infarction. Images are viewed by comparing sternum and rib uptake with that seen in the myocardium. This type of imaging also can be used to assess graft patency after coronary artery bypass. Certain characteristics of the images obtained have been linked with various prognostic values but await confirmation in comparative and long-term prognostic trials.

Other technetium-labeled agents used include technetium-*t*-butyl isonitrile (^{99m}Tc-TIBI); technetium-carboxy isopropyl isonitrile (^{99m}Tc-CPI); technetium-sestamibi, also known as methoxy-isobutyl isonitrile (Tc-MIBI); and technetium-teboroxime. Technetium-sestamibi has a similar myocardial uptake pattern to thallium and produces similar results but with improved image quality because it generates a much higher photon yield. This is now popular as an alternative perfusion imaging agent to thallium. Technetium-teboroxime is still primarily an investigational agent. The main advantage of the newer technetium compounds is the lack of redistribution perfusion, allowing for delayed imaging. This is particularly useful in acute clinical settings; the radiopharmaceutical can be injected during the acute event and imaging undertaken when the patient is more stable.

Thallium Scanning

Thallium is a potassium analog taken up into normal myocardium by passive diffusion and possibly by active transport via the Na^+-K^+-adenosine triphosphatase (ATPase) pump. Uptake depends on regional blood flow and in a linear fashion up to very high blood flow rates. It is used primarily for the analysis of coronary and myocardial perfusion. High thallium uptake occurs in perfused myocardium; in ischemic myocardium, uptake is reduced significantly. Scans taken during acute ischemia or following infarction show areas of poor or nil distribution of thallium corresponding to the site of ischemia. A scan repeated 4 to 6 hours after the initial scan may show a redistribution of the thallium into areas that previously had little to no thallium uptake. These defects are referred to as *partial defects,* demonstrating areas hypoperfused during "stress" but viable myocardium at rest. Redistribution occurs because there is delayed washout of thallium from poorly perfused myocardium, resulting in less contrast between the density of thallium in different areas of the heart. This gives the appearance of "redistribution" of the radionuclide into the previously ischemic area. To enhance evaluation of potential partial defects, a second injection of thallium can be used. Areas of nil distribution are called *cold spots* or *fixed defects* and reflect infarcted myocardium.

Thallium scanning with the aid of computer analysis segregates the images into anatomic regions and specifically localizes areas of dead or necrotic myocardial tissue. In conjunction with echocardiography or single-photon emission computed tomography (SPECT), thallium scans can correlate areas of abnormal wall motion with areas of poor perfusion. Sensitivity and specificity of thallium scanning to detect IHD disease are comparable with those of ETT (75% and 80%, respectively). When used in conjunction with exercise ECG, sensitivity increases to approximately 80%. Thallium scanning also can be used in conjunction with ETT to allow detection of lower levels of ischemia than may be determined from ECG abnormalities or patient symptoms. Thallium is injected at the peak of the ETT, and exercise continues for another 30 to 60 seconds, when the initial images are taken. Repeat images are taken at 3 to 4 hours.

Thallium scanning is useful in patients with atypical chest pain and ambiguous or false-positive ETT to determine if IHD is the cause of symptoms and the ETT abnormalities. Thallium scanning is also used for postoperative evaluation of revascularization or angioplasty procedures and for preoperative evaluation for prognostic stratification for persons with IHD. A normal thallium scan heralds a benign outcome, even in patients who have angiographically evident CAD. The finding of redistribution is a marker of jeopardized but viable myocardium that has important prognostic value. Major cardiac events such as myocardial infarction in patients with normal ^{201}Tl studies average less than 1% per year. The best predictor of coronary events, which correlates thallium scans with clinical significance, is the number of myocardial segments with transient (redistribution) defects.

A number of other radiopharmaceuticals have found some use in cardiovascular testing, such as labeled antimyosin antibodies. Theoretically, these antibodies should be more specific markers of myocyte necrosis. The currently used antibodies are a murine Fab fragment. Phase I, II, and III trials suggest that these are highly specific for irreversibly injured myocytes, but they have limitations in terms of pharmacokinetic properties. Uptake into myocardial tissues is very slow, with a prolonged blood pool activity seen for at least 24 hours. In clinical use, the antibody is given within 24 hours of the infarction, and planar or SPECT imaging is undertaken 24 to 48 hours later. Despite the supposed specificity of the antibody to myosin, localization is more dependent on blood flow than on myosin concentration, so measurement of infarction size is not as accurate as expected. Another investigational agent, [^{123}I]phenylpentadecanoic acid, is able to assess both myocardial perfusion and metabolism by virtue of its affinity for fatty acid metabolism.

Pharmacologic Stress Testing

❾ Pharmacologic stress testing is an alternative to ETT and ETT with thallium in patients who are unable or unwilling to undergo ETT.[43,44] Additionally, pharmacologic stress testing is now used more than 50% of the time to assess coronary perfusion. The pharmacologic agent produces stress by a hyperemic (vasodilator) response or by increasing myocardial oxygen demand (heart rate and myocardial contractility). Agents currently used include dipyridamole and adenosine (hyperemic stress) and dobutamine (myocardial stress). Pharmacologic stress tests can be linked to various imaging techniques such as thallium planar scanning, SPECT, MRI, and echocardiography. Dobutamine is linked most frequently to echocardiography, allowing quantification of wall motion abnormalities, which correlate well with areas of ischemia.

The principle of dipyridamole and adenosine thallium imaging is related to their coronary arteriolar vasodilator properties. Dipyridamole inhibits adenosine cellular reuptake, resulting in increased concentrations of adenosine in the blood and tissues. Adenosine is a potent coronary artery vasodilator and can increase perfusion four to five times over baseline. Areas distal to a coronary artery obstruction will show a relative hypoperfusion compared with normal coronary arteries because there is reduced perfusion pressure as a consequence of preferential perfusion of normal segments over stenotic segments. Acutely, these areas will appear as cold spots, but on the redistribution scans, the defects will fill, indicating viable but jeopardized myocardium.

Dipyridamole is given intravenously in a dose of 0.142 mg/kg per minute over 4 minutes. This dose has been shown to increase baseline coronary blood flow in the normal tissues up to four to five times over control. Some studies have used doses up to 0.84 mg/kg to enhance the vasodilator response. At the higher dose, acute adverse effects such as chest pain are more common. Adenosine for stress testing is an unlabeled use of this drug. Adenosine is given over 6 minutes at a dose of 0.140 mcg/kg per minute. At the end of infusion (dipyridamole) or after 3 minutes (adenosine), a 2.5- to 4-mCi dose of thallium is given. The maximum effect of dipyridamole occurs at 5 to 7 minutes and adenosine at approximately 30 seconds after the end of infusion. Imaging follows immediately and can be repeated at 24 hours (thallium scanning) to heighten the redistribution defects from fixed or partial defects.

Like exercise thallium scanning, dipyridamole and adenosine scanning or echocardiography is used to detect IHD, evaluate the prognosis of patients with known disease, assess patients after myocardial infarction, and as a risk-stratification method prior to vascular, cardiac, and noncardiac surgery. Pharmacologic stress testing evaluates wall motion abnormalities and perfusion defects under stress and has been shown in numerous studies to have comparable sensitivity and specificity with the traditional ETT. Using planar scanning and dipyridamole, sensitivity to detect IHD ranges from 67% to 95% with a 67% to 100% specificity. A summary of 13 studies in almost 900 patients gave a pooled sensitivity of 85% and specificity of 87%. SPECT scanning has at least comparable sensitivity and slightly lower specificity to planar imaging but produces higher-quality imaging, which may enhance quantitative interpretation.

Dipyridamole testing is safe and effective in the elderly and in those with unstable angina immediately after myocardial infarction (within days). It also may be used to assess the status of revascularization procedures.[43] As a prognostic test, dipyridamole testing is very useful. In several studies, abnormal scans have shown about a 10-fold increase in event rates over 1 to 2 years of followup. Abnormal scans also have been shown to be an independent risk factor for myocardial infarction and death with a relative risk ratio of 3.1. Reversible defects correlate best with events, with one study demonstrating a 4.41 relative risk ratio for cardiac events.

Adverse effects with dipyridamole thallium testing are minimal, the main adverse effects being chest pain (with or without ischemic changes on the ECG), headache, dizziness, and nausea. Adverse effects are related to the increased adenosine activity and can be ameliorated by xanthine compounds because they are direct competitive antagonists of adenosine. Caffeine products must be avoided for about 24 hours prior to the test. Adenosine is associated with a higher incidence of adverse effects (80% versus 50%), but these are very transient, and some studies have shown that patients prefer it over dipyridamole. Both agents are relatively contraindicated in patients with a history of bronchospasm.

Dobutamine, a synthetic catecholamine, raises heart rate and cardiac output, which increases myocardial oxygen demand. Ischemia develops in areas where stenosis prevents the increase in oxygen demand from being met with increased blood flow. Ischemia is detected by the ECHO as regional wall motion abnormalities or with thallium scanning.

Dobutamine, when used as a stress test, is given in doses of 10 to 40 mcg/kg per minute.[44] The dose is titrated at 3-minute intervals in increments of 10 mcg/kg per minute. If thallium is used, it is given 2 to 3 minutes before the end of infusion. Atropine 0.5 to 1 mg may be given to augment the heart rate response to 85% of the patient's calculated maximum. ECG and blood pressure are recorded continuously throughout the test, and ECHO recordings are made during the last minute of each dose level and during recovery.

β-Blocker and calcium channel blocker therapy may interfere with the heart rate response to dobutamine stress tests and is recommended to be discontinued prior to the test. Dobutamine stress testing is relatively well tolerated. Reasons to discontinue the test include development of severe chest pain, extensive new wall motion abnormalities, ST-segment elevation and depression suggestive of significant ischemia, tachyarrhythmias, and symptomatic reductions in blood pressure.[45] β-Blockers can be used to reverse most adverse effects if they persist. Dobutamine stress tests are contraindicated in patients with aortic stenosis, uncontrolled hypertension, and severe ventricular arrhythmias. Ventricular fibrillation and myocardial infarction occur at a rate of approximately 0.05%.

Dobutamine stress testing has been studied as a diagnostic, prognostic, and therapy assessment tool after myocardial infarction and for unstable and chronic angina. One study compared dobutamine, dipyridamole, and ETT with coronary angiography for diagnostic accuracy in patients with IHD and showed an overall accuracy of 87% for ETT, 82% for dobutamine, and 77% for dipyridamole. A recent review of 14 studies of 942 patients for the detection of IHD with dobutamine stress testing calculated the sensitivity to be approximately 80% (70% to 100%) with a 75% (64% to 100%) specificity. Sensitivity is highest for detection of three-vessel disease (92%). Dobutamine-sestamibi stress testing seems to be less sensitive than thallium even for multivessel disease. Comparative studies with ETT and dipyridamole echocardiography show dobutamine to be more sensitive. After myocardial infarction, dobutamine stress testing identifies patients at high risk of subsequent cardiac events. For patients with suspected or known IHD, a positive dobutamine stress test is an independent predictor of cardiac events, and a negative test affords protection from cardiac death.[46]

The current 2006 guidelines on the use of these tests in clinical practice are rather brief, only to say that cardiac imaging is currently undergoing rapid evolution. The use of these types of test in intermediate to high risk patients are markedly increasing. The identification of asymptomatic intermediate-risk patients (10% to 20% risk of cardiovascular death/myocardial infarction in 10 years) is still undergoing considerable debate. The clinical treatment of these patients with atherosclerosis *must* include appropriate risk factor treatment according to existing AHA guidelines. Patients with high-risk findings of cardiovascular disease may require more invasive testing but global risk reduction will still be required before and after there testing or invasive treatment if essential.[47]

COMPUTED TOMOGRAPHY

CT scanning is becoming more popular as a primary screening procedure in the evaluation of CVD and function because it provides similar information as other diagnostic procedures (e.g., catheterization, echocardiography) and is less expensive and less invasive than a routine heart catheterization. In recent years, advancement in technology has considerably enhanced definition and spatial resolution of all cardiac structures that are useful in evaluation of many specific areas, such as coronary arteries, aortic and pericardial disease, and paracardiac and cardiac masses. Very accurate determination of chamber volume and size and mass calculations of myocardial wall thickness can be obtained from CT scanning than with other methods such as echocardiography or angiography. Additionally, CT scanning acquires three-dimensional images.[48] New techniques such as ultrafast CT (cine-CT) scanning have significantly improved problems with cardiac motion that distorted conventional CT images. In cine-CT scanning, complete tomograms are assembled within one cardiac cycle (50 msec), thus providing real-time images. For ultrafast CT scanners, a set event within the cardiac cycle (determined by ECG) usually is used as initiator for imaging to ensure standardization. Conventional CT scanning requires that images be correlated with the cardiac cycle by gating the CT to the ECG. Cine-CT scans examine the heart at 10 to 14 tomographic levels in <10-mm slices. The resolution has improved considerably in the last few years as a result of advances in many areas of computer science and now 64-section multidetector CT scans are significantly better.

Although still in its infancy, cine-CT scanning has matured significantly and is now being used as a screening tool for evaluating the risk of significant obstructive CAD and as a diagnostic tool for CAD in limited centers. Recent AHA/ACC guidelines address the current state of practice with this methodology. The CT scan will show localized areas of infarction and abnormal perfusion and allows quantification of the extent and density of coronary artery calcification.[49] Cine-CT scanning is more sensitive and specific than fluoroscopy in identifying the extent and density of coronary artery calcification. The calcium score (calcium density and volume of calcium) in patients older than 30 to 70 years with known CAD is significantly higher than in subjects with no CAD and appears to correlate well with the degree of coronary artery occlusion (Table 13–15).[50]

New CT scanning may be more definitive and accurate in the diagnosis of aortic dissection and evaluation of the pericardium than TTE but in many expert centers, TEE maybe as good. Currently 3D echocardiography can add other important information to a critical patient's case, for example, valvular leaks and wall motion changes. Diagnostic accuracy of aortic dissections with CT scanning is >90%. CT scanning affords definition of the

TABLE 13-15 ACCF/AHA 2007 Clinical Expert Consensus Document on Coronary Artery Calcium Scoring By Computed Tomography—Conclusions

1. What is the role of coronary calcium measurement by coronary CT scanning in asymptomatic patients with intermediate CHD risk (between 10% and 20% 10-year risk of estimated coronary events)?

The Committee judged that it may be reasonable to consider use of CAC measurement in such patients based on available evidence that demonstrates incremental risk prediction information in this selected (intermediate-risk) patient group. This conclusion is based on the possibility that such patients might be reclassified to a higher risk status based on high CAC score, and subsequent patient management may be modified.

2. What is the role of coronary calcium measurement by CT scan in patients with low CHD risk (below 10% 10-year risk of estimated CHD events)?

The Committee does not recommend use of CAC measurement in this selected patient group. This patient group is similar to the "population screening" scenario, and the Committee does not recommend screening of the general population using CAC measurement.

3. What is the role of coronary calcium measurement by fast CT scan in asymptomatic patients with high CHD risk (greater than 20% estimated 10-year risk of estimated CHD events, or established coronary disease, or other high-risk diagnoses)?

The Committee does not advise CAC measurement in this selected patient stratum as they are already judged to be candidates for intensive risk-reducing therapies based on current NCEP guidelines.

4. Is the evidence strong enough to reduce the treatment intensity in patients with calcium score = 0 in patients who are considered intermediate risk before coronary calcium score?

No evidence is available that allows the Committee to make a consensus judgment on this question. Accordingly, the Committee felt that current standard recommendations for treatment of intermediate risk patients should apply in this setting.

5. Is there evidence that coronary calcium measurement is better than other potentially competing tests in intermediate risk patients for modifying cardiovascular disease risk estimate?

In general, CAC measurement has not been compared to alternative approaches to risk assessment in head-to-head studies. The question cannot be adequately answered from available data.

6. Should there be additional cardiac testing when a patient is found to have high coronary calcium score (e.g., CAC is greater than 400)?

Current clinical practice guidelines indicate that patients classified as high risk based on high-risk factor burden or existence of known high-risk disease states (e.g., diabetes) are regarded as candidates for intensive preventive therapies (medical treatments). There is no clear evidence that additional noninvasive testing in this clear patient population will result in more appropriate selection of treatments.

7. Is there a role for CAC testing in patients with atypical cardiac symptoms?

Evidence indicates that patients considered to be at low risk of coronary disease by virtue of atypical cardiac symptoms may benefit from CAC testing to help in ruling out the presence of obstructive coronary disease. Other competing approaches are available, and most of these competing modalities have not been compared head-to-head with CAC.

8. Can coronary calcium data collected to date be generalized to specific patient populations (women, African American men)?

CAC data are strongest for Caucasian, non-Hispanic men. The Committee recommends caution in extrapolating CAC data derived from studies in white men to women and to ethnic minorities.

9. What is the appropriate followup when an incidental finding in the lungs or other noncardiac tissues is found on a fast coronary CT study?

Current radiology guidelines should be considered when determining need for followup of incidental findings on a fast CT study, such as that which was recently published to guide followup of small pulmonary nodules.

CAC, coronary artery calcium; CHD, coronary heart disease; CT, computed tomography; NCEP, National Cholesterol Education Program.

Greenland, Bonow RO, Brundage BH, et al. ACCF/AHA 2007 clinical expert consensus document on coronary artery calcium scoring by computed tomography in global cardiovascular risk assessment and in evaluation of patients with chest pain. J AM Coll Cardiol 2007;49:378–402.

edges of the intimal flap of the dissection, and true and false channels can be seen. It also demarcates the components of the myocardial wall from the inner endocardial wall through to the epicardial surface and pericardium, allowing visualization of abnormalities, such as aneurysms and thrombin. Detection of the presence of a thrombus on a CT scan is comparable in accuracy with 2D echocardiography. The pericardium appears as a distinct entity and can be evaluated for thickening and calcification. CT scanning is the most sensitive technique to differentiate types of pericarditis and estimate pericardial fluid volume. Compared with echocardiography, CT scanning is equivocal to define loculated and hemorrhagic effusions. Important advances in 3D echocardiography is currently making significant advancement as we have seen with new CT scanners.

In the evaluation of cardiac masses, CT scanning shows the mass as a distinct space-occupying entity. Tissue density differentiation as seen on a CT scan allows characterization of density, aiding in determination of the nature of masses. Masses as small as 0.5 to 1 cm can be identified on CT scans.

Like radionuclide assessment, contrast angiography, and echocardiography, CT scanning can be used to calculate ejection fraction, left ventricular volume, and stroke volume. The blood pool is defined with intravenous iodinated contrast material. Ventricular volumes, ejection fraction, and stroke volume are determined directly from the blood pool on each image. Values obtained with CT scanning are more accurate and reproducible than those obtained on angiography and ECHO. The three-dimensional image of a CT scan also allows determination of the extent and distribution of LVH in patients with hypertrophic or congestive cardiomyopathy.

CT scanning has proven to be an effective noninvasive method to visualize congenital heart disease, but its role is challenged by the higher-resolution capacity of MRI.[50] For measuring parameters in some congenital disorders, such as evaluation of ventricular function and estimation of the volume of cardiac shunts, CT scanning still remains an important choice. As patients have more procedures related to implanted metallic devices, CT scanning is a very important option and newer CT scanners are making major strides in many areas of congenital heart disease.

A few practical considerations when one considers CT for evaluating the coronary arteries. Diagnostic quality imaging may require in most cases the patient to have normal sinus rhythm, and a targeted heart rate of less than 65 beats per minute during image acquisition. The patient's heart rate should be measured during a breath-holding test to determine whether the administration of a β-blocker is necessary. If the heart rate drops after inspiration breath holding by 10 beats per minute, the study should be of good quality. However, sometimes short-acting β-blockers are needed to reduce heart rates to below 65 beats per minute.[51]

Recently published guidelines from the AHA[52] on the assessment of coronary artery disease by cardiac computed tomography have an excellent review of the topic with a wonderful reference section. Table 13–16 is an overview of current considerations for scanning. Most expert panels generally agree that patients with a prior probability of a coronary event in the intermediate range (>6% in 10 years but <20% in 10 years), a calcium score of >100 would yield a posttest probability >2% per year in the majority of patients. This would place the patient in the range of a coronary heart disease risk equivalent population and within a level requiring secondary prevention strategies. Table 13–17 describes the American College of Cardiology Foundation (ACCF) results of appropriate use of cardiac computed tomography in cardiovascular disease from the Appropriateness Criteria Working Group.[53]

In summary, CT scanning, especially cine-CT scanning, is a rapidly evolving technique for evaluation of CVD. It remains an expensive alternative to other methodologies in many instances, but the high resolution and spatial capabilities mean that CT scanning offers unique properties. It is important to remember that CT scanning radiation dosage on average is three times more than a routine heart catheterization. Current coronary angiography has a mean effective radiation dosage of approximately 5 mSv (millisievert) and cardiac CT varies between 6.9 and 20 mSv depending on the configuration.[54,55]

TABLE 13-16 Criteria for Cardiac Computed Tomography (CCT) and Cardiac Magnetic Resonance (CMR) ACCF/ACR/SCCT/SCMR/ASNC/NASCI/SCAI/SIR 2006 Appropriateness

Appropriate test for specific indication (Score 7–9)
Detection of CAD: Symptomatic
Intermediate pretest probability of CAD
ECG uninterpretable *or* unable to exercise
Evaluation of Intracardiac Structures (Use of CT Angiogram)
Evaluation of suspected coronary anomalies
Acute Chest Pain (Use of CT Angiogram)
Intermediate pretest probability of CAD
No ECG changes and serial enzymes negative
Morphology (Use of CT Angiogram)
Assessment of complex congenital heart disease including anomalies of coronary circulation, great vessels, and cardiac chambers and valves
Evaluation of coronary arteries in patients with new onset heart failure to assess etiology.
Evaluation of Intra- and Extracardiac Structures (Use of Cardiac CT)
Evaluation of cardiac mass (suspected tumor or thrombus)
Patients with technically limited images from echocardiogram, MRI, or TEE
Evaluation of pericardial conditions (pericardial mass, constrictive pericarditis, or complications of cardiac surgery)
Patients with technically limited images from echocardiogram, MRI, or TEE
Evaluation of pulmonary vein anatomy prior to invasive radiofrequency ablation for atrial fibrillation
Noninvasive coronary vein mapping prior to placement of biventricular pacemaker
Noninvasive coronary arterial mapping, including internal mammary artery prior to repeat cardiac surgical revascularization
Evaluation of Aortic and Pulmonary Disease (Use of CT Angiogram[a])
Evaluation of suspected aortic dissection or thoracic aortic aneurysm
Evaluation of suspected pulmonary embolism
Uncertain for specific indication (Score 4–6)
Inappropriate test for that indication (Score 1-3)

CAD, coronary artery disease; ECG, electrocardiogram; MRI, magnetic resonance imaging; TEE, transesophageal echocardiography.

[a]Nongated, CT angiogram which has a sufficiently large field of view for these specific indications.

Hendel (Guidelines). JACC 2007;48:1475. Summary of Table 11–20.

POSITRON EMISSION TOMOGRAPHY

PET is a relatively new modality for diagnostic imaging in CVD medicine.[56,57] PET has found a niche to characterize myocardial physiologic and metabolic activity, perfusion, and viability. PET can measure regional myocardial uptake of exogenous glucose and fatty acids, quantitate free fatty acid metabolism, define perfused myocardium energy source(s), and evaluate myocardial chemoreceptor sites.[61] Although many other techniques can be used similarly to evaluate myocardial function, PET images are superior in definition. The primary advantages of PET are its noninvasive nature, the ability to do repeat scans within a short period of time, such as before and after percutaneous transluminal coronary angioplasty (PTCA), and the reproducibility of images over time. PET is very expensive because of the need for onsite cyclotrons for many of the radiotracers, and there is limited availability of sites that offer the technique. Cheaper forms of PET-like scanning are in development, but image resolution is lower.

PET uses positron-emitting isotopes such as oxygen-15, nitrogen-13, carbon-11, and fluoride-18. These are incorporated into sub-

TABLE 13-17 Interpretation and Recommendations for CT Heart Scanning and CACP Scoring

Negative test result
A negative test (score = 0) makes the presence of atherosclerotic plaque, including unstable or vulnerable plaque, highly unlikely.
A negative test (score = 0) makes the presence of significant luminal obstructive disease highly unlikely (negative predictive power by EBCT on the order of 95% to 99%).
A negative test is consistent with a low risk (0.1% per year) of a cardiovascular event in the next 2 to 5 years.
Positive test result
A positive test (CAC 0) confirms the presence of a coronary atherosclerotic plaque.
The greater the amount of coronary calcium, the greater the atherosclerotic burden in men and women, irrespective of age.
The total amount of coronary calcium correlates best with the total amount of atherosclerotic plaque, although the true atherosclerotic burden is underestimated.
High score
A high calcium score (an Agatston score >100) is consistent with a high risk of a cardiac event within the next 2 to 5 years (2% annual risk).
Risk prediction
Coronary artery calcium measurement can improve risk prediction in conventional intermediate-risk patients, and CACP scanning should be considered in individuals at intermediate risk for a coronary event (1.0% per year to 2.0% per year) for clinical decision making with regard to refinement of risk assessment.
Decisions for further testing (such as stress testing or cardiac catheterization) beyond assistance in risk stratification in patients with a positive CACP score cannot be made on the basis of coronary calcium scores alone, as calcium score correlates poorly with stenosis severity in a given individual and should be based upon clinical history and other conventional clinical criteria.

CACP, coronary artery calcified plaque; CAC, coronary artery calcium; CT, computed tomography; EBCT, electron-beam computed tomography.

stances such as water, glucose analogs, or fatty acids, the metabolic substrates for myocardial tissue. For myocardial perfusion studies, rubidium-82 (^{82}Rb), nitrogen-13 ammonia ([^{13}N]H_3), and $^{15}O_2$-labeled water are used. For myocardial substrate metabolism studies, [^{11}C]palmitate, [^{11}C]acetate, and [^{18}F]2-deoxyglucose (FDG) are used. All these substances have very short half-lives (<10 minutes). In the fasting state, perfused myocardium primarily uses fatty acids as energy source. Postprandially, glucose is the preferred substrate. Ischemic myocardium primarily metabolizes glucose because mitochondrial fatty acid oxidation is impaired. Hence, with PET using either a fatty acid or glucose substrate, ischemic versus nonischemic areas can be defined. Frequently, PET is used in conjunction with pharmacologic stress testing to provoke ischemia, with images obtained before and after stress application.

Uptake of ^{82}Rb occurs via the Na^+-K^+-ATPase pump and occurs preferentially in viable tissue. Net uptake into tissue resolving from an ischemic insult and infarcted tissue is reduced. With a half-life of 1.26 minutes, serial images of myocardial perfusion can be taken as frequently as every 5 minutes, and a dobutamine stress test is completed within 45 minutes. Comparative studies with ETT, SPECT, and stress echocardiography show PET to be more accurate in the detection of IHD. The substrate [^{13}N]H_3 rapidly crosses capillary membranes and is trapped in the myocardium by glutamate–glutamine reactions. This product produces high-contrast images with a sensitivity of 88% to 97% and a specificity of 90% to 100% to detect IHD. $^{15}O_2$-labeled water has a high extraction ratio into myocardial tissue, which appears to be independent of blood flow or the metabolic state of the myocardium. $^{15}O_2$-labeled water studies are done in conjunction with [^{15}O]carbon monoxide (labels red blood cells in the vascular space) studies to help eliminate some of the background activity that occurs as a result of the high extraction ratio.[58]

Tracers used for assessment of myocardial metabolism are selected based on the type of metabolism of interest: FDG traces glucose metabolism, [^{11}C]palmitate traces mitochondrial fatty acid metabolism, and [^{11}C]acetate is an indirect marker for myocardial oxygen consumption, allowing assessment of ventricular performance. [^{11}C]Palmitate is a useful marker for normal myocardial oxygen consumption because baseline energy needs of the myocardium are met through fatty acid oxidation. Clearance of [^{11}C]palmitate is biexponential, and studies in animals and in healthy men show clearance to be proportional to cardiac workload and myocardial oxygen consumption. In acute ischemia, the first component of clearance is reduced and the second is increased. The use of [^{11}C]palmitate to assess myocardial metabolism in ischemic tissue is limited because there is altered transport and storage of the compound and significant back diffusion of the agent into the vascular space.

FDG accumulates in the heart proportional to glucose use by the myocardial cell and so is a marker of cell viability. FDG studies help to identify the affected vascular bed and allow evaluation as to whether angioplasty or surgery might be used. Detection of hibernating myocardium is possible because it predominantly uses glucose and can be seen readily on PET scans. Patients with a significant degree of jeopardized or hibernating myocardium identified on PET scanning then could be candidates for revascularization procedures. In contrast, a perfusion study would not show as good differentiation of infarcted versus hibernating tissue, and revascularization may not be considered. In studies of recovery of left ventricular function following revascularization, PET has a positive predictive value of 72% and a negative predictive value of 83%. PET with FDG has been used in the assessment of cardiomyopathies. In ischemic cardiomyopathy, discrete regional ischemia is seen as a patchy, nonhomogeneous uptake of the tracers; dilated cardiomyopathies show global decreased uptake of tracers.

In CAD, PET is used to assess and follow the physiologic significance of stenotic lesions. After infarction, PET myocardial substrate metabolism studies are used to evaluate the amount and activity of viable tissue around the infarcted area and the site and extent of infarction. Myocardial perfusion studies with PET identify more accurately the viable and nonviable myocardium compared with technetium and thallium. PET also quantifies regional myocardial perfusion more accurately than other modalities. When linked with physiologic or pharmacologic stress tests, PET enables evaluation of the myocardium under stress conditions. Studies in patients with more than 50% stenosis on angiography suggest that dipyridamole stress SPECT and [^{13}N]ammonia PET are comparable tests to assess coronary artery perfusion, with respective sensitivities of 98% and 96% and specificities of 88% and 81%. SPECT analysis using FDG compared with PET with FDG shows comparable accuracy for the detection of CAD. Comparative studies with SPECT thallium in conjunction with bicycle ergometer or dipyridamole versus PET perfusion scanning showed comparative sensitivities (76% to 79%) but improved specificity (90% versus 82%, $p < 0.005$).[58]

The future of PET appears promising. Improved tomographic scanners, development of new radiopharmaceuticals, and improved understanding of substrate metabolism and its relationship to myocardial tissue viability will provide new dimensions to assess and evaluate myocardial function. Research enterprises are developing agents to label receptors as a tool to determine cardiovascular physiology and how altered receptor function, biochemical abnormalities, substrate metabolism, or other as yet unrecognized abnormalities impair cardiac function. It continues to be used mostly to answer research questions than in clinical practice settings. A few specialized, large centers do offer PET scanning.

CARDIAC CATHETERIZATION AND ANGIOGRAPHY[59]

❹ Development of the cardiac catheterization technique was a major milestone in the diagnosis and management of CVD because it provided a physiologic and anatomic approach to assess patency of coronary vessels and hemodynamic parameters of cardiac function. Cardiac catheterization is the technique used to gain vascular access to the coronary arteries by intravascular catheters and heart chambers. Once cardiac catheterization is complete, other diagnostic and therapeutic procedures, such as angiography, ventriculography, and PTCA, and drug administration (e.g., thrombolytics) may be undertaken. Following interventional procedures such as PTCA, catheterization with angiography can be used to evaluate efficacy of the intervention. In recurrent clinical syndromes, following a procedure, catheterization is used to help delineate a new management strategy. Catheterization is also now used commonly with PTCA and/or drug therapy in the management of acute coronary syndromes.

Additionally, catheterization allows assessment of valvular function and computation of various cardiac performance parameters such as cardiac output, stroke volume, systemic vascular resistance, cardiac chamber pressures, and blood flow. It also allows for placement of cardiac pacemakers. Drug administration during cardiac catheterization is used primarily for assessment of end points in clinical trials (e.g., thrombolytics to assess coronary artery patency), for management of events (e.g., chest pain) during catheterization, or for diagnostic purposes (e.g., ergonovine to evaluate coronary spasm). Further applications of cardiac catheterization include aortic root angiography, pulmonary angiography, retrieval of foreign bodies, and atherectomy.[60]

More than 1 million cardiac catheterizations are performed in the United States each year, making it the second most frequent in-hospital procedure. Images obtained during catheterization are stored on 35-mm cineradiographic film or are digitized, allowing comparison of studies at a later date. The ACC/AHA guidelines on angiography and PTCA describe the classes I, II, and III indications for each of these procedures; examples are given in Tables 13–18 and 13–19.[63] The guidelines for angiography, PTCA, and catheterization also include recommendations regarding technique, procedures, facilities, personnel, and training.

The cardiac catheterization procedure requires vascular access, usually obtained percutaneously at brachial or femoral arteries or veins. Left-sided catheterization provides access to the aorta, left ventricle, and left atrium. Right-sided catheterization enables the right side of the heart, coronary sinus, pulmonary arteries, and pulmonary wedge position to be reached. Left-sided catheterization is used for coronary angiography and ventriculography, whereas right-sided catheterization is used for determination of cardiac performance parameters.

Prior to an elective procedure, the patient is given nothing by mouth (after midnight) except for oral medications. It is not necessary to stop any medications except warfarin prior to catheterization. Patients receiving warfarin may be transitioned to low-molecular-weight or unfractionated heparin or anticoagulation may be discontinued depending on the clinical scenario about 3 days prior to the procedure. Heparin products are stopped about 6 hours before the procedure to allow normalization of coagulation. There are no data to support low-molecular-weight heparin during catheterization procedures because its longer half-life may increase the risk of intra- and postprocedural bleeding. Patients who require anticoagulation prior to angiography (e.g., those with acute coronary syndromes) usually are treated with unfractionated heparin or low-molecular-weight heparin.

Patients frequently develop chest pain and/or vasospasm during introduction and manipulation of catheters and injection of angiographic dyes. Nitroglycerin/nitroprusside and/or morphine may be given for chest pain. Nitroglycerin also is used to prevent vasospasm and is given sublingually or by intravenous infusion. The use of nitroprusside has increased in recent years because it is a direct smooth muscle vasodilator. Sedatives, such as midazolam and other short-acting benzodiazepines, frequently are given to ensure patient comfort and safety, but the patient is awake and aware of the procedure. Patient cooperation is necessary to obtain the angiographic views and assess symptoms. The patient is required to remain still for about 6 to 8 hours to reduce the risk of bleeding from the catheter entry site(s). Depending on the procedure, patients may be discharged the same day or within 24 hours, if stable.

Heparin products are used during procedures such as angiography, left-sided heart catheterization, and PTCA to prevent thrombotic complications. Depending on the procedure undertaken,

TABLE 13-18 Recommendations for Coronary Angiography in Patients with Known or Suspected Coronary Artery Disease Who Are Currently Asymptomatic or Have Stable Angina

Class I

1. Canadian Cardiovascular Society (CCS) class III and class IV angina on medical treatment. (*Level of Evidence: B*)
2. High-risk criteria on noninvasive testing regardless of anginal severity. (*Level of Evidence: A*)
3. Patients who have been successfully resuscitated from sudden cardiac death or have sustained (>30 seconds) monomorphic ventricular tachycardia or nonsustained (<30 seconds) polymorphic ventricular tachycardia. (*Level of Evidence: B*)

Class IIa

1. CCS class III or IV angina, which improves to class I or II with medical therapy. (*Level of Evidence: C*)
2. Serial noninvasive testing with identical testing protocols, at the same level of medical therapy, showing progressively worsening abnormalities. (*Level of Evidence: C*)
3. Patients with angina and suspected coronary disease who, because of disability, illness, or physical challenge, cannot be adequately risk stratified by other means. (*Level of Evidence: C*)
4. CCS class I or II angina with intolerance to adequate medical therapy or with failure to respond, or patients who have recurrence of symptoms during adequate medical therapy as defined above. (*Level of Evidence: C*)
5. Individuals whose occupation involves the safety of others (e.g., pilots, bus drivers, etc.) who have abnormal but not high-risk stress test results or multiple clinical features that suggest high risk. (*Level of Evidence: C*)

Class III

1. Angina in patients who prefer to avoid revascularization even though it might be appropriate. (*Level of Evidence: C*)
2. Angina in patients who are not candidates for coronary revascularization or in whom revascularization is not likely to improve quality or duration of life. (*Level of Evidence: C*)
3. As a screening test for coronary artery disease in asymptomatic patients. (*Level of Evidence: C*)
4. After coronary artery bypass grafting or angioplasty when there is no evidence of ischemia on noninvasive testing, unless there is informed consent for research purposes. (*Level of Evidence: C*)
5. Coronary calcification on fluoroscopy, electron-beam computed tomography, or other screening tests without criteria listed above. (*Level of Evidence: C*)

Scanlon PJ, Faxon DP, Audet A-M, et al. ACC/AHA Guidelines for Coronary Angiography: Executive Summary and Recommendations. Circulation 1999;99:2345–2357. ©American Heart Association, Inc.

TABLE 13-19 Recommendations for Coronary Angiography in Patients with Nonspecific Chest Pain

Class I

High-risk findings on noninvasive testing. (*Level of Evidence: B*)

Class IIa

None.

Class IIb

Patients with recurrent hospitalizations for chest pain who have abnormal (but not high-risk) or equivocal findings on noninvasive testing. (*Level of Evidence: B*)

Class III

All other patients with nonspecific chest pain. (*Level of Evidence: C*)

Scanlon PJ, Faxon DP, Audet A-M, et al. ACC/AHA Guidelines for Coronary Angiography: Executive Summary and Recommendations. Circulation 1999;99:2345–2357. ©American Heart Association, Inc.

heparin is either discontinued almost immediately following the procedure or continued for 12 to 24 hours. Heparin administration during the procedure is measured with the activated clotting time, not the partial thromboplastin time. For patients undergoing percutaneous coronary intervention, aspirin, and clopidogrel are used prior to and following the procedure. Despite the invasive nature of the procedure, there are no data to support the need for prophylactic antibiotics in patients at risk for bacterial endocarditis because of valvular prostheses or a prior history of rheumatic fever. At present, the infectious risk of this procedure is extremely low. With the advent of classes IIb/IIIa receptor antagonists such as tirofiban, eptifibatide, and abciximab, which improve short- and long-term coronary artery patency rates with high-risk percutaneous coronary intervention, patients who receive a stent also will receive one of these agents prior to, during, and/or after the procedure. Abciximab is usually preferred.

During the procedure, hemodynamic parameters, blood pressure, and heart rate are monitored continuously. ECG monitoring and intermittent 12-lead ECGs are also maintained. Measurements taken during catheterization are obtained only after hemodynamic stabilization: at baseline, following catheter movement, or during pharmacologic intervention. Information obtained during catheterization is in real time and is assumed to reflect the ongoing status of the coronary circulation. Procedurally related vasospasm may be misleading because the catheter itself is a powerful stimulus for spasm.

Complications associated with cardiac catheterization procedures and attending angiographic or interventional activities are related to the expertise and experience of the operator, with case load being a good indicator of the latter. The incidence of significant complications related to catheterization with angiography is reported to be less than 2%, with mortality approximately 0.11%. Patient factors such as hemodynamic stability and renal function increase risk. There are no absolute contraindications to coronary angiography, and the relative contraindications are not well substantiated (Table 13–20). In essence, clinical stability of the patient and potential benefit of the procedure in terms of future patient management predicate the importance of relative contraindications. Complication rates, especially those of a thrombotic nature, increase with the dwell time of the catheters, duration of catheterization, catheter type, and operator technique. Bleeding complications can be reduced by ensuring that patients have normal coagulation studies prior to the procedure and remain at bedrest for several hours after the procedure, and that the nursing staff undertakes good care of the catheter entry and exit sites. In the event of bleeding complications, direct pressure is required with sandbags, followed by emergency surgery if there is no resolution, to prevent further complications. Heart perforation is an uncommon but potentially lethal complication requiring emergency surgical intervention. Other complications, such as a vagal reflex with hypotension, bradycardia, and nausea, can occur. These occur most frequently in conjunction with patient anxiety and can be prevented or treated with atropine. An increased predisposition to myocardial infarction during and after the procedure is seen in patients with unstable angina, recent subendocardial infarction, and type 1 diabetes mellitus. After catheterization, patients may have elevated creatine phosphokinase and troponins as a consequence of tissue damage during the procedure. There is some controversy as to how to interpret these values with respect to what they indicate regarding myocardial damage. Acute closure of a coronary vessel or myocardial ischemia is managed by return to the catheterization laboratory or cardiac surgery. All facilities should be in close liaison with a cardiothoracic surgery unit.

TABLE 13-20 Contraindications of Cardiac Catheterization and Other Procedures[a]

Recent stroke	Patient noncompliance[b]
Advanced physiologic age	Digoxin intoxication
Severe anemia	Anaphylaxis to radiographic dyes
Severe hypertension	Active infection
Active gastrointestinal bleed	Severe electrolyte imbalances
Fever	Unstable condition
Other comorbid illnesses, e.g., COPD[c,d]	

COPD, chronic obstructive pulmonary disease; PTCA, percutaneous transluminal coronary angioplasty.

[a]Primarily contraindications to procedures such as arteriography and PTCA.

[b]Patient not willing to undergo further treatment (e.g., surgery based on results of catheterization).

[c]Disease states that may prohibit or increase risk of other interventions (e.g., surgery).

[d]Patients in whom emergency cardiac surgery would pose a high risk (e.g., during acute asthma or acute exacerbation of COPD).

Angiography, which accompanies most cardiac catheterization procedures, is defined as the "radiographic visualization of coronary vessels after injection of radiopaque contrast medium." Despite the expanding role of cardiac catheterization, angiography is used most frequently to describe the presence and extent of CAD and to allow planning for medical or surgical intervention. Cardiac catheterization with angiography is the "gold standard" in the diagnosis and assessment of CAD, against which all new invasive and noninvasive tests are measured. Unlike most other procedures, angiography determines the morphology of a stenotic lesion and the degree of luminal obstruction. However, this does not relate well to physiologic or functional significance of the lesion.[59] For example, a 50% luminal occlusion not considered significant by radiologic standards may still be the lesion producing symptomatic chest pain, and a diabetic patient with significant microvascular CAD may appear to have unaffected larger arteries at angiography and yet still be at risk of a cardiac event. Angiography also assesses the presence of collateral circulation and dynamic abnormalities such as vasospasm.

The extent of disease by angiography is defined as the number of vessels, and the vessels affected are named. Angiography is able to detect lesions that occlude the vessel by as little as 20%. Occlusions of 75% or more are almost always seen on angiography. Significant narrowing is usually assumed to be 50% or more, although some studies use 70% narrowing as the cutoff point. The lesion can be measured in several ways. Considerable controversy exists as to the best methodology. During angiography, the lesion is compared visually with surrounding vessels. Inherent difficulties include individual evaluator variability and also the assumption that surrounding vessels are normal. Calipers can be used to document physical size, but generally, the degree of stenosis is reported as a percentage of narrowing. Various grading scales, such as the coronary artery score and myocardial jeopardy scores, are used, and these scores predict long-term outcomes. Coronary artery lesions most prone to rupture and thrombosis are those with 40% to 60% narrowing, so lesions with less than 50% narrowing are not benign.

Multiple views are required to obtain a good image of the vessel; the right anterior oblique planes are used most commonly (two views at 90° to each other). Lesions may be described as concentric and smooth (simple lesions) or eccentric and broad with a rough surface (complicated lesions). The number of lesions is also considered of importance to the severity and prognosis of IHD, although there is considerable variation in the accuracy of such predictions because angiographic and pathologic correlation of lesions is imperfect. The occurrence of spasm, variants in anatomy, and collateral filling also complicate interpretation of the angiogram.

Angiographic films are used to plan interventions, in particular coronary artery bypass grafting and percutaneous coronary intervention. They are also used during both surgery and percutaneous coronary intervention to guide the procedure. Ventriculographic studies may be performed during cardiac catheterization to obtain information about the contours of the heart and to assess global and segmental function. Regional wall motion, filling defects, and the

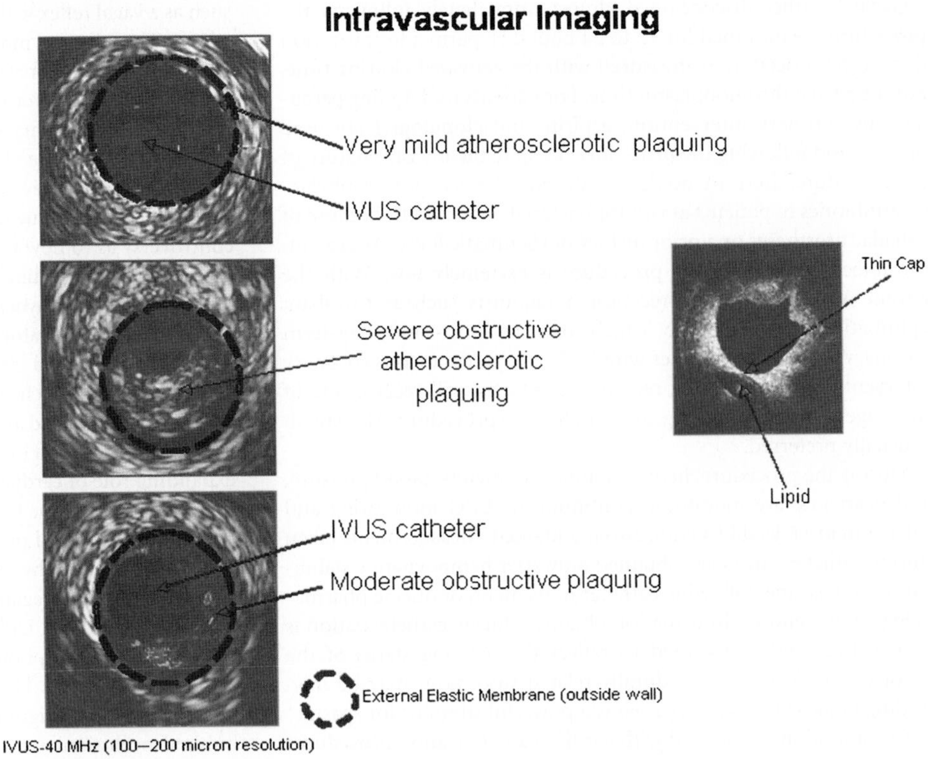

FIGURE 13-9. Intravascular ultrasound (IVUS) imaging demonstrating mild to severe atherosclerosis. Optical coherence tomography demonstrating a lipid pool inside of a plaque.

presence of mural thrombi also may be visualized. During this procedure, radiopaque dye is injected into the heart chambers, and serial films are taken to follow the dye passage. Left ventricular ventriculography is a routine part of left-sided catheterization unless ventricular function information is already available from other noninvasive studies or there are specific contraindications to the procedure.

Cardiac performance is also best assessed during catheterization procedures as direct visualization of performance along with calculated parameters that can be obtained simultaneously and represent real-time values. Measured and observed parameters obtained during catheterization are used to determine cardiac performance. Contractility, as judged by wall motion and ejection fraction, can be used to assess global cardiac performance and to plan and evaluate or assess therapy.

Invasive cardiology is growing rapidly not only in terms of the numbers of patients undergoing such procedures but also in terms of the diversity of procedures. The development of electrophysiologic studies for the assessment and treatment of arrhythmias was made possible because of catheterization. The diversity of techniques is "limited only by the imagination of the physician and inventiveness of the microtechnologist."

INTRAVASCULAR ULTRASOUND

Intravascular ultrasound (IVUS) is a procedure that uses a very small ultrasound transducer on the tip of a coronary catheter to construct detailed images of the inner wall of a coronary artery. It combines braided polyethylene catheter technology with miniaturized ultrasound transducers that can be inserted into a variety of vascular beds within the body, including the coronary artery vasculature.[60–63] Catheter configurations vary and may include over-the-wire, monorail, and fixed-guidewire tip configurations, resulting in different torqueability, steerability, and pushability characteristics for each type of catheter. There are two basic types of transducers: the solid-state phased array and a rotating mechanical transducer. In general, the phased-array transducers are smaller and may be mounted on more flexible catheters so that smaller vessels (such as coronary arteries) can be visualized, but they require a more complex system for image reconstruction and show more artifacts in imaging. Recently, new software packages have allowed detailed images identifying calcium, fibrofatty, and lipid plaques. This could be a major advance in IVUS clinical use (Fig. 13–9).

In contrast to angiography, IVUS provides quantitative information from within the vessel on diameter, circumference, luminal diameter, plaque volume, and percent stenosis. Qualitative information regarding the amount of plaque stenosis, plaque composition (e.g., calcific, fibrous, or fatty plaque), and the presence of plaque versus thrombus, thrombus versus tumor, and aneurysm and hematoma can be provided by IVUS. IVUS is also used as a therapeutic adjunct with PTCA, atherectomy, stent or graft placement, and fibrinolysis, although routine use may not be justified. These combination procedures may be monitored in real time as the procedure (e.g., atherectomy) is being performed. In current trials, IVUS has been very helpful in evaluation of disease progression or regression. Many current trials are underway to test medication for atherosclerosis regression, plaque morphology changes and other.[66]

Another new development in imaging the inner wall of the coronary is the recently developed, intravascular optical coherence tomography providing high-resolution, cross-sectional images of tissue with an axial resolution of 10 microns and a lateral resolution of 20 microns.[63] Optical coherence tomography images of human coronary atherosclerotic plaques are much more structurally detailed than IVUS.[63] Clinically, the detection of thin fibrous caps (vulnerable atheromas) (<65 microns) is below the resolution of the current 40-MHz IVUS (100 to 200 microns).[60] A summary of tests used in cardiovascular medicine is provided in Appendices 13–1 and 13–2.

REFERENCES

1. Myerburg RJ, Kessler KM, Castellanos A. Sudden cardiac death: Epidemiology, transient risk, and intervention assessment. Ann Intern Med 1993;119:1187–1197.
2. Rosamond,W, Flegal, K Friday, G Furie, K, et al. Heart Association Statistics Committee and Stroke Statistics Subcommittee Heart Dis-

ease and Stroke Statistics—2007 update: A report from the American Heart Association. Circulation 2007;115;69-171.

3. Venkat Narayan KM, Boyle JP, Geiss LS, Saaddine JB, Thompson TJ. Impact of recent increase in incidence on future diabetes burden: U.S., 2005–2050. Diabetes Care 2006;29:2114–2116.
4. Hurst W, Alexander RW, Schlant RC, Fuster Valentin. The Heart, Arteries and Veins, 10th ed. New York: McGraw-Hill, 2002.
5. Chiuve SE, McCullough ML, Sacks FM, Rimm EB. Healthy lifestyle factors in the primary prevention of coronary heart disease among men benefits among users and nonusers of lipid-lowering and antihypertensive medications. Circulation 2006;114:160–167.
6. Li J, Hansen D, Mortensen PB, Olsen J. Myocardial infarction in parents who lost a child a nationwide prospective cohort study in Denmark. Circulation 2002;106:1634–1639.
7. Sackett DL, Haynes RB, Guyatt GH, Tugwell P. Clinical Epidemiology, A Basic Science for Clinical Medicine. Boston: Little Brown, 1991:20.
8. Braunwald E. Physical examination. In: Braunwald E, ed. Heart Disease: A Textbook of Cardiovascular Medicine, 4th ed. Philadelphia: WB Saunders, 1992:13–42.
9. Come PC, Lee RT, Braunwald E. Noninvasive methods of cardiac examination. In: Isselbacher KJ, Braunwald E, Wilson JD, et al. eds. Harrison's Principles of Internal Medicine, 13th ed. New York: McGraw-Hill, 1994:966–972.
10. O'Rourke RA, Braunwald E. Physical examination of the cardiovascular system. In: Fauci AS, Braunwald E, Isselbacher KJ, et al. eds. Harrison's Principles of Internal Medicine, 14th ed. New York: McGraw-Hill, 1998:1231–1237.
11. Hirsch T, Haskal ZJ, Hertzer NR. ACC/AHA 2005 guidelines for the management of patients with peripheral arterial. J Am Coll Cardiol 2006;47:1–192.
12. Hirsch AT, Criqui MH, Treat-Jacobson D, et al. Peripheral arterial disease detection, awareness, and treatment in primary care. JAMA. 2001;286:1317-1324.
13. Becker GJ, McClenny TE, Kovacs ME, Raabe RD, Katzen BT. The importance of increasing public and physician awareness of peripheral arterial disease. J Vasc Interv Radiol 2002;13:7–11.
14. Faxon DP, Creager MA. Atherosclerotic Vascular Disease Conference: Executive Summary: Atherosclerotic Vascular Disease Conference Proceeding for Healthcare Professionals From a Special Writing Group of the American Heart Association Circulation 2004;109:2595–2604.
15. Garland JL, Wolfson AB. Routine admission electrocardiography in emergency department patients. Ann Emerg Med 1994;23:275–280.
16. Zimetbaum PJ, Josephson ME. Use of the electrocardiogram in acute myocardial infarction. N Engl J Med 2003;348:933–940.
17. Bernstein SJ, Hilborne LH, Leape LL, et al. The appropriateness of use of cardiovascular procedures in women and men. Arch Intern Med 1994;1554:2759–2765.
18. Zimetbaum PJ, Josephson ME. Use of the electrocardiogram in acute myocardial infarction. N Engl J Med 2003;348:933–940.
19. Fisch C. Evolution of the clinical electrocardiogram. J Am Coll Cardiol 1989;14:1127–1138.
20. Davis D. How to Quickly and Accurately Master ECG Interpretation, 2nd ed. Philadelphia: JB Lippincott, 1992:89–95, 235–273.
21. Garland JL, Wolfson AB. Routine admission electrocardiography in emergency department patients. Ann Emerg Med 1994;23:275–280.
22. Reiter MJ, Karagounis LA, Mann De, et al. Reproducibility of drug efficacy predictions by Holter monitoring in the Electrophysiologic Study Versus Electrocardiographic Monitoring (ESVEM) trial. Am J Cardiol 1997;79:315–322.
23. ACC Expert Consensus Document. Signal-averaged electrocardiography. J Am Coll Cardiol 1996;27:238–249.
24. Kadish AH, Buxton AE, Kennedy HL, et al. ACC/AHA clinical competence statement on electrocardiography and ambulatory electrocardiography: A report of the American College of Cardiology/American Heart Association/American College of Physicians-American Society of Internal Medicine Task Force on Clinical Competence (ACC/AHA Committee to Develop a Clinical Competence Statement on Electrocardiography and Ambulatory Electrocardiography). Circulation 2001;104:3169–3178.
25. Linzer M, Yang EH, Estes M, et al. Diagnosing syncope: 1. Value of history, physical examination and electrocardiography. Ann Intern Med 1997;126:989–996.
26. Fowler-Brown A, Pignone M, Pletcher M, et al. Exercise tolerance testing to screen for coronary heart disease: A systematic review for the technical support for the U.S. Preventive Services Task Force. Ann Intern Med 2004;140:W9–W24.
27. Gibbons RJ, Balady GJ, Bricker JT, Chaitman BR. ACC/AHA 2002 Guideline Update for the Management of Patients With Chronic Stable Angina. 2002, *http://www.americanheart.org/presenter.jhtml?identifier=3006769.*
28. Chaitman B. Exercise stress testing. In: Braunwald E, ed. Heart Disease: A Textbook of Cardiovascular Medicine, 4th ed. Philadelphia: WB Saunders, 1992:161–179.
29. Mark D. Prognostic value of a treadmill exercise score in outpatients with suspected coronary artery disease. N Engl J Med 1991;325:849–853.
30. Snader CE, Marwick TH, Pashkow FJ, Harvey SA, Thomas JD, Lauer MS. Importance of estimated functional capacity as a predictor of all-cause mortality among patients referred for exercise thallium single-photon emission computed tomography: Report of 3,400, patients from a single center. J Am Coll Cardiol 1997;30:641– 648.
31. Cheitlin MD, Armstrong WF, Aurigemma GP, et al. ACC/AHA/ASE 2003, guideline update for the clinical application of echocardiography—Summary article: A report of the American College of Cardiology/American Heart Association Task Force on Practice Guidelines (ACC/AHA/ASE Committee to Update the 1997 Guidelines on the Clinical Application of Echocardiography). Circulation 2003;108:1146–1162.
32. Mark D. Prognostic value of a treadmill exercise score in outpatients with suspected coronary artery disease. N Engl J Med 1991;325:849–853.
33. Gibbons RJ, Balady GJ, Bricker JT, Chaitman BR. ACC/AHA 2002 Guideline Update for Exercise Testing. 2002, *http://www.americanheart.org/presenter.jhtml?identifier=3004540.*
34. Feigenbaum H. Echocardiography. In: Braunwald E, ed. Heart Disease: A Textbook of Cardiovascular Medicine, 4th ed. Philadelphia: WB Saunders, 1992:64–115.
35. Birmingham GD, Rahko PS, Ballantyne F III. Improved detection of infective endocarditis with transesophageal echocardiography. Am Heart J 1992;123:774–781.
36. Shively BK, Gurule FT, Roldan CA, et al. Diagnostic value of transesophageal compared with transthoracic echocardiography in infective endocarditis. J Am Coll Cardiol 1991;18:391–397.
37. Seward JB, Khandheria BK, Oh JK, et al. Critical appraisal of transesophageal echocardiography: Limitations, pitfalls, and complications. J Am Soc Echocardiogr 1992;5:288–305.
38. Shively BK, Gurule FT, Roldan CA, et al. Diagnostic value of transesophageal compared with transthoracic echocardiography in infective endocarditis. J Am Coll Cardiol 1991;18:391–397.
39. Cerqueira MD, Lawrence A. Nuclear cardiology update. Radiol Clin North Am 2001;39:931–946.
40. Sabharwal NK, Lahiri A. Role of myocardial perfusion imaging for risk stratification in suspected or known coronary artery disease. Heart 2003;89:1291–1297.
41. Cheitlin MD, Antman EM, Smith SC, Armstrong WF. ACC/AHA/ASE 2003 Guideline Update for the Clinical Application of Echocardiography. 2003, *http://www.americanheart.org/presenter.jhtml?identifier=3014402.*
42. Gibbons RJ, Eckel RH, Jacobs AK. The utilization of cardiac imaging. Circulation 2006;113:1715.
43. Travain MI, Wexler JP. Pharmacological stress testing. Semin Nucl Med 1999;29:298–318.
44. Beleslin BD, Ostojic M, Stepanovic J, et al. Stress echocardiography in the detection of myocardial ischemia: Head to toe comparison of exercise, dobutamine, and dipyridamole test. Circulation 1994;90:1168–1176.
45. Greco CA, Salustri A, Seccareccia F, et al. Prognostic value of dobutamine echocardiography early after uncomplicated acute myocardial infarction: A comparison with exercise electrocardiography. J Am Coll Cardiol 1997;29:261–267.
46. Sabharwal NK, Lahiri A. Role of myocardial perfusion imaging for risk stratification in suspected or known coronary artery disease. Heart 2003;89:1291–1297.
47. Gibbons RJ, Eckel RH. The Utilization of Cardiac Imaging 2006. 2006, *http://www.americanheart.org/presenter.jhtml?identifier=3004557.*
48. Thompson BH, Stanford W. Evaluation of cardiac function with ultrafast computed tomography. Radiol Clin North Am 1995;32:537–554.

49. Lazem F, Barbir M, Banner N, et al. Coronary calcification detected by ultrafast computed tomography is a predictor of cardiac events in heart transplant recipients. Transplant Proc 1997;29:572–575.
50. Ganz W, Serafini A, Lerner D, et al. Cardiovascular magnetic resonance imaging goes beyond anatomy. Crit Rev Diagn Imaging 1995;36:479–503.
51. Shim SS, Kim Y, Lim SM. Improvement of image quality with betablocker premedication on ECGgated 16-MDCT coronary angiography. AJR Am J Roentgenol 2005;184:649–654.
52. Budoff MJ, Achenbach S, Blumenthal RS, et al. Assessment of coronary artery disease by cardiac computed tomography. Circulation 2006;114:1761–1791.
53. Hendel RC, Douglas PS, Peterson ED, et al. ACCF/ACR/SCCT/SCMR/ASNC/NASCI/SCAI/SIR 2006 appropriateness criteria for cardiac computed tomography and cardiac magnetic resonance imaging: a report of the American College of Cardiology Foundation Quality Strategic Directions Committee Appropriateness Criteria Working Group, American College of Radiology, Society of Cardiovascular Computed Tomography, Society for Cardiovascular Magnetic Resonance, American Society of Nuclear Cardiology, North American Society for Cardiac Imaging, Society for Cardiovascular Angiography and Interventions, and Society of Interventional Radiology. J. Am Coll. Cardiol 2006;48;1475–1497.
54. Udo Hoffmann,, Antonio J. Pena, Ricardo C. Cury. Cardiac CT in emergency department patients with acute chest pain. Radiographics 2006;26:963–979.
55. Globits S, Higgins CB. Assessment of valvular heart disease by magnetic resonance imaging. Am Heart J 1995;129:369–381.
56. Schwaiger M, Muzik O. Assessment of myocardial perfusion by perfusion emission tomography. Am J Cardiol 1991;67:35D–43D.
57. Schelbert HR. Metabolic imaging to assess myocardial viability. J Nucl Med 1994;35(Suppl):8S–14S.
58. Schwaiger M, Hutchins G. Quantification of regional myocardial perfusion by PET. Rationale and first clinical results. Eur Heart J 1995;16(Suppl J):84–91.
59. Smith SC Jr, Feldman TE. ACC/AHA/SCAI 2005 guideline update for percutaneous coronary intervention. Circulation 2006;113:156–175.
60. Gorlin R. Perspectives on invasive cardiology: The 24th Louis F. Bishop lecture. J Am Coll Cardiol 1994;23:525–532.
61. Nair A, Kuban BD, Tuzcu EM. Coronary plaque classification with intravascular ultrasound radiofrequency data analysis. Circulation 2002;106:2200–2206.
62. Nicholls SJ, Tuzcu EM, Sipahi I, Schoenhagen P, Nissen SE. Intravascular ultrasound in cardiovascular medicine. Circulation 2006;114:55–59.
63. Elliott MR, Thrush AJ. Measurement of resolution in intravascular ultrasound images. Physiol. Meas 1996;17, 259–265.
64. Kawasaki M, Bouma BE, Bressner J, et al. Diagnostic accuracy of optical coherence tomography and integrated backscatter intravascular ultrasound images for tissue characterization of human coronary plaques. J Am Coll Cardiol 2006;48:81–88.

Appendix 13-1

Types of Tests Used to Evaluate the Cardiovascular System

	Cardiac Function[a]			
	Myocardial Perfusion	***Pump***	***Electrical Rhythm***	***Anatomy***
Type of test	Stress tests Nuclear imaging Angiography Echocardiography	Angiography MUGA Echocardiography	ECG Electrophysiologic studies Holter monitoring Angioscopy	Echocardiography Angiography Intravascular ultrasound
Parameters evaluated	Coronary anatomy and blood flow Myocardial perfusion	Cardiac output Ejection fraction Valvular function Shunts	Rhythm Rate Conduction pathways	Chamber size Wall motion Valve function Valve structure Pericardium Coronary anatomy

ECG, electrocardiogram; MUGA, multigated acquisition.
[a]Not all tests for any one cardiac function are used to evaluate all parameters listed.

Appendix 13-2

Types of Tests for Various Cardiac Diseases or Features

Feature/Disorder	**CXR**	**Echo**	**Angiography**	**Nuclear Scan**	**CT**	**MRI**	**ET**	**ECG**	**PET**
Ischemic	–	+++	++++	+++	++/++[a]	++	++	++	+++
Valvular	+	++++	+++	+	+++	+++	++	+	+
Congenital	++	++++	+++	+	+++	++++	+	+	+
Anatomy	+	+++	++	+	+++	++++	–	+	+
Cardiomyopathy	+	++++	+++	++	+++	+++	–	–	++
Pericardial	+	++++	++	–	++++	++++	–	±	–
Endocarditis	–	++++[b]	+	–	++	+++	–	±	–
Masses	–	++++	+	–	+++	+++	–	–	+
Metabolism	–	–	–	+	–	–	–	–	++++
Graft patency	–	±	+++	++	+	++	++	+	+++
CA anatomy	–	–	++++	++	+	++	++	+	+
Ventricular function	–	++++	+++	++	+++	+++	+	–	++

CA, coronary artery; CT, computed tomography; CXR, chest radiograph; ECG, electrocardiogram; echo, echocardiography; ET, exercise testing; PET, positron emission tomography.
[a]Ultrafast or cine-CT may be very useful in detecting ischemia based on calcium disposition.
[b]Transesophageal echocardiography is superior to transthoracic echocardiography.

CHAPTER 14 Cardiopulmonary Arrest

JEFFREY F. BARLETTA AND JEFFREY L. WILT

KEY CONCEPTS

1. High-quality cardiopulmonary resuscitation (CPR) with minimal interruptions in chest compressions should be emphasized in all patients following cardiac arrest.
2. Chest compressions before a defibrillation attempt might be warranted especially with cardiac arrests that are not witnessed.
3. The purpose of using vasopressors following cardiac arrest is to increase both coronary and cerebral perfusion pressures.
4. Either epinephrine or vasopressin is an appropriate drug of first choice in patients with ventricular fibrillation (VF)/pulseless ventricular tachycardia (PVT).
5. Amiodarone is preferred over lidocaine as the antiarrhythmic drug of choice in patients with VF/PVT.
6. Therapy for pulseless electrical activity (PEA) or asystole is aimed at identifying the precipitating cause of the arrest.
7. Intraosseous administration is the preferred alternative for drug delivery if intravenous access cannot be obtained.

INTRODUCTION

Cardiopulmonary arrest is the abrupt cessation of spontaneous and effective ventilation and circulation following a cardiac or respiratory event.[1] CPR provides artificial ventilation and circulation until it is possible to provide advanced cardiac life support (ACLS) and reestablish spontaneous circulation. In the United States, there are more than 460,000 victims of sudden cardiac arrest each year with most occurring outside the hospital.[2–4] The annual incidence of sudden cardiac arrest has been estimated to be approximately 0.55 per 1,000 population and in the United States, sudden cardiac death represents up to 15% of total mortality.[5–7]

Early attempts at resuscitation date back to the biblical era.[8] Modern-day resuscitation began in the late 1950s when it was discovered that expired air delivered via a mouth-to-mouth technique can maintain adequate oxygenation of blood.[9] Later, in 1960, Kouwenhoven and colleagues described "closed chest cardiac massage," and together with mouth-to-mouth ventilation, modern-day CPR was born.[10]

Learning objectives, review questions, and other resources can be found at **www.pharmacotherapyonline.com.**

EPIDEMIOLOGY

In an adult patient, cardiopulmonary arrest usually results from the development of an arrhythmia.[11] Most cardiac arrests take place outside the hospital, and most patients have underlying acute or chronic heart disease.[6] In more than two-thirds of patients, cardiac arrest occurs as the first manifested clinical event with no preceding symptoms or warning.[6,12] Although the most common arrhythmia is either VF or PVT, the number of patients with out-of-hospital cardiac arrests presenting with VF as the initial rhythm has changed dramatically.[4,13] In one study, the number of patients with VF was 61% in 1980 compared with only 41% in 2000, a reduction of greater than 30%.[13] A similar trend was noted with in-hospital cardiac arrest as one study reported the number of patients presenting with VF or PVT as the initial rhythm to be only 23%.[14] Hospital survival for in-hospital cardiac arrest related to VF or PVT is approximately 36% with 75% having a good neurologic outcome.[14] Survival for out-of-hospital cardiac arrest caused by VF or PVT is 25% to 40%, with higher survival rates being observed in communities that have a rapid response system.[6,15,16]

In contrast to adult patients, only 15% of pediatric patients present with VF or PVT as the initial rhythm.[2] This is probably because most pediatric arrests are respiratory-related as opposed to the primary cardiac etiology seen in adult patients. Unfortunately, survival following pediatric out-of-hospital cardiopulmonary arrest ranges only from 2% to 10%, with most survivors having a poor neurologic status.[2]

ETIOLOGY

The most common cause of cardiopulmonary arrest in adult patients is an acute myocardial infarction (MI) or pulmonary embolism (PE) representing more than 70% of victims.[17] In pediatric patients, conversely, cardiopulmonary arrest is often the terminal event of progressive shock or respiratory failure.[2] The cause of cardiac arrest varies with age, the underlying health of the child, and the location of the event. Out-of-hospital arrests frequently are associated with events such as trauma, sudden infant death syndrome, drowning, poisoning, choking, severe asthma, and pneumonia.[3] In-hospital pediatric arrests are associated with sepsis, respiratory failure, drug toxicity, metabolic disorders, and arrhythmias. Pediatric out-of-hospital arrest generally presents with hypoxia and hypercarbia progressing to respiratory arrest and bradycardia and finally to asystolic cardiac arrest.

PATHOPHYSIOLOGY OF CPR

There are two proposed theories describing the mechanism of blood flow during CPR.[1,18,19] The first theory, known as the cardiac pump theory, states that the active compression of the heart between the sternum and vertebrae creates an "artificial systole" in which intraventricular pressure increases, the atrioventricular valves close, the aortic valve opens, and blood is forced out of the ventricles. When ventricular compression ends, the decline in intraventricular pressure causes the mitral and tricuspid valves to open, and ventricular filling begins. The second, more recent theory is the thoracic pump theory. The basis for this theory is the belief that blood flow results from intrathoracic pressure alterations induced by chest compressions. During compression or systole, a pressure gradient develops between the intrathoracic arteries and the extrathoracic veins, causing forward blood flow from the lungs into the systemic circulation. The heart merely acts as a passive conduit for flow. After compression ends, or diastole, intrathoracic pressure declines, and blood flow returns to the lungs.

The concept of cough CPR supports the importance of changes in intrathoracic pressure as a means of generating forward blood flow.[18,19] During vigorous coughing, intrathoracic pressures increase secondary to contractions of the diaphragm, abdominal muscles, and intracostal muscles. These pressure changes occur without direct chest compression and are sufficient to maintain consciousness. The observation that cough alone can maintain consciousness led many investigators to question the cardiac pump theory and accept the thoracic pump theory. In reality, it is likely that both models apply to the mechanism of blood flow during CPR.[19]

CLINICAL PRESENTATION

Symptoms

- Anxiety, change in mental status or unconscious
- Cold, clammy extremities
- Dyspnea, shortness of breath or no respiration
- Chest pain
- Diaphoresis
- Nausea and vomiting

Signs

- Hypotension
- Tachycardia, bradycardia, irregular or no pulse
- Cyanosis
- Hypothermia
- Distant or absent heart and lung sounds

TREATMENT

Cardiopulmonary Resuscitation

■ DESIRED OUTCOME

The goal of CPR is the return of spontaneous circulation (ROSC), with effective perfusion (and similarly, ventilation) as quickly as possible to minimize hypoxic damage to vital organs. It is not sufficient to restore spontaneous circulation if the patient is left neurologically devastated or incurs severe morbidity in the process. Factors proven to enhance survival to hospital discharge include the occurrence of a witnessed arrest, rapid implementation of bystander CPR, presence of VF as the initial rhythm, and early defibrillation therapy for VF.[4,20] In one report, the rate of survival to hospital discharge was 74% when defibrillation was performed within 3 minutes of a witnessed cardiac arrest compared with 49% when defibrillation was performed after 3 minutes ($P = 0.02$).[21]

Several patient-specific factors exist that can affect resuscitation survival, but few have been evaluated in clinical trials. In one study, a 3% decrease in survival was noted for each 1-year increment in age.[22] Other proposed risk factors include concomitant diseases, initial pH, duration of resuscitation, and end-tidal carbon dioxide.[11]

■ GENERAL APPROACH TO TREATMENT

National conferences and organized committees have played a major role in encouraging widespread competency in CPR technique. The first national conference took place in 1966 and recommended the training of healthcare professionals in the techniques of CPR.[8] Since then, the American Heart Association (AHA) has organized seven additional national conferences to update philosophies for providing CPR and emergency cardiovascular care (ECC) to the general population. The most recent conference was held in 2005, which provides the latest set of recommendations for CPR and ECC.[2]

The Guidelines 2005 Conference recommendations were built on the same edifice that led to the ECC 2000 guidelines in that they are internationally developed as well as evidence-based. The classification system used was consistent with that used by the AHA/American College of Cardiology for evidence-based guidelines [i.e., class I through class III or indeterminate (Table 14–1)]. These guidelines differ from previous years although, as they have been streamlined to simplify the treatment algorithms, to reduce the amount of information clinicians need to learn, and to clarify the most important issues. Additionally, a new process for disclosure and conflicts of interest was implemented.

The AHA continues to use the "chain of survival" to highlight the treatment approach and illustrate the importance of a timely response.[2] Based on the concept that "a chain is only as strong as its weakest link," each element in the chain is essential for a successful resuscitation outcome. The four links of the chain of survival are as follows:

1. Early recognition of the emergency and activation of emergency medical services (EMS)
2. Early bystander basic life support (BLS) and CPR
3. Early delivery of a shock with a defibrillator
4. Early ACLS followed by postresuscitation care delivered by healthcare professionals

Although all four links of the chain of survival are important, the most crucial may be the first three, particularly early CPR.[2] Cardiopulmonary resuscitation provides critical blood flow to the heart and brain, prolongs the time VF is present (prior to the deterioration to asystole), and increases the likelihood that a shock will terminate VF resulting in a rhythm compatible with life.[2] In one study of out-of-hospital cardiac arrest, early recognition of cardiac arrest (odds ratio [OR] 4.4, 95% confidence interval [CI] 3.1–6.4), early CPR (OR 3.7, 95% CI 2.5–5.4), and defibrillation within 8 minutes (OR 3.4, 95% CI 1.4–8.4) were associated with an increase in survival to hospital discharge.[20] Advanced cardiac life support, conversely, did not improve survival (OR 1.1, 95% CI 0.8–1.5). ❶ Henceforth, the guidelines for CPR and ECC emphasize the provision of high-quality CPR with minimal interruptions in chest compressions.[2] The use of drug therapy as part of ACLS, however, has evolved to a minimal role because survival to hospital discharge does not appear to be impacted.

GENERAL MANAGEMENT OF CARDIAC ARREST

■ BASIC LIFE SUPPORT

The general management of cardiac arrest is based on algorithms developed by the AHA, and are published for widespread dissemi-

TABLE 14-1 Evidence-Based Treatment Recommendations

Recommendations	Recommendation (Grades)
Immediate bystander CPR High-quality CPR should be performed with minimal interruption in chest compressions and defibrillation as soon as it can be accomplished.	Class I
Epinephrine 1 mg IV/IO should be administered every 3 to 5 minutes in patients with VF, PVT, PEA, or asystole	Class IIb
Vasopressin 40 units IV/IO can replace either the first or second dose of epinephrine in patients with VF, PVT, or asystole. There is insufficient evidence to recommend either for or against its use in PEA.	Class indeterminate
Amiodarone 300 mg IV/IO can be followed by 150 mg IV/IO in patients with VF/PVT unresponsive to CPR, shock, and a vasopressor.	Class IIb
Lidocaine Lidocaine can be considered an alternative to amiodarone in patients with VF/PVT. The initial dose is 1 to 1.5 mg/kg IV. Additional doses of 0.5 to 0.75 mg/kg can be administered at 5 to 10 minute intervals to a maximum dose of 3 mg/kg if VF/PVT persists.	Class indeterminate
Magnesium Magnesium is recommended for VF/PVT that is caused by torsade de pointes. 1 to 2 g diluted in 10 mL D5W should be administered IV/IO push over 5 to 20 minutes. Clinical studies have not demonstrated a benefit when magnesium was routinely administered during CPR when torsade de pointes was not present.	Class IIa
Fibrinolysis Thrombolytics should be considered on a case-by-case basis when pulmonary embolism is suspected.	Class IIa
Hypothermia Hypothermia should be implemented in unconscious adult patients with ROSC after out-of-hospital cardiac arrest when the initial rhythm was VF. These patients should be cooled to 32°C (89.6°F) to 34°C (93.2°F) for 12 to 24 hours.	Class IIa
Hypothermia may be beneficial for patients with non-VF arrest out-of-hospital or for in-hospital cardiac arrest.	Class IIb
Atropine Atropine 1 mg IV/IO every 3 to 5 minutes (maximum total of 3 doses or 3 mg) can be considered for patients with asystole or PEA.	Class indeterminate

CPR, cardiopulmonary resuscitation; D5W, 5% dextrose in water; IO, intraosseous; IV, intravenous; PEA, pulseless electrical activity; PVT, pulseless ventricular tachycardia; ROSC, return of spontaneous circulation; VF, ventricular fibrillation.

Key for evidence-based classifications[2]:

Class I: High-level prospective studies support the action or therapy and the benefit substantially outweighs the potential for harm. The treatment should be administered.

Class IIa: The weight of evidence supports the action or therapy, and the therapy is considered acceptable and useful. It is reasonable to administer the treatment.

Class IIb: The evidence documented only short-term benefits, or positive results were documented with lower levels of evidence. Class IIb recommendations can be considered either optional or recommended by experts despite the absence of high-level supporting evidence.

Class III: The risk outweighs the benefit for a particular treatment. The treatment should not be administered and can be harmful.

Class indeterminate: This is either a continuing area of research or an area where research is just beginning. No recommendation (either for or against) can be made.

nation.[2] The initial algorithm is BLS, and the first action is to determine responsiveness of the patient. If there is no response, the rescuer should immediately activate the emergency medical response team, and obtain an automated external defibrillator (AED) if one is available. Next, the victim's airway should be opened, with an assessment of effective breathing. If the victim is not breathing, then two rescue breaths should be administered. Subsequent to this, the rescuer should determine if there is an effective pulse. If there is an effective pulse, then rescue breathing with frequent assessments of effective circulation should be continued until help arrives. If there is no pulse, then chest compressions need to be immediately instituted. The recommended rate is 100 beats/min, with cycles of 30 compressions followed by 2 rescue breaths. The 2005 guidelines for CPR and ECC stress that there should be minimal interruptions in chest compressions. If there is no AED available, then cycles of compressions/breaths should continue, with pulse checks every 2 minutes (5 cycles) until help arrives or the patient regains spontaneous circulation. If there is an AED available, then the rhythm should be checked to determine if defibrillation is advised. If so, then one shock should be delivered with the immediate resumption of chest compressions/rescue breaths. After five cycles, the rhythm should be reevaluated to determine the need for defibrillation. This algorithm should be repeated until help arrives, or the rhythm is no longer "shockable." If the rhythm is not shockable, then chest compressions/rescue breath cycles should be continued until help arrives, or the victim recovers spontaneous circulation (Fig. 14–1).

■ ADVANCED CARDIAC LIFE SUPPORT

Once ACLS providers arrive, then further definitive therapy is given. If the rhythm is not shockable, then it is likely to be either asystole or pulseless electrical activity (PEA) (Fig. 14–2). The general management of these rhythms is CPR and pharmacologic therapy as listed below. For PEA, the rescuer must consider reversible causes (Table 14–2). If the person is in VF or PVT, then one shock should be delivered (appropriate to the available electrical device), with the immediate resumption of 30 compressions and 2 breaths for 5 cycles prior to rechecking the rhythm or pulse. If there is still a shockable rhythm, then one shock should be delivered and at this time pharmacologic intervention can be considered. After the first unsuccessful shock, vasopressors are the initially recommended pharmacologic intervention (before or after the second shock), and after the second unsuccessful shock, antiarrhythmics can be considered (before or after the third shock). Five cycles of chest compressions/breaths should be performed in between attempts at defibrillation. This algorithm will repeat until either a pulse is obtained with effective circulation, the rhythm changes, or the patient expires. For completeness, please refer to the guidelines published by the AHA.[2]

VENTRICULAR FIBRILLATION/ VENTRICULAR TACHYCARDIA

■ NONPHARMACOLOGIC THERAPY

Electrical defibrillation is the only effective method of restoring a perfusing cardiac rhythm, therefore it is a crucial link in the "chain of survival" especially for a witnessed arrest.[2] The probability of successful defibrillation is directly related to the time interval between the onset of VF and the delivery of the first shock.[2] Generally, with each passing minute, the rate of survival decreases by 8% to 10% when CPR is not provided.[23] In one study, a 23% relative improvement in survival was observed with each 1-minute reduction in the time to defibrillation (OR 0.77, 95% CI 0.73–0.81).[24]

❷ Although early defibrillation is crucial for survival following cardiac arrest, several studies have suggested that CPR prior to defibrillation can lead to more successful outcomes.[23] One study (published after the 2005 guidelines) cites the concept of "cardiocerebral" resuscitation, based on applying appropriate cardiac resuscitation principles to the three phases of cardiac arrest: First, the "electrical" phase (0–4 minutes) when defibrillation is most likely to

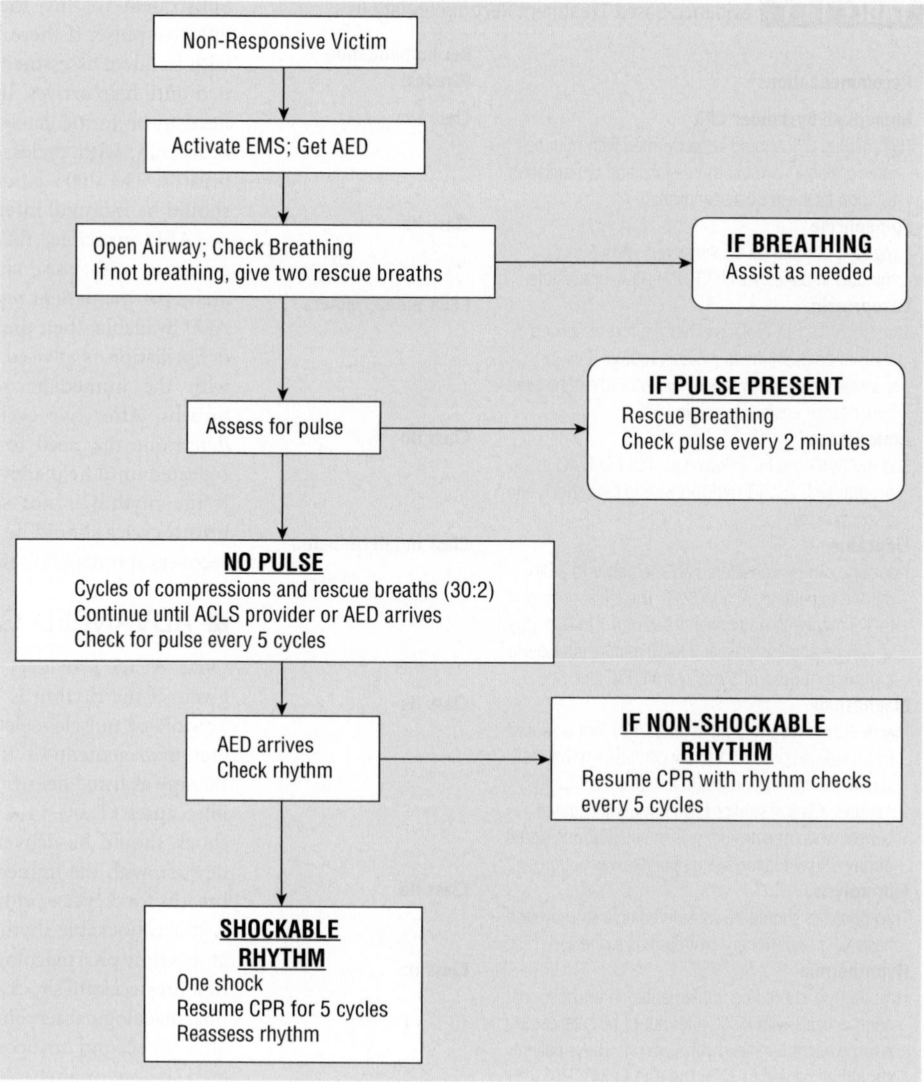

FIGURE 14-1. Treatment algorithm for adult cardiopulmonary arrest. (BLS, basic life support.)

be effective; second, the "circulatory" phase (4–10 minutes or longer) where adequate coronary or cerebral perfusion prior to defibrillation is likely to be helpful; and, third, the "metabolic" phase (greater than 10 minutes) in which survival is very low, and hypothermia is likely to be the most beneficial approach.[23,25] Using a protocol where each defibrillation, including the first, was preceded by 200 uninterrupted chest compressions, an increase in total survival (57% [19/33] vs. 20% [18/92], $P = 0.001$) and neurologically normal survival (48% [16/33] vs. 15% [14/92], $P = 0.001$) was noted compared to standard CPR practices.[25]

Other clinical trials have evaluated the impact of delaying defibrillation to allow for CPR in patients with out-of-hospital VF.[26,27] In one trial, the provision of roughly 90 seconds of CPR prior to defibrillation was associated with an increased rate of hospital survival (compared with a historical control group) when response intervals were 4 minutes or longer (27% vs. 17%; $P < 0.007$).[26] In a second trial, hospital survival rates were higher in patients with response intervals greater than 5 minutes when 3 minutes of CPR was administered prior to defibrillation (22% vs. 4%; $P = 0.006$).[27]

Collectively, these trials support the theory of a three-phase time-sensitive model for resuscitation after cardiac arrest mentioned above. Successful defibrillation most likely will occur when cardiac arrest victims are in the electrical phase because there is enough tissue oxygenation still present to support metabolic demands. Conversely, when cardiac arrest victims are in the circulatory phase, global ischemia has already occurred, and immediate defibrillation could lead to asystole. It can be more important to first provide some blood flow and cardiac perfusion via CPR to "flush out" the deleterious metabolic factors that have accumulated during ischemia.[23] Because of this, the recent guidelines offer that EMS personnel can give 2 minutes of chest compressions prior to attempting defibrillation. Recommendations are similar for victims in the metabolic phase recognizing the likelihood of achieving ROSC, however, is drastically lower. Further trials are needed to evaluate this resuscitation technique.[25]

As opposed to the previous guidelines, where "stacked," multiple shocks were initially given, persons in VF or PVT should receive electrical defibrillation with one shock.[2] The defibrillation attempt should be with 360 joules (monophasic defibrillator) or 150 to 200 joules (biphasic defibrillator). Automatic external defibrillators are reliable, computerized defibrillators that can be useful for both healthcare providers and lay personnel. These devices are effective, easy to use, and have led to the development of public access defibrillation programs in many communities.[15,28] When an arrest is witnessed, and AED is immediately available, it should be used as soon as possible. However, CPR should be started immediately (after EMS activation), as the AED is being prepared. If early CPR is provided to a witnessed VF arrest, and defibrillation is able to be provided within 3 to 5 minutes, survival rates have been reported to be has high as 41% to 74%.[2,15,21,29–31]

After defibrillation is attempted, CPR should be immediately restarted and continued for 2 minutes without checking a pulse.

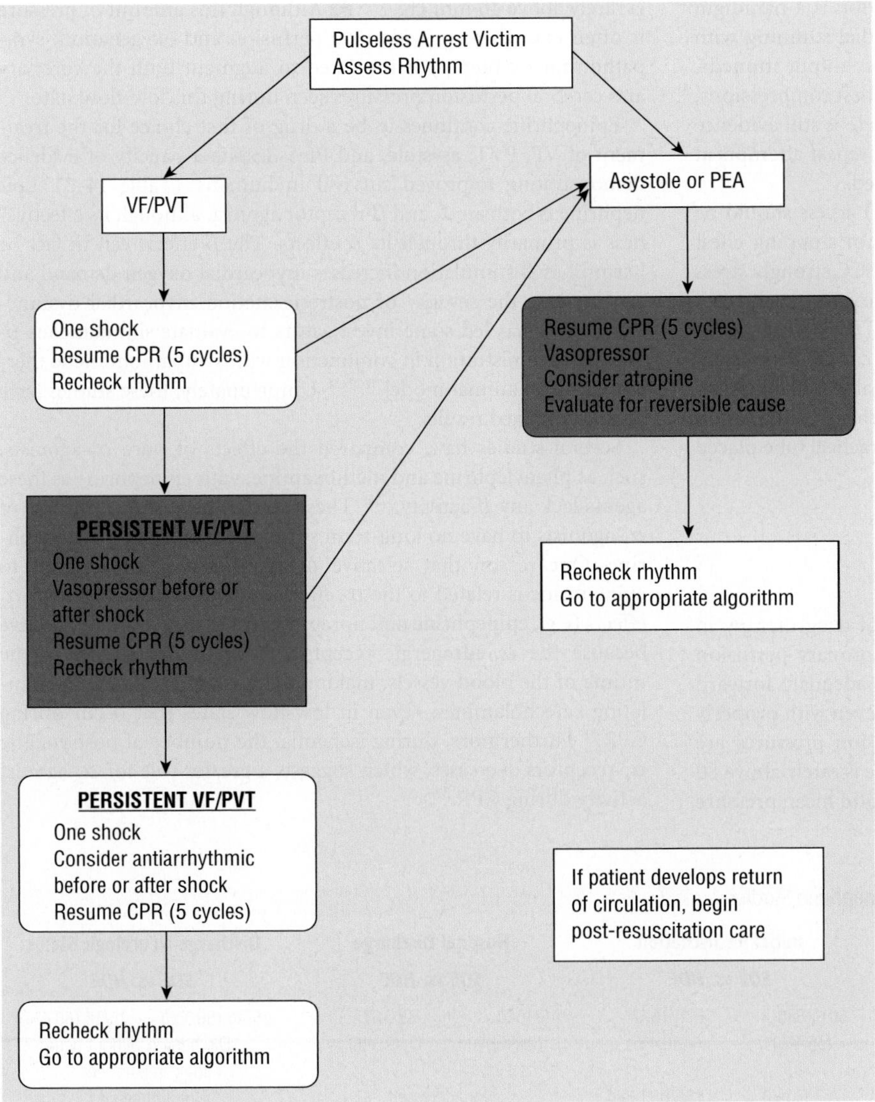

FIGURE 14-2. Treatment algorithm for adult cardiopulmonary arrest. (ACLS, advanced cardiac life support.)

TABLE 14-2 Potentially Reversible Causes of PEA and Asystole (Think: 6 H's; 6 T's)

Condition	Clues	Treatment
Hypovolemia	History, flat neck veins	Intravenous fluids
Hypoxia	Cyanosis, blood gases, airway problems	Ventilation, oxygen
Hydrogen ion (acidosis)	History of bicarbonate-responsive preexisting acidosis	Sodium bicarbonate, hyperventilation
Hyper (Hypo) kalemia	History of renal failure, diabetes, recent dialysis, dialysis fistulas, medications	Calcium chloride, insulin, glucose, sodium bicarbonate, sodium polystyrene sulfonate, dialysis
Hypothermia	History of exposure to cold, central body temperature	Rewarming, oxygen, intravenous fluids
Hypoglycemia	History of diabetes	Glucose infusion
Toxin (Drug overdose)	Bradycardia, history of ingestion, empty bottles at the scene, pupils, neurologic exam	Drug screens, intubation, lavage, activated charcoal
Tamponade (Cardiac)	History (trauma, renal failure, thoracic malignancy), no pulse with CPR, vein distension, impending tamponade-tachycardia, hypotension, low pulse pressure changing to sudden bradycardia as terminal event	Pericardiocentesis
Tension pneumothorax	History (asthma, ventilator, chronic obstructive pulmonary disease, trauma), no pulse with CPR, neck vein distension, tracheal deviation	Needle decompression
Thrombosis, coronary	History, ECG, enzymes	Thrombolytics, oxygen, nitroglycerin, heparin, aspirin, morphine
Thrombosis, pulmonary	History, no pulse with CPR, distended neck veins	Pulmonary arteriogram, surgical embolectomy, thrombolytics
Trauma	History, examination	Volume infusion, intracranial pressure monitoring, bleeding control, surgical intervention

CPR, cardiopulmonary resuscitation; ECG, electrocardiogram; PEA, pulseless electrical activity.
Data from American Heart Association[2] and Ornato and Peberdy.[4]

The omission of the pulse check after defibrillation is a paradigm shift in the algorithm, and is related to myocardial stunning with resultant poor perfusion and diminished cardiac output immediately after electrical therapy.[2] After 2 minutes of chest compressions, the rhythm and pulse should be rechecked. If there is still evidence of VF or PVT, then pharmacologic therapy with repeat attempts at single-discharge defibrillation should be attempted.

Endotracheal intubation and intravenous (IV) access should be obtained when feasible, but not at the expense of stopping chest compressions. The 2005 guidelines for CPR and ECC strongly stress the need for uninterrupted CPR.[2] Once an airway is achieved, patients should be ventilated with 100% oxygen. The recent guidelines suggest that lower tidal volumes and rates can be beneficial.[2] There are several airway adjuncts that are potentially available, such as laryngeal mask airways and esophageal-tracheal combination tubes. However, the definitive airway is an endotracheal tube placed with direct laryngoscopy.

■ PHARMACOLOGIC THERAPY

Sympathomimetics

The use of sympathomimetics is a major part of drug therapy in CPR. Animal studies have demonstrated that coronary perfusion pressures above 30 mm Hg are associated with adequate forward blood flow and improved survival.[32] In humans, even with properly performed chest compressions, coronary perfusion pressures are only 10 to 15 mm Hg, the systolic arterial pressure is rarely above 80 mm Hg, the diastolic pressure is low, and the carotid mean pressure is rarely above 40 mm Hg.[2,33] ❸ Although this amount of pressure is often enough to provide vital perfusion and oxygenation, sympathomimetic therapy is indicated to augment both the coronary and cerebral perfusion pressures seen during this low-flow state.

Epinephrine continues to be a drug of first choice for the treatment of VF, PVT, asystole, and PEA despite a paucity of evidence demonstrating improved survival in humans[2] (Table 14–3). Epinephrine is both an α- and β-receptor agonist, although its effectiveness is primarily through its α effects. The β effects can in fact be harmful as β-stimulation increases myocardial oxygen demand and can increase the severity of postresuscitation myocardial dysfunction.[34] This has led some investigators to evaluate simultaneous β-blocker administration in conjunction with sympathomimetic therapy using an animal model.[32,35,36] Unfortunately, these studies have produced mixed results.

Several studies have compared the effects of pure α_1-agonists, such as phenylephrine and methoxamine, with epinephrine as these agents lack any β-activity.[37,38] These studies have shown the use of α_1-agonists to have no long-term survival advantage over epinephrine. One reason that selective α_1-agonists are not superior to epinephrine is related to the α_2 effects. Agents that have potent α_2 effects (e.g., epinephrine and norepinephrine) can be more effective because the α_2-adrenergic receptors lie extrajunctionally in the intima of the blood vessels, making them more accessible to circulating catecholamines—even in low-flow states that occur during CPR.[38] Furthermore, during ischemia, the number of postsynaptic α_1-receptors decreases, which suggests a greater role for α_2-agonist activity during CPR.[39]

TABLE 14-3 Summary of Adult High-Dose Epinephrine Studies

	Epinephrine Dosing			Initial Resuscitation		Hospital Discharge		Discharge Neurologic Status	
Author	***Design***	***SDE vs. HDE***	***N***	***SDE vs. HDE***		***SDE vs. HDE***		***SDE vs. HDE***	
Gueugniaud et al., 1998	P, MC, R, DB	1 mg vs. 5 mg, up to 15 doses	3327	601/1650 (36.4%)	678/1677[a] (40.4%)	46/1650 (2.8%)	38/1677 (2.3%)	26/46 (56.5%)	26/38 (68.4%) Discharged without neurologic impairment
Sherman et al., 1997	P, MC, R, DB	0.01 mg/kg vs. 0.1 mg/kg, up to 4 doses	140	7/62 (11%)	15/78 (19%)	Not addressed		Not addressed	
Choux et al., 1995	P, R, DB	1 mg vs. 5 mg, up to 15 doses	536	85/265 (32%)	96/271 (35.5%)	20/54 (37%)	23/63[b] (35.4%)	GCS ≥9 (at day 3): 4/20 EEG normal (at day 3): 1/20	3/23 3/23
Lipman et al., 1993	P, R, DB	1 mg vs. 10 mg, up to 3 doses	35	11/16 (69%)	15/19 (79%)	1/16 (6.3%)	0/19 (0%)	Not addressed	
Stiell et al.,1992	P, R, DB	1 mg vs. 7 mg, up to 5 doses	650	76/333 (23%)	56/317 (18%)	16/333 (5%)	10/317 (3%)	94%	90% Remained in their best CPC on discharge
Brown et al., 1992	P, MC, R, DB	0.02 mg/kg vs. 0.2 mg/kg for the first dose	1280	190/632 (30%)	217/648 (33%)	26/632 (4%)	31/648 (5%)	92%	94% Conscious at discharge (CPC = 1–3)
Callaham et al., 1992	P, R, DB	1 mg vs. 15 mg, up to 3 doses	556	22/270 (8%)	37/286[a] (13%)	3/270 (1.2%)	5/286 (1.7%)	2.3%	3.2 Mean CPC score
Lindner et al., 1991	P, R, DB	1 mg vs. 5 mg for the first dose	68	6/40 (15%)	16/28[a] (57%)	2/40 (5%)	4/28 (14%)	Not addressed	
Callaham et al., 1991	Ret	HDE: ≥50 mcg/kg or total dose >2.8 mcg/kg/min	68	Not addressed		11/35 (31%)	6/33 (18.2%)	Intact: 8/11 vs. 4/6 Impaired: 2/11 vs. 2/6 Vegetative: 1/11 vs. 0/6	

CPC, cerebral performance category; DB, double-blind; EEG, electroencephalogram; GCS, Glasgow Coma Scale; HDE, high-dose epinephrine; MC, multicenter; P, prospective; R, randomized; Ret, retrospective; SDE, standard dose epinephrine.

[a] $P < 0.05$.

[b] Number of patients admitted to the hospital alive on day 3.

Data from Brown et al.,[49] Calaham et al.,[50] Choux et al.,[51] Gueugniaud et al.,[52] Lipman et al.,[53] Sherman et al.,[54] and Stiell et al.[55]

Several investigators have compared norepinephrine with epinephrine in both human and animal models.[33,40–43] Norepinephrine is a potent α-agonist (both α_1 and α_2) but also has β_1-agonist effects. In the only large-scale randomized, double-blind, prospective trial that compared norepinephrine with epinephrine in the prehospital cardiac arrest setting, there were no significant differences in ROSC (norepinephrine, 13% [35:260] vs. epinephrine, 8% [22:270]; P = 0.19), hospital admission (norepinephrine, 13% [36:260] vs. epinephrine, 10% [27:270]; P = 0.37), or discharge (norepinephrine, 2.6% [7:260] vs. epinephrine, 1.2% [3:270]; P = 0.37).[41] A second, smaller study demonstrated higher resuscitation rates with norepinephrine compared to epinephrine (64% [16:25] vs. 32% [8:25]) but no significant difference in hospital discharge.[42] Consequently, epinephrine remains the first-line sympathomimetic for CPR.

The recommended dose for epinephrine is 1 mg administered by intravenous (IV) or by intraosseous (IO) injection every 3 to 5 minutes.[2] This epinephrine dose was derived from animal studies (0.1 mg/kg in a 10-kg dog) and equates to approximately 0.015 mg/kg for a 70-kg human.[44] Both animal and human studies have demonstrated a positive dose-response relationship with epinephrine suggesting that higher doses might be necessary to improve hemodynamics and achieve successful resuscitation.[45–48] These results, however, have not been replicated in human studies[41,49–56] (see Table 14–3). Collectively, these studies have shown that high-dose epinephrine can increase the initial resuscitation success rate, but that overall survival is not significantly different. The discrepancy between animal and human studies can be caused by the fact that most victims of cardiac arrest have coronary artery disease, a condition not present in an animal model. In a human model, however, atherosclerotic plaques can aggravate the balance between myocardial oxygen supply and demand. Moreover, the interval from arrest to treatment in animal studies is shorter than the interval frequently reported in human studies. Because time to CPR and defibrillation are crucial variables for success, prolonging this time period can lower resuscitation rates.

Vasopressin

Vasopressin, also known as *antidiuretic hormone*, is a potent, nonadrenergic vasoconstrictor that increases blood pressure and systemic vascular resistance. Although it acts on various receptors throughout the body, its vasoconstrictive properties are caused primarily by its effects on the V_1 receptor.[57] Measurement of vasopressin levels in patients undergoing CPR has shown a high correlation between the levels of endogenous vasopressin released and the potential for ROSC.[58] In fact, in one study, plasma vasopressin concentrations were approximately three times as high in survivors compared with nonsurvivors, suggesting that vasopressin is released as an adjunct vasopressor to epinephrine in life-threatening events such as cardiac arrest.[59]

Vasopressin may have several advantages over epinephrine. First, the metabolic acidosis that frequently accompanies cardiopulmonary arrest can blunt the vasoconstrictive effect of adrenergic agents such as epinephrine. This effect does not occur with vasopressin. Second, the stimulation of β-receptors caused by epinephrine can increase myocardial oxygen demand and complicate the postresuscitative phase of CPR. Because vasopressin does not act on β-receptors, this effect does not occur with its use. Vasopressin also can have a beneficial effect on renal blood flow by stimulating V_2 receptors in the kidney, causing vasodilation and increased water reabsorption. With regard to splanchnic blood flow, however, vasopressin has a detrimental effect when compared to epinephrine.[60]

Clinical experience with vasopressin in humans is limited, and comparative trials evaluating vasopressin and epinephrine have produced mixed results[57] (Table 14–4). Potential reasons include the setting in which cardiac arrest was evaluated (in-hospital versus out-of-hospital), variability in the quality of CPR performed, the average time from collapse to study drug administration, and the number of patients presenting with VF as the initial rhythm.

In the largest comparative trial with vasopressin and epinephrine for out-of-hospital cardiac arrest conducted to date, no significant differences were noted in ROSC, hospital admission rate, or discharge rate.[61] Furthermore, when patients were stratified according to their initial presenting rhythm, no significant differences were noted for patients with VF or PEA. Interestingly, patients with asystole had a significantly higher rate of hospital admission (29% vs. 20%; P = 0.02) and discharge (4.7% vs. 1.5%; P = 0.04) when vasopressin was administered compared with epinephrine. In addition, a subgroup analysis of 732 patients who required additional

TABLE 14-4 Summary of Adult Vasopressin Comparative Trials

						Initial Resuscitation		Hospital Discharge	
Author	**Design**	**Setting**	**Initial Rhythm**	**Intervention[a]**	***N***	***Vasopressin***	***Epinephrine***	***Vasopressin***	***Epinephrine***
Lindner, et al., 1997	P, R, DB	Out-of-hospital	VF: 100%	Vasopressin 40 units vs. Epinephrine 1 mg for initial drug treatment	40	16/20 (80%)	11/20 (55%)	8/20 (40%)	3/20 (15%)
Stiell, et al., 2001	P, R, TB, MC	In-hospital	VF/PVT: 21% PEA: 48% Asystole: 31%	Vasopressin 40 units vs. Epinephrine 1 mg for initial drug treatment	200	62/104 (60%)	57/96 (59%)	12/104 (12%)	13/96 (14%)
Wenzel, et al., 2004	P, R, DB, MC	Out-of-hospital	VF/PVT: 40% PEA: 16% Asystole: 45%	Vasopressin 40 units vs. Epinephrine 1 mg for 2 doses as initial drug treatment	1186	145/589 (25%)	167/597 (28%)	57/578 (10%)	58/588 (10%)
Guyette, et al., 2004	Ret	Out-of-hospital	VF/PVT: 27% PEA: 17% Asystole: 51%	Epinephrine vs. Epinephrine + vasopressin	298	16/37[b] (43%)	58/231[b] (25%)	NR	NR
Grmec, et al., 2006	P, O with Ret control	Out-of-hospital	VF/PVT: 100%	Epinephrine 1 mg vs. Vasopressin 40 units initially vs. Vasopressin 40 units after 3 doses of epinephrine 1 mg	109	Initial therapy: 17/27 (63%)[b] Delayed therapy: 19/31 (61%)[b]	23/51 (45%)[b]	Initial therapy: 7/27 (26%) Delayed therapy: 8/31 (26%)	10/51 (20%)

DB, double-blind; MC, multicenter; O, observational; P, prospective; PEA, pulseless electrical activity; PVT, pulseless ventricular tachycardia; R, randomized; Ret, retrospective; TB, triple-blind; VF, ventricular fibrillation.
[a]All study groups received epinephrine following the initial study drug.
[b]P < 0.05.
Data from Wenzel et al.,[61] Guyette, et al.,[109] Lindner et al.,[110] Stiell et al.,[111] and Grmec, et al.[112]

epinephrine therapy despite the two doses of study drug revealed significant benefits in ROSC (37% vs. 26%; $P = 0.002$), hospital admission rate (26% vs. 16%; $P = 0.002$), and discharge rate (6.2% vs. 1.7%; $P = 0.002$) with vasopressin. There was a trend, however, toward a poorer neurologic state or coma among the patients who survived to discharge and received vasopressin.

The effectiveness of vasopressin for cardiac arrest has also been evaluated in a systematic review/meta-analysis.[62] No significant differences were noted between vasopressin and epinephrine in failure of ROSC (relative risk [RR] 0.81, 95% CI 0.58–1.12), death before hospital admission (RR 0.72, 95% CI 0.38–1.39), death within 24 hours (RR 0.74, 95% CI 0.38–1.43) or death before hospital discharge (RR 0.96, 95% CI 0.87–1.05). Similarly, no differences were noted in death before hospital discharge when patients were stratified according to their initial rhythm (VF/PVT, RR 0.97, 95% CI 0.79–1.19; PEA, RR 1.02, 95% CI 0.95–1.10; asystole, RR 0.97, 95% CI 0.94–1.00).

❹ Overall, these studies suggest that vasopressin is effective as part of ACLS following cardiac arrest, but its superiority to epinephrine remains questionable. Vasopressin can be more beneficial when used for out-of-hospital cardiac arrests, arrests secondary to asystole, or situations when the effect of catecholamines may be diminished because of profound acidosis than when it is used for in-hospital cardiac arrest secondary to VF or PVT. Further research is needed to define the role of vasopressin in cardiac arrest.

Antiarrhythmics

The purpose of antiarrhythmic drug therapy following unsuccessful defibrillation and vasopressor administration is to prevent the development or recurrence of VF and PVT by raising the fibrillation threshold. Clinical evidence demonstrating improved survival to hospital discharge, however, is lacking. As the role of antiarrhythmics during CPR remains limited, only two individual agents are currently recommended in the 2005 guidelines for CPR and ECC: amiodarone and lidocaine.

The use of lidocaine has been beneficial in animal studies and in patients with arrhythmias following an acute myocardial infarction, but its benefit in cardiac arrest remains questionable. In the only published case-control trial where patients were classified according to whether they received lidocaine, no significant difference was noted in ROSC, admission to the hospital, or survival to hospital discharge between groups.[63] Similarly, a prospective study comparing the effectiveness of lidocaine with that of standard-dose epinephrine showed not only a lack of benefit with lidocaine but also a higher tendency to promote asystole.[64] In contrast, a retrospective analysis in patients with VF indicated that lidocaine was associated with a higher rate of ROSC and hospitalization ($P < 0.01$) but not an increase in the hospital discharge rate.[65]

Amiodarone is classified as a class III antiarrhythmic but possesses electrophysiologic characteristics of all four Vaughan Williams classifications. The most frequent adverse effect is hypotension, which has occurred in approximately 20% of clinical trials. This hypotension appears to be related to the diluent used for the amiodarone solution (i.e., polysorbate 80) and the rate of IV administration. An aqueous formulation is available, which has not been associated with these deleterious effects.[66]

In a large, randomized, double-blind trial in out-of-hospital cardiac arrest secondary to VF or PVT, patients were randomized to receive either amiodarone 300 mg or placebo.[67] Recipients of amiodarone were more likely to be resuscitated and survive to hospital admission than were recipients of placebo (44% and 34%, respectively; $P = 0.03$) for a relative improvement of 29%. There was no difference in survival to hospital discharge for those patients who received amiodarone compared to placebo (13.4% vs. 13.2%, respectively; P = not significant). This was the first trial to demonstrate the benefit of an antiarrhythmic agent over placebo in patients with out-of-hospital cardiac arrest.

A subsequent trial compared amiodarone 5 mg/kg with lidocaine 1.5 mg/kg in patients with out-of-hospital cardiac arrest caused by VF.[68] In this trial, amiodarone was associated with a relative improvement of 90% in survival to hospital admission compared with lidocaine (22.8% vs. 12%; OR 2.17, 95% CI 1.21–3.83; $P = 0.009$). Similar to the previous trial, there was no difference in survival to hospital discharge (amiodarone, 5% vs. lidocaine, 3%; $P = 0.34$).

Amiodarone and lidocaine have also been compared following in-hospital cardiac arrest secondary to VF or PVT. In a multicentered, retrospective review, 194 patients who received amiodarone ($n = 74$), lidocaine ($n = 79$), or both ($n = 41$) were evaluated.[69] The rate of survival at 24 hours was 55%, 63%, and 50% for patients receiving amiodarone, lidocaine, or both, respectively ($P = 0.39$). There was no difference in survival to hospital discharge (39% for amiodarone, 45% for lidocaine, and 42% for patients receiving both agents; $P = 0.72$). After adjusting for multiple covariates, Cox regression analysis revealed higher mortality for those patients who received amiodarone (as opposed to lidocaine) (survival to 24 hours: hazard ratio 3.15, 95% CI 1.68–5.92, $P < 0.001$; survival to hospital discharge: hazard ratio 3.25, 95% CI 1.22–8.65, $P = 0.02$) and in those patients with VF/PVT as the initial rhythm (as opposed to bradycardia followed by VF/PVT) (survival to 24 hours: hazard ratio 3.36, 95% CI 1.98–5.71, $P < 0.001$; survival to hospital discharge: hazard ratio 3.6, 95% CI 1.2–10.6, $P = 0.021$). The mean initial dose of amiodarone, however, was 190 mg, and only 25% of patients received the recommended dose of 300 mg. Additionally, the time to first dose of antiarrhythmic was significantly longer in the amiodarone group than in the lidocaine group (14 minutes vs. 6 minutes, $P < 0.001$) Although these differences could have biased the results in favor of lidocaine, they provide a "real-world" experience with the use of amiodarone. Further large-scale trials are needed to determine the preferred antiarrhythmic for both in-hospital and out-of-hospital cardiac arrest. ❺ In the meantime, amiodarone remains the preferred antiarrhythmic during cardiac arrest according to the 2005 guidelines for CPR and ECC with lidocaine considered as an alternative.[2]

Thrombolytics

Because most cardiac arrests are related to either MI or PE, several investigators have evaluated the role of thrombolytics during CPR. Several studies have demonstrated successful use of thrombolytics, but few have shown improvements to hospital discharge[70–76] (Table 14–5). Of note, an increase in bleeding, which is especially concerning in the setting of traumatic or prolonged CPR, has not been noted. Thrombolytics, therefore, should be considered on a case-by-case basis when PE is suspected.[2] A large, international, multicentered, randomized controlled trial is currently underway to better address the efficacy and safety of thrombolytic therapy during CPR.[17]

Magnesium

Although severe hypomagnesemia has been associated with VF/PVT, clinical trials have not demonstrated any benefit with the routine administration of magnesium during a cardiac arrest. Two observation trials, however, have shown an improvement in ROSC in patients with arrests associated with torsade de pointes.[2] Therefore, magnesium administration should be limited to these patients.

■ POSTRESUSCITATIVE CARE

Therapeutic Hypothermia

Restoration of blood flow following cardiac arrest can lead to several chemical cascades and destructive enzymatic reactions that can result in cerebral injury. These reactions include free-radical production,

TABLE 14-5 Summary of Adult Thrombolytic Comparative Trials

Author	Design	Drug Studied	N	Initial Resuscitation: Thrombolytic	Initial Resuscitation: No Thrombolytic	Hospital Discharge: Thrombolytic	Hospital Discharge: No Thrombolytic	Major Bleeding: Thrombolytic	Major Bleeding: No Thrombolytic
Kurkciyan, et al., 2000	Ret	t-PA 100 mg	42	17/21[a] (81%)	9/21[a] (43%)	2/21 (10%)	1/21 (5%)	5/21 (24%)	NA
Bottiger, et al., 2001	P, NR, PC	t-PA 50 mg, up to 2 doses	90	27/40[a] (68%)	22/50[a] (44%)	6/40 (15%)	4/50 (8%)	2/40 (5%)	0/50 (0%)
Ruiz-Bailen, et al., 2001	Ret	SK (3%) t-PA (94%) Other (3%)	303	22/67[a] (33%)	144/236[a] (61%)	12/67[a] (18%)	109/236[a] (46%)	5/67 (7%)	2/236 (1%)
Lederer, et al., 2001	Ret	t-PA	324	76/108[a] (70%)	110/214[a] (51%)	27/108[a] (25%)	33/214[a] (15%)	6/45 (13%)	7/46 (15%)
Abu-Laban, et al., 2002	P, R, MC, PC	t-PA 100 mg	233	25/117 (21%)	27/116 (23%)	1/117 (1%)	0/116 (0%)	2/117 (2%)	0/116 (0%)
Janata et al., 2003	Ret	t-PA 0.6–1 mg/kg (100 mg max)	66	24/36 (67%)	13/30 (43%)	7/36 (19%)	2/30 (7%)	9/36 (25%)	3/30 (10%)
Fatovich, et al., 2004	P, R, DB, PC	Tenecteplase 50 mg	35	8/19[a] (42%)	1/16[a] (6%)	1/19 (5%)	1/16 (6%)	0	0
Stadlbauer, et al., 2006	Ret	Tenecteplase or reteplase	1186	44/99[a] (46%)	355/1087[a] (33%)	14/99 (14%)	101/1067 (10%)	0	NA

DB, double-blind; MC, multicentered; NA, not available; NR, non-randomized; P, prospective; PC, placebo controlled; R, randomized; Ret, retrospective; SK, streptokinase; t-PA, tissue plasminogen activator.
[a]$P < 0.05$
Data from Abu-Laban et al.,[70] Bottiger et al.,[71] Fatovich et al.,[72] Janata et al.,[73] Kurkciyan et al.,[74] Lederer et al.,[75] Ruiz-Bailen et al.,[76] and Stadlbauer et al.[113]

excitatory amino acid release, and calcium shifts, leading to mitochondrial damage and apoptosis (programmed cell death).[77] Hypothermia can protect from cerebral injury by suppressing these chemical reactions, thereby reducing the production of free radicals. Various animal models have demonstrated improved functional recovery and reduced cerebral deficits with the induction of mild therapeutic hypothermia.[77] Clinical trials in humans have shown similar results.[78,79]

One trial was conducted in nine centers in five European countries.[78] In this study, patients who had been resuscitated after cardiac arrest caused by VF but remained comatose were assigned randomly to undergo therapeutic hypothermia, targeting a temperature of 32°C (89.6°F) to 34°C (93.2°F), for 24 hours. The primary end point was neurologic outcome within 6 months of cardiac arrest. Secondary end points were mortality (within 6 months) and complication rate within 7 days. A favorable neurologic outcome was achieved in 55% of patients in the hypothermia group as opposed to 39% in the normothermia group ($P = 0.009$). Additionally, mortality rates were improved significantly in the hypothermia group (41% vs. 55%; $P = 0.02$). Based on this difference, seven patients would need to be treated with hypothermia to prevent one death. The rate of complications (e.g., bleeding, pneumonia, sepsis, and renal failure) did not differ between the two groups (73% for the hypothermia group and 70% for the normothermia group; $P = 0.70$).

A second trial was conducted in four hospitals in Melbourne, Australia.[79] Entry criteria were similar to the previous trial, but the target temperature for hypothermia was 33°C (91.4°F), which was maintained for 12 hours. The primary outcome measure was survival to hospital discharge with good neurologic function. Forty-nine percent of patients in the hypothermia group had good neurologic function on discharge (to either home or a rehabilitation facility) compared with 26% of patients in the normothermia group ($P = 0.046$). Mortality rates were similar between the two groups (51% for the hypothermia group and 68% for the normothermia group; $P = 0.145$). Hypothermia was associated with a lower cardiac index, higher systemic vascular resistance, and hyperglycemia. It is important to note that only 8% of patients with cardiac arrest were selected for therapeutic hypothermia in these two studies. Thus, further research needs to focus on the subset of arrest patients who are most likely to benefit from this strategy.

In light of these trials, unconscious adult patients with spontaneous circulation after out-of-hospital cardiac arrest should be cooled to 32°C (89.6°F) to 34°C (93.2°F) for 12 to 24 hours when the initial rhythm is VF.[2,77] Such cooling also can be of benefit for other rhythms or in-hospital cardiac arrests. There is insufficient evidence to make a recommendation on the use of therapeutic hypothermia in children, however, an evaluation in neonates with asphyxiation suggested that hypothermia in this select population may be beneficial.[80]

Hypothermia must be used with caution, however, as there are several complications that can develop. Coagulopathy, dysrhythmias, hyperglycemia, increased incidence of pneumonia, as well as sepsis have been described.[79,81] Further research is needed in this area.

Glucose Control

Electrolyte abnormalities are frequent after cardiac arrest, and can be very deleterious to outcome. Although no controlled evidence exists regarding glucose control post–cardiac arrest, there is growing consensus among critical care practitioners that tight glucose control improves outcome among critically ill patients. Studies have documented increased survival, as well as less infectious complications using insulin drips to obtain tight glucose control (i.e., 80 to 110 mg/dL).[82] Because hyperglycemia is common after cardiac arrest, it would seem reasonable for post-arrest providers to maintain normoglycemia, albeit further study is warranted to determine the role of tight glycemic control in these patients.

Cardiovascular Perfusion

The patient who has achieved ROSC often has myocardial stunning/dysfunction, either caused by reperfusion injury or the direct effects of defibrillation.[2] Postresuscitation support involves adequate fluid and vasopressor support in order to maintain sufficient cardiac output with acceptable organ perfusion. Evaluation should thus include electrocardiographic and echocardiographic analysis. Patients often develop a delayed vasodilatation that is responsive to fluids and vasoactive support. Invasive monitoring can be required; however the optimal target numbers for either mean arterial pressure or hemodynamic indices have not been ascertained. It is also unclear whether antiarrhythmics are beneficial in the post-arrest timeframe, despite the fact that many arrests are precipitated by dysrhythmias. Relative adrenal insufficiency has also been shown to develop in the post-arrest period, but adrenal replacement has not been shown to date to be efficacious. However, again borrowing on critical care literature in sepsis, adrenal replacement in the correct situation has been shown to be beneficial.[83] Whether or not this is true in post–cardiac arrest requires further study.

NON-VF/PVT RHYTHMS: PEA AND ASYSTOLE

■ NONPHARMACOLOGIC THERAPY

Pulseless electrical activity is defined as the absence of a detectable pulse and the presence of some type of electrical activity other than VF or PVT. Several studies have documented that patients with PEA actually have mechanical cardiac contractions, but they are too weak to produce a palpable pulse or blood pressure. Asystole is defined as the presence of a flat line on the electrocardiogram (ECG) monitor. Although PEA is still classified as a "rhythm of survival," the success rate of treatment is much lower than the rates seen with VF/PVT.[14] PEA is often caused by treatable conditions, and the resuscitation team needs to identify and correct these conditions emergently if the resuscitation is to be successful. The rate of survival among patients with out-of-hospital cardiac arrest secondary to asystole is 1% to 2% but can be up to 10% in patients with in-hospital arrest.[13,14,20] Successful treatment of both PEA and asystole depends almost entirely on diagnosis of the underlying cause (see Table 14–2). ❻ The algorithm for treatment of PEA is the same as the treatment of asystole. Both conditions require CPR, airway control, and IV access. Asystole should be reconfirmed by checking a second lead on the cardiac monitor. Defibrillation should be avoided in patients with asystole because the parasympathetic discharge that occurs with defibrillation can reduce the chance of ROSC and worsen the chance of survival. The emphasis in resuscitation is good quality CPR without interruption and to try to identify a correctable cause. If available, transcutaneous pacing can be attempted. Asystole often represents confirmation of death rather than a rhythm to be treated; therefore, withdrawal of efforts must be strongly considered if there is not a rapid ROSC.[2]

Much like VF/PVT, there is an interest in hypothermia in these post-arrest patients. Metabolic parameters (e.g., lactate and oxygen [O_2] extraction) have been shown to be improved when post-arrest comatose adults survived their arrest and were treated with hypothermia.[84] Further studies are warranted in this area.

■ PHARMACOLOGIC THERAPY

The primary pharmacologic agents used in the treatment of asystole are vasopressors (i.e., epinephrine and vasopressin) and atropine. Studies comparing epinephrine and vasopressin in patients with PEA and asystole have not demonstrated an advantage with one agent over the other. In one large trial of patients with out-of-hospital cardiac arrest, a post hoc, subgroup analysis was conducted for those patients with asystole.[61] In these patients, ROSC was 16% with vasopressin and 17% with epinephrine (OR 1.00, 95% CI 0.7–1.6; $P = 0.87$), survival to hospital admission was 29% with vasopressin and 20% with epinephrine (OR 0.6, 95% CI 0.4–0.9, $P = 0.02$) and survival to hospital discharge was 4.7% with vasopressin and 1.5% with epinephrine (OR 0.3, 95% CI 0.1–1.0, $P = 0.04$). An increase in intact neurologic survival, however, was not noted. In contrast, 40% (8/20) of patients who received vasopressin and subsequently required additional treatment with epinephrine were discharged in a coma or vegetative state compared to 0% (0/5) of patients who received epinephrine only ($P = 0.14$). Nevertheless, vasopressin can be substituted for the first or second dose of epinephrine in patients with asystole.[2] There is insufficient data to recommend for or against its use in PEA. Epinephrine should be administered similarly to its use in VF/PVT; that is, 1 mg every 3 to 5 minutes.

Atropine is an antimuscarinic agent that blocks the depressant effect of acetylcholine on both the sinus and atrioventricular nodes, thus decreasing parasympathetic tone. During asystole, parasympathetic tone may increase because of the vagal stimulation that occurs secondary to intubation, the effects of hypoxia and acidosis, or alterations in the balance of parasympathetic and sympathetic control.[85] Unfortunately, there are no prospective controlled trials showing benefit from atropine for the treatment of asystole or PEA.

Earlier small observational reports found some response to atropine in asystole or pulseless idioventricular rhythm but little evidence to suggest that long-term outcomes were altered.[86] In one retrospective case-control study, a success rate of 14% (6:43) was noted with atropine compared with to a 0% (0:41) rate with a control but no patients survived to hospital discharge.[86] In a second retrospective study, asystole was terminated in only 4 of 22 patients (18%) when atropine was administered.[87] Once again, none survived to hospital discharge. Finally, a third retrospective review evaluated 101 patients who received atropine for asystole.[88] Twenty-four patients (24%) survived 24 hours after resuscitation. It is unclear how many survived to hospital discharge. These results show that although atropine can achieve ROSC in some instances, asystolic arrest is almost always fatal. Given the relative safety of atropine, the ease of administration, low cost, and theoretical advantages, atropine should be considered for asystole or PEA.[2] The beneficial effects, however, are limited.

■ ACID/BASE MANAGEMENT

Acidosis seen during cardiac arrest is the result of decreased blood flow and inadequate ventilation. Chest compressions generate approximately 20% to 30% of normal cardiac output, leading to inadequate organ perfusion, tissue hypoxia, and metabolic acidosis. In addition, the lack of ventilation causes retention of carbon dioxide, leading to respiratory acidosis. This combined acidosis produces not only reduced myocardial contractility and negative inotropic effect, but also the appearance of arrhythmias because of a lower fibrillation threshold. In early cardiac arrest, adequate alveolar ventilation is the mainstay of control to limit the accumulation of carbon dioxide and control the acid–base imbalance.[2] With arrests of long duration, buffer therapy is often considered, however, few data supports its use during cardiac arrest.

Although sodium bicarbonate was once given routinely to reduce the detrimental effects associated with acidosis (e.g., reduced myocardial contractility), enhance the effect of epinephrine, and improve the rate of defibrillation, there are few clinical data supporting its use.[89] In fact, sodium bicarbonate can have some detrimental effects.[89,90] The effect of sodium bicarbonate can be described by the following reaction:

$$[HCO_3^-] + [H^+] \leftrightarrow [H_2CO_3] \leftrightarrow [H_2O] + [CO_2]$$

When sodium bicarbonate is added to an acidic environment, this reaction will shift to the right, thereby increasing tissue and venous hypercarbia. The carbon dioxide generated by this reaction will diffuse into the cell and decrease intracellular pH. The accumulation of intracellular carbon dioxide, specifically within the myocardium, is inversely correlated with coronary perfusion pressure produced by CPR. Intracellular acidosis also will decrease myocardial contractility, further complicating the low-flow state associated with CPR.[89] Furthermore, treatment with sodium bicarbonate often overcorrects extracellular pH because sodium bicarbonate has a greater effect when the pH is closer to normal.[90] The induced alkalosis, causes an increase in the affinity of oxygen to hemoglobin ("left shift"), thus interfering with oxygen release into the tissues.

Sodium bicarbonate can be used in special circumstances (i.e., underlying metabolic acidosis, hyperkalemia, salicylate overdose, or tricyclic antidepressant overdose), however, the dosage should be guided by laboratory analysis if possible. There has been clinical interest in other buffering agents (an equimolar mixture of sodium bicarbonate and sodium carbonate [Carbicarb]; tris(hydroxymethyl aminomethane [THAM]; a mixture of THAM, acetate, sodium bicarbonate, and phosphate [Tribonat]) as they have shown less potential for the adverse effects seen with sodium bicarbonate.[2] However, there is a dearth of clinical experience with these agents, and outcome studies are not available.

MODIFICATIONS FOR SPECIAL SITUATIONS

■ DROWNING

Drowning is a process resulting in primary respiratory impairment from immersion in a liquid. It is a common, preventable cause of morbidity and mortality. The most important inciting event is the hypoxia induced by submersion. Thus, early care of the drowning patient includes immediate rescue breathing, even before he or she is removed from the water. This is performed much in the same way as for other victims of cardiac arrest. Prompt initiation of this therapy increases chance of survival.[91] Once victims are removed from the water, immediate chest compressions should be started if they are pulseless. Drowning victims can present with any of the pulseless rhythms; standard guidelines need to be followed for therapy of these rhythms.

■ HYPOTHERMIA

Unintentional hypothermia (as opposed to the therapeutic hypothermia used post-arrest, described above) is defined by a body temperature <30°C (86°F), and is associated with marked derangements in body function. Because it can depress virtually every body system, including pulse and respiration, the patient may appear to be dead on the initial evaluation. Hypothermia can lead to benefit on brain recovery after cardiac arrest (discussed earlier), thus aggressive intervention is clearly indicated when there is a hypothermic arrest victim.

If the patient still has a perfusing rhythm, therapy is mainly based on rewarming techniques. For mild hypothermia (i.e., >34°C [>93.2°F]), passive rewarming is recommended. For moderate hypothermia (i.e., 30°C to 34°C [86°F to 93.2°F]), active external rewarming is recommended, and for severe hypothermia (i.e., <30°C [<86°F]) active internal rewarming is recommended. These patients need to be manipulated very gently as VF is sometimes precipitated by movement.[92]

If the patient is in cardiac arrest, then the standard BLS algorithm should be followed. However, there are some modifications that the rescuer needs to consider. The rescuer should evaluate for respiration and pulse for a longer time frame, as these can be slow or very difficult to realize. If there is no breathing, then rescue breaths should ensue. If there is any doubt about the presence of a pulse, then chest compressions should be started immediately. If the patient is in VF or PVT then electrical therapy should be given in a standard manner. However, the hypothermic heart may be less responsive to medications or defibrillation, and thus there have been worries about the optimal temperature at which to start defibrillation attempts.[2] There are no published consensus guidelines regarding this. Immediately after defibrillation, CPR should resume as in the standard manner. During CPR, continued attempts at rewarming are of paramount importance. Included in this concept is preventing further heat loss (i.e., removal of wet clothing, protection from the environment, etc.). Patients often require significant volume challenges during the rewarming process. The use of steroids, antibiotics, and barbiturates has been proposed, but none of these agents have ever been shown to increase survival rates.[2]

It is debatable when to stop resuscitative efforts in the hypothermic patient. Many authors have proposed that a patient should not be pronounced until the core temperature has been restored to near normal.[2] Once the patient is in the hospital, it is still the judgment of the treating physician when efforts should be terminated.

■ PREGNANCY

Pregnancy is a unique situation in that survival of both the fetus and the mother depend on CPR. The best hope for survival of the fetus is maternal survival. Because of the gravid uterus, resuscitation needs to be modified. Because the vena cava and aorta can be obstructed by a uterus of approximately 20 weeks of gestation or later, it is appropriate to position the patient approximately 15 to 30 degrees back from the left lateral decubitus position, or to pull the uterus to the side.[93]

Airway control is important in the pregnant patient. The airway may be smaller because of the hormonal changes and edema that accompany pregnancy. Similarly, because of increased intraabdominal pressure exerted by the uterus, as well as hormonal changes that change the resting state of the gastroesophageal sphincter, clinicians need to be acutely aware of the increased risk of aspiration. Because of this, cricoid pressure needs to be maintained continuously during airway manipulation. The rescuer may need to give smaller tidal volumes than normal because of the diaphragm elevation that accompanies the later stages of pregnancy. Similarly, circulatory support also has to be adjusted. In particular, chest compressions need to be administered slightly above the center of the sternum to adjust for the anatomic changes of the pregnant uterus.[2]

In an arrest situation during pregnancy the ACLS provider needs to follow the standard guidelines, including the same use of defibrillation and medications. Although it is true that vasoactive agents, such as epinephrine, can diminish uterine blood flow, safer alternatives do not exist.[2]

Although etiologies of arrest in pregnancy are often the same as in the nonpregnant patient, there are several unique situations that need to be considered in the differential diagnosis of a pregnancy arrest. These include: excess magnesium sulfate institution (i.e., iatrogenic from treating eclampsia) in which case the therapeutic administration of calcium gluconate can be lifesaving; amniotic embolism, which is associated with complete cardiovascular collapse during labor and delivery (cardiopulmonary bypass has been reportedly successful in salvaging this condition); preeclampsia/eclampsia developing after 20 weeks of gestation producing hypertension and multiple organ dysfunction; as well as vascular events including acute coronary syndromes and acute pulmonary embolism.[94,95]

It is paramount to remember that unless circulation is restored to the mother, both the mother and the fetus will succumb especially if standard therapy is not used correctly and promptly. Because of this the resuscitation leader should consider the need for emergent hysterotomy (i.e., Cesarean delivery) and delivery as soon as the arrest happens. The best survival reported for infants >24 weeks of gestation happens when delivery occurs no more than 5 minutes after the arrest of the mother.[2,96]

■ TRAUMA

Cardiac resuscitation of the trauma arrest patient is basically performed with the same guidelines as any other arrest. There are some specific etiologies to rapidly consider however, as the survival of an out-of-hospital cardiac arrest caused by trauma is rare.[2] The rescuer needs to consider airway obstruction, pneumothorax, tracheobronchial injury, cardiac or large arterial injury, cardiac tamponade, severe head injury with secondary cardiac collapse, and other injuries specific to the particular trauma.[2] The best survival seems to be in young patients with treatable penetrating injuries.

Trauma patients often suffer head or cervical injuries; thus cervical spine precautions should be used in these patients. A jaw thrust maneuver is the preferred way to open the airway, with in-line stabilization during attempts at advanced airway placement.[2] The rescuer must be vigilant for the development of tension pneumothorax during ventilation. Inadequate ventilation of one side is usually caused by tube malposition, tension pneumothorax, or hemothorax. These conditions are usually treated by medical personnel at the hospital after transport.

Chest compressions should be performed in a standard manner. Any visible hemorrhage should be controlled with direct pressure. Fluid resuscitation is done with a goal of adequate blood pressure and organ perfusion. The specific details of fluid resuscitation are highly controversial however, and the optimal volume infusion for trauma resuscitation is a subject of ongoing debate.

Open thoracotomy for trauma-induced arrest has been performed in many instances. For penetrating chest trauma patients who arrest immediately before arrival or in the emergency department, open thoracotomy can allow relief of tamponade, control of major vessel hemorrhage, or direct repair of cardiac insult.[97] In the case of blunt trauma however, open thoracotomy does not improve outcome.

For definitive post-arrest care, trauma patients should be rapidly transferred to a facility with expertise in the provision of trauma care.

■ ELECTRICAL SHOCK

There are many etiologies of electrical shock injuries, from lightning strike (mortality estimated to be 30%, with 70% of survivors sustaining significant morbidity) to high-tension current, to household current.[98,99] The severity of injury depends on the site, type of current, duration of contact, pathway, and the magnitude of delivered electricity.

Cardiac arrest is common in electrical injury caused by current passing through the heart during the "vulnerable period" of the cardiac cycle. In large-current events, such as lightning strike, the heart undergoes massive depolarization simultaneously.[100] Sometimes the intrinsic pacemaker can restore an organized cardiac electrical cycle, but because of injury to other muscles, specifically the thoracic musculature, the patient cannot retain or sustain viable circulation because of the lack of ventilation and oxygenation.[101]

When approaching a victim of electrocution, the rescuer must first be certain of his or her own safety. Thereafter, standard BLS, prompt CPR, and ACLS when available is indicated. Electric shock is often associated with multiple trauma, including spinal injury, multiple injuries to the skeletal muscles, as well as fractures. These factors need to be evaluated by the resuscitation team.

Airway control can be difficult because of the edema that often accompanies such injuries; thus an advanced airway early in the treatment process is recommended.[2] With soft tissue swelling, there is often a need for aggressive fluid resuscitation in these patients. The underlying tissue, or visceral organ damage, is often worse than the external appearance. It is usually recommended that these patients be transferred to centers with expertise in dealing with these types of injuries.

GUIDELINES FOR DRUG ADMINISTRATION

The routes of administration that are available for drug delivery during CPR include IV (both central and peripheral access), IO, and endotracheal. The chosen route represents a compromise between the availability of access and their apparent efficacy in introducing the drug into the central circulation. When selecting a route for drug administration, it is of utmost importance to minimize any interruptions in chest compressions during CPR.

Central venous access will result in a faster and higher peak drug concentration than peripheral access, but central line access is not needed in most resuscitation attempts. If a central line is already present, however, it should be the access site of choice. Central lines located above the diaphragm are preferable to those located below the diaphragm because of poor blood flow during CPR.[102] If IV access (either central or peripheral) has not been established a large peripheral venous catheter should be inserted. Peripheral drug administration yields a peak concentration in the major systemic arteries in roughly 1.5 to 3 minutes but circulation time can be shortened by up to 40% if the drug is followed by a 20-mL fluid bolus with elevation of the extremity.[102]

❼ The 2005 guidelines for CPR and ECC now recommend IO administration as the preferred alternative if IV administration cannot be achieved.[2] Drug administration using the IO route is as quick and effective as drug administration via central access and superior to that achieved with peripheral access. Several studies have documented the effectiveness and safety of this administration route in both adults and children.[2] Potential anatomic sites for insertion for an IO needle are the distal tibia, the proximal tibia, and the distal femur.[103] Intraosseous infusion devices are available that allow for rapid insertion (i.e., within 90 seconds) and are easy to use.[104]

In the event that neither IV nor IO access can be established, then a few drugs can be administered endotracheally. These drugs are atropine, lidocaine, epinephrine, naloxone, and vasopressin.[2] Medications administered through the endotracheal route, however, will have both a lower and delayed peak concentration than when they are administered by the IV or IO routes.[2] Furthermore, clinical trials have failed to demonstrate any benefit with using the endotracheal route.[105,106] In fact, one clinical trial noted lower rates of ROSC (15% [15:101] vs. 27% [134:495], $P \leq 0.01$), hospital admission (9% [9:101] vs. 20% [97:495], $P \leq 0.02$), and hospital discharge (0% [0:101] vs. 5% [27:495], $P \leq 0.02$) with endotracheal drug administration compared to IV.[106] Currently, the recommended endotracheal dose is 2 to 2.5 times larger than the IV/IO dose.[2] Given the unpredictable absorption and the lack of clinical effectiveness, however, either the IV or IO routes are preferred.

ETHICAL AND ECONOMIC CONSIDERATIONS

The primary objective of CPR is to obtain neurologic survival. Because this is often unobtainable, many healthcare professionals are attempting to identify patients unlikely to benefit from cardiac resuscitation. One difficulty in accomplishing this task is defining medical futility. The two major determinants of medical futility are length of life and quality of life.[2] An intervention that cannot increase length or quality of life is considered futile. Key factors in CPR are the disease underlying the cardiac arrest and the expected state of health after resuscitation. One important question that is debated often is how low should the chance of survival be before medical therapy is considered futile? Is the chance of 1 or 2 months of life for a patient an acceptable goal? These are important questions that must be addressed when determining resuscitation status. Ethically, healthcare providers are obligated to respect patient autonomy, which is easiest in the arrest situation if the patient has an advance directive. If the patient loses the ability to make informed decisions regarding medical care, then a spouse or a designated healthcare advocate must act as a surrogate decision maker, invoking what has been termed substituted judgment: following the predetermined wishes of the patient.

Unfortunately, there is no scientific evidence or scoring system that can predict the outcome following CPR. Therefore, all patients in cardiac arrest should receive resuscitation unless the patient has a "do not attempt resuscitation" (DNAR) order, signs of irreversible death, or vital organ function deterioration that makes it impossible to expect any benefit from CPR—despite maximum therapy.[2] Withholding CPR attempts in these futile cases not only would decrease the number of patients left in a vegetative state with poor neurologic status but also would improve the cost-effectiveness of CPR programs. CPR is of minimal economic benefit if the only outcome following ROSC is a prolonged, expensive hospital stay.

The decision to terminate resuscitative efforts usually rests with the treating medical team in the hospital. This is often based on many factors, including time to CPR, time of CPR, time to ROSC, premorbid conditions, and so forth. None of these is clearly predictive of outcome however. In a prehospital arrest, it is the duty of the treating team to provide BLS and ACLS unless there is clear evidence of death (i.e., signs of rigor mortis), the provision of CPR would place the rescuer at personal risk, or there is clear evidence of a DNAR order.

CLINICAL CONTROVERSIES

Some clinicians feel that vasopressin should be the vasopressor of first choice in patients with VF/PVT although others prefer epinephrine.

Although amiodarone is considered the preferred antiarrhythmic in patients with VF/PVT, there is conflicting data regarding its effect on outcome when compared to lidocaine.

Some clinicians feel that CPR should be performed before defibrillation is attempted in patients who have had an unwitnessed arrest. Others feel that defibrillation should be attempted as soon as possible.

EVALUATION OF THERAPEUTIC OUTCOMES

To measure the success of resuscitation outcomes, therapeutic outcome monitoring should occur both during the resuscitation attempt and in the postresuscitation phase. The optimal outcome following CPR is an awake, responsive, spontaneously breathing patient. Patients must remain neurologically intact with minimal morbidity following the resuscitation if it is to be truly classified as a success.

Unfortunately, there are no reliable criteria for clinicians to use to gauge the efficacy of CPR. Nonetheless, heart rate, cardiac rhythm, and blood pressure should be assessed and documented throughout the resuscitation attempt and subsequent to each intervention. Coronary perfusion pressure (CPP; CPP is the aortic diastolic pressure minus right atrial diastolic pressure) should be assessed in patients for whom intraarterial monitoring is in place. Determination of the presence or absence of a pulse is paramount to deciding which interventions are appropriate. Palpating a pulse to determine the efficacy of blood flow during CPR, however, has not been shown to be useful.

End-tidal carbon dioxide monitoring is a safe and effective method to assess cardiac output during CPR and has been associated with ROSC.[2] The main determinant for carbon dioxide excretion is the rate of delivery from the peripheral sites (where it's produced) to the lungs. Increasing cardiac output (through effective CPR), will yield higher end-tidal carbon dioxide levels as delivery of carbon dioxide to the lungs increases.

Clinicians should also consider the precipitating cause of the cardiac arrest, such as an MI, electrolyte imbalance, or primary arrhythmia. Pre-arrest status should be carefully reviewed, particularly if the patient was receiving drug therapy. Altered cardiac, hepatic, and renal function resulting from ischemic damage during the cardiopulmonary arrest warrant special attention and can require advanced care. Neurologic function should be assessed by means of the Cerebral Performance Category and the Glasgow Coma Scale.[107,108] Nonresponse to an array of suitable interventions can indicate that resuscitation is impossible.

ABBREVIATIONS

ACLS: advanced cardiac life support
AHA: American Heart Association
BLS: basic life support
CPP: coronary perfusion pressure
CPR: cardiopulmonary resuscitation
ECC: emergency cardiovascular care
EMS: emergency medical services
IO: intraosseous
IV: intravenous
MI: myocardial infarction
PEA: pulseless electrical activity
PE: pulmonary embolism
ROSC: return of spontaneous circulation
PVT: pulseless ventricular tachycardia
VF: ventricular fibrillation

REFERENCES

1. Niemann JT. Cardiopulmonary resuscitation. *N Engl J Med* 1992;327(15):1075–1080.
2. American Heart Association. 2005 American Heart Association guidelines for cardiopulmonary resuscitation and emergency cardiovascular care. *Circulation* 2005;112(24 suppl):IV1–203.
3. Centers for Disease Control and Prevention, National Centers for Injury Prevention and Control. Web-based Injury Statistics Query and Reporting System (WISQARS), 2005, *www.cdc.gov/ncipc/wisqars.*
4. Ornato JP, Peberdy MA. Prehospital and emergency department care to preserve neurologic function during and following cardiopulmonary resuscitation. *Neurol Clin* 2006;24(1):23–39.
5. Vaillancourt C, Stiell IG. Cardiac arrest care and emergency medical services in Canada. *Can J Cardiol* 2004;20(11):1081–1090.
6. Podrid PJ, Myerburg RJ. Epidemiology and stratification of risk for sudden cardiac death. *Clin Cardiol* 2005;28(11 suppl 1):I3–11.
7. Rea TD, Eisenberg MS, Sinibaldi G, White RD. Incidence of EMS-treated out-of-hospital cardiac arrest in the United States. *Resuscitation* 2004;63(1):17–24.
8. Paraskos JA. History of CPR and the role of the national conference. *Ann Emerg Med* 1993;22(2 pt 2):275–280.
9. Safar P, Escarraga LA, Elam JO. A comparison of the mouth-to-mouth and mouth-to-airway methods of artificial respiration with the chest-pressure arm-lift methods. *N Engl J Med* 1958;258(14):671–677.
10. Kouwenhoven WB, Jude JR, Knickerbocker GG. Closed-chest cardiac massage. *JAMA* 1960;173:1064–1067.
11. Thel MC, O'Connor CM. Cardiopulmonary resuscitation: Historical perspective to recent investigations. *Am Heart J* 1999;137(1):39–48.
12. Myerburg RJ, Castellanos A. Emerging paradigms of the epidemiology and demographics of sudden cardiac arrest. *Heart Rhythm* 2006;3(2):235–239.
13. Cobb LA, Fahrenbruch CE, Olsufka M, Copass MK. Changing incidence of out-of-hospital ventricular fibrillation, 1980–2000. *JAMA* 2002;288(23):3008–3013.
14. Nadkarni VM, Larkin GL, Peberdy MA, et al. First documented rhythm and clinical outcome from in-hospital cardiac arrest among children and adults. *JAMA* 2006;295(1):50–57.
15. White RD, Hankins DG, Bugliosi TF. Seven years' experience with early defibrillation by police and paramedics in an emergency medical services system. *Resuscitation* 1998;39(3):145–151.

16. Stiell IG, Wells GA, Field BJ, et al. Improved out-of-hospital cardiac arrest survival through the inexpensive optimization of an existing defibrillation program: OPALS study phase II. Ontario Prehospital Advanced Life Support. *JAMA* 1999;281(13):1175–1181.
17. Spohr F, Arntz HR, Bluhmki E, et al. International multicentre trial protocol to assess the efficacy and safety of tenecteplase during cardiopulmonary resuscitation in patients with out-of-hospital cardiac arrest: The Thrombolysis in Cardiac Arrest (TROICA) Study. *Eur J Clin Invest* 2005;35(5):315–323.
18. Chandra NC. Mechanisms of blood flow during CPR. *Ann Emerg Med* 1993;22(2 pt 2):281–288.
19. Tucker KJ, Savitt MA, Idris A, Redberg RF. Cardiopulmonary resuscitation. Historical perspectives, physiology, and future directions. *Arch Intern Med* 1994;154(19):2141–2150.
20. Stiell IG, Wells GA, Field B, et al. Advanced cardiac life support in out-of-hospital cardiac arrest. *N Engl J Med* 2004;351(7):647–656.
21. Valenzuela TD, Roe DJ, Nichol G, et al. Outcomes of rapid defibrillation by security officers after cardiac arrest in casinos. *N Engl J Med* 2000;343(17):1206–1209.
22. Rea TD, Eisenberg MS, Becker LJ, et al. Temporal trends in sudden cardiac arrest: A 25-year emergency medical services perspective. *Circulation* 2003;107(22):2780–2785.
23. Weisfeldt ML, Becker LB. Resuscitation after cardiac arrest: A 3-phase time-sensitive model. *JAMA* 2002;288(23):3035–3038.
24. De Maio VJ, Stiell IG, Wells GA, Spaite DW. Optimal defibrillation response intervals for maximum out-of-hospital cardiac arrest survival rates. *Ann Emerg Med* 2003;42(2):242–250.
25. Kellum MJ, Kennedy KW, Ewy GA. Cardiocerebral resuscitation improves survival of patients with out-of-hospital cardiac arrest. *Am J Med* 2006;119(4):335–340.
26. Cobb LA, Fahrenbruch CE, Walsh TR, et al. Influence of cardiopulmonary resuscitation prior to defibrillation in patients with out-of-hospital ventricular fibrillation. *JAMA* 1999;281(13):1182–1188.
27. Wik L, Hansen TB, Fylling F, et al. Delaying defibrillation to give basic cardiopulmonary resuscitation to patients with out-of-hospital ventricular fibrillation: A randomized trial. *JAMA* 2003;289(11):1389–1395.

Davis EA, Mosesso VN, Jr. Performance of police first responders in utilizing automated external defibrillation on victims of sudden cardiac arrest. *Prehosp Emerg Care* 1998;2(2):101–107.

Caffrey SL, Willoughby PJ, Pepe PE, Becker LB. Public use of automated external defibrillators. *N Engl J Med* 2002;347(16):1242–1247.

White RD, Bunch TJ, Hankins DG. Evolution of a community-wide early defibrillation programme experience over 13 years using police/fire personnel and paramedics as responders. *Resuscitation* 2005;65(3):279–283.

31. White RD, Russell JK. Refibrillation, resuscitation and survival in out-of-hospital sudden cardiac arrest victims treated with biphasic automated external defibrillators. *Resuscitation* 2002;55(1):17–23.
32. Hilwig RW, Kern KB, Berg RA, et al. Catecholamines in cardiac arrest: Role of alpha agonists, beta-adrenergic blockers and high-dose epinephrine. *Resuscitation* 2000;47(2):203–208.
33. Robinson LA, Brown CG, Jenkins J, et al. The effect of norepinephrine versus epinephrine on myocardial hemodynamics during CPR. *Ann Emerg Med* 1989;18(4):336–340.
34. Zhong JQ, Dorian P. Epinephrine and vasopressin during cardiopulmonary resuscitation. *Resuscitation* 2005;66(3):263–269.
35. Cammarata G, Weil MH, Sun S, et al. Beta1-adrenergic blockade during cardiopulmonary resuscitation improves survival. *Crit Care Med* 2004;32(9 suppl):S440–443.
36. Ditchey RV, Lindenfeld J. Failure of epinephrine to improve the balance between myocardial oxygen supply and demand during closed-chest resuscitation in dogs. *Circulation* 1988;78(2):382–389.
37. Holmes HR, Babbs CF, Voorhees WD, et al. Influence of adrenergic drugs upon vital organ perfusion during CPR. *Crit Care Med* 1980;8(3):137–140.
38. Ornato JP. Use of adrenergic agonists during CPR in adults. *Ann Emerg Med* 1993;22(2 pt 2):411–S416.
39. Brown C, Wiklund L, Bar-Joseph G, et al. Future directions for resuscitation research. IV. Innovative advanced life support pharmacology. *Resuscitation,* 1996;33(2):163–177.
40. Brown CG, Robinson LA, Jenkins J, et al. The effect of norepinephrine versus epinephrine on regional cerebral blood flow during cardiopulmonary resuscitation. *Am J Emerg Med* 1989;7(3):278–282.
41. Callaham M, Madsen CD, Barton CW, et al. A randomized clinical trial of high-dose epinephrine and norepinephrine vs standard-dose epinephrine in prehospital cardiac arrest. *JAMA* 1992;268(19):2667–2672.
42. Lindner KH, Ahnefeld FW, Grunert A. Epinephrine versus norepinephrine in prehospital ventricular fibrillation. *Am J Cardiol* 1991;67(5):427–428.
43. Lindner KH, Ahnefeld FW, Schuermann W, Bowdler IM. Epinephrine and norepinephrine in cardiopulmonary resuscitation. Effects on myocardial oxygen delivery and consumption. *Chest* 1990;97(6):1458–1462.
44. Redding JS, Pearson JW. Evaluation of drugs for cardiac resuscitation. *Anesthesiology* 1963;24:203–207.
45. Brown CG, Werman HA, Davis EA, et al. Comparative effect of graded doses of epinephrine on regional brain blood flow during CPR in a swine model. *Ann Emerg Med* 1986;15(10):1138–1144.
46. Brunette DD, Jameson SJ. Comparison of standard versus high-dose epinephrine in the resuscitation of cardiac arrest in dogs. *Ann Emerg Med* 1990;19(1):8–11.
47. Gonzalez ER, Ornato JP, Garnett AR, et al. Dose-dependent vasopressor response to epinephrine during CPR in human beings. *Ann Emerg Med* 1989;18(9):920–926.
48. Kosnik JW, Jackson RE, Keats S, et al. Dose-related response of centrally administered epinephrine on the change in aortic diastolic pressure during closed-chest massage in dogs. *Ann Emerg Med* 1985;14(3):204–208.
49. Brown CG, Martin DR, Pepe PE, et al. A comparison of standard-dose and high-dose epinephrine in cardiac arrest outside the hospital. The Multicenter High-Dose Epinephrine Study Group. *N Engl J Med* 1992;327(15):1051–1055.
50. Callaham M, Barton CW, Kayser S. Potential complications of high-dose epinephrine therapy in patients resuscitated from cardiac arrest. *JAMA* 1991;265(9):1117–1122.
51. Choux C, Gueugniaud PY, Barbieux A, et al. Standard doses versus repeated high doses of epinephrine in cardiac arrest outside the hospital. *Resuscitation* 1995;29(1):3–9.
52. Gueugniaud PY, Mols P, Goldstein P, et al. A comparison of repeated high doses and repeated standard doses of epinephrine for cardiac arrest outside the hospital. European Epinephrine Study Group. *N Engl J Med* 1998;339(22):1595–1601.
53. Lipman J, Wilson W, Kobilski S, et al. High-dose adrenaline in adult in-hospital asystolic cardiopulmonary resuscitation: A double-blind randomised trial. *Anaesth Intensive Care* 1993;21(2):192–196.
54. Sherman BW, Munger MA, Foulke GE, et al. High-dose versus standard-dose epinephrine treatment of cardiac arrest after failure of standard therapy. *Pharmacotherapy* 1997;17(2):242–247.
55. Stiell IG, Hebert PC, Weitzman BN, et al. High-dose epinephrine in adult cardiac arrest. *N Engl J Med* 1992;327(15):1045–1050.
56. Lindner KH, Ahnefeld FW, Prengel AW. Comparison of standard and high-dose adrenaline in the resuscitation of asystole and electromechanical dissociation. *Acta Anaesthesiol Scand* 1991;35(3):253–256.
57. Miano TA, Crouch MA. Evolving role of vasopressin in the treatment of cardiac arrest. *Pharmacotherapy* 2006;26(6):828–839.
58. Babbs CF, Berg RA, Kette F, et al. Use of pressors in the treatment of cardiac arrest. *Ann Emerg Med* 2001;37(4 suppl):S152–S162.
59. Lindner KH, Strohmenger HU, Ensinger H, et al. Stress hormone response during and after cardiopulmonary resuscitation. *Anesthesiology* 1992;77(4):662–668.
60. Voelckel WG, Lindner KH, Wenzel V, et al. Effects of vasopressin and epinephrine on splanchnic blood flow and renal function during and after cardiopulmonary resuscitation in pigs. *Crit Care Med* 2000;28(4):1083–1088.
61. Wenzel V, Krismer AC, Arntz HR, et al. A comparison of vasopressin and epinephrine for out-of-hospital cardiopulmonary resuscitation. *N Engl J Med* 2004;350(2):105–113.
62. Aung K, Htay T. Vasopressin for cardiac arrest: A systematic review and meta-analysis. *Arch Intern Med* 2005;165(1):17–24.
63. Harrison EE. Lidocaine in prehospital countershock refractory ventricular fibrillation. *Ann Emerg Med* 1981;10(8):420–423.
64. Weaver WD, Fahrenbruch CE, Johnson DD, et al. Effect of epinephrine and lidocaine therapy on outcome after cardiac arrest due to ventricular fibrillation. *Circulation* 1990;82(6):2027–2034.
65. Herlitz J, Ekstrom L, Wennerblom B, et al. Lidocaine in out-of-hospital ventricular fibrillation. Does it improve survival? *Resuscitation* 1997;33(3):199–205.

66. Gallik DM, Singer I, Meissner MD, et al. Hemodynamic and surface electrocardiographic effects of a new aqueous formulation of intravenous amiodarone. *Am J Cardiol* 2002;90(9):964–968.
67. Kudenchuk PJ, Cobb LA, Copass MK, et al. Amiodarone for resuscitation after out-of-hospital cardiac arrest due to ventricular fibrillation. *N Engl J Med* 1999;341(12):871–878.
68. Dorian P, Cass D, Schwartz B, et al. Amiodarone as compared with lidocaine for shock-resistant ventricular fibrillation. *N Engl J Med* 2002;346(12):884–890.
69. Rea RS, Kane-Gill SL, Rudis MI, et al. Comparing intravenous amiodarone or lidocaine, or both, outcomes for inpatients with pulseless ventricular arrhythmias. *Crit Care Med* 2006;34(6):1617–1623.
70. Abu-Laban RB, Christenson JM, Innes GD, et al. Tissue plasminogen activator in cardiac arrest with pulseless electrical activity. *N Engl J Med* 2002;346(20):1522–1528.
71. Bottiger BW, Bode C, Kern S, et al. Efficacy and safety of thrombolytic therapy after initially unsuccessful cardiopulmonary resuscitation: A prospective clinical trial. *Lancet* 2001;357(9268):1583–1585.
72. Fatovich DM, Dobb GJ, Clugston RA. A pilot randomised trial of thrombolysis in cardiac arrest (The TICA trial). *Resuscitation* 2004;61(3):309–313.
73. Janata K, Holzer M, Kurkciyan I, et al. Major bleeding complications in cardiopulmonary resuscitation: The place of thrombolytic therapy in cardiac arrest due to massive pulmonary embolism. *Resuscitation* 2003;57(1):49–55.
74. Kurkciyan I, Meron G, Sterz F, et al. Pulmonary embolism as a cause of cardiac arrest: Presentation and outcome. *Arch Intern Med* 2000;160(10):1529–1535.
75. Lederer W, Lichtenberger C, Pechlaner C, et al. Recombinant tissue plasminogen activator during cardiopulmonary resuscitation in 108 patients with out-of-hospital cardiac arrest. *Resuscitation* 2001;50(1):71–76.
76. Ruiz-Bailen M, Aguayo de Hoyos E, Serrano-Corcoles MC, et al. Efficacy of thrombolysis in patients with acute myocardial infarction requiring cardiopulmonary resuscitation. *Intensive Care Med* 2001;27(6):1050–1057.
77. Nolan JP, Morley PT, Vanden Hoek TL, et al. Therapeutic hypothermia after cardiac arrest: An advisory statement by the advanced life support task force of the International Liaison Committee on Resuscitation. *Circulation* 2003;108(1):118–121.
78. Mild therapeutic hypothermia to improve the neurologic outcome after cardiac arrest. *N Engl J Med* 2002;346(8):549–556.
79. Bernard SA, Gray TW, Buist MD, et al. Treatment of comatose survivors of out-of-hospital cardiac arrest with induced hypothermia. *N Engl J Med* 2002;346(8):557–563.
80. Shankaran S, Laptook AR, Ehrenkranz RA, et al. Whole-body hypothermia for neonates with hypoxic-ischemic encephalopathy. *N Engl J Med* 2005;353(15):1574–1584.
81. Bunch TJ, White RD, Gersh BJ, et al. Long-term outcomes of out-of-hospital cardiac arrest after successful early defibrillation. *N Engl J Med* 2003;348(26):2626–2633.
82. van den Berghe G, Wouters P, Weekers F, et al. Intensive insulin therapy in the critically ill patients. *N Engl J Med* 2001;345(19):1359–1367.
83. Annane D, Sebille V, Charpentier C, et al. Effect of treatment with low doses of hydrocortisone and fludrocortisone on mortality in patients with septic shock. *JAMA* 2002;288(7):862–871.
84. Hachimi-Idrissi S, Corne L, Ebinger G, et al. Mild hypothermia induced by a helmet device: A clinical feasibility study. *Resuscitation* 2001;51(3):275–281.
85. Gonzalez ER. Pharmacologic controversies in CPR. *Ann Emerg Med* 1993;22(2 pt 2):317–323.
86. Stueven HA, Tonsfeldt DJ, Thompson BM, et al. Atropine in asystole: Human studies. *Ann Emerg Med* 1984;13(9 pt 2):815–817.
87. Ornato JP, Gonzales ER, Morkunas AR, et al. Treatment of presumed asystole during pre-hospital cardiac arrest: Superiority of electrical countershock. *Am J Emerg Med* 1985;3(5):395–399.
88. Tortolani AJ, Risucci DA, Powell SR, Dixon R. In-hospital cardiopulmonary resuscitation during asystole. Therapeutic factors associated with 24-hour survival. *Chest* 1989;96(3):622–626.
89. Levy MM. An evidence-based evaluation of the use of sodium bicarbonate during cardiopulmonary resuscitation. *Crit Care Clin* 1998;14(3):457–483.
90. Bjerneroth G. Tribonat—A comprehensive summary of its properties. *Crit Care Med* 1999;27(5):1009–1013.
91. Kyriacou DN, Arcinue EL, Peek C, Kraus JF. Effect of immediate resuscitation on children with submersion injury. *Pediatrics* 1994;94(2 pt 1):137–142.
92. Schneider SM. Hypothermia: From recognition to rewarming. *Emerg Med Rep* 1992;13:1–20.
93. Goodwin AP, Pearce AJ. The human wedge. A manoeuvre to relieve aortocaval compression during resuscitation in late pregnancy. *Anaesthesia* 1992;47(5):433–434.
94. Munro PT. Management of eclampsia in the accident and emergency department. *J Accid Emerg Med* 2000;17(1):7–11.
95. Stanten RD, Iverson LI, Daugharty TM, et al. Amniotic fluid embolism causing catastrophic pulmonary vasoconstriction: Diagnosis by transesophageal echocardiogram and treatment by cardiopulmonary bypass. *Obstet Gynecol* 2003;102(3):496–498.
96. Boyd R, Teece S. Towards evidence based emergency medicine: Best BETs from the Manchester Royal Infirmary. Perimortem caesarean section. *Emerg Med J* 2002;19(4):324–325.
97. Working Group, Ad Hoc Subcommittee on Outcomes, American College of Surgeons-Committee on Trauma. Practice management guidelines for emergency department thoracotomy. *J Am Coll Surg* 2001;193(3):303–309.
98. Cooper MA. Lightning injuries: Prognostic signs for death. *Ann Emerg Med* 1980;9(3):134–138.
99. Stewart CE. When lightning strikes. *Emerg Med Serv* 2000;29(3):57–67; quiz 103.
100. Browne BJ, Gaasch WR. Electrical injuries and lightning. *Emerg Med Clin North Am* 1992;10(2):211–229.
101. Milzman DP, Moskowitz L, Hardel M. Lightning strikes at a mass gathering. *South Med J* 1999;92(7):708–710.
102. Vincent R. Drugs in modern resuscitation. *Br J Anaesth* 1997;79(2):188–197.
103. West VL. Alternate routes of administration. *J Intraven Nurs* 1998;21(4):221–231.
104. Calkins MD, Fitzgerald G, Bentley TB, Burris D. Intraosseous infusion devices: A comparison for potential use in special operations. *J Trauma* 2000;48(6):1068–1074.
105. Niemann JT, Stratton SJ. Endotracheal versus intravenous epinephrine and atropine in out-of-hospital "primary" and postcountershock asystole. *Crit Care Med* 2000;28(6):1815–1819.
106. Niemann JT, Stratton SJ, Cruz B, Lewis RJ. Endotracheal drug administration during out-of-hospital resuscitation: Where are the survivors? *Resuscitation* 2002;53(2):153–157.
107. Jennett B, Bond M. Assessment of outcome after severe brain damage. *Lancet* 1975;1(7905):480–484.
108. Jennett B, Teasdale G. Aspects of coma after severe head injury. *Lancet* 1977;1(8017):878–881.
109. Guyette FX, Guimond GE, Hostler D, Callaway CW. Vasopressin administered with epinephrine is associated with a return of a pulse in out-of-hospital cardiac arrest. *Resuscitation* 2004;63(3):277–282.
110. Lindner KH, Dirks B, Strohmenger HU, et al. Randomised comparison of epinephrine and vasopressin in patients with out-of-hospital ventricular fibrillation. *Lancet* 1997;349(9051):535–537.
111. Stiell IG, Hebert PC, Wells GA, et al. Vasopressin versus epinephrine for inhospital cardiac arrest: A randomised controlled trial. *Lancet* 2001;358(9276):105–109.
112. Grmec S, Mally S. Vasopressin improves outcome in out-of-hospital cardiopulmonary resuscitation of ventricular fibrillation and pulseless ventricular tachycardia: A observational cohort study. *Crit Care* 2006;10(1):R13–R20.
113. Stadlbauer KH, Krismer AC, Arntz HR, et al. Effects of thrombolysis during out-of-hospital cardiopulmonary resuscitation. *Am J Cardiol* 2006;97(3):305–308.

CHAPTER 15

Hypertension

JOSEPH J. SASEEN AND ERIC J. MACLAUGHLIN

KEY CONCEPTS

1. The risk of cardiovascular (CV) morbidity and mortality is directly correlated with blood pressure (BP). Even patients with prehypertension have an increased risk of CV disease.

2. Outcome trials have shown that antihypertensive drug therapy substantially reduces the risks of CV events and death in patients with hypertension.

3. Essential hypertension is usually an asymptomatic condition. A diagnosis cannot be made based on one elevated BP measurement. Elevated values from the average of two or more measurements on two or more clinical encounters are needed to diagnose hypertension.

4. The overall goal of treating hypertension is to reduce hypertension-associated morbidity and mortality from CV events. The selection of specific drug therapy is based on evidence that demonstrates CV risk reduction.

5. A goal BP of less than 140/90 mm Hg is appropriate for general prevention of CV events or CV disease. However, achieving BP of less than 130/80 mm Hg goal is recommended in patients with diabetes, significant chronic kidney disease, known coronary artery disease (myocardial infarction, stable angina, unstable angina), noncoronary atherosclerotic vascular disease (ischemic stroke, transient ischemic attack, peripheral arterial disease, abdominal aortic aneurism), or a 10% or greater 10-year risk of fatal coronary heart disease or nonfatal myocardial infarction based on Framingham risk scoring. Patients with left ventricular dysfunction (systolic heart failure) have a BP goal of less than 120/80 mm Hg.

6. Lifestyle modifications should be prescribed in all patients with hypertension and prehypertension. However, they should never be used as a replacement for antihypertensive drug therapy in patients with hypertension, especially patients with additional CV risk factors.

7. Thiazide-type diuretics have traditionally been classified as first-line agents for treating most patients with hypertension. This recommendation is supported by clinical trials showing reduced CV morbidity and mortality with thiazide diuretic therapy. Comparative data from the landmark Antihypertensive and Lipid-Lowering Treatment to Prevent Heart Attack Trial (ALLHAT) confirm the first-line role of thiazide-type diuretics.

8. An angiotensin-converting enzyme (ACE) inhibitor, angiotensin II receptor blocker (ARB), or calcium channel blocker (CCB) may be used as first-line agents in patients without compelling indications. Clinical trials have demonstrated that these agents reduce the risk of CV events when used to treat hypertension.

9. β-Blockers do not reduce CV events to the extent that thiazide-type diuretics, ACE inhibitors, ARBs, or CCBs do when used as the primary antihypertensive agent in patients with hypertension but without a compelling indication for β-blocker therapy.

10. Compelling indications are comorbid conditions where specific drug therapies have been shown in outcome trials to provide unique long-term benefits (reducing the risk of CV events).

11. Patients with diabetes are at very high risk for CV events. All patients with diabetes and hypertension should be managed with either an ACE inhibitor or an ARB. These are typically in combination with one or more other antihypertensive agents because multiple agents frequently are needed to lower BP to less than 130/80 mm Hg.

12. Older patients with isolated systolic hypertension are often at risk for orthostatic hypotension when antihypertensive drug therapy is started, particularly with diuretics, ACE inhibitors, and ARBs. Although overall treatment should be the same, low initial doses should be used and dosage titrations should be gradual to minimize risk of orthostatic hypotension.

13. Alternative antihypertensive agents have not been proven to reduce the risk of CV events compared with first-line antihypertensive agents. They should be used primarily in combination with first-line agents to provide additional BP lowering.

14. Hypertensive urgency is ideally managed by adjusting maintenance therapy (adding a new antihypertensive and/or increasing the dose of a present medication). This provides a gradual reduction in BP, which is a safer treatment approach than very rapid reductions in BP.

15. Most patients require combination therapy to achieve goal BP values. Combination regimens should include a diuretic, preferably a thiazide-type. If a diuretic was not the first drug used, it should be the second drug add-on therapy for most patients.

16. Patients have resistant hypertension when they fail to attain goal BP values while adherent with an appropriate three drug-regimen. This three-drug regimen must include full doses and include a diuretic.

Learning objectives, review questions, and other resources can be found at **www.pharmacotherapyonline.com.**

Hypertension is a common disease that is simply defined as persistently elevated arterial blood pressure (BP). Although elevated BP was perceived to be "essential" for adequate perfusion of essential organs during the early and middle 1900s, it is now identified as one of the most significant risk factors for cardiovascular (CV) disease. Increasing awareness and diagnosis of hypertension, and improving control of BP with appropriate treatment, are considered critical public health initiatives to reduce CV morbidity and mortality.

The Seventh Report of the Joint National Committee on the Detection, Evaluation, and Treatment of High Blood Pressure (JNC7) is the most prominent evidence-based clinical guideline in the United States for the management of hypertension,[1] supplemented by the 2007 American Heart Association (AHA) Scientific Statement on the treatment of hypertension.[2] This chapter reviews relevant components of these guidelines and additional evidence from clinical trials, with a focus on the pharmacotherapy of hypertension. Data from the National Health and Nutrition Examination Survey from 1999 to 2000 indicate that of the population of Americans with hypertension, 68.9% are aware that they have hypertension, only 58.4% are on some form of antihypertensive treatment, and only 34% of all patients have controlled BP.[3] Therefore, there are ample opportunities for clinicians to improve the care of patients with hypertension.

EPIDEMIOLOGY

Approximately 31% of the population (72 million Americans) have high BP (≥140/90 mm Hg).[4] The percentage of men with high BP is higher than that of women before the age of 45 years, but between the ages of 45 and 54 years the percentage is slightly higher with women.[4] After age 55 years, a much higher percentage of women have high BP than men.[4] Prevalence rates are highest in non-Hispanic blacks (33.5%) followed by non-Hispanic whites (28.9%) and Mexican Americans (20.7%).[3]

BP values increase with age, and hypertension (persistently elevated BP values) is very common in the elderly. The lifetime risk of developing hypertension among those 55 years of age and older who are normotensive is 90%.[1] Most patients have prehypertension before they are diagnosed with hypertension, with most diagnoses occurring between the third and fifth decades of life. In the population age ≥60 years, the prevalence of hypertension in 2000 was estimated at 65.4%, which is significantly higher than the 57.9% prevalence estimated in 1988.[3]

ETIOLOGY

In most patients, hypertension results from an unknown pathophysiologic etiology (*essential or primary hypertension*). This form of hypertension cannot be cured, but it can be controlled. A small percentage of patients have a specific cause of their hypertension (*secondary hypertension*). There are many potential secondary causes that are either concurrent medical conditions or are endogenously induced. If the cause can be identified, hypertension in these patients has the potential to be cured.

ESSENTIAL HYPERTENSION

More than 90% of individuals with hypertension have essential hypertension.[1] Numerous mechanisms have been identified that may contribute to the pathogenesis of this form of hypertension, so identifying the exact underlying abnormality is not possible. Genetic factors may play an important role in the development of essential hypertension. There are monogenic and polygenic forms of BP dysregulation that may be responsible for essential hypertension.[5] Many of these genetic traits feature genes that affect sodium balance, but genetic mutations altering urinary kallikrein excretion, nitric oxide release, and excretion of aldosterone, other adrenal steroids, and angiotensinogen are also documented.[5] In the future, identifying individuals with these genetic traits could lead to alternative approaches to preventing or treating hypertension; however, this is not currently recommended.

SECONDARY HYPERTENSION

Fewer than 10% of patients have secondary hypertension where either a comorbid disease or drug is responsible for elevating BP (Table 15–1).[1,6] In most of these cases, renal dysfunction resulting from severe chronic kidney disease or renovascular disease is the most common secondary cause. Certain drugs, either directly or indirectly, can cause hypertension or exacerbate hypertension by increasing BP. Table 15–1 lists the most common agents. Some of these agents are herbal products. Although these are not technically drugs, they have been identified as secondary causes. When a secondary cause is identified, removing the offending agent (when feasible) or treating/correcting the underlying comorbid condition should be the first step in management.

PATHOPHYSIOLOGY[5,7]

Multiple factors that control BP are potential contributing components in the development of essential hypertension. These include malfunctions in either humoral (i.e., the renin–angiotensin–aldosterone system [RAAS]) or vasodepressor mechanisms, abnormal

TABLE 15-1 Secondary Causes of Hypertension

Diseases	Drugs Associated with Hypertension in Humans[a]
Chronic kidney disease	**Prescription drugs**
Cushing's syndrome	• Adrenal steroids (e.g., prednisone, fludrocortisone, triamcinolone)
Coarctation of the aorta	• Amphetamines/anorexiants (e.g., phendimetrazine, phentermine, sibutramine)
Obstructive sleep apnea	• Antivascular endothelin growth factor agents (bevacizumab, sorafenib, sunitinib), estrogens (usually oral contraceptives)
Parathyroid disease	• Calcineurin inhibitors (cyclosporine and tracolimus)
Pheochromocytoma	• Decongestants (phenylpropanolamine and analogs)
Primary aldosteronism	• Erythropoiesis stimulating agents (erythropoietin and darbepoietin)
Renovascular disease	• Nonsteroidal antiinflammatory drugs, cyclooxygenase-2 inhibitors
Thyroid disease	• Others: venlafaxine, bromocriptine, bupropion, buspirone, carbamazepine, clozapine, desulfrane, ketamine, metoclopramide
	Situations: β-blocker or centrally acting α-agonists (when abruptly discontinued); β-blocker without α-blocker first when treating pheochromocytoma
	Street drugs and other natural products
	Cocaine and cocaine withdrawal
	Ephedra alkaloids (e.g., Ma-huang), "herbal ecstasy," other phenylpropanolamine analogs[a]
	Nicotine withdrawal, anabolic steroids, narcotic withdrawal, methylphenidate, phencyclidine, ketamine, ergotamine and other ergot-containing herbal products, St. John's wort
	Food substances
	Sodium
	Ethanol
	Licorice
	Tyramine-containing foods if taking a monoamine oxidase inhibitor

[a]Agents of most clinical importance.

Data from Kaplan NM, Kaplan's Clinical Hypertension. 8th ed. Philadelphia, PA: Lippincott Williams & Wilkins, 2002:1–550.

neuronal mechanisms, defects in peripheral autoregulation, and disturbances in sodium, calcium, and natriuretic hormones. Many of these factors are cumulatively affected by the multifaceted RAAS, which ultimately regulates arterial BP. It is probable that none of these factors is solely responsible for essential hypertension; however, most antihypertensives specifically target these mechanisms and components of the RAAS.

ARTERIAL BLOOD PRESSURE

Arterial BP is the pressure in the arterial wall measured in millimeters of mercury (mm Hg). The two typical arterial BP values are *systolic BP* (SBP) and *diastolic BP* (DBP). SBP is achieved during cardiac contraction and represents the peak value. DBP is achieved after contraction when the cardiac chambers are filling, and represents the nadir value. The difference between SBP and DBP is called the pulse pressure and is a measure of arterial wall tension. Mean arterial pressure is the average pressure throughout the cardiac cycle of contraction. It is sometimes used clinically to represent overall arterial BP, especially in hypertensive emergency. During a cardiac cycle, two-thirds of the time is spent in diastole and one-third in systole. Consequently, the mean arterial pressure can be estimated by using the following equation:

$$\text{mean arterial pressure} = (\text{SBP} \times 1/3) + (\text{DBP} \times 2/3)$$

Arterial BP is hemodynamically generated by the interplay between blood flow and the resistance to blood flow. It is mathematically defined as the product of cardiac output and total peripheral resistance according to the following equation:

$$\text{BP} = \text{cardiac output} \times \text{total peripheral resistance}$$

Cardiac output is the major determinant of SBP, whereas total peripheral resistance largely determines DBP. In turn, cardiac output is a function of stroke volume, heart rate, and venous capacitance. Table 15–2 lists physiologic causes of increased cardiac output and total peripheral resistance and correlates them to potential mechanisms of pathogenesis.

Under normal physiologic conditions, arterial BP fluctuates throughout the day. It typically follows a circadian rhythm, where it decreases to its lowest daily values during sleep. This is followed by a sharp rise starting a few hours prior to awakening with the highest values occurring midmorning. BP is also increased acutely during physical activity or emotional stress.

TABLE 15-2 Potential Mechanisms of Pathogenesis

Blood pressure is the mathematical product of cardiac output and peripheral resistance. Elevated blood pressure can result from increased cardiac output and/or increased total peripheral resistance.	
Increased cardiac output	Increased cardiac preload: • Increased fluid volume from excess sodium intake or renal sodium retention (from reduced number of nephrons or decreased glomerular filtration) Venous constriction: • Excess stimulation of the RAAS • Sympathetic nervous system overactivity
Increased peripheral resistance	Functional vascular constriction: • Excess stimulation of the RAAS • Sympathetic nervous system overactivity • Genetic alterations of cell membranes • Endothelial-derived factors Structural vascular hypertrophy: • Excess stimulation of the RAAS • Sympathetic nervous system overactivity • Genetic alterations of cell membranes • Endothelial-derived factors • Hyperinsulinemia resulting from obesity or the metabolic syndrome

RAAS, renin–angiotensin–aldosterone system.

TABLE 15-3 Classification of Blood Pressure in Adults (Age ≥18 Years)[a]

Classification	Systolic Blood Pressure (mm Hg)		Diastolic Blood Pressure (mm Hg)
Normal	<120	and	<80
Prehypertension[b]	120–139	or	80–89
Stage 1 hypertension	140–159	or	90–99
Stage 2 hypertension	≥160	or	≥100

[a]Classification determined based on the average of two or more properly measured seated blood pressure measurements from two or more clinical encounters. If systolic and diastolic blood pressure values yield different classifications, the highest category is used for the purpose of determining a classification.

[b]For patients with diabetes mellitus, significant chronic kidney disease, known coronary artery disease (myocardial infarction, stable angina, unstable angina), noncoronary atherosclerotic vascular disease (ischemic stroke, transient ischemic attack, peripheral arterial disease, abdominial aortic aneurism), or a Framingham risk score of 10% or greater, values ≥130/80 mm Hg are considered above goal; patients with left ventricular dysfuction have a blood pressure goal of less than 120/80 mm Hg.

Classification

The JNC7 classification of BP in adults (age ≥18 years) is based on the average of two or more properly measured BP readings from two or more clinical encounters (Table 15–3).[1] It includes four categories: normal, prehypertension, stage 1 hypertension, and stage 2 hypertension. Prehypertension is not considered a disease category, but identifies patients whose BP is likely to increase into the classification of hypertension in the future.

Hypertensive crises are clinical situations where BP values are very elevated, typically greater than 180/120 mm Hg.[7] They are categorized as either a *hypertensive emergency* or *hypertensive urgency*. Hypertensive emergencies are extreme elevations in BP that are accompanied by acute or progressing target-organ damage. Hypertensive urgencies are high elevations in BP without acute or progressing target-organ injury. Recommendations for managing hypertensive crises are described later in this chapter.

❶ Cardiovascular Risk and Blood Pressure

Epidemiologic data clearly indicate a strong correlation between BP and CV morbidity and mortality.[8] Risk of stroke, myocardial infarction, angina, heart failure, kidney failure, or early death from a CV cause are directly correlated with BP. Starting at a BP of 115/75 mm Hg, risk of CV disease doubles with every 20/10 mm Hg increase.[1] Even patients with prehypertension have an increased risk of CV disease.

❷ Treating patients with hypertension with antihypertensive drug therapy provides significant benefits. Large-scale, placebo-controlled, outcome trials show that the increased risks of CV events and death associated with elevated BP are reduced substantially by antihypertensive drug therapy.[9–12]

SBP is a stronger predictor of CV disease than DBP in adults ≥50 years of age and is the most important clinical BP parameter for most patients.[1] Patients with DBP values less than 90 mm Hg and SBP values ≥140 mm Hg have *isolated systolic hypertension*. Isolated systolic hypertension is believed to result from pathophysiologic changes in the arterial vasculature consistent with aging. These changes decrease the compliance of the arterial wall and portend an increased risk of CV morbidity and mortality. Pulse pressure is the difference between the SBP and the DBP. It is believed to reflect extent of atherosclerotic disease in the elderly and is a measure of increased arterial stiffness. Higher pulse pressure values are correlated with an increased risk of CV mortality, especially in those with isolated systolic hypertension.

HUMORAL MECHANISMS

Several humoral abnormalities may be involved in the development of essential hypertension. These abnormalities may involve the RAAS, natriuretic hormones, and hyperinsulinemia.

The Renin–Angiotensin–Aldosterone System

The RAAS is a complex endogenous system that is involved with most regulatory components of arterial BP. Activation and regulation are primarily governed by the kidney (Fig. 15–1). The RAAS regulates sodium, potassium, and fluid balance. Consequently, this system significantly influences vascular tone and sympathetic nervous system activity and is the most influential contributor to the homeostatic regulation of BP.

Renin is an enzyme that is stored in the juxtaglomerular cells, which are located in the afferent arterioles of the kidney. The release of renin is modulated by several factors: intrarenal factors (e.g., renal perfusion pressure, catecholamines, angiotensin II), and extrarenal factors (e.g., sodium, chloride, and potassium).

Juxtaglomerular cells function as a baroreceptor-sensing device. Decreased renal artery pressure and kidney blood flow are sensed by these cells and stimulate secretion of renin. The juxtaglomerular apparatus also includes a group of specialized distal tubule cells referred to collectively as the *macula densa.* A decrease in sodium and chloride delivered to the distal tubule stimulates renin release. Catecholamines increase renin release probably by directly stimulating sympathetic nerves on the afferent arterioles that in turn activate the juxtaglomerular cells. Decreased serum potassium and/or intracellular calcium are detected by the juxtaglomerular cells resulting in renin secretion.

Renin catalyzes the conversion of angiotensinogen to angiotensin I in the blood. Angiotensin I is then converted to angiotensin II by angiotensin-converting enzyme (ACE). After binding to specific receptors (classified as either AT_1 or AT_2 subtypes), angiotensin II exerts biologic effects in several tissues. The AT_1 receptor is located in brain, kidney, myocardium, peripheral vasculature, and the adrenal glands. These receptors mediate most responses that are critical to CV and kidney function. The AT_2 receptor is located in adrenal medullary tissue, uterus, and brain. Stimulation of the AT_2 receptor does not influence BP regulation.

Circulating angiotensin II can elevate BP through pressor and volume effects. Pressor effects include direct vasoconstriction, stimulation of catecholamine release from the adrenal medulla, and centrally mediated increases in sympathetic nervous system activity. Angiotensin II also stimulates aldosterone synthesis from the adrenal cortex. This leads to sodium and water reabsorption that increases plasma volume, total peripheral resistance, and ultimately BP. Aldosterone also has a deleterious role in the pathophysiology of other CV diseases (heart failure, myocardial infarction [MI] and kidney dis-

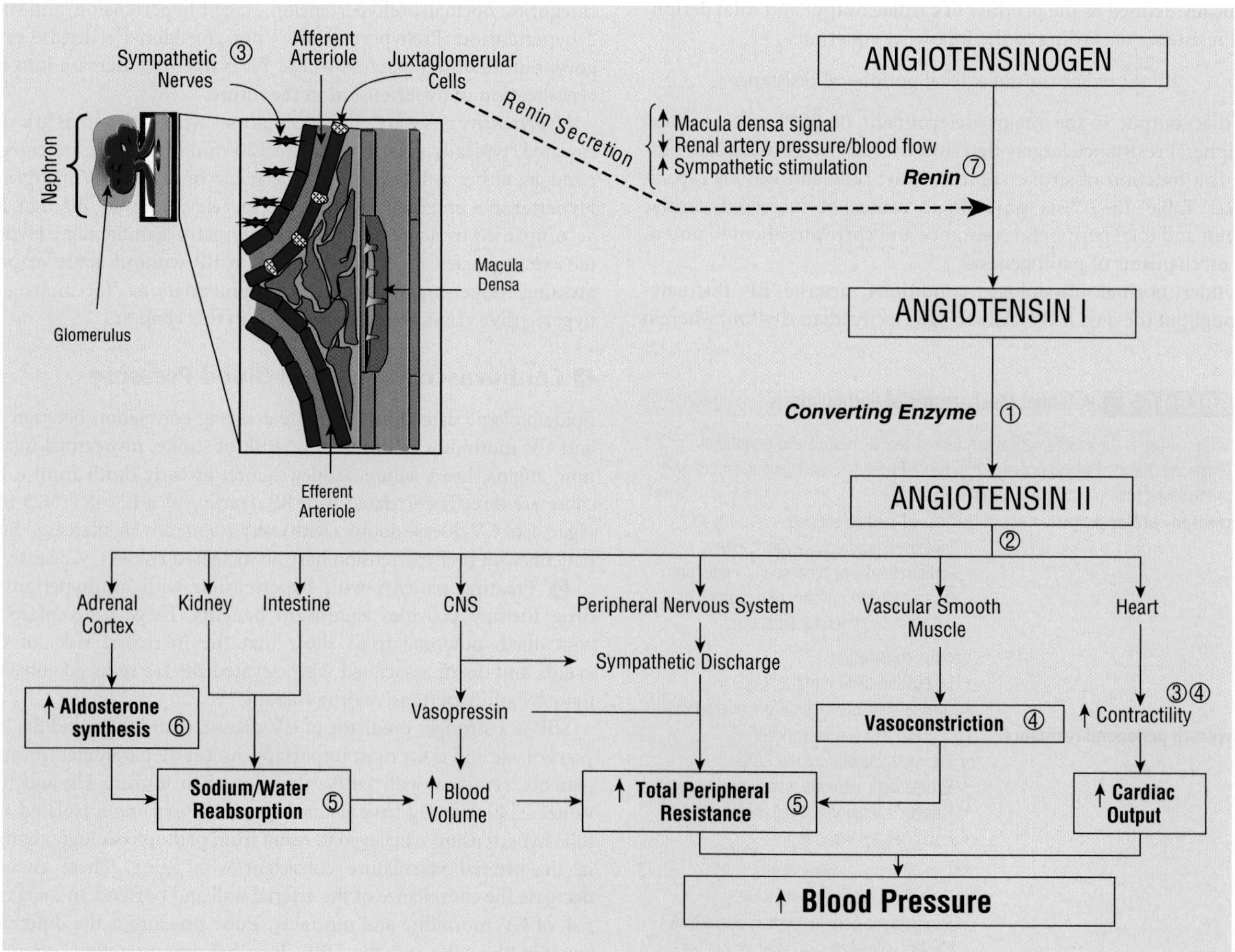

FIGURE 15-1. Diagram representing the renin–angiotensin–aldosterone system. The interrelationship between the kidney, angiotensin II, and regulation of blood pressure are depicted. There are three major regulators of renin secretion from the juxtaglomerular cells in this system. The primary sites of action for major antihypertensive agents are included. (①, angiotensin-converting enzyme inhibitors; ②, angiotensin II receptor blockers; ③, β-blockers; ④, calcium channel blockers; ⑤, diuretics; ⑥, aldosterone antagonists; ⑦, direct renin inhibitor; CNS, central nervous system.)

ease) by promoting tissue remodeling leading to myocardial fibrosis and vascular dysfunction. Clearly, any disturbance in the body that leads to activation of the RAAS could explain chronic hypertension.

The heart and brain contain a local RAAS. In the heart, angiotensin II is also generated by a second enzyme, angiotensin I convertase (human chymase). This enzyme is not blocked by ACE inhibition. Activation of the myocardial RAAS increases cardiac contractility and stimulates cardiac hypertrophy. In the brain, angiotensin II modulates the production and release of hypothalamic and pituitary hormones, and enhances sympathetic outflow from the medulla oblongata.

Peripheral tissues can locally generate biologically active angiotensin peptides, which may explain the increased vascular resistance seen in hypertension. Some evidence suggests that angiotensin produced by local tissue may interact with other humoral regulators and endothelium-derived growth factors to stimulate vascular smooth muscle growth and metabolism. These angiotensin peptides may, in fact, instigate increased vascular resistance in low plasma renin forms of hypertension. Components of the tissue RAAS may also be responsible for the long-term hypertrophic abnormalities seen with hypertension (left ventricular hypertrophy, vascular smooth muscle hypertrophy, and glomerular hypertrophy).

Natriuretic Hormone

Natriuretic hormone inhibits sodium and potassium-adenosine triphosphatase and thus interferes with sodium transport across cell membranes. Inherited defects in the kidney's ability to eliminate sodium can cause an increased blood volume. A compensatory increase in the concentration of circulating natriuretic hormone theoretically could increase urinary excretion of sodium and water. However, this same hormone is also thought to block the active transport of sodium out of arteriolar smooth muscle cells. The increased intracellular sodium concentration ultimately would increase vascular tone and BP.

Insulin Resistance and Hyperinsulinemia

The development of hypertension and associated metabolic abnormalities is referred to as the metabolic syndrome.[13] Hypothetically, increased insulin concentrations may lead to hypertension because of increased renal sodium retention and enhanced sympathetic nervous system activity. Moreover, insulin has growth hormone-like actions that can induce hypertrophy of vascular smooth muscle cells. Insulin also may elevate BP by increasing intracellular calcium, which leads to increased vascular resistance. The exact mechanism by which insulin resistance and hyperinsulinemia occur in hypertension is unknown. However, this association is strong because many of the criteria used to define this population (elevated BP, abdominal obesity, dyslipidemia, and elevated fasting glucose) are often present in patients with hypertension.[13]

NEURONAL REGULATION

Central and autonomic nervous systems are intricately involved in the regulation of arterial BP. A number of receptors that either enhance or inhibit norepinephrine release are located on the presynaptic surface of sympathetic terminals. The α and β presynaptic receptors play a role in negative and positive feedback to the norepinephrine-containing vesicles located near the neuronal ending. Stimulation of presynaptic α-receptors (α_2) exerts a negative inhibition on norepinephrine release. Stimulation of presynaptic β-receptors facilitates norepinephrine release.

Sympathetic neuronal fibers located on the surface of effector cells innervate the α- and β-receptors. Stimulation of postsynaptic α-receptors (α_1) on arterioles and venules results in vasoconstriction. There are two types of postsynaptic β-receptors, β_1 and β_2. Both are present in all tissue innervated by the sympathetic nervous system. However, in some tissues β_1-receptors predominate and in other tissues β_2-receptors predominate. Stimulation of β_1-receptors in the heart results in an increase in heart rate and contractility, whereas stimulation of β_2-receptors in the arterioles and venules causes vasodilation.

The baroreceptor reflex system is the major negative-feedback mechanism that controls sympathetic activity. Baroreceptors are nerve endings lying in the walls of large arteries, especially in the carotid arteries and aortic arch. Changes in arterial pressure rapidly activate baroreceptors that then transmit impulses to the brainstem through the ninth cranial nerve and vagus nerves. In this reflex system, a decrease in arterial BP stimulates baroreceptors, causing reflex vasoconstriction and increased heart rate and force of cardiac contraction. These baroreceptor reflex mechanisms may be blunted (less responsive to changes in BP) in the elderly and those with diabetes.

Stimulation of certain areas within the central nervous system (nucleus tractus solitarius, vagal nuclei, vasomotor center, and the area postrema) can either increase or decrease BP. For example, α_2-adrenergic stimulation within the central nervous system decreases BP through an inhibitory effect on the vasomotor center. However, angiotensin II increases sympathetic outflow from the vasomotor center, which increases BP.

The purpose of these neuronal mechanisms is to regulate BP and maintain homeostasis. Pathologic disturbances in any of the four major components (autonomic nerve fibers, adrenergic receptors, baroreceptors, or central nervous system) could conceivably lead to chronically elevated BP. These systems are physiologically interrelated. A defect in one component may alter normal function in another, and such cumulative abnormalities may then explain the development of essential hypertension.

PERIPHERAL AUTOREGULATORY COMPONENTS

Abnormalities in renal or tissue autoregulatory systems could cause hypertension. It is possible that a renal defect in sodium excretion may first develop, which can then cause resetting of tissue autoregulatory processes resulting in a higher arterial BP. The kidney usually maintains normal BP through a volume-pressure adaptive mechanism. When BP drops, the kidneys respond by increasing retention of sodium and water. These changes lead to plasma volume expansion that increases BP. Conversely, when BP rises above normal, renal sodium and water excretion are increased to reduce plasma volume and cardiac output. This ultimately will maintain homeostatic BP conditions.

Local autoregulatory processes maintain adequate tissue oxygenation. When tissue oxygen demand is normal to low, the local arteriolar bed remains relatively vasoconstricted. However, increases in metabolic demand trigger arteriolar vasodilation that lowers peripheral vascular resistance and increases blood flow and oxygen delivery through autoregulation.

Intrinsic defects in these renal adaptive mechanisms could lead to plasma volume expansion and increased blood flow to peripheral tissues, even when BP is normal. Local tissue autoregulatory processes that vasoconstrict would then be activated to offset the increased blood flow. This effect would result in increased peripheral vascular resistance, and if sustained, would also result in thickening of the arteriolar walls. This pathophysiologic component is plausible because increased total peripheral resistance is a common underlying finding in patients with essential hypertension.

VASCULAR ENDOTHELIAL MECHANISMS

Vascular endothelium and smooth muscle play important roles in regulating blood vessel tone and BP. These regulating functions are mediated through vasoactive substances that are synthesized by endothelial cells. It has been postulated that a deficiency in the local synthesis of vasodilating substances (prostacyclin and bradykinin) or excess vasoconstricting substances (angiotensin II and endothelin I) contribute to essential hypertension, atherosclerosis, and other CV diseases.

Nitric oxide is produced in the endothelium, relaxes the vascular epithelium, and is a very potent vasodilator. The nitric oxide system is an important regulator of arterial BP. Patients with hypertension may have an intrinsic deficiency in nitric oxide, resulting in inadequate vasodilation.

ELECTROLYTES AND OTHER CHEMICALS

Epidemiologic and clinical data have associated excess sodium intake with hypertension. Population-based studies indicate that high salt diets are associated with a high prevalence of stroke and hypertension. Conversely, low salt diets are associated with a low prevalence of hypertension. Clinical studies consistently show that dietary sodium restriction lowers BP in many (but not all) patients with elevated BP. The exact mechanisms by which excess sodium leads to hypertension are unknown. However, they may be linked to increased circulating natriuretic hormones, which would inhibit intracellular sodium transport causing increased vascular reactivity and increased BP.

Altered calcium homeostasis also may play an important role in the pathogenesis of hypertension. A lack of dietary calcium hypothetically can disturb the balance between intracellular and extracellular calcium, resulting in an increased intracellular calcium concentration. This imbalance can alter vascular smooth muscle function by increasing peripheral vascular resistance. Some studies show that dietary calcium supplementation results in a modest BP reduction in patients with hypertension.

The role of potassium fluctuations is also inadequately understood. Potassium depletion may increase peripheral vascular resistance, but the clinical significance of small serum potassium concentration changes is unclear. Furthermore, data demonstrating reduced CV risk with dietary potassium supplementation is very limited.

CLINICAL PRESENTATION

CLINICAL PRESENTATION OF HYPERTENSION

General

- The patient may appear very healthy, or may have the presence of additional CV risk factors:
  - Age (≥55 years for men and 65 years for women)
  - Diabetes mellitus
  - Dyslipidemia (elevated low-density lipoprotein-cholesterol, total cholesterol, and/or triglycerides; low high-density lipoprotein-cholesterol)
  - Microalbuminuria
  - Family history of premature CV disease
  - Obesity (body mass index ≥30 kg/m^2)
  - Physical inactivity
  - Tobacco use

Symptoms

- Most patients are asymptomatic.

Signs

- Previous BP values in the prehypertension or hypertension category.

Laboratory Tests

- Blood urea nitrogen/serum creatinine, fasting lipid panel, fasting blood glucose, serum electrolytes, spot urine albumin-to-creatinine ratio. The patient may have normal values and still have hypertension. However, some may have abnormal values consistent with either additional CV risk factors or hypertension-related damage.

Other Diagnostic Tests

- 12-lead electrocardiogram (to detect left ventricular hypertrophy), estimated glomerular filtration rate (using Modification of Diet in Renal Disease equation).
- 10-year risk of fatal coronary heart disease or non-fatal myocardial infarction, based on Framingham scoring.

Target-Organ Damage

- The patient may have a previous medical history or diagnostic findings that indicate the presence of hypertension-related target-organ damage:
- Brain (stroke, transient ischemic attack)
- Eyes (retinopathy)
- Heart (left ventricular hypertrophy, angina or prior MI, prior coronary revascularization, heart failure)
- Kidney (chronic kidney disease)
- Peripheral vasculature (peripheral arterial disease)

❸ DIAGNOSTIC CONSIDERATIONS

Hypertension is termed the "silent killer" because most patients do not have symptoms. The primary physical finding is elevated BP. The diagnosis of hypertension cannot be made based on one elevated BP measurement. The average of two or more measurements taken during two or more clinical encounters should be used to diagnose hypertension.[1] Thereafter, this BP average can be used to establish a diagnosis, and then classify the stage of hypertension present using Table 15–3.

Measuring Blood Pressure

Indirect measurement of BP using a sphygmomanometer is a common routine medical screening tool that should be conducted at every healthcare encounter.[1]

Sphygmomanometry—American Heart Association Procedure[14] The appropriate procedure to measure BP has been described by the AHA.[14] It is imperative that the measurement equipment (inflation cuff, stethoscope, manometer) meet certain national standards to ensure maximum quality and precision with the ascultatory measurement of BP.

The AHA stepwise technique is recommended:

- Patients should refrain from nicotine or caffeine ingestion for 30 minutes and be seated with the lower back supported in a chair and with their bare arm supported and resting near heart level. Feet should be flat on the floor (with legs not crossed). Measuring BP in the supine or standing position may be required under special circumstances (suspected orthostatic hypotension, volume depletion, or dehydration). The measurement environment should be relatively quiet and provide privacy.
- Measurement should begin only after a 5-minute period of rest.
- A properly sized cuff (pediatric, small, regular, large, or extra large) should be used. If the cuff is too small, the measured BP can be overestimated. The inflatable rubber bladder inside the cuff should encircle at least 80% of the arm of the upper arm in length and 40% in width.

- The palpatory method should be used to estimate the SBP:
  - Place the cuff on the upper arm 2 to 3 cm above the antecubital fossa and attach it to the manometer (either a mercury or aneroid)
  - Close the inflation valve with the thumb and index finger, and inflate the cuff to 70 mm Hg
  - Simultaneously palpate the radial pulse with the index and middle fingers of the opposite hand
  - Inflate in increments of 10 mm Hg by pumping the inflation bulb (as it is resting in the palm of your hand) with the pinky, ring, and middle fingers (the last three) until the radial pulse disappears
  - Note the pressure at which radial pulse disappears; this is the estimated SBP
  - Release pressure from the cuff by turning the valve counter-clockwise
- The bell (not the diaphragm) of the stethoscope should be placed on the skin of the antecubital fossa, directly over where the brachial artery is palpated. The stethoscope earpieces should be inserted appropriately. The valve should be closed with the cuff then inflated rapidly to about 30 mm Hg above the estimated SBP from the palpatory method. The value should be only slightly opened to release pressure at a very slow rate of 2 to 3 mm Hg per second.
- The clinician should listen for Korotkoff sounds with the stethoscope. The first phase of Korotkoff sounds are the initial presence of clear tapping sounds. Note the pressure at the first recognition of these sounds. This is the SBP. As pressure continues to deflate, note the pressure when all sounds disappear (also known as the fifth Korotkoff phase). This is the DBP.
- Measurements should be taken to the nearest 2 mm Hg.
- A second measurement should be obtained after a minimum of 1 minute, and the average should be documented. If these values differ by more than 5 mm Hg, additional measurements should be collected and averaged.
- Neither the patient nor the observer should talk during measurement.
- At the first visit, BP should be measured in both arms. When consistent interarm differences exist, the higher number should be used for diagnostic and treatment purposes.

It is recommended that the stethoscope bell, rather than the diaphragm, be used for measurement, although some studies suggest little difference between two.[14] Low-frequency Korotkoff sounds, however, may not be heard clearly and accurately with the diaphragm. This is especially problematic in patients with faint or "distant" sounds.

Inaccuracies with indirect measurements result from inherent biologic variability of BP, inaccuracies related to suboptimal technique, and the white coat effect.[14] Variations in BP occur with environmental temperature, the time of day and year, meals, physical activity, posture, alcohol, nicotine, and emotions. In the clinic setting, standard BP measurement procedures (e.g., appropriate rest period, poor technique, minimal number of measurements) are often not followed, which results in poor estimation of true BP. Approximately 15% to 20% of patients have *white coat hypertension,* where BP values rise in a clinical setting but return to normal in nonclinical environments using home or ambulatory BP measurements.[14] Interestingly, the rise in BP dissipates gradually over several hours after leaving the clinical setting. It may or may not be precipitated by other stresses in the patient's daily life.

CLINICAL CONTROVERSY

Aggressive treatment of white coat hypertension is controversial. However, patients with white coat hypertension may have increased CV risk compared with those without such BP changes.[15]

Several additional factors can result in erroneous BP measurements. *Pseudohypertension* is a falsely elevated BP measurement. It may be seen in the elderly, those with long-standing diabetes, or in those with chronic kidney disease caused by rigid, calcified brachial arteries.[14] In these patients, the true arterial BP when measured directly with intraarterial measurement (the most accurate measurement of BP) is much lower than that measured using the indirect cuff method. The Osler maneuver can be used to test for pseudohypertension. In this maneuver, the BP cuff is inflated above peak SBP. If the radial artery remains palpable, the patient has a positive Osler sign (rigid artery), which may indicate pseudohypertension.

Elderly patients with a wide pulse pressure may have an auscultatory gap which can lead to underestimated SBP or overestimated DBP measurements.[14] In this situation, as the cuff pressure falls from the true SBP value, the Korotkoff sound may disappear (indicating a false DBP measurement), reappear (a false SBP measurement), and then disappear again at the true DBP value. This is often identified by using the palpatory method to estimate SBP and then inflating the cuff an additional 30 mm Hg above this estimate because the "gap" is usually less than 30 mm Hg. When an auscultatory gap is present, Korotkoff sounds are usually heard when pressure in the cuff first starts to decrease after inflation. This may be eliminated by raising the arm overhead for 30 seconds before bringing it to the proper position and inflating the cuff. This maneuver decreases the intravascular volume and improves inflow thereby allowing Korotkoff sounds to be heard.[14]

Patients with irregular ventricular heart rates (e.g., atrial fibrillation, atrial flutter) may have misleading BP values when measured indirectly. In this situation, SBP and DBP values may vary from one heartbeat to the next.

Ambulatory and Self Blood Pressure Monitoring

Ambulatory BP monitoring using an automated device can document BP at frequent time intervals (e.g., every 15 to 30 minutes) throughout a 24-hour period.[14] Ambulatory BP values are usually lower than clinic-measured values. The upper limit for normal ambulatory BP is 140/90 mm Hg during the day, 125/75 mm Hg at night, and 135/85 mm Hg during 24 hours. Home BP measurements are collected by patients, preferably in the morning, using home monitoring devices. Either of these may be warranted in patients with suspected white coat hypertension (without hypertension-related target-organ damage) to differentiate white coat from essential hypertension.[1] Moreover, ambulatory BP monitoring may be helpful in patients with apparent drug resistance, hypotensive symptoms while on antihypertensive therapy, episodic hypertension (e.g., white coat hypertension), autonomic dysfunction, and to identify "nondippers" whose BP does not decrease by >10% during sleep and which may portend increased risk of BP-related complications.[1,14]

Some data suggest that 24-hour and home BP measurements correlate better with CV risk than do conventional office-based BP measurements.[14,16] However, one controlled study found that ambulatory BP and self BP monitoring are complementary to conventional clinic-based measurements.[17] Limitations of these measurements that may prohibit routine use of such technology include lack of validated devices, complexity of use, costs, and lack of prospective outcomes data describing normal ranges for these measurements. Although self-monitoring of BP at home is less complicated and less costly than ambulatory monitoring, patients may omit or fabricate readings. Thus, devices that have a memory or printouts are recommended.[14]

CLINICAL EVALUATION

Frequently, the only sign of essential hypertension is elevated BP. The rest of the physical examination may be completely normal. However, a complete medical evaluation (a comprehensive medical history, physical examination, and laboratory and/or diagnostic tests) is recommended after diagnosis to (a) identify secondary causes, (b) identify other CV risk factors or comorbid conditions that may define prognosis and/or guide therapy, and (c) assess for the presence or absence of hypertension-associated target-organ damage.[1] All patients with hypertension should have the following measured prior to initiating therapy: 12-lead electrocardiogram; spot urine albumin-to-creatinine ratio; blood glucose and hematocrit; serum potassium, creatinine (with estimated glomerular filtration rate [GFR]), and calcium; and a fasting lipid panel.[1,18] For patients without a history of coronary artery disease, noncoronary atherosclerotic vascular disease (also referred to as coronary artery disease risk equivalents), left ventricular dysfunction, or diabetes, it is also important to estimate a 10-year risk of fatal coronary heart disease or nonfatal myocardial infarction using Framingham Risk scoring (*http://www.nhlbi.nih.gov/guidelines/cholesterol/risk_tbl.htm*).[2]

Secondary Causes

Table 15–1 lists the most common secondary causes of hypertension. A complete medical evaluation may provide clues for identifying secondary hypertension.

Patients with secondary hypertension may complain of symptoms suggestive of the underlying disorder, but some are asymptomatic. Patients with pheochromocytoma may have a history of paroxysmal headaches, sweating, tachycardia, and palpitations. Over half of these patients suffer from episodes of orthostatic hypotension. In primary aldosteronism, symptoms related to hypokalemia usually include muscle cramps and muscle weakness. Patients with Cushing's syndrome may complain of weight gain, polyuria, edema, menstrual irregularities, recurrent acne, or muscular weakness and have several classic physical features (e.g., moon face, buffalo hump, hirsutism, abdominal striae). Patients with coarctation of the aorta may have diminished or even absent femoral pulses, and patients with renal artery stenosis may have an abdominal systolic–diastolic bruit.

Routine laboratory tests may also help identify secondary hypertension. Baseline hypokalemia may suggest mineralocorticoid-induced hypertension. Protein, blood cells, and casts in the urine may indicate renovascular disease. Some laboratory tests are used specifically to diagnose secondary hypertension. These include plasma norepinephrine and urinary metanephrine for pheochromocytoma, plasma and urinary aldosterone concentrations for primary aldosteronism, and plasma renin activity, captopril stimulation test, and renal artery angiography for renovascular disease.

Certain medications and herbal products can result in drug-induced hypertension (see Table 15–1). For some patients, the addition of these agents can be the cause of hypertension or can exacerbate underlying hypertension. Identifying a temporal relationship between starting the suspected agent and developing elevated BP is most suggestive of drug-induced BP elevation.

NATURAL COURSE OF DISEASE

Essential hypertension is usually preceded by elevated BP values that are in the prehypertension category. BP values may fluctuate between elevated and normal levels for an extended period of time. These changes may begin as early as the second decade of life. During this stage, many patients have a hyperdynamic circulation with increased cardiac output and normal or even low peripheral vascular resistance. As the disease progresses, peripheral vascular resistance increases, and BP elevation is sustained to the point where essential hypertension is diagnosed.

Target-Organ Damage

Target-organ damage (see Clinical Presentation of Hypertension above) can develop as a complication of hypertension. The primary organs involved are the eye, brain, heart, kidneys, and peripheral blood vessels. Clinical CV events (e.g., MI, stroke, kidney failure) are clinical end points of target-organ damage and are the primary causes of CV morbidity and mortality in patients with hypertension. The probability of CV events and CV morbidity and mortality in patients with hypertension is directly correlated with the severity of BP elevation and additional CV risk factors.

Hypertension accelerates atherosclerosis and stimulates left ventricular and vascular hypertrophy. These pathologic changes are thought to be secondary to both a chronic pressure overload and a variety of nonhemodynamic stimuli. Some of the nonhemodynamic disturbances that have been implicated in these effects include the adrenergic system, RAAS, increased synthesis and secretion of endothelin I, and a decreased production of prostacyclin and nitric oxide. Accelerated atherogenesis in hypertension is accompanied by proliferation of smooth muscle cells, lipid infiltration into the vascular endothelium, and an enhancement of vascular calcium accumulation.

Cerebrovascular disease is a consequence of hypertension. A neurologic assessment can detect either gross neurologic deficits or a slight hemiparesis with some incoordination and hyperreflexia that are indicative of cerebrovascular disease. Stroke can result from lacunar infarcts caused by thrombotic occlusion of small vessels or intracerebral hemorrhage resulting from ruptured microaneurysms. Transient ischemic attacks secondary to atherosclerotic disease in the carotid arteries are possible long-term complications of hypertension.

Retinopathies can occur in hypertension and may manifest as a variety of different findings. A funduscopic examination can detect hypertensive retinopathy and can be categorized according to the Keith-Wagener-Barker retinopathy classification. Retinopathy manifests as arteriolar narrowing, focal arteriolar constrictions, arteriovenous crossing changes (nicking), retinal hemorrhages and exudates, and disk edema. Accelerated arteriosclerosis, a long-term consequence of essential hypertension, can cause nonspecific changes such as increased light reflex, increased tortuosity of vessels, and arteriovenous nicking. Focal arteriolar narrowing, retinal infarcts, and flame-shaped hemorrhages usually are suggestive of accelerated or malignant phase of hypertension. Papilledema is swelling of the optic disk and is caused by a breakdown in autoregulation of capillary blood flow in the presence of high pressure. It is usually only present in hypertensive emergencies.

Heart disease is the best identified form of target-organ damage. A thorough cardiac and pulmonary examination can identify cardiopulmonary abnormalities. Clinical manifestations include left ventricular hypertrophy, coronary heart disease (angina, prior MI, and prior coronary revascularization), and heart failure. These complications may lead to cardiac arrhythmias, angina, MI, and sudden death. Coronary disease (also called coronary heart disease or coronary artery disease) and associated CV events are the most common causes of death in patients with hypertension.

The kidney damage caused by hypertension is characterized pathologically by hyaline arteriosclerosis, hyperplastic arteriosclerosis, arteriolar hypertrophy, fibrinoid necrosis, and atheroma of the major renal arteries. Glomerular hyperfiltration and intraglomerular hypertension are early stages of hypertensive nephropathy. Microalbuminuria is followed by a gradual decline in renal function. The primary renal complication in hypertension is nephrosclerosis, which is secondary to arteriosclerosis. Atheromatous disease of a major renal artery may give rise to renal artery stenosis. Although overt kidney failure is an uncommon complication of essential hypertension, it is an important cause of end-stage kidney disease, especially in African Americans, Hispanics, and Native Americans. It is not completely understood why these ethnic groups are more at risk for kidney decline than other ethnic groups.

The peripheral vasculature is a target organ. Physical examination of the vascular system can detect evidence of atherosclerosis, which may present as arterial bruits (aortic, abdominal, or peripheral), distended veins, diminished or absent peripheral arterial pulses, or lower-extremity edema. Peripheral arterial disease is a clinical condition that can result from atherosclerosis, which is accelerated in hypertension. Other CV risk factors (e.g., smoking) can increase the likelihood of peripheral arterial disease as well as all other forms of target-organ damage.

TREATMENT

Hypertension

■ DESIRED OUTCOMES

❹ Overall Goal of Therapy

The overall goal of treating hypertension is to reduce hypertension-associated morbidity and mortality.[1] This morbidity and mortality is related to target-organ damage (e.g., CV events, heart failure, and kidney disease). Reducing risk remains the primary purpose of hypertension therapy and the specific choice of drug therapy is significantly influenced by evidence demonstrating such risk reduction.

❺ Surrogate Goal of Therapy

Treating patients with hypertension to achieve a desired target BP value is simply a surrogate goal of therapy. Reducing BP to goal does not guarantee that target-organ damage will not occur. However, attaining goal BP values is associated with lower risk of CV disease and target-organ damage.[1,19] Targeting a goal BP value is a tool that clinicians can easily use to evaluate response to therapy and is the primary method used to determine the need for titration and regimen modification.

Most patients have a goal BP of less than 140/90 mm Hg for the general prevention of CV events or CV disease (e.g., coronary artery disease).[1,2] However, this goal is lowered to less than 130/80 mm Hg for patients with diabetes, significant chronic kidney disease, known coronary artery disease (myocardial infarction, stable angina, unstable angina), noncoronary atherosclerotic vascular disease (ischemic stroke, transient ischemic attack, peripheral arterial disease, abdominal aortic aneurism), or a 10% or greater 10-year risk of fatal coronary heart disease or nonfatal myocardial infarction based on Framingham risk scoring (*http://www.nhlbi.nih.gov/guidelines/cholesterol/risk_tbl.htm*).[2] Moreover, patients with left ventricular dysfunction (heart failure) have a BP goal of less than 120/80 mm Hg.[2]

GOAL BLOOD PRESSURE VALUES RECOMMENDED BY THE AMERICAN HEART ASSOCIATION IN 2007[2]

• Most patients for general prevention	<140/90 mm Hg
• Patients with diabetes (referred to as coronary artery disease risk equivalent), significantchronic kidney disease, known coronary artery disease (myocardial infarction, stable angina, unstable angina), noncoronary atherosclerotic vascular disease (ischemic stroke, transient ischemic attack, peripheral arterial disease, abdominal aortic aneurism [referred to as coronary artery disease risk equivalents]), or a Framingham risk score of 10% or greater	<130/80 mm Hg
• Patients with left ventricular dysfunction (heart failure)	<120/80 mm Hg

Significant chronic kidney disease is considered to be moderate-to-severe chronic kidney disease, defined as estimated GFR <60 mL/min/1.73 m^2 (correlating to a serum creatinine >1.3 mg/dL in women and >1.5 in men) or albuminuria (>300 mg/day or >200 mg/g creatinine).

Framingham risk score is calculated using the risk calculator available at *http://www.nhlbi.nih.gov/guidelines/cholesterol/risk_tbl.htm*

Some clinicians advocate attaining BP goal values that are lower than what is recommended as a modality to further reduce CV risk following the myth that "lower is better." Contrary to this, a *J-curve hypothesis,* where lowering BP too much might increase the risk of CV events, has been described.[20] However, these data are based off of observational studies and cannot establish a cause-and-effect relationship because of confounding variables.

Lower goal BP values have been evaluated prospectively in the Hypertension Optimal Treatment (HOT) trial.[19] In this study, more than 18,700 patients were randomized to target DBP values of 90 mm Hg or less, 85 mm Hg or less, or 80 mm Hg or less. Although the actual DBP values achieved were 85.2, 83.2, and 81.1 mm Hg, respectively, the risk of major CV events was the lowest with a BP of 139/83 mm Hg, and the lowest risk of stroke was with a BP of 142/80 mm Hg. Risk of events in subjects with either diabetes or ischemic heart disease were lowest at DBP values of less than 80 mm Hg. No J-curve relationship was seen.

CLINICAL CONTROVERSY

There is increasing evidence suggesting that ambulatory BP measurements may be more accurate and better predict target-organ damage than manual BP measurements using a sphygmomanometer in a clinic setting (considered the gold standard).[14] Studies document that large numbers of individuals may be misdiagnosed or misclassified based on clinic BP measurements as a result of a variety of factors such as poor technique, daily variability of BP, and white coat hypertension. Validated ambulatory BP monitoring may obviate some of these factors, but their role in the routine management of hypertension is unclear.

■ AVOIDING CLINICAL INERTIA

Although hypertension is one of the most common medical conditions, BP control rates are poor. Many patients, especially older patients, with hypertension are at goal DBP values but continue to have elevated SBP values. It has been estimated that of the hypertensive population that is treated, yet not controlled, 76.9% have SBP ≥140 mm Hg with DBP values less than 90 mm Hg.[21] For most patients with hypertension, attaining the SBP goal almost always assures achievement of the DBP goal. When coupled with the fact that SBP is a better predictor of CV risk than DBP, SBP must be used as the primary clinical marker of disease control in hypertension.

Clinical inertia in hypertension has been defined as an office visit at which no therapeutic move was made to lower BP in a patient with uncontrolled hypertension.[22] Clinical inertia is not the entire reason why most patients with hypertension do not have at-goal BP values. However, it is certainly a major reason that can be simply remedied through more aggressive treatment with drug therapy. This can involve initiating, titrating, or changing drug therapy.

■ GENERAL APPROACH TO TREATMENT

After a definitive diagnosis of hypertension is made, most patients should be placed on both lifestyle modifications and drug therapy concurrently. Lifestyle modification alone is considered appropriate therapy for patients with prehypertension. However, lifestyle modi-

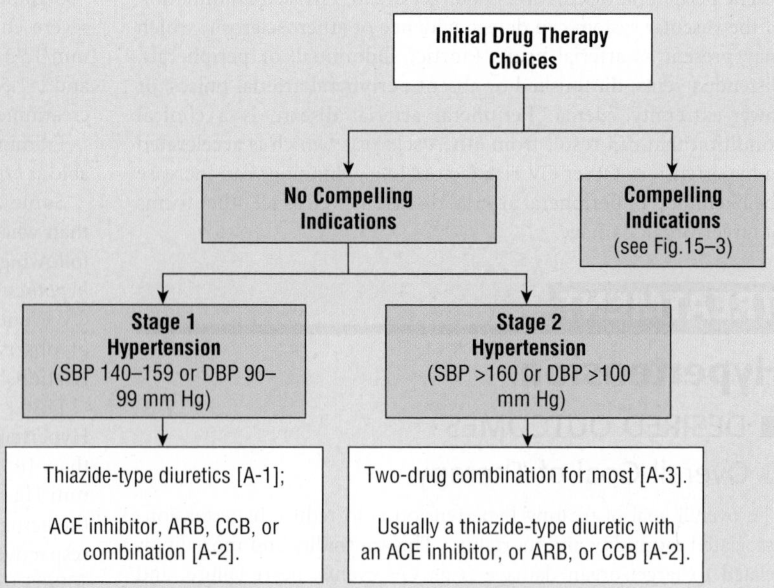

FIGURE 15-2. Algorithm for treatment of hypertension. Drug therapy recommendations are graded with strength of recommendation and quality of evidence in brackets. Strength of recommendations: A, B, C = good, moderate, and poor evidence to support recommendation, respectively. Quality of evidence: 1 = Evidence from more than 1 properly randomized, controlled trial. 2 = Evidence from at least one well-designed clinical trial with randomization; from cohort or case-controlled analytic studies; or dramatic results from uncontrolled experiments or subgroup analyses. 3 = Evidence from opinions of respected authorities, based on clinical experience, descriptive studies, or reports of expert communities. (ACE, angiotensin-converting enzyme; ARB, angiotensin receptor blocker; CCB, calcium channel blocker; DBP, diastolic blood pressure; SBP, systolic blood pressure.) *(Adapted from references 1 and 2.)*

fications alone are not considered adequate for patients with hypertension and additional CV risk factors, especially patients with BP goals of less than 130/80 mm Hg (e.g., diabetes, coronary artery disease, chronic kidney disease) or less than 120/80 mm Hg (i.e., left ventricular dysfunction), who have not attained this goal BP.

The choice of initial drug therapy depends on the degree of BP elevation and presence of compelling indications (see Patients with Compelling Indications section). Most patients with stage 1 hypertension should be initially treated with a thiazide-type diuretic, ACE inhibitor, ARB, or CCB. For patients with more severe BP elevation (stage 2 hypertension), combination drug therapy, with one of the agents being preferably a thiazide type-diuretic, is recommended. Figure 15–2 outlines this general approach. There are six compelling indications where specific antihypertensive drug classes have evidence showing unique benefits in patients with the compelling indication (Fig. 15–3).

■ ❻ NONPHARMACOLOGIC THERAPY

All patients with prehypertension and hypertension should be prescribed lifestyle modifications. Table 15–4 lists modifications that lower BP. These approaches are recommended by the JNC7 and the AHA.[1,23] They can provide small to moderate reductions in SBP. Aside from lowering BP in patients with known hypertension, lifestyle modification can decrease the progression to hypertension in patients with prehypertension BP values.[23] In a portion of patients with hypertension that have relatively good BP control while on single antihypertensive drug therapy, sodium reduction and weight loss may allow withdrawal of drug therapy.[24]

A sensible dietary program is one that is designed to reduce weight gradually, for overweight and obese patients, and one that restricts sodium intake with only moderate alcohol consumption. Successful implementation of dietary lifestyle modifications by clinicians requires aggressive promotion through reasonable patient education, encouragement, and continued reinforcement. Patients may better understand the rationale for dietary intervention in hypertension if they are provided the following observations and facts[23]:

1. Hypertension is two to three times more likely in overweight than in lean persons.
2. More than 60% of patients with hypertension are overweight.
3. As little as 10 pounds of weight loss can decrease BP significantly in overweight patients.
4. Abdominal obesity is associated with the metabolic syndrome, which is a precursor to diabetes, dyslipidemia, and, ultimately, CV disease.[13]
5. Diets rich in fruits and vegetables and low in saturated fat lower BP in patients with hypertension.
6. Most people experience some degree of SBP reduction with sodium restriction.

The Dietary Approaches to Stop Hypertension (DASH) eating plan is a diet that is rich in fruits, vegetables, and low-fat dairy products with a reduced content of saturated and total fat. It is advocated by the JNC7 as a reasonable and feasible diet that is proven to lower BP. Intake of sodium should be minimized as much as possible, ideally to 1.5 g/day, although an interim goal of less than 2.3 g/day may be reasonable considering the difficulty in achieving these low intakes. Patients should be aware of the multiple sources of dietary sodium (e.g., processed foods, soups, table salt) so that they may follow these recommendations. Potassium intake should be encouraged through fruits and vegetables with high content (ideally 4.7 g/day) in those with normal kidney function. Excessive alcohol use can either cause or worsen hypertension. Patients with hypertension who drink alcoholic beverages should restrict their daily intake (see Table 15–4). Patients should be counseled that 1 drink is equivalent to 1.5 oz of 80-proof distilled spirits (e.g., whiskey), a 5 oz glass of wine (12%), or 12 oz of beer.[23]

Carefully designed programs of physical activity can lower BP. Regular physical activity for at least 30 minutes most days of the week is recommended for all adults, with at least 60 minutes recommended for adults attempting to lose weight or maintain weight loss.[25] Studies show that aerobic exercise can reduce BP, even in the absence of weight loss. Patients should consult their physicians before starting an exercise program, especially those with CV and/or target-organ disease.

Cigarette smoking is a major, independent, modifiable risk factor for CV disease. Patients with hypertension who smoke should be thoroughly counseled regarding the additional health risks that result from smoking. Moreover, the potential benefits that cessation can provide should be explained to encourage cessation. Several smoking-cessation programs, pharmacotherapy options, and aids are available to assist patients.

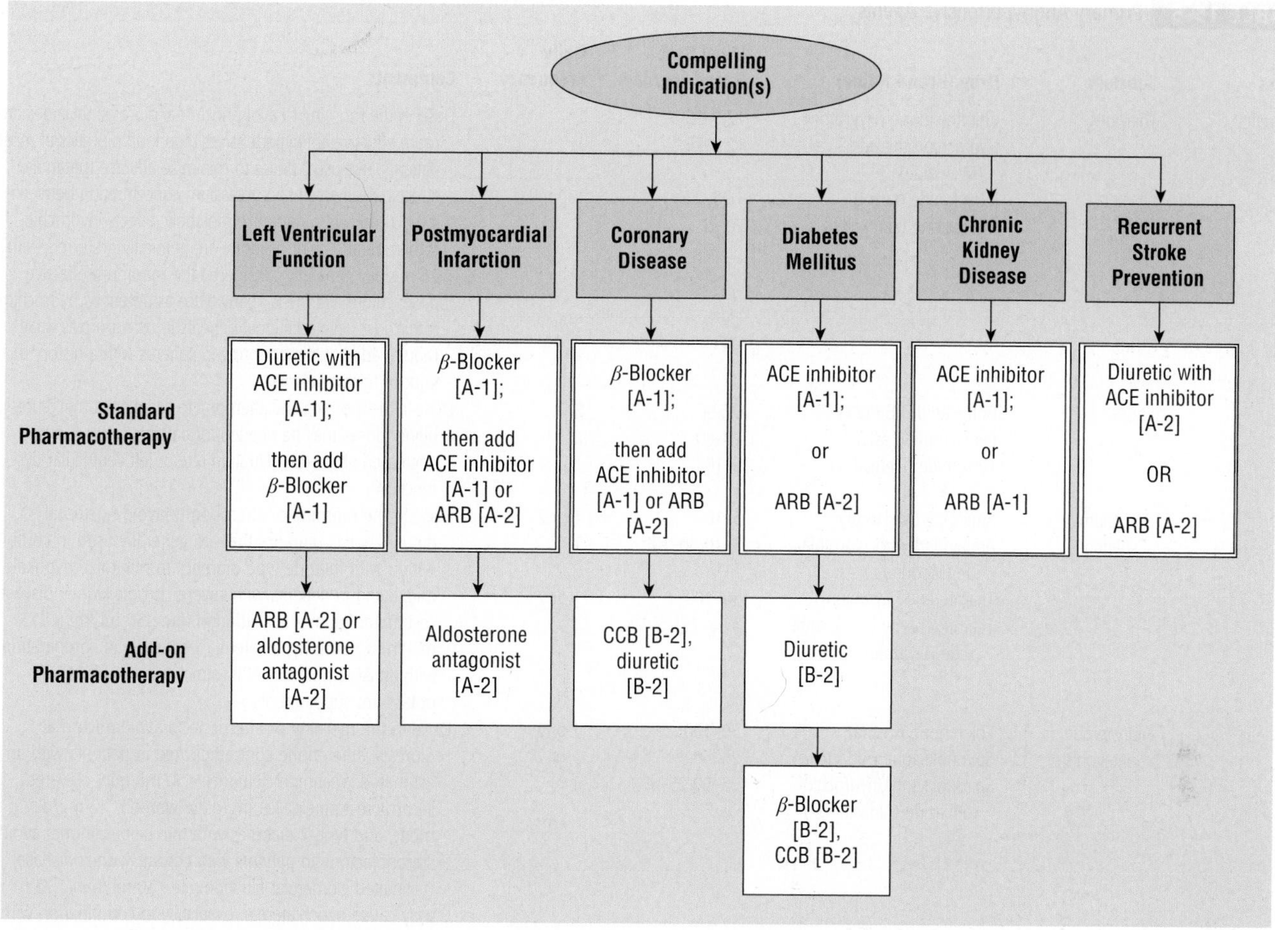

FIGURE 15-3. Compelling indications for individual drug classes. Compelling indications for specific drugs are evidence-based recommendations from outcome studies or existing clinical guidelines. The order of drug therapies serves as a general guidance that should be balanced with clinical judgment and patient response; however, standard pharmacotherapy should be considered first-line recommendations, preferably in the order depicted. Add-on pharmacotherapy recommendations then are intended to be used to further reduce risk of cardiovascular events and to lower blood pressure to goal values. Blood pressure control should be managed concurrently with the compelling indication. Drug therapy recommendations are graded with strength of recommendation and quality of evidence in brackets. Strength of recommendations: A, B, C = good, moderate, and poor evidence to support recommendation, respectively. Quality of evidence: 1 = Evidence from more than one properly randomized, controlled trial. 2 = Evidence from at least one well-designed clinical trial with randomization; from cohort or case-controlled analytic studies or multiple time series; or dramatic results from uncontrolled experiments or subgroup analyses. 3 = Evidence from opinions of respected authorities, based on clinical experience, descriptive studies, or reports of expert communities. (ACE, angiotensin-converting enzyme; ARB, angiotensin receptor blocker; CCB, calcium channel blocker.) *(Adapted from references 1, 2, 58, and 74.)*

■ PHARMACOTHERAPY

A diuretic (primarily a thiazide-type), ACE inhibitor, angiotensin II receptor blocker (ARB), or calcium channel blocker (CCB) are considered primary antihypertensive agents that are acceptable first-line options (Table 15–5). These agents should be used to treat the majority of patients with hypertension because evidence from outcomes data have demonstrated CV risk reduction benefits with these classes. Several have subclasses where significant differences in mechanism of action, clinical use, side effects, or evidence from outcomes studies exist. β-Blockers are effective antihypertensive agents that previously were considered primary agents. They are now preferred either to treat a specific compelling indication, or in combination with one of the aforementioned primary antihypertensive agents for

TABLE 15-4 Lifestyle Modifications to Prevent and Manage Hypertension

Modification	Recommendation	Approximate Systolic Blood Pressure Reduction (mm Hg)[a]
Weight loss	Maintain normal body weight (body mass index 18.5–24.9 kg/m^2)	5–20 per 10-kg weight loss
DASH-type dietary patterns	Consume a diet rich in fruits, vegetables, and low-fat dairy products with a reduced content of saturated and total fat	8–14
Reduced salt intake	Reduce daily dietary sodium intake as much as possible, ideally to ≈65 mmol/day (1.5 g/day sodium, or 3.8 g/day sodium chloride)	2–8
Physical activity	Regular aerobic physical activity (at least 30 min/day, most days of the week)	4–9
Moderation of alcohol intake	Limit consumption to ≤2 drinks/day in men and ≤1 drink/day in women and lighter-weight persons	2–4

DASH, Dietary Approaches to Stop Hypertension.
[a]Effects of implementing these modifications are time and dose dependent and could be greater for some patients.
Data from Chobanian et al.,[1] and Kostis et al.[24]

TABLE 15-5 Primary Antihypertensive Agents

Class	Subclass	Drug (Brand Name)	Usual Dose Range (mg/day)	Daily Frequency	Comments
Diuretics	Thiazides	Chlorthalidone (Hygroton)	12.5–25	1	Dose in the morning to avoid nocturnal diuresis; thiazides are more effective antihypertensives than loop diuretics in most patients; use usual doses to minimize adverse metabolic effects; ideally maintain potassium concentration between 4.0–5.0 mEq/L to minimize metabolic effects; hydrochlorothiazide and chlorthalidone are generally preferred, with 25 mg/day generally considered the maximum effective dose; chlorthalidone is nearly twice as potent as hydrochlorothiazide; have additional benefits in osteoporosis; may require additional monitoring in patients with a history of gout or hyperglycemia
		Hydrochlorothiazide (Microzide)	12.5–25	1	
		Indapamide (Lozol)	1.25–2.5	1	
		Metolazone (Zaroxolyn)	2.5–5	1	
	Loops	Bumetanide (Bumex)	0.5–4	2	Dose in the morning and afternoon to avoid nocturnal diuresis; higher doses may be needed for patients with severely decreased glomerular filtration rate or left ventricular dysfunction
		Furosemide (Lasix)	20–80	2	
		Torsemide (Demadex)	5–10	1	
	Potassium sparing	Amiloride (Midamor)	5–10	1 or 2	Dose in the morning or afternoon to avoid nocturnal diuresis; weak diuretics that are generally used in combination with thiazide-type diuretics to minimize hypokalemia; avoid in patients with severe chronic kidney disease (estimated glomerular filtration rate <30 mL/min/1.73 m^2); may cause hyperkalemia, especially in combination with an ACE inhibitor, ARB, direct renin inhibitor or potassium supplements
		Amiloride/hydrochlorothiazide (Moduretic)	5–10/50–100	1	
		Triamterene (Dyrenium)	50–100	1 or 2	
		Triamterene/hydrochlorothiazide (Dyazide)	37.5–75/25–50	1	
	Aldosterone antagonists	Eplerenone (Inspra)	50–100	1 or 2	Dose in the morning or afternoon to avoid nocturnal diuresis; eplerenone contraindicated in patients with an estimated creatinine clearance <50 mL/min, elevated serum creatinine (>1.8 mg/dL in women, >2 mg/dL in men), and type 2 diabetes with microalbuminuria; avoid spironolactone in patients with chronic kidney disease (estimated glomerular filtration rate <30 mL/min/1.73 m^2); may cause hyperkalemia, especially in combination with an ACE inhibitor, ARB, direct renin inhibitor or potassium supplements
		Spironolactone (Aldactone)	25–50	1 or 2	
		Spironolactone/hydrochlorothiazide (Aldactazide)	25–50/25–50	1	
ACE inhibitors		Benazepril (Lotensin)	10–40	1 or 2	Starting dose may be reduced 50% in patients who are on a diuretic, are volume depleted, or are very elderly because of risks of hypotension; may cause hyperkalemia in patients with chronic kidney disease or in those receiving potassium-sparing diuretics, aldosterone antagonists, ARB, or direct renin inhibitors; can cause acute kidney failure in patients with severe bilateral renal artery stenosis or severe stenosis in artery to solitary kidney; do not use in pregnancy or in patients with a history of angioedema
		Captopril (Capoten)	25–150	2 or 3	
		Enalapril (Vasotec)	5–40	1 or 2	
		Fosinopril (Monopril)	10–40	1	
		Lisinopril (Prinivil, Zestril)	10–40	1	
		Moexipril (Univasc)	7.5–30	1 or 2	
		Perindopril (Aceon)	4–16	1	
		Quinapril (Accupril)	10–80	1 or 2	
		Ramipril (Altace)	2.5–10	1 or 2	
		Trandolapril (Mavik)	1–4	1	
ARBs		Candesartan (Atacand)	8–32	1 or 2	Starting dose may be reduced 50% in patients who are on a diuretic, are volume depleted, or are very elderly because of risks of hypotension; may cause hyperkalemia in patients with chronic kidney disease or in those receiving potassium-sparing diuretics, aldosterone antagonists, ACE inhibitors, or direct renin inhibitor; can cause acute kidney failure in patients with severe bilateral renal artery stenosis or severe stenosis in artery to solitary kidney; do not cause a dry cough like ACE inhibitors may; do not use in pregnancy
		Eprosartan (Teveten)	600–800	1 or 2	
		Irbesartan (Avapro)	150–300	1	
		Losartan (Cozaar)	50–100	1 or 2	
		Olmesartan (Benicar)	20–40	1	
		Telmisartan (Micardis)	20–80	1	
		Valsartan (Diovan)	80–320	1	
Calcium channel blockers	Dihydropyridines	Amlodipine (Norvasc)	2.5–10	1	Short-acting dihydropyridines should be avoided, especially immediate-release nifedipine and nicardipine; dihydropyridines are more potent peripheral vasodilators than nondihydropyridines and may cause more reflex sympathetic discharge (tachycardia), dizziness, headache, flushing, and peripheral edema; have additional benefits in Raynaud's syndrome
		Felodipine (Plendil)	5–20	1	
		Isradipine (DynaCirc)	5–10	2	
		Isradipine SR (DynaCirc SR)	5–20	1	
		Nicardipine SR (Cardene SR)	60–120	2	
		Nifedipine long-acting (Adalat CC, Procardia XL)	30–90	1	
		Nisoldipine (Sular)	10–40	1	

(continued)

TABLE 15-5 Primary Antihypertensive Agents (continued)

Class	Subclass	Drug (Brand Name)	Usual Dose Range (mg/day)	Daily Frequency	Comments
	Nondihydropyridines	Diltiazem SR (Cardizem SR)	180–360	2	Extended-release and sustained-release products are preferred for hypertension; these agents block slow channels in the heart and reduce heart rate; may produce heart block, especially in combination with β-blockers; these products are not AB rated as interchangeable on a equipotent mg-per-mg basis because of different release mechanisms and different bioavailability parameters; Cardizem LA, Covera HS, and Verelan PM have delayed drug release for several hours after dosing; when dosed in the evening can provide chronotherapeutic drug delivery starting shortly before patients awake from sleep; have additional benefits in patients with atrial tachyarrhythmia
		Diltiazem SR (Cardizem CD, Cartia XT, Dilacor XR, Diltia XT, Tiazac, Taztia XT)	120–480	1	
		Diltiazem ER (Cardizem LA)	120–540	1 (morning or evening)	
		Verapamil SR (Calan SR, Isoptin SR, Verelan)	180–480	1 or 2	
		Verapamil ER (Covera HS)	180–420	1 (in the evening)	
		Verapamil oral drug absorption system ER (Verelan PM)	100–400	1 (in the evening)	
β-Blockers	Cardioselective	Atenolol (Tenormin)	25–100	1	Abrupt discontinuation may cause re-bound hypertension; inhibit β_1-receptors at low to moderate dose, higher doses also block β_2-receptors; may exacerbate asthma when selectivity is lost; have additional benefits in patients with atrial tachyarrhythmia or preoperative hypertension
		Betaxolol (Kerlone)	5–20	1	
		Bisoprolol (Zebeta)	2.5–10	1	
		Metoprolol tartrate (Lopressor)	100–400	2	
		Metoprolol succinate (Toprol XL)	50–200	1	
	Nonselective	Nadolol (Corgard)	40–120	1	Abrupt discontinuation may cause rebound hypertension; inhibit β_1- and β_2-receptors at all doses; can exacerbate asthma; have additional benefits in patients with essential tremor, migraine headache, thyrotoxicosis
		Propranolol (Inderal)	160–480	2	
		Propranolol long-acting (Inderal LA, InnoPran XL)	80–320	1	
		Timolol (Blocadren)	10–40	1	
	Intrinsic sympathomimetic activity	Acebutolol (Sectral)	200–800	2	Abrupt discontinuation may cause rebound hypertension; partially stimulate β-receptors while blocking against additional stimulation; no clear advantage for these agents; contraindicated in patients with coronary disease or post-myocardial infarction
		Carteolol (Cartrol)	2.5–10	1	
		Penbutolol (Levatol)	10–40	1	
		Pindolol (Visken)	10–60	2	
	Mixed α- and β-blockers	Carvedilol (Coreg)	12.5–50	2	Abrupt discontinuation may cause rebound hypertension; additional α-blockade produces more orthostatic hypotension
		Carvedilol phosphate (Coreg CR)	20–80	1	
		Labetalol (Normodyne, Trandate)	200–800	2	

ACE, angiotensin-converting enzyme; ARB, angiotensin receptor blocker; ER, extended-release; SR, sustained-release.

patients without a compelling indication. Other antihypertensive drug classes are considered alternative drug classes that may be used in select patients after primary agents (Table 15–6).

CLINICAL CONTROVERSY

Prehypertension is a BP classification that identifies patients who do not have hypertension, but are at risk for developing it. The Trial of Preventing Hypertension (TROPHY) showed that treating patients with prehypertension with the ARB candesartan decreased progression to stage 1 hypertension.[26] However, it is not known whether managing prehypertension with antihypertensive drug therapy, in addition to lifestyle modifications, decreases CV events or whether this treatment approach is cost-effective.

❼ Thiazide-Type Diuretics as Traditional First-Line Therapy for Most Patients

JNC7 guidelines recommend thiazide-type diuretics whenever possible, as first-line therapy for most patients, which is consistent with the traditional pharmacotherapy of hypertension.[1] However, AHA guidelines do not recommend thiazide-type diuretics as preferred over an ACE inhibitor, ARB, or CCB for first-line therapy. Figure 15–2 displays the algorithm for the treatment of hypertension. This recommendation is specifically for patients without compelling indications and is based on best available evidence demonstrating reductions in CV morbidity and mortality.

Landmark placebo-controlled clinical trials—SHEP (Systolic Hypertension in the Elderly Program),[9] STOP (Swedish Trial in Old Patients),[10] and MRC (Medical Research Council)[11]—showed significant reductions in stroke, MI, all-cause CV disease, and mortality with thiazide-type diuretic-based therapy versus placebo. These trials allowed for β-blockers as add-on therapy for BP control. Newer agents (ACE inhibitors, ARBs, and CCBs) were not available at the time of these studies. However, subsequent clinical trials have compared these newer antihypertensive agents to thiazide-type diuretics.[27–32] These data show similar effects, but most trials used a prospective open-label, blinded end point study methodology that is not double-blinded and limited their ability to prove equivalence of newer drugs to diuretics. Other prospective trials have compared different primary antihypertensive agents to each other.[29,33,34] Although these studies used head-to-head comparisons, they did not use a thiazide-type diuretic as their comparator treatment. Consequently, their results cannot be easily used to justify an antihypertensive drug class other than a thiazide-type diuretic as first-line therapy.

The ALLHAT Study[30] The result of the Antihypertensive and Lipid-Lowering Treatment to Prevent Heart Attack Trial (ALLHAT) was the deciding evidence that the JNC7 used to justify thiazide-type diuretics as first-line therapy.[30] It was designed to test the hypothesis that newer antihypertensive agents (an α-blocker, ACE inhibitor, or dihydropyridine CCB) would be superior to thiazide-type diuretic-based therapy. The primary objective was to compare the combined end point of fatal coronary heart disease and nonfatal MI. Other hypertension-related complications (e.g., heart failure,

TABLE 15-6 Alternative Antihypertensive Agents

Class	Drug (Brand Name)	Usual Dose Range (mg/day)	Daily Frequency	Comments
α_1-Blockers	Doxazosin (Cardura)	1–8	1	First dose should be given at bedtime; counsel patients to rise from a sitting or laying position slowly to minimize risk of orthostatic hypotension; have additional benefits in men with benign prostatic hyperplasia
	Prazosin (Minipress)	2–20	2 or 3	
	Terazosin (Hytrin)	1–20	1 or 2	
Direct renin inhibitor	Aliskiren (Tekturna)	150–300	1	May cause hyperkalemia in patients with chronic kidney diease and diabetes or in those receiving a potassium-sparing diuretic, aldosterone antagonist, ACE inhibitor, or ARB; may cause acute kidney failure in patients with severe bilateral renal artery stenosis or severe stenosis in artery to solitary kidney; do not use in pregnancy
Central α_2-agonists	Clonidine (Catapres)	0.1–0.8	2	Abrupt discontinuation may cause rebound hypertension; most effective if used with a diuretic to diminish fluid retention; clonidine patch is replaced once per week; not recommended in very elderly
	Clonidine patch (Catapres-TTS)	0.1–0.3	1 weekly	
	Methyldopa (Aldomet)	250–1000	2	
Peripheral adrenergic antagonist	Reserpine (generic only)	0.05–0.25		A very useful agent that has been used in many of the major clinical trials; should be used with a diuretic to diminish fluid retention
Direct arterial vasodilators	Minoxidil (Loniten)	10–40	1 or 2	Should be used with diuretic and β-blocker to diminish fluid retention and reflex tachycardia
	Hydralazine (Apresoline)	20–100	2 to 4	

ACE, angiotensin-converting enzyme; ARB, angiotensin receptor blocker.

stroke) were evaluated as secondary end points. This was the largest hypertension trial ever conducted and included 42,418 patients ages 55 and older with hypertension and one additional CV risk factor. This prospective, double-blind trial randomized patients to chlorthalidone-, amlodipine-, doxazosin-, or lisinopril-based therapy for a mean of 4.9 years.

The doxazosin arm was terminated early when a significantly higher risk of heart failure versus chlorthalidone was observed.[35] The other arms were continued as scheduled and no significant differences in the primary end point were seen between the chlorthalidone and lisinopril or amlodipine treatment groups. However, chlorthalidone had statistically fewer secondary end points than amlodipine (heart failure) and lisinopril (combined CV disease, heart failure, and stroke). The study conclusions were that chlorthalidone-based therapy was superior in preventing one or more major forms of CV disease and was less expensive than amlodipine or lisinopril-based therapy.

ALLHAT was designed as a superiority study with the hypothesis that amlodipine, doxazosin, and lisinopril would be better than chlorthalidone.[36] It did not prove this hypothesis because the primary end point was no different between chlorthalidone, amlodipine, and lisinopril. Many subgroup analyses of specific populations (e.g., black patients, chronic kidney disease, diabetes) from the ALLHAT have been conducted to assess response in certain unique patient populations.[37–39] Surprisingly, none of these analyses demonstrated superior CV event reductions with lisinopril or amlodipine versus chlorthalidone. Overall, thiazide-type diuretics remain unsurpassed in their ability to reduce CV morbidity and mortality in most patients.

Most patients require two or more agents to control BP. Therefore, a thiazide-type diuretic should be one of these agents unless contraindicated.

❽ Other First-Line Treatment Options for Most Patients

Clinical trials data cumulatively demonstrate that ACE inhibitor-, CCB-, or ARB-based antihypertensive therapy reduces CV events. These agents may be used in patients without compelling indications, similarly to thiazide-type diuretics, as first-line therapy. The Blood Pressure Lowering Treatment Trialists' Collaboration evaluated the incidence of major CV events and death among different antihypertensive drug classes from 29 major randomized trials in 162,341 patients.[40] In placebo-controlled trials, the incidences of major CV events were significantly lower with ACE inhibitor- and CCB-based regimens than with placebo. Although there were differences in the incidences of certain CV events in some comparisons (e.g., stroke was lower with diuretic- or CCB-based regiments versus ACE inhibitor-based regimens), there were no differences in total major CV events when ACE inhibitors, CCBs, or diuretics were compared to each other. In studies evaluating ARB-based therapy to control regimens, the incidence of major CV events was lower with ARB-based regimens. However, the control regimens used in these comparisons included both active antihypertensive drug therapies and placebo.

Data from meta-analyses may not be as influential as data from well-designed, prospective, randomized, controlled trials (e.g., the ALLHAT). However, they provide clinically useful data that support using ACE inhibitor-, CCB-, or ARB-based treatment for hypertension as first-line therapy. Clinicians can use meta-analyses data as supporting evidence when selecting an alternative first-line antihypertensive regimen for hypertension in most patients, in addition to the 2007 AHA recommendations.[41]

Other major consensus guidelines recommend multiple first-line options for treating hypertension in most patients. The 2007 European Society of Hypertension–European Society of Cardiology guidelines and the 2006 United Kingdom's National Institute for Health and the Clinical Excellence guidelines list more than one drug therapy option as an acceptable first-line treatment approach.[42,43] The European Society of Hypertension–European Society of Cardiology guidelines are founded on the principle that CV risk reduction is a function of BP control that is largely independent of specific antihypertensives.[42] The United Kingdom guidelines stratify patients based on age and race; they recommend an ACE inhibitor first-line for patients younger than age 55 years, and either a CCB or thiazide-type diuretic first-line for patients age 55 years or older and for black patients.[43]

❾ β-Blockers versus Other First-Line Drug Therapies

Clinical trials data cumulatively suggests that β-blockers may not reduce CV events to the extent that ACE inhibitors, CCBs, or ARBs do. These data are from three meta-analyses of clinical trials evaluating β-blocker–based therapy for hypertension.[44–47] Overall, these analyses demonstrated fewer reductions in CV events with β-blocker–based antihypertensive therapy compared mostly with ACE inhibitor- and CCB-based therapy. Although comparative data with ARB-based therapy are more limited, a similar trend was observed.

Meta-analyses data evaluating β-blockers and their ability to reduce CV events have limitations. Most studies that were included used atenolol as the β-blocker studied. Thus it is possible that atenolol is the only β-blocker that does not reduce risk of CV events as well as the other primary antihypertensive drug classes. However, it is acceptable to extrapolate these findings to the β-blocker drug class in general. Interestingly, the 2006 United Kingdom guidelines recommend a β-blocker only after other primary antihypertensive agents (thiazide-type diuretics, CCBs, ACE inhibitors, or ARBs) have been used. These findings also call in question the validity of results from prominent prospective, controlled clinical trials evaluating antihypertensive drug therapy that use β-blocker–based therapy, especially atenolol, as the primary comparator.[29,34,47]

β-Blocker therapy in patients without compelling indications still has a prominent role in the management of hypertension. It is important for clinicians to remember that β-blocker–based antihypertensive therapy does not increase risk of CV events; β-blocker–based therapy reduces risk of CV events compared to no antihypertensive therapy. Using a β-blocker as a primary antihypertensive agent is optimal when a thiazide-type diuretic, ACE inhibitor, ARB, or CCB cannot be used as the primary agent. Additionally, using a β-blocker in a young patient with hypertension that is thought to have high adrenergic drive, as evidenced by an elevated heart rate, may still be clinically reasonable.[46] β-Blockers still have an important role as an alternative add-on agent to reduce BP in patients with hypertension but without compelling indications.

⑩ Patients with Compelling Indications[1]

The JNC7 report identifies six compelling indications. Compelling indications represent specific comorbid conditions where evidence from clinical trials supports using specific antihypertensive classes to treat both the compelling indication and hypertension (see Fig. 15–3). Data from these clinical trials demonstrate a reduction in CV morbidity and/or mortality that justifies use in patients with hypertension and with such a compelling indication. Some compelling indications include recommendations that are provided by other national treatment guidelines, or from newer clinical trials, which are complementary to the JNC7 guidelines.

Left Ventricular Dysfunction: Systolic Heart Failure[48] Five drug classes are listed as compelling indications for heart failure. These recommendations specifically refer to left ventricular dysfunction (also known as systolic heart failure), where the primary physiologic abnormality is decreased cardiac output. ACE inhibitor with diuretic therapy is recommended as the first-line regimen of choice. ACE inhibitor therapy is recommended based on numerous outcome studies showing reduced CV morbidity and mortality[48]; diuretics are also a part of this first-line regimen because they provide symptomatic relief of edema by inducing diuresis. Loop diuretics are often needed, especially in patients with more advanced disease. Patients with left ventricular dysfunction have a BP goal of less than 120/80 mm Hg, so multiple drug therapies are typically needed.

Evidence from clinical trials shows that ACE inhibitors significantly modify disease progression by reducing morbidity and mortality. Although left ventricular dysfunction was the primary disease in these studies, ACE inhibitor therapy will also control BP. ACE inhibitors should be started with low-doses in patients with heart failure, especially those in acute exacerbation. Heart failure induces a compensatory high renin condition, and starting ACE inhibitors under these conditions can cause a pronounced first-dose effect and possible orthostatic hypotension.

β-Blocker therapy is appropriate to further modify disease in left ventricular dysfunction, and is a component of this first-line regimen (standard therapy) for these patients. In patients on an initial regimen of diuretics and ACE inhibitors, β blockers reduce CV morbidity and mortality.[49,50] It is of paramount importance that β-blockers be dosed appropriately because of the risk of inducing an acute exacerbation of heart failure. They must be started in very low doses, doses much lower than that used to treat hypertension, and titrated slowly to high-doses based on tolerability. Bisoprolol, carvedilol, and metoprolol succinate are the only β-blockers proven to be beneficial in left ventricular dysfunction.[48]

After diuretics, ACE inhibitors, and β-blockers (collectively considered standard therapy), other agents may be added to further reduce CV morbidity and mortality, and reduce BP if needed. Early data suggested that ARBs may be better than ACE inhibitors in left ventricular dysfunction.[51] However, when directly compared in a well-designed prospective trial, ACE inhibitors were found to be better.[52] ARBs are acceptable as an alternative therapy for patients who cannot tolerate ACE inhibitors, and possibly as add-on therapy to those already on a standard three-drug regimen based on data from the CHARM (Candesartan in Heart Failure: Assessment of Reduction in Mortality and Morbidity) studies.[53,54]

The addition of aldosterone antagonists can reduce CV morbidity and mortality in left ventricular dysfunction.[55,56] Spironolactone has been studied in severe left ventricular dysfunction and has shown benefit in addition to diuretic and ACE inhibitor therapy.[55] Eplerenone has been studied in patients with symptomatic left ventricular dysfunction within 3 to 14 days after an acute MI in addition to standard therapy.[56] An aldosterone antagonist may be considered in addition to a diuretic, ACE inhibitor or ARB, and β-blocker. It is not currently recommended to use both an aldosterone inhibitor and an ARB as add-on therapy to a standard therapy, because of the potential increase in risk of severe hyperkalemia.[48]

Post-Myocardial Infarction[57] β-Blocker (those without intrinsic sympathomimetic activity [ISA]) and ACE inhibitor therapy are recommended in the AHA/American College of Cardiology and JNC7 guidelines.[1,2,57] β-Blockers decrease cardiac adrenergic stimulation and reduce the risk of a subsequent MI or sudden cardiac death, as demonstrated in clinical trials. ACE inhibitors improve cardiac remodeling, cardiac function, and reduce CV events post-MI. These two drug classes, with β-blockers first, are considered the first drugs of choice for patients who have experienced a MI. One study, the Valsartan in Acute Myocardial Infarction Trial (VALLIANT), demonstrated that ARB therapy is similar to ACE inhibitor therapy in patients post-MI with left ventricular dysfunction.[58] However, ARBs are considered alternatives to ACE inhibitors in post-MI patients with left ventricular dysfunction. These patients have coronary artery disease, and have a BP goal of less than 130/80 mm Hg. Framingham risk scoring is not needed.

Eplerenone reduces CV morbidity and mortality in patients soon after an acute MI (within 3 to 14 days).[56] However, this supporting evidence was in patients with symptoms of acute left ventricular dysfunction. Considering that this drug has the propensity to cause significant hyperkalemia and the patient population studied, eplerenone should only be used in selected patients following a MI with very diligent monitoring of potassium.

Coronary Artery Disease[57,59] Chronic stable angina and acute coronary syndrome (unstable angina and acute MI) are forms of coronary disease (also called coronary artery disease or ischemic heart disease). This compelling indication is also referred to as high coronary disease risk and high CV disease risk in the JNC7 report.[1] These are the most common forms of hypertension-associated target-organ disease. β-Blocker therapy has the most evidence demonstrating benefits in these patients. β-Blockers (those without ISA) are first-line therapy in chronic stable angina and have the ability to reduce BP, improve myocardial oxygen consumption and decrease demand. These patients have coronary artery disease, and have a BP goal of less than 130/80 mm Hg. Framingham risk scoring is not needed.

Long-acting CCBs are either alternatives (the nondihydropyridine CCBs diltiazem and verapamil) or add-on therapy (dihydropyridine CCBs) to β-blockers in chronic stable angina.[59] The International Verapamil-Trandolapril Study (INVEST) demonstrated no difference in CV risk reduction when β-blocker–based therapy was compared to nondihydropyridine CCB-based therapy in this population.[60] Nonetheless, the preponderance of data are with β-blockers and they remain therapy of choice.[1,2,57,59]

For acute coronary syndromes (ST-elevation MI and unstable angina/non–ST-segment MI), first-line therapy should consist of a β-blocker and ACE inhibitor.[61,62] This regimen will lower BP, control acute ischemia, and reduce CV risk.

CCBs (especially nondihydropyridine CCBs) and β-blockers provide antiischemic effects; they lower BP and reduce myocardial oxygen demand in patients with hypertension and coronary disease. However, cardiac stimulation may occur with dihydropyridine CCBs or β-blockers with ISA, making these agents less desirable. Consequently, β-blockers with ISA should be avoided, nondihydropyridines CCBs should be alternatives to β-blockers, and dihydropyridines should be add-on therapy to β-blockers.

Once ischemic symptoms are controlled with β-blocker and/or CCB therapy, other antihypertensive drugs can be added to provide additional CV risk reduction. Clinical trials have demonstrated that the addition of an ACE inhibitor, or alternatively an ARB further reduces risk CV events in patients with chronic stable angina.[63] Thiazide-type diuretics can be added thereafter to provide additional BP lowering and to further reduce CV risk. Neither ACE inhibitors, nor thiazide-type diuretics provide anti-ischemic effects.

There has been concern that overtreating high BP in patients with coronary artery disease may bring about more harm than good (termed the *J-curve phenomenon*). Coronary blood flow occurs during diastole and the rate of flow is directly influenced by the DBP. Therefore, excessively reducing DBP may compromise coronary perfusion, especially in patients with fixed coronary artery stenosis, and lead to myocardial infarction. This concern has been theoretical based on retrospective analyses, and prospective studies have not found a J-curve until DBPs were very low (<60 mm Hg).

Diabetes Mellitus[1,64–67] The primary cause of mortality in diabetes is CV disease, and hypertension management is a very important risk-reduction strategy. The BP goal in diabetes is less than 130/80 mm Hg. Diabetes is considered a coronary artery disease risk equivalent and Framingham risk scoring is not needed. Five antihypertensive agents have evidence supporting their compelling indications in diabetes (see Fig. 15–3). All of these agents have been shown to reduce CV events in patients with diabetes. However, risk reduction may not be equal when comparing these agents.

⓫ All patients with diabetes and hypertension should be treated with either an ACE inhibitor or an ARB.[64] Pharmacologically, both of these agents should provide nephroprotection as a result of vasodilation in the efferent arteriole of the kidney. Moreover, ACE inhibitors have overwhelming data demonstrating CV risk reduction in patients with established forms of heart disease. Evidence from outcome studies have demonstrated reductions in both CV risk (mostly with ACE inhibitors) and reduction in risk of progressive kidney dysfunction (mostly with ARBs) in patients with diabetes.[64] There is controversy surrounding which agent is better because data support both drug classes. Nonetheless, either drug class should be used to control BP as one of the drugs in the antihypertensive regimen for patients with diabetes because multiple agents are often needed to attain goal BP values.

A thiazide-type diuretic is recommended as the second agent to lower BP and provide additional CV risk-reduction. A subgroup analysis of patients with diabetes from the ALLHAT trial showed no difference in long term risk of CV events in the chlorthalidone and lisinopril treatment groups.[38] Therefore, some argue that thiazide-type diuretics, used in low-doses, are equally effective in patients with hypertension and diabetes. Nonetheless, the entire body of evidence evaluating pharmacotherapy in patients with hypertension and diabetes, and consensus guidelines, support an ACE inhibitor or ARB first-line, with a thiazide-type diuretic as add-on therapy.[1,64,65]

CCBs are useful add-on agents for BP control in patients with diabetes. Several studies have compared an ACE inhibitor with either a dihydropyridine CCB or a β-blocker. In the studies comparing a dihydropyridine with an ACE inhibitor, the ACE inhibitor group had significantly lower rates of CV end points, including MIs and all CV events.[67] These data do not suggest that CCBs are harmful in diabetic patients, but indicate that they are not as protective as ACE inhibitors. Although data are limited, nondihydropyridine CCBs (diltiazem and verapamil) appear to have more renal protective effects than the dihydropyridines.[65]

β-Blockers reduce CV risk in patients with diabetes. These agents should be used when needed as add-on therapy with other standard agents, or to treat another compelling indication (e.g., post-MI). β-Blockers have been shown in at least one study to be as effective as ACE inhibitors in protection against morbidity and mortality in patients with diabetes.[66]

β-Blockers (especially nonselective agents) may mask the signs and symptoms of hypoglycemia in patients with tightly controlled diabetes because most of the symptoms of hypoglycemia (i.e., tremor, tachycardia, and palpitations) are mediated through the sympathetic nervous system. Sweating, a cholinergically mediated symptom of hypoglycemia, should still occur during a hypoglycemic episode despite β-blocker therapy. Patients may also have a delay in hypoglycemia recovery time because compensatory recovery mechanisms need the catecholamine inputs that are antagonized by β-blocker therapy. Finally, unopposed α-receptor stimulation during the acute hypoglycemic recovery phase (as a consequence of endogenous epinephrine release intended to reverse hypoglycemia) may result in acutely elevated BP because of vasoconstriction. Despite these potential problems, β-blockers can be safely used in patients with diabetes.

Based on the weight of all evidence, ACE inhibitors or ARBs are preferred first-line agents for treating patients with hypertension and diabetes. The need for combination therapy should be anticipated, and thiazide-type diuretics should be the second agent added. Based on scientific evidence, β-blockers and CCBs are useful evidence-based agents in this population, but are considered add-on therapies to the aforementioned agents.

Chronic Kidney Disease[68] Patients with hypertension may develop damage to either the renal tissue (parenchyma) or the renal arteries. Chronic kidney disease initially presents as microalbuminuria (30 to 299 mcg/mg albumin-to-creatinine ratio on a spot urine sample or ≥30 mg albumin in a 24-hour urine collection) that can progress to overt kidney failure. The rate of kidney function deterioration is accelerated when both hypertension and diabetes are present. Once patients have an estimated GFR of less than 60 mL/min/1.73 m^2 or albuminuria, they have significant chronic kidney disease and the risk of CV disease and progression to severe chronic kidney disease increases.[1] Strict BP control to a goal of less than 130/80 mm Hg can slow the decline in kidney function. Although this strict BP goal is recommended in significant chronic kidney disease, long-term benefits of this lower BP goal have mostly been demonstrated in patients with both significant chronic kidney disease and diabetes.[69] This strict control often requires two or more antihypertensive agents.

In addition to lowering BP, ACE inhibitors and ARBs reduce intraglomerular pressure, which can theoretically provide additional benefits by further reducing the decline in kidney function. ACE inhibitors and ARBs have been shown to reduce progression of chronic kidney disease in diabetes[64] and in those without diabetes.[65,70] It is difficult to differentiate whether the kidney protection benefits are from RAAS blockade or BP lowering. A recent meta-analysis failed to demonstrate any unique long-term kidney-protective effects of RAAS-blocking drugs compared with other antihypertensive drugs.[71] Moreover, a subgroup analysis of patients from the ALLHAT stratified by different baseline GFR values also did not show a difference in long-term outcomes with chlorthalidone versus lisinopril.[37] Nonetheless, consensus guidelines recommend either an ACE inhibitor or ARB as first-line therapy to control BP and preserve kidney function in chronic kidney disease.

Some data indicate that the combination of an ACE inhibitor with an ARB may be more effective than either agent alone.[72] However, routine use of this combination in all patients with chronic kidney disease is controversial. Because these patients typically require multiple antihypertensive agents, diuretics and a third antihypertensive drug class (e.g., β-blocker, CCB) are often needed.

CLINICAL CONTROVERSY

Thiazide-type diuretics traditionally have been viewed as less effective than loop diuretics in patients with severe chronic kidney disease. Some clinicians routinely replace thiazide-type diuretics with a loop diuretic in patients who have estimated creatinine clearances below 30 mL/min. However, limited data demonstrate that the antihypertensive effects of hydrochlorothiazide are equal to that of furosemide in patients with chronic renal failure and hypertension.[73]

Patients may rarely experience acute kidney failure when given an ACE inhibitor or ARB. The potential to produce acute kidney failure is particularly problematic in patients with bilateral renal artery stenosis or a solitary functioning kidney with stenosis. Patients with renal artery stenosis are usually older, and the condition is more common in patients with diabetes and in those who smoke. Patients with renal artery stenosis do not necessarily have evidence of kidney disease unless sophisticated tests are performed. Evaluating kidney function shortly after starting the drug can minimize this risk.

Recurrent Stroke Prevention Ischemic stroke is considered target-organ damage caused by hypertension. Attaining goal BP values in patients who have experienced a stroke, or a transient ischemic attack, is considered a primary modality to reduce risk of a second stroke. In general, these patients have noncoronary atherosclerotic vascular disease, are considered a coronary artery disease risk equivalent, and have a BP goal of less than 130/80 mm Hg. However, BP lowering should only be attempted after patients have stabilized following an acute cerebrovascular event. One clinical trial, PROGRESS (Perindopril Protection Against Recurrent Stroke Study), showed that the incidence of recurrent stroke in patients with a history of ischemic stroke can be reduced when a thiazide-type diuretic is used in combination with an ACE inhibitor.[31] Reduction in recurrent stroke was seen with this combination therapy, even in those who had BP values less than 140/90 mm Hg. Recurrent stroke was not reduced with ACE inhibitor monotherapy in the PROGRESS, it was only reduced when the thiazide-type diuretic was added.

Reductions in risk of recurrent stroke have also been seen with ARBs.[74] In another clinical trial, the MOSES (Morbidity and Mortality After Stroke, Eprosartan Compared with Nitrendipine for Secondary Prevention), patients with a history of stroke or transient ischemic attack had a lower risk of a recurrent stoke when treated with ARB-based therapy compared to dihydropyridine CCB-based therapy. Therefore, both an ACE inhibitor with a thiazide-type diuretic,[1,75] or ARB-based therapy are evidence-based antihypertensive regimens for patients with a history of cerebrovascular disease, specifically ischemic stroke or transient ischemic attack, to prevent recurrent stroke. These recommendations do not apply to patients with a history of hemorrhagic stroke.

Alternative Drug Treatments

It is necessary to use other agents such as α-blockers, central α_2-agonists, a direct renin inhibitor, adrenergic inhibitors, and vasodilators in some patients. Although these agents are potent, many of them have a much greater incidence of adverse effects. Moreover, they do not have compelling outcomes data showing reduced morbidity and mortality in hypertension. They are generally reserved for patients with resistant hypertension, and should only be used as add-on therapy with other primary antihypertensive agents.

Special Populations[1]

Selection of drug therapy should follow the guidelines provided by the JNC7, which are summarized in Figures 15–2 and 15–3. These should be maintained as the guiding principles of drug therapy. However, there are some patient populations where the approach to drug therapy may be slightly different or necessitate tailored dosing strategies. In some cases this is because other agents have unique properties that benefit a coexisting condition, but may not be based on evidence from outcomes studies in hypertension.

Hypertension in Older People Hypertension often presents as isolated systolic hypertension in the elderly. Epidemiologic data indicate that CV morbidity and mortality are more closely related to SBP than to DBP in patients ages 50 years and older, so this population is at high risk for hypertension-related target-organ damage.[1] Although several placebo-controlled trials have specifically demonstrated risk reduction in this form of hypertension, many older people with hypertension are either not treated, or treated yet not controlled.[21]

The SHEP was a landmark, double-blind, placebo-controlled trial that evaluated chlorthalidone-based treatment (with atenolol or reserpine as add-on therapy) for isolated systolic hypertension.[9] A 36% reduction in total stroke, a 27% reduction in coronary artery disease, and 55% reduction in heart failure were demonstrated versus placebo. The Syst-Eur (Systolic Hypertension in Europe) was another placebo-controlled trial that evaluated treatment with a long-acting dihydropyridine CCB.[12] Treatment resulted in a 42% reduction in stroke, 26% reduction in coronary artery disease, and 29% reduction in heart failure. These data clearly demonstrate reductions in CV morbidity and mortality in older patients with isolated systolic hypertension, especially with thiazide-type diuretics and long-acting dihydropyridine CCBs.

The very-elderly population (age ≥80 years) has been underrepresented in clinical trials, including the SHEP and Syst-Eur studies. This population often is not treated to goal either because of a fear of lowering BP too much or because of limited data demonstrating benefit. The best available data in the very elderly comes from meta-analyses.[76,77] Although these data do not show reductions in mortality, they consistently show fewer strokes with antihypertensive drug therapy. However, care should be taken that BP not be excessively lowered in this population, as it this is associated with increased risk of mortality.[78] The HYVET (Hypertension in the Very Elderly Trial), a prospective controlled clinical trial was recently stopped early due to significant reductions in stroke and total mortality with antihypertensive treatment in the very elderly versus placebo.[79]

Thiazide-type diuretics or β-blockers have been compared with either ACE inhibitors or CCBs in elderly patients with either systolic or diastolic hypertension or both.[80] In the Swedish Trial in Old Patients with Hypertension-2 (STOP-2) study, no significant differences were seen between conventional drugs and either ACE inhibitors or CCBs. However, there were significantly fewer MIs and cases of heart failure in the ACE inhibitor group compared with the CCB group. These data suggest that overall treatment may be more important than specific antihypertensive agents in this population.

Elderly patients are more sensitive to volume depletion and sympathetic inhibition than younger individuals. This may lead to orthostatic hypotension (see Patients at Risk for Orthostatic Hypotension below). In the elderly, this can increase the risk of falls as a consequence of the associated dizziness and risk of fainting. Centrally acting agents and α-blockers should generally be avoided or used with caution in the elderly because they are frequently associated with dizziness and postural hypotension. Diuretics and ACE inhibitors provide significant benefits and can safely be used in the elderly, but smaller-than-usual initial doses might be needed.

The JNC7 and AHA goal BP recommendations are independent of age.[1,2] Age-adjusted goals are inappropriate. Moreover, treatment of hypertension in older patients should follow the same principles that are outlined for general care of hypertension. However, initial drug doses may be lower, and dosage titrations should occur over a longer period of time to minimize the risk of hypotension. An interim goal of a SBP of below 160 mm Hg may be necessary for those with very high initial SBP, but the ultimate goal should still be less than 140 mm Hg, less than 130 mm Hg, or less than 120 mm Hg, depending on CV risk and comorbid conditions of the patient.

⓬ Patients at Risk for Orthostatic Hypotension *Orthostatic hypotension* is a significant drop in BP when standing and can be associated with dizziness and/or fainting. It is defined as a SBP decrease of greater than 20 mm Hg or DBP decrease of greater than 10 mm Hg when changing from supine to standing.[1] Older patients (especially those with isolated systolic hypotension), patients with diabetes, severe volume depletion, baroreflex dysfunction, autonomic insufficiency, and use of venodilators (α-blockers, mixed α/β-blockers, nitrates, and phosphodiesterase inhibitors) all increase risk of orthostatic hypotension. In patients with these risks, antihypertensive agents should be started in low doses, especially diuretics, ACE inhibitors, and ARBs.

Hypertension in Children and Adolescents[81] Detecting hypertension in children requires special attention to BP measurement, and is defined as SBP and/or DBP that is greater than 95th percentile for sex, age, and height on at least three occasions.[81] BP between the 90th and 95th percentile, or equal to or greater than 120/80 mm Hg in adolescents, is considered prehypertension. Hypertensive children often have a family history of high BP, and many are overweight, predisposing them to insulin resistance and associated CV disease. Unlike hypertension in adults, secondary hypertension is more common in children and adolescents. An appropriate workup for secondary causes is essential if elevated BP is identified. Kidney disease (e.g., pyelonephritis, glomerulonephritis) is the most common cause of secondary hypertension in children. Coarctation of the aorta can also produce secondary hypertension. Medical or surgical management of the underlying disorder usually normalizes BP.

Nonpharmacologic treatment, particularly weight loss in those who are overweight, is the cornerstone of therapy for essential hypertension in children.[81] The goal is to reduce the BP to below the 95th percentile for sex, age, and height, or below the 90th percentile if concurrent conditions, such as chronic kidney disease, diabetes, or target-organ damage, are present. ACE inhibitors, ARBs, β-blockers, CCBs, and thiazide-type diuretics are all acceptable choices in children. ACE inhibitors, ARBs, and direct renin inhibitors are contraindicated in sexually active girls because of potential teratogenic effect, and in those who might have bilateral renal artery stenosis or unilateral stenosis in a solitary kidney. As with adults, consideration for initial agents should be based on the presence of compelling indications or concurrent conditions that may warrant their use (e.g., ACE inhibitor or ARB for those with diabetes or microalbuminuria).

Pregnancy[1,82] Hypertension during pregnancy is a major cause of maternal and neonatal morbidity and mortality. Hypertension during pregnancy is categorized as preeclampsia, eclampsia, gestational, chronic, and superimposition of preeclampsia on chronic hypertension. Preeclampsia, defined as a elevated BP greater than or equal to 140/90 mm Hg that appears after 20 weeks gestation accompanied by new-onset proteinuria (≥300 mg/24 hours), can lead to life-threatening complications for both mother and fetus. Eclampsia, the onset of convulsions in preeclampsia, is a medical emergency. Gestational hypertension is defined as new-onset hypertension arising after midpregnancy in the absence of proteinuria, and chronic hypertension is elevated BP that is noted before the pregnancy began. It is controversial whether treating elevated BP in patients with chronic hypertension in pregnancy is beneficial. However, women with chronic hypertension prior to pregnancy are at increased risk of a number of complications, including superimposed preeclampsia, preterm delivery, fetal growth restriction or demise, placental abruption, heart failure, and acute kidney failure.[82]

Definitive treatment of preeclampsia is delivery. Delivery is indicated if pending or frank eclampsia is present. Otherwise, management consists of restricting activity, bedrest, and close monitoring. Salt restriction, or any other measures that contract blood volume, should not be employed. Antihypertensive agents are used prior to induction of labor if DBP is greater than 105 to 110 mm Hg with a target DBP of 95 to 105 mm Hg. Intravenous hydralazine is most commonly used, and intravenous labetalol is also effective. Immediate-release oral nifedipine has been used, but it is not approved by the Food and Drug Administration (FDA) for hypertension and untoward fetal and maternal effects (hypotension with fetal distress) have been reported.

Many agents can be used to treat chronic hypertension in pregnancy (Table 15–7). Unfortunately, there is little consensus and few data regarding the most appropriate therapy in pregnancy. Methyldopa is still considered the drug of choice.[1] Data indicate that uteroplacental blood flow and fetal hemodynamics are stable with methyldopa. Moreover, it is viewed as very safe, based on long-term followup data (7.5 years) that has not demonstrated adverse effects on childhood development. β-Blockers, labetalol and CCBs are also reasonable alternatives. ACE inhibitors and ARBs are known teratogens and are absolutely contraindicated.[83]Aliskiren also should not be used in pregnancy.

African Americans[1,84] Hypertension affects African American patients at a disproportionately higher rate, and hypertension-related target-organ damage is more prevalent than in other populations. Reasons for these differences are not fully understood, but may be related to differences in electrolyte homeostasis, GFR, sodium excretion and transport mechanisms, plasma renin activity, and BP response to plasma volume expansion.

African Americans have an increased need for combination therapy to attain and maintain BP goals.[84] The Hypertension in African American Working Group of the International Society on Hypertension in Blacks has published treatment guidelines that are similar to the JNC7.[84] Lifestyle modifications are recommended to

TABLE 15-7 Treatment of Chronic Hypertension in Pregnancy

Drug/Class	Comments
Methyldopa	Preferred agent based on long-term followup data supporting safety
β-Blockers	Generally safe, but intrauterine growth retardation reported
Labetalol	Increasingly preferred over methyldopa because of fewer side effects
Clonidine	Limited data available
Calcium channel blockers	Limited data available; no increase in major teratogenicity with exposure
Diuretics	Not first-line agents but probably safe in low doses if used chronically prior to conception
Angiotensin-converting enzyme inhibitors, angiotensin II receptor blockers and direct renin inhibitors	Contraindicated; major teratogenicity reported with exposure (fetal toxicity and death)

augment drug therapy. They also support thiazide-type diuretics as first-line for most patients and selecting specific drug therapy to treat compelling indications, if present. These guidelines aggressively promote combination therapy. They recommend starting with two drugs in patients with SBP values ≥15 mm Hg from goal. This aggressive approach is reasonable considering that overall goal BP attainment rates are low in African Americans.

BP-lowering effects of antihypertensive classes varies in African Americans. Thiazide diuretics and CCBs seem to be particularly effective at lowering BP in African Americans. When either of these two classes (especially thiazides) is used in combination with a β-blocker, ACE inhibitor, or ARB, antihypertensive response is significantly increased. This may be a result of the low renin pattern of hypertension, which can result in less BP lowering with β-blockers, ACE inhibitors, or ARBs when used as monotherapy compared to the effect in white patients. Interestingly, African Americans have a higher risk of angioedema and cough from ACE inhibitors than do whites.[84]

Despite potential differences in antihypertensive effects, drug therapy selection should be based on evidence. Thiazide-type diuretics are first-line agents based on the preponderance of evidence. A subgroup analysis of African American patients from the ALLHAT also supports the first-line role of thiazide-type diuretics in treating African American patients with hypertension.[39] These agents just so happen to also be very effective at controlling BP in this population. ACE inhibitors, ARBs, and CCBs may also be used as first-line options. Other drug therapies should be used if a compelling indication is present, even if the antihypertensive effect may not be as great as with another drug class (e.g., a β-blocker is first-line therapy for BP control in an African American patient who is post-MI).

Other Concomitant Conditions

Most patients with hypertension have some other coexisting condition(s) that may influence selection or use of drug therapy. The influence of concomitant conditions should only be complementary to, and never in replacement of, drug therapy choices indicated by compelling indications. Under some circumstances, these are helpful in deciding on a particular antihypertensive agent when more than one antihypertensive class is recommended. In some cases, an agent should be avoided because it may aggravate a concomitant disorder. In other cases, an antihypertensive can be used to treat hypertension, a compelling indication, and another concomitant condition.

Pulmonary Disease and Peripheral Arterial Disease[85] β-Blockers, especially nonselective agents, have been generally avoided in patients with hypertension and reactive airway disease (asthma or chronic obstructive pulmonary disease with a reversible obstructive component) because of a fear of inducing bronchospasm. This precaution is more of a myth than a fact. Data suggests that cardioselective β-blockers can safely be used in patients with asthma or chronic obstructive pulmonary disease.[86] Consequently, cardioselective β-blockers should be used to treat a compelling indication (i.e., post-MI, coronary disease, or heart failure) in patients with reactive airway disease.

Peripheral arterial disease, noncoronary atherosclerotic vascular disease, is a coronary artery disease risk equivalent. The 2007 AHA guidelines now recommend a BP goal of less than 130/80 mm Hg in this population. ACE inhibitors may be ideal in patients with symptomatic lower-extremity peripheral arterial disease who also have hypertension, as they decrease CV events in these patients.[85] CCBs may also be beneficial because of their vasodilatory effects on the peripheral arteries. β-Blockers have traditionally been considered problematic in patients with peripheral arterial disease because of possible decreased peripheral blood flow secondary to unopposed stimulation of α-receptors that results in vasoconstriction. However, β-blockers are not contraindicated in peripheral arterial disease and have not been shown to adversely affect walking capability.[85]

Dyslipidemia Dyslipidemia is considered a major CV risk factor. Controlling dyslipidemia is important to the overall care of patients with hypertension. Thiazide-type diuretics and β-blockers without ISA may adversely affect serum cholesterol values, although these effects generally are transient and of no clinical consequence.[87] α-Blockers have favorable effects (decreased low-density lipoprotein cholesterol and increased high-density lipoprotein cholesterol). However, because data from the ALLHAT show that α-blocker therapy does not reduce CV risk as much as thiazide-type diuretic therapy, this benefit is not clinically applicable.[35]

Metabolic Syndrome[13,88,89] Metabolic syndrome is a cluster of multiple cardiometabolic risk factors. It was most recently defined as the presence of three of the following five criteria: abdominal obesity (waist circumference >40 inches in men, >35 inches in women), elevated triglycerides (≥150 mg/dL or receiving drug treatment for elevated triglycerides), low high-density lipoprotein cholesterol (<40 mg/dL in men, <50 mg/dL in women or receiving drug treatment for low high-density lipoprotein), elevated BP (≥130/≥85 mm Hg or receiving drug treatment for high BP), and elevated fasting blood glucose (≥100 mg/dL or receiving drug treatment for elevated glucose).[13]

Regardless of the debate regarding whether or not metabolic syndrome is a true "disease," it is widely accepted that patients with metabolic syndrome are at significant increased risk of developing CV disease and/or type 2 diabetes. Using an ACE inhibitor or ARB to treat patients with hypertension and the metabolic syndrome, especially patients with elevated fasting glucose but not yet type 2 diabetes, may be beneficial. A recent meta-analysis demonstrated that ARBs and ACE inhibitors are less likely then β-blockers or thiazide-diuretics to be associated with progression to new-onset type 2 diabetes.[89] However, studies specifically evaluating the most effective antihypertensive regimen in patients with metabolic syndrome have not been done. In addition, an ALLHAT subgroup analysis of patients with impaired fasting glucose showed that CV events were reduced more with chlorthalidone compared to lisinopril.[38] Thus, thiazides-type diuretics can be used in patients with metabolic syndrome, similar to ACE inhibitors, ARBs, or CCBs. In patients with elevated fasting glucose, or any patient at risk for developing type 2 diabetes, close monitoring of serum potassium should occur when treated with thiazide-type diuretics. If hypokalemia develops, or even subclinical hypokalemia (serum potassium within the normal range, but at the low end of the normal range), in thiazide treated patients, the risk of developing type 2 diabetes significantly increases.[90] Therefore, treatment of thiazide-induced hypokalemia, or even subclinical hypokalemia, should be considered to maintain serum potassium in the mid to high end of the normal range (e.g., 4.0–5.0 mEq/L). This may reverse thiazide-induced glucose intolerance or possibly prevent onset of type 2 diabetes. This can be accomplished though the addition of an ACE inhibitor, ARB, or potassium sparing diuretic, or with potassium supplementation for cases of more severe hypokalemia.

Erectile Dysfunction[91] Most antihypertensive agents are associated with erectile dysfunction in men. However, it is not clear if erectile dysfunction associated with antihypertensive treatment is solely a result of drug therapy or is a symptom of underlying CV disease. Traditionally, β-blockers have been labeled as agents that significantly cause sexual dysfunction, and many practitioners have avoided prescribing them as a result. However, data supporting this notion are limited. A systematic review of 15 studies involving 35,000 patients assessing β-blocker use for MI, heart failure, and hypertension found only a very slight increased risk erectile dysfunction.[92] In addition, prospective long-term data from the TOMHS (Treatment of Mild Hypertension Study) show no difference in the incidence of erectile dysfunction between diuretics and β-blockers versus ACE inhibitors and CCBs.[93] Centrally acting agents are associated with higher rates of sexual dysfunction and should be avoided in men with erectile dysfunction.

Hypertensive men frequently have atherosclerotic vascular disease, which frequently results in erectile dysfunction. Consequently, erectile dysfunction may be mostly associated with chronic arterial changes resulting from elevated BP and lack of control may increase the risk of erectile dysfunction. These changes are even more pronounced in hypertensive men with diabetes.

Erectile dysfunction in hypertension may be an important marker for CV disease. A study of men prospectively screened for erectile dysfunction after being referred for nuclear stress test imaging showed that erectile dysfunction was a stronger predictor of severe coronary heart disease than traditional risk factors (age, smoking, hypertension, diabetes, and dyslipidemia).[94]

Individual Antihypertensive Agents[1,7]

Diuretics[9–11,30] Diuretics, preferably a thiazide, are first-line agents for hypertension.[1,2] The best available evidence justifying this recommendation is from ALLHAT.[30] Moreover, when combination therapy is needed in hypertension to control BP, a diuretic is recommended to be one of the agents used.[1] There are four subclasses of diuretics that are used in the treatment of hypertension: thiazides, loops, potassium-sparing agents, and aldosterone antagonists (see Table 15–5). Potassium-sparing diuretics are weak antihypertensive agents but provide an additive effect when used in combination with a thiazide or loop diuretic. Moreover, they counteract the potassium- and magnesium-losing properties of the other diuretic agents and possible glucose intolerance. Aldosterone antagonists (spironolactone and eplerenone) may be technically considered potassium-sparing agents, but are more potent antihypertensives. However, they are viewed by the JNC7 as an independent class because of evidence supporting compelling indications.

The exact hypotensive mechanisms of action of diuretics are multifaceted. The drop in BP seen when diuretics are first started is caused by an initial diuresis. Diuresis causes reductions in plasma and stroke volume, which decreases cardiac output and BP. This initial drop in cardiac output causes a compensatory increase in peripheral vascular resistance. With chronic diuretic therapy, extracellular fluid and plasma volume return to near pretreatment values. However, peripheral vascular resistance decreases to values that are lower than the pretreatment baseline. This reduction in peripheral vascular resistance is responsible for chronic antihypertensive effects.

Thiazide-type diuretics have additional actions that may further explain their antihypertensive effects. Thiazides mobilize sodium and water from arteriolar walls. This effect would lessen the amount of physical encroachment on the lumen of the vessel created by excessive accumulation of intracellular fluid. As the diameter of the lumen relaxes and increases, there is less resistance to the flow of blood and peripheral vascular resistance further drops. High dietary sodium intake can blunt this effect and a low salt intake can enhance this effect. Thiazides are also postulated to cause direct relaxation of vascular smooth muscle.

Thiazides are the preferred type of diuretic for treating hypertension. In patients requiring diuresis to treat concurrent edema, such as in heart failure, a loop diuretic should be considered. Diuretics should ideally be dosed in the morning if given once daily, and in the morning and afternoon when dosed twice daily to minimize risk of nocturnal diuresis. However, with chronic use, thiazide-type diuretics, potassium sparing diuretics, and aldosterone antagonists rarely cause a pronounced diuresis.

The major pharmacokinetic differences between the various thiazide-type diuretics are serum half-life and duration of diuretic effect. The clinical relevance of these differences is unknown because the serum half-life of most antihypertensive agents does not correlate with the hypotensive duration of action. Moreover, diuretics lower BP primarily through extrarenal mechanisms. Hydrochlorothiazide and chlorthalidone are the two most frequently used thiazide diuretics in landmark clinical trials that have demonstrated reduced morbidity and mortality. These agents are not equipotent on a milligram-per-milligram basis; chlorthalidone is 1.5 to 2.0 times more potent than hydrochlorothiazide.[95] This is attributed to a longer half-life (45 to 60 hours vs. 8 to 15 hours) and longer duration of effect (48 to 72 hours vs. 16 to 24 hours) with chlorthalidone. These differences in BP lowering do not appear to result in differences in CV outcomes. A small meta-analysis of five outcome-based clinical trials evaluating CV events suggests there is no difference in long-term CV outcomes with chlorthalidone compared with other thiazide-type diuretics, including hydrochlorothiazide.[96] It is well accepted that CV benefits in hypertension apply to all thiazide-type diuretics, and benefits are considered a class effect.[2]

Diuretics are very effective in lowering BP when used in combination with most other antihypertensives. This additive response is explained by two independent pharmacodynamic effects. First, when two drugs cause the same overall pharmacologic effect (BP lowering) through different mechanisms of action, their combination usually results in an additive or synergistic effect. This is especially relevant when a β-blocker, ACE inhibitor, or ARB is indicated in an African American, but does not elicit sufficient antihypertensive effect. Adding a diuretic in this situation can often significantly lower BP. Second, a compensatory increase in sodium and fluid retention may be seen with antihypertensive agents. This problem is counteracted with the concurrent use of a diuretic.

Side effects of thiazide-type diuretics include hypokalemia, hypomagnesemia, hypercalcemia, hyperuricemia, hyperglycemia, dyslipidemia, and sexual dysfunction. Many of these side effects were identified when high-doses of thiazides were used in the past (e.g., hydrochlorothiazide 100 mg/day). Current guidelines recommend limiting the dose of hydrochlorothiazide or chlorthalidone to 12.5 to 25 mg/day, which markedly reduces the risk for most metabolic side effects. Loop diuretics may cause the same side effects, although the effect on serum lipids and glucose is not as significant, and hypocalcemia may occur.

Hypokalemia and hypomagnesemia may cause muscle fatigue or cramps. However, serious cardiac arrhythmias can occur in patients with severe hypokalemia and hypomagnesemia. Patients at greatest risk for this are patients with left ventricular hypertrophy, coronary disease, post-MI, a history of arrhythmia, or those concurrently receiving digoxin. Low-dose therapy (i.e., 25 mg hydrochlorothiazide or 12.5 mg chlorthalidone daily) rarely causes significant electrolyte disturbances. Efforts should be made to keep potassium in the therapeutic range by careful monitoring.

Diuretic-induced hyperuricemia can precipitate gout. This side effect may be especially problematic in patients with a previous history of gout and with thiazide-type diuretics. However, acute gout is unlikely in patients with no previous history of gout. If gout does occur in a patient who requires diuretic therapy, allopurinol can be given to prevent gout and will not compromise the antihypertensive effects of the diuretic. High doses of thiazide-type and loop diuretics may increase fasting glucose and serum cholesterol values. Diligent monitoring and treatment of diuretic-induced hypokalemia, even if subclinical, will lessen the associated increase in fasting glucose, and perhaps onset of type 2 diabetes.[90]

Potassium-sparing diuretics can cause hyperkalemia, especially in patients with chronic kidney disease or diabetes and in patients receiving concurrent treatment with an ACE inhibitor, nonsteroidal antiinflammatory drugs, or potassium supplements. Hyperkalemia is especially problematic for the newest aldosterone antagonist eplerenone. This agent is a very selective aldosterone antagonist, and its propensity to cause hyperkalemia is greater than with the other potassium sparing agents, and even spironolactone. Because of this increased risk of hyperkalemia, eplerenone is contraindicated in patients with impaired kidney function or type 2 diabetes with proteinuria (see Table 15–5). Although spironolactone may cause gynecomastia in up to 10% of patients, this occurs rarely with eplerenone.

Diuretics can be used safely with most other agents. However, concurrent administration with lithium may result in increased lithium serum concentrations. This interaction can predispose patients to lithium toxicity.

ACE Inhibitors[27,32,80] ACE inhibitors are a first-line agents for hypertension.[1,2] The ALLHAT demonstrated less heart failure and stroke with chlorthalidone than with lisinopril.[30] However, other outcome studies have demonstrated similar, if not better outcomes with ACE inhibitors than with thiazide diuretics.[27,32]

ACE facilitates production of angiotensin II which has a major role in arterial BP regulation as depicted in Fig. 15–1. ACE is distributed in many tissues and is present in several different cell types, but its principal location is in endothelial cells. Thus the major site for angiotensin II production is in the blood vessels, not the kidney. ACE inhibitors block the ACE (also termed *bradykinase*), thus inhibiting conversion of angiotensin I to angiotensin II. Angiotensin II is a potent vasoconstrictor that also stimulates aldosterone secretion, causing an increase in sodium and water reabsorption with accompanying potassium loss. By blocking the ACE, vasodilation and a decrease in aldosterone occur. ACE inhibitors also block degradation of bradykinin and stimulate the synthesis of other vasodilating substances (prostaglandin E_2 and prostacyclin). The observation that ACE inhibitors lower BP in patients with normal plasma renin activity suggests that bradykinin and perhaps tissue production of ACE are important in hypertension. Increased bradykinin enhances the BP-lowering effects of ACE inhibitors, but also is responsible for the side effect of dry cough. ACE inhibitors effectively prevent or regress left ventricular hypertrophy by reducing the direct stimulation by angiotensin II on myocardial cells.

There are many evidence-based uses for ACE inhibitors (see Fig. 15–3). ACE inhibitors reduce CV morbidity and mortality in patients with left ventricular dysfunction,[48] and decrease progression of chronic kidney disease.[65] They should be first-line as disease modifying therapy in all of these patients unless absolutely contraindicated. ACE inhibitors, or ARBs in certain patients, are first-line in patients with diabetes and hypertension because of demonstrated CV disease and kidney benefits. A regimen including an ACE inhibitor with a thiazide-type diuretic is considered first-line in recurrent stroke prevention base on proven benefits from the PROGRESS trial showing reduced risk of secondary stroke.[31] In combination with β-blocker therapy, evidence shows that ACE inhibitors further reduce CV risk in coronary disease, and in patients post-MI.[57,59,61,62] These benefits of ACE inhibitors occur in patients with atherosclerotic vascular even in the absence of left ventricular systolic dysfunction or heart failure, and have the potential to reduce the development of new-onset type 2 diabetes.[63]

There are 10 ACE inhibitors on the U.S. market (see Table 15–5). All except captopril, which has a much shorter half-life than the others, can be dosed once daily; captopril is dosed two or three times daily. In some patients, especially when higher doses are used, twice daily dosing is needed to maintain 24-hour effects with enalapril, benazepril, moexipril, quinapril, and ramipril. The absorption of captopril, but not other ACE inhibitors, is reduced when given with food.

ACE inhibitors are well tolerated,[98] but are not absent of side effects. ACE inhibitors decrease aldosterone and can increase serum potassium concentrations. Although this increase is usually small, and beneficial in thiazide-treated patients, hyperkalemia is possible. Patients with chronic kidney disease or those on concomitant nonsteroidal antiinflammatory drugs, potassium supplements, or potassium-sparing diuretics are at risk for hyperkalemia. Judicious monitoring of serum potassium and creatinine values within 4 weeks of starting or increasing the dose of an ACE inhibitor can often identify these abnormalities before they evolve into serious hyperkalemia.

A worrisome adverse effect of ACE inhibitor is acute kidney failure. Fortunately, this serious adverse effect is rare, occurring in less than 1% of patients. Preexisting kidney disease increases the risk of this side effect. Bilateral renal artery stenosis or unilateral stenosis of a solitary functioning kidney render patients dependent on the vasoconstrictive effect of angiotensin II on the efferent arteriole of the kidney, thus explaining why these patients are particularly susceptible to acute kidney failure from ACE inhibitors. Slowly titrating the dose of ACE inhibitor and judicious kidney function monitoring can minimize risk and allow for early detection of those with renal artery stenosis.

It is important to note that GFR decreases in patients treated with ACE inhibitors or ARBs.[65] This is attributed to the inhibition of angiotensin II vasoconstriction on the efferent arteriole. This decrease in GFR often increases serum creatinine, and small increases should be anticipated when monitoring patients on ACE inhibitors. Modest elevations of either up to a 35% (for baseline creatinine values less than or equal to 3 mg/dL) or absolute increases less than 1 mg/dL, do not warrant changes.[65] If larger increases occur, ACE inhibitor therapy should be stopped or the dose reduced.

Angioedema is a serious potential complication of ACE inhibitor therapy. It occurs in less than 1% of the population, and is more likely in African Americans and smokers. Symptoms include lip and tongue swelling and possibly difficulty breathing. Drug discontinuation is needed for ACE inhibitor-associated angioedema. However, angioedema associated with laryngeal edema and/or pulmonary symptoms occasionally occurs and requires treatment with epinephrine, corticosteroids, antihistamines and/or emergent intubations to support respiration. A history of angioedema, even if not from an ACE inhibitor, precludes use of another ACE inhibitor (it is a contraindication). Cross-reactivity between ACE inhibitors and ARBs is small, but has been reported.[53,99] An ARB can be used in a patient with a history of ACE inhibitor-induced angioedema when there is a compelling indication for an ARB with careful monitoring for a repeat occurrence of angioedema.

A persistent dry cough develops in up to 20% of patients, and is pharmacologically explained by the inhibition of bradykinin breakdown. This cough does not cause clinical illness, but is annoying to patients. It should be clearly differentiated from a wet cough because of pulmonary edema, which may be a sign of uncontrolled heart failure versus an ACE inhibitor-induced cough.

ACE inhibitors, in addition to ARBs, are absolutely contraindicated in pregnancy.[1,83] Female patients of child-bearing age should be counseled regarding effective forms of birth control as ACE inhibitors are associated major congenital malformations when exposed in the first trimester and fetopathy (group of conditions that includes renal failure, renal dysplasia, hypotension, oligohydramnios, pulmonary hypotension, hypocalvaria, and death) when exposed in the second and third trimester.[83] Similar to diuretics, ACE inhibitors can increase lithium serum concentrations in patients on lithium therapy. Concurrent use of an ACE with a potassium-sparing diuretic (including aldosterone antagonists), potassium supplements, or an ARB may result in excessive increases in potassium.

Starting doses of ACE inhibitors should be low, with even lower doses in patients at risk for orthostatic hypotension, or severe renal dysfunction (e.g., elderly, chronic kidney disease). Acute hypotension may occur at the onset of ACE inhibitor therapy. Patients who are sodium or volume depleted, in heart failure exacerbation, very elderly, or on concurrent vasodilators or diuretics are at high risk for this effect. It is important to start with half the normal dose of an ACE inhibitor for all patients with these risk factors, and use slow dose titration.

Angiotensin Receptor Blockers ARBs are first-line agents for hypertension.[1,2] Angiotensin II is generated by two enzymatic pathways: the RAAS, which involves ACE, and an alternative pathway that uses other enzymes such as chymases (also known as "tissue ACE"). ACE inhibitors inhibit only the effects of angiotensin II produced through the RAAS, whereas ARBs inhibit angiotensin II from all pathways. It is unclear how these differences affect tissue concentrations of ACE. ACE inhibitors only partially block the effects of angiotensin II, though the clinical significance of this is not known.

ARBs directly block the angiotensin II receptor subtype 1 receptor that mediates the known effects of angiotensin II in humans: vasoconstriction, aldosterone release, sympathetic activation, antidiuretic hormone release, and constriction of the efferent arterioles of the glomerulus. Because they do not block the angiotensin II receptor subtype 2 receptor, the beneficial effects of angiotensin II receptor subtype 2 stimulation (vasodilation, tissue repair, and inhibition of cell growth) remain intact when ARBs are used. Unlike ACE inhibitors, ARBs do not block the breakdown of bradykinin. Therefore, some of the beneficial effects of bradykinin, such as vasodilation (which can enhance treatment of left ventricular dysfuntion), regression of myocyte hypertrophy and fibrosis, and increased levels of tissue plasminogen activator, are not present with ARB therapy.

ARBs have outcomes data showing long-term reductions in progression of target-organ damage in patients with hypertension and certain compelling indications. In patients with type 2 diabetes and nephropathy, progression of nephropathy has been shown to be significantly reduced with ARB therapy.[64] Some benefits appear to be independent of BP lowering, suggesting that the pharmacologic effects of ARBs on the efferent arteriole may result in progression of kidney disease. For patients with left ventricular dysfunction, the CHARM studies showed that ARB therapy reduces risk of CV events when added to a stable regimen of a diuretic, ACE inhibitor, and β-blocker, or as alternative therapy in ACE-intolerant patients.[53,54] Importantly, the ELITE (Evaluation of Losartan in the Elderly) studies show that losartan is not superior to captopril in left ventricular dysfunction when compared head-to-head.[51,52] One outcome study, the VALLIANT, also showed that an ARBs can reduce CV events in patients post-MI with left ventricular dysfunction, but would be used mostly as an alternative to an ACE inhibitor for this use.[58]

ARBs have been compared head-to-head with CCBs. The MOSES demonstrated that eprosartan reduces the occurrence of recurrent stroke more than nitrendipine does in patients with a past medical history of cerebrovascular disease.[74] Using nitrendipine was a reasonable comparator because the Syst-Eur had already demonstrated that nitrendipine reduces the occurrence of CV events, particularly stroke, in older patients with isolated systolic hypertension.[12] These data support the common notion that ARBs may have cerebroprotective effects that may explain CV event reductions. Another outcome study, the VALUE (Valsartan Long-term Use Evaluation) trial, showed that valsartan-based therapy is equivalent to amlodipine-based therapy for the primary composite outcome of first CV event in patients with hypertension and additional CV risk factors.[33] However, occurrence of certain components of the primary end point (stroke and MI) and new-onset type 2 diabetes was lower in the valsartan group. Although patients treated with amlodipine had slightly lower mean BP values than valsartan treated patients, there was no difference in the primary end point.

Data from pooled analyses and direct comparisons have demonstrated that ARBs have a fairly flat dose–response curve, suggesting that increasing the dose above low or moderate doses is unlikely to result in a large degree of BP lowering.[98] The addition of low doses of a thiazide-type diuretic to an ARB significantly increases antihypertensive efficacy. Similar to ACE inhibitors, most ARBs have long enough half-lives to allow for once-daily dosing. However, candesartan, eprosartan, losartan, and valsartan have the shortest half-lives and may require twice-daily dosing for sustained BP lowering.

ARBs have the lowest incidence of side effects compared to other antihypertensive agents.[98] Because they do not affect bradykinin, they do not have the potential to illicit a dry cough like ACE inhibitors. Although these drugs have been termed "ACE inhibitors without the cough," pharmacologic differences highlight that they could have very different effects on vascular smooth muscle and myocardial tissue that can correlate to different effects on target-organ damage and CV risk reduction when compared with ACE inhibitors. It is possible that their effects may be superior to ACE inhibitors in patients with type 2 diabetic nephropathy, but may be inferior to ACE inhibitors in patients with more advanced heart disease (e.g., heart failure, post-MI). Unfortunately, there are no direct comparisons looking at long-term effects in patients with just hypertension. Regardless, their role in patients with type 2 diabetic nephropathy is well established and they also are very reasonable alternatives in patients requiring an ACE inhibitor but who experience intolerable side effects.

CLINICAL CONTROVERSY

Data demonstrates that risk of CV events is further reduced when an ARB is added to an ACE inhibitor in patients with left ventricular dysfunction. Other data support this combination in patients with severe forms of nephrotic syndrome. However, using the combination of an ACE with an ARB has not been well studied as a standard treatment regimen in hypertension and incurs a significantly higher risk of side effects (e.g., hyperkalemia).[100]

Like ACE inhibitors, ARBs may cause renal insufficiency, hyperkalemia, and orthostatic hypotension. The same precautions that apply to ACE inhibitors for patients with suspected bilateral renal artery stenosis, those on drugs that can raise potassium, and those on drugs that increase risk of hypotension apply to ARBs. ARBs can be used with caution in patients with a history of angioedema, but unlike ACE inhibitors are not contraindicated. Angioedema is also less likely to occur than with ACE inhibitors, but cross-reactivity has been reported.[53,99] An ARB should only be used in a patient with a history of ACE inhibitor-induced angioedema when there is a compelling indication for an ARB with careful monitoring for a repeat occurrence of angioedema. ARBs should not be used in pregnancy.[83]

Calcium Channel Blockers[12,27] CCBs, both dihydropyridine CCBs and nondihydropyridine CCBs, are first-line agents for hypertension.[1,2] They have compelling indications in coronary disease and in diabetes. However, with these compelling indications, they are essentially in addition to, or in replacement of, other antihypertensive drug classes.

Previous data indicated that dihydropyridine CCBs may not provide as much protection against CV events when compared with conventional therapy (diuretics and β-blockers) or ACE inhibitors in uncomplicated hypertension.[27] However, newer data shows that CCBs are likely to be as effective at lowering CV events as other agents. In ALLHAT there was no difference in the primary outcome between chlorthalidone and amlodipine, and only the secondary outcome of heart failure was higher with amlodipine.[30] A subgroup analysis of ALLHAT directly compared amlodipine to lisinopril and demonstrated that there was no difference in the primary outcome.[101] As discussed previously, the VALUE study also showed no difference in the primary outcome of first CV event in high-risk patients between valsartan and amlodipine.[33]

There may be differences in CV event reduction between dihydropyridine CCBs and nondihydropyridine CCBs. In patients with hypertension and diabetes, dihydropyridine CCBs appear to be less cardioprotective than ACE inhibitors.[64] Studies with the nondihydropyridine CCBs (diltiazem and verapamil) are limited, but the NORDIL (Nordic Diltiazem) study found diltiazem to be equivalent to diuretics and β-blockers in reducing CV events.[27] It is possible that these differences (beneficial with diltiazem and neutral with dihydropyridines) may relate to the sympathetic stimulation that can occur with dihydropyridines.

Dihydropyridine CCBs are very effective in older patients with isolated systolic hypertension. The Syst-Eur demonstrated that a long-acting dihydropyridine CCB reduced the risk of CV events markedly in isolated systolic hypertension.[12] A long-acting dihydropyridine CCB should be strongly considered in isolated systolic hypertension.

Contraction of cardiac and smooth muscle cells requires an increase in free intracellular calcium concentrations from the extracellular fluid. When cardiac or vascular smooth muscle is stimulated, voltage-sensitive channels in the cell membrane are opened, allowing calcium to enter the cells. The influx of extracellular calcium into the cell releases stored calcium from the sarcoplasmic reticulum. As intracellular free calcium concentration increases, it binds to a protein, calmodulin, which then activates myosin kinase enabling myosin to interact with actin to induce contraction. CCBs work by inhibiting influx of calcium across the cell membrane. There are two types of voltage-gated calcium channels: a high-voltage channel (L type) and a low-voltage channel (T type). Currently available CCBs only block the L-type channel, which leads to coronary and peripheral vasodilation.

The two subclasses of CCBs, dihydropyridines and nondihydropyridines (see Table 15–5) are pharmacologically very different from each other. Antihypertensive effectiveness is similar with both subclasses, but they differ in other pharmacodynamic effects. Nondihydropyridines decrease heart rate and slow atrioventricular nodal conduction. Similar to β-blockers, these drugs may also treat supraventricular tachyarrhythmias (e.g., atrial fibrillation). Verapamil produces negative inotropic and chronotropic effects that are responsible for its propensity to precipitate or cause systolic heart failure in high-risk patients. Diltiazem also has these effects but to a lesser extent than verapamil. All CCBs (except amlodipine and felodipine) have negative inotropic effects. Dihydropyridines may cause a baroreceptor-mediated reflex tachycardia because of their potent peripheral vasodilating effects. This effect appears to be more pronounced with the first generation dihydropyridines (e.g., nifedipine) and is significantly diminished with the newer agents (e.g., amlodipine) and when given in sustained-release dosage forms. Dihydropyridines do not alter conduction through the atrioventricular node and thus are not effective agents in supraventricular tachyarrhythmias.

Among dihydropyridines, short-acting nifedipine may rarely cause an increase in the frequency, intensity, and duration of angina in association with acute hypotension. This effect is most likely due to a reflex sympathetic stimulation, and is likely obviated by using sustained-release formulations of nifedipine. For this reason, all other dihydropyridines have an intrinsically long-half-life or are provided in sustained release formulations. Immediate-release nifedipine has been associated with an increased incidence of adverse CV effects, is not approved for treatment of hypertension, and should not be used to treat hypertension. Other side effects with dihydropyridines include dizziness, flushing, headache, gingival hyperplasia, and peripheral edema. Side effects caused by vasodilation, such as dizziness, flushing, headache, and peripheral edema, occur more frequently with all dihydropyridines than with the nondihydropyridines because they are less-potent vasodilators.

Diltiazem and verapamil can cause cardiac conduction abnormalities such as bradycardia or atrioventricular block. These problems occur mostly with high-doses or when used in patients with preexisting abnormalities in the cardiac conduction system. Heart failure has been reported in otherwise healthy patients as a consequence of negative inotropic effects. Both drugs can cause anorexia, nausea, peripheral edema, and hypotension. Verapamil causes constipation in approximately 7% of patients. This side effect also occurs with diltiazem, but to a lesser extent.

Verapamil and to a lesser extent diltiazem, can cause drug interactions because of their ability to inhibit the cytochrome P450 3A4 isoenzyme system. This inhibition can increase serum concentrations of other drugs that are metabolized by this isoenzyme system (e.g., cyclosporine, digoxin, lovastatin, simvastatin, tacrolimus, theophylline). Verapamil and diltiazem should be given very cautiously with a β-blocker because there is an increased risk of heart block with these combinations. When a CCB is needed in combination with a β-blocker for BP lowering, a dihydropyridine should be selected, because it will not increase risk of heart block. The hepatic metabolism of CCBs, especially felodipine, nicardipine, nifedipine, and nisoldipine, may be inhibited by ingesting large quantities of grapefruit juice (≥1 quart daily).

Many different formulations of verapamil and diltiazem are currently available (see Table 15–5). Although certain sustained-release verapamil and diltiazem products may contain the same active drug (e.g., Calan SR and Verelan), they are usually not AB rated by the FDA as interchangeable on a mg-per-mg basis because of different biopharmaceutical release mechanisms. However, the clinical significance of these differences is likely negligible.

Two sustained-release verapamil products (Covera HS and Verelan PM) and one diltiazem product (Cardizem LA) are chronotherapeutically designed to target the circadian BP rhythm. These agents are primarily dosed in the evening (with the exception of Cardizem LA which may be dosed in the morning or evening) so that drug is released during the early morning hours when BP first starts to increase. The rationale behind chronotherapy in hypertension is that blunting the early morning BP surge may result in greater reductions in CV events than conventional dosing of regular antihypertensive products in the morning. However, evidence from the CONVINCE (Controlled Onset Verapamil Investigation of Cardiovascular End Points) trial showed that chronotherapeutic verapamil was similar, but not better than, a thiazide-type diuretic/β-blocker–based regimen with respect to CV events.[28]

β-Blockers[27,28,48,59,62] β-Blockers have been used in several large outcome trials in hypertension. However, in most of these trials, a thiazide-type diuretic was the primary agents with a β-blocker added on for additional BP lowering. Therefore, β-blockers are now only considered appropriate first-line agents to treat specific compelling indications (post-MI, coronary disease). They also are evidence-based as additional therapy for other compelling indications (heart failure and diabetes). Numerous trials have shown reduced CV risk when β-blockers are used following an MI, during an acute coronary syndrome, or in chronic stable angina. Although once considered contraindicated in heart failure, multiple studies have shown that carvedilol and metoprolol succinate reduce mortality in patients with left ventricular dysfunction who are treated with a diuretic and ACE inhibitor.

For patients with hypertension but without compelling indications, other primary agents (thiazide-type diuretics, ACE inhibitors, ARBs, and CCBs) should be used as the initial first-line agent before β-blockers. While this may be surprising to experienced clinicians, this recommendation is consistent with the 2007 AHA guidelines, the 2007 European Society of Hypertension guidelines, and the 2006 United Kingdom's National Institute for Health and the Clinical Excellence guidelines.[2,92,93] It is based on meta-analyses data that suggest β-blocker–based therapy may not reduce CV events as well as these other agents when used as the initial drug to treat patients with hypertension and without a compelling indication for a β-blocker.

Several mechanisms of action have been proposed for β-blockers, but none of them alone is consistently associated with a reduction in arterial BP. β-Blockers have negative chronotropic and inotropic cardiac effects that reduce cardiac output and explains some of the antihypertensive effect. However, cardiac output falls equally in patients treated with β-blockers regardless of BP lowering.

β-Adrenoceptors are located on the surface membranes of juxtaglomerular cells, and β-blockers inhibit these receptors and thus the release of renin. However, there is a weak association between plasma renin and antihypertensive efficacy of β-blocker therapy. Some patients with low plasma renin concentrations do respond to β-blockers. Therefore, additional mechanisms must also account for the antihypertensive effect of β-blockers. However, the ability of β-blockers to reduce plasma renin and thus angiotensin II concentrations may play a major role in their ability to reduce CV risk.

There are important pharmacodynamic and pharmacokinetic differences among β-blockers, but all agents provide a similar degree of BP lowering. There are two pharmacodynamic properties of the β-blockers that differentiate this class: cardioselectivity and ISA. β-Blockers that possess a greater affinity for β_1-receptors than β_2-receptors are *cardioselective.*

The β_1- and β_2-adrenoceptors are distributed throughout the body, but they concentrate differently in certain organs and tissues. There is a preponderance of β_1-receptors in the heart and kidney, and a preponderance of β_2-receptors in the lungs, liver, pancreas, and arteriolar smooth muscle. β_1-Receptor stimulation increases heart rate, contractility, and renin release. β_2-Receptor stimulation results in bronchodilation and vasodilation. Cardioselective β-blockers are not likely to provoke bronchospasm and vasoconstriction. Insulin secretion and glycogenolysis are mediated by β_2-receptors. Blocking β_2-receptors may reduce these processes and cause hyperglycemia or blunt recovery from hypoglycemia.

Cardioselective β-blockers (e.g., atenolol, metoprolol) have clinically significant advantages over nonselective β-blockers (e.g., propranolol, nadolol), and are generally preferred to treat hypertension. Cardioselective agents are safer than nonselective agents in patients with asthma or diabetes. However, cardioselectivity is a dose-dependent phenomenon; at higher doses, cardioselective agents lose their relative selectivity for β_1-receptors and block β_2-receptors as effectively as they block β_1-receptors. The dose at which cardioselectivity is lost varies from patient to patient.

Some β-blockers (e.g., acebutolol, pindolol) have ISA and act as partial β-receptor agonists. When they bind to the β-receptor, they stimulate it, but far less than a pure β-agonist. If sympathetic tone is low, as it is during resting states, β-receptors are partially stimulated by ISA β-blockers. Therefore, resting heart rate, cardiac output, and peripheral blood flow are not reduced when these type of β-blockers are used. Theoretically, ISA agents would appear to have advantages over β-blockers in certain patients with heart failure, or sinus bradycardia. Unfortunately, they do not appear to reduce CV events as well as other β-blockers. In fact, they may increase risk post-MI or in those with coronary disease. Thus, agents with ISA are rarely needed and have little to no clinical utility.

Pharmacokinetic differences among β-blockers relate to first-pass metabolism, route of elimination, degree of lipophilicity, and serum half-lives. Propranolol and metoprolol undergo extensive first-pass metabolism, so the dose needed to attain β-blockade with either drug varies from patient to patient. Atenolol and nadolol have are renally excreted. The dose of these agents may need to be reduced in patients with moderate to severe chronic kidney disease.

β-Blockers, especially those with highly lipophilic properties, penetrate the central nervous system penetration and may cause other effects. Propranolol is the most lipophilic drug and atenolol is the least lipophilic. It is unclear whether higher lipophilicity is associated with more central nervous system side effects (dizziness, drowsiness). However, the lipophilic properties can provide better effects for non-CV conditions such as migraine headache prevention, essential tremor, and thyrotoxicosis. BP lowering is equal among β-blockers regardless of lipophilicity.

CLINICAL CONTROVERSY

Many of the clinical trials included in the meta-analyses data that suggest β-blocker–based therapy may not reduce CV events as well as these other agents used atenolol dosed once daily.[44–47] Atenolol has a half life of 6 to 7 hours and is nearly always dosed once daily, whereas immediate-release forms of carvedilol and metoprolol tartrate have 6- to 10- and 3- to 7-hour half-lives respectively, and are always dosed at least twice daily. Consequently, it is possible that these findings might only apply to atenolol and also that these findings may be a result of using atenolol once daily instead of twice daily.

Most side effects of β-blockers are an extension of their ability to antagonize β-adrenoceptors. β-Blockade in the myocardium can be associated with bradycardia, atrioventricular conduction abnormalities (e.g., second- or third-degree heart block), and the development of acute heart failure. The decreases in heart rate may actually benefit certain patients with atrial arrhythmias (atrial fibrillation, atrial flutter) and hypertension by both providing rate control and BP lowering. β-Blockers usually only produce heart failure if they are used in high initial doses in patients with preexisting left ventricular dysfunction or if started in these patients during an acute heart failure exacerbation. Blocking β_2-receptors in arteriolar smooth muscle may cause cold extremities and may aggravate peripheral arterial disease or Raynaud's phenomenon as a result of decreased peripheral blood flow. In addition, there is an increase of sympathetic tone during periods of hypoglycemia that may result in an increase in BP because of unopposed α-receptor-mediated vasoconstriction.

Abrupt cessation of β-blocker therapy can produce unstable angina, MI, or even death in patients with coronary disease. Abrupt cessation may also lead to rebound hypertension (a sudden increase in BP to above pretreatment values). To avoid this, β-blockers should always be tapered gradually over 1 to 2 weeks before eventually discontinuing the drug. This acute withdrawal syndrome is believed to be secondary to progression of underlying coronary disease and hypersensitivity of β-adrenergic receptors as a result of upregulation. In patients without coronary disease, abrupt discontinuation may present as tachycardia, sweating, and generalized malaise, in addition to increased BP.

Like diuretics, β-blockers have been shown to increase serum cholesterol and glucose values, but these effects are transient and of questionable clinical significance. In patients with diabetes or dyslipidemia, the reduction in CV events was as great with β-blockers as with an ACE inhibitor in the United Kingdom Prospective Diabetes Study,[66] and far superior to placebo in the SHEP trial.[9] In the GEMENI (Glycemic Effects in Diabetes Mellitus: Carvedilol-Metoprolol Comparison in Hypertension) trial, patients with diabetes and hypertension who were randomized to metoprolol had an increase in hemoglobin A_{1c} values, whereas patients randomized to carvedilol did not.[102] This suggests that mixed α- and β-blocking effects of carvedilol may be preferential to metoprolol in patients with uncontrolled diabetes. However, differences in hemoglobin A_{1c} values were too small to make this application clinically relevant in all patients with diabetes that need treatment with a β-blocker.

β-Blockers can slightly increase serum triglycerides and decrease high-density lipoprotein cholesterol. β-Blockers with α-blocking properties produce no changes in these lipid values. Because these are of questionable clinical significance, cardioselective agents, which have less overall side effects, remain the β-blockers of choice for most patients.

⑬ Alternative Agents The primary role of an alternative antihypertensive agent is to provide additional BP lowering in patients who are already treated with an agent from a drug class proven to reduce CV events (diuretics, ACE inhibitors, ARBs, CCBs, or even β-blockers).

α_1-Blockers.[35] Prazosin, terazosin, and doxazosin are selective α_1-receptor blockers. They work in the peripheral vasculature and inhibit the uptake of catecholamines in smooth muscle cells resulting in vasodilation and BP lowering.

Doxazosin was one of the original treatment arms of the ALLHAT. However, it was stopped prematurely when statistically more secondary end points of stoke, heart failure, and CV events were seen with doxazosin compared with chlorthalidone.[35] There were no differences in the primary end point of fatal coronary heart disease and nonfatal MI. These data suggest that thiazide-type diuretics are superior to α_1-blockers in preventing CV events in patients with hypertension. Therefore, α_1-blockers are alternative agents that should be used in combination with primary antihypertensive agents.

α_1-Blockers can provide symptomatic benefits in men with benign prostatic hypertrophy. These agents block postsynaptic α_1-adrenergic receptors located on the prostate capsule, causing relaxation and decreased resistance to urinary outflow. However, when used to lower BP, they should only be in addition to primary antihypertensive agents.

A potentially severe side effect of α_1-blockers is a "first-dose" phenomenon that is characterized by transient dizziness or faintness, palpitations, and even syncope within 1 to 3 hours of the first dose. This adverse reaction can also happen after dose increases. These episodes are accompanied by orthostatic hypotension and can be obviated by taking the first dose and subsequent first increased doses at bedtime. Because orthostatic hypotension and dizziness may persist with chronic administration, these agents should be used cautiously in elderly patients. Even though antihypertensive effects are achieved through a peripheral α_1-receptor antagonism, these agents cross the blood–brain barrier and may cause central nervous system side effects. α_1-Blockers also may cause priapism. Sodium and water retention can occur with chronic administration. Consequently, these agents are most effective when given in combination with a diuretic to maintain antihypertensive efficacy and minimize potential edema.

Aliskiren.[103,104] Aliskiren is the first oral agent within a new antihypertensive drug class that directly inhibits renin.[103] This drug blocks the RAAS at its point of activation, which results in reduced plasma renin activity and BP lowering. It has a 24-hour half-life, is primarily eliminated through biliary excretion unchanged, and provides 24-hour antihypertensive effects with once-daily dosing.

The exact role of this drug class in the management of hypertension is unclear. Aliskiren is approved as monotherapy or in combination therapy. However, because of the lack of long-term studies evaluating CV event reduction and significant drug cost compared to generic agents with outcomes data, it should clearly be used as an alternative therapy for the treatment of hypertension. Studies evaluating the ability of aliskiren to lower CV events and decrease progression of diabetic nephropathy are planned to start in 2007, but will not be completed for many years. Aliskiren provides BP reductions comparable to an ACE inhibitor, ARB, or CCB. It also has additive antihypertensive effects when used in combination with thiazides, ACE inhibitors, ARBs, or a CCB, although its effectiveness in combination with maximum doses of ACE inhibitors has not been adequately studied.

Many of the cautions and adverse effects seen with ACE inhibitors and ARBs apply to direct renin inhibitors (i.e., aliskiren). Aliskiren should never be used in pregnancy because of the known teratogenic effects of using other drugs that block the RAAS system. Angioedema has also been reported in patients treated with aliskiren. Increases in serum creatinine and serum potassium values have been observed. The mechanisms of these adverse effects are likely similar to those with ACE inhibitors and ARBs. It is reasonable to use similar monitoring strategies by measuring serum creatinine and serum potassium in patients treated with aliskiren. This is particularly important in patients treated with the combination of aliskiren and an ACE inhibitor or an ARB who are at higher risk for hyperkalemia (e.g., chronic kidney disease).

Central α_2-Agonists. Clonidine, guanabenz, guanfacine, and methyldopa lower BP primarily by stimulating α_2-adrenergic receptors in the brain. This stimulation reduces sympathetic outflow from the vasomotor center in the brain and increases vagal tone. It is also believed that peripheral stimulation of presynaptic α_2-receptors may further reduce sympathetic tone. Reduced sympathetic activity together with enhanced parasympathetic activity can decrease heart rate, cardiac output, total peripheral resistance, plasma renin activity, and baroreceptor reflexes. Clonidine is often used in resistant hypertension, and methyldopa is a first-line agent for pregnancy-induced hypertension.

Chronic use of centrally acting α_2-agonists results in sodium and water retention. As with other centrally acting antihypertensives, depression can occur, especially with high doses. The incidence of orthostatic hypotension and dizziness is high, so they should be used very cautiously in the elderly. Lastly, clonidine has a relatively high incidence of anticholinergic side effects (sedation, dry mouth, constipation, urinary retention, and blurred vision). Thus it should generally be avoided for chronic antihypertensive therapy in the elderly.

Abrupt cessation of central α_2-agonists may lead to rebound hypertension. This effect is thought to be secondary to a compensatory increase in norepinephrine release after abrupt discontinuation. In addition, other effects such as nervousness, agitation, headache, and tremor can also occur, which may be exacerbated by concomitant β-blocker use, particularly with clonidine. Thus, if clonidine is to be continued it should be tapered. In patients who are receiving concomitant β-blocker therapy, the β-blocker should be gradually discontinued first several days before gradual discontinuation of clonidine.

Methyldopa can cause hepatitis or hemolytic anemia, although this is rare. Transient elevations in serum hepatic transaminases are occasionally seen with methyldopa therapy but are clinically irrelevant unless they are greater than three times the upper limit of normal. Methyldopa should be quickly discontinued if persistent increases in serum hepatic transaminases or alkaline phosphatase are detected because this may indicate the onset of a fulminate life-threatening hepatitis. A Coombs-positive hemolytic anemia occurs in less than 1% of patients receiving methyldopa, although 20% of patients exhibit a positive direct Coombs test without anemia. For these reasons, methyldopa has limited use in routine management of hypertension except in pregnancy.

Reserpine. Reserpine lowers BP by depleting norepinephrine from sympathetic nerve endings, and blocking transport of norepinephrine into its storage granules. Norepinephrine release into the synapse following nerve stimulation is reduced and results in reduced sympathetic tone, peripheral vascular resistance, and BP. Reserpine also depletes catecholamines in the brain and the myocardium.

Reserpine has a slow onset of action and long-half life that allows for once-daily dosing. However, it may take 2 to 6 weeks before the maximal antihypertensive effect is seen. Because reserpine can cause significant sodium and water retention, it should only be given in combination with a diuretic (preferably a thiazide). Reserpine's strong inhibition of sympathetic activity results in increased parasympathetic activity. This effect explains why side effects such as nasal stuffiness, increased gastric acid secretion, diarrhea, and bradycardia can occur. Depression has been reported, which is a consequence of central nervous system depletion of catecholamines and serotonin. The initial reports of depression with reserpine were in the 1950s and are inconsistent with current definitions of depression. Regardless, reserpine-induced depression is dose-related. Moreover, very high doses (above 1 mg daily) were frequently used in the 1950s, resulting in more depression. When reserpine is used in doses between 0.05 and 0.25 mg daily (recommended doses), the rate of depression is equal to that seen with β-blockers, diuretics, or placebo.[9]

Reserpine was used as a third-line agent in many of the landmark clinical trials that have documented the benefit in treating hypertension, including the VA Cooperative trials and most importantly, the SHEP trial.[9] An analysis of the SHEP data found that reserpine was very well tolerated.

Direct Arterial Vasodilators. Hydralazine and minoxidil directly relax arteriolar smooth muscle resulting in vasodilation and BP lowering. Both agents cause potent reductions in perfusion pressure that activates the baroreceptor reflexes. Activation of baroreceptors results in a compensatory increase in sympathetic outflow, which leads to an increase in heart rate, cardiac output, and renin release. Consequently, tachyphylaxis can develop resulting in a loss of hypotensive effect with continued use. This compensatory baroreceptor response can be counteracted by concurrent use of a β-blocker.

All patients receiving hydralazine or minoxidil long-term for hypertension should first receive both a diuretic and a β-blocker. Direct arterial vasodilators can precipitate angina in patients with underlying coronary disease unless the baroreceptor reflex mechanism is completely blocked with a β-blocker. Nondihydropyridine CCBs can be used as an alternative to β-blockers in these patients, but a β-blocker is preferred. The side effect of sodium and water retention is significant with these drugs, and is minimized by using a diuretic concomitantly.

One side effect unique to hydralazine is a dose-dependent drug-induced lupus-like syndrome. Hydralazine is eliminated by hepatic *N*-acetyltransferase. This enzyme displays genetic polymorphism, and "slow acetylators" are especially prone to develop drug-induced lupus with hydralazine. This syndrome is more common in women and is reversible upon discontinuation. Drug-induced lupus may be avoided by using less than 200 mg of hydralazine daily. Other side effects of hydralazine include dermatitis, drug fever, peripheral neuropathy, hepatitis, and vascular headaches. For these reasons, hydralazine has limited usefulness in the treatment of hypertension. However, it is still especially useful in patients with severe chronic kidney disease and in kidney failure.

Because minoxidil is a more potent vasodilator than hydralazine, the compensatory increases in heart rate, cardiac output, renin release, and sodium retention are even more dramatic. Sodium and water retention can be so severe with minoxidil that heart failure can be precipitated. It is even more important to coadminister a β-blocker and a diuretic with minoxidil. A loop diuretic is often more effective than a thiazide in patients treated with minoxidil. A troublesome side effect of minoxidil is hypertrichosis (hirsutism), presenting as increased hair growth on the face, arms, back, and chest. This usually ceases when the drug is discontinued. Minoxidil is reserved for very-difficult-to-control hypertension and in patients requiring hydralazine who experience drug-induced lupus.

Other Agents. Guanethidine and guanadrel are postganglionic sympathetic inhibitors. Because of significant complications, these drugs have little to no role in the management of hypertension. They deplete norepinephrine from postganglionic sympathetic nerve terminals and inhibit the release of norepinephrine in response to sympathetic nerve stimulation, resulting in reduced cardiac output and peripheral vascular resistance. Orthostatic hypotension is common because reflex-mediated vasoconstriction is blocked. Long-term norepinephrine depletion leads to postsynaptic receptor supersensitivity. Consequently, concomitant use of sympathomimetics or tricyclic antidepressants may provoke hypertensive crisis. Erectile dysfunction, diarrhea, and weight gain are also common.

Agents in Development.[104] Darusentan, clevidipine, and nebivolol are new agents under study that provide significant reductions in BP and may be approved for hypertension in the near future. Darusentan is an endothelin (A) selective endothelin receptor antagonist. There currently are no antihypertensive agents available that target the endothelin receptor. If this agent is approved, it will likely be used in patients with resistant hypertension. Nebivolol is a "third-generation" cardioselective β-blocker. It produces vasodilation and improves endothelial function via the L-arginine–nitric oxide pathway. Clevidipine is an ultrashort-acting, vascular-selective, dihydropyridine calcium antagonist. It is being developed for intravenous use in patients with hypertensive crisis.

PHARMACOECONOMIC CONSIDERATIONS

The cost of effectively treating hypertension is substantial. However, these costs can be offset by savings that would be realized by reducing CV morbidity and mortality. Cost related to treating target-organ damage (e.g., MI, end-stage kidney failure) can drastically increase healthcare costs. The cost per life-year saved from treating hypertension is estimated to be $40,000 for younger adults and even less for older adults.[105] Treatments that cost less than $50,000 per quality-adjusted life-year saved generally are considered favorable by health economists.

In a cost-minimization study that included the cost of drug acquisition, supplemental drugs, laboratory tests, clinic visits, and complications, the total costs of treating hypertension with either a diuretic, ACE-inhibitor, or CCB was under $1,500.[106] Another cost-minimization analysis found that 86 middle-age or 29 elderly patients with hypertension would need to be treated to prevent 1 MI, stroke, or death.[107]

A comparative analysis of 133,624 patients with hypertension ages 65 and older from a state prescription drug-assistance program demonstrated that 40% of patients were prescribed pharmacotherapy that was not necessarily recommended by the JNC7 guidelines recommendations.[108] If these 40% had drug-therapy modifications made to follow evidence-based treatment, a reduction in costs of $11.6 million would have been realized in the 2001 calendar year based on discounted prices. This was projected to increase to $20.5 million using usual Medicaid pricing limits.

Thus it is crucial to identify ways to control the cost of care without increasing the morbidity and mortality associated with uncontrolled hypertension. Using evidence-based pharmacotherapy will save costs not only by using the most effective agents. Thiazide-type diuretics are first-line treatment options in most patients without compelling indications, and are very inexpensive. Just using thiazides, either as monotherapy or in combination, is appropriate under almost all circumstances and aspects of hypertension management. When needed, using other generic primary antihypertensive agents that can be administered once daily should be considered.

HYPERTENSIVE URGENCIES AND EMERGENCIES[1,7]

Both hypertensive urgencies and emergencies are characterized by the presence of very elevated BP—greater than 180/120 mm Hg.

However, the need for urgent or emergent antihypertensive therapy should be determined based on the presence of acute or immediately progressing target-organ injury, but not elevated BP alone. Urgencies are not associated with acute or immediately progressing target-organ injury, whereas emergencies are. Examples of acute target-organ injury include encephalopathy, intracranial hemorrhage, acute left ventricular failure with pulmonary edema, dissecting aortic aneurysm, unstable angina, and eclampsia or severe hypertension during pregnancy.

⓮ Hypertensive Urgency

A common error with treating hypertensive urgency is initiating overly aggressive antihypertensive therapy. This treatment likely has been caused by the classification terminology "urgency." Hypertensive urgencies are ideally managed by adjusting maintenance therapy by adding a new antihypertensive and/or increasing the dose of a present medication. This is the preferred approach to these patients as it provides a more gradual reduction in BP. Very rapid reductions in BP to goal values should be discouraged because of potential risks. Because autoregulation of blood flow in patients with hypertension occurs at a much higher range of pressure than in normotensive persons, the inherent risks of reducing BP too precipitously include cerebrovascular accidents, MI, and acute kidney failure. Hypertensive urgency requires BP reductions with oral antihypertensive agents to stage 1 values over a period of several hours to several days. All patients with hypertensive urgency should be reevaluated within 7 days (preferably after 1 to 3 days).

Acute administration of a short-acting oral antihypertensive (captopril, clonidine or labetalol) followed by careful observation for several hours to assure a gradual reduction in BP is an option for hypertensive urgency. However, there are no data supporting this approach as being absolutely needed. Oral captopril is one of the agents of choice and can be used in doses of 25 to 50 mg at 1- to 2-hour intervals. The onset of action of oral captopril is 15 to 30 minutes, and a marked fall in BP is unlikely to occur if no hypotensive response is observed within 30 to 60 minutes. For patients with hypertensive rebound following withdrawal of clonidine, 0.2 mg clonidine can be given initially, followed by 0.2 mg hourly until the DBP falls below 110 mm Hg or a total of 0.7 mg clonidine has been administered. A single dose may be all that is necessary. Labetalol can be given in a dose of 200 to 400 mg, followed by additional doses every 2 to 3 hours.

Oral or sublingual immediate-release nifedipine for acute BP lowering is dangerous. This approach produces a rapid reduction in BP. Use of immediate-release and should never be used for hypertensive urgencies because of reports of severe adverse events such nifedipine as MIs and strokes.[109]

Hypertensive Emergency

Hypertensive emergencies are those rare situations that require immediate BP reduction to limit new or progressing target-organ damage (see Arterial Blood Pressure: Classification above). Hypertensive emergencies require parenteral therapy, at least initially, with one of the agents listed in Table 15–8. The goal in hypertensive emergencies is not to lower BP to less than 140/90 mm Hg; rather, a reduction in mean arterial pressure of up to 25% within minutes to hours is the initial target. If then stable, BP can be reduced to 160/100–110 mm Hg within the next 2 to 6 hours. Precipitous drops in BP may lead to end-organ ischemia or infarction. If patients tolerate this reduction, additional gradual reductions toward goal BP values can be attempted after 24 to 48 hours. The exception to this guideline is for patients with an acute ischemic stroke where maintaining an elevated BP is needed for a much longer period of time.

The clinical situation should dictate which intravenous medication is used to treat hypertensive emergencies. Regardless, therapy should be provided in a hospital or emergency room setting with intraarticular BP monitoring. Table 15–8 lists special indications for agents that can be used. Some of these agents are discussed in further detail below.

Nitroprusside is widely considered the agent of choice for most cases, but can be problematic in patients with chronic kidney disease. It is a direct-acting vasodilator that decreases peripheral vascular resistance but does not increase cardiac output unless left ventricular failure is present. Nitroprusside can be given to treat most hypertensive emergencies, but in aortic dissection, propranolol should be given first to prevent reflex sympathetic activation. Nitroprusside is

TABLE 15-8 Parenteral Antihypertensive Agents for Hypertensive Emergency

Drug	Dose	Onset (min)	Duration (min)	Adverse Effects	Special Indications
Sodium nitroprusside	0.25–10 mcg/kg/min intravenous infusion (requires special delivery system)	Immediate	1–2	Nausea, vomiting, muscle twitching, sweating, thiocyanate and cyanide intoxication	Most hypertensive emergencies; caution with high intracranial pressure, azotemia, or in chronic kidney disease
Nicardipine hydrochloride	5–15 mg/h intravenous	5–10	15–30; may exceed 240	Tachycardia, headache, flushing, local phlebitis	Most hypertensive emergencies except acute heart failure; caution with coronary ischemia
Fenoldopam mesylate	0.1–0.3 mcg/kg/min intravenous infusion	<5	30	Tachycardia, headache, nausea, flushing	Most hypertensive emergencies; caution with glaucoma
Nitroglycerin	5–100 mcg/min intravenous infusion	2–5	5–10	Headache, vomiting, methemoglobinemia, tolerance with prolonged use	Coronary ischemia
Hydralazine hydrochloride	12–20 mg intravenous 10–50 mg intramuscular	10–20 20–30	60–240 240–360	Tachycardia, flushing, headache vomiting, aggravation of angina	Eclampsia
Labetalol hydrochloride	20–80 mg intravenous bolus every 10 min; 0.5–2.0 mg/min intravenous infusion	5–10	180–360	Vomiting, scalp tingling, bronchoconstriction, dizziness, nausea, heart block, orthostatic hypotension	Most hypertensive emergencies except acute heart failure
Esmolol hydrochloride	250–500 mcg/kg/min intravenous bolus, then 50–100 mcg/kg/min intravenous infusion; may repeat bolus after 5 minutes or increase infusion to 300 mcg/min	1–2	10–20	Hypotension, nausea, asthma, first-degree heart block, heart failure	Aortic dissection; perioperative

metabolized to cyanide and then to thiocyanate, which is eliminated by the kidneys. Therefore, serum thiocyanate levels should be monitored when infusions are continued longer than 72 hours. Nitroprusside should be discontinued if the concentration exceeds 12 mg/dL. The risk of thiocyanate accumulation and toxicity is increased in patients with impaired kidney function.

Intravenous nitroglycerin dilates both arterioles and venous capacitance vessels, thereby reducing both cardiac afterload and preload which can decrease myocardial oxygen demand. It also dilates collateral coronary blood vessels and improves perfusion to ischemic myocardium. These properties make intravenous nitroglycerin ideal for the management of hypertensive emergency in the presence of myocardial ischemia. Intravenous nitroglycerin is associated with tolerance when used over 24 to 48 hours, and can cause severe headache.

Fenoldopam and nicardipine are newer and more expensive alternative agents. Fenoldopam is a dopamine-1 agonist. It can improve renal blood flow and may be especially useful in patients with kidney insufficiency. Nicardipine provides arterial vasodilation, and can treat cardiac ischemia similar to nitroglycerin, but may provide more predictable reductions in BP.

The hypotensive response of hydralazine is less predictable than with other parenteral agents. Consequently, its major role is in the treatment of eclampsia or hypertensive encephalopathy associated with renal insufficiency.

EVALUATION OF THERAPEUTIC OUTCOMES

ACHIEVING GOALS

The most important strategy to prevent CV morbidity and mortality in hypertension is BP control to goal values. Routine goal BP values should be attained in elderly patients and in those with isolated systolic hypertension, but actual BP lowering can occur at a very gradual pace over a period of several months to avoid orthostatic hypotension. Modifying other CV risk factors (e.g., smoking, dyslipidemia, and diabetes) is also important.

⓯ COMBINATION ANTIHYPERTENSIVE THERAPY

Starting therapy with a combination of two drugs is recommended in patients who are far from their BP goal, for patients where goal achievement may be difficult (e.g., those with BP goals of less than 130/80 mm Hg, African Americans), and in patients with multiple compelling indications for different antihypertensive agents. Moreover, combination therapy is often needed to control BP and most patients require two or more agents.[1,21,42,65]

Combination regimens for hypertension should ideally include a diuretic, preferably a thiazide-type. This method will provide additional BP lowering as most patients respond well to a combination regimen that includes a diuretic. Clinicians should anticipate the need for three drugs to control BP in patients with aggressive BP goals of <130/80 mm Hg.[65] Using low-dose combinations also provides greater reductions in BP compared to high doses of single agents, with fewer drug-related side effects.[98]

Diuretics, when combined with several agents (especially an ACE inhibitor, ARB or β-blocker), can result in additive antihypertensive effects. BP lowering from certain antihypertensive agents can activate the RAAS as a compensatory mechanism to counteract BP changes, and regulate fluid loss. Most alternative antihypertensive agents (i.e., reserpine, arterial vasodilators, and centrally acting agents) need to be given with a diuretic to avoid sodium and water retention.

Many fixed-dose combination products are commercially available (Table 15–9). Most of these products contain a thiazide-type diuretic and have multiple dose strengths available. Individual dose titration is more complicated with fixed-dose combination products, but this strategy can reduce the number of daily tablets/capsules and can simplify regimens to improve adherence. This alone may increase the likelihood of achieving or maintaining goal BP values.

TABLE 15-9 Fixed-Dose Combination Products

Combination	Drugs (Brand Name)	Strengths (mg/mg)	Daily Frequency
ACE inhibitor with a thiazide diuretic	Benazepril/hydrochlorothiazide (Lotensin HCT)	5/6.25, 10/12.5, 20/12.5, 20/25	1
	Captopril/hydrochlorothiazide (Capozide)	25/15, 25/25, 50/15, 50/25	1 to 3
	Enalapril/hydrochlorothiazide (Vaseretic)	5/12.5, 10/25	1
	Lisinopril/hydrochlorothiazide (Prinzide, Zestoretic)	10/12.5, 20/12.5, 20/25	1
	Moexipril/hydrochlorothiazide (Uniretic)	7.5/12.5, 15/25	1 or 2
	Quinapril/hydrochlorothiazide (Accuretic)	10/12.5, 20/12.5, 20/25	1
ARB with a thiazide diuretic	Candesartan/hydrochlorothiazide (Atacand HCT)	600/12.5, 600/25	1
	Eprosartan/hydrochlorothiazide (Teveten HCT)	16/12.5, 32/12.5	1
	Irbesartan/hydrochlorothiazide (Avalide)	75/12.5, 150/12.5, 300/12.5	1
	Losartan/hydrochlorothiazide (Hyzaar)	50/12.5, 100/25	1
	Olmesartan/hydrochlorothiazide (Benicar HCT)	20/12.5, 40/12.5, 40/25	1
	Telmisartan/hydrochlorothiazide (Micardis HCT)	40/12.5, 80/12.5	1
	Valsartan/hydrochlorothiazide (Diovan HCT)	80/12.5, 160/12.5	1
β-Blocker with a thiazide diuretic	Atenolol/chlorthalidone (Tenoretic)	50/25, 100/25	1
	Bisoprolol/hydrochlorothiazide (Ziac)	2.5/6.25, 5/6.25, 10/6.25	1
	Propranolol/hydrochlorothiazide (Inderide)	40/25, 80/25	2
	Propranolol LA/hydrochlorothiazide (Inderide LA)	80/50, 120/50, 160/50	1
	Metoprolol/hydrochlorothiazide (Lopressor HCT)	50/25, 100/25	1 or 2
	Nadolol/bendroflumethiazide (Corzide)	40/5, 80/5	1
	Timolol/hydrochlorothiazide (Timolide)	10/25	1 or 2
ACE inhibitor with calcium channel blocker	Amlodipine/benazepril (Lotrel)	2.5/10, 5/10, 10/20	1
	Enalapril/pelodipine (Lexxel)	5/5	1
	Trandolapril/verapamil (Tarka)	2/180, 1/240, 2/240, 4/240	1 or 2
ARB with calcium channel blocker	Valsartan/amlodipine (Exforge)	5/160, 10/160, 5/320, 10/320	1
	Olmesartan/amlodipine (AZOR)	5/20, 10/20, 5/40, 10/40	1

ACE, angiotensin-converting enzyme; ARB, angiotensin receptor blocker.

TABLE 15-10 Causes of Resistant Hypertension

Improper blood pressure measurement
Volume overload
- Excess sodium intake
- Volume retention from kidney disease
- Inadequate diuretic therapy

Drug-induced or other causes
- Nonadherence
- Inadequate doses
- Agents listed in Table 15-1

Associated conditions
- Obesity, excess alcohol intake

Secondary hypertension

⓰ RESISTANT HYPERTENSION

Resistant hypertension is the failure to achieve goal BP in patients who are adhering to full doses of an appropriate three-drug regimen that includes a diuretic.[1] Patients with newly diagnosed hypertension or who are not receiving drug therapy should not be considered to have resistant hypertension.[110] Difficult-to-control hypertension is persistently elevated BP despite treatment with two or three drugs that does not meet the criteria for resistant hypertension (e.g., maximum doses that includes a diuretic).

Table 15–10 lists several causes of resistant hypertension. Volume overload is a common cause, thus highlighting the importance of diuretic therapy in the management of hypertension. In addition, nonadherence to drug therapy and lifestyle modifications plays an important role. Patients should be closely evaluated to see if any of these causes can be reversed. If nothing is identified, the principle of drug therapy selection from the JNC7 and AHA guidelines should still apply. Compelling indications, if present, should guide selection assuming these patients are on a diuretic.

Medications that have additive or synergistic effects when given in combination should ideally be used. In patients with severe chronic kidney disease (e.g., estimated GFR <30 mL/min 1.73 m^2), a loop diuretic might be considered over a thiazide.

CLINICAL MONITORING

Routine ongoing monitoring to assess disease progression, the desired effects of antihypertensive therapy (efficacy), and undesired adverse side effects (toxicity) is needed in all patients treated with antihypertensive drug therapy.

Disease Progression

Patients should be monitored for signs and symptoms of progressive target-organ disease (see Table 15–1). A careful history for chest pain (or pressure), palpitations, dizziness, dyspnea, orthopnea, headache, sudden change in vision, one-sided weakness, slurred speech, and loss of balance should be taken to assess for the presence of hypertensive complications. Other clinical monitoring parameters that may be used to assess target-organ disease include funduscopic changes on eye examination, left ventricular hypertrophy on electrocardiogram, proteinuria, and changes in kidney function. These parameters should be monitored periodically because any sign of deterioration requires immediate assessment and followup.

Efficacy

Clinic-based BP monitoring remains the standard for managing hypertension. BP response should be evaluated 2 to 4 weeks after initiating or making changes in therapy. Once goal BP values are attained, assuming no signs or symptoms of acute target-organ disease are present, BP monitoring can be done every 3 to 6 months. More frequent evaluations are required in patients with a history of poor control, nonadherence, progressive target-organ damage, or symptoms of adverse drug effects.

Self-measurements of BP or automatic ambulatory BP monitoring can be useful clinically to establish effective 24-hour control. This type of monitoring may become the standard of care in the future, but the JNC7 and AHA recommends that ambulatory BP monitoring only be used in select situations such as suspected white coat hypertension. If patients are measuring their BP at home, it is important that they measure during the early morning hours for most days, and then at different times of the day on alternative days of the week. Additionally, patients should be instructed to measure BP two to three times each time they measure BP, and to document all values accurately.

Toxicity

Patients should be monitored routinely for adverse drug effects (Table 15–11). Monitoring should typically occur 2 to 4 weeks after starting a new agent or dose increases, and then every 6 to 12 months in stable patients. Additional monitoring may be needed for other concomitant diseases if present (e.g., diabetes, dyslipidemia, gout). Moreover, patients treated with an aldosterone antagonist (eplerenone or spironolactone), should have potassium concentrations and kidney function assessed within 3 days and again at 1 week after initiation to detect potential hyperkalemia.[48] The occurrence of an adverse drug event may require dosage reduction or substitution with an alternative antihypertensive agent.

ADHERENCE

Lack of persistence with hypertension treatment is a major problem in the United States and is associated with significant increases in costs as a result of development of complications. Because hypertension is a relatively asymptomatic disease, poor adherence is frequent, particularly in patients newly treated. It has been estimated that only up to 50% of patients with newly diagnosed hypertension are continuing treatment at 1 year.[111] Therefore, it is imperative to assess patient adherence on a regular basis.

Identification of nonadherence should be followed up with appropriate patient education, counseling, and intervention. Once-daily regimens are preferred in most patients to improve adherence. Although some may believe that aggressive treatment may negatively impact quality of life and thus adherence, several studies have found that most patients actually feel better once their BP is controlled. Patients on antihypertensive therapy should be questioned periodically about changes in their general health perception, energy level, physical functioning, and overall satisfaction with treatment. Lifestyle modifications should always be recommended to provide additional BP lowering and other potential health benefits. Persistence with lifestyle modifications should be continually encouraged in patients engaging in such endeavors.

TABLE 15-11 Select Monitoring for Antihypertensive Pharmacotherapy

Class	Parameters
Diuretics	Blood pressure, blood urea nitrogen (BUN)/serum creatinine, serum electrolytes (potassium, magnesium, sodium), uric acid (for thiazides)
Aldosterone antagonists	Blood pressure, BUN/serum creatinine, serum potassium
Angiotensin-converting enzyme inhibitors	Blood pressure, BUN/serum creatinine, serum potassium
Angiotensin receptor blockers	Blood pressure, BUN/serum creatinine, serum potassium
Calcium channel blockers	Blood pressure; heart rate
β-Blockers	Blood pressure, heart rate

CONCLUSIONS

Hypertension is a very common medical condition in the United States. Treatment of patients with hypertension should include both lifestyle modifications and pharmacotherapy. Outcome-based studies have definitively demonstrated that treating hypertension reduces the risk of CV events and subsequently reduces morbidity and mortality. Moreover, evidence evaluating individual drug classes has resulted in an evidence-based approach to selecting pharmacotherapy in an individual patient, which is outlined in the JNC7 and 2007 AHA guidelines. Diuretics, ACE inhibitors, ARBs, and CCBs are all first-line agents. However, diuretics, specifically thiazide-type diuretics, are unsurpassed in their ability to reduce risk of CV events in hypertension based on an extensive body of supportive evidence. If patients with hypertension have a comorbid condition that is considered a compelling indication, a different set of drugs may be recommended for first-line therapy. Data suggests that using a β-blocker as the primary agent to treat patients with hypertension, without the presence of a compelling indication, may not be as beneficial on reducing risk of CV events compared to diuretic-, ACE inhibitor-, ARB-, or CCB-based therapy. Therefore, β-blockers are not first-line therapy options unless an appropriate compelling indication is present.

An often overlooked concept in managing hypertension is to treat patients to a goal BP value. In addition to selecting the most appropriate agent, attaining a goal BP is also of paramount importance to ensure maximum reduction in risk for CV events is provided. A BP goal of less than 140/90 mm Hg is recommended for general prevention of CV events or disease; however, this goal is less than 130/80 mm Hg for patients with diabetes, significant chronic kidney disease, coronary artery disease, noncoronary atherosclerotic vascular disease or a Framingham risk score of 10% or greater, and is less than 120/80 mm Hg for patients with left ventricular dysfunction (i.e., systolic heart failure). Most patients with hypertension require more than one pharmacologic agent to attain goal BP values; therefore, combination therapy is often needed.

ABBREVIATIONS

ACE: angiotensin-converting enzyme

ARB: angiotensin II receptor blocker

AHA: American Heart Association

BP: blood pressure

CCB: calcium channel blocker

CV: cardiovascular

DBP: diastolic blood pressure

GFR: glomerular filtration rate

ISA: intrinsic sympathomimetic activity

JNC 7: Seventh report of the Joint National Committee on Prevention, Detection, Evaluation, and Treatment of High Blood Pressure

MI: myocardial infarction

RAAS: renin-angiotensin aldosterone system

SBP: systolic blood pressure

REFERENCES

1. Chobanian AV, Bakris GL, Black HR, et al. Seventh report of the Joint National Committee on Prevention, Detection, Evaluation, and Treatment of High Blood Pressure. Hypertension 2003;42(6):1206–1252.
2. Rosendorff C, Black HR, Cannon CP, et al. Treatment of hypertension in the prevention and management of ischemic heart disease: A scientific statement from the American Heart Association Council for High Blood Pressure Research and the Councils on Clinical Cardiology and Epidemiology and Prevention. Circulation 2007;115(21):2761–2788.
3. Hajjar I, Kotchen TA. Trends in prevalence, awareness, treatment, and control of hypertension in the United States, 1988–2000. JAMA 2003;290(2):199–206.
4. Thom T, Haase N, Rosamond W, et al. Heart disease and stroke statistics—2006 update: A report from the American Heart Association Statistics Committee and Stroke Statistics Subcommittee. Circulation 2006;113(6):e85–e151.
5. Staessen JA, Wang J, Bianchi G, Birkenhager WH. Essential hypertension. Lancet 2003;361(9369):1629–1641.
6. Saseen JJ. Hypertension. In: Tisdale JE, Miller DA, eds. Drug-Induced Diseases: Prevention, Detection, and Management. Bethesda, MD: American Society of Health-Systems Pharmacists, 2005.
7. Kaplan NM. Kaplan's Clinical Hypertension, 8th ed. Philadelphia: Lippincott Williams & Wilkins, 2002:1–550.
8. MacMahon S, Peto R, Cutler J, et al. Blood pressure, stroke, and coronary heart disease. Part 1: Prolonged differences in blood pressure: Prospective observational studies corrected for the regression dilution bias. Lancet 1990;335(8692):765–774.
9. SHEP Cooperative Research Group. Prevention of stroke by antihypertensive drug treatment in older persons with isolated systolic hypertension. Final results of the Systolic Hypertension in the Elderly Program (SHEP). JAMA 1991;265(24):3255–3264.
10. Dahlof B, Lindholm LH, Hansson L, et al. Morbidity and mortality in the Swedish Trial in Old Patients with Hypertension (STOP-Hypertension). Lancet 1991;338(8778):1281–1285.
11. MRC Working Party. Medical Research Council trial of treatment of hypertension in older adults: Principal results. BMJ 1992;304(6824):405–412.
12. Staessen JA, Fagard R, Thijs L, et al. Randomised double-blind comparison of placebo and active treatment for older patients with isolated systolic hypertension. The Systolic Hypertension in Europe (Syst-Eur) Trial Investigators. Lancet 1997;350(9080):757–764.
13. Grundy SM, Cleeman JI, Daniels SR, et al. Diagnosis and management of the metabolic syndrome. An American Heart Association/National Heart, Lung, and Blood Institute Scientific Statement. Executive summary. Circulation 2005;112(17):2735–2752.
14. Pickering TG, Hall JE, Appel LJ, et al. Recommendations for blood pressure measurement in humans and experimental animals: Part 1: Blood pressure measurement in humans: A statement for professionals from the Subcommittee of Professional and Public Education of the American Heart Association Council on High Blood Pressure Research. Circulation 2005;111(5):697–716.
15. Glen SK, Elliott HL, Curzio JL, et al. White-coat hypertension as a cause of cardiovascular dysfunction. Lancet 1996;348(9028):654–657.
16. Bobrie G, Chatellier G, Genes N, et al. Cardiovascular prognosis of "masked hypertension" detected by blood pressure self-measurement in elderly treated hypertensive patients. JAMA 2004;291(11):1342–1349.
17. Staessen JA, Den Hond E, Celis H, et al. Antihypertensive treatment based on blood pressure measurement at home or in the physician's office: A randomized controlled trial. JAMA 2004;291(8):955–964.
18. Brosius FC 3rd, Hostetter TH, Kelepouris E, et al. Detection of chronic kidney disease in patients with or at increased risk of cardiovascular disease: A science advisory from the American Heart Association Kidney and Cardiovascular Disease Council; the Councils on High Blood Pressure Research, Cardiovascular Disease in the Young, and Epidemiology and Prevention; and the Quality of Care and Outcomes Research Interdisciplinary Working Group: Developed in collaboration with the National Kidney Foundation. Circulation 2006;114(10):1083–1087.
19. Hansson L, Zanchetti A, Carruthers SG, et al. Effects of intensive blood-pressure lowering and low-dose aspirin in patients with hypertension: Principal results of the Hypertension Optimal Treatment (HOT) randomised trial. HOT Study Group. Lancet 1998;351(9118):1755–1762.
20. Farnett L, Mulrow CD, Linn WD, et al. The J-curve phenomenon and the treatment of hypertension. Is there a point beyond which pressure reduction is dangerous? JAMA 1991;265(4):489–495.
21. Hyman DJ, Pavlik VN. Characteristics of patients with uncontrolled hypertension in the United States. N Engl J Med 2001;345(7):479–486.
22. O'Connor PJ. Overcome clinical inertia to control systolic blood pressure. Arch Intern Med 2003;163(22):2677–2678.

23. Appel LJ, Brands MW, Daniels SR, et al. Dietary approaches to prevent and treat hypertension: A scientific statement from the American Heart Association. Hypertension 2006;47(2):296–308.
24. Kostis JB, Wilson AC, Shindler DM, et al. Persistence of normotension after discontinuation of lifestyle intervention in the trial of TONE. Trial of Nonpharmacologic Interventions in the Elderly. Am J Hypertens 2002;15(8):732–734.
25. Lichtenstein AH, Appel LJ, Brands M, et al. Diet and lifestyle recommendations revision 2006: A scientific statement from the American Heart Association Nutrition Committee. Circulation 2006;114(1):82–96.
26. Julius S, Nesbitt SD, Egan BM, et al. Feasibility of treating prehypertension with an angiotensin-receptor blocker. N Engl J Med 2006;354(16):1685–1697.
27. Saseen JJ, MacLaughlin EJ, Westfall JM. Treatment of uncomplicated hypertension: Are ACE inhibitors and calcium channel blockers as effective as diuretics and beta-blockers? J Am Board Fam Pract 2003;16(2):156–164.
28. Black HR, Elliott WJ, Grandits G, et al. Principal results of the Controlled Onset Verapamil Investigation of Cardiovascular End Points (CONVINCE) trial. JAMA 2003;289(16):2073–2082.
29. Dahlof B, Devereux RB, Kjeldsen SE, et al. Cardiovascular morbidity and mortality in the Losartan Intervention For Endpoint reduction in hypertension study (LIFE): A randomised trial against atenolol. Lancet 2002;359(9311):995–1003.
30. ALLHAT Officers and Coordinators for the ALLHAT Collaborative Research Group. Major outcomes in high-risk hypertensive patients randomized to angiotensin-converting enzyme inhibitor or calcium channel blocker vs diuretic: The Antihypertensive and Lipid-Lowering Treatment to Prevent Heart Attack Trial (ALLHAT). JAMA 2002;288(23):2981–2997.
31. PROGRESS Collaborative Group. Randomised trial of a perindopril-based blood-pressure-lowering regimen among 6,105 individuals with previous stroke or transient ischaemic attack. Lancet 2001;358(9287):1033–1041.
32. Wing LM, Reid CM, Ryan P, et al. A comparison of outcomes with angiotensin-converting--enzyme inhibitors and diuretics for hypertension in the elderly. N Engl J Med 2003;348(7):583–592.
33. Julius S, Kjeldsen SE, Weber M, et al. Outcomes in hypertensive patients at high cardiovascular risk treated with regimens based on valsartan or amlodipine: The VALUE randomised trial. Lancet 2004;363(9426):2022–2031.
34. Dahlof B, Sever PS, Poulter NR, et al. Prevention of cardiovascular events with an antihypertensive regimen of amlodipine adding perindopril as required versus atenolol adding bendroflumethiazide as required, in the Anglo-Scandinavian Cardiac Outcomes Trial–Blood Pressure Lowering Arm (ASCOT-BPLA): A multicentre randomised controlled trial. Lancet 2005;366(9489):895–906.
35. ALLHAT officers and coordinators for the ALLHAT Collaborative Research Group. Diuretic versus alpha-blocker as first-step antihypertensive therapy: Final results from the Antihypertensive and Lipid-Lowering Treatment to Prevent Heart Attack Trial (ALLHAT). Hypertension 2003;42(3):239–246.
36. Davis BR, Cutler JA, Gordon DJ, et al. Rationale and design for the Antihypertensive and Lipid Lowering Treatment to Prevent Heart Attack Trial (ALLHAT). ALLHAT Research Group. Am J Hypertens 1996;9(4 Pt 1):342–360.
37. Rahman M, Pressel S, Davis BR, et al. Renal outcomes in high-risk hypertensive patients treated with an angiotensin-converting enzyme inhibitor or a calcium channel blocker vs a diuretic: A report from the Antihypertensive and Lipid-Lowering Treatment to Prevent Heart Attack Trial (ALLHAT). Arch Intern Med 2005;165(8):936–946.
38. Whelton PK, Barzilay J, Cushman WC, et al. Clinical outcomes in antihypertensive treatment of type 2 diabetes, impaired fasting glucose concentration, and normoglycemia: Antihypertensive and Lipid-Lowering Treatment to Prevent Heart Attack Trial (ALLHAT). Arch Intern Med 2005;165(12):1401–1409.
39. Wright JT Jr, Dunn JK, Cutler JA, et al. Outcomes in hypertensive black and nonblack patients treated with chlorthalidone, amlodipine, and lisinopril. JAMA 2005;293(13):1595–1608.
40. Turnbull F. Effects of different blood-pressure-lowering regimens on major cardiovascular events: Results of prospectively-designed overviews of randomised trials. Lancet 2003;362(9395):1527–1535.
41. Rosamond W, Flegal K, Friday G, et al. Heart disease and stroke statistics—2007 update: A report from the American Heart Association Statistics Committee and Stroke Statistics Subcommittee. Circulation 2007;115(5):e69–e171.
42. 2007 Guidelines for the management of arterial hypertension. The Task Force for the Managment of Arterial Hypertension of the European Society of Hypertension (ESH) and of the European Society of Cardiology (ESC). J Hypertens 2007;25:1105–1187.
43. National Collaborating Centre for Chronic Conditions. Hypertension: Management of Hypertension in Adults in Primary Care: Partial Update. London: Royal College of Physicians, 2006.
44. Carlberg B, Samuelsson O, Lindholm LH. Atenolol in hypertension: Is it a wise choice? Lancet 2004;364(9446):1684–1689.
45. Lindholm LH, Carlberg B, Samuelsson O. Should beta blockers remain first choice in the treatment of primary hypertension? A meta-analysis. Lancet 2005;366(9496):1545–1553.
46. Khan N, McAlister FA. Re-examining the efficacy of beta-blockers for the treatment of hypertension: A meta-analysis. CMAJ 2006;174(12):1737–1742.
47. Wiysonge C, Bradley H, Mayosi B, et al. Beta-blockers for hypertension. Cochrane Database Syst Rev 2007;(1):CD002003.
48. Hunt SA. ACC/AHA 2005 guideline update for the diagnosis and management of chronic heart failure in the adult: A report of the American College of Cardiology/American Heart Association Task Force on Practice Guidelines (Writing Committee to Update the 2001 Guidelines for the Evaluation and Management of Heart Failure). J Am Coll Cardiol 2005;46(6):e1–e82.
49. Merit-HF Study Group. Effect of metoprolol CR/XL in chronic heart failure: Metoprolol CR/XL Randomised Intervention Trial in Congestive Heart Failure (MERIT-HF). Lancet 1999;353(9169):2001–2007.
50. Packer M, Coats AJ, Fowler MB, et al. Effect of carvedilol on survival in severe chronic heart failure. N Engl J Med 2001;344(22):1651–1658.
51. Pitt B, Segal R, Martinez FA, et al. Randomised trial of losartan versus captopril in patients over 65 with heart failure (Evaluation of Losartan in the Elderly Study, ELITE). Lancet 1997;349(9054):747–752.
52. Pitt B, Poole-Wilson PA, Segal R, et al. Effect of losartan compared with captopril on mortality in patients with symptomatic heart failure: Randomised trial—The Losartan Heart Failure Survival Study ELITE II. Lancet 2000;355(9215):1582–1587.
53. Granger CB, McMurray JJ, Yusuf S, et al. Effects of candesartan in patients with chronic heart failure and reduced left-ventricular systolic function intolerant to angiotensin-converting-enzyme inhibitors: The CHARM-Alternative trial. Lancet 2003;362(9386):772–776.
54. McMurray JJ, Ostergren J, Swedberg K, et al. Effects of candesartan in patients with chronic heart failure and reduced left-ventricular systolic function taking angiotensin-converting-enzyme inhibitors: The CHARM-Added trial. Lancet 2003;362(9386):767–771.
55. Pitt B, Zannad F, Remme WJ, et al. The effect of spironolactone on morbidity and mortality in patients with severe heart failure. Randomized Aldactone Evaluation Study Investigators. N Engl J Med 1999;341(10):709–717.
56. Pitt B, Remme W, Zannad F, et al. Eplerenone, a selective aldosterone blocker, in patients with left ventricular dysfunction after myocardial infarction. N Engl J Med 2003;348(14):1309–1321.
57. Smith SC, Jr., Allen J, Blair SN, et al. AHA/ACC guidelines for secondary prevention for patients with coronary and other atherosclerotic vascular disease: 2006 update endorsed by the National Heart, Lung, and Blood Institute. J Am Coll Cardiol 2006;47(10):2130–2139.
58. Pfeffer MA, McMurray JJ, Velazquez EJ, et al. Valsartan, captopril, or both in myocardial infarction complicated by heart failure, left ventricular dysfunction, or both. N Engl J Med 2003;349(20):1893–1906.
59. Fraker TO Jr, Fihn SD, writing on behalf of the 2002 Chronic Stable Angina Writing Committee. 2007 Chronic angina focused updated of the ACC/AHA 2002 guidelines for the managment of patients with chronic stable angina: A report of the American College of Cardiology/American Heart Association Task Force on Practice Guidelines Writing Group to Develop the Focused Update of the 2002 guidelines of the managment of patients with chronic stable angina. Circulation 2007; 116:Dec.
60. Pepine CJ, Handberg EM, Cooper-DeHoff RM, et al. A calcium antagonist vs a non-calcium antagonist hypertension treatment strategy for patients with coronary artery disease. The International Verapamil-Trandolapril Study (INVEST): A randomized controlled trial. JAMA 2003;290(21):2805–2816.

61. Antman EM, Anbe DT, Armstrong PW, et al. ACC/AHA guidelines for the management of patients with ST-elevation myocardial infarction—Executive summary: A report of the American College of Cardiology/American Heart Association Task Force on Practice Guidelines (Writing Committee to Revise the 1999 Guidelines for the Management of Patients with Acute Myocardial Infarction). Circulation 2004;110(5):588–636.
62. Braunwald E, Antman EM, Beasley JW, et al. ACC/AHA 2002 guideline update for the management of patients with unstable angina and non-ST-segment elevation myocardial infarction—Summary article: A report of the American College of Cardiology/American Heart Association task force on practice guidelines (Committee on the Management of Patients With Unstable Angina). J Am Coll Cardiol 2002;40(7):1366–1374.
63. Dagenais GR, Pogue J, Fox K, et al. Angiotensin-converting-enzyme inhibitors in stable vascular disease without left ventricular systolic dysfunction or heart failure: A combined analysis of three trials. Lancet 2006;368(9535):581–588.
64. American Diabetes Association. Standards of medical care in diabetes—2007. Diabetes Care 2006;30(Suppl 1):S4–S41.
65. Bakris GL, Williams M, Dworkin L, et al. Preserving renal function in adults with hypertension and diabetes: A consensus approach. National Kidney Foundation Hypertension and Diabetes Executive Committees Working Group. Am J Kidney Dis 2000;36(3):646–661.
66. UK Prospective Diabetes Study Group. Efficacy of atenolol and captopril in reducing risk of macrovascular and microvascular complications in type 2 diabetes: UKPDS 39. BMJ 1998;317(7160):713–720.
67. Pahor M, Psaty BM, Alderman MH, et al. Therapeutic benefits of ACE inhibitors and other antihypertensive drugs in patients with type 2 diabetes. Diabetes Care 2000;23(7):888–892.
68. National Kidney Foundation. K/DOQI clinical practice guidelines on hypertension and antihypertensive agents in chronic kidney disease. Am J Kidney Dis 2004;43(5 Suppl 1):S1–S290.
69. Ruggenenti P, Perna A, Loriga G, et al. Blood-pressure control for renoprotection in patients with non-diabetic chronic renal disease (REIN-2): Multicentre, randomised controlled trial. Lancet 2005;365(9463):939–946.
70. Wright JT Jr, Bakris G, Greene T, et al. Effect of blood pressure lowering and antihypertensive drug class on progression of hypertensive kidney disease: Results from the AASK trial. JAMA 2002;288(19):2421–2431.
71. Casas JP, Chua W, Loukogeorgakis S, et al. Effect of inhibitors of the renin–angiotensin system and other antihypertensive drugs on renal outcomes: Systematic review and meta-analysis. Lancet 2005;366(9502):2026–2033.
72. Nakao N, Yoshimura A, Morita H, et al. Combination treatment of angiotensin-II receptor blocker and angiotensin-converting-enzyme inhibitor in non-diabetic renal disease (COOPERATE): A randomised controlled trial. Lancet 2003;361(9352):117–124.
73. Dussol B, Moussi-Frances J, Morange S, et al. A randomized trial of furosemide vs hydrochlorothiazide in patients with chronic renal failure and hypertension. Nephrol Dial Transplant 2005;20(2):349–353.
74. Schrader J, Luders S, Kulschewski A, et al. Morbidity and mortality after stroke, eprosartan compared with nitrendipine for secondary prevention: Principal results of a prospective randomized controlled study (MOSES). Stroke 2005;36(6):1218–1226.
75. Sacco RL, Adams R, Albers G, et al. Guidelines for prevention of stroke in patients with ischemic stroke or transient ischemic attack: A statement for healthcare professionals from the American Heart Association/American Stroke Association Council on Stroke: Co-sponsored by the Council on Cardiovascular Radiology and Intervention: The American Academy of Neurology affirms the value of this guideline. Circulation 2006;113(10):e409–449.
76. Gueyffier F, Bulpitt C, Boissel JP, et al. Antihypertensive drugs in very old people: A subgroup meta-analysis of randomised controlled trials. INDANA Group. Lancet 1999;353(9155):793–796.
77. Staessen JA, Gasowski J, Wang JG, et al. Risks of untreated and treated isolated systolic hypertension in the elderly: Meta-analysis of outcome trials. Lancet 2000;355(9207):865–872.
78. Rastas S, Pirttila T, Viramo P, et al. Association between blood pressure and survival over 9 years in a general population aged 85 and older. J Am Geriatr Soc 2006;54(6):912–918.
79. Bulpitt CJ, Beckett NS, Cooke J, et al. Results of the pilot study for the Hypertension in the Very Elderly Trial. J Hypertens 2003;21(12):2409–2417.
80. Hansson L, Lindholm LH, Ekbom T, et al. Randomised trial of old and new antihypertensive drugs in elderly patients: Cardiovascular mortality and morbidity the Swedish Trial in Old Patients with Hypertension-2 study. Lancet 1999;354(9192):1751–1756.
81. National High Blood Pressure Education Program Working Group on High Blood Pressure in Children and Adolescents. The fourth report on the diagnosis, evaluation, and treatment of high blood pressure in children and adolescents. Pediatrics 2004;114(2 Suppl 4th Report):555–576.
82. Roberts JM, Pearson G, Cutler J, Lindheimer M. Summary of the NHLBI Working Group on Research on Hypertension During Pregnancy. Hypertension 2003;41(3):437–445.
83. Cooper WO, Hernandez-Diaz S, Arbogast PG, et al. Major congenital malformations after first-trimester exposure to ACE inhibitors. N Engl J Med 2006;354(23):2443–2451.
84. Douglas JG, Bakris GL, Epstein M, et al. Management of high blood pressure in African Americans: Consensus statement of the Hypertension in African Americans Working Group of the International Society on Hypertension in Blacks. Arch Intern Med 2003;163(5):525–541.
85. Hirsch AT, Haskal ZJ, Hertzer NR, et al. ACC/AHA 2005 Practice guidelines for the management of patients with peripheral arterial disease (lower extremity, renal, mesenteric, and abdominal aortic): A collaborative report from the American Association for Vascular Surgery/Society for Vascular Surgery, Society for Cardiovascular Angiography and Interventions, Society for Vascular Medicine and Biology, Society of Interventional Radiology, and the ACC/AHA Task Force on Practice Guidelines (Writing Committee to Develop Guidelines for the Management of Patients With Peripheral Arterial Disease): Endorsed by the American Association of Cardiovascular and Pulmonary Rehabilitation; National Heart, Lung, and Blood Institute; Society for Vascular Nursing; TransAtlantic Inter-Society Consensus; and Vascular Disease Foundation. Circulation 2006;113(11):e463–e654.
86. Salpeter SR, Ormiston TM, Salpeter EE. Cardioselective beta-blockers in patients with reactive airway disease: A meta-analysis. Ann Intern Med 2002;137(9):715–725.
87. Lakshman MR, Reda DJ, Materson BJ, et al. Diuretics and beta-blockers do not have adverse effects at 1 year on plasma lipid and lipoprotein profiles in men with hypertension. Department of Veterans Affairs Cooperative Study Group on Antihypertensive Agents. Arch Intern Med 1999;159(6):551–558.
88. Eckel RH, Kahn R, Robertson RM, Rizza RA. Preventing cardiovascular disease and diabetes: A call to action from the American Diabetes Association and the American Heart Association. Diabetes Care 2006;29(7):1697–1699.
89. Elliot WJ, Meyer PM. Incident diabetes in clinical trials of antihypertensive drugs: A network analysis. Lancet 2007;369:201–207.
90. Zillich AJ, Garg J, Basu S, et al. Thiazide diuretics, potassium, and the development of diabetes. Hypertension 2006;48:219–224.
91. Barksdale JD, Gardner SF. The impact of first-line antihypertensive drugs on erectile dysfunction. Pharmacotherapy 1999;19(5):573–581.
92. Ko DT, Hebert PR, Coffey CS, et al. Beta-blocker therapy and symptoms of depression, fatigue, and sexual dysfunction. JAMA 2002;288(3):351–357.
93. Grimm RH Jr, Grandits GA, Prineas RJ, et al. Long-term effects on sexual function of five antihypertensive drugs and nutritional hygienic treatment in hypertensive men and women. Treatment of Mild Hypertension Study (TOMHS). Hypertension 1997;29(1 Pt 1):8–14.
94. Min JK, Williams KA, Okwuosa TM, et al. Prediction of coronary heart disease by erectile dysfunction in men referred for nuclear stress testing. Arch Intern Med 2006;166(2):201–206.
95. Carter BL, Ernst ME, Cohen JD. Hydrochlorothiazide versus chlorthalidone: Evidence supporting their interchangeability. Hypertension 2004;43(1):4–9.
96. Psaty BM, Lumley T, Furberg CD. Meta-analysis of health outcomes of chlorthalidone-based vs nonchlorthalidone-based low-dose diuretic therapies. JAMA 2004;292(1):43–44.
97. Grimm RH, Jr., Flack JM, Grandits GA, et al. Long-term effects on plasma lipids of diet and drugs to treat hypertension. Treatment of Mild Hypertension Study (TOMHS) Research Group. JAMA 1996;275(20):1549–1556.
98. Law MR, Wald NJ, Morris JK, Jordan RE. Value of low dose combination treatment with blood pressure lowering drugs: Analysis of 354 randomised trials. BMJ 2003;326(7404):1427.

99. Cicardi M, Zingale LC, Bergamaschini L, Agostoni A. Angioedema associated with angiotensin-converting enzyme inhibitor use: Outcome after switching to a different treatment. Arch Intern Med 2004;164(8):910–913.
100. Phillips CO, Kashani A, Ko DK, et al. Adverse effects of combination angiotensin II receptor blockers plus angiotensin–converting enzyme inhibitors for left ventricular dysfunction. Arch Intern Med 2007; 167(18):1930–1936.
101. Leenen FH, Nwachuku CE, Black HR, et al. Clinical events in high-risk hypertensive patients randomly assigned to calcium channel blocker versus angiotensin-converting enzyme inhibitor in the antihypertensive and lipid-lowering treatment to prevent heart attack trial. Hypertension 2006;48(3):374–384.
102. Bakris GL, Fonseca V, Katholi RE, et al. Metabolic effects of carvedilol vs metoprolol in patients with type 2 diabetes mellitus and hypertension: A randomized controlled trial. JAMA 2004;292(18):2227–2236.
103. Staessen JA, Li Y, Richart T. Oral renin inhibitors. Lancet 2006;368 (9545):1449–1456.
104. Gradman AH, Vivas Y. New drugs for hypertension: What do they offer? Curr Hypertens Rep 2006;8(5):425–432.
105. Edelson JT, Weinstein MC, Tosteson AN, et al. Long-term cost-effectiveness of various initial monotherapies for mild to moderate hypertension. JAMA 1990;263(3):407–413.
106. Hilleman DE, Mohiuddin SM, Lucas BD, Jr, et al. Cost-minimization analysis of initial antihypertensive therapy in patients with mild-to-moderate essential diastolic hypertension. Clin Ther 1994;16(1):88–102, discussion 187.
107. Pearce KA, Furberg CD, Psaty BM, Kirk J. Cost-minimization and the number needed to treat in uncomplicated hypertension. Am J Hypertens 1998;11(5):618–629.
108. Fischer MA, Avorn J. Economic implications of evidence-based prescribing on hypertension: Can better care cost less? JAMA 2004;291(15):1850–1856.
109. Grossman E, Messerli FH, Grodzicki T, Kowey P. Should a moratorium be placed on sublingual nifedipine capsules given for hypertensive emergencies and pseudoemergencies? JAMA 1996;276(16):1328–1331.
110. Moser M, Setaro JF. Clinical practice. Resistant or difficult-to-control hypertension. N Engl J Med 2006;355(4):385–392.
111. Degli Esposti L, Valpiani G. Pharmacoeconomic burden of undertreating hypertension. Pharmacoeconomics 2004;22(14):907–928.

CHAPTER 16 Heart Failure

ROBERT B. PARKER, JO E. RODGERS, AND LARISA H. CAVALLARI

KEY CONCEPTS

1. Heart failure is a clinical syndrome caused by the inability of the heart to pump sufficient blood to meet the metabolic needs of the body. Heart failure can result from any disorder that reduces ventricular filling (diastolic dysfunction) and/or myocardial contractility (systolic dysfunction). The leading causes of heart failure are coronary artery disease and hypertension. The primary manifestations of the syndrome are dyspnea, fatigue, and fluid retention.

2. Heart failure is a progressive disorder that begins with myocardial injury. In response to the injury, a number of compensatory responses are activated in an attempt to maintain adequate cardiac output, including activation of the sympathetic nervous system (SNS) and the renin–angiotensin–aldosterone system (RAAS), resulting in vasoconstriction and sodium and water retention, as well as ventricular hypertrophy/remodeling. These compensatory mechanisms are responsible for the symptoms of heart failure and contribute to disease progression.

3. Our current understanding of heart failure pathophysiology is best described by the neurohormonal model. Activation of endogenous neurohormones, including norepinephrine, angiotensin II, aldosterone, vasopressin, and numerous proinflammatory cytokines, plays an important role in ventricular remodeling and the subsequent progression of heart failure. Importantly, pharmacotherapy targeted at antagonizing this neurohormonal activation has slowed the progression of heart failure and improved survival.

4. Most patients with symptomatic heart failure should be routinely treated with an angiotensin-converting enzyme (ACE) inhibitor, a β-blocker, and a diuretic. The benefits of these medications on slowing heart failure progression, reducing morbidity and mortality, and improving symptoms are clearly established. Patients should be treated with a diuretic if there is evidence of fluid retention. Treatment with digoxin may also be considered to improve symptoms and reduce hospitalizations.

5. In patients with heart failure, ACE inhibitors improve survival, slow disease progression, reduce hospitalizations, and improve quality of life. The doses for these agents should be targeted at those shown in clinical trials to improve survival. When ACE inhibitors are contraindicated or not tolerated, an angiotensin II receptor blocker or the combination of hydralazine and isosorbide dinitrate are reasonable alternatives. Patients with asymptomatic left ventricular dysfunction and/or a previous myocardial infarction (stage B of the American College of Cardiologists/American Heart Association [ACC/AHA] classification scheme) should also receive ACE inhibitors, with the goal of preventing symptomatic heart failure and reducing mortality.

6. The β-blockers carvedilol, metoprolol CR/XL, and bisoprolol prolong survival, decrease hospitalizations and the need for transplantation, and cause "reverse remodeling" of the left ventricle. These agents are recommended for all patients with a reduced left ventricular ejection fraction. Therapy must be instituted at low doses, with slow upward titration to the target dose.

7. Although chronic diuretic therapy frequently is used in heart failure patients, it is not mandatory. Diuretic therapy along with sodium restriction is required only in those patients with peripheral edema and/or pulmonary congestion. Many patients will need continued diuretic therapy to maintain euvolemia after fluid overload is resolved.

8. Digoxin does not improve survival in patients with heart failure but does provide symptomatic benefits. Digoxin doses should be adjusted to achieve plasma concentrations of 0.5 to 1.0 ng/mL; higher plasma concentrations are not associated with additional benefits but may be associated with increased risk of toxicity.

9. Aldosterone antagonism with low-dose spironolactone reduces mortality in patients with New York Heart Association (NYHA) classes III and IV heart failure and thus should be strongly considered in these patients, provided that potassium and renal function can be carefully monitored. Aldosterone antagonists should also be considered soon after myocardial infarction in patients with left ventricular dysfunction and either heart failure or diabetes.

10. The combination of hydralazine and nitrates improves the composite end point of mortality, hospitalizations for heart failure, and quality of life in African Americans who receive standard therapy. The addition of hydralazine and nitrates is reasonable in patients with persistent symptoms despite optimized therapy with an ACE inhibitor (or angiotensin receptor blocker) and β-blocker.

11. No therapy for acute decompensated heart failure studied to date has been shown conclusively to influence mortality. Treatment goals are directed toward restoration of systemic oxygen transport and tissue perfusion, relief of pulmonary edema, and limitation of further cardiac damage. Maximizing oral therapy and using combinations of short-acting intravenous medica-

Learning objectives, review questions, and other resources can be found at **www.pharmacotherapyonline.com.**

tions with different cardiovascular actions are often needed to optimize cardiac output, relieve pulmonary edema, and limit myocardial ischemia. Invasive hemodynamic monitoring may be required to provide immediate feedback on treatment efficacy and adverse effects.

⓬ Pharmacists should play an important role as part of a multidisciplinary team to optimize therapy in heart failure. The pharmacist should be responsible for such activities as optimizing regimens for heart failure drug therapy (namely, ensuring that appropriate drugs at appropriate doses are used), educating patients about the importance of adherence to their heart failure regimen (including pharmacologic and dietary interventions), screening for drugs that may exacerbate or worsen heart failure, and monitoring for adverse drug effects and drug interactions.

❶ ❷ Heart failure is a progressive clinical syndrome that can result from any disorder that impairs the ability of the ventricle to fill with or eject blood, thus rendering the heart unable to pump blood at a rate sufficient to meet the metabolic demands of the body.[1] Heart failure is the final common pathway for numerous cardiac disorders including those affecting the pericardium, heart valves, and myocardium. Diseases that adversely affect ventricular diastole (filling), ventricular systole (contraction), or both can lead to heart failure. For many years it was believed that reduced myocardial contractility, or systolic dysfunction (i.e., reduced left ventricular ejection fraction [LVEF]), was the sole disturbance in cardiac function responsible for heart failure. However, it is now recognized that large numbers of patients with the heart failure syndrome have relatively normal systolic function (i.e., normal LVEF). This is now referred to as heart failure with preserved LVEF and is believed to be primarily caused by diastolic dysfunction of the heart.[1] Recent estimates suggest 20% to 60% of patients with heart failure have preserved LVEF with disturbances in relaxation (lusitropic) properties of the heart, or diastolic dysfunction.[2] However, regardless of the etiology of heart failure, the underlying pathophysiologic process and principal clinical manifestations (fatigue, dyspnea, and volume overload) are similar and appear to be independent of the initial cause. Historically, this disorder was commonly referred to as *congestive heart failure*; the preferred nomenclature is now *heart failure* because a patient can have the clinical syndrome of heart failure without having symptoms of congestion. This chapter focuses on treatment of patients with systolic dysfunction (with or without concurrent diastolic dysfunction), whereas Chap. 20 focuses on the treatment of heart failure with preserved LVEF (diastolic dysfunction).

EPIDEMIOLOGY

Heart failure is an epidemic public health problem in the United States. Approximately 5 million Americans have heart failure with an additional 550,000 cases diagnosed each year. Unlike most other cardiovascular diseases, the incidence, prevalence, and hospitalization rates associated with heart failure are increasing and are expected to continue to increase over the next few decades as the population ages. A large majority of patients with heart failure are elderly, with multiple comorbid conditions that influence morbidity and mortality.[3,4] The incidence of heart failure doubles with each decade of life and affects nearly 10% of individuals older than age 75 years. Heart failure is more common in men than in women until age 65 years, reflecting the greater incidence of coronary artery disease in men.[4] As such, improved survival of patients after myocardial infarction is a likely contributor to the increased incidence and prevalence of heart failure.[3] Recent results from the Framingham Heart Study showed that the incidence of heart failure in men has not changed over the last 40 years, but has decreased by approximately one-third in women.[5] These differences in heart failure incidence may be a result of sex-based differences in the cause of heart failure as myocardial infarction is the leading cause in men, whereas hypertension is the leading etiology in women.

Heart failure is the most common hospital discharge diagnosis in individuals older than age 65 years. Annual hospital discharges for heart failure now total more than 1 million, a 174% increase over the last two decades.[4] Heart failure also has a tremendous economic impact, which is expected to increase markedly as the baby boom generation ages. Current estimates suggest annual expenditures for heart failure of approximately $33 billion, with the majority of these costs spent on hospitalized patients.[4] Thus, heart failure is a major medical problem, with substantial economic impact that is expected to become even more significant as the population ages.

Despite prodigious advances in our understanding of the etiology, pathophysiology, and pharmacotherapy of heart failure, the prognosis for patients with this disorder remains grim. Although the mortality rates have declined over the last 50 years, the overall 5-year survival remains approximately 50% for all patients with a diagnosis of heart failure, with mortality increasing with symptom severity.[5] For heart failure patients younger than age 65 years, 80% of men and 70% of women will die within 8 years. Death is classified as sudden in approximately 40% of patients,[1,6] implicating serious ventricular arrhythmias as the underlying cause in many patients with heart failure. Factors affecting the prognosis of patients with heart failure include, but are not limited to, age, gender, LVEF, renal function, blood pressure, heart failure etiology, and drug or device therapy. Recent models incorporating these and other factors enable clinicians to develop reliable estimates of an individual patient's prognosis.[7]

ETIOLOGY

❶ ❷ Heart failure can result from any disorder that affects the ability of the heart to contract (systolic function) and/or relax (diastolic dysfunction); Table 16–1 lists the common causes of heart failure.[8] Heart failure with impaired systolic function (i.e., reduced LVEF) is the classic, more familiar form of the disorder, but current estimates suggest up to 50% of patients with heart failure have preserved left ventricular systolic function with presumed diastolic dysfunction.[2] In contrast to systolic heart failure that is usually caused by previous myocardial infarction (MI), patients with preserved LVEF typically are elderly, female, obese, and have hypertension, atrial fibrillation, or diabetes.[2] Recent data indicate that survival

TABLE 16-1 Causes of Heart Failure

Systolic dysfunction (decreased contractility)
• Reduction in muscle mass (e.g., myocardial infarction)
• Dilated cardiomyopathies
• Ventricular hypertrophy
• Pressure overload (e.g., systemic or pulmonary hypertension, aortic or pulmonic valve stenosis)
• Volume overload (e.g., valvular regurgitation, shunts, high-output states)
Diastolic dysfunction (restriction in ventricular filling)
• Increased ventricular stiffness
• Ventricular hypertrophy (e.g., hypertrophic cardiomyopathy, other examples above)
• Infiltrative myocardial diseases (e.g., amyloidosis, sarcoidosis, endomyocardial fibrosis)
• Myocardial ischemia and infarction
• Mitral or tricuspid valve stenosis
• Pericardial disease (e.g., pericarditis, pericardial tamponade)

Data from Colucci W, Braunwald E. Pathophysiology of heart failure. In: Zipes DP, Libby P, Bonow RO, Braunwald E, eds. Heart Disease: A Textbook of Cardiovascular Medicine, 7th ed. Philadelphia: Elsevier Saunders, 2005:509–538.

is similar in patients with impaired or preserved LVEF.[2] Frequently, systolic and diastolic dysfunction coexist. The common cardiovascular diseases, such as MI and hypertension, can cause both systolic and diastolic dysfunction; thus many patients have heart failure as a result of reduced myocardial contractility and abnormal ventricular filling. Heart failure with preserved LVEF is discussed in Chap. 20.

❶ Coronary artery disease is the most common cause of systolic heart failure, accounting for nearly 70% of cases.[3] Myocardial infarction leads to reduction in muscle mass as a consequence of death of affected myocardial cells. The degree to which contractility is impaired will depend on the size of the infarction. In an attempt to maintain cardiac output, the surviving myocardium undergoes a compensatory remodeling, thus beginning the maladaptive process that initiates the heart failure syndrome and leads to further injury to the heart. This is discussed in greater detail in Pathophysiology below. Myocardial ischemia and infarction also affect the diastolic properties of the heart by increasing ventricular stiffness and slowing ventricular relaxation. Thus, myocardial infarction frequently results in systolic and diastolic dysfunction.

Impaired systolic function is a cardinal feature of dilated cardiomyopathies. Although the cause of reduced contractility frequently is unknown, abnormalities such as interstitial fibrosis, cellular infiltrates, cellular hypertrophy, and myocardial cell degeneration are seen commonly on histologic examination. Genetic causes of dilated cardiomyopathies may also occur.[9]

Pressure or volume overload causes ventricular hypertrophy, which attempts to return contractility to a near-normal state. If the pressure or volume overload persists, the remodeling process results in alterations in the geometry of the hypertrophied myocardial cells and is accompanied by increased collagen deposition in the extracellular matrix. Thus, both systolic and diastolic function may be impaired.[8] Examples of pressure overload include systemic or pulmonary hypertension and aortic or pulmonic valve stenosis.

Hypertension remains an important cause and/or contributor to heart failure in many patients, particularly women, the elderly, and African Americans.[1] The role of hypertension should not be underestimated because hypertension is an important risk factor for ischemic heart disease and thus is also present in a high percentage of the patients with this disorder. Volume overload may occur in the presence of valvular regurgitation, shunts, or high-output states such as anemia or pregnancy. Table 16–1 lists less-common causes of diastolic dysfunction, which include infiltrative myocardial diseases, mitral or tricuspid valve stenosis, and pericardial disease.

Because ischemic heart disease and/or hypertension contribute so significantly to the development of heart failure in the majority of patients, it is important to emphasize that heart failure is a largely preventable disorder. Thus, control of blood pressure and appropriate management of other risk factors for cardiovascular disease (e.g., smoking cessation, treatment of lipid disorders, diabetes management, dietary modification) are important strategies for clinicians to implement to reduce their patients' risk of heart failure.

PATHOPHYSIOLOGY

NORMAL CARDIAC FUNCTION

To understand the pathophysiologic processes in heart failure, a basic understanding of normal cardiac function is necessary. *Cardiac output* (CO) is defined as the volume of blood ejected per unit time (L/min) and is the product of heart rate (HR) and stroke volume (SV):

$$CO = HR \times SV$$

The relationship between CO and mean arterial pressure (MAP) is:

$$MAP = CO \times \text{systemic vascular resistance (SVR)}$$

Heart rate is controlled by the autonomic nervous system. Stroke volume, or the volume of blood ejected during systole, depends on preload, afterload, and contractility.[8] As defined by the Frank-Starling mechanism, the ability of the heart to alter the force of contraction depends on changes in preload. As myocardial sarcomere length is stretched, the number of cross-bridges between thick and thin myofilaments increases, resulting in an increase in the force of contraction. The length of the sarcomere is determined primarily by the volume of blood in the ventricle; therefore, left ventricular end-diastolic volume is the primary determinant of preload. In normal hearts, the preload response is the primary compensatory mechanism such that a small increase in end-diastolic volume results in a large increase in cardiac output. Because of the relationship between pressure and volume in the heart, left ventricular end-diastolic pressure is often used in the clinical setting to estimate preload. The hemodynamic measurement used to estimate left ventricular end-diastolic pressure is the pulmonary artery occlusion pressure (PAOP). Afterload is a more complex physiologic concept that can be viewed pragmatically as the sum of forces preventing active forward ejection of blood by the ventricle. Major components of global ventricular afterload are ejection impedance, wall tension, and regional wall geometry. In patients with left ventricular systolic dysfunction, an inverse relationship exists between afterload (or SVR) and stroke volume such that increasing afterload causes a decrease in stroke volume (Fig. 16–1). Contractility is the intrinsic property of cardiac muscle describing fiber shortening and tension development.

COMPENSATORY MECHANISMS IN HEART FAILURE

❷ Heart failure is a progressive disorder initiated by an event that impairs the ability of the heart to contract and/or relax. The index event may have an acute onset, as with myocardial infarction, or the onset may be slow, as with long-standing hypertension. Regardless of the index event, the decrease in the heart's pumping capacity results in the heart having to rely on compensatory responses to maintain an adequate cardiac output.[10] These compensatory responses include (a) tachycardia and increased contractility through sympathetic nervous system (SNS) activation, (b) the Frank-Starling mechanism, whereby an increase in preload results in an increase in stroke volume, (c) vasoconstriction, and (d) ventricular hypertrophy and remodeling. These compensatory responses are intended to be short-term responses to maintain circulatory homeostasis after acute reductions in blood pressure or renal perfusion. However, the

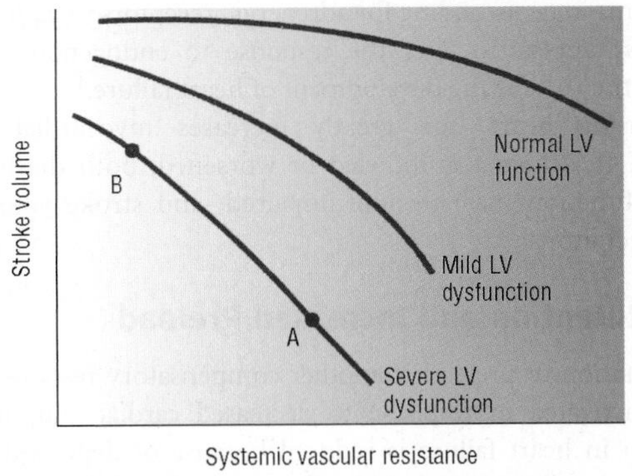

FIGURE 16-1. Relationship between stroke volume and systemic vascular resistance. In an individual with normal left ventricular (LV) function, increasing systemic vascular resistance has little effect on stroke volume. As the extent of LV dysfunction increases, the negative, inverse relationship between stroke volume and systemic vascular resistance becomes more important *(B to A)*.

TABLE 16-2 Beneficial and Detrimental Effects of the Compensatory Responses in Heart Failure

Compensatory Response	Beneficial Effects of Compensation	Detrimental Effects of Compensation
Increased preload (through Na^+ and water retention)	Optimize stroke volume via Frank-Starling mechanism	Pulmonary and systemic congestion and edema formation Increased MVO_2
Vasoconstriction	Maintain BP in face of reduced CO Shunt blood from nonessential organs to brain and heart	Increased MVO_2 Increased afterload decreases stroke volume and further activates the compensatory responses
Tachycardia and increased contractility (because of SNS activation)	Helps maintain CO	Increased MVO_2 Shortened diastolic filling time β_1-receptor downregulation, decreased receptor sensitivity Precipitation of ventricular arrhythmias Increased risk of myocardial cell death
Ventricular hypertrophy and remodeling	Helps maintain CO Reduces myocardial wall stress Decreases MVO_2	Diastolic dysfunction Systolic dysfunction Increased risk of myocardial cell death Increased risk of myocardial ischemia Increased arrhythmia risk Fibrosis

BP, blood pressure; CO, cardiac output; MVO_2, myocardial oxygen demand; SNS, sympathetic nervous system.

persistent decline in cardiac output in heart failure results in long-term activation of these compensatory responses resulting in the complex functional, structural, biochemical, and molecular changes important for the development and progression of heart failure. The beneficial and detrimental effects of these compensatory responses are described below and are summarized in Table 16–2.

Tachycardia and Increased Contractility

The change in heart rate and contractility that rapidly occurs in response to a drop in cardiac output is primarily a result of release of norepinephrine (NE) from adrenergic nerve terminals, although parasympathetic nervous system activity is also diminished. Cardiac output increases with heart rate until diastolic filling becomes compromised, which in the normal heart is at 170 to 200 beats per minute. Loss of atrial contribution to ventricular filling also can occur (atrial fibrillation, ventricular tachycardia), reducing ventricular performance even more. Because ionized calcium is sequestered into the sarcoplasmic reticulum and pumped out of the cardiac myocyte during diastole, shortened diastolic time also results in a higher average intracellular calcium concentration during diastole, increasing actin–myosin interaction, augmenting the active resistance to fibril stretch, and reducing lusitropy. Conversely, the higher average calcium concentration translates into greater filament interaction during systole, generating more tension.[8] In addition, polymorphisms in genes coding for adrenergic receptors (e.g., β_1 and α_{2c} receptors) appear to alter the response to endogenous NE and increase the risk for the development of heart failure.[11]

Increasing heart rate greatly increases myocardial oxygen demand. If ischemia is induced or worsened, both diastolic and systolic function may become impaired, and stroke volume can drop precipitously.

Fluid Retention and Increased Preload

Augmentation of preload is another compensatory response that is rapidly activated in response to decreased cardiac output. Renal perfusion in heart failure is reduced because of depressed cardiac output and redistribution of blood away from nonvital organs. The kidney interprets the reduced perfusion as an ineffective blood volume, resulting in activation of the renin–angiotensin–aldosterone system (RAAS) in an attempt to maintain blood pressure and increase renal sodium and water retention. Reduced renal perfusion and increased sympathetic tone also stimulate renin release from juxtaglomerular cells in the kidney. As shown in Fig. 16–2, renin is responsible for conversion of angiotensinogen to angiotensin I. Angiotensin I is converted to angiotensin II by angiotensin-converting enzyme (ACE). Angiotensin II may also be generated via non–ACE-dependent pathways. Angiotensin II feeds back on the adrenal gland to stimulate aldosterone release, thereby providing an additional mechanism for sodium and water retention in the kidney. As intravascular volume increases secondary to sodium and water retention, left ventricular volume and pressure (preload) increase, sarcomeres are stretched, and the force of contraction is enhanced.[8] While the preload response is the primary compensatory mechanism in normal hearts, the chronically failing heart usually has exhausted its preload reserve.[8] As shown in Fig. 16–3, increases in preload will increase stroke volume only to a certain point. Once the flat portion of the curve is reached, further increases in preload will only lead to pulmonary or systemic congestion, a detrimental result.[8] Figure 16–3 also shows that the curve is flatter in patients with left ventricular dysfunction. Consequently, a given increase in preload in a patient with heart failure will produce a smaller increment in stroke volume than in an individual with normal ventricular function.

Vasoconstriction and Increased Afterload

Vasoconstriction occurs in patients with heart failure to help redistribute blood flow away from nonessential organs to coronary and cerebral circulations to support blood pressure, which may be reduced secondary to a decrease in cardiac output (mean arterial pressure = CO × SVR).[8] A number of neurohormones likely contribute to the vasoconstriction, including NE, angiotensin II, endothelin-1, and arginine vasopressin (AVP).[8] Vasoconstriction impedes forward ejection of blood from the ventricle, further depressing cardiac output and heightening the compensatory responses. Because the failing ventricle usually has exhausted its preload reserve (unless the patient is intravascularly depleted), its performance is exquisitely sensitive to changes in afterload (see Fig. 16–1). Thus, increases in afterload often potentiate a vicious cycle of continued worsening and downward spiraling of the heart failure state.

Ventricular Hypertrophy and Remodeling[8,10]

❸ Although the signs and symptoms of heart failure are closely associated with the items described above, the progression of heart failure appears to be independent of the patient's hemodynamic status. It is now recognized that ventricular hypertrophy and

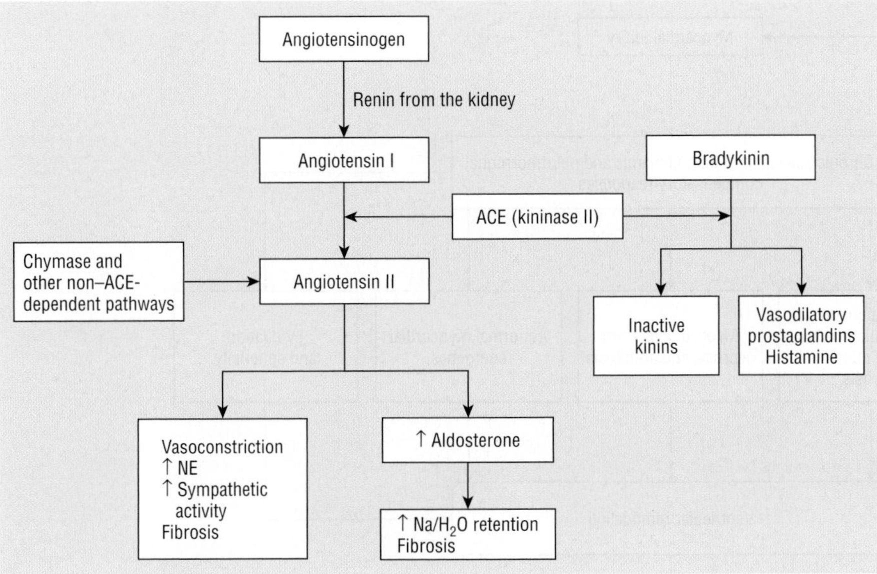

FIGURE 16-2. Physiology of the renin–angiotensin–aldosterone system. Renin produces angiotensin I from angiotensinogen. Angiotensin I is cleaved to angiotensin II by angiotensin-converting enzyme (ACE). Angiotensin II has a number of physiologic actions that are detrimental in heart failure. Note that angiotensin II can be produced in a number of tissues, including the heart, independent of ACE activity. ACE is also responsible for the breakdown of bradykinin. Inhibition of ACE results in accumulation of bradykinin that, in turn, enhances the production of vasodilatory prostaglandins. (NE, norepinephrine.)

remodeling are key components in the pathogenesis of progressive myocardial failure. *Ventricular hypertrophy* is a term used to describe an increase in ventricular muscle mass. *Cardiac* or *ventricular remodeling* is a broader term describing changes in both myocardial cells and extracellular matrix that result in changes in the size, shape, structure, and function of the heart. Ventricular hypertrophy and remodeling can occur in association with any condition that causes myocardial injury including MI, cardiomyopathy, hypertension, and valvular heart disease.

Cardiac remodeling is a complex process that affects the heart at the molecular and cellular levels. Figure 16–4 shows key elements in the process. Collectively, these events result in progressive changes in myocardial structure and function such as cardiac hypertrophy, myocyte loss, and alterations in the extracellular matrix. The progression of the remodeling process leads to reductions in myocardial systolic and/or diastolic function that, in turn, result in further myocardial injury, perpetuating the remodeling process and the decline in ventricular dysfunction. Angiotensin II, NE, endothelin, aldosterone, vasopressin and numerous inflammatory cytokines, as well as substances under investigation, that are activated both systemically and locally in the heart play an important role in initiating the signal–transduction cascade responsible for ventricular remodeling. Although these mediators produce deleterious effects on the heart, their increased circulating and tissue concentrations also serve as an important reminder that heart failure is a systemic, as well as cardiac, disorder.

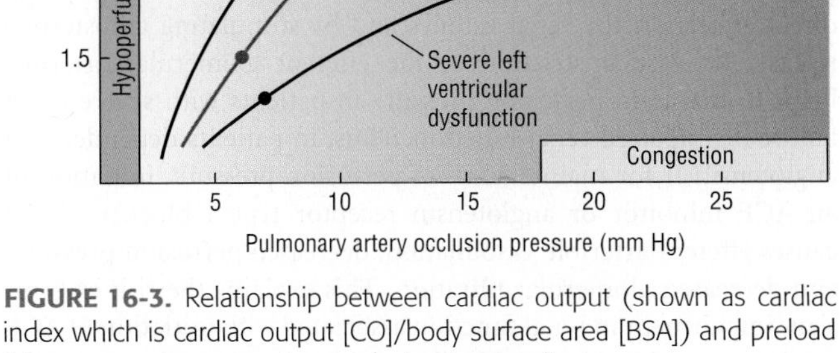

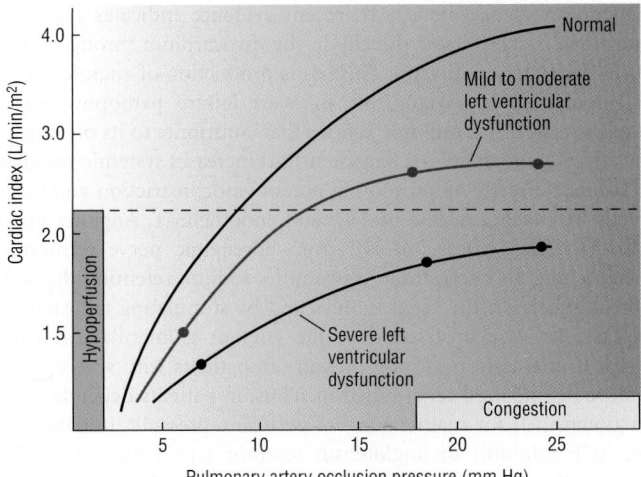

FIGURE 16-3. Relationship between cardiac output (shown as cardiac index which is cardiac output [CO]/body surface area [BSA]) and preload (shown as pulmonary artery occlusion pressure).

Pressure overload (and probably hormonal activation) associated with hypertension produces a concentric hypertrophy (increase in the ventricular wall thickness without chamber enlargement). Conversely, eccentric left ventricular hypertrophy (myocyte lengthening with increased chamber size with minimal increase in wall thickness) characterizes the hypertrophy seen in patients with systolic dysfunction or previous MI. As the myocytes undergo change, so do various components of the extracellular matrix. For example, there is evidence for collagen degradation, which may lead to slippage of myocytes, fibroblast proliferation, and increased fibrillar collagen synthesis, resulting in fibrosis and stiffening of the entire myocardium. Thus, a number of important ventricular changes that occur with remodeling include changes in the geometry of the heart from elliptical to spherical, increases in ventricular mass (from myocyte hypertrophy), and changes in ventricular composition (especially the extracellular matrix) and volumes, all of which likely contribute to the impairment of cardiac function. If the event that produces cardiac injury is acute (e.g., MI), the ventricular remodeling process begins immediately. However, it is the progressive nature of this process that results in continual worsening of the heart failure state, and thus is now the major focus for identification of therapeutic targets. In fact, it is believed that all the heart failure therapies that are associated with decreased mortality and/or slowing the progression of the disease produce this effect largely through their ability to slow or reverse the ventricular remodeling process, a process often referred to as *reverse remodeling*. Thus, although ventricular hypertrophy and remodeling may have some beneficial effects by helping maintain cardiac output, they also are believed to play an essential role in the progressive nature of heart failure.

THE NEUROHORMONAL MODEL OF HEART FAILURE AND THERAPEUTIC INSIGHTS IT PROVIDES[8,10]

❷ ❸ Over the years, several different paradigms have guided our understanding of the pathophysiology and treatment of heart failure. The early paradigm is often called the *cardiorenal model*, where the problem was viewed as excess sodium and water retention, and diuretic therapy was the main therapeutic approach. The next para-

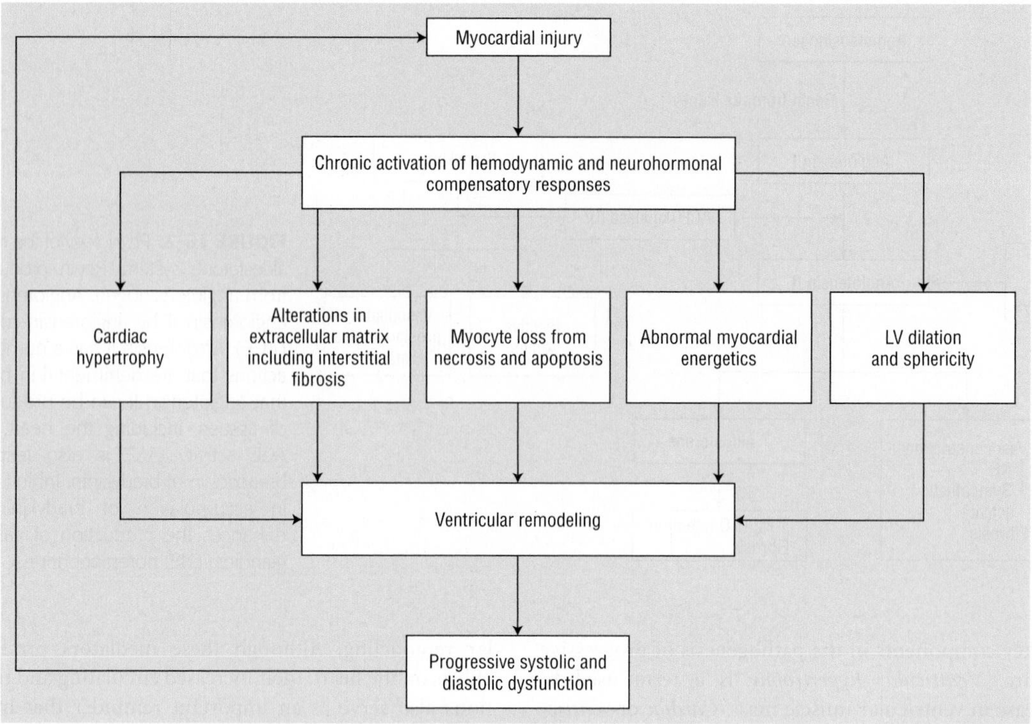

FIGURE 16-4. Key components of the pathophysiology of cardiac remodeling. Myocardial injury (e.g., myocardial infarction) results in the activation of a number of hemodynamic and neurohormonal compensatory responses in an attempt to maintain circulatory homeostasis. Chronic activation of the neurohormonal systems results in a cascade of events that affect the myocardium at the molecular and cellular levels. These events lead to the changes in ventricular size, shape, structure, and function known as ventricular remodeling. The alterations in ventricular function result in further deterioration in cardiac systolic and diastolic function which further promotes the remodeling process. (LV, left ventricle.)

digm was the *cardiocirculatory model,* which focused on impaired cardiac output (viewed as being a result of both reduced pumping capacity of the heart and systemic vasoconstriction). This paradigm focused on positive inotropes and, later, vasodilators as the primary therapies to overcome reductions in cardiac output. Although the therapeutic approaches associated with these paradigms provided some symptomatic benefits to patients with heart failure, they did little to slow progression of the disease. In fact, the detrimental effects of positive inotropic drugs on survival highlighted the inadequacy of the cardiocirculatory model to explain the progressive nature of heart failure. The first studies with ACE inhibitors were initiated with the thought that they might be effective because of their balanced (arterial and venous) vasodilation. Subsequent realization that ACE inhibitors were providing benefit beyond their vasodilating effects, followed by the positive results with β-adrenergic receptor blockers and aldosterone antagonists, has led to the current paradigm used to describe heart failure: the *neurohormonal model.* This model recognizes that there is an initiating event (e.g., MI, long-standing hypertension) that leads to decreased cardiac output and begins the "heart failure state," but then the problem moves beyond the heart, and it essentially becomes a systemic disease whose progression is mediated largely by neurohormones and autocrine/paracrine factors. Although the former paradigms still guide us to some extent in the symptomatic management of the disease (e.g., diuretics and digoxin), it is the latter paradigm that helps us understand disease progression and, more importantly, the ways to slow disease progression. In the sections that follow, important neurohormones and autocrine/paracrine factors are described with respect to their role in heart failure and its progression. The benefits of current and investigational drug therapies can be better understood through a solid understanding of the neurohormones they regulate/affect. Although the neurohormonal model provides a logical framework for our current understanding of heart failure progression and the role of various medications in attenuating this progression, it must be emphasized that this model does not completely explain heart failure progression. For example, drug therapies that target the neurohormonal perturbations in heart failure usually only slow the progressive nature of the disorder rather than completely stop it. Ongoing research will likely identify additional targets for drug therapy.

Angiotensin II[10]

Of the neurohormones and autocrine/paracrine factors that play an important role in the pathophysiology of heart failure, angiotensin II is probably the best understood. Although circulating angiotensin II produced from ACE activity is the most familiar route for generation of angiotensin II, recent evidence indicates that this hormone is synthesized directly in the myocardium through non–ACE-dependent pathways. This tissue production of angiotensin II also plays an important role in heart failure pathophysiology. Angiotensin II has multiple actions that contribute to its detrimental effects in heart failure. Angiotensin II increases systemic vascular resistance directly by promoting potent vasoconstriction and indirectly by causing release of AVP and endothelin-1. Angiotensin II also facilitates release of NE from adrenergic nerve terminals, heightening SNS activation. It promotes sodium retention through direct effects on the renal tubules and by stimulating aldosterone release. Its vasoconstriction of the efferent glomerular arteriole helps to maintain perfusion pressure in patients with severe heart failure or impaired renal function. Thus, in patients dependent on angiotensin II for maintenance of perfusion pressure, initiation of an ACE inhibitor or angiotensin receptor type I blocker (ARB) causes efferent arteriole vasodilation, decreased perfusion pressure, and decreased glomerular filtration. This explains the risk of transient impairment in renal function associated with initiation of ACE inhibitor or ARB therapy. Finally, angiotensin II, and many of the neurohormones released in response to angiotensin II, play a central role in stimulating ventricular hypertrophy, remodeling, myocyte apoptosis (programmed cell death), oxidative stress, inflammation, and alterations in the extracellular matrix. Clinical data suggest that blocking angiotensin II-mediated effects contributes substantially to the prolonged survival of ACE inhibitor- and ARB-treated heart failure patients.[12,13] The favorable effects of ACE inhibitors and ARBs on hemodynamics, symptoms, quality of life, and survival in heart failure highlight the importance of angiotensin II in the pathophysiology of heart failure.

Norepinephrine[8,10]

Many of the detrimental effects of NE in heart failure are described above. It plays a central role in the tachycardia, vasoconstriction, and increased contractility observed in heart failure. Plasma NE concentrations are elevated in correlation with the degree of heart failure, and patients with the highest plasma NE concentrations have the poorest prognosis. In addition to the detrimental effects described, excessive SNS activation causes downregulation of β_1-receptors, with a subsequent loss of sensitivity to receptor stimulation. Evidence suggests that genetic variations in the β_1- and α_{2c}-receptors, which are targets for NE's actions, may modify the extent of receptor downregulation and increase the risk of heart failure.[11] Excess catecholamines increase the risk of arrhythmias and can cause myocardial cell loss by stimulating both necrosis and apoptosis. Finally, NE contributes to ventricular hypertrophy and remodeling. The detrimental effects of SNS activation are further highlighted by the clinical trials of chronic therapy with β-agonists, phosphodiesterase inhibitors, and other drugs that cause SNS activation, as they have been shown uniformly to increase mortality in heart failure. Conversely, β-blockers, ACE inhibitors, and digoxin all help to decrease SNS activation through various mechanisms, and are beneficial in heart failure. Thus, it is clear that NE plays a critical role in the pathophysiology of the heart failure state.

Aldosterone[14,15]

Aldosterone-mediated sodium retention and its key role in volume overload and edema has long been recognized as an important component of the heart failure syndrome. Circulating aldosterone is increased in heart failure as a consequence of stimulation of its synthesis and release from the adrenal cortex by angiotensin II and because of decreased hepatic clearance secondary to reduced hepatic perfusion. Although its enhancement of sodium retention is an important component of heart failure symptoms, recent studies indicate direct effects of aldosterone on the heart that may be even more important in heart failure pathophysiology. Chief among these is the ability of aldosterone to produce interstitial cardiac fibrosis through increased collagen deposition in the extracellular matrix of the heart. This cardiac fibrosis may decrease systolic function, and also impair diastolic function by increasing the stiffness of the myocardium. Current research shows that extraadrenal production of aldosterone in the heart, kidneys, and vascular smooth muscle also contributes to the progressive nature of heart failure through target organ fibrosis and vascular remodeling. Induction of a systemic proinflammatory state and increased oxidative stress are other important direct detrimental actions of aldosterone. Aldosterone also may increase the risk of ventricular arrhythmias through a number of mechanisms, including creation of reentrant circuits as a result of fibrosis, inhibition of cardiac NE reuptake, depletion of intracellular potassium and magnesium, and impairment of parasympathetic traffic. Recent studies demonstrate that the aldosterone antagonists spironolactone[16] and eplerenone[17] produce significant reductions in mortality in patients with heart failure, without appreciable effects on diuresis or hemodynamics, providing substantial evidence that the direct cardiac effects of aldosterone play an important role in heart failure pathophysiology.

Natriuretic Peptides[18]

The natriuretic peptide family has three members, atrial natriuretic peptide, B-type natriuretic peptide (BNP), and C-type natriuretic peptide. Atrial natriuretic peptide is stored mainly in the right atrium, whereas BNP is found primarily in the ventricles. Both are released in response to pressure or volume overload. C-type natriuretic peptide is found mainly in the brain and has very low plasma concentrations. Atrial natriuretic peptide and BNP plasma concentrations are elevated in patients with heart failure and are thought to balance the effects of the renin–angiotensin system by causing natriuresis, diuresis, vasodilation, decreased aldosterone release, decreased hypertrophy, and inhibition of the SNS and RAAS.

The development of easily performed commercial assays for BNP and the related biologically inactive peptide, N-terminal prohormone BNP, resulted in significant attention to the role of these peptides as a biomarker for prognostic, diagnostic, and therapeutic use. In patients with chronic heart failure, the degree of elevation in BNP levels is closely associated with increased mortality, risk of sudden death, symptoms, and hospital readmission. Current data indicate BNP is more sensitive than NE for predicting morbidity and mortality in heart failure patients. Accurate diagnosis of acute decompensated heart failure in acute care settings is often difficult because many of the symptoms (e.g., dyspnea) mimic those of other disorders, such as pulmonary disease or obesity. The best-established clinical application of BNP testing is in the urgent care setting where the BNP assay is useful when combined with clinical evaluation for discriminating dyspnea secondary to heart failure from other causes. The BNP assay may also be useful in the diagnosis of heart failure in the outpatient setting and used as a marker to guide titration of heart failure drug therapy. However, the usefulness of the assay in these situations remains uncertain and the results of ongoing studies may help clarify the role of BNP testing in these patients. Finally, administration of recombinant human BNP (nesiritide) for short-term management of acute heart failure resulted in hemodynamic and symptomatic improvement, further supporting the role of BNP in heart failure pathophysiology.

Arginine Vasopressin[19]

AVP is a pituitary peptide hormone that plays an important role in regulation of renal water and solute excretion. AVP secretion is directly linked to changes in plasma osmolality, thus attempting to maintain body fluid homeostasis. The physiologic effects of AVP are mediated through the V_{1a} and V_2 receptors. V_{1a} receptors are located in vascular smooth muscle and in myocytes where AVP stimulation results in vasoconstriction and increased cardiac contractility, respectively. V_2 receptors are located in the collecting duct of the kidney where AVP stimulation causes reabsorption of free water.

Plasma concentrations of AVP are elevated in patients with heart failure supporting current research that indicates AVP plays a role in the pathophysiology of heart failure. Important effects associated with increased circulating AVP concentrations include (a) increased renal free water reabsorption in the face of plasma hypoosmolality resulting in volume overload and hyponatremia; (b) increased arterial vasoconstriction which contributes to reduced cardiac output; and (c) stimulation of remodeling by cardiac hypertrophy and extracellular matrix collagen deposition.

Given the importance of AVP in heart failure, recent efforts have focused on the development of AVP antagonist drugs for treatment of acute and chronic heart failure. By blocking the AVP receptor, these agents primarily increase free water excretion (i.e., an "aquaretic" effect). The oral V_2 receptor antagonist tolvaptan increased serum sodium and urine output without affecting heart rate, blood pressure, renal function, or other electrolytes in patients hospitalized for hyponatremia from various causes (hyponatremia due to heart failure in approximately 33% of patients).[20] In another clinical trial, the addition of oral tolvaptan to diuretic therapy in patients hospitalized for worsening heart failure had no effect on mortality or the composite end point of cardiovascular death or hospitalization for heart failure.[21] However, tolvaptan did produce short-term reductions in body weight, edema, and patient-assessed dyspnea without causing any serious adverse events.[22] These results suggest that AVP antagonists may be useful in the treatment of heart failure patients with volume overload. Unlike diuretics, they appear to reduce excess fluid volume without affecting hemodynamics, renal function, or electrolytes. Thus, these agents may offer a new therapeutic approach to currently available drug therapies.

Other Circulating Mediators[23]

In addition to neurohormones, several proinflammatory cytokines are under extensive investigation for their role in heart failure pathophysiology. Tumor necrosis factor-α (TNF-α), interleukin (IL)-6 -6), and IL-1β have all been shown to be elevated in heart failure, with a direct relationship between the degree of elevation and the severity of heart failure. Of these cytokines, TNF-α is best studied for its pathophysiologic role in heart failure. TNF-α produces multiple deleterious actions including negative inotropic effects, uncoupling α-adrenergic receptors from adenylyl cyclase (thus reducing β-receptor-mediated responses), increasing myocardial cell apoptosis, and stimulating remodeling via several mechanisms. Although these findings clearly implicate a role for TNF-α in the pathophysiology of heart failure, clinical trials evaluating anti–TNF-α therapies (e.g., etanercept and infliximab) have been disappointing, with no improvement in outcomes demonstrated.

The endothelin peptides are potent vasoconstrictors that may be involved in heart failure pathophysiology through a number of mechanisms. Endothelin-1, the best characterized of these peptides, is synthesized by endothelial and vascular smooth muscle cells with the release of endothelin-1 enhanced by NE, angiotensin II, and inflammatory cytokines. Like other peptides and hormones described earlier, endothelin-1 plasma concentrations are elevated in heart failure and are correlated directly with the severity of hemodynamic abnormality, symptoms, and mortality. Its arterial and venous constrictive effects increase preload and afterload, and its vasoconstriction of both efferent and afferent renal arterioles may decrease renal plasma flow and induce sodium retention. Endothelin-1 has direct cardiotoxic and arrhythmogenic effects and is a potent stimulator of cardiac myocyte hypertrophy. The putative role of endothelin in heart failure led to the development of a number of endothelin-receptor antagonists. Although these agents improved hemodynamics, no benefit on morbidity or mortality has been demonstrated and further clinical development is unlikely.

The role of inflammation and endothelial dysfunction has generated significant interest in the use of statins in patients with heart failure. In addition to lowering cholesterol and reducing the risk of death and other atherosclerotic vascular diseases, the proposed pleiotropic effects (e.g., antiinflammatory, improved endothelial function, promotion of angiogenesis) may be beneficial in heart failure.[24] Although some observational studies and short-term prospective clinical trials indicate beneficial effects, others have failed to demonstrate significant improvement with statin therapy. Ongoing trials to assess effects on mortality will help clarify the role of statin therapy.

FACTORS PRECIPITATING/EXACERBATING HEART FAILURE

Although significant advancements have been made in treatment, symptom exacerbations, to the point that hospitalization is required, are a common and growing problem in patients with heart failure. Hospitalization for heart failure exacerbation consumes large amounts of healthcare dollars and significantly impairs the patient's quality of life, thus there is great interest in identifying, and then remedying, factors that increase the risk of decompensation. In patients with heart failure, appropriate therapy can often maintain them in a "compensated" state, indicating that they are relatively symptom-free. However, there are many aggravating or precipitating factors that may cause a previously compensated patient to develop worsened symptoms necessitating hospitalization. Factors that may precipitate or exacerbate heart failure typically do so by one or more of the following mechanisms: (a) negative inotropic effects; (b) direct cardiotoxicity; or (c) increased sodium and/or water retention (Table 16–3). The resulting symptoms are typically those associated with volume overload, but in more severe cases hypoperfusion may also be present.

TABLE 16-3 Drugs That May Precipitate or Exacerbate Heart Failure

Negative inotropic effect
Antiarrhythmics (e.g., disopyramide, flecainide, propafenone, and others)
β-Blockers (e.g., propranolol, metoprolol, atenolol, and others)
Calcium channel blockers (e.g., verapamil, diltiazem)
Itraconazole
Terbinafine
Cardiotoxic
Doxorubicin
Daunomycin
Cyclophosphamide
Trastuzumab
Imatinib
Ethanol
Amphetamines (e.g., cocaine, methamphetamine)
Sodium and water retention
Nonsteroidal antiinflammatory drugs
Cyclooxygenase-2 inhibitors
Rosiglitazone and pioglitazone
Glucocorticoids
Androgens and estrogens
Salicylates (high dose)
Sodium-containing drugs (e.g., carbenicillin disodium, ticarcillin disodium)

Noncompliance with prescribed heart failure medications or with dietary recommendations (e.g., sodium intake and fluid restriction) are common causes of heart failure exacerbation.[25] For example, 43% of patients admitted with an acute decompensation of chronic heart failure were assessed as having dietary sodium excess, 34% had excess fluid intake (defined as >2.5 L/day), and approximately 24% had drug noncompliance that may have contributed to their decompensation (although not necessarily defined as the primary cause of decompensation).

Cardiac events may also precipitate heart failure exacerbations. Myocardial ischemia and infarction are potentially reversible causes that must be carefully considered because nearly 70% of heart failure patients have coronary artery disease. It should be noted that myocardial ischemia can either be a cause or consequence of heart failure decompensation. Revascularization should be considered in appropriate patients. Atrial fibrillation occurs in up to 30% of patients with heart failure, and is associated with increased morbidity and mortality.[26,27] Atrial fibrillation can exacerbate heart failure through rapid ventricular response and loss of atrial contribution to ventricular filling. Conversely, heart failure can precipitate atrial fibrillation by worsening atrial distension resulting from ventricular volume overload. Control of ventricular response, maintenance of sinus rhythm in appropriate patients, and prevention of thromboembolism are important elements in the treatment of heart failure patients with atrial fibrillation.

A number of noncardiac events may also be associated with heart failure decompensation. Pulmonary infections frequently cause worsening of heart failure. Many of these events would be preventable with more widespread use of the pneumococcal and influenza vaccines. Recent studies suggest that anemia occurs frequently in patients with heart failure and that it is an independent predictor of death and hospitalization for heart failure, regardless of left ventricular systolic function.[28] The exact cause of anemia in heart failure patients is uncertain but likely involves reduced response to erythropoietin, the presence of inhibitors to hematopoiesis, and/or impaired iron supply. Correction of anemia with erythropoietin analogs is associated with improved symptoms and exercise capacity but some have expressed concern that raising hemoglobin concentrations may increase the risk of thromboembolism or other cardiovascular events. Therefore, the results of ongoing clinical trials evaluating survival are needed to determine the role of this therapy in heart failure.

⓬ What should be evident is that many of the precipitating factors are preventable, particularly through appropriate pharmacist intervention. Specifically, patient education and counseling by a pharmacist should help to decrease the most common reason for heart failure exacerbation: noncompliance with dietary sodium and water restrictions, drug therapy, or both. Pharmacists also should be able to identify and address inadequate heart failure therapy, poorly controlled hypertension, and administration of drugs that may worsen heart failure (see Table 16–3). Use of medications such as antiarrhythmic agents and selected calcium channel blockers are important precipitants of exacerbations. It should be noted that the cyclooxygenase-2 (COX-2) inhibitor celecoxib and nonsteroidal antiinflammatory drugs (NSAIDs) have similar effects on renal function.[29] Thus, both NSAIDs and COX-2 inhibitors should be used judiciously in heart failure patients. The thiazolidinedione hypoglycemic drugs, rosiglitazone and pioglitazone, are associated with the development of weight gain and edema that may exacerbate heart failure. Current guidelines indicate these agents should not be used in patients with New York Heart Association (NYHA) class III or IV heart failure and recent evidence suggests rosiglitazone may increase the risk of myocardial infarction.[1,30,31] It can be argued that heart failure exacerbations caused by noncompliance, inadequate/inappropriate drug therapy, and poorly controlled hypertension are all preventable and amenable to pharmacist intervention. Thus the value of the pharmacist's role in careful and repeated education of patients and in monitoring of the drug regimen should not be underestimated. Attention to these factors may make an important contribution to reducing the risk of hospitalization and improving the patient's quality of life.

CLINICAL PRESENTATION[32]

SIGNS AND SYMPTOMS

❷ The primary manifestations of heart failure are dyspnea and fatigue, which lead to exercise intolerance, and fluid overload, that can result in pulmonary congestion and peripheral edema. The presence of these signs and symptoms may vary considerably from patient to patient, such that some patients have dyspnea but no signs of fluid retention whereas others may have marked volume overload with few complaints of dyspnea or fatigue. However, many patients may have both dyspnea and volume overload. Clinicians should remember that symptom severity often does not correlate with the degree of left ventricle dysfunction. Patients with a low LVEF (less than 20% to 25%) may be asymptomatic, whereas patients with preserved LVEF may have significant symptoms. It is also important to note that symptoms can vary considerably over time in a given patient. Historically, signs and symptoms are classified as being a result of left ventricular (pulmonary congestion) or right ventricular failure (systemic congestion). Although most patients initially have left ventricular failure, the ventricles share a septal wall, and because left ventricular failure increases the workload of the right ventricle, both ventricles eventually fail and contribute to the heart failure syndrome. Because of the complex nature of this syndrome, it has become exceedingly more difficult to attribute a specific sign or symptom as caused by either right or left ventricular failure. Therefore, the numerous signs and symptoms associated with this disorder are collectively attributed to heart failure, rather than due to dysfunction of a specific ventricle.

CLINICAL PRESENTATION OF HEART FAILURE

General

- Patient presentation may range from asymptomatic to cardiogenic shock

Symptoms

- Dyspnea, particularly on exertion
- Orthopnea
- Paroxysmal nocturnal dyspnea
- Exercise intolerance
- Tachypnea
- Cough
- Fatigue
- Nocturia
- Hemoptysis
- Abdominal pain
- Anorexia
- Nausea
- Bloating
- Poor appetite, early satiety
- Ascites
- Mental status changes

Signs

- Pulmonary rales
- Pulmonary edema
- S_3 gallop
- Cool extremities
- Pleural effusion
- Cheyne-Stokes respiration
- Tachycardia
- Narrow pulse pressure
- Cardiomegaly
- Peripheral edema
- Jugular venous distension
- Hepatojugular reflux
- Hepatomegaly

Laboratory Tests

- BNP >100 pg/mL
- Electrocardiogram may be normal or it could show numerous abnormalities including acute ST-T–wave changes from myocardial ischemia, atrial fibrillation, bradycardia, left ventricular hypertrophy
- Serum creatinine may be increased because of hypoperfusion. Preexisting renal dysfunction can contribute to volume overload.

- Complete blood count useful to determine if heart failure is a result of reduced oxygen-carrying capacity
- Chest radiography is useful for detection of cardiac enlargement, pulmonary edema, and pleural effusions
- Echocardiogram assesses left ventricle size, valve function, pericardial effusion, wall motion abnormalities, and ejection fraction
- Hyponatremia, serum sodium <130 mEq/L, is associated with reduced survival and may indicate worsening volume overload and/or disease progression

Pulmonary congestion arises as the left ventricle fails and is unable to accept and eject the increased blood volume that is delivered to it. Consequently, pulmonary venous and capillary pressures rise, leading to interstitial and bronchial edema, increased airway resistance, and dyspnea. The associated signs and symptoms may include (a) dyspnea (with or without exertion), (b) orthopnea, (c) paroxysmal nocturnal dyspnea, and (d) pulmonary edema. Exertional dyspnea occurs when there is a reduction in the level of exertion that causes breathlessness. This is typically described as more breathlessness than was associated previously with a specific activity (e.g., vacuuming, stair climbing). As heart failure progresses, many patients eventually have dyspnea at rest.

Orthopnea is dyspnea that occurs with assumption of the supine position. It occurs within minutes of recumbency and is a result of reduced pooling of blood in the lower extremities and abdomen. Orthopnea is relieved almost immediately by sitting upright and typically is prevented by elevating the head with pillows. An increase in the number of pillows required to prevent orthopnea (e.g., a change from "two-pillow" to "three-pillow" orthopnea) suggests worsening heart failure. Attacks of paroxysmal nocturnal dyspnea typically occur after 2 to 4 hours of sleep; the patient awakens from sleep with a sense of suffocation. The attacks are caused by severe pulmonary and bronchial congestion, leading to shortness of breath and wheezing. The reasons these attacks occur at night are unclear but may include (a) reduced pooling of blood in the lower extremities and abdomen (as with orthopnea), (b) slow resorption of interstitial fluid from sites of dependent edema, (c) normal reduction in sympathetic activity that occurs with sleep (e.g., less support for the failing ventricle), and (d) normal depression in respiratory drive that occurs with sleep.

Rales (crackling sounds heard on auscultation) are present in the lung bases as a result of transudation of fluid into alveoli. The rales typically are bibasilar, but if heard unilaterally, they are usually right-sided. Rales are not present in most patients with chronic heart failure even though there is volume overload. This is thought to be a consequence of a compensatory increase in lymphatic drainage. Detection of rales is usually indicative of a rapid onset of worsening heart failure rather than the amount of excess fluid volume. A third heart sound, or S_3 gallop, is heard frequently in patients with left ventricular failure and may be caused by elevated atrial pressure and altered distensibility of the ventricle.

Pulmonary edema is the most severe form of pulmonary congestion, and is caused by accumulation of fluid in the interstitial spaces and alveoli. In heart failure patients, it is the result of increased pulmonary venous pressure. The patient experiences extreme breathlessness and anxiety and may cough pink, frothy sputum. Pulmonary edema can be terrifying for the patient, causing a feeling of suffocation or drowning. Patients with pulmonary edema may also report any of the above mentioned signs or symptoms of pulmonary congestion.

Systemic congestion is associated with a number of signs and symptoms. Jugular venous distension (JVD) is the simplest and most reliable sign of fluid overload. Examination of the right internal jugular vein with the patient at a 45° angle is the preferred method for assessing JVD. The presence of JVD more than 4 cm above the sternal angle suggests systemic venous congestion. In patients with mild systemic congestion, JVD may be absent at rest, but application of pressure to the abdomen will cause an elevation of JVD (hepatojugular reflux).

Peripheral edema is a cardinal finding in heart failure. Edema usually occurs in dependent parts of the body, and thus is seen as ankle or pedal edema in ambulatory patients, although it may be manifested as sacral edema in bedridden patients. Adults typically have a 10-lb fluid weight gain before trace peripheral edema is evident; therefore, patients with acute decompensated heart failure may have no clinical evidence of systemic congestion except weight gain. Consequently, body weight is the best short-term end point for evaluating fluid status. Nonfluid weight gain or loss of muscle mass as a result of cardiac cachexia are potential confounders for long-term use of weight as a marker for fluid status. Ascites is another common sign of systemic congestion.

Heart failure patients may exhibit signs and symptoms of low cardiac output alone or in addition to volume overload. The primary complaint associated with such poor perfusion is fatigue. Patients may also complain of poor appetite or early satiety because of limited perfusion of the gastrointestinal tract. Conversely, patients with such gastrointestinal complaints may simply be experiencing gut edema. More subjective measures of low cardiac output include worsening renal function, cool extremities, and narrow pulse pressure.

DIAGNOSIS[1]

No single test is available to confirm the diagnosis of heart failure. Because the syndrome of heart failure can be caused or worsened by multiple cardiac and noncardiac disorders, accurate diagnosis is essential for development of therapeutic strategies. Heart failure is often initially suspected in a patient based on their symptoms. These will often include dyspnea, exercise intolerance, fatigue, and/or fluid retention. However, it must be emphasized that signs and symptoms lack sensitivity for diagnosing heart failure since these symptoms are frequently found with many other disorders. Even in patients with known heart failure, there is poor correlation between the presence or severity of symptoms and hemodynamic abnormality.

A complete history and physical examination targeted at identifying cardiac or noncardiac disorders or behaviors that may cause or hasten heart failure development or progression are essential in the initial evaluation of a symptomatic patient. A careful medication history should also be obtained with a focus on use of ethanol, tobacco, illicit drugs (e.g., cocaine or methamphetamine), vitamins and supplements (including herbal or "natural" supplements), NSAIDs, and antineoplastic agents (anthracyclines, cyclophosphamide, trastuzumab, imatinib). Particular attention should be paid to cardiovascular risk factors and to other disorders that can cause or exacerbate heart failure. Because coronary artery disease is the cause of heart failure in nearly 70% of patients, careful attention and evaluation of the possibility of coronary disease is essential, especially in men. If coronary artery disease is detected, appropriate revascularization procedures may then be considered. The patient's volume status should be documented by assessing the body weight, JVD, and presence or absence of pulmonary congestion and peripheral edema. Laboratory testing may assist in identification of disorders that cause or worsen heart failure. The initial evaluation should include a complete blood count, serum electrolytes (including calcium and magnesium), tests of renal and hepatic function, urinalysis, lipid profile, hemoglobin A_{1c}, thyroid function tests, chest radiography, and 12-lead electrocardiogram (ECG). There are no specific ECG findings associated with heart failure, but findings may help detect coronary artery disease or conduction abnormali-

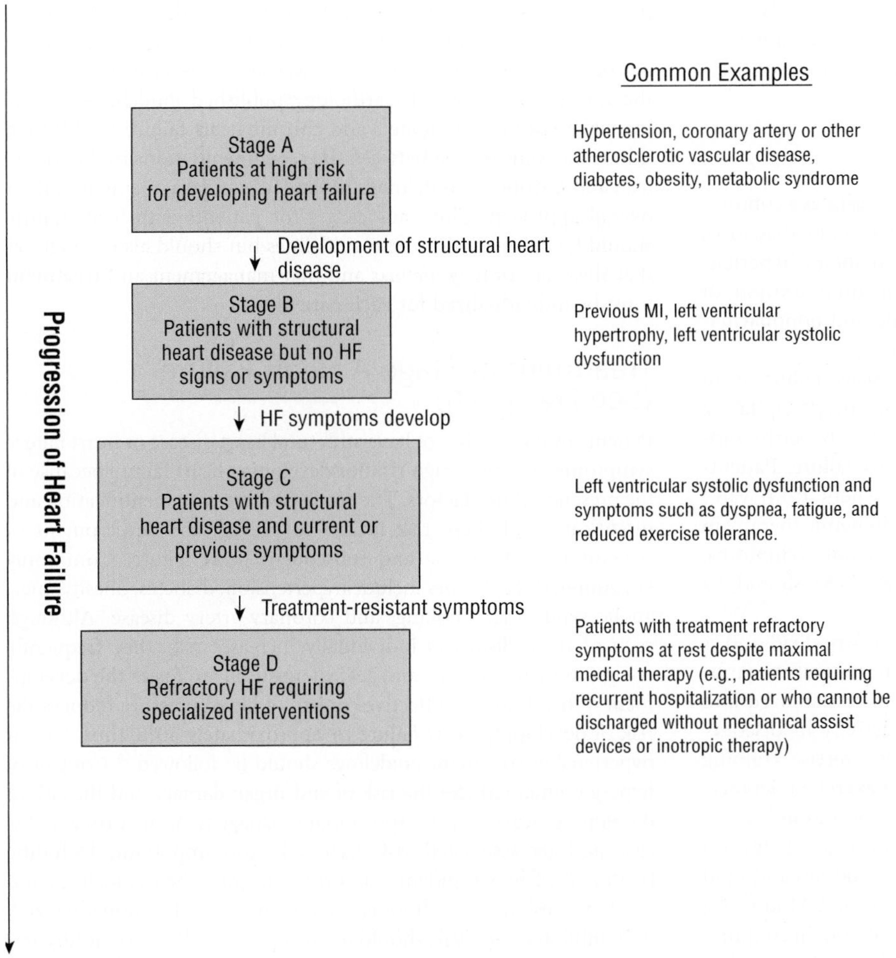

FIGURE 16-5. ACC/AHA heart failure staging system. (HF, heart failure; MI, myocardial infarction.) *(Adapted with permission from Circulation 2005;112:154–234.)*

ties that could affect prognosis and guide treatment decisions. Measurement of BNP may also assist in differentiating dyspnea caused by heart failure from other causes.[18]

Although the history, physical examination, and laboratory tests can provide important clues to the underlying cause of heart failure, the echocardiogram is the single most useful test in the evaluation of a patient with heart failure. The echocardiogram is used to evaluate abnormalities in the pericardium, myocardium, or heart valves and to quantify the LVEF to determine if systolic or diastolic dysfunction is present.

TREATMENT

Chronic Heart Failure

■ DESIRED OUTCOMES

The goals of therapy in management of chronic heart failure are to improve the patient's quality of life; relieve or reduce symptoms; prevent or minimize hospitalizations for exacerbations of heart failure; slow progression of the disease process; and prolong survival. Although these goals are still important, identification of risk factors for heart failure development and recognition of its progressive nature have led to increased emphasis on preventing the development of this disorder. With this in mind, the American College of Cardiology/American Heart Association (ACC/AHA) guidelines for the evaluation and management of chronic heart failure use a staging system that recognizes not only the evolution and progression of the disorder, but also emphasizes risk factor modification and preventive treatment strategies.[1] The system is comprised of four stages (Fig. 16–5). This staging system differs from the NYHA functional classification (Table 16–4) with which most clinicians are familiar. The NYHA system is primarily intended to classify *symptomatic* heart failure according to the clinician's subjective evaluation and does not recognize preventive measures or the progression of the disorder. A patient's symptoms can change frequently over a short period of time as a result of changes in, medications, diet, or intercurrent illnesses. For example, a patient with NYHA class IV symptoms with marked volume overload could rapidly improve to class II or III with aggressive diuretic therapy. In spite of these limitations, this system can be useful for monitoring patients and is widely used in heart failure studies. In contrast, and consistent with the progressive nature of heart failure, a patient's ACC/AHA heart failure stage could not improve (e.g., go from stage C to stage B) even though the

TABLE 16-4 New York Heart Association Functional Classification

Functional class	
I	Patients with cardiac disease but without limitations of physical activity. Ordinary physical activity does not cause undue fatigue, dyspnea, or palpitation.
II	Patients with cardiac disease that results in slight limitations of physical activity. Ordinary physical activity results in fatigue, palpitation, dyspnea, or angina.
III	Patients with cardiac disease that results in marked limitation of physical activity. Although patients are comfortable at rest, less-than-ordinary activity will lead to symptoms.
IV	Patients with cardiac disease that results in an inability to carry on physical activity without discomfort. Symptoms of congestive heart failure are present even at rest. With any physical activity, increased discomfort is experienced.

patient's symptoms could fluctuate from NYHA class IV to class I. In addition, the ACC/AHA staging system provides a more comprehensive framework for evaluation, prevention, and treatment of heart failure.

■ GENERAL MEASURES

The complexity of the heart failure syndrome necessitates a comprehensive approach to management that includes accurate diagnosis, identification and treatment of risk factors (e.g., diabetes, hypertension, coronary artery disease), elimination or minimization of precipitating factors, appropriate pharmacologic and nonpharmacologic therapy, and close monitoring and followup.

The first step in management of chronic heart failure is to determine the etiology (see Table 16–1) and/or any precipitating factors. Treatment of underlying disorders, such as hyperthyroidism, may obviate the need for treatment of heart failure. Patients with valvular diseases may derive significant benefit from valve replacement or repair. Revascularization or antiischemic therapy in patients with coronary disease may reduce heart failure symptoms. Drugs that aggravate heart failure (see Table 16–3) should be discontinued if possible.

Restriction of physical activity reduces cardiac workload and is recommended for virtually all patients with acute congestive symptoms. However, once the patient's symptoms have stabilized and excess fluid is removed, restrictions on physical activity are discouraged. In fact, current guidelines indicate that exercise training programs in stable heart failure patients improve exercise tolerance, functional capacity, and may slow heart failure progression.[1]

Because a major compensatory response in heart failure is sodium and water retention, restriction of dietary sodium and fluid intake are important nonpharmacologic interventions. Mild (<3 g per day) to moderate (<2 g per day) sodium restriction, in conjunction with daily measurement of weight, should be implemented to minimize volume retention and allow use of lower and safer diuretic doses. The typical American diet contains 3 to 6 g of sodium per day so most patients would need to reduce their intake by approximately 50%. This can often be accomplished by not adding salt to prepared foods and eliminating foods high in sodium (e.g., salt-cured meats, salted snack foods, pickles, soups, delicatessen meats, and processed foods). In patients with hyponatremia (serum Na <130 mEq/L) or those with persistent volume retention despite high diuretic doses and sodium restriction, daily fluid intake should be limited to 2 L per day from all sources.

Other important general measures include patient and family counseling on the signs and symptoms of heart failure, detailed instructions on the importance of appropriate medication use and compliance, and the need for close monitoring and followup to reinforce compliance and minimize the risk of heart failure exacerbations and subsequent hospitalization.

■ GENERAL APPROACH TO TREATMENT

❹ Current ACC/AHA treatment guidelines are organized around the four identified stages of heart failure and the treatment recommendations are summarized below (Figs. 16–6 and 16–7).[1] This staging system emphasizes the progressive nature of the disorder and targets treatment to prevent and/or slow the progression of heart failure. Clinicians are reminded that, in addition to the ACC/AHA, other cardiology professional societies have developed guidelines for evaluation and treatment of heart failure. The Heart Failure Society of America (HFSA) issued practice guidelines in 2006.[33] The HFSA and ACC/AHA guidelines are very similar with regard to care and treatment of patients with chronic heart failure. In addition, the HFSA guidelines provide a thorough discussion of other areas including acute decompensated heart failure, heart failure with preserved LVEF, and management of patients with heart failure and a number of comorbid diseases. The HFSA guidelines will be periodically updated on the HFSA website (*www.hfsa.org*). Finally, the European Society of Cardiology published guidelines for the management of both acute[34] and chronic heart failure.[35] Although minor differences exist between the recommendations in the American and European guidelines, they are in general agreement in their overall approach. Clinicians caring for patients with heart failure should be familiar with these guidelines but should also remember that these are only *guidelines* and that management and treatment must be individualized for each patient.

Treatment of Stage A Heart Failure (See Fig. 16–6)

Patients in stage A do not have structural heart disease or heart failure symptoms but are at high risk for developing heart failure because of the presence of risk factors. The emphasis here is on identification and modification of these risk factors to prevent the development of structural heart disease and subsequent heart failure. Commonly encountered risk factors include hypertension, diabetes, obesity, metabolic syndrome, smoking, and coronary artery disease. Although each of these disorders individually increases risk, they frequently coexist in many patients and act synergistically to foster the development of heart failure. Effective control of blood pressure reduces the risk of developing heart failure by approximately 50%, thus current hypertension treatment guidelines should be followed.[36] Control of hyperglycemia reduces the risk of end-organ damage and the risk of developing heart failure. Appropriate management of coronary disease and its associated risk factors is also important, including treatment of hyperlipidemia according to published guidelines and smoking cessation.[37] Although treatment must be individualized, ACE inhibitors or ARBs should be strongly considered for antihypertensive therapy in patients with multiple vascular risk factors.[1] Diuretics and β-blockers may also useful in this setting.

Treatment of Stage B Heart Failure (See Fig. 16–6)

Patients in stage B have structural heart disease, but do not have heart failure symptoms. This group includes patients with left ventricular hypertrophy, recent or remote MI, valvular disease, or reduced LVEF (less than 40%). These individuals are at risk for developing heart failure and treatment is targeted at minimizing additional injury and preventing or slowing the remodeling process. In addition to the treatment measures outlined in stage A, ACE inhibitors and β-blockers are important components of therapy. Patients with a previous MI should receive both ACE inhibitors and β-blockers, regardless of the LVEF.[1] Similarly, patients with a reduced LVEF should also receive both these agents, whether or not they have had a MI.[1] ARBs are an effective alternative in patients intolerant to ACE inhibitors.[1]

Treatment of Stage C Heart Failure (See Fig. 16–7)

❹ ❺ ❻ ❼ Patients with structural heart disease and previous or current heart failure symptoms are classified in stage C. In addition to treatments in stages A and B, most patients in stage C should be routinely treated with three medications: a diuretic, an ACE inhibitor, and a β-blocker (see Drug Therapies for Routine Use below). The benefits of these medications on slowing heart failure progression, reducing morbidity and mortality, and improving symptoms are clearly established. Aldosterone receptor antagonists, ARBs, digoxin, and hydralazine-isosorbide dinitrate are also useful in selected patients. Nonpharmacologic therapy with devices such as an implantable cardiac-defibrillator (ICD) or cardiac resynchroni-

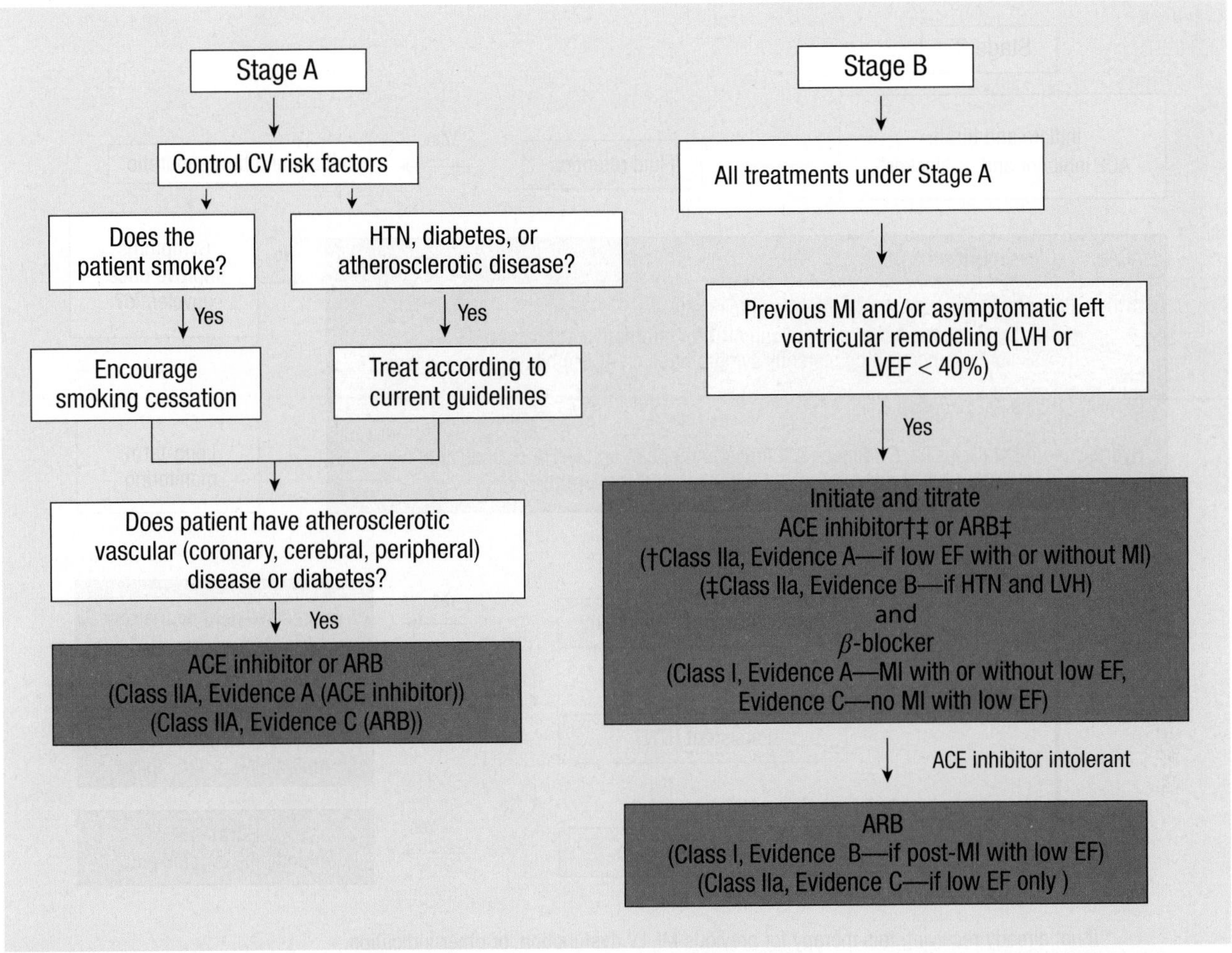

FIGURE 16-6. Treatment algorithm for patients with ACC/AHA stages A and B heart failure. (ACE, angiotensin-converting enzyme; ARB, angiotensin receptor blocker; CV, cardiovascular; EF, ejection fraction; HTN, hypertension; LVEF, left ventricular ejection fraction; LVH, left ventricular hypertrophy; MI, myocardial infarction.) *(Adapted with permission from Circulation 2005;112:154–234.)*

zation therapy (CRT) with a biventricular pacemaker is also indicated in certain patients in stage C (see Nonpharmacologic Therapy below). Other general measures are also important, including moderate sodium restriction, daily weight measurement, immunization against influenza and pneumococcus, modest physical activity, and avoidance of medications that can exacerbate heart failure. Recent evidence suggests that careful followup and patient education that reinforces dietary and medication compliance can prevent clinical deterioration and reduce hospitalization.[1]

Treatment of Stage D Heart Failure

Stage D heart failure includes patients with symptoms at rest that are refractory despite maximal medical therapy. This includes patients who undergo recurrent hospitalizations or who cannot be discharged from the hospital without special interventions. These individuals have the most advanced form of heart failure and should be considered for specialized therapies including mechanical circulatory support, continuous intravenous positive inotropic therapy, cardiac transplantation, or hospice care. The approach to treatment of patients with stage D heart failure is discussed in more detail in Acute Decompensated Heart Failure below.

■ NONPHARMACOLOGIC THERAPY

Sudden cardiac death, primarily as a consequence of ventricular tachycardia and fibrillation, is responsible for 40% to 50% of the mortality in heart failure patients. In general, patients in the earlier stages of heart failure with milder symptoms are more likely to die from sudden death, whereas death from pump failure is more frequent in those with advanced heart failure. Many of these patients have complex and frequent ventricular ectopic beats, although it remains unknown whether these ectopic beats contribute to the risk of malignant arrhythmias or merely serve as markers for individuals at higher risk for sudden death. Drugs that attenuate disease progression such as β-blockers and aldosterone antagonists reduce the risk of sudden death. However, empiric treatment with class I antiarrhythmic agents, although they can suppress ventricular ectopic beats, adversely affect survival.[38] The role of the ICD compared to amiodarone for primary prevention of sudden death was evaluated in Sudden Cardiac Death in Heart Failure Trial (SCD-HeFT). Placement of an ICD was superior to amiodarone or placebo for reducing mortality in patients with NYHA class II or III heart failure and LVEF ≤35%, regardless of the etiology of heart failure.[39] Importantly, this study also found that amiodarone had no benefit compared to placebo and thus this drug, because of its multiple adverse effects, drug interactions, and lack of effect on mortality, should not be used for primary prevention of sudden death. However, because of the neutral effects of amiodarone on survival, it is often used in heart failure patients with atrial fibrillation to maintain sinus rhythm and/or to prevent ICD discharges. In cardiac arrest survivors with a reduced LVEF, the ICD is superior to antiarrhythmic drug therapy for improving survival.[40] Thus, the ACC/AHA guidelines recommend the ICD for both primary and secondary prevention to improve survival in patients with current or previous heart failure symptoms and reduced LVEF. Chapter 19 thoroughly reviews ICD therapy.

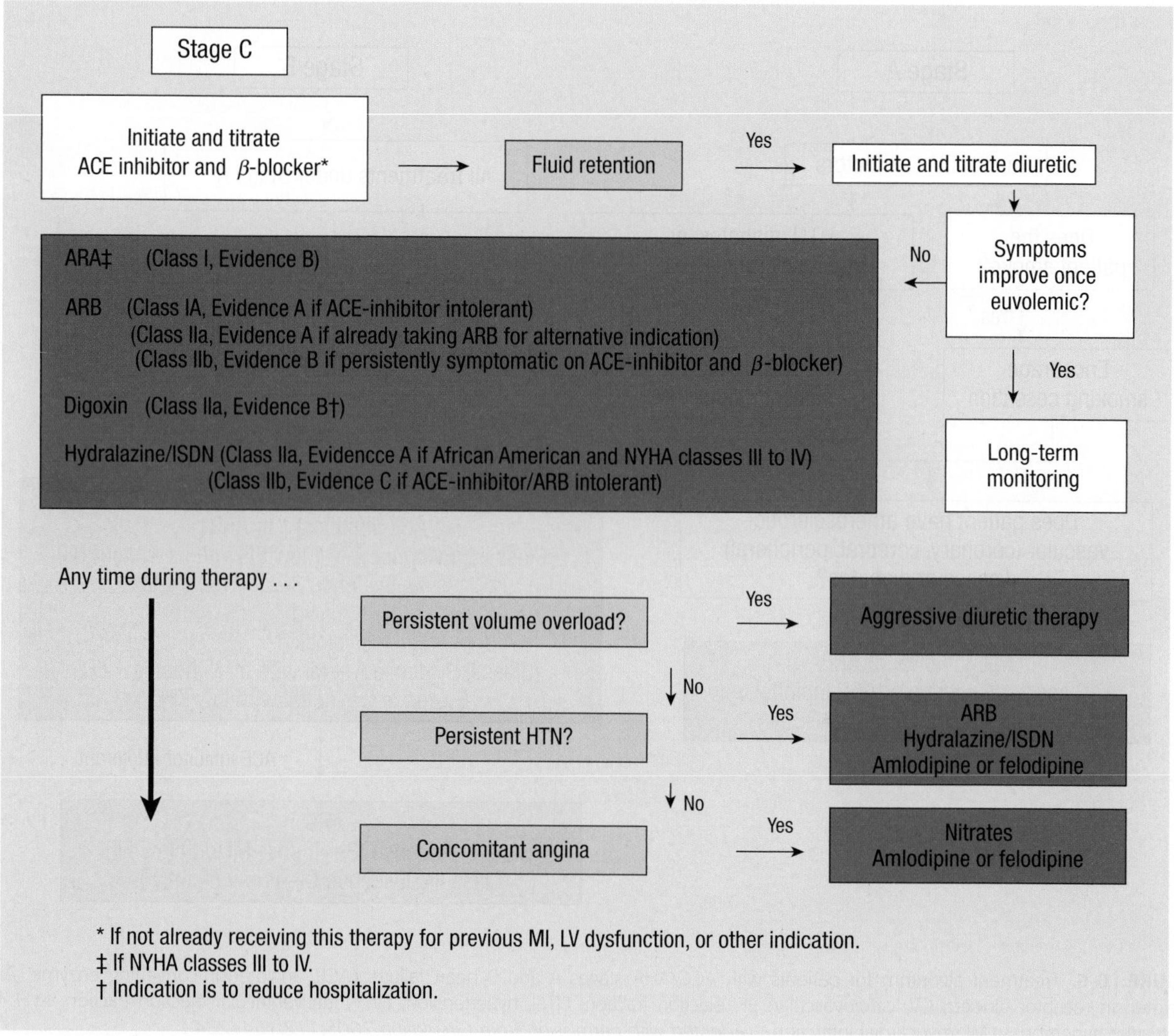

FIGURE 16-7. Treatment algorithm for patients with ACC/AHA stage C heart failure. (ACE, angiotensin-converting enzyme; ARA, aldosterone receptor antagonist; ARB, angiotensin receptor blocker; HTN, hypertension; ISDN, isosorbide dinitrate; LV, left ventricle; MI, myocardial infarction.) *(Adapted with permission from Circulation 2005;112:154–234.)*

Recent studies demonstrate that CRT offers a promising approach to selected patients with chronic heart failure.[41,42] Delayed electrical activation of the left ventricle, characterized on the ECG by a QRS duration that exceeds 120 msec, occurs in approximately one-third of patients with moderate to severe systolic heart failure. Because the left and right ventricles normally activate simultaneously, this delay results in asynchronous contraction of the ventricles, which contributes to the hemodynamic abnormalities of heart failure. Implantation of a specialized biventricular pacemaker to restore synchronous activation of the ventricles can improve ventricular contraction and hemodynamics. Recent trials show improvements in exercise capacity, NYHA classification, quality of life, hemodynamic function, hospitalizations, and mortality with CRT.[41,42] A CRT is currently indicated only in NYHA classes III to IV patients receiving optimal medical therapy and with a QRS duration ≥120 msec and LVEF ≤35%. Combined CRT and ICD devices are available and can be used if the patient meets the indications for both devices.

■ PHARMACOLOGIC THERAPY

Drug Therapies for Routine Use

❹ ❺ ❻ ❼ ❽ ❾ Figure 16–7 is a treatment algorithm for management of patients with reduced LVEF and current or prior heart failure symptoms (i.e., stage C). In general, these patients should receive combined therapy with an ACE inhibitor or ARB and a β-blocker, plus a diuretic if there is evidence of fluid retention. Initiation of digoxin therapy can be considered at any time for symptom reduction, to decrease hospitalizations, or slow ventricular response in patients with concomitant atrial fibrillation. An aldosterone receptor antagonist should also be considered in selected patients.[1]

❼ **Diuretics**[43,44] The compensatory mechanisms in heart failure stimulate excessive sodium and water retention, often leading to pulmonary and systemic congestion. Diuretic therapy, in addition to sodium restriction, is recommended in all patients with clinical evidence of fluid retention. Once fluid overload has been resolved, many patients require chronic diuretic therapy to maintain euvolemia. Among the drugs used to manage heart failure, diuretics are the most rapid in producing symptomatic benefits. Because diuretics do not alter disease progression or prolong survival, they are not considered mandatory therapy. Thus patients who do not have fluid retention would not require diuretic therapy.

The primary goal of diuretic therapy is to reduce symptoms associated with fluid retention, improve exercise tolerance and quality of life, and reduce hospitalizations from heart failure. They accomplish this by decreasing pulmonary and peripheral edema through reduction of preload. Although preload is a determinant of cardiac output, the Frank-Starling curve (see Fig. 16–3) shows that patients with congestive symptoms have reached the flat portion of the curve. A reduction in preload improves symptoms but has little effect on the patient's stroke volume or cardiac output until the steep portion of the curve is reached. However, diuretic therapy must be used judiciously because overdiuresis can lead to a reduction in cardiac output and symptoms of dehydration.

Diuretic therapy is usually initiated in low doses in the outpatient setting, with dosage adjustments based on symptom assessment and daily body weight. Change in body weight is a sensitive marker of fluid retention or loss, and it is recommended that patients monitor their status by taking daily morning body weights. Patients who gain a pound per day for several consecutive days, or 3 to 5 lb in a week, should contact their healthcare provider for instructions (which often will be to increase the diuretic dose temporarily). Such action often will allow patients to prevent a decompensation that requires hospitalization. One study demonstrated a significant reduction in emergency department visits with a protocol that directed patients to self-adjust their diuretic dose based on changes in heart failure symptoms and daily body weight.[45] Hypotension or worsening renal function (e.g., increases in serum creatinine) may be indicative of volume depletion and necessitate a reduction in the diuretic dose. Assessing for volume depletion is particularly important before ACE inhibitor or β-blocker initiation or dose up-titration as overdiuresis may predispose patients to hypotension and other adverse effects with increases in ACE inhibitor or β-blocker doses.

Thiazide Diuretics. Thiazide diuretics such as hydrochlorothiazide block sodium and chloride reabsorption in the distal convoluted tubule (approximately 5% to 8% of filtered sodium). Consequently, the thiazides are relatively weak diuretics and infrequently are used alone in heart failure. However, as reviewed in Treatment: Acute Decompensated Heart Failure below, under Diuretic Resistance, thiazides or the thiazide-like diuretic metolazone can be used in combination with loop diuretics to promote a very effective diuresis. In addition, thiazide diuretics may be preferred in patients with only mild fluid retention and elevated blood pressure because of their more persistent antihypertensive effects compared to loop diuretics.

Loop Diuretics. Loop diuretics are usually necessary to restore and maintain euvolemia in heart failure. They act by inhibiting a Na-K-^{2}Cl transporter in the thick ascending limb of the loop of Henle, where 20% to 25% of filtered sodium normally is reabsorbed. Because loop diuretics are highly bound to plasma proteins, they are not highly filtered at the glomerulus. They reach the tubular lumen by active transport via the organic acid transport pathway. Competitors for this pathway (probenecid or organic by-products of uremia) can inhibit delivery of loop diuretics to their site of action and decrease effectiveness. Loop diuretics also induce a prostaglandin-mediated increase in renal blood flow, which contributes to their natriuretic effect. Coadministration of NSAIDs blocks this prostaglandin-mediated effect and can diminish diuretic efficacy. Excessive dietary sodium intake may also reduce the efficacy of loop diuretics. Unlike thiazides, loop diuretics maintain their effectiveness in the presence of impaired renal function, although higher doses may be necessary to obtain adequate delivery of the drug to the site of action.

Heart failure is one of the disease states in which the maximal response to loop diuretics is reduced. This is believed to result from a decrease in the rate of diuretic absorption and/or increased proximal or distal tubule reabsorption of sodium, possibly due to increased activity of the Na-K-^{2}Cl transporter.[43] As a consequence, doses above the recommended ceiling doses produce no additional diuresis. Thus, once the ceiling dose is reached, it is recommended to give the diuretic more frequently for additional effect rather than

TABLE 16-5 Loop Diuretics—Use in Heart Failure

	Furosemide	Bumetanide	Torsemide
Usual daily dose (oral)	20–160 mg/day	0.5–4 mg/day	10–80 mg/day
Ceiling dose[a]			
Normal renal function	80–160 mg	1–2 mg	20–40 mg
CL_{cr} - 20–50 mL/min	160 mg	2 mg	40 mg
CL_{cr} <20 mL/min	400 mg	8–10 mg	100 mg
Bioavailability	10%–100% average: 50%	80%–90%	80%–100%
Affected by food	Yes	Yes	No
Half-life	0.3–3.4 h	0.3–1.5 h	3–4 h

CL_{cr}, creatine clearance.
[a]Ceiling dose: single dose above which additional response is unlikely to be observed.
Adapted from Am J Med Sci 2000;319:38–50.

to give progressively higher doses. The appropriate chronic dose is that which maintains the patient at a stable dry weight without symptoms of dyspnea. Table 16–5 lists ranges of doses of loop diuretics and recommended ceiling doses.

❺ ACE Inhibitors ACE inhibitors are the cornerstone of pharmacotherapy for patients with heart failure. By blocking the conversion of angiotensin I to angiotensin II by ACE, the production of angiotensin II and, in turn, aldosterone is decreased, but not completely eliminated.[13] This decrease in angiotensin II and aldosterone attenuates many of the deleterious effects of these neurohormones, including ventricular remodeling, myocardial fibrosis, myocyte apoptosis, cardiac hypertrophy, norepinephrine release, vasoconstriction, and sodium and water retention.[13] Thus, ACE inhibitor therapy plays an important role in preventing RAAS-mediated progressive worsening of myocardial function. The endogenous vasodilator bradykinin, which is inactivated by ACE, is also increased by ACE inhibitors, along with the release of vasodilatory prostaglandins and histamine.[13] The precise contribution of the effects of ACE inhibitors on bradykinin and vasodilatory prostaglandins is unclear. However, the persistence of clinical benefits with ACE inhibitors despite angiotensin II and aldosterone levels returning to pretreatment levels suggests this is a potentially important effect.[13]

Numerous placebo-controlled clinical trials involving more than 7,000 patients with reduced LVEF have documented the favorable effects of ACE inhibitor therapy on symptoms, NYHA functional classification, clinical status, exercise tolerance, and quality of life.[13] When compared with placebo, patients treated with ACE inhibitors have fewer treatment failures, hospitalizations, and increases in diuretic dosages.[13]

More importantly, these trials show that ACE inhibitors improve survival by 20% to 30% compared to placebo.[13] In addition, the Studies of Left Ventricular Dysfunction (SOLVD) Prevention and Treatment trials indicate the survival benefit is maintained long-term (12 years) in patients who were treated with enalapril.[46] In addition to improving survival, ACE inhibitors also reduce the combined risk of death or hospitalization, slow the progression of heart failure, and reduce the rates of reinfarction.[13] The benefits of ACE inhibitor therapy are independent of the etiology of heart failure (ischemic versus nonischemic) and are observed in patients with mild, moderate, or severe symptoms.

The most common cause of heart failure is ischemic heart disease, where MI results in loss of myocytes, followed by ventricular dilation and remodeling. Captopril, ramipril, and trandolapril all benefit post-MI patients, whether they are initiated early (within 36 hours) and continued for 4 to 6 weeks or started later and administered for several years.[13] Collectively, these studies indicate that ACE inhibitors after MI improve overall survival, decrease development of severe heart failure, and reduce reinfarction and heart failure hospitalization rates.[13] The benefit occurs within the first few days of therapy and persists during long-term treatment. The effects are most pronounced in higher-risk patients, such as those with symptomatic heart failure or reduced LVEF, with 20% to 30% reductions in mortality reported in these patients.[13] Post-MI patients without heart failure symptoms or decreases in LVEF (stage B) should also receive ACE inhibitors to prevent the development of heart failure and to reduce mortality.[1,13,47]

In addition to their benefits in patients with established heart failure, ACE inhibitors also are effective for preventing the development of heart failure and reducing cardiovascular risk. Enalapril decreases the risk of hospitalization for worsening heart failure and reduces the composite end point of death and heart failure hospitalization in patients with asymptomatic left ventricular dysfunction.[48] The development of diabetes mellitus, an important risk factor for cardiovascular disease that also increases morbidity and mortality in heart failure patients, is reduced by enalapril in patients with chronic heart failure.[49] In patients with established atherosclerotic vascular disease (e.g., coronary, cerebral, or peripheral circulations) and normal LVEF, ACE inhibitors reduce the development of new-onset heart failure and diabetes, cardiovascular death, overall mortality, MI, and stroke.[50]

The clear benefit of ACE inhibitors is evident in the Joint Commission for Accreditation of Healthcare Organizations (JCAHO) and Centers for Medicare and Medicaid Services (CMS) selection of ACE inhibitor use in patients with heart failure and decreased LVEF as a key quality measure. Despite the overwhelming benefit demonstrated with these agents, there is substantial evidence that they are underused and underdosed.[51,52] These data indicate that significant numbers of heart failure patients do not receive ACE inhibitors, and of those who are receiving these agents, many are taking lower-than-recommended doses.[52] Also, for patients receiving an ACE inhibitor at hospital discharge, use significantly decreases over time and patients who were not prescribed ACE inhibitors at discharge were unlikely to have therapy initiated in the outpatient setting.[51] The most common reasons cited for underuse or underdosing are concerns about safety and adverse reactions to ACE inhibitors, especially in patients with underlying renal dysfunction or hypotension. The use of ACE inhibitors in patients with renal insufficiency is particularly relevant because it is present in 25% to 50% of heart failure patients and is associated with an increased risk of mortality.[53] Several recent studies in different patient populations, including post-MI patients with decreased left ventricular function and patients with stable coronary artery disease and preserved left ventricular function, indicate that ACE inhibitors may be more effective in those patients with renal insufficiency.[54–56] Because many heart failure patients have concomitant disorders (e.g., diabetes, hypertension, previous MI) that also may be favorably affected by ACE inhibitors, renal dysfunction should not be an absolute contraindication to ACE inhibitor use in patients with left ventricular dysfunction. However, these patients should be monitored carefully for the development of worsening renal function and/or hyperkalemia with special attention to risk factors associated with this complication of ACE inhibitor therapy.[1]

An important practical consideration is determining the proper dose of an ACE inhibitor. The ability to achieve target doses shown to be effective in clinical trials is often limited by hypotension and/or a decline in renal function. Clinical trials establishing the efficacy of these agents titrated drug doses to a predetermined target rather than according to therapeutic response. Although data on the dose-dependent effects of ACE inhibitors in patients with heart failure are limited, higher doses may reduce the risk of hospitalization compared to lower doses, but there do not appear to be significant differences in mortality.[57] In many positive trials of other heart failure therapies (e.g., β-blockers, aldosterone antagonists), intermediate ACE inhibitor doses were generally used as background therapy. These results emphasize that clinicians should attempt to use ACE inhibitor doses proven beneficial in clinical trials, but if these doses are not tolerated, lower doses can be used with the knowledge that there are likely only small differences in mortality outcomes between the high and low doses. Also, initiation of β-blocker therapy should not be delayed until target ACE inhibitor doses are achieved as the addition of a β-blocker is proven to reduce mortality, whereas that is not the case with increasing ACE inhibitor doses.

In summary, the evidence that ACE inhibitors improve symptoms, slow disease progression, and decrease mortality in patients with heart failure and reduced LVEF (stage C) is unequivocal. Current guidelines indicate these patients should receive ACE inhibitors, unless contraindications are present.[1] Moreover, ACE inhibitors should also be used to prevent the development of heart failure in at-risk patients (i.e., stages A and B).[1]

❻ β-Blockers There is overwhelming evidence from multiple randomized, placebo-controlled clinical trials that β-blockers reduce morbidity and mortality in patients with heart failure. As such, the ACC/AHA guidelines on the management of heart failure recommend that β-blockers should be used in all stable patients with heart failure and a reduced left ventricular ejection fraction in the absence of contraindications or a clear history of β-blocker intolerance.[1] Patients should receive a β-blocker even if their symptoms are mild or well controlled with diuretic and ACE inhibitor therapy. Importantly, it is not essential that ACE inhibitor doses be optimized before a β-blocker is started because the addition of a β-blocker is likely to be of greater benefit than an increase in ACE inhibitor dose.[1] β-Blockers are also recommended for asymptomatic patients with a reduced left ventricular ejection fraction (stage B) to decrease the risk of progression to heart failure.

β-Blockers have been studied in more than 20,000 patients with heart failure in placebo-controlled trials. Three β-blockers have been shown to significantly reduce mortality compared to placebo: carvedilol, metoprolol controlled-release/extended-release (CR/XL), and bisoprolol. Each was studied in a large population with the primary end point of mortality. Carvedilol was the first β-blocker shown to improve survival in heart failure. In the U.S. Carvedilol Heart Failure Study, 1,094 patients were randomized to carvedilol or placebo in addition to standard therapy, including an ACE inhibitor, digoxin, and diuretic. The study was stopped early because of a 65% reduction in the risk of death with carvedilol.[58] Nearly 4,000 patients were randomized to metoprolol CR/XL (Toprol-XL) or placebo in the Metoprolol CR/XL Randomized Intervention Trial in Congestive Heart Failure (MERIT-HF), the largest β-blocker mortality trial to date.[59] This trial was also stopped early because of a significant survival benefit with β-blockade. Specifically, metoprolol was associated with a 34% reduction in total mortality, a 41% reduction in sudden death, and a 49% reduction in death from worsening heart failure. Bisoprolol was studied in more than 2,600 patients enrolled in the Cardiac Insufficiency Bisoprolol Study (CIBIS) II.[60] The study was also stopped prematurely because of a 34% reduction in total mortality with bisoprolol compared to placebo. Bisoprolol was also associated with a 44% reduction in sudden death and a 26% reduction in death because of worsening heart failure. Multiple post-hoc subgroup analyses of data from the MERIT-HF and CIBIS II trials suggest that the benefits of β-blockade occur regardless of heart failure etiology or disease severity.

The majority of participants in MERIT-HF and CIBIS II had either class II or class III heart failure, and β-blockers became standard therapy in patients with class II or III disease after these trials were published. However, the efficacy and safety of β-blockers in patients with class IV heart failure were unclear until publication of the Carvedilol, Prospective, Randomized, Cumulative Survival (COPERNICUS) trial.[61] This trial randomized nearly 2,300 clinically stable patients who had symptoms at rest or with minimal exertion to carvedilol or placebo. Like the other studies, COPERNICUS was stopped prematurely after carvedilol produced a 35% relative reduction in mortality. Carvedilol was well tolerated in this population, with fewer participants receiving carvedilol compared to placebo requiring permanent discontinuation of study medication.

Data supporting the use of β-blockers in asymptomatic patients with left ventricular systolic dysfunction (stage B) come from a study of carvedilol in post-MI patients with a decreased LVEF.[62] While the primary end point of all-cause mortality or hospital admission for cardiovascular problems was similar in the carvedilol and placebo groups, carvedilol significantly reduced all-cause mortality alone compared to placebo. Cardiovascular mortality and nonfatal MI were also lower among carvedilol-treated patients.

In addition to improving survival, β-blockers improve multiple other end points. All the large clinical trials demonstrated 15% to 20% reductions in all-cause hospitalization and 25% to 35% reductions in hospitalizations for worsening heart failure with β-blocker therapy.[60,63,64] Studies also show consistent improvements in left ventricular systolic function with β-blockers, with increases in LVEF of 5 to 10 units (e.g., from an ejection fraction of 20% to 25% or 30%) after several weeks to months of therapy. β-Blockers have also been shown to decrease ventricular mass, improve the sphericity of the ventricle, and reduce systolic and diastolic volumes (left ventricular end-systolic volume and left ventricular end-diastolic volume).[65,66] These effects are often collectively called *reverse remodeling,* referring to the fact that they return the heart toward more normal size, shape, and function.

The effects of β-blockers on symptoms and exercise tolerance varies among studies. Many studies show improvements in NYHA functional class, patient symptom scores, or quality-of-life assessments (such as the Minnesota Living with Heart Failure Questionnaire), and exercise performance, as assessed by the 6-minute walk test.[63–65] Other investigators find significant reductions in mortality with β-blockers but no significant improvement in symptoms.[67] As such, it is important to educate patients that β-blocker therapy is expected to positively influence disease progression and survival even if there is little to no symptomatic improvement.

The majority of participants in β-blocker trials were on ACE inhibitors at baseline as the benefits of ACE inhibitors were proven prior to β-blocker trials. Whether the strategy of starting a β-blocker prior to an ACE inhibitor is safe and effective has been debated. This issue was addressed in CIBIS III, in which patients with mild to moderate symptoms were randomized to initial therapy with either bisoprolol or enalapril.[68] The two strategies produced similar rates of death or hospitalization. However, the trial failed to satisfy the prespecified statistical criterion for noninferiority of initial therapy with a β-blocker compared to an ACE inhibitor. In the absence of more compelling evidence, ACE inhibitors should be started first in most patients. Initiating a β-blocker first may be advantageous for patients with evidence of excessive SNS activity (e.g., tachycardia) and may also be appropriate for patients whose renal function or potassium concentrations preclude starting an ACE inhibitor at that time. However, the risk for decompensation during β-blocker initiation may be greater in the absence of preexisting ACE inhibitor therapy, and careful monitoring is essential.

The mechanism by which β-blockers exert their therapeutic benefit is unclear. β-Blockers antagonize the detrimental effects of the SNS described earlier in the chapter. To this end, potential mechanisms to explain the favorable effects of β-blockers in heart failure include antiarrhythmic effects, attenuating or reversing ventricular remodeling, decreasing myocyte death from catecholamine-induced necrosis or apoptosis, preventing fetal gene expression, improving left ventricular systolic function, decreasing heart rate and ventricular wall stress thereby reducing myocardial oxygen demand, and inhibiting plasma renin release.[1]

Components that are critical for successful β-blocker therapy include appropriate patient selection, drug initiation and titration, and patient education. β-Blockers should be initiated in stable patients who have no or minimal evidence of fluid overload.[1] Although β-blockers are typically started in the outpatient setting, there are data indicating that initiation of a β-blocker prior to discharge in patients who are hospitalized for decompensated heart failure increases β-blocker usage compared with outpatient initiation without increasing the risk of serious adverse effects.[69] However, β-blockers should not be started in patients who are hospitalized in the intensive care unit or recently required intravenous inotropic support. In unstable patients, other heart failure therapy should be optimized and then β-blocker therapy reevaluated once stability is achieved.

Initiation of a β-blocker at normal doses in patients with heart failure may to lead to symptomatic worsening or acute decompensation owing to the drug's negative inotropic effect. For this reason, β-blockers are listed as drugs that may exacerbate or worsen heart failure (see Table 16–3). To minimize the likelihood for acute decompensation, β-blockers should be started in very low doses with slow upward dose titration. Table 16–6 describes the starting and target doses. Of note, the smallest commercially available tablet of bisoprolol is a scored 5-mg tablet. Because the recommended starting dose of 1.25 mg/day is not readily available, bisoprolol is the least commonly used of the three agents and, in fact, is not approved by the Food and Drug Administration (FDA) for use in heart failure. Thus, therapy is generally limited to either carvedilol or metoprolol CR/XL, and there is no compelling evidence that one drug is superior to the other. A controlled-release formulation of carvedilol (carvedilol CR) that allows once-daily dosing was recently FDA-approved, and pharmacokinetic studies demonstrate similar degrees of drug exposure with the controlled- and immediate-release formations of the drug.[70] Carvedilol CR should be considered in patients with difficulty maintaining adherence to the immediate-release formulation.

β-Blocker doses should be doubled no more often than every 2 weeks, as tolerated, until the target or maximally tolerated dose is reached. Target doses are those associated with reductions in mortality in placebo-controlled clinical trials. It is important to make every effort to titrate doses up to target whenever possible in order to provide maximal survival benefits. In addition, there is evidence that response to β-blockers is dose dependent, with greater reductions in hospitalization rates and improvements in LVEF at higher doses. However, even low doses appear to prolong survival compared to placebo, and thus, any dose of β-blocker is likely to provide some benefit.[71] Data with metoprolol suggest that heart rate may serve as a guide to the degree of β-blockade and that lower β-blocker doses might be considered reasonable if the reduction in heart rate indicates a good response to β-blocker therapy.[71]

Good communication between the patient and healthcare provider(s) is particularly important for successful therapy. Patients

TABLE 16-6 Initial and Target Doses for β-Blockers Used in Treatment of Heart Failure

Drug	Initial Dose[a]	Target Dose
Bisoprolol[b]	1.25 mg daily	10 mg daily
Carvedilol[b]	3.125 mg bid	25 mg bid[c]
Metoprolol succinate CR/XL[b]	12.5-25 mg daily[d]	200 mg daily

[a]Doses should be doubled approximately every 2 weeks, or as tolerated by the patient, until the highest tolerated or target dose is reached.
[b]Regimens proven in large trials to reduce mortality.
[c]Target dose for patients who weigh >85 kg is 50 mg bid.
[d]In Metroprolol CR/XL Randomized Intervention Trial in Congestive Heart Failure (MERIT-HF), the majority of class II patients were given 25 mg daily, whereas the majority of class III patients were given 12.5 mg daily as their starting dose.

should understand that dose up-titration is a long, gradual process and that achieving the target dose is important to maximize the benefits of therapy. Patients should also be aware that response to therapy may be delayed and that heart failure symptoms may actually worsen during the initiation period. In the event of worsening symptoms, patients who understand the potential benefits of long-term β-blocker therapy may be more likely to continue treatment.

In summary, the data provide clear evidence that β-blockers slow disease progression, decrease hospitalizations, and improve survival in heart failure. β-Blockers have also been shown to improve quality of life in many patients with heart failure, although this is not a universal finding. Based on these data, β-blockers are recommended as standard therapy for all patients with systolic dysfunction, regardless of the severity of their symptoms. Clinical trial experience shows that target β-blocker doses can be achieved in the majority of patients provided that appropriate initiation, titration, and education are implemented.

Drug Therapies to Consider for Selected Patients

5 Angiotensin II Receptor Blockers The use of ARBs in heart failure has generated great interest and controversy.[72] The crucial role of the RAAS in heart failure development and progression is well established, as are the benefits of inhibiting this system with ACE inhibitors. Although ACE inhibitors decrease angiotensin II production in the short-term, these agents do not completely suppress generation of this hormone. With chronic administration of ACE inhibitors, *ACE escape*, characterized by increases in circulating angiotensin II and aldosterone, often occurs.[12,73] In addition, angiotensin II can be formed in a number of tissues, including the heart, through non–ACE-dependent pathways (e.g., chymase, cathepsin, and kallikrein).[12] Therefore, blockade of the detrimental effects of angiotensin II by ACE inhibition is incomplete. In addition, troublesome adverse effects of ACE inhibitors such as cough are linked to accumulation of bradykinin.[13] The ARBs block the angiotensin II receptor subtype 1 (AT_1), preventing the deleterious effects of angiotensin II, regardless of its origin. Because ARBs do not inhibit the ACE enzyme, these agents do not appear to affect bradykinin.[12,73] By inhibiting both the formation of angiotensin II and its effects on the AT_1 receptor, combination therapy with an ACE inhibitor plus an ARB offers a theoretical advantage over either agent used alone through more complete blockade of the deleterious effects of angiotensin II. Also, by directly blocking AT_1 receptors, ARBs would allow unopposed stimulation of AT_2 receptors, causing vasodilation and inhibition of ventricular remodeling.[12] Because bradykinin-related adverse effects of ACE inhibitors such as angioedema and cough lead to drug discontinuation in some patients, the potential for an ARB to produce similar clinical benefits with fewer side effects is of great interest. Whether ARBs add incremental benefit to current established therapies or are superior (or equivalent) to ACE inhibitors is the focus of several clinical trials.[72]

Although a number of ARBs are currently available, the primary clinical trials supporting the use of these agents in heart failure used either valsartan or candesartan.[72] The Valsartan Heart Failure Trial (Val-HeFT) evaluated whether the addition of valsartan to standard background heart failure therapy (which included an ACE inhibitor in 93% and a β-blocker in 35% of patients) improved survival.[74] The addition of valsartan had no effect on all-cause mortality but produced a 13% reduction in morbidity and mortality (principally as a result of reductions in heart failure hospitalizations). Subgroup analysis showed that the benefits were greatest in those patients not receiving background ACE inhibitor therapy. Based on these results, valsartan is now approved for use in patients with NYHA classes II to IV heart failure. The Valsartan in Acute Myocardial Infarction (VALIANT) trial compared the effect of valsartan, captopril, and the combination of the two agents in post-MI patients with symptomatic heart failure, reduced left ventricular systolic function, or both, in a noninferiority trial design.[47] The primary end point of total mortality occurred in 19.3% of patients receiving valsartan and captopril, 19.5% of captopril-treated patients, and 19.9% of the valsartan group. Thus, in this high-risk post-MI population, valsartan was as effective as captopril in reducing the risk of death, but combination therapy only increased the risk of adverse effects and did not improve survival compared to monotherapy with either agent. Based on these findings, valsartan is now approved for use in post-MI patients with left ventricular failure or left ventricular dysfunction.

The Candesartan in Heart Failure: Assessment of Reduction in Mortality and Morbidity (CHARM) trials were designed as three studies to compare candesartan with placebo in patients with symptomatic heart failure (Table 16–7).[75] Both the CHARM-Added (patients receiving background ACE-inhibitor therapy)[76] and CHARM-Alternative (patients intolerant of ACE-inhibitor therapy)[77] trials found significant reductions in the primary end point of cardiovascular death or hospitalization for heart failure in patients receiving candesartan, although the benefit was modest in CHARM-Added. No significant benefit of candesartan was observed in CHARM-Preserved (patients with LVEF >40%).[78] Overall, candesartan was well tolerated but its use was associated with an increased risk of hypotension, hyperkalemia, and renal dysfunction. On the basis of these results, candesartan is now approved for use in heart failure.

Although ACE inhibitors remain first-line therapy in patients with stage C heart failure and reduced LVEF, the current ACC/AHA guidelines recommend the use of ARBs in patients who are unable to tolerate ACE inhibitors.[1] Similarly, ARBs are alternatives to ACE inhibitors in patients with stages A and B heart failure.[1] Cough and angioedema are the most common causes of ACE inhibitor intolerance. Caution should be exercised when ARBs are used in patients with angioedema from ACE inhibitors as some cross-reactivity has been reported.[77,79] ARBs are not an alternative in patients with hypotension, hyperkalemia, or renal insufficiency secondary to ACE inhibitors because they are as likely to cause these adverse effects. Also, the combined use of ACE inhibitors, ARBs, and aldosterone

TABLE 16-7 Clinical Trials of Candesartan in Heart Failure

Trial	Drug	Patient Population	Primary End Point	Results (%) Drug	Results (%) Placebo	Adjusted Hazard Ratio	*P* Value
CHARM-Added	Candesartan vs. placebo	Symptomatic HF and EF ≤40% on ACE inhibitors	CV death or hospital admission for HF	37.9	42.3	0.85	0.01
CHARM-Alternative	Candesartan vs. placebo	Symptomatic HF and EF ≤40%, ACE-inhibitor intolerant	CV death or hospital admission for HF	33.0	40.0	0.70	<0.0001
CHARM-Preserved	Candesartan vs. placebo	Symptomatic HF and EF ≤40%	CV death or hospital admission for HF	22.0	24.3	0.86	0.051
CHARM-Overall	Candesartan vs. placebo	Combined from above 3 trials	All-cause mortality	23.0	25	0.90	0.032

ACE, angiotensin-converting enzyme; CHARM, Candesartan in Heart Failure: Assessment of Reduction in Mortality and Morbidity trial; CV, cardiovascular; EF, ejection fraction; HF, heart failure.

antagonists is not recommended because of the increased risk of renal dysfunction and hyperkalemia.[1] The specific drugs and doses proven to be effective in clinical trials should be used.

The role of ARBs as an adjunct to ACE inhibitors remains controversial. The CHARM-Added trial found the addition of candesartan to ACE inhibitor and β-blocker therapy produced incremental reductions in cardiovascular death and hospitalizations for heart failure, but did not improve overall survival.[76] In contrast, neither the VALIANT nor the Val-HeFT trials found additional benefit from the addition of valsartan to ACE-inhibitor treatment.[47,74] These results suggest the addition of an ARB to optimal heart failure therapy (ACE inhibitors, β-blockers, diuretics, etc.) offers, at best, marginal benefits with increased risk of adverse effects. The current guidelines indicate that the addition of an ARB can be considered in patients who remain symptomatic despite receiving conventional heart failure pharmacotherapy. Some clinicians suggest that the addition of an aldosterone antagonist to ACE inhibitor and β-blocker therapy is preferred over that of an ARB. The proven survival benefit of aldosterone antagonists in patients with NYHA classes III to IV heart failure (Randomized Aldactone Evaluation Study [RALES] trial) and in post-MI patients with left ventricular systolic dysfunction (Eplerenone Post-Acute Myocardial Infarction Heart Failure Efficacy and Survival Study [EPHESUS] trial), as discussed in the following section, supports this approach.[16,17]

⑨ Aldosterone Antagonists Spironolactone and eplerenone are aldosterone antagonists that work by blocking the mineralocorticoid receptor, the target site for aldosterone. In the kidney, aldosterone antagonists inhibit sodium reabsorption and potassium excretion. Although the diuretic effects with low doses of aldosterone antagonists are minimal, the potassium-sparing effects can have significant consequences as discussed below. In the heart, aldosterone antagonists inhibit cardiac extracellular matrix and collagen deposition, thereby attenuating cardiac fibrosis and ventricular remodeling.[80] Spironolactone also interacts with androgen and progesterone receptors, which may lead to gynecomastia and other sexual side effects in some patients. Such adverse effects are less frequent with eplerenone owing to its low affinity for the progesterone and androgen receptors.

Evidence that ACE inhibitors incompletely suppress aldosterone provided the impetus for examining the benefits of adding an aldosterone antagonist to ACE inhibitor therapy.[81] RALES randomized more than 1,600 patients with current or recent class IV heart failure to aldosterone blockade with spironolactone 25 mg/day or placebo.[16] Patients were also treated with standard therapy, usually including an ACE inhibitor, loop diuretic, and digoxin. Those with a serum creatinine concentration above 2.5 mg/dL or a serum potassium concentration above 5 mEq/L were excluded. The study was stopped prematurely after an average followup of 24 months because of a significant 30% reduction in the primary end point of total mortality with spironolactone. Spironolactone reduced mortality as a consequence of both progressive heart failure and sudden cardiac death. Spironolactone also produced a 35% reduction in hospitalizations for worsening heart failure and significant symptomatic improvement, as assessed by changes in NYHA functional class. The low dose of spironolactone was well tolerated in RALES. The most common adverse effect was gynecomastia, which occurred in 10% of men on spironolactone, compared to 1% of men on placebo, and led to treatment discontinuation in 2% of patients. There were statistically (but not clinically) significant increases in serum creatinine (by 0.05 to 0.10 mg/dL) and potassium concentrations (by 0.30 mEq/L) with spironolactone. The incidence of serious hyperkalemia (>6 mEq/L) was minimal and did not differ between spironolactone- and placebo-treated groups.

More recently, the EPHESUS trial evaluated the effect of selective antagonism of the mineralocorticoid receptor with eplerenone in patients with left ventricular dysfunction after MI.[17] To be eligible for study participation, patients had to have either evidence of heart failure or diabetes. More than 6,600 patients were randomized within 3 to 14 days of MI to eplerenone, titrated to 50 mg/day, or placebo in addition to standard therapy, which usually included an ACE inhibitor, β-blocker, aspirin, and diuretics. As occurred in RALES, patients with serum creatinine concentrations greater than 2.5 mg/dL or serum potassium concentrations greater than 5 mEq/L were excluded. Treatment with eplerenone was associated with a significant 15% relative reduction in the risk for death from any cause and a 15% reduction in the risk of hospitalization from heart failure. Serious hyperkalemia occurred in 5.5% of eplerenone-treated patients and 3.9% of placebo-treated patients. Eplerenone was not associated with gynecomastia.

The benefits of aldosterone antagonists in heart failure are not just a result of the inhibition of aldosterone's actions in the heart resulting in inhibition of aldosterone-mediated cardiac fibrosis and ventricular remodeling. Recent evidence points to an important role of aldosterone antagonists in attenuating the systemic proinflammatory state and oxidative stress caused by aldosterone.[14,80] And while spironolactone historically has been viewed as a diuretic, this is believed to contribute little to its benefits in heart failure, in part, because the doses used have minimal diuretic effect.[16] Thus, as with ACE inhibitors and β-blockers, the data on aldosterone antagonists also support the neurohormonal model of heart failure.

The clinical trial data suggest that the use of aldosterone antagonists in heart failure is associated with minimal risk. However, data from clinical practice suggest otherwise. In particular, an observational study of approximately 1.3 million elderly patients in the Ontario Drug Benefit Program found that the spironolactone prescription rate increased approximately fourfold immediately after the publication of RALES.[82] The increase in the prescription rate was accompanied by nearly threefold increases in the rate of hospital admissions and the rate of death related to hyperkalemia. Further evidence of spironolactone-induced hyperkalemia comes from small case series showing that 25% to 35% of patients treated outside the controlled clinical trial setting develop hyperkalemia (>5 mEq/L) and that 10% to 12% develop serious hyperkalemia.[83,84]

Potential factors contributing to the high incidence of hyperkalemia in clinical practice include the initiation of aldosterone antagonists in patients with impaired renal function or high potassium concentrations and the failure to decrease or stop potassium supplements when starting aldosterone antagonists. Other risk factors for hyperkalemia include diabetes, older age, inadequate laboratory monitoring, and concomitant use of high-dose ACE inhibitors, β-blockers, NSAIDs, or cyclooxygenase-2 inhibitors. The ACC/AHA recently recommended strategies to minimize the risk for hyperkalemia with aldosterone antagonists in heart failure.[1] Table 16–8 summarizes these strategies. Chief among these recommendations is to avoid aldosterone antagonists in patients with renal dysfunction. It is important to emphasize here that serum creatinine may overestimate renal function in the elderly and in patients with decreased muscle mass, in whom creatinine clearance should serve as a guide for the appropriateness of aldosterone antagonist therapy. The risk for hyperkalemia is dose dependent, and the morbidity and mortality reductions with aldosterone antagonists in clinical trials occurred at low doses (i.e., spironolactone 25 mg/day and eplerenone 50 mg/day). Therefore, the doses of aldosterone antagonists should be limited to those associated with beneficial effects so as to decrease the risk for hyperkalemia.

Only 10% of RALES participants were taking β-blockers at baseline because the benefits of β-blockers in heart failure were not appreciated fully at the time the trial began.[16] β-Blockers inhibit plasma renin release and may provide additional suppression of the renin–angiotensin–aldosterone system when used with ACE inhib-

TABLE 16-8 Recommended Strategies for Reducing the Risk for Hyperkalemia with Aldosterone Antagonists

- Avoid starting aldosterone antagonists in patients with any of the following:
  - Serum creatinine concentration >2.0 in women or >2.5 mg/dL in men or a creatinine clearance <30 mL/min
  - Recent worsening of renal function
  - Serum potassium concentration ≥5.0 mEq/L
  - History of severe hyperkalemia
- Start with low doses (12.5 mg/day for spironolactone and 25 mg/day for eplerenone), especially in the elderly and in those with diabetes or a creatinine clearance <50 mL/min
- Decrease or discontinue potassium supplements when starting an aldosterone antagonist
- Avoid concomitant use of NSAIDs or COX-2 inhibitors
- Avoid concomitant use of high-dose ACE inhibitors or ARBs
- Avoid triple therapy with an ACE inhibitor, ARB, and aldosterone antagonist
- Monitor serum potassium concentrations and renal function within 3 days and 1 week after the initiation or dose titration of an aldosterone antagonist or any other medication that could affect potassium homeostasis; thereafter, potassium concentrations and renal function should be monitored monthly for the first 3 months, and then every 3 months
- If potassium exceeds 5.5 mg/dL at any point during therapy, discontinue any potassium supplementation or, in the absence of potassium supplements, reduce or stop aldosterone antagonist therapy
- Counsel patients to
  - Limit intake of high-potassium-containing foods and salt substitutes
  - Avoid the use of over-the-counter nonsteroidal antiinflammatory drugs
  - Temporarily discontinue aldosterone antagonist therapy if diarrhea develops or diuretic therapy is interrupted

ACE, angiotensin-converting enzyme; ARB, angiotensin receptor blocker; COX, cyclooxygenase; NSAIDs, nonsteroidal antiinflammatory drugs.
Adapted from Hunt SA, Abraham WT, Chin MH et al. Circulation 2005;112:e154–235.

itors. Thus, there has been some speculation about whether spironolactone will provide further benefit in patients receiving both ACE inhibitors and β-blockers. However, data from EPHESUS provide some clarity to this issue, as the majority of EPHESUS participants were on β-blockers at baseline and the trial still demonstrated significant reductions in mortality with the addition of eplerenone.[17]

Current guidelines state that it is reasonable to add an aldosterone antagonist to standard therapy in select patients provided that potassium and renal function can be carefully monitored.[1] Based on data from RALES and EPHESUS, low-dose aldosterone antagonists may be appropriate for two groups of patients: those with moderately severe to severe heart failure who are receiving standard therapy and those with left ventricular dysfunction early after MI.[1] For patients who fall outside the populations studied in these clinical trials, there are no clear guidelines on aldosterone antagonist use. Trials to address the efficacy of aldosterone antagonism in patients with mild to moderate heart failure symptoms or in patients with preserved left ventricular systolic function are ongoing. Although there are currently no data on the use of aldosterone antagonists in patients with class I, class II, or stable class III heart failure, it might be reasonable to consider their use in these patients who require potassium supplementation. The premise for use in this setting would be that it might be possible to reduce or eliminate potassium supplementation while potentially providing additional benefit with respect to altering the disease course.

9 Digoxin In 1785, William Withering was the first to report extensively on the use of foxglove (*Digitalis purpurea*) for the treatment of dropsy (i.e., edema). Although digitalis glycosides have been in clinical use for more than 200 years, not until the 1920s were they clearly demonstrated to have a positive inotropic effect on the heart. Furthermore, it was not until the late 1980s that clinical trials were conducted to critically evaluate the role of digoxin in the therapy of chronic heart failure. The results of the Digitalis Investigational Group (DIG) trial helped clarify the role of digoxin in this setting.[85] The view of digoxin has also shifted over the past decade. Although it was historically considered useful in heart failure because of its positive inotropic effects, it now seems clear that its real benefits in heart failure are related to its neurohormonal modulating effects.

The efficacy of digoxin in patients with heart failure and supraventricular tachyarrhythmias such as atrial fibrillation is well established and widely accepted. Its role in heart failure patients with normal sinus rhythm has been considerably more controversial. Until the 1980s, most data supporting efficacy of digoxin in these patients came from anecdotal evidence and seriously flawed or uncontrolled studies. Since then, a number of clinical trials have shown that digoxin improves LVEF, quality of life, exercise tolerance, and heart failure symptoms.[86,87] However, these studies involved small numbers of patients followed for short time periods with many of the patients being withdrawn from preexisting digoxin treatment upon entering the trial. Although these trials demonstrated hemodynamic and symptomatic improvement in heart failure patients receiving digoxin, an unresolved issue was the unknown effect of digoxin on mortality. This was of particular concern given the increased mortality seen with other positive inotropic drugs, and finally led to organization and performance of the DIG trial to determine the effects of digoxin on survival in patients with heart failure in sinus rhythm.[85]

The DIG trial was a double-blind, randomized, placebo-controlled trial with the primary end point of all-cause mortality.[85] Patients (n = 6,800) with heart failure symptoms and an ejection fraction of 45% or less were eligible and were followed for a mean of 37 months. Most patients received background therapy with diuretics and ACE inhibitors. The mean serum digoxin concentration achieved was 0.8 ng/mL after 12 months of therapy. No significant difference in all-cause mortality was found between patients receiving digoxin and placebo (34.8% and 35.1%, respectively). A trend toward lower mortality as a consequence of worsening heart failure was observed in the digoxin group, although this was offset by a trend toward an increased mortality from other cardiovascular causes (presumably arrhythmias) in patients receiving digoxin. Hospitalizations for worsening heart failure were reduced 28% by digoxin compared to placebo ($P <$ 0.001), whereas hospitalizations for other cardiovascular causes were increased in the digoxin group. In all, 64.3% of digoxin-treated patients were hospitalized compared to 67.1% of patients receiving placebo ($P = 0.006$). Therefore, DIG is the first trial to show that a positive inotropic agent does not increase mortality and actually decreases morbidity in patients with heart failure.

Although digoxin does not improve survival in heart failure patients, multiple post-hoc analyses of data from studies evaluating the effect of digoxin withdrawal have helped clarify the role of digoxin use for patients in sinus rhythm.[86] Collectively, these studies suggested the drug produces important symptomatic benefits and that digoxin withdrawal increased the risk of treatment failure and deterioration of exercise capacity and ejection fraction. Furthermore, the risk of symptomatic exacerbation of heart failure after digoxin discontinuation was highest in patients with the most severe symptoms.[86] Based on this evidence, digoxin can be beneficial in patients with symptomatic or stage C heart failure and reduced LVEF in addition to standard therapy to reduce heart failure hospitalizations. Furthermore, digoxin should not be used in patients with a normal LVEF, sinus rhythm, and no history of heart failure symptoms, because the risk is not balanced by any known benefit.[1]

Two retrospective analyses of the combined PROVED/RADIANCE database[88] and the DIG Trial database[89] offer additional insights into the clinical benefit of low serum digoxin concentrations. While all patients in the Prospective Randomized Study of Ventricular Failure and Efficacy of Digoxin (PROVED) and Randomized Assessment of Digoxin on Inhibitors of the Angiotensin

Converting Enzyme (RADIANCE) trials who continued to take digoxin did significantly better than those who were withdrawn, those who had plasma digoxin concentrations between 0.5 and 0.9 ng/mL were just as likely to be free of worsening heart failure as those with higher plasma concentrations. Retrospective analysis of the DIG trial database suggests that a serum digoxin concentration of 0.5 to 0.8 ng/mL may be associated with a reduction in mortality, whereas higher concentrations may increase mortality.[89] In another post-hoc analysis of the DIG trial, digoxin therapy was associated with an increased risk of death in women, but not in men.[90] This finding was refuted in another analysis of the same data which demonstrated that a beneficial effect of digoxin was evident at serum concentrations from 0.5 to 0.9 ng/mL, whereas serum concentrations greater than or equal to 1.2 ng/mL were harmful.[91] More recently, the most comprehensive reanalysis of the DIG trial database found that serum concentrations of 0.5 to 0.9 ng/mL were associated with lower mortality, all-cause hospitalizations, and heart failure hospitalizations, whereas serum concentrations greater than or equal to 1 ng/mL were associated with lower heart failure hospitalizations with no effect on mortality. Serum concentrations of 0.5 to 0.9 ng/mL had no interaction with LVEF greater than 45% or gender.[92] Of the 7,788 patients randomized in the DIG trial, 988 patients had a LVEF greater than 45%; digoxin had no effect on mortality or hospitalization in these patients.[93]

These results suggest that most of the benefit from digoxin is achieved at low plasma concentrations and little additional effect is achieved with higher doses. Thus, for most patients, the target digoxin plasma concentration should be 0.5 to 1.0 ng/mL. This more conservative target would also be expected to decrease the risk of adverse effects from digoxin toxicity; in fact, more recent assessment of the rate of digoxin toxicity suggests a significant decline in the overall incidence.[94] In most patients with normal renal function, this plasma concentration range can be achieved with a daily dose of 0.125 mg. Patients with decreased renal function, the elderly, and those who are receiving interacting drugs (e.g., amiodarone) should receive 0.125 mg every other day. In patients with atrial fibrillation and a rapid ventricular response, the historic practice of increasing digoxin doses (and concentrations) until rate control is achieved is no longer recommended. Digoxin alone is often ineffective to control ventricular response in patients with atrial fibrillation and increasing the dose only increases the risk of toxicity. Digoxin combined with a β-blocker or amiodarone is superior to either agent alone for controlling ventricular response in patients with atrial fibrillation and heart failure.[95] Consequently, target digoxin plasma concentrations are the same regardless of whether the patient is in sinus rhythm or atrial fibrillation. Several equations and nomograms have been proposed to estimate digoxin maintenance doses based on estimated renal function for a particular patient and population pharmacokinetic parameters. These methods are extensively reviewed elsewhere.[96] Recently, investigators developed a digoxin dosing nomogram that targets a lower digoxin plasma concentration.[97] In the absence of supraventricular tachyarrhythmias, a loading dose is not indicated because digoxin is a mild inotropic agent that will produce gradual effects over several hours, even after loading.

Digoxin's place in the pharmacotherapy of chronic heart failure can be summarized for two patient groups. In patients with heart failure and supraventricular tachyarrhythmias such as atrial fibrillation, it should be considered early in therapy to help control ventricular response rate. For patients in normal sinus rhythm, although digoxin does not improve survival, its effects on symptom reduction and clinical outcomes are evident in patients with mild to severe heart failure. Consequently, it should be used in conjunction with other standard heart failure therapies, including diuretics, ACE inhibitors, and β-blockers, in patients with symptomatic heart failure to reduce hospitalizations.

⑩ Nitrates and Hydralazine Nitrates and hydralazine were combined originally in the treatment of heart failure because of their complementary hemodynamic actions. Nitrates, by serving as nitric oxide donors, activate guanylate cyclase to increase cyclic guanosine monophosphate in vascular smooth muscle. This results in venodilation and reductions in preload. Hydralazine is a direct-acting vasodilator that acts predominantly on arterial smooth muscle to reduce SVR and increase stroke volume and cardiac output (see Fig. 16–1). Hydralazine also has antioxidant properties and appears to prevent nitrate tolerance.[98] Evidence also suggests that the combination of hydralazine and nitrates may exert beneficial effects beyond their hemodynamic actions by interfering with the biochemical processes associated with heart failure progression.[1,99]

The efficacy of the combination of hydralazine and isosorbide dinitrate (ISDN) was evaluated in three large, randomized heart failure trials. The first trial predated the use of ACE inhibitors and β-blockers in heart failure and found that the combination of hydralazine 75 mg and ISDN 40 mg, each given four times daily, reduced mortality in patients receiving diuretics and digoxin compared to placebo.[100] However, a subsequent trial comparing the combination with an ACE inhibitor demonstrated greater mortality reduction with the ACE inhibitor.[101] Post-hoc analysis of these trials suggested that the combination of hydralazine and ISDN was particularly effective in African Americans, and led to examining the efficacy of adding the combination to standard therapy in this racial group.

The African American Heart Failure Trial (A-HeFT) randomized 1,050 self-identified African Americans with class III or IV heart failure to hydralazine plus ISDN or placebo, each in addition to standard therapy, usually including an ACE inhibitor (or ARB), β-blocker, and diuretic, with or without digoxin and spironolactone.[99] The trial used a fixed dose combination product, BiDil®, that contains hydralazine 37.5 mg and ISDN 20 mg. Therapy was initiated as a single tablet given three times daily, then titrated to two tablets (hydralazine 75 mg/ISDN 40 mg) three times daily if tolerated. The trial was terminated early after a mean followup of 10 months because of a significant (43%) reduction in all-cause mortality in patients receiving hydralazine/ISDN compared to placebo. The primary composite end point of mortality, hospitalizations for heart failure, and quality of life was also significantly improved with the combination product. Based on these results, BiDil® was approved by the FDA to treat heart failure exclusively in African Americans.

The mechanism for the beneficial effects of hydralazine/ISDN is believed to relate to an increase in nitric oxide bioavailability secondary to nitric oxide donation from ISDN and a hydralazine-mediated reduction in oxidative stress.[98] Nitric oxide attenuates myocardial remodeling and may play a protective role in heart failure.[102] It is suggested that African Americans have less nitric oxide than do non-African Americans, and thus, may derive particular benefit from therapy that enhances nitric oxide bioavailability. Whether the benefits of adding hydralazine/ISDN to standard therapy extend to non-African Americans remains to be determined.

Guidelines from the Heart Failure Society of America recommend the addition of hydralazine and ISDN as part of standard therapy, including ACE inhibitors, in African Americans with moderately severe to severe heart failure.[33] The addition of hydralazine and ISDN is also reasonable in patients of other ethnicities who continue to have symptoms despite optimized therapy with an ACE inhibitor (or ARB) and β-blocker.[1] For patients who are unable to tolerate an ACE inhibitor because of cough or angioedema, an ARB is recommended as the first-line alternative.[1] Hydralazine and ISDN is appropriate as first-line therapy in patients unable to tolerate either an ACE inhibitor or ARB because of renal insufficiency, hyperkalemia, or possibly hypotension.

There are several potential obstacles to successful therapy with hydralazine and ISDN in heart failure. First is the need for frequent dosing, with the fixed-dose combination dosed three times daily and the individual drugs dosed four times daily in clinical trials. Second, adverse effects are common with hydralazine/ISDN, with headache, dizziness, and gastrointestinal distress occurring more frequently with hydralazine/ISDN than with placebo in clinical trials.[99,100] A third potential obstacle is the increased cost of the fixed-dose combination product compared to the individual drugs purchased separately, which may preclude the use of the combination product in some patients. Treatment with the two separate drugs rather than the combination product may compromise adherence to therapy. Thus, if therapy with hydralazine and ISDN is deemed appropriate, patients may need continual reinforcement to maintain good medication adherence, especially if the individual drugs are used. It is important to recognize that none of the above trials incorporated a nitrate-free interval in the dosing regimen.

Treatment of Concomitant Disorders

Heart failure is often accompanied by other disorders whose natural history or therapy may affect morbidity and mortality. In selected patients, optimal management of these concomitant disorders may have a profound impact on heart failure symptoms and outcomes.

Hypertension Although ischemic heart disease has replaced hypertension as the most common cause of heart failure, still nearly two-thirds of heart failure patients have current hypertension or a previous history of hypertension.[1] Hypertension can contribute directly to the development of heart failure and also contributes indirectly by increasing the risk of coronary artery disease. Pharmacotherapy of hypertension in patients with heart failure should initially involve agents that can treat both disorders such as ACE inhibitors, β-blockers, and diuretics. If control of hypertension is not achieved after optimizing treatment with these agents, the addition of an ARB, aldosterone antagonist, isosorbide dinitrate/hydralazine, or a second-generation calcium channel blocker such as amlodipine (or possibly felodipine) should be considered. Medications that should be avoided include the calcium channel blockers with negative inotropic effects (e.g., verapamil, diltiazem, and most dihydropyridines) and direct-acting vasodilators (e.g., minoxidil) that cause sodium retention.

Angina Coronary artery disease is the most common heart failure etiology. Consequently, appropriate management of coronary disease and its risk factors is an important strategy for the prevention and treatment of heart failure. Coronary revascularization should be strongly considered in patients with both heart failure and angina.[1] Pharmacotherapy of angina in patients with heart failure should use drugs that can successfully treat both disorders. Nitrates and β-blockers are effective antianginal agents and are the preferred agents for patients with both disorders as they may improve hemodynamics and clinical outcomes.[1] It should be noted that the antianginal effectiveness of these agents may be significantly limited if fluid retention is not controlled with diuretics. Similar to their use in hypertension, both amlodipine and felodipine appear to be safe to use in this setting. Optimization of other treatments for secondary prevention of coronary and other atherosclerotic vascular disease should also be considered.[37] Although their precise role in the treatment of heart failure awaits the results of additional studies, initial evidence suggests statins might decrease the risk of heart failure hospitalizations and death, regardless of heart failure etiology.[24]

Atrial Fibrillation Atrial fibrillation is the most frequently encountered arrhythmia and it is commonly found in patients with heart failure, affecting 10% to 30% of patients.[1] The high incidence of atrial fibrillation in the heart failure population is not surprising as each of these two disorders predisposes to the other and they share many risk factors, including coronary artery disease and hypertension. The presence of atrial fibrillation in patients with heart failure is associated with a worse long-term prognosis.[1] The combination of atrial fibrillation and heart failure may exert a number of detrimental effects, including increased risk of thromboembolism secondary to stasis of blood in the atria, a reduction in cardiac output because of loss of the atrial contribution to ventricular filling, and hemodynamic compromise from the rapid ventricular response. Moreover, heart failure exacerbations and atrial fibrillation are closely linked and it is often difficult to determine which disorder caused the other. For example, worsening heart failure results in volume overload which, in turn, causes atrial distension and increases the risk of atrial fibrillation. Similarly, atrial fibrillation with a rapid ventricular response can reduce cardiac output and lead to heart failure exacerbation. Thus, optimal management of both conditions is required with careful attention paid to control of ventricular response and anticoagulation for stroke prevention (see Chap. 19).[95]

Recent studies suggest that ACE inhibitors, ARBs, and β-blockers decrease the incidence of atrial fibrillation in patients with heart failure, providing further support for their use in these patients.[103,104] Digoxin is frequently used to slow ventricular response in patients with heart failure and atrial fibrillation. However, it is more effective at rest than with exercise and it does not affect the progression of heart failure. β-Blockers are more effective than digoxin and have the added benefits of improving morbidity and mortality. Combination therapy with digoxin and a β-blocker may be more effective for rate control than either agent used alone. Calcium channel blockers with negative inotropic effects, such as verapamil or diltiazem, should be avoided. Amiodarone is a reasonable alternative for rate control in those patients who are not responding to digoxin and/or β-blockers or who have contraindications to these agents.[95] Appropriate selection of antithrombotic therapy that considers the presence of risk factors for thromboembolism in an individual patient is also required.[95]

Because of the close association between atrial fibrillation, heart failure exacerbations, and hospitalizations, many clinicians prefer maintenance of sinus rhythm with antiarrhythmic drugs to the rate-control approach in the treatment of patients with both disorders. However, it must be noted that the benefits of restoring and maintaining sinus rhythm remain unclear in this population and is not without risk. Although the Atrial Fibrillation Follow-up Investigation of Rhythm Management (AFFIRM) study showed no difference in outcomes between the rhythm control and rate control approaches, less than 10% of the patients in this study had significant left ventricular dysfunction.[105] Several ongoing clinical trials should help clarify the best approach to these difficult-to-manage patients. In general, amiodarone is the preferred agent if the rhythm control approach is taken. Although it has many noncardiac toxicities, amiodarone does not have cardiodepressant or significant proarrhythmic effects and appears to be safe in heart failure. Dofetilide also appears to be safe and effective in this population. Class I antiarrhythmics should be avoided.[95]

Diabetes Diabetes is highly prevalent in the heart failure population, with current estimates indicating it is present in approximately one-third of heart failure patients.[30,106] As an important risk factor for coronary artery disease, diabetes directly contributes to the development of heart failure. Importantly though, diabetes is a risk factor for heart failure independent of coronary artery disease or hypertension, is associated with hastened heart failure progression, and is a significant predictor of mortality in patients with heart failure.[106]

Pharmacotherapy of diabetes in heart failure patients is complicated by concerns about adverse effects associated with metformin and the thiazolidinedione (TZD) drugs (rosiglitazone and pioglitazone). The beneficial effects of these agents on glucose control and cardiovascular risk factors lead to their widespread use in patients with heart failure in spite of the warnings in the product labeling against their use.[106] The metformin product labeling states that it is contraindicated for use in patients with heart failure requiring pharmacologic treatment because of the purported risk of lactic acidosis. However, data from retrospective analyses involving more than 3,000 patients suggest that metformin is safe (no reports of lactic acidosis) in patients with heart failure.[107] In addition, these reports show that metformin treatment is associated with decreased mortality and hospitalizations compared to conventional antihyperglycemic therapy.[107] Consequently, some clinicians suggest that the contraindication to metformin use in heart failure should be reexamined. However, the lack of prospective data about the safety and efficacy of metformin in patients with heart failure indicates that if the drug is used, it should be used cautiously with careful monitoring of volume status and renal function. Although the mechanism(s) are presently unclear, the TZDs are associated with weight gain, peripheral edema, and heart failure. The TZD package insert indicates these agents should not be used in patients with class III or IV heart failure because they may cause intravascular volume expansion and heart failure exacerbation. Most clinical trials with these drugs excluded patients with moderate to severe heart failure, thus the evidence supporting this precaution comes mainly from retrospective analyses and case reports. Because of the potential risk, a recent consensus statement indicates TZDs should not be used in patients with NYHA class III or class IV heart failure.[30] TZDs should be used cautiously in patients with class I or II symptoms, with close observation needed to detect weight gain, edema formation, or heart failure exacerbation.[30]

Drug Class Information

7 Diuretics[44] Loop diuretics, as described earlier, represent the typical diuretic therapy for patients with heart failure because of their potency and, as such, are the only diuretics discussed here. There are currently three loop diuretics available that are used routinely: furosemide, bumetanide, and torsemide. They share many similarities in their pharmacodynamics, with their differences being largely pharmacokinetic in nature. Table 16–5 shows the relevant information on the loop diuretics. Following oral administration, the peak effect with all the agents occurs in 30 to 90 minutes, with duration of 2 to 3 hours (slightly longer for torsemide). Following intravenous administration, the diuretic effect begins within minutes. All three drugs are highly (>95%) bound to serum albumin and enter the nephron by active secretion in the proximal tubule. The magnitude of effect is determined by the peak concentration achieved in the nephron, and there is a threshold concentration that must be achieved before any diuresis is seen.

The biggest difference between the agents is bioavailability. Bioavailability of bumetanide and torsemide is essentially complete (80% to 100%), whereas furosemide bioavailability exhibits marked intra- and interpatient variability. Furosemide bioavailability ranges from 10% to 100%, with an average of 50%. Thus, if bioequivalent intravenous and oral doses are desired, oral furosemide doses should be approximately double that of the intravenous dose, whereas intravenous and oral doses are the same for torsemide and bumetanide. Coadministration of furosemide and bumetanide with food can decrease bioavailability significantly, whereas food has no effect on bioavailability of torsemide. The intraabdominal congestion that can occur in heart failure also may slow the rate (and thus decrease the peak concentration) of furosemide, which can reduce the diuretic's efficacy. Thus furosemide is most problematic with respect to rate and extent of absorption and the factors that influence it, whereas torsemide has the least-variable bioavailability.

Recent data suggest that these differences in bioavailability and variability may have clinical implications. For example, several studies suggest that torsemide is absorbed reliably and is associated with better outcomes than the more variably absorbed furosemide.[108,109] Torsemide is preferred in patients with persistent fluid retention despite high doses of other loop diuretics. And while the costs of torsemide exceed those of furosemide, pharmacoeconomic analyses suggest that the costs of care are similar or less with torsemide.[109] These data require confirmation in controlled, double-blinded clinical trials but provide preliminary evidence that the more reliably absorbed loop diuretics may be superior to furosemide.

The loop diuretics exhibit a ceiling effect in heart failure, meaning that once the ceiling dose is reached, no additional response is achieved by increasing the dose. Thus, when this dose is reached, additional diuresis is achieved by giving the drug more often (twice daily or occasionally three times daily) or by giving combination diuretic therapy. Table 16–5 lists the ceiling doses. Multiple daily dosing achieves a more sustained diuresis throughout the day. When dosed two or three times daily, the first dose is usually given first thing in the morning and the final dose in late afternoon/early evening.

Diuretics cause a variety of metabolic abnormalities, with severity related to the potency of the diuretic. Chapter 15 has a detailed discussion on the adverse effects of diuretic therapy. Hypokalemia is the most common metabolic disturbance with thiazide and loop diuretics, which in heart failure patients may be exacerbated by hyperaldosteronism. Hypokalemia increases the risk for ventricular arrhythmias in heart failure and is especially worrisome in patients receiving digoxin. Hypokalemia is often accompanied by hypomagnesemia. Because adequate magnesium is necessary for entry of potassium into the cell, cosupplementation with both magnesium and potassium may be necessary to correct the hypokalemia. Concomitant ACE inhibitor (or ARB) and/or aldosterone antagonist therapy may help to minimize diuretic-induced hypokalemia because these drugs tend to increase serum potassium concentration through their inhibitory effect on aldosterone secretion. Nonetheless, the serum potassium concentration should be monitored closely in heart failure patients and supplemented appropriately when needed. In addition to metabolic abnormalities, a recent post-hoc analysis of the DIG trial suggested that chronic diuretic use was associated with increased risk of mortality and hospitalization.[110] These findings must be interpreted with caution because this trial was not designed to evaluate outcomes associated with diuretic therapy. However, they do serve to remind clinicians of the importance of appropriate patient selection and monitoring when using diuretic therapy.

5 Angiotensin-Converting Enzyme Inhibitors A number of ACE inhibitors are available currently in the United States; Table 16–9 summarizes those commonly used in the treatment of patients with heart failure. Although ACE inhibitors vary in their chemical structure (e.g., sulfhydryl- vs. non–sulfhydryl-containing agents) and tissue affinity, the major differences in the ACE inhibitors are not in these pharmacologic properties but in their pharmacokinetic properties.[13] Although it appears that mortality reduction with ACE inhibitors is probably a drug class effect, not all ACE inhibitors that are FDA approved for treatment of heart failure have been evaluated for their effects on mortality in heart failure. Thus it seems most prudent to use those agents that have been documented to reduce morbidity and mortality because the dose required for this effect has been documented.[1] Table 16–9 also summarizes the target doses for survival benefit.

To minimize the risk of hypotension and renal insufficiency, ACE inhibitor therapy should be started with low doses followed by gradual titration to the target doses as tolerated.[1] Asymptomatic hypotension should not be considered a contraindication to initiation of an ACE inhibitor although initiation or dose increases in patients with systolic blood pressures less than 90 to 100 mm Hg should be done cautiously. Renal function and serum potassium

TABLE 16-9 Angiotensin-Converting Enzyme Inhibitors Routinely Used for the Treatment of Heart Failure

Generic Name	Brand Name	Initial Dose	Target Dosing–Survival Benefit[a]	Prodrug	Elimination[b]
Captopril	Capoten	6.25 mg tid	50 mg tid	No	Renal
Enalapril	Vasotec	2.5–5 mg bid	10 mg bid	Yes	Renal
Lisinopril	Zestril, Prinivil	2.5–5 mg daily	20–40 mg daily[c]	No	Renal
Quinapril	Accupril	10 mg bid	20–40 mg bid[d]	Yes	Renal
Ramipril	Altace	1.25–2.5 mg bid	5 mg bid	Yes	Renal
Fosinopril	Monopril	5-10 mg daily	40 mg daily[d]	Yes	Renal/hepatic
Trandolapril	Mavik	0.5–1 mg daily	4 mg daily	Yes	Renal/hepatic
Perindopril	Aceon	2 mg daily	8–16 mg daily[d]	Yes	Renal/hepatic

[a]Target doses associated with survival benefits in clinical trials.
[b]Primary route of elimination.
[c]Note that in the Assessment of Treatment with Lisinopril and Survival (ATLAS) trial (Circulation 1999;100:2312–2318), no significant difference in mortality was found between low dose (~5 mg/day) and high dose (~35 mg/day) lisinopril therapy.
[d]Effects on mortality have not been evaluated.

should be evaluated within 1 to 2 weeks after therapy is started with subsequent periodic assessments, especially after dose increases. Careful attention to appropriate doses of diuretics is important as fluid overload may blunt the beneficial effects of ACE inhibitors and overdiuresis increases the risk of hypotension and renal insufficiency. After titration of the drug to the target dose, most patients tolerate chronic therapy with few complications. Although symptoms may improve within a few days of initiating therapy, it may take weeks to months before the full benefits are apparent. Even if symptoms do not improve, long-term ACE inhibitor therapy should be continued to reduce the risk of mortality and hospitalization.

Because ACE inhibitors were the first agents to show improvements in heart failure survival and were frequently used as background therapy in clinical trials of other medications, they are often used as the initial therapy in patients with left ventricular systolic function. Traditionally, after titration of the ACE inhibitor dose, the addition of β-blockers was considered. The expected ACE inhibitor-mediated decrease in blood pressure made some clinicians reluctant to initiate β-blocker therapy. Because of the impressive benefits of β-blockers, initiation of β-blocker therapy should not be delayed in patients who fail to reach target ACE inhibitor doses.[1] Because activation of the SNS occurs before that of the RAAS and is an important stimulus for RAAS activation, there is debate over whether ACE inhibitors or β-blockers should be used as initial therapy. The results of the previously discussed CIBIS III trial did not provide compelling evidence to support initiation of β-blockers prior to ACE inhibitors.[68] Consequently, in most patients, ACE inhibitors should be the initial therapy, but it is important to remember that the greatest benefit is seen when both an ACE inhibitor and β-blocker are used.

Because of the high prevalence of coronary artery disease in patients with heart failure, aspirin is frequently coadministered with ACE inhibitors. Several retrospective cohort analyses suggest that aspirin may attenuate the hemodynamic and mortality benefits of ACE inhibitors.[111] The postulated mechanism of this interaction involves opposing effects on synthesis of vasodilatory prostaglandins. The ACE inhibitor–mediated increase in bradykinin increases the synthesis of vasodilatory prostaglandins that have favorable hemodynamic benefits in heart failure. Because of aspirin's effect on prostaglandin synthesis, this potentially beneficial action of ACE inhibitors may be negated. However, in contrast with studies that showed an ACE inhibitor-aspirin interaction, other investigators have found no interaction, even in patients without coronary artery disease or with impaired renal function.[111,112] Because there is no prospective evidence confirming an interaction between these agents, it is currently recommended that the decision to use each of these medications be made based on whether an individual patient has indications for each drug. Use of aspirin doses of 160 mg per day or less should be considered.

Adverse Effects. The primary adverse effects of ACE inhibitor therapy are secondary to their major pharmacologic effects of suppressing angiotensin II and increasing bradykinin. The reductions in angiotensin II are associated with hypotension and functional renal insufficiency which are the most common adverse effects observed with ACE inhibitors. Hypotension may be asymptomatic or manifested as dizziness, lightheadedness, presyncope, or syncope. It occurs most commonly early in therapy or after an increase in dose, although it may occur at any time during treatment. Risk factors for hypotension include hyponatremia (serum sodium <130 mEq/L), hypovolemia, and overdiuresis.[1] The occurrence of hypotension may be minimized by initiating therapy with lower ACE inhibitor doses and/or temporarily withholding or reducing the dose of diuretic, and liberalizing salt and fluid intake.[1] An often overlooked solution to hypotension is to space the administration times of vasoactive medications (e.g., diuretics and β-blockers) throughout the day so that these medications are not all administered at or near the same time. Many patients who experience symptomatic hypotension early in therapy are still good candidates for long-term treatment if risk factors for low blood pressure are addressed.

Functional renal insufficiency is manifested as increases in serum creatinine and blood urea nitrogen. As cardiac output and renal blood flow decline, renal perfusion is maintained by the vasoconstrictor effect of angiotensin II on the efferent arteriole. Patients most dependent on this system for maintenance of renal perfusion (and therefore most likely to develop functional renal insufficiency with ACE inhibitors) are those with severe heart failure, hypotension, hyponatremia, volume depletion, bilateral renal artery stenosis, and concomitant use of NSAIDs.[113] Sodium depletion, usually secondary to diuretic therapy, is the most important factor in the development of functional renal insufficiency with ACE inhibitor therapy. Renal insufficiency therefore can be minimized in many cases by reduction in diuretic dosage or liberalization of sodium intake. Increases in serum creatinine of 10% to 20% from baseline are commonly observed after initiation of ACE inhibitor therapy. In some patients, the serum creatinine will return to baseline levels without a reduction in ACE inhibitor dose.[113] Increases in serum creatinine of >0.5 mg/dL if the baseline creatinine is <2.0 mg/dL or >1.0 mg/dL if the creatinine is >2.0 mg/dL, should prompt clinicians to reconsider ACE therapy and evaluate potential causes for the abrupt decline in renal function.[113] Because renal dysfunction with ACE inhibitors is secondary to alterations in renal hemodynamics, it is almost always reversible upon discontinuation of the drug.[113]

Careful dose titration can minimize the risks of hypotension and transient worsening of renal function. Thus usual initial doses should be about one-fourth the final target dose with slow upward dose titration over several days based on blood pressure and serum creatinine. In certain patients, especially those hospitalized patients who seem to be at high risk for hypotension or worsening of renal function, it also may be advisable to initiate therapy with a short-acting agent such as captopril. This will help minimize the duration of adverse effects should they occur. Once stabilized on ACE inhibitor therapy with captopril, the patient can then be switched to a longer-half-life drug.

Retention of potassium with ACE inhibitor therapy can occur and is caused by the reduced feedback of angiotensin II to stimulate aldosterone release. Hyperkalemia is most likely to occur in patients with renal insufficiency and in those taking concomitant potassium supplements, potassium-containing salt substitutes, or potassium-sparing diuretic therapy (including an aldosterone antagonist), especially if they have diabetes.[113] The more widespread use of aldosterone antagonists (e.g., spironolactone) in patients with heart failure may increase the risk of hyperkalemia.[82]

ACE inhibitors are also associated with other important adverse effects. A dry, hacking cough occurs with a similar frequency (5% to 15% of patients) with all the agents and is related to bradykinin accumulation. The cough is usually nonproductive, occurs within the first few months of therapy, resolves within 1 to 2 weeks of drug discontinuation, and reappears with rechallenge. Because cough occurs in up to 40% of patients with heart failure, independent of ACE inhibitor use, it is important to rule out other potential causes of cough, such as pulmonary congestion. Because cough is a bradykinin-mediated effect, replacement of ACE inhibitor therapy with an ARB would be reasonable in those patients who cannot tolerate the cough. Angioedema is a rare, but potentially life-threatening complication that is also believed to be related to bradykinin accumulation. It may occur more frequently in African Americans than in other populations.[1] Use of ACE inhibitors is contraindicated in patients with a history of angioedema. ARBs may be an alternative therapy in patients with ACE inhibitor-induced angioedema, although caution is advised as rare cross-reactivity is reported.[1,77,79] ACE inhibitors are contraindicated during the second and third trimesters of pregnancy because of the increased risk of fetal renal failure, intrauterine growth retardation, and other congenital defects. A recent analysis using a Medicaid database of nearly 30,000 patients suggests that first trimester use of ACE inhibitors should also be avoided as the risk of major congenital defects was increased 2.7-fold in infants exposed to these agents during the first trimester.[114]

❺ Angiotensin II Receptor Blockers Although ACE inhibitors remain the agents of first choice to treat stage C heart failure with reduced LVEF, ARBs approved for the treatment of heart failure are now the recommended alternatives in patients who are unable to tolerate an ACE inhibitor.[1] Although seven ARBs are currently on the market, only two, candesartan and valsartan, are approved for the treatment of heart failure. The use of these two agents is supported by clinical trial data that document a target dose associated with improved survival and other important outcomes in patients with decreased LVEF.[47,74,75] Thus, candesartan or valsartan are the preferred agents in patients with heart failure, whether used alone or in combination with ACE inhibitors. ARBs are also alternative to ACE inhibitors in patients with stages A or B heart failure.[1]

The clinical use of ARBs is also similar to that of ACE inhibitors. Therapy should be initiated at low doses (candesartan 4 to 8 mg once daily; valsartan 20 to 40 mg twice daily) and then titrated to target doses (candesartan 32 mg once daily; valsartan 160 mg twice daily).[1] Blood pressure, renal function, and serum potassium should be evaluated within 1 to 2 weeks after initiation of therapy and after increases in dose and these end points used to guide subsequent dose changes. It is not necessary to reach target ARB doses before adding a β-blocker.

Adverse Effects. The ARBs have a low incidence of adverse effects. Because they do not affect bradykinin, they are not associated with cough and have a lower risk of angioedema than ACE inhibitors. However, because of reports of recurrences of ACE inhibitor-related angioedema after ARB administration, ARBs should be used cautiously in any patient with a history of angioedema.[77,79] The major adverse effects are related to suppression of the RAAS. The incidence and risk factors for developing hypotension, decreases in renal function, and hyperkalemia with the ARBs is similar to that of ACE inhibitors.[12] Thus, ARBs are not alternatives in patients who develop these complications from ACE inhibitors. Careful monitoring is required when an ARB is used with another inhibitor of the RAAS (e.g., ACE inhibitor or aldosterone antagonist) as this combination increases the risk of these adverse effects. Similar to the ACE inhibitors, the ARBs are contraindicated in the second and third trimesters of pregnancy and should be avoided in the first trimester because of increased risk of fetal/neonatal morbidity and mortality. Neither candesartan nor valsartan are metabolized by the cytochrome P450 (CYP) system, so no pharmacokinetic drug–drug interactions with these agents are expected.

❻ β-Blockers Metoprolol CR/XL, carvedilol, and bisoprolol are the only β-blockers shown to reduce mortality in large heart failure trials. Metoprolol and bisoprolol selectively block the β_1-receptor, whereas carvedilol blocks the β_1, β_2, and α_1-receptors and also possesses antioxidant effects. Although there is no clear evidence that these pharmacologic differences result in differences in efficacy among agents, they may aid in selection of a specific agent. For example, carvedilol is expected to have greater antihypertensive effects than the other agents because of its α-receptor blocking properties and may be preferred in patients with poorly controlled blood pressure. Conversely, metoprolol or bisoprolol may be preferred in patients with low blood pressure or dizziness and in patients with significant airway disease.

Bisoprolol is eliminated approximately 50% by renal elimination, whereas metoprolol and carvedilol are essentially completely metabolized and undergo extensive hepatic first-pass metabolism. Both metoprolol and carvedilol are also substrates for the CYP2D6, which is known to be polymorphic. The 7% of the white population and 1% to 2% of the Asian American and African American populations who are CYP2D6-poor metabolizers would be expected to have higher plasma concentrations than anticipated at the usual doses of carvedilol and metoprolol. However, given that β-blockers have a wide therapeutic index, it is unclear whether the poor metabolizer phenotype would result in more pronounced hemodynamic effects.

There is fairly strong evidence that benefits of β-blockers in heart failure are not a class effect. Specifically, in a study powered for mortality reduction, there was no difference in survival between the nonselective β-blocker bucindolol and placebo.[115] Although there has been considerable debate over why bucindolol failed to provide a survival benefit, it may be related to the drug's ancillary properties or differences among β-blocker trials in the characteristics of study participants. These data emphasize the importance of confining β-blocker use to one of the agents with proven survival benefits, especially given the diversity among β-blockers in their receptor sensitivities and ancillary properties.

There has been much debate over whether one β-blocker is superior to another. Specifically, it has been hypothesized that nonselective blockade with carvedilol might produce greater benefits than β_1-selective blockade. This hypothesis is based on observations that the β_1-receptor is downregulated, and the β_2- and α_1-receptors account for a larger proportion of total cardiac adrenergic receptors in the failing heart. Only one trial with a mortality end point has provided a head-to-head comparison of carvedilol and a β_1-selective blocker. The Carvedilol or Metoprolol European Trial

(COMET) compared carvedilol 25 mg twice daily and immediate-release metoprolol 50 mg twice daily and found a significant 17% lower mortality rate in patients treated with carvedilol.[116] However, concerns regarding the formulation and dose of metoprolol used in COMET limit the conclusions that can be drawn from these findings. Specifically, the study used the immediate-release formulation of metoprolol (metoprolol tartrate) not the sustained-release formation (metoprolol succinate) shown to reduce mortality compared to placebo.[59] The efficacy of the immediate-release formulation in reducing mortality in heart failure has not been proven. Metoprolol CR/XL provides more consistent plasma concentrations over a 24-hour period and appears to provide more favorable effects on heart rate variability, autonomic balance, and blood pressure, suggesting that this formulation might be superior to immediate-release metoprolol.[117] The target dose of metoprolol also differed between COMET and MERIT-HF. The target dose in COMET was 100 mg/day (50 mg twice daily), whereas the target dose of metoprolol in MERIT-HF was 200 mg/day. Many question whether the degree of β-blockade achieved in COMET with immediate-release metoprolol 50 mg twice daily is comparable to that achieved with metoprolol CR/XL 200 mg/day in MERIT-HF or carvedilol 25 mg twice daily in COMET. Thus, the debate over β-blocker superiority continues, and although some clinicians would argue superiority of carvedilol, it seems clear that what is most important is that one of the three β-blockers proven to reduce mortality is used.

Adverse Effects. Possible adverse effects with β-blocker use in heart failure include bradycardia or heart block, hypotension, fatigue, impaired glycemic control in diabetic patients, bronchospasm in patients with asthma, and worsening heart failure. Clinicians should monitor vital signs and carefully assess for signs and symptoms of worsening heart failure during β-blocker initiation and up-titration. Hypotension is more common with carvedilol because of its α_1-receptor–blocking properties. Bradycardia and hypotension generally are asymptomatic and require no intervention; however, β-blocker dose reduction is warranted in symptomatic patients. Fatigue usually resolves after several weeks of therapy, but sometimes requires dose reduction. In diabetic patients, β-blockers may worsen glucose tolerance and can mask the tachycardia and tremor (but not sweating) that accompany hypoglycemia. In addition, nonselective agents such as carvedilol may prolong insulin-induced hypoglycemia and slow recovery from a hypoglycemic episode. Despite this, there is evidence that carvedilol produces better glycemic control in diabetic patients compared to immediate-release metoprolol and may improve insulin sensitivity.[118] Diabetic patients should be warned of these potential adverse effects, and blood glucose should be monitored with initiation, adjustment, and discontinuation of β-blocker therapy. Adjustment of hypoglycemic therapy may be necessary with concomitant β-blocker use in diabetics.

Up-titration should be avoided if the patient experiences signs of worsening heart failure, including volume overload and poor perfusion. Fluid overload may be asymptomatic and manifest solely as an increase in body weight. Mild fluid overload may be managed by intensifying diuretic therapy. The treatment of moderate to severe congestion is discussed in the section on acute decompensated heart failure. Once the patient has been stabilized, dose titration may continue as tolerated until the target or highest tolerated dose is reached.

Absolute contraindications to β-blocker use include uncontrolled bronchospastic disease, symptomatic bradycardia, advanced heart block without a pacemaker, and acute decompensated heart failure. However, β-blockers may be tried with caution in patients with asymptomatic bradycardia or well-controlled asthma. Particular caution is warranted in patients with marked bradycardia (<55 beats/min) or hypotension (systolic blood pressure <80 mm Hg). Importantly, concerns of masking symptoms of hypoglycemia or worsening glycemic control should not preclude β-blockers use in patients with diabetes. Indeed, post-hoc analysis of heart failure trials shows that β-blockers are well tolerated and significantly reduce morbidity and mortality in patients with diabetes and heart failure.[119] β-Blockers should be used cautiously in patients with diabetes and recurrent hypoglycemia.

Digoxin Digoxin exerts its positive inotropic effect by binding to sodium- and potassium-activated adenosine triphosphatase (Na-K-ATPase or sodium pump). Inhibition of Na-K-ATPase decreases outward transport of sodium and leads to increased intracellular sodium concentrations. Higher intracellular sodium concentrations favor calcium entry and reduce calcium extrusion from the cell through effects on the sodium–calcium exchanger. The result is increased storage of intracellular calcium in the sarcoplasmic reticulum, and with each action potential, a greater release of calcium to activate contractile elements. Digoxin also has beneficial neurohormonal actions. These effects occur at low plasma concentrations, where little inotropic effect is seen, and are independent of inotropic activity. Unlike other positive inotropes that increase intracellular cyclic adenosine monophosphate (cAMP), digoxin attenuates the excessive SNS activation present in heart failure patients. Although the precise mechanism is unknown, a digoxin-mediated reduction in central sympathetic outflow and improvement in impaired baroreceptor function appear to play an important role. Because mortality and progression of heart failure are linked to the extent of SNS activation, these sympathoinhibitory effects may be an important component of the clinical response to the drug. Chronic heart failure is also marked by autonomic dysfunction, most notably suppression of the parasympathetic (vagal) system. Digoxin increases parasympathetic activity in heart failure patients and leads to a decrease in heart rate, thus enhancing diastolic filling. The vagal effects also result in slowed conduction and prolongation of atrioventricular node refractoriness, thus slowing the ventricular response in patients with atrial fibrillation. Because atrial fibrillation is a common complication of heart failure, the combined positive inotropic, neurohormonal, and negative chronotropic effects of digoxin can be particularly beneficial for such patients. The overall response to digoxin is usually an increase in cardiac index and a decrease in PAOP with relatively little change in arterial blood pressure.[86,87,96]

Pharmacokinetics. Numerous studies of digoxin pharmacokinetics have been published; Table 16–10 summarizes them. Digoxin

TABLE 16-10 Clinical Pharmacokinetics of Digoxin

Oral bioavailability	
Tablets	0.5–0.9 (0.65)[a]
Elixir	0.75–0.85 (0.80)
Capsules	0.9–1.0 (0.95)
Onset of action	
Oral	1.5–6 h
Intravenous	15–30 min
Peak effect	
Oral	4–6 h
Intravenous	1.5–4 h
Terminal half-life	
Normal renal function	36 h
Anuric patients	5 days
Volume of distribution at steady state	7.3 L/kg
Fraction unbound in plasma	0.75–0.80
Fraction excreted unchanged in urine	0.65–0.70

[a]Range and mean value in parentheses.

Data from Schentag JJ, Bang AJ, Kozinski-Tober JL. Digoxin. In: Burton ME, Shaw LM, Schentag JJ, Evans WE, eds. Applied Pharmacokinetics and Pharmacodynamics: Principles of Therapeutic Drug Monitoring, 4th ed. Baltimore: Lippincott Williams & Wilkins, 2006:410–439.

TABLE 16-11 Digoxin Drug Interactions

Drugs	Mechanism/Effect	Suggested Clinical Management
Amiodarone	Inhibits P-glycoprotein resulting in decrease in renal and nonrenal clearance; can increase SDC by 70%–100%	Monitor SDC and adverse effects; anticipate the need to reduce the dose by 50%
Antacids	Concurrent administration may decrease digoxin bioavailability by 20%–35%	Space doses at least 2 h apart or avoid concurrent use if possible
Cholestyramine, colestipol	Bind digoxin in gut and decrease bioavailability 20%–35%; may also decrease enterohepatic recycling	Space doses at least 2 h apart or avoid concurrent colestipol use if possible
Diuretics	Thiazides or loop diuretics may cause hypokalemia and hypomagnesemia, thereby increasing the risk of digitalis toxicity	Monitor and replace electrolytes if necessary
Erythromycin, clarithromycin, tetracycline	Alter gut bacterial flora; bioavailability and SDC increase 40%–100% in approximately 10% of patients who extensively metabolize digoxin in the gut; may also be caused by inhibition of P-glycoprotein by macrolides	Monitor SDC and anticipate the need to reduce the dose; avoid concurrent use if possible
Ketoconazole, itraconazole	Decrease in renal and nonrenal clearance by inhibition of P-glycoprotein; SDC may increase by 50%–100%	Monitor SDC and anticipate the need to reduce the dose by 50%
Kaolin-pectin	Large dose (30–60 mL) may decrease digoxin bioavailability by approximately 60%	Space doses at least 2 h apart or avoid concurrent use if possible
Metoclopramide	Increase in gut mobility may decrease bioavailability of slow dissolving tablets; unknown significance	Effect is minimized by administration of digoxin capsules
Neomycin, sulfasalazine	Decrease in bioavailability by 20%–25% sulfasalazine	Space doses at least 2 h apart or avoid concurrent use if possible
Propafenone	Decrease in renal clearance; SDC may increase 30%–40%	Monitor SDC and anticipate the need to reduce the dose
Quinidine	Inhibits P-glycoprotein resulting in decrease in renal and nonrenal clearance; also displacement of digoxin from tissue-binding sites with decrease in the volume of distribution; SDC generally increases about twofold	Monitor SDC and adverse effects; anticipate the need to reduce dose by 50%
Spironolactone	Decrease in renal and nonrenal clearance; also interference with some digoxin assays thus increasing apparent SDC	Monitor SDC and anticipate the need to reduce dose; check assay for interference
Verapamil	Inhibits P-glycoprotein resulting in decrease in renal and nonrenal clearance, SDC may increase 70%–100%	Monitor SDC and anticipate the need to reduce the dose by 50%; consider using another calcium channel blocker

SDC, serum digoxin concentration.

has a large volume of distribution and is extensively bound to various tissues, most notably to Na-K-ATPase in skeletal and cardiac muscles. Because it does not distribute appreciably to body fat, loading doses of digoxin (when necessary) should be calculated based on estimates of lean body weight. There is a long "distribution phase" after administration of oral or intravenous digoxin, resulting in a lag time before maximum pharmacologic response is observed (Table 16–10). Transiently elevated serum digoxin concentrations during the distribution phase are not associated with increased therapeutic or adverse effects, although they can mislead the clinician who is unaware of the timing of blood sampling relative to the previous digoxin dose. Consequently, blood samples for measurement of serum digoxin concentrations should be collected at least 6 hours, and preferably 12 hours or more, after the last dose.

In patients with normal renal function, 60% to 80% of a dose of digoxin is eliminated unchanged in urine via glomerular filtration and tubular secretion. The terminal half-life of digoxin is approximately 1.5 days in subjects with normal renal function but approximately 5 days in anuric patients (see Table 16–10). Recent evidence indicates that the drug efflux transporter P-glycoprotein plays an important role in the bioavailability, renal and nonrenal clearance, and drug interactions with digoxin. Table 16–11 summarizes clinically important pharmacokinetic/pharmacodynamic drug interactions. An extensive review of the pharmacokinetics and pharmacodynamics of digoxin is available.[96]

Adverse Effects. Although digoxin can produce a variety of cardiac and noncardiac adverse effects, it is usually well tolerated by most patients (Table 16–12).[86,87] Noncardiac adverse effects frequently involve the CNS or gastrointestinal systems but also may be nonspecific (e.g., fatigue or weakness). Cardiac manifestations include numerous different arrhythmias that are believed to be caused by multiple electrophysiologic effects (Table 16–12). Cardiac arrhythmias may be the first evidence of toxicity in a patient (before any noncardiac symptoms occur). Rhythm disturbances are of particular concern because patients with chronic heart failure are already at increased risk for sudden cardiac death, presumably as a consequence of ventricular arrhythmias. Patients who are at increased risk of toxicity include those with impaired renal function, decreased lean body mass, the elderly, and those taking interacting drugs. Hypokalemia, hypomagnesemia, and hypercalcemia will predispose patients to cardiac manifestations of digoxin toxicity. Thus, concomitant therapy with diuretics may lead to electrolyte abnormalities and increase the likelihood of cardiac arrhythmias. Similarly, hypothyroidism, myocardial ischemia, and acidosis will also increase the risk of cardiac adverse effects. Although digoxin toxicity is commonly associated with plasma concentrations greater than 2 ng/mL, clinicians should remember that digoxin toxicity is based on the presence of symptoms rather than a specific plasma concentration.[96] Usual treatment of digoxin toxicity

TABLE 16-12 Signs and Symptoms of Digoxin Toxicity

Noncardiac (mostly CNS) adverse effects
Anorexia, nausea, vomiting, abdominal pain
Visual disturbances
Halos, photophobia, problems with color perception (i.e., red-green or yellow-green vision), scotomata
Fatigue, weakness, dizziness, headache, neuralgia, confusion, delirium, psychosis
Cardiac adverse effects[a,b]
Ventricular arrhythmias
Premature ventricular depolarizations, bigeminy, trigeminy, ventricular tachycardia, ventricular fibrillation
Atrioventricular (AV) block
First degree, second degree (Mobitz type I), third degree
AV junctional escape rhythms, junctional tachycardia
Atrial arrhythmias with slowed AV conduction or AV block
Particularly paroxysmal atrial tachycardia with AV block
Sinus bradycardia

[a]Some adverse effects may be difficult to distinguish from the signs/symptoms of heart failure.
[b]Digoxin toxicity has been associated with almost every known rhythm abnormality (only the more common manifestations are listed).
Reprinted and adapted from Prog Cardiovasc Dis, Vol. 44, Eichorn EJ, Gheorghiade M, Pages 251–266, Copyright 2002, with permission from Elsevier.

includes drug withdrawal or dose reduction and treatment of cardiac arrhythmias and electrolyte abnormalities. In patients with life-threatening digoxin toxicity, purified digoxin-specific Fab antibody fragments should be administered. Serum digoxin concentrations will not be reliable until the antidote has been eliminated from the body.[87]

TREATMENT

Acute Decompensated Heart Failure

⓫ As discussed previously, the number of patients with heart failure is substantial and continues to increase. Although mortality from heart failure has improved, the growing number of patients with the disorder and the progressive nature of the syndrome have led to substantial increases in hospitalizations for heart failure.[4] Recent data indicate approximately 1 million patients are hospitalized annually for heart failure, resulting in significant morbidity, mortality, and consumption of large quantities of healthcare resources.[4] Inpatient admission for heart failure exacerbations is associated with an increased risk of subsequent hospitalization and decreased survival.[120] The economic impact of heart failure is considerable with cost driven primarily by hospitalization and inpatient care.[4]

A number of descriptive terms have been used to characterize patients with worsening heart failure requiring hospitalization. Patients with persistent symptoms or *refractory* heart failure requiring specialized interventions despite optimal standard therapy such as ACE inhibitors and β-blockers are classified as stage D in the ACC/AHA classification scheme. These patients typically fall into the category of NYHA class III or IV heart failure, with symptoms upon minimal exertion or at rest.[1] The terms *decompensated heart failure* or *exacerbation of heart failure* refer to those patients with new or worsening signs or symptoms, which are usually caused by volume overload and/or hypoperfusion and lead to additional medical care, such as emergency room visits and hospitalizations. The term *acute* heart failure may be misleading as it more often refers to the patient with a sudden onset of signs or symptoms of heart failure in the setting of previously normal cardiac function. This section of the chapter focuses on the management of patients with acute decompensated heart failure. Clinical syndromes within decompensated heart failure include systemic volume overload, low output, and acute pulmonary edema. It is important to recognize that such patients may present with impaired or preserved left ventricular function and a variety of etiologies may be responsible for the primary disease process. The clinical course of heart failure manifests as periods of relative stability with an increasing frequency in episodes of decompensation as the underlying disease progresses.[121]

Despite the considerable morbidity and mortality associated with decompensated heart failure, the first randomized placebo-controlled trials in this patient population were published in 2002.[122,123] In addition, it was not until recently that guidelines were generated focusing specifically on managing decompensated heart failure. Currently, the ACC/AHA guidelines focus a portion of their recommendations for chronic heart failure on the decompensated patient, but the HFSA and the European Society of Cardiology have published separate guidelines for evaluating and treating decompensated heart failure.[1,34,124] Because available drug therapies differ between Europe and the United States, the HFSA guidelines are the focus of the remainder of this chapter.

■ PATHOPHYSIOLOGY AND CLINICAL PRESENTATION

Patients requiring intensive therapy for decompensated heart failure may have a variety of underlying etiologies and clinical presentations. Patients with worsening chronic heart failure associated with reduced or preserved left ventricular function comprise approximately 70% of heart failure hospital admissions. These patients can become refractory to available oral therapy and decompensate following a relatively mild insult (e.g., dietary indiscretion), medical noncompliance, or a noncardiac concurrent illness (e.g., infection). A new cardiac event, such as recurrent MI, atrial fibrillation, myocarditis, or acute valvular insufficiency also can cause a stable patient to decompensate. Secondly, de novo heart failure may occur following a large myocardial infarction or sudden increase in blood pressure in the setting of left ventricular dysfunction and represents approximately 25% of admissions. A third group of patients with severe left ventricular systolic dysfunction associated with progressive worsening of cardiac output and refractoriness to therapy represents approximately 5% of heart failure admissions.[125] Additional insight into the clinical characteristics of decompensated heart failure patients unexpectedly indicates that a high percentage of patients present with hypertension and preserved systolic function.[126]

Several studies provide a better understanding of the prognostic factors associated with decompensated heart failure. Data from the Acute Decompensated Heart Failure Registry (ADHERE), a registry of hospitalized patients with a primary diagnosis of decompensated heart failure, found blood urea nitrogen greater than or equal to 43 mg/dL to be the best individual predictor of in-hospital mortality, followed by systolic blood pressure less than 115 mm Hg and then by serum creatinine greater than or equal to 2.75 mg/dL. Using these three parameters, patients were identified as low, intermediate, high, and very high risk with an in-hospital mortality of 2%, 6%, 13%, and 20%, respectively.[127] Additional studies confirm an increase in in-hospital mortality in patients with low systolic blood pressure and worsening renal function on admission.[128,129] Hyponatremia, elevations in troponin I, ischemic etiology, and poor functional capacity are additional negative prognostic factors.[125]

■ GENERAL APPROACH TO TREATMENT

⓫ The overall goals of therapy in the patient with decompensated heart failure are to relieve congestive symptoms or optimize volume status, as well as treat symptoms of low cardiac output, so that the patient can be discharged in a compensated state on oral drug therapy. Although diuretic, vasodilator, and positive inotrope therapy can be very effective at achieving these goals, their efficacy must be balanced against the potential for serious toxicity. Thus, another important goal is to minimize the risks of pharmacologic therapy. Maintenance of vital organ perfusion to preserve renal function and prevention of additional myocardial injury, diuretic-induced electrolyte depletion, hypotension from vasodilators, and myocardial ischemia and arrhythmias from positive inotropes are all important goals.

In addition, all patients should be evaluated for potential etiologies and precipitating factors, including atrial fibrillation and other arrhythmias, worsening hypertension, myocardial ischemia or infarction, anemia, hypothyroidism or hyperthyroidism, and other causes. Medications, including noncardiac medications, which may worsen cardiac function, should also be considered as precipitating or contributing factors. Patients who may benefit from revascularization should also be identified. Prior to discharge, optimization of chronic oral therapy and patient education are critical to preventing future hospitalizations. When available and appropriate, patients should be referred to a heart failure disease management program.[124] A careful history and physical examination are key components in the diagnosis of decompensated heart failure. The history should focus on the potential etiologies of heart failure, the presence of any precipitating factors, onset, duration, and severity of symptoms, and a careful medication history. Current guidelines recommend making the diagnosis of decompensated heart failure based primarily on signs and symptoms.[124] With congestion representing the more common presentation of heart failure, orthopnea is the main symptom of fluid overload that best correlates with elevated pulmonary pressures.[129] Important elements of the physical examination include assessment of vital signs and weight, cardiac auscultation for heart sounds and murmurs, pulmonary exam for the presence of rales, and evaluation for the presence of peripheral edema. The jugular venous pressure is the most reliable indicator of the patient's volume status and should be carefully evaluated on admission and closely followed during hospitalization as an indicator of the efficacy of diuretic therapy.[129] An S_3 gallop also represents ventricular filling and has high diagnostic specificity for heart failure decompensation. Other physical findings, such as pulmonary crackles and lower-extremity edema, have low specificity and sensitivity for the diagnosis of decompensated heart failure.[124] The development of a bedside assay for plasma BNP has focused considerable attention on the use of BNP as an aid in the diagnosis of suspected heart failure. Plasma BNP is positively correlated with the degree of left ventricular dysfunction and heart failure and this assay is now frequently used in acute care settings to assist in the differential diagnosis of dyspnea (heart failure vs. asthma, chronic obstructive pulmonary disease, or infection). A low BNP concentration has a 96% predictive value for excluding heart failure as an etiology when evaluating patients presenting with dyspnea. In addition, an elevated prehospital discharge BNP concentration is associated with an increased risk of worse long-term outcome. It is important to note that any disease process that increases right heart pressures will elevate BNP, including pulmonary emboli, chronic obstructive lung disease, and primary pulmonary hypertension. Also, BNP levels may be mildly increased with increasing age, female gender, and renal dysfunction, whereas concentrations may be lower with obesity.[129] Additional research will better characterize the role of BNP measurement in the diagnosis and treatment of heart failure. When the diagnosis of decompensated heart failure is uncertain, current guidelines recommend obtaining a BNP concentration in conjunction with assessing signs and symptoms.

Hospitalization *should occur* or *should be considered* depending on each patient's presenting symptoms and physical examination. Table 16–13 describes the clinical presentation of patients in whom hospitalization should occur or should be considered. Most patients do not require admission to an intensive care unit and are admitted to a monitored unit or general medical floor. Admission to an intensive care unit may be required if the patient experiences hemodynamic instability requiring frequent monitoring of vital signs, invasive hemodynamic monitoring, or rapid titration of intravenous medications with concurrent monitoring to assure safe and effective outcomes.

The first step in the management of decompensated heart failure is to ascertain that optimal treatment with oral medications has been achieved. If fluid retention is evident on physical examination, aggressive diuresis should be accomplished. Although increasing the dose of oral diuretic may be effective in some cases, the use of intravenous diuretics frequently is necessary. Every effort should be made to optimally treat the patient with an ACE inhibitor. β-Blocker therapy should generally be continued during the hospital admission unless recent dose initiation or up-titration was responsible for the decompensated state. In such cases, β-blocker therapy may need to be temporarily held or dose reduced. Appropriateness of initiating this therapy prior to hospital discharge will be discussed later in this chapter. Discontinuation of ACE inhibitor or β-blocker therapy occasionally may be necessary in the setting of cardiogenic shock or symptomatic hypotension. Certain therapies may also need to be temporarily held in the setting of renal dysfunction, especially in the setting of oliguria or hyperkalemia (e.g., ACE inhibitor, ARB, and/or aldosterone antagonist) or elevated serum digoxin concentrations. Most patients should be receiving digoxin at a low dose prescribed to achieve a trough serum concentration of 0.5 to 1.0 ng/mL.[1]

TABLE 16-13 Recommendations for Hospitalizing Patients Presenting with Acute Decompensated Heart Failure

Recommendation	Clinical Circumstances
Hospitalization recommended	Evidence of severely decompensated heart failure, including • Hypotension • Worsening renal function • Altered mentation Dyspnea at rest • Typically reflected by resting tachypnea • Less commonly reflected by oxygen saturation <90% Hemodynamically significant arrhythmia • Including new onset of rapid atrial fibrillation Acute coronary syndromes
Hospitalization should be considered	Worsened congestion • Even without dyspnea • Typically reflected by a weight gain of ≥5 kg Signs and symptoms of pulmonary or systemic congestion • Even in the absence of weight gain Major electrolyte disturbance Associated comorbid conditions • Pneumonia • Pulmonary embolus • Diabetic ketoacidosis • Symptoms suggestive of transient ischemic accident or stroke Repeated implantable cardioverter-defibrillator firings Previously undiagnosed heart failure with signs and symptoms of systemic or pulmonary congestion

Adapted from Adams KF, Lindenfield J, Arnold JMO, et al. HFSA 2006 comprehensive heart failure practice guidelines. J Card Fail 2006;12:e1–e122.

There are two general approaches to maximize therapy in the decompensated heart failure patient. One is to use simple clinical parameters (signs and symptoms, blood pressure, renal function) and the second is to use invasive hemodynamic monitoring in addition to these clinical parameters. In all decompensated heart failure patients, close monitoring is essential for assuring optimal response to therapy while avoiding adverse effects. Daily monitoring should include weight, strict fluid intake and output, and heart failure signs and symptoms to assess clinical efficacy of drug therapy. Foley catheter placement is not recommended unless close monitoring of urine output is needed. As safety end points, monitoring for electrolyte depletion, symptomatic hypotension, and renal dysfunction should be assessed frequently. Although many of the above parameters may be monitored daily, some will need to be monitored more frequently as dictated by the patient's clinical status. Vital signs should be assessed multiple times throughout the day at a frequency that is appropriate for a given patients' level of stability. Orthostatic blood pressure should be assessed at least once daily.[124] Table 16–14 summarizes the recommendations for monitoring.

■ PRINCIPLES OF THERAPY BASED ON CLINICAL PRESENTATION

Appropriate medical management of the patient presenting with decompensated heart failure is aided by determination of whether the patient has signs and symptoms of fluid overload ("wet" heart failure) or low cardiac output ("dry" heart failure).[129,130] As previously discussed, most patients present with *fluid overload* (or the "wet" profile). Symptoms consistent with pulmonary congestion include orthopnea and dyspnea with minimal exertion and those of systemic congestion include gastrointestinal discomfort, ascites, and peripheral edema. Patients with no or minimal fluid overload (or the "dry" category of decompensated heart failure) may have symptoms that

TABLE 16-14 Monitoring Recommendations for Patients Hospitalized with Acute Decompensated Heart Failure

Value	Frequency	Specifics
Weight	At least daily	Determine after voiding in the morning Account for possible increased food intake as a result of improved appetite
Fluid intake/output	At least daily	Strict documentation necessary
Vital signs	More than daily	Including orthostatic blood pressure
Signs	At least daily	Edema, acites, pulmonary rales, hepatomegaly, increased jugular venous pressure, hepatojugular reflux, liver tenderness
Symptoms	At least daily	Orthopnea, paroxysmal nocturnal dyspnea, nocturnal cough, dyspnea, fatigue
Electrolytes	At least daily	Potassium, magnesium, sodium
Renal function	At least daily	blood urea nitrogen, serum creatinine

Adapted from Adams KF, Lindenfield J, Arnold JMO, et al. HFSA 2006 comprehensive heart failure practice guidelines. J Card Fail 2006;12:e1–e122.

are more difficult to distinguish. This is a syndrome of *low cardiac output* and is characterized principally by extreme fatigue and tiredness as well as other symptoms not commonly attributed to cardiac causes such as poor appetite, nausea, and early satiety. It is important to recognize that gastrointestinal symptoms may be associated with congestion rather than low cardiac output to the gastrointestinal tract. Moreover, these patients frequently exhibit worsening renal function and a decline in serum sodium level. Many patients will present with signs and symptoms of both types of advanced heart failure. In these patients, low-output symptoms may not be obvious until congestion is optimally treated. Figure 16–8 outlines a suggested treatment approach based on whether the patient has signs and symptoms of fluid overload and/or low cardiac output.

■ PRINCIPLES OF THERAPY BASED ON HEMODYNAMIC SUBSETS

Patients with decompensated heart failure may have critically reduced cardiac output, usually with low arterial blood pressure and systemic hypoperfusion resulting in organ system dysfunction (i.e., cardiogenic shock). They also may have pulmonary edema with hypoxemia, respiratory acidosis, and markedly increased work of breathing. With cardiopulmonary support, response to interventions should be assessed promptly to allow for timely adjustments in treatment. Because cardiopulmonary support must be instituted and adjusted rapidly, immediate assessment of the results of an intervention limits risks and makes adjustments in therapy more prompt. ECG monitoring, continuous pulse oximetry, urine flow monitoring, and automated blood pressure recording are now the minimal noninvasive standard of care for critically ill patients with cardiopulmonary decompensation. Peripheral or femoral arterial catheters may be used for continuous and accurate assessment of arterial pressure.

Hemodynamic Monitoring

The role of invasive hemodynamic monitoring for improving outcomes in patients with decompensated heart failure remains controversial. The Evaluation Study of Congestive Heart Failure and Pulmonary Artery Catheterization Effectiveness (ESCAPE) trial assessed the role of invasive hemodynamic monitoring in the management of patients hospitalized for heart failure. The use of a pulmonary artery catheter had no impact on survival after hospital discharge.[131] It is important to note that patients with a clear indication for pulmonary artery catheter were excluded from this trial. Thus, the routine use of invasive monitoring is not recommended. However, invasive hemodynamic monitoring often provides essential information necessary to achieve optimal drug therapy in patients with a confusing or complicated clinical picture and during dose titration of rapidly acting medications. And thus, such monitoring should be considered in patients who are refractory to initial therapy, whose volume status is unclear, or who has clinically significant hypotension such as a systolic blood pressure less than 80 mm Hg, or worsening renal function despite therapy. Such monitoring is required to document adequate hemodynamic response to inotropic therapy prior to committing to chronic outpatient inotropic therapy.[124] Finally, assessment of hemodynamic parameters is required to document adequate reversal of pulmonary hypertension prior to cardiac transplantation.[129]

Invasive hemodynamic monitoring is usually performed with a flow-directed pulmonary artery or Swan-Ganz catheter placed percutaneously through a central vein and advanced through the right side of the heart and into the pulmonary artery. Inflation of a balloon proximal to the end port allows the catheter to "wedge," yielding the PAOP, which estimates the pulmonary venous (left atrial) pressure and, in the absence of intracardiac shunt, mitral valve disease or pulmonary disease, the left ventricular diastolic pressure. Additionally, cardiac output may be measured and systemic vascular resistance (SVR) calculated. Table 16–15 lists the normal values for hemodynamic parameters.

In addition to the clinical presentation, invasive hemodynamic monitoring helps in the selection of appropriate medical therapy as well as in the classification of patients into specific subsets. These *hemodynamic subsets* were first proposed for patients with left ventricular dysfunction following an acute MI but also are applicable to patients with acute or severe heart failure from other causes (Fig. 16–9).[132] This hemodynamic classification has four subsets and is based on a cardiac index above or below 2.2 L/min/m^2 and a PAOP above or below 18 mm Hg. Figure 16–10 is a treatment algorithm based on hemodynamic subsets. In addition to using the above profiles or categories to stratify patients with decompensated heart failure, these four hemodynamic profiles are predictive for outcome with patients in the wet-warm profile having a twofold greater risk of death and those in the wet-cold profile having a 2.5-fold increased risk of death at 1 year compared to dry-warm patients.[129]

Subset I Patients in hemodynamic subset I have a cardiac index and PAOP within generally acceptable ranges and have the lowest mortality of any subset. These patients do not need immediate specific interventions other than maximizing oral therapy and monitoring. It should be emphasized that patients with significant left ventricular dysfunction may still present in subset I because normal compensatory mechanisms and/or appropriate drug therapy may at least partially correct an otherwise abnormal hemodynamic profile.

Subset II As shown in Fig. 16–9, patients in subset II have an adequate cardiac index but a PAOP greater than 18 mm Hg. These patients are likely to have pulmonary congestion (i.e., "wet" heart failure) secondary to increased hydrostatic pressure in the pulmonary capillaries but no evidence of peripheral hypoperfusion. The primary goal of therapy in these patients is to reduce pulmonary congestion by lowering PAOP which is associated with improved outcomes. Accordingly, the therapeutic goal in this setting is to reduce filling pressures without reducing cardiac output, increasing heart rate, or further activating neurohormones. And thus, it is critically important that PAOP not be decreased excessively so as to cause a significant decrease in cardiac index. Although the normal range of PAOP is 5 to 12 mm Hg for individuals without cardiac dysfunction, higher pressures of 15 to 18 mm Hg frequently are necessary for heart failure patients to optimize cardiac index while avoiding pulmonary congestion. Generally, the PAOP can be low-

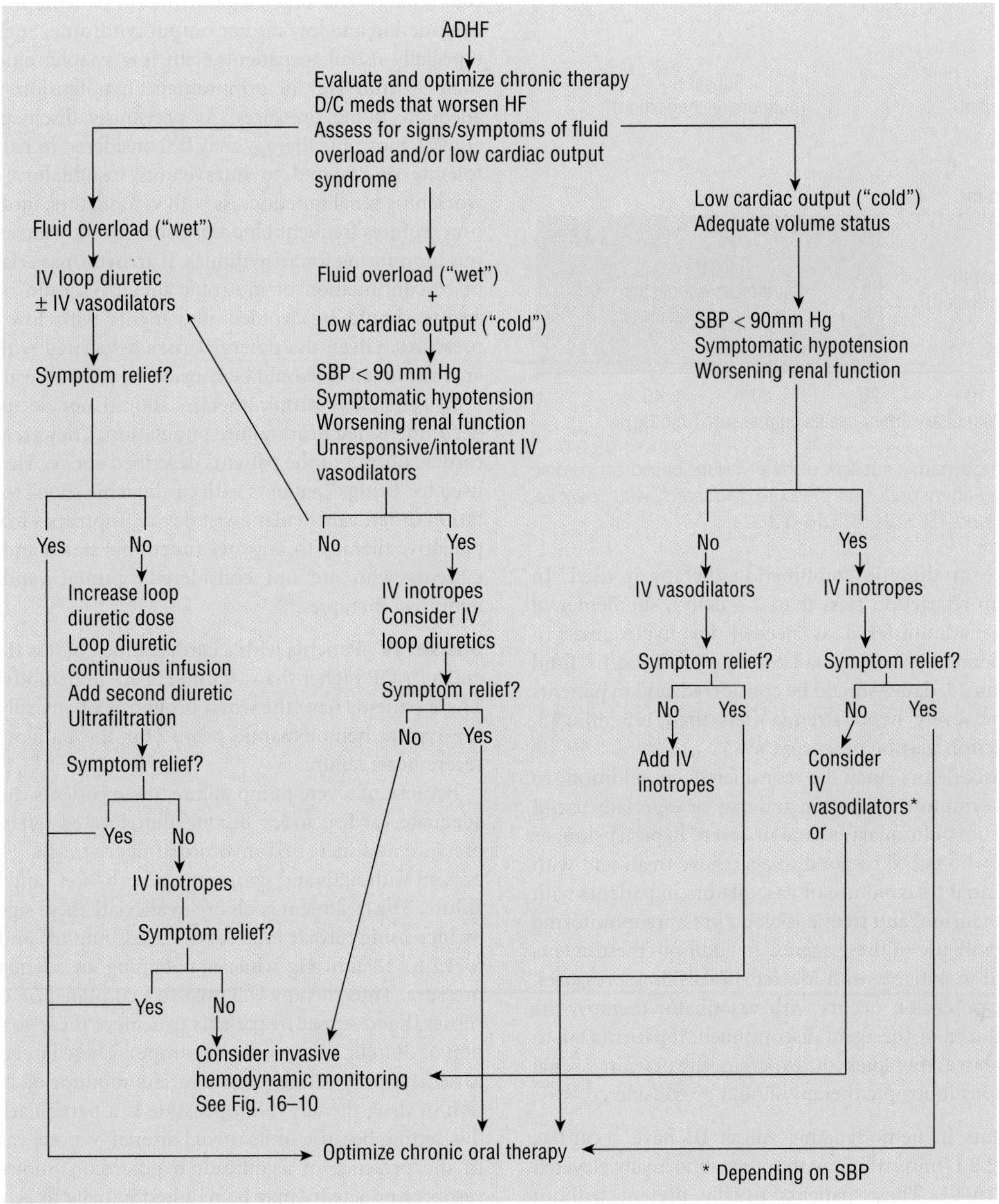

FIGURE 16-8. General treatment algorithm for acute decompensated heart failure (ADHF) based on clinical presentation. IV vasodilators that may be used include nitroglycerin, nesiritide, or nitroprusside. Metolazone or spironolactone may be added if the patient fails to respond to loop diuretics and a second diuretic is required. IV inotropes that may be used include dobutamine or milrinone. (D/C, discontinue; HF, heart failure; SBP, systolic blood pressure.) *(Reprinted and adapted from J Cardiac Fail, Vol. 12, Pages e1–e122, Copyright 2006, with permission from Elsevier.)*

TABLE 16-15 Hemodynamic Monitoring: Normal Values

Central venous (right atrial) pressure, mean	<5 mm Hg
Right ventricular pressure	25/0 mm Hg
Pulmonary artery pressure	25/10 mm Hg
Pulmonary artery pressure, mean	<18 mm Hg
Pulmonary artery occlusion pressure, mean	<12 mm Hg
Systemic arterial pressure	120/80 mm Hg
Mean arterial pressure	90–110 mm Hg
Cardiac index	2.8–4.2 L/min/m^2
Stroke volume index	30–65 mL/b/m^2
Systemic vascular resistance	900–1,400 dyne.sec.cm^{-5}
Pulmonary vascular resistance	150–250 dyne.sec.cm^{-5}
Arterial oxygen content	20 mL/dL
Mixed venous oxygen content	15 mL/dL
Arteriovenous oxygen content difference	3–5 mL/dL

ered to the range of 15 to 18 mm Hg with relatively little decrease in cardiac index because the Frank-Starling curve is flatter at higher PAOP values, particularly in patients with heart failure. Intravenous administration of agents that reduce preload (i.e., loop diuretics, nitroglycerin, or nesiritide) is the most appropriate acute therapy to achieve the therapeutic goal for patients in subset II. These agents will produce a very rapid decrease in preload, although signs and symptoms of pulmonary congestion may take longer to resolve.

Current guidelines recommend loop diuretics as first-line therapy for management of heart failure patients admitted with fluid overload and that such agents should typically be administered intravenously. The rate of diuresis should achieve a desirable volume status without causing a rapid reduction in intravascular volume resulting in symptomatic hypotension or renal dysfunction. Electrolyte depletion should be monitored for closely, especially

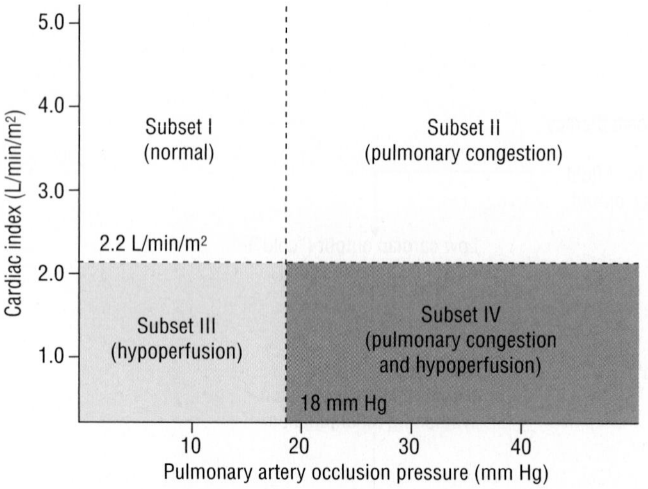

FIGURE 16-9. Hemodynamic subsets of heart failure based on cardiac index and pulmonary artery occlusion pressure. *(Adapted with permission from N Engl J Med 1976;295:1356–1362.)*

when a high dose or diuretic combination therapy is used. In addition to sodium restriction (less than 2 g daily), supplemental oxygen should be administered as needed for hypoxemia. In patients with moderate hyponatremia (less than 130 mEq/L), fluid restriction (less than 2 L daily) should be considered, and in patients with worsening or severe hyponatremia (less than 125 mEq/L), stricter fluid restriction may be necessary.[124]

Intravenous vasodilators may be considered in addition to diuretics for rapid symptom resolution and may be especially useful in patients with acute pulmonary edema or severe hypertension, as well as in patients who fail to respond to aggressive treatment with diuretics. It is essential to avoid use of vasodilators in patients with symptomatic hypotension, and frequent blood pressure monitoring is essential for the safe use of these agents. In addition, these agents should not be used in patients with low left-heart filling pressures. If symptomatic hypotension occurs with vasodilator therapy, the dose should be reduced or the agent discontinued. If patients fail to respond to the above therapies or experience worsening renal function, intravenous inotropic therapy should be considered.[124]

Subset III Patients in hemodynamic subset III have a cardiac index of less than 2.2 L/min/m^2 but without an abnormally elevated PAOP (see Fig. 16–9). These patients usually present without evidence of pulmonary congestion, but the low cardiac index results in signs and symptoms of peripheral hypoperfusion (i.e., decreased urine output, weakness, peripheral vasoconstriction, weak pulses). The mortality rate of subset III patients is reported to be four times higher than that of patients without hypoperfusion.[132] Although the treatment goal is to alleviate signs and symptoms of hypoperfusion by increasing cardiac index and perfusion to essential organs, therapy will differ among patients. If the PAOP is significantly below 15 mm Hg, initial therapy will be to administer intravenous fluids to provide a more optimal left ventricular filling pressure of 15 to 18 mm Hg and consequently improve cardiac index. When there is only mild left ventricular dysfunction, intravenous fluid administration may be all that is necessary to achieve a cardiac index above 2.2 L/min/m^2. However, many patients will have significant left ventricular dysfunction and a depressed Frank-Starling relationship despite adequate preload (i.e., PAOP of 15 to 18 mm Hg). In these patients, intravenously administered positive inotropic agents (e.g., dobutamine, milrinone) and/or arterial vasodilators (e.g., nitroprusside or nitroglycerin) are often necessary to achieve an adequate cardiac index. It is noteworthy that some positive inotropic medications also will have arterial vasodilating activity (see specific drug classes that follow).

Current guidelines recommend intravenous inotropes for symptom relief or end-organ dysfunction in patients with left ventricular dysfunction and low cardiac output syndrome. Such therapy may be especially useful in patients with low systolic blood pressure (less than 90 mm Hg) or symptomatic hypotension in the setting of adequate filling pressures. As previously discussed (see Subset II above), inotropic therapy may be considered in patients who do not tolerate or respond to intravenous vasodilators or patients with worsening renal function. As with vasodilators, inotrope administration requires frequent blood pressure monitoring as well as continuous monitoring for arrhythmias. If arrhythmias arise, dose reduction or discontinuation of inotropic therapy should occur. Also, these agents should be avoided in patients with low left-heart filling pressures. Given the potential risks associated with inotropic therapy, vasodilators should be considered prior to using inotropes.[124]

In general, inotropic therapy should not be used in the broad decompensated heart failure population. They are useful to increase cardiac output in the patients described above. These agents may be used to "bridge" patients with cardiogenic shock to heart transplantation or left ventricular assist device. Inotropes may also be used as palliative therapy to improve functional status and quality of life in patients who are not considered optimal candidates for these definitive therapies.[124]

Subset IV Patients with a cardiac index of less than 2.2 L/min/m^2 and a PAOP higher than 18 mm Hg are in hemodynamic subset IV. These patients have the worst prognosis of any subset and illustrate the typical hemodynamic profile for the patient hospitalized for severe heart failure.

Because of severe pump failure, these patients cannot maintain an adequate cardiac index despite the elevated left ventricular filling pressure and increased myocardial fiber stretch. These patients will present with signs and symptoms of both "wet" and low-output heart failure. The treatment goals are to alleviate these signs and symptoms by increasing cardiac index above 2.2 L/min/m^2 and reducing PAOP to 15 to 18 mm Hg while maintaining an adequate mean arterial pressure. Thus therapy will involve a combination of agents used for subset II and subset III patients to achieve these goals (i.e., combination of diuretic plus positive inotrope). These targets may be difficult to achieve and will necessitate careful monitoring and individualization of drug therapy. Nitroprusside is a particularly useful agent in this setting because of its mixed arterial–venous vasodilating effects. In the presence of significant hypotension, inotropic agents with vasopressor activity may be required initially to achieve an adequate perfusion pressure to essential organs and can then be combined, if necessary, with diuretics and/or vasodilators to obtain the desired hemodynamic effects and clinical response.

■ PHARMACOLOGIC THERAPY OF ACUTE DECOMPENSATED HEART FAILURE

⓫ Unfortunately, the treatment of decompensated heart failure has not improved substantially in the past decade in large part because of the lack of clinical trial data in this population. The pharmacotherapeutic agents used to treat patients with decompensated heart failure rarely, if ever, produce a single cardiovascular action. Even when intended for a single purpose (e.g., a positive inotrope), other drug effects (tachycardia, vasodilation, or vasoconstriction) may either add to the therapeutic effect or cause adverse events that negate or even outweigh the intended therapeutic benefit. It often can be difficult to anticipate how an individual patient will respond to a given intervention. For this reason, hemodynamic monitoring can be useful, and many drugs are considered first-line therapy due in part to their short half-lives and ease of titration. The description of expected drug actions outlined below should be viewed as a general guide to the clinician, who must continuously reassess the

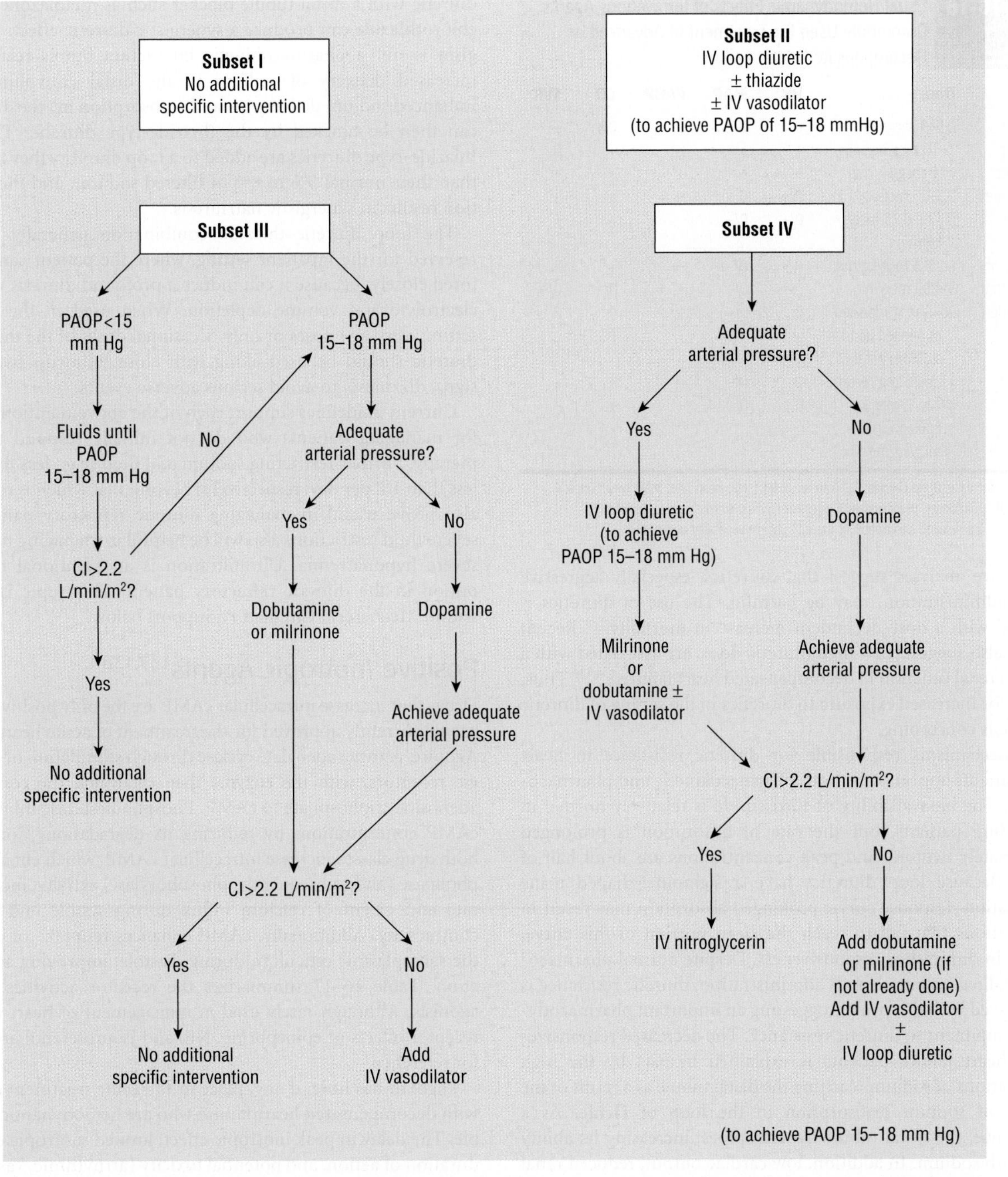

FIGURE 16-10. General treatment algorithm for patients with advanced/decompensated heart failure based on hemodynamic monitoring and hemodynamic subsets. IV vasodilators that may be used include nitroglycerin, nesiritide, or nitroprusside. See text for details. (CI, cardiac index; PAOP, pulmonary artery occlusive pressure.)

patient for desired outcomes. Table 16–16 contains a summary of the expected hemodynamic effects of the various drugs discussed below (see also Chap. 25).

Diuretics[44,133,134]

Intravenous loop diuretics, including furosemide, bumetanide, and torsemide, are used in the management of decompensated heart failure, with furosemide being the most widely studied and used agent in this setting. Bolus administration of diuretics decreases preload within 5 to 15 minutes by functional venodilation and later (>20 minutes) via sodium and water excretion, thereby improving pulmonary congestion. However, the acute reduction in venous return may severely compromise effective preload in patients with significant diastolic dysfunction or intravascular depletion. This results in a reflex increase in sympathetic activation, renin release, NE, and AVP elevations and the expected consequences of arteriolar and coronary constriction, tachycardia, and increased PAOP and myocardial oxygen consumption. Unlike arterial dilators and positive inotropic agents, diuretics do not cause an upward shift in the Frank-Starling curve or increase cardiac index significantly in most patients (see Table 16–16). Excessive preload reduction with diuretics can lead to a decline in cardiac output (see Fig. 16–3). Consequently, diuretics must be used judiciously to obtain the desired improvement in symptoms of congestion while avoiding a reduction in cardiac output, symptomatic hypotension, or worsening renal function. Although counterintuitive, renal function may also improve in the setting of diuresis.

Diuretic Resistance Occasionally, patients respond poorly to large doses of loop diuretics, and heart failure is the most common clinical setting in which diuretic resistance is observed. Data from

TABLE 16-16 Usual Hemodynamic Effects of Intravenous Agents Commonly Used for Treatment of Advanced or Decompensated Heart Failure[a]

Drug	Dose	HR	MAP	PAOP	CO	SVR
Dopamine	0.5–3 mcg/kg/min	0	0	0	0/+	–
Dopamine	3–10 mcg/kg/min	+	+	0	+	0
Dopamine	>10 mcg/kg/min	+	+	+	+	+
Dobutamine	2.5–20 mcg/kg/min	0/+	0	–	+	–
Milrinone	0.375–0.75 mcg/kg/min	0/+	0/–	–	+	–
Nitroprusside	0.25–3 mcg/kg/min	0/+	0/–	–	+	–
Nitroglycerin	5–200 mcg/min	0/+	0/–	–	0/+	0/–
Furosemide	20–80 mg, repeated as needed up to six times per day	0	0/–	–	0	0
Enalaprilat	1.25–2.5 mg q6-8h	0	0/–	–	+	+
Nesiritide	bolus: 2 mcg/kg; infusion 0.01 mcg/kg/min 0	0	0/–	–	+	–

+, increase; –, decrease; 0, no change; CO, cardiac output; HR, heart rate; MAP, mean arterial pressure; PAOP, pulmonary artery occlusion pressure; SVR, systemic vascular resistance.
[a]See text for a more detailed description of the interpatient variability in response.

retrospective analyses suggest that diuretics, especially aggressive diuretic administration, may be harmful. The use of diuretics is associated with a dose-dependent increase in mortality.[135] Recent evidence also suggests that high diuretic doses are associated with a decline in renal function in decompensated heart failure.[134,136] Thus, the need for increased exposure to diuretics in the setting of diuretic resistance is concerning.

The mechanisms responsible for diuretic resistance in heart failure patients appear to be both pharmacokinetic and pharmacodynamic. The bioavailability of furosemide is relatively normal in heart failure patients, but the rate of absorption is prolonged approximately twofold, and peak concentrations are about half of normal. Because loop diuretics have a sigmoidal-shaped urine concentration–response curve, prolonged absorption may result in concentrations that fail to reach the steep portion of this curve, resulting in diminished responsiveness. Despite normal pharmacokinetics following intravenous administration, diuretic resistance is also observed with this route, suggesting an important pharmacodynamic component to diuretic resistance. The decreased responsiveness in heart failure patients is explained in part by the high concentrations of sodium reaching the distal tubule as a result of the blockade of sodium reabsorption in the loop of Henle. As a consequence, the distal tubule hypertrophies, increasing its ability to reabsorb sodium. In addition, low cardiac output, reduced renal perfusion, and subsequent decreased delivery of drug to the kidney may also contribute to resistance.

Several maneuvers can be attempted to overcome diuretic resistance. Treatment of heart failure with other agents (e.g., positive inotropes or afterload reducers) may improve diuresis by increasing cardiac output and renal perfusion. Administration of low doses of dopamine with the hope of enhancing diuresis is also a common practice. However, data suggest that addition of dopamine to furosemide provides no additional diuresis.[124] Larger intravenous bolus doses of diuretics may achieve concentrations closer to the top of the concentration–response curve, or a continuous intravenous infusion may be used to maintain more constant concentrations in the steep portion of the concentration–response curve. Studies of continuous-infusion furosemide suggest a greater natriuretic effect and no difference in metabolic adverse effects when compared with the same total daily dose given by intravenous bolus.[124] Continuous infusions also may limit adverse hemodynamic events.

Another approach to improving diuresis is addition of a second diuretic with a different mechanism of action. Combining a loop diuretic with a distal tubule blocker such as metolazone or hydrochlorothiazide can produce a synergistic diuretic effect. The synergism is not a pharmacokinetic interaction but is related to the increased delivery of sodium to the distal convoluted tubule. Enhanced sodium delivery to (and reabsorption in) the distal tubule can then be blocked by the thiazide-type diuretic. Thus, when thiazide-type diuretics are added to a loop diuretic, they block more than their normal 5% to 8% of filtered sodium, and the combination results in synergistic natriuresis.

The loop diuretic–thiazide combination generally should be reserved for the inpatient setting, where the patient can be monitored closely, because it can induce a profound diuresis with severe electrolyte and volume depletion. When used in the outpatient setting, very low doses or only occasional doses of the thiazide-type diuretic should be used along with close followup (weight, vital signs, dizziness) to avoid serious adverse events.

Current guidelines support each of the above mentioned options for managing patients who do not initially respond to diuretic therapy. Further restricting sodium and fluid (e.g., less than 1 g and less than 1 L per day, respectively) beyond that which is routine may also prove useful in managing diuretic refractory patients. Such severe fluid restrictions also will be helpful in managing moderate to severe hyponatremia. Ultrafiltration is an additional therapeutic option in the diuretic refractory patient. This topic is discussed within Mechanical Circulatory Support below.

Positive Inotropic Agents[137,138]

Drugs that increase intracellular cAMP are the only positive inotropic agents currently approved for the treatment of acute heart failure. β-Agonists activate adenylate cyclase through stimulation of β-adrenergic receptors, with the enzyme then catalyzing the conversion of adenosine triphosphate to cAMP. Phosphodiesterase inhibitors raise cAMP concentrations by reducing its degradation. Consequently, both drug classes increase intracellular cAMP, which enhances phospholipase (and, subsequently, phosphorylase) activity, increasing the rate and extent of calcium influx during systole and enhancing contractility. Additionally, cAMP enhances reuptake of calcium by the sarcoplasmic reticulum during diastole, improving active relaxation. Table 16–17 summarizes the receptor activities of the β-agonists. Although rarely used in management of heart failure, the receptor effects of epinephrine, NE, and isoproterenol are provided for reference.

Digoxin has little, if any, place in the acute treatment of patients with decompensated heart failure who are hemodynamically unstable. The delay in peak inotropic effect, limited inotropic effect, long duration of action, and potential toxicity (arrhythmic, vasoconstrictive, neurologic) are disadvantages in the acute setting. However, in patients with acute decompensation who are taking digoxin as part of their chronic therapy, it is generally unnecessary to adjust the dose or discontinue its use unless changes in renal function increase the risk of toxicity.

Although a number of parenteral agents have been used for the treatment of patients with decompensated heart failure, dobutamine and milrinone have emerged as the two drugs most commonly

TABLE 16-17 Relative Effects of Adrenergic Drugs on Receptors

Drug	α_1	β_1	β_2	$Dopamine_1$
Norepinephrine	++++	++++	0	0
Epinephrine	++++	++++	++	0
Dopamine[a]	++++	++++	++	++
Isoproterenol	0	++++	++++	0
Dobutamine[b]	+	++++	++	0

[a]See text for a more detailed description of the dose-dependent hemodynamic effects.
[b]Combined effects of the commercially available racemic mixture (see text).

administered. These drugs differ in their mechanism of action and resulting pharmacologic effects and provide advantages and disadvantages in any given patient.

Dobutamine Dobutamine, a synthetic catecholamine, is a β_1- and β_2-receptor agonist with some α_1-agonist effects (see Table 16–17). Unlike dopamine, dobutamine does not cause release of NE from nerve terminals. The overall hemodynamic effects of dobutamine are the result of its effects on adrenergic receptors and reflex-mediated actions. Its β_2-receptor-mediated effects are greater than those of dopamine, and β_2-receptor-mediated vasodilation will tend to offset some of the α_1-receptor-mediated vasoconstriction. Thus the net vascular effect is usually vasodilation. The positive inotropy is primarily a β_1-receptor mediated effect. Cardiac β_1-receptor stimulation by dobutamine causes an increase in contractility but generally no significant change in heart rate and may provide an explanation for the apparently more modest chronotropic actions of dobutamine compared with dopamine.

The overall hemodynamic effects of dobutamine are those of a potent inotropic agent with vasodilating action. Initial doses of 2.5 to 5 mcg/kg per minute can be increased progressively to 20 mcg/kg/min based on clinical and hemodynamic responses. The onset of action is within minutes; however, peak effects may take 10 minutes to become evident. Dobutamine has a half-life of 2 minutes. Cardiac index is increased because of inotropic stimulation, arterial vasodilation, and a variable increase in heart rate. Because of the offsetting changes in arteriolar resistance and cardiac index, dobutamine usually will cause relatively little change in mean arterial pressure although these effects may be variable. This is compared with the more consistent increase observed with dopamine. Dobutamine's vasodilating action usually can decrease PAOP, making it particularly useful in the presence of low cardiac index and an elevated left ventricular filling pressure, or detrimental in the presence of a reduced filling pressure. Unfortunately, an increase in oxygen consumption with dobutamine has been demonstrated in patients with both ischemic and nonischemic cardiomyopathy. The major adverse effect of dobutamine is tachycardia. Although concern over attenuation of dobutamine's hemodynamic effects has been raised with prolonged administration, some effect is likely still retained. And thus, dobutamine dose should be tapered rather than abruptly discontinued.

In some patients, dobutamine (or milrinone) dose reduction or discontinuation results in acute decompensation and these patients may then require placement of an indwelling intravenous catheter for continuous therapy. This approach may be used to "bridge" patients awaiting cardiac transplantation, and may also be used to facilitate the discharge of patients who are not transplant candidates, but who cannot be weaned from inotrope therapy. In this latter group, the use of continuous outpatient dobutamine therapy is for palliative use only and should only be considered after multiple unsuccessful attempts to maximize oral therapy and discontinue inotrope therapy. Although effective for symptom palliation, it should be realized that the risk of mortality is likely increased. In contrast, the use of regularly scheduled intermittent dobutamine infusions at home or in an outpatient clinic is not recommended in the current guidelines.[124]

Milrinone Milrinone is a bipyridine derivative that inhibits phosphodiesterase III, an enzyme responsible for the breakdown of cAMP to adenosine monophosphate. Milrinone has supplanted the use of amrinone, the prototype drug for milrinone, because of the more frequent occurrence of thrombocytopenia with amrinone. Both positive inotropic and arterial and venous vasodilating effects contribute to the therapeutic response in heart failure patients; hence milrinone has been referred to as an *inodilator*. The relative balance of these pharmacologic effects may vary with dose and underlying cardiovascular pathology.

During intravenous administration, there is an increase in stroke volume (and, therefore, cardiac output) with little change in heart rate (see Table 16–16). Despite the increase in cardiac index, mean arterial pressure may remain constant as a result of a concomitant decrease in arteriolar resistance. In contrast, the vasodilating effects may predominate and lead to a decrease in blood pressure and a reflex tachycardia. Like dobutamine, milrinone lowers PAOP by venodilation and thus is particularly useful in patients with a low cardiac index and an elevated left ventricular filling pressure. Such a reduction in preload, however, can be hazardous for patients without excessive filling pressure (especially those with symptoms of "dry" heart failure), leading to a decrease in cardiac index. Such an effect would blunt the improvement in cardiac output that would otherwise be produced by the positive inotropic and arterial dilating actions. Milrinone should be used cautiously as a single agent in severely hypotensive heart failure patients because it will not increase, and may even decrease, arterial blood pressure. The results of controlled studies comparing dobutamine with milrinone indicate that these agents produce generally similar hemodynamic effects. A clinically insignificant but greater increase in heart rate with dobutamine is the most consistent difference in these studies.

Milrinone has a longer terminal elimination half-life than adrenergic agonists. The average milrinone half-life in healthy subjects is about 1 hour and approximately 3 hours in patients with heart failure. This long elimination half-life may be a disadvantage in this patient population because a loading dose may be necessary to obtain a prompt initial response, minute-to-minute titrations in dose cannot be made based on response, and adverse effects (arrhythmias or hypotension) will persist longer after drug discontinuation. The usual loading dose for milrinone is 50 mcg/kg administered over 10 minutes. However, if rapid hemodynamic changes are unnecessary, the loading dose should be eliminated because of the risk of hypotension. Thus, most patients are simply started on the maintenance infusion without a preceding bolus dose. The maintenance infusion for milrinone is 0.25 mcg/kg/min (up to 0.75 mcg/kg/min). Milrinone is excreted unchanged in urine, and thus, its infusion rate should be decreased by 50% to 70% in patients with significant renal impairment.

The most notable adverse events associated with milrinone are arrhythmia, hypotension, and thrombocytopenia. Although the incidence of thrombocytopenia associated with milrinone therapy is rare, patients should still have platelet counts determined before and during therapy.

The combination of dobutamine and milrinone is expected to produce additive effects on cardiac index and PAOP reduction, suggesting this regimen as an option in patients who have dose-limiting adverse effects with either class of drugs. It is unclear, however, if this combination provides a therapeutic advantage over the combination of a positive inotrope and a traditional pure vasodilator such as nitroprusside.

One study with milrinone points out the risk associated with routine administration of inotropic therapy to a broad population of patients admitted to the hospital with an acute exacerbation of heart failure. Although this approach is not supported by clinical trial data, many patients without signs or symptoms of hypoperfusion receive milrinone or other inotropic therapy with the belief that the hemodynamic effects may shorten hospitalization and improve clinical outcomes. Designed to evaluate this strategy, the Outcomes of a Prospective Trial of Intravenous Milrinone for Exacerbations of Chronic Heart Failure (OPTIME-CHF) trial was a randomized, double-blind trial comparing the effects of milrinone and placebo in patients hospitalized with an acute exacerbation of chronic heart failure who, in the investigator's opinion, did not require inotropic therapy.[122] The 949 patients received a 48-hour infusion of milrinone 0.5 mcg/kg/min with no loading dose or placebo. No difference between milrinone and placebo was found in the primary end point of the number of days patients were hospitalized for cardiovascular causes within 60 days of randomization. However, adverse events were more common in the milrinone group. Sustained hypotension requiring intervention (10.7% vs. 3.2%; $P < 0.001$) and new onset of atrial fibrillation or flutter (4.6% vs. 1.5%; $P = 0.004$) occurred more frequently in patients receiving milrinone.

Recently, data from the ADHERE Registry (n = 15,230) was used to compare in-hospital mortality with intravenous nitroglycerin, nesiritide, milrinone, and dobutamine. After adjusting for baseline parameters that predict in-hospital mortality, both dobutamine- and milrinone-treated patients had a higher in-hospital mortality when compared to patients receiving either nitroglycerin or nesiritide ($P < 0.005$). There was no difference in in-hospital mortality between nitroglycerin- and nesiritide-treated patients ($P = 0.58$). In-hospital mortality was higher in patients receiving dobutamine compared to milrinone ($P = 0.027$).[139]

These results add to the growing concern about the use of inotropic drugs in patients with decompensated heart failure and strongly suggest that milrinone, and probably other inotropes, should not be routinely used for the treatment of acute heart failure exacerbations. Although the routine use of milrinone should be discouraged, clinicians should be aware that inotropic therapy may be needed in selected patients such as those with low cardiac output states with organ hypoperfusion or with cardiogenic shock. Generally, milrinone should be considered for patients who are receiving chronic β-blocker therapy because its positive inotropic effect does not involve stimulation of β-receptors. In contrast to dobutamine, milrinone's positive hemodynamic effects persist despite concomitant β-blocker therapy.

Dopamine Although dopamine generally should be avoided in the treatment of decompensated heart failure, the only clinical scenario where its pharmacologic actions may be preferable to dobutamine or milrinone is in the patient with marked systemic hypotension or cardiogenic shock in the face of elevated ventricular filling pressures, where dopamine in doses greater than 5 mcg/kg per minute may be necessary to raise central aortic pressure. However, there are no data to support this commonly employed practice.

Dopamine, the endogenous precursor of NE, exerts its effects by directly stimulating adrenergic receptors, as well as causing release of NE from adrenergic nerve terminals. Dopamine produces dose-dependent hemodynamic effects because of its relative affinity for α_1-, β_1-, β_2-, and D_1- (vascular dopaminergic) receptors (see Table 16–17). The following dose-dependent actions are intended as a general guide to the clinician.

Positive inotropic effects mediated primarily by β_1-receptors become more prominent with dopamine doses of 2 to 5 mcg/kg/min. Cardiac index is increased because of an increase in stroke volume and a variable increase in heart rate, which is partially dose dependent. There is usually little change in SVR, presumably because neither vasodilation (D_1- and β_2-receptor mediated) nor vasoconstriction (α_1-receptor mediated) predominates. At doses between 5 and 10 mcg/kg/min, chronotropic and α_1-receptor–mediated vasoconstricting effects become more prominent. Mean arterial pressure usually increases because of an increase in both cardiac index and SVR (see Table 16–16). The vasoconstricting effects of higher doses could indirectly limit the increase in cardiac index by increasing afterload and PAOP, thus complicating the management of patients with preexisting high afterload. In such patients, alternative agents (dobutamine, milrinone) or the addition of diuretics and/or vasodilators may be necessary.

Dopamine, particularly at higher doses, may alter several parameters that increase myocardial oxygen demand (increased heart rate, contractility, and systolic pressure) and potentially decrease myocardial blood flow (coronary vasoconstriction and increased wall tension), worsening ischemia in some patients with coronary disease. As with dobutamine and milrinone, arrhythmogenesis is also more common at higher doses.

Vasodilators[134,140]

Activation of the SNS, the RAAS, AVP, and other mediators all cause vasoconstriction and increased SVR. In patients with heart failure, stroke volume varies inversely with SVR such that an increase in peripheral resistance leads to a severe decline in stroke volume and cardiac output (see Fig. 16–1).

Vasodilators typically are described by their prominent site of action (arterial or venous). Arterial vasodilators act as impedance-reducing agents, reducing afterload and a reflexive increase in cardiac output. Venodilators act as preload reducers by increasing venous capacitance, reducing symptoms of pulmonary congestion in patients with high cardiac filling pressures. Mixed vasodilators act on both resistance and capacitance vessels, reducing congestive symptoms while increasing cardiac output. Nitroprusside, nitroglycerin, and nesiritide are the most commonly used intravenous vasodilating agents in decompensated heart failure.

Nitroprusside Sodium nitroprusside, a mixed arterial–venous vasodilator, acts on vascular smooth muscle, increasing synthesis of nitric oxide to produce its balanced vasodilating action. As such, it both increases cardiac index and decreases venous pressure. Nitroprusside's effects on these parameters are qualitatively similar to those produced by dobutamine and phosphodiesterase inhibitors, despite the fact that it has no direct inotropic activity (see Table 16–16). However, nitroprusside generally causes a greater decrease in PAOP, SVR, and blood pressure than these agents. Mean arterial pressure may remain fairly constant but often decreases depending on the relative increase in cardiac output and reduction in arteriolar tone. Hypotension is an important dose-limiting adverse effect of nitroprusside and other vasodilators. Consequently, this drug is used primarily in patients who have a significantly elevated SVR and often requires invasive hemodynamic monitoring.

Patients with normal left ventricular function will not have an increase in stroke volume when SVR falls because the normal ventricle is fairly insensitive to small changes in afterload. Consequently, these patients experience a significant decrease in blood pressure after administration of arterial vasodilators. This explains why nitroprusside is a potent antihypertensive agent in patients without heart failure but causes less hypotension and reflex tachycardia in patients with left ventricular dysfunction. Nonetheless, even a modest increase in heart rate could have adverse consequences in patients with underlying ischemic heart disease and/or resting tachycardia, and close monitoring is necessary during therapy.

Nitroprusside has been studied extensively and shown to be effective in the short-term management of patients with severe heart failure in a variety of settings (i.e., acute MI, valvular regurgitation, after coronary bypass surgery, decompensated chronic heart failure). Generally, nitroprusside will not worsen, and may improve, the balance between myocardial oxygen demand and supply. This is mainly a result of a decrease in oxygen demand caused by the lowering of left ventricular wall tension and a possible increase in subendocardial blood flow resulting from decreased left ventricular end-diastolic pressure. However, an excessive decrease in systemic arterial pressure can reduce coronary perfusion and worsen ischemia, leading to increased risk of coronary steal.

Nitroprusside has a rapid onset of action and a duration of action of less than 10 minutes, necessitating its administration by continuous intravenous infusion. This allows for precise dose titration based on measured clinical and hemodynamic parameters. It, like other vasodilators used in heart failure, should be initiated at a low dose (0.1 to 0.2 mcg/kg/min) to avoid excessive hypotension and then increased by small increments (0.1 to 0.2 mcg/kg/min) every 5 to 10 minutes as needed and tolerated. Effective doses usually range from 0.5 to 3.0 mcg/kg/min. A rebound phenomenon has been reported after abrupt withdrawal of nitroprusside in patients with heart failure and is apparently caused by reflex neurohormonal activation during therapy. If renal perfusion pressure is compromised by the drug, salt and water retention can contribute to volume expansion and tachyphylaxis; this is seen typically only in patients with chronic hypertension, baseline azotemia, or when therapeutic augmentation of cardiac output during therapy is minimal. When stopping nitroprusside and switching to oral drugs, it is usually advisable to taper doses slowly. Nitroprusside can cause cyanide and thiocyanate toxicity, but these are very unlikely when doses less than 3 mcg/kg/min are administered for less than 3 days, except in patients with a serum creatinine level greater than 3 mg/dL.

Given the potent pulmonary vasodilatory effects of nitroprusside as well as its short half-life, this agent is frequently used to determine reversibility of pulmonary hypertension in patients being assessed for heart transplantation. This is the most common use of nitroprusside for the management of decompensated heart failure.

Nitroglycerin Intravenous nitroglycerin is often considered the preferred agent for preload reduction in patients with severe heart failure. Because of its short half-life, intravenous nitroglycerin is administered by continuous infusion. Its major hemodynamic actions are reductions in preload and PAOP via functional venodilation and mild arterial vasodilation that is particularly evident in patients with heart failure and elevated SVR or when given in doses approaching 200 mcg/min (see Table 16–16). Intravenous nitroglycerin is used primarily as a preload reducer for patients with pulmonary congestion. In higher doses, nitroglycerin displays potent coronary vasodilating properties and beneficial effects on myocardial oxygen demand and supply, making it the vasodilator of choice for patients with severe heart failure and ischemic heart disease.

Nitroglycerin should be initiated at a dose of 5 to 10 mcg/min (0.1 mcg/kg/min) and increased every 5 to 10 minutes as necessary and tolerated. Hypotension and an excessive decrease in PAOP are important dose-limiting side effects. Maintenance doses usually vary from 35 to 200 mcg/min (0.5 to 3.0 mcg/kg/min). Tolerance to the hemodynamic effects of nitroglycerin may develop over 12 to 72 hours of continuous administration, but some patients have a sustained response. Neither nitroglycerin nor nitroprusside should be used in the presence of elevated intracranial pressure because either may worsen cerebral edema in this setting.

Nesiritide Nesiritide is the first new drug approved for the treatment of decompensated heart failure since milrinone. Manufactured by recombinant techniques, it is identical to the endogenous human BNP secreted by the ventricular myocardium in response to volume overload. Exogenous administration of nesiritide mimics the vasodilatory and natriuretic actions of the endogenous peptide by stimulating the natriuretic peptide receptor A which leads to increased levels of cyclic guanosine monophosphate in target tissues. Nesiritide produces dose-dependent venous and arterial vasodilation, increases in cardiac output, natriuresis, and diuresis, and decreases cardiac filling pressures, SNS and RAAS activity. Unlike nitroglycerin or dobutamine, tolerance does not develop to nesiritide's pharmacologic actions. It does not affect cAMP or stimulate β-receptors, mechanisms that are thought to contribute to the myocardial toxicity associated with the positive inotropic drugs. Thus, nesiritide does not have the proarrhythmic effects associated with dobutamine. Nesiritide is eliminated by several pathways including the natriuretic peptide receptor C on target tissues, proteolytic cleavage by neutral endopeptidase, and renal filtration. Its elimination half-life of 18 minutes is considerably longer than that of other vasodilators or β-agonists.

The Vasodilation in the Management of Acute CHF (VMAC) trial was a randomized, double-blind trial that compared the effects of nesiritide, IV nitroglycerin, and placebo in patients with decompensated heart failure and dyspnea who were receiving standard background therapy.[123] Patients received pulmonary artery catheterization at the discretion of the investigators. The primary end points were the patient's self-assessment of dyspnea (all patients) and the change in PAOP at 3 hours after the start of the study drug infusion (only in patients with a pulmonary artery catheter) compared to placebo. Although nesiritide reduced dyspnea at 3 hours compared to placebo, no difference between nesiritide and nitroglycerin was found.

The precise role of nesiritide in the pharmacotherapy of decompensated heart failure remains controversial. Some of this controversy centers on the marginal lack of improvement in mortality or other clinical outcomes with nesiritide compared to nitroglycerin (or nitroprusside) balanced against nesiritide's significantly greater costs (~$450 for a 24-hour nesiritide infusion compared to $10 to $15 for nitroglycerin). In addition, two recent meta-analyses suggest an increased risk of worsening renal function, as well as an increase in mortality with nesiritide.[141,142] The authors of these studies concluded that these finding are hypothesis generating and should be further investigated. More recently, the safety of nesiritide in 303 patients with a low LVEF (<40%) who were undergoing coronary artery bypass surgery was evaluated in the multicenter, randomized, placebo-controlled Nesiritide Administered Peri-Anesthesia in Patients Undergoing Cardiac Surgery (NAPA) study.[143] Patients received intravenous nesiritide 0.01 mcg/kg/min or placebo in the perianesthesia period and the infusion continued for 24 to 96 hours at the investigator's discretion. Serum creatinine increased and glomerular filtration rate decreased after surgery compared with preoperative values in both treatment groups. However, the changes in creatinine and glomerular filtration rate were significantly greater in placebo-treated patients. In contrast, the mean hospital length of stay was significantly shorter and the 180-day mortality rate was significantly lower in the nesiritide group. To clarify these issues about the safety and efficacy of nesiritide, its manufacturer is conducting an additional prospective randomized controlled trial.

■ MECHANICAL CIRCULATORY SUPPORT[144]

Intraaortic Balloon Pump

The intraaortic balloon pump (IABP) is a frequently used form of mechanical circulatory assistance and typically is employed in patients with advanced heart failure who do not respond adequately to drug therapy, such as those with intractable myocardial ischemia or patients in cardiogenic shock. The IABP consists of a polyethylene balloon mounted on a catheter that is usually inserted percutaneously into the femoral artery and the balloon is then advanced into the descending thoracic aorta. During counterpulsation, the balloon is synchronized with the ECG so that it inflates during diastole and displaces aortic blood thus increasing aortic diastolic pressure and coronary perfusion. The balloon deflates just prior to the opening of the aortic valve during systole and causes a sudden decrease in aortic pressure, allowing the left ventricle to pump against reduced arterial impedance. IABP support results in increased cardiac index, coronary artery perfusion, and myocardial oxygen supply accompanied by decreased myocardial oxygen demand. Thus, it is particularly useful for short-term use in patients with decompensated heart failure in the setting of myocardial ischemia (evolving infarction, patients awaiting emergency coronary bypass surgery). It is also used in hemodynamically unstable patients who are unresponsive to inotropic therapy to stabilize them prior to insertion of a left ventricular assist device that will serve as a bridge to transplantation. Generally, intravenous vasodilators and inotropic agents are used in conjunction with the IABP to maximize hemodynamic and clinical benefits.

Ventricular Assist Devices

A number of ventricular assist devices are available or under investigation. These pumps are surgically implanted and assist, or in some cases replace, the pumping functions of the right and/or left ventricles. A left ventricular assist device (LVAD) removes blood directly from the left ventricle or the left atrium and pumps it to the aorta. The right ventricular assist device works similar to the LVAD and may be used alone or in conjunction with the LVAD.

LVADs can be used in the short-term (days to a couple of weeks) for temporary stabilization of a patient awaiting an intervention to correct the underlying cardiac dysfunction. Alternatively, these devices can be used in the long-term (several months to a couple of years) as a bridge to heart transplantation. More recently, permanent device implantation has become an option for patients who are not heart transplantation candidates.

The REMATCH (Randomized Evaluation of Mechanical Assistance for the Treatment of Congestive Heart Failure) trial randomized 129 patients with decompensated heart failure to LVAD or optimal medical therapy. LVAD patients experienced improved 2-year survival; however, only 23% of these patients were alive at 2 years, compared to only 8% in the medically managed group.[145] The REMATCH trial was responsible for the approval of the use of these devices as "destination" therapy, destination being the last therapeutic option for a given patient. It also raised awareness regarding some of the limitations of these devices. Complications with LVADs include bleeding, air embolism, and right ventricular failure, as well as those complications associated with a major surgical procedure, including infection. In addition, these pumps can cause hemolysis, thrombosis, renal and hepatic dysfunction, and arrhythmias. Finally, device malfunction may occur. Controversy exists regarding the cost of such procedures given the already significant economic impact of this disease state on the healthcare system. Although only a small number of patients were studied, recent research suggests that prolonged unloading of the left ventricle with an LVAD in combination with drug therapy to induce reverse remodeling can produce sustained recovery in left ventricle function and amelioration of symptoms.[146]

For complete heart replacement therapy, the total artificial heart systems continue to be investigated; however, embolic complications, as well as the large size of the currently available systems, are limiting their use. Inserted percutaneously, catheter-based LVADs are a more recent advancement. Although these small pumps may offer an advantage as they avoid the need for open-heart surgery, the technology is still in developmental stages.

Ultrafiltration

Renal dysfunction often occurs in the setting of decompensated heart failure, and thus, renal replacement therapy may be necessary. Ultrafiltration provides an additional modality for fluid removal by rapidly removing salt and water (up to 500 mL/h) in a predictable manner. It reduces PAOP and increases cardiac output and diuresis without adversely affecting blood pressure, heart rate, or renal function. Also, ultrafiltration is proposed to be safer than diuretics because removal of sodium and water is isotonic. Potential candidates for ultrafiltration include patients with diuretic resistance, renal impairment with diuretic administration, and renal impairment despite inotropic therapy. Complications of ultrafiltration include those associated with central venous access, such as infection, as well as those associated with rapid volume removal and intravascular depletion. Electrolyte depletion is not significant, but still requires close monitoring.

Small studies suggest that ultrafiltration is an effective method to remove fluid in heart failure patients and that early initiation prior to intravenous diuretics is effective and safe in reducing hospital length of stay and readmission in diuretic resistant patients. Recently, the Ultrafiltration versus IV Diuretics for Patients Hospitalized for Acute Decompensated Congestive Heart Failure (UNLOAD) trial investigated the effects of early ultrafiltration alone compared to intravenous diuretics alone in 200 patients hospitalized for decompensated heart failure and evidence of fluid overload. The primary end point of weight loss after 48 hours was significantly greater in the ultrafiltration group (5.0 kg) than in the diuretic group (3.1 kg). There was no significant difference between the two treatment groups in the dyspnea score at 48 hours, another primary end point. Compared with the diuretic group, the net fluid loss was significantly greater in the ultrafiltration group (4.6 L vs. 3.3 L) after 48 hours. After 90 days, the incidence and duration of rehospitalization and the incidence of unscheduled office or emergency department visits were significantly lower in patients who were treated using ultrafiltration than in patients who were treated with intravenous diuretics.[147]

■ SURGICAL THERAPY

Orthotopic cardiac transplantation remains the best therapeutic option for patients with chronic, irreversible NYHA class IV heart failure, with a 10-year survival of approximately 50% in well-selected patients.[148] Unfortunately, the shortage of acceptable donor hearts has resulted in long waiting times for transplantation, with many patients succumbing to their disease prior to transplantation. Another large percentage of patients are rejected from consideration for transplantation because of age, concurrent illnesses, psychosocial factors, and other reasons. See Chap. 92 for additional details on cardiac transplantation. The shortage of donor hearts has prompted development of new surgical techniques, including ventricular aneurysm resection, mitral valve repair, and myocardial cell transplantation, which have resulted in variable degrees of symptomatic improvement. Further development of these and other techniques may offer additional options in patients who are not transplantation candidates.

■ PREPARATION FOR HOSPITAL DISCHARGE

For patients who are hospitalized with decompensated heart failure, all factors contributing to decompensation should be addressed. Patients should be near if not at optimal fluid status, transitioned from intravenous to oral diuretic therapy. Both the patient and family should receive appropriate education (see details below). Chronic drug therapy should be optimized and appropriate followup clinic appointments scheduled. Typically, patients should be seen in the clinic in 7 to 10 days following hospital discharge. For patients with recurrent hospital admissions, additional discharge criteria should be considered (Table 16–18).[124]

Patient education is essential in the discharge process and should be multidisciplinary involving input from dietitians, pharmacists, and other healthcare providers. Teaching should promote self-care by incorporating identification of specific positive and negative behaviors. By having a better understand of the key concepts of the disease and its management, patient self-care should improve and future hospitalizations may be avoided.[124]

Although all patients should benefit from education, those with more severe symptoms (NYHA class III or IV) require the most intensive counseling. During a hospitalization, only essential education is recommended, which should be supplemented within a couple of weeks after discharge in the clinic setting. Patients recently hospitalized for heart failure should be considered for referral to a disease-management program.

TABLE 16-18 Discharge Criteria for Patients with Heart Failure

Recommended for all heart failure patients	• Exacerbating factors addressed • At least near-optimal volume status achieved • Transition from intravenous to oral diuretic successfully completed • Patient and family education completed • At least near-optimal pharmacologic therapy achieved • Followup clinic visit scheduled, usually for 7–10 days after discharge
Should be considered for patients with advanced heart failure or recurrent admissions for heart failure	• Oral medication regimen stable for 24 hours • No intravenous vasodilator or inotropic agent for 24 hours • Ambulation before discharge to assess functional capacity after therapy • Plans for postdischarge management (scale present in home, visiting nurse or telephone followup generally no longer than 3 days after discharge) • Referral for disease management

Adapted from Adams KF, Lindenfield J, Arnold JMO, et al. HFSA 2006 comprehensive heart failure practice guidelines. J Card Fail 2006;12:e1–e122.

For patients with end-stage disease, quality of life and prognosis should be discussed with the patient and caregivers. The patient's clinical status should be optimally managed prior to discussing end-of-life care. If possible, this discussion should occur while the patient is still able to participate in the decision-making process. End-of-life care should be considered in patients with persistent symptoms at rest despite multiple attempts to optimize therapy as evidenced by frequent hospitalizations (three or more per year), ongoing limited quality of life, requiring intermittent or continuous intravenous therapy, or consideration of assist devices as destination therapy. In such cases, inactivation of an ICD should be discussed and patients may be considered for hospice services.[124] Integration of a palliative care approach may be necessary. As clinical status deteriorates and medical therapies become ineffective, healthcare providers should transition from focusing on mortality reduction to palliative care.[149]

■ PHARMACOECONOMIC CONSIDERATIONS

Heart failure imposes a tremendous economic burden on the healthcare system. In patients older than age 65 years, it is the most common reason for hospitalization, with hospital admission rates for this disorder continuing to increase. Heart failure is also associated with unacceptably high readmission rates during the 3 to 6 months after initial discharge. Current estimates of costs of heart failure treatment in the United States approach $30 billion with most of the costs associated with hospitalization.[1,4] The prevalence of heart failure and the costs associated with patient care are expected to increase as the population ages and as survival from ischemic heart disease is improved. Thus approaches to improve the quality and cost-effectiveness of care for these patients may have a significant impact on healthcare costs.

Studies to assess the cost-effectiveness of drug therapy for heart failure were recently reviewed.[150] Many studies provide direct cost estimates, demonstrating an economic value when employing standard heart failure therapies, specifically ACE inhibitors, β-blockers, and digoxin. Much of the economic benefit of these therapies is a result of a reduction in hospitalization. While the clinical and economic benefits of these therapies are well-recognized, standard heart failure therapies are often underprescribed. A recent study found that more optimal use of evidence-based therapies with a 10% increase in the use of ACE inhibitors, β-blockers, digoxin, and spironolactone would result in cost savings as a consequence of a reduction in hospitalization.[151] In addition, prescribing optimal doses that approach target doses shown in clinical trials to affect outcomes would have a similar impact. For example, patients receiving high doses versus low doses of ACE inhibitors experienced cost saving as a consequence of fewer heart failure hospitalizations.[152]

More recent pharmacoeconomic studies have focused on the impact of newer heart failure therapies or those used as alternatives to standard therapy. ARBs have been shown to be cost effective in patients not receiving ACE inhibitors.[153] Eplerenone is a cost-effective therapy in patients with post-MI heart failure.[154] Fixed-dose combination hydralazine and isosorbide dinitrate is cost-effective in black patients with severe heart failure.[155] Other cost-effective studies have focused on device therapy. Prophylactic ICD implantation in heart failure patients with systolic dysfunction is cost-effective.[156] Although cost-effectiveness of CRT has been suggested, it was found to be sensitive to changes in several key variables. Thus investigators cautioned that such therapy should not be considered in patients with any comorbid illnesses that may shorten life expectancy.[157] Finally, LVADs as a bridge to heart transplantation were found to be cost-ineffective unless costs associated with their implantation decrease or their clinical benefits increase.[158]

As the management of heart failure has become increasingly complex, the development of disease-management programs approaches that use multidisciplinary teams has been studied extensively. These programs use several broad approaches, including heart failure specialty clinics and/or home-based interventions. Most are multidisciplinary and may include physicians, advanced practice nurses, dieticians, and pharmacists. In general, the programs focus on optimization of drug and nondrug therapy, patient and family education and counseling, exercise and dietary advice, intense followup by telephone or home visits, and monitoring and management of signs and symptoms of decompensation. In general, multidisciplinary disease management programs reduce heart failure and all-cause hospitalizations, mortality, and costs.[159]

⓬ Pharmacists can play an important role in the multidisciplinary team management of heart failure.[160,161] Compared to conventional treatment, pharmacist interventions, that included medication evaluation and therapeutic recommendations, patient education, and followup telephone monitoring, reduced hospitalizations for heart failure. Adherence to guideline-recommended therapy was also improved by pharmacist intervention. A recent study found that pharmacist intervention improved medication adherence and reduced emergency department visits and hospitalizations in low-income patients with heart failure.[162] Thus, the role and cost benefits of pharmacist involvement in the multidisciplinary care of heart failure patients are now apparent and should include optimizing doses of heart failure drug therapy, screening for drugs that exacerbate heart failure, monitoring for adverse drug effects and drug interactions, educating patients, and patient followup.

■ CURRENT CONTROVERSIES

1. For patients with chronic heart failure who remain symptomatic despite standard therapy (ACE inhibitor, β-blocker, diuretic, digoxin), which additive therapy should be used is uncertain. Agents that can be considered are aldosterone antagonists, ARBs, or hydralazine/nitrates. Drug selection should be based on patient-specific criteria (e.g., renal function, ethnicity) that will influence the benefits and risks of each agent.
2. The African American Heart Failure Trial confirmed that the addition of a fixed-dose combination of isosorbide dinitrate and hydralazine to standard background therapy improved survival in African American patients with heart failure. Whether isosorbide/hydralazine is beneficial in non-African American patients is unknown.
3. The optimal pharmacotherapy for patients with acute decompensated heart failure who are refractory to diuretic therapy is controversial. Recent meta-analyses suggest that nesiritide use

is associated with worsening renal function and increased mortality. However, the safety of other vasodilators, such as nitroglycerin or nitroprusside, is not well established and the use of positive inotropes is associated with poor outcomes.

EVALUATION OF THERAPEUTIC OUTCOMES

CHRONIC HEART FAILURE

Although mortality is an important end point, it does not give a complete measure of the overall effects of the disease on patient outcomes because many patients are hospitalized repeatedly for heart failure exacerbations and continue to survive. Thus some of the more important therapeutic outcomes in heart failure management, such as prolonged survival or prevention or slowing of the progression of heart failure, cannot be quantified in an individual patient. However, after appropriate diagnostic evaluation to determine the etiology of heart failure, ongoing clinical assessment of patients typically focuses on three general areas: (a) evaluation of functional capacity, (b) evaluation of volume status, and (c) laboratory evaluation.

The evaluation of functional capacity should focus on the presence and severity of symptoms the patient experiences during activities of daily living and how their symptoms affect these activities. Questions directed toward the patient's ability to perform specific activities may be more informative than general questions about what symptoms the patient may be experiencing. For example, ask patients if they can participate in exercise, climb stairs, get dressed without stopping, check the mail, or clean the house. Another important component of assessment of functional capacity is to ask patients what activities they would like to do but are now unable to perform.

Assessment of volume status is a vital component of the ongoing care of patients with heart failure. This evaluation provides the clinician important information about the adequacy of diuretic therapy. Because the cardinal signs and symptoms of heart failure are caused by excess fluid retention, the efficacy of diuretic treatment is readily evaluated by the disappearance of these signs and symptoms. The physical examination is the primary method for the evaluation of fluid retention and specific attention should be focused on the patient's body weight, extent of jugular venous distension, presence of hepatojugular reflux, presence and severity of pulmonary congestion, and peripheral edema. Specifically, in a patient with pulmonary congestion, monitoring is indicated for resolution of rales and pulmonary edema and improvement or resolution of dyspnea on exertion, orthopnea, and paroxysmal nocturnal dyspnea. For patients with systemic congestion, a decrease or disappearance of peripheral edema, jugular venous distension, and hepatojugular reflux is sought. Other therapeutic outcomes include an improvement in exercise tolerance and fatigue, decreased nocturia, and a decrease in heart rate. Clinicians also will want to monitor blood pressure and ensure that the patient does not develop symptomatic hypotension as a result of drug therapy. Body weight is a sensitive marker of fluid loss or retention, and patients should be counseled to weigh themselves daily, reporting changes to their healthcare provider so that adjustments can be made in diuretic doses. It should be noted, particularly with β-blocker therapy, that symptoms may worsen initially and that it may take weeks to months of treatment before patients notice improvement in symptoms. Also, patients and healthcare providers should be aware that heart failure progression may be slowed even though symptoms have not resolved.

Routine monitoring of serum electrolytes and renal function is required in patients with heart failure. Assessment of serum potassium is especially important because hypokalemia is a common adverse effect of diuretic therapy and is associated with an increased risk of arrhythmias and digoxin toxicity. Serum potassium monitoring is also required because of the risk of hyperkalemia associated with ACE inhibitors, ARBs, and aldosterone antagonists. A serum potassium ≥4.0 mEq/L should be maintained with some evidence suggesting it should be ≥4.5 mEq/L.[163] Assessment of renal function (blood urea nitrogen and serum creatinine) is also an important end point for monitoring diuretic and ACE inhibitor therapy. Common causes of worsening renal function in patients with heart failure include overdiuresis, adverse effects of ACE inhibitor or ARB therapy, and hypoperfusion.

ACUTE DECOMPENSATED HEART FAILURE

Assessment of adequacy of therapy in the acute decompensated heart failure patient can be separated into two general categories: initial improvement of physiologic parameters and safe discharge from the intensive care unit following conversion to a chronic oral therapeutic regimen. Both goals must be achieved because hemodynamic improvement has not correlated with prolonged symptom improvement or enhanced survival.

Initial stabilization requires achievement of adequate arterial oxygen saturation and content. Cardiac index and blood pressure must be sufficient to ensure adequate organ perfusion, as assessed by alert mental status, creatinine clearance sufficient to prevent metabolic azotemic complications, hepatic function adequate to maintain synthetic and excretory functions, a stable heart rate and rhythm (predominately sinus rhythm, rate-stabilized atrial fibrillation or flutter, or paced rhythm), absence of ongoing myocardial ischemia or infarction, skeletal muscle and skin blood flow sufficient to prevent ischemic injury, and normal arterial pH (7.34 to 7.47) with a normal serum lactate concentration. Although these goals are achieved most often with a cardiac index greater than 2.2 L/min/m^2, a mean arterial blood pressure greater than 60 mm Hg, and a PAOP of 15 mm Hg or greater, the absolute values are highly variable and depend on chronicity of illness, efficacy of chronic compensatory mechanisms, previous chronic therapy, and concurrent illness.

Discharge from the intensive care unit requires maintenance of the preceding parameters in the absence of ongoing intravenous infusion therapy, mechanical circulatory support, or positive-pressure ventilation. Some patients may achieve this goal with markedly lower blood pressure or higher filling pressure than suggested earlier; hence numerical goals cannot always be substituted for clinical status. Nonpharmacologic treatments aimed at the precipitants of a patient's heart failure exacerbation include permanent pacing, CRT with or without ICD, coronary angioplasty or valvuloplasty, pericardial drainage, cardiac surgery (coronary bypass, valve replacement or reconstruction, closure of intracardiac shunts), or even cardiac transplantation, to achieve initial stabilization, definitive therapy, or both.

ABBREVIATIONS

ACE: angiotensin-converting enzyme

ARB: angiotensin receptor blocker

AVP: arginine vasopressin

BNP: B-type natriuretic peptide

cAMP: cyclic adenosine monophosphate

COX-2: cyclooxygenase-2

CRT: cardiac resynchronization therapy

HFSA: Heart Failure Society of America

IABP: intraaortic balloon pump

ICD: implantable cardioverter-defibrillator

JVD: jugular venous distension

LVAD: left ventricular assist device

LVEF: left ventricular ejection fraction

MI: myocardial infarction

NE: norepinephrine

NSAID: nonsteroidal antiinflammatory drug

NYHA: New York Heart Association

PAOP: pulmonary artery occlusion pressure

RAAS: renin–angiotensin–aldosterone system

SNS: sympathetic nervous system

SVR: systemic vascular resistance

TNF-α: tumor necrosis factor-α

TZD: thiazolidinedione

REFERENCES

1. Hunt SA, Abraham WT, Chin MH, et al. ACC/AHA 2005 guideline update for the diagnosis and management of chronic heart failure in the adult: A report of the American College of Cardiology/American Heart Association Task Force on Practice Guidelines (Writing Committee to Update the 2001 Guidelines for the Evaluation and Management of Heart Failure): Developed in collaboration with the American College of Chest Physicians and the International Society for Heart and Lung Transplantation: Endorsed by the Heart Rhythm Society. Circulation 2005;112:e154–e235.
2. Owan TE, Hodge DO, Herges RM, et al. Trends in prevalence and outcome of heart failure with preserved ejection fraction. N Engl J Med 2006;355:251–259.
3. Gheorghiade M, Sopko G, De Luca L, et al. Navigating the crossroads of coronary artery disease and heart failure. Circulation 2006;114:1202–1213.
4. Rosamond W, Flegal K, Friday G, et al. Heart disease and stroke statistics—2007 update: A report from the American Heart Association Statistics Committee and Stroke Statistics Subcommittee. Circulation 2007;115:e69–e171.
5. Levy D, Kenchaiah S, Larson MG, et al. Long-term trends in the incidence of and survival with heart failure. N Engl J Med 2002;347:1397–1402.
6. Jessup M, Brozena S. Heart failure. N Engl J Med 2003;348:2007–2018.
7. Levy WC, Mozaffarian D, Linker DT, et al. The Seattle Heart Failure Model: Prediction of survival in heart failure. Circulation 2006;113:1424–1433.
8. Colucci W, Braunwald E. Pathophysiology of heart failure. In: Zipes DP, Libby P, Bonow RO, Braunwald E, eds. Heart Disease: A Textbook of Cardiovascular Medicine, 7th ed. Philadelphia: Elsevier Saunders, 2005:509–538.
9. Richard P, Villard E, Charron P, Isnard R. The genetic bases of cardiomyopathies. J Am Coll Cardiol 2006;48:A79–A89.
10. Mann DL, Bristow MR. Mechanisms and models in heart failure: The biomechanical model and beyond. Circulation 2005;111:2837–2849.
11. Small KM, Wagoner LE, Levin AM, et al. Synergistic polymorphisms of beta$_1$- and alpha$_{2C}$-adrenergic receptors and the risk of congestive heart failure. N Engl J Med 2002;347:1135–1142.
12. Patterson JH. Angiotensin II receptor blockers in heart failure. Pharmacotherapy 2003;23:173–182.
13. Wong J, Patel RA, Kowey PR. The clinical use of angiotensin-converting enzyme inhibitors. Prog Cardiovasc Dis 2004;47:116–130.
14. Weber KT. The proinflammatory heart failure phenotype: A case of integrative physiology. Am J Med Sci 2005;330:219–226.
15. Weber KT. Aldosterone in congestive heart failure. N Engl J Med 2001;345:1689–1697.
16. Pitt B, Zannad F, Remme WJ, et al. The effect of spironolactone on morbidity and mortality in patients with severe heart failure. Randomized Aldactone Evaluation Study Investigators. N Engl J Med 1999;341:709–717.
17. Pitt B, Remme W, Zannad F, et al. Eplerenone, a selective aldosterone blocker, in patients with left ventricular dysfunction after myocardial infarction. N Engl J Med 2003;348:1309–1321.
18. Felker GM, Petersen JW, Mark DB. Natriuretic peptides in the diagnosis and management of heart failure. CMAJ 2006;175:611–617.
19. Greenberg A, Verbalis JG. Vasopressin receptor antagonists. Kidney Int 2006;69:2124–2130.
20. Schrier RW, Gross P, Gheorghiade M, et al. Tolvaptan, a selective oral vasopressin V2-receptor antagonist, for hyponatremia. N Engl J Med 2006;355:2099–2112.
21. Konstam MA, Gheorghiade M, Burnett JC Jr, et al. Effects of oral tolvaptan in patients hospitalized for worsening heart failure: The EVEREST Outcome Trial. JAMA 2007;297:1319–1331.
22. Gheorghiade M, Konstam MA, Burnett JC, Jr, et al. Short-term clinical effects of tolvaptan, an oral vasopressin antagonist, in patients hospitalized for heart failure: The EVEREST Clinical Status Trials. JAMA 2007;297:1332–1343.
23. Mann DL. Inflammatory mediators and the failing heart: Past, present, and the foreseeable future. Circ Res 2002;91:988–998.
24. Laufs U, Custodis F, Bohm M. HMG-CoA reductase inhibitors in chronic heart failure: Potential mechanisms of benefit and risk. Drugs 2006;66:145–154.
25. Tsuyuki RT, McKelvie RS, Arnold JM, et al. Acute precipitants of congestive heart failure exacerbations. Arch Intern Med 2001;161:2337–2342.
26. Wang TJ, Larson MG, Levy D, et al. Temporal relations of atrial fibrillation and congestive heart failure and their joint influence on mortality: The Framingham Heart Study. Circulation 2003;107:2920–2925.
27. Olsson LG, Swedberg K, Ducharme A, et al. Atrial fibrillation and risk of clinical events in chronic heart failure with and without left ventricular systolic dysfunction: Results from the Candesartan in Heart Failure Assessment of Reduction in Mortality and Morbidity (CHARM) program. J Am Coll Cardiol 2006;47:1997–2004.
28. Go AS, Yang J, Ackerson LM, et al. Hemoglobin level, chronic kidney disease, and the risks of death and hospitalization in adults with chronic heart failure: The Anemia in Chronic Heart Failure: Outcomes and Resource Utilization (ANCHOR) Study. Circulation 2006;113:2713–2723.
29. Bleumink GS, Feenstra J, Sturkenboom MC, Stricker BH. Nonsteroidal anti-inflammatory drugs and heart failure. Drugs 2003;63:525–534.
30. Nesto RW, Bell D, Bonow RO, et al. Thiazolidinedione use, fluid retention, and congestive heart failure: A consensus statement from the American Heart Association and American Diabetes Association. Circulation 2003;108:2941–2948.
31. Nissen SE, Wolski K. Effect of rosiglitazone on the risk of myocardial infarction and death from cardiovascular causes. N Engl J Med 2007;356:2457–2471.
32. Givertz M, Colucci W, Braunwald E. Clinical aspects of heart failure: High-output failure, pulmonary edema. In: Zipes DP, Libby P, Bonow RO, Braunwald E, eds. Heart Disease: A Textbook of Cardiovascular Medicine, 7th ed. Philadelphia: Elsevier Saunders, 2005:539–568.
33. Adams K, Lindenfeld J, Arnold J, et al. Executive summary: HFSA 2006 comprehensive heart failure practice guideline. J Card Fail 2006;12:10–38.
34. Nieminen MS, Bohm M, Cowie MR, et al. Executive summary of the guidelines on the diagnosis and treatment of acute heart failure: The Task Force on Acute Heart Failure of the European Society of Cardiology. Eur Heart J 2005;26:384–416.
35. Swedberg K, Cleland J, Dargie H, et al. Guidelines for the diagnosis and treatment of chronic heart failure: Executive summary (update 2005): The Task Force for the Diagnosis and Treatment of Chronic Heart Failure of the European Society of Cardiology. Eur Heart J 2005;26:1115–1140.
36. Chobanian AV, Bakris GL, Black HR, et al. The Seventh Report of the Joint National Committee on Prevention, Detection, Evaluation, and Treatment of High Blood Pressure: The JNC 7 report. JAMA 2003;289:2560–2572.
37. Smith SC Jr, Allen J, Blair SN, et al. AHA/ACC guidelines for secondary prevention for patients with coronary and other atherosclerotic vascular disease: 2006 update: Endorsed by the National Heart, Lung, and Blood Institute. Circulation 2006;113:2363–2372.
38. Echt DS, Liebson PR, Mitchell LB, et al. Mortality and morbidity in patients receiving encainide, flecainide, or placebo. The Cardiac Arrhythmia Suppression Trial. N Engl J Med 1991;324:781–788.
39. Bardy GH, Lee KL, Mark DB, et al. Amiodarone or an implantable cardioverter-defibrillator for congestive heart failure. N Engl J Med 2005;352:225–237.
40. DiMarco JP. Implantable cardioverter-defibrillators. N Engl J Med 2003;349:1836–1847.
41. Bristow MR, Saxon LA, Boehmer J, et al. Cardiac-resynchronization therapy with or without an implantable defibrillator in advanced chronic heart failure. N Engl J Med 2004;350:2140–2150.

42. Abraham WT. Cardiac resynchronization therapy. Prog Cardiovasc Dis 2006;48:232–238.
43. Shankar SS, Brater DC. Loop diuretics: From the Na-K-2Cl transporter to clinical use. Am J Physiol Renal Physiol 2003;284:F11–F21.
44. Brater DC. Pharmacology of diuretics. Am J Med Sci 2000;319:38–50.
45. Prasun MA, Kocheril AG, Klass PH, et al. The effects of a sliding scale diuretic titration protocol in patients with heart failure. J Cardiovasc Nurs 2005;20:62–70.
46. Jong P, Yusuf S, Rousseau MF, et al. Effect of enalapril on 12-year survival and life expectancy in patients with left ventricular systolic dysfunction: A follow-up study. Lancet 2003;361:1843–1848.
47. Pfeffer MA, McMurray JJ, Velazquez EJ, et al. Valsartan, captopril, or both in myocardial infarction complicated by heart failure, left ventricular dysfunction, or both. N Engl J Med 2003;349:1893–1906.
48. Dries DL, Strong MH, Cooper RS, Drazner MH. Efficacy of angiotensin-converting enzyme inhibition in reducing progression from asymptomatic left ventricular dysfunction to symptomatic heart failure in black and white patients. J Am Coll Cardiol 2002;40:311–317.
49. Vermes E, Ducharme A, Bourassa MG, et al. Enalapril reduces the incidence of diabetes in patients with chronic heart failure: Insight from the Studies of Left Ventricular Dysfunction (SOLVD). Circulation 2003;107:1291–1296.
50. Dagenais GR, Pogue J, Fox K, et al. Angiotensin-converting-enzyme inhibitors in stable vascular disease without left ventricular systolic dysfunction or heart failure: A combined analysis of three trials. Lancet 2006;368:581–588.
51. Butler J, Arbogast PG, Daugherty J, et al. Outpatient utilization of angiotensin-converting enzyme inhibitors among heart failure patients after hospital discharge. J Am Coll Cardiol 2004;43:2036–2043.
52. Stafford RS, Radley DC. The underutilization of cardiac medications of proven benefit, 1990 to 2002. J Am Coll Cardiol 2003;41:56–61.
53. Smith GL, Lichtman JH, Bracken MB, et al. Renal impairment and outcomes in heart failure: Systematic review and meta-analysis. J Am Coll Cardiol 2006;47:1987–1996.
54. Frances CD, Noguchi H, Massie BM, et al. Are we inhibited? Renal insufficiency should not preclude the use of ACE inhibitors for patients with myocardial infarction and depressed left ventricular function. Arch Intern Med 2000;160:2645–2650.
55. Solomon SD, Rice MM, K AJ, et al. Renal function and effectiveness of angiotensin-converting enzyme inhibitor therapy in patients with chronic stable coronary disease in the Prevention of Events with ACE Inhibition (PEACE) trial. Circulation 2006;114:26–31.
56. Tokmakova MP, Skali H, Kenchaiah S, et al. Chronic kidney disease, cardiovascular risk, and response to angiotensin-converting enzyme inhibition after myocardial infarction: The Survival And Ventricular Enlargement (SAVE) study. Circulation 2004;110:3667–3673.
57. Packer M, Poole-Wilson PA, Armstrong PW, et al. Comparative effects of low and high doses of the angiotensin-converting enzyme inhibitor, lisinopril, on morbidity and mortality in chronic heart failure. ATLAS Study Group. Circulation 1999;100:2312–2318.
58. Packer M, Bristow MR, Cohn JN, et al. The effect of carvedilol on morbidity and mortality in patients with chronic heart failure. U.S. Carvedilol Heart Failure Study Group. N Engl J Med 1996;334:1349–1355.
59. Effect of metoprolol CR/XL in chronic heart failure: Metoprolol CR/XL Randomised Intervention Trial in Congestive Heart Failure (MERIT-HF). Lancet 1999;353:2001–2007.
60. The Cardiac Insufficiency Bisoprolol Study II (CIBIS-II): A randomised trial. Lancet 1999;353:9–13.
61. Packer M, Coats AJ, Fowler MB, et al. Effect of carvedilol on survival in severe chronic heart failure. N Engl J Med 2001;344:1651–1658.
62. Dargie HJ. Effect of carvedilol on outcome after myocardial infarction in patients with left-ventricular dysfunction: The CAPRICORN randomised trial. Lancet 2001;357:1385–1390.
63. Packer M, Fowler MB, Roecker EB, et al. Effect of carvedilol on the morbidity of patients with severe chronic heart failure: Results of the carvedilol prospective randomized cumulative survival (COPERNICUS) study. Circulation 2002;106:2194–2199.
64. Hjalmarson A, Goldstein S, Fagerberg B, et al. Effects of controlled-release metoprolol on total mortality, hospitalizations, and well-being in patients with heart failure: The Metoprolol CR/XL Randomized Intervention Trial in Congestive Heart Failure (MERIT-HF). MERIT-HF Study Group. JAMA 2000;283:1295–1302.
65. Kukin ML, Kalman J, Charney RH, et al. Prospective, randomized comparison of effect of long-term treatment with metoprolol or carvedilol on symptoms, exercise, ejection fraction, and oxidative stress in heart failure. Circulation 1999;99:2645–2651.
66. Metra M, Nodari S, Parrinello G, et al. Marked improvement in left ventricular ejection fraction during long-term beta-blockade in patients with chronic heart failure: Clinical correlates and prognostic significance. Am Heart J 2003;145:292–299.
67. Bristow MR, Gilbert EM, Abraham WT, et al. Carvedilol produces dose-related improvements in left ventricular function and survival in subjects with chronic heart failure. MOCHA Investigators. Circulation 1996;94:2807–2816.
68. Willenheimer R, van Veldhuisen DJ, Silke B, et al. Effect on survival and hospitalization of initiating treatment for chronic heart failure with bisoprolol followed by enalapril, as compared with the opposite sequence: Results of the randomized Cardiac Insufficiency Bisoprolol Study (CIBIS) III. Circulation 2005;112:2426–2435.
69. Gattis WA, O'Connor CM, Gallup DS, et al. Predischarge initiation of carvedilol in patients hospitalized for decompensated heart failure: Results of the Initiation Management Predischarge: Process for Assessment of Carvedilol Therapy in Heart Failure (IMPACT-HF) trial. J Am Coll Cardiol 2004;43:1534–1541.
70. Packer M. Controlled-release carvedilol: A concluding perspective. Am J Cardiol 2006;98:67–69.
71. Wikstrand J, Hjalmarson A, Waagstein F, et al. Dose of metoprolol CR/XL and clinical outcomes in patients with heart failure: Analysis of the experience in Metoprolol CR/XL Randomized Intervention Trial in Chronic Heart Failure (MERIT-HF). J Am Coll Cardiol 2002;40:491–498.
72. Bhatia V, Bhatia R, Mathew B. Angiotensin receptor blockers in congestive heart failure: Evidence, concerns, and controversies. Cardiol Rev 2005;13:297–303.
73. Coats AJ. Angiotensin type-1 receptor blockers in heart failure. Prog Cardiovasc Dis 2002;44:231–242.
74. Cohn JN, Tognoni G. A randomized trial of the angiotensin-receptor blocker valsartan in chronic heart failure. N Engl J Med 2001;345:1667–1675.
75. Pfeffer MA, Swedberg K, Granger CB, et al. Effects of candesartan on mortality and morbidity in patients with chronic heart failure: The CHARM-Overall programme. Lancet 2003;362:759–766.
76. McMurray JJ, Ostergren J, Swedberg K, et al. Effects of candesartan in patients with chronic heart failure and reduced left-ventricular systolic function taking angiotensin-converting-enzyme inhibitors: The CHARM-Added trial. Lancet 2003;362:767–771.
77. Granger CB, McMurray JJ, Yusuf S, et al. Effects of candesartan in patients with chronic heart failure and reduced left-ventricular systolic function intolerant to angiotensin-converting-enzyme inhibitors: The CHARM-Alternative trial. Lancet 2003;362:772–776.
78. Yusuf S, Pfeffer MA, Swedberg K, et al. Effects of candesartan in patients with chronic heart failure and preserved left-ventricular ejection fraction: The CHARM-Preserved Trial. Lancet 2003;362:777–781.
79. Cicardi M, Zingale LC, Bergamaschini L, Agostoni A. Angioedema associated with angiotensin-converting enzyme inhibitor use: Outcome after switching to a different treatment. Arch Intern Med 2004;164:910–913.
80. Zannad F, Dousset B, Alla F. Treatment of congestive heart failure: Interfering the aldosterone-cardiac extracellular matrix relationship. Hypertension 2001;38:1227–1232.
81. Struthers AD. The clinical implications of aldosterone escape in congestive heart failure. Eur J Heart Fail 2004;6:539–545.
82. Juurlink DN, Mamdani MM, Lee DS, et al. Rates of hyperkalemia after publication of the Randomized Aldactone Evaluation Study. N Engl J Med 2004;351:543–551.
83. Bozkurt B, Agoston I, Knowlton AA. Complications of inappropriate use of spironolactone in heart failure: When an old medicine spirals out of new guidelines. J Am Coll Cardiol 2003;41:211–214.
84. Svensson M, Gustafsson F, Galatius S, et al. How prevalent is hyperkalemia and renal dysfunction during treatment with spironolactone in patients with congestive heart failure? J Card Fail 2004;10:297–303.
85. The Digitalis Investigation Group. The effect of digoxin on mortality and morbidity in patients with heart failure. N Engl J Med 1997;336:525–533.
86. Eichhorn EJ, Gheorghiade M. Digoxin. Prog Cardiovasc Dis 2002;44:251–266.

87. Gheorghiade M, van Veldhuisen DJ, Colucci WS. Contemporary use of digoxin in the management of cardiovascular disorders. Circulation 2006;113:2556–2564.
88. Adams KF, Gheorghiade M, Uretsky BF, et al. Clinical benefits of low serum digoxin concentrations in heart failure. J Am Coll Cardiol 2002;39:946–953.
89. Rathore SS, Curtis JP, Wang Y, et al. Association of serum digoxin concentration and outcomes in patients with heart failure. JAMA 2003;289:871–878.
90. Rathore SS, Wang Y, Krumholz HM. Sex-based differences in the effect of digoxin for the treatment of heart failure. N Engl J Med 2002;347:1403–1411.
91. Adams KF Jr, Patterson JH, Gattis WA, et al. Relationship of serum digoxin concentration to mortality and morbidity in women in the digitalis investigation group trial: A retrospective analysis. J Am Coll Cardiol 2005;46:497–504.
92. Ahmed A, Rich MW, Love TE, et al. Digoxin and reduction in mortality and hospitalization in heart failure: A comprehensive post hoc analysis of the DIG trial. Eur Heart J 2006;27:178–186.
93. Ahmed A, Rich MW, Fleg JL, et al. Effects of digoxin on morbidity and mortality in diastolic heart failure: The ancillary digitalis investigation group trial. Circulation 2006;114:397–403.
94. Bauman JL, Didomenico RJ, Galanter WL. Mechanisms, manifestations, and management of digoxin toxicity in the modern era. Am J Cardiovasc Drugs 2006;6:77–86.
95. Fuster V, Ryden LE, Cannom DS, et al. ACC/AHA/ESC 2006 guidelines for the management of patients with atrial fibrillation: A report of the American College of Cardiology/American Heart Association Task Force on Practice Guidelines and the European Society of Cardiology Committee for Practice Guidelines (Writing Committee to Revise the 2001 Guidelines for the Management of Patients With Atrial Fibrillation): Developed in collaboration with the European Heart Rhythm Association and the Heart Rhythm Society. Circulation 2006;114:e257–e354.
96. Schentag J, Bang A, Kozinski-Tober J. Digoxin. In: Burton M, Shaw L, Schentag J, Evans W, eds. Applied Pharmacokinetics and Pharmacodynamics, 4th ed. Baltimore: Lippincott Williams & Wilkins, 2006:411–439.
97. Bauman JL, DiDomenico RJ, Viana M, Fitch M. A method of determining the dose of digoxin for heart failure in the modern era. Arch Intern Med 2006;166:2539–2545.
98. Daiber A, Mulsch A, Hink U, et al. The oxidative stress concept of nitrate tolerance and the antioxidant properties of hydralazine. Am J Cardiol 2005;96:25i–36i.
99. Taylor AL, Ziesche S, Yancy C, et al. Combination of isosorbide dinitrate and hydralazine in blacks with heart failure. N Engl J Med 2004;351:2049–2057.
100. Cohn JN, Archibald DG, Ziesche S, et al. Effect of vasodilator therapy on mortality in chronic congestive heart failure. Results of a Veterans Administration Cooperative Study. N Engl J Med 1986;314:1547–1552.
101. Cohn JN, Johnson G, Ziesche S, et al. A comparison of enalapril with hydralazine-isosorbide dinitrate in the treatment of chronic congestive heart failure. N Engl J Med 1991;325:303–310.
102. Prabhu SD. Nitric oxide protects against pathological ventricular remodeling: Reconsideration of the role of NO in the failing heart. Circ Res 2004;94:1155–1157.
103. Anand K, Mooss AN, Hee TT, Mohiuddin SM. Meta-analysis: Inhibition of renin-angiotensin system prevents new-onset atrial fibrillation. Am Heart J 2006;152:217–222.
104. Nasr IA, Bouzamondo A, Hulot JS, et al. Prevention of atrial fibrillation onset by beta-blocker treatment in heart failure: A meta-analysis. Eur Heart J 2007;28:457–462.
105. Wyse DG, Waldo AL, DiMarco JP, et al. A comparison of rate control and rhythm control in patients with atrial fibrillation. N Engl J Med 2002;347:1825–1833.
106. Masoudi FA, Inzucchi SE. Diabetes mellitus and heart failure: Epidemiology, mechanisms, and pharmacotherapy. Am J Cardiol 2007;99:113B–132B.
107. Roberts F, Ryan GJ. The safety of metformin in heart failure. Ann Pharmacother 2007;41:642–646.
108. Murray MD, Deer MM, Ferguson JA, et al. Open-label randomized trial of torsemide compared with furosemide therapy for patients with heart failure. Am J Med 2001;111:513–520.
109. Young M, Plosker GL. Torasemide: A pharmacoeconomic review of its use in chronic heart failure. Pharmacoeconomics 2001;19:679–703.
110. Ahmed A, Husain A, Love TE, et al. Heart failure, chronic diuretic use, and increase in mortality and hospitalization: An observational study using propensity score methods. Eur Heart J 2006;27:1431–1439.
111. Teo KK, Yusuf S, Pfeffer M, et al. Effects of long-term treatment with angiotensin-converting-enzyme inhibitors in the presence or absence of aspirin: A systematic review. Lancet 2002;360:1037–1043.
112. McAlister FA, Ghali WA, Gong Y, et al. Aspirin use and outcomes in a community-based cohort of 7352 patients discharged after first hospitalization for heart failure. Circulation 2006;113:2572–2578.
113. Schoolwerth AC, Sica DA, Ballermann BJ, Wilcox CS. Renal considerations in angiotensin converting enzyme inhibitor therapy: A statement for healthcare professionals from the Council on the Kidney in Cardiovascular Disease and the Council for High Blood Pressure Research of the American Heart Association. Circulation 2001;104:1985–1991.
114. Cooper WO, Hernandez-Diaz S, Arbogast PG, et al. Major congenital malformations after first-trimester exposure to ACE inhibitors. N Engl J Med 2006;354:2443–2451.
115. A trial of the beta-blocker bucindolol in patients with advanced chronic heart failure. N Engl J Med 2001;344:1659–1667.
116. Poole-Wilson PA, Swedberg K, Cleland JG, et al. Comparison of carvedilol and metoprolol on clinical outcomes in patients with chronic heart failure in the Carvedilol or Metoprolol European Trial (COMET): Randomised controlled trial. Lancet 2003;362:7–13.
117. Aquilante CL, Terra SG, Schofield RS, et al. Sustained restoration of autonomic balance with long- but not short-acting metoprolol in patients with heart failure. J Card Fail 2006;12:171–176.
118. Bakris GL, Fonseca V, Katholi RE, et al. Metabolic effects of carvedilol vs metoprolol in patients with type 2 diabetes mellitus and hypertension: A randomized controlled trial. JAMA 2004;292:2227–2236.
119. Deedwania PC, Giles TD, Klibaner M, et al. Efficacy, safety and tolerability of metoprolol CR/XL in patients with diabetes and chronic heart failure: Experiences from MERIT-HF. Am Heart J 2005;149:159–167.
120. Mehra MR. Optimizing outcomes in the patient with acute decompensated heart failure. Am Heart J 2006;151:571–579.
121. Felker GM, Adams KF Jr, Konstam MA, et al. The problem of decompensated heart failure: Nomenclature, classification, and risk stratification. Am Heart J 2003;145:S18–S25.
122. Cuffe MS, Califf RM, Adams KF, et al. Short-term intravenous milrinone for acute exacerbation of chronic heart failure: A randomized controlled trial. JAMA 2002;287:1541–1547.
123. The VMAC Investigators. Intravenous nesiritide vs nitroglycerin for treatment of decompensated congestive heart failure: A randomized controlled trial. JAMA 2002;287:1531–1540.
124. Adams KF, Lindenfeld J, Arnold JMO, et al. Evaluation and management of patients with acute decompensated heart failure. J Card Fail 2006;12:e86–e103.
125. Gheorghiade M, Zannad F, Sopko G, et al. Acute heart failure syndromes: Current state and framework for future research. Circulation 2005;112:3958–3968.
126. Adams KF Jr, Fonarow GC, Emerman CL, et al. Characteristics and outcomes of patients hospitalized for heart failure in the United States: Rationale, design, and preliminary observations from the first 100,000 cases in the Acute Decompensated Heart Failure National Registry (ADHERE). Am Heart J 2005;149:209–216.
127. Fonarow GC, Adams KF Jr, Abraham WT, et al. Risk stratification for in-hospital mortality in acutely decompensated heart failure: Classification and regression tree analysis. JAMA 2005;293:572–580.
128. Gheorghiade M, Abraham WT, Albert NM, et al. Systolic blood pressure at admission, clinical characteristics, and outcomes in patients hospitalized with acute heart failure. JAMA 2006;296:2217–2226.
129. Nohria A, Mielniczuk LM, Stevenson LW. Evaluation and monitoring of patients with acute heart failure syndromes. Am J Cardiol 2005;96:32G-40G.
130. Nohria A, Lewis E, Stevenson LW. Medical management of advanced heart failure. JAMA 2002;287:628–640.
131. Binanay C, Califf RM, Hasselblad V, et al. Evaluation study of congestive heart failure and pulmonary artery catheterization effectiveness: The ESCAPE trial. JAMA 2005;294:1625–1633.
132. Forrester JS, Diamond G, Chatterjee K, Swan HJC. Medical therapy of acute myocardial infarction by application of hemodynamic subsets. N Engl J Med 1976;295:1356–1362.

133. Brater DC. Diuretic therapy in congestive heart failure. Congest Heart Fail 2000;6:197–210.
134. Stough WG, O'Connor CM, Gheorghiade M. Overview of current noninodilator therapies for acute heart failure syndromes. Am J Cardiol 2005;96:41G–46G.
135. Eshaghian S, Horwich TB, Fonarow GC. Relation of loop diuretic dose to mortality in advanced heart failure. Am J Cardiol 2006;97:1759–1764.
136. Butler J, Forman DE, Abraham WT, et al. Relationship between heart failure treatment and development of worsening renal function among hospitalized patients. Am Heart J 2004;147:331–338.
137. Bayram M, De Luca L, Massie MB, Gheorghiade M. Reassessment of dobutamine, dopamine, and milrinone in the management of acute heart failure syndromes. Am J Cardiol 2005;96:47G–58G.
138. Lehtonen LA, Antila S, Pentikainen PJ. Pharmacokinetics and pharmacodynamics of intravenous inotropic agents. Clin Pharmacokinet 2004;43:187–203.
139. Abraham WT, Adams KF, Fonarow GC, et al. In-hospital mortality in patients with acute decompensated heart failure requiring intravenous vasoactive medications: An analysis from the Acute Decompensated Heart Failure National Registry (ADHERE). J Am Coll Cardiol 2005;46:57–64.
140. Dorsch MP, Rodgers JE. Nesiritide: Harmful or harmless? Pharmacotherapy 2006;26:1465–1478.
141. Sackner-Bernstein JD, Skopicki HA, Aaronson KD. Risk of worsening renal function with nesiritide in patients with acutely decompensated heart failure. Circulation 2005;111:1487–1491.
142. Sackner-Bernstein JD, Kowalski M, Fox M, Aaronson K. Short-term risk of death after treatment with nesiritide for decompensated heart failure: A pooled analysis of randomized controlled trials. JAMA 2005;293:1900–1905.
143. Mentzer RM Jr, Oz MC, Sladen RN, et al. Effects of perioperative nesiritide in patients with left ventricular dysfunction undergoing cardiac surgery: The NAPA Trial. J Am Coll Cardiol 2007;49:716–726.
144. Boehmer JP, Popjes E. Cardiac failure: Mechanical support strategies. Crit Care Med 2006;34:S268–S277.
145. Rose EA, Gelijns AC, Moskowitz AJ, et al. Long-term mechanical left ventricular assistance for end-stage heart failure. N Engl J Med 2001;345:1435–1443.
146. Birks EJ, Tansley PD, Hardy J, et al. Left ventricular assist device and drug therapy for the reversal of heart failure. N Engl J Med 2006;355:1873–1884.
147. Costanzo MR, Guglin ME, Saltzberg MT, et al. Ultrafiltration versus intravenous diuretics for patients hospitalized for acute decompensated heart failure. J Am Coll Cardiol 2007;49:675–683.
148. Taylor DO, Edwards LB, Boucek MM, et al. Registry of the International Society for Heart and Lung Transplantation: Twenty-third official adult heart transplantation report—2006. J Heart Lung Transplant 2006;25:869–879.
149. Hauptman PJ, Havranek EP. Integrating palliative care into heart failure care. Arch Intern Med 2005;165:374–378.
150. Lee WC, Chavez YE, Baker T, Luce BR. Economic burden of heart failure: A summary of recent literature. Heart Lung 2004;33:362–371.
151. Shibata MC, Nilsson C, Hervas-Malo M, et al. Economic implications of treatment guidelines for congestive heart failure. Can J Cardiol 2005;21:1301–1306.
152. Schwartz JS, Wang YR, Cleland JG, et al. High- versus low-dose angiotensin converting enzyme inhibitor therapy in the treatment of heart failure: An economic analysis of the Assessment of Treatment with Lisinopril and Survival (ATLAS) trial. Am J Manag Care 2003;9:417–424.
153. Smith DG, Cerulli A, Frech FH. Use of valsartan for the treatment of heart-failure patients not receiving ACE inhibitors: A budget impact analysis. Clin Ther 2005;27:951–959.
154. Croom KF, Plosker GL. Eplerenone: A pharmacoeconomic review of its use in patients with post-myocardial infarction heart failure. Pharmacoeconomics 2005;23:1057–1072.
155. Angus DC, Linde-Zwirble WT, Tam SW, et al. Cost-effectiveness of fixed-dose combination of isosorbide dinitrate and hydralazine therapy for blacks with heart failure. Circulation 2005;112:3745–3753.
156. Sanders GD, Hlatky MA, Owens DK. Cost-effectiveness of implantable cardioverter-defibrillators. N Engl J Med 2005;353:1471–1480.
157. Feldman AM, de Lissovoy G, Bristow MR, et al. Cost effectiveness of cardiac resynchronization therapy in the Comparison of Medical Therapy, Pacing, and Defibrillation in Heart Failure (COMPANION) trial. J Am Coll Cardiol 2005;46:2311–2321.
158. Clegg AJ, Scott DA, Loveman E, et al. Clinical and cost-effectiveness of left ventricular assist devices as a bridge to heart transplantation for people with end-stage heart failure: A systematic review and economic evaluation. Eur Heart J 2006;27:2929–2938.
159. Holland R, Battersby J, Harvey I, et al. Systematic review of multidisciplinary interventions in heart failure. Heart 2005;91:899–906.
160. Gattis WA, Hasselblad V, Whellan DJ, O'Connor CM. Reduction in heart failure events by the addition of a clinical pharmacist to the heart failure management team. Arch Intern Med 1999;159:1939–1945.
161. Whellan DJ, Gaulden L, Gattis WA, et al. The benefit of implementing a heart failure disease management program. Arch Intern Med 2001;161:2223–2228.
162. Murray M, Young J, Hoke S, et al. Pharmacist intervention to improve medication adherence in heart failure. A randomized trial. Ann Intern Med 2007;146:714–725.
163. Macdonald JE, Struthers AD. What is the optimal serum potassium level in cardiovascular patients? J Am Coll Cardiol 2004;43:155–161.

CHAPTER 17

Ischemic Heart Disease

ROBERT L. TALBERT

KEY CONCEPTS

1. Ischemic heart disease (IHD) is primarily caused by coronary atherosclerotic plaque formation that leads to an imbalance between oxygen supply and demand resulting in myocardial ischemia.

2. Chest pain is the cardinal symptom of myocardial ischemia caused by coronary artery disease (CAD).

3. Risk factor identification and modification are important interventions for individual patients with known or suspected IHD and as a population-based policy to reduce the impact of this disease.

4. Major risk factors that can be altered include dyslipidemia (high total and low-density lipoprotein cholesterol, low high-density lipoprotein cholesterol, and high triglycerides), smoking, glycemic control in diabetes mellitus, hypertension, and adoption of therapeutic lifestyle changes (exercise, weight reduction and reduced cholesterol and fat in the diet). Reduction in inflammation may also play an important role.

5. Most patients with CAD should be receiving antiplatelet therapy. Chronic stable angina should be managed initially with β-blockers because they provide better symptomatic control, at least as well as nitrates or calcium channel blockers, and decrease the risk of recurrent myocardial infarction and CAD mortality.

6. Nitroglycerin and other nitrate products are useful for prophylaxis of angina when patients are undertaking activities know to provoke angina; however, when angina is occurring on a regular, routine basis, chronic prophylactic therapy should be instituted.

7. Although calcium channel blockers are effective as monotherapy, they are generally used in combination with β-blockers or as monotherapy if patients are intolerant of β-blockers; most patients with moderate to severe angina will require two drugs to control their symptoms. Ranolazine is a second-line drug to be used with β-blockers and certain calcium channel blockers.

8. Pharmacologic management is as effective as revascularization (percutaneous transluminal coronary angioplasty, coronary artery bypass graft, etc.) if one or two vessels are involved and there are no differences in survival, recurrent myocardial infarction, or other measures of effectiveness.

9. Multivessel involvement, especially if the patient has left main coronary artery disease or left main equivalent disease, or two- to three-vessel involvement with significant left ventricular dysfunction is best managed with revascularization.

10. Percutaneous transluminal coronary angioplasty and coronary artery bypass graft produce similar results overall but certain patient subsets (e.g., diabetics) should have coronary artery bypass grafting done.

11. The clinical performance measures for chronic stable CAD recommended by the American College of Cardiology and the American Heart Association include blood pressure measurement, lipid profile, symptom and activity assessment, smoking cessation, antiplatelet therapy, drug therapy for lowering low-density lipoprotein cholesterol, β-blocker therapy for prior myocardial infarction, angiotensin-converting enzyme inhibitor therapy, and screening for diabetes.

Learning objectives, review questions, and other resources can be found at **www.pharmacotherapyonline.com.**

Ischemic heart disease (IHD) caused by atherosclerosis of the epicardial vessels leading to coronary heart disease (CHD) is the main etiology of IHD. This process begins early in life, often not being clinically manifest until the middle-aged years and beyond. IHD may present as an acute coronary syndrome (acute coronary syndrome includes unstable angina, non–ST-segment elevation myocardial infarction or ST-segment elevation myocardial infarction; see Chap. 18), chronic stable exertional angina pectoris, and ischemia without clinical symptoms. Coronary artery vasospasm (variant or Prinzmetal angina) produces similar symptoms but is not caused by atherosclerosis. Other manifestations of atherosclerosis include heart failure, arrhythmias, cerebrovascular disease (stroke), and peripheral vascular disease. The American Heart Association, the American College of Cardiology, and the European Society of Cardiology have published management guidelines for stable and unstable angina.[1–3]

EPIDEMIOLOGY

The American Heart Association (AHA) estimates that 79,400,000 American adults have one or more types of cardiovascular disease (CVD) based on data from 1999 through 2004.[4] Nearly 2,400 Americans die of CVD each day, or an average of 1 death every 33 seconds. In 2004, the death rates from CVD were 448.9 (per 100,000) for black males, 335.7 for white males, 331.6 for black females, and 239.3 for white females.[4] CHD was responsible for 52% of deaths from CVD. Men die earlier from IHD and acute myocardial infarction than women, and aging of both sexes is associated with a higher incidence of these afflictions. The disparity in mortality from IHD between men and women decreases with aging, being about four to five times more common in men from the age of the mid-30s to a preponderance of female deaths in the very elderly.

The syndrome of angina pectoris is reported to occur with an average annual incidence rate (number of new cases per time period/

total number of persons in the population for the same time period) of approximately 1.5% (range: 0.1 to 5/1,000) depending on the patient's age, gender, and risk-factor profile.[5] The presenting manifestation in women is more commonly angina, whereas men more frequently have myocardial infarction as the initial event. Estimates of the incidence and prevalence of angina are not entirely accurate because of waxing and waning of symptoms; angina may disappear in up to 30% of patients with angina that is less severe and of recent onset.

Data from the Framingham study show that the prevalence in a 1970 cohort followed for 10 years was approximately 1.5% for women and 4.3% for men ages 50 to 59 years at inception.[5] The annual rate of new episodes of angina range from 28.3 to 33 per 1,000 population for nonblack men, 22.4 to 39.5 for black men, 14.1 to 22.9 for nonblack women, and 15.3 to 35.9 for black women in the age range of 65 to 84 years or older.[4] AHA estimates that the prevalence of angina was 8.9 million in 2004.[4] Other interesting trends noted included a 21% decline in the incidence of cardiovascular disease in women, but only a 6% decline in men over two cohorts from 1950 and 1970. Cardiovascular mortality was reduced by 59% in women and 53% in men from the same cohorts. The risk of developing ischemic heart disease is not the same worldwide. Countries such as Japan and France are on the low end of the spectrum, whereas Finland, Northern Ireland, Scotland, and South Africa have very high rates of IHD.[6,7]

Angina may be classified according to symptom severity, disability induced, or a specific activity scale (Tables 17–1 and 17–2). The specific activity scale developed by Goldman and coworkers[8] may be preferable because it has been shown to be equal to or better than the New York Heart Association or Canadian Cardiovascular Society functional classifications for reproducibility and provides better agreement with exercise treadmill testing.

TABLE 17-1 Criteria for Determination of the Specific Activity Scale Functional Class

	Any Yes	No
1. Can you walk down a flight of steps without stopping (4.5–5.2 MET)?	Go to 2	Go to 4
2. Can you carry anything up a flight of 8 steps without stopping (5–5.5 MET)? Or can you: a. Have sexual intercourse without stopping (5–5.2 MET) b. Garden, rake, weed (5.6 MET) c. Roller skate, dance foxtrot (5–6 MET) d. Walk at a 4-miles/h rate on level ground (5–6 MET)	Go to 3	Class III
3. Can you carry at least 24 lb up 8 steps (10 MET)? Or can you: a. Carry objects that weigh at least 80 lb (18 MET) b. Do outdoor work, shovel snow, spade soil (7 MET) c. Do recreational activities such as skiing, basketball, touch football, squash, handball (7–10 MET) d. Jog/walk 5 miles/h (9 MET)	Class I	Class II
4. Can you shower without stopping (3.6–4.2 MET)? Or can you: a. Strip and make bed (3.9–5 MET) b. Mop floors (4.2 MET) c. Hang washed clothes (4.4 MET) d. Clean windows (3.7 MET) e. Walk 2.5 miles/h (3–3.5 MET) f. Bowl (3–4.4 MET) g. Play golf, walk and carry clubs (4.5 MET) h. Push a power lawnmower (4 MET)	Class III	Go to 5
5. Can you dress without stopping because of symptoms (2–2.3 MET)?	Class III	Class IV

MET, metabolic equivalents of activity.

From Goldman L, Hashimoto B, Cook F, et al. Comparative reproducibility and validity of systems for assessing cardiovascular functional class: Advantages of a new specific activity scale. Circulation 1981;64:1228, with permission.

TABLE 17-2 Grading of Angina Pectoris by the Canadian Cardiovascular Society Classification System

Class	Description of Stage
Class I	Ordinary physical activity does not cause angina, such as walking, climbing stairs. Angina occurs with strenuous, rapid, or prolonged exertion at work or recreation.
Class II	Slight limitation or ordinary activity. Angina occurs on walking or climbing stairs rapidly, walking uphill, walking or stair climbing after meals, or in cold, or in wind, or under emotional stress, or only during the few hours after wakening. Walking more than 2 blocks on the level and climbing more than 1 flight of ordinary stairs at a normal pace and in normal condition.
Class III	Marked limitations of ordinary physical activity. Angina occurs on walking 1 to 2 blocks on the level and climbing 1 flight of stairs in normal conditions and at a normal pace.
Class IV	Inability to carry on any physical activity without discomfort–anginal symptoms may be present at rest.

From Campeau L. Grading of angina [letter]. Circulation 1976;54:522–523, with permission.

An important determinate of outcome for the angina patient is the number of vessels obstructed. Twelve-year survival from the Coronary Artery Surgery Study (CASS) for patients with zero-, one-, two-, and three-vessel disease was 88%, 74%, 59%, and 40%, respectively.[9] Other factors that increase the risk of death in medically managed patients include the presence of heart failure (or markers such as poor ventricular wall motion and low ejection fraction), smoking, left main or left main equivalent coronary artery disease, diabetes, and prior myocardial infarction. Twelve-year survival for patients with at least one diseased vessel and ejection fractions in the ranges of ≥50%, 35% to 49%, and 0% to 34% is 73%, 54%, and 21%, respectively. Of particular note, patients with left main coronary artery disease (or left main equivalent) are at extremely high risk and constitute a unique group for therapeutic consideration.[10] In the CASS, at 15 years of followup, 37% of the surgery group and 27% of the medical group are surviving; median survival is 13.3 years versus 6.7 years, respectively (P <0.0001). If systolic function was normal, then median survival and percent surviving were not different between the surgery and medical groups (median survival of about 15 years). Patients screened but not randomized to CASS had similar survival rates, suggesting that results from randomized patients may be applicable to more generalized populations as a measure of external reliability.

ETIOLOGY AND PATHOPHYSIOLOGY

The pathophysiology that underlies this disease process is dynamic, evolutionary, and complex. An understanding of the determinants of myocardial oxygen demand (MVO_2), regulation of coronary blood flow, the effects of ischemia on the mechanical and metabolic function of the myocardium, and how ischemia is recognized are important to understanding the rationale for the selection and use of pharmacotherapy for IHD.

❶ Ischemia may be defined as lack of oxygen and decreased or no blood flow in the myocardium. In contrast, anoxia, defined as the absence of oxygen to the myocardium, results in continued perfusion with washout of acid by-products of glycolysis, thereby preserving the mechanical and metabolic status of the heart to a greater extent than does ischemia for short periods of time.

DETERMINANTS OF OXYGEN DEMAND

The major determinants of MVO_2 are (a) heart rate, (b) contractility, and (c) intramyocardial wall tension during systole. Overall, intramyocardial wall tension is thought to be the most important among these three factors. As the consequences of IHD are a result of increased demand in the face of a fixed supply of oxygen in most situations, alterations in MVO_2 are critically important in producing ischemia and for interventions intended to alleviate ischemia. MVO_2 cannot be directly measured in patients; however, an indirect assessment that correlates reasonably well with MVO_2 as determined in experimental animal models is the tension–time index. This is a measure of the area under the curve of the left ventricular (LV) pressure curve. Tension in the ventricle wall is a function of the radius of the LV and intraventricular pressure. These factors are related through the Laplace law, which states that wall stress is related directly to the product of intraventricular pressure and internal radius and inversely to wall thickness multiplied by a factor of two. Increasing systemic blood pressure or ventricular dilation would increase wall tension and oxygen demand whereas ventricular hypertrophy would tend to minimize increasing MVO_2. Clinical application of these principles has led to the use of the double product (DP), which is heart rate (HR) multiplied by systolic blood pressure (SBP) ($DP = HR \times SBP$). Although this is a clinically useful indirect estimate of MVO_2, it does not consider changes in contractility (an independent variable), and because only changes in pressure are considered with the double product, volume loading of the LV and increased MVO_2 related to ventricular dilation are underestimated.

REGULATION OF CORONARY BLOOD FLOW

Although coronary blood flow is influenced by multiple factors, the caliber of the resistance vessels delivering blood to the myocardium and MVO_2 are the prime determinants in the occurrence of ischemia. The anatomy of the vascular bed will affect oxygen supply and, subsequently, myocardial metabolism and mechanical function.

Anatomic Factors

The normal coronary system (Fig. 17–1 illustrates normal anatomy) consists of large epicardial or surface vessels (R1) that normally offer little intrinsic resistance to myocardial flow and intramyocardial arteries and arterioles (R2), which branch into a dense capillary network (about 4,000 capillaries per mm^2) to supply basal blood flow of 60 to 90 mL/min per 100 g of myocardium. R1 and R2 are in series and total resistance is the algebraic sum; however, under normal circumstances, the resistance in R2 is much greater. Myocardial blood flow is inversely related to arteriolar resistance and directly related to the coronary driving pressure. The arterioles dynamically alter their intrinsic tone in response to demands for oxygen and other factors, and as a result, myocardial oxygen delivery and myocardial oxygen demand are tightly coupled in a rapidly responsive system.

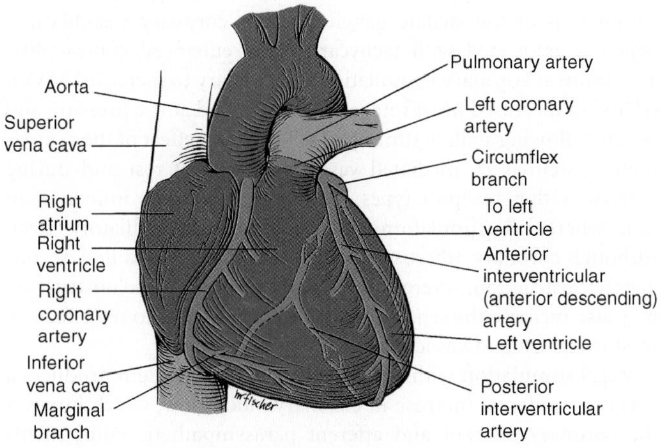

FIGURE 17-1. Coronary anatomy. *(From Tintinalli JE, Kelen GD, Stapczynski JR, eds. Tintinalli's Emergency Medicine: A Comprehensive Study Guide, 6th ed. New York: McGraw-Hill, 2004:344.)*

Atherosclerotic lesions encroaching on the luminal cross-sectional area of the larger epicardial vessels (R1) transform the relationships among R1, R2, and blood flow. As resistance increases in R1 owing to occlusion, R2 can vasodilate to maintain coronary blood flow. This response is inadequate with greater degrees of obstruction, and the coronary flow reserve afforded by R2 vasodilation is insufficient to meet oxygen demand (also referred to as autoregulation). The extent of functional obstruction is important in the limitation of coronary blood flow, and the presence of relatively severe stenosis (>70%) may provoke ischemia and symptoms at rest, whereas less-severe stenosis may allow a reserve of coronary blood flow for exertion.[11]

The diameter of the lesion impeding blood flow through a vessel is important, but other factors such as length of the lesion and the influence of pressure drop across an area of stenosis also affect coronary blood flow and function of the collateral circulation. Resistance to flow in a vessel is directly related to length of the obstructing lesion, but resistance is inversely related to the diameter of the vessel to the fourth power. Consequently, diameter is much more important. As blood flows across a stenotic lesion the pressure drops (energy losses) as a result of friction between blood and the lesion and to the abrupt turbulent expansion as blood emerges from the stenosis. This pressure drop is dynamic and directly related to flow giving rise to a resistance that is not fixed, but rather fluctuates, as flow is changed. This relationship can dramatically affect collateral blood flow and its response to exercise, resulting in what has been called "coronary steal." A similar situation may also occur when the epicardial or subepicardial vessels "steal" blood flow from the endocardium in the presence of a stenotic lesion.

Large and small coronary arteries may undergo dynamic changes in coronary vascular resistance and coronary blood flow. Dynamic coronary obstruction can occur in normal vessels and vessels with stenosis in which vasomotion or spasm may be superimposed on a fixed stenosis. Although it is possible that these changes may be "active" in small coronary arteries, it is also possible that the observed changes may reflect collapse owing to poststenotic intraluminal pressure drop or increased intramyocardial compressive forces associated with inadequate ventricular relaxation.

Collateral blood flow exists to a certain extent from birth as native collaterals, but persisting ischemia may promote collateral growth as developed collaterals. These two types of collaterals differ in anatomy and in their ability to regulate coronary blood flow. Collateral development is dependent on the severity of obstruction, the presence of various growth factors (basic fibroblast growth factor [β-FGF] and vascular endothelial growth factor), endogenous vasodilators (e.g., nitrous oxide, prostacyclin), hormones such as estrogen, and, potentially, exercise. Collateral development is highly species dependent and this should be considered when reading experimental literature.

Metabolic Regulation

Coronary blood flow is closely tied to the oxygen needs of the heart. Changes in oxygen balance lead to very rapid changes in coronary blood flow. Although a number of mediators may contribute to these changes, the most important ones are likely to be adenosine, other nucleotides, nitric oxide, prostaglandins, CO_2, and H^+. Adenosine, which is formed from adenosine triphosphate and adenosine monophosphate under conditions of ischemia and stress, is a potent vasodilator that links decreased perfusion to metabolically induced vasodilation or "reactive hyperemia." The synthesis and release of adenosine into coronary sinus venous effluent occurs within seconds after coronary artery occlusion, and approximately 30% of the hyperemic response can be blocked by metabolic blockers of adenosine.[12]

Endothelial Control of Coronary Vascular Tone

The vascular endothelium, a single-cell tissue with an enormous surface area separating the blood from vascular smooth muscle of the artery wall, is capable of a broad range of metabolic functions. The endothelium functions as a protective surface for the artery wall, and as long as it remains intact and functional, it promotes vascular smooth muscle relaxation and inhibits thrombogenesis and atherosclerotic plaque formation; damaged endothelium reacts to numerous stimuli with vasoconstriction, thrombosis, and plaque formation. The vascular endothelium of the coronary arteries synthesizes large molecules such as fibronectin, interleukin-1, tissue plasminogen activator, and various growth factors. Small molecules that are also produced include prostacyclin, platelet-activating factor, endothelin-1, and endothelium-derived relaxing factor (EDRF) that is now characterized as nitric oxide. EDRF is synthesized from 1-arginine via nitric oxide synthase and released by shear force on the endothelium, as well as through interaction with many biochemical stimuli such as acetylcholine, histamine, arginine, catecholamines, arachidonic acid, adenosine diphosphate, endothelin-1, bradykinin, serotonin, and thrombin.[12] EDRF or nitric oxide then causes relaxation of the underlying smooth muscle and may be thought of as a paracrine homeopathic defense mechanism against noxious stimuli. Denudation or loss of the vascular endothelium results in loss of EDRF and this protective mechanism. Loss of the endothelial cell layer and function may occur secondary to physical disruption (percutaneous transluminal angioplasty [PTCA]), factors impinging from the vascular side (cyanide from smoke), or disruption of the intimal–medial layers (oxidized low-density lipoprotein). Impaired endothelial function may be related to the development of premature atherosclerosis based on recent family studies.[13]

Factors Extrinsic to the Vascular Bed

Blood flow to the coronary arteries arises from orifices located immediately distal to the aorta valve. Perfusion pressure is equal to the difference between the aortic pressure at an instantaneous point in time minus the intramyocardial pressure. Coronary vascular resistance is influenced by phasic systolic compression of the vascular bed. Consequently, the driving force for perfusion is not constant throughout the cardiac cycle. Opening of the aortic valve may also lead to a Venturi effect, which can slightly decrease perfusion pressure. If perfusion pressure is elevated for a period of time, coronary vascular resistance declines and blood flow increases; however, continued perfusion pressure increases lead, within limits, to a return of coronary blood flow back toward baseline levels through autoregulation.

Alterations in intramyocardial wall tension throughout the cardiac cycle will also impose significant changes in coronary blood flow. Diastole is the period during which coronary artery filling can occur as a result of these pressure differences and little or no coronary blood flow occurs to the left ventricle during systole. The extent of pressure development in the ventricle and heart rate have a major effect on the development of wall tension, time for diastolic coronary artery filling, and myocardial oxygen demand.

Under normal conditions, the average global distribution of blood flow between the epicardial and endocardial layer is about 1:1 at rest and remains approximately even during exercise secondary to autoregulatory changes. Regional disparity of blood flow distribution does exist normally, and these disparities are magnified in the presence of diseased coronary arteries and with increased cardiac work as the vasodilator reserve in the resistance vessels of the subendocardium layers is exhausted. Factors that favor a reduction in subendocardial blood flow include decreased perfusion pressure because of decreased diastolic blood pressure or coronary artery obstruction by atherosclerotic plaques with or without vasomotion, abbreviation of diastole (increased heart rate), and increased intraventricular diastolic pressure (e.g., valvular obstruction to flow).

Extravascular resistance may decrease coronary blood flow, primarily during systole. This effect is much more pronounced in the left ventricle compared with the right ventricle. When the effect of increased contractility is separated from the effect of ventricular pressure, approximately 75% of extravascular resistance is accounted for by passive stretch in equilibrium with ventricular pressure whereas only 25% results from active myocardial contraction.

Factors Intrinsic to the Vascular Bed

Metabolic factors, myogenic responses, neural reflexes, and humoral substances within the vascular bed of the coronary circulation function in an orchestrated fashion to maintain relative consistency in blood flow to the myocardium in the face of imposed changes in perfusion pressures. Autoregulation, mediated primarily through the effects of myogenic responses and metabolic factors, is thought to be responsible for maintaining regional blood flow in a narrow range while systemic pressure varies over a range of approximately 50 to 150 mm Hg.

Myogenic control (also known as the Bayliss effect) of coronary artery tone occurs when the vessel is stretched secondary to an increase in pressure and contracts to return blood flow to normal. It is thought that the myogenic response to stretching in coronary arteries is a modest one and that metabolic factors such as nitric oxide play a much larger role in autoregulation.

There are three well-studied metabolic factors that have the ability to modify coronary artery resistance and blood flow at the local level. Basal coronary blood flow meets oxygen demands of 8 to 10 mL/min per 100 g of myocardium with essentially complete extraction of oxygen from the blood. As cardiac output or mean arterial blood pressure increases, the increased demand for oxygen is met by increasing blood flow because little additional oxygen is available from hemoglobin. Decreased oxygen availability causes vasodilation of vascular smooth muscle and relaxation of precapillary sphincters, which increase tissue oxygen and help maintain blood flow on a regional basis.

At perfusion pressures below 60 mm Hg, as the coronary arteries are maximally dilated and the buffering effect of autoregulation has reached its capacity, further reduction in coronary blood flow will decrease perfusion pressure and tissue oxygenation. It is thought that autoregulation works more efficiently in the epicardial layers than in subendocardial layers, and this may contribute to coronary steal.

Neural components that participate in the regulation of coronary blood flow include the sympathetic nervous system, the parasympathetic nervous system, coronary reflexes, and possibly, central control of coronary blood flow. Within the sympathetic system, stimulation of the stellate ganglion elicits coronary vasodilation, which is associated with tachycardia and enhanced contractility. This indirect coronary vasodilation is secondary to increased MVO_2 related to increased heart rate, contractility, and aortic pressure and occurs following stellate stimulation. The direct effect of the sympathetic system is α_1-mediated vasoconstriction at rest and during exercise. Other receptor types, α_2 and β_1, have little influence on tone, whereas β_2 stimulation produces a modest vasodilatory effect. Although coronary atherosclerosis may decrease blood flow secondary to obstruction, severe coronary atherosclerosis and obstruction may also increase the sensitivity of coronary arteries to the effects of α_1 stimulation and vasoconstriction.

Vagal stimulation within the parasympathetic system produces a small to moderate increase in coronary blood flow, which involves the coronary efferent and afferent parasympathetic components (Bezold-Jarisch reflex). Indirectly, vasoconstriction may result, with vagal stimulation as the result of bradycardia and decreased contractility reducing myocardial oxygen demand.

Coronary reflexes have an undetermined role in the regulation of coronary blood flow. Based on experimental data, coronary reflexes that may be important include the baroreceptor, the chemoreceptor, Bezold-Jarisch reflex, and the pulmonary inhalation reflex.

Factors Limiting Coronary Perfusion

During exercise and pacing, as MVO_2 increases, coronary vascular resistance can be reduced to approximately 25% of basal values, which results in a four- to fivefold increase in coronary blood flow. The cross-sectional area can be reduced by approximately 80% prior to any mechanical or biochemical changes in the myocardium, reflecting a margin of safety for coronary blood flow. The extent of cross-sectional obstruction, the length of the lesion, lesion composition, and the geometry of the obstructing lesion can each affect flow across coronary arteries with atherosclerosis. The Bernoulli theorem states that the pressure drop across a lesion is directly related to the length of the lesion and inversely related to the radius of the lesion to the fourth power; critical stenosis occurs when the obstructing lesion encroaches on the luminal diameter and exceeds 70%. Lesions creating an obstruction of 50% to 70% may reduce blood flow; however, these obstructions are not consistent and vasospasm and thrombosis superimposed on a "noncritical" lesion may lead to clinical events such as myocardial infarction.[14] If the lesion enlarges from 80% to 90%, resistance in that vessel is tripled. Coronary reserve is diminished at approximately 85% obstruction owing to vasoconstriction. Exaggerated responsiveness can be seen when coronary stenosis reaches this critical level and the role of vasoactive substances such as prostaglandins, thromboxanes, and serotonin may play more of a role in the regulation of coronary vascular tone and thrombosis.

Little reserve exists for coronary blood flow and a relatively small reduction of 10% to 20% results in decreased myocardial fiber shortening as the first evidence for abnormal function. The subendocardial layers are affected to a greater extent than the epicardium by ischemia, considering changes in fiber shortening, arteriovenous (AV) difference in oxygen saturation, and lactate production. A reduction of 80% gives rise to akinesis and a 95% reduction of coronary blood flow produces dyskinesis during contraction of the ventricles. Although these abnormalities of contraction are associated with transient impaired function, depletion of high-energy phosphate compounds and ultrastructural changes may last for days, even after transient ischemia; this is referred to as "stunned myocardium." Chronic hypoperfusion may lead to "hibernation," in which ventricular function is impaired over longer time intervals. Hibernating myocardium can be differentiated from necrosis with various techniques (see Chap. 13) and revascularization of hibernating myocardium is useful in improving ventricular function. Regional loss of contractility may impose a burden on the remaining myocardial tissue, resulting in heart failure, increased MVO_2, and rapid depletion of blood flow reserve. Consequently, zones of tissue with marginal blood flow may develop in a lateral or transmural fashion; such development puts this tissue at risk for more severe damage if the ischemic episode persists or becomes more severe. Nonischemic areas of myocardium may compensate for the severely ischemic and border zones of ischemia by developing more tension than usual in an attempt to maintain cardiac output. At the cellular level, ischemia and the attendant acidosis are thought to alter calcium release from storage sites such as the sarcolemma and the sarcoplasmic reticulum, as well as inhibiting the binding of calcium to troponin, thereby impairing the association of actin and myosin. The clinical correlates of these cellular biochemical events leading to the development of left ventricle or right ventricle dysfunction include an S_3, dyspnea, orthopnea, tachycardia, fluctuating blood pressure, transient murmurs, and mitral or tricuspid regurgitation.

Calcium accumulation and overload secondary to ischemia impairs ventricular relaxation as well as contraction. This is apparently a result of impaired calcium uptake after systole from the myofilaments, leading to a less negative decline of the pressure in the ventricle over time. Impaired relaxation is associated with enhanced diastolic stiffness, decreased rate of wall thinning, and slowed pressure decay, producing an upward shift in the ventricular pressure–volume relationship; put more simply, MVO_2 is likely to be increased secondary to increased wall tension. Impairment of both diastolic and systolic function leads to elevation of the filling pressure of the left ventricle.

CLINICAL PRESENTATION AND DIAGNOSIS OF ANGINA

General

- Many episodes of ischemia do not cause symptoms of angina (silent ischemia)
- Patients often have a reproducible pattern of pain or other symptoms which appear after specific amount of exertion
- Increased frequency, severity, duration, or symptoms at rest suggest an unstable angina pattern and the patient should seek help immediately

Symptoms

- ❷ Sensation of pressure or burning over the sternum or near it, often but not always radiating to the left jaw, shoulder and arm; also chest tightness, shortness of breath
- Pain usually lasts from 0.5 to 30 minutes, often with a visceral quality (deep location)
- Precipitating factors include exercise, cold environment, walking after a meal, emotional upset, fright, anger, and coitus
- Relief occurs with rest and nitroglycerin

Signs

- Abnormal precordial (over the heart) systolic bulge
- Abnormal heart sounds

Laboratory Tests

- Typically, no laboratory tests are abnormal; however, if the patient has intermediate to high-risk features for unstable angina, electrocardiographic changes and serum troponin, or creatine kinase may become abnormal (Table 17–3)
- Patients are likely to have laboratory test abnormalities for the risk factors for IHD such as elevated total and low-density lipoprotein cholesterol, low high-density lipoprotein cholesterol, impaired fasting glucose or elevated glucose, high blood pressure, elevated C-reactive protein, and abnormal renal function. Hemoglobin should be checked to make sure the patient is not anemic.

Other Diagnostic Tests (See Chap. 13)

- A resting electrocardiogram followed by an exercise tolerance test are usually the first tests done in stable patients. A chest radiograph should be done if the patient has heart failure symptoms. Cardiac imaging using radioisotopes to detect ischemic myocardium and measure ventricular function are commonly done when revascularization is being considered. Echocardiography may also be used to assess ventricular wall motion at rest or during stress. Cardiac catheterization and coronary arteriography are used to determine coronary artery anatomy and if the patient would benefit from angioplasty, coronary artery bypass surgery or other revascularization procedures. Coronary artery calcium may be useful in detecting early disease.

TABLE 17-3 Short-Term Risk of Death or Nonfatal Myocardial Infarction in Patients with Unstable Angina

Feature	High Risk (At least 1 of the following features must be present)	Intermediate Risk (No high-risk feature but must have 1 of the following)	Low Risk (No high- or intermediate-risk feature but may have any of the following)
History	Accelerating tempo of ischemic symptoms in preceding 48 h	Prior MI, peripheral or cerebrovascular disease, or CABG, prior aspirin use	
Character of pain	Prolonged ongoing (>20 min), rest pain	Prolonged (>20 min), rest angina, now resolved, with moderate or high likelihood of CAD	New-onset CCS class III or IV angina in the past 2 weeks without prolonged (>20 min) rest pain but with moderate or high likelihood of CAD
Clinical findings	Pulmonary edema, most likely caused by ischemia New or worsening MR murmur S_3 or new/worsening rales Hypotension, bradycardia, tachycardia Age >75 y		
ECG	Angina at rest with transient ST-segment changes >0.05 mV Bundle-branch block, new or presumed new	T-wave inversions >0.2 mV Pathologic Q waves	Normal or unchanged ECG during an episode of chest discomfort
Cardiac markers	Markedly elevated (e.g., TnT or TnI >0.1 ng/mL)	Slightly elevated (e.g., TnT >0.01 but <0.1 ng/mL)	Normal

CABG, coronary artery bypass grafting; CAD, coronary artery disease; CCS, Canadian Cardiovascular Society; ECG, electrocardiogram; MI, myocardial infarction; MR, mitral regurgitation; TnI, troponin; TnT, troponin T.

CLINICAL PRESENTATION AND DIAGNOSIS

Important aspects of the clinical history for chest pain for patients with angina include the nature or quality of the pain, precipitating factors, duration, pain radiation, and the response to nitroglycerin or rest. Because there can be considerable variation in the manifestations of angina, it is more accurate to refer to these symptoms as an anginal syndrome. For some patients with significant coronary disease, their presenting symptoms may differ from the classical symptoms, yet the symptoms are a result of ischemic pain, and these are often referred to as anginal equivalents. Obtaining an accurate and detailed family history is useful in placing symptoms in perspective. Significant positive information includes premature coronary heart disease (<55 years of age in men and <65 years of age in women) as manifested as fatal and nonfatal myocardial infarction (MI), stroke, and peripheral vascular disease, as well as other risk factors such as hypertension, smoking, familial lipid disorders, and diabetes mellitus. Typical pain radiation patterns include anterior chest pain (96%), left upper arm pain (83.7%), left lower arm pain (29.3%), and neck pain at some time (22%). Pain from other areas is less common. Ischemia detected by electrocardiogram (ECG) monitoring is more likely to be detected in the morning hours (6 AM to 12 noon) than other periods throughout the day. Patients suffering from variant or Prinzmetal angina secondary to coronary spasm are more likely to experience pain at rest and in the early morning hours. Prinzmetal anginal pain is not usually brought on by exertion or emotional stress, nor is it relieved by rest, and the ECG pattern is that of current injury with ST elevation rather than depression.

It is also important to differentiate the pattern of pain for stable angina from that of unstable angina. Unstable angina may be stratified into categories of risk ranging from high to low (see Table 17–3).[15] Ischemia may also be painless or "silent" in 60% to 100% of patients, depending on the series cited and the patient population.[16] In patients with myocardial ischemia, approximately 70% of the episodes of documented ischemia are painless as determined by ambulatory ECG monitoring, and the ST segment changes associated with these episodes can be ST elevation or depression. The mechanism of silent ischemia is unclear, but studies show that patients not experiencing pain have altered pain perception, with the threshold and tolerance for pain being higher than that of patients who have pain more frequently. Although patients with diabetes tend to have more extensive coronary disease than those without diabetes and may suffer from autonomic neuropathy, asymptomatic ischemia is not more prevalent based on the Asymptomatic Cardiac Ischemia Pilot (ACIP) study.[17] Altered endorphin release is a plausible explanation, but investigations with naloxone to block endorphins do not consistently show altered pain thresholds to various stimuli compared with patients with symptomatic ischemia and patients with asymptomatic ischemia do not necessarily have impaired somatic pain sensitivity.[18] Alternatively, adenosine and substance P release during ischemia and mechanical stretch on coronary arteries may play a role in the perception of pain.

Lastly, it should be recognized that the threshold for pain caused by exertion is fixed in some patients and variable in others and that the amount of exercise or stress necessary to provoke symptoms can change over time. A fixed threshold for the induction of pain or ECG evidence of ischemia means these indicators of ischemia occur at the same, or nearly so, double rate–pressure product (systolic blood pressure × heart rate). This is apparently a consequence of at least two factors. Over long periods of time, atherosclerosis may progress, leading to more severe stenosis, reduced oxygen supply, and less of an increase in demand to precipitate ischemic symptoms. Once stenotic lesions reach a critical level of approximately 80% or greater, vasomotion, vasospasm, and thrombotic occlusion become significant factors impairing blood flow to the myocardium. Consequently, anatomic considerations and vasoactive substances may interact to provide an environment amenable to changing thresholds for the production of angina.

There appears to be little relationship between the historical features of angina and the severity or extent of coronary artery vessel involvement. Therefore, one may speculate that severe symptoms might be associated with multivessel disease, but no predictive markers exist on a routine basis.

Chest pain may resemble pain arising from a variety of noncardiac sources and the differential diagnosis of anginal pain from other etiologies may be quite difficult based on history alone. Table 17–4 outlines other common problems that may present with episodic chest pain. Although much less common, nonatherosclerotic etiologies of coronary artery disease do exist and should be excluded with appropriate tests. The clinical classification of chest pain encompasses typical angina including (a) substernal chest pain with a characteristic quality and duration that is (b) provoked by exertion or emotional stress and (c) relieved by rest or nitroglycerin); atypical angina (meets two of the characteristics for typical angina); and noncardiac chest pain (meets ≤1 of the typical angina characteristics).[2,3]

There are few signs apparent on physical examination to indicate the presence of coronary artery disease and usually only the cardio-

TABLE 17-4 Differential Diagnosis of Episodic Chest Pain Resembling Angina Pectoris

	Duration	Quality	Provocation	Relief	Location	Comment
Effort angina	5–15 min	Visceral (pressure)	During effort or emotion	Rest, NTG	Substernal, radiates	First episode vivid
Rest angina	5–15 min	Visceral (pressure)	Spontaneous (? with exercise)	NTG	Substernal, radiates	Often nocturnal
Mitral prolapse	Min–hours	Superficial (rarely visceral)	Spontaneous (no pattern)	Time	Left anterior	No pattern, variable
Esophageal reflux	10 min–1 h	Visceral	Spontaneous, cold liquids, exercise, lying down	Foods, antacids, H_2 blockers, proton pump inhibitors, NTG	Substernal, radiates	Mimics angina
Peptic ulcer	Hours	Visceral, burning	Lack of food, "acid" foods	Foods, antacids, H_2 blockers, proton pump inhibitors	Epigastric, substernal	
Biliary disease	Hours	Visceral (wax and wane)	Spontaneous, food	Time, analgesia	Epigastric, radiates	Colic
Cervical disk	Variable (gradually subsides)	Superficial	Head and neck, movement and palpation	Time, analgesia	Arm, neck	Not relieved by rest
Hyperventilation	2–3 min	Visceral	Emotion, tachypnea	Stimulus removed	Substernal	Facial paraesthesia
Musculoskeletal	Variable	Superficial	Movement, palpation	Time, analgesia	Multiple	Tenderness
Pulmonary	30 min	Visceral (pressure)	Often spontaneous	Rest, time bronchodilator	Substernal	Dyspneic

NTG, nitroglycerin.

vascular system reveals any useful information. Elevated heart rate or blood pressure can yield an increased double product and may be associated with angina, and it would be important to correct extreme tachycardia or hypertension if present. Other noncardiac physical findings that suggest that significant cardiovascular disease may be associated with angina include abdominal aortic aneurysms or peripheral vascular disease. Table 17–5 lists the cardiac examination findings in coronary artery disease. During an angina attack these findings may appear or become more prominent, making them more valuable if present.

TABLE 17-5 Cardiac Findings in Patients with Coronary Artery Disease

Sign	Clinical Significance	Frequency
Abnormal precordial systolic bulge	Left ventricular wall motion abnormality	Not usually present unless patient has sustained a prior MI (especially anterior wall) or is experiencing angina at time of examination
Decreased intensity of S_1	Decrease in left ventricular contractility	Difficult to evaluate in resting state, but can be commonly demonstrated during angina
Paradoxical splitting of S_2	Left ventricular wall motion abnormality	Very uncommon but occasionally noted during angina
S_3 (ventricular gallop)	Increased left ventricular diastolic pressure, with or without clinical CHF	Not usually present unless patient sustained extensive MI; may occasionally be present during angina
S_4 (atrial gallop)	Reduced ventricular compliance ("stiff heart")	Common; very common in patients who have sustained a prior MI as well as during angina
Apical systolic murmur (in absence of rheumatic mitral regurgitation or Barlow syndrome)	Papillary muscle dysfunction	Not usually present unless patient has sustained prior MI
Diastolic murmur (in absence of aortic regurgitation)	Coronary artery stenosis	Rare

CHF, congestive heart failure; MI, myocardial infarction; S_1, first heart sound; S_2, second heart sound; S_3, third heart sound; S_4, fourth heart sound.

From Cohn PF, ed. Diagnosis and Therapy of Coronary Artery Disease, 2d ed. Boston: Martinus Nijhoff, 1985:101, with permission.

In addition to screening for CVD risk factors (see Table 23–7), other recommended tests include hemoglobin, fasting glucose, fasting lipoprotein panel, resting ECG, and chest radiograph in patients with signs or symptoms of heart failure, valvular heart disease, pericardial disease, or aortic dissection/aneurysm.[2] Hemoglobin is assessed to insure adequate oxygen carrying capacity. Fasting glucose determinations to exclude diabetes and glucose monitoring for concurrent diabetes should be performed routinely. Lipids are assessed total-, low-density lipoprotein (LDL)- and high-density lipoprotein (HDL)-cholesterol and triglycerides (see Chap. 23).[19] Other risk factors that may be important for some patients include C-reactive protein, homocysteine level, evidence of chlamydia infection, and elevations in lipoprotein(a), fibrinogen, and plasminogen activator inhibitor.[20,21] Cardiac enzymes should all be normal in stable angina. Troponin T or I, myoglobin, or creatinine phosphokinase-MB (myocardial band) isoform may be elevated in patients with unstable angina, and interventions such as anticoagulation or antiplatelet therapy reduce cardiac end points when these markers for injury are elevated (see Table 17–3).[22]

Patients presenting with chest pain are stratified into chronic stable angina or having features of intermediate or high-risk unstable angina (Fig. 17–2 and see Table 17–3). These features include rest pain lasting longer than 20 minutes, age older than 65 years, ST- and T-wave changes and pulmonary edema. Patients with acute coronary syndrome (unstable angina, non–ST-segment elevation acute myocardial infarction and ST-segment elevation acute myocardial infarction) are managed differently than chronic stable angina.

DIAGNOSTIC TESTS

See also Chap. 13.

Electrocardiogram

The ECG is normal in about one-half of patients with angina who are not experiencing an acute attack. Typical ST-T–wave changes include depression, T-wave inversion, and ST-segment elevation. Forms of ischemia other than exertional angina may have ECG manifestations that are different; variant angina is associated with ST-segment elevation, whereas silent ischemia may produce elevation or depression. Significant ischemia is associated with ST-segment depression of greater than 2 mm, exertional hypotension, and reduced exercise tolerance.

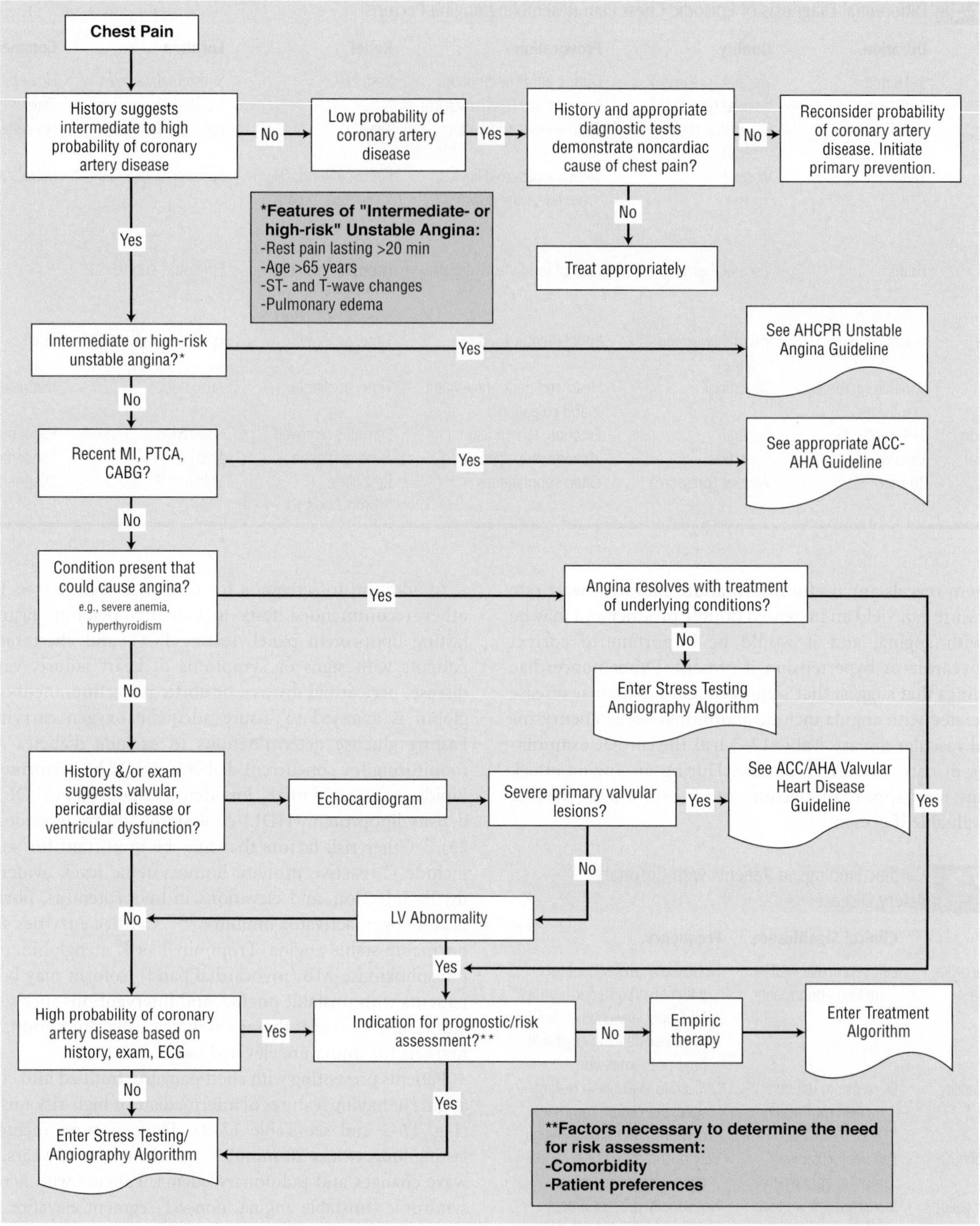

FIGURE 17-2. Clinical assessment. (ACC/AHA, American College of Cardiologists/American Heart Association; AHCPR, Agency for Health Care Policy and Research; CABG, coronary artery bypass graft; ECG, electrocardiogram; LV, left ventricular; MI, myocardial infarction; PTCA, percutaneous transluminal coronary angioplasty.)

Exercise Tolerance Testing[23]

Exercise tolerance (stress) testing (ETT) is recommended for patients with intermediate pretest probability of coronary artery disease (CAD) based on age, gender, and symptoms, including those with complete right bundle-branch block or <1 mm of rest ST depression (Fig. 17–3). Although ETT is insensitive for predicting coronary artery anatomy, it does correlate well with outcome, such as the likelihood of progressing to angina, the occurrence of acute MI, and cardiovascular death. Ischemic ST depression that occurs during ETT is an independent risk factor for cardiac events and cardiovascular mortality. Thallium (^{201}Tl) myocardial perfusion scintigraphy may be used in conjunction with ETT to detect reversible and irreversible defects in blood flow to the myocardium because it is more sensitive than ETT.

Cardiac Imaging

Radionuclide angiocardiography (performed with technetium-99m, a radioisotope) is used to measure ejection fraction, regional ventricular performance, cardiac output, ventricular volumes, valvular regurgitation, asynchrony or wall motion abnormalities, and intracardiac shunts.[24] Technetium pyrophosphate scans are used routinely for detection and quantification of acute myocardial infarction. Positron emission tomography is useful for quantifying ischemia with metabolically important substrates such as oxygen,

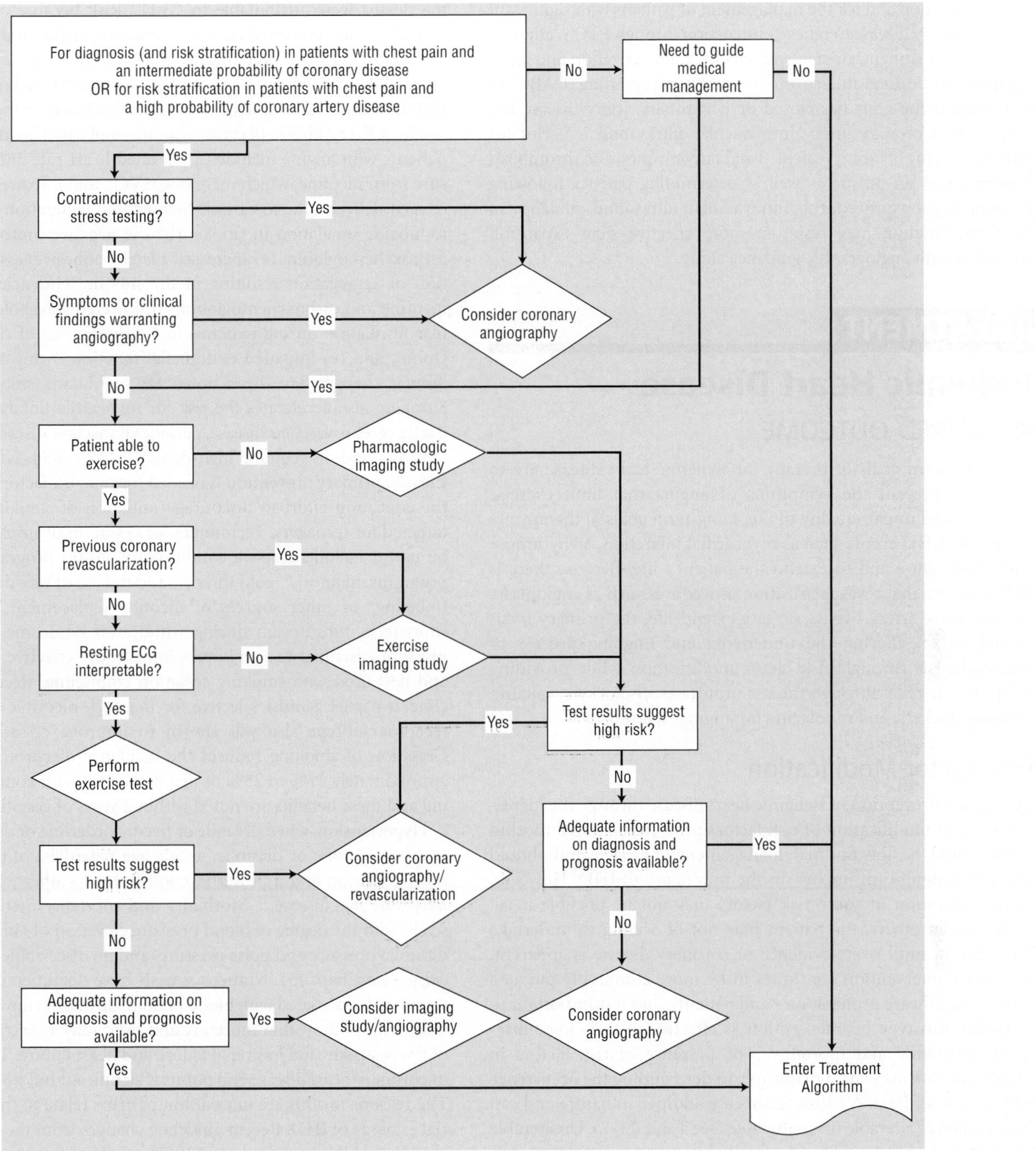

FIGURE 17-3. Stress testing/angiography algorithm. (ECG, electrocardiogram.)

carbon, and nitrogen. Other metabolic probes use radiolabeled fatty acids and glucose to study metabolic processes that may be deranged during ischemia in animals and for investigative purposes in man.

A new method using ultrarapid computerized tomography (spiral CT, ultrafast CT, electron-beam CT) minimizes artifact caused by motion of the heart during contraction and relaxation and provides a semiquantitative assessment of calcium content in coronary arteries.[25] Calcium scores >150 provide a sensitivity of 74% and specificity of 89%; consequently, this method may be cost-effective compared with ETT.

Echocardiography

Echocardiography is useful if patients have history or physical examination suggestive of valvular, pericardial disease or ventricular dysfunction. For patients unable to exercise, pharmacologic stress echocardiography (dobutamine, dipyridamole, or adenosine) or pacing may be done to identify abnormalities during stress.

Cardiac Catheterization and Coronary Arteriography

Cardiac catheterization and angiography in patients with suspected coronary artery disease are used diagnostically to document the presence and severity of disease, as well as for prognostic purposes. High-risk features during ETT suggesting the need for coronary angiography include early and significant (≥2 mm) changes on the ECG during ETT as well as multiple lead involvement, prolonged recovery from ischemia, low workload performance, abnormal blood pressure response (reduction in blood pressure), or ventricular arrhythmias. Multiple defects with thallium scans as well as lung uptake during exercise or postexercise ventricular cavity dilation are also high-risk indications for catheterization. Interventional catheterization is used for thrombolytic therapy in patients with acute myocardial infarction and for the management of patients with significant coronary artery disease to relieve obstruction through PTCA, atherectomy, laser treatment, or stent placement. Catheterization and angiography may be done after coronary artery bypass grafting (CABG) to determine if the graft has closed or if coronary artery disease has progressed. Coronary artery intravascular ultrasound is useful for directly imaging anatomy, calcified and fatty plaques, and thrombosis superimposed on plaque as well as determining patency following revascularization procedures. Intravascular ultrasound guidance of stent implantation may result in more effective stent expansion compared with angiographic guidance alone.[26]

TREATMENT

Ischemic Heart Disease

■ DESIRED OUTCOME

The short-term goals of therapy for ischemic heart disease are to reduce or prevent the symptoms of angina that limit exercise capability and impair quality of life. Long-term goals of therapy are to prevent CHD events such as myocardial infarction, arrhythmias, and heart failure and to extend the patient's life. Because there is little evidence that revascularization procedures such as angioplasty and coronary artery bypass surgery extend life, the primary focus should be on altering the underlying and ongoing process of atherosclerosis through risk factor modification while providing symptomatic relief through the use of nitrates, β-blockers, calcium channel blockers, and ranolazine for anginal symptoms.

Risk Factor Modification

❸ Primary prevention of ischemic heart disease through the identification and modification of risk factors prior to the initial morbid event would be the optimal management approach and should result in a significant impact on the prevalence of IHD. However, early recognition of some risk factors may not be possible in all cases, and in others, the patient may not be willing to undertake intervention until overt evidence of coronary disease is apparent. Secondary intervention continues to be more commonly pursued by both healthcare professionals and patients, and it is important to recognize this type of intervention as effective in reducing subsequent morbidity and mortality. The presence of risk factors in individual patients plays a major role in determining the occurrence and severity of IHD.[19,27] Risk factors are additive in nature and can be classified as alterable or unalterable (see Table 23–7). Unalterable risk factors include gender; age; family history or genetic composition; environmental influences such as climate, air pollution, trace metal composition of drinking water; and to some extent, diabetes mellitus. Improved glycemic control reduces the microvascular complications of diabetes mellitus (see Chap. 77) and reduces coronary end points; however, based on the Diabetes Control and Complications study, the reduction was impressive (40 vs. 23 major events) but not significant because the trial was underpowered to detect these changes.[28] ❹ Risk factors that can be altered include smoking, hypertension, hyperlipidemia, obesity, sedentary lifestyle, hyperuricemia, psychosocial factors such as stress and type A behavior patterns, and the use of certain drugs that may be detrimental, including progestins, corticosteroids, and cyclosporine.

Cigarette smoking is common. The Centers for Disease Control and Prevention estimates that 45.1 million people are current smokers (23.9% men; 18.1% women) in this country, and the risk for CHD is increased by about 1.8 in active smokers and by about 1.3 for passive or environmental smoke exposure.[29] From 1997 to 2001 437,902 Americans died from smoking-related illnesses and 34.7% of the deaths were attributable to CVD.[4] Risk because of smoking is related to the number of cigarettes smoked per day and the duration of smoking. Passive smoking in angina pectoris patients decreases exercise time.[6] Pipe and cigar smokers are at increased risk compared with nonsmokers, but their risk is somewhat less than that of cigarette smokers.[30] The direct effects of cigarette smoke that are detrimental to patients with angina include (a) elevated heart rate and blood pressure from nicotine, which increases MVO_2, and impaired myocardial oxygen delivery due to carboxyhemoglobin generation from carbon monoxide inhalation in smoke; (b) the negative inotropic effect of carboxyhemoglobin; (c) increased platelet adhesiveness and promotion of aggregation resulting in thrombotic tendencies because of nicotine and carboxyhemoglobin; (d) lowered threshold for ventricular fibrillation during ischemia as a consequence of carboxyhemoglobin; and (e) impaired endothelial function owing to smoking.[31] Similar changes have been noted for marihuana smoking as well. Smoking also accelerates the risk for myocardial infarction, sudden death, cerebrovascular disease, peripheral vascular disease, and hypertension, and it reduces high-density lipoprotein concentrations. Clearly, primary prevention is needed for this risk factor and much of the education effort to discourage initiation of smoking should be targeted for teenagers. Techniques for cessation of smoking that may be useful include aversive conditioning, group programs, self-help programs, hypnosis, "cold turkey," and the use of nicotine substitutes (lobeline) or other sources of nicotine replacement products for short-term substitution during withdrawal syndrome. The antidepressant sustained-release bupropion is more effective than placebo and best used with smoking cessation counseling. Recently, varenicline, a partial agonist selective for the $\alpha_4\beta_2$ nicotinic acetylcholine receptor subtype also was shown to improve cessation rates.[32,33] Cessation of smoking reduces the incidence of coronary events to approximately 15% to 25% of that associated with continued smoking and these benefits are noted within 2 years of cessation.[34]

Hypertension, whether labile or fixed, borderline or definite, casual or basal, systolic or diastolic, at any age regardless of gender, is the most common and a powerful contributor to atherosclerotic coronary vascular disease.[35] Morbidity and mortality increase progressively with the degree of blood pressure elevation of either systolic or diastolic pressure and pulse pressure, and no discernible critical value exists (see Chap. 15). Numerous trials have documented the reduction in risk associated with blood pressure lowering; however, most of these studies show that mortality and morbidity reduction is a result of fewer strokes and less renal failure and heart failure. The reduction in coronary heart disease end points is significant but not as dramatic. The reasons for this are unclear but perhaps relate to the multifactorial etiology of IHD. Recent guideline changes from the AHA recommend goal blood pressure of <130/80 mm Hg for patients with stable angina, unstable angina, non–ST-segment myocardial infarction, ST-segment myocardial infarction and <120/80 mm Hg in patients with left ventricular dysfunction.[36]

Hypercholesterolemia is a significant cardiovascular risk factor, and risk is directly related to the degree of cholesterol elevation.[19,27] As with hypertension, there is no critical value that defines risk, but rather, risk is incrementally related to the degree of elevation and the presence of other risk factors (see Chap. 23 for a detailed discussion). A fasting lipoprotein panel should be obtained in all patients with known CAD. Chapter 23 discusses the goals for total-, LDL-, and HDL-cholesterol and triglycerides. All patients should undertake therapeutic lifestyle changes. Reductions in LDL-cholesterol for primary prevention and secondary intervention have been shown to reduce total and CAD mortality and stroke as well as the need for interventions such as PTCA and CABG. Supplemental vitamin E or other antioxidants reduce the susceptibility of LDL-cholesterol to oxidation, but clinical trial data fail to show any benefit with supplementation.[37]

The prevalence of overweight and obesity, defined as a body mass index (weight in kilograms divided by height in meters squared) of ≥25 kg/m^2 and ≥30 kg/m,^{2} respectively, are estimated to occur in 66.3% and 32.2% of the U.S. population. Body mass index is associated with an increased mortality ratio compared with individuals of normal body weight, and the objective for patients with IHD is to maintain or reduce to a normal body weight.[4] This may be accomplished through dietary modification, exercise, pharmacologic therapy, or surgical therapy. Frequently associated with obesity is a sedentary lifestyle, and inactivity may contribute to higher blood pressure, elevated blood lipid levels, and insulin resistance associated with glucose intolerance in diabetics (insulin resistance or metabolic syndrome). Exercise to the level of about 300 kcal three times a week is useful in improving maximal oxygen uptake, improving cardiorespiratory efficiency, promoting collateral artery formation, and promoting potential alterations in the risk of ventricular fibrillation, coronary thrombosis, and improved tolerance to stress. Epidemiologic studies have found that mortality is directly related to resting heart rate and a low heart rate difference between resting and maximal exercise heart rate, and inversely related to exercise heart rate. A regular exercise program has been shown to reduce all-cause and cardiac mortality.[38]

Competitiveness, intense striving for achievement, easily provoked hostility, a sense of urgency about doing things quickly and being punctual, impatience, abrupt and rapid speech and gestures, and concentration on self-selected goals to the point of not perceiving and attending to other aspects of the environment are traits that characterize the behavioral pattern known as the type A or coronary prone personality. Although the issue is somewhat controversial, type A individuals may have increased cardiovascular risk with risk ratios ranging from insignificant to three times that of a matched population. Psychological stress and type D personality have been associated with adverse cardiac prognosis, but little is known about their relative effect on the pathogenesis of CHD. "Type D" refers to the tendency to experience negative emotions and to inhibit the expression of these emotions in social interactions. The mechanism by which personality affects the cardiovascular system is not understood, but may reflect the activity of the sympathetic system and enhanced responsiveness of other stress hormones when compared with non-type A personalities.

Alcohol ingestion in small to moderate amounts (<40 g/day of pure ethanol) reduces the risk of coronary heart disease; however, consumption of large amounts (>50 g/day) or binge drinking of alcohol is associated with increased mortality from stroke, cancer, vehicular accidents, and cirrhosis.[39,40] There appears to be a differential effect depending on race with an inverse relationship between ethanol consumption in whites but a direct relationship in Blacks between consumption and CAD risk. The mechanisms for the presumed protective effects of alcohol are not known but the effects may be related to increased high-density lipoprotein levels, impaired platelet function, or associations between the amount of alcohol ingested and personality type. Whatever the relationship, it is well to remember that alcohol drinking is implicated in more than 40% of all fatal automobile accidents and consumption of alcohol predisposes to hepatic cirrhosis, the sixth to seventh most common cause of death in middle age adults in the United States. With this in mind, it seems illogical to suggest alcohol ingestion as a prophylactic measure for coronary disease but rather to advise moderation of alcohol consumption, if it is the preference of the individual.

Thiazide diuretics elevate serum cholesterol and triglyceride levels whereas β-blockers tend to lower HDL and raise LDL slightly; however, a direct association between these drugs and cardiovascular risk is tenuous and based on aggregating results rather than randomized clinical trials. Conjugated equine estrogen alone or in combination with progestin lowers LDL and raises HDL based on the Postmenopausal Estrogen/Progestin Interventions (PEPI) study.[41] Unfortunately, the Heart and Estrogen/Progestin Replacement Study (HERS) trial showed no benefit of hormone replacement therapy for secondary intervention and an increased risk for thromboembolism.[42] In secondary intervention, hormone replacement therapy or estrogen alone in women after hysterectomy, HERS found that hormonal therapy health risks exceeded benefits as well.[43] Unopposed estrogen is the optimal regimen for elevation of HDL, but the high rate of endometrial hyperplasia restricts use to women without a uterus. In women with a uterus, estrogen with cyclic medroxyprogesterone has the most favorable effect on HDL and no excess risk of endometrial hyperplasia. Use of oral contraceptives in women who smoke and are older than age 35 years increases the risk of MI, stroke, and venous thromboembolism by threefold or greater. Alternative forms of contraception and cessation of smoking should be promoted in these patients. The risk for nonsmoking oral contraceptive users younger than age 35 years is very small. The relative risk of breast cancer is increased, but in the absence of risk factors for breast cancer, the relative risk is approximately 1.3 (30% increase). Coffee consumption is also linked to coronary heart disease and caffeine does transiently elevate blood pressure; however, the overall risk, if any, appears to be low and may be related to genetic makeup.[44] Although thiazide diuretics and β-blockers (nonselective without intrinsic sympathomimetic activity) may elevate both cholesterol and triglycerides by some 10% to 20%, and these effects may be detrimental, no objective evidence exists from prospective well-controlled studies to support avoiding these drugs at this time. This controversy is most pertinent in the treatment of mild hypertension and it is discussed in greater detail in Chap. 15.

TREATMENT

Stable Exertional Angina Pectoris

Table 17–6 lists the American College of Cardiology and American Heart Association's evidence-grading recommendations.

The current national guidelines recommend that all patients be given the following unless contraindications exist: (a) aspirin (Class I, Level A); (b) β-blockers with prior MI (Class I, Level A); (c) angiotensin-converting enzyme inhibitor (ACEI) to patients with CAD and

TABLE 17-6 The American College of Cardiology and American Heart Association Evidence Grading System

Recommendation Class		Level of Evidence	
I	Conditions for which there is evidence or general agreement that a given procedure or treatment is useful and effective	A	Data derived from multiple randomized clinical trials with large numbers of patients
II	Conditions for which there is conflicting evidence or a divergence of opinion about the usefulness/efficacy of a given procedure or treatment is useful and effective	B	Data derived from a limited number of randomized trials with small numbers of patients, careful analyses of nonrandomized studies, or observational registries
IIa	Weight of evidence/opinion is in favor or usefulness/efficacy	C	Expert consensus was the primary basis for the recommendation
IIb	Usefulness/efficacy is less-well established by evidence/opinion		
III	Conditions for which there is evidence or general agreement that a given procedure or treatment is not useful/effective and in some cases may be harmful		

diabetes or LV systolic dysfunction (Class I, Level A); (d) LDL-lowering therapy with CAD and LDL >130 mg/dL (Class I, Level A) (target LDL <100 mg/dL; <70 mg/dL in patients with CHD and multiple risk factors is reasonable)[27]; (e) sublingual nitroglycerin or immediate relief of angina (Class I, Level B); (f) calcium antagonists or long-acting nitrates for reduction of symptoms when β-blockers are contraindicated (Class I, Level B); (g) calcium antagonists or long-acting nitrates in combination with β-blockers when initial treatment with β-blockers is unsuccessful (Class I, Level C); (h) calcium antagonists or long-acting nitrates are recommended as a substitute for β-blockers if initial treatment with β-blockers leads to unacceptable side effects (Class I, Level A). Clopidogrel may be substituted for when aspirin is absolutely contraindicated (Class IIa, Level B) and long-acting nondihydropyridine calcium antagonists used instead of β-blockers as initial therapy (Class IIa, Level B). ACEIs are recommended in patients with CAD or other vascular disease (Class IIa, Level B). Angiotensin receptor antagonists are not mentioned in these guidelines but substitution for ACEI intolerance is reasonable. Low-intensity anticoagulation with warfarin, in addition to aspirin is recommended, but bleeding would be increased (Class IIb, Level B).[2] Therapies to be avoided include dipyridamole (Class III, Level B) and chelation therapy (Class III, Level B). Ranolazine is not addressed in these guidelines because it was released after their publication. In the European Society of Cardiology guidelines, it has a Class IIb, Level B recommendation.

After assessing and manipulating the alterable risk factors as discussed previously, the next intervention that could be undertaken is the institution of a regular exercise program. Training is possible in many patients with angina and the observed benefits include decreased heart rate and systolic blood pressure, as well as increased ejection fraction and duration of exercise. Although the mechanism of these effects has been debated, improved overall cardiovascular and muscular condition are probably most important. Improved production of nitric oxide and coronary vasomotion may account partially for the beneficial effects of exercise. The intensity of exercise influences training and more vigorous programs provide better overall results.[38] Obviously, an exercise program should be undertaken with caution and in a graded fashion with adequate supervision.

❺ Chronic prophylactic therapy for patients with more than one angina episode per day may also be instituted with β-adrenergic blocking agents, and in many instances β-blockers may be preferable because of less-frequent dosing and other properties inherent in β-blockade (e.g., potential cardioprotective effects, antiarrhythmic effects, lack of tolerance, and antihypertensive effects), as well as their antianginal effects and documented protective effects in post-MI patients.[2] Patients who continue to smoke have reduced antianginal efficacy of β-blockers. This may be a result of enhanced hepatic metabolism of drugs that are eliminated through this route or related to the effects of smoking on MVO_2 and oxygenation.[45] The one characteristic that is relevant is the duration of effect on the double product. β-Blockers with longer half-lives (e.g., nadolol) are more likely to affect the double product for a longer period of time and require fewer doses per day. The choice of β-blocker for angina rests on choosing the appropriate dose to achieve the goals outlined for heart rate and double product, and choosing an agent that is well tolerated by individual patients and cost. Selective use may incorporate ancillary properties but these are secondary considerations in overall drug product selection. Patients most likely to respond well to β-blockade are those who have a high resting heart rate and those who have a relatively fixed anginal threshold. In other words, their symptoms appear at the same level of exercise or workload on a consistent basis. Symptoms appearing with variable work loads suggest fluctuations in myocardial oxygen supply, perhaps due to coronary artery vasomotion, and these patients are more likely to respond to calcium channel antagonists.

❻ Nitrate therapy should be the first step in managing acute attacks for patients with chronic stable angina if the attacks are infrequent (i.e., a few times per month) or for prophylaxis of symptoms when undertaking activities known to precipitate attacks. In general, if angina occurs no more often than once every few days, then sublingual nitroglycerin tablets or spray or buccal products may be sufficient to allow the patient to maintain an adequate lifestyle. For episodes of "first-effort" angina occurring in a predictable fashion, nitroglycerin may be used in a prophylactic manner with the patient taking 0.3 to 0.4 mg sublingually about 5 minutes prior to the anticipated time of activity. Nitroglycerin spray may be useful when inadequate saliva is produced to rapidly dissolve sublingual nitroglycerin or if a patient has difficulty opening the container. Most patients have a response that lasts about 30 minutes or so, but this is subject to interindividual variability. When angina occurs more frequently than once a day, a chronic prophylactic regimen using β-blockers as the first line of therapy should be considered (Fig. 17–4 illustrates the stable angina algorithm). Chronic prophylactic therapy with long-acting forms of nitroglycerin (oral or transdermal), isosorbide dinitrate, 5-mononitrate, and pentaerythritol trinitrate may be effective; however, the development of tolerance is a major limiting step in their continued effectiveness. Because long-acting nitrates are not as effective as β-blockers and do not have beneficial effects, monotherapy with nitrates should not be first-line therapy unless β-blockers and calcium channel blockers are contraindicated or not tolerated. As described previously, providing a nitrate-free interval of 8 hours per day or longer appears to be the most promising approach to maintaining the efficacy of chronic nitrate therapy. Recent investigations into the mechanisms of nitrate tolerance have shown in normal volunteers that treatment with isosorbide mononitrate for 7 days resulted in tolerance as well as endothelial dysfunction, which is thought to be a consequence of reactive oxygen species generated during bioactivation of high-potency nitrates.[46,47] Oral administration of nitrates is susceptible to a saturable first-pass effect; consequently, larger doses can produce a measurable hemodynamic effect and dose titration should be based on these changes in the double product. There are few well-controlled studies that compare oral or sublingual nitrate efficacy, and the choice among these products should be based on familiarity with the preparation, cost, and patient acceptance.

❼ Calcium channel antagonists have the potential advantage of improving coronary blood flow through coronary artery vasodilation as well as decreasing MVO_2 and may be used instead of β-blockers for chronic prophylactic therapy; however, in chronic stable angina, comparative trials of long-acting calcium channel blockers with β-blockers do not show significant differences in response.[48,49] They are as effective as β-blockers and are most useful in patients who have a variable threshold for exertional angina. Calcium antagonists may provide better skeletal muscle oxygenation, resulting in decreased fatigue and better exercise tolerance. Additionally, if contraindications exist to β-blocker therapy, calcium antagonists can be safely used in many patients. The available calcium channel blockers appear to have similar efficacy in the management of chronic stable angina. Differences in their electrophysiology, peripheral and central hemodynamic effects, and adverse-effect profiles are useful in selecting the appropriate agent. Patients with conduction abnormalities and moderate to severe LV dysfunction (ejection fraction <35%) should not be treated with verapamil, whereas amlodipine may be safely used in many of these patients. Diltiazem has significant effects on the AV node and can produce heart block in patients with preexisting conduction disease or when other drugs with effects on conduction, such as digoxin or β-blockers, are used concurrently. Nifedipine may cause excessive heart rate elevation, especially if the patient is not receiving a β-blocker, and this may offset the beneficial effect it has on MVO_2. Gingival hyperplasia has also been reported

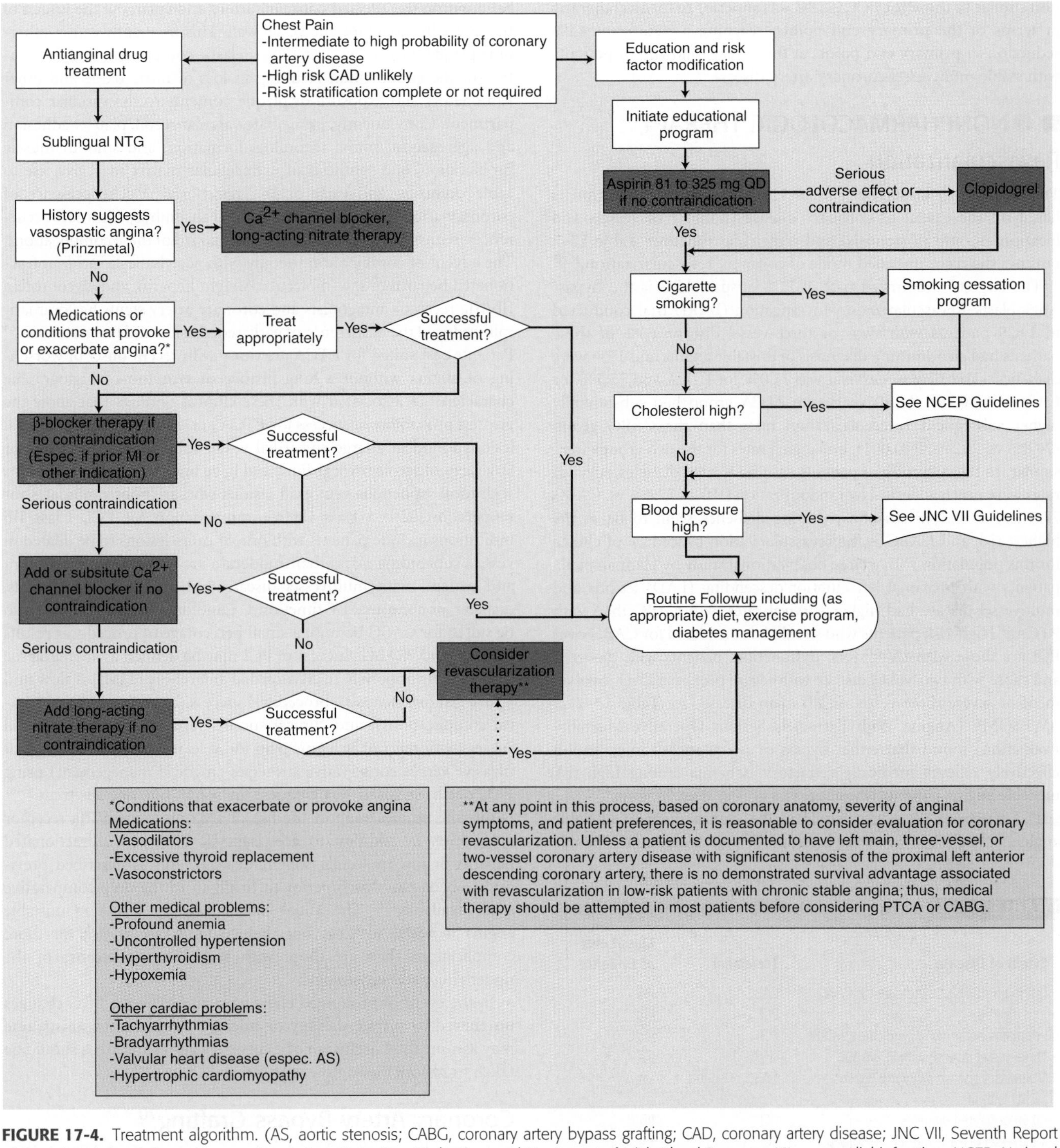

FIGURE 17-4. Treatment algorithm. (AS, aortic stenosis; CABG, coronary artery bypass grafting; CAD, coronary artery disease; JNC VII, Seventh Report of the Joint National Committee on Prevention, Detection, Evaluation, and Treatment of High Blood Pressure; MI, myocardial infarction; NCEP, National Cholesterol Education Program; NTG, nitroglycerin; PTCA, percutaneous transluminal coronary angioplasty; QD, every day.)

with nifedipine, and some dental authorities say this may be seen in as many as 20% of patients on nifedipine. Case control studies with calcium blockers suggest an increased risk for MI and cancer.[50,51] The relationship to cancer appears to be weak to nonexistent whereas the risk for MI is probably real and related to the type of drug used and relationship to recent MI. Immediate-release formulations of calcium blockers can activate the sympathetic nervous system and in patients with recent MI or significant coronary disease, may induce ischemia. This effect has not been shown for longer-acting products. The hemodynamic effect of calcium antagonists is complementary to β-blockade and, consequently, combination therapy is rational but clinical trial data do not support the notion that combination therapy is always more effective.[48,52]

Although revascularization (see below) would seem to provide better symptomatic relief and improved survival rates, recent randomized trials have shown no advantage of angioplasty or surgery over medical therapy in patients with stable coronary artery disease.[53,54] In the Clinical Outcomes Utilizing Revascularization and Aggressive Drug Evaluation (COURAGE) trial, the 4.6-year cumulative primary event rates (death from any cause and nonfatal myocardial infarction) were 19.0% in the percutaneous coronary intervention (PCI) group and 18.5% in the medical therapy group (hazard ratio for the PCI group, 1.05; 95% confidence interval [CI], 0.87 to 1.27; $P = 0.62$).[53] The Medicine, Angioplasty, or Surgery Study (MASS II) found medical therapy was associated with an incidence of long-term events and rate of additional revascularization similar to those for PCI. CABG was superior to medical therapy in terms of the primary end points, reaching a significant 44% reduction in primary end points at the 5-year followup of patients with stable multivessel coronary artery disease.[54]

■ 8 NONPHARMACOLOGIC THERAPY

Revascularization

The decision to undertake PCI or CABG for revascularization is based on the extent of coronary disease (number of vessels and location/amount of stenosis) and ventricular function. Table 17–7 outlines the recommended mode of coronary revascularization.[15,55]

The largest randomized trial of PCI versus CABG is the Bypass Angioplasty Revascularization Investigation (BARI) trial conducted in 1,829 patients with two- or three-vessel disease; 64% of these patients had an admitting diagnosis of unstable angina and 19% were diabetic.[56] The 10-year survival was 71.0% for PTCA and 73.5% for CABG (P= 0.18). At 10 years, the PTCA group had substantially higher subsequent revascularization rates than the CABG group (76.8% vs. 20.3%, P<0.001), but angina rates for the two groups were similar. In the subgroup of patients with no treated diabetes, survival rates were nearly identical by randomization (PTCA 77.0% vs. CABG 77.3%, P = 0.59).[57] Insulin-requiring diabetics seem to be at the highest risk and CABG is the revascularization procedure of choice for this population.[58] In a large observational study by Hannan et al., patients with proximal left anterior descending (LAD) lesions and multivessel disease had higher survival rates with CABG than with PTCA.[59] High-risk patients who should be considered for CABG over PCI are those with LV systolic dysfunction, patients with diabetes, and those with two-vessel disease with severe proximal LAD involvement or severe three-vessel or left main disease (see Table 17–7).[15] AWESOME (Angina With Extremely Serious Operative Mortality Evaluation) found that either bypass or percutaneous intervention effectively relieves medically refractory ischemia among high-risk unstable angina patients whose age was greater than 70 years.[60]

PCI has been used successfully in the management of unstable angina.[55,61] PTCA involves the insertion of a guidewire and inflatable balloon into the affected coronary artery and enlarging the lumen of the artery by stretching the vessel wall. This frequently causes atheroma plaque fracture by stretching inelastic components and denudation of the endothelium resulting in loss of nitric oxide and other vasodilators and exposure of plaque contents to the vascular compartment. Consequently, immediate vascular recoil, platelet adhesion and aggregation, mural thrombus formation, and smooth muscle proliferation, and synthesis of extracellular matrix may give rise to acute occlusion and early or late restenosis.[62,63] The presence of coronary artery spasm and intraluminal thrombus, common occurrences in unstable angina, increases the hazard of these complications. The advent of combination therapy with acetylsalicylic acid, unfractionated heparin or low-molecular-weight heparin, and glycoprotein IIb/IIIa receptor antagonists and coronary artery stents has dramatically reduced the occurrence of early reocclusion and late restenosis.[64] Patients best suited for PTCA are those with recent onset of worsening of angina without a long history of symptoms. Angiographic characteristics associated with these clinical findings that allow the greatest probability of success for PTCA are severe, discrete, proximal lesions found in a large epicardial vessel subtending a moderate or large area of viable myocardium and have high-risk features. Patients with focal saphenous vein graft lesions who are poor candidates for reoperation have a class IIa recommendation for PCI. Class IIb indications include patients with one or more lesions to be dilated in vessels subtending a less-than-moderate area of viable myocardium and patients with multivessel disease and proximal LAD lesions, diabetes, or abnormal LV function.[65] Candidates for PTCA must also be suited for CABG because a small percentage of procedures results in emergency CABG. Success of PCI may be defined as angiographic success (Thrombolysis In Myocardial Infarction [TIMI] 3 flow and <20% residual stenosis), procedural success (lack of in-hospital clinical complications), and clinical success (anatomic and procedural success with relief of ischemic pain for at least 6 months). In trials of invasive versus conservative strategies (medical management) using PCI, death or MI is less frequent in some, but not all, trials.[66–69] Numerous studies support the use of glycoprotein IIb/IIIa receptor antagonists in addition to acetylsalicylic acid and unfractionated heparin or low-molecular-weight heparin, and as described previously, abciximab was superior to tirofiban in the only comparative study available.[15,65] The initial success rate for PTCA in unstable angina is ~80% to 90%, but these patients are at risk for more complications than are those with stable angina because of the underlying pathophysiology.

In the event of prolonged chest pain and ischemic ECG changes unrelieved by nitrate therapy or calcium channel antagonists, one may assume total occlusion of a coronary vessel and steps should be taken to restore blood flow with either PCI or CABG.

TABLE 17-7 Recommended Mode of Coronary Revascularization

Extent of Disease	Treatment	Class/Level of Evidence
Left main disease,[a] candidate for CABG	CABG	I/A
	PCI	III/C
Left main disease, not a candidate for CABG	PCI	IIb/C
Three-vessel disease with EF <0.50	CABG	I/A
Multivessel disease including proximal LAD with EF	CABG	I/A
<0.50 or treated diabetes	PCI	IIb/B
Multivessel disease with EF >0.50 and without diabetes	PCI	I/A
One- or two-vessel disease without proximal LAD but with large areas of myocardial ischemia or high-risk criteria on noninvasive testing (see text)	CABG or PCI	I/B
One-vessel disease with proximal LAD	CBAG or PCI	IIa/B
One- or two-vessel disease without proximal LAD with small area of ischemia or no ischemia on noninvasive testing	CABG or PCI	III/C
Insignificant coronary stenosis	CABG or PCI	III/C

CABG, coronary artery bypass grafting; EF, ejection fraction; LAD, left anterior descending coronary artery; PCI, percutaneous coronary intervention.

[a]≥50% diameter stenosis.

From Braunwald E, Antman EM, Beasley JW, et al. ACC/AHA guidelines for the management of patients with unstable angina and non–ST-segment elevation myocardial infarction: A report of the American College of Cardiology/American Heart Association Task Force on Practice Guidelines (Committee on the Management of Patients with Unstable Angina). J Am Coll Cardiol 2000;36:970–1062, with permission.

Coronary Artery Bypass Grafting[70]

Following the introduction of saphenous vein graft replacement for the severely occluded coronary arteries by Favorolo and Garrett in 1967, CABG became an accepted and commonly used approach for the management of IHD. The objectives in performing CABG are twofold: (a) to reduce the number of symptomatic anginal attacks not controlled with medical management or PCI and improve the lifestyle of the patient, and (b) to reduce the mortality associated with coronary artery disease. Surgery is effective in providing pain relief in large numbers of patients, with approximately 70% to 95% being pain-free at 1 year and 46% to 55% being pain-free at 5 years. This compares favorably with medical management, with which only approximately 30% are free of symptoms at 5 years. Mortality at 10 years from the largest published studies is 26.4% with CABG and 30.5% with medical management (P = 0.03) but there are significant differences based on subgroup analysis (e.g., left main disease vs. one-vessel disease without a proximal LAD lesion).[71] The second objective is met in certain patients and was addressed in three large, well-controlled trials of bypass surgery. These three studies, the Veterans Administration, European Cooperative Surgery Study, and the CASS, are not directly comparable because the inclusion and exclusion criteria for entry into each study were different and patients were followed for different periods of time. They have also been criticized for not being representative of the population that may be candidates for surgery, lacking women or late-middle aged or elderly patients, and for crossover of medically managed patients to the surgical group. A major change in medical practice that influences the interpretation of these older studies is the common procedure of stent placement at the time of angioplasty.[72] There are about 20 different types of stents available and their use is associated with greater luminal diameter after angioplasty, fewer acute reocclusions and less restenosis after stent placement. Consequently, the validity of generalizing the results from these studies to routine practice has been questioned, but these studies are useful for providing a basis for decisions concerning surgery. Current class I recommendations for CABG in asymptomatic or mild angina patient includes significant (>50%) left main coronary artery stenosis, left main equivalent (≥70% stenosis of the proximal LAD and proximal left circumflex artery), and three-vessel disease, especially in patients with a LV ejection fraction <0.50.[71] Class IIa recommendations for CABG are proximal LAD stenosis with one- or two-vessel disease and class IIb recommendations for one- or two-vessel disease not involving the proximal LAD. In stable angina, class I recommendations are the same as for mild angina with the following additions: one- or two-vessel disease without significant proximal LAD stenosis, but with a large area of viable myocardium and high-risk criteria in noninvasive testing; disabling angina despite maximal medical therapy, when surgery can be performed with acceptable risk. Class IIb recommendations in stable angina include proximal LAD stenosis with one-vessel disease and one- or two-vessel disease without significant proximal LAD stenosis but with a moderate area of viable myocardium and ischemia on noninvasive testing. The indications for CABG in unstable angina/non–ST-segment elevation myocardial infarction were described previously. In ST-segment MI, CABG is indicated for ongoing ischemia/infarction not responsive to maximal medical therapy (class IIb).

In patients with poor LV function CABG is indicated for the same indications as in mild angina for class I. Class IIa recommendations include poor LV function with significant viable, noncontracting, revascularizable myocardium without any of the aforementioned anatomic patterns (e.g., left main disease). CABG is useful in patients with life-threatening ventricular arrhythmia in the presence of left main disease, three-vessel disease (class I) and in bypassable one- or two-vessel disease causing life-threatening ventricular arrhythmias and proximal LAD disease with one- or two-vessel disease (class IIa).

CABG may also be used for patients who have failed PTCA if there is ongoing ischemia or threatened occlusion with significant myocardium at risk and in patients with hemodynamic compromise (class I). Class IIa recommendations for failed PTCA include a foreign body in a crucial anatomic position and hemodynamic compromise in patient with impairment of the coagulation system and without a previous sternotomy. CABG may be repeated in patients with a previous CABG if disabling angina exists despite maximal noninvasive therapy (class I) and if a large area of myocardium is threatened and is subtended by bypassable distal vessels (class IIa).

The need for nitrates and β-blockers is clearly reduced by surgery, with only 30% of CABG patients requiring chronic medication, whereas 70% of their medical counterparts received anginal drugs. CASS showed that employment status after surgery was more dependent on the pretreatment status than an effect induced by the treatment arm, and that approximately 70% of patients are employed before and after surgery. Recent followup analyses of these studies suggest that patients who have diabetes or peripheral vascular disease, who are African Americans, or who continue to smoke are at high risk for CAD events, and diabetics, in particular, are more likely to have a better outcome with CABG than PTCA.[56,73,74] The overall benefit noted after CABG is similar in men and women, and elderly patients appear to have outcomes similar to younger patients.

Operative mortality is reported to range from 1% to 3% and is related to the number of vessels involved and preoperative ventricular function. Patients in CASS with one-, two-, or three-vessel disease had operative mortalities of 1.4%, 2.1%, and 2.8%, respectively. The relationship to left ventricular ejection fraction follows a similar trend with ejection fractions of greater than 50%, 20% to 40%, and less than 20% having operative mortality rates of 1.9%, 4.4%, and 6.7%, respectively. Perioperative infarction averages 5% depending on the sensitivity of the method for assessment, and the occurrence of an infarct reduces long-term survival. Neurologic dysfunction is relatively common postoperatively in CABG patients (~6%), but many of the deficits are clinically insignificant and resolve with time. Fatal brain damage occurs in 0.3% to 0.7%, stroke in approximately 5%, and ophthalmologic defects in 25%, but only 3% have clinically apparent field defects. Peripheral nerve lesions (12%) and brachial plexopathy (7%) are also reported to occur. Other complications include constrictive pericarditis (0.2%), cellulitis at the site of vein graft, and mediastinal infections (1% to 4%).

Graft patency influences the success for symptom control, and survival and the mechanism for early graft occlusion is probably different from that associated with late closure. Early occlusion is related to platelet adhesion and aggregation whereas late occlusion may be related to endothelial proliferation and progression of atherosclerosis. Patency of grafts early on after the CABG are reported to range from 88% to 97% in at least one graft and 58% to 81% in all grafts at 1 year. Long-term patency based on the CASS Montreal Heart Institute experience suggests that 60% to 67% of all grafts remain patent at 5 to 11 years. Antiplatelet therapy has been demonstrated to improve early and late patency rates and should probably be used in all patients who do not have any contraindications. Aspirin with or without other antiplatelet agents (clopidogrel) reduces the late development of vein-graft occlusions. Late graft closure is related to elevated lipid levels and the progression of atherosclerosis in the grafted vessels as well as the native circulation. Elevation of very-low-density lipoprotein, LDL, and LDL apolipoprotein B is correlated to disease progression and graft closure. Aggressive lipid lowering can stabilize the progression of CAD and may induce regression in selected coronary artery segments within a patient following CABG. Cessation of smoking is an important preoperative and postoperative objective as well as in the management of other coronary risk factors (e.g., hypertension) and institution of a supervised, daily exercise program is recommended. Internal mammary artery grafts should be used for revascularizing the left anterior descending artery system when possible owing to better graft survival and clinical outcomes.

Valvular heart disease can coexist with coronary heart disease, although this is relatively uncommon with rheumatic valve disease, usually the mitral valve, and more common with aortic stenosis and regurgitation. Angina may occur in 35% to 65% of patients with aortic stenosis or regurgitation, and if severe, may be the cause of angina in the absence of coronary artery disease. Patients being evaluated for possible CABG should also be evaluated for valvular disease to determine if valve replacement needs to be performed along with bypass grafting.

Percutaneous Transluminal Coronary Angioplasty[55]

Since the introduction into clinical cardiology of PTCA by Gruentzig in 1977, this procedure has gained rapid acceptance as a safe and effective means of managing coronary artery disease. It is estimated that more than 750,000 PCI procedures are done each year in this country and 525,000 of them are PTCA. The proposed mechanisms of reduced stenosis with PTCA include (a) compression and redistribution of the atherosclerotic plaque; (b) embolization of plaque contents; (c) aneurysm formation; and (d) disruption of the plaque and arterial wall with distortion and tearing of the intima and media, which leads to denudation of the endothelium, platelet adhesion and aggregation, thrombus formation, and smooth muscle proliferation. Of these mechanisms, the last one is felt to be the most important, but the others may contribute to opening of the lesions in some situations.

❾ The indications for PTCA have been provided by the American College of Cardiology/American Heart Association (ACC/AHA) and now span single or multivessel disease, as well as asymptomatic and symptomatic patients (Table 17–8).[55] In addition to providing recommendations for which type of patients are appropriate for PTCA, the guidelines also provide recommendations for the volume of procedures, the use of intravascular ultrasound, and surgery backup when PTCA is being considered. ❿ PTCA generally is not useful if only a small area of viable myocardium is at risk, or when ischemia cannot be demonstrated, borderline (<50%) stenosis or lesions that are difficult to dilate are present, or the patient were at high risk for morbidity or mortality or both (e.g., left main or equivalent disease or three-vessel disease). PTCA alone or when used in conjunction or sequentially with thrombolysis for acute myocardial infarction is discussed in Chap. 18. Stent placement accompanies balloon angioplasty in approximately 80% of cases in the United States. Table 17–8 lists the current recommendations for PCI based on class of angina.

Assessment of outcome with PCI can be based on several angiographic, procedural, and clinical outcomes, as discussed previously. The success of PCI is dependent on the experience of the operator (high volume, better outcome), on complicating factors for the patient (including the number of vessels to be dilated), and on technical advances in the equipment used (e.g., steerable and low-profile catheters). The acute success rate for opening of uncomplicated stenotic lesions ranges from 96% to 99% with the combined balloon/device/pharmacologic approach in experienced hands, and angina is decreased or eliminated in approximately 80% of cases. The success rate totally occluded lesions is somewhat less (~65%). Mortality at 1 year is 1% for single-vessel disease and 2.5% for multivessel involvement, reflecting the good prognosis associated with this degree of coronary artery disease. At 10 years, survival is 95% for single-vessel disease and 81% for multivessel disease.[75] Most patients remain event-free (no death, MI, or CABG) for an extended period. Symptomatic status, as measured by the New York Heart Association classification, is improved in many patients. Restenosis is noted in 32% to 40% after balloon angioplasty at 6 months, and half of these patients will have symptoms associated with restenosis.[75] A few late restenotic events occur, but most restenosis occurs within the first 6 months. Anatomic factors that predict restenosis include lesions >20 mm in length, excessive tortuosity of the proximal segment, extremely angulated segments (>90°), total occlusions >3 months old and and/or bridging collaterals, inability to protect major side branches, and degenerated vein grafts with friable lesions. Clinical factors that predict worse outcome include diabetes, advanced age, female gender, unstable angina, heart failure and multivessel disease. A four-variable scoring system that predicts cardiovascular collapse for failed PTCA includes percentage of myocardium at risk (e.g., >50% viable myocardium at risk and LV ejection fraction <25%), preangioplasty percent diameter stenosis, multivessel CAD, and diffuse disease in the dilated segment or a high myocardial jeopardy score.[65] Strut thickness of the stent influences restenosis as well and thicker struts are associated with angiographic and clinical restenosis.[76]

The overall complication rate ranges from 2% to 21%, depending on the lesion type.[77] Coronary occlusion, dissection, or spasm occurs in 4% to 8% of patients, whereas ST-segment elevation MI occurs in 1.6% to 4.8%.[65] Prolonged angina and ventricular tachycardia or fibrillation occurs in 6.9% and 2.3%, respectively. In-hospital mortality ranges from 0.7% to 2.5% overall, and high-risk events for mortality includes ventricular arrhythmias and myocardial infarction. The frequency of urgent CABG because of complications ranges from 0.4% to 5.8%.[65]

Table 17–9 outlines current AHA/ACC recommendations for antithrombotic therapy in PCI.[55,78] Antiplatelet therapy with acetylsalicylic acid 80 to 325 mg/day given at least 2 hours prior to angioplasty is currently recommended. If patients are sensitive to acetylsalicylic acid, clopidogrel or ticlopidine are acceptable alternatives. Most centers now use clopidogrel because of adverse effects (described in Chap. 18) and prolonged time to onset for ticlopidine. In elective settings, clopidogrel should be started at least 72 hours in advance of the procedure to allow for maximal antiplatelet effects. Alternatively, a loading dose of clopidogrel (300 to 600 mg) or ticlopidine (500 mg) may be given to achieve a more rapid antiplatelet effect.[79] The combination of acetylsalicylic acid plus clopidogrel is currently recommended for patients undergoing angioplasty and stenting, and this combination is safer and superior to antiplatelet therapy plus anticoagulation with warfarin-like drugs.[80] Followup for up to 4 years from the ISAR (Intracoronary Stenting and Antithrombotic Regimen) trial shows that the benefit of combined antiplatelet therapy evident after 30 days is maintained after 4 years.[81] Aspirin is an incomplete inhibitor of platelet aggregation; combination therapy of acetylsalicylic acid plus a glycoprotein (GP) IIb/IIIa receptor antagonist for PCI shows a relative risk reduction of 37.5% for death and nonfatal MI at 30 days, favoring GP IIb/IIIa receptor antagonists over placebo (absolute rates of 5.5% vs. 8.9% based on PCI trials. As discussed in Chap. 18, high-risk patients and those having a stent placed are most likely to benefit from GP IIb/IIIa receptor antagonist use. Patients presenting with elevated cardiac biomarkers are also more likely to receive benefit from GP IIb/IIIa receptor antagonists than patients with normal levels of biomarkers.[82] In the only comparative trial, abciximab was superior to tirofiban.[83]

During PTCA patients are usually heparinized to prevent immediate thrombus formation at the site of arterial injury and on coronary guidewires and catheters; anticoagulation is continued for up to 24 hours. The intensity of anticoagulation is monitored using the activated clotting time and the targeted range for activated clotting time is 250 to 300 seconds (HemoTec device) in the absence of GP IIb/IIIa receptor antagonist use.[65] When GP IIb/IIIa receptor antagonists are not used, unfractionated heparin is given as an IV bolus of 70 to 100 international units/kg to achieve a target activated clotting time of 200 seconds. The loading dose is lowered to 50 to 70 international units/kg when GP IIb/IIIa receptor antagonists are given. Target activated clotting time for eptifibatide and tirofiban is <300 seconds during angioplasty; post-procedure unfractionated heparin infusions are not recommended during GP IIb/IIIa receptor antagonist therapy. Mechanisms that result in restenosis include acute lumen loss owing to "recoil," mural thrombosis formation, and smooth muscle cell proliferation with synthesis of extracellular matrix.[84] Approaches to prevent restenosis may be aimed at altering the underlying mechanisms. Recoil and loss of luminal diameter may be reduced by the use of stent placement; however, this beneficial effect is offset by an increased number of vascular complications. Cracking of the plaque leads to severe damage to the arterial wall, exposure of collagen, and endothelial dysfunction. These factors promote mural thrombi, and the propensity for thrombus formation is related, in part, to the composition of the plaque as well as the depth of injury. Combination therapy with acetylsalicylic acid, heparin and GP IIb/IIIa receptor antagonists is recommended to minimize acute occlusion and numerous clinical

TABLE 17-8 Percutaneous Coronary Intervention Based on Angina Class

Patients with Asymptomatic Ischemia or Canadian Cardiovascular Society (CCS) Class I or II Angina		
Class I Patients who do not have treated diabetes with asymptomatic ischemia or mild angina with 1 or more significant lesions in 1 or 2 coronary arteries suitable for PCI with a high likelihood of success and low risk of morbidity and mortality. The vessels to be dilated must subtend a large area of viable myocardium. *(Level of Evidence: B)*	**Class IIa** 1. PCI is reasonable in patients with asymptomatic ischemia or CCS class I or II angina and with 1 or more significant lesions in 1 or 2 coronary arteries suitable for PCI with a high likelihood of success and a low risk of morbidity and mortality. The vessels to be dilated must subtend a moderate to large area of viable myocardium or be associated with a moderate to severe degree of ischemia on noninvasive testing. *(Level of Evidence: B)*	Phrasing has been changed to reflect current terminology. The recommendation and all of those that follow in Section 5 have been reworded to be consistent with the CCS classification system of angina. This recommendation has been changed to class IIa to reflect the published data and Writing Committee consensus that not all patients in this clinical category must have PCI performed.
Class IIa 1. The same clinical and anatomic requirements as for Class I, except the myocardial area at risk is of moderate size or the patient has treated diabetes. *(Level of Evidence: B)*		This recommendation has been merged with other class IIa recommendations of this section, and the phrasing has been changed to reflect current terminology.
	2. PCI is reasonable for patients with asymptomatic ischemia or CCS class I or II angina, and recurrent stenosis after PCI with a large area of viable myocardium or high-risk criteria on noninvasive testing. *(Level of Evidence: C)*	This is a new recommendation dealing with the management of recurrent stenosis after PCI among patients with asymptomatic ischemia or class I or II angina.
	3. Use of PCI is reasonable in patients with symptomatic ischemia or CCS class I or II angina with significant left main CAD (greater than 50% diameter stenosis) who are candidates for revascularization but are not eligible for CABG. *(Level of Evidence: B)*	This recommendation for PCI among patients who are eligible for CABG who have significant left main disease has been added to reflect the favorable results noted by several trials with PCI.
Class IIb Patients with asymptomatic ischemia or mild angina with greater than or equal to 3 coronary arteries suitable for PCI with a high likelihood of success and a low risk of morbidity and mortality. The vessels to be dilated must subtend at least a moderate area of viable myocardium. In the physician's judgment, there should be evidence of myocardial ischemia by ECG exercise testing, stress nuclear imaging, stress echocardiography or ambulatory ECG monitoring or intracoronary physiologic measurements. *(Level of Evidence: B)*		This recommendation has been eliminated and replaced by the following 2 recommendations. For each, the phrasing has been constructed to reflect current terminology.
	Class IIb 1. The effectiveness of PCI for patients with asymptomatic ischemia or CCS class I or II angina who have 2- or 3-vessel disease with significant proximal LAD CAD who are otherwise eligible for CABG with 1 arterial conduit and who have treated diabetes or abnormal LV function is not well established. *(Level of Evidence: B)*	Phrasing has been changed to reflect current terminology. Among patients who are eligible, CABG with 1 arterial conduit is generally preferred for treatment of multivessel disease with significant proximal LAD obstruction in patients with treated diabetes and/or abnormal OV function.
	2. PCI might be considered for patients with asymptomatic ischemia or CCS class I or II angina with nonproximal LAD CAD that subtends a moderate area of viable myocardium and demonstrates ischemia on noninvasive testing. *(Level of Evidence: C)*	Phrasing has been changed to reflect current terminology. PCI might be considered in this clinical setting.
Class III Patients with asymptomatic ischemia or mild angina who do not meet the criteria as listed under Class I or Class II and who have: a. Only a small area of viable myocardium at risk b. No objective evidence of ischemia c. Lesions that have a low likelihood of successful dilation d. Mild symptoms that are unlikely to be due to myocardial ischemia e. Factors associated with increased risk of morbidity or mortality f. Left main disease g. Insignificant disease less than 50% *(Level of Evidence: C)*	**Class III** PCI is not recommended in patients with asymptomatic ischemia or CCS class I or II angina who do not meet the criteria as listed under the class II recommendations or who have 1 or more of the following: a. Only a small area of viable myocardium at risk *(Level of Evidence: C)* b. No objective evidence of ischemia *(Level of Evidence: C)* c. Lesions that have a low likelihood of successful dilation *(Level of Evidence: C)* d. Mild symptoms that are unlikely to be due to myocardial ischemia *(Level of Evidence: C)* e. Factors associated with increased risk of morbidity or mortality *(Level of Evidence: C)* f. Left main disease and eligibility for CABG *(Level of Evidence: C)* g. Insignificant disease (less than 50% coronary stenosis) *(Level of Evidence: C)*	Phrasing has been changed to reflect current terminology. Recommendation has been reworded to be consistent with CCS classification system for angina. Level of evidence has been added for each subgroup.

(continued)

TABLE 17-8 Percutaneous Coronary Intervention Based on Angina Class (continued)

Patients with CCS Class III Angina		
Class I	**Class IIa**	
Patient with 1 or more significant lesions in 1 or more coronary arteries suitable for PCI with a high likelihood of success and low risk of morbidity or mortality. The vessel(s) to be dilated must subtend a moderate or large area of viable myocardium and high risk. *(Level of Evidence: B)*	1. It is reasonable that PCI be performed in patients with CCS class III angina and single-vessel or multivessel CAD who are undergoing medical therapy and who have 1 or more significant lesions in 1 or more coronary arteries suitable for PCI with a high likelihood of success and low risk of morbidity or mortality. *(Level of Evidence: B)*	Phrasing has been changed to reflect current terminology. Recommendation has been reworded to be consistent with CCS classification system for angina. The recommendation class has been changed to IIa to reflect published data and Writing Committee consensus. Criteria regarding viable and high-risk myocardium have been deleted from this commendation.
Class IIa		
Patients with focal saphenous vein graft lesions or multiple stenoses who are poor candidates for reoperative surgery. *(Level of Evidence: C)*	2. It is reasonable that PCI be performed in patients with CCS class III angina with single-vessel or multivessel CAD who are undergoing medical therapy with focal saphenous vein graft lesions or multiple stenoses who are poor candidates for reoperative surgery. *(Level of Evidence: C)*	Phrasing has been changed to reflect current terminology.
	3. Use of PCI is reasonable in patients with CCS class III angina with significant left main CAD (greater than 50% diameter stenosis) who are candidates for revascularization but are not eligible for CABG. *(Level of Evidence: B)*	This recommendation for PCI among patients with significant left main disease who are not eligible for CABG has been added to reflect the favorable results noted by several trials with PCI.
Class IIb	**Class IIb**	
Patient has 1 or more lesions to be dilated with reduced likelihood of success of the vessel(s) subtend a less than moderate area of viable myocardium. Patients with 2- or 3-vessel disease, with significant proximal LAD CAD and treated diabetes or abnormal LV function. *(Level of Evidence: B)*	1. PCI may be considered in patients with CCS class III angina with single-vessel or multivessel CAD who are undergoing medical therapy and who have 1 or more lesions to be dilated with a reduced likelihood of success. *(Level of Evidence: B)*	Phrasing has been changed to reflect current terminology. The 2001 recommendation has been split into 2 separate recommendations.
	2. PCI may be considered in patients with CCS class III angina and no evidence of ischemia on noninvasive testing or who are undergoing medical therapy and have 2- or 3-vessel CAD with significant proximal LAD CAD and treated diabetes or abnormal LV function. *(Level of Evidence: B)*	Phrasing has been changed to reflect current terminology. The use of noninvasive testing to evaluate for evidence of ischemia has been added.
Class III	**Class III**	
Patient has no evidence of myocardial injury or ischemia on objective testing and has not had a trial of medical therapy, or has a. Only a small area of myocardium at risk b. All lesions or the culprit lesion to be dilated with morphology with a low likelihood of success c. A high risk of procedure-related morbidity or mortality. *(Level of Evidence: C)* 2. Patients with insignificant coronary stenosis (e.g., less than 50% diameter). *(Level of Evidence: C)* 3. Patients with significant left main CAD who are candidates for CABG. *(Level of Evidence: B)*	PCI is not recommended for patients with CCS class III angina with single-vessel or multivessel CAD, no evidence of myocardial injury or ischemia on objective testing, and no trial of medical therapy, or who have 1 of the following: a. Only a small area of myocardium at risk *(Level of Evidence: C)* b. All lesions or the culprit lesion to be dilated with morphology that conveys a low likelihood of success *(Level of Evidence: C)* c. A high risk of procedure-related morbidity or mortality *(Level of Evidence: C)* d. Insignificant disease (less than 50% coronary stenosis) *(Level of Evidence: C)* e. Significant left main CAD and candidacy for CABG *(Level of Evidence: C)*	Phrasing has been changed to reflect current terminology. Class II recommendations #2 and #3 from the 2001 guidelines have been merged into this recommendation.

CAEBG, coronary artery bypass graft; CAD, coronary artery disease; ECG, electrocardiograpy; LAD, left anterior descending; LV, left ventricle; OV, outflow volume; PCI, percutaneous coronary intervention.
From Smith SC Jr, Feldman TE, Hirshfeld JW Jr, et al. ACC/AHA/SCAI 2005 guideline update for percutaneous coronary intervention–Summary article: A report of the American College of Cardiology/American Heart Association Task Force on Practice Guidelines (ACC/AHA/SCAI Writing Committee to Update the 2001 Guidelines for Percutaneous Coronary Intervention). Circulation 2006;113:156–175.

trials document the efficacy of this combined approach.[55,78] Bivalirudin is a specific and reversible direct thrombin inhibitor that is indicated for use as an anticoagulant in patients with unstable angina undergoing PTCA. Bivalirudin is comparable to heparin in preventing thrombosis and may be associated with less bleeding.[85–87] Chapter 18 has a more complete discussion of antithrombotic therapy.

Alternatives to PTCA include directional coronary atherectomy (DCA), excimer laser, rotational atherectomy (rotablator), and intracoronary stents, or some combination of these interventions.[88] Based on randomized trials, DCA produces greater initial luminal diameter but results in a higher rate of post-procedure complications, such as non–Q-wave MI and death, and is more expensive. Consequently, PTCA is considered to be superior to DCA for most patients. Tissue debulking with DCA is useful for in-stent restenosis, particularly for diabetic patients.[89] The use of abciximab may improve these results.[90] Excimer laser angioplasty followed by balloon angioplasty or rotational atherectomy provides no benefit additional to balloon angioplasty alone.[91]

TABLE 17-9 Pharmacologic Management of Percutaneous Coronary Intervention

Antiplatelet and antithrombotic adjuctive therapies for PCI–oral antiplatelet therapy	
Class I	
1. Patients already taking daily chronic aspirin therapy should take 75 to 325 mg of aspirin before the PCI procedure is performed. *(Level of Evidence: A)*	A daily dose of 75 mg of aspirin has been shown to result in improved cardiovascular outcomes similar to daily doses of 325 mg but with fewer bleeding complications.
2. Patients not already taking daily chronic aspirin therapy should be given 300 to 325 mg of aspirin at least 2 hours and preferably 24 hours before the PCI procedure is performed. *(Level of Evidence: C)*	Higher doses of aspirin are recommended for patients not already taking aspirin therapy immediately before PCI procedures.
3. After the PCI procedure, in patients with neither aspirin resistance, allergy, nor increased risk of bleeding, aspirin 325 mg daily should be given for at least 1 month after bare-metal stent implantation, 3 months after sirolimus-eluting stent implantation, and 6 months after paclitaxel-eluting stent implantation, after which daily chronic aspirin use should be continued indefinitely at a dose of 75 to 162 mg. *(Level of Evidence: B)*	The doses and duration of aspirin therapy recommended herein and derived from those used for US Food and Drug Administration approval of the specific stent types noted in the recommendation. Daily chronic aspirin therapy is based on recommendations in the *ACC/AHA Guidelines for the Management of Patents with ST-Elevation Myocardial Infarction* and evidence indicating that aspiring therapy in dosages as low as 75 mg per day yields outcomes similar to those achieved with 325 mg per day but with fewer side effects.
4. A loading dose of clopidogrel should be administered before PCI is performed. *(Level of Evidence: A)* An oral loading dose of 300 mg, administered at least 6 hours before the procedure, has the best established evidence of efficacy. *(Level of Evidence: B)*	Clopidogrel is an important adjunctive therapy for patients undergoing PCI with stent placement. The best evidence of efficacy exists for 300 mg given at lest 6 hours before PCI is performed.
5. In patients who have undergone PCI, clopidogrel 75 mg daily should be given for at least 1 month after bare-metal stent implantation (unless the patient is at increased risk for bleeding; then it should be given for a minimum of 2 weeks), 3 months after sirolimus stent implantation, and 6 months after paclitaxel stent implantation, and ideally u to 12 months in patients who are not at high risk of bleeding. *(Level of Evidence: B)*	Clopidogrel therapy in the dosage of 75 mg daily should be given after stent placement to all patients. The duration of therapy varies for each stent and is based on data from clinical trails used for U.S. Food and Drug Administration approval of that stent.
Class IIa	
1. If clopidogrel is given at the time of procedure, supplementation with GP IIb/IIIa receptor antagonists can be beneficial to facilitate earlier platelet inhibition than with clopidogrel alone. *(Level of Evidence: B)*	When clopidogrel is given at the time of a PCI procedure, supplementation with glycoprotein IIb/IIIa receptor antagonists can be beneficial, especially among high-risk patients.
2. For patients with an absolute contraindication to aspirin, it is reasonable to give a 300-mg loading dose of clopidogrel, administered at least 6 hours before PCI, and/or GP IIb/IIIa antagonists, administered at the time of PCI. *(Level of Evidence: C)*	A significant number of patients will have resistance to aspirin. The strongest evidence for clopidogrel benefit exists for doses of 300 mg given at least 6 hours before the procedure.
3. When a loading dose of clopidogrel is administered, a regimen of greater than 300 mg is reasonable to achieve higher levels of antiplatelet activity more rapidly, but the efficacy and safety compared with a 300-mg loading dose are less established. *(Level of Evidence: C)*	Many patients receive clopidogrel therapy at the time of PCI in dosages greater than 600 mg. Although more pronounced inhibition of platelet function has been demonstrated for doses of clopidogrel greater than 300 mg, the safety of these higher doses and their benefits on clinical outcome are not fully established.
4. It is reasonable that patients undergoing brachytherapy be given daily clopidogrel 75 mg indefinitely and daily aspirin 75 to 325 mg indefinitely unless there is significant risk for bleeding. *(Level of Evidence: C)*	Subacute or later thrombosis has been observed in patients undergoing brachytherapy, and for this reason long-term antiplatelet therapy is recommended.
Class IIb	
In patients in whom subacute thrombosis may be catastrophic or lethal (unprotected left main, bifurcating left main, or last patent coronary vessel), platelet aggregation studies may be considered and the dose of clopidogrel increased to 150 mg per day if less than 505 inhibition of platelet aggregation is demonstrated. *(Level of Evidence: C)*	Clopidogrel resistance is a significant problem, and owing to its contribution to catastrophic clinical outcomes, the Writing Committee recommends studies be performed with increases in clopidogrel dose being recommended for use in those with higher-risk lesions.
Glycoprotein IIb/IIIa inhibitors	
Class I	
In patients with UA/NSTEMI undergoing PCI without clopidogrel administration, a C IIb/IIIa inhibitor (abciximab, eptifibatide, or tirofiban) should be administered. *(Level of Evidence: A)* It is acceptable to administer the GP IIb/IIIa inhibitor before performance of the diagnostic angiogram ("upstream treatment") or just before PCI ("in-lab treatment").	This recommendation and phrasing are compatible with the *ACC/AHA 2002 Guideline Update for the Management of Patients With Unstable Angina and Non–ST-Segment Myocardial Infarction* and current evidence from randomized clinical trials. The benefits of GP IIb/IIa inhibition are especially efficacious when clopidogrel is not given.
Class IIa	
1. In patients with UA/NSTEMI undergoing PCI with clopidogrel administration, it is reasonable to administer a GP IIb/IIIa inhibitor (abciximab, eptifibatide, or tirofiban). *(Level of Evidence: B)* It is acceptable to administer the GP IIb/IIIa inhibitor before performance of the diagnostic angiogram ("upstream treatment") or just before PCI ("in-lab treatment").	
2. In patients with STEMI undergoing PCI, it is reasonable to administer abciximab as early as possible. *(Level of Evidence: B)*	Recommendation has been added for consistency with the *ACC/AHA Guidelines for the Management of Patients With ST-Elevation Myocardial Infarction*.
3. In patients undergoing elective PCI with stent placement, it is reasonable to administer a GP IIb/IIIa inhibitor (abciximab, epitifibatide, or tirofiban). *(Level of Evidence: B)*	Phrasing has been changed to reflect current terminology, especially in a high-risk patient.
Class IIb	
In patients with STEMI undergoing PCI, treatment with eptifibatide or tirofiban may be considered. *(Level of Evidence: C)*	Recommendation has been added for consistency with the *ACC/AHA Guidelines for the Management of Patients With ST-Elevation Myocardial Infarction*.
Antithrombotic therapy	
Unfractionated heparin, low-molecular-weight heparin, and bivalirudin	
Class I	
1. Unfractionated heparin should be administered to patients undergoing PCI. *(Level of Evidence: C)*	Phrasing has been changed to reflect current terminology.
2. For patients with heparin-induced thrombocytopenia, it is recommended that bivalirudin or argatroban be used to replace heparin. *(Level of Evidence: B)*	Bivalirudin and argatroban are established therapies in place of heparin among patients with heparin-induced thrombocytopenia.

(continued)

TABLE 17-9 Pharmacologic Management of Percutaneous Coronary Intervention (continued)

Class IIa	
1. It is reasonable to use bivalirudin as an alternative to unfractionated heparin and glycoprotein IIb/IIIa antagonists in low-risk patients undergoing elective PCI. *(Level of Evidence: B)*	New recommendation is based on data from a clinical trial (REPLACE-2) indicating bivalirudin is an acceptable alternative to heparin and GP IIb/IIIa antagonists in low-risk patients undergoing PCI.
2. Low-molecular-weight heparin is a reasonable alternative to unfractionated heparin in patients with UA/NSTEMI undergoing PCI. *(Level of Evidence: B)*	Recommendation from the *ACC/AHA 2002 Guideline Update for the Management of Patients with Unstable Angina and Non–ST-Segment Myocardial Infarction* has been approved by this Writing Committee and included in these guidelines for consistency.
Class IIb	
Low-molecular-weight heparin may be considered as an alternative to unfractionated heparin in patients with STEMI undergoing PCI. *(Level of Evidence: B)*	Recommendation from the *ACC/AHA Guidelines for the Management of Patients With ST-Elevation Myocardial Infarction* has been approved by this Writing Committee and included in these guidelines for consistency.

GP, glycoprotein; NSTEMI, non–ST-segment elevation myocardial infarction; PCU, percutaneous coronary intervention; STEMI, ST-segment elevation myocardial infarction; UA, unstable angina.
From Smith SC Jr, Feldman TE, Hirshfeld JW Jr, et al. ACC/AHA/SCAI 2005 guideline update for percutaneous coronary intervention–Summary article: A report of the American College of Cardiology/American Heart Association Task Force on Practice Guidelines (ACC/AHA/SCAI Writing Committee to Update the 2001 Guidelines for Percutaneous Coronary Intervention). Circulation 2006;113:156–175.

When medical therapy, PTCA, and CABG have been compared, low-risk patients with single-vessel coronary artery disease and normal left ventricular function had greater alleviation of symptoms with PTCA than with medical treatment; mortality rates and rates of myocardial infarction were unchanged. In high-risk patients (risk was defined by severity of ischemia, number of diseased vessels, and presence of left ventricular dysfunction), improvement of survival was greater with CABG than with medical therapy. In moderate-risk patients with multivessel coronary artery disease (most had two-vessel disease and normal left ventricular function), PTCA and CABG produced equivalent mortality rates and rates of myocardial infarction.

The development of drug-eluting stents has changed the natural course of stent thrombosis when compared to bare-metal stents that have existed for a longer period of time. Currently there are two types of drug-eluting stents available: (sirolimus (Cypher) and paclitaxel (Taxus). Soon after the introduction of bare-metal stents, it became apparent that early stent thrombosis (≤30 days) was an uncommon but serious complication of therapy.[92–95] Stent thrombosis is an infrequent but severe complication of both bare-metal stents and drug-eluting stents but there is no apparent difference in overall stent thrombosis frequency at 4 years of followup, but the time course appears to be different. Although there is a relative numeric excess of stent thrombosis late after drug-eluting stents implantation, no differences in death or death and infarction have been observed. Target lesion revascularization is needed less often with drug-eluting stents than with bare-metal stents. Implantation of drug-eluting stents outside of approved indications is probably related to the occurrence of late stent thrombosis. Longer-term followup with larger subsets of patients (i.e., lesion number, type and location, and patient comorbidities) is needed to fully understand this issue and the evolution of newer platforms for drug delivery will likely alter the natural history of drug-eluting stent thrombosis. A very important consideration is the use of combination antiplatelet therapy (aspirin + clopidogrel) for at least 1 year following implantation.[96] Patients who are hyporesponsive to clopidogrel may be treated with 150 mg/day rather than 75 mg/day.[94]

PHARMACOLOGIC THERAPY

Historically, approximately 30% of anginal syndrome symptoms have responded regardless of which therapy was instituted. These observations stem from two problems inherent in clinical trials undertaken to assess the efficacy of any therapy for angina: (a) adequate trial design incorporating appropriate controls and washout periods, and (b) assessment of treatment effects using objective measures of efficacy, including improvement in exercise performance, resting and ambulatory ECG improvement in ischemic changes, or other objective tests to address other aspects of myocardial function or metabolism. The use of pain episode frequency and nitroglycerin consumption is subjective, and their use as sole measures of efficacy should be avoided. Objective assessment using ETT has shown that placebo does not provide improvement in patients with exertional angina, substantiating this as a valid means to assess efficacy.

β-Adrenergic–Blocking Agents[97]

Decreased heart rate, decreased contractility, and a slight to moderate decrease in blood pressure with β-adrenergic receptor antagonism reduce MVO_2. The predominant receptor type in the heart is the β_1-receptor, and competitive blockade minimizes the influence of endogenous catecholamines on the chronotropic and inotropic state of the myocardium. These beneficial effects may be countered to some degree with increased ventricular volume and ejection time seen with β-blockade; however, the overall effect of β-blockers in patients with effort-induced angina is a reduction in oxygen demand (Table 17–10). The β-blockers do not improve oxygen supply, and in certain instances, unopposed α-adrenergic stimulation following the use of β-blockers may lead to coronary vasoconstriction. For patients with chronic exertional stable angina, β-blockers improve symptoms approximately 80% of the time and objective measures of efficacy demonstrate improved exercise duration and delay in the time at which ST-segment changes and initial or limiting symptoms occur. β-Blockers do not alter the rate–pressure product (double product) for maximal exercise, therefore substantiating reduced demand rather than improved supply as the major consequence of their actions. Reflex tachycardia from nitrate therapy can be blunted with β-blocker therapy, making this a common and useful combination. Although β-blockade may decrease exercise capacity in healthy individuals or in patients with hypertension, it may allow angina patients previously limited by symptoms to perform more exercise and ultimately improve overall cardiovascular performance through a training effect. Ideal candidates for β-blockers include patients in whom physical

TABLE 17-10 Effect of Drug Therapy on Myocardial Oxygen Demand[a]

			LV Wall Tension	
	Heart Rate	**Myocardial Contractility**	***Systolic Pressure***	***LV Volume***
Nitrates	⇓	0	⇓	⇓⇓
β-Blockers	⇓⇓	⇓	⇓	⇓
Nifedipine	⇓	0 or ⇓	⇓⇓	0 or ⇓
Verapamil	⇓	⇓	⇓	0 or ⇓
Diltiazem	⇓⇓	0 or ⇓	⇓	0 or ⇓

LV, left ventricular.
[a]Calcium channel antagonists and nitrates also may increase myocardial oxygen supply through coronary vasodilation. Diastolic function also may be improved with verapamil, nifedipine, and perhaps, diltiazem. These effects may vary from those indicated in the table depending on individual patient baseline hemodynamics.

activity figures prominently in their anginal attacks, those who have coexistent hypertension, those with a history of supraventricular arrhythmias or post-MI angina, and those who have a component of anxiety associated with angina.[3] β-Blockers may also be safely used in angina and heart failure as described in Chap. 16.

Pertinent pharmacokinetics for the β-blockers include half-life and route elimination, which are reviewed in Chap. 15. Drugs with longer half-lives need to be dosed less frequently than drugs with shorter half-lives; however, disparity exists between half-life and duration of action for several β-blockers (e.g., metoprolol), which may reflect attenuation of the central nervous system-mediated effects on the sympathetic system, as well as the direct effects of this category on heart rate and contractility. Renal and hepatic dysfunction can affect the disposition of β-blockers, but these agents are dosed to effect, either hemodynamic or symptomatic, and route of elimination is not a major consideration in drug selection.

Guidelines for the use of β-blockers in treating angina include the objective of lowering resting heart rate to 50 to 60 beats per minute and limiting maximal exercise heart rate to about 100 beats per minute or less. It has also been suggested that exercise heart rate should be no more than about 20 beats per minute or a 10% increment over resting heart rate with modest exercise. Because β-blockade is competitive and circulating catecholamine concentrations vary depending on the intensity of exercise and other factors, and cholinergic tone may be important in controlling heart rate in some patients, these guidelines are general in nature. These effects are generally dose and plasma concentration related, and for propranolol, plasma concentrations of 30 ng/mL are needed for a 25% reduction of anginal frequency. Initial doses of β-blockers should be at the lower end of the usual dosing range and titrated to response as indicated above.

Although there is little evidence to suggest superiority of any β-blocker, the duration of β-blockade is dependent partially on the half-life of the agent used, and agents with longer half-lives may be dosed less frequently. Of note, propranolol may be dosed twice a day in most patients with angina and the efficacy is similar to that seen with more frequent dosing. The ancillary property of membrane stabilizing activity is irrelevant in the treatment of angina, and intrinsic sympathomimetic activity appears to be detrimental in rest or severe angina because the reduction in heart rate would be minimized, therefore limiting a reduction in MVO_2. Cardioselective β-blockers may be used in some patients to minimize adverse effects such as bronchospasm in asthma, intermittent claudication, and sexual dysfunction. A common misunderstanding is that β-blockers are not well tolerated in peripheral arterial disease but, in fact, their use is associated with a reduction in death and improved quality of life.[98] It should be remembered that cardioselectivity is a relative property and the use of larger doses (e.g., metoprolol 200 mg/day) is associated with the loss of selectivity and with adverse effects. Post-acute-MI patients with angina are particularly good candidates for β-blockade, both because anginal symptoms may be treated and the risk of post-MI reinfarction reduced, and because mortality has been demonstrated with timolol, propranolol, and metoprolol (see Chap. 15). Combined β- (nonselective) and α-blockade with labetalol may be useful in some patients with marginal LV reserve, and fewer deleterious effects on coronary blood flow are seen when compared with other β-blockers.

Extension of pharmacologic effect is the underlying reason for many of the adverse effects seen with β-blockade. Hypotension, decompensated heart failure, bradycardia and heart block, bronchospasm, and altered glucose metabolism are directly related to β-adrenoreceptor antagonism. Patients with preexisting left ventricular systolic decompensated and heart failure and the use of other negative inotropic agents are most prone to developing overt heart failure, and in the absence of these, heart failure is uncommon (less than 5%). Other drugs that depress conduction are additive to β-blockade, and intrinsic conduction system disease predisposes the patient to conduction abnormalities. Altered glucose metabolism is most likely to be seen in insulin-dependent diabetics, and β-blockade obscures the symptoms of hypoglycemia except for sweating. β-Blockers may also aggravate the lipid abnormalities seen in patients with diabetes; however, these changes are dose related, are more common with normal baseline lipids than dyslipidemia, and may be of short-term significance only. One of the more common reasons for discontinuation of β-blocker therapy is related to central nervous system adverse effects of fatigue, malaise, and depression. Cognition changes seen with β-blockers are usually minimal and comparable to other categories of drugs based on studies done in hypertension.[99,100] Abrupt withdrawal of β-blocker therapy in patients with angina has been associated with increased severity and number of pain episodes and myocardial infarction. The mechanism of this effect is unknown but may be related to increased receptor sensitivity or disease progression during therapy, which becomes apparent following discontinuation of β-blockade. In any event, tapering of β-blocker therapy over about 2 days should minimize the risk of withdrawal reactions for those patients in whom therapy is being discontinued.

β-Adrenoreceptor blockade is effective in chronic exertional angina as monotherapy and in combination with nitrates and/or calcium channel antagonists. β-Blockers should be the first-line drug in chronic angina that requires daily maintenance therapy because β-blockers are more effective in reducing episodes of silent ischemia, reducing early morning peak of ischemic activity, and improving mortality after Q-wave MI than nitrates or calcium channel blockers (see Fig. 17–4).[3] If β-blockers are ineffective or not tolerated, then monotherapy with a calcium channel blocker or combination therapy if monotherapy is ineffective may be instituted. Patients with severe angina, rest angina, or variant angina (i.e., a component of coronary artery spasm) may be better treated with calcium channel blockers or long-acting nitrates.

Nitrates[101,102]

Nitroglycerin has a well-documented role in the alleviation of acute anginal attacks when used as rapidly absorbed and readily available preparations by the oral and intravenous routes (Table 17–11; see also Fig. 17–4). Sublingual, buccal, or spray products are the products of choice for this indication. Prevention of symptoms may be accomplished by the prophylactic use of oral or transdermal products; however, recent concern has been expressed over the long-term efficacy of many of these preparations and the development of tolerance.[46,47]

Nitrates have multiple potential mechanisms of action, and for a given patient it is not always clear which of these is most important. In general, the major action appears to be indirectly mediated

TABLE 17-11 Nitrate Products

Product	Onset (min)	Duration	Initial Dose
Nitroglycerin			
IV	1–2	3–5 min	5 mcg/min
Sublingual/lingual	1–3	30–60 min	0.3 mg
Oral	40	3–6 h	2.5–9 mg tid
Ointment	20–60	2–8 h	0.5–1 in
Patch	40–60	>8 h	1 patch
Erythritol tetranitrate	5–30	4–6 h	5–10 mg tid
Pentaerythritol tetranitrate	30	4–8 h	10–20 mg tid
Isosorbide dinitrate			
Sublingual/chewable	2–5	1–2 h	2.5–5 mg tid
Oral	20–40	4–6 h	5–20 mg tid
Isosorbide mononitrate	30–60	6–8 h	20 mg daily, bid[a]

[a]Product dependent.

through a reduction of myocardial oxygen demand secondary to venodilation and arterial–arteriolar dilation, leading to a reduction in wall stress from reduced ventricular volume and pressure (see Table 17–10). Systemic venodilation also promotes increased flow to deep myocardial muscle by reducing the gradient between intraventricular pressure and coronary arteriolar (R2) pressure. Direct actions on the coronary circulation include dilation of large and small intramural coronary arteries, collateral dilation, coronary artery stenosis dilation, abolition of normal tone in narrowed vessels, and relief of spasm; these actions occur even if the endothelium is denuded or dysfunctional. It is likely that depending on the underlying pathophysiology, different mechanisms become operative. For example, in the presence of a 60% to 70% stenosis, venodilation with MVO_2 reduction is most important; however, with higher grade lesions, direct effects on the coronary circulation and vessel tone are the predominant effects. Nitroglycerin and pentaerythritol tetranitrate in low doses are bioactivated by mitochondrial aldehyde dehydrogenase to nitrite or denitrated metabolites, which require further activation by cytochrome oxidase or acidic disproportionation in the inner membrane space, finally yielding nitric oxide. Nitric oxide activates soluble guanylate cyclase to increase intracellular concentrations of cyclic guanosine monophosphate (GMP) resulting in vasorelaxation.[47] In contrast, isosorbide dinitrate (ISDN) and isosorbide mononitrate (ISMN) are bioactivated via P450 enzymes to nitric oxide. At higher concentrations, nitroglycerin and pentaerythritol tetranitrate may also be bioactivated to nitric oxide via P450 enzymes. Increased cyclic GMP induces a sequence of protein phosphorylation associated with reduced intracellular calcium release from the sarcoplasmic reticulum or reduced permeability to extracellular calcium and, consequently, smooth muscle relaxation. Oxidative stress within the mitochondria causes inactivation of mitochondrial aldehyde dehydrogenase, leading to impaired bioactivation of nitroglycerin during prolonged treatment.[103,104] Thomas et al. performed a study in normal volunteers to evaluate the effect of ISMN 120 mg/day given for 7 days on endothelial function. They found that ISMN impaired endothelial function suggesting a role for oxygen free radicals and nitrate induced abnormalities in endothelial-dependent vasomotor responses that were reversed with a vitamin C infusion of 24 mg/min given for 15 minutes.[46] Furthermore, ISDN impairs flow-mediated dilation and carotid intimal-media thickness after 3 months of treatment.[105] These deleterious changes in endothelial function, intima-media thickness and the occurrence of tolerance suggest that the role of nitrates in IHD may be changing.

Pharmacokinetic characteristics common to the organic nitrates used for angina include a large first-pass effect of hepatic metabolism, short to very short half-lives (except for isosorbide mononitrate), large volumes of distribution, high clearance rates, and large interindividual variations in plasma or blood concentrations. Pharmacodynamic–pharmacokinetic relationships for the entire class remain poorly defined, presumably because of methodologic difficulty in characterizing the parent drug and metabolite concentrations at or within vascular smooth muscle and secondary to counterregulatory or adaptive mechanisms from the drug's effects, as well as the occurrence of tolerance. Nitroglycerin is extracted by a variety of tissues and metabolized locally; differential extraction and metabolite generation occur depending on the tissue site. There are also numerous technical problems limiting the generation of reliable pharmacokinetic parameter estimates including the following: assay sensitivity; arterial–venous extraction gradients and therefore extrahepatic metabolism; in vitro degradation; drug adsorption to polyvinyl chloride tubing and syringes; potentially saturable metabolism; accumulation of metabolites (some of which are active) with multiple doses; postural and exercise-induced changes in pharmacokinetics; a variety of variables associated with transdermal delivery including the delivery system (matrix, membrane-limited, ointment), vehicle used, the surface area and thickness of application, the site application, and other skin variables (temperature, moisture content).

Nitroglycerin concentrations are affected by the route of administration, with the highest concentrations usually obtained with intravenous administration, the lowest seen with lower oral doses. Peak concentrations with sublingual nitroglycerin appear within 2 to 4 minutes, with the oral route producing peaks at about 15 to 30 minutes and by the transdermal route at 1 to 2 hours. The half-life of nitroglycerin is 1 to 5 minutes regardless of route; hence the potential advantage of sustained-release and transdermal products. Transdermal nitroglycerin does produce sufficient concentrations for acute hemodynamic effects to occur and these concentrations are maintained for long intervals; however, the hemodynamic and antianginal effects are minimal after 1 week or less with chronic, continuous (24 h/day) therapy.

ISDN is metabolized to isosorbide 2-mono- and 5-mononitrate (ISMN). ISMN is well absorbed and has a half-life of about 5 hours and may be given once or twice daily depending on the product chosen. Multiple, larger doses of ISDN lead to disproportionate increases in the area under the plasma time profile, suggesting that metabolic pathways are being saturated or that metabolite accumulation may influence the disposition of ISDN. Little pharmacokinetic information is available for other nitrate compounds.

Nitrate therapy may be used to terminate an acute anginal attack, to prevent effort or stress-induced attacks, or for long-term prophylaxis, usually in combination with β-blockers or calcium channel blockers. Sublingual nitroglycerin 0.3 to 0.4 mg will relieve pain in approximately 75% of patients within 3 minutes, with another 15% becoming pain free in 5 to 15 minutes. Pain persisting beyond about 20 to 30 minutes following the use of two or three nitroglycerin tablets is suggestive of acute coronary syndrome and the patient should be instructed to seek emergency aid. Patients should be instructed to keep nitroglycerin in the original, tightly closed glass container and to avoid mixing with other medication, because mixing may reduce nitroglycerin adsorption and vaporization. Additional counseling should include the facts that nitroglycerin is not an analgesic but rather it partially corrects the underlying problem and that repeated use is not harmful or addicting. Patients should also be aware that enhanced venous pooling in the sitting or standing positions may improve the effect, as well as the symptoms of postural hypotension, and that inadequate saliva may slow or prevent tablet disintegration and dissolution. An acceptable, albeit expensive, alternative is lingual spray, which may be more convenient and has a shelf-life of 3 years, compared with 6 months or so for some forms of nitroglycerin tablets.

Chewable, oral, and transdermal products are acceptable for the long-term prophylaxis of angina; however, considerable controversy surrounds their use and it appears that the development of tolerance or adaptive mechanisms limits the efficacy of all chronic nitrate therapies regardless of route. Dosing of the longer-acting preparations should be adjusted to provide a hemodynamic response and, as an example, may require doses of oral ISDN ranging from 10 to 60 mg as often as every 3 to 4 hours owing to tolerance or first-pass metabolism, and similar large doses are required for other products. Nitroglycerin ointment has a duration of up to 6 hours, but it is difficult to apply in a cosmetically acceptable fashion over a consistent surface area, and response varies depending on the epidermal thickness, vascularity, and amount of hair. Percutaneous adsorption of nitroglycerin ointment may occur unintentionally if someone other than the patient applies the ointment, and limiting exposure through the use of gloves or some other means is advisable. Peripheral edema may also impair the response to nitroglycerin because venodilation cannot increase capacitance to a maximum and pooling may be reduced. Transdermal patch delivery systems were approved on the basis of sustained and equivalent plasma concentrations to other forms of therapy. Trials required by the Food and Drug Administration using transdermal patches as a continuous 24-hour delivery system revealed a lack of efficacy for improved exercise tolerance. Subsequently, large, randomized, double-blind, placebo-controlled trials of intermittent (10 to 12 hours on; 12 to 14 hours off) transdermal nitroglycerin therapy in chronic stable angina demonstrated modest but significant improvement in exercise time after 4 weeks for the highest doses at 8 to 12 hours after patch placement.[106] Subjective assessment methods for nitrate effects include reduction in the number of painful episodes and the amount of nitroglycerin consumed. Objective assessment includes the resolution of ECG changes at rest, during exercise, or with ambulatory ECG monitoring. Because nitrates work primarily through a reduction in MVO_2, the double product can be used to optimize the dose of sublingual and oral nitrate products. It is important to realize that reflex tachycardia may offset the beneficial reduction in systolic blood pressure and calculation of the observed changes is necessary. The double product is best assessed in the sitting position and at intervals of 5 to 10 minutes and 30 to 60 minutes following sublingual and oral therapy, respectively. Owing to the placebo effect, unpredictable and variable course of angina, numerous pharmacologic effects of nitroglycerin, diurnal variation in pain patterns, stringent investigative protocols, and interindividual sensitivity to nitroglycerin, assessment with transdermal and sustained-release products is difficult. ETT provides valuable information concerning efficacy and mechanism of action for nitrates but its use is usually reserved for clinical investigation rather than routine patient care. Most ETT studies have shown nitrates to delay the onset of ischemia (ST-segment changes or initial chest discomfort) at submaximal exercise but that the threshold for maximal exercise is unaltered, suggesting a reduction in oxygen demand rather than an improved oxygen supply. More sophisticated studies of myocardial function, such as wall motion abnormalities and myocardial metabolism, could be used to document efficacy; however, these studies are generally only for investigative purposes.

Adverse effects of nitrates are related most commonly to an extension of their pharmacologic effects and include postural hypotension with associated central nervous system symptoms, headaches and flushing secondary to vasodilation, and occasional nausea from smooth muscle relaxation. If hypotension is excessive, coronary and cerebral filling may be compromised, leading to myocardial infarction and stroke. Although reflex tachycardia is most common, bradycardia with nitroglycerin has been reported. Other noncardiovascular adverse effects include rash with all products, but particularly with transdermal nitroglycerin, the production of methemoglobinemia with high doses given for extended periods, and measurable concentrations of ethanol (intoxication has been reported) and propylene glycol (found in the diluent) with intravenous nitroglycerin.

Tolerance with nitrate therapy was first described in 1867 with the initial experience using amyl nitrate for angina and later widely recognized in munitions workers who underwent withdrawal reactions during periods of absence from exposure. Tolerance to nitrates is associated with a reduction in tissue cyclic GMP, which results from decreased production (guanylate cyclase) and increased breakdown via cyclic GMP-phosphodiesterase and increased superoxide levels. One proposed mechanism for the lack of cyclic GMP is lack of conversion of organic nitrates to nitric oxide as described previously.[47,97]

Most of the published information from controlled trials examining nitrate tolerance have been done with either ISDN or transdermal nitroglycerin, and these studies demonstrate the development of tolerance within as little as 24 hours of therapy. Although the onset of tolerance is rapid, the offset may be just as rapid, and one alternative-dosing strategy to circumvent or minimize tolerance is to provide a daily nitrate-free interval of 6 to 8 hours. Studies with a variety of nitrate preparations and dosing schedules demonstrate that this approach is useful and the nitrate-free interval should be a minimum of 8 hours, and perhaps 12 hours for even better effects.[97] Another concern for intermittent transdermal nitrate therapy is the occurrence of rebound ischemia during the nitrate-free interval. Freedman et al.[107] found more silent ischemia during the patch-free interval during a randomized, double-blind, placebo-controlled trial than during the placebo patch phase, although others have not noted this effect. ISDN, for example, should not be used more often than three times per day if tolerance is to be avoided. Interestingly, hemodynamic tolerance does not always coincide with antianginal efficacy, but this is not well studied.

Nitrates may be combined with other drugs for anginal therapy including β-adrenergic-blocking agents and calcium channel antagonists. These combinations are usually instituted for chronic prophylactic therapy based on complementary or offsetting mechanisms of action (see Table 17–10). Combination therapy is generally used in patients with more frequent symptoms or with symptoms that are not responding to β-blockers alone (nitrates plus β-blockers or calcium blockers), in patients intolerant of β-blockers or calcium channel blockers, and in patients having an element of vasospasm leading to decreased supply (nitrates plus calcium blockers).[108] Modulation of calcium entry into vascular smooth muscle and myocardium as well as a variety of other tissues is the principal action of the calcium antagonists. The cellular mechanism of these drugs is incompletely understood and it differs among the available classes of the phenylalkylamines (verapamil-like), dihydropyridines (nifedipine-like), benzothiazepines (diltiazem-like), bepridil, and a recent class referred to as T-channel blockers. Receptor-operated channels stimulated by norepinephrine and other neurotransmitters, and potential-dependent channels activated by membrane depolarization, control the entry of calcium, and, consequently, the cytosolic concentration of calcium responsible for activation of actin–myosin complex leading to contraction of vascular smooth muscle and myocardium. In the myocardium, calcium entry triggers the release of intracellular stores of calcium to increase cytosolic calcium, whereas in smooth muscle, calcium derived from the extracellular fluid may do this directly. Binding proteins within the cell, calmodulin and troponin, after binding with calcium, participate in phosphorylation reactions leading to contraction. Decreased calcium availability, through the actions of calcium antagonists, inhibits these reactions.

Direct actions of the calcium antagonists include vasodilation of systemic arterioles and coronary arteries, leading to a reduction of arterial pressure and coronary vascular resistance, as well as depression of the myocardial contractility and conduction velocity of the sinoatrial and atrioventricular nodes (see Chap. 19). Reflex β-adrenergic stimulation overcomes much of the negative inotropic effect, and depression of contractility becomes clinically apparent only in the presence of LV dysfunction and when other negative inotropic drugs are used concurrently. Verapamil and diltiazem cause less peripheral vasodilation than nifedipine, and, consequently, the risk of myocardial depression is greater with these two agents. Conduction through the AV node is predictably depressed with verapamil and diltiazem, and they must be used cautiously in patients with preexisting conduction abnormalities or in the presence of other drugs with negative chronotropic properties. MVO_2 is reduced with all of the calcium channel antagonists because of reduced wall tension secondary to reduced arterial pressure and, to a minor extent, depressed contractility (see Table 17–10). Heart rate changes are dependent on the drug used and the state of the conduction system. Nifedipine generally increases heart rate or causes no change, whereas either no change or decreased heart rate is seen with verapamil and diltiazem because of the interaction of these direct and indirect effects. In contrast to the β-blockers, calcium channel antagonists have the potential to improve coronary blood flow through areas of fixed coronary obstruction and by inhibiting coronary artery vasomotion and vasospasm. Beneficial redistribution of blood flow from well-perfused myocardium to ischemic areas and from epicardium to endocardium may also contribute to improvement in ischemic symptoms. Overall, the benefit provided by calcium channel antagonists is related to reduced MVO_2 rather than improved oxygen supply, based on lack of alteration in the rate pressure product at maximal exercise in most studies performed to date. However, as coronary artery disease progresses and vasospasm becomes superimposed on critical stenotic lesions, improved oxygen supply through coronary vasodilation may become more important.

Absorption of the calcium channel antagonists is characterized by excellent absorption and large, variable, first-pass metabolism resulting in oral bioavailability ranging from approximately 20% to 50% or greater for diltiazem, nicardipine, nifedipine, verapamil, felodipine, and isradipine. Amlodipine has a range of bioavailability of approximately 60% to 80%. Saturation of this effect may occur with verapamil and diltiazem, resulting in greater amounts of drug being absorbed with chronic dosing. Nifedipine may have slow or fast absorption patterns, and the ingestion of food delays and impairs its absorption as well as potential enhanced absorption in elderly patients. This variability in absorption produces fluctuation in the hemodynamic response with nifedipine. Sublingual nifedipine is frequently used to provide a more rapid response; however, the rationale for this application is suspect because little nifedipine is absorbed from the buccal mucosa and the swallowed drug is responsible for the observed plasma concentrations. Absorption of verapamil in sustained-release products may be influenced by food, and when used in the fasted state, dose dumping may occur, resulting in high peak concentrations with some products. The approved sustained-release products for nifedipine, verapamil, and diltiazem are approved primarily for the treatment of hypertension (see Chap. 15). The presence of severe liver disease (e.g., alcoholic liver disease with cirrhosis) reduces the first-pass metabolism of verapamil, and this shunting of drug around the liver gives rise to higher plasma concentrations and lower dose requirements in these patients. Interestingly, this effect appears to be stereoselective for the more active isomer of verapamil. Verapamil may also reduce liver blood flow; however, evidence for this reduction is based primarily on animal experiments. Few data are available regarding the influence of liver disease on the kinetics of calcium blockers; however, these drugs undergo extensive hepatic metabolism with little unchanged drug being renally excreted, and liver disease can be expected to alter the pharmacokinetics. Nifedipine has no active metabolites whereas norverapamil possesses 20% or less activity of the parent compound. Desacetyl-diltiazem has not been studied in man, but canine studies suggest its potency ranges from 100% to 40% of the parent compound for various cardiovascular effects; the clinical importance of these observations remains to be determined. With chronic dosing of verapamil and diltiazem, apparent saturation of metabolism occurs, producing higher plasma concentrations of each drug than those seen with single-dose administration. Consequently, the elimination half-life for verapamil is prolonged, and less-frequent dosing intervals may be used in some patients. The elimination half-life for diltiazem is also somewhat prolonged and the half-life of desacetyl-diltiazem is longer than that of the parent drug, but it is not clear if less-frequent dosing may be used. Bepridil also undergoes hepatic elimination and an active metabolite, 4-hydroxyphenyl bepridil, is produced; the parent compound has a long half-life of 30 to 40 hours. Nifedipine does not accumulate with chronic dosing; however, it is eliminated via oxidative pathways that may be polymorphic, and slow and fast metabolizers have been described for nifedipine. Most of the calcium channel blockers are eliminated via cytochrome (CYP) 3A4 and other CYP isoenzymes and many inhibit CYP3A4 activity as well.[109] Renal insufficiency has little or no effect on the pharmacokinetics of these three drugs. Although disease alterations in kinetics have been described, the most important quantitative alteration is the influence of liver disease on bioavailability and elimination that reduce the clearance of verapamil and diltiazem, and dosing in this population should be done with caution. Altered protein binding because of renal disease, decreased protein concentration, or increased α_1-acid glycoprotein has been noted, but the clinical import of these changes is unknown.

Good candidates for calcium channel blockers in angina include patients with contraindications or intolerance of β-blockers, coexisting conduction system disease (except for verapamil and diltiazem), patients with Prinzmetal angina (vasospastic or variable threshold angina), the presence of peripheral vascular disease, severe ventricular dysfunction (amlodipine is probably the calcium channel blocker of choice and others need to be used with caution if the ejection fraction is <40%), and concurrent hypertension.

Ranolazine is a new drug for angina that has a unique mechanism of action which is unlike that of any other drug used to alter the relationship between oxygen supply and demand. Ranolazine reduces calcium overload in the ischemic myocyte through inhibition of the late sodium current (I_{Na}). Myocardial ischemia produces a cascade of complex ionic exchanges that can result in intracellular acidosis, excess cytosolic Ca^{2+}, myocardial cellular dysfunction, and, if sustained, cell injury and death. Activation of the adenosine triphosphate-dependent K^+ current during ischemia results in a strong efflux of K^+ ions from myocytes. Sodium channels are activated on depolarization, leading to a rapid influx of sodium into the cells. The inactivation of I_{Na} has a fast component that lasts a few milliseconds and a slowly inactivating component that can last hundreds of milliseconds.[110] Ranolazine is a relatively selective inhibitor for late I_{Na}. In isolated ventricular myocytes in which the late I_{Na} was pathologically augmented, ranolazine prevented or reversed the induced mechanical dysfunction, as well as ameliorated abnormalities of ventricular repolarization. Ranolazine does not affect heart rate, inotropic state, or hemodynamic state or increase coronary blood flow.

Ranolazine is extensively metabolized via CYP450 3A and potent inhibitors of 3A increase the plasma concentration by a factor of about three. Ketoconazole, diltiazem and verapamil should not be coadministered with ranolazine. Absorption from the gut is quite variable and the apparent half-life is 7 hours. Steady state is reached after 3 days of twice-daily dosing. Ranolazine is indicated for the treatment of chronic angina and because it prolongs the QT interval, it should be reserved for patients who have not achieved an adequate response with other antianginal agents. Contraindications include preexisting QT interval prolongation, hepatic impairment, concurrent QT interval-prolonging drugs, and moderately potent to potent concurrent 3A inhibitors. QT prolongation occurs in a dose-dependent fashion with ranolazine with an average increase of 6 milliseconds but 5% of the population has QT_c prolongation of 15 milliseconds. Baseline and followup ECGs should be obtained to evaluate effects of the QT interval. In controlled trials, the most common adverse reactions are dizziness, headache, constipation and nausea. Ranolazine should be started at 500 mg twice daily and increased to 1,000 mg twice daily as needed based on symptoms.[111]

Based on randomized, placebo-controlled trials, the improvement in exercise time is a modest increase of 15 to about 45 seconds compared with placebo.[112,113] In a large acute coronary syndrome trial, ranolazine reduced recurrent ischemia but did not improve the primary efficacy end point of the composite of cardiovascular death, MI, or recurrent ischemia.[114]

Investigational Agents

Therapeutic angiogenesis aims to deliver an angiogenic growth factor or cytokine to the myocardium to stimulate collateral blood vessel growth throughout the ischemic tissue. The angiogenic factor may be administered as a recombinant protein or as a transgene within a plasmid or gene-transfer vector. An example of this approach is the intracoronary administration of the adenoviral gene for fibroblast growth factor (Ad5FGF-4) to determine if therapeutic angiogenesis could improve myocardial perfusion compared with placebo.[115] In this study of 52 patients with stable angina and reversible ischemia, Ad5FGF-4 decreased ischemic defect by 21% (P <0.001) as determined by single-photon emission computed tomography imaging.[115] More trials are needed before angiogenesis becomes a standard therapy.[116]

TREATMENT

Coronary Artery Spasm and Variant Angina Pectoris (Prinzmetal Angina)[117]

Prinzmetal, in his original description of variant angina pectoris, noted the waxing and waning course of this syndrome associated with ST-segment elevation and that it most commonly resolves without progression to MI. Patients who develop variant angina are usually younger, have fewer coronary risk factors but more commonly smoke than patients with chronic stable angina. Hyperventilation, exercise, and exposure to cold may precipitate variant angina attacks, or there may be no apparent precipitating cause. The onset of chest discomfort is usually in the early morning hours. The exact cause of variant angina is not well understood, but may be an imbalance between endothelium-produced vasodilator factors (prostacyclin, nitric oxide) and vasoconstrictor factors (e.g., endothelin, angiotensin II) as well as an imbalance of autonomic control characterized by parasympathetic dominance or inflammation may also play a role.[118,119] More recently there have been a number potential common adrenoreceptor polymorphisms that may predispose patients to developing vasospasm.[120,121]

The diagnosis of variant angina is based on ST-segment elevation during transient chest discomfort (usually at rest) that resolves when the chest discomfort diminishes in patients who have normal or nonobstructive coronary lesions. In the absence of ST-segment elevation, provocative test using ergonovine, acetylcholine, or methacholine may be used to precipitate coronary artery spasm, ST-segment elevation and typical symptoms. Nitrates and calcium antagonists should be withdrawn prior to provocative testing. Provocative testing should not be used in patients with high-grade lesions. Hyperventilation may also be used to provoke spasm and patients who positive a hyperventilation test are more likely to have higher frequency of attacks, multivessel disease, and a high degree of AV block or ventricular tachycardia.

Optimization of therapy includes dose titration using sufficiently high doses to obtain clinical efficacy without unacceptable adverse effects in individual patients. All patients should be treated for acute attacks and maintained on prophylactic treatment for 6 to 12 months following the initial episode. The occurrence of serious arrhythmias during attacks is associated with a greater risk of sudden death, and these patients should be treated more aggressively and for prolonged periods. Patients without arrhythmias who become asymptomatic and remain so for several months after treatment has been instituted, withdrawal of therapy may be safe after first ascertaining that disease activity is quiescent. Aggravating factors such as alcohol or cocaine use or cigarette smoking should be eliminated when instituting treatment.

Nitrates have been the mainstay of therapy for the acute attacks of variant angina and coronary artery spasm for many years. Most patients respond rapidly to sublingual nitroglycerin or isosorbide dinitrate; however, intravenous and intracoronary nitroglycerin may be very useful for patients who do not respond to sublingual preparations. In particular, vasospasm provoked by ergonovine may require intracoronary nitroglycerin. Although studies with nitrates generally show them to be efficacious, high does are often required and it is unclear if they reduce mortality. Because calcium antagonists may be more effective, have few serious adverse effects in effective doses, and can be given less frequently than nitrates, some consider them the agents of choice for variant angina.

Nifedipine, verapamil, and diltiazem are all equally effective as single agents for the initial management of variant angina and coronary artery spasm. Dose titration is important to maximize the response with calcium antagonists. Comparative trials are few in number and do not reveal significant differences among these three drugs for variant angina. Patients unresponsive to calcium antagonists alone, may have nitrates added. Combination therapy with nifedipine–diltiazem or nifedipine–verapamil is reported to be useful for patients who are unresponsive to single-drug regimens. Although this is probably rational as at the cellular level the drugs have different receptors, the combination of verapamil–diltiazem should be used cautiously owing to their potential additive effects on contractility and conduction.

β-Adrenergic blockade has little or no role in the management of variant angina according to most authorities.[122] Although not all studies report increased painful episodes of variant angina with the addition of β-blockers, they may induce coronary vasoconstriction and prolong ischemia, as documented by continuous ECG monitoring. Other approaches to therapy attempting to modify sympathetic/parasympathetic tone include α-antagonists, anticholinergics, plexectomy, surgical interruption of the sympathetic innervation of the heart, thromboxane receptor antagonism, prostacyclin, lipoxygenase inhibition, and ticlopidine but these drugs or procedures do not occupy a major place in therapy at the present time.

TREATMENT

Silent Ischemia[16]

The objective in the treatment of silent myocardial ischemia is to reduce the total number of ischemic episodes, both symptomatic and asymptomatic, regardless of the direction of ST-segment shift. The incidence of silent ischemia in the general, asymptomatic population is unknown. Significant day-to-day variability in the number of episodes, the duration of ischemia, and the amount of ST-segment deviation complicates both the understanding of this process and the utility of various therapeutic interventions. Silent ischemia in patients with known CAD is common (~80% of all ischemic episodes) and associated with the extent of disease as well as a high risk for myocardial infarction and sudden death when compared with symptomatic episodes of ischemia. Although the underlying mechanisms for silent ischemia are continuing to be defined, increased physical activity, activation of the sympathetic nervous system, increased cortisol secretion, increased coronary artery tone, and enhanced platelet aggregation as a result of endothelia dysfunction leading to intermittent coronary obstruction may be additive in lowering the threshold for ischemia. Platelet aggregability is increased in the morning hours (7 AM to 11 AM), corresponding to circadian rhythms noted for the peak frequency of ischemia, acute myocardial infarction, and sudden death. Silent ischemia is associated with ST-segment elevation or depression and frequently occurs without antecedent changes in heart rate or blood pressure, suggesting that this form of ischemia is a result of primary reduction in oxygen supply. Silent ischemia is classified into class I, patients who do not experience angina at any time, and class II, patients who have both asymptomatic and symptomatic ischemia. Patients with silent ischemia have a defective warning system for angina pain that may encourage excessive myocardial demand. Regardless of the exact mechanism, there is increasing concern that painless ischemia carries considerable risk for myocardial perfusion defects, detrimental hemodynamic changes, arrhythmogenesis, and sudden death. Silent ischemia is associated with reduced survival and increased need for PTCA and CABG, as well as increased risk of acute MI.[123] Because it is apparently very common in some settings, major emphasis should be placed on its management. Although a consensus has not been reached for the most appropriate method of detecting and quantifying the magnitude of silent ischemia, ambulatory electrocardiogram monitoring is thought by many to be the most useful tool at the present time.

The initial step in management is to modify the major risk factors for IHD, hypertension, hypercholesterolemia, and smoking, and data from the Multiple Risk Factor Intervention Trial (MRFIT) show these interventions to be useful in patients with silent ischemia. In a subset of the study population who had abnormal baseline exercise ECG responses, the special intervention group had a 57% reduction in coronary heart disease death (22.2/1,000 vs. 51.8/1,000) and a reduction in sudden death resulting from cessation of smoking and lowering of blood pressure and cholesterol when compared with the usual-care group.

ACIP, a randomized trial of medical therapy versus revascularization (PTCA or CABG), at the 2-year followup demonstrated that total mortality was 6.6% in the angina-guided strategy (i.e., therapy based on symptoms), 4.4% in the ischemia-guided strategy (based on ECG changes), and 1.1% in the revascularization strategy ($P < 0.02$). The rate of death or myocardial infarction was 12.1% in the angina-guided strategy, 8.8% in the ischemia-guided strategy, and 4.7% in the revascularization strategy ($P < 0.04$).[124] The rate of death, myocardial infarction, or recurrent cardiac hospitalization was 41.8% in the angina-guided strategy, 38.5% in the ischemia-guided strategy, and 23.1% in the revascularization strategy ($P < 0.001$). Post-MI patients and those with a high level of sympathetic nervous system activity are perhaps the best candidates for β-blocker therapy.

Calcium channel antagonists alone and in combination are effective in reducing symptomatic and asymptomatic ischemia; however, they do not interrupt the diurnal surge in ischemia observed on ambulatory monitoring and, in general, are somewhat less effective than β-blockers for silent ischemia.[125,126] Nifedipine in particular seems to provide less protection and provides wide fluctuations in response, with approximate reductions in the number of episodes ranging from 0% to 93% and in duration from 23% to 65% unless combined with β-blockers. Fewer studies are available with other calcium blockers and comparative trials are uncommon. Earlier studies showed that combination therapy with calcium and β-blockers provides a better response than calcium blockers and nitrates or monotherapy.[127,128]

Swiss Interventional Study on Silent Ischemia Type II (SWISSI II), a randomized, unblinded, controlled trial of PCI in patients with silent ischemia after acute MI, found that PCI, compared with antiischemic drug therapy, reduced the long-term risk of major cardiac events with better preservation of ventricular function than did medical therapy.[129]

PHARMACOECONOMIC CONSIDERATIONS

Pharmacoeconomic studies have been performed primarily in patients with acute coronary syndromes and only with low-molecular-weight heparins, GP IIb/IIIa receptor antagonists, and statins.[130] Most of the studies on low-molecular-weight heparins have been cost-minimization analyses that focused on enoxaparin sodium, because this is the only low-molecular-weight heparin proven to be superior to unfractionated heparin. Several analyses show that, compared with unfractionated heparin plus aspirin, enoxaparin sodium provides cost savings both during hospitalization (30 days) and at 1-year followup. These cost savings are mainly attributable to fewer cardiac interventions, shorter hospital stays, and lower administrative costs. Indeed, the clinical and economic advantages of enoxaparin sodium have led to its recommendation in recent guidelines as the antithrombotic agent of choice for coronary artery disease. Most of the economic analyses of GP IIb/IIIa inhibitors have been cost-effectiveness analyses.[131] Such analyses indicate that the high acquisition costs of these drugs may be at least partially offset by reductions in other costs if a noninvasive approach to risk stratification is used. Furthermore, use of GP IIb/IIIa inhibitors appears to give favorable cost-effectiveness ratios compared with other accepted therapies, such as fibrin-specific thrombolytic therapy, in the cardiovascular field, particularly in high-risk patients and those undergoing percutaneous coronary intervention. However, more comprehensive economic data on the GP IIb/IIIa inhibitors are needed. Bivalirudin combined with provisional glycoprotein IIb/IIIa inhibitors appears to be an acceptable alternative to the standard of care and is superior to unfractionated heparin alone in PCI and is considered to be cost-effective.[132]

Atorvastatin when used in acute coronary syndrome reduces events, which offsets the upfront acquisition costs.[131] The total expected cost was $1,573.83 per patient in the placebo cohort and $1,709.39 per patient in the atorvastatin cohort, resulting in an incremental cost of $135.56 per patient in the atorvastatin group. The cost per event avoided was $3,536.95. A third of the cost of atorvastatin treatment was offset within 16 weeks by the cost savings resulting from the reduction in the number of events in the atorvastatin cohort compared with the placebo cohort. Other analyses of statins have found this class to be cost-effective, especially in patients who are at higher risk of an ischemic event.[133]

Aspirin and clopidogrel have been evaluated for secondary prevention of CHD, and although aspirin is very cost-effective, clopidogrel is only cost-effective for patients who cannot take aspirin.[134]

CLINICAL CONTROVERSIES

Once patients with angina develop symptoms sufficient for pharmacologic therapy on a daily basis, the initial prophylactic therapy recommended is a β-blocker. There is a paucity of comparative, long-term clinical trials of β-blockade versus calcium channel blockers to determine which is superior for survival benefit. β-Blockers are recommended first-line therapy because of their efficacy in post-MI patients and favorable adverse effect profile.

Recent developments in the understanding of bioactivation of organic nitrates have given rise to concern over endothelial dysfunction induced by nitrates when administered long-term. Not all nitrate products are activated via the same mechanisms and this may impact how effective individual drugs are in long-term treatment.

In stable CAD, medical management has been reported to produce outcomes similar to revascularization and these findings may have a significant impact on how healthcare resources are used in the future.

EVALUATION OF THERAPEUTIC OUTCOMES

Improved symptoms of angina, improved cardiac performance and improvement in risk factors may all be used to assess the outcome of treatment of IHD and angina. Symptomatic improvement in exercise capacity (longer duration) or fewer symptoms at the same level of exercise is subjective evidence that therapy is working. Once patients have been optimized on medical therapy, symptoms should improve over 2 to 4 weeks and remain stable until their disease progresses. There are several instruments (e.g., Seattle angina questionnaire, specific activity scale [see Table 17–1], Canadian classification system [see Table 17–2]) that could be used improve the reproducibility of symptom assessment.[2] If the patient is doing well, then no other assessment may be necessary. Objective assessment is obtained through increase exercise duration on ETT and the absence of ischemic changes on ECG or deleterious hemodynamic changes. Echocardiography and cardiac imaging may also be used, however, due to their expense, they are only used if a patient is not doing well to determine if revascularization or other measures should be undertaken. Coronary angiography may be used to assess the extent of stenosis or re-stenosis after angioplasty or CABG. Table 17–12 outlines the performance measurement set recommended by the ACC/AHA.

TABLE 17-12 American College of Cardiology, American Heart Association, and Physician Consortium for Performance Improvement Chronic Stable Coronary Artery Disease Core Physician Performance Measurement Set[a]

	Clinical Recommendations
Blood pressure measurement	A blood pressure ready is recommended at every visit. Recommended blood pressure management targets are ≤130 mm Hg systolic *(Class I Recommendation, Level A Evidence)* and ≤85 mm Hg diastolic in patient with CAD coexisting condition (e.g., diabetes, heart failure, or renal failure) and <140/90 mm Hg in patient with CAD and no coexisting condition.
Lipid profile	A lipid profile is recommended and should include total cholesterol, high-density lipoprotein cholesterol (HDL-C), low-density lipoprotein cholesterol (LDL-C), and triglycerides. *(Class I Recommendation, Level C Evidence)*
Symptom and activity assessment	Regular assessment of patients' anginal symptoms and levels of activity is recommended. (Serves as a basis for treatment modification.)
Smoking cessation	Smoking status should be determined and smoking cessation counseling and interventions are recommended. *(Class I Recommendation, Level B Evidence)*
Antiplatelet therapy *Denominator exclusion* Documentation of medical reason(s)[b] for not prescribing antiplatelet therapy; documentation of patient reason(s)[c] for not prescribing antiplatelet therapy	Routine use of aspirin is recommended in the absence of contraindications. If contraindications exist, other antiplatelet therapies may be substituted. *(Class I Recommendation, Level A Evidence)*
Drug therapy for lowering LCL-cholesterol *Denominator exclusion* Documentation that a statin was not indicated;[e] documentation of medical reason(s)[b] for not prescribing a statin; documentation of patient reason(s)[c] for not prescribing statin	The LCL-C treatment goal is <100 mg/dL. Persons with established coronary heart disease (CHD) who have a baseline LCL-C ≥130 mg/dL should be started on a cholesterol-lowering drug simultaneously with therapeutic lifestyle changes and control of nonlipid risk factors. *(Class I Recommendation, Level A Evidence)*
β-Blocker therapy—prior myocardial infarction (MI) *Denominator inclusion* Prior MI *Denominator exclusion* Documentation that a β-blocker was not indicated; documentation of medical reason(s)[b] for not prescribing a β-blocker; documentation of patient reason(s)[c] for not prescribing a β-blocker	β-Blocker therapy is recommended for all patients with prior MI in the absence of contraindications. *(Class I Recommendation, Level A Evidence)*
ACE inhibitor therapy *Denominator inclusion* Patient with CAD who also has diabetes and/or left ventricular systolic dysfunction (LVSD) (left ventricular ejection fraction [LVEF] <40% or moderately or severely depressed left ventricular systolic function) *Denominator exclusion* Documentation that ACE inhibitor was not indicated (e.g., patients on angiotensin receptor blockers [ARB]); documentation of medical reason(s)[b] for not prescribing ACE inhibitor; documentation of patient reason(s)[c] for not prescribing ACE inhibitor	ACE inhibitor use is recommended in all patients with CAD who also have diabetes and/or LVSD *(Class I Recommendation, Level A Evidence)* ACE inhibitor use is also recommended in patients with CAD or other vascular disease *(Class IIa Recommendation, Level B Evidence)*
Screening for diabetes[f] *Denominator exclusion* Patients with documented diabetes	Screening for diabetes is recommended in patients who are considered high risk (e.g., CAD) *(Class I Recommendation, Level A Evidence)*

ACE, angiotensin-converting enzyme; CAD, coronary artery disease; MI, myocardial infarction.
[a]Refers to all patients diagnosed with CAD
[b]Medical reasons for not prescribing **antiplatelet therapy** (aspirin, clopidogrel, or combination of aspirin and dipyridamole): active bleeding in the previous 6 months with required hospitalization and/or transfusion(s), patient on other antiplately therapy, etc.
Medical reasons for not prescribing a **statin**: clinical judgement, documented LCL-C <130 mg/dL, etc.
Medical reasons for not prescribing a **β-blocker**: bradycardia (defined as heart rate <50 beats/min without β-blocker therapy), history of class IV (congestive) heart failure, history of second- or third-degree atrioventricular block without permanent pacemaker, etc.
Medical reasons for not prescribing **ACE inhibitor (ACEI)**: allergy, angioedema caused by ACEI, anuric rental failure caused by ACEI, pregnancy, moderate or severe aortic stenosis, etc.
[c]Patient reasons for not prescribing antiplatelet therapy, statin, β-blocker, or ACEI: economic, social, and/or religious, etc.
[d]Antiplatelet therapy may include aspirin, clopidogrel, or combination of aspirin and dipyridamole.
[e]Not indicated for a stat refers to LCL-C <100 mg/dL.
[f]Test measure.
[g]Screening for diabetes is usually done by fasting blood glucose or 2-hour glucose tolerance testing. Clinical recommendations indicate screening should be considered at 3-year intervals.

ABBREVIATIONS

ACC: American College of Cardiology
ACEI: angiotensin-converting enzyme inhibitor
ACIP: Asymptomatic Cardiac Ischemia Pilot
AHA: American Heart Association
AV: arteriovenous
CABG: coronary artery bypass grafting
CAD: coronary artery disease
CASS: Coronary Artery Surgery Study
CHD: coronary heart disease
CT: computed tomography
CVD: cardiovascular disease
DCA: directional coronary atherectomy
ECG: electrocardiogram
EDRF: endothelium-derived relaxing factor
ETT: exercise tolerance (stress) testing
GMP: guanosine monophosphate
HDL: high-density lipoprotein
HERS: Heart Estrogen/Progestin Replacement Study
IHD: ischemic heart disease
I_{Na}: late sodium current
ISDN: isosorbide dinitrate
ISMN: isosorbide mononitrate
LAD: left anterior descending
LDL: low-density lipoprotein
LV: left ventricle
MI: myocardial infarction
MVO_2: myocardial oxygen demand
PCI: primary coronary intervention
PTCA: percutaneous transluminal angioplasty
R1: resistance 1-large epicardial or surface vessels
R2: resistance 2-intramyocardial arteries and arterioles

REFERENCES

1. Fraker TD Jr, Fihn SD, writing on behalf of the 2002 Chronic Stable Angina Writing Committee. 2007 chronic angina focused update of the ACC/AHA 2002 guidelines for the management of patients with chronic stable angina: a report of the American College of Cardiology/American Heart Association Task Force on Practice Guidelines Writing Group to Develop the Focused Update of the 2002 guidelines for the management of patients with chronic stable angina. Circulation 2007;116:2762–2772.
2. Gibbons RJ, Abrams J, Chatterjee K, et al. ACC/AHA 2002 guideline update for the management of patients with chronic stable angina—Summary article: A report of the American College of Cardiology/American Heart Association Task Force on Practice Guidelines (Committee on the Management of Patients with Chronic Stable Angina). Circulation 2003;107:149–158.
3. Fox K, Garcia MA, Ardissino D, et al. Guidelines on the management of stable angina pectoris: Executive summary: The Task Force on the Management of Stable Angina Pectoris of the European Society of Cardiology. Eur Heart J 2006;27:1341–1381.
4. Rosamond W, Flegal K, Friday G, et al. Heart disease and stroke statistics—2007 update: A report from the American Heart Association Statistics Committee and Stroke Statistics Subcommittee. Circulation 2007;115:69–171.
5. Sytkowski PA, D'Agostino RB, Belanger A, Kannel WB. Sex and time trends in cardiovascular disease incidence and mortality: The Framingham Heart Study, 1950–1989. Am J Epidemiol 1996;143:338–350.
6. Menotti A, Keys A, Blackburn H, et al. Comparison of multivariate predictive power of major risk factors for coronary heart diseases in different countries: Results from eight nations of the Seven Countries Study, 25-year follow-up. J Cardiovasc Risk 1996;3:69–75.
7. Keys A. Mediterranean diet and public health: Personal reflections. Am J Clin Nutr 1995;61:1321S–1323S.
8. Goldman L, Hashimoto B, Cook F, et al. Comparative reproducibility and validity of systems for assessing cardiovascular functional class: Advantages of a new specific activity scale. Circulation 1981;64:1227–1234.
9. Emond M, Mock MB, Davis KB, et al. Long-term survival of medically treated patients in the Coronary Artery Surgery Study (CASS) Registry. Circulation 1994;90:2645–2657.
10. Caracciolo EA, Davis KB, Sopko G, et al. Comparison of surgical and medical group survival in patients with left main coronary artery disease. Long-term CASS experience. Circulation 1995;91:2325–2334.
11. Epstein SE CRI, Talbot TL. Hemodynamic principles in the control of coronary blood flow. Am J Cardiol 1985;56:4E–10E.
12. Gielen S, Schuler G, Hambrecht R. Exercise training in coronary artery disease and coronary vasomotion. Circulation 2001;103:E1–E6.
13. Wassmann S, Faul A, Hennen B, Scheller B, Bohm M, Nickenig G. Rapid effect of 3-hydroxy-3-methylglutaryl coenzyme a reductase inhibition on coronary endothelial function. Circ Res, 2003;93:e98–e103.
14. Libby P. Coronary artery injury and the biology of atherosclerosis: Inflammation, thrombosis, and stabilization. Am J Cardiol 2000;86:3J–8J.
15. Braunwald E, Antman EM, Beasley JW, et al. ACC/AHA guidelines for the management of patients with unstable angina and non-ST-segment elevation myocardial infarction: Executive summary and recommendations. A report of the American College of Cardiology/American Heart Association task force on practice guidelines (committee on the management of patients with unstable angina). Circulation 2000;102:1193–1209.
16. Cohn PF. A new look at benefits of drug therapy in silent myocardial ischemia. Eur Heart J 2007;28:2053–2054.
17. Caracciolo EA, Chaitman BR, Forman SA, et al. Diabetics with coronary disease have a prevalence of asymptomatic ischemia during exercise treadmill testing and ambulatory ischemia monitoring similar to that of nondiabetic patients. An ACIP database study. ACIP Investigators. Asymptomatic Cardiac Ischemia Pilot Investigators. Circulation 1996;93:2097–2105.
18. Glusman M, Coromilas J, Clark WC, et al. Pain sensitivity in silent myocardial ischemia. Pain 1996;64:477–483.
19. Panel E. Executive summary of the third report of the National Cholesterol Education Program (NCEP) Expert Panel on Detection, Evaluation, and Treatment of High Blood Cholesterol in Adults (ATP III). JAMA 2001;285:2486–2497.
20. Hoeg JM. Evaluating coronary heart disease risk. Tiles in the mosaic. JAMA 1997;277:1387–1390.
21. Ridker PM, Morrow DA. C-reactive protein, inflammation, and coronary risk. Cardiol Clin, 2003;21:315–325.
22. O'Rourke RA, Hochman JS, Cohen MC, Lucore CL, Popma JJ, Cannon CP. New approaches to diagnosis and management of unstable angina and non-ST-segment elevation myocardial infarction. Arch Intern Med 2001;161:674–682.
23. Gibbons RJ, Balady GJ, Bricker JT, et al. ACC/AHA 2002 guideline update for exercise testing: Summary article: A report of the American College of Cardiology/American Heart Association Task Force on Practice Guidelines (Committee to Update the 1997 Exercise Testing Guidelines). Circulation 2002;106:1883–1892.
24. Klocke FJ, Baird MG, Lorell BH, et al. ACC/AHA/ASNC guidelines for the clinical use of cardiac radionuclide imaging—Executive summary: A report of the American College of Cardiology/American Heart Association Task Force on Practice Guidelines (ACC/AHA/ASNC Committee to Revise the 1995 Guidelines for the Clinical Use of Cardiac Radionuclide Imaging). J Am Coll Cardiol 2003;42:1318–1333.
25. Raggi P, Callister TQ, Cooil B, Russo DJ, Lippolis NJ, Patterson RE. Evaluation of chest pain in patients with low to intermediate pretest probability of coronary artery disease by electron beam computed tomography. Am J Cardiol 2000;85:283–288.

26. Fitzgerald PJ, Oshima A, Hayase M, et al. Final results of the Can Routine Ultrasound Influence Stent Expansion (CRUISE) study. Circulation 2000;102:523–530.
27. Grundy SM, Cleeman JI, Merz CN, et al. Implications of recent clinical trials for the National Cholesterol Education Program Adult Treatment Panel III guidelines. [erratum appears in Circulation, 2004;110(6):763]. Circulation 2004;110:227–239.
28. Anonymous. Effect of intensive diabetes management on macrovascular events and risk factors in the Diabetes Control and Complications Trial. Am J Cardiol 1995;75:894–903.
29. Smith CJ, Fischer TH, Sears SB. Environmental tobacco smoke, cardiovascular disease, and the nonlinear dose-response hypothesis. Toxicol Sci 2000;54:462–472.
30. Wald NJ, Watt HC. Prospective study of effect of switching from cigarettes to pipes or cigars on mortality from three smoking related diseases [see comments]. BMJ 1997;314:1860–1863.
31. Vogel RA. Coronary risk factors, endothelial function, and atherosclerosis: A review. Clin Cardiol 1997;20:426–432.
32. Tonstad S, Tonnesen P, Hajek P, et al. Effect of maintenance therapy with varenicline on smoking cessation: A randomized controlled trial [see comment]. JAMA 2006;296:64–71.
33. Oncken C, Gonzales D, Nides M, et al. Efficacy and safety of the novel selective nicotinic acetylcholine receptor partial agonist, varenicline, for smoking cessation [see comment]. Arch Intern Med 2006;166:1571–1577.
34. Russell LB, Carson JL, Taylor WC, Milan E, Dey A, Jagannathan R. Modeling all-cause mortality: Projections of the impact of smoking cessation based on the NHEFS. NHANES I Epidemiologic Follow-up Study. Am J Public Health 1998;88:630–636.
35. Kannel WB. Blood pressure as a cardiovascular risk factor: Prevention and treatment. JAMA 1996;275:1571–1576.
36. Rosendorff C, Black HR, Cannon CP, et al. Treatment of hypertension in the prevention and management of ischemic heart disease: A scientific statement from the American Heart Association Council for High Blood Pressure Research and the Councils on Clinical Cardiology and Epidemiology and Prevention. Circulation 2007;115:2761–2788.
37. Bleys J, Miller ER 3rd, Pastor-Barriuso R, Appel LJ, Guallar E. Vitamin-mineral supplementation and the progression of atherosclerosis: A meta-analysis of randomized controlled trials [see comment]. Am J Clin Nutr 2006;84:880–887.
38. Taylor RS, Brown A, Ebrahim S, et al. Exercise-based rehabilitation for patients with coronary heart disease: Systematic review and meta-analysis of randomized controlled trials [see comment]. Am J Med 2004;116:682–692.
39. Fuchs FD, Chambless LE, Folsom AR, et al. Association between alcoholic beverage consumption and incidence of coronary heart disease in whites and blacks: The Atherosclerosis Risk in Communities Study. Am J Epidemiol 2004;160:466–474.
40. Britton A, Marmot M. Different measures of alcohol consumption and risk of coronary heart disease and all-cause mortality: 11-year follow-up of the Whitehall II Cohort Study. Addiction 2004;99:109–116.
41. Subbiah MT. Mechanisms of cardioprotection by estrogens. Proc Soc Exp Biol Med 1998;217:23–29.
42. Hulley S, Grady D, Bush T, et al. Randomized trial of estrogen plus progestin for secondary prevention of coronary heart disease in postmenopausal women. Heart and Estrogen/progestin Replacement Study (HERS) Research Group. JAMA 1998;280:605–613.
43. Rossouw JE, Anderson GL, Prentice RL, et al. Risks and benefits of estrogen plus progestin in healthy postmenopausal women: Principal results From the Women's Health Initiative randomized controlled trial [see comment] [summary for patients in CMAJ 2002;167(4):377–378]. JAMA, 2002;288:321–333.
44. Cornelis MC, El-Sohemy A. Coffee, caffeine, and coronary heart disease. Curr Opin Lipidol 2007;18:13–19.
45. Kroon LA. Drug interactions and smoking: Raising awareness for acute and critical care providers. Crit Care Nurs Clin North Am 2006;18:53–62.
46. Thomas GR, DiFabio JM, Gori T, Parker JD. Once daily therapy with isosorbide-5-mononitrate causes endothelial dysfunction in humans: Evidence of a free-radical-mediated mechanism [see comment]. J Am Coll Cardiol 2007;49:1289–1295.
47. Munzel T, Wenzel P, Daiber A. Do we still need organic nitrates [comment]? J Am Coll Cardiol 2007;49:1296–1298.
48. Pehrsson SK, Ringqvist I, Ekdahl S, Karlson BW, Ulvenstam G, Persson S. Monotherapy with amlodipine or atenolol versus their combination in stable angina pectoris. Clin Cardiol 2000;23:763–770.
49. Verdecchia P, Reboldi G, Angeli F, et al. Angiotensin-converting enzyme inhibitors and calcium channel blockers for coronary heart disease and stroke prevention [see comment]. Hypertension 2005;46:386–392.
50. Howes LG, Edwards CT. Calcium antagonists and cancer. Is there really a link? Drug Saf 1998;18:1–7.
51. Opie LH, Yusuf S, Kubler W. Current status of safety and efficacy of calcium channel blockers in cardiovascular diseases: A critical analysis based on 100 studies. Prog Cardiovasc Dis 2000;43:171–196.
52. Knight CJ, Fox KM. Amlodipine versus diltiazem as additional anti-anginal treatment to atenolol. Centralised European Studies in Angina Research (CESAR) Investigators. Am J Cardiol 1998;81:133–136.
53. Boden WE, O'Rourke RA, Teo KK, et al. Optimal medical therapy with or without PCI for stable coronary disease [see comment]. N Engl J Med 2007;356:1503–1516.
54. Hueb W, Lopes NH, Gersh BJ, et al. Five-year follow-up of the Medicine, Angioplasty, or Surgery Study (MASS II): A randomized controlled clinical trial of 3 therapeutic strategies for multivessel coronary artery disease [see comment]. Circulation 2007;115:1082–1089.
55. Smith SC Jr, Feldman TE, Hirshfeld JW Jr, et al. ACC/AHA/SCAI 2005 guideline update for percutaneous coronary intervention: A report of the American College of Cardiology/American Heart Association Task Force on Practice Guidelines (ACC/AHA/SCAI Writing Committee to Update 2001 Guidelines for Percutaneous Coronary Intervention). Circulation 2006;113:e166–e286.
56. Anonymous. Seven-year outcome in the Bypass Angioplasty Revascularization Investigation (BARI) by treatment and diabetic status. J Am Coll Cardiol 2000;35:1122–1129.
57. Investigators B. The final 10-year follow-up results from the BARI randomized trial. J Am Coll Cardiol 2007;49:1600–1606.
58. Weintraub WS, Stein B, Kosinski A, et al. Outcome of coronary bypass surgery versus coronary angioplasty in diabetic patients with multivessel coronary artery disease. J Am Coll Cardiol 1998;31:10–19.
59. Hannan EL, Racz MJ, McCallister BD, et al. A comparison of three-year survival after coronary artery bypass graft surgery and percutaneous transluminal coronary angioplasty. J Am Coll Cardiol 1999;33:63–72.
60. Ramanathan KB, Weiman DS, Sacks J, et al. Percutaneous intervention versus coronary bypass surgery for patients older than 70 years of age with high-risk unstable angina. Ann Thorac Surg 2005;80:1340–1346.
61. Janzon M, Levin LA, Swahn E. Invasive treatment in unstable coronary artery disease promotes health-related quality of life: Results from the FRISC II trial [see comment]. Am Heart J 2004;148:114–121.
62. Kaluza GL, Mazur W, Raizner AE. Basic science review: Radiotherapy for prevention of restenosis. Catheter Cardiovasc Interv 2001;52:518–529.
63. Cutlip DE. Stent thrombosis: Historical perspectives and current trends. J Thromb Thrombolysis 2000;10:89–101.
64. Levine GN, Berger PB, Cohen DJ, et al. Newer pharmacotherapy in patients undergoing percutaneous coronary interventions: A guide for pharmacists and other health care professionals. Pharmacotherapy 2006;26:1537–1556.
65. Smith SC Jr, Dove JT, Jacobs AK, et al. ACC/AHA guidelines for percutaneous coronary intervention (revision of the 1993 PTCA guidelines)—Executive summary: A report of the American College of Cardiology/American Heart Association task force on practice guidelines (Committee to revise the 1993 guidelines for percutaneous transluminal coronary angioplasty) endorsed by the Society for Cardiac Angiography and Interventions. Circulation 2001;103:3019–3041.
66. Williams DO, Braunwald E, Thompson B, Sharaf BL, Buller CE, Knatterud GL. Results of percutaneous transluminal coronary angioplasty in unstable angina and non-Q-wave myocardial infarction. Observations from the TIMI IIIB Trial. Circulation 1996;94:2749–2755.
67. Pepine CJ. An ischemia-guided approach for risk stratification in patients with acute coronary syndromes. Am J Cardiol 2000;86:27M–35M.
68. Boden WE, O'Rourke RA, Crawford MH, et al. Outcomes in patients with acute non–Q-wave myocardial infarction randomly assigned to an invasive as compared with a conservative management strategy. Veterans Affairs Non-Q-Wave Infarction Strategies in Hospital (VANQWISH) Trial Investigators. N Engl J Med 1998;338:1785–1792.

69. Anonymous. Invasive compared with non-invasive treatment in unstable coronary-artery disease: FRISC II prospective randomised multicentre study. FRagmin and Fast Revascularisation during InStability in Coronary artery disease Investigators. Lancet 1999;354:708–715.
70. Eagle KA, Guyton RA, Davidoff R, et al. ACC/AHA 2004 guideline update for coronary artery bypass graft surgery: Summary article: A report of the American College of Cardiology/American Heart Association Task Force on Practice Guidelines (Committee to Update the 1999 Guidelines for Coronary Artery Bypass Graft Surgery) [erratum appears in Circulation, 2005;111(15):2014]. Circulation 2004;110:1168–1176.
71. Eagle KA, Guyton RA, Davidoff R, et al. ACC/AHA guidelines for coronary artery bypass graft surgery: Executive summary and recommendations: A report of the American College of Cardiology/American Heart Association Task Force on Practice Guidelines (Committee to Revise the 1991 Guidelines for Coronary Artery Bypass Graft Surgery). Circulation 1999;100:1464–1480.
72. Colombo A, Tobis J. Techniques in Coronary Artery Stenting. London, England: Martin Dunitz, 2000:1–422.
73. Jacobs AK, Kelsey SF, Brooks MM, et al. Better outcome for women compared with men undergoing coronary revascularization: A report from the bypass angioplasty revascularization investigation (BARI). Circulation 1998;98:1279–1285.
74. Taylor HA Jr, Mickel MC, Chaitman BR, Sopko G, Cutter GR, Rogers WJ. Long-term survival of African Americans in the Coronary Artery Surgery Study (CASS). J Am Coll Cardiol 1997;29:358–364.
75. Smith SC Jr, Dove JT, Jacobs AK, et al. ACC/AHA guidelines of percutaneous coronary interventions (revision of the 1993 PTCA guidelines)—Executive summary. A report of the American College of Cardiology/American Heart Association Task Force on Practice Guidelines (Committee to Revise the 1993 Guidelines for Percutaneous Transluminal Coronary Angioplasty). J Am Coll Cardiol, 2001;37:2215–2239.
76. Kastrati A, Mehilli J, Dirschinger J, et al. Intracoronary stenting and angiographic results. Strut thickness effect on restenosis outcome (ISAR-STEREO) trial. Circulation 2001;103:2816–2821.
77. Keelan ET, Nunez BD, Grill DE, Berger PB, Holmes DR Jr, Bell MR. Comparison of immediate and long-term outcome of coronary angioplasty performed for unstable angina and rest pain in men and women. Mayo Clin Proc 1997;72:5–12.
78. Spinler SA. Managing acute coronary syndrome: Evidence-based approaches. Am J Health Syst Pharm 2007;64:1432–1434.
79. Bertrand ME, Rupprecht HJ, Urban P, Gershlick AH, et al. Double-blind study of the safety of clopidogrel with and without a loading dose in combination with aspirin compared with ticlopidine in combination with aspirin after coronary stenting: The clopidogrel aspirin stent international cooperative study (CLASSICS). Circulation 2000;102:624–629.
80. Schomig A, Neumann FJ, Walter H, et al. Coronary stent placement in patients with acute myocardial infarction: Comparison of clinical and angiographic outcome after randomization to antiplatelet or anticoagulant therapy. J Am Coll Cardiol 1997;29:28–34.
81. Schuhlen H, Kastrati A, Pache J, Dirschinger J, Schomig A. Sustained benefit over four years from an initial combined antiplatelet regimen after coronary stent placement in the ISAR trial. Intracoronary Stenting and Antithrombotic Regimen. Am J Cardiol 2001;87:397–400.
82. Heeschen C, van Den Brand MJ, Hamm CW, Simoons ML. Angiographic findings in patients with refractory unstable angina according to troponin T status. Circulation 1999;100:1509–1514.
83. Topol EJ, Moliterno D, Herrmann HC, et al. Comparison of two platelet glycoprotein IIb/IIIa inhibitors, tirofiban and abciximab, for the prevention of ischemic events with percutaneous coronary revascularization. N Engl J Med 2001;344:1888–18894.
84. Landzberg BR, Frishman WH, Lerrick K. Pathophysiology and pharmacological approaches for prevention of coronary artery restenosis following coronary artery balloon angioplasty and related procedures. Prog Cardiovasc Dis 1997;39:361–398.
85. Stone GW, White HD, Ohman EM, et al. Bivalirudin in patients with acute coronary syndromes undergoing percutaneous coronary intervention: A subgroup analysis from the Acute Catheterization and Urgent Intervention Triage strategy (ACUITY) trial [see comment]. Lancet 2007;369:907–919.
86. Cohen DJ, Lincoff AM, Lavelle TA, et al. Economic evaluation of bivalirudin with provisional glycoprotein IIB/IIIA inhibition versus heparin with routine glycoprotein IIB/IIIA inhibition for percutaneous coronary intervention: Results from the REPLACE-2 trial [see comment]. J Am Coll Cardiol 2004;44:1792–1800.
87. Lincoff AM, Kleiman NS, Kereiakes DJ, et al. Long-term efficacy of bivalirudin and provisional glycoprotein IIb/IIIa blockade vs heparin and planned glycoprotein IIb/IIIa blockade during percutaneous coronary revascularization: REPLACE-2 randomized trial [erratum appears in JAMA 2006;296(1):46]. JAMA 2004;292:696–703.
88. Ellis SG, Holmes DR Jr, eds. Strategic Approaches in Coronary Interventional. Philadelphia: Lippincott Williams & Wilkins, 1999:1–622.
89. Moustapha A, Assali AR, Sdringola S, et al. Percutaneous and surgical interventions for in-stent restenosis: Long-term outcomes and effect of diabetes mellitus. J Am Coll Cardiol 2001;37:1877–1882.
90. Ghaffari S, Kereiakes DJ, Lincoff AM, et al. Platelet glycoprotein IIb/IIIa receptor blockade with abciximab reduces ischemic complications in patients undergoing directional coronary atherectomy. EPILOG Investigators. Evaluation of PTCA to Improve Long-term Outcome by c7E3 GP IIb/IIIa Receptor Blockade. Am J Cardiol 1998;82:7–12.
91. Appelman YE, Piek JJ, van der Wall EE, et al. Evaluation of the long-term functional outcome assessed by myocardial perfusion scintigraphy following excimer laser angioplasty compared to balloon angioplasty in longer coronary lesions. Int J Card Imaging 2000;16:267–277.
92. Kaul S, Shah PK, Diamond GA. As time goes by: Current status and future directions in the controversy over stenting. J Am Coll Cardiol 2007;50:128–137.
93. Jaffe R, Strauss BH. Late and very late thrombosis of drug-eluting stents: Evolving concepts and perspectives. J Am Coll Cardiol 2007;50:119–127.
94. Holmes DR Jr, Kereiakes DJ, Laskey WK, et al. Thrombosis and drug-eluting stents: An objective appraisal. J Am Coll Cardiol 2007;50:109–118.
95. Luscher TF, Steffel J, Eberli FR, et al. Drug-eluting stent and coronary thrombosis: Biological mechanisms and clinical implications. Circulation 2007;115:1051–1058.
96. Grines CL, Bonow RO, Casey DE Jr, et al. Prevention of premature discontinuation of dual antiplatelet therapy in patients with coronary artery stents: A science advisory from the American Heart Association, American College of Cardiology, Society for Cardiovascular Angiography and Interventions, American College of Surgeons, and American Dental Association, with representation from the American College of Physicians. J Am Coll Cardiol 2007;49:734–739.
97. Abrams J. Clinical practice. Chronic stable angina [see comment] [erratum appears in N Engl J Med 2005;353(25):2728]. N Engl J Med 2005;352:2524–2533.
98. Feringa HH, van Waning VH, Bax JJ, et al. Cardioprotective medication is associated with improved survival in patients with peripheral arterial disease. J Am Coll Cardiol 2006;47:1182–1187.
99. Prince MJ, Bird AS, Blizard RA, Mann AH. Is the cognitive function of older patients affected by antihypertensive treatment? Results from 54 months of the Medical Research Council's trial of hypertension in older adults. BMJ 1996;312:801–805.
100. Rosenthal J, Bahrmann H, Benkert K, et al. Analysis of adverse effects among patients with essential hypertension receiving an ACE inhibitor or a beta-blocker. Cardiology 1996;87:409–414.
101. Darius H. Role of nitrates for the therapy of coronary artery disease patients in the years beyond 2000. J Cardiovasc Pharmacol 1999;34:S15–S20; discussion S29–S31.
102. Thadani U. Oral nitrates: More than symptomatic therapy in coronary artery disease? Cardiovasc Drugs Ther 1997;11:213–218.
103. Chen Z, Stamler JS. Bioactivation of nitroglycerin by the mitochondrial aldehyde dehydrogenase. Trends Cardiovasc Med 2006;16:259–265.
104. Sydow K, Daiber A, Oelze M, et al. Central role of mitochondrial aldehyde dehydrogenase and reactive oxygen species in nitroglycerin tolerance and cross-tolerance [see comment]. J Clin Invest 2004;113:482–489.
105. Sekiya M, Sato M, Funada J, Ohtani T, Akutsu H, Watanabe K. Effects of the long-term administration of nicorandil on vascular endothelial function and the progression of arteriosclerosis. J Cardiovasc Pharmacol 2005;46:63–67.
106. Parker JO, Amies MH, Hawkinson RW, et al. Intermittent transdermal nitroglycerin therapy in angina pectoris. Clinically effective without tolerance or rebound. Minitran Efficacy Study Group. Circulation 1995;91:1368–1374.

107. Freedman SB, Daxini BV, Noyce D, Kelly DT. Intermittent transdermal nitrates do not improve ischemia in patients taking beta-blockers or calcium antagonists: Potential role of rebound ischemia during the nitrate-free period. J Am Coll Cardiol 1995;25:349–355.
108. Ajani AE, Yan BP. The mystery of coronary artery spasm. Heart Lung Circ 2007;16:10–15.
109. Katoh M, Nakajima M, Shimada N, Yamazaki H, Yokoi T. Inhibition of human cytochrome P450 enzymes by 1,4-dihydropyridine calcium antagonists: Prediction of in vivo drug-drug interactions. Eur J Clin Pharmacol 2000;55:843–852.
110. Chaitman BR. Ranolazine for the treatment of chronic angina and potential use in other cardiovascular conditions. Circulation 2006;113:2462–2472.
111. Cheng JW. Ranolazine for the management of coronary artery disease. Clin Ther 2006;28:1996–2007.
112. Chaitman BR, Pepine CJ, Parker JO, et al. Effects of ranolazine with atenolol, amlodipine, or diltiazem on exercise tolerance and angina frequency in patients with severe chronic angina: A randomized controlled trial [see comment]. JAMA 2004;291:309–316.
113. Chaitman BR, Skettino SL, Parker JO, et al. Anti-ischemic effects and long-term survival during ranolazine monotherapy in patients with chronic severe angina. J Am Coll Cardiol 2004;43:1375–1382.
114. Morrow DA, Scirica BM, Karwatowska-Prokopczuk E, et al. Effects of ranolazine on recurrent cardiovascular events in patients with non-ST-elevation acute coronary syndromes: The MERLIN-TIMI 36 randomized trial [see comment]. JAMA 2007;297:1775–1783.
115. Grines CL, Watkins MW, Mahmarian JJ, et al. A randomized, double-blind, placebo-controlled trial of Ad5FGF-4 gene therapy and its effect on myocardial perfusion in patients with stable angina. J Am Coll Cardiol 2003;42:1339–1347.
116. Abo-Auda W, Benza RL. Therapeutic angiogenesis: Review of current concepts and future directions. J Heart Lung Transplant 2003;22:370–382.
117. Lanza GA, Sestito A, Sgueglia GA, et al. Current clinical features, diagnostic assessment and prognostic determinants of patients with variant angina. Int J Cardiol 2007;118:41–47.
118. Sakata K, Miura F, Sugino H, et al. Assessment of regional sympathetic nerve activity in vasospastic angina: Analysis of iodine 123-labeled metaiodobenzylguanidine scintigraphy. Am Heart J 1997;133:484–489.
119. Hung MJ, Cherng WJ, Yang NI, Cheng CW, Li LF. Relation of high-sensitivity C-reactive protein level with coronary vasospastic angina pectoris in patients without hemodynamically significant coronary artery disease. Am J Cardiol 2005;96:1484–1490.
120. Mishra PK. Variations in presentation and various options in management of variant angina. Eur J Cardiothorac Surg 2006;29:748–759.
121. Park JS, Zhang SY, Jo SH, et al. Common adrenergic receptor polymorphisms as novel risk factors for vasospastic angina. Am Heart J 2006;151:864–869.
122. Lanza GA, Pedrotti P, Pasceri V, Lucente M, Crea F, Maseri A. Autonomic changes associated with spontaneous coronary spasm in patients with variant angina. J Am Coll Cardiol 1996;28:1249–1256.
123. Conti CR, Geller NL, Knatterud GL, et al. Anginal status and prediction of cardiac events in patients enrolled in the asymptomatic cardiac ischemia pilot (ACIP) study. ACIP investigators. Am J Cardiol 1997;79:889–892.
124. Davies RF, Goldberg AD, Forman S, et al. Asymptomatic Cardiac Ischemia Pilot (ACIP) study two-year follow-up: Outcomes of patients randomized to initial strategies of medical therapy versus revascularization [see comments]. Circulation 1997;95:2037–2043.
125. Singh N, Mironov D, Goodman S, Morgan CD, Langer A. Treatment of silent ischemia in unstable angina: A randomized comparison of sustained-release verapamil versus metoprolol. Clin Cardiol 1995;18:653–658.
126. Dwivedi SK, Saran RK, Mittal S, Gupta R, Narain VS, Puri VK. Silent ischemic interval on exercise test is a predictor to drug therapy: A randomized crossover trial of metoprolol versus diltiazem in stable angina. Clin Cardiol 2001;24:45–49.
127. Pratt CM, McMahon RP, Goldstein S, et al. Comparison of subgroups assigned to medical regimens used to suppress cardiac ischemia (the Asymptomatic Cardiac Ischemia Pilot [ACIP] Study). Am J Cardiol 1996;77:1302–1309.
128. Davies RF, Habibi H, Klinke WP, et al. Effect of amlodipine, atenolol and their combination on myocardial ischemia during treadmill exercise and ambulatory monitoring. Canadian Amlodipine/Atenolol in Silent Ischemia Study (CASIS) Investigators. J Am Coll Cardiol 1995;25:619–625.
129. Erne P, Schoenenberger AW, Burckhardt D, et al. Effects of percutaneous coronary interventions in silent ischemia after myocardial infarction: The SWISSI II randomized controlled trial. JAMA 2007;297:1985–1991.
130. Bosanquet N, Jonsson B, Fox KA. Costs and cost effectiveness of low molecular weight heparins and platelet glycoprotein IIb/IIIa inhibitors: In the management of acute coronary syndromes. Pharmacoeconomics 2003;21:1135–1152.
131. Plosker GL, Ibbotson T. Eptifibatide: A pharmacoeconomic review of its use in percutaneous coronary intervention and acute coronary syndromes. Pharmacoeconomics 2003;21:885–912.
132. Caron MF, McKendall GR. Bivalirudin in percutaneous coronary intervention. Am J Health Syst Pharm 2003;60:1841–1849.
133. Hay JW, Yu WM, Ashraf T. Pharmacoeconomics of lipid-lowering agents for primary and secondary prevention of coronary artery disease. Pharmacoeconomics 1999;15:47–74.
134. Lamotte M, Annemans L, Evers T, Kubin M. A multi-country economic evaluation of low-dose aspirin in the primary prevention of cardiovascular disease. Pharmacoeconomics 2006;24:155–169.

CHAPTER 18 Acute Coronary Syndromes

SARAH A. SPINLER AND SIMON DE DENUS

KEY CONCEPTS

1. The cause of an acute coronary syndrome (ACS) is erosion or rupture of an atherosclerotic plaque with subsequent platelet adherence, activation, aggregation, and activation of the clotting cascade. Ultimately, a clot composed of fibrin and platelets forms.
2. The American Heart Association and the American College of Cardiology recommend strategies or guidelines for the care of patients with ST-segment elevation and non–ST-segment elevation ACS.
3. Patients with ischemic chest discomfort and suspected ACS are risk stratified based on a 12-lead electrocardiogram, medical history, signs and symptoms, and results of creatine kinase myocardial band (CK MB) and troponin biochemical marker tests.
4. The diagnosis of myocardial infarction is confirmed based on the results of the CK MB and troponin tests.
5. Early reperfusion therapy with either primary percutaneous coronary intervention or administration of a fibrinolytic agent is the recommended therapy for patients presenting with ST-segment elevation ACS.
6. In addition to reperfusion therapy, all patients with ST-segment elevation ACS and without contraindications should receive pharmacotherapy within the first day of hospitalization and preferably in the emergency department, consisting of intranasal oxygen (if oxygen saturation is low), aspirin, clopidogrel, sublingual nitroglycerin, oral β-blockers, and either unfractionated heparin or enoxaparin. Intravenous β-blockers and nitroglycerin should be given to selected patients.
7. High-risk patients with non–ST-segment elevation ACS should undergo early coronary angiography and revascularization with either percutaneous coronary intervention or coronary artery bypass graft surgery.
8. In the absence of contraindications, all patients with non–ST-segment elevation ACS should be treated in the emergency department with intranasal oxygen (if oxygen saturation is low), aspirin, sublingual nitroglycerin, oral β-blockers, and an anticoagulant (unfractionated heparin, enoxaparin, fondaparinux, or bivalirudin). Most patients should receive additional therapy with clopidogrel. High-risk patients also should receive a glycoprotein IIb/IIIa receptor blocker. Intravenous β-blockers and nitroglycerin should be given to selected patients.
9. Following myocardial infarction, all patients, in the absence of contraindications, should receive indefinite therapy with aspirin, a β-blocker, and an angiotensin-converting enzyme inhibitor for secondary prevention of death, stroke, and recurrent infarction. Most patients are given a statin to reduce the low-density-lipoprotein cholesterol level to less than 70 to 100 mg/dL. Administration of clopidogrel should be considered for most patients, but the level of the recommendation and duration of therapy depend on the diagnosis, the method of reperfusion used, and the risk of bleeding. Anticoagulation with warfarin should be considered for patients at high risk for death, reinfarction, or stroke.

Learning objectives, review questions, and other resources can be found at **www.pharmacotherapyonline.com.**

Since the early 1900s, cardiovascular disease (CVD) has been the leading cause of death in the United States. Acute coronary syndromes (ACSs), including unstable angina and myocardial infarction (MI), are forms of coronary heart disease (CHD) that constitute the most common cause of CVD death.[1] **1** The cause of an ACS is erosion or rupture of an atherosclerotic plaque with subsequent platelet adherence, activation, aggregation, and activation of the clotting cascade. Ultimately, a clot composed of fibrin and platelets forms. Correspondingly, pharmacotherapy of ACS has advanced to include combinations of fibrinolytics, antiplatelets, and anticoagulants, with more traditional therapies such as nitrates and β-adrenergic blockers. Pharmacotherapy is integrated with reperfusion therapy and revascularization of the culprit coronary artery through interventional means such as percutaneous coronary intervention (PCI) and coronary artery bypass graft (CABG) surgery. **2** The American Heart Association (AHA) and the American College of Cardiology (ACC) recommend strategies or guidelines for the care of patients with ST-segment elevation (STE) and non–ST-segment elevation (NSTE) ACS. These joint practice guidelines are based on a review of available clinical evidence, have graded recommendations based on the weight and quality of evidence, and are updated periodically. The guidelines form the cornerstone for quality patient care of the ACS patient.[2,3]

EPIDEMIOLOGY

Each year more than 1.5 million Americans will experience an ACS, and 220,000 will die of an MI.[1] In the United States, more than 7.6 million living persons have survived an MI.[1] Chest discomfort is the second most frequent reason for patient presentation to emergency departments. Up to 5.6 million (~5.1%) emergency department visits are linked to chest discomfort and possible ACS.[2,4] CHD is the leading cause of premature chronic disability in the United States. The cost of CHD is high, with direct and indirect costs estimated at $151.6 billion for 2007.[1] The median length of hospital stay for MI in 1999 was 4.3 days[1] but decreased to a median of 3.3 days in 2006.[5]

Much of the epidemiologic data regarding ACS treatment and survival come from the National Registry of Myocardial Infarction (NRMI), the Global Registry of Acute Coronary Events (GRACE), and statistical summaries of U.S. hospital discharges prepared by the AHA. In-hospital death rates are approximately 4.6% for patients with STE ACS but are lower (2.2%) for patients with NSTE ACS.[6] Patients with STEMI who are treated with reperfusion therapy, either fibrinolytics or primary PCI, have lower mortality rates than patients treated without reperfusion. Reperfusion rates and mortality rates are higher in the elderly and in women. For example, the mortality rate is 19% in elderly patients who were eligible for reperfusion therapy but did not receive it compared to 10.5% in patients who did.[7] In women, the mortality rate is 18% for those eligible for reperfusion therapy but did not receive it compared to 9.3% for those who do not.[7] In the first year after MI, 23% of women and 18% of men will die, most from recurrent infarction.[1] At 1 year, rates of mortality and reinfarction between STE and NSTE MI are similar.

The rate of developing heart failure during hospitalization for ACS is declining rapidly. Compared to data from 1999, the incidence of in-hospital heart failure in patients with STEMI declined from 19.5% to 11% and that for patients with NSTE ACS declined from 13% to 6.1%.[6] In-hospital death rates for patients who present with or develop heart failure are more than threefold higher than for those who do not.[6]

Because reinfarction and death are major outcomes following ACS, therapeutic strategies to reduce morbidity and mortality, particularly use of coronary angiography, revascularization, and pharmacotherapy, will have a significant impact on the social and economic burden of CHD in the United States.

ETIOLOGY

This section discusses the formation of atherosclerotic plaques, the underlying cause of coronary artery disease (CAD), and ACS in most patients. The process of atherosclerosis starts early in life. Although atherosclerosis once was considered only a disease of cholesterol excess, it now is clear that inflammation also plays a central role in the genesis, progression, and complication of the disease.[8] In the earliest stage of atherosclerosis—endothelial dysfunction—induction and/or repression of several genes occurs in response to sheer stress of the blood flowing over the atherosclerotic plaque on the endothelial lining of the artery. In response to gene induction and repression, the endothelial cells decrease synthesis of nitric oxide, increase oxidation of lipoproteins and facilitate their entry into the arterial wall, promote the adherence of monocytes to the vessel wall and deposition of extracellular matrix, cause smooth muscle cell proliferation, and release local vasoconstrictor and prothrombotic substances into the blood; each action has a subsequent inflammatory response.[9] Taken together, all these factors contribute to the evolution of endothelial dysfunction to the formation of fatty streaks in the coronary arteries and eventually to atherosclerotic plaques. Therefore, the endothelium serves as an important autocrine and paracrine organ in the development of atherosclerosis.

A number of factors are directly responsible for the development and progression of endothelial dysfunction and atherosclerosis, including hypertension, age, male gender, tobacco use, diabetes mellitus, obesity, and dyslipidemias.[1]

PATHOPHYSIOLOGY

SPECTRUM OF ACS

Acute coronary syndromes (ACSs) is a term that includes all clinical syndromes compatible with acute myocardial ischemia resulting from an imbalance between myocardial oxygen demand and supply.[3] In contrast to stable angina, an ACS results primarily from diminished myocardial blood flow secondary to an occlusive or partially occlusive coronary artery thrombus. ACSs are classified according to electrocardiographic (ECG) changes into STE ACS, also called STEMI, and NSTE ACS, which includes NSTE MI and unstable angina (Fig. 18–1).[10] Approximately 21% of patients presenting with ACS have STEMI.[1] NSTE MI differs from unstable angina in that ischemia is severe enough to produce myocardial necrosis, resulting in the release of a detectable amount of biochemical markers, mainly troponin I or T, and creatine kinase myocardial band (CK MB) from the necrotic myocytes into the bloodstream.[3] The clinical significance of serum biochemical markers is discussed in greater detail in the Clinical Presentation and Biochemical Markers sections of this chapter. Following an STEMI, pathologic Q waves are seen frequently on the ECG; such an ECG manifestation is seen less commonly in patients with NSTE MI.[7] The presence of Q waves usually indicates transmural MI. Non–Q-wave MI, which is predominantly seen in NSTE MI, is limited to the subendocardial myocardium.[2]

PLAQUE RUPTURE AND CLOT FORMATION

❶ The predominant cause of ACS in more than 90% of patients is atheromatous plaque rupture, fissuring, or erosion of an unstable atherosclerotic plaque. Plaques that encompass less than 50% of the coronary lumen are more likely to rupture than those that occlude 70% to 90% of the coronary artery.[3] Such stable 70% to 90% stenoses of the coronary artery are characteristic of stable angina and tend to have a small lipid core, a thick fibrous cap, more calcification, and less compensatory enlargement.[8] Plaques that are more susceptible to rupture are characterized by an eccentric shape, thin fibrous cap (particularly in the shoulder region of the plaque), large fatty core, high content in inflammatory cells such as macrophages and lymphocytes, limited amounts of smooth muscle, and significant compensatory enlargement. Compensatory enlargement is the growth of the lesion pushing the vessel outward rather than inward plaque growth. Therefore, compensatory enlargement may result in underestimation of the atherosclerotic stenosis as measured by coronary angiography. Inflammatory cells promote thinning of the fibrous cap through the release of proteolytic enzymes, particularly matrix metalloproteinases.[8]

Following plaque rupture, a partially occlusive or completely occlusive thrombus—a clot—forms on top of the ruptured plaque. The thrombogenic contents of the plaque are exposed to blood elements. Exposure of collagen and tissue factor induces platelet adhesion and activation, which promote the release of platelet-derived vasoactive substances, including adenosine diphosphate (ADP) and thromboxane A_2.[11] These substances produce vasoconstriction and potentiate platelet activation. Furthermore, during platelet activation, the conformation of the glycoprotein (GP) IIb/IIIa surface receptors of platelets changes such that platelets cross-link to each other via fibrinogen bridges. This process is considered the final common pathway of platelet aggregation. Other substances known to promote platelet aggregation include serotonin, thrombin, and epinephrine.[8] Inclusion of platelets gives the clot a white appearance. Simultaneously, the extrinsic coagulation cascade pathway is activated as a result of exposure of blood components to the thrombogenic lipid core and endothelium, which are rich in tissue factor. This leads to the production of thrombin (factor IIa), which converts fibrinogen to fibrin through enzymatic activity.[11] Fibrin stabilizes the clot and traps red blood cells, giving the clot a red appearance. Therefore, the clot is composed of both cross-linked platelets and fibrin strands.[11] Although patients with an ACS more commonly present with a single, ruptured atherosclerotic plaque in one major coronary artery, they also may present with more than one ruptured plaque and multiple active lesions in more than one coronary artery, which predispose patients to a worse prognosis.[8]

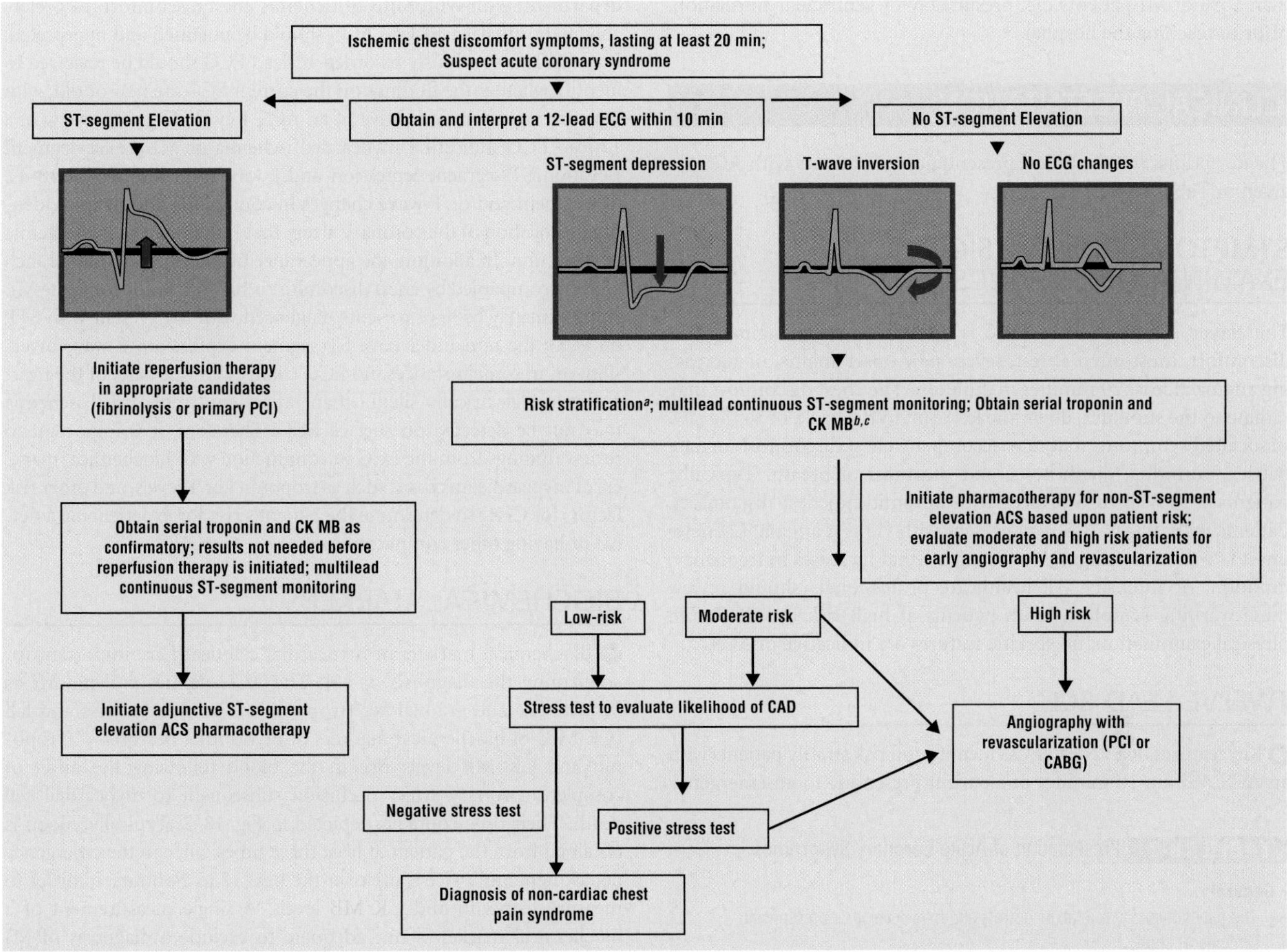

FIGURE 18-1. Evaluation of the acute coronary syndrome patient. (ACS, acute coronary syndrome; CABG, coronary artery bypass graft surgery; CAD, coronary artery disease; CK MB, creatine kinase myocardial band; ECG, electrocardiogram; PCI, percutaneous coronary intervention.) [a]As described in Table 18–2. [b]Positive, above the myocardial infarction (MI) decision limit. [c]"Negative," below the MI decision limit. *(Reprinted with permission from the American College of Clinical Pharmacy. Spinler SA. Acute coronary syndromes. In: Dunsworth TS, Richardson MM, Cheng JWM, et al., eds. Pharmacotherapy Self-Assessment Program, 6th ed. Cardiology II module. Kansas City: American College of Clinical Pharmacy, 2007:69–70.)*

A thrombus containing more platelets than fibrin, or a "white" clot, generally produces an incomplete occlusion of the coronary lumen and is more common in NSTE ACS. In patients presenting with STE ACS, the vessel generally is completely occluded by a "red" clot, which contains larger amounts of fibrin and red blood cells but a smaller amount of platelets compared with a "white" clot.[2] As discussed later in Treatment of Acute Coronary Syndromes, the composition of the clot influences the selection of the combinations of antithrombotic agents used for treatment of STE and NSTE ACS. Finally, myocardial ischemia can result from downstream embolization of microthrombi and produce ischemia with eventual necrosis.[2]

VENTRICULAR REMODELING FOLLOWING AN ACUTE MI

Ventricular remodeling is a process that occurs in several cardiovascular conditions, including heart failure, and following an MI. It is characterized by changes in the size, shape, and function of the left ventricle (LV) of both the infarcted area and the remaining ventricle, ultimately leading to cardiac failure.[12] Because heart failure is one of the principal causes of mortality and morbidity following an MI, preventing ventricular remodeling is an important therapeutic goal.[12]

Many factors contribute to ventricular remodeling, including neurohormonal factors (e.g., activation of the renin-angiotensin-aldosterone and sympathetic nervous systems), hemodynamic factors, mechanical factors, changes in gene expression, and modifications in myocardial matrix metalloproteinase activity and their inhibitors.[13,14] This process affects both cardiomyocytes (cardiomyocyte hypertrophy, loss of cardiomyocytes) and the extracellular matrix (increased interstitial fibrosis), thereby promoting both systolic and diastolic dysfunction.[14]

Angiotensin-converting enzyme (ACE) inhibitors, β-blockers, and aldosterone antagonists are agents that slow down or reverse ventricular remodeling through neurohormonal blockage and/or through improvement in hemodynamics (decreasing preload or afterload).[12] These agents also improve survival (discussed in more detail in the Secondary Prevention Following MI section of this chapter). This effect underlines the importance of the remodeling process and the urgency of preventing, halting, or reversing the process in patients who have experienced an MI.

COMPLICATIONS

This chapter focuses on management of the uncomplicated ACS patient. However, it is important for clinicians to recognize complications of MI because they are associated with increased mortality. The most serious complication is cardiogenic shock, which occurs in approximately 5% to 6% of patients presenting with STEMI and in less than 2% of those presenting with NSTE ACS.[9,15] Mortality in cardiogenic shock patients with MI is high, approaching 60%.[16] Other complications that may result from MI are heart failure, valvular dysfunction, ventricular and atrial tachyarrhythmias, bradycardia, heart block, pericarditis, stroke secondary to LV thrombus embolization, venous thromboembolism, and LV free-wall rupture.[17] More than 25% of MI patients die, presumably of ventricular fibrillation, prior to reaching the hospital.[18]

CLINICAL PRESENTATION

The key points in the clinical presentation of patients with ACS are given in Table 18–1.

SYMPTOMS AND PHYSICAL EXAMINATION FINDINGS

The classic symptom of an ACS is midline anterior anginal chest discomfort, most often at rest, severe new-onset angina, or increasing angina at least 20 minutes in duration. The chest discomfort may radiate to the shoulder, down the left arm, to the back, or to the jaw. Associated symptoms that may accompany chest discomfort include nausea, vomiting, diaphoresis, and shortness of breath. Typically, patients with STE ACS present with unremitting chest discomfort. Patients with NSTE ACS may present with (1) rest angina, (2) new-onset (<2 months) angina, or (3) angina that increases in frequency, duration, or intensity. All healthcare professionals should review these warning symptoms with patients at high risk for CHD. On physical examination, no specific features are indicative of ACS.

TWELVE-LEAD ECG

❸ Key features of a 12-lead ECG identify and risk stratify patients with an ACS. Within 10 minutes of a patient presenting to an emergency department with symptoms of ischemic chest discomfort (or preferably prehospital), a 12-lead ECG should be obtained and interpreted. If available, a previously recorded 12-lead ECG should be reviewed to identify whether the findings on the current ECG are new or old, with new findings more indicative of an ACS. Key findings on review of a 12-lead ECG indicating myocardial ischemia or MI are ST-segment elevation, ST-segment depression, and T-wave inversion (see Fig. 18–1). ST-segment and/or T-wave changes in contiguous leads help to identify the location of the coronary artery that is the cause of the ischemia or infarction. In addition, the appearance of a new left bundle-branch block accompanied by chest discomfort is highly specific for acute MI. Approximately 65% of patients diagnosed with MI present with STE on ECG; the remainder have ST-segment depression, T-wave inversion, or, in some instances, no ECG changes.[5] Some parts of the heart are more "electrically silent" than others, and myocardial ischemia may not be detected on surface ECG. Therefore, it is important to review findings from the ECG in conjunction with biochemical markers of myocardial necrosis, such as troponin I or T levels, and other risk factors for CHD to determine the patient's risk for experiencing a new MI or having other complications.

TABLE 18-1 Presentation of Acute Coronary Syndromes

General
• The patient typically is in acute distress and may develop or present with cardiogenic shock.
Symptoms
• The classic symptom of ACS is midline anterior chest discomfort. Accompanying symptoms may include arm, back or jaw pain, nausea, vomiting, or shortness of breath.
• Patients less likely to present with classic symptoms include elderly patients, diabetic patients, and women.
Signs
• No signs are classic for ACS.
• However, patients with ACS may present with signs of acute heart failure, including jugular venous distension, rales, and S_3 sound on auscultation.
• Patients may present with arrhythmias and therefore may have tachycardia, bradycardia, or heart block.
Laboratory tests
• Troponin I or T and creatine kinase MB are measured.
• Blood chemistry tests are performed with particular attention to potassium and magnesium, which may affect heart rhythm, and glucose, which when elevated places the patient at higher risk for morbidity and mortality.
• Serum creatinine level is measured to identify patients who may need dosing adjustments for some pharmacotherapy and patients who are at high risk for morbidity and mortality.
• Baseline complete blood count and coagulation tests (activated partial thromboplastin time and international normalized ratio) should be obtained because most patients will receive antithrombotic therapy, which increases the risk for bleeding.
• Fasting lipid panel is obtained.
Other diagnostic tests
• The 12-lead electrocardiogram is the first step in management. Patients are risk stratified into two groups: ST-segment elevation ACS and suspected non–ST-segment elevation ACS.
• During hospitalization, measurement of left ventricular function, such as an echocardiogram, is performed to identify patients with low ejection fractions (<40%) who are at high risk for death following hospital discharge.
• Selected low-risk patients may undergo early stress testing.

ACS, acute coronary syndrome.

BIOCHEMICAL MARKERS

❹ Biochemical markers of myocardial cell death are important for confirming the diagnosis of MI. The ACC defines *evolving MI* as "typical rise and gradual fall (troponin) or more rapid rise and fall (CK MB) of biochemical markers of myocardial necrosis."[19] Troponin and CK MB levels rise in the blood following the onset of complete coronary artery occlusion subsequent to myocardial cell death. Their time course is depicted in Fig. 18–2. Typically, blood is obtained from the patient at least three times, once in the emergency department and twice more over the next 12 to 24 hours, in order to measure troponin and CK MB levels. A single measurement of a biochemical marker is not adequate to exclude a diagnosis of MI because up to 15% of values that initially were below the level of detection (a negative test) are above the level of detection (a positive test) in the subsequent hours. An MI is identified if at least one troponin value is greater than the MI decision limit (set by the hospital laboratory) or two CK MB results are greater than the MI decision limit (set by the hospital laboratory). These are termed *positive* biochemical markers for MI. Although troponins and CK MB appear in the blood within 6 hours of infarction, troponins stay elevated in the blood for up to 10 days, whereas CK MB returns to normal values within 48 hours. Therefore, if a patient is admitted with elevated troponin and CK MB concentrations and several days later experiences recurrent chest discomfort, the troponin will be less sensitive for detecting new myocardial damage because the level still is elevated from the earlier event. If early reinfarction is suspected, CK MB concentration determination is the preferred diagnostic test.[19] Biochemical markers, such as troponin measurements, that are below the detectable limit of hospital laboratories are termed *negative,* and the diagnosis of MI is excluded.

RISK STRATIFICATION

Patient signs and symptoms, medical history, ECG, and troponin or CK MB determinations are used to stratify patients as having low, medium, or high risk of death or MI or likelihood of not responding to pharmacotherapy and requiring urgent coronary angiography and PCI. Initial treatment according to risk stratification is depicted in Fig. 18–1. Patients with STE ACS are at the highest risk of death. Initial treatment of STE ACS should proceed without evaluation of troponin or CK MB levels because these patients have a greater than 97% chance of having an MI subsequently diagnosed with biochemical markers. The ACC/AHA defines a target time to initiate reperfu-

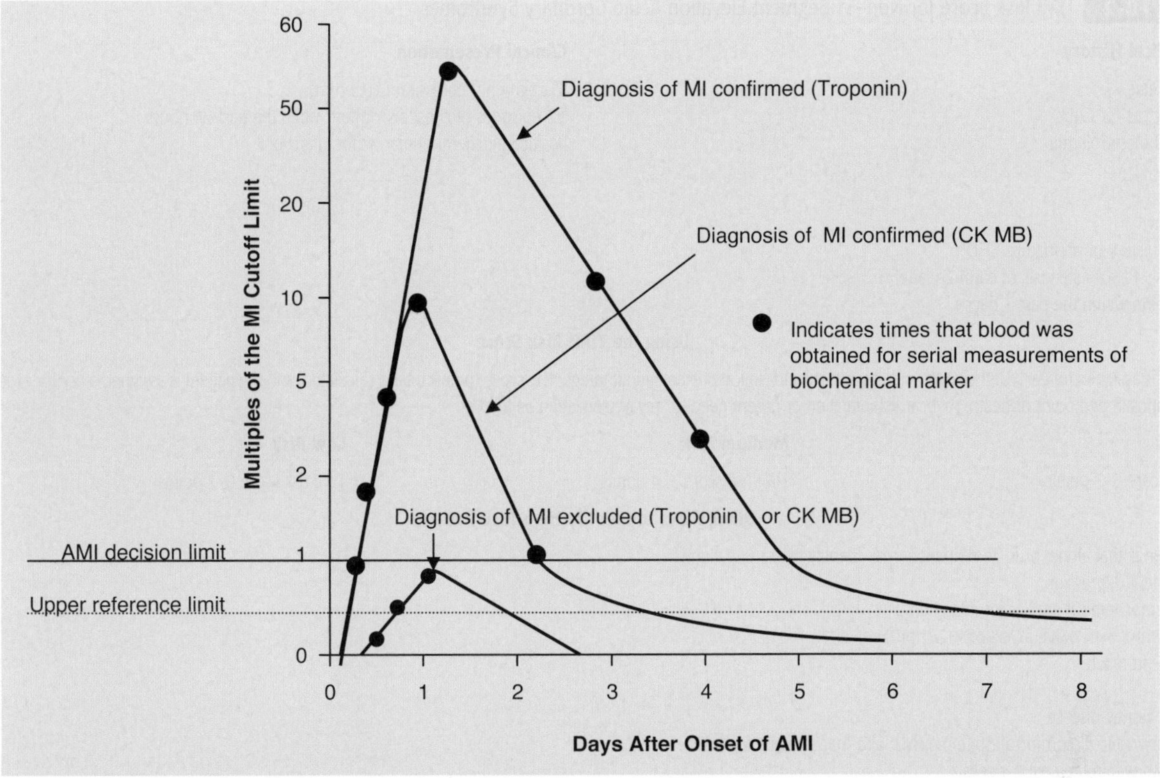

FIGURE 18-2. Biochemical markers in suspected acute coronary syndrome. (AMI, acute myocardial infarction; CK MB, creatine kinase myocardial band; MI, myocardial infarction.)

sion treatment for STEMI within 30 minutes of hospital presentation for fibrinolytics and within no more than 90 minutes from presentation for primary PCI.[3] The sooner the infarct-related coronary artery is opened in these patients, the lower is their mortality and the greater is the amount of preserved myocardium.[20,21] While all patients should be evaluated for reperfusion therapy, not all patients may be eligible. Indications and contraindications for fibrinolytic therapy as well as eligibility criteria for primary PCI are described in the treatment section of this chapter. In the United States in 2006, approximately 83% of *eligible* patients presenting to the hospital with STEMI underwent reperfusion therapy; 62% of the patients were treated with primary PCI, 17% fibrinolysis alone, 1% fibrinolysis followed by immediate PCI, and 2% immediate CABG surgery.[5] However, more than 40% of patients with STEMI present too late for reperfusion therapy (>12 hours since onset of symptoms).[22,23] In addition, fewer than 25% of hospitals in the United States are equipped to perform primary PCI,[24] and approximately 5% to 6% of patients present with at least one contraindication to fibrinolysis.[23,25] Unfortunately, 17% of patients *eligible* for reperfusion therapy consisting of either fibrinolysis or primary PCI do not receive it, suggesting a need for more thorough patient evaluation and treatment triage.[5]

If patients are not eligible for reperfusion therapy, additional pharmacotherapy for STE patients should be initiated in the emergency department, and patients should be transferred to the coronary intensive care unit.

Risk stratification of the patient with NSTE ACS is more complex because in-hospital outcomes for this group of patients vary, with reported rates of death of 0% to 12%, reinfarction 0% to 3%, and recurrent severe ischemia 5% to 20%.[26] Not all patients who present with suspected NSTE ACS have CAD. Some eventually are diagnosed with nonischemic chest discomfort. Additional information regarding risk stratification of NSTE ACS is presented in the General Approach to Treatment section.

Newer markers that identify patients at high risk of mortality or reinfarction that are under development but have not yet been incorporated into routine patient care include C-reactive protein,[27] a maker of vascular inflammation; elevated serum creatinine or reduced creatinine clearance,[28] and brain (B-type) natriuretic peptide (BNP),[29] which is released predominately from ventricular myocytes in response to cell stretch as the infarct remodels. Dialysis patients have a 1-year mortality rate of greater than 40% following a first MI.[28]

TREATMENT

Acute Coronary Syndromes

■ DESIRED OUTCOMES

The short-term goals of treatment for the ACS patient are as follows:

1. Early restoration of blood flow to the infarct-related artery to prevent infarct expansion (in the case of MI) or prevent complete occlusion and MI (in unstable angina)
2. Prevention of death and other complications
3. Prevention of coronary artery reocclusion
4. Relief of ischemic chest discomfort
5. Maintenance of normoglycemia

■ GENERAL APPROACH TO TREATMENT

Selecting evidence-based therapies described in the ACC/AHA guidelines for patients without contraindications results in lower mortality.[30,31] General treatment measures for all STE ACSs and high- and intermediate-risk NSTE ACS patients include admission to hospital, oxygen administration (if oxygen saturation is low, i.e., <90%), continuous multilead ST-segment monitoring for arrhythmias and ischemia, glycemic control, frequent measurement of vital signs, bedrest for 12 hours in hemodynamically stable patients, avoidance of Valsalva maneuver (prescribe stool softeners routinely), and pain relief.

TABLE 18-2 TIMI Risk Score for Non–ST-Segment Elevation Acute Coronary Syndromes

Past Medical History	Clinical Presentation
Age ≥65 years	ST-segment depression (≥0.5 mm)
≥3 Risk factors for CAD	≥2 episodes of chest discomfort within the past 24 hours
Hypercholesterolemia	Positive biochemical marker for infarction[a]
HTN	
TM	
Smoking	
Family history of premature CHD[b]	
Known CAD (≥50% stenosis of coronary artery)	
Use of aspirin within the past 7 days	

Using the TIMI Risk Score

One point is assigned for each of the seven medical history and clinical presentation findings. The score (point) total is calculated, and the patient is assigned a risk for experiencing the composite end point of death, myocardial infarction or urgent need for revascularization as follows:

High Risk	Medium Risk	Low Risk
TIMI risk score 5–7 points	TIMI risk score 3–4 points	TIMI risk score 0–2 points

Other Ways to Identify High-Risk Patients

Other findings that alone, or in combination, may identify high-risk patients:

- ST-segment depression
- Positive biochemical marker for infarction
- Deep symmetric T-wave inversions (≥2 mm)
- Acute heart failure
- DM
- Chronic kidney disease
- Refractory chest discomfort despite maximal pharmacotherapy for ACS
- Recent MI within the past 2 weeks

ACS, acute coronary syndromes; CAD, coronary artery disease; CHD, coronary heart disease; DM, diabetes mellitus; HTN, hypertension; MI, myocardial infarction; TIMI, Thrombolysis in Myocardial Infarction

[a]A positive biochemical marker for infarction is a value of troponin I, troponin T, or creatinine kinase MB greater than the MI detection limit.

[b]As defined in Chapter 23.

From Anderson et al.[2] *and Eagle et al.*[31]

Because risk varies and resources are limited, triage and treatment of patients according to their risk category are important. Initial approaches to treatment of STE and NSTE ACS patients are outlined in Fig. 18–1.[2,3,10] Patients with STE ACS are at high risk of death, and efforts to reestablish coronary perfusion should be initiated immediately. Reperfusion therapy should be considered immediately and adjunctive pharmacotherapy initiated.[3]

Features identifying low-, moderate-, and high-risk NSTE ACS patients are listed in Table 18–2.[2,30] Patients at low risk for death, MI, or the need for urgent coronary artery revascularization typically are evaluated in the emergency department, where serial biochemical marker tests are obtained. If these test results are negative, the patient may be admitted to a general medical floor with ECG telemetry monitoring for ischemic changes and arrhythmias, undergo a noninvasive stress test, or be discharged from the emergency department. Moderate- and high-risk patients are admitted to a coronary intensive care unit, an intensive care step-down unit, or a general medical floor in the hospital depending on the patient's symptoms and perceived level of risk. High-risk patients should undergo early coronary angiography (within 24–48 hours) and revascularization (with PCI or CABG) if a significant coronary artery stenosis is found[2] (see Fig. 18–1 and Table 18–2). Moderate-risk patients with positive biochemical markers for infarction typically also undergo angiography and revascularization during hospital admission. Moderate-risk patients with negative biochemical markers for infarction also may undergo angiography and revascularization or first undergo a noninvasive stress test; only selected patients with a positive stress test proceed to angiography. Following risk stratification, pharmacotherapy for NSTE ACS is initiated.

■ NONPHARMACOLOGIC THERAPY

Primary PCI for STE ACS

❺ Either fibrinolysis or immediate primary PCI is the treatment of choice for reestablishing coronary artery blood flow in patients with STE ACS when the patient presents within 3 hours of symptom onset and both options are available at the institution. For primary PCI, the patient is taken from the emergency department to the cardiac catheterization laboratory and undergoes coronary angiography with either balloon angioplasty or placement of a bare-metal or drug-eluting intracoronary stent. Additional details regarding angioplasty and intracoronary stenting are provided in Chapter 17. Results from a meta-analysis of trials comparing fibrinolysis with primary PCI indicate a lower mortality rate with primary PCI.[20] One reason for the superiority of primary PCI compared with fibrinolysis is that more than 90% of occluded infarct-related coronary arteries are opened with primary PCI compared with less than 60% of coronary arteries with currently available fibrinolytics.[3,32] In addition, the intracranial hemorrhage (ICH) and major bleeding risks from primary PCI are lower than following fibrinolysis. An invasive strategy of primary PCI is generally preferred for patients presenting to institutions where skilled interventional cardiologists and a catheterization laboratory are immediately available, patients with cardiogenic shock, patients with contraindications to fibrinolytics, and patients presenting with symptom onset greater than 3 hours.[3] A quality performance measure in the care of patients with STEMI is the time from hospital presentation to the time that the occluded artery is opened with PCI. This "door-to-primary PCI time" should be 90 minutes or less (Table 18–3).[3,10,33] In 2006, the median time to primary PCI in the United States was 86 minutes, and only 55% of patients met the performance measure target of 90 minutes or less, suggesting that slightly less than half of the primary PCIs occur more than 90 minutes after hospital presentation.[5] Unfortunately, most hospitals do not have interventional cardiology services capable of performing primary PCI 24 hours per day.

PCI during hospitalization for STEMI also may be appropriate for other patients following STEMI, such as those in whom fibrinolysis is not successful (termed *rescue* PCI), those presenting later in cardiogenic shock, patients with life-threatening ventricular arrhythmias, and those with persistent rest ischemia or signs of ischemia on stress

TABLE 18-3 2006 American College of Cardiology/American Heart Association ST-Segment Elevation and Non–ST-Segment Elevation Myocardial Infarction Performance Measures

Performance Measure	Description
1. Aspirin upon arrival	STEMI and NSTE MI patients without aspirin contraindications who received aspirin within 24 hours before or after hospital arrival
2. Aspirin prescribed at hospital discharge	STEMI and NSTE MI patients without aspirin contraindications who are prescribed aspirin at hospital discharge
3. β-Blocker upon hospital arrival	β-Blocker STEMI and NSTE MI patients without β-blocker contraindications who received a β-blocker within 24 hours after hospital arrival
4. β-Blocker prescribed at hospital discharge	STEMI and NSTE MI patients without β-blocker contraindications who are prescribed a β-blocker at hospital discharge
5. LDL cholesterol assessment	STEMI and NSTE MI patients with documentation of LDL cholesterol level in the hospital record or documentation that LDL cholesterol testing was done during the hospital stay or is planned for after hospital discharge
6. Lipid-lowering therapy at hospital discharge	STEMI and NSTE MI patients with elevated LDL cholesterol (≥100 mg/dL or narrative equivalent[a]) who are prescribed lipid-lowering medicine at hospital discharge
7. ACE inhibitor or ARB for LVSD at discharge	STEMI and NSTE MI patients with LVSD and without ACE inhibitor and ARB contraindications who are prescribed an ACE inhibitor or ARB at hospital discharge
8. Time to fibrinolytic therapy	Median time from arrival to administration of fibrinolytic therapy in patients with STE or LBBB on the ECG performed closest to hospital arrival time
	STEMI or LBBB patients receiving fibrinolytic therapy during the hospital stay and having a time from hospital arrival to fibrinolysis of 30 minutes or less
9. Time to PCI	Median time from arrival to PCI in patients with STE or LBBB on the ECG performed closest to hospital arrival time
	STEMI or LBBB patients receiving PCI during the hospital stay with a time from hospital arrival to PCI of 90 minutes or less
10. Reperfusion therapy	STEMI patients with STE on the ECG performed closest to the arrival who receive fibrinolytic therapy or primary PCI
11. Adult smoking cessation advice counseling	STEMI and NSTE MI patients with a history of smoking cigarettes who are given smoking cessation advice or counseling during hospital stay

[a]Mention in the patient's medical record of elevated LDL cholesterol if not measured.

ACE, angiotensin-converting enzyme; ARB, angiotensin receptor blocker; ECG, electrocardiogram; LDL, low-density lipoprotein; LBBB, left bundle-branch block; LVSD, left ventricular systolic dysfunction; cholesterol; MI, myocardial infarction; NSTE, non–ST-segment elevation; PCI, percutaneous coronary intervention; STE, ST-segment elevation.

Reproduced with permission ACC/AHA Clinical Performance Measures for Adults with ST-Elevation and Non-ST-Elevation Myocardial Infarction. ©2006, American Heart Association, Inc.

testing following MI.[3,32] A randomized study established that rescue PCI was superior to repeated fibrinolytic administration or conservative management and resulted in fewer cardiac and cerebrovascular events.[34] The strategy of routine angiography and revascularization performed in all STE patients later during hospitalization was controversial for almost more than a decade, but data from the Occluded Artery Trial (OAT)[35] demonstrated that routine angiography followed by PCI in stable patients 3 to 28 days post-MI, without recurrent unprovoked ischemia or ischemia induced by stress testing, was not beneficial in reducing mortality or heart failure and may increase the risk of recurrent MI.[35] Therefore, routine *late* restoration of antegrade coronary artery blood flow should not be performed.

PCI in NSTE ACS

❻ The most recent NSTE ACS ACC/AHA clinical practice guidelines recommend early coronary angiography with either PCI or CABG revascularization as an early treatment for high-risk NSTE ACS patients, and that such an approach be considered in patients at moderate risk.[2,32] Several clinical trials support an "early invasive strategy" with PCI or CABG versus a "medical stabilization management strategy" whereby coronary angiography with revascularization is reserved for patients with symptoms refractory to pharmacotherapy and patients with signs of ischemia on stress testing. An early invasive approach results in fewer MIs, hospital readmissions for recurrent ACS, and less need for additional revascularization procedures over the next year following hospitalization.[36] In addition, an early invasive strategy is less costly than the conservative medical stabilization approach.[37]

Additional Testing and Risk Stratification

At some point during hospitalization but prior to discharge, patients with MI should undergo evaluation of LV function for the purpose of risk stratification.[2,3,33] The most common form of LV function measurement is echocardiography to calculate the patient's left ventricular ejection fraction (LVEF). LV function is the single best predictor of mortality following MI. Patients with LVEF less than 40% are at highest risk of death. Patients with ventricular fibrillation or sustained ventricular tachycardia more than 2 days following MI and those with LVEF <30% measured at least 1 month following STEMI and 3 months after coronary artery revascularization with either PCI or CABG benefit from placement of an implantable cardioverter-defibrillator (ICD).[3] The Multicenter Automatic Defibrillator Implantation Trial II (MADIT II) demonstrated a 29% reduction in mortality in patients with a history of MI, low LVEF, and no history of symptomatic ventricular arrhythmias who underwent prophylactic placement of an ICD.[38] Additional discussion of the role of ICDs in the management of high-risk patients and those with ventricular arrhythmias can be found in Chapter 19.

Predischarge stress testing (see Fig. 18–1) may be indicated for moderate- or low-risk patients in order to determine which patients would benefit from coronary angiography to establish the diagnosis of CAD and for patients following MI to predict intermediate- and long-term risk of recurrent MI and death.[39] In most cases, patients with a positive stress test indicating coronary ischemia then undergo coronary angiography and subsequent revascularization of significantly occluded coronary arteries. Exercise stress testing, most often with the addition of a radionuclide imaging agent, is preferred over nonpharmacologic stress testing because it evaluates the workload achieved with exercise as well as the occurrence of ischemia. If a patient has a negative exercise stress test for ischemia, the patient is at low risk for subsequent CHD events. Therefore, exercise stress testing has high negative predictive value. Additional discussion of the types of stress testing can be found in Chapter 13.

For patients admitted to the hospital for ACS, a fasting lipid panel should be drawn within the first 24 hours of hospitalization because, after that period, values for cholesterol, an acute-phase reactant, may be falsely low.[33] Initiation of pharmacotherapy with a statin is common for all ACS patients.

■ EARLY PHARMACOTHERAPY FOR STE ACS

Pharmacotherapy for early treatment of STE ACS is outlined in Fig. 18–3.[2,3,10,40] ❼ According to the ACC/AHA STE ACS practice guidelines, early pharmacotherapy of STE ACS should include intranasal oxygen (if oxygen saturation is <90%), sublingual (SL) nitroglycerin

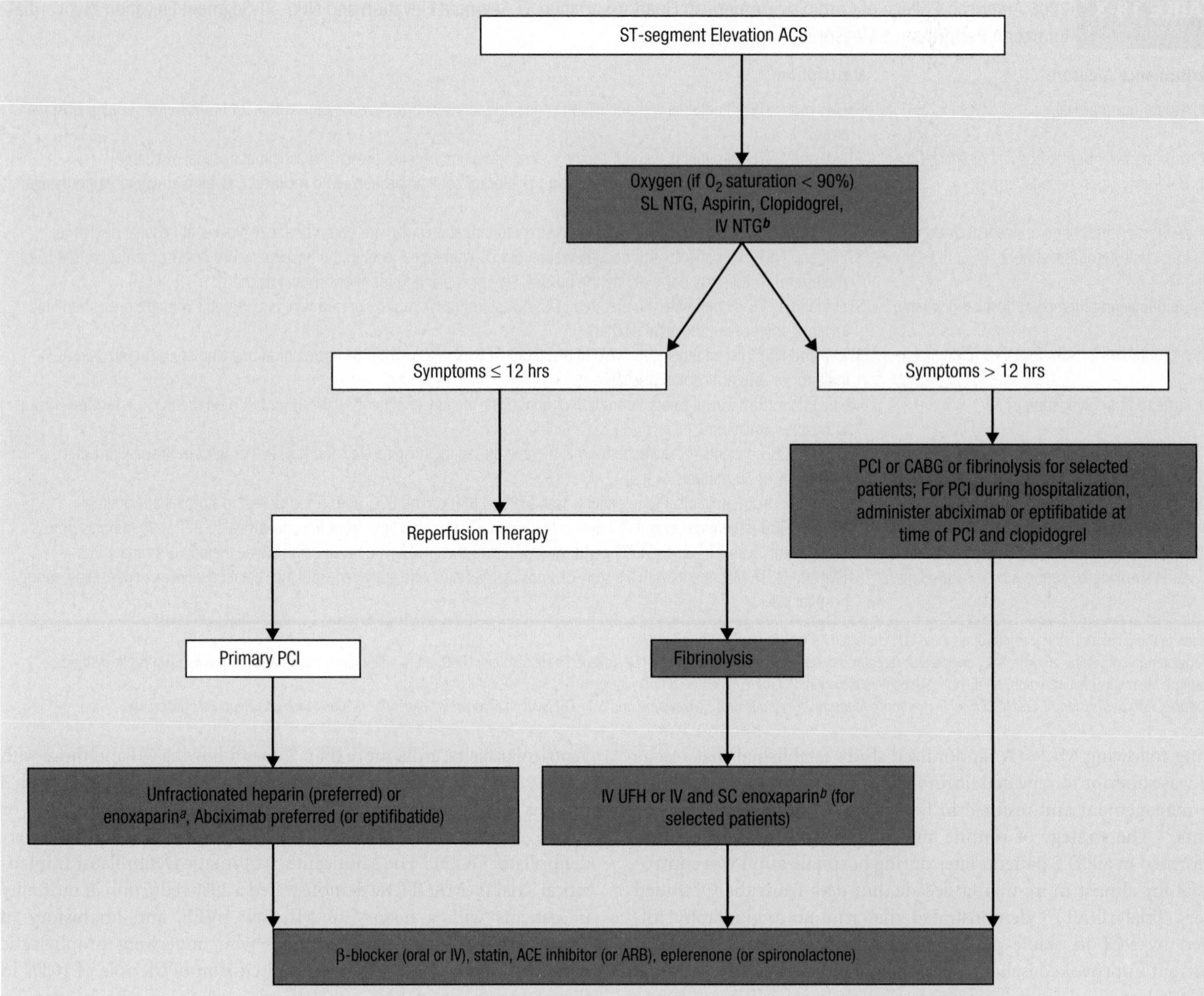

FIGURE 18-3. Initial pharmacotherapy for ST-segment elevation acute coronary syndromes. (ACE, angiotensin-converting enzyme; ACS, acute coronary syndrome; ARB, angiotensin receptor blocker; CABG, coronary artery bypass graft surgery; IV, intravenous; NTG, nitroglycerin; PCI, percutaneous coronary intervention; SC, subcutaneous; SL, sublingual; UFH, unfractionated heparin.) [a]Although recommended by the 2004 American College of Cardiology and American Heart Association practice guidelines, no dose recommendation is given. [b]See Table 18–4 for dosing and specific types of patients who should not receive enoxaparin or IV NTG.) *(Reprinted with permission from the American College of Clinical Pharmacy. Spinler SA. Acute coronary syndromes. In: Dunsworth TS, Richardson MM, Cheng JWM, et al., eds. Pharmacotherapy Self-Assessment Program, 6th ed. Cardiology II module. Kansas City: American College of Clinical Pharmacy, 2007:69–70.)*

(NTG), aspirin, a β-blocker, unfractionated heparin (UFH) or enoxaparin, and fibrinolysis in eligible candidates. Morphine is administered to patients with refractory angina as an analgesic and a venodilator that lowers preload. These agents should be administered early, while the patient is still in the emergency department. An ACE inhibitor should be started within 24 hours of presentation, particularly in patients with LVEF ≤40%, signs of heart failure, or an anterior wall MI, in the absence of contraindications. Intravenous (IV) NTG and β-blockers should be administered to selected patients without contraindications as described in Table 18–4. Dosing and contraindications for SL and IV NTG, aspirin, β-blockers, UFH, enoxaparin, ACE inhibitors, and fibrinolytics are listed in Table 18–4.[2,3,10,32,40]

Fibrinolytic Therapy

Administration of a fibrinolytic agent is indicated in patients with STE ACS who present to the hospital within 12 hours of onset of chest discomfort and have at least 1 mm of STE in two or more contiguous ECG leads or a new left bundle-branch block.[3] Fibrinolytic therapy also should be considered in patients presenting within 12–24 hours of onset of chest discomfort and have persistent symptoms of ischemia and at least 1 mm of STE in two or more contiguous leads. The mortality benefit of fibrinolysis is highest with early administration and diminishes after 12 hours. Fibrinolytic therapy is preferred over primary PCI in patients who present within 3 hours of symptom onset if primary PCI will be delayed, because a delay in access to a cardiac catheterization laboratory or a delay in obtaining patient vascular access would result in a "door-to-primary PCI" delay greater than 90 minutes.[3] Other indications and contraindications for fibrinolysis are listed in Table 18–5.[3] It is not necessary to obtain the results of biochemical markers before initiating fibrinolytic therapy. Because administration of fibrinolytics results in clot lysis, patients at high risk for major bleeding, including those with ICH, have either relative or absolute contraindications. Patients presenting with an absolute contraindication likely will not receive fibrinolytic therapy, and primary PCI is preferred. Patients with a relative contraindication can receive fibrinolytic therapy if the perceived risk of death from the MI is higher than the risk of major hemorrhage. For every 1,000 patients with anterior wall MI, treatment with fibrinolysis saves 37 lives compared with placebo. For patients with inferior wall MI, who

TABLE 18-4 Evidence-Based Pharmacotherapy for ST-Segment Elevation and Non–ST-Segment Elevation Acute Coronary Syndrome

Drug	Clinical Condition and ACC/AHA Guideline Recommendation[a]	Contraindications[b]	Dose and Duration of Therapy
Aspirin	STEMI, class I recommendation for all patients NSTE ACS, class I recommendation for all patients	Hypersensitivity Active bleeding Severe bleeding risk	162–325 mg orally once on hospital day 1 75–162 mg once daily orally starting hospital day 2 and continued indefinitely in patients not receiving an intracoronary stent 162–325 mg once daily orally for a minimum of 30 days in patients undergoing PCI receiving a bare metal stent, 3 months with a sirolimus-eluting stent and 6 months with a paclitaxel-eluting stent, followed by 75–162 mg once daily orally thereafter Continue indefinitely
Clopidogrel	STEMI, class I recommendation in patients allergic to aspirin NSTE ACS, class I recommendation for all hospitalized patients in whom a noninterventional approach is planned In PCI in STE and NSTE ACS, class I recommendations In STEMI with fibrinolytics, large randomized trial data published after 2004 guidelines	Hypersensitivity Active bleeding Severe bleeding risk	300 mg (class I recommendation) to 600 mg (class IIa recommendation in NSTE ACS) loading dose on hospital day 1 followed by a maintenance dose of 75 mg po once daily starting on hospital day 2; consider omitting the loading dose in patients >75 years old when given with fibrinolytics Administer indefinitely in patients with aspirin allergy (class I recommendation) Administer at least 9 months in patients with NSTE ACS who are managed medically (class I recommendation). For post-PCI stented patients, administer at least 12 months (AHA Science Advisory)
Unfractionated heparin (UFH)	STEMI, class I recommendation in patients undergoing PCI, and for patients treated with alteplase, reteplase, or tenecteplase, class IIa recommendation for patients not treated with fibrinolytic therapy NSTE ACS, class I recommendation in combination with aspirin PCI, class I recommendation (NSTE ACS and STEMI)	Active bleeding History of heparin-induced thrombocytopenia Severe bleeding risk Recent stroke	For STEMI, administer 60 units/kg IV bolus (maximum 4000 units) followed by a constant IV infusion at 12 units/kg/h (maximum 1000 units/h) For NSTE ACS, administer 60–70 units/kg IV bolus (maximum 5000 units) followed by a constant IV infusion at 12–15 units/kg/h (maximum 1000 units/h) Titrated to maintain an aPTT of 1.5–2.5 times control for NSTE ACS and 50–70 seconds for STEMI First aPTT should be measured at 4–6 hours for NSTE ACS and STE ACS in patients not treated with fibrinolytics First aPTT should be measured at 3 hours in patients with STE ACS who are treated with fibrinolytics Continue for at least 48 hours or until the end of PCI
Low-molecular weight heparin	STEMI class IIb recommendation (and a large randomized trial) for patients treated with fibrinolytics and class IIa for patients not undergoing reperfusion therapy NSTE ACS, class I recommendation For PCI, class IIa recommendation as an alternative to UFH in patients with NSTE ACS For primary PCI in STEMI, class IIb recommendation as an alternative to UFH	Active bleeding History of heparin-induced thrombocytopenia Severe bleeding risk Recent stroke Avoid enoxaparin if CrCl <15 mL/min Avoid dalteparin if CrCl <30 mL/min Avoid if CABG surgery	Enoxaparin 1 mg/kg SC every 12 hours for patients with NSTE ACS (CrCl ≥30 mL/min) Enoxaparin 1 mg/kg SC every 24 hours (CrCl 15–29 mL/min) for NSTE ACS or STEMI Dalteparin 120 IU/kg SC every 12 hours for patients with NSTE ACS (maximum single dose) For patients undergoing PCI following initiation of SC enoxaparin for NSTE ACS, a supplemental 0.3 mg/kg IV dose of enoxaparin should be administered at the time of PCI if the last dose of SC enoxaparin was given 8–12 hours prior to PCI For patients with STEMI receiving fibrinolytics: Age <75 years: administer enoxaparin 30-mg IV bolus followed immediately by 1 mg/kg SC every 12 hours (first two doses administer maximum of 100 mg for patients for weighing >100 kg) For patients ≥75 yrs old with STEMI: administer enoxaparin 0.75 mg/kg SC every 12 hours (first two doses administer maximum of 75 mg for patients weighing >75 kg) Continue throughout hospitalization or up to 8 days for STEMI Continue for hospital stay or until the end of PCI for NSTE ACS
Bivalirudin	NSTE ACS class I recommendation for early invasive strategy	Active bleeding Severe bleeding risk	For NSTE ACS, administer 0.1 mg/kg IV bolus followed by 0.25 mg/kg/h infusion For PCI, administer a second bolus of 0.5 mg/kg IV and increase infusion rate to 1.75 mg/kg/h Discontinue at end of PCI or continue for up to 4 hours
Fondaparinux	NSTE ACS, class I recommendation Dosing information based on dose administered in OASIS-5 and OASIS-6 trials	Active bleeding Severe bleeding risk SCr ≥3.0 mg/dL	For STEMI, 2.5-mg IV bolus followed by 2.5 mg SC once daily starting on hospital day 2 For NSTE ACS, 2.5 mg SC once daily For PCI, administer UFH 50–60 units/kg UFH (strategy not rigorously tested in clinical trials) Continue until hospital discharge

(continued)

TABLE 18-4 Evidence-Based Pharmacotherapy for ST-Segment Elevation and Non–ST-Segment Elevation Acute Coronary Syndrome (continued)

Drug	Clinical Condition and ACC/AHA Guideline Recommendation[a]	Contraindications[b]	Dose and Duration of Therapy
Fibrinolytic therapy	STEMI, class I recommendation for patients presenting within 12 hours after onset of symptoms, class IIa in patients presenting between 12 and 24 hours after the onset of symptoms with continuing signs of ischemia NSTE ACS, class III recommendation	Any prior intracranial hemorrhage Known structural cerebrovascular lesions such as arteriovenous malformation Known intracranial malignant neoplasm Ischemic stroke within 3 months Active bleeding (excluding menses) Significant closed head or facial trauma within 3 months	Streptokinase: 1.5 million units IV over 60 minutes Alteplase: 15-mg IV bolus followed by 0.75 mg/kg IV over 30 minutes (maximum 50 mg) followed by 0.5 mg/kg (maximum 35 mg) over 60 minutes (maximum dose 100 mg) Reteplase: 10 units IV × 2, 30 minutes apart Tenecteplase: <60 kg = 30-mg IV bolus 60–69.9 kg = 35-mg IV bolus 70–79.9 kg = 40-mg IV bolus
Glycoprotein IIb/IIIa receptor blockers	NSTE ACS, class IIa recommendation for either tirofiban or eptifibatide for patients with continuing ischemia, elevated troponin, or other high-risk features, class I recommendation for patients undergoing PCI, class IIb recommendation for patients without high-risk features who are not undergoing PCI STEMI, class IIa for abciximab for primary PCI and class IIb for either tirofiban or eptifibatide for primary PCI	Active bleeding Thrombocytopenia Prior stroke	**Drug** / **Dose for PCI** / **Dose for NSTE ACS with/without PCI** / **Dose adjustment for renal insufficiency** Abciximab / 0.25 mg/kg IV bolus followed by 0.125 mcg/kg/min (maximum 10 mcg/min) for 12 hours / Not recommended / None Eptifibatide / 180 mcg/kg IV bolus × 2, 10 minutes apart with an infusion of 2 mcg/kg/min for 18–24 hours / 180 mcg/kg IV bolus followed by an infusion of 2 mcg/kg/min for 18–24 hours / Reduce maintenance infusion to 1 mcg/kg/min for patients with CrCl <50 mL/min; not studied in patients with serum creatinine >4.0 mg/dL; patients weighing ≥121 kg should receive a maximum infusion rate of 22.6 mg per bolus and a maximum infusion rate of 15 mg/h Tirofiban / Not FDA approved / 0.4 mg/kg IV bolus administered over 30 minutes followed by an infusion of 0.1 mcg/kg/min for 18–24 hours / Reduce maintenance infusion to 0.05 mcg/kg/min for patients with CrCl <30 mL/min
Nitroglycerin	STEMI and NSTE ACS, class I indication in patients with persistent ischemia, symptoms of acute heart failure, or signs of hypertension	SBP <90 mm Hg HR <50 beats/min Right ventricular infarction Sildenafil or vardenafil within 24 hours or tadalafil within 48 hours	0.4 mg SL, repeated every 5 minutes × 3 doses 5–10 mcg/min IV infusion titrated up to 200 mcg/min until relief of symptoms or limiting side-effects (headache) with a SBP <90 mm Hg or >30% below starting mean arterial pressure levels if significant hypertension is present) Topical patches or oral nitrates and acceptable alternatives for patients without ongoing or refractory symptoms Discontinue if SBP drops >30 mm Hg below baseline SBP Continue IV infusion for 24–48 hours
β-Blockers[c]	STEMI and NSTE ACS, oral β-blockers, class I recommendation in all patients without contraindications, class IIa recommendation for IV β-blockers for patients with hypertension	PR ECG segment >0.24 second 2nd-degree or 3rd-degree atrioventricular heart block HR <60 beats per min	Target resting HR of 50–60 beats/min Metoprolol 5 mg slow IV push (over 1–2 minutes), repeated every 5 minutes for a total of 15 mg followed in 15–30 minutes by 25–50 mg by mouth every 6 hours; if a very conservative regimen is desired, initial doses can be reduced to 1–2 mg Propranolol 0.5–1 mg IV dose followed in 1–2 hours by 40–80 mg by mouth every 6–8 hours

(continued)

TABLE 18-4 Evidence-Based Pharmacotherapy for ST-Segment Elevation and Non–ST-Segment Elevation Acute Coronary Syndrome (continued)

Drug	Clinical Condition and ACC/AHA Guideline Recommendation[a]	Contraindications[b]	Dose and Duration of Therapy
		SBP <90 mm Hg Shock Signs and symptoms of heart failure Severe reactive airway disease	Atenolol 5-mg IV dose followed in 5 minutes by a second 5-mg IV dose for a total of 10 mg followed in 1–2 hours by 50–100 mg by mouth once daily Initial IV therapy can be omitted and initial doses of oral therapy started Continue oral β-blocker indefinitely
Calcium channel blockers	STEMI, class IIa recommendation and NSTE ACS, class I recommendation for patients with ongoing ischemia who are already taking adequate doses of nitrates and β-blockers For STEMI (diltiazem, verapamil, or amlodipine) For NSTE ACS, class I recommendation for diltiazem or verapamil for continuing ischemia in patients with a contraindication to a β-blocker; class IIa recommendation for patients with continuing ischemia who do not have a contraindication to a β-blocker; class IIb recommendation instead of a β-blocker	Pulmonary edema Evidence of left ventricular dysfunction SBP <100 mm Hg PR ECG segment >0.24 second for verapamil and diltiazem 2nd- or 3rd-degree atrioventricular heart block for verapamil or diltiazem HR <60 beats/min for diltiazem or verapamil	Diltiazem 120–360 mg sustained release orally once daily Verapamil 180–480 mg sustained release orally once daily Nifedipine 30–90 mg sustained release orally once daily Amlodipine 5–10 mg orally once daily Continue indefinitely if contraindication to oral β-blocker persists
ACE inhibitors	STEMI and NSTE ACS, class I recommendation within the first 24 hours after hospital presentation for patients with clinical signs of heart failure or left ventricular EF <40% in the absence of contraindications class IIa recommendation for all other patients in the absence of contraindications STEMI and NSTE MI, class I recommendation for late hospital care and post-discharge care for patients with left ventricular EF <40%, diabetes mellitus, or chronic kidney disease Indicated indefinitely for all patients with EF <40%, class I recommendation	SBP <100 mm Hg History of intolerance to an ACE inhibitor Bilateral renal artery stenosis Serum potassium >5.5 mEq/L Acute renal failure Pregnancy	**Drug** / **Initial Dose** / **Target Dose** Captopril / 6.25–12.5 mg / 50 mg twice daily orally to 50 mg three times daily Enalapril / 2.5–5.0 mg / 10 mg twice daily orally Lisinopril / 2.5–5.0 mg / 10–20 mg once daily orally Ramipril / 1.25–2.5 mg / 5 mg twice daily or 10 mg once daily orally Trandolapril / 1.0 / 4 mg once daily orally Continue indefinitely
Angiotensin receptor blockers	STEMI and NSTE ACS, class I recommendation in patients with an indication for an ACE inhibitor and a history of ACE inhibitor intolerance <40% STEMI and NSTE MI, class I recommendation for late hospital care and post-discharge care for patients with a history of ACE inhibitor intolerance STEMI and NSTE MI, class IIa recommendation as an alternative to an ACE inhibitor in patients presenting with signs of heart failure or left ventricular EF <40% STEMI and NSTE MI, class IIb recommendation added to an ACE inhibitor for long-term management of symptomatic heart failure in patients with left ventricular ejection fraction <40%	SBP <100 mm Hg Bilateral renal artery stenosis Serum potassium >5.5 mg/dL Acute renal failure Pregnancy	**Drug** / **Initial Dose** / **Target Dose** Candesartan / 4–8 mg / 32 mg once daily orally Valsartan / 40 mg / 160 mg twice daily orally Continue indefinitely
Aldosterone antagonists	STEMI and NSTE MI, class I recommendation for patients with EF ≤40% and either diabetes mellitus or heart failure symptoms who are already receiving an ACE inhibitor	Hypotension Hyperkalemia, serum potassium >5.0 mEq/L SCr >2.5 mg/dL	**Drug** / **Initial Dose** / **Maximum Dose** Eplerenone / 25 mg / 50 mg once daily orally Spironolactone / 12.5 mg / 25–50 mg once daily orally Continue indefinitely

(continued)

TABLE 18-4 Evidence-Based Pharmacotherapy for ST-segment Elevation and Non–ST-segment Elevation Acute Coronary Syndrome (continued)

Drug	Clinical Condition and ACC/AHA Guideline Recommendation[a]	Contraindications[b]	Dose and Duration of Therapy
Morphine sulfate	STE and NSTE ACS, class IIa recommendation for patients whose symptoms are not relieved after three serial SL nitroglycerin tablets or whose symptoms recur with adequate antiischemic therapy	Hypotension Respiratory depression Confusion Obtundation	2–5 mg IV bolus dose Can be repeated every 5–30 minutes as needed to relieve symptoms and maintain patient comfort

[a]Class I recommendations are conditions for which there is evidence and/or general agreement that a given procedure or treatment is useful and effective. Class II recommendations are those conditions for which there is conflicting evidence and/or divergence of opinion about the usefulness/efficacy of a procedure or treatment. For Class IIa recommendations, the weight of the evidence/opinion is in favor of usefulness/efficacy. Class IIb recommendations are those for which usefulness/efficacy is less well established by evidence/opinion. Class III recommendations are those for which the procedure or treatment is not useful and may be harmful.
[b]Allergy or prior intolerance contraindication for all categories of drugs listed.
[c]Choice of specific agent is not as important as ensuring that appropriate candidates receive this therapy. If there are concerns about patient intolerance due to existing pulmonary disease, especially asthma, selection should favor a short-acting agent, such as propranolol or metoprolol or the ultrashort-acting agent esmolol. Mild wheezing or a history of chronic obstructive pulmonary disease should prompt a trial of a short-acting agent at a reduced dose (e.g., 2.5-mg IV metoprolol, 12.5-mg oral metoprolol, or 25 mcg/kg/min esmolol as initial doses) rather than complete avoidance of β-blocker therapy.
ACC, American College of Cardiology; ACE, angiotensin-converting enzyme; AHA, American Heart Association; ACS, acute coronary syndrome; ACUITY, Acute Catheterization and Urgent Intervention Triage Strategy; CABGF, coronary artery bypass graft; CrCl, creatinine clearance; ECG, electrocardiogram; EF, ejection fraction; HR, heart rate; IV, intravenous; MI, myocardial infarction; NSTE, non–ST-segment elevation; OASIS, Organization to Assess Strategies in Acute Ischemic Syndromes; PCI, percutaneous coronary intervention; SBP, systolic blood pressure; SC, subcutaneous; SCr, serum creatinine; SL, sublingual; STE, ST-segment elevation.
Data from references 2, 3, 10, 32, 55, and 108.

generally have smaller MIs and are at lower risk of death, treatment with fibrinolysis saves eight lives per 1,000 patients treated.[20]

Fibrinolytic therapy is controversial in patients older than 75 years. More than 60% of all MI deaths occur in this group. Benefit in terms of absolute mortality reduction compared with placebo varies from approximately 1% to 9%, with some observational studies suggesting higher mortality in the very elderly treated with fibrinolysis compared with no fibrinolysis. Stroke rates also grow in number with increasing patient age. The ICH rate is approximately 1% in younger patients versus 2% to 3% in older patients. There is no excess risk of stroke in patients younger than 55 years, whereas patients older than 75 years experience more than eight strokes per 1,000 patients treated.[20] However, the ACC/AHA practice guidelines recommend use of fibrinolytics in this age group, provided the patient has no contraindications.[3] A 1% absolute mortality benefit is believed to be clinically significant, and the benefit in terms of lives saved per 1,000 patients treated has been reported to range from 10 to 80 in patients older than 75 years.[20] An AHA Scientific Statement concluded that a mortality benefit with fibrinolysis compared with no reperfusion was demonstrated in patients up to age 85 years and includes deaths related to ICH, stroke, and shock, which all are higher in the elderly compared to younger patients.[41] Careful attention to correct dosing of UFH and enoxaparin can reduce ICH and bleeding rates.[41] Because older patients may have cognitive impairment, careful history taking and assessment weighing the bleeding risk versus the benefit must be performed prior to administration of fibrinolysis.

The comparative pharmacology of commonly prescribed fibrinolytics is given in Table 18–6.[42] According to the ACC/AHA STE ACS practice guidelines, a more fibrin-specific agent, such as alteplase, reteplase, or tenecteplase, is preferred over a non–fibrin-specific agent, such as streptokinase.[3] Early administration of more fibrin-specific fibrinolytics opens a greater percentage of infarct arteries. Because an early open artery results in smaller infarcts, administration of fibrin-specific agents should result in lower mortality. This concept has been termed the *open-artery hypothesis.* In a large clinical trial, administration of alteplase reduced mortality by 1% (absolute reduction) and costs about $30,000 per year of life saved compared with streptokinase.[43] Two other trials that compared alteplase with reteplase and alteplase with tenecteplase found similar mortality between agents.[44,45] Therefore, alteplase, reteplase, or tenecteplase is acceptable as a first-line agent. Most hospitals have at least two of these agents on their formulary. Most often, formulary decisions are based on the frequency of use of fibrinolytics for other approved indications, such as ischemic stroke or pulmonary embolism, with alteplase having the most indications of the fibrin-specific agents. Administration considerations also guide formulary decision making and choice for patient treatment, with tenecteplase given as a single, weight-based dose and reteplase given as two fixed doses without weight adjustment. Therefore, both tenecteplase and reteplase are easier to administer than alteplase.

TABLE 18-5 Indications and Contraindications to Fibrinolytic Therapy According to ACC/AHA Guidelines for Management of Patients with ST-Segment Elevation Myocardial Infarction

Indications
1. Ischemic chest discomfort at least 20 minutes in duration but ≤12 hours since symptom onset
and
ST-segment elevation of at least 1 mm in height in ≤2 contiguous leads or
New or presumed new left bundle-branch block
2. Ongoing ischemic chest discomfort at least 20 minutes in duration 12–24 hours since symptom onset
and
ST-segment elevation of at least 1 mm in height in ≥2 contiguous leads
Absolute contraindications
Active internal bleeding (not including menses)
Previous intracranial hemorrhage at any time; ischemic stroke within 3 months
Known intracranial neoplasm
Known structural vascular lesion (e.g., arteriovenous malformation)
Suspected aortic dissection
Significant closed head or facial trauma within 3 months
Relative contraindications
Severe, uncontrolled hypertension on presentation (blood pressure >180/110 mm Hg)
History of prior ischemic stroke >3 months, dementia, or known intracranial pathology not covered above under absolute contraindications
Current use of anticoagulants
Known bleeding diathesis
Traumatic or prolonged (>10 minutes) CPR or major surgery (<3 weeks)
Noncompressible vascular puncture (e.g., a recent liver biopsy or carotid artery puncture)
Recent (within 2–4 weeks) internal bleeding
For streptokinase administration, previous streptokinase use (>5 days) or prior allergic reactions
Pregnancy
Active peptic ulcer
History of severe, chronic poorly controlled hypertension

CPR, cardiopulmonary resuscitation.
Data from Antman EM, Anbe DT, Armstrong PW, Bates ER, et al. ACC/AHA guidelines for the management of patients with ST-elevation myocardial infarction: Executive summary. A report of the American College of Cardiology/American Heart Association Task Force on Practice Guidelines (Committee to revise the 1999 Guidelines for the Management of Patients with Acute Myocardial Infarction). Circulation 2004;110:588–636..

TABLE 18-6 Comparison Between Fibrinolytic Agents

Agent	Fibrin Specificity	TIMI-3 Blood Flow Complete Perfusion at 90 Minutes	Systemic Bleeding Risk/ ICH Risk	Administration	Average Wholesale Price	Other Approved Uses
Streptokinase (Streptase)	+	35%	+++/+	Infusion over 60 minutes	$563	Pulmonary embolism, deep-vein thrombosis, clearance of an occluded arteriovenous catheter, intrapleural administration for clearance of pulmonary effusion
Alteplase (rt-PA) (Activase)	+++	50%–60%	++/++	Bolus followed by infusions over 90 minutes, weight-based dosing	$3,826	Pulmonary embolism, acute ischemic stroke, clearance of an occluded arteriovenous catheter
Reteplase (rPA) (Retavase)	++	50%–60%	++/++	Two bolus doses, 30 minutes apart	$2,896	
Tenecteplase (TNK-tPA) (TNKase)	++++	50%–60%	+/++	Single bolus dose, weight-based dosing	$2,918	

ICH, intracranial hemorrhage; TIMI, Thrombolysis in Myocardial Blood Flow (TIMI-3 blood flow indicates complete perfusion of the infarct artery).
Adapted from Spinler.[10]

ICH and major bleeding are the most serious side effects of fibrinolytic agents (see Table 18–6). The risk of ICH is higher with fibrin-specific agents than with streptokinase. Models for use in clinical practice are available to predict an individual patient's risk of ICH following administration of a fibrinolytic.[3] The risk of systemic bleeding other than ICH is higher with streptokinase than with other, more fibrin-specific agents.[43]

The percentage of eligible patients who receive reperfusion therapy is another quality performance measure of care in patients with STEMI (see Table 18–3).[33] The "door-to-needle time," which is the time from hospital arrival to start of fibrinolytic therapy, is another quality performance measure (see Table 18–3).[33] Although the ACC/AHA guidelines recommend a door-to-needle time of less than 30 minutes, the median administration time in the United States in 2006 was 30 minutes, with only 50% of patients meeting the quality performance measure target of less than 30 minutes.[5] Therefore, healthcare professionals should work to shorten fibrinolytic administration times.

Aspirin

Based on several randomized trials, aspirin has become the preferred antiplatelet agent for treatment of all ACSs.[2,3] Early aspirin administration to all patients without contraindications within the first 24 hours of hospital admission is a quality care indicator (see Table 18–3).[33] The antiplatelet effects of aspirin are mediated by inhibition of thromboxane A_2 synthesis through irreversible inhibition of platelet cyclooxygenase-1 (COX-1).[46] Following administration of a non–enteric-coated formulation, aspirin rapidly (<10 minutes) inhibits thromboxane A_2 production in the platelets. Aspirin also has antiinflammatory actions, which decrease C-reactive protein and may contribute to its effectiveness in ACS.[46] In patients undergoing PCI, aspirin prevents acute thrombotic occlusion during the procedure.

The Second International Study of Infarct Survival (ISIS-2), which studied the impact of streptokinase and aspirin (162.5 mg/day) either alone or in combination, is a landmark clinical trial that convincingly demonstrated the value of aspirin in patients with STE ACS.[47] In this trial (n = 17,187), patients who received aspirin demonstrated a lower risk of 35-day vascular mortality compared with placebo (9.4% vs 11.8%; P <0.0001). Use of aspirin was not associated with an increase in major bleeding, although the incidence of minor bleeding was increased. The combination of aspirin and streptokinase reduced mortality compared with placebo as well as compared with either agent alone, thereby highlighting the additive effects of combination antithrombotic therapy.

In patients experiencing an ACS, an initial dose equal to greater than 160 mg nonenteric aspirin is necessary to achieve rapid platelet inhibition (see Table 18–4).[46,47] This first dose can be chewed in order to achieve high blood concentrations and rapid platelet inhibition.[2,3] The notion of chewing aspirin came from use of an enteric-coated formulation of aspirin in the ISIS-2 trial in order to break the enteric coating to ensure more rapid effect.[47] Current data suggest that although an initial dose of 160 to 325 mg is required, long-term therapy with doses of 75 to 150 mg daily are as effective as higher doses and, therefore,[48] a daily maintenance dose of 75 to 160 mg is recommended in most patients to inhibit the 10% of the total platelet pool that is regenerated daily.[2,49] Whether these lower doses are as effective as a dose of 325 mg daily in patients undergoing intracoronary stent placement remains uncertain. Current AHA/ACC guidelines recommend the use of 162–325 mg daily for 1 month after placement of a bare-metal stent, 3 months after placement of a sirolimus-coated stent, and 6 months after placement of a paclitaxel-coated stent, after which a daily aspirin dose of 75 to 162 mg should be used indefinitely.[40] Therefore, although the risk of major bleeding, particularly gastrointestinal bleeding, appears to be reduced by using lower doses of aspirin, low-dose aspirin, taken chronically, is not free of adverse effects.[49,50] Patients should be counseled on the potential risk of bleeding.

The ACC/AHA STE ACS guidelines specifically recommend that ibuprofen not be administered on a regular basis for pain relief concurrently with aspirin due to a reported drug interaction with aspirin whereby ibuprofen blocks aspirin's antiplatelet effects.[3] Theoretically, such a risk is also possible with other nonsteroidal antiinflammatory drugs (NSAIDs), although these theoretical drug interactions remain to be clearly established. Finally, although some concern has been voiced regarding the possible increased risk of hemorrhagic stroke in patients taking aspirin, this risk appears to be very small and is outweighed by the benefit in reducing the risk of ischemic stroke and other vascular events.[48] The risk of hemorrhagic stroke appears to be minimal in patients with adequate blood pressure control,[20] and there are no specific contraindications to antiplatelet therapy in hypertensive patients presenting with ACS.[51] Aspirin therapy should be continued indefinitely.[3]

Thienopyridines

Although aspirin is effective in the setting of ACS, it is a relatively weak platelet inhibitor that blocks platelet aggregation through only one pathway. The thienopyridines clopidogrel and ticlopidine are antiplatelet agents that mediate their antiplatelet effects through a blockade of ADP $P2Y_{12}$ receptors on platelets.[2] Because ticlopidine is associated with the occurrence of neutropenia that requires frequent monitoring of the complete blood count during the first 3 months of use,[52] clopidogrel is the preferred thienopyridine for ACS and PCI patients[40] (see Table 18–4).

The AHA/ACC guidelines currently recommend clopidogrel as an alternative to aspirin in patients who have an allergy to aspirin.[2,3] The updated recommendations from these professional associations, expected in 2007, are likely to extend the recommendation regarding the use of clopidogrel to include most patients with STE ACS. A trial of more than 45,000 patients with STE ACS showed that early therapy with clopidogrel 75 mg once daily (started within 24 hours of hospital presentation), added to aspirin for the duration of hospitalization (average 15 days) or up to 28 days, reduced mortality and reinfarction compared to placebo in patients treated with medical therapy, including fibrinolytics, without increasing the risk of major bleeding.[53] Another smaller study showed that clopidogrel added to aspirin reduced the composite rate of 30-day death, MI, or stroke by 20% in patients ages 18 to 75 years with STE ACS treated with fibrinolytics. Clopidogrel or placebo was administered as an initial dose of 300 mg orally on day 1, followed by 75 mg daily. Angiography was encouraged as early as hospital day 2, and patients undergoing PCI at the time of angiography continued on open-label clopidogrel at a 300-mg loading dose followed by 75 mg once daily for the duration of the study. Patients who did not undergo revascularization received clopidogrel up to the time of discharge or hospital day 8. At the time of angiography, more open infarct arteries were present in the clopidogrel-treated patients.[54] Based on current data, therefore, clopidogrel (either 75 mg or 300 mg on day 1 followed by 75 mg once daily) should be given for at least 14 to 28 days in addition to aspirin in patients treated by fibrinolytics and in those receiving no revascularization therapy with either PCI or CABG surgery. The safety of the 300-mg loading dose has not been evaluated in patients older than over 75 years receiving a fibrinolytic.

Clopidogrel is recommended in addition to aspirin in patients undergoing primary PCI. For primary PCI, clopidogrel is administered as a 300-mg loading dose, followed by 75 mg once daily, in combination with aspirin 325 mg once daily, to prevent subacute stent thrombosis and long-term events cardiovascular CV events.[2,32,40] Alternatively, an initial dose of 600 mg can be considered, although the clinical efficacy and safety of this dose is under investigation.[40] The duration of clopidogrel therapy depends on the type of stent implemented (either a bare-metal stent or a drug-eluting stent; see Table 18–4), the patient's presentation (ACS vs stable angina), and the patient's risk of bleeding.[55,56]

The most frequent side effects of clopidogrel are nausea, vomiting, and diarrhea, which occur in approximately 5% of patients. Rarely, thrombotic thrombocytopenic purpura has been reported with clopidogrel.[52] The most serious side effect of clopidogrel is bleeding (see Early Pharmacotherapy for NSTE ACS below).

GP IIb/IIIa Receptor Inhibitors

Abciximab is a first-line GP IIb/IIIa receptor inhibitor for patients undergoing primary PCI[3,32,40,57] who have not received fibrinolytics. It should not be administered for medical management of patients with STE ACS who will not be undergoing PCI. Abciximab is preferred over eptifibatide and tirofiban in this setting because abciximab is the most common GP IIb/IIIa receptor inhibitor studied in primary PCI trials.[3,32,40,57] Abciximab, in combination with aspirin, a thienopyridine, and UFH (administered as an infusion for the duration of the procedure) reduced mortality and reinfarction without increasing the risk of major bleeding in a meta-analysis of primary PCI clinical trials.[57]

Dosing and contraindications for abciximab are listed in Table 18–4. GP IIb/IIIa receptor inhibitors block the final common pathway of platelet aggregation, namely, cross-linking of platelets by fibrinogen bridges between the GP IIb/IIIa receptors on the platelet surface. Abciximab typically is initiated at the time of PCI, and the infusion is continued for 12 hours. Administration of a GP IIb/IIIa receptor inhibitor may increase the risk of bleeding, especially if it is given in the setting of recent (<4 hours) administration of fibrinolytic therapy.[57–59] An immune-mediated thrombocytopenia occurs in approximately 5% of patients.[60]

Some trials suggest that early administration of abciximab results in early opening of the coronary artery, making primary PCI easier for the interventional cardiologist. Clinical trials performed to date suggest that the combination of early administration of a reduced dose of a fibrinolytic agent in combination with abciximab does not reduce mortality and increases the risk of bleeding, including ICH, in elderly patients with STE ACS.[57–59] Additional clinical trials of combined antithrombotic therapy for STE PCI patients are ongoing.

Anticoagulants

Options for anticoagulant therapy for patients with STE ACS are outlined in Fig. 18–3 and Table 18–4. UFH, administered as an IV bolus followed by a continuous infusion, is a first-line anticoagulant for treatment of patients with STE ACS, both for medical therapy and for patients undergoing PCI.[3,40] UFH binds to antithrombin and then inhibits the activity of clotting factors Xa and IIa (thrombin). Anticoagulant therapy should be initiated in the emergency department and continued for at least 48 hours in selected patients who will be bridged over to receive chronic warfarin anticoagulation following acute MI.[3] If a patient undergoes PCI, UFH is discontinued immediately after the procedure. UFH dosing is listed in Table 18–4. The dose of UFH infusion is adjusted frequently to a target activated partial thromboplastin time (aPTT; see Table 18–4). When coadministered with a fibrinolytic, aPTTs above the target range are associated with an increased rate of bleeding, whereas aPTTs below the target range are associated with increased mortality and reinfarction.[61]

For more than 40 years UFH has been the traditional anticoagulant administered to patients with STE ACS for prevention of infarct artery reocclusion. Other beneficial effects of anticoagulation in patients with ACS are prevention of cardioembolic stroke and venous thromboembolism.[3] When a fibrinolytic agent is administered, UFH is given concomitantly with alteplase, reteplase, and tenecteplase. UFH is not administered to patients receiving the non–fibrin-selective agent streptokinase because no benefit of combined therapy has been be demonstrated.[62] Rates of reinfarction are higher if UFH is not given in combination with fibrin-selective agents.[62] UFH currently is the preferred anticoagulant in patients undergoing primary PCI.[32,40]

Besides bleeding, the most frequent adverse effect of UFH is the immune-mediated clotting disorder heparin-induced thrombocytopenia (see Chapter 21), which occurs in up to 5% of patients treated with UFH. Heparin-induced thrombocytopenia is less common in patients receiving low-molecular-weight heparins (LMWHs).[3,40] Because randomized controlled clinical trials comparing UFH to placebo are lacking, no conclusive data support a benefit of UFH over placebo in reducing mortality or reinfarction in STE ACS.[63] On the contrary, the results of a meta-analysis of more than 7,500 patients suggests that LMWHs reduce both mortality and reinfarction compared to placebo.[63]

LMWHs, like UFH, bind to antithrombin and inhibit both factor Xa and IIa. However, because their composition is mostly short saccharide chain lengths, they preferentially inhibit factor Xa over factor IIa, which requires larger chain lengths for binding and inhibition. Although the possible superiority of LMWHs, particularly enoxaparin, has been suggested by many small trials,[63] their relative benefits have been properly compared only recently in the Enoxaparin and Thrombolysis Reperfusion for Acute Myocardial Infarction Treatment (ExTRACT)-Thrombolysis in Myocardial Infarction (TIMI) 25 trial.[64] In this large trial, enoxaparin administered for a median of 7 days significantly reduced the risk of death or nonfatal MI compared to UFH administered for a median of 2 days (see Table 18–4). The benefit, although modest, was already apparent after 48 hours of treatment. Enoxaparin use was associated with a small (2.1% vs 1.4%) but significant increased risk of major bleeding. Whether the observed benefits and increase in bleeding observed in this trial can be solely attributed to the pharmacokinetic and pharmacodynamic differences between UFH and enoxaparin or the longer duration of treatment in the enoxaparin group is uncertain. Although the bleeding rates were increased in patients older than 75 years compared to younger patients, the rates of major bleeding between enoxaparin and UFH use were similar in the older patient subgroup.[65] Therefore, enoxaparin can be considered a valuable anticoagulant in the context of STEMI. Enoxaparin has not been studied in the setting of primary PCI.

Fondaparinux is an indirect-acting specific inhibitor of factor Xa that has recently been studied in the setting of STE ACS. Unlike UFH and LMWHs, fondaparinux does not cause heparin-induced thrombocytopenia. In the Sixth Organization for the Assessment of Strategies for Ischemic Syndromes (OASIS 6) trial, fondaparinux administered for a median of 8 days had similar efficacy and safety as UFH administered for a median of 2 days in patients receiving fibrinolytic therapy with alteplase, reteplase, or tenecteplase (see Table 18–4 for dosing).[66] A small reduction in mortality was observed in patients treated with fondaparinux versus placebo in patients treated with streptokinase or receiving no fibrinolytic therapy. No benefit of fondaparinux was observed in the subgroup of patients undergoing PCI during hospitalization.[66] Because of the lack of benefit of in the fondaparinux compared to UFH group as well as in the subgroup of patients undergoing PCI, coupled with the relatively long duration of administration, fondaparinux likely will not be used widely in practice for treatment of STEMI in the United States.

Nitrates

Nitrates promote the release of nitric oxide from the endothelium, which results in venous and arterial vasodilation at higher doses. Venodilation lowers preload and myocardial oxygen demand. Arterial vasodilation may lower blood pressure, thus reducing myocardial oxygen demand. Arterial vasodilation relieves coronary artery vasospasm, dilating coronary arteries to improve myocardial blood flow and oxygenation. One SL NTG tablet (0.4 mg) should be administered every 5 minutes for up to three doses to relieve myocardial ischemia. If patients have previously been prescribed SL NTG and ischemic chest discomfort persists for more than 5 minutes after the first dose, the patient should be instructed to contact emergency medical services before self-administering subsequent doses in order to activate emergency care sooner. IV NTG is indicated in patients with ACS who do not have a contraindication and who have persistent ischemic symptoms, heart failure, or uncontrolled blood pressure. It should be continued for approximately 24 hours after ischemia is relieved (see Table 18–4).[3] Importantly, other lifesaving therapies, such as ACE inhibitors or β-blockers, should not be withheld for nitrates use because the mortality benefit of nitrates is unproven. Nitrates play a limited role in the treatment of ACS patients, with two large, randomized clinical trials failing to show a mortality benefit for IV followed by oral nitrate therapy in patients with acute MI.[67,68] The most significant adverse effects of nitrates are tachycardia, flushing, headache, and hypotension. Nitrate administration is contraindicated in patients who have received oral phosphodiesterase-5 inhibitors, such as sildenafil and vardenafil, within the past 24 hours and tadalafil within the past 48 hours.

β-Blockers

A β-blocker should be administered early in the care of patients with STE ACS and continued indefinitely. Early administration of a β-blocker within the first 24 hours of hospitalization in patients lacking a contraindication is a quality care indicator (see Table 18–3).[33] In ACS, the benefit of β-blockers results mainly from the competitive blockade of β_1-adrenergic receptors located on the myocardium. β_1-blockade produces a reduction in heart rate, myocardial contractility, and blood pressure, decreasing myocardial oxygen demand. In addition, the reduction in heart rate increases diastolic time, thus improving ventricular filling and coronary artery perfusion.[69] As a result of these effects, β-blockers reduce the risk for recurrent ischemic, infarct size, risk of reinfarction, and occurrence of ventricular arrhythmias in the hours and days following MI.[69]

Landmark clinical trials have established the role of early β-blocker therapy in reducing MI mortality. Most of these trials were performed in the 1970s and 1980s before routine use of early reperfusion therapy.[70–73] However, data regarding the acute benefit of β-blockers in MI in the reperfusion era are derived mainly from a large clinical trial reported in 2005. The trial suggests that although initiating IV followed by oral β-blockers early in the course of STEMI was associated with a lower risk of reinfarction or ventricular fibrillation, there may be an early risk of cardiogenic shock, especially in patients presenting with pulmonary congestion or systolic blood pressure $<$120 mm Hg.[74] Therefore, the use of β-blockers, particularly when administered IV, should be limited to patients who are hemodynamically stable and who do not demonstrate any signs or symptoms of decompensated heart failure. Careful assessment for signs of hypotension and heart failure should be performed following β-blocker initiation and prior to any dose titration. Early administration of β-blockers (to patients without contraindications) within the first 24 hours of hospital admission is a quality performance measure (see Table 18–3).[3,33] The AHA and ACC now are reevaluating this recommendation given the results of the aforementioned trial. Current AHA guidelines for the management of hypertension in the setting of ACS suggest that β-blockers should be delayed in patients with hemodynamic instability or shock until resolution of heart failure symptoms and hypotension.[51]

The most serious side effects of β-blocker administration early in ACS are hypotension, acute heart failure, bradycardia, and heart block. Although initial acute administration of β-blockers is not appropriate for patients who present with decompensated heart failure, initiation of β-blockers can be attempted before hospital discharge in most patients following treatment of acute heart failure. It cannot be overemphasized that diabetes mellitus does not constitute a contraindication to β-blockers. Although the use of β-blockers may mask symptoms of hypoglycemia, except sweating, diabetics greatly benefit from β-blocker administration because they are at high risk for recurrent events.[69] In patients in whom a major concern exists regarding a possible intolerance to β-blockers, such as patients with bronchospastic pulmonary disease, a short-acting β-blocker, such as metoprolol or esmolol, initially should be administered IV.[69] β-Blockers are continued indefinitely.[3]

Calcium Channel Blockers

Administration of calcium channel blockers in the setting of STE ACS is reserved for patients who have contraindications to β-blockers and is given for relief of ischemic symptoms.[3] In patients prescribed calcium channel blockers for treatment of hypertension who are not receiving β-blockers and who do not have a contraindication to β-blockers, the calcium channel blocker should be discontinued and a β-blocker initiated. Calcium channel blockers inhibit calcium influx into myocardial and vascular smooth muscle cells, causing vasodilation. Although all calcium channel blockers produce coronary vasodilation and decrease blood pressure, other effects are more heterogeneous between agents. Dihydropyridine calcium channel blockers (e.g., amlodipine, felodipine, and nifedipine) primarily produce their antiischemic effects through peripheral vasodilation, with no clinical effects on atrioventricular nodal conduction and heart rate. Diltiazem and verapamil, on the other hand, have additional antiischemic effects by reducing contractility and atrioventricular nodal conduction and slowing heart rate.[75]

Current data suggest little benefit on clinical outcomes beyond symptom relief for calcium channel blockers in the setting of ACS.[76,77] Moreover, the use of first-generation short-acting dihydropyridines, such as nifedipine, should be avoided because they appear to worsen outcomes through their negative inotropic effects, induction of reflex sympathetic activation, tachycardia, and increased myocardial ischemia.[75] Therefore, the role of verapamil or diltiazem appears to be limited to relief of ischemia-related symptoms or control of heart rate in patients with supraventricular arrhythmias for whom β-blockers are contraindicated or ineffective.[2,3]

Adverse effects and contraindications of calcium channel blockers are listed in Table 18–4. Verapamil, diltiazem, and first-generation dihydropyridines also should be avoided in patients with decompensated heart failure or LV dysfunction because these drugs can worsen heart failure and potentially increase mortality secondary to their negative inotropic effects. In patients with heart failure requiring treatment with a calcium channel blocker, amlodipine is the preferred agent.[77,78]

Two groups of patients may benefit from calcium channel blockers as opposed to β-blockers as initial therapy. Cocaine-induced ACS and variant (or Prinzmetal) angina are two conditions in which coronary vasospasm plays an important role.[2,3,75] Calcium channel blockers and/or NTG generally are considered the agents of choice in these patients because they can reverse coronary spasm by inducing smooth muscle relaxation in the coronary arteries. In contrast, β-blockers generally should be avoided in these patients unless they have uncontrolled sinus tachycardia (>100 beats/min) or severe uncontrolled hypertension following cocaine use because β-blockers actually may worsen vasospasm through an unopposed β_2-blocking effect on the smooth muscle cells.[2]

■ EARLY PHARMACOTHERAPY FOR NSTE ACS

In general, early pharmacotherapy for NSTE ACS (see Fig. 18–4) is similar to that for STE ACS with three exceptions:

1. Fibrinolytic therapy is not administered.
2. GP IIb/IIIa receptor blockers are administered to high-risk patients.
3. There are no standard quality performance measures for patients with NSTE ACS with unstable angina (not diagnosed with MI).

8 According to the ACC/AHA NSTE ACS practice guidelines, early pharmacotherapy for NSTE ACS should include intranasal

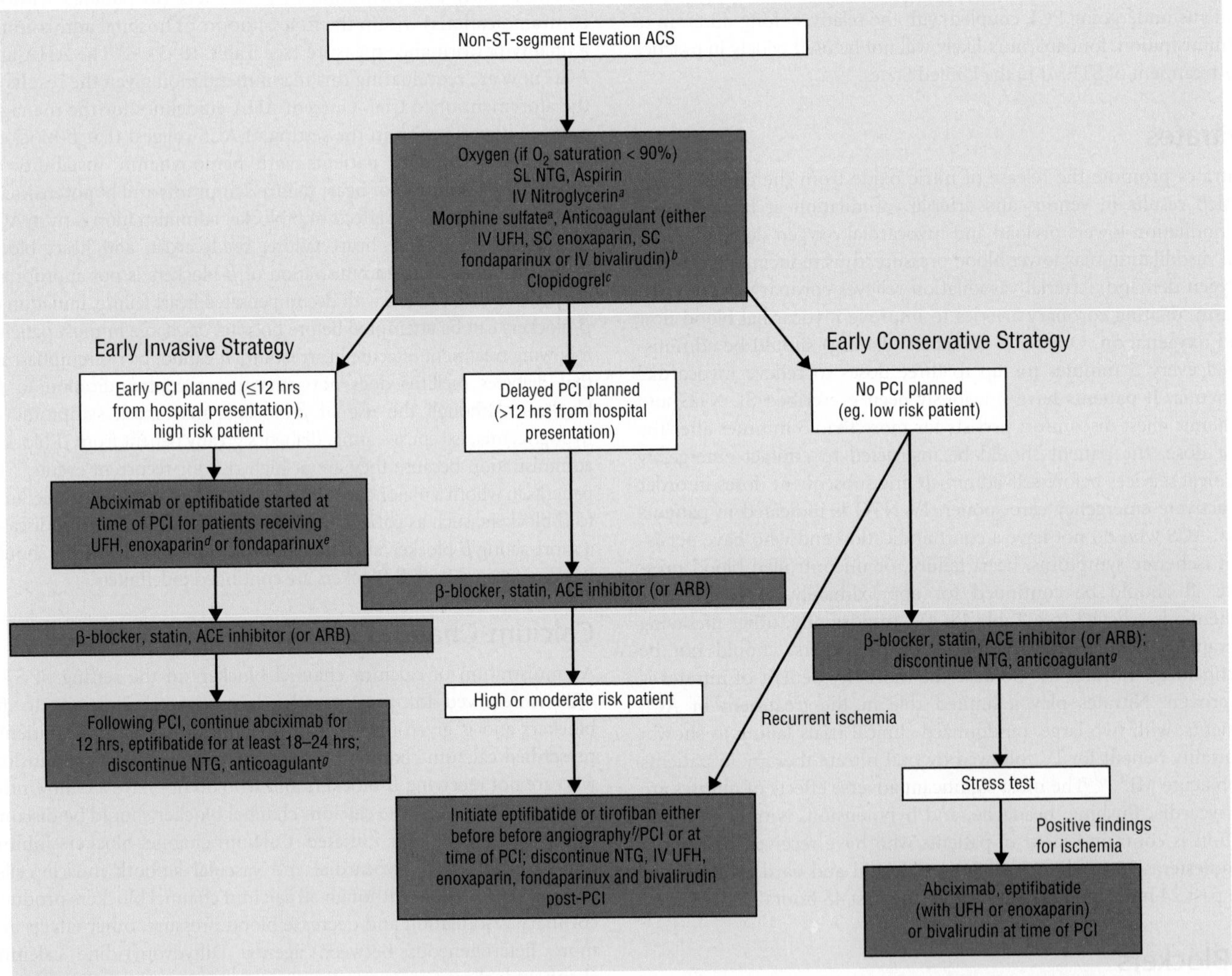

FIGURE 18-4. Initial pharmacotherapy for non–ST-segment elevation acute coronary syndrome. (ACE, angiotensin-converting enzyme; ARB, angiotensin receptor blocker; ACS, acute coronary syndrome; CABG, coronary artery bypass graft surgery; IV, intravenous; NTG, nitroglycerin; PCI, percutaneous coronary intervention; SC, subcutaneous; SL, sublingual; UFH, unfractionated heparin.) [a]For selected patients, see Table 18–4. [b]Enoxaparin, UFH, fondaparinux, or bivalirudin for early invasive strategy; enoxaparin or fondaparinux preferred if no angiography/PCI planned but UFH acceptable; fondaparinux preferred if high risk for bleeding; UFH preferred anticoagulant for patients undergoing CABG. [c]In patients unlikely to undergo CABG. [d]May require an IV supplemental dose; see Table 18–4. [e]Requires supplemental UFH bolus for PCI; see Table 18–4. [f]For signs and symptoms of recurrent ischemia. [g]SC enoxaparin or UFH can be continued at a lower dose for venous thromboembolism prophylaxis. *(Adapted with permission from the American College of Clinical Pharmacy. Spinler SA. Acute coronary syndromes. In: Dunsworth TS, Richardson MM, Cheng JWM, et al., eds. Pharmacotherapy Self-Assessment Program, 6th ed. Cardiology II module. Kansas City: American College of Clinical Pharmacy, 2007: 69–70.)*

oxygen (if oxygen saturation is <90%), SL NTG, aspirin, an oral β-blocker (IV β-blocker optional), and an anticoagulant (UFH, LMWH [enoxaparin], fondaparinux, or bivalirudin). Morphine is also administered to patients with refractory angina, as described previously in Early Pharmacotherapy for STE ACS. IV NTG should be administered in selected patients without contraindications as described in Table 18–4. These agents should be administered early, while the patient is still in the emergency department. Dosing and contraindications for SL and IV NTG, aspirin, β-blockers, UFH, and enoxaparin are listed in Table 18–4.[2,3,10]

Fibrinolytic Therapy

Fibrinolytic therapy is not indicated in any patient with NSTE ACS, even those who have positive biochemical markers (e.g., troponin) that indicate infarction. Because the risk of death from MI is lower in patients with NSTE ACS whereas the risk for life-threatening adverse effects, such as ICH, with fibrinolytics is similar between patients with STE and NSTE ACS, the risks of fibrinolytic therapy outweigh the benefit for NSTE ACS patients. In fact, increased mortality has been reported with fibrinolytics compared with controls in clinical trials where fibrinolytics have been administered to patients with NSTE ACS (patients with normal or ST-segment depression ECGs).[20]

Aspirin

Aspirin reduces the risk of death or developing MI by about 50% (compared with no antiplatelet therapy) in patients with NSTE ACS.[49] Therefore, aspirin remains the cornerstone of early treatment for all ACSs. Dosing of aspirin for NSTE ACS is the same as that for STE ACS (see Table 18–4). Aspirin is continued indefinitely.

Thienopyridines

For patients with NSTE ACS, the addition of clopidogrel started on the first day of hospitalization as a 300- to 600-mg loading dose followed the next day by 75 mg/day orally is recommended for most patients.[2] Although the use of aspirin in ACS is the mainstay of antiplatelet therapy, morbidity and mortality following an ACS remain high. Researchers explored whether combining two oral antiplatelet agents with different mechanisms of action, aspirin and clopidogrel, would result in additional clinical benefit over using aspirin alone. Efficacy and safety of this dual antiplatelet therapy were demonstrated in the Clopidogrel in Unstable Angina to Prevent Recurrent Events (CURE) trial.[79,80] In CURE, 12,562 patients with unstable angina or an NSTE MI and new ECG changes consistent with ischemia or positive cardiac markers were randomized to a loading dose of clopidogrel 300 mg, followed by a daily dose of 75 mg or placebo in addition to aspirin for a mean duration of 9 months. Clopidogrel reduced the combined risk of death from cardiovascular causes, nonfatal MI, or stroke from 11.4% to 9.4% compared with placebo, mainly through a reduction in the risk of MI. Cardiovascular mortality was similar between groups. Results from a second trial in PCI patients, the Clopidogrel for the Reduction of Events During Observation (CREDO) trial,[81] in which patients were treated with long-term clopidogrel (1 year), demonstrated a lower risk of death, MI, or stroke compared with patients who received only 28 days of clopidogrel (8.5% vs 11.5%; $P = 0.02$). However, the interpretation of this study is limited in that the control group did not receive a loading dose of clopidogrel on the first day. According to the ACC/AHA 2007 guidelines, clopidogrel is indicated for up to 12 months in NSTE ACS patients, with a minimum duration of treatment of 1 month after placement of a bare-metal stent and 12 months after placement of a sirolimus or paclitaxel coated stent.[2,55] Whether or not treatment with clopidogrel should be extended to more than 1 year is questionable based on recent a large, randomized trial.[82]

The major concern when combining two antiplatelet agents is the increased risk of bleeding. In CURE, the risk of major bleeding was increased in patients who received clopidogrel plus aspirin compared with aspirin alone (3.7% vs 2.7%; $P = 0.001$).[79] A post hoc analysis of CURE revealed that the rate of major bleeding depended on the dose of aspirin and showed that doses ≤100 mg daily reduced the risk of bleeding with similar efficacy compared with higher doses.[83] The recommendation to use a lower dose of aspirin with clopidogrel is also supported by the results of a recent systematic review of clinical trials that found no benefit to aspirin as a sole antiplatelet agent for chronic treatment in doses greater than 75 to 81 mg.[48] However, administration of a 325-mg dose of aspirin with clopidogrel is recommended for patients with recent intracoronary stent placement (see Early Pharmacotherapy for STE ACS) to prevent stent thrombosis.[40]

In patients undergoing CABG, major bleeding was increased in those who underwent the procedure within 5 days of clopidogrel discontinuation (9.6% vs 6.3%; $P = 0.06$) but not in those in whom clopidogrel was discontinued more than 5 days before the procedure.[79] Aspirin was continued up to and after CABG. Therefore, in patients scheduled for CABG, clopidogrel should be withheld at least 5 days and preferably 7 days before the procedure.[2]

The timing of initiation of clopidogrel in patients presenting with NSTE ACS is controversial. Although clopidogrel should be initiated as soon as possible in patients being treated with a noninterventional strategy or in patients who have a contraindication to aspirin, the need to delay CABG for 5 to 7 days following clopidogrel has led many to suggest that clopidogrel administration should be delayed until coronary angiography is performed and the need for CABG is excluded. This is particularly relevant in centers where the waiting time for CABG is less than 5 days. However, existing data also suggest that early treatment with clopidogrel before angiography is performed reduces the number of cardiovascular events following the procedure.[81] Therefore, others have advocated the expanded use of early clopidogrel in all patients experiencing a NSTE ACS.

GP IIb/IIIa Receptor Inhibitors

Administration of tirofiban or eptifibatide is recommended for high-risk NSTE ACS patients as medical therapy without planned revascularization, and administration of either abciximab or eptifibatide is recommended for NSTE ACS patients undergoing PCI. Administration of tirofiban or eptifibatide is also indicated in patients with continued or recurrent ischemia despite treatment with aspirin, clopidogrel, and an anticoagulant.[2] The pharmacologic similarities and differences between GP IIb/IIIa receptor inhibitors are reviewed in Chapter 17. As discussed in Chapter 17, the benefits of GP IIb/IIIa receptor inhibitors in PCI is well established, and they are considered first-line agents for reducing the risk of reinfarction and the need for repeat PCI.[2,32,40]

Two large clinical trials highlight the role of GP IIb/IIIa receptor inhibitors in the setting of NSTE ACS and PCI. In the Platelet Glycoprotein IIb/IIIa in Unstable Angina: Receptor Suppression Using Integrilin Therapy (PURSUIT) trial (n = 10,948), eptifibatide added to aspirin and UFH and continued for 48 to 96 hours reduced the combined end point of death or MI at 30 days (14.2% vs 15.7%) compared with aspirin and UFH alone.[84] In the Platelet Receptor Inhibition in Ischemic Syndrome Management in Patients Limited by Unstable Signs and Symptoms (PRISM-PLUS) study (n = 1,915), tirofiban added to aspirin and UFH and continued for up to 72 hours reduced the rate of death, MI, or refractory ischemia at 7 days compared with aspirin and UFH alone.[85] However, in these and other trials of GP IIb/IIIa inhibitors for NSTE ACS, the benefit was mostly limited to patients undergoing PCI and not those treated without interventional therapy.[86] Therefore, medical therapy with GP IIb/IIIa receptor inhibitors is reserved for higher-risk patients, such as those with positive troponin or ST-segment depression, and patients who have continued or recurrent ischemia despite other antithrombotic therapy.[2,32,40] Patients undergoing PCI in these trials received several hours to days of pretreatment with the GP IIb/IIIa receptor inhibitor before proceeding to PCI.

The role of GP IIb/IIIa receptor antagonists in patients with NSTE ACS undergoing PCI also was evaluated in two large clinical trials that used GP IIb/IIIa receptor inhibitors initiated at the time of PCI. In the Enhanced Suppression of the Platelet IIb/IIIa Receptor with Integrilin Therapy (ESPRIT) trial (n = 1,024), eptifibatide in combination with aspirin and UFH reduced the rate of death or MI up to 1 year in patients undergoing PCI.[87] The benefits of treatment in the ACS subgroup were more pronounced compared with the stable angina subgroup, thereby establishing a role for eptifibatide in ACS PCI patients.

Only one trial has compared two GP IIb/IIIa receptor inhibitors with each other. In the Do Tirofiban and ReoPro Give Similar Efficacy Outcomes Trial (TARGET), tirofiban, at a different dose from that used in the PRISM-PLUS study, was compared with abciximab in patients undergoing PCI.[88,89] In the subgroup of patients with ACS, there was a statistically significant reduction in the composite end point of death, nonfatal MI, or need for repeat PCI at 30 days in patients randomized to receive abciximab compared with tirofiban (6.3% vs 9.3%).[89] Although the numerical benefit of a 3% absolute risk reduction was maintained at 6 months, it approached but was no longer statistically significant (hazard ratio 1.19, abciximab better than tirofiban, 95% confidence internal 0.99–1.42).[89] Following TARGET, the dose of tirofiban that was used in that trial has been shown to be ineffective at inhibiting platelet aggregation during the PCI procedure.[90] Therefore, tirofiban cannot be recommended for PCI unless the patient has been treated with tirofiban for several hours to days prior to PCI and adequate inhibition of platelet aggregation can be ensured. If a GP IIb/IIIa receptor inhibitor is initiated while the patient is undergoing the procedure, abciximab or eptifibatide should be used. Importantly, in patients with NSTE ACS undergoing PCI, use of clopidogrel does not obviate the need for a GP IIb/IIIa inhibitor.[91]

As emphasized in the ACC/AHA guidelines,[2] the benefits of GP IIb/IIIa inhibitors are greater in patients undergoing PCI. A meta-analysis estimated that 30 adverse outcomes (either death or MI) are prevented for every 1,000 patients treated with a GP IIb/IIIa inhibitor before PCI, whereas only four events are prevented for medical management of patients with NSTE ACS using GP IIb/IIIa inhibitors without PCI.[92] This translates into a number needed to treat (NNT) of 32 patients to prevent one event if a GP IIb/IIIa inhibitor is administered before PCI and 250 patients to prevent one event if it is administered as medical therapy without PCI.[92]

Doses and contraindications to GP IIb/IIIa receptor blockers are listed in Table 18–4, and common adverse effects are described in the preceding section. Administration of IV GP IIb/IIIa receptor inhibitor in combination with aspirin and either UFH or enoxaparin results in major bleeding rates of 0.4% to 10.6%[84,85] but no increased risk of ICH in the absence of concomitant fibrinolytic treatment. Some studies suggest that although the risk of minor bleeding is higher, the risk of major bleeding with a GP IIb/IIIa inhibitor is similar to placebo in patients treated with UFH who undergo PCI.[85,91] Risk factors that increase the chance of bleeding with a GP IIb/IIIa inhibitor include female gender, older age, and reduced renal function.[93] Older patients, especially women, are more likely to receive an excessive dose of a GP IIb/IIIa inhibitor, which can result in bleeding.[94] Because both eptifibatide and tirofiban require dose reductions for patients with renal insufficiency (see Table 18–4), careful attention to calculating creatinine clearance and dose adjustment is required for these agents. The risk of thrombocytopenia with tirofiban and eptifibatide appears to be lower than that with abciximab. Bleeding risks appear similar among agents.

CLINICAL CONTROVERSIES

A recent noninferiority study comparing early "upstream" administration of a GP IIb/IIIa inhibitor versus delayed selective therapy at the time of PCI in patients with NSTE ACS showed no statistical difference in ischemic events but more bleeding events when a GP IIb/IIIa inhibitor (with either UFH or enoxaparin) was administered prior to angiography.[95] Ninety-eight percent of patients in the upstream arm received a GP IIb/IIIa inhibitor, but only 56% of patients received one in the selective arm, mostly because no PCI was performed and therefore a GP IIb/IIIa inhibitor was no longer indicated. The median duration of administration of a GP IIb/IIIa inhibitor prior to PCI in the upstream arm was short, only 4 hours, as were the overall median durations of administration in both groups, 18 hours in the upstream arm and 13 hours in the selective arm, indicating that statistical power may not have been sufficient. Because the difference in duration of administration between the two groups was small, some question whether this study was a true comparison of early versus deferred treatment. Therefore, although a GP IIb/IIIa inhibitor may be used in patients with NSTE ACS the timing of administration, whether given early or deferred and used selectively at the time of angiography is controversial.

Anticoagulants

The recommendations for anticoagulants in the 2007 NSTE ACS ACC/AHA guidelines are guided by the results of recent clinical trials.[2] For patients undergoing planned early angiography and revascularization with PCI, UFH, LMWH, fondaparinux, or bivalirudin should be administered to patients with NSTE ACS.[2] Because more data support the use of enoxaparin,[2] it is the preferred LMWH for ACS. Therapy should be continued for up at least 48 hours for UFH, until the patient is discharged from the hospital for either enoxaparin or fondaparinux or a maxiumum of 8 days, and until the end of PCI or angiography procedure (or up to 42 hours following PCI) for bivalirudin.[2] UFH is the preferred anticoagulant following angiography in patients subsequently undergoing CABG during the same hospitalization.[2] In patients in whom an initial conservative strategy is planned (i.e., are not anticipated to receive angiography and revascularization), enoxaparin, UFH, or fondaparinux is recommended.[2] For patients presenting with NSTE ACS in whom cardiologists suspect a high risk for bleeding while receiving an anticoagulant, fondaparinux is the preferred anticoagulant recommended by the ACC/AHA NSTA ACS guidelines.[2] In patients initiating warfarin therapy, UFH or LMWHs should be continued until the international normalized ratio (INR) with warfarin is in the therapeutic range.

Data supporting the addition of UFH to aspirin stems from a meta-analysis of six randomized trials demonstrating a 33% reduction in the risk of death or MI at 6 weeks with UFH plus aspirin compared with aspirin alone.[96] One trial compared the LMWH dalteparin plus aspirin with aspirin alone and found a 60% reduction in death or MI at 6 days.[97] Three clinical trials have compared UFH with LMWHs for medical management of NSTE ACS.[98–100] Two trials with a total of approximately 7,000 patients demonstrated a 15% reduction in the composite end point of death, MI, or recurrent ischemia with enoxaparin compared with UFH.[98,99] One trial of dalteparin in approximately 1,400 patients demonstrated similar outcomes between dalteparin and UFH.[100] The results from these trials also showed no increased risk of major bleeding with LMWHs compared with UFH.[98–100] Minor bleeding, mostly injection-site hematomas, was increased because the LMWHs are given by subcutaneous injection, whereas UFH was administered by continuous infusion.[98–100] Because of a reduction in event rates compared with UFH, enoxaparin was mentioned as "preferred" over UFH in the ACC/AHA clinical practice guidelines.[2]

Previously, lack of data with LMWHs in NSTE ACS patients undergoing PCI has limited their use in this setting. Traditionally, interventional cardiologists monitor the degree of anticoagulation of UFH using the activated clotting time (ACT) in the cardiac catheterization laboratory. Because LMWHs have only a small effect on increasing the ACT owing to their preferential effect on activated factor X inhibition, the ACT cannot be used to monitor LMWH efficacy or toxicity. One large clinical trial of enoxaparin compared with UFH in this setting found similar efficacy with a higher risk of major bleeding with enoxaparin (9.1% vs 7.6%; $P = 0.008$).[101] The authors concluded that use of enoxaparin resulted in a similar reduction in death or MI compared to UFH. This trial was confounded by a large number of patients who received both UFH and enoxaparin either prior to randomization or during PCI. A subgroup analysis of patients receiving only consistent therapy with either enoxaparin or UFH throughout the study demonstrated an 18% reduction in 30-day death or MI with enoxaparin ($P = 0.004$), but still with an increased risk of bleeding with enoxaparin compared to UFH.[102] Switching between UFH and enoxaparin should be avoided.

The risk of major bleeding with UFH or LMWHs is higher in patients undergoing angiography because of an associated risk of hematoma at the femoral access site. The risk of heparin-induced thrombocytopenia is lower in some, but not all, clinical trials with LMWHs compared with UFH.

Because LMWHs are eliminated renally and patients with renal insufficiency generally are excluded from clinical trials, some practice protocols recommend UFH for patients with creatinine clearance rates less than 30 mL/min. (Creatinine clearance is calculated based on total patient body weight.) However, although recommendations for dosing adjustment of enoxaparin in patients with creatinine clearances between 10 and 30 mL/min are listed in the product manufacturer's label, the safety and efficacy of LMWH in this patient population remain vastly understudied (see Table 18–4). Administration of LMWHs should be avoided in dialysis patients with ACS. UFH is monitored and the dose adjusted to a target aPTT, whereas LMWHs are administered by a fixed, weight-based dose. Other dosing information and contraindications are listed in Table 18–4.

In OASIS-5, the largest NSTE ACS trial performed to date (N = 20,078), a low dose of fondaparinux, 2.5 mg administered once daily subcutaneously, was compared to the usual NSTE ACS dose of enoxaparin, 1 mg/kg administered every 12 hours.[103] Fondaparinux was found to be noninferior to enoxaparin with respect to the clinical end point of 9-day death, MI, or refractory ischemia (5.8% vs 5.7%, hazard ratio 1.01, 95% confidence interval 0.90–1.13). Fondaparinux also reduced the rate of major bleeding compared to enoxaparin (2.2% vs 4.1%, $P < 0.001$). At 30 days, mortality was lower in fondaparinux-treated patients (8.0 vs 8.6%, hazard ratio 0.83, 95% confidence interval 0.71–0.97), and the investigators suggested that the excess mortality observed in enoxaparin-treated patients was related to bleeding events. The major limitation of OASIS-5 is that only 30% of patients underwent PCI. In addition, the duration of study drug administration (median ≈5 days) was longer than usual in the United States, which may have increased bleeding events. Supplemental doses of UFH were administered to patients randomized to enoxaparin who underwent PCI. For patients randomized to fondaparinux who underwent PCI, the protocol was changed. The original protocol specified that IV fondaparinux be administered to patients undergoing PCI. When this practice was associated with catheter thrombosis, the protocol was changed to recommend administration of supplemental UFH (see Table 18–4 for recommendations) to fondaparinux-treated patients undergoing PCI. As a result, interventional cardiologists may be reluctant to use low-dose fondaparinux in patients undergoing PCI.

Bivalirudin is an IV direct thrombin inhibitor that has been compared to the combination of a heparin, either UFH or enoxaparin, with a GP IIb/IIIa inhibitor in patients with NSTE ACS. Potential advantages of direct thrombin inhibitors over UFH are that they bind to and inhibit clot-bound thrombin in addition to circulating thrombin, and they have no significant binding to plasma proteins so they have a more predictable anticoagulant response. In addition, because thrombin is a potent stimulus for platelet aggregation, direct thrombin inhibitors have antiplatelet as well as anticoagulant activity. Like lepirudin, bivalirudin exhibits bivalent binding to thrombin, that is, it binds to both the active site and exosite-1, although argatroban binds to only to the active site. Unlike lepirudin, both argatroban and bivalirudin exhibit reversible binding to thrombin, whereas lepirudin binds irreversibly. After bivalirudin binds to thrombin, thrombin cleaves a bivalirudin Arg3–Pro4 bond, reexposing the thrombin catalytic site.[104] Thus, bivalirudin provides consistent anticoagulation when administered as an IV bolus and infusion, but its activity is short lived when the drug is discontinued. These potential advantages suggest that bivalirudin may have similar or superior efficacy and fewer bleeding complications compared to traditional anticoagulants.

In the Acute Catheterization and Urgent Intervention Triage Strategy (ACUITY) trial, 13,819 patients with NSTE ACS at moderate to high risk of death or MI (expected to undergo coronary angiography within the first 48–72 hours of hospital admission) were randomized to one of three antithrombotic treatment strategies: (1) heparin (UFH or enoxaparin) plus a GP IIb/IIIa inhibitor, (2) bivalirudin plus GP IIb/IIIa inhibitor, or (3) bivalirudin alone in a noninferiority trial (see Table 18–4 for dosing).[104] The primary end point was "net clinical outcome" at 30 days, which was a quadruple end point consisting of the composite ischemic end point (death, MI, or unplanned revascularization for ischemia) plus non-CABG major bleeding. The results of the quadruple end point were that bivalirudin alone was noninferior to bivalirudin plus a GP IIb/IIIa inhibitor and superior to heparin plus a GP IIb/IIIa inhibitor. The benefit of bivalirudin alone was that it reduced the rate of major bleeding by 47% compared to heparin plus a GP IIb/IIIa receptor inhibitor. Although numerically higher in the bivalirudin group, the ischemic end points were not statistically different between the groups.[105]

With similar efficacy and a lower bleeding rate, on the surface bivalirudin alone appears the preferred therapy. However, several issues surround the study design and application to practice. The main issue surrounds the noninferiority margin of 25% used in the trial. This means that bivalirudin could be 25% "worse" than heparin plus GP IIb/IIIa inhibitor treatment and still be called "noninferior." In fact, the upper boundary of the 95% confidence interval for the ischemic composite end point comparing bivalirudin alone with heparin plus a GP IIb/IIIa inhibitor was 1.24.[105] Other contemporary NSTE ACS trials, such as SYNERGY (Superior Yield of the New Strategy of Enoxaparin, Revascularization, and Glycoprotein Inhibitors), have used lower margins. More than 60% of patients received on average more than 14 hours of prerandomized treatment prior to study enrollment and were "crossed over" to study medications.[105] Study medications were administered for a median duration of less than 6 hours before coronary angiography and PCI, and the overall duration of study drug administration was less than 18 hours because most study drugs were discontinued after angiography.[105] Therefore, although patients were randomized, there was potential for the prerandomization therapy to impact study outcomes. Some have questioned whether the short duration of treatment was long enough to impact outcomes. Therefore, although bivalirudin is a choice for higher-risk patients anticipated to undergo angiography and PCI, it was not given a "preferred" recommendation in the 2007 NSTE ACS guidelines.

Because a variety of anticoagulants are recommended by the guidelines, practitioners should be familiar with the study designs, patient demographics, and results for recent NSTE ACS studies and develop protocols for dosing each agent that is on the hospital formulary.

Nitrates

In patients with ischemic chest discomfort, SL NTG 0.4 mg every 5 minutes for a total of three doses should be administered. IV NTG should be administered to all patients with NSTE ACS who have persistent ischemia, heart failure symptoms, or hypertension in the absence of contraindications (see Table 18–4).[2] The mechanism of action, dosing, contraindications, and adverse effects are the same as described in the section on Early Pharmacotherapy for STE ACS above. IV NTG typically is continued for approximately 24 hours following ischemia relief. The mechanism of action, dosing, contraindications, and adverse effects are the same as described in the section on Early Pharmacotherapy for STE ACS above.

β-Blockers

Oral β-blockers should be administered to all patients with NSTE ACS in the absence of contraindications.[2] IV β-blockers should be considered in hemodynamically stable patients who present with persistent ischemia, hypertension, or tachycardia. The mechanism of action, dosing, contraindications, and adverse effects are the same as described in the section on Early Pharmacotherapy for STE ACS above. β-Blockers are continued indefinitely.

Calcium Channel Blockers

Calcium channel blockers should not be administered to most patients with ACS.[2] Their role is a second-line treatment for patients with certain contraindications to β-blockers (as described in Table 18–4) and those with continued ischemia despite β-blocker and nitrate therapy. They are a first-line therapy for patients with Prinzmetal vasospastic angina and those with cocaine-associated ACS. Administration of amlodipine, diltiazem, or verapamil is preferred.[2] Agent selection based on heart rate and LV dysfunction (diltiazem and verapamil contraindicated in patients with bradycardia, heart block, or systolic heart failure) is described in more detail in the section on Early Pharmacotherapy for STE ACS above. Dosing and contraindications are described in Table 18–4.

Glycemic Control

Numerous guidelines and standards address the management of diabetes mellitus in the outpatient setting, but only recently has sufficient evidence warranted the development of standards of care to optimize inpatient glycemic control for hospitalized individuals with diabetes or illness-induced hyperglycemia. A joint practice guideline from the American Diabetes Association and the American College of Endocrinology recommends that the blood glucose level in critically ill patients, such as those with ACS, be kept as close as possible to 110 mg/dL (6.1 mmol/L).[106] This is supported by the 2004 ACC/AHA STEMI guidelines that recommend normalization of blood glucose during the first 24 to 48 hours of care.[3] Elevated blood glucose levels are associated with higher mortality rates and larger infarct size in patients with acute MI.[106] Beneficial outcomes associated with "tight" glucose control include reductions in the development of renal dysfunction, infections, and length of mechanical ventilation.[3,106] A meta-analysis of 35 clinical trials found a 15% reduction in mortality.[107] IV insulin infusions are commonly administered to critically ill patients hospitalized in the intensive care unit to maintain euglycemia.[3] Additional information on management of hyperglycemia in the hospitalized patient can be found in Chapter 77.

■ SECONDARY PREVENTION FOLLOWING MI

The long-term goals following MI are as follow:

1. Control modifiable CHD risk factors
2. Prevent development of systolic heart failure
3. Prevent recurrent MI and stroke
4. Prevent death, including sudden cardiac death

❾ Pharmacotherapy that has been proven to decrease mortality, heart failure, reinfarction, or stroke should be initiated prior to hospital discharge for secondary prevention. Guidelines from the ACC/AHA suggest that following MI from either STE or NSTE ACS, patients should receive indefinite treatment with aspirin, a β-blocker, and an ACE inhibitor.[2,3,108] All patients should receive SL NTG or lingual spray and instructions for use in case of recurrent ischemic chest discomfort.[2] Clopidogrel should be considered for most patients, but the duration of therapy is individualized according to the type of ACS and whether the patient is treated medically or undergoes intracoronary stent implantation.[2] All patients should receive annual influenza vaccination.[108,109] Selected patients (described below in Anticoagulation) also should be treated with long-term warfarin anticoagulation. Newer therapies include eplerenone, an aldosterone antagonist for heart failure. For all ACS patients, treatment and control of modifiable risk factors, such as hypertension, dyslipidemia, and diabetes mellitus, are essential. Most patients with CHD will require drug therapy for dyslipidemia, usually with a statin (hydroxymethylglutaryl coenzyme A reductase inhibitor). Benefits and adverse effects of long-term treatment with these medications are discussed in more detail below.

Aspirin

Aspirin decreases the risk of death, recurrent MI, and stroke following MI. An aspirin prescription at hospital discharge is a quality care indicator in MI patients (see Table 18–3).[33] The clinical value of aspirin in secondary prevention of ACS and other vascular diseases was demonstrated in a large number of clinical trials. Following an MI, aspirin is expected to prevent 36 vascular events per 1,000 patients treated for 2 years.[46] Because the benefit of antiplatelet agents appears to be sustained for at least 2 years following an MI,[49] aspirin should be given indefinitely to all patients, or clopidogrel to patients with a contraindication to aspirin.[2,3]

The risk of major bleeding from chronic aspirin therapy is approximately 2% and is dose related. Although high doses of aspirin (>325 mg daily) are well established to have a higher risk of bleeding compared to lower doses, whether dose of 75 to 100 mg daily have a lower bleeding risk than doses >100 to 325 mg daily remains controversial.[48,50] After an initial dose of 325 mg, chronic therapy with aspirin should be 75 to 81 mg once daily. The exception is patients in the setting of recent intracoronary stent placement for whom the AHA/ACC recommend 162–325 mg of aspirin once daily for at least 30 days following placement of a bare-metal stent, 3 months after a sirolimus-coated stent, and 6 months after a paclitaxel-coated, followed thereafter by a daily dose of 75 to 162 mg.[40]

In order to minimize the risk of bleeding, use of aspirin with other agents that can induce bleeding, including clopidogrel and warfarin, should be avoided, unless the combination is clinically indicated and the increased risk of bleeding has been considered in evaluating the potential benefit of using such a combination.

Other gastrointestinal disturbances, including dyspepsia and nausea, are infrequent when low-dose aspirin is used.[46]

Thienopyridines

For patients with NSTE ACS, clopidogrel decreases the risk of developing death, MI, or stroke. The benefit derives primarily from reducing the rate of MI.[79] Most patients with NSTE ACS should receive clopidogrel, in addition to aspirin, for up to 12 months.[2,108] For patients with an STEMI treated medically without revascularization including PCI or CABG, clopidogrel can be given for 14 to 28 days.[53,54] In patients in whom an intracoronary stent has been implanted, clopidogrel can be continued for up to 12 months in patients at low risk for bleeding, with a minimum duration of treatment contingent upon the type of stent placed.[2,48]

The most common adverse effects in patients receiving clopidogrel are rash (5%) and gastrointestinal upset (3%).[79]

Anticoagulation

Warfarin should be considered in selected patients following an ACS, including patients with an LV thrombus, patients demonstrating extensive ventricular wall-motion abnormalities on cardiac echocardiogram, and patients with a history of thromboembolic disease or chronic atrial fibrillation.[3] A more detailed discussion regarding the use of warfarin is given in Chapter 21.

Because of the importance of thrombus formation in the pathophysiology of ACS and the findings from several studies suggesting residual thrombus at the site of plaque rupture even months following an MI, anticoagulants, primarily warfarin, have been the subject of many clinical trials of patients after an ACS. These trials have produced varying and inconsistent results. Because the intensity of anticoagulation varied among these trials, it is important to take into consideration the intensity of the anticoagulation when interpreting the results of these trials.

Data from two large, randomized trials demonstrate that use of low, fixed-dose warfarin (mean INR 1.4) combined with aspirin[110] or of low-intensity anticoagulation (mean INR 1.8) monotherapy[111] provided no significant clinical benefit compared with aspirin monotherapy but significantly increased the risk of major bleeding. Therefore, warfarin therapy targeted to INR <2 cannot be recommended for secondary prevention of CHD events following MI.

Subsequently, in two other large, randomized trials, a strategy of combining intermediate-intensity anticoagulation (target INR 2–2.5) with low-dose aspirin reduced the combined end point of death, MI, or stroke in patients following MI compared with aspirin alone. The Antithrombotics in Secondary Prevention of Events in Coronary Thrombosis-2 (ASPECT-2)[112] and the Warfarin-Aspirin Re-Infarction Study (WARIS II)[113] reported that warfarin alone targeted to a high-intensity INR and medium-intensity warfarin plus low-dose aspirin were superior to aspirin alone in preventing the combined end point of death, MI, or stroke. The target INR in the high-intensity warfarin monotherapy group was 3 to 4[111] and 2.8 to 4.2,[113] respectively. The target INR in the more effective medium-intensity warfarin and low-dose aspirin group was 2 to 2.5 in both trials. No significant differences in efficacy were observed between the combination of medium-intensity anticoagulation and low-dose aspirin and monotherapy with high-intensity anticoagulation. A meta-analysis of 14 clinical trials in more than 25,000 patients following either STE or NSTE MI found that the addition of warfarin (target INR of 2 to 3) to aspirin reduced the risk of death, MI or stroke, whereas the addition of warfarin with a target INR outside this target was of no benefit.[114] Nonetheless, this benefit was obtained at the cost of doubling the risk of major bleeding.[114]

Many consider this net benefit to be small in comparison with the large management issues related to warfarin therapy, such as INR monitoring and drug interactions. In the meta-analysis described above,[114] the NNT to prevent one event was 33, whereas the number needed to harm (NNH) was 100. In addition, WARIS II and ASPECT-2 were conducted in the Netherlands and in Norway, two countries renowned for the quality of their anticoagulation programs and clinics, thereby limiting generalization of the findings. Furthermore, a large proportion of ACS patients in North America undergo coronary revascularization with subsequent intracoronary stent implementation for which patients require a combination of aspirin and clopidogrel to prevent stent thrombosis, a platelet-dependent phenomenon that warfarin does not effectively prevent.[115] Therefore, because of the complexity of managing current anticoagulants, use of warfarin is unlikely to gain wide acceptance (see Clinical Controversies). Despite the superiority of warfarin plus aspirin over aspirin alone, warfarin currently is not recommended as a preferred regimen by any professional association practice guidelines in the absence of the conditions for selected patients outlined previously.

CLINICAL CONTROVERSIES

No prospective, randomized trials have evaluated whether the addition of warfarin to aspirin plus clopidogrel therapy is safe or effective. However, the combination is used in select patients in practice. Clinical situations in which aspirin, clopidogrel, and warfarin can be used together include placement of an intracoronary stent (where aspirin and clopidogrel are indicated) in patients with an indication for anticoagulant therapy including atrial fibrillation, acute deep vein thrombosis, presence of a mechanical heart valve, and MI with a low EF. In such cases, the duration of use of this triple antithrombotic drug combination should be minimized and the INR monitored closely. The most recent guidelines from the ACC/AHA recommend a lower target INR of 2.0 to 2.5 in patients receiving this combination, but no prospective randomized trials have been reported.[2]

β-Blockers, Nitrates, and Calcium Channel Blockers

Current treatment guidelines recommend that, following an ACS, patients should receive a β-blocker indefinitely,[2,3,107] whether or not they have residual symptoms of angina.[116] β-Blocker prescription at hospital discharge in the absence of contraindications is a quality performance measure (see Table 18–3).[33] Overwhelming data support the use of β-blockers in patients with a previous MI. Data from a systematic review of long-term trials of patients with recent MI demonstrate that the NNT for 1 year with a β-blocker to prevent one death is only 84 patients.[116] Because the benefit from β-blockers appears to be maintained for at least 6 years following an MI,[117] it is recommended that all patients receive β-blockers indefinitely in the absence of contraindications or intolerance.[2,3] Currently, no data support the superiority of one β-blocker over another. Although β-blockers with intrinsic sympathomimetic actvity are generally not recommended, one study of modest size showed that acebutolol, a β-blocker with intrinsic sympathomimetic activity, was beneficial following MI.[118]

Although β-blockers should be avoided in patients with decompensated heart failure from LV systolic dysfunction complicating an MI, clinical trial data suggest that initiation of β-blockers prior to hospital discharge is safe in these patients once heart failure symptoms have resolved.[119] These patients actually may benefit more than those without LV dysfunction.[120]

Despite the overwhelming benefit demonstrated in clinical trials, β-blockers are still widely underused, perhaps because clinicians fear that patients will experience adverse reactions, including depression, fatigue, and sexual dysfunction. A systematic review of 15 trials that included more than 35,000 patients demonstrated that withholding β-blocker therapy in such a group was unfounded because β-blockers do not significantly increase the risk of depression and only modestly increase the risk of fatigue and sexual dysfunction.[121]

In patients who cannot tolerate or have a contraindication to a β-blocker, a calcium channel blocker can be used to prevent anginal symptoms but should not be used routinely in the absence of such symptoms.[2,3,122] Finally, all patients should be prescribed short-acting SL NTG or lingual NTG spray to relieve any anginal symptoms when necessary and should be instructed on its use.[2,3] Chronic long-acting nitrate therapy has not been shown to reduce CHD events following MI. Therefore, IV NTG is not followed routinely by chronic, long-acting oral nitrate therapy in ACS patients who have undergone revascularization unless they have chronic stable angina or significant coronary stenoses that were not revascularized.[122]

ACE Inhibitors and Angiotensin Receptor Blockers

ACE inhibitors should be initiated in all patients following MI to reduce mortality, decrease reinfarction, and prevent development of heart failure.[2,3,108] Dosing and contraindications are described in Table 18–4. The benefit of ACE inhibitors in patients with MI most likely derives from their ability to prevent cardiac remodeling. Other proposed mechanisms include improvement in endothelial function, reduction in atrial and ventricular arrhythmias, and promotion of angiogenesis, leading to a reduction in ischemic events. The largest reduction in mortality is observed for patients with LV dysfunction (low LVEF) or heart failure symptoms. Use of ACE inhibitors in relatively unselected patients without a contraindication to ACE inhibitors can be expected to save five lives per 1,000 patients treated for 30 days.[123] Long-term studies in patients with LV systolic dysfunction with or without heart failure symptoms demonstrate greater benefit because mortality reductions are larger (23.4% vs 29.1%; $P < 0.0001$) such that only 17 patients need treatment to prevent one death, with 57 lives saved for every 1,000 patients treated.[124] ACE inhibitor prescription at hospital discharge following MI, in the absence of contraindications, to patients with depressed LV function (EF <40%) currently is a quality care indicator, and plans are being made to make administration of an ACE inhibitor in all patients without contraindications a quality care indicator (see Table 18–3).[33]

Early initiation (within 24 hours) of an *oral* ACE inhibitor appears to be crucial during an acute MI because 40% of the 30-day survival benefit is observed during the first day, 45% from days 2 to 7, and approximately only 15% from days 8 to 30.[123] However, current data do not support the early administration of *IV* ACE inhibitors in patients experiencing an MI because mortality may be increased.[125] Hypotension should be avoided because coronary artery filling may be compromised. Because the benefits of ACE inhibitor administration have been documented for up to 12 years following therapy for 2 to 4 years post- MI in patients with LV dysfunction,[124,126] administration should continue indefinitely.

Additional data suggest that most patients with CAD, not just ACS or heart failure, benefit from an ACE inhibitor. In the Heart Outcome Prevention Evaluation (HOPE) trial, ramipril significantly reduced the risk of death, MI, or stroke in high-risk patients aged 55 years or older with chronic CAD or with diabetes and one cardiovascular risk factor.[127] The European Trial on Reduction of Cardiac Events with Perindopril in Stable Coronary Artery Disease (EUROPA) extended the benefit of chronic therapy with ACE inhibitors, in this case perindopril, to patients with stable CAD at moderate risk for cardiovascular events.[128] However, a trial of low-risk patients with stable CAD and normal LV function has suggested that the benefit of ACE inhibitors may not extend to these populations.[129] Importantly, in this trial, patients were treated more aggressively with both medical therapy and revascularization than in HOPE and EUROPA, and risk factors were more optimally managed. Recent AHA/ACC guidelines on secondary prevention of coronary and other vascular diseases have highlighted that although an ACE inhibitor should be started and continued indefinitely in all patients with LVEF ≤40% and in those with hypertension, diabetes, or chronic kidney disease, unless contraindicated, and that these agents should be considered for all other patients, use of ACE inhibitors may be considered optional in low-risk patients with normal LVEF in whom cardiovascular risk factors are well controlled and revascularization has been performed.[108] Therefore, although all patients with an ACS initially should be treated with an ACE inhibitor, it may be appropriate to reevaluate their long-term use in selected low-risk individuals who may want to limit the number of medications they receive.

Many patients cannot tolerate chronic ACE inhibitor therapy secondary to adverse effects outlined in the next paragraph. However, trials have documented that the angiotensin receptor blockers (ARBs) candesartan and valsartan improve clinical outcomes in patients with heart failure.[130,131] Therefore, either an ACE inhibitor or candesartan or valsartan is an acceptable choice for chronic therapy for patients with a low EF and heart failure following MI. Because more than five different ACE inhibitors have proven benefits in MI but only two ARBs have been studied, the benefits of ACE inhibitors are generally considered a class effect while the benefits of ARBs are still under study. ACE inhibitor prescription (or alternatively an ARB) at hospital discharge following MI, in the absence of contraindications, to patients with depressed LV function (EF <40%) currently is a quality performance measure,[33] and plans are being made to make administration of an ACE inhibitor in all patients without contraindications a quality care measure.

Besides hypotension, the most frequent adverse reaction to an ACE inhibitor is cough, which may occur in up to 30% of patients. Patients with ACE inhibitor cough and either clinical signs of heart failure or LVEF <40% can be prescribed an ARB.[3] Other less common but more serious adverse effects of ACE inhibitors and ARBs include acute renal failure and hyperkalemia. Although the incidence of angioedema appears higher in patients receiving ACE inhibitors (0.1%–1.0% with ACE inhibitor), ARBs also have been associated with angioedema, including recurrent angioedema in patients with a history of angioedema while receiving an ACE inhibitor.[132] Therefore, although ARBs are not contraindicated, the severity of angioedema while receiving an ACE inhibitor (e.g., tongue or laryngeal edema necessitating intubation and mechanical ventilation) should be considered before starting an ARB in a patient with prior ACE inhibitor-associated angioedema.

Although some data have suggested that aspirin use may decrease the benefits of ACE inhibitor treatment, a systematic review of more than 20,000 patients demonstrated that ACE inhibitors improve outcome irrespective of treatment with aspirin.[133]

Aldosterone Antagonists

Administration of an aldosterone antagonist, either eplerenone or spironolactone, should be considered within the first 2 weeks following MI in all patients already receiving an ACE inhibitor who have EF ≤40% and either heart failure symptoms or a diagnosis of diabetes mellitus to reduce mortality.[3,108] Aldosterone plays an important role in heart failure and MI because it promotes vascular and myocardial fibrosis, endothelial dysfunction, hypertension, LV hypertrophy, sodium retention, potassium and magnesium loss, and arrhythmias. Experimental and human studies have shown that aldosterone blockers attenuate these adverse effects.[134] As discussed in Chapter 16, the benefit of aldosterone blockade in patients with stable, severe heart failure was highlighted in the Randomized Aldactone Evaluation Study (RALES), in which spironolactone decreased the risk of all-cause mortality.[135]

Eplerenone, like spironolactone, is an aldosterone blocker that blocks the mineralocorticoid receptor. In contrast to spironolactone, eplerenone has no effect on the progesterone or androgen receptor, thereby minimizing the risk of gynecomastia, sexual dysfunction, and menstrual irregularities.[134] The Eplerenone Post-Acute Myocardial Infarction Heart Failure Efficacy and Survival Study (EPHESUS) evaluated the effect of aldosterone antagonism in patients with an MI complicated by heart failure or LV dysfunction. Patients ($n = 6{,}642$) were randomized 3 to 14 days following the MI to eplerenone or placebo.[136] Eplerenone significantly reduced the risk of mortality (14.4% vs 16.7%; $P = 0.008$). Data from EPHESUS suggest that eplerenone reduced mortality from sudden death, heart failure, and MI. Eplerenone also reduced the risk of hospitalizations for heart failure. Most patients in EPHESUS also were being treated with aspirin, a β-blocker, and an ACE inhibitor. Approximately half the patients were also receiving a statin. Therefore, the mortality reduction observed was in addition to that resulting from standard therapy for secondary CHD prevention. These benefits were obtained at the expense of an increased risk of severe hyperkalemia (5.5% vs 3.9%; $P = 0.002$), defined as a potassium concentration ≥6 mEq/L. Patients with serum creatinine concentration >2.5 mg/dL or serum potassium concentration >5 mEq/L at baseline were excluded. The risk of hyperkalemia was particularly alarming in patients with creatinine clearance <50 mL/min. This highlights the importance of close monitoring of potassium levels and renal function in patients being treated with eplerenone. No increase in gynecomastia, breast pain, or impotence was noted.

The results from EPHESUS have raised the question of which aldosterone blocker, spironolactone or eplerenone, should be used preferentially. Currently, no data support that the more selective but more expensive eplerenone is superior to, or should be preferred to, the less expensive generic spironolactone unless a patient has experienced gynecomastia, breast pain, or impotence while receiving spironolactone. Finally, it should be noted that hyperkalemia is just as likely to appear with both these agents.

Lipid-Lowering Agents

Overwhelming data now support the benefits of statins in patients with CAD for the prevention of total mortality, cardiovascular mortality, and stroke. According to the National Cholesterol Education Program (NCEP) Adult Treatment Panel recommendations, all patients with CAD should receive dietary counseling and pharmacologic therapy in order to reach a low-density lipoprotein (LDL) cholesterol concentration <100 mg/dL, with statins the preferred agents for lowering LDL cholesterol.[108,137,138] Although the primary effect of statins is to decrease LDL cholesterol, statins are believed to produce many non–lipid-lowering or "pleiotropic" effects. These effects, which include improvement in endothelial dysfunction, antiinflammatory and antithrombotic properties, and decreased matrix metalloproteinase activity, may be relevant in patients experiencing an ACS and result in short-term (<1 year) benefit. In a meta-analysis of randomized, controlled clinical trials of almost 18,000 patients with recent ACS (<14 days), statin therapy reduced mortality by 19%, with benefits observed after approximately 4 months of treatment.[139]

Newer recommendations from the NCEP give an optional goal of LDL cholesterol <70 mg/dL for secondary prevention.[2,138] This recommendation is based upon a large clinical trial evaluating recurrence of major cardiovascular events in patients with a history of an ACS occurring within the past 10 days. This trial documented the benefit of lowering LDL cholesterol to, on average, 62 mg/dL, with 80 mg of atorvastatin compared to 95 mg/dL in patients treated with pravastatin 40 mg daily.[140] Whether a statin should be used routinely in all patients irrespective of their baseline LDL cholesterol level is currently being investigated, but preliminary data from the Heart Protection Study suggest that patients benefit from statin therapy irrespective of their baseline LDL cholesterol level.[141] The 2007 ACC/AHA NSTE ACS guidelines recommend statin therapy, in addition to diet, for all ACS patients, regardless of LDL cholesterol level, although the exact target LDL, if the patient's LDL cholesterol at hospital presentation is already <70 mg/dL is not stated.[2]

A fibrate or niacin should be considered in selective patients with a low high-density lipoprotein (HDL) cholesterol concentration (<40 mg/dL) and/or a high triglyceride level (>200 mg/dL).[2,108,137] In a large, randomized trial of men with established CAD and low levels of HDL cholesterol, use of gemfibrozil (600 mg twice daily) significantly decreased the risk of nonfatal MI or death from coronary causes.[142] No such benefit was observed with fenofibrate in a large multicenter primary and secondary prevention study in patients with diabetes mellitus.[143] Due to the increased risk of myopathy, gemfibrozil is not recommended in patients receiving a statin.[144]

Additional discussion, dosing, monitoring, and adverse effects of using lipid-lowering drugs for secondary prevention can be found in Chapter 23.

Fish Oils (Marine-Derived ω-3 Fatty Acids)

Eicosapentaenoic acid (EPA) and docosahexaenoic acid (DHA) are ω-3 polyunsaturated fatty acids that are most abundant in fatty fish such as sardines, salmon, and mackerel. Epidemiologic and randomized trials have demonstrated that a diet high in EPA plus DHA or supplementation with these fish oils reduces the risk of cardiovascular mortality, reinfarction, and stroke in patients who have experienced an MI.[145] Although the exact mechanism responsible for the beneficial effects of ω-3 fatty acids has not been clearly elucidated, potential mechanisms include triglyceride-lowering effects, antithrombotic effects, retardation in the progression of atherosclerosis, endothelial relaxation, mild antihypertensive effects, and reduction in ventricular arrhythmias.[145]

The Gruppo Italiano per lo Studio della Sopravvivenza nell'Infarcto (GISSI)-Prevenzione trial, the largest randomized trial of fish oils published to date, evaluated the effects of open-label EPA plus DHA (Lovaza) in 11,324 patients with recent MI who were randomized to receive 850 to 882 mg/day of n-3 polyunsaturated fatty acid (EPA plus DHA) at an EPA/DHA ratio of 1.2:1, 300 mg of vitamin E, both, or neither.[146,147] Use of EPA plus DHA reduced the risk of death, nonfatal acute MI, or nonfatal stroke, whereas use of vitamin E had no significant impact on this combined clinical end point. Therefore, based on current data, the AHA recommends that CHD patients consume approximately 1 g EPA plus DHA per day, preferably from oily fish.[108,145] Because oil content in fish varies, the number of 6-oz servings of fish that would need to be consumed to provide 7 g EPA plus DHA per week varies from approximately four to more than 14 for secondary prevention. The average diet only contains one tenth to one fifth the recommended amount.[145] Supplements could be considered in selected patients who do not eat fish, have limited access to fish, or who cannot afford to purchase fish. Approximately three 1-g fish oil capsules per day should be consumed to provide 1 g of ω-3 fatty acids, depending on the brand of supplement.[145] Alternatively, the prescription drug Lovaza can be used at a dose of 1 g/day. Finally, current guidelines suggest that higher doses of EPA plus DHA (2–4 g/day) can be considered for the management of hypertriglyceridemia.[2,108,145] Adverse effects from fish oils include fishy aftertaste, nausea, and diarrhea.[145]

Other Modifiable Risk Factors

Smoking cessation, control of hypertension, weight loss, and tight glucose control for patients with diabetes mellitus, in addition to treatment of dyslipidemia, are important treatments for secondary prevention of CHD events.[3,108] All patients with CAD should receive annual influenza vaccination.[108,109] Influenza-related deaths are highest among patients with CVD compared to patients with other medical conditions.[109] Randomized controlled clinical trials have shown that annual influenza vaccination reduces cardiovascular mortality and MI.[109] Smoking cessation is accompanied by a significant reduction in all-cause mortality in patients with CAD.[148] Smoking cessation counseling at the time of discharge following MI is a quality care indicator (see Table 18–3).[33] Use of nicotine patches or gum or of bupropion alone or in combination with nicotine patches should be considered in appropriate patients.[3] Following MI, hypertension should be strictly controlled to a target blood pressure <130/80 and even lower, and to <120/80 in patients with LV dysfunction according to recently published guidelines from AHA.[51] Patients who are overweight should be educated on the importance of regular exercise, healthy eating habits, and of reaching and maintaining an ideal weight.[149] Finally, because diabetics have up to a fourfold increased risk of mortality compared with nondiabetics, the importance of tight glucose control, as well as other CHD risk factor modification, cannot be understated.[150]

Therapies Not Useful and Potentially Harmful following MI

Administration of hormone-replacement therapy to all women following MI does not prevent recurrent CHD events and may be harmful.[151,152] According to the NSTE and NSTE ACS guidelines, postmenopausal women already taking estrogen plus progestin should not continue, especially while at bedrest in hospital, because of an increased risk of venous thromboembolism.[2,3] The U.S. Preventative Services Task Force as well as the ACC/AHA have concluded that the administration of vitamins A, C, or E, multivitamins with vitamins B_6, B_{12}, folic acid, or a combination of antioxidants for secondary prevention are ineffective following MI.[2,146,153–157] Furthermore, they caution against the use of β-carotene supplementation, particularly in heavy smokers, because of an apparent increased risk of lung cancer.[154] A stepped-care approach using acetaminophen, small doses of narcotics, and nonacetylated salicylates are preferable to COX-2–selective NSAIDs for treatment of chronic musculoskeletal pain. Use of the nonselective NSAID naproxen is recommended over more COX-2–selective agents, which have been associated with risks for MI.[2]

ADHERENCE TO THERAPY

Medication noncompliance poses a problem in patients following ACS. Medication discontinuation has been associated with an increased risk of cardiovascular events and mortality in patients with various types of CVD.[158–160] In clinical trials, poor adherence is associated with poor outcome, regardless of treatment assignment,[160] highlighting that this behavior may be related with other health-related behaviors in patients. Increased adherence to statins and β-blockers has been associated with lower long-term mortality.[161]

The discontinuation of clopidogrel may be particularly problematic in patients treated with a drug-eluting stent,[162] because this action places the patient at increased risk for stent thrombosis.[55] Current data suggest that long-term adherence and persistence to statins in patients with an ACS and in patients with chronic CAD is variable.[163–166] Early initiation of statins in patients with ACS appears to increase long-term adherence with statin therapy, which should result in clinical benefit.[139] Therefore, statin therapy initiation should not be delayed in patients with an ACS, and statins should be prescribed at or prior to discharge in most patients.

Several clinical trials have documented the value of a pharmacist in the management of improving adherence and persistence to medication, which in turn can significantly improve the treatment of risk factors such as hypertension, heart failure, and dyslipidemia.[167,168]

TABLE 18-7 Therapeutic Drug Monitoring for Adverse Effects of Pharmacotherapy for Acute Coronary Syndromes

Drug	Adverse Effects	Monitoring
Aspirin	Dyspepsia, bleeding, gastritis	Clinical signs of bleeding,[a] gastrointestinal upset; baseline CBC and platelet count; CBC platelet count every 6 months
Clopidogrel	Bleeding, TTP (rare), diarrhea, rash	Clinical signs of bleeding[a]; baseline CBC and platelet count; CBC and platelet count every 6 months following hospital discharge
Unfractionated heparin	Bleeding, heparin-induced thrombocytopenia	Clinical signs of bleeding[a]; baseline CBC, platelet count, aPTT and INR; aPTT every 6 hours until target then every 24 hours; daily CBC; platelet count every 2 days (minimum, preferably every day)
Low-molecular-weight heparins (enoxaparin and dalteparin)	Bleeding, heparin-induced thrombocytopenia	Clinical signs of bleeding[a]; baseline CBC, platelet count, SCr, aPTT and INR; daily CBC, platelet count every 2–3 days (minimum, preferably every day); SCr daily
Fondaparinux	Bleeding	Clinical signs of bleeding,[a] baseline CBC, platelet count, INR, SCr, and aPTT; daily CBC and SCr
Bivalirudin	Bleeding	Clinical signs of bleeding,[a] baseline CBC, platelet count, INR, SCr, and aPTT; daily CBC and SCr
Fibrinolytics	Bleeding, especially intracranial hemorrhage	Clinical signs of bleeding,[a] baseline CBC, platelet count, INR, and aPTT; mental status every 2 hours for signs of intracranial hemorrhage; daily CBC
Glycoprotein IIb/IIIa receptor blockers	Bleeding, acute profound thrombocytopenia	Clinical signs of bleeding,[a] baseline CBC and platelet count; daily CBC; platelet count at 4 hours after initiation then daily
Intravenous nitrates	Hypotension, flushing, headache, tachycardia	BP and HR every 2 hours
β-Blockers	Hypotension, bradycardia, heart block, bronchospasm, heart failure, fatigue, depression, sexual dysfunction, nightmares, masking hypoglycemia symptoms in diabetic patients	BP, RR, HR, 12-lead ECG, and clinical signs of heart failure every 5 minutes during bolus intravenous dosing; BP, RR, HR, and clinical signs of heart failure every shift during oral administration during hospitalization, then BP and HR every 6 months following hospital discharge
Diltiazem or verapamil	Hypotension, bradycardia, heart block, heart failure, gingival hyperplasia, constipation	BP and HR and signs of clinical heart failure every shift during oral administration during hospitalization, then every 6 months following hospital discharge; dental examination and teeth cleaning every 6 months
Amlodipine	Hypotension, dependent peripheral edema, gingival hyperplasia	BP every shift during hospitalization, then every 6 months following hospital discharge; dental examination and teeth cleaning every 6 months
Angiotensin-converting enzyme (ACE) inhibitors and angiotensin receptor blockers (ARBs)	Hypotension, cough (with ACE inhibitors), hyperkalemia, prerenal azotemia, angioedema (ACE inhibitors >ARBs)	BP every 2 hours × 3 for first dose, then shift during oral administration during hospitalization, then once every 6 months following hospital discharge; baseline SCr and potassium; daily SCr and potassium while hospitalized, then every 6 months (or 1–2 weeks after each outpatient dose titration); closer monitoring required in selected patients (e.g., those taking spironolactone or eplerenone or with renal insufficiency); counsel patient on throat, tongue, and facial swelling
Aldosterone antagonists	Hypotension, hyperkalemia, prerenal azotemia	BP and HR every shift during oral administration during hospitalization, then once every 6 months; baseline SCr and serum potassium concentration; SCr and potassium at 48 hours, monthly for 3 months then every 3 months thereafter
Statins	Myalgia, myopathy, elevated LFTs, rhabdomyolysis, teratogenic in first trimester	Baseline LFTs, then repeat LFTs at 6 weeks and when patient titrated to target maintenance dose; if LFTs >3 times upper limit of normal, decrease dose or discontinue; if myalgia and/or brown urine, monitor creatine kinase for rhabdomyolysis
Morphine sulfate	Hypotension, respiratory depression	BP and RR 5 minutes after each bolus dose

[a]Clinical signs of bleeding include bloody stools, melena, hematuria, hematemesis, and bruising and oozing from arterial or venous puncture sites.

aPTT, activated partial thromboplastin time; BP, blood pressure; CBC, complete blood count; ECG, electrocardiogram; HR, heart rate; INR, international normalized ratio; LFT, liver function test; RR, respiratory rate; SCr, serum creatinine, TTP, thrombotic thrombocytopenic purpura.

PHARMACOECONOMIC CONSIDERATIONS

The risks of CHD events, such as death, recurrent MI, and stroke, are higher for patients with established CHD and a history of MI than for patients with no known CHD. Because the costs for chronic preventative pharmacotherapy are the same for primary and secondary prevention while the risk of events is higher with secondary prevention, secondary prevention is more cost effective than primary prevention of CHD.[169] Pharmacotherapy, which has demonstrated cost effectiveness in preventing death in ACS and post-MI patient, includes fibrinolytics ($2,000–$33,000 cost per year of life saved),[169,170] aspirin,[171] GP IIb/IIIa receptor blockers ($13,700–$16,500 per year of life added),[172] β-blockers (<$5,000–$15,000 cost per year of life saved),[173] ACE inhibitors ($3,000–$5,000 cost per year of life saved),[174,175] eplerenone ($15,300–$32,400 per life year gained),[176] statins ($4,500– $9,500 per year of life saved),[177] gemfibrozil ($17,000 per year of life saved),[178] and fish oil.[179] Because cost-effectiveness ratios less than $50,000 per added life-year are considered economically attractive from a societal perspective,[169] pharmacotherapy for ACS and secondary prevention are standards of care because of their efficacy and cost attractiveness to payors.

EVALUATION OF THERAPEUTIC OUTCOMES

The monitoring parameters for *efficacy* of nonpharmacologic and pharmacotherapy for both STE and NSTE ACS are similar:

- Relief of ischemic discomfort
- Return of ECG changes to baseline
- Absence or resolution of heart failure signs

Monitoring parameters for recognition and prevention of *adverse effects* from ACS pharmacotherapy are given in Table 18–7. In general, the most common adverse reactions to ACS therapies are hypotension and bleeding. Treatment for bleeding and hypotension involves discontinuation of the offending agent(s) until symptoms resolve. Severe bleeding resulting in hypotension secondary to hypovolemia may require blood transfusion.

CONCLUSIONS

The AHA and ACC published evidence-based practice guidelines for the treatment of patients with STE and NSTE ACS. Mainstays of therapy include risk stratification, primary PCI for STE ACS, and early angiography and revascularization with either PCI or CABG for patients with NSTE ACS at high risk for MI and death. Pharmacotherapy for acute treatment includes SL NTG, antiplatelets, anticoagulants, and β-blockers. Insulin infusions can be administered to maintain euglycemia in patients with diabetes mellitus. Pharmacotherapy for secondary prevention of recurrent ACS, MI, and CHD death includes aspirin, clopidogrel, lipid-lowering therapy (statin preferred), β-blockers and either an ACE inhibitor or an ARB. Ensuring selection of evidence-based therapies in all patients without contraindications results in lower mortality. Pharmacists have an important role in encouraging patient adherence and persistence to pharmacotherapy.

In January 2008, the AHA/ACC published an update to the 2004 STE MI guidelines. (Antman EM, Hand M, Armstrong PW, et al. 2007 focused update of the ACC/AHA 2004 guidelines for the management of patients with ST-elevation myocardial infarction: A report of the American College of Cardiology/American Heart Association Task Force on Practice Guidelines. Circulation 2008 Jan 15;117(2):296-329.) The most significant changes in this guideline compared to the 2004 guidelines are:

1. Emphasis on oral beta-blocker therapy administered within the first 24 hours with monitoring for hemodynamic instability (hypotension and bradycardia) rather than immediate therapy with intravenous beta-blocker (Class I recommendation).
2. Reinforcement of a short time to reperfusion (Class I recommendations)
   a. If a patient arrives at a hospital capable of performing primary PCI, the hospital arrival-to-balloon time for PCI should be within 90 minutes.
   b. If a patient arrives at a hospital that is not capable of performing primary PCI, the door-to-needle time for initiation of fibrinolytic therapy should be within 30 minutes.
   c. If a patient arrives at a hospital that is not capable of performing primary PCI, the patient can be transferred to a hospital that can perform primary PCI if there is a contraindication to fibrinolysis and PCI can be initiated at the receiving hospital within 90 minutes of arrival at the first hospital or if fibrinolysis was administered but was not successful at opening the coronary artery.
3. A PCI performed after successful fibrinolysis therapy (i.e. facilitated PCI) is associated with excess bleeding, stroke, and mortality risk, and is not recommended (Class III recommendation).
4. Either enoxaparin, UFH, or fondaparinux may be administered in combination with a fibrinolytic agent (Grade I recommendation).
5. For patients undergoing PCI, either UFH, enoxaparin, or fondaparinux in combination with UFH may be administered (Class I recommendations) as fondaparinux alone is associated with PCI-related catheter thrombosis (Class III recommendation).
6. Clopidogrel 75 mg daily (Class I recommendation) should be administered to all patients regardless of whether or not they undergo reperfusion therapy and should be continued for at least 14 days (Class I recommendation) and up to one year (Class IIa recommendation).
7. A loading dose of clopidogrel of 300 mg may be administered as the initial dose (Class IIa recommendation).
8. In patients who do not undergo reperfusion therapy, it is reasonable to administer anticoagulant therapy for the duration of hospitalization, up to 8 days (Class IIa recommendation).
9. In patients requiring warfarin for clinical indications such as atrial fibrillation, atrial flutter, or presence of LV thrombus who also receive clopidogrel and aspirin, it is recommended that the INR be maintained at 2.0 to 2.5 and that a lower dose of aspirin be used, 75 mg to 81 mg (Class I recommendation).
10. Nonselective nonsteroidal antiinflammatory agents (except aspirin) as well as COX-2 selecting antiinflammatory agents should be discontinued at the time of STE MI secondary to increased risk of mortality, reinfarction, heart failure, and myocardial rupture (Class III recommendation).

ABBREVIATIONS

ACC: American College of Cardiology

ACE: angiotensin-converting enzyme

ACS: acute coronary syndrome

ACT: activated clotting time

ACUITY: Acute Catheterization and Urgent Intervention Triage Strategy

ADP: adenosine diphosphate

AHA: American Heart Association

aPTT: activated partial thromboplastin time

ARB: angiotensin receptor blocker

ASPECT: Antithrombotics in Secondary Prevention of Events in Coronary Thrombosis

BNP: brain (B-type) natriuretic peptide

CABG: coronary artery bypass graft

CHD: coronary heart disease

CK: creatine kinase

CREDO: Clopidogrel for the Reduction of Events During Observation

CURE: Clopidogrel in Unstable Angina to Prevent Recurrent Events

CVD: cardiovascular disease

DHA: docosahexaenoic acid

ECG: electrocardiogram

EF: ejection fraction

EPA: eicosapentaenoic acid

EPHESUS: Eplerenone Post-Acute Myocardial Infarction Heart Failure Efficacy and Survival Study

ESPRIT: Enhanced Suppression of the Platelet IIb/IIIa Receptor with Integrilin Therapy

EUROPA: European Trial on Reduction of Cardiac Events with Perindopril in Stable Coronary Artery Disease

ExTRACT: Enoxaparin and Thrombolysis Reperfusion for Acute Myocardial Infarction Treatment

GRACE: Global Registry of Acute Coronary Events

GUSTO: Global Use of Strategies to Open Occluded Arteries

HOPE: Heart Outcomes Prevention Evaluation

ICH: intracranial hemorrhage

INR: international normalized ratio

ISIS-2: Second International Study of Infarct Survival

IV: intravenous

LDL: low-density lipoprotein

LMWH: low-molecular-weight heparin

LV: left ventricular

LVEF: left ventricular ejection fraction

MADIT: Multicenter Automatic Defibrillator Implantation Trial

MB: myocardial band

MI: myocardial infarction

NCEP: National Cholesterol Education Program

NNH: number need to harm

NNT: number needed to treat

NRMI: National Registry of Myocardial Infarction

NSAID: nonsteroidal antiinflammatory drug

NSTE: non–ST-segment elevation

NTG: nitroglycerin

OASIS: Organization for the Assessment of Strategies for Ischemic Syndromes

OAT: Occluded Artery Trial

PCI: percutaneous coronary intervention

PRISM-PLUS: Platelet Receptor Inhibition in Ischemic Syndrome Management in Patients Limited by Unstable Signs and Symptoms

PURSUIT: Platelet Glycoprotein IIb/IIIa in Unstable Angina: Receptor Suppression Using Integrilin Therapy

RALES: Randomized Aldactone Evaluation Study

SL: sublingual

STE: ST-segment elevation

TARGET: Do Tirofiban and ReoPro Give Similar Efficacy Outcomes Trial

TIMI: Thrombolysis in Myocardial Infarction

UFH: unfractionated heparin

WARIS: Warfarin Re-Infarction Study

REFERENCES

1. American Heart Association. Heart Disease and Stroke Statistics—2007, Update. Dallas, TX: American Heart Association, 2007.
2. Anderson JL, Adams CD, Antman EM, et al. ACC/AHA 2007, guidelines for the management of patients with unstable angina/non ST-elevation myocardial infarction: A report of the American College of Cardiology/American Heart Association Task Force on Practice Guidelines (Writing Committee to Revise the 2002 Guidelines for the Management of Patients With Unstable Angina/Non ST-Elevation Myocardial Infarction): Developed in collaboration with the American College of Emergency Physicians, the Society for Cardiovascular Angiography and Interventions, and the Society of Thoracic Surgeons: Endorsed by the American Association of Cardiovascular and Pulmonary Rehabilitation and the Society for Academic Emergency Medicine. Circulation 2007;116:803–877.
3. Antman EM, Anbe DT, Armstrong PW, Bates ER, et al. ACC/AHA guidelines for the management of patients with ST-elevation myocardial infarction: Executive summary. A report of the American College of Cardiology/American Heart Association Task Force on Practice Guidelines (Committee to revise the 1999 Guidelines for the Management of Patients with Acute Myocardial Infarction). Circulation 2004;110:588–636.
4. Centers for Disease Control: Advance Data from Vital and Health Statistics: National Hospital Ambulatory Medical Care Survey: 2002 Emergency Department Summary. *http://www.cdc.gov/nchs/data/ad/ad340.pdf*
5. National Registry of Myocardial Infarction 5. *http://nrmi.org/index.html.*
6. Fox KAA, Steg PG, Eagle KA, et al. Decline in rates of death and heart failure in acute coronary syndromes, 1999–2006. JAMA 2007;297:1892–1900.
7. Gibson CM. NRMI and current treatment patterns for ST-elevation myocardial infarction. Am Heart J 2004;148(5 Suppl):S29–S33.
8. Libby P, Theroux P. Pathophysiology of coronary artery disease. Circulation 2005;111:3481–3488.
9. Fuster V, Moreno PR, Fayad ZA, et al. Atherothrombosis and high-risk plaque: Part I. evolving concepts. J Am Coll Cardiol 2005;46:937–954.
10. Spinler SA. Acute coronary syndromes. In: Dunsworth TS, Richardson MM, Cheng JWM, eds. Pharmacotherapy Self-Assessment Program, Book 1, Cardiology, 6th ed. Kansas City: American College of Clinical Pharmacy, 2007:59–83.
11. Ruberg FL, Leopold JA, Loscalzo J. Atherothrombosis: Plaque instability and thrombogenesis. Prog Cardiovasc Dis 2003;44:381–394.
12. St John Sutton M, Ferrari VA. Prevention of left ventricular remodeling after myocardial infarction. Curr Treat Options Cardiovasc Med 2002;4:97–108.
13. Opie LH, Commerford PJ, Gersh BJ, Pfeffer MA. Controversies in ventricular remodeling. Lancet 2006;367:356–367.
14. Mann DL. Mechanisms and models in heart failure: A combinatorial approach. Circulation 1999;100:999–1008.
15. Babaev A, Frederick PD, Pasta DJ, et al. Trends in management and outcomes of patients with acute myocardial infarction complicated by cardiogenic shock. JAMA 2005;294:448–454.
16. Goldberg RJ, Gore JM, Thompson CA, Gurwitz JH. Recent magnitude of and temporal trends (1994–1997) in the incidence and hospital death rates of cardiogenic shock complicating acute myocardial infarction: The second National Registry of Myocardial Infarction. Am Heart J 2001;141:65–72.
17. Lavie CJ, Gersh BJ. Mechanical and electrical complications of acute myocardial infarction. Mayo Clin Proc 1990;65:709–730. Erratum in Mayo Clin Proc 1990;65:1032.
18. Rosamond,W, Flegal, K Friday, G Furie, K, et al. Heart Association Statistics Committee and Stroke Statistics Subcommittee Heart Disease and Stroke Statistics—2007 Update: A report from the American Heart Association. Circulation 2007;115;169–171.
19. The Joint European Society of Cardiology/American College of Cardiology Committee. Myocardial infarction redefined: A consensus document of the joint European Society of Cardiology/American College of

Cardiology Committee for the Redefinition of Myocardial Infarction. J Am Coll Cardiol 2000;36:959–969.
20. Fibrinolytic Therapy Trialists' (FTT) Collaborative Group. Indications for fibrinolytic therapy in suspected myocardial infarction: Collaborative overview of early mortality and major morbidity results from all randomized trials of more than 1000 patients. Lancet 1994;343:311–322.
21. Berger P, Ellis SG, Holmes DR Jr, et al. Relationship between delay in performing direct coronary angioplasty and early clinical outcome in patients with acute myocardial infarction: Results from the Global Use of Strategies to Open Occluded Arteries in Acute Coronary Syndromes (GUSTO-IIb) trial. Circulation 1999;100:14–20.
22. Cohen M, Gensini GF, Maritz F, et al. TETAMI Investigators. Prospective evaluation of clinical outcomes after acute ST-elevation myocardial infarction in patients who are ineligible for reperfusion therapy: Preliminary results from the TETAMI registry and randomized trial. Circulation 2003;108(16 Suppl I):III14–III21.
23. Eagle KA, Goodman, SG, Avezum A, et al. Practice variation and missed opportunities for reperfusion in ST-segment-elevation myocardial infarction: Findings from the Global Registry of Acute Coronary Events (GRACE). Lancet 2002;359:373–377.
24. Jacobs A. Regionalized care for patients with ST-elevation myocardial infarction: It's closer than you think. Circulation 2006;113:1159–1161.
25. Svilaas T, Zijlstra F. The benefit of an invasive approach in thrombolysis-ineligible patients with acute myocardial infarction. Am J Med 2005;118:123–125.
26. Steg PG, Goldberg RJ, Gore JM, et al. Baseline characteristics, management practices, and in-hospital outcomes of patients hospitalized with acute coronary syndromes in the Global Registry of Acute Coronary Events (GRACE). Am J Cardiol 2002;90:358–363.
27. Anwaruddin S, Askari A, Topol EJ. Redefining risk in acute coronary syndromes using molecular medicine. J Am Coll Cardiol 2007;49:279–289.
28. Townsend R. Cardiac mortality in chronic kidney disease: A clearer perspective. Ann Intern Med 2002;137:615–616.
29. de Lemos JA, Morrow DA. Use of natriuretic peptides in clinical decision-making for patients with non-ST-elevation acute coronary syndromes. Am Heart J 2007;153:450–453.
30. Peterson ED, Roe MT, Muglund J, et al. Association between hospital process performance and outcomes among patients with acute coronary syndromes. JAMA 2006;295:1912–1920.
31. Eagle KA, Montoye CK, Riba AL, et al. Guideline-based standardized care is associated with substantially lower mortality in Medicare patients with acute myocardial infarction: The American College of Cardiology's Guidelines Applied in Practice (GAP) Projects in Michigan. J Am Coll Cardiol 2005;46:1242–1248.
32. Smith SC Jr, Feldman TE, Hirshfeld JW Jr, et al. ACC/AHA/SCAI 2005 guideline update for percutaneous coronary intervention: A report of the American College of Cardiology/American Heart Association Task Force on Practice Guidelines (ACC/AHA/SCAI Writing Committee to Update 2001 Guidelines for Percutaneous Coronary Intervention). Circulation 2006;113:e166–e286.
33. Krumholz HM, Anderson JL, Brooks NH, et al. ACC/AHA clinical performance measures for adults with ST-elevation and non-ST-elevation myocardial infarction: A report of the American College of Cardiology/American Heart Association Task Force on Performance Measures (Writing Committee to Develop Performance Measures on ST-Elevation and Non-ST-Elevation Myocardial Infarction). J Am Coll Cardiol 2006;47:236–265.
34. Gershlick AH, Stephens-Lloyd A, Hughes S, et al. Rescue angioplasty after failed thrombolytic therapy for acute myocardial infarction. N Engl J Med 2005;353:2758–2768.
35. Hochman JS, Lamas GA, Buller CE, et al. Coronary intervention for persistent occlusion after myocardial infarction. N Engl J Med 2006;355:2395–2407.
36. Bavry DA, Kumbhan DJ, Rassi AN, et al. Benefit of early invasive therapy in acute coronary syndromes: A meta-analysis of contemporary, randomized clinical trials. J Am Coll Cardiol 2006;48:1319–1325.
37. Mahoney M, Jurkovitz CT, Chu H, et al. Cost and cost-effectiveness of an early invasive vs conservative strategy for the treatment of unstable angina and non-ST-segment elevation myocardial infarction. JAMA 2002;288:1851–1858.
38. Moss AJ, Zareba W, Hall WJ. Prophylactic implantation of a defibrillator in patients with myocardial infarction and reduced ejection fraction. N Engl J Med 2002;346:877–883.
39. Bertrand ME, Simoons ML, Fox KAA. Management of acute coronary syndromes in patients presenting without persistent ST-segment elevation. The Task Force on the Management of Acute Coronary Syndromes of the European Society of Cardiology. Eur Heart J 2002;23: 1809–1840.
40. Levine GL, Berger PB, Cohen DJ, et al. Newer pharmacotherapy in patients undergoing percutaneous coronary interventions: A guide for pharmacists and other health care professionals. Pharmacotherapy 2006;26:1537–1556.
41. Alexander KP, Newby K, Armstrong PW, et al. Acute coronary syndromes in the elderly, Part II: ST-segment-elevation myocardial infarction. A scientific statement for healthcare professionals from the American Heart Association Council on Clinical Cardiology. Circulation 2007;115:2570–2589.
42. Spinler SA. Acute coronary syndromes. In: Shumock GT, Brundage DM, Chapman MM, et al., eds. Pharmacotherapy Self-Assessment Program, Book 1: Cardiovascular I, Cardiovascular II, 5th ed. Kansas City: American College of Clinical Pharmacy, 2004:1–40.
43. The Global Use of Strategies to Open Occluded Coronary Arteries (GUSTO) Investigators. An international randomized trial comparing four thrombolytic strategies for acute myocardial infarction. N Engl J Med 1993;329:673–682.
44. The Global Use of Strategies to Open Occluded Coronary Arteries (GUSTO III) Investigators. A comparison of reteplase with alteplase for acute myocardial infarction. N Engl J Med 1997;337:1118–1123.
45. Assessment of the Safety and Efficacy of a New Thrombolytic (ASSENT-2) Investigators. Single-bolus tenecteplase compared with front-loaded alteplase in acute myocardial infarction: The ASSENT-2 double-blind, randomized trial. Lancet 2001;354:716–722.
46. Awtry EH, Loscalzo J. Aspirin. Circulation 2000;101:1206–1218.
47. ISIS-2 (Second International Study of Infarct Survival) Collaborative Group). Randomised trial of intravenous streptokinase, oral aspirin, both, or neither among 17,187 cases of suspected acute myocardial infarction: ISIS-2. Lancet 1988;2:349–360.
48. Campbell CL, Smyth S, Montalescot G, Steinhubl SR. Aspirin dose for the prevention of cardiovascular disease. JAMA 2007;297:2018–2024.
49. Antiplatelet Trialists' Collaboration. Collaborative meta-analysis of randomised trials of antiplatelet therapy for prevention of death, myocardial infarction, and stroke in high risk patients. Br Med J 2002;324:71–86.
50. Serebruany VL, Steinhubl SR, Berger PB, et al. Analysis of risk of bleeding complications after different doses of aspirin in 193,036 patients enrolled in 31 randomized controlled trials. Am J Cardiol 2005;95:1218–1222.
51. Rosendorff C, Black HR, Cannon CP, et al. Treatment of hypertension in the prevention and management of ischemic heart disease: A scientific statement from the American Heart Association Council for High Blood Pressure Research and the Councils on Clinical Cardiology and Epidemiology and Prevention. Circulation 2007;115:2761–2788.
52. Bertrand ME, Rupprecht HJ, Urban P, et al. Double-blind study of the safety of clopidogrel with and without a loading dose in combination with aspirin compared with ticlopidine in combination with aspirin after coronary stenting: The clopidogrel aspirin stent international cooperative study (CLASSICS). Circulation 2000;102:624–629.
53. Chen ZM, Jiang XL, Chen YP, et al. Addition of clopidogrel to aspirin in 45,852 patients with acute myocardial infarction: Randomised placebo-controlled trial. Lancet 2005;366:1607–1621.
54. Sabatine MS, Cannon CP, Gibson CM, et al. Addition of clopidogrel to aspirin and fibrinolytic therapy for myocardial infarction with ST-segment elevation. N Engl J Med 2005;352:1179–1189.
55. Grines CL, Bonow RO, Casey DE, et al. Prevention of premature discontinuation of dual antiplatelet therapy in patients with coronary artery stents: A science advisory from the American Heart Association, American College of Cardiology, Society for Cardiovascular Angiography and Interventions, American College of Surgeons, and American Dental Association, with representation from the American College of Physicians. J Am Dent Assoc 2007;138:652–655.
56. Einstein EL, Anstrom KJ, Kong DF, et al. Clopidogrel use and long-term clinical outcomes after drug-eluting stent implantation. JAMA 2007;297:159–168.
57. De Luca G, Suryapranata H, Stone GW, et al. Abciximab as adjunctive therapy to reperfusion in acute ST-segment elevation myocardial infarction: A meta-analysis of randomized trials. JAMA 2005;293:1759–1765.

58. The GUSTO V Investigators. Reperfusion therapy for acute myocardial infarction with fibrinolytic therapy or combination reduced fibrinolytic therapy and platelet glycoprotein IIb/IIIa inhibition: The GUSTO V randomised trial. Lancet 2001;357:1905–1914.
59. The Assessment of the Safety and Efficacy of a New Thrombolytic Regimen (ASSENT) 3 Investigators. Efficacy and safety of tenecteplase in combination with enoxaparin, abciximab, or unfractionated heparin: The ASSENT-3 randomised trial in acute myocardial infarction. Lancet 2001;358:605–613.
60. Dasgupta H, Blankenship JC, Wood C, et al. Thrombocytopenia complicating treatment with intravenous glycoprotein IIb/IIIa receptor inhibitors: A pooled analysis. Am Heart J 2000;140:206–211.
61. Granger CB, Hirsh J, Califf RM, et al. Activated partial thromboplastin time and outcome after thrombolytic therapy for acute myocardial infarction. Circulation 1996;93:870–878.
62. Gruppo Italiano per Lo Studio della Sopravvivenza Nell'infarcto Myiocardio. GISSI-2: A factorial randomised trial of alteplase versus streptokinase and heparin versus no heparin among 12,490 patients with acute myocardial infarction. Lancet 1990;336:65–71.
63. Eikelboom JW, Quinlan DJ, Mehta SR, et al. Unfractionated and low-molecular-weight heparin as adjuncts to thrombolysis in aspirin-treated patients with ST-Elevation acute myocardial infarction: A meta-analysis of the randomized trials. Circulation 2005;112:3855–3867.
64. Antman EM, Morrow DA, McCabe CH, et al. Enoxaparin versus unfractionated heparin with fibrinolysis for ST-elevation myocardial infarction. N Engl J Med 2006;354:1477–1488.
65. White HD, Braunwald E, Murphy SA, et al. Enoxaparin vs. unfractionated heparin with fibrinolysis for ST-elevation myocardial infarction in elderly and younger patients: Results from ExTRACT-TIMI 25. Eur Heart J 2007;28:1066–1071.
66. Yusuf S, Mehta SR, Chrolavicius S, et al. Effects of fondaparinux on mortality and reinfarction in patients with acute ST-segment elevation myocardial infarction: The OASIS-6 randomized trial. JAMA 2006; 295:1519–1530.
67. Gruppo Italiano per Lo Studio della Sopravvivenza Nell'infarcto Myiocardio. GISSI-3: Effects of lisinopril and transdermal glyceryl trinitrate singly and together on 6-week mortality and ventricular function after acute myocardial infarction. Lancet 1994;343:1115–1122.
68. ISIS-4 (Fourth International Study of Infarct Survival Collaborative Group). ISIS-4: A randomised factorial trial assessing early oral captopril, oral mononitrate, and intravenous magnesium sulphate in 58,050 patients with suspected acute myocardial infarction. Lancet 1995;345:669–685.
69. Gheorghiade M, Goldstein S. β-Blockers in the post-myocardial infarction patient. Circulation 2002;106:394–398.
70. First International Study of Infarct Survival Collaborative Group. Randomised trial of intravenous atenolol among 16,027 cases of suspected acute myocardial infarction: ISIS-1. Lancet 1986;2:57–661.
71. Metoprolol in acute myocardial infarction (MIAMI). A randomised, placebo-controlled international trial. Eur Heart J 1985;6:199–226.
72. Hjalmarson A, Herlitz J, Homberg S, et al. The Goteborg metoprolol trial. Effects on mortality and morbidity in acute myocardial infarction. Circulation 1983;67(6 Pt 2):I26–I32.
73. Goldstein S. Propranolol therapy in patients with acute myocardial infarction: The Beta-Blocker Heart Attack Trial. Circulation 1983;67(6 Pt 2):I53–I57.
74. Chen Z, Pan HC, Chen YP, et al. Early intravenous then oral metoprolol in 45,852 patients with acute myocardial infarction: Randomised placebo-controlled trial. Lancet 2005;366:1622–1632.
75. Abernethy DR, Schwartz JB. Calcium-antagonist drugs. N Engl J Med 1999;341:1447–1457.
76. Boden WE, van Gilst WH, Scheldewaert RG, et al. Diltiazem in acute myocardial infarction treated with thrombolytic agents: A randomised, placebo-controlled trial. Incomplete Infarction Trial of European Research Collaborators Evaluating Prognosis post-Thrombolysis (INTERCEPT). Lancet 2000;355:1751–1756.
77. Pitt B, Byington RP, Furberg CD, et al. Effect of amlodipine on the progression of atherosclerosis and the occurrence of clinical events. PREVENT Investigators. Circulation 2000;102:1503–1510.
78. Packer M, O'Connor CM, Ghali JK, et al. Effect of amlodipine on morbidity and mortality in severe chronic heart failure: Prospective Randomized Amlodipine Survival Evaluation Study Group. N Engl J Med 1996;335:1107–1114.
79. Yusuf S, Zhao F, Meta SR, et al. Effects of clopidogrel in addition to aspirin in patients with acute coronary syndromes without ST-segment elevation. N Engl J Med 2001;345:494–502.
80. Mehta SR, Yusuf S, Peters RJ, et al. Effects of pretreatment with clopidogrel and aspirin followed by long-term therapy in patients undergoing percutaneous coronary intervention: The PCI-CURE study. Lancet 2001;358:527–533.
81. Steinhubl SR, Berger PB, Mann JT 3d, et al. Early and sustained dual oral antiplatelet therapy following percutaneous coronary intervention: A randomized, controlled trial. JAMA 2002;288:2411–2420.
82. Bhatt DL, Fox KA, Hacke W, et al. Clopidogrel and aspirin versus aspirin alone for the prevention of atherothrombotic events. N Engl J Med 2006;354:1706–1717.
83. Peters RJ, Mehta SR, Fox KA, et al. Effects of aspirin dose when used alone or in combination with clopidogrel in patients with acute coronary syndromes: Observations from the clopidogrel in unstable angina to prevent recurrent events (CURE) study. Circulation 2003;108:1682–1687.
84. The PURSUIT Trial Investigators. Inhibition of platelet glycoprotein IIb/IIIa with eptifibatide in patients with acute coronary syndromes. N Engl J Med 1998;339:436–443.
85. Platelet Receptor Inhibition in Ischemic Syndrome Management in Patients Limited by Unstable Signs and Symptoms (PRISM-PLUS) Study Investigators. Inhibition of the platelet glycoprotein IIb/IIIa receptor with tirofiban in unstable angina and non-Q-wave myocardial infarction. N Engl J Med 1998;338:1488–1497.
86. Boersma E, Harrington RA, Moliterno DJ, et al. Platelet glycoprotein IIb/IIIa inhibitors in acute coronary syndromes: A meta-analysis of all major randomised clinical trials. Lancet 2002;359:189–198. Erratum in Lancet 2002;359:2120.
87. O'Shea JC, Buller CE, Cantor WJ, et al. Long-term efficacy of platelet glycoprotein IIb/IIIa integrin blockade with eptifibatide in coronary stent intervention. JAMA 2002;287:618–621.
88. Topol EJ, Moliterno DJ, Herrmann HC, et al. Comparison of two platelet glycoprotein IIb/IIIa inhibitors tirofiban and abciximab for the prevention of ischemic events with percutaneous coronary revascularization. N Engl J Med 2001;344:1888–1894.
89. Moliterno DJ, Yakubov SJ, DiBattiste PM, et al. Outcomes at 6 months for the direct comparison of tirofiban and abciximab during percutaneous coronary revascularization with stent placement: The TARGET follow-up study. Lancet 2002;360:355–360.
90. Soffer D, Moussa I, Karatepe M, et al. Suboptimal inhibition of platelet aggregation following tirofiban bolus in patients undergoing percutaneous coronary intervention for unstable angina pectoris. Am J Cardiol 2003;91:872–875.
91. Kastrati A, Mehilli J, Neumann FJ, et al. Abciximab in patients with acute coronary syndromes undergoing percutaneous coronary intervention after clopidogrel pretreatment: The ISAR-REACT 2 randomized trial. JAMA 2006;295:1531–1538.
92. Roffi M, Chew DP, Mukherjee D, et al. Platelet glycoprotein IIb/IIIa inhibitors in acute coronary syndromes: A meta-analysis of all major randomised clinical trials. Eur Heart J 2002;23:1408–1411.
93. Alexander KP, Chen AY, Newby K, et al. Sex differences in major bleeding with GP IIb/IIIa inhibitors: Results from the CRUSADE (Can Rapid Risk Stratification of Unstable Angina Patients Suppress Adverse Outcomes with Early Implementation of the ACC/AHA Guidelines) Initiative. Circulation 2006;114:1380–1387.
94. Alexander KP, Chen AY, Roe MT, et al. Excess dosing of antiplatelet and antithrombin agents in the treatment of non-ST-segment elevation acute coronary syndromes. JAMA 2005;294:3108–3116.
95. Stone GW, Bertrand ME, Moses JW, et al. Routine upstream initiation vs deferred selective use of glycoprotein IIb/IIIa inhibitors in acute coronary syndromes: The ACUITY Timing trial. JAMA 2007;297:591–602.
96. Oler A, Whooley MA, Oler J. Grady D. Adding heparin to aspirin reduces the incidence of myocardial infarction and death in patients with unstable angina: A meta-analysis. JAMA 1996;276:811–815.
97. Fragmin During Instability in Coronary Artery Disease Study Group. Low-molecular-weight heparin during instability in coronary artery disease. Lancet 1996;347:561–568.
98. Klein W, Buchwald A, Hillis SE, et al. Comparison of low-molecular-weight heparin with unfractionated heparin acutely and with placebo for 6 weeks in the management of unstable coronary artery disease:

Fragmin in Unstable Coronary Artery Disease Study (FRIC). Circulation 1997;96:61–68.
99. Antman EM, McCabe CH, Gurfinkle EP, et al. Enoxaparin prevents deaths and cardiac ischemic events in unstable angina/non-Q-wave myocardial infarction: Results of the Thrombolysis in Myocardial Infarction (TIMI 11B) trial. Circulation 1999;100:1593–1601.
100. Cohen M, Demers C, Gurfinkle EP, et al. A comparison of low-molecular-weight heparin with unfractionated heparin for unstable coronary artery disease. N Engl J Med 1997;337:447–452.
101. Ferguson JJ, Califf RM, Antman EM, et al. The Synergy Trial Investigators. Enoxaparin versus unfractionated heparin in high-risk patients with non-ST-segment elevation acute coronary syndromes managed with an intended early invasive strategy. JAMA 2004;292:45–54.
102. Cohen M, Mahaffey KW, Pollack CV Jr, et al. A subgroup analysis of the impact of prerandomization antithrombin therapy on outcomes in the SYNERGY trial: Enoxaparin versus unfractionated heparin in non-ST-segment elevation acute coronary syndromes. J Am Coll Cardiol 2006;48:1346–1354.
103. Yusuf S, Mehta SR, Chrolavicius S, et al. Comparison of fondaparinux and enoxaparin in acute coronary syndromes. N Engl J Med 2006;354:1464–1476.
104. Weitz JI, Hirsh J, Samama MM. New anticoagulant drugs: The Seventh ACCP Conference on Antithrombotic and Thrombolytic Therapy. Chest 2004;126(Suppl):265S-286S.
105. Stone GW, McLaurin BT, Cox DA, et al. Bivalirudin for patients with acute coronary syndromes. N Engl J Med 2006;355:2203–2216.
106. ACE/ADA Task Force on Inpatient Diabetes. American College of Endocrinology and American Diabetes Association Consensus statement on inpatient diabetes and glycemic control: A call to action. Diabetes Care 2006;29:1955–1962.
107. Pittas AG, Siegel RD, Lau J. Insulin therapy for critically ill hospitalized patients: A meta-analysis of randomized controlled trials. Arch Intern Med 2004;164:2005–2011.
108. Smith SC, Allen J, Blair SN, et al. AHA/ACC guidelines for secondary prevention for patients with coronary and other atherosclerotic vascular disease: 2006 update: Endorsed by the National Heart Lung and Blood Institute. J Am Coll Cardiol 2006;47:2130–2139.
109. Davis MM, Taubert K, Benin AL, et al. Influenza vaccination as secondary prevention for cardiovascular disease: A science advisory from the American Heart Association/American College of Cardiology. J Am Coll Cardiol 2006;48:1498–1502.
110. Coumadin Aspirin Reinfarction Study (CARS) Investigators. Randomised, double-blind trial of fixed low-dose warfarin with aspirin after myocardial infarction. Lancet 1997;350:389–396.
111. Fiore LD, Ezekowitz MD, Brophy MT, et al. Department of Veterans Affairs Cooperative Studies Program Clinical Trial comparing combined warfarin and aspirin with aspirin alone in survivors of acute myocardial infarction: Primary results of the CHAMP study. Circulation 2002;105:557–563.
112. van Es RF, Jonker JJ, Verheugt FW, et al. Aspirin and Coumadin after acute coronary syndromes (the ASPECT-2 study): A randomised, controlled trial. Lancet 2002;360:109–113.
113. Hurlen M, Abdelnoor M, Smith P, et al. Warfarin, aspirin, or both after myocardial infarction. N Engl J Med 2002;347:969–974.
114. Andreotti F, Testa L, Biondi-Zocca GG, Crea F. Aspirin plus warfarin compared to aspirin alone after acute coronary syndromes: An updated and comprehensive meta-analysis of 25,307 patients. Eur Heart J 2006;27:519–526.
115. Leon MB, Baim DS, Popma JJ, et al. Clinical trial comparing three antithrombotic-drug regimens after coronary-artery stenting. Stent Anticoagulation Restenosis Study Investigators. N Engl J Med 1998;339:1665–1671.
116. Freemantle N, Cleland J, Young P, et al. β-Blockade after myocardial infarction: Systematic review and meta regression analysis. Br Med J 1999;318:1730–1737.
117. Pedersen TR. Six-year follow-up of the Norwegian Multicenter Study on Timolol after Acute Myocardial Infarction. N Engl J Med 1985;313:1055–1058.
118. Cucherat M, Boissel JP, Leizorovicz A. Persistent reduction of mortality for five years after one year of acebutolol treatment initiated during acute myocardial infarction. The APSI Investigators. Acebutolol et Prevention Secondaire de l'Infarctus. Am J Cardiol 1997;79:587–589.
119. Dargie HJ. Effect of carvedilol on outcome after myocardial infarction in patients with left-ventricular dysfunction: The CAPRICORN randomised trial. Lancet 2001;357:1385–1390.
120. Houghton T, Freemantle N, Cleland JG, et al. Are beta-blockers effective in patients who develop heart failure soon after myocardial infarction? A meta-regression analysis of randomised trials. Eur J Heart Fail 2000;2:333–340.
121. Ko DT, Hebert PR, Coffey CS, et al. Beta-blocker therapy and symptoms of depression, fatigue, and sexual dysfunction. JAMA 2002;288:351–357.
122. Gibbons RJ, Abrams J, Chatterjee K, et al. ACC/AHA 2002 guideline update for the management of patients with chronic stable angina: Summary article. A report of the American College of Cardiology/American Heart Association Task Force on Practice Guidelines (Committee on the Management of Patients With Chronic Stable Angina). J Am Coll Cardiol 2003;41:159–168.
123. ACE Inhibitor Myocardial Infarction Collaborative Group. Indications for ACE inhibitors in the early treatment of acute myocardial infarction: Systematic overview of individual data from 100,000 patients in randomized trials. Circulation 1998;97:2202–2212.
124. Flather MD, Yusuf S, Kober L, et al. Long-term ACE inhibitor therapy in patients with heart failure or left ventricular dysfunction: A systematic overview of data from individual patients. ACE Inhibitor Myocardial Infarction Collaborative Group. Lancet 2000;355:1575–1581.
125. Swedberg K, Held P, Kjekshus J, et al. Effects of the early administration of enalapril on mortality in patients with acute myocardial infarction: Results of the Cooperative New Scandinavian Enalapril Survival Study II (CONSENSUS II). N Engl J Med 1992;327:678–684.
126. Buch P, Rasmussen PS, Abildstrom AZ, et al. The long-term impact of the angiotensin-converting enzyme inhibitor trandolapril on mortality and hospital admissions in patients with left ventricular dysfunction after a myocardial infarction: Follow-up to 12 years. Eur Heart J 2005;26:145–152.
127. Yusuf S, Sleight P, Pogue J, et al. Effects of an angiotensin-converting enzyme inhibitor, ramipril, on cardiovascular events in high-risk patients. The Heart Outcomes Prevention Evaluation Study Investigators. N Engl J Med 2000;342:145–153.
128. Fox KM. Efficacy of perindopril in reduction of cardiovascular events among patients with stable coronary artery disease: Randomised, double-blind, placebo-controlled, multicentre trial (the EUROPA study). Lancet 2003;362:782–788.
129. Braunwald E, Domanski MJ, Fowler SE, et al. Angiotensin-converting-enzyme inhibition in stable coronary artery disease. N Engl J Med 2004;351:2058–2068.
130. Pfeffer MA, McMurray JJV, Velazquez EJ, et al. Valsartan, captopril, or both in myocardial infarction complicated by heart failure, left ventricular dysfunction, or both. N Engl J Med 2003;349:1893–1906.
131. Granger CB, McMurray JV, Yusuf S, et al., eds. CHARM Investigators and Committees. Effects of candesartan in patients with chronic heart failure and reduced left-ventricular systolic function intolerant to angiotensin-converting-enzyme inhibitors: CHARM Alternative trial. Lancet 2004;362:772–776.
132. Warner KK, Visconti JA, Tschampel MM. Angiotensin II receptor blockers in patients with ACE inhibitor-induced angioedema. Ann Pharmacother 2000;34:526–528.
133. Teo KK, Yusuf S, Pfeffer M, et al. Effects of long-term treatment with angiotensin-converting enzyme inhibitors in the presence or absence of aspirin: A systematic review. Lancet 2002;360:1037–1043.
134. Zillich AJ, Carter BL. Eplerenone: A novel selective aldosterone blocker. Ann Pharmacother 2002;36:1567–1576.
135. Pitt B, Zannad F, Remme WJ, et al. The effect of spironolactone on morbidity and mortality in patients with severe heart failure. Randomized Aldactone Evaluation Study Investigators. N Engl J Med 1999;341:709–717.
136 Pitt B, Remme W, Zannad F, et al. Eplerenone, a selective aldosterone blocker in patients with left ventricular dysfunction after myocardial infarction. N Engl J Med 2003;348:1309–1321.
137. Executive Summary of the Third Report of the National Cholesterol Education Program (NCEP) Expert Panel on Detection, Evaluation, and Treatment of High Blood Cholesterol in Adults (Adult Treatment Panel III). JAMA 2001;285:2486–2497.
138. Grundy SM, Cleeman JI, Bairey Merz, CN, et al., eds. Coordinating Committee of the National Cholesterol Education Program, Endorsed by the National Heart, Lung, and Blood Institute, American College of Cardiology Foundation, and American Heart Association. Implications of

Recent Clinical Trials for the National Cholesterol Education Program Adult Treatment Panel III Guidelines. Circulation 2004;110:227–239.

139. Hulten E, Jackson JL, Douglas K, et al. The effect of early, intensive statin therapy on acute coronary syndrome: A meta-analysis of randomized controlled trials. Arch Intern Med 2006;166:1814–1821.
140. Cannon CP, Braunwald E, McCabe CH, et al. Pravastatin or Atorvastatin Evaluation and Infection Therapy: Thrombolysis in Myocardial Infarction 22 Investigators. Intensive versus moderate lipid lowering with statins after acute coronary syndromes. N Engl J Med 2004;350:1495–1504.
141. Anonymous. MRC/BHF Heart Protection Study of cholesterol lowering with simvastatin in 20,536 high-risk individuals: A randomised placebo-controlled trial. Lancet 2002;360:7–22.
142 Rubins HB, Robins SJ, Collins D, et al. Gemfibrozil for the secondary prevention of coronary heart disease in men with low levels of high-density lipoprotein cholesterol. Veterans Affairs High-Density Lipoprotein Cholesterol Intervention Trial Study Group. N Engl J Med 1999;341:410–418.
143. Keech A, Simes RJ, Barter P, et al. Effects of long-term fenofibrate therapy on cardiovascular events in 9795 people with type 2 diabetes mellitus (the FIELD study): Randomised controlled trial. Lancet 2005;366:1849–1861.
144. Mcpherson R, Frohlich J, Fodor G, et al. Canadian Cardiovascular Society position statement—Recommendations for the diagnosis and treatment of dyslipidemia and prevention of cardiovascular disease. Can J Cardiol 2006;22:913–927.
145. Kris-Etherton PM, Harris WS, Appel LJ. Fish consumption, fish oil, omega-3 fatty acids, and cardiovascular disease. Circulation 2002; 106:2747–2757.
146. Gruppo Italiano per lo Studio della Sopravvivenza nell'infarcto miocardio. Dietary supplementation with n-3 fatty acids and vitamin E after myocardial infarction: Results of GISSI-Prevenzione trial. Lancet 1999;354:447–455.
147. Bays H. Fish oil composition of Omacor and the GISSI trial. Am J Cardiol 2007;99:1483–1484.
148. Critchley JA, Capewell S. Mortality risk reduction associated with smoking cessation in patients with coronary heart disease: A systematic review. JAMA 2003;290:86–97.
149. Thompson PD, Bucner D, Pina IL, et al. Exercise and physical activity in the prevention and treatment of atherosclerotic cardiovascular disease: A statement from the Council on Clinical Cardiology (Subcommittee on Exercise, Rehabilitation and Prevention) and the Council on Nutrition, Physical Activity, and Metabolism (Subcommittee on Physical Activity). Circulation 2003;107:3109–3116.
150. Rydén L, Standl E, Bartnik M, et al. Guidelines on diabetes, prediabetes, and cardiovascular disease: Executive summary. The Task Force on Diabetes and Cardiovascular Disease of the European Society of Cardiology (ESC) and the European Association for the Study of Diabetes (EASD). Eur Heart J 2007;28:88–136.
151. Hulley S, Grady D, Bush T, et al. Randomized trial of estrogen plus progestin for secondary prevention of coronary heart disease in postmenopausal women. JAMA 1998;280:605–613.
152. Writing Group for the Women's Health Initiative Investigators. Risks and benefits of estrogen plus progestin in health postmenopausal women: Principal results from the Women's Health Initiative Randomized Controlled Trial. JAMA 2002;288:321–333.
153. The Heart Outcomes Prevention Evaluation Study Investigators. Vitamin E supplementation and cardiovascular risk in high-risk patients. N Engl J Med 2000;342:154–160.
154. U.S. Preventive Services Task Force. Routine vitamin supplementation to prevent cancer and cardiovascular disease: Recommendations and rationale. Ann Intern Med 2003;139:51–55.
155. Bonaa KH, Njolstad I, Ueland PM, et al. Homocysteine lowering and cardiovascular events after acute myocardial infarction. N Engl J Med 2006;354:1578–1588.
156. Lonn E, Bosch J, Yusuf S, et al. Effects of long-term vitamin E supplementation on cardiovascular events and cancer: A randomized controlled trial. JAMA 2005;293:1338–1347.
157. Kris-Etherton PM, Lichtenstein AH, Howard BV. Antioxidant vitamins and cardiovascular disease. Circulation 2004;110:637–641.
158. Ho PM, Spertus JA, Masoudi FA, et al. Impact of medication therapy discontinuation on mortality after myocardial infarction. Arch Intern Med 2006;166:1842–1847.
159. Biondi-Zoccai GG, Lotrionte M, Agostoni P, et al. A systematic review and meta-analysis on the hazards of discontinuing or not adhering to aspirin among 50,279 patients at risk for coronary artery disease. Eur Heart J 2006;27:2667–2674.
160. Granger BB, Swedberg K, Ekman I, et al. Adherence to candesartan and placebo and outcomes in chronic heart failure in the CHARM programme: Double-blind, randomised, controlled clinical trial. Lancet 2005;366:1989–1991.
161. Rasmussen JN, Chong A, Alter DA. Relationship between adherence to evidence-based pharmacotherapy and long-term mortality after acute myocardial infarction. JAMA 2007;297:177–186.
162. Spertus JA, Kettelkamp R, Vance C, et al. Prevalence, predictors, and outcomes of premature discontinuation of thienopyridine therapy after drug-eluting stent placement: Results from the PREMIER registry. Circulation 2006;113:2803–2809.
163. Muhlestein JB, Horne BD, Bair TL, et al. Usefulness of in-hospital prescription of statin agents after angiographic diagnosis of coronary artery disease in improving continued compliance and reduced mortality. Am J Cardiol 2001;87:257–261.
164. Jackevicius CA, Mamdani M, Tu JV. Adherence with statin therapy in elderly patients with and without acute coronary syndromes. JAMA 2002;288:462–467.
165. Lachaine J, Rinfret S, Merikle EP, Terride JE. Persistence and adherence to cholesterol lowering agents: Evidence from Regie de l'Assurance Maladie du Quebec data. Am Heart J 2006;152:164–169.
166. Kulkarni SP, Alexander KP, Lytle B, et al. Long-term adherence with cardiovascular drug regimens. Am Heart J 2006;151:185–191.
167. Murray MD, Young J, Hoke S, et al. Pharmacist intervention to improve medication adherence in heart failure: A randomized trial. Ann Intern Med 2007;146:714–725.
168. Lee JK, Grace KA, Taylor AJ. Effect of a pharmacy care program on medication adherence and persistence, blood pressure, and low-density lipoprotein cholesterol: A randomized controlled trial. JAMA 2006;296:2563–2571.
169. Mark DB. Medical economics in cardiovascular medicine. In: Topol EJ, Califf RM, Isner J, et al., eds. Textbook of Cardiovascular Medicine. Philadelphia: Lippincott Williams & Wilkins, 2003:957–979.
170. Hlatky MA, Califf RM, Naylor CD, et al. Cost effectiveness of thrombolytic therapy with tissue plasminogen activator as compared with streptokinase for acute myocardial infarction. N Engl J Med 1996;332:1418–1424.
171. Eccles M, Freemantle N, Mason J, et al. North of England evidence based guideline development project: Guideline on the use of aspirin as secondary prophylaxis for vascular disease in primary care. Br Med J 1998;316:1303–1309.
172. Mark DB, Harrington RA, Lincoff AM, et al. Cost effectiveness of platelet glycoprotein IIb/IIIa inhibition with eptifibatide in patients with non-ST-segment-elevation acute coronary syndromes. Circulation 2000;101:366–371.
173. Phillips KA, Shlipak MG, Coxson P, et al. Health and economic benefits of increased beta-blocker use following myocardial infarction. JAMA 2001;284:2748–2754.
174. McMurray JJ, McGuire A, Davie AP, Hughs D. Cost-effectiveness of different ACE inhibitor treatment scenarios post-myocardial infarction. Eur Heart J 1997;18:1411–1415.
175. Franzosi MG, Maggioni AP, Santoro E. Cost-effective analysis of early lisinopril use with acute myocardial infarction: Results from GISSI-3 trial. Pharmacoeconomics 1998;13:337–346.
176. Weintraub WS, Zhang Z, Mahoney EM, et al. Cost-effectiveness of eplerenone compared with placebo in patients with myocardial infarction complicated by left ventricular dysfunction and heart failure. Circulation 2005;11:1106–1113.
177. Grover SA, Coupal L, Paquet S, Zowall H. Cost-effectiveness of 3-hydroxy-3-methylglutaryl-coenzyme A reductase inhibitors in the secondary prevention of cardiovascular disease: Forecasting the incremental benefits of preventing coronary and cerebrovascular events. Arch Intern Med 1999;159:593–600.
178. Nyman JA, Martinson MS, Nelson D, et al. Cost-effectiveness of gemfibrozil for coronary heart disease patients with low levels of high-density lipoprotein cholesterol: The Department of Veterans Affairs High-Density Lipoprotein Cholesterol Intervention Trial. Arch Intern Med 2002;162:177–182.
179. Franzosi MG, Brunetti M, Marchioli R, et al. Cost-effectiveness analysis of n-3 polyunsaturated fatty acids (PUFA) after myocardial infarction: Results from Gruppo Italiano per lo Studio della Sopravvivenza nell'Infarcto (GISSI)-Prevenzione Trial. Pharmacoeconomics 2001:19:411–420.

CHAPTER 19

The Arrhythmias

CYNTHIA A. SANOSKI, MARIEKE DEKKER SCHOEN, AND JERRY L. BAUMAN

KEY CONCEPTS

1. The use of antiarrhythmic drugs in the United States has declined because of major trials that show increased mortality with their use in several clinical situations, the realization of proarrhythmia as a significant side effect and the advancing technology of nondrug therapies such as ablation and the implantable cardioverter-defibrillator (ICD).

2. Antiarrhythmic drugs frequently cause side effects and are complex in their pharmacokinetic characteristics. The therapeutic range of these agents provide only a rough guide to modifying treatment; it is preferable to attempt to define an individual's effective (or target) concentration and match that during long-term therapy.

3. The most commonly prescribed antiarrhythmic drug is now amiodarone. This agent is effective in terminating and preventing a wide variety of symptomatic supraventricular and ventricular tachycardias. However, because this antiarrhythmic drug is plagued by frequent side effects, it requires close monitoring. The most concerning toxicity is pulmonary fibrosis; side-effect profiles of the intravenous (IV) (acute, short-term) and oral (chronic, long-term) forms differ substantially.

4. In patients with atrial fibrillation (AF), therapy is traditionally aimed at controlling ventricular response (digoxin, nondihydropyridine calcium channel blockers [CCBs], β-blockers), preventing thromboembolic complications (warfarin, aspirin), and restoring and maintaining sinus rhythm (antiarrhythmic drugs, direct-current cardioversion [DCC]). Studies show there is no need to aggressively pursue strategies to maintain sinus rhythm (i.e., long-term antiarrhythmic drugs); rate control alone (leaving the patient in AF) is often sufficient in patients who can tolerate it. Nonetheless, it is not uncommon for patients to have remaining troublesome symptoms with the rate-control strategy alone, necessitating oral antiarrhythmic drug therapy.

5. Paroxysmal supraventricular tachycardia (PSVT) is usually a result of reentry in or proximal to the atrioventricular (AV) node or AV reentry incorporating an extranodal pathway; common tachycardias can be terminated acutely with AV nodal-blocking agents such as adenosine, and recurrences can be prevented by ablation with radiofrequency current.

6. Patients with Wolff-Parkinson-White (WPW) Syndrome may have several different tachycardias that are acutely treated by different strategies: orthodromic reentry (adenosine), antidromic reentry (adenosine or procainamide), and AF (procainamide or amiodarone). Atrioventricular nodal-blocking drugs are contraindicated in patients with WPW and AF.

7. Because of the results of the Cardiac Arrhythmia Suppression Trial (CAST) and other trials, antiarrhythmic drugs (with the exception of β-blockers) should not be routinely used in patients with prior myocardial infarction (MI) or left ventricular (LV) dysfunction and minor ventricular rhythm disturbances (e.g., premature ventricular complexes [PVCs]).

8. Patients with hemodynamically significant ventricular tachycardia (VT) or ventricular fibrillation (VF) not associated with an acute MI who are successfully resuscitated (electrical cardioversion, vasopressors, amiodarone) are at high risk for sudden cardiac death (SCD) and should receive an ICD ("secondary prevention").

9. Implantation of an ICD should be considered for the primary prevention of SCD in certain high-risk patient populations. High-risk patients include those with a history of MI and LV dysfunction (regardless of whether they have inducible sustained ventricular arrhythmias), as well as those with New York Heart Association (NYHA) class II or III heart failure (HF) as a result of either ischemic or nonischemic causes.

10. Life-threatening ventricular proarrhythmia generally takes two forms: sinusoidal or incessant monomorphic VT (type Ic antiarrhythmic drugs) and torsade de pointes (TdP) (type Ia or III antiarrhythmic drugs and many other noncardiac drugs).

Learning objectives, review questions, and other resources can be found at **www.pharmacotherapyonline.com.**

The heart has two basic properties, namely an electrical property and a mechanical property. The synchronous interaction between these two properties is complex, precise, and relatively enduring. The study of the electrical properties of the heart has grown at a steady rate, interrupted by periodic salvos of scientific breakthroughs. Einthoven's pioneering work allowed graphic electrical tracings of cardiac rhythm and probably represents the first of these breakthroughs. This discovery (of the surface electrocardiogram [ECG]) has remained the cornerstone of diagnostic tools for cardiac rhythm disturbances. Since then, intracardiac recordings and programmed cardiac stimulation have advanced our understanding of arrhythmias, and microelectrode, voltage-clamping, and patch-clamping techniques have allowed considerable insight into the electrophysiologic actions and mechanisms of antiarrhythmic drugs. Certainly, the new era of molecular biology and mapping of the human genome promises even greater insights into mechanisms (and potential therapies) of arrhythmias. Noteworthy in this regard is the discovery of genetic abnormalities in the ion channels that control electrical repolarization (heritable long QT syndrome) or depolarization (Brugada syndrome).

The clinical use of drug therapy started with the use of digitalis and then quinidine, followed somewhat later by a surge of new agents in the 1980s. A theme of drug discovery during this decade was initially to find orally absorbed lidocaine-congeners (such as mexiletine and tocainide); later, the emphasis was on drugs with extremely potent effects on conduction (i.e., flecainide-like agents). The most recent focus of investigational antiarrhythmic drugs are the potassium channel blockers, with dofetilide being the most recently approved in the United States. Previously, there was some expectation that advances in antiarrhythmic drug discovery would lead to a highly effective and nontoxic agent that would be effective for a majority of patients (i.e., the so-called magic bullet). Instead, significant problems with drug toxicity and proarrhythmia have resulted in a decline in the overall volume of antiarrhythmic drug usage in the United States since 1989. ❶ The other phenomenon, which has significantly contributed to the decline in antiarrhythmic drug usage, is the development of extremely effective nondrug therapies. Technical advances have made it possible to permanently interrupt reentry circuits with radiofrequency ablation, which renders long-term antiarrhythmic drug use unnecessary in certain arrhythmias. Furthermore, the impressive survival data associated with the use of ICDs for the primary and secondary prevention of SCD has led most clinicians to choose "device" therapy as the first-line treatment for patients who are at high-risk for life-threatening ventricular arrhythmias. Both of these nondrug therapies have become increasingly popular for the management of arrhythmias so that the potential proarrhythmic effects and organ toxicities associated with antiarrhythmic drugs can be avoided. What does the future hold for the use of antiarrhythmic drugs? Certainly new knowledge and technologic advances have forced investigators and clinicians to rethink the concept of traditional membrane-active drugs. Although some degree of enthusiasm exists for some of the newer or investigational agents, the overall impact of these drugs has yet to be determined.

This chapter reviews the principles involved in both normal and abnormal cardiac conduction and addresses the pathophysiology and treatment of the more commonly encountered arrhythmias. Certainly, many volumes of complete text could be (and have been) devoted to basic and clinical electrophysiology. Consequently, this chapter briefly addresses those principles necessary for clinicians.

ARRHYTHMOGENESIS

NORMAL CONDUCTION

Electrical activity is initiated by the sinoatrial (SA) node and moves through cardiac tissue by a tree-like conduction network. The SA node initiates cardiac rhythm under normal circumstances because this tissue possesses the highest degree of automaticity or rate of spontaneous impulse generation. The degree of automaticity of the SA node is largely influenced by the autonomic nervous system in that both cholinergic and sympathetic innervations control sinus rate. Most tissues within the conduction system also possess varying degrees of inherent automatic properties. However, the rates of spontaneous impulse generation of these tissues are less than that of the SA node. Thus these latent automatic pacemakers are continuously overdriven by impulses arising from the SA node (primary pacemaker) and do not become clinically apparent.

From the SA node, electrical activity moves in a wave front through an atrial specialized conducting system and eventually gains entrance to the ventricle via the atrioventricular (AV) node and a large bundle of conducting tissue referred to as the bundle of His. Aside from this AV nodal–Hisian pathway, a fibrous AV ring that will not permit electrical stimulation separates the atria and ventricles. The conducting tissues bridging the atria and ventricles are referred to as the junctional areas. Again, this area of tissue (junction) is largely influenced by autonomic input, and possesses a relatively high degree of inherent automaticity (about 40 beats/min, less than that of the SA node). From the bundle of His, the cardiac conduction system bifurcates into several (usually three) bundle branches: one right bundle and two left bundles. These bundle branches further arborize into a conduction network referred to as the Purkinje system. The conduction system as a whole innervates the mechanical myocardium and serves to initiate excitation–contraction coupling and the contractile process. After a cell or group of cells within the heart is electrically stimulated, a brief period of time follows in which those cells cannot again be excited. This time period is referred to as the refractory period. As the electrical wavefront moves down the conduction system, the impulse eventually encounters tissue refractory to stimulation (recently excited) and subsequently dies out. The SA node subsequently recovers, fires spontaneously, and begins the process again.

Prior to cellular excitation, an electrical gradient exists between the inside and the outside of the cell membrane. At this time the cell is polarized. In atrial and ventricular conducting tissue, the intracellular space is approximately 80 to 90 mV negative with respect to the extracellular environment. The electrical gradient just prior to excitation is referred to as resting membrane potential (RMP) and is the result of differences in ion concentrations between the inside and the outside of the cell. At RMP, the cell is polarized primarily by the action of active membrane ion pumps, the most notable of these being the sodium-potassium pump. For example, this specific pump (in addition to other systems) attempts to maintain the intracellular sodium concentration at 5 to 15 mEq/L and the extracellular sodium concentration at 135 to 142 mEq/L; the intracellular potassium concentration at 135 to 140 mEq/L and the extracellular potassium concentration at 3 to 5 mEq/L. The RMP can be calculated by using the Nernst equation:

$$\text{RMP} = 61.5 \log \left(\frac{[\text{K}^+] \text{ outside}}{[\text{K}^+] \text{ inside}} \right)$$

Electrical stimulation (or depolarization) of the cell will result in changes in membrane potential over time or a characteristic action potential curve (Fig. 19–1). The action potential curve results from the transmembrane movement of specific ions and is divided into different phases. Phase 0 or initial, rapid depolarization of atrial and ventricular tissues is caused by an abrupt increase in the permeability of the membrane to sodium influx. This rapid depolarization more than equilibrates (overshoots) the electrical potential, resulting in a brief initial repolarization or phase 1. Phase 1 (initial depolarization) is caused by a transient and active potassium efflux (i.e., the I_{Kto} current). Calcium begins to move into the intracellular space at about -60 mV (during phase 0) causing a slower depolarization. Calcium influx continues throughout phase 2 of the action potential (plateau phase) and is balanced to some degree by potassium efflux. Calcium entrance (only through L channels in myocardial tissue) distinguishes cardiac conducting cells from nerve tissue, and provides the critical ionic link to excitation-contraction coupling and the mechanical properties of the heart as a pump (see Chap. 16). The membrane remains permeable to potassium efflux during phase 3, resulting in cellular repolarization. Phase 4 of the action potential is the gradual depolarization of the cell and is related to a constant sodium leak into the intracellular space balanced by a decreasing (over time) efflux of potassium. The slope of phase 4 depolarization determines, in large part, the automatic properties of the cell. As the cell is slowly depolarized during phase 4, an abrupt increase in sodium permeability occurs, allowing the rapid cellular depolarization of phase 0. The juncture of phase 4 and phase 0 where rapid sodium influx is initiated

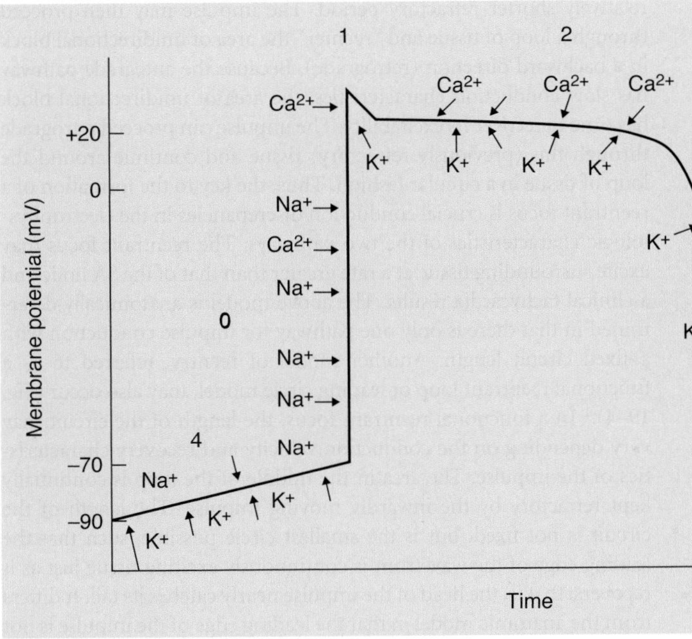

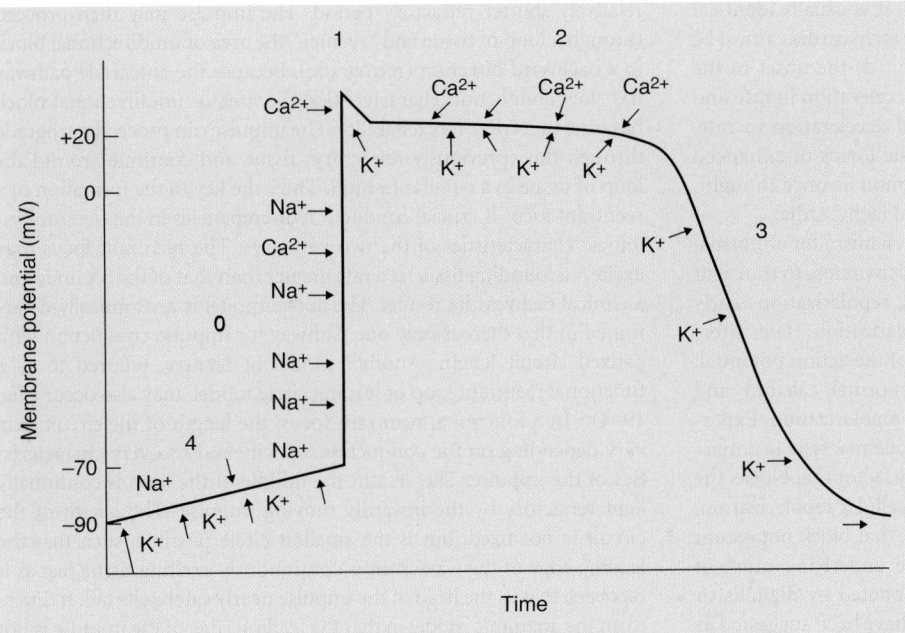

FIGURE 19-1. Purkinje fiber action potential showing specific ion flux responsible for the change in membrane potential. Ions outside of the line (e.g., sodium) move from the extracellular space to the intracellular space and ions on the inside of the line (e.g., potassium) move from the inside of the cell to the outside. Below the line is the corresponding ventricular excitation and recovery from the surface ECG. One can see that excessive sodium channel block from drugs may lead to QRS prolongation and excessive potassium channel block from drugs may lead to QT prolongation.

is referred to the threshold potential of the cell. The level of threshold potential also regulates the degree of cellular automaticity.

Not all cells in the cardiac conduction system rely on sodium influx for initial depolarization. Some tissues depolarize in response to a slower inward ionic current caused by calcium influx. These "calcium-dependent" tissues are found primarily in the SA and AV nodes (both L and T channels) and possess distinct conduction properties in comparison to "sodium-dependent" fibers. Calcium-dependent cells generally have a less-negative RMP (-40 to -60 mV) and a slower conduction velocity. Furthermore, in calcium-dependent tissues, recovery of excitability outlasts full repolarization, whereas in sodium-dependent tissue, recovery is prompt after repolarization. These two types of electrical fibers also differ dramatically in how drugs modify their conduction properties.

Ion conductance across the lipid bilayer of the cell membrane occurs via the formation of membrane pores or "channels" (Fig. 19–2). Selective ion channels probably form in response to specific electrical potential differences between the inside and the outside of the cell (voltage dependence). The membrane itself is composed of both organized and disorganized lipids and phospholipids in a dynamic sol-gel matrix. During ion flux and electrical excitation, changes in this sol-gel equilibrium occur and permit the formation of activated ion channels. Besides channel formation and membrane composition, intrachannel proteins or phospholipids, referred to as gates also regulate the transmembrane movement of ions. These gates are thought to be positioned strategically within the channel to modulate ion flow (Fig. 19–2). Each ion channel conceptually has two types of gates: an activation gate and an inactivation gate. The activation gate opens during depolarization to allow the ion current to enter or exit from the cell, and the inactivation gate later closes to stop ion movement. When the cell is in a rested state, the activation gates are closed and the inactivation gates are open. The activation gates then open to allow ion movement through the channel, and the inactivation gates later close to stop ion conductance. Thus, the cell cycles between three states: resting, activated or open, and inactivated or closed. Activation of SA and AV nodal tissue is dependent on a slow depolarizing current through calcium channels and gates, whereas the activation of atrial and ventricular tissue is dependent on a rapid depolarizing current through sodium channels and gates.

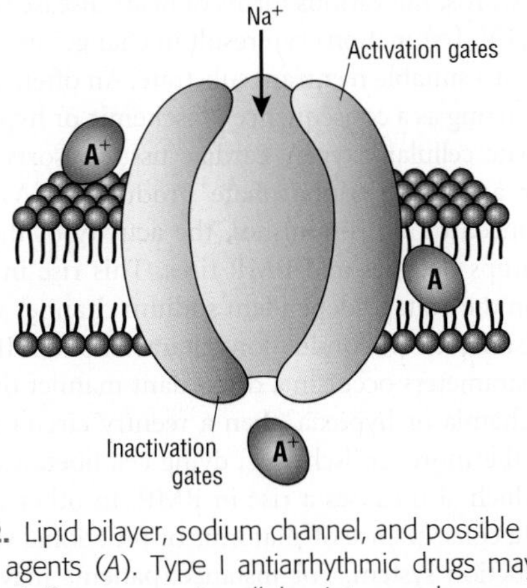

FIGURE 19-2. Lipid bilayer, sodium channel, and possible sites of action of the type I agents (*A*). Type I antiarrhythmic drugs may theoretically inhibit sodium influx at an extracellular, intramembrane, or intracellular receptor site. However, all approved agents appear to block sodium conductance at a single receptor site by gaining entrance to the interior of the channel from an intracellular route. Active ionized drugs block the channel predominantly during the activated or inactivated state and bind and unbind with specific time constants (described as fast on-off, slow on-off, and intermediate).

ABNORMAL CONDUCTION

The mechanisms of tachyarrhythmias have been classically divided into two general categories: those resulting from an abnormality in impulse generation or "automatic" tachycardias and those resulting from an abnormality in impulse conduction or "reentrant" tachycardias.

Automatic tachycardias depend upon spontaneous impulse generation in latent pacemakers and may be a result of several different mechanisms. Experimentally, chemicals, such as digitalis glycosides or catecholamines, and conditions, such as hypoxemia, electrolyte abnormalities (e.g., hypokalemia), and fiber stretch (cardiac dilation), may lead to an increased slope of phase 4 depolarization in cardiac tissues other than the SA node. These factors, which experimentally lead to abnormal automaticity, are also known to be arrhythmogenic in clinical situations. The increased slope of phase 4 causes heightened automaticity of these tissues and competition with the SA node for dominance of cardiac rhythm. If the rate of spontaneous impulse generation of the abnormally automatic tissue exceeds that of the SA node, then an automatic tachycardia may result. Automatic tachycardias have the following characteristics: (a) the onset of the tachycardia is unrelated to an initiating event such as a premature beat; (b) the initiating beat is usually identical to subsequent beats of the tachycardia; (c) the tachycardia cannot be initiated by programmed cardiac stimulation; (d) the onset of the tachycardia is usually preceded by a gradual acceleration in rate and termination is usually preceded by a gradual deceleration in rate. Clinical tachycardias resulting from the classic forms of enhanced automaticity described above are not as common as once thought. Examples are sinus tachycardia and junctional tachycardia.

Triggered automaticity is also a possible mechanism for abnormal impulse generation. Briefly, triggered automaticity refers to transient membrane depolarizations that occur during repolarization (early after-depolarizations [EADs]) or after repolarization (late after-depolarizations [LADs]) but prior to phase 4 of the action potential. After-depolarizations may be related to abnormal calcium and sodium influx during or just after full cellular repolarization. Experimentally, EADs may be precipitated by hypokalemia, type Ia antiarrhythmic drugs, or slow stimulation rates—any factor that blocks the ion channels (e.g., potassium) responsible for cellular repolarization. Early after-depolarizations provoked by drugs that block potassium conductance and delay repolarization are the underlying cause of TdP. Late after-depolarizations may be precipitated by digitalis or catecholamines and suppressed by CCBs, and have been suggested as the mechanism for multifocal atrial tachycardia, digitalis-induced tachycardias and exercise-provoked VT. Triggered automatic rhythms possess some of the characteristics of automatic tachycardias and some of the characteristics of reentrant tachycardias (described below).

As previously mentioned, the impulse originating from the SA node in an individual with sinus rhythm eventually meets previously excited and thus refractory tissue. Reentry is a concept that involves indefinite propagation of the impulse and continued activation of previously refractory tissue. There are three conduction requirements for the formation of a viable reentrant focus: two pathways for impulse conduction; an area of unidirectional block (prolonged refractoriness) in one of these pathways; and slow conduction in the other pathway (Fig. 19–3). Usually a critically timed premature beat initiates reentry. This premature impulse enters both conduction pathways but encounters refractory tissue in one of the pathways at the area of unidirectional block. The impulse dies out because it is still refractory from the previous (sinus) impulse. Although it fails to propagate in one pathway, the impulse may still proceed in a forward direction (antegrade) through the other pathway because of this pathway's relatively shorter refractory period. The impulse may then proceed through a loop of tissue and "reenter" the area of unidirectional block in a backward direction (retrograde). Because the antegrade pathway has slow conduction characteristics, the area of unidirectional block has time to recover its excitability. The impulse can proceed retrograde through this (previously refractory) tissue and continue around the loop of tissue in a circular fashion. Thus, the key to the formation of a reentrant focus is crucial conduction discrepancies in the electrophysiologic characteristics of the two pathways. The reentrant focus may excite surrounding tissue at a rate greater than that of the SA node and a clinical tachycardia results. The above model is anatomically determined in that there is only one pathway for impulse conduction with a fixed circuit length. Another model of reentry, referred to as a functional reentrant loop or leading circle model, may also occur (Fig. 19–4).[1] In a functional reentrant focus, the length of the circuit may vary depending on the conduction velocity and recovery characteristics of the impulse. The area in the middle of the loop is continually kept refractory by the inwardly moving impulse. The length of the circuit is not fixed, but is the smallest circle possible, such that the leading edge of the wavefront is continuously exciting tissue just as it recovers; that is, the head of the impulse nearly catches its tail. It differs from the anatomic model in that the leading edge of the impulse is not preceded by an excitable gap of tissue, and it does not have an obstacle in the middle or a fixed anatomic circuit. Clinically, many reentrant foci probably have both anatomic and functional characteristics. In the figure 8 model, a zone of unidirectional block is present; allowing for two impulse loops that join and reenter the area of block in a retrograde fashion to form a pretzel-shaped reentrant circuit. This model combines functional characteristics with an excitable gap. All of these theoretical models require a critical balance of refractoriness and conduction velocity within the circuit and as such have helped to explain the effects of drugs on terminating, modifying, and causing cardiac rhythm disturbances.

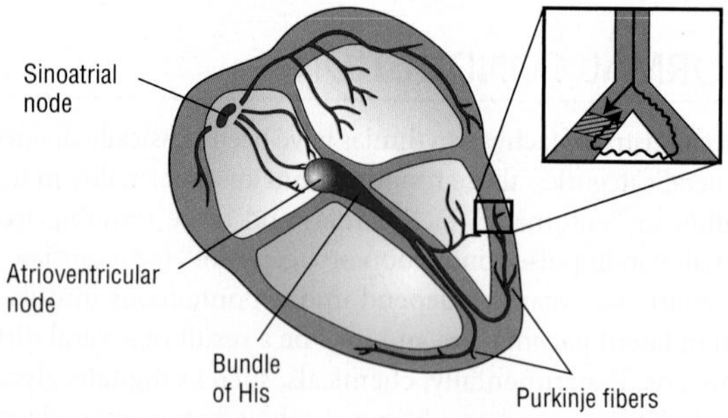

FIGURE 19-3. Conduction system of the heart. The magnified portion shows a bifurcation of a Purkinje fiber traditionally explained as the etiology of reentrant ventricular tachycardia. A premature impulse travels to the fiber, damaged by heart disease or ischemia. It encounters a zone of prolonged refractoriness (area of unidirectional block; *cross-hatched area*) but fails to propagate because it remains refractory to stimulation from the previous impulse. However, the impulse may slowly travel *(squiggly line)* through the other portion of the Purkinje twig and will "reenter" the cross-hatched area if the refractory period is concluded and it is now excitable. Thus, the premature impulse never meets refractory tissue; circus movement ensues. If this site stimulates the surrounding ventricle repetitively, clinical reentrant ventricular tachycardia results.

What causes reentry to become clinically manifest? Reentrant foci may occur at any level of the conduction system: within the branches of the specialized atrial conduction system, the Purkinje network, and even within portions of the SA and AV nodes. The anatomy of the Purkinje system appears to provide a suitable substrate for the formation of microreentrant loops and is often used as a model to facilitate the understanding of reentry concepts (see Fig. 19–4). Of course, because reentry does not usually occur in normal, healthy conduction tissue, various forms of heart disease or conduction abnormalities must usually be present before reentry becomes manifest. In other words, the various forms of heart disease (e.g., ischemic heart disease, LV dysfunction) can result in changes in conduction in the pathways of a suitable reentrant substrate. An often-used example is reentry occurring as a consequence of ischemic or hypoxic damage: with inadequate cellular oxygen, cardiac tissue resorts to anaerobic glycolysis for adenosine triphosphate production. As high-energy phosphate concentration diminishes, the activity of the transmembrane ion pumps declines and RMP rises. This rise in RMP causes inactivation in the voltage-dependent sodium channel and the tissue begins to assume slow conduction characteristics. If changes in conduction parameters occur in a discordant manner due to varying degrees of ischemia or hypoxia, then a reentry circuit may become manifest. Furthermore, an ischemic, dying cell liberates intracellular potassium, which also causes a rise in RMP. In other cases, reentry may occur as a consequence of anatomic or functional variants in the normal conduction system. For instance, patients may possess two (instead of one) conduction pathways near or within the AV node, or have an anomalous extranodal AV pathway that possesses different electrophysiologic characteristics from the normal AV nodal pathway. Reentry in these cases may occur within the AV node or encompass both atrial and ventricular tissue. Reentrant tachycardias have the following characteristics: (a) the onset of the tachycardia is

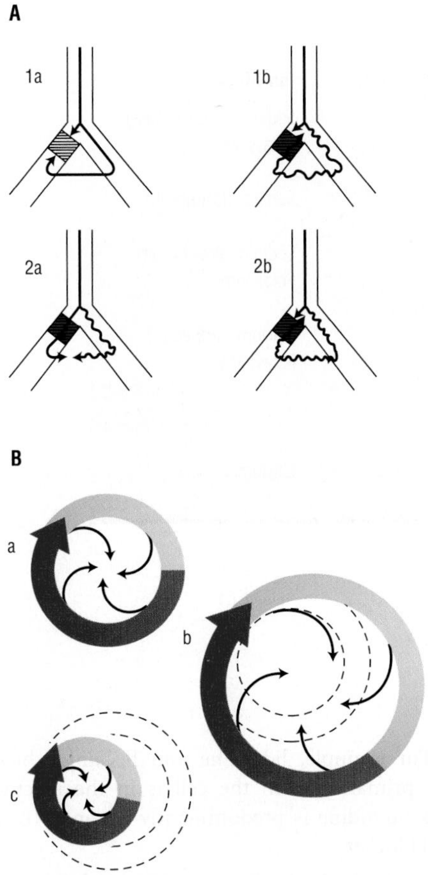

FIGURE 19-4. *A.* Possible mechanism of proarrhythmia in the anatomic model of reentry. *(1a)* Nonviable reentrant loop due to bidirectional block *(shaded area)*. *(1b)* Instance where a drug slows conduction velocity without significantly prolonging the refractory period. The impulse is now able to reenter the area of unidirectional block *(shaded area)* because slowed conduction through the contralateral limb allows recovery of the block. A new reentrant tachycardia may result. *(2a)* Nonviable reentrant loop due to a lack of a unidirectional block. *(2b)* Instance where a drug prolongs the refractory period without significantly slowing conduction velocity. The impulse moving antegrade meets refractory tissue *(shaded area)* allowing for unidirectional block. A new reentrant tachycardia may result. *B.* Mechanism of reentry and proarrhythmia. *(a)* Functionally determined *(leading circle)* reentrant circuit. This model should be contrasted with anatomic reentry; here the circuit is not fixed (it does not necessarily move around an anatomic obstacle) and there is no excitable gap. All tissue inside is held continuously refractory. *(b)* Instance where a drug prolongs the refractory period without significantly slowing conduction velocity. The tachycardia may terminate or slow in rate as shown as a consequence of a greater circuit length. The *dashed lines* represent the original reentrant circuit prior to drug treatment. *(c)* Instance where a drug slows conduction velocity without significantly prolonging the refractory period (i.e., type Ic agents) and accelerates the tachycardia. The tachycardia rate may increase (proarrhythmia) as shown as a consequence of a shorter circuit length. The dashed lines represent the original reentrant circuit prior to drug treatment. *(From McCollam PL, Parker RB, Beckman KJ, et al. Proarrhythmia: A paradoxic response to antiarrhythmic agents. Pharmacotherapy 1989;9:146, with permission.)*

usually related to an initiating event (i.e., premature beat), (b) the initiating beat is usually different in morphology from subsequent beats of the tachycardia, (c) the initiation of the tachycardia is usually possible with programmed cardiac stimulation, and (d) the initiation and termination of the tachycardia is usually abrupt without an acceleration or deceleration phase. There are many examples of reentrant tachycardias including AF, atrial flutter, AV nodal or AV reentrant tachycardia, and recurrent VT.

ANTIARRHYTHMIC DRUGS

In a theoretical sense, drugs may have antiarrhythmic activity by directly altering conduction in several ways. First, a drug may depress the automatic properties of abnormal pacemaker cells. An agent may do this by decreasing the slope of phase 4 depolarization and/or by elevating threshold potential. If the rate of spontaneous impulse generation of the abnormally automatic foci becomes less than that of the SA node, normal cardiac rhythm can be restored. Second, drugs may alter the conduction characteristics of the pathways of a reentrant loop.[1,2] An agent may facilitate conduction (shorten refractoriness) in the area of unidirectional block, allowing antegrade conduction to proceed. On the other hand, an antiarrhythmic may further depress conduction (prolong refractoriness) in either the area of unidirectional block or in the pathway with slowed conduction and a relatively shorter refractory period. If refractoriness is prolonged in the area of unidirectional block, retrograde propagation of the impulse is not permitted, causing a "bidirectional" block. In the anatomic model, if refractoriness is prolonged in the pathway with slow conduction, antegrade conduction of the impulse is not permitted through this route. In either case, drugs that reduce the discordance and cause uniformity in conduction properties of the two pathways may suppress the reentrant substrate. In the functionally determined model, if refractoriness is prolonged without significantly slowing conduction velocity, the tachycardia may terminate or slow in rate as a consequence of a greater circuit length (see Fig. 19–4). There are other theoretical ways to stop reentry: a drug may eliminate the critically timed premature impulse that triggers reentry; a drug may slow conduction velocity to such an extent that conduction is extinguished; or a drug may reverse the underlying form of heart disease that was responsible for the conduction abnormalities that led to the arrhythmia (i.e., "reverse remodeling").

Antiarrhythmic drugs have specific electrophysiologic actions that alter cardiac conduction in patients with or without heart disease. These actions form the basis of grouping antiarrhythmics into specific categories based upon their electrophysiologic actions *in vitro*. Vaughan Williams proposed the most frequently used classification system (Table 19–1).[2] This classification has been criticized because (a) it is incomplete and does not allow for the classification of agents such as digoxin or adenosine; (b) it is not pure and many agents have properties of more than one class of drugs; (c) it does not incorporate drug characteristics such as mechanisms of tachycardia termination/prevention, clinical indications, or side effects; and (d) agents become "labeled" within a class although they may be distinct in many regards.[3] These criticisms formed the basis for an attempt to reclassify antiarrhythmic agents based upon a variety of basic and clinical characteristics (called the Sicilian Gambit[3]). Nonetheless, the Vaughan Williams classification remains the most frequently used despite many proposed modifications and alternative systems.

The type Ia antiarrhythmic drugs—quinidine, procainamide, and disopyramide—slow conduction velocity, prolong refractoriness, and decrease the automatic properties of sodium-dependent (normal and diseased) conduction tissue. Although type Ia agents are primarily considered sodium channel blockers, their electrophysiologic actions can also be attributed to blockade of potassium channels. In reentrant tachycardias, these drugs generally depress conduction and prolong refractoriness, theoretically transforming the area of unidirectional block into a bidirectional block. Clinically, type Ia drugs are broad-spectrum antiarrhythmics that are effective for both supraventricular and ventricular arrhythmias.

The type Ib antiarrhythmic drugs—lidocaine and phenytoin—were historically categorized separately from quinidine-like drugs. This was a result of early work demonstrating that lidocaine had distinctly different electrophysiologic actions. In normal tissue models, lidocaine generally facilitates actions on cardiac conduction by

TABLE 19-1 Classification of Antiarrhythmic Drugs

Type	Drug	Conduction Velocity[a]	Refractory Period	Automaticity	Ion Block
Ia	Quinidine Procainamide Disopyramide	↓	↑	↓	Sodium (intermediate) Potassium
Ib	Lidocaine Mexiletine	0/↓	↓	↓	Sodium (fast on-off)
Ic	Flecainide Propafenone[b] Moricizine[c]	↓↓	0	↓	Sodium (slow on-off) Potassium[d]
II[e]	β-blockers	↓	↑	↓	Calcium (indirect)
III	Amiodarone[f] Dofetilide Sotalol[b] Ibutilide	0	↑↑	0	Potassium
IV[e]	Verapamil Diltiazem	↓	↑	↓	Calcium

AV, atrioventricular; SA, sinoatrial.
[a]Variables for normal tissue models in ventricular tissue.
[b]Also has type II, β-blocking actions.
[c]Classification controversial.
[d]Not clinically manifest.
[e]Variables for SA and AV nodal tissue only.
[f]Also has sodium, calcium, and β-blocking actions; see Table 19–2.

shortening refractoriness and having little effect on conduction velocity. Thus, it was postulated that these agents could improve antegrade conduction, eliminating the area of unidirectional block. Of course, arrhythmias do not usually arise from normal tissue, leading investigators to study the actions of lidocaine and phenytoin in ischemic and hypoxic tissue models. Interestingly, studies have shown these drugs to possess type Ia quinidine-like properties in diseased tissues. Therefore, it is probable that lidocaine acts in clinical tachycardias in a similar fashion to the type Ia drugs (i.e., prolong refractoriness in diseased ischemic tissues leading to bidirectional block in a reentrant circuit). Lidocaine and similar agents have accentuated effects in ischemic tissue caused by the local acidosis and potassium shifts that occur during cellular hypoxia. Changes in pH alter the time that local anesthetics occupy the sodium channel receptor, thereby affecting the agent's electrophysiologic actions. In addition, the intracellular acidosis that ensues as a consequence of ischemia could cause lidocaine to become "trapped" within the cell, allowing increased access to the receptor. The type Ib agents are considerably more effective in ventricular arrhythmias than supraventricular arrhythmias. As a group these drugs are relatively weak sodium channel antagonists (at normal stimulation rates).

The type Ic antiarrhythmic drugs include propafenone, flecainide, and moricizine. These agents are extremely potent sodium blockers, profoundly slowing conduction velocity while leaving refractoriness relatively unaltered. The type Ic drugs theoretically eliminate reentry by slowing conduction to a point where the impulse is extinguished and cannot propagate further. Although the type Ic drugs are effective for both ventricular and supraventricular arrhythmias, their use for ventricular arrhythmias has been limited by the risk of proarrhythmia.

Type I agents are grouped together because of their common action in blocking sodium conductance. The receptor site for these antiarrhythmics is probably inside the sodium channel so that, in effect, the drug plugs the pore. The agent may gain access to the receptor either via the intracellular space through the membrane lipid bilayer or directly through the channel. Several principles are inherent in antiarrhythmic sodium channel receptor theories[4]:

1. Type I antiarrhythmics have predominant affinity for a particular state of the channel (e.g., during activation or inactivation). For example, lidocaine and flecainide block sodium current primarily when the cell is in the inactivated state, whereas quinidine is predominantly an open (or activated)-channel blocker.
2. Type I antiarrhythmics have specific binding and unbinding characteristics to the receptor. For example, lidocaine binds to and dissociates from the channel receptor quickly (termed "fast on-off") but flecainide has very "slow on-off" properties. This explains why flecainide has such potent effects on slowing ventricular conduction whereas lidocaine has little effect on normal tissue (at normal heart rates). In general the type Ic antiarrhythmics are slow on-off, the type Ib antiarrhythmics are fast on-off, and the type Ia antiarrhythmics are intermediate in their binding kinetics.
3. Type I antiarrhythmics possess rate dependence (i.e., sodium channel blockade and slowed conduction are greatest at fast heart rates and least during bradycardia). For slow on-off drugs, sodium channel blockade is evident at normal rates (60 to 100 beats/min) but for fast on-off agents, slowed conduction is only apparent at rapid rates of stimulation.
4. Type I antiarrhythmics (except phenytoin) are weak bases with a pK_a >7.0 and block the sodium channel in their ionized form. Consequently, pH will alter these actions: acidosis accentuates and alkalosis diminishes sodium channel blockade.
5. Type I antiarrhythmics appear to share a single receptor site in the sodium channel. It should be noted, however, that a number of type I antiarrhythmics have other electrophysiologic properties. For instance, quinidine has potent potassium channel blocking activity (manifest predominantly at low concentrations) as does *N*-acetylprocainamide (manifest predominantly at high concentrations), the primary metabolite of procainamide. Additionally propafenone has β-blocking actions.

These principles are important in understanding additive drug combinations (e.g., quinidine and mexiletine), antagonistic combinations (e.g., flecainide and lidocaine), and potential antidotes to excess sodium channel blockade (sodium bicarbonate or propranolol). They also explain a number of clinical observations, such as why lidocaine-like drugs are relatively ineffective for supraventricular tachycardia. The type Ib antiarrhythmics are fast on-off, inactivated sodium blockers; atrial cells, however, have a very brief inactivated phase relative to ventricular tissue.

The β-blockers are classified as type II antiarrhythmic drugs. For the most part, the clinically relevant acute antiarrhythmic mechanisms of the β-blockers result from their antiadrenergic actions. Because the SA and AV nodes are heavily influenced by adrenergic innervation, β-blockers would be most useful in tachycardias in which these nodal tissues are abnormally automatic or are a portion of a reentrant loop. These agents are also helpful in slowing ventricular response in atrial tachycardias (e.g., AF) by their effects on the AV node. Furthermore, some tachycardias are exercise-related or precipitated by states of high sympathetic tone (perhaps through triggered activity), and β-blockers may be useful in these instances. β-adrenergic stimulation results in increased conduction velocity, shortened refractoriness, and increased automaticity of the nodal tissues; β-blockers will antagonize these effects. Propranolol is often noted to have "local anesthetic" or quinidine-like activity; however, suprapharmacologic concentrations are usually required to elicit this action. In the nodal tissues, β-blockers interfere with calcium entry into the cell by altering catecholamine-dependent channel integrity and gating kinetics. In sodium-dependent atrial and ventricular tissue, β-blockers shorten repolarization somewhat, but otherwise have little direct effect. The antiarrhythmic properties of β-blockers observed with long-term, chronic therapy in patients with heart disease are less well understood. Although it is clear that β-blockers decrease the likelihood of SCD (presumably arrhythmic death) after myocardial infarction (MI), the mechanism for this benefit remains unclear but may relate to the complex interplay of changes in sympathetic tone, damaged myocardium, and ventricular conduction. In patients with HF, drugs such as β-blockers, angiotensin-converting enzyme inhibitors, and angiotensin II receptor blockers may prevent arrhythmias such as AF by attenuating the structural remodeling process in the myocardium and subsequently improving ventricular performance over time.[5,6]

The type III antiarrhythmic drugs include those agents that specifically prolong refractoriness in atrial and ventricular tissue. This class includes very different drugs: bretylium, amiodarone, sotalol, ibutilide, and dofetilide; they share the common effect of delaying repolarization by blocking potassium channels. While rarely used, bretylium has complex pharmacology: in addition to blocking potassium channels and delaying repolarization, it first releases then depletes catecholamines. Bretylium increases the VF threshold and seems to have selective antifibrillatory but not antitachycardic effects. In other words, bretylium can be effective in VF, whereas it is often ineffective in VT.

In contrast, amiodarone and sotalol are effective in most supraventricular and ventricular tachycardias. Amiodarone displays electrophysiologic characteristics of all the classes within the Vaughan Williams scheme; it is a sodium channel blocker with relatively fast on-off kinetics, has noncompetitive, nonselective β-blocking actions, blocks potassium channels and also has a small degree of calcium antagonist activity (Table 19–2). At normal heart rates and with chronic use, its predominant effect is to prolong repolarization. Upon IV administration, its onset is relatively quick (unlike the oral form) and β-blockade predominates initially. Theoretically, amiodarone, like type I agents, may interrupt the reentrant substrate by transforming an area of unidirectional block into an area of bidirectional block. However, electrophysiologic studies using programmed cardiac stimulation imply that amiodarone may leave the reentrant loop intact. In addition, the potent β-blocking properties of amiodarone may contribute significantly to both its acute and chronic efficacy. The impressive effectiveness of amiodarone coupled with its low proarrhythmic potential has challenged the notion that selective ion channel blockade by antiarrhythmic agents is preferable. Sotalol is a potent inhibitor of outward potassium movement during repolarization and also possesses nonselective β-blocking actions. Unlike amiodarone and sotalol, ibutilide and dofetilide are only used for the treatment of supraventricular arrhythmias. Both ibutilide (only available IV) and dofetilide (only available orally) can be used for the acute conversion of AF or atrial flutter to sinus rhythm. Dofetilide can also be used to maintain sinus rhythm in patients with AF or atrial flutter of longer than 1 week's duration who have been converted to sinus rhythm. Both of these agents are structurally similar to sotalol and exert their electrophysiologic effects by blocking the rapid component of the delayed potassium rectifier current (I_{Kr}).

There are a number of different potassium channels which function during normal conduction; all approved type III antiarrhythmic drugs inhibit the delayed rectifier current (I_K) responsible for phases 2 and 3 repolarization. Subcurrents make up I_K; an ultrarapid component (I_{Kur}), a rapid component (I_{Kr}), and the slow component (I_{Ks}). *N*-acetylprocainamide, sotalol, ibutilide, and dofetilide selectively block I_{Kr}, whereas amiodarone and azimilide (investigational) block both I_{Kr} and I_{Ks}. New drugs that selectively block I_{Kur} (found predominantly in the atrium but not ventricle) are being investigated for supraventricular arrhythmias. The clinical relevance of selectively blocking components of the delayed rectifier current remains to be determined. Potassium current blockers (particularly those with selective I_{Kr} blocking properties) display "reverse use dependence" (i.e., their effects on repolarization are greatest at low heart rates). Sotalol and drugs like it also appear to be much more effective in preventing VF (in dog models) than the traditional sodium channel blockers. They also decrease defibrillation threshold in contrast to type I agents, which tend to increase this parameter. This could be important in patients with ICDs, as concurrent therapy with type I drugs may require more energy for successful cardioversion or may render the ICD ineffective in terminating the ventricular tachyarrhythmia. The Achilles' heel of all type III agents is an extension of their underlying ionic mechanism (i.e., by blocking potassium channels and delaying repolarization, they may also cause proarrhythmia in the form of TdP by provoking EADs).

TABLE 19-2 Time Course and Electrophysiologic Effects of Amiodarone

				IV		Oral	
Class	**Mechanism**	**EP**	**ECG**	***Min-Hrs***	***Hrs-Days***	***Days-Wks***	***Wks-Mos***
Type I	Na^+ block	↑ HV	↑ QRS	0	+	+	++
Type II	β-block	↑ AH	↑ PR ↓ HR	++	++	++	++
Type III	K^+ block	↑ VERP ↑ AERP	↑ QT	0	+	++	++++
Type IV	Ca^{2+} block[a]	↑ AH	↑ PR	+	+	+	+

[a]Rate-dependent.

AERP, atrial effective refractory period; AH, atria-His interval; ECG, electrocardiographic effects; EP, electrophysiologic actions; HR, heart rate; HV, His-ventricle interval; VERP, ventricular effective refractory period.

The nondihydropyridine CCBs—verapamil and diltiazem—comprise the type IV antiarrhythmic category. At least two types of calcium channels are operative in SA and AV nodal tissues: an L-type channel and a T-type channel. Both L-channel blockers (verapamil and diltiazem) and selective T-channel blockers (mibefradil—previously approved but withdrawn from the market) will slow conduction, prolong refractoriness, and decrease automaticity (e.g., due to EADs or LADs) of the calcium-dependent tissue in the SA and AV nodes. Therefore, these agents are effective in automatic or reentrant tachycardias, which arise from or use the SA or AV nodes. In supraventricular arrhythmias (e.g., AF), these drugs can slow ventricular response by slowing AV nodal conduction. Furthermore, because calcium entry seems to be integral to exercise-related tachycardias and/or tachycardias caused by some forms of triggered automaticity, these agents may be effective in the treatment of these types of arrhythmias. In all likelihood, verapamil and diltiazem work at different receptor sites because of their dissimilar chemical structures and pharmacologic actions. Calcium channel blockers can slightly shorten repolarization in normal sodium-dependent tissue, but otherwise have little effect. The dihydropyridine CCBs (e.g., nifedipine) do not have significant antiarrhythmic activity because a reflex increase in sympathetic tone caused by vasodilation counteracts their direct negative dromotropic action.

All antiarrhythmic agents currently available have an impressive side-effect profile (Table 19–3). A considerable percentage of patients cannot tolerate long-term therapy with these drugs and chances are good that an agent will have to be discontinued because of side effects. ❷ In one trial,[7] more than 50% of patients had to discontinue long-term procainamide (mostly because of a lupus-like syndrome) after MI. In another study,[8] disopyramide caused anticholinergic side effects in approximately 70% of patients. Flecainide, propafenone, and disopyramide may precipitate congestive HF in a significant number of patients with underlying LV systolic dysfunction; consequently, these drugs should be avoided in this patient population.[9] The type Ib agents, such as tocainide and mexiletine, cause neurologic and/or gastrointestinal toxicity in a high percentage of patients. Tocainide, specifically, has been reported to cause both pulmonary fibrosis and leukopenia, the significance of which came to light after its approval by the Food and Drug Administration; it has now been withdrawn from the market and is currently unavailable. One of the most frightening adverse effects related to antiarrhythmic drugs is the aggravation of underlying ventricular arrhythmias or the precipitation of new (and life-threatening) ventricular arrhythmias.[10]

Amiodarone has assumed a prominent place in the treatment of both chronic and acute supraventricular and ventricular arrhythmias and is now the most commonly prescribed antiarrhythmic drug.[11] Once considered a drug of last resort, it is now the first drug considered in many symptomatic tachycardias. Yet amiodarone is a peculiar and complex drug, displaying unusual pharmacologic effects, pharmacokinetics, dosing schemes, and multiorgan side effects. Amiodarone has an extremely long elimination half-life and large volume of distribution; consequently, its onset of action with the oral form is delayed (days to weeks) despite a loading regimen and its effects persist long (months) after discontinuation. Amiodarone inhibits P-glycoprotein and most cytochrome P450 (CYP) enzymes, resulting in the potential for numerous drug interactions (e.g., it will cause digoxin levels to approximately double and one must reduce the maintenance dose of warfarin by one-third to one-half). Acute administration of amiodarone is usually well-tolerated by patients, but severe organ toxicities may result with chronic use. Severe bradycardia (sometimes requiring pacing to allow the patient to remain on amiodarone), hyper- and hypothyroidism, photosensitivity, and a blue-gray skin discoloration on exposed areas are common. Fulminant hepatitis (uncommon) and pulmonary fibrosis (5% to 10% of patients) have caused death.[12,13] Although amiodarone can cause corneal microdeposits (which usually do not affect vision) in virtually every patient, it has also been associated with the development of optic neuropathy/neuritis, which can lead to blindness. All of these side effects mandate close and continued monitoring (liver enzymes, thyroid function tests, eye exams, chest radiographs, pulmonary function tests) and have led to a proliferation of "amiodarone clinics" designed just for patients receiving this agent on a chronic basis (Table 19–4). ❸[14]

TABLE 19-3 Side Effects of Antiarrhythmic Drugs

Quinidine	Cinchonism, diarrhea, abdominal cramps, nausea, vomiting, hypotension, TdP, aggravation of underlying HF, conduction disturbances or ventricular arrhythmias, fever, hepatitis, thrombocytopenia, hemolytic anemia
Procainamide	Systemic lupus erythematosus, diarrhea, nausea, vomiting, TdP, aggravation of underlying HF, conduction disturbances or ventricular arrhythmias, agranulocytosis
Disopyramide	Anticholinergic symptoms (dry mouth, urinary retention, constipation, blurred vision), nausea, anorexia, TdP, HF, aggravation of underlying conduction disturbances and/or ventricular arrhythmias
Lidocaine	Dizziness, sedation, slurred speech, blurred vision, paresthesia, muscle twitching, confusion, nausea, vomiting, seizures, psychosis, sinus arrest, aggravation of underlying conduction disturbances
Mexiletine	Dizziness, sedation, anxiety, confusion, paresthesia, tremor, ataxia, blurred vision, nausea, vomiting, anorexia, aggravation of underlying conduction disturbances or ventricular arrhythmias
Moricizine	Dizziness, headache, fatigue, insomnia, nausea, diarrhea, blurred vision, aggravation of underlying conduction disturbances or ventricular arrhythmias
Flecainide	Blurred vision, dizziness, dyspnea, headache, tremor, nausea, aggravation of underlying HF, conduction disturbances or ventricular arrhythmias
Propafenone	Dizziness, fatigue, bronchospasm, headache, taste disturbances, nausea, vomiting, bradycardia or AV block, aggravation of underlying HF, conduction disturbances or ventricular arrhythmias
Amiodarone	Tremor, ataxia, paresthesia, insomnia, corneal microdeposits, optic neuropathy/neuritis, nausea, vomiting, anorexia, constipation, TdP (<1%), bradycardia or AV block (IV and oral use), pulmonary fibrosis, liver function test abnormalities, hepatitis, hypothyroidism, hyperthyroidism, photosensitivity, blue-gray skin discoloration, hypotension (IV use), phlebitis (IV use)
Dofetilide	Headache, dizziness, TdP
Ibutilide	Headache, TdP, hypotension
Sotalol	Dizziness, weakness, fatigue, nausea, vomiting, diarrhea, bradycardia, TdP, bronchospasm, aggravation of underlying HF

AV, atrioventricular; HF, heart failure; IV, intravenous; TdP, torsades de pointes.

Table 19–5 summarizes the pharmacokinetics of the antiarrhythmic agents and Table 19–6 lists recommended dosages of the oral dosage forms. Table 19–7 lists the dosing recommendations for the corresponding IV forms.

SUPRAVENTRICULAR ARRHYTHMIAS

The common supraventricular tachycardias that often require drug treatment are (a) AF or atrial flutter, (b) PSVT, and (c) automatic atrial tachycardias. Other common supraventricular arrhythmias that usually do not require drug therapy include premature atrial complexes, wandering atrial pacemaker, sinus arrhythmia, and sinus tachycardia. As an example, premature atrial complexes rarely cause symptoms, never cause hemodynamic compromise, and therefore drug therapy is usually not indicated. Likewise, sinus tachycardia is usually the result of underlying metabolic or hemodynamic disorders (e.g., infection, dehydration, hypotension) and therapy should be directed at the underlying cause, not the tachycardia per se. Of course,

TABLE 19-4 Amiodarone Monitoring

Side Effect	Monitoring Recommendations	Management of Side Effect
Pulmonary fibrosis	Chest radiograph (baseline, then every 12 months) Pulmonary function tests (if symptomatic)	Discontinue amiodarone immediately; initiate corticosteroid therapy
Hypothyroidism	Thyroid function tests (baseline, then every 6 months)	Thyroid hormone supplementation (e.g., levothyroxine)
Hyperthyroidism	Thyroid function tests (baseline, then every 6 months)	Antithyroid drugs
Optic neuritis/neuropathy	Ophthalmologic examination (baseline, then every 12 months)	Discontinue amiodarone immediately
Corneal microdeposits	Slit-lamp examination (routine monitoring not necessary)	No treatment necessary
Increased LFTs	LFTs (baseline, then every 6 months)	Consider lowering the dose or discontinuing amiodarone if LFTs >3× normal
Bradycardia/heart block	ECG (baseline, then every 3–6 months)	Lower the dose, if possible, or discontinue amiodarone if severe
Tremors, ataxia, peripheral neuropathy	History/physical examination (each office visit)	Lower the dose, if possible, or discontinue amiodarone if severe
Photosensitivity/blue-gray skin discoloration	History/physical examination (each office visit)	Advise patients to wear sunblock while outdoors

ECG, electrocardiogram; LFTs, liver function tests.

TABLE 19-5 Pharmacokinetics of Antiarrhythmic Drugss

Drug	Bioavailability (%)	Primary Route of Elimination[a]	Substrate[b]	Inhibitor[b]	$V_{D\,ss}$ (L/kg)	Protein Binding (%)	$t_{1/2}$[c]	Therapeutic Range (mg/L)
Quinidine	70–80	H	CYP3A4 (M) CYP2C9	CYP2D6 (S) CYP3A4 (S) CYP2C9 P-GP	2.0–3.5	80–90	5–9 h	2–6
Procainamide	75–95	H/R	NAT CYP2D6 (M)	–	1.5–3.0	10–20	5–6 h (SAs) 2–3 h (FAs)	4–15
Disopyramide	70–95	H/R	CYP3A4 (M)	–	0.8–2.0	50–80	4–8 h	2–6
Lidocaine	–	H	CYP3A4 (M) CYP2D6 (M) CYP1A2 CYP2C9	CYP1A2 (S) CYP2D6 CYP3A4	1–2	65–75	1–3 h	1.5–5.0
Mexiletine	80–95	H	CYP2D6 (M) CYP1A2 (M)	CYP1A2 (S)	5–12	60–75	12–20 h (PMs) 7–11 h (EMs)	0.8–2.0
Moricizine	34–38	H	CYP3A4 (M)	–	6–11	92–95	2–4 h	–
Flecainide	90-95	H/R	CYP2D6 (M) CYP1A2	CYP2D6	8–10	35–45	14–20 h (PMs) 10–14 h (EMs)	0.2–1.0
Propafenone[d]	11–39	H	CYP2D6 (M) CYP1A2 CYP2D6	CYP1A2 CYP2D6	2.5–4.0	85–95	10–25 h (PMs) 3–7 h (EMs)	–
Amiodarone	22–88	H	CYP3A4 (M) CYP1A2 CYP2C19 CYP2D6	CYP2C9 CYP2D6 CYP3A4 CYP1A2 CYP2C19 P-GP	70–150	95–99	15–100 d	1.0–2.5
Sotalol	90–95	R	–	–	1.2–2.4	30–40	10–20 h	–
Dofetilide	85–95	R/H	CYP3A4	–	2.5–3.5	60–70	6–10 h	–
Ibutilide	–	H	–	–	6–12	40–50	3–6 h	–
Verapamil	20–40	H	CYP3A4 (M) CYP1A2 CYP2C9	CYP3A4 CYP1A2 CYP2C9 CYP2D6 P-GP	1.5–5.0	95–99	4–12 h	–
Diltiazem	35–50	H	CYP3A4 (M) CYP2C9 CYP2D6	CYP3A4 CYP2C9 CYP2D6 P-GP	3–5	70–85	4–10 h	–

[a]H, hepatic; R, renal.
[b]CYP, cytochrome P450 isoenzyme; M, major; NAT, *N*-acetyltransferase; P-GP, P-glycoprotein; S, strong.
[c]EMs, extensive metabolizers; FAs, fast acetylators; PMs, poor metabolizers; SAs, slow acetylators.
[d]Variables for parent compound (not 5-OH-propafenone).

TABLE 19-6 Typical Maintenance Doses of Oral Antiarrhythmic Drugs

Drug	Dose	Dose Adjusted
Quinidine	200–300 mg sulfate salt q 6 h 324–648 gluconate salt q 8–12 h	HEP, age >60 yr
Procainamide	500–1,000 mg q 6 h (Pronestyl SR) 1,000–2,000 mg q 12 h (Procanbid)	HEP, REN[a]
Disopyramide	100–150 mg q 6 h 200–300 mg q 12 h (SR form)	HEP, REN
Mexiletine	200–300 mg q 8 h	HEP
Flecainide	50–150 mg q 8 h	HEP, REN
Propafenone	150–300 mg q 8 h	HEP
Moricizine	200 mg q 8 h	HEP, REN
Sotalol	80–160 mg q 12 h	REN[b]
Dofetilide	500 mcg q 12 h	REN[c]
Amiodarone	400 mg two to three times daily until 10 g total, then 200–400 mg daily[d]	

HEP, hepatic disease; REN, renal dysfunction; SR, sustained release.
[a]Accumulation of parent compound or metabolite (e.g., NAPA) may occur.
[b]Should not be used for atrial fibrillation when creatinine clearance <40 mL/min.
[c]Dose should be based upon creatinine clearance; should not be used when creatinine clearance <20 mL/min.
[d]Usual maintenance dose for atrial fibrillation is 200 mg/day (may further decrease dose to 100 mg/day with long-term use if patient clinically stable in order to decrease risk of toxicity); usual maintenance dose for ventricular arrhythmias is 300–400 mg/day.

there are exceptions to these suggestions. For example, sinus tachycardia may be deleterious in patients after cardiac surgery or MI. In another unusual tachycardia termed *nonparoxysmal sinus tachycardia*, chronically elevated heart rates may cause alterations in LV function. In both of these instances, antiarrhythmic drugs, such as β-blockers, may be indicated. Stated in another way, although many arrhythmias generally do not require therapy, clinical judgment and patient-specific variables play an important role in this decision. Nevertheless, for the purpose of this discussion, only the tachycardias usually requiring antiarrhythmic drug therapy, as listed above, are addressed.

CLINICAL PRESENTATION: SUPRAVENTRICULAR TACHYCARDIA

Atrial Fibrillation/Flutter

General

- These rhythms are usually not directly life-threatening nor do they generally cause hemodynamic collapse or syncope; 1:1 atrial flutter (ventricular response ~300 beats/min) is an exception. Also, patients with underlying forms of heart disease that are heavily reliant on atrial contraction to maintain adequate cardiac output (e.g., mitral stenosis, obstructive cardiomyopathy) display more severe symptoms of AF or atrial flutter.

Symptoms

- Most often, patients complain of rapid heart rate/palpitations and/or worsening symptoms of HF (shortness of breath, fatigue). Medical emergencies are severe HF (i.e., pulmonary edema, hypotension) or AF occurring in the setting of acute MI.

Diagnostic Tests/Signs (ECG; See Text for Details)

- Atrial fibrillation is an irregularly, irregular supraventricular rhythm with no discernible, consistent atrial activity (P waves). Ventricular response is usually 120 to 180 beats/min and the pulse is irregular. Atrial flutter is (usually) a regular supraventricular rhythm with characteristic flutter waves (or sawtooth pattern) reflecting more organized atrial activity. Commonly, the ventricular rate is in factors of 300 beats/min (e.g., 150, 100, or 75 beats/min).

Paroxysmal Supraventricular Tachycardia caused by Reentry

General

- These rhythms can be transient, resulting in little, if any, symptoms.

Symptoms

- Patients frequently complain of intermittent episodes of rapid heart rate/palpitations that abruptly start and stop, usually without provocation (but occasionally as a result of exercise). Severe symptoms include syncope. Often (in particular, those with AV nodal reentry), patients complain of a chest pressure or neck sensation. This is caused by simultaneous AV contraction with the right atrium contracting against a closed tricuspid valve. Life-threatening symptoms (syncope, hemodynamic collapse) are associated with an extremely rapid heart rate (e.g., >200 beats/min) and AF associated with an accessory AV pathway.

Diagnostic Tests/Signs (ECG; See Text for Details)

- Most commonly, PSVT is a rapid, narrow QRS tachycardia (regular in rhythm) that starts and stops abruptly. Atrial activity, although present, is difficult to ascertain on surface ECG because P waves are "buried" on the QRS or T wave.

ATRIAL FIBRILLATION AND ATRIAL FLUTTER

Mechanisms and Background

Atrial fibrillation and atrial flutter are common supraventricular tachycardias. These tachycardias occur more often in men and the

TABLE 19-7 Intravenous Antiarrhythmic Dosing

Drug	Clinical Situation	Dose
Amiodarone	Pulseless VT/VF	300 mg IV/IO push (can give additional 150 mg IV/IO push if persistent VT/VF), followed by infusion of 1 mg/min for 6 h, then 0.5 mg/min
	Stable VT (with a pulse)	150 mg IV over 10 min, followed by infusion of 1 mg/min for 6 h, then 0.5 mg/min
	AF (termination)	5 mg/kg IV over 30 min, followed by infusion of 1 mg/min for 6 h, then 0.5 mg/min
Diltiazem	PSVT; AF (rate control)	0.25 mg/kg IV over 2 min (may repeat with 0.35 mg/kg IV over 2 min), followed by infusion of 5–15 mg/h
Ibutilide	AF (termination)	1 mg IV over 10 min (may repeat if needed)
Lidocaine	Pulseless VT/VF	1–1.5 mg/kg IV/IO push (can give additional 0.5–0.75 mg/kg IV/IO push every 5–10 min if persistent VT/VF [maximum cumulative dose = 3 mg/kg]), followed by infusion of 1–4 mg/min (1–2 mg/min if liver disease or HF)
	Stable VT (with a pulse)	1–1.5 mg/kg IV push (can give additional 0.5–0.75 mg/kg IV push every 5–10 min if persistent VT [maximum cumulative dose = 3 mg/kg]), followed by infusion of 1–4 mg/min (1–2 mg/min if liver disease or HF)
Procainamide	AF (termination); stable VT (with a pulse)	15–18 mg/kg IV over 60 min, followed by infusion of 1–4 mg/min
Verapamil	PSVT; AF (rate control)	2.5–5 mg IV over 2 min (may repeat up to maximum cumulative dose of 20 mg); can follow with infusion of 2.5–10 mg/h

AF, atrial fibrillation; IO, intraosseous; IV, intravenous; PSVT, paroxysmal supraventricular tachycardia; VF, ventricular fibrillation; VT, ventricular tachycardia.

elderly. In the general population, the overall prevalence of AF is 0.4% to 1% and this increases with age (e.g., approximately an 8% prevalence in patients >80 years old).[15] The prevalence of AF also appears to increase as patients develop more severe HF, increasing from 4% in asymptomatic NYHA functional class I patients to 50% in patients with NYHA functional class IV HF.[15]

Atrial flutter and AF may present as a chronic, established tachycardia, an acute tachycardia, or a self-terminating, paroxysmal form. The following semantics and definitions are sometimes used specifically for AF:[15,16] acute AF (onset within 48 hours); paroxysmal AF (terminates spontaneously in <7 days); recurrent AF (two or more episodes); persistent AF (duration >7 days and does not terminate spontaneously); and permanent AF (does not terminate with attempts at pharmacologic or electrical cardioversion). Atrial fibrillation is characterized as an extremely rapid (atrial rate of 400 to 600 beats/min) and disorganized atrial activation. With this disorganized atrial activity, there is a loss of the contribution of synchronized atrial contraction (atrial kick) to forward cardiac output. Supraventricular impulses penetrate the AV conduction system in variable degrees resulting in an irregular activation of the ventricles and an *irregularly, irregular* pulse. The AV junction will not conduct most of the supraventricular impulses causing ventricular response to be considerably slower (120 to 180 beats/min) than the atrial rate. It is sometimes stated that "AF begets AF"; that is, the arrhythmia tends to perpetuate itself. Long episodes are more difficult to terminate perhaps because of tachycardia-induced changes in atrial function (mechanical and/or electrical "remodeling").

Atrial flutter occurs less frequently than AF, but is similar in its precipitating factors, consequences, and drug therapy approach. This arrhythmia is characterized by rapid (270 to 330 atrial beats/min) but regular atrial activation. The slower and regular electrical activity results in a regular ventricular response that is in approximate factors of 300 beats/min (i.e., 1:1 AV conduction = ventricular rate of 300 beats/min; 2:1 AV conduction = ventricular rate of 150 beats/min; 3:1 AV conduction = ventricular rate of 100 beats/min). Atrial flutter may occur in two distinct forms (type I and type II). Type I flutter is the more common classic form with atrial rates of approximately 300 beats/min and the typical "sawtooth" pattern of atrial activation as shown by the surface ECG. Type II flutter tends to be faster, being somewhat of a hybrid between classic atrial flutter and AF. Although the ventricular response usually has a regular pattern, atrial flutter with varying degrees of AV block or that occur with episodes of AF ("fib-flutter") can cause an irregular ventricular rate.

It is generally accepted that the predominant mechanism of AF and atrial flutter is reentry. Atrial fibrillation appears to result from multiple atrial reentrant loops (or wavelets) while atrial flutter is caused by a single, dominant, reentrant substrate (counterclockwise circus movement in the right atrium around the tricuspid annulus). Atrial fibrillation or flutter usually occurs in association with various forms of structural heart disease that cause atrial distension, including myocardial ischemia or infarction, hypertensive heart disease, valvular disorders such as mitral stenosis or mitral insufficiency, congenital abnormalities such as septal defects, dilated or hypertrophic cardiomyopathy, and obesity. Disorders that cause right atrial stretch and are associated with AF or atrial flutter include acute pulmonary embolus and chronic lung disease resulting in pulmonary hypertension and cor pulmonale. Atrial fibrillation may also occur in association with states of high adrenergic tone such as thyrotoxicosis, surgery, alcohol withdrawal, sepsis, and excessive physical exertion. Atrial fibrillation that develops in the absence of clinical, electrocardiographic, radiographic, and echocardiographic evidence of structural heart disease is defined as lone AF. Other states in which patients are predisposed to episodes of AF are the presence of an anomalous AV pathway (i.e., Kent bundle) and sinus node dysfunction (i.e., tachy-brady or sick sinus syndrome).

Patients with AF or artrial flutter may experience the entire range of symptoms associated with other supraventricular tachycardias, although syncope as a presenting symptom is uncommon. Because atrial kick is lost with the onset of AF, patients with LV systolic or diastolic dysfunction may develop worsening signs and symptoms of HF as they often depend on the contribution of their atrial kick to maintain an adequate cardiac output. Thromboembolic events, resulting from atrial stasis and poorly adherent mural thrombi, are an additional complication of AF. Of course, the most devastating complication in this regard is the occurrence of an embolic stroke. Approximately 15% of all strokes in the United States can be attributed to AF.[17] The average rate of ischemic stroke in patients with AF who are not receiving antithrombotic therapy is approximately 5% per year.[17,18] Stroke can precede the onset of documented AF, probably as a result of undetected paroxysms prior to the onset of established AF. The risk of stroke significantly increases with age, with the annual attributable risk increasing from 1.5% in individuals ages 50 to 59 years to almost 24% in those ages 80 to 89 years of age.[17] Patients with concomitant AF and rheumatic heart disease are at particularly high risk for stroke, with their risk being increased 17-fold compared to patients in sinus rhythm.[17] Other risk factors for stroke identified from recent trials are previous ischemic stroke, transient ischemic attack, or other systemic embolic event; moderate or severe LV systolic dysfunction and/or congestive HF; hypertension; and diabetes.[17] Younger patients (age <65 years) with AF in whom precipitating factors cannot be identified (i.e., lone AF) are considered to be at low risk for stroke.[17] The risk of stroke in patients with only atrial flutter has been traditionally believed to be low, prompting some to recommend only aspirin for prevention of thromboembolism in this particular patient population. However, because patients with atrial flutter may also intermittently have episodes of AF, this patient population also may be at risk for a thromboembolic event. Although the role of antithrombotic therapy in patients with atrial flutter has not been adequately studied in clinical trials, the most recent guidelines suggest that the same risk stratification scheme and antithrombotic recommendations used in patients with AF also be applied to those with atrial flutter.[17]

Management

The traditional approach to the treatment of AF can be organized into several sequential goals: (a) First, evaluate the need for acute treatment (usually the administration of drugs that slow ventricular rate). (b) Next, contemplate methods to restore sinus rhythm taking into consideration the risks (e.g., thromboembolism). (c) Last, consider ways to prevent the long-term complications of AF such as arrhythmia recurrences and thromboembolism. ❹ One of the biggest controversies in the management of AF is whether or not the restoration and maintenance of sinus rhythm is a desirable goal for all patients with AF. A review of the management of AF/atrial flutter, including a discussion of this controversy follows, organized according to the goals outlined above. Figure 19–5 shows an algorithm for the management of AF and atrial flutter. In addition, Table 19–8 summarizes the recommendations for pharmacologically controlling ventricular rate and restoring and maintaining sinus rhythm from the most recent AF guidelines developed by the American College of Cardiology (ACC)/American Heart Association (AHA)/European Society of Cardiology (ESC).[15]

Acute Treatment First, consider the patient with new-onset, symptomatic AF or atrial flutter. Although uncommon, patients may present with signs and/or symptoms of hemodynamic instability (e.g., severe hypotension, angina, or pulmonary edema), which qualifies as a medical emergency. In these situations, DCC is indicated as first-line therapy in an attempt to immediately restore sinus rhythm (without regard to the risk of thromboembolism).

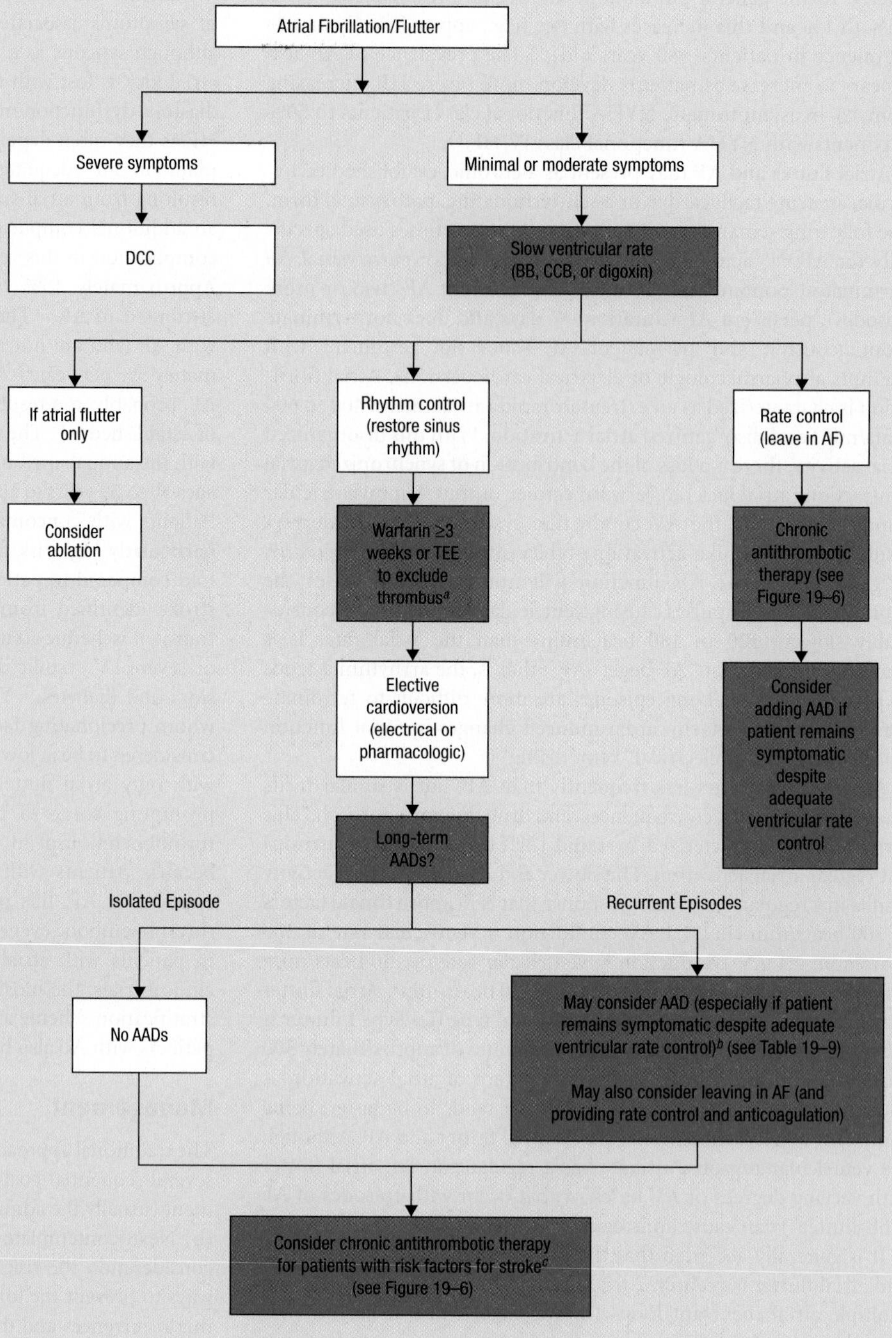

FIGURE 19-5. Algorithm for the treatment of atrial fibrillation and atrial flutter. [a]If AF <48 hours, anticoagulation prior to cardioversion is unnecessary; may consider TEE if patient has risk factors for stroke. [b]Ablation may be considered for patients who fail or do not tolerate ≥1 AAD. [c]Chronic antithrombotic therapy should be considered in all patients with AF and risk factors for stroke regardless of whether or not they remain in sinus rhythm. (AAD, antiarrhythmic drug; AF, atrial fibrillation; BB, β-blocker; CCB, calcium channel blocker [i.e., verapamil or diltiazem]; DCC, direct-current cardioversion; TEE, transesophageal echocardiogram.)

Atrial flutter often requires relatively low energy levels of countershock (i.e., 50 joules), whereas AF often requires higher energy levels (i.e., greater than 200 joules).

If patients are hemodynamically stable, there is no emergent need to restore sinus rhythm. Instead, the focus should be directed toward controlling the patient's ventricular rate. Achieving adequate ventricular rate control should be a treatment goal for all patients with AF. To achieve this goal, drugs that slow conduction and increase refractoriness in the AV node (e.g., β-blockers, nondihydropyridine CCBs, or digoxin) should be used as initial therapy. Although loading dosages of digoxin have been historically recommended as first-line treatment to slow ventricular rate, use of this drug for achieving ventricular rate control, especially in patients with normal LV systolic function (left ventricular ejection fraction [LVEF] >40%) has declined.[11] In this patient population, IV β-blockers (propranolol, metoprolol, esmolol), diltiazem, or verapamil is preferred. A few of the potential reasons for the declining use of digoxin in this patient population are its relatively slow onset and its inability to control the heart rate during exercise. Although an initial decrease in the ventricular rate can sometimes be observed within 1 hour of IV administration, full control (heart rate <80 beats/min at rest and <100 beats/min during exercise) is usually not achieved for 24 to 48 hours. In addition, digoxin tends to be ineffective for controlling ventricular rate under conditions of increased sympathetic tone (i.e., surgery, thyrotoxicosis) because it slows AV nodal conduction primarily through vagotonic mechanisms. In contrast, IV β-blockers and nondihydropyridine CCBs have a relatively quick onset and can effectively control the ventricular rate at rest and during exercise. β-blockers are also effective for controlling ventricular rate under conditions of increased sympathetic tone.

Based on the most recent guidelines for the treatment of AF, the selection of a drug to control ventricular rate in the acute setting should be primarily based on the patient's LV function.[15] In patients with normal LV function (LVEF >40%), IV β-blockers, diltiazem, or verapamil is recommended as first-line therapy to control ventricular rate.[15] All of these agents have proven efficacy in controlling the

TABLE 19-8 Evidence-Based Pharmacologic Treatment Recommendations for Controlling Ventricular Rate, Restoring Sinus Rhythm, and Maintaining Sinus Rhythm in Patients with Atrial Fibrillation

Treatment Recommendations	ACC/AHA/ESC Guideline Recommendation
Ventricular rate control (acute setting)	
In the absence of an accessory pathway, IV β-blockers, or IV nondihydropyridine CCBs are recommended for patients without hypotension or HF.	Class I
In the absence of an accessory pathway, IV digoxin or IV amiodarone is recommended for patients with HF.	Class I
IV amiodarone can be used to control the ventricular rate in patients who are refractory to or have contraindications to IV β-blockers, nondihydropyridine CCBs, or digoxin.	Class IIa
IV procainamide or ibutilide is a reasonable alternative in patients with an accessory pathway when DCC is not necessary.	Class IIa
IV procainamide, ibutilide, or amiodarone may be considered for hemodynamically stable patients with an accessory pathway.	Class IIb
IV nondihydropyridine CCBs are not recommended in patients with decompensated HF.	Class III
Ventricular rate control (chronic setting)	
Oral digoxin is effective for controlling the ventricular rate at rest in patients with HF or LV dysfunction, and in those who are sedentary.	Class I
Combination therapy with oral digoxin and either an oral β-blocker or nondihydropyridine CCB is reasonable to control the ventricular rate both at rest and during exercise.	Class IIa
Oral amiodarone can be used when the ventricular rate cannot be adequately controlled at rest and during exercise with an oral β-blocker, nondihydropyridine CCB, and/or digoxin.	Class IIb
Digoxin should not be used as the only agent for controlling the ventricular rate in patients with paroxysmal AF.	Class III
Restoration of sinus rhythm	
Flecainide, dofetilide, propafenone, or ibutilide is recommended for pharmacologic cardioversion of AF.	Class I
Amiodarone is a reasonable option for pharmacologic cardioversion of AF.	Class IIa
The "pill-in-the-pocket" approach (see text) can be used to terminate persistent AF on an outpatient basis once the treatment has been used safely in the hospital, in patients without sinus or AV node dysfunction, bundle-branch block, QT interval prolongation, Brugada syndrome, or structural heart disease (Note: AV node must be adequately blocked before initiating this therapy.)	Class IIa
Amiodarone can be used on an outpatient basis in patients with paroxysmal or persistent AF when rapid restoration of sinus rhythm is not necessary.	Class IIa
Quinidine or procainamide might be considered for pharmacologic cardioversion of AF, but their efficacy is not well established.	Class IIb
Digoxin and sotalol should not be used for pharmacologic cardioversion of AF (may be harmful).	Class III
Quinidine, procainamide, disopyramide, and dofetilide should not be initiated on an outpatient basis	Class III
Maintenance of sinus rhythm	
Antiarrhythmic therapy can be useful for maintaining sinus rhythm and preventing tachycardia-induced cardiomyopathy.	Class IIa
Outpatient initiation of antiarrhythmic therapy is reasonable in patients without structural heart disease.	Class IIa
Propafenone or flecainide may be initiated on an outpatient basis in patients with paroxysmal AF who have no structural heart disease and are in sinus rhythm at the time therapy is initiated.	Class IIa
Sotalol may be initiated on an outpatient basis in patients without structural heart disease, QT interval prolongation, electrolyte abnormalities, or other risk factors for proarrhythmia.	Class IIa
An antiarrhythmic drug should not be used when patients have risk factors for proarrhythmia with that particular agent.	Class III
Antiarrhythmic therapy is not recommended in patients with sinus or AV node dysfunction unless a pacemaker is present.	Class III

ACC, American College of Cardiology; AF, atrial fibrillation; AHA, American Heart Association; AV, atrioventricular; CCB, calcium channel blocker; DCC, direct-current cardioversion; ESC, European Society of Cardiology; HF, heart failure; IV, intravenous; LV, left ventricular.
Adapted from reference 15.

ventricular rate in patients with AF. Propranolol and metoprolol can be administered as intermittent IV boluses, whereas esmolol (because of its very short half-life of 5 to 10 minutes) must be administered as a series of loading doses followed by a continuous infusion. Likewise, because control of ventricular rate can be transient with a single bolus, verapamil or diltiazem can be given as an initial IV bolus followed by a continuous infusion.[19] These continuous infusions can be adjusted in monitored settings to the desired ventricular response (e.g., acutely <100 beats/min). In situations where AF or atrial flutter is precipitated by states of increased adrenergic tone, IV β-blockers can be highly effective and should be considered first.

In patients with LV dysfunction (LVEF ≤40%), IV diltiazem or verapamil should be avoided because of their potent negative inotropic effects. Intravenous β-blockers should be used with caution in this patient population and should be avoided if patients are in the midst of an episode of decompensated HF. In those patients who are having an exacerbation of HF symptoms, IV administration of either digoxin or amiodarone should be used as first-line therapy to achieve ventricular rate control.[15] Intravenous amiodarone can also be used in patients who are refractory to or have contraindications to β-blockers, nondihydropyridine CCBs, and digoxin.[15] However, clinicians should be aware that the use of amiodarone for controlling ventricular rate may also stimulate the conversion of AF to sinus rhythm, and place the patient at risk for a thromboembolic event, especially if the AF is at least 48 hours or of unknown duration.

Patients may present with a slow ventricular response (in the absence of AV nodal-blocking drugs) and thus, do not require therapy with β-blockers, nondihydropyridine CCBs, or digoxin. This type of presentation should alert the clinician to the possibility of preexisting SA or AV nodal conduction disease such as sick sinus syndrome. In these patients, DCC should not be attempted without a temporary pacemaker in place.

Restoration of Sinus Rhythm? After treatment with AV nodal-blocking agents and a subsequent decrease in the ventricular rate, the patient should be evaluated for the possibility of restoring sinus rhythm if AF persists. Within the context of this evaluation, several factors should be considered. First, many patients spontaneously convert to sinus rhythm without intervention, obviating therapy needed to achieve this goal. For instance, AF occurs frequently as a complication of cardiac surgery and often spontaneously reverts to sinus rhythm without therapy. Second, restoring sinus rhythm is not a necessary or realistic goal in some patients. To date, a total of five clinical trials (Pharmacological Intervention in Atrial Fibrillation [PIAF], Rate Control versus Electrical Cardioversion for Persistent Atrial Fibrillation [RACE], Atrial Fibrillation Follow-up Investigation of Rhythm Management [AFFIRM], Strategies of Treatment of Atrial Fibrillation [STAF], and How to Treat Chronic Atrial Fibrillation [HOT-CAFE]), have been published that have shed some light on this particular issue.[20–24] Of these, the AFFIRM is the largest study to compare the effects of a rate-control (controlling ventricular rate; patient remains in AF) and rhythm-control (restoring and maintaining sinus rhythm) strategy in patients with AF.[22] In the AFFIRM trial, patients with AF and at least one risk factor for stroke were randomized to either a rate-control or rhythm-control group. Rate-control treatment involved AV nodal-blocking drugs (digoxin, β-blockers, and/or CCBs) first, then nondrug treatment (AV nodal ablation with pacemaker implantation), if necessary. All patients in this group were anticoagulated with warfarin to achieve an international normalized ratio (INR) of 2.0 to 3.0. In the rhythm-control group, type I or type III antiarrhythmic drugs were used to maintain sinus rhythm. The choice of antiarrhythmic therapy was left up to each patient's physician; however, by the end of the trial, more than 60% of patients had received at least one trial of amiodarone and approximately 40% of patients had received at least one trial of sotalol. In this group, anticoagulation was encouraged but could be discontinued if sinus rhythm had been maintained for at least 4 weeks. After a mean follow-up period of 3.5 years, overall mortality was not statistically different between the two strategies but tended ($P = 0.08$) to be higher in the rhythm-control group. The results of the PIAF, RACE, STAF, and HOT-CAFE trials were consistent with those of the AFFIRM trial.[20,21,23,24] In addition, a recently published meta-analysis of the data from all of these trials demonstrated no significant difference in overall mortality between rate-control and rhythm-control strategies, which persisted even when the results from the AFFIRM trial were excluded from this analysis.[25] Overall, the results of these trials collectively demonstrate that a rate-control strategy is a viable alternative to a rhythm-control strategy in patients with persistent AF.

Clearly, these important findings temper the old approach of aggressively attempting to maintain sinus rhythm. Because a rhythm-control strategy does not confer any advantage over a rate-control strategy in the management of AF, it now remains acceptable to allow patients to remain in AF, while being chronically treated with AV nodal-blocking agents to achieve adequate ventricular rate control (e.g., heart rate <80 beats/min at rest and <100 beats/min during exercise). ❹ Overall, the selection of an AV nodal-blocking agent to control ventricular rate in the chronic setting should be primarily based on the patient's LV function.[15] In patients with normal LV function (LVEF >40%), oral β-blockers, diltiazem, or verapamil are preferred over digoxin because of their relatively quick onset and maintained efficacy during exercise. When adequate ventricular rate control cannot be achieved with one of these agents, the addition of digoxin may provide an additive lowering of the heart rate. If adequate ventricular rate control during rest and exercise cannot be achieved with β-blockers, nondihydropyridine CCBs, and/or digoxin, oral amiodarone can be used as alternative therapy to control the heart rate.[15] Verapamil and diltiazem should not be used in patients with LV dysfunction (LVEF ≤40%). Instead, β-blockers (i.e., metoprolol, carvedilol, or bisoprolol) and digoxin are preferred in these patients, as these agents are also concomitantly used to treat chronic HF; if possible, β-blockers should be considered over digoxin in this situation because of their survival benefits in patients with LV systolic dysfunction. If patients are having an episode of decompensated HF, digoxin is preferred as first-line therapy to achieve ventricular rate control. Occasionally, patients may be encountered who are highly refractory to AV nodal-blocking agents (including combination drug therapy) and continue to have a rapid ventricular rate. In this situation, aggressive attempts to lower the heart rate are necessary as chronic tachycardia can result in a progressive decline in LV function causing so-called *tachycardia-induced cardiomyopathy*. Hence, in drug-refractory patients, ablation or modification of the AV node by a transvenous catheter delivering radiofrequency current is indicated.[15,26] This procedure often completely blocks conduction from the atrium to the ventricle, requiring the concurrent implantation of a permanent pacemaker with a ventricular lead. Regardless of the situation, if the decision is made to allow a patient to remain in AF, consideration must be given to selecting the most appropriate antithrombotic therapy for these patients as they continue to be at risk for thromboembolic complications (see below).

Because a rate-control strategy is now considered a reasonable approach for the chronic management of AF, the question that remains to be answered is, "In which patients should restoration of sinus rhythm be considered?" Given the results of the AFFIRM trial, this decision should be left to clinical judgment but one could imagine that several groups of patients should undergo electrical or pharmacologic cardioversion. They include those patients who are judged to have a relatively low chance of recurrence (e.g., first episode of lone AF in young individuals, transient states of high sympathetic tone) and those with troublesome symptoms despite adequate ventricular rate control. In the former patient population, chronic antiarrhythmic therapy is usually not needed since the AF is often self-limiting.

In those patients in whom it is decided to restore sinus rhythm, one must consider that this very act (regardless of whether an electrical or pharmacologic method is chosen) places the patient at risk for a thromboembolic event. The reason for this is that the return of sinus rhythm restores effective contraction in the atria, which may dislodge poorly adherent thrombi. Administering antithrombotic therapy prior to cardioversion not only prevents clot growth and the formation of new thrombi but also allows existing thrombi to become organized and well-adherent to the atrial wall. It is a generally accepted principle that patients become at increased risk of thrombus formation and a subsequent embolic event if the duration of the AF exceeds 48 hours. Therefore, it is vital for clinicians to estimate the duration of the patient's AF, so that appropriate antithrombotic therapy can be administered prior to cardioversion, if needed. According to the most recent guidelines derived from the Seventh American College of Chest Physicians Consensus Conference on Antithrombotic Therapy, patients with AF for longer than 48 hours or an unknown duration should receive warfarin treatment (target INR 2.5; range: 2.0 to 3.0) for at least 3 weeks prior to cardioversion.[17] The common clinical scenario is to discharge the patient from the hospital, monitor them on an ambulatory basis, and readmit for elective cardioversion after this time period. After restoration of sinus rhythm, full atrial contraction does not occur immediately. Rather, it returns gradually to a maximum contractile force over a 3- to 4-week period. Consequently, warfarin should be continued for at least 4 weeks after effective cardioversion and return of sinus rhythm. To shorten the time to cardioversion, these patients may alternatively undergo transesophageal echocardiography (TEE) to provide guidance regarding the need for antithrombotic therapy prior to cardioversion. If no thrombus is noted on TEE, then these patients can be cardioverted without the mandatory 3 weeks of warfarin pretreatment. However, IV unfractionated heparin should still be administered during the TEE and cardioversion procedures to prevent the formation of thrombi during the pericardioversion and postcardioversion periods. After effective cardioversion and return of sinus rhythm, these patients should receive 4 weeks of warfarin therapy, as their atria may still be mechanically stunned during this period. If the TEE performed prior to cardioversion reveals thrombus, patients should then be anticoagulated indefinitely, and cardioversion should not be attempted until there is absence of thrombus on repeat TEE. Overall, the use of TEE in this manner has been compared to the conventional 3 weeks of anticoagulation before cardioversion in patients with AF.[27] In this large, multicenter, randomized trial, the incidence of thromboembolic events was not different between the two strategies, but bleeding episodes were higher in the "3 weeks of warfarin" group. Patients in the TEE strategy group had a higher success rate of achieving sinus rhythm, probably because it's more difficult to terminate AF the longer a patient remains in it (i.e., "AF begets AF").

In patients with AF that is less than 48 hours in duration, anticoagulation prior to cardioversion is unnecessary because there has not been sufficient time to form atrial thrombi.[17] However, it is recommended that these patients should receive either IV unfractionated heparin or a low-molecular-weight heparin (subcutaneously at treatment doses) at presentation prior to cardioversion. If these patients have risk factors for stroke, a TEE could alternatively be performed prior to cardioversion to exclude the presence of thrombus. Patients with AF that is less than 48 hours in duration do not require the 4 weeks of postcardioversion anticoagulation therapy unless they have risk factors for stroke or if the AF recurs.

After prior anticoagulation or TEE, the methods available to restore sinus rhythm can be considered. There are two methods of restoring sinus rhythm in patients with AF or atrial flutter: pharmacologic cardioversion and DCC. Which of these is the method of choice is generally a matter of clinical preference. The disadvantages of pharmacologic cardioversion are the risk of significant side effects (e.g., drug-induced TdP),[28] the inconvenience of drug–drug interactions (e.g., digoxin–amiodarone), and the fact that drugs are generally less effective when compared to DCC. The advantages of DCC are that it is quick and more often successful (80% to 90% success rate). The disadvantages of DCC are the need for prior sedation/anesthesia and a risk (albeit small) of serious complications such as sinus arrest or ventricular arrhythmias. Contrary to past beliefs, DCC carries very little risk in patients who are receiving digoxin and have no evidence of digitalis toxicity.

Nonetheless, despite the relatively high success rate associated with DCC, some clinicians elect to use antiarrhythmic drugs first, then resort to DCC in the event that these agents fail. Pharmacologic cardioversion appears to be most effective when initiated within 7 days after the onset of AF.[15] According to the most recent treatment guidelines for AF, there is relatively strong evidence for efficacy of the type III pure I_K blockers (ibutilide and dofetilide), the type Ic antiarrhythmics (e.g., flecainide and propafenone), and amiodarone (oral or IV).[15] Type Ia antiarrhythmics have limited efficacy in this setting. Sotalol is not effective for cardioversion of paroxysmal or persistent AF. Single, oral loading doses of propafenone (600 mg) and flecainide (300 mg) are effective compared to placebo for conversion of recent-onset AF and provide a simple regimen.[29] A method called the "pill-in-the-pocket" approach was recently endorsed by the treatment guidelines.[15] With this method, outpatient, patient-controlled self-administration of a single, oral loading dose of either flecainide or propafenone can be a relatively safe and effective approach for the termination of recent-onset AF in a selected patient population that does not have sinus or AV node dysfunction, bundle-branch block, QT interval prolongation, Brugada syndrome, or structural heart disease.[30] In addition, this treatment regimen should only be considered in patients who have been successfully cardioverted with these drugs on an inpatient basis. In patients with AF that is longer than 7 days in duration, only dofetilide, amiodarone, and ibutilide have proven efficacy for cardioversion.[15] The types Ia and Ic antiarrhythmics have limited efficacy in this setting.

Overall, when considering pharmacologic cardioversion, the selection of an antiarrhythmic drug should be based on whether the patient has structural heart disease (e.g., LV dysfunction, coronary artery disease, valvular heart disease, LV hypertrophy).[15] In the absence of any type of structural heart disease, the use of a single, oral loading dose of flecainide or propafenone is a reasonable approach for cardioversion; the "pill-in-the-pocket" approach should only be used in select patients (see above). Ibutilide can also be used as an alternative agent in this patient population; however, this agent can only be administered in the hospital because it is only available in IV form. In patients with underlying structural heart disease, these antiarrhythmics should be avoided because of the increased risk of proarrhythmia, and amiodarone or dofetilide should be used instead. Although amiodarone can be administered safely on an outpatient basis because of its low proarrhythmic potential, dofetilide can only be initiated in the hospital. Additionally, it should be remembered that a patient's ventricular rate should be adequately controlled with AV nodal-blocking drugs prior to administering a type Ic (or Ia) antiarrhythmic for cardioversion. The types Ia and Ic agents may paradoxically increase ventricular response. Traditionally, this observation has been attributed to the vagolytic action of these drugs despite the fact that only disopyramide displays significant anticholinergic side effects. Therefore, a more likely alternative explanation exists: all of these agents slow atrial conduction, decreasing the number of impulses reaching the AV node; as a result, the AV node paradoxically allows more impulses to gain entrance to the ventricular conduction system (increasing ventricular rate).

Long-Term Complications There are two forms of therapy that the clinician must consider in each patient: long-term antithrombotic therapy to prevent stroke, and long-term antiarrhythmic drugs to prevent recurrences of AF. Consider the issue of antithrombotic therapy first. In the past, patients with AF were not routinely anticoagulated (unless there was a history of stroke or concurrent mitral valve disease) because it was believed that the risk of warfarin exceeded its potential (though unknown) benefit. In the past several years, a large number of randomized, placebo-controlled trials designed to evaluate this issue have been published. All possess relatively similar findings and many were terminated prematurely because of a significant effect in the treatment group (warfarin). In all, these studies culminated in the following recommendations from the Seventh American College of Chest Physicians Consensus Conference on Antithrombotic Therapy for patients with paroxysmal, persistent, or permanent AF[17]: warfarin (target INR: 2.5; range: 2.0 to 3.0) should be prescribed to all patients who are at high risk for stroke (rheumatic mitral valve disease; previous ischemic stroke, transient ischemic attack, or other systemic embolic event; age >75 years; moderate or severe LV systolic dysfunction and/or congestive HF; hypertension; or prosthetic heart valve); those at intermediate risk (age 65 to 75 years with none of the above high-risk factors) should receive either warfarin (target INR: 2.5; range: 2.0 to 3.0) or aspirin 325 mg/day; and those at low risk (age <65 years with none of the above high-risk factors) should receive aspirin 325 mg/day. In the intermediate-risk group, the decision of whether to use warfarin or aspirin should be based on such factors as the patient's risk for bleeding, patient preference, potential drug interactions with warfarin, and the availability of an appropriate monitoring system for warfarin therapy. Although it was previously an acceptable practice to continue antithrombotic therapy for only 4 weeks after successful cardioversion (with the belief that a patient's risk for thromboembolism had abated since they were in sinus rhythm), recent data from the PIAF, RACE, AFFIRM, STAF, and HOT-CAFE trials strongly suggest that patients with AF and other risk factors for stroke continue to be at risk for stroke even when maintained in sinus rhythm.[20–24] It is possible that these patients may be having undetected episodes of paroxysmal AF, placing them at risk for stroke. Consequently, the updated treatment guidelines for AF recommend that chronic antithrombotic therapy be considered for all patients with AF and risk factors for stroke regardless of whether or not they remain in sinus rhythm.[15] Figure 19–6 is an algorithm for preventing thromboembolism in patients with AF.

The second form of chronic therapy to be considered is antiarrhythmic drugs to prevent recurrences of AF. With some exceptions (e.g., postoperative situations or transient states of high sympathetic tone), AF often recurs after initial cardioversion because most patients have irreversible, underlying heart or lung disease. Large atrial size, poor LV function, and the presence of long-standing AF are factors that make the restoration and maintenance of sinus

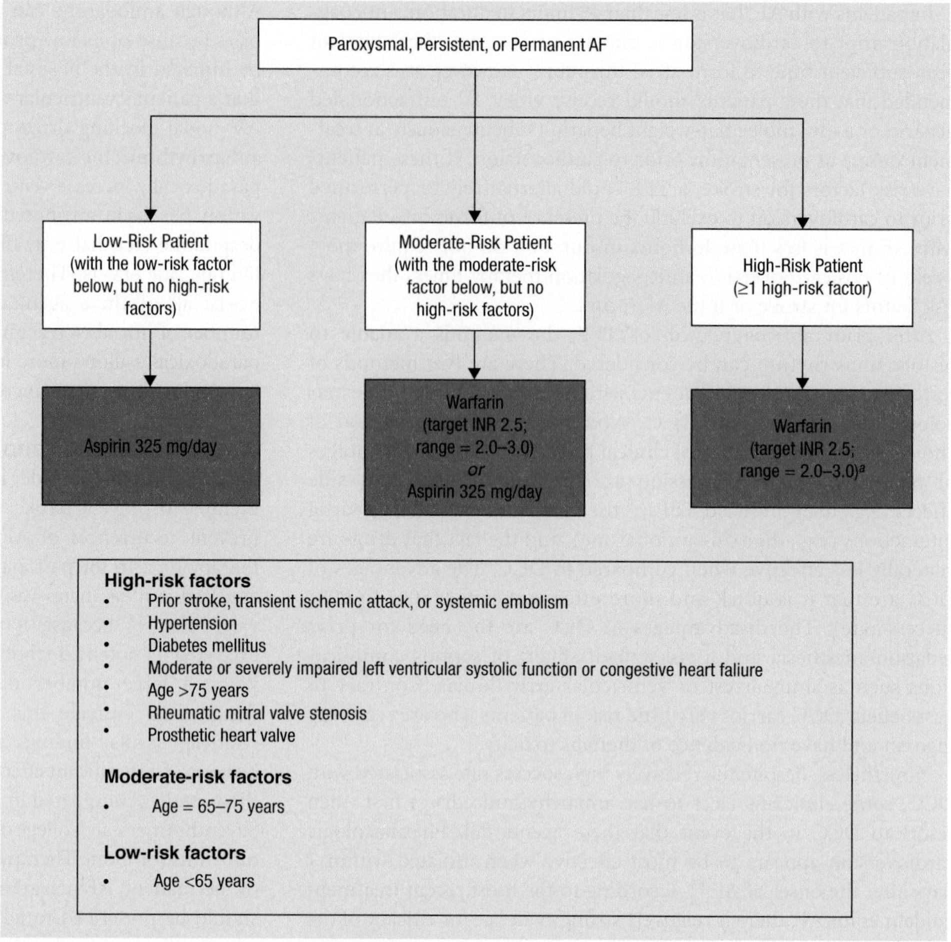

FIGURE 19-6. Algorithm for the prevention of thromboembolism in paroxysmal, persistent, or permanent atrial fibrillation. [a]The target INR for patients with prosthetic heart valves should be based upon the type of valve that is present. (AF, atrial fibrillation; INR, international normalized ratio.)

rhythm difficult if not impossible. Nevertheless, historically, many clinicians have aggressively attempted to maintain sinus rhythm by prescribing oral antiarrhythmic drugs (usually quinidine) to prevent these recurrences despite the fact that only small studies with conflicting results existed evaluating this approach. To evaluate the efficacy of quinidine in preventing AF, a well-known meta-analysis of the existing literature was completed.[31] This meta-analysis demonstrated that indeed more patients remain in sinus rhythm with quinidine therapy (compared to placebo); however, approximately 50% have recurrences of AF within a year despite quinidine. However, this reported effectiveness was at the cost of an associated increase in mortality (presumably due, in part, to proarrhythmia) in the quinidine-treated patients. These disturbing results (published soon after the CAST[32]) became widely quoted and highly visible, making clinicians question the wisdom of long-term prevention of recurrences of AF with antiarrhythmic drugs. Although the results were questioned because some of the reported causes of death in the treated patients could not be directly attributed to quinidine, subsequent studies[33] tended to support the findings of the meta-analysis.

These results coupled with the recent findings of the PIAF, RACE, AFFIRM, STAF, and HOT-CAFE trials question the need to use antiarrhythmic drugs to prevent recurrences of AF.[20–24] Perhaps this practice should now be totally abandoned, allowing patients to remain in AF once recurrences happen and only using strategies to control rate and prevent thromboembolism. Although it is true that these data have certainly led to a less-aggressive approach, patients with paroxysmal AF who continue to have intolerable symptoms during recurrences do require antiarrhythmic drugs to prevent these symptomatic attacks.

According to the recent treatment guidelines for AF, the type Ic or type III antiarrhythmic drugs are reasonable to consider to maintain patients in sinus rhythm (Table 19–9).[15] The role of the type Ia antiarrhythmic drugs for maintenance of sinus rhythm has been deemphasized throughout these updated guidelines as they are considered less effective or incompletely studied compared to the type Ic and type III agents. Realistically, however, these agents can still be considered as last-line therapy in patients without structural heart disease and in patients with hypertension (without significant LV hypertrophy) or coronary artery disease (with normal LV systolic function).

TABLE 19-9 Guidelines for Selecting Antiarrhythmic Drug Therapy for Maintenance of Sinus Rhythm in Patients with Recurrent Paroxysmal or Recurrent Persistent Atrial Fibrillation

No structural heart disease[a]
- First line: flecainide, propafenone, or sotalol
- Second line: amiodarone or dofetilide (catheter ablation could also be considered as an alternative to antiarrhythmic therapy)

Heart failure[a]
- First line: amiodarone or dofetilide
- Second line: catheter ablation

Coronary artery disease[a]
- First line: sotalol (to be used only if patients have normal LV systolic function)
- Second line: amiodarone or dofetilide (catheter ablation could also be considered as an alternative to antiarrhythmic therapy)

Hypertension[a]
- Presence of significant LVH
  - First line: amiodarone
  - Second line: catheter ablation
- Absence of significant LVH:
  - First line: flecainide, propafenone, or sotalol
  - Second line: amiodarone or dofetilide (catheter ablation could also be considered as an alternative to antiarrhythmic therapy)

LV, left ventricular; LVH, left ventricular hypertrophy.
[a]Drugs are listed alphabetically and not in order of suggested use.

The type Ic antiarrhythmics, flecainide and propafenone, are effective for maintaining sinus rhythm. However, because of the increased risk for proarrhythmia, these drugs should be avoided in patients with structural heart disease.

Although all of the oral type III antiarrhythmic drugs have demonstrated efficacy in preventing recurrences of AF, amiodarone is clearly the most effective agent and is now the most frequently chosen despite its impressive organ toxicity.[11] Since 2000, the superiority of amiodarone over other antiarrhythmics for maintaining patients in sinus rhythm has been demonstrated in a number of clinical trials. In the Canadian Trial of Atrial Fibrillation, amiodarone was significantly more effective than sotalol or propafenone in maintaining sinus rhythm in patients with persistent or paroxysmal AF.[34] Furthermore, in a substudy of the AFFIRM trial, amiodarone appeared to be the most effective antiarrhythmic agent of those used in the study.[35] In the more recently published Sotalol Amiodarone Atrial Fibrillation Efficacy Trial, amiodarone and sotalol were equally effective at converting AF to sinus rhythm.[36] However, amiodarone was significantly more effective than sotalol at maintaining sinus rhythm in all patient subgroups, except for those with ischemic heart disease where the efficacy of these two drugs was comparable.

Although sotalol is not effective for conversion of AF, it is an effective agent for maintaining sinus rhythm. Sotalol has been shown to be at least as effective as quinidine or propafenone in preventing recurrences of AF.[34,37] However, treatment with either quinidine or sotalol is associated with a similar incidence of TdP. Because this form of proarrhythmia primarily occurs with higher doses of sotalol (quinidine usually causes TdP at low or therapeutic concentrations), it may be more easily predicted and therefore avoided. Nonetheless, sotalol may increase mortality in patients with AF similar to quinidine; however, this requires further study.[38]

Dofetilide is effective in preventing recurrences of AF[39] but has not been directly compared with either amiodarone or sotalol. In a large, multicenter trial,[40] dofetilide (dose adjusted for renal function and QT interval) was more effective than placebo in maintaining sinus rhythm (approximately 35% to 50% at 1 year). The efficacy of dofetilide for the maintenance of sinus rhythm has also specifically been demonstrated in patients with LV dysfunction.[41] Like sotalol and quinidine, dofetilide also has significant potential to cause TdP (in a dose-related fashion).

Overall, the use of antiarrhythmic drug therapy to maintain sinus rhythm is reasonable to consider in patients with recurrent paroxysmal or persistent AF who develop intolerable symptoms during episodes of AF. As with cardioversion, the selection of an antiarrhythmic drug for maintaining sinus rhythm should be based on whether the patient has structural heart disease.[15] For those patients with no underlying structural heart disease, flecainide, propafenone, or sotalol should be considered initially because they have the most optimal long-term safety profile. However, amiodarone or dofetilide could be used as alternative therapy if the patient fails or does not tolerate one of these initial antiarrhythmic drugs. In the presence of structural heart disease, flecainide and propafenone, should be avoided because of the risk of proarrhythmia. If LV dysfunction is present (LVEF ≤40%), amiodarone should be considered the antiarrhythmic of choice. Dofetilide can be used as an alternative if patients develop intolerable side effects with amiodarone. In patients with coronary artery disease, sotalol can be used initially, provided that the patient's LV function is normal. Amiodarone or dofetilide could be used as an alternative therapy if the patient fails or does not tolerate sotalol. The presence of LV hypertrophy may predispose the myocardium to proarrhythmic events. Because of its low proarrhythmic potential, amiodarone should be considered first-line therapy in these patients.

Nondrug forms of therapy, designed to maintain sinus rhythm are becoming increasingly popular treatment options for patients with AF or atrial flutter. For patients who have "pure" (i.e., not associated with concurrent AF) type I atrial flutter, ablation of the reentrant substrate with radiofrequency current is highly effective (~80%)[42] and can be considered first-line treatment of atrial flutter to prevent recurrences.[43] For patients with AF, an innovative surgical procedure, referred to as the "maze" operation, has been used for more than a decade.[44] Because of its highly complex and invasive nature, the maze procedure is often reserved for highly drug-refractory patients. Over the past several years, most of the emerging data in the literature regarding nondrug treatment of AF have primarily focused on the safety and efficacy of catheter ablation techniques. Patients with AF have been found to have arrhythmogenic foci that occur in atrial tissue near and within the pulmonary veins. During the ablation procedure, radiofrequency energy can be delivered to these areas in an attempt to abolish the foci. Historically, this procedure was often considered last-line therapy for patients who had failed all antiarrhythmic drugs, including amiodarone. However, in some of the recent trials, the use of catheter ablation in patients with AF has been associated with a significant reduction in recurrent episodes of AF and an improvement in quality of life when compared with antiarrhythmic drug therapy.[45,46] There is even some evidence[47] to suggest that this procedure may be superior to antiarrhythmic drugs as first-line therapy of symptomatic AF; however, these results will have to be validated in larger trials. Based on this recent data, the guidelines now recommend that catheter ablation be considered as a reasonable treatment alternative for patients with symptomatic episodes of recurrent AF who fail or do not tolerate at least one antiarrhythmic drug.[15] This procedure is not without its risks, as major complications, such as pulmonary vein stenosis, thromboembolic events, cardiac tamponade, and new atrial flutter, have been reported in up to 6% of patients.[48]

PAROXYSMAL SUPRAVENTRICULAR TACHYCARDIA CAUSED BY REENTRY

Paroxysmal supraventricular tachycardia arising by reentrant mechanisms includes those arrhythmias caused by AV nodal reentry, AV reentry incorporating an anomalous AV pathway, SA nodal reentry, and intraatrial reentry. Atrioventricular nodal reentry and AV reentry are by far the most common of these tachycardias. ❺

Mechanisms

The underlying substrate of AV nodal reentry is the functional division of the AV node into two (or more) longitudinal conduction pathways or "dual" AV nodal pathways.[49] Most clinicians now believe that there are not two distinct anatomic pathways inside the AV node itself; rather, it is likely that a fan-like network of perinodal fibers inserts into the AV node and represents the second pathway. The two pathways possess key differences in conduction characteristics: one is a fast conducting pathway with a relatively long refractory period (fast pathway), and the other is a slower conducting pathway with a shorter refractory period (slow pathway). The presence of dual pathways does not necessarily imply that the patient will have clinical PSVT. In fact, it is estimated that between 10% and 50% of patients have discernible dual pathways but the incidence of PSVT is considerably lower.[49] Sustenance of the tachycardia depends on the critical electrophysiologic discrepancies and the ability of one pathway (usually the slow) to allow repetitive antegrade conduction, and the ability of the other pathway (usually the fast) to allow repetitive retrograde conduction. During sinus rhythm, a patient with dual pathways conducts supraventricular impulses antegrade through both pathways. Electrical activity reaches the distal common pathway at the level of or above the His bundle and continues to depolarize the ventricles in an antegrade direction. Conduction proceeds via the two pathways but reaches the distal common pathway first through the

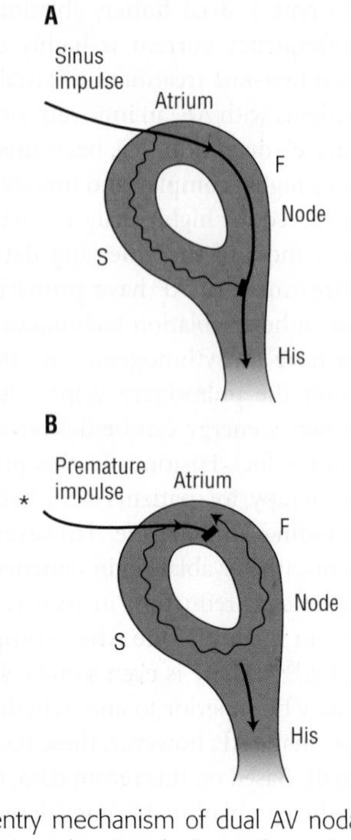

FIGURE 19-7. Reentry mechanism of dual AV nodal pathway PSVT. *A.* Sinus rhythm: The impulse travels from the atrium through the fast pathway *(F)* and then to the His-Purkinje system *(His)*. The impulse also travels through the slow pathway *(S)* but is stopped when refractory tissue is encountered. *B.* Dual AV nodal reentry: A critically timed premature impulse (*) is stopped in the fast pathway (because of prolonged refractoriness) but is able to travel antegrade down the slow pathway and retrograde through the fast pathway.

fast AV nodal route (Fig. 19–7). For this reason, a short PR interval is sometimes observed during sinus rhythm.

Paroxysmal supraventricular tachycardia caused by AV nodal reentry may occur by the following sequence of events. The occurrence of an appropriately timed premature impulse penetrates the AV node, but is blocked in the fast pathway that is still refractory from the previous beat. However, the slow pathway, which has a shorter refractory period, permits antegrade conduction of the premature impulse. By the time the impulse has reached the distal common pathway, the fast pathway has recovered its excitability and now will permit retrograde conduction. The impulse reaches the common proximal pathway, preceded by an excitable gap of tissue, and reenters the slow pathway. A reentrant circuit that does not require atrial or ventricular tissue is completed within (or nearly so) the AV node, and a tachycardia is thereby initiated (see Fig. 19–7). The common form of this tachycardia uses the slow pathway for antegrade conduction and the fast pathway for retrograde conduction; an uncommon form exists in which the reentrant impulse travels in the opposite direction.

Atrioventricular reentrant tachycardia depends upon the presence of an anomalous, or accessory, extranodal pathway that bypasses the normal AV conduction pathway. Several different types of accessory pathways have been described, depending on the specific anatomic areas they connect (e.g., AV bundles or nodoventricular tracts); some are also referred to as eponyms, such as the Kent bundle. A Kent bundle is an extranodal AV connection that is associated with WPW syndrome. During sinus rhythm (Fig. 19–8), patients with WPW syndrome depolarize the ventricles simultaneously through both AV pathways (AV nodal pathway and the Kent bundle), creating a fusion pattern on the early portion of the QRS complex (delta wave). The degree of ventricular "preexcitation" depends on the contribution of antegrade ventricular activation through the accessory pathway. Patients may have an accessory pathway that is not evident on ECG, which is referred to as a "concealed" Kent bundle. These concealed

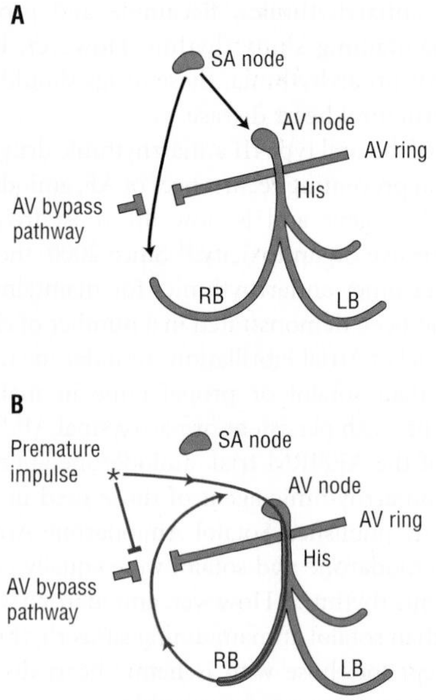

FIGURE 19-8. Reentry mechanism for AV accessory pathway PSVT in Wolff-Parkinson-White syndrome. *A.* Sinus rhythm: The impulse travels from the atrium to the ventricle by two pathways—the AV node and an accessory bypass pathway. *B.* AV reentry: A critically timed premature impulse (*) is stopped in the Kent bundle (because of prolonged refractoriness) but travels antegrade through the AV node and retrograde through the Kent bundle. (AV, atrioventricular; His, His-Purkinje system; LB, left bundle-branch; RB, right bundle-branch; SA, sinoatrial.)

accessory pathways are often incapable of antegrade conduction and can only accept electrical stimulation in a retrograde fashion. The electrocardiographic expression of preexcitation (delta wave) depends on the location of the accessory pathway, the distance from the wavefront of sinus activation and the conduction characteristics of the various structures involved. It should be noted that (similar to patients with dual AV nodal pathways) not all patients with preexcitation with an accessory AV pathway are capable of having clinical PSVT.

Patients with an accessory AV pathway may have three forms of supraventricular tachycardia: orthodromic reentry, antidromic reentry, and/or AF or atrial flutter. Atrioventricular reentrant PSVT usually occurs by the following sequence of events. Analogous to AV nodal reentry, two pathways (the normal AV nodal pathway and the accessory AV pathway) exist that have different electrophysiologic characteristics. The AV nodal pathway usually has a relatively slower conduction velocity and shorter refractory period, and the accessory pathway has a faster conduction velocity and a longer refractory period. A critically timed premature impulse may be blocked in the accessory pathway because this area is still refractory from the previous sinus beat. However, the AV nodal pathway, with a relatively shorter refractory period, may accept antegrade conduction of the premature impulse. Meanwhile, the accessory pathway may recover its excitability and now allow retrograde conduction. A macroreentrant tachycardia is thereby initiated in which the antegrade pathway is the AV nodal pathway; the distal common pathway is the ventricle; the retrograde pathway the accessory pathway; and the proximal common pathway is the atrium (see Fig. 19–8). This sequence of events (down the node, up the Kent bundle), termed *orthodromic PSVT*, is the common variety of reentry in patients with an accessory AV pathway, resulting in a narrow QRS tachycardia. In the uncommon variety, conduction proceeds in the opposite direction (down the Kent bundle, up the node), resulting in a wide QRS tachycardia, which is termed *antidromic PSVT*. Patients with WPW syndrome can have a third type of tachycardia, namely AF. The occurrence of AF in the setting of an accessory AV pathway (i.e., WPW syndrome) can be extremely serious and has been documented. As AF is an extremely rapid atrial tachycardia, conduction can proceed down the accessory AV pathway, resulting in a very fast ventricular response or even VF. Unlike the AV nodal pathway, the refractory period of the accessory bundle shortens in response to rapid stimulation rates.

Sinus node reentry and intraatrial reentry occur less commonly and are not as well-described as AV nodal reentry and AV reentry. Aside from a characteristic abrupt onset and termination, coupled with subtle changes in P-wave morphology, these tachycardias can be difficult to diagnose. Electrophysiologic studies may be necessary to determine the ultimate mechanism of the PSVT.

Management

Both pharmacologic and nonpharmacologic methods have been used to treat patients with PSVT. Drugs used in the treatment of PSVT can be divided into three broad categories: (a) those that directly or indirectly increase vagal tone to the AV node (e.g., digoxin); (b) those that depress conduction through slow, calcium-dependent tissue (e.g., adenosine, β-blockers, and CCBs); and (c) those that depress conduction through fast, sodium-dependent tissue (e.g., quinidine, procainamide, disopyramide, and flecainide). Drugs within these categories alter the electrophysiologic characteristics of the reentrant substrate so that PSVT cannot be sustained.[50,51] In PSVT caused by AV nodal reentry, type I antiarrhythmic drugs, such as procainamide, act primarily on the retrograde fast pathway. Digoxin and β-blockers may work on either the retrograde fast or the antegrade slow limb. Verapamil, diltiazem, and adenosine prolong conduction time and increase refractoriness primarily in the slow antegrade pathway of the reentrant loop. In PSVT caused by AV reentry incorporating an extranodal pathway, type I drugs increase refractoriness in the fast accessory pathway or within the His-Purkinje system. β-blockers, digoxin, adenosine, and verapamil all act by their effects on the AV nodal (antegrade, slow) portion of the reentrant circuit. Regardless of the mechanism, treatment measures are directed at first terminating an acute episode of PSVT and then preventing symptomatic recurrences of the arrhythmia.

For those patients with PSVT who present with severe symptoms (syncope, near syncope, angina, or severe HF), synchronized DCC is the treatment of choice. Even at low energy levels (such as 25 joules), DCC is almost always effective in quickly restoring sinus rhythm and correcting symptomatic hypotension. Patients with only mild to moderate symptoms usually do not require DCC and nondrug measures that increase vagal tone to the AV node can be used initially. Unilateral carotid sinus massage, Valsalva maneuver, ice water facial immersion, induced retching, and other more elaborate vagomimetic measures are often successful in terminating PSVT, although carotid massage and Valsalva maneuver are the simplest, least obtrusive, and most frequently used of these techniques.

In the event that vagal maneuvers fail (approximately 80% of acute episodes) in those patients with tolerable symptoms, drug therapy is the next option. Figure 19–9 shows a therapeutic approach to the acute treatment of the different forms of reentrant PSVT. ❻ This approach is based on analysis of the electrocardiographic characteristics of the rhythm because PSVT is not always discernible from other

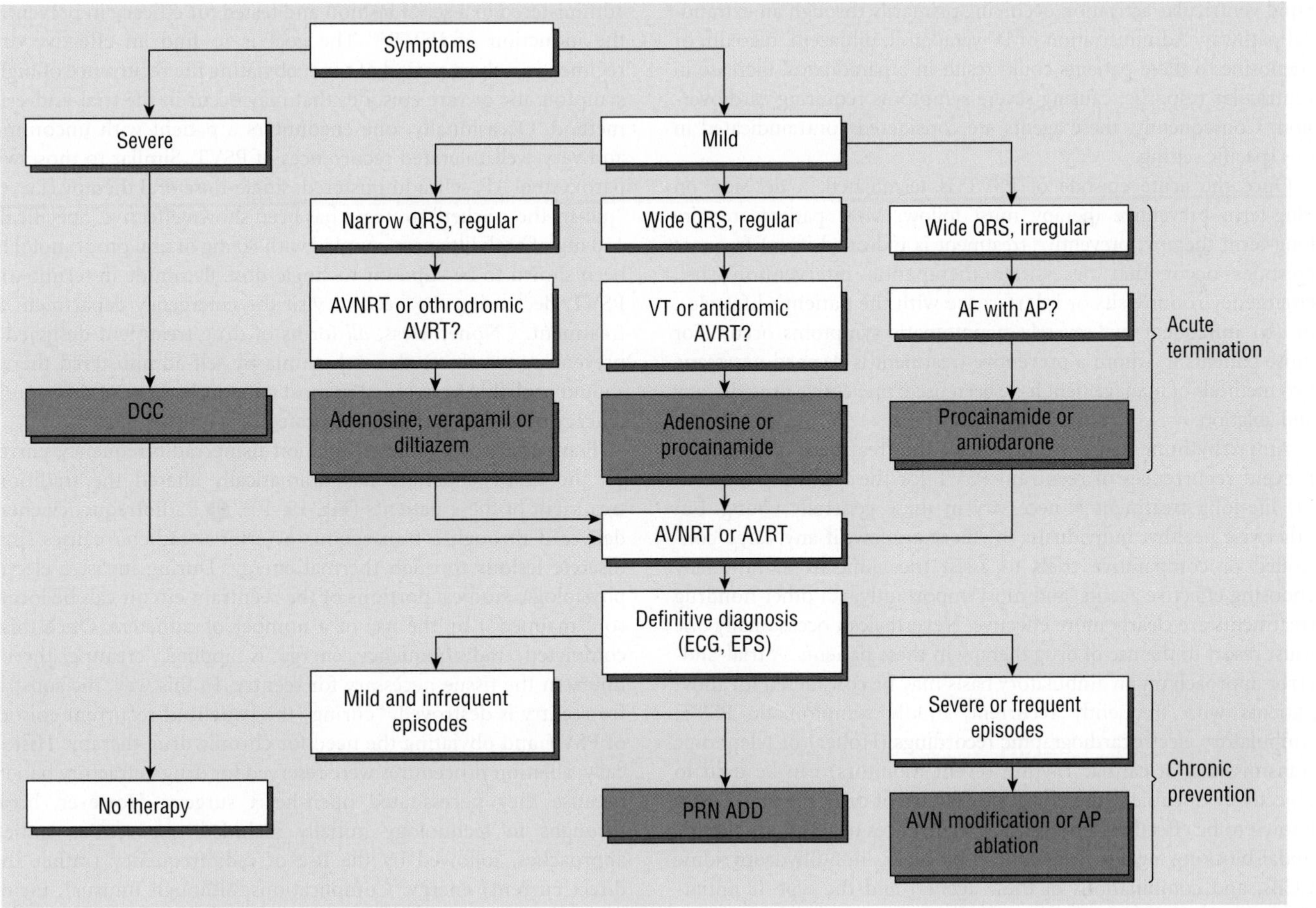

FIGURE 19-9. Algorithm for the treatment of acute *(top portion)* paroxysmal supraventricular tachycardia and chronic prevention of recurrences *(bottom portion)*. *Note:* For empiric bridge therapy prior to radiofrequency ablation procedures, calcium channel blockers (or other AV nodal blockers) should not be used if the patient has AV reentry with an accessory pathway. (AAD, antiarrhythmic drugs; AF, atrial fibrillation; AP, accessory pathway; AV, atrioventricular; AVN, atrioventricular nodal; AVNRT, atrioventricular nodal reentrant tachycardia; AVRT, atrioventricular reentrant tachycardia; DCC, direct current cardioversion; ECG, electrocardiographic monitoring; EPS, electrophysiologic studies; PRN, as needed; VT, ventricular tachycardia.)

arrhythmias, and some forms of PSVT require different treatment. In patients with a narrow QRS, regular arrhythmia (AV nodal reentry or orthodromic AV reentry), IV verapamil (5 to 10 mg), IV diltiazem (15 to 25 mg), or adenosine (6 to 12 mg) are all equally efficacious. Approximately 80% to 90% of PSVT episodes will revert to sinus rhythm within 5 minutes of IV verapamil, diltiazem, or adenosine therapy.[52] Both verapamil and diltiazem have the advantage in terms of cost, being available in generic formulations; whereas adenosine (although it has a higher frequency of side effects) may be safer because of its ultrashort duration of action. Adenosine should not be used in patients with severe asthma because of the potential risk of bronchospasm. The most recent guidelines for cardiopulmonary resuscitation (CPR) and emergency cardiovascular care from the AHA,[53] and practice guidelines from the ACC/AHA/ESC,[43] promote adenosine as the drug of first choice in patients with PSVT. ❺ These recommendations are particularly important when treating a patient who presents with a wide QRS, regular tachycardia that may be VT or PSVT (antidromic AV reentry or as a result of aberrancy). Because of its short duration of action (seconds), adenosine will not cause the severe and prolonged hemodynamic compromise seen in patients with VT who were mistakenly treated with verapamil and suffer from its negative inotropic effects and vasodilator properties.[54] If, in fact, the arrhythmia is PSVT, adenosine will likely terminate it. An alternative treatment for this type of patient is IV procainamide, which works on the fast, sodium-dependent extranodal pathway, and is also effective for VT. Likewise, IV procainamide, or perhaps amiodarone (particularly in patients with LV dysfunction), should be used for the patient who presents with a wide QRS, irregular arrhythmia that is hemodynamically stable.[53] This rhythm could represent AF with rapid ventricular activation occurring primarily through an extranodal pathway. Administration of IV verapamil, diltiazem, digoxin, or adenosine to these patients could result in a paradoxical increase in ventricular response, causing severe symptoms requiring cardioversion. Consequently, these agents are considered contraindicated in this specific setting.

Once the acute episode of PSVT is terminated, a decision on long-term preventive therapy must follow. Most patients require long-term therapy; preventive treatment is indicated if: (a) frequent episodes occur that necessitate therapeutic intervention (i.e., emergency room visits or interference with the patient's lifestyle), or (b) infrequent but severely symptomatic symptoms occur. For those patients in whom a preventive treatment is deemed necessary, two methods of management have been used: preventive drug therapy and ablation.

Antiarrhythmic drugs are no longer the treatment of choice to prevent recurrences of reentrant PSVT for the following reasons: (a) life-long treatment is necessary in these generally young, but otherwise healthy, individuals; (b) there are few, if any, large controlled or comparative trials to assist the clinician in rationally choosing effective agents, and most importantly; (c) other nondrug treatments are clearly more effective. Nevertheless, occasionally one must resort to the use of drug therapy in these patients. A trial-and-error approach on an ambulatory basis may be considered for those patients with frequently recurrent, mildly symptomatic PSVT. Ambulatory electrocardiographic recordings (Holter) or telephonic transmissions of cardiac rhythm (event monitors) can be used to objectively document the efficacy or failure of drug therapy. Drugs known to be effective in preventing recurrences of PSVT are the AV nodal-blocking agents (digoxin, β-blockers, nondihydropyridine CCBs, and combinations of these agents) and the type Ic antiarrhythmic drugs (flecainide, propafenone). Agents such as quinidine, disopyramide, amiodarone, and dofetilide, although effective in some patients, should be discouraged because of the risk of toxicity with long-term treatment. One concept that can serve as an aid to arriving at an effective regimen is that there are patterns of drug response in patients with PSVT; in other words, the tachycardia behaves as if it has a "weak link." Patients who respond to agents that act on one limb of the reentrant loop are less likely to respond to drugs that block conduction on the other limb. For instance, in a patient with AV nodal reentry, one may first choose a nondihydropyridine CCB or β-blocker (to affect the antegrade, slow pathway). If symptomatic recurrences are subsequently documented, it may be prudent to switch to a type Ic agent (to affect the retrograde, fast pathway) in an attempt to find the weak link or susceptible pathway. Patients with evidence of preexcitation (delta waves during sinus rhythm) should not be treated with only AV nodal-blocking agents. If AF were to occur, these agents would facilitate rapid conduction over the accessory pathway. The trial-and-error method for determining drug effectiveness in this setting has inherent shortcomings. If the PSVT episodes are infrequent, a considerable time period may be consumed before an effective regimen is realized, or if the patient has moderate to severe symptoms associated with PSVT, he/she may experience several troublesome episodes before the correct agent is identified. Consequently, a method of serial testing of antiarrhythmic agents by invasive electrophysiologic techniques has been used to determine effective long-term therapy in those patients with sporadic and/or symptomatic PSVT and this method represents another strategy to find an effective antiarrhythmic regimen. Using this method, the patient's clinical tachycardia is replicated in the laboratory by inserting appropriately timed, premature extra stimuli via a transvenous right-heart catheter. The patient is first studied off of antiarrhythmic therapy; induction of the tachycardia by premature stimuli by programmed stimulation serves as a control study. Then, over a period of several days, specific drugs are administered in a serial fashion and tested for efficacy in preventing the induction of PSVT.[50] The goal is to find an effective drug regimen in a short period of time, obviating the recurrence of highly symptomatic or rare episodes that may occur in the trial-and-error method. Occasionally, one encounters a patient with uncommon and very-well-tolerated recurrences of PSVT. Similar to those with paroxysmal AF, self-administered, single-dose oral therapy (i.e., the "pill-in-the-pocket" strategy) has been shown effective. Specifically, 120 mg of oral diltiazem coupled with 80 mg of oral propranolol has been shown to be superior to single-dose flecainide in terminating PSVT, decreasing the need to visit the emergency department for treatment.[55] Nonetheless, *all* forms of drug treatment designed to prevent or terminate the arrhythmia by self-administered therapy should probably be avoided in most patients because of the superior efficacy of nondrug treatment strategies.

Transcutaneous catheter ablation using radiofrequency current on the PSVT substrate has dramatically altered the traditional treatment of these patients (Fig. 19–10). ❺ Radiofrequency energy delivered through a transvenous or arterial catheter causes small, discrete lesions through thermal energy. During invasive electrophysiologic studies, portions of the reentrant circuit can be located (or "mapped") by the use of a number of catheters. Once this is completed, radiofrequency energy is applied, creating thermal injury in the tissue necessary for reentry. In this way, the substrate for reentry is destroyed, "curing" the patient of recurrent episodes of PSVT and obviating the need for chronic drug therapy. Historically, ablation procedures were reserved for drug-refractory patients because they necessitated open-heart surgery. However, breakthroughs in technology initially included transvenous catheter approaches, followed by the use of radiofrequency (rather than direct current) energy. Complications, although unusual, include tamponade, pericarditis, valvular insufficiency, and AV block. Radiofrequency ablation is highly effective, preventing the recurrences of PSVT in 85% to 98% of patients.[56,57] The procedure was originally used in patients with WPW syndrome.[56] In these patients, the extranodal pathway is most often located at the left lateral free

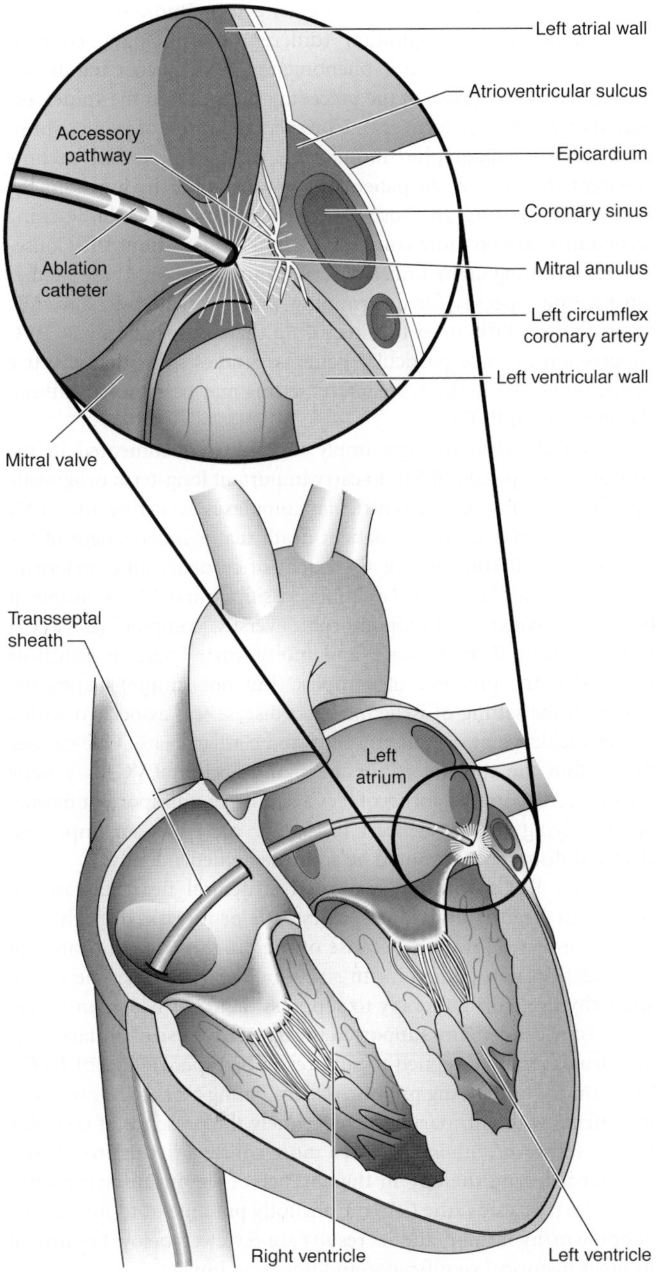

FIGURE 19-10. Drawing showing catheter placement for radiofrequency ablation of a left lateral free wall accessory pathway. Here, a venous (atrial) transseptal puncture to gain access to the Kent bundle is shown; a retrograde arterial approach has also been used. *(From Lerman BB, Basson CT. High risk patients with ventricular preexcitation: A pendulum in motion. N Engl J Med 2003;349:1787–1789, with permission.)*

wall of the left ventricle (Fig. 19–10). After the pathway is located, the catheter is put as close to the site as possible and radiofrequency current is applied to make small burns in the tissue. Ablation of the extranodal connection occurs promptly and evidence of preexcitation (delta waves) disappears. Thereafter, a similar approach was developed for patients with AV nodal reentry, placing the catheter in the coronary sinus, proximal to the AV node.[57] The preferred method in these individuals is to apply small amounts of radiofrequency current to the slow pathway of the reentrant circuit in order to modify its properties enough so that PSVT can not recur.

It has been suggested that *all* patients with symptomatic PSVT undergo radiofrequency catheter ablation.[58] This is because it is highly effective and curative, rarely results in complications, and obviates the need for chronic antiarrhythmic drug therapy. In other words, it should be considered in *any* patient who would previously be considered for chronic antiarrhythmic drug treatment. Radiofrequency ablation is also a cost-effective approach (in the long-term) because, if effective, the costs of drugs and repeated hospital visits are avoided. In one cost-effectiveness analysis, radiofrequency ablation improved quality of life and reduced lifetime medical expenditures by nearly $30,000 compared to chronic drug treatment.[59]

AUTOMATIC ATRIAL TACHYCARDIAS

Automatic atrial tachycardias, such as multifocal atrial tachycardia, appear to arise from supraventricular foci that have enhanced automatic properties.[60] It is presumed that multifocal atrial tachycardia is the result of multiple ectopic atrial pacemakers, which account for the variable and differing P-wave morphology. In unifocal atrial tachycardia (more often referred to as ectopic atrial tachycardia), a single P-wave morphology, different from that of sinus rhythm, is recorded. In either case, the underlying, precipitating disorder present in the majority (60% to 80%) of these patients is severe pulmonary disease. Other disease states associated with these arrhythmias include acute infection (pneumonia and sepsis) and dilated congestive cardiomyopathy. It should be noted that young patients without associated precipitating factors might rarely present with rapid atrial tachycardias from unknown etiologies. In these cases, long-standing tachycardias cause the cardiomyopathic state. Effective treatment of the tachycardia may result in reversal of the LV dysfunction. Traditionally, many factors (i.e., electrolyte disturbances, hypoxia, catecholamines, and tissue stretch) may cause an elevated slope of phase 4 depolarization and theoretically result in abnormal heightened automaticity. Noteworthy is that many of these factors are often clinically present in patients with concurrent pulmonary disease and automatic atrial tachycardia. However, it appears that triggered activity (i.e., LADs) is a more likely mechanism in the genesis of these tachycardias. Atrial tachycardias with AV block or a slow ventricular response should alert the clinician to the possibility of digitalis toxicity.

The first step in the treatment of automatic atrial tachycardia is to correct the underlying, precipitating factors.[60] One should ensure proper oxygenation and ventilation and correct acid–base or electrolyte disturbances. These measures alone may result in the return of sinus rhythm, but in some cases, the tachycardia will persist. Patients with an asymptomatic atrial tachycardia and a relatively slow ventricular rate usually require no drug therapy. In symptomatic patients, medical therapy can be tailored to either control ventricular rate or to restore sinus rhythm. Type I antiarrhythmic drugs, such as procainamide and quinidine, are only occasionally effective in restoring sinus rhythm, and are usually not considered first-line therapy. Direct-current cardioversion is ineffective in restoring sinus rhythm, and the use of programmed stimulation will not replicate the clinical tachycardia; consequently, serial drug testing is of no value. The use of IV β-blockers to slow ventricular rate is usually contraindicated because of the frequent coexistence of bronchospastic pulmonary disease or decompensated HF. Digoxin has been used but is controversial because of its ability to increase the automatic properties of atrial tissue and the high sympathetic state of these patients frequently overrides the vagotonic effects of digoxin, rendering it ineffective. Nondihydropyridine CCBs, such as verapamil, are most effective and are now considered first-line drug therapy.[61] Interestingly, verapamil seems to decrease ventricular rate by altering atrial automaticity, not by slowing AV nodal conduction.[61] Intravenous magnesium (independent of serum magnesium) can also be effective, but high doses are required and its effects are transient, rendering it impractical.[60] Both verapamil and parenteral magnesium probably act by suppressing calcium-mediated LADs.

CLINICAL PRESENTATION: VENTRICULAR ARRHYTHMIAS

Premature Ventricular Contractions

- Premature ventricular contractions are non-life-threatening and usually asymptomatic. Occasionally, patients will complain of palpitations or uncomfortable heart beats. Since the PVC, by definition, occurs early and the ventricle contracts when it is incompletely filled, patients do not feel the PVC. Rather, the next beat (after the PVC and a compensatory pause) is usually responsible for the patient's symptoms.

Ventricular Tachycardia

- The symptoms of VT (monomorphic VT or TdP), if prolonged (i.e., sustained), can vary from nearly completely asymptomatic to pulseless, hemodynamic collapse. Fast heart rates and underlying poor LV function will result in more severe symptoms. Symptoms of nonsustained, self-terminating VT also correlate with duration of episodes (e.g., patients with 15-second episodes will be more symptomatic than those with 3-beat episodes).

Ventricular Fibrillation

- By definition, VF results in hemodynamic collapse, syncope, and cardiac arrest. Cardiac output and blood pressure are not recordable.

VENTRICULAR ARRHYTHMIAS

The common ventricular arrhythmias include: (a) PVCs, (b) VT, and (c) VF. These arrhythmias may result in a wide variety of symptoms. Premature ventricular complexes often cause no symptoms or only mild palpitations. Ventricular tachycardia may be a life-threatening situation associated with hemodynamic collapse or may be totally asymptomatic. Ventricular fibrillation, by definition, is an acute medical emergency necessitating CPR.

PREMATURE VENTRICULAR COMPLEXES AND PREVENTION OF SUDDEN CARDIAC DEATH

Premature ventricular complexes are very common ventricular rhythm disturbances that occur in patients with or without structural heart disease. Experimental models show that premature ventricular depolarizations may be elicited by abnormal automaticity, triggered activity, or by reentrant mechanisms. It is well known that PVCs are commonly observed in apparently healthy individuals; in these patients, the PVCs seem to have little if any prognostic significance. Premature ventricular contractions occur more frequently and in more complex forms in patients with structural heart disease than in healthy individuals. The prognostic meaning of PVCs has been well studied in patients with MI (acute or remote) with several consistent themes. Patients with some forms of PVCs are at higher risk for "sudden death" than if they did not have these minor rhythm disturbances. Sudden cardiac death can be defined as unexpected death occurring in a patient within 1 hour of experiencing symptoms. Studies of patients who experienced SCD (and happened to be wearing an electrocardiographic monitor at the time) often demonstrate the cause to be VF preceded by a short run of VT and frequent PVCs.[62] Therein lies the basis of the so-called "PVC hypothesis" (i.e., preventing more minor arrhythmias, such as PVCs, may prevent the occurrence of SCD).

Significance

Historically, investigators promoted the concept that patients in the acute phase of MI may have types of PVCs that are predictive of VF and SCD. These types of PVCs were referred to as "warning arrhythmias" and included frequent ventricular ectopy (more than 5 beats/min), multiform configuration (different morphology), couplets (two in a row), and R-on-T phenomenon (PVCs occurring during the repolarization phase of the preceding sinus beat in the vulnerable period of ventricular recovery). However, as a result of using continuous electrocardiographic monitoring techniques, it has become apparent that almost all patients have warning arrhythmias in the acute infarct setting. In those patients who experience VF, warning arrhythmias are no more common than in those without VF. Consequently, warning arrhythmias observed during acute MI are neither sensitive nor specific for determining which patients will have VF. Thus, there is little need to direct drug therapy specifically at PVC suppression in these particular patients. Studies show that effective prevention of VF in the acute infarct setting may be achieved without the abolition of PVCs.

Conversely, data strongly imply that PVCs documented in the convalescence period of MI do carry important long-term prognostic significance.[63] Premature ventricular complexes occurring after a MI seem to be a risk factor for patient death that is independent of the degree of LV dysfunction or the extent of coronary atherosclerosis. Ruberman et al.[63] employed a simple classification of PVCs: simple or benign (infrequent and monomorphic) versus "complex" (≥5 PVCs/min, couplets, R-on-T beats, and multiform). These investigators found that the presence of complex (but not simple) ventricular ectopy in the setting of ischemic heart disease was associated with a higher incidence of overall mortality and cardiac death. One can see that within the controversy of the significance of PVCs is a basic question: Are complex forms of PVCs simply an unimportant marker of underlying structural heart disease or are PVCs an important electrical disorder that should be addressed independently?

Because PVCs without associated structural heart disease, in apparently healthy individuals, carry little or no risk, drug therapy is unnecessary. However, because of the prognostic significance of complex PVCs in patients with structural heart disease, the use of antiarrhythmic drug therapy to suppress them has been controversial. Historically, many supported the aggressive use of antiarrhythmic drug therapy designed to suppress a high percentage of PVCs, based on the underlying premise of eliminating a risk factor for SCD in patients with coronary disease (namely the presence of complex PVCs). However, others favored a more conservative approach and disregarded drug therapy in the absence of significant symptoms. An important study, the CAST,[32] abruptly put an end to this debate in noteworthy fashion and its results are reviewed below because of its great historical significance and lingering impact.

The Cardiac Arrhythmia Suppression Trial

The CAST[32,64] was initiated by the National Institutes of Health in 1987 to determine if suppression of ventricular ectopy with encainide, flecainide, or moricizine could decrease the incidence of death from arrhythmia in patients who had suffered a MI. ❼ Entrance criteria included documented MI between 6 days and 2 years prior to enrollment, and ≥6 PVCs per hour (associated with no or minimal symptoms) without runs of VT greater than 15 beats in length. Also, patients were required to have a LVEF ≤55% if recruited within 90 days of MI or ≤40% if recruited 90 days or more after infarction. Patients with a LVEF <30% were randomized only to encainide or moricizine. Patients were randomized to receive drug therapy or placebo after demonstrating PVC suppression with one of the agents. The drug and dose were determined during an open-label, dose-titration phase that preceded randomization.

In April 1989, a routine, preliminary review of the study by the Safety and Monitoring Board revealed alarming results and the study was interrupted. The results showed that compared to placebo, treatment with encainide or flecainide was associated with a significantly higher rate of total mortality and death due to arrhyth-

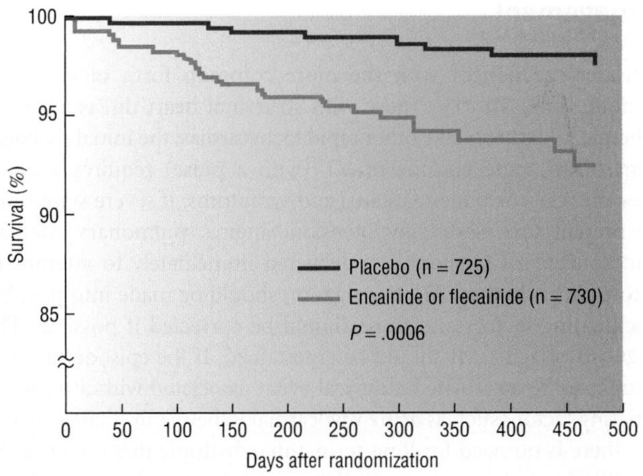

FIGURE 19-11. Life table curves from the Cardiac Arrhythmia Suppression Trial (CAST), specifically for patients receiving encainide or flecainide *(lighter line)* and matching placebo *(darker line)*. Note the divergent slopes of each line, implying a sustained risk of death (presumed proarrhythmia). *(From The CAST Investigators. Preliminary report: Effect of encainide and flecainide on mortality in a randomized trial of arrhythmia suppression after myocardial infarction. N Engl J Med 1989;321:406–412, with permission.)*

mia, presumably caused by proarrhythmia (Fig. 19–11). Analysis of the moricizine arm indicated neither harm nor benefit from this therapy; therefore, only this portion of the study was allowed to continue as CAST II.[64] However, in July 1991, CAST II was also prematurely stopped because there was a trend toward an increase in mortality in moricizine-treated patients. This increase in mortality was primarily observed during the initiation of moricizine therapy (dose-titration phase) but not during the chronic treatment phase. The overall results of the two CASTs conclusively prove that that the use of antiarrhythmic drug therapy (beyond the general use of β-blocking agents) to suppress PVCs in patients after a MI does not improve survival and is most likely detrimental. These studies also put into perspective the risk associated with the use of antiarrhythmic therapy and the need to carefully select only those patients with a defined therapeutic benefit.

Even though the CAST was conducted nearly 2 decades ago, it is considered one of the most important trials ever undertaken and has had a tremendous influence on the overall approach to the treatment of arrhythmias, as well as a far-reaching impact on new drug development. The results of the CAST have clearly had a negative influence on the long-term use of all antiarrhythmics, causing a broad skepticism in the risk-versus-benefit analysis of this class of drugs. Consequently, pharmaceutical companies have shifted their drug discovery and investigative efforts away from potent sodium channel blockers. As immediate fallout, encainide was withdrawn from the market, and another type Ic agent, indecainide, was not even brought to market despite approval by the Food and Drug Administration. The findings of the CAST also provided additional fuel for the pursuit of nondrug therapies for arrhythmias, such as ablation and implantable devices.

Despite the discouraging results of the CAST, post-MI patients with complex ventricular ectopy remain at risk for death. Other drugs, besides the type Ic agents, have been studied, including sotalol. Sotalol is marketed as a racemic mixture of a *d* and *l* isomer: both are type III potassium blockers but the *l* isomer has β-blocking actions. Chronic therapy with *d*-sotalol was studied in patients with remote MI complicated by complex ectopy in the Survival With Oral *d*-Sotalol trial.[65] Unlike the CAST, *d*-sotalol treatment was not designed to cause PVC suppression, yet (like the CAST) the trial was halted prematurely because of excessive mortality in the treatment arm. Again, the presumed reason for this observation was *d*-sotalol–related proarrhythmia. Currently, only two antiarrhythmic drugs have been shown *not* to increase mortality with long-term use: amiodarone and dofetilide. A number of trials[66,67] have shown amiodarone to decrease the incidence of sudden (or arrhythmic) death, but not total mortality, in post-MI patients with complex ventricular ectopy. A meta-analysis of all trials (6,553 combined patients) demonstrated a reduction in total mortality (by 13%) with long-term amiodarone therapy.[68] It is unclear if these findings can be attributed to one property (e.g., β-blocking) or a combination of amiodarone's complex pharmacologic effects on conduction. Noteworthy is that in two major studies, patients treated with amiodarone *and* a β-blocker generally did better than when no β-blocker was used.[66,67] Clearly, because of its impressive adverse effect profile and its inability to improve survival, amiodarone cannot routinely be recommended in patients with heart disease such as remote MI and complex PVCs. Two randomized, controlled trials[69,70] showed that chronic therapy with dofetilide has no effect on overall mortality in patients who have suffered MI with LV dysfunction. Dofetilide (not approved for prevention of sudden death) caused TdP in approximately 5% of patients, necessitating a protocol amendment with dosage adjustments during both trials (particularly in those with renal disease because its primary route of elimination is through the kidney).

How should the clinician approach the patient with documented asymptomatic PVCs? Clearly, attempts to suppress asymptomatic PVCs should not be made with any antiarrhythmic drug. Indeed, those patients who are at risk for arrhythmic death (recent MI, LV dysfunction, complex PVCs) should not be routinely given *any* type I or III antiarrhythmic agent.[71] If these patients have symptomatic PVCs, chronic drug therapy should be limited to the use of β-blockers. The use of β-blockers in post-MI patients is associated with a decrease in the incidence of total mortality and SCD, especially in the presence of LV dysfunction. These agents can also be used in patients without underlying structural heart disease to suppress symptomatic PVCs. 7

VENTRICULAR TACHYCARDIA

Mechanisms and Types of VT

Ventricular tachycardia is a wide QRS tachycardia that may acutely occur as a result of metabolic abnormalities, ischemia, or drug toxicity, or chronically recur as a paroxysmal form. On electrocardiographic inspection, VT may appear as either repetitive monomorphic or polymorphic ventricular complexes. The definition of VT is three or more consecutive PVCs occurring at a rate greater than 100 beats/min. An acute episode of VT may be precipitated by severe electrolyte abnormalities (hypokalemia), hypoxemia, or digitalis toxicity, or (most commonly) may occur during an acute MI or ischemia complicated by HF. In these cases, correction of the underlying precipitating factors will usually prevent further recurrences of VT. As an example, if VT occurs during the first 24 hours of an acute MI, it will probably not reappear on a chronic basis after the infarcted area has been reperfused or healed with scar formation. This form of acute VT may be caused by a transient reentrant mechanism within temporarily ischemic or dying ventricular tissue. In contrast, some patients have a chronic recurrent form of VT that is almost always associated with some type of underlying structural heart disease. Common examples are paroxysmal VT associated with idiopathic dilated cardiomyopathy or remote MI with a LV aneurysm. Indeed, severe LV dysfunction and aneurysm formation are risk factors for the development of VT on a recurrent basis after MI. In chronic, recurrent VT, microreentry within the distal Purkinje network is presumed to be responsible for the underlying substrate in a large majority of patients (see Fig. 19–3). Theoretically, electrophysiologic discrepancies occur as a result of structural damage and heart disease within the ventricular conducting system. The reentrant circuit may possess both anatomically determined and functional properties coursing through normal tissue, damaged (but not dead) tissue and islands of necrosed tissue. In a minority of patients, macro-reentrant circuits may be responsible for recurrent VT, including reentry incorporating the bundle branches.

Patients with acute VT associated with a precipitating factor often suffer severe symptoms, requiring immediate treatment measures. Chronic recurrent VT may also cause severe hemodynamic compromise, but may also be associated with only mild symptoms, which are generally well tolerated. Sustained VT is that which requires therapeutic intervention to restore a stable rhythm or persists for a relatively long time (usually longer than 30 seconds). Nonsustained VT is that which self-terminates after a brief duration (usually less than 30 seconds). If the patient has VT more frequently than sinus rhythm (i.e., VT is the dominant rhythm), this is referred to as incessant VT. In monomorphic VT, the QRS complexes are similar in morphologic characteristics from beat to beat. In polymorphic VT, the QRS complexes vary in shape between beats. A characteristic type of polymorphic VT, in which the QRS complexes appear to undulate around a central axis and is associated with evidence of delayed ventricular repolarization (long QT interval or prominent U waves), is referred to as TdP.

Most but not all forms of recurrent VT occur in patients with extensive structural heart disease. Ventricular tachycardia occurring in a patient without structural heart disease is sometimes referred to as "idiopathic VT" and may take several forms.[72–74] Fascicular tachycardia arises from a fascicle of the left bundle branch (usually posterior) and is usually not associated with severe underlying structural heart disease. In distinct contrast to the common form of recurrent VT associated with extensive structural heart disease, nondihydropyridine CCBs (but not adenosine) are effective in terminating an acute episode of fascicular VT. Ventricular outflow tract tachycardia (usually originating from the right ventricular outflow tract) originates from near the pulmonic valve (or uncommonly the aortic valve) and also occurs in patients with normal LV function without discernible cardiac disease.[74] Unlike other forms of VT, right ventricular outflow tract tachycardia often terminates with adenosine and may be prevented with β-blockers and/or nondihydropyridine CCBs.

Some unusual forms of VT are congenital or heritable (Table 19–10). Torsade de pointes can be associated with heritable defects in the flux of ions that govern ventricular repolarization. Although nine syndromes and genetic mutations have been described, the more common examples are long QT syndrome 1 (depressed I_{Ks}), long QT syndrome 2 (depressed I_{Kr}), and long QT syndrome 3 (enhanced inward sodium ion flux during repolarization).[75,76] Polymorphic VT (without a long QT interval) or VF may also occur as a result of a heritable defect in the sodium channel. This is the case in Brugada syndrome, described as a typical ECG pattern (ST-segment elevation in leads V_1 to V_3) in sinus rhythm associated with SCD, commonly in males of Asian descent.[77] It is estimated that Brugada syndrome accounts for approximately 40% of all cases of VF in patients without heart disease.

Management

Consider the patient with the more common form of sustained monomorphic VT (i.e., those with structural heart disease, usually ischemic in nature). Like other rapid tachycardias, the initial management of an acute episode of VT (with a pulse) requires a quick assessment of the patient's status and symptoms. If severe symptoms are present (i.e., severe hypotension, angina, pulmonary edema), synchronized DCC should be delivered immediately to attempt to restore sinus rhythm. An investigation should be made into possible precipitating factors and these should be corrected if possible. The diagnosis of acute MI should be entertained. If the episode of VT is thought to be an isolated electrical event associated with a transient initiating factor (such as acute myocardial ischemia or digitalis toxicity), there is no need for long-term antiarrhythmic therapy once the precipitating factors are corrected (e.g., an infarct has been reperfused and healed and the patient is stable). Nevertheless, the patient should be monitored closely for possible recurrences of VT.

Patients presenting with an acute episode of VT (with a pulse) associated with only mild symptoms can be initially treated with antiarrhythmic drugs (synchronized DCC should be readily available). The reader is referred to the most recent guidelines for CPR and emergency cardiovascular care put forth by the AHA.[53] Intravenous amiodarone is now recommended as first-line antiarrhythmic therapy in this situation. Intravenous procainamide or lidocaine are suitable alternatives, although in one small study comparing these two agents, procainamide was shown to be superior in terminating VT.[78] Synchronized DCC should be delivered if the patient's status deteriorates, VT degenerates to VF (would be unsynchronized in this situation), or drug therapy fails.

Once an acute episode of sustained VT has been successfully terminated by electrical or pharmacologic means and an acute MI has been ruled out, the possibility of a patient having recurrent episodes of VT should be considered. Evidence for the possibility of VT recurrence can often be gleaned from invasive electrophysiologic studies using programmed ventricular stimulation. The management of the patient with chronic, recurrent, sustained VT deserves considerable attention. Because these patients are at extremely high risk for death, trial-and-error attempts to find effective therapy are unwarranted. To gain some objective evidence of a response to a specific antiarrhythmic regimen, serial testing of these drugs using the following two surrogate end points has been used: (a) inability to induce sustained VT with programmed extrastimuli by invasive electrophysiologic studies and (b) suppression of ventricular ectopic beats by serial 24-hour continuous electrocardiographic (Holter) monitoring. These two strategies have been compared[79,80] but largely abandoned for several reasons. First, the yield for finding an effective drug is low. For instance, sustained monomorphic VT can be rendered noninducible or nonsustained by programmed stimulation protocols in only 20% to 25% of patients. Therefore, the clinician frequently must search for other therapeutic options or settle for other treatment end

TABLE 19-10 Heritable Polymorphic Ventricular Tachycardia

Syndrome	Channel Defect	Mutant Gene	Characteristics	Treatment
$LQTS_1$	$\downarrow I_{Ks}$	KVLQT1	SCD/TdP with exercise	BB/ICD
$LQTS_2$	$\downarrow I_{Kr}$	HERG	SCD/TdP with arousal	BB/ICD
$LQTS_3$	$\uparrow I_{Na}^+$ during plateau/ repolarization	SCN5A	SCD/TdP at rest/sleep	Flecainide Mexiletine/ICD
Brugada	$\downarrow I_{Na}^+$	SCN5A	SCD/PMVT or VF at rest/sleep in Asian males	ICD/quinidine

BB, β-blocker; ICD, implantable cardioverter-defibrillator; LQTS, long QT syndrome; PMVT, polymorphic ventricular tachycardia; SCD, sudden death; TdP, torsade de pointes; VF, ventricular fibrillation.

Note: LQTS can be provoked by potassium channel blockers (e.g., quinidine, sotalol) and Brugada syndrome can be provoked by potent sodium channel blockers (e.g., cocaine, flecainide). $LQTS_3$ and Brugada syndrome may coexist.

points such as slower and more tolerable inducible VT. Second, amiodarone is clearly the most effective (approximately 50% effective after 2 years) agent in patients with recurrent VT; however, electrophysiologic drug testing does not necessarily predict the clinical efficacy of amiodarone. Patients may have continued inducibility of VT on amiodarone despite long-term success. Indeed, empiric amiodarone has been compared to therapy (with other agents) guided by electrophysiologic testing in patients at high risk for recurrent VT.[81] In this trial, amiodarone therapy without invasive testing was superior in preventing SCD and recurrences of severe ventricular arrhythmias at all time points. Third, the recurrence rate of life-threatening VT is high (20% to 50% per year depending on the drug chosen), regardless of the method of acute drug testing. Fourth, is the substantial side-effect profile of the type I and type III antiarrhythmic agents referred to previously. Lastly, and perhaps most importantly, is the impressive demonstrated effectiveness of nondrug approaches to the treatment of recurrent VT/VF.[82] For instance, some forms of recurrent VT are amenable to catheter ablation therapy using radiofrequency current. This approach is highly effective (approximately 90%) in idiopathic VT (right ventricular outflow tract or fascicular VT), but less so in recurrent VT associated with a cardiomyopathic process or remote MI with LV aneurysm. In the latter patients, ablation is usually regarded as second-line therapy after other methods have failed.

The Implantable Cardioverter-Defibrillator The introduction of and advances in the ICD (Fig. 19–12) have obviated the need for serial drug testing (by invasive or noninvasive methods).[83] ❽ Numerous advancements in device technology have allowed the ICD to become smaller, less invasive to implant, and programmable. Early ICDs required a thoracotomy to place the generator in the abdomen, whereas with the newer, smaller models, the leads are implanted transvenously with the generator placed into the pectoral region in a manner similar to cardiac pacemakers. Modern ICDs now employ a "tiered-therapy approach" meaning that overdrive pacing (i.e., antitachycardia pacing) can be attempted first to terminate the tachyarrhythmia (no painful shock delivered), followed by low-energy cardioversion, and, finally, by painful, high-energy defibrillation

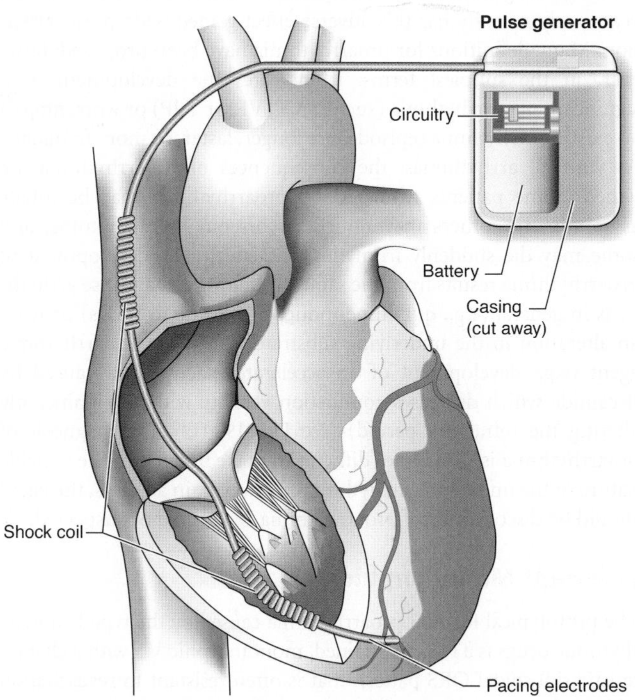

FIGURE 19-12. Drawing showing implantable cardioverter defibrillator. *(From reference 83 with permission.)*

shocks. In addition, backup antibradycardia pacing and extended battery lives have made these newer devices much more attractive. All models store recordings during delivery of pacing shocks; this is extremely important in discerning appropriate from inappropriate shocks (i.e., delivers shock for AF with rapid ventricular rate) and in documenting true recurrences of the patient's tachycardia.

Although the ICD is a highly effective method for preventing SCD due to recurrent VT or VF,[84] several problems remain. First, the device itself, implantation procedure, electrophysiologic studies, hospitalization, and physician fees are costly. Given that the indications for receiving an ICD have significantly expanded over the past several years, the total cost associated with the implantation of this device is likely to place a great burden on the healthcare system. Second, many patients (as high as 70% of patients) end up receiving antiarrhythmic drugs (usually amiodarone or sotalol) in addition to the ICD.[85,86] Antiarrhythmic drugs can be initiated in these patients for a number of reasons, including: (a) decreasing the frequency of VT/VF episodes to subsequently reduce the frequency of appropriate shocks; (b) reducing the rate of VT so that it can be terminated with antitachycardia pacing; and (c) decreasing episodes of supraventricular arrhythmias (e.g., AF, atrial flutter) that may trigger inappropriate shocks. As result of these potential benefits, the concomitant use of antiarrhythmic drugs can minimize patient discomfort and prolong the battery life of the ICD. The decision to initiate concomitant antiarrhythmic therapy should be individualized, with treatment usually being reserved for those with frequent shocks because of VT or AF. If antiarrhythmic drugs are added to ICD therapy, one should note that many agents alter defibrillation thresholds; consequently, the device should be reprogrammed to account for this alteration.[87]

Secondary Prevention of Sudden Cardiac Death Over the past decade, numerous trials have established the ICD as a superior treatment over antiarrhythmic therapy not only for the secondary prevention of SCD in patients who have been resuscitated from cardiac arrest or had sustained VT ("secondary prevention"), but also for the prevention of an initial episode of SCD in certain high-risk patient populations ("primary prevention"). With regard to the use of ICDs for secondary prevention, the results of three trials, the Antiarrhythmics Versus Implantable Defibrillators (AVID), Cardiac Arrest Study Hamburg (CASH), and Canadian Implantable Defibrillator Study (CIDS), definitively support this device as first-line therapy in this patient population.[88–90] Of these, the AVID trial was the largest, randomizing more than 1,000 patients with resuscitated VF, sustained VT with syncope, or hemodynamically significant sustained VT (with LVEF ≤40%) to either an ICD or antiarrhythmic drugs (~95% receiving amiodarone at discharge).[88] The trial was stopped early because of a demonstrated superiority of the ICD; patients in the ICD group had a better overall survival when compared to those in the antiarrhythmic drug group (75% vs. 64%, respectively, at 3 years). Although they were smaller trials, both CASH and CIDS demonstrated the efficacy of an ICD compared with amiodarone in patients with a history of sustained VT or VF, with the ICD reducing overall mortality by 20% to 25%.[89,90] Despite the high costs, the results of AVID, CASH, and CIDS provide strong support for the aggressive use of the ICD in patients who are at high risk for recurrent, life-threatening ventricular arrhythmias. Implantation of an ICD can be cost-effective, particularly in patients with poor LV function. Although nearly all clinicians now consider the ICD as first-line treatment for secondary prevention of SCD, there is at least one possible patient group that may do as well with antiarrhythmic drug therapy alone. In the AVID trial, there was no difference in survival between ICD and antiarrhytmic drug treatment in patients with mild LV dysfunction (LVEF >35%), which suggests that long-term amiodarone therapy may be appropriate to use in this lower-risk patient population.[88] However, because this data was obtained from a post-hoc analysis, additional trials need to be performed to confirm these findings.

Primary Prevention of Sudden Cardiac Death Over the past decade, the above trials have established the ICD as an effective treatment for the secondary prevention of SCD in patients who have previously suffered a documented episode of VT or VF. Most of the studies that have been performed in the past several years have focused on the efficacy of the ICD for primary prevention in patients deemed to be at high risk for SCD.[91–94]

One of the patient populations that appears to be at high risk for a first episode of SCD are those with a prior MI, LV dysfunction, and nonsustained VT. The use of antiarrhythmic drugs to prevent SCD in this high-risk group has been significantly limited by the results of the CAST and other similar trials that have collectively demonstrated that these drugs may actually increase the risk of mortality in these patients. As a result of these trials, clinicians have sought a more clearly defined strategy for risk stratification in these patients before initiating drug therapy.

Traditionally, there are three strategies to approach the treatment of nonsustained VT: (a) conservative (i.e., no antiarrhythmic drug treatment beyond β-blockers), (b) empiric amiodarone, and (c) aggressive (i.e., electrophysiologic studies with possible insertion of an ICD) (Fig. 19–13). ⑨ A number of early studies[95,96] suggested that tests such as electrophysiologic studies could be used to determine long-term risk in patients with nonsustained VT. For instance, Wilbur et al.[95] demonstrated that post-MI patients with nonsustained VT and inducible sustained VT after programmed stimulation were at increased risk for subsequent VT/VF or SCD compared to those in whom sustained VT could not be induced. These data provided the basis for the Multicenter Automatic Defibrillator Implantation Trial (MADIT) and the Multicenter Unsustained Tachycardia Trial (MUSTT).[91,92] The MADIT was the first of these trials to be conducted to evaluate the efficacy of ICD therapy in this high-risk patient population. Specifically, this trial randomized patients with a previous MI, LVEF ≤36%, asymptomatic nonsustained VT, and inducible VT that was not suppressed with the use of IV procainamide to receive an ICD or conventional medical therapy (74% of patients in this particular group received amiodarone).[91] This trial was terminated prematurely after a significant survival benefit was detected in the ICD group. The findings of the MADIT were subsequently supported by those of the MUSTT. In the MUSTT, patients with a history of MI, LVEF ≤40%, asymptomatic nonsustained VT, and inducible sustained VT were randomized to the conservative approach (no antiarrhythmic drug therapy beyond β-blockers) or electrophysiologically-guided therapy (antiarrhythmic drugs and/or ICD).[92] The results showed that the conservative approach had a significantly higher event rate (cardiac arrest or death from arrhythmia). However, when the results of the electrophysiologically-guided group were further stratified, those receiving only antiarrhythmic drugs (no ICD) were no different in terms of outcomes than those who received no treatment. In other words, only those treated with an ICD had a significantly lower event rate and greater survival. One problem with the MUSTT, however, is that because of when the trial was initiated (1989), nearly 50% of patients received type I antiarrhythmic drugs or drugs that are now known not to improve survival in patients with coronary artery disease, LV dysfunction, and ventricular arrhythmias; only 10% of patients received the most effective agent in this setting, amiodarone. Based on the results of the MADIT and MUSTT, it is reasonable for patients with coronary artery disease, LV dysfunction, and nonsustained VT to undergo electrophysiologic testing;[97] that is, invasive electrophysiologic studies with programmed stimulation are used to determine risk and guide subsequent therapy. If these patients do not have inducible sustained VT/VF, chronic antiarrhythmic drug therapy is unnecessary; however, if these patients do have inducible sustained VT/VF, implantation of an ICD is warranted.

Although the MADIT and MUSTT provided clinicians with important information regarding risk stratification, both of these trials targeted patients who had a history of nonsustained VT. The results of two landmark trials, the MADIT II and Sudden Cardiac Death in Heart Failure Trial (SCD-HeFT), have provided clinicians with additional information regarding the treatment of other groups of high-risk patients who have no prior history of ventricular arrhythmia (see Fig. 19–13).[93,94] In the MADIT II, patients with a prior MI and LVEF ≤30% were randomized to receive either an ICD or conventional therapy (routine post-MI and HF therapy).[93] Neither a history of ventricular arrhythmia nor electrophysiologic testing was required for inclusion in this study. Patients in the ICD group experienced a significant reduction in mortality when compared to the conventional therapy group; the reduction in mortality in the ICD group was primarily due to a reduction in arrhythmic death. Whereas the MADIT, MUSTT, and MADIT II limited enrollment to patients with ischemic cardiomyopathy, the SCD-HeFT is the largest trial, to date, to evaluate the efficacy of an ICD in a nonischemic HF population. In this trial, patients with NYHA class II or III HF (of either ischemic or nonischemic etiology) and LVEF ≤35% were randomized to receive placebo, amiodarone, or an ICD.[94] All patients were treated with appropriate HF therapies, as indicated. Implantation of an ICD resulted in a significantly lower mortality rate compared to treatment with either placebo or amiodarone (there was no difference between placebo and amiodarone). The survival benefits of the ICD were observed regardless of the etiology of the HF.

Overall, as the ICD trials have evolved over the past decade, the indications for implanting these devices have significantly expanded (Table 19–11).[97] Based on the results of the MUSTT, MADIT, MADIT II, and SCD-HeFT, many patients will be eligible for an ICD. ⑨ In fact, just based on the results of the MADIT II and SCD-HeFT alone, it is estimated that an additional 500,000 Medicare beneficiaries will now qualify for implantation of an ICD for primary prevention of SCD.

VENTRICULAR PROARRHYTHMIA

All antiarrhythmic agents have the potential to aggravate existing arrhythmias or to cause new arrhythmias. It is believed that antiarrhythmic drugs may cause proarrhythmia in 5% to 20% of patients.[10] Although drug-induced arrhythmias have been recognized for several years, only recently has this adverse effect gained widespread attention. Many definitions for proarrhythmia have been proposed; however, in the simplest terms, it indicates the development of a significant new arrhythmia (such as VT, VF, or TdP) or worsening of an existing arrhythmia (episodes are longer, faster, or more frequent). As with all arrhythmias, the consequences of proarrhythmia are varied. Some patients who develop proarrhythmia may be totally asymptomatic, others may notice a worsening of symptoms, and some may die suddenly from this side effect. The development of proarrhythmia results from the same mechanisms that cause arrhythmias in general (e.g., quinidine-induced TdP due to EADs) or from an alteration in the underlying substrate due to the antiarrhythmic agent (e.g., development of an accelerated tachycardia caused by flecainide which decreases conduction velocity without significantly altering the refractory period) (see Fig. 19–4).[10] The diagnosis of proarrhythmia is sometimes difficult to make because of the variable nature of the underlying arrhythmias. However, in all cases, the agent should be discontinued if proarrhythmia is detected or suspected.

Incessant Monomorphic VT

The prototypical form of proarrhythmia caused by the type Ic antiarrhythmic drugs is a rapid, sustained, monomorphic VT with a characteristic sinusoidal QRS pattern that is often resistant to resuscitation with cardioversion or overdrive pacing. ⑩ It is sometimes referred to as sinusoidal or incessant VT and is the result of excessive sodium

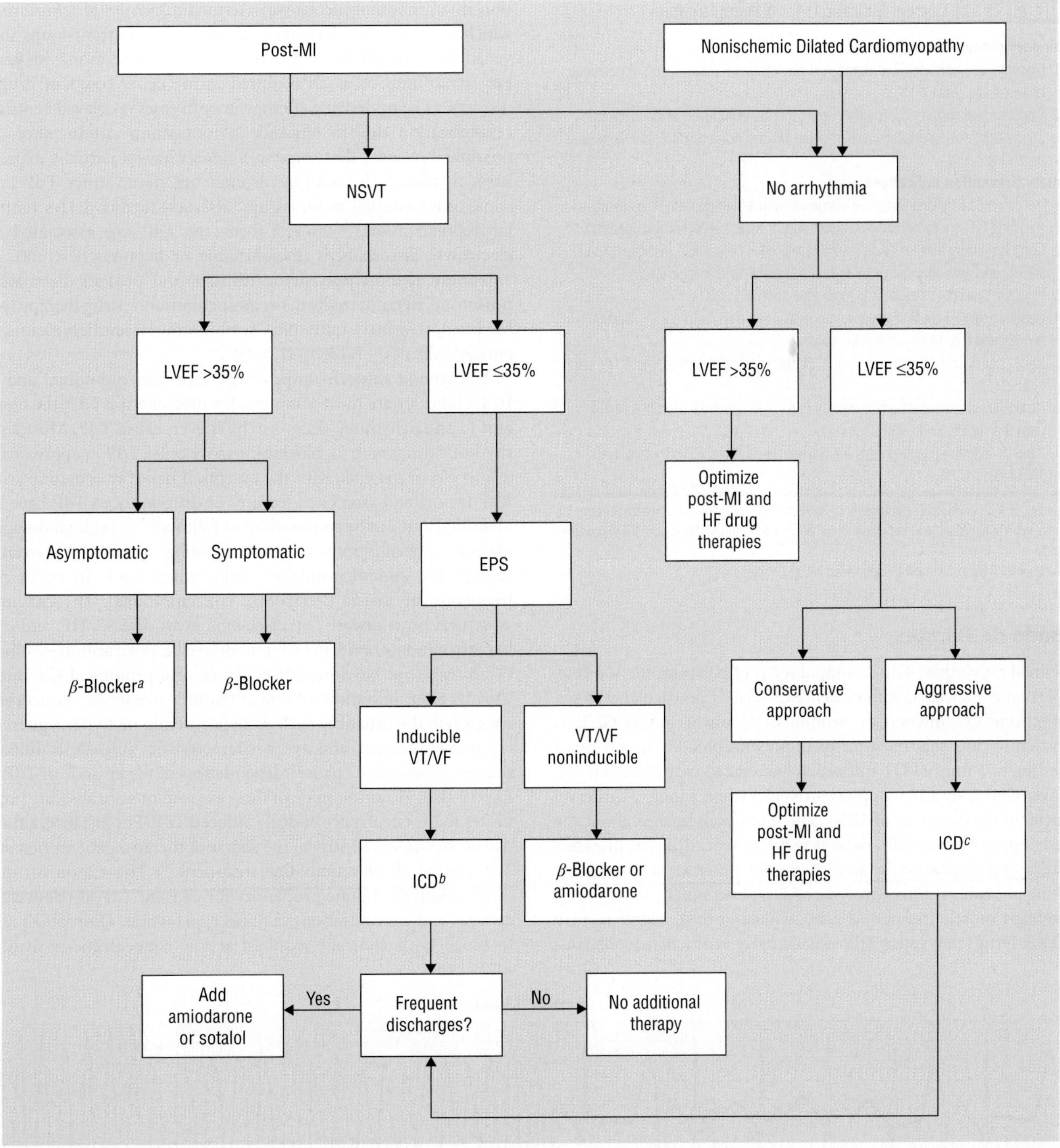

FIGURE 19-13. Algorithm for the primary prevention of sudden cardiac death in patients with a history of myocardial infarction or with a nonischemic dilated cardiomyopathy. [a]In these patients, the β-blocker is being used to reduce post-MI mortality. [b]Patients should be >40 days post-MI prior to insertion of ICD. [c]Patients with an ischemic cardiomyopathy should be >40 days post-MI prior to insertion of ICD. (EPS, electrophysiologic study; HF, heart failure; ICD, implantable cardioverter-defibrillator; LVEF, left ventricular ejection fraction; MI, myocardial infarction; NSVT, nonsustained VT; VF, ventricular fibrillation; VT, ventricular tachycardia.)

channel blockade and slowed conduction. Sinusoidal VT caused by the type Ic drugs was thought to occur within the first several days of drug initiation; however, the results of the CAST indicate that the risk for this type of proarrhythmia may exist as long as the agent is continued. Factors that definitely predispose a patient to this form of proarrhythmia are: (a) the presence of underlying ventricular arrhythmias, (b) ischemic heart disease, and (c) LV dysfunction. Provocation of proarrhythmia by the type Ic drugs is sometimes reported during exercise, which is most likely a result of augmented slowed conduction at rapid heart rates (i.e., rate-dependent sodium blockade). The incidence of proarrhythmia caused by type Ic drugs is greatest in patients with all three risk factors (approximately 10% to 20%) and extremely uncommon in those without risks, such as patients with supraventricular tachycardias and normal LV function. In one study, in patients with risk factors, the incidence of death due to proarrhythmia from encainide and flecainide was approximately the same as the chance of long-term effectiveness![98] Other factors that have a less well-defined association with proarrhythmia are elevated antiarrhythmic serum concentrations and rapid dosage escalation. It has been proposed that the presence of underlying ventricular conduction delays may also pose a risk for proarrhythmia. As mentioned earlier, this arrhythmia is resistant to resuscitation; however, some have had success with lidocaine (competes for sodium channel receptor) or sodium bicarbonate (reverses the excessive sodium channel blockade).

TABLE 19-11 Current Indications for ICD Implantation

Secondary prevention indications
1. Documented episode of cardiac arrest caused by VF (not a result of transient or reversible cause)[a]
2. Documented sustained VT, either spontaneous or induced at electrophysiologic study, not associated with an acute MI and not a result of transient or reversible cause
Primary prevention indications
1. Documented familial or inherited conditions with a high-risk of life-threatening VT (i.e., long QT syndrome, Brugada syndrome, or hypertrophic cardiomyopathy)
2. Coronary artery disease (with prior MI >40 days before ICD insertion), LVEF ≤35%, and sustained VT or VF induced at electrophysiologic study[a]
3. Prior MI (>40 days before ICD insertion) and LVEF ≤30%
4. Ischemic dilated cardiomyopathy, prior MI (>40 days before ICD insertion), NYHA class II or III HF, and LVEF ≤35%
5. Nonischemic dilated cardiomyopathy (>9 months), NYHA class II or III HF, and LVEF ≤35%
6. Nonischemic dilated cardiomyopathy (>3 months but <9 months), NYHA class II or III HF, and LVEF ≤35%
7. Patients meeting requirements for cardiac resynchronization therapy with NYHA class IV HF

HF, heart failure; ICD, implantable cardioverter-defibrillator; LVEF, left ventricular ejection fraction; MI, myocardial infarction; NYHA, New York Heart Association; VF, ventricular fibrillation; VT, ventricular tachycardia.

[a]The electrophysiologic study must be performed >4 weeks after the MI.

Torsade de Pointes

As defined previously, TdP is a rapid form of polymorphic VT (Fig. 19–14) that is associated with evidence of delayed ventricular repolarization (long QT interval or prominent U waves) on ECG. It is important to note that most forms of polymorphic VT occurring in the setting of a normal QT interval are similar to monomorphic VT in terms of etiology and treatment strategies (thus, a long QT interval is crucial to the diagnosis of TdP). Much has been learned about the underlying etiology of TdP. Basic defects (genetic, drugs or diseases) that delay repolarization by influencing ion movement (usually by blocking potassium efflux) provoke EADs, preferentially in cells deep in the heart muscle (termed *M cells*), which, in turn, trigger reentry and TdP. Drugs that cause TdP usually delay ventricular repolarization in an inhomogeneous way (termed *dispersion of refractoriness*), which facilitates the formation of multiple reentrant loops in the ventricle.[99] Torsade de pointes may occur in association with hereditary syndromes or as an acquired form (i.e., a result of drugs or diseases). The underlying etiology in both cases is delayed ventricular repolarization due to blockade of potassium conductance. It is possible, however, that some individuals have a partially expressed form of these congenital syndromes but never suffer TdP unless some other external factor (drugs, diseases) further delays ventricular repolarization. Acquired forms of TdP are associated with electrolyte disturbances (hypokalemia or hypomagnesemia), subarachnoid hemorrhage, myocarditis, liquid protein diets, arsenic poisoning, hypothyroidism, or, most commonly, drug therapy (notably phenothiazines, antibiotics, antihistamines, antidepressants, and antiarrhythmics) (Table 19–12). ⑩

The type Ia antiarrhythmic drugs (especially quinidine) and type III I_{Kr} blockers are most notorious for precipitating TdP; the types Ib and Ic antiarrhythmic drugs rarely, if ever, cause TdP. Most antiarrhythmic drugs with I_{Kr} blocking activity cause TdP in approximately 2% to 4% of patients, with the exception being amiodarone (<1%). Risk factors and associated features of drug-induced TdP have been identified and can be summarized as follows[28,100]: (a) high dosages or plasma concentrations of the offending agent ("dose-related") (except for quinidine-induced TdP, which tends to occur more frequently at low-to-therapeutic concentrations); (b) concurrent structural heart disease (e.g., ischemic heart disease, HF, and/or LV hypertrophy); (c) evidence of mild delayed repolarization (prolonged QT interval) at baseline; (d) evidence of a prolonged QT interval shortly after initiation of the offending agent; (e) concomitant electrolyte disturbances such as hypokalemia or hypomagnesemia; (f) female gender; and (g) a characteristic long–short initiating sequence (so-called "pause" dependence) of the episode of TdP (see Fig. 19–14). However, none of these associations are absolute prerequisites to the occurrence of drug-induced TdP. For instance, although usually documented early in the course of therapy, patients may suffer TdP during chronic quinidine treatment.[101] The reason for quinidine's relatively unique propensity for causing TdP at relatively low dosages and concentrations requires explanation. Quinidine's ability to block I_{Kr} is clinically manifest at low concentrations; at higher

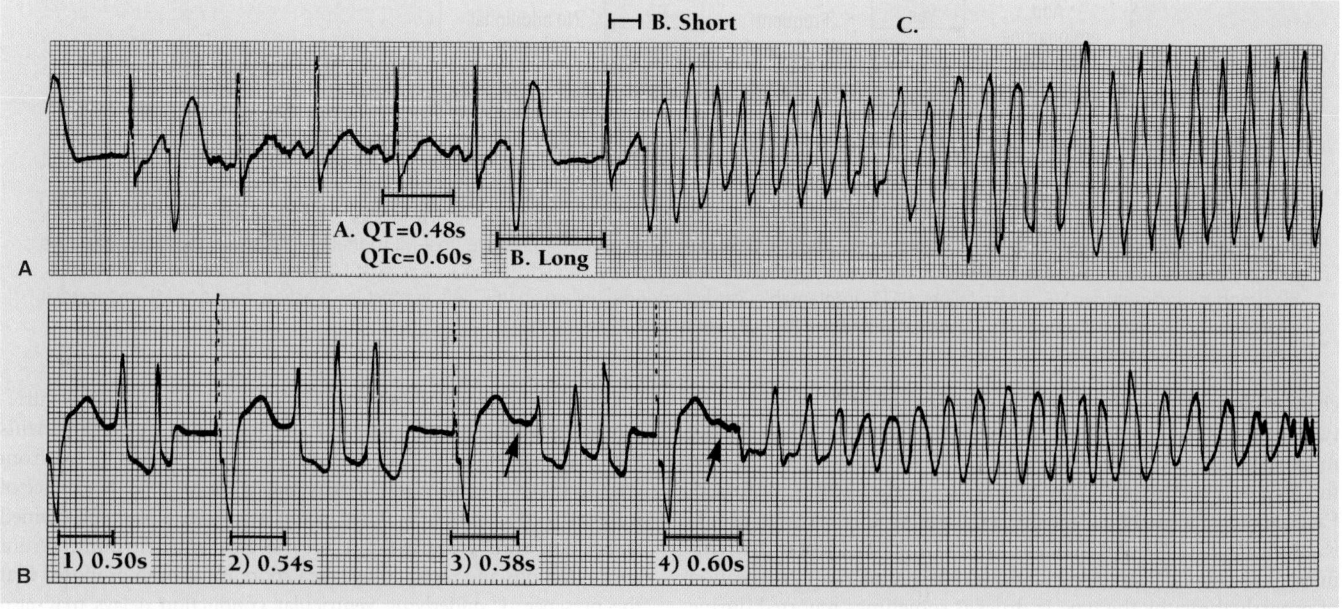

FIGURE 19-14. Torsade de pointes caused by quinidine. Note the presence of a couplet and two triplets following each extra systolic pause. The pause gets progressively longer until it is long enough to result in an episode of sustained torsade de pointes. Also, as the pause lengthens, discernible U waves (labeled ↑) (EADs?) begin to appear. The amplitude of the U wave is somewhat greater with the longest pause. *(From Bauman JL. Drug safety: Cardiac arrhythmias. Antihistamine update symposium. Hosp Med 1995;31:24, with permission.)*

concentrations its sodium-blocking properties predominate. Other agents that block I_{Kr} usually do so in a concentration-dependent fashion. The observation that most patients who suffer drug-induced TdP have evidence of mildly delayed repolarization (long QT intervals) even before they are prescribed the offending agent has stimulated a search for a potential genetically linked risk. Could it be that patients with drug-induced TdP have a partially expressed form of the congenital long QT syndrome? Indeed, it does appear that at least some of these patients with acquired drug-induced TdP appear to possess mutations of genes that encode for I_{Kr} or I_{Ks}.[100]

The common underlying electrophysiologic cause of TdP is a delay in ventricular repolarization (provoking EADs), which usually results from inhibition (drug-induced or genetic) of I_K current and manifests as QT interval prolongation on the ECG. Therefore, the extent of QT interval prolongation has been used as a measurement of risk of TdP; however, considerable controversy exists. Amiodarone, for example, commonly causes significant QT prolongation but is a relatively infrequent cause of TdP. Nonetheless, the QT interval should be measured and monitored in all patients prescribed drugs that have a high potential for causing TdP (see Table 19–12). Patients with a baseline QT_c interval (QT interval corrected for heart rate) >450 msec should not be given these agents; an increase in the QT_c interval to ≥560 msec after the initiation of the drug is an indication to discontinue the agent or, at least, to reduce its dosage and carefully observe and monitor. The QT_c interval can be calculated using Bazett's formula: $QT_c = QT\ measured/\sqrt{R\text{-}R\ interval}$.

Drug-induced TdP has become an extremely visible hazard plaguing new drugs, sometimes resulting in public health disasters. For instance, six drugs (cisapride, astemizole, terodiline, levomethadyl, grepafloxacin, and terfenadine) have been withdrawn from the market in the United States because of TdP. One of the most visible and striking examples was with regard to the popular nonsedating antihistamine, terfenadine. Terfenadine is a potent I_{Kr} blocker but is rapidly metabolized by CYP3A4 to an active moiety (fexofenadine) that is not associated with delayed repolarization. Consequently, in the presence of drugs that block the CYP3A4 isoenzyme (e.g., ketoconazole, erythromycin, diltiazem), accumulation of the parent compound, terfenadine, causes clinically significant blockade of I_{Kr} that could result in TdP and even death.[102] Because of experiences like this, all new drug entities under investigation are screened for their ability to block I_K and cause significant QT prolongation.

Acute treatment of TdP is different than treatment for the more common acute monomorphic VT. For an acute episode of TdP, most patients will require and respond to DCC. However, TdP tends to be paroxysmal in nature and often will rapidly recur after DCC. Therefore, after the initial restoration of a stable rhythm, therapy designed to prevent recurrences of TdP should be instituted. Drugs that further prolong repolarization such as IV procainamide are absolutely contraindicated. Lidocaine is usually ineffective. Although there are no true efficacy trials, IV magnesium sulfate, by suppressing EADs, is now considered the drug of choice in preventing recurrences of TdP.[103] If IV magnesium sulfate is ineffective, treatment strategies designed to increase heart rate, shorten ventricular repolarization, and prevent the pause dependency should be initiated. Either temporary transvenous pacing (105 to 120 beats/min) or pharmacologic pacing (isoproterenol or epinephrine infusion) can be initiated for this purpose. All agents that prolong QT interval should be discontinued and exacerbating factors (such as hypokalemia or hypomagnesemia) should be corrected.

TABLE 19-12 Potential Causes of QT Prolongation and Torsade de Pointes

Conditions
Congenital long QT syndromes
Myocarditis
Myocardial ischemia/infarction
Heart failure
Severe bradycardia (<50 beats/min)
Hypokalemia
Severe hypothermia
Hypomagnesemia
Severe starvation/liquid-protein diets
Subarachnoid hemorrhage
Drugs
Antiarrhythmic drugs
Quinidine
Procainamide (also *N*-acetylprocainamide)
Disopyramide
Amiodarone
Dofetilide
Sotalol
Ibutilide
Bepridil[a]
Psychotropics
Phenothiazines (e.g. thioridazine, mesoridazine, chlorpromazine)
Tricyclic and tetracyclic antidepressants
Haloperidol/droperidol
Pimozide
Atypical antipsychotics (e.g. quetiapine, ziprasidone)
Toxins
Organophosphate insecticides
Arsenic
Antihistamines
Terfenadine[a]
Astemizole[a]
Antibiotics
Pentamidine
Macrolides (erythromycin and clarithromycin)
Trimethoprim-sulfamethoxazole
Fluoroquinolones (grepafloxacin,[a] sparfloxacin,[a] moxifloxacin, gatifloxacin, gemifloxacin)
Voriconazole
Pain
Methadone
Levomethadyl[a]
Miscellaneous
Liquid-protein diets[b]
Corticosteroids[b]
Diuretics[b]
Quinine
Chloroquine
Chloral hydrate
Cisapride[a]
Terodiline[a]
Tacrolimus

[a]Withdrawn from market because of torsade de pointes.
[b]More than likely a result of severe electrolyte imbalance.
Note: For a complete list, see *www.qtdrugs.org*.

VENTRICULAR FIBRILLATION

Background and Prevention

Ventricular fibrillation is electrical anarchy of the ventricle resulting in no cardiac output and cardiovascular collapse. Death will ensue rapidly if effective treatment measures are not taken. Patients who die abruptly (within 1 hour of initial symptoms) and unexpectedly (i.e., "sudden death") usually have VF recorded at the time of death.[61] Sudden cardiac death accounts for about 330,000 deaths per year in the United States. Sudden cardiac death occurs most commonly in patients with ischemic heart disease and primary myocardial disease associated with LV dysfunction; it occurs less commonly in those with WPW syndrome or mitral valve prolapse, and occasionally in those without associated heart disease (e.g., Brugada syndrome). Patients who have SCD (not associated with acute MI) but survive because of appropriate CPR, often have inducible sustained VT and/or VF during electrophysiologic studies. These individuals are at high risk for the recurrence of VT and/or VF.

In contrast, patients who have VF associated with acute MI (i.e., within the first 24 hours after symptoms) usually have little risk of recurrence. Of all patients who die as a result of an acute MI, approximately 50% die suddenly prior to hospitalization. Ventricular fibrillation associated with acute MI can be subdivided into two types: primary VF and complicated or secondary VF. Primary VF occurs in an uncomplicated MI not associated with HF; secondary VF occurs in an MI complicated by HF. The time course, incidence, mechanisms, treatment, and complications of these two forms of VF are different. For example, approximately 2% to 6% of patients with acute MI suffer primary VF within 24 hours of chest pain, but the risk of VF declines rapidly over time and is nearly zero after the initial 24-hour period. Complicated or secondary VF does not follow such a predictable time course and may occur in the late infarction period. The premise of prophylactic antiarrhythmic drugs administered to all patients with uncomplicated MI is based on (a) the inability to predict which patients are at risk for primary VF and (b) the predictable time course of primary VF (in contrast to complicated VF). Of the prophylactic therapies used, lidocaine has been the most widely debated and studied. Lie et al.[104] performed the classic study showing the effectiveness of lidocaine in preventing primary VF. Although lidocaine significantly reduced the incidence of VF compared to placebo, there was no significant difference in mortality due to VF between the groups. This data, along with the effectiveness of rapidly instituted DCC in modern coronary care units with sophisticated monitoring techniques, have caused most to reject the notion of prophylactic lidocaine administration for all patients with uncomplicated MI. In support of this, two meta-analyses[105,106] concluded against the routine use of prophylactic lidocaine because of a possible increase in mortality in lidocaine-treated patients[105] as well as the declining incidence of primary VF documented in recent years (probably a result of the more aggressive and rapid use of β-blockers, thrombolytics, and percutaneous intervention for the treatment of acute coronary syndromes).[106]

The use of IV magnesium sulfate has also been entertained for the prevention of VF during the acute infarct period. Small trials implying its effectiveness were subsequently incorporated into a meta-analysis.[107] This meta-analysis found a decrease in the incidence of VT/VF and a reduction in total mortality with magnesium therapy. A subsequent large multicenter trial[108] found similar results, although most of the reduction in mortality was (surprisingly) attributed to HF deaths rather than to deaths caused by ventricular arrhythmia. These results would lead one to conclude that magnesium sulfate should be routinely administered to patients with suspected MI because of its ease of administration and safety. However, data from another large trial apparently has verified no such effectiveness of magnesium therapy in this setting.[109] Hence, prophylactic magnesium cannot be recommended. Indeed, no therapy (lidocaine, magnesium, or other antiarrhythmic drugs) has shown a conclusive benefit to prevent VF in the acute infarct period and no form of therapy can be recommended at this time.

Acute Management

A patient with pulseless VT or VF (with or without associated myocardial ischemia) should be managed according to the most recent AHA guidelines for CPR and emergency cardiovascular care.[53] To summarize, in patients with an unwitnessed arrest, five cycles (or 2 minutes) of CPR (one cycle of CPR = 30 chest compressions followed by 2 breaths) should be given before defibrillation. When the arrest is witnessed, and a defibrillator is readily available, defibrillation should be instituted immediately after two rescue breaths are provided; in these patients, there is no need for an initial period of CPR. Because of the increased availability of biphasic defibrillators which have a higher first-shock efficacy than monophasic defibrillators, delivery of only one shock at a time is recommended. For biphasic defibrillators, the dose of the shock to be used is device-specific; however, 200 joules can be used as the default if the effective dose range of the device is unknown. For all subsequent shocks, the initial dose or a higher dose can be used. If a monophasic defibrillator is used, 360 joules should be used for the initial as well as all subsequent shocks. After delivery of the initial shock, five cycles of CPR should be delivered, followed by a check of the patient's pulse and rhythm. If pulseless VT/VF is still present, another shock can be delivered, followed by five cycles of CPR. This general sequence of providing shocks followed by CPR can be followed as long as the patient remains in pulseless VT/VF.

Although there is very little, if any, evidence that demonstrates an increased survival rate with either vasopressor or antiarrhythmic agents in patients with pulseless VT/VF, these drugs still continue to play a role in the management of these ventricular arrhythmias.[53] To minimize interruptions in chest compressions, any vasopressor or antiarrhythmic administered during the course of the cardiac arrest should be given during CPR either before or after a shock. With regard to vasopressor therapy, either epinephrine or vasopressin can be administered if pulseless VT/VF persists after delivery of one or two shocks plus CPR. More specifically, epinephrine can be administered every 3 to 5 minutes while the patient remains in pulseless VT/VF. Alternatively, one dose of vasopressin can be given to replace either the first or second dose of epinephrine. In a recent comparative trial, patients with out-of-hospital cardiac arrest (60% with asystole or pulseless electrical activity, 40% with VF) were randomized to receive up to two doses of either vasopressin or epinephrine, followed by an additional dose of epinephrine if a stable rhythm was not restored.[110] Overall, no significant differences were observed between the treatment groups with regard to the end points of survival to hospital admission or survival to hospital discharge (in patients with asystole, however, vasopressin was superior for both of these end points).

If pulseless VT/VF persists after delivery of two or three shocks plus CPR and after administration of a vasopressor, antiarrhythmic therapy can then be initiated.[53] It appears clear from the most recent AHA guidelines for CPR and emergency cardiovascular care that IV amiodarone continues to be the antiarrhythmic drug of first choice in patients with pulseless VT/VF. Amiodarone's status as the first-line antiarrhythmic drug during pulseless VT/VF (and lidocaine's resulting role as second-line antiarrhythmic therapy) is the result of (a) a lack of data demonstrating the effectiveness of other antiarrhythmic agents; (b) the Amiodarone in Out-of-Hospital Resuscitation of Refractory Sustained Ventricular Tachyarrhythmias (ARREST) trial;[111] and (c) the Amiodarone versus Lidocaine in Prehospital Ventricular Fibrillation Evaluation (ALIVE) trial.[112] In the ARREST trial,[111] significantly more patients with out-of-hospital pulseless VT/VF who received 300 mg of IV amiodarone survived to hospital admission than did a corresponding placebo group. Noteworthy was that survival to hospital discharge was no different between the groups (although the study was not powered to determine this end point). In the ALIVE trial,[112] IV amiodarone was significantly more effective than lidocaine in increasing survival to hospital admission in patients with out-of-hospital VF. Again, there were no differences in survival to hospital discharge between the groups. Nonetheless, the results of these trials stimulated a change (away from lidocaine and toward amiodarone) in the treatment of pulseless VT/VF. In the event that a patient remains in pulseless VT/VF despite the administration of IV amiodarone and/or lidocaine, it is interesting to note that IV procainamide is no longer recommended in the treatment algorithm because of limited evidence and the need for a prolonged infusion.[53]

Once the patient is successfully resuscitated, antiarrhythmics should be continued until the patient's rhythm and overall status is stable. If the episode of pulseless VT/VF was associated with acute ischemia, long-term antiarrhythmic drugs are probably unnecessary provided that the patient undergoes successful revascularization; however, the patient should be monitored closely for recurrence of VT and/or VF. If, on the other hand, the pulseless VT/VF was not associated with acute MI (or a known precipitating factor), the patient should undergo ICD implantation.

BRADYARRHYTHMIAS

SINUS NODE DYSFUNCTION

The previous sections reviewed the pathophysiology and treatment of tachyarrhythmias, and this section serves to briefly consider the bradyarrhythmias. For the most part, the symptoms of bradyarrhythmias result from a decline in cardiac output. Because cardiac output decreases as heart rate decreases (to a point), patients with bradyarrhythmias may experience symptoms in association with hypotension, such as dizziness, syncope, fatigue, and confusion. If LV dysfunction exists, patients may experience worsening HF symptoms. Except in the case of recurrent syncope, symptoms associated with bradyarrhythmias are often subtle and nonspecific.

SINUS BRADYCARDIA

Sinus bradyarrhythmias (heart rate <60 beats/min) is a common finding, especially in young, athletically active individuals, and usually is neither symptomatic nor requires therapeutic intervention. On the other hand, some patients, particularly the elderly, have sinus node dysfunction. This may be the result of underlying structural heart disease and the normal aging process which, over time, attenuate SA nodal function. Sick sinus syndrome refers to this process resulting in symptomatic sinus bradycardia and/or periods of sinus arrest.[113,114] Sinus node dysfunction is usually reflective of diffuse conduction disease, and accompanying AV block is relatively common. Furthermore, symptomatic bradyarrhythmias may be accompanied by alternating periods of paroxysmal tachycardias such as AF. In this instance, AF sometimes presents with a rather slow ventricular response (in the absence of AV nodal blocking drugs) because of diffuse conduction disease. The occurrence of alternating bradyarrhythmias and tachyarrhythmias is referred to as the "tachy-brady syndrome." The occurrence of paroxysmal AF in a patient with sinus node dysfunction may be a result of underlying structural heart disease with atrial dysfunction or to atrial escape in response to reduced sinus node automaticity. In fact, because the rate of impulse generation by the sinus node is generally depressed or may fail altogether, other automatic pacemakers within the conduction system may "rescue" the sinus node. These rescue rhythms often present as paroxysmal atrial rhythms (e.g., AF) or as a junctional escape rhythm.

The treatment of sinus node dysfunction involves the elimination of symptomatic bradycardia and the possibility of managing alternating tachycardias such as AF. In general, the long-term therapy of choice is a permanent ventricular pacemaker. Dual-chamber, rate-adaptive chronic pacing clearly improves symptoms and overall quality of life and decreases the incidence of paroxysmal AF and systemic embolism.[113] Drugs that are commonly employed to treat supraventricular tachycardias should be used with caution, if at all, in the absence of a functioning pacemaker. Antiarrhythmic drugs prescribed to prevent recurrences of AF may also suppress the escape or rescue rhythms that appear in severe sinus bradycardia or sinus arrest. In this way, these drugs may transform an asymptomatic patient with bradycardia into a symptomatic one. It is also important to remember that the addition of type I antiarrhythmic agents can affect pacemaker threshold and result in loss of capture if the pacemaker is not appropriately interrogated and adjusted.[87] Other drugs that depress SA or AV nodal function, such as β-blockers and nondihydropyridine CCBs, may also significantly exacerbate bradycardia. Even agents with indirect sympatholytic actions, such as methyldopa and clonidine, may worsen sinus node dysfunction. The use of digoxin in these patients is controversial, but in most cases, it can be used safely.

Other Causes

Another reason for paroxysmal bradycardia and sinus arrest that is not directly due to sinus node dysfunction is carotid-sinus hypersensitivity.[115,116] Again, this syndrome occurs commonly in the aged with underlying structural heart disease, and may precipitate falls and hip fractures. Symptoms occur when the carotid sinus is stimulated, resulting in an accentuated baroreceptor reflex. Often, however, symptoms are not well correlated with the obvious physical manipulation of the carotid sinus (in the lateral neck region). Patients may experience intermittent episodes of dizziness or syncope because of sinus arrest caused by increased vagal tone and sympathetic withdrawal (the cardioinhibitory type), a drop in systemic blood pressure caused by sympathetic withdrawal (the vasodepressor type), or both (mixed cardioinhibitory and vasodepressor types). The diagnosis can be confirmed by performing carotid-sinus massage with electrocardiographic and blood pressure monitoring in controlled conditions. Symptomatic carotid-sinus hypersensitivity should also be treated with permanent pacemaker therapy.[115] However, some patients, particularly those with a significant vasodepressor component, still experience syncope or dizziness. The choice of definitive drug therapy in this situation is marred by the lack of controlled trials although α-adrenergic stimulants such as midodrine are often tried in addition to the pacemaker.[116]

Vasovagal syndrome, by causing bradycardia, sinus arrest, and/or hypotension, is the cause of syncope in many patients who present with recurrent fainting of unknown origin.[117–119] By history, many individuals can recount rare instances of fainting spells at times of duress or fear. These are most often caused by vasovagal syncope. However, some have extremely frequent, unexpected syncopal episodes that interfere with the patient's quality of life and cause physical danger (sometimes referred to as neurocardiogenic syncope syndrome or malignant vasovagal syndrome). Vasovagal syncope is presumed to be a neurally mediated, paradoxical reaction involving stimulation of cardiac mechanoreceptors (i.e., Bezold-Jarisch reflex). Forceful contraction of the ventricle (e.g., as with adrenergic stimulation) coupled with low ventricular volumes (e.g., with upright posture or dehydration) provide a powerful stimulus for cardiac mechanoreceptors. Syncope results from the spontaneous development of transient hypotension (sympathetic withdrawal) and bradycardia (vagotonia). However, the true mechanism of vasovagal syncope remains to be definitively determined. For instance, patients with denervated hearts (e.g., heart transplant recipients) can still experience this form of syncope. This observation has led some to question the ultimate role of the Bezold-Jarisch reflex in these patients. Regardless, patients believed to have frequent episodes of vasovagal syncope have been evaluated and diagnosed using the upright body-tilt test,[121] a potent stimulus for the development of vasovagal symptoms. Although commonly used, the sensitivity and reproducibility of this test has been questioned.[120]

Traditionally, oral β-blockers, such as metoprolol, were frequently chosen as the drugs of choice in preventing episodes of vasovagal syncope. Although these agents may seem inappropriate to treat a syndrome resulting from vasodilation and bradycardia, the therapeutic approach is designed to block an inappropriate vasovagal reaction (i.e., they inhibit the sympathetic surge that causes forceful ventricular contraction and precedes the onset of hypotension and bradycardia). To most clinicians' surprise, most controlled trials of the use of β-blockers in patients with severe vasovagal syncope have shown no effect compared to placebo in preventing syncopal episodes.[122] Some trials have suggested that β-blockers are more effective and should be used in older patients (>40 years of age) with vasovagal syncope rather than the relatively young.[123] Other drugs that have been used successfully (with or without β-blockers) include mineralocorticoids as volume expanders (fludrocortisone), anticholinergic agents (scopolamine patches, disopyramide), α-adrenergic agonists (midodrine), adenosine analogs (theophylline, dipyridamole), and selective serotonin receptor antagonists (sertraline, paroxetine).[124] Permanent pacing has been used for patients with malignant vasovagal syncope but its routine use is controversial. Chronic pacing has been used with some success but should be reserved for drug-refractory patients.[118,119] Because of the questionable effectiveness of β-blockers and the paucity of controlled or comparative trials, there is not a true drug of choice for severe vasovagal syncope and clinicians are left with choosing agents and judging clinical effectiveness in individual patients on a case-by-case basis.

ATRIOVENTRICULAR BLOCK

Conduction delay or block may occur in any area of the AV conduction system: the AV node, the His bundle, or the bundle branches. Atrioventricular block is usually categorized into three different types based on ECG findings (Table 19–13). First-degree AV block is 1:1 AV conduction with a prolonged PR interval. Second-degree AV block is divided into two forms: Mobitz I AV block (Wenckebach periodicity) is less than 1:1 AV conduction with progressively lengthening PR intervals until a ventricular complex is dropped; Mobitz II AV block is intermittently dropped ventricular beats in a random fashion without progressive PR lengthening. Third-degree AV block is complete heart block where AV conduction is totally absent (AV dissociation). By using intracardiac His bundle ECGs, the actual site of conduction delay/block can be correlated to the above diagnosis. First-degree AV block usually represents prolonged conduction in the AV node. Mobitz I, second-degree AV block is also usually caused by prolonged conduction in the AV node. Indeed, Wenckebach periodicity is a normal AV nodal response to rapid supraventricular stimulation or high vagal tone. In contrast, Mobitz II AV block is usually caused by conduction disease below the AV node (i.e., His bundle). Third-degree AV block may be caused by disease at any level of the AV conduction system: complete AV nodal block, His bundle block, or trifascicular block. In this situation, the ventricle beats independently of the atria (AV dissociation), and the rate of ventricular activation and QRS configuration are determined by the site of AV block. The usual degree of automaticity of ventricular pacemakers progressively declines as impulses move down the conduction system. Therefore, the ventricular escape rate in cases of trifascicular block will be significantly less than complete AV nodal block.

Atrioventricular block may be found in patients without underlying structural heart disease such as trained athletes or during sleep when vagal tone is high. Also, AV block may be transient where the underlying etiology is reversible such as in myocarditis, myocardial ischemia, after cardiovascular surgery, or during drug therapy. β-blockers, digoxin, or nondihydropyridine CCBs may cause AV block, primarily in the AV nodal area. Type I antiarrhythmic agents may exacerbate conduction delays below the level of the AV node (sodium-dependent tissue). In other cases, AV block may be irreversible, such as that caused by acute MI, rare degenerative diseases, primary myocardial disease, or congenital forms.

If patients with Mobitz II AV block or third-degree AV block develop signs or symptoms of poor perfusion (e.g., altered mental status, chest pain, hypotension, shock) associated with bradycardia or AV block, transcutaneous pacing should be initiated immediately.[53,125] Intravenous atropine (0.5 mg given every 3 to 5 minutes, up to 3 mg total dose) should be given as the leads for pacing are being placed. Drugs such as atropine will facilitate the effectiveness of transcutaneous pacing. In the past, isoproterenol infusion was frequently chosen for this purpose but is now not recommended because of its vasodilating properties and its ability to increase myocardial oxygen consumption (particularly during acute MI). If patients do not respond to atropine, transcutaneous pacing is usually indicated. Sympathomimetic infusions such as epinephrine (2 to 10 mcg/min) or dopamine (2 to 10 mcg/kg/min) can also be used in the event of atropine failure and are particularly effective in sinus bradycardia/arrest and AV nodal block. These agents usually do not help when the site of AV block is below the AV node (e.g., Mobitz II or trifascicular AV block). If patients with bradycardia or AV block present with signs and symptoms of adequate perfusion, no therapy other than close observation is recommended.

Patients with chronic symptomatic AV block should be treated with the insertion of a permanent pacemaker. Patients without symptoms can sometimes be followed closely without the need for a pacemaker. The reader is referred for more detail to the national consensus guidelines for pacemaker implantation, which were last updated in 2002.[125] Because symptoms often correlate with the ventricular rate and the ventricular rate corresponds to the site of block, pacemaker therapy is usually necessary in distal AV blocks such as those occurring in the His bundle or the bundle branches. Patients with acute MI and evidence of new AV block or conduction disturbances will often require the insertion of a temporary transvenous pacemaker. Atrioventricular block more commonly occurs as a complication of inferior wall infarcts because of high vagal innervation at this site, and the coronary blood flow to the nodal areas usually supplies the inferior wall. However, the AV block may only be transient, obviating the need for permanent pacing. In patients with chronic AV conduction disturbances, intracardiac recordings (His bundle ECGs) are sometimes used to document the actual site of block and define the potential need for and specific type of pacemaker therapy.

TABLE 19-13 Forms of Atrioventricular Block

Type	Criteria	Site of Block
First-degree block	Prolonged PR interval (>0.2 sec); 1:1 AV conduction	Usually AVN
Second-degree block		
Mobitz I	Progressive PR prolongation until QRS is dropped; <1:1 AV conduction	AVN
Mobitz II	Random nonconducted beats (absence of QRS); <1:1 AV conduction	Below AVN
Third-degree block	AV dissociation Absence of AV conduction	AVN or below

AV, atrioventricular; AVN, atrioventricular node.

EVALUATION OF THERAPEUTIC AND ECONOMIC OUTCOMES

Generally, patients who suffer from tachyarrhythmias can be monitored for one or several possible therapeutic outcomes. Obviously, the presence or recurrence of any arrhythmia can be documented by electrocardiographic means (e.g., surface ECG, Holter monitor, or event monitor). Furthermore, patients may experience a decrease in blood pressure that may result in symptoms ranging from lightheadedness to abrupt syncope, depending on the rate of the arrhythmia and the status of the underlying heart disease. For some patients, the potential alteration in hemodynamics may result in death if the arrhythmia is not detected and treated immediately. Besides these clinical outcomes, many patients with tachyarrhythmias experience alterations in quality of life as a result of recurrent symptoms of the

TABLE 19-14 Arrhythmia Outcomes

Mortality
Total, all-cause
Arrhythmic death (i.e., sudden cardiac death)
Recurrences documented by electrocardiogram
Time to recurrence
Frequency of recurrences
Tolerance
Symptoms
Blood pressure
Rate of tachycardia
Surrogate markers of efficacy such as:
Number of premature ventricular contractions/day
Inducibility of tachycardia with programmed stimulation
Necessity of nondrug interventions (e.g., ICD)
ICD shocks
Side effects of drugs/treatment complications
Quality of life
Economics
Outcomes specific to tachycardia (e.g., systemic embolism in atrial fibrillation)

ICD, implantable cardioverter-defibrillator.

arrhythmia or from side effects of therapy. And, finally, there are the economic considerations of medical or surgical intervention, continued medical care, and chronic drug or nondrug treatment.[126,127] Most of the studies are limited to the use of nondrug therapies such as the ICD or radiofrequency ablation.[43,97] Because that technology is rapidly evolving, what is not very cost-effective now, indeed may be cost-effective in the next several years. For example, original cost-effectiveness analysis of the ICD showed it to be highly sensitive to the life of the generator, yet newer-generation devices have made significant advances in not only the size, but also with regard to battery life. More recent data on the effect of the ICD on mortality coupled with the declining costs of an ICD imply that the device is indeed cost-effective in certain subsets of patients, not unlike well-proven drug therapies used for other disorders.[97] Other nondrug treatments, such as radiofrequency ablation, for PSVT not only improve quality of life, but also save money on medical expenditures compared to chronic drug therapy.[43]

There are some therapeutic outcomes that are unique to certain arrhythmias. For instance, patients with AF or atrial flutter need to be monitored for thromboembolism and for complications of anticoagulation therapy (bleeding, drug interactions) prescribed to prevent thromboembolic events. However, the most important monitoring parameters for most patients fall into the following categories: (a) mortality (total and arrhythmic), (b) arrhythmia recurrence (duration, frequency, symptoms), (c) hemodynamic consequences (heart rate, blood pressure, symptoms), and (d) treatment complications (need for alternative or additional drugs, devices, surgery) (Table 19–14). When evaluating the arrhythmia literature, care should be taken to consider real outcomes. For example, total mortality is more meaningful than only SCD rates; it is possible an intervention prevents arrhythmic death but patients die from other causes, leaving all-cause mortality unaltered. Likewise, surrogate markers of drug efficacy (e.g., noninducible tachycardia, suppression of minor arrhythmias) should be judged with a degree of skepticism. One should ask: Did the treatment make patients live longer (reduce mortality)? Did it make them feel better (improve humanistic outcomes or quality of life)? Was it economically worth it (cost-effective)?

ABBREVIATIONS

ACC: American College of Cardiology

AF: atrial fibrillation

AFFIRM: Atrial Fibrillation Follow-up Investigation of Rhythm Management

AHA: American Heart Association

ALIVE: Amiodarone versus Lidocaine in Prehospital Ventricular Fibrillation Evaluation

ARREST: Amiodarone in Out-of-Hospital Resuscitation of Refractory Sustained Ventricular Tachycardia trial

AV: atrioventricular

AVID: Antiarrhythmics Versus Implantable Defibrillators trial

CASH: Cardiac Arrest Study Hamburg

CAST: Cardiac Arrhythmia Suppression Trial

CCB: calcium channel blocker

CIDS: Canadian Implantable Defibrillator Study

CPR: cardiopulmonary resuscitation

CYP: cytochrome P450

DCC: direct-current cardioversion

EADs: early after-depolarizations

ECG: electrocardiogram

ESC: European Society of Cardiology

HF: heart failure

HOT-CAFE: How to Treat Chronic Atrial Fibrillation trial

ICD: implantable cardioverter-defibrillator

INR: international normalized ratio

IV: intravenous

LADs: late after-depolarizations

LV: left ventricular

LVEF: left ventricular ejection fraction

MADIT: Multicenter Automatic Defibrillator Implantation Trial

MI: myocardial infarction

MUSTT: Multicenter Unsustained Tachycardia Trial

NYHA: New York Heart Association

PIAF: Pharmacological Intervention in Atrial Fibrillation trial

PSVT: paroxysmal supraventricular tachycardia

PVCs: premature ventricular complexes

RACE: Rate Control versus Electrical Cardioversion for Persistent Atrial Fibrillation trial

RMP: resting membrane potential

SA: sinoatrial

SCD: sudden cardiac death

SCD-HeFT: Sudden Cardiac Death in Heart Failure Trial

STAF: Strategies of Treatment of Atrial Fibrillation trial

TdP: torsade de pointes

TEE: transesophageal echocardiography

VF: ventricular fibrillation

VT: ventricular tachycardia

WPW: Wolff-Parkinson-White syndrome

REFERENCES

1. Alice MA, Bonke FIM, Schopman FJG. Circus movement in rabbit atrial muscle as a mechanism of tachycardia III. The "leading circle" concept: A new model of circus movement in cardiac tissue without the involvement of an anatomic obstacle. Circ Res 1977;41:9-18.
2. Vaughan Williams EM. A classification of antiarrhythmic actions reassessed after a decade of new drugs. J Clin Pharmacol 1984;24: 129-147.

3. Working Group on Arrhythmias of the European Society of Cardiology. The Sicilian Gambit. A new approach to the classification of antiarrhythmic drugs based upon their actions on arrhythmogenic mechanisms. Circulation 1991;84:1831–1851.
4. Hondeghem LM, Katzung BG. Antiarrhythmic agents: The modulated receptor mechanism of action of sodium and calcium channel-blocking drugs. Annu Rev Pharmacol Toxicol 1984;24:387–423.
5. MERIT-HF Study Group. Effect of metoprolol CR/XL in chronic heart failure: Metoprolol CR/XL randomized intervention trial in congestive heart failure (MERIT-HF). Lancet 1999;353:2001–2007.
6. Healey JS, Morillo CA, Connolly SJ. Role of the renin-angiotensin-aldosterone system in atrial fibrillation and cardiac remodeling. Curr Opin Cardiol 2005;20:31–37.
7. Kosowsky BD, Taylor J, Lown B, et al. Long-term procaine amide following acute myocardial infarction. Circulation 1973;47:1204–1210.
8. Bauman JL, Gallastegui J, Strasberg B, et al. Long-term therapy with disopyramide phosphate: Side effects and effectiveness. Am Heart J 1986;111:654–660.
9. Podrid PJ, Schoeneburger A, Lown B. Congestive heart failure caused by oral disopyramide. N Engl J Med 1980;302:614–617.
10. McCollam PL, Parker RB, Beckman KJ, et al. Proarrhythmia: A paradoxic response to antiarrhythmic agents. Pharmacotherapy 1989;9:144–153.
11. Fang MC, Stafford RS, Ruskin JN, et al. National trends in antiarrhythmic and antithrombotic medication use in atrial fibrillation. Arch Intern Med 2004;164:55–60.
12. Dusman RE, Stanton MS, Miles WM, et al. Clinical features of amiodarone-induced pulmonary toxicity. Circulation 1990;82:51–59.
13. Podrid PJ. Amiodarone: Reevaluation of an old drug. Ann Intern Med 1995;122:689–700.
14. Sanoski C, Schoen MD, Gonzalez RD, et al. Rational, development and outcomes of a multidisciplinary clinic for patients receiving chronic oral amiodarone. Pharmacotherapy 1998;18:1465–1515.
15. Fuster V, Rydén LE, Cannom DS, et al. ACC/AHA/ESC 2006 guidelines for the management of patients with atrial fibrillation: A report of the American College of Cardiology/American Heart Association Task Force on Practice Guidelines and the European Society of Cardiology Committee for Practice Guidelines (Writing Committee to Revise the 2001 Guidelines for the Management of Patients with Atrial Fibrillation). J Am Coll Cardiol 2006;48:e149–e246.
16. Levy S, Camm AJ, Saksena S, et al. International consensus on nomenclature and classification of atrial fibrillation. A collaborative project of the Working Group on Arrhythmias and the Working Group on Cardiac Pacing of the European Society of Cardiology and the North American Society of Pacing and Electrophysiology. Europace 2003;5:119–122.
17. Singer DE, Albers GW, Dalen JE, et al. Antithrombotic therapy in atrial fibrillation: The Seventh ACCP Conference on Antithrombotic and Thrombolytic Therapy. Chest 2004;126(Suppl):429S–456S.
18. Atrial Fibrillation Investigators. Risk factors for stroke and efficacy of antithrombotic therapy in atrial fibrillation. Analysis of pooled data from five randomized controlled trials. Arch Intern Med 1994;154:1449–1457.
19. Phillips BG, Gandhi AJ, Sanoski CA, et al. Comparison of intravenous diltiazem and verapamil for the acute treatment of atrial fibrillation and flutter. Pharmacotherapy 1997;17:1238–1245.
20. Hohnloser SH, Kuck KH, Lilienthal J. Rhythm or rate control in atrial fibrillation—Pharmacological Intervention in Atrial Fibrillation (PIAF): A randomised trial. Lancet 2000;356:1789–1794.
21. Van Gelder IC, Hagens VE, Bosker HA, et al. The Rate Control Versus Electrical Cardioversion for Persistent Atrial Fibrillation Study Group. A comparison of rate control and rhythm control in patients with recurrent persistent atrial fibrillation. N Engl J Med 2002;347:1834–1840.
22. The Atrial Fibrillation Follow-up Investigation of Rhythm Management (AFFIRM) Investigators. A comparison of rate control and rhythm control in patients with atrial fibrillation. N Engl J Med 2003;347:1825–1833.
23. Carlsson J, Miketic S, Windeler J, et al. Randomized trial of rate-control versus rhythm-control in persistent atrial fibrillation: The Strategies of Treatment of Atrial Fibrillation (STAF) study. J Am Coll Cardiol 2003;41:1690–1696.
24. Opolski G, Torbicki A, Kosior DA, et al. Rate control vs rhythm control in patients with nonvalvular persistent atrial fibrillation: The results of the Polish How to Treat Chronic Atrial Fibrillation (HOT CAFE) Study. Chest 2004;126:476–486.
25. de Denus S, Sanoski CA, Carlsson J, Opolski G, Spinler SA. Rate vs rhythm control in patients with atrial fibrillation: A meta-analysis. Arch Intern Med 2005;165:258–262.
26. Feld GK, Fleck P, Fujimura O, et al. Control of rapid ventricular response by radiofrequency catheter modification of the atrioventricular node in patients with medically refractory atrial fibrillation. Circulation 1994;90:2299–2307.
27. Klein AL, Grimm RA, Murray D, et al. Use of transesophageal echocardiography to guide cardioversion in patients with atrial fibrillation. N Engl J Med 2001;344:1411–1420.
28. Bauman JL, Bauernfeind RA, Hoff JV, et al. Torsade de pointes due to quinidine: Observations in 31 patients. Am Heart J 1984;107:425-430.
29. Slavik RS, Tisdale JE, Borzak S. Pharmacologic conversion of atrial fibrillation: A systematic review of available evidence. Prog Cardiovasc Dis 2001;44:121–152.
30. Alboni P, Botto GL, Baldi N, et al. Outpatient treatment of recent-onset atrial fibrillation with the "pill-in-the-pocket" approach. N Engl J Med 2004;351:2384–2391.
31. Coplen SE, Antman EM, Berlin JA, et al. Efficacy and safety of quinidine therapy for maintenance of sinus rhythm after cardioversion: A meta-analysis of randomized control trials. Circulation 1990;82:1106-1116.
32. Echt DS, Liebson PR, Mitchell B, et al. Mortality and morbidity in patients receiving encainide, flecainide, or placebo. The cardiac arrhythmia suppression trial. N Engl J Med 1991;324:781-788.
33. Flaker GC, Blackshear JL, McBride R, et al. Antiarrhythmic drug therapy and cardiac mortality in atrial fibrillation. J Am Coll Cardiol 1992;20:527–532.
34. Roy D, Talajic M, Dorian P, et al. Amiodarone to prevent recurrence of atrial fibrillation. Canadian Trial of Atrial Fibrillation Investigators. N Engl J Med 2000;324(13):913–920.
35. AFFIRM First Antiarrhythmic Drug Substudy Investigators. Maintenance of sinus rhythm in patients with atrial fibrillation: An AFFIRM substudy of the first antiarrhythmic drug. J Am Coll Cardiol 2003;42:20–29.
36. Singh BN, Singh SN, Reda DJ, et al. Amiodarone versus sotalol for atrial fibrillation. N Engl J Med 2005;352:1861–1872.
37. Juul-Moller S, Edvardsson N, Rehnqvist-Ahlberg N. Sotalol versus quinidine for the maintenance of sinus rhythm after direct current conversion of atrial fibrillation. Circulation 1990;82:1932–1939.
38. Southworth MR, Zarembski D, Viana M, Bauman JL. Comparison of sotalol versus quinidine for maintenance of normal sinus rhythm in patients with chronic atrial fibrillation. Am J Cardiol 1999;83:1629–1632.
39. Pedersen OD, Bagger H, Keller N, et al. Efficacy of dofetilide in the treatment of atrial fibrillation-flutter in patients with reduced left ventricular function, A Danish Investigation of Arrhythmia and Mortality ON Dofetilide (DIAMOND) Substudy. Circulation 2001;104:292–296.
40. Singh S, Zoble RG, Yellen L, et al. Efficacy and safety of oral dofetilide in converting and maintaining sinus rhythm in patients with chronic atrial fibrillation or atrial flutter. The Symptomatic Atrial Fibrillation Investigative Research on Dofetilide (SAFIRE-D) Study. Circulation 2000;102:2385–2390.
41. Pedersen OD, Bagger H, Keller N, et al. Efficacy of dofetilide in the treatment of atrial fibrillation-flutter in patients with reduced left ventricular function: A Danish investigations of arrhythmia and mortality on dofetilide (DIAMOND) substudy. Circulation 2001;104:292–296.
42. Fischer B, Haissaguerre M, Garrigues S, et al. Radiofrequency catheter ablation of common atrial flutter in 80 patients. J Am Coll Cardiol 1995;25:1365–1372.
43. Blomstrom-Lundgrist C, Scheimanman MM, Aliot EM, et al. ACC/AHA/ESC Guidelines for the management of patients with supraventricular arrhythmias. A report of the American College of Cardiology/American Heart Association Task Force and the European Society of Cardiology Committee for Practice Guidelines. J Am Coll Cardiol 2003;42:1493–1531.
44. Cox JL, Schuessler RB, Loppas DG, Boineau JP. An 8 1/2 year clinical experience with surgery for atrial fibrillation. Ann Surg 1996;224:267–275.
45. Pappone C, Rosanio S, Augello G, et al. Mortality, morbidity, and quality of life after circumferential pulmonary vein ablation for atrial fibrillation: Outcomes from a controlled nonrandomized long-term study. J Am Coll Cardiol 2003;42:185–197.

46. Oral H, Pappone C, Chugh A, et al. Circumferential pulmonary-vein ablation for chronic atrial fibrillation. N Engl J Med 2006;354:934–941.
47. Wazni OM, Marrouche NF, Martin DO, et al. Radiofrequency ablation vs antiarrhythmic drugs as first-line treatment of symptomatic atrial fibrillation: A randomized trial. JAMA 2005;293:2634–2640.
48. Cappato R, Calkins H, Chen SA, et al. Worldwide survey on the methods, efficacy, and safety of catheter ablation for human atrial fibrillation. Circulation 2005;111:1100–1105.
49. Sung RJ, Lauer MR, Chun H. Atrioventricular Node Reentry: Current concepts and new perspectives. Pacing Clin Electrophysiol 1994;17:1413–1430.
50. Bauernfeind RA, Wyndham CR, Dhingra RC, et al. Serial electrophysiologic testing of multiple drugs in patients with atrioventricular nodal reentrant paroxysmal tachycardia. Circulation 1980;62:1341–1349.
51. Wu D, Amat-Y-Leon F, Simpson R, et al. Electrophysiological studies with multiple drugs in patients with atrioventricular reentrant tachycardias utilizing an extra nodal pathway. Circulation 1977;56:727-736.
52. DiMarco JP, Miles W, Akhtar M, et al. Adenosine for paroxysmal supraventricular tachycardia: Dose ranging and comparison with verapamil. Assessment in placebo-controlled, multicenter trials. Ann Intern Med 1990;1113:104–110.
53. 2005 American Heart Association guidelines for cardiopulmonary resuscitation and emergency cardiovascular care. Circulation 2005;112(Suppl 1):IV-1–IV-211.
54. Rankin AC, McGovern BA. Adenosine or verapamil for the acute treatment of supraventricular tachycardia? Ann Intern Med 1991;114:513-515.
55. Alboni P, Tomasi C, Menozzi C, et al. Efficacy and safety of out-of-hospital self-administered single-dose oral drug treatment in the management of infrequent, well-tolerated paroxysmal supraventricular tachycardia. J Am Coll Cardiol 2001;37:548–553.
56. Jackman WM, Wang Z, Friday KJ, et al. Catheter ablation of accessory atrioventricular pathways (Wolff-Parkinson-White syndrome) by radiofrequency current. N Engl J Med 1991;324:1605–1611.
57. Jackman WM, Beckman KJ, McClelland JH, et al. Treatment of supraventricular tachycardia due to atrioventricular nodal reentry by radiofrequency catheter ablation of slow pathway conduction. N Engl J Med 1992;327:313–318.
58. Scheinman MM. Radiofrequency catheter ablation for patients with supraventricular tachycardia. Pacing Clin Electrophysiol 1993;16:671–679.
59. Cheng CH, Sanders GD, Hlatky MA, et al. Cost effectiveness of radiofrequency ablation for supraventricular tachycardia. Ann Intern Med 2000;133:864–876.
60. McCord J, Borzak S. Multifocal atrial tachycardia. Chest 1998;113:203–209.
61. Levine JH, Michael JR, Guarnier T. Treatment of multifocal atrial tachycardia with verapamil. N Engl J Med 1985;312:21–25.
62. Bayes deLuna A, Coumel P, LeClercq IF. Ambulatory sudden cardiac death: Mechanisms of production of fatal arrhythmia on the basis of data from 157 cases. Am Heart J 1989;117:151–159.
63. Ruberman W, Weinblatt E, Goldberg JD, et al. Ventricular premature beats and mortality after myocardial infarction. N Engl J Med 1977;297:750–757.
64. The Cardiac Arrhythmia Suppression Trial II Investigators. Effect of the antiarrhythmic agent moricizine on survival after myocardial infarction. N Engl J Med 1992;327:227–233.
65. Waldo AL, Camm AJ, deRuyter H, et al. Effect of *d*-sotalol on mortality in patients with left ventricular dysfunction and remote myocardial infarction. Lancet 1996;348:7–12.
66. Julian DG, Camm AJ, Frangin G, et al. Randomized trial of effect of amiodarone on mortality in patients with left ventricular dysfunction after recent myocardial infarction: EMIAT. Lancet 1997;349:667–674.
67. Cairns JA, Connolly SJ, Roberts R, et al. Randomized trial of outcome after myocardial infarction in patients with frequent or repetitive ventricular premature depolarizations: CAMIAT. Lancet 1997;349:675–682.
68. Amiodarone Trials Meta-Analysis Investigators. Effect of prophylactic amiodarone on mortality after acute myocardial infarction and in congestive heart failure: Meta-analysis of individual data from 6,500 patients in randomized trials. Lancet 1997;350:1417–1424.
69. Torp-Pederson C, Moller M, Bloch-Thomsen PE, et al. Dofetilide in patients with congestive heart failure and left ventricular dysfunction. N Engl J Med 1999;341:857–865.
70. Kober L, Block-Thomsen PE, Moller M, et al. Effect of dofetilide in patients with recent myocardial infarction and left ventricular dysfunction: A randomized trial. Lancet 2000;356:2052–2058.
71. Hilleman DE, Bauman JL. Role of antiarrhythmic therapy in patients at risk for sudden cardiac death: An evidence-based review. Pharmacotherapy 2001;21:556–575.
72. Edhouse J, Morris F. Broad Complex Tachycardia—Part 1. BMJ 2002;312:719–722.
73. Edhouse J, Morris F. Broad Complex Tachycardia—Part II. BMJ 2002;324:776–779.
74. Cole CR, Marrouche NF, Natale A. Evaluation and management of ventricular outflow tract tachycardias. Card Electrophysiol Rev 2002;6:442–447.
75. Modell SM, Lehmann MH. The long QT syndrome family of cardiac ion channelopathies: A HuGE review. Genet Med 2006;8:143–155.
76. Keating MT, Sanguinetti MC, Molecular and cellular mechanisms of cardiac arrhythmias. Cell 2001;104:569–580.
77. Antzelevitch C, Brugada P, Brugada J, et al. Brugada Syndrome: 1992–2002: A historical perspective. J Am Coll Cardiol 2003;41:1665–1671.
78. Gorgels A, van den Dool A, Hofs A, et al. Comparison of procainamide and lidocaine in terminating sustained monomorphic ventricular tachycardia. Am J Cardiol 1996;78:43–46.
79. Mason JW and the Electrophysiologic Study versus Electrocardiographic Monitoring Investigators. A comparison of electrophysiologic testing with Holter monitoring to predict antiarrhythmic drug efficacy for ventricular tachyarrhythmias. N Engl J Med 1993;329:445–451.
80. Mason JW and the Electrophysiologic Study versus Electrocardiographic Monitoring Investigators. A comparison of seven antiarrhythmic drugs in patients with ventricular tachyarrhythmias. N Engl J Med 1993;329:452–458.
81. The Cascade Investigators. Randomized antiarrhythmic drug therapy in survivors of cardiac arrest (the CASCADE Study). Am J Cardiol 1993;72:280–287.
82. Zipes DP. Cardiac electrophysiology: Promises and contributions. J Am Coll Cardiol 1989;13:1329–1352.
83. DiMarco JP. Implantable Cardioverter-defibrillators. N Engl J Med 2003;349:1836–1847.
84. Powell AC, Fuchs T, Finklestein DM, et al. Influence of implantable cardioverter-defibrillators on long-term prognosis of survivors of out-of-hospital cardiac arrest. Circulation 1993;88:1083–1092.
85. Pacifico A, Hohnloser SH, Williams JH, et al. Prevention of implantable-defibrillator shocks by treatment with sotalol. N Engl J Med 1999;340:1855–1862.
86. Connolly SJ, Dorian P, Roberts RS, et al. Comparison of beta-blockers, amiodarone plus beta-blockers, or sotalol for prevention of shocks from implantable cardioverter defibrillators: The OPTIC Study: A randomized trial. JAMA 2006;295:165–171.
87. Tworek DA, Nazari J, Ezri M, Bauman JL. Interference by antiarrhythmic agents with the function of electrical cardiac devices. Clin Pharm 1992;11:48–56.
88. Moss AJ, Hall WJ, Cannom DS, et al. Improved survival with an implanted defibrillator in patients with coronary disease at high risk for ventricular arrhythmia. N Engl J Med 1996;335:1933–1940.
89. Connolly SJ, Gene M, Roberts TS, et al. Cardiac Implantable Defibrillator Study (CIDS): A randomized trial of the implantable cardioverter-defibrillator against amiodarone. Circulation 2000;101:1297–1302.
90. Kuck KH, Cappato R, Siebels J, et al. Randomized comparison of antiarrhythmic drug therapy with implantable defibrillators in patients resuscitated from cardiac arrest: The Cardiac Arrest Study Hamburg (CASH). Circulation 2000;102:748–754.
91. Moss AJ, Hall WJ, Cannom DS, et al. Improved survival with an implanted defibrillator in patients with coronary disease at high risk for ventricular arrhythmia. N Engl J Med 1996;335:1933–1940.
92. Buxton AE, Lee KL, Fisher JD, et al. . A randomized study of the prevention of sudden death in patients with coronary artery disease. N Engl J Med 1999;341:1882–1890.
93. Moss AJ, Zareba W, Hall WJ, et al. Prophylactic implantation of a defibrillator in patients with myocardial infarction and reduced ejection fraction. N Engl J Med 2002;346:877–883.
94. Bardy GH, Lee KL, Mark DB, et al. Amiodarone or an implantable cardioverter-defibrillator for congestive heart failure. N Engl J Med 2005;352:225–237.

95. Wilber DJ, Olshansky B, Moran JF, et al. Electrophysiological testing and nonsustained VT. Use and limitations in patients with coronary artery disease and impaired ventricular function. Circulation 1990;82:350–358.
96. Buxton AE, Leek KL, DiCarlo L, et al. Electrophysiologic testing to identify patients with coronary artery disease who are at risk for sudden death. Multicenter Unsustained Tachycardia trial. N Engl J Med 2000;342:1937–1945.
97. Zipes DP, Camm AJ, Borggrefe M, et al. ACC/AHA/ESC 2006 guidelines for management of patients with ventricular arrhythmias and the prevention of sudden cardiac death—Executive summary: A report of the American College of Cardiology/American Heart Association Task Force and the European Society of Cardiology Committee for Practice Guidelines (Writing Committee to Develop Guidelines for Management of Patients with Ventricular Arrhythmias and the Prevention of Sudden Cardiac Death). Circulation 2006;114:1–45.
98. Herre JM, Titus C, Oeff M, et al. Inefficacy and proarrhythmic effects of flecainide and encainide for sustained ventricular tachycardia and ventricular fibrillation. Ann Intern Med 1990;113:671–676.
99. Antzelevitch C. Heterogeneity of cellular repolarization in LQTS. The role of M cells. Eur Heart J 2001;3:K2–K16.
100. Roden DM. Long Qt syndrome: Reduced repolarization reserve and the genetic link. J Intern Med 2006;259:59–69.
101. Oberg KC, O'Toole MF, Gallastegui JL, Bauman JL. "Late" proarrhythmia due to quinidine. Am J Cardiol 1994;74:192–194.
102. Bauman JL. The role of pharmacokinetics, drug interactions and pharmacogenetics in the acquired long QT syndrome. Eur Heart J 2001;3:K93-K100.
103. Tzivoni D, Banai S, Schuger C, et al. Treatment of torsade de pointes with magnesium sulfate. Circulation 1987;77:392–397.
104. Lie KI, Wellens HJJ, Van Capelle FJ. Lidocaine in the prevention of primary ventricular fibrillation. N Engl J Med 1974;291:1324–1326.
105. MacMahon S, Collin R, Peto R, et al. Effects of prophylactic lidocaine in suspected acute myocardial infarction. An overview of results from the randomized controlled trials. JAMA 1988;260:1910–1916.
106. Antman EM, Berlin JA. Declining incidence of ventricular fibrillation in myocardial infarction. Implications for the prophylactic use of lidocaine. Circulation 1992;86:764–773.
107. Horner SM. Efficacy of intravenous magnesium in acute myocardial infarction in reducing arrhythmias and mortality. Meta-analysis of magnesium in acute myocardial infarction. Circulation 1992;86:774–779.
108. Woods KL, Fletcher S, Roffe C, Haider Y. A randomized trial of intravenous magnesium sulfate in suspected acute myocardial infarction: Results of the second Leicester Intravenous Magnesium Intervention Trial (LIMIT-2). Lancet 1992;339:1553–1558.
109. Sleight P. Vasodilators after myocardial infarction—ISIS IV. Am J Hypertens 1994;7:1025–1055.
110. Wenzel V, Krismer AC, Arnz R, et al. A comparison of vasopressin and epinephrine for out-of-hospital cardiopulmonary resuscitation. N Engl J Med 2004;350:105–113.
111. Kudenchuk PJ, Cobb LA, Copass MK, et al. Amiodarone for resuscitation after out-of-hospital cardiac arrest due to ventricular fibrillation. N Engl J Med 1999;341:871–878.
112. Dorian P, Schwartz B, Cooper R, et al. Amiodarone as compared with lidocaine for shock-resistant ventricular fibrillation. N Engl J Med 2002;346:884–890.
113. Task Force on Syncope, European Society of Cardiology. Guidelines on the management (diagnosis and treatment) of syncope—Update 2004. Europace 2004;6:467–537.
114. Sneddon JF, Camm AJ. Sinus node disease. Current concepts in diagnosis and therapy. Drugs 1992;44:728–737.
115. Sugrue DD, Gersh BJ, Holmes DR, et al. Symptomatic "isolated" carotid sinus hypersensitivity: Natural history and results of treatment with anticholinergic drugs or pacemaker. J Am Coll Cardiol 1986;7:158–162.
116. Strasberg B, Sagie A, Erdman S, et al. Carotid sinus hypersensitivity and the carotid sinus syndrome. Prog Cardiovasc Dis 1989;31:379–391.
117. Zagga M, Massumi A. Neurally mediated syncope. Tex Heart Inst J 2000;27:268–272.
118. Grubb BP. Neurocardiogenic syncope and related disorders of orthostatic intolerance. Circulation 2005;111:2997–3006.
119. Grubb BP. Neurocardiogenic syncope. N Engl J Med 2005;352:1004–1010.
120. Milstein S, Reyes WJ, Benditt DG. Upright body tilt for evaluation of patients with recurrent, unexplained syncope. Pacing Clin Electrophysiol 1989;12:117–124.
121. Almquist A, Goldenberg I, Milstein S. Provocation of bradycardia and hypotension by isoproterenol and upright posture in patients with unexplained syncope. N Engl J Med 1990;320:346-351.
122. Brignole M. Randomized clinical trials of neurally mediated syncope. J Cardiovasc Electrophysiol 2003;14(Suppl):S64–S69.
123. Sheldon R, Connolly S, Rose S, for the POST Investigators. Prevention of Syncope Trial (POST). A randomized, placebo-controlled study of metoprolol in the prevention of vasovagal syncope. Circulation 2006;113:1164–1170.
124. Bloomfield DM. Strategy for the management of vasovagal syncope. Drugs Aging 2002;19:179–202.
125. Gregoratos G, Abrams J, Epstein AE. ACC/AHA/NASPE 2002 guideline update for implantation of cardiac pacemakers and antiarrhythmic devices: Summary article. A report of the American College of Cardiology/American Heart Association Task Force on Practice Guidelines (ACC/AHA/NASPE Committee to Update the 1998 Pacemaker Guidelines). Circulation 2002;106:2145–2161.
126. Kupersmith J, Holmes-Novner M, Hogan A, et al. Cost-effectiveness analysis in heart disease, Part I. General principles. Prog Cardiovasc Dis 1994;37:161–184.
127. Kupersmith J, Holmes-Novner M, Hogan A, et al. Cost-effectiveness analysis in heart disease, Part III. Ischemia, congestive heart failure, and arrhythmias. Prog Cardiovasc Dis 1995;37:307–346.

CHAPTER 20 Diastolic Heart Failure and the Cardiomyopathies

JEAN M. NAPPI AND ROBERT L. PAGE, II

KEY CONCEPTS

1. Diastolic heart failure is a frequent cause of heart failure (prevalence 35% to 50%) and has a significant effect on mortality (25% to 35% 5-year mortality rate) and morbidity (50% 1-year readmission rate).
2. Hypertension is a common cause of diastolic heart failure.
3. The diagnosis of diastolic heart failure can be made when a patient has both (a) symptoms and signs of congestive heart failure on physical examination and (b) preserved left ventricular (LV) function.
4. Treatment should be targeted at symptom reduction, causal clinical disease, and underlying basic mechanisms. Patients with diastolic heart failure may be treated differently than those with systolic dysfunction.
5. Symptom-targeted therapy includes decreasing pulmonary venous pressure, maintaining atrial contraction and atrioventricular synchrony, and reducing heart rate. Exercise tolerance is increased by reducing exercise-induced increases in blood pressure and heart rate.
6. Disease-targeted therapy includes preventing or treating myocardial ischemia and preventing or regressing LV hypertrophy.
7. Future directions may include modifying neurohormonal activation, inhibiting endothelin, and altering intracellular mechanisms and extracellular matrix structures.
8. Treatment strategies for patients with hypertrophic cardiomyopathy (HCM) are aimed at improving symptoms and preventing sudden cardiac death.
9. Patients with HCM who are at high risk for sudden cardiac death should receive an implantable cardioverter-defibrillator.
10. Patients with HCM who are symptomatic may benefit from β-blockade or verapamil.
11. Antibiotic prophylaxis for endocarditis is appropriate for HCM patients with evidence of outflow obstruction.

Learning objectives, review questions, and other resources can be found at **www.pharmacotherapyonline.com.**

DIASTOLIC HEART FAILURE

Heart failure (HF) may be caused by a primary abnormality in systolic function, diastolic function, or both. Making the distinction is important because the prevalence, prognosis, and treatment of HF may be quite different depending on whether the predominant mechanism causing the symptoms is systolic or diastolic dysfunction. Clinical studies have reported that up to 74% of patients with HF have preserved left ventricular (LV) ejection fraction (EF), variably defined as exceeding 40%, 45%, or 50%.[1–3] When patients with preserved EF exhibit symptoms consistent with effort intolerance and dyspnea, especially in the presence of venous congestion and edema, the term *diastolic heart failure* (DHF) is used.[4] Despite recognition of its importance, no strong consensus exists regarding appropriate terminology for this syndrome; therefore, the terms DHF and HF with preserved EF may be used synonymously.

DHF can be defined as a condition in which myocardial relaxation and filling are impaired and incomplete. The ventricle is unable to accept an adequate volume of blood from the venous system, does not fill at low pressure, and/or is unable to maintain normal stroke volume. In its most severe form, DHF results in overt symptoms of HF. In modest DHF, symptoms of dyspnea and fatigue occur only during stress or activity, when heart rate and/or end-diastolic volume increase. In its mildest form, DHF can be manifested as a slow or delayed pattern of relaxation and filling with little or no elevation in diastolic pressure and few or no cardiac symptoms. The congestive symptoms that occur with DHF are a manifestation of increased pulmonary venous pressures. DHF is caused by impaired myocardial relaxation and/or increased diastolic stiffness. When HF is caused by a predominant abnormality in diastolic function, the ventricular chamber is not enlarged, and EF may normal or even elevated.[5] Figure 20–1 shows the pressure–volume relationship in a patient with normal versus abnormal diastolic function. Changes in the myocardium are associated with a shift upward and to the left of the

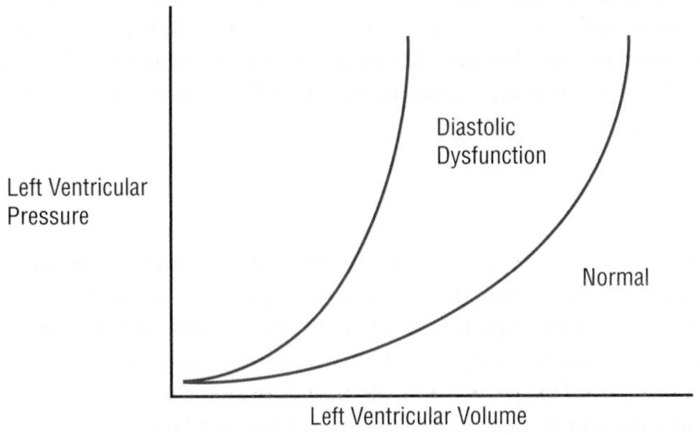

FIGURE 20-1. Diastolic pressure–volume relationship in a normal patient *(right trace)* and a patient with diastolic dysfunction *(left trace)*.

pressure–volume curve so that for any increase in LV volume, diastolic pressure rises to a much greater level than normally would occur. Clinically, patients present with reduced exercise tolerance and dyspnea when they have elevated LV diastolic pressures. Patients with DHF have a predominant abnormality in diastolic function, whereas patients with systolic heart failure (SHF) have a predominant abnormality in systolic function of the LV.[6]

EPIDEMIOLOGY

❶ Recent studies suggest that as many as half of patients presenting with overt HF have preserved EF.[7,8] The prevalence of DHF depends on a number of determinants: patient age, patient gender, study design, particular population under consideration, and EF. It is important to recognize that these determinants are not independent but interdependent. The most important determinant appears to be patient age. DHF is relatively uncommon in young and middle-aged patients. The prevalence of DHF increases with age, approximating 15% in patients younger than 60 years, 35% in patients between 60 and 70 years, and 50% in patients older than 70 years. Prospective community-based studies showed that in patients older than 70 years, the prevalence of DHF approaches 50%.[9,10] As the proportion of the population older than 65 years continues to grow, it has been estimated that DHF may eventually become the most common form of HF.[11]

ETIOLOGY

❷ Several disorders can impair ventricular function and play a role in the development of DHF. DHF is seen often in patients with hypertension, coronary artery disease (CAD), valvular heart disease, atrial fibrillation, diabetes, and hypertrophic cardiomyopathies.[11–13] Hypertension is the most common underlying cardiovascular disorder in patients with DHF.[14] There are several proposed mechanisms by which hypertension may impair diastolic function. Hypertension can alter diastolic function through its effects on (a) wall tension, (b) myocardial hypertrophy and fibrosis, (c) small-vessel structure and function, and (d) by predisposing to epicardial CAD. An association between impaired LV filling and subnormal high-energy phosphate metabolism has been shown in hypertensive patients, even in the absence of left ventricular hypertrophy (LVH).[15]

LVH plays a central role in the adaptation of the myocardium to pressure overload. Severe and long-standing pressure overload has been associated with phenotypic alterations at the myocyte level, which differs from the physiologic hypertrophy seen in athletes.[16] Long-term chronic pressure overload stimulates cardiac growth and collagen production, which lead to an increase in myocardial mass and structural remodeling. The results of these changes are an increase in myocardial stiffness and a decrease in diastolic filling.

Diastolic dysfunction has been reported to be present in 90% of patients with CAD.[17] Patients with CAD, such as those with (a) exercise-induced ischemia but normal function at rest, (b) myocardial stunning, and (c) previous myocardial infarction (MI), all may exhibit signs of diastolic dysfunction.

PATHOPHYSIOLOGY

The pathologic disease processes that cause DHF include myocardial ischemia with or without epicardial CAD, pressure overload hypertrophy, and genetic hypertrophy. Hypertrophy consequent to the physiologic adaptation to pregnancy, hypertrophy that occurs in athletes, and volume-overload hypertrophy do not cause abnormalities in diastolic function and do not result in the development of DHF.

Hypertrophic cardiomyopathy (HCM) is a prototype for DHF. The grossly thickened myocardium, structural changes, and interstitial fibrosis severely alter the passive elastic properties of the myocardium. Patients with HCM and LV outflow obstruction are sensitive to small changes in volume such that a small decrease in filling pressure can lead to a decrease in LV end-diastolic volume and a dramatic fall in stroke volume and cardiac output.

TABLE 20-1 Potential Pathologic Mechanisms of Diastolic Heart Failure

Mechanisms directly affecting myocardial tissue	
Cardiomyocyte	Increased intracellular calcium, producing calcium overload
	Myofilaments
	Increased troponin C calcium binding and increased myofilament calcium sensitivity
	Cytoskeleton
	Changes in cytoskeletal proteins
	Energetics
	Decrease in ATP availability, leading to decreased rate or extent of actomyosin dissociation
Extracellular matrix	Increased content of fibrillar collagen
	Thickening of existing fibrillar collagen
	Decreased MMP and/or increased TIMP
Neurohormones	Increased renin–angiotensin–aldosterone
	Increased endothelin
Extramyocardial mechanisms	
Increased hemodynamic load: preload or afterload	
Increased heterogeneity	
Systemic neurohormones	Increased levels of angiotensin II
Pericardium	Pericardium may have a constraining effect as LV filling pressure and end-diastolic volume increase

ATP, adenosine triphosphate; LV, left ventricular; MMP, matrix metalloproteinase; TIMP, tissue inhibitor of MMP.

The basic mechanisms by which pressure-overload hypertrophy and genetic hypertrophy cause DHF include extramyocardial factors and factors intrinsic to the myocardium, which include changes in the cardiac muscle cell and in the extracellular matrix that surrounds the cardiomyocyte (Table 20–1).[18,19] Intracellular processes, such as changes in calcium homeostasis, contractile and noncontractile proteins, energetics, and the cytoskeleton, contribute to abnormalities in myocardial relaxation and stiffness. Changes in the extracellular matrix, particularly changes in fibrillar collagen, alter relaxation and stiffness. In addition to the cardiomyocyte and the extracellular matrix, local myocardial neuroendocrine activation can impair relaxation and increase stiffness. Activation of neurohormones such as the renin–angiotensin–aldosterone system may act directly to alter diastolic properties or act indirectly by altering calcium homeostasis. Finally, extramyocardial changes in loading conditions and changes in heterogeneity occur in hypertrophied ventricles and contribute to changes in relaxation and stiffness so that even when the myocardium itself is normal, changes in these extramyocardial factors can cause abnormalities in diastolic function.[19]

Myocardial ischemia, particularly in the subendocardial region, is common when ventricular hypertrophy is present. Slow or delayed myocardial relaxation and perivascular fibrosis can adversely affect coronary blood flow and coronary blood flow reserve. This may contribute to the development of myocardial ischemia and sudden death.[20,21] Therefore, myocardial ischemia may be part of the clinical syndrome of DHF even if no epicardial CAD is present.

Endothelial dysfunction is associated with the progression of myocardial diastolic dysfunction in patients with CAD.[22] Both in the acute manifestation of myocardial ischemia and within the chronic consequences of myocardial fibrosis, epicardial CAD is frequently the underlying pathologic cause of DHF.[23] Myocardial ischemia caused by either an acute decrease in supply or an increase in demand (exercise and tachycardia) results in impaired relaxation and an acute increase in myocardial stiffness.[5,15] Chronic coronary occlusions may result in myocardial fibrosis, remodeling, and DHF. It is clear that the same basic mechanisms causing diastolic dysfunction in the presence of pressure-overload hypertrophy also underlie changes produced by CAD.

DIAGNOSIS

❸ The criteria used to make the diagnosis of DHF remain controversial. However, making an accurate diagnosis is extremely important. Guidelines from the European Society of Cardiology (ESC) propose that three requirements must be present to make the diagnosis of DHF: (a) symptoms or signs of HF, (b) normal or only mildly abnormal systolic function (EF exceeding 45% to 50%), and (c) abnormal diastolic function (e.g., abnormal relaxation, filling, distensibility, or stiffness).[24] The first two requirements appear to be well justified; the third requirement may not be.[6]

CLINICAL PRESENTATION OF DIASTOLIC DYSFUNCTION

General

- The majority of patients do not show symptoms at rest but in response to stress conditions. Symptoms may be induced or worsened by physical exercise but also by events such as anemia, fever, tachycardia, and systemic pathologies.

Symptoms

- The patient may complain of exertional dyspnea, orthopnea, paroxysmal dyspnea, and exercise intolerance.

Signs

- Pulmonary congestion (rales)
- Exaggerated rise in blood pressure and heart rate in response to exercise
- Presence of an S4 gallop

Laboratory Tests

- B-type natriuretic peptide and N-terminal pro–B-type natriuretic peptide will be elevated.

Other Diagnostic Tests

- Two-dimensional echocardiography will show a normal or elevated ejection fraction, normal or decreased cardiac output, and LVH and/or concentric remodeling.
- Doppler echocardiography will show elevated pulmonary venous pressures.
- Chest radiography will show pulmonary congestion.
- Electrocardiography may reflect LVH.

Vasan and Levy proposed criteria for DHF according to the degree of diagnostic certainty.[25] Three conditions would be met for a definite diagnosis of DHF: (a) definitive evidence of HF, (b) objective evidence of normal LV systolic function within 72 hours of a HF event, and (c) objective evidence of LV diastolic dysfunction. If the third criterion is lacking, then the patient would have *probable* DHF. If the objective evidence for normal systolic function is not apparent at the time of the HF event and there is no conclusive information on LV dysfunction, then the patient would be classified as having *possible* DHF.

With few exceptions, DHF cannot be distinguished from SHF on the basis of the history, physical examination, chest x-ray, and electrocardiogram (ECG) alone. The frequency with which patients have symptoms of HF and signs of HF on physical examination or chest x-ray is not dependent on whether they have SHF or DHF.[21] Patients with DHF are often elderly, hypertensive females.[1] In one study, patients with DHF had a higher prevalence of hypertension with higher systolic, diastolic, and pulse pressures when compared with control patients and patients with SHF.[26]

The data from a number of studies demonstrate that signs and symptoms of HF do not predict EF. In contrast, they do predict the presence of increased LV diastolic pressure. The question then becomes whether the increase in LV diastolic pressure occurs in association with normal LV volume and EF, as would occur in DHF, or whether the increase in LV diastolic pressure occurs in association with an increased LV volume and decreased EF, as would occur with SHF. Therefore, determining whether HF is caused by systolic or diastolic dysfunction requires some estimate of LV size and EF. These measurements can be made using echocardiography, radionuclide ventriculography, or contrast ventriculography. When a patient presents with dyspnea, pulmonary rales, and radiographic evidence of pulmonary venous hypertension, the detection of normal LV end-diastolic volume and normal EF supports the diagnosis of DHF. Conditions such as mitral stenosis, pulmonary disease, sleep apnea, anemia, cirrhosis, hypothyroidism, and drug-induced fluid retention must be ruled out because they can cause similar symptoms.[27]

B-type natriuretic peptide (BNP) and its biologically inactive fragment N-terminal proBNP (NT-proBNP) are cardiac neurohormones secreted from the myocardium in response to increases in ventricular volume and pressure. Both are used as an aid in the differential diagnosis of dyspnea. The Breathing Not Properly study evaluated 452 patients with echocardiography within 30 days of an emergency department visit. Of the 452 patients, 165 (36.5%) had EF >45% (mean EF 59%).[28] In these patients with preserved EF who had been admitted to the hospital for dyspnea, BNP levels were significantly lower than those found in patients with SHF (413 versus 821 pg/mL). However, there was considerable overlap in the BNP levels in patients with DHF compared with those without HF, making BNP levels less useful. Furthermore, the sensitivity, specificity, and predictive accuracy of BNP levels in DHF are limited in part because BNP is altered by age, adiposity, gender, and other factors. Similar findings have been documented with NT-proBNP. In a study of 68 symptomatic patients with isolated DHF (EF >50%), NT-proBNP was significantly increased in patients with isolated DHF and correlated with disease severity. Compared to conventional echocardiography, Doppler imaging, and heart catheterization, NT-proBNP exhibited the best negative predictive value for detection of DFH.[29]

PROGNOSIS

The prognosis in patients with DHF, although less ominous than in patients with SHF, is worse than that of age-matched control patients. The 5-year mortality of these patients approximates 25%, although mortality rates as high as 13% over a 6-month period have been reported.[1,7] In comparison, the annual mortality of patients with SHF approximates 10% to 15%, whereas age-matched control mortality approaches 1%. However, in a population-based cohort study of 2,802 patients with HF, no significant difference was demonstrated in the adjusted 1-year mortality rate for patients with EF <40% compared to those with EF >50%.[30] Unfortunately, compared to SHF, little improvement in the survival rate among patients with DHF has been seen.[11]

In patients with DHF, the prognosis is also affected by the clinical pathologic etiology causing the disease. When patients with CAD are excluded, the annual mortality for DHF approximates 2% to 3%. In addition to the clinical pathologic etiology causing HF, other predictors of mortality include impaired renal function ≤60 mL/min/m^2, worse functional class (New York Heart Association [NYHA] class III–IV), male gender, and older age >74 years).[31,32]

The mode of death appears similar in patients with systolic versus diastolic HF. Sudden death and death from progressive pump failure occurred with equal frequency in patients with SHF versus those with DHF. Morbidity also is similar between patients with SHF and DHF. The 1-year hospital readmission rate can approach 50%, thereby placing significant expenditures on healthcare resources. However, compared to patients with SHF, those with DHF appear to have a higher risk of nonfatal MI and stroke.[12,30]

TREATMENT

Diastolic Heart Failure

The general principles used to guide the treatment of SHF are based on numerous large, randomized, double-blind, multicenter trials. Until recently, no such randomized trials had been performed in patients with DHF. Consequently, the guidelines for the management of DHF are based primarily on clinical investigations in relatively small groups of patients, clinical experience, and concepts based on the knowledge and understanding of the pathophysiology of the disease process. The treatment regimen outlined in Table 20–2 applies to patients with DHF who have clear manifestations of congestion either at rest or with exertion. Whether treatment of asymptomatic diastolic dysfunction confers any benefit has not been examined.

■ DESIRED OUTCOME

❹ Treatment should be targeted at reducing symptoms, principally those of increased pulmonary venous pressure. Treatment should include decreasing diastolic pressure by decreasing LV volume, maintaining atrial contraction, and reducing heart rate without reducing cardiac output. Second, treatment should be targeted at the pathologic diseases that cause DHF. For example, CAD, hypertensive heart disease, and aortic stenosis provide relatively specific therapeutic targets, such as lowering blood pressure, inducing LVH regression, performing aortic valve replacement, and treating ischemia by increasing myocardial blood flow and reducing myocardial oxygen demand. Third, treatment should be targeted at the underlying mechanisms that are altered by the disease processes just mentioned.[33]

■ NONPHARMACOLOGIC THERAPY

Diet and Lifestyle

The initial effort in the treatment of DHF is aimed at decreasing symptoms. The first step in this effort is to decrease pulmonary congestion by decreasing LV volume using sodium and fluid restriction. A low-sodium diet (≤2 g/day) and moderate fluid restriction will help to prevent volume overload. Both sodium and fluid restriction must be done with care. Excessive restriction can lead to hypotension, low-output state, and/or renal insufficiency. Daily weights may help to assess volume status. Dietary and lifestyle factors that decrease the risk of development of epicardial CAD and high blood pressure should be encouraged.[24]

Exercise

Moderate aerobic exercise to improve cardiovascular conditioning is beneficial to maintain a slower heart rate, improve cardiac reserve, and maintain skeletal muscle function. Isometric exercise should be avoided.[34]

Interventional/Surgical Procedures

An important step in symptom-targeted therapy that acts to decrease pulmonary venous pressures is to maintain atrial contraction and atrioventricular (AV) synchrony. Maintaining atrial contraction and AV synchrony is important both in preserving normal cardiac output and in keeping LV diastolic pressure low. Chemical or electrical cardioversion of persistent atrial tachyarrhythmias will decrease diastolic pressure, increase cardiac output, and resolve pulmonary edema. An AV sequential pacemaker should be used to treat bradyarrhythmias in patients requiring pacing.

Therapy also should be aimed at preventing or treating the underlying pathologic cause of DHF. Aortic valve replacement should be performed in symptomatic patients with pressure-overload hypertrophy caused by aortic stenosis. Revascularization should be performed in selected patients with DHF caused by CAD-induced myocardial ischemia. In addition, myocardial oxygen consumption and myocardial blood flow should be increased using medical treatment, including nitrates, β-blockers, and calcium channel blockers.[23]

Indications for Hospitalization

Patients with DHF may present with an acute onset of pulmonary edema. A number of potential causes for the acute decompensation of these patients include volume overload, uncontrolled hypertension, acute myocardial ischemia, progressive valvular disease (aortic stenosis), and new-onset or uncontrolled tachyarrhythmias. Treatment strategies for these patients eventually may include the need for surgery, as in the case of valvular disease.

The initial management focuses on relieving pulmonary congestion and maintaining oxygenation. Intravenous diuretic agents and nesiritide for patients are effective for volume overload. Caution

TABLE 20-2 Targeted Approach to Treatment of Diastolic Heart Failure

Symptom-targeted treatment		
Decrease pulmonary venous pressure	Reduce left ventricular volume	Diuretics, nitrates, salt restriction
	Maintain atrial contraction	Cardioversion of atrial fibrillation
	Reduce heart rate	β-Blockers, diltiazem, verapamil
Improve exercise tolerance	As above	
Use positive inotropic agents with caution		
Disease-targeted treatment		
Prevent/treat myocardial ischemia		β-Blockers, diltiazem, verapamil, nitrates
Prevent/regress ventricular hypertrophy		Antihypertensive therapy
Mechanism-targeted treatment		
Modify myocardial and extramyocardial mechanisms		Possibly ACE inhibitors or angiotensin receptor blockers, diuretics, spironolactone
Modify intracellular and extracellular mechanisms		Possibly ACE inhibitors or angiotensin receptor blockers, spironolactone

ACE, angiotensin-converting enzyme.

must be exercised to avoid overdiuresis or excessive lowering of LV end-diastolic volume, which can lead to a decrease in stroke volume. Morphine and nitroglycerin also are effective in reducing LV end-diastolic pressure.[35]

■ PHARMACOLOGIC TREATMENT

Drug Treatments of First Choice

With a few notable exceptions, many of the drugs used to treat SHF are the same as those used to treat DHF. However, the rationale for their use, the pathophysiologic process that is being altered by the drug, and the dosing regimen may be entirely different depending on whether the patient has SHF or DHF. For example, β-blockers are recommended for the treatment of both SHF and DHF. In DHF, however, β-blockers are used to decrease heart rate, increase diastolic duration, and modify the hemodynamic response to exercise. In SHF, β-blockers are used in the long run to increase inotropic state and modify LV remodeling. Diuretics also are used in the treatment of both SHF and DHF. However, the doses of diuretics used to treat DHF are in general much smaller than the doses used to treat SHF. Antagonists of the renin–angiotensin–aldosterone system are useful in lowering blood pressure and reducing LVH. Some drugs, however, are used only to treat either SHF or DHF but not both. Calcium channel blockers such as diltiazem, nifedipine, and verapamil have little utility in the treatment of SHF. In contrast, each of these drugs has been proposed as being useful in the treatment of DHF.

Published Guidelines

Much less objective information on the treatment of DHF is available. This relative paucity of objective information is reflected in guidelines for the diagnosis and management of HF published from the American College of Cardiology (ACC)/American Heart Association (AHA), the ESC, and the Heart Failure Society of America (HFSA).[24,36,37] In general, all three guidelines recommend treating comorbid conditions by controlling heart rate and blood pressure, alleviating causes of myocardial ischemia, reducing volume, and restoring and maintaining sinus rhythm. Table 20–3 summarizes the therapeutic recommendations from the HFSA.

General Information

Although dozens of trials evaluating pharmacologic therapy have been conducted in patients with SHF, few trials have focused on patients with isolated DHF. In fact, most published HF trials have specifically excluded patients with preserved EF. A few published large clinical studies and several trials examining various agents in the treatment of DHF are underway (Table 20–4). With these studies and others that currently are under development, an effective treatment for DHF will be defined more completely.

Alternative Drug Treatment

As a result of the controversy regarding the diagnosis of DHF, the development and design of large clinical trials have been hindered. At this time, most antihypertensive agents would be acceptable forms of therapy for hypertensive heart disease, with the exception of α-blockers (e.g., doxazosin). In the Antihypertensive and Lipid-Lowering Treatment to Prevent Heart Attack Trial (ALLHAT), the doxazosin treatment arm was dropped because patients randomized to doxazosin had an increased risk for developing HF and stroke compared with the chlorthalidone arm.[38]

Special Populations

DHF is associated with hypertension and aging, making it a common diagnosis in elderly white women. Because these women often are frail and have low muscle mass, their creatinine clearance and renal function may be compromised. Special care must be taken when selecting and titrating doses of drugs, monitoring levels of serum creatinine and electrolytes, and using diuretics, angiotensin-converting enzyme (ACE) inhibitors, and angiotensin receptor blockers.[39]

Diabetes is often a comorbid condition in patients with HF. Because the thiazolidinediones (pioglitazone and rosiglitazone) are associated with fluid retention, caution is warranted when initiating these drugs in

TABLE 20-3 Evidence-Based Pharmacotherapy for Diastolic Heart Failure

Recommendations	Recommendation Grade[a]
Diuretics	
• A loop and a thiazide diuretic should be considered for patients with volume overload. However, with more severe volume overload or inadequate response to a thiazide, a loop diuretic should be implemented. Caution is warranted not to lower preload excessively, which may reduce stroke volume and cardiac output.	C
ACE inhibitors	
• ACE inhibitors should be considered in all patients.	C
• ACE inhibitors should be considered in all patients who have symptomatic atherosclerotic cardiovascular disease or diabetes and one additional risk factor.	C
Angiotensin receptor blockers	
• Angiotensin receptor blockers should be considered in all patients.	B
• In patients who are intolerant of ACE inhibitors, an angiotensin receptor blocker can be considered an alternative.	C
β-Blockers	
• β-Blockers should be considered in patients with one or more of the following conditions:	
Myocardial infarction	A
Hypertension	B
Atrial fibrillation requiring ventricular rate control.	B
Calcium channel blockers	
• In patients with atrial fibrillation warranting ventricular rate control who either are intolerant to or have not responded to a β-blocker, diltiazem or verapamil should be considered.	C
• A nondihydropyridine or dihydropyridine calcium channel blocker can be considered for symptom-limiting angina.	A
• A nondihydropyridine or dihydropyridine calcium channel blocker can be considered for hypertension; however, amlodipine is recommended.	C

[a]Strength of recommendations: A, randomized controlled clinical trials; B, cohort and case control studies based upon observations from observational studies or registries, post hoc, subgroup, and meta-analysis; C, expert opinion, epidemiologic findings from observational studies, and safety findings from large-scale use.
ACE, angiotensin-converting enzyme.
Data from Heart Failure Society of America.[36]

TABLE 20-4 Completed and Ongoing Large Clinical Trials for Diastolic Heart Failure

Trial (No. of Patients)	Treatment	Inclusion Criteria	Primary End Point	Results
DIG Ancillary Study[30] (n = 988)	Digoxin vs placebo for a mean of 37 months. Patients received ACE inhibitor (86%) and diuretics (85%).	EF >45%, NYHA II–IV, normal sinus rhythm	Composite of HF hospitalization or HF mortality	No significant difference was found in the primary end point between treatment groups (HR = 0.82, P = 0.136). Digoxin had no effect on all-cause mortality or cause-specific mortality or on all-cause or CV hospitalization. Compared to placebo, digoxin use was associated with a trend toward a reduction in HF hospitalizations (HR = 0.79, P = 0.094) and an increase in unstable angina admissions (HR = 1.37, P = 0.061).
CHARM-Preserved[13] (n = 3,023)	Candesartan vs placebo for a mean of 36.6 months. Patients continued their background HF medications: ACE inhibitor (19%), β-blocker (55%), diuretics (75%), spironolactone (11%).	EF >40%, NYHA II–IV, ≥1 hospitalization for CV reason	Composite of CV mortality or HF hospitalization	No significant difference was found in the primary end point between treatment groups (adjusted HR = 0.86, P = 0.051) or in CV deaths (adjusted HR = 0.95, P = 0.635). Compared to placebo, candesartan use was associated with fewer HF admissions (P = 0.017), lower incidence of new diabetes (HR = 0.60, P = 0.005), and a reduction in the composite of CV death, HF hospitalization, nonfatal MI, and nonfatal stroke (adjusted HR = 0.91, P = 0.037).
PEP-CHF[46] (n = 850)	Perindopril vs placebo for a mean of 2.1 years.	Clinical criteria for HF, EF ≥40%, age ≥70 years	Composite of total mortality and HF hospitalization	At 1 year and at study completion, no significant difference was found in the primary end point between treatment groups (HR = 0.69, P = 0.055; HR = 0.70, P = 0.545). In a subgroup analysis, patients ≤75 years of age (HR = 0.29, P = 0.035) and with a history of MI (HR = 0.38, P = 0.004) showed a reduction in the primary end point. Compared to placebo, perindopril use at 1 year was associated with fewer unplanned hospital admissions (HR = 0.63, P = 0.033), greater improvements in exercise tolerance (P = 0.011), and improvement in NYHA class (P = 0.030).
I-Preserve[65] (n = 4,100)	Irbesartan vs placebo for 2 years. ACE inhibitor can be used for any indication other than HTN.	Clinical criteria for HF or hospitalized within 6 months for HF, age ≥60 years, NYHA II–IV, EF ≥45%	Composite of all-cause mortality or CV hospitalization	Expected to be completed in 2007
TOPCAT[65] (n = 4,500)	Spironolactone vs placebo for 2 years.	Clinical criteria for HF, age ≥50 years, EF ≥45%, ≥1 hospitalization for HF, controlled SBP	CV mortality, aborted cardiac arrest, HF hospitalization	Expected to be completed in 2011

Trials: CHARM, Candesartan in Heart Failure: Assessment of Reduction in Mortality and Morbidity; DIG, Digitalis Investigational Group; I-Preserve, Irbesartan in Heart Failure with Preserved EF; PEP-CHF, Perindopril for Elderly Persons with Chronic Heart Failure; TOPCAT, Trial of Aldosterone Antagonist Therapy in Adults with Preserved Ejection Fraction Congestive Heart Failure.
ACE, angiotensin-converting enzyme; CV, cardiovascular; EF, ejection fraction; HF, heart failure; HR, hazard ratio; HTN, hypertension; MI, myocardial infarction; NYHA, New York Heart Association; SBP, systolic blood pressure.

patients with a history of DHF. Thiazolidinediones should be discontinued in patients with symptoms related to volume overload.[3,37]

■ DRUG CLASS INFORMATION

Diuretics

❺ Diuretics can provide symptom-targeted therapy by decreasing systemic and LV volume. By decreasing LV diastolic volumes, LV pressures slide down the curvilinear diastolic pressure–volume relationship toward a lower, less steep portion of the curve. As pressure throughout diastole falls, mean diastolic pressure, pulmonary capillary wedge pressure, and pulmonary venous pressure fall. These agents effectively reduce the central blood volume and lower diastolic pressures, thus alleviating the symptoms of the congestive state. Diuretics can provide disease-targeted therapy by decreasing blood pressure and favorably affecting the myocardial oxygen supply-versus-demand ratio. Lower LV diastolic pressures may increase subendocardial blood flow, preventing or alleviating the imbalance between myocardial oxygen supply and demand (see Fig. 20–1). Diuretics alone and especially in combination with other antihypertensive drugs are an effective approach to therapy.

Treatment with diuretics should be initiated at low doses in order to avoid hypotension and fatigue. Hypotension can be a significant problem in the treatment of DHF because these patients have a very steep LV diastolic pressure–volume curve such that a small change in volume causes a large change in filling pressure and cardiac output. After the acute treatment of DHF has been completed, long-term treatment should include small-to-moderate doses of diuretics (furosemide 20 to 40 mg/day orally or hydrochlorothiazide 12.5 to 25 mg/day orally). If prompt and sustained diuresis is not achieved, the dosage of a single diuretic should be increased, or a loop and thiazide or thiazide-like diuretic should be used in combination. Aldosterone antagonists such as spironolactone and eplerenone may be especially effective for long-term use because of their potassium-sparing effects and because their antagonism of renin–angiotensin–aldosterone system activation may alter intramyocardial and extramyocardial mechanisms causing abnormalities in diastolic function.[40] Thiazide diuretics generally are ineffective as diuretics in patients with a creatinine clearance <30 mL/min.

Excessive diuresis may result in hypotension, low-output syndrome, and worsening renal insufficiency. In some cases, loop diuretics may be withdrawn safely from elderly patients without any worsening of HF symptoms and with improvement in symptoms of orthostatic hypotension.[41] Electrolyte imbalances, including hypokalemia and hypomagnesemia, are common with diuretics. Carbohydrate intolerance and hyperuricemia are dose-related adverse drug reactions seen with thiazide diuretics. Spironolactone can cause hyperkalemia and gynecomastia. Eplerenone may be used as an alternative to spironolactone in patients who complain of gynecomastia. In general, diuretic agents are very cost-effective agents in the management of DHF.

Nitrates

❻ Similar to diuretics, nitrates can provide symptom-targeted therapy by acting to decrease LV volume by increasing venous capacitance. In addition, nitrates can provide disease-targeted therapy by providing antiischemic effects in patients with DHF due to CAD.

Like diuretics, therapy should be initiated at low doses in order to avoid hypotension. Isosorbide dinitrate 10 mg three or four times daily, isosorbide mononitrate (Imdur) 30 mg/day, nitroglycerin paste 0.5 to 1 inch every 4 to 6 hours, and nitroglycerin patch 0.1 to 0.2 mg/h applied each day are common initial doses. Doses can be increased during long-term therapy and titrated against symptoms. Nitrate tolerance has not been studied in this patient population but probably occurs (for more detail regarding nitrate tolerance, see Chap. 17). Similar to diuretics, nitrates can cause hypotension and a low-output syndrome. Headaches are common but may be less frequent with continued use.

Sublingual nitroglycerin tablets or nitroglycerin spray may be used for patients who develop shortness of breath with mild exercise, and they can be used much in the same way as in patients with ischemic symptoms. Nitroglycerin will decrease LV end-diastolic volume, resulting in relief of breathlessness.

β-Adrenergic Blockers

β-Blockers can provide symptom-targeted therapy by decreasing heart rate and can provide disease-targeted therapy by treating high blood pressure and CAD. By decreasing heart rate and increasing the duration of diastole, β-blockers can help to lower and maintain low pulmonary venous pressures. Tachycardia is poorly tolerated in patients with DHF for several reasons. First, rapid heart rates cause an increase in myocardial oxygen demand and a decrease in coronary perfusion time. This rapid rate can promote ischemic diastolic dysfunction even in the absence of epicardial CAD, especially in patients with LVH. Second, incomplete relaxation between cardiac cycles may result in an increase in diastolic pressure relative to volume. Thus, LV distensibility is reduced. Third, a rapid rate reduces diastolic filling time and ventricular filling. Fourth, hearts with diastolic dysfunction exhibit a flat or even negative relaxation rate versus frequency relationship. Thus, as heart rate increases in these hearts, relaxation does not become augmented and may become slower and incomplete, causing diastolic pressures, especially early in diastole, to increase.[9] For these and other reasons, most clinicians use β-blockers (and calcium channel blockers) to prevent excessive tachycardia and produce a relative bradycardia in patients with diastolic dysfunction. However, excessive bradycardia can result in a fall of cardiac output despite an increase in LV filling. Such considerations underscore the need for individualizing therapeutic interventions that affect heart rate. Although the optimal heart rate must be individualized, an initial goal might be a resting heart rate of approximately 60 beats/min with a blunted exercise-induced increase in heart rate not to exceed 110 beats/min.[9]

No evidence suggests a specific therapeutic advantage of one β-blocker over another. Selective and nonselective β-blockers appear equally effective in DHF. In general, it is not necessary to start the drug at an extremely low dose and titrate the β-blocker in a slow, progressive fashion in DHF, as it is in SHF. Because the population is older, it is prudent to start with a moderate dose of β-blockers, such as metoprolol tartrate 25 mg twice daily, metoprolol succinate 25 mg daily, atenolol 25 mg daily, or carvedilol 3.125 mg twice daily and titrate to a higher dose with a treatment target of a heart rate of approximately 60 beats/min.

Prinzmetal vasospastic angina, occlusive peripheral vascular disease, type 1 diabetes mellitus that is prone to hypoglycemia, severe heart block, and excessive bradycardia are contraindications to β-blockers. β-Blockers may be considered in patients with reactive airway disease or asymptomatic bradycardia but should be used with extreme caution. The main side effects of β-blockers are depression, fatigue, bradycardia, bronchospasm, and impotence. Many of the β-blockers are eliminated via hepatic metabolism and may be affected by other drugs that either inhibit (e.g., cimetidine and verapamil) or enhance (e.g., barbiturates) hepatic enzymes. Because the doses are titrated to patient response, these interactions are managed easily.

Calcium Channel Blockers

Calcium channel blockers can provide symptom-targeted treatment by decreasing heart rate and increasing exercise tolerance. They can provide disease-targeted treatment by treating high blood pressure and CAD. However, the beneficial effect of these agents on exercise tolerance is not always paralleled by improved LV diastolic function or increased relaxation rate. Nonetheless, a number of small clinical trials have shown that the use of these agents results in both short-term and long-term improvement in exercise capacity in patients with DHF.[33,36]

Of the calcium channel blockers, the nondihydropyridines (verapamil and diltiazem) are the most effective because they lower heart rate in addition to lowering blood pressure.[42] Sustained-release nifedipine, because of its strong vasodilator properties, tends to cause hypotension and reflex tachycardia. In addition, nifedipine causes peripheral edema. These characteristics make it less useful in DHF. Amlodipine may be effective because it reduces blood pressure. Initial doses are verapamil 120 to 240 mg/day, diltiazem 90 to 120 mg/day, and amlodipine 2.5 mg/day.

Heart block is a contraindication for the nondihydropyridines. The most common side effects are bradycardia and heart block (for the nondihydropyridines). Peripheral edema and headache also are common. Nondihydropyridines exacerbate the bradycardic effects of β-blockers, and verapamil raises digoxin serum concentrations by 70%. Diltiazem raises cyclosporine, tacrolimus, and sirolimus serum concentrations. Intravenous calcium salts inhibit the pharmacologic effect of calcium channel blockers. Generic formulations or similar products, but not necessarily generic equivalents to the original brand names, are available for some of the calcium channel blockers.

Neurohormonal Antagonists

❼ Both basic and clinical studies suggest that DHF is associated with activation of systemic and local cardiac neuroendocrine systems such as the renin–angiotensin–aldosterone system. One mechanism causing fluid retention and the increases in central and systemic volume in patients with DHF is activation of these neuroendocrine systems. Therefore, treatment of DHF should include agents such as ACE inhibitors, angiotensin receptor blockers, and aldosterone antagonists that attenuate the fluid retention caused by neuroendocrine activation. In addition to promoting fluid retention, neuroendocrine activation can have direct effects on cellular and extracellular mechanisms that contribute to the development of DHF. Modulation of neuroendocrine activation may provide mechanism-targeted treatment by decreasing fibroblast activity and interstitial fibrosis, improving intracellular calcium handling, and decreasing myocardial stiffness. Finally, renin–angiotensin–aldosterone system antagonists provide disease-targeted treatment by treating hypertension.[43]

The mechanisms that evoke activation of the neuroendocrine system remain incompletely understood in patients with DHF. A number of factors have been suggested. Myocardial ischemia, uncontrolled hypertension, and excessive dietary sodium or sodium-retaining medications may contribute to neuroendocrine activation. Limited distensibility of the atria may attenuate the secretion of atrial natriuretic factor and thereby reduce its diuretic effect. In others, low systemic vascular resistance and/or low arterial pressure may contribute to an increase in renin–angiotensin–aldosterone system activation and salt and water retention. Elevated venous pressure may cause renal sodium retention directly. The reduction in blood volume that follows the use of diuretics triggers an increase in sympathetic tone and further activation of the renin–angiotensin–aldosterone system. Such neurohormonal activation can lead to vasoconstriction and a worsening of the congestive state. Some vasodilators, particularly nitrates and pure arteriolar vasodilators, evoke a similar response. By contrast, ACE inhibitors, aldosterone antagonists, and β-blockers blunt neurohormonal activation and decrease the salt and water retention that complicates the treatment of HF.

Angiotensin-Converting Enzyme Inhibitors

ACE inhibitors can provide symptom-targeted treatment by decreasing LV volume and directly improving relaxation. They can provide disease-targeted treatment by treating high blood pressure, preventing LVH, promoting regression, and preventing fibrosis. Treatment of high blood pressure with ACE inhibitors has been shown to normalize load, prevent and/or regress LVH, correct the abnormality in intracellular processes, and modify the extracellular matrix response.[43] ACE inhibitors may reduce the incidence of HF by 23% among patients with CAD and preserved EF.[44]

A small, prospective, double-blind, randomized trial compared lisinopril with hydrochlorothiazide in 35 patients with primary hypertension, LVH, and LV diastolic dysfunction.[45] After 6 months of therapy, lisinopril caused regression of myocardial fibrosis and improved LV diastolic function, although LVH was unchanged. However, the largest study, the Perindopril for Elderly Persons with Chronic Heart Failure (PEP-CHF) trial, failed to find a significant effect on clinical outcomes at 1 year in patients with DHF who received perindopril (see Table 20–4). Based on these limited data, it appears that ACE inhibitors may improve HF symptomatology and exercise capacity while not impacting mortality.[46]

At this time, no evidence suggests an advantage of one ACE inhibitor over another. Their effects appear to be a class effect. Initial doses should be small to moderate in order to avoid hypotension, especially if the patient examination does not indicate volume overload. Examples of initial starting doses are captopril 6.25 mg three times daily, enalapril 2.5 mg/day, or lisinopril 2.5 mg/day.

Severe renal failure, history of angioedema, and pregnancy are contraindications to ACE inhibitors. Hyperkalemia, persistent cough, hypotension, taste disturbances, and worsening renal function are common side effects but are managed by decreasing the dose or discontinuing the drug.

Angiotensin Receptor Blockers

Angiotensin receptor blockers can provide symptom-targeted treatment by decreasing LV pressure, decreasing LV volume, and increasing exercise tolerance. They can provide disease-targeted treatment by lowering blood pressure. The Candesartan in Heart Failure: Assessment of Reduction in Mortality and Morbidity (CHARM)-Preserved trial (see Table 20–4) was the first large prospective study to demonstrate the benefits of an angiotensin receptor blocker in patients with preserved EF currently receiving usual treatment.[13] However, 22% of candesartan-treated patients discontinued therapy because of hypotension ($P = 0.009$), increased serum creatinine ($P = 0.0005$), and hyperkalemia ($P = 0.029$).

Presently, no angiotensin receptor blocker has yet been shown to have any major advantage over another. Initial doses of candesartan start at 4 mg/day, irbesartan 150 mg/day, losartan 25 mg/day, telmisartan 40 mg/day, and valsartan 80 mg/day. As with the ACE inhibitors, angiotensin receptor blockers are contraindicated in pregnancy. The side effects of angiotensin receptor blockers are similar to those of ACE inhibitors, but they are not associated with persistent cough.

Aldosterone Antagonists

Aldosterone antagonists can provide improved myocardial functioning by decreasing LV volume and chamber stiffness.[47,48] They can provide disease-targeted treatment by decreasing the fibrosis that accompanies LVH. An analysis of the Randomized Aldactone Evaluation Study (RALES) found that spironolactone significantly decreased the levels of serum markers for cardiac collagen turnover. The benefit from spironolactone was seen in patients with higher levels of collagen synthesis markers. This was the first study to show that serum levels of markers of cardiac collagen synthesis were associated with a poor clinical outcome and could be decreased with spironolactone. This property distinguishes spironolactone from other diuretics that have no effect on myocardial necrosis or collagen turnover.

Like other diuretics, spironolactone should be initiated at a low dose and increased to treat symptoms. Spironolactone may be initiated at doses of 12.5 to 25 mg/day. Spironolactone should be avoided in patients severe renal failure. Hyperkalemia and gynecomastia are the most common side effects. Eplerenone is a viable alternative to spironolactone in patients complaining of sex hormone–related side effects and may be initiated at 25 mg/day.[40]

Positive Inotropic Agents

Positive inotropic agents, such as β-agonists and phosphodiesterase inhibitors, generally are not used in the treatment of patients with isolated DHF because LV EF is preserved and there appears to be little potential for a beneficial effect. Positive inotropic agents have the potential to worsen DHF by adversely affecting energetics, inducing ischemia, raising heart rate, and inducing arrhythmias.[9] In contrast to long-term use, positive inotropic drugs may be beneficial in the short-term treatment of pulmonary edema associated with DHF. These agents can enhance sarcoplasmic reticular function, promote more rapid and complete relaxation, increase splanchnic blood flow, increase venous capacitance, and facilitate diuresis.[9] However, these agents should be used with caution, if they are used at all, because the risk-to-benefit ratio is not clearly established.

Digitalis Derivatives

Digoxin, by inhibiting the Na^+,K^+-adenosine triphosphatase (ATPase) pump, augments intracellular calcium and thereby augments contractile state. In this manner, digoxin produces an increase in systolic energy demands while adding to a relative calcium overload in diastole. These effects may not be apparent clinically under many circumstances, but during hemodynamic stress or ischemia, digoxin may promote or contribute to diastolic dysfunction.[9] However, based on the data from the Digitalis Investigational Group (DIG) Ancillary Study (see Table 20–4), it appears that digoxin has, at most, a very limited role in the management of patients with DHF in normal sinus rhythm.[49]

TABLE 20-5 Characteristics of the Cardiomyopathies

	Dilated	Hypertrophic	Restrictive
Myocardial mass	↑→ ↑↑	↑↑↑	nl→↑
Ventricular cavity size	↑↑↑↑↑	↓↓→nl	nl→↓
Contractile function	↓↓↓	↑↑→	nl→↓
LV filling pressure	↑↑	nl→↑	↑
Chest x-ray film	Moderate to marked cardiac enlargement	Mild to moderate cardiac enlargement	Mild cardiac enlargement
Electrocardiogram	ST-segment and T-wave abnormalities	ST-segment and T-wave abnormalities, LV hypertrophy	Low voltage, conduction defects
Echocardiogram	LV dilation and dysfunction	Asymmetric septal hypertrophy, systolic anterior motion of the mitral valve	Increased LV wall thickness possible
Radionuclide studies	LV dilatation and dysfunction	Vigorous systolic function	Normal systolic function

↑, increased; ↓, decreased; LV, left ventricular; nl, normal.

PHARMACOECONOMIC CONSIDERATIONS

Frequent admission to the hospital is common in patients with DHF. Unfortunately, there are no pharmacoeconomic data associated with the only large clinical outcome trial (CHARM-Preserved) published to date. Because DHF is primarily a disease of the elderly, comorbid conditions will create challenges in any trial designed. At the present time, cost to the patient should be considered because adherence to an antihypertensive regimen is paramount to a beneficial outcome.

CLINICAL CONTROVERSIES

- Digoxin may increase hospitalizations for unstable angina in patients with DHF and normal sinus rhythm.
- Drugs that antagonize the renin–angiotensin–aldosterone system may be the preferred antihypertensive drugs for patients with DHF.

EVALUATION OF THERAPEUTIC OUTCOMES

The end points used in assessing effective therapies for DHF include mortality, hospitalization for worsening HF, functional status or quality-of-life indicators, and cost. Other end points may target underlying mechanisms of disease, such as calcium homeostasis or regression of fibrosis. A number of clinical trials addressing this important clinical problem are underway.

CARDIOMYOPATHIES

Diastolic dysfunction plays a role in the presentation of some types of cardiomyopathy. Over the past decade, the terminology and classification used for the cardiomyopathies have been confusing because of overlap among the diseases and/or classification schemes. In 2006, the ACC/AHA suggested a broader definition for the cardiomyopathies. The expert panel defined the cardiomyopathies as "a heterogeneous group of diseases of the myocardium associated with mechanical and/or electrical dysfunction that usually (but not invariably) exhibit inappropriate ventricular hypertrophy or dilation and are due to variety of causes that frequently are genetic. Cardiomyopathies either are confined to the heart (*primary* cardiomyopathy) or are part of generalized systemic disorders (*secondary* cardiomyopathy), often leading to cardiovascular death or progressive HF-related disability."[50]

The *primary* cardiomyopathies are further divided into genetic, mixed (genetic and nongenetic), and acquired. Endocrine conditions, inflammation, metabolic disorders, infiltrative diseases, and toxins are a few of the causative factors of secondary cardiomyopathy.[50] It is important to note that this new contemporary classification does not include pathologic myocardial processes that are a direct result of other cardiovascular conditions such as valvular heart disease, hypertension, and CAD. Therefore, the commonly used term "ischemic cardiomyopathy" is not considered a "true" cardiomyopathy.

Frequently, a specific etiology is not evident. Therefore, another commonly used categorization of the cardiomyopathies is based on the structural and/or functional abnormalities present. The three groups of primary cardiomyopathies usually are described as dilated, hypertrophic, and restrictive. An understanding of the pathophysiologic basis for each type of cardiomyopathy leads to a rational selection of drug therapy or other treatment modality. The characteristics for each of the types of cardiomyopathy are listed in Table 20–5. The distinction among the cardiomyopathies is not absolute, and there is some overlap in the functional abnormalities.

In dilated cardiomyopathy, the cardinal feature is ventricular chamber enlargement. Systolic function is abnormal with normal LV wall thickness, leading to a decreased cardiac output. In patients with HCM, the ventricular cavity is not dilated, but the ventricular muscle mass is increased, existing in the absence of known causes of LVH. Ventricular cavity size is normal or decreased, and systolic function often is preserved. Patients with HCM may have an obstructive or nonobstructive form. Patients with restrictive cardiomyopathy have inadequate ventricular compliance causing diastolic dysfunction as a result of endocardial and/or myocardial disease. The clinical presentation is similar to that of constrictive pericarditis.

HYPERTROPHIC CARDIOMYOPATHY

HCM is a primary, genetic cardiomyopathy that is inherited as an autosomal dominant trait caused by mutations in any of 10 genes. The distribution of the hypertrophy usually is asymmetric, meaning that segments of the LV are thickened to varying degrees. There also may be enlargement of the atria, thickening of the mitral valve leaflets, and fibrotic areas within the ventricular wall. In the past, the terms of *idiopathic hypertrophic subaortic stenosis* and *hypertrophic obstructive cardiomyopathy* were used to describe patients with HCM with an outflow obstruction. These terms are used less frequently now because they overemphasize the obstructive component of the disease, which is present in a minority of patients.[50]

Epidemiology

Recent epidemiologic investigations estimate the prevalence of phenotypically expressed HCM in the general adult population to be approximately 0.2% (1:500), making it the most frequently occurring cardiomyopathy. HCM is the most common genetic cardiovascular disease. However, many individuals have a mutant gene but go undetected.[51]

Etiology

The genetic predisposition to HCM is thought to be an autosomal dominant trait with variable penetrance. Because of the wide variability of presentation, not all cases in a family may be detected.

HCM usually is caused by mutations in the genes for β-myosin heavy chain, myosin-binding protein C, and cardiac troponin T.[52]

Pathophysiology

HCM appears to have several different pathophysiologic mechanisms leading to similar clinical manifestations, although the prognoses for patients will vary. The pathophysiology of HCM is a complex relationship among several factors, including (a) asymmetric LVH, (b) diastolic dysfunction, (c) dynamic obstruction of the outflow tract, and (d) myocardial ischemia. Each of these components contributes to the overall presentation of the patient to a varying degree.[51,52]

Left Ventricular Hypertrophy The hypertrophy seen in HCM usually is diffuse and involves the septum and LV anterolateral free wall to a greater degree than the posterior segment. Asymmetric septal hypertrophy is a sensitive marker for HCM but is not specific for this disorder. In patients with outflow obstruction, the basal septum usually is markedly thickened at the level of the mitral valve. In patients with nonobstructive HCM, the outflow tract is larger, and the septal hypertrophy that occurs has a more distal or apical distribution.[53]

Cellular disorganization is a common histologic finding in HCM. Morphologic abnormalities are found at the gross, microscopic, and ultrastructural levels. The disarray of myocytes may contribute to diastolic and systolic dysfunction, as well as serving as a nidus for ventricular arrhythmias. The degree of LVH is associated with a worse clinical course. The presence of hypertrophy correlates directly with myocardial infarction, HF, stroke, and ventricular arrhythmias. Spirito and Autore[51] found that the magnitude of LVH was directly related to the risk of sudden cardiac death.

Diastolic Dysfunction Diastolic dysfunction is the most common abnormality found in patients with HCM. Approximately 80% of patients exhibit symptoms associated with diastolic dysfunction. Studies of the LV led to the realization that diastolic dysfunction is the result of abnormalities in relaxation, distensibility (compliance), and filling. The abnormalities of diastolic function can be both regional and global and lead to an incoordination of contraction and relaxation. β-Adrenergic stimulation can aggravate these abnormalities, whereas β-receptor blockade may diminish them.[52]

Abnormalities in filling are also associated with changes in chamber stiffness that occur in HCM. This stiffness may be the result of myocardial fibrosis, cellular disorganization, or increased myocardial mass. The decreased distensibility leads to an abnormally steep slope of the diastolic pressure–volume curve such that an increase in LV volume results in a disproportionate increase in diastolic pressure.

Myocardial relaxation is an energy-dependent process that is sensitive to episodes of ischemia. Diastolic resequestration of calcium ions by the sarcoplasmic reticulum is an energy-dependent process. In the event of ischemia, the sequestration of calcium is inhibited, allowing the calcium to continue its interaction with the myofibrillar contractile proteins. Calcium channel blockers have been used with some success in patients with diastolic dysfunction.[54]

Systolic Function and Outflow Tract Obstruction Abnormalities of systolic function also occur in patients with HCM. The hypertrophied LV may cause a powerful but sometimes uncoordinated contraction presumably as a result of the abnormal architecture of the myocardium. The increase in LV wall thickness results in decreased wall stress during systole. Therefore, the LV contracts against a decreased afterload so that the LV is described as being *hyperdynamic*. EF often is increased.

Considerable controversy has surrounded the issue of the importance of outflow tract obstruction in conjunction with HCM. The presence of a gradient (the systolic pressure difference between the body and the outflow tract of the LV) is indicative of a dynamic obstruction of the LV outflow tract. Outflow tract gradients occur in approximately 25% of patients with HCM.[50] The obstruction that occurs usually shows spontaneous variability and may be reduced by interventions that decrease myocardial contractility. The gradient can be augmented by factors that increase contractility (Table 20–6).[54] LV outflow tract obstruction at rest has been found to be a predictor of progression to severe HF symptoms, stroke, and death.[55]

TABLE 20-6 Factors Known to Affect Outflow Gradients in Hypertrophic Cardiomyopathy

Factors that diminish gradients
Decreasing myocardial contractility
β-Blocking drugs
Verapamil
Increasing ventricular volume
Increasing arterial pressure
Factors that enhance gradients
Increasing myocardial contractility
Exercise
Inotropic agents
Decreasing ventricular volume
Decreasing arterial pressure

Myocardial Ischemia Chest pain in the absence of CAD is a common symptom of patients with HCM. However, it is appropriate to consider typical CAD in any patient with HCM if they have the usual risk factors for atherosclerosis.[50,54,56] Several mechanisms are proposed for the myocardial ischemia seen in this patient population. There may be inadequate capillary density in relation to the increased LV muscle mass. The small intramural coronary arteries may be abnormally narrowed or excessively compressed during systole. Impaired relaxation during diastole may inhibit blood flow to the subendocardium. Once myocardial ischemia develops, further increases in LV filling pressure may occur, which, in turn, lead to more ischemia. Repeated episodes of ischemia may be responsible for progressive myocyte loss and fibrosis. The subendocardium is at greatest risk for ischemic damage because of the lower capillary density and higher oxygen demand secondary to wall tension.[54]

Diagnosis

Making the diagnosis of HCM may be difficult because the disorder may be confused with CAD, aortic stenosis, or mitral regurgitation. Patients with HCM can be young and physically active. The physical signs of the cardiac examination depend on the presence of a systolic pressure gradient within the LV. If a gradient is present, a late-onset systolic murmur is heard often. The murmur is intensified by standing and the Valsalva maneuver and lessened with squatting or handgrip. Very rarely, some patients develop an end-stage LV dilation and a declining LV EF, which often are confused with idiopathic dilated cardiomyopathy.

Echocardiography is used to confirm the diagnosis. The diagnosis of HCM is made with two-dimensional echocardiography, with the usual criterion of LV wall thickness ≥15 mm. Magnetic resonance imaging of the entire LV may add valuable information, especially if the echocardiogram is of suboptimal quality.[50,56]

The development of or increase in a murmur suggests progression of disease, but disappearance of a murmur does not imply improvement. In fact, disappearance of a murmur may herald further impairment of systolic function. Some patients will progress to CHF a result of atrial fibrillation, mitral regurgitation, or myocardial infarction. If SHF develops, the patient has a poor prognosis.

Contemporary methods of diagnosis consist of genotype assessment. Genetic testing allows for a definitive diagnosis and precise identification of mutations in myocardial sarcomere proteins. Unfortunately, screening for more than 200 mutations in multiple genes is complex, time consuming, costly, and restricted to a small number of research laboratories. Furthermore, genetic screening identifies gene variants in only 50% to 60% of patients. Based on these limitations, genotype assessment has not become a standard part of routine clinical evaluation.[50,51]

CLINICAL PRESENTATION OF HYPERTROPHIC CARDIOMYOPATHY

General

- The clinical presentation varies widely, ranging from no symptoms to severe symptoms of angina, HF, and/or sudden death. The severity of symptoms corresponds to the degree of LVH, but this relationship is not absolute.

Symptoms

- The patient may complain of dyspnea, chest pain, fatigue, palpitations, presyncope, and syncope.

Signs

- Systolic murmur

Other Diagnostic Tests

- Echocardiography will show increased myocardial mass.
- Electrocardiography will reveal LVH with or without ST-segment and T-wave abnormalities.

Prognosis

The clinical course for a patient with HCM should be viewed in terms of the specific subtypes of the disease spectrum. Patients fall into one of several relatively discrete pathways: (a) high risk for sudden death; (b) symptoms of DHF, including syncope; (c) progression toward advanced end-stage HF; and (d) atrial fibrillation and its sequelae. Of major concern is the incidence of sudden cardiac death among patients with HCM. Approximately 10% to 20% of HCM patients are at increased risk for sudden death. The mechanism responsible for sudden cardiac death is thought to be related to an electrically unstable myocardium leading to complex ventricular arrhythmias. Less often, sudden death may be the result of hemodynamic changes. The onset of atrial fibrillation in the face of severe LV diastolic dysfunction may result in a significant decrease in stroke volume. This decrease in cardiac output could lead acute LV failure, MI, or sudden death. Sudden death can be a complication, especially in young athletes with HCM. It is recommended that young patients with HCM refrain from competitive athletics.[50,56]

Quantification of the risk of sudden death remains elusive for patients with HCM. The clinical markers associated with an increased risk for sudden death (Table 20–7) have a high negative predictive value. The absence of all these markers can be used to develop a profile for a patient at low risk for sudden death. The magnitude of hypertrophy appears to be a strong predictor, with the cumulative risk nearly zero for patients with a wall thickness ≤19 mm. Young patients with severe hypertrophy (wall thickness >30 mm) are at high risk for sudden death even if they are asymptomatic. A high LV outflow tract pressure gradient ≥30 mm Hg is a strong predictor for older patients.[57] Presentation of HCM in the latter decades of life is common. Patients who present with HCM at an advanced age of 65 years or older usually have a prognosis that is no different from that of age- and gender-matched controls. Elderly patients with HCM tend to have mild degrees of LVH, and their symptoms are not severe.[58] Because systolic hypertension and diastolic HF are common in the elderly, the diagnosis of HCM may be challenging. However, marked LVH out of proportion to blood pressure, unusual patterns of LVH, or an outflow obstruction at rest strongly suggests HCM.[50]

TABLE 20-7 Risk Factors Associated with Sudden Cardiac Death in Hypertrophic Cardiomyopathy

Major risk factors
Prior cardiac arrest
Spontaneous sustained ventricular tachycardia
Positive family history of premature death
Multiple syncopal or near-syncopal episodes, especially if associated with exertion
Multiple and repetitive or prolonged episodes of nonsustained ventricular tachycardia
Marked left ventricular hypertrophy ≥30 mm
Hypotensive blood pressure response to exercise
Potential individual risk factors
Atrial fibrillation
Myocardial ischemia
Left ventricular outflow obstruction
Identification of a malignant genotype
Intense (competitive) physical exertion

Data from Zipes et al.[62]

TREATMENT

Hypertrophic Cardiomyopathy

DESIRED OUTCOMES

Because no known means are available for preventing HCM, the focus must be on methods to minimize the consequences of the disorder.

GENERAL APPROACH TO TREATMENT

8 The treatment of HCM is designed to reduce symptoms, improve exercise tolerance, retard disease progression, and improve prognosis. Agents that decrease contractility, improve diastolic dysfunction, reduce ischemia, and suppress arrhythmias have been used with some success (Fig. 20–2). In 2003, the ACC in conjunction with the ESC published a consensus document on HCM.[59]

NONPHARMACOLOGIC THERAPY

Surgical treatment generally is reserved for patients who are refractory to medical management, have an outflow gradient ≥50 mm Hg, a very thick ventricular septum, and high LV pressures. Surgical intervention is designed to relieve the outflow obstruction and the elevated LV pressures. The surgeon accomplishes this by performing a myectomy (i.e., removal of excess tissue). The procedure results in a reduction in LV filling pressures and a long-term improvement in symptoms. However, early mortality rates of up to 5% have been reported.[52,59] Other complications may include septal perforation and late occurrence of HF.

The results of uncontrolled studies suggested that dual-chamber pacing decreased LV outflow gradients and improved symptoms. Subsequent controlled trials were not able to replicate the initial findings but demonstrated more modest improvement. Consequently, the ACC/AHA and the North American Society of Pacing and Electrophysiology have issued guidelines suggesting pacing for severely symptomatic patients who have not responded to medical management (class IIb recommendation, or one in which the efficacy is less well established by evidence).[60]

Ablation of the myocardium using alcohol is another alternative to surgery. Septal ablation with alcohol results in the same type of outcomes as seen with myectomy. Long-term followup is limited because this procedure has been used for less than a decade. Because it is a percutaneous procedure (similar to cardiac catheterizations), it is being performed more frequently than myectomy. There is some concern that the risk for arrhythmia-related cardiac events may increase following alcohol ablation. Long-term followup is needed to assess this risk. Complete heart block is a common complication of septal ablation (14% in one case series) and requires a permanent pacemaker if it occurs.[52,59]

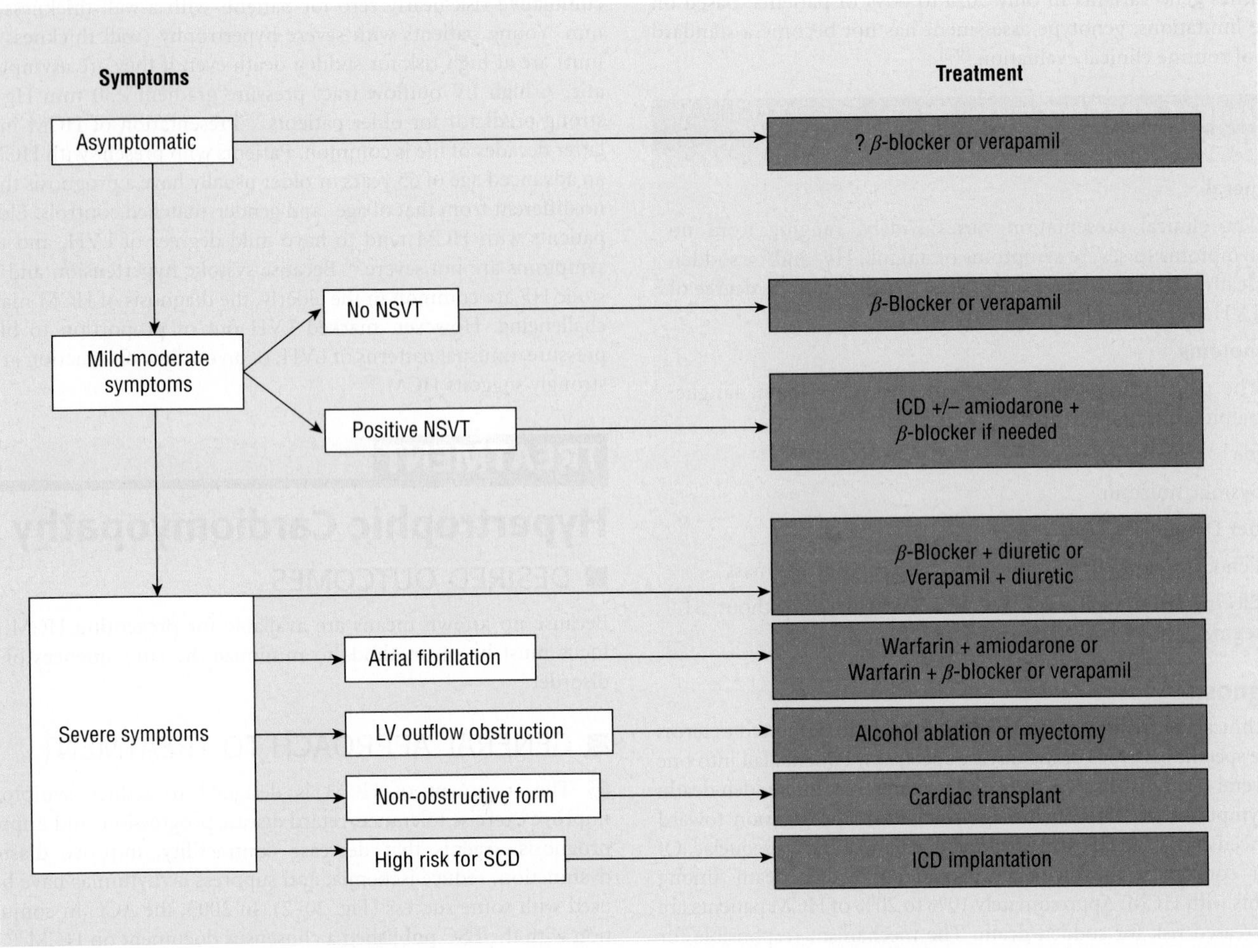

FIGURE 20-2. Treatment algorithm for hypertrophic cardiomyopathy. (ICD, implantable cardioverter-defibrillator; LV, left ventricular; NSVT, nonsustained ventricular tachycardia; SCD, sudden cardiac death; ?, questionable role.)

■ IMPLANTABLE CARDIOVERTER-DEFIBRILLATOR

9 Sudden death is the most worrisome outcome of HCM, and the implantable cardioverter-defibrillator (ICD) is the most effective therapy for prevention of sudden death.[61] It is difficult to know when to implant an ICD, especially in a young patient diagnosed with HCM. Patients who are candidates for an ICD for primary prevention will be young and relatively asymptomatic. In 2006, the ACC/AHA with the ESC published updated guidelines designating the ICD for primary prevention of sudden death (class IIa recommendation or one in which the weight of the evidence or opinion favors efficacy). These guidelines stipulate that patients should exhibit one or more major risk factors for sudden death (see Table 20–7), currently be receiving chronic medical therapy, and have a reasonable survival with good functional status at 1 year. For secondary prevention following cardiac arrest, ICD placement is considered a class I recommendation, where there is evidence or general agreement that the procedure is beneficial.[60] Conducting a clinical trial to provide evidence for a higher-level recommendation for primary prevention is unlikely to occur.[61]

■ PHARMACOLOGIC THERAPY

β-Adrenergic Blockers

10 β-Blocking agents have been used in obstructive and nonobstructive forms of HCM since the 1960s. Approximately one third to half of patients with angina, dyspnea, light-headedness, or syncope will have a favorable response to these agents.[54] Doses up to 480 mg/day of propranolol or its equivalent are used. Resting heart rate should be 60 beats/min, and the maximum exercise heart rate should be <120 beats/min. The mechanism by which β-blockade is beneficial is by inhibiting sympathetic stimulation of the heart. Myocardial oxygen demand is reduced by decreasing heart rate, LV contractility, and myocardial wall stress during systole. Outflow tract obstruction may be minimized with β-blockade, especially under conditions of stress or exercise, when sympathetic stimulation is high.

Calcium Channel Blockers

Patients who have an inadequate response to β-blockade may respond to verapamil.[51] Doses of verapamil up to 480 mg/day have beneficial effects on symptoms.[59] Calcium channel blockers may be of benefit to patients with HCM for several reasons. Increased calcium concentrations have been shown to play a role in prolonging ventricular depolarization, as well as the duration of isometric contraction and relaxation. Patients with HCM have a hyperdynamic ventricle in systole and delayed relaxation and decreased compliance during diastole. Calcium channel blockers decrease the myocardial oxygen demand, resulting in an improved balance between oxygen supply and demand; therefore, diastolic function may be improved.

Most patients with HCM who have been treated with a calcium channel blocker have received verapamil, although others also have been used. Intravenous verapamil has been noted to acutely reduce the outflow tract gradient in patients with obstructive HCM. The mechanism may be a decrease in systolic function as well as an increase in LV volumes as a result of enhanced LV diastolic filling.

The adverse effects associated with use of verapamil include constipation, sinus nodal blockade, prolongation of the PR interval,

AV dissociation, hypotension, and pulmonary congestion.[54] The risks may outweigh the benefits in patients with (a) a markedly elevated pulmonary capillary wedge pressure or pulmonary artery occlusion pressure, (b) a history of paroxysmal nocturnal dyspnea or orthopnea, (c) sick sinus syndrome or significant AV nodal disease in the absence of a permanent pacemaker, (d) low systolic blood pressure, and (e) a substantial outflow gradient. Verapamil should be avoided in patients with HF as a result of systolic dysfunction.[59] There is no evidence that either β-blockade or verapamil protects the patient from sudden cardiac death.

Studies using other calcium channel blockers are limited. Improvement in diastolic dysfunction may occur, but the dihydropyridines may cause a reflex increase in heart rate or hypotension or worsen the outflow tract gradient.

Antiarrhythmic Agents

Disopyramide has been used for treating both the supraventricular and ventricular arrhythmias occurring in patients with HCM. In addition, the negative inotropic effect and the ability to increase peripheral vascular resistance attributed to disopyramide have been used to reduce outflow tract obstruction. The anticholinergic side effects (blurred vision, dry mouth, and urinary retention) make disopyramide a problematic agent for long-term therapy in some patients. The QT interval on the ECG should be monitored in patients on disopyramide.[59]

The role of amiodarone for the prevention of sudden death in patients with HCM has been questionable. A few nonrandomized studies have suggested a protective effect, whereas others demonstrate only symptomatic improvement. Nonetheless, the 2006 ACC/AHA/ESC give amiodarone a class IIb recommendation for primary prophylaxis against sudden death in patients with HCM when ICD placement is not feasible and who demonstrate one or more major risk factors for sudden death (see Table 20–7). Furthermore, in patients with HCM who are not candidates for ICD placement and have suffered a cardiac arrest, amiodarone therapy is considered the preferred treatment (class I recommendation).[62]

A significant number of patients with HCM develop atrial fibrillation. Amiodarone is one of the most effective agents available to maintain normal sinus rhythm in these patients. For patients in chronic atrial fibrillation requiring rate control, a β-blocker or verapamil may be used. Anticoagulation should be considered because these patients are at risk for systemic embolization and stroke. If amiodarone is added to the therapy of a patient already receiving warfarin, the prothrombin time or international normalized ratio will be increased and should be monitored closely.[51]

Other Drugs

⓫ There is a small risk for bacterial endocarditis in HCM patients with LV outflow obstruction under resting conditions and in those with intrinsic mitral valve disease. Patients undergoing dental or selected surgical procedures that cause bloodborne bacteremia should receive appropriate antibiotic therapy. The administration of nitroglycerin and digoxin generally is discouraged in the presence of LV outflow obstruction.[59]

CLINICAL CONTROVERSY

Some clinicians believe that ACE inhibitors have no role in the management of HCM with LV outflow obstruction. Others believe that ACE inhibitors may be beneficial by limiting hypertrophy.

Evaluation of Therapeutic Outcomes

The goal of treatment of patients with HCM is primarily to reduce their symptoms of dyspnea and exercise intolerance. Either β-blocker or calcium channel blockers can be used. If a β-blocker is chosen, it is best to use an agent that does not have intrinsic sympathomimetic activity. The dose should be maximized. If the patient does not tolerate a β-blocker or has a contraindication to use of a β-blocker, then verapamil can be tried. Patients should be monitored for resolution of symptoms and an increase in exercise tolerance. Resolution of symptoms may take months to occur. In addition, both β-blockers and calcium channel blockers may cause hypotension and conduction abnormalities. β-Blockers may worsen pulmonary function. If dyspnea continues with maximal doses of a β-blocker or calcium channel blocker, a diuretic agent or a nitrate may be added with caution. Patients who are at high risk for sudden cardiac death should be considered candidates for an ICD.

For patients with significant obstruction to LV outflow who do not respond to medical management, a surgical approach may be necessary. Septal myectomy and alcohol ablation have been used. These approaches generally are reserved for patients who have an outflow gradient >50 mm Hg and/or severe symptoms and who have not responded an adequate trial of medical therapy.

RESTRICTIVE CARDIOMYOPATHY

Restrictive cardiomyopathy is primarily an abnormality of diastolic function that results in impaired filling and increases in ventricular end-diastolic pressures with normal or decreased diastolic volume. It is associated with normal systolic function early in the course of the disease but a decrease in systolic function later in the disease process. Either one or both of the ventricles may be affected; therefore, restrictive cardiomyopathy may present as either left- or right-sided HF.[50]

CLINICAL PRESENTATION OF RESTRICTIVE CARDIOMYOPATHY

General

- The majority of patients remain asymptomatic but experience symptoms during exercise or vigorous activity.

Symptoms

- The patient may complain of dyspnea, orthopnea, fatigue, edema, ascites, or chest pain.

Signs

- Significant jugular venous distension
- Mitral and/or tricuspid regurgitant murmurs
- Thromboembolic complications
- Kussmaul sign may be present

Laboratory Tests

- BNP and N-proBNP levels will be elevated.

Other Diagnostic Tests

- ECG may reflect atrial arrhythmias, tachybrady syndrome, or conduction abnormalities.
- Echocardiography may reveal small ventricles and dilated atria.

Epidemiology and Etiology

Restrictive cardiomyopathy is the type of cardiomyopathy encountered least frequently in western countries. Because restrictive cardiomyopathy is rare, the natural course of the disease is not well characterized, and reports on prognosis have been highly variable. Restrictive cardiomyopathies may be classified as either myocardial or endomyocardial. The myocardial types may be noninfiltrative, infiltrative, or storage diseases. The endomyocardial types are due to endomyocardial fibrosis, hypereosinophilic syndrome, carcinoid heart disease, metastatic cancers, radiation, and anthracycline toxicity or secondary to drugs known to cause fibrosis.[54]

Restrictive myocardial disease may result from several local or systemic disorders. Amyloidosis, hemochromatosis, scleroderma, carcinoid, sarcoidosis, diabetes, pseudoxanthoma elasticum, and endomyocardial fibrosis have been known to cause restrictive cardiomyopathy. The most common cause of restrictive cardiomyopathy in the industrialized world is amyloidosis, whereas endomyocardial fibrosis is a common cause in tropical areas of the world. There may be a genetic predisposition to idiopathic restrictive cardiomyopathy.[54]

The cause of the disease, the severity of HF symptoms, and the presence of cardiac thrombi and arrhythmias are factors that affect long-term survival. Children diagnosed with restrictive cardiomyopathy have a worse prognosis than do adults and should be considered for early cardiac transplantation.[63]

Pathophysiology

The major hemodynamic abnormality in restrictive cardiomyopathy is a limitation in ventricular filling leading to increased filling pressures. The cavity size and wall thickness of the ventricles usually are normal. Atrial dimensions often are increased. Thrombi are found frequently in the cardiac chambers. Patients have signs and symptoms consistent with HF. The abnormality is similar to that seen in pericardial disease causing constriction or tamponade.

Diagnosis

The diagnosis of restrictive cardiomyopathy should be considered in any patient who presents with signs and symptoms of HF but has only mild cardiomegaly. Differentiation from constrictive pericarditis is important because pericardectomy is an effective form of treatment of constrictive pericarditis. Recent studies have focused on using BNP as a potential noninvasive marker for differentiation of the two conditions.[64]

TREATMENT

Restrictive Cardiomyopathy

The treatment of restrictive cardiomyopathy is complex because of the heterogeneity of the pathophysiologic abnormalities. Diuretics are used for the symptoms of venous congestion in the presence of restrictive cardiomyopathy, but caution is advised because these patients require high filling pressures to maintain an adequate stroke volume and cardiac output. Hypotension and hypoperfusion may occur as a result of excessive use of diuretics. Because systolic function often is normal, digoxin is of little benefit and may be proarrhythmic. Amiodarone can be used to maintain normal sinus rhythm in patients who have episodes of atrial fibrillation. Anticoagulation is needed to decrease the risk of systemic embolization, particularly in patients with atrial fibrillation, valvular regurgitation, and low cardiac output. In the case of hemochromatosis, chelation therapy and/or repeated phlebotomy may be of benefit. Treatment with corticosteroids and cytotoxic drugs has been used with some success in the early phase of endomyocardial fibrosis and eosinophilic cardiomyopathy.[54]

Evaluation of Therapeutic Outcomes

The first step in assessing and treating a patient with restrictive cardiomyopathy is to rule out constrictive pericarditis because the two conditions have a similar presentation. Patients with constrictive pericarditis are treated easily with surgery, whereas patients with restrictive cardiomyopathy undergo a varied approach to therapy depending on the etiology of their disorder. The treatment is aimed at relieving the symptoms associated with high filling pressures. This is achieved generally through the use of diuretics. Diuretic therapy should be initiated with low doses. Normalization of filling pressures is not possible or desirable. Patients' symptoms should be monitored for improvement. Excessive diuresis will result in inadequate cardiac output. Chelation therapy has been advocated for patients with hemochromatosis. Prednisone has been suggested for patients with sarcoidosis. There is no curative treatment for restrictive cardiomyopathy.

ABBREVIATIONS

ACC: American College of Cardiology

ACE: angiotensin-converting enzyme

AHA: American Heart Association

ALLHAT: antihypertensive and lipid-lowering treatment to prevent heart attack trial

AV: atrioventricular

BNP: B-type natriuretic peptide

CAD: coronary artery disease

CHARM: candesartan in heart failure: assessment of reduction in mortality and morbidity

DHF: diastolic heart failure

DIG: Digitalis Investigational Group

ECG: electrocardiogram

EF: ejection fraction

ESC: European Society of Cardiology

HCM: hypertrophic cardiomyopathy

HF: heart failure

HFSA: Heart Failure Society of America

HR: hazard ratio

ICD: implantable cardioverter-defibrillator

I-Preserve: irbesartan in heart failure with preserved ejection fraction

LV: left ventricular

LVH: left ventricular hypertrophy

MI: myocardial infarction

MMP: matrix metalloproteinase

NT-proBNP: N-terminal proBNP

NYHA: New York Heart Association

PEP-CHF: perindopril for elderly persons with chronic heart failure

RALES: randomized aldactone evaluation study

SBP: systolic blood pressure

SHF: systolic heart failure

TOPCAT: trial of aldosterone antagonist therapy in adults with preserved ejection

REFERENCES

1. Owan TE, Redfield MM. Epidemiology of diastolic heart failure. Prog Cardiovasc Dis 2005;47:320–332.
2. Brutsaert DL, De Keulenaer GW. Diastolic heart failure: A myth. Curr Opin Cardiol 2006;21:240–248.
3. Executive summary: HFSA 2006 Comprehensive Heart Failure Practice Guideline. J Card Fail 2006;12:10–38.
4. Zile MR, Brutsaert DL. New concepts in diastolic dysfunction and diastolic heart failure: Part I. diagnosis, prognosis, and measurements of diastolic function. Circulation 2002;105:1387–1393.

5. Leite-Moreira AF. Current perspectives in diastolic dysfunction and diastolic heart failure. Heart 2006;92:712–718.
6. Zile MR. Heart failure with preserved ejection fraction: Is this diastolic heart failure? J Am Coll Cardiol 2003;41:1519–1522.
7. Smith GL, Masoudi FA, Vaccarino V, et al. Outcomes in heart failure patients with preserved ejection fraction: Mortality, readmission, and functional decline. J Am Coll Cardiol 2003;41:1510–1518.
8. Fonarow GC, Adams KF Jr, Abraham WT, et al. Risk stratification for in-hospital mortality in acutely decompensated heart failure: Classification and regression tree analysis. JAMA 2005;293:572–580.
9. Zile MR. Diastolic heart failure. Diagnosis, prognosis, treatment. Minerva Cardioangiol 2003;51:131–142.
10. Redfield MM, Jacobsen SJ, Burnett JC Jr, et al. Burden of systolic and diastolic ventricular dysfunction in the community: Appreciating the scope of the heart failure epidemic. JAMA 2003;289:194–202.
11. Owan TE, Hodge DO, Herges RM, et al. Trends in prevalence and outcome of heart failure with preserved ejection fraction. N Engl J Med 2006;355:251–259.
12. Franklin KM, Aurigemma GP. Prognosis in diastolic heart failure. Prog Cardiovasc Dis 2005;47:333–339.
13. Yusuf S, Pfeffer MA, Swedberg K, et al. Effects of candesartan in patients with chronic heart failure and preserved left-ventricular ejection fraction: The CHARM-Preserved Trial. Lancet 2003;362:777–781.
14. Yamamoto K, Wilson DJ, Canzanello VJ, Redfield MM. Left ventricular diastolic dysfunction in patients with hypertension and preserved systolic function. Mayo Clin Proc 2000;75:148–155.
15. Galderisi M. Diastolic dysfunction and diastolic heart failure: Diagnostic, prognostic and therapeutic aspects. Cardiovasc Ultrasound 2005;3:1–14.
16. Neilan TG, Yoerger DM, Douglas PS, et al. Persistent and reversible cardiac dysfunction among amateur marathon runners. Eur Heart J 2006;27:1079–1084.
17. Mandinov L, Eberli FR, Seiler C, Hess OM. Diastolic heart failure. Cardiovasc Res 2000;45:813–825.
18. Ahmed SH, Clark LL, Pennington WR, et al. Matrix metalloproteinases/tissue inhibitors of metalloproteinases: Relationship between changes in proteolytic determinants of matrix composition and structural, functional, and clinical manifestations of hypertensive heart disease. Circulation 2006;113:2089–2096.
19. Zile MR, Brutsaert DL. New concepts in diastolic dysfunction and diastolic heart failure: Part II. causal mechanisms and treatment. Circulation 2002;105:1503–1508.
20. Cecchi F, Olivotto I, Gistri R, et al. Coronary microvascular dysfunction and prognosis in hypertrophic cardiomyopathy. N Engl J Med 2003;349:1027–1035.
21. Torosoff M, Philbin EF. Improving outcomes in diastolic heart failure. Techniques to evaluate underlying causes and target therapy. Postgrad Med 2003;113:51–58.
22. Ma LN, Zhao SP, Gao M, et al. Endothelial dysfunction associated with left ventricular diastolic dysfunction in patients with coronary heart disease. Int J Cardiol 2000;72:275–279.
23. Colucci WS, Braunwald E. Pathophysiology of heart failure. In: Zipes DP, Libby P, Bonow RO, Braunwald E, eds. Braunwald's Heart Disease, 7th ed. Philadelphia: Elsevier Saunders, 2005:509–538.
24. Swedberg K, Cleland J, Dargie H, Drexler H, et al. Guidelines for the diagnosis and treatment of chronic heart failure: Executive summary (update 2005): The Task Force for the Diagnosis and Treatment of Chronic Heart Failure of the European Society of Cardiology. Eur Heart J 2005;26:1115–1140.
25. Vasan RS, Levy D. Defining diastolic heart failure: A call for standardized diagnostic criteria. Circulation 2000;101:2118–2121.
26. Kitzman DW, Little WC, Brubaker PH, et al. Pathophysiological characterization of isolated diastolic heart failure in comparison to systolic heart failure. JAMA 2002;288:2144–2150.
27. Massie BM. Natriuretic peptide measurements for the diagnosis of "nonsystolic" heart failure: Good news and bad. J Am Coll Cardiol 2003;41:2018–2021.
28. Maisel AS, McCord J, Nowak RM, et al. Bedside B-type natriuretic peptide in the emergency diagnosis of heart failure with reduced or preserved ejection fraction. Results from the Breathing Not Properly Multinational Study. J Am Coll Cardiol 2003;41:2010–2017.
29. Tschope C, Kasner M, Westermann D, Gaub R, Poller WC, Schultheiss HP. The role of NT-proBNP in the diagnostics of isolated diastolic dysfunction: Correlation with echocardiographic and invasive measurements. Eur Heart J 2005;26:2277–2284.
30. Bhatia RS, Tu JV, Lee DS, et al. Outcome of heart failure with preserved ejection fraction in a population-based study. N Engl J Med 2006;355:260–269.
31. Deswal A, Bozkurt B. Comparison of morbidity in women versus men with heart failure and preserved ejection fraction. Am J Cardiol 2006;97:1228–1231.
32. Jones RC, Francis GS, Lauer MS. Predictors of mortality in patients with heart failure and preserved systolic function in the Digitalis Investigation Group trial. J Am Coll Cardiol 2004;44:1025–1029.
33. Little WC, Brucks S. Therapy for diastolic heart failure. Prog Cardiovasc Dis 2005;47:380–388.
34. Pina IL, Apstein CS, Balady GJ, et al. Exercise and heart failure: A statement from the American Heart Association Committee on exercise, rehabilitation, and prevention. Circulation 2003;107:1210–1225.
35. Gaasch WH, Zile MR. Left ventricular diastolic dysfunction and diastolic heart failure. Annu Rev Med 2004;55:373–394.
36. Heart Failure Society of America. Evaluation and management of patients with heart failure and preserved left ventricular ejection fraction. J Card Fail 2006;12:e80–e85.
37. Hunt SA. ACC/AHA 2005 guideline update for the diagnosis and management of chronic heart failure in the adult: A report of the American College of Cardiology/American Heart Association Task Force on Practice Guidelines (Writing Committee to Update the 2001 Guidelines for the Evaluation and Management of Heart Failure). J Am Coll Cardiol 2005;46:e1–e82.
38. Major cardiovascular events in hypertensive patients randomized to doxazosin vs chlorthalidone: The Antihypertensive and Lipid-Lowering Treatment to Prevent Heart Attack Trial (ALLHAT). ALLHAT Collaborative Research Group. JAMA 2000;283:1967–1975.
39. Banerjee P, Clark AL, Cleland JG. Diastolic heart failure: A difficult problem in the elderly. Am J Geriatr Cardiol 2004;13:16–21.
40. Davis KL, Nappi JM. The cardiovascular effects of eplerenone, a selective aldosterone-receptor antagonist. Clin Ther 2003;25:2647–2668.
41. van Kraaij DJ, Jansen RW, Bouwels LH, Gribnau FW, Hoefnagels WH. Furosemide withdrawal in elderly heart failure patients with preserved left ventricular systolic function. Am J Cardiol 2000;85:1461–1466.
42. Lefrandt JD, Heitmann J, Sevre K, et al. Contrasting effects of verapamil and amlodipine on cardiovascular stress responses in hypertension. Br J Clin Pharmacol 2001;52:687–692.
43. Hogg K, McMurray J. Neurohumoral pathways in heart failure with preserved systolic function. Prog Cardiovasc Dis 2005;47:357–366.
44. Baker DW. Prevention of heart failure. J Card Fail 2002;8:333–346.
45. Brilla CG, Funck RC, Rupp H. Lisinopril-mediated regression of myocardial fibrosis in patients with hypertensive heart disease. Circulation 2000;102:1388–1393.
46. Cleland J, Tendera M, Adamus J, et al. The perindopril in elderly people with chronic heart failure (PEP-CHF) study. Eur Heart J 2006;27:2338–2345.
47. Mottram PM, Haluska B, Leano R, et al. Effect of aldosterone antagonism on myocardial dysfunction in hypertensive patients with diastolic heart failure. Circulation 2004;110:558–565.
48. Roongsritong C, Sutthiwan P, Bradley J, et al. Spironolactone improves diastolic function in the elderly. Clin Cardiol 2005;28:484–487.
49. Ahmed A, Rich MW, Fleg JL, et al. Effects of digoxin on morbidity and mortality in diastolic heart failure: The ancillary digitalis investigation group trial. Circulation 2006;114:397–403.
50. Maron BJ, Towbin JA, Thiene G, et al. Contemporary definitions and classification of the cardiomyopathies: An American Heart Association Scientific Statement from the Council on Clinical Cardiology, Heart Failure and Transplantation Committee; Quality of Care and Outcomes Research and Functional Genomics and Translational Biology Interdisciplinary Working Groups; and Council on Epidemiology and Prevention. Circulation 2006;113:1807–1816.
51. Spirito P, Autore C. Management of hypertrophic cardiomyopathy. BMJ 2006;332:1251–1255.
52. Roberts R, Sigwart U. Current concepts of the pathogenesis and treatment of hypertrophic cardiomyopathy. Circulation 2005;112:293–296.
53. Poliac LC, Barron ME, Maron BJ. Hypertrophic cardiomyopathy. Anesthesiology 2006;104:183–192.

54. Wynne J, Braunwald E. The cardiomyopathies. In: Zipes DP, Libby P, Bonow RO, Braunwald E, eds. Braunwald's Heart Disease, 7th ed. Philadelphia: Elsevier Saunders, 2005:1659–1696.
55. Maron MS, Olivotto I, Betocchi S, et al. Effect of left ventricular outflow tract obstruction on clinical outcome in hypertrophic cardiomyopathy. N Engl J Med 2003;348:295–303.
56. Ho CY, Seidman CE. A contemporary approach to hypertrophic cardiomyopathy. Circulation 2006;113:e858–e862.
57. Klein GJ, Krahn AD, Skanes AC, et al. Primary prophylaxis of sudden death in hypertrophic cardiomyopathy, arrhythmogenic right ventricular cardiomyopathy, and dilated cardiomyopathy. J Cardiovasc Electrophysiol 2005;16(Suppl 1):S28–S34.
58. Maron BJ, Casey SA, Hauser RG, Aeppli DM. Clinical course of hypertrophic cardiomyopathy with survival to advanced age. J Am Coll Cardiol 2003;42:882–888.
59. Maron BJ, McKenna WJ, Danielson GK, et al. American College of Cardiology/European Society of Cardiology clinical expert consensus document on hypertrophic cardiomyopathy. A report of the American College of Cardiology Foundation Task Force on Clinical Expert Consensus Documents and the European Society of Cardiology Committee for Practice Guidelines. J Am Coll Cardiol 2003;42:1687–1713.
60. Gregoratos G, Abrams J, Epstein AE, et al. ACC/AHA/NASPE 2002 guideline update for implantation of cardiac pacemakers and antiarrhythmia devices: Summary article: A report of the American College of Cardiology/American Heart Association Task Force on Practice Guidelines (ACC/AHA/NASPE Committee to Update the 1998 Pacemaker Guidelines). Circulation 2002;106:2145–2161.
61. Maron BJ, Estes NA 3rd, Maron MS, et al. Primary prevention of sudden death as a novel treatment strategy in hypertrophic cardiomyopathy. Circulation 2003;107:2872–2875.
62. Zipes DP, Camm AJ, Borggrefe M, Buxton AE, et al. ACC/AHA/ESC 2006 guidelines for management of patients with ventricular arrhythmias and the prevention of sudden cardiac death: A report of the American College of Cardiology/American Heart Association Task Force and the European Society of Cardiology Committee for Practice Guidelines (writing committee to develop Guidelines for management of patients with ventricular arrhythmias and the prevention of sudden cardiac death): Developed in collaboration with the European Heart Rhythm Association and the Heart Rhythm Society. Circulation 2006;114:e385–e484.
63. Weller RJ, Weintraub R, Addonizio LJ, et al. Outcome of idiopathic restrictive cardiomyopathy in children. Am J Cardiol 2002;90:501–506.
64. Leya FS, Arab D, Joyal D, et al. The efficacy of brain natriuretic peptide levels in differentiating constrictive pericarditis from restrictive cardiomyopathy. J Am Coll Cardiol 2005;45:1900–1902.
65. Massie BM, Fabi MR. Clinical trials in diastolic heart failure. Prog Cardiovasc Dis 2005;47:389–395.

CHAPTER 21

Venous Thromboembolism

STUART T. HAINES, DANIEL M. WITT, AND EDITH A. NUTESCU

KEY CONCEPTS

1. The risk of venous thromboembolism (VTE) is related to several easily identifiable factors, including age, major surgery (particularly orthopedic procedures of the lower extremities), previous VTE, trauma, malignancy, and hypercoagulable states. These risks are additive.
2. The diagnosis of VTE must be confirmed by objective testing.
3. Antithrombotic therapies require meticulous and systematic monitoring as well as ongoing patient education. Well-organized anticoagulation management services improve the quality of patient care and reduce overall cost.
4. Bleeding is the most common adverse effect associated with anticoagulant drugs. A patient's risk of major hemorrhage is related to the intensity and stability of therapy, concurrent drug use, history of gastrointestinal bleeding, risk of falls, recent surgery or trauma, and age.
5. At the time of hospital admission, all patients should receive prophylaxis against venous thromboembolism that corresponds to their level of risk. Prophylaxis should be continued throughout the period of risk.
6. In the absence of contraindications, the treatment of VTE should initially include a rapid-acting anticoagulant (e.g., unfractionated heparin, low-molecular-weight heparin, or fondaparinux) overlapped with warfarin for at least 5 days and until the patient's international normalized ratio is greater than 2.0. Anticoagulation therapy should be continued for a minimum of 3 months. The duration of anticoagulation therapy should be based on the patient's risk of VTE recurrence and major bleeding.
7. Most patients with an uncomplicated deep vein thrombosis, with or without pulmonary embolism, can be safely treated as an outpatient.

Venous thromboembolism (VTE) is a potentially fatal disorder and a significant national health problem in our aging society.[1,2] Although it can strike young, otherwise healthy adults, it most frequently occurs in patients who sustain multiple trauma, undergo major surgery, are immobile for a lengthy period of time, or have a hypercoagulable disorder. Resulting from clot formation within the venous circulation (Fig. 21–1), VTE is manifested as deep vein thrombosis (DVT) and pulmonary embolism (PE). Death from PE can occur within minutes after the onset of symptoms, before effective treatment can be given.

Learning objectives, review questions, and other resources can be found at **www.pharmacotherapyonline.com.**

Unfortunately, the disease is often clinically silent, and the first manifestation may be sudden death. In some case series, 80% of patients who died suddenly had some evidence of PE at the time of autopsy.[3] Beyond the symptoms produced by the acute event, the long-term sequelae of VTE, such as the postthrombotic syndrome and recurrent thromboembolic events, also cause substantial pain and suffering.[1]

The treatment of VTE is fraught with substantial risks.[4] Antithrombotic drugs require precise dosing and meticulous monitoring.[5–7] Systematic approaches to drug therapy management substantially reduce the risks, but bleeding remains an all too common and serious complication of administering antithrombotic drugs.[7,8] Consequently, the prevention of VTE in at-risk patients is paramount to improving outcomes.[3] When there is a suspicion of VTE, the rapid and accurate diagnosis of the disorder is critical to making appropriate treatment decisions.[9] The optimal use of antithrombotic drugs requires not only an in-depth knowledge of their pharmacology and pharmacokinetic properties, but also a comprehensive approach to patient management.[5]

EPIDEMIOLOGY

The true incidence of VTE in the general population is unknown, because a substantial portion of patients, perhaps more than 50%, have clinically silent disease. An estimated 2 million people in the United States develop VTE each year; 600,000 are hospitalized, and 60,000 die.[2] The estimated annual direct medical costs of managing the disease are well over $1 billion and growing. The best available data indicate the age-adjusted annual incidence of symptomatic VTE in whites to be 117 per 100,000 population.[10] The incidence of VTE nearly doubles in each decade of life over the age of 50 years and is slightly higher in men. The age-adjusted incidence of PE has declined slightly in recent years, presumably because of heightened awareness of VTE, effective prevention strategies, early diagnosis, and prompt treatment. However, as the population ages, the total number of cases of DVT and PE continues to climb.

Relatively little is known about the risk of VTE in ethnic populations. African Americans appear to be at somewhat higher risk of VTE than are Americans of predominantly European ancestry, whereas Hispanic Americans may be at slightly lower risk.[11] Asian Americans and Pacific Islanders appear to have a strikingly low incidence of VTE.

The incidence of VTE in specific high-risk patient populations has been extensively studied.[3] Patients who sustain multiple traumas or undergo an orthopedic procedure involving a lower extremity are at particularly high risk, with the incidence of VTE often exceeding

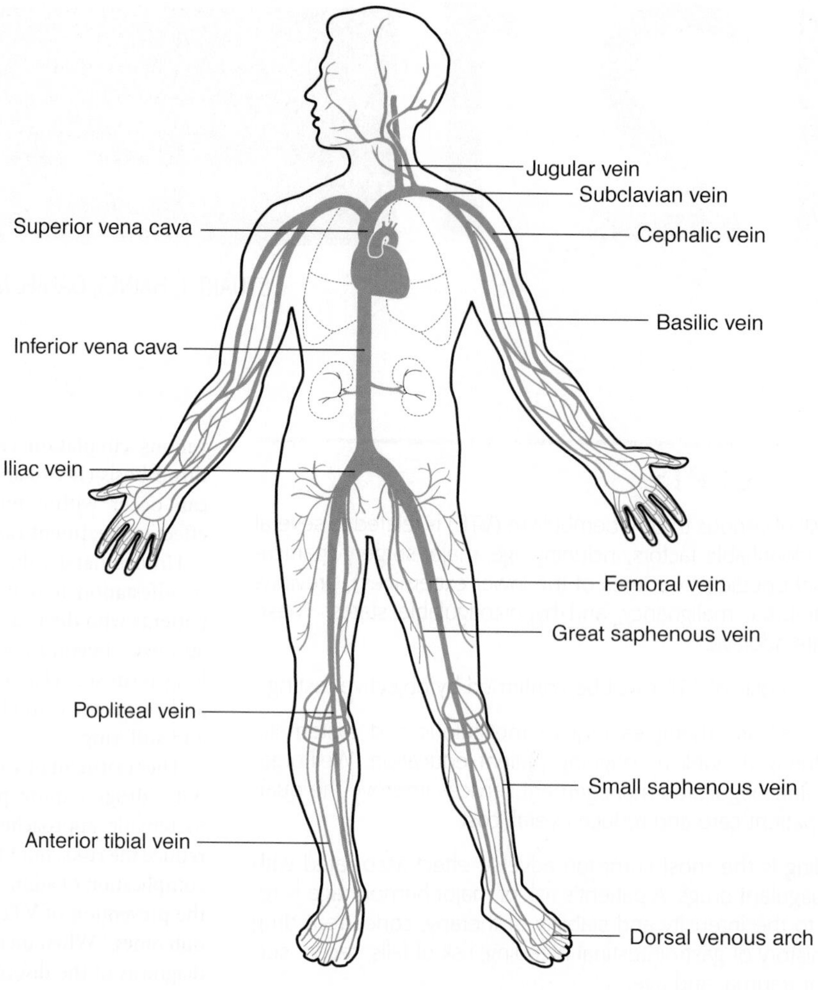

FIGURE 21-1. Venous circulation.

50% in the absence of effective prophylaxis. Among those undergoing major surgeries other than procedures involving the lower extremities, the incidence of VTE is 20% to 40% when one or more other risk factors are present, such as age older than 60 years. The long-term incidence of VTE among patients who have a prior history of VTE and who have metastatic cancer is extremely high.[12,13] Likewise, the incidence of VTE after a myocardial infarction, stroke, and spinal cord injury is high.[3] Several disorders of hypercoagulability have also been linked to a high lifetime incidence of VTE.[3,14]

ETIOLOGY

❶ A number of factors increase the risk of developing VTE (Table 21–1). These risk factors are additive and can be easily identified in clinical practice. A prior history of VTE is perhaps the strongest risk factor for recurrent VTE, presumably because of the destruction of venous valves and obstruction of blood flow caused by the initial event.[15] Rapid blood flow has an inhibitory effect on thrombus formation, but a slow rate of flow reduces the clearance and dilution of activated clotting factors in the zone of injury and slows the influx of regulatory substances. Stasis of blood tips the delicate balance of procoagulation and anticoagulation in favor of thrombogenesis. The rate of blood flow in the venous circulation, particularly in the deep veins of the lower extremities, is relatively slow. Valves in the deep veins of the legs, as well as contraction of the calf and thigh muscles, facilitate the flow of blood back to the heart and lungs; thus, damage to the venous valves and prolonged periods of immobility result in venous stasis. Vessel obstruction, either from external compression or a thrombus, also promotes clot propagation. Reduced venous blood flow explains, at least in part, why numerous medical conditions and surgical procedures are associated with an increased risk of VTE (Table 21–1). Greater-than-normal blood viscosity, seen in myeloproliferative disorders like polycythemia vera, for example, may also contribute to slowed blood flow and thrombus formation.

A growing list of hereditary deficiencies, gene mutations, and acquired diseases have been linked to hypercoagulability (see Table 21–1).[12–14] Activated protein C resistance is the most common genetic disorder of hypercoagulability, with a prevalence rate approaching 5% among community-dwelling whites, and a rate as high as 40% among those who suffer an idiopathic DVT or who have a strong family history of VTE. Although these patients have normal plasma concentrations of protein C, they often have a mutation on factor V that renders it resistant to degradation by activated protein C. This mutation is known as factor V Leiden, named after the city of Leiden, Holland, where the defect was initially reported. The prothrombin G20210A mutation also appears to be a relatively common defect, occurring in as many as 3% of healthy individuals of southern European descent and 16% of those with an idiopathic DVT. Although less common, inherited deficiencies of the natural anticoagulants protein C, protein S, and antithrombin place patients at a high lifetime risk for VTE. Conversely, excessively high concentrations of factors VIII, IX, and XI also increase the risk of VTE. Given the prevalence of these inherited abnormalities in the general population, some patients have multiple genetic defects that have additive effects in terms of increasing the lifetime thrombotic risk.

Acquired disorders of hypercoagulability may result from malignancy, the presence of antiphospholipid antibodies, and estrogen use.[12–15] The strong link between cancer and thrombosis has been recognized since the late 1800s.[13] Tumor cells secrete a number of

TABLE 21-1 Risk Factors for Venous Thromboembolism

Risk Factor	Example
Age	Risk doubles with each decade after age 50 y
History of VTE	Strongest known risk factor of DVT and PE
Venous stasis	Major medical illness (e.g., CHF, status post-MI)
	Major surgery (e.g., general anesthesia >30 minutes)
	Paralysis (e.g., status post-stroke, spinal cord injury)
	Polycythemia vera
	Obesity
	Varicose veins
Vascular injury	Major orthopedic surgery (e.g., knee and hip replacement)
	Trauma (especially fractures of the pelvis, hip, or leg)
	Indwelling venous catheters
Hypercoagulable states	Malignancy, diagnosed or occult
	Activated protein C resistance/factor V Leiden
	Prothrombin (G20210A) gene mutation
	Protein C deficiency
	Protein S deficiency
	Antithrombin deficiency
	Factor VIII excess (>90th percentile)
	Factor XI excess (>90th percentile)
	Antiphospholipid antibodies
	Dysfibrinogenemia
	Hyperhomocysteinemia
	Plasminogen activator inhibitor-1 excess
	Inflammatory bowel disease
	Nephrotic syndrome
	Pregnancy/postpartum
Drug therapy	Estrogen-containing contraception
	Estrogen replacement therapy
	Selective estrogen receptor modulators
	Heparin-induced thrombocytopenia

CHF, congestive heart failure; DVT, deep vein thrombosis; MI, myocardial infarction; PE, pulmonary embolism; VTE, venous thromboembolism.

From Geerts et al., Thomas, and Federman and Kirsner.[3,14,111]

procoagulant substances that activate the coagulation cascade. Furthermore, patients with cancer often have suppressed levels of protein C, protein S, and antithrombin. It has been postulated that cancer cells use thrombotic mechanisms to recruit a blood supply (angiogenesis), metastasize, and create a barrier against host defense mechanisms. Antiphospholipid antibodies, most commonly found in patients with autoimmune disorders such as systemic lupus erythematosus and inflammatory bowel disease, can cause venous and arterial thrombosis.[14] These antibodies are also associated with repeated pregnancy loss presumably caused by placental thrombosis. The precise mechanism by which the antiphospholipid antibodies provoke thrombosis is unclear, but they appear to activate the coagulation cascade and platelets, as well as to inhibit the anticoagulant activity of proteins C and S. Estrogen-containing contraception, estrogen replacement therapy, and the selective estrogen receptor modulators are all linked to venous thrombosis.[16] Women with an underlying disorder of hypercoagulability are at particularly high risk of developing venous thrombosis while taking estrogens. Although the mechanisms are not clearly understood, estrogens increase serum clotting factor concentrations and induce activated protein C resistance. Increased serum estrogen concentrations may explain, in part, the increased risk of VTE observed during pregnancy and the immediate postpartum period.[17]

PATHOPHYSIOLOGY

The arrest of bleeding following vascular injury (hemostasis) is essential to life.[18,19] Within the vascular system, blood remains in a fluid state, transporting oxygen, nutrients, plasma proteins, and waste. With vascular injury, a dynamic series of reactions involving a complex interplay of thrombogenic and antithrombotic stimuli result in the local formation of a hemostatic plug that seals the vessel wall and prevents further blood loss (Figs. 21–2, 21–3, and 21–4). A disruption of this delicate system of checks and balances may lead to inappropriate clot formation within the blood vessel that subsequently obstructs blood flow or embolizes to a distant vascular bed. In the late 1800s, Dr. Rudolf Virchow, a German pathologist, recognized the role played by blood vessels, circulating elements in the blood, and the speed of blood flow in the regulation of clot formation (Table 21–2). Alterations in any one of these elements, known today as Virchow's triad, may lead to pathologic clot formation.

Under normal circumstances, the endothelial cells that form the intima of vessels maintain blood flow by producing a number of substances that inhibit platelet adherence, prevent the activation of the coagulation cascade, and facilitate fibrinolysis.[18,19] Vascular injury can expose the subendothelium (see Fig. 21–3). Platelets readily adhere to the subendothelium, using glycoprotein Ib receptors found on their surfaces and facilitated by von Willebrand factor. This causes platelets to become activated, releasing a number of procoagulant substances into the local circulation that stimulate platelets to expose glycoprotein IIb/IIIa receptors. These receptors allow the platelets to adhere to one another, resulting in platelet aggregation. In addition, the damaged vascular tissue releases tissue factor, also known as tissue thromboplastin, which activates the extrinsic pathway of the coagulation cascade (see Fig. 21–4).

The coagulation cascade is a stepwise series of enzymatic reactions that result in the formation of a fibrin mesh.[18,19] Clotting factors circulate in the blood in inactive forms. Specific stimuli convert an inactive precursor into an active form that, in turn, converts the next precursor in the sequence. It was once believed that all clotting factors were proteolytic enzymes, known as zymogens. It is now known that factors V and VIII have no enzymatic activity themselves, but rather serve as cofactors that greatly accelerate the enzymatic activity of their respective partners. The final steps in the cascade are the conversion of prothrombin to thrombin and fibrinogen to fibrin. Thrombin plays a key role in the coagulation cascade; it is responsible not only for the production of fibrin, but also for the conversion of factors V and VIII to their active forms, creating a positive feedback loop that greatly accelerates the production of more thrombin. Additionally, thrombin enhances platelet aggregation through its interactions with the glycoprotein IIb/IIIa receptor.

Traditionally, the coagulation cascade has been divided into three distinct parts: the intrinsic, extrinsic, and common pathways (see Fig. 21–4).[18,19] This artificial division is somewhat misleading, as there are numerous interactions between the three pathways. The extrinsic pathway, sometimes referred to as the tissue factor pathway, appears to be the principal mechanism that triggers the coagulation cascade. Tissue factor, released from the subendothelium, forms a complex with factor VIIa. The factor VIIa–tissue factor complex activates factor X in the common pathway and factor IX in the intrinsic pathway. The intrinsic pathway plays a key role in the propagation of clot formation. The activation and inhibition of factor X in the common pathway is a key step in the regulation of clot formation. With its cofactor, factor Va, factor Xa converts prothrombin (II) to thrombin (IIa), which then cleaves fibrinogen to form fibrin monomers. Finally, as the fibrin monomers reach a critical concentration, they begin to precipitate and polymerize to form fibrin strands. Factor XIIIa covalently bonds these strands to one another.

Normally, a number of tempering mechanisms control coagulation (see Table 21–2 and Fig. 21–2).[18,19] Without effective self-regulation, the coagulation cascade would proceed unabated until all the clotting factors and platelets were consumed. The intact endothelium adjacent to the damaged tissue actively secretes several anti-

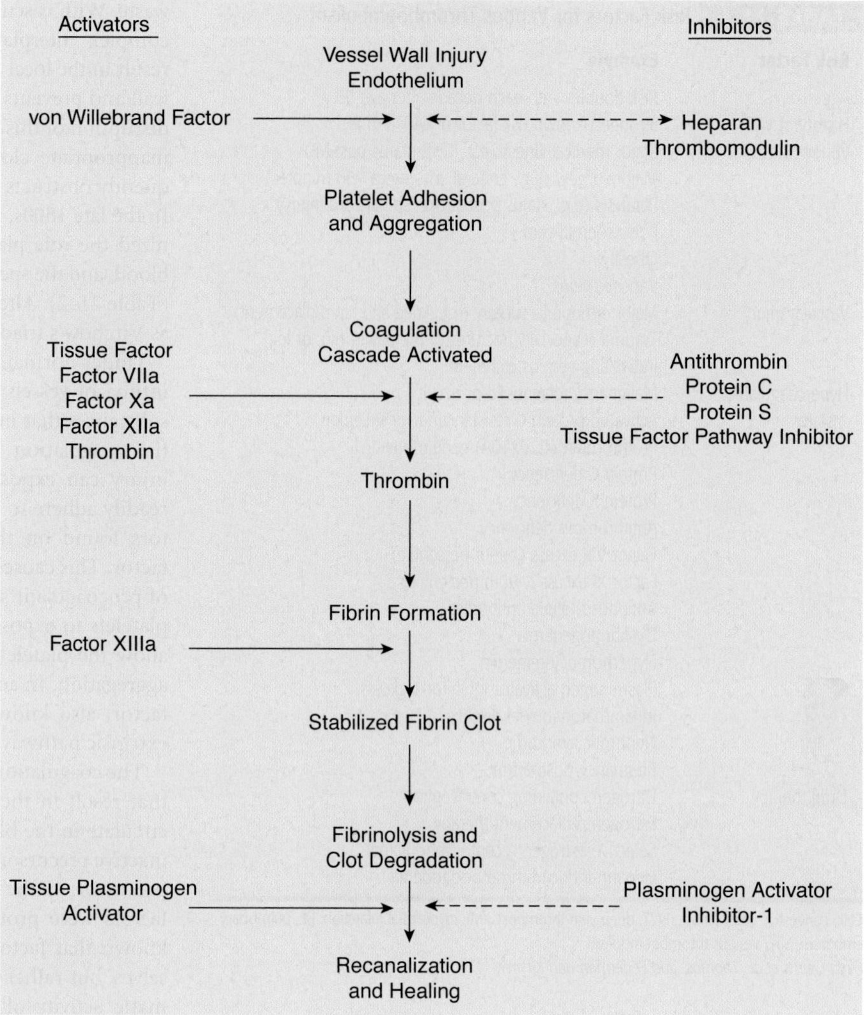

FIGURE 21-2. Hemostasis and thrombosis.

thrombotic substances. As its name implies, thrombomodulin modulates thrombin activity by converting protein C to its active form. When joined with its cofactor protein S, protein C enzymatically inactivates factors Va and VIIIa. Activated protein C also stimulates the release of tissue plasminogen activator. Antithrombin is a circulating protein that inhibits thrombin and factor Xa. Heparan sulfate, a heparin-like compound secreted by endothelial cells, exponentially accelerates antithrombin activity. By a similar mechanism, heparin cofactor II also inhibits thrombin. Tissue factor pathway inhibitor plays an important role by regulating the initiation of the coagulation cascade. When these self-regulatory mechanisms are intact, the formation of the fibrin clot is limited to the zone of tissue injury. However, disruptions in the system, so-called hypercoagulable states, often result in thrombosis.

The fibrinolytic protein plasmin degrades the fibrin mesh into soluble end products collectively known as fibrin split products or fibrin degradation products.[18,19] The fibrinolytic system is also under the control of a series of stimulatory and inhibitory substances. Tissue plasminogen activator and urokinase plasminogen activator convert plasminogen to plasmin. Plasminogen activator inhibitor-1 inhibits the plasminogen activators, and α_2-antiplasmin inhibits plasmin activity. Aberrations in the fibrinolytic system have also been linked to hypercoagulability.

CLINICAL PRESENTATION AND DIAGNOSIS

Although a thrombus can form in any part of the venous circulation, the majority begin in the lower extremities. Once formed, a venous thrombus may either (a) remain asymptomatic, (b) spontaneously lyse, (c) obstruct the venous circulation, (d) propagate into more proximal veins, (e) embolize, or (f) act in any combination of these ways.[20] The majority of patients with VTE never develop symptoms from the acute event.[21] However, even those who experience no symptoms may suffer long-term consequences, such as the postthrombotic syndrome and recurrent VTE. Even when symptoms of DVT or PE are present (Tables 21–3 and 21–4), they are nonspecific.[1] It is extremely difficult to distinguish VTE from other disorders, and additional objective tests are required to confirm or exclude the diagnosis. Patients with DVT frequently present with unilateral leg pain and swelling. The postthrombotic syndrome, a long-term complication of DVT caused by damage to the venous valves, can produce symptoms very similar to those of an acute thrombotic event including chronic lower-extremity swelling, pain, tenderness, skin discoloration, and ulceration. Symptomatic PE often produces dyspnea, tachypnea, and tachycardia. Hemoptysis, while distressing, occurs in less than one-third of patients. Cardiovascular collapse, characterized by cyanosis, shock, and oliguria, is an ominous sign.

❷ Given that VTE can be debilitating or fatal, it is important to treat it quickly and aggressively.[9] Conversely, because major bleeding induced by antithrombotic drugs can be equally harmful, it is important to avoid treatment when the diagnosis is not a reasonable certainty. Assessment of the patient's status should focus on the search for risk factors in the patient's medical history (see Table 21–1). Venous thrombosis is uncommon in the absence of risk factors, and the effects of these risks are additive. Even in the presence of mild, seemingly inconsequential symptoms, VTE should be strongly suspected in those with multiple risk factors.

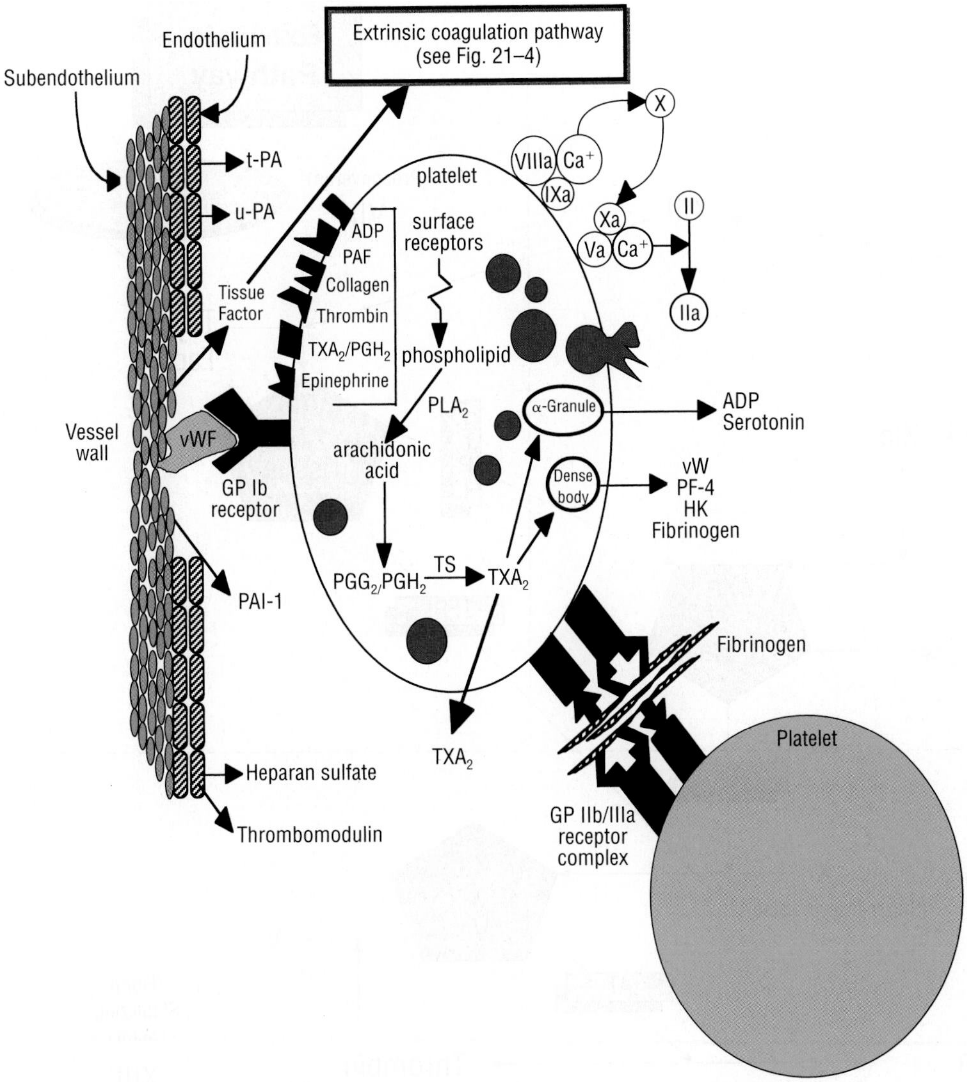

FIGURE 21-3. Vascular injury and thrombosis. (ADP, adenosine diphosphate; CO, cyclooxygenase; GP Ib, glycoprotein Ib; GP IIb/IIa, glycoprotein IIb/IIa; HK, high-molecular-weight kininogen; PAF, platelet-activating factor; PAI-1, plasminogen activator inhibitor; PF-4, platelet factor-4; PGG/PGH, prostaglandins; PGI, prostacyclin; PLA, phospholipase A; TS, thromboxane synthetase; TXA_2, thromboxane A_2; t-PA, tissue plasmogen activator; u-PA, urokinase plasmogen activator; vWF, von Willebrand factor.)

Because radiographic contrast studies are the most accurate and reliable methods for the diagnosis of VTE, they are considered the gold standards in clinical trials.[9] Contrast venography allows visualization of the entire venous system in the lower extremity and abdomen. Pulmonary angiography allows the visualization of the pulmonary arteries. The diagnosis of VTE can be made if there is a persistent intraluminal filling defect observed on multiple radiographic films. Contrast studies are expensive, invasive procedures that are technically difficult to perform and evaluate. Severely ill patients often are unable to tolerate the procedure, and many develop hypotension and cardiac arrhythmias. Furthermore, the contrast medium is irritating to vessel walls and toxic to the kidneys. For these reasons, noninvasive tests, such as ultrasonography, computed tomography scans, and the ventilation–perfusion scan, are frequently used in clinical practice for the initial evaluation of patients with suspected VTE.[1]

D-dimer is a simple blood test frequently used in the diagnostic evaluation of patients suspected to have VTE.[9] D-dimer is a degradation product of a fibrin blood clot and levels of D-dimer are significantly elevated in patients with acute thrombosis. Although the D-dimer test is a very sensitive marker of clot formation, it is not sufficiently specific. A variety of conditions can cause elevations of serum D-dimer, including recent surgery or trauma, pregnancy, and cancer. Therefore, a negative test can help to "rule out" a DVT or PE but a positive test should not be used to "rule in" the diagnosis.

Clinical assessment significantly improves the diagnostic accuracy of noninvasive tests such as ultrasonography, ventilation–perfusion scanning, and D-dimer.[1,9] Simple assessment checklists can be used to determine if a patient has a high, moderate, or low probability of a DVT or PE (Table 21–5). Patients with a high pretest probability of VTE have a greater than 60% chance of having VTE, compared with only 5% for the low pretest probability group. Clinical assessment can rule in or out the diagnosis of VTE with reasonable certainty when the results are consistent with those of a noninvasive test.[9] For example, in patients with a high or moderate pretest probability of VTE and an abnormal lower-extremity ultrasonogram, the diagnosis of VTE can be reasonably concluded. In patients with a low pretest probability of VTE and a negative D-dimer test, the diagnosis of VTE can be excluded. However, if the results of the clinical assessment and the ultrasonogram are discordant, venography should be performed to make the definitive diagnosis.

PHARMACOLOGIC AGENTS USED IN THE MANAGEMENT OF VENOUS THROMBOEMBOLISM

UNFRACTIONATED HEPARIN

Unfractionated heparin (UFH) has been used for the prevention and treatment of thrombosis for decades. Commercially available UFH preparations are derived from bovine lung or porcine intestinal mucosa. Although some differences exist between the two sources, no differences in antithrombotic activity have been demon-

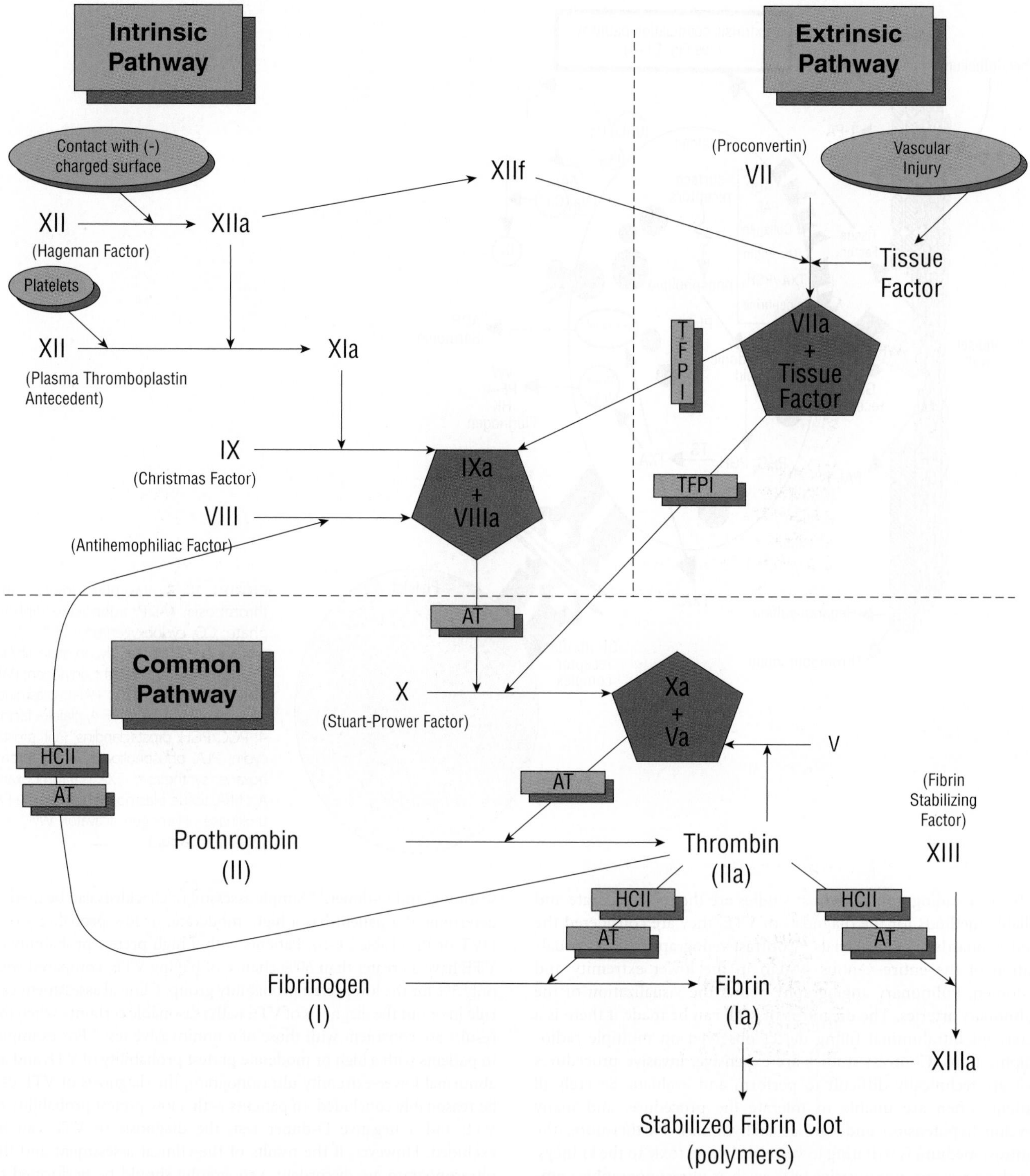

FIGURE 21-4. Coagulation cascade. (AT, antithrombin; HCII, heparin cofactor II; TFPI, tissue factor pathway inhibitor.)

strated. Today, UFH and the low-molecular-weight heparins (LMWHs) are the most commonly used therapies for the acute treatment of arterial and venous thrombosis.[22]

Pharmacology

Unfractionated heparin is a heterogeneous mixture of sulfated glycosaminoglycans of variable lengths and pharmacologic properties (Table 21–6). Each heparin molecule is composed of repetitive units of D-glycosamine and uronic acid. The molecular weight of UFH molecules ranges from 3,000 to 30,000 daltons, with a mean of 15,000 daltons. The anticoagulant profile and clearance of each UFH molecule varies based on its length. The smaller chains are cleared less rapidly than their longer counterparts.[22]

The anticoagulant effect of UFH is mediated through a specific pentasaccharide sequence on the heparin molecule that binds to antithrombin, provoking a conformational change (Fig. 21–5). Only one-third of the UFH molecules possess the unique pentasaccharide sequence with affinity for antithrombin. The UFH–antithrombin complex is 100 to 1,000 times more potent as an anticoagulant compared to antithrombin alone. Antithrombin inhibits the activity of several clotting factors including IXa, Xa,

TABLE 21-2 Factors Regulating Hemostasis and Thrombosi

	Thrombogenic	Antithrombotic
Vessel wall	Exposed subendothelium	Heparan sulfate
	Tissue factor	Dermatan sulfate
	Plasminogen activator inhibitor-1	Thrombomodulin
		Tissue plasminogen activator
		Urokinase Plasminogen Activator
Circulating elements	Platelets	Antithrombin
	Platelet activating factor	Heparin cofactor II
	The clotting factors	Protein C
	Prothrombin (factor II)	Protein S
	Fibrinogen (factor I)	Plasminogen
	von Willebrand factor	Tissue factor pathway inhibitor
	α_2-Antiplasmin	Proteolytic enzymes
Blood flow	Slow rate of flow	Fast rate of flow
	Turbulent flow	Laminar flow

XIIa, and thrombin (see Fig. 21–4). Through its action on thrombin, the UFH–antithrombin complex also inhibits the thrombin-induced activation of factors V and VIII.[22] Unfractionated heparin prevents the growth and propagation of a formed thrombus and allows the patient's own thrombolytic system to degrade the clot.

Factors IIa (thrombin) and Xa are the most sensitive to inhibition by the UFH–antithrombin complex. To inactivate thrombin, the heparin molecule must form a ternary complex bridging between antithrombin and thrombin (see Fig. 21–5). Only molecules that contain more than 18 saccharides are able to bind to both antithrombin and thrombin simultaneously. Smaller heparin molecules cannot facilitate the interaction between antithrombin and thrombin. In contrast, the inactivation of factor Xa does not require UFH to form a bridge with antithrombin. It only requires that UFH bind to antithrombin using the specific pentasaccharide sequence. Heparin molecules with as few as 5 saccharide units are able to catalyze the

TABLE 21-3 Clinical Presentation of Deep Vein Thrombosis

General

Venous thromboembolism most commonly develops in patients with identifiable risk factors (see Table 21–2) during or following a hospitalization. Many, perhaps the majority, of patients have asymptomatic disease. Patients may die suddenly of pulmonary embolism.

Symptoms

The patient may complain of leg swelling, pain, or warmth. Symptoms are nonspecific and objective testing must be performed to establish the diagnosis.

Signs

The patient's superficial veins may be dilated and a "palpable cord" may be felt in the affected leg.

The patient may experience pain in back of the knee when the examiner dorsiflexes the foot of the affected leg (known as Homans sign).

Laboratory tests

Serum concentrations of D-dimer, a byproduct of thrombin generation, is usually elevated.

The patient may have an elevated erythrocyte sedimentation rate and white blood cell count.

Diagnostic tests

Duplex ultrasonography is the most commonly used test to diagnosis deep vein thrombosis. It is a noninvasive test that can measure the rate and direction of blood flow and visualize clot formation in proximal veins of the legs. It cannot reliably detect small blood clots in distal veins. Coupled with a careful clinical assessment, it can rule in or out the diagnosis in the majority of cases.

Venography (also known as phlebography) is the gold standard for the diagnosis of deep vein thrombosis. However, it is an invasive test that involves injection of radiopaque contrast dye into a foot vein. It is expensive and can cause anaphylaxis and nephrotoxicity.

TABLE 21-4 Clinical Presentation of Pulmonary Embolism

General

Pulmonary embolism (PE) most commonly develops in patients with risk factors for venous thromboembolism (see Table 21–2) during or following a hospitalization. Although many patients develop a symptomatic deep vein thrombosis prior to developing a PE, many do not. Patients may die suddenly before effective treatment can be initiated.

Symptoms

The patient may complain of cough, chest pain, chest tightness, shortness of breath, or palpitation. The patient may spit or cough up blood (hemoptysis). When PE is massive, the patient may complain of dizziness or lightheadedness. Symptoms may be confused for a myocardial infarction, requiring objective testing to establish the diagnosis.

Signs

The patient may have tachypnea (increased respiratory rate) and tachycardia (increased heart rate). The patient may appear diaphoretic (sweaty). The patient's neck veins may be distended. In massive PE, the patient may appear cyanotic and may become hypotensive. In such cases, oxygen saturation by pulse oximetry or arterial blood gas will likely indicate that the patient is hypoxic. In the worse cases, the patient may go into circulatory shock and die within minutes.

Laboratory tests

Serum concentrations of D-dimer, a byproduct of thrombin generation, is usually elevated.

The patient may have an elevated erythrocyte sedimentation rate and white blood cell count.

Diagnostic tests

Ventilation–perfusion (V/Q) and computerized tomography (CT) scans are the most commonly used tests to diagnosis PE. A V/Q scan measures the distribution of blood and air flow in the lungs. When there is a large mismatch between blood and air flow in one area of the lung, there is a high probability that the patient has a PE. Spiral CT scans can detect emboli in the pulmonary arteries.

Pulmonary angiography is the gold standard for the diagnosis of PE. However, it is an invasive test that involves injection of radiopaque contrast dye into the pulmonary artery. The test is expensive and associated with a significant risk of mortality.

TABLE 21-5 Clinical Assessment Models for Deep Vein Thrombosis and Pulmonary Embolism

Pretest Probability of Deep Vein Thrombosis

Clinical feature	Score
Tenderness along entire deep vein system	1.0
Swelling of the entire leg	1.0
Greater than 3 cm difference in calf circumference	1.0
Pitting edema	1.0
Collateral superficial veins	1.0
Risk factors present:	
Active cancer	1.0
Prolonged immobility or paralysis	1.0
Recent surgery or major medical illness	1.0
Alternative diagnosis likely (ruptured Baker cyst, rheumatoid arthritis, superficial thrombophlebitis, or infective cellulitis)	−2.0

Score ≥3 = high probability; 1–2 = moderate probability; ≤0 = low probability

Pretest Probability of Pulmonary Embolism

Clinical feature	Score
Deep vein thrombosis suspected	
Clinical features of deep vein thrombosis	3.0
Recent prolonged immobility or surgery	1.5
Active cancer	1.0
History of deep vein thrombosis or pulmonary embolism	1.5
Hemoptysis	1.0
Resting heart rate >100 beats/min	1.5
No alternative explanation for acute shortness of breath or chest pain	3.0

Score ≥6 = high probability; 2–6 = moderate probability; ≤1.5 = low probability

From Wells et al.[9]

TABLE 21-6 Comparison of the Chemical and Pharmacokinetic Properties of Antithrombotic Drugs Used for Venous Thrombosis

Agent	FDA-Approved	Method of Preparation	Mean Molecular Weight (Daltons)	Plasma Half-Life	Anti-Xa: Anti-IIa Activity	Bioavailability
Unfractionated heparin	Yes	Extracted from porcine gut mucosa or beef lung	≈15,000	30–90 min (dose dependent)	1:1	SC: 30–70% (dose dependent)
Low molecular weight heparins						
Ardeparin (Normiflo)	Yes (no longer marketed in U.S.)	Peroxidative depolymerization	≈6,000	200 min	1.9:1	SC: 90%
Dalteparin (Fragmin)	Yes	Nitrous acid depolymerization	≈6,000	119–139 min	2.7:1	SC: 87%
Enoxaparin (Lovenox)	Yes	Benzoylation and alkaline depolymerization	≈4,200	129–180 min	3.8:1	SC: 92%
Nadroparin (Fraxiparine)	No (Available in Canada and Mexico)	Nitrous acid depolymerization	≈4,500	132–162 min	3.6:1	SC: 99%
Tinzaparin (Innohep)	Yes	Heparinase digestion	≈4,500	111–234 min	2.8:1	SC: 90%
Heparinoid						
Danaparoid (Orgaran)	Yes (no longer marketed in U.S.)	Extracted from porcine gut mucosa	≈6,500	22–24 h	20:1	SC: 95%
Anti–factor Xa inhibitors						
Fondaparinux (Arixtra)	Yes	Synthetic	1,728	15–18 h	100% anti-Xa	SC: 100%
Idraparinux (SanOrg 34006)	No	Synthetic	≈1,700	≈80 h	100% anti-Xa	SC: 100%
Direct thrombin inhibitors						
Argatroban (Argatroban)	Yes	Synthetic	509	30–50 min	100% anti-IIa	
Bivalirudin (Angiomax)	Yes	Semisynthetic	2,180	25 min	100% anti-IIa	
Desirudin (Iprivask)	Yes	Recombinant DNA technology	6,964	120 min	100% anti-IIa	SC: >90%
Lepirudin (Refludan)	Yes	Recombinant DNA technology	6,980	80 min	100% anti-IIa	SC: 70%
Dabigatran	No	Synthetic	471	14 h	100% anti-IIa	Oral: 7%
Vitamin K antagonists						
Warfarin (Coumadin)	Yes	Synthetic	330	40 h	1:1	Oral: 90–100%

SC, subcutaneous.

From Haines and Bussey and Nutescu et al.[19,46]

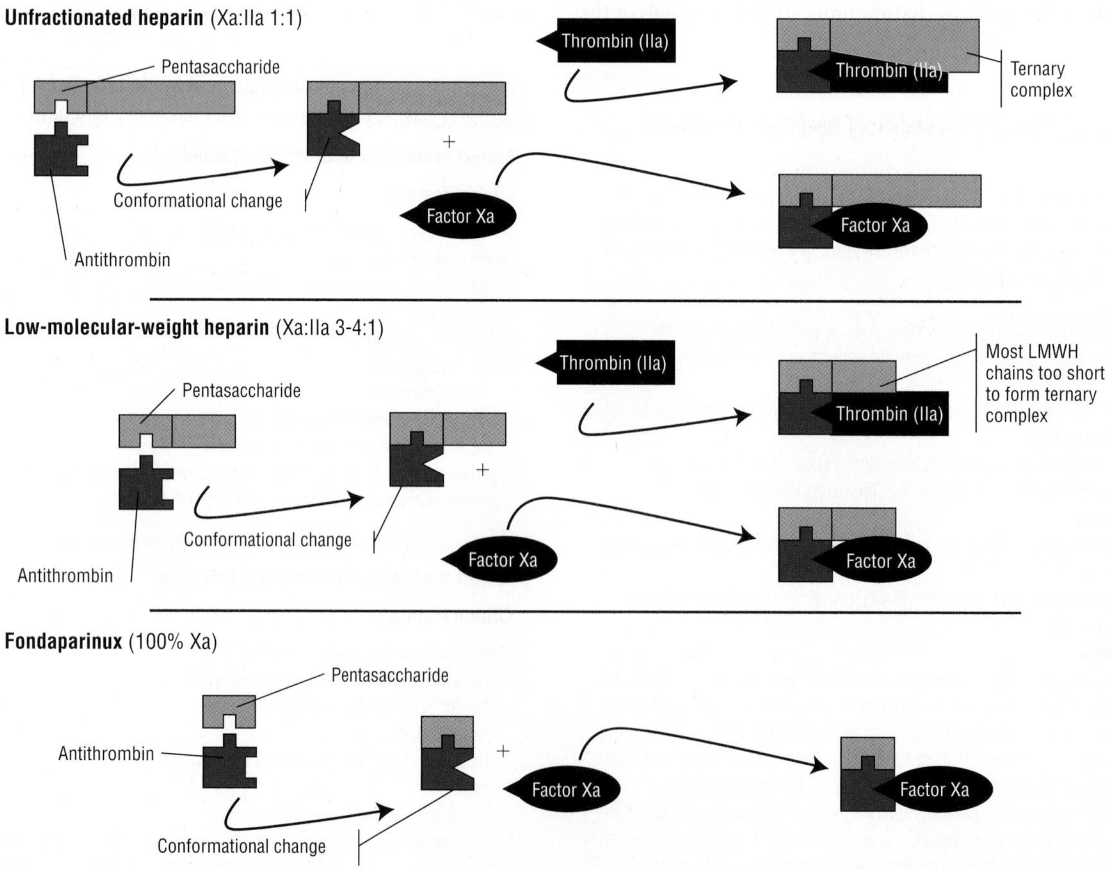

FIGURE 21-5. Pharmacologic activity of unfractionated heparin, low-molecular-weight heparins (LMWHs), and fondaparinux.

inhibition of factor Xa. Heparin uncouples from antithrombin after it has produced its effect and quickly recouples with another antithrombin molecule. Because of its relatively large size, the UFH–antithrombin complex is incapable of inactivating thrombin or factor Xa within a formed clot or bound to surfaces. At high doses, UFH also binds to heparin cofactor II, further inhibiting the activity of thrombin. UFH increases the release of tissue factor pathway inhibitor from vascular endothelium, augmenting its inhibitory effect on factor Xa. UFH, especially high-molecular-weight heparin fractions, also binds to platelets and inhibits platelet aggregation.[22]

Pharmacokinetics

Unfractionated heparin is not reliably absorbed when taken orally as a result of its large molecular size and anionic structure. The bioavailability and biologic activity of UFH is limited by its propensity to bind to plasma proteins, platelet factor-4 (PF-4), macrophages, fibrinogen, lipoproteins, and endothelial cells.[22] This may explain the substantial inter- and intrapatient variability observed in the anticoagulation response to UFH.[22]

The subcutaneous bioavailability of UFH is dose dependent and ranges from 30% at low doses to as much as 70% at high doses. Higher doses presumably saturate protein-binding sites, thereby permitting a larger proportion to reach the systemic circulation. The onset of anticoagulant effect is usually evident 1 to 2 hours after subcutaneous injection and peaks at 3 hours.[22] When UFH is administered via the IV route, a continuous infusion is preferable. Intermittent IV boluses produce relatively high peaks in anticoagulation activity and have been associated with a greater risk of major bleeding.[22] Intramuscular administration is discouraged because of erratic absorption and risk of large hematoma formation.

Unfractionated heparin has a dose-dependent half-life of approximately 30 to 90 minutes, but may be prolonged to as much as 150 minutes when given in high doses to some patients. There are two primary mechanisms for the elimination of UFH. The relative contribution of each mechanism to the total clearance of heparin is related to the dose and size of the UFH molecules. One mechanism is a rapid, but saturable zero-order process. Heparinases and desulfatases enzymatically inactivate heparin molecules bound to endothelial cells and macrophages, reducing them to smaller and less-sulfated molecules. Heparin is also eliminated renally. This first-order process is slower and nonsaturable. Low doses of UFH are cleared principally by the saturable, rapid, zero-order mechanism, whereas the renal route predominates at very high doses. With typical therapeutic regimens, a combination of the two mechanisms are used to eliminate UFH with the saturable mechanism predominating. Renal and hepatic dysfunction reduces the rate of clearance of UFH. Patients with active thrombosis may eliminate UFH more rapidly, possibly because of increased binding to acute phase reactants.[22]

Dose and Administration

The dose and route of administration for UFH are based on the indication, the therapeutic goals, and the patient's individual response to therapy. The dose of UFH is expressed in units of activity. The number of units per milligram is variable and depends on the manufacturing process. For the prevention of VTE, UFH is given by subcutaneous injection in the abdominal fat layer over the iliac crest. The typical dose for prophylaxis is 5,000 units every 8 to 12 hours. When immediate and full anticoagulation is required, a weight-based IV bolus dose followed by a continuous infusion is preferred (Table 21–7).[22] Subcutaneous UFH (initial dose of 333 units/kg followed by 250 units/kg every 12 hours) also provides adequate therapeutic anticoagulation for the treatment of acute VTE.[23]

TABLE 21-7 Weight-Based[a] Dosing for Unfractionated Heparin Administered by Continuous Intravenous Infusion

Indication	Initial Loading Dose	Initial Infusion Rate
Deep venous thrombosis/pulmonary embolism	80–100 units/kg	17–20 units/kg/h
	Maximum = 10,000 units	Maximum = 2,300 units/h
Activated Partial Thromboplastin Time (seconds)	**Maintenance Infusion Rate**	
	Dose adjustment	
<37 (or >12 s below institution-specific therapeutic range)	80 units/kg bolus then increase infusion by 4 units/kg/h	
37–47 (or 1–12 s below institution-specific therapeutic range)	40 units/kg bolus then increase infusion by 2 units/kg/h	
48–71 (within institution-specific therapeutic range)	No change	
72–93 (or 1–22 s above institution-specific therapeutic range)	Decrease infusion by 2 units/kg/h	
>93 (or >22 s above institution-specific therapeutic range)	Hold infusion for 1 h then decrease by 3 units/kg/h	

[a]Use actual body weight for all calculations. Adjusted body weight may be used for obese patients (>130% of ideal body weight).

From Hirsh and Raschke.[22]

Therapeutic Monitoring

❸ Administration of UFH has traditionally required close monitoring because of the unpredictable anticoagulant patient response.[22] Several tests are available to monitor UFH therapy including whole blood clotting time, activated partial thromboplastin time (aPTT), activated clotting time (ACT), antifactor Xa activity, and plasma heparin concentrations. The aPTT is the most widely used test to determine the degree of anticoagulation. The therapeutic range of aPTT has traditionally been considered to be 1.5 to 2.5 times the mean normal control value.[22] Many currently available aPTT reagents do not accurately measure the response to heparin within this fixed therapeutic range; thus, the use of a fixed aPTT therapeutic range of 1.5 to 2.5 times the control represents a subtherapeutic dose of UFH in many instances.[22] Because of substantial interlaboratory variability in the aPTT, an institution-specific aPTT therapeutic range that correlates with a plasma heparin concentration of 0.3 to 0.7 units/mL by an amidolytic antifactor Xa assay should be established.[22]

Although most experts advocate using the aPTT to monitor UFH provided that institution-specific therapeutic ranges are defined, the use of aPTT has several limitations. First, preanalytical variables such as reagent sensitivity, temperature, phlebotomy methods, and hemodilution may result in aPTT results that do not correlate with the in vivo level of heparin anticoagulation present.[22] Second, the aPTT response exhibits diurnal variation, with a peak response occurring around 3 AM during continuous IV infusion. Adjusting infusion rates in response to this diurnal variation could lead to subsequent over- or underdosing.[24] Third, the aPTT is prolonged beyond measurable limits when the heparin concentration exceeds 1 unit/mL; consequently, the aPTT is unsuitable for monitoring heparin therapy in patients who require doses of heparin that will produce serum concentrations >1 unit/mL. The ACT is the most suitable assay when high doses of heparin are used, especially during coronary angioplasty or coronary bypass surgery.[25] Fourth, the lower-weight heparin fragments accumulate but have little effect on the aPTT in vivo.[22] Lastly, the data supporting the currently recommended heparin concentration therapeutic range is not derived from scientifically rigorous research.

The aPTT should be measured prior to the initiation of therapy to determine the patient's baseline. When administered by IV

TABLE 21-8 Risk Factors for Major Bleeding While Taking Anticoagulation Therapy

Anticoagulation intensity (e.g., international normalized ratio >4.0)
Initiation of therapy (first few days and weeks)
Unstable anticoagulation response
Age >65 years
Concurrent antiplatelet drug use
Concurrent nonsteroidal antiinflammatory drug use
History of gastrointestinal bleeding
Recent surgery or trauma
High risk for fall/trauma
Heavy alcohol use
Renal failure
Cerebrovascular disease
Malignancy

Data from Levine MN, Raskob G, Beyth RJ, et al. Hemorrhagic complications of anticoagulant treatment: The Seventh ACCP Conference on Antithrombotic and Thrombolytic Therapy. Chest 2004;126:287S–310S.

TABLE 21-9 Contraindications to Anticoagulation Therapy

General
Active bleeding
Hemophilia or other hemorrhagic tendencies
Severe liver disease with elevated baseline PT
Severe thrombocytopenia (platelet count <20,000)
Malignant hypertension
Inability to meticulously supervise and monitor treatment
Product-specific contraindications
Argatroban
Hypersensitivity to argatroban
Bivalirudin
Hypersensitivity to bivalirubin
Fondaparinux
Hypersensitivity to fondaparinux
Severe renal insufficiency (creatinine clearance <30 mL/min)
Body weight <50 kg
Bacterial endocarditis
Thrombocytopenia with a positive in vitro test for anti-platelet antibodies in the presence of fondaparinux
Lepirudin
Hypersensitivity to hirudins
LMWHs
Hypersensitivity to LMWH, UFH, pork products, methylparaben, or propylparaben
History of HIT or suspected HIT
UFH
Hypersensitivity to UFH
History of HIT
Warfarin
Hypersensitivity to warfarin
Pregnancy
History of warfarin-induced skin necrosis
Inability to obtain followup PT/INR measurements
Inappropriate medication use or lifestyle behaviors

HIT, heparin-induced thrombocytopenia; INR, international normalized ratio; LMWH, low-molecular-weight heparin; PT, prothrombin time; UFH, unfractionated heparin.

infusion, the response to therapy should be measured 6 hours after the initiation of therapy or a dose change. This is usually sufficient time for heparin to reach steady state. The dose of heparin should be promptly adjusted based on the patient's response and the institution-specific therapeutic range (see Table 21–7).[22]

Some patients with acute VTE and myocardial infarction have a diminished response to UFH (so-called heparin resistance), presumably because of variations in the plasma concentrations of heparin-binding proteins. Some patients are reported to have acute elevations in factor VIII, preventing the prolongation of the aPTT by UFH. In some cases, antithrombin deficiency might be the culprit. The possibility of this phenomenon should be suspected in patients who require more than 40,000 units of UFH per 24-hour period. The recommended management of patients with "heparin resistance" is to adjust the UFH dose based on antifactor Xa concentrations.[22]

Adverse Effects

❹ Bleeding is the primary adverse effect associated with all anticoagulant drugs (Table 21–8).[4] There is not solid evidence linking supratherapeutic aPTT values and the risk for bleeding in patients receiving UFH. The risk for bleeding is more closely related to underlying risk factors than to high aPTT values.[24] Therefore, UFH should not be administered to patients with contraindications to anticoagulation therapy (Table 21–9). Low-dose subcutaneous UFH is associated with a minimal risk of major bleeding. The rates of major bleeding for patients with VTE receiving full therapeutic doses of UFH via IV infusion for 5 to 10 days range from 2% to 4% and the rate of fatal bleeding ranges from approximately 0% to 2%.[4] The presence of concomitant bleeding risks such as thrombocytopenia, the use other antithrombotic therapy, and a preexisting source of bleeding increase the risk of UFH-induced hemorrhage. The risk of bleeding also increases with age. Recent surgery, hemostatic defects, heavy alcohol consumption, renal failure, peptic ulcers, and neoplasms also increase the risk of major bleeding while receiving UFH.[4]

Anatomic sites commonly associated with UFH-related bleeding include the gastrointestinal and urinary tracts, as well as soft tissues. Minor bleeding, such as epistaxis, gingival bleeding, and prolonged bleeding from cuts and scrapes, is frequently reported. Bruising from minor trauma and at the sites of subcutaneous injections and venous access is also common. Local irritation, mild pain, erythema, histamine-like reactions, and hematoma can occur during UFH administration. Even small amounts of bleeding into critical sites such as the central nervous system (CNS) or the structures of the eye can cause catastrophic consequences.

Thrombocytopenia, defined as a platelet count less than 150,000, is common with UFH therapy.[26] Up to 30% of patients have some appreciable decline in their platelet count. Two distinct clinical presentations for thrombocytopenia can occur during heparin therapy. Heparin-associated thrombocytopenia (HAT) is a benign, transient, and mild phenomena, generally occurring within the first few days of treatment in the heparin-naive patient. Platelet counts rarely drop below 100,000 in patients with HAT, and recover with continued therapy. Conversely, heparin-induced thrombocytopenia (HIT) is a serious drug-induced problem requiring immediate intervention (see Heparin-Induced Thrombocytopenia below). A baseline platelet count should be obtained before UFH therapy is initiated. If the patient has received UFH within the previous 100 days, or if previous UFH exposure is uncertain, a repeat platelet count should be performed within 24 hours.[26] Monitoring platelet counts every other day for 14 days or until UFH therapy is stopped, whichever occurs first, is recommended for patients who are receiving therapeutic doses of UFH.[26]

Long-term UFH has been reported to cause alopecia, priapism, and suppressed aldosterone synthesis with subsequent hyperkalemia. The use of UFH in doses ≥20,000 units/day for more than 6 months, especially during pregnancy, is associated with significant bone loss and may lead to osteoporosis.[24] Few drug interactions are reported with UFH. Concurrent use with other antithrombotic drugs, thrombolytics, and antiplatelet agents increases the risk of bleeding, however.

Management of Bleeding and Excessive Anticoagulation

Hemorrhage can occur at any site in patients receiving UFH and close monitoring for signs and symptoms of bleeding is crucial.[4,22]

In addition to an appropriate coagulation study to measure the response to UFH, it is necessary to regularly monitor hemoglobin, hematocrit, and blood pressure. Bleeding can produce a wide variety of symptoms, depending on the site of hemorrhage. Symptoms can include severe headache, joint pain, chest pain, abdominal pain, swelling, tarry stools, frank hematuria, or the passage of bright red blood through the rectum. Life-threatening bleeding, either as a consequence of a significant volume loss or because of the location (e.g., bleeding into a critical space), must be recognized swiftly and immediately treated. Critical areas include intracranial, pericardial, and intraocular sites, as well as the adrenal glands.

When major bleeding occurs, UFH should be immediately discontinued and the underlying source of bleeding should be identified and treated. Intravenous protamine sulfate, given in a dose of 1 mg per 100 units of UFH up to a maximum of 50 mg, can be administered to reverse the anticoagulant effects of UFH. Protamine sulfate has intrinsic anticoagulation activity, but when administered with UFH, it forms a stable salt that results in the loss of anticoagulation activity of both drugs. Protamine sulfate neutralizes UFH in 5 minutes, and its activity persists for 2 hours. It should be given by slow IV infusion over 10 minutes.[22] In cases of large heparin overdoses or in patients with renal failure, a "rebound" effect may occur with a return of some anticoagulant activity several hours after the administration of protamine sulfate. Therefore, the patient's coagulation status should be closely monitored. Multiple doses of protamine sulfate may be necessary if hemorrhage continues.

Use in Special Populations

Heparin-related compounds such as UFH or LMWH are the anticoagulants of choice during pregnancy.[27] Because UFH does not cross the placenta, it is not associated with teratogenicity or fetal bleeding complications.[27] UFH should be used cautiously during the last trimester of pregnancy and the peripartum period because of the risk of maternal hemorrhage. Induction of labor is advisable so that UFH can be discontinued prior to delivery to minimize the risk for excessive bleeding during delivery. Long-term use of UFH during pregnancy may result in bone loss and increased risk for osteoporosis-related fractures.[27] Unfractionated heparin is not excreted in breast milk and is considered safe to use by women who are breast-feeding.[27]

Advances in tertiary care for pediatric patients have resulted in increasing numbers of children requiring antithrombotic therapy, and UFH is commonly used in this setting.[28] For the treatment of acute thrombosis in children, the dosage of UFH is an initial loading dose of 75 to 100 units/kg over 10 minutes followed by a maintenance dose of 28 units/kg/h for infants up to 12 months of age and 20 units/kg/h for children 1 year old and older.[28]

LOW-MOLECULAR-WEIGHT HEPARINS

Produced by either chemical or enzymatic depolymerization (see Table 21–6), LMWHs are fragments of UFH. They are heterogeneous mixtures of sulfated glycosaminoglycans with approximately one-third the molecular weight of UFH. Although all the LMWHs share similarities in their mechanisms of action with UFH, their molecular weight distributions vary, resulting in differences in their activity against factor Xa and thrombin, affinity for plasma proteins, propensity to release tissue factor pathway inhibitor, and duration of activity.[22] The mean molecular weight of the LMWHs is product specific. These agents have several advantages over UFH, including (a) predictable anticoagulation dose response, (b) improved subcutaneous bioavailability, (c) dose-independent clearance, (d) longer biologic half-life, (e) lower incidence of thrombocytopenia, and (f) a reduced need for routine laboratory monitoring.[22]

Currently, there are three LMWH products available in the United States. The usefulness of LMWHs has been extensively evaluated for a wide array of indications, including the treatment of acute coronary syndromes, DVT, and PE, as well as for the prevention of VTE in several high-risk populations. The FDA-approved indications and doses for the LMWHs are product specific (Table 21–10). The

TABLE 21-10 Indications and Doses for Low-Molecular-Weight Heparins

Indications	Enoxaparin	Dalteparin	Tinzaparin
Hip-replacement surgery (prophylaxis)	30 mg SC q 12 h initiated 12–24 h after surgery *or* 40 mg SC q 24 h initiated 12 h prior to surgery[a] Extended prophylaxis may be given for up to 3 weeks[a]	2,500 units SC given 2 h prior to surgery, followed by 2,500 international units the evening after surgery and at least 6 h after first dose, then 5,000 international units SC q 24 h[a] *or* 5,000 international units SC q 24 h initiated the evening prior to surgery[a]	75 units/kg SC q 24 h initiated the evening prior to surgery or 12 h after surgery *or* 4,500 unit SC q 24 h initiated 12 h prior to surgery
Knee-replacement surgery (prophylaxis)	30 mg SC q 12 h initiated 12–24 h prior to surgery[a]		75 units/kg SC q 24 h initiated the evening prior to surgery or 12 h after surgery
Abdominal surgery (prophylaxis)	40 mg SC q 24 h initiated 2 h prior to surgery[a]	2,500 units SC q 24 h initiated 1–2 h prior to surgery[a] Patients with malignancy: 5,000 units SC the evening prior surgery then 5,000 units SC q 24 h[a] *or* 2,500 units SC 1–2 h prior to surgery then 2,500 units 12 h after surgery followed by 5,000 units SC q 24 h[a]	3,500 unit SC q 24 h initiated 1–2 h prior to surgery
Acute medical illness (prophylaxis)	40 mg SC q 24 h[a]	2,500 units SC q 24 h	
Trauma (prophylaxis)	30 mg SC q 12 h starting 12–36 h after injury		
Deep vein thrombosis treatment (with or without pulmonary embolism)	1 mg/kg SC q 12 h[a] *or* 1.5 mg/kg SC q 24 h[a]	100 units/kg SC q 12 h *or* 200 units/kg SC q 24 h	175 units/kg SC q 24 h[a]
Unstable angina or non–Q-wave myocardial infarction	1 mg/kg SC q 12 h[a]	100 units/kg SC q 12 h[a] (maximum dose 10,000 units)	

[a]FDA approved dose for indication.
Data from Geerts WH, Pineo GF, Heit JA, et al. Prevention of venous thromboembolism. ACCP Conference on Antithrombotic and Thrombolytic Therapy. Chest 2004;126:338S–400S.[3]

LMWHs have largely replaced UFH for the prevention and treatment of VTE in some hospitals. However, institutional resources and individual patient needs should determine their precise role in the management of VTE.

Pharmacology

The LMWHs prevent the growth and propagation of formed thrombi. Like UFH, the LMWHs enhance and accelerate the activity of antithrombin through binding to a specific pentasaccharide sequence. Fewer than one-third of LMWH molecules contain the specific sequence necessary to interact with antithrombin. The principal difference in the pharmacologic activity of the LMWHs and UFH is their relative inhibition of factor Xa and thrombin. Because of their smaller chain length, the LMWHs have limited activity against thrombin (see Fig. 21–6). Fewer than 50% of the LMWH molecules have the requisite chain length to simultaneously bind antithrombin and thrombin. For this reason, the LMWHs have proportionally greater antifactor Xa activity. The ratio of antifactor Xa-to-IIa activity varies between 5.3:1 and 1.9:1. By comparison, UFH has an antifactor Xa-to-IIa activity ratio of 1:1. Like UFH, the LMWHs cause the endothelium to release tissue factor pathway inhibitor, which is believed to enhance the inhibition of factor Xa and to inactivate factor VIIa.[22]

Pharmacokinetics

Compared with UFH, the LMWHs have a more predictable anticoagulation response. The improved pharmacokinetic profile of LMWHs is the result of reduced binding to proteins and cells.[22] The bioavailability of LMWHs approaches 100% when administered subcutaneously, whereas the absorption of UFH is relatively poor and erratic. The subcutaneous bioavailability of the available LMWH products differs only slightly. The peak anticoagulation effect is seen in 3 to 5 hours.[22]

The renal route is the predominant mode of elimination for the LMWHs. Consequently, their biologic half-life may be prolonged in patients with renal impairment. Longer heparin chains bind to macrophages and are rapidly degraded. Therefore, antifactor Xa activity, which is mediated by smaller heparin molecules, persists longer than antithrombin activity. The plasma half-life of the LMWH preparations is two to four times longer than UFH. The clearance of LMWHs is independent of dose.[22]

Dosing and Administration

The LMWHs are given in fixed or weight-based doses based on the product and indication (see Table 21–10).[22] Doses should be based on actual body weight and studies in obese patients indicate that full weight-based doses do not lead to elevated LMWH concentrations when compared with normal subjects; consequently, capping of the dose is not recommended.[24] The dose for enoxaparin is expressed in milligrams, whereas dalteparin and tinzaparin are expressed in units of antifactor Xa activity. Although they can be given by continuous intravenous infusion, the LMWHs are generally given by subcutaneous injection in the abdominal area or the upper outer part of the thigh while the patient is in a supine position. The clinician or patient pinches a layer of skin between the thumb and forefinger, and then introduces the entire length of the needle into a skin fold at a 90° angle. Injection sites should be alternated between right and left sides. Following subcutaneous administration, the drug is absorbed slowly, resulting in sustained antithrombotic activity over several hours.

The dosing interval for the LMWHs is every 12 or 24 hours depending on the indication and product. Larger doses are given once daily and produce significantly higher peak plasma concentrations. Given that the elimination half-life of the LMWHs is prolonged in patients with severe renal impairment, high doses may lead to a significant accumulation in these patients. The enoxaparin dose should be reduced and the dosing interval extended to once daily in patients with creatinine clearance <30 mL/min.[29] The pharmacokinetics of dalteparin and tinzaparin are less-well characterized in patients with renal insufficiency, but some studies suggest that there is a lower degree of accumulation. Data on the use of LMWH in patients with end-stage renal disease receiving hemodialysis is very limited, thus UFH should be recommended for these patients. Given that few published data are available regarding the use of LMWHs in the setting of renal insufficiency, some experts recommend measuring antifactor Xa activity if therapy is continued for more than a few days.

For the prevention of VTE, the LMWHs have been studied in a variety of high-risk circumstances, including orthopedic surgery, abdominal surgery, acute spinal cord injury, neurosurgery, multiple trauma, and critical illness.[3] The effectiveness of the LMWHs has been extensively evaluated for the treatment of VTE in hospitalized patients and used in the outpatient management of DVT.[2] They are also a reasonable alternative to warfarin therapy in circumstances when a prothrombin time (PT)/international normalized ratio (INR) can not be routinely obtained.

Therapeutic Monitoring

Because the LMWHs achieve predictable anticoagulant response when given subcutaneously, routine laboratory monitoring is unnecessary to guide the dosing of these agents. The PT, the ACT, and the aPTT are minimally affected by LMWHs.[22] Prior to initiation of LMWH, a baseline PT/INR, aPTT, complete blood cell count with platelet count, and serum creatinine should be obtained. Most experts recommend monitoring the complete blood cell count every 5 to 10 days during the first 2 weeks of LMWH therapy and every 2 to 4 weeks thereafter.

Although several methods to monitor LMWHs have been explored, measurement of antifactor Xa activity has been the most widely used method in clinical practice. Routine antifactor Xa activity measurement is unnecessary in patients whose condition is stable and uncomplicated.[22] Although very limited data support the use of laboratory monitoring to guide LMWH therapy, measuring antifactor Xa activity may be helpful in patients who have significant renal impairment (e.g., creatinine clearance <30 mL/min), weigh less than 50 kg, are morbidly obese, or require prolonged therapy (e.g., longer than 14 days). Periodic antifactor Xa activity monitoring may also be useful in women treated with a LMWH during pregnancy because of changing pharmacokinetic variables (e.g., volume of distribution and renal function).[27] Patients who are at very high risk of bleeding or thrombotic recurrence may also benefit from antifactor Xa monitoring to avoid periods of over- or underanticoagulation. Because newborns and pediatric patients have unpredictable pharmacokinetic profiles, they may require monitoring to ensure adequate therapy.

When antifactor Xa activity is used to monitor LMWH therapy, the sample should be drawn after steady state has been achieved (after the second or third dose) and approximately 4 hours after the subcutaneous injection, during the peak period of antifactor Xa activity.[22] A calibrated LMWH heparin should be used to establish the standard curve for the assay. The therapeutic range for antifactor Xa activity is not well defined and as of this writing has not been clearly correlated with efficacy or the risk of bleeding.[30] For the treatment of VTE, an acceptable target range for the peak level is 0.5 to 1.0 units/mL and for the prevention of VTE an acceptable target range for the peak level is 0.2 to 0.4 units/mL.

Adverse Effects

As with UFH, bleeding is the most common adverse effect of the LMWHs.[4] Although not consistently demonstrated in clinical trials, the frequency of major bleeding is purported to be less with the LMWHs than with UFH.[22] This difference may be partly a result of their reduced effects on platelet function, endothelial cells, and microvascular permeability. The incidence of major bleeding reported in clinical trials is less than 3% and varies among the LMWH preparations, their indication for use, patient population, and dose administered. Minor bleeding, particularly at the site of injection, occurs frequently with LMWH use. Several cases of epidural and spinal hematoma resulting in long-term or permanent paralysis have been reported with the use of enoxaparin during spinal and epidural anesthesia or spinal puncture.[29] The risk of these events is higher with the use of indwelling epidural catheters and concomitant use of drugs that affect hemostasis. Epidural catheters should be removed only after a minimum of 12 hours has elapsed after the last dose of the LMWH, and any subsequent dose should be given at least 2 hours later.

Although there is no proven method for reversing LMWH, if major bleeding does occur in a patient receiving an LMWH, it is recommended that IV protamine sulfate be administered.[22] However, because of its limited binding to the shorter LMWH chains, protamine sulfate cannot completely neutralize the anticoagulant effects of LMWH. When given in equimolar concentrations, protamine sulfate neutralizes an estimated 60% to 75% of the antithrombotic activity of LMWH. The recommended dose of protamine sulfate is 1 mg/1 mg of enoxaparin or 1 mg/100 antifactor Xa units of dalteparin or tinzaparin administered in the previous 8 hours. If the LMWH dose was given in the previous 8 to 12 hours, a 0.5-mg dose of protamine should be given for every 100 antifactor Xa units. The use of protamine sulfate is not recommended if the LMWH was administered more than 12 hours earlier.[22]

Although thrombocytopenia can occur with the use of a LMWH, the incidence of HIT is substantially lower than that observed with the use of UFH.[22,26] The explanation may lie in the reduced propensity of the LMWHs to bind to platelets and PF-4. Because the LMWHs exhibit nearly 100% cross-reactivity with heparin antibodies in vitro, the LMWHs should be avoided in patients with an established diagnosis or history of HIT.[26] Platelet counts must be periodically monitored in all patients who are receiving a LMWH, and thrombocytopenia of any degree should be promptly evaluated.

The risk of osteoporosis appears to be substantially lower with the LMWHs than with UFH. The LMWHs have not caused appreciable changes in bone mineral density after several months of use.[27] They have been used in a limited number of patients with established heparin-induced osteoporosis. Although these reports are promising, it cannot be concluded that the LMWHs have no effect on bone formation until well-designed clinical trials are available.

Use in Special Populations

There is growing experience with the use of LMWHs during pregnancy.[27] The LMWHs do not cross the placenta. According to the results of a few large case series, the LMWH appear to be relatively safe to use during pregnancy and are an attractive alternative to UFH when long-term anticoagulation therapy is required. Furthermore, the LMWHs do not appear to affect bone formation.[27] Dalteparin, enoxaparin, and tinzaparin are classified as FDA pregnancy category B. The LMWHs are becoming the preferred agents in pediatric populations despite the fact that the safety and effectiveness of the LMWHs to treat VTE in children and infants has not been extensively studied.[28] Weight-based LMWH doses provide a less-predictable anticoagulant response in children compared to adults.[28] For enoxaparin, suggested therapeutic doses are 1.5 mg/kg every 12 hours for infants <2 months old and 1.0 mg/kg every 12 hours for those >2 months old. The suggested dose for dalteparin is 86 to 172 units/kg every 24 hours, keeping in mind that neonates appear to require higher doses/kg than older children or adults.[28] Until more data are available, it is prudent to periodically monitor antifactor Xa activity in these special populations during long-term use.

FONDAPARINUX

Pharmacology

Fondaparinux, also known as pentasaccharide, is a synthetic molecule consisting of the five critical saccharide units that bind specifically, but reversibly, to antithrombin (see Fig. 21–5).[19] Fondaparinux is the first in a class of anticoagulants that selectively inhibits factor Xa activity.[31] Similar to UFH and the LMWHs, fondaparinux prevents thrombus generation and clot formation by indirectly inhibiting factor Xa activity through its interaction with antithrombin. When fondaparinux binds to antithrombin it causes a permanent conformational change in antithrombin's active site and catalyzes antifactor Xa activity by about 300-fold. Fondaparinux is not destroyed during this process and is released to bind many other antithrombin molecules.[31] Unlike UFH and LMWH, fondaparinux has no direct effect on thrombin activity at therapeutic plasma concentrations.[19] Selective inhibition of factor Xa may provide more efficient control over fibrin generation while preserving thrombin's regulatory functions in the control of hemostasis. Fondaparinux has no known effect on platelet function.[19]

Pharmacokinetics

Fondaparinux is rapidly and completely absorbed following subcutaneous administration (absolute bioavailability 100%). Peak plasma concentrations are achieved in approximately 2 hours after a single dose and 3 hours with repeated once-daily dosing. It is distributed primarily in blood. At therapeutic concentrations, fondaparinux is highly and specifically bound to antithrombin.[31] It does not bind to red blood cells or other plasma proteins including albumin, glycoprotein, platelets, or PF-4.[19] Fondaparinux is primarily eliminated unchanged in the urine. It is contraindicated in patients with severe renal function impairment (creatinine clearance <30 mL/min) because of an increased risk for bleeding. The terminal elimination half-life is 17 to 21 hours and is independent of the patient's age or sex.[32] The anticoagulant effect of fondaparinux persists for 2 to 4 days following discontinuation of the drug in patients with normal renal function. Fondaparinux has no known pharmacokinetic drug interactions. However, concurrent use with other antithrombotic agents increases the risk of hemorrhage.

Dose and Administration

Fondaparinux is FDA-approved for the prevention of VTE following orthopedic (hip fracture, hip replacement, and knee replacement) surgery and for the treatment of DVT and PE.[32] In the setting of VTE prevention, the dose of fondaparinux is 2.5 mg injected subcutaneously once daily starting 6 to 8 hours following surgery. It is important to avoid initiating fondaparinux too soon because there is a significant relationship between the timing of the first dose and the risk of major bleeding complications. Patients who weigh less than 50 kg should not be given fondaparinux for VTE prophylaxis. The usual duration of therapy is 5 to 9 days, but may be given as extended prophylaxis following hospital discharge for up to 21 days.[33] Fondaparinux has been evaluated for the treatment of DVT and PE in two phase III clinical trials.[19] For the treatment of DVT or PE, the dose of fondaparinux is 7.5 mg given subcutaneously once daily. Patients who weight more than 100 kg should be given 10 mg once daily and those who weigh less than 50 kg should receive only 5 mg daily.[32]

Similar to the LMWHs, fondaparinux is administered into the fatty tissue of the abdominal wall. Patients should be instructed to pinch a fold of skin at the injection site and hold it throughout the injection. The needle should be inserted at a 90° angle. Injection sites should be alternated from side to side.[32]

Therapeutic Monitoring

A complete blood cell count should be measured at baseline and monitored periodically to detect the possibility of occult bleeding.[32] Baseline kidney function should be determined and monitored closely in patients at risk of developing renal failure. Fondaparinux should be discontinued if the creatinine clearance drops below 30 mL/min. Signs and symptoms of bleeding should be monitored daily, particularly in patients with a baseline creatinine clearance between 30 and 50 mL/min. If neuraxial anesthesia has been used, patients should be closely monitored for signs and symptoms of neurologic impairment.

Fondaparinux does not alter coagulation tests such as the aPTT and PT. The role of antifactor Xa monitoring during fondaparinux is not well defined. Patients receiving fondaparinux therapy do not require routine coagulation testing.

Adverse Effects

The primary adverse effect associated with fondaparinux therapy is bleeding.[32] The rate of major bleeding in the VTE prophylaxis trials was approximately 2% to 3%. Because the risk of major bleeding appears to be related to weight, in patients who weigh less than 50 kg, fondaparinux is contraindicated for VTE prophylaxis and the treatment dose is only 5 mg every 24 hours. Similar to UFH and the LMWHs, fondaparinux should be used with extreme caution in patients with neuraxial anesthesia or following a spinal puncture because of the risk for spinal or epidural hematoma formation. Unlike UFH and the LMWHs, fondaparinux does not cause heparin-induced thrombocytopenia and does not produce cross-sensitivity in vitro.[19] A specific antidote to reverse the antithrombotic activity of fondaparinux is not currently available, but several potential products have been evaluated.[31]

Use in Special Populations

Fondaparinux has been used safely in elderly patients but the risk of major bleeding increases with age (1.8% in patients <65 years of age, 2.2% in patients age 65 to 74 years, and 2.7% in patients age 75 years or older).[32] This is an important consideration because many patients who undergo orthopedic surgery are elderly. Elderly patients are also more likely to have decreased renal function and careful assessment of renal status should be conducted prior to initiating therapy. Fondaparinux is contraindicated in patients with a creatinine clearance less than 30 mL/min.

Fondaparinux is a pregnancy category B drug.[32] However, there is very limited information regarding fondaparinux use during pregnancy. The drug is excreted in the milk of lactating rats, but excretion in human milk is unknown. Until more data becomes available, UFH and LMWH should remain the agents of choice during pregnancy. Fondaparinux use in pediatric populations has not been studied.

IDRAPARINUX

Idraparinux is an analog of fondaparinux that has very long duration of effect (see Table 21–6) and was developed to be administered once weekly by subcutaneous injection. Idraparinux is currently undergoing phase III clinical trials evaluating its usefulness for both the acute and long-term management of VTE.[34]

DIRECT THROMBIN INHIBITORS

In recent years, research has focused on the development of direct thrombin inhibitors (DTIs) that may offer benefits over traditional agents in the treatment and prevention of various thrombotic disorders. The DTIs have been studied for many indications such as HIT, prophylaxis and treatment of VTE, acute coronary syndromes with and without percutaneous transluminal coronary angioplasty, and nonvalvular atrial fibrillation. Currently four parenteral agents—lepirudin, desirudin, bivalirudin, and argatroban—are approved for use in the United States, and several oral compounds are in various phases of clinical development (Table 21–11).[19,35,36]

Pharmacology and Pharmacokinetics

The direct thrombin inhibitors, as their name implies, directly interact with the thrombin molecule (Fig. 21–6). The agents in this class differ in terms of their molecular weight, chemical structure, and binding to the thrombin molecule. Unlike UFH, LMWH, and fondaparinux, DTIs do not require a cofactor (antithrombin) to exert their antithrombotic activity. They are capable of inhibiting

TABLE 21-11 Pharmacologic and Clinical Properties of Direct Thrombin Inhibitors

	Lepirudin	Desirudin	Bivalirudin	Argatroban	Dabigatran[a]
Route of administration	IV or SC	IV or SC	IV	IV	PO
Indication	Treatment of thrombosis in patients with HIT	DVT prevention after THA (not available in the U.S.)	Patients with UA undergoing PTCA; PCI with provisional use of GPI	Treatment of thrombosis in patients with HIT; patients at risk for HIT undergoing PCI	Investigational for VTE prevention and treatment, and stroke prevention in AF
Binding to thrombin	Irreversible catalytic site and exosite-1	Irreversible catalytic site and exosite-1	Partially Reversible catalytic site and exosite-1	Reversible catalytic site	Reversible catalytic site
Monitoring	aPTT (IV) S_{cr}/Cl_{cr}	aPTT (IV) S_{cr}/Cl_{cr}	aPTT/ACT S_{cr}/Cl_{cr}	aPTT/ACT Liver function	[b]S_{cr}/Cl_{cr} Effect on liver function unclear at this time
Clearance	Renal	Renal	Enzymatic (80)% and Renal (20%)	Hepatic	Renal
Antibody development	Antihirudin antibodies in up to 60% of patients	Possible; lower incidence than with lepirudin	May cross-react with antihirudin antibodies	No	Unknown
Effect on INR	Slight increase	Slight increase	Slight increase	Increase	Unpredictable and variable

ACT, activated clotting time; AF, atrial fibrillation; aPTT, activated partial thromboplastin time; bid, twice daily; Cl_{cr}, creatinine clearance; DVT, deep vein thrombosis; GPI, glycoprotein IIb/IIIa inhibitor; HIT, heparin induced thrombocytopenia; INR, international normalized ratio; IV, intravenous ; PCI, percutaneous coronary intervention; PO, oral ; PTCA, percutaneous transluminal coronary angioplasty; qd, daily; SC, subcutaneous; S_{cr}, serum creatinine; THA, total hip arthroplasty; UA, unstable angina; VTE, venous thromboembolism.

[a]Investigational.

[b]Routine monitoring of anticoagulant effect may not be necessary.

From Nutescu et al.[35]

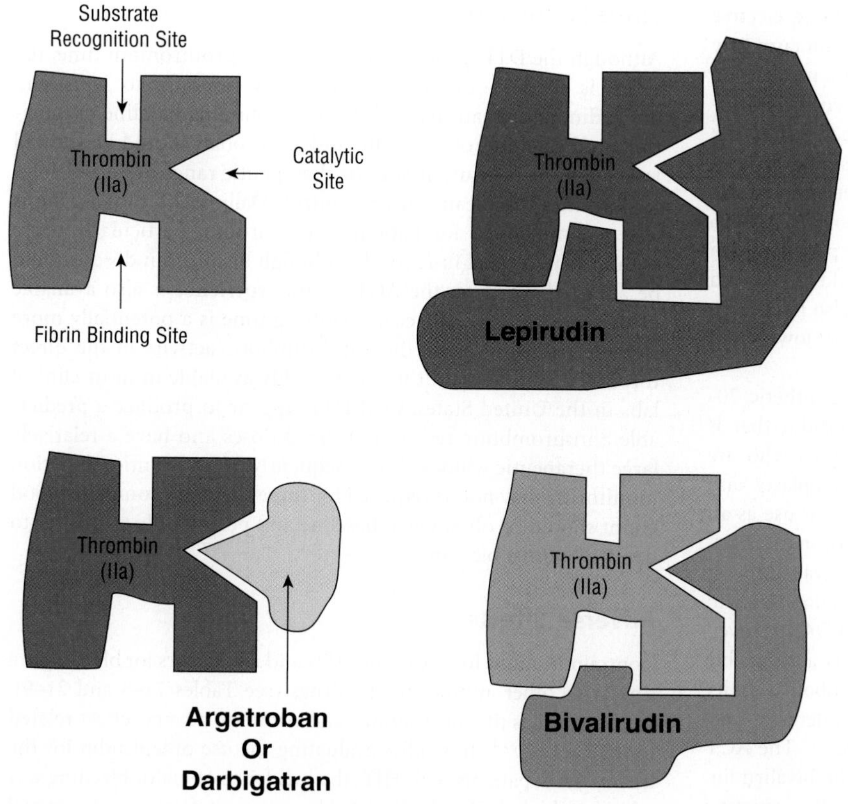

FIGURE 21-6. Pharmacologic activity of lepirudin, bivalirudin, argatroban, and dabigatran.

both circulating and clot-bound thrombin, a potential advantage over UFH and LMWH. Furthermore, DTIs do not induce immune-mediated thrombocytopenia and are widely used for the treatment of HIT.[19,35,36]

Hirudin, the prototype of this class, is a 65-amino-acid polypeptide (7,000 Da) that was originally isolated from the salivary secretions of the medicinal leech (*Hirudo medicinalis*). Although not commercially available, the discovery of hirudin led to the development of derivatives such as lepirudin and desirudin via recombinant DNA technology. The hirudins (lepirudin, desirudin, and bivalirudin) form a stoichiometric and very slowly reversible complex by binding to both the active site and exosite-1 of the thrombin molecule (see Fig. 21–6). Because of this bivalent bond, hirudins are considered the most potent inhibitors of thrombin.[19,35,36]

Lepirudin, a recombinant analogue of hirudin, is a 65-amino-acid polypeptide that is administered parenterally, either by continuous IV infusion or subcutaneous injection.[19,37] It is indicated for anticoagulation in patients with HIT and associated thrombosis so as to prevent further thromboembolic complications. Research is also being conducted on the use of lepirudin for other indications, such as acute coronary syndromes and VTE. Because of the strong, almost irreversible bond between lepirudin and thrombin, lepirudin is associated with bleeding complications.[37] The primary route of elimination for lepirudin is through renal excretion, and systemic clearance is directly proportional to the glomerular filtration rate. Lepirudin has a terminal half-life of 1.3 hours in young healthy volunteers. In patients with marked renal insufficiency (Cl_{cr} <15 mL/min) and on hemodialysis, elimination half-lives are prolonged up to 2 days.[36] Thus, dose adjustment is required in the setting of impaired renal function, a potential disadvantage of this agent (Table 21–12). Many patients develop antibodies to lepirudin. Up to 60% of patients treated with lepirudin for 10 days or more will develop antibodies. This may increase the anticoagulant effect of lepirudin, possibly as a result of delayed renal elimination of active lepirudin–antihirudin complexes. Consequently, strict monitoring of aPTT is necessary during prolonged therapy.[19,35] Because fatal anaphylaxis has been reported in patients who developed antibodies, patients should not be treated with lepirudin more than once.[38]

Desirudin, also a recombinant hirudin analogue, is administered by subcutaneous injection and approved by the FDA in 2003 for the

TABLE 21-12 Dosing Considerations for Direct Thrombin Inhibitors in Patients with Renal and Hepatic Dysfunction

	Renal Impairment	Hepatic Impairment
Lepirudin	Bolus: 0.2 mg/kg (bolus dose is should be avoided in patients with renal impairment) Infusion: Cl_{cr} 45–60 mL/min: 0.075 mg/kg/h Cl_{cr} 30–44 mL/min: 0.045 mg/kg/h Cl_{cr} 15–29 mL/min: 0.0225 mg/kg/h Cl_{cr}<15 mL/min: no bolus; avoid or stop infusion HD: stop infusion & additional IV bolus doses of 0.1 mg/kg every other day should be considered if the aPTT ratio falls below 1.5	Dose adjustment not required
Desirudin	Cl_{cr} 31–60 mL/min: 5mg SC q 12 h Cl_{cr} <30 mL/min: 1.7 mg SC q 12 h	Dose adjustment not required
Bivalirudin	Bolus: no dose adjustment Infusion: Cl_{cr} <30: 1 mg/kg/h HD: 0.25 mg/kg/h	Dose adjustment not required
Argatroban	Dose adjustment not required	Initiate at 0.5 mcg/kg/min then titrate to aPTT 1.5–3.0 × baseline
Dabigatran	Dose adjustment will be required; degree of dose decrease not defined at this time.	Unclear at this time

aPTT, activated partial thromboplastin time; Cl_{cr}, creatinine clearance; HD, hemodialysis; SC, subcutaneous.
From Nutescu et al.[35]

prevention of venous thrombosis in patients undergoing elective hip surgery.[39] Although approved for use, the agent is not currently commercially available in the United States. For acute myocardial infarction and unstable angina, desirudin has been given via continuous IV infusion.[35,40] Desirudin has a terminal elimination half-life after subcutaneous dosing of approximately 2 hours, and 80% to 90% of the elimination is by renal clearance and metabolism. The total urinary excretion of unchanged drug amounts to 40% to 50% of the administered dose. Similar to lepirudin, in patients with moderate to severe renal impairment, the dosage should be reduced (see Table 21–12). Although antihirudin antibodies also have been documented with desirudin, the incidence appears to be lower than with lepirudin.[35,41]

Bivalirudin, formerly known as Hirulog, is a semisynthetic 20-amino-acid polypeptide analogue of recombinant hirudin that is FDA approved for use in patients with unstable angina who are undergoing percutaneous transluminal coronary angioplasty and with provisional use of glycoprotein IIb/IIIa inhibitor for use as an anticoagulant in patients undergoing percutaneous coronary intervention.[42] Recent reports also support the use of bivalirudin in patients with acute ST elevation myocardial infarction and in patients with HIT, although the agent is not currently FDA approved for these indications. Unlike lepirudin, bivalirudin is a reversible inhibitor of thrombin and provides transient antithrombotic activity with an estimated 20- to 30-minute half-life. This difference may reduce the risk of bleeding and antibody production.[35,43] The ACT can be used to monitor the anticoagulant effect of bivalirudin. Therapeutic ACT levels are achieved within 5 minutes after initiating bivalirudin therapy, and ACT levels return to subtherapeutic levels within 1 hour of discontinuing the infusion. The aPTT test has also been used to monitor the anticoagulant effect of bivalirudin in patients with HIT. Bivalirudin is mostly cleared by proteolytic cleavage and by hepatic metabolism, with approximately 20% eliminated renally. The manufacturer recommends reducing the dose by 20% to 60% in patients with renal impairment and monitoring the ACT closely (see Table 21–12).[35,43]

Argatroban differs from the hirudins in that it is a small, synthetic molecule derived from arginine that reversibly binds only to the active catalytic site of thrombin. Its small size relative to other DTIs enables it to inhibit both clot-bound and soluble thrombin, offering a potential therapeutic advantage over other agents in its class.[26,44] Argatroban is primarily eliminated by hydroxylation and aromatization in the liver to inactive metabolites. A small percentage is excreted unchanged in the bile. The elimination half-life is 39 to 51 minutes, but extends to approximately 181 minutes in hepatic impairment. Dose adjustment is required in patients with hepatic impairment (see Table 21–12). The aPTT and ACT can be used to monitor the anticoagulant effect of argatroban. It is FDA approved for the prophylaxis or treatment of thrombosis in patients with HIT, and also as an anticoagulant in patients with HIT, or at risk of HIT, who are undergoing percutaneous coronary intervention.[35,45]

Oral Direct Thrombin Inhibitors

Recent progress has also been made in the development of oral DTIs. These agents appear promising and offer various advantages such as oral administration, predictable pharmacokinetics and pharmacodynamics, a broad therapeutic window, no routine laboratory monitoring, no significant drug interactions, and fixed-dose administration. Several of these compounds are being investigated with dabigatran etexilate being in most advanced phases of clinical development. A previous agent of the class (ximelagatran) was denied FDA approval because of concerns of drug-induced liver toxicity. The first safe, oral DTI to make it to the U.S. market has the potential to revolutionize the provision of antithrombotic therapy.[35,36]

Therapeutic Monitoring

Although the DTIs produce changes in the prothrombin time, the aPTT is used to monitor the patient's response to lepirudin, desirudin, and argatroban.[19,35,40] After obtaining baseline coagulation studies, doses of lepirudin and argatroban should be titrated to achieve the institution-specific therapeutic range or an aPTT 1.5 to 3.0 times the mean normal control. Daily aPTT monitoring is also recommended for patients on desirudin, particularly those with impaired renal function.[41] Although bivalirudin doses should be adjusted based on the ACT, some experience is also available using the aPTT.[42,43] The ecarin clotting time is a potentially more suitable test to measure the antithrombotic activity of the direct thrombin inhibitors, but it is not readily available in most clinical labs in the United States. Oral DTIs appear to produce a predictable antithrombotic response in fixed doses and have a relatively large therapeutic window.[35] Consequently, routine anticoagulation monitoring may not be required for these agents. A complete blood count should be obtained at baseline and periodically thereafter to detect potential bleeding.

Adverse Effects

Contraindications for use of the DTIs and risk factors for bleeding are similar to other antithrombotic drugs (see Tables 21–8 and 21–9). Hemorrhage is the most serious and common adverse effect related to the DTIs.[19,35,40] In studies evaluating the use of lepirudin for the treatment of patients with HIT, the incidence of major bleeding was relatively high (13% to 17%).[37] However, no fatal or intracranial bleeding events occurred. A slightly lower rate of major hemorrhage was reported in HIT trials using argatroban (approximately 5%) and, similarly, there were no reports of fatal or intracranial bleeding.[45] Bleeding complications with desirudin were similar to enoxaparin in a trial of patients undergoing elective hip surgery. Serious bleeding occurred in less than 1% of all patients in the trial.[41] Minor bleeding and small reductions in red blood cell counts occurred relatively frequently but typically did not require drug discontinuation. There are no known agents that reverse the activity of the DTIs. Nonhemorrhagic effects such as fever, nausea, vomiting, and allergic reactions occur infrequently.

Drug–Drug and Drug–Food Interactions

The concurrent use of DTIs and thrombolytic agents substantially increases the bleeding risk, particularly intracranial hemorrhage, and should be undertaken with great caution. Warfarin and antiplatelet agents can be concurrently initiated with these agents. Because the DTIs prolong the PT and INR, close monitoring for bleeding complications is required. Few pharmacokinetic drug interactions with this class of agents are known. Drugs that alter renal function could prolong lepirudin, desirudin, and bivalirudin activity. Drugs that inhibit liver enzymes have the potential to interact with argatroban.[46]

Use in Special Populations

Lepirudin, bivalirudin, and argatroban are classified by the FDA as pregnancy category B drugs but they should be used cautiously in women of child bearing age because experience is very limited.[37,42,45] Desirudin is classified as pregnancy category C with no controlled trials in pregnant women.[41] Lepirudin and argatroban have been evaluated in a very small number of children. Dosing requirements can vary widely in pediatric patients, thus product-specific dosing guidelines and monitoring should be followed.[47] Critically ill patients and patients with renal or hepatic impairment will require dosage adjustments according to the specific DTI used, and lower initiation doses are recommended (see Table 21–12).[48]

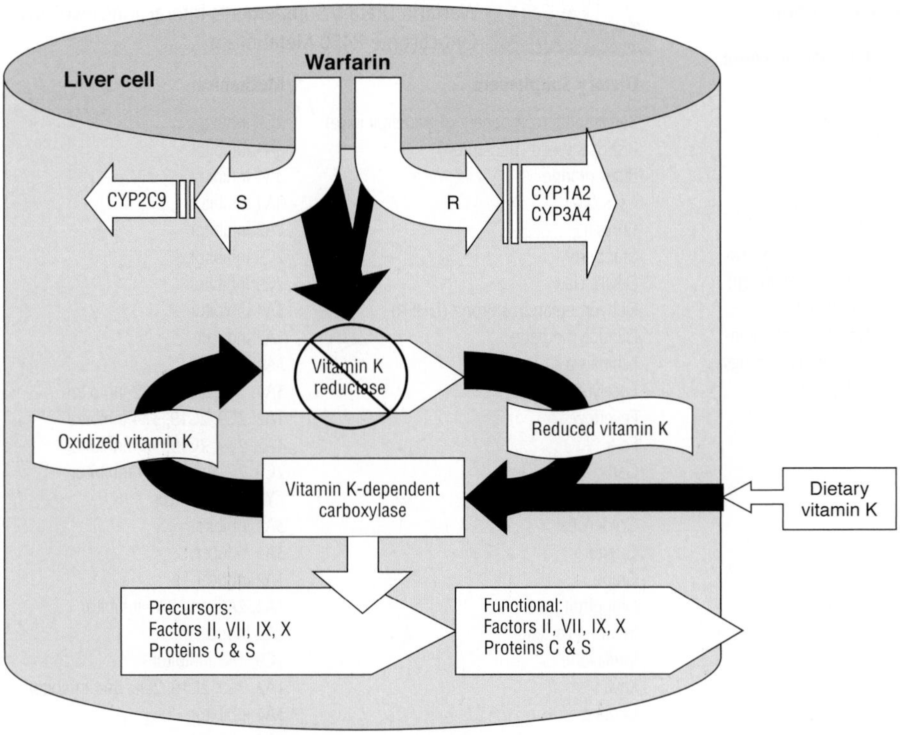

FIGURE 21-7. Pharmacologic activity and metabolism of warfarin.

WARFARIN

The most widely prescribed anticoagulant in North American is warfarin sodium (Coumadin). It was serendipitously discovered in the early 1940s at the University of Wisconsin after hemorrhagic deaths occurred in cattle eating spoiled sweet clover. Warfarin is the anticoagulant of choice when long-term or extended anticoagulation is indicated. Warfarin is FDA-approved for the prevention and treatment of VTE, as well as for the prevention of thromboembolic complications associated with atrial fibrillation, heart valve replacement, and myocardial infarction. Because of its narrow therapeutic index, predisposition to drug and food interactions, and propensity to cause hemorrhage, warfarin requires continuous patient monitoring and education to achieve optimal outcomes.[5]

Pharmacology

Warfarin exerts its anticoagulation effect by inhibiting the enzymes responsible for the cyclic interconversion of vitamin K in the liver (Fig. 21–7). Reduced vitamin K is a cofactor required for the carboxylation of the vitamin K-dependent coagulation proteins, namely factors II (prothrombin), VII, IX, and X, as well as the endogenous anticoagulant proteins C and S. Carboxylation of the N-terminal region of these proteins in the liver is required for biologic activity. By inhibiting the supply of vitamin K to serve as a cofactor in the production of these proteins, warfarin indirectly slows their rate of synthesis. Warfarin has no direct effect on previously circulating clotting factors or previously formed thrombus.[5,6] The time required for warfarin to achieve its pharmacologic effect is dependant on the elimination half-lives of the coagulation proteins (Table 21–13). Given that prothrombin has a 2- to 3-day half-life, warfarin's full antithrombotic effect is not achieved for 8 to 15 days after the initiation of therapy. By suppressing the production of clotting factors, warfarin prevents the initial formation and propagation of thrombus.[5,46]

Pharmacokinetics

Commercially available warfarin is a racemic mixture of *R* and *S* isomers. The *S* isomer is 2 to 5 times more potent that the *R* isomer. Warfarin is rapidly and extensively absorbed from the gastrointestinal tract and reaches peak plasma concentration in approximately 90 minutes with a bioavailability of greater than 90% following oral administration. In plasma, both the *R* and *S* isomers are extensively (97% to 99%) bound to albumin.[5,46] Warfarin undergoes stereoselective metabolism via cytochrome P450 (CYP) 1A2, 2C9, 2C19, 2C8, 2C18, and 3A4 isoenzymes in the liver (see Fig. 21–7). The pharmacokinetic parameters of warfarin, particularly hepatic metabolism, vary substantially between individuals leading to large interpatient differences in dose requirements. Genetic variations in the 2C9 isoenzyme and vitamin K epoxide reductase (VKOR) have been shown to correlate with warfarin dose requirements.[49,50] Given the relatively greater potency of *S*-warfarin, coadministration of drugs that induce or inhibit the CYP2C isoenzymes are more likely to cause a clinically significant interaction.[5] These and other pharmacokinetic variations in warfarin metabolism likely explain the large interpatient dose–response seen with warfarin in clinical practice.

Dosing and Administration

The dose of warfarin is patient-specific based on the desired intensity of anticoagulation and the patient's individual response.[5,6] There is tremendous interpatient variability with regard to the pharmacodynamic response and pharmacokinetic disposition of warfarin. In addition, there is significant intrapatient variability in these parameters over time. Therefore, the dose of warfarin must be based on continual clinical and laboratory monitoring. At the

TABLE 21-13 Biologic Half-Life of Vitamin K-Dependent Coagulation Proteins

Protein	Half-Life (hours)
Prothrombin (factor II)	60–100
Factor VII	6–8
Factor IX	20–30
Factor X	24–40
Protein C	8–10
Protein S	40–60

From Haines and Bussey.[19]

TABLE 21-14 Clinically Important Warfarin Drug Interactions

Increase Anticoagulation Effect (↑INR)	Decrease Anticoagulation Effect (↓INR)	Increase Bleeding Risk
Acetminophen	Amobarbital	Argatroban
Alcohol binge	Butabarbital	Aspirin
Allopurinol	Carbamazepine	Clopidogrel
Amiodarone	Cholestyramine	Danaparoid
Cephalosporins (with NMTT side chain)	Dicloxacillin	Dipyridamole
Chloral hydrate	Griseofulvin	Unfractionated/low-molecular-weight heparins
Cimetidine	Nafcillin	Nonsteroidal antiinflammatory drugs
Ciprofloxacin	Phenobarbital	Ticlopidine
Clofibrate	Phenytoin	
Chloramphenicol	Primidone	
Danazol	Rifampin	
Disulfuram	Rifabutin	
Doxycycline	Secobarbital	
Erythromycin	Sucralfate	
Fenofibrate	Vitamin K	
Fluconazole		
Fluorouracil		
Fluoxetine		
Fluvoxamine		
Gemfibrozil		
Influenza vaccine		
Isoniazid		
Itraconazole		
Lovastatin		
Moxalactam		
Metronidazole		
Miconazole		
Neomycin		
Norfloxacin		
Ofloxacin		
Omeprazole		
Phenylbutazone		
Piroxicam		
Propafenone		
Propoxyphene		
Quinidine		
Sertraline		
Sulfamethoxazole		
Sulfinpyrazone		
Tamoxifen		
Testosterone		
Vitamin E		
Zafirlukast		

INR, international normalized ratio; NMTT, *N*-methylthiotetrazole.
From Holbrook et al.[63]

TABLE 21-15 Warfarin Dietary Supplements Interactions Involving Cytochrome P450 Metabolism

Dietary Supplement	Mechanism
Bergamottin (component of grapefruit juice)	2C9 inhibitor
Bishop's weed (Bergapten)	3A4 inhibitor
Bitter orange	3A4 Inhibitor
Cat's claw	3A4 inhibitor
Chrysin	1A2 inhibitor
Cranberry	2C9 inhibitor
Devil's claw	2C9 Inhibitor
Dehydroepiandrosterone (DHEA)	3A4 inhibitor
Diindolymethane	1A2 inducer
Echinacea	3A4 inhibitor
Eucalyptus	3A4, 2C9, 2C19, 1A2 inhibitor
Feverfew	1A2, 2C9, 2C19, 3A4 inhibitor
Fo-ti	1A2, 2C9, 2C19, 3A4 inhibitor
Garlic	2C9, 2C19, and 3A4 inhibitor
Ginseng	CYP P450 inducer
Goldenseal	3A4 inhibitor
Guggul	3A4 inducer
Grape	1A2 inducer
Grapefruit juice	1A2, 2A6, and 3A4 inhibitor
Indole-3-carbinol	1A2 Inducer
Ipriflavone	2C9, 1A2 inhibitor
Kava	1A2, 2C9, 2C19, 2D6, 3A4 inhibitor
Licorice	3A4 inhibitor
Lime	3A4 inhibitor
Limonene	2C9, 2C19 substrate, and 2C9 inducer
Lycium (Chinese wolfberry)	2C9 inhibitor
Milk thistle	2C9 and 3A4 inhibitor
Peppermint	1A2, 2C9, 2C19, 3A4 inhibitor
Red clover	1A2, 2C9, 2C19, 3A4 inhibitor
Resveratrol	1A, 2E1 3A4 inhibitor
St. John's wort	1A2, 2C9, 3A4 inducer
Sulforaphane	1A2 inhibitor
Valerian	3A4 inhibitor
Wild cherry	3A4 inhibitor

From Nutescu et al.[64]

initiation of therapy, it is difficult to predict the specific dose that an individual will require. Warfarin dosing algorithms that incorporate pharmacogenetic information regarding CYP2C9 and VKOR polymorphisms are currently being evaluated. The usefulness of pharmacogenetic information in managing patients is not yet known.

Although the average weekly dose of warfarin is between 25 mg and 55 mg, some patient-related variables are associated with lower than usual dose requirement including: advanced age (>65 years old), elevated baseline INR, poor nutritional status, liver disease, hyperthyroidism, genetic polymorphisms in CYP2C9 and VKOR, and concurrent use of medications known to enhance the effect of warfarin (Table 21–14).[5,6] Prior to initiating therapy, the clinician should screen for the presence of contraindications to anticoagulation therapy and risk factors for major bleeding (see Tables 21–8 and 21–9). It is essential to collect a complete medication history, including the use of herbal and nutritional products (Tables 21–15 and 21–16).

CLINICAL CONTROVERSY

Some clinicians recommend that warfarin therapy be started using no more than 5 mg daily based on evidence that the majority of patients will achieve a therapeutic INR by day 5. Furthermore, some patients become excessively anticoagulated when higher doses are used. However, some clinicians recommend initiating warfarin therapy with 10 mg daily because a therapeutic INR is achieved 1 day sooner, thereby facilitating earlier hospital discharge and more rapid discontinuation of LMWH therapy. In addition, they argue, there is no evidence that bleeding complications occur more frequently when a higher initial dose is used.

There is some controversy regarding the optimal dosing regimen when initiating warfarin therapy.[5,51,52] To achieve a therapeutic INR in the least amount of time, some clinicians have used relatively high doses of warfarin (10 or 15 mg) and then adjusted the dose based on the patient's response. Studies in patients with atrial fibrillation that compared a 5-mg initial dose to a 10-mg dose questioned this practice.[53] Although a 10-mg dose produced a more rapid response in the INR, many patients subsequently became excessively anticoagulated. However, a more recent study in patients with acute venous thrombosis demonstrated that 10-mg initial doses can be used safely when the subsequent INR response is monitored appropriately.[51]

Although data on the optimal induction regimen is conflicting, there is a pharmacodynamic rationale for avoiding doses larger than

TABLE 21-16 Dietary Supplements That Can Affect Platelet Function and Anticoagulation Status

Agent	Mechanism	Comments
Bladderwrack	Has anticoagulant effects	Increased risk of bleeding or bruising
Boldo	Constituents may have antiplatelet effects	Increased risk of bleeding or bruising
Bromelain	Decreased platelet aggregation	Increased risk of bleeding or bruising
Burdock	Decreased platelet aggregation by inhibiting platelet activation factor	Increased risk of bleeding or bruising
Caffeine	May have antiplatelet activity; not reported in humans	Increased risk of bleeding or bruising; found in black tea, green tea, guarana, mate, oolong tea
Clove	Eugenol has antiplatelet activity	Increased risk of bleeding or bruising
Cod liver oil	May inhibit platelet aggregation	Increased risk of bleeding or bruising; avoid concomitant use
Coltsfoot	May inhibit platelet aggregation	Increased risk of bleeding or bruising; avoid concomitant use
Danshen	Decreased platelet aggregation; may also have antithrombotic effects	Increased risk of bleeding or bruising; avoid concomitant use
Dong quai	May inhibit platelet aggregation	Increased risk of bleeding or bruising
Fenugreek	Constituents may have antiplatelet effects; concentration may not be clinically significant	Increased risk of bleeding or bruising
Fish oil	Has antiplatelet effects	Increased risk of bleeding or bruising
Flax seed	Decreased platelet aggregation and increased bleeding time	Increased risk of bleeding or bruising
Gamma linolenic acid (GLA)	Has anticoagulant effects	Increased risk of bleeding or bruising; found in borage and evening primrose oil
Garlic	Has anticoagulant effects and may inhibit platelet aggregation	Increased risk of bleeding or bruising
Ginger	Inhibit thromboxane synthetase and decrease platelet aggregation	Increased risk of bleeding or bruising
Ginkgo	Decreased platelet aggregation; ginkgolide B, a component of ginkgo, is a potent inhibitor of PAF	Increased risk of bleeding or bruising
Ginseng, panax	Components may decrease platelet aggregation through PAF antagonism; not shown in humans	Increased risk of bleeding or bruising; use with caution until more is known.
Ginseng, Siberian	A component, dihydroxybenzoic acid, may inhibit platelet aggregation	Increased risk of bleeding or bruising
Melatonin	Unknown; might increase the anticoagulant or antiplatelet effect; decreased prothrombin activity observed	Increased risk of bleeding or bruising
Nattokinase	Has thrombolytic activity	Increased risk of bleeding or bruising
Onion	Decreased platelet aggregation	Increased risk of bleeding or bruising
Pantethine	Decreased platelet aggregation	Increased risk of bleeding or bruising
Policosanol	Inhibits platelet aggregation	Increased risk of bleeding or bruising
Poplar	Contains salicylates and may cause decreased platelet aggregation	Increased risk of bleeding or bruising
Resveratrol	Has antiplatelet effects	Increased risk of bleeding or bruising
Sea buckthorn	Inhibits platelet aggregation	Increased risk of bleeding or bruising
Turmeric	Decreased platelet aggregation; has antiplatelet effects	Increased risk of bleeding or bruising
Vinpocetine	Has antiplatelet effects	Increased risk of bleeding or bruising
Vitamin E	Inhibits platelet aggregation and antagonizes the effects of vitamin K-dependent clotting factors	Dose dependent and significant with doses greater than 800 units per day; advise patients to avoid high doses of vitamin E; increased risk of bleeding or bruising
Willow bark	Decreased platelet aggregation; has antiplatelet effects but less than aspirin	Increased risk of bleeding or bruising

PAF, platelet activating factor.
From Nutescu et al.[64]

10 mg.[5] Large doses result in a more rapid depression in factor VII concentrations.[53] This early response to therapy may give the clinician a false impression that a therapeutic INR has been achieved after only 2 or 3 days. It is important to remember that patients are not truly anticoagulated at this point because a significant reduction in prothrombin concentrations requires at least 5 days to occur. Large doses may also increase the theoretical risk for early thrombotic complications, such as warfarin-induced skin necrosis. After the initiation of warfarin therapy protein C becomes rapidly depleted, but prothrombin concentrations will remain near normal for several days. If protein C concentrations are severely suppressed relative to prothrombin, there is a potential for inducing a hypercoagulable state.

For most patients, initiating therapy with 5 mg daily and adjusting the dose based on the INR response will produce therapeutic INRs in 4 to 5 days (Fig. 21–8). Lower or higher starting doses may be acceptable based on patient-related factors and how quickly followup laboratory monitoring can be performed. Several dosing nomograms have been developed and prospectively evaluated.[5,51,54] For patients with acute venous thrombosis, UFH, LMWH, or fondaparinux should be overlapped with warfarin therapy for at least 5 days regardless of whether the target INR has been achieved earlier.[2]

Warfarin therapy can be safely initiated on an outpatient basis provided there is no urgent need for anticoagulation (i.e., prevention of venous thrombosis). Given that laboratory monitoring is performed less frequently in the outpatient setting, warfarin therapy should be undertaken a bit more cautiously. In most circumstances, the initial dose should not exceed the anticipated maintenance dose. The response to therapy should be measured every 3 to 5 days until stabilized. The full antithrombotic effect may require up to 15 days to be achieved.[5,46]

When adjusting the dose of warfarin, the clinician should allow sufficient time for changes in the INR to occur. In general, dose changes should not be made more frequently than every 3 days. Doses should be adjusted by calculating the weekly dose and reducing or increasing the weekly dose by 5% to 25%. The effect of a small dose change may not become evident for 5 to 7 days. Patients should not have followup INR tests sooner than anticipated changes are likely to occur.[5]

Therapeutic Monitoring

Warfarin requires frequent laboratory monitoring to ensure optimal therapeutic outcomes and minimize bleeding complications.

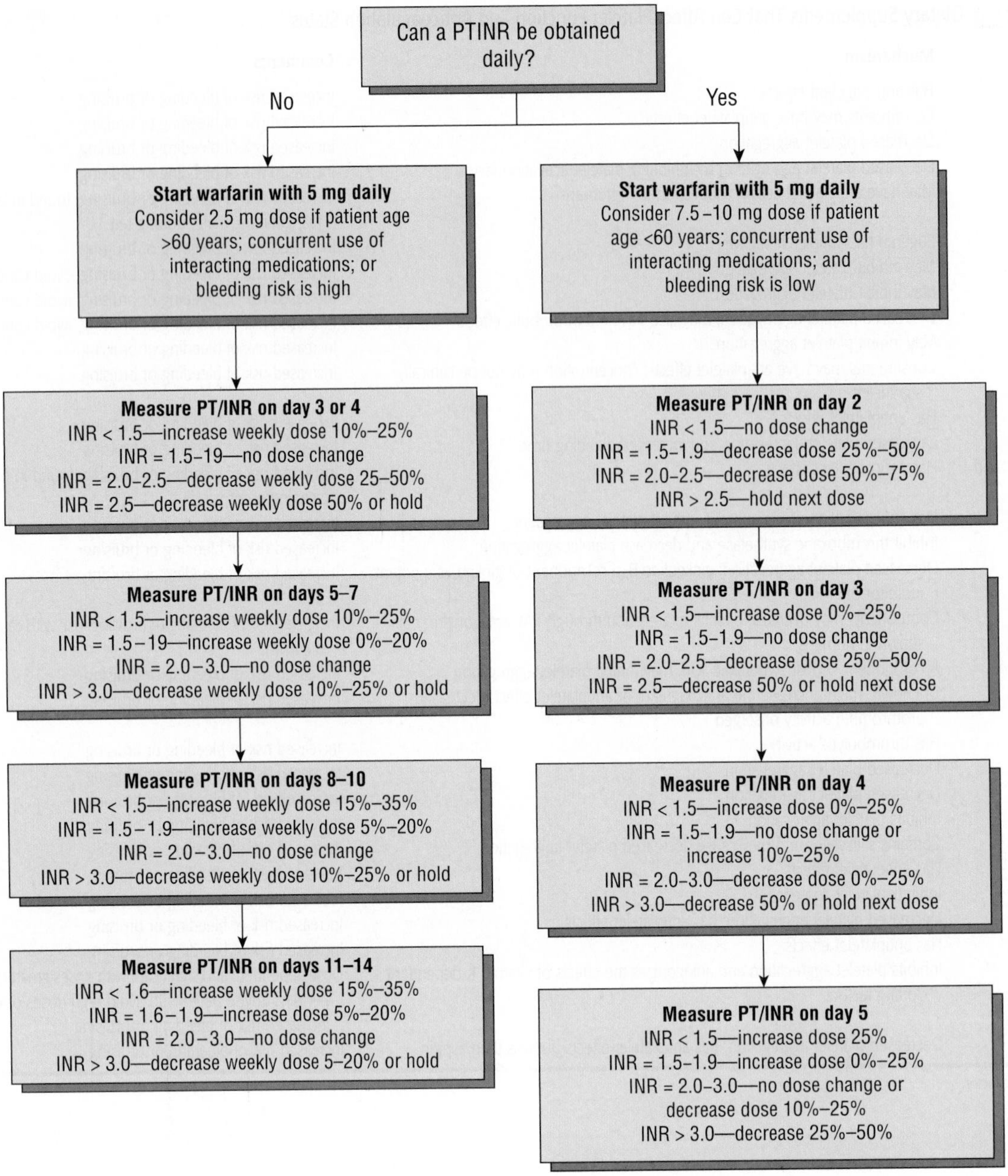

FIGURE 21-8. Initiation of warfarin therapy. (INR, international normalized ratio; PT, prothrombin time.)

The prothrombin time (PT), also known as the protime and one-step Quick test, has been used for decades to monitor the anticoagulation effects of warfarin.[5,55] The PT measures the biologic activity of factors II, VII, and X activity and correlates well to warfarin's anticoagulation effect. The test is performed by measuring the time required for clot formation after adding calcium and thromboplastin to citrated plasma. Several thromboplastins are commercially available and are extracted from mammalian tissue rich in tissue factor (e.g., rabbit brain) or produced from recombinant human tissue factor. Although an effective tool for monitoring warfarin therapy, the PT is problematic to interpret because there is wide variability in the sensitivity of thromboplastin reagents. Given the same blood sample, different thromboplastins will produce substantially different results that may prompt clinicians to make potentially inappropriate dosing decisions. The World Health Organization (WHO) addressed the need for standardization in the late 1970s by developing a reference thromboplastin and recommending the use of the INR to monitor warfarin therapy. The INR corrects for differences in thromboplastin reagents through the following formula:

$$\text{INR} = \left(\frac{\text{PT}^{\text{Patient}}}{\text{PT}^{\text{Control}}}\right)^{\text{ISI}}$$

The International Sensitivity Index (ISI) is a measure of the thromboplastin's responsiveness compared to the WHO reference standard. Each thromboplastin reagent manufactured has an ISI value that should be used to calculate the INR. Although the INR system has a number of potential problems, it is currently the best means available to interpret the PT and the preferred method for monitoring oral anticoagulation therapy.

The recommended target INR and goal range is based on the therapeutic indication.[5,55] For most indications, the target INR is 2.5 with an acceptable range of 2.0 to 3.0. The target INR is higher for some patients with mechanical prosthetic heart valves (target INR = 3.0, range 2.5 to 3.5). A baseline PT and complete blood cell count should be obtained prior to initiating warfarin therapy. In patients with an acute thromboembolic event, a PT should be measured minimally every 3 days during the first week of therapy. In this situation, UFH or LMWH therapy should be continued for at least

TABLE 21-17 Vitamin K Content of Select Foods[a]

Very High (>200 mcg)	High (100–200 mcg)	Medium (50–100 mcg)	Low (<50 mcg)
Brussel sprouts	Basil	Apple, green	Apple, red
Chickpea	Broccoli	Asparagus	Avocado
Collard greens	Chive	Cabbage	Beans
Coriander	Coleslaw	Cauliflower	Breads, grains
Endive	Cucumber (with peel)	Mayonnaise	Carrot
Kale	Canola oil	Nuts, pistachio	Cereal
Lettuce, red leaf	Green onion/scallion	Squash, summer	Celery
Parsley	Lettuce, butterhead		Coffee
Spinach	Mustard greens		Corn
Swiss chard	Soybean oil		Cucumber (without peel)
Tea, green			Dairy products
Tea, black			Eggs
Turnip greens			Fruit (varies)
Watercress			Lettuce, iceberg
			Meats, fish, poultry
			Pasta
			Peanuts
			Peas
			Potato
			Rice
			Tomato

[a]Approximate amount of vitamin K per 100 g (3.5 oz) serving.
From Booth and Centurelli.[112]

5 days and until the INR is greater than 2.0 and stable. The concurrent use of antithrombotic drugs with warfarin may prolong the prothrombin time slightly. Once the patient's dose–response is established, an INR should be determined every 7 to 14 days until it stabilizes and optimally every 4 weeks thereafter.[2,5,6]

At each encounter, patients should be meticulously questioned regarding their medication use and symptoms related to bleeding and thromboembolic complications. Any changes in medications, including changes in dose as well as non-prescription drug and dietary supplement use, should be carefully explored (see Tables 21–14, 21–15, and 21–16). Dietary intake of vitamin K rich foods should also be evaluated (Table 21–17).

Anticoagulation therapy management services can improve the care of patients who take warfarin therapy by providing structured, comprehensive patient education and evaluation.[5] When staffed by experienced and knowledgeable practitioners, anticoagulation management services improve the safety and effectiveness of warfarin therapy compared to "usual" medical care. Anticoagulation patient management services lower the overall cost of care by reducing the frequency of major bleeding and recurrent thromboembolic events.[7,56]

Portable prothrombin time monitoring devices have enhanced patient management. Not only do these devices permit clinicians to do "real-time" therapeutic drug monitoring, but they enable patients to engage in self-testing at home.[57,58] Self-monitoring, in its simplest form, requires the patient to report their test results to a healthcare professional. In such arrangements, the clinician continues to make warfarin dosing decisions. Highly motivated and sophisticated patients can be trained to manage themselves, independently altering the dose of warfarin therapy based on their INR results. Patients who engage in INR self-monitoring and warfarin self-management report high levels of satisfaction with care and maintain the INR within the therapeutic range more frequently than those managed by "usual care." Home INR testing and self-management are clearly not for everyone, however. It requires careful patient selection and considerable education. Unfortunately, PT monitoring systems remain relatively expensive and are rarely covered by medical insurance.

Adverse Effects

Warfarin's primary adverse effect is bleeding.[4] Hemorrhagic complications, ranging from mild to life-threatening, can occur at any site in the body. Although warfarin is not believed to cause bleeding per se, it can "unmask" an existing lesion or enable a massive hemorrhage from an ordinarily minor bleeding source. The gastrointestinal tract is the most frequent site of bleeding. Bruising on the arms and legs is commonplace, but a painful hematoma may necessitate the temporary discontinuation of therapy. Intracranial hemorrhage is the most serious and feared complication related to warfarin therapy, often resulting in permanent disability or death.

The annual incidence of major bleeding ranges from 1% in highly selected patient populations who are carefully managed, to greater than 10% in patients managed in less-structured environments, according to some studies.[4,5] There are no universally accepted criteria for defining a bleeding event as major or minor. Most studies have defined major bleeding as any bleeding event that required hospitalization, transfusion of 2 or more units of blood or plasma, or that led to a greater than 2 g/dL drop in hemoglobin concentration. Bleeding that does not meet the criteria for a major hemorrhage is generally considered to be a minor. Minor bleeding is very common. Few studies have prospectively evaluated the incidence of minor bleeding but it is likely to be greater than 15% annually even in the most expertly managed patients.[4,5]

Several risk factors for bleeding while taking anticoagulation therapy have been identified (see Table 21–8). Intensity of anticoagulation therapy appears to be the most powerful risk factor. Patients whose target INR is greater than 3.0 have twice the incidence of major bleeding compared to those with a target of 2.5. The risk of intracranial hemorrhage increases significantly when the INR remains greater than 4.0 for prolonged periods of time especially in the elderly. Patients given low-intensity warfarin therapy (goal INR 1.3 to 1.9) may have a lower incidence of bleeding, but this level of anticoagulation is insufficient protection against thrombosis for most indications. Wide variability in the anticoagulation response, as seen in patients with very unstable INR values, also appears to be associated with an increased risk of bleeding. The risk of hemorrhage is greatest during the first few weeks of therapy; however, bleeding can occur at any time and the cumulative incidence steadily increases over time.[4,5]

Nonhemorrhagic adverse effects associated with warfarin are uncommon, but can be serious when they do occur.[5,6] The "purple toe syndrome," manifested as a purplish discoloration of the toes, is an extremely rare event reported in a small percentage of patients receiving warfarin. The etiology of this unusual phenomenon is unknown, but is thought to be the result of cholesterol microembolization into the arterial circulation of the toes.

Warfarin-induced skin necrosis is an uncommon but very serious dermatologic reaction that is manifested by a painful maculopapular rash and ecchymosis or purpura that subsequently progresses to necrotic gangrene.[59] It most frequently appears in areas of the body rich in subcutaneous fat, such as the breasts, thighs, buttocks, and abdomen. The incidence of warfarin-induced skin necrosis is less than 0.1%. It is occurs most commonly in middle-aged women who are being treated for acute venous thrombosis. Although symptoms generally appear during the first week of therapy, it has been reported in a small number of patients who had taken warfarin for months and even years. The pathogenesis of warfarin-induced skin necrosis is not clearly understood. Many believe imbalances between procoagulant and anticoagulant proteins that occur early in the course of warfarin therapy resulting in capillary thrombosis and secondary hemorrhages. The observation that patients with proteins C or S deficiency appear to be at greater risk for warfarin-induced skin necrosis supports this theory. Warfarin-induced skin necrosis has also been reported in patients with other disorders of hypercoagulability, such as antithrombin deficiency and antiphospholipid antibodies. Patients who receive large "loading" doses of warfarin may also be at greater risk. It is recommended that heparin therapy be overlapped for a minimum of 7 days when initiating therapy in any patient suspected to have a hypercoagulable state or who has a strong family history of venous thrombosis. If the diagnosis of skin necrosis is suspected, warfarin therapy should be immediately discontinued, vitamin K administered, and full-dose UFH or LMWH therapy initiated. Warfarin therapy should be restarted with extreme caution in patients with a history of skin necrosis, if at all.

Gastrointestinal side effects of warfarin therapy are uncommon and usually self-limited. Because warfarin interferes with vitamin K metabolism, there has been some theoretical concern that it may adversely affect bone formation and cause osteoporosis with long-term use. In one recent analysis, long-term use of warfarin was associated with osteoporotic fractures, in men with atrial fibrillation.[60]

Management of Bleeding and Excessive Anticoagulation

Specific recommendations for the management of patients with an elevated INR are published by the American College of Chest Physicians (ACCP) Consensus Conference on Antithrombotic Therapy (Fig. 21–9).[5] Patients with a mildly elevated INR (3.5 to 5.0) should be examined for signs and symptoms of bleeding, as well as factors that increase bleeding risk. In this circumstance, either reducing the dose of warfarin or holding one or two doses will safely manage most patients. When a swift reduction in an elevated INR is required, oral or intravenous vitamin K_1 (phytonadione) can be given.[5,61] In the absence of major bleeding, the oral route of administration is preferred. While the IV route produces a more rapid reversal, it is associated with rare but serious anaphylactoid reactions. If the INR is between 5 and 9, doses of warfarin should be withheld and may be combined with a low dose of oral vitamin K (≤5 mg). Low doses of oral vitamin K will consistently reduce the INR within 24 hours without making the patient refractory to warfarin therapy. Overcorrection of the INR in the patient who is not bleeding is unnecessary but common. Simply withholding warfarin will result in correction of INRs between 5 and 9 within 48 to 72 hours in most patients.[62] The decision to administer vitamin K should be individualized based on the patient's bleeding risk and the underlying indication for anticoagulation therapy. Vitamin K should be used with caution in patients at high risk of recurrent thromboembolism because of the possibility of INR overcorrection. Conversely, simply withholding warfarin therapy may not lower a high INR quickly enough in patients at high risk for developing bleeding complications. If the INR is greater than 9, a 5-mg oral dose of vitamin K is recommended. High doses of vitamin K (e.g., 10 mg) are associated with prolonged resistance to warfarin and the occurrence of thromboembolic complications. In the event of a serious or life-threatening bleed, intravenous vitamin K should be administered as well as fresh-frozen plasma, clotting factor concentrates, or recombinant FVII.

Drug–Drug and Drug–Food Interactions

The pharmacokinetic and pharmacodynamic properties of warfarin, coupled with its narrow therapeutic index, predispose this agent to numerous clinically important food and drug interactions (see Tables 21–14, 21–15, 21–16, and 21–17).[5,63,64] Vitamin K can reverse warfarin's pharmacologic activity, and many foods contain sufficient vitamin K to reduce the anticoagulation effect of warfarin if a patient consumes them in large portions or repetitively within a short period of time.[64] Patients should be given a list of vitamin K-rich foods and instructed to maintain a relatively consistent intake. It is important to stress consistency and moderation rather than absolute abstinence. Abrupt changes in vitamin K intake should be considered when unexplained changes in the INR occur. Alternative sources of vitamin K, such as multivitamins and nutritional supplements (e.g., Sustacal and Ensure) should also be considered. Patients who require parenteral nutrition should not receive a weekly bolus dose of vitamin K if they are taking warfarin therapy.

Pharmacokinetic drug interactions with warfarin are primarily a result of alterations in hepatic metabolism or binding to plasma proteins. Drugs that inhibit or induce the CYP2C9, CYP1A2, and CYP3A4 isoenzymes have the greatest potential to significantly alter the response to warfarin therapy. Protein-binding displacement interactions can also occur. However, in the absence of hepatic disease or a diminished capacity to metabolize warfarin, changes in protein binding result in only transient changes in the INR. Drugs that alter hemostasis, platelet function, or the clearance of clotting factors (e.g., thyroid hormone replacement) can alter the response to warfarin therapy or increase the risk of bleeding by pharmacodynamic mechanisms.[5,63]

The explosive increase in the use of herbal and alternative therapies in North America has raised concern regarding their potential to interact with warfarin therapy.[64] All patients on warfarin therapy should be questioned regarding the use of herbal drugs and dietary supplements. Clinicians should advise patients on warfarin therapy to seek information about potential interactions with warfarin whenever they start to take a new drug product, whether it is prescribed or purchased over the counter. If there is a known drug interaction or doubt about its potential to alter the response to warfarin, more frequent INR testing following the initiation of the new agent is prudent.

Use in Special Populations

In the absence of a clear and compelling indication, warfarin should not be used during pregnancy because of the potential for fetal hemorrhage and teratogenic complications.[27] Warfarin crosses the placenta and is associated with several embryopathies, particularly CNS abnormalities, that have occurred throughout gestation. The FDA has designated warfarin a pregnancy category X agent. As UFH and the LMWHs are large molecules that do not cross the placental

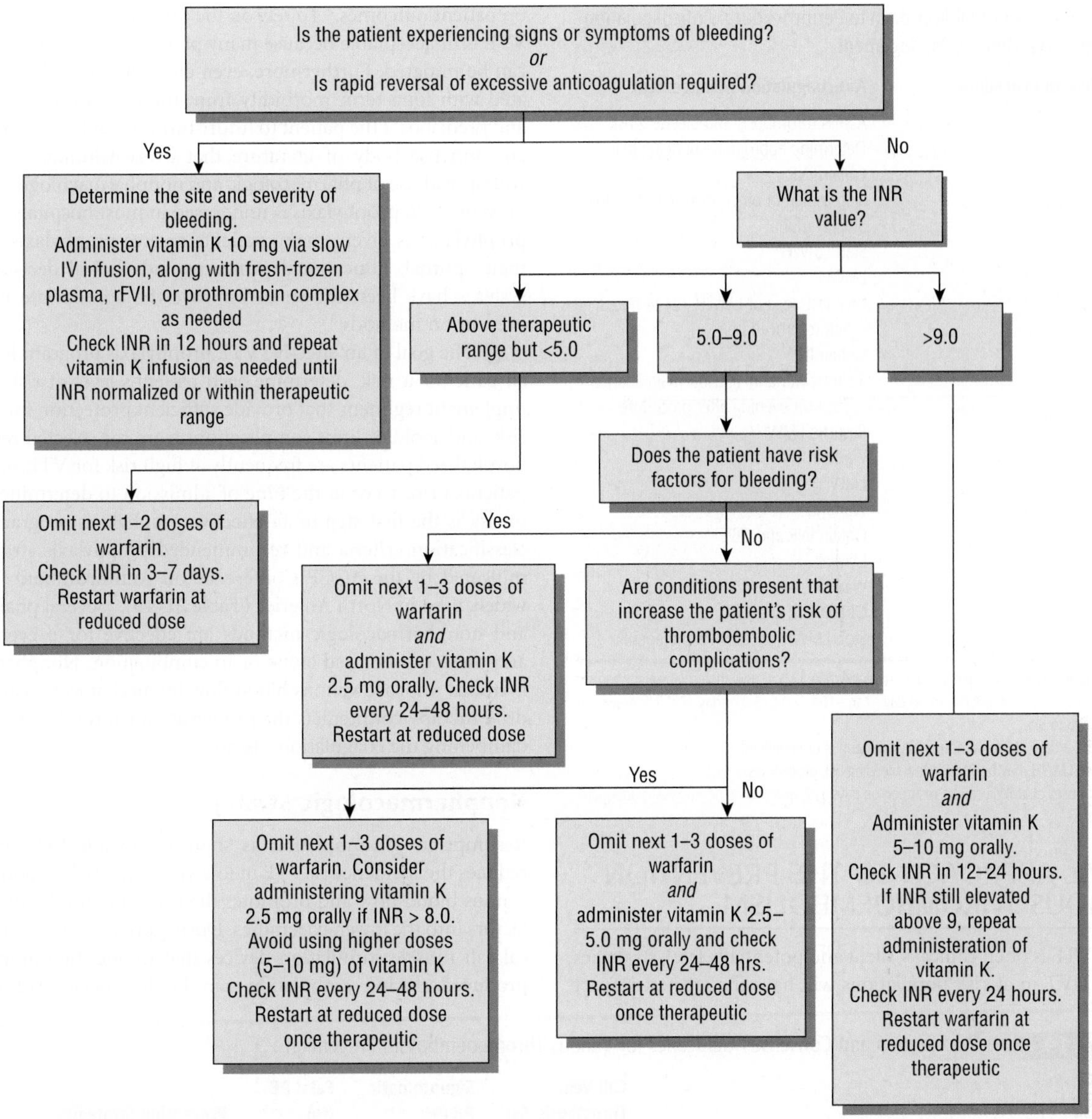

FIGURE 21-9. Management of an elevated international normalized ratio (INR) in patients taking warfarin. Dose reductions should be made by determining the weekly warfarin dose and reducing the weekly dose by 10% to 25% based on degree of INR elevation. Conditions that increase the risk of thromboembolic complications include history of hypercoagulability disorders (e.g., protein C or S deficiency, presence of antiphospholipid antibodies, antithrombin deficiency, activated protein C resistance), arterial or venous thrombosis within the previous month, thromboembolism associated with malignancy, and mechanical mitral valve in conjunction with atrial fibrillation, previous stroke, poor ventricular function, or coexisting mechanical aortic valve. (INR, international normalized ratio; rFVII, recombinant factor VII.)

barrier, they are considered the drugs of choice for anticoagulation during pregnancy. Warfarin is excreted into the breast milk in very low concentrations and is generally considered safe to use by women who are breast-feeding.

Patients scheduled to undergo major surgery or other invasive procedures often require temporary discontinuation of warfarin therapy.[5] The decision to withhold warfarin therapy should be based on the type of surgical procedure being performed and the patient's risk of bleeding and thromboembolism. Warfarin therapy should generally not be discontinued in patients undergoing minimally invasive procedures such as dental work.[5,65] If the bleeding risk from the procedure is considerable, warfarin should be stopped 4 to 5 days prior to the procedure in order to allow the INR to return to near-normal values. Alternatively, warfarin can be stopped and a low dose (2.5 mg) of oral vitamin K may be given 2 days prior to the procedure.[5] Patients at moderate or high risk of thromboembolism (i.e., DVT or PE in the previous month) should be given so-called bridge therapy with UFH or a LMWH before and/or after the procedure (Table 21–18).

Warfarin use among elderly patients is increasingly common. Although the drug has been extensively studied in this population, some debate still remains regarding the relative risks of warfarin therapy in the elderly.[5,6] Data supporting the notion that age increases hemorrhagic risk are somewhat conflicting. Age greater than 75 years is associated with an increased risk of intracranial hemorrhage, but the overall incidence of major bleeding is similar to younger users. Elderly patients may be more prone to excessive anticoagulation as a consequence of nutritional deficiencies, comorbidities, and multiple-drug interactions. Furthermore, they are often at greater risk of falls. Although they often derive the greatest benefit from anticoagulation therapy, elderly patients should be monitored with greater vigilance, and warfarin dose changes should be made more cautiously.

TABLE 21-18 General Approach to Periprocedural Anticoagulation Therapy Management

Days Relative to Procedure	Anticoagulation Management
−7 to −10	Assess thrombosis and bleeding risk Determine appropriate bridging plan Obtain INR
−7	Stop aspirin or other antiplatelet therapy
−6 or −5	Stop Warfarin[a]
−4 or −3	Start LMWH[b]
−2	LMWH
−1	Give last dose of LMWH 12–24 hours before procedure Obtain INR
0 = Surgery	Resume warfarin[c] at usual maintenance dose on evening after procedure
+ 1	Resume LMWH[d] Warfarin
+2 to + 3	LMWH[d] Warfarin Obtain INR and CBC
+4 to +5	LMWH Warfarin Obtain INR and CBC
> +6	Stop LMWH once INR is therapeutic

CBC, complete blood count; INR, international normalized ratio; LMWH, low-molecular-weight heparin.
[a]Warfarin stopped on day −5 if INR drawn on day −7 to −10 is 2.0 to 3.0 or day −6 if INR drawn on day −7 to −10 is 2.5 to 3.5.
[b]LMWH is initiated 2 days (36 to 48 hours) after warfarin is discontinued.
[c]Prophylactic dose LMWH may be used in low bleeding-risk procedures.
[d]Full (treatment) doses of LMWH can be resumed on days 1, 2, and 3 once hemostasis is adequate.
From Ansell et al.[5]

GENERAL APPROACH TO THE PREVENTION OF VENOUS THROMBOEMBOLISM

Given that VTE is often clinically silent and potentially fatal, strategies to prevent DVT in at-risk populations will have the greatest impact on patient outcomes.[3] To rely on the early diagnosis and treatment of VTE is unacceptable because many patients will die before treatment can be initiated. Furthermore, even clinically silent disease is associated with long-term morbidity from the postthrombotic syndrome and predisposes the patient to future thromboembolic events. Despite an immense body of literature that overwhelmingly supports the widespread use of pharmacologic and nonpharmacologic strategies to prevent VTE, prophylaxis is underused in most hospitals. Even when prophylaxis is given, many patients receive prophylaxis that is less than optimal. Educational programs and clinical decision support systems have been shown to improve the appropriate use of VTE prevention methods.[3]

❺ The goal of an effective VTE prophylaxis program is to identify all patients at risk, determine each patient's level of risk, select and implement regimens that provide sufficient protection for the level of risk, and avoid or limit complications from the selected regimens. As hospitalized patients are frequently at high risk for VTE, screening all patients prior to or at the time of admission to determine their level of risk is the first step in an effective prophylaxis program. The risk classification criteria and recommended prophylaxis strategies promulgated by the ACCP Conference on Antithrombotic Therapy is widely used in North America (Table 21–19).[3] Several pharmacologic and nonpharmacologic methods are effective for preventing VTE, and these can be used alone or in combination. Nonpharmacologic methods improve venous blood flow by mechanical means, whereas drug therapy counteracts the propensity for thrombus formation by dampening the coagulation cascade.

Nonpharmacologic Strategies

Resumption of ambulation as soon as possible following surgery reduces the incidence of VTE in low-risk patients.[3] Walking increases venous blood flow and promotes the flow of natural antithrombotic factors into the lower extremities. During prolonged surgeries, electrical calf muscle stimulation devices that mimic the pumping action produced during ambulation can be beneficial. Although these

TABLE 21-19 Risk Classification and Consensus Guidelines for Venous Thromboembolism Prevention

Level of Risk	Calf Vein Thrombosis (%)	Symptomatic PE (%)	Fatal PE (%)	Prevention Strategies
Low				
Minor surgery, age <40 years, and no clinical risk factors	2	0.2	0.002	Ambulation
Moderate	10–20	1–2	0.1–0.4	UFH 5,000 units SC q 12 h
Major or minor surgery, age 40–60 years, and no clinical risk factors				Dalteparin 2,500 units SC q 24 h
Major surgery, age <40 years, and no clinic risk factors				Enoxaparin 40 mg SC q 24 h
Minor surgery, with clinical risk factor(s)				Tinzaparin 3,500 units SC q 24 h
Acutely ill (e.g., MI, ischemic stroke, CHF exacerbation), and no clinical risk factors				IPC Graduated compression stockings
High				
Major surgery, age >60 years, and no clinical risk factors	20–40	2–4	0.4–1.0	UFH 5,000 units SC q 8 h
Major surgery, age 40–60 years, with clinical risk factor(s)				Dalteparin 5,000 units SC q 24 h
Acutely ill (e.g., MI, ischemic stroke, CHF exacerbation), with risk factor(s)				Enoxaparin 40 mg SC q 24 h Fondaparinux 2.5 mg SC q 24 h Tinzaparin 75 units/kg SC q 24 h IPC
Highest				
Major lower-extremity orthopedic surgery	40–80	4–10	0.2–5	Adjusted dose UFH SC q 8 h (aPTT >36 s)
Hip fracture				Dalteparin 5,000 units SC q 24 h
Multiple trauma				Desirudin 15 mg SC q 12 h
Major surgery, age >40 years, and prior history of VTE				Enoxaparin 30 mg SC q 12 h
Major surgery, age >40 years, and malignancy				Fondaparinux 2.5 mg SC q 24 h
Major surgery, age >40 years, and hypercoagulable state				Tinzaparin 75 units/kg SC q 24 h
Spinal cord injury or stroke with limb paralysis				Warfarin (INR = 2.0–3.0) IPC with UFH 5,000 units SC q 8 h

aPTT, activated partial thromboplastin time; CHF, congestive heart failure; INR, international normalized ratio; IPC, intermittent pneumatic compression; MI, myocardial infarction; SC, subcutaneous; UFH, unfractionated heparin; VTE, venous thromboembolism.
From Geerts et al.[3]

devices can reduce the risk of DVT by more than 50%, their use is painful, and they can be used only when the patient is under general anesthesia. Continuous passive motion devices and plantar compression systems are also available but their effectiveness is uncertain.

Graduated compression stockings reduce the incidence of VTE by approximately 60% following general surgery, neurosurgery, and stroke.[3,66] Compression stockings work by increasing the velocity of venous blood flow. They apply a graded amount of pressure, with the greatest amount of pressure applied at the ankle. Inexpensive and safe, they are an excellent choice when pharmacologic interventions are either contraindicated or difficult to monitor adequately. When combined with pharmacologic interventions, graduated compression stockings have an additive effect. Some patients are unable to wear compression stockings because of the size or shape of their legs, however.

Similar to graduated compression stockings, intermittent pneumatic compression (IPC) devices increase the velocity of blood flow in the lower extremities.[3,67] The technique involves the sequential inflation of a series of cuffs wrapped around the patient's legs. Using graded pressure, the cuffs inflate in 1- to 2-minute cycles continually throughout the day from the ankles to the thighs. IPC reduces the risk of VTE by more than 60% following general surgery, neurosurgery, and orthopedic surgery.[3] There is some theoretical concern that external compression may dislodge a previously formed clot.[68] Although IPC is well tolerated and safe to use in patients who have contraindications to pharmacologic therapies, it does have a few drawbacks. It is more expensive than the use of graduated compression stockings, it is a relatively cumbersome technique, and some patients may have difficulty sleeping while using it.[3] Like graduated compression hose, IPC can increase the effectiveness of pharmacologic prophylaxis.

Inferior vena cava (IVC) filters, also known as Greenfield filters, provide short-term protection against PE in very-high-risk patients by preventing the embolization of a thrombus formed in the lower extremities into the pulmonary circulation.[3,69,70] Percutaneous insertion of a filter into the IVC is a minimally invasive procedure performed via fluoroscopy. Despite the widespread use of IVC filters, there are very limited data regarding their effectiveness and long-term safety. The evidence suggests that IVC filters, particularly in the absence of effective antithrombotic therapy, increase the long-term risk of recurrent DVT. In the only randomized clinical trial examining the short- and long-term effectiveness of the filters in patients with a documented proximal DVT, treatment with IVC filters in combination with anticoagulation therapy reduced the risk of pulmonary embolism by more than 75% during the first 12 days following insertion.[70] However, this benefit was not sustained during 2 years of followup and the long-term risk of recurrent deep vein thrombosis was nearly twofold higher in those who received a filter. Although IVC filters can reduce the short-term risk of PE in patients who are at highest risk, they should be reserved for patients in whom other prophylactic strategies cannot be used. Furthermore, to reduce the long-term risk of VTE in association with IVC filters, pharmacologic prophylaxis is necessary, and warfarin therapy should begin as soon as the patient is able to tolerate it.

Pharmacologic Strategies

Several pharmacologic interventions have been extensively evaluated in numerous randomized clinical trials.[3] Appropriately selected drug therapies can dramatically reduce the incidence of VTE following hip replacement, knee replacement, general surgery, myocardial infarction, and ischemic stroke (see Table 21–19). The choice of agent and dose to use for VTE prevention must be based on the patient's level of risk for thrombosis and bleeding complications, as well as cost and the availability of an adequate drug therapy monitoring system.

Most randomized controlled trials fail to show a significant benefit from aspirin therapy in the prevention of VTE.[3] The ACCP Consensus Conference continues to recommend against the use of aspirin as the primary method of VTE prophylaxis. Antiplatelet drugs clearly reduce the risk of coronary artery and cerebrovascular events in patients with arterial disease, but aspirin produces a very modest reduction in VTE following orthopedic surgeries of the lower extremities. The relative contribution of platelets in the pathogenesis of venous thrombosis compared with that of arterial thrombosis can explain the reason for this difference. Venous thrombosis results primarily from venous stasis, while arterial thrombosis is most often the result of vascular wall injury.

CLINICAL CONTROVERSY

In a series of large, well-designed phase III clinical trials, fondaparinux was superior to enoxaparin for the prevention of VTE in patients who were undergoing lower-extremity orthopedic surgery. However, the rate of symptomatic pulmonary embolism and death was not different between the two treatments in any of these studies. Furthermore, fondaparinux has not been compared to warfarin for the prevention of VTE in high-risk patients. Based on these findings, some experts contend that fondaparinux offers no clinical advantages over enoxaparin or warfarin. In addition, although there was no difference in the risk of major hemorrhage seen in the clinical trials when compared to enoxaparin, some clinicians worry about the potential for bleeding with fondaparinux because it has a long half-life and it cannot be reversed with protamine sulfate. Despite these concerns, some experts believe fondaparinux should be used preferentially because asymptomatic DVTs and PEs may increase the future risk of recurrent thrombotic events and the postthrombotic syndrome.

The most extensively studied agents for the prevention of VTE are UFH, the LMWHs, and fondaparinux.[3,71] The LMWHs and fondaparinux provide superior protection against VTE when compared to low-dose UFH.[3,71] Their more predictable absorption when given by subcutaneous injection may be the explanation. Even so, UFH remains a highly effective, cost-conscious choice for many patient populations, provided that it is given in the appropriate dose (see Table 21–19). Low-dose UFH (5,000 units every 12 hours or every 8 hours) given subcutaneously reduces the risk of VTE by 55% to 70% in patients undergoing a wide range of general surgical procedures and following a myocardial infarction or stroke. For the prevention of VTE following hip and knee replacement surgery, the effectiveness of low-dose UFH is considerably lower.[3] Adjusted-dose UFH therapy provided subcutaneously, which requires dose adjustments to maintain the aPTT at the high end of the normal range, appears to be substantially more effective than low-dose UFH in the highest-risk patient populations. However, adjusted-dose UFH has been studied in only a few relatively small clinical trials and requires frequent laboratory monitoring. The LMWHs and fondaparinux appear to provide a high degree of protection against VTE in most high-risk populations. The appropriate prophylactic dose for each LMWH product is indication specific (see Table 21–10). There is no evidence that one LMWH is superior to another for the prevention of VTE. Fondaparinux was significantly more effective than enoxaparin in several clinical trials that enrolled patients undergoing high risk orthopedic procedures but has not been shown to reduce the incidence of symptomatic PE or mortality.[71] To provide optimal protection, some experts believe that the LMWHs should be initiated prior to surgery.[3,72]

Warfarin is a commonly used option for the prevention of VTE following orthopedic surgeries of the lower extremities.[3] The evidence is equivocal regarding the relative effectiveness of warfarin compared to the LMWHs for the prevention of clinically important VTE events in the highest risk populations. When used to prevent VTE, the dose of warfarin should be adjusted to maintain an INR between 2.0 and 3.0; however, some orthopedic surgeons favor lower initial INR goal ranges (e.g., 1.5 to 2.5) because of fear of bleeding at the surgical site. Oral administration and low drug cost give warfarin some advantages over the LMWHs and fondaparinux. However, warfarin does not achieve its full antithrombotic effect for several days, requires frequent monitoring and periodic dosage adjustments, and carries a substantial risk of major bleeding. For these reasons, warfarin is reserved for the highest-risk patients. Furthermore, warfarin should be recommended only when a well-developed monitoring system is available.[5]

The optimal duration for VTE prophylaxis following surgery is not well established.[3,73] Prophylaxis should be given throughout the period of risk. For general surgical procedures and medical conditions, once the patient is able to ambulate regularly and other risk factors are no longer present, prophylaxis can be discontinued. Because of the relatively high incidence of VTE in the first month following hospital discharge among patients who have undergone a lower extremity orthopedic procedure, extended prophylaxis following hospital discharge with either a LMWH, fondaparinux, or warfarin appears to be beneficial. Most clinical trials support the use of antithrombotic therapy for 21 to 35 days following total hip replacement and hip fracture repair surgeries.[33,74,75]

Pharmacoeconomic Considerations

Only a handful of studies have formally evaluated the cost-effectiveness of VTE prevention strategies. The acquisition costs of graduated compression stockings, heparin, and warfarin are considerably less than those of the LMWHs and fondaparinux. However, the acquisition cost for drug therapy is relatively small when compared with the overall cost of care.[76] Economic analyses must take into account the efficacy of the strategy, treatment complications, and monitoring costs.

The determination of the cost-effectiveness of VTE prophylaxis is based on the premise that a reduction in future VTE events will reduce overall healthcare costs.[77] Furthermore, the incremental cost per patient will decrease proportionally with an increase in the frequency of VTE in the population. Stated another way, the cost of providing prophylaxis to 1,000 patients will decline as the incidence of VTE in the given population increases. Consequently, more expensive and effective strategies become more cost-effective in higher-risk populations. In populations at low risk for VTE, early ambulation appears to be the most cost-effective strategy. In populations at moderate risk, the use of graduated compression stockings, the least expensive intervention, results in a lower overall cost of care, whereas low-dose UFH is estimated to increase the cost $50 (in 1990 dollars) per patient when compared with no prophylaxis.[78] This compares favorably with the incremental costs associated with other routinely employed preventative measures. Although LMWH provides slightly greater reductions in the risk of VTE in patients who are at moderate risk of VTE, the additional cost is estimated to be $107 (in 1999 dollars) per patient when compared to low-dose UFH.[79] Whether universal use of LMWH in moderate-risk patients is a cost-effective strategy remains controversial.

In high-risk patients, the cost-effectiveness of prevention is far greater because the incidence of VTE is higher. Following hip replacement surgery, regardless of the strategy selected, prophylaxis saves money when compared with no prophylaxis.[77] The LMWHs and fondaparinux slightly increase the total mean cost of care after total hip and knee replacement when compared with low-dose UFH and warfarin.[80,81] However, because of their superior effectiveness, the LMWHs have a significantly lower cost per DVT and PE avoided.[77] Based on typical drug-acquisition costs, LMWH and fondaparinux appear to be cost-effective choices in the highest-risk patient populations.[82]

GENERAL APPROACH TO THE TREATMENT OF VENOUS THROMBOEMBOLISM

❻ Before initiating anticoagulation therapy for the treatment of VTE, it is imperative to establish an accurate diagnosis; thus preventing unnecessary risk and expense to the patient.[83] Anticoagulation therapy remains the mainstay of treatment for VTE. DVT and PE are manifestations of the same disease process and are treated similarly.[2] Full "therapeutic" doses of antithrombotic drugs prevent thrombus extension and embolization as well as reduce the risk of long-term sequelae such as the postthrombotic syndrome, pulmonary hypertension, and recurrent thromboembolism.[2,84] The standard approach is to initiate therapy with UFH by continuous IV infusion or a LMWH or fondaparinux by subcutaneous injection and to make the transition to warfarin for maintenance therapy (Table 21–20 and Fig. 21–10). In rare circumstances, elimination of the obstructing thrombus is warranted and the use of venous thrombectomy or thrombolysis can be considered.[2] Inferior vena

TABLE 21-20 Consensus Guidelines for Venous Thromboembolism Treatment

	Recommendation	Grade[a]
Acute anticoagulation	Acute treatment of DVT or PE should be with LMWH, fondaparinux, intravenous UFH, or adjusted-dose subcutaneous UFH	1A
	The dose of UFH should be sufficient to prolong the aPTT to a range that corresponds to a plasma heparin level of 0.2 to 0.4 international units/mL by protamine titration or an anti-Xa level of 0.3 to 0.6 international units/mL	1C+
	LMWH and fondaparinux are preferred over UFH	2B
	A LMWH is preferred in patients with cancer	1A
Duration of acute treatment	Treatment with UFH, LMWH, or fondaparinux should be overlapped with warfarin for at least 5 days and can be stopped when the INR is >2.0; most patients should have warfarin started at the same time as UFH, LMWH, or fondaparinux	1A
	Patients with cancer should be treated with a LMWH for at least 6 months	1A
	A longer period of heparin therapy (approximately 10 days) is recommended for massive PE or severe iliofemoral thrombosis	1C
Long-term anticoagulation	Oral anticoagulation therapy (target INR 2.5, range: 2.0 to 3.0) should be continued for at least 3 months; if oral anticoagulation therapy is contraindicated (e.g., pregnancy), a treatment dose of LMWH or adjusted-dose UFH should be used	1A
	Patients with an idiopathic VTE, an inherited disorder of hypercoagulability, or antiphospholipid antibodies should be treated indefinitely (at least 2.5 years)	1A
	Patients with continuing risk factors (e.g., malignancy, immobility) should be treated for *at least* 12 months	1C

aPTT, activated partial thromboplastin time; DVT, deep vein thrombosis; INR, international normalized ratio; LMWH, low-molecular-weight heparin; PE, pulmonary embolism; UFH, unfractionated heparin; VTE, venous thromboembolism.

[a]Refers to grade of recommendation (1A, strong recommendation applying to most patients without reservation; 1C, intermediate-strength recommendation that may change when stronger evidence becomes available; 1C+, strong recommendation that applies to most patients in most circumstances; 2B, weak recommendation where alternative approaches likely to be better for some patients under some circumstances).

From Buller et al.[2]

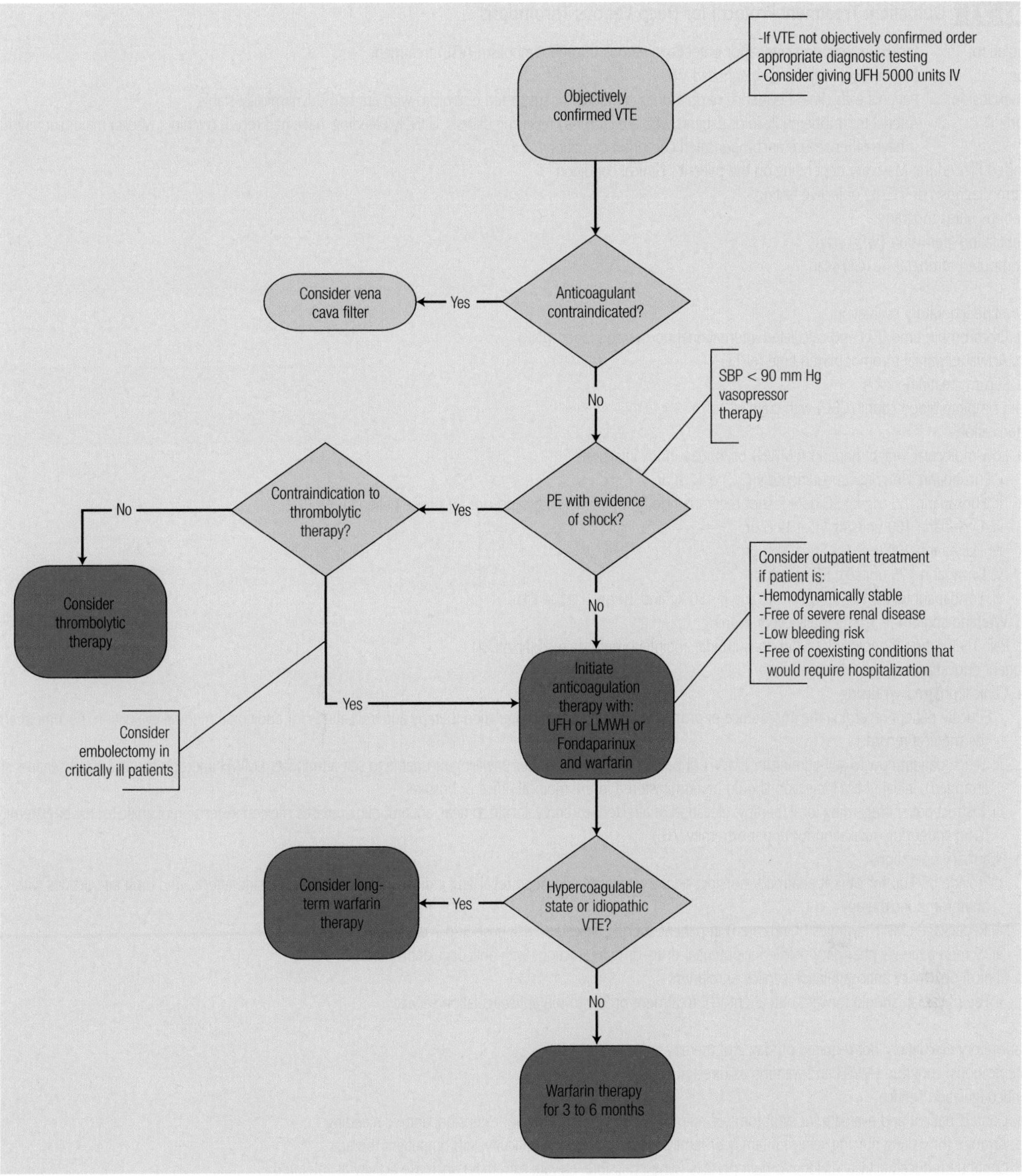

FIGURE 21-10. Treatment of venous thromboembolism (VTE). (LMWH, low-molecular-weight heparin; PE, pulmonary embolism; SBP, systolic blood pressure; UFH, unfractionated heparin.)

cava interruption with a filter is also an option in those with contraindications to anticoagulation therapy or in whom anticoagulant therapy has failed.

Once the diagnosis of VTE has been objectively confirmed (see Clinical Presentation and Diagnosis below), anticoagulant therapy with either UFH, LMWH, or fondaparinux should be instituted as soon as possible. LMWHs and fondaparinux are highly effective and can be administered in the outpatient setting. The decision to initiate therapy with a LMWH or fondaparinux on an outpatient basis should be based on institutional resources and patient specific variables (Table 21–21). ❼

UNFRACTIONATED HEPARIN

The parenteral administration of UFH followed by warfarin has been the conventional treatment of patients with VTE for decades. Although UFH can be given by either subcutaneous or IV injection, continuous IV infusion has been preferred because of improved dosing precision (see Table 21–7).[2] When UFH is administered by IV infusion, the aPTT or a suitable coagulation study should be used to monitor the anticoagulant effect.[24] The infusion rate should be adjusted to maintain an appropriate range corresponding to a heparin concentration of 0.3 to 0.7 international units/mL anti-Xa activity by the amidolytic assay. Weight-based dosing of UFH achieves a therapeutic aPTT in the vast majority of patients in the first 24 hours (see Table 21–7).[22] Failure to give a sufficient dose of IV UFH has been shown to increase the risk of VTE recurrence not only during the initial treatment but also during long-term therapy.[24] Intravenous UFH requires hospitalization with frequent monitoring and dose adjustment. Well organized inpatient anticoagulation management services have been shown to improve patient care by increasing the proportion of aPTT values in the therapeutic

TABLE 21-21 Outpatient Treatment Protocol for Deep Venous Thrombosis

Target Population: Inclusion/exclusion criteria for outpatient venous thromboembolism (VTE) treatment
- Inclusion: Patients with objectively diagnosed VTE
- Relative exclusion: Patients with clinical evidence of pulmonary embolus or suspected embolism who are hemodynamically stable
- Exclusion: Arterial thromboembolism or patients who are currently receiving dialysis, actively bleeding, have had recent (within 2 weeks) major surgery/trauma, or have other severe uncompensated comorbid conditions

Recommended Procedure: May vary depending on the patient's clinical condition

A. Confirm diagnosis of VTE by objective testing
   1. Venous ultrasonogram
   2. Ventilation–perfusion (V/Q) scan
   3. Computed tomography (CT) scan

B. Day 1
   1. Baseline laboratory evaluation
      a. Prothrombin time (PT) and calculated international normalized ration (INR)
      b. Activated partial thromboplastin time (aPTT)
      c. Serum creatinine (Scr)
      d. Complete blood count (CBC) with platelets
   2. Medication
      a. Low-molecular-weight heparin (LMWH) or fondaparinux injections
         i. Enoxaparin 1 mg/kg subcutaneously (SC) q 12 h or
         ii. Enoxaparin 1.5 mg/kg SC q 24 h (not recommended for patients with cancer or for obese patients)
         iii. Dalteparin 100 units/kg SC q 12 h or
         iv. Dalteparin 200 units/kg SC q 24 h or
         v. Tinzaparin 175 units/kg SC q 24 h or
         vi. Fondaparinux 7.5 mg SC q 24 h (5 mg if <50 kg and 10 mg if >100 kg)
      b. Warfarin sodium 5–10 mg orally every evening
      c. Pain medication if necessary (avoid nonsteroidal antiinflammatory drugs [NSAIDs])
   3. Patient education
      a. Clinical pharmacy/nursing
         i. Educate patient regarding the importance of proper monitoring of anticoagulation therapy and indications for additional medical evaluation; document activities in the medical record
         ii. Teach patient how to self-administer LMWH (if patient or family member unwilling or unable to self-administer LMWH injection, visiting nurse services should be arranged); initial LMWH injection should be administered in the medical office or hospital
         iii. Instruct patient regarding local therapy: elevation of affected extremity; localized heat, antiembolic exercises (flexion–extension of ankle for lower-extremity VTE, or hand squeezing–relaxation for upper-extremity VTE)
      b. Pharmacy operations
         i. Provide backup for clinical pharmacy/nursing; reinforce patient education regarding indication, use, monitoring, side effects, and drug interactions with antithrombotic therapy
         ii. Repackage LMWH syringes (if indicated) in patient-specific doses and dispense 5 to 7 days of therapy
         iii. Screen patient's pharmacy profile for potential drug–drug interactions with anticoagulation therapy
      c. Clinical pharmacy anticoagulation service enrollment
         i. The physician should forward outpatient VTE treatment orders to the anticoagulation service

C. Day 2
   1. Laboratory evaluation: not required on day 2 of therapy
   2. Medications: continue LMWH and warfarin as directed
   3. Anticoagulation service
      a. Contact patient and evaluate for symptoms of pulmonary embolism (PE), clot extension, and/or bleeding
      b. Arrange for visiting nursing service if family or family member is having difficulty with outpatient therapy
      c. Continue reduced activity as long as pain persists (when possible, elevate extremity); increase activity as tolerated
      d. Document activities in medical record

D. Day 3
   1. Laboratory evaluation: check INR
   2. Medications: continue LMWH and warfarin directed
   3. Anticoagulation service
      a. Contact patient and evaluate for symptoms of PE, clot extension, and/or bleeding
      b. Interpret results of INR and adjust dose of warfarin to achieve a target INR of 2.5
      c. Patient activity: continue reduced activity as long as pain persists (when possible, elevate extremity); increase activity as tolerated
      d. Document activities in medical record

E. Day 4
   1. Laboratory evaluation: check INR
   2. Medications: continue LMWH and warfarin as directed
   3. Anticoagulation service
      a. Contact patient and evaluate for symptoms of PE, clot extensions, and/or bleeding
      b. Interpret results of INR and adjust dose of warfarin to achieve a target INR of 2.5
      c. Patient activity: no restrictions; if pain increases, contact anticoagulation service or provider
      d. Document activities in medical record

(continued)

TABLE 21-21 Outpatient Treatment Protocol for Deep Venous Thrombosis (continued)

F. Day 5
1. Laboratory evaluation: check INR and CBC with platelets
2. Medications: continue LMWH if indicated and warfarin as directed
3. Anticoagulation service
   a. Contact patient and evaluate for symptoms of PE, clot extension, and/or bleeding
   b. Interpret results of INR and adjust does of warfarin to achieve a target INR of 2.5
   c. Patient activity: no restriction; if pain increases, contact primary care provider
   d. Document activities in medical record

range, reducing the length of hospital stay, and lowering total hospital costs when compared to usual care.[8] However, despite the widespread use of weight-based dosing protocols, some patients still fail to achieve an adequate response to UFH therapy.[24] There is also evidence that UFH does not prevent thrombus progression in some patients with DVT, and rebound thrombin generation has been observed when UFH is discontinued abruptly.[24] These limitations of traditional IV UFH in the acute treatment of VTE have led to the investigation of alternative approaches.

LOW-MOLECULAR-WEIGHT HEPARIN

Because of their improved pharmacokinetic and pharmacodynamic profile as well as ease of use, the LMWHs have replaced UFH for the treatment of VTE in many institutions. The LMWHs given subcutaneously in fixed, weight-based doses (see Table 21–10) are at least as effective as UFH given IV for the treatment of VTE.[2] A number of meta-analyses comparing LMWH to UFH in the treatment of venous thromboembolism have been conducted. These analyses demonstrate no differences in clinically important end points, including recurrent DVT, PE, major or minor bleeding, and thrombocytopenia.[2] Surprisingly, patients who received LMWH had a significantly lower mortality rate. The reduction in mortality was primarily seen in patients with cancer.[2] The explanation for this survival advantage is unknown. There appears to be no difference in the risk of recurrent VTE between patients who are treated on an inpatient or outpatient basis with a LMWH for DVT.[85] However, outpatient treatment was associated with a slightly greater risk of major bleeding indicating the need for close monitoring when LMWH is given in this setting. There appears to be no difference in the efficacy or safety of once-daily versus twice-daily dosing regimens.[2] However, a subgroup analysis in one study suggested that patients with cancer and obese patients have higher recurrence rates with once-daily enoxaparin.[86]

Given the predictable response and the reduced need for laboratory monitoring with LMWH, stable patients with DVT who have normal vital signs, low bleeding risk and no other comorbid conditions requiring hospitalization can be discharged early or treated entirely on an outpatient basis (see Table 21–21).[87] The efficacy and safety of LMWH in the home-based treatment of proximal DVT was initially established in large clinical studies.[87,88] The results of randomized controlled clinical trials, as well as the experience of several successful outpatient DVT treatment programs in a variety of health-care settings, have led to an increased acceptance for outpatient management. Indeed, surveys of patients who received outpatient DVT treatment indicate a high degree of satisfaction and comfort, with 91% expressing satisfaction with home treatment.[87]

Patients presenting with PE and no evidence of hemodynamic instability are at low risk of subsequent morbidity and mortality. Evidence exists suggesting that patients with submassive PE who are hemodynamically stable can be managed safely as outpatients with LMWH or fondaparinux.[24] However, hemodynamically unstable patients with PE should generally be admitted and treated with either intravenous UFH, LMWH, or fondaparinux. If thrombolytic therapy or embolectomy is anticipated, UFH, which can be rapidly reversed, is preferred.[89] Patients with PE who present with shock have the highest risk of mortality and require aggressive interventions such as volume expansion, vasopressor therapy, intubation and mechanical ventilation in addition to antithrombotic therapy.[90]

Not all patients are appropriate candidates for outpatient DVT treatment. At a minimum, patients with objectively diagnosed DVT must be reliable or have adequate caregiver support.[87] Patients and their caregivers must be willing and active participants in the outpatient management of DVT (Table 21–22). Patients who are unable to manage or who decline at-home treatment should be admitted to the hospital. These patients may subsequently opt for early discharge on LMWH. Daily patient contact either in person or via telephone is essential to identify potential complications and to address questions and concerns promptly. During daily contacts patients must be asked about symptoms that may indicate bleeding, thrombus extension, and PE.[87] Once acute treatment with a LMWH or fondaparinux has been transitioned to long-term warfarin therapy (approximately 5 to 10 days), patient contact can occur less frequently.

FONDAPARINUX

Two clinical trials have shown fondaparinux to be a safe and effective alternative to enoxaparin and intravenous UFH for the treatment of VTE.[91,92] In the Mondial Assessment of Thromboembolism Treatment Initiated by Synthetic Pentasaccharide with Symptomatic Endpoints-Deep Venous Thrombosis (MATISSE-DVT) trial, a fixed-dose regimen of fondaparinux (7.5 mg q 24 h) given by subcutaneous injection was compared to the standard weight-adjusted dosing of enoxaparin (1 mg/kg q 12 h) for the acute treatment DVT followed by 3 months of warfarin therapy.[91] In the MATISSE-PE trial, fondaparinux (7.5 mg subcutaneously [SC] q 24 h) was compared to UFH administered by IV infusion.[92] In both trials, the dose of fondaparinux was increased to 10 mg SC every 24 hours for patients who weighed more than 100 kg and reduced to 5 mg SC every 24 hours for those who weighed less than 50 kg. Fondaparinux received FDA approval for the acute treatment of DVT and PE in 2004.[32]

WARFARIN

Warfarin monotherapy is an unacceptable choice for the acute treatment of VTE because it does not produce a rapid anticoagulation effect and is associated high incidence of recurrent thromboembolism. However, warfarin is very effective in the long-term management of VTE and should be started concurrently with rapid acting injectable anticoagulant therapy.[2] The rapid acting injectable anticoagulant should overlap with warfarin therapy for at least 5 days and until a therapeutic INR has been achieved. The initial dose of warfarin should be 5 to 10 mg (see Fig. 21–8) and periodically adjusted to achieve and maintain an INR between 2.0 and 3.0.

The appropriate duration of warfarin maintenance therapy requires careful consideration of the circumstances surrounding the initial thromboembolic event, the presence of ongoing thromboembolic risk factors, and the risk of bleeding.[2,93] A major consideration

TABLE 21-22 Patient Education for Outpatient Deep Vein Thrombosis Therapy

General information regarding DVT and the goals of treatment
- Anticoagulant medications (injections and warfarin tablets) have been prescribed to prevent the blood clot from growing larger so that the body can begin to dissolve the clot
- Your body may be able to completely dissolve the clot, but in some cases the clot never goes completely away; even with adequate anticoagulation therapy, some people will have chronic pain and swelling in the affected extremity; people who have had one clot are at increased risk of having future clots
- Warfarin tablets take several days to begin to work; LMWH injections work right away so at first LMWH injections and warfarin tablets are used together
- When the warfarin has become effective, you will be able to stop the LMWH injections; you will continue to take warfarin tablets for 3 to 6 months or longer to prevent blood clots from returning
- It is important for you to administer your LMWH or fondaparinux and warfarin exactly as directed

Subcutaneous injection technique
- You must learn to give yourself a subcutaneous injection of LMWH or fondaparinux; alternatively, you may have a family member or visiting nurse give it to you
- If your LMWH or fondaparinux syringes were filled by the manufacturer, they can be stored at room temperature; if your syringes were filled by the pharmacy, they should be stored in the refrigerator; if you were instructed to fill your own syringes, you should prepare the syringe immediately prior to injecting its contents
- If you see a bubble in the syringe, do not try to get it out, you may accidentally squirt out part of your dose
- Choose an injection site on your abdomen; clean the area with alcohol, then position an uncapped syringe at a 90-degree angle; pinch the skin, stick the needle in as far as it will go and gently but firmly push the plunger down; this will inject the medicine into the skin; when all the medication has been injected, remove the needle and dispose of it in an appropriate container
- You will likely experience a burning sensation when the medication is injected; this will go away after a few minutes
- Rotate injection sites from side to side, do not inject into the same site more than once; avoid the area around your navel; do not inject into any bruises

Blood test monitoring
- Regular blood tests are required to make sure your medication is working properly
- The prothrombin time tells how quickly your blood forms a clot; it is used to tell how well warfarin is working
- The INR is a way to standardize the prothrombin time between laboratories; your goal INR range is between 2.0 and 3.0; if your INR is less than 2.0, you are at higher risk for clotting, if your INR is greater than 3.0, you are at higher risk for bleeding; your dose of warfarin will be adjusted based on the results of this test
- You need to have a complete blood count test both before you begin therapy and after you have been on LMWH or fondaparinux for about 5 days; this will help detect internal bleeding and the occurrence of a rare side effect of heparin therapy that can decrease a component of your blood called platelets

Warfarin information
- Each strength of warfarin has a unique color; each time you refill your prescription, make sure your new tablets are the same color you have been taking; if they are not the same color, ask your pharmacist why
- Warfarin should be taken at approximately the same time each day
- The most common and serious side effect of warfarin is bleeding; you should be careful to avoid situations or activities that increase your risk of injury; apply direct pressure to control bleeding from superficial cuts
- Warfarin has many drug interactions; always check with your provider before taking any new medications (including over-the-counter medications and dietary supplements)
- Foods rich in vitamin K (green leafy vegetables, etc.) may interfere with warfarin; you do not need to avoid foods rich in vitamin K, but you should try to maintain consistent dietary habits
- Alcohol can increase your risk for bleeding and interfere with warfarin therapy; drink alcohol in moderation (1 to 2 drinks per day); avoid binge drinking

Contact your provider if you experience
- Persistent bleeding from a cut or scrape
- Blood in your urine
- Blood in your stool
- Persistent nose bleeding
- Increased swelling or pain in your affected extremity

Go to the emergency department if you experience
- Shortness of breath
- Chest pain
- Coughing up blood
- Black tarry-appearing stool
- Severe headache of sudden onset
- Slurred speech

DVT, deep vein thrombosis; INR, international normalized ratio; LMWH, low-molecular-weight heparin.

in determining the risk of recurrent VTE once anticoagulation therapy is stopped is whether the initial thrombotic event was associated with a major transient or reversible risk factor (e.g., within 3 months of surgery with general anesthesia, plaster cast immobilization of a leg, or hospitalization). For patients in this situation, the risk of recurrence is relatively small, approximately 3% in the first year and approximately 10% over 5 years, and only 3 months of oral anticoagulation treatment is warranted.[93] For VTE associated with a minor transient or reversible risk factor (e.g., within 6 weeks of initiation of estrogen therapy, air travel lasting >10 hours, pregnancy, or less marked leg injuries or immobilization) 3 months of oral anticoagulation therapy is reasonable, but some experts prefer 6 months of treatment.[93]

Patients with unprovoked (idiopathic) VTE have a recurrence risk of approximately 10% in the first year and approximately 30% over 5 years. These patients should be considered for indefinite oral anticoagulation therapy if possible, but should receive at least 6 to 12 months of therapy.[2] Factors that may lead to the decision to stop oral anticoagulation therapy after 6 to 12 months include noncompliance with warfarin therapy, initial clot although idiopathic was isolated in calf veins, or a moderate to high risk of bleeding.[93] Risk factors for bleeding include age >65 years, previous stroke, history of bleeding (e.g., gastrointestinal), active peptic ulcer disease, renal impairment, anemia, thrombocytopenia, liver disease, diabetes mellitus, concurrent antiplatelet use, noncompliance, and the presence of a structural lesion (e.g., tumor, recent surgery) expected to be associated with bleeding. Presence of one to two bleeding risk factors suggests moderate bleeding risk while three or more risk factors suggest a high bleeding risk.[93]

Increasingly, patients with VTE are being tested for hereditary and acquired hypercoagulable states (thrombophilia). With the exception of individuals with the antiphospholipid antibody syndrome, homozygotes for the factor V Leiden mutation, and heterozygotes with both the factor V Leiden and prothrombin 20210 gene mutations, the presence of thrombophilia does not appear to confer a clinically important risk for VTE recurrence.[93] Indefinite or life-long anticoagulation therapy should be considered for those patients with recurrent VTE events or one of the thrombophilias known to impart a high life-time risk of thrombosis. Otherwise decisions regarding duration of therapy should be guided by the presence or absence of transient VTE risk factors.[93] The decision to continue anticoagulation therapy indefinitely should be reassessed annually. Patients should be involved in any decision to continue anticoagulation therapy with consideration given to the patient's long-term prognosis, risk of bleeding, ability to adhere to anticoagulation therapy instructions, financial resources, lifestyle, and quality of life. When the benefits of continued anticoagulation therapy no longer outweigh the risks, therapy should be discontinued.[93]

THROMBOLYSIS AND THROMBECTOMY

Most cases of VTE require only anticoagulation therapy. In some cases, however, removal of the occluding thrombus by either pharmacologic or surgical means may be warranted.[2] There is a relative paucity of data supporting either thrombolysis or thrombectomy in the routine management of VTE, and more study is clearly needed to clarify their precise role.

Thrombolytic agents are proteolytic enzymes that enhance the conversion of plasminogen to plasmin which subsequently degrades the fibrin matrix. Thrombolytic therapy for DVT was once believed to improve long-term outcomes by preventing the postthrombotic syndrome. Indeed, thrombolytic therapy improves venous patency. However, clinical trials have failed to demonstrate any sustained benefit from the routine use of thrombolytic therapy and the evidence that thrombolytic therapy is superior to anticoagulation therapy alone in preventing the postthrombotic syndrome is uncertain.[2] Patients who present with massive DVT and limb gangrene despite anticoagulation therapy are candidates for thrombolysis (Table 21–23).[2] Some authorities recommend thrombolytic treatment for patients with massive iliofemoral VTE who are at low risk for bleeding. Catheter-directed instillation of a thrombolytic agent directly into the clot is increasingly being used. The risk of bleeding associated with catheter-directed drug administration appears to be less than systemic administration. Prospective clinical trials are necessary to clarify the clinical utility of catheter-directed thrombolysis in the treatment of DVT but most experts recommend against its routine use.[2]

In the management of acute PE, alteplase, streptokinase, and urokinase have all been shown to restore pulmonary artery patency more rapidly than UFH alone. However, this early benefit does not improve long-term patient outcomes. One week following acute treatment, clot lysis and vessel patency are similar with or without thrombolytic therapy. Thrombolytic therapy has never been shown to improve morbidity or mortality, but is associated with a substantial risk of hemorrhage.[2] For this reason, patients being considered for thrombolytic therapy should be screened carefully for contraindications relating to bleeding risk.[89] Admittedly, clinical trials to date have been underpowered to detect a benefit from thrombolytic therapy. The association of thrombolytic therapy with hemorrhage is particularly problematic because PE frequently occurs following a surgical procedure when the risk of bleeding is high. Given the relative lack of data to support their routine use, thrombolytic agents should be reserved for those patients with PE who are most likely to benefit (see Table 21–23). Patients who have hemodynamic compromise as evidenced by significant hypotension (systolic blood pressure 90 mm Hg or less) or severe right ventricular strain because of a large clot burden may benefit from thrombolytic therapy.[2] Five percent to 10% of patients diagnosed with a PE present with shock. Mortality among these patients is as high as 50%, thus justifying the risks

TABLE 21-23 Thrombolysis for the Treatment of Venous Thromboembolism

- Thrombolytic therapy should be reserved for patients who present with shock, hypotension, right ventricular strain, or massive DVT with limb gangrene
- Diagnosis must be objectively confirmed before initiating thrombolytic therapy
- Thrombolytic therapy is most effective when administered as soon as possible after PE diagnosis, but benefit may extend up to 14 days after symptom onset
- Approved PE thrombolytic regimens
  - Streptokinase 250,000 units intravenously over 30 minutes followed by 100,000 units/h for 24 hours[a]
  - Urokinase 4,400 units/kg intravenously over 10 minutes followed by 4,400 units/kg/h for 12 to 24 hours[a]
  - Alteplase 100 mg intravenously over 2 hours
- Factors that increase the risk of bleeding must be evaluated before thrombolytic therapy is initiated (i.e., recent surgery, trauma or internal bleeding, uncontrolled hypertension, recent stroke or intracranial hemorrhage)
- Baseline labs should include CBC and blood typing in case transfusion is needed
- UFH should not be used during thrombolytic therapy; the aPTT nor any other anticoagulation parameter should not be monitored during the thrombolytic infusion
- aPTT should be measured following the completion of thrombolytic therapy
  - If aPTT less than 2.5 times control value, UFH infusion should be started and adjusted to maintain aPTT in therapeutic range
  - If aPTT greater than 2.5 times control value, remeasure every 2 to 4 hours and start UFH infusion when aPTT is less than 2.5
- Avoid phlebotomy, arterial puncture, and other invasive procedures during thrombolytic therapy to minimize the risk of bleeding

aPTT, activated partial thromboplastin time; CBC, complete blood cell count; DVT, deep vein thrombosis; PE, pulmonary embolism; UFH, unfractionated heparin.
[a]Two hour infusions of streptokinase and urokinase are as effective and safe as alteplase.

associated with thrombolytic therapy. Although thrombolytic therapy for patients with massive PE manifested by shock and cardiovascular collapse is considered the standard of care, only one trial has demonstrated a mortality benefit.[90]

A significant number of hemodynamically stable patients with PE have evidence of right ventricular dysfunction and appear to be at higher risk for recurrent PE and death when treated with heparin alone. Some experts believe that thrombolytic therapy is beneficial in patients with evidence of right ventricular dysfunction because it restores pulmonary blood flow and reduces pulmonary artery pressure. However, convincing data are lacking.[89]

Although it is an uncommon choice, venous thrombectomy is a reasonable approach to remove a massive obstructive thrombus in a patient with significant iliofemoral venous thrombosis, particularly if the patient is either not a candidate for or has not responded to thrombolysis.[2] In cases of chronic PE—where persistent emboli produce progressive pulmonary hypertension, hypoxemia, and right-sided heart failure—surgical embolectomy offers greater benefit than anticoagulants and may be the treatment of choice if performed by an experienced surgical team.[2] The surgical technique has been refined over the past 20 years. The procedure uses a balloon catheter to extract the thrombus while the patient is under general anesthesia. Fluoroscopy and venography guide the procedure. Balloon angioplasty, with or without stent placement, can be used if a focal iliac vein stenosis is discovered. Full-dose anticoagulation therapy is essential during the entire operative and postoperative period. These patients need indefinite oral anticoagulation therapy targeted to an INR of 2.5 (range 2.0 to 3.0).[2]

VENA CAVA INTERRUPTION

Anticoagulation therapy is the accepted standard for treating DVT and PE. However, an IVC filter may be indicated in special situations when anticoagulants are ineffective or unsafe, including in (a) patients with an absolute contraindication to anticoagulation therapy because of active bleeding or anticipated bleeding from a predisposing lesion; (b) patients with a massive PE who survives but in whom recurrent embolism might be fatal; and (c) patients who have recurrent VTE despite adequate anticoagulation therapy.[2] Interruption of the IVC can be accomplished with an occlusive filter, often called a Greenfield filter, inserted percutaneously through the femoral or jugular vein and advanced into place using fluoroscopic guidance, usually below the renal veins. There is little evidence to support the widespread use of vena cava filters. Vena cava filters reduce the risk of PE in the short-term, but also appear to increase the long-term risk for recurrent DVT presumably as a consequence of the accumulation of thrombus on the filter, which may partially occlude the vena cava, resulting in venous stasis.[2] Data from the International Cooperative Pulmonary Embolism Registry have documented a reduction in 90-day mortality associated with IVC filters, but this observation was not confirmed in a randomized study of filter placement where all patients were treated with anticoagulants.[2,89] Whether patients with permanent IVC filters should receive anticoagulant therapy remains unresolved but many clinicians opt to resume warfarin therapy as soon as possible and continue it indefinitely.[2] Given these concerns, retrievable filters that can be removed after the period of greatest risk for PE have been developed and have been suggested for use in patients with transient contraindications to anticoagulation therapy.[89]

ANCILLARY THERAPY

In addition to anticoagulant therapy for patients with proximal DVT, wearing graduated compression stockings can reduce the risk of developing the postthrombotic syndrome by as much as 50%.[94] To be effective, graduated compression stockings must fit properly and provide adequate pressure at the ankle (30 to 40 mm Hg). The discomfort associated with wearing properly fitted stockings along with the expense and unflattering cosmetic appeal makes routine use of compression stockings undesirable for many patients.

During the acute phase of DVT, antiembolic leg exercise may also be useful. To perform the exercise, patients should elevate the legs above the hips (7° to 10°) with feet supported. The patient then flexes one foot at a time back and forth for 3 to 5 minutes or until the calf muscle group is fatigued. This exercise should be repeated 4 to 6 times daily. Patients should also be instructed not to remain in a sitting position for more than 20 minutes without ambulating briefly or stretching the leg for a few minutes.

Strict bedrest was traditionally recommended following acute DVT based on the assumption that leg movement would dislodge the clot, resulting in PE. However, the evidence contradicts this assumption. Ambulation in conjunction with graduated compression stockings results in faster reduction in pain and swelling with no apparent increase in the rate of clot embolization.[95] Patients should be encouraged to ambulate as much as their symptoms permit. If pain and swelling increase with ambulation, the patient should be instructed to lie down and elevate the affected leg until symptoms subside.

TREATMENT OF VENOUS THROMBOEMBOLISM IN SPECIAL POPULATIONS

Pregnancy

The use of anticoagulation therapy for the treatment of DVT or PE in pregnant women is common.[27] UFH and LMWH are the preferred anticoagulants for use during pregnancy (Table 21–24). They do not cross the placenta and evidence suggests they are safe for the fetus.[27] Warfarin should be avoided because it crosses the placenta and can produce fetal bleeding, central nervous system abnormalities, and embryopathy. The direct thrombin inhibitors also cross the placenta. To date, fondaparinux has not been formally evaluated in pregnant patients.

TABLE 21-24 Unfractionated and Low-Molecular-Weight Heparin Use during Pregnancy

Acute treatment	LMWH • Enoxaparin 1 mg/kg SC q 12 h or 1.5 mg/kg q 24 h *or* • Dalteparin 100 U/kg SC q 12 h or 200 U/kg q 24 h *or* • Tinzaparin 175 U/kg SC q 24 h *or* UFH • Initiate using weight-based intravenous therapy and adjust dose to achieve therapeutic anti-Xa level for at least 5 days • Transition to SC adjusted-dose UFH administered q 8–12 h with midinterval anti-Xa activity in the therapeutic range[a]
Long-term treatment[b]	LMWH Maintain initial LMWH dose regimen throughout pregnancy *or* Alter LMWH dose in proportion to any weight change (usually gain) *or* Obtain monthly anti-Xa level measurements 4 to 6 hours after morning dose and adjust LMWH dose based on anti-Xa level (target = 0.5 to 1.2 units/mL if twice daily dosing; 1.0 to 2.0 units/mL if once-daily dosing) *or* UFH Obtain monthly anti-Xa level at the midpoint of the dosing interval and adjust UFH dose to achieve an anti-Xa level of 0.3 to 0.7 units/mL
Issues at time of delivery	Elective induction of labor • Discontinue UFH or LMWH 24 hours prior to induction • Initiate therapeutic doses of UFH by IV infusion and discontinue 4 to 6 hours prior to expected time of delivery if risk of recurrent VTE is deemed high Spontaneous labor • For LMWH, if there is a reasonable expectation that significant anticoagulant effect will be present at time of delivery (a) epidural should be avoided, and (b) reversal with protamine sulfate may be considered • For UFH, monitor the aPTT and reverse with protamine sulfate if aPTT is prolonged near the time of delivery Postpartum • Commence UFH or LMWH as soon as safely possible (usually 12 hours following delivery) • Concurrently initiate warfarin therapy and discontinue UFH or LMWH when the INR is 2.0 or greater • Continue anticoagulants for at least 4 weeks following delivery • Warfarin can be safely used by women who are breast-feeding

aPTT, activated partial thromboplastin time; INR, international normalized ratio; IV, intravenous; LMWH, low-molecular-weight heparin; SC, subcutaneously; UFH, unfractionated heparin; VTE, venous thromboembolism.

[a]Anti-Xa monitoring preferred as the relationship between aPTT and heparin levels differs in pregnant compared to nonpregnant patients.

[b]As pregnancy progresses the volume of distribution of LMWH changes, glomerular filtration rate increases, and most women gain weight.

From Bates et al. and Ginsberg and Bates.[27,113]

Long-term UFH therapy has been linked to significant bone loss and osteoporosis, requires multiple daily injections, and must be monitored frequently (every 1 to 2 weeks) throughout pregnancy. Because of these limitations, many experts recommend the use of LMWH over UFH throughout pregnancy.[27]

Pediatric Patients

Although seen far more frequently in adults, VTE in children has become increasing common secondary to prematurity, cancer, trauma, surgery, congenital heart disease, and systemic lupus erythematosus. Children often develop DVTs associated with an indwelling central venous catheter. In contrast to adults, children rarely develop idiopathic VTE.[28]

Anticoagulation with UFH and warfarin remains the most frequently used approach for the treatment of VTE in pediatric patients. The recommended target aPTT and INR ranges as well as the duration of therapy are extrapolated from clinical trials in adults. The recommended initial bolus dose of UFH is 75 to 100 units/kg given intravenously over 10 minutes followed by a maintenance infusion of 28 units/kg/h for infants 2 to 12 months of age and 20 unit/kg/h for children age 1 year or older. Subsequent adjustments should be made every 4 to 6 hours to maintain the aPTT within the institution-specific therapeutic range. The usual warfarin starting dose is 0.2 mg/kg with a maximum of 10 mg.[28] Infants require higher doses of warfarin per kg to maintain a target INR of 2.0 to 3.0 compared to teenagers and adults (mean dose 0.33 mg/kg, 0.09 mg/g, and 0.04 to 0.08 mg/kg, respectively). The INR target range is 2.0 to 3.0. Frequent INR monitoring and warfarin dose adjustments are typically required. When compared to adults, only 10% to 20% of pediatric patients can be safely monitored once monthly. Obtaining coagulation monitoring tests in pediatric patients is problematic because many have poor or nonexistent venous access. To address this problem, many clinicians recommend using fingerstick blood samples with a portable point-of-care monitor. Because LMWHs have low drug-interaction potential, are less likely to cause HIT or osteoporosis, and require less-frequent laboratory testing, they are an attractive alternative in pediatric patients.[28] Enoxaparin, dalteparin, tinzaparin, and reviparin have been evaluated in pediatric patients. Most experts recommend that anti-Xa activity be monitored and the dose adjusted to maintain antifactor Xa levels between 0.5 and 1.0 units/mL. Compared to adults, children younger than 2 to 3 years of age or who weigh less than 5 kg have higher per-kilogram dose requirements to achieve a "therapeutic" response. The doses of LMWH for older children are generally similar to the weight-adjusted doses used in adults.[28] Warfarin can be initiated concurrently with UFH or LMWH therapy. Therapy should be overlapped for a minimum of 5 days and until the INR is therapeutic. Warfarin should be continued for at least 3 months. Thrombolysis and thrombectomy have been successfully employed in pediatric patients but published data are very limited.

Patients with Cancer

VTE is a frequent complication of malignancy. Furthermore, compared to patients without cancer, the rate of recurrent VTE in patients with cancer is threefold higher and the risk of bleeding is two- to sixfold higher.[34] Warfarin therapy in cancer patients is often complicated by drug interactions (e.g., chemotherapy and antibiotics) and the need to frequently interrupt therapy for invasive procedures (e.g., thoracentesis, percutaneous biopsies, and abdominal paracentesis). Maintaining stable INR control is more difficult in this patient population because of nausea, anorexia, and vomiting.[34]

CLINICAL CONTROVERSY

Evidence suggests that LMWH administered for 3 to 6 months after a DVT or PE is more effective than warfarin in preventing recurrent VTE events in patients with cancer. Despite the fact that current consensus guidelines recommend the use of a LMWH over warfarin for the long-term treatment of VTE in cancer patients, many practitioners still prefer the use of warfarin in these patients.

Randomized trials provide evidence that long-term LMWH therapy for VTE in cancer patients significantly decreases the rate of recurrent VTE without increasing bleeding risks compared to traditional therapy with oral anticoagulants.[34] In one relatively small study in cancer patients with VTE, fixed-dose SC enoxaparin for 3 months appeared to be more effective than conventional warfarin therapy, with only 10.5% of enoxaparin-treated patient compared to 21% of warfarin-treated patients reaching the composite outcome of major bleeding and recurrent VTE ($p = 0.09$).[96] In the Comparison of LMWH versus Oral Anticoagulation Therapy for the Prevention of Recurrent Venous Thrombosis (CLOT) trial, continuous treatment with dalteparin for 6 months (200 units/kg SC every day for 1 month followed by 150 units/kg every day thereafter) was compared to conventional therapy with dalteparin followed by warfarin in cancer patients following an acute VTE.[97] The probability of recurrent VTE was reduced by nearly 50% in the long-term dalteparin treatment group, from 17.4% to 8.8% ($p = 0.0017$). There was no difference in the rate of major bleeding. Although this provides compelling data that cancer patients should be given LMWH instead of warfarin for the long-term treatment of VTE, the economic implications of this strategy have not yet been evaluated. In the absence of insurance coverage to offset the relatively high cost of long-term LMWH therapy, most patients are unable to afford it.

For patients with VTE and cancer who do receive LMWH, therapy should continue for at least the first 3 to 6 months of long-term treatment, at which time further LMWH can be considered or warfarin therapy can be substituted.[2] Anticoagulation therapy should continue for as long as the cancer is "active" and while the patient is receiving antitumor therapy.[34] A risk-to-benefit assessment should be performed on a regular basis and the overall clinical status of the patient should be considered, along with the risk for bleeding, quality of life, and life expectancy.[34] Many patients with terminal cancer receiving palliative care prefer LMWH over warfarin.[98] Consideration should be given to stopping anticoagulant therapy even in the presence of active cancer for patients who are at very high risk of bleeding complications.[93]

PHARMACOECONOMIC CONSIDERATIONS

Hospitalization is the main cost driver in the management of VTE.[88] Although the drug acquisition cost for the LMWHs and fondaparinux are substantially higher than UFH, avoiding hospitalization dramatically decreases the overall costs of DVT treatment. A number of cost-effectiveness analyses using decision modeling suggest that the treatment of DVT with LMWHs is more cost effective than the treatment with UFH in both inpatient and outpatient settings.[99] Based on this decision model, the LMWHs will reduce overall healthcare cost if as few as 8% of patients are treated entirely on an outpatients basis or 13% of patients are discharged from hospital early.

Despite the substantial cost savings stemming from outpatient DVT treatment from the perspective of the insurer, the reality is that some patients are unable to afford LMWH or fondaparinux prescriptions and are therefore denied outpatient treatment. The results of a recent study may provide a therapeutic option for patients in this situation. The objective of this trial was to determine if fixed-dose, weight-adjusted, subcutaneous UFH is as effective and safe as LMWH for the treatment of VTE.[23] Eligible patients were randomized to receive either UFH administered subcutaneously as an initial dose of 333 units/kg, followed by a fixed dose of 250 units/kg every 12 hours or a weight-based dose of LMWH. Both treatments could be administered at home and both were overlapped with warfarin therapy in the traditional manner. End points included recurrent VTE within 3 months and major bleeding within 10 days of study entry. The groups did not differ significantly in either of the study end points and treatment was administered completely at home in 72% of the UFH group and in 68% of the LMWH group. Further evidence is required to confirm these results; however, this lower cost option may facilitate the outpatient treatment of VTE for selected patients who otherwise would not have been able to afford it.

HEPARIN-INDUCED THROMBOCYTOPENIA

HIT is an uncommon but extremely serious adverse effect associated with heparin use.[26] The immune-mediated platelet activation and thrombin generation seen during HIT can lead to severe and unusual thrombotic complications. Morbidity and mortality associated with HIT is disturbingly high—up to 50% of patients who develop the disorder will suffer a thrombotic complication or die within 30 days in the absence of treatment. The diagnosis of HIT is based on laboratory findings that confirm heparin antibody formation and platelet activation (Table 21–25). To prevent the thrombotic complications associated with HIT, prompt discontinuation of heparin and initiation of an alternative anticoagulant therapy is imperative.

ETIOLOGY AND PATHOPHYSIOLOGY OF HIT

Two types of thrombocytopenia associated with heparin use have been described.[100] As many as 25% of patients receiving heparin therapy develop a benign, mild reduction in platelet counts referred to as non–immune-mediated heparin-associated thrombocytopenia (previously called HIT type 1). HAT produces a transient fall in platelet count that occurs early, typically between days 2 and 4, during the course of therapy. The degree of thrombocytopenia is usually mild, with platelet counts rarely going below 100,000. It is not necessary to discontinue heparin therapy in these patients as platelet counts generally rebound to baseline values despite continued use. The exact mechanism of HAT is unknown; however, it may be the result of platelet aggregation, a dilutional effect, or diminished platelet production often seen in acutely ill patients. No clinical sequelae are associated with this benign phenomenon.

The second type of thrombocytopenia associated with heparin use is known as immune-mediated HIT (formally known as HIT type 2).[38,100] HIT is a severe pathologic adverse effect of heparin with a significant potential to cause thrombotic complications (see Table 21–25). The time course and magnitude of thrombocytopenia associated with HIT differs from that of HAT. Platelets counts typically begin to fall days 5 to 10 following initiation of heparin and reach a nadir by days 7 to 14. The development of thrombocytopenia can be delayed (delayed-onset HIT) up to 20 days, and begin several days after heparin has been stopped in patients naive to heparin therapy. Conversely, so-called rapid-onset HIT can occur rapidly and abruptly (within 24 hours following heparin initiation) in patients with a recent exposure to heparin (i.e., previous 3 months).[26] Platelet counts commonly fall below 150,000 mm^3 but rarely nadir as low as 20,000 mm.[3] In some cases, overt thrombocytopenia may not occur, but a drop in platelet count greater than 50% from baseline is considered indicative of HIT.

The frequency of immune-mediated HIT is most powerfully related to the duration and type of heparin used and to a lesser extent the dose and route of administration.[26,38]The incidence of HIT associated with intravenous full dose UFH given for prolonged periods is significantly higher than that of low-dose subcutaneous UFH or LMWHs. The estimated overall incidence of HIT after 5 days of UFH use is 1% to 3% but the cumulative incidence may be as high as 6% after 14 days of continuous intravenous use. The incidence of HIT with low dose subcutaneous UFH in medical patients has been reported to be approximately 1%.[101] Low-molecular-weight heparins are associated with a significantly lower risk of HIT (<1%).[26] The incidence of HIT is higher with bovine UFH versus porcine UFH. In addition, the HIT risk varies with the exposed patient population: surgical patients > medical patients > pregnant patients.[26,102]

The pathogenesis of HIT involves an immunoglobulin mediated response to the heparin molecule leading to platelet activation and thrombin generation (Fig. 21–11).[38,100] With platelet activation there is release of PF-4 from platelet granules. Heparin binds to PF-4 forming a negatively charged polysaccharide molecule that is highly antigenic and stimulates the production of immunoglobulin (Ig) G antibodies. Although heparin-induced antibody formation occurs in 10% to 20% of patients treated with heparin, the vast majority of these patients never develop HIT. In patients who develop HIT, the heparin–PF-4–IgG complexes bind to the Fc receptor on platelets, leading to further platelet activation and the release of PF-4 and procoagulant microparticles from platelet granules. In addition, PF-4 and heparin-like molecules bind to the surface of endothelial cells resulting in antibody-induced endothelial cell damage and the release of tissue factor. The net result of this cascade of events is an increased risk of thrombotic events secondary to platelet activation, endothelial damage, and thrombin generation despite moderate to severe thrombocytopenia. Antibodies to the heparin/PF-4 complex are transient, and they have been reported to disappear from the circulation within a median of 85 days.[26,38]

TABLE 21-25 Presentation of Heparin-Induced Thrombocytopenia

General
Venous thromboembolism is the most common presentation of heparin-induced thrombocytopenia (HIT), although arterial events (e.g., myocardial infarction, stroke) can occur. HIT should be suspected if a patient develops a deep vein thrombosis or pulmonary embolism while or soon after receiving unfractionated heparin.
Symptoms and signs
Thromboembolic events secondary to HIT produce the same signs and symptoms as those of other etiologies (see Presentation of Deep Venous Thrombosis and Pulmonary Embolism).
Laboratory tests
The patient's platelets count will typically be below 150,000/mm^3 or drop more than 50% from baseline. The platelet count usually drops after 5 to 10 days of unfractionated heparin therapy, but may drop sooner if the patient has received heparin in the past 3 months.
Other diagnostic tests
An enzyme-linked immunoabsorbent assay (ELISA) for the presence of antibodies to the heparin–PF4 complex should be performed to confirm the diagnosis. Functional assays, including the heparin-induced platelet activation assay (HIPAA), the serotonin release assay (SRA), or the platelet-aggregation assay (PAA), may also be performed to confirm the diagnosis.

CLINICAL PRESENTATION AND DIAGNOSIS OF HIT

Thrombotic complications are the most common clinical sequelae of HIT (see Table 21–25).[26,38] The incidence of thrombosis can be as high as 50% in those patients with laboratory-confirmed immune-mediated thrombocytopenia. Thrombosis may occur in patients with seemingly mild thrombocytopenia but platelet counts invariably have dropped more than 50% from baseline. This syndrome is poorly recognized and many, perhaps most, patients diagnosed with HIT initially presented with thrombosis. Even among those who are diagnosed prior to the development of thrombosis, the prognosis is poor. In patients diagnosed with HIT without thrombosis and managed only by discontinuation of UFH, the risk of symptomatic thrombosis is 25% to 50%, and fatal thrombosis is 5%.[26,38]

The thrombotic risk is 30 times higher in patients with HIT as compared to control populations.[101] Venous thrombosis is the most common thrombotic complication associated with HIT and the majority of patients develop proximal DVT. PE occurs in 25% of patients with thrombotic complications and contributes signifi-

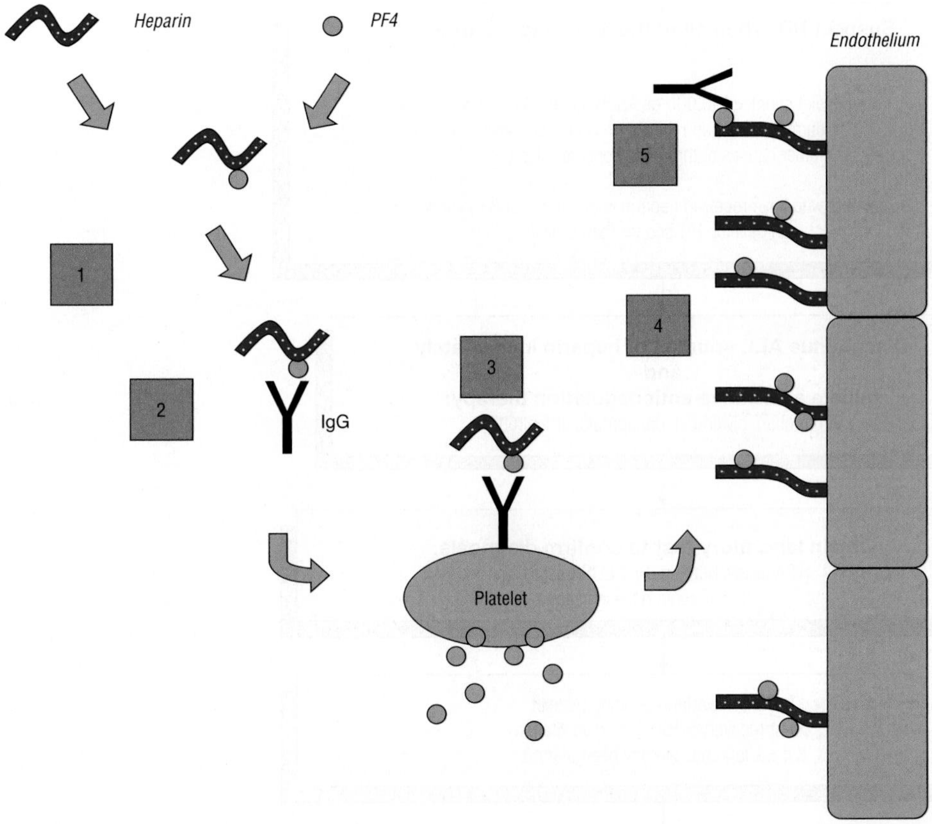

FIGURE 21-11. Pathogenesis of heparin-induced thrombocytopenia. (IgG, immunoglobulin G; PF4, platelet factor-4.)

cantly to mortality. Arterial thrombosis occurs less commonly.[26,100] Limb artery occlusion, stroke, and myocardial infarction are the most commonly reported arterial events. HIT has also been linked with atypical manifestations such as skin necrosis, venous limb gangrene, and anaphylactic-type reactions after IV bolus of UFH. Heparin-induced skin lesions occur in 10% to 20% of patients with HIT. Lesions range from painful, localized erythematous plaques to widespread dermal necrosis. Amputation in such cases is frequently required. Mortality from HIT may be as high as 50% in patients with acute thrombosis. The relatively high frequency of thrombotic complications and poor outcomes associated with HIT emphasize the need for prompt recognition and diagnosis.[26,38]

The diagnosis of immune-mediated HIT is made based on clinical findings supplemented by laboratory tests confirming the presence of antibodies to heparin or platelet activation induced by heparin.[26,38] While thrombocytopenia is the most common initial event suggesting the diagnosis of HIT, clinicians should evaluate all the potential causes. New thrombosis shortly after the development of thrombocytopenia is a distinguishing feature in nearly half of all patients with HIT. The time course and magnitude of thrombocytopenia are the features distinguishing immune-mediated HIT from HAT. Acute thrombosis and skin lesions may also occur prior to the development of overt thrombocytopenia. HIT should immediately be suspected when these events occur in any patient on UFH or LMWH therapy.[26,38]

Laboratory testing must be performed to confirm the diagnosis of HIT.[26,100,103] Laboratory testing is very helpful in patients with only mild to moderate thrombocytopenia in whom HIT is suspected. Two types of assays are available to detect the presence of heparin antibodies. Platelet activation assays, also known as functional assays, confirm in vitro platelet activation in the presence of therapeutic heparin levels. Functional assays include the heparin-induced platelet-activation assay, the serotonin release assay, and the platelet-aggregation assay. The heparin-induced platelet-activation assay and serotonin release assay tests have higher sensitivity and specificity than the platelet-aggregation assay but are technically more difficult to perform. Antigen assays that detect the presence of specific antibodies against the heparin–PF-4 complex using enzyme-linked immunosorbent assays are also available. These tests have reasonably high sensitivity and specificity. The optimal test for laboratory confirmation of immune-mediated HIT is unclear. The most readily available test with the greatest sensitivity and specificity should be used. The combined use of functional and enzyme-linked immunosorbent assays may reduce false-negative results. When results of one test are negative or indeterminate in patients suspected of HIT, another test should be considered.

GENERAL APPROACHES TO THE TREATMENT OF HIT

The goal of therapy in patients with HIT is to reduce the thrombosis risk by decreasing thrombin generation and platelet activation. The ACCP Consensus Conference on Antithrombotic Therapy has established recommendations for the treatment of HIT.[26] Once the diagnosis of HIT is established or strongly suspected, *all* sources of heparin, including heparin flushes, should be discontinued and an alternative anticoagulant agent should be initiated (Fig. 21–12).[26,38] Even in the absence of thrombosis, patients with HIT are at extremely high risk for developing serious thrombotic complications without treatment. Because the time required for diagnostic laboratory results to be reported can be prolonged, it is crucial that alternate anticoagulant agents be initiated in a timely fashion to prevent new thrombosis. Anticoagulant agents that rapidly inhibit thrombin activity and are devoid of significant cross-reactivity with heparin–PF-4 antibodies are the drugs of choice for the management of HIT (Table 21–26).[26,38] In cases of severe or life-threatening thrombosis, surgical extraction of thrombi may be required. Limited data exists regarding the use of thrombolytic therapy (see Table 21–23) in severe HIT with thrombosis. The use of warfarin for long-term anticoagulation in patients with HIT and thrombosis

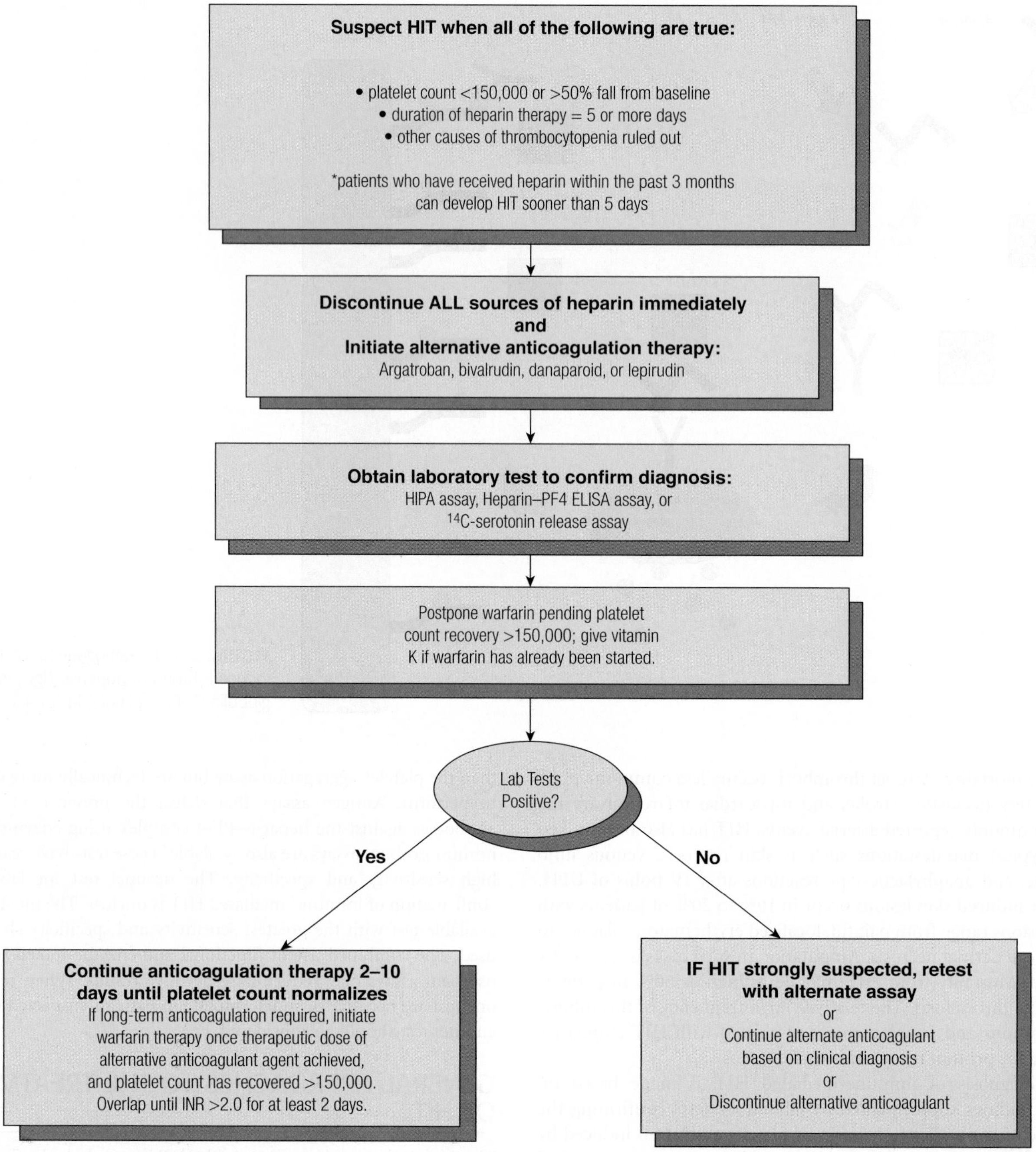

FIGURE 21-12. Treatment of heparin-induced thrombocytopenia (HIT). (HIPA assay, heparin-induced platelet activation assay; ELISA, enzyme-linked immunosorbent assay; INR, international normalized ratio.)

is recommended, but warfarin should only be initiated after substantial platelet count recovery has been documented (e.g., >150,000/mm^3) In addition, great care with dosing must be taken when initiating warfarin in these patients, as the risk of inducing further thrombosis secondary to inhibition of proteins C and S is possible.[26]

PHARMACOLOGIC TREATMENT OPTIONS

DTIs are the drugs of choice for the treatment of HIT with or without thrombosis (see Table 21–26).[26] Three DTIs are currently available in the United States for the treatment of patients with HIT—lepirudin, argatroban, and bivalirudin—but only the first two are FDA approved for this indication. For the treatment of HIT, lepirudin and argatroban are administered by intravenous infusion and should be titrated based on aPTT testing. The comparative efficacy of these agents has not been formally evaluated, and they are considered equally suitable for the initial treatment of HIT. Some clinicians prefer argatroban because it has a shorter half-life, modest bleeding risk, and lower cost when compared to lepirudin.[104] Because of a short-half life, low immunogenicity, minimal effect on INR, and enzymatic metabolism, bivalirudin appears to be a promising alternative for treatment of HIT. However, to date efficacy data is only based on case series.[43] Given fondaparinux is devoid of in vitro cross-reactivity to HIT antibodies, does not interfere with PT/INR measurement, and has enjoyed favorable experience in HIT in a few case reports, it is a promising alternative for the management of HIT.[105] Patient-related factors, such as the presence of renal or hepatic dysfunction, drug-specific features such as prior exposure to lepirudin, as well as institutional preference, availability, and cost should be used to determine the most appropriate agent. The LMWHs are not recommended for use in HIT because they have nearly 100% cross reactivity with heparin-antibodies by in vitro testing.[26,38]

TABLE 21-26 Recommended Dose and Monitoring Parameters for Direct Thrombin Inhibitors to Treat Heparin-Induced Thrombocytopenia

Agent	Dose	Monitoring Parameters	Clinical Considerations
Lepirudin	0.4 mg/kg (up to 110 kg) slow IV bolus[a] (can also be given without bolus), followed by 0.15 mg/kg/h (up to 110 kg) IV infusion[b]	Obtain baseline PT, aPTT, CBC, S_{cr}. Check aPTT 2 hours after initiation and each dose change and adjust dose to achieve aPTT 1.5–2.5 times control. Once stabile, monitor aPTT q 12 h.	Dose must be reduced in patients with renal impairment; avoiding the bolus dose may reduce the risk of accumulation and may reduce the risk of anaphylaxis; antihirudin antibodies can occur in 40%–60% of patients and can lead to reduced clearance. Concomitant warfarin requires dose adjustment.
Argatroban	2 mcg/kg/min continuous IV infusion (no bolus); maximum infusion 10 mcg/kg/min	Obtain baseline PT, aPTT, CBC. Monitor aPTT 2 hours after initiation and each dose change and adjust dose to achieve aPTT of 1.5–3 times control (maximum 100 s).	Dose reduction is necessary for those patients with hepatic impairment and in critically ill; will cause significant elevation in PT/INR; concurrent warfarin therapy requires special management (when INR >4, argatroban therapy should be withheld and the INR rechecked to determine if it is therapeutic).
Bivalirudin	0.15–0.20 mg/kg/h IV infusion (no bolus); approved dose for PCI: 0.75 mg IV bolus, followed by 1.75 mg/kg/h infusion up to 4 hours	Obtain baseline PT, aPTT, CBC, S_{cr}. Check aPTT 2 hours after initiation and adjust dose to achieve aPTT 1.5–2.5 times control.	Not FDA approved for treatment of HIT.

aPTT, activated partial thromboplastin time; CBC, complete blood cell count; HIT, heparin-induced thrombocytopenia; INR, international normalized ratio; IV, intravenous; PCI, percutaneous coronary intervention; PT, prothrombin time; S_{cr}, serum creatinine.

[a]Bolus dose is not advised in patients with renal impairement.

[b]Dose in isolated HIT: no bolus, 0.1 mg/kg/h infusion with aPTT adjusted to 1.5–2.0 times control.

The use of warfarin during the initial treatment of HIT is potentially dangerous.[26,38] The rapid reduction in protein C concentrations induced early in the course of warfarin therapy further increases the risk thrombosis in patients with HIT. This concern is supported by the observation that several patients with HIT have developed venous limb gangrene and warfarin-induced skin necrosis when treated with warfarin. Patients with venous limb gangrene had relatively high INRs after the initiation of warfarin therapy and presumably had rapid depletion of protein C but persisting thrombin generation. Therefore, warfarin is contraindicated as monotherapy for the initial treatment of patients diagnosed with HIT. However, patients with HIT and thrombosis requiring long-term anticoagulation can be treated with warfarin if therapy is appropriately timed and carefully initiated. A conservative approach is to withhold warfarin until the patient is stabilized and platelet counts have substantially recovered at least above 100,000 mm^3, and preferably above 150,000 mm^3. If warfarin has already been initiated when HIT is diagnosed, reversing therapy with vitamin K (5 to 10 mg either IV or oral) is recommended. This may prevent the development of further thrombotic adverse events caused by protein C depletion. Warfarin can be reinitiated once platelet counts have been recovered (>150,000 mm^3) but it should be overlapped with a direct thrombin inhibitor for a minimum of 5 days and until the full anticoagulant effect of warfarin has been achieved (i.e., INR within the therapeutic range for at least 2 consecutive days). Initial doses of warfarin greater than 5 mg should be strictly avoided in these patients.[26,38]

The management of pregnant patients with a history of HIT whom requires anticoagulation therapy presents a challenge. Both UFH and LMWH are the anticoagulants of choice for pregnant patients requiring anticoagulation therapy.[27] Women who develop HIT during pregnancy or who have a recent history of HIT (e.g., less than 3 months) cannot use UFH or LMWH safely. Limited evidence exists for the use of DTIs in pregnancy. Lepirudin is known to cross the placenta, however case reports suggest it may be safe for the management of HIT with thrombosis in pregnancy.[106] Danaparoid, a low-molecular-weight heparinoid not available in the United States, does not cross the placenta and it has also been investigated as a potential anticoagulant option in pregnant patients with HIT.[27] Limited case reports suggest that fondaparinux may also be a future potential alternative in pregnant patients.[107]

EVALUATION OF THERAPEUTIC OUTCOMES

The appropriate duration of therapy in patients with HIT will depend on whether the patient had a thrombotic event. Patients with HIT without thrombosis should be continued on therapeutic doses of an alternative anticoagulant agent until the platelet counts have normalized. Platelet counts should be monitored frequently, and patients should be watched closely for the development of new thrombosis after starting an alternate anticoagulant. Patients with thrombosis, either at the time of presentation or following the diagnosis of HIT, should receive therapy with an alternative anticoagulant such as lepirudin or argatroban followed by a transition to warfarin after the platelet count has recovered to >150,000 mm^3. Warfarin therapy is usually continued for at least 6 months, or longer if indicated. The initial anticoagulant used should be continued until the INR is stable and therapeutic for more than two consecutive days. In addition, it is important to clearly document the occurrence of immune-mediated HIT in the patient's medical record and educate the patient regarding this adverse effect. Future use of UFH, particularly in the next 3 to 6 months, should be strictly avoided. As PF-4–heparin antibodies are transient and usually cleared within 3 months, patients with a history of HIT should be tested for HIT antibodies prior to any future use of UFH. Although there are few data regarding the use if UFH in patients with a remote history of HIT, these patients should receive alternative anticoagulant agents for most indications until more rigorous data are available.[26,38]

NATIONAL QUALITY INITIATIVES

Venous thromboembolism is the most common preventable cause of hospital death in the United States and nearly two-thirds of all VTE events are related to hospitalization.[2] Furthermore, PE is the third most common cause of hospital-related deaths in the United States (300,000 fatalities annually). Survivors of VTE are at-risk for recurrence and other serious long-term complications, including post-thrombotic syndrome and chronic pulmonary hypertension. The estimated annual direct medical costs of managing the disease are well over $1 billion. Although VTE is often clinically silent, with as many as 25% of cases presenting as sudden death from PE, needless mortality and morbidity occur as a result of underdiagnosis and underuse of

TABLE 21-27 Organizations Monitoring Quality Care

The Joint Commission
www.jointcommission.org
A not-for-profit healthcare accreditation organization that issues performance-based standards and assesses organizational compliance to improve patient safety and quality of care.
Leapfrog Group
www.leapfroggroup.org
An initiative of healthcare purchasing organizations seeking improvements in safety, quality, and affordability of healthcare, with funding from the Business Roundtable, Robert Wood Johnson Foundation, and member organizations.
National Quality Forum
www.qualityforum.org
A not-for-profit that develops and implements national strategies for healthcare quality measurement and reporting.

prophylaxis. Despite the fact that several clinical interventions are known to be effective in preventing and treating VTE, only one-third of all patients who are at risk for VTE and who are appropriate candidates actually receive prophylaxis.[108] Although preventing VTE is a significant patient safety issue, there is little public awareness of the life-threatening nature of DVT and PE. A survey conducted on behalf of the American Public Health Association suggests that 75% of Americans have little or no awareness of DVT, and less than one-half of respondents could identify any risk factors associated with its development.[109] Recognizing the lack of public awareness, several organizations have focused on increasing consumer knowledge of the risks, signs, and symptoms of VTE through increased media visibility.

Given the number and variety of clinical conditions or circumstances that place individuals at risk for VTE, improvements in VTE prevention and care have the potential to benefit many patients. Over the past decade, the focus on quality health care has been emphasized by the call to accountability through the Joint Commission's Agenda for Change, the Institute of Medicine's report on medical errors, the National Quality Forum's endorsed safe practices, the Leapfrog Group, and the demand for value by healthcare consumers (Table 21–27).[108,110] Despite widespread national efforts to educate healthcare professionals about VTE prevention and treatment and the publication of numerous clinical guidelines, VTE prevention measures are not widely or consistently used. Therefore, wide variation in the prevention and treatment of VTE persists. Given the mortality and morbidity attributed to VTE, the need for standards of care is compelling. The National Quality Forum (NQF) is developing national consensus standards for VTE prevention and treatment that will be applicable to a variety of healthcare settings.[108] The outcomes of this effort will provide a framework for measuring the effective screening, prevention, and treatment of VTE. NQF's recommendations include developing organizational policies that address staff education, treatment protocols, and adherence measurements to improve VTE prevention in the hospital. The ultimate goal of the NQF consensus standards is to facilitate early promulgation of VTE policies, risk assessment, prophylaxis, diagnosis and treatment services as well as patient education and organizational accountability. To that end, the Joint Commission is developing performance measures to enforce the NQF's recommendations.[108,110] Four major domains have been identified: risk assessment, prevention, diagnosis, and treatment. Ten proposed measures have been selected for testing using a multiphased testing approach (Table 21–28).

Hopefully, through the concerted efforts of government and accrediting agencies working with hospitals and other healthcare institutions, the incidence of DVT and PE will begin to fall. Systematic approaches to this problem are needed at every level, starting with increased public and health practitioner awareness, continuing with the uniform use of effective prophylactic strategies in patients at risk, and concluding with greater accountability with precise quality measurements.

TABLE 21-28 The Joint Commission's Proposed Performance Measures for the Prevention and Treatment of Venous Thrombosis

Number	Description of Proposed Performance Measure
1	Documentation of Venous Thromboembolism Risk Assessment/Prophylaxis within 24 Hours of Hospital Admission
2	Documentation of Venous Thromboembolism Risk Assessment/Prophylaxis within 24 Hours of Transfer to ICU
3	Documentation of Inferior Vena Cava Filter Indication
4	Venous Thromboembolism Patients with Overlap of Parenteral and Warfarin Anticoagulation Therapy
5	Venous Thromboembolism Patients Receiving Unfractionated Heparin with Platelet Count Monitoring
6	Venous Thromboembolism Patients with Renal Insufficiency that Received Reduced/Discontinued Anticoagulation Therapy
7	Venous Thromboembolism Patients Receiving Unfractionated Heparin Management by Nomogram/Protocol
8	Venous Thromboembolism Discharge Instructions
9	Venous Thromboembolism Patients with International Normalized Ratio >6 After Initiation of Warfarin Therapy
10	Incidence of Potentially Preventable Hospital-Acquired Venous Thromboembolism

From The Joint Commission.[110]

CLINICAL CONTROVERSY

For the treatment of an acute VTE, LMWHs should be dosed based on the patient's actual (or total) body weight. Efficacy and safety data from clinical trials indicate that obese patients should be given full therapeutic doses based on the patient's actual (or total) body weight are used. Dose adjustments or dosing "caps" are not recommended in obese patients. Despite these data, some clinicians only use LMWH doses up to 150 mg (or 150 international units) per dose even if the patient's actual body weight is higher then 150 kg.

ABBREVIATIONS

ACCP: American College of Chest Physicians
DTI: direct thrombin inhibitor
DVT: deep vein thrombosis
FDA: Food and Drug Administration
HIT: heparin-induced thrombocytopenia
INR: international normalized ratio
IPC: Intermittent Pneumatic Compression
IV: intravenous
LMWH: low-molecular-weight heparin
aPTT: activated partial thromboplastin time
PE: pulmonary embolism
PF-4: platelet factor-4
PT: prothrombin time
SC: subcutaneous
UFH: unfractionated heparin
VTE: venous thromboembolism

REFERENCES

1. Turpie AGG, Chin BSP, Lip GYH. Venous thromboembolism: Pathophysiology, clinical features, and prevention. BMJ 2002;325:887–890.

2. Buller HR, Agnelli G, Hull RD, Hyers TM, Prins MH, Raskob GE. Antithrombotic therapy for venous thromboembolic disease: The Seventh ACCP Conference on Antithrombotic and Thrombolytic Therapy. Chest 2004;126:401S–428S.
3. Geerts WH, Pineo GF, Heit JA, et al. Prevention of venous thromboembolism. The Seventh ACCP Conference on Antithrombotic and Thrombolytic Therapy. Chest 2004;126:338S–400S.
4. Levine MN, Raskob G, Beyth RJ, Kearon C, Schulman S. Hemorrhagic complications of anticoagulant treatment: The Seventh ACCP Conference on Antithrombotic and Thrombolytic Therapy. Chest 2004;126:287S–310S.
5. Ansell J, Hirsh J, Poller L, Bussey H, Jacobson A, Hylek E. The pharmacology and management of the vitamin K antagonists: The Seventh ACCP Conference on Antithrombotic and Thrombolytic Therapy. Chest 2004;126:204S–233S.
6. Hirsh J, Fuster V, Ansell J, Halperin JL. American Heart Association/American College of Cardiology Foundation Guide to Warfarin Therapy. Circulation 2003;107:1692–1711.
7. Chiquette E, Amato MG, Bussey HI. Comparison of an anticoagulation clinic with usual medical care: Anticoagulation control, patient outcomes, and health care costs. Arch Intern Med 1998;158:1641–1647.
8. Mamdani MM, Racine E, McCreadie S, et al. Clinical and economic effectiveness of an inpatient anticoagulation service. Pharmacotherapy 1999;19:1064–1074.
9. Wells PS, Anderson DR, Ginsberg J. Assessment of deep vein thrombosis or pulmonary embolism by the combined use of clinical model and noninvasive tests. Semin Thromb Hemost 2000;26:643–656.
10. Silverstein MD, Heit JA, Mohr DN, Petterson TM, WM OF, Melton LJ 3rd. Trends in the incidence of deep vein thrombosis and pulmonary embolism: A 25-year population-based study. Arch Intern Med 1998;158:585–593.
11. White RH, Zhou H, Romano PS. Incidence of idiopathic deep venous thrombosis and secondary thromboembolism among ethnic groups in California. Ann Intern Med 1998;128:737–740.
12. Heit JA, Mohr DN, Silverstein MD, Petterson TM, O'Fallon WM, Melton LJ 3rd. Predictors of recurrence after deep vein thrombosis and pulmonary embolism. A population-based cohort study. Arch Intern Med 2000;160:761–768.
13. Levitan N, Dowlati A, Remick SC, et al. Rates of initial and recurrent thromboembolic disease among patients with malignancy versus those without malignancy. Risk analysis using Medicare claims data. Medicine (Baltimore) 1999;78:285–291.
14. Thomas RH. Hypercoagulability syndromes. Arch Intern Med 2001; 161:2433–2439.
15. Hansson PO, Sorbo J, Eriksson H. Recurrent venous thromboembolism after deep vein thrombosis: Incidence and risk factors. Arch Intern Med 2000;160:769–774.
16. Rosendaal FR, Helmerhorst FM, Vandenbroucke JP. Female hormones and thrombosis. Arterioscler Thromb Vasc Biol 2002;22:201–210.
17. Bates SM, Greer IA, Hirsh J, Ginsberg JS. Use of antithrombotic agents during pregnancy. Chest 2004;126:627S–44S.
18. Dahlback B. Blood coagulation. Lancet 2000;355:1627–1632.
19. Haines ST, Bussey HI. Thrombosis and the pharmacology of antithrombotic agents. Ann Pharmaco 1995;29:892–905.
20. Kearon C, O'Donnell M, Linkins LA, et al. Natural history of venous thromboembolism. Circulation 2003;107:I-22–I-30.
21. Meignan M, Rosso J, Gauthier H, et al. Systematic lung scans reveal a high frequency of silent pulmonary embolism in patients with proximal deep venous thrombosis. Arch Intern Med 2000;160:159–164.
22. Hirsh J, Raschke R. Heparin and low-molecular-weight heparin. The Seventh ACCP Conference on Antithrombotic and Thrombolytic Therapy. Chest 2004;126:188S–203S.
23. Kearon C, Ginsberg JS, Julian JA, et al. Comparison of fixed-dose weight-adjusted unfractionated heparin and low-molecular-weight heparin for acute treatment of venous thromboembolism. JAMA 2006;296:935–942.
24. Hull RD, Pineo GF. Heparin and low-molecular-weight heparin therapy for venous thromboembolism: Will unfractionated heparin survive? Semin Thromb Hemost 2004;30:11–23.
25. Popma JJ, Berger P, Ohman EM, Harrington RA, Grines C, Weitz JI. Antithrombotic therapy during percutaneous coronary intervention. Chest 2004;126:576S-599S.
26. Warkentin TE, Greinacher A. Heparin-induced thrombocytopenia: Recognition, treatment, and prevention: The Seventh ACCP Conference on Antithrombotic and Thrombolytic Therapy. Chest 2004;126: 311S–337S.
27. Bates SM, Greer IA, Hirsh J, Ginsberg JS. Use of antithrombotic agents during pregnancy: The Seventh ACCP Conference on Antithrombotic and Thrombolytic Therapy. Chest 2004;126:627S–644S.
28. Monagle P, Chan A, Massicotte P, Chalmers E, Michelson AD. Antithrombotic therapy in children. Chest 2004;126:645S–687S.
29. Lovenox prescribing information. Aventis Pharmaceuticals. November 2005, *http://products.sanofi-aventis.us/lovenox/lovenox.html.*
30. Rosenbloom D, Ginsberg JS. Arguments against monitoring levels of anti-factor Xa in conjunction with low-molecular-weight heparin therapy. Can J Hosp Pharm 2002;55:15–19.
31. Keam SJ, Goa KL. Fondaparinux sodium. Drugs 2002;62:1673–1685.
32. Arixtra prescribing information. GlaxoSmithKline. October 2005, *http://us.gsk.com/products/assets/us_arixtra.pdf.*
33. Eriksson BI, Lassen MR. Duration of prophylaxis against venous thromboembolism with fondaparinux after hip fracture surgery: A multicenter, randomized, placebo-controlled, double-blind study. Arch Intern Med 2003;163:1337–1342.
34. van Gogh Investigators. Buller HR, Cohen AT, Davidson B, et al. Idraparinux versus standard therapy for venous thromboembolic disease. N Engl J Med 2007;357:1094–1104.
35. Nutescu EA, Shapiro NL, Chevalier A. New anticoagulant agents: Direct thrombin inhibitors. Clin Geriatr Med 2006;22:33–56, viii.
36. Nutescu EA, Wittkowsky AK. Direct thrombin inhibitors for anticoagulation. Ann Pharmacother 2004;38:99–109.
37. Refludan prescribing information. Berlex Laboratories. October 2004, *http://www.refludan.com/product/index.htm.*
38. Arepally GM, Ortel TL. Clinical practice. Heparin-induced thrombocytopenia. N Engl J Med 2006;355:809–817.
39. Revasc/Iprivask (Desirudin). Canyon Pharmaceuticals. 2006, *http://www.canyonpharma.com/desirudin.html.*
40. Frenkel EP, Shen YM, Haley BB. The direct thrombin inhibitors: Their role and use for rational anticoagulation. Hematol Oncol Clin North Am 2005;19:119–45, vi–vii.
41. Matheson AJ, Goa KL. Desirudin: A review of its use in the management of thrombotic disorders. Drugs 2000;60:679–700.
42. Angiomax prescribing information. The Medicines Company. December 2005, *http://www.angiomax.com/Files/SalesAidRef/PI.pdf.*
43. Seybert AL, Coons JC, Zerumsky K. Treatment of heparin-induced thrombocytopenia: Is there a role for bivalirudin? Pharmacotherapy 2006;26:229–241.
44. Serebruany MV, Malinin AI, Serebruany VL. Argatroban, a direct thrombin inhibitor for heparin-induced thrombocytopaenia: Present and future perspectives. Expert Opin Pharmacother 2006;7:81–89.
45. Argatroban prescribing information. SmithKline Glaxo. July 2005, *http://us.gsk.com/products/assets/us_argatroban.pdf.*
46. Nutescu EA, Shapiro NL, Chevalier A, Amin AN. A pharmacologic overview of current and emerging anticoagulants. Cleve Clin J Med 2005;2006;72(Suppl 1):S2–S6.
47. Hursting MJ, Dubb J, Verme-Gibboney CN. Argatroban anticoagulation in pediatric patients: A literature analysis. J Pediatr Hematol Oncol 2006;28:4–10.
48. Kiser TH, Fish DN. Evaluation of bivalirudin treatment for heparin-induced thrombocytopenia in critically ill patients with hepatic and/or renal dysfunction. Pharmacotherapy 2006;26:452–460.
49. Sconce EA, Khan TI, Wynne HA, et al. The impact of CYP2C9 and VKORC1 genetic polymorphism and patient characteristics upon warfarin dose requirements: Proposal for a new dosing regimen. Blood 2005;106:2329–2333.
50. Takahashi H, Wilkinson GR, Nutescu EA, et al. Different contributions of polymorphisms in VKORC1 and CYP2C9 to intra- and inter-population differences in maintenance dose of warfarin in Japanese, Caucasians and African-Americans. Pharmacogenet Genomics 2006; 16:101–110.
51. Kovacs MJ, Rodger M, Anderson DR, et al. Comparison of 10-mg and 5-mg warfarin initiation nomograms together with low-molecular-weight heparin for outpatient treatment of acute venous thromboembolism. A randomized, double-blind, controlled trial. Ann Intern Med 2003;138:714–719.

52. Roberts GW, Helboe T, Nielsen CB, et al. Assessment of an age-adjusted warfarin initiation protocol. Ann Pharmacother 2003;37:799–803.
53. Crowther MA, Ginsberg JB, Kearon C, et al. A randomized trial comparing 5-mg and 10-mg warfarin loading doses. Arch Intern Med 1999;159:46–48.
54. Pengo V, Biasiolo A, Pegoraro C. A simple scheme to initiate oral anticoagulant treatment in outpatients with nonrheumatic atrial fibrillation. Am J Cardiol 2001;88:1214–1216.
55. Fairweather RB, Ansell J, van den Besselaar AM, et al. College of American Pathologists Conference XXXI on laboratory monitoring of anticoagulant therapy. Laboratory monitoring of oral anticoagulant therapy. Arch Pathol Lab Med 1998;122:768–781.
56. Witt DM, Sadler MA, Shanahan RL, Mazzoli G, Tillman DJ. Effect of a centralized clinical pharmacy anticoagulation service on the outcomes of anticoagulation therapy. Chest 2005;127:1515–1522.
57. Heneghan C, Alonso-Coello P, Garcia-Alamino JM, Perera R, Meats E, Glasziou P. Self-monitoring of oral anticoagulation: A systematic review and meta-analysis. Lancet 2006;367:404–411.
58. Nutescu EA. Point of care monitors for oral anticoagulant therapy. Semin Thromb Hemost 2004;30:697–702.
59. Chan YC, Valenti D, Mansfield AO, Stansby G. Warfarin induced skin necrosis. Br J Surg 2000;87:266–272.
60. Gage BF, Birman-Deych E, Radford MJ, Nilasena DS, Binder EF. Risk of osteoporotic fracture in elderly patients taking warfarin: Results from the National Registry of Atrial Fibrillation 2. Arch Intern Med 2006;166:241–246.
61. Crowther MA, Douketis JD, Schnurr T, et al. Oral vitamin K lowers the international normalized ratio more rapidly than subcutaneous vitamin K in the treatment of warfarin-associated coagulopathy. A randomized, controlled trial. Ann Intern Med 2002;137:251–254.
62. Patel RJ, Witt DM, Saseen JJ, Tillman DJ, Wilkinson DS. Randomized, placebo-controlled trial of oral phytonadione for excessive anticoagulation. Pharmacotherapy 2000;20:1159–1166.
63. Holbrook AM, Pereira JA, Labiris R, et al. Systematic overview of warfarin and its drug and food interactions. Arch Intern Med 2005;165:1095–1106.
64. Nutescu EA, Shapiro NL, Ibrahim S, West P. Warfarin and its interactions with foods, herbs and other dietary supplements. Expert Opin Drug Saf 2006;5:433–451.
65. Dunn AS, Turpie AG. Perioperative management of patients receiving oral anticoagulants: A systematic review. Arch Intern Med 2003;163:901–908.
66. Agu O, Hamilton G, Baker D. Graduated compression stockings in the prevention of venous thromboembolism. Br J Surg 1999;86:992–1004.
67. Hooker JA, Lachiewicz PF, Kelley SS. Efficacy of prophylaxis against thromboembolism with intermittent pneumatic compression after primary and revision total hip arthroplasty. J Bone Joint Surg Am 1999;81:690–696.
68. Siddiqui AU, Buchman TG, Hotchkiss RS. Pulmonary embolism as a consequence of applying sequential compression device on legs in a patient asymptomatic of deep vein thrombosis. Anesthesiology 2000;92:880–882.
69. Velmahos GC, Kern J, Chan LS, Oder D, Murray JA, Shekelle P. Prevention of venous thromboembolism after injury: An evidence-based report—part II. analysis of risk factors and evaluation of the role of vena caval filters. J Trauma 2000;49:140–144.
70. Decousus H, Leizorovicz A, Parent F, et al. A clinical trial of vena caval filters in the prevention of pulmonary embolism in patients with proximal deep-vein thrombosis. N Engl J Med 1998;1998:409–415.
71. Turpie AG, Bauer KA, Eriksson BI, Lassen MR. Fondaparinux vs enoxaparin for the prevention of venous thromboembolism in major orthopedic surgery: A meta-analysis of 4 randomized double-blind studies. Arch Intern Med 2002;162:1833–1840.
72. Hull RD, Brant RF, Pineo GF, Stein PD, Raskob GE, Valentine KA. Preoperative vs postoperative initiation of low-molecular-weight heparin prophylaxis against venous thromboembolism in patients undergoing elective hip replacement. Arch Intern Med 1999;159:137–141.
73. Eikelboom JW, Quinlan DJ, Douketis JD. Extended-duration prophylaxis against venous thromboembolism after total hip or knee replacement: A meta-analysis of the randomised trials. Lancet 2001;358:9–15.
74. Heit JA, Elliott CG, Trowbridge AA, Morrey BF, Gent M, Hirsh J. Ardeparin sodium for extended out-of-hospital prophylaxis against venous thromboembolism after total hip or knee replacement. A randomized, double-blind, placebo-controlled trial. Ann Intern Med 2000;132:853–861.
75. Prandoni P, Bruchi O, Sabbion P, et al. Prolonged thromboprophylaxis with oral anticoagulants after total hip arthroplasty: A prospective controlled randomized study. Arch Intern Med 2002;162:1966–1971.
76. MacDougall DA, Feliu AI, Boccuzzi SJ, Lin J. Economic burden of deep-vein thrombosis, pulmonary embolism, and post-thrombotic syndrome. Am J Health Syst Pharm 2006;63(Suppl 6):S5–S15.
77. Davidson BL, Sullivan SD, Kahn SR, Borris L, Bossuyt P, Raskob G. The economics of venous thromboembolism prophylaxis: A primer for clinicians. Chest 2003;124:393S–396S.
78. Corditz GA. Cost-effectiveness of prevention. In: Bergqvist D, Comerota A, Nicolaides AN, Scurr JH, eds. Prevention of Venous Thromboembolism. London: Med-Orion, 1994:403–420.
79. Etchells E, McLeod RS, Geerts W, Barton P, Detsky AS. Economic analysis of low-dose heparin vs the low-molecular-weight heparin enoxaparin for prevention of venous thromboembolism after colorectal surgery. Arch Intern Med 1999;159:1221–1228.
80. Hawkins DW, Langley PC, Krueger KP. Pharmacoeconomic model of enoxaparin versus heparin for prevention of deep vein thrombosis after total hip replacement. Am J Health Syst Pharm 1997;54:1185–1190.
81. Gordois A, Posnett J, Borris L, et al. The cost-effectiveness of fondaparinux compared with enoxaparin as prophylaxis against thromboembolism following major orthopedic surgery. J Thromb Haemost 2003;1:2167–2174.
82. Wade WE, Spruill WJ, Leslie RB. Cost analysis: Fondaparinux versus preoperative and postoperative enoxaparin as venous thromboembolic event prophylaxis in elective hip arthroplasty. Am J Orthop 2003;32:201–205.
83. Merli G. Anticoagulants in the treatment of deep vein thrombosis. Am J Med 2005;118:13S-20S.
84. Turpie AGG, Chin BSP, Lip GYH. Venous thromboembolism: Treatment strategies. BMJ 2002;325:948–950.
85. Dolovich L, Ginsberg JS, Douketis J, et al. A meta-analysis comparing low-molecular-weight heparins with unfractionated heparin in the treatment of venous thromboembolism. Arch Intern Med 2000;160:181–188.
86. Merli GJ, Spiro TE, Olson C, et al. Subcutaneous enoxaparin once or twice daily compared with intravenous unfractionated heparin for treatment of venous thromboembolic disease. Ann Intern Med 2001;134:191–202.
87. American Society of Health-System Pharmacists. ASHP therapeutic position statement on the use of low-molecular-weight heparins for adult outpatient treatment of acute deep-vein thrombosis. Am J Health Syst Pharm 2004;61:1950–1955.
88. Tillman DJ, Charland SL, Witt DM. Effectiveness and economic impact associated with a program for outpatient management of acute deep vein thrombosis in a group model health maintenance organization. Arch Intern Med 2000;160:2926–2932.
89. Piazza G, Goldhaber SZ. Acute pulmonary embolism. Part II. Treatment and prophylaxis. Circulation 2006;114:e42-e7.
90. Wood KE. Major pulmonary embolism: Review of a pathophysiologic approach to the golden hour of hemodynamically significant pulmonary embolism. Chest 2002;121:877–905.
91. Buller HR, Davidson BL, Decousus H, et al. Fondaparinux or enoxaparin for the initial treatment of symptomatic deep venous thrombosis: A randomized trial. Ann Intern Med 2004;140:867–873.
92. Buller HR, Davidson BL, Decousus H, et al. Subcutaneous fondaparinux versus intravenous unfractionated heparin in the initial treatment of pulmonary embolism. N Engl J Med 2003;349:1695–1702.
93. Kearon C. Long-term management of patients after venous thromboembolism. Circulation 2004;110(Suppl I):I-10–I-8.
94. Prandoni P, Lensing AWA, Prins MH, et al. Below-knee elastic compression stockings to prevent the post-thrombotic syndrome. Ann Intern Med 2004;141:249–256.
95. Aldrich D, Hunt DP. When can the patient with deep venous thrombosis begin to ambulate? Phys Ther 2004;84:268–273.
96. Meyer G, Marjanovic Z, Valcke J, et al. Comparison of low-molecular-weight heparin and warfarin for the secondary prevention of venous thromboembolism in patients with cancer: A randomized controlled study. Arch Intern Med 2002;162:1729–1735.
97. Lee AY, Levine MN, Baker RI, et al. Low-molecular-weight heparin versus a coumarin for the prevention of recurrent venous thromboembolism in patients with cancer. N Engl J Med 2003;349:677–681.

98. Noble SIR, Finlay IG. Is long-term low-molecular-weight heparin acceptable to palliative care patients in the treatment of cancer related venous thromboembolism? a qualitative study. Palliat Med 2005;19: 197–201.
99. Gould MK, Dembitzer AD, Sanders GD, Garber AM. Low-molecular-weight heparins compared with unfractionated heparin for treatment of acute deep venous thrombosis. A cost-effectiveness analysis. Ann Intern Med 1999;130:789–799.
100. Kelton JG. The pathophysiology of heparin-induced thrombocytopenia: Biological basis for treatment. Chest 2005;127:9S–20S.
101. Girolami B, Prandoni P, Stefani PM, et al. The incidence of heparin-induced thrombocytopenia in hospitalized medical patients treated with subcutaneous unfractionated heparin: A prospective cohort study. Blood 2003;101:2955–2959.
102. Warkentin TE. Heparin-induced thrombocytopenia: Diagnosis and management. Circulation 2004;110:e454–e458.
103. Warkentin TE. New approaches to the diagnosis of heparin-induced thrombocytopenia. Chest 2005;127:35S–45S.
104. Lewis BE, Wallis DE, Hursting MJ, Levine RL, Leya F. Effects of argatroban therapy, demographic variables, and platelet count on thrombotic risks in heparin-induced thrombocytopenia. Chest 2006;129:1407–1416.
105. Efird LE, Kockler DR. Fondaparinux for thromboembolic treatment and prophylaxis of heparin-induced thrombocytopenia. Ann Pharmacother 2006;40:1383–1387.
106. Messmore H, Jeske W, Wehrmacher W, Walenga J. Benefit-risk assessment of treatments for heparin-induced thrombocytopenia. Drug Saf 2003;26:625–641.
107. Mazzolai L, Hohlfeld P, Spertini F, Hayoz D, Schapira M, Duchosal MA. Fondaparinux is a safe alternative in case of heparin intolerance during pregnancy. Blood 2006;108:1569–1570.
108. National Quality Forum Project Brief: National Voluntary Consensus Standards for the Prevention and Care of Venous Thromboembolism, Including Deep-Vein Thrombosis and Pulmonary Embolism. January 2006, *www.qualityforum.org/txDVTprojectsummaryFINAL.pdfM.*
109. American Public Health Association. Deep-Vein Thrombosis: Advancing Awareness to Protect Patient Lives. White Paper, Public Health Leadership Conference on Deep-Vein Thrombosis. January 2003, *www.apha.org/news/press/2003/DVT_whitepaper.pdf.*
110. The Joint Commission. National Consensus Standards on the Prevention and Care of Venous Thromboembolism. *http://www.jointcommission.org/PerformanceMeasurement/PerformanceMeasurement/VTE.htm.* Published December 5, 2007.
111. Federman DG, Kirsner RS. An update on hypercoagulable disorders. Arch Intern Med 2001;161:1051–1056.
112. Booth SL, Centurelli MA. Vitamin K. A practical guide to the dietary management of patients on warfarin. Nutr Rev 1999;57:288–296.
113. Ginsberg JS, Bates SM. Management of venous thromboembolism during pregnancy. J Thromb Haemost 2003;1:1435–1442.

CHAPTER 22

Stroke

SUSAN C. FAGAN AND DAVID C. HESS

KEY CONCEPTS

1. Stroke is one of the leading killers of individuals worldwide.
2. Stroke can be either ischemic (88%) or hemorrhagic (12%).
3. Transient ischemic attacks (TIAs) require urgent intervention to reduce the risk of stroke, which is known to be highest in the first few days after TIA.
4. Carotid endarterectomy should be performed in ischemic stroke patients with 70% to 99% stenosis of the ipsilateral carotid artery, provided that it is done in an experienced center.
5. Early reperfusion (<3 hours from onset) with tissue plasminogen activator (t-PA) has been shown to reduce the ultimate disability caused by ischemic stroke.
6. Antiplatelet therapy is the cornerstone of antithrombotic therapy for the secondary prevention of ischemic stroke.
7. Warfarin is the drug of choice for secondary prevention of cardioembolic stroke.
8. Blood pressure lowering is effective in both the primary and secondary prevention of both ischemic and hemorrhagic stroke regardless of blood pressure.
9. Blood pressure lowering in the acute stroke period (first 7 days) can result in decreased cerebral blood flow and worsened symptoms.
10. Statin therapy is recommended for all ischemic stroke patients, regardless of baseline cholesterol, to reduce recurrent vascular events.

❶ Stroke is the second leading killer worldwide and the third leading cause of death in the United States, behind cardiovascular disease and all cancers. Despite improvements in the stroke mortality rates in the second half of the 20th century, stroke occurs in more than 700,000 individuals per year and results in 150,000 deaths.[1] Recent advances in our knowledge of the pathophysiology of stroke and efforts to organize stroke care have led to evidence-based recommendations on the management of the stroke patient.

Learning objectives, review questions, and other resources can be found at **www.pharmacotherapyonline.com.**

EPIDEMIOLOGY

There are currently 4.6 million stroke survivors in the United States, and stroke is the leading cause of adult disability.[1] Approximately 20% of patients in nursing homes have had a stroke,[2] and stroke is also a leading diagnosis in inpatient rehabilitation. Owing in part to the need for these expensive posthospitalization care environments, stroke is also one of the most expensive diseases in the United States, with annual costs greater than $50 billion.[1] Current projections are that death caused by stroke will increase exponentially in the next 30 years owing to aging of the population and our inability to control risk factors.[3]

Stroke risk is increased above that of the general population in elderly male individuals and in African Americans.[1] In addition, geographic disparity in stroke incidence exists, such that several areas of the southeastern United States have stroke mortality rates more than twice that of the national average.[4] This phenomenon, originally describing areas of the coastal Carolinas and Georgia, has been named the "Stroke Belt."

ETIOLOGY AND CLASSIFICATION

❷ Stroke can be either ischemic or hemorrhagic (88% and 12%, respectively, of all strokes in the 2006 American Heart Association report).[1] A classification of stroke by mechanism is given in Fig. 22–1. Hemorrhagic strokes include subarachnoid hemorrhage, intracerebral hemorrhage, and subdural hematomas. Subarachnoid hemorrhage occurs when blood enters the subarachnoid space (where cerebrospinal fluid is housed) owing to either trauma, rupture of an intracranial aneurysm, or rupture of an arteriovenous malformation (AVM). By contrast, intracerebral hemorrhage occurs when a blood vessel ruptures within the brain parenchyma itself, resulting in the formation of a hematoma. These types of hemorrhages very often are associated with uncontrolled high blood pressure and sometimes antithrombotic or thrombolytic therapy. Subdural hematomas refer to collections of blood below the dura (covering of the brain), and they are caused most often by trauma. Hemorrhagic stroke, although less common, is significantly more lethal than ischemic stroke, with 30-day case-fatality rates that are two to six times higher.[5,6]

Ischemic strokes are caused either by local thrombus formation or by embolic phenomenon, resulting in occlusion of a cerebral artery. Atherosclerosis, particularly of the cerebral vasculature, is a causative factor in most cases of ischemic stroke, although 30% are cryptogenic. Emboli can arise either from intra- or extracranial arteries (including the aortic arch) or, as is the case in 20% of all ischemic strokes, the heart. Cardiogenic embolism is presumed to have occurred if the patient has concomitant atrial fibrillation, valvular heart disease, or any other condition of the heart that can lead to clot formation.[7] Distinguishing between cardiogenic embolism and other causes of ischemic stroke is important in determining long-term pharmacotherapy in a given patient.

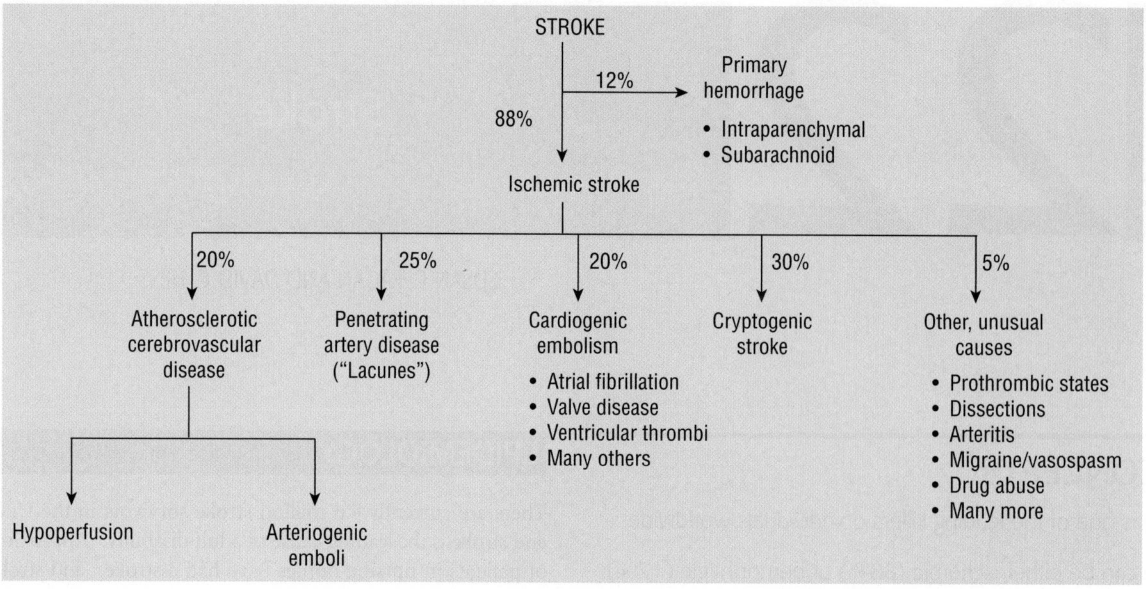

FIGURE 22-1. A classification of stroke by mechanism with estimates of the frequency of various categories of abnormalities. Approximately 30% of ischemic strokes are cryptogenic.

RISK FACTORS

Risk factors for stroke can be subdivided into nonmodifiable, modifiable, and potentially modifiable. In addition, risk factors can be either well documented or less well documented.[8] The main risk factors of stroke are listed in Table 22–1. Recommendations for risk factor reduction aggressively target the modifiable, well-documented risk factors, even in individuals with nonmodifiable risk.[8] The nonmodifiable risk factors are age, race, sex, low birth weight, and family history.

TABLE 22-1 Risk Factors for Ischemic Stroke

Nonmodifiable risk factors or risk markers
Age
Gender
Race
Family history of stroke
Low birth weight
Modifiable, well-documented
Hypertension–single most important risk factor for ischemic stroke
Atrial fibrillation–most important and treatable cardiac cause of stroke
Other cardiac diseases
Diabetes–independent risk factor
Dyslipidemia
Cigarette smoking
Alcohol
Sickle cell disease
Asymptomatic carotid stenosis
Postmenopausal hormone therapy
Lifestyle factors–associated with stroke risk
Obesity
Physical inactivity
Diet
Potentially modifiable, less-well documented
Oral contraceptives
Migraine
Drug and alcohol abuse
Hemostatic and inflammatory factors–fibrinogen linked to increased risk
Homocysteine
Sleep disordered breathing

Adapted from Goldstein LB, Adams R, Alberts MJ, et al. Primary prevention of ischemic stroke: A guideline from the American Heart Association/American Stroke Association Stroke Council: Cosponsored by the Atherosclerotic Peripheral Vascular Disease Interdisciplinary Working Group; Cardiovascular Nursing Council; Clinical Cardiology Council; Nutrition, Physical Activity, and Metabolism Council; and the Quality of Care and Outcomes Research Interdisciplinary Working Group. Stroke 2006;37:1583–1633.

An individual's risk of having a stroke increases substantially as he or she ages, with a doubling of risk for each decade older than 55 years of age. African Americans, Asian-Pacific Islanders, and Hispanics experience higher death rates than their Caucasian counterparts.[1,4] Men are at a higher risk of stroke than women when matched for age, but women who suffer from a stroke are more likely to die from it.[1]

The most common modifiable, well-documented risk factors for stroke include hypertension, cigarette smoking, diabetes, atrial fibrillation, and dyslipidemia. The treatment of hypertension, beginning in the mid-20th century, is thought to be primarily responsible for the drastic reduction in stroke death rates between 1950 and 1980 in the United States.[4] A second very important risk factor for stroke is cardiac disease. Patients with coronary artery disease, congestive heart failure, left ventricular hypertrophy, and especially atrial fibrillation are at increased risk of stroke.[8,9] In fact, the presence of atrial fibrillation is one of the most potent risk factors for ischemic stroke, with stroke rates from 5% to 20% per year depending on the patient's comorbid conditions.[10,11] Other known risk factors for atherosclerosis are also known to place patients at risk of stroke. Diabetes mellitus, dyslipidemia, and cigarette smoking are known atherogenic states that lead to cerebrovascular disease and ischemic stroke.[8,9,12]

PATHOPHYSIOLOGY

ISCHEMIC STROKE

In carotid atherosclerosis, progressive accumulation of lipids and inflammatory cells in the intima of the affected arteries, combined with hypertrophy of arterial smooth muscle cells, results in plaque formation. Eventually, sheer stress may result in plaque rupture, collagen exposure, platelet aggregation, and clot formation. The clot can remain in the vessel, causing local occlusion, or travel distally as an embolism, eventually lodging downstream in a cerebral vessel. In the case of cardiogenic embolism, stasis of blood in the atria or ventricles of the heart leads to the formation of local clots that can become dislodged and travel directly through the aorta to the cerebral circulation. The final result of both thrombus formation and embolism is an arterial occlusion, decreasing cerebral blood flow and causing ischemia distal to the occlusion.[13]

Normal cerebral blood flow averages 50 mL/100 g per minute, and this is maintained over a wide range of blood pressures (mean arterial pressures of 50 to 150 mm Hg) by a process called *cerebral autoregu-*

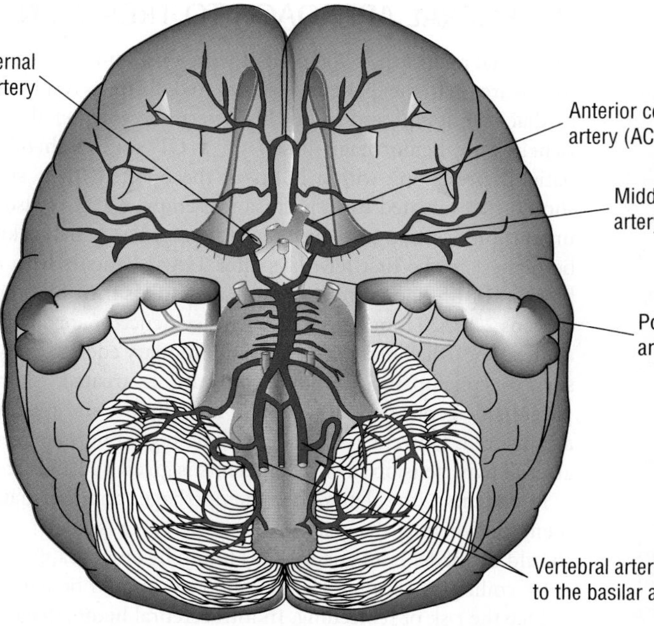

FIGURE 22-2. Main arterial blood supply to the brain.

lation. Cerebral blood vessels dilate and constrict in response to changes in blood pressure, but this process can be impaired by atherosclerosis and acute injury, such as stroke. When local cerebral blood flow decreases below 20 mL/100 g per minute, ischemia ensues, and when further reductions below 12 mL/100 g per minute persist, irreversible damage to the brain occurs, and this is called *infarction.* Tissue that is ischemic but maintains membrane integrity is referred to as the ischemic *penumbra* because it usually surrounds the infarct core. This penumbra is potentially salvageable through therapeutic intervention.

Reduction in the provision of nutrients to the ischemic cell eventually leads to depletion of the high-energy phosphates (e.g., adenosine triphosphate [ATP]) necessary for the maintenance of membrane integrity. Subsequently, extracellular potassium accumulates at the same time that sodium and water are sequestered intracellularly, leading to cell swelling and eventual lysis. Electrolyte imbalance also leads to depolarization of the cell and influx of calcium into the cell. The increase in intracellular calcium results in the activation of lipases, proteases, and endonucleases and the release of free fatty acids from membrane phospholipids. The depolarization of the neuron leads to the release of excitatory amino acids, such as glutamate and aspartate, that perpetuate the neuronal damage when released in excess. The accumulation of free fatty acids, including arachidonic acid, results in the formation of prostaglandins, leukotrienes, and free radicals. In ischemia, the magnitude of free-radical production overwhelms normal scavenging systems, leaving these reactive molecules to attack cell membranes and contribute to the mounting intracellular acidosis. All these events occur within 2 to 3 hours of the onset of ischemia and contribute to the ultimate cell death.[13]

Later targets for intervention in the pathophysiologic process involved after cerebral ischemia include the influx of activated inflammatory cells, starting from 2 hours after the onset of ischemia and lasting for several days. Also, the initiation of apoptosis, or programmed cell death, is thought to occur many hours after the acute insult and can interfere with recovery and repair of brain tissue.[14]

HEMORRHAGIC STROKE

The pathophysiology of hemorrhagic stroke is not as well studied as that of ischemic stroke. However, it is known that the presence of blood in the brain parenchyma causes damage to the surrounding tissue through the mechanical effect it produces (mass effect) and the neurotoxicity of the blood components and their degradation products.[5] Approximately 30% of intracerebral hemorrhages continue to enlarge over the first 24 hours, most within 4 hours, and clot volume is the most important predictor of outcome, regardless of location.[15] Hemorrhage volumes >60 mL are associated with 71% to 93% mortality at 30 days.[5,6] Much of the early mortality of hemorrhagic stroke (up to 50% at 30 days) is caused by the abrupt increase in intracranial pressure that can lead to herniation and death.[1] There is also evidence to support that both early and late edema contributes to worsened outcome after intracerebral hemorrhage.[6]

CLINICAL PRESENTATION (INCLUDING DIAGNOSTIC CONSIDERATIONS)

Stroke is a term used to describe an abrupt-onset focal neurologic deficit that lasts at least 24 hours and is of presumed vascular origin. A TIA is the same but lasts less than 24 hours and usually less than 30 minutes. The abrupt onset and the duration of the symptoms are determined through the history. The use of sensitive imaging techniques (magnetic resonance imaging [MRI]) has revealed that symptoms lasting more than 1 hour and less than 24 hours, although technically TIAs, are associated with infarction, making TIA and minor stroke clinically indistinguishable. The location of the central nervous system injury and its reference to a specific arterial distribution in the brain are determined through the neurologic examination and confirmed by imaging studies such as computed tomography (CT) scanning and MRI. The main arterial supply to the brain is illustrated in Fig. 22–2. Further diagnostic tests are performed to identify the cause of the patient's stroke and to design appropriate therapeutic strategies to prevent further events.[16]

CLINICAL PRESENTATION OF STROKE

General

- The patient may not be able to reliably report the history owing to cognitive or language deficits. A reliable history may have to come from a family member or another witness.

Symptoms

- The patient may complain of weakness on one side of the body, inability to speak, loss of vision, vertigo, or falling. Ischemic stroke is not usually painful, but patients may complain of headache, and with hemorrhagic stroke, it can be very severe.

Signs

- Patients usually have multiple signs of neurologic dysfunction, and the specific deficits are determined by the area of the brain involved.
- Hemi- or monoparesis occurs commonly, as does a hemisensory deficit.
- Patients with vertigo and double vision are likely to have posterior circulation involvement.
- Aphasia is seen commonly in patients with anterior circulation strokes.
- Patients also may suffer from dysarthria, visual field defects, and altered levels of consciousness.

Laboratory Tests

- Tests for hypercoagulable states (protein C deficiency, antiphospholipid antibody) should be done only when the cause of the stroke cannot be determined based on the presence of well-known risk factors for stroke. Protein C, protein S, and antithrombin III are best measured in the "steady state," not in the acute stage. Antiphospholipid antibodies as measured by anticardiolipin antibodies, β_2-glycoprotein I, and lupus anticoagulant screen are of higher yield than protein C, protein S, and antithrombin III but should be reserved for patients who are young (<50 years of age), have had multiple venous/arterial thrombotic events, or have livedo reticularis (a skin rash).

Other Diagnostic Tests

- CT scan of the head will reveal an area of hyperintensity (white) in the area of hemorrhage and will be normal or hypointense (dark) in the area of infarction. The CT scan may take 24 hours (and rarely longer) to reveal the area of infarction.
- MRI of the head will reveal areas of ischemia with higher resolution and earlier than the CT scan. Diffusion-weighted imaging (DWI) will reveal an evolving infarct within minutes.
- Carotid Doppler (CD) studies will determine whether the patient has a high degree of stenosis in the carotid arteries supplying blood to the brain (extracranial disease).
- An electrocardiogram (ECG) will determine whether the patient has atrial fibrillation, a potent etiologic factor for stroke.
- Transthoracic echocardiography (TTE) will determine whether valve abnormalities or wall-motion abnormalities are sources of emboli to the brain. A "bubble test" can be done to look for an intraatrial shunt indicating an atrial septal defect or a patent foramen ovale.
- Transesophageal echocardiography (TEE) is a more sensitive test for thrombus in the left atrium. It is effective at examining the aortic arch for atheroma, a potential source of emboli.
- Transcranial Doppler (TCD) will determine whether the patient is likely to have intracranial stenosis (e.g., middle cerebral artery stenosis).

TREATMENT

Stroke

DESIRED OUTCOME

The goals of treatment of acute stroke are (1) to reduce the ongoing neurologic injury and decrease mortality and long-term disability, (2) prevent complications secondary to immobility and neurologic dysfunction, and (3) prevent stroke recurrence.[17–19] Primary prevention of stroke is reviewed elsewhere.[8]

GENERAL APPROACH TO TREATMENT

The initial approach to the patient with a presumed acute stroke is to ensure that the patient is supported from a respiratory and cardiac standpoint and to quickly determine whether the lesion is ischemic or hemorrhagic-based on a CT scan. Ischemic stroke patients presenting within hours of the onset of their symptoms should be evaluated for reperfusion therapy. ❸ TIAs also require urgent intervention to reduce the risk of stroke, which is known to be highest in the first few days after TIA.[20] Patients with elevated blood pressure should remain untreated unless their blood pressure exceeds 220/120 mm Hg, or they have evidence of aortic dissection, acute myocardial infarction (AMI), pulmonary edema, or hypertensive encephalopathy. If blood pressure is treated, short-acting parenteral agents, such as labetalol, nicardipine, and nitroprusside, are favored. Current recommendations regarding management of arterial hypertension in stroke patients is given in Table 22–2.[17–19]

In patients with subarachnoid hemorrhage , an immediate assessment of whether the patient has a berry or saccular aneurysm should be made. If an aneurysm is found by angiography, endovascular coiling or clipping via a craniotomy should be performed to reduce the risk of rebleeding. In intracerebral hemorrhage, patients may require external ventricular drainage (EVD) if there is intraventricular blood and evolving hydrocephalus (enlargement of the ventricles). Once the patient is out of the hyperacute phase, attention is placed on preventing worsening, minimizing complications, and instituting appropriate secondary prevention strategies. The acute phase of the stroke includes the first week after the event.[17]

NONPHARMACOLOGIC THERAPY

Ischemic Stroke

Surgical interventions in the acute ischemic stroke patient are limited. In certain cases of ischemic cerebral edema owing to a large infarction, craniectomy to release some of the rising pressure has been tried. In cases of significant swelling associated with a cerebellar infarction, surgical decompression can be lifesaving. Beyond surgical intervention, however, the use of an organized, multidisciplinary approach to stroke care that includes early rehabilitation has been shown to be very effective in reducing the ultimate disability owing to ischemic stroke. In fact, the use of "stroke units" has been associated with outcomes similar to those achieved with early thrombolysis when compared with usual care.[17]

❹ In secondary prevention, carotid endarterectomy of an ulcerated and/or stenotic carotid artery is a very effective way to reduce stroke incidence and recurrence in appropriate patients and in centers where the operative morbidity and mortality are low. In fact, in ischemic stroke patients with 70% to 99% stenosis of an ipsilateral internal carotid artery, recurrent stroke risk can be reduced by up to 48% compared with medical therapy alone when combined

TABLE 22-2 Blood Pressure Treatment Guidelines in Acute Ischemic Stroke Patients

Treatment	Received t-PA	Did Not Receive t-PA
None	<180/105	<220/120
Labetalol IV[a] or Nicardipine IV[b]	180–230/105–120	>220/121–140
Nitroprusside[c]	Diastolic >140	Diastolic >140

t-PA, tissue plasminogen activator.

[a]Labetalol IV = 10–20 mg, doubled every 10–20 minutes, to a maximum of 300 mg. Also can use an infusion of 2–8 mg/min.

[b]Nicardipine IV = infusion starting at 5 mg/h up to 15 mg/h.

[c]Nitroprusside IV = infusion starting at 0.5 mcg/kg/min, with continuous arterial blood pressure monitoring.

Adapted from Adams HP, del Zoppo G, Alberts MJ, et al. Stroke 2007;38:1655–1711.

with aspirin 325 mg daily.[21] In patients in whom the risk of endarterectomy is thought to be excessive, carotid stenting can be effective in reducing recurrent stroke risk but is less invasive.[22] Carotid stenting is still considered investigational, however, and issues remain regarding the optimal methods and patients for this procedure.

Hemorrhagic Stroke

In patients with subarachnoid hemorrhage owing to a ruptured intracranial aneurysm or an AVM, surgical intervention to either clip or ablate the offending vascular abnormality substantially reduces mortality owing to rebleeding.[23] In the case of primary intracerebral hemorrhage, however, the benefits of surgery are less well documented. Although many patients undergo surgical treatment of intracerebral hematomas, the procedures have not been studied adequately in clinical trials.[5,15] Insertion of EVD for hydrocephalus and subsequent monitoring of intracranial pressure are done commonly and are the least invasive of the procedures done in these patients. Surgical decompression of a hematoma is more controversial, except when it is a last option in a life-threatening situation. Guidelines have been developed for the use of surgical intervention in the treatment of intracerebral hemorrhage, but they are limited in their impact by the lack of clinical trial data to support them.[15]

■ PHARMACOLOGIC THERAPY

Ischemic Stroke

Drug Treatments of First Choice: Published Guidelines

The Stroke Council of the American Stroke Association has created and published guidelines that address the management of acute ischemic stroke.[17] In general, the only two pharmacologic agents recommended with a grade A recommendation are intravenous t-PA within 3 hours of onset and aspirin within 48 hours of onset.

❺ Early reperfusion (<3 hours from onset) with intravenous t-PA has been shown to reduce the ultimate disability caused by ischemic stroke.[24] Caution must be exercised when using this therapy, and adherence to a strict protocol is essential to achieving positive outcomes.[17] The essentials of the treatment protocol can be summarized as (1) stroke team activation, (2) onset of symptoms within 3 hours, (3) CT scan to rule out hemorrhage, (4) meet inclusion and exclusion criteria (Table 22–3), (5) administer t-PA 0.9 mg/kg over 1 hour, with 10% given as initial bolus over 1 minute, (6) avoid antithrombotic (anticoagulant or antiplatelet) therapy for 24 hours, and (7) monitor the patient closely for response and hemorrhage.[17]

Early aspirin therapy also has been shown to reduce long-term death and disability[25,26] but should never be given within 24 hours of the administration of t-PA because it can increase the risk of bleeding in such patients.[17]

The American Heart Association/American Stroke Association (AHA/ASA) guidelines address all pharmacotherapy used in the secondary prevention of ischemic stroke and are updated every 3 years.[27] It is clear that antiplatelet therapy is the cornerstone of antithrombotic therapy for the secondary prevention of ischemic stroke and should be used in noncardioembolic strokes. All three currently used agents, aspirin, clopidogrel, and extended-release dipyridamole plus aspirin (ERDP-ASA), are considered first-line antiplatelet agents by the American College of Chest Physicians (ACCP). In patients with atrial fibrillation and a presumed cardiac source of embolism, warfarin is the antithrombotic agent of first choice. Other pharmacotherapy recommended for secondary prevention of stroke include blood pressure lowering and statin therapy. Current recommendations regarding the acute treatment and secondary prevention of stroke are given in Table 22–4.

TABLE 22-3 Inclusion and Exclusion Criteria for Alteplase Use in Acute Ischemic Stroke

Inclusion criteria (all YES boxes must be checked before treatment)

YES

- ☐ Age 18 years or older
- ☐ Clinical diagnosis of ischemic stroke causing a measurable neurologic deficit
- ☐ Time of symptom onset well established to be less than 180 minutes before treatment would begin

Exclusion criteria (all NO boxes must be checked before treatment)

NO

- ☐ Evidence of intracranial hemorrhage on noncontrast head CT
- ☐ Only minor or rapidly improving stroke symptoms
- ☐ High clinical suspicion of subarachnoid hemorrhage even with normal CT
- ☐ Active internal bleeding (e.g., GI/GU bleeding within 21 days)
- ☐ Known bleeding diathesis, including but not limited to platelet count <100,000/mm³
- ☐ Patient has received heparin within 48 hours and had an elevated APTT
- ☐ Recent use of anticoagulant (e.g., warfarin) and elevated PT (>15 second)/INR
- ☐ Intracranial surgery, serious head trauma, or previous stroke within 3 months
- ☐ Major surgery or serious trauma within 14 days
- ☐ Recent arterial puncture at noncompressible site
- ☐ Lumbar puncture within 7 days
- ☐ History of intracranial hemorrhage, arteriovenous malformation, or aneurysm
- ☐ Witnessed seizure at stroke onset
- ☐ Recent acute myocardial infarction
- ☐ SBP >185 mm Hg or DBP >110 mm Hg at time of treatment

APTT, activated partial thromboplastin time; CT, computed tomography; DBP, diastolic blood pressure; GI, gastrointestinal; GU, genitourinary; INR, international normalized ratio; PT, prothrombin time; SBP, systolic blood pressure.

TABLE 22-4 Recommendations for Pharmacotherapy of Ischemic Stroke

	Recommendation	Evidence[a]
Acute treatment	t-PA 0.9 mg/kg IV[7,17] (maximum 90 kg) over 1 hour in selected patients within 3 hours of onset	IA
	ASA 160–325 mg daily[7,17] started within 48 hours of onset	IA
Secondary prevention		
Noncardioembolic	Antiplatelet therapy	IA
	Aspirin 50–325 mg daily[7,27]	IIa A (all three as initial options)
	Clopidogrel 75 mg daily[7,27]	IIb B (over aspirin)
	Aspirin 25 mg + extended-release dipyridamole 200 mg twice daily[7,27]	IIa A (over aspirin)
Cardioembolic (esp. atrial fibrillation)	Warfarin (INR = 2.5)[7,27]	IA
All	Antihypertensive treatment[27]	IA
Previously hypertensive	ACE inhibitor + diuretic[27]	IA
Previously normotensive	ACE inhibitor + diuretic[27]	IIa B
Dyslipidemic	Statin[27]	IA
Normal lipids	Statin[27]	IIa B

ACE, angiotensin-converting enzymes; ASA, aspirin; INR, international normalized ratio; t-PA, tissue plasminogen activator.

[a]Classes and levels of evidence: I—evidence or general agreement that useful and effective; II—conflicting evidence about the usefulness; IIa—weight of evidence in favor of the treatment; IIb—usefulness less well established; III—not useful and maybe harmful. Levels of evidence: A—multiple randomized clinical trials; B—a single randomized trial or nonrandomized studies; C—expert opinion or case studies.[25] (Level A in reference 7—t-PA recommendation—does not require multiple trials, just randomized, well-controlled clinical trial.)

Data from Albers et al.,[7] Adams et al.,[17] and Sacco et al.[27]

■ GENERAL INFORMATION REGARDING SAFETY AND EFFICACY (INCLUDING PIVOTAL CLINICAL TRIALS)

t-PA

The effectiveness of IV t-PA in the treatment of ischemic stroke was demonstrated in the National Institutes of Neurologic Disorders and Stroke (NINDS) Recombinant Tissue-Type Plasminogen Activator (rt-PA) Stroke Trial, published in 1995.[24] In 624 patients treated in equal numbers with either t-PA 0.9 mg/kg IV or placebo within 3 hours of the onset of their neurologic symptoms, 39% of the treated patients achieved an "excellent outcome" at 3 months compared with 26% of the placebo patients. An "excellent outcome" was defined as minimal or no disability by several different neurologic scales. This beneficial effect was reported despite a 10-fold increase in the risk of symptomatic intracerebral hemorrhage in the t-PA-treated patients (0.6% vs. 6.4%). Overall mortality was not different between the two groups (17% with t-PA and 21% with placebo). Patients with very severe symptoms at baseline (National Institutes of Health Stroke Scale [NIHSS] >20) and early ischemic changes on CT scan were shown to be at highest risk for the development of symptomatic intracranial hemorrhage. Even in patients at highest risk for bleeding, however, those receiving t-PA had better outcomes at 90 days than those who received placebo.[24] The publication of the NINDS trial results significantly changed the way in which acute stroke is managed in the community, promoting the development of acute stroke teams and emphasis on the early diagnosis and treatment of acute stroke. Prospectively collected data, even from the best centers, report between 3% and 8.5% of ischemic stroke patients in the United States receive t-PA, primarily owing to failure of patients to present in time to facilities equipped to administer the therapy safely.[28] Hemorrhage rates associated with t-PA use in the community have been reported to be similar to those reported in the NINDS trial (5%),[29] but significantly higher rates (up to 15%) have been reported when a strict protocol is not followed.[30]

Aspirin

The use of early aspirin to reduce long-term death and disability owing to ischemic stroke is supported by two large, randomized clinical trials. In the International Stroke Trial (IST),[26] aspirin 300 mg/day significantly reduced stroke recurrence within the first 2 weeks without effect on early mortality, resulting in a significant decrease in death and dependency at 6 months. In the Chinese Acute Stroke Trial (CAST),[25] aspirin 160 mg/day reduced the risk of recurrence and death in the first 28 days, but long-term death and disability were not different than with placebo. In both trials, a small but significant increase in hemorrhagic transformation of the infarction was demonstrated. Overall, the beneficial effects of early aspirin have been embraced and adopted into clinical guidelines.

Antiplatelet Agents

All patients who have had an acute ischemic stroke or TIA should receive long-term antithrombotic therapy for secondary prevention.[27] ❻ In patients with noncardioembolic stroke, this will be some form of antiplatelet therapy. In a recent meta-analysis, the overall benefit of antiplatelet therapy in patients with atherothrombotic disorders was estimated to be 22%.[31] Aspirin is the best-studied of the available agents and, until recently, was considered the sole first-line agent. However, published literature has supported the use of clopidogrel and the combination product ERDP-ASA as additional first-line agents in secondary stroke prevention.

The efficacy of clopidogrel as an antiplatelet agent in atherothrombotic disorders was demonstrated in the Clopidogrel versus Aspirin in Patients at Risk of Ischemic Events (CAPRIE) trial.[32] In this study of more than 19,000 patients with a history of either myocardial infarction (MI), stroke, or peripheral arterial disease (PAD), clopidogrel 75 mg/day was compared with aspirin 325 mg/day for its ability to decrease MI, stroke, or cardiovascular death. In the final analysis, clopidogrel was slightly (8% relative risk reduction [RRR]) more effective than aspirin (P = 0.043) and had a similar incidence of adverse effects. It is not associated with the blood dyscrasias (neutropenia) common with its congener, ticlopidine, and is used widely in patients with atherosclerosis.

In the European Stroke Prevention Study 2 (ESPS-2), aspirin 25 mg and extended-release dipyridamole (ERDP) 200 mg twice daily were compared alone and in combination with placebo for their ability to reduce recurrent stroke over a 2-year period.[33] In a total of more than 6,600 patients, all three treatment groups were shown to be superior to placebo—aspirin alone, 18% RRR; ERDP alone, 16% RRR; and the combination, 37% RRR. Importantly, this study was the first to show a significant benefit of combination antiplatelet therapy in stroke prevention, with the combination demonstrating a significant advantage over the aspirin-alone group (23% RRR; P = 0.006) and the ERDP-alone group (24% RRR; P = 0.002). Headache resulting in discontinuation occurred in approximately 15% of the ERDP groups (four times more common than in the placebo group), and the aspirin-treated patients, even at the low dose of 50 mg/day, experienced significantly more bleeding than the other groups. The combination of aspirin 25 mg and ERDP 200 mg twice daily is a highly effective treatment to prevent recurrence in patients with stroke or TIA. The European/Australasian Stroke Prevention in Reversible Ischemia Trial (ESPRIT) confirmed the results of ESPS-2, in that the combination of dipyridamole (83% extended release) and aspirin (30–325 mg daily) was more effective than aspirin alone in reducing recurrent stroke.[34] Headache was an important cause of discontinuation in the ESPRIT trial, further stressing the importance of monitoring and education in these patients. No data exist on the ability of this combination to reduce MI and/or cardiovascular death in patients with other indications for antiplatelet therapy.

Warfarin

❼ Warfarin is the most effective treatment for the prevention of stroke in patients with atrial fibrillation.[10,11,35,36] In patients with atrial fibrillation and a recent history of stroke or TIA, the risk of recurrence places these patients in one of the highest risk categories known. In the European Atrial Fibrillation Trial (EAFT), 669 patients with nonvalvular atrial fibrillation (NVAF) and a prior stroke or TIA were randomized to either warfarin (international normalized ratio [INR] = 2.5–4), aspirin 300 mg/day, or placebo. Patients in the placebo group experienced stroke, MI, or vascular death at a rate of 17% per year compared with 8% per year in the warfarin group and 15% per year in the aspirin group. This represents a 53% reduction in risk with anticoagulation.[10] Subsequent studies in the primary prevention of stroke in patients with NVAF have demonstrated that targeting an international normalization ratio (INR) of 2.5 prevents stroke with the lowest bleeding risk (Stroke Prevention in Atrial Fibrillation [SPAF III]); therefore, a target INR of 2.5 is recommended in the secondary prevention of stroke.[11,35,36]

Use of warfarin in the secondary prevention of noncardioembolic stroke was addressed in the Warfarin Aspirin Recurrent Stroke Study.[37] In 2,206 patients with recent stroke, warfarin (INR = 1.4–2.8) was not superior to aspirin 325 mg/day in the prevention of recurrent events. Further data from the Warfarin-Aspirin in Intracranial Disease (WASID) trial demonstrated that aspirin therapy was as effective and safer than warfarin in patients with intracranial stenosis.[38] These studies led most clinicians to abandon the practice of using warfarin in all but patients with cardioembolic sources of emboli, mainly atrial fibrillation.

Blood Pressure Lowering

8 Elevated blood pressure is very common in ischemic stroke patients, and treatment of hypertension in these patients is associated with a decreased risk of stroke recurrence.[39] In the Perindopril pROtection aGainst REcurrent Stroke Study (PROGRESS), a multinational stroke population (40% Asian) was randomized to receive either blood pressure lowering with the angiotensin-converting enzyme (ACE) inhibitor perindopril (with or without the thiazide diuretic indapamide) or placebo.[40] Treated patients achieved an overall 9 points systolic and 4 points diastolic mm Hg blood pressure reduction, and this was associated with a 28% reduction in stroke recurrence. In the patients who received the combination treatment (clinician's discretion), the average blood pressure lowering achieved was 12 systolic and 5 diastolic mm Hg, and this was associated with an even larger reduction in stroke recurrence (43%). Similar results were achieved in patients with and without hypertension. Based on the results of this study and other evidence of the tolerability and vascular protective properties of the ACE inhibitors, the Seventh Report of the Joint National Committee on Prevention, Detection, Evaluation, and Treatment of High Blood Pressure (JNC7) and the AHA/ASA guidelines recommend an ACE inhibitor and a diuretic for the reduction of blood pressure in patients with stroke or TIA.[27,41] 9 Blood pressure lowering in the acute stroke period (first 7 days) can result in decreased cerebral blood flow and worsened symptoms; therefore, recommendations are limited to patients out of the acute stroke period.[27]

Statins

10 The statins have been shown to reduce the risk of stroke by approximately 30% in patients with coronary artery disease and elevated plasma lipids.[42–44] The National Cholesterol Education Program (NCEP) considers ischemic stroke or TIA to be a coronary "equivalent" and has recommended the use of statins to achieve a low-density lipoprotein (LDL) concentration of less than 100 mg/dL.[45] When the Heart Protection Study was published, it provided evidence that simvastatin 40 mg/day reduced stroke risk in high-risk individuals (including patients with prior stroke) by 25% ($P < 0.0001$), even in patients with LDL concentrations of less than 116 mg/dL.[46] The investigators also showed that this practice is extremely safe, with an excess incidence of myopathy of 0.01%. The Stroke Prevention by Aggressive Reduction in Cholesterol (SPARCL) study went one step further by demonstrating, in stroke patients, that atorvastatin 80 mg daily reduced the risk of recurrent stroke by 16% and coronary events by 42% while causing an increase in liver enzymes, but no increase in myopathy.[47] Statin therapy is an effective way to reduce stroke risk and should be considered in all ischemic stroke patients. Whether high-dose statin therapy is prescribed should be determined in the individual patient by a careful weighing of the benefits against the potential increase in adverse events.

Heparin for Prophylaxis of Deep-Vein Thrombosis (DVT)

The use of low-molecular-weight heparins or low-dose subcutaneous unfractionated heparin (5,000 units twice daily) can be recommended for the prevention of DVT in hospitalized patients with decreased mobility owing to their stroke and should be used in all but the most minor strokes.[7,17]

■ ALTERNATIVE DRUG TREATMENTS

Aspirin Plus Clopidogrel

In the Management of ATherothrombosis with Clopidogrel in High-risk patients (MATCH) study, clopidogrel in combination with aspirin 75 mg daily was no better than clopidogrel alone in secondary stroke prevention.[48] However, the combination has been studied in patients with acute coronary syndromes and patients undergoing percutaneous coronary interventions and shown to be significantly more effective than aspirin alone in reducing MI, stroke, and cardiovascular death.[49,50] Also, when clopidogrel was used with aspirin, the risk of life-threatening bleeding increased from 1.3% to 2.6%.[48] In the Clopidogrel for High Atherothrombotic Risk and Ischemic Stabilization, Management and Avoidance (CHARISMA) trial, the combination was again found to significantly increase serious bleeding in a high risk atherosclerosis population (clinically evident disease or multiple risk factors) with no consistent benefit in terms of preventing vascular events, when compared to aspirin alone.[51] This combination can only be recommended in patients with a recent history of MI or coronary stent placement and only with ultra–low-dose aspirin to minimize bleeding risk.[52]

Angiotensin II Receptor Blockers

Angiotensin II receptor blockers (ARBs) also have been shown to reduce the risk of stroke. In the Losortan Intervention For Endpoint Reduction in Hypertension (LIFE) study, losartan and metoprolol were compared for their ability to reduce blood pressure and prevent cardiovascular events in a group of severely hypertensive patients.[53] Despite similar reductions in blood pressure of approximately 30/16 mm Hg, the losartan group experienced a 24% reduction in the risk of stroke. In a similar study comparing eprosartan to nitrendipine, the ARB eprosartan was superior to the calcium channel blocker in reducing recurrent stroke risk, when equal blood pressure lowering was achieved.[54] The ARBs should be considered in patients unable to tolerate ACE inhibitors for blood pressure lowering after acute ischemic stroke.

Heparins

The use of full-dose unfractionated heparin in the acute stroke period has never been proven to positively affect stroke outcome, and it significantly increases the risk of intracerebral hemorrhage.[7,17] Trials of low-molecular-weight heparins or heparinoids have been largely negative and do not support their routine use in stroke patients.[55–57] Other potential but unproven uses for treatment doses of either unfractionated or low-molecular-weight heparins include bridge therapy in patients being initiated on warfarin, carotid dissection, or continuous worsening of ischemia despite adequate antiplatelet therapy.[7]

■ DRUG CLASS INFORMATION

Aspirin

Aspirin exerts its antiplatelet effect by irreversibly inhibiting cyclooxygenase, which, in platelets, prevents conversion of arachidonic acid to thromboxane A_2 (TXA_2), which is a powerful vasoconstrictor and stimulator of platelet aggregation. Platelets remain impaired for their life span (5 to 7 days) after exposure to aspirin. Aspirin also inhibits prostacyclin (PGI_2) activity in the smooth muscle of vascular walls. PGI_2 inhibits platelet aggregation, and the vascular endothelium can synthesize prostacyclin such that the platelet antiaggregating effect is maintained. The suppression of PGI_2 production by aspirin has been found to be dose- and duration-related; the higher the dose, the longer the cyclooxygenase production is suppressed. Therefore, the lower the aspirin dose, the less effect on PGI_2.[7] The optimal dose of aspirin is still under study, but it should be the dose that inhibits TXA_2 with the least amount of PGI_2 inhibition. It has been shown that an aspirin dose of 325 mg/day will inhibit TXA_2 but will not significantly inhibit PGI_2 production. There is probably a point at which lower doses of aspirin do not completely block TXA_2, and recent studies indicate that the lowest effective dose may be in the range of 50 mg/day.[58] Upper gastrointestinal (GI) discomfort and bleeding are the most common adverse effects of aspirin and have been shown to be dose-related. The highest rates of GI bleeding (5%) have been reported in patients receiving 1,200 mg/day as compared with rates of 2% in patients taking the more commonly prescribed, 300 mg/day. Upper GI symptoms are much more common than frank bleeding, however, with 40% of patients affected at 1,200 mg/day and 25% at 300 mg/day.[59] In the ESPS-2 study, even 50 mg/day of aspirin was associated with a twofold increase in bleeding over the placebo group.[33]

Low doses (<100 mg) of aspirin quickly inhibit cyclooxygenase in all the platelets in the circulation. Therefore, the onset of the antiplatelet effect of aspirin is less than 60 minutes.[60] It has been reported, however, that some patients either have or develop "aspirin resistance" and can require higher doses to achieve the desired antiplatelet effect.[61] Despite this, routine testing for aspirin resistance is not recommended. It was observed recently that administration of ibuprofen prior to the administration of a daily aspirin dose prohibits the aspirin from binding irreversibly to the cyclooxygenase and can decrease its antiplatelet effect.[62] Current recommendations are to administer aspirin at least 2 hours before ibuprofen or to wait at least 4 hours after an ibuprofen dose.

Extended-Release Dipyridamole Plus Aspirin

Early studies of the role of dipyridamole in stroke prevention failed to show a benefit over that realized by aspirin alone. Dipyridamole, in high doses, is thought to inhibit platelet aggregation by inhibiting phosphodiesterase, leading to accumulation of cyclic adenosine monophosphate (cAMP) and cyclic guanosine monophosphate (cGMP) intracellularly, which prevent platelet activation. In addition, dipyridamole also enhances the antithrombotic potential of the vascular wall.[63] The ESPS-2 demonstrated the efficacy of high-dose extended-release dipyridamole alone and in combination with aspirin in secondary stroke prevention.[33] This was the first study to demonstrate the benefits of combination antiplatelet therapy in stroke prevention (the combination was significantly more effective than either agent alone). The extended-release formulation of dipyridamole is important in that it allows twice-daily administration and higher doses to be tolerated in patients. The use of immediate-release generic dipyridamole in combination with regular aspirin, in order to reduce costs, is unproven and should be discouraged.

In the ESPS-2, 25% of the patients who received combination dipyridamole and aspirin discontinued the therapy early, and the rate of discontinuation owing to headache was more than three times as common (10%) as in the aspirin-alone group (3%). Other reasons for discontinuation were GI problems. Slow initiation of ERDP-ASA at one capsule at bedtime daily for 2 or 3 days can be tried in order to lessen headache symptoms. The headache caused by ERDP-ASA is mostly self-limiting and decreases after several days.[64]

Clopidogrel

Clopidogrel has a unique platelet antiaggregatory effect in that it is an inhibitor of the adenosine diphosphate (ADP) pathway of platelet aggregation and inhibits known stimuli to platelet aggregation.[7,32] This effect causes an alteration of the platelet membrane and interference with the membrane-fibrinogenic interaction leading to a blocking of the platelet glycoprotein IIb/IIIa receptor. A time lag of 3 to 7 days before the antiplatelet effect is maximal should be expected. The tolerability of clopidogrel 75 mg/day is at least as good as medium-dose (325 mg/day) aspirin, and GI bleeding is less.[32] Clopidogrel is associated with an increased risk of diarrhea and rash, but discontinuation rates owing to adverse effects are similar to those with aspirin 325 mg/day (5.3% to 6%, respectively).[32] There is no excess neutropenia in patients taking clopidogrel, and rates of thrombotic thrombocytopenic purpura probably are no greater than background rates.[65]

Clopidogrel is a thienopyridine prodrug and needs to be biotransformed by the liver to an active metabolite. Evidence suggests that the enzyme responsible for the conversion is human cytochrome P450 3A4 (CYP3A4) and that the platelet effects of clopidogrel can be diminished in patients receiving agents that inhibit this enzyme.[66] Although high doses of the lipophilic statins atorvastatin and simvastatin can diminish the effectiveness of clopidogrel to inhibit platelet aggregation in vitro, there does not appear to be any adverse effect on atherothrombotic event rates.[67] Concomitant administration of clopidogrel with lipophilic statins is often recommended.

■ INVESTIGATIONAL STRATEGIES

Reperfusion

Various investigations aimed at shortening the time required to open the occluded cerebral artery and preserve its patency are underway in acute ischemic stroke patients.[68] Strategies being tried include longer-acting fibrinolytic agents, intraarterial fibrinolysis with t-PA and other agents, and endovascular clot removal using mechanical and laser-guided approaches. In addition, investigators are trying to identify, using sensitive MRI techniques, which patients benefit from reperfusion at time points outside the approved 3-hour time window. Undoubtedly, efforts to reperfuse the ischemic brain will continue to be explored, so more patients will be eligible for this therapy.

Neuroprotection and Neurorestoration

Although many different neuroprotective agents have been studied in clinical trials of acute ischemic stroke, most have been unsuccessful.[69] A promising nonpharmacologic strategy that has been shown to provide neuroprotection in patients has been hypothermia.[70] Currently, clinical trials are underway to optimize the mechanism of cooling the ischemic brain (intravascular coils versus surface cooling) and rewarming the patient after hypothermia. Despite discouraging results in previous attempts, however, there is still great interest in developing pharmacologic agents that provide neuroprotection. Some of the most promising agents include free-radical scavengers (NXY-059),[71] anti-inflammatory agents, and agents with multiple proposed mechanisms of protection (e.g., albumin infusions).[72] In addition, hope still exists that clinicians will be able to enhance the reparative process of the brain (neurorestoration) through targeted neurorehabilitation and the use of neural and cell transplantation.[73]

HEMORRHAGIC STROKE

There are currently no standard pharmacologic strategies for treating intracerebral hemorrhage (ICH).[15] The use of hemostatic agents (e.g., factor VII) in the hyperacute phase (<4 hours from onset) can reduce hematoma growth, but no improvement in outcomes has been demonstrated.[74] Medical guidelines for the management of blood pressure, raised intracranial pressure, and other medical complications of ICH are those required for the management of any acutely ill patient in a neurointensive care unit.

Subarachnoid hemorrhage (SAH) owing to aneurysm rupture is associated with a high incidence of delayed cerebral ischemia (DCI) in the 2 weeks following the bleeding episode. Vasospasm of the cerebral vasculature is thought to be responsible for DCI and occurs between 4 and 21 days after the bleed, peaking at days 5 through 9.[23] The calcium channel blocker nimodipine is recommended to reduce the incidence and severity of neurologic deficits owing to DCI. Nimodipine at a dose of 60 mg every 4 hours should be initiated on diagnosis and continued for 21 days in all SAH patients. Administration of nimodipine therapy is complicated by a fairly high incidence of hypotension. This can be managed by reducing the dosing interval to 30 mg every 2 hours (same daily dose), reducing the total daily dose (30 mg every 4 hours), and maintaining intravascular volume and pressor therapy.[23]

PHARMACOECONOMIC CONSIDERATIONS

Although t-PA is expensive, when the total healthcare costs are factored in, savings can accrue to the healthcare system as a direct result of appropriate t-PA therapy.[75] It has been estimated that, at a rate of $600 per patient treated, annual cost savings of $15 and $22 million could be realized by increasing national t-PA use to 4% and 6%, respectively (from the current 2%).[76]

In antithrombotic prophylaxis for atrial fibrillation, warfarin therapy was evaluated using quality-adjusted life-years (QALYs) saved.[77] It was found that in patients with atrial fibrillation and one additional risk factor, warfarin therapy cost $8,000 per QALY saved. In high-risk patients, those with atrial fibrillation and two or more risk factors, warfarin use was estimated to save $6,200 in costs from stroke and TIA. Costs of monitoring and hemorrhages from warfarin were estimated to be $5,500, thus showing a positive savings from warfarin use. Those without risk factors were much more costly to treat at an estimated $370,000 per QALY saved when compared with aspirin treatment. Warfarin is cost-effective in high-risk patients, particularly if the hemorrhagic side effects are lower relative to the stroke risk. For comparison purposes, hypertension screening is estimated to cost $10,000 to $50,000 per QALY saved. A Swedish study reported the cost-effectiveness of primary stroke prevention in atrial fibrillation patients with oral anticoagulants or aspirin based on four published clinical trials.[78] The authors found that the total cost per stroke prevented was a $16 savings if the intracerebral bleeding was 0.3% and $43 if the bleeding rate was 2%. At a bleeding complication rate of 1.3%, warfarin would prevent 1,000 strokes per year and save approximately $29 million. The cost-effectiveness of the various first-line antiplatelet agents have been compared as well.[79] Without a doubt, aspirin, owing to its extremely low acquisition cost (pennies daily), is cost saving. In other words, it reduces costs at the same time as saving QALYs. The use of clopidogrel or ERDP-ASA is associated with higher efficacy but significantly greater costs as well (up to $3 daily). Despite this, both options have been deemed "cost-effective" when administered to a 65-year-old patient with a history of stroke or TIA for the prevention of recurrence. In a recent analysis, ERDP-ASA was associated with $5,000 to $15,000 per QALY (adjusted for the acquisition cost) and clopidogrel was $26,580 per QALY. Any cost per QALY less than $50,000 is thought to be "cost-effective."[79] These estimates are extremely dependent on the assumptions made in the model. Cost-effectiveness in an individual patient is much more difficult to discern.

Primary prevention strategies that address the risk factors for ischemic stroke can be powerful in reducing the costs of stroke. Many of the stroke risk factors can be modified and some eliminated at very low costs (lifestyle changes), therefore developing risk-factor-reduction strategies can be the most cost-effective measure of all. More research is needed in identifying the cost-effectiveness of other forms of acute stroke treatment.

CLINICAL CONTROVERSIES

The use of full-dose unfractionated heparin in the management of acute ischemic stroke remains controversial despite years of debate and a lack of evidence supporting its use. Proponents of the therapy cite strong anecdotal evidence of positive responses in selected patients who have never been studied in clinical trials.

The use of intracranial angioplasty and stenting is strongly supported in the few institutions where the technology exists. Whether these procedures should be attempted in patients outside clinical trials remains controversial.

The use of surgical evacuation of intracranial hemorrhage with and without instillation of fibrinolytic agents is controversial. Although fervently pursued in select centers and countries, indications and outcomes are not known. Results of ongoing clinical trials can assist in settling this controversy.

EVALUATION OF THERAPEUTIC OUTCOMES

MONITORING OF THE PHARMACEUTICAL CARE PLAN

Patients with acute stroke should be monitored intensely for the development of neurologic worsening (recurrence or extension), complications (thromboembolism or infection), or adverse effects from pharmacologic or nonpharmacologic interventions. The most common reasons for deterioration in a stroke patient are (1) exten-

TABLE 22-5 Monitoring the Hospitalized Acute Stroke Patient

	Treatment	Parameter(s)	Frequency	Comments
Ischemic stroke	t-PA	BP, neurologic function, bleeding	Every 15 minutes × 1 hour; every 0.5 h × 6 h; every 1 hour × 17 hour; every shift after	
	Aspirin	Bleeding	Daily	
	Clopidogrel	Bleeding	Daily	
	ERDP/ASA	Headache, bleeding	Daily	Headache usually transient (2–3 days) and may respond to simple analgesics
	Warfarin	Bleeding, INR, Hb/Hct	INR daily × 3 days; weekly until stable; monthly	
Hemorrhagic stroke		BP, neurologic function, ICP	Every 2 hours in ICU	Many patients require intervention with short-acting agents to reduce BP to <180 mm Hg systolic
	Nimodipine (for SAH)	BP, neurologic function, fluid status	Every 2 hours in ICU	
All		Temperature, CBC	Temp. every 8 hours; CBC daily	For infectious complications such as UTI or pneumonia
		Pain (calf or chest)	Every 8 hours	For DVT, MI, acute headache
		Electrolytes and ECG	Up to daily	For fluid and electrolyte imbalances, cardiac rhythm abnormalities
	Heparins for DVT prophylaxis	Bleeding, platelets	Bleeding daily, platelets if suspected thrombocytopenia	

BP, blood pressure; CBC, complete blood count; DVT, deep-vein thrombosis; ECG, electrocardiography, ERDP-ASA, extended-release dipyridamole plus aspirin; Hb/Hct, hemoglobin/hematocrit; ICP, intracranial pressure; ICU, intensive care unit; MI, myocardial infarction; SAH, subarachnoid hemorrhage.

sion of the original lesion—ischemic or hemorrhagic—in the brain, (2) development of cerebral edema and raised intracranial pressure, (3) hypertensive emergency, (4) infection (urinary and respiratory most common), (5) venous thromboembolism (deep venous thrombosis and pulmonary embolism), (6) electrolyte abnormalities and cardiac rhythm disturbances (can be associated with brain injury), and (7) recurrent stroke.

The approach to monitoring the stroke patient is summarized in Table 22–5. Customization of the plan should be made for each patient based on his or her comorbidities and ongoing disease processes.

ABBREVIATIONS

ACE: angiotensin-converting enzyme
ADP: adenosine diphosphate
ARB: angiotensin II receptor blocker
ATP: adenosine triphosphate
AVM: arteriovenous malformation
cAMP: cyclic adenosine monophosphate
CAST: Chinese Acute Stroke Trial
CD: carotid Doppler
cGMP: cyclic guanosine monophosphate
CT scan: computed tomographic scan
CYP3A4: cytochrome P450 3A4
DCI: delayed cerebral ischemia
EAFT: European Atrial Fibrillation Trial
ECG: electrocardiogram
ERDP-ASA: extended-release dipyridamole plus aspirin
GI: gastrointestinal
ICH: intracerebral hemorrhage
INR: international normalized ratio
IST: International Stroke Trial
JNC: Joint National Committee
LDL: low-density lipoprotein
MI: myocardial infarction
MRI: magnetic resonance imaging
NCEP: National Cholesterol Education Program
NIHSS: National Institutes of Health Stroke Scale
NINDS: National Institute of Neurologic Disorders and Stroke
NVAF: nonvalvular atrial fibrillation
PAD: peripheral arterial disease
PGI_2: prostacyclin
QALY: quality-adjusted life-year
RRR: relative risk reduction
SAH: subarachnoid hemorrhage
TCD: transcranial Doppler
TIA: transient ischemic attack
TXA_2: thromboxane A_2
t-PA: tissue plasminogen activator

REFERENCES

1. Thon T, Haase N, Rosamond W, et al. Heart disease and stroke statistics—2006 update: A report from the American Heart Association Statistics Committee and Stroke Statistics Subcommittee. Circulation 2006;113:85–151.
2. Quilliam BJ, Lapane KL. Clinical correlates and drug treatment of residents with stroke in long-term care. Stroke 2001;32:1385–1393.
3. Elkins JS, Johnston SC. Thirty-year projections for deaths from ischemic stroke in the United States. Stroke 2003;34:2109–2113.
4. Cooper R, Cutler J, Desvigne-Nickens P, et al. Trends and disparities in coronary heart disease, stroke, and other cardiovascular diseases in the United States: Findings of the National Conference on Cardiovascular Disease Prevention. Circulation 2000;102:3137–3147.
5. Juvela S, Kase CS. Advances in intracerebral hemorrhage management. Stroke 2006;37:301–304.
6. Badjatia N, Rosand J. Intracerebral hemorrhage. Neurologist 2005; 11(6):311–324.
7. Albers GW, Amerenco P, Easton JD, et al. Antithrombotic and thrombolytic therapy for ischemic stroke: The seventh ACCP Conference on Antithrombotic and Thrombolytic Therapy. Chest 2004;126(3 suppl):483S–512S.
8. Goldstein LB, Adams R, Alberts MJ, et al. Primary prevention of ischemic stroke. A Guideline from the American Heart Association/American Stroke Association Stroke Council: Cosponsored by the Atherosclerotic Peripheral Vascular Disease Interdisciplinary Working Group; Cardiovascular Nursing Council; Clinical Cardiology Council; Nutrition, Physical Activity, and Metabolism Council; and the Quality of Care and Outcomes Research Interdisciplinary Working Group. Stroke 2006;37:1583–1633.
9. Helgason CM, Wolf PA. American Heart Association Prevention Conference IV. Prevention and rehabilitation of stroke. Circulation 1997;96:701–707.
10. European Atrial Fibrillation Trial Study Group. Secondary prevention in nonrheumatic atrial fibrillation after transient ischaemic attack or minor stroke. Lancet 1993;342:1255–1262.
11. Hart RG, Halperin JL, Pearce LA, et al. Lessons from the stroke prevention in atrial fibrillation trials. Ann Intern Med 2003;138:831–838.
12. Wolf PA. Fifty years at Framingham: Contributions to stroke epidemiology. Adv Neurol 2003;92:165–172.
13. Dirnagl U, Iadecola C, Moskowitz MA. Pathobiology of ischemic stroke: An integrated view. Trends Neurosci 1999;22:391–397.
14. Feuerstein GZ, Wang X. New opportunities for stroke prevention and therapeutics: A hope from anti-inflammatory drugs? In: Feuerstein GZ, ed. Inflammation and Stroke. Basel: Birkhauser-Verlag, 2001:3–10.
15. Broderick J, Connelly S, Feldman E, et al. Guidelines for the management of spontaneous intracerebral hemorrhage in adults: 2007 Update. Stroke 2007;38:2001–2023.
16. Greenberg DA, Aminoff MJ, Simon RP, eds. Stroke. In: Clinical Neurology, 5th ed. New York: McGraw-Hill, 2002:282–316.
17. Adams HP Jr, del Zoppo G, Alberts MJ, et al. Guidelines for the early managment of adults with ischemic stroke: A guideline from the American Heart Association. Stroke 2007;38:1655–1711.
18. Khaja AM, Grotta JC. Established treatments for acute ischemic stroke. Lancet 2007;369:319–330.
19. Goldstein LB. Acute ischemic stroke treatment in 2007. Circulation 2007;116:1504–1514.
20. Johnston SC, Nguyen-Huynh MN, Schwartz ME, et al. National Stroke Association guidelines for the management of transient ischemic attacks. Ann Neurol 2006;60(3):301–313.
21. Cina CA, Clase CM, Haynes RB. Carotid endarterectomy for symptomatic carotid stenosis (Cochrane Review on CD-ROM). Oxford: Cochrane Library Update Software, 2001; issue 1.
22. Narins CR, Illig KA. Patient selection for carotid stenting versus endarterectomy: A systemic review. J Vasc Surg 2006;44:661–672.
23. Miller J, Diringer M. Management of aneurysmal subarachnoid hemorrhage. Neurol Clin 1995;13:451–478.
24. The National Institute of Neurological Disorders and Stroke rt-PA Stroke Study Group. Tissue plasminogen activator for acute ischemic stroke. N Engl J Med 1995;333:1581–1587.
25. Chinese Acute Stroke Trial (CAST) Collaborative Group. CAST: A randomized, placebo-controlled trial of early aspirin use in 20,000 patients with acute ischemic stroke. Lancet 1997;349:1641–1649.
26. International Stroke Trial Collaborative Group. The International Stroke Trial (IST): A randomized trial of aspirin, subcutaneous hep-

arin, both, or neither among 19,435 patients with acute ischemic stroke. Lancet 1997;349:1560–1581.

27. Sacco RL, Adams R, Albers G, et al. Guidelines for prevention of stroke in patients with ischemic stroke or transient ischemic attack. A statement for health care professionals from the American Heart Association/American Stroke Association Council on Stroke. Stroke 2006;37:577–617.
28. The Paul Coverdell Prototype Registries Writing Group. Acute stroke care in the U.S. Results from four pilot prototypes of the Paul Coverdell National Acute Stroke Registry. Stroke 2005;36:1232–1240.
29. Albers GW, Bates VE, Clark WM, et al. Intravenous tissue-type plasminogen activator for treatment of acute stroke: The Standard Treatment with Alteplase to Reverse Stroke (STARS) study. JAMA 2000;283:1145–1150.
30. Katzan IL, Furlan AJ, Lloyd LE, et al. Use of tissue-type plasminogen activator for acute ischemic stroke: The Cleveland area experience. JAMA 2000;283:1189–1191.
31. Antithrombotic Trialists' Collaboration. Collaborative meta-analysis of randomized trials of antiplatelet therapy for prevention of death, myocardial infarction, and stroke in high risk patients. BMJ 2002;324:71–86.
32. CAPRIE Steering Committee. A randomized, blinded trial of clopidogrel versus aspirin in patients at risk of ischaemic events (CAPRIE). Lancet 1995;348:1329–1339.
33. Diener HC, Cunha L, Forbes C, et al. European Stroke Prevention Study 2: Dipyridamole and acetylsalicylic acid in the secondary prevention of stroke. J Neurol Sci 1996;143:1–13.
34. ESPRIT Study Group. Aspirin plus dipyridamole versus aspirin alone after cerebral ischaemia of arterial origin (ESPRIT): Randomized controlled trial. Lancet 2006;367:1665–1673.
35. American Society of Health-System Pharmacists. ASHP therapeutics position statement on antithrombotic therapy in chronic atrial fibrillation. Am J Health Syst Pharm 1998;55:376–381.
36. Hart RG, Benevente O, McBride R, Pearce LA. Antithrombotic therapy to prevent stroke in patients with atrial fibrillation: A meta-analysis. Ann Intern Med 1999;131:492–501.
37. Mohr JP, Thompson JLP, Lazar RM, et al. A comparison of warfarin and aspirin for the prevention of recurrent ischemic stroke. N Engl J Med 2001;345:1444–1451.
38. Chimowitz MI, Lynn MJ, Howlett-Smith H, et al. Comparison of warfarin and aspirin for symptomatic intracranial arterial stenosis. N Engl J Med 2005;352:1305–1316.
39. Gueyffer F, Boissel JP, Bouttie F, et al. for the INDANA Project Collaborators. Effect of antihypertensive treatment in patients having already suffered from stroke: Gathering of the evidence. Stroke 1997;28:2557–2562.
40. PROGRESS Collaborative Group. Randomized trial of perindopril-based blood-pressure-lowering regimen among 6105 individuals with previous stroke or transient ischaemic attack. Lancet 2001;358:1033–1041.
41. Chobanian AV, Bakris GL, Black HR, et al. The Seventh Report of the Joint National Committee on Prevention, Detection, Evaluation, and Treatment of High Blood Pressure. The JNC7 Report. JAMA 2003;289(19):2560–2572.
42. Hebert PR, Gaziano JM, Chan KS, Hennekens CH. Cholesterol lowering with statin drugs, risk of stroke, and total mortality: An overview of randomized trials. JAMA 1997;278:313–321.
43. Scandinavian Simvastatin Survival Study Group. Randomized trial of cholesterol lowering in 4444 patients with coronary heart disease: The Scandinavian Simvastatin Survival Study (4S). Lancet 1994;344:1383–1389.
44. Byrington RP, Davis BR, Plehn JF, et al. Reduction of stroke events with pravastatin: The Prospective Pravastatin Pooling (PPP) Project. Circulation 2001;103:387–392.
45. Executive Summary of the Third Report of the National Cholesterol Education Program (NCEP) Expert Panel on Detection, Evaluation, and Treatment of High Blood Cholesterol in Adults (Adult Treatment Panel III). JAMA 2001;285:2486–2497.
46. Heart Protection Study Collaborative Group. MRC/BHF Heart Protection Study of cholesterol lowering with simvastatin in 20,536 high-risk individuals: A randomized, placebo-control trial. Lancet 2002;360:7–22.
47. The Stroke Prevention by Aggressive Reduction in Cholesterol Levels (SPARCL) Investigators. High-dose atorvastatin after stroke or transient ischemic attack. N Engl J Med 2006;355:549–559.
48. Diener HC, Bogousslavsky J, Brass LM, et al. Aspirin and clopidogrel compared with clopidogrel alone after recent ischemic stroke or transient ischaemic attack in high-risk patients (MATCH): Randomized, double-blind, placebo-controlled trial. Lancet 2004;364:331–337.
49. Yusuf S, Zhao F, Mehta SR, et al. Effects of clopidogrel in addition to aspirin in patients with acute coronary syndromes without ST-segment elevation. N Engl J Med 2001;54:1022–1028.
50. Steinhubl SR, Berger PB, Mann JT, et al. Early and sustained dual oral antiplatelet therapy following percutaneous coronary intervention: A randomized, controlled trial. JAMA 2002;288:2411–2420.
51. Bhatt DL, Fox KAA, Hacke W, et al. Clopidogrel and aspirin versus aspirin alone for the prevention of atherothrombotic events. N Engl J Med 2006;354:1706–1717.
52. Peters RJG, Mehta SR, Fox KAA, et al. Effects of aspirin dose when used alone or in combination with clopidogrel in patients with acute coronary syndromes: Observations from the clopidogrel in unstable angina to prevent recurrent events (CURE) study. Circulation 2003;108:1682–1687.
53. Dahlof B, Devereux RB, Kjeldsen SE, et al. Cardiovascular morbidity and mortality in the Losartan Intervention for Endpoint Reduction in Hypertension Study (LIFE). Lancet 2002;359:995–1003.
54. Schrader J, Luders S, Kulschewski A, et al. Morbidity and mortality after stroke, eprosartan compared with nitrendipine for secondary prevention. Principal results of a prospective randomized controlled study (MOSES). Stroke 2005;36:1218–1226.
55. The Publications Committee for the Trial of ORG 10172 in Acute Stroke Treatment (TOAST) Investigators. Low-molecular-weight heparinoid, ORG 10172 (danaparoid), and outcome after acute ischemic stroke: a randomized, controlled trial. JAMA 1998;279:1265–1272.
56. Bath PM, Lidenstrom E, Boysen G, et al. Tinzaparin in acute ischaemic stroke (TAIST): A randomized, aspirin-controlled trial. Lancet 2001;358:702–710.
57. Berge E, Abdelnoor M, Nakstad PH, et al. Low-molecular-weight heparin versus aspirin in patients with acute ischaemic stroke and atrial fibrillation: A double-blind, randomised study. HAEST Study Group. Heparin in Acute Embolic Stroke Trial. Lancet 2000;355:1205–1210.
58. Food and Drug Administration. FDA Approves New Prescribed Uses for Aspirin. FDA Talk Paper. 1998;T98–76, *www.fda.gov/bbs/topics/ANSWERS/ANS00919.html.*
59. Farrell B, Godwin J, Richards S, Warlow C. The United Kingdom transient ischaemic attack (UK-TIA) aspirin trial: Final results. J Neurol Neurosurg Psychiatry 1991;54:1044–1054.
60. Serebruany VL, Malinin AI, Sane DC. Rapid platelet inhibition after a single capsule of Aggrenox: Challenging a conventional full-dose aspirin antiplatelet advantage? Am J Hematol 2003;72:280–281.
61. Eikelboom JW, Hankey GJ. Aspirin resistance: A new independent predictor of vascular events? J Am Coll Cardiol 2003;41:966–968.
62. Catella-Lawson F, Reilly MP, Kapoor SC, et al. Cyclooxygenase inhibitors and the antiplatelet effects of aspirin. N Engl J Med 2001;345:1809–1817.
63. Eisert WG. Near-field amplification of antithrombotic effects of dipyridamole through vessel wall cells. Neurology 2001;57(suppl 2):S20–23.
64. Theis JG, Deichsel G, Marshall S. Rapid development of tolerance to dipyridamole-associated headaches. Br J Clin Pharm 1999;48:750–755.
65. Bennett CL, Connors JM, Carwile JM, et al. Thrombotic thrombocytopenic purpura associated with clopidogrel. N Engl J Med 2000;342:1773–1777.
66. Lau WC, Waskell LA, Watkins PB, et al. Atorvastatin reduces the ability of clopidogrel to inhibit platelet aggregation: A new drug-drug interaction. Circulation 2003;107:32–37.
67. Saw J, Steinhubl SR, Berger PB, et al. Lack of adverse clopidogrel-atorvastatin clinical interaction from secondary analysis of a randomized, placebo-controlled clopidogrel trial. Circulation 2003;108:921–924.
68. Broderick JP, Hacke W. Treatment of acute ischemic stroke: I. Recanalization strategies. Circulation 2002;106:1563–1569.
69. Kidwell CS, Liebeskind DS, Starkman S, Saver JL. Trends in acute ischemic stroke trials through the 20th century. Stroke 2001;32:1349–1359.
70. Broderick JP, Hacke W. Treatment of acute ischemic stroke: II. Neuroprotection and medical management. Circulation 2002;106:1736–1740.
71. Lees KR, Zivin JA, Ashwood T, et al. NXY-059 for acute ischemic stroke. N Engl J Med 2006:354:588–600.

72. Gladstone DJ, Black SE, Hakim AM. Toward wisdom from failure: Lessons from neuroprotective stroke trials and new therapeutic directions. Stroke 2002;33:2123–2136.
73. Kondziolka D, Wechsler L, Goldstein S, et al. Transplantation of cultured human neuronal cells for patients with stroke. Neurology 2000;55:565–569.
74. Mayer SA, Brun NC, Begtrup K, et al. Recombinant activated factor VII for acute intracerebral hemorrhage. N Engl J Med 2005;352:777–785.
75. Fagan SC, Morgenstein LB, Peitta A, et al. Cost effectiveness of tissue plasminogen activate for acute ischemic stroke. Neurology 1998;50:883–890.
76. Demaerschalk BM, Yip TR. Economic benefit of increasing utilization of intravenous tissue plasminogen activator for acute ischemic stroke in the United States. Stroke 2005;36:2500–2503.
77. Gage BF, Cardinalli AB, Albers GW, Owens DK. Cost-effectiveness of warfarin and aspirin for prophylaxis of stroke in patients with nonvalvular atrial fibrillation. JAMA 1995;274:1839–1845.
78. Gustafsson C, Asplund K, Britton M, et al. Cost-effectiveness of stroke prevention in atrial fibrillation. BMJ 1992;305:1457–1460.
79. Sarasin FP, Gaspoz JM, Bournameaux H. Cost-effectiveness of new antiplatelet regimens used as secondary prevention of stroke or transient ischemic attack. Arch Intern Med 2000;160:2773–2778.

CHAPTER 23

Hyperlipidemia

ROBERT L. TALBERT

KEY CONCEPTS

1. Hypercholesterolemia, elevated low-density lipoprotein (LDL) levels, and low high-density lipoprotein (HDL) levels are unequivocally linked to increased risk for coronary heart disease and cerebrovascular morbidity and mortality. LDL is the primary target.
2. Multiple genetic abnormalities and environmental factors are involved in clinical lipid abnormalities, and routinely used clinical laboratory measurements do not define the underlying abnormalities.
3. Initial therapy for any lipoprotein disorder is therapeutic lifestyle changes with restricted intake of total and saturated fat and cholesterol and a modest increase in polyunsaturated fat intake along with a program of regular exercise and weight reduction if needed.
4. If pharmacologic therapy is insufficient after therapeutic lifestyle changes, lipid-lowering agents should be chosen based on the specific lipoprotein disorder presentation and the severity of the lipid abnormality.
5. Considering compliance, adverse effects, and effectiveness, for patients with hypercholesterolemia statins are the drugs of choice because they are the most potent form of monotherapy and are cost effective in patients with known coronary artery disease or multiple risk factors and in high-risk primary prevention patients.
6. Patients who do not respond to statin monotherapy can be treated with combination therapy for hypercholesterolemia but should be monitored closely because of an increased risk for adverse effects and drug interactions.
7. Hypertriglyceridemia usually responds well to niacin, gemfibrozil, and fenofibrate. High-dose niacin should be used cautiously in diabetics because of worsening glycemic control. Statins lower triglycerides to a variable extent depending on baseline triglyceride concentration and statin potency.
8. Low high-density lipoprotein-cholesterol (HDL-C) levels are addressed with lifestyle modifications, such as smoking cessation and increased exercise. Niacin, gemfibrozil, and fenofibrate can significantly increase HDL-C.
9. Lipid-lowering therapy is generally considered cost effective, particularly in secondary intervention and high-risk patients.
10. Decreasing elevated total cholesterol and low-density lipoprotein cholesterol (LDL-C) levels reduce coronary heart disease mortality and total mortality; increasing HDL reduces coronary heart disease events as well. Aggressive treatment of hypercholesterolemia results in fewer patients progressing to myocardial infarction, angina, and stroke and reduces the need for interventions such as coronary artery bypass graft and percutaneous transluminal coronary angioplasty.

Learning objectives, review questions,
and other resources can be found at
www.pharmacotherapyonline.com.

Cholesterol, triglycerides, and phospholipids are the major lipids in the body. They are transported as complexes of lipid and proteins known as *lipoproteins*. Plasma lipoproteins are spherical particles with surfaces that consist largely of phospholipid, free cholesterol, and protein and cores composed mostly of triglyceride and cholesterol ester (Fig. 23–1). The three major classes of lipoproteins in serum are low-density lipoproteins (LDLs), high-density lipoproteins (HDLs), and very-low-density lipoproteins (VLDLs). VLDL is carried in the circulation as triglyceride and can be estimated by dividing the triglyceride concentration by five. Intermediate-density lipoprotein (IDL) resides between VLDL and LDL and is included in the LDL measurement in routine clinical measurement. Abnormalities of plasma lipoproteins can result in a predisposition to coronary, cerebrovascular, and peripheral vascular arterial disease and constitutes one of the major risk factors for coronary heart disease (CHD). Accumulating evidence over the last decades had linked elevated total cholesterol and low-density lipoprotein-cholesterol (LDL-C) levels and reduced HDL levels to the development of CHD. Premature coronary atherosclerosis, leading to the manifestations of ischemic heart disease (see Chap. 17), is the most common and significant consequence of dyslipidemia. The National Cholesterol Education Program (NCEP) Adult Treatment Panel III (ATP III) published its third report summarizing these data and giving recommendations for the management of hypercholesterolemia in adults.[1,2] This report and the later update modify earlier recommendations and provide a new way of risk-stratifying patients based on multiple risk factors, the presence of diabetes, and the metabolic syndrome. The American Heart Association (AHA) also provides guidelines for primary and secondary prevention of CHD.[3,4]

Total cholesterol and LDL-C increase throughout life in men and women, representing an atherogenic pattern characteristic of westernized society diets.[5] Based on the National Health and Nutrition Examination Survey (NHANES 1999–2004) and ATP III guidelines, slightly more than 50% or nearly 105 million American adults older than 20 years have total cholesterol levels ≥200 mg/dL.[6] More than half of individuals at borderline to high risk remain unaware that they have hypercholesterolemia, and fewer than half of highest-risk persons (those with symptomatic CHD) are receiving lipid-lowering

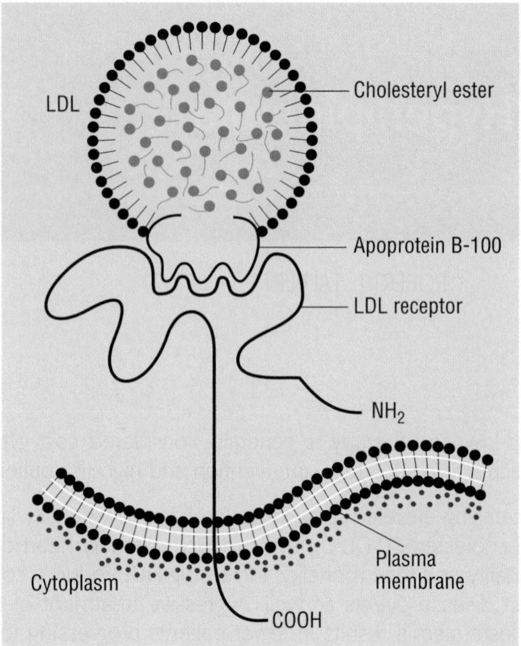

FIGURE 23-1. Diagrammatic representation of the structure of low-density lipoprotein (LDL), the LDL receptor, and the binding of LDL to the receptor via apolipoprotein B-100. *(From Ganong WF. Review of Medical Physiology, 22nd ed. New York: McGraw-Hill, 2005:303.)*

treatment. Approximately one third of treated patients are achieving their LDL goal; fewer than 20% of CHD patients are at their LDL goal.[6,7] Changes in the NCEP guidelines have increased the number of persons eligible for therapeutic lifestyle changes (TLC) or lipid-lowering therapy by millions. NCEP estimates that only 26% of patients have an optimal LDL-C (<100 mg/dL) and that large numbers of patients either are untreated or undertreated.[1] Unfortunately, those patients at highest risk are less likely to be treated to desirable levels of LDL.[8] Although these numbers seem staggering in their enormity, substantial progress has been made, and the number of Americans with a desirable blood cholesterol level (<200 mg/dL) has risen to 49% from 45% from the earlier survey (1976–1980), whereas the average total cholesterol in the United States has fallen from 220 mg/dL in 1960–1962 to 203 mg/dL in 2002.[9] Patients who are at risk but who have not yet experienced their first cardiovascular or cerebrovascular event (e.g., myocardial infarction [MI]) are termed *primary prevention* patients, whereas those with manifest vascular disease are termed *secondary intervention* patients.

❶ Data from the Framingham study and from other studies demonstrate that the risk for developing cardiovascular disease is related to the degree of total cholesterol and LDL elevation in a graded, continuous fashion.[10,11] Hypercholesterolemia is additive to the other nonlipid risk factors for CHD, including cigarette smoking, hypertension, diabetes, low HDL levels, and electrocardiographic abnormalities. The presence of established CHD or prior MI increases the risk of MI five to seven times that seen in men or women without CHD, and LDL level is a significant predictor of subsequent morbidity and mortality. Approximately 50% of all MIs and at least 70% of CHD deaths occur in patients with known CHD; therefore, these patients should be targeted for screening, identification, and treatment. Unfortunately, the identification of patients at high risk because of hypercholesterolemia or other lipid disorders is too frequently overlooked because blood lipid levels are not always evaluated in this population even after an event such as MI.

A comparison of the United States to other countries shows similar relationships between total cholesterol, LDL, and an inverse relationship with HDL to coronary artery disease (CAD) mortality.[10] On a positive note, the U.S. mortality rate is midway among the countries studied. The United States has shown the greatest decline in CAD mortality (35%–40%) in men and women over the last 10 years compared to other countries. A decline in the prevalence of hypercholesterolemia in certain segments of the U.S. population parallels these trends in mortality.[1] LDL and the ratio of LDL to HDL also have been used to assess risk, but their use adds little information to total cholesterol alone unless HDL is abnormally high or low. HDL transports cholesterol from lipid-laden foam cells to the liver. HDL has been shown to be protective for the occurrence of CHD, and an inverse relationship exists between CHD and HDL levels.[12]

VLDL, the major lipoprotein associated with triglycerides, is enriched with cholesterol esters. It is smaller, denser, and more atherogenic than less-dense VLDL. Routine measurement of triglycerides cannot distinguish between the types of VLDL present in plasma. Elevation of triglyceride-rich lipoproteins is associated with low HDL, and this ratio predicts increased risk. The 8-year follow-up of the Copenhagen male study found a clear gradient of risk for ischemic heart disease with increasing triglyceride levels within each level of high-density lipoprotein-cholesterol (HDL-C). Compared to the lowest tertile of triglyceride concentrations, the highest tertile had 2.2 relative risk for ischemic heart disease, and the relationship extended across all concentrations of HDL.[13] The Helsinki Heart Study showed that hypertriglyceridemia and low HDL are associated with obesity (body mass index [BMI] >26 kg/m^2), smoking, sedentary lifestyle, blood pressure ≥140/90 mm Hg, and blood glucose >4.4 mmol/L, and that the benefit of gemfibrozil (risk reduction 68%, P <0.03) was largely confined to overweight subjects.[14] Hypertriglyceridemia in certain instances (e.g., diabetes mellitus, nephrotic syndrome, chronic renal disease, and perhaps in women) is associated with increased cardiovascular risk. This is thought to be a consequence of the presence of atherogenic lipoproteins and of hypertriglyceridemia being a marker for them, as triglycerides usually are not independently predictive for CHD.[15]

LIPOPROTEIN METABOLISM AND TRANSPORT

As the major plasma lipids, cholesterol and triglycerides are essential substrates for cell membrane formation and hormone synthesis, and they provide a source of free fatty acids.[16] Dyslipidemia can be defined as elevated total cholesterol, LDL-C, or triglycerides level, low HDL-C concentration, or some combination of these abnormalities. Lipids, which are water immiscible, are not present in free form in the plasma but rather circulate as lipoproteins. Hyperlipoproteinemia refers to an increased concentration of the lipoprotein macromolecules that transport lipids in the plasma. The density of plasma lipoproteins is determined by their relative content of protein and lipid. Density, composition, size, and electrophoretic mobility divide lipoproteins into four classes (Table 23–1).

LDL is further divided into LDL$_1$ (or IDL; density 1.006–1.019 g/mL) and LDL$_2$ (1.019–1.063 g/mL). LDL$_2$ is the major LDL component in plasma; it carries 60% to 70% of the total serum cholesterol. HDL has been subdivided into HDL$_2$ (density 1.063–1.125 g/mL) and HDL$_3$ (1.125–1.21 g/mL). Fluctuations in HDL usually are caused by alterations in the levels of HDL$_2$. HDL normally carries approximately 20% to 30% of the total cholesterol. VLDL also has been subdivided into three classes, and it carries approximately 10% to 15% of serum cholesterol and most of the triglyceride in the fasting state. VLDL is the precursor for LDL, and VLDL remnants also may be atherogenic. Table 23–2 lists the characteristics of the protein constituent of lipoproteins known as *apolipoproteins*. The structure of LDL, the LDL receptor, and the binding of LDL to the receptor via apolipoprotein B-100 is shown in Fig. 23–1.

TABLE 23-1 Composition of Lipoprotein Isolated from Normal Subjects

			Composition (Weight %)				
					Cholesterol		
Lipoprotein Class	**Density Range (g/mL)**	**Diameter (nm)**	***Protein***	***Triglyceride***	***Free***	***Ester***	***Phospholipid***
Chylomicrons	<0.94	75–1200	1–2	80–95	1–3	2–4	3–9
VLDL	0.94–1.006	30–80	6–10	55–80	4–8	16–22	10–20
LDL	1.006–1.063	18–25	18–22	5–15	6–8	45–50	18–24
HDL	1.063–1.21	5–12	45–55	5–10	3–5	15–20	20–30

HDL, high-density lipoprotein; LDL, low-density lipoprotein; VLDL, very-low-density lipoprotein.

Chylomicrons are large triglyceride-rich particles that contain apolipoproteins B-48, B-100, and E. They are formed from dietary fat solubilized by bile salts in intestinal mucosal cells. Chylomicrons normally are not present in the plasma after a fast of 12 to 14 hours. They are catabolized by lipoprotein lipase (LPL), which is activated by apolipoprotein C-II and in the vascular endothelium and hepatic lipase to form chylomicron remnants. The remnants that contain apolipoprotein E (Fig. 23–2) are taken up by the "remnant receptor," which may be an LDL receptor–related protein, in the liver. Free cholesterol is liberated intracellularly after attachment to the remnant receptor. Chylomicrons also function to deliver dietary triglyceride to skeletal muscle and adipose tissue. During the catabolism of nascent chylomicrons to remnants, triglyceride is converted to free fatty acids and apolipoproteins A-I, A-II, A-IV (free in plasma), C-I, C-II, and C-III, and phospholipids are transferred to HDL. Apolipoproteins E and C-II are transferred to chylomicrons from HDL and eventually back through these metabolic events. Hepatic VLDL synthesis is regulated in part by diet and hormones and is inhibited by uptake of chylomicron remnants in the liver. VLDL is secreted from the liver and serially converted via LPL to IDL and finally to LDL. VLDL receptors are found in adipose tissue and muscle and bear close homology to the structure of LDL receptors.

LDL, the major cholesterol transport lipoprotein, basically has only apolipoprotein B-100. It is mostly derived from VLDL catabolism and cellular synthesis. When normal subjects fast and consume a low-fat diet, most cholesterol is synthesized and used in the extrahepatic organs; most of the cholesterol carried by LDL is taken up by the liver for catabolism. In patients with homozygous familial hypercholesterolemia, enhanced synthesis of LDL may occur because LDL clearance is reduced as a consequence of the lack of LDL receptors. LDL is catabolized through interaction of cell surface receptors found on liver, adrenal, and peripheral cells (including fibroblasts and smooth muscle cells). These cells recognize apolipoprotein B-100 on LDL, and, after binding to a receptor on the cell membrane, LDL is internalized and degraded. In the normal fasting state, approximately 70% of LDL is cleared through the receptor-dependent mechanism, although this is highly dependent on the availability and type of saturated and monosaturated or polyunsaturated fat from dietary sources. Ingestion of cholesterol and saturated fatty acids such as C12:0, C14:0, and C16:0 is associated with reduced LDL receptor activity, increased LDL production rate, and elevated LDL plasma concentration. Receptor-independent mechanisms are also involved to a lesser extent in the catabolism of LDL, and these receptors are present in many tissues but are most active in animals in the adrenals and ovary. Increased intracellular cholesterol resulting from LDL catabolism inhibits the activity of 3-hydroxy-3-methylglutaryl-coenzyme A (HMG-CoA) reductase, the rate-limiting enzyme for intracellular cholesterol biosynthesis (Fig. 23–3). Additional consequences of increased intracellular cholesterol include reduced synthesis of LDL receptors, which limits subsequent cholesterol uptake from the plasma, and accelerated activity of acyl-coenzyme A:cholesterol acyltransferase (ACAT) to facilitate cholesterol storage within cells. LDL-C also may be excreted into bile and become part of the enterohepatic pool or may be lost in the stool.

TABLE 23-2 Characteristics and Functions of Apolipoproteins

Apolipoprotein	Lipoprotein Density Class	Approximate Plasma Concentration (mg/dL)	Approximate Molecular Weight (kDa)	Reported Functions	Major Site of Synthesis
A-I	Chylomicrons, HDL	120	28	Cofactor with LCAT, structural protein on HDL, ligand for HDL receptor	Liver, intestine
A-II	Chylomicrons, HDL	35	17	Structural protein for HDL, ligand for HDL receptor	Liver
A-IV	Chylomicrons, 1.21B	15	46	Possibly facilitates transfer of other apolipoproteins between HDL and chylomicrons	Intestine
Lp(a)	LDL, HDL	10	500±	Bound to B-100, high homology with plasminogen, may prevent LDL uptake by B, E receptor	Liver
B-100	VLDL, LDL, IDL	100	540	Necessary for assembly and secretion of VLDL from liver, structural protein of VLDL, IDL, LDL, ligand for LDL receptor	Liver
B-48	Chylomicrons	Trace	264	Necessary for assembly and secretion of chylomicrons from small intestine	Intestine
C-I	Chylomicrons, VLDL, HDL	7	6.6	Cofactor with LCAT; may inhibit hepatic uptake of chylomicron and VLDL remnants	Liver
C-II	Chylomicrons, VLDL, HDL	4	8.9	Activator of LPL	Liver
C-III	Chylomicrons, VLDL, HDL	13	8.8	Inhibitor with LPL; may inhibit hepatic uptake of chylomicron and VLDL remnants	Liver
D	HDL	6	32	?	?
E2-E4	Chylomicrons, VLDL, HDL	5	34	Ligand for several lipoproteins to LDL receptor, LRP and possibly to a separate hepatic apolipoprotein E receptor	Liver

IDL, intermediate-density lipoprotein; LCAT, lecithin-cholesterol acyltransferase; LRP, LDL receptor–related protein. Other abbreviations are in Table 23–1.

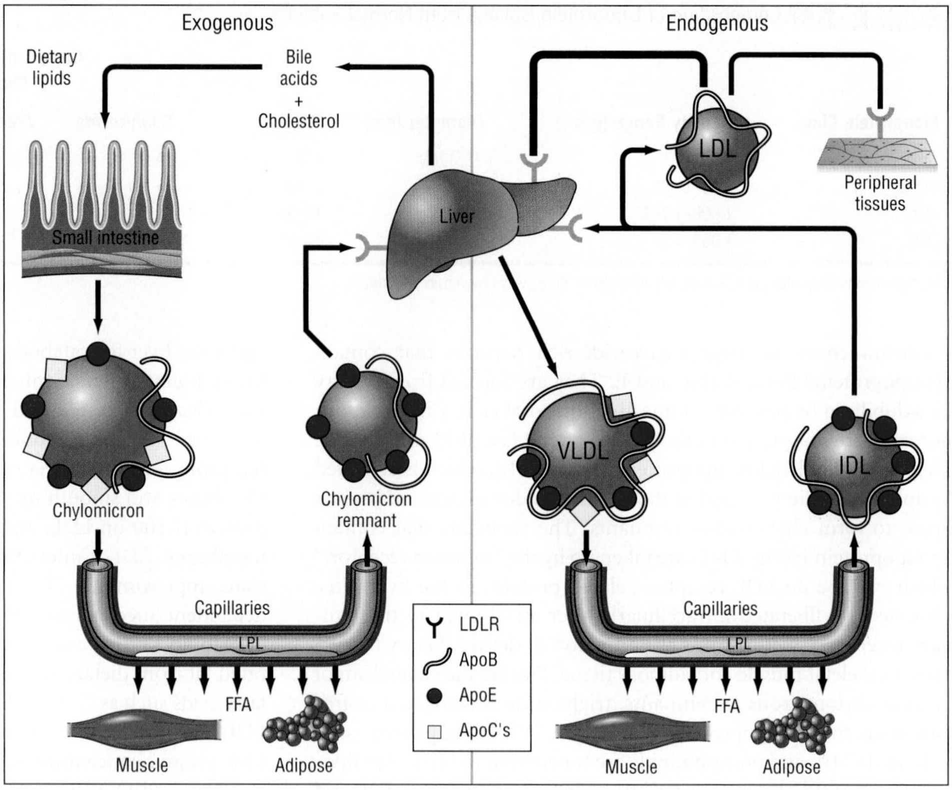

FIGURE 23-2. Simplified diagram of lipoprotein systems for transporting lipids in humans. In the exogenous system, chylomicrons rich in triglycerides of dietary origin are converted to chylomicron remnants rich in cholesteryl esters by the action of lipoprotein lipase (LPL). In the endogenous system, very-low-density lipoproteins (VLDL) rich in triglycerides are secreted by the liver and converted to intermediate-density lipoproteins (IDL) and then to low-density lipoproteins (LDL) rich in cholesteryl esters. Some of the LDLs enter the subendothelial space of arteries, are oxidized, and then are taken up by macrophages, which become foam cells. The letters on the chylomicrons, chylomicron remnants, VLDL, IDL, and LDL identify the primary apoproteins (ApoB, ApoC, ApoE) found in them. (LDLR, low-density lipoprotein receptor.) *(From Kasper DL, Braunwald E, Fauci AS, et al., eds. Harrison's Principles of Internal Medicine, 16th ed. New York, McGraw-Hill, 2005, p. 2289.)*

Lipoprotein(a) is a cholesterol-rich lipoprotein similar in composition and density to LDL and with close homology to fibrinogen. It is reported to be an important independent risk factor for the development of premature cardiovascular disease.

Nascent HDL is derived from liver and gut synthesis primarily in the form of apolipoprotein A-I phospholipid discs.[12] Esterification of free cholesterol in nascent HDL and from peripheral tissues to cholesteryl esters by lecithin-cholesterol acyltransferase (LCAT) results in the production of HDL_3. Further addition of tissue cholesterol to HDL_3 results in the formation of HDL_2. HDL_2 can also be formed from remodeling of chylomicrons and VLDL catabolism. HDL_2 can be converted back to HDL_3 by the action of hepatic lipase and by the transfer of cholesteryl esters to the liver, LDL, and VLDL. Apolipoprotein A-I production is increased by estrogens, leading to higher HDL levels in women and in individuals receiving estrogen. Transfer of excess cholesterol from peripheral tissues by HDL is called *reverse cholesterol transport.* Putative HDL receptors in peripheral cells facilitate the uptake of cholesterol by HDL, which transfers cholesterol to either VLDL and LDL or to the liver for secretion into bile or conversion into bile acids. These processes rid peripheral tissue (e.g., coronary arteries) of excessive amounts of cholesterol and account for some of the protective effects noted with increasing HDL in women and other factors that elevate HDL levels. Variants of the cholesterol ester transfer protein (CETP) have been demonstrated in humans, and the B1B1 genotype is associated with lower HDL and progression of coronary atherosclerosis. Inhibition of CETP leads to elevations in HDL. However, CETP inhibitors tested in clinical trials did not induce regression of atherosclerotic plaque and were associated with higher blood pressure and CHD events.[17–19]

The "response-to-injury" hypothesis states that risk factors such as oxidized LDL, mechanical injury to the endothelium (e.g., percutaneous transluminal angioplasty), excessive homocysteine, immunologic attack, and infection-induced (e.g., *Chlamydia,* herpes simplex virus 1) changes in endothelial and intimal function lead to endothelial dysfunction and a series of cellular interactions that culminate in atherosclerosis. C-reactive protein is an acute phase reactant and a marker for inflammation; it may be useful in identifying patients at risk for developing CAD.[20] The eventual outcomes of this atherogenic cascade are clinical events such as angina, MI, arrhythmias, stroke, peripheral arterial disease, abdominal aortic aneurysm, and sudden death. Atherosclerotic lesions are thought to arise from transport and retention of plasma LDL-C through the endothelial cell layer into the extracellular matrix of the subendothelial space. Once in the artery wall, LDL is chemically modified through oxidation and nonenzymatic glycation. Mildly oxidized LDL then recruits monocytes into the artery wall, and the monocytes become transformed into macrophages. Macrophages have tremendous potential for accelerating LDL oxidation and apolipoprotein B accumulation and altering the receptor-mediated uptake of LDL into the artery wall from the usual LDL receptor to a "scavenger receptor" not regulated by cell content of cholesterol. Oxidized LDL increases plasminogen inhibitor levels (promotion of coagulation), induces expression of endothelin (vasoconstrictive substance), inhibits expression of nitric oxide (a vasodilator and platelet inhibitor), and is toxic to macrophages if highly oxidized. As oxidation of biologically active lipids proceeds, other lipids such as lysophosphatidylcholine, hydroperoxides, aldehydic breakdown products of fatty acids, and oxysterol are formed and continue the reaction within the tissue. These events lead to a massive accumulation of cholesterol. The cholesterol-laden cells are called *foam cells,* which are the earliest recognized cells of the arterial fatty streak.

Oxidized LDL provokes an inflammatory response that is mediated by a number of chemoattractants and cytokines. Examples that appear to be involved at different stages of lesion development include monocyte chemoattractant protein 1 (MCP-1); monocyte colony stimulating factor (M-CSF); *gro;* vascular cell adhesion molecule (VCAM-1); E-selectin (endothelial-leukocyte adhesion molecule [ELAM]-1); intercellular adhesion molecule (ICAM-1); platelet-derived growth factor (PDGF); vascular endothelial growth factor (VEGF); transforming growth factors (TGF-α and TGF-β); interleukin (IL)-1 and IL-6; and the ratio of IL-10 and IL-12. Some of these factors (e.g., MCP-1 and M-CSF) appear to participate early in the

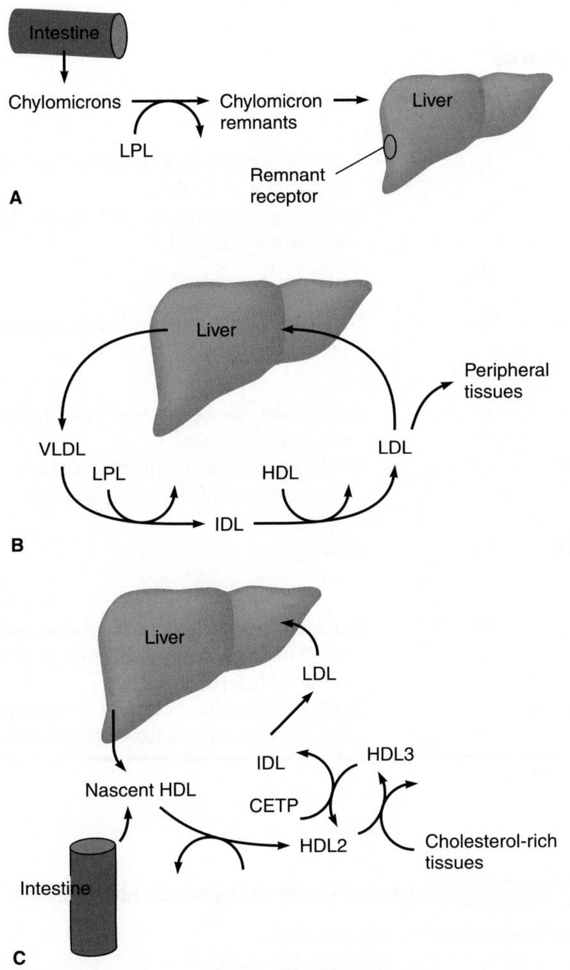

FIGURE 23-3. Biosynthetic pathway for cholesterol. The rate-limiting enzyme in this pathway is 3-hydroxy-3-methylglutaryl coenzyme A reductase (HMG-CoA reductase). (CETP, cholesterol ester transfer protein; HDL, high-density lipoprotein; IDL, intermediate-density lipoprotein; LDL, low-density lipoprotein; LPL, lipoprotein lipase; VLDL, very-low-density lipoprotein.) *(Modified from Breslow JL. Genetic basis of lipoprotein disorders. J Clin Invest 1989; 84:373.)*

process of monocyte–macrophage attachment and transmigration across the endothelium, whereas others (PDGF and VCAM-1) promote later lesion growth.[18] Based on murine model studies, the extent of oxidation and the inflammatory response is under genetic control of a major gene termed *Ath*-1. The process of aging may lead to lipoproteins that are more susceptible to oxidation and have longer resident time in the vascular compartment. Two proteins associated with HDL (apolipoprotein J and paraxonase) appear to play important roles in minimizing oxidation of LDL-C.[21,22] Increased recognition of the role of these growth regulatory molecules provides the possibility of future directions for antagonists to regulatory molecules such as PDGF, TGF-β, and the interleukins. Repeated injury and repair within an atherosclerotic plaque eventually leads to the formation of a fibrous cap that protects the underlying core of lipids, collagen, calcium, and inflammatory cells such as T-lymphocytes. Maintenance of the fibrous plaque is critical to preventing plaque rupture and subsequent coronary thrombosis. An imbalance between plaque synthesis and degradation may lead to a weakened or vulnerable plaque prone to rupture. The fibrous cap may become weakened through decreased synthesis of the extracellular matrix or increased degradation of the matrix. The cytokine interferon-γ, produced by T lymphocytes, inhibits the ability of smooth muscle cells to synthesize collagen, a structurally important component of the fibrous cap. A family of enzymes known as *matrix metalloproteinases* can degrade all major constituents of the vascular extracellular matrix: collagen, elastin, and proteoglycans.[23]

TABLE 23-3 Fredrickson-Levy-Lees Classification of Hyperlipoproteinemia

Type	Lipoprotein Elevation
I	Chylomicrons
IIa	LDL
IIb	LDL + VLDL
III	IDL (LDL_1)
IV	VLDL
V	VLDL + Chylomicrons

IDL, intermediate-density lipoprotein; LDL, low-density lipoprotein; VLDL, very-low-density lipoprotein.

Lipoprotein disorders are classified into six categories, which are commonly used for phenotypical description of dyslipidemia (Table 23–3). ❷ Specific genetic defects with disrupted protein, cell, and organ function give rise to several disorders within each family of lipoproteins (Table 23–4). An elevated cholesterol level does not necessarily equate with familial hypercholesterolemia or type IIa, as cholesterol may be elevated in other lipoprotein disorders and the lipoprotein pattern does not describe the underlying genetic defect. The preceding discussion focused on primary or genetic dyslipoproteinemia; however, secondary forms exist, and several drugs may elevate lipid levels (Table 23–5). The secondary forms of hyperlipidemia initially should be managed by correcting the underlying abnormality, including modification of drug therapy when appropriate.

Familial hypercholesterolemia is characterized by (a) selective elevation in the plasma level of LDL, (b) deposition of LDL-derived cholesterol in tendons (xanthomas) and arteries (atheromas), and (c) inheritance as an autosomal dominant trait with homozygotes more severely affected than heterozygotes. Homozygotes (prevalence 1:1,000,000) have severe hypercholesterolemia (650–1,000 mg/dL), with early appearance of cutaneous xanthomas and fatal CHD generally before age 20 years. The primary defect in familial hypercholesterolemia is the inability to bind LDL to the LDL receptor or, rarely, a defect of internalizing the LDL receptor complex into the cell after normal binding. Homozygotes have essentially no functional LDL receptors. This leads to lack of LDL degradation by cells and unregulated biosynthesis of cholesterol, with total cholesterol and LDL-C inversely proportional to the deficit in LDL receptors. Heterozygotes have only about half the normal number of LDL receptors, total cholesterol levels in the range from 300 to 600 mg/dL and cardiovascular events beginning in the third and fourth decades of life.

Familial LPL deficiency is a rare, autosomal recessive trait characterized by massive accumulation of chylomicrons and corresponding increase in plasma triglycerides or a type I lipoprotein pattern. VLDL concentration is normal. Presenting manifestations include repeated attacks of pancreatitis and abdominal pain, eruptive cutaneous xanthomatosis, and hepatosplenomegaly beginning in childhood. Symptom severity is proportional to dietary fat intake and consequently to the elevation of chylomicrons. LPL is normally released from vascular endothelium or by heparin and hydrolyzes chylomicrons and VLDL (see Fig. 23–2). Diagnosis is based on low or absent enzyme activity with normal human plasma or apolipoprotein C-II, a cofactor of the enzyme. Accelerated atherosclerosis is not associated with the disease. Abdominal pain, pancreatitis, eruptive xanthomas, and peripheral polyneuropathy characterize type V (VLDL and chylomicrons). Symptoms may occur in childhood, but usually the disorder is expressed at a later age. The risk of atherosclerosis is increased with the disorder. Patients commonly are obese, hyperuricemic, and diabetic, and alcohol intake, exogenous estrogens, and renal insufficiency tend to be exacerbating factors.

Patients with familial type III hyperlipoproteinemia (also called *dysbetalipoproteinemia*, *broad-band*, or *β-VLDL*) develop the fol-

TABLE 23-4 Lipoprotein Disorders

Lipid Phenotype	Plasma Lipid Levels [mmol/L (mg/dL)]	Lipoproteins *Elevated*	Lipoproteins *Phenotype*	Clinical Signs
Isolated hypercholesterolemia				
Familial hypercholesterolemia	Heterozygotes TC = 7–13 (275–500)	LDL	IIa	Usually develop xanthomas in adulthood and vascular disease at 30–50 years
	Homozygotes TC >13 (>500)	LDL	IIa	Usually develop xanthomas in adulthood and vascular disease in childhood
Familial defective Apo B-100	Heterozygotes TC = 7–13 (275–500)	LDL	IIa	
Polygenic hypercholesterolemia	TC = 6.5–9 (250–350)	LDL	IIa	Usually asymptomatic until vascular disease develops; no xanthomas
Isolated hypertriglyceridemia				
Familial hypertriglyceridemia	TG = 2.8–8.5 (250–750)	VLDL	IV	Asymptomatic; may be associated with increased risk of vascular disease
Familial LPL deficiency	TG >8.5 (750)	Chylomicrons, VLDL	I, V	May be asymptomatic; may be associated with pancreatitis, abdominal pain, hepatosplenomegaly
Familial Apo C-II deficiency	TG >8.5 (>750)	Chylomicrons, VLDL	I, V	As above
Hypertriglyceridemia and hypercholesterolemia				
Combined hyperlipidemia	TG = 2.8–8.5 (250–750) TC = 6.5–13 (250–500)	VLDL, LDL	IIb	Usually asymptomatic until vascular disease develops; familial form may present as isolated high TG or isolated high LDL cholesterol
Dysbetalipoproteinemia	TG = 2.8–8.5 (250–750); TC = 6.5–13 (250–500)	VLDL, IDL; LDL normal	III	Usually asymptomatic until vascular disease develops; may have palmar or tuboeruptive xanthomas

Apo, apolipoprotein; LPL, lipoprotein lipase; TC, total cholesterol; TG, triglycerides. Other abbreviations as in Table 23–1.

lowing clinical features after age 20 years: xanthoma striata palmaris (yellow discolorations of the palmar and digital creases); tuberous or tuberoeruptive xanthomas (bulbous cutaneous xanthomas); and severe atherosclerosis involving the coronary arteries, internal carotids, and abdominal aorta. A defective structure of apolipoprotein E does not allow normal hepatic surface receptor binding of remnant particles derived from chylomicrons and VLDL (known as IDL). Aggravating factors such as obesity, diabetes, and pregnancy may promote overproduction of apolipoprotein B–containing lipoproteins. Although homozygosity for the defective allele (E_2/E_2) is common (1:100), only 1 in 10,000 express the full-blown picture, and interaction with other genetic or environmental factors, or both, is needed to produce clinical disease.

Familial combined hyperlipidemia is characterized by elevations in total cholesterol and triglycerides, decreased HDL, increased apolipoprotein B, and small, dense LDL.[24] It is associated with premature CHD and may be difficult to diagnose because lipid levels do not consistently display the same pattern.

Type IV hyperlipoproteinemia is common and occurs in adults, primarily in patients who are obese, diabetic, and hyperuricemic and do not have xanthomas. It may be secondary to alcohol ingestion and can be aggravated by stress, progestins, oral contraceptives, thiazides, or β-blockers. Two genetic patterns that occur in type IV hyperlipoproteinemia are familial hypertriglyceridemia, which does not carry a great risk for premature CAD, and familial combined hyperlipidemia, which is associated with increased risk for cardiovascular disease.

Rare forms of lipoprotein disorders include hypobetalipoproteinemia, abetalipoproteinemia, Tangier disease, LCAT deficiency (fish eye disease), cerebrotendinous xanthomatosis, and sitosterolemia. Most of these rare lipoprotein disorders do not result in premature atherosclerosis, with the exceptions of familial LCAT deficiency, cerebrotendinous xanthomatosis, and sitosterolemia with xanthomatosis. Treatment consists of dietary restriction of plant sterols (sitosterolemia with xanthomatosis) and chenodeoxycholic acid (cerebrotendinous xanthomatosis), or, potentially, blood transfusion (LCAT deficiency).

TABLE 23-5 Secondary Causes of Lipoprotein Abnormalities

Hypercholesterolemia	Hypothyroidism Obstructive liver disease Nephrotic syndrome Anorexia nervosa Acute intermittent porphyria Drugs: progestins, thiazide diuretics, glucocorticoids, β-blockers, isotretinoin, protease inhibitors, cyclosporine, mirtazapine, sirolimus
Hypertriglyceridemia	Obesity Diabetes mellitus Lipodystrophy Glycogen storage disease Ileal bypass surgery Sepsis Pregnancy Acute hepatitis Systemic lupus erythematous Monoclonal gammopathy: multiple myeloma, lymphoma Drugs: Alcohol, estrogens, isotretinoin, β-blockers, glucocorticoids, bile acid resins, thiazides; asparaginase, interferons, azole antifungals, mirtazapine, anabolic steroids, sirolimus, bexarotene
Hypocholesterolemia	Malnutrition Malabsorption Myeloproliferative diseases Chronic infectious diseases: acquired immune deficiency syndrome, tuberculosis Monoclonal gammopathy Chronic liver disease
Low high-density lipoprotein	Malnutrition Obesity Drugs: non-ISA β-blockers, anabolic steroids, probucol, isotretinoin, progestins

ISA, intrinsic sympathomimic activity.

CLINICAL PRESENTATION

General

- Most patients are asymptomatic for many years before disease is clinically evident
- Patients with the metabolic syndrome may have three or more of the following: abdominal obesity, atherogenic dyslipidemia, increased blood pressure, insulin resistance with or without glucose intolerance, prothrombotic state, or proinflammatory state

Symptoms

- None to severe chest pain, palpitations, sweating, anxiety, shortness of breath, loss of consciousness or difficulty with speech or movement, abdominal pain, sudden death

Signs

- None to severe abdominal pain, pancreatitis, eruptive xanthomas, peripheral polyneuropathy, high blood pressure, body mass index >30 kg/m^2 or waist size >40 inches in men (35 inches in women)

Laboratory Tests

- Elevations in total cholesterol, LDL, triglycerides, apolipoprotein B, C-reactive protein
- Low HDL

Other Diagnostic Tests

- Lipoprotein(a), homocysteine, serum amyloid A, small dense LDL (pattern B), HDL subclassification, apolipoprotein E isoforms, apolipoprotein A-1, fibrinogen, folate, *Chlamydia pneumoniae* titer, lipoprotein-associated phospholipase A_2, omega-3 index[25]
- Various screening tests for manifestations of vascular disease (ankle–brachial index, exercise testing, magnetic resonance imaging) and diabetes (fasting glucose, oral glucose tolerance test)

PATIENT EVALUATION

A fasting lipoprotein profile including total cholesterol, LDL-C, HDL-C, and triglycerides should be measured in all adults 20 years and older at least once every 5 years.[1] If the profile is obtained in the nonfasted state, only total cholesterol and HDL-C will be usable because LDL-C usually is a calculated value. If total cholesterol is ≥200 mg/dL or HDL-C is <40 mg/dL, a followup fasting lipoprotein profile should be obtained. After a lipid abnormality is confirmed (Table 23–6), major components of the evaluation are the history (including age, gender, and, if female, menstrual and hormone replacement status), physical examination, and laboratory investigations. A complete history and physical examination should assess (a) presence or absence of cardiovascular risk factors (Table 23–7) or definite cardiovascular disease in the individual; (b) family history of premature cardiovascular disease or lipid disorders; (c) presence or absence of secondary causes of lipid abnormalities, including concurrent medications (see Table 23–5); and (d) presence or absence of xanthomas or abdominal pain, or history of pancreatitis, renal or hepatic disease, peripheral vascular disease, abdominal aortic aneurysm, or cerebral vascular disease (carotid bruits, stroke, or transient ischemic attack). In an important change in the ATP III guidelines, diabetes mellitus is regarded as a CHD risk equivalent.[1] The presence of diabetes in patients without known CHD is associated with the same level of risk as in patients without diabetes but with confirmed CHD.[26,27] ATP III identifies four categories of risk that modify the goals and modalities of LDL-lowering therapy (Table 23–8).[2] The highest category is known CHD or CHD risk equivalents, which is defined as the risk for major coronary events equal to or greater than established CHD, that is, >20% per 10 years (2% per year). The next category is moderately high risk, consisting of patients with multiple (2+) risk factors in which 10-year risk for CHD is 10% to 20%. Moderate risk is defined as ≥2 risk factors and a 10-year risk of ≥10%. The lowest risk category is persons with a risk factor of 0 to 1. Risk is estimated from Framingham risk scores[28] and is estimated based on the patient's age, LDL-C or total cholesterol level, blood pressure, presence of diabetes, and smoking status (Table 23–7). This approach for a single patient is referred to as a *case finding* or *patient-based approach*, whereas large-scale screening and recommendations for the general populace, health care providers, and the food industry are called a *population-based approach*.

Measurement of plasma cholesterol (which is approximately 3% lower than serum determinations), triglyceride, and HDL-C levels after a fast of 12 hour or longer is important, as triglycerides may be elevated in nonfasted individuals; total cholesterol is only modestly affected by fasting. Analytic and biologic variability can have a major impact on the measurement and interpretation of cholesterol level (or any other laboratory test). Analytic variability can be minimized through the use of adequate quality control procedures, including internal training, routine calibration and monitoring, and external proficiency testing. Even with these measures, the coefficient of variability in the best procedures can acceptably be up to 5%, and,

TABLE 23-6 Classification of Total, LDL, and HDL Cholesterol, and Triglycerides

Total cholesterol	
<200	Desirable
200–239	Borderline high
≥240	High
LDL cholesterol	
<100	Optimal
100–129	Near or above optimal
130–159	Borderline high
160–189	High
≥190	Very high
HDL cholesterol	
<40	Low
≥60 mg/dL	High
Triglycerides	
<150	Normal
150–199	Borderline high
200–499	High
≥500	Very high

All values are given in milligrams per deciliters.
HDL, high-density lipoprotein; LDL, low-density lipoprotein.

TABLE 23-7 Major Risk Factors (Exclusive of LDL Cholesterol) That Modify LDL Goals[a]

Age
- Men: ≥45 years
- Women: ≥55 years or premature menopause without estrogen replacement therapy

Family history of premature CHD (definite myocardial infarction or sudden death before age 55 years in father or other male first-degree relative, or before age 65 years in mother or other female first-degree relative)

Cigarette smoking

Hypertension (≥140/90 mm Hg or taking antihypertensive medication)

Low HDL cholesterol (<40 mg/dL)[b]

HDL, high-density lipoprotein; LDL, low-density lipoprotein.
[a]Diabetes is regarded as a coronary heart disease (CHD) risk equivalent.
[b]HDL cholesterol ≥60 mg/dL counts as a "negative" risk factor; its presence removes one risk factor from the total count.

TABLE 23-8 LDL Cholesterol Goals and Cutpoints for Therapeutic Lifestyle Changes and Drug Therapy in Different Risk Categories

Risk Category	LDL Goal (mg/dL)	LDL Level at Which to Initiate TLC (mg/dL)	LDL Level at Which to Consider Drug Therapy (mg/dL)
High risk: CHD or CHD risk equivalents (10-year risk >20%)	<100 (optional goal: <70)	≥100	≥100 (<100 mg/dL; consider drug options)[a]
Moderately high risk: 2+ risk factors (10-year risk >10%–20%)	<130	≥130	≥130 (100–129: consider drug options)
Moderate risk: 2+ risk factors (10-year risk <10%)	<130	≥130	≥160
Lower risk: 0–1 risk factor[b]	<160	≥160	≥190 (160–189: LDL-lowering drug optional)

CHD, coronary heart disease; LDL, low-density lipoprotein.

[a]Some authorities recommend use of LDL-lowering drugs in this category if LDL cholesterol <100 mg/dL cannot be achieved by therapeutic lifestyle changes (TLC). Others prefer to use drugs that primarily modify triglycerides and high-density lipoprotein, e.g., nicotinic acid or fibrates. Clinical judgement also may call for deferring drug therapy in this subcategory.

[b]Almost all people with 0–1 risk factor have a 10-year risk <10%; thus, 10-year risk assessment in people with 0–1 risk factor is not necessary.

when combined with average biologic variability, total variability may be as high as approximately 22%. Analytic variability with desktop equipment generally is greater in the fingerstick capillary blood methods, usually yielding measurements less than those from a clinical laboratory; this technology should be considered for use only as a screening method. Reliance on desktop methods can result in misclassification of 7% to 14% of patients if capillary blood is used. Two determinations, 1 to 8 weeks apart, with the patient on a stable diet and weight and in the absence of acute illness, are recommended to minimize variability and obtain a reliable baseline.[1] If total cholesterol is >200 mg/dL, a second determination is recommended, and if the values are more than 30 mg/dL apart, the average of three values should be used. Familiarity with the method and quality control procedures used by local laboratories are essential for interpretation of reported values. If the physical examination and history are insufficient to diagnose a familial disorder, then agarose-gel lipoprotein electrophoresis is useful to determine which class of lipoproteins is affected. If triglyceride levels are <400 mg/dL and neither type III hyperlipidemia nor chylomicrons are detected by electrophoresis, then VLDL and LDL concentrations can be calculated as follows: VLDL = Triglycerides/5; LDL = Total cholesterol – (VLDL + HDL).

Because total cholesterol is composed of cholesterol derived from LDL, VLDL, and HDL, determination of HDL is useful when total plasma cholesterol is elevated. HDL may be elevated by moderate alcohol ingestion (fewer than two drinks per day), physical exercise, smoking cessation, weight loss, oral contraceptives, phenytoin, and terbutaline. Smoking, obesity, a sedentary lifestyle, and use of drugs such as β-blockers lower HDL. Only exercise and smoking cessation can be recommended as interventions for low HDL concentrations. Niacin and gemfibrozil increase HDL concentrations.

The range of lipid concentrations represents a population mean ±2 SD and does not define the risk of disease. Reference values for plasma total, LDL, and HDL-C concentrations for men and women, as well as various ethnic groups, are available from the NHANES III.[5] Levels of Cholesterol and triglycerides increase throughout life until about the fifth decade for men and the sixth decade for women. Past these ages, total cholesterol and LDL plateau and fall slightly. HDL tends to fall slightly with time and more rapidly after menopause in women. Institution of a population-based approach for cholesterol reduction should shift the entire curve to the left, and the potential reduction in cardiovascular mortality would be proportional to mean reductions at any cholesterol concentration.

Based on a careful review of the experimental pathologic, genetic, and epidemiologic evidence relating to the relationship between blood cholesterol levels and CHD, the adult treatment panel III of the NCEP recommends use of a fasting lipoprotein profile and risk factor assessment in the initial classification of adults.[1,29] If total cholesterol is <200 mg/dL, then the patient has a *desirable blood cholesterol level* (Table 23–6). Cholesterol levels between 200 and 239 mg/dL are classified as *borderline–high blood cholesterol levels,* and assessment of risk factors (Table 23–7) is needed to more clearly define disease risk. Blood cholesterol levels ≥240 mg/dL are classified as *high blood cholesterol levels.* If total cholesterol is <200 mg/dL and HDL is >40 mg/dL, no further followup is recommended for patients without known CHD who have fewer than two risk factors. In patients with evidence of CHD or other clinical atherosclerotic disease, the LDL goal is <100 mg/dL, and most patients will require diet and/or drug intervention. In patients with very high risk (known CHD and multiple risk factors), the LDL goal may be set <70 mg/dL based on evidence from newer studies.[29] Decisions regarding classification and management are based on the LDL-C levels listed in Table 23–8. An increasing number of persons have the metabolic syndrome, which is characterized by abdominal obesity, atherogenic dyslipidemia (elevated triglycerides, small LDL particles, low HDL-C), increased blood pressure, insulin resistance (with or without glucose intolerance), and prothrombotic and proinflammatory states. ATP III recognizes the metabolic syndrome as a secondary target of risk reduction therapy after LDL-C has been addressed, and, if the metabolic syndrome is present, the patient is considered to have a CHD risk equivalent. Other lipid targets include non-HDL goals for patients with triglycerides >200 mg/dL. Non-HDL is calculated by subtracting HDL from total cholesterol, and the targets are 30 mg/dL greater than for LDL at each risk stratum. Non-HDL takes into consideration atherogenic particles such as remnant lipoproteins and IDL, which are not measured in routine clinical laboratory testing.[30] HDL raising has potential benefit, but the current guidelines do not set any specific goals, and evidence in support of aggressively increasing HDL levels is modest.[31]

The Expert Panel on Children and Adolescents of the NCEP recommends screening of higher-risk children (positive family history or parental high blood cholesterol ≥240 mg/dL).[32,33] The rationale for this approach is based partly on the recognition that atherosclerosis begins in the childhood and adolescent years, as documented in the Pathobiologic Determinants of Atherosclerosis in Youth (PDAY) and the Bogalusa studies.[34] Similarly, if children with high blood lipids or lipoprotein levels are identified but the levels in the parents are unknown, the parents should be screened because they likely are at high risk. Racial and gender differences do exist in the determination of lipoprotein fractions and should be considered in screening. Use of the serum cholesterol level alone may be of insufficient specificity or sensitivity, depending on the cut points used in screening, and other discretionary factors, such as hypertension, smoking, obesity, high-fat diet, and use of cholesterol-raising medication, may be needed to correctly identify children at risk. Presently, children older than 10 years are candidates for drug therapy if a trial of diet (6 months to 1 year) proves to be inadequate and LDL-C remains >190 mg/dL, or >160 mg/dL if two or more risk factors or CHD is present in the child or adolescent, or if patient has a history of premature CHD. The Dietary Intervention Study in

Children (DISC) found that a fat-restricted diet in pubertal children modestly lowered LDL-C and maintained psychologic well-being, and that dietary changes are acceptable to children.[35,36] Although bile acid sequestrants have been the recommended drugs for this population, clinical trials now demonstrate that statin therapy is effective and well tolerated in pediatric populations.[37,38] The long-term consequences of drug therapy in this population are unknown. In special instances, familial hypercholesterolemia (particularly the homozygous form) or the existence of CHD or two or more risk factors in the child prompts earlier institution of drug therapy after a trial of dietary intervention.

TREATMENT

DESIRED OUTCOMES

The goals of therapy expressed as LDL-C levels and the level of initiation of TLC and drug therapy are given in Tables 23–8 and 23–9 for adults and children, respectively. Although these goals are surrogate end points, the primary reason for instituting TLC and drug therapy is to reduce the risk of first events or recurrent events such as MI, angina, heart failure, ischemic stroke, and other forms of peripheral arterial disease, such as carotid stenosis and abdominal aortic aneurysm.

GENERAL APPROACH[1]

Establishing targeted changes and outcomes with consistent reinforcement of goals and measures at followup visits to attain goals are important to reduce barriers for optimizing TLC and pharmacologic therapy. ❸ TLC should be implemented in all patients prior to considering drug therapy. The components of TLC include reduced intake of saturated fats and cholesterol, dietary options to reduce LDL, such as consumption of plant stanols and sterols and soluble fiber, weight reduction, and increased physical activity. In general, physical activity of moderate intensity 30 minutes per day for most days of the week should be encouraged.[39,40] Patients with known CAD or who are at high risk should be evaluated before they undertake vigorous exercise. Weight and BMI should be determined at each visit, and lifestyle patterns to induce a weight loss of 10% should be discussed with persons who are overweight. All patients should be counseled to stop smoking and to meet the Joint National Committee VII guidelines for control of hypertension.

NONPHARMACOLOGIC THERAPY

Individualized dietary counseling that provides acceptable substitutions for unhealthy foods and ongoing reinforcement by a registered dietitian are necessary for maximal effect. The objectives of dietary therapy are to progressively decrease the intake of total fat, saturated fatty acids (i.e., saturated fat), and cholesterol and to achieve a desirable body weight. Typical American diets now include 13% to 20% of total calories from saturated fat and cholesterol intake of 350 to 450 mg/day, both in excess of a "heart healthy" diet for normal Americans, let alone patients with a lipid disorder. Excessive dietary intake of cholesterol and saturated fatty acids leads to decreased hepatic clearance of LDL and deposition of LDL and oxidized LDL in peripheral tissues. The targeted saturated fatty acids have carbon chain lengths of 12 (lauric acid), 14 (myristic acid), and 16 (palmitic acid). The rationale for using a nutritionally balanced, low-fat, low-cholesterol diet for treatment of hypercholesterolemia is based on the following principles: (a) it represents a reasonable extension of the diet recommended for the general public; (b) it progressively decreases the major cholesterol-raising constituent of the diet; (c) it precludes large intakes of polyunsaturated fats; and (d) it facilitates weight reduction by removing foods of high caloric density.[41–44]

Dietary expertise in providing a wide range of options and suggestions in food preparation can make the difference between a good and an inadequate response to diet. Information on eating out in a healthy fashion and advice for shopping are important factors for success in diet therapy. An example is awareness of products with misleading labels, such as coffee creamers that state they contain "no cholesterol" when they may contain hydrogenated (saturated) fats or oils (e.g., palmitic acid, palm kernel oil, or coconut oil), which makes them undesirable because of their saturated fat content. Variations in polyunsaturated and saturated fat and cholesterol intake influence the LDL concentration, but the amount of cholesterol has been found to have a greater effect than the proportion of polyunsaturated or saturated fat. There were racial differences in elevation of LDL, with diets high in saturated fat consumed more by whites than by other racial groups. The isomeric form of fatty acids is important.[41] Fatty acids with the *cis* configuration are the preferred substrate for the ACAT reaction and significantly increase hepatic LDL receptor clearance while reducing LDL-C production rate. The *trans* isomeric form cannot be used by ACAT and is biologically inactive, with no effect on LDL concentration.

Ideally, therapeutic TLC, including reduced intake of saturated fats and cholesterol, increased stanol/sterol and fiber intake, weight reduction, and increased physical activity, should be used to attain lower LDL-C and to achieve reductions in CHD risk (Table 23–10). TLC may obviate the need for drug therapy, augment LDL-lowering drug therapy, and allow for lower doses. Weight control plus increased physical activity reduce risk beyond LDL-C lowering, are the primary management approach for the metabolic syndrome, raise HDL, and reduce non-HDL-C.[45,46] Many persons should be given a 3-month trial (two visits 6 weeks apart) of dietary therapy and TLC before advancing to drug therapy unless patients are at very high risk (severe hypercholesterolemia, known CHD, CHD risk equivalents, multiple risk factors, strong family history). Although changes in blood lipid levels may change before 3 months, adoption

TABLE 23-9 Classification of Lipid Levels in Children and Adolescents (Age <20 Years)

	Desirable (mg/dL)	Borderline (mg/dL)	Undesirable (mg/dL)
Total cholesterol	<170	170–199	≥200
LDL cholesterol	<110	110–129	≥130
HDL cholesterol	>45	25–45	<35
Triglycerides	<125	NA	≥125

HDL, high-density lipoprotein; LDL, low-density lipoprotein; NA, not applicable.
From Davis et al.[33]

TABLE 23-10 Macronutrient Recommendations for the Therapeutic Lifestyle Changes Diet

Component[a]	Recommended Intake
Total fat	25%–35% of total calories
Saturated fat	Less than 7% of total calories
Polyunsaturated fat	Up to 10% of total calories
Monounsaturated fat	Up to 20% of total calories
Carbohydrates[b]	50%–60% of total calories
Cholesterol	<200 mg/day
Dietary fiber	20–30 g/day
Plant sterols	2 g/day
Protein	Approximately 15% of total calories
Total calories	To achieve and maintain desirable body weight

[a]Calories from alcohol not included.
[b]Carbohydrates should derive from foods rich in complex carbohydrates, such as whole grains, fruits, and vegetables.

of a different eating pattern may require a longer period of time. It is important to involve all family members, especially if the patient is not the primary person preparing food. The NCEP and AHA both have excellent Internet-based resources to aid patients in altering their diet in a culturally sensitive manner (*http://www.americanheart.org/presenter.jhtml?identifier=1200009*; *http://www.nhlbi.nih.gov/health/index.htm*). If all of the recommended dietary changes from NCEP were made, the estimated reduction, on average, in LDL would range from 20% to 30%.[1] Adherence to diet and interindividual variability in macronutrient intake influence the eventual LDL level achieved. Based on the NHANES data, less than half of patients who should be instructed on heart healthy diet receive any dietary instructions.

Other dietary interventions or diet supplements may be useful in certain patients with lipid disorders. Increased intake of soluble fiber in the form of oat bran, pectins, certain gums, and psyllium products can result in useful adjunctive reductions in total cholesterol and LDL-C, but these dietary alterations or supplements should not be substituted for more active forms of treatment. Total daily fiber intake should be about 20–30 g/day, with about 25% or 6 g/day, being soluble fiber.[1] Studies with psyllium seed in doses of 10 to 15 g/day show reductions in total cholesterol and LDL-C ranging from approximately 5% to 20%.[47,48] They have little or no effect on HDL-C or triglyceride concentrations. These products also may be useful in managing constipation associated with the bile acid sequestrants. Psyllium binds cholesterol in the gut but also reduces hepatic production and clearance. Fish oil supplementation provides an increased amount of the omega-3 polyunsaturated fatty acids, such as eicosapentaenoic acid and docosahexaenoic acid. In epidemiologic studies, ingestion of large amounts of cold-water oily fish was associated with a reduction in CHD risk, but whether the same advantage is conferred with commercially prepared fish oil products is unclear. Each 20 g/day ingestion of fish lowers CHD risk by 7%, and eating fish at least once weekly should reduce CHD mortality.[49] Fish oil supplementation has a fairly large effect in reducing triglycerides and VLDL-C, but it either has no effect on total cholesterol and LDL-C or may cause elevations in these fractions. Other actions of fish oil may account for their protective effects. These effects include quantitative and qualitative alterations in the synthesis of prostanoid substances, changes in immune function and cellular proliferation, and potential antioxidative actions.[50] Responses noted with fish oil are discussed in Pharmacologic Therapy below.[51]

Fat substitutes such as olestra (sucrose polyester, Olean, Procter and Gamble), a mixture of hexa-esters, hepta-esters, and octa-esters formed from the reaction of sucrose with long-chain fatty acids, are approved by the Food and Drug Administration (FDA) as a nondigestible, nonabsorbable, noncaloric fat substitute for snack foods. Olestra is heat stable, so it can be used in the preparation of fried and baked foods, an advantage over several other fat substitutes. It is similar in composition to triglycerides, but olestra is not hydrolyzed in the gastrointestinal tract by pancreatic lipase and, consequently, is not taken up by the intestinal mucosa. The principal adverse effects associated with olestra use are bloating, flatulence, diarrhea, and "anal leakage." Because of the ability of olestra to solubilize lipophilic substances, there has been concern over potential drug interactions in which lipophilic drugs (e.g., digitoxin, cyclosporine, or colchicine) or vitamins (A, D, E, and K) are solubilized in olestra and excreted in the feces.

Studies have demonstrated the LDL-lowering effect of plant sterols, which are isolated from soybean and tall pine-tree oils. Ingestion of 2 to 3 g/day will reduce LDL by 6% to 15%.[1] Plant sterols can be esterified to unsaturated fatty acids (creating sterol esters) to increase lipid solubility. Hydrogenating sterols produces plant stanols and, with esterification, stanol esters. The efficacies of plant sterols and stanols are considered comparable. Because lipids are needed to solubilize stanol/sterol esters, they usually are available in commercial margarines. The presence of plant stanols/sterols is listed on the food label. When margarine products are used, persons must be advised to adjust caloric intake to account for the calories contained in the products. For example, Benecol (McNeil) is a butter-like spread that contains a plant stanol ester, an ingredient that can lower cholesterol, which is derived from plant stanols found naturally in small amounts in foods such as wheat, rye, and corn.[52] In August 2007, the FDA issued a warning about the consumption of red yeast rice and products containing red yeast rice/policosonal. These products contained lovastatin, which could interact with other drugs and would have the same toxicity of statins but would not be recognized by the consumer. The reduction in LDL with their use is minimal.[53]

Drug therapy is indicated after an adequate trial of TLC changes as outlined in Tables 23–8 and 23–9.

■ PHARMACOLOGIC THERAPY

Numerous randomized, double-blinded clinical trials have demonstrated that reduction of LDL reduces CHD event rates in primary prevention, secondary intervention, and angiographic trials.[54] Generally speaking, for every 1% reduction in LDL, there is a 1% reduction in CHD event rates.[1] However, if treatment extends beyond the typical duration of a clinical trial (2–5 years), the accumulated benefit could be greater. A 1% elevation of HDL results in an approximately 2% reduction in CHD events.[12,55] Of interest, angiographic trials, which typically cause small changes in luminal diameter (i.e., approximately 0.04-mm difference in change between placebo and active treatment), result in fewer clinical events, such as MI, and a decreased need for revascularization. These unexpected findings suggest that plaque size and luminal encroachment by plaque may be less important than the effects of cholesterol lowering on activity in the plaque and endothelial dysfunction. These studies provide a strong rationale for attempting to lower plasma cholesterol and LDL in patients with hypercholesterolemia.

❹ Although many efficacious lipid-lowering drugs exist, none is effective for all lipoprotein disorders, and all such agents are associated with some adverse effects.[56] Lipid-lowering drugs can be broadly divided into agents that decrease the synthesis of VLDL and LDL, agents that enhance VLDL clearance, agents that enhance LDL catabolism, agents that decrease cholesterol absorption, agents that elevate HDL, or some combination of these characteristics (Table 23–11). Table 23–12 lists recommended drugs of choice for each lipoprotein phenotype and alternate agents. Table 23–13 lists available products and their doses.

Treatment of type I hyperlipoproteinemia is directed toward reducing the levels of chylomicrons derived from dietary fat, with subsequent reduction in plasma triglycerides. Total daily fat intake should be no more than 10–25 g/day, or approximately 15% of total calories. Secondary causes of hypertriglyceridemia (see Table 23–5) should be excluded. Any underlying disorder should be treated appropriately. Type V hyperlipoproteinemia also requires stringent restriction of the fat component of dietary intake; in addition, drug therapy is indicated (as outlined in Table 23–12) if the response to diet alone is inadequate. Medium-chain triglycerides, which are absorbed without chylomicron formation, can be used as a dietary supplement for caloric intake if needed for types I and V. Hepatic fibrosis has been reported with medium-chain triglycerides. Omega-3 fatty acids may be useful for patients with LPL deficiency. In patients with apolipoprotein C-II deficiency, infusion of plasma may normalize plasma triglyceride levels.

Primary hypercholesterolemia (familial hypercholesterolemia, familial combined hyperlipidemia, type IIa hyperlipoproteinemia) is treated with bile acid resins (BARs) or sequestrants (colestipol, cholestyramine, and colesevelam), HMG-CoA reductase inhibitors

TABLE 23-11 Effects of Drug Therapy on Lipids and Lipoproteins

Drug	Mechanism of Action	Effects on Lipids	Effects on Lipoproteins	Comment
Cholestyramine, colestipol, colesevelam	↑ LDL catabolism ↓ Cholesterol absorption	↓ Cholesterol	↓ LDL ↑ VLDL	Problem with compliance; binds many coadministered acidic drugs
Niacin	↓ LDL and VLDL synthesis	↓ Triglyceride ↓ Cholesterol	↓ VLDL ↓ LDL ↑ HDL	Problems with patient acceptance; good in combination with bile acid resins; extended-release niacin causes less flushing and is less hepatotoxic than sustained-release form
Gemfibrozil, fenofibrate, clofibrate	↑ VLDL clearance ↓ VLDL synthesis	↓ Triglycercide ↓ Cholesterol	↓ VLDL ↓ LDL ↑ HDL	Clofibrate causes cholesterol gallstones; modest LDL lowering; raises HDL; gemfibrozil inhibits glucuronidation of simvastatin, lovastatin, atorvastatin
Lovastatin, pravastatin, simvastatin, fluvastatin, atorvastatin, rosuvastatin	↑ LDL catabolism; inhibit LDL synthesis	↓ Cholesterol	↓ LDL	Highly effective in heterozygous familial hypercholesterolemia and in combination with other agents
Ezetimibe	Blocks cholesterol absorption across the intestinal border	↓ Cholesterol	↓ LDL	Few adverse effects; effects additive to other drugs

HDL, high-density lipoprotein; LDL, low-density lipoprotein; VLDL, very-low-density lipoprotein.

(statins), niacin, or ezetimibe. ❺ Of these choices, statins are first choice because they are the most potent LDL-lowering agents. Statins interrupt the conversion of HMG-CoA to mevalonate, the rate-limiting step in de novo cholesterol biosynthesis, by inhibiting HMG-CoA reductase (see Fig. 23–3). Currently available products include lovastatin, pravastatin, simvastatin, fluvastatin, and atorvastatin. Rosuvastatin is the most potent statin currently on the market. Table 23–14 lists the pharmacokinetic properties of the statins.[57] The plasma half-lives of all the statins are reported to be short, except for atorvastatin and rosuvastatin, which may account for their potency. In the Comparative Dose Efficacy Study of Atorvastatin Versus Simvastatin, Pravastatin, Lovastatin, and Fluvastatin in Patients with Hypercholesterolemia (CURVES), the largest head-to-head comparison of statins, atorvastatin was found to be the most potent drug for lowering total cholesterol and LDL-C, with reductions in LDL-C of 38%, 46%, 51%, and 54% for the 10-, 20-, 40-, and 80-mg doses, respectively.[58] Metabolic studies of statin use in normal volunteers and patients with hypercholesterolemia suggest reduced synthesis of LDL-C as well as enhanced catabolism of LDL mediated through LDL receptors as the principal mechanisms for lipid-lowering effects. Total cholesterol and LDL-C are reduced in a dose-related fashion by at least 30% on average when added to dietary therapy, with the effects more pronounced in nonfamilial than in familial hypercholesterolemia. ❻ Combination therapy with bile acid sequestrants and lovastatin is rational: LDL receptor numbers are increased, leading to greater degradation of LDL-C; intracellular synthesis of cholesterol is inhibited; and enterohepatic recycling of bile acids is interrupted. Combination therapy with a statin pulse ezetimibe also is rational because ezetimibe inhibits cholesterol absorption across the gut border and adds 12% to 20% further reduction when combined with a statin or other drugs.[59] Elevation of serum transaminase levels (primarily alanine aminotransferase) to more than three times the upper limit of normal occurs in approximately 1.3% of patients taking moderate to high doses of statins; serious muscle toxicity occurs in <0.6% of patients.[60] Meta-analysis of placebo-controlled studies with statins demonstrated a low risk of abnormal alanine aminotransferase or creatine kinase (CK) and a low risk of myopathy without or with rhadomyolysis.[61] Lens opacities have been reported with lovastatin. However, in the age groups studied, these abnormalities are common and tend to wax and wane with time irrespective of drug therapy, and no statistical association is known to exist. As a category of monotherapy, the HMG-CoA reductase inhibitors are the most potent total cholesterol and LDL-C-lowering agents and are among the best tolerated.[60,61] In an analysis of more than 75,000 patients allocated to statins in clinical trials, Alsheikh-Ali et al.[62] found that risk of statin-associated elevated liver enzymes or rhabdomyolysis was not related to the magnitude of LDL-C lowering. A highly significant inverse relationship between achieved LDL-C levels and rates of newly diagnosed cancer was observed ($R^2 = 0.43$, $P = 0.009$).[62] The WHO Foundation Collaborating Centre for International Drug Monitoring has issued a report suggesting that a rare relationship may exist between statin use and the onset of upper motor neuron diseases such as amyotrophic lateral sclerosis, but this association remains uncertain.[63] Numerous pharmacokinetic and pharmacodynamic differences among statins and patients give rise to variable responses to therapy.[64]

TABLE 23-12 Lipoprotein Phenotype and Recommended Drug Treatment

Lipoprotein Type	Drug of Choice	Combination Therapy
I	Not indicated	–
IIa	Statins	Niacin or BAR
	Cholestyramine or colestipol	Statins or niacin
	Niacin	Statins or BAR Ezetimibe
IIb	Statins	BAR, fibrates,[b] or niacin
	Fibrates	Statins, niacin, BAR[a]
	Niacin	Statins or fibrates Ezetimibe
III	Fibrates	Statins or niacin
	Niacin	Statins or fibrates Ezetimibe
IV	Fibrates	Niacin
	Niacin	Fibrates
V	Fibrates	Niacin
	Niacin	Fish oils

[a]Bile acid resins (BARs) are not used as first-line therapy if triglycerides are elevated at baseline because hypertriglyceridemia may worsen with BAR alone.
[b]Fibrates includes gemfibrozil or fenofibrate.

The primary action of BAR is binding bile acids in the intestinal lumen, with concurrent interruption of enterohepatic circulation of bile acids and markedly increased excretion of acidic steroids in the feces. This action decreases the bile acid pool size and stimulates hepatic synthesis of bile acids from cholesterol. Depletion of the hepatic pool of cholesterol results in increased cholesterol biosynthesis and increased number of LDL receptors on the hepatocyte membrane. The increased number of receptors stimulates catabolism from plasma and lowers LDL levels. BAR also reduces CETP, which correlates with total cholesterol and LDL-C concentrations, perhaps by interfering with hepatic microsomal cholesterol content; however,

TABLE 23-13 Comparison of Drugs Used in the Treatment of Hyperlipidemia

Drug	Manufacturer	Dosage Forms	Usual Daily Dose	Maximum Daily Dose
Cholestyramine (Questran)	BMS	Bulk powder/4-g packets	8 g tid	32 g
Cholestyramine (Questran Light)	BMS	Bulk powder/4-g packets		
Cholestyramine (Cholybar)	Parke-Davis	4-g resin per bar		
Colestipol hydrochloride (Colestid)	Upjohn	Bulk powder/5-g packets	10 g bid	30 g
Colesevelam (WelChol)	Sankyo	625-mg tablets	1,875 mg bid	4,375 mg
Niacin	Various	50-, 100-, 250-, 500-mg tablets; 125-, 250-, 500-mg capsules	2 g tid	9 g
Extended-release niacin (Niaspan)	Kos	500, 750, 1,000 mg tablets	500 mg	2,000 mg
Extended-release niacin + lovastatin (Advicor)[a]	Kos	Niacin/lovastatin 500-mg/20-mg tablets Niacin/lovastatin 750-mg/20-mg tablets Niacin/lovastatin 1,000-mg/20-mg	Niacin/lovastatin 500 mg/20 mg	Niacin/lovastatin 1,000 mg/ 20 mg tablets
Clofibrate	Banner Pharmacaps, USL Pharma	500-mg capsules	1 g bid	2 g
Fenofibrate (TriCor and others)	Abbott, various	67-, 134-, 200-mg capsules (micronized); 54-,160-mg tablets; 40-, 120-mg tablets; 50-, 160-mg tablets	54 mg or 67 mg	201 mg
Gemfibrozil (Lopid)	Parke-Davis	300-mg capsules	600 mg bid	1.5 g
Lovastatin (Mevacor)	MSD	20-, 40-mg tablets	20–40 mg	80 mg
Pravastatin (Pravachol)	Bristol-Myers Squibb	10-, 20-mg tablets	10–20 mg	40 mg
Simvastatin (Zocor)	MSD	5-, 10-, 20-, 40- and 80-mg tablets	10–20 mg	80 mg
Atorvastatin (Lipitor)	Pfizer	10-mg tablets	10 mg	80 mg
Rosuvastatin (Crestor)	Astra-Zeneca	5- and 10-mg tablets	5 mg	40 mg
Ezetimibe (Zetia)	MSD	10-mg tablets	10 mg	10 mg
Atorvastatin/amlodipine (Caduet)	Pfizer	Atorvastatin/amlodipine 10 mg/5 mg Atorvastatin/amlodipine 20 mg/5 mg Atorvastatin/amlodipine 40 mg/5 mg Atorvastatin/amlodipine 80 mg/5 mg Atorvastatin/amlodipine 10 mg/10 mg Atorvastatin/amlodipine 20 mg/10 mg Atorvastatin/amlodipine 40 mg/10 mg Atorvastatin/amlodipine 80 mg/10 mg	Atorvastatin/amlodipine 10 mg/5 mg	Atorvastatin/amlodipine 80 mg/10 mg
Pravastatin/aspirin (Pravigard PAC)	BMS	Pravastatin/aspirin 20 mg/81 mg Pravastatin/aspirin 20 mg/325 mg Pravastatin/aspirin 40 mg/81 mg Pravastatin/aspirin 40 mg/325 mg Pravastatin/aspirin 80 mg/81 mg Pravastatin/aspirin 80 mg/325 mg		
Simvastatin/ezetimibe (Vytorin)	Merck/Schering-Plough	Simvastatin/ezetimibe 10 mg/10 mg Simvastatin/ezetimibe 20 mg/10 mg Simvastatin/ezetimibe 40 mg/10 mg	Simvastatin/ezetimibe 20 mg/ 10 mg	Simvastatin/ezetimibe 40 mg/10 mg
ω-3 Acid ethyl esters (Lovaza)	Reliant	Eicosapentaenoic acid (EPA) 465 mg, docosahexaenoic acid (DHA) 375 mg	Four 1-g capsules QD or two 1-g capsules bid	Four 1-g capsules QD or two 1-g capsules bid

BMS, Bristol-Myers Squibb; MSD, Merck Sharp & Dohme.

Probucol is no longer on the market in the United States. Gemfibrozil, fenofibrate, and lovastatin are available as generic products.

[a]Manufacturer does not recommend use of the fixed combination as initial therapy for primary hypercholesterolemia or mixed dyslipidemia. It is specifically indicated for patients receiving lovastatin alone plus diet who require an additional reduction in triglyceride levels or increase in HDL-cholesterol levels; it also is indicated for those treated with niacin alone who require additional decreases in LDL cholesterol.

this effect is not as great as with statins.[65] BARs are generally ineffective in patients with homozygous familial hypercholesterolemia because these individuals genetically lack the ability to increase synthesis of LDL receptors. The increase in hepatic cholesterol biosynthesis may be paralleled by increased hepatic VLDL production; consequently, BARs may aggravate hypertriglyceridemia in patients with combined hyperlipidemia. Gastrointestinal complaints of constipation, bloating, epigastric fullness, nausea, and flatulence are most commonly reported.[1] With intensive education, patients can learn to tolerate resins on a long-term basis, as evidenced in clinical trials by adherence to active drug regimens. In routine clinical practice, at least 40% of patients discontinue therapy within 1 year, but adherence rates can be improved with pharmacist interventions.[66,67] Adverse effects can be managed by increasing fluid intake, modifying the diet

TABLE 23-14 Pharmacokinetics of the Statins

Parameter	Lovastatin	Simvastatin	Pravastatin	Fluvastatin	Atorvastatin	Rosuvastatin
Isoenzyme	3A4	3A4	None	2C9	3A4	2C9/2C19
Lipophilic	Yes	Yes	No	Yes	Yes	No
Protein binding (%)	>95	95–98	~50	>90	96	88
Active metabolites	Yes	Yes	No	No	Yes	Yes
Elimination half-life (h)	3	2	1.8	1.2	7–14	13–20

Isoenzyme refers to the specific isoenzyme in the cytochrome P450 system, which is responsible for the metabolism of each drug. Pharmacokinetic parameters in this table are based on studies and reviews presented in the literature.

to increase bulk, and using stool softeners. The other major limiting complaint with BARs is their gritty texture and bulk. This problem can be minimized by mixing the powder with orange drink or juice. Tablet forms of bile acid sequestrants should help to improve compliance with this form of therapy, whereas the bar does not improve compliance.[68] Other potential adverse effects include impaired absorption of fat-soluble vitamins A, D, E, and K; hypernatremia and hyperchloremia; gastrointestinal obstruction; and reduced bioavailability of acidic drugs such as coumarin anticoagulants, digitoxin, nicotinic acid, thyroxine, acetaminophen, hydrocortisone, hydrochlorothiazide, loperamide, and possibly iron. Hyperchloremic metabolic acidosis, hypernatremia, and gastrointestinal obstruction have been reported to occur almost exclusively in children, and malabsorption of fat-soluble vitamins probably is most common with high doses (e.g., 30 g/day of cholestyramine) of the BARs. Drug interactions can be avoided by alternating administration times, with an interval of at least 6 hours between the BAR and other drugs. Colestipol and cholestyramine have comparable side effects; however, colestipol may have better palatability because it is odorless and tasteless. Colesevelam is the newest BAR, and total and LDL-C reduction are dose related. Adverse effects are qualitatively similar to those occurring with the older BARs but may occur less often. Because of adverse effects that occur commonly with BARs at higher doses, BARs are increasingly used in combination with other drugs because low doses are tolerated well, and the BARs work in complementary fashion with other agents.

Niacin (nicotinic acid) can be used for treatment of primary hypercholesterolemia in combination with bile acid sequestrants or as monotherapy for this and other disorders (Table 23–12). Niacin reduces hepatic synthesis of VLDL, which in turn leads to reduced synthesis of LDL. Factors responsible for decreased VLDL production include inhibition of lipolysis with decreased free fatty acids in plasma, decreased hepatic esterification of triglycerides, and a possible direct effect on hepatic production of apolipoprotein B.[69] The complementary action of niacin and bile acid sequestrants in increasing catabolism and decreasing LDL synthesis may account for the additive effects of this combination in patients with hyperlipidemia. Niacin also increases HDL by reducing its catabolism. Niacin selectively decreases hepatic removal of HDL apolipoprotein A-I but not removal of cholesterol esters, thereby increasing the capacity of retained apolipoprotein A-I to augment reverse cholesterol transport in isolated hepatic cells. Niacin is used principally for treatment of mixed hyperlipemia or as a second-line agent in combination therapy for hypercholesterolemia. It is considered the first-line agent or an alternative for treatment of hypertriglyceridemia and diabetic dyslipidemia.[70,71] Numerous smaller trials suggest that lower doses of niacin can be combined with statins or gemfibrozil to minimize adverse effects and maximize response. These combinations require careful monitoring because interactions occur.

Many adverse drug reactions occur commonly with niacin use, but most of the symptoms and biochemical abnormalities do not require discontinuation of therapy. Cutaneous flushing and itching appear to be prostaglandin mediated and can be reduced by aspirin 325 mg given shortly before niacin ingestion.[1,72] Flushing seems to be related to rising plasma concentrations of niacin; taking the dose with meals and slowly titrating the dose upward may minimize these effects. Laropiprant is a selective antagonist of the prostaglandin D_2 receptor subtype 1 (DP1), which may mediate niacin-induced vasodilation. Coadministration of laropiprant 30, 100, and 300 mg with extended-release (ER) niacin significantly lowered flushing symptom scores (by at least 50%) and significantly reduced malar skin blood flow measured by laser Doppler perfusion imaging.[73] Gastrointestinal intolerance and flushing are common problems. Acanthosis nigricans, a darkening of the skin in skinfold areas and an external marker of insulin resistance, may be seen with high doses of niacin. Sustained-release products may minimize these complaints in some patients, but controlled trials with regular-release products do not demonstrate much difference between sustained- and regular-release products. The only legend form of niacin, Niaspan (Kos), is an extended-release form of niacin with pharmacokinetics intermediate between instant and sustained-release products, which are sold as food supplements rather than legend products. In controlled trials, Niaspan is reported to have fewer dermatologic reactions and a low risk for hepatoxicity. Niaspan in combination with statins produces large reductions in LDL and increases in HDL.[74] Potentially important laboratory abnormalities occurring with niacin therapy include elevated liver function tests, hyperuricemia, and hyperglycemia. Experience with niacin in diabetes suggests that some diabetic patients do not have worsened glycemic control with dose-titration and sustained-release products.[75] With doses less than 3 g/day, the degree of liver function test elevation generally is not marked and often is transient, and a temporary reduction in dosage frequently corrects the problem. Niacin-associated hepatitis is more common with sustained-release preparations, and their use should be restricted to patients intolerant of regular-release products.[75,76] Sustained-release products often are more expensive and, given the lack of data on reduced adverse effects and increased incidence of hepatitis, regular-release products should always be used first. Preexisting gout and diabetes may be exacerbated by niacin; patients with these conditions should be monitored more closely and their medication titrated appropriately. Patients with well-controlled diabetes mellitus type 2 do not have significant changes in glycemic control with niacin doses up to 2 g/day.[76] Niacin is contraindicated in patients with active liver disease. Dry eyes and other ophthalmologic complaints are occasionally noted. Concomitant alcohol and hot drinks may magnify flushing and pruritus with niacin and should be avoided at the time of ingestion. Nicotinamide should not be used for treatment of hyperlipidemia because it does not effectively lower cholesterol or triglyceride levels.

Combined hyperlipoproteinemia (type IIb) can be treated with statins, niacin, or gemfibrozil to lower LDL-C without elevating VLDL and triglycerides. Niacin is the most effective agent and can be combined with a bile acid sequestrant. BARs alone for treatment of this disorder may elevate VLDL and triglycerides, and their use as single agents for treatment of combined hyperlipoproteinemia should be avoided. Fibric acid (gemfibrozil, fenofibrate) monotherapy is effective in reducing VLDL, but a reciprocal rise in LDL may occur, and total cholesterol values may remain relatively unchanged. Gemfibrozil reduces synthesis of VLDL and, to a lesser extent, apolipoprotein B, with a concurrent increase in the rate of removal of triglyceride-rich lipoproteins from plasma. Plasma HDL concentrations may rise 10% to 15% or more with fibrates. Ezetimibe also can be used in combination therapy for type IIb disease. Gastrointestinal complaints with fibric acid derivatives occur in 3% to 5% of patients, rash in 2%, dizziness in 2.4%, and transient elevations in transaminase levels and alkaline phosphatase in 4.5% and 1.3%, respectively.[77] Gemfibrozil and fenofibrate may enhance the formation of gallstones associated with an increase in the lithogenic index; however, the rate is low (0.5%–7%) and similar to that seen with placebo in the Helsinki Heart Study.[77] Fibric acid derivatives may potentiate the effects of oral anticoagulants, so prothrombin time and international normalized ratio should be monitored very closely when this combination is used.

Type III hyperlipoproteinemia can be treated with fibric acid derivatives or niacin. Although fibric acid derivatives have been suggested as the drugs of choice for treatment of this disorder, the lack of data from major studies on hypercholesterolemia supporting their efficacy in altering cardiovascular mortality and the numerous, well-documented serious adverse effects occurring with their use make niacin a reasonable consideration. Gemfibrozil increases the activity of LPL and reduces the synthesis or secretion of VLDL from the liver into the plasma. A myositis syndrome of myalgia, weakness, stiffness, malaise, and elevations in creatinine phosphokinase and aspartate aminotransaminase is seen with the fibric acid derivatives and seems to be more common in patients with renal insufficiency.[77] Enhanced hypoglycemic effects are reported to occur when fibric acid derivative are given to patients taking sulfonylurea compounds, but the mechanisms for these interactions are not well understood.

Three fibric acid derivatives (clofibrate, gemfibrozil, and fenofibrate) are approved for use in the United States. Gemfibrozil and fenofibrate are used much more commonly than clofibrate. All reduce LDL-C by 20% to 25% in patients with heterozygous familial hypercholesterolemia. The response of LDL-C, HDL-C, and triglycerides to this category of drug is highly dependent on the specific lipoprotein type (e.g., type IIa vs IIb) and the baseline triglyceride concentration.[78]

As a potential alternative therapy for this phenotype, numerous epidemiologic and normal volunteer studies have found that diets high in omega-3 polyunsaturated fatty acids (from fish oil), mostly commonly eicosapentaenoic acid, reduce cholesterol, triglycerides, LDL-C, and very-low-density lipoprotein cholesterol (VLDLC) and may elevate HDL-C.[51] The effects of fish oil on lipoprotein metabolism are mediated by a reduction in VLDL production and suppression of VLDL apolipoprotein B. In patients with hypertriglyceridemia (either phenotype type IIb or V), a diet high in omega-3 fatty acids given for 4 weeks reduced cholesterol 27% and 45% and triglyceride 64% and 79% in the type IIb and type V patients, respectively.[49] A diet high in eicosapentaenoic acid given to hyperlipidemic hemodialysis patients resulted in significant decreases in cholesterol and triglycerides for as long as 13 weeks. Fish oil supplementation may be most useful in patients with hypertriglyceridemia; however, its role in treatment is not well defined. Potential complications of fish oil supplementation, such as thrombocytopenia and bleeding disorders, have been noted, especially with high doses (eicosapentaenoic acid 15–30 g/day). Well-controlled trials are needed to determine if fish oils are safe and effective before their use can be broadly recommended. Based a meta-analysis, fish consumption lowers the risk of CHD, but nutraceuticals have not been adequately tested.[49] A prescription form of concentrated fish oil, Lovaza, has become available.[51] This product lowers triglycerides by 14% to 30% and raises HDL by approximately 10%, depending on baseline values.

Combination drug therapy may be considered after adequate trials of monotherapy and for patients who are documented as compliant to the prescribed regimen. Two or three lipoprotein profiles at 6-week intervals should confirm lack of response prior to initiation of combination therapy. Cholestyramine can be added for patients with fasting hypertriglyceridemia but should not be used as the initial drug because triglycerides are likely to increase. Contraindications to, and drug interactions with, combined therapy should be carefully screened. Consideration should be given to the extra cost of drug product and monitoring that may be required. In general, a statin and a BAR or niacin with a BAR provide the greatest reduction in total cholesterol and LDL-C. Regimens intended to increase HDL levels should include either gemfibrozil or niacin, bearing in mind that statins combined with either of these drugs may result in a greater incidence of hepatotoxicity or myositis. This is particularly important for statins that are eliminated via cytochrome 3A4 or through glucuronidation.[57] Familial combined hyperlipidemia may respond better to a fibric acid and a statin than to a fibric acid and a BAR.[79]

Severe forms of hypercholesterolemia, such as familial hypercholesterolemia, familial defective apolipoprotein B-100, severe polygenic hypercholesterolemia, familial combined hyperlipidemia, and familial dysbetalipoproteinemia (type III), may require more intensive therapy. In particular, patients with familial hypercholesterolemia often require combination therapy (two or three drugs) and are managed with surgical therapy (partial ileal bypass), plasmapheresis (LDL apheresis), and liver transplantation (to replace LDL receptors).

■ HYPERTRIGLYCERIDEMIA

It is important to remember that lipoprotein pattern types I, III, IV, and V are associated with hypertriglyceridemia, and that these primary lipoprotein disorders and underlying diseases should be excluded prior to implementing therapy (see Table 23–5). A family history positive for CHD is important in identifying patients at risk for premature atherosclerosis.[80,81] If a patient with CHD has elevated triglycerides, the associated abnormality probably is a contributing factor to CHD and should be treated.[29]

High serum triglycerides (see Tables 21–6 and 21–12) should be treated by achieving desirable body weight, consumption of a diet low in saturated fat and cholesterol, regular exercise, smoking cessation, and restriction of alcohol (in selected patients). ATP III identifies the sum of LDL and VLDL (termed *non-HDC* [total cholesterol – HDL]) as a secondary target of therapy in persons with high triglycerides (≥200 mg/dL).[1,29] This approach is used when triglycerides are >200 mg/dL and accounts for atherogenic particles carried in VLDL and remnant particles. The goal for non-HDL in persons with high serum triglycerides can be set 30 mg/dL higher than that for LDL on the premise that VLDL ≤30 mg/dL is normal. ❼ In patients with borderline-high triglycerides but accompanying risk factors for established CHD disease, family history of premature CHD, concomitant LDL elevation or low HDL, and genetic forms of hypertriglyceridemia associated with CHD (familial dysbetalipoproteinemia, familial combined hyperlipidemia), drug therapy with niacin should be considered. Niacin can be used cautiously in diabetics based on the results of the Arterial Disease Multiple Intervention Trial (ADMIT), which found triglycerides were reduced by 23%, HDL-C increased by 29%, glucose increased only slightly (mean 8.7 mg/dL), and hemoglobin A_{1c} did not change.[82] Alternative therapies include gemfibrozil, statins, and fish oil.[81,83,84] Fibrates may increase LDL, and their use in borderline–high triglyceridemia requires careful monitoring to detect this deleterious change in lipid profile. Statins also can be used because they provide modest reductions in triglycerides and modest elevations in HDL. Higher doses of statins may reduce HDL as well as LDL and triglycerides, with the amount of reduction related to the baseline concentration and dose.[81,84] In this situation, the goal of therapy is to lower triglycerides and VLDL particles that may be atherogenic, increase HDL, and reduce LDL.

Very high triglycerides are associated with pancreatitis and other consequences of the chylomicron syndrome. At this level of triglycerides elevation, a genetic form of hypertriglyceridemia often coexists with other causes of elevated triglycerides, such as diabetes. Dietary fat restriction (10%–20% of calories as fat), weight loss, alcohol restriction, and treatment of the coexisting disorder are the basic elements of management. Drugs useful for treatment of hypertriglyceridemia include gemfibrozil, niacin, and higher-potency statins (atorvastatin, rosuvastatin, and simvastatin). Gemfibrozil is the preferred drug in diabetics because of the effect of niacin on glycemic control unless the newer extended-release forms are used. Fenofibrate may be preferred in combination with statin therapy because it does not impair glucuronidation and minimizes potential drug interactions. Successful treatment is defined as a reduction in triglycerides <500 mg/dL.[1]

■ LOW HDL-C

Low HDL is a strong independent risk predictor of CHD. ATP III redefined low HDL-C as <40 mg/dL but specified no goal for HDL-C raising.[1] Low HDL may be a consequence of insulin resistance, physical inactivity, type 2 diabetes mellitus, cigarette smoking, very high carbohydrate intake, and certain drugs (see Table 23–5). ❽ In low HDL, the primary target remains LDL according to ATP III, but emphasis shifts to weight reduction, increased physical activity, smoking cessation, and, if drug therapy is required, fibric acid derivatives and niacin. Niacin has the potential for the greatest increase in HDL, and the effect is more pronounced with regular or immediate-release forms than with sustained-release forms.[85]

DIABETIC DYSLIPIDEMIA

Diabetic dyslipidemia is characterized by hypertriglyceridemia, low HDL, and LDL that is minimally elevated. Small, dense LDL (pattern B) in diabetes is more atherogenic than larger, more buoyant forms of LDL (pattern A). Routine lipoprotein profiles do not differentiate between pattern A and pattern B.[86–88] Diabetes in ATP III is a CHD risk equivalent. The primary target is LDL, and the goal of treatment is to lower LDL-C to <100 mg/dL.[1] When LDL is >130 mg/dL, most patients require simultaneous therapeutic lifestyle changes and drug therapy. When LDL-C is between 100 and 129 mg/dL, intensifying glycemic control, options include adding drugs for the atherogenic dyslipidemia (fibric acid derivatives, niacin), and intensifying LDL-C-lowering therapy. Because the primary target is LDL-C in patients with diabetic dyslipidemia, statins are considered by many to be the initial drugs of choice.[1,29] The relative risk reduction for CHD in diabetics versus nondiabetics was greater in several trials, including the West of Scotland Coronary Prevention Study (37% vs 20%),[89] Air Force/Texas Coronary Atherosclerosis Prevention Study (AFCAPS/TexCAPS; 43% vs 36%),[90] Cholesterol and Recurrent Events (CARE) trial (25% vs 23%),[91] and Scandinavian Simvastatin Survival Study (4S; 55% vs 32%).[92] All statins are fairly comparable in triglyceride lowering, and because statins differ in potency for LDL reduction, a ratio of LDL reduction to triglyceride reduction can be applied. Statin therapy may protect against the development of diabetes.[26] The most recent trial of LDL lowering in type 2 diabetes mellitus is the Collaborative Atorvastatin Diabetes Study (CARDS).[93] This was a randomized, double-blinded placebo comparison of atorvastatin 10 mg/day versus placebo in 2,838 diabetes to reduce first CHD events. Baseline LDL was 118 mg/dL, and with atorvastatin LDL fell by 46 mg/dL. The primary end point, a composite of acute CHD death, nonfatal MI, hospitalized unstable angina, resuscitated cardiac arrest, coronary revascularization, or stroke, was reduced by 37%. This study suggests that all diabetics should have LDL much lower than 100 mg/dL, and these results are consistent with the Heart Protection Study analysis of diabetic patients.[94]

According to the Diabetes Atherosclerosis Intervention Study (DAIS), fenofibrate reduced angiographic progression of CAD in type 2 diabetics.[95] Fewer CHD events were seen with fenofibrate compared with placebo, but the difference was not significant. Fibric acids principally lower VLDL and triglycerides while increasing HDL, with only modest lowering of total cholesterol and LDL-C. Fibric acid derivatives may increase LDL levels. In contrast to niacin, fibric acid derivatives tend to improve glucose tolerance, with the greatest effect seen with bezafibrate. The Helsinki Heart Study found gemfibrozil was most effective for diabetic dyslipidemia.[96] Although the effect of statins on triglycerides and HDL abnormalities commonly seen in patients with diabetes is less than with fibric acids, the subgroup analyses cited earlier suggest that these drugs significantly reduce CHD risk. Cholestyramine in diabetic patients may result in lower LDL levels but may increase VLDL and triglyceride levels, which already are commonly elevated in diabetes. Resins may aggravate constipation, which is common in diabetics. As demonstrated in ADMIT and in the Assessment of Diabetes Control and Evaluation of the Efficacy of Niaspan Trial (ADVENT), immediate-release and extended-release niacin are highly effective in raising HDL and lowering triglycerides and LDL.[82,97]

SPECIAL CONSIDERATIONS

Elderly

Hypercholesterolemia is an independent risk factor for CHD in the elderly (>65 years old) as it is in younger patients. The attributable risk, which is the difference in absolute rates of CHD between segments of the population with higher or lower serum cholesterol levels, increases with age. Older patients potentially benefit to a greater extent from cholesterol lowering than do younger patients. Data from studies of elderly men in a variety of settings are consistent with a relative risk of at least 1.5 in the highest compared to the lowest quartile of cholesterol levels.[98,99] Treatment of hypercholesterolemia in the elderly may result in reduction of absolute risk comparable to that obtained in younger persons.[1] Subgroup analyses of the West of Scotland (primary) and 4S (secondary) intervention studies show that elderly patients had lower CHD risk reduction (relative risk reduction 27% and 29%, respectively) compared to younger patients (relative risk reduction 40% and 39%, respectively).[89,100] The Framingham study suggests that elderly women are at higher risk because of high blood cholesterol levels, but no other large studies included women, and the risks or benefits from cholesterol reduction are not well defined. Primary prevention in younger patients requires approximately 2 years before reduction in CHD risk is apparent, and this lag time should be taken into consideration during patient selection for therapy. Relative risk of nonlipid CHD risk factors does not decline with aging, and aggressive management of modifiable nonlipid risk factors is important in older patients. High-risk elderly patients are less likely to be prescribed statins, and their potent benefits are not realized.[101] Because most women with CHD are elderly and at risk for osteoporosis, they are logical candidates for diet therapy with consideration of calcium intake consistent with osteoporosis prevention, exercise, and perhaps estrogen replacement therapy. Evidence suggests that statins reduce the risk of osteoporosis; however, data from various studies are conflicting.[102]

Drug therapy in principle differs little between older and younger patients, and older patients respond as well as younger patients to lipid-lowering drugs.[103,104] Based on the Heart Protection Study, which comprised more elderly patients than any other trial, simvastatin 40 mg/day reduced the CHD event rate in patients older than 70 years the same as in younger patients.[105] The gain in life expectancy may be small, depending on the patient's age at the start of treatment and the magnitude of cholesterol reduction.[82] Changes in body composition, renal function, and other physiologic changes of aging may make older patients more susceptible to adverse effects of lipid-lowering drug therapy. In particular, older patients are more likely to have constipation (BARs), skin and eye changes (niacin), gout (niacin), gallstones (fibric acid derivatives), and bone/joint disorders (fibric acid derivatives, statins). Therapy should be started with lower doses and titrated up slowly to minimize adverse effects.

Women

Cholesterol is an important determinant of CHD in women, but the relationship is not as strong as that seen in men. HDL may be a more important predictor of disease in women.[4] LDL and HDL genetic regulation in women and men does not appear to be different. Based on the Nurses' Health Study, obesity is an important determinant of CHD in women, with a relative risk of 3.3 in the highest Quetelet index (weight in kilograms divided by the square of the height in meters) compared to the lowest category (i.e., <21 vs ≥29); low HDL levels usually accompany obesity.[106] No major differences exist in the influence of exercise, alcohol ingestion, and smoking on lipid levels between men and women. Women in the highest tertile of cholesterol appear to be more responsive to dietary therapy than women in the lower tertiles and more responsive than predicted using formulas based on men.

Based on the Heart and Estrogen/Progestin Replacement Study (HERS)[107] and the Women's Health Initiative (WHI) trial,[108–110] published national guidelines recommended similar types of lifestyle and risk factor goals and interventions as recommended by NCEP for the entire population.[4] Hormone therapy may continue to have a role for treatment of postmenopausal symptoms; however, a notable exception is hormone replacement therapy and heart protection. Combined estrogen plus progestin hormone therapy for prevention of cardiovascular disease should not be initiated in postmenopausal women. Combined estrogen plus progestin hormone therapy for prevention of cardiovascular disease should not be continued in postmenopausal women. Other forms of menopausal hormone therapy (e.g., unopposed estrogen) for prevention of cardiovascular disease should not be initiated or continued in postmenopausal women pending the results of ongoing trials. Results of the Women's International Study of Long Duration Oestrogen after Menopause (WISDOM) confirm the lack of benefit seen in HERS and WHI.[111] In a post hoc analysis of the WHI, women who initiated hormone therapy closer to menopause tended to have a reduced CHD risk compared with the increased CHD risk in women more distant from menopause, but this trend did not meet statistical signifance.[108]

Cholesterol and triglyceride levels rise progressively throughout pregnancy, with an average increment in cholesterol of 30 to 40 mg/dL occurring around weeks 36 to 39. Triglyceride levels may increase by as much as 150 mg/dL. Drug therapy is not instituted, nor is it usually continued during pregnancy. If the patient is very high risk, a bile acid resin may be considered because no systemic drug exposure occurs.[1] Statins are category X and are contraindicated. Ezetimibe might be an alternative because it is a category C drug (animal studies have shown that the drug exerts teratogenic and embryocidal effects, no adequate and well-controlled studies in pregnant women are available, or no studies are available in either animals or pregnant women). Dietary therapy is the mainstay of treatment, with emphasis on maintaining a nutritionally balanced diet per the needs of pregnancy.

Children

Drug therapy in children is not recommended until they are 10 years and older, and the guidelines for institution of therapy and the goals of therapy are different from those in adults (see Table 23–9).[33] Younger children are generally managed with therapeutic lifestyle changes until after age 2 years.[1,44] In the past bile acid sequestrants were recommended as first-line therapy, but evidence now shows that statins are safe and effective in children and provide greater lipid lowering than BAR.[38,112,113] Severe forms of hypercholesterolemia (e.g., familial hypercholesterolemia) may require more aggressive treatment.

■ CONCURRENT DISEASE STATES

Nephrotic syndrome, end-stage renal disease and nephrotic syndrome, and hypertension compound the risk of dyslipidemia and may present difficult-to-treat lipid abnormalities. Abnormalities of lipoprotein metabolism in the nephrotic syndrome include elevated total and LDL-C, lipoprotein(a), VLDL, and triglycerides. The ratio of apolipoprotein C-III to apolipoprotein C-II is elevated, consistent with greater LPL inhibitor activity, and the extent of hypoalbuminemia is correlated with dyslipidemia. The basic abnormality appears to be overproduction of LDL apolipoprotein B from VLDL rather than reduced clearance of LDL-C and related proteins. Protein restriction and a "vegan" diet corrects lipid abnormalities to some extent. Statins have been shown to be effective in reducing elevated total cholesterol and LDL-C in the nephrotic syndrome, although the levels do not usually return to normal.[114] Fibric acid derivatives and statins reduce small, dense LDL-C by different mechanisms, suggesting a potential role for combination therapy in optimizing the lowering of small, dense LDL-C and remnant lipoproteins. Statins appear to be safe and effective in renal insufficiency and may alter the natural course of declining renal function.[115–119]

Renal insufficiency without proteinuria leads to hypertriglyceridemia, slightly elevated total cholesterol and LDL-C (particularly with chronic ambulatory peritoneal dialysis), and low HDL levels (especially during hemodialysis). These abnormalities are thought to be caused by a deficiency in apolipoprotein C-II, perhaps as a result of sustained use of heparin during hemodialysis and depletion of LPL, carbohydrate-induced obesity and hypertriglyceridemia, loss of carnitine during hemodialysis, use of acetate buffer (acetate is a precursor to fatty acid synthesis) during hemodialysis, and decreased LCAT activity during hemodialysis. Dialysis does not correct the lipid abnormalities. Renal transplantation may correct lipid abnormalities in some patients; however, use of transplantation-related medications, such as corticosteroids, cyclosporine, and certain antihypertensive agents (see Chaps. 15 and 92), may aggravate the lipid abnormalities in other patients. Cyclosporine interferes with the metabolism of statins metabolized by cytochrome P450 3A4 (Table 23–14), and patients must be observed closely for myositis and worsening renal function. Of interest, correction of lipid abnormalities may improve renal hemodynamics. Pravastatin and fluvastatin may be safer than other statins, but this must be validated in larger, long-term trials. Diet will modify lipoprotein levels, and polyunsaturated fatty acids may have a role in impeding the progression of renal disease as well as the cardiovascular complications. Bile acid sequestrants do not correct the lipid abnormalities seen in renal insufficiency. Lovastatin or its active metabolite may accumulate in renal insufficiency, and lower doses of reductase inhibitors should be used to avoid adverse effects. Gemfibrozil can be used with caution; its pharmacokinetics are unchanged and it lowers triglycerides and increases HDL.[120] Statins (simvastatin, lovastatin and atorvastatin) and fibric acid derivatives may increase the risk of severe myopathy, and attention to symptoms of myositis is needed. Niacin may be useful in nondiabetic patients with renal insufficiency.

Hypertensive patients have a greater-than-expected prevalence of high blood cholesterol levels; conversely, patients with hypercholesterolemia have a higher than expected prevalence of hypertension caused by the metabolic syndrome. Recommendations for management of hypertension in patients with hypercholesterolemia include avoiding use of drugs that elevate cholesterol, such as diuretics and β-blockers, and using agents that either are lipid neutral or may reduce cholesterol slightly (see Chap. 15).[1] Bile acid sequestrants may bind to thiazide diuretics and some β-blockers and may interfere with their absorption. Reactions may be avoided by giving the antihypertensive 1 hour before or 4 hours after the resin. Niacin may magnify the hypotensive effects of vasodilators.

■ PHARMACOECONOMIC CONSIDERATIONS

The clinical benefits of lipid-lowering therapy for primary and secondary intervention are well established based on the results of studies showing a reduction in CHD morbidity and mortality.[121,122] The balance of benefits and costs has been examined in a few studies.[82,95] The cost per year of life saved has been estimated to range from less than $10,000 to more than $1 million dollars, depending on the presence or absence of CHD, patient's age, baseline total or LDL-C level, reduction in cholesterol, and number of risk factors present. ❾ Intervention with statin therapy in general is cost effective in patients with known CHD, with CHD risk equivalents, or with a 10-year risk of 10% to 20%. Other types of therapy may be cost effective if certain assumptions concerning compliance and efficacy are met. Based on 4S, the range for secondary intervention is $3,800 for a 70-year-old man with a high cholesterol level to $27,400 per year of life gained for a middle-aged woman with an average cholesterol level.[123] In contrast, primary prevention in men based on the West of Scotland trial averages about $35,000 per year of life gained.[124] These studies demonstrate that primary and secondary intervention are well within the accepted boundary of less than $50,000 for a medical intervention to be considered cost effective. Based on the specific lipoprotein phenotype, fibric acid derivatives, niacin, or combination therapy of statins plus BAR may be cost effective. Cost effectiveness is maximized by treating high-risk patients and those with established CHD.

Specialty lipid clinics have become increasingly popular, and many use pharmacists to provide direct patient care in this setting. An interesting analysis showed that a specialty clinic may be more expensive ($659 ± $43 vs $477 ± $42 per patient, $P < 0.001$) than usual care. However, the overall cost effectiveness is improved when expressed as program costs per unit (mmol/L) reduction in the LDL-C, a measure of cost effectiveness that was significantly lower for specialized care ($758 ± $58 vs $1,058 ± $70, $P = 0.002$) because more patients achieve their targeted goal.[125] Project ImPACT (Improve Persistence and Compliance with Therapy) demonstrated that pharmacists, working collaboratively with patients and physicians, can improve persistence and compliance, and that nearly two thirds of patients achieved their NCEP lipid goal.[126] Other programs showed similar trends.[67,127,128]

■ OTHER THERAPIES

Partial ileal bypass has been used for treatment of severe heterozygous and homozygous familial hypercholesterolemia; however, it is ineffective in the latter case. Ileal bypass removes the site of bile acid reabsorption, depleting the bile acid pool and increasing the catabolism of cholesterol. The Program on the Surgical Control of the Hyperlipidemias (POSCH), a randomized trial of diet versus surgery, reported that total cholesterol and LDL-C were decreased (23.3% and 37.7%, respectively) and HDL increased (4.3%) in patients who had undergone ileal bypass for hypercholesterolemia.[97] Surgery delayed overall death by nearly 3 years ($P = 0.032$) and delayed CHD mortality by nearly 4 years ($P = 0.046$) compared to the control group. Revascularization procedures were delayed by an average of 7 years ($P < 0.001$). Postsurgery diarrhea was more common in the surgical group, as were the rates of kidney stones (4% vs 0.4%), gallstones (10% vs 2%), and bowel obstruction (13.5% vs 3.6%).

Portacaval shunts have been used to decrease the formation of LDL-C, with reported reductions of 10% to 20%. Plasma exchange combined with niacin was found to reduce plasma cholesterol levels by approximately 50% over 5 years in patients with homozygous familial hypercholesterolemia, and coronary atherosclerosis did not progress as documented by angiography. LDL apheresis (i.e., selective removal of LDL-C via a filtering system) plus statin therapy is effective in lowering LDL-C and appears to affect the progression of vascular disease. Combined liver and heart transplantation in patients with homozygous familial hypercholesterolemia reduced total cholesterol and LDL-C concentrations from approximately 1,100 and 900 mg/dL before surgery to approximately 300 and 185 mg/dL after surgery, respectively. Liver transplantation replaced the missing LDL receptors, enhanced catabolism, and reduced lipoprotein synthesis in this patient population.

■ SUMMARY OF MAJOR STUDIES

⑩ Primary and secondary prevention diet and drug trials have been performed to determine whether lowering cholesterol levels will prevent CHD. These trials are summarized in Tables 23–15 and 23–16. A number of earlier angiographic studies demonstrated that cholesterol reduction led to regression of atherosclerosis and plaque stabilization. Most of the primary and secondary studies were double blinded, randomized, and placebo controlled, lasted for at least 5 years, and had sufficient patient numbers to be meaningful. Exceptions to these qualifications were seen in the early studies, such as the Newcastle and Edinburgh trials, which were small and generally did not show much benefit; and the Coronary Drug Project (CDP), using dextrothyroxine, which was terminated early because of observed adverse effects on CHD mortality. The Helsinki Heart Study, using gemfibrozil, resulted in a reduction in nonfatal MI, which was the primary contributor to reduced CHD incidence (Table 23–15).[14]

Total cholesterol and LDL-C were reduced an average of 13.4% and 20.3%, respectively, by cholestyramine in the Lipid Research Clinics Coronary Primary Prevention Trial (LRC-CPPT). The reduction of lipid levels was related to the amount of drug ingested (5.4% reduction in total cholesterol with 1–2 packets vs 19.0% reduction with ≥5 packets).[129] The prescribed dose of cholestyramine was 24 g (or 6 packets) per day. The cholestyramine group experienced a 19% reduction in risk ($P < 0.05$) of the primary end point of definite CHD death and/or definite nonfatal MI, reflecting a 24% reduction in definite CHD death and a 19% reduction in nonfatal MI. Other end points of new positive exercise tests, angina, and coronary bypass surgery were reduced by 25%, 20%, and 21%, respectively. Death from all causes was

TABLE 23-15 Primary Prevention Trials with Lipid-Lowering Drugs

Trial	Followup (y)	N	Treatment	Control Events	Treatment Events	*P* Value	RRR	ARR	NNT
AFCAPS/TexCAPS	5	6,605	Lovastatin 20–40 mg	5.5%	3.5%	<0.001	36.4%	2.0%	50
Helsinki	5	4,081	Gemfibrozil 1,200 mg	4.1%	2.7%	<0.02	34.0%	1.4%	71
LRC-CPPT	7.4	3,806	Cholestyramine 24 g	9.8%	8.1%	<0.05	17.3%	1.7%	59
Oslo	5	1,232	Diet + smoking cessation	4.2%	2.5%	0.03	40.5%	1.7%	59
WOSCOPS	4.9	6,595	Pravastatin 40 mg	7.8%	5.5%	<0.001	29.5%	2.3%	43
ALLHAT	4.8	10,355	Usual care Pravastatin 40 mg	10.4%	9.3%	0.16	9.0%	1.1%	91
WHI	5.2	16,608	Usual care Diet, CEE 0.625 mg + MPA 2.5 mg	1.5%	1.9%	0.05	1.29[a]	0.4%	200[b]
WHI	5.2	16,608	Usual care Diet, CEE 0.625 mg	3.7%	3.3%	NS	9.0%	0.4%	250
CARDS	4	2,838	Atorvastatin 10 mg	9.0%	5.8%	0.001	37.0%	3.2%	32

AFCAPS/TexCAPS, Air Force/Texas Coronary Atherosclerosis Prevention Study (Downs et al., 1998); ALLHAT, Antihypertensive and Lipid-Lowering Treatment to Prevent Heart Attack Trial; approximately 13%–15% of patients had a history of coronary heart disease (CHD); events are CHD events only; ARR, absolute risk reduction; CARDS, Collaborative Atorvastatin Diabetes Study (presented at the 2004 American Diabetes Association meeting); CEE, conjugated equine estrogen; Helsinki, Helsinki Heart Study (Frick et al., 1987); LRC-CPPT, Lipid Research Clinics Coronary Primary Prevention Trial (Insull et al., 1984); MPA, medroxyprogesterone acetate; NA, not available; NNT, number needed to treat; Oslo, Oslo Study (Hjermann et al., 1988); RRR, relative risk reduction; WHI, Women's Health Initiative; WOSCOPS, West of Scotland Coronary Prevention Study (Shepherd et al., 1995).

[a]Hazard ratio. Risk of coronary heart disease was increased by 29%.

[b]Number needed to harm as CEE + MPA was worse than placebo.

TABLE 23-16 Secondary Prevention Trials with Lipid Lowering Drugs

Trial	Followup (y)	N	Treatment	Control Events	Treatment Events	*P* Value	RRR	ARR	NNT
VA-HIT	5.1	2,531	Gemfibrozil 1,200 mg	23.7%	17.3%	0.006	22%	4.4%	23
AVERT	1.5	341	Atorvastatin 80 mg	21%	13.0%	0.048	38%	8%	12
CARE	5	4,159	Pravastatin 40 mg	13.2%	10.2%	0.003	22.7%	3.0%	33
CDP	5	8,341	Niacin 3 g + clofibrate 1.8 g	20.9%	20.6%	NS	1.4%	0.3%	333
HERS	4.1	2,673	Estrogen 0.625 mg + progestin 2.5 mg	12.7%	12.5%	0.91	1.6%	0.2%	500
LIPID	7.4	3,806	Pravastatin 40 mg	9.8%	8.1%	<0.05	17.3%	1.7%	59
4S	5	4,444	Simvastatin 20 mg	11.5%	8.2%	0.0003	28.7%	3.3%	30
WHO	5.3	15,745	Clofibrate 1.6 g	3.9%	3.1%	<0.005	20.5%	0.8%	125
BIP	6.2	3,090	Placebo Bezafibrate 400 mg	15.0%	13.6%	0.26	9.3%	1.4%	72
TIMI-22	2	4,162	Pravastatin 40 mg Atorvastatin 80 mg	26.3% (P)	22.4% (A)	0.005	16%	3.9%	26
HPS	5	20,536	Simvastatin 40 mg	14.7%	12.9%	0.003	13%	1.8%	56
MIRACL		3,086	Atorvastatin 80 mg	17.4%	14.8%	0.048	16%	2.6%	39
PROSPER	3	5,804	Pravastatin 40 mg	16.2%	14.1%	0.014	24%	2.1%	48
SPARCL	4.0	4,731	Atorvastatin 80 mg	13.1%	11.2%	0.03	16%	2.2%	46
TNT	4.9	10,001	Atorvastatin 10 mg vs 80 mg	10.9%	8.7%	<0.001	22%	2.2%	46

4S, Scandinavian Simvastatin Survival Study (Pederson et al., 1994); ARR, absolute risk reduction; AVERT, Atorvastatin Versus Revascularization Treatments; BIP, Bezafibrate Infarction Prevention; CARE, Cholesterol and Recurrent Events (Melendez et al., 1996); CDP, Coronary Drug Project (Berge et al., 1975); HERS, Heart and Estrogen Replacement Study (Hulley et al., 1998); HPS, Heart Protection Study; results expressed as all-cause mortality (HPS Collaborative Group, 2002); LIPID, Long-Term Intervention with Pravastatin in Ischaemic Disease Study (MacMahon et al., 1995); MIRACL, Myocardial Ischemia Reduction with Aggressive Cholesterol Lowering (Schwartz et al., 2001); NNT, number needed to treat; PROSPER, prospective study of pravastatin in the elderly at risk; RRR, relative risk reduction; SPARCL, Stroke Prevention by Aggressive Reduction in Cholesterol Levels; TIMI-22, Thrombolysis in Myocardial Infarction study 22; also known as the PROVE-IT trial (Cannon et al., 2004); TNT, treatment to new targets; VA-HIT, Veterans Administration-High-Density Lipoprotein Cholestol (HDL-C) Intervention Trial; WHO, World Health Organization (Committee of Principal Investigators, 1978).

not significantly reduced by cholestyramine secondary to more accidents and violence in this group. The mean falls in total cholesterol and LDL-C in the cholestyramine group were 8% and 12% relative to levels in placebo-treated men, providing evidence that for every 1% reduction in cholesterol, a 2% decline in CHD mortality can be realized.

AFCAPS/TexCAPS was a primary prevention trial conducted in 6,605 men and women aged 57 to 63 years with average total cholesterol (<221 mg/dL) and LDL (<150 mg/dL) who were treated with lovastatin 20 to 40 mg/day for 5.2 years. The study showed a 37% reduction ($P < 0.001$) in the risk for first acute major coronary event (fatal or nonfatal MI, unstable angina, or sudden cardiac death).[90] The need for revascularization procedures was reduced by 33% ($P < 0.001$). The implications of this trial are enormous; based on these results, millions of "normal" people potentially could benefit from lipid lowering with statins. The number of patients who need to be treated (Table 23–15) for primary prevention ranged from 43 in the West of Scotland trial to 71 in the Helsinki Heart Study. This range is within the typical boundary used for treatment decisions and described previously; cost effectiveness is achieved routinely in patients with moderate to high risk. The Antihypertensive and Lipid-Lowering Treatment to Prevent Heart Attack Trial—Lipid Lowering Trial (ALLHAT-LLT) tested pravastatin 40 mg/day versus placebo in hypertensive patients with at least one CHD risk factor. Pravastatin did not reduce either all-cause mortality or CHD significantly compared with usual care in older participants with well-controlled hypertension and moderately elevated LDL-C. The results may be due to the modest differential in total cholesterol (9.6%) and LDL-C (16.7%) between pravastatin and usual care compared with prior statin trials supporting cardiovascular disease prevention.[130] The long-awaited WHI trial proved to be disappointing, showing no beneficial effects on CHD event reduction in the hormone replacement arm (conjugated equine estrogens + medroxyprogesterone) or the conjugated equine estrogens alone arm compared to placebo.[107,109] Women did experience greater risk for thromboembolism, a slight increase in breast cancer, and a reduced risk of hip fracture. Consequently, hormone replacement therapy can no longer be recommended for cardiovascular protection.[4] In the WISDOM trial, comparison of hormone therapy (n = 2,196) versus placebo (n = 2,189) revealed a significant increase in the number of major cardiovascular events (7 vs 0, $P = 0.016$) and venous thromboembolism (22 vs 3, hazard ratio 7.36, 95% confidence interval 2.20–24.60), confirming the findings of HERS and WHI. There were no statistically significant differences in the numbers of breast or other cancers, cerebrovascular events, fractures, and overall death.[111]

In the CDP, niacin significantly reduced definite nonfatal MI compared to placebo (10.1% vs 13.9%), whereas clofibrate did not reduce death from any cause or nonfatal or fatal MI during the 5-year followup.[131]

One of the most important studies published is 4S, a secondary intervention trial with a large number of patients.[132] Simvastatin 20–40 mg/day reduced LDL-C by 35% and reduced the risk of death from any cause by 30%. Coronary deaths were reduced with simvastatin (relative risk 0.58, confidence interval 0.46–0.73). Therapy was shown to be effective in women (18%–19% of patients enrolled) and in the elderly (≥60 years). The relative risk of death or major coronary event was reduced to a greater extent in the elderly than in younger patients. Death from noncardiovascular causes was similar for simvastatin and placebo (2.1% and 2.2%, respectively). The survival curves for simvastatin and placebo began to separate at 1 year and became more divergent with additional followup. 4S clearly demonstrates the benefit of cholesterol lowering and placates long-held fears of death from non-CHD causes. The Long-Term Intervention with Pravastatin in Ischemic Disease (LIPID) study (N = 7,498 men and 1,516 women) investigated the effect of pravastatin therapy over 6 years on CHD mortality in patients with prior MI or unstable angina and mean cholesterol level of 219 mg/dL.[133] Pravastatin reduced the risk of CHD mortality by 24% (8.3% vs 6.4%, $P = 0.0004$) and total mortality by 23% (14.1% vs 11.0%, $P = 0.00002$), reduced stroke by 20% (4.3% vs 3.5%, $P = 0.22$), and reduced the need for coronary artery bypass graft surgery (11.3% vs 8.9%, $P = 0.0001$) and percutaneous transluminal coronary angioplasty (5.3% vs 4.4%, $P = 0.04$).

The Veterans Administration High-Density Lipoprotein Intervention trial (VA-HIT) was a double-blinded trial that compared gemfibrozil (1,200 mg/day) with placebo in 2,531 men with CHD, HDL-C level ≤40 mg/dL, and LDL-C level ≤140 mg/dL.[134] The primary study outcome was nonfatal MI or death from coronary causes. Median followup was 5.1 years. At 1 year, mean HDL-C level was 6% higher, mean triglyceride level was 31% lower, and mean total cholesterol level was 4% lower in the gemfibrozil group than in the placebo group. LDL-C levels did not differ significantly between groups. A primary event occurred in 21.7% of the patients assigned to placebo and in 17.3% of the patients assigned to gemfibrozil. The overall reduction in the risk of an event was 4.4 percentage points, and the reduction in relative risk was 22% (P = 0.006). This trial presents the strongest evidence to date that raising HDL-C and lowering triglycerides levels reduce risk for CHD.

The Atorvastatin Versus Revascularization Treatment (AVERT) trial compared atorvastatin 80 mg/day with percutaneous transluminal coronary angioplasty.[135] The followup period was 18 months. Of the patients who received aggressive lipid-lowering treatment with atorvastatin, 13% had ischemic events compared to 21% of patients who underwent angioplasty. Thus, the incidence of ischemic events was 36% lower in the atorvastatin group over an 18-month period (P = 0.048, which was not statistically significant after adjustment for interim analyses). This reduction in events was the result of a smaller number of angioplasty procedures, coronary artery bypass operations, and hospitalizations for worsening angina (the most common end point). Compared to the patients who were treated with angioplasty and usual care, the patients who received atorvastatin had a significantly longer time to the first ischemic event (P = 0.03). In low-risk patients with stable CAD, aggressive lipid-lowering therapy is at least as effective as angioplasty and usual care in reducing the incidence of ischemic events.

The Prospective Study of Pravastatin in the Elderly at Risk (PROSPER) investigates men and women in the age range from 70 to 82 years at risk for cardiovascular disease and found that pravastatin 40 mg/day reduced CHD events by 24%, with no effect on cognitive function.[136] The more recent Thrombolysis in Myocardial Infarction 22 (TIMI-22) study (also known as PROVE-IT [Pravastatin or Atorvastatin Evaluation and Infection Therapy]), enrolled 4,162 patients who had been hospitalized for an acute coronary syndrome within the preceding 10 days and compared pravastatin 40 mg/day (standard therapy) with atorvastatin 80 mg/day (intensive therapy).[137] An intensive lipid-lowering statin regimen with atorvastatin 80 mg/day provided greater protection against death or major cardiovascular events than did a standard regimen. This study clearly points to "lower is better" for LDL concentration and likely will lead to revision in guideline goals to lower LDL levels. The Treating to New Targets (TNT) study assessed the efficacy and safety of lowering LDL-C levels to <100 mg/dL (2.6 mmol/L) in patients with stable CHD.[138,139] Intensive lipid-lowering therapy with atorvastatin 80 mg/day in patients with stable CHD provided significant clinical benefit beyond than treatment with atorvastatin 10 mg/day, providing additional evidence that intensive lipid lowering brings greater benefits.

Statins reduce the incidence of strokes among patients at increased risk for cardiovascular disease. Whether statins reduce the risk of stroke after a recent stroke or transient ischemic attack (TIA) was addressed by Stroke Prevention by Aggressive Reduction in Cholesterol Levels (SPARCL). During a median followup of 4.9 years, 265 patients (11.2%) who received atorvastatin 80 mg/day and 311 patients (13.1%) who received placebo had a fatal or nonfatal stroke (5-year absolute reduction in risk 2.2%, adjusted hazard ratio 0.84, 95% confidence interval 0.71–0.99, P = 0.03; unadjusted P = 0.05).[140]

CLINICAL CONTROVERSIES

The CETP inhibitor torcetrapib was associated with a substantial increase in HDL-C and decrease in LDL-C. It also was associated with an increase in blood pressure and no significant decrease in the progression of coronary atherosclerosis. The lack of efficacy may be related to the mechanism of action of this drug class or to molecule-specific adverse effects. Other means of raising HDL-C (HDL mimetics, which include apolipoprotein A-I mutants and peptide mimetics of apolipoprotein A-I and HDL Milano A, a synthetic form of HDL) still hold hope of HDL modification leading to a reduction in clinical events.

The enzyme ACAT esterifies cholesterol in a variety of tissues. In some animal models, ACAT inhibitors have antiatherosclerotic effects. However, when tested in clinical trials, ACAT inhibition was not an effective strategy for limiting atherosclerosis and may promote atherogenesis.[141]

Statins differ in their pharmacokinetic properties and in pleiotropic effects (i.e., nonlipid lowering). The contribution of lipid lowering alone (a class effect) versus other effects (antiinflammatory, antithrombotic) is controversial.

Proteinuria has been associated with high-dose rosuvastatin therapy (40 mg/day), but a review of a clinical trial database revealed an increase in the estimated glomerular filtration rate for rosuvastatin-treated patients that was consistent across all major demographic and clinical subgroups of interest, including patients with baseline proteinuria, patients with baseline estimated glomerular filtration rate <60 mL/min/1.73 m^2, and patients with hypertension and/or diabetes.[142]

The role of nontraditional risk factors (high-sensitivity C-reactive protein, homocysteine) is being studied and may lead to recommendations for the use of these tests in patient evaluation.

EVALUATION OF THERAPEUTIC OUTCOMES

Short-term evaluation of therapy for hyperlipidemia is based on response to diet and drug treatment as measured in the clinical laboratory by total cholesterol, LDL-C, HDL-C, and triglycerides for patients being treated for primary intervention, as well as on response to secondary intervention. The followup interval is dependent on the severity of illness, and patients with known CAD or multiple risk factors should be monitored more closely. Less commonly used laboratory measurements include C-reactive protein, homocysteine, apolipoprotein B, and lipoprotein(a) levels. Because many patients being treated for primary hyperlipidemia have no symptoms and may not have any clinical manifestations of a genetic lipid disorder such as xanthomas or eruptions, monitoring and outcome are solely laboratory based. In patients treated for secondary intervention, symptoms of atherosclerotic cardiovascular disease (e.g., angina or intermittent claudication) may improve over months to years. In patients have xanthomas or other external manifestations of hyperlipidemia, the lesions should regress with therapy. Lipid measurements should be obtained in the fasted state to minimize interference from chylomicrons. Once the patient is stable, monitoring is needed at intervals of 6 months to 1 year. The goals for LDL-C and HDL-C are listed in Tables 23–8 and 23–9.

Patients with multiple risk factors and established CHD should be monitored and evaluated for progress in managing their other risk factors, such as hypertension, smoking cessation, exercise and weight control, and glycemic control if diabetic. The goals are to maintain blood pressure <130/80 mm Hg, especially for patients with diabetes or renal insufficiency, stop smoking, maintain an ideal body weight, exercise for at least 20 minutes per day at least three times per week, and keep plasma glucose concentration <100 mg/dL (threshold for glucose intolerance). Invasive evaluation, such as cardiac catheterization, is useful in patients with established CHD and typically is used for planning revascularization rather than monitoring of lipid-lowering therapy.

Evaluation of dietary therapy is part of the outcome evaluation for treating hyperlipidemia, and the assistance of a dietitian is recommended. Use of diet diaries and recall survey instruments enables systematic collection of information about diet and may improve patient adherence to dietary recommendations. Patients undergoing resin therapy should have a fasting lipoprotein profile checked every 4 to 8 weeks until a stable dose is achieved; triglycerides should be checked at stable dose to ensure levels have not increased. Niacin requires baseline liver function tests, and uric acid and glucose concentrations; repeat tests are appropriate at doses of 1,000–1,500 mg/day. Myopathy or diabetes-like symptoms should be investigated and may require CK or glucose determinations; more frequent monitoring in diabetics may be necessary. A fasting lipoprotein profile 4 to 8 weeks after the initial dose or after dose changes with statins is appropriate. Liver function tests should be obtained at baseline and periodically thereafter based on package insert information; recognized experts believe that monitoring for hepatotoxicity and myopathy should be symptom triggered.[56,61] Ezetimibe requires little specific monitoring.

REFERENCES

1. Expert Panel on Detection E, and Treatment of High Blood Cholesterol in Adults. Executive summary of the third report of the National Cholesterol Education Program (NCEP) Expert Panel on Detection, Evaluation and Treatment of High Blood Cholesterol in Adults (Adult Treatment Panel III). JAMA 2001;285:2486–2497.
2. Grundy SM, Cleeman JI, Merz CN, et al. Implications of recent clinical trials for the National Cholesterol Education Program Adult Treatment Panel III guidelines [published erratum appears in Circulation 2004;110:763]. Circulation 2004;110:227–239.
3. Smith SC Jr, Allen J, Blair SN, et al. AHA/ACC guidelines for secondary prevention for patients with coronary and other atherosclerotic vascular disease: 2006 update: Endorsed by the National Heart, Lung, and Blood Institute [erratum appears in Circulation 2006;113:e847]. Circulation 2006;113:2363–2372.
4. Mosca L, Banka CL, Benjamin EJ, et al. Evidence-based guidelines for cardiovascular disease prevention in women: 2007 update. Circulation 2007;115:1481–1501.
5. Ford ES, Mokdad AH, Giles WH, Mensah GA. Serum total cholesterol concentrations and awareness, treatment, and control of hypercholesterolemia among US adults: Findings from the National Health and Nutrition Examination Survey, 1999 to 2000. Circulation 2003;107:2185–2189.
6. Rosamond W, Flegal K, Friday G, et al. Heart disease and stroke statistics—2007 update: A report from the American Heart Association Statistics Committee and Stroke Statistics Subcommittee. Circulation 2007;115:6.
7. Arnett DK, Jacobs DR Jr, Luepker RV, Blackburn H, Armstrong C, Claas SA. Twenty-year trends in serum cholesterol, hypercholesterolemia, and cholesterol medication use: The Minnesota Heart Survey, 1980–1982 to 2000–2002. Circulation 2005;112:3884–3891.
8. Foley KA, Denke MA, Kamal-Bahl S, et al. The impact of physician attitudes and beliefs on treatment decisions: Lipid therapy in high-risk patients. Med Care 2006;44:421–428.
9. Carroll MD, Lacher DA, Sorlie PD, et al. Trends in serum lipids and lipoproteins of adults, 1960–2002. JAMA 2005;294:1773–1781.
10. Menotti A, Lanti M, Nedeljkovic S, Nissinen A, Kafatos A, Kromhout D. The relationship of age, blood pressure, serum cholesterol and smoking habits with the risk of typical and atypical coronary heart disease death in the European cohorts of the Seven Countries Study. Int J Cardiol 2006;106:157–163.
11. Kannel WB. Range of serum cholesterol values in the population developing coronary artery disease. Am J Cardiol 1995;76:69C77C.
12. Rader DJ. Mechanisms of disease: HDL metabolism as a target for novel therapies. Nat Clin Pract Cardiovasc Med 2007;4:102–109.
13. Jeppesen J, Hein HO, Suadicani P, Gyntelberg F. Triglyceride concentration and ischemic heart disease: An eight-year follow-up in the Copenhagen Male Study. Circulation 1998;97:1029–1036.
14. Huttunen JK, Manninen V, Manttari M, et al. The Helsinki Heart Study: Central findings and clinical implications. Ann Med 1991;23:155–159.
15. Austin MA, McKnight B, Edwards KL, et al. Cardiovascular disease mortality in familial forms of hypertriglyceridemia: A 20-year prospective study. Circulation 2000;101:2777–2782.
16. Ganong WF. Pathophysiology of Disease: An Introduction to Clinical Medicine, 5th ed. In: McPhee SJ, Ganong WF, eds. New York: McGraw Hill, 2006, *www.accessmedicine.com/content.aspx?aID=2088359*.
17. Nissen SE, Tardif JC, Nicholls SJ, et al. Effect of torcetrapib on the progression of coronary atherosclerosis. N Engl J Med 2007;356:1304–1316.
18. Libby P, Aikawa M, Jain MK. Vascular endothelium and atherosclerosis. Handbook Exp Pharmacol 2006;176:285–306.
19. Miller DT, Ridker PM, Libby P, Kwiatkowski DJ. Atherosclerosis: The path from genomics to therapeutics. J Am Coll Cardiol 2007;49:1589–1599.
20. Ridker PM, Cannon CP, Morrow D, et al. C-reactive protein levels and outcomes after statin therapy. N Engl J Med 2005;352:20–28.
21. Kujiraoka T, Hattori H, Miwa Y, et al. Serum apolipoprotein j in health, coronary heart disease and type 2 diabetes mellitus. J Atheroscler Thromb 2006;13:314–322.
22. Lavie L, Vishnevsky A, Lavie P. Evidence for lipid peroxidation in obstructive sleep apnea. Sleep 2004;27:123–128.
23. Huang CY, Wu TC, Lin WT, et al. Effects of simvastatin withdrawal on serum matrix metalloproteinases in hypercholesterolaemic patients. Eur J Clin Invest 2006;36:76–84.
24. Suviolahti E, Lilja HE, Pajukanta P. Unraveling the complex genetics of familial combined hyperlipidemia. Ann Med 2006;38:337–351.
25. Harris WS, von Schacky C. The omega-3 index: A new risk factor for death from coronary heart disease. Prevent Med 2004;39:212–220.
26. Buse JB, Ginsberg HN, Bakris GL, et al. Primary prevention of cardiovascular diseases in people with diabetes mellitus: A scientific statement from the American Heart Association and the American Diabetes Association. Diabetes Care 2007;30:162–172.
27. Grundy SM, Cleeman JI, Daniels SR, et al. Diagnosis and management of the metabolic syndrome: An American Heart Association/National Heart, Lung, and Blood Institute Scientific Statement [erratum appears in Circulation 2005;112:e297]. Circulation 2005;112:2735–2752.
28. Grundy SM, Pasternak R, Greenland P, Smith S Jr, Fuster V. AHA/ACC scientific statement: Assessment of cardiovascular risk by use of multiple-risk-factor assessment equations: A statement for healthcare professionals from the American Heart Association and the American College of Cardiology. J Am Coll Cardiol 1999;34:1348–1359.
29. Grundy SM, Cleeman JI, Merz CN, et al. A summary of implications of recent clinical trials for the National Cholesterol Education Program Adult Treatment Panel III guidelines. Arterioscler Thromb Vasc Biol 2004;24:1329–1330.
30. Grundy SM, Cleeman JI, Merz CN, et al. Implications of recent clinical trials for the National Cholesterol Education Program Adult Treatment Panel III Guidelines. J Am Coll Cardiol 2004;44:720–732.
31. Singh IM, Shishehbor MH, Ansell BJ. High density lipoprotein as a therapeutic target. A systematic review. JAMA 2007;298:786–798.
32. American Academy of Pediatrics. Committee on North American Academy of Pediatrics. Committee on Nutrition. Cholesterol in childhood. Pediatrics 1998;101:141–147.
33. Davis V, Schatz D, Winter W. Pediatric lipid disorders in clinical practice. eMedicine 2006, *http://www.emedicine.com/ped/topic2787.htm #section~pictures*.
34. Strong JP, Malcom GT, Oalmann MC, Wissler RW. The PDAY Study: Natural history, risk factors, and pathobiology. Pathobiological Determinants of Atherosclerosis in Youth. Ann N Y Acad Sci 1997;811:226–235.
35. Lauer RM, Obarzanek E, Hunsberger SA, et al. Efficacy and safety of lowering dietary intake of total fat, saturated fat, and cholesterol in children with elevated LDL cholesterol: The Dietary Intervention Study in Children. Am J Clin Nutr 2000;72:1332S–1342S.
36. Van Horn L, Obarzanek E, Friedman LA, Gernhofer N, Barton B. Children's adaptations to a fat-reduced diet: The Dietary Intervention Study in Children (DISC). Pediatrics 2005;115:1723–1733.
37. McCrindle BW, Ose L, Marais AD. Efficacy and safety of atorvastatin in children and adolescents with familial hypercholesterolemia or severe hyperlipidemia: A multicenter, randomized, placebo-controlled trial. J Pediatr 2003;143:74–80.
38. Wiegman A, Hutten BA, de Groot E, et al. Efficacy and safety of statin therapy in children with familial hypercholesterolemia: A randomized controlled trial. JAMA 2004;292:331–337.
39. Trejo-Gutierrez JF, Fletcher G. Impact of exercise on blood lipids and lipoproteins. J Clin Lipidol 2007;1:175–181.
40. Williams MA, Haskell WL, Ades PA, et al. Resistance exercise in individuals with and without cardiovascular disease: 2007 update: A scientific statement from the American Heart Association Council on Clinical Cardiology and Council on Nutrition, Physical Activity, and Metabolism. Circulation 2007;116:572–584.
41. Eckel RH, Borra S, Lichtenstein AH, Yin-Piazza SY, Trans Fat Conference Planning Group. Understanding the complexity of trans fatty acid

reduction in the American diet: American Heart Association Trans Fat Conference 2006: Report of the Trans Fat Conference Planning Group. Circulation 2007;115:2231–2246.

42. American Heart Association Nutrition C, Lichtenstein AH, Appel LJ, et al. Diet and lifestyle recommendations revision 2006: A scientific statement from the American Heart Association Nutrition Committee [erratum appears in Circulation 2006;114:e27]. Circulation 2006;114:82–96.
43. Sacks FM, Lichtenstein A, Van Horn L, et al. Soy protein, isoflavones, and cardiovascular health: An American Heart Association Science Advisory for professionals from the Nutrition Committee. Circulation 2006;113:1034–1044.
44. Gidding SS, Dennison BA, Birch LL, et al. Dietary recommendations for children and adolescents: A guide for practitioners: Consensus statement from the American Heart Association [erratum appears in Circulation 2005;112:2375]. Circulation 2005;112:2061–2075.
45. Grundy SM, Cleeman JI, Daniels SR, et al. Diagnosis and management of the metabolic syndrome: An American Heart Association/National Heart, Lung, and Blood Institute scientific statement. Curr Opin Cardiol 2006;21:1–6.
46. Assmann G, Guerra R, Fox G, et al. Harmonizing the definition of the metabolic syndrome: Comparison of the criteria of the Adult Treatment Panel III and the International Diabetes Federation in United States American and European populations. Am J Cardiol 2007;99:541–548.
47. Shrestha S, Volek JS, Udani J, et al. A combination therapy including psyllium and plant sterols lowers LDL cholesterol by modifying lipoprotein metabolism in hypercholesterolemic individuals. J Nutr 2006;136:2492–2497.
48. Petchetti L, Frishman WH, Petrillo R, Raju K. Nutriceuticals in cardiovascular disease: Psyllium. Cardiol Rev 2007;15:116–122.
49. He K, Song Y, Davigius ML, et al. Accumulated evidence on fish consumption and coronary heart disease mortality: A meta-analysis of cohort studies. Circulation 2004;109:2705–2711.
50. von Schacky C, Harris WS. Cardiovascular benefits of omega-3 fatty acids. Cardiovasc Res 2007;73:310–315.
51. McKenney JM, Sica D. Role of prescription omega-3 fatty acids in the treatment of hypertriglyceridemia. Pharmacotherapy 2007;27:715–728.
52. Bhattacharya S. Therapy and clinical trials: Plant sterols and stanols in management of hypercholesterolemia: Where are we now? Curr Opin Lipidol 2006;17:98–100.
53. Berthold HK, Unverdorben S, Degenhardt R, Bulitta M, Gouni-Berthold I. Effect of policosanol on lipid levels among patients with hypercholesterolemia or combined hyperlipidemia: A randomized controlled trial. JAMA 2006;295:2262–2269.
54. Baigent C, Keech A, Kearney PM, et al. Efficacy and safety of cholesterol-lowering treatment: Prospective meta-analysis of data from 90,056 participants in 14 randomised trials of statins. Lancet 2005;366:1267–1278.
55. Link JJ, Rohatgi A, de Lemos JA. HDL cholesterol: Physiology, pathophysiology, and management. Curr Probl Cardiol 2007;32:268–314.
56. McKenney JM. Introduction. Report of the National Lipid Association's Safety Task Force: The nonstatins. Am J Cardiol 2007;99:1C–58C.
57. Shitara Y, Sugiyama Y. Pharmacokinetic and pharmacodynamic alterations of 3-hydroxy-3-methylglutaryl coenzyme A (HMG-CoA) reductase inhibitors: Drug-drug interactions and interindividual differences in transporter and metabolic enzyme functions. Pharmacol Ther 2006; 112:71–105.
58. Jones P, Kafonek S, Laurora I, Hunninghake D. Comparative dose efficacy study of atorvastatin versus simvastatin, pravastatin, lovastatin, and fluvastatin in patients with hypercholesterolemia. (The CURVES Study). Am J Cardiol 1998;81:582–587.
59. Robinson JG, Davidson MH. Combination therapy with ezetimibe and simvastatin to achieve aggressive LDL reduction. Exp Rev Cardiovasc Ther 2006;4:461–476.
60. Davidson MH, Robinson JG. Safety of aggressive lipid management. J Am Coll Cardiol 2007;49:1753–1762.
61. McKenney JM, Davidson MH, Jacobson TA, Guyton JR, National Lipid Association Statin Safety Assessment Task Force. Final conclusions and recommendations of the National Lipid Association Statin Safety Assessment Task Force. Am J Cardiol 2006;97:17.
62. Alsheikh-Ali AA, Maddukuri PV, Han H, Karas RH. Effect of the magnitude of lipid lowering on risk of elevated liver enzymes, rhabdomyolysis, and cancer: Insights from large randomized statin trials. J Am Coll Cardiol 2007;50:409–418.
63. Edwards IR, Star K, Kiuru A. Statins, neuromuscular degenerative disease and an amyotrophic lateral sclerosis-like syndrome: An analysis of individual case safety reports from vigibase. Drug Saf 2007;30:515–525.
64. Mangravite LM, Thorn CF, Krauss RM. Clinical implications of pharmacogenomics of statin treatment. Pharmacogenomics J 2006;6:360–374.
65. McPherson R. Comparative effects of simvastatin and cholestyramine on plasma lipoproteins and CETP in humans. Can J Clin Pharmacol 1999;6:85–90.
66. Tsuyuki RT, Bungard RJ. Poor adherence with hypolipidemic drugs: A lost opportunity. Pharmacotherapy 2001;21:576–582.
67. Tsuyuki RT, Olson KL, Dubyk AM, Schindel TJ, Johnson JA. Effect of community pharmacist intervention on cholesterol levels in patients at high risk of cardiovascular events: The Second Study of Cardiovascular Risk Intervention by Pharmacists (SCRIP-plus). Am J Med 2004;116:130–133.
68. McCrindle BW, O'Neill MB, Cullen-Dean G, Helden E. Acceptability and compliance with two forms of cholestyramine in the treatment of hypercholesterolemia in children: A randomized, crossover trial. J Pediatr 1997;130:266–273.
69. Zhang Y, Schmidt RJ, Foxworthy P, et al. Niacin mediates lipolysis in adipose tissue through its G-protein coupled receptor HM74A. Biochem Biophys Res Commun 2005;334:729–732.
70. Carlson LA. Nicotinic acid: The broad-spectrum lipid drug. A 50th anniversary review. J Intern Med 2005;258:94–114.
71. Shepherd J, Betteridge J, Van Gaal L, European Consensus P. Nicotinic acid in the management of dyslipidaemia associated with diabetes and metabolic syndrome: A position paper developed by a European Consensus Panel. Curr Med Res Opin 2005;21:665–682.
72. Stern RH. The role of nicotinic acid metabolites in flushing and hepatoxicity. J Clin Lipidol 2007;1:191–193.
73. Lai E, De Lepeleire I, Crumley TM, et al. Suppression of niacin-induced vasodilation with an antagonist to prostaglandin D2 receptor subtype 1. Clin Pharmacol Ther 2007;81:849–857.
74. McKenney JM, Jones PH, Bays HE, et al. Comparative effects on lipid levels of combination therapy with a statin and extended-release niacin or ezetimibe versus a statin alone (the COMPELL study). Atherosclerosis 2007;192:432–437.
75. McKenney J. Niacin for dyslipidemia: Considerations in product selection. Am J Health Syst Pharm 2003;60:995–1005.
76. Guyton JR, Bays HE. Safety considerations with niacin therapy. Am J Cardiol 2007;99:19.
77. Davidson MH, Armani A, McKenney JM, Jacobson TA. Safety considerations with fibrate therapy. Am J Cardiol 2007;99:19.
78. Sveger T, Flodmark CE, Nordborg K, Nilsson-Ehle P, Borgfors N. Hereditary dyslipidaemias and combined risk factors in children with a family history of premature coronary artery disease. Arch Dis Child 2000;82:292–296.
79. Grundy SM, Vega GL, Yuan Z, Battisti WP, Brady WE, Palmisano J. Effectiveness and tolerability of simvastatin plus fenofibrate for combined hyperlipidemia (the SAFARI trial) [erratum appears in Am J Cardiol 2006;98:427–428]. Am J Cardiol 2005;95:462–468.
80. Capell WH, Eckel RH. Treatment of hypertriglyceridemia. Curr Diabetes Rep 2006;6:230–240.
81. Yuan G, Al-Shali KZ, Hegele RA. Hypertriglyceridemia: Its etiology, effects and treatment. CMAJ 2007;176:1113–1120.
82. Elam MB, Hunninghake DB, Davis KB, et al. Effect of niacin on lipid and lipoprotein levels and glycemic control in patients with diabetes and peripheral arterial disease: The ADMIT study: A randomized trial. Arterial Disease Multiple Intervention Trial. JAMA 2000;284:1263–1270.
83. McKenney JM, Sica D. Prescription omega-3 fatty acids for the treatment of hypertriglyceridemia. Am J Health Syst Pharm 2007;64:595–605.
84. Oh RC, Lanier JB. Management of hypertriglyceridemia. Am Fam Physician 2007;75:1365–1371.
85. McKenney J. New perspectives on the use of niacin in the treatment of lipid disorders. Arch Intern Med 2004;164:697–705.
86. Gadi R, Samaha FF. Dyslipidemia in type 2 diabetes mellitus. Curr Diabetes Rep 2007;7:228–234.
87. Tan KC. Management of dyslipidemia in the metabolic syndrome. Cardiovasc Hematol Disord Drug Targets 2007;7:99–108.

88. Garg A, Simha V. Update on dyslipidemia. J Clin Endocrinol Metab 2007;92:1581–1589.
89. Shepherd J, Cobbe SM, Ford I, et al. Prevention of coronary heart disease with pravastatin in men with hypercholesterolemia. West of Scotland Coronary Prevention Study Group. N Engl J Med 1995;333:1301–1307.
90. Downs JRMD, Clearfield MDO, Weis SDO, et al. Primary prevention of acute coronary events with lovastatin in men and women with average cholesterol levels: Results of AFCAPS/TexCAPS. JAMA May 1998;279:1615–1622.
91. Sacks FM, Pfeffer MA, Moye LA, et al. The effect of pravastatin on coronary events after myocardial infarction in patients with average cholesterol levels. N Engl J Med 1996;335:1001–1009.
92. Anonymous. Design and baseline results of the Scandinavian Simvastatin Survival Study of patients with stable angina and/or previous myocardial infarction. Am J Cardiol 1993;71:393–400.
93. Colhoun HM, Betteridge DJ, Durrington PN, et al. Primary prevention of cardiovascular disease with atorvastatin in type 2 diabetes in the Collaborative Atorvastatin Diabetes Study (CARDS): Multicentre randomised placebo-controlled trial. Lancet 2004;364:685–696.
94. Collins R, Armitage J, Parish S, Sleight P, Peto R, Heart Protection Study Collaborative Group. Effects of cholesterol-lowering with simvastatin on stroke and other major vascular events in 20536 people with cerebrovascular disease or other high-risk conditions. Lancet 2004;363:757–767.
95. Anonymous. Effect of fenofibrate on progression of coronary-artery disease in type 2 diabetes: The Diabetes Atherosclerosis Intervention Study, a randomised study. Lancet 2001;357:905–910.
96. Backes JM, Gibson CA, Ruisinger JF, Moriarty PM. Fibrates: What have we learned in the past 40 years? Pharmacotherapy 2007;27:412–424.
97. Grundy SM, Vega GL, McGovern ME, et al. Efficacy, safety, and tolerability of once-daily niacin for the treatment of dyslipidemia associated with type 2 diabetes: Results of the assessment of diabetes control and evaluation of the efficacy of Niaspan trial. Arch Intern Med 2002;162:1568–1576.
98. Davidson MH, Kurlandsky SB, Kleinpell RM, Maki KC. Lipid management and the elderly. Prevent Cardiol 2003;6:128–133.
99. Mazza A, Tikhonoff V, Schiavon L, Casiglia E. Triglycerides + high-density-lipoprotein-cholesterol dyslipidaemia, a coronary risk factor in elderly women: The CArdiovascular STudy in the ELderly. Intern Med J 2005;35:604–610.
100. Anonymous. Randomised trial of cholesterol lowering in 4444 patients with coronary heart disease: The Scandinavian Simvastatin Survival Study (4S). Lancet 1994;344:1383–1389.
101. Berger AK, Duval SJ, Armstrong C, Jacobs DR Jr, Luepker RV. Contemporary diagnosis and management of hypercholesterolemia in elderly acute myocardial infarction patients: A population-based study. Am J Geriatr Cardiol 2007;16:15–23.
102. Hatzigeorgiou C, Jackson JL. Hydroxymethylglutaryl-coenzyme A reductase inhibitors and osteoporosis: A meta-analysis. Osteoporos Int 2005;16:990–998.
103. Blue Cross Blue Shield A, Technology Evaluation C. Special report: The efficacy and safety of statins in the elderly. Technology Evaluation Center Assessment Program. Executive Summary 2007;21:1–3.
104. Anonymous. Pravastatin benefits elderly patients: Results of PROSPER study. Cardiovasc J S Afr 2003;14:48.
105. Heart Protection Study Collaborative Group. MRC/BHF Heart Protection Study of cholesterol lowering with simvastatin in 20,536 high-risk individuals: A randomised placebo-controlled trial [summary for patients in Curr Cardiol Rep 2002;4:486–7]. Lancet 2002;360:7–22.
106. Abate N. Obesity and cardiovascular disease. Pathogenetic role of the metabolic syndrome and therapeutic implications. J Diabetes Complicat 2000;14:154–174.
107. Hulley S, Grady D, Bush T, et al. Randomized trial of estrogen plus progestin for secondary prevention of coronary heart disease in postmenopausal women. Heart and Estrogen/progestin Replacement Study (HERS) Research Group. JAMA 1998;280:605–613.
108. Rossouw JE, Prentice RL, Manson JE, et al. Postmenopausal hormone therapy and risk of cardiovascular disease by age and years since menopause. JAMA 2007;297:1465–1477.
109. Anderson GL, Limacher M, Assaf AR, et al. Effects of conjugated equine estrogen in postmenopausal women with hysterectomy: The Women's Health Initiative randomized controlled trial. JAMA 2004;291:1701–1712.
110. Wassertheil-Smoller S, Hendrix SL, Limacher M, et al. Effect of estrogen plus progestin on stroke in postmenopausal women: The Women's Health Initiative: A randomized trial. JAMA 2003;289:2673–2684.
111. Vickers MR, MacLennan AH, Lawton B, et al. Main morbidities recorded in the Women's International Study of Long Duration Oestrogen after Menopause (WISDOM): A randomised controlled trial of hormone replacement therapy in postmenopausal women. BMJ 2007;335:239.
112. Clauss SB, Holmes KW, Hopkins P, et al. Efficacy and safety of lovastatin therapy in adolescent girls with heterozygous familial hypercholesterolemia. Pediatrics 2005;116:682–688.
113. de Jongh S, Ose L, Szamosi T, et al. Efficacy and safety of statin therapy in children with familial hypercholesterolemia: A randomized, double-blind, placebo-controlled trial with simvastatin. Circulation 2002;106:2231–2237.
114. Toto RD, Grundy SM, Vega GL. Pravastatin treatment of very low density, intermediate density and low density lipoproteins in hypercholesterolemia and combined hyperlipidemia secondary to the nephrotic syndrome. Am J Nephrol 2000;20:12–17.
115. Campese VM, Park J. HMG-CoA reductase inhibitors and the kidney. Kidney Int 2007;71:1215–1222.
116. Kwan BC, Kronenberg F, Beddhu S, Cheung AK. Lipoprotein metabolism and lipid management in chronic kidney disease. J Am Soc Nephrol 2007;18:1246–1261.
117. Baber U, Toto RD, de Lemos JA. Statins and cardiovascular risk reduction in patients with chronic kidney disease and end-stage renal failure. Am Heart J 2007;153:471–477.
118. Ozsoy RC, van Leuven SI, Kastelein JJ, Arisz L, Koopman MG. The dyslipidemia of chronic renal disease: Effects of statin therapy. Curr Opin Lipidol 2006;17:659–666.
119. D'Amico G. Statins and renal diseases: From primary prevention to renal replacement therapy. J Am Soc Nephrol 2006;17.
120. Samuelsson O, Attman PO, Knight-Gibson C, et al. Effect of gemfibrozil on lipoprotein abnormalities in chronic renal insufficiency: A controlled study in human chronic renal disease. Nephron 1997;75:286–294.
121. Peterson AM, McGhan WF. Pharmacoeconomic impact of non-compliance with statins. Pharmacoeconomics 2005;23:13–25.
122. Tarraga-Lopez PJ, Celada-Rodriguez A, Cerdan-Oliver M, et al. A pharmacoeconomic evaluation of statins in the treatment of hypercholesterolaemia in the primary care setting in Spain [erratum appears in Pharmacoeconomics 2006;24:106]. Pharmacoeconomics 2005;23:275–287.
123. Johannesson M, Jonsson B, Kjekshus J, Olsson AG, Pedersen TR, Wedel H. Cost effectiveness of simvastatin treatment to lower cholesterol levels in patients with coronary heart disease. Scandinavian Simvastatin Survival Study Group. N Engl J Med 1997;336:332–336.
124. Caro J, Klittich W, McGuire A, et al. The West of Scotland coronary prevention study: Economic benefit analysis of primary prevention with pravastatin. BMJ 1997;315:1577–1582.
125. Schectman G, Wolff N, Byrd JC, Hiatt JG, Hartz A. Physician extenders for cost-effective management of hypercholesterolemia. J Gen Intern Med 1996;11:277–286.
126. Bluml BM, McKenney JM, Cziraky MJ. Pharmaceutical care services and results in project ImPACT: Hyperlipidemia. J Am Pharm Assoc 2000;40:157–165.
127. Charrois TL, Johnson JA, Blitz S, Tsuyuki RT. Relationship between number, timing, and type of pharmacist interventions and patient outcomes. Am J Health Syst Pharm 2005;62:1798–1801.
128. Yamada C, Johnson JA, Robertson P, Pearson G, Tsuyuki RT. Long-term impact of a community pharmacist intervention on cholesterol levels in patients at high risk for cardiovascular events: Extended follow-up of the second study of cardiovascular risk intervention by pharmacists (SCRIP-plus). Pharmacotherapy 2005;25:110–115.
129. Anonymous. The Lipid Research Clinics Coronary Primary Prevention Trial results. I. Reduction in incidence of coronary heart disease. JAMA 1984;251:351–364.
130. ALLHAT Officers and Coordinators for the ALLHAT Collaborative Research Group. The Antihypertensive and Lipid-Lowering Treatment to Prevent Heart Attack Trial. Major outcomes in moderately hypercholesterolemic, hypertensive patients randomized to pravastatin vs usual

care: The Antihypertensive and Lipid-Lowering Treatment to Prevent Heart Attack Trial (ALLHAT-LLT). JAMA 2002;288:2998–3007.

131. Canner PL, Berge KG, Wenger NK, et al. Fifteen year mortality in Coronary Drug Project patients: Long-term benefit with niacin. J Am Coll Cardiol 1986;8:1245–1255.
132. Strandberg TE, Pyorala K, Cook TJ, et al. Mortality and incidence of cancer during 10-year follow-up of the Scandinavian Simvastatin Survival Study (4S). Lancet 2004;364:771–777.
133. Tonkin AM, Colquhoun D, Emberson J, et al. Effects of pravastatin in 3260 patients with unstable angina: Results from the LIPID study. Lancet 2000;356:1871–1875.
134. Rubins HB, Robins SJ, Collins D. The Veterans Affairs High-Density Lipoprotein Intervention Trial: Baseline characteristics of normocholesterolemic men with coronary artery disease and low levels of high-density lipoprotein cholesterol. Veterans Affairs Cooperative Studies Program High-Density Lipoprotein Intervention Trial Study Group. Am J Cardiol 1996;78:572–575.
135. Pitt B, Waters D, Brown WV, et al. Aggressive lipid-lowering therapy compared with angioplasty in stable coronary artery disease. Atorvastatin versus Revascularization Treatment Investigators. N Engl J Med 1999;341:70–76.
136. Shepherd J, Blauw GJ, Murphy MB, et al. Pravastatin in elderly individuals at risk of vascular disease (PROSPER): A randomised controlled trial. Lancet 2002;360:1623–1630.
137. Cannon CP, Braunwald E, McCabe CH, et al. Intensive versus moderate lipid lowering with statins after acute coronary syndromes [erratum appears in N Engl J Med 2006;354:778]. N Engl J Med 2004;350:1495–1504.
138. LaRosa JC, Grundy SM, Waters DD, et al. Intensive lipid lowering with atorvastatin in patients with stable coronary disease. N Engl J Med 2005;352:1425–1435.
139. Waters DD, LaRosa JC, Barter P, et al. Effects of high-dose atorvastatin on cerebrovascular events in patients with stable coronary disease in the TNT (Treating to New Targets) study. J Am Coll Cardiol 2006;48:1793–1799.
140. Amarenco P, Bogousslavsky J, Callahan A 3rd, et al. High-dose atorvastatin after stroke or transient ischemic attack. N Engl J Med 2006;355:549–559.
141. Nissen SE, Tuzcu EM, Brewer HB, et al. Effect of ACAT inhibition on the progression of coronary atherosclerosis [erratum appears in N Engl J Med 2006;355:638]. N Engl J Med 2006;354:1253–1263.
142. Vidt DG, Harris S, McTaggart F, Ditmarsch M, Sager PT, Sorof JM. Effect of short-term rosuvastatin treatment on estimated glomerular filtration rate. Am J Cardiol 2006;97:1602–1606.

CHAPTER 24 Peripheral Arterial Disease

BARBARA J. HOEBEN AND ROBERT L. TALBERT

KEY CONCEPTS

1. The prevalence of peripheral arterial disease is dependent upon patient age and the presence of traditional risk factors for cardiovascular disease. Many patients are undiagnosed and are at substantial risk for coronary and cerebrovascular events.

2. The clinical presentation of peripheral arterial disease is variable and includes a range of symptoms. The two most common characteristics of peripheral arterial disease are intermittent claudication and pain at rest in the lower extremities.

3. The ankle–brachial index (ABI) is a simple, noninvasive, quantitative test that has proved to be a highly sensitive and specific tool in the diagnosis of peripheral arterial disease.

4. As with any atherosclerotic condition, several risk factors play an important role in the morbidity and mortality of peripheral vascular disease. Many of these risk factors can be modified with the help of various nonpharmacologic and pharmacologic interventions.

5. Nonpharmacologic interventions, such as smoking cessation and walking exercise programs, can positively impact several of the pathophysiologic abnormalities present in patients with peripheral arterial disease.

6. Data proving that antiplatelet therapies can prevent or delay the progression of peripheral arterial disease are unavailable. However, aspirin therapy has repeatedly been proven to significantly reduce serious vascular events in these "high-risk" patients and, in the absence of contraindications, is highly recommended.

7. Patients who continue to experience severe intermittent claudication even after implementation of appropriate exercise therapy and therapeutic lifestyle changes may benefit from additional pharmacologic therapy with cilostazol.

Peripheral arterial disease (PAD), the most common form of peripheral vascular disease, is a manifestation of progressive narrowing of the arteries due to atherosclerosis.[1] PAD is associated with elevated risk of morbidity and mortality from cardiovascular disease (CVD), even in the absence of a history of acute myocardial infarction, stroke, or other manifestations of CVD.[1–3] Patients with PAD have approximately the same relative risk of death from CVD as do patients with a history of coronary or cerebrovascular disease, and PAD should be considered a surrogate marker of subclinical coronary artery disease (CAD) and other vascular territories.[1,4,5] Treatment of PAD focuses on decreasing the functional impairment caused by symptoms of intermittent claudication through nonpharmacologic and pharmacologic therapy and minimizing the impact of other cardiovascular risk factors.[6]

Learning objectives, review questions, and other resources can be found at **www.pharmacotherapyonline.com.**

EPIDEMIOLOGY

1 Using the definition of an ankle–brachial index (ABI) <0.9 in either leg, the National Health and Nutrition Examination Survey (NHANES) found a 4.3% prevalence of PAD among adults age 40 years and older in the United States.[2] The prevalence of PAD is highly dependent on patient age, being infrequent in younger individuals and common in older individuals (Fig. 24–1). In age- and gender-adjusted logistic regression analyses, black race/ethnicity (odds ratio [OR] 2.83), current smoking (OR 4.46), diabetes (OR 2.71), hypertension (OR 1.75), hypercholesterolemia (OR 1.68), and impaired renal function (estimated glomerular filtration rate <60 mL/min/1.73 m^2; OR 2.00) were associated with more prevalent PAD.[2,7] Individuals with PAD are more likely to have a self-reported history of any CAD or CVD but, interestingly, no association with elevated body mass index. The reported relative risk of death from CVD in patients with PAD ranges from 2 to 5.1 in those with or without CVD and 2.9 to 5.7 in those with known CVD.[8] CVD accounts for 75% of all deaths in patients with PAD.[9] The risk of death is approximately the same in men and women and is elevated even in asymptomatic patients. Annual mortality is 25% in patients with critical leg ischemia who have the lowest ABI values.[10]

More than five million (estimated range four to seven million) adults age 40 years and older have PAD. Ninety-five percent of individuals with PAD have at least one cardiovascular risk factor; the majority of patients have multiple risk factors for CVD.[2] Based on the PAD Awareness, Risk, and Treatment: New Resources for Survival

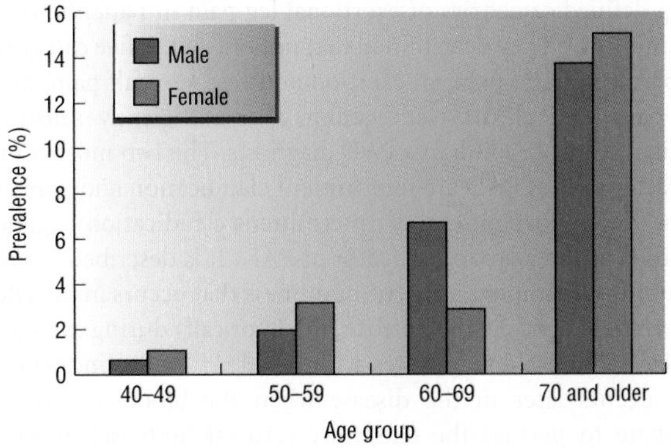

FIGURE 24-1. Prevalence of peripheral arterial disease by age and gender.

(PARTNERS) program, the prevalence of PAD seen in primary care practices is high, yet physician awareness of the PAD diagnosis is relatively low.[11] In this cross-sectional study, PAD was detected in 29% of 6,979 patients. Eighty-three percent of the patients were aware of their diagnosis compared to only 49% of their physicians. The reason for this observation is that patient self-report of symptoms and use of questionnaires for detecting PAD are not sufficiently sensitive and specific to reproducibly diagnosis PAD, and the cardinal symptom of PAD—intermittent claudication—is present in the minority of patients (1%–27%).[8,12,13] A simple ABI measurement will identify a large number of patients with previously unrecognized PAD. Atherosclerosis risk factors were highly prevalent in PAD patients, but these patients received less intensive treatment for lipid disorders and hypertension and were prescribed antiplatelet therapy less frequently than were patients with CVD. These results demonstrate that underdiagnosis of PAD in primary care practice may be a barrier to effective secondary prevention of the high ischemic cardiovascular risk associated with PAD.[11] Because of the systemic nature of atherosclerosis and the high risk of ischemic events, patients with PAD should be considered for secondary prevention strategies, including aggressive modification of risk factors and antiplatelet drug therapy.[8,14–16]

TABLE 24-1 Clinical Presentation of Peripheral Arterial Disease

General
• Patients with PAD are likely to be 40 years of age and older with hypertension, hypercholesterolemia, diabetes, impaired renal function, a history of coronary artery disease or cardiovascular disease, and/or a history of smoking.
Signs and symptoms
• The clinical presentation of PAD is variable and includes symptoms ranging from no symptoms at all (typically early in the disease) to pain and discomfort.
• The two most common characteristics of PAD are intermittent claudication and pain at rest in the lower extremities.
• Intermittent claudication is generally regarded as the primary indicator of PAD. It has been described as fatigue, discomfort, cramping, pain, or numbness in the affected extremities (typically the buttock, thigh, or calf) during exercise and resolves within a few minutes with rest.
• Physical examination may reveal nonspecific signs of decreased blood flow to the extremities (e.g., cool skin temperature, shiny skin, thickened toenails, lack of hair on the calf, feet, and/or toes).
Laboratory tests
• None specific to PAD.
Other diagnostic tests
• The ankle–brachial is a simple, noninvasive, quantitative test that has been proven to be a highly sensitive and specific (≥90%) tool in the diagnosis of PAD.

PAD, peripheral arterial disease.
Data from references 2, 7, 12, 19–26, 28, 30, 31, and 78.

ETIOLOGY AND PATHOPHYSIOLOGY

PAD is most commonly a manifestation of systemic atherosclerosis in which the arterial lumen of the lower extremities becomes progressively occluded by atherosclerotic plaque.[9] The major risk factors for development of atherosclerosis are older age (>40 years), cigarette smoking, diabetes mellitus, hypercholesterolemia, hypertension, and hyperhomocysteinemia.[8,9,12] The arteries most commonly involved, in order of occurrence, are the femoropopliteal–tibial, aortoiliac, carotid and vertebral, splenic and renal, and brachiocephalic.[17] Familial hypercholesterolemia leading to hypercholesterolemia and elevated low-density lipoprotein (LDL) levels is associated with accelerated development of atherosclerosis earlier and with more severe symptoms (e.g., intermittent claudication) and abnormal blood flow studies compared to controls.[18] Intima–media thickness can be used as a surrogate phenotype for cardiovascular risk in familial hypercholesterolemia. Carotid and/or femoral artery atherosclerosis results in increased intima–media thickness and is correlated to cardiovascular risk in patients with familial hypercholesterolemia compared with normolipidemic individuals.

CLINICAL PRESENTATION AND DIAGNOSIS

❷ The clinical presentation of PAD is variable, ranging from no symptoms at all (typically early in the disease) to symptoms of pain and discomfort (Table 24–1). This finding was illustrated in a study by Wang et al.,[19] who attempted to aid the diagnosis of PAD by using defined categories of exertional leg pain in patients with and without PAD. They determined that not one of the five categories of leg pain (no pain, pain on exertion and rest, noncalf pain, atypical calf pain, and classic claudication) was sufficiently sensitive or specific to enable a link to a PAD diagnosis. The two most common characteristics of PAD are intermittent claudication and pain at rest in the lower extremities.[19–22] Intermittent claudication is generally regarded as the primary indicator of PAD. It is described as fatigue, discomfort, cramping, pain, or numbness that occurs in the affected extremities (typically the buttock, thigh, or calf) during exercise and resolves within a few minutes with rest.[20,21,23–25] Resting pain typically occurs later in the disease when the blood supply is not adequate to perfuse the extremity (critical limb ischemia). This condition most often is felt at night in the feet (typically the toes or heel) while the patient is lying in bed.[20–22]

As with any good medical encounter, obtaining a detailed patient history of symptoms and atherosclerosis risk factors (e.g., smoking, hypertension, hyperlipidemia, and diabetes) can be helpful in making the diagnosis of PAD. Unfortunately, as illustrated by the PARTNERS program, providers who rely on a history alone will miss approximately 85% to 90% of patients with PAD.[23] Therefore, physical examination of the patient is vital to proper diagnosis. Requesting that the patient remove socks and shoes may reveal nonspecific signs of decreased blood flow to the extremities (e.g., cool skin temperature, shiny skin, thickened toenails, lack of hair on the calf, feet, and/ or toes) or, in severe cases, visible sores or ulcers that are slow to heal or even black in appearance.[12,20–22,26–28]

An important criterion for accurate diagnosis of PAD is exclusion of other conditions having similar signs and symptoms. Differential diagnosis should rule out other neurologic conditions (e.g., peripheral neuropathy), musculoskeletal conditions (e.g., restless leg syndrome or spinal stenosis), inflammatory conditions (e.g., arthritis), and vascular conditions (e.g., deep-vein thrombosis or venous congestion), which may mimic PAD.[12,21,25,28,29]

❸ The ABI is a simple, noninvasive, quantitative test that has proved to be a highly sensitive and specific (≥90%) tool in the diagnosis of PAD.[23,30,31] For measurement of the ABI, the patient lies in the supine position as systolic blood pressure is measured at the brachial arteries on both arms and the dorsalis pedis and posterior tibial arteries of the legs using a standard sphygmomanometer and a continuous-wave Doppler device. The pressures obtained at the dorsalis pedis and posterior tibial arteries are averaged and divided by the mean measurement taken at the left and right brachial arteries.[8,26,32,33] ABI = 1 is considered normal, whereas ABI <0.9 is consistent with PAD. ABI from 0.7 to 0.9 correlates with mild PAD, 0.4 to 0.7 indicates moderate disease, and <0.4 indicates severe PAD.[9,24,32] In addition to providing diagnostic information, the ABI measurement has been shown to be a strong predictor of future cardiovascular events associated with PAD.[34] The ABI can be useful after an exercise tolerance test (e.g., 5 minutes on a treadmill or 30 to 50 repetitions of heel raises). Patients with PAD will demonstrate a significant drop in ABI after exercise, but their pain will be normal or unchanged. ABI can rule out PAD and suggest alternate diagnoses.[9,12,24,26] Not only is ABI an effective diagnostic tool, but a systematic review determined that ABI has high specificity for predicting future cardiovascular outcomes (incident coronary heart diseases, incident stroke, and cardiovascular mortality).[35]

Other noninvasive tools are available for diagnosis of PAD. One study has suggested a calculation that takes into consideration the patient's history of acute myocardial infarction and the number of auscultated and palpated posterior tibial arteries.[36,37] Magnetic resonance angiography can be used to examine the presence and location of significant stenosis, or lack thereof, and is a reasonable option in patients who are being considered for surgical revascularization.[38] Similarly, computed tomographic angiography can be used to determine the presence of significant stenosis and soft-tissue diagnostic information that may be associated with PAD (e.g., aneurysms).[38] However, because ABI is a sufficient means of diagnosis, arteriography is not necessary or encouraged.[20,25,31]

TREATMENT

Peripheral Arterial Disease

■ GOALS OF TREATMENT

PAD is caused by atherosclerotic plaque formation in the arteries that results in decreased blood flow to the legs. Several of the treatment goals for patients with PAD involve the reduction of confounding variables that contribute to the disease process, progress, and eventual outcome. Specific goals should include increasing maximal walking distance, duration of walking, and amount of pain-free walking; and improving control of comorbid conditions that contribute to morbidity (e.g., hypertension, hyperlipidemia, and diabetes), resulting in improvement in overall quality of life and reduction in cardiovascular complications and death.

■ GENERAL APPROACH TO TREATMENT

❹ As with any atherosclerotic condition, several risk factors play an important role in the morbidity and mortality of PAD. Many of these risk factors can be modified with the help of various nonpharmacologic and pharmacologic interventions.

■ NONPHARMACOLOGIC THERAPY

Smoking Cessation

❺ Cigarette smoking not only increases the risk of developing PAD and other cardiovascular disorders, but the duration and quantity smoked can negatively impact disease progression (i.e., increase the risk of amputation) and increase mortality.[8,29,34,39–43] As a result, providers must advise patients to quit and should offer nonpharmacologic and pharmacologic means to aid patients in that goal. Numerous studies have proved the effectiveness of individual or group behavior modification therapy with or without the addition of certain antidepressants (e.g., bupropion) or nicotine replacement therapies (e.g., gum or patches). Reassessment of smoking status and progress encouragement at each visit can help reemphasize to the patient the vital importance of this lifestyle change.

Exercise

❺ Walking exercise programs for patients with PAD have been proven to result in increased walking duration and distance, increased pain-free walking, and delayed onset of claudication by 179%.[14,27,29,40,41,44–48] Walking, or any aerobic exercise program conducted under the supervision of a healthcare provider, can positively impact several of the pathophysiologic abnormalities present in patients with PAD. Benefits of exercise programs include improving diabetes and lipid management, reducing weight, improving blood viscosity and flow, and reducing blood pressure.[6] The American College of Cardiology/American Heart Association Guidelines for the Management of PAD recommend supervised exercise training for patients with intermittent claudication, for a minimum of 30–45 minutes, performed at least three times per week.[38] A prospective, observational study has concluded that PAD patients with higher physical activity (as measured with a vertical accelerometer) have reduced mortality and cardiovascular events compared to those with low physical activity, regardless of confounders.[49] Exercise treadmill walking testing should be repeated at regular intervals (i.e., quarterly to biannually) to assess improvement or decline in walking duration and distance as well as time to pain onset while performing this activity. The type of aerobic activity recommended, as well as the duration and frequency of the activity, should be individually designed on a patient-to-patient basis.

Revascularization Therapy

Various surgical procedures are available for patients with severe, debilitating claudication who have attempted, and failed, other means of nonpharmacologic and pharmacologic therapy. The TransAtlantic Inter-Society Consensus (TASC) document on PAD provides clear recommendations for invasive therapy.[27] First, the patient must have a lack of adequate response to exercise therapy and risk factor modification. Second, the patient must have severe disability from intermittent claudication resulting in impairment of daily activities. Third, a thorough evaluation of the risks versus benefits of an invasive intervention must be preformed, including probability of success, anticipated future course of the disease if intervention is not performed, and evaluation of concomitant disease states.[27] Although the TASC is clear that revascularization is mostly reserved for those who do not respond to conservative therapy consisting of risk factor modification, exercise, and pharmacologic therapy, revascularization does have a role in patients with favorable anatomy, whose lifestyle and/or job performance are compromised and who have a favorable risk-to-benefit ratio based on procedural risk.[12] The decision to attempt percutaneous revascularization often is made with the guidance of diagnostic angiography. Angiography can help to identify the location and size of lesions and provide valuable information regarding the likelihood of success with surgical revascularization.[27]

Percutaneous transluminal angioplasty (PTA) is an example of an invasive treatment of PAD. A randomized controlled clinical trial by Whyman et al.[50] determined that in a 2-year postintervention, PTA outcomes on maximum walking distance and ABI were not significantly different than outcomes in patients who had received only daily low-dose ASA ($P > 0.05$). Nevertheless, patients who had received PTA had significantly fewer occluded arteries ($P = 0.003$), but the true clinical significance of this finding was not realized in the time allotted for the study. PTA typically is reserved for patients whose lifestyle and/or job performance are compromised secondary to claudication despite adequate pharmacologic interventions and exercise.[12,38]

Stent placement in PAD patients has been an area of study and controversy. A meta-analysis examining the use of stent placement versus PTA for treatment of aortoiliac occlusive disease determined that although stent placement and PTA yielded similar complication and mortality rates, posttreatment ABI was more improved with stents (0.87 with PTA and 0.76 with stents, $P < 0.03$) and the risk of long-term failure was 39% less with stent placement.[51] However, other studies have not demonstrated improvement in patency rates in peripheral arteries versus PTA alone.[20] The TASC document provides specific recommendations for PTA, with or without stenting, depending on the how diffuse the disease process is, the number and size of the lesions, and the location of the lesions.[27]

For patients with severe intermittent claudication resulting in critical leg ischemia, physicians may need to discuss alternate surgical interventions, including aortofemoral bypass, femoropopliteal bypass, or even amputation.[20,21,40]

PHARMACOLOGIC THERAPY

Hypertension

Hypertension is a major risk factor for PAD and can lead to acute myocardial infarction, stroke, heart failure, and death.[14] Current guidelines recommend that the treatment goal for blood pressure in patients with PAD mirror those in patients with documented CVD: 130/85 mm Hg.[14,39] Although, the Heart Outcomes Prevention Evaluation (HOPE) study demonstrated that angiotensin-converting enzyme inhibitors reduced not only blood pressure but other cardiovascular events (e.g., acute myocardial infarction, stroke, and death) in high-risk patients, including those with PAD, no specific class of antihypertensives is recommended over another for treatment of hypertension in patients with PAD. Therefore, selection of drug therapy for hypertension should be made on the basis of comorbid disease states, drug costs and availability, drug allergies, or other possible limiting factors. For example, patients with documented CAD may receive a dual benefit by the selection of a β-blocker, whereas patients with concomitant Raynaud phenomenon may benefit from calcium channel blockers.[14,39,52] Dosing, monitoring guidelines, and contraindications for specific agents are discussed in Chapter 15.

Hyperlipidemia

Although a reduction in lipid levels can reduce the progression of PAD and the severity of claudication, the current recommendations for management of hyperlipidemia in patients with PAD are based on only a few small studies and sub hoc analyses from larger trials.[8,39,53,54] The Expert Panel on Detection, Evaluation, and Treatment of High Blood Cholesterol in Adults (Adult Treatment Panel III) considers PAD to be in the category of highest risk, or a coronary heart disease risk equivalent. Therefore, the Expert Panel recommends that LDL levels be maintained at <100 mg/dL and non–high-density lipoprotein (HDL) levels (total cholesterol – HDL cholesterol) maintained at <130 mg/dL.[53] Results of clinical trials conducted since issuance of the Expert Panel recommendation, specifically the Heart Protection Study (HPS)[55] and the Pravastatin or Atorvastatin Evaluation and Infection—Thrombolysis in Myocardial Infarction (PROVE IT)[56] trial, have led many clinical experts to now recommend an LDL goal of <70 mg/dL for additional retardation of atherosclerotic plaque formation in persons considered to be at very high risk, including patients with PAD.[20] Regardless of the goal LDL level chosen, initiation of patient therapeutic lifestyle changes (e.g., reduction in consumption of saturated fat, weight reduction, and increased physical activity) is vital to achieving these recommendations.[16,53] Unfortunately, in many cases, therapeutic lifestyle changes alone will not achieve the desired goals.

Several options are available for initiating drug therapy to lower LDL levels in patients with PAD. Statins, bile acid sequestrants, and nicotinic acid all are effective treatment options. However, statins are the preferred starting agent in this patient population.[23,40,53,55] As proven in the HPS, simvastatin demonstrated potent action in reducing LDL and also provided a significant reduction in cardiovascular events overall (e.g., acute myocardial infarction, stroke, and death).[55] If an increase in HDL levels also is necessary, niacin should be considered alone or in combination with a statin without the fear of worsening glucose metabolism, as previously believed.[8,21,29,52,57] Dosing, monitoring guidelines, and contraindications for specific agents are discussed in Chapter 23.

Diabetes Mellitus

A meta-analysis of more than 95,000 diabetic patients provided additional support for the accepted premise that glycemic control serves as a risk factor for CVD.[58] The analysis demonstrated an increasing risk of death from cardiovascular events as blood glucose concentrations increased, with the same relationship observed even at levels below the threshold of clinically defined diabetes mellitus. This relationship is just one illustration of the criticality of good glycemic control. Due to the high prevalence of PAD among diabetic patients, the American Diabetes Association recommends ABI screening for PAD in all diabetics older than 50 years.[59] Because of the presence of peripheral neuropathy, patients with diabetes may be less likely to experience or report symptoms of PAD, and the first sign may be as drastic as the appearance of a gangrenous foot ulcer. Therefore, although a lack of randomized controlled studies illustrates that the degree of glycemic control is predictive of the extent of PAD present, it is widely recommended that all patients with concomitant diabetes and PAD maintain good glycemic control, as evidenced by a hemoglobin A_{1c} level <7%.[8,27,29,39,41,59,60] This recommendation is supported by a prospective cohort study of 1,894 diabetic patients. The study demonstrated that patients with poor glucose control (hemoglobin A_{1c} >7.5%) were five times more likely to develop intermittent claudication and to be hospitalized for PAD compared to patients with hemoglobin A_{1c} <6%.[61] Despite this finding, a study by Rehring et al.[62] of 365 patients with known PAD and concomitant diabetes showed that only 45.8% of these patients had hemoglobin A_{1c} <7%. Oral antidiabetic agents, insulin regimens, and other pharmacologic and nonpharmacologic strategies for reducing the risk of complications associated with diabetes mellitus are discussed at length in Chapter 77.

ANTIPLATELET DRUG THERAPY (TABLE 24–2)

Aspirin

❻ By far, the most compelling evidence for the use of any pharmacologic agent in patients with PAD can be found for aspirin (acetylsalicylic acid [ASA]). The Antithrombotic Trialists' Collaboration (ATC) conducted a meta-analysis of 195 randomized trials, composed of more than 135,000 patients at high risk for occlusive arterial disease. The ATC concluded that low-dose ASA (75–160 mg) and medium-dose ASA (160–325 mg/day) led to a significant reduction in serious vascular events (12%) in "high-risk" patients, such as those with PAD.[63] The ATC also noted in this analysis that the risk of major extracranial bleed was similar between low-dose and medium-dose regimens.

Tran and Anand[64] conducted a systematic review of the literature in an effort to summarize the best evidence for oral antiplatelet therapy in patients with cerebrovascular disease, CAD, and PAD. This review included 111 trials (42 of which included patients with PAD, n = 9,214) and concluded that patients with PAD should use ASA (160–325 mg/day) or clopidogrel (75 mg/day) when ASA is not tolerated or contraindicated.[64,65] This is in concordance with the recommendations of the Seventh American College of Chest Physicians (ACCP) Conference on Antithrombotic and Thrombolytic Therapy, which recommends lifelong ASA (75–325 mg/day) over clopidogrel, ticlopidine, and no antithrombotic therapy in patients with PAD.[66] Unfortunately, no data from large clinical randomized trials have yet shown that ASA, or any other antiplatelet therapy, actually can prevent or delay the progression of PAD.[66]

ASA + Dipyridamole Extended-Release (Aggrenox)

The ATC also examined the use of dipyridamole extended-release (Aggrenox) in combination with ASA in "high-risk" patients, such as those with PAD. The meta-analysis of 25 trials (which included more than 10,000 patients) concluded that the addition of dipyridamole to aspirin led to a further reduction in serious vascular events over ASA

TABLE 24-2 Pharmacotherapy Options for Patients with Peripheral Arterial Disease

Agent	Daily Dose (Oral)	Mechanism of Action	Side Effects	Contraindications	Level of Evidence[b]
Aspirin	81–325 mg	Irreversibly inhibits prostaglandin cyclooxygenase in platelets, prevents formation of thromboxane A_2	Gastrointestinal upset and/or bleeding	Active bleeding; hemophilia; thrombocytopenia	With coronary or cerebrovascular (grade 1A), without (grade 1C+)
Dipyridamole extended-release (Aggrenox)	400 mg (+ aspirin 50 mg)	May act by inhibiting platelet aggregation (complete mechanism of action unknown)	Angina, dyspnea, hypotension, headache, dizziness	Active bleeding; coronary artery disease ("coronary steal syndrome")	Recommendation for use not specified in report
Cilostazol (Pletal)[a]	100 mg bid	Phosphodiesterase inhibitor, suppresses platelet aggregation; direct artery vasodilator	Fever from infection, tachycardia	All congestive heart failure patients (decreased survival)	With intermittent claudication (grade 2A)
Clopidogrel (Plavix)	75 mg	Inhibits binding of ADP analogues to its platelet receptor, causing irreversible inhibition of platelets	Chest pain, purpura generalized pain, rash	Active pathologic bleeding (e.g., peptic ulcer, intracranial hemorrhage)	Recommend clopidogrel over no antiplatelet therapy (grade 1C+)
Pentoxifylline (Trental)	1.2 g	Alters red blood cell flexibility; decreases platelet adhesion; reduces blood viscosity; decreases fibrinogen concentration	Dyspnea, nausea, vomiting, headache, dizziness	Recent retinal or cerebral hemorrhage; active bleeding	Not recommended in patients with intermittent claudication (grade 1B)
Ticlopidine (Ticlid)	500 mg	Inhibits binding of ADP analogues to its platelet receptor, causing irreversible inhibition of platelets	Leukopenia; rash; thrombocytopenia; neutropenia, agranulocytosis; aplastic anemia	Active bleeding, hemophilia; thrombocytopenia	Clopidogrel recommended over ticlopidine (grade 1C+)

[a]Cilostazol should be used in combination with antiplatelet therapy.
[b]Grades of recommendation for antithrombotic and thrombolytic therapy are part of the Seventh ACCP Conference on Antithrombotic and Thrombolytic Therapy.
Data from references 5, 22, 29, 30, 63, 65, 66, and 79–83.

alone (6%); however, this reduction did not reach statistical significance ($P = 0.32$).[63,64] Also to be taken into consideration is that most of the reduction in nonfatal stroke in this analysis came from one trial, and these data have not been replicated in other studies.[63,65,67] The addition of dipyridamole to ASA may cause an increased risk of bleeding and gastrointestinal side effects compared to placebo, so the combination should not be used in patients with CAD.[67]

Clopidogrel (Plavix)

The ATC meta-analysis also reviewed the effectiveness of clopidogrel 75 mg/day in "high-risk" patients, including those with PAD. The ATC concluded that although clopidogrel was able to reduce serious vascular events by 10%, this was significantly less than the reduction seen with ASA (12%, $P = 0.03$) described previously.[63] Included in the meta-analysis was the report from the Clopidogrel versus ASA in Patients at Risk of Ischemic Events (CAPRIE) trial, which concluded that clopidogrel 75 mg/day was more effective than ASA 325 mg/day in preventing vascular events in "high-risk" patients. In comparison to ASA therapy, the clopidogrel regimen resulted in an overall reduction in ischemic stroke, myocardial infarction, or vascular death from 5.83% to 5.32% ($P = 0.043$). This difference was even more pronounced in the subgroup analysis of PAD patients, in which clopidogrel therapy led to a significant reduction of 4.86% versus 3.71% in the ASA group ($P = 0.0028$).[5,30,34] It must be noted that clopidogrel is significantly more expensive than ASA therapy, not only in terms of drug costs but also in cost of physician visits because clopidogrel is a prescription-only medication. For all these reasons, the current recommendations list clopidogrel as a first-line agent, but only in cases where ASA therapy is either not tolerated or contraindicated.[63,65]

Ticlopidine (Ticlid)

Although ticlopidine has the same mechanism of action as clopidogrel and possesses a similar molecular structure, the results of clinical trials investigating the two agents are strikingly different.[22] The Swedish Ticlopidine Multicenter Study (STIMS) had determined that ticlopidine therapy (500 mg/day) reduced total mortality in patients with intermittent claudication in comparison to placebo ($P = 0.015$).[22,68,69] However, the once promising results seen with ticlopidine therapy now have been overshadowed by the severe hematologic side effects unique to this agent. Ticlopidine has a black box warning from the Food and Drug Administration (FDA) warning providers that use of this agent can cause neutropenia/agranulocytosis, thrombotic thrombocytopenic purpura, and aplastic anemia.[70] Other agents, namely clopidogrel, are now used instead of ticlopidine.[8,29,41]

■ INTERMITTENT CLAUDICATION (TABLE 24–2)

Cilostazol (Pletal)

7 In a head-to-head, randomized, placebo-controlled study of 698 patients with moderate-to-severe claudication, Dawson et al.[71] assigned patients to cilostazol (100 mg twice daily), pentoxifylline (400 mg three times daily), or placebo in an effort to improve maximal walking distance. After 24 weeks, the cilostazol group demonstrated a 54% mean increase in distance versus pentoxifylline, which demonstrated only a 30% mean increase ($P < 0.001$).[71] Similarly, a meta-analysis of eight randomized, double-blind, placebo-controlled, parallel-design trials supported this conclusion, with a reported increase in maximal walking distance and pain-free walking distance with cilostazol at doses of 50 mg and 100 mg twice daily ($P < 0.05$ for all) over placebo.[72] Regrettably, improvement in walking distance has appeared to come with a price (in addition to the high drug cost); cilostazol has a black box warning from the FDA warning providers not to use this medication in patients with PAD and coexisting heart failure.[39] However, the Seventh ACCP Conference on Antithrombotic and Thrombolytic Therapy does suggest the use of this agent in patients with PAD who are not candidates for surgical interventions to improve severe intermittent claudication that persists even after implementation of appropriate exercise therapy and therapeutic lifestyle changes.[66]

Pentoxifylline (Trental)

Unlike cilostazol, pentoxifylline has produced less promising results in clinical trials, as illustrated by the randomized, placebo-controlled trial by Dawson et al.[71] Not only did cilostazol outperform pentoxifylline with regard to improvement in walking distance, but the improvement seen with pentoxifylline was no different from placebo ($P = 0.82$).[71] This nonsignificant improvement in walking distance has been observed in other studies as well.[8,73] Meanwhile, other meta-analyses of pentoxifylline in comparison to placebo for improvement of maximal walking distance have shown minimal improvement over placebo, but the average effects were relatively small.[8,74–77] For these reasons, the Seventh ACCP Conference on Antithrombotic and Thrombolytic Therapy does not recommend the use of this agent.[66]

EVALUATION OF THERAPEUTIC OUTCOMES

It is vital that the physician counsel the patient on the evaluation measures that will be used to monitor the outcomes of therapeutic interventions for PAD. Various laboratory measurements will assess patient progress in glycemic control (i.e., hemoglobin A_{1c}) and lipid management (i.e., total cholesterol, LDL, HDL, and non-HDL cholesterol). Blood pressure measurements obtained in the clinic and by patient home monitoring can assess the effectiveness of antihypertensive therapy. Exercise treadmill walking testing should be repeated at regular intervals (i.e., quarterly to biannually) to assess improvement or decline in walking duration and distance, as well as the time to pain onset while performing this activity. Repeat ABI measurements should be assessed at each patient visit to determine if the disease process has stabilized or progressed. Most importantly to many patients, simple concern and questioning about improvements to their daily quality of life will highlight the physician's concern for their well-being and aid in the patient's overall general state of health.

ABBREVIATIONS

ABI: ankle–brachial index

ACCP: American College of Chest Physicians

ASA: acetylsalicylic acid (aspirin)

ATC: Antithrombotic Trialists' Collaboration

CAD: coronary artery disease

CVD: cardiovascular disease

FDA: Food and Drug Administration

HOPE: Heart Outcomes Prevention Evaluation (study)

HPS: Heart Protection Study

NHANES: National Health and Nutrition Examination Survey

OR: odds ratio

PAD: peripheral arterial disease

PARTNERS: PAD Awareness, Risk, and Treatment: New Resources for Survival

PTA: percutaneous transluminal angioplasty

STIMS: Swedish Ticlopidine Multicenter Study

TASC: TransAtlantic Inter-Society Consensus

REFERENCES

1. Hiatt WR. Sounding the PAD alarm. GPs can diagnose peripheral artery disease with a simple ankle-and-arm blood pressure test. Health News 2004;10:4.
2. Selvin E, Erlinger TP. Prevalence of and risk factors for peripheral arterial disease in the United States. Results from the National Health and Nutrition Examination Survey 1999–2000. Circulation 2004;110:738–743.
3. Golomb BA, Dang TT, Criqui MH. Peripheral arterial disease: Morbidity and mortality implications. Circulation 2006;114:688–699.
4. Newman AB, Shemanski L, Manolio TA, et al. Ankle-arm index as a predictor of cardiovascular disease and mortality in the Cardiovascular Health Study. The Cardiovascular Health Study Group. Arterioscler Thromb Vasc Biol 1999;19:538–545.
5. CAPRIE Steering Committee. A randomised, blinded, trial of clopidogrel versus aspirin in patients at risk of ischaemic events (CAPRIE). CAPRIE Steering Committee. Lancet 1996;348:1329–1339.
6. Stewart KJ, Hiatt WR, Regensteiner JG, Hirsch AT. Exercise training for claudication. N Engl J Med 2002;347:1941–1951.
7. O'Hare AM, Glidden DV, Fox CS, Hsu CY. High prevalence of peripheral arterial disease in persons with renal insufficiency: Results from the National Health and Nutrition Examination Survey 1999–2000. Circulation 2004;109:320–323.
8. Hiatt WR. Medical treatment of peripheral arterial disease and claudication. N Engl J Med 2001;344:1608–1621.
9. Mohler ER 3rd. Peripheral arterial disease. Identification and implications. Arch Intern Med 2003;163:2306–2314.
10. Dormandy JA, Murray GD. The fate of the claudicant—A prospective study of 1969 claudicants. Eur J Vasc Surg 1991;5:131–133.
11. Hirsch AT, Hiatt WR, Committee PS. PAD awareness, risk, and treatment: New resources for survival—The USA PARTNERS program. Vasc Med 2001;6(3 Suppl):9–12.
12. White C. Intermittent claudication. N Engl J Med 2007;356:1241–1250.
13. McDermott MM, Kerwin DR, Liu K, et al. Prevalence and significance of unrecognized lower extremity peripheral arterial disease in general medicine practice. J Gen Intern Med 2001;16:384–390.
14. Chobanian AV, Bakris GL, Black HR, et al. The Seventh Report of the Joint National Committee on Prevention, Detection, Evaluation, and Treatment of High Blood Pressure: The JNC 7 Report. JAMA 2003;289:2560–2571.
15. National Cholesterol Education Program Expert Panel on Detection Evaluation and Treatment of High Blood Cholesterol in Adults. Third Report of the National Cholesterol Education Program (NCEP) Expert Panel on Detection, Evaluation, and Treatment of High Blood Cholesterol in Adults (Adult Treatment Panel III) final report. Circulation 2002;106:3143–3421.
16. Grundy S, Cleeman J, Merz CB, et al. Implications of recent clinical trials for the National Cholesterol Education Program Adult Treatment Panel III Guidelines. Circulation 2004;110:227–239.
17. Jackson M, Clagett G. Antithrombotic therapy in peripheral arterial occlusive disease. Chest 2001;119(Suppl):283S–299S.
18. Hutter C, Austin M, Humphries S. Familial hypercholesterolemia, peripheral arterial disease, and stroke: A HuGE minireview. Am J Epidemiol 2004;160:430–435.
19. Wang JC, Criqui MH, Denenberg JO, McDermott MM, Golomb BA, Fronek A. Exertional leg pain in patients with and without peripheral arterial disease. Circulation 2005;112:3501–3508.
20. Hirsch AT, Haskal ZJ, Hertzer NR, et al., ACC/AHA 2005 Practice Guidelines for the management of patients with peripheral arterial disease (lower extremity, renal, mesenteric, and abdominal aortic): A collaborative report from the American Association for Vascular Surgery/Society for Vascular Surgery, Society for Cardiovascular Angiography and Interventions, Society for Vascular Medicine and Biology, Society of Interventional Radiology, and the ACC/AHA Task Force on Practice Guidelines (Writing Committee to Develop Guidelines for the Management of Patients with Peripheral Arterial Disease): Endorsed by the American Association of Cardiovascular and Pulmonary Rehabilitation; National Heart, Lung, and Blood Institute; Society for Vascular Nursing; TransAtlantic Inter-Society Consensus; and Vascular Disease Foundation. Circulation 2006;113(11):e463–654.
21. Hiatt W, Nehler MR, eds. Peripheral Arterial Disease, 4th ed. New York: Spring-Verlag, 2003.
22. Hiatt WR. Preventing atherothrombotic events in peripheral arterial disease: The use of antiplatelet therapy. J Intern Med 2002;251:193–206.
23. Hirsch AT, Criqui MH, Treat-Jacobson D, et al. Peripheral arterial disease detection, awareness, and treatment in primary care. JAMA 2001;286:1317–1324.
24. Dormandy JA, Rutherford RB. Management of peripheral arterial disease (PAD). TASC Working Group. TransAtlantic Inter-Society Concensus (TASC). J Vasc Surg 2000;31(1 Pt 2):S1–S296.
25. Carman TL, Fernandez BB, Jr. A primary care approach to the patient with claudication. Am Fam Physician 2000;61:1027–1032, 1034.

26. Schmieder FA, Comerota AJ. Intermittent claudication: Magnitude of the problem, patient evaluation, and therapeutic strategies. Am J Cardiol 2001;87(12A):3D–13D.
27. TransAtlantic Inter-Society Consensus (TASC) Working Group. Management of peripheral arterial disease (PAD). TransAtlantic Inter-Society Consensus (TASC). Section B. intermittent claudication. Eur J Vasc Endovasc Surg 2000;19(Suppl A):S47–S114.
28. Sontheimer DL. Peripheral vascular disease: Diagnosis and treatment. Am Fam Physician 2006;73:1971–1976.
29. Gey DC, Lesho EP, Manngold J. Management of peripheral arterial disease. Am Fam Physician 2004;69:525–532.
30. Aronow WS. Management of peripheral arterial disease of the lower extremities in elderly patients. J Gerontol Series A Biol Sci Med Sci 2004;59:172–177.
31. Criqui MH. Systemic atherosclerosis risk and the mandate for intervention in atherosclerotic peripheral arterial disease. Am J Cardiol 2001;88(7B):43J–47J.
32. McDermott MM, Greenland P, Liu K, et al. The ankle brachial index is associated with leg function and physical activity: The Walking and Leg Circulation Study. Ann Intern Med 2002;136:873–883.
33. McDermott MM, Criqui MH, Liu K, et al. Lower ankle/brachial index, as calculated by averaging the dorsalis pedis and posterior tibial arterial pressures, and association with leg functioning in peripheral arterial disease. J Vasc Surg 2000;32:1164–1171.
34. Belch JJ, Topol EJ, Agnelli G, et al. Critical issues in peripheral arterial disease detection and management: A call to action. Arch Intern Med 2003;163:884–892.
35. Doobay AV, Anand SS. Sensitivity and specificity of the ankle-brachial index to predict future cardiovascular outcomes: A systematic review. Arterioscler Thromb Vasc Biol 2005;25:1463–1469.
36. Farkouh ME. Improving the clinical examination for a low ankle-brachial index. Int J Angiol 2002;11:41–45.
37. Khan NA, Rahim SA, Anand SS, Simel DL, Panju A. Does the clinical examination predict lower extremity peripheral arterial disease? JAMA 2006;295:536–546.
38. Hirsch AT, Haskal ZJ, Hertzer NR, et al. ACC/AHA guidelines for the management of patients with peripheral arterial disease (lower extremity, renal, mesenteric, and abdominal aortic): Executive summary: A collaborative report from the American Association for Vascular Surgery/ Society for Vascular Surgery, Society for Vascular Medicine and Biology, Society of Interventional Radiology, and the ACC/AHA Task Force on Practice Guidelines (Writing Committee to Develop Guidelines for the Management of Patients with Peripheral Arterial Disease [Lower Extremity, Renal, Mesenteric, and Abdominal Aortic]). J Am Coll Cardiol 2006;46:1239–1312.
39. Hiatt WR. Pharmacologic therapy for peripheral arterial disease and claudication. J Vasc Surg 2002;36:1283–1291.
40. Burns P, Gough S, Bradbury AW. Management of peripheral arterial disease in primary care. BMJ 2003;326:584–588.
41. Regensteiner JG, Hiatt WR. Current medical therapies for patients with peripheral arterial disease: A critical review. Am J Med 2002;112:49–57.
42. Kannel WB, Shurtleff D. National Heart and Lung Institute, National Institutes of Health. The Framingham Study: Cigarettes and the development of intermittent claudication. Geriatrics 1973;28:61–68.
43. Tierney S, Fennessy F, Hayes DB. ABC of arterial and vascular disease: Secondary prevention of peripheral vascular disease. BMJ 2000;320:1262–1265.
44. Gardner AW, Katzel LI, Sorkin JD, Goldberg AP. Effects of long-term exercise rehabilitation on claudication distances in patients with peripheral arterial disease: A randomized controlled trial. J Cardiopulm Rehabil 2002;22:192–198.
45. Gardner AW, Katzel LI, Sorkin JD, et al. Exercise rehabilitation improves functional outcomes and peripheral circulation in patients with intermittent claudication: A randomized controlled trial. J Am Geriatr Soc 2001;49:755–762.
46. Langbein WE, Collins EG, Orebaugh C, et al. Increasing exercise tolerance of persons limited by claudication pain using polestriding. J Vasc Surg 2002;35:887–893.
47. Falcone RA, Hirsch AT, Regensteiner JG, et al. Peripheral arterial disease rehabilitation: A review. J Cardiopulm Rehabil 2003;23:170–175.
48. Tan KH, De Cossart L, Edwards PR. Exercise training and peripheral vascular disease. Br J Surg 2000;87:553–562.
49. Garg PK, Tian L, Criqui MH, et al. Physical activity during daily life and mortality in patients with peripheral arterial disease. Circulation 2006;114:242–248.
50. Whyman MR, Fowkes FG, Kerracher EM, et al. Is intermittent claudication improved by percutaneous transluminal angioplasty? A randomized controlled trial. J Vasc Surg 1997;26:551–557.
51. Bosch J, Hunink M. Meta-analysis of the results of percutaneous transluminal angioplasty and stent placement for aortoiliac occlusive disease [published erratum appears in Radiology 1997;205:584]. Radiology 1997;204:87–96.
52. McDermott MM. Peripheral arterial disease: Epidemiology and drug therapy. Am J Geriatr Cardiol 2002;11:258–266.
53. National Cholesterol Education Program Expert Panel on Detection Evaluation and Treatment of High Blood Cholesterol in Adults. Executive Summary of the Third Report of the National Cholesterol Education Program (NCEP) Expert Panel on Detection, Evaluation, and Treatment of High Blood Cholesterol in Adults (Adult Treatment Panel III). JAMA 2001;285:2486–2497.
54. Leng GC, Price JF, Jepson RG. Lipid-lowering for lower limb atherosclerosis. Cochrane Database Syst Rev 2000;2:CD000123.
55. MRC/BHF Heart Protection Study of cholesterol lowering with simvastatin in 20536 high-risk individuals: A randomised placebo-controlled trial. Lancet 2002;360:7–22.
56. Cannon CP, Braunwald E, McCabe CH, et al. Intensive versus moderate lipid lowering with statins after acute coronary syndromes. N Engl J Med 2004;350:1495–1504.
57. Elam MB, Hunninghake DB, Davis KB, et al. Effect of niacin on lipid and lipoprotein levels and glycemic control in patients with diabetes and peripheral arterial disease: The ADMIT study: A randomized trial. JAMA 2000;284:1263–1270.
58. Coutinho M, Gerstein H, Wang Y, Yusuf S. The relationship between glucose and incident cardiovascular events. A metaregression analysis of published data from 20 studies of 95,783 individuals followed for 12.4 years. Diabetes Care 1999;22:233–240.
59. American Diabetes Association. Peripheral arterial disease in people with diabetes. Diabetes Care 2003;26:3333–3341.
60. Creager MA, Luscher TF, Cosentino F, Beckman JA. Diabetes and vascular disease: Pathophysiology, clinical consequences, and medical therapy: Part I. Circulation 2003;108:1527–1532.
61. Selvin E, Wattanakit K, Steffes MW, Coresh J, Sharrett AR. HbA1c and peripheral arterial disease in diabetes: The atherosclerosis risk in communities study. Diabetes Care 2006;29:877–882.
62. Rehring TF, Sandhoff BG, Stolcpart RS, Merenich JA, Hollis HW Jr. Atherosclerotic risk factor control in patients with peripheral arterial disease. J Vasc Surg 2005;41:816–822.
63. Antithrombotic Trialists' Collaboration. Collaborative meta-analysis of randomised trials of antiplatelet therapy for prevention of death, myocardial infarction, and stroke in high risk patients. BMJ 2002;324:71–86.
64. Tran H, Anand SS. Oral antiplatelet therapy in cerebrovascular disease, coronary artery disease, and peripheral arterial disease. JAMA 2004;292:1867–1874.
65. Moore TD, Linn WD, O'Rourke RA. Hot Topic: Current Evidence for the Use of Antiplatelet Therapy in Cerebrovascular Disease, Coronary Artery Disease, and Peripheral Arterial Disease. New York: McGraw-Hill, 2004.
66. Clagett GP, Sobel M, Jackson MR, Lip GYH, Tangelder M, Verhaeghe R. Antithrombotic therapy in peripheral arterial occlusive disease: The Seventh ACCP Conference on Antithrombotic and Thrombolytic Therapy. Chest 2004;126(3 Suppl):609S–626S.
67. Diener HC, Cunha L, Forbes C, Sivenius J, Smets P, Lowenthal A. European Stroke Prevention Study 2. Dipyridamole and acetylsalicylic acid in the secondary prevention of stroke. J Neurol Sci 1996;143:1–13.
68. Janzon L. The STIMS trial: The ticlopidine experience and its clinical applications. Swedish Ticlopidine Multicenter Study. Vasc Med 1996;1:141–143.
69. Janzon L, Bergqvist D, Boberg J, et al. Prevention of myocardial infarction and stroke in patients with intermittent claudication; effects of ticlopidine. Results from STIMS, the Swedish Ticlopidine Multicentre Study. [published erratum appears in J Intern Med 1990;228:659]. J Intern Med 1990;227:301–308.
70. Ticlid (ticlopidine hydrochloride) tablets. Roche Laboratories, Nutley, NJ, March 2001.

71. Dawson DL, Cutler BS, Hiatt WR, et al. A comparison of cilostazol and pentoxifylline for treating intermittent claudication. Am J Med 2000;109:523–530.
72. Thompson PD, Zimet R, Forbes WP, Zhang P. Meta-analysis of results from eight randomized, placebo-controlled trials on the effect of cilostazol on patients with intermittent claudication. Am J Cardiol 2002;90:1314–1319.
73. Lindgarde F, Jelnes R, Bjorkman H, et al. Conservative drug treatment in patients with moderately severe chronic occlusive peripheral arterial disease. Scandinavian Study Group. Circulation 1989;80:1549–1556.
74. Girolami B, Bernardi E, Prins MH, et al. Treatment of intermittent claudication with physical training, smoking cessation, pentoxifylline, or nafronyl: A meta-analysis. Arch Intern Med 1999;159:337–345.
75. Radack K, Wyderski RJ. Conservative management of intermittent claudication. Ann Intern Med 1990;113:135–146.
76. Ernst E. Pentoxifylline for intermittent claudication. A critical review. Angiology 1994;45:339–345.
77. Hood SC, Moher D, Barber GG. Management of intermittent claudication with pentoxifylline: Meta-analysis of randomized controlled trials. CMAJ 1996;155:1053–1059.
78. Mannava K, Money SR. Current management of peripheral arterial occlusive disease: A review of pharmacologic agents and other interventions. Am J Cardio Drugs 2007;7(1);59–66.
79. Plavix package insert. Bristol-Myers Squibb/Sanofi Pharmaceuticals Partnership, New York, NY, February 2006.
80. "S" Monographs; Salicylates (Systemic); Aspirin. In: Group UDE, ed. USP DI® Drug Information for the Health Care Professional, 26th ed. Taunton, MA: Micromedex, 2006.
81. "D" Monographs; Dipyridamole (Systemic). In: Group UDE, ed. USP DI® Drug Information for the Health Care Professional, 26th ed. Taunton, MA: Micromedex, 2006.
82. "P" Monographs; Pentoxifylline (Systemic). In: Group UDE, ed. USP DI® Drug Information for the Health Care Professional, 26th ed. Taunton, MA: Micromedex, 2006.
83. "C" Monographs; Cilostazol (Systemic). In: Group UDE, ed. USP DI® Drug Information for the Health Care Professional, 26th ed. Taunton, MA: Micromedex, 2006.
84. Guyatt G, Schunemann HJ, Cook D, Jaeschke R, Pauker S. Applying the grades of recommendation for antithrombotic and thrombolytic therapy: The Seventh ACCP Conference on Antithrombotic and Thrombolytic Therapy. Chest 2004;126(3 Suppl):179S–187S.

CHAPTER 25

Use of Vasopressors and Inotropes in the Pharmacotherapy of Shock

ROBERT MACLAREN, MARIA I. RUDIS, AND JOSEPH F. DASTA

KEY CONCEPTS

1. Continuous hemodynamic monitoring with an arterial catheter or a central venous catheter capable of measuring mixed venous oxygen saturation (Svo_2) or central venous oxygen saturation ($Scvo_2$) should be used early and throughout the course of septic shock to assess intravascular fluid status and ventricular filling pressures, determine cardiac output (CO), and monitor arterial and venous oxygenation. They can be used for monitoring the response to drug therapy and guiding dosage titration.

2. Early goal-directed therapy with aggressive fluid resuscitation in the emergency department within the first 6 hours of presentation improves survival of patients with sepsis and septic shock.

3. Derangements in adrenergic receptor sensitivity or activity frequently result in resistance to catecholamine vasopressor and inotropic therapy in critically ill patients. These changes may be a function of endogenous catecholamine concentrations, dosage/duration of exposure to and type of exogenously administered vasopressors, stage of septic shock, preexisting illness, and other factors.

4. In refractory septic shock, rational use of vasopressor or inotropic agents should be guided by receptor activity, pharmacologic and pharmacokinetic characteristics, and regional and systemic hemodynamic effects of the drug and should be tailored to the patient's physiologic needs. Pharmacologically sound combinations of vasopressor and/or inotrope agents should be initiated early to optimize and facilitate rapid response.

5. Goals of therapy with vasopressors and inotropes should be predetermined and should optimize regional perfusion to tissues (e.g., cardiac, renal, mesenteric, and periphery). This can be accomplished by continuous or intermittent measurements. $Svo_2/Scvo_2$ >70% should be maintained. Arbitrarily targeting vasopressor and inotrope therapy to supranormal values of global oxygen-transport variables cannot be recommended because of lack of clear benefit and possible increased morbidity.

6. Much higher dosages of all vasopressors and inotropes than traditionally recommended are required to improve hemodynamic and oxygen-transport variables in patients with septic shock.

7. Dose titration and monitoring of vasopressor and inotropic therapy should be guided by the "best clinical response" while observing for and minimizing evidence of myocardial ischemia (e.g., tachydysrhythmias, electrocardiographic changes), renal (decreased glomerular filtration rate and/or urine production), splanchnic/gastric [low intramucosal pH, bowel ischemia], or peripheral (cold extremities) hypoperfusion, and worsening of partial pressure of arterial oxygen (Pao_2), pulmonary artery occlusive pressure, and other hemodynamic variables.

8. First-line therapy of septic shock is aggressive volume resuscitation with crystalloid or colloid types of fluids. Dopamine or norepinephrine typically is used as the initial vasopressor agent for hemodynamic support. Dopamine is limited by its ability to increase CO and complications of tachycardia, tachydysrhythmias, increase in pulmonary artery occlusive pressure, and decrease in splanchnic oxygen use. Low-dose dopamine should not be used to prevent renal failure. Norepinephrine may achieve greater hemodynamic response than dopamine and is less likely to cause tachydysrhythmias and a decrease in splanchnic oxygen utilization.

9. Phenylephrine may be a particularly useful alternative in patients who cannot tolerate tachycardia or tachydysrhythmia with dopamine or norepinephrine or in patients with known underlying myocardial dysfunction.

10. Epinephrine appears to be effective as a single agent and as an add-on agent. It is particularly useful in the young, in patients with otherwise healthy myocardium, and potentially in patients when used early in the course of treatment. However, because epinephrine causes a significant, yet transient, increase in lactate and worsening of splanchnic oxygen utilization, it is not the agent of first choice in patients with septic shock. It should be used cautiously in patients with a history of coronary artery disease or underlying cardiac disturbances.

11. Therapy with vasopressors and inotropes is continued until the myocardial depression and vascular hyporesponsiveness of septic shock improve, usually measured in hours to days. Discontinuation of vasopressor or inotropic therapy should be executed slowly; therapy should be "weaned" to avoid a precipitous worsening in regional and systemic hemodynamics.

12. Vasopressin produces vasoconstriction independent of adrenergic receptors and reduces the doses of catecholamine vasopressors. Replacement doses of vasopressin (0.01–0.04 units/min) can be considered in patients with septic shock refractory to catecholamine vasopressors despite adequate fluid resuscitation. Vasopressin may enhance urine production. Given the current data, corticosteroids can be administered to patients with septic shock when adrenal insufficiency is present or when vasopressors have been administered for prolonged periods without evidence of dose reduction.

Learning objectives, review questions, and other resources can be found at **www.pharmacotherapyonline.com.**

TABLE 25-1 Hemodynamic and Oxygen-Transport Monitoring Parameters

Parameter	Normal Value[a]
Blood pressure (systolic/diastolic)	100–130/70–85 mm Hg
Mean arterial pressure (MAP)	80–100 mm Hg
Pulmonary artery pressure (PAP)	25/10 mm Hg
Mean pulmonary artery pressure (MPAP)	12–15 mm Hg
Central venous pressure (CVP)	8–12 mm Hg
Pulmonary artery occlusive pressure (PAOP)	12–15 mm Hg
Heart rate (HR)	60–80 beats/min
Cardiac output (CO)	4–7 L/min
Cardiac index (CI)	2.8–3.6 L/min/m^2
Stroke volume index (SVI)	30–50 mL/m^2
Systemic vascular resistance index (SVRI)	1,300–2,100 dyne • s/m^2 • cm^5
Pulmonary vascular resistance index (PVRI)	45–225 dyne • s/m^2 • cm^5
Arterial oxygen saturation (Sao_2)	97% (range 95%–100%)
Mixed venous oxygen saturation (Svo_2)	70%–75%
Arterial oxygen content (Cao_2)	20.1 vol% (range 19–21)
Venous oxygen content (Cvo_2)	15.5 vol% (range 11.5–16.5)
Oxygen content difference ($C[a-v]O_2$)	5 vol% (range 4–6)
Oxygen consumption index (Vo_2)	131 mL/min/m^2 (range 100–180)
Oxygen delivery index (Do_2)	578 mL/min/m^2 (range 370–730)
Oxygen extraction ratio (O_2ER)	25% (range 22–30)
Intramucosal pH (pHi)	7.40 (range 7.35–7.45)
Index (I)	Parameter indexed to body surface area

[a]Normal values may not be the same as values needed to optimize the management of a critically ill patient.

Shock is an acute, generalized state of inadequate perfusion of critical organs that can produce serious pathophysiologic consequences, including death, when therapy is not optimal. Shock is defined as systolic blood pressure <90 mm Hg or reduction of at least 40 mm Hg from baseline with perfusion abnormalities despite adequate fluid resuscitation.[1] At one time, mortality from septic or cardiogenic shock exceeded 70%.[1] Currently, 10% to 30% of patients with severe sepsis are admitted to hospitals, and 8.6% of patients experience cardiogenic shock following an acute ST-segment elevation myocardial infarction.[1–3] Mortality rates for shock of either cause are at least 30% to 50% despite enhanced treatment modalities and sophisticated monitoring techniques.[1–3] This chapter reviews the theory and current status of hemodynamic monitoring and presents an update on the optimal use of inotropes and vasopressor drugs in shock states, specifically septic shock.[3–10]

Hemodynamic and perfusion monitoring can be categorized into two broad areas: global and regional monitoring. Global parameters, such as systemic blood pressure and pulse oximetry, assess perfusion and oxygen utilization of the entire body. Regional monitoring techniques, such as tonometry, focus on oxygen flow and subsequent changes in metabolism of individual organs and tissues. Normal values for commonly monitored parameters are listed in Table 25–1. Evidence-based goals of therapy are listed in Table 25–2.[3–10] The adequacy of regional perfusion can be assessed by indices of specific organ perfusion, although none of these indices alone is a reliable indicator of adequate resuscitation. These measurements include coagulation abnormalities (disseminated intravascular coagulation), altered renal function with reduced urine production or increased serum concentrations of blood urea nitrogen and creatinine, altered

TABLE 25-2 Evidence-Based Treatment Recommendations for Management of Severe Sepsis or Septic Shock

Recommendations	Grade
An arterial catheter should be placed as soon as practical to monitor blood pressure in all patients with septic shock requiring vasopressors.	E
Resuscitation of tissue hypoperfusion from severe sepsis or septic shock should begin as soon as the syndrome is recognized. An elevated serum lactate concentration identifies tissue hypoperfusion in patients at risk who are not hypotensive. During the first 6 hours of resuscitation, goals should include all of the following: (1) CVP 8–12 mm Hg, (2) MAP ≥65 mm Hg, (3) urine production ≥0.5 mL/kg/h, and (4) Svo_2 or $Scvo_2$ ≥70%.	B
Fluid resuscitation should be the initial step in hemodynamic support of septic shock.	B
Fluid resuscitation may consist of natural or artificial colloids or crystalloids. No evidence supports one type of fluid over another.	C
Fluid challenge in patients with suspected hypovolemia or inadequate arterial circulation can be administered at a rate of 500–1,000 mL of crystalloid or 300–500 mL of colloid over 30 minutes and repeated based upon response (blood pressure and/or urine production) and tolerance (intravascular volume overload).	E
When an appropriate fluid challenge fails to restore adequate blood pressure and organ perfusion, vasopressor therapy should begin. Vasopressor therapy also may be required transiently to sustain life and maintain perfusion in the face of life-threatening hypotension, even when a fluid challenge is in progress and when hypovolemia has not yet been corrected.	E
Either dopamine or norepinephrine is effective for increasing arterial blood pressure, and either can be used as a first-line vasopressor agent to correct hypotension in septic shock. Dopamine raises CO more than norepinephrine, but its use may be limited by tachycardia. Norepinephrine may be the more effective vasopressor.	C
The combination of norepinephrine and dobutamine is superior to dopamine in the treatment of septic shock.	D
Phenylephrine is an alternative for increasing blood pressure, especially in the setting of tachyarrhythmias.	D
Epinephrine can be considered for refractory hypotension, but adverse effects, including decreased mesenteric perfusion, are common.	D
Low-dose dopamine should *not* be used for renal protection or to maintain renal function during sepsis.	B
Vasopressin can be considered in patients with refractory shock despite adequate fluid resuscitation and administration of high-dose catecholamine vasopressor. It should be administered as hormone replacement at doses of 0.01–0.04 units/min.	C
A strategy of increasing cardiac index to achieve supranormal Do_2 is *not* recommended.	A
Dobutamine can be used to increase CO in the presence of low cardiac index or low Svo_2 or $Scvo_2$ despite adequate fluid administration. If used in the presence of low blood pressure, it should be combined with vasopressor therapy. Dobutamine may cause tachycardia.	C
Intravenous corticosteroid therapy at hormone replacement doses (200–300 mg/d of hydrocortisone or equivalent corticosteroid dose) for 7 days can be used in septic shock when hypotension is present despite adequate fluid resuscitation and vasopressor therapy.	C
Daily corticosteroid doses >300 mg/d of hydrocortisone (or equivalent corticosteroid dose) should *not* be used for treating septic shock.	A
ACTH-250 mcg stimulation test should be used to identify adrenal insufficiency (≤9 mcg/dL increase in cortisol concentration 30–60 minutes after ACTH). Corticosteroid therapy should be initiated before stimulation test results are known. Corticosteroid therapy should be discontinued when adrenal insufficiency is absent (>9 mcg/dL increase in cortisol concentration 30–60 minutes after ACTH).	E
Once tissue hypoperfusion has resolved and in the absence of extenuating circumstances, such as significant coronary artery disease or acute hemorrhage, red blood cell transfusions should occur when hemoglobin decreases below 7 g/dL.	B

ACTH, adrenocorticotropic hormone; CO, cardiac output; CVP, central venous pressure; Do_2, oxygen delivery; MAP, mean arterial pressure; $Scvo_2$, central-venous oxygen saturation; Svo_2, mixed venous oxygen saturation. Strength of recommendations: A, supported by at least two large, randomized trials with clear-cut results (low risk of false-positive error or false-negative error); B, supported by one large, randomized trial with clear-cut results (low risk of false-positive error or false-negative error); C, supported by small, randomized trials with uncertain results (moderate-to-high risk of false-positive error or false-negative error); D, supported by at least one nonrandomized investigation with contemporaneous controls; E, supported by nonrandomized investigations with historical controls, case series, or expert opinion.
Based on data from references 4–7.

hepatic parenchymal function with increased serum concentrations of transaminases and bilirubin, altered gastrointestinal perfusion manifested by ileus and diminished bowel sounds, cardiac ischemia with elevated troponin levels and electrocardiographic changes, and altered sensorium.

GLOBAL PERFUSION MONITORING

ARTERIAL BLOOD PRESSURE MEASUREMENT

Mean arterial blood pressure (MAP) is the product of cardiac output (CO) and systemic vascular resistance (SVR). Conditions that may lower blood pressure in critically ill patients include cardiac failure (etiology may be myocardial infarction, arrhythmia, acute heart failure, or valvular disease) and hypovolemia (etiology may be hemorrhage, intractable diarrhea, or heat stroke) by lowering CO and vasodilation (etiology may be sepsis, drugs, anaphylaxis, acute hepatic failure, or neurotrauma) by lowering SVR. Arterial blood pressure is the end point of therapy; however, restoration of adequate pressure is the primary criterion of effectiveness.[4] Profound hypotension (MAP <50 mm Hg) is associated with a pressure-dependent decrease in coronary and cerebral blood flow and may rapidly produce myocardial and cerebral ischemia. Arterial blood pressure can be determined by noninvasive and invasive methods. All noninvasive blood pressure monitoring techniques depend on the use of an occluding cuff. Systolic and diastolic blood pressures are further determined by auscultation, palpation (systolic pressure only), oscillometry, or Doppler technique (systolic pressures are most reliable). Auscultation is the most commonly used method outside the intensive care unit (ICU). Its use, however, is limited in patients with hypovolemia, hypothermia, or cardiogenic shock when pulses or Korotkoff sounds may be difficult to hear. Similar constraints exist for the palpation and oscillometric methods. However, oscillometry is preferred in edematous patients. Oscillometry measures blood pressure by sensing arterial blood pressure changes, or oscillations, against an inflated cuff. Rapid changes in oscillation amplitude correspond to systolic and diastolic pressure. It is the only noninvasive method to measure MAP even in low-flow states and lends itself to automatic cycling and serial measurements (every 1–3 minutes) that do not require operator intervention, a key component in ICU monitoring. The use of narrow cuffs or cuffs applied too loosely can result in falsely high readings, whereas wide cuffs may produce falsely low readings.[6,8] Fingertip devices offer another avenue for continuous indirect blood pressure measurement, but their accuracy in ICU patients may be significantly diminished by concurrent administration of vasoactive drugs.

❶ The use of invasive arterial catheters makes possible the continuous measurement of MAP as well as procurement of blood samples for blood gas monitoring. The radial artery is the most commonly used vessel, but the dorsalis pedis, femoral, brachial, and axillary arteries and the umbilical artery in the newborn also can be accessed. This method of blood pressure monitoring is the standard technique used in the ICU against which all other methods are compared. Major complications of peripheral artery catheterization include infection and distal ischemia. Acute distal ischemia and catheter-related bacteremia occur in <1% of catheter insertions. This translates to 2.9% of bloodstream infections per 1,000 catheter-days.[11] Ischemia is most common in patients with multiple or prolonged arterial cannulations, hypertension, or vasopressor therapy.[6] Invasive techniques are labor intensive, require aseptic techniques, and offer potential sources of equipment errors, such as length and quality of tubing, air bubbles, stopcocks, thrombus formation, tube kinking, and transducer placement. Hypertension, advanced age, and atherosclerosis also may affect the accuracy of invasive blood pressure readings.[7]

CENTRAL VENOUS CATHETER

❶ The central venous catheter is used to measure the central venous pressure (CVP), to obtain venous blood gas samples, and to administer drugs or fluids directly to the central circulation. A triple-lumen catheter frequently is used, whereby drugs with known incompatibility can be administered. Blood volume, venous wall compliance, right-sided cardiac function, intraabdominal and intrathoracic pressures, and vasopressor therapy affect CVP. The CVP is not a reliable estimate of blood volume but can be used to qualitatively assess blood volume changes in patients during the early phases of fluid resuscitation. The goal of fluid administration is to maintain the CVP at 8 to 12 mm Hg, but values of 15 mm Hg may be targeted in mechanically ventilated patients to account for increased intrathoracic pressures.[5,6] Sustained elevated pressures may be indicative of fluid overloading. Few data support the use of CVP monitoring in the ICU. However, initial reports in septic patients suggest that CVP monitoring of fluid therapy during shock was associated with a 50% reduction in mortality.[8]

PULMONARY ARTERY CATHETER

❶ Pulmonary artery catheterization, introduced in 1970, is routinely performed in many ICUs. With this catheter, the practitioner can obtain multiple cardiovascular parameters, including CVP, pulmonary artery pressure, pulmonary artery occlusive pressures (PAOP), CO, and SVR. Mixed venous blood samples from the pulmonary artery also can be obtained. In an effort to reduce blood loss from samples, many clinicians use special pulmonary artery catheters, called *fiberoptic catheters,* which measure mixed venous oxygen saturation ($S\bar{v}O_2$). Trends in venous oxygen saturation can be observed and necessary action taken, if needed. Most important, inflation of the balloon at the catheter tip occludes the pulmonary artery, isolates the distal catheter tip from the right side of the heart, and allows the user to measure the PAOP, an approximate measure of the left ventricular end-diastolic volume and a major determinant of left ventricular preload. Some centers use a new pulmonary artery catheter capable of continuously measuring the right ventricular end-diastolic volume index. The right ventricular end-diastolic volume index may be a better predictor of CO than PAOP, but its clinical utility during shock remains to be studied. Ideally, the pulmonary artery catheter should be positioned fluoroscopically; however, satisfactory placement also may be obtained by observing pulmonary artery pressure readings and electrocardiographic waveforms during catheter advancement. Proper positioning in the lower lung (zone 3) is essential to measure PAOP and to prevent distal pulmonary artery collapse. Poor wedging may be caused by catheter migration, patient movement, mechanical ventilation, or eccentric balloon inflation. Pulmonary artery catheters equipped with a distal thermistor also allow measurement of CO by thermodilution. Rapid injection of saline or dextrose solutions via the right atrial port allows complete mixing of blood with injectate, and the resulting change in blood temperature is measured in the pulmonary artery. From the temperature change, the patient's CO can be calculated. Newer pulmonary artery catheters contain a temperature coil that intermittently warms the blood in the right ventricle for near-continuous CO measurement. Significant tricuspid regurgitation, an intracardiac shunt, and significant positive end-expiratory pressure decrease the validity of CO measurements. The most common complications of pulmonary artery catheterization include mural thrombus formation (14%–91%), transient ventricular tachydysrhythmias (11%–63%), pulmonary infarction (1%–7%), pulmonary artery rupture (0.06%–2.0%), and sepsis (0.3%–0.5%).[12] Most pulmonary artery catheters are heparin bonded, and the relative risk (RR) of infection is 2.6 per 1,000 patient-days, similar to the risk with central venous catheters of 2.3

per 1,000 patient-days.[11] Despite its ubiquitous use, much controversy surrounds the utility and safety of the pulmonary artery catheter, including issues surrounding correct placement and impact of the device on patient outcome.[13] As a result, recommendations have been made to standardize and monitor clinician education on proper use of the catheter (see *www.pacep.org*), to conduct clinical trials assessing the safety and efficacy of the catheter, and to evaluate new device technology on patient outcome.[12] The most recent guidelines suggest a careful evaluation of the indications and the risk of placing a pulmonary artery catheter for resuscitation of critically ill patients.[14]

❶ The optimal PAOP needs to be individualized for each patient. Administering a fluid bolus followed by simultaneous PAOP and CO measurements with the goal of increasing the PAOP until CO does not change can be accomplished and is based on Starling's law of the heart. However, clinical experience suggests that most patients have an optimal response to PAOP values in the range from 12 to 15 mm Hg.

CLINICAL CONTROVERSY: CVP VERSUS PAOP

Limited data are available comparing the use of CVP and PAOP for guiding therapy in patients in shock. The results of a study of patients with acute respiratory distress syndrome suggest CVP and PAOP are equivalent in terms of clinical outcomes, including mortality.[15] Therefore, a pulmonary artery catheter should be inserted when hemodynamic data are needed that cannot be obtained from a central venous catheter or when the validity of measurements from the central venous catheter is questionable.

OXYGEN TENSION AND SATURATION MONITORING

Partial pressure of arterial oxygen (PaO_2) and arterial oxygen saturation (SaO_2) can be measured subjectively by assessing capillary refill or invasively by obtaining an arterial blood sample. Arterial blood gases measured by conventional arterial sampling are considered standard, but their accuracy and usefulness are affected by poor sampling techniques, transportation and analysis delays, analyzer accuracy, sample cellular metabolism, and inability to trend results. Indwelling fiberoptic and electrochemical systems allow continuous monitoring and trend analyses of blood pH, PaO_2, and partial pressure of arterial carbon dioxide ($PaCO_2$) while decreasing patient blood loss from less frequent sampling. Unfortunately, studies evaluating the in vitro accuracy of these devices may not apply to the ICU environment. The indwelling sensors may exhibit lower PaO_2, higher $PaCO_2$, and lower pH than central arterial blood when peripheral flow is diminished. Furthermore, sensor contact with blood vessel wall and vigorous arterial line flushing diminish sensor accuracy.

❶ SvO_2 depends on CO, oxygen demand, hemoglobin, and SaO_2. It can be measured in patients using a pulmonary artery catheter. Initially, critically ill septic patients may present with a low SvO_2 value (<70%) indicating high extraction of oxygen by tissues and lack of adequate oxygen delivery (DO_2, or DO_2I, indexed to body surface area) to tissues. In patients with sepsis and other conditions who present with a low SvO_2 value, rapid intervention should be undertaken to increase DO_2 to tissues, with the goal of obtaining SvO_2 >70%.[16] The length of time SvO_2 is <70% is associated with mortality.[17] As sepsis worsens, however, SvO_2 often is >70%. This occurs because of a maldistribution of blood flow and a lack of extraction of oxygen in the arteriolar beds.

❶ Central venous oxygen saturation ($ScvO_2$) is a less invasive measure of venous oxygen saturation because the catheter is placed at the junction of the inferior and superior venae cavae rather than at the pulmonary artery. It is as accurate as SvO_2 but provides slightly higher normal values.[18,19] Although controversial, many clinicians use these measurements interchangeably. Concentrations of $ScvO_2$ <70% reliably indicate inadequate oxygenation in shock states and detect subclinical ("cryptic") shock much earlier than hypotension.[18] Targeting fluid and hemodynamic resuscitation to achieve $ScvO_2$ >70% is a sensitive indicator and measure of the extent of global tissue hypoxia, as well as a determinant of the adequacy of hemodynamic resuscitation.[18] Targeting resuscitation to achieve $ScvO_2$ >70% is associated with improved survival in patients with sepsis and septic shock.[19]

OXYGEN DELIVERY AND CONSUMPTION

The concept of tissue oxygen debt as a determinant of organ damage in critical illness was proposed in the 1970s. In normal individuals, oxygen consumption (VO_2 or VO_2I, indexed to body surface area) depends on DO_2 (or DO_2I) up to a certain critical level (VO_2 flow dependency). At this point, tissue oxygen requirements apparently are satisfied, and further increases in DO_2 will not alter VO_2 (VO_2 flow independency). Although animal models of sepsis have substantiated this relationship, studies in critically ill humans show a continuous, pathologic dependence relationship of VO_2 with DO_2. Furthermore, ICU survivors exhibited higher DO_2 and VO_2 values than did nonsurvivors. This finding became the basis for targeting supranormal DO_2 and VO_2 values in the treatment of ICU patients.[8] However, a meta-analysis of randomized clinical trials involving 1,016 adult ICU patients failed to show that achievement of this goal improved patient mortality.[20] This may have been due in part to the heterogeneous nature of the ICU patients studied, lack of study blinding, crossover patients (control patients who achieve supranormal DO_2 and VO_2 values by themselves), or lack of adequate control of cointerventions.

The debate continues in more homogeneous patient populations. In high-risk surgical patients, supranormal DO_2 values decreased mortality.[21,22] Two randomized studies published after the meta-analysis further evaluated the effect of increasing DO_2I values to >600 $mL/m^2/min$ in a homogeneous population of elderly surgical patients with systemic inflammatory response syndrome, sepsis, severe sepsis, or septic shock, with conflicting results. In one study, among patients between 50 and 75 years of age the intervention group had a significant increase in survival at 24 hours (21% vs 52%; $P = 0.01$) compared with the control group.[21] This benefit was not seen in patients older than 75 years. The authors suggested that the combination of increasing DO_2 and maintaining the oxygen extraction ratio (O_2ER) at <25% without a changing VO_2 may be helpful in maintaining or improving the body's reserve in meeting the oxygen demands. This may be particularly true in older patients who have a lower baseline VO_2. In the second study, the same intervention revealed a significant reduction in 60-day survival (15.7% vs 50%; $P <0.05$) in high-risk elderly surgical patients randomized to supranormal DO_2 goals.[22] Thus, whether supranormal DO_2 is beneficial and whether the mechanism of benefit of supranormal DO_2 in these patients is prevention and reversal of tissue hypoxia remain unclear. A review of alternative potential mechanisms of beneficial effect of supranormal DO_2 suggests that catecholamines exert antiinflammatory actions by modulating cytokine response.[23] In general, catecholamines inhibit the production of inflammatory cytokines (e.g., interleukin [IL]-6, tumor necrosis factor [TNF]-α) and may enhance synthesis of antiinflammatory cytokine (e.g., IL-4 and IL-10).[23] The actions of epinephrine on these cytokines are blocked by propranolol and thus are mediated by adrenergic β-receptors. These data must be interpreted with caution because most studies used animal or cell models of sepsis, pretreated patients with vasopressors prior to endotoxin infusion, and used doses that may not always be clinically relevant. Another problem with therapy directed to achieve supranormal oxygen transport values is that the apparent linear relationship between DO_2 and VO_2 has been questioned because both share variables, and this *mathematical cou-*

pling can produce artifactual relationships between variables. The DO_2 and VO_2 indexed parameters are calculated as follows:

$$DO_2 = CI \times CaO_2$$

$$VO_2 = CI \times (CaO_2 - CvO_2),$$

where CI = cardiac index, CaO_2 = arterial oxygen content determined by hemoglobin concentration and SaO_2, and CvO_2 = mixed venous oxygen content determined by hemoglobin concentration and SvO_2.

However, variable relationships between DO_2 and VO_2 have been observed when VO_2 was measured independently by indirect calorimetry. Therefore, a linear relationship between DO_2 and VO_2 may be the result of mathematical coupling or flow-dependent VO_2. Currently available data do not support the concept that patient outcome or survival is altered by treatment measures directed toward achieving supranormal DO_2 and VO_2 values.[20] In fact, a consensus conference concluded that although pulmonary artery catheterization is useful for guiding therapy, routinely increasing cardiac index to predetermined supranormal values does not improve outcome.[4] Furthermore, achievement of a supranormal DO_2 does not ensure parallel improvements in regional blood flow and oxygenation.[19] The VO_2/DO_2 ratio, or O_2ER, can be used to assess adequacy of perfusion and metabolic response. Patients who are able to increase VO_2 when DO_2 is increased show improved survival. However, low VO_2 and O_2ER values are indicative of poor oxygen utilization and lead to greater mortality.[20] Another approach that may decrease the effect of mathematical coupling and provide individualized therapy may lie in titrated therapy, with sequential measurements of DO_2 and VO_2 to achieve VO_2 flow independency along with normalization of blood lactate and hemodynamic parameters.

❷ The most recent data regarding goal-directed therapy in the hemodynamic support of sepsis relates to the importance of achieving predetermined parameters early in the management of sepsis. In a meta-analysis of early (defined as 8–12 hours postoperatively or before the development of organ failure) versus late (defined as after onset of organ failure) resuscitative efforts in patients stratified according to severity of illness (determined by control group mortality >20% [12 studies] or <15% [9 studies]) and targeting supranormal oxygen-transport variables, the data suggest that timing of resuscitation matters.[24] Early goal-directed therapy reduced mortality and the development of organ failure in patients who were more severely ill and when therapeutic interventions produced differences in DO_2. Moreover, outcome was not improved significantly in less severely ill patients (control group mortality <15% and normal DO_2 values as goals) or when therapy did not improve DO_2.[23]

❷ In a prospective, randomized controlled trial of sepsis, Rivers et al.[19] demonstrated a significant reduction in mortality (30.5% versus 46.5%; $P < 0.001$) in patients with severe sepsis and septic shock randomized to receive therapy based on goal-directed hemodynamic end points that were achieved within 6 hours of hospital presentation. They used a strategy of serial administering (1) fluids rapidly to achieve CVP 8–12 mm Hg, (2) vasopressor agents to achieve MAP at least 65 mm Hg, (3) red blood cell transfusion to maintain hematocrit >30%, and (4) dobutamine to achieve $ScvO_2$ >70%. This approach demonstrates the benefits of initiating therapy early in the course of sepsis and directs therapy toward clearly defined goals in a consistent manner. The results of this study cannot delineate which end point or combination of end points was most beneficial, so until proven otherwise, clinicians should direct therapy to achieve all the hemodynamic goals of this study. In addition, whether these goals must be maintained after resuscitation is unknown. Therefore, after resuscitation and assuming patients do not have coronary artery disease, red blood cell transfusions should be administered in patients with hemoglobin <7 g/dL to maintain a hemoglobin concentration 7–9 g/dL (or hematocrit approximately 21%–27%).[4,5] Several observational studies have shown that improvement of organ function within the first 24 hours of therapy with maintenance of hemodynamic variables for at least 48 hours with goals similar to those in the study by Rivers et al. is associated with improved survival.[17,25] The results of several before and after evaluations of protocols or order sets designed to achieve the hemodynamic end points of early goal-directed therapy show that implementation is easily accomplished, and patient outcomes, including survival, are improved.[26–28] Therefore, healthcare facilities should implement strategies to achieve early goal-directed therapy using the predefined hemodynamic variables of the study by Rivers et al. Directing therapy to increase the goal MAP from 65 to 85 mm Hg with higher doses of vasopressor agents does not confer additional improvement in organ function.[29]

BLOOD LACTATE

Lactate is a metabolic product of pyruvate. Its production is increased under anaerobic conditions, such as may occur during shock. Blood lactate concentrations are used as a diagnostic and prognostic tool in sepsis; they also are used to measure the repayment of oxygen debt to tissues.[16] It is a useful tool in combination with DO_2 and VO_2 because these measures change independently of one another. Serial lactate concentrations may show better correlation with outcome than oxygen transport parameters and may be superior to hemodynamic markers in determining adequacy of restoration of systemic oxygenation.[16] However, several caveats guide the use of lactate concentrations in septic patients.[6] First, lactate may accumulate in patients with other conditions, such as significant hepatic dysfunction or acute respiratory distress syndrome, who are not in shock. Second, both well-perfused and poorly perfused tissues contribute to arterial and mixed venous lactate concentrations and therefore are not reflective of regional perfusion. Third, although increased lactate concentrations have been correlated with increased mortality, the utility of blood lactate measurements in guiding therapy has not been clearly demonstrated. Fourth, elevated lactate concentrations may result from cellular metabolic failure rather than global hypoperfusion in shock. Serial blood lactate measurements are more useful than single isolated measurements.

REGIONAL PERFUSION MONITORING

GASTROINTESTINAL TONOMETRY

Blood pressures, CO, blood lactate, and global oxygen homeostasis parameters do not offer information about the function of individual organs. Organ-specific hypoxia may be evident by coagulopathy as indicated by thrombocytopenia (platelet count <100,000/L and/or prolonged clotting times [international normalized ratio >1.5 or activated partial thromboplastin time at least 1.5-fold the upper limit of normal]), impaired renal function with urine production <0.5 mL/kg/h and/or increased serum concentrations of blood urea nitrogen and creatinine, altered hepatic function with substantially increased serum concentrations of transaminases and bilirubin, altered gastrointestinal perfusion manifested by ileus and diminished bowel sounds, cardiac ischemia with elevated troponin levels and electrocardiogram changes, and altered sensorium.[4–10] Objective measurement of regional perfusion to detect inadequate tissue oxygenation has focused on the splanchnic circulation, which is sensitive to changes in blood flow and oxygenation for several reasons. First, the normally large majority of blood flow to the gut mucosa is redistributed toward the serosa and muscularis. Second, the gut may have a higher critical DO_2 threshold than other organs. Third, the tip of the villus has a countercurrent oxygen-exchange mechanism, rendering it highly sensitive to alterations in regional blood flow and oxygenation.[16]

Gastric tonometry measures gut luminal partial pressure of carbon dioxide (P_{CO_2}) at equilibrium by placing a saline- or air-filled gas-permeable balloon in the gastric lumen. Assuming that CO_2 permeates freely among tissues and that the arterial bicarbonate (HCO_3^-) concentration is equal to that of the gut mucosa, the intramucosal pH (pHi) may be calculated using the Henderson-Hasselbalch equation:

$$pHi = 6.1 \log (HCO_3^-)\ 0.03 \times P_{CO_2}$$

Increases in mucosal P_{CO_2} and calculated decreases in pHi are associated with mucosal hypoperfusion and perhaps increased mortality.[30] Calculation of pHi can be confounded by increases in luminal P_{CO_2}, such as may occur when buffering antacids are used. Histamine$_2$-receptor antagonists or proton pump inhibitors can be used instead. The presence of respiratory acid–base disorders; systemic bicarbonate administration; arterial blood gas measurement errors; or enteral feeding products, blood, or stool in the gut may confound pHi determinations.[6] As a result, many clinicians believe that the change in gastric mucosal P_{CO_2} may be more accurate than pHi.[6] Furthermore, because mucosal P_{CO_2} is influenced by arterial P_{CO_2}, the consensus is that the mucosal–arterial P_{CO_2} difference (P_{CO_2} gap) likely is the optimal measurement.[30] Gastric tonometry can be performed using either a saline- or air-filled balloon. The time delay (30 minutes) associated with equilibration of saline inside the balloon makes this method inconvenient for routine bedside monitoring. An air-filled balloon requires a shorter equilibrium time, is simpler to use, and is equally accurate.[31] However, the clinical utility of gastric tonometry remains uncertain. Clinical trials of pHi-directed therapy have not shown consistently that gastric tonometry reduces mortality in critically ill patients.[30] In a study of 28 patients with septic shock, gastric tonometry measurements were not beneficial during initial resuscitation; however, after stabilization, pHi, mucosal P_{CO_2}, and P_{CO_2} gap were independent predictors of hospital mortality.[32]

Evidence suggests that the most proximal part of the gastrointestinal tract, the sublingual mucosa, may be an acceptable location for monitoring regional perfusion and P_{CO_2}. Sublingual capnometry is noninvasive, is not technically complex, and provides results within minutes.[33] The device consists of a disposable sublingual carbon dioxide pressure (P_{slCO_2}) sensor, a fiberoptic cable that connects the disposable sensor to a blood gas analyzer, and a blood gas monitoring instrument. A small study of 22 critically ill patients with and without sepsis and septic shock attempted to validate the usefulness of sublingual capnography.[34] The study measured simultaneous gastric and sublingual P_{CO_2} along with traditional hemodynamic parameters. P_{slCO_2} correlated well with mucosal P_{CO_2}; however, the initial sublingual-to-arterial P_{CO_2} gap was a better predictor of mortality than the mucosal-to-arterial P_{CO_2} gap. Another small study of 18 patients with septic shock also found significant correlation between gastric and sublingual P_{CO_2}, but enhancement of DO_2 with dobutamine better correlated with the decrease in P_{slCO_2} gap than gastric P_{CO_2} gap.[35] These pilot studies must be expanded before this technology becomes part of routine practice, but it offers the possibility of noninvasively measurement of regional perfusion.

MYOCARDIAL DYSFUNCTION

Although loss of vascular tone is the hallmark of septic shock, myocardial dysfunction characterized by transient impairment of contractility is a recognized complication. The range of left ventricular ejection fraction (LVEF) upon presentation is wide, but approximately 35% of patients with septic shock have left ventricular hypokineses (mean ejection fraction 38% ± 17%) and low CO.[36] Because LVEF also is affected by preload and afterload, the low SVR of septic shock may mask depressed myocardial contractility that may be revealed upon restoration of MAP by administration of fluid and vasopressors. Cardiac troponin release in septic patients occurs in the absence of flow-limiting disease, likely due to a loss in membrane integrity with subsequent leakage or microvascular thrombosis. Elevation of cardiac troponin concentrations in patients with sepsis indicates left ventricular dysfunction and portends a poor prognosis.[37] Early recognition of myocardial dysfunction is crucial for administration of appropriate therapy. In the absence of other mechanisms for assessing cardiac function, echocardiographic findings and troponin concentrations may help guide and monitor therapy. Whereas cardiac troponins may be integrated into the monitoring of myocardial dysfunction to identify patients requiring aggressive therapy, natriuretic peptides have not been shown to correlate with LVEF and should not be routinely monitored.[37]

VASOPRESSORS AND INOTROPES

❺ Vasopressors and inotropes in patients with septic shock are required when volume resuscitation fails to maintain adequate blood pressure (MAP 65 mm Hg) and organs and tissues remain hypoperfused despite optimizing CVP to 8 to 12 mm Hg or PAOP to 12 to 15 mm Hg. However, vasopressors may be needed temporarily to treat life-threatening hypotension when filling pressures are inadequate despite aggressive fluid resuscitation.[4] Inotropes are frequently used to optimize cardiac function in cases of cardiogenic shock.[3] The clinician must decide on the choice of agent, therapeutic end points, and safe and effective doses of vasopressors and inotropes to be used. This section reviews adrenergic receptor pharmacology, exogenous catecholamine use, and alterations in receptor function in critically ill patients. It also provides guidelines for the clinical use of adrenergic agents, optimization of pharmacotherapeutic outcomes, and minimization of adverse effects in critically ill patients with septic shock. Therapies of hypovolemic shock and cardiogenic shock are discussed in other chapters.

Of note, agents other than catecholamines have been used as inotropes and vasopressors in shock states. They include phosphodiesterase III inhibitors, naloxone, nitric oxide synthase (NOS) inhibitors, and calcium sensitizers. This chapter focuses on catecholamines. Vasopressin and corticosteroids, as they relate to septic shock, also are emphasized because they have pharmacologic interactions with catecholamines, possess hemodynamic effects, and are frequently used.

CATECHOLAMINE RECEPTOR PHARMACOLOGY

❹ Comparative receptor activity of endogenous and exogenously administered catecholamines is summarized in Table 25–3.[3–10] Endogenous catecholamines are responsible for regulation of vascular and bronchiolar smooth muscle tone and myocardial contractility. These effects are mediated by sympathetic adrenergic receptors of the autonomic nervous system located in the vasculature, myocardium, and bronchioles. Postsynaptic adrenoceptors are located at or near the synaptic junction. These receptors can be activated by naturally circulating or exogenous catecholamines (e.g., norepinephrine, epinephrine, and phenylephrine), whereas presynaptic adrenoceptors are stimulated by locally released neurotransmitters (e.g., norepinephrine) and are controlled by a negative feedback mechanism.

The signal transduction pathways associated with catecholamine- and vasopressin-induced effects in the heart and blood vessels are illustrated in Fig. 25–1. Agonists of β-adrenoceptors and dopamine (D_1) receptors stimulate adenylate cyclase by a G-protein (G_s)–dependent mechanism (Fig. 25–1, top). Adenylate cyclase generates cyclic adenosine monophosphate (cAMP) from adenosine triphosphate (ATP). cAMP-Dependent protein kinase A, which is activated by elevations in intracellular cAMP, phosphorylates target proteins to modify cellular function. Through these mechanisms, β_1-adrenocep-

TABLE 25-3 Adrenergic, Dopaminergic, and Vasopressin Receptor Pharmacology and Organ Distribution

Effector Organ	Receptor Subtype	Physiologic Response
Heart		
Sinoatrial node	β_1, β_2	Increased heart rate
Atria	β_1, β_2	Increased contractility Increased conduction velocity
Atrioventricular node	β_1, β_2	Increased automaticity Increased conduction velocity
His-Purkinje system	β_1, β_2	Increased automaticity Increased conduction velocity
Ventricles	β_1, β_2	Increased contractility Increased conduction velocity Increased automaticity Increased rate idioventricular pacemaker cells
Arterioles		
Coronary	α_1, α_2, V1; β_2, D_1, V_2 (via NO)	Constriction; dilation
Skin and mucosa	α_1, α_2, V_1	Constriction
Skeletal muscle	α_1, V_1; β_2	Constriction; dilation
Cerebral	α_1, V_1; V_2 (via NO)	Constriction (slight); dilation
Pulmonary	α_1; β_2, V_2 (via NO)	Constriction; dilation
Abdominal viscera (mesentery)	α_1, V_1; β_2, D_1	Constriction; dilation
Renal	α_1, α_2, V_1; β_1, β_2, D_1	Constriction; dilation
Veins (systemic)	α_1, α_2; β_2	Constriction; dilation
Lungs		
Tracheal/bronchial smooth muscle	β_2	Relaxation
Bronchial glands	α_1; β_2	Decreased; increased secretion
Stomach		
Motility and tone	α_1, α_2, β_1, β_2	Decreased (usually)
Sphincter	α_1	Contraction (usually)
Secretions	α_2	Inhibition
Intestine		
Motility and tone	α_1, α_2, β_1, β_2; V_1	Decreased (usually); Increased?
Sphincters	α_1	Contraction
Secretions	α_2	Inhibition
Kidney		
Renin secretion	α_1; β_1	Decreased; Increased
Reabsorption of water	V_2	Increased
Skeletal muscle	β_2	Increased contractility, glycogenesis, K^+ uptake
Liver	α_1, β_2	Glycogenolysis and gluconeogenesis
Fat cells	α_1, β_1, β_2	Lipolysis (thermogenesis)

D, dopamine; NO, nitric oxide; V, vasopressin.
Based on data from references 4–7, 42, 45, and 46.

tor activation exerts positive inotropic and chronotropic effects in the heart, and β_2-adrenoceptor and D_1-receptor activation induces vascular smooth muscle relaxation. Agonists of α_1-adrenoceptors or vasopressin $(V)_1$ receptors stimulate phospholipase C-β (PLC-β) through a G-protein (G_q)–dependent process (Fig. 25–1, bottom). PLC-β produces inositol trisphosphate and diacylglycerol from cell membrane phosphatidylinositol bisphosphate. Diacylglycerol activates protein kinase C, an enzyme that phosphorylates several key proteins (e.g., extracellular signal-regulated kinases, c-Jun NH2-terminal kinases, and mitogen-activated protein kinases) that modify cellular function (e.g., hypertrophy). Inositol trisphosphate elicits the release of calcium from intracellular stores, such as the sarcoplasmic reticulum. Calcium forms a complex with calmodulin, which then activates calcium–calmodulin-dependent protein kinases (CaMK). CaMKs phosphorylate target proteins to alter cellular function. Myosin light-chain kinase is an example of a CaMK. Its action of phosphorylating myosin light chain leads to vascular smooth muscle contraction.

The normal heart contains primarily postsynaptic β_1-receptors, which when stimulated cause increased rate and force of contraction. This effect is mediated by activation of adenylate cyclase and subsequent generation and accumulation of cAMP. Stimulation of postsynaptic cardiac α_1-receptors causes a significant increase in contractility without an increase in rate, an effect mediated by PLC rather than adenylate cyclase. The increased contractility is more pronounced at lower heart rates and has a slower onset and longer duration in comparison with β_1-mediated inotropic response. Presynaptic α_2-adrenoceptors also are found in the heart and appear to be activated by norepinephrine released by the sympathetic nerve itself. Their activation inhibits further norepinephrine release from the nerve terminal.

Both presynaptic and postsynaptic adrenoceptors are present in the vasculature. Postsynaptic α_1- and α_2-receptors mediate vasoconstriction, whereas postsynaptic β_2-receptors induce vasodilation. Presynaptic α_2-receptors inhibit norepinephrine release in the vasculature, also promoting vasodilation. Presynaptic β_1-adrenoceptors promote neurotransmitter release. Stimulation of peripheral D_1-receptors produces renal, coronary, and mesenteric vasodilation and a natriuretic response. Stimulation of D_2-receptors inhibits norepinephrine release from sympathetic nerve endings, sequesters prolactin and aldosterone, and may induce nausea and vomiting. D_1- and D_2-receptor stimulation also suppresses peristalsis and may precipitate ileus.[3–9]

ALTERED ADRENOCEPTOR FUNCTION: IMPLICATIONS FOR CRITICALLY ILL PATIENTS

❸ Most of the work describing receptor function and associated clinical pharmacology has been performed in either animal models or human volunteers. In critically ill septic patients, derangements in adrenergic receptor activity may result in resistance to exogenously administered catecholamine.[38–43] This "desensitization" frequently is characterized by myocardial and vascular hyporesponsiveness to high dosages of inotropes and vasopressor agents. Prolonged exposure of vascular endothelial tissue to vasopressor drugs (α-adrenergic agonists) or endogenous catecholamines may promote additional receptor downregulation. Increased endogenous catecholamine concentrations have been reported in endotoxemic and other critically ill patients, suggesting an acquired adrenergic receptor defect and desensitization of adrenergic receptors and alteration in voltage-sensitive calcium channels.[38–42] The problem in critically ill patients may be related to decreased receptor activity or density. However, in patients with septic shock, catecholamine concentrations are even higher, so abnormalities in adrenergic receptor function are greater, with associated reductions in the concentrations of intracellular signal transduction mediators. The worsened receptor abnormality may be explained by defects distal to the receptor site, such as uncoupling of adrenergic receptors from adenylate cyclase or PLC, or dysfunction in the regulatory G-protein unit of signal transduction pathways.[38–42]

In addition to catecholamines, circulating inflammatory cytokines may be partly responsible for distal alterations. Macrophage-derived IL-1 and TNF-α produce impaired coupling of β-adrenoceptors to adenylate cyclase.[38,39] Patients with septic shock have exhibited impaired β-adrenergic receptor stimulation of cAMP associated with myocardial hyporesponsiveness to various vasopressors and inotropes.[38,39] However, increased chronotropic sensitivity to β-adrenergic stimulation with hypersensitivity of the adenylate cyclase system to isoproterenol stimulation also has been reported in animal models of bacteremia and endotoxemia. In the presence of intrinsic myocardial dysfunction and increased metabolic demands, this dysfunctional adrenergic system is incapable of mobilizing functional cardiac reserve to maintain adequate myocardial performance.[38–40]

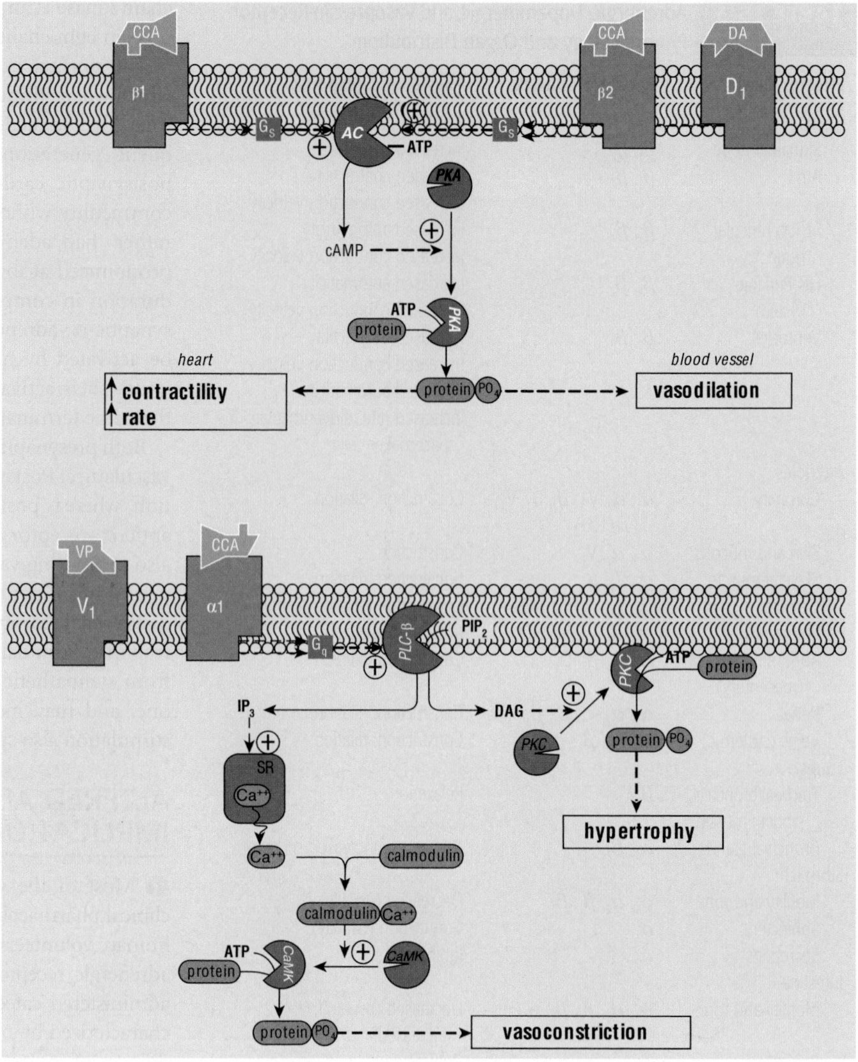

FIGURE 25-1. Signal transduction pathways in heart and blood vessels. *Top.* Catecholamine (CCA)-induced effects mediated in heart (β_1) or vascular smooth muscle (β_2, D_1). (AC, adenylate cyclase; ATP, adenosine triphosphate; cAMP, cyclic adenosine monophosphate; PKA, cAMP-dependent protein kinase; +, stimulation.) *Bottom.* CCA (α_1) and vasopressin (VP)-induced actions in vascular smooth muscle. (Ca^{++}, calcium ion; CaMK, calcium/calmodulin-dependent protein kinase; DAG, diacylglycerol; IP_3, inositol trisphosphate; PIP_2, phosphatidylinositol bisphosphate; PKC, protein kinase C; PLC-β, phospholipase C-β; SR, sarcoplasmic reticulum.) These pathways have been extensively simplified, and denoted cellular effects represent one of many produced. *(Figure based on data from references 4–6, 10, 42, 44, 45, and 89.)*

IL-1 and TNF-α have been shown to suppress gene expression of α_1-adrenoceptors, resulting in fewer receptor proteins.[40] Overproduction of nitric oxide (NO) by inducible nitric oxide synthase (iNOS) directly contributes to vasodilation by cyclic guanosine monophosphate–mediated smooth muscle relaxation. NO indirectly produces vasodilation by combining with superoxide to form peroxynitrite, a highly toxic reactive species that causes endothelial dysfunction, uncoupling of α_1-adrenoceptors to PLC, and deactivation of catecholamines.[41,42] The result of sepsis-induced inflammation is a system that promotes adrenergic receptor dysfunction to accentuate vasodilation and shock.

❹ Functional α_1-adrenergic receptor changes occur at various stages of sepsis; thus, adrenoceptor sensitivity may be time dependent during progression of sepsis to septic shock. The findings are not always consistent in various animal models of sepsis and in critically ill septic patients. Time-dependent alterations in the production of NO, a potent vasodilator, may explain the apparent differences in vascular reactivity to phenylephrine during the phases of endotoxemia.[43] This finding suggests that the clinical response to vasopressor and possibly inotropic agents is variable during the stages of hemodynamic, myocardial, and peripheral vascular derangements of septic shock. In contrast, in critically ill septic patients in the ICU (24–48 hours from hospital admission), β-adrenergic receptor changes already were present, although the progression of desensitization of receptors earlier in sepsis was not quantified.[39] In summary, α- and β-adrenergic receptor derangements may vary among patients and during each bacteremic insult; therefore, doses of catecholamines vary among patients and during the insult. For these reasons, these drugs should be dosed to clinical end points and not to arbitrary maximal doses.

VASOPRESSIN AND CORTISOL: IMPLICATIONS ON CATECHOLAMINES

⓬ Endogenous arginine vasopressin, a peptide hormone also known as antidiuretic hormone, is important for osmoregulation under normal physiologic conditions. Vasopressin is produced in the hypothalamus, stored in the posterior pituitary, and released from magnocellular neurons of the hypothalamus.[44,45] Increased serum osmolality and hypovolemia are the major stimuli for vasopressin release.[44,45] Other stimuli commonly associated with shock are dopamine, histamine, angiotensin II, prostaglandins, pain, hypoxia, acidosis, hypotension, hypercarbia, and α_1-adrenergic receptor stimulation. Vasopressin release is inhibited by NO, natriuretic peptides, γ-aminobutyric acid, β-adrenergic receptor stimulation, and α_2-adrenergic receptor stimulation.[44,45]

Vasopressin has minimal to no inotropic or chronotropic effects. Vasopressin-induced vasoconstriction occurs through a variety of direct and indirect mechanisms.[44,45] Stimulation of vascular V_1 receptors causes vasoconstriction by receptor-coupled activation of PLC and calcium release from intracellular stores via secondary messengers similar to α_1-adrenergic stimulation. Vasopressin also directly inhibits vascular potassium-sensitive ATP channels to activate vascular calcium channels independent of V_1 receptors (Fig. 25–1). V_1-

receptor stimulation inhibits the actions of IL-1β and thereby facilitates vasoconstriction. Vasopressin also increases the activity of adrenergic receptors. The greatest vasoconstriction occurs in the skin and soft tissue, skeletal muscle, fat tissue, pancreas, and thyroid gland.

V_2 receptors located in the kidneys are responsible for the antidiuretic properties of vasopressin.[44,45] Stimulation of V_2 receptors facilitates integration of aquaporins into the luminal cell membrane of distal tubules and collecting duct capillaries to increase permeability and thus retain intravascular volume. However, vasopressin stimulation of V_1 receptors causes vasoconstriction of efferent arterioles and relative vasodilation of afferent arterioles to increase glomerular perfusion pressure and filtration rate to enhance urine production.

Vasopressin rapidly increases serum cortisol concentration by stimulating V_3 receptors in the pituitary gland to enhance the release of adrenocorticotropic hormone (ACTH).[44,45] Cortisol helps regulate the proinflammatory state associated with sepsis and increases blood pressure through several mechanisms, including inhibition of iNOS to reduce NO production, reversal of adrenergic receptor desensitization, and increased intravascular volume through retention of sodium and water.

Normal serum vasopressin concentrations are <4 pg/mL.[44,45] Serum vasopressin concentrations are elevated with hypotension. Vasopressin response in septic shock is biphasic. During the first 8 hours of septic shock requiring catecholamine adrenergic therapy, serum concentrations of vasopressin are appropriately high to help maintain blood pressure and organ perfusion. Thereafter, serum vasopressin concentrations decline dramatically over the next 96 hours to physiologically normal but inappropriately low values, resulting in a state of "relative deficiency." In contrast, serum vasopressin concentrations remain elevated in patients with cardiogenic shock, requiring at least 1 day of hemodynamic support with catecholamine agents. Administration of vasopressin at 0.01 to 0.06 units/min produces concentrations similar to those observed in early septic shock and other hypotensive states; however, vasopressin concentrations do not correlate with blood pressure.

The mechanism of vasopressin insufficiency in septic shock is not well understood. Neurohypophyseal stores in the posterior lobe of the pituitary gland are depleted during septic shock, likely as a result of excessive and continuous baroreceptor stimulation that eventually exhausts the limited vasopressin secretory stores. In addition, secretion of vasopressin is inhibited by enhanced endothelial production of NO, high circulating concentrations of adrenergic agonists (both endogenous and exogenous), and tonic inhibition by stretch receptors in response to volume replacement and mechanical ventilation.

As with vasopressin, during sepsis a state of "relative adrenal insufficiency" is produced by continuous activation of the hypothalamic–pituitary–adrenal axis by IL-1, IL-6, and TNF-α that causes depletion of cortisol in the adrenal glands.[46] Administration of corticosteroids has been shown to improve arterial pressure while minimizing the dose of catecholamine vasopressors.[47,48] Current proposed mechanisms of the vasoconstrictor effect of corticosteroids include increasing the number and stimulating the function of α_1- and β-adrenergic receptors and attenuating the production of inflammatory mediators responsible for vasodilation.

⓬ The use of corticosteroids for treatment of septic shock has been a topic of controversy for many years. Meta-analyses of early studies of steroids in patients with sepsis demonstrated a lack of benefit and potential harm in sepsis and septic shock.[49,50] Interest in corticosteroid use is renewed because of the increased awareness of adrenocortical insufficiency in critically ill patients with septic shock.[46] Relative adrenal insufficiency has been defined as a poor adrenal response (<9 mcg/dL [250 nmol/L] irrespective of the initial serum cortisol level) to a dose of synthetic ACTH, indicating a low functional reserve of the adrenal cortex.[51] Although absolute insufficiency is rare, relative adrenocortical insufficiency in the presence of normal or high cortisol concentrations at baseline is present in 30% to 50% of patients with septic shock and is associated with a poor outcome.[46,51]

CLINICAL CONTROVERSY: DIAGNOSING RELATIVE ADRENAL INSUFFICIENCY

The diagnosis of relative adrenal insufficiency in septic shock is based on serum cortisol concentration(s) rather than clinical parameters. Some leading experts suggest defining adrenal insufficiency as a random cortisol concentration <15 to 25 mcg/dL, irrespective of ACTH testing results because the test dose of ACTH may cause sufficient cortisol production in patients with mild-to-moderate adrenal insufficiency. In the only study to correlate mortality with adrenal response, an elevated random cortisol concentration (>34 mcg/dL) was an independent predictor of mortality.[51] The predictive value of mortality further increased if ACTH response was <9 mcg/dL, suggesting that the risk of mortality is greatest in situations of adrenal gland "fatigue" (i.e., degree of stress is not matched by sufficient cortisol production by the adrenal glands despite operating at maximal functional capacity).

CLINICAL PHARMACOLOGY OF VASOPRESSORS AND INOTROPES

❹ ⓬ The receptor selectivity of clinically used, catecholamine-based vasopressors and inotropes and hemodynamic effects are listed in Table 25–4. In general, these drugs are rapid acting, with short durations of action. As such, these drugs are given as continuous infusions and titrated rapidly to predetermined effects. Vasopressin is administered as a replacement dose of 0.01 to 0.04 units/min and should not be titrated. Careful monitoring and calculation of infusion rates are advised for all vasopressors because dosing adjustments are made frequently, and varying admixtures and concentrations are used in volume-restricted patients.

❽ Dopamine is often considered a first-line initial therapy in patients with septic shock because it increases blood pressure by increasing myocardial contractility and vasoconstriction.[4–10] Dopamine has been described as having dose-related receptor activity at D_1-, D_2-, β_1-, and α_1-receptors (Table 25–4). Unfortunately, this dose–response relationship has not been confirmed in critically ill patients. In patients with septic shock, great overlap of hemodynamic effects occurs, even at doses as low as 3 mcg/kg/min.[52] Tachydysrhythmias are common due to the release of endogenous norepinephrine by dopamine entering the sympathetic nerve terminal. Dopamine may increase PAOP through pulmonary vasoconstriction.[6,7] This drug also may depress ventilation and worsen hypoxemia in patients dependent on the hypoxic ventilatory drive.

Dobutamine, a synthetic catecholamine, is primarily a selective β_1-agonist with mild β_2- and vascular α_1-activity, resulting in strong positive inotropic activity without concomitant vasoconstriction. In comparison with dopamine, dobutamine produces a larger increase in CO and is less arrhythmogenic.[7,40] α_1-Adrenoceptors in the heart are directly stimulated by the (–) isomer of dobutamine, but β_1- and β_2-activity resides in the (+) isomer.[7,40] This finding suggests that the strong inotropic action of dobutamine is a function of its structure, the additive effect of cardiac α_1- and β_1-agonist activity, and a relatively weak chronotropic effect limited to the (+) isomer action on the β-receptors. Clinically, β_2-induced vasodilation and the increased myocardial contractility with subsequent reflex reduction in sympathetic tone lead to a decrease in SVR. Dobutamine is used optimally for patients in low CO states with high filling pressures or in those in cardiogenic shock; however, vasopressors may be needed to counteract arterial vasodilation.

TABLE 25-4 Receptor Pharmacology of Selected Inotropic and Vasopressor Agents Used in Septic Shock[a]

Agent	α_1	α_2	β_1	β_2	D	V_1	V_2
Dobutamine (0.5–4 mg/mL D_5W or NS)							
2–10 mcg/kg/min	+	0	++++	++	0	0	0
>10–20 mcg/kg/min	++	0	++++	+++	0	0	0
Dopamine (0.8–3.2 mg/mL D_5W or NS)							
1–3 mcg/kg/min	0	0	+	0	++++	0	0
3–10 mcg/kg/min	0/+	0	++++	+	++++	0	0
>10–20 mcg/kg/min	+++	0	++++	+	0	0	0
Epinephrine (0.008–0.016 mg/mL D_5W or NS)							
0.01–0.05 mcg/kg/min	++	++	++++	+++	0	0	0
0.05–3 mcg/kg/min	++++	++++	+++	+	0	0	0
Norepinephrine (0.016–0.064 mg/mL D_5W)							
0.02–3 mcg/kg/min	+++	+++	+++	+/++	0	0	0
Phenylephrine (0.1–0.4 mg/mL D_5W or NS)							
0.5–9 mcg/kg/min	+++	+	+	0	0	0	0
Vasopressin (0.8 units/mL D_5W or NS)							
0.01–0.04 units/min	0	0	0	0	0	+++	+++

[a]Activity ranges from no activity (0) to maximal (++++) activity.
D, dopamine; D_5W, dextrose 5% in water; NS, normal saline; V, vasopressin.
Based on data from references 4–7, 42, 45, and 46.

❽ Norepinephrine is a combined α- and β-agonist that produces vasoconstriction primarily via its more prominent α-effects on all vascular beds, thus increasing SVR. Norepinephrine administration generally produces either no change or some increase in CO.[53,54] In addition to dopamine, norepinephrine is considered an option for initial vasopressor therapy for septic shock.

❾ Phenylephrine is a pure α_1-agonist and is believed to increase blood pressure through vasoconstriction. Given the presence of cardiac α_1-receptors, phenylephrine also may increase contractility and CO.[55] It is a therapeutic option in hypotensive patients experiencing a tachyarrhythmia when a vasopressor with minimal to no β_1-agonist activity is indicated.

❿ Epinephrine exerts combined α- and β-agonist effects. At the high epinephrine infusion rates used for patients with septic shock, predominantly α-adrenergic effects are seen, and SVR and MAP are increased. Epinephrine traditionally has been reserved as the vasopressor of last resort due to peripheral vasoconstriction, particularly in the splanchnic and renal beds.[42,56,57]

⓬ Unlike adrenergic receptor agonists, the vasoconstrictive effects of vasopressin are preserved during hypoxia and severe acidosis. Several small studies have evaluated short-term infusions of vasopressin at doses <0.08 units/min as add-on therapy to patients requiring catecholamine adrenergic agents.[44,45] The results show that initiating vasopressin in patients with septic shock increases SVR and arterial blood pressure to reduce the dose requirements of catecholamine adrenergic agents. These effects are rapid and sustained. Vasopressin causes vasodilation in the cerebral, pulmonary, coronary, and selected renal vascular beds by enhancing endothelial NO release through V_1-receptor stimulation in these tissues.[44] Organ-specific vasodilation reduces pulmonary artery pressure and may preserve cardiac and renal function. Several studies have shown substantial enhancement of urine production, likely due to increased glomerular filtration rate. At doses exceeding 0.04 units/min, vasopressin was associated with ischemia of the mesenteric mucosa, skin, and myocardium; elevated hepatic transaminases and bilirubin concentrations; hyponatremia; and thrombocytopenia. Limiting the dose to a maximum of 0.04 units/min may minimize the development of adverse effects.

CLINICAL APPLICATION

Vasopressors and Inotropes

❺ ❽ Initial hemodynamic therapy for septic shock is administration of intravenous fluid (20–40 mL/kg), with the goal of attaining CVP of 8 to 12 mm Hg.[4–10] Crystalloid fluids (e.g., normal saline, Ringer lactate solution) and colloid fluids (e.g., albumin, hetastarch, dextrans, blood products) are considered equivalent for shock resuscitation. Crystalloid fluids are generally preferred unless patients are at risk for adverse events from redistribution of intravenous fluids to extravascular tissues and/or are fluid restricted (e.g., patients with renal dysfunction, decompensated heart failure, ascites compromising diaphragmatic function).

Traditional vasopressors and inotropes used for hemodynamic support of patients with hypotension refractory to fluid administration include dopamine, dobutamine, epinephrine, norepinephrine, and phenylephrine. Optimizing MAP to 65 mm Hg as the goal of vasopressor therapy does not uniformly correlate with decreased mortality in patients with septic shock.[19,20] Historically, significant concerns about the adverse effects of vasopressors limited their use. The past focus of achieving supranormal oxygen-transport variables also has yielded poor results in patients with septic shock.[20] In fact, normalization of systemic DO_2 and VO_2, whether spontaneously or with intervention, is associated with improved outcome and is not dependent on administration of vasopressor agents. Part of the inability to detect an improvement with vasopressor or inotropic therapies may result from the limited ability to quantify regional tissue perfusion. However, use of early goal-directed therapy to $ScvO_2$ >70% has been shown to reduce mortality in patients with sepsis and septic shock.[19]

❻ ❼ Dosage titration and monitoring of vasopressor and inotropic therapy should be guided by the "best clinical response" and the goals of early goal-directed therapy.[4–10,19] Dopamine or norepinephrine is considered the agent of choice as initial vasopressor therapy. Norepinephrine may be added in cases where suboptimal response is obtained from dopamine but adding dopamine to norepinephrine does not provide a hemodynamic benefit. Phenylephrine may be tried as the initial vasopressor in cases of severe tachydysrhythmias. Regardless of which vasopressor is chosen, low doses are initiated and titrated rapidly (usually every 5–15 minutes) to clinical response. Clinically effective dosing of vasopressors and inotropes in septic shock often requires doses much larger than recommended by most references. These large infusion rates must be tempered with the development of adverse effects. The goal is to use the minimally effective infusion rate while minimizing evidence of myocardial ischemia (e.g., tachydysrhythmias, electrocardiographic changes), renal (decreased glomerular filtration rate and/or urine output), splanchnic/gastric (low pHi, bowel ischemia), or peripheral (cold extremities) hypoperfusion, and worsening PaO_2, PAOP, and other hemodynamic variables.

⑪ Therapy with catecholamine vasopressors and inotropes is continued until the myocardial depression and vascular hyporesponsiveness (i.e., blood pressure) of septic shock improve, usually measured in hours to days. Discontinuation of vasopressor or inotropic therapy should be executed slowly; therapy should be "weaned" to avoid a precipitous worsening in regional and systemic hemodynamics. Careful monitoring of global and regional end points also should be geared toward discontinuation of vasopressors and inotropes as soon as the patient is hemodynamically stable. This requires moment-by-moment observation. Because vasopressors and inotropes often are started while the patient is not yet optimally volume resuscitated, clinicians should reevaluate intravascular volume status continuously so that the patient can be weaned from the vasopressor as soon as possible. Doses should be titrated carefully downward approximately every 10 minutes to determine if the patient can tolerate gradual withdrawal and eventual discontinuation of the vasopressor and/or inotrope. Discontinuation of agents may occur only minutes to hours after their initiation, or it may take days to weeks. Septic shock requiring vasopressor and/or inotropic support usually resolves within 1 week.

Vasopressin

⑫ At present, vasopressin therapy should not be initiated as first-line therapy. Lauzier et al. randomized 23 hyperdynamic septic shock patients to initial therapy with vasopressin 0.04 to 0.20 units/min or norepinephrine 0.1 to 2.8 mcg/kg/min for 48 hours to achieve MAP of 70 mm Hg.[58] Both agents increased MAP over 48 hours, but norepinephrine achieved the desired MAP significantly faster, and norepinephrine was required in 36% of the vasopressin patients. One patient who received vasopressin developed acute coronary syndrome with dose-dependent electrocardiographic changes. Additional studies are needed to determine the optimal dose, duration, and place in therapy of vasopressin relative to adrenergic agents. In addition, no randomized, blinded, placebo-controlled trials have shown improvement in long-term outcomes such as mortality and length of hospital stay. The preliminary results (not yet published at the time this chapter was prepared) of a randomized, double-blind study of 800 patients with septic shock requiring catecholamine vasopressors showed that 28-day mortality rates were similar when vasopressin 0.01 to 0.03 units/min or norepinephrine was added to traditional therapy (see *www.utoronto.ca/criticalcare/Research/VASST.shtml*). Until further safety data and larger efficacy trials are completed, vasopressin is not recommended as a replacement for norepinephrine or dopamine in patients with septic shock but may be considered in patients who are refractory to catecholamine vasopressors despite adequate fluid resuscitation. If used, vasopressin should be administered in doses not exceeding 0.01 to 0.04 units/min.[44,45] Use of vasopressin for reducing the dose of adrenergic agents can be considered, but the risks must be considered prior to initiating therapy.

CLINICAL CONTROVERSY: VASOPRESSIN

Adding vasopressin reduces the dose of traditional catecholamine therapies and is associated with improved renal function. However, the occurrence of ischemic events to digits and splanchnic circulation may be increased with vasopressin. Therefore, the lowest possible dose should be implemented if vasopressin is used.

Corticosteroids

⑫ Since the two meta-analyses reported in 1995,[49,50] several randomized controlled trials of low-dose corticosteroids in vasopressor-dependent septic shock patients have been published.[46–48] These studies used moderate physiologic doses (200–300 mg/day) of hydrocortisone. A meta-analysis of five studies (n = 465) showed that steroid therapy was associated with an overall improvement in survival rate (RR 1.23, 95% confidence interval [CI] 1.01–1.50; $P = 0.036$) and shock reversal (RR 1.71, 95% CI 1.29–2.26; $P < 0.001$).[47] These effects were beneficial in both responders and nonresponders to ACTH stimulation testing ($P = 0.63$ and $P = 0.75$, respectively). These studies also showed that low-dose corticosteroid administration improves hemodynamics and reduces the duration of vasopressor support. All these studies differ from earlier studies in that steroids were administered at lower total doses (hydrocortisone equivalents: 1,209 mg vs 23,975 mg; $P = 0.01$) starting later in septic shock (23 hours vs <2 hours; $P = 0.02$) for longer courses (6 days vs 1 day; $P = 0.01$) to patients with higher control group mortality rates (mean 57% vs 34%; $P = 0.06$) who were more likely to be vasopressor dependent (100% vs 65%; $P = 0.03$). The relationship between corticosteroid dose and survival was linear, with survival benefit at low doses ($P = 0.02$). Another meta-analysis of 16 trials (n = 2,063) found similar results with long-term administration of corticosteroids associated with lower mortality in hospital (RR 0.83, 95% CI 0.70–0.97; $P = 0.02$) and at 28 days (RR 0.80, 95% CI 0.67–0.95; $P = 0.02$) and greater shock reversal at 7 days (RR 1.22, 95% CI 1.06–1.40; $P = 0.006$).[48] Combining all corticosteroid studies did not reveal an increased risk for adverse events, including gastrointestinal hemorrhage (RR 1.16, 95% CI 0.82–0.1.65; $P = 0.4$), superinfections (RR 0.93, 95% CI 0.73–1.18; $P = 0.54$), and hyperglycemia (RR 1.22, 95% CI 0.84–1.78; $P = 0.30$). Of note, the results of both meta-analyses were heavily driven by data supplied by one study.[59] Annane et al.[59] randomized 300 patients with septic shock within 8 hours of hypotension to placebo or a daily combination of hydrocortisone 50 mg IV every 6 hours and fludrocortisone 0.05 mg enterally for 7 days. Similar to the meta-analyses, use of hydrocortisone reduced 28-day mortality (odds ratio [OR] 0.65, 95% CI 0.39–1.07; $P = 0.09$), but all the benefit was seen in patients with adrenal insufficiency (OR 0.54, 95% CI 0.31–0.97; $P = 0.04$). The placebo group was more likely to continually require vasopressor therapy (hazard ratio [HR] 1.54, 95% CI 1.10–12.16; $P = 0.01$), but differences between groups were exhibited only in patients with adrenal insufficiency (HR 1.91, 95% CI 1.29–2.84; $P = 0.001$). Approximately 76% of patients were deemed adrenally insufficient. Only one study has been published since the most recent meta-analyses.[60] Oppert et al.[60] randomized 41 patients with septic shock within 4 hours of hypotension to placebo or continuous infusion hydrocortisone and found that patients treated with hydrocortisone required shorter therapy with vasopressors (53 hours vs 120 hours; $P < 0.02$). This effect was more pronounced in patients with adrenal insufficiency but still was evident in those with adrenal reserve. Of note, serum concentrations of the inflammatory cytokine IL-6 were significantly reduced with hydrocortisone, and this finding was equally apparent irrespective of adrenal function.

Given the current data, corticosteroids can be administered to patients with septic shock and adrenal insufficiency.[46] In the absence of adrenal function assessment, corticosteroids can be considered in cases of refractory shock, as approximately 75% of these patients have insufficient adrenal reserve.[59] Use of vasopressors for prolonged periods without evidence of dose reduction also warrants corticosteroid administration. Whenever corticosteroids are used for septic shock, a daily dose equivalent to 200 to 300 mg hydrocortisone should be continued for 7 days. At the time this chapter was prepared, the results of a randomized study of 499 patients with severe sepsis were released (not yet published) and showed that 28-day mortality rates were similar amongst patients with and without adrenal insufficiency (defined by an ACTH response of less than 9 mcg/dL) and that hydrocortisone did not alter mortality but did shorten the length of time patients required vasopressors by 2 to 3 days (see *www.esicm.org/PAGE_corticus*).

CLINICAL CONTROVERSY: CORTICOSTEROID THERAPY

Low-dose corticosteroid therapy for 7 days in patients with septic shock improves outcomes when adrenal insufficiency is present. Several questions surround the application of corticosteroid therapy in septic patients, including use in patients with sepsis but without shock, use when sufficient adrenal reserve is present, use when patients were taking corticosteroids prior to ICU admission, most effective dose and duration, use of corticosteroids other than hydrocortisone, and need for coadministration of fludrocortisone.

Adverse Effects

4 Catecholamine vasopressors may result in adverse peripheral vasoconstrictive, metabolic, and dysrhythmogenic effects that limit or outweigh their positive effects on the central circulation.[8,40,42] Norepinephrine, phenylephrine, and epinephrine can produce lactic acidosis secondary to excessive constriction in peripheral arterioles or enhanced glycogenolysis, or as a result of mobilization of lactate from peripheral tissues as a result of improved oxygenation. Additionally, excessive peripheral vasoconstriction may cause ischemia or necrosis of already poorly perfused tissues such as the skin and the mesenteric and splanchnic circulations.[42,56,57,61] Some of these profound vasoconstrictive effects have been compounded by the use of epinephrine and phenylephrine in patients with septic shock who are significantly hypovolemic. These agents are used in the context of late septic shock, where hypotension is refractory to less selective vasoconstrictors (e.g., norepinephrine or dopamine) such that very large doses of epinephrine or phenylephrine are required but provide little or no benefit. Myocardial ischemia and dysrhythmias may occur in patients with coronary artery disease, atherosclerosis, cardiomyopathies, left ventricular hypertrophy, congestive heart failure, or underlying dysrhythmias because of their inability to tolerate β_1 cardiac stimulation that mediates increases in CO. However, the effect usually is opposite in healthy myocardium and in young patients. β_1 Cardiac stimulation is well tolerated, ventricular filling pressures decrease, and CO and DO_2 increase, with a resulting increase in peripheral perfusion. The dysrhythmogenic potential of the catecholamine vasopressors includes a variety of resulting atrial and ventricular arrhythmias. Sympathomimetic vasopressors also have been found to possess immunomodulatory actions, primarily mediated by β_2-adrenergic actions (e.g., epinephrine) because almost all immune cells express this receptor.[42] The actions include downregulating expression of proinflammatory cytokines such as TNF-α by neutrophils, suppression of oxygen free radical production from neutrophils, and direct proapoptotic effects. Dopamine suppresses prolactin secretion from the anterior pituitary gland, which may lead to reduced T-cell responsiveness.[42] These effects may be either beneficial or deleterious by dampening harmful effects of oxygen free radical–mediated tissue injury or by reducing neutrophilic defense against bacteria.

Vasopressor catecholamines have the potential to cause extravasation-associated tissue damage if infusions infiltrate during peripheral administration. In the event of infiltration, an α-receptor antagonist such as phentolamine (10 mg in 10 mL saline) should be injected intradermally to reverse local vasoconstriction, with administration of vasopressor drugs into a large central vein.

Dopamine

Dopamine frequently is the initial vasopressor used for patients with septic shock.[4–10] Doses of 5 to 10 mcg/kg/min are initiated to improve MAP. Most studies of patients with septic shock have shown that dopamine at these doses increases the cardiac index by improving contractility and heart rate, primarily from its β_1 effects. It increases MAP and SVR as a result of both increased CO and, at higher doses (>10 mcg/kg/min), its α_1 effects.

6 8 The clinical utility of dopamine as a vasopressor in the setting of septic shock is limited because large doses frequently are necessary to maintain CO and MAP. At doses exceeding 20 mcg/kg/min, further improvement in cardiac performance and regional hemodynamics is limited. Its clinical use frequently is hampered by tachycardia and tachydysrhythmias, which may lead to myocardial ischemia. Although tachydysrhythmias theoretically should not be expected to occur until administration of dopamine 5 to 10 mcg/kg/min, these β_1 effects are observed with doses as low as 3 mcg/kg/min. They seem to be more prevalent in patients who are inadequately resuscitated (hypovolemic), in the elderly, in those with preexisting or concurrent cardiac ischemia or dysrhythmias, and in patients currently receiving other dysrhythmogenic agents, including vasopressors and inotropes.

8 Dopamine increases PAOP and pulmonary shunting to decrease PaO_2.[42] The increase in PAOP may be due to changes in diastolic volumes from decreased cardiac compliance or increased venous return to the heart by α-adrenergic receptor–mediated venoconstriction. This may affect gas exchange and decrease PaO_2. The increase in pulmonary shunting also may result from acute enhancement of pulmonary blood flow to nonhomogeneous lung regions. Thus, dopamine should be used with caution in patients with elevated preload because the drug may worsen pulmonary edema. In the instance of high filling pressures, tachycardia, or tachydysrhythmias, dopamine should be replaced by another vasopressor and/or inotrope such as norepinephrine, dobutamine, phenylephrine, or epinephrine, depending on the desired effect.

The effect of dopamine on global oxygen-transport variables parallels the hemodynamic effects. Although dopamine improves global DO_2 in septic patients, it may compromise O_2ER in the splanchnic and mesenteric circulations by α_1-mediated vasoconstriction. Splanchnic blood flow and DO_2 increase with dopamine, but with no preferential increase in splanchnic perfusion as a fraction of CO and systemic increases in DO_2.[62,63] Indeed, large doses of dopamine worsen pHi and the PCO_2 gap.[64,65] This is reflected by a decrease or lack of change in regional VO_2 and a decrease in tissue O_2ER.[61] Dopamine at low or pressor doses directly impedes gastric motility in critical illness[66] and may aggravate gut ischemia in septic shock.[67,68] Similar to high-dose administration, low-dose dopamine increases splanchnic blood flow but lowers splanchnic VO_2 in sepsis.[68] Therefore, dopamine at all doses impairs hepatosplanchnic metabolism despite an increase in regional perfusion. Lastly, immune suppression of T-cell proliferation and inhibited secretion of growth and thyroid hormones and prolactin are other potentially clinically significant unwanted neuroendocrine effects of dopamine.

8 Currently, insufficient evidence promotes the use of dopamine as a first-line agent because regional hemodynamics, oxygen-transport variables, and functional parameters of improved organ perfusion are not consistently enhanced in a sustained manner and may be negatively impaired. The negative findings of low-dose dopamine use (see Low-Dose Dopamine below) and the deleterious effects of inotropic and vasopressor doses of dopamine on regional hemodynamics and oxygen transport raise controversy over whether dopamine should be considered the first-line vasopressor agent in patients with severe sepsis or septic shock.[4,6–8] The results of an observational study found dopamine use was an independent factor associated with ICU mortality in all 1,058 patients with shock (OR 1.67, 95% CI 1.19–2.35; $P = 0.003$) and the subgroup of 462 patients with septic shock (OR 2.05, 95% CI 1.25–3.37; $P = 0.005$).[69] Until dopamine is found to have definitive deleterious clinical outcomes compared to other vasopressors, empirical use of dopamine in a hypotensive patient in whom a pulmonary arterial catheter has not been inserted and in

whom the cause of hypotension—low CO or vasodilation—is yet undetermined still may be reasonable.[3,5,9,10] In addition, unlike other vasopressor agents, dopamine is available as premixed ready-to-use solutions of various concentrations that can be stored in automated distribution systems for rapid initiation.

Low-Dose Dopamine

In the critical care setting, low doses (1–3 mcg/kg/min) of dopamine once were advocated for use in patients with septic shock receiving vasopressors with or without oliguria. The goal of this therapy is to minimize or reverse renal vasoconstriction caused by other pressors, to prevent oliguric renal failure, or to convert oliguric to nonoliguric renal failure. At low dosages, dopamine has been shown to increase urine production as a result of enhanced renal blood flow from its D_1-receptor–mediated vasodilation, its D_2-receptor–mediated natriuretic effects (inhibition of Na^+/K^+ ATP of renal tubular cells), or its β_1-receptor–mediated increase in cardiac index.[70,71] In healthy subjects, the addition of dopamine to incremental doses of norepinephrine may blunt norepinephrine-induced renal vasoconstriction, thereby maintaining renal blood flow, natriuresis, urine production, and glomerular filtration.[52] These effects also have been observed during the course of dopamine administration in oliguric[62] and nonoliguric[57,63,70] patients with septic shock. For this reason, low doses of dopamine sometimes are added to other vasopressors (e.g., norepinephrine).

Tolerance to the vasodilatory effects of dopamine after 24 to 48 hours is evident in nonoliguric patients with sepsis syndrome and has been reported in other conditions.[72,73] The lack of response to dopamine in patients with septic shock receiving vasopressors and the tolerance to low-dose dopamine that develops in responders may be explained in part by time- and disease-dependent desensitization of the dopamine receptors[72,73]; this may not occur in patients with sepsis syndrome[72] or in normal volunteers.[52] Furthermore, differences in the extent of preexisting vasodilation and the pathophysiology of renal dysfunction in oliguric and septic shock patients may contribute to the inconsistent responses to administration of low doses of dopamine. A paucity of evidence suggests that the etiology of acute renal failure from sepsis is due to efferent arteriole vasodilation and that potential beneficial outcomes with dopamine, and other vasopressors, are due to enhanced CO.[74,75] Enhanced urine production has been shown to occur in hyperdynamic shock with use of agents that constrict the efferent arteriole such as vasopressin and norepinephrine; however, delineating the effects of improved arterial blood pressure and CO associated with these agents from regional renal effects is difficult.[44,45,64,65,76]

Two studies have settled the debate surrounding low-dose dopamine. Friedrich et al.[77] performed a meta-analysis to determine if low-dose dopamine reduces mortality or the need for dialysis in patients with critical illness. Among 61 clinical trials (n = 3,359), low-dose dopamine had no effect on mortality (RR 0.96, 95% CI 0.78–1.19), need for dialysis (RR 0.93, 95% CI 0.76–1.15), or occurrence of adverse events (RR 1.13, 95% CI 0.90–1.41). Low-dose dopamine improved urine production by 24% (CI 14%–35%) on the first day of therapy but failed to maintain this effect on days 2 and 3. No improvements in serum creatinine concentration (4% relative increase, 95% CI 1%–7%) and measured creatinine clearance (6% relative increase, 95% CI 1%–11%) occurred. One adequately designed prospective, controlled trial has been conducted with low-dose dopamine in critically ill patients.[78] This study was cited in the meta-analysis by Friedrich et al. Bellomo et al.[78] randomized 328 critically ill patients with early renal dysfunction to either low-dose dopamine (2 mcg/kg/min) or placebo and found no differences in peak serum creatinine concentration (245 ± 144 μmol/l vs 249 ± 147 μmol/l), increase in serum creatinine concentration (62 ± 107 μmol/L vs 66 ± 108 μmol/L), need for renal replacement therapies (27.7% vs 24.5%), and urine production at any time point. On the basis of available evidence, low-dose dopamine for treatment or prevention of acute renal failure cannot be justified and should be eliminated from routine clinical use.[74,75]

Norepinephrine

Norepinephrine was first used 3 decades ago for treatment of hypotensive states prior to the development of the synthetic catecholamines dopamine and dobutamine. Traditionally, norepinephrine was viewed as causing significant peripheral tissue vasoconstriction, which could selectively impair regional blood flow and thus DO_2 to the renal and splanchnic beds. However, clinical studies of norepinephrine now support the primary use of norepinephrine to restore blood pressure in septic shock.[53,79] Several retrospective analyses have demonstrated improved MAP and mortality in ICU patients with severe hypotension treated with norepinephrine either as first-line therapy or after therapeutic failure with fluid resuscitation and dopamine treatment.[6] However, in patients with increased sequential organ failure assessment scores and associated multiorgan failure, treatment with norepinephrine no longer offered an advantage. Early aggressive vasopressor support may be key to a positive outcome in septic shock. Use of norepinephrine as first-line therapy may be more rational because norepinephrine is more potent than dopamine and is more effective in increasing MAP. It has combined strong α_1-activity and less potent β_1-agonist effects while maintaining weak vasodilatory effects of β_2-receptor stimulation. In clinical practice, however, norepinephrine often is initiated after vasopressor doses of dopamine (4–20 mcg/kg/min) alone or in combination with dobutamine (5 mcg/kg/min) fail to achieve desired goals.[4–10] Doses of dopamine and dobutamine are kept constant or stopped; in some instances, dopamine is kept at low doses for purported renal protection.

❼ Norepinephrine infusions can be titrated to preset goals of MAP (usually at least 65 mm Hg), improvement in peripheral perfusion (to restore urine production or decrease blood lactate), and/or achievement of desired oxygen-transport variables while not compromising the cardiac index. Norepinephrine 0.01 to 2 mcg/kg/min reliably and predictably improves hemodynamic parameters to "normal" or "supranormal" values in most patients with septic shock. As with ❻ other vasopressors, norepinephrine doses exceeding those recommended by most references frequently are needed in critically ill patients with septic shock to achieve predetermined goals. A significant increase in MAP generally is caused by an increase in SVR. In contrast to dopamine, heart rate generally does not increase significantly with norepinephrine because of diminished stimulation of cardiac β_1-receptors in septic shock and reflex bradycardia from increased SVR.[54,80] In a study of 10 patients with septic shock in whom norepinephrine doses were increased to 23, 31, and 47 mcg/min to maintain MAPs of 65, 75, and 85 mm Hg, mean heart rates were 95, 101, and 105 beats/min, respectively.[54] The increasing doses of norepinephrine required for the three levels of MAP resulted in a progressive increase in the cardiac index (mean values 4.7, 5.3, and 5.5 L/m²/min, respectively).[54] Others have demonstrated no change or a minor increase in the cardiac index with norepinephrine in patients with septic shock.[53] In contrast to dopamine, norepinephrine does not influence PAOP.[81]

The effect of norepinephrine on oxygen transport parameters is variable and depends on baseline values and concurrently administered vasoactive agents. In most studies of norepinephrine alone, either an increase or no change in DO_2 is seen with no change in O_2ER, particularly when mean DO_2 values were "supranormal" prior to therapy.[61,64,65] Norepinephrine has demonstrated either no effect or improvement in PCO_2 gap and pHi.[61,65] Splanchnic blood flow and fractional blood flow are higher with norepinephrine than either dopamine or epinephrine despite higher CO with the two latter agents.[61,81,82]

In a randomized study of 32 septic shock patients unresponsive to volume resuscitation, Martin et al.[76] found norepinephrine alone was superior to dopamine in achieving and maintaining preset hemodynamic (MAP of at least 80 mm Hg) and oxygen-transport variables for at least 6 hours (93% vs 31% of patients, $P < 0.001$). Of the 11 patients who did not respond to dopamine, 10 achieved the desired hemodynamic goal when norepinephrine was added. The authors suggested that differences between the two agents resulted from norepinephrine's combined increase in $V\text{O}_2$ and decrease in lactate concentrations due to reversal of splanchnic ischemia and efficient hepatic clearance of lactate or a preferential increase in $D\text{O}_2$ to areas of greatest oxygen demand, thus optimizing O_2ER.

The same investigators showed in a prospective, observational cohort study of 97 adult patients with septic shock that use of norepinephrine to provide hemodynamic support was associated with a significant decrease in mortality (day 7: 28% vs 40%, $P < 0.005$; day 28: 55% vs 82%, $P < 0.001$; at hospital discharge: 62% vs 84%, $P < 0.001$).[79] Using stepwise logistic regression analysis, norepinephrine was found to be the only factor associated with significantly improved survival ($P = 0.03$). Despite the drawback of lack of randomization, this study is the first to demonstrate a survival benefit with any vasopressor. In an interventional study, Martin et al.[53] showed that addition of norepinephrine in patients with dobutamine-resistant septic shock resulted in significant improvements (40%) in the cardiac index and stroke volume index during a 4 hour study period. This occurred despite an increase in left ventricular afterload, suggesting that either a positive inotropic effect or the correction of systemic hypotension was responsible. The authors further speculated that older patients may benefit from a combined α- and β-vasopressor versus a pure β-agonist given the higher incidence of coronary disease and compromised ventricles in this patient population. By virtue of restored MAP and hence coronary perfusion, cardiac index is increased in older patients, whereas in younger patients with less coronary artery disease and a higher cardiac index at baseline, norepinephrine acts primarily as a vasopressor. In younger patients in this study, norepinephrine did not significantly increase the cardiac index or stroke volume index.

Whereas the effects of norepinephrine on MAP, SVR, cardiac index, and heart rate appear to be desirable and more predictable, the effect of norepinephrine on urine production may depend on concurrently administered vasoactive agents.[6,81] The results of many studies are difficult to interpret because of concurrent inotropic support with dobutamine and dopamine or low doses of dopamine precluding the attribution of any beneficial effects to norepinephrine alone. In the randomized study of norepinephrine and dopamine by Martin et al.,[76] urine production increased with norepinephrine but not with dopamine (22 ± 7 mL/h to 189 ± 52 mL/h vs 24 ± 6 mL/h to 8.2 ± 10 mL/h; , $P < 0.001$). Adding norepinephrine to the dopamine group increased urine production to 107 ± 125 mL/h. An increase in urine production may be due to increased renal perfusion pressure secondary to elevated MAP from improved CO and SVR or the localized vasoconstrictive effect of norepinephrine in the kidney (greater vasoconstriction of the efferent arteriole than the afferent arteriole) to increase the glomerular filtration rate.

Taken together, these data suggest that norepinephrine should be repositioned as the vasopressor of choice in patients in septic shock because of its multiple benefits: (1) norepinephrine may decrease mortality in septic shock, (2) it reverses inappropriate vasodilation and low global oxygen extraction, (3) it attenuates myocardial depression at unchanged or increased CO and increased coronary blood flow, (4) it improves renal perfusion pressure and renal filtration, (5) it enhances splanchnic perfusion, and (6) it is less likely than other vasopressors to cause tachycardias and tachydysrhythmias.[79,80,83]

Dobutamine

Dobutamine is an inotrope with vasodilatory properties (a "inodilator"). It is used for treatment of septic and cardiogenic shock to increase the cardiac index, typically by 25% to 50%. In septic shock, LVEF and right ventricular function are depressed despite a high cardiac index, whereas ventricular volumes and compliance are increased. Stroke index is maintained by an increased heart rate and ventricular dilation. In survivors, myocardial depression is reversible and normalizes 5 to 10 days after onset of sepsis.[7] Dobutamine has been shown to increase stroke index, left ventricular stroke work index, and thus cardiac index and $D\text{O}_2$ without increasing PAOP in septic shock in animals, in human volunteers, and in controlled studies of human septic shock.[7] The ability of dobutamine to enhance cardiac index and $D\text{O}_2$ during septic shock appears to be related to its chronotropic effect.[84]

Most prospective, randomized controlled studies of therapy directed toward achieving supranormal hemodynamic variables with dobutamine were performed in surgical and medical ICU patients with septic shock refractory to concurrently administered vasopressors (dopamine and/or norepinephrine).[7] The achievement of supranormal oxygen transport values with dobutamine is of little value compared with treatment to normal values. In addition, administration of dobutamine to achieve these high values has resulted in an unchanged or increased mortality rate and/or a greater incidence of adverse effects,[85] with the exception of a study of older, nonseptic, high-risk surgical patients.[22] Results in medical and surgical patients may differ because of differences in time of starting dobutamine infusion, duration of the infusion, and dosages administered. Among critically ill, high-risk trauma and surgical patients receiving dobutamine, subgroups of patients with septic shock (6%–34%) have small and insignificant changes in $D\text{O}_2$, $V\text{O}_2$, O_2ER, and cardiac index.[86] The lack of response may be related to late treatment (>72 hours after surgery) resulting in irreversible changes due to hypoperfusion and hypoxia. In a group of medical patients, the lack of sustained effect may have been attributed to the fact that very large doses were needed to achieve the desired effects over a longer treatment period (72 hours). The requirement for vasopressor support with dopamine may have decreased O_2ER and negated the beneficial effects of increased delivery with dobutamine. O_2ER, mixed venous oxygen tension, and relative changes in SVR were not reported. In populations of medical and surgical patients, dobutamine did not increase the likelihood of patients achieving supranormal oxygen-transport variables. Continuation of dobutamine until death or resolution of acute illness resulted in increased mortality despite an increase in the mean area under the $D\text{O}_2$ curve.[85] This is explained in part by the fact that no change in $V\text{O}_2$ was seen, and thus O_2ER decreased. Also, much higher doses of dobutamine were used in this study compared with the previous study (5–200 mcg/kg/min vs 5–20 mcg/kg/min). Seventeen of the 50 patients in the experimental group received dobutamine 50 mcg/kg/min or more at some time during the study. Despite these high doses, 35 (70%) of 50 patients were unable to achieve the predetermined goals. In fact, dose increments of dobutamine were limited by complications in half of the dobutamine patients in the treatment group, with occurrence of tachycardia, ischemic changes on electrocardiogram, hypertension, and tachydysrhythmias despite the absence of preexisting cardiac abnormalities.[85]

Studies have focused on the effects of dobutamine on gastric mucosal flow and the splanchnic circulation. The addition of dobutamine to norepinephrine or epinephrine improves gastric mucosal perfusion without increasing the cardiac index.[87,88] This is consistent with findings that dobutamine may improve pHi and mucosal perfusion in septic patients.[89] The addition of dobutamine to norepinephrine or epinephrine treatment has been shown to improve gastric mucosal perfusion as measured by improvements in pHi, arterial lactate concentrations, and $P\text{CO}_2$ gap.[88,90–92] These findings likely relate to blood flow redistribution toward gastric mucosa.[89] This effect may be due to either an increase in the fraction of CO distributed to the global hepatosplanchnic blood flow[87] and/

or a redistribution of blood flow within gastric wall layers toward mucosal by "stealing" blood away from the muscularis potentially as a result of the greater β_2-mediated vasodilation attributable to norepinephrine. This hypothesis is supported by four other investigations,[90–93] including one showing that sublingual microcirculation improved after dobutamine was given to vasopressor-dependent septic shock patients.[93] The changes in capillary perfusion were unrelated to arterial pressure or cardiac index.[93]

In many of these studies, a constant dose of dobutamine (usually 5 mcg/kg/min) was added to norepinephrine or epinephrine and compared with either vasopressor alone to determine comparative effects on systemic and regional hemodynamics and oxygen-transport variables.[88,90–92] At the same increase in MAP, no significant difference in the systemic hemodynamic variables was observed between treatment groups. The combination of dobutamine and norepinephrine results in a lower increase in heart rate compared with use of other vasopressors alone. There is no difference in DO_2I between groups. Arterial lactate concentrations decrease significantly with norepinephrine and dobutamine compared with dopamine and epinephrine infusions. Norepinephrine and dobutamine infusion is associated with a higher pHi compared with epinephrine infusion, but the differences are not statistically different. The difference between gastric and arterial PCO_2 with norepinephrine and dobutamine tends to be lower compared with values obtained with dopamine, epinephrine, and norepinephrine alone. Therefore, for the same level of MAP as the therapeutic goal in patients with septic shock, gastric mucosal perfusion and tissue oxygen utilization are most improved with norepinephrine and dobutamine.

❻ Dobutamine should be started at dosages ranging from 2.5 to 5 mcg/kg/min. In a study of early goal-directed therapy, dobutamine was administered to 13.7% of patients within 6 hours of resuscitation to achieve $ScvO_2$ >70%.[19] Although a dose response may be seen, evidence now suggests that doses >5 mcg/kg/min may provide limited beneficial effects on oxygen transport values and hemodynamics and may increase adverse cardiac effects.[93] If given to patients who are intravascularly depleted, dobutamine will result in hypotension and a reflexive tachycardia. Pathophysiologic factors influence dosing requirements and pharmacokinetic parameters over the time course of the illness and the duration of the infusion. Decreases in PaO_2, as well as myocardial adverse effects such as tachycardia, ischemic changes on electrocardiogram, tachydysrhythmias, and hypotension, are seen.[85,89] Thus, infusion rates should be guided by clinical end points and SvO_2/$ScvO_2$. Dobutamine, like other inotropes, usually is given until improvement in myocardial function with resolution of the septic episode or dose-limiting side effects are observed.

Phenylephrine

❻ Despite its purported use in refractory septic shock, little information is available regarding the clinical efficacy of phenylephrine. Nevertheless, it is an attractive agent for use in sepsis because of its selective α-agonism with primarily vascular effects. It is generally initiated at dosages of 0.5 mcg/kg/min and can be titrated every 5 to 15 minutes to desired effects.

Three clinical trials have evaluated phenylephrine use in 38 patients with septic shock. Phenylephrine (0.5–9 mcg/kg/min), used alone or in combination with dobutamine or low doses of dopamine, improves blood pressure and myocardial performance in fluid-resuscitated septic patients.[94] Incremental doses of phenylephrine administered over 3 hours result in linear dose-related increases in MAP, SVR, heart rate, and stroke index when administered alone as a single agent in stable, nonhypotensive but hyperdynamic, volume-resuscitated surgical ICU patients. In septic shock, phenylephrine did not impair the cardiac index, PAOP, or peripheral perfusion.[55,95] Phenylephrine administration improves myocardial performance in hyperdynamic, normotensive septic patients but worsens myocardial performance in cardiac controls.[94] In sepsis, phenylephrine improves MAP by increasing the cardiac index through enhanced venous return to the heart (increase in CVP and stroke index) and by acting as a positive inotrope. In cardiac patients, myocardial performance worsens as a result of a decrease in the cardiac index and an increase in SVR.

In septic shock, phenylephrine appears to increase global tissue oxygen use, although information regarding the relationship of the oxygen-transport variables with increases in MAP and cardiac index is conflicting.[55,95] Increases in VO_2 appear to be dissociated from DO_2, representing an increase in O_2ER as the cardiac index remains unchanged. Increases in VO_2 may result from redistribution of blood flow to previously underperfused areas, improving oxygen use as a result of changes in MAP and SVR. With phenylephrine administration, no organ dysfunction was documented, and evidence of globally improved peripheral tissue perfusion was observed as lactic acid concentration fell or remained unchanged and urine production increased significantly at increased or maximal VO_2. An increased O_2ER may contribute to improved tissue use.[55,95] In one small study, measured DO_2 and VO_2 values paralleled MAP in most patients.[95] As with epinephrine, phenylephrine dosages (1.3–3.7 mcg/kg/min) required to achieve goals of therapy were significantly higher than dosages traditionally recommended for use. When phenylephrine (0.5 mcg/kg/min) was titrated to a plateau in VO_2 or the appearance of adverse cardiac effects, both DO_2 and VO_2 increased at least 15%. When combined with dobutamine, phenylephrine resulted in a more consistent and statistically significant increase in both DO_2 and VO_2. However, these observations may be biased because baseline DO_2 and VO_2 values were somewhat higher in patients who did not require dobutamine (5/11 patients). In a second study, use of phenylephrine as a single agent without another cardiotonic agent was evaluated in 10 septic, hyperdynamic surgical ICU patients.[55] Eight patients had a clinically significant increase (at least 15%) in VO_2 with variable doses of phenylephrine, whereas DO_2 increased in only three patients. Phenylephrine predictably increased MAP but not VO_2 in a dose-dependent fashion in the surgical patient population.

Few data regarding the effect of phenylephrine on regional hemodynamics and oxygen-transport variables are available. When phenylephrine replaced norepinephrine in patients with septic shock, phenylephrine selectively reduced splanchnic blood flow and thus splanchnic DO_2 and splanchnic lactate uptake rate without changing the overall splanchnic VO_2.[96] Because all these parameters normalized when norepinephrine was reinstated, these data suggest that exogenous β-adrenergic stimulation (norepinephrine) may determine hepatosplanchnic perfusion and oxygen availability but not utilization in septic shock. This study also demonstrated that although the phenylephrine-induced reduction in splanchnic DO_2 reduced the de novo synthesis of glucose (a highly oxygen-dependent pathway in the periportal region), it did not affect the formation of monoethylglycinexylidide, a metabolite of lidocaine (a cytochrome P450–dependent pathway in the perivenous region). This finding demonstrates the heterogeneity of metabolic function in different areas of the liver.

The available data on hemodynamics, oxygen-transport variables, and mortality with phenylephrine in septic shock patients may not be generalizable because of the small numbers of patients evaluated. Adverse effects, such as tachydysrhythmias, are notably infrequent with phenylephrine, particularly when it is used as a single agent or at higher doses, because phenylephrine does not exert any activity on β_1-adrenergic receptors. Whether the beneficial effects can be sustained with longer administrations of phenylephrine is unclear.[55] In an experimental animal model, however, sustained endotoxemia (48 hours) did not result in desensitization of α_1-adrenergic responsiveness when phenylephrine was used.[43] Other mechanisms may be responsible for the ineffectiveness (9) of vasopressors during advanced sepsis. Phenylephrine may be a particularly useful alternative in patients who cannot tolerate tachycardia or tachydysrhythmias with use of dopamine or norepinephrine, in patients with known underlying myocardial dysfunction, and in patients who are refractory to dopamine or norepinephrine (because of β-adrenergic receptor desensitization). As with other vasopressors, phenylephrine is continued until resolution of the hemodynamic instability associated with the septic episode and is weaned when patients are clinically stable.

Epinephrine

(10) By convention, epinephrine has been reserved as a last-line agent for hemodynamic support of sepsis. Few objective data evaluating its comparative efficacy in early sepsis are available; most studies have examined the effects of epinephrine in refractory septic shock.[89] Despite this lack of data, epinephrine is an acceptable choice as a single agent because of its combined vasoconstrictor and inotropic effects. (9) Epinephrine infusion rates of 0.04 to 1 mcg/kg/min alone increase hemodynamic and oxygen-transport variables to "supranormal" values without adverse effects in septic patients without coronary artery disease. Among 69 patients evaluated in five studies, epinephrine alone or combined with either dobutamine or low doses of dopamine achieved the desired outcomes.[89] Large doses (0.5–1 mcg/kg/min) often were required when epinephrine was added to other agents. Smaller doses (0.10–0.50 mcg/kg/min) are effective if dobutamine and dopamine infusions are kept constant, potentially as a result of less exposure to β-receptor stimulation and thus less receptor desensitization. The same holds true when epinephrine is used as a first-line agent and when it is used in younger patients. A linear dose–response curve is seen, with rapid improvement of hemodynamic variables and DO_2. Although DO_2 increases mainly as a function of consistent increases in the cardiac index and a more variable increase in (10) SVR, VO_2 may not increase, and O_2ER may fall. A transient fall in pHi may be seen during epinephrine administration, and the impairment in gastric mucosal perfusion can be counteracted in part by dobutamine. Furthermore, lactate concentrations may rise during the first few hours of epinephrine therapy but normalize over the ensuing 24 hours in survivors.[89] The increase in lactate may be a result of worsened DO_2 to the liver (and subsequent anaerobic metabolism) or to the hepatosplanchnic circulation or, alternately, may be due to a direct increase in calorigenesis and breakdown of glycogen and lactate production as a result of epinephrine. However, evidence suggests that epinephrine, in contrast to dopamine, increases the proportion of total CO delivered to the splanchnic circulation, although VO_2 is not increased sufficiently to increase O_2ER. In contrast, when epinephrine is compared with a short infusion (2 hours) of a combination of norepinephrine and dobutamine, epinephrine preferentially decreases splanchnic DO_2, worsens pHi, and increases systemic lactate concentration without increasing VO_2. Methodologic limitations of many of these studies included nonrandomized crossover periods, potentially leading to pharmacologic carryover; failure of patients to achieve a steady state before crossover; and use of time-dependent response measures. Also unclear is whether patients were comparable at baseline—that is, whether they had received the same or other vasoactive agents before the study period and for how long.[89]

(10) Because data on the effects of vasopressors on splanchnic circulation in humans are limited and are confounded by the concurrent use of multiple agents, De Backer et al.[61] conducted a study in which regional hemodynamic effects of three catecholamine vasopressors were evaluated individually in septic shock patients. A sample of 20 patients with septic shock was divided into two groups: a moderate shock group, in which the MAP was at least 65 mm Hg with dopamine doses between 10 and 20 mcg/kg/min, and a severe group, in which MAP was <65 mm Hg. After a stable dose of dopamine, patients were randomized to either norepinephrine or epinephrine initially and then the other agent after a period of at least 45 minutes with each agent. Systemic and regional measurements were taken for each drug. Minimal differences between agents were noted for moderate shock. However, in the severe shock group, epinephrine resulted in higher DO_2 and VO_2 but lower absolute and fractional splanchnic blood flow. Although the PCO_2 gap was not different, indocyanine green clearance was lower with epinephrine compared with norepinephrine. No detrimental effects on splanchnic circulation were found with dopamine. This study concluded that epinephrine titrated to blood pressure in patients with severe septic shock causes deterioration in splanchnic circulation and induces changes in splanchnic metabolism. Given that these changes are likely deleterious, high-dose epinephrine should be avoided in severe septic shock patients.[61]

Four studies have compared epinephrine with either norepinephrine alone or norepinephrine in combination with dobutamine to determine their comparative effects on systemic and regional hemodynamics and oxygen-transport variables.[87,90–92] Two randomized studies compared the effects of epinephrine with the combination of norepinephrine and dobutamine on gastric perfusion, systemic and pulmonary hemodynamics, hepatic function, and blood gases in a total of 52 patients with septic shock.[90,91] Epinephrine or norepinephrine was started at a dose of 0.1 mcg/kg/min and titrated rapidly to achieve MAP of 70 to 80 mm Hg. Dobutamine was infused continuously at 5 mcg/kg/min. At the same increase in MAP, no significant differences in the systemic or pulmonary hemodynamic and blood gas variables were observed between treatment groups. Epinephrine tended to induce greater increases in the cardiac index and oxygen transport compared with norepinephrine and dobutamine. Epinephrine also significantly increased gastric mucosal blood flow compared with norepinephrine and dobutamine without modifying clearance of indocyanine green. The effects seen with epinephrine most likely were the result of an increase in the cardiac index. In the short term, however, epinephrine was associated with increased lactate concentrations, decreased pHi, and widened PCO_2 gap. All these variables improved in the group that received norepinephrine and dobutamine.

The two other studies are prospective, randomized crossover studies performed in dopamine-resistant, volume-replete patients with septic shock.[87,92] The design and results of the two studies are similar. Dopamine, epinephrine, norepinephrine, and norepinephrine plus dobutamine were adjusted to a MAP of 70 mm Hg. Epinephrine and the combination of norepinephrine and dobutamine both produced a significant increase in heart rate compared with norepinephrine alone. Epinephrine also significantly increased the cardiac index and DO_2 compared with norepinephrine alone as well as with norepinephrine and dobutamine. For the same level of MAP, epinephrine and the combination of norepinephrine and dobutamine induced a greater increase in mucosal perfusion than did norepinephrine alone, but the same ratio between gastric mucosal perfusion and DO_2 was observed with norepinephrine and dobutamine and with epinephrine or norepinephrine alone. However, O_2ER values were lower with epinephrine infusion compared with the other three groups. Arterial lactate concentrations decreased significantly with norepinephrine and dobutamine as compared with dopamine and epinephrine infusions. In addition, pHi and PCO_2 improved more with norepinephrine and dobutamine than with epinephrine or norepinephrine alone, but the differences were not statistically different. These results can be explained by the vasodilatory effect of dobutamine on gastric mucosal microcirculation resulting in a redistribution of blood flow toward the mucosa.[87] The results of these studies suggest that epinephrine has deleterious effects on regional hemodynamics and oxygen utilization. Of all the vasopressors, epinephrine exhibits the most pronounced capacity to induce hyperglycemia by increased gluconeogenesis and glycogenolysis with α-mediated suppression of insulin secretion.[42] The increase in lactate concentrations with epinephrine may be secondary to exaggerated aerobic glycolysis rather than anaerobic metabolism from decreased oxygen utilization.

❻ It is important to note that despite the large doses used in all the studies discussed, clinically important dysrhythmias or cardiac ischemia were reported rarely in patients of any age or underlying cardiac status. Nevertheless, caution must be exercised before considering epinephrine for managing hypoperfusion in hypodynamic patients with coronary artery disease, in whom ischemia, chest pain, and myocardial infarction may result. Based on the current evidence, epinephrine should be avoided in septic shock. Although it effectively increases CO and DO_2, it has deleterious effects on the splanchnic circulation. If it is used as a second-line agent in septic shock, factors that may influence successful therapy with epinephrine include the time from onset of septic shock to effective therapy and the age of the population.

Vasopressin

⓬ Studies involving vasopressin infusion for management of septic shock show rapid and sustained improvement in hemodynamic parameters. These effects are evident with administration of doses not exceeding 0.08 units/min. Administration of doses >0.04 units/min and 0.05 units/min are associated with negative changes in CO and mesenteric mucosal perfusion, respectively. The reduction in CO likely is the result of lowered stroke volume.[44] The studies that reported cardiac function indicate patients had adequate CO prior to initiating vasopressin therapy. Therefore, vasopressin use in septic shock patients with cardiac dysfunction warrants extreme caution. Cardiac ischemia appears to be a rare occurrence and may be related to administration of doses >0.05 units/min.[44]

Mesenteric ischemia associated with vasopressin may be clinically relevant. Two studies demonstrated increased hepatic transaminases and total bilirubin concentrations during vasopressin therapy, suggesting impaired hepatic blood flow or a direct effect on excretory hepatic function.[42,44] Three prospective studies of a total of 30 patients with septic shock requiring moderate-to-high doses of norepinephrine found that pHi and PCO_2 gap rapidly worsened after vasopressin at doses of 0.04 to 1.8 units/min was added, despite increased splanchnic blood flow and fractional blood flow.[97–99] Two randomized studies demonstrated contrasting results, likely because of their study designs.[100,101] Dunser et al.[100] randomized 48 patients with vasodilatory shock to norepinephrine alone or norepinephrine with vasopressin 0.07 units/min for 48 hours. The PCO_2 gap rose after 1 hour in the norepinephrine group and then stabilized, whereas the combination induced a progressive rise in the PCO_2 gap and reached the same values as norepinephrine alone at 48 hours.[100] Patel et al. [101] randomized 24 septic shock patients requiring high-dose norepinephrine to 4 hours of additional norepinephrine or vasopressin at a median dose of 0.06 units/min. The PCO_2 gap remained unaltered in both groups. Differences between studies may reflect the time of initiation relative to onset of shock, the stage of shock, and study duration. It is not surprising that even replacement doses of vasopressin in septic shock are associated with mesenteric mucosal hypoperfusion because mesenteric vasoconstriction occurs at vasopressin serum concentrations as low as 10 pg/dL, and the effect is dose dependent.[44] Of concern is the additive effective with norepinephrine despite substantially reduced doses of norepinephrine when vasopressin is initiated.[97–99] Although controversial, the degree of hypoperfusion with vasopressin may be greater than with norepinephrine alone[44] unless the dose of norepinephrine is markedly increased to maintain adequate arterial blood pressure. Vasopressin's strongest vasoconstrictive action occurs in the skin and soft tissues, skeletal muscles, and fat tissues. As a result, ischemic skin lesions have been observed in several studies, with an occurrence rate as high as 30% after vasopressin was added to norepinephrine-resistant shock.[44,101]

Although vasopressin may have deleterious effects on mesenteric and skin perfusion, studies report vasodilation of cerebral, pulmonary, coronary, and some renal vasculature beds. The clinical outcomes associated with selective vasodilation are not yet determined except for enhanced urine production in patients not anuric at baseline.[44,100] Whereas V_2 stimulation promotes water retention from the distal tubules and collecting ducts, V_1 receptors cause vasoconstriction of efferent arterioles and relative vasodilation of afferent arterioles to increase glomerular perfusion pressure and filtration rate, enhancing urine production. Animal data suggest that urine production is not increased with even higher vasopressin doses, likely because of relative vasoconstriction of the afferent arteriole to reduce glomerular filtration rate.[44] In the studies reporting benefit, the maximum dose used was 0.08 units/min.[44]

In order to minimize the potential for adverse events and maximize the beneficial effects, vasopressin doses should be limited to 0.04 units/min. Most studies initiated vasopressin as add-on therapy to one or two catecholamine adrenergic agents rather than as first-line therapy or salvage therapy. The results of these studies showed that vasopressin markedly reduced the requirements for adrenergic agents, but few studies demonstrated complete discontinuation of these therapies. Therefore, vasopressin should be used only if response to one or two adrenergic agents is inadequate or as a method for reducing the dose of these therapies. Increased arterial pressure should be evident within the first hour of vasopressin therapy, at which time the dose(s) of adrenergic agent(s) should be reduced while maintaining blood pressure. This method should help limit the degree of ischemia.

Most studies evaluated vasopressin use for <48 hours, and several studies reported difficulty discontinuing vasopressin therapy. Whether additional benefits, deleterious effects, or tolerance is observed with longer infusions remains unclear. Because vasopressin is being used to replace a physiologic deficiency, it stands to reason that the requirement for vasopressin will subside with reversal of the septic process. Attempts to discontinue vasopressin should occur when the dose(s) of adrenergic agent(s) has been minimized (e.g., dopamine ≤5 mcg/kg/min, norepinephrine ≤0.1 mcg/kg/min, phenylephrine ≤1 mcg/kg/min, epinephrine ≤0.15 mcg/kg/min). At present, vasopressin should not be initiated as first-line therapy or added to existing therapy solely because a patient is septic.

Corticosteroids

⓬ Corticosteroids can be initiated in cases of septic shock when adrenal insufficiency is present or when weaning of vasopressor therapy proves futile.[46] Adverse events are few because corticosteroids are administered for a finite period of time, usually 7 days. Acutely, elevated serum concentrations of blood urea nitrogen, white blood cell count, and glucose occur. Although long-term administration of corticosteroids is associated with several chronic disease states, a meta-analysis did not show an increase in adverse events, including gastrointestinal hemorrhage and infections (RR 0.93, 95% CI 0.73–1.18; $P = 0.54$), impacting critically ill patients.[48] Therefore, therapy of septic shock with corticosteroids improves hemodynamic variables and lowers catecholamine vasopressor dosages with minimal to no effect on patient safety.

EXPERIMENTAL THERAPIES

NITRIC OXIDE SYNTHASE INHIBITORS

NO is a short-acting, potent vasodilator derived from enzymatic oxidation of arginine. Its production is under control of NOS. This enzyme is present (expressed) in two forms: a constitutive form (ecNOS) and an inducible form (iNOS). Small amounts of NO normally are produced by the vascular endothelium under the control of ecNOS for physiologic control of vascular tone and blood flow distribution. Under pathophysiologic conditions such as stimulation by lipopolysaccharide or cytokines, iNOS becomes diffusely expressed, producing large amounts of NO. The latter has been implicated in the cardiovascular failure of septic shock.[102–104]

Pharmacologic inhibition of NO production has been investigated as an adjunct to standard therapies of septic shock. L-Arginine analogs such as monomethyl-L-arginine (L-NMMA) and L-arginine-methyl-ester (L-NAME) are competitive inhibitors of NOS and have been shown to increase blood pressure, partially restore vascular reactivity, and reduce vasopressor use.[102–104] However, because these arginine analogs nonselectively block ecNOS and iNOS, their use has been associated with extensive vasoconstriction, decreased CO, and regional hypoperfusion, thus promoting organ failure and mortality.[102–104] Some *S*-substituted thiourea derivatives have demonstrated, both in vitro and in vivo (rodent), dose-dependent selectivity for iNOS inhibition, but the clinical application must be evaluated. A phase I/IIa clinical trial of septic shock patients is underway (see *www.medinox.com*).

METHYLENE BLUE

Methylene blue counteracts ecNOS, iNOS, and soluble guanylate cyclase to reduce serum concentrations of NO and cyclic guanosine monophosphate. Despite these effects, methylene blue does not alter the expression of inflammatory cytokines.[105] Clinically, methylene blue at doses of 0.25 to 3 mg/kg/h increases SVR, MAP, myocardial contractility, and DO_2 in septic shock patients refractory to vasopressors.[105–108] Additional studies are needed before methylene blue can be recommended; at present it has been used only for salvage therapy.

TERLIPRESSIN

Terlipressin, an investigational prodrug that is converted into lysine vasopressin, has been used in septic shock patients.[109] This drug has a half-life of 6 hours and acts via vascular V_1 receptors and renal tubular V_2 receptors.[110] In one report, terlipressin 1 mg was given intravenously to 15 patients with norepinephrine-resistant septic shock.[110] Terlipressin increased MAP at 30 minutes, and the effect lasted for 24 hours. Despite a decrease in CO, terlipressin increased gastric mucosal perfusion, urine production, and creatinine clearance. An open-label study randomized 20 septic shock patients after fluid resuscitation to terlipressin 1 mg or norepinephrine after fluid resuscitation.[111] Despite significant decreases in heart rate, cardiac index, and DO_2I with terlipressin, blood pressure was increased to a greater extent than with norepinephrine.[111] Both agents improved urine production and decreased serum lactate concentration. These preliminary findings suggest that a clinical trial evaluating mortality as well as hemodynamic effects should be conducted.

LEVOSIMENDAN

Levosimendan is a novel inotropic and vasodilator calcium-sensitizing drug. In acute decompensated heart failure, it improves cardiac contractility by sensitizing troponin C to calcium. A blinded study randomized 28 septic shock patients with left ventricular dysfunction despite at least 48 hours of conventional therapy that included dobutamine to levosimendan 0.2 mcg/kg/min or dobutamine 5 mcg/kg/min for 24 hours.[112] At the same MAP, levosimendan decreased PAOP, increased LVEF and cardiac index, improved PCO_2 gap, and enhanced urine production. Additional clinical trials of levosimendan in septic shock are needed.

DOPEXAMINE AND ISOPROTERENOL

Dopexamine is a structural and synthetic analog of dopamine that exerts systemic vasodilation through stimulation of β_2-adrenoceptors and peripheral D_1 and D_2 receptors and weak inotropic properties through stimulation of β_1-adrenoceptors. It has been used in patients with acute heart failure and septic shock. Similar to dobutamine, dopexamine is administered in combination with a vasopressor agent in septic shock. In small studies of septic shock, dopexamine produced a dose-related (range 2–6 mcg/kg/min) increase in cardiac index, stroke volume, and heart rate, as well as a decrease in SVR over the course of 0.5 to 1 hour while the dosages of other vasopressors were kept constant.[113–118] The increase in myocardial oxygen demand is less than with dopamine, but tachycardia and tachydysrhythmia may lead to myocardial ischemia, especially when ischemic heart disease is present. Global oxygen-transport variables are similar to those of dopamine: DO_2 increases but VO_2 increases insufficiently, resulting in impaired O_2ER. The combined β_2-adrenoceptors and peripheral D_1 agonistic effects of dopexamine should improve distribution of blood flow. However, the results of studies of dopexamine use in septic shock failed to show preferential increase in splanchnic blood flow.[115–118] In fact, gastric pHi was lowered. When administered over 7 days, dopexamine had no impact on gastrointestinal barrier and renal function.[118] Therefore, initial data do not support a role for dopexamine in improving regional hemodynamics and blood flow, but studies continue to investigate dopexamine as an alternative therapy for septic shock.

Isoproterenol is a synthetic catecholamine that stimulates only β_1- and β_2-adrenoceptors to produce vasodilatory and inotropic effects. Although not thought of as a traditional agent for managing septic shock, isoproterenol has received attention because of the concepts of early goal-directed therapy.[19] The strong β-adrenergic effects of isoproterenol make it a potential alternative to dobutamine for optimizing DO_2 in patients with low SvO_2 despite use of other therapies (e.g., fluid resuscitation, vasopressors, red blood cell transfusion). A study of 14 patients with septic shock and SvO_2 <70% despite volume administration, norepinephrine, and red blood cell transfusion showed that adding isoproterenol over a 12-hour period increased SvO_2, cardiac index, and stroke index without increasing heart rate or causing myocardial ischemia.[119] Although these results are intriguing, additional studies are needed to define the role of isoproterenol, especially considering that dobutamine has become standard therapy for early goal-directed therapy. At present, isoproterenol is an agent of last resort.

OTHER THERAPIES

As with vasopressin and cortisol, critical illness impairs hypothalamic–pituitary function, producing relative deficiencies of triiodothyronine (T_3) and thyroxine (T_4). This condition, referred to as *euthyroid sick syndrome*, may contribute to hypotension.[120] Concentrations of thyrotropin-releasing hormone and thyroid-stimulating hormone are inappropriately low. Measured concentrations of free T_3 and T_4 may be low or normal, but synthesis is consistently impaired. Only scant data regarding the replacement of these hormones in critically ill patients are available, and the results are variable depending on the extent of additional hormone replacement (growth hormone, gonadotropin-releasing hormone, leptin, insulin, thyrotropin-releasing hormone, and thyroid-stimulating hormone). Given the data for replacing vasopressin and cortisol in septic shock, it is reasonable to assume that one day a "thyroid replacement" regimen will be offered as an adjunctive treatment to vasopressors.

Drotrecogin alfa (activated) or activated protein C has been established as a treatment of severe sepsis because it reduces mortality when used early in patients with at least two organ dysfunctions or an

Acute Physiology and Chronic Health Evaluation (APACHE) II score of 25.[121] Drotrecogin alfa (activated) promotes fibrinolysis, inhibits coagulation, and modulates inflammation. Animal studies suggest that inhibition of TNF-α and inactivation of iNOS by drotrecogin alfa (activated) prevents endotoxin-induced hypotension. A study of 22 septic shock patients treated with drotrecogin alfa (activated) showed that the norepinephrine dose decreased 33% over 24 hours.[122] In contrast, the norepinephrine dose increased 38% in the matched control group despite MAP values similar to the drotrecogin alfa (activated) group. Although these results deserve further investigation, drotrecogin alfa (activated) likely will never be administered solely for hemodynamic support of septic shock patients because it is an expensive agent with concerns of hemorrhage as a side effect. Ultimately, patients who "qualify" for drotrecogin alfa (activated) will receive it irrespective of hemodynamic effect.

GENERAL CONCLUSIONS AND RECOMMENDATIONS

The choice of vasopressor or inotropic agent in septic shock should be made according to the needs of the patient (Fig. 25–2). The traditional algorithm suggests a stepwise approach, first using dopamine and then norepinephrine. Dobutamine is added for low CO states or to optimize $Svo_2/Scvo_2$. Occasionally, epinephrine and phenylephrine are used when necessary. Although this approach is empirical, it is used broadly in clinical practice and has been justified by the desire to avoid strong vasoconstriction and by the sense of safety resulting from graded doses of dopamine. This dose–response relationship, however, has never been established in critically ill patients. In addition, observations of improved outcomes with norepinephrine and decreased regional perfusion with dopamine are calling into question the use of dopamine as a first-line agent. Although goal-directed therapies to supranormal values cannot be recommended, developing a strategy to titrate therapy early in the course of illness to predetermined values is an acceptable approach. For all catecholamine vasopressors, doses higher than recommended traditionally are required for goal-directed therapy to MAP and for normalization of oxygen-transport variables, Do_2, and Vo_2. Attainment of supranormal Do_2 and Vo_2 values is difficult in most patients, even when large doses are used. Patients who develop supranormal Do_2 and Vo_2 values have lower mortality, but whether this effect is achieved intrinsically or with exogenous administration of vasopressors/inotropes appears inconsequential. Therefore, goal-directed therapy to supranormal oxygen-transport variables cannot be recommended because little or no benefit has been demonstrated. Further work is required to better elucidate the differential effects of vasopressors on regional hemodynamic and oxygen-transport values as measures of local tissue perfusion.

The algorithmic approach (Fig. 25–2) we recommend for use of vasopressors and inotropes in the hemodynamic support of critically ill septic patients is consistent with the recommendations made in the Surviving Sepsis Campaign[5] and the American College of Critical Care Medicine's guidelines to the hemodynamic support of adult patients with sepsis (Table 25–2).[4,6] Although difficult to demonstrate, true differences in clinical outcomes as a result of differences in

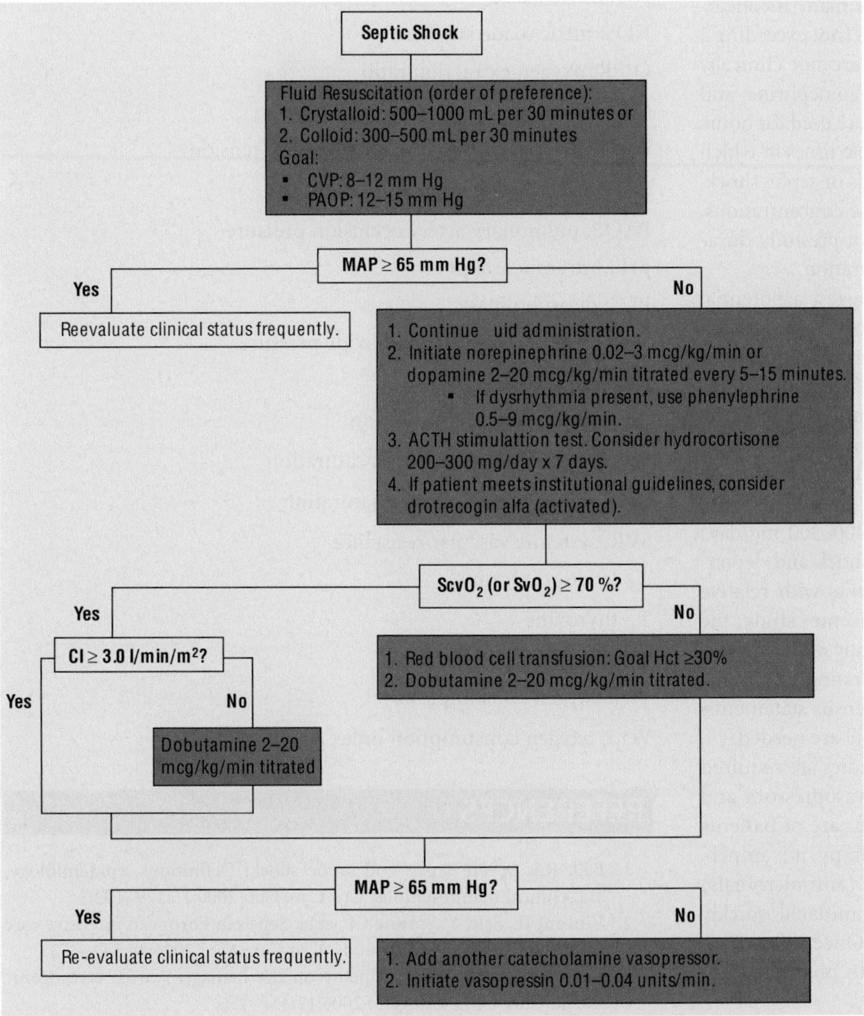

FIGURE 25-2. Algorithmic approach to resuscitative management of septic shock. Algorithmic approach is intended to be used in conjunction with clinical judgment, hemodynamic monitoring parameters, and therapy end points, as discussed in the text. (ACTH, adrenocorticotropic hormone; CI, cardiac index; CVP, central venous pressure; Hct, hematocrit; MAP, mean arterial pressure; PAOP, pulmonary artery occlusive pressure; $Scvo_2$, central venous oxygen saturation; Svo_2, mixed venous oxygen saturation.) *(Figure based on data from references 4–6 and 19.)*

the pharmacologic activity of vasopressors and inotropes may exist. For example, evidence suggests that norepinephrine, when used appropriately with fluid replenishment, is safe and effective in treating septic shock; it decreases mortality, particularly when started early in the course of septic shock. It is effective in optimizing hemodynamic variables and improving systemic and regional (e.g., renal, gastric mucosal, and splanchnic) perfusion. Epinephrine causes a greater increase in the cardiac index and DO_2 and increases gastric mucosal flow but may not preserve splanchnic circulation adequately. Epinephrine may cause a short-lived increase in lactic acid that resolves in 24 hours, and no difference in clinical outcome has been documented. Epinephrine may be particularly useful when used earlier in the course of septic shock in young patients and in those with no known cardiac abnormalities. Unlike epinephrine, dopamine does not increase the proportion of CO that preferentially goes to the splanchnic circulation. The ability of dopamine to increase CO by no more than 35% accompanied by a tachycardia or tachydysrhythmias limits its utility. Dopamine, as opposed to norepinephrine, has been shown to worsen splanchnic VO_2 and O_2ER and is of limited value in improving urine production. Low-dose dopamine has not been shown consistently to increase the glomerular filtration rate, does not prevent renal failure, and actually worsens splanchnic tissue oxygen utilization. Low-dose dopamine should not be used. Phenylephrine should be used when a pure vasoconstrictor is desired in patients who may not require or cannot tolerate the β-effects of dopamine or norepinephrine with or without dobutamine. In patients with a high filling pressure and hypotension, the combination of phenylephrine and dobutamine may be useful.

Shortcomings of study methodology prevent the establishment of definitive conclusions. As a consequence, published guidelines for the management of severe sepsis and septic shock have many inconclusive recommendations (Table 25–2). Short infusions (not exceeding 2 hours) during studies may show differences that are not clinically significant after 24 hours, as demonstrated for epinephrine and dobutamine. Clinically, vasopressors and inotropes are used for hours to days. Possible confounding factors are the variable times at which studies are initiated with respect to the stage of sepsis or septic shock, the inherent differences in circulating catecholamine concentrations, changes in receptor activity, as well as differences in prestudy duration and type of exogenous catecholamine administration.

Initial uncontrolled studies with vasopressin suggest a potential role in the management of vasopressor-refractory septic shock patients, although further data are needed. Vasopressin appears to reduce the requirements of adrenergic agents, but few studies demonstrate complete discontinuation of these therapies. Therefore, vasopressin should be used only if response to one or two adrenergic agents is inadequate or as a method for reducing the dose of these therapies. Close monitoring of ischemic events is needed. Data indicate that moderate doses of hydrocortisone (200–300 mg/day) administered over 5 to 7 days may reverse septic shock and dependency on vasopressor agents, particularly in patients with relative adrenal insufficiency. As a result of a recent multicenter study, the presence of adrenal insufficiency to indicate therapy with corticosteroids is controversial and the authors believe testing of adrenal function will not be recommended in future consensus statements. Data on optimal dosing and definitive outcomes still are needed.

Further pharmacotherapeutic and outcomes studies are required to elucidate the place in therapy of individual vasopressors and inotropes or their combinations in the supportive care of patients with bacteremia or septic shock. As supportive therapy, it is imperative that primary therapy aimed at the source of (antimicrobials) and consequences of (anticytokines) infection be initiated quickly to afford the patient the best chance of survival. Once this goal is accomplished, we will need to direct our efforts to pharmacoeconomics and the cost effectiveness of these therapies.

ABBREVIATIONS

ACTH: adrenocorticotropic hormone

APACHE: Acute Physiology and Chronic Health Evaluation

ATP: adenosine triphosphate

CaMK: calcium/calmodulin-dependent protein kinase

cAMP: cyclic adenosine monophosphate

CaO_2: arterial oxygen content

CI: confidence interval

CO: cardiac output

CvO_2: venous oxygen content

CVP: central venous pressure

DO_2: oxygen delivery

DO_2I: oxygen delivery index

ecNOS: constitutive nitric oxide synthase

HR: hazard ratio

ICU: intensive care unit

IL: interleukin

iNOS: inducible nitric oxide synthase

L-NAME: L-arginine-methylester

L-NMMA: monomethyl-L-arginine

LVEF: left ventricular ejection fraction

MAP: mean arterial pressure

NO: nitric oxide

NOS: nitric oxide synthase

O_2ER: oxygen extraction ratio

OR: odds ratio

$PaCO_2$: arterial carbon dioxide pressure (tension)

PaO_2: arterial oxygen pressure (tension)

PAOP: pulmonary artery occlusion pressure

pHi: intramucosal pH

PLC: phospholipase

$PslCO_2$: sublingual carbon dioxide pressure

RR: relative risk

SaO_2: arterial oxygen saturation

$ScvO_2$: central venous oxygen saturation

SvO_2: mixed venous oxygen saturation

SVR: systemic vascular resistance

T_3: triiodothyronine

T_4: thyroxine

TNF: tumor necrosis factor

VO_2: oxygen consumption

VO_2I: oxygen consumption index

REFERENCES

1. Balk RA. Severe sepsis and septic shock: Definitions, epidemiology, and clinical manifestations. Crit Care Clin 2000;16:179–192.
2. Vincent JL, Sakr Y, Sprung CL, et al. Sepsis in European intensive care unit: Results of the SOAP study. Crit Care Med 2006;34:344–353.
3. Mann HJ, Nolan PE Jr. Update on the management of cardiogenic shock. Curr Opin Crit Care 2006;12:431–436.

4. Hollenberg SM, Ahrens TS, Annane D, et al. Practice parameters for hemodynamic support of sepsis in adult patients in sepsis. Crit Care Med 2004;32:1928–1948.
5. Dellinger RP, Carlet JM, Masur H, et al. Surviving sepsis campaign guidelines for management of severe sepsis and septic shock. Crit Care Med 2004;32:858–873.
6. Beale RJ, Hollenberg SM, Vincent JL, et al. Vasopressor and inotropic support in septic shock: An evidence-based review. Crit Care Med 2004;32(Suppl):S455–S465.
7. Dellinger RP. Cardiovascular management of septic shock. Crit Care Med 2003;32:946–955.
8. Rudis MI, Rowland KL. Current concepts in severe sepsis and septic shock. J Pharm Practice 2005;18:351–362.
9. Holmes CL. Vasoactive drugs in the intensive care unit. Curr Opin Crit Care 2005;11:413–417.
10. Balk RA. Optimum treatment of severe sepsis and septic shock: Evidence in support of the recommendations. Dis Mon 2004;50:163–213.
11. O'Grady N, Alexander M, Dellinger E, et al. Guidelines for the prevention of intravascular catheter-related infections. Clin Infect Dis 2002;35:1281–1307.
12. Bernard GR, Sopko G, Cerra F, et al. Pulmonary artery catheterization and clinical outcomes: National Heart, Lung, and Blood Institute and Food and Drug Administration Workshop Report. Consensus Statement. JAMA 2000;283:2568–2572.
13. Prentice D, Ahrens T. Controversies in the use of the pulmonary artery catheter. J Cardiovasc Nurs 2001;15:1–5.
14. Practice guidelines for pulmonary artery catheterization: An updated report by the American Society of Anesthesiologists Task Force on Pulmonary Artery Catheterization. Anesthesiology 2003;99:988–1014.
15. The National Heart, Lung, and Blood Institute Acute Respiratory Distress Syndrome (ARDS) Clinical Trials Network. Pulmonary-artery central venous catheter to guide treatment of acute lung injury. N Engl J Med 2006;354:2213–2224.
16. Vincent JL. Hemodynamic support in septic shock. Intensive Care Med 2001;27:S80–S92.
17. Varpula M, Tallgren M, Saukkonen K, et al. Hemodynamic variables related to outcome in septic shock. Intensive Care Med 2005;31:1066–1071.
18. Varpula M, Karlsson S, Ruokonen E, et al. Mixed venous oxygen saturation cannot be estimated by central venous oxygen saturation in septic shock. Intensive Care Med 2006;32:1336–1343.
19. Rivers E, Nguyen B, Havstad S, et al. Early goal-directed therapy in the treatment of severe sepsis and septic shock. N Engl J Med 2001;345:1368–1377.
20. Heyland DK, Cook DJ, King D, et al. Maximizing oxygen delivery in critically ill patients: A methodologic appraisal of the evidence. Crit Care Med 1996;24:517–524.
21. Yu M, Burchell S, Hasaniya NW, et al. Relationship of mortality to increasing oxygen delivery in patients 50 years of age: A prospective, randomized trial. Crit Care Med 1998;26:1011–1019.
22. Lobo SM, Salgado PF, Castillo VG, et al. Effects of maximizing oxygen delivery on morbidity and mortality in high-risk surgical patients. Crit Care Med 2000;28:3396–3404.
23. Uusaro A, Russell JA. Could anti-inflammatory actions of catecholamines explain the possible beneficial effects of supranormal oxygen delivery in critically ill surgical patients? Intensive Care Med 2000;26:299–304.
24. Kern JW, Shoemaker WC. Meta-analysis of hemodynamic optimization in high-risk patients. Crit Care Med 2002;30:1686–1692.
25. Levy MM, Macias WL, Vincent JL, et al. Early changes in organ function predict eventual survival in severe sepsis. Crit Care Med 2005;33:2194–2201.
26. Kortgen A, Neiderprum P, Bauer M. Implementation of an evidence-based standard operating procedure and outcome in septic shock. Crit Care Med 2006;34:943–949.
27. Micek ST, Roubinian N, Heuring T, et al. Before–after study of a standardized hospital order set for the management of septic shock. Crit Care Med 2006;34:2707–2713.
28. Shapiro NI, Howell MD, Talmor D, et al. Implementation and outcomes of the multiple urgent sepsis therapies (MUST) protocol. Crit Care Med 2006;34:1025–1032.
29. Bourgoin A, Leone M, Delmas A, et al. Increasing mean arterial pressure in patients with septic shock: Effects on oxygen variables and renal function. Crit Care Med 2005;33:780–786.
30. Chapman MV, Mythen MG, Webb AR, Vincent JL. Report from the meeting: Gastrointestinal tonometry: State of the art, 22–23 May 1998 London, UK. Intensive Care Med 2000;26:613–622.
31. Barry B, Mallick A, Hartley G, et al. Comparison of air tonometry with gastric tonometry using saline and other equilibrating fluids: An in vivo and in vitro study. Intensive Care Med 1998;24:777–784.
32. Poeze M, Solberg BCJ, Greve JWM, et al. Monitoring global volume-related hemodynamic or regional variables after initial resuscitation: What is a better predictor of outcomes in critically ill septic patients? Crit Care Med 2005;33:5494–5500.
33. Boswell SA, Scalea TM. Sublingual capnometry: An alternative to gastric tonometry for the management of shock resuscitation. AACN Clin Issues 2003;14:176–184.
34. Marik PE. Sublingual capnography: A clinical validation study. Chest 2001;120:923–927.
35. Creteur J, De Backer D, Sakr Y, et al. Sublingual capnometry tracks microcirculatory changes in septic patients. Intensive Care Med 2006;32:516–523.
36. Price S, Nicol E, Gibson DG, et al. Echocardiography in the critically ill: Current and potential roles. Intensive Care Med 2006;32:48–59.
37. Maeder M, Fehr T, Rickli H, et al. Sepsis-associated myocardial dysfunction: Diagnostic and prognostic impact of cardiac troponins and natriuretic peptides. Chest 2006;129:1349–1366.
38. Bernardin G, Kisoka RL, Delporte C, et al. Impairment of β-adrenergic signaling in healthy peripheral blood mononuclear cells exposed to serum from patients with septic shock: Involvement of the inhibitory pathway of adenylyl cyclase stimulation. Shock 2003;19:108–112.
39. Bernardin G, Strosberg AD, Bernard A, et al. β-Adrenergic receptor–dependent and –independent stimulation of adenylate cyclase is impaired during severe sepsis in humans. Intensive Care Med 1998;24:1315–1322.
40. Dunser M, Wenzel V, Mayr A, et al. Management of vasodilatory shock. Drugs 2003;63:237–256.
41. Bucher M, Kees F, Taeger K, et al. Cytokines down-regulate α_1-adrenergic receptor expression during endotoxemia. Crit Care Med 2003;31:566–571.
42. Asfar P, Hauser B, Radermacher P, et al. Catecholamines and vasopressin during critical illness. Crit Care Clin 2006;22:131–149.
43. Dickerson RN, Lima JJ, Kuhl DA, et al. Effect of sustained endotoxemia on α_1-adrenergic responsiveness in parenterally fed rats. Pharmacotherapy 1998;18:170–174.
44. Obritsch M, Bestul D, Jung R, et al. The role of vasopressin in vasodilatory septic shock. Pharmacotherapy 2004;24:1050–1063.
45. Vincent JL. Vasopressin in hypotensive and shock states. Crit Care Clin 2006;22:187–197.
46. MacLaren R, Jung R. Stress-dose corticosteroid therapy for sepsis and acute lung injury or acute respiratory distress syndrome in critically ill adults. Pharmacotherapy 2002;22:1140–1156.
47. Minneci PC, Deans KJ, Banks SM, et al. Meta-analysis: The effect of steroids on survival and shock during sepsis depends on the dose. Ann Intern Med 2004;141:47–56.
48. Annane D, Bellissant E, Bollaert PE, et al. Corticosteroids for treating severe sepsis and septic shock. Cochrane Database Syst Rev 2004;1:CD002243.
49. Lefering LR, Neugebauer EAM. Steroids controversy in sepsis and septic shock: A meta-analysis. Crit Care Med 1995;23:1294–1303.
50. Cronin L, Cook DJ, Carlet J, et al. Corticosteroid treatment for sepsis: A critical appraisal and meta-analysis. Crit Care Med 1995;23:1430–1439.
51. Ananne D, Sebille V, Troche G, et al. A 3-level prognostic classification in septic shock based on cortisol levels and cortisol response to corticotropin. JAMA 2000;283:1038–1045.
52. Richer M, Robert S, Lebel M. Renal hemodynamics during norepinephrine and low-dose dopamine infusions in man. Crit Care Med 1996;24:1150–1156.
53. Martin C, Viviand X, Arnaud S, et al. Effects of norepinephrine plus dobutamine or norepinephrine alone on left ventricular performance of septic shock patients. Crit Care Med 1999;27:1708–1713.
54. LeDoux D, Astiz ME, Carpati CM, Rackow EC. Effects of perfusion pressure on tissue perfusion in septic shock. Crit Care Med 2000;28:2729–2732.
55. Flancbaum L, Dick M, Dasta J, et al. A dose-response study of phenylephrine in critically ill, septic surgical patients. Eur J Clin Pharmacol 1997;51:461–465.

56. Woolsey CA, Coopersmith CM. Vasoactive drugs and the gut: Is there anything new? Curr Opin Crit Care 2006;12:155–159.
57. Day NP, Phu NH, Mai NT, et al. Effects of dopamine and epinephrine infusions on renal hemodynamics in severe malaria and severe sepsis. Crit Care Med 2000;28:1353–1362.
58. Lauzier F, Levy B, Lamarre P, et al. Vasopressin or norepinephrine in early hyperdynamic septic shock: A randomized clinical trial. Intensive Care Med 2006;32:1782–1789.
59. Annane D, Sebille V, Charpentier C, et al. Effect of treatment with low doses of hydrocortisone and fludrocortisone on mortality in patients with septic shock. JAMA 2002;288:862–871.
60. Oppert M, Schindler R, Husung C, et al. Low-dose hydrocortisone improves shock reversal and reduces cytokine levels in early hyperdynamic septic shock. Crit Care Med 2005;33:2457–2464.
61. De Backer D, Creteur J, Silva E, Vincent JL. Effects of dopamine, norepinephrine, and epinephrine on the splanchnic circulation in septic shock: Which is best? Crit Care Med 2003;31:1659–1667.
62. Meier-Hellmann A, Bredle DL, Specht M, et al. The effects of low-dose dopamine on splanchnic blood flow and oxygen uptake in patients with septic shock. Intensive Care Med 1997;23:31–37.
63. Olson D, Pohlman A, Hall JB. Administration of low-dose dopamine to nonoliguric patients with sepsis syndrome does not raise intramucosal gastric pH nor improve creatinine clearance. Am J Respir Crit Care Med 1996;154:1664–1670.
64. Ruokonen E, Takala J, Kari A, et al. Regional blood flow and oxygen transport in septic shock. Crit Care Med 1993;21:1296–1303.
65. Marik PE, Mohedin M. The contrasting effects of dopamine and norepinephrine on systemic and splanchnic oxygen utilization in hyperdynamic sepsis. JAMA 1994;272:1354–1357.
66. Dive A, Foret F, Jamart J, et al. Effect of dopamine on gastrointestinal motility during critical illness. Intensive Care Med 2000;26:901–907.
67. Yu M. A peek at renal blood flow, renal function, and oxygen consumption with epinephrine and dopamine therapy. Crit Care Med 2000;28:1661–1663.
68. Jakob SM, Ruokonen E, Takala J. Effects of dopamine on systemic and regional blood flow and metabolism in septic and cardiac surgery patients. Shock 2002;18:8–13.
69. Sakr Y, Reinhart K, Vincent JL, et al. Does dopamine administration in shock influence outcome? Results of the sepsis occurrence in acutely ill patients (SOAP) study. Crit Care Med 2006;34:589–597.
70. Girbes AR, Patten MT, McCloskey BV, et al. The renal and neurohumoral effects of the addition of low-dose dopamine in septic critically ill patients. Intensive Care Med 2000;26:1685–1689.
71. Ichai C, Soubielle J, Carles M, et al. Comparison of the renal effects of low to high doses of dopamine and dobutamine in critically ill patients: A single-blind randomized study. Crit Care Med 2000;28:921–928.
72. Lherm T, Troche G, Rossignol M, et al. Renal effects of low-dose dopamine in patients with sepsis syndrome or septic shock treated with catecholamines. Intensive Care Med 1996;22:213–219.
73. Ichai C, Passeron C, Carles M, et al. Prolonged low-dose dopamine infusion induces a transient improvement in renal function in hemodynamically stable, critically ill patients: A single-blind, prospective, controlled study. Crit Care Med 2000;28:1329–1335.
74. Bellomo R, Bonventre J, Macias W, et al. Management of early acute renal failure: Focus on post-injury prevention. Curr Opin Crit Care 2005;11:542–547.
75. Schrier RW, Wang W. Acute renal failure and sepsis. N Engl J Med 2004;351:159–169.
76. Martin C, Papazian L, Perrin G, et al. Norepinephrine or dopamine for the treatment of hyperdynamic septic shock? Chest 1993;103:1826–1831.
77. Friedrich JO, Adhikari N, Herridge MS, et al. Meta-analysis: Low-dose dopamine increases urine output but does not prevent renal dysfunction or death. Ann Intern Med 2005;142:510–524.
78. Bellomo R, Chapman M, Finfer S, et al. Low-dose dopamine in patients with early renal dysfunction: A placebo-controlled randomized trial. Australian and New Zealand Intensive Care Society (ANZICS) Clinical Trials Group. Lancet 2000;356:2139–2143.
79. Martin C, Viviand X, Leone M, Thirion X. Effect of norepinephrine on the outcome of septic shock. Crit Care Med 2000;28:2758–2765.
80. Groeneveld AB, Girbes AR, Thijs LG. Treating septic shock with norepinephrine. Crit Care Med 1999;27:2022–2023.
81. Redl-Wenzl EM, Armbruster C, Edelmann G, et al. The effects of norepinephrine on hemodynamics and renal function in severe septic shock states. Intensive Care Med 1993;19:151–154.
82. Guerin JP, Levraut J, Samat-Long C, et al. Effects of dopamine and norepinephrine on systemic and hepatosplanchnic hemodynamics, oxygen exchange, and energy balance in vasoplegic septic patients. Shock 2005;23:18–24.
83. Sharma VK, Dellinger RP. The International Sepsis Forum's controversies in sepsis: My initial vasopressor agent in septic shock is norepinephrine rather than dopamine. Crit Care 2003;7:3–5.
84. Jellema WT, Groeneveld J, Wesseling KH, et al. Heterogeneity and prediction of hemodynamic responses to dobutamine in patients with septic shock. Crit Care Med 2006;34:2392–2398.
85. Hayes MA, Timmins AC, Yau EH, et al. Elevation of systemic oxygen delivery in the treatment of critically ill patients. N Engl J Med 1994;330:1717–1722.
86. Shoemaker WC, Appel PL, Kram HB. Oxygen transport measurements to evaluate tissue perfusion and titrate therapy: Dobutamine and dopamine effects. Crit Care Med 1991;19:672–688.
87. Duranteau J, Sitbon P, Teboul JL, et al. Effects of epinephrine, norepinephrine, or the combination of norepinephrine and dobutamine on gastric mucosa in septic shock. Crit Care Med 1999;27:893–900.
88. Reinelt H, Radermacher P, Fischer G, et al. Effects of a dobutamine-induced increase in splanchnic blood flow on hepatic metabolic activity in patients with septic shock. Anesthesiology 1997;86:818–824.
89. Rudis MI, Chant C. Update on vasopressors and inotropes in septic shock. J Pharm Practice 2001;15:124–134.
90. Levy B, Bollaert PE, Charpentier C, et al. Comparison of norepinephrine and dobutamine to epinephrine for hemodynamics, lactate metabolism, and gastric tonometry variables in septic shock: A prospective, randomized study. Intensive Care Med 1997;23:282–287.
91. Seguin P, Bellissant E, Le Tulzo Y, et al. Effects of epinephrine compared with the combination of dobutamine and norepinephrine on gastric perfusion in septic shock. Clin Pharmacol Ther 2002;71:381–388.
92. Zhou SX, Qiu HB, Huang YZ, et al. Effects of norepinephrine, epinephrine, and norepinephrine-dobutamine on systemic and gastric mucosal oxygenation in septic shock. Acta Pharmacol Sin 2002;23:654–658.
93. De Backer D, Creteur J, Dubois MJ, et al. The effects of dobutamine on microcirculatory alterations in patients with septic shock are independent of it systemic effects. Crit Care Med 2006;34:403–408.
94. Yamazaki T, Shimada Y, Taenaka N, et al. Circulatory responses to afterloading with phenylephrine in hyperdynamic sepsis. Crit Care Med 1982;10:432–435.
95. Gregory JS, Bonfiglio MF, Dasta JF, et al. Experience with phenylephrine as a component of the pharmacologic support of septic shock. Crit Care Med 1991;19:1395–1400.
96. Reinelt H, Radermacher P, Kiefer P, et al. Impact of exogenous β-adrenergic receptor stimulation on hepatosplanchnic oxygen kinetics and metabolic activity in septic shock. Crit Care Med 1999;27:325–331.
97. Bracco DC, Revelly JP. Systemic and splanchnic haemodynamic effects of vasopressin administration in vasodilatory shock. Intensive Care Med 2001;27:S138.
98. Klinzing S, Simon M, Reinhart K, et al. High-dose vasopressin is not superior to norepinephrine in septic shock. Crit Care Med 2003;31:2646–2650.
99. Van Haren FMP, Rozendaal FW, Van der Hoeven G. The effect of vasopressin on gastric perfusion in catecholamine-dependent patients in septic shock. Chest 2003;124:2256–2260.
100. Dunser MW, Mayr AJ, Ulmer H, et al. Arginine vasopressin in advanced vasodilatory shock: A prospective, randomized, controlled study. Circulation 2003;107:2313–2319.
101. Patel BM, Chittock DR, Russell JA, et al. Beneficial effects of short-term vasopressin infusion during severe septic shock. Anesthesiol 2002;96:576–582.
102. Watson D, Grover R, Anzueto A, et al. Cardiovascular effects of the nitric oxide synthase inhibitor NG-methyl-L-arginine hydrochloride (546C88) in patients with septic shock: Results of a randomized, double-blind, placebo-controlled multicenter study (study no. 144-002). Crit Care Med 2004;32:13–20.
103. Lopez A, Lorente JA, Steingrub J, et al. Multiple-center, randomized, placebo-controlled, double-blind study of the nitric oxide synthase

inhibitor 546C88: Effect on survival in patients with septic shock. Crit Care Med 2004;32:21–30.
104. Bakker J, Grover R, McLuckie A, et al. Administration of the nitric oxide synthase inhibitor NG-methyl-L-arginine hydrochloride (546C88) by intravenous infusion for up to 72 hours can promote the resolution of shock in patients with severe sepsis: Results of a randomized, double-blind, placebo-controlled multicenter study (study no. 144-002). Crit Care Med 2004;32:1–12.
105. Park BK, Shim TS, Lim CM, et al. The effects of methylene blue on hemodynamic parameters and cytokine levels in refractory septic shock. Korean J Intern Med 2005;20:123–128.
106. Kirov MY, Evgenov OV, Evgenov NV, et al. Infusion of methylene blue in human septic shock: A pilot, randomized, controlled study. Crit Care Med 2001;29:1860–1867.
107. Donati A, Conti G, Loggi S, et al. Does methylene blue administration to septic shock patients affect vascular permeability and blood volume? Crit Care Med 2002;30:2271–2277.
108. Memis D, Karamanlioglu B, Yuksel M, et al. The influence of methylene blue infusion on cytokine levels during severe sepsis. Anaesth Intensive Care 2002;30:755–762.
109. O'Brien A, Clapp L, Singer M. Terlipressin for norepinephrine-resistant septic shock. Lancet 2002;359:1209–1210.
110. Morelli A, Rocco M, Conti G, et al. Effects of terlipressin on systemic and regional haemodynamics in catecholamine-treated hyperkinetic septic shock. Intensive Care Med 2004;30:597–604.
111. Albanese J, Leone M, Delmas A, et al. Terlipressin or norepinephrine in hyperdynamic septic shock: A prospective, randomized study. Crit Care Med 2005;33:1897–1902.
112. Morelli A, De Castro S, Teboul JL, et al. Effects of levosimendan on systemic and regional hemodynamics in septic myocardial depression. Intensive Care Med 2005;31:628–644.
113. Hannemann L, Reinhart K, Meier-Hellmann A, et al. Dopexamine hydrochloride in septic shock. Chest 1996;109:756–760.
114. Smithies M, Yee TH, Jackson L, et al. Protecting the gut and the liver in the critically ill: Effects of dopexamine. Crit Care Med 1994;22:789–795.
115. Kiefer P, Tugtekin I, Wiedeck H, et al. Effect of a dopexamine-induced increase in cardiac index on splanchnic hemodynamics in septic shock. Am J Respir Crit Care Med 2000;161:775–779.
116. Seguin P, Laviolle B, Guinet P, et al. Dopexamine and norepinephrine versus epinephrine on gastric perfusion in patients with septic shock: A randomized study [NCT00134212]. Crit Care 2006;10:R32.
117. Meier-Hellmann A, Bredle DL, Specht M, et al. Dopexamine increased splanchnic blood flow but decreases gastric mucosal pH in severe septic patients treated with dobutamine. Crit Care Med 1999;27:2166–2171.
118. Ralph CJ, Tanser SJ, Macnaughton PD, et al. A randomized controlled trial investigating the effects of dopexamine on gastrointestinal function and organ dysfunction in the critically ill. Intensive Care Med 2002;28:884–890.
119. Leone M, Boyadjiev I, Boulos E, et al. A reappraisal of isoproterenol in goal-directed therapy of septic shock. Shock 2006;26:353–357.
120. De Groot LJ. Non-thyroidal illness syndrome is a manifestation of hypothalamic-pituitary dysfunction, and in view of current evidence, should be treated with appropriate replacement therapies. Crit Care Clin 2006;22:57–86.
121. Bernard GR, Vincent JL, Laterre PF, et al. Efficacy and safety of recombinant human activated protein C for severe sepsis. N Engl J Med 2001;344:699–709.
122. Monnet X, Lamia B, Anguel N, et al. Rapid and beneficial hemodynamic effects of activated protein C in septic shock patients. Intensive Care Med 2005;31:1573–1576.

CHAPTER 26

Hypovolemic Shock

BRIAN L. ERSTAD

KEY CONCEPTS

1. Plasma does not have to be lost from the body for hypovolemic shock to occur.
2. Patients may die of hypovolemic shock despite having normal serum electrolyte concentrations.
3. Although the Starling equation of fluid transport is useful for understanding the factors involved in fluid shifting between compartments, it is not a practical tool for use in the clinical setting.
4. Patients may have complications and death as a result of reperfusion injury as well as the initial insult.
5. The clinical presentation of patients with hypovolemic shock can vary substantially depending on concomitant disease states, medications, and cause of hypovolemia.
6. The initial monitoring of a patient with suspected volume depletion always should include vital signs, urine output, mental status, and physical examination.
7. The need for intravenous (versus oral) rehydration in children often is overestimated.
8. Crystalloid (sodium-containing) solutions should be used for most forms of circulatory insufficiency that are associated with hemodynamic instability.
9. Crystalloid solutions are preferred over colloid solutions for circulatory insufficiency as a result of decreased plasma volume.
10. With adequate fluid administration, vasoactive medications usually are not needed for the patient with circulatory insufficiency as a result of decreased plasma volume.

This chapter discusses the assessment and management of hypovolemic shock. Spinal shock resulting from loss of sympathetic activity and anaphylactic shock resulting from increased vascular permeability often are considered separately from hypovolemic shock because fluid loss from the body is not necessary for their occurrence. Although these forms of shock are not discussed in detail, it is important to note that the initial therapy for both is the same as for hypovolemic shock (i.e., adequate volume replacement) because circulating volume is decreased. In this regard, adequate fluid resuscitation to maintain circulating blood volume is a common principle in managing all forms of shock.

Learning objectives, review questions, and other resources can be found at **www.pharmacotherapyonline.com.**

EPIDEMIOLOGY

Because shock is not a reportable category by state and federal agencies that track causes of death, the incidence is unknown. Estimates of deaths due to shock are complicated by differences in definitions and classification systems. Part of the problem is defining when progressive circulatory insufficiency results in the loss of normal compensatory responses by the body, which could reverse the processes leading to irreversible organ dysfunction. This loss of appropriate compensation varies from patient to patient and is not always readily apparent during the initial patient presentation. Therefore, forms of hypovolemic shock, such as hemorrhagic shock, are subsumed by more readily identifiable categories of death, such as accidental injuries and homicides. Crude and conservative estimates of death due to hypovolemic shock are available for some of its forms. At least 100,000 deaths each year in the United States are due to perioperative bleeding,[1] and approximately 5,000 deaths are due to hyperthermia and dehydration associated with heat exposure.[2] The figures are much higher when considered on a global basis. For example, electrolyte depletion and dehydration due to diarrheal disease result in approximately two million deaths each year in children younger than 5 years.[3] The most liberal estimates of death include all causes of circulatory failure (i.e., the last stage of shock).

ETIOLOGY

1 Hypovolemic shock may result from blood loss (plasma and red blood cells) due to trauma, surgery, or internal hemorrhage or from plasma loss due to fluid sequestered within the body or lost from the body (Table 26–1). In some cases, such as in postoperative patients, a number of these problems occur at the same time. For example, a patient may have blood loss secondary to trauma or surgery, with additional fluid being third spaced (e.g., as tissue edema in the gastrointestinal tract with a concomitant ileus) and lost through a

TABLE 26-1 Causes of Hypovolemic Shock[a]

Decreased blood (plasma + red blood cells) volume
External: Surgery or trauma
Internal (e.g., gastrointestinal bleeding)
Decreased plasma volume
External: Losses from urine, gastrointestinal tract (e.g., vomiting, nasogastric suctioning, fistula, diarrhea), lungs, or skin (including thermal injury)
Internal (decreased oncotic pressure or increased capillary permeability): fluid accumulation in bowel, peritoneal or pleural cavities

[a]Shock may result from various combinations of blood and plasma volume losses listed (i.e., causes are not mutually exclusive).

high-output gastrointestinal fistula postoperatively. As this example of third-spaced fluid indicates, fluid (i.e., plasma) does not have to be lost from the body for a person to develop hypovolemic shock, although the fistula output would clearly aggravate the situation. Approximately 20 L of fluid is secreted and reabsorbed daily in the gastrointestinal tract, so it is not surprising that volume loss could be substantial depending on the location of the fistula and function of the tract preceding the fistula.

Dehydration may result from primary water deficiency, usually because of decreased intake, but in some instances (e.g., diabetes insipidus) may result from increased losses of water. With most forms of dehydration, such as those caused by diarrheal disease and heat-related illness, a combination of inadequate intake and higher than normal losses occurs. In general, the term *dehydration* implies intracellular and interstitial fluid depletion, in contrast to *volume depletion,* which implies extracellular, and particularly intravascular, sodium and water loss. In the case of primary water deficit, cell dehydration occurs. Initially, the patient may be thirsty and possibly have some mental status changes, such as confusion. If cellular dehydration occurs slowly, intracellular substances, referred to as *idiogenic osmols,* develop that limit progressive complications (e.g., cerebral edema or coma). Death due to primary water deficit, if it occurs, is usually a result of delayed circulatory failure. With combined water and salt deficiencies, such as might occur with gastrointestinal (e.g., diarrhea) and skin losses (e.g., heat stroke), interstitial and intravascular depletion is an early occurrence. Fortunately, dehydration is relatively easy to prevent with routine vigilance and water replacement compared with some of the other causes of shock.

PATHOPHYSIOLOGY

❷ Hypovolemic shock often is described in terms of monitoring parameters such as lowered blood pressure, but patients with shock may die despite normal surrogate markers of circulatory insufficiency. Therefore, an appropriate definition should mention the underlying problem, which is inadequate tissue perfusion resulting from circulatory failure. In the case of hypovolemic shock, the cause of the altered perfusion is fluid (or volume) depletion resulting from trauma, surgery, thermal injury, or some form of dehydration. Figure 26–1 provides a simplified view of the pathophysiology of circulatory insufficiency. Cell damage and death may occur from the primary insult or from reperfusion injury. The latter problem is associated most frequently with trauma and blood loss that cause the release of a multitude of mediators of inflammation and injury that have complex interactions. Cells have varying responses to hypoxia, ranging from astrocytes that quit functioning almost immediately to hepatic cells that may function for several hours after injury.[4] Left unmitigated, cell death occurs.

The body attempts to compensate for volume depletion beginning with autoregulatory changes involving smaller blood vessels. When the cause of circulatory insufficiency continues unabated, local mechanisms eventually fail to provide adequate compensation, and macrocirculatory changes ensue. Approximately 75% of blood volume is contained in venous capacitance vessels, with gravity being the major impedance to flow back to the heart.[4] With increasing volume depletion, blood flow to the heart (preload) is decreased, with subsequent activation of baroreceptors and chemoreceptors leading to sympathetic discharge. Also, fluid shifting from the interstitial space to the intravascular space occurs through a phenomenon known as *transcapillary refill,* and hormones (e.g., adrenocorticotropic hormone, angiotensin, catecholamines, and vasopressin) that cause sodium and water retention by the kidneys are released. The phenomenon of transcapillary refill means that the body can have fluid losses exceeding normal plasma volume. These responses cause alterations in stroke volume, heart rate, and peripheral vascular resistance so that blood pressure and hence tissue perfusion can be maintained.

The microcirculatory changes associated with shock are complex and difficult to study. Although some mediators such as endothelin-1 cause vasoconstriction, other mediators, such as adenosine and nitric oxide, yield vasodilation.[5] These changes result in hypoperfusion or hyperperfusion depending on the area. As these microcirculatory changes fail to maintain adequate organ perfusion, more widespread sympathetic nervous system activation and vasoconstriction ensue. Failure to respond to sympathetic stimulation and fluid administration is indicative of the vasodilation that occurs in the final phase of circulatory failure leading to death.

The factors involved in fluid shifting between the intravascular and interstitial spaces are described by the modified Starling equation:

$$J_V = K_{f,c}\,[(P_c - P_t) - [\sigma(\pi_c - \pi_t)]$$

where J_V = net transvascular flow rate (cannot be measured in the clinical setting)

$K_{f,c}$ = capillary filtration coefficient for fluids (cannot be measured in the clinical setting)

P_c = capillary hydrostatic pressure (indirectly estimated in the clinical setting, e.g., pulmonary artery occlusive pressure)

P_t = tissue hydrostatic pressure (cannot be measured in the clinical setting)

σ = reflection coefficient for proteins (cannot be measured in the clinical setting)

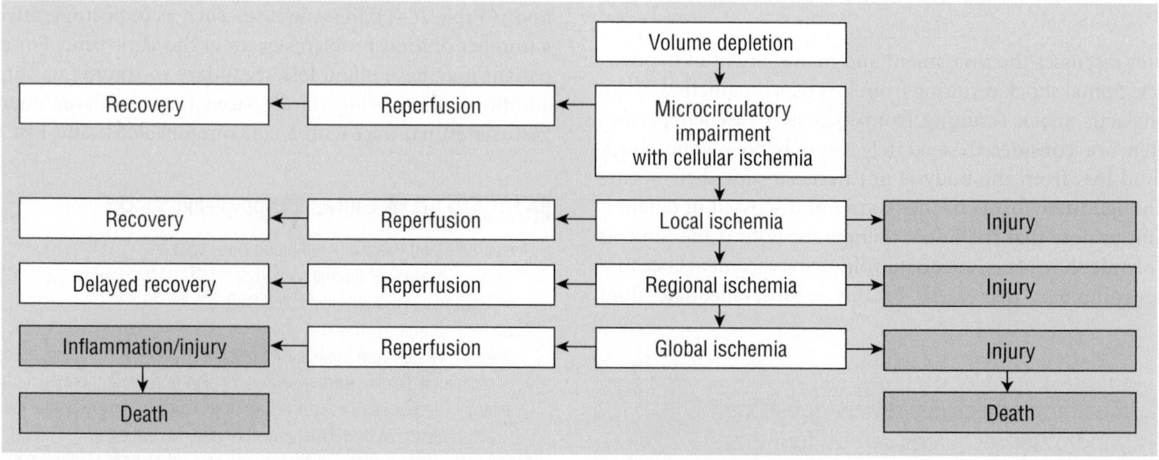

FIGURE 26-1. Pathophysiology of circulatory insufficiency.

π_c = plasma colloid osmotic pressure (not usually measured in the clinical setting, but technology is available)

π_t = tissue colloid osmotic pressure (cannot be measured in the clinical setting)

Proteins act as oncotic agents in each of these spaces to attract fluid, whereas hydrostatic forces push fluid into or out of the vessels. The equation has distinct permeability values for water and protein because each crosses the vascular membrane at a different rate. The values for the variables listed in the equation are not the same for capillaries in all parts of the body. For example, on a scale from 0 to 1 with 0 being free passage of protein and 1 being impermeable to protein, the typical value for the reflection coefficient in most capillaries is >0.9. However, in the pulmonary capillaries the value is closer to 0.7 and approaches 0 in inflammatory states associated with increased capillary permeability.[6] As the value approaches 0, the capillaries are freely permeable not only to the usual fluid and electrolytes but to plasma proteins such as albumin. Because albumin accounts for approximately 80% of the plasma oncotic pressure, its free passage into the interstitial space effectively negates its intravascular oncotic benefit. ❸ Although the Starling equation is useful to practitioners in terms of understanding the factors involved in fluid shifting between compartments, the rate and direction of transvascular flow cannot be calculated accurately in the clinical setting because most factors cannot be measured directly and the values for the factors vary in different capillaries in the body.

The body's compensatory mechanisms may have beneficial and harmful consequences. For example, cardiac output can be increased substantially by increases in stroke volume or heart rate. Although this may be useful for providing blood flow to inadequately perfused tissues, it may cause large increases in oxygen consumption by the heart that could aggravate preexisting ischemia in patients with underlying coronary artery disease (CAD). Another example is the sympathetic nervous system–mediated vasoconstriction that causes blood to shift from the skin, skeletal muscle, and some internal organs such as the kidneys and gastrointestinal tract to organs (e.g., heart and brain) that are less tolerant of inadequate flow. If the vasoconstriction continues unabated, the hypoperfused organs eventually become damaged. Figure 26–2 provides an overview of the compensatory changes that occur with a loss of circulating blood volume.

❹ In addition to the more acute implications of hypovolemia and attendant complications, reperfusion damage is likely to occur particularly after prolonged resuscitation attempts. In addition to oxygen free radical damage of cell membranes, a number of cellular (e.g., white blood cells and platelets) and humoral (e.g., procoagulants, anticoagulants, complement, and kinins) components are activated, causing the release of other inflammatory mediators.[5] The resulting reperfusion injury may range from readily reversible organ dysfunction to multiple-organ failure and death.

Although the basic pathophysiology is similar for the various causes of hypovolemic shock, there are unique considerations relative to each. For example, whereas isolated head injuries associated with trauma typically do not result in substantial blood loss or shock, pelvic fractures may sequester several liters of blood as hematoma formation.[5] Patients with traumatic or thermal injuries, as well as postoperative patients, may have substantial fluid accumulation in sites where the fluid cannot be readily transferred back into blood vessels (i.e., third-spaced fluid) for maintaining pressure. With these types of injuries, prompt control of compressible bleeding sources with rapid patient transfer to the hospital for definitive treatment may preclude the cascade of events leading to shock. Indeed, with trauma patients, a "scoop and run" approach that places a priority on rapid transport to a hospital is used by most urban hospitals.

In the case of hemorrhagic shock, prompt attention must be given to cell as well as plasma losses. Red blood cells lost during the bleeding episode may lead to ischemic damage in vital organs.

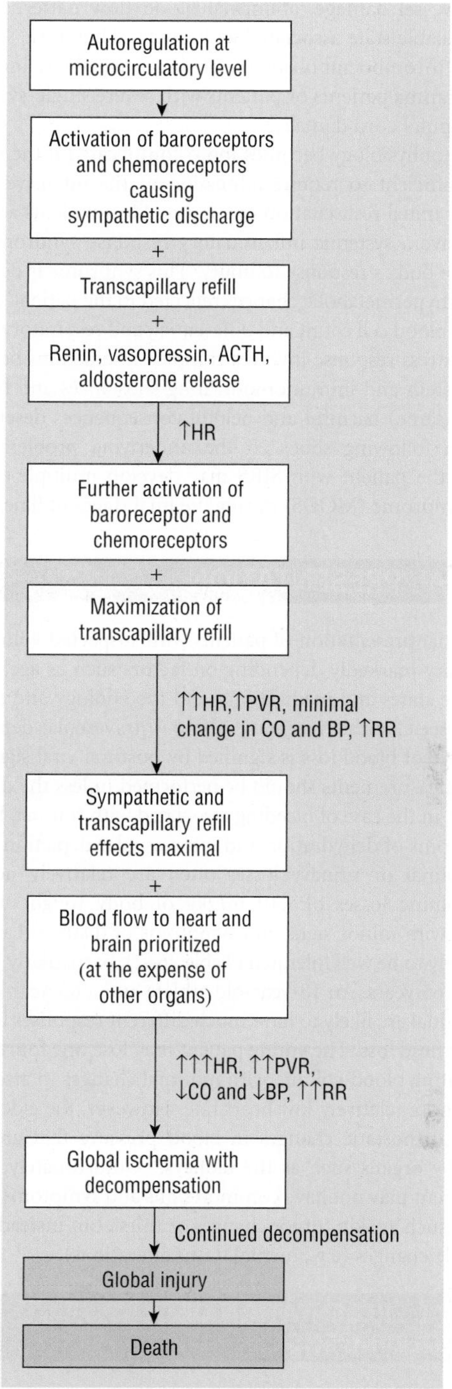

FIGURE 26-2. Activation of compensatory mechanisms with loss of circulatory volume. Certain stages may be absent depending on a number of factors, such as age, preexisting disease states, and cause of circulatory insufficiency. (ACTH, corticotropin; BP, blood pressure; CO, cardiac output; HR, heart rate; PVR, peripheral vascular resistance; RR, respiratory rate.)

Packed red blood cell transfusions may be needed to increase the oxygen-carrying capacity of the blood because oxygen transport is a function not only of cardiac output but also of hemoglobin concentration and saturation and of hemoglobin affinity for oxygen.

Clotting factors and platelets are also lost in hemorrhage. The resulting bleeding problems may be aggravated by the dilutional effect of fluid resuscitation on clotting factor activity. Fresh-frozen plasma that contains necessary clotting factors and platelets is often needed in massive blood loss to restore adequate coagulation. On the other hand, trauma patients are at increased risk for deep vein thrombosis and pulmonary embolism caused by multiple factors, including vessel damage, abnormal blood flow patterns, and the hypercoagulable state associated with injury. Therefore, some form of venous thromboembolism prophylaxis usually is indicated in multiple-trauma patients or patients with severe single-system injuries (e.g., spinal cord damage).

The pathophysiology becomes more complicated if the severity of shock is sufficient to require admission to the intensive care unit (ICU) after initial resuscitation or surgery. Most patients admitted to the ICU have a systemic inflammatory response syndrome (SIRS), which is the body's response to injury. This syndrome is defined by a number of hypermetabolic changes reflected in the patient's temperature, white blood cell count and differential, and respiratory and heart rates. The stress response involves complex interactions between the nervous system and immunomodulating substances and has similar (if not the same) harmful and helpful consequences described with reperfusion following shock. If the underlying problems are left untreated, the patient with SIRS may develop multiple-organ dysfunction syndrome (MODS) during the final stages of illness.

CLINICAL PRESENTATION

❺ The initial presentation of patients with suspected volume depletion can vary markedly depending on factors such as age, concomitant disease states and medications, and the etiology and rapidity of depletion (see Clinical Presentation box). Intravascular depletion as a consequence of blood loss is signified by postural vital sign changes, and such measurements should be performed unless the diagnosis is obvious, as in the case of bleeding associated with trauma. Early signs and symptoms of dehydration and intravascular depletion caused by gastrointestinal or urinary losses often are relatively nonspecific. Plasma volume losses of <10 mL/kg of body weight usually are associated with minor signs and symptoms of distress. Larger losses are not likely to be well tolerated (Table 26–2), particularly in patients older than 65 years. An 18-year-old athlete and a 65-year-old sedentary individual are likely to have much different responses to a similar amount of fluid loss. The young patient may lose one fourth of his or her circulating blood volume with minimal changes in arterial blood pressure and a relatively low heart rate. However, the elderly patient may have orthostatic changes in blood pressure that are not well tolerated by organs such as the kidneys.[4] Unfortunately, this same elderly patient may not have common signs and symptoms of volume depletion, such as skin turgor changes or thirst, but instead may have more subtle changes (e.g., mental status alterations).

CLINICAL PRESENTATION OF HYPOVOLEMIC SHOCK

General

- The initial presentation of adult patients with suspected volume depletion could vary markedly depending on factors such as age, concomitant disease states and medications, and the etiology and rapidity of depletion.
- Plasma volume losses of <10 mL/kg of body weight usually are associated with minor signs and symptoms of distress.

Symptoms

- Patients may present with thirst, nausea, anxiousness, weakness, light-headedness, and dizziness.
- Patients may report scanty urine output and dark-yellow urine.

Signs

With more severe volume loss:

- Patients would have marked increases in heart rate (e.g., >120 beats/min) and respiratory rate (e.g., >30 breaths/min).
- Blood pressure would be decreased (e.g., systolic blood pressure <90 mm Hg).
- Mental status changes or unconsciousness may occur.
- Agitation may be present if the patient is conscious.
- Body temperature would be low or normal [e.g., 36° to 37°C (96.8° to 98.6°F)] in the absence of concomitant infection.

Laboratory Tests

- Sodium and chloride concentrations usually are high with acute depletion but may be low or normal depending on type of fluid intake.
- The ratio of blood urea nitrogen (BUN) to creatinine is likely to be elevated initially, but the creatinine level would increase as renal dysfunction occurs.
- The complete blood count should be normal in the absence of concomitant disease states such as infection; in hemorrhagic shock, the red cell count, hemoglobin, and hematocrit would decrease over time.
- With more severe volume depletion, other organs may become dysfunctional, which may be reflected in laboratory testing (e.g., elevated transaminase levels with hepatic dysfunction).

Other Diagnostic Tests

- Urine output would be decreased to <0.5 to 1 mL/h.

The diagnosis of dehydration and intravascular depletion in children is complicated by difficulties in obtaining an accurate history. However, some excellent resources are available for healthcare providers, such as the Centers for Disease Control and Prevention (CDC) guidelines (*www.CDC.gov*), which discuss the evaluation and management of diarrhea in patients of all ages. In younger children, parental observations are important for estimating fluid deficits and deciding whether hospitalization is necessary. Fortunately, prospective data suggest that parental histories are predictive of acidosis and the need for hospitalization.[7] ❻ Regardless of patient age or preexisting conditions, the initial monitoring of a patient with suspected volume depletion should include the following noninvasive parame-

TABLE 26-2 Acute Circulatory Insufficiency: Initial Presentation and Therapy[a]

	Mild	Severe
Plasma/blood loss	10 mL/kg adult 20 mL/kg child	30 mL/kg adult 35 mL/kg child
Mental status/level of consciousness	None–small changes (e.g., anxious, irritable)	Marked changes (e.g., confusion to unconsciousness)
Vital signs/orthostatic changes	Minor changes	Marked changes
Therapy	20 mL/kg lactated Ringer IV[a] over 10–15 min Unlikely to need blood cell replacement even if hemorrhagic loss	Lactated Ringer IV as rapidly as possible until response in adult, then decrease rate of infusion 20 mL/kg lactated Ringer IV in child (repeat quickly if minimal response); likely to need blood cell replacement and surgery if hemorrhagic

[a]Patients may have intermediate degrees of volume loss in addition to those listed, but the amount of loss often is difficult to quantify. The presentations may also vary greatly in patients with similar amounts of loss (young athlete vs sedentary, elderly person). In patients particularly prone to complications associated with fluid overload, the fluid can be administered in multiple smaller boluses titrated to clinical response. See text for a more in-depth discussion of some of the guidelines in this table.

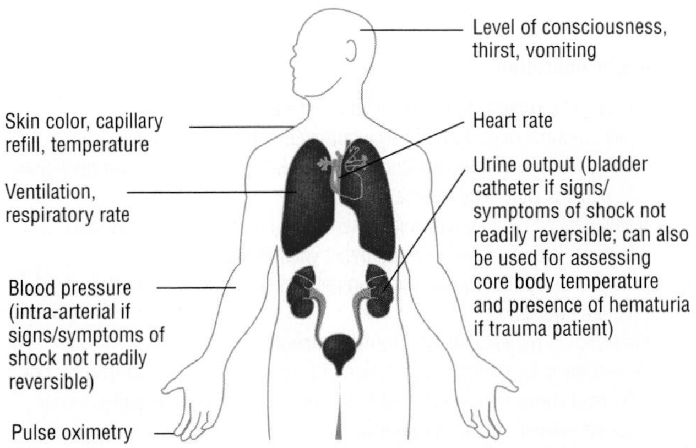

FIGURE 26-3. Noninvasive assessment of circulatory insufficiency.

ters: vital signs, urine output, mental status, and physical examination (Fig. 26–3).

Although the presenting signs and symptoms of circulatory insufficiency are variable, patients usually have decreased blood pressure, increased heart and respiratory rates, and a normal or low–normal temperature (e.g., 36° to 37°C [96.8° to 98.6°F]) in the absence of infection, exposure to extremes of temperature, and medications that impair thermoregulation. As mentioned earlier, recordings of vital signs must be interpreted in light of known or suspected baseline conditions. For example, alcohol, β-blockers, butyrophenones such as haloperidol, diuretics, and medications with anticholinergic effects may impair thermoregulation.[8] Medications such as β-blockers and calcium channel blockers may alter resting blood pressure and heart rate, as well as the subsequent response to therapeutic interventions.

Although a blood pressure reading of 110/70 mm Hg (systolic/diastolic) may be acceptable in many patients, it may be inadequate in a patient with preexisting hypertension who normally has a blood pressure of 170/105 mm Hg. At the other extreme, patients with very low blood pressure may have inaudible or inaccurate determinations with cuff (sphygmomanometric) measurements. Chapter 15 details blood pressure measurement (e.g., cuff size, position). In this case, intraarterial monitoring is indicated. As a noninvasive tool, the respiratory rate may correlate better than the heart rate with volume loss, but respiratory rate often is not used.[4] The respiratory rate may be elevated because of anxiety or as a compensatory mechanism for the metabolic acidosis caused by lactic acidosis associated with poor tissue perfusion.

Although the kidneys continually produce urine, the bladder stores the urine for intermittent elimination. For the initial diagnosis and management of acute circulatory insufficiency, a catheter can be inserted into the bladder for measuring urine output. In contrast to thirst, which is a relatively insensitive indicator of volume depletion, urine output is generally diminished with inadequate fluid administration and increases with appropriate resuscitation. This presumes, of course, that acute renal failure or medications such as diuretics are not altering the expected response. Adults should produce at least 0.5 to 1 mL/kg/h of urine, whereas children up to 12 years of age should produce at least 1 mL/kg/h (2 mL/kg/h if younger than 1 year).

Mental status changes associated with volume depletion, if present, may range from subtle fluctuations in mood to unconsciousness. Although the latter finding typically is indicative of more severe depletion, less dramatic findings should not be interpreted as indicating mild fluid deficits. Losses of 4 L of plasma volume may be associated only with lassitude in an otherwise healthy adult patient.[4] Similar interpretation difficulties must be considered when performing the initial physical examination. An orderly progression from warm, reddish skin with appropriate capillary refill (rapid return of blood flow to the extremity after removal of compression) to cold, cyanotic discoloration with impaired refill may not occur. Also, dry mucous membranes in elderly patients may be caused by mouth breathing or medications and not by fluid depletion.

TREATMENT

Hypovolemic Shock

DESIRED OUTCOME

The desired outcomes of therapy for circulatory insufficiency that has led to hypovolemic shock are to prevent further progression of the disease with subsequent organ damage and, to the extent possible, to reverse organ dysfunction that has already taken place.

GENERAL APPROACH TO TREATMENT

Milder forms of volume depletion may be managed in outpatient settings. For example, supplemental fluids can be added to the usual estimated daily requirements of 30 to 35 mL/kg in patients older than 12 years with dehydration. Commercially available carbohydrate/electrolyte drinks generally are more palatable than water and may promote earlier recovery. The rationale for combining carbohydrates with sodium is based on the cotransport absorption mechanism in the intestinal tract. With diarrheal states in particular, sodium absorption is impaired. Because water follows sodium, the diarrhea is likely to continue despite oral crystalloid fluid administration until the intestinal pathology resolves. However, when dextrose and sodium are combined in 1:1 equimolar amounts, both are absorbed via the cotransport mechanism, which also allows for absorption of water. This concept forms the basis for the World Health Organization's (WHO) oral rehydration solution, which contains 75 mmol/L of dextrose, 75 mmol/L of sodium, 20 mmol/L of potassium, 65 mmol/L of chloride, and 10 mmol/L of citrate for a total osmolarity of 245 mOsm/L.[3] Commercially available over-the-counter rehydration drinks for children in the United States also have an osmolarity of approximately 250 mOsm/L but typically contain 50 mEq/L or less of sodium, and the dextrose-to-sodium ratio often is 3:1. How these differences between commercially available formulations and the WHO rehydration formula might affect hospitalization rates is unclear, but attempts to alter the commercially available products to make them more consistent with the WHO formula are not recommended.[3] Improper home mixing of a previous WHO formulation led to cases of hypernatremia.[9] Outpatient rehydration of children usually is recommended for those with uncomplicated (e.g., vomiting less than 48 hours) acute gastroenteritis and relatively mild dehydration after the exclusion of more severe illnesses such as bowel obstruction. ❼ The need for intravenous (IV) rehydration often is overestimated. Randomized studies conducted in pediatric emergency departments have found oral rehydration to be at least as effective as IV rehydration,[10,11] and in one study children receiving oral rehydration for acute gastroenteritis had shorter lengths of stay than those receiving IV rehydration (225 versus 358 minutes; $P < 0.01$). Furthermore, there was a trend toward decreased hospital admissions in the oral compared with the IV rehydration group (11% versus 25%; $P = 0.2$).[11]

Hospitalization is indicated for more severe forms of circulatory insufficiency. If access to the circulatory system for administration of fluids and medication was not obtained prior to hospitalization, this should be a priority. Venous access generally is obtained during the preliminary examination process that includes the ABCs of life support (i.e., airway, breathing, and circulation), assessment of vital signs and mental status, and determination of urine output after

TABLE 26-3 Fluid Distribution and Major Indications[a]

Fluid	Intracellular	Interstitial	Intravascular	Major Indication
Normal saline or lactated Ringer	None	750 mL	250 mL	Intravascular repletion in symptomatic patients
3% sodium chloride	→	750 mL+	250 mL+	Small amounts (e.g., 250 mL) by intermittent infusion have been used in conjunction with normal saline or lactated Ringer for intravascular depletion in patients with head trauma
5% dextrose/0.45% sodium chloride	333 mL	500 mL	167 mL	Maintenance fluid in euvolemic or dehydrated (sodium and water loss) patients with mild signs/symptoms of volume depletion
5% dextrose	667 mL	250 mL	83 mL	Dehydration (primarily water loss) in patients with mild signs/symptoms of volume depletion
5% albumin	None	None	1,000 mL[b]	Intravascular repletion in symptomatic patients
25% albumin	→	→	1,000 mL+++[b]	Usually given by intermittent infusion of small volumes (e.g., 50–100 mL) or by continuous infusion titrated to response in hypovolemic patients with excess interstitial fluid accumulation

[a]Based on administration of 1 L of each solution *for comparative purposes only*. This amount of fluid, particularly for 3% saline and 25% albumin, would be inappropriate and likely harmful if given over a short period of time. Numbers are approximations; arrows indicate direction of fluid shift and plus signs indicate fluid pulled from other compartments.
[b]After distribution and attainment of steady-state conditions, 60% of albumin (and associated fluid) is in interstitial compartment and 40% is in intravascular compartment.

catheterization. Whenever large-volume fluid resuscitation is expected, as in hemorrhagic shock, at least two IV catheters are desirable. Because flow is a function of tubing length and catheter diameter, large-bore peripheral IV lines are preferred over longer central lines. Unfortunately, vascular access in some patients may be problematic, and other routes (e.g., intraosseous infusion in children) may be necessary. One interesting method of fluid administration that has been investigated in elderly patients is subcutaneous infusion, or hypodermoclysis. This route of administration is not used commonly, probably because of concerns of adverse effects that were found in early studies that used excessively hypotonic or hypertonic solutions. Although alternative methods of fluid administration, such as hypodermoclysis, are desirable, well-conducted trials are needed before such methods can be recommended for routine use.

■ PHARMACOLOGIC THERAPY

❽ Dextrose-in-water solutions may be appropriate for uncomplicated dehydration caused by water deprivation, but crystalloid (sodium-containing) solutions should be used for forms of circulatory insufficiency that are associated with hemodynamic instability. In the latter situation, IV solutions with sodium concentrations approximating normal serum sodium values usually are indicated because they cause more expansion of the intravascular and interstitial spaces compared with dextrose solutions (Table 26–3). Lactated Ringer and normal saline solutions are examples of such crystalloid solutions, although lactated Ringer solution is typically the preferred solution for major bleeding because it is unlikely to cause the hyperchloremic metabolic acidosis that is seen with infusion of large amounts of normal saline (Table 26–4). A "large" amount of fluid does not mean a single bolus volume typically used as fluid challenge in a critically ill patient. An isolated bolus (e.g., 250 to 500 mL) in a young adult trauma patient is unlikely to cause a substantial change in blood pressure or acid–base balance.[12] Therefore, multiple fluid boluses usually are needed in such patients to achieve hemodynamic stability in the perioperative period.

Although lactated Ringer solution does contain lactate, it does not cause substantial elevations in circulating lactate concentrations when used as a resuscitation solution.[13] Once adequate plasma volume has been restored by fluid administration, the body can readily clear the blood of the excess lactate that has accumulated from both anaerobic metabolism and from lactated Ringer solution. However, blood samples for lactate determinations drawn through catheters (arterial and venous) that have not been cleared appropriately may have spurious increases or decreases in lactate concentrations because of retained lactated Ringer and nonlactated solutions (e.g., varying concentrations of dextrose-in-water or sodium chloride), respectively.[14] Therefore, blood samples for lactate concentration determinations should be drawn from a catheter that has been cleared adequately (e.g., 5 mL) of infusate after temporarily stopping the fluid infusion.

A number of pharmacologic therapies show promise in animal models of shock, but few demonstrate success in subsequent trials involving patients with shock. In large part this is a result of the lack of acceptable animal models of shock that mimic the pathophysiology of patients.[15] In cases in which a relevant animal model is available, care must be taken when extrapolating the information to forms of shock other than the one under study. This may be the problem with naloxone, which has been shown to raise blood pressure in some studies of shock but not in others. In light of the lack of other demonstrated pharmaceutical interventions, fluids remain the mainstay of therapy, although their use is not devoid of controversy.

Larger-molecular-weight solutions (i.e., >30,000) known as *colloids* have been recommended in conjunction with or as replacements for crystalloid solutions. Examples of colloids used as plasma expanders include albumin, hetastarch, and dextran. Albumin is known as a *monodisperse colloid* because all its molecules are of the same molecular size and weight (~67,000), whereas hetastarch and dextran solutions are *polydisperse compounds* with molecules of varying molecular size that are roughly proportional to molecular weight [*average* molecular weights of 450,000 (range 10,000 to 1 million) for hetastarch, 40,000 (range 10,000 to 90,000) for dextran 40, or 70,000 to 75,000 (range 20,000 to 200,000) for dextran 70 or dextran 75, respectively]. In light of these differences, colloid

TABLE 26-4 Adverse Effects of Plasma Expanders: Crystalloids

Normal saline
- Primarily extensions of pharmacologic actions (e.g., fluid overload, dilutional coagulopathy)
- Hyperchloremic metabolic acidosis (has 154 mEq/L of chloride)
- Hypernatremia (has 154 mEq/L of sodium)

Lactated ringer
- Primarily extensions of pharmacologic actions (e.g., fluid overload, dilutional coagulopathy)
- Hyponatremia (has 130 mEq/L of sodium)
- Aggravation of preexisting hyperkalemia (has 4 mEq/L of potassium)

Hypertonic saline
- Primarily extensions of pharmacologic actions (e.g., fluid overload, dilutional coagulopathy; intracellular volume depletion)
- Hypernatremia (has 513 mEq/L of sodium)
- Hyperchloremia (has 513 mEq/L of chloride)

comparisons are based on weight-averaged [(number of molecules at each weight × particle weight)/total weight of all molecules] or number-averaged (arithmetic mean of all particles weights) molecular weight.[16] The size and weight differences of the colloids have important implications for the distribution of the products because lower-molecular-weight substances are retained in the intravascular space for a shorter period of time as a result of more rapid leakage across the vessel membrane. The theoretical usefulness of colloids is based on their increased molecular weight (average molecular weight in the case of hetastarch and dextran) that corresponds to increased intravascular retention time in the absence of increased capillary permeability compared with crystalloids. Even in patients with intact capillary permeability, the colloid molecules eventually will leak through the membrane. In the case of albumin with a distribution half-life of 15 hours in normal subjects, approximately 60% of administered albumin molecules (and associated fluid) would be shifted to the interstitial space within 3 to 5 days of exogenous administration. In patients with altered permeability (e.g., acute respiratory distress syndrome), the leakage of albumin from the intravascular to the interstitial space may occur within hours, not days.

Albumin is available in 5% and 25% concentrations. Plasma protein fraction has oncotic actions similar to a 5% albumin solution, which is not surprising because albumin is the predominant protein in this product. When given in equipotent amounts, albumin is much more costly than crystalloid solutions. Additionally, the 5% and 25% albumin solutions typically are priced such that no cost savings is associated with dilution of the 25% product to make a 5% concentration. In general, dilution should be avoided because of the possibility of preparation errors; cases of hemolysis and death have occurred when 25% albumin was inappropriately diluted with sterile water for injection, causing a dramatic lowering of effective osmolarity. The 5% albumin solution is relatively *iso-oncotic,* which means that it does not pull fluid into the compartment in which it is contained. In contrast, 25% albumin is referred to as *hyperoncotic* albumin because it tends to pull fluid into the compartment containing the albumin molecules. In general, the 5% albumin solution is used for hypovolemic states. The 25% solution should not be used for acute circulatory insufficiency unless it is used in combination with other fluids or it is being used in patients with excess total body water but intravascular depletion as a means of pulling fluid into the intravascular space. An example of the latter condition is cirrhosis with ascites in which total body water is substantially increased, but the patient is hypotensive as a consequence of lack of intravascular volume. This use of hyperoncotic albumin presumes that there is evidence of adverse effects associated with the excess water (e.g., interstitial fluid accumulation in the lungs) and that the albumin remains in the intravascular space long enough to be of benefit. Albumin has a variety of other functions, such as binding properties, inflammatory gene modification, and antioxidant and free radical scavenging effects, which have been used to justify its administration. Although appealing theoretically, improved patient outcomes related to these properties have not been documented in adequately powered, randomized, controlled trials.

Hetastarch 6% has comparable plasma expansion to a 5% albumin solution but usually is less expensive, which accounts for much of its use. Most of the trials comparing albumin with hetastarch for volume expansion have found no significant differences in clinically important outcomes (e.g., mortality). Few trials have directly compared hetastarch with crystalloid solutions for intravascular expansion. Although hetastarch often is stated as being contraindicated in bleeding disorders, it has been most studied in patients with blood loss (e.g., trauma and perioperative patients). Hetastarch should be avoided in situations where short-term impairments in hemostasis could have dire consequences, such as in patients undergoing cardiopulmonary bypass surgery and patients with intracranial bleeding. Hetastarch may aggravate bleeding through mechanisms specific to this colloid (e.g., decreased factor VIII activity). These mechanisms have not been well elucidated and often are difficult to distinguish from the dilutional effects on clotting factors caused by all plasma expanders. Hetastarch may cause elevations in serum amylase concentrations but does not cause pancreatitis.

Dextran 40, dextran 70, and dextran 75 are available for use as plasma expanders in the United States. The numbers refer to the average molecular weight of the solutions. In general, dextran solutions are not used as often as albumin or hetastarch solutions for plasma expansion, possibly because of concerns related to aggravation of bleeding (i.e., anticoagulant actions related to inhibiting stasis of microcirculation) and anaphylaxis that is more likely to occur with the higher-molecular-weight solutions. However, both these concerns can be reduced if proper attention is paid to patient selection and, in the case of bleeding, published dosing guidelines with regard to the amounts of these products that should be infused. There are few comparative trials involving the dextran solutions, but the intravascular expansion within hours after infusion is approximately equal to the amount of dextran infused.

The crystalloid versus colloid debate was intensified when a metaanalysis by the well-respected Cochrane group found an overall increase in mortality associated with albumin using pooled results of randomized investigations.[17] The metaanalysis involved 30 randomized trials with 1,419 patients (relative risk of death with albumin versus no administration or crystalloid administration 1.68, 95% confidence interval 1.26 to 2.23). For hypovolemia (caused by blood loss in the majority of studies), the risk of death associated with albumin administration was not quite statistically significant (relative risk 1.46, 95% confidence interval 0.97 to 2.22). However, with the notable exception of trauma patients, a subsequent and more comprehensive systematic review did not find increased mortality attributable to albumin.[18] Furthermore, a landmark investigation involving almost 7,000 critically ill patients (conducted after the previously mentioned metaanalyses) did not find statistically significant differences in 28-day mortality between patients resuscitated with either normal saline or 4% albumin.[19] As in the previous meta-analysis, there was a trend toward increased mortality in patients with trauma, particularly in a subset of patients with traumatic brain injury. This multicenter, randomized, double-blind investigation, referred to as the Saline versus Albumin Fluid Evaluation (SAFE) study, involved a heterogeneous group of ICU patients and was not sufficiently powered to look at various subsets, so clinicians must be cautious when extrapolating the results to more specific patient populations. With this caution in mind, this trial provides strong evidence that crystalloid solutions should be considered first-line therapy in patients with hypovolemic shock.

■ SPECIAL POPULATIONS

Trauma/Perioperative Patients

The need for immediate treatment of hemorrhagic circulatory insufficiency with plasma expanders (i.e., crystalloids or colloids) seems obvious, but no large, well-controlled trials conducted in humans have supported this practice. To the contrary, evidence suggests that fluid resuscitation beyond minimal levels (i.e., mean arterial pressure >40 to 60 mm Hg) is harmful. One prospective study involving 598 adult patients with gunshot or stab wound injuries to the torso and systolic blood pressure measurements of 90 mm Hg or less found that delayed fluid resuscitation until operation was associated with increased survival and discharge from the hospital ($P = 0.04$).[20] Since concerns were expressed about the comparability of the immediate and delayed resuscitation groups, particularly because true randomization did not take place, a followup randomized trial was conducted to verify the findings. There were no differences in survival (four deaths in each group) in the second trial regardless of whether systolic blood pressure was titrated to >100 mm Hg or to 70 mm Hg.[21] Both studies were conducted in populated urban areas with approximately 2 hours from the time of injury to operation. Therefore, the results may not be applicable to rural areas with extended transport times. There also is a concern in applying the results of these investigations to patients with certain kinds of single-system injuries, particularly head trauma, where cerebral perfusion pressure is of primary importance. Although the applicability of these studies to other populations and settings is debatable, the *presumption* of benefits from immediate plasma expansion in all preoperative patients with circulatory insufficiency caused by hemorrhage is no longer valid. Instead, the initial priority should be surgical control of the bleeding source.

Despite the studies suggesting that vigorous prehospital resuscitation is not helpful and possibly is harmful, hypertonic solutions have several characteristics that make them attractive for acute resuscitation. The intravascular and interstitial expansion resulting from administration of these solutions is much greater than the volume infused by emergency personnel.

CLINICAL CONTROVERSY

Some clinicians believe that hypertonic solutions should be used for resuscitation of patients with head injuries who have concomitant circulatory insufficiency.

By causing redistribution (i.e., pulling fluid) from the intracellular space, hypertonic solutions cause rapid expansion of the intravascular compartment, which is essential for vital organ perfusion. In head-injured patients, it has been postulated that this redistribution should decrease intracranial pressure because the vessels of the brain are more impermeable to sodium ions than are vessels in other areas of the body. Additionally, hypertonic saline solutions have beneficial immunomodulating actions when compared with more isotonic solutions in experiments with animals, although these actions have not always translated into similar beneficial effects in patients.[22]

Potential dosing and administration errors and related adverse events can occur when hypertonic saline is ordered and administered by clinicians relatively unfamiliar with its use. Potential adverse events include cellular crenation and damage caused by the dramatic fluid shifts associated with hypernatremia, hyperchloremic metabolic acidosis from hyperchloremia, and peripheral vein destruction from high osmolality. In the limited number of studies conducted in humans to date, such adverse effects have been uncommon and apparently of little clinical importance.[23,24]

Unfortunately, beneficial outcome data attributable to administration of these hypertonic solutions are lacking. Most of these studies were conducted in prehospital and emergency department settings using 250 mL of 7.5% sodium chloride with or without 6% dextran 70. A metaanalysis of randomized, controlled trials found no statistical difference between the survival rates of patients receiving the hypertonic saline solutions and those receiving standard isotonic crystalloid solutions.[25] Additionally, a subsequent double-blind, randomized controlled trial involving 229 patients with hypotension and severe brain injury demonstrated no significant differences in neurologic function at 6 months when 250 mL of 7.5% saline or lactated Ringer solution was administered as part of a prehospital resuscitation regimen.[26] Part of the explanation for this finding may be related to supplemental crystalloid fluids that were given routinely to patients in both the treatment and control groups, which probably would increase the number of patients needed to demonstrate a statistically significant difference in mortality. Until the concerns regarding efficacy and toxicity of these solutions have been resolved, normal saline could be considered an alternative for head-injured patients when a hypertonic solution is desirable because it contains 154 mmol/L of both sodium and chloride. Given their relatively poor intravascular expansion and association with poor outcome in animal models of closed head injury, hypotonic solutions should be avoided in this population.[27]

In addition to crystalloid solutions, colloids have been used for plasma expansion in patients with hemorrhagic circulatory insufficiency. In the United States, albumin and starch (i.e., hetastarch) derivatives are used most commonly, although dextran solutions also are available commercially.

CLINICAL CONTROVERSY

Some clinicians believe that colloid solutions have advantages beyond crystalloid solutions that justify their use for patients with hypovolemic shock.

The major theoretical advantage of these compounds is their prolonged intravascular retention time compared with crystalloid solutions. In contrast to isotonic crystalloid solutions that have substantial interstitial distribution within minutes of IV administration, colloids remain in the intravascular space for hours or days, depending on factors such as capillary permeability.

The colloids, particularly albumin, are expensive solutions. Therefore, it is difficult to justify the additional cost of colloidal products unless the benefit-to-risk ratio is substantially greater than that associated with inexpensive crystalloid solutions. This does not appear to be the case based on randomized, controlled studies and metaanalyses comparing colloid and crystalloid solutions for acute circulatory insufficiency. Because other colloids, such as hetastarch, almost always have been compared with albumin and not with crystalloid solutions in published clinical studies (with no clinically important differences found), there is no reason to suspect that these other colloids have any unique advantages as volume expanders. Adverse effects associated with colloids appear to be uncommon and generally are extensions of their pharmacologic activity (Table 26–5), ❾ but this is also true of crystalloids. The benefit-to-risk ratio appears to be similar for colloids and crystalloids; thus, based on cost, crystalloids are preferred for initial treatment of circulatory insufficiency.

The preceding discussion dealt primarily with acute circulatory insufficiency, but there are other considerations with regard to fluid replacement in elective surgical procedures. Preoperative fluid deficits in patients undergoing minor procedures may be associated with increased perioperative morbidity, some of which (e.g., drowsiness, dizziness) may be reduced by appropriate fluid administration prior to surgery.[28] However, care must be taken to avoid overhydration in the perioperative period because excess fluid will lead to weight gain and decreased pulmonary function. Some evidence suggests that fluid restriction on the day of surgery may reduce postoperative morbidity in patients undergoing major surgical procedures. In one randomized, multicenter trial, use of a restricted intraoperative and postoperative IV fluid protocol led to significantly fewer cardiopulmonary (7% versus 24%; $P = 0.007$) and wound (16% versus 31%; $P = 0.04$) complications.[29] As the preceding discussion indicates, the benefits and risks of fluid administration in the perioperative period are not just a function of too little or too much fluid but involve other patient- and procedure-related issues.

Another consideration in the patient with injuries or surgery is the potential need for blood product administration (Table 26–6) to replace oxygen-carrying and clotting functions. Although a small group of trauma patients respond to the initial fluid bolus and remain stable, most patients respond initially and then deteriorate.

TABLE 26-5 Adverse Effects of Plasma Expanders: Colloids

Albumin
Primarily extensions of pharmacologic actions (e.g., fluid overload; dilutional coagulopathy)
Amino acid profile and catabolism alterations (clinical significance?); potential protein overload if given with exogenous protein (e.g., parenteral nutrition)
Anaphylactoid/anaphylaxis reactions (life-threatening reactions rare; higher in patients with immunoglobulin A deficiency)
Infectious complications (all reported cases have been associated with improper handling by manufacturer or institution; no reported cases of human immunodeficiency virus or hepatitis transmission)
Interactions with medications and nutrients (clinical significance varies)
Metal loading, particularly aluminum (long-term administration in patients with renal failure)
Negative inotropic effect; reductions in ionized calcium concentrations (not well documented)
Pyrogenic reactions (not well documented)
Hetastarch
Primarily extensions of pharmacologic actions (e.g., fluid overload, dilutional coagulopathy)
Bleeding (decreases factor VIII/C activity; not recommended in patients at high risk for bleeding or in patients with severe bleeding conditions such as subarachnoid hemorrhage)
Macroamylase formation may cause elevation in blood amylase that leads to inaccurate diagnosis of pancreatitis
Anaphylactoid/anaphylaxis reactions
Pruritus (particularly when large amounts are given; may take months to resolve)
Dextrans
Primarily extensions of pharmacologic actions (e.g., fluid overload, dilutional coagulopathy)
Anaphylactoid/anaphylaxis reactions (increased incidence of anaphylaxis with increased molecular weight)
Bleeding (sometimes used for anticoagulant activity, so not recommended for patients with severe bleeding)

The latter patients, as well as patients undergoing blood loss associated with surgery, frequently need blood components such as packed red blood cells. In the case of the latter component, red blood cells contain hemoglobin that delivers oxygen to tissues. Neither crystalloids nor colloids perform this function.

Administration of excessive blood products may be counterproductive. In the case of red blood cells, attempts to raise the hematocrit to high–normal or supranormal concentrations may decrease oxygen delivery by increasing blood viscosity. Although there is no optimal hematocrit value for all patients, a minimum hematocrit concentration of 30% (equivalent to a hemoglobin concentration of 10 Gm/dl) traditionally has been used as the threshold for transfusion, particularly in patients at risk for ischemia, such as those with CAD. Use of a more liberal transfusion strategy has been called into question with the publication of a randomized, multicenter trial involving critically ill patients that found 30-day mortality to be similar whether patients were transfused at a hemoglobin concentration of 7 or 10 g/dL (18.7% versus 23.3%, respectively; $P = 0.11$).[30] The mortality during hospitalization was significantly lower in the restrictive group (22.2% versus 28.1%; $P = 0.05$). Although the investigators were cautious about extrapolating the results of this investigation to patients with myocardial ischemia, the study does question the use of a liberal transfusion strategy for critically ill patients.

Blood products are not risk-free. There is the rare but important risk of virus transmission [e.g., human immunodeficiency virus (HIV), hepatitis]. Citrate that is added to stored blood to prevent coagulation may bind to calcium, resulting in hypocalcemia, although potassium and phosphate concentrations often are elevated in stored blood, particularly when hemolysis has occurred during storage. Other issues that must be considered with blood product administration include monitoring for transfusion-related reactions and attention to appropriate warming, particularly when large volumes are given to pediatric patients, because hypothermia is associated with increased fluid requirements and mortality.

The periodic shortages, high costs, and adverse effect concerns related to blood products have prompted investigations of alternative "bloodless" strategies. In addition to the use of more restrictive transfusion thresholds, as mentioned previously, these strategies have included hemoglobin-based oxygen carriers and perfluorocarbon compounds to deliver oxygen to tissues. Other strategies have aimed at reducing blood loss through the use of improved procedural and surgical techniques, as well as the administration of hemostatic medications.

TABLE 26-6 General Indications for Blood Products in Acute Circulatory Insufficiency Due to Hemorrhage[a]

Packed red blood cells
Increase oxygen-carrying capacity of blood: Usually indicated in patients with continued deterioration after volume replacement or obvious exsanguination; must be warmed, particularly when used in children
Fresh-frozen plasma
Replacement of clotting factors: Generally overused; indicated if ongoing hemorrhage in patients with PT/PTT >1.5 times normal, severe hepatic disease, or other bleeding diathesis
Platelets
Used for bleeding due to severe thrombocytopenia (i.e., platelet count <10,000 mcL) or rapidly dropping platelet counts as would occur with massive bleeding
Other products
With the exception of recombinant activated factor VII, which is currently undergoing trials for use in life-threatening hemorrhage unresponsive to traditional blood product administration, components such as cryoprecipitate and factor VIII are generally not indicated in acute hemorrhage but rather are used after specific deficiencies are identified

[a]Although whole blood can be used for large-volume blood loss, most hospitals use component therapy, and use crystalloids or colloids for plasma expansion.
PT, prothrombin time; PTT, partial thromboplastin time.

Patients with Thermal Injuries

There are a number of formulas for estimating fluid requirements in thermally injured patients, but there is little reason to choose one over another based on well-controlled studies. In general, the amount of loss corresponds to the size of the thermal injury. Approximately 3 to 4 mL/kg of isotonic fluid (lactated Ringer solution) for each percent burn can be used for calculating the expected fluid requirements for the first 24 hours after the burn. For example, a 60-kg person with 30% body surface area (BSA) burns is expected to require 5,400 to 7,200 mL of fluid over the initial 24 hours. Regardless of the calculated deficit, fluids should be administered until adequate tissue perfusion has been documented or adverse effects (e.g., pulmonary edema) occur. Crystalloids are preferred as initial therapy for burn victims because there is no substantial evidence that colloids mobilize edematous fluid, and there is a theoretical concern that extravascular fluid accumulation might be prolonged by the oncotic actions of albumin and other colloid products that have leaked through vessel walls.[31] Additionally, there is no evidence that colloids reduce mortality in patients with thermal injuries.[17] Some novel therapies for thermal resuscitation are currently under study. For example, in a prospective study involving patients with >30% BSA burns, antioxidant therapy with extremely high doses on IV vitamin C (66 mg/kg/h for 24 hours) reduced resuscitation fluid requirements and wound edema.[32] The proposed mechanism is reduction in free radical–induced increases in capillary permeability.

CLINICAL CONTROVERSY

The appropriate use of invasive hemodynamic monitoring tools, such as right-sided heart catheterization in patients with hypovolemic shock, is controversial.

■ ONGOING MONITORING

One form of monitoring that may take place in the emergency and operating rooms, as well as in the ICU, requires placement of a central venous pressure (CVP) line. Monitoring of CVP provides the clinician with a somewhat insensitive yet useful estimate of the relationship between increased right atrial pressure and cardiac output. A protocol that used a particular type of central catheter to perform continuous monitoring of central venous oxygen saturation in conjunction with so-called goal-directed therapy in the first 6 hours of patient arrival in an urban emergency department resulted in decreased mortality compared to standard monitoring (30.5% vs. 46.5%, $P = 0.009$).[33] However, the patients in this study had severe sepsis and septic shock, so the results might not be applicable to other forms of shock with different pathophysiologic considerations. For example, in hemorrhagic shock due to trauma, the most important intervention is surgical control of bleeding, and anything that delays this control is likely to increase, not decrease, mortality. Until additional studies have been performed, it would be premature to recommend goal-directed therapy with the associated central venous monitoring in patients with nonseptic forms of shock, particularly shock due to blood loss. The monitoring of patients with various forms of hypovolemic shock becomes more controversial once initial stabilization has been achieved and the patient has been transferred to an ICU. This is particularly true with regard to the value of right-sided heart catheterization (also known as pulmonary artery or Swan-Ganz catheterization). Clearly, some form of intensive monitoring is important because patients in the postresuscitation phase of hypovolemic shock are at risk for various complications secondary to ischemia. A more complete discussion of invasive and noninvasive hemodynamic monitoring is given in Chapter 25.

A number of laboratory tests are indicated for subacute monitoring of shock in the ICU setting. These include a renal battery for assessing possible electrolyte alterations and kidney perfusion (e.g., BUN and creatinine). Among other things, a complete blood count will enable assessment of possible infection (white blood cell count), oxygen-carrying capacity of the blood (hemoglobin, hematocrit), and ongoing bleeding (hemoglobin, hematocrit, and platelet count). The prothrombin time (PT) and partial thromboplastin time (PTT) will give an indication of the ability of the blood to clot because, in the case of hemorrhagic shock, clotting factors are lost and diluted. An increasing lactate concentration (arterial, mixed venous, or central venous), an increasing arterial base deficit, or a decreasing bicarbonate concentration are consistent with inadequate perfusion leading to anaerobic metabolism with accumulation of lactic acid. Although the value of these surrogate markers for improving patient outcomes is more controversial, they are considered traditional end points of resuscitation in certain populations such as trauma patients.[34] Other tests may be indicated if organ dysfunction is likely. For example, when blood flow to the liver is interrupted because of sustained hypotension, a condition known as *shock liver* may occur. In this condition, the levels of transaminases on a liver panel may be markedly elevated in the first couple of days after marked hypotension, although the concentrations should decrease over time.[4] Along with laboratory testing, a more extensive history can be obtained during the subacute monitoring period.

The value of pulmonary artery catheters has been debated hotly since their introduction. Such catheters are placed to obtain various oxygen-transport variables, some of which cannot be determined reliably from peripheral or other central vessels. The debate was intensified when early studies suggested improved outcomes when cardiac output and other oxygen-transport variables were raised to supranormal levels, the monitoring of which required placement of a pulmonary artery catheter. Subsequent studies using similar monitoring parameters associated with pulmonary artery catheterization gave conflicting results.[35]

The controversy led to consensus conferences and workshops, the development of organizational guidelines, and the publication of a metaanalysis (which found a statistically significant reduction in *morbidity* using pulmonary artery catheters to guide therapy).[36] Ultimately, a large randomized, controlled trial involving pulmonary artery catheters was conducted in high-risk surgical patients.[37] The trial involved 1,994 patients. The mortality was almost identical for the catheter and control groups (7.8% versus 7.7%, 95% confidence interval 2.3 to 2.5). There were no episodes of pulmonary embolism in the catheter group and eight episodes in the control group ($P = 0.004$). This trial is important not only because of the implications for high-risk surgical patients but also because it allows conduction of future trials in other patient populations without some of the ethical issues raised about such trials in the past.

Part of the concern regarding pulmonary artery catheterization relates to interpretation of its results by inexperienced practitioners. Studies in both Europe and the United States found that one of two physicians incorrectly interpreted a tracing from a pulmonary artery catheter.[38] This could explain some of the results of studies finding no benefits to pulmonary artery catheterization or, in some cases, worse outcomes in the pulmonary artery catheterization group by actions taken as a result of inaccurate measurements or misinterpretation of information obtained from the monitoring process.

Complications related to pulmonary artery catheter insertion, maintenance, and removal include damage to vessels and organs during insertion, arrhythmias, infections, and thromboembolic damage. To avoid the complications associated with pulmonary artery catheterization, other less invasive tools were developed to obtain similar information. For example, cardiac output determinations have been made by Doppler, bioimpedance, dye, and ionic dilution techniques, although such measurements would not provide other data that are obtained routinely with pulmonary artery catheters (e.g., left-sided heart filling pressure). Additionally, advances in pulmonary artery catheter technology that expand the information obtained from such monitoring (e.g., mixed venous oxyhemoglobin) are under investigation. However, given the lack of well-defined outcome data associated with pulmonary artery catheterization, its use is best reserved for complicated cases of shock not responding to conventional fluid and medication therapies.

Commonly measured and calculated hemodynamic and oxygen-transport indices associated with invasive monitoring are primarily global indicators of tissue perfusion. Attempts have been made to find regional and local indicators of hypoperfusion so that circulatory insufficiency could be treated before overt shock occurs. One focus of recent research has been monitoring modalities involving the gastrointestinal tract.

Although the literature is fairly consistent concerning low gastric intramucosal pH (pHi) values being predictive of death, pHi-guided therapy to decrease mortality has not been demonstrated.[39] Additionally, a number of technical considerations remain to be resolved when using pHi or, more recently, capnometry (luminal $P\text{CO}_2$ tonometry) for monitoring and therapy. Despite these concerns, measures of regional tissue oxygenation continue to be investigated through a variety of novel monitoring techniques.

In addition to regional monitoring of tissue perfusion, local methods of monitoring are being studied. For example, subcutaneous measurement of tissue oxygen pressure shows promise in preliminary investigations. Regional and local measurements likely will not replace more global indicators of perfusion; rather, the methods will complement each other.

■ ONGOING MANAGEMENT

Proper attention to plasma expansion must be continued into the intraoperative and postoperative periods. A number of neurohormonal changes take place that affect urine output, and patients may have substantial third spacing of fluid depending on the operation and preexisting conditions. Furthermore, postoperative patients are prone to hyponatremia from renal generation of electrolyte-free water and from antidiuretic hormone release.[40] As in acute resuscitation, the administration of hypotonic solutions in the perioperative period does not prevent the decrease in extracellular volume that often occurs. Therefore, although excess fluid administration is to be avoided in the perioperative setting, isotonic crystalloid solutions should be used when fluids are indicated to prevent intravascular depletion and circulatory insufficiency.

Of the randomized studies comparing albumin with crystalloid solutions in the perioperative period, the majority found no statistically significant differences between groups.[41] Any significant differences found involved isolated hemodynamic or respiratory variables with no obvious clinical correlates (e.g., duration of mechanical ventilation). Therefore, albumin and other colloids cannot be recommended for the prevention or initial treatment of circulatory insufficiency, although their use may be appropriate in patients who are not responding to crystalloids and are developing problems such as interstitial fluid accumulation. Practice guidelines published by a consortium of academic medical centers reflect this recommendation, but colloids continue to be used widely.[42]

In general, medications are not indicated in the initial therapy of hypovolemic shock. With hypovolemia, the body's natural response is to increase cardiac output and to constrict blood vessels to maintain blood pressure. There is no reason why most patients should need ⑩ inotropic or vasoactive agents, assuming that fluid therapy is adequate. For that matter, there is no evidence that these medications improve outcome in patients with hypovolemic shock. However, once the cause of acute circulatory insufficiency has been stopped or treated and fluids have been optimized, some patients continue to have signs and symptoms of inadequate tissue perfusion. This may be caused by reperfusion injury. Although the search for a cryptogenic source (e.g., intraabdominal bleeding in a trauma patient) should continue, the clinician may need to administer medications to improve perfusion.

Pressor agents such as norepinephrine and high-dose dopamine are to be avoided, if possible, because they may increase blood pressure at the expense of peripheral tissue ischemia. Some sources use stronger language and state that vasopressors are contraindicated in certain forms of shock (e.g., hemorrhagic). This does not help the clinician who is treating a patient with unstable blood pressure despite massive fluid replacement and increasing interstitial fluid accumulation. In such situations, inotropic agents such as dobutamine are preferred if blood pressure is adequate (e.g., systolic blood pressure ≥90 mm Hg) because they should not aggravate the existing vasoconstriction. The inotropic agents are justified by presumed inadequate cardiac output for the specific situation, although the measured values may be in the normal range.[4]

When pressure cannot be maintained with inotropic agents or when inotropic agents with vasodilatory properties cannot be used because of

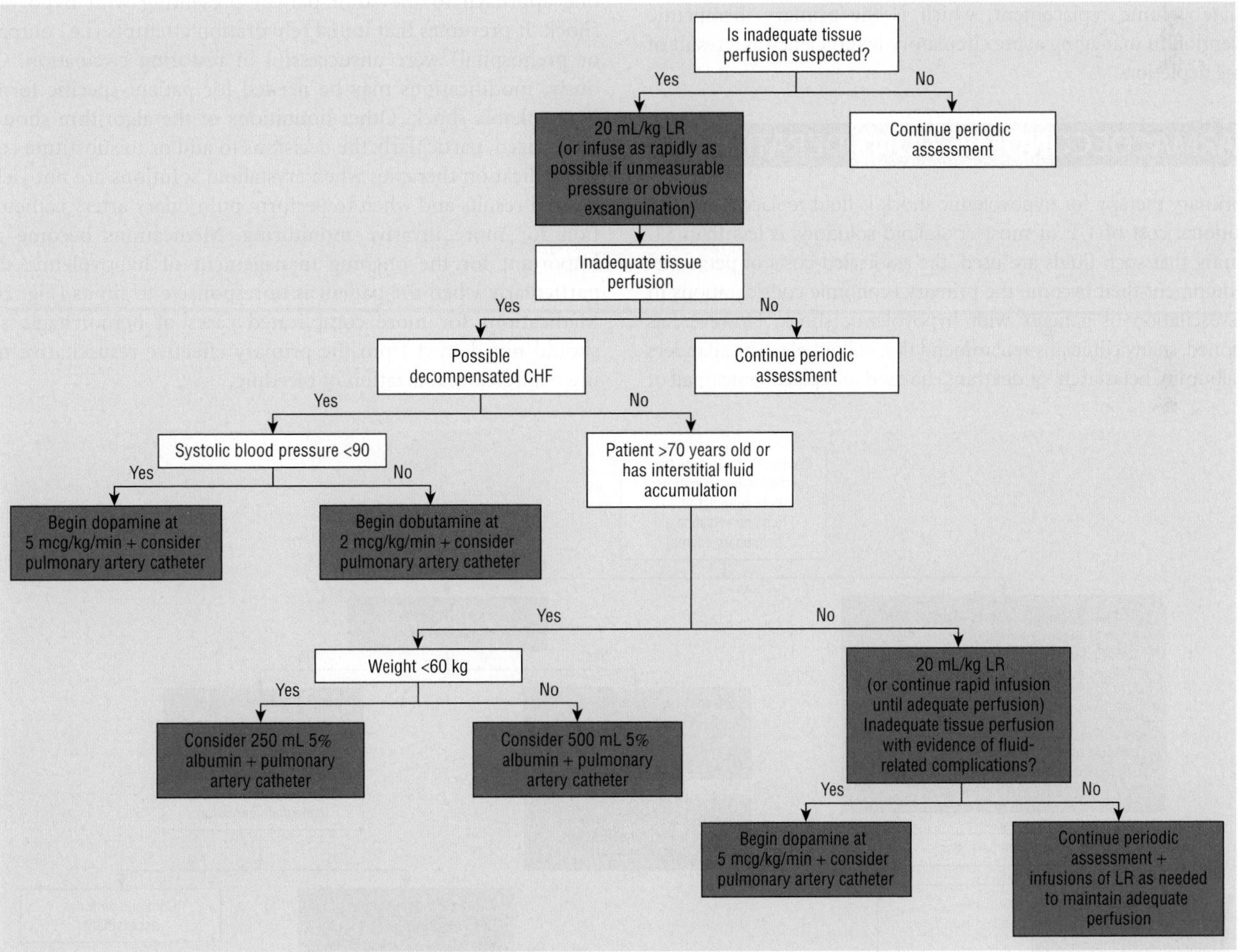

FIGURE 26-4. Hypovolemia protocol for adults. This protocol is not intended to replace or delay therapies such as surgical intervention or blood products for restoring oxygen-carrying capacity or hemostasis. If available, some measurements can be used in addition to those listed in the algorithm, such as mean arterial pressure or pulmonary artery catheter recordings. The latter can be used to assist in medication choices (e.g., agents with primary pressor effects may be desirable in patients with normal cardiac outputs, whereas dopamine or dobutamine may be indicated in patients with suboptimal cardiac outputs). Lower maximal doses of the medications in this algorithm should be considered when pulmonary artery catheterization is not available. Colloids that can be substituted for albumin are hetastarch 6% and dextran 40. See text for an in-depth discussion of these and other issues involved in this protocol. (CHF, congestive heart failure; LR, lactated Ringer solution.)

inadequate blood pressure concerns, pressors may be required as a last resort. In general, the need for pressors is predictive of the development of MODS and increased length of hospital stay.[43] Although the response to pressor agents may be variable in hypovolemic shock, there does not appear to be resistance as a consequence of altered receptor response, as is sometimes seen in patients with septic shock.[4] Potent vasoconstrictors such as norepinephrine and phenylephrine should be given through central veins because of the possibility of extravasation and necrosis with peripheral administration.

In managing patients with hypovolemic shock, the clinician must be aware of potential adverse effects of medications being used for supportive care purposes. For example, some patients are particularly susceptible to the histamine release associated with morphine and may have substantial decreases in blood pressure. Propofol is commonly used for sedation in the ICU, but it may cause substantial decreases in blood pressure. The initial dose of propofol probably should be decreased by at least 50% in patients with hemorrhagic shock who have recently been resuscitated and by at least 80% (if it is given at all) in patients who may not be fully resuscitated.[44]

A number of interesting treatments for shock are under investigation, including autotransfusion for removing harmful cytokines from the body. Various alternatives to conventional blood components also are being studied, such as stroma-free hemoglobin and perfluorocarbon compounds, as virus-free alternatives to red blood cell transfusion. Hopefully, these methods will be useful adjuncts to adequate volume replacement, which is the primary therapeutic intervention in managing acute circulatory insufficiency as a result of volume depletion.

PHARMACOECONOMIC CONSIDERATIONS

The primary therapy for hypovolemic shock is fluid replacement. The institutional cost of 1 L of most crystalloid solutions is less than $1. Assuming that such fluids are used, the associated costs of personnel and equipment then become the primary economic considerations in the resuscitation of patients with hypovolemic shock. However, as mentioned, many clinicians recommend that colloid plasma expanders (e.g., albumin, hetastarch, or dextrans) be used to replace some or all of the standard crystalloid solutions. Although the costs of these solutions vary depending on contractual arrangements, as might occur with purchasing groups, in general, albumin solutions are more expensive than hetastarch and dextran products. All these solutions are markedly more costly than crystalloid solutions; in some cases, the differences are 50- to 100-fold, even when used in equipotent amounts.

The only trial that investigated albumin use on a large-scale basis was an observational study involving 15 academic medical centers in the United States. Based on previously published guidelines, 62% of albumin use was defined as inappropriate, at a cost of $124,939.[45] Presuming equal efficacy and toxicity (as available studies indicate) between crystalloid and colloid solutions, cost-minimization analysis clearly indicates the economic advantages of the crystalloids.

Because medications are not simply alternatives to crystalloids but rather are used when crystalloid therapy has been optimized, there is little reason to compare medication and fluid therapies from an economic perspective. Furthermore, there are no economic comparisons of the various inotropic and vasopressor medications used in the treatment of hypovolemic shock.

EVALUATION OF THERAPEUTIC OUTCOMES

Figure 26–4 is an algorithm that summarizes many of the treatment principles discussed in this chapter. The algorithm is an example of one approach to the adult patient presenting with hypovolemic shock. It presumes that initial rehydration attempts (i.e., outpatient or prehospital) were unsuccessful in restoring circulation. Obviously, modifications may be needed for patient-specific forms of hypovolemic shock. Other limitations of the algorithm should be recognized, particularly the decisions to add or to substitute colloid or medication therapies when crystalloid solutions are not yielding desired results and when to perform pulmonary artery catheterization for more invasive monitoring. Medications become more important for the ongoing management of hypovolemic shock, particularly when the patient is unresponsive to fluids (Fig. 26–5). Medications for more complicated cases of hemorrhagic shock should not detract from the primary effective resuscitative measure—surgical stabilization of bleeding.

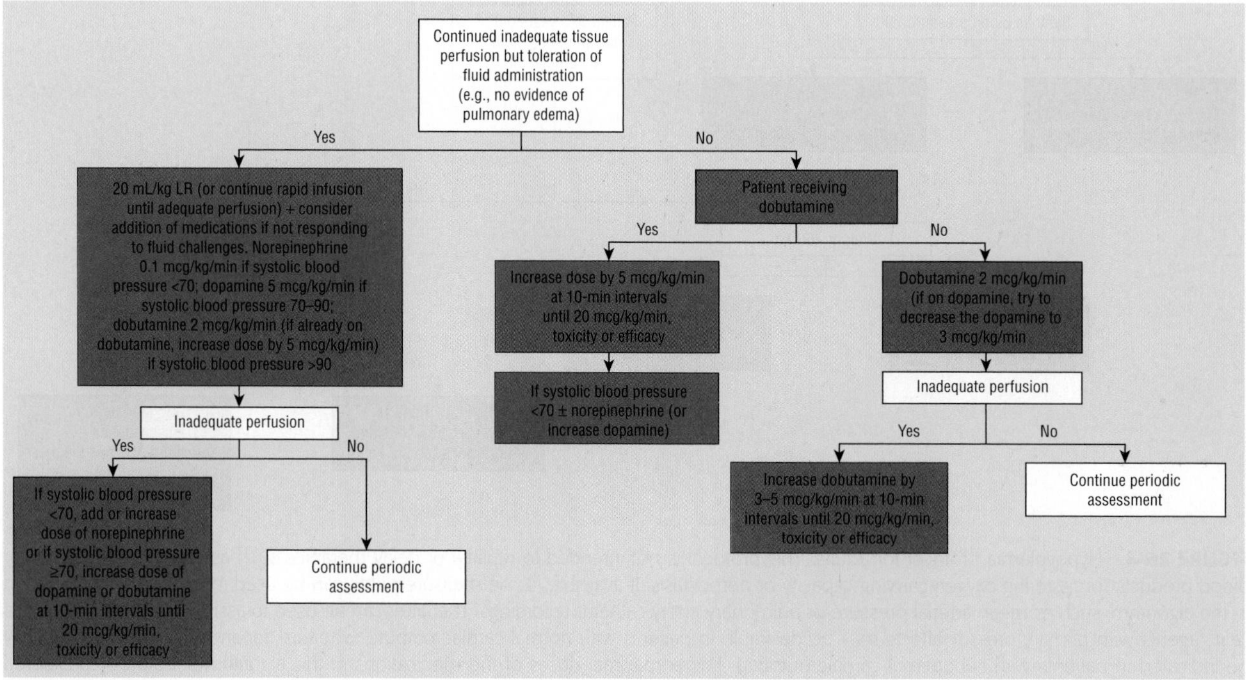

FIGURE 26-5. Ongoing management of inadequate tissue perfusion. (LR, lactated Ringer solution.)

ABBREVIATIONS

BSA: body surface area
CAD: coronary artery disease
CDC: Centers for Disease Control and Prevention
CVP: central venous pressure
ICU: intensive care unit
MODS: multiple-organ dysfunction syndrome
pHi: gastric intramucosal pH
PT: prothrombin time
PTT: partial thromboplastin time
SIRS: systemic inflammatory response syndrome
WHO: World Health Organization

REFERENCES

1. Dutton RP. Initial resuscitation of the hemorrhaging patient. In: Spiess BD, Spence RK, Shander A, eds. Perioperative Transfusion Medicine, 2nd ed. Philadelphia: Lippincott Williams & Wilkins, 2006:289–299.
2. Anonymous. Heat-related mortality—Arizona, 1993–2002, and United States, 1979–2002. MMWR Weekly 2005;54:628–630.
3. Duggan C, Fontaine O, Pierce NF, et al. Scientific rationale for a change in the composition of oral rehydration solution. JAMA 2004;291:2628–2635.
4. Ramsay G, Boom S. Pathophysiology and management of shock. In: Cuschieri A, Giles GR, Moossa AR, eds. Essential Surgical Practice, 3rd ed. Oxford, UK: Butterworth-Heinemann, 1995:72–89.
5. Marzi I. Hemorrhagic shock: Update in pathophysiology and therapy. Acta Anaesthesiol Scand 1997;111(Suppl):42–44.
6. Vercueil A, Grocott MPW, Mythen MG. Physiology, pharmacology, and rationale for colloid administration for the maintenance of effective hemodynamic stability in critically ill patients. Trans Med Rev 2005;19:93–109.
7. Porter SC, Fleisher GR, Kohane IS, Mandl KD. The value of parental report for diagnosis and management of dehydration in the emergency department. Ann Emerg Med 2003;41:196–205.
8. Anonymous. Prevention and treatment of heat injury. Med Lett 2003;45:58–60.
9. Nalin DR, Hirschhorn N, Greenough W, et al. Clinical concerns about reduced-osmolarity oral rehydration solution. JAMA 2004:291:2632–2635.
10. Spandorfer PR, Alessandrini EA, Joffe MD, et al. Oral versus intravenous rehydration of moderately dehydrated children: a randomized, controlled trial. Pediatrics 2005;115:295–301.
11. Atherly-John YC, Cunningham SJ, Crain EF. A randomized trial of oral vs intravenous rehydration in a pediatric emergency department. Arch Pediatr Adolesc Med 2002;156:1240–1243.
12. Axler OA, Tousiganant C, Thompson CR, et al. Small hemodynamic effect of typical rapid volume infusions in critically ill patients. Crit Care Med 1997;25:965–970.
13. Didwania A, Miller J, Kassel D, et al. Effect of intravenous lactated Ringer solution infusion on the circulating lactate concentration: Results of a prospective, randomized, double-blind, placebo-controlled trial. Crit Care Med 1997;25:1851–1854.
14. Jackson EV, Wiese J, Sigal B, et al. Effects of crystalloid solutions on circulating lactate concentrations: 1. Implications for the proper handling of blood specimens obtained in critically ill patients. Crit Care Med 1996;24:1840–1846.
15. Deitch EA. Animal models of sepsis and shock: A review and lessons learned. Shock 1998;9:1–11.
16. Grocott MPW, Mythen MG, Gan TJ. Perioperative fluid management and clinical outcomes in adults. Anesth Analg 2005;100:1093–1106.
17. Cochrane Injuries Group Albumin Reviewers. Human albumin administration in critically ill patients: Systematic review of randomized controlled trials. BMJ 1998;317:235–240.
18. Choi PTL, Yip G, Quinonez LG, Cook DJ. Crystalloids vs. colloids in fluid resuscitation: A systematic review. Crit Care Med 1999;27:200–210.
19. The SAFE Study Investigators. A comparison of albumin and saline for fluid resuscitation in the intensive care unit. N Engl J Med 2004;350:2247–2256.
20. Bickell WH, Wall MJ, Pepe PE, et al. Immediate versus delayed fluid resuscitation for hypotensive patients with penetrating torso injuries. N Engl J Med 1994;331:1105–1109.
21. Dutton RP, Mackenzie CF, Scalea TM. Hypotensive resuscitation during active hemorrhage: Impact on in-hospital mortality. J Trauma 2002;52:1141–1146.
22. Kolsen-Petersen JA, Nielsen JD, Tonnesen EM. Effect of hypertonic saline infusion on postoperative cellular outcome. Anesthesiology 2004;100:1108–1118.
23. Vassar MJ, Fischer RP, O'Brien PE, et al. A multicenter trial for resuscitation of injured patients with 7.5% sodium chloride: The effect of added dextran 70. Arch Surg 1993;128:1003–1013.
24. Suarez JI, Qureshi AI, Bhardwa A, et al. Treatment of refractory intracranial hypertension with 23.4% saline. Crit Care Med 1998;26:1118–1122.
25 Wade CE, Kramer GC, Grady JJ, et al. Efficacy of hypertonic 7.5% saline and 6% dextran-70 in treating trauma: A meta-analysis of controlled studies. Surgery 1997;122:609–616.
26. Cooper DJ, Myles PS, McDermott FT, et al. Prehospital hypertonic saline resuscitation of patients with hypotension and severe traumatic brain injury. JAMA 2004;291:1350–1357.
27. Gurevich B, Talmore D, Artru AA, et al. Brain edema, hemorrhagic necrosis volume, and neurological status with rapid infusion of 0.45% saline or 5% dextrose in 0.9% saline after closed head trauma in rats. Anesth Analg 1997;84:554–559.
28. Holte K, Klarskov B, Christensen DS, et al. Liberal versus restrictive fluid administration to improve recovery after laparoscopic cholecystectomy. Ann Surg 2004;240:892–899.
29. Brandstrup B, Tonnesen H, Beier-Holgersen R, et al. Effects of intravenous fluid restriction on postoperative complications: Comparison of two perioperative fluid regimens. Ann Surg 2003;238:641–648.
30. Hebert PC, Wells G, Blajchman MA, et al. A multicenter, randomized, controlled clinical trial of transfusion requirements in critical care. N Engl J Med 1999;340:409–417.
31. Zdolsek HJ, Lisander B, Jones AW, Sjoberg F. Albumin supplementation during the first week after a burn does not mobilise tissue oedema in humans. Intensive Care Med 2001;27:844–852.
32. Tanaka J, Matsuda T, Miyagantani Y, et al. Reduction of resuscitation fluid volumes in severely burned patients using ascorbic acid administration. Arch Surg 2000;135:326–331.
33. Rivers E, Nguyen B, Havstad S, et al. Early goal-directed therapy in the treatment of severe sepsis and septic-shock. N Engl J Med 2001;345:1368–1377.
34. Bilkovski RN, Rivers EP, Horst HM. Targeted resuscitation strategies after injury. Curr Opin Crit Care 2004;10:529–538.
35. Yu M. Oxygen transport optimization. New Horiz 1999;7:46–53.
36. Ivanov R, Allen J, Calvin JE. The incidence of major morbidity in critically ill patients managed with pulmonary artery catheters: A meta-analysis. Crit Care Med 2000;28:615–619.
37. Sandham JD, Hull RD, Brant RF, et al. A randomized, controlled trial of the use of pulmonary-artery catheters in high-risk surgical patients. N Engl J Med 2003;348:5–14.
38. Ginosar Y, Thijs LG, Sprung CL. Raising the standard of hemodynamic monitoring: Targeting the practice or the practitioner? Crit Care Med 1997;25:209–211.
39. Gomersall CD, Joynt GM, Freebairn RC, et al. Resuscitation of critically ill patients based on the results of gastric tonometry: A prospective, randomized, controlled trial. Crit Care Med 2000;28:607–614.
40. Steele A, Gowrishankar M, Abrahamson S, et al. Postoperative hyponatremia despite near-isotonic saline infusion: A phenomenon of desalination. Ann Intern Med 1997;126:20–25.
41. Erstad BL. Concerns with defining appropriate uses of albumin by meta-analysis. Am J Health Syst Pharm 1999;56:1451–1454.
42. Fox DL, Vermeulen LC. UHC Technology Assessment: Albumin, Nonprotein Colloid, and Crystalloid Solutions. Oak Brook, IL: University Health System Consortium, 2000.
43. Goncalves JA, Hydo LJ, Barie PS. Factors influencing outcome of prolonged norepinephrine therapy for shock in critical surgical illness. Shock 1998;10:231–236.
44. Shafer SL. Shock values. Anesthesiology 2004;101:567–568.
45. Yim JM, Vermeulen LC, Erstad BL, et al. Albumin and nonprotein colloid solution use in US academic health centers. Arch Intern Med 1995;155:2450–2455.

SECTION 3
RESPIRATORY DISORDERS

CHAPTER 27 Introduction to Pulmonary Function Testing

JAY I. PETERS AND STEPHANIE M. LEVINE

KEY CONCEPTS

1. Normal ventilation–perfusion ratio. The function of the lungs is to maintain Pa_{O_2} and Pa_{CO_2} within normal ranges. This goal is accomplished by matching 1 mL mixed venous blood with 1 mL fresh air ($\dot{V}/\dot{Q} = 1$). Normally, ventilation ($\dot{V}$) is less than perfusion ($\dot{Q}$), and $\dot{V}/\dot{Q}$ ratio is 0.8.

2. The air in the lung is divided into four compartments: tidal volume—air exhaled during quiet breathing; inspiratory reserve volume—maximal air inhaled above tidal volume; expiratory reserve volume—maximum air exhaled below tidal volume; and residual volume—air remaining in the lung after maximal exhalation. The sum of all four components is the total lung capacity.

3. Obstructive lung disease is defined as an inability to get air out of the lung. It is identified on spirometry when FEV_1/FVC (force expiratory volume in the first second of expiration/forced vital capacity [total amount of air that can be exhaled during a forced exhalation]) is <70% to 75%.

4. Reversible airway obstruction is common in asthma and chronic obstructive pulmonary disease. An increase in FEV_1 of 12% (and >0.2 L in adults) after an inhaled β-agonist suggests an acute bronchodilator response.

5. Restrictive lung disease is defined as an inability to get air into the lung and is best defined as a reduction in total lung capacity. It is suspected when FVC is low and FEV_1/FVC is normal.

6. Restrictive lung disease can be produced by a number of defects, such as increased elastic recoil (interstitial lung disease), respiratory muscle weakness (myasthenia gravis), mechanical restrictions (pleural effusion or kyphoscoliosis), and poor effort.

The primary function of the respiratory system is to maintain normality of arterial blood gases, that is, arterial pressure of oxygen (Pa_{O_2}) and arterial pressure of carbon dioxide (Pa_{CO_2}). To achieve this goal, several processes must be accomplished, including alveolar ventilation, pulmonary perfusion, ventilation–perfusion matching, and gas transfer across the alveolar–capillary membrane. Alveolar ventilation is achieved by the cyclic process of air movement in and out of the lung. During inspiration, the inspiratory muscle contracts and generates negative pressure in the pleural space. This pressure gradient between the mouth and the alveoli draws fresh air (tidal volume) into the lung. Approximately one third of the inspired gas stays in the conducting airways (dead space), and two thirds reaches the alveoli.

Learning objectives, review questions, and other resources can be found at **www.pharmacotherapyonline.com.**

(1) The human lung contains a series of branching, progressively tapering airways that originate at the glottis and terminate in a matrix of thin-walled alveoli. Coursing through this matrix of alveoli is a rich network of capillaries that originates from the pulmonary arterioles and terminates in the pulmonary venules. The adequacy of respiration in each gas exchange unit depends on the opposition of a thin film of mixed venous blood with just the right amount of fresh alveolar gas. During "ideal" gas exchange, blood flow and ventilation are uniform; accordingly, there is no alveolar–arterial difference (or gradient) in the partial pressure of oxygen [$P(A\text{–}a)O_2$, sometimes called the A–a gradient]. However, gas exchange is not perfect, even in the normal lung. Normally, alveolar ventilation is less than pulmonary blood flow, and the overall ventilation–perfusion ratio is 0.8 (not 1.0).

Normal expiration is a passive process, and when the inspiratory muscles end their contraction, the elastic recoil of the lung pulls the lung back to its original size and shape. This process makes the alveolar pressure positive relative to the pressure at the mouth, and air flows out of the lung. During inspiration, the respiratory muscles must overcome the elastic properties of the lung (elastic recoil) and the resistance to airflow by the airways. During expiration, the flow of air is determined primarily by the elastic recoil and airway resistance.

Different pulmonary function tests (PFTs) are used to evaluate the physiologic processes of the respiratory system. Physiologic abnormalities that can be measured by pulmonary function testing include obstruction to airflow, restriction of lung size, and decrease in transfer of gas across the alveolar–capillary membrane. Abnormal values on PFTs are outside the range of values obtained from a group of normal individuals matched according to age, height, sex, and race. A PFT is labeled abnormal when the results fall outside the range in which 95% of people the same age, height, and sex would be found (95% confidence interval). This definition is arbitrary and may misclassify a small percentage of normal individuals as having lung dysfunction; it also may miss patients with mild pulmonary disease. Therefore, clinical correlation and serial pulmonary function testing may be necessary for optimal interpretation of PFTs.

Potential uses of pulmonary function testing include evaluation of patients with known or suspected lung disease; evaluation of symptoms such as chronic cough, dyspnea, or chest tightness; monitoring of the effects of exposure to dust, chemicals, or pulmonary toxic drugs; risk stratification prior to surgery; monitoring of the effectiveness of therapeutic interventions; and objective assessment of impairment or disability.[1]

DEFINITIONS OF LUNG VOLUMES AND EXPIRATORY FLOWS

❷ The air within the lung at the end of a forced inspiration can be divided into four compartments or lung volumes (Fig. 27–1). The volume of air exhaled during normal quiet breathing is the *tidal volume* (VT). The maximal volume of air inhaled above tidal volume is the *inspiratory reserve volume* (IRV), and the maximal air exhaled below tidal volume is the *expiratory reserve volume* (ERV). The *residual volume* (RV) is the amount of air remaining in the lungs after a maximal exhalation.

The combinations or sums of two or more lung volumes are termed *capacities* (Fig. 27–1). *Vital capacity* (VC) is the maximal amount of air that can be exhaled after a maximal inspiration. It is equal to the sum of IRV, VT, and ERV. When measured on a forced expiration, it is called the *forced vital capacity* (FVC). When measured over an exhalation of at least 30 seconds, it is called the *slow vital capacity* (SVC). The VC is approximately 75% of the *total lung capacity* (TLC), and when the SVC is within the normal range, a significant restrictive disorder is unlikely. Normally, the values for SVC and FVC are very similar unless airway obstruction is present.

TLC is the volume of air in the lung after the maximal inspiration and is the sum of the four primary lung volumes (IRV, VT, ERV, and RV). Its measurement is difficult because the amount of air remaining in the chest after maximal exhalation (RV) must be measured by indirect methods. The definition of restrictive lung disease is based on a reduction in TLC (i.e., an inability to get air into the lung or restriction to air movement on inhalation).

The *functional residual capacity* (FRC) is the volume of air remaining in the lungs at the end of a quiet expiration. FRC is the normal resting position of the lung; it occurs when there is no contraction of either inspiratory or expiratory muscles and normally is 40% of TLC. *Inspiratory capacity* (IC) is the maximal volume of air that can be inhaled from the end of a quiet expiration and is the sum of VT and IRV.

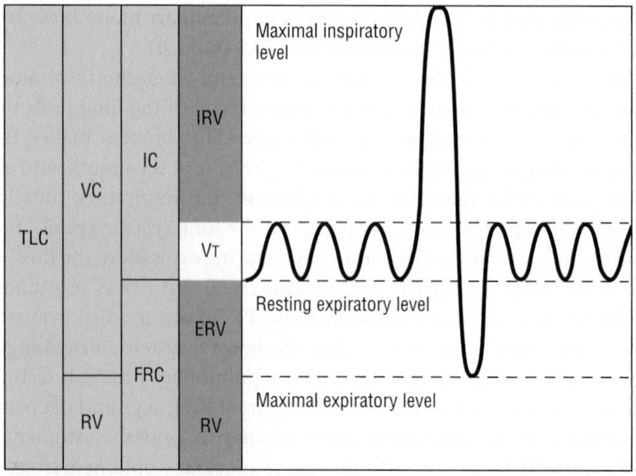

FIGURE 27-1. Lung volumes and capacities. (ERV, expiratory reserve volume; FRC, functional residual capacity; IC, inspiratory capacity; IRV, inspiratory reserve volume; RV, residual volume; TLC, total lung capacity; VC, vital capacity; VT, tidal volume.)

FVC, which represents the total amount of air that can be exhaled, can be expressed as a series of timed volumes. The *forced expiratory volume in the first second of expiration* (FEV_1) is the volume of air exhaled during the first second of the FVC maneuver. Although FEV_1 is a volume, it conveys information on obstruction because it is measured over a known time interval. FEV_1 depends on the volume of air within the lung and the effort during exhalation; therefore, it can be diminished by a decrease in TLC or by a lack of effort. A more sensitive way to measure obstruction is to express FEV_1 as a ratio of FVC. This ratio is independent of the patient's size or TLC; therefore, FEV_1/FVC is a specific measure of airway obstruction with or without restriction. Normally, this ratio is ≥75%, and any value <70% to 75% suggests obstruction.

Because *flow* is defined as the change in volume with time, forced expiratory flow can be determined graphically by dividing the volume change by the time change. The *forced expiratory flow* (FEF) *during 25% to 75% of FVC* ($FEF_{25\%–75\%}$) represents the mean flow during the middle half of the FVC. $FEF_{25\%–75\%}$, formerly called the *maximal midexpiratory flow*, is reported frequently in the assessment of small airways. The 95% confidence limit is so wide that $FEF_{25\%–75\%}$ has limited utility in the early diagnosis of small airways disease in an individual subject. The *peak expiratory flow* (PEF), also called *maximum forced expiratory flow* (FEFmax), is the maximum flow obtained during FVC. This measurement is used often in the outpatient management of asthma because it can be measured with inexpensive peak flowmeters.

All lung volumes and flows are compared to normal values obtained from healthy subjects. There are significant ethnic and racial variations in normal values, and all PFTs should report that race/ethnic adjustment factors have been used. The 2005 American Thoracic Society–European Respiratory Society (ATS–ERS) guidelines for interpretation of PFT results recommend that, for spirometry in the United States, the National Health and Nutrition Examination Survey (NHANES) III reference be used for subjects aged 8 to 80 years and the Wang equation used in subjects younger than 8 years.[2]

SPIROMETRY/FLOW–VOLUME LOOP

Spirometry is the most widely available and useful PFT. It takes only 15 to 20 minutes, carries no risks, and provides information about obstructive and restrictive disease. Spirometry allows for measurement of all lung volumes and capacities except RV, FRC, and TLC; it also allows assessment of FEV_1 and $FEF_{25\%–75\%}$. Spirometry measurements can be reported in two different formats—standard spirometry (Fig. 27–2) and the flow–volume loop (Fig. 27–3). In stan-

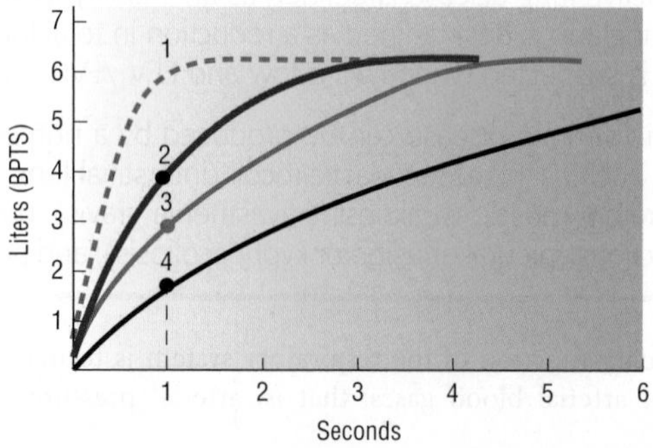

FIGURE 27-2. Standard spirometry. Curve 1 is for a normal subject with normal FEV_1; curve 2 is for a patient with mild airways obstruction; curve 3 is for a patient with moderate airways obstruction; curve 4 is for a patient with severe airways obstruction. (BPTS, body temperature saturated with water vapor.)

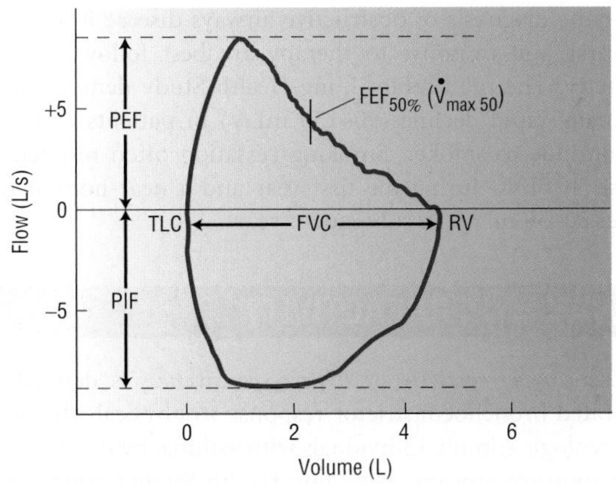

FIGURE 27-3. Normal flow–volume loop. Flows are measured on the vertical (y) axis, and lung volumes are measured on the horizontal (x) axis. Forced vital capacity (FVC) can be read from the tracing as the maximal horizontal deflection. Instantaneous flow ($\dot{V}_{max}$) at any point in FVC also can be measured directly. ($FEF_{50\%}$, forced expiratory flow at 50% of forced vital capacity; PEF, peak expiratory flow; PIF, peak inspiratory flow; RV, residual volume; TLC, total lung capacity.)

dard spirometry, the volumes are recorded on the vertical (y) axis and the time on the horizontal (x) axis. In flow–volume loops, volume is plotted on the horizontal (x) axis, and flow (derived from volume/time) is plotted on the vertical (y) axis. The shape of the flow–volume loop can be helpful in differentiating obstructive and restrictive defects and in diagnosing upper airway obstruction (Fig. 27–4). This curve gives a visual representation of obstruction because the expiratory descent becomes more concave with worsening obstruction.

LUNG VOLUMES

Spirometry measures three of the four basic lung volumes but cannot measure RV. RV must be measured to determine TLC. TLC should be measured anytime VC is reduced. In the setting of chronic obstructive pulmonary disease (COPD) and a low VC, measurement of TLC can help to determine the presence of a superimposed restrictive disorder. The four methods for measuring TLC are helium dilution, nitrogen washout, body plethysmography, and chest x-ray

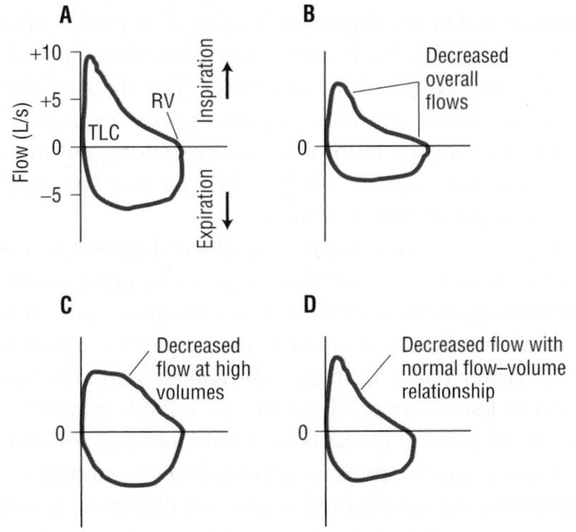

FIGURE 27-4. *A.* Flow–volume loop depicting mild obstruction characterized by decrease flow at low lung volumes. *B.* Moderate airflow obstruction characterized by a more concave curve. *C.* Variable intrathoracic obstruction in which peak flow is decreased at higher lung volumes with normalization of curve at lower lung volumes. *D.* Restrictive lung disease with a curve that is decreased in width but with a normal shape. (RV, residual volume; TLC, total lung capacity.)

measurement (planimetry). The first two methods are called *dilution techniques* and only measure lung volumes in communication with the upper airway. In patients with airway obstruction who have trapped air, dilution techniques will underestimate the actual volume of the lungs. Planimetry measures the circumference of the lungs on the posteroanterior view and lateral views of a chest x-ray film and estimates the total lung volume.

Body plethysmography, or body box, is the most accurate technique for lung volume determinations. It measures all the air in the lungs, including trapped air. The principle of the measurement of the body box is Boyle's gas law ($P_1V_1 = P_2V_2$): A volume of gas in a closed system varies inversely with the pressure applied to it. The changes in alveolar pressure are measured at the mouth, as well as pressure changes in the body box. The volume of the body box is known. Lung volumes can be determined measuring the changes in pressures caused by panting against a closed shutter.[2] Measurement of lung volumes provides useful information about elastic recoil of the lungs. If elastic recoil is increased (as in interstitial lung disease), lung volumes (TLC) are reduced. When elastic recoil is reduced (as in emphysema), lung volumes are increased.

CARBON MONOXIDE DIFFUSING CAPACITY

The diffusing capacity of the lungs (DL) is a measurement of the ability of a gas to diffuse across the alveolar–capillary membrane. Carbon monoxide is the usual test gas because normally it is not present in the lungs and is much more soluble in blood than in lung tissue. When the diffusing capacity is determined with carbon monoxide, the test is called the *diffusing capacity of lung for carbon monoxide* (DLCO). Because DLCO is directly related to alveolar volume (VA), it frequently is normalized to the value DL/VA, which allows for its interpretation in the presence of abnormal lung volumes (e.g., after surgical lung resection).

The diffusing capacity will be reduced in all clinical situations where gas transfer from the alveoli to capillary blood is impaired.[3] Common conditions that reduce DLCO include lung resection, emphysema (loss of functioning alveolar–capillary units), and interstitial lung disease (thickening of the alveolar–capillary membrane). Normal PFTs with reduced DLCO should suggest the possibility of pulmonary vascular disease (e.g., pulmonary embolus) but also can be seen with anemia, early interstitial lung disease, and mild *Pneumocystis carinii* pneumonia (PCP) infection in patients with acquired immune deficiency syndrome.

OBSTRUCTIVE LUNG DISEASE

❸ Obstructive lung disease implies a reduced capacity to get air through the conducting airways and out of the lungs. This reduction in airflow may be caused by a decrease in the diameter of the airways (bronchospasm), a loss of their integrity (bronchomalacia), or a reduction in elastic recoil (emphysema) with a resulting decrease in driving pressure. The most common diseases associated with obstructive pulmonary functions are asthma, emphysema, and chronic bronchitis; however, bronchiectasis, infiltration of the bronchial wall by tumor or granuloma, aspiration of a foreign body, and bronchiolitis also cause obstructive PFTs. The standard test used to evaluate airway obstruction is the forced expiratory spirogram.

Standard spirometry and flow–volume loop measurements include many variables; however, according to ATS guidelines, the diagnosis of obstructive and restrictive ventilatory defects should be made using the basic measurements of spirometry.[3] A reduction in FEV_1 (with normal FVC) establishes the diagnosis of obstruction. When both FEV_1 and FVC are reduced, FEV_1 cannot be used to assess airway obstruction because such patients may have either obstruction or restriction. In restrictive lung disease, the patient has an inability to get air into the lung, which results in a reduction of all expiratory volumes (FEV_1, FVC, and SVC). In obstructed patients, a better measurement is the ratio FEV_1/FVC. Patients with restrictive lung disease have reduced FEV_1 and use of reduced FVC, but FEV_1/FVC remains normal. Although a normal FEV_1/FVC ratio is >70% to 75%, the ratio is age dependent, and slightly lower values may be normal in older patients. Younger children have increased lung elastic recoil and may have higher ratios. Children with asthma often have FEV_1/FVC >90% despite obstructive lung disease. In children, the improvement in FEV_1 after use of an inhaled bronchodilator often is the only way to document mild-to-moderate obstructive lung disease. Caution should be used in interpreting obstruction when FEV_1/FVC is below normal, but FEV_1 and FVC both are within the normal range because this pattern can be seen with healthy, athletic subjects. In screening spirometry performed in office practice, FEV_6 (forced expiratory volume in 6 seconds) can be used in place of FVC. FEV_6 is a more reproducible number when obtained by less skilled personnel. The measurement of $FEF_{25\%-75\%}$ also is abnormal in patients with obstructive airways disease. In general, this test has so much variability that it adds little to the measurement of FEV_1 and FEV_1/FVC. $FEF_{25\%-75\%}$ has been of value in monitoring lung transplant patients for graft rejection,[4] and a reduced value may be an early indicator of acute rejection.

Although there is no standardization for interpretation of severity of obstruction, most pulmonary laboratories state that FEV_1/FVC <70% of the predicted value is diagnostic for obstruction, and the degree of obstruction then is based on the percent predicted of FEV_1. FEV_1 <60% of the predicted value is moderate obstruction, and <40% of the predicted value is severe obstruction. In patients with obstruction, a dose of a bronchodilator (e.g., albuterol or isoproterenol) by metered-dose inhaler is given during the initial examination. An increase in FEV_1 of >12% and >0.2 L suggests an acute bronchodilator response.[3] Because bronchodilator responsiveness is variable over time, the lack of an acute bronchodilator response should not preclude a 6- to 8-week trial of bronchodilators and/or corticosteroids.

Although all patients with obstructive lung disease of any etiology will have reduced flow rates on forced exhalation, the pattern on PFTs may be helpful in differentiating among the various etiologies (Table 27–1). Asthma is characterized by variable obstruction that often improves or resolves with appropriate therapy. Because asthma is an inflammatory disorder of the airways (predominantly large airways), DLCO is normal. Most patients with acute asthma have a bronchodilator response >15% to 20%; however, this response is also seen in 20% of patients with COPD. These patients are said to have asthmatic bronchitis. Chronic bronchitis may be limited to the airways, but the vast majority of patients with chronic bronchitis and airway obstruction have a mixture of bronchitis and emphysema and have a reduction in DLCO. Therefore, DLCO is the best PFT for separating asthma from COPD.

TABLE 27-1 Specific Patterns of Pulmonary Function in Patients with Chronic Obstructive Pulmonary Disease

		COPD	
	Asthma	***Chronic Bronchitis***	***Emphysema***
Decreased FEV_1	++++	++++	++++
Decreased FEV_1/FVC	++++	++++	++++
Increased airway resistance	++++	++++	+
Decreased D_{LCO}	–	–/++[a]	++++
Response to bronchodilators	++++	+[b]	–[b]

D_{LCO}, diffusing capacity of carbon monoxide; FEV_1, forced expiratory volume in the first second of expiration; FVC, forced vital capacity.

[a]Most smokers with chronic bronchitis have reduced D_{LCO}.

[b]Twenty percent of patients with chronic obstructive pulmonary disease (COPD) have a large (++++) bronchodilator response.

After the diagnosis of obstructive airways disease is established, the course and response to therapy are best followed by serial spirometry. The multicenter Lung Health Study demonstrated an abnormally rapid decline (90–150 mL/y) in patients with COPD who continue to smoke.[5] Smoking cessation often resulted in an increase in FEV_1 during the first year and a near-normal rate of decline (30–50 mL/y) in subsequent years.

AIRWAY HYPERREACTIVITY

❹ *Airway hyperreactivity* or *hyperresponsiveness* is defined as an exaggerated bronchoconstrictor response to physical, chemical, or pharmacologic stimuli. Individuals with asthma, by definition, have hyperresponsive airways. The Lung Health Study Group observed nonspecific hyperresponsiveness in a significant number of patients with COPD. This group of patients with airway hyperreactivity appears to have a worse prognosis and an accelerated rate of decline in FEV_1.[6]

Some patients with asthma (especially cough-variant asthma) present with no history of wheezing and normal PFTs. The diagnosis of asthma still can be established by demonstrating hyperresponsiveness to provocative agents. The two agents used most widely in clinical practice are methacholine and histamine. Other agents used for bronchial provocation include distilled water, cold air, and exercise. During a typical bronchoprovocation test, baseline FEV_1 is measured after inhalation of isotonic saline, then increasing doses of methacholine are given at set intervals. Hyperresponsiveness is defined as a decline in FEV_1 ≥20% and reversibility of obstruction to bronchodilators. The result can best be expressed as the provocative concentration needed to cause a 20% fall in FEV_1 (PC_{20}). A test is considered positive if either methacholine or histamine demonstrates a PC_{20} for FEV_1 ≤8 mg/mL or <60 to 80 cumulative breath units.[7] This test is used most frequently to establish a diagnosis of asthma in patients with normal PFTs, but it also may be useful in following patients with occupational asthma, establishing the severity of asthma, and assessing the response to treatment.

UPPER AIRWAY OBSTRUCTION

Obstruction of airflow by abnormalities in the upper airway often goes undiagnosed or misdiagnosed because of improper interpretation of PFTs. Patients have obstructive physiology and often are misclassified as having asthma or COPD. The shape of the flow–volume loop, which includes inspiratory and expiratory flow–volume curves, and the ratio of forced expiratory and inspiratory flow at 50% of vital capacity ($FEF_{50\%}/FIF_{50\%}$) may be useful in the diagnosis of upper airway obstruction.[8]

The shape of the flow–volume curve differs depending on whether the obstruction is fixed or variable (Fig. 27–5). Fixed lesions, as in strictures from previous intubations or tracheostomy, cause a uniform caliber of airway during inspiration and expiration. With variable lesions, the airway caliber changes with changes in intrathoracic pressure. Variable lesions are subclassified into variable intrathoracic and variable extrathoracic. If the lesion is intrathoracic, as with tumors of the trachea, the negative pressure generated during inspiration opens the obstruction, whereas the positive pressure during expiration worsens the obstruction. If the lesion is a variable extrathoracic obstruction, as with vocal cord dysfunction, the negative pressure within the airways will pull the vocal cord toward the midline and potentiate the obstruction. In this case, there will be a plateau on the inspiratory limb of the flow–volume loop, and $FEF_{50\%}/FIF_{50\%}$ will be >1. Typical flow–volume curves from upper airway obstruction are shown in Fig. 27–4.

Another test used to distinguish upper airway obstruction from COPD and asthma is $FEV_1/FEV_{0.5}$ (FEV at 0.5 second). This ratio

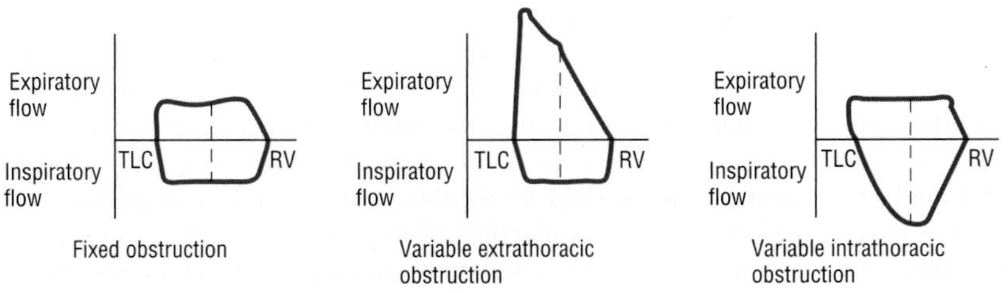

FIGURE 27-5. Maximum expiratory flow–volume curves from patients with fixed obstruction, variable extrathoracic obstruction, and variable intrathoracic obstruction. (RV, residual volume; TLC, total lung capacity.)

usually is >1.5 in patients with upper airway obstruction.[9] This is so because $FEV_{0.5}$ is proportionately more reduced in upper airway obstruction because forced expiration measured at 0.5 second better reflects obstruction at high lung volumes. The abnormality seen on the flow–volume loop has been referred to as "straightening" of the curve during early expiration.

RESTRICTIVE LUNG DISEASE

❺ *Restrictive lung disease* is defined as an inability to get air into the lungs and to maintain normal lung volumes. Restrictive lung disease reduces all the subdivisions of lung volumes (IRV, VT, ERV, and RV) without reducing airflow. Patients have normal airway resistance and FEV_1/FVC >75%.

Although *restriction* could be defined as a reduction in vital capacity (VC or FVC) with normal FEV_1/FVC, poor effort also will reduce FVC with normal FEV_1/FVC. A reduction in TLC is the most accurate measurement of restrictive lung function. TLC can be measured by various techniques. The gas dilution methods (e.g., helium dilution and nitrogen washout) are unable to measure gas trapped in cysts or bullae and may underestimate the true lung volume. Therefore, TLC is best measured by plethysmography. Most restrictive lung disease is associated with impairment or destruction of the alveolar–capillary membrane; therefore, DLCO is reduced in most patients with restrictive lung disease. The reduction in DLCO may occur prior to a reduction in lung volumes and is used as a marker of early interstitial (restrictive) lung disease. DLCO may be abnormal even with a normal chest x-ray film, and thin-cut computed tomographic scans of the chest may be required to diagnose early interstitial lung disease. Because peribronchiolar inflammation and fibrosis occur in patients with restrictive parenchymal lung disease, $FEF_{25\%-75\%}$ may be reduced and fail to respond to bronchodilators.

The severity of restrictive disease has not been standardized; however, many laboratories classify patients with reduced TLC as mild (TLC ≤80%), moderate (TLC ≤65%), or severe (TLC ≤50%). These definitions are completely arbitrary because a patient with obstructive lung disease may start with TLC 120% and subsequently develop a moderately severe restrictive lung disease while maintaining TLC within the normal range. On flow–volume loop, patients with restrictive disease have normal-shaped curves with a reduction in the height and width of the curve because peak expiratory flow rate and VC both depend on the amount of air within the lung prior to performance of expiratory maneuvers (Fig. 27–3).

❻ Restrictive lung function can be produced by increased elastic recoil of the lung parenchyma (interstitial lung disease), respiratory muscle weakness, mechanical restrictions (chest wall deformities), and/or poor effort. Table 27–2 lists common causes of restrictive lung disease.

Restrictive lung function from parenchymal lung disease usually can be differentiated from processes causing mechanical restriction as a result of chest bellows malfunction (Table 27–3). Restrictive parenchymal diseases are associated with a reduction in alveolar volume and an increase in lung elastic recoil. All lung volumes, as well as DLCO, are reduced. RV/TLC (normal ≤30%) and measurements of maximal inspiratory pressure (normal = –75 cm H_2O in males, –50 cm H_2O in females) remain normal. In addition, patients exhibit mild resting hypoxemia that worsens with exercise. Monitoring gas exchange during exercise may be the most sensitive test for detecting progression of interstitial lung disease.[10]

Mechanical restriction caused by chest bellows malfunction may result from chest wall or skeletal deformity, loss of neuromuscular function, fibrosis of the pleural space, and abdominal overdistension causing upward displacement of the diaphragm, as well as decreased diaphragm movement. The most common pulmonary function pattern seen in these patients is a decrease in TLC and VC with only a slight decrease in RV. RV is maintained in these diseases because lung compliance remains normal. DLCO is normal or only minimally reduced, and DLCO/VA (corrected for alveolar volume) is normal. RV/TLC often is increased in patients with restrictive chest bellows disease. Patients with neuromuscular disease have reduced respiratory muscle function with a reduction in maximal inspiratory pressure.

PULMONARY GAS EXCHANGE

The essential function of the lungs is to maintain blood gas homeostasis. Arterial blood gas measurement plays an important role in

TABLE 27-2 Causes of Restrictive Lung Disease

Interstitial lung diseases	Chest wall diseases
Idiopathic pulmonary fibrosis	Kyphoscoliosis
Sarcoidosis	Ankylosing spondylitis
Collagen vascular disease	Neuromuscular disease
Pneumoconiosis	Miscellaneous causes
Drug-induced lung disease	Obesity
Pulmonary edema	Pregnancy
Infiltrative lung diseases	Ascites
Granulomatosis	Paralyzed diaphragm
Tumor	Lung resection
Pleural diseases	
Pleural effusion	
Fibrothorax	
Pneumothorax	

TABLE 27-3 Patterns of Pulmonary Function

	Obstructive Lung Disease		Restrictive Lung Disease	
	Asthma	*COPD*	*Parenchymal Disease*	*Chest Bellows Disease*
FVC	Nl or I	Nl or I	D	D
FEV_1	D	D	D	D
FEV_1/FVC	<75%	<75%	≥75%	≥75%
TLC	Nl or I	Nl or I	D	D
RV/TLC	Nl or I	Nl or I	Nl	I
Airway resistance	I	I	Nl	Nl
DLCO	Nl	D	D	Nl

D, decreased; I, increased; Nl, normal.

the diagnosis and management of patients with pulmonary disease and should be ordered whenever hypoxemia, hypercapnia (CO_2 retention), and/or acid–base disorders are suspected clinically. Every time arterial blood gas determinations are ordered, the A–a gradient (difference between partial pressure of oxygen in the alveolus and partial pressure of oxygen in arterial blood) should be calculated. This is accomplished by computer on all automated blood gas machines, and a normal $P(A–a)O_2$ can be approximated for sea-level breathing room air by multiplying the age by 0.3. The presence of hypoxemia with a normal A–a gradient usually implies alveolar hypoventilation (e.g., sedative overdose). Most patients develop hypoxemia secondary to mismatching of ventilation and perfusion, and $P(A–a)O_2$ will be significantly elevated.

Oxygen saturation as measured by pulse oximetry (SpO_2) is widely used in clinical practice for monitoring arterial saturation. A pulse oximeter is a small battery-operated device that is placed on the finger or the earlobe. The device emits and reads the reflected light from capillary blood, and estimates the saturation. Although SpO_2 is clinically very useful, SpO_2 is only an estimate of arterial saturation. Actual arterial oxygen saturation (SaO_2) can be ± 2% to 4% of the oximetric reading. The error may be even greater with saturation <88%. Pulse oximeters do not measure carboxyhemoglobin, and SpO_2 may be overestimated significantly in patients with smoke inhalation or in recent smokers. An initial validation of pulse oximetry with direct measurement of SaO_2 is recommended in any critically ill patient.

EXERCISE TESTING

Cardiopulmonary exercise testing allows for assessment of multiple organs involved in exercise and has benefits over assessment of either the cardiac system or pulmonary system alone. The major indications for exercise testing are dyspnea on exertion, evaluation of exercise-induced bronchospasm, and suspected arterial desaturation during exercise.[11–14] Exercise testing also can be useful in the evaluation of ventilatory or cardiovascular limitations to work, assessment of general fitness or conditioning, evaluation of disability, establishment of safe levels for exercise, evaluation of drug therapy, determining the need and liter flow for supplemental oxygen therapy during exercise, assessment of the effects of a rehabilitation program, and preoperative assessment before lung resection.[11–14]

Tests for general fitness include the 6-minute walking distance and the Harvard step test.[11,13–15] For the 6-minute walking distance, the subject simply walks a predetermined route or circuit as fast as possible for 6 minutes. The subject is allowed to stop and rest, but the clock continues to run. The greater the distance covered, the better are the patient's general fitness and exercise tolerance. For the Harvard step test, the subject steps up and down on a 20-inch step at a set rate for 5 minutes. A 1-minute rest period is followed by measurement of the subject's recovery heart rate. The lower the recovery heart rate, the better is the subject's general fitness.

Exercise testing sometimes is performed to determine if exercise results in arterial oxygen desaturation (SaO_2 <90%).[12,13] The test may be useful for quantifying the level of exertion the patient can perform during the activities of daily living as well as determining appropriate levels of supplemental oxygen therapy. Typically, this test is done using a treadmill or cycle ergometer. A baseline measurement of arterial blood gas values or pulse oximetry is followed by up to 6 minutes of exercise, during which time the patient is monitored for oxygen desaturation using pulse oximetry. If significant desaturation occurs (saturation ≤88%–90%), the test is terminated. In the event of oxygen desaturation, the test can be repeated to determine the level of supplemental oxygen therapy needed to compensate for the desaturation that otherwise would occur.

When more formal exercise testing is needed for some of the indications previously listed (e.g., dyspnea evaluation, evaluation of ventilatory or cardiovascular limitations to work, evaluation of disability and preoperative assessment before lung resection), exercise tolerance tests or cardiopulmonary stress testing can be performed. Tests include measurement of oxygen consumption ($\dot{V}O_2$), carbon dioxide production ($\dot{V}CO_2$), minute volume ($\dot{V}E$), VT, respiratory rate, SpO_2, heart rate, blood pressure, and recording or monitoring of the electrocardiogram. During exercise, $\dot{V}O_2$ increases with workload in a linear fashion until a maximum oxygen consumption level ($\dot{V}O_2max$) is reached. Consequently, $\dot{V}O_2max$ is a measure of an individual's muscular work capacity.[11–13] Normal $\dot{V}O_2max$ is approximately 1,700 mL/min for a sedentary person and up to 5,800 mL/min for a trained athelete.[13] This compares with a resting $\dot{V}O_2$ of approximately 250 mL/min. Ventilatory equivalents for oxygen, carbon dioxide, and O_2 pulse are often calculated. Ventilatory equivalent for oxygen is a measure of the efficiency of the ventilatory pump at various workloads[11,13,14] and is calculated as follows:

$$\text{Ventilatory equivalent for } O_2 = \dot{V}e/\dot{V}O_2.$$

A normal ventilatory equivalent for oxygen is 20 to 30.[11,13]

O_2 pulse is an estimate of oxygen consumption per cardiac cycle and can be decreased with cardiac problems. O_2 pulse can be calculated as follows:

$$O_2 \text{ pulse} = (\dot{V}O_2 \text{ [in L/min]} \times 1{,}000)/\text{Heart rate}.$$

TABLE 27-4 Indications and Contraindications for Exercise Testing

Indications
Dyspnea upon exertion
Exercise-induced bronchospasm
Suspected arterial desaturation with exercise
Evaluation of ventilatory limitations to exercise
Evaluation of cardiac limitations to exercise
Assessment of general fitness or conditioning
Evaluation of cardiopulmonary disability
Establishment of safe levels for exercise
Evaluation of drug therapy
Determining appropriate use of supplemental oxygen therapy
Establishing an exercise prescription for a rehabilitation program
Assessment of the effect of a rehabilitation program
Evaluation of specific disease states or conditions (e.g., asthma, chronic obstructive pulmonary disease [COPD], interstitial lung disease, pulmonary vascular disorders, coronary artery disease, other vascular disorders, neuromuscular disorders, obesity, anxiety-induced hyperventilation)
Assessment before resection
Assessment before lung volume reduction surgery or lung transplantation
Contraindications
PaO_2 <40 mm Hg on room air
$PaCO_2$ >70 mm Hg
FEV_1 <30% of predicted
Recent (within 4 weeks) myocardial infarction
Unstable angina pectoris
Second- or third-degree heart block
Rapid ventricular/atrial arrhythmias
Orthopedic impairment
Severe aortic stenosis
Congestive heart failure
Uncontrolled hypertension
Limiting neurologic disorders
Dissecting/ventricular aneurysms
Severe pulmonary hypertension
Thrombophlebitis or intracardiac thrombi
Recent systemic or pulmonary embolus
Acute pericarditis

TABLE 27-5 Typical Findings during Maximum Exercise with Poor Conditioning, Pulmonary Limitations to Exercise, and Cardiac Limitations to Exercise

Test Parameter	Poor Conditioning	Pulmonary Limitation	Cardiac Limitation
$\dot{V}O_2$max	↓	↓	↓
SpO_2	N	↓	N
O_2 pulse	N or ↓	N or ↓	↓
Anaerobic threshold	↓ or N	↓ or N	↓
Ventilatory reserve[a] (MVV − VEmax)	N	↓	N or ↑

[a]Ventilatory reserve = Maximum voluntary ventilation (MVV) − Minute volume during maximum exercise (VEmax).
N, normal.
Adapted from Madama VE. Pulmonary Function Testing and Cardiopulmonary Stress Testing. Albany, NY: Delmar, 1993.

A normal O_2 pulse is 2.5 to 4.0 mL per beat at rest and increases to 10 to 15 mL per beat during strenuous exercise.[11,13]

The anaerobic threshold is the point during strenuous exercise at which anaerobic metabolism and lactic acid production begin.[11,13,14] $\dot{V}CO_2$max increases with exercise at about the same rate as $\dot{V}O_2$ until the subject's anaerobic threshold is reached. From that point on, $\dot{V}CO_2$ increases faster than $\dot{V}O_2$, and this change can be used to estimate the anaerobic threshold. A breath-by-breath plot of the ventilatory equivalents for O_2 and CO_2 also can be used to determine the anaerobic threshold. Anaerobic threshold is a measure of fitness in normal subjects, and aerobic training can delay the anaerobic threshold.[11,13]

For exercise tolerance testing, the patient typically is subjected to either a constant workload (steady-state tests) or an increasing workload (progressive multistage tests) using a cycle ergometer or treadmill.[11,13] With progressive multistage tests, the patient exercises to exhaustion or the occurrence of an adverse reaction, at which point the test is stopped. Safety during exercise testing is of major importance, and rigorous guidelines for termination of the test should be followed. Both types of tests can be used to determine $\dot{V}O_2$max. A limit to exercise, as indicated by a decrease in $\dot{V}O_2$max, can result from (1) poor conditioning, (2) pulmonary limitation, (3) cardiac limitation, or (4) poor effort. In the case of poor conditioning, SpO_2 and O_2 pulse will be normal. With a pulmonary limitation to exercise, SpO_2 will be reduced, and O_2 pulse will be normal. With a cardiac limitation to exercise, SpO_2 will be normal, and O_2 pulse will be reduced. Table 27–4 summarizes the indications and contraindications for exercise testing. Table 27–5 summarizes the findings during maximum exercise associated with poor conditioning, pulmonary limitations to exercise, and cardiac limitations to exercise.

ABBREVIATIONS

COPD: chronic obstructive pulmonary disease

DL: diffusing capacity of lung

DLCO: diffusing capacity of lung for carbon monoxide

ERV: expiratory reserve volume

FEF: forced expiratory flow

$FEF_{25\%-75\%}$: forced expiratory flow during 25% to 75% of forced vital capacity

$FEF_{50\%}$: forced expiratory flow at 50% of forced vital capacity

FEFmax: maximum forced expiratory flow

$FEV_{0.5}$: forced expiratory volume at 0.5 second

FEV_1: forced expiratory volume in first second of expiration

FEV_6: forced expiratory volume in 6 seconds

$FIF_{50\%}$: forced inspiratory flow at 50% of forced vital capacity

FRC: functional residual capacity

FVC: forced vital capacity

IC: inspiratory capacity

IRV: inspiratory reserve volume

$P_1V_1 = P_2V_2$: Boyle's gas law

$P(A-a)O_2$: alveolar–arterial difference in partial pressure of oxygen

$PaCO_2$: arterial partial pressure of carbon dioxide

PaO_2: arterial partial pressure of oxygen

PC_{20}: provocative concentration needed to cause a 20% fall in FEV_1

PCP: *Pneumocystis carinii* pneumonia

PFT: pulmonary function test

PO_2: partial pressure of oxygen

RV: residual volume

SaO_2: arterial oxygen saturation

SpO_2: oxygen saturation as measured by pulse oximetry

SVC: slow vital capacity

TLC: total lung capacity

VA: alveolar volume

VC: vital capacity

VT: tidal volume

REFERENCES

1. Renzessi AA Jr, Bleeker, ER, Eppler, GR, et al. Evaluation of impairment/disability secondary to respiratory disorders. Am Rev Respir Dis 1986;133:1205–1209.
2. Pelligrino R, Viegi G, Brusasco V, et al. Series ATS/ERS Task Force: Standardization of lung function testing; interpretative strategies for lung function tests. Eur Respir J 2005;26:319–338.
3. Crapo RO, Hankinson JL, Irvin C, et al. American Thoracic Society statement: Standardization of spirometry—1994 update. Am J Respir Crit Care Med 1995;152:1107–1136.
4. Levine SM, Peters JI, Jenkinson SG. Lung transplantation and lung volume reduction surgery. In: George RB, Light RW, Matthaw MA, eds. Chest Medicine: Essentials of Pulmonary and Critical Care Medicine, 4th ed. Philadelphia: Lippincott Williams & Wilkins, 2000:208–232.
5. Anthonisen NR, Connett JE, Kiley JP, et al. Effects of smoking intervention and the use of an inhaled anticholinergic bronchodilator on the rate of decline of FEV_1: The Lung Health Study. JAMA 1994;272:1497–1505.
6. Tashkin DP, Altose MD, Bleeker ER, et al. The Lung Health Study: Airway responsiveness to inhaled methacholine in smokers with mild to moderate airflow limitation. Am Rev Respir Dis 1992;145:301–310.
7. Crapo RO, Casaburi R, Coates AL, et al. American Thoracic Society statement: Guidelines for methacholine and exercise challenge testing—1999. Am J Respir Crit Care Med 2000;161:309–329.
8. Aboussouan LS, Stoller JK. Diagnosis and management of upper airway obstruction. Clin Chest Med 1994;15:35–53.
9. Bright P, Miller MR, Franklyn JA, et al. The use of a neural network to detect upper airway obstruction caused by goiter. Am J Respir Crit Care Med 1998;157:1885–1891.
10. Leith DE, Brown R. ERS/ATS Workshop Series: Human lung volumes and the mechanisms that set them. Eur Respir J 1999;13:468–472.
11. Wasserman K, Hansen JE, Sue DY, Stringer WW, Whipp BJ. Principles of Exercise Testing and Interpretation: Including Pathophysiology and Clinical Applications, 4th ed. Philadelphia: Lippincott Williams & Wilkins, 2004.

12. Ruppel GE. Manual of Pulmonary Function Testing. St. Louis: Mosby, 1994.
13. ATS/ACCP statement on cardiopulmonary exercise testing. Am J Respir Crit Care Med 2003;167:211–277.
14. Weisman IM, Zeballos RJ. Clinical exercise testing. Clin Chest Med 2001;22:679–701.
15. ATS Statement: Guidelines for the six-minute walk test. Am J Respir Crit Care Med 2002;166:111–117.

CHAPTER 28 Asthma

H. WILLIAM KELLY AND CHRISTINE A. SORKNESS

KEY CONCEPTS

1. Asthma is a disease of increasing prevalence that is a result of genetic predisposition and environmental interactions; it is one of the most common chronic diseases of childhood.
2. Asthma is primarily a chronic inflammatory disease of the airways of the lung for which there is no known cure or primary prevention; the immunohistopathologic features include cell infiltration by neutrophils, eosinophils, T-helper type 2 lymphocytes, mast cells, and epithelial cells.
3. Asthma is characterized by either the intermittent or persistent presence of highly variable degrees of airflow obstruction from airway wall inflammation and bronchial smooth muscle constriction; in some patients, persistent changes in airway structure occur.
4. The inflammatory process in asthma is treated most effectively with corticosteroids, with the inhaled corticosteroids having the greatest efficacy and safety profile for long-term management.
5. Bronchial smooth muscle constriction is prevented or treated most effectively with inhaled β_2-adrenergic receptor agonists.
6. Variability in response to medications requires individualization of therapy within existing evidence-based guidelines for management.
7. Ongoing patient education, for a partnership in asthma care, is essential for optimal patient outcomes and includes trigger avoidance and self-management techniques.

Asthma has been known since antiquity, yet it is a disease that still defies precise definition. The word *asthma* is of Greek origin and means "panting." More than 2,000 years ago, Hippocrates used the word *asthma* to describe episodic shortness of breath; however, the first detailed clinical description of the asthmatic patient was made by Aretaeus in the second century.[1] An expert panel of the National Institutes of Health, the National Asthma Education and Prevention Program (NAEPP), has provided the following working definition of asthma[2]:

Asthma is a chronic inflammatory disorder of the airways in which many cells and cellular elements play a role: in particular, mast cells, eosinophils, T-lymphocytes, macrophages, neutrophils, and epithelial cells. In susceptible individuals, this inflammation causes recurrent episodes of wheezing, breathlessness, chest tightness, and coughing, particularly at night or in the early morning. These episodes are usually associated with widespread but variable airflow obstruction that is often reversible either spontaneously or with treatment. The inflammation also causes an associated increase in the existing bronchial hyperresponsiveness (BHR) to a variety of stimuli. Reversibility of airflow limitation may be incomplete in some patients with asthma.

This definition encompasses the important heterogeneity of the clinical presentation of asthma by describing the scientific and clinically accepted characteristics of asthma.

Learning objectives, review questions, and other resources can be found at **www.pharmacotherapyonline.com.**

EPIDEMIOLOGY

1 An estimated 20.5 million persons in the United States have asthma (approximately 7% of the population).[3] Asthma is the most common chronic disease among children in the United States, with approximately 6.5 million children affected. The prevalence of asthma in the United States and worldwide has continued to increase. The prevalence rate is highest in children 5–17 years at 9.6%.[3] In the United States, as in other Western industrialized countries, the prevalence of asthma has reached epidemic proportions. Asthma accounts for 1.6% of all ambulatory care visits (13.7 million physician office visits and 1.0 million hospital outpatient visits) and results in more than 497,000 hospitalizations and 1.8 million emergency department visits per year.[3] Although asthma is the third leading cause of preventable hospitalization in the United States, hospitalizations for asthma have decreased only slightly over the past 10 years to 17 per 10,000 population.[4] Children younger than 15 years of age have the highest rate of hospitalization at 31 per 10,000 population. Asthma accounts for more than 10 million missed school days per year.[3] The prevalence of disabling asthma in children has increased 232% over the past 20 years compared with a 113% increase from all other chronic conditions in childhood.[4] In young children (0 to 10 years of age), the risk of asthma is greater in boys than in girls, becomes about equal during puberty, and then is greater in women than in men.[3]

Ethnic minorities continue to share the burden of asthma disproportionately. African Americans have a higher prevalence than whites, but this appears to be a result of urbanization and not race or socioeconomic status.[4] African Americans are three times as likely to be hospitalized and approximately 2.5 times more likely to die from asthma.[3] In addition, African Americans and Puerto Ricans living in inner cities are four times more likely to experience emergency department visits than whites.[3] These patterns are likely a result of poor access to care as Hispanics in general have a lower prevalence than African Americans or whites.

The estimated direct medical cost of asthma in the United States in 2004 was $11.5 billion.[3] The societal burden of asthma (indirect medical expenditures) in the United States was $4.6 billion. Prescription drugs were the largest single direct medical expenditure at $5 billion, however, the combined costs of emergency care of acute asthma exacerbations makes up 36% of direct medical costs.[3] Almost $1.5 billion of indirect costs were a result of school days lost, and lost productivity secondary to asthma mortality cost $1.7 billion.

The natural history of asthma is still not well defined. Although asthma can occur at any time, it is principally a pediatric disease, with most patients being diagnosed by 5 years of age and up to 50% of children having symptoms by 2 years of age.[2] Between 30% and 70% of children with asthma will improve markedly or become symptom-free by early adulthood; chronic disease persists in approximately 30% to 40% of patients, and generally 20% or less develop severe chronic disease.[2] Atopic status is the strongest indicator of persistence into adulthood, although initial severity also predicts severity as an adult.[5] Other predictors of persistent adult asthma include onset during school age and presence of BHR. Diminished lung growth may occur in children with uncontrolled severe asthma but does not appear to occur in children with mild to moderate asthma.[6] Most of the deficits in lung function growth occur in children whose symptoms begin during the first 3 years of life.[6]

In adults, most longitudinal studies have suggested a more rapid rate of decline in lung function in asthmatics than in normal volunteers, primarily reflected in forced expiratory volume in 1 second (FEV_1).[5] However, the annual decline in FEV_1 is less than in smokers or in patients with a diagnosis of emphysema. In general, individuals with less-frequent asthma attacks and normal lung function on initial assessment have higher remission rates, whereas smokers have the lowest remission and highest relapse rates.[5] The level of BHR tends to predict the rate of decline in FEV_1, with a greater decline with high levels of BHR.[6] Thus airways obstruction in asthma not only may become irreversible but also may worsen over time owing to airway remodeling (see below Remodeling of the Airway section).[7] Many elderly patients with asthma have irreversible airways obstruction.[5] However, most patients do not die from long-term progression of their disease and their life span is not different from that of the general population.[5]

Although the prevalence of asthma is increasing in the United States, measures of significant morbidity (hospital admissions) and mortality from acute exacerbations of asthma have reached plateaus and have been slightly decreasing the past few years.[3] Asthma results in a little more than 4,000 deaths per year.[3] Despite the relatively low number of asthma deaths, 80% to 90% are preventable.[2,8] Most deaths from asthma occur outside the hospital, and death is rare after hospitalization. The most common cause of death from asthma is inadequate assessment of the severity of airways obstruction by the patient or physician and inadequate therapy. The most common cause of death in hospitalized patients is also inadequate or inappropriate therapy. Thus the key to prevention of death from asthma, as advocated by the NAEPP, is education.[6]

ETIOLOGY

❶ Asthma is at least a partially heritable complex syndrome that requires a gene-by-environment interaction for phenotypic expression. Epidemiologic studies strongly support the concept of a genetic predisposition to the development of asthma, yet the picture remains complex and incomplete.[9] Genetic factors account for 35% to 70% of the susceptibility. Asthma represents a complex genetic disorder in that the asthma phenotype is likely a result of polygenic inheritance or different combinations of genes. Initial searches focused on establishing links between atopy (genetically determined state of hypersensitivity to environmental allergens) and asthma, but more recent genome-wide searches have found linkages with genes for metalloproteinases (e.g., *ADAM33*).[10,11] Thus, although genetic predisposition to atopy is a significant risk factor for developing asthma, not all atopic individuals develop asthma, nor do all asthmatics exhibit atopy.

❶ Environmental risk factors for the development of asthma include socioeconomic status, family size, exposure to secondhand tobacco smoke in infancy and in utero, allergen exposure, urbanization, and decreased exposure to common childhood infectious agents.[12] The "hygiene hypothesis" proposes that genetically susceptible individuals develop allergies and asthma by allowing the allergic immunologic system (T-helper cell type 2 [TH_2]-lymphocytes) to develop instead of the immunologic system used to fight infections (T-helper cell type 1 [TH_1]-lymphocytes), and is being used to explain the increase of asthma in Western countries.[6,12] The first 2 years of life appear to be most important for the exposures to produce an alteration in the immune response system. Support for the hygiene hypothesis for asthma comes from studies demonstrating a lower risk for asthma in children who live on farms and are exposed to high levels of bacteria, in those with a large number of siblings, in those with early enrollment into child care, in those with exposure to cats and dogs early in life, or in those with exposure to fewer antibiotics.[10,12]

Risk factors for early (<3 years of age) recurrent wheezing associated with viral infections include low birth weight, male gender, and parental smoking. However, this early pattern is a result of smaller airways, and these risk factors are not necessarily risk factors for asthma in later life.[7] Atopy is the predominant risk factor for children to have continued asthma.[7] Asthma can occur in adults later in life. Occupational asthma in previously healthy individuals emphasizes the effect of environment on the development of asthma.[13] The heterogeneity of the asthma phenotype appears most obvious when listing the diverse triggers of bronchospasm in asthmatic subjects (Table 28–1).[2,6] The various triggers have relative degrees of importance from patient to patient. This variety should serve as ample evidence that asthma is likely to be as complex genetically.

Environmental exposures are the most important precipitants of severe asthma exacerbations (see Table 28–1).[2,6] Epidemics of severe asthma in cities have followed exposures to high concentrations of aeroallergens.[2] Viral respiratory tract infections remain the single most significant precipitant of severe asthma in children, and are an important trigger in adults as well.[2,6] Other possible factors include air pollution, sinusitis, food preservatives, and drugs.

TABLE 28-1 List of Agents and Events Triggering Asthma

Respiratory infection
Respiratory syncytial virus (RSV), rhinovirus, influenza, parainfluenza, *Mycoplasma pneumonia*
Allergens
Airborne pollens (grass, trees, weeds), house-dust mites, animal danders, cockroaches, fungal spores
Environment
Cold air, fog, ozone, sulfur dioxide, nitrogen dioxide, tobacco smoke, wood smoke
Emotions
Anxiety, stress, laughter
Exercise
Particularly in cold, dry climate
Drugs/preservatives
Aspirin, nonsteroidal antiinflammatory drugs (cyclooxygenase inhibitors), sulfites, benzalkonium chloride, nonselective β-blockers
Occupational stimuli
Bakers (flour dust); farmers (hay mold); spice and enzyme workers; printers (arabic gum); chemical workers (azo dyes, anthraquinone, ethylenediamine, toluene diisocyanates, polyvinyl chloride); plastics, rubber, and wood workers (formaldehyde, western cedar, dimethylethanolamine, anhydrides)

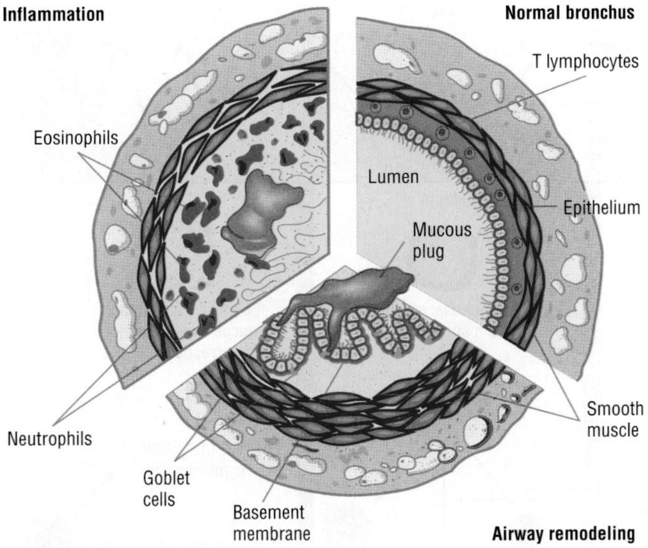

FIGURE 28-1. Representative illustration of the pathology found in the asthmatic bronchus compared with a normal bronchus *(upper right)*. Each section demonstrates how the lumen is narrowed. Hypertrophy of the basement membrane, mucus plugging, smooth muscle hypertrophy, and constriction contribute *(lower section)*. Inflammatory cells infiltrate, producing submucosal edema, and epithelial desquamation fills the airway lumen with cellular debris and exposes the airway smooth muscle to other mediators *(upper left)*.

PATHOPHYSIOLOGY

❷ The major characteristics of asthma include a variable degree of airflow obstruction (related to bronchospasm, edema, and hypersecretion), BHR, and airways inflammation (Fig. 28–1). Evidence of inflammation arose from the studies of nonspecific BHR, bronchoalveolar lavage, bronchial biopsies, and induced sputum, as well as from postmortem observations of patients with asthma who died from an attack of asthma or from other causes. To understand the pathogenetic mechanisms that underlie the many variants of asthma, it is critical to identify factors that initiate, intensify, and modulate the inflammatory response of the airways and to determine how these immunologic and biologic processes produce the characteristic airways abnormalities. Immune responses mediated by immunoglobulin (Ig) E antibodies are of foremost importance.

ACUTE INFLAMMATION

Inhaled allergen challenge models contribute most to our understanding of acute inflammation in asthma.[14] Inhaled allergen challenge in allergic patients leads to an early phase allergic reaction that, in some cases, may be followed by a late-phase reaction. The activation of cells bearing allergen-specific IgE initiates the early phase reaction. It is characterized primarily by the rapid activation of airway mast cells and macrophages. The activated cells rapidly release proinflammatory mediators such as histamine, eicosanoids, and reactive oxygen species that induce contraction of airway smooth muscle, mucus secretion, and vasodilation.[14] The bronchial microcirculation has an essential role in this inflammatory process. Inflammatory mediators induce microvascular leakage with exudation of plasma in the airways.[14] Acute plasma protein leakage induces a thickened, engorged, and edematous airway wall and a consequent narrowing of the airway lumen. Plasma exudation may compromise epithelial integrity, and the presence of plasma in the lumen may reduce mucus clearance.[14] Plasma proteins also may promote the formation of exudative plugs mixed with mucus and inflammatory and epithelial cells. Together these effects contribute to airflow obstruction (see Fig. 28–1).

The late-phase inflammatory reaction occurs 6 to 9 hours after allergen provocation and involves the recruitment and activation of eosinophils, CD4+ T cells, basophils, neutrophils, and macrophages.[14] There is selective retention of airway T cells, the expression of adhesion molecules, and the release of selected proinflammatory mediators and cytokines involved in the recruitment and activation of inflammatory cells.[14] The activation of T cells after allergen challenge leads to the release of TH_2-like cytokines that may be a key mechanism of the late-phase response.[14] The release of preformed cytokines by mast cells is the likely initial trigger for the early recruitment of cells. This cell type may recruit and induce the more persistent involvement by T cells.[14] The enhancement of nonspecific BHR usually can be demonstrated after the late-phase reaction but not after the early phase reaction following allergen or occupational challenge.

CHRONIC INFLAMMATION

Airways inflammation has been demonstrated in all forms of asthma, and an association between the extent of inflammation and the clinical severity of asthma has been demonstrated in selected studies.[7,15] It is accepted that both central and peripheral airways are inflamed.

In asthma, all cells of the airways are involved and become activated (Fig. 28–2). Included are eosinophils, T cells, mast cells, macrophages, epithelial cells, fibroblasts, and bronchial smooth muscle cells. These cells also regulate airway inflammation and initiate the process of remodeling by the release of cytokines and growth factors.[15]

Epithelial Cells

Bronchial epithelial cells traditionally have been considered as a barrier, participating in mucociliary clearance and removal of noxious agents. However, epithelial cells also participate in inflammation by the release of eicosanoids, peptidases, matrix proteins, cytokines, and nitric oxide (NO). Epithelial cells can be activated by IgE-dependent mechanisms, viruses, pollutants, or histamine. In asthma, especially fatal asthma, extensive epithelial shedding occurs. The functional consequences of epithelial shedding may include heightened airways responsiveness, altered permeability of the airway mucosa, depletion of epithelial-derived relaxant factors, and loss of enzymes responsible for degrading proinflammatory neuropeptides. The integrity of airway epithelium may influence the sensitivity of the airways to various provocative stimuli. Epithelial cells also may be important in the regulation of airway remodeling and fibrosis.[15,16]

Eosinophils

Eosinophils play an effector role in asthma by release of proinflammatory mediators, cytotoxic mediators, and cytokines.[15] Circulating eosinophils migrate to the airways by cell rolling, through interactions with selectins, and eventually adhere to the endothelium through the binding of integrins to adhesion proteins (vascular cell adhesion molecule 1 [VCAM-1] and intercellular adhesion molecule 1 [ICAM-1]). As eosinophils enter the matrix of the membrane, their survival is prolonged by interleukin (IL)-5 and granulocyte-macrophage colony-stimulating factor (GM-CSF). On activation, eosinophils release inflammatory mediators such as leukotrienes and granule proteins to injure airway tissue.[15]

Lymphocytes

Mucosal biopsy specimens from patients with asthma contain lymphocytes, many of which express surface markers of inflammation. There are two types of T-helper CD4+ cells. TH_1 cells produce IL-2 and interferon-γ (INF-γ), both essential for cellular defense mechanisms. TH_2 cells produce cytokines (IL-4, -5, and -13)

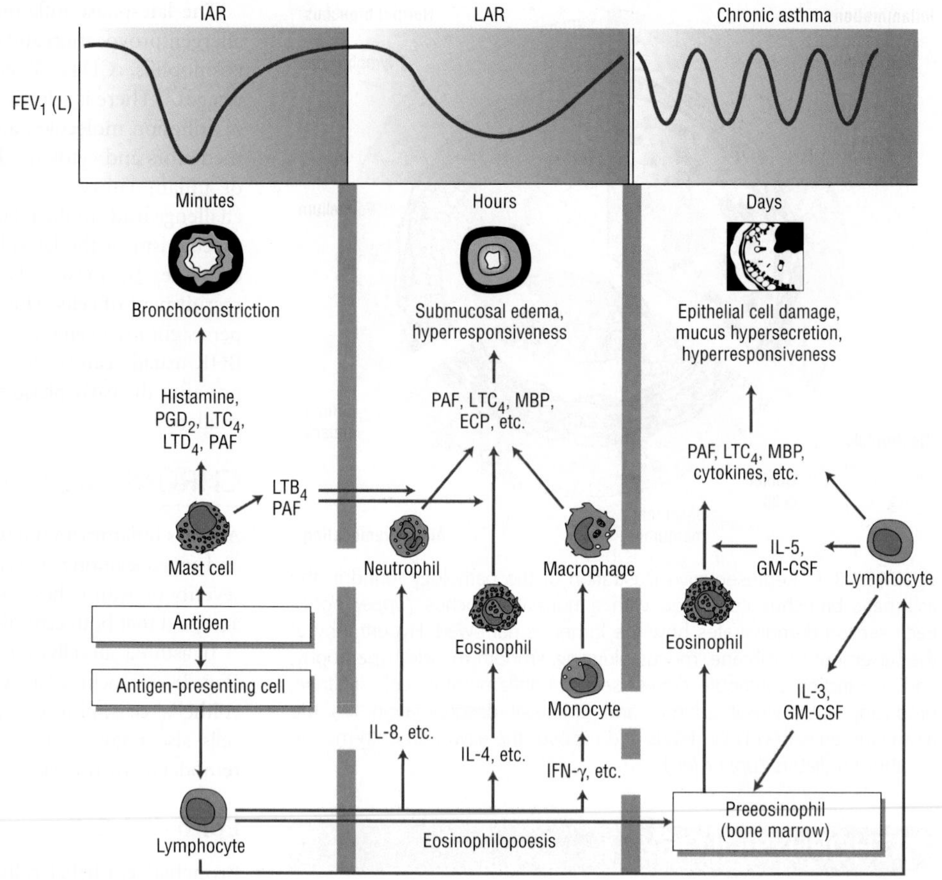

FIGURE 28-2. Diagrammatic presentation of the relationship between inflammatory cells, lipid and preformed mediators, inflammatory cytokines, and proposed pathogenesis and clinical presentation in asthma. See text for details. (ECP, eosinophil cationic protein; GM-CSF, granulocyte-macrophage colony-stimulating factor; IAR, immediate asthmatic reaction; IFN, interferon; IL, interleukin; LAR, late asthmatic response; LT, leukotriene; MBP, major basis protein; PAF, platelet-activating factor; PG, prostaglandin.)

that mediate allergic inflammation. It is known that TH_1 cytokines inhibit the production of TH_2 cytokines, and vice versa. It is hypothesized that allergic asthmatic inflammation results from a TH_2-mediated mechanism (an imbalance between TH_1 and TH_2 cells).[15]

TH_1 and TH_2 Cell Imbalance

It has been postulated that the TH_1/TH_2 imbalance contributes to the cause and evolution of atopic diseases, including asthma. The T-cell population in the cord blood of newborn infants is skewed toward a TH_2 phenotype.[7,15] The extent of the imbalance between TH_1 and TH_2 cells (as indicated by diminished INF-γ production) during the neonatal phase may predict the subsequent development of allergic disease, asthma, or both. It has been suggested that infants at high risk of asthma and allergies should be exposed to stimuli that upregulate TH_1-mediated responses in order to restore the balance during a critical time in the development of the immune system and the lung.[7]

The basic premise of the hygiene hypothesis is that the newborn's immune system is skewed toward TH_2 cells and needs timely and appropriate environmental stimuli to create a balanced immune response. Factors that enhance TH_1-mediated responses include infection with *Mycobacterium tuberculosis,* measles virus, and hepatitis A virus; increased exposure to infections through contact with older siblings; attendance at day care during the first 6 months of life; and a reduction in the production of INF-γ. Restoration of the balance between TH_1 and TH_2 cells may be impeded by frequent administration of oral antibiotics, with concomitant alterations in gastrointestinal flora. Other factors favoring the TH_2 phenotype include Western lifestyle, urban environment, diet, and sensitization to house-dust mites and cockroaches. Immune "imprinting" may begin in utero by transplacental transfer of allergens and cytokines.

Mast Cells

Mast cell degranulation is important in the initiation of immediate responses following exposure to allergens.[2] Mast cells are found throughout the walls of the respiratory tract, and increased numbers of these cells (three- to fivefold) have been described in the airways of asthmatics with an allergic component. Once binding of allergen to cell-bound IgE occurs, mediators such as histamine; eosinophil and neutrophil chemotactic factors; leukotrienes (LTs) C_4, D_4, and E_4; prostaglandins; platelet-activating factor; and others are released from mast cells (see Fig. 28–2). Histologic examination has revealed decreased numbers of granulated mast cells in the airways of patients who have died from acute asthma attacks, suggesting that mast cell degranulation is a contributing factor in the progression of the disease. Sensitized mast cells also may be activated by osmotic stimuli to account for exercise-induced bronchospasm (EIB).[15]

Alveolar Macrophages

The primary function of alveolar macrophages in the normal airway is to serve as "scavengers," engulfing and digesting bacteria and other foreign materials. They are found in large and small airways, ideally located for affecting the asthmatic response. A number of mediators produced and released by macrophages have been identified, including platelet-activating factor, LTB_4, LTC_4, and LTD_4.[15] Additionally, alveolar macrophages are able to produce neutrophil chemotactic factor and eosinophil chemotactic factor, which, in turn, amplify the inflammatory process.

Neutrophils

The role of neutrophils in the pathogenesis of asthma remains somewhat unclear because they normally may be present in the airways and usually do not infiltrate tissues showing chronic allergic inflammation despite the potential to participate in late-phase inflammatory reactions. However, high numbers of neutrophils have been reported to be present in the airways of patients who died from sudden-onset fatal asthma[7] and in those with severe disease.[16] This suggests that neutrophils may play a pivotal role in the disease process, at least in some patients with long-standing or corticosteroid-dependent asthma.[16] The neutrophil also can be a source for a variety of mediators, including platelet-activating factor, prostaglandins, thromboxanes, and leukotrienes, that contribute to BHR and airway inflammation.

Fibroblasts and Myofibroblasts

Fibroblasts are found frequently in connective tissue. Human lung fibroblasts may behave as inflammatory cells on activation by IL-4 and IL-13. The myofibroblast may contribute to the regulation of inflammation via the release of cytokines and to tissue remodeling. In asthma, myofibroblasts are increased in numbers beneath the reticular basement membrane, and there is an association between their numbers and the thickness of the reticular basement membrane.[16]

Inflammatory Mediators

Associated with asthma for many years, histamine is capable of inducing smooth muscle constriction and bronchospasm and is thought to play a role in mucosal edema and mucus secretion.[2] Lung mast cells are an important source of histamine. The release of histamine can be stimulated by exposure of the airways to a variety of factors, including physical stimuli (such as exercise) and relevant allergens.[2] Histamine is involved in acute bronchospasm following allergen exposure; however, other mediators, such as leukotrienes, are also involved.

Besides histamine release, mast cell degranulation releases interleukins, proteases, and other enzymes that activate the production of other mediators of inflammation. Several classes of important mediators, including arachidonic acid and its metabolites (i.e., prostaglandins, LTs, and platelet-activating factor), are derived from cell membrane phospholipids.

Once arachidonic acid is released, it can be metabolized by the enzyme cyclooxygenase to form prostaglandins. Although prostaglandin D_2 is a potent bronchoconstricting agent, it is unlikely to produce sustained effects and its role in asthma remains to be determined. Similarly, prostaglandin $F_{2\alpha}$ is a potent bronchoconstrictor in patients with asthma and can enhance the effects of histamine.[2] However, its pathophysiologic role in asthma is unclear. Another cyclooxygenase product, prostacyclin (prostaglandin I_2), is known to be produced in the lung and may contribute to inflammation and edema owing to its effects as a vasodilator.

Thromboxane A_2 is produced by alveolar macrophages, fibroblasts, epithelial cells, neutrophils, and platelets within the lung.[15] Indirect evidence from animal models suggests that thromboxane A_2 may have several effects, including bronchoconstriction, involvement in the late asthmatic response, and involvement in the development of airway inflammation and BHR.

The 5-lipoxygenase pathway of arachidonic acid metabolism is responsible for the production of the *cysteinyl leukotrienes.*[15] LTC_4, LTD_4, and LTE_4 are released during inflammatory processes in the lung. LTD_4 and LTE_4 share a common receptor (LTD_4 receptor) that, when stimulated, produces bronchospasm, mucus secretion, microvascular permeability, and airway edema, whereas LTB_4 is involved with granulocyte chemotaxis.

Thought to be produced by macrophages, eosinophils, and neutrophils within the lung, platelet-activating factor is involved in the mediation of bronchospasm, sustained induction of BHR, edema formation, and chemotaxis of eosinophils.[15]

Adhesion Molecules

An important step in the inflammatory process is the adhesion of the various cells to each other and the tissue matrix to facilitate infiltration and migration of these cells to the site of inflammation. To promote this, cell membranes express a number of glycoproteins, or adhesion molecules. Adhesion molecules have additional functions involved in the inflammatory process aside from promoting cell adhesion, including activation of cells and cell–cell communication, and promoting cellular migration and infiltration.[2] The many adhesion molecules are divided into families on the basis of their chemical structure. These families are the integrins, cadherins, immunoglobulin supergene family, selectins, vascular adressins, and carbohydrate ligands.[15] Those thought to be important in inflammation include the integrins, immunoglobulin supergene family, selectins, and carbohydrate ligands, including ICAM-1 and VCAM-1.[15] Adhesion molecules are found on a variety of cells, such as neutrophils, monocytes, lymphocytes, basophils, eosinophils, granulocytes, platelets, endothelial cells, and epithelial cells, and can be expressed or activated by the many inflammatory mediators present in asthma.[15]

CLINICAL CONSEQUENCES OF CHRONIC INFLAMMATION

Chronic inflammation is associated with nonspecific BHR and increases the risk of asthma exacerbations. Exacerbations are characterized by increased symptoms and worsening airways obstruction over a period of days or even weeks, and rarely hours. Hyperresponsiveness of the airways to physical, chemical, and pharmacologic stimuli is a hallmark of asthma.[2] BHR also occurs in some patients with chronic bronchitis and allergic rhinitis.[2] Normal healthy subjects also may develop a transient BHR after viral respiratory infections or exposure to ozone. However, the degree of BHR is quantitatively greater in asthmatic patients than in other groups. Bronchial responsiveness of the general population fits a unimodal distribution that is skewed toward increased reactivity. Patients with clinical asthma represent the extreme end of the distribution. The degree of BHR within asthmatics correlates with the clinical course of their disease and medication requirement necessary to control symptoms.[2] Patients with mild symptoms or in remission demonstrate lower levels of responsiveness, although still greater than the normal population.

Our current understanding recognizes that the increased BHR seen in asthma is at least in part owing to an inflammatory response within the airways. Early investigations found correlations with inflammatory cells in bronchoalveolar lavage fluids and degree of BHR.[2] Newer evidence suggests that airways remodeling, subepithelial fibrosis, or collagen deposition also correlates with BHR.[16] Although the precise link is unknown, BHR is in part related to the extent of inflammation in the airways.

REMODELING OF THE AIRWAYS

Acute inflammation is a beneficial, nonspecific response of tissues to injury and generally leads to repair and restoration of the normal structure and function. In contrast, asthma represents a chronic inflammatory process of the airways followed by healing. The end result may be an altered structure referred to as a *remodeling of the airways.*[16] Repair involves replacement of injured tissue by parenchymal cells of the same type and replacement by connective tissue and its maturation into scar tissue. In asthma, the repair process can be followed by complete or altered restitution of airways structure and function, presenting as fibrosis and an increase in smooth muscle and mucus gland mass.[16]

The precise mechanisms of remodeling of the airways are under intense study. Airways remodeling is of concern because it may represent an irreversible process that can have more serious sequelae such as the development of chronic obstructive pulmonary disease.[2] Observations in children with asthma indicate that some loss of lung function may occur during the first 5 years of life.[7] Of greatest concern is that no current therapies have been shown to alter either early decreased lung growth or later increased loss of lung function.

MUCUS PRODUCTION

The mucociliary system is the lung's primary defense mechanism against irritants and infectious agents. Mucus, composed of 95% water and 5% glycoproteins, is produced by bronchial epithelial glands and goblet cells.[7] The lining of the airways consists of a continuous aqueous layer controlled by active ion transport across the epithelium in which water moves toward the lumen along the concentration gradient. Catecholamines and vagal stimulation enhance the ion transport and fluid movement. Mucus transport depends on the viscoelastic properties of the mucus. Mucus that is either too watery or too viscous will not be transported optimally. The exudative inflammatory process and sloughing of epithelial cells into the airway lumen impair mucociliary transport. The bronchial glands are increased in size and the goblet cells are increased in size and number in asthma. Expectorated mucus from patients with asthma tends to have a high viscosity. The mucus plugs in the airways of patients who died in status asthmaticus are tenacious and tend to be connected by mucous strands to the goblet cells. Asthmatic airways also may become plugged with casts consisting of epithelial and inflammatory cells. Although it is tempting to speculate that death from asthma attacks is a result of the mucus plugging resulting in irreversible obstruction, there is no direct evidence for this. Autopsies of asthmatics who died from other causes have shown similar pathology. In addition, some subjects who have died of sudden severe asthma did not show the characteristic mucus plugging on necropsy.[7]

AIRWAY SMOOTH MUSCLE

The smooth muscle of the airways does not form a uniform coat around the airways but is wrapped around in a connecting network best described as a spiral arrangement.[15] The muscle contraction displays a sphincteric action that is capable of completely occluding the airway lumen. The airway smooth muscle extends from the trachea through the respiratory bronchioles. When expressed as a percentage of wall thickness, the smooth muscle represents 5% of the large central airways and up to 20% of the wall thickness in the bronchioles. Total smooth muscle mass decreases rapidly past the terminal bronchioles to the alveoli, so the contribution of smooth muscle tone to airway diameter in this region is relatively small. In the large airways of asthmatics, smooth muscle may account for 11% of the wall thickness. It is possible that the increased smooth muscle mass of the asthmatic airways is important in magnifying and maintaining BHR in chronic asthma. However, it appears that the hypertrophy and hyperplasia are secondary processes caused by chronic inflammation and are not the primary cause of BHR.[7]

NEURAL CONTROL/NEUROGENIC INFLAMMATION

The airway is innervated by parasympathetic, sympathetic, and nonadrenergic inhibitory nerves.[2] Parasympathetic innervation of the smooth muscle consists of efferent motor fibers in the vagus nerves and sensory afferent fibers in the vagus and other nerves.[15] The normal resting tone of human airway smooth muscle is maintained by vagal efferent activity. Maximum bronchoconstriction mediated by vagal stimulation occurs in the small bronchi and is absent in the small bronchioles. The nonmyelinated C fibers of the afferent system lie immediately beneath the tight junctions between epithelial cells lining the airway lumen.[15] These endings probably represent the irritant receptors of the airways. Stimulation of these irritant receptors by mechanical stimulation, chemical and particulate irritants, and pharmacologic agents such as histamine produces reflex bronchoconstriction.[15]

The nonadrenergic noncholinergic (NANC) nervous system has been described in the trachea and bronchi. Substance P, neurokinin A, neurokinin B, and vasoactive intestinal peptide are the best-characterized neurotransmitters in the NANC nervous system.[15] Vasoactive intestinal peptide is an inhibitory neurotransmitter in the system. Inflammatory cells in asthma can release peptidases that can degrade vasoactive intestinal peptide, producing exaggerated reflex cholinergic bronchoconstriction. NANC excitatory neuropeptides such as substance P and neurokinin A are released by stimulation of C-fiber sensory nerve endings. The NANC system may play an important role in amplifying inflammation in asthma by releasing NO.

NITRIC OXIDE

NO is produced by cells within the respiratory tract. It has been thought to be a neurotransmitter of the NANC nervous system.[17] Endogenous NO is generated from the amino acid L-arginine by the enzyme NO synthase.[17] There are three isoforms of NO synthase. One isoform is induced in response to proinflammatory cytokines, inducible NO synthase, in airway epithelial cells and inflammatory cells of asthmatic airways.[17] NO produces smooth muscle relaxation in the vasculature and bronchials; however, it appears to amplify the inflammatory process and is unlikely to be of therapeutic benefit. Recent investigations measuring the fraction of exhaled NO (FeNO) concentrations have suggested that it may be a useful measure of ongoing lower airways inflammation in patients with asthma and for guiding asthma therapy.[17]

CLINICAL PRESENTATION

CHRONIC ASTHMA

❸ Classic asthma is characterized by episodic dyspnea associated with wheezing; however, the clinical presentation of asthma is as diverse as the number of triggering events (see Clinical Presentation: Chronic Ambulatory Asthma). Although wheezing is the characteristic symptom of asthma, the medical literature is replete with the warning that "not all that wheezes is asthma." A wheeze is a high-pitched, whistling sound created by turbulent airflow through an obstructed airway, so any condition that produces significant obstruction can result in wheezing as a symptom. In addition, "all of asthma does not wheeze" is an equally justifiable warning. Patients may present with a chronic persistent cough as their only symptom.[2]

CLINICAL PRESENTATION: CHRONIC AMBULATORY ASTHMA

General

- Asthma is a disease of exacerbation and remission, so the patient may not have any signs or symptoms at the time of examination.

Symptoms

- The patient may complain of episodes of dyspnea, chest tightness, coughing (particularly at night), wheezing, or a whistling sound when breathing. These often occur in association with exercise, but also occur spontaneously or in association with known allergens.

Signs

- Expiratory wheezing on auscultation, dry hacking cough, or signs of atopy (allergic rhinitis and/or eczema) may occur.

Laboratory

- Spirometry demonstrates obstruction (reduced FEV_1/FVC) with reversibility following inhaled β_2-agonist administration (at least a 12% improvement in FEV_1).

Other Diagnostic Tests

- A fall in FEV_1 of at least 15% following 6 minutes of near maximal exercise. Elevated eosinophil count and IgE concentration in blood. Elevated FeNO (greater than 20 parts per billion in children younger than 12 years of age, and greater than 25 parts per billion in adults). Positive methacholine challenge (PC_{20} FEV_1 less than 12.5 mg/mL).

There is no single test that can diagnose asthma. The diagnosis is based primarily on a good history (Table 28–2).[2,6] The patient may have a family history of allergy or asthma or have symptoms of allergic rhinitis.[2] Reversibility of airways obstruction following administration of an inhaled short-acting β_2-agonist provides confirmation but is not by itself diagnostic. Patients with normal values of spirometry can be challenged by exercise or substances that produce bronchoconstriction, such as methacholine, to determine if they have hyperresponsive airways, but again, positive challenges are not diagnostic. Newer tests of inflammation in the airways such as induced sputum eosinophil counts and FeNO measurements are consistent with but not diagnostic of asthma.

Asthma has a widely variable presentation from chronic daily symptoms to only intermittent symptoms. The intervals between symptoms can be days, weeks, months, or years. Asthma also can vary as to its severity, the intrinsic intensity of the disease process. Severity is most easily and directly measured in a patient who is not currently receiving asthma treatment. The NAEPP has provided a means of classifying asthma severity that is broken down into two domains: impairment and risk.[6] This classification system is individualized for three age groups (0 to 4 years, 5 to 11 years, and ≥12 years) and summarized in Table 28–3. The intermittent and/or chronic nature of symptoms does not necessarily determine the severity of symptoms during exacerbations. The severity is determined by lung function, symptoms, nighttime awakenings, and interference with normal activity prior to therapy. Patients can present with a range from intermittent symptoms that require no medications or only occasional use of short-acting inhaled β_2-agonists to severe persistent asthma symptoms despite receiving multiple medications.

TABLE 28-2 Sample Questions[a] for the Diagnosis and Initial Assessment of Asthma

A "yes" answer to any question suggests that an asthma diagnosis is likely. In the past 12 months…

- Have you had a sudden severe episode or recurrent episodes of coughing, wheezing (high-pitched whistling sounds when breathing out), chest tightness, or shortness of breath?
- Have you had colds that "go to the chest" or that take more than 10 days to get over?
- Have you had coughing, wheezing, or shortness of breath during a particular season or time of the year?
- Have you had coughing, wheezing, or shortness of breath in certain places or when exposed to certain things (e.g., animals, tobacco smoke, perfumes)?
- Have you used any medications that help you breathe better? How often?
- Are your symptoms relieved when the medications are used?

In the past 4 weeks, have you had coughing, wheezing, or shortness of breath…

- At night that has awakened you?
- Upon awakening?
- After running, moderate exercise, or other physical activity?

[a]These questions are recommended by the National Asthma Education and Prevention Program but have not been formally validated.

SEVERE ACUTE ASTHMA

Uncontrolled asthma, with its inherent variability, can progress to an acute state where inflammation, airways edema, excessive accumulation of mucus, and severe bronchospasm result in a profound airways narrowing that is poorly responsive to usual bronchodilator therapy (see Clinical Presentation: Severe Acute Asthma).[2,6] Although this progression is the most common scenario, some patients experience rapid onset or hyperacute attacks.[2,6] Hyperacute attacks are associated with neutrophilic as opposed to eosinophilic infiltration and resolve rapidly with bronchodilator therapy, suggesting that smooth muscle spasm is the major pathogenic mechanism.[6] In most cases, emergency department visits for severe acute asthma represent the failure of an adequate therapeutic regimen for persistent asthma. Underuse of antiinflammatory drugs and excessive reliance on short-acting inhaled β_2-agonists are the major risk factors for severe exacerbations.[2] A blunted perception of airway obstruction may predispose certain individuals to fatal asthma attacks.[2]

CLINICAL PRESENTATION: SEVERE ACUTE ASTHMA

General

- An episode can progress over several days or hours (usual scenario) or can progress rapidly over 1 to 2 hours.

Symptoms

- The patient is anxious in acute distress and complains of severe dyspnea, shortness of breath, chest tightness, or burning. The patient is only able to say a few words with each breath. Symptoms are unresponsive to usual measures (inhaled short-acting β_2-agonist administration).

Signs

- Signs include expiratory and inspiratory wheezing on auscultation (breath sounds may be diminished with very severe obstruction), dry hacking cough, tachypnea, tachycardia, pale or cyanotic skin, hyperinflated chest with intercostal and supraclavicular retractions, and hypoxic seizures if very severe.

Laboratory

- PEF and/or FEV_1 less than 50% of normal predicted values. Decreased arterial oxygen (PaO_2), and O_2 saturations by pulse oximetry (SaO_2 less than 90% on room air is severe). Decreased arterial or capillary CO_2 if mild, but in the normal range or increased in moderate to severe obstruction.

Other Diagnostic Tests

- Blood gases to assess metabolic acidosis (lactic acidosis) in severe obstruction. Complete blood count if there are signs of infection (fever and purulent sputum). Serum electrolytes as therapy with β_2-agonist and corticosteroids can lower serum potassium and magnesium and increase glucose. Chest radiograph if signs of consolidation on auscultation.

EXERCISE-INDUCED BRONCHOSPASM

During vigorous exercise, pulmonary functions (FEV_1 and peak expiratory flow [PEF]) in patients with asthma increase during the first few minutes but then begin to decrease after 6 to 8 minutes (Fig. 28–3).[2] EIB is defined as a drop in FEV_1 of greater than 15% of baseline (preexercise value).[2] Most studies suggest that many patients with persistent asthma experience EIB.[2] The exact pathogenesis of EIB is unknown, but heat loss and/or water loss from the central airways

TABLE 28-3 Classifying Asthma Severity for Patients Who Are Not Currently Taking Long-Term Control Medications

	Children 0–4 Years and 5–11 Years of Age				
			Persistent		
	Components	**Intermittent**	***Mild***	***Moderate***	***Severe***
Impairment	Symptoms	≤2 days/week	>2 days/week but not daily	Daily	Throughout the day
	Nighttime awakenings (0–4 years)	0	Once or twice per month	Three to four times per month	> once per week
	(5–11 years)	≤ twice per month	Three to four times per month	> once per week, but not nightly	Often seven times per week
	SABA use for symptom control	≤2 days/week	>2 days/week but not daily	Daily	Several times per day
	Interference with normal activity	None	Minor limitation	Some limitation	Extremely limited
	Lung function	FEV_1 >80%	FEV_1 >80%	FEV_1 60%–80%	FEV_1 <60%
	(5–11 years)	FEV_1/FVC >85%	FEV_1/FVC >80%	FEV_1/FVC 75%–80%	FEV_1/FVC <75%
Risk	**Exacerbations**	**Intermittent**	**Persistent**		
	(0–4 years)	0–1/year	≥2 in 6 months or ≥4 wheezing episodes/1 year lasting >1day		
	(5–11 years)	0–2/year	>2 in 1 year →		
	Recommended step for initiating treatment	Step 1	Step 2	Step 3 and consider short course of systemic oral corticosteroids	
	Youths ≥12 Years of Age and Adults				
			Persistent		
	Components	**Intermittent**	***Mild***	***Moderate***	***Severe***
Impairment	Symptoms	≤2 days/week	>2 days/week but not daily	Daily	Throughout the day
	Nighttime awakenings	≤ twice per month	Three to four times per month	> once per week, but not nightly	Often seven times per week
	SABA use for symptom control	≤2 days/week	>2 days/week but not > once per day	Daily	Several times per day
	Interference with normal activity	None	Minor limitation	Some limitation	Extremely limited
	Lung function (Normal FEV_1/FVC: age 8–19 y 85%; 20–39 y 80%; 40–59 y 75%; 60–80 y 70%)	FEV_1 >80% FEV_1/FVC normal	FEV_1 >80% FEV_1/FVC normal	FEV_1 60%–80% FEV_1/FVC reduced 5%	FEV_1 <60% FEV_1/FVC reduced >5%
Risk	**Exacerbations**	**Intermittent**	**Persistent**		
		0–2/year	>2 in 1 year →		
	Recommended step for initiating treatment	Step 1	Step 2	Step 3 and consider short course of systemic oral corticosteroids	Step 4 or 5

FEV_1, force expiratory volume in the first second of expiration; FVC, forced vital capacity; SABA, short-acting β-antagonist.

appears to play an important role.[18] EIB is provoked more easily in cold, dry air, and warm, humid air can blunt or block it.[18] A number of studies have demonstrated increased plasma histamine, cysteinyl leukotrienes, prostaglandins, and tryptase concentrations during EIB, suggesting a role for mast cell degranulation.[18]

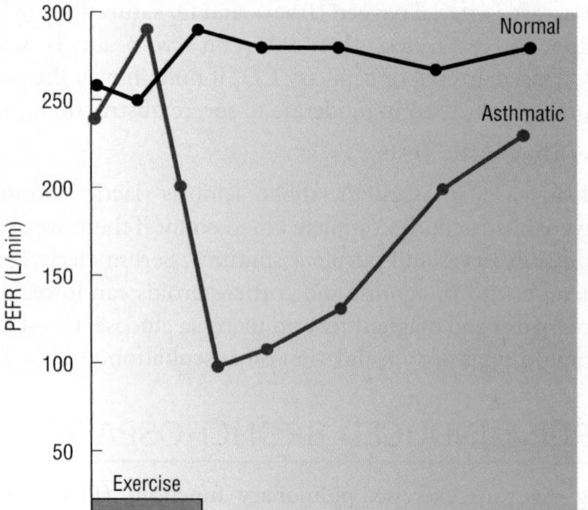

FIGURE 28-3. Typical responses to exercise in a normal subject and an asthmatic subject. Note the initial bronchodilation. (PEFR, peak expiratory flow rate.)

A refractory period following EIB lasts up to 3 hours after exercise. During this period, repeat exercise of the same intensity produces either no decrease in pulmonary function or a drop of less than 50% of the initial response.[18] This refractory period is thought to be caused by an acute depletion of mast cell mediators and time required for their repletion. Patients with known refractoriness to exercise will still respond to histamine, so acute hyporesponsiveness of airway smooth muscle does not appear to be a factor.[18]

Exercise-induced bronchospasm is believed to be a reflection of the increased BHR of asthmatics. A correlation, though not perfect, exists between EIB and reactivity to histamine and methacholine.[18] Other patient groups with BHR (e.g., after viral infection, cystic fibrosis, or allergic rhinitis) show bronchoconstriction after exercise to a lesser degree (5% to 10% drop) than patients with asthma (20% to 40% drops).[18] Patients will not always demonstrate the same sensitivity. During periods of remission, they often have a decreased sensitivity to the same degree of exercise. Finally, a number of children and adults with EIB are otherwise normal, without symptoms or abnormal pulmonary function except in association with exercise.[2] Elite athletes have a higher prevalence of EIB than the general population.[18]

NOCTURNAL ASTHMA

❸ Worsening of asthma during sleep is referred to as *nocturnal asthma*. Patients with nocturnal asthma exhibit significant falls in pulmonary function between bedtime and awakening.[2,8] Typically, their lung function reaches a nadir at 3 to 4 AM. Although the pathogenesis of this phenomenon is unknown, it is associated with diurnal patterns of endogenous cortisol secretion and circulating epinephrine.[8] Direct evidence for an inflammatory component to nocturnal asthma includes increased circulating histamine and activated eosinophils and leukotriene excretion at night associated with increased hyperresponsiveness to methacholine.[8]

Numerous other factors that may affect nocturnal worsening of asthma, including allergies and improper environmental control, gastroesophageal reflux, obstructive sleep apnea, and sinusitis, also must be considered when evaluating these patients.[2,6] Most experts consider nocturnal asthma to be a sign of inadequately treated persistent asthma.[2,8] Awakening from nocturnal asthma is a sensitive indicator of both severity and asthma control.[6]

FACTORS CONTRIBUTING TO ASTHMA SEVERITY

VIRAL RESPIRATORY INFECTIONS

Viral respiratory infections are primarily responsible for exacerbations of asthma, particularly in children younger than age 10 years.[6] Infants are particularly susceptible to airways obstruction and wheezing with viral infections because of their small airways. The most common cause of exacerbations in both children and adults is the common rhinovirus.[6] Other viruses isolated include respiratory syncytial virus, parainfluenza virus, coronavirus, and influenza viruses. The inflammatory response to viral infection is thought to be associated directly with the increasing BHR. Certain viruses (respiratory syncytial virus and parainfluenza virus) are capable of inducing specific IgE antibodies, and rhinovirus can activate eosinophils directly in asthmatics. The increase in asthma symptoms and BHR that occurs may last for days or weeks following resolution of the symptoms of the viral infection. Recent evidence does not support a beneficial effect of influenza vaccine for preventing asthma exacerbations from subsequent influenza infections.[19]

ENVIRONMENTAL AND OCCUPATIONAL FACTORS

Table 28–1 lists the agents, events, and mechanisms that are known to trigger asthma.[2,8] The general mechanisms are unknown but presumably are the result of epithelial damage and inflammation in the airway mucosa. Ozone and sulfur dioxide, common components of air pollution, have been used to induce BHR in animals. Exposure to 0.2 parts per million ozone for 2 to 3 hours can induce bronchoconstriction and increase BHR in asthmatics.[2,8] Sulfur dioxide in the ambient atmosphere is highly irritating. It presumably induces bronchoconstriction through mast cell or irritant-receptor involvement.[8] Asthma produced by repeated prolonged exposure to industrial inhalants is a significant health problem. It has been estimated that occupational asthma accounts for 2% of all asthmatic persons.[13] Persons with occupational asthma have the typical symptoms of asthma with cough, dyspnea, and wheeze. Typically, the symptoms are related to work and improve on weekends and during vacations.[13] In some instances, symptoms may persist even after termination of exposure.[13]

STRESS, DEPRESSION, AND PSYCHOSOCIAL FACTORS IN ASTHMA

Observational studies demonstrate an association between increased stress and worsening asthma, but the role is not clearly defined.[6] Bronchoconstriction from psychological factors appears to be mediated primarily through excess parasympathetic input. Atropine has been shown to block experimental psychogenic bronchoconstriction. It is most important to emphasize to both patients and parents that asthma is not an emotional disease; however, coping skills may benefit the patient who becomes emotionally distraught during an asthma attack.

RHINITIS AND SINUSITIS

Disorders of the upper respiratory tract, particularly rhinitis and sinusitis, have been linked with asthma for many years. As many as 40% to 50% of asthmatics have abnormal sinus radiographs.[2] However, chronic sinusitis may just represent a nonbacterial coexisting condition with allergic asthmatics because the histologic changes in the paranasal sinuses are similar to those seen in the lung and nose.[2] Treatment of upper airway disease may optimize overall asthma control. The mechanism by which sinusitis aggravates asthma is unknown. The treatment of allergic rhinitis with inhaled corticosteroids and cromolyn but not antihistamines will reduce BHR in asthmatic patients.[2] It has been postulated that transport of mucus chemotactic factors and inflammatory mediators from nasal passages during allergic rhinitis into the lung may accentuate BHR.

GASTROESOPHAGEAL REFLUX DISEASE

Symptoms of gastroesophageal reflux disease are common in both children and adults who have asthma.[6] Nocturnal asthma may be associated with nighttime reflux.[8] Reflux of acidic gastric contents into the esophagus is thought to initiate a vagally mediated reflex bronchoconstriction.[8] Also of concern is that most medications that decrease airways smooth muscle tone also have a relaxant effect on gastroesophageal sphincter tone. Although a systematic review concluded there was no significant improvement in asthma symptoms from medical management of gastroesophageal reflux disease, the standard approach is to initiate standard antireflux therapy in those patients who are exhibiting symptoms of reflux (particularly with nocturnal asthma) and observe the asthma symptoms.[2,20]

FEMALE HORMONES AND ASTHMA

Premenstrual worsening of asthma has been reported in as many as 30% to 40% of women in some studies, whereas worsening of pulmonary functions has been reported even in women who are unaware of worsening symptoms.[21] The pathophysiology is uncertain because estrogen replacement in postmenopausal women worsens asthma, whereas estradiol and progesterone administration have been variably reported to improve or have no effect on asthma in women with premenstrual asthma.[21] The clinical significance of menstruation-related asthma is still unclear because some studies report that up to 50% of emergency department visits by women were premenstrual, whereas others report no association with menstrual phase.[21,22] Studies indicate that, in general, BHR and symptoms improve in asthmatics during pregnancy.[8,21]

FOODS, DRUGS, AND ADDITIVES

There is no documentation in the literature of food allergens as triggers for asthma.[8] However, additives, specifically sulfites used as preservatives, can trigger life-threatening asthma exacerbations. Beer, wine, dried fruit, and open salad bars in particular have high concentrations of metabisulfites.[2] Severe oral corticosteroid-dependent patients should be warned about ingesting foods processed with sulfites. Another additive producing bronchospasm is benzalkonium chloride, which is found as a preservative in some nebulizer solutions of antiasthmatic drugs.[23]

Aspirin and other nonsteroidal antiinflammatory drugs can precipitate an attack in up to 20% of adults and 5% of children with asthma.[24] The mechanism is related to cyclooxygenase inhibition, and

5-lipoxygenase inhibition can alter dose–response but cannot completely block the symptoms.[24] The prevalence increases with age and severity of asthma.[6] The greatest frequency occurs in severe corticosteroid-dependent asthmatics in their fourth and fifth decades who also have perennial rhinitis and nasal polyposis (presence of several polyps).[24] Other drugs that do not precipitate bronchospasm but which prevent its reversal are the nonselective β-blocking agents.[2,6]

TREATMENT

Asthma

■ AEROSOL THERAPY FOR ASTHMA

❹ ❺ Aerosol delivery of drugs for asthma has the advantage of being site-specific and thus enhancing the therapeutic ratio.[2,25] Inhalation of short-acting β_2-agonists provides more rapid bronchodilation than either parenteral or oral administration, as well as the greatest degree of protection against EIB and other challenges.[2] Inhaled corticosteroids have been developed with rapid oral and systemic clearance to enhance lung activity and reduce systemic activity. Specific agents (e.g., cromolyn, nedocromil, formoterol, salmeterol, and ipratropium) are only effective by inhalation.[25] The international ban on the production and use of chlorofluorocarbons, has resulted in the ongoing development of new devices for delivering topically active medication.[2,25] Consequently, an understanding of aerosol drug delivery is essential to optimal asthma therapy. Table 28–4 lists the factors determining lung deposition of therapeutic aerosols.

Device Determinants of Delivery

Devices used to generate therapeutic aerosols include jet nebulizers, ultrasonic nebulizers, metered-dose inhalers (MDIs), and dry-powder inhalers (DPIs). The single most important device factor determining the site of aerosol deposition is particle size.[25] Devices for delivering therapeutic aerosols generate particles with aerodynamic diameters from 0.5 to 35 microns.[25] Particles larger than 10 microns deposit in the oropharynx, particles between 5 and 10 microns deposit in the trachea and large bronchi, particles 1 to 5 microns in size reach the lower airways, and particles smaller than 0.5 microns act as a gas and are exhaled. In asthma, the airways, not the alveoli, are the target for delivery. Respirable particles are deposited in the airways by three mechanisms: (a) inertial impaction, (b) gravitational sedimentation, and (c) Brownian diffusion.[25] The first two mechanisms are the most important for therapeutic aerosols and probably are the only factors that can be manipulated by patients.

Each delivery device within a classification generates specific aerosol characteristics, so extrapolation of delivery data from one device cannot be done for the other devices in the class. For instance, MDIs can deliver 5% to 50% of the actuated dose; DPIs, 10% to 30% of the labeled dose; and nebulizers, 2% to 15% of the starting dose.[25] Unlike nebulizers, MDIs and DPIs are portable and convenient. MDIs consist of a pressurized canister with a metering valve; the canister contains active drug, low-vapor-pressure propellants such as chlorofluorocarbon or hydrofluoroalkane (HFA), cosolvents, and/or surfactants.[25] With any change in these components, the Food and Drug Administration (FDA) considers it to be a new drug that requires stability, safety, and efficacy studies prior to approval. The drug is either in solution or a suspended micronized powder. To disperse the suspension for accurate delivery, the canister must be shaken. The metering chamber measures a liquid volume; consequently, the device must be held with the valve stem facing downward so that the chamber is covered with liquid (Fig. 28–4).[25] When the canister is actuated, the device releases the propellant and drug in a forceful spray whose particles are large (mass median aerodynamic diameter [MMAD] = 45 microns; Fig. 28–4).[25]As evaporation occurs, the particle size is reduced to a final MMAD of 0.5 to 5.5 microns depending on the MDI. The aerosol cloud of a chlorofluorocarbon-propelled MDI extends at least 10 inches beyond the MDI at the lowest MMAD, and that of an HFA-propelled MDI extends about 6 inches.[25]

The breath-actuated MDI Autohaler, is cocked with a lever to "load" the dose of medication, a baffle is opened by inspiratory pressure, and the dose is expelled from the canister metering chamber.[25] Although the need for hand–lung coordination for proper actuation is reduced significantly with breath-actuated MDIs, these devices do not allow the use of a spacer device.

Spacer devices are used frequently with a MDI to decrease oropharyngeal deposition and enhance lung delivery.[2,6] However, not all spacer devices produce similar effects. The design of spacers varies from simple, open-ended tubes that separate the MDI from the mouth to holding chambers with one-way valves (valved hold-

TABLE 28-4 Factors Determining Lung Deposition of Aerosols

Device	Device Factors	Patient Factors
Metered-dose inhaler (MDI)	Canister held inverted Formulation (CFC, HFA, solution, suspension) Actuator cleanliness Addition of a spacer device	Inspiratory flow (slow, deep) Breath-holding Coordinating actuation with inhalation Priming and shaking the device
Dry-powder inhaler (DPI)	Device cleanliness Resistance to inhalation Humidity	Inspiratory flow (deep, forceful) Tilting head back Maintaining parallel to ground once activated
Jet nebulizer (small volume)	Volume fill (3–6 mL) Gas flow (6–12 L/min) Dead-space volume Open versus closed system Thumb-activating valve Mouthpiece versus face mask	Inspiratory flow (slow, deep) Breath-holding Tapping nebulizer
Ultrasonic nebulizer	Volume fill Not effective for suspensions Mouthpiece versus face mask	Inspiratory flow (slow, deep) Breath-holding Tapping nebulizer
Spacer device	Volume (≥650 mL) One-way valves Holding chamber versus open-ended Metal versus plastic Mouthpiece versus face mask	Inspiratory flow (slow, deep) Time between actuation and inhalation (<5 s) Cleaning with detergent to reduce static Multiple actuations decrease delivery Coordination of actuation and inhalation for the simple open-tube spacers

CFC, chlorofluorocarbon; HFA, hydrofluoroalkane.

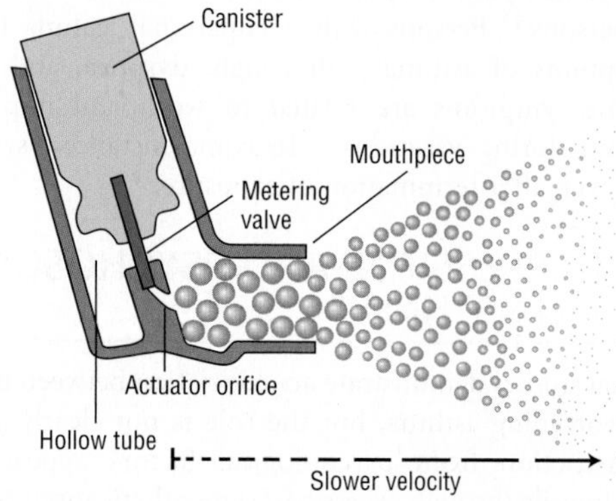

FIGURE 28-4. Illustration of a metered-dose inhaler demonstrating the particle size difference as the aerosol cloud extends outward.

ing chambers [VHCs]) that open during inhalation (the preferred system). A VHC allows evaporation of the propellant prior to inhalation permitting a greater number of drug particles to achieve a respirable droplet size. It also allows inhalation after actuation of the device, obviating the need for good hand–lung coordination.[25] Additionally, the large particles that normally would deposit in the oropharynx "rain out" in the spacer.[25] All the available spacers significantly reduce oropharyngeal deposition from MDIs, with the VHCs being superior to the open-ended tubes.[25] This reduction in oropharyngeal deposition is an important factor in reducing local adverse effects (i.e., hoarseness and thrush) from inhaled corticosteroids.[25] The change in lung delivery depends on both the MDI and the drug, where one spacer device may enhance delivery with one MDI preparation and decrease delivery with others.[25] The use of VHCs is less likely to enhance delivery from HFA propelled MDIs. Finally, over time, holding chambers can build up static electricity that attracts small particles to the sides of the chamber, significantly reducing aerosol availability. It is recommended that some spacers be washed weekly with household detergent, with a single rinse, and allowed to drip dry.[25]

Dry, micronized powders can be inhaled directly into the lung. A number of DPIs are now available for use in the United States, and others are under development.[25] Currently, there are no generic DPIs as each drug plus device has its own patent. Each DPI has unique characteristics with advantages and disadvantages (Table 28–5). The primary advantage of DPIs is that they are breath-actuated and require minimal hand–lung coordination, making it easier to teach patients proper technique.[25] Some DPIs are more flow-dependent than others.[25] Thus, similar to MDIs and spacers, delivery data from one DPI cannot be extrapolated to another.

Nebulizers come in two basic types: the jet nebulizer and the ultrasonic nebulizer. Jet nebulizers produce an aerosol from a liquid solution or suspension placed in a cup. A tube connected to a stream of compressed air or oxygen flows up through the bottom and draws the liquid up an adjacent open-ended tube.[25] The air and liquid strike a baffle, creating a droplet cloud that is then inhaled.[25] Ultrasonic nebulizers produce an aerosol by vibrating liquid lying above a transducer at speeds of about 1 mHz.[25] Both produce similar degrees of lung deposition, with the exception that ultrasonic nebulizers are ineffective for nebulizing micronized suspensions.[25] The aerosol output and lung delivery vary significantly among the commercially available jet nebulizers even when operated in the same manner.[25] Increasing fill volume will increase the total amount of drug delivered; however, it also will take longer for the patient to nebulize the dose.[25] The MMAD of the droplets is related directly to the gas flow, with flows of 5 to 12 L/min providing an aerosol cloud with a MMAD of 4 to 8 microns for most jet nebulizers.[25] Each jet nebulizer comes with its optimal operating instructions.

Patient Determinants of Delivery (See Table 28–4)

❻ ❼ The most important patient factor determining aerosol deposition is inspiratory flow.[2,25] High inspiratory flows increase the degree of deposition owing to impaction of particles of any size, thereby increasing deposition centrally (i.e., throat and large airways) and decreasing peripheral deposition. Use of a VHC will enhance the clinical efficacy in patients with poor hand–lung coordination but may offer no advantage in patients who can use an MDI optimally alone.[25] Optimal inspiratory flow for most MDIs is slow and deep (approximately 30 L/min or 5 seconds for a full inhalation).[2] In general, DPIs require higher inspiratory flows (≥60 L/min) and a change in inhalation technique (i.e., deep, forceful inspiration) for optimal dispersion of the powder, which, in turn, increases the amount of drug delivered to the larger central airways.[25] However, this difference in delivery may not produce clinically significant differences.[25] Patients should be cautioned not to exhale into DPIs because this causes loss of dose and moistens the dry powder, causing aggregation into larger particles. Patient factors that cannot be controlled include interpatient variability in airway geometry (particularly the differences between children and adults)[25] and the effects of bronchospasm, edema, and mucus hypersecretion. Mild obstruction increases aerosol deposition; however, severe obstruction probably leads to increased central deposition from impac-

TABLE 28-5 Characteristics of Various Inhalation Devices

Device	Drugs	Breath-Activated	Dose Counter	Other Excipients	Disadvantages
CFC MDI	All classes	No	No	Propellants, surfactants	Requires coordination of actuation and inhalation Large pharyngeal deposition Difficult to teach
HFA MDI	Albuterol Levalbuterol Corticosteroids	No No No	No/Yes No No	Propellants, surfactants, cosolvents	Same as CFC MDI
Autohaler MDI	Pirbuterol	Yes	No	CFC propellant, surfactant	Requires rapid inhalation to activate
MDI plus holding chamber	All classes	No	No		More expensive than MDI alone; less portable; some payers will not pay; inconsistent effect on delivery
Jet nebulizers	All classes	No	–	Preservatives in some solutions	Significant interbrand variability; expensive and time-consuming; less efficient than MDIs; contamination possible; preparations may be light- and temperature-sensitive (short shelf-life)
Ultrasonic nebulizer	Cromolyn solution short-acting β_2-agonist solutions	No	–	Preservatives in some solutions	Same as for jet nebulizers plus cannot be used for suspensions
Turbuhaler	Budesonide	Yes	Indicator for last 20 doses	No	Requires high inspiratory flow (60 L/min). Pharyngeal deposition; not approved for <6 years of age
Diskus	Fluticasone Salmeterol Fluticasone/salmeterol	Yes	Yes	Lactose filler	Not approved for <4 years of age
Aerolizer	Formoterol	Yes	–	Lactose filler	Single-dose capsules; not approved for <5 years of age Requires high inspiratory flow (≥60 L/min)
Twisthaler	Mometasone	Yes	Yes	Lactose filler	Not approved for <12 years of age

CFC, chlorofluorocarbon; HFA, hydrofluoroalkane; MDI, metered-dose inhaler.

Steps for Using Your Inhaler

Please demonstrate your inhaler technique at every visit.

1. Remove the cap and hold inhaler upright.
2. Shake the inhaler.
3. Tilt your head back slightly and breathe out slowly.
4. Position the inhaler in one of the following ways (A or B is optimal, but C is acceptable for those who have difficulty with A or B. C is required for breath-activated inhalers):

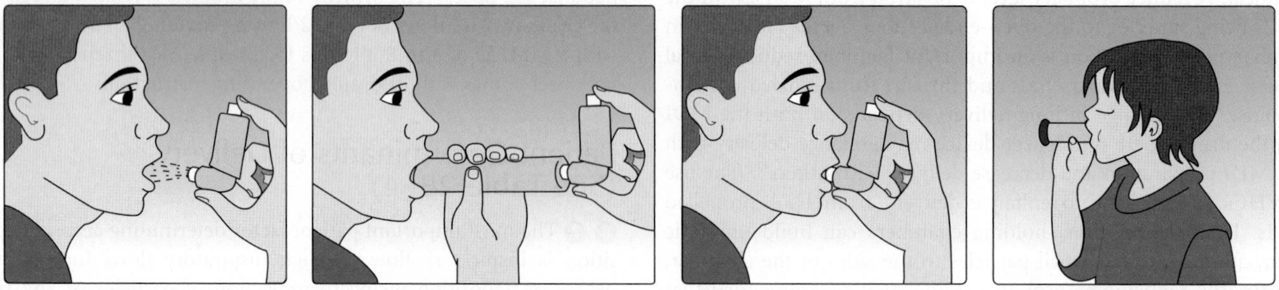

A Open mouth with inhaler 1 to 2 inches away.

B Use spacer/holding chamber (that is recommended especially for young children and for people using corticosteroids).

C In the mouth. Do not use for corticosteroids.

D NOTE: Inhaled dry powder capsules require a different inhalation technique. To use a dry powder inhaler, it is important to close the mouth tightly around the mouthpiece of the inhaler and to inhale rapidly.

5. Press down on the inhaler to release medication as you start to breathe in slowly.
6. Breathe in slowly (3 to 5 seconds).
7. Hold your breath for 10 seconds to allow the medicine to reach deeply into your lungs.
8. Repeat puff as directed. Waiting 1 minute between puffs may permit second puff to penetrate your lungs better.
9. Spacers/holding chambers are useful for all patients. They are particularly recommended for young children and older adults and for use with corticosteroids.

Avoid common inhaler mistakes. Follow these inhaler tips:

- Breathe out *before* pressing your inhaler.
- Inhale *slowly.*
- Breathe in through your mouth, not your nose.
- Press down on your inhaler at the *start* of inhalation (or within the first second of inhalation).
- Keep inhaling as you press down on inhaler.
- Press your inhaler only *once* while you are inhaling (one breath for each puff).
- Make sure you breathe in evenly and deeply.

NOTE: Other inhalers are becoming available in addition to those illustrated above. Different types of inhalers require different techniques.

FIGURE 28-5. Instructions for inhaler use from the National Asthma Education and Prevention Program Expert Panel Report 2. *(Adapted from reference 2.)*

tion.[25] The absolute delivery to the lung is not as important as consistency of delivery, assuming that a sufficient dose to produce the desired therapeutic effect is achieved. No single inhalation device is the best for all patients. Table 28–5 lists the differing characteristics of inhalation devices.

Appropriate inhalation technique is essential to achieve optimal drug delivery and therapeutic effect.[2,8] Figure 28–5 illustrates the components of appropriate technique. Approximately 50% to 80% of a dose from MDIs and DPIs impacts on the oropharynx and is then swallowed; the rest is either left in the device or exhaled.[25] It is important that actuation occurs during inhalation, although the time during inspiration is unimportant.[2,25] Although radiolabeled studies with chlorofluorocarbon-propelled MDIs indicate improved delivery by holding the actuator 2 to 3 cm in front of an open mouth to allow more evaporation and less impaction, physiologic studies with bronchodilators have failed to document an advantage for this method.[2,25] Many patients do not use their MDIs optimally, and patient instruction with demonstration is the most effective means of improving inhaler technique.[2,25] Even with instruction, up to 30% of patients, particularly young children and the elderly, cannot master the use of an MDI. For these patients, attachment of a VHC to the MDI or use of a breath-actuated MDI can improve efficacy significantly.[2,25] Mouth rinsing following treatment with MDI- and DPI-inhaled corticosteroids is important to minimize local effects and oral absorption.[2,25]

Delivery from high-resistance DPIs is more flow-dependent than from low-resistance DPIs. Thus younger children, and possibly elderly adults, will have more variability in delivery from high-resistance devices.[25] Most children who are younger than 4 years of age cannot generate a sufficient inspiratory flow to use DPIs. Young children (age <4 years) and infants generally require the use of a face mask attached to either an MDI plus VHC or to a nebulizer. The use of a face mask results in a reduction in lung delivery because of the portion of the aerosol inhaled nasally so the doses of drugs used in these patients is often not decreased from that of older children.

TREATMENT

Severe Acute Asthma

The primary goal is prevention of life-threatening asthma by early recognition of signs of deterioration and early intervention. As such, the principal goals of treatment include[2]

- Correction of significant hypoxemia
- Rapid reversal of airflow obstruction
- Reduction of the likelihood of relapse of the exacerbation or future recurrence of severe airflow obstruction
- Development of a written asthma action plan in case of a further exacerbation

These goals are best achieved by early initiation or intensification of treatment and close monitoring of objective measures of oxygenation and lung function.[2] Early response to treatment as measured by the improvement in FEV_1 at 30 minutes following inhaled β_2-agonists is the best predictor of outcome.[2,8] Providing adequate oxygen supplementation to maintain oxygen (O_2) saturations above 90% (or above 95% in pregnant women and those who have coexistent heart disease) is essential. In children younger than 6 years of age, in whom lung function measures are difficult to obtain, a combination of objective (e.g., oxygen saturation, capillary CO_2, respiratory rate, and heart rate) and subjective measures may be used to assess severity.[2,8]

The primary therapy of acute exacerbations is pharmacologic, which includes inhaled short-acting β_2-agonists and, depending on the severity, systemic corticosteroids, inhaled ipratropium and O_2 (Figs. 28–6 and 28–7).[6] It is important that therapy not be delayed, so the history and physical examination should be obtained while initial therapy is being provided. Patients at risk for life-threatening exacerbations require special attention. Risk factors include a history of previous severe asthma exacerbations (e.g., hospitalizations, intubations, or hypoxic seizures); difficulty perceiving asthma symptoms or severity of exacerbations; comorbidities (e.g., cardiac disease, other chronic lung disease, illicit drug use, or major psychosocial/psychiatric history); use of more than two canisters per month of short-acting inhaled β_2-agonists; and current intake of oral corticosteroids or recent withdrawal from oral corticosteroids.[6]

A complete blood count may be appropriate for patients with fever or purulent sputum, but modest leukocytosis is common in asthma exacerbations as a consequence of viral infection or secondary to corticosteroid administration. Chest radiography is not recommended for routine assessment but should be obtained for patients suspected of a complicating cardiopulmonary process or another pulmonary process (pneumothorax or pulmonary consolidation).[2] Serum electrolytes should be monitored if high-dose continuous-inhaled or systemic β_2-agonists are to be used because they can produce transient decreases in potassium, magnesium, and phosphate.[26] Measurement of serum electrolytes is also prudent in patients who take diuretics regularly, and in patients with coexistent cardiovascular disease. The combination of high-dose β_2-agonists and systemic corticosteroids occasionally may result in excessive elevations of glucose.[26]

Initial response should be achieved within minutes, and most patients experience significant improvement within the first 30 to 60 minutes of therapy, with most patients doubling their FEV_1 or PEF.[27] In patients ultimately admitted to the hospital, only a 10% to 20% predicted improvement is seen within the first 2 hours. Hypoxemia, primarily a result of ventilation–perfusion mismatch, is immediately correctable by low-flow oxygen.[2] While reversal of lung function into the normal range may take 12 to 24 hours, complete restoration takes much longer—up to 3 to 7 days.[8,26] A strategy to prevent recurrence, such as systemic corticosteroids and symptom or PEF monitoring, should be used.[2,8] It is essential to provide the patient with a self-management plan that includes a written action plan for dealing with exacerbations. Patients who are at risk for severe exacerbations should be taught how to use a peak-flow meter and to monitor morning peak flows at home.[2,8] In young children, an increased respiratory rate, increased heart rate, and inability to speak more than one or two words between breaths are signs of severe obstruction.[2] Oxygen saturations by pulse oximetry and peak flows should be measured in all patients who are not completely responding to initial intensive inhaled β_2-agonist therapy. Initially, on admission, the peak flows or clinical symptoms should be monitored every 2 to 4 hours. Prior to discharge from the emergency department or hospital, the patient should be given a sufficient supply of prednisone, taught the purpose of the medications and proper inhaler technique, and referred to

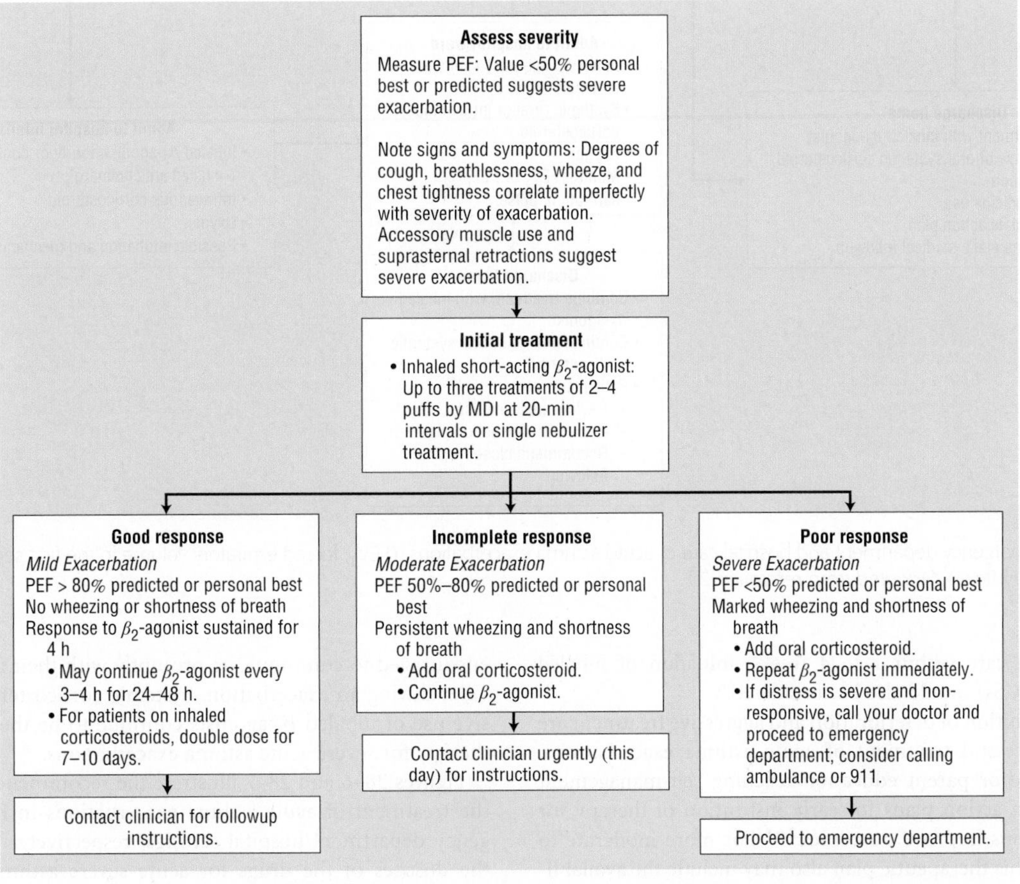

FIGURE 28-6. Home management of acute asthma exacerbation. Patients at risk for asthma-related death should receive immediate clinical attention after initial treatment. Additional therapy may be required. (MDI, metered-dose inhaler; PEF, peak expiratory flow.) *(Adapted from reference 2.)*

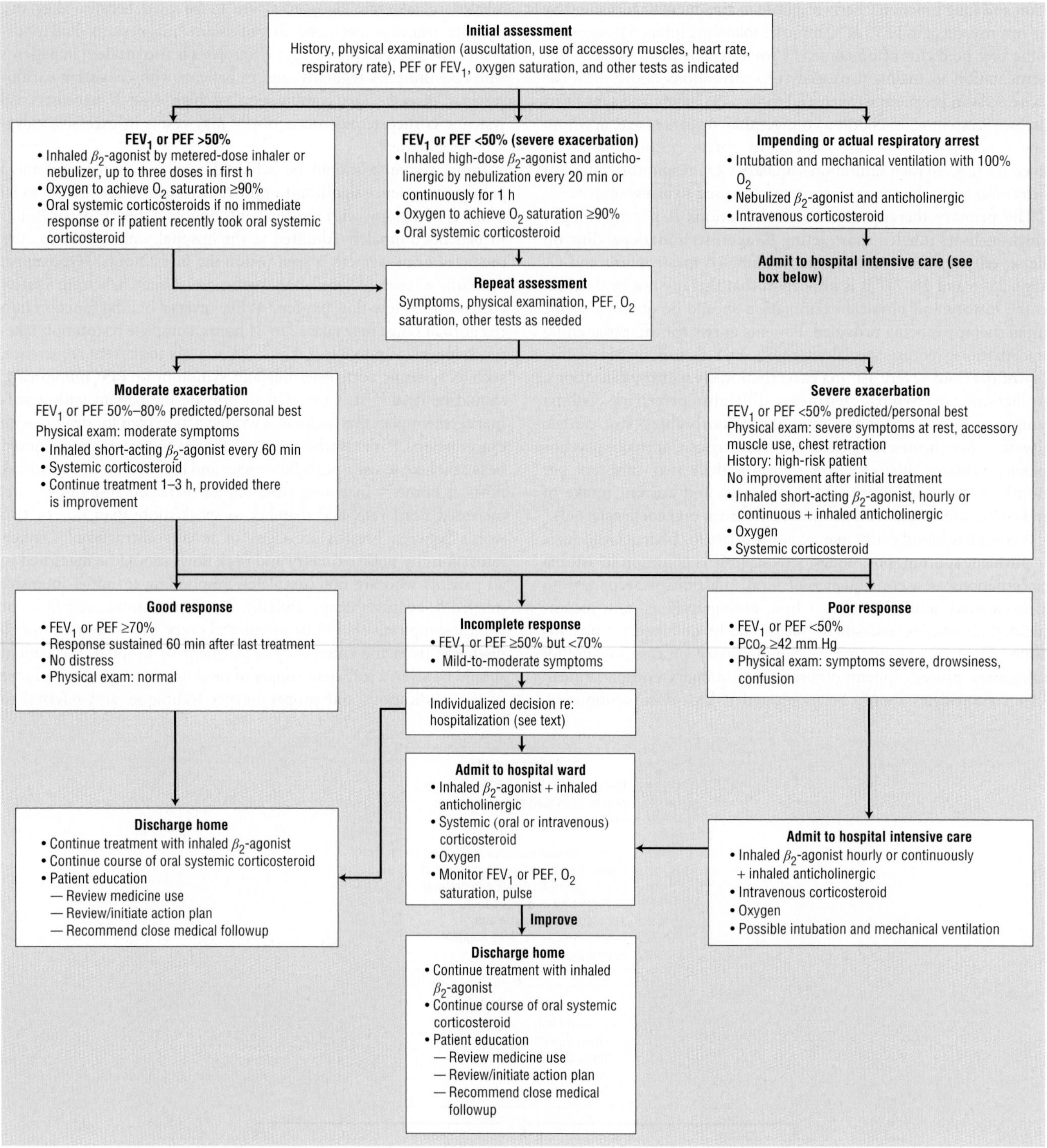

FIGURE 28-7. Emergency department and hospital care of acute asthma exacerbations. (FEV_1, forced expiratory volume in the first second of expiration; PEF, peak expiratory flow.) *(Adapted from reference 2.)*

followup asthma care within 1 to 4 weeks; initiation of inhaled corticosteroids (ICSs) should also be considered.[6]

❼ Early recognition of deterioration and aggressive treatment are the keys to successful treatment of acute asthma exacerbations. Thus patient and/or parent education teaching self-management skills and written action plans for early institution of therapy for acute exacerbations improve outcomes.[2,6,8] For more moderate to severe patients, this therapeutic plan also may include the availability of oral prednisone to begin at home.[2] Easy access by telephone to healthcare providers is also needed. Because of the rapid progression to severe asthma that can occur, patients and parents should be encouraged to communicate promptly with their asthma care provider during an exacerbation. Systemic corticosteroids and aggressive use of inhaled β_2-agonists continue to be the cornerstones of therapy for severe acute asthma exacerbations.[2,6]

Figures 28–6 and 28–7 illustrate the recommended therapies for the treatment of acute asthma exacerbations in home and emergency department/hospital settings, respectively.[2] Table 28–6 lists the dosages of the drugs for acute severe asthma.[2,6] Institutions should strongly consider developing critical pathways/treatment algorithms for their emergency departments because their implementation improves outcomes and decreases the cost of care.[28]

TABLE 28-6 Dosages of Drugs of Acute Severe Exacerbations of Asthma in the Emergency Department or Hospital

	Dosages		
Medications	***>6 Years Old***	***≤6 Years Old***	***Comments***
Inhaled β-agonists			
Albuterol nebulizer solution (5 mg/mL)	2.5–5 mg every 20 min for 3 doses, then 2.5–10 mg every 1–4 h as needed, or 10–15 mg/h continuously	0.15 mg/kg (minimum dose 2.5 mg) every 20 min for 3 doses, then 0.15–0.3 mg/kg up to 10 mg every 1–4 h as needed, or 0.5 mg/kg/h by continuous nebulization	Only selective β_2-agonists are recommended; for optimal delivery, dilute aerosols to minimum of 4 mL at gas flow of 6–8 L/min
Albuterol MDI (90 mcg/puff)	4–8 puffs every 30 min up to 4 h, then every 1–4 h as needed	4–8 puffs every 20 min for 3 doses, then every 1–4 h as needed	In patients in severe distress, nebulization is preferred; use holding-chamber-type spacer
Levalbuterol nebulizer solution	Give at one-half the mg dose of albuterol above	Give at one-half the mg dose of albuterol above	The single isomer of albuterol is likely to be twice as potent on a mg basis
Levalbuterol MDI (45 mcg/puff)	Give at one-half the mg dose of albuterol above	Give at one-half the mg dose of albuterol above	
Pirbuterol MDI (200 mcg/puff)	See albuterol dose	See albuterol dose; one-half as potent as albuterol on a mcg basis	Has not been studied in acute severe asthma
Systemic β-agonists			
Epinephrine 1:1000 (1 mg/mL)	0.3–0.5 mg every 20 min for 3 doses subcutaneously	0.01 mg/kg up to 0.5 mg every 20 min for 3 doses subcutaneously	No proven advantage of systemic therapy over aerosol
Terbutaline (1 mg/mL)	0.25 mg every 20 min for 3 doses subcutaneously	0.01 mg/kg every 20 min for 3 doses, then every 2–6 h as needed subcutaneously	Not recommended
Anticholinergics			
Ipratropium bromide nebulizer solution (0.25 mg/mL)	500 mcg every 30 min for 3 doses, then every 2–4 h as needed	250 mcg every 20 min for 3 doses, then 250 mcg every 2–4 h	May mix in same nebulizer with albuterol; do not use as first-line therapy; only add to β_2-agonist therapy
Ipratropium bromide MDI (17 mcg/puff)	4–8 puffs as needed every 2–4 h	4–8 puffs as needed every 2–4 h	Not recommended because dose in inhaler is low and has not been studied in acute asthma
Corticosteroids			
Prednisone, methylprednisolone, prednisolone	60–80 mg in 3 or 4 divided doses for 48 h, then 30–40 mg/day until PEF reaches 70% of personal best	1 mg/kg every 6 h for 48 h, then 1–2 mg/kg/day in 2 divided doses until PEF is 70% of normal predicted	For outpatient "burst" use 1–2 mg/kg/day, maximum 60 mg, for 3–7 days; it is unnecessary to taper course

FEV_1, forced expiratory volume in the first second of expiration; MDI, metered-dose inhaler; PEF, peak expiratory flow.

Note: No advantage has been found for very-high-dose corticosteroids in acute severe asthma, nor is there any advantage for intravenous administration over oral therapy. The usual regimen is to continue the frequent multiple daily dosing until the patient achieves an FEV1 or PEF of 50% of personal best or normal predicted value and then lower the dose to twice-daily dosing. This usually occurs within 48 hours. The final duration of therapy following a hospitalization or emergency department visit may be from 7 to 14 days. If patient is then started on inhaled corticosteroids, studies indicate there is no need to taper the systemic steroid dose. If the followup therapy is to be given once daily, studies indicate there may be an advantage to giving the single daily dose in the afternoon at around 3 pm.

NONPHARMACOLOGIC AND ANCILLARY THERAPY

Infants and young children may be mildly dehydrated owing to increased insensible loss, vomiting, and decreased intake.[2] Unless dehydration has occurred, increased fluid therapy is not indicated in acute asthma management because the capillary leak from cytokines and increased negative intrathoracic pressures may promote edema in the airways.[2] Correction of significant dehydration is always indicated, and the urine specific gravity may help to guide therapy in young children, in whom the state of hydration may be difficult to determine.[2] Chest physical therapy and mucolytics are not recommended in the therapy of acute asthma.[6] Sedatives should not be given because anxiety may be a sign of hypoxemia, which could be worsened by central nervous system depressants. Antibiotics also are not indicated routinely because viral respiratory tract infections are the primary cause of asthma exacerbations.[2,8] Antibiotics should be reserved for patients who have signs and symptoms of pneumonia (e.g., fever, pulmonary consolidation, and purulent sputum from polymorphonuclear leukocytes). *Mycoplasma* and *Chlamydia* are infrequent causes of severe asthma exacerbations but should be considered in patients with high oxygen requirements.[8]

Respiratory failure or impending respiratory failure as measured by rising $Pa{CO_2}$ (>45 mm Hg) or failure to correct hypoxemia with supplemental oxygen therapy is treated with intubation and mechanical ventilation. To prevent barotrauma and pneumothoraces from excess positive pressure, it is recommended that controlled hypoventilation or permissive hypercapnia be used (correcting the hypoxemia, $Pa{O_2}$ >60 mm Hg, but allowing the $Pa{CO_2}$ to rise to the high 60 mm Hg range).

PHARMACOTHERAPY

β_2-Agonists

❹ The short-acting inhaled β_2-agonists are the most effective bronchodilators and the treatment of first choice for the management of severe acute asthma.[2,8,26] Up to 66% of adults presenting to an emergency department require only three doses of 2.5-mg nebulized albuterol to be discharged.[27] Most well-controlled clinical trials have demonstrated equal to greater efficacy and greater safety of aerosolized β_2-agonists over systemic administration regardless of the severity of obstruction.[2,26] Systemic adverse effects, hypokalemia, hyperglycemia, tachycardia, and cardiac dysrhythmias are more pronounced in patients receiving systemic β_2-agonist therapy. Children younger than 2 years of age achieve clinically significant responses from nebulized albuterol.[2,29] Effective doses of aerosolized β_2-agonists can be delivered successfully through mechanical ventilator circuits to infants, children, and adults in respiratory failure secondary to severe airways obstruction.[29]

Frequent administration of inhaled β_2-agonists (every 20 minutes or continuous nebulization) is superior to the same dosage administered at 1-hour intervals.[30] In the subset of more severely obstructed patients, continuous nebulization decreases the hospital admission rate, provides greater improvement in the FEV_1 and PEF, and reduces duration of hospitalization when compared with intermittent (hourly) nebulized albuterol in the same total dose.[30] Thus continuous nebulization is recommended for patients having an unsatisfactory response (achieving less than 50% of normal FEV_1 or PEF) following the initial three doses (every 20 minutes) of aerosolized β_2-agonists and potentially for patients presenting initially with PEF or FEV_1 values of less than 30% of predicted normal.[2,30]

The doses of inhaled β_2-agonists for severe acute asthma (see Table 28–6) have been derived empirically. The β_2-agonists follow a log-linear dose–response curve.[31] In addition, the dose–response curve is shifted to the right by more severe bronchospasm or by increased concentrations of bronchospastic mediators, which is characteristic of functional antagonists.[31] The ability to increase the dose of the short-acting aerosolized β_2-agonists by as much as 5- to 10-fold over doses producing adequate bronchodilation in chronic stable asthmatics is what contributes to their efficacy in reversing the bronchospasm of acute severe asthma. The nebulizer dose of inhaled β_2-agonists for children often is listed on a weight basis (milligrams per kilogram). However, a fixed minimal dose (2.5 mg albuterol or equivalent), as opposed to a weight-adjusted dose, is more appropriate in younger children because children younger than 5 years of age receive a lower lung dose.[25] Adults dosed on a weight basis demonstrate excessive cardiac stimulation, so they have fixed maximal doses (see Table 28–6).[29] Initial doses of inhaled β_2-agonists can produce vasodilation, worsening ventilation–perfusion mismatch, slightly lowering oxygen saturation or PaO_2.[26] High-doses of inhaled β_2-agonists can produce a decrease in serum potassium concentration, an increase in heart rate, and an increase in serum glucose concentration. However, both children and adults receiving continuously nebulized β_2-agonists have demonstrated decreased heart rates as their lung function improves.[30] Thus, an elevated heart rate is not an indication to use lower doses or to avoid using inhaled β_2-agonists.

Some controversy exists concerning the most cost-effective delivery system (MDI plus VHC vs. nebulization) to be used in treating severe acute asthma in the emergency department and hospital (see Clinical Controversies below).[25,29] The DPIs are currently not indicated for the treatment of severe acute asthma exacerbations because of the higher inspiratory flows required for adequate delivery.[25]

Corticosteroids

Systemic corticosteroids are indicated in all patients with acute severe asthma not responding completely to initial inhaled β_2-agonist administration (every 20 minutes for three to four doses).[2] Intravenous therapy offers no therapeutic advantage over oral administration.[26,32] This therapy usually is continued until hospital discharge. Tapering the dose in acute asthma following discharge from the hospital appears unnecessary, provided that patients are prescribed inhaled corticosteroids for outpatient therapy.[2] Most patients achieve 70% of predicted normal FEV_1 within 48 hours and 80% of predicted by 6 days after plateauing by day 3. Thus maintaining systemic corticosteroid courses for 10 to 14 days may be unnecessarily long in some patients. Indeed, many patients not admitted to the hospital respond to 3- to 5-day courses of systemic corticosteroids. Short courses of oral prednisone (3 to 10 days) have been effective in preventing hospitalizations in infants and young children.[2] It is recommended that a full dose of the corticosteroid be continued until the patient's peak flow reaches 70% of predicted normal or personal best.[2]

Multiple daily dosing of systemic corticosteroids for the initial therapy of acute asthma exacerbations appears warranted because receptor-binding affinities of lung corticosteroid receptors are decreased in the face of airway inflammation.[32] However, patients with less-severe exacerbations may be treated adequately with once-daily administration. High-dose and very-high-pulse-dose corticosteroid regimens do not enhance the outcomes in severe acute asthma but are associated with a higher likelihood of side effects.[32]

Studies of ICSs in acute exacerbations of asthma have provided conflicting results. Studies have demonstrated both greater and lesser efficacy than standard doses of oral corticosteroids.[32] Currently, there is insufficient evidence supporting efficacy in the emergency department setting, although continued research appears warranted.[32] There is evidence that prescribing ICSs on discharge from the emergency department reduces the risk of relapse.[32] This policy seems like a reasonable recommendation because inflammation is the underlying cause of deterioration in most cases.[6]

Anticholinergics

Inhaled ipratropium bromide produces a further improvement in lung function of 10% to 15% over inhaled β_2-agonists alone. In children and adults, multiple-dose ipratropium bromide added to initial therapy also produced a reduced hospitalization rate in the subset of patients with an FEV_1 of less than 30% of predicted at baseline.[33] Ipratropium bromide, a quaternary amine, is poorly absorbed and produces minimal or no systemic effects. Care should be used when administering ipratropium bromide by nebulizer. If a tight mask or mouthpiece is not used, the ipratropium bromide that deposits in the eyes may produce pupillary dilation and difficulty in accommodation. Ipratropium bromide is not a vasodilator, so unlike β_2-agonists it will not worsen ventilation–perfusion mismatch.[26]

Alternative Therapies

The emergency department use of aminophylline, a moderate bronchodilator, for acute asthma has not been recommended for a number of years.[2] Clinical trials of aminophylline in adults and children hospitalized with acute asthma have not reported sufficient evidence of efficacy (improvement in lung function and reduced hospital stay) but have reported an increased risk of adverse effects.[34] Adverse effects of theophylline include nausea and vomiting and potentiation of the cardiac effects of the inhaled β_2-agonists.

Magnesium sulfate is a moderately potent bronchodilator, producing relaxation of smooth muscle and central nervous system depression.[35] The use of intravenous magnesium sulfate in patients presenting to the emergency department is controversial (see Clinical Controversies below).[35,36] The adverse effects of magnesium sulfate include hypotension, facial flushing, sweating, nausea, loss of deep tendon reflexes, and respiratory depression.[35] Some patients have required dopamine to treat the hypotension.

Helium is an inert gas of low density with no pharmacologic properties that can lower resistance to gas flow and increase ventilation because the low density decreases the pressure gradient needed to achieve a given level of turbulent flow, converting turbulent flow to laminar flow.[2] Helium is given as a mixture of helium and oxygen (heliox), usually 60% to 70% helium with 30% to 40% oxygen.[37] As with a number of experimental approaches, heliox was reported to be efficacious in initial nonrandomized clinical trials. However, the small number of randomized, controlled trials completed to date have failed to document efficacy.[37] Although heliox is free of adverse effects, its use is limited to patients with a low inspired oxygen requirement because the decrease in density generally is insignificant clinically with less than 60% helium.[37]

The inhalational anesthetics halothane, isoflurane, and enflurane all have been reported to have a positive effect in children and adults with severe asthma that is unresponsive to standard medical therapy.[2] The proposed mechanisms for inhalational anesthetics include direct action on bronchial smooth muscle, inhibition of airway reflexes, attenuation of histamine-induced bronchospasm, and interaction with β_2-adrenergic receptors.[2] Well-controlled trials with these agents have not been completed. Potential adverse effects include myocardial depression, vasodilation, arrhythmias, and depression of mucociliary function. In addition, the practical problem of delivery and scavenging these agents in the intensive care environment as opposed to the operating room is a concern. The use of volatile anesthetics cannot be recommended based on insufficient evidence of efficacy.

Ketamine has been recommended for rapid induction of anesthesia in patients with asthma who require intubation and mechanical ventilation.[2] Ketamine is thought to produce bronchodilation from a combination of an increase in circulating catecholamines, direct

TABLE 28-7 Pharmacologic Responses to Sympathomimetic Agonists

Tissue	Receptor Type	Response
Airways	β_2	Smooth muscle relaxation (bronchodilation), increased ciliary beat, increased serous secretion, and inhibition of mast cell degranulation
	α	Smooth muscle contraction (bronchoconstriction?)
Heart	β_1	Inotropic and chronotropic
	β_2	Chronotropic
Vasculature	β_2	Vasodilation, decrease microvascular leakage
	α	Vasoconstriction
Skeletal	β_2	Increased neuromuscular transmission (tremor and increased strength of contraction)
Uterus	β_2	Relaxation (tocolysis)
Metabolic	α, β_1	Glycogenolysis, lipolysis
	β_2	Gluconeogenesis, hypokalemia, increased lactate production

smooth muscle relaxation, and inhibition of vagal flow.[2] Anecdotal reports have suggested that ketamine is useful as a short-term adjunct in severe acute asthma; controlled trials have not provided sufficient evidence of efficacy, however. Ketamine has several significant adverse effects, including the anesthesia emergence reaction, which can alter mood and cause delirium. These emergence phenomena occur in at least 25% of patients older than 16 years of age; the incidence seems to be much lower in younger patients.[2] Other risks include an increase in heart rate, arterial blood pressure, and cerebral blood flow because of its sympathetic effects.[26]

SPECIAL POPULATIONS

6 Infants and children younger than 4 years of age may be at greater risk of respiratory failure than older children and adults. Although treated with the same drugs, these younger children require the use of a facemask as opposed to a mouthpiece for delivery of aerosolized medication. Use of the facemask reduces delivery of drug to the lung by one-half so that a minimal dose is recommended as opposed to a weight-adjusted dose.[25,29] The facemask should be sized appropriately and should fit snugly over the nose and mouth. Use of the "blow-by" method, where the respiratory therapist or parent places the mask or extension tubing near the child's nose and mouth, should be discouraged because holding the mask as few as 2 cm from the patient's face reduces lung delivery of the aerosol by 80%.[25]

DRUG CLASS INFORMATION

Short-Acting β_2-Agonists

5 6 The β_2-agonists are the most effective bronchodilators available. The β_2-adrenergic receptors are transmembrane proteins consisting of clusters of seven helices of amino acids that form the ligand-binding core.[31] The human β_2-adrenergic receptors are polymorphic in structure, with the most common polymorphisms in the amino terminus of the receptor at amino acid positions 16 (encoding either arginine [Arg] or glycine [Gly]) and 27 (encoding either glutamine [Gln] or glutamic acid [Glu]).[38] Some of the polymorphisms determine responsiveness to β_2-agonists, whereas others may act as disease modifiers (see Treatment section on Chronic Asthma, Clinical Controversy below).[38] Stimulation of β_2-adrenergic receptor activates cytoplasmic G proteins, which, in turn, activate adenylyl cyclase to produce cyclic adenosine monophosphate (cAMP), generally thought to be responsible for the bulk of activity through activation of various proteins by cAMP-dependent protein kinase A.[31] This activation, in turn, decreases unbound intracellular calcium, producing smooth muscle relaxation, mast cell membrane stabilization, and skeletal muscle stimulation.[31] Despite the fact that β_2-agonists are potent inhibitors of mast cell degranulation in vitro, they do not inhibit the late asthmatic response to allergen challenge or the subsequent bronchial hyperresponsiveness.[2,31] Long-term administration of β_2-agonists does not reduce BHR, confirming a lack of significant antiinflammatory activity.[31] β_2-Adrenergic stimulation also activates Na^+-K^+-ATPase, produces gluconeogenesis, and enhances insulin secretion, resulting in a mild to moderate decrease in serum potassium concentration by driving potassium intracellularly.[31] The chronotropic response to β_2-agonists is mediated in part by baroreceptor reflex mechanisms as a result of the drop in blood pressure from vascular smooth muscle relaxation, as well as by direct stimulation of cardiac β_2-receptors and some β_1 stimulation at high concentrations.[31] Table 28–7 lists the pharmacologic effects of adrenergic receptor stimulation. Because β_1-receptor stimulation produces excessive cardiac stimulation, resulting in cardiac arrhythmias, and because the inotropic effect enhancing myocardial oxygen consumption leads to myocardial necrosis, there is no rationale for using non–β_2-selective agonists in the treatment of asthma.[31]

Table 28–8 compares the various β-adrenergic agonists used in asthma in terms of selectivity, potency, oral activity, and duration of action. The β_2-agonists are functional or physiologic antagonists in that they relax airway smooth muscle regardless of the mechanism for constriction.[31] When administered in equipotent doses, all the short-acting drugs produce the same intensity of response; the only differences are in duration of action and cardiac toxicity.[2,31] The catecholamine derivatives all have the disadvantage of rapid inactivation of their 3,4-hydroxyl catechol group from catechol-O-methyltransferase found in the gastrointestinal tract, rendering them orally inactive. In addition, catecholamines are taken up rapidly into tissues by secondary uptake mechanisms that limit their receptor occupancy and thus have a shorter duration of action.[31] All the β_2-agonists are more bronchoselective when administered by the aerosol route. Aerosol administration of the short-acting β_2-agonists provides more rapid response and greater protection against

TABLE 28-8 Relative Selectivity, Potency, and Duration of Action of the β-Adrenergic Agonists

Agent	Selectivity β_1	Selectivity β_2	Potency, β_2[a]	Duration of Action[b]: Bronchodilation (h)	Duration of Action[b]: Protection (h)[c]	Oral Activity
Isoproterenol	++++	++++	1	0.5–2	0.5–1	No
Metaproterenol	+++	+++	15	3–4	1–2	Yes
Albuterol	+	++++	2	4–8	2–4	Yes
Pirbuterol	+	++++	5	4–8	2–4	Yes
Terbutaline	+	++++	4	4–8	2–4	Yes
Formoterol	+	++++	0.12	≥12	6–12	Yes
Salmeterol	+	++++	0.5	≥12	6–12	No

[a]Relative molar potency to isoproterenol: 15 = lowest potency.
[b]Median durations with the highest value after a single dose and lowest after chronic administration.
[c]Protection refers to the prevention of bronchoconstriction induced by exercise or nonspecific bronchial challenges.

provocations that induce bronchospasm such as exercise and allergen challenges than does systemic administration.[25] Differences in myocardial effects are discernible between selective and nonselective agents even when administered as aerosols, particularly at the higher doses used for severe acute asthma. The β_2-agonists also differ in efficacy or ability to activate the β_2-adrenergic receptors. Full agonists include the catecholamines, metaproterenol, and formoterol.[31] Partial agonists include albuterol, terbutaline, pirbuterol, and salmeterol.[31] The principal differences between full and partial agonists are that full agonists require a lower fraction of receptor occupancy to produce their maximum effect and more easily produce receptor desensitization.[38] However, these differences have not been proven to be clinically significant.

All synthetic β_2-agonists are 1:1 racemic mixtures of two mirror images (enantiomers) owing to an asymmetric or chiral carbon.[38] Because most physiologic functions (receptor occupancy and activation and enzymatic metabolism) are stereoselective, the (*R*)-enantiomers of the β_2-agonists are the most pharmacologically active isomer.[38] Although it was initially thought that the (*S*)-enantiomers were essentially inactive owing to the 100- to 1,000-fold potency difference between the enantiomers, studies in animal models and isolated in vitro tissue preparations have suggested that the (*S*)-enantiomer of albuterol may be proinflammatory and could induce BHR.[38] However, evidence that this occurs consistently in humans or is clinically relevant is lacking.[38] The pharmacokinetics also are stereoselective, although not predictable. (*R*)-Albuterol is metabolized more rapidly than (*S*)-albuterol, which could lead to accumulation of (*S*)-albuterol with continued dosing.[38] This accumulation is more exaggerated with oral dosing, as would be expected from a drug with a high first-pass effect.[31] On the other hand, (*S*)-terbutaline is eliminated more rapidly than (*R*)-terbutaline.[38]

Both the intensity and duration of response are dose-dependent, and more importantly, the dose–response relationship is dynamic.[31] At increasing levels of baseline bronchoconstriction (irrespective of the stimulus), the dose-response curve is shifted to the right, and the duration of bronchodilation is decreased.[31] This shift is reflected in the need for higher, more frequent doses in acute asthma exacerbations; the duration of protection against significant provocation is much less than the duration of bronchodilation in chronic stable asthma (see Table 28–8).[31]

Chronic administration of β_2-agonists leads to downregulation (decreased number of β_2-receptors) and a decreased binding affinity for these receptors.[31] Systemic corticosteroid therapy can both prevent and partially reverse this phenomenon.[2,31] However, the use of inhaled corticosteroids appears to have minimal ability to prevent tolerance to β_2-agonists.[31] The homozygous Gly-16 form of the receptor downregulates to a much greater extent compared with the homozygous Arg-16 form of the receptor with heterozygous Arg-16/Gly-16 intermediately desensitized.[38] On the other hand, glutamate substitution at codon 27 (Glu-27) protects against downregulation compared with the glutamine form (Gln-27) of the receptor.[38] However, the Gly-16 overcomes any protective effect of Glu-27.[38] Tolerance primarily reduces duration of bronchodilation as opposed to peak response although that can occur as well. A significantly greater tolerance develops in other tissues (e.g., lymphocytes and cardiac and skeletal muscle) compared with the lung primarily as a result of the surplus β_2 receptors found in respiratory smooth muscle.[31] Tolerance to the extrapulmonary effects (cardiac stimulation and hypokalemia) may account for a lack of significant cardiac effects with retention of the bronchodilator response despite chronic inhaled β_2-agonist therapy, whereas tolerance to mast cell stabilization may be a drawback to chronic use.[31] Thus, chronic β_2-agonist administration produces a tolerance of minimal clinical significance that is overcome easily by increasing the dose or by administering corticosteroids.[2,31,38] Most of the tolerance occurs within a week of regular administration and does not worsen with continued administration. As would be expected from a receptor phenomenon, tolerance is a cross-tolerance to all β_2-agonists.[31] Whether or not regular use of short-acting inhaled β_2-agonists produces worsening of asthma in a subset of patients remains controversial (see Treatment section on Chronic Asthma, Clinical Controversy below), but it does not appear to occur in the entire population.[38] Regular treatment with short-acting β_2-agonists can increase BHR and in homozygous Arg-16 patients reduced morning PEF and increased exacerbations.[38] Regular treatment (four times daily) does not improve symptom control over as-needed use.[2,8]

In conclusion, the inhaled short-acting selective β_2-agonists are indicated for the treatment of intermittent episodes of bronchospasm. They are the first treatment of choice for acute severe asthma and exercise-induced bronchospasm.[2,8,31] They inhibit EIB in a dose-dependent fashion and provide complete protection for a 2-hour period following inhalation with varying levels of patient-dependent protection over 4 hours.[31] Although the regular administration of β_2-agonists slightly decreases the effect, two inhalations prior to exercise still essentially blocks exercise-induced bronchospasm completely (1% versus 5% drop in FEV_1).[38]

Systemic Corticosteroids

❹ The corticosteroids are the most effective antiinflammatories available to treat asthma.[2,6,8] Actions useful in treating asthma include (a) increasing the number of β_2-adrenergic receptors and improving the receptor responsiveness to β_2-adrenergic stimulation, (b) reducing mucus production and hypersecretion, (c) reducing BHR, and (d) reducing airway edema and exudation.[7,8] The glucocorticoid receptor is found in the cytoplasm of most cells throughout the body, explaining the multiple effects of systemic corticosteroids. Although there is no difference between the glucocorticoid receptors found throughout the body, genetic differences between glucocorticoid receptors from different individuals may determine some of the variations in response.[39] The corticosteroids are lipophilic, readily cross the cell membrane, and combine with the glucocorticoid receptor. The activated complex then enters the nucleus, where it acts as a transcription factor leading to gene activation or suppression.[40] This leads to specific messenger ribonucleic acid (mRNA) production, resulting in increased production of antiinflammatory mediators; suppression of several proinflammatory cytokines such as IL-1, GM-CSF, IL-3, IL-4, IL-5, IL-6, and IL-8, reducing inflammatory cell activation, recruitment, and infiltration; and decreasing vascular permeability.[40] In addition, the activated glucocorticoid receptor complex can act directly with cytoplasmic transcription factors, nuclear factor κB, and activating protein 1 to prevent the action of proinflammatory cytokines on the cell.[40]

Owing to the mechanism that modifies gene expression, the time required to see the particular effect depends on the time required for new protein synthesis, decreased formation of the particular mediator, and resolution of the inflammatory response.[40] Generally, the cellular and biochemical effects are immediate, but varying amounts of time are required to produce a clinical response. β_2-Receptor density increases within 4 hours of corticosteroid administration.[40] Improved responsiveness to β_2-agonists occurs within 2 hours.[40] In severe acute asthma, 4 to 12 hours may be required before any clinical response is noted.[32,40] Reversal of seasonally increased BHR requires at least 1 week of therapy.[40] The chronic use of corticosteroids does not induce a state of corticosteroid dependence. Nor is there evidence of tolerance produced by chronic administration.

Table 28–9 compares the corticosteroids used in asthma.[39–41] Besides acute severe asthma, systemic corticosteroids are also recommended for the treatment of impending episodes of severe asthma unresponsive to bronchodilator therapy.[2,6,8] The effects of corticosteroids in asthma

TABLE 28-9 Pharmacodynamic/Pharmacokinetic Comparison of the Corticosteroids

Systemic	Antiinflammatory Potency	Mineralcorticoid Potency	Duration of Biologic Activity (h)	Elimination Half-Life (h)	
Hydrocortisone	1	1.0	8–12	1.5–2.0	
Prednisone	4	0.8	12–36	2.5–3.5	
Methylprednisolone	5	0.5	12–36	3.3	
Dexamethasone	25	0	36–54	3.4–4.0	
ICS	**Receptor Binding Affinity**	**Topical Skin Blanching**	**Oral Bioavailability (%)**	**Systemic Clearance (L/h)**	**Half-Life (h) IV/ Inhaled**
BDP/BMP[b]	0.4/13.5	600/400	15–20	UK	0.5/1.5–6.5
BUD	9.4	980	11	55–84	2.8/2.0
CIC/des-CIC[b]	0.12/12.0	UK	<1/<1	152/228	(0.36/3.4)/UK
FLU	1.8	330	20	58	1.6/1.6
FP	18	1200	≤1	66	7.8/14.4
MF	27[a]	UK	<1	53	5.8/UK
TAA	3.6	330	23	45–69	2.0/3.6

BDP, beclomethasone dipropionate; BMP, beclomethasone 17-monopropionate; BUD, budesonide; CIC, ciclesonide; des-CIC, des-ciclesonide; FLU, flunisolide; FP, fluticasone propionate; MF, mometasone furoate; TAA, triamcinolone acetonide; UK, unknown.

Note: Receptor binding affinities and topical skin blanching are relative to dexamethasone equal to 1.

[a]MF studied in a different receptor system. Value estimated from relative values of BDP, TAA, and FP in that system.

[b]BDP and CIC are prodrugs that are activated in the lung to their active metabolites BMP and des-CIC respectively.

are dose and duration dependent. This pattern is true for the adverse effects as well (Table 28–10). The clinician must continually balance the toxicity of chronic systemic corticosteroid therapy with control of asthma symptoms. Because short-term (1 to 2 weeks) high-dose corticosteroids (1 to 2 mg/kg per day of prednisone) do not produce serious toxicities, the ideal use is to administer the systemic corticosteroids in a short "burst" and then to maintain the patient on appropriate long-term control therapy with ICSs (discussed below under Inhaled Corticosteroids).[2,8] In general, therapy for more than 5 days at doses that exceed the usual physiologic endogenous cortisol production will cause temporary aberration in adrenal cortisol release.[39] However, this hypothalamic–pituitary–adrenal axis suppression is short-lived (1 to 3 days) and readily reversible following short bursts (10 days or less) of pharmacologic doses.[40] A maximum number of short bursts that a patient can receive probably exists, after which chronic corticosteroid side effects occur. Patients receiving at least eight bursts (≥10 days each) have a similar decrease in trabecular bone density as patients on daily or alternate-day corticosteroids over 1 year.[40] Children who received four or more bursts of prednisone exhibited a subnormal response to hypoglycemic stress or adrenocorticotropic hormone administration.[40] Very short courses (3 to 5 days) have been effective in reducing hospitalization from acute exacerbations.[2,8] Use of the shorter-acting corticosteroids, such as prednisone, produces less adrenal suppression than the longer-acting dexamethasone.[40]

Anticholinergics

The anticholinergic agents have a long history of use for asthma, but they do not have an FDA-approved indication for asthma.[2,42] Anticholinergics are competitive inhibitors of muscarinic receptors.[42] Unlike β_2-agonists, they are not functional antagonists; they only reverse cholinergic-mediated bronchoconstriction. Normal bronchial tone is maintained through parasympathetic innervation of the airways via the vagus nerve.[42] A number of the triggers and mediators of asthma (i.e., histamine, prostaglandins, sulfur dioxide, exercise, and allergens) produce bronchoconstriction in part through vagal reflex mechanisms.[42] Studies of asthmatics consistently demonstrate that anticholinergics are effective bronchodilators, although not as effective as β_2-agonists. Anticholinergics attenuate but do not block allergen-induced asthma in a dose-dependent fashion and have no effect on BHR.[42] Anticholinergics attenuate but do not block EIB.[43]

TABLE 28-10 Adverse Effects of Chronic Systemic Glucocorticoid Administration

Hypothalamic–pituitary–adrenal suppression	Hypertension
Growth retardation	Skin striae
Skeletal muscle myopathy	Impaired wound healing
Osteoporosis/fractures	Inhibition of leukocyte and monocyte function
Aseptic necrosis of bone	Subcutaneous tissue atrophy
Pancreatitis	Glaucoma
Pseudotumor cerebri	Posterior subcapsular cataracts
Psychiatric disturbances	Moon facies
Sodium and water retention	Central redistribution of fat
Hypokalemia/hyperglycemia	

Ipratropium bromide is a nonselective muscarinic receptor blocker, and blockade of inhibitory muscarinic receptors theoretically could result in an increased release of acetylcholine and overcome the block on the smooth muscle receptors (M_3).[42] Only the quaternary ammonium derivatives such as ipratropium bromide should be used because they have the advantage of poor absorption across mucosae and the blood–brain barrier. This results in negligible systemic effects with a prolonged local effect (i.e., bronchodilation). In addition, the quaternary compounds do not appear to produce a decrease in mucociliary clearance.[42] Ipratropium bromide has a duration of action of 4 to 8 hours. Both intensity and duration of action are dose-dependent. Tiotropium bromide, a new long-acting inhaled anticholinergic, has a duration of 24 hours. Time to reach maximum bronchodilation for ipratropium is considerably slower than from aerosolized short-acting β_2-agonists (30 to 60 minutes vs. 5 to 10 minutes). However, this is of little clinical consequence because some bronchodilation is seen within 30 seconds, 50% of maximum response occurs within 3 minutes.[42] Ipratropium bromide is only indicated as adjunctive therapy in severe acute asthma not completely responsive to β_2-agonists alone because it does not improve outcomes in chronic asthma.[2,8] Tiotropium has not been studied in asthma.

PHARMACOECONOMICS

The number of emergency department visits for asthma exceeds the number of hospitalizations by approximately four times, yet the annual expenditure for emergency department visits ($518 million) is significantly less than the estimated $2.7 billion spent on inpatient hospital services for patients with acute severe asthma.[3] Thus, reducing the number of patients requiring hospitalizations is a primary goal of therapy. Because the primary drugs used to treat severe acute asthma are available generically, drug costs account for only a small portion of the overall costs of care. Few of the therapies used in the management of acute severe asthma have been evaluated formally for their pharmacoeconomic impact. One evaluation based on a meta-analysis of inhaled anticholinergics added to short-acting inhaled β_2-agonists in children with acute severe asthma suggested that this approach was cost-effective and would reduce overall costs by reducing hospitalizations.[44] In children with acute severe asthma admitted to an intensive care unit, the use of continuously nebulized albuterol resulted in a decreased cost of care compared with intermittent nebulization.[30]

CLINICAL CONTROVERSIES

Some clinicians believe that intravenous magnesium sulfate is effective for the treatment of severe acute asthma unresponsive to standard doses of inhaled β_2-agonists in the emergency department. This is based on subset analyses of two studies showing that patients with the most severe obstruction following initial inhaled β_2-agonists decreased hospitalizations with magnesium treatment compared with placebo.[35] However, the subset with severe obstruction is the one demonstrating an improved response to the addition of ipratropium bromide and continuous nebulization of inhaled β_2-agonists. In addition a large, randomized trial failed to confirm a decreased hospitalization even in the severe group. The new NAEPP[6] and the Global Initiative for Asthma guidelines state that it can be considered for use in patients with severe episodes with a poor response to initial inhaled β_2-agonists.[8]

Numerous studies show that the inhaled β_2-agonists administered by MDI plus VHC provide a similar outcome in severe acute asthma as administration by jet nebulizers.[29] Proponents of administration by MDI plus VHC argue that it is more cost-effective and so should replace nebulizer therapy. However, appropriate cost analyses have yet to be performed.[25] Nor have there been comparisons in the most severe subsets, where combination therapy and continuous nebulization are recommended.[25] Current practice should be based on the comfort level of the clinical staff until sufficient data are available to warrant a wholesale recommendation of one method.[29]

EVALUATION OF THERAPEUTIC OUTCOMES

Figures 28–6 and 28–7 provide the monitoring parameters for severe acute asthma. Lung function, either spirometry or peak flows, should be monitored 5 to 10 minutes after each treatment.[2] Oxygen saturations can be easily monitored continuously with pulse oximetry. For young children and infants, pulse oximetry, lung auscultation, and observation of the presence of supraclavicular retractions is useful.[2,26] The majority of patients will respond within the first hour of initial inhaled β_2-agonists regardless of history of home administration of drug.[26] Patients not achieving an initial response should be monitored every 0.5 to 1 hour. Depending on whether there is a standard emergency department or a special unit for severe acute asthma, the decision to admit to the hospital should be made within 4 to 6 hours of entry to the emergency department.[26] The mean duration of hospitalization following admission is 2 to 3 days. Frequency of monitoring depends on the severity of the exacerbation. With mild exacerbations, monitor lung function every 2 to 3 hours; with severe exacerbations, monitor every 30 minutes to 1 hour.

TREATMENT

Chronic Asthma

The diagnosis of chronic asthma is made primarily by history and confirmatory spirometry (see Clinical Presentation above).[2,6] The NAEPP has provided a list of questions that would lead to the diagnosis of asthma (see Table 28–2).[2,6] In the older child and adult patient in whom spirometric evaluations can be performed, failure of pulmonary functions to improve acutely does not necessarily rule out asthma. Patients with long-standing disease or substantial inflammation may require an intensive, prolonged course of bronchodilators and glucocorticoids before reversibility is detected.[2,8] If baseline spirometry is normal, challenge testing with exercise, histamine, or methacholine can be used to elicit BHR.[2] Patients with significant symptoms and/or an FEV_1 of less than 65% of predicted normal should not be challenged. Studies for atopy, such as serum IgE and sputum and blood eosinophil determinations, are unnecessary to make the diagnosis of asthma, but they may help differentiate asthma from chronic bronchitis in adults. Clinically, this distinction is often difficult to make. Some patients with chronic bronchitis may have a reversible component, and some patients with long-standing severe chronic asthma may have significant irreversible damage and obstruction. Very high peripheral blood eosinophil counts may point to the diagnosis of allergic bronchopulmonary aspergillosis or other hypereosinophilic syndromes.[8] Skin testing is of no value in diagnosing asthma but is useful in identifying triggers.[2] In small infants unable to perform spirometry, the diagnosis is more difficult. They may demonstrate hyperinflation on the chest roentgenogram.[2] Radiologic examination is helpful in ruling out other causes of wheezing (e.g., foreign-body aspiration, parenchymal lung disease, cardiac disease, and congenital anomalies).[2] In place of pulmonary functions, the parents should be given a diary card to record symptoms and precipitating events.

■ GOALS FOR MANAGING ASTHMA LONG TERM

The NAEPP has provided key points for managing asthma long term.[6] The goal for therapy is to control asthma by:

Reducing impairment

1. Prevent chronic and troublesome symptoms (e.g., coughing or breathlessness in the daytime, in the night, or after exertion)
2. Require infrequent use (≤2 days a week) of inhaled short-acting β_2-agonist for quick relief of symptoms[2] (not including prevention of EIB)
3. Maintain (near-) normal pulmonary function
4. Maintain normal activity levels (including exercise and other activity and attendance at work or school)
5. Meet patients' and families' expectations of and satisfaction with care

Reducing risk

1. Prevent recurrent exacerbations of asthma and minimize the need for visits or hospitalizations
2. Prevent loss of lung function; for children, prevent reduced lung growth
3. Minimal or no adverse effects of therapy

■ NONPHARMACOLOGIC THERAPY

Although the mainstay of the management of asthma is pharmacologic therapy, it is likely to fail without concurrent attention to relevant environmental control and management of comorbid conditions. Figure 28–8 depicts the stepwise approach for managing asthma recommended in the newest update by the NAEPP.[6] It is important to note that the nonpharmacologic aspects of therapy are incorporated into the steps. The guidelines were designed to give primary healthcare providers a framework with which to develop the proper approach to the individualized therapy of patients. The heterogeneity of asthma demands an individualized approach to therapy with the basic goals of therapy as primary outcome measures.[2,6]

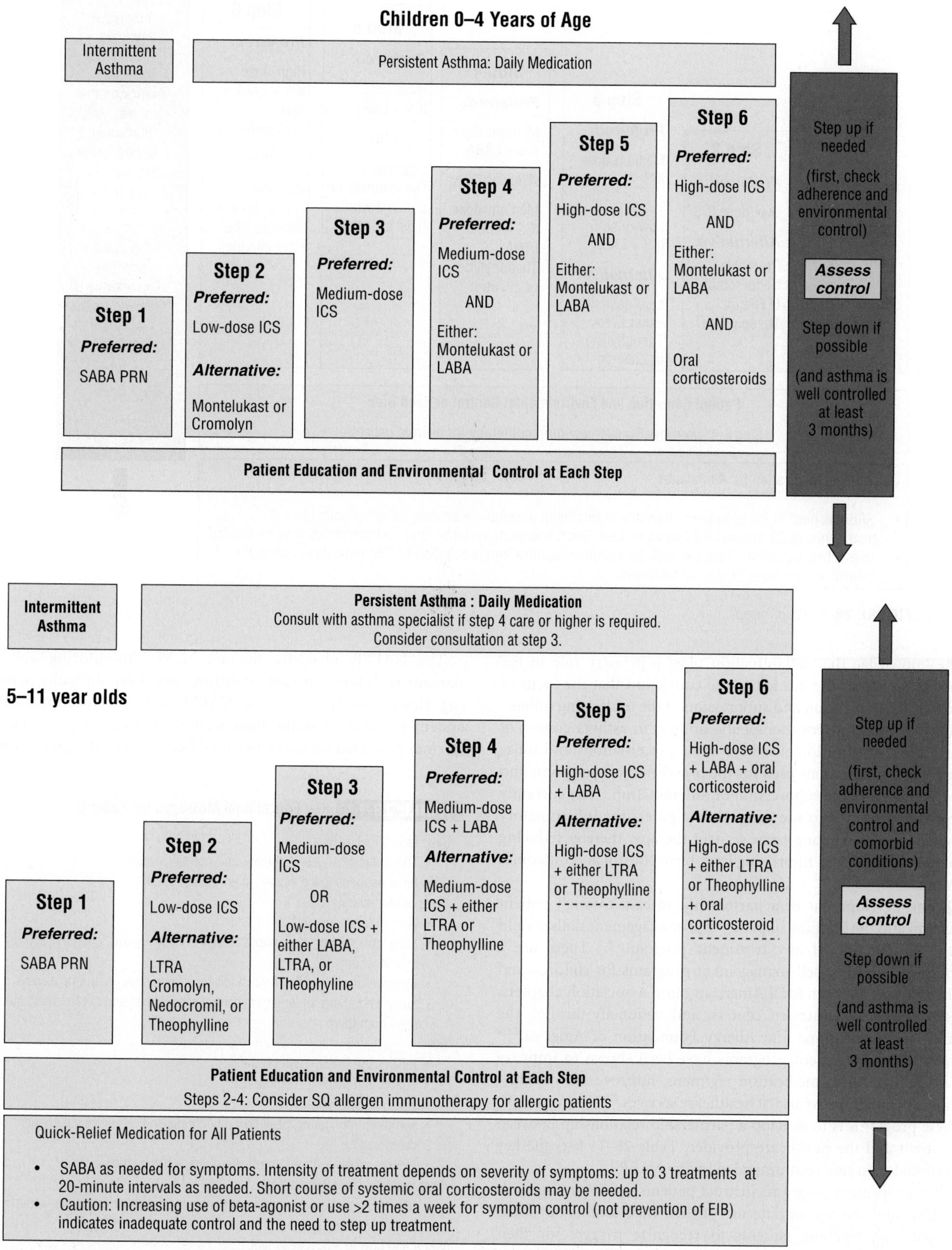

FIGURE 28-8. Stepwise approach for managing asthma in adults and children. (ICS, inhaled corticosteroid; LABA, long-acting β-agonist; LTRA, leukotriene receptor antagonist; PRN, as needed; SABA, short-acting β-agonist.) *(Adapted from reference 6.)*

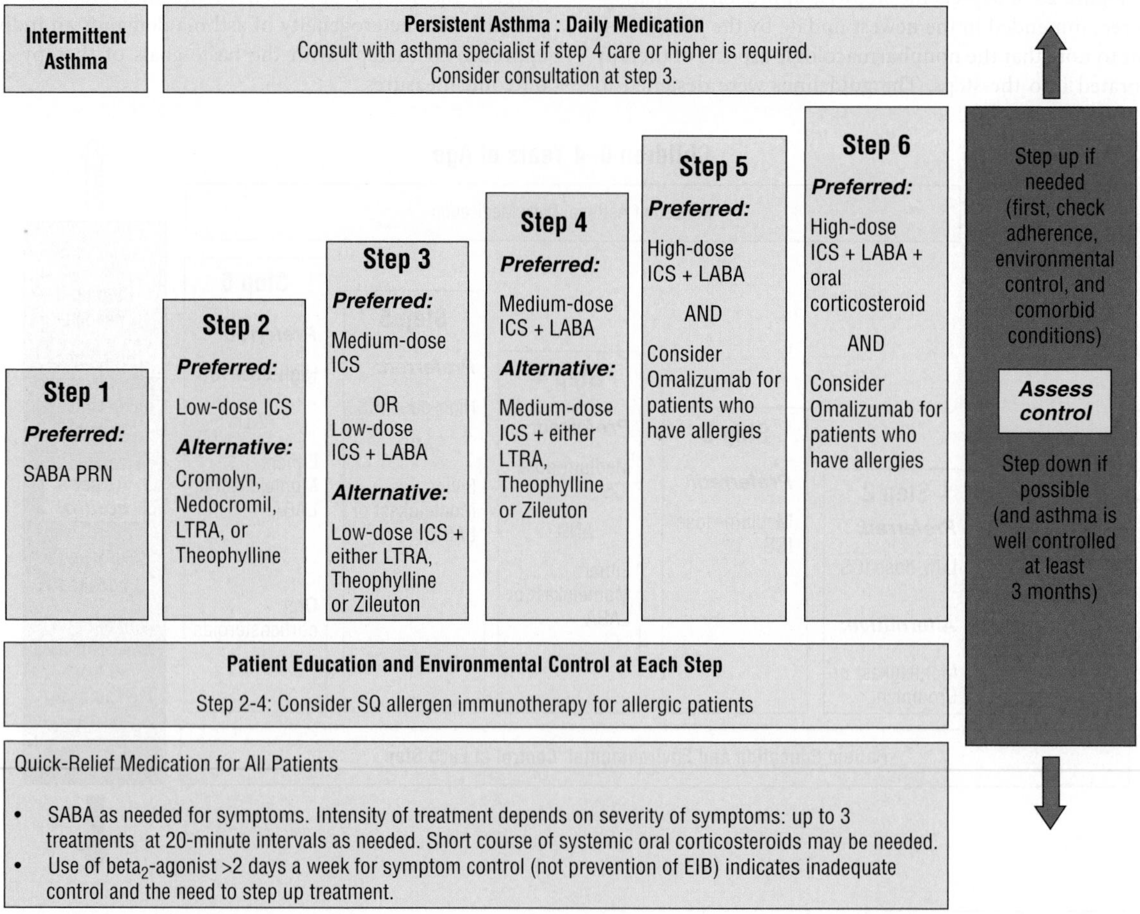

FIGURE 28-8. *(continued)*

The knowledge that inflammation plays a primary role in the pathogenesis of asthma has led to the conviction that the focus of therapy is the prevention and suppression of the underlying inflammation.[2,6,8] Thus current therapeutic options in asthma consist of acute reliever medications used for acute exacerbations and long-term control medications used for the prevention of symptoms and exacerbations and the suppression of inflammation.[2] The currently accepted approach is to use drugs that suppress the inflammatory response as primary long-term control therapy, thereby reducing the degree of BHR and improving long-term control and outcomes in asthma.[2,6,8]

❼ The development of a partnership in care through patient education and the teaching of patient self-management skills should be the cornerstone of any treatment program.[2,6,8] There are a number of published self-management programs for children and adults available through local American Lung Association chapters, as well as asthma treatment centers, and nationally through the NAEPP and the Asthma and Allergy Foundation of America.[2,6,8] Asthma self-management programs have been shown to improve patient adherence to medication regimens, improve self-management skills, and improve use of healthcare services.[2,6,8] The objective of these programs is to develop a partnership relationship between the patient and the healthcare provider. Table 28–11 lists the key educational messages recommended by the NAEPP.[6]

Self-management programs instruct patients in the pathogenesis of asthma and the appropriate use of their medications but focus principally on teaching patients to recognize triggers for their asthma and how to recognize early signs of deterioration. Home PEF monitoring is part of some programs.[2,8] However, routine PEF monitoring in and of itself does not improve patient outcomes.[6]

The NAEPP advocates the use of PEF monitoring only for patients with severe persistent asthma who have difficulty perceiving airway obstruction.[2] The NAEPP also has recommended a system based on a traffic light scenario (based on percentage of normal predicted values or personal best values): the green zone is

TABLE 28-11 Key Educational Messages for Patients

Basic facts about asthma
• The contrast between asthmatic and normal airways
• What happens to the airways in an asthma attack
Roles of medications
• How medications work
• Long-term control: medications that prevent symptoms, often by reducing inflammation
• Quick relief: short-acting bronchodilator relaxes muscles around airways
• Stress importance of long-term-control medications and not to expect quick relief from them
Skills
• Inhaler use (patient demonstrate)
• Spacer and holding chamber use
• Use of the nebulizer
• Symptom monitoring, peak flow monitoring, and recognizing early signs of deterioration
• How to assess asthma control after therapy has begun
Environmental control measures
• Identifying and avoiding environmental precipitants or exposures, including tobacco smoke
When and how to adjust treatment
• Using written action plan
• Responding to changes in asthma control

equal to 80% to 100%, the yellow zone is equal to 50% to 79%, and the red zone is less than 50%. The yellow zone is cautionary and requires increasing as-needed bronchodilator use and possibly beginning prednisone if not improved, whereas the red zone warrants contacting the patient's healthcare provider.[2]

Patient education is essential before monitoring can be effective. Patient education has proved successful regardless of the health professional who provided the information (physician, nurse, or pharmacist). The NAEPP advocates significant involvement of all points of patient care in the educational process. The provision of written action plans enhances the success of education and is considered an essential component of care.[2,6] Samples of clinically tested written action plans are available from the NAEPP guidelines and other sources.[2,6]

In patients with known allergic triggers for their asthma, allergen avoidance has resulted in an improvement in symptoms, a reduction in medication use, and a decrease in BHR.[2,6] A comprehensive approach to environmental control is advocated. For example, for patients with house-dust mite allergy, removing carpeting from bedrooms, washing sheets in hot water (>54.4°C [130°F]), and using special dust-proof pillow and mattress covers can reduce symptoms and need for medications.[2,6] Obvious environmental triggers (e.g., animal dander, cockroaches), if the patient is sensitive, should be avoided. Evidence for home air-filtering systems and chemicals for killing house-dust mites is limited.[6] Immunotherapy (allergy shots) with single antigens particularly, has been beneficial and may be considered in patients with persistent asthma with documented sensitivity.[6] Immunotherapy with multiple antigens has been less effective.

Patients who smoke should be encouraged to stop. Parents of children with asthma should stop or at least not smoke around their children.[2,6,8]

■ PHARMACOLOGIC THERAPY

Figure 28–8 illustrates the current NAEPP recommendations for therapy of persistent asthma.[6] Therapy should be adjusted based on control status of the patient (refer to Evaluation of Asthma Control section). Regardless of the long-term therapy, all patients need to have quick-relief medication in the form of short-acting inhaled β_2-agonists available for acute symptoms. The ICSs are considered the preferred long-term control therapy for persistent asthma in all patients because of their potency and consistent effectiveness.[6,8] Low- to medium-dose ICSs reduce BHR, improve lung function, and reduce severe exacerbations leading to emergency department visits and hospitalizations. They are more effective than cromolyn, nedocromil, theophylline, or the leukotriene receptor antagonists.[6] In addition, the ICSs are the only therapy that reduces the risk of dying from asthma.[45] In the low to medium doses recommended by the NAEPP guidelines (Table 28–12), ICSs are safe for long-term administration (see Drug Class Information, Inhaled Corticosteroids below).[6,39] The ICSs do not appear to reduce airway remodeling and loss of lung function found in some patients with persistent asthma. The ICSs do not enhance lung growth in children with asthma, prevent the development of asthma in high risk infants, or induce remission of asthma as BHR and other measures of inflammation return to pretreatment levels on discontinuation of therapy.[46,47] The sensitivity and consequent clinical response to ICSs can vary among patients.[6]

Although studies of the alternative long-term control therapies (e.g., cromolyn, leukotriene receptor antagonists, nedocromil, and theophylline) demonstrate improvement in symptoms, lung function, and as-needed short-acting inhaled β_2-agonist use, they do not reduce BHR, suggesting minimal antiinflammatory activity.[6] The evidence suggests minimal to no differences in efficacy between these alternatives. Consequently, the NAEPP lists them in alphabetical order to show no preference for one over the other.[6]

For those patients who are inadequately controlled on low-dose ICSs, either an increased dose of the ICS or the combination of ICS and long-acting inhaled β_2-agonist (LABA) is the next step to gain control of more moderate persistent asthma.[6,8] Alternatives could be the addition of leukotriene modifiers or theophylline to ICSs.[6,8] The addition of theophylline or leukotriene modifiers to ICSs is no more

TABLE 28-12 Available Inhaled Corticosteroid Products, Lung Delivery, and Comparative Daily Dosages

Inhaled Corticosteroids	Product	Lung Delivery[a]
Beclomethasone dipropionate (BDP)	40 and 80 mcg/actuation HFA MDI, 120 actuations	55–60%
Budesonide (BUD)	200 mcg/dose DPI, Turbuhaler, 200 doses	32% (16–59%)
	200 and 500-mcg ampules, 2 mL each	6%
Flunisolide (FLU)	250 mcg/actuation CFC MDI, 100 actuations	20%
	80 mcg/actuation HFA MDI, 120 actuations	68%
Fluticasone propionate (FP)	44, 110, and 220 mcg/actuation HFA MDI, 120 actuations	20–25%
	50 mcg/dose DPI, Diskus, 60 doses	15%
Mometasone furoate (MF)	200 and 400 mcg/dose DPI, Twisthaler, 14, 30, 60, and 120 doses	11%
Triamcinolone acetonide (TAA)	75 mcg/actuation CFC MDI, 240 actuations with spacer	22%

Comparative Daily Dosages (mcg) of Inhaled Corticosteroids

	Low Daily Dose Child[b]/Adult	***Medium DailyDose Child[b]/Adult***	***High Daily Dose Child[b]/Adult***
BDP			
HFA MDI	80–160/80–240	>160–320/>240–480	>320/>480
BUD			
DPI	200–400/200–600	>400–800/>600–1,200	>800/>1,200
Nebules	500/UK	1,000/UK	2,000/UK
FLU			
CFC MDI	500–750/500–1,000	1,000–1,250/1,000–2,000	>1,250/>2,000
HFA MDI	160/320	320/320–640	≥640/>640
FP			
HFA MDI	88–176/88–264	176–352/264–440	>352/>440
DPIs	100–200/100–300	200–400/300–500	>400/>500
MF, DPI	UK/200	UK/400	UK/>400
TAA, CFC MDI	300–600/300–750	600–900/750–1,500	>900/>1,500

[a]Lung delivery from in vivo radiolabel scintigraphy or pharmacokinetic studies.
[b]5–11 years of age.
CFC, chlorofluorocarbon; DPI, dry-powder inhaler; HFA, hydrofluoroalkane; MDI, metered-dose inhaler; UK, unknown.

effective than doubling the dose of the ICS.[6] The combination of ICS/LABA is more effective at reducing severe asthma exacerbations than doubling the dose of ICS in moderate persistent asthma; increasing the dose of ICSs fourfold also will result in a significant reduction in exacerbations.[48–50] However, doses of ICSs in the high range significantly enhance the risk of toxicity. Thus, high doses of ICSs plus LABA are reserved for patients with severe persistent asthma.[6]

Although the addition of a third controller medication is often used clinically in patients with severe, persistent asthma uncontrolled on high-dose ICS/LABA, there are few studies evaluating this practice.[6] Leukotriene receptor antagonists or theophylline added to high-dose combination ICS/LABA do not improve outcomes.[6] Omalizumab, a recombinant anti-IgE has demonstrated significant activity in these severe, uncontrolled patients.[51] Thus adult patients with severe, persistent, uncontrolled asthma and atopy would be candidates for omalizumab therapy.

■ SPECIAL POPULATIONS

❻ Children 4 years of age and younger have not been studied adequately. Thus, many of the recommendations in this age group are based on extrapolation of data from older children and adults.[6] The studies of ICSs in this younger group demonstrate improvement in symptoms, as needed bronchodilator use and exacerbations. The nebulized suspension of budesonide gained FDA approval from three pivotal efficacy and safety trials.[6] The FDA approval for montelukast in children younger than age 6 years was based on safety and pharmacokinetic studies establishing doses but not on efficacy although improvement in symptoms and as needed bronchodilators was noted.[6] Cromolyn nebulizer solution was approved down to 2 years based upon efficacy, however, not all trials of cromolyn, particularly when administered by MDI plus VHC, in this younger group have demonstrated efficacy.[6] Theophylline has not been evaluated adequately, except for pharmacokinetics.[6] Combination therapy of any kind has not been studied except for a small number of patients down to 4 years of age on ICS/LABA.[6]

The FDA approval of the fluticasone/salmeterol DPI 100/50 in patients 4 to 11 years of age was largely based on extrapolation of efficacy data from patients older than 12 years of age and by a single safety and efficacy study in children with asthma aged 4 to 11 years. In children 5 to 11 years old, the ICS/LABA combination has not been shown to decrease exacerbations compared to medium-dose ICS as in adults although impairment domains improved. The only study of the addition of montelukast to ICS showed minimal improvement in PEF and as-needed albuterol use. Thus combination therapy has been inadequately studied in this population.

Owing to the increased risk of osteoporosis in the elderly, patients requiring high doses of ICSs should have their bone mineral density determinations followed and appropriate therapies for prevention of osteoporosis instituted.[39]

Asthma affects 7% of pregnant women, making it potentially the most common serious medical condition to complicate pregnancy.[52] Maternal asthma has been reported to increase the risk of perinatal mortality, preeclampsia, preterm birth, and low-birth-weight infants.[52] More severe asthma is associated with increased risks, whereas better-controlled asthma is associated with decreased risks. A systematic review of the evidence on the safety of asthma medications has been conducted by drug class.[52] This review concluded that it is safer for pregnant women with asthma to be treated with effective medications than for them to have exacerbations.[52] Proper monitoring and control of asthma should enable a woman with asthma to maintain a normal pregnancy with little or no risk to mother or her fetus.

A stepwise approach to managing asthma during pregnancy and lactation has been published, with low-dose ICSs recommended as preferred treatment for mild persistent asthma with the addition of a LABA if not adequately controlled.[52] Budesonide is considered the preferred ICS to initiate because it has the greatest amount of safety data.[52] Albuterol is considered the preferred rescue therapy.[52]

■ DRUG CLASS INFORMATION

Inhaled Corticosteroids

The mechanism of action of the corticosteroids was reviewed under Systemic Corticosteroids above. The principal advantage of the ICSs is their high topical potency to reduce inflammation in the lung and low systemic activity.[39–41] The ICSs have high antiinflammatory potency, approximately 1,000-fold greater than endogenous cortisol, and differ from each other by as much as 4- to 6-fold.[41] However, potency differences, which are simply a measure of binding affinity to the receptor, can be overcome simply by giving different microgram dosages of drug. Aerosol delivery of the preparations is remarkably variable, ranging from 10% to 60% of the nominal dose (i.e., that dose which leaves an actuator for an MDI or, in the case of a DPI, that which is released on actuation of the inhaler).[25,41] Different devices for the same chemical entity may result in twofold differences in delivery, such as with fluticasone propionate and budesonide, or as much as eightfold with beclomethasone dipropionate preparations.[39] Thus the delivery method can make a significant difference in the relative comparable dose.[2,6]

Table 28–12 lists and compares the ICSs, beclomethasone dipropionate, budesonide, flunisolide, fluticasone propionate, mometasone furoate, and triamcinolone acetonide, which are currently available for use, and ciclesonide, which is undergoing clinical trials. The ICSs have pharmacokinetic differences that result in different topical/systemic activity.[44,45] Most evidence is consistent with log-linear dose–response curves for both indirect and direct responses.[39] The log-linear nature of the dose–response curve for corticosteroid activity raises the issue of how much of a difference in dose (or lung delivery) or potency is detectable. The measures used to assess efficacy (lung function, BHR, symptoms, and as-needed, short-acting, inhaled β_2-agonist use) are downstream events from the antiinflammatory activity.[39] In general, it takes a fourfold difference in potency or dose to detect clinically significant differences in efficacy. The table of comparable doses (see Table 28–12) is based on extensive clinical trial data.[6] Clinically comparable doses take into consideration drug potency differences as well as device delivery differences.

Because the glucocorticoid receptors within the various tissues are the same, differences in the pharmacokinetic profile are required to produce differences in the topical–systemic effect ratio (therapeutic index).[39] Pharmacokinetic properties that enhance improved topical selectivity include rapid systemic clearance, poor oral bioavailability, and long residence time in the lung.[39,41] Owing to their high lipophilicity, systemic clearance of the available ICSs is very rapid, approaching the rate of liver blood flow, with the exception of ciclesonide, which is inactivated by blood esterases.[41] However, the ICSs differ markedly in their oral bioavailability, although they all undergo rather extensive first-pass metabolism to less active substances when absorbed (see Table 28–9).[41] The ICSs produce dose-dependent systemic effects from a combination of the orally absorbed fraction and the fraction absorbed from the lung (Table 28–13).[39,41] Essentially all the drug that reaches the lung is absorbed systemically; thus a slow absorption from the lung results in an apparent long elimination half-life and enhances topical selectivity by lowering the systemic concentration.[41] The potential advantage of the drugs with low oral bioavailability is obviated by using a spacer device with the MDI for the drugs with higher oral bioavailability because appropriate spacers reduce the oral dose by 80%.[25] The use of VHCs also can increase systemic activity by increasing lung delivery of drugs not absorbed significantly orally.[39] If this increase in lung deposition is twofold or less, it will increase systemic activity without producing a clinically important

TABLE 28-13 Effects of Inhaled Corticosteroids

Beneficial Effects	Potential Adverse Effects
Decrease eosinophil numbers	Growth retardation, skeletal muscle myopathy
Decrease mast cell numbers	Osteoporosis, fractures, and aseptic necrosis of hip
Decrease T-lymphocyte cytokine production	Posterior subcapsular cataract formation and glaucoma
Inhibit transcription of inflammatory genes in airway epithelium	Adrenal axis suppression, immunosuppression
Reduce endothelial cell leak	Impaired wound healing, easy bruising, skin striae
Upregulate β_2-receptor production	Hyperglycemia/hypokalemia, hypertension
Reduce airway epithelial subbasement membrane thickening	Psychiatric disturbances

increase in efficacy, thus decreasing the therapeutic index.[39] Mouth rinsing and spitting also will reduce the oral availability and are particularly useful for DPI devices.[2,25]

The response to ICSs is somewhat delayed. Most patients' symptoms will improve in the first 1 to 2 weeks of therapy and will reach maximum improvement in 4 to 8 weeks.[53] Improvement in baseline FEV_1 and PEFs may require 3 to 6 weeks for maximum improvement, whereas improvement in BHR requires 2 to 3 weeks and approaches maximum in 1 to 3 months but may continue to improve over 1 year.[53] Most of the improvement in these parameters occurs at low to medium doses, and there is a large variability in response, with 10% of patients not demonstrating an improvement in either parameter.[53] Whether these nonresponders also show no improvement in rates of exacerbations is unknown. Maximum decrease in FeNO occurs within 2 to 3 weeks.[54] Sensitivity to exercise challenge decreases after 4 weeks of therapy.[18,53] Although single doses do not inhibit the immediate asthmatic response to antigen challenge, continued therapy for 1 week partially suppresses the response. These two latter effects are likely caused by a reduction in mucosal mast cells.[53]

Local adverse effects from ICSs include oropharyngeal candidiasis and dysphonia that are dose-dependent. The dysphonia (reported in 5% to 50% of patients) appears to be caused by a local corticosteroid-induced myopathy of the vocal cords.[2] The use of a spacer device with MDIs can decrease oropharyngeal deposition and thus decrease the incidence and severity of local side effects.[25,53] There is less data on the use of spacers with ICS HFA MDIs. In infants who require delivery through a facemask, the parent should clean the nasal-perioral area with a damp cloth following each treatment to prevent topical candidal infections.

Systemic adverse effects can occur with any of the ICSs given in a sufficiently high dose.[39] Long-term adverse effects of greatest concern include growth suppression in children, osteoporosis, cataracts, dermal thinning, and adrenal insufficiency and crisis.[39,53] Of these, only growth retardation occurs in low to medium doses. However, the growth reduction appears to be transient in that growth velocity is reduced in the first 6 months to 1 year of therapy and then returns to normal.[6,39] The effect is small (1 to 2 cm total) and not cumulative, and current studies suggest that attainment of predicted adult height is not affected.[6,39] The suppression of the hypothalamic–pituitary–adrenal axis and decreased bone mineralization are dose-dependent and do not appear to be significant clinically except at high doses.[39] The risks of these adverse effects are all dose-dependent and depend on the therapeutic index of each ICS and its delivery device. The effect of delivery device is illustrated by fluticasone propionate, which has both the greatest therapeutic index when administered by DPI and the lowest therapeutic index when administered by MDI plus VHC.[39] Some of the ICSs including fluticasone propionate, budesonide and mometasone are metabolized in the gastrointestinal tract and liver by cytochrome P450 (CYP) 3A4 isoenzymes. Potent inhibitors of CYP3A4, such as ritonavir and ketoconazole, have the potential for increasing systemic concentrations of these ICSs by increasing oral availability and decreasing systemic clearance. Some cases of clinically significant Cushing syndrome and secondary adrenal insufficiency have been reported.[41]

Most patients with moderate disease can be controlled with twice-daily dosing of most ICSs.[6,8,53] Twice-daily dosing produces less thrush than three- to four-times-daily dosing regimens. In milder asthma, once-daily dosing is often sufficient to maintain control.[53] Some of the newer products have gained once-daily dosing indications, particularly in mild asthma once initial control is established.[41] There does not appear to be any specific pharmacologic or pharmacokinetic aspect of the ICSs that allows for once-daily dosing because all the agents studied (both the older low-potency and newer high-potency ICSs) have been effective, provided that patients had relatively mild to moderate asthma.[39,53] Patients with more severe asthma require multiple daily dosing. The inflammatory response of asthma inhibits steroid-receptor binding.[53] This provides strong theoretical evidence for initially beginning patients on higher and more frequent doses and then tapering down once control has been achieved. Once asthma is controlled, many patients are able to reduce the ICS dose and maintain control.[53]

Long-Acting Inhaled β_2-Agonists

The two LABAs, formoterol and salmeterol, provide long-lasting bronchodilation (12 or more hours) when administered as aerosols (see Table 28–8).[30] Unlike the more water-soluble short-acting β_2-agonists, the long-acting agents are lipid soluble, readily partitioning into the outer phospholipid layer of the cell membrane.[30] Salmeterol is more β_2-selective than albuterol and more bronchoselective by virtue of its property of remaining in the lung tissue cell membrane, which produces its longer duration.[30] However, both formoterol and salmeterol will produce dose-dependent systemic β_2-agonist effects.[30]

The principal differences between formoterol and salmeterol are that formoterol has a more rapid onset of action (similar to that of albuterol) and formoterol is a full agonist, whereas salmeterol is a partial agonist. These differences are unlikely to produce clinically significant differences because both are recommended for chronic therapy only in combination with ICSs.[6] They are available singly and as fixed-dose combinations with ICSs. Patients should be warned to not use salmeterol for acute relief of asthma because it can take up to 20 minutes for onset and 1 to 4 hours for maximum bronchodilation following inhalation.[2,6] Formoterol also does not have approved FDA labeling for acute relief. Patients need to be counseled to continue to use their short-acting inhaled β_2-agonists for acute exacerbations while receiving the LABAs.

The LABAs are the preferred adjunctive therapy to ICSs in children ≥12 years of age and in adults for step 3, and in children 5 to 11 years of age for steps 4 and 5.[6] Combination treatment with ICS/LABA provides greater asthma control than increasing the dose of ICS alone while at the same time reducing the frequency and perhaps the severity of exacerbations.[48–50] Because they are devoid of antiinflammatory activity, LABAs should not be used as monotherapy for asthma. Recent evidence suggests that patients treated with LABA monotherapy added to usual therapy are at an increased risk for severe, life-threatening exacerbations and asthma-related death.[55,56] This risk may be greater in African American patients. Whether this risk is obviated by concomitant ICS use is unknown at this time but preliminary evidence does not support an increased risk of severe, life-threatening exacerbations in patients receiving LABAs in combination with ICSs.[57,58]

As with short-acting β_2-agonists, tolerance is produced with chronic administration of LABAs. Long-term trials show no diminution in bronchodilator response, but do show a partial loss of the bronchoprotective effect against methacholine, histamine, and exercise challenge.[58] In particular, the duration of protection against EIB following a single dose of salmeterol is up to 9 hours but is reduced to less than 4 hours following regular treatment.[58] Following regular treatment with salmeterol and formoterol, decreased protection against nonspecific bronchoprovocation with methacholine also occurs, although it provides greater protection than placebo.[58] Responsiveness to short-acting β_2-agonists is reported to be slightly decreased but easily overcome by increasing the dose (by approximately 1 puff) following chronic therapy with LABAs.[58]

There is ample evidence that the use of a LABA in combination with ICS therapy does not mask inflammation.[57] A meta-analysis of studies comparing the addition of salmeterol to ICS therapy versus at least a doubling of ICS dose demonstrates that rather than increasing asthma exacerbations, the number of these events was reduced.[48] As stated previously LABAs added to ICS in children improve impairment but have yet to be adequately studied for reducing exacerbations over ICS alone.[59]

Methylxanthines

Methylxanthines have been used for asthma therapy for more than 50 years but their use in recent years has declined markedly owing to the high risk of severe life-threatening toxicity and numerous drug interactions, as well as decreased efficacy when compared with ICSs and LABAs. Theophylline, the primary methylxanthine of interest, is a moderately potent bronchodilator with mild antiinflammatory properties.[2,8] Like the β_2-agonists, the methylxanthines are functional antagonists of bronchospasm; however, their clinical usefulness is limited by their low therapeutic index.[2] Theophylline as a sustained-release product is the preferred oral preparation, whereas its complex with ethylenediamine (aminophylline) is the preferred injectable product because of increased solubility.[60]

The mechanism by which theophylline produces bronchodilation appears to be through nonselective phosphodiesterase inhibition.[60] Inhibition of phosphodiesterase results in increased cAMP and cyclic guanosine monophosphate concentrations. The phosphodiesterase isoenzymes currently thought to be important for theophylline's clinical effects are isoenzymes III, predominant in airway smooth muscle, and IV, important in inflammatory cell regulation such as mast cells, neutrophils, eosinophils, and T lymphocytes.[60] Selective phosphodiesterase isoenzyme IV inhibitors, however, have no significant effects in clinical asthma. Theophylline is a competitive antagonist of adenosine and stimulates endogenous catecholamine release.[60] These latter two effects are important determinants of toxic symptoms of excess theophylline.[60]

Theophylline has a log-linear dose–response curve.[60] Most chronic stable asthmatics will obtain significant bronchodilation when the serum theophylline concentration reaches 5 mcg/mL, and most patients will have no toxic symptoms with serum concentrations of less than 15 mcg/mL.[6,60] The percentage of patients experiencing adverse effects increases sharply as concentrations exceed 15 mcg/mL. As with the β_2-agonists, the dose–response curves for smooth muscle relaxation by theophylline are dynamic and shifted to the right in the face of increasing contractile stimuli.[60] This probably explains theophylline's relative lack of bronchodilatory effect in acute severe asthma.[6,60] The severity of theophylline's toxicity precludes even doubling the usual dosage. Toxicities include caffeine-like effects of nausea, vomiting, tachycardia, jitteriness, and difficulty sleeping to more severe toxicities such as cardiac tachyarrhythmias and seizures. Death has occurred in children receiving their usual doses of theophylline during acute systemic viral illnesses.[60]

Routine monitoring of serum concentrations is essential for the safe and effective use of theophylline.[6] Theophylline is eliminated primarily by metabolism via the hepatic cytochrome P450 mixed-function oxidase microsomal enzymes (primarily the CYP1A2 and CYP3A3 isozymes), with 10% or less excreted unchanged in the kidney.[60] Theophylline clearance is age-dependent, with 1- to 9-year-olds having the highest systemic clearances and therefore requiring the largest dosages (on a weight basis). However, even within the same age groups, theophylline clearance can vary two- to threefold.[60] Figure 28–9 gives a dosing and monitoring schedule for theophylline. Table 28–14 lists factors that affect theophylline's hepatic metabolism.[2] Only drugs or diseases that produce a 20% or greater inhibition or a 50% or greater induction of theophylline metabolism are likely to result in clinically significant interactions.[60]

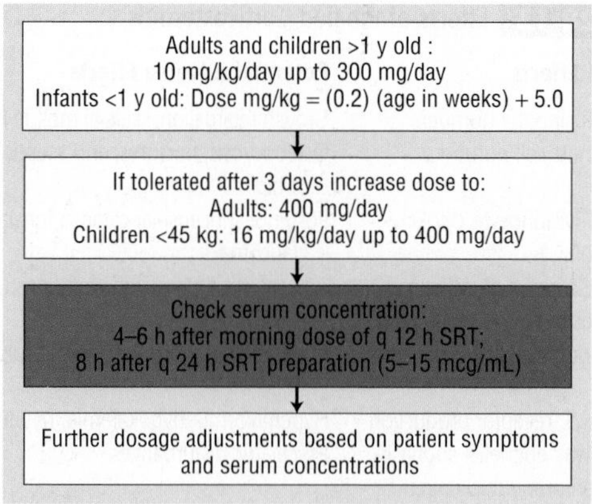

FIGURE 28-9. Algorithm for slow titration of theophylline dosage and guide for final dosage adjustment based on serum theophylline concentration measurement. For infants younger than 1 year of age, the initial daily dosage can be calculated by the following regression equation: Dose (mg/kg) = (0.2) (age in weeks) + 5.0. Whenever side effects occur, dosage should be reduced to a previously tolerated lower dose. (SRT, sustained-release theophylline.)

Sustained-release theophylline is less effective than ICSs and no more effective than oral sustained-release β_2-agonists, cromolyn, or leukotriene antagonists.[6] The addition of theophylline to ICSs is similar to doubling the dose of the ICS and is less effective overall than the LABAs as adjunctive therapy.[6]

Cromolyn Sodium and Nedocromil Sodium

Cromolyn sodium and nedocromil sodium are pharmacologically similar.[2] They are classified as mast cell stabilizers, and the principal difference appears to be potency, with 4 mg nedocromil by MDI equivalent to 10 mg cromolyn.[2,61] However, there is no apparent difference in the clinical efficacy between these two drugs.[2] They inhibit the early and late asthmatic response to allergen challenge, as well inhibit EIB.[2,8] Treatment prevents the usual rise in bronchial hyperresponsiveness with specific pollen seasons, but long-term treatment produces minimal to no change in baseline bronchial

TABLE 28-14 Factors Affecting Theophylline Clearance

Decreased Clearance	% Decrease	Increased Clearance	% Increase
Cimetidine	−25 to −60	Rifampin	+53
Macrolides: erythromycin, clarithromycin	−25 to −50	Carbamazepine	+50
		Phenobarbital	+34
		Phenytoin	+70
Allopurinol	−20	Charcoal-broiled meat	+30
Propranolol	−30		
Quinolones: ciprofloxacin, enoxacin, pefloxacin	−20 to −50	High-protein diet	+25
		Smoking	+40
Interferon	−50	Sulfinpyrazone	+22
Thiabendazole	−65	Moricizine	+50
Ticlopidine	−25	Aminoglutethimide	+50
Zileuton	−35		
Systemic viral illness	−10 to −50		

hyperresponsiveness.[6,61] They inhibit neurally mediated bronchoconstriction, through C-fiber sensory nerve stimulation in the airways, although neither drug has a bronchodilatory effect.[61]

Cromolyn and nedocromil are only effective by inhalation and are available as MDIs, whereas cromolyn also is available as a nebulizer solution. The pharmacokinetics of both drugs are very similar. They are not bioavailable orally, but the portion of the dose that reaches the lung is absorbed completely.[61] Absorption from the airway is significantly slower than elimination (hours versus minutes). The short duration in the lung likely limits their efficacy. Both the intensity and duration of protection against various challenges are dose-dependent.[61] Higher doses produce greater and more prolonged protection.

Both drugs are remarkably nontoxic. No evidence of mutagenesis or teratogenesis has been found for cromolyn. Cough and wheeze have been reported following inhalation of each, and bad taste and headache following nedocromil are reported.[2] The taste from nedocromil is sufficiently bad in some patients (approximately 20%) to preclude them from taking the drug.[61] Tolerance to cromolyn or nedocromil has not been demonstrated. Neither are ICS-sparing agents.

Cromolyn and nedocromil are no more or less effective than theophylline or the leukotriene antagonists for persistent asthma.[6] Neither cromolyn nor nedocromil is as effective as the ICSs for controlling persistent asthma.[6,46] Neither is as effective as the inhaled β_2-agonists for preventing EIB but can be used in conjunction for patients not responding completely to the inhaled β_2-agonists.[43]

Most patients will experience an improvement in 1 to 2 weeks, but it may take longer to achieve maximum benefit. Patients initially should receive cromolyn or nedocromil four times daily, and then only after stabilization of symptoms may the frequency be reduced to two times daily for nedocromil and three times daily for cromolyn. Only the nebulizer solution should be used for children younger than 5 years of age.[6]

Leukotriene Modifiers

Two clinically distinct cysteinyl leukotriene receptor antagonists (zafirlukast and montelukast) and one 5-lipoxygenase inhibitor (zileuton) have been available in the United States since 1996 for both children and adults with persistent asthma.[62] In challenge studies, they reduce allergen-, exercise-, cold air hyperventilation-, irritant-, and aspirin-induced asthma.[63] Clinical use of zileuton is limited because of the potential for elevated liver enzymes (especially in the first 3 months of therapy), and the potential inhibition of drugs metabolized by the CYP3A4 isoenzymes.[62,63]

In clinical trials, the LTD_4 receptor antagonists (zafirlukast and montelukast) have demonstrated efficacy in adults and children with persistent asthma. These drugs improve pulmonary function tests (FEV_1 and PEF), decrease nocturnal awakenings and β_2-agonist use, and improve asthma symptoms.[62,63] A major advantage is that they are effective orally, administered once or twice a day, and contribute to patient adherence and satisfaction with therapy.[62] However, they are less effective in asthma than low doses of ICSs.[64,65] It is not yet possible to predict which patients respond best to leukotriene modifiers, although there is some evidence that patients with aspirin-sensitive asthma do well, as predicted by studies showing increased cysteinyl leukotriene production in these patients.[63] It is possible that genetic polymorphisms in the 5-lipooxygenase or LTC_4 synthase pathways or in cys-LT_1 receptors might predict better responders in the future.[63] Antileukotrienes also have modest efficacy in allergic rhinitis.

In general, the LTD_4 receptor antagonists are well tolerated and do not appear to have serious class-specific effects.[6] An idiosyncratic syndrome similar to the Churg-Strauss syndrome, with marked circulating eosinophilia, heart failure, and associated eosinophilic vasculitis, has been reported in a small number of patients treated with zafirlukast or montelukast.[6] The majority of these patients had been receiving high-dose inhaled or oral corticosteroids and were able to reduce the dose as a consequence of the LTD_4 receptor antagonists. It is unclear whether the increased reports are a result of increased case findings among patients with asthma prescribed a new drug or whether the syndrome is related to corticosteroid dose reduction or an idiosyncratic effect of leukotriene modifiers in general. Whatever the cause, it appears to be a rare syndrome, with an estimated incidence of fewer than 1 case per 15,000 to 20,000 patient-years of treatment.[6] Montelukast has been prescribed widely worldwide owing to its approval for use in young children. Churg-Strauss syndrome has not been reported in children, and the drug has been very well tolerated and palatable.[6] Recent reports of fatal hepatic failure associated with zafirlukast have prompted a warning for patients to be made aware of signs and symptoms of hepatic dysfunction.

Zileuton can be administered four times daily or twice daily as controlled release tablets.[6] Efficacy data is more limited, liver function monitoring is recommended, and drug interactions are reported with warfarin and theophylline.

Combination Controller Therapy: ICS/LABA versus ICS/Leukotriene Receptor Agonists

Whereas ICS therapy is considered the most effective antiinflammatory treatment, in cases of moderate to severe persistent asthma, the addition of a second long-term control medication to ICS therapy is one recommended treatment option. Single inhaler combination products containing fluticasone propionate and salmeterol or budesonide and formoterol are commercially available and there likely will be more in the future. The inhalers, both DPIs and MDIs, contain varied doses of the ICSs and a fixed dose of the respective LABAs. The pivotal trials for gaining FDA approval of fixed-dose combinations require that the combination demonstrate greater efficacy than either component alone. Importantly, the addition of a LABA allows reduction in ICS dosage by 50% in most patients with persistent asthma.[48,50] Furthermore, combination therapy is more effective than higher-dose ICS alone in reducing asthma exacerbations in patients with persistent asthma.[6,50] The ability to detect deteriorating asthma and the severity of exacerbation were similar between groups. Leukotriene receptor agonists also are successful as additive therapy in patients inadequately controlled on ICS alone and as ICS-sparing therapy.[6] However, the magnitude of these benefits is less than those reported with the addition of LABAs.[6,49]

Anti-IgE (Omalizumab)

Omalizumab is a recombinant anti-IgE antibody approved for the treatment of allergic asthma not well controlled by oral corticosteroids or ICSs.[66] Omalizumab is a composite of 95% human and 5% antihuman murine IgE sequences. The mouse protein becomes part of the receptor complex and thus is shielded from exposure to the immune system, lowering the risk for an anaphylactic response.[66] Omalizumab binds to the Fc portion of the IgE antibody, preventing the binding of IgE to its high-affinity receptor (FcεRI) on mast cells and basophils. The decreased binding of IgE on the surface of mast cells leads to a decrease in the release of mediators in response to allergen exposure. Omalizumab also decreases FcεRI expression on basophils and airway submucosal cells.

Omalizumab is administered subcutaneously and has a slow absorption rate; peak serum concentration is achieved in 3 to 14 days.[66] It is eliminated primarily through the reticuloendothelial system and has an elimination half-life of 17 to 22 days; serum free IgE levels return to baseline in about 3 weeks.[66] It should be administered under medical observation with drugs for treating anaphylaxis available.

The dosage of omalizumab is determined by the patient's baseline total serum IgE level (international units per milliliter) and body weight (kilograms).[66] Doses range from 150 to 375 mg and are given at either 2- or 4-week intervals. No further adjustments for variations in total serum IgE are required, and patients receive a consistent dose for the duration of treatment.[66] Omalizumab is approved for patients older than 12 years of age who have allergic asthma.[66] Clinical trials in 5- to 12-year-olds are ongoing. Because of its significant cost, it is only indicated as step 5 or 6 care for patients who have allergies and severe persistent asthma that is inadequately controlled with the combination of high-dose ICS/LABA.[6] It is the only adjunctive therapy that has demonstrated improved outcomes in patients uncontrolled on ICS/LABA and has allowed oral corticosteroid reduction in a number of studies.[6,66] However, recent postmarketing surveillance suggests that omalizumab therapy is associated with a 0.1% rate of anaphylaxis, prompting an FDA warning that patients should remain in the physician's office for a reasonable period of time past the injection because 70% of reactions occur within 2 hours. In addition, patients should be counseled on the signs and symptoms of anaphylaxis because some reactions have occurred up to 24 hours following an injection.[6]

MISCELLANEOUS THERAPIES (IMMUNOMODULATORS)

The following therapies have been loosely categorized by the NAEPP with omalizumab as immunomodulators because they either affect the immune system or have antiinflammatory properties. Many have been used experimentally in severe persistent uncontrolled asthma for years to try to avoid or lower oral corticosteroid dosages.

Low-dose methotrexate (15 mg/week) used for inflammatory diseases, psoriatic and rheumatoid arthritis, and polymyositis has been used to reduce the systemic steroid dose in patients with severe steroid-dependent asthma.[67] Double-blind, placebo-controlled trials have given decidedly mixed results, with half the studies showing no effect.[68] A recent meta-analysis determined that there was insufficient evidence to support its use, particularly in light of the risk for severe side effects.[67] Methotrexate inhibits chemotaxis of neutrophils, inhibits leukotriene B_4-induced adherence to endothelium, and inhibits the proinflammatory activity of IL-1. Low-dose weekly methotrexate is associated with hepatotoxicity and pulmonary fibrosis.[67] The NAEPP has concluded that it should not be used chronic asthma.[6]

A number of the drugs with antiinflammatory or immunomodulatory activity such as hydroxychloroquine, dapsone, gold, intravenous γ-globulin, cyclosporine, and colchicine have been studied in severe steroid-dependent asthma with mixed and limited results.[6,68] Routine use is not recommended.[6]

FUTURE THERAPIES

Agents that are now in development for asthma focus on the treatment of allergic inflammation.[68,69] Examples include inhibitors of eosinophilic inflammation, drugs that may inhibit allergen presentation, and inhibitors of TH_2 cells. Multiple cytokines have been implicated in allergic inflammation, and several possible inhibiting approaches are being explored. These range from drugs that inhibit cytokine synthesis (cyclosporine A and tacrolimus), humanized blocking antibodies to cytokines or their receptors, soluble receptors to mop up secreted cytokines, receptor antagonists, and drugs that block the signal-transduction pathways activated by cytokines.[68] Specifically, humanized monoclonal antibodies to IL-5 and nebulized soluble IL-4 receptors have been tested but have been disappointing to date.[68,69]

PHARMACOECONOMIC CONSIDERATIONS

Of the estimated $11.5 billion cost of asthma in the United States in 2004, direct medical expenditure accounted for 60% of the total, with emergency care (emergency department and inpatient hospital care) reaching $2.5 billion.[3] A cost-of-illness approach takes in all measurable costs; both indirect costs or costs to society and direct medical costs are considered. Using this approach, indirect costs, such as lost work and death, accounted for two-thirds of total expenditures per patient. Although prescription drugs were the largest single direct medical expenditure at $5 billion, an increase in these costs secondary to improved patient adherence could significantly reduce other costs because of school days lost and lost productivity secondary to asthma morbidity and mortality.

The medication cost increase over the past 10 years resulted from a doubling of prescribed medications, as well as a 169% increase in unit cost per medication, presumably as a result of a shift to more expensive antiinflammatory drugs consistent with the recommendations of the NAEPP guidelines.[2] Asthma severity obviously has an impact on cost of care. Studies from health maintenance organizations suggest that up to 45% of the cost of asthma is accrued by 10% of the patients, primarily as a result of emergency care.[70]

Numerous studies demonstrate the cost-effectiveness of patient education programs for asthma, particularly those providing guided self-management.[70] Several studies report positive results from pharmacist interventions reducing overall cost of care.[70] Similar studies demonstrate the cost-effectiveness of specialist care compared with generalist care. However, the results of these trials may be confounded by changes in prescribing as part of the overall program. Indeed, use of ICSs reduces both morbidity, particularly hospitalizations, and mortality in asthma patients.[6,53,71]

The NAEPP recommendations provide numerous alternatives for long-term controllers in mild to moderate persistent asthma, and few studies have compared their relative cost-effectiveness. This is important because outside the realm of randomized clinical trials that evaluate efficacy, other factors such as concern about adverse effects and adherence to therapy may alter the overall clinical effectiveness. Use of ICSs in children has produced a cost of $9.45 per symptom-free day gained, and in adults a cost of $5.00 per symptom-free day.[70] Retrospective analyses of large managed-care-linked pharmacy claims and healthcare utilization databases has allowed direct comparisons of the various long-term controllers in a general population to assess clinical effectiveness and cost-effectiveness. These studies have confirmed comparative randomized clinical trials showing ICSs to be significantly more cost-effective than leukotriene antagonists despite slightly better compliance with the leukotriene antagonists.[72,73] In addition, the combination of ICSs/LABA lowers healthcare use and total healthcare costs compared with the combination of a leukotriene antagonist and an ICS.[74]

CLINICAL CONTROVERSY

The potential for chronic use of inhaled β_2-agonists to worsen asthma has been a concern for more than 30 years. Large multicenter, double-blind, placebo-controlled trials with both mild and moderate persistent asthma did not show that regular administration of short-acting inhaled β_2-agonists worsened asthma. However, studies that have genotyped patients at the β-receptor suggest that homozygous Arg-16 patients (who make up approximately 16% of the population) are predisposed to worsening asthma with regular administration as measured by lower morning PEFs.[58] This phenomenon does not appear to occur with as-needed therapy with short-acting β_2-agonists. It is yet unknown if regular treatment with LABAs produces similar effects as retrospective analyses have not shown worsening of asthma or whether concurrent use of ICS is protective. These patients still respond acutely to the β_2-agonists, so whether they should avoid all β_2-agonists is speculative. Because the regular use of short-acting inhaled β_2-agonists does not improve control of symptoms, they should be used only as needed for symptoms.[6,58]

EVALUATION OF ASTHMA CONTROL

Control of asthma is defined as reducing both impairment and risk domains. The stepwise approach to therapy should be used to achieve and maintain this control. Figure 28–8 outlines the steps of care appropriate to the three age ranges of asthma. Depending on the severity of the patient's asthma, compromises from the ideal control are made, and the best possible outcome, balancing disease control and possible adverse effects from the drugs, is attempted. Regular followup contact is essential (at 1- to 6-month intervals, depending on control). A 3-month interval of well-controlled asthma should be considered if a step-down is anticipated.

Components of evaluations control include symptoms, nighttime awakenings, interference with normal activities, pulmonary function, quality of life, exacerbations, adherence, treatment-related adverse effects, and satisfaction with care. The categories of well-controlled, not well-controlled, and very poorly controlled are recommended.[6] Validated questionnaires such as the Asthma Therapy Assessment Questionnaire (ATAQ), the Asthma Control Questionnaire (ACQ), and the Asthma Control Test (ACT) can be regularly administered. The NAEPP minimally recommends spirometric tests at initial assessment, after treatment is initiated, and then every 1 to 2 years. In moderate to severe persistent asthma, peak-flow monitoring is recommended. Peak flow monitoring should also be considered for patients who are poor symptom perceivers and for those with a history of severe exacerbations. Patients also should be asked about exercise tolerance. All patients on inhaled drugs should have their inhalation delivery technique evaluated periodically—monthly initially, and then every 3 to 6 months. Before step-up in therapy, adherence, environmental control, and comorbid conditions should be reviewed.

Following initiation of antiinflammatory therapy or an increase in dosage, most patients should begin experiencing a decrease in symptoms in 1 to 2 weeks and achieve maximum symptomatic improvement within 4 to 8 weeks. The use of higher doses or more potent ICS agents may accelerate the process. Improvement in FEV_1 and PEF should follow a similar time frame; however, a decrease in BHR, as measured by morning PEF, PEF variability, and exercise tolerance, may take longer and improve over 1 to 3 months.[2] Patients should be informed that following a viral respiratory infection, they may experience increased exercise intolerance for up to 4 weeks.

Initial visits with the patient should focus on the patient's concerns, expectations, and goals of treatment. Basic education should focus on asthma as a chronic lung disease, the types of medications, and how they are to be used. Inhaler technique is taught, as is when to seek medical advice. Written action plans should be provided. Either peak-flow-based or symptom-based self-monitoring can be effective, if taught and followed correctly.[6] The first followup visit should be in 2 to 6 weeks, to evaluate control. At that time, the educational messages of the first visit should be repeated, as well as questions about the patient's current medications, adherence, and any difficulties related to the therapy.

CONCLUSIONS

Asthma is a complicated disease with a multitude of clinical presentations. The exact defect in asthma has not been defined, and it may be that asthma is a common presentation of a heterogeneous group of diseases. Asthma is defined and characterized by excessive reactivity of the bronchial tree to a wide variety of noxious stimuli. The reaction is characterized by bronchospasm, excessive mucus production, and inflammation. The central role of inflammation in inducing and maintaining BHR is now becoming widely appreciated and studied. The goal of asthma therapy is to normalize, as much as possible, the patient's life and prevent chronic irreversible lung changes. Drugs are the mainstay of asthma therapy. The goal of drug therapy is to use the minimum amount of medications possible to completely control the disease. In chronic asthma, therapy should be aimed at both bronchospasm and inflammation so as to produce the best results. Patients should be followed and monitored diligently for toxicities. Although death from asthma is an uncommon event, the most common cause of death is underassessment of the severity of obstruction either by the patient or by the clinician; the next common cause is undertreatment. A cornerstone of any therapy is education and the realization that most asthma deaths are avoidable.

ABBREVIATIONS

Arg: arginine

BHR: bronchial hyperresponsiveness

cAMP: cyclic adenosine monophosphate

CYP: cytochrome P450

DPI: dry-powder inhaler

EIB: exercise-induced bronchospasm

FeNO: fraction of exhaled nitric oxide

FEV_1: forced expiratory volume in 1 second

Gln: glutamine

Glu: glutamic acid

Gly: glycine

GM-CSF: granulocyte-macrophage colony-stimulating factor

HFA: hydrofluoroalkane

ICAM-1: intercellular adhesion molecule 1

ICS: inhaled corticosteroids

IgE: immunoglobulin E

IL: interleukin

LABA: long-acting β-agonists

LT: leukotriene

MDI: metered-dose inhaler

MMAD: mass median aerodynamic diameter

NAEPP: National Asthma Education and Prevention Program

NANC: nonadrenergic, noncholinergic

NO: nitric oxide

PEF: peak expiratory flow

VCAM-1: vascular cell adhesion molecule 1

REFERENCES

1. Rosenblatt MB. History of bronchial asthma. In: Weiss EB, Segal MS, Stein M, eds. Bronchial Asthma: Mechanisms and Therapeutics, 2d ed. Boston, Little, Brown, 1976:5–17.
2. NHLBI, National Asthma Education and Prevention Program, Expert Panel Report 2. Guidelines for the Diagnosis and Management of Asthma. NIH Publication No. 97–4051. Bethesda, MD: U.S. Department of Health and Human Services, 1997.
3. American Lung Association. Trends in asthma morbidity and mortality. American Lung Association Epidemiology & Statistics Unit Research and Program Services. July 2006, *http://www.lungusa.org.*
4. Kelly HW. Asthma. In: Cosby AG, Greenberg RE, Southward LH, Weitzman M eds. About Children: An Authoritative Resource on the State of Childhood Today. American Academy of Pediatrics, 2005:114–117.

5. Reed CE. The natural history of asthma. J Allergy Clin Immunol 2006;118:543–548.
6. National Institutes of Health, National Heart, Lung, and Blood Institute. National Asthma Education and Prevention Program. Full Report of the Expert Panel: Guidelines for the diagnosis and management of asthma (EPR-3) 2007. 2007, *http://www.nhlbi.nih.gov/guidelines/asthma.*
7. Bousquet J, Jeffery PK, Busse WW, et al. Asthma: From bronchoconstriction to airways inflammation and remodeling. Am J Respir Crit Care Med 2000;161:1720–1745.
8. National Institutes of Health, National Heart, Lung, and Blood Institute. Global Initiative for Asthma (GINA). Global Strategy for Asthma Management and Prevention Revised (2002). NHLBI/WHO Workshop Report. NIH publication No. 02–3659. Bethesda, MD: U.S. Department of Health and Human Services, 2002.
9. Ober C. Perspectives on the past decade of asthma genetics. J Allergy Clin Immunol 2005;116(2):274–278.
10. Holgate ST. Genetic and environmental interaction in allergy and asthma. J Allergy Clin Immunol 1999;104(6):1139–1146.
11. Van Eerdewegh P, Little RD, Dupuis J, et al. Association of the *ADAM33* gene with asthma and bronchial hyperresponsiveness. Nature 2002;418:426–430.
12. von Mutius E. The environmental predictors of allergic disease. J Allergy Clin Immunol 2000;105:9–19.
13. Malo J-L, Chan-Yeung M. Occupational asthma. J Allergy Clin Immunol 2001;108:317–328.
14. Kay AB. Allergy and allergic diseases: First of two parts. N Engl J Med 2001;344:30–37.
15. Busse WW, Lemanske RF Jr. Asthma. N Engl J Med 2001;344:350–362.
16. Holgate ST, Polosa R. The mechanisms, diagnosis, and management of severe asthma in adults. Lancet 2006;368(9537):780–793.
17. Smith AD, Cowan JO, Brassett KP, Herbison GP, Taylor DR. Use of exhaled nitric oxide measurements to guide treatment in chronic asthma. N Engl J Med 2005;352:2163–2173.
18. Anderson SD. How does exercise cause asthma attacks? Curr Opin Allergy Clin Immunol 2006;6:37–42.
19. Cates CJ, Jefferson TO, Bara AI, Rowe BH. Vaccines for preventing influenza in people with asthma. Cochrane Database Syst Rev 2004(2):CD000364.
20 Gibson PG, Henry RL, Coughlan JL. Gastro-oesophageal reflux treatment for asthma in adults and children. Cochrane Database Syst Rev 2003(2):CD001496.
21. Haggerty CL, Ness RB, Kelsey S, Waterer GW. The impact of estrogen and progesterone on asthma. Ann Allergy Asthma Immunol 2003;90:284–291.
22. Brenner BE, Holmes T M, Mazal B, Camargo CA Jr. Relation between phase of the menstrual cycle and asthma presentations in the emergency department. Thorax 2005;60:806–809.
23. Beasely R, Burgess C, Holt S. Call for a worldwide withdrawal of benzalkonium chloride from nebulizer solutions. J Allergy Clin Immunol 2001;107:222–223.
24. Jenkins C, Costello J, Hodge L. Systematic review of the prevalence of aspirin induced asthma and its implications for clinical practice. BMJ 2004;328(7437):434–440.
25. Dolovich MA, MacIntyre NR, Dhand R, et al. Consensus conference on aerosols and delivery devices. Respir Care 2000;45:588–776.
26. McFadden ER Jr. Acute severe asthma. Am J Respir Crit Care Med 2003;168:740–759.
27. Strauss L, Hejal R, Galan G, et al. Observations on the effects of aerosolized albuterol in acute asthma. Am J Respir Crit Care Med 1997;155:454–458.
28. McFadden Jr ER, Elsanadi N, Dixon L, Takacs M, Deal EC, Boyd KK, et al. Protocol therapy for acute asthma: Therapeutic benefits and cost savings. Am J Med 1995;99:651–661.
29. Dolovich MB, Ahrens RC, Hess DR, et al. Device selection and outcomes of aerosol therapy: Evidence-based guidelines. Chest 2005;127:335–371.
30. Camargo CA Jr, Spooner CH, Rowe BH. Continuous versus intermittent β-agonists in the treatment of acute asthma . Cochrane Database Syst Rev 2003;4:CD001115.
31. Nelson HS. β-adrenergic bronchodilators. N Engl J Med 1995;333:499–506.
32. Rowe BH, Edmonds ML, Spooner CH, Diner B, Camargo CA Jr. Corticosteroid therapy for acute asthma. Respir Med 2004;98:275–284.
33. Rodrigo GJ, Castro-Rodriguez JA. Anticholinergics in the treatment of children and adults with acute asthma: A systematic review with meta-analysis. Thorax 2005;60:740–746.
34. Parameswaran K, Belda J, Rowe BH. Addition of intravenous aminophylline to β_2-agonists in adults with acute asthma. Cochrane Database Syst Rev 2000(4):CD002742.
35. Rowe BH, Bretzlaff JA, Bourdon C, et al. Intravenous magnesium sulfate treatment for acute asthma in the emergency department: A systematic review of the literature. Ann Emerg Med 2000;36:181–190.
36. Silverman RA, Osborn H, Runge J, et al. IV magnesium sulfate in the treatment of acute severe asthma: A multicenter randomized controlled trial. Chest 2002:122:489–497.
37. Rodrigo GJ, Rodrigo C, Pollack CV, Rowe B. Use of helium-oxygen mixtures in the treatment of acute asthma: A systematic review. Chest 2003;123:891–896.
38. Kelly HW. What is new with the β_2 agonists: Issues in the management of asthma. Ann Pharmacother 2005;39:931–938.
39. Kelly HW. Potential adverse effects of the inhaled corticosteroids. J Allergy Clin Immunol 2003;112:469–478.
40. Green RH, Wardlaw AJ. Systemic corticosteroids in asthma. In: Li JT, ed. Pharmacotherapy of Asthma. New York: Taylor and Francis, 2006:233–262.
41. Winkler J, Hochhaus G, Derendorf H. How the lung handles drugs: Pharmacokinetics and pharmacodynamics of inhaled corticosteroids. Proc Am Thorac Soc 2004;1:356–363.
42. Gross NJ. Anticholinergic bronchodilators. In: Li JT, ed. Pharmacotherapy of Asthma. New York: Taylor and Francis, 2006:65–82.
43. Spooner CH, Spooner GR, Rowe BH. Mast-cell stabilising agents to prevent exercise-induced bronchoconstriction. Cochrane Database Syst Rev 2003;(4):CD002307.
44. Lord J, Ducharme FM, Stamp RJ, et al. Cost-effectiveness analysis of inhaled anticholinergics for acute childhood and adolescent asthma. BMJ 1999;319:1470–1471.
45. Suissa S, Ernst P, Benayoun S, et al. Low-dose inhaled corticosteroids and the prevention of death from asthma. N Engl J Med 2000;343:332–336.
46. Childhood Asthma Management Program Research Group. Long-term effects of budesonide or nedocromil in children with asthma. N Engl J Med 2000;343:1054–1063.
47. Guilbert TW, Morgan WJ, Zeiger RS, et al. Long-term inhaled corticosteroids in preschool children at high risk for asthma. N Engl J Med 2006;354:1985–1997.
48. Greenstone I, Ni CM, Masse V, et al. Combination of inhaled long-acting β_2-agonists and inhaled steroids versus higher dose of inhaled steroids in children and adults with persistent asthma. Cochrane Database Syst Rev 2005;4:CD005533.
49. Sin DD, Man J, Sharpe H, Gan WQ, Man SFP. Pharmacological management to reduce exacerbations in adults with asthma: A systematic review and meta-analysis. JAMA 2004;292:367–376.
50. Masoli M, Weatherall M, Holt S, Beasley R. Moderate dose inhaled corticosteroids plus salmeterol versus higher doses of inhaled corticosteroids in symptomatic asthma. Thorax 2005;60:730–734.
51. D'Amato GD, Buschioni E, Oldani V, Canonica W. Treating moderate-to-severe allergic asthma with a recombinant humanized anti-IgE monoclonal antibody (omalizumab). Treat Respir Med 2006;5(6):393–398.
52. National Institutes of Health, National Heart, Lung and Blood Institute. NAEPP Expert Panel Report Managing Asthma During Pregnancy: Recommendations for Pharmacologic Treatment—Update 2004. NIH Publication No. 04–5246. March 2004.
53. Masoli M, Shirtcliffe P, Weatherall M, Holt S, Beasley R. Inhaled corticosteroid therapy in the management of asthma in adults. In: Li JT, ed. Pharmacotherapy of Asthma. New York: Taylor and Francis, 2006:83–115.
54. Kharitonov SA, Barnes PJ. Exhaled markers of pulmonary disease. Am J Respir Crit Care Med 2001;163:1693–1722.
55. Nelson HS, Weiss ST, Bleecker ER, Yancey SW, Dorinsky PM. The Salmeterol Multicenter Asthma Research Trial: A comparison of usual pharmacotherapy for asthma or usual pharmacotherapy plus salmeterol. Chest 2006;129:15–26.
56. US Food and Drug Administration. Medical officer review. Provided for meeting of Pulmonary-Allergy Drugs Advisory Committee, July 13, 2005. *http://www.fda.gov/ohrms/dockets/ac/05/briefing/.*
57. Nelson HS. Is there a problem with inhaled long-acting β-adrenergic agonists. J Allergy Clin Immunol 2006;117:3–16.

58. Kelly HW. Risk versus benefit considerations for the β_2-agonists. Pharmacotherapy 2006;26:164S–174S.
59. Bisgaard H. Effect of long-acting β_2-agonists on exacerbation rates of asthma in children. Pediatr Pulmonol 2003;36:391–398.
60. Blake K. Theophylline. In: Murphy SA, Kelly HW, eds. Pediatric Asthma. New York: Marcel Dekker, 1999:363–431.
61. Lowery M, Kelly KJ. Cromolyn and nedocromil. In: Li JT, ed. Pharmacotherapy of Asthma. New York: Taylor and Francis, 2006:195–231.
62. Sorkness CA. Leukotriene receptor antagonists in the treatment of asthma. Pharmacotherapy 2001;21:34S–37S.
63. Drazen JM, Israel E, O'Byrne PM. Treatment of asthma with drugs modifying the leukotriene pathway. N Engl J Med 1999;340:197–206.
64. Busse W, Raphael GD, Galant S, et al. Low-dose fluticasone propionate compared with montelukast for first-line treatment of persistent asthma: A randomized clinical trial. J Allergy Clin Immunol 2001;107:461–468.
65. Sorkness CA, Lemanske RF Jr, Mauger DT, et al. Long-term comparison of 3 controller regimens for mild-moderate persistent childhood asthma. The Pediatric Asthma Controller Trial. J Allergy Clin Immunol 2007;119(1):64–72.
66. Strunk RC, Bloomberg GR. Omalizumab for asthma. N Engl J Med 2006;354:2689–2695.
67. Davies H, Olson L, Gibson P. Methotrexate as a steroid sparing agent for asthma in adults. Cochrane Database Syst Rev 2000(2):CD000391.
68. Barnes PJ. New directions in allergic diseases: Mechanism based anti-inflammatory therapies. J Allergy Clin Immunol 2000;106:5–16.
69. Hendeles L, Asmus M, Chesrown S. Evaluation of cytokine modulators for asthma. Paediatr Respir Rev 2003;4(Suppl 1):S105–S110.
70. National Asthma Education and Prevention Program. Task force report on the cost effectiveness, quality of care, and financing of asthma care. Am J Respir Crit Care Med 1996;154(Suppl):S81–S130.
71. Donahue JG, Weiss ST, Livingston JM, et al. Inhaled steroids and the risk of hospitalization for asthma. JAMA 1997;277:887–891.
72. Stempel DA, Meyer JW, Stanford RH, Yancey SW. One-year claims analysis comparing inhaled fluticasone propionate with zafirlukast for the treatment of asthma. J Allergy Clin Immunol 2001;107:94–98.
73. Stempel DA, Mauskopf J, McLaughlin T, et al. Comparison of asthma costs in patients starting fluticasone propionate compared to patients starting montelukast. Respir Med 2001;95:227–234.
74. Stempel DA, O'Donnell JC, Meyer JW. Inhaled corticosteroids plus salmeterol or montelukast: Effects on resource utilization and costs. J Allergy Clin Immunol 2002;109:433–439.

CHAPTER 29

Chronic Obstructive Pulmonary Disease

DENNIS M. WILLIAMS AND SHARYA V. BOURDET

KEY CONCEPTS

1. Chronic obstructive pulmonary disease (COPD) is a progressive disease characterized by airflow limitation that is not fully reversible and is associated with an abnormal inflammatory response of the lungs to noxious particles or gases.
2. COPD is historically described as either *chronic bronchitis* or *emphysema*. Chronic bronchitis is defined in clinical terms, whereas emphysema is defined in terms of anatomic pathology. Because most patients exhibit some features of each disease, the appropriate emphasis of COPD pathophysiology is on small airway disease and parenchymal damage that contributes to chronic airflow limitation.
3. Mortality from COPD has increased steadily over the past three decades; it currently is the fourth leading cause of death in the United States.
4. The primary cause of COPD is cigarette smoking. Other risks include a genetic predisposition, environmental exposures (including occupational dusts and chemicals), and air pollution.
5. Smoking cessation is the only management strategy proven to slow progression of COPD.
6. Oxygen therapy has been shown to reduce mortality in selected patients with COPD. Oxygen therapy is indicated for patients with a resting Pa_{O_2} (partial pressure alveolar oxygen) of less than 55 mm Hg or a Pa_{O_2} of less than 60 mm Hg and evidence of right-sided heart failure, polycythemia, or impaired neurologic function.
7. Bronchodilators represent the mainstay of drug therapy for COPD. Pharmacotherapy is used to relieve patient symptoms and improve quality of life. Guidelines recommend short-acting bronchodilators as initial therapy for patients with mild or intermittent symptoms
8. For the patient who experiences chronic symptoms, long-acting bronchodilators are appropriate. Either a β_2-agonist or an anticholinergic offers significant benefits. Combining long-acting bronchodilators is recommended if necessary despite limited data.
9. The role of inhaled corticosteroid therapy in COPD is controversial. International guidelines suggest that patients with severe COPD and frequent exacerbations may benefit from inhaled corticosteroids.
10. Acute exacerbations of COPD have a significant impact on disease progression and mortality. Treatment of acute exacerbations includes intensification of bronchodilator therapy and a short course of systemic corticosteroids.
11. Antimicrobial therapy should be used during acute exacerbations of COPD if the patient exhibits at least two of the following: increased dyspnea, increased sputum volume, and increased sputum purulence.

Learning objectives, review questions,
and other resources can be found at
www.pharmacotherapyonline.com.

Chronic obstructive pulmonary disease (COPD) is a common chronic disease of the airways characterized by the gradual and progressive loss of lung function. The prevalence and mortality of COPD have increased substantially over the past two decades. Currently, COPD is the fourth leading cause of death in the United States.

Although national guidelines for COPD management have been available for nearly two decades, questions were raised concerning their quality and supporting evidence. To standardize the care of patients with COPD and present evidence-based recommendations, the National Heart, Lung, and Blood Institute and the World Health Organization launched the Global Initiative for Chronic Obstructive Lung Disease (GOLD) in 2001.[1] This report was updated most recently in 2006. The goals of the GOLD organization are to increase awareness of COPD and reduce morbidity and mortality associated with the disease. International guidelines have also been developed through a collaborative effort of the American Thoracic Society and the European Respiratory Society and are widely available.[2] These two guidelines are generally concordant in their recommendations.

1 A consensus definition recognizes COPD as a disease characterized by airflow limitation that is not fully reversible. The airflow limitation is usually both progressive and associated with an abnormal inflammatory response of the lungs to noxious particles or gases.[2] Although COPD primarily affects the lungs, it also is associated with significant consequences. Finally, COPD is preventable and treatable.

For many years, clinicians and researchers have exhibited a nihilistic attitude toward the value of treatments for COPD. This was based on the paucity of effective therapies, the destructive nature of the condition, and the fact that the common etiology is cigarette smoking, a modifiable health risk. Currently, there is renewed interest in evaluating the value of treatments and prevention based on the availability of new therapeutic options for pharmacotherapy and guidelines based on evidence.[3] Support for renewed optimism is also reflected in the availability of research funding to improve understanding about this disease and its management. This includes National Heart, Lung, and Blood Institute funding of Specialized Centers of Clinically Oriented Research programs in COPD, whose objective is to promote multidisciplinary research on clinically relevant questions enabling basic science findings to be more rapidly applied to clinical problems.[4]

❷ The most common conditions comprising COPD are chronic bronchitis and emphysema. Chronic bronchitis is associated with chronic or recurrent excessive mucus secretion into the bronchial tree with cough that is present on most days for at least 3 months of the year for at least 2 consecutive years in a patient in whom other causes of chronic cough have been excluded.[2] Although chronic bronchitis is defined in clinical terms, emphysema is defined in terms of anatomic pathology. Emphysema historically was defined on histologic examination at autopsy. Because this histologic definition is of limited clinical value, emphysema also has been defined as abnormal permanent enlargement of the airspaces distal to the terminal bronchioles accompanied by destruction of their walls yet without obvious fibrosis.[2]

Current guidelines have moved away from chronic bronchitis and emphysema as descriptive subsets of COPD. This is based on the observation that the majority of COPD is caused by a common risk factor (cigarette smoking), and most patients exhibit features of both chronic bronchitis and emphysema. Therefore, emphasis is currently placed on the pathophysiologic features of small airways disease and parenchymal destruction as contributors to chronic airflow limitation. Most patients with COPD demonstrate features of both problems. Chronic inflammation affects the integrity of the airways and causes damage and destruction of the parenchymal structures. The underlying problem is persistent exposure to noxious particles or gases that sustain the inflammatory response. The airways of the lung and the parenchyma are both susceptible to inflammation and the result is chronic airflow limitation that characterizes COPD (Fig. 29–1).

EPIDEMIOLOGY

The true prevalence of COPD is likely underreported. Data from the National Health Interview Survey in 2001 indicate that 12.1 million people older than age 25 years in the United States have COPD.[5] More than 9 million of these individuals have chronic bronchitis; the remainder have emphysema or a combination of both diseases. According to national surveys, the true prevalence of people with symptoms of chronic airflow obstruction may exceed 24 million.[6] The burden may be even greater because more than one-third of adults in the United States reported respiratory complaints compatible with symptomatic COPD in some surveys.[7]

❸ COPD is the fourth leading cause of death in the United States, exceeded only by cancer, heart disease, and cerebrovascular accidents. In 2004, COPD accounted for 123,884 deaths in the United States.[8] It is the only leading cause of death to increase over the last 30 years and is projected to be the third leading cause by 2020.[9] Overall, the mortality rate is higher in males; however, the female death rate has doubled over the last 25 years, and the number of female deaths has exceeded male deaths since 2000. The mortality rate is higher in whites than in blacks.[9]

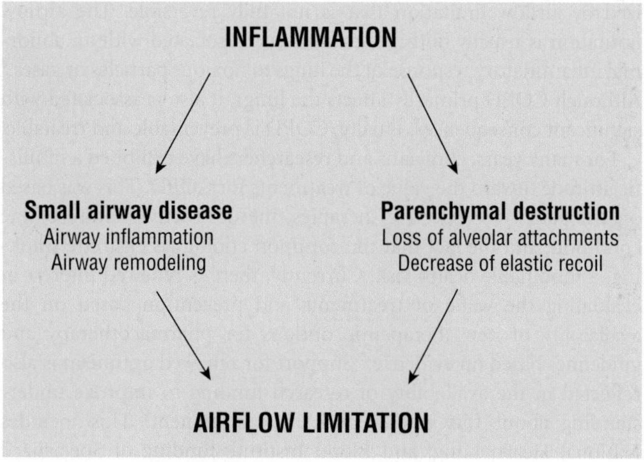

FIGURE 29-1. Mechanisms for developing chronic airflow limitation in chronic obstructive pulmonary disease. *(From reference 1.)*

Cigarette smoking is the primary cause of COPD and although the prevalence of cigarette smoking has declined compared with 1965, approximately 25% of individuals in the United States currently smoke. The trend of increasing COPD mortality likely reflects the long latency period between smoking exposure and complications associated with COPD.

Although the mortality of COPD is significant, morbidity associated with the disease also has a significant impact on patients, their families, and the healthcare system. COPD represents the second leading cause of disability in the United States. In the last 20 years, COPD has been responsible for nearly 50 million hospital visits nationwide.[10] In recent years, a diagnosis of COPD accounts for more than 15 million physician office visits, 1.5 million emergency room visits, and 700,000 hospitalizations annually. A survey by the American Lung Association revealed that among COPD patients, 51% reported that their condition limits their ability to work, 70% were limited in normal physical activity, 56% were limited in performing household chores, and 50% reported that sleep was affected adversely.[11]

The economic impact of COPD continues to increase as well. It was estimated at $23 billion in 2000 and rose to $37.2 billion in 2004, including $20.9 billion in direct costs and $16.3 billion in indirect morbidity and mortality costs.[9,12] By 2020, COPD will be the fifth most burdensome disease, as measured by disability-adjusted life years lost as a consequence of illness.

ETIOLOGY

❹ Although cigarette smoking is the primary modifiable risk factor for the development of COPD, the disease can be attributed to a combination of risk factors that results in lung injury and tissue destruction. Smokers are 12 to 13 times more likely to die from COPD than nonsmokers.[13] Risk factors can be divided into host factors and environmental factors (Table 29–1), and commonly, the interaction between these risks leads to expression of the disease. Host factors, such as genetic predisposition, may not be modifiable but are important for identifying patients at high risk of developing the disease.

Environmental factors, such as tobacco smoke and occupational dust and chemicals, are modifiable factors that, if avoided, may reduce the risk of disease development. Environmental exposures associated with COPD are particles that are inhaled by the individual and result in inflammation and cell injury. Exposure to multiple environmental toxins increases the risk of COPD. Thus, the total burden of inhaled particles (e.g., cigarette smoke as well as occupational and environmental particles and pollutants) can play a significant role in the development of COPD. In such cases, it is helpful to assess an individual's total burden of inhaled particles. For example, an individual who smokes and works in a textile factory has a higher total burden of inhaled particles than an individual who smokes and has no occupational exposure.

TABLE 29-1 Risk Factors for Development of Chronic Obstructive Pulmonary Disease

Exposures	Host Factors
Environmental tobacco smoke	Genetic predisposition (α_1-antitrypsin)
Occupational dusts and chemicals	Airway hyperresponsiveness
Air pollution	Impaired lung growth

Cigarette smoking is the most common risk factor and accounts for 85% to 90% of cases of COPD.[1] Components of tobacco smoke activate inflammatory cells, which produce and release the inflammatory mediators characteristic of COPD. Although the risk is lower in pipe and cigar smokers, it is still higher than in nonsmokers. Age of starting, total pack-years, and current smoking status are predictive of COPD mortality.

However, only 15% to 20% of all smokers go on to develop COPD, and not all smokers who have equivalent smoking histories develop the same degree of pulmonary impairment, suggesting that other host and environmental factors contribute to the degree of lung dysfunction. Nevertheless, the rate of loss of lung function is determined primarily by smoking status and history.[2] Children and spouses of smokers are also at increased risk of developing significant pulmonary dysfunction by passive smoking, also known as *environmental tobacco smoke* or *secondhand smoke.*

Occupational exposures are also important risk factors for COPD and, in nonindustrialized countries, may be more common than cigarette smoking. These exposures include dust and chemicals such as vapors, irritants, and fumes. Reduced lung function and deaths from COPD are higher for individuals who work in gold and coal mining, in the glass or ceramic industries with exposure to silica dust, and in jobs that expose them to cotton dust or grain dust, toluene diisocyanate, or asbestos. Other occupational risk factors include chronic exposure to open cooking or heating fires.

It is unclear whether or not air pollution alone is a significant risk factor for the development of COPD in smokers and nonsmokers with normal lung function. However, in individuals with existing pulmonary dysfunction, significant air pollution worsens symptoms. As evidence for this, emergency department visits are increased during higher-intensity periods of air pollution.

Individuals exposed to the same environmental risk factors do not have the same chance of developing COPD, suggesting that host factors play an important role in pathogenesis.[1,2] While many not yet identified genes may influence the risk of developing COPD, the best documented genetic factor is a hereditary deficiency of α_1-antitrypsin (AAT). AAT-associated emphysema is an example of a pure genetic disorder inherited in an autosomal recessive pattern. Some researchers sometimes describe inheritance as autosomal codominant because heterozygotes can also have decreased concentrations of AAT enzyme.[14] The consequences of AAT deficiency are discussed in Pathophysiology below as protease-antiprotease imbalance. True AAT deficiency accounts for less than 1% of COPD cases.[2]

AAT is a 42-kDa plasma protein that is synthesized in hepatocytes. A primary role of AAT is to protect cells, especially those in the lung, from destruction by elastase released by neutrophils. In fact, AAT may be responsible for 90% of the inhibition of this destructive enzyme.[15] In individuals with the most common allele (M), plasma levels of AAT are approximately 20 to 50 micromolars (100 to 350 mg/dL). The protective effect of AAT in the lungs is significantly diminished when plasma levels are less than 11 micromolars (80 mg/dL).[15] AAT is an acute-phase reactant, and the serum concentration can be quite variable.

Several types of AAT deficiency have been identified and are caused by mutations in the AAT gene. Two main gene variants, S and Z, have been identified. In patients who are homozygous with the S variant, AAT levels are at least 60% of those of normal individuals. These patients usually do not have an increased risk of COPD compared with normal individuals. Patients with homozygous Z deficiency (ZZ), represent 95% of clinical cases of AAT-associated emphysema[14] and have AAT levels that are 10% of those of normal individuals, whereas patients with heterozygous Z variant (SZ) have levels closer to 40% of those of normal individuals. Homozygous Z patients have a higher risk of developing COPD than do heterozygous Z patients. A history of cigarette smoking increases this risk. A small number of patients have a null, null phenotype and are at high risk for developing emphysema because they produce virtually no AAT.

Patients with AAT deficiency develop COPD at an early age (20 to 50 years) primarily owing to an accelerated decline in lung function. Compared with an average annual decline in forced expiratory volume in 1 second (FEV_1) of 25 mL/year in healthy nonsmokers, patients with homozygous Z deficiency have been reported to have declines of 54 mL/year for nonsmokers and 108 mL/year for current smokers. Effective diagnosis is dependent on clinical suspicion, diagnostic testing of serum concentrations, and genotype confirmation.[14] Patients developing COPD at an early age or those with a strong family history of COPD should be screened for AAT deficiency. If the concentration is low, genotype testing (DNA) should be performed.

Two additional host factors that may influence the risk of COPD include airway hyperresponsiveness and lung growth. Individuals with airway hyperresponsiveness to various inhaled particles may have an accelerated decline in lung function compared with those without airway hyperresponsiveness. Additionally, individuals who do not attain maximal lung growth owing to low birth weight, prematurity at birth, or childhood illnesses may be at risk for COPD in the future.[1]

PATHOPHYSIOLOGY

COPD is characterized by chronic inflammatory changes that lead to destructive changes and the development of chronic airflow limitation. The inflammatory process is widespread and involves not only the airways but also extends to the pulmonary vasculature and lung parenchyma. The inflammation of COPD is often referred to as neutrophilic in nature, but macrophages and CD8+ lymphocytes also play major roles.[16–18] The inflammatory cells release a variety of chemical mediators, of which tumor necrosis factor-α, interleukin (IL-8), and leukotriene (LT) B_4 play major roles.[1,19] The actions of these cells and mediators are complementary and redundant, leading to the widespread destructive changes. The stimulus for activation of inflammatory cells and mediators is an exposure to noxious particles and gas through inhalation. The most common etiologic factor is exposure to environmental tobacco smoke, although other chronic inhalational exposures can lead to similar inflammatory changes.

Other processes that have been proposed to play a major role in the pathogenesis of COPD include oxidative stress and an imbalance between aggressive and protective defense systems in the lungs (proteases and antiproteases).[16] These processes may be the result of ongoing inflammation or occur as a result of environmental pressures and exposures (Fig. 29–2).

An altered interaction between oxidants and antioxidants present in the airways is responsible for the increased oxidative stress present in COPD. Increases in markers (e.g., hydrogen peroxide and nitric oxide) of oxidants are seen in the epithelial lining fluid.[1] The increased oxidants generated by cigarette smoke react with and damage various proteins and lipids, leading to cell and tissue damage. Oxidants also promote inflammation directly and exacerbate the protease-antiprotease imbalance by inhibiting antiprotease activity.

The consequences of an imbalance between proteases and antiproteases in the lungs was described over 40 years ago when the hereditary deficiency of the protective antiprotease AAT was discovered to result in an increased risk of developing emphysema prematurely. This enzyme (AAT) is responsible for inhibiting several protease enzymes, including neutrophil elastase. In the presence of unopposed activity, elastase attacks elastin, a major component of alveolar walls.[1]

In the inherited form of emphysema, there is an absolute deficiency of AAT. In cigarette smoking-associated emphysema, the

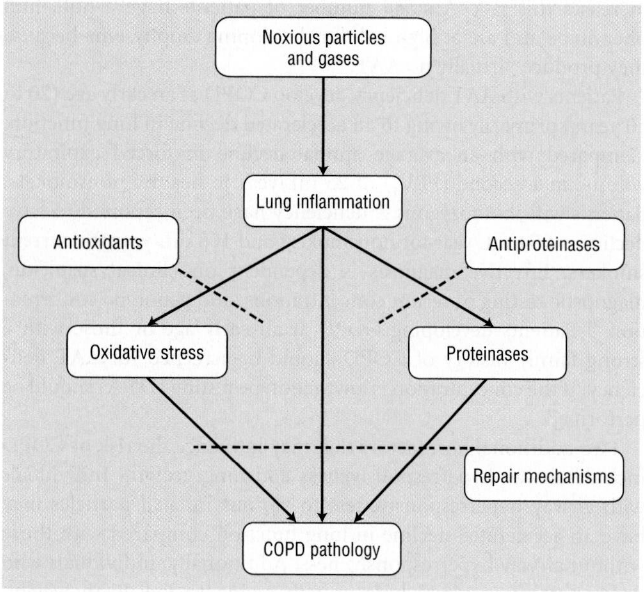

FIGURE 29-2. Pathogenesis of chronic obstructive pulmonary disease (COPD). *(From reference 1.)*

imbalance is likely associated with increased protease activity or reduced activity of antiproteases. Activated inflammatory cells release several proteases other than AAT, including cathepsins and metalloproteinases. In addition, oxidative stress reduces antiprotease (or protective) activity.

It is helpful to differentiate inflammation occurring in COPD from that present in asthma because the response to antiinflammatory therapy differs. The inflammatory cells that predominate differ between the two conditions, with neutrophils playing a major role in COPD and eosinophils and mast cells in asthma. Mediators of inflammation also differ with LTB_4, IL-8, and tumor necrosis factor-α predominating in COPD, compared with LTD_4, IL-4, and IL-5 among the numerous mediators modulating inflammation in asthma.[1] Table 29–2 summarizes the characteristics of inflammation for the two diseases.

Pathologic changes of COPD are widespread, affecting large and small airways, lung parenchyma, and the pulmonary vasculature.[1] An inflammatory exudate is often present that leads to an increase in the number and size of goblet cells and mucus glands. Mucus secretion is increased, and ciliary motility is impaired. There is also a thickening of smooth muscle and connective tissue in the airways. Inflammation is present in central and peripheral airways. The chronic inflammation results in a repeated injury and repair process that leads to scarring and fibrosis. Diffuse airway narrowing is present and is more prominent in smaller peripheral airways. The decrease in FEV_1 is attributed to the presence of inflammation in the airways while the blood gas abnormalities result from impaired gas transfer due to parenchymal damage.

Parenchymal changes affect the gas-exchanging units of the lungs, including the alveoli and pulmonary capillaries. The distribution of destructive changes varies depending on the etiology. Most commonly, smoking-related disease results in centrilobular emphysema that primarily affects respiratory bronchioles. Panlobular emphysema is seen in AAT deficiency and extends to the alveolar ducts and sacs.

The vascular changes of COPD include a thickening of pulmonary vessels and often are present early in the disease. Increased pulmonary pressures early in the disease are caused by hypoxic vasoconstriction of pulmonary arteries. If persistent, the presence of chronic inflammation may lead to endothelial dysfunction of the pulmonary arteries. Later, structural changes lead to an increase in pulmonary pressures, especially during exercise. In severe COPD, secondary pulmonary hypertension leads to the development of right-sided heart failure.

Mucus hypersecretion is present early in the course of the disease and is associated with an increased number and size of mucus-producing cells. The presence of chronic inflammation perpetuates the process, although the resulting airflow obstruction and chronic airflow limitation may be reversible or irreversible. Table 29–3 summarizes the various causes of airflow obstruction.

Recently, there has been interest in the role of thoracic overinflation as it relates to the pathophysiology of COPD. Chronic airflow obstruction leads to air trapping which results in thoracic hyperinflation that can be detected on chest radiograph. This problem results in several dynamic changes in the chest, including flattening of diaphragmatic muscles. Under normal circumstances, the diaphragms are dome-shaped muscles tethered at the base of the lungs. When the diaphragm contracts, the muscle becomes shorter and flatter, which creates the negative inspiratory force through which air flows into the lung during inspiration. In the presence of thoracic hyperinflation, the diaphragmatic muscle is placed at a disadvantage and is a less-efficient muscle of ventilation. The increased work required by diaphragmatic contractions predisposes the patient to muscle fatigue especially during periods of exacerbations.

The other consequence of thoracic hyperinflation is a change in lung volumes. In patients with COPD who exhibit thoracic hyperinflation there is an increase in the functional residual capacity which is the amount of air left in the lung after exhalation at rest. Therefore, these patients are breathing at higher lung volumes which perturbs gas exchange. In addition, the increased functional residual capacity limits the inspiratory reserve capacity which is the amount of air that

TABLE 29-2 Features of Inflammation in Chronic Obstructive Pulmonary Disease (COPD) Compared with Asthma

	COPD	Asthma
Cells	Neutrophils	Eosinophils
	Large increase in macrophages	Small increase in macrophages
	Increase in CD8+ T lymphocytes	Increase in CD4+ TH_2 lymphocytes
		Activation of mast cells
Mediators	LTB_4	LTD_4
	IL-8	IL-4, IL-5
	TNF-α	(Plus many others)
Consequences	Squamous metaplasia of epithelium	Fragile epithelium
	Parenchymal destruction	Thickening of basement membrane
	Mucus metaplasia	Mucus metaplasia
	Glandular enlargement	Glandular enlargement
Response to treatment	Glucocorticosteroids have variable effect	Glucocorticosteroids inhibit inflammation

IL, interleukin; LT, leukotriene; TH, T-helper; TNF, tumor necrosis factor.
From reference 1.

TABLE 29-3 Etiology of Airflow Limitation in Chronic Obstructive Pulmonary Disease

Reversible
Presence of mucus and inflammatory cells and mediators in bronchial secretions
Bronchial smooth muscle contraction in peripheral and central airways
Dynamic hyperinflation during exercise
Irreversible
Fibrosis and narrowing of airways
Reduced elastic recoil with loss of alveolar surface area
Destruction of alveolar support with reduced patency of small airways

the patient can inhale to fill the lungs. The increased functional residual capacity also limits the duration of inhalation time and this has been associated with an increase in dyspnea complaints by patients.[20] Drug therapy for COPD, especially bronchodilators, can reduce thoracic hyperinflation by reducing airflow obstruction. This may partially explain the improvement in symptoms reported by patients with COPD despite minimal improvements in lung function with drug therapy.

Airflow limitation is assessed through spirometry, which represents the "gold standard" for diagnosing and monitoring COPD. The hallmark of COPD is a reduction in the ratio of FEV_1 to forced vital capacity (FVC) to less than 70%.[1,2] The FEV_1 generally is reduced, except in very mild disease, and the rate of FEV_1 decline is greater in COPD patients compared with normal subjects.

The impact of the numerous pathologic changes in the lung perturbs the normal gas-exchange and protective functions of the lung. Ultimately, these are exhibited through the common symptoms of COPD, including dyspnea and a chronic cough productive of sputum. As the disease progresses, abnormalities in gas exchange lead to hypoxemia and/or hypercapnia; although there often is not a strong relationship between pulmonary function and arterial blood gas results.

Significant changes in arterial blood gases usually are not present until the FEV_1 is less than 1 L.[1] In these patients, hypoxemia and hypercapnia can become chronic problems. Initially, when hypoxemia is present, it usually is associated with exercise. However, as the disease progresses, hypoxemia at rest develops. Patients with severe COPD can have a low arterial oxygen tension (PaO_2 = 45 to 60 mm Hg) and an elevated arterial carbon dioxide tension ($PaCO_2$ = 50 to 60 mm Hg). The hypoxemia is attributed to hypoventilation ($\dot{V}$) of lung tissue relative to perfusion ($\dot{Q}$) of the area. This low $\dot{V}/\dot{Q}$ ratio will progress over a period of several years, resulting in a consistent decline in the PaO_2. Some COPD patients lose the ability to increase the rate or depth of respiration in response to persistent hypercapnia. Although this is not completely understood, the decreased ventilatory drive may be a result of abnormal peripheral or central respiratory receptors responses. This relative hypoventilation subsequently leads to hypercapnia. In this case, the central respiratory response to a chronically increased $PaCO_2$ can be blunted. These changes in PaO_2 and $PaCO_2$ are subtle and progress over a period of many years; as a result, the pH usually is nearly normal because the kidneys compensate by retaining bicarbonate. If acute respiratory distress develops, such as might be seen in pneumonia or a COPD exacerbation with impending respiratory failure, the $PaCO_2$ may rise sharply, and the patient presents with an uncompensated respiratory acidosis.

The consequences of long-standing COPD and chronic hypoxemia include the development of secondary pulmonary hypertension that progresses slowly if appropriate treatment of COPD is not initiated. Pulmonary hypertension is the most common cardiovascular complication of COPD and can result in cor pulmonale, or right-sided heart failure.[21]

The elevated pulmonary artery pressures are attributed to vasoconstriction (in response to chronic hypoxemia), vascular remodeling, and loss of pulmonary capillary beds. If elevated pulmonary pressures are sustained, cor pulmonale can develop, characterized by hypertrophy of the right ventricle in response to increases in pulmonary vascular resistance.

The risks of cor pulmonale include venous stasis with the potential for thrombosis and pulmonary embolism. Another important systemic consequence of COPD is a loss of skeletal muscle mass and general decline in the overall health status.

Although airway inflammation is prominent in patients with COPD, there is also evidence of systemic inflammation.[22] The systemic manifestations can have devastating effects on overall health status and comorbidities. These include cardiovascular events associated with ischemia, cachexia, and muscle wasting. There is some interest in the role of measuring C-reactive protein as a parameter to assess systemic inflammation and its impact on COPD severity; however, it is premature to recommend this strategy currently.[23]

PATHOPHYSIOLOGY OF EXACERBATION

The natural history of COPD is characterized by recurrent exacerbations associated with increased symptoms and a decline in overall health status. An exacerbation is defined as a change in the patient's baseline symptoms (dyspnea, cough, or sputum production) beyond day-to-day variability sufficient to warrant a change in management.[1,2] Exacerbations have a significant impact on the natural course of COPD and occur more frequently in patients with more severe chronic disease. Because many patients experience chronic symptoms, the diagnosis of an exacerbation is based, in part, on subjective measures and clinical judgment. Repeated exacerbations, especially those requiring hospitalization, are associated with an increased mortality risk.

There are limited data about pathology during exacerbations owing to the nature of the disease and the condition of patients; however, inflammatory mediators including neutrophils and eosinophils are increased in the sputum. Chronic airflow limitation is a feature of COPD and may not change remarkably even during an exacerbation.[1] The lung hyperinflation present chronic COPD is worsened during an exacerbation which contributes to worsening dyspnea and poor gas exchange.

The primary physiologic change is often a worsening of arterial blood gas results owing to poor gas exchange and increased muscle fatigue. In a patient experiencing a severe exacerbation, profound hypoxemia and hypercapnia can be accompanied by respiratory acidosis and respiratory failure.

CLINICAL PRESENTATION

The diagnosis of COPD is made based on the patient's symptoms, including cough, sputum production, and dyspnea, and a history of exposure to risk factors such as tobacco smoke and occupational exposures. Patients may have these symptoms for several years before dyspnea develops and often will not seek medical attention until dyspnea is significant. A diagnosis of COPD should be considered in any patient who presents with chronic cough, sputum production, or dyspnea and who has risk factors for the disease.

The presence of airflow limitation should be confirmed with spirometry. Spirometry represents a comprehensive assessment of lung volumes and capacities. The hallmark of COPD is an FEV_1:FVC ratio of less than 70%, which indicates airway obstruction, and a postbronchodilator FEV_1 of less than 80% of predicted confirms the presence of airflow limitation that is not fully reversible.[1] An improvement in FEV_1 of less than 12% following inhalation of a rapid-acting bronchodilator is considered to be evidence of irreversible airflow obstruction. Reversibility of airflow limitation is measured by a bronchodilator challenge, which is described in Table 29–4. Although a low peak expiratory flow is consistent with COPD, the use of peak expiratory flow measurements is inadequate for the diagnosis of COPD owing to low specificity and the high degree of effort dependence. Chapter 27 has a comprehensive discussion of spirometry.

Spirometry combined with a physical examination improves the diagnostic accuracy of COPD.[7] Spirometry is also used to determine the severity of the disease, along with an assessment of symptoms and the presence of complications. A primary benefit of spirometry is to identify individuals who might benefit from pharmacotherapy to reduce exacerbations. Currently, the GOLD consensus guidelines suggest a four-stage classification system (Table 29–5).

TABLE 29-4 Procedures for Reversibility Testing

Preparation
Tests should be performed when patients are clinically stable and free from respiratory infection.
Patients should not have taken inhaled short-acting bronchodilators in the previous 6 hours, long-acting β-agonists in the previous 12 hours, or sustained-release theophylline in the previous 24 hours.
Spirometry
FEV_1 should be measured before bronchodilator is given.
Bronchodilators can be given by either metered-dose inhaler or nebulization.
Usual doses are 400 mcg of β-agonist, up to 160 mcg of anticholinergic, or the two combined.
FEV1 should be measured 10–15 minutes after the β-agonist or 30–45 minutes after combination is given.
Results
An increase in FEV_1 that is both greater than 200 mL and 12% above the prebronchodilator FEV_1 is considered significant.

FEV_1, forced expiratory volume in the first second of expiration.
From reference 1.

The 2006 GOLD guidelines were modified to remove the stage 0 category for COPD classification. Patients at risk (stage 0) have normal spirometry but experience chronic symptoms of cough or sputum production and a history of exposure to risk factors. This change was made because of inadequate evidence to identify patients who might progress to stage 1 disease. Patients in the remaining four stages of classification all exhibit the hallmark finding of airflow obstruction, that is, a reduction in the FEV_1:FVC ratio to less than 70%. FVC is the total amount of air exhaled after a maximal inhalation. The extent of reduction in FEV_1 further defines the patient with mild, moderate, severe, or very severe disease.[1]

Spirometry is the primary tool in classifying COPD according to severity. However, two other factors that influence disease severity, survival, and health-related quality are life are body mass index (BMI) and dyspnea.[2] A low BMI is a systemic consequence of chronic COPD and a BMI of less than 21 kg/m^2 is associated with increased mortality.[24]

Dyspnea is often the most troublesome complaint for the patient with COPD. Dyspnea can impair exercise performance and functional capacity and is frequently associated with depression and anxiety. Together, these have a significant effect on health related quality of life.[20] As a subjective symptom, dyspnea is often difficult for the clinician to assess. Various tools are available to evaluate the severity of dyspnea. A version of the Medical Research Council scale, modified by the American Thoracic Society, is commonly employed and categorizes dyspnea grades from 0 to 4 (Table 29–6).[25]

TABLE 29-5 Classification of Chronic Obstructive Pulmonary Disease Severity

Stage I: mild
$FEV_1/FVC < 70\%$
$FEV_1 \geq 80\%$
With or without symptoms
Stage II: moderate
$FEV_1/FVC < 70\%$
$50\% < FEV_1 < 80\%$
With or without symptoms
Stage III: severe
$FEV_1/FVC < 70\%$
$30\% < FEV_1 < 50\%$
With or without symptoms
Stage IV: very severe
$FEV_1/FVC < 70\%$
$FEV_1 < 30\%$ or $< 50\%$ with presence of chronic respiratory failure or right heart failure

FEV_1, forced expiratory volume in the first second of expiration; FVC, forced vital capacity.
From reference 1.

TABLE 29-6 Modified Medical Research Council (MRC) Dyspnea Scale

Grade 0	No dyspnea	Not troubled by breathlessness except with strenuous exercise
Grade 1	Slight dyspnea	Troubled by shortness of breath when hurrying on a level surface or walking up a slight hill
Grade 2	Moderate dyspnea	Walks slower than normal based on age on a level surface due to breathlessness or has to stop for breath when walking on level surface at own pace
Grade 3	Severe dyspnea	Stops for breath after walking 100 yards or after a few minutes on a level surface
Grade 4	Very severe dyspnea	Too breathless to leave the house or becomes breathless while dressing or undressing

From reference 2.

Although a physical examination is appropriate in the diagnosis and assessment of COPD, most patients who present in the milder stages of COPD will have a normal physical examination. In later stages of the disease, when airflow limitation is severe, patients may have cyanosis of mucosal membranes, development of "barrel chest" because of hyperinflation of the lungs, an increased respiratory rate and shallow breathing, and changes in breathing mechanics such as pursing of the lips to help with expiration or use of accessory respiratory muscles.

CLINICAL PRESENTATION

Symptoms

- Chronic cough
- Sputum production
- Dyspnea

Exposure to Risk Factors

- Tobacco smoke
- α_1-Antitrypsin deficiency
- Occupational hazards

Physical Examination

- Cyanosis of mucosal membranes
- Barrel chest
- Increased resting respiratory rate
- Shallow breathing
- Pursed lips during expiration
- Use of accessory respiratory muscles

Diagnostic Tests

- Spirometry with reversibility testing
- Radiograph of chest
- Arterial blood gas (not routine)

FEATURES OF CHRONIC OBSTRUCTIVE PULMONARY DISEASE EXACERBATION

Symptoms

- Increased sputum volume
- Acutely worsening dyspnea
- Chest tightness
- Presence of purulent sputum
- Increased need for bronchodilators
- Malaise, fatigue
- Decreased exercise tolerance

Physical Examination
- Fever
- Wheezing, decreased breath sounds

Diagnostic Tests
- Sputum sample for Gram stain and culture
- Chest radiograph to evaluate for new infiltrates

PROGNOSIS

For the patient with COPD, the combination of impaired lung function and recurrent exacerbations promote a clinical scenario characterized by dyspnea, reduced exercise tolerance and physical activity, and deconditioning. These factors lead to disease progression, poor quality of life, possible disability, and premature mortality.[26] COPD is ultimately a fatal disease if it progresses and advanced directives and end-of-life care options are appropriate to consider.

The FEV_1 is the most important prognostic indicator in a patient with COPD. The average rate of decline of FEV_1 is the most useful objective measure to assess the course of COPD. The average rate of decline in FEV_1 for healthy, nonsmoking patients owing to age alone is 25 to 30 mL/year. The rate of decline for smokers is steeper, especially for heavy smokers compared with light smokers. The decline in pulmonary function is a steady curvilinear path. The more severely diminished the FEV_1 at diagnosis; the steeper is the rate of decline. Greater numbers of years of smoking and number of cigarettes smoked also correlate with a steeper decline in pulmonary function.[27] Conversely, the rate of decline of blood gases has not been shown to be a useful parameter to assess progression of the disease. Patients with COPD should have spirometry performed at least annually to assess disease progression.

The survival rate of patients with COPD is highly correlated to the initial level of impairment in the FEV_1 and to age. Other, less-important factors include degree of reversibility with bronchodilators, resting pulse, perceived physical disability, diffusing capacity of lung for carbon monoxide (D_{LCO}), cor pulmonale, and blood gas abnormalities. A rapid decline in pulmonary function tests indicates a poor prognosis. Median survival is approximately 10 years when the FEV_1 is 1.4 L, 4 years when the FEV_1 is 1.0 L, and about 2 years when the FEV_1 is 0.5 L.

Although arterial blood gas (ABG) measurements are important, they do not carry the prognostic value of pulmonary function tests. Measurement of ABGs is more useful in patients with severe disease and is recommended for all patients with an FEV_1 of less than 40% of predicted or those with signs of respiratory failure or right-sided heart failure.[1]

It is important to recognize that patients with COPD die from a variety of causes, not only respiratory failure. Cardiovascular complications, as well as lung cancer, are the leading causes of death in patients with COPD.[28,29]

CLINICAL PRESENTATION OF CHRONIC OBSTRUCTIVE PULMONARY DISEASE EXACERBATION

Because of the subjective nature of defining an exacerbation of COPD, the criteria used among clinicians varies widely; however, most rely on a change in one or more of the following clinical findings: worsening symptoms of dyspnea, increase in sputum volume, or increase in sputum purulence. Acute exacerbations have a significant impact of the economics of treating COPD as well, estimated at 35% to 45% of the total costs of the disease in some settings.[30]

With an exacerbation, patients using rapid-acting bronchodilators may report an increase in the frequency of use. Exacerbations are commonly staged as mild, moderate, or severe according to the criteria summarized in Table 29–7.[31]

TABLE 29-7 Staging Acute Exacerbations of Chronic Obstructive Pulmonary Disease[a]

Mild (type 1)	One cardinal symptom[a] plus at least one of the following: URTI within 5 days, fever without other explanation, increased wheezing, increased cough, increase in respiratory or heart rate >20% above baseline
Moderate (type 2)	Two cardinal symptoms[a]
Severe (type 3)	Three cardinal symptoms[a]

URTI, upper respiratory tract infection.
[a]Cardinal symptoms include worsening of dyspnea, increase in sputum volume, and increase in sputum purulence.

An important complication of a severe exacerbation is acute respiratory failure. In the emergency department or hospital, an ABG usually is obtained to assess the severity of an exacerbation. The diagnosis of acute respiratory failure in COPD is made on the basis of an acute change in the ABGs. Defining acute respiratory failure as a PaO_2 of less than 50 mm Hg or a $PaCO_2$ of greater than 50 mm Hg often may be incorrect and inadequate because these values may not represent a significant change from a patient's baseline values. A more precise definition is an acute drop in PaO_2 of 10 to 15 mm Hg or any acute increase in $PaCO_2$ that decreases the serum pH to 7.3 or less. Additional acute clinical manifestations of respiratory failure include restlessness, confusion, tachycardia, diaphoresis, cyanosis, hypotension, irregular breathing, miosis, and unconsciousness.

PROGNOSIS

COPD exacerbations are associated with significant morbidity and mortality. While mild exacerbations may be managed at home, mortality rates are higher for patients admitted to the hospital. In one study of patients hospitalized with COPD exacerbations, in-hospital mortality was 6% to 8%.[32] Many patients experiencing an exacerbation do not have a return to their baseline clinical status for several weeks, significantly affecting their quality of life. Additionally, as many as half the patients originally hospitalized for an exacerbation are readmitted within 6 months.[33]

It is now evident that acute exacerbations of COPD have a tremendous impact on disease progression and ultimate mortality. For exacerbations requiring hospitalizations, mortality rates range from 22% to 43% after 1 year, and 36 to 49% in 2 years.[32,34,35]

TREATMENT

Chronic Obstructive Pulmonary Disease

■ DESIRED OUTCOMES

Given the nature of COPD, a major focus in healthcare should be on prevention. However, in patients with a diagnosis of COPD, the primary goal is to prevent or minimize progression. Table 29–8 lists specific management goals. The primary goal of pharmacotherapy has been relief of symptoms, including dyspnea. More recently, however, there has been increased interest in the value of therapeutic interventions that reduce exacerbation frequency and severity, as well as reduce mortality.

Optimally, these goals can be accomplished with minimal risks or side effects. The therapy of the patient with COPD is multifaceted and includes pharmacologic and nonpharmacologic strategies. Appropriate measures of effectiveness of the management plan include continued smoking cessation, symptom improvement, reduction in FEV_1

TABLE 29-8 Goals of Chronic Obstructive Pulmonary Disease Management

Prevent disease progression
Relieve symptoms
Improve exercise tolerance
Improve overall health status
Prevent and treat exacerbations
Prevent and treat complications
Reduce morbidity and mortality

decline, reduction in the number of exacerbations, improvements in physical and psychological well-being, and reduction in mortality, hospitalizations, and days lost from work.

Unfortunately, most treatments for COPD have not been shown to improve survival or to slow the progressive decline in lung function. However, many therapies do improve pulmonary function and quality of life and reduce exacerbations and duration of hospitalization. Several disease-specific quality-of-life measures are available to assess the overall efficacies of therapies for COPD, including the Chronic Respiratory Questionnaire and the St. George's Respiratory Questionnaire. These questionnaires measure the impact of various therapies on such disease variables as severity of dyspnea and level of activity; they do not measure impact of therapies on survival. Whereas early studies of COPD therapies focused primarily on improvements in pulmonary function measurements such as FEV_1, there is a trend toward greater use of these disease-specific quality-of-life measures to evaluate the benefits of therapy on larger clinical outcomes.

■ GENERAL APPROACH TO TREATMENT

To be effective, the clinician should address four primary components of management: assess and monitor the condition; avoidance of or reduced exposure to risk factors; manage stable disease; and treat exacerbations. These components are addressed through a variety of nonpharmacologic and pharmacologic approaches.

■ NONPHARMACOLOGIC THERAPY

Patients with COPD should receive education about their disease, treatment plans, and strategies to slow progression and prevent complications.[1] Advice and counseling about smoking cessation are essential, if applicable. Because the natural course of the disease leads to respiratory failure, the clinician should address end-of-life decisions and advanced directives prospectively with the patient and family.[36]

Smoking Cessation

❺ A primary component of COPD management is avoidance of or reduced exposure to risk factors. Exposure to environmental tobacco smoke is a major risk factor, and smoking cessation is the most effective strategy to reduce the risk of developing COPD and to slow or stop disease progression. The cost-effectiveness of smoking-cessation interventions compares favorably with interventions made for other major chronic diseases.[37] The importance of smoking cessation cannot be overemphasized. Smoking cessation leads to decreased symptomatology and slows the rate of decline of pulmonary function even after significant abnormalities in pulmonary function tests have been detected (FEV_1:FVC <60%).[27] As confirmed by the Lung Health Study, smoking cessation is the only intervention proven at this time to affect long-term decline in FEV_1 and slow the progression of COPD.[28] In this 5-year prospective trial, smokers with early COPD were randomly assigned to one of three groups: smoking-cessation intervention plus inhaled ipratropium three times a day, smoking-cessation intervention alone, or no intervention. During an 11-year followup, the rate of decline in FEV_1 among subjects who continued to smoke was more than twice the rate in sustained quitters. Smokers who underwent smoking-cessation intervention had fewer respiratory symptoms and a smaller annual decline in FEV_1 compared with smokers who had no intervention. However, this study also demonstrated the difficulty in achieving and sustaining successful smoking cessation.

Tobacco cessation has mortality benefits beyond those related to COPD. A followup analysis of the Lung Health Study data conducted more than 14 years later demonstrated an 18% reduction in all-cause mortality in patients who received the intervention compared to usual care.[29] Intervention patients had lower death rates as a consequence of coronary artery disease (the leading cause of mortality), cardiovascular diseases, and lung cancer, although no category reached clinical significance.

Every clinician has a responsibility to assist smokers in smoking-cessation efforts. A clinical practice guideline for treating tobacco dependence from the U.S. Public Health Service was updated in 2000.[38] Table 29–9 summarizes the major findings and recommendations of that report. In 2004, a report from the Surgeon General on the health consequences of smoking broadened the scope of the detrimental effects of cigarette smoking, indicating that "Smoking harms nearly every organ of the body, causing many diseases and reducing the health of smokers in general."[13]

All clinicians should take an active role in assisting patients with tobacco dependence in order to reduce the burden on the individual, the individual's family, and the healthcare system. It is estimated that more than 75% of smokers want to quit and that one-third have made a serious effort. Yet complete and permanent tobacco cessation is difficult.[28] Counseling that is provided by clinicians is associated with greater success rates than self-initiated efforts.[38]

The U.S. Public Health Service guidelines recommend that clinicians take a comprehensive approach to smoking-cessation counseling. Advice should be given to smokers even if they have no symptoms of smoking-related disease or if they are receiving care for reasons unrelated to smoking. Clinicians should be persistent in their efforts because relapse is common among smokers owing to the chronic nature of dependence. Brief interventions (3 minutes) of counseling are proven effective. However, it must be recognized that the patient must be ready to stop smoking because there are several stages of decision making. Based on this, a five-step intervention program is proposed (Table 29–10).

TABLE 29-9 Treating Tobacco Use and Dependence: Public Health Service Report (2000) Major Findings and Recommendations

Tobacco dependence should be recognized as a chronic condition requiring repeated treatment until permanent abstinence is achieved.
Effective treatments for tobacco dependence are available and should be offered to all tobacco users.
Clinicians and healthcare systems should ensure mechanisms to identify, document, and treat all tobacco users in the system.
Brief treatment interventions for tobacco dependence should be offered to all tobacco users at a minimum.
There is a strong dose–response relationship between the intensity of tobacco dependence counseling and its effectiveness.
The most effective types of counseling and behavioral therapies are (a) practical counseling employing problem-solving and skills training, (b) social support as part of treatment, and (c) social support outside of treatment.
Numerous pharmacotherapies are effective for smoking cessation and should be offered in the absence of contraindications. These include sustained-release bupropion, nicotine gum, nicotine inhaler, nicotine nasal spray, nicotine patch, and varenicline.
Tobacco dependence treatments are effective and cost-effective compared with other medical and disease-prevention measures.

TABLE 29-10 Five-Step Strategy for Smoking-Cessation Program (5 A's)

Ask	Use systematic approach to identify all tobacco users.
Advise	Urge all tobacco users to quit.
Assess	Determine willingness to make a cessation attempt.
Assist	Provide support for the patient to quit smoking.
Arrange	Schedule followup and monitor for continued abstinence.

There is strong evidence to support the use of pharmacotherapy to assist in smoking cessation. In fact, it should be offered to most patients as part of a cessation attempt. In general, available therapies will double the effectiveness of a cessation effort. Table 29–11 lists first-line agents. The usual duration of therapy is 8 to 12 weeks, although some individuals may require longer courses of treatment. Precautions to consider before using bupropion include a history of seizures or an eating disorder. Nicotine-replacement therapies are contraindicated in patients with unstable coronary artery disease, active peptic ulcers, or recent myocardial infarction or stroke. Nicotine patch, bupropion, and the combination of bupropion and the nicotine patch were compared with placebo in a controlled trial.[39] The treatment groups that received bupropion had higher rates of smoking cessation than the groups that received placebo or the nicotine patch. The addition of the nicotine patch to bupropion slightly improved the smoking-cessation rate compared with bupropion monotherapy. Recently, a new agent became available to assist in tobacco cessation attempts. Varenicline is a nicotine acetylcholine receptor partial agonist that has shown benefit in tobacco cessation.[40] Varenicline relieves physical withdrawal symptoms and reduces the rewarding properties of nicotine. Nausea and headache are the most frequent complaints associated with varenicline. Currently, varenicline has not been studied in combination with other tobacco cessation therapies. Second-line agents, such as clonidine and nortriptyline, a tricyclic antidepressant, are less effective or associated with greater side effects; however, they may be useful in selected clinical situations.

Behavioral modification techniques or other forms of psychotherapy also may be helpful in assisting in smoking cessation. Programs that address the many issues associated with smoking (i.e., learned behaviors, environmental influences, and chemical dependence) using a team approach are more likely to be successful. The role of alternative medicine therapies in smoking cessation is controversial. Hypnosis may aid in improving abstinence rates when added to a smoking-cessation program but appears to give little benefit when used alone. Acupuncture has not been shown to contribute to smoking cessation and is not recommended.[2]

Pulmonary Rehabilitation

Exercise training is beneficial in the treatment of COPD to improve exercise tolerance and to reduce symptoms of dyspnea and fatigue.[1] Pulmonary rehabilitation programs are an integral component in the management of COPD and should include exercise training along with smoking cessation, breathing exercises, optimal medical treatment, psychosocial support, and health education. High-intensity training (70% maximal workload) is possible even in advanced COPD patients, and the level of intensity improves peripheral muscle and ventilatory function. Studies have demonstrated that pulmonary rehabilitation with exercise three to seven times per week can produce long-term improvement in activities of daily living, quality of life, exercise tolerance, and dyspnea in patients with moderate to severe COPD.[41] Improvements in dyspnea can be achieved without concomitant improvements in spirometry. Programs using less-intensive exercise regimens (two times per week) are not beneficial.[42]

Immunizations

Vaccines can be considered as pharmacologic agents; however, their role is described here in reducing risk factors for COPD exacerbations. Because influenza is a common complication in COPD that can lead to exacerbations and respiratory failure, an annual vaccination with the inactivated intramuscular influenza vaccine is recommended. Immunization against influenza can reduce serious illness and death by 50% in COPD patients.[43] Influenza vaccine should be administered in the fall of each year (October and November) during regular medical visits or at vaccination clinics. There are few contraindications to influenza vaccine except for a patient with a serious allergy to eggs. An oral antiinfluenza agents (oseltamivir) can be considered for patients with COPD during an outbreak for patients who have not been immunized; however, this therapy is less effective and causes more side effects.[44]

The polyvalent pneumococcal vaccine, administered one time, is widely recommended for people from 2 to 64 years of age who have chronic lung disease and for all people older than age 65 years. Thus COPD patients at any age are candidates for vaccination. Although evidence for the benefit of the pneumococcal vaccine in COPD is not strong, the argument for continued use is that the current vaccine provides coverage for 85% of pneumococcal strains causing invasive disease and the increasing rate of resistance of pneumococcus to selected antibiotics. Currently, administering the vaccine remains the standard of practice and is recommended by the Centers for Disease Control and Prevention and the American Lung Association. Repeated vaccination with the 23-valent product is not recommended for patients ages 2 to 64 years with chronic lung disease; however, revaccination is recommended for patients older than 65 years of age if the first vaccination was more than 5 years earlier and the patient was younger than age 65 years. The GOLD guidelines recommend pneumococcal vaccine for all COPD patients age 65 years and older and for patients younger than age 65 years only if the FEV_1 is less than 40% of predicted.[45,46]

Long-Term Oxygen Therapy

❻ The use of supplemental oxygen therapy increases survival in COPD patients with chronic hypoxemia. Although long-term oxygen has been used for many years in patients with advanced COPD, it was not until 1980 that data became available documenting its benefits. At that time, the Nocturnal Oxygen Therapy Trial Group published its data comparing nocturnal oxygen therapy (12 h/day) with continuous oxygen therapy (average of 20 h/day).[47] Among patients who were followed for at least 12 months, the results revealed a mortality rate in the nocturnal oxygen therapy group that

TABLE 29-11 First-Line Pharmacotherapies for Smoking Cessation

Agent	Usual Dose	Duration	Common Complaints
Bupropion SR	150 mg orally daily for 3 days, then twice daily	12 weeks, up to 6 months	Insomnia, dry mouth
Nicotine gum	2–4 mg gum prn, up to 24 pieces daily	12 weeks	Sore mouth, dyspepsias
Nicotine inhaler	6–16 cartridges daily	Up to 6 months	Sore mouth and throat
Nicotine nasal spray	8–40 doses daily	3 to 6 months	Nasal irritation
Nicotine patches	Various, 7–21 mg every 24 hours	Up to 8 weeks	Skin reaction, insomnia
Varenicline	0.5 mg daily for 3 days, then 0.5 mg twice daily for 4 days, then 1 mg twice daily	12 weeks	Nausea, sleep disturbances

was nearly double that of the continuous oxygen therapy group (51% versus 26%). Statistical estimates of the continuous oxygen therapy group suggest that continuous oxygen therapy may have added 3.25 years to a COPD patient's life. Additional data from the Nocturnal Oxygen Therapy Trial Group revealed that continuous oxygen therapy patients had fewer (but statistically insignificant) hospitalizations, improved quality of life and neuropsychological function, reduced hematocrit, and decreased pulmonary vascular resistance.[47]

The decline in mortality with oxygen therapy was further substantiated in 1981 in a study by the British Medical Research Council that compared 15 h/day of oxygen versus no supplemental oxygen in COPD patients.[48] Patients receiving oxygen therapy for at least part of the day had lower rates of mortality than those not receiving oxygen. Long-term oxygen therapy provides even more benefit in terms of survival after at least 5 years of use, and it improves the quality of life of these patients by increasing walking distance and neuropsychological condition and reducing time spent in the hospital.[49] Before patients are considered for long-term oxygen therapy, they should be stabilized in the outpatient setting, and pharmacotherapy should be optimized. Once this is accomplished, long-term oxygen therapy should be instituted if either of two conditions exists: (a) a resting Pa_{O_2} of less than 55 mm Hg or (b) evidence of right-sided heart failure, polycythemia, or impaired neuropsychiatric function with a Pa_{O_2} of less than 60 mm Hg.

The most practical means of administering long-term oxygen is with the nasal cannula, at 1 to 2 L/min which provides 24% to 28% oxygen. The goal is to raise the Pa_{O_2} above 60 mm Hg. Patient education about flow rates and avoidance of flames (i.e., smoking) is of the utmost importance.

There are three different ways to deliver oxygen, including (a) in liquid reservoirs, (b) compressed into a cylinder, and (c) via an oxygen concentrator. Although conventional liquid oxygen and compressed oxygen are quite bulky, smaller, portable tanks are available to permit greater patient mobility. Oxygen concentrator devices separate nitrogen from room air and concentrate oxygen. These are the most convenient and the least-expensive method of oxygen delivery. Oxygen-conservation devices are available that allow oxygen to flow only during inspiration, making the supply last longer. These may be particularly useful to prolong the oxygen supply for mobile patients using portable cylinders. However, the devices are bulky and subject to failure.

Adjunctive Therapies

In addition to supplemental oxygen, adjunctive therapies to consider as part of a pulmonary rehabilitation program are psychoeducational care and nutritional support. Psychoeducational care (such as relaxation) has been associated with improvement in the functioning and well-being of adults with COPD.[1,2] The role of nutritional support in patients with COPD is controversial. Several studies have shown an association between malnutrition, low BMI, and impaired pulmonary status among patients with COPD. However, a meta-analysis suggests that the effect of nutritional support on outcomes in COPD is small and not associated with improved anthropometric measures, lung function, or functional exercise capacity.[50]

■ PHARMACOLOGIC THERAPY

In contrast to the survival benefit conferred by supplemental oxygen therapy, there is no medication available for the treatment of COPD that has been shown to modify the progressive decline in lung function or prolong survival.[1] Thus a primary goal of pharmacotherapy is to control patient symptoms and reduce complications, including the frequency and severity of exacerbations and improving the overall the health status and exercise tolerance of the patient.

International guidelines recommend a stepwise approach to the use of pharmacotherapy based on disease severity,[1,2] which is determined by the extent of airflow limitation and degree of symptoms. The impact of recurrent exacerbations on disease progression is increasingly recognized as an important factor and should be considered. The primary goals of pharmacotherapy are to control symptoms (including dyspnea), reduce exacerbations, and improve exercise tolerance and health status. Currently, there is inadequate evidence to support the use of more aggressive pharmacotherapy early in the course of disease, although data from ongoing trials may provide answers.

❼ Pharmacotherapy focuses on the use of bronchodilators to control symptoms. There are several classes of bronchodilators to choose from, and no single class has been proven to provide superior benefit over other available agents. The initial and subsequent choice of medications should be based on the specific clinical situation and patient characteristics. Medications can be used as needed or on a scheduled basis depending on the clinical situation, and additional therapies should be added in a stepwise manner depending on the response and severity of disease. Considerations should be given to individual patient response, tolerability, adherence, and economic factors. A stepwise approach to the management of COPD has been proposed based on the stage of disease severity (Fig. 29–3).

❽ According to the guidelines, patients with intermittent symptoms should be treated with short-acting bronchodilators. When symptoms become more persistent, long-acting bronchodilators should be initiated. For patients with an FEV_1 less than 50% and who experience frequent exacerbations, inhaled corticosteroids should be considered. Short-acting bronchodilators relieve symptoms and increase exercise tolerance. Long-acting bronchodilators relieve symptoms, reduce exacerbation frequency, and improve quality of life and health status. Patients have a variety of choices in using inhalational therapies, including metered dose inhalers (MDIs), dry powder inhalers (DPIs), or nebulizers. There is not a clear advantage of one delivery method over another and it is recommended that patient-specific factors and preferences should be considered in selecting the device.[51]

Bronchodilators

Bronchodilator classes available for the treatment of COPD include β_2-agonists, anticholinergics, and methylxanthines. There is no clear benefit to one agent or class over others, although inhaled therapy generally is preferred. In general, it can be more difficult for patients with COPD to use inhalation devices effectively compared with other populations owing to advanced age and the presence of other comorbidities. Clinicians should advise, counsel, and observe patient technique with the devices frequently and consistently.

Bronchodilators generally work by reducing the tone of airway smooth muscle (relaxation), thus minimizing airflow limitation. In patients with COPD, the clinical benefits of bronchodilators include increased exercise capacity, decreased air trapping in the lungs, and relief of symptoms such as dyspnea. However, use of bronchodilators may not be associated with significant improvements in pulmonary function measurements such as FEV_1. In general, side effects of bronchodilator medications are related to their pharmacologic effects and are dose-dependent. Because COPD patients are older and more likely to have comorbid conditions, the risk for side effects and drug interactions is higher compared with patients with asthma.

Short-Acting Bronchodilators The initial therapy for COPD patients who experience symptoms intermittently are short-acting bronchodilators. Among these agents, the choices are a short-acting β_2-agonist or an anticholinergic. Either class of agents has a relatively rapid onset on action, relieves symptoms, and improves exercise tolerance and lung function. In general, both classes are equally effective.

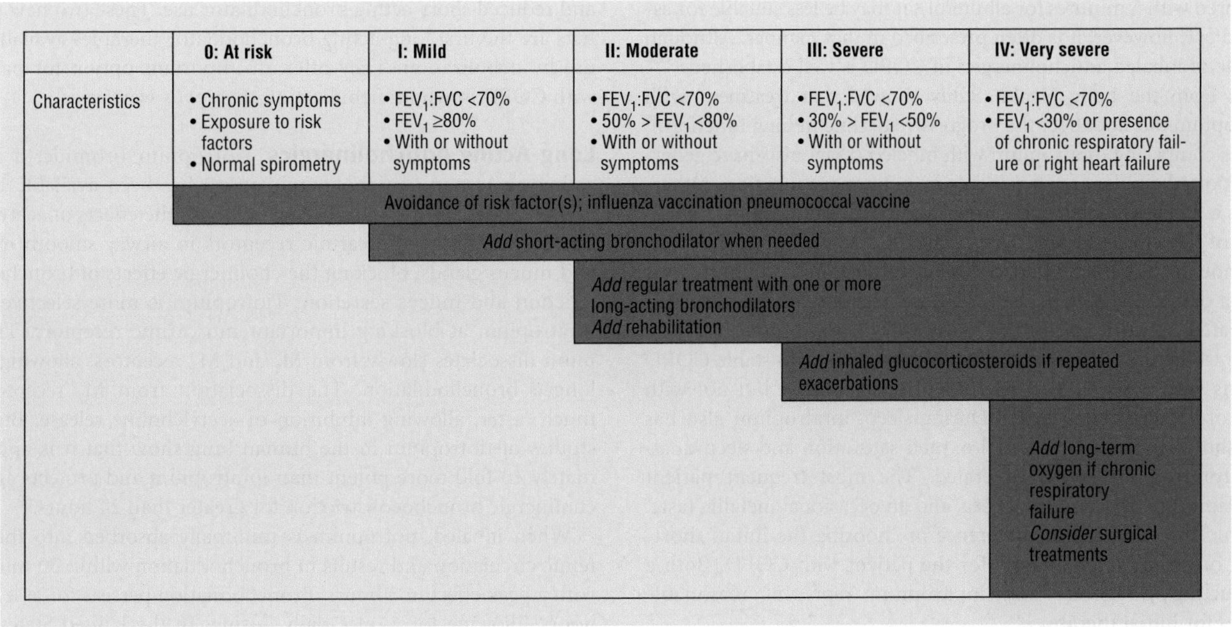
0: At risk
I: Mild
II: Moderate
III: Severe
IV: Very severe
Characteristics
• Chronic symptoms • Exposure to risk factors • Normal spirometry
• FEV1:FVC <70% • FEV1 ≥80% • With or without symptoms
• FEV1:FVC <70% • 50% > FEV1 <80% • With or without symptoms
• FEV1:FVC <70% • 30% > FEV1 <50% • With or without symptoms
• FEV1:FVC <70% • FEV1 <30% or presence of chronic respiratory failure or right heart failure
Avoidance of risk factor(s); influenza vaccination pneumococcal vaccine
Add short-acting bronchodilator when needed
Add regular treatment with one or more long-acting bronchodilators
Add rehabilitation
Add inhaled glucocorticosteroids if repeated exacerbations
Add long-term oxygen if chronic respiratory failure
Consider surgical treatments

FIGURE 29-3. Recommended therapy of stable chronic obstructive pulmonary disease. (FEV_1, forced expiratory volume in the first second of expiration; FVC, forced vital capacity.) *(From reference 1.)*

Short-Acting Sympathomimetics (β_2-Agonists) A number of sympathomimetic agents are available in the United States. They vary in selectivity, route of administration, and duration of action. In COPD management, sympathomimetic agents with β_2-selectivity, or β_2-agonists, should be used as bronchodilators. β_2-Agonists cause bronchodilation by stimulating the enzyme adenyl cyclase to increase the formation of cyclic adenosine monophosphate. Cyclic adenosine monophosphate is responsible for mediating relaxation of bronchial smooth muscle, leading to bronchodilation. In addition, it may improve mucociliary clearance. Although shorter-acting and less-selective β-agonists are still used widely (e.g., metaproterenol, isoetharine, isoproterenol, and epinephrine), they should not be used owing to their shorter duration of action and increased cardiostimulatory effects. Short-acting, selective β_2-agonists such as albuterol, levalbuterol, and pirbuterol, are preferred for therapy.

Sympathomimetics are available in inhaled, oral, and parenteral dosage forms. The preferred route of administration is by inhalation. The use of oral and parenteral β-agonists in COPD is discouraged because they are no more effective than a properly used MDI or DPI, and the incidence of systemic adverse effects such as tachycardia and hand tremor is greater. Administration of β_2-agonists in the outpatient and emergency room settings via inhalers (MDIs or DPIs) is at least as effective as nebulization therapy and usually favored for reasons of cost and convenience.[51] Chapter 28 includes a complete description of the devices used for delivering aerosolized medication and a comparison β_2-agonist therapies.

Albuterol is the most frequently used β_2-agonist. It is available as an oral and inhaled preparation. Albuterol is a racemic mixture of (*R*)-albuterol that is responsible for the bronchodilator effect and (*S*)-albuterol that has no therapeutic effect. (*S*)-Albuterol is considered by some clinicians to be inert, whereas others believe that it may be implicated in worsening airway inflammation and antagonizing the response to (*R*)-albuterol. Levalbuterol is a single-isomer formulation of (*R*)-albuterol. A retrospective evaluation of levalbuterol versus albuterol use in patients with asthma and COPD concluded that levalbuterol offered significant advantages over albuterol for hospitalized patients.[52] Other clinicians feel that there are no significant differences between the products and that the use of levalbuterol is not justified owing to its higher acquisition cost.[53] The effects of a single dose of levalbuterol have been compared with those of albuterol and ipratropium plus albuterol in patients with COPD. No significant differences in pulmonary function improvements or adverse effects were noted.[54]

In COPD patients, β_2-agonists exert a rapid onset of effect, although the response generally is less than that seen in asthma. Short-acting inhaled β_2-agonists cause only a small improvement in FEV_1 acutely but may improve respiratory symptoms and exercise tolerance despite the small improvement in spirometric measurements.[55] Patients with COPD can use quick-onset β_2-agonists as needed for relief of symptoms or on a scheduled basis to prevent or reduce symptoms. The duration of action of short-acting β_2-agonists is 4 to 6 hours.

Short-Acting Anticholinergics When given by inhalation, anticholinergics such as ipratropium or atropine produce bronchodilation by competitively inhibiting cholinergic receptors in bronchial smooth muscle. This activity blocks acetylcholine, with the net effect being a reduction in cyclic guanosine monophosphate, which normally acts to constrict bronchial smooth muscle. Muscarinic receptors on airway smooth muscle include M_1, M_2, and M_3 subtypes. Activation of M_1 and M_3 receptors by acetylcholine results in bronchoconstriction; however, activation of M_2 receptors inhibits further acetylcholine release.

Ipratropium is the primary short-acting anticholinergic agent used for COPD in the United States. Atropine has a tertiary structure and is absorbed readily across the oral and respiratory mucosa, whereas ipratropium has a quaternary structure that is absorbed poorly. The lack of systemic absorption of ipratropium greatly diminishes the anticholinergic side effects such as blurred vision, urinary retention, nausea, and tachycardia associated with atropine. Ipratropium bromide is available as a MDI and a solution for inhalation. The MDI was recently reformulated with an hydrofluoroalkane propellant and delivers 17 mcg per puff. Ipratropium is also available as a MDI in combination with albuterol and as a solution for nebulization at 200 mcg/mL. It provides a peak effect in 1.5 to 2 hours and has a duration of effect of 4 to 6 hours. Ipratropium has a slower onset of action and a more prolonged bronchodilator effect compared with standard β_2-agonists. Because of the slower onset of effect (15 to 20 minutes compared with 5 minutes for albuterol), it may be less suitable for as-needed use; however, it is often prescribed in that manner. Although the role of inhaled anticholinergics in COPD is well established,[56–58] results from the Lung Health Study showed that treatment with ipratropium did not affect the progressive decline in lung function.[28] Studies comparing ipratropium with inhaled β_2-agonists have generally reported similar improvements in pulmonary function. Others report a modest benefit with ipratropium, including a lower incidence of side effects such as tachycardia.[56,57]

Although the recommended dose of ipratropium is 2 puffs four times a day, there is evidence for a dose–response, so the dose can be titrated upward, often to 24 puffs a day. Ipratropium has been shown to increase maximum exercise performance in stable COPD patients with doses of 8 to 12 puffs prior to exercise but not with doses of 4 puffs or fewer.[58,59] During sleep, ipratropium also has been shown to improve arterial oxygen saturation and sleep quality.[60] Ipratropium is well tolerated. The most frequent patient complaints are dry mouth, nausea, and an occasional metallic taste.

Clinicians differ about preference in choosing the initial short-acting bronchodilator therapy for the patient with COPD. Both a short-acting β_2-agonist and ipratropium represent reasonable choices for initial therapy.

Long-Acting Bronchodilators For patients with moderate to severe COPD who experience symptoms on a regular and consistent basis, or in whom short-acting therapies do not provide adequate relief, long-acting bronchodilator therapies are the recommended treatment. Long-acting, inhaled bronchodilator therapy can be administered as a β_2-agonist or an anticholinergic. Long-acting bronchodilators provide similar benefits to short-acting agents. In addition, they reduce exacerbation frequency and improve quality of life.

Long-Acting, Inhaled β_2-Agonists Long-acting, inhaled β_2-agonists offer the convenience and benefit of a long duration of action for patients with persistent symptoms. Both salmeterol and formoterol are dosed every 12 hours and provide sustained bronchodilation. Formoterol has an onset of action similar to albuterol (less than 5 minutes), whereas salmeterol has a slower onset (15 to 20 minutes); however, neither agent is recommended for acute relief of symptoms. The clinical benefits of long-acting inhaled β_2-agonists compared to short-acting therapies include similar or superior improvements in lung function and symptoms, as well as reduced exacerbation rates.[61–63] The use of the long-acting agents should be considered for patients with frequent and persistent symptoms. When patients require short-acting β_2-agonists on a scheduled basis, long-acting agents, such as formoterol and salmeterol, are more convenient based on dosing frequency, but are also more expensive.

Long-acting β-agonists are also useful to reduce nocturnal symptoms and improve quality of life. When compared to short-acting bronchodilators or theophylline, both salmeterol and formoterol improve lung function, symptoms, exacerbation frequency and quality of life.[64] These benefits are apparent even in patients with poorly reversible lung function and are related to improvements in inspiratory capacity.[65] Both salmeterol and formoterol have been compared to ipratropium. In separate studies, each agent improved FEV_1 compared to ipratropium and, in addition, the long-acting bronchodilator was more effective for other selected outcomes (e.g., prolonged time to exacerbation for salmeterol while formoterol reduced symptoms and rescue inhaler use).[66,67]

In 2007, two new long-acting, inhaled β-agonists became available in the United States. Formoterol and arformoterol are unique in that they are the first long-acting β-agonists available as nebulized solutions. When arformoterol was compared to salmeterol (administered by MDI) in a 12-week study, both treatments increased the trough FEV_1.[68] Arfomoterol also improved peak flows and reduced short-acting bronchodilator use. These two new products are the first long-acting bronchodilator therapies available for use by nebulization. They offer an important option for patients with COPD in whom nebulization therapy is warranted.

Long-Acting Anticholinergics Tiotropium bromide, a long-acting quaternary anticholinergic agent, has been available in the United States since 2004. This agent blocks the effects of acetylcholine by binding to muscarinic receptors in airway smooth muscle and mucus glands, blocking the cholinergic effects of bronchoconstriction and mucus secretion. Tiotropium is more selective than ipratropium at blocking important muscarinic receptors. Tiotropium dissociates slowly from M_1 and M_3 receptors, allowing prolonged bronchodilation. The dissociation from M_2 receptors is much faster, allowing inhibition of acetylcholine release. Binding studies of tiotropium in the human lung show that it is approximately 10-fold more potent than ipratropium and protects against cholinergic bronchoconstriction for greater than 24 hours.[69]

When inhaled, tiotropium is minimally absorbed into the systemic circulation and results in bronchodilation within 30 minutes, with a peak effect in 3 hours. Bronchodilation persists for at least 24 hours, allowing for a once-daily dosing. In the United States, it is delivered via the HandiHaler, a single-load, dry-powder, breath-actuated device. Because it acts locally, tiotropium is well tolerated, with the most common complaint being a dry mouth. Other anticholinergic side effects that are reported include constipation, urinary retention, tachycardia, blurred vision, and precipitation of narrow-angle glaucoma symptoms.

The benefits of tiotropium have been evaluated in numerous trials of patients with COPD. Similar to long-acting β-agonists, tiotropium improves lung function and, dyspnea, exacerbation frequency, and health-related quality of life.[70] The tolerance that is demonstrated with chronic use of β-agonists does not occur with tiotropium therapy, as improvements in lung function are sustained with long-term therapy.[71]

There is a large body of evidence supporting the use of tiotropium as a long-acting bronchodilator for COPD patients. Benefits have been demonstrated compared to placebo[72] and to ipratropium.[73] Equivalent or superior effects have been proven compared to long-acting β-agonist therapy.[72] Tiotropium therapy is associated with a decreased risk of exacerbations compared to placebo or ipratropium, and equal or superior efficacy compared to long-acting β-agonists.[74]

Tiotropium was evaluated as an addition to standard COPD medications in a 1-year, placebo-controlled, double-blind study involving more than 900 subjects. Tiotropium 18 mcg/day improved the FEV_1 response an average of 12% (trough) to 22% (peak) when added to standard therapy.[70]

The efficacy and safety of tiotropium administered via a DPI was compared with ipratropium administered four times daily by MDI in a multicenter, double-blind study that followed patients for 1 year.[73] Patients who received once-daily tiotropium demonstrated significantly greater improvements in lung function and selected quality-of-life scores, decreased dyspnea, and fewer exacerbations compared with patients who received ipratropium. There were no differences in side effects between the two agents.

As a long-acting bronchodilator, tiotropium is an option to consider in addition to long-acting inhaled β_2-agonists for COPD management. Once-daily tiotropium has been compared with twice-daily salmeterol in two placebo-controlled trials of 6 months' duration. Tiotropium reduced asthma exacerbations and hospital admissions and improved quality of life, whereas both active treatments improved lung function and reduced dyspnea.[72] In another 6-month randomized, controlled trial of patients with COPD, patients were randomized to receive either tiotropium once daily by DPI, salmeterol twice daily by MDI, or placebo.[75] Patients receiving tiotropium had greater improvements in trough FEV_1 and dyspnea scores than those receiving salmeterol. Patients also were more likely to have improvements in quality-of-life indicators with tiotropium than with salmeterol. However, no differences in frequency of exacerbations were noted among the three groups.

These data offer some promise about the long term benefit of tiotropium on slowing the progressive decline in lung function, although this claim is premature. A major clinical trial evaluating the benefit of long-term treatment is currently ongoing. This trial is evaluating the long-term benefits of tiotropium in the treatment of COPD, including the effects on FEV_1 decline, exacerbation frequency, and overall mortality. The results of the UPLIFT (Understanding the Potential Long-Term Impacts on Function with Tiotropium) trial are anticipated in 2008.[76]

The potential benefit of tiotropium therapy in augmenting pulmonary rehabilitation has been evaluated. The basis for this combination is that tiotropium can improve ventilatory mechanics and allow greater participation in exercise and muscle training. Tiotropium therapy combined with pulmonary rehabilitation improved exercise endurance and health status, and reduced dyspnea compared to pulmonary rehabilitation alone.[77] The effects were sustained for three months after the pulmonary rehabilitation program was complete.

Combination Anticholinergics and β-Agonists Combination regimens of bronchodilators are used often in the treatment of COPD, especially as the disease progresses and symptoms worsen over time. Combining bronchodilators with different mechanisms of action allows the lowest possible effective doses to be used and reduces potential adverse effects from individual agents.[1] Combinations of both short- and long-acting β_2-agonists with ipratropium have been shown to provide added symptomatic relief and improvements in pulmonary function.[78–80]

A combination of albuterol and ipratropium (Combivent) is available as a MDI in the United States for chronic maintenance therapy of COPD. This product offers the obvious convenience of two classes of bronchodilators in a single inhaler.

Although clinical practice guidelines recommend that combinations of long-acting bronchodilators are appropriate in patients who do not receive adequate benefit from a single agent, data to support the use of these combinations have been lacking. These approaches have been the focus of more recent research. Future combination inhalation products may contain long-acting β_2-agonists with tiotropium to reduce the need for frequent dosing. In a preliminary single-dose study, the combination of tiotropium and formoterol resulted in a faster and greater improvement in FEV_1 compared with either treatment alone.[81] In another trial, 95 subjects received either tiotropium 18 mcg or tiotropium plus formoterol 12 mcg, either once or twice daily. All patients received each therapy for 2 weeks each in an open-label crossover design. Both combination regimens improved lung function and reduced rescue therapy use compared to tiotropium alone.[82]

Methylxanthines Methylxanthines, including theophylline and aminophylline, have been available for the treatment of COPD for at least five decades and at one time were considered first-line therapy. However, with the availability of long-acting inhaled β_2-agonists and inhaled anticholinergics, the role of methylxanthine therapy is significantly limited. Inhaled bronchodilator therapy is preferred for COPD. Because of the risk for drug interactions and the significant intrapatient and interpatient variability in dosage requirements, theophylline therapy generally is considered in patients who are intolerant or unable to use an inhaled bronchodilator. Theophylline is still an alternative to commonly used inhaled therapies partially because of the potential for multiple mechanisms (bronchodilation and antiinflammatory) and the possible benefit that systemic administration may exert on peripheral airways.[83]

The methylxanthines may produce bronchodilation through numerous mechanisms, including (a) inhibition of phosphodiesterase, thereby increasing cyclic adenosine monophosphate levels, (b) inhibition of calcium ion influx into smooth muscle, (c) prostaglandin antagonism, (d) stimulation of endogenous catecholamines, (e) adenosine receptor antagonism, and (f) inhibition of release of mediators from mast cells and leukocytes.[84]

Chronic theophylline use in patients with COPD has been shown to exert improvements in lung function, including vital capacity, FEV_1, minute ventilation, and gas exchange.[83] Subjectively, theophylline has been shown to reduce dyspnea, increase exercise tolerance, and improve respiratory drive in COPD patients.[83,84] Other nonpulmonary effects of theophylline that may contribute to improved overall functional capacity in patients with COPD include improved cardiac function and decreased pulmonary artery pressure.

Although theophylline is available in a variety of oral dosage forms, sustained-release preparations are most appropriate for the long-term management of COPD. These products have the advantages of improving patient compliance and achieving more consistent serum concentrations over rapid-release theophylline and aminophylline preparations. However, caution must be used in switching from one sustained-release preparation to another because there are considerable variations in sustained-release characteristics.[84] Aside from intravenous aminophylline, there is no need to use any of the various salts forms of theophylline.

Regular use of methylxanthines has not been shown to have either a beneficial or a detrimental effect on the progression of COPD. However, methylxanthines may be added to the treatment plan of patients who have not achieved an optimal clinical response to ipratropium and an inhaled β_2-agonist. Studies suggest that adding theophylline to a combination of albuterol and ipratropium provides added benefit for stable COPD patients, supporting the hypothesis that there is a synergistic bronchodilator effect.[85–87] The efficacy of combination therapy with salmeterol and theophylline for patients with COPD was reported to improve pulmonary function and reduce dyspnea better than either treatment alone.[88] Combination treatment also was associated with a reduced number of exacerbations only when compared with the theophylline group, suggesting that the salmeterol component was responsible for this beneficial effect.

As is the case with other bronchodilator therapy, parameters other than objective measurements, such as FEV_1, should be monitored to assess efficacy of theophylline in COPD. Subjective parameters, such as perceived improvements in symptoms of dyspnea, and exercise tolerance, become increasingly important in assessing the acceptability of methylxanthines for COPD patients. Although objective improvement may be minimal, patients may experience an improvement in clinical symptoms, and thus benefit to the individual may be meaningful.

Theophylline's role in COPD is as maintenance therapy in the nonacutely ill patient. Therapy can be initiated at 200 mg twice daily and titrated upward every 3 to 5 days to the target dose. Most patients required daily doses of 400 to 900 mg. Dosage adjustments generally should be made based on serum concentration results. Traditionally, the therapeutic range of theophylline was identified as 10 to 20 mcg/mL; however, because of the frequency of dose-related side effects and the relatively minor benefit of higher concentrations, a more conservative therapeutic range of 8 to 15 mcg/mL often is targeted. This is especially preferable in the elderly. When concentrations are measured, trough measurements are most appropriate.

Once a dose is established, serum concentrations should be monitored once or twice a year unless the patient's disease worsens, medications that interfere with theophylline metabolism are added to therapy, or toxicity is suspected. The most common side effects of theophylline therapy are related to the gastrointestinal system, the cardiovascular system, and the central nervous system. Side effects are dose-related; however, there is overlap in side effects between the therapeutic and toxic ranges. Minor side effects include dyspepsia, nausea, vomiting, diarrhea, headache, dizziness, and tachycardia. More serious toxicities, especially at toxic concentrations, include arrhythmias and seizures.

Factors that decrease theophylline clearance and lead to reduced maintenance-dose requirements include advanced age, bacterial or viral pneumonia, left or right ventricular failure, liver dysfunction, hypoxemia from acute decompensation, and use of drugs such as cimetidine, macrolides, and fluoroquinolone antibiotics. Factors that may enhance theophylline clearance and result in the need for higher maintenance doses include tobacco and marijuana smoking, hyperthyroidism, and the use of such drugs as phenytoin, phenobarbital, and rifampin.

In summary, there are decades of experience with theophylline and other methylxanthine products in the management of patients with COPD. However, inhalation therapy is currently preferred based on superior efficacy and safety, as well as ease of use by the clinician. Theophylline is a challenging medication to dose, monitor, and manage because of the significant intrapatient and interpatient variability in pharmacokinetics and the potential for drug interactions and toxicities.

Corticosteroids

❾ Corticosteroid therapy has been studied and debated in COPD therapy for half a century; however, owing to the poor risk-to-benefit ratio, chronic systemic corticosteroid therapy should be avoided if possible.[1] Because of the potential role of inflammation in the pathogenesis of the disease, clinicians hoped that corticosteroids would be promising agents in COPD management. However, their use continues to be debated, especially in the management of stable COPD.

The antiinflammatory mechanisms whereby corticosteroids exert their beneficial effect in COPD include (a) reduction in capillary permeability to decrease mucus, (b) inhibition of release of proteolytic enzymes from leukocytes, and (c) inhibition of prostaglandins. Unfortunately, the clinical benefits of systemic corticosteroid therapy in the chronic management of COPD are often not evident, and the risk of toxicity is extensive and far-reaching. Currently, the appropriate situations to consider corticosteroids in COPD include (a) short-term systemic use for acute exacerbations and (b) inhalation therapy for chronic stable COPD.

The role of oral steroid use in chronic stable COPD patients was evaluated in a meta-analysis over a decade ago.[89] Investigators concluded that only a small fraction (10%) of COPD patients treated with steroids showed clinically significant improvement in baseline FEV_1 (increase of 20%) compared with those treated with placebo. While a small number of COPD patients are considered responders to oral steroids, many of these patients actually may have an asthmatic, or reversible, component to their disease. The best predictors for response to oral steroids is the presence of eosinophils on sputum examination (≥3%) and a significant response on pulmonary function tests to sympathomimetics.[90] Both the presence of eosinophils in sputum and the responsiveness to sympathomimetics suggest an asthmatic component to the disease process and thus may explain the clinical benefit seen with steroids.

Long-term adverse effects associated with systemic corticosteroid therapy include osteoporosis, muscular atrophy, thinning of the skin, development of cataracts, and adrenal suppression and insufficiency. The risks associated with long-term steroid therapy are much greater than the clinical benefits. If a decision to treat with long-term systemic corticosteroids is made, the lowest possible effective dose should be given once per day in the morning to minimize the risk of adrenal suppression. If therapy with oral agents is required, an alternate-day schedule should be used.

Previously, a common clinical practice was to administer a short course (2 weeks) of oral corticosteroids as a trial to predict which patients would benefit from chronic oral or inhaled corticosteroids. There is now sufficient evidence suggesting that this practice is not effective in predicting a long-term response to inhaled corticosteroid and should not be recommended.[91]

The use of chronic inhaled corticosteroid therapy has been of interest for the past decade. Their use has been common despite the lack of firm evidence about significant clinical benefit until recently. Inhaled corticosteroids have an improved risk-to-benefit ratio compared with systemic corticosteroid therapy. Using the model for asthma, it was hoped that the inhalation of potent corticosteroid would result in high local efficacy and limited systemic exposure and toxicity. In the latter part of the 1990s, several large international trials were initiated to evaluate the effect on inhaled corticosteroids in COPD. Unfortunately, the results of these major clinical trials failed to demonstrate any benefit from chronic treatment with inhaled corticosteroids in modifying long-term decline in lung function that is characteristic of COPD. Therefore, the role of inhaled corticosteroids in COPD continues to be debated in the literature, unlike asthma, where their use is clearly advocated. Much of the debate centers on the appropriate outcome measures in this population of patients.

During the last decade, several studies of inhaled corticosteroids in COPD were designed to detect a benefit on slowing the progressive loss of lung function, but the results were disappointing.[92–98] None of the large national or international trials were able to demonstrate a benefit of high-dose inhaled corticosteroid therapy on this primary outcome. However, inhaled corticosteroids are associated with other important benefits in some patients, including a decrease in exacerbation frequency and improvements in overall health status.[94,98,99] Clinicians continue to debate the most appropriate and relevant outcome measure to evaluate in COPD studies. Based on the results of clinical trials, consensus guidelines suggest that inhaled corticosteroid therapy should be considered for symptomatic patients with stage III or IV disease (FEV_1 <50%) who experience repeated exacerbations.[1,2] These are the patients who demonstrated benefit in clinical trials and in whom a trial of inhaled corticosteroid therapy is warranted. There are also data from epidemiologic studies that suggest that chronic treatment with inhaled corticosteroids is associated with a lower risk of rehospitalization for a broader group of patients with COPD. Thus the debate about the appropriate role for this antiinflammatory therapy continues.

A meta-analysis evaluating randomized clinical trials involving inhaled corticosteroids in patients COPD indicated that treatment was associated with a relative risk reduction in exacerbation frequency of 33%. The report indicated that 12 patients would require treatment for 20.8 months to prevent one exacerbation episode. The benefit was evident for patients with moderate to severe COPD.[100] This meta-analysis did not detect a mortality benefit.

Other investigators have reported a reduction in mortality in patients with COPD who were treated with inhaled corticosteroids. In an epidemiologic study of a Canadian database, patient mortality 3 months to 1 year following a hospitalization for a COPD exacerbation was evaluated in patients who received inhaled corticosteroids in the first 3 months compared to those who did not. For patients older than 65 years of age, inhaled corticosteroid therapy reduced mortality by 25%. Much of the mortality reduction was reflected in deaths from cardiovascular causes. Conversely, patients who received only bronchodilator therapy trended toward higher mortality rates, although not significant.[101] A pooled analysis of seven large trials also concluded that inhaled corticosteroids reduced all-cause mortality in COPD patients.[102]

Currently, the recommended role of inhaled corticosteroid therapy is for COPD patients with moderate to severe airflow obstruction

(FEV_1 <50% predicted), and who experience frequent exacerbations despite bronchodilator therapy. The initial hope that treatment with inhaled corticosteroids would prevent or slow the progressive decline in FEV_1 remains unproven; however, it is often argued that additional important outcomes in patients with COPD include relief of symptoms, fewer and less-severe exacerbations, and improved quality of life.[103] The role of inhaled corticosteroids in prolonging survival of patients with COPD has been widely debated in recent years. Investigators have reported mixed success and studies are confounded by small sample size and differences in study design.[104]

Although a dose–response relationship for inhaled corticosteroids has not been demonstrated in COPD, the major clinical trials employed moderate to high doses for treatment. Side effects of inhaled corticosteroids are relatively mild compared with the toxicity from systemic therapy. Hoarseness, sore throat, oral candidiasis, and skin bruising have been reported in the clinical trials. Severe side effects, such as adrenal suppression, osteoporosis, and cataract formation, have been reported less frequently than with systemic corticosteroids, but clinicians should monitor patients who are receiving high-dose chronic therapy.[105,106]

There is evidence supporting a dose relationship between inhaled corticosteroid use and the risk of fractures. In a cohort of more than 1,600 subjects with a diagnosis of asthma or COPD (mean age: 80 years), the risk of a fracture was 2.53 times higher (confidence interval: 1.65 to 3.89) in those receiving a mean daily dose of inhaled corticosteroid of 601 mcg or greater.[107] However, the data are conflicting about this issue. A meta-analysis found no evidence supporting an increased risk of fractures or decreased bone mineral density with chronic inhaled corticosteroid use.[108] It appears prudent to suggest that, to minimize the risk of fracture, patients should be treated with the lowest effective dose of inhaled corticosteroids.[109] It may also be helpful to recommend adequate intake of calcium and vitamin D, and possibly periodic bone mineral density testing.

Combination Therapy: Bronchodilators and Inhaled Corticosteroids

Following the disappointing results of chronic inhaled corticosteroid studies and the progressive decline in lung function, investigators became interested in the combination of potent antiinflammatory therapies and long-acting bronchodilators. Subsequently, several studies have shown an additive benefit with long-acting bronchodilators.[110–113] In various studies, combination therapy with salmeterol plus fluticasone or formoterol plus budesonide was associated with greater improvements in clinical outcomes such as FEV_1, health status, and frequency of exacerbations compared with inhaled corticosteroids or long-acting bronchodilators alone. The availability of combination inhalers (e.g., salmeterol plus fluticasone) makes administration of both inhaled corticosteroids and long-acting bronchodilators more convenient for patients and decreases the total number of inhalations needed daily. Therefore, there is growing evidence that inhaled corticosteroid and long-acting β-agonist combinations improve lung function, as well as reduce symptoms of dyspnea and exacerbation frequency.[112–114]

The combination of a long-acting β-agonist and inhaled corticosteroid has been compared to the long-acting β-agonist therapy alone. In a study involving nearly 1,000 patients with severe but stable COPD, subjects received either salmeterol 50 mcg/fluticasone 500 mcg twice daily or salmeterol 50 mcg twice daily for 44 weeks. Exacerbation frequency was significantly lower in the combination group (334 versus 464 episodes) which corresponded to a 35% reduction in the annualized rate. The time to the first exacerbation was also delayed with the combination therapy.[115] One finding of concern reported in this trial was the increased number of pneumonia cases in patients receiving combination therapy compared to salmeterol alone. There were 23 cases reported, compared with 7 in the salmeterol group.[115] An increase in the risk for pneumonia was also reported in the Towards a Revolution in COPD Health (TORCH) study.[116] This finding requires further investigation.

The largest prospective study to date is referred to as the TORCH study.[116] This trial consisted of 6,112 patients who received one of four treatments for 3 years. Treatment groups were placebo, salmeterol 50 mcg twice daily, fluticasone 500 mcg twice daily, or the combination of salmeterol and fluticasone in a single inhaler. The primary outcome was death from any cause and secondary outcomes were exacerbation rates, lung function, and health status. None of the active treatments differed significantly from placebo, although the combination of salmeterol and fluticasone trended toward fewer deaths ($p = 0.052$). The combination also reduced exacerbation rates, and improved lung function and health status compared to the other treatments. Exacerbation rates were also significantly reduced with combination therapy compared to either single agent alone. Both treatment groups that included fluticasone had higher rates of pneumonia. Although this study did not reflect a mortality benefit, the authors indicated the risk of death was reduced by 17.5% with the combination and that the number needed to treat for 1 year to provide a benefit was 4.

Combinations of Long-Acting Bronchodilators Compared to Long-Acting Bronchodilators Plus Inhaled Corticosteroids The combination of salmeterol and tiotropium has also been evaluated in a short-term crossover study involving only 22 subjects who received either salmeterol (50 mcg twice daily) plus fluticasone (500 mcg twice daily), fluticasone plus tiotropium (18 mcg once daily), or fluticasone, salmeterol, and tiotropium for 1 week. The triple combination provided a significant benefit of improved lung function compared to either of the dual treatments in subjects with moderate to severe COPD.[117] The benefit of triple therapy was evaluated in a 1-year randomized, double-blind, placebo control study involving 449 subjects with moderate to severe COPD. Treatment consisted of either tiotropium, tiotropium plus salmeterol, or tiotropium, salmeterol and fluticasone.[118] There was no difference between treatments for the primary outcome of percentage of patients experiencing an exacerbation requiring systemic corticosteroids or antibiotics. The triple-drug regimen improved lung function, quality of life, and reduced hospitalization compared to tiotropium alone, whereas two-drug therapy did not offer any benefit in lung function improvement or hospitalization rates compared to the single agent. Another small study evaluated the addition of tiotropium for 1 month to a regimen of an inhaled corticosteroid and a long-acting β-agonist.[119] The addition of tiotropium improved lung function and quality-of-life scores, apparently by improving dynamics of lung capacity (inspiratory capacity). These effects were reversed when tiotropium therapy was discontinued. These data involving combinations of long acting bronchodilators are limited and preliminary. More research is required and should include other outcome parameters including relief of symptoms, exacerbation rates and quality of life. Larger sample sizes and longer durations will provide insight into the value of combinations.

α_1-Antitrypsin Replacement Therapy

In patients with inherited AAT deficiency-associated emphysema, treatment focuses on reduction of risk factors such as smoking, symptomatic treatment with bronchodilators, and augmentation therapy with replacement AAT. Based on knowledge about the relationship between serum concentrations of AAT and the risk of developing emphysema, the rationale for augmentation therapy is to maintain serum concentrations above the protective threshold throughout the dosing interval.[120] Indirect evidence of AAT activity in the interstitium of the lung has been demonstrated by measuring concentrations of the enzyme in epithelial lining fluid obtained during bronchoalveolar lavage. Augmentation therapy consists of weekly infusions of pooled human AAT to maintain AAT plasma levels greater than 10 micromolars. Much of the data supporting the use of AAT replacement is based on evidence of biochemical efficacy (e.g., administering the product and demonstrating protective serum concentrations of AAT).

Clinical evidence for slowing lung function decline or improving outcomes with augmentation therapy is sparse. Stated challenges to performing randomized clinical trials include the large sample size and long duration of followup required, and the expense of conducting such a trial. One observational study followed patients in the National Registry of Severe AAT Deficiency over a period of several years and documented clinical outcomes. In this study, patients who received weekly augmentation therapy with purified AAT had slower declines in FEV_1 and decreased mortality compared with patients who never received augmentation therapy.[121] However, this was an observational study of patients, not a randomized, placebo-controlled trial, and so direct cause-and-effect relationships cannot be concluded. One randomized, placebo-controlled study of patients with severe AAT deficiency (ZZ phenotype) did show a significant reduction in lung tissue loss and destruction as measured by computed tomographic scan in patients receiving augmentation therapy.[122] Other measures of lung function and mortality were not recorded.

The recommended dosing regimen for replacement AAT is 60 mg/kg administered intravenously once a week at a rate of 0.08 mL/kg per minute, adjusted to patient tolerance. It has been estimated that this form of augmentation therapy will cost more than $54,000 annually.[123] In the absence of alternative treatments, it is difficult to assess cost-effectiveness using conventional criteria. There have been repeated problems with supply of this biologic replacement therapy (derived from pooled blood donors) related to production difficulty and contamination issues. Currently, there are three products available (Prolastin [Bayer], Aralast [Baxter], and Zemaira [ZLB Behring]), which should minimize this problem in the future. Drug development research continues in the area of recombinant products and inhalational therapy.

The safety of AAT replacement therapy has been recently evaluated in two large observational studies. In the most recent study, 174 patients (n = 747) reported 720 adverse events, classified as severe in 8.8% of cases and moderate in 72.4% of cases.[124] Common complaints included headache, dizziness, nausea, dyspnea, and fever. The overall rate of adverse events was low (i.e., two events over 5 years).

TREATMENT

Chronic Obstructive Pulmonary Disease Exacerbation

■ DESIRED OUTCOMES

⑩ The goals of therapy for patients experiencing exacerbations of COPD are (a) prevention of hospitalization or reduction in hospital stay, (b) prevention of acute respiratory failure and death, and (c) resolution of exacerbation symptoms and a return to baseline clinical status and quality of life. Acute exacerbations can range from mild to severe. Factors that influence the severity, and subsequently the level of care required, include the severity of airflow limitation, presence of comorbidities and the history of previous exacerbations. Table 29–12 includes factors that warrant treatment in the hospital.

Table 29–13 summarizes the various therapeutic options for exacerbation management. Pharmacotherapy consists of intensification of bronchodilator therapy and a short course of systemic corticosteroids. Antimicrobial therapy is indicated in the presence of selected symptoms. As the frequency and severity of exacerbations are closely related to each patient's overall health status, all patients should receive optimal chronic treatment, including smoking cessation, appropriate pharmacologic therapy, and preventative therapy such as vaccinations.

TABLE 29-12 Factors Favoring Hospitalization for Treatment of Chronic Obstructive Pulmonary Disease Exacerbation

Presence of high risk comorbidity (e.g., pneumonia, arrhythmia, congestive heart failure, diabetes, renal or hepatic failure)
Suboptimal response to outpatient management
Marked worsening of dyspnea
Inability to eat or sleep because of symptoms
Worsening hypoxemia or hypercapnia
Mental status changes
Lack of home support for care
Uncertain diagnosis

Modified from the American Thoracic Society.
Adapted from reference 2.

■ NONPHARMACOLOGIC THERAPY

Controlled Oxygen Therapy

Oxygen therapy should be considered for any patient with hypoxemia during an exacerbation. Caution must be used, however, because many patients with COPD rely on mild hypoxemia to trigger their drive to breathe. In normal, healthy individuals, the drive to breathe is triggered by carbon dioxide accumulation. In patients with COPD who retain carbon dioxide as a result of their disease progression, hypoxemia rather than hypercapnia becomes the main trigger for their respiratory drive. Overly aggressive administration of oxygen to patients with chronic hypercapnia may result in respiratory depression and respiratory failure. Oxygen therapy should be used to achieve a PaO_2 of greater than 60 mm Hg or oxygen saturation of greater than 90%. However, an ABG should be obtained after oxygen initiation to monitor carbon dioxide retention owing to hypoventilation.

Noninvasive Mechanical Ventilation

Noninvasive positive-pressure ventilation (NPPV) provides ventilatory support with oxygen and pressurized airflow using a face or nasal mask with a tight seal but without endotracheal intubation. Numerous

TABLE 29-13 Therapeutic Options for Acute Exacerbations of Chronic Obstructive Pulmonary Disease

Therapy	Comments
Antibiotics	Recommended if two or more of the following are present: Increased dyspnea Increased sputum production Increased sputum purulence
Corticosteroids	Oral or intravenous therapy may be used. If intravenous is used, it should be changed to oral after improvement in pulmonary status. If continued longer than 14 days, then the dose should be tapered to avoid hypothalamic–pituitary–adrenal axis suppression.
Bronchodilators	Metered-dose inhalers and dry-powder inhalers equal in efficacy to nebulization. β-Agonists also may increase mucociliary clearance. Long-acting β-agonists should not be used for quick relief of symptoms or on an as-needed basis.
Controlled oxygen therapy	Titrate oxygen to desired oxygen saturation (>90%). Monitor arterial blood gas for development of hypercapnia.
Noninvasive mechanical ventilation	Consider for patients with acute respiratory failure. Not appropriate for patients with altered mental status, severe acidosis, respiratory arrest, or cardiovascular instability.

trials have reported the benefits of NPPV in patients with acute respiratory failure caused by COPD exacerbations. In one meta-analysis of eight studies, NPPV was associated with lower mortality, lower intubation rates, shorter hospital stays, and greater improvements in serum pH in 1 hour when compared with treatment with usual care alone.[125] The benefits seen with NPPV generally can be attributed to a reduction in the complications that often arise with invasive mechanical ventilation. Not all patients with COPD exacerbations are appropriate candidates for NPPV. Patients with altered mental status may not be able to protect their airway and thus may be at increased risk for aspiration. Patients with severe acidosis (pH <7.25), respiratory arrest, or cardiovascular instability should not be considered for NPPV. Patients failing a trial of NPPV or those considered poor candidates may be considered for intubation and mechanical ventilation.

PHARMACOLOGIC THERAPY

Bronchodilators

During exacerbations, intensification of bronchodilator regimens is used commonly. The doses and frequency of bronchodilators are increased to provide symptomatic relief. Short-acting β_2-agonists are preferred owing to rapid onset of action. Anticholinergic agents may be added if symptoms persist despite increased doses of β_2-agonists. In fact, combinations of these agents are employed often, although data are lacking about the benefit versus higher doses of one agent. Bronchodilators may be administered via MDIs or nebulization with equal efficacy. Nebulization may be considered for patients with severe dyspnea who are unable to hold their breath after actuation of an MDI. Clinical evidence supporting the use of theophylline during exacerbations is lacking, and thus theophylline generally should be avoided. However, addition of one of these agents may be considered for patients not responding to other therapies. The risk of adverse effects such as cardiac arrhythmias should be considered and serum levels monitored closely.

Corticosteroids

Until recently, the literature supporting the use of corticosteroids in acute exacerbations of COPD was sparse. However, since 1996, five studies have been performed that document the value of systemic corticosteroids in exacerbations of COPD.[126–130] The Systemic Corticosteroids in Chronic Obstructive Pulmonary Disease Exacerbations (SCCOPE) trial evaluated three groups of patients hospitalized for exacerbations of COPD.[126] The first group received an 8-week course of corticosteroids given as methylprednisolone 125 mg intravenously every 6 hours for 72 hours, followed by once-daily oral prednisone (60 mg on days 4 through 7; 40 mg on days 8 through 11; 20 mg on days 12 through 43; 10 mg on days 44 through 50; and 5 mg on days 51 through 57). The second group received a 2-week course given as methylprednisolone 125 mg intravenously every 6 hours for 72 hours, followed by oral prednisone (60 mg on days 5 through 7; 40 mg on days 8 through 11; and 20 mg on days 12 through 15) and placebo on days 16 through 57. The third group received placebo for all 57 days of study. Rates of treatment failure and hospital stay were significantly higher in the placebo group than in either treatment group at 30 and 90 days. Groups randomized to corticosteroid treatment also had a significantly shorter length of hospital stay than did the placebo group. The 8-week regimen was not found to be superior to the 2-week regimen. Significant treatment benefits were no longer evident at 6 months.

Davies et al.[127] evaluated the oral use of corticosteroids in hospitalized patients with acute exacerbations of COPD. Patients received either 30 mg/day oral prednisolone or placebo for 14 days. Patients who were treated with corticosteroids had a significantly more rapid improvement in FEV_1 and a shorter hospital stay than did patients who received placebo. There was no significant difference between groups at 6-week followup.

In total, results from these trials suggest that patients with acute exacerbations of COPD should receive a short course of intravenous or oral corticosteroids. However, because of the large variability in dosage ranges, the optimal dose and duration of corticosteroid treatment are not known. It appears that short courses (9 to 14 days) are as effective as longer courses and have a lower risk of associated adverse effects owing to less time of exposure. Several trials used high initial doses of steroids before tapering to a lower maintenance dose. Adverse effects such as hyperglycemia, insomnia, and hallucinations may occur at higher doses. Depending on the clinical status of the patient, treatment may be initiated at a lower dose or tapered more quickly if these effects occur. It appears that a regimen of prednisone 40 mg orally daily (or equivalent) for 10 to 14 days can be effective for most patients.[131] If steroid treatment is continued for longer than 2 weeks, a tapering oral schedule should be employed to avoid signs of hypothalamic–pituitary–adrenal axis suppression.

Antimicrobial Therapy

⓫ Most acute exacerbations of COPD are thought to be caused by viral or bacterial infections. However, as many as 30% of exacerbations are caused by unknown factors.[1] A meta-analysis of nine studies evaluating the effectiveness of antibiotics in treating exacerbations of COPD determined that patients receiving antibiotics had a greater improvement in peak expiratory flow rate than those who did not.[132]

This meta-analysis concluded that antibiotics are of most benefit and should be initiated if at least two of the following three symptoms are present: increased dyspnea, increased sputum volume, and increased sputum purulence. The utility of sputum Gram stain and culture is questionable because some patients have chronic bacterial colonization of the bronchial tree between exacerbations.

The emergence of drug-resistant organisms has mandated that antibiotic regimens be chosen judiciously. Selection of empirical antimicrobial therapy should be based on the most likely organism(s) thought to be responsible for the infection based on the individual patient profile. The most common organisms for any acute exacerbation of COPD are *Haemophilus influenzae, Moraxella catarrhalis, Streptococcus pneumoniae,* and *Haemophilus parainfluenzae.* More virulent bacteria may be present in patients with more complicated acute exacerbations of COPD, including drug-resistant pneumococci, β-lactamase–producing *H. influenzae* and *M. catarrhalis,* and enteric gram-negative organisms, including *Pseudomonas aeruginosa.* Table 29–14 summarizes recommended antimicrobial therapy for exacerbations of COPD and the most common organisms based on patient presentation.[133]

Therapy with antibiotics generally should be continued for at least 7 to 10 days. Studies evaluating shorter treatment courses (usually 5 days) with the fluoroquinolones, second- and third-generation cephalosporins, and macrolide antimicrobials have demonstrated comparable efficacy with the longer treatment regimens.[134] If the patient deteriorates or does not improve as anticipated, hospitalization may be necessary, and more aggressive attempts should be made to identify potential pathogens responsible for the exacerbation.

COMPLICATIONS

Cor Pulmonale

Cor pulmonale is right-sided heart failure secondary to pulmonary hypertension. Long-term oxygen therapy and diuretics have been the mainstays of therapy for cor pulmonale. Increasing the PaO_2 above 60 mm Hg with supplemental oxygen therapy decreases pulmonary hypertension and thus decreases the force against which the right ventricle has to work. Although diuretics may help decrease fluid overload, caution should be used because patients with significant

TABLE 29-14 Recommended Antimicrobial Therapy in Acute Exacerbations of Chronic Obstructive Pulmonary Disease

Patient Characteristics	Likely Pathogens	Recommended Therapy
Uncomplicated exacerbations <4 exacerbations per year No comorbid illness FEV_1 >50% of predicted	*Streptococcus pneumoniae* *Haemophilus influenzae* *Moraxella catarrhalis* *Haemophilus parainfluenzae* Resistance uncommon	Macrolide (azithromycin, clarithromycin) Second- or third-generation cephalosporin Doxycycline Therapies not recommended[a]: TMP-SMX, amoxicillin, first-generation cephalosporins, and erythromycin
Complicated exacerbations Age ≥65 years >4 exacerbations per year FEV_1 <50% but >35% of predicted	As above plus drug-resistant pneumococci, β-lactamase–producing *H. influenzae* and *M. catarrhalis*	Amoxicillin/clavulanate Fluoroquinolone with enhanced pneumococcal activity (levofloxacin, gemifloxacin, moxifloxacin)
Complicated exacerbations with risk of *Pseudomonas aeruginosa*	Some enteric gram-negatives	Fluoroquinolone with enhanced pneumococcal and *P. aeruginosa* activity (levofloxacin)
Chronic bronchial sepsis[b] Need for chronic corticosteroid therapy Resident of nursing home >4 exacerbations per year FEV_1 >35% of predicted	As above plus *P. aeruginosa*	IV therapy if required: β-lactamase–resistant penicillin with antipseudomonal activity Third- or fourth-generation cephalosporin with antipseudomonal activity

FEV_1, forced expiratory volume in the first second of expiration; TMP-SMX, trimethoprim-sulfamethoxazole.
[a]TMP-SMX should not be used because of increasing pneumococcal resistance; amoxicillin and first-generation cephalosporins are not recommended because of β-lactamase susceptibility; and erythromycin is not recommended because of insufficient activity against *H. influenzae*.
[b]In sepsis, double antipseudomonal coverage should be considered (e.g., addition of aminoglycoside).
Modified and updated from reference 1.

right-sided heart failure are highly dependent on preload for cardiac output. Consequently, the decision to use diuretics must be based on a risk-to-benefit ratio. Digitalis glycosides have no role in the treatment of cor pulmonale.

Other pharmacologic agents that have been investigated to treat cor pulmonale include hydralazine, calcium channel blockers, angiotensin-converting enzyme inhibitors, and angiotensin II antagonists. However, there is insufficient evidence to offer guidelines for the role of these agents in COPD patients with cor pulmonale.

Polycythemia

Polycythemia secondary to chronic hypoxemia in COPD patients can be improved by either oxygen therapy or periodic phlebotomy if oxygen therapy alone is not sufficient. Continuous oxygen therapy was shown by the Nocturnal Oxygen Therapy Trial Group to reduce hematocrit values in treated patients.[31] Acute phlebotomy is indicated if the hematocrit is above 55% to 60% and the patient is experiencing central nervous system effects suggestive of sludging from high blood viscosity. Long-term oxygen then can be used to maintain a lower hematocrit.

OTHER PHARMACOLOGIC CONSIDERATIONS

A number of other treatments have been explored over the years. Among these therapies, there is either insufficient evidence to warrant recommending their use, or they have been proven to not be beneficial in the management of COPD. A brief summary is provided because the clinician likely will encounter patients who are receiving or inquire about these treatments.

Suppressive Antimicrobial Agents

Because COPD patients often are colonized with bacteria and experience recurrent exacerbations of their condition, a common practice employed in the past has been the use of low-dose antimicrobial therapy as preventative or prophylaxis against these acute exacerbations. However, clinical studies over the past 40 years have failed to demonstrate any benefit from this practice.[1] The role of antimicrobial therapy is limited to acute exacerbations of COPD meeting specific criteria.

Expectorants and Mucolytics

Adequate water intake generally is acceptable to maintain hydration and assist in the removal of airway sections. Beyond this, the regular use of mucolytics or expectorants for COPD patients has no proven benefit.[135] This includes the use of saturated solutions of potassium iodide, ammonium chloride, acetylcysteine, and guaifenesin. In 2007, the FDA announced its intention to take action against several companies marketing unapproved timed-released formulations of guaifenesin. Two formulations are approved by the FDA (Humibid and Mucinex); however, data are lacking on their benefit.

Narcotics

Systemic (oral and parenteral) opioids, especially morphine, can relieve dyspnea in patients with endstage COPD. Nebulized therapy is sometimes used in clinical practice although data about clinical benefit are lacking.[136] Opioids should be used carefully, if at all, to avoid adverse effects on ventilatory drive.

Respiratory Stimulants

There is no role for respiratory stimulants in the long-term management of COPD.[1] Agents that have shown some usefulness in the acute setting include almitrine and doxapram. However, amiltrine is available only in Europe, and its usefulness is limited by neurotoxicity. Doxapram is available for intravenous use only and may be no better than intermittent NPPV.

SURGICAL INTERVENTION

Various surgical options have been employed in the management of COPD. These include bullectomy, lung volume reduction surgery (LVRS), and lung transplantation. Bullectomy has been performed for many years and may be useful when large bullae (>1 cm) are noted on computed tomographic scan. The presence of bullae may contribute to complaints of dyspnea and their removal can improve lung function and reduce symptoms, although there is no evidence of a mortality benefit. Because of the prevalence of COPD, it is the most frequent indication for lung transplantation. Intervention is considered when predicted survival is less than 2 years, FEV_1 is <25% predicted, and hypoxemia, hypercapnia, and pulmonary hypertension exists despite medical management.[2] Experience to date shows 2-year survival of 65% to 90%, and 5-year survival of 41% to 53%.

Recent trials have evaluated the effect of bilateral LVRS for management of severe COPD. Short-term trials comparing the effects of pulmonary rehabilitation plus LVRS with pulmonary rehabilitation alone reported that the combination of treatments resulted in greater improvements in lung function, gas exchange, and quality of life at 3 months. Only recently have data evaluating the long-term effect of LVRS compared with pulmonary rehabilitation been published. The National Emphysema Treatment Trial, a prospective, randomized trial evaluating the long-term effects of LVRS plus pulmonary rehabilitation compared with pulmonary rehabilitation alone, followed 1,218 patients for 3 years.[137] The primary end points for the study were mortality and maximal exercise capacity 2 years after randomization. Secondary end points included pulmonary function, distance walked in 6 minutes, and quality-of-life measurements. At an interim analysis, patients with an FEV_1 of less than 20% of predicted or a carbon monoxide diffusing capacity of less than 20% of predicted were noted to be at high risk of death after surgery and subsequently were excluded from the study. Results of the study showed no mortality benefit with LVRS compared with pulmonary rehabilitation alone. Patients undergoing surgery had improved exercise capacity, lung function, and quality of life at 2 years, but these patients also had a higher risk of short-term morbidity and mortality associated with the surgery. A subgroup analysis of the study noted that patients with predominately upper-lobe emphysema and low exercise capacity undergoing surgery had lower mortality rates at 2 years compared with patients treated with medical therapy alone. Because of the costs and risks associated with LVRS, more studies are needed to better determine the ideal surgical candidates and identify subgroups of patients who would benefit most from surgery.

■ DIETARY SUPPLEMENTS

There is increasing interest in the role of antioxidants, including vitamins E and C and β-carotene, in reducing the frequency of exacerbations. It is postulated that they may be beneficial in COPD as a result of an imbalance between oxidants and antioxidants that has been considered in the pathogenesis of smoking-induced lung disease. However, there is no good evidence that antioxidant therapies improve COPD symptoms or slow disease progression.

■ INVESTIGATIONAL THERAPIES

Based on the knowledge about the importance of neutrophilic inflammation in COPD and potential therapeutic benefit of inhibition of neutrophil activity, a number of antiinflammatory compounds are being explored. Specifically, agents inhibiting leukotriene B_4, neutrophil elastase, and phosphodiesterases currently are being evaluated. To date, studies evaluating leukotriene-modifying therapies have been disappointing. Further studies are needed to evaluate the clinical benefit of such inhibitors in patients with COPD.

Phosphodiesterase-4 is the major phosphodiesterase found in airway smooth muscle cells and inflammatory cells and is responsible for degrading cyclic adenosine monophosphate. Inhibition of phosphodiesterase-4 results in relaxation of airway smooth muscle cells and decreased activity of inflammatory cells and mediators such as tumor necrosis factor-α and interleukin-8. Two phosphodiesterase-4 inhibitors have reached clinical trials—cilomilast and roflumilast. Cilomilast has been evaluated in several human trials and has been shown to improve expiratory airflow as measured by FEV_1 in patients with COPD when given at a dose of 15 mg twice daily for 6 weeks. To date, the results of clinical trials investigating these agents have been modest. Future studies of these agents should evaluate effects on other clinical outcomes such as health status, exacerbation frequency, and progression of disease.

Neutrophil elastase is implicated in the induction of bronchial disease, causing structural changes in lungs, impairment of mucociliary clearance, and impairment of host defenses. Protease inhibitors, namely, inhibitors of neutrophil elastase, are being investigated currently for the treatment of COPD.

Results have been disappointing in evaluating the benefit of infliximab, a tumor necrosis factor-α blocker, in treating COPD. A total of 234 patients with moderate to severe COPD received either infliximab 3 mg/kg or 5 mg/kg, or placebo at baseline, 2, 6, 12, 18, and 24 weeks. Subjects completed a quality-of-life questionnaire (Chronic Respiratory Questionnaire) during treatment and out to 44 weeks. There were no differences on the Chronic Respiratory Questionnaire, or on any secondary end points, including lung function, exercise capacity, or exacerbation rates. The discontinuation rate as a consequence of adverse events was high (20% to 27%) in the active-treatment group.[138]

PHARMACOECONOMIC CONSIDERATIONS

The overall cost of therapy is an important consideration in contemporary medical practice. Meaningful cost analysis goes beyond the cost of the medication itself and incorporates the impact of a given therapeutic agent on overall healthcare cost. Because of the relative lack of benefit among objective outcome measures in COPD clinical trials, pharmacoeconomic studies can be useful in decision making about pharmacotherapy options. Pharmacoeconomic analyses in COPD, although limited, are available regarding antibiotic use in acute exacerbations and some therapies for management of chronic stable COPD.

The costs of managing an acute exacerbation of COPD in the ambulatory setting was evaluated in more than 2,400 patients. Subjects were followed for 1 month following the diagnosis of the exacerbation. The overall relapse rate was 21%, with 31% and 16% of subjects requiring care in the emergency department and hospital, respectively. The overall costs for exacerbation treatment averaged $159, with 58% attributed to hospitalization.[139] These authors concluded that a significant cost savings would result from improving the successful ambulatory management of acute exacerbations.

Grossman et al. conducted a trial investigating the use of aggressive antimicrobial therapy (ciprofloxacin), comparing it with usual antibiotic therapy (defined as any nonquinolone) in the treatment of acute exacerbations of COPD.[140] Overall, the results indicated no preference for either treatment arm. However, in patients who were categorized as high risk (severe underlying lung disease, more than four exacerbations per year, duration of bronchitis longer than 10 years, elderly, significant comorbid illness), the use of aggressive antibiotic therapy was associated with improved clinical outcome, higher quality of life, and fewer costs. The results of this study are consistent with Table 29–14, which suggests that higher-risk patients are likely to have more resistant strains of organisms and thus require more aggressive antimicrobial treatment.

Friedman et al. conducted a post hoc pharmacoeconomic evaluation of two multicenter, randomized trials comparing the combination of ipratropium and albuterol with both drugs used as monotherapy.[141] Patients who received a combination of ipratropium and albuterol had lower rates of exacerbations, lower overall treatment costs, and improved cost-effectiveness compared with either drug used alone. With the introduction of new bronchodilator therapies, and with no clearly consistent advantage of one class of agents over another, pharmacoeconomic analyses may be useful for clinicians in determining the most appropriate therapy for their patients.

CLINICAL CONTROVERSIES

Albuterol is one of the most commonly prescribed medications in the United States. Albuterol is a 50/50 racemic mixture of (*R*)-albuterol and (*S*)-albuterol, with the (*R*)-isomer responsible for all the therapeutic effect. A single-isomer product, levalbuterol, claims clinical superiority based on the absence of the (*S*)-isomer, which may have detrimental effects in the airway and antagonistic effects on the active isomer. However, the acquisition cost of levalbuterol is significantly higher than that of generic albuterol. The advantages of using the single-isomer product in clinical practice are not clear and require further investigation.

A combination product of a long-acting inhaled β-agonist (salmeterol) and an inhaled corticosteroid agent (fluticasone) is one of the most commonly prescribed medications for lung disease, including COPD. However, in expert guidelines, inhaled corticosteroids are indicated only for patients with more severe disease who experience frequent exacerbations. Many patients now receiving therapy with the combination inhaler may be candidates for bronchodilator therapy alone, although the benefit of inhaled corticosteroids continues to be a focus of clinical research, including the potential for a mortality benefit.

The role of systemic corticosteroids for acute exacerbations of COPD has been clarified in recent years. However, the appropriate dosage regimen is not well established. Regimens range from initial high doses (methylprednisolone 125 mg every 6 hours) to more conservative dosing (prednisone 40 to 60 mg/day). Consensus guidelines indicate that bronchodilator therapy is the focus of pharmacotherapy for COPD. However, there is no clear choice for the initial agent. For patients with daily but not persistent symptoms, either ipratropium or albuterol offers advantages as initial therapy. Both also have limitations if chosen as the initial therapy.

International guidelines recommend long-acting bronchodilator therapy in patients with moderate to very severe disease, or who when symptoms are not adequately managed with short-acting agents or as needed therapy. When response to a single long-acting bronchodilator is not optimal, guidelines recommend the use of combinations. However, data are lacking presently about the therapeutic benefit of combinations of long-acting bronchodilators and this approach is associated with substantial costs.

EVALUATION OF THERAPEUTIC OUTCOMES

To evaluate therapeutic outcomes of COPD effectively, the practitioner must first delineate between chronic stable COPD and acute exacerbations. In chronic stable COPD, pulmonary function tests should be assessed periodically and with any therapy addition, change in dose, or deletion of therapy. Because objective improvements often are minimal, subjective assessments are important. Other outcome parameters are commonly evaluated, including dyspnea score, quality-of-life assessments, and exacerbation rates, including visits to the emergency department or hospitalization. In acute exacerbations of COPD, white blood cell count, vital signs, chest radiography, and changes in frequency of dyspnea, sputum volume, and sputum purulence should be assessed at the onset and throughout treatment of an exacerbation. In more severe exacerbations, ABGs and oxygen saturation also should be monitored. As with any drug therapy, patient adherence to therapeutic regimens, side effects, potential drug interactions, and subjective measures of quality of life also must be evaluated.

END-OF-LIFE CARE

Based on the natural course of COPD, characterized by the progressive decline in lung function, and development of complications, consideration should be given to end-of-life decisions and advanced directives.[142] Factors associated with expected mortality within 1 year have been identified and include older age, diagnosis of depression, declining overall health status, hypercapnia, an FEV_1 of less than 30% predicted, ability to walk only a few steps without resting, more than one emergent hospitalization in the past year, and the presence of comorbidities, including congestive heart failure. An effective strategy to discuss end-of-life care involves the patient's participation in identifying advanced directives. Patients should be assured that symptoms, including pain, will be managed, and their dignity will be preserved. Specific issues that should be addressed include location and provider for terminal care, desires to use or withhold mechanical ventilation, and involvement of other family members in decisions on behalf of the patient.

ABBREVIATIONS

AAT: α_1-antitrypsin

BMI: body mass index

COPD: chronic obstructive pulmonary disease

DPI: dry-powder inhaler

FEV_1: forced expiratory volume in the first second of expiration

FVC: forced vital capacity

GOLD: Global Initiative for Chronic Obstructive Lung Disease

LVRS: lung volume reduction surgery

MDI: metered-dose inhaler

NPPV: noninvasive positive-pressure ventilation

PaO_2: pressure exerted by oxygen gas in arterial blood

$PaCO_2$: pressure exerted by carbon dioxide gas in arterial blood

REFERENCES

1. Global Initiative for Chronic Obstructive Lung Disease. Global Strategy for the Diagnosis, Management and Prevention of Chronic Obstructive Pulmonary Disease. NHLBI/WHO workshop report. Bethesda, MD: National Heart, Lung and Blood Institute, April 2001; Updated November 2006. Available at *http://www.goldcopd.com/*.
2. Celli BR, MacNee W, ATS/ERS Task Force. Standards for the diagnosis and treatment of patients with COPD. A summary of the ATS/ERS position paper. Eur Respir J 2004;23:932–946. Full report accessible at *http://www.thoracic.org*.
3. Rabe KF. Guidelines for chronic obstructive pulmonary disease treatment and issues of implementation. Proc Am Thorac Soc 2006;3:641–644.
4. SCCOR in Chronic Obstructive Pulmonary Disease (COPD). RFA Number: RFA-HL-05–008. Available at *http://grants.nih.gov/grants/guide/RFA-files/RFA-HL-05-008.html*.
5. National Center for Health Statistics. National Health Interview Survey. Hyattsville, MD: U.S. Department of Health and Human Services, CDC, NCHS, 2001. Available at *www.cdc.gov/nchs/nhis.htm*.
6. Mannino DM, Homa DM, Akinbami LJ, et al. Chronic obstructive pulmonary disease surveillance—United States, 1971–2000. MMWR Surveill Summ 2002;51:1–16.
7. Wilt TJ, Niewoehner D, Kim C, et al. Use of Spirometry for Case Finding, Diagnosis, and Management of Chronic Obstructive Pulmonary Disease. (COPD). Evidence Report #121. AHRQ Publication 05-E017–1. Washington, DC: Agency for Healthcare Research and Quality, 2005.

8. Minino AM, Heron MP, Smith BL. Deaths: Preliminary Data for 2004. National Vital Statistics Reports, 2006;54 (19). Hyattsville, MD: National Center for Health Statistics.
9. Chronic Obstructive Pulmonary Disease: Data Fact Sheet. NIH Publication 03–5529. Bethesda, MD: U.S. Department of Health and Human Services, National Institutes of Health, NHLBI, 2003.
10. Holguin F, Folch E, Redd SC, Mannino DM. Comorbidity and mortality in COPD-related hospitalizations in the United States, 1979–2001. Chest 2005;128:2005–2011.
11. Confronting COPD in America, Glaxo Smith Kline 1997–2007. Available at *http://www.copdinamerica.com*.
12. National Institutes of Health. NHLBI Morbidity & Mortality: 2004 Chart Book on Cardiovascular, Lung & Blood Diseases. 2004, *http://www.nhlbi.nih.gov/resources/docs/cht-book.htm*.
13. The Health Consequences of Smoking: A Report of the Surgeon General, 2004. Centers for Diseass Control. Available at *http://www.cdc.gov/tobacco/data-statistics/sgr/sgr_2004/index.htm*.
14. Sandford AJ, Silverman EK. Chronic obstructive pulmonary disease. 1: Susceptibility factors for COPD the genotype-environment interaction. Thorax 2002;57(8):736–741.
15. Carrel RW, Lomas DA. Alpha-1 antitrypsin deficiency: A model for conformational diseases. N Engl J Med 2002;346(1):45–53.
16. Barnes PJ. Chronic obstructive pulmonary disease. N Engl J Med 2000;343:269–280.
17. Stockley RA. Neutrophils and the pathogenesis of COPD. Chest 2002;121:151S–155S.
18. Hogg JC. Pathophysiology of airflow limitation in chronic obstructive pulmonary disease. Lancet 2004;364:709–721.
19. Hill AT, Bayley D, Stockely RA. The interrelationship of sputum inflammatory markers in patients with chronic bronchitis. Am J Respir Crit Care Med 1999;160:893–898.
20. Ries AL. Impact of chronic obstructive pulmonary disease on quality of life: The role of dyspnea. Am J Med 2006;119 (10A):s12–s20.
21. MacNee W. Pathophysiology of cor pulmonale in chronic obstructive pulmonary disease, part 2. Am J Respir Crit Care Med 1994;150:1158–1168.
22. Sin DD, Man SF. Why are patients with chronic obstructive pulmonary disease at increased risk of cardiovascular disease? The potential role of systemic inflammation in chronic obstructive pulmonary disease. Circulation 2003;107:1514–1519.
23. Rodriguez-Roisin R. Toward a consensus definition for COPD exacerbations. Chest 2000;117(Suppl 2):398S–401S.
24. Landbo C, Prescott E, Lange P, Vestbo J, Almdal TP. Prognostic value of nutritional status in chronic obstructive pulmonary disease. Am J Respir Crit Care Med 1999;160:1856–1861.
25. Ferris BG. Epidemiology standardization project (American Thoracic Society). Am Rev Respir Dis 1978;118:1–120.
26. Anzueto A. Clinical course of chronic obstructive pulmonary disease: Review of therapeutic interventions. Am J Med 2006;119(10A):s46–s53.
27. Celli BR. The importance of spirometry in COPD and asthma. Chest 2000;117:15S–19S.
28. Anthonisen NR, Connett JE, Kiley JP, et al. Effects of smoking intervention and the use of an inhaled anticholinergic bronchodilator on the rate of decline of FEV_1: The Lung Health Study. JAMA 1994;272:1497–1505.
29. Anthonisen NR, Skeans MA, Wise RA, Manfreda J, Kanner RE, Connett JE. The effects of a smoking cessation intervention on 14.5 year mortality: A randomized clinical trial. Ann Intern Med 2005;142:233–239.
30. Andersson F, Borg S, Janson S-A, et al. The costs of exacerbations in chronic obstructive pulmonary disease (COPD). Respir Med 2002;96:700–708.
31. Anthonisen NR, Manfreda J, Warren CPW, et al. Antibiotic therapy in exacerbations of chronic obstructive pulmonary disease. Ann Intern Med 1987;106:196–204.
32. Groenewegen KH, Schols AMW, Wouters EFM. Mortality and mortality-related factors after hospitalization for acute exacerbation of COPD. Chest 2003;124:459–467.
33. Bach PB, Brown C, Gelfand SE, McCrory DC. Management of acute exacerbations of chronic obstructive pulmonary disease: A summary and appraisal of published evidence. Ann Intern Med 2001;134:600–620.
34. Almagro P, Calbo E, Ochoa de Echaguen A, et al. Mortality after hospitalization for COPD. Chest 2002;121:1441–1448.
35. Connors AF, Dawson NV, Thomas C, et al. Outcomes following acute exacerbation of severe chronic obstructive disease. Am J Respir Crit Care Med 1996;154:959–967.
36. Heffner JE, Fahy B, Hilling L, Barbieri C. Outcomes of advanced directive education of pulmonary rehabilitation patients. Am J Respir Crit Care Med 1997;155:1055–1059.
37. Parrott S, Godfrey C, Raw M, et al. Guidance for commissioners on the cost-effectiveness of smoking cessation interventions. Health International Authority. Thorax 1998;53(Suppl 5):S1–S38.
38. The Tobacco Use and Dependence Clinical Practice Guideline Panel, Staff, and Consortium Representatives. A clinical practice guideline for treating tobacco use and dependence. JAMA 2000;283:244–254. Available at: *http://www.cdc.gov/tobacco/sgr/sgr_2004/pdf/executivesummary.pdf.*
39. Jorenby DE, Leischow SJ, Nides MA, et al. A controlled trial of sustained-release bupropion, a nicotine patch or both for smoking cessation. N Engl J Med 1999;340:685–691.
40. Tonstad S, Tonnesen P, Hajek P, et al. Effect of maintenance therapy with varenicline on smoking cessation: A randomized controlled trial. JAMA 2006;296(1):64–71.
41. American Thoracic Society. Pulmonary rehabilitation-1999: Official statement of the American Thoracic Society. Am J Respir Crit Care Med 1999;159:1666–1682.
42. Ringbaek TJ, Broendum L, Hemmingsen K, et al. Rehabilitation of patients with chronic obstructive pulmonary disease: Exercise twice a week is not sufficient! Respir Med 2000;94:150–154.
43. Nichol KL, Margolis KL, Wourenma J, Von Sternberg T. The efficacy and cost effectiveness of vaccination against influenza among elderly persons living in the community. N Engl J Med 1994;331:778–784.
44. Centers for Disease Control and Prevention. Prevention and control of influenza: Recommendations of the Advisor Committee on Immunization Practices (ACIP). Morbidity Mortality Weekly Report 2006;55:1–42.
45. Jackson LA, Neuzil KM, Yu O, et al. Effectiveness of pneumococcal polysaccharide vaccine in older adults. N Engl J Med 2003;348(18):1747–1755.
46. Alfageme I, Vazquez R, Reyes N, et al. Clinical efficacy of anti-pneumococcal vaccination in patients with COPD. Thorax 2006;61:189–195.
47. Nocturnal Oxygen Therapy Trial Group. Continuous or nocturnal oxygen therapy in hypoxemic chronic obstructive lung disease. Ann Intern Med 1980;93:391–398.
48. Medical Research Council Working Party. Long-term domiciliary oxygen therapy in chronic hypoxic cor pulmonale complicating chronic bronchitis and emphysema. Lancet 1981;1:681–685.
49. O'Donohue WJ. Home oxygen therapy. Med Clin North Am 1996;80:611–622.
50. Ferreira IM, Brooks D, Lacasse Y, et al. Nutritional support for individuals with COPD. A meta-analysis. Chest 2000;117:672–678.
51. Dolovich MB, Ahrens RC, Hess DR, et al. Device selection and outcomes of aerosol therapy: Evidence-based guidelines. Chest 2005;127:335–271.
52. Truitt T, Witko J, Halpern M. Levalbuterol compared to racemic albuterol: Efficacy and outcomes in patients hospitalized with COPD or asthma. Chest 2003;123:128–135.
53. Asmus MJ, Hendeles L. Levalbuterol nebulizer solution: Is it worth five times the cost of albuterol? Pharmacotherapy 2000;20:123–129.
54. Datta D, Vitale A, Lahiri B, ZuWallack R. An evaluation of nebulized levalbuterol in stable COPD. Chest 2003;124:844–849.
55. O'Donnel DE, Lam M, Webb KA. Measurement of symptoms, lung hyperinflation, and endurance during exercise in chronic obstructive pulmonary disease. Am J Respir Crit Care Med 1998;158:1557–1565.
56. Friedman M. A multicenter study of nebulized bronchodilator solutions in chronic obstructive pulmonary disease. Am J Med 1996;100(Suppl 1A):30S–39S.
57. Wiggins J. The role of anticholinergics in "stable" chronic obstructive pulmonary disease: Unanswered questions. Respiration 1994;61:303–304.
58. Ikeda A, Nishimura K, Koyama H, et al. Dose-response study of ipratropium bromide aerosol on maximum exercise performance in stable patients with chronic obstructive pulmonary disease. Thorax 1996;51:48–53.
59. Tsukino M, Nishimura K, Ikeda A, et al. Effects of theophylline and ipratropium bromide on exercise performance in patients with stable chronic obstructive pulmonary disease. Thorax 1998;53:269–273.
60. Martin RJ, Bartelson BL, Smith P, et al. Effect of ipratropium bromide treatment on oxygen saturation and sleep quality in COPD. Chest 1999;115:1338–1345.

61. Mahler DA, Donohue JF, Barbee RA, et al. Efficacy of salmeterol xinafoate in the treatment of COPD. Chest 1999;115:957–965.
62. Rennard SI, Anderson W, ZuWallack R, et al. Use of a long-acting β_2-agonist, salmeterol xinafoate, in patients with chronic obstructive pulmonary disease. Am J Respir Crit Care Med 2001;163:1087–1092.
63. van Noord JA, Smeets JJ, Raaijmakers JAM, et al. Salmeterol versus formoterol in patients with moderately severe asthma: Onset and duration of action. Eur Respir J 1996;9:1684–1688.
64. Dougherty JA, Didur BL, Aboussouan LS. Long-acting inhaled beta$_2$ agonists for stable COPD. Ann Pharmacother 2003;37:1247–1255.
65. Bouros D, Kottakis J, LeGros V, Overend T, Della Cioppa G, Siafakas N. Effects of formoterol and salmeterol on resting inspiratory capacity in COPD patients with poor FEV$_1$ reversibility. Curr Med Res Opin 2004;20:581–586.
66. Rennard, SI, Anderson W, ZuWallack R, et al. Use of a long-acting inhaled beta 2 adrenergic agonist, salmeterol xinafoate, in patients with chronic obstructive pulmonary disease. Am J Respir Crit Care Med 2001;163:1087–1092.
67. Dahl R, Greefhorst LAPM, Nowak D, et al. Inhaled formoterol dry powder versus ipratropium bromide in chronic obstructive pulmonary disease. Am J Respir Crit Care Med 2001;164:778–784.
68. Baumgartner RA, Hanania NA, Calhoun WJ, Sahn SA, Sciarappa K, Hanrahan JP. Nebulized arformoterol in patients with COPD. A 12-week, multicenter, randomized, double-blind, double-dummy, placebo and active-controlled trial. Clin Ther 2007;29(2):261–278.
69. Barnes PJ. The pharmacological properties of tiotropium. Chest 2000;117:63S–66S.
70. Casaburi R, Mayler DA, Jones PW, et al. A long-term evaluation of once-daily inhaled ipratropium in chronic obstructive pulmonary disease. Eur Respir J 2002;19:217–224.
71. Anzueto A, Tashkin D, Menjoge S, Kesten S. One year analysis of longitudinal changes in spirometry in patients with COPD receiving tiotropium. Pulm Pharmacol Ther 2005;18:75–81.
72. Brusasco V, Hodder R, Miravitlles M, Korducki L, Towse L, Kesten S. Health outcomes following treatment for six months with once daily tiotropium compared with twice daily salmeterol in patients with COPD. Thorax 2003;58:399–404.
73. Vincken W, van Noord JA, Greefhorst APM, et al. Improved health outcomes in patients with COPD during one year treatment with tiotropium. Eur Respir J 2002;19:209–216.
74. Barr RG, Bourbeau J, Camargo CA Jr, Ram FSF. Tiotropium for stable chronic obstructive pulmonary disease: A meta-analysis. Thorax 2006;61(10):854–862.
75. Donohue JF, van Noord JA, Bateman ED, et al. A 6-month placebo-controlled study comparing lung function and health status changes in COPD patients treated with tiotropium or salmeterol. Chest 2002;122:47–55.
76. Decramer M, Celli B, Tashkin DP, et al. Clinical trial design considerations in assessing long-term functional impacts of tiotropium in COPD. The UPLIFT trial. COPD 2004;1:303–312.
77. Casiburi R, Kukafka D, Cooper CB, Witek TJ Jr, Kesten S. Improvement in exercise tolerance with the combination of tiotropium and pulmonary rehabilitation in patients with COPD. Chest 2005;127:809–817.
78. van Noord JA, de Munck DRAJ, Bantje TA, et al. Long-term treatment of chronic obstructive pulmonary disease with salmeterol and the additive effect of ipratropium. Eur Respir J 2000;15:880–885.
79. Combivent Inhalation Aerosol Study Group. In chronic obstructive pulmonary disease, a combination of ipratropium and albuterol is more effective than either agent alone. Chest 1994;105:1411–1419.
80. D'Urzo AD, De Salvo MC, Ramirez-Rivera A, et al. In patients with COPD, treatment with a combination of formoterol and ipratropium is more effective than a combination of salbutamol and ipratropium. Chest 2001;119:1347–1356.
81. Cazzola M, Marco FD, Santus P, et al. The pharmacodynamic effects of single inhaled doses of formoterol, tiotropium and their combination in patients with COPD. Pulm Pharmacol Ther 2004;17:35–39.
82. van Noord JA, Aumann JL, Janssens E, et al. Effects of tiotropium with and without formoterol on airflow obstruction and resting hyperinflation in patients with COPD. Chest 2006;129:509–517.
83. Barnes PJ. Theophylline in chronic obstructive pulmonary disease: New horizons. Proc Am Thorac Soc 2005;2:334–339.
84. Barnes PJ. Theophylline: New perspectives for and old drug. Am J Respir Crit Care Med 2003;167:813–818.
85. Man GC, Chapman KR, Ali SH, Darke AC. Sleep quality and nocturnal respiratory function with once-daily theophylline (Uniphyl) and inhaled salbutamol in patients with COPD. Chest 1996;110:648–653.
86. Nishimura K, Koyama H, Ikeda A, et al. The additive effect of theophylline on a high-dose combination of inhaled salbutamol and ipratropium bromide in stable COPD. Chest 1995;107:718–723.
87. Karpel JP, Kotch A, Zinny M, et al. A comparison of inhaled ipratropium, oral theophylline plus inhaled beta agonist, and the combination of all three in patients with COPD. Chest 1994;105:1089–1094.
88. ZuWallack RL, Mahler DA, Reilly D, et al. Salmeterol plus theophylline combination therapy in the treatment of COPD. Chest 2001;119:1661–1670.
89. Callahan CM, Dittus RS, Katz BP. Oral corticosteroid therapy for patients with stable chronic obstructive pulmonary disease: A meta-analysis. Ann Intern Med 1991;114:216–223.
90. Pizzichini E, Pizzichini MM, Gibson P, et al. Sputum eosinophilia predicts benefit from prednisone in smokers with chronic obstructive bronchitis. Am J Respir Crit Care Med 1998;158:1511–1517.
91. Senderovitz T, Vestbo J, Frandsen J, et al. Steroid reversibility test followed by inhaled budesonide or placebo in outpatients with stable chronic obstructive pulmonary disease. The Danish Society of Respiratory Medicine. Respir Med 1999;93:715–718.
92. Pauwels RA, Claes-Goran L, Latinen LA, et al. Long-term treatment with inhaled budesonide in persons with mild chronic obstructive pulmonary disease who continue smoking. N Engl J Med 1999;340:1948–1953.
93. Vestbo J, Sorenson T, Lange P, et al. Long-term effect of inhaled budesonide in mild and moderate chronic obstructive pulmonary disease: A randomized, controlled trial. Lancet 1999;353:1819–1823.
94. Burge PS, Calverley PM, Jones PW, et al. Randomised, double-blind, placebo-controlled study of fluticasone propionate in patients with moderate to severe chronic obstructive pulmonary disease: The ISOLDE trial. BMJ 2000;320:1297–1303.
95. Nishimura K, Koyama H, Ikeda A, et al. The effect of high-dose inhaled beclomethasone dipropionate in patients with stable COPD. Chest 1999;115:31–37.
96. Weir DC, Bale GA, Bright P, Sherwood Burge P. A double-blind placebo-controlled study of the effect of inhaled beclomethasone dipropionate for 2 years in patients with nonasthmatic chronic obstructive pulmonary disease. Clin Exp Allergy 1999;29(Suppl 2):125–128.
97. Paggiaro PL, Dahle R, Bakran I, et al. Multicentre, randomized, placebo-controlled trial of inhaled fluticasone propionate in patients with chronic obstructive pulmonary disease. International COPD Study Group. Lancet 1998;351:773–780.
98. The Lung Health Study Research Group. Effect of inhaled triamcinolone on the decline in pulmonary function in chronic obstructive pulmonary disease. N Engl J Med 2000;343:1902–1909.
99. Sutherland ER, Allmers H, Ayas NT, Venn AJ, Martin RJ. Inhaled corticosteroids reduce the progression of airflow limitation in chronic obstructive pulmonary disease: A meta-analysis. Thorax 2003;58:937–941.
100. Gartlehner G, Hansen RA, Carson SS, Lohr KN. Efficacy and safety of inhaled corticosteroids in patients with COPD. a systematic review and meta-analysis of health outcomes. Ann Fam Med 2006;4:253–262.
101. Macie C, Wooldrage K, Manfreda J, Anthonisen NR. Inhaled corticosteroids and mortality in COPD. Chest 2006;130:640–646.
102. Sin DD, Wu L, Anderson JA, et al. Inhaled corticosteroids and mortality in chronic obstructive pulmonary disease. Thorax 2005;60:992–997.
103. Mapel DW, Hurley JS, Roblin D, et al. Survival of COPD patients using inhaled corticosteroids and long-acting beta agonists. Respir Med 2006;100:595–609.
104. Samet JM. Inhaled corticosteroids and chronic obstructive pulmonary disease: New and improved evidence? Am J Respir Crit Care Med 2005;172:407–408.
105. Lipworth BJ. Systemic adverse effects of inhaled corticosteroid therapy: A systematic review and meta-analysis. Arch Intern Med 1999;159:941–955.
106. van Grunsven PM, van Schayck CP, Derenne JP, et al. Long-term effects of inhaled corticosteroids in chronic obstructive pulmonary disease: A meta-analysis. Thorax 1999;54:7–14.

107. Hubbard R, Tatterfield A, Smith C, et al. Use of inhaled corticosteroids and the risk of fracture. Chest 2006;130:1082–1088.
108. Jones A, Fay JK, Burr M, et al. Inhaled corticosteroid effects on bone metabolism in asthma and mild chronic obstructive pulmonary disease. Cochrane Database Syst Rev 2002;CD003537.
109. Decramer M, Ferguson G. Clinical Safety of long acting beta2 agonists and inhaled corticosteroid combination therapy in COPD. COPD 2006;3:163–171.
110. Calverly P, Pauwels R, Vestbo, J, et al. Combined salmeterol and fluticasone in the treatment of chronic obstructive pulmonary disease: A randomized, controlled trial. Lancet 2003;361:449–456.
111. Szafranski W, Cukier A, Ramirez A, et al. Efficacy and safety of budesonide/formoterol in the management of chronic obstructive pulmonary disease. Eur Respir J 2003;21:74–81.
112. Mahler DA, Wire P, Horstman D, et al. Effectiveness of fluticasone propionate and salmeterol combination delivered via the Diskus device in the treatment of chronic obstructive pulmonary disease. Am J Respir Crit Care Med 2002;166:1084–1091.
113. Hanania NA, Darken P, Horstman D, et al. Efficacy and safety of fluticasone propionate (250 mcg) and salmeterol (50 mcg) combined in the Diskus inhaler for the treatment of COPD. Chest 2003;124:834–843.
114. Calverley PM, Boonsawat W, Cseke Z, Zhong N, Peterson S, Olsson H. Maintenance therapy with budesonide and formoterol in chronic obstructive pulmonary disease. Eur Respir J 2003;22:912–919.
115. Kardos P, Wencker M, Glaab T, Vogelmeier C. Impact of salmeterol/fluticasone propionate versus salmeterol on exacerbations in severe chronic obstructive pulmonary disease. Am J Respir Crit Care Med 2007;175:144–149.
116. Calverley PMA, Anderson JA, Celli B, et al. Salmeterol and fluticasone propionate and survival in chronic obstructive pulmonary disease. N Engl J Med 2007;356:775–789.
117. Baloria VA, Vialrino PC. Bronchodilator efficacy of combined salmeterol and tiotropium in patients with chronic obstructive pulmonary disease. Arch Bronchoneumol 2005;41:130–134.
118. Aaron SD, Vandemheen KL, Fergusson D, et al. Tiotropium in combination with placebo, salmeterol or fluticasone-salmeterol for treatment of chronic obstructive pulmonary disease. Ann Intern Med 2007;146:545–555.
119. Perng DW, Wu CC, Su KC, Lee YC, Perng RP, Tao CW. Additive benefits of tiotropium in COPD patients treated with long-acting beta2 agonists and corticosteroids. Respirology 2006;11:598–602.
120. Juvelekian GS, Stoller JK. Augmentation therapy for alpha 1 antitrypsin deficiency. Drugs 2004;64(16):1743–1756.
121. Alpha-1-Antitrypsin Deficiency Registry Study Group. Survival and FEV_1 decline in individuals with severe deficiency of alpha-1-antitrypsin. Am J Respir Crit Care Med 1998;158:49–59.
122. Dirksen A, Dijkman JH, Madsen F, et al. A randomized clinical trial of alpha-1-antitrypsin augmentation therapy. Am J Respir Crit Care Med 1999;160:1468–1472.
123. Gildea TR, Shermock KM, Singer ME, et al. Cost-effectiveness analysis of augmentation therapy for severe alpha 1 antitrypsin deficiency. Am J Respir Crit Care Med 2003;167(10):1387–1392.
124. Stoller JK, Fallat R, Schluchter MD, et al. Augmentation therapy with alpha 1 antitrypsin: Patterns of use and adverse events. Chest 2003;123(5):1425–1434.
125. Lightowler JV, Wedzicha JA, Elliott MW, et al. Noninvasive positive pressure ventilation to treat respiratory failure resulting from exacerbations of chronic obstructive pulmonary disease: Cochrane systemic review and meta-analysis. BMJ 2003;326:185–189.
126. Niewoehner DE, Erbland ML, Deupree RH, et al. Effect of systemic glucocorticoids on exacerbations of chronic obstructive pulmonary disease. Department of Veterans Affairs Cooperative Study Group. N Engl J Med 1999;340:1941–1947.
127. Davies L, Angus RM, Calverley PMA. Oral corticosteroids in patients admitted to hospital with exacerbations of chronic obstructive pulmonary disease: A prospective, randomised, controlled trial. Lancet 1999;354:456–460.
128. Thompson WH, Nielson CP, Carvalho P, et al. Controlled trial of oral prednisone in outpatients with acute COPD exacerbation. Am J Respir Crit Care Med 1996;154:407–412.
129. Sayiner A, Aytemur ZA, Cirit M, et al. Systemic glucocorticoids in severe exacerbations of COPD. Chest 2001;119:726–730.
130. Aaron SD, Vandemheen KL, Hebert P, et al. Outpatient oral prednisone after emergency treatment of chronic obstructive pulmonary disease. N Engl J Med 2003;348:2618–2625.
131. Vondracek SF, Hemstreet BA. Is there an optimal corticosteroid regimen for the management of an acute exacerbation of chronic obstructive pulmonary disease? Pharmacotherapy 2006;26(4):522–532.
132. Saint S, Bent S, Vittinghoff E, Grady D. Antibiotics in chronic obstructive pulmonary disease exacerbations: A meta-analysis. JAMA 1995;273:957–960.
133. Niederman MS. Antibiotic therapy for exacerbations of chronic bronchitis. Semin Respir Infect 2000;15:59–70.
134. Chodosh S, DeAbate C, Haverstock D, et al. Short-course moxifloxacin therapy for treatment of acute bacterial exacerbations of chronic bronchitis. Respir Med 2000;94:18–27.
135. Poole PJ, Black PN. Mucolytic agents for chronic bronchitis or chronic obstructive pulmonary disease. Cochrane Database Syst Rev 1998, Issue 4. Art No. CD001287. Available at *www.cochrane.org/reviews/en/aboo1287.html.*
136. Jenning AL, Davies AN, Higgins JP, Gibbs JS, Broadley KE. A systematic review of the use of opioids in the management of dyspnea. Thorax 2002;57(11):939–944.
137. National Emphysema Treatment Trial Research Group. N Engl J Med 2003;348:2059–2073.
138. Rennard SI, Fogarty C, Kelsen S, et al. The safety and efficacy of infliximab in moderate to severe chronic obstructive pulmonary disease. Am J Respir Crit Care Med 2007;175:926–934.
139. Miravitlles M, Murio C, Guerrero T, Gisbert R. Pharmacoeconomic evaluation of acute exacerbations of chronic bronchitis and COPD. Chest 2002;121:1449–1455.
140. Grossman RF, Mukerjee J, Vaughan D, et al. A one-year community-based health economic study of ciprofloxacin versus usual antibiotic treatment in acute exacerbations of chronic bronchitis. Chest 1998;113:131–141.
141. Friedman M, Serby CW, Menjoge SS, et al. Pharmacoeconomic evaluation of a combination of ipratropium plus albuterol compared with ipratropium alone and albuterol alone in COPD. Chest 1999;115:635–641.
142. Hansen-Flashen J. Chronic obstructive pulmonary disease: The last year of life. Respir Care 2004;49:90–97.

CHAPTER 30

Pulmonary Hypertension

ROBERT L. TALBERT, REBECCA BOUDREAUX, AND REBECCA L. OWENS

KEY CONCEPTS

1. Pulmonary arterial hypertension (PAH) may be defined as a mean pulmonary artery pressure (PAPm) ≥25 mm Hg at rest with a pulmonary wedge pressure (also known as pulmonary artery occlusion pressure) ≤15 mm Hg measured by cardiac catheterization.
2. Idiopathic PAH (IPAH) is one of the most common forms of PAH. Fortunately, it is generally more responsive to therapy than secondary forms of PAH.
3. PAH is uncommon but increasing in prevalence.
4. The underlying cause of PAH is a complicated amalgam of endothelial cell dysfunction, a procoagulant state, platelet activation, constricting factors, loss of relaxing factors, cellular proliferation, hypertrophy, fibrosis and inflammation
5. PAH presents with exertional dyspnea, fatigue, weakness, complaints of general exertion intolerance, dyspnea at rest as the disease progresses, anginal chest pain, syncope.
6. Right-heart catheterization provides important prognostic information and can be used to assess pulmonary vasoreactivity prior to initiating therapy.
7. The goals of treatment are alleviation of symptoms, improvement in the quality of life, prevention of disease progression, and improvement in survival.
8. The general principle of PAH treatment is to attempt to correct the imbalance between vasoconstriction and vasodilation and prevent adverse thrombotic events to improve oxygenation and quality of life.
9. Nonpharmacologic therapy is frequently used to address comorbid conditions that often accompany PAH.
10. General care interventions in PAH include oral anticoagulants, diuretics, oxygen, and digoxin.
11. A small number of patients with IPAH who demonstrate a favorable response to acute vasodilator testing will do well with calcium channel blockers.
12. Sildenafil is a potent and highly specific phosphodiesterase-5 inhibitor that has been shown to reduce PAPm and improve functional class.
13. Prostacyclin analogs such as epoprostenol, treprostinil and iloprost induce potent vasodilation of all vascular beds.
14. Endothelin antagonists, bosentan and ambrisentan, improve exercise capacity, hemodynamics, and functional class in PAH.
15. Combination therapy in PAH may address more than one mechanism causing this disease. Combination therapy in uncontrolled trials has provided additional benefit (but at the risk of increased side effects).

WWW

The complete chapter, learning objectives, and other resources can be found at **www.pharmacotherapyonline.com.**

(1) Pulmonary arterial hypertension (PAH) may be defined as a mean pulmonary artery pressure (PAPm) ≥25 mm Hg at rest with a pulmonary wedge pressure (also known as pulmonary artery occlusion pressure) ≤15 mm Hg measured by cardiac catheterization.[1] PAH is a disorder that may occur either in the setting of a variety of underlying medical conditions or as a disease that uniquely affects the pulmonary circulation. Historically, medical treatment of PAH has been difficult. Idiopathic PAH (IPAH) was formerly known as primary pulmonary hypertension and carried a poor prognosis (medial survival 2.8 years) through the mid-1980s.[2] Prior to the availability of disease-specific or targeted drug therapy for IPAH, survival rates for 1, 3, and 5 years were 68%, 48%, and 34%, respectively.[3] Others have found similar survival rates in registry studies.[4,5] Since then a number of new therapeutic options have been developed which address this difficult to treat disease. (2) PAH may be classified into several types depending on etiology and diseases. Several sets of guidelines exist to aid clinicians in diagnosis and management of PAH.[1,2,6–9]

EPIDEMIOLOGY

(3) The prevalence of PAH is estimated to be 50,000 to 100,000 individuals in the United States.[6] Unfortunately, only 15,000 to 20,000 of the afflicted patients have an established diagnosis of PAH and are currently receiving treatment. In a French registry study of more than 600 patients with PAH, Humbert et al. found that the most common cause of PAH was IPAH (approximately 40%) followed by PAH associated with connective tissue diseases (15.3%), congenital heart disease (11.3%), portal hypertension (10.4%), and familial PAH (FPAH) (3.9%).[5] Based on autopsy findings, PAH was found to occur in 0.13% of all patients autopsied and was more commonly found if patients had cirrhosis (0.73%).[7] (Through extrapolation of these autopsy findings to the entire U.S. population, there may be well over 1 million individuals with PAH in this country.)

CHAPTER 31 Drug-Induced Pulmonary Diseases

HENGAMEH H. RAISSY, MICHELLE HARKINS, AND PATRICIA L. MARSHIK

KEY CONCEPTS

1. Select populations may be more susceptible to toxicities associated with specific agents.
2. Primary treatment is discontinuation of the offending agent and supportive care.

The manifestations of drug-induced pulmonary diseases span the entire spectrum of pathophysiologic conditions of the respiratory tract. As with most drug-induced diseases, the pathologic changes are nonspecific. Therefore, the diagnosis is often difficult and, in most cases, is based on exclusion of all other possible causes. In addition, the true incidence of drug-induced pulmonary disease is difficult to assess as a result of the pathologic nonspecificity and the interaction between the underlying disease state and the drugs.

Considering the physiologic and metabolic capacity of the lung, it is surprising that drug-induced pulmonary disease is not more common. The lung is the only organ of the body that receives the entire circulation. In addition, the lung contains a heterogeneous population of cells capable of various metabolic functions, including *N*-alkylation, *N*-dealkylation, *N*-oxidation, reduction of *N*-oxides, and *C*-hydroxylation.

Evaluation of epidemiologic studies on adverse drug reactions provides a perspective on the importance of drug-induced pulmonary disease. In a 2-year prospective survey of a community-based general practice, 41% of 817 patients experienced adverse drug reactions.[1] Four patients, or 0.5% of the total respondents, experienced adverse respiratory symptoms. Respiratory symptoms occurred in 1.2% of patients experiencing adverse drug reactions. In a recent retrospective analysis of clinical case series in France, 898 patients had reported drug allergy, with a bronchospasm incidence of 6.9%. When these patients were rechallenged with the suspected drug, only 241 (17.6%) tested positive. The incidence of bronchospasm in patients with positive provocation test was 7.9%.[2]

Adverse pulmonary reactions are uncommon in the general population but are among the most serious reactions, often requiring intervention. In a study of 270 adverse reactions leading to hospitalization from two populations, 3.0% were respiratory in nature.[3] Of the reactions considered to be life-threatening, 12.3% were respiratory. An early report on death caused by drug reactions from the Boston Collaborative Drug Surveillance Program indicated that 7 of 27 drug-induced deaths were respiratory in nature.[4] This was confirmed in a followup study in which 6 of 24 drug-induced deaths were respiratory in nature.[5]

Learning objectives, review questions, and other resources can be found at **www.pharmacotherapyonline.com.**

DRUG-INDUCED APNEA

Apnea may be induced by central nervous system depression or respiratory neuromuscular blockade (Table 31–1). Patients with chronic obstructive airway disease, alveolar hypoventilation, and chronic carbon dioxide retention have an exaggerated respiratory depressant response to narcotic analgesics and sedatives. In addition, the injudicious administration of oxygen in patients with carbon dioxide retention can worsen ventilation-perfusion mismatching, producing apnea.[6] Although the benzodiazepines are touted as causing less respiratory depression than barbiturates, they may produce a profound additive or synergistic effect when taken in combination with other respiratory depressants. Combining intravenous diazepam with phenobarbital to stop seizures in an emergency department frequently results in admissions to an intensive care unit for a short period of assisted mechanical ventilation, regardless of the drug administration rate. Too rapid intravenous administration of any of the benzodiazepines, even without coadministration of other respiratory depressants, will result in apnea. The risk appears to be the same for the various available agents (diazepam, lorazepam, and midazolam). Respiratory depression and arrests resulting in death and hypoxic encephalopathy have occurred following rapid intravenous administration of midazolam for conscious sedation prior to medical procedures. (1) This has been reported more commonly in the elderly and the chronically debilitated or in combination with opioid analgesics. Concurrent use of inhibitors of cytochrome P450 3A4 with benzodiazepines are likely to lead to greater risk of respiratory depression.

(1) Prolonged apnea may follow administration of any of the neuromuscular blocking agents used for surgery, particularly in patients with hepatic or renal dysfunction. In addition, persistent neuromuscular blockade and muscle weakness have been reported in critically ill patients who are receiving neuromuscular blockers continuously for more than 2 days to facilitate mechanical ventilation.[7] This has resulted in delayed weaning from mechanical ventilation and prolonged intensive care unit stays. The prolonged neuromuscular blockade has been confined principally to pancuronium and vecuronium in patients with renal disease. Both agents have pharmacologic active metabolites that are excreted renally. The persistent muscular weakness is less-well defined but appears to represent an acute myopathy.[7] High-dose corticosteroids appear to produce a synergistic effect, supported by animal studies showing that corticosteroids at dosages ≥2 mg/kg per day of prednisone produce atrophy in denervated muscle.[8] The fluorinated corticosteroids (e.g., triamcinolone) appear to be more myopathic.[9] Dose-dependent respiratory muscle weakness has been reported in chronic obstructive pulmonary disease (COPD) and asthma patients receiving repeated short courses of oral prednisone in the previous 6 months.[10]

TABLE 31-1 Drugs That Induce Apnea

	Relative Frequency of Reactions
Central nervous system depression	
Narcotic analgesics	F
Barbiturates	F
Benzodiazepines	F
Other sedatives and hypnotics	I
Tricyclic antidepressants	R
Phenothiazines	R
Ketamine	R
Promazine	R
Anesthetics	R
Antihistamines	R
Alcohol	I
Fenfluramine	R
l-Dopa	R
Oxygen	R
Respiratory muscle dysfunction	
Aminoglycoside antibiotics	I
Polymyxin antibiotics	I
Neuromuscular blockers	I
Quinine	R
Digitalis	R
Myopathy	
Corticosteroids	F
Diuretics	I
Aminocaproic acid	R
Clofibrate	R

F, Freguent; I, infrequent; R, rare.

Respiratory failure has been known to occur following local spinal anesthesia. Apnea from respiratory paralysis and rapid respiratory muscle fatigue has followed the administration of polymyxin and aminoglycoside antibiotics.[6] The mechanism appears to be related to the complexation of calcium and its depletion at the myoneural junction. Intravenous calcium chloride has been variably effective in reversing the paralysis.[6] The aminoglycosides competitively block neuromuscular junctions. This has resulted in life-threatening apnea when neomycin, gentamicin, streptomycin, or bacitracin has been ❶ administered into the peritoneal and pleural cavities.[6] The aminoglycosides will produce an additive blockade and ventilatory paralysis with curare or succinylcholine and in patients with myasthenia gravis or myasthenic syndromes.[6] Intravenous administration of aminoglycosides has resulted in respiratory failure in babies with infantile ❷ botulism. Treatment consists of ventilatory support and administration of an anticholinesterase agent (neostigmine or edrophonium).[6]

DRUG-INDUCED BRONCHOSPASM

Bronchoconstriction is the most common drug-induced respiratory problem. Bronchospasm can be induced by a wide variety of drugs through a number of disparate pathophysiologic mechanisms ❶ (Table 31–2). Regardless of the pathophysiologic mechanism, drug-induced bronchospasm is almost exclusively a problem of patients with preexisting bronchial hyperreactivity (e.g., asthma, chronic obstructive lung disease).[11] By definition, all patients with nonspecific bronchial hyperreactivity will experience bronchospasm if given sufficiently high doses of cholinergic or anticholinesterase agents. Severe asthmatics with a high degree of bronchial reactivity may wheeze following the inhalation of a number of particulate substances, such as the lactose in dry-powder inhalers and inhaled corticosteroids, presumably through direct stimulation of the central airway irritant receptors. Other pharmacologic mechanisms for inducing bronchospasm include β_2-receptor blockade and nonimmunologic histamine release from mast cells and basophils.[11] A large number of agents are capable of producing bronchospasm through immunoglobulin (Ig) E-mediated reactions.[11] These drugs can become a significant occupational hazard for pharmacists, nurses, and pharmaceutical industry workers.[11]

TABLE 31-2 Drugs That Induce Bronchospasm

	Relative Frequency of Reactions
Anaphylaxis (IgE-mediated)	
Penicillins	F
Sulfonamides	F
Serum	F
Cephalosporins	F
Bromelin	R
Cimetidine	R
Papain	F
Pancreatic extract	I
Psyllium	I
Subtilase	I
Tetracyclines	I
Allergen extracts	I
Ll-Asparaginase	F
Pyrazolone analgesics	I
Direct airway irritation	
Acetate	R
Bisulfite	F
Cromolyn	R
Smoke	F
N-acetylcysteine	F
Inhaled steroids	I
Precipitating IgG antibodies	
β-Methyldopa	R
Carbamazepine	R
Spiramycin	R
Cyclooxygenase inhibition	
Aspirin/nonsteroidal antiinflammatory drugs	F
Phenylbutazone	I
Acetaminophen	R
Anaphylactoid mast-cell degranulation	
Narcotic analgesics	I
Ethylenediamine	R
Iodinated-radiocontrast media	F
Platinum	R
Local anesthetics	I
Steroidal anesthetics	I
Iron–dextran complex	I
Pancuronium bromide	R
Benzalkonium chloride	I
Pharmacologic effects	
α-Adrenergic receptor blockers	I–F
Cholinergic stimulants	I
Anticholinesterases	R
β-Adrenergic agonists	R
Ethylenediamine tetraacetic acid	R
Unknown mechanisms	
Angiotensin-converting enzyme inhibitors	I
Anticholinergics	R
Hydrocortisone	R
Isoproterenol	R
Monosodium glutamate	I
Piperazine	R
Tartrazine	R
Sulfinpyrazone	R
Zinostatin	R
Losartan	R

F, frequent; I, infrequent; R, rare.

Epidemiologic studies demonstrate an increase in the prevalence of asthma and COPD with increased use of acetaminophen. The use of aspirin or ibuprofen is not associated with asthma or COPD. The acetaminophen–asthma/COPD association may be explained by reduction of glutathione, an endogenous antioxidant enzyme in the airway epithelial lining fluid, with high doses of acetaminophen resulting in oxidant damage in the lung.[12]

ASPIRIN-INDUCED BRONCHOSPASM

Aspirin sensitivity or intolerance occurs in 4% to 20% of all asthmatics.[13] The frequency of aspirin-induced bronchospasm increases with age. Patients older than age 40 years have a frequency approximately four times that of patients younger than 20 years.[13] The frequency increases to 14% to 23% in patients with nasal polyps.[13] Women predominate over men, and there is no evidence for a genetic or familial predisposition.[14]

The classic description of the aspirin-intolerant asthmatic includes the triad of severe asthma, nasal polyps, and aspirin intolerance. The typical patient experiences intense vasomotor rhinitis, which may or may not be associated with aspirin exposure, beginning during the third or fourth decade of life.[15] Over a period of months, nasal polyps begin to appear, followed by severe asthma exacerbated by aspirin. Bronchospasm typically begins within minutes to hours following ingestion of aspirin and is associated with rhinorrhea, flushing of the head and neck, and conjunctivitis.[15] The reactions are severe and often life-threatening.

All aspirin-sensitive asthmatics do not fit the classic "aspirin triad" picture, and not all patients with asthma and nasal polyps develop sensitivity to aspirin.[14] In most cases, aspirin-sensitive asthmatics are clinically indistinguishable from the general population of asthmatics except for their intolerance to aspirin and other nonsteroidal antiinflammatory drugs (NSAIDs). Aspirin-induced asthmatics are not at higher risk of having fatal asthma if aspirin and other NSAIDs are avoided.[16]

Diagnosis of aspirin-induced asthma requires a detailed medical history. The definitive diagnosis is made by aspirin provocation tests, which may be done via different routes.[14,17] An oral provocation test is used commonly where threshold doses of aspirin induce a positive reaction measured by a drop in forced expiratory volume in the first second of expiration (FEV_1) and/or the presence of symptoms.[17,18] A nasal provocation test is done by the application of one dose of lysine-aspirin, and aspirin sensitivity is manifested with clinical symptoms of watery discharge and a significant fall in inspiratory nasal flow.[17,18] When lysine-aspirin bronchoprovocation was compared with oral aspirin provocation, both methods were equally sensitive.[19]

PATHOGENESIS

Aspirin-induced asthma is correctly classified as an idiosyncratic reaction in that the pathogenesis is still unknown. Patients with aspirin intolerance have increased plasma histamine concentrations after ingestion of aspirin and elevated peripheral eosinophil counts.[14,15] All attempts to define an immunologic mechanism have been unsuccessful. Chemically similar drugs such as salicylamide and choline salicylate do not cross-react, whereas a large number of chemically dissimilar NSAIDs do produce reactions.[14,15] Table 31–3 lists the analgesics that do and do not cross-react with aspirin.

The currently accepted hypothesis of aspirin-induced asthma is that aspirin intolerance is integrally related to inhibition of cyclooxygenase. This is supported by the following evidence: (a) All NSAIDs that inhibit cyclooxygenase produce reactions, (b) the degree of cross-reactivity is proportional to the potency of cyclooxygenase inhibition, and (c) each patient with aspirin sensitivity has a threshold dose for precipitating bronchospasm that is specific for the degree of cyclooxygenase inhibition produced, and once established, the dose of another cyclooxygenase inhibitor needed to induce bronchospasm can be estimated.[15]

TABLE 31-3 Tolerance of Antiinflammatory and Analgesic Drugs in Aspirin-Induced Asthma

Cross-Reactive Drugs	Drugs with No Cross-Reactivity
Diclofenac	Acetaminophen[a]
Diflunisal	Benzydamine
Fenoprofen	Chloroquine
Flufenamic acid	Choline salicylate
Flurbiprofen	Corticosteroids
Hydrocortisone hemisuccinate	Dextropropoxyphene
Ibuprofen	Phenacetin[a]
Indomethacin	Salicylamide
Ketoprofen	Sodium salicylate
Mefenamic acid	
Naproxen	
Noramidopyrine	
Oxyphenbutazone	
Phenylbutazone	
Piroxicam	
Sulindac	
Sulfinpyrazone	
Tartrazine	
Tolmetin	

[a]A very small percentage (5%) of aspirin-sensitive patients react to acetaminophen and phenacetin.

The mechanism by which cyclooxygenase inhibition produces bronchospasm in susceptible individuals is unknown. Arachidonic acid metabolism through the 5-lipoxygenase pathway may lead to the excess production of leukotrienes C_4 and D_4.[16] Leukotrienes C_4, D_4, and E_4 produce bronchospasm and promote histamine release from mast cells.[15] The precise mechanism by which augmented leukotriene production occurs is unknown, and available hypotheses do not explain why only a small number of asthmatic patients react to aspirin and NSAIDs.

DESENSITIZATION

Patients with aspirin sensitivity can be desensitized. The ease of desensitization correlates with the sensitivity of the patient.[15] Highly sensitive patients who react initially to less than 100 mg aspirin require multiple rechallenges to produce desensitization.[14] Desensitization usually persists for 2 to 5 days following discontinuance, with full sensitivity reestablished within 7 days.[14] Cross-desensitization has been established between aspirin and all NSAIDs tested to date. Because patients may experience life-threatening reactions, desensitization should be attempted only in a controlled environment by personnel with expertise in handling these patients. In addition, there are reports of patients who have failed to maintain a desensitized state despite continued aspirin administration.[14] In one open followup trial in 172 aspirin-sensitive asthmatics who had undergone desensitization and continued daily aspirin treatment (1,300 mg/day) an improvement in nasal-sinus and asthma symptoms occurred after 6 months of treatment, which persisted up to 5 years.[20]

CROSS-SENSITIVITY WITH FOOD AND DRUG ADDITIVES

❶ Up to 80% of aspirin-sensitive asthmatics will have an adverse reaction to the yellow azo dye tartrazine (FD&C Yellow No. 5), which is used widely for coloring foods, drinks, drugs, and cosmetics.[13] However, the studies reporting high cross-reactivity were poorly controlled and often used only subjective criteria.[13,21] In double-blind, placebo-controlled trials using pulmonary function testing, sensitivity to tartrazine has proved to be a rare event.[21] Tartrazine sensitivity appears to occur only in aspirin-intolerant patients at a prevalence of 2%.[21] Although rare, owing to the severity of reaction and widespread use of tartrazine, the U.S. Food and Drug Administration (FDA) requires labeling for the products containing this dye.[22] The likely mechanism is dose-related histamine release, and the clinical presentation is the same as the reaction to aspirin in aspirin-sensitive patients.[22]

Reactions to other azo dyes, monosodium glutamate, parabens, and nonazo dyes have been reported much less frequently than reactions to tartrazine and have been equally difficult to confirm with controlled challenges.[21] Positive reactions to sodium benzoate, a food preservative, have been reported in as many as 23% of aspirin-sensitive individuals.[13] Acetaminophen is a weak inhibitor of cyclooxygenase. As such, approximately 5% of aspirin-sensitive asthmatics will experience reactions to acetaminophen.[13] Most aspirin-sensitive asthmatics can use acetaminophen as a safe alternative to aspirin. There is a growing body of evidence that selective cyclooxygenase-2 inhibitors may be used safely in aspirin-sensitive patients,[23–26] but long-term studies with these agents should be undertaken to confirm their safe use in aspirin-sensitive patients. At this point, the package inserts of these agents state that they are contraindicated for aspirin-sensitive asthmatics.[23–26] Sporadic cases of worsening bronchospasm and anaphylaxis have been reported in aspirin-sensitive asthmatics receiving intravenous hydrocortisone succinate, but such reactions have not been reported with use of other corticosteroids.[14] It is not known whether it is the hydrocortisone or the succinate that is the problem.

TREATMENT

Aspirin-Sensitive Asthma

❷ Therapy of aspirin-sensitive asthmatics takes one of two general approaches: desensitization or avoidance. Avoidance of triggering substances seldom alters the clinical course of patients' asthma. The therapy of asthma has been nonspecific; however, in theory, 5-lipoxygenase inhibitors such as zileuton or leukotriene antagonists should provide specific therapy. A few studies have investigated use of leukotriene modifiers to prevent aspirin-induced bronchospasm in aspirin-sensitive asthmatic patients.[27–29] Pretreatment with zileuton in eight aspirin-sensitive asthmatic patients protected them from the same threshold-provoking doses of aspirin.[27] However, larger, escalating doses of aspirin above the threshold challenge doses were not examined in this study. Furthermore, when doses of aspirin were escalated above the threshold provocative doses, zileuton did not prevent formation of leukotrienes.[28] In a similar study, pretreatment with montelukast 10 mg/day did not protect patients when aspirin doses were increased above their threshold doses.[29] In another study, the mean provoking dose of aspirin did not differ in the asthmatics who were taking leukotriene modifiers and the control group (60.4 mg vs. 70.3 mg, respectively).[30] Although initial studies suggested that leukotriene modifiers blocked aspirin-induced reactions, it is now apparent that they merely shift the dose–response curve to the right, leaving the patient at risk at higher doses. Thus even patients who might benefit from leukotriene modifiers should avoid aspirin and all NSAIDs. A case of ibuprofen 400-mg–induced asthma was reported in an asthmatic patient on zafirlukast 20 mg twice daily.[31] Furthermore, most of the challenge studies are based on incremental doses of aspirin or NSAIDs, and exposure of patients to full clinical doses of aspirin or NSAIDs can overcome the antagonistic effect of leukotriene modifiers. The respiratory symptoms can be decreased but not prevented by pretreatment with antihistamines, cromolyn, and nedocromil.[14,32] The long-term asthma control of patients with aspirin sensitivity does not differ from that for other asthmatics. There is no evidence to support that aspirin-sensitive asthmatics respond better to leukotriene modifiers. In a double-blind, randomized, placebo-controlled study, aspirin-sensitive asthmatic patients on montelukast showed a 10% improvement in FEV_1 compared with the placebo group.[33] Similar results were reported when montelukast was compared with placebo in patients with intermittent or persistent asthma.[34]

β-BLOCKERS

❶ β-Adrenergic receptor blockers comprise the other large class of drugs that can be hazardous to a person with asthma. Even the more cardioselective agents such as acebutolol, atenolol, and metoprolol have been reported to cause asthma attacks.[11] Patients with asthma may take nonselective and β_1-selective blockers without incident for long periods; however, the occasional report of fatal asthma attacks resistant to therapy with β-agonists should provide ample warning of the dangers inherent in β-blocker therapy.[11]

If a patient with bronchial hyperreactivity requires β-blocker therapy, one of the selective β_1-blockers (e.g., acebutolol, atenolol, metoprolol, or pindolol) should be used at the lowest possible dose. Celiprolol and betaxolol appear to possess greater cardioselectivity than currently marketed drugs.[35,36] Fatal status asthmaticus has occurred with the topical administration of the nonselective timolol maleate ophthalmic solution for the treatment of open-angle glaucoma.[37] Early investigations with ophthalmic betaxolol suggest that it is well tolerated even in timolol-sensitive asthmatics.[38,39]

SULFITES

Severe, life-threatening asthmatic reactions following consumption of restaurant meals and wine have occurred secondary to ingestion of the food preservative potassium metabisulfite.[21] Sulfites have been used for centuries as preservatives in wine and food. As antioxidants, they prevent fermentation of wine and discoloration of fruits and vegetables caused by contaminating bacteria.[40] Previously, sulfites had been given "generally recognized as safe" status by the FDA. Sensitive patients react to concentrations ranging from 5 to 100 mg, amounts that are consumed routinely by anyone eating in restaurants. Consumption of sulfites in U.S. diets is estimated to be 2 to 3 mg/day in the home with 5 to 10 mg per 30 mL of beer or wine consumed.[21] Anaphylactic or anaphylactoid reactions to sulfites in nonasthmatics are extremely rare. In the general asthmatic population, reactions to sulfites are ❶ uncommon. Approximately 5% of steroid-dependent asthmatics demonstrate sensitivity to sulfiting agents, but the prevalence is only around 1% in non–steroid-dependent asthmatic patients.[40]

MECHANISM

Three different mechanisms have been proposed to explain the reaction to sulfites in asthmatic patients.[40] The first is explained by the inhalation of sulfur dioxide, which produces bronchoconstriction in all asthmatics through direct stimulation of afferent parasympathetic irritant receptors. Furthermore, inhalation of atropine or the ingestion of doxepin protects sulfite-sensitive patients from reacting to the ingestion of sulfites. The second theory, IgE-mediated reaction, is supported by reported cases of sulfite-sensitive anaphylaxis reaction in patients with positive sulfite skin test. Finally, a reduced concentration of sulfite oxidase enzyme (the enzyme that catalyzes oxidation of sulfites to sulfates) compared with normal individuals has been demonstrated in a group of sulfite-sensitive asthmatics.

A number of pharmacologic agents contain sulfites as preservatives and antioxidants. The FDA now requires warning labels on drugs containing sulfites. Most manufacturers of drugs for the treatment of asthma have discontinued the use of sulfites. In addition, labeling is required on packaged foods that contain sulfites at 10 parts per million or more, and sulfiting agents are no longer allowed on fresh fruits and vegetables (excluding potatoes) intended for sale.

Pretreatment with cromolyn, anticholinergics, and cyanocobalamin have protected sulfite-sensitive patients.[40,41] Presumably, pharmacologic doses of vitamin B_{12} catalyze the nonenzymatic oxidation of sulfite to sulfate.

OTHER PRESERVATIVES

Both ethylenediamine tetraacetic acid (EDTA) and benzalkonium chloride, used as stabilizing and bacteriostatic agents, respectively, can produce bronchoconstriction.[42] In addition to producing bronchoconstriction, EDTA potentiates the bronchial responsiveness to histamine.[42] These effects presumably are mediated through calcium chelation by EDTA. Benzalkonium chloride is more potent than EDTA, and its mechanism appears to be a result of mast cell degranulation and stimulation of irritant C fibers in the airways.[42]

The bronchoconstriction from benzalkonium chloride can be blocked by cromolyn but not the anticholinergic ipratropium bromide.[43] Benzalkonium chloride is found in the commercial multiple-dose nebulizer preparations of ipratropium bromide and beclomethasone dipropionate marketed in the United Kingdom and Europe and is presumed to be in part responsible for paradoxical wheezing following administration of these agents.[42–44] Benzalkonium chloride is also found in albuterol nebulizer solutions marketed in the United States and has been implicated as a possible cause of paradoxical wheezing in infants receiving this preparation.[42] The effect of these agents on FEV_1 when used in the amount administered for treatment of acute asthma was evaluated in subjects with stable asthma.[45] Patients were assigned randomly to inhale up to four 600-mcg nebulized doses of EDTA and benzalkonium chloride and normal saline. The change in FEV_1 was not different between EDTA and the placebo group; however, benzalkonium chloride was associated with a statistically significant decrease in FEV_1 compared with placebo. It is important to consider that these agents are always used in combination with bronchodilators and β_2-agonists, which are potent mast cell stabilizers, and the anecdotal reports have not yet been confirmed with controlled investigations.[42,43]

CONTRAST MEDIA

Iodinated radiocontrast materials are the most common cause of anaphylactoid reactions producing bronchospasm.[46] Chapter 91 discusses this topic.

NATURAL RUBBER LATEX ALLERGY

Allergy to natural rubber latex, first reported in 1989 in the United States, is a common cause of occupational allergy for healthcare workers.[47] Natural rubber is a processed plant product from the commercial rubber tree, *Hevea brasiliensis.*[48] Latex allergens are proteins found in both raw latex and the extracts used in finished rubber products. Latex gloves are the largest single source of exposure to the protein allergens.[48]

❶ The reported prevalence of latex allergy depends on the sample population. In the general population, latex allergy is less than 1%; however, the prevalence increases in healthcare workers to 5% to 15%.[48] Risk factors for latex allergy include frequent exposure to rubber gloves, history of atopic disease, and presence or history of hand dermatitis. Patients with spina bifida are at an increased risk of latex allergy, with an incidence of 24% to 60% as a result of early and repeated exposure to rubber devices during the surgical procedures.[48]

Clinical manifestations of latex allergy range from contact dermatitis and urticaria, rhinitis and asthma, and reported cases of anaphylaxis.[47,48] The early manifestation of rubber allergy is contact urticaria, which is an IgE-mediated reaction to rubber proteins following direct contact with the medical devices: mainly rubber gloves.[48] Contact dermatitis may occur within 1 to 2 days. Contact dermatitis is a cell-mediated delayed-type hypersensitivity reaction to the additive chemical component of rubber products.[48] Rhinitis and asthma may follow inhalation of allergens by cornstarch powder used to coat the latex gloves. Asthma caused by occupational exposure is seen mostly in atopic patients with histories of seasonal and perennial allergies and asthma.[48] Isolated cases of wheezing secondary to latex exposure in patients without a history of asthma have also been reported.[48]

The diagnosis of latex allergy is based on the presence of latex-specific IgE, as well as symptoms consistent with IgE-mediated ❷ reactions.[49] The mainstay of therapy for latex allergy is avoidance. The FDA requires appropriate labeling for all medical devices containing natural rubber latex to ensure avoidance and a latex-free environment. The role of pretreatment with antihistamines, corticosteroids, and allergen immunotherapy remains to be determined.[48,49] Two randomized, placebo-controlled clinical trials have evaluated the role of specific immunotherapy in the treatment of latex allergy.[50,51] Although both studies showed an improvement of cutaneous and rhinitis reactions, systemic reactions were observed, and bronchoconstriction did not improve. At this time, immunotherapy remains investigational for the treatment of latex allergy.

ANGIOTENSIN-CONVERTING ENZYME INHIBITOR–INDUCED COUGH

❶ Cough has become a well-recognized side effect of angiotensin-converting enzyme (ACE) inhibitor therapy. According to spontaneous reporting by patients, cough occurs in 1% to 10% of patients receiving ACE inhibitors, with a preponderance of females. In a retrospective analysis, 14.6% of women had cough compared with 6.0% of the men on ACE inhibitors. It is suggested that women have a lower cough threshold, resulting in their reporting this adverse effect more commonly than men.[52] Studies specifically evaluating cough caused by ACE inhibitors report a prevalence of 19% to 25%.[53,54] Patients receiving ACE inhibitors had a 2.3 times greater likelihood of developing cough than a similar group of patients receiving diuretics.[53] Patients with hyperreactive airways do not appear to be at greater risk.[54] African Americans and Chinese have a higher incidence of cough.[52] When different disease states were compared, 26% of patients with heart failure had ACE inhibitor-induced cough compared with 14% of those with hypertension.[52] Cough can occur with all ACE inhibitors.[55]

The cough typically is dry and nonproductive, persistent, and not paroxysmal.[55] The severity of cough varies from a "tickle" to a debilitating cough with insomnia and vomiting. The cough can begin within 3 days or have a delayed onset of up to 12 months following initiation of ACE inhibitor therapy.[55] The cough remits within 1 to 4 days of discontinuing therapy but (rarely) can last up to 4 weeks and recur with rechallenge.[55] Patients should be given a 4-day withdrawal to determine if the cough is induced by ACE inhibitors. The chest radiograph is normal, as are pulmonary function tests (spirometry and diffusing capacity). Bronchial hyperreactivity, as measured by histamine and methacholine provocation, may be worsened in patients with underlying bronchial hyperreactivity such as asthma and chronic bronchitis. However, bronchial hyperreactivity is not induced in others.[55,56] The cough reflex to capsaicin is enhanced but not to nebulized distilled water or citric acid.[55]

The mechanism of ACE inhibitor–induced cough is still unknown. ACE is a nonspecific enzyme that also catalyzes the hydrolysis of bradykinin and substance P (see Chap. 15) that produce or facilitate inflammation and stimulate lung irritant receptors.[55] ACE inhibitors also may induce cyclooxygenase to cause the production of prostaglandins. NSAIDs, benzonatate, inhaled bupivacaine, theophylline, baclofen, thromboxane A_2 synthase inhibitor,[52,57] and cromolyn sodium all have been used to suppress or inhibit ACE inhibitor-induced cough.[55,58] The cough generally is unresponsive to cough suppressants or bronchodilator therapy. No long-term trials evaluating different treatment options for ACE inhibitor-induced cough exist. Cromolyn sodium may be considered first because it is the ❷ most studied agent and has minimal toxicity.[52] The preferred therapy is withdrawal of the ACE inhibitor and replacement with an alternative antihypertensive agent. Owing to their decrease in ACE inhibitor-induced side effects, angiotensin II receptor antagonists often are recommended in place of an ACE inhibitor; however, there are rare reports of this agent inducing bronchospasm.[59] The clinical trials suggest that angiotensin II receptor antagonists have the same incidence of cough as placebo. Furthermore, when angiotensin II receptor antagonists were compared with ACE inhibitors, cough occurred much less frequently. Reduction in the incidence of cough with angiotensin II receptor antagonists is likely caused by the lack of effect on clearance of bradykinin and substance P.[60] The use of alternative therapies to treat ACE inhibitor-induced cough generally is not recommended.[55]

PULMONARY EDEMA

Pulmonary edema may result from the failure of any of a number of homeostatic mechanisms. The most common cause of pulmonary edema is an increase in capillary hydrostatic pressure because of left ventricular failure. Excessive fluid administration in compensated and decompensated heart failure patients is the most frequent cause of iatrogenic pulmonary edema. Besides hydrostatic forces, other homeostatic mechanisms that may be disrupted include the osmotic and oncotic pressures in the vasculature, the integrity of the alveolar epithelium, interstitial pulmonary pressure, and the interstitial lymph flow.[6] The edema fluid in cardiogenic pulmonary edema contains a low amount of protein, whereas noncardiogenic pulmonary edema fluid has a high protein concentration.[6] This indicates that noncardiogenic pulmonary edema results primarily from disruption of the alveolar epithelium.

The clinical presentation of pulmonary edema includes persistent cough, tachypnea, dyspnea, tachycardia, rales on auscultation, hypoxemia from ventilation–perfusion imbalance and intrapulmonary shunting, widespread fluffy infiltrates on chest roentgenogram, and decreased lung compliance (stiff lungs). Noncardiogenic pulmonary edema may progress to hemorrhage; cellular debris collects in the alveoli, followed by hyperplasia and fibrosis with a residual restrictive mechanical defect.[6]

NARCOTIC-INDUCED PULMONARY EDEMA

The most common drug-induced noncardiogenic pulmonary edema is produced by the narcotic analgesics (Table 31–4).[6] Narcotic-induced pulmonary edema is associated most commonly with intravenous heroin use but also has occurred with morphine, methadone, meperidine, and propoxyphene use.[6,61] There also have been a few reported cases associated with the use of the opiate antagonist naloxone and nalmefene, a long-acting opioid antagonist.[62,63] The mechanism is unknown but may be related to hypoxemia similar to the neurogenic pulmonary edema associated with cerebral tumors or trauma or a direct toxic effect on the alveolar capillary membrane.[61] Initially thought to occur only with overdoses, most evidence now supports the theory that narcotic-induced pulmonary edema is an idiosyncratic reaction to moderate as well as high narcotic doses.[61]

Patients with pulmonary edema may be comatose with depressed respirations or dyspnea and tachypnea. They may or may not have other signs of narcotic overdose. Symptomology varies from cough and mild crepitations on auscultation with characteristic radiologic findings to severe cyanosis and hypoxemia, even with supplemental oxygen. Symptoms may appear within minutes of intravenous administration but may take up to 2 hours to occur, particularly following oral methadone.[61] Hemodynamic studies in the first 24 hours have demonstrated normal pulmonary capillary wedge pressures in the presence of pulmonary edema.

TABLE 31-4 Drugs That Induce Pulmonary Edema

	Relative Frequency of Reactions
Cardiogenic pulmonary edema	
Excessive intravenous fluids	F
Blood and plasma transfusions	F
Corticosteroids	F
Phenylbutazone	R
Sodium diatrizoate	R
Hypertonic intrathecal saline	R
β_2-Adrenergic agonists	I
Noncardiogenic pulmonary edema	
Heroin	F
Methadone	I
Morphine	I
Oxygen	I
Propoxyphene	R
Ethchlorvynol	R
Chlordiazepoxide	R
Salicylate	R
Hydrochlorothiazide	R
Triamterene + hydrochlorothiazide	R
Leukoagglutinin reactions	R
Iron–dextran complex	R
Methotrexate	R
Cytosine arabinoside	R
Nitrofurantoin	R
Dextran 40	R
Fluorescein	R
Amitriptyline	R
Colchicine	R
Nitrogen mustard	R
Epinephrine	R
Metaraminol	R
Bleomycin	R
Iodide	R
Cyclophosphamide	R
VM-26	R

F, frequent; I, infrequent; R, rare.

Clinical symptoms generally improve within 24 to 48 hours and radiologic clearing occurs in 2 to 5 days, but abnormalities in pulmonary function tests may persist for 10 to 12 weeks. Therapy consists of naloxone administration, supplemental oxygen, and ventilatory support if required. Mortality is less than 1%.[61]

Cough has been reported with intravenous administration of fentanyl.[64] A cohort of 1,311 adult patients undergoing elective surgery had 120 patients with vigorous cough within 20 seconds after administration of fentanyl.[64] The cough was associated with young age and absence of cigarette smoking.[64] Among anesthetic factors, it was associated with the absence of epidurally administered lidocaine and the absence of a priming dose of vecuronium.[64] A history of asthma or COPD had no predictive effect.[64] Further clinical trials are required to understand the mechanism of paradoxical cough with fentanyl and to identify the means to prevent it.

OTHER DRUGS THAT CAUSE PULMONARY EDEMA

A paradoxical pulmonary edema has been reported in a few patients following hydrochlorothiazide ingestion but not any other benzthiazide diuretic.[6] Acute pulmonary edema rarely has followed the injection of high concentrations of contrast medium into the pulmonary circulation during angiocardiography.[6] Rare occurrences of pulmonary edema have followed the intravenous administration of bleomycin, cyclophosphamide, and vinblastine.[6]

The selective β_2-adrenergic agonists terbutaline and ritodrine have been reported to induce pulmonary edema when used as tocolytics.[6] This disorder commonly occurs 48 to 72 hours after tocolytic therapy.[63] This has never occurred with their use in asthma patients, even in inadvertent overdosage. This reaction may result from excess fluid administration used to prevent the hypotension from β_2-mediated vasodilation or the particular hemodynamics of pregnancy. In a review of 330 patients who received tocolytic therapy and were monitored closely for their fluid status, no episode of pulmonary edema was reported.[63]

Interleukin-2, a cytokine used alone or in combination with cytotoxic drugs, has been reported to induce pulmonary edema. Although other cytokines have been associated with pulmonary edema, the problem is most significant with interleukin-2. A weight gain of 2 kg has been reported after treatment with interleukin-2.[63]

Pulmonary edema has occurred occasionally with salicylate overdoses. The serum salicylate concentrations are often greater than 45 mg/dL, and the patients have other signs of toxicity, although some cases have been associated with concentrations in the usual therapeutic range.[61]

PULMONARY EOSINOPHILIA

Pulmonary infiltrates with eosinophilia (Loeffler syndrome) are associated with nitrofurantoin, *para*-aminosalicylic acid, methotrexate, sulfonamides, tetracycline, chlorpropamide, phenytoin, NSAIDs, and imipramine (Table 31–5).[6,65] The disorder is characterized by fever, nonproductive cough, dyspnea, cyanosis, bilateral pulmonary infiltrates, and eosinophilia in the blood.[6] Lung biopsy has revealed perivasculitis with infiltration of eosinophils, macrophages, and proteinaceous edema fluid in the alveoli. The symptoms and eosinophilia generally respond rapidly to withdrawal of the offending drug.

Sulfonamides were first reported as causative agents in users of sulfanilamide vaginal cream.[6] *para*-Aminosalicylic acid frequently produced the syndrome in tuberculosis patients being treated with this agent.[6] There are nine reported cases associated with sulfasalazine use in inflammatory bowel disease.[65] The drug associated most frequently with this syndrome is nitrofurantoin.[6,61] Nitrofurantoin-induced lung disorders appear to be more common in postmenopausal women.[61] Lung reactions made up 43% of 921 adverse reactions to nitrofurantoin reported to the Swedish Adverse Drug Reaction Committee between 1966 and 1976.[65] No apparent correlation exists between duration of drug exposure and severity or reversibility of the reaction.[65] Most cases occur within 1 month of therapy. Typical symptoms include fever, tachypnea, dyspnea, dry cough, and, less commonly, pleuritic chest pain. Radiographic findings include bilateral interstitial infiltrates, predominant in the bases and pleural effusions 25% of the time. Although there are anecdotal reports that steroids are beneficial, the usual rapid improvement following discontinuation of the drugs brings the usefulness of steroids into question. Complete recovery usually occurs within 15 days of withdrawal.

A few cases of pulmonary eosinophilia have been reported in asthmatics treated with cromolyn.[6,65] The significance of this is unknown in light of the occasional spontaneous occurrence of pulmonary eosinophilia in asthmatic patients. Cases of acute pneumonitis and eosinophilia have been reported to occur with phenytoin and carbamazepine therapy.[65] Patients have had other symptoms of hypersensitivity, including fever and rashes. The symptoms of dyspnea and cough subside following discontinuation of the drug.

TABLE 31-5 Drugs That Induce Pulmonary Infiltrates with Eosinophilia (Loeffler Syndrome)

Drug	Relative Frequency of Reactions	Drug	Relative Frequency of Reactions
Nitrofurantoin	F2	Tetracycline	R
para-Aminosalicylic acid	F	Procarbazine	R
Sulfonamides	I	Cromolyn	R
Penicillins	I	Niridazole	R
Methotrexate	I	Gold salts	R
Imipramine	I	Chlorpromazine	R
Chlorpropamide	R	Naproxen	R
Carbamazepine	R	Sulindac	R
Phenytoin	R	Ibuprofen	R
Mephenesin	R		

F, frequent; I, infrequent; R, rare.

OXYGEN TOXICITY

Because of the similarity to pulmonary fibrosis, oxygen-induced lung toxicity is reviewed briefly. More extensive reviews on this topic have been published.[66,67]

The earliest manifestation of oxygen toxicity is substernal pleuritic pain from tracheobronchitis.[67] The onset of toxicity follows an asymptomatic period and presents as cough, chest pain, and dyspnea. Early symptoms usually are masked in ventilator-dependent patients. The first noted physiologic change is a decrease in pulmonary compliance caused by reversible atelectasis. Then decreases in vital capacity occur, followed by progressive abnormalities in carbon monoxide diffusing capacity.[67] Decreased inspiratory flow rates, reflected in the need for high inspiratory pressures in ventilator-dependent patients, occur as the fractional concentration of inspired oxygen requirement increases. The lungs become progressively stiffer as the ability to oxygenate becomes more compromised.

The fraction of inspired oxygen and duration of exposure are both important determinants of the severity of lung damage. Normal human volunteers can tolerate 100% oxygen at sea level for 24 to 48 hours with minimal to no damage.[66] Oxygen concentrations of less than 50% are well tolerated even for extended periods. Inspired oxygen concentrations between 50% and 100% carry a substantial risk of lung damage, and the duration required is inversely proportional to the fraction of inspired oxygen.[66] Underlying disease states may alter this relationship. Lung damage may not be lasting and may improve months to years after the exposure.[68,69]

Oxygen-induced lung damage generally is separated into the acute exudative phase and the subacute or chronic proliferative phase. The acute phase consists of perivascular, peribronchiolar, interstitial, and alveolar edema with alveolar hemorrhage and necrosis of pulmonary endothelium and type I epithelial cells.[66] The proliferative phase consists of resorption of the exudates and hyperplasia of interstitial and type II alveolar lining cells. Collagen and elastin deposition in the interstitium of alveolar walls then leads to thickening of the gas-exchange area and the fibrosis.[66]

The biochemical mechanism of the tissue damage during hyperoxia is the increased production of highly reactive, partially reduced oxygen metabolites (Fig. 31–1).[67] These oxidants normally are produced in small quantities during cellular respiration and include the superoxide anion, hydrogen peroxide, the hydroxyl radical, singlet oxygen, and hypochlorous acid.[67] Oxygen free radicals normally are formed in phagocytic cells to kill invading microorganisms, but they also are toxic to normal cell components. The oxidants produce toxicity through destructive redox reactions with protein sulfhydryl groups, membrane lipids, and nucleic acids.[67]

The oxidants are products of normal cellular respiration that are normally counterbalanced by an antioxidant defense system that prevents tissue destruction. The antioxidants include superoxide dismutase, catalase, glutathione peroxidase, ceruloplasmin, and

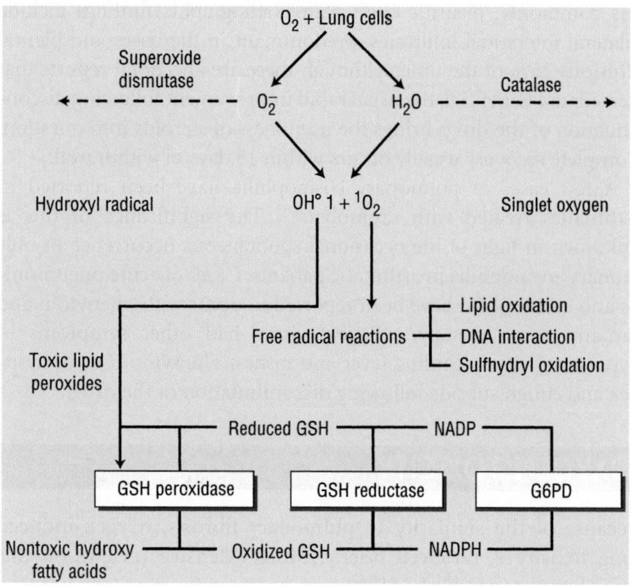

FIGURE 31-1. Schematic of the interaction of oxygen radicals and the antioxidant system. (GSH, glutathione; G6PD, glucose-6-phosphate dehydrogenase; NADP, nicotinamide-adenine dinucleotide phosphate; NADPH, reduced NADP.)

α-tocopherol (vitamin E). Antioxidants are ubiquitous in the body. Hyperoxia produces toxicity by overwhelming the antioxidant system. There is experimental evidence that a number of drugs and chemicals produce lung toxicity through increasing production of oxidants (e.g., bleomycin, cyclophosphamide, nitrofurantoin, and paraquat) and/or by inhibiting the antioxidant system (e.g., carmustine, cyclophosphamide, and nitrofurantoin).[70,71]

PULMONARY FIBROSIS

A large number of drugs are associated with chronic pulmonary fibrosis with or without a preceding acute pneumonitis (Table 31–6). The cancer chemotherapeutic agents make up the largest group and have been the subject of numerous reviews.[70,71] Although the mechanisms by which all the drugs produce pneumonitis and/or fibrosis are not known, the clinical syndrome, pulmonary function abnormalities, and histopathology present a relatively homogeneous pattern.[70] The histopathologic picture closely resembles oxidant lung damage, and in some experimental cases, oxygen enhances the pulmonary injury.[61] Although the terms *pulmonary fibrosis* or *interstitial pneumonitis* have been used widely to describe pneumonia after bone marrow transplantation, in 1991, a National Institutes of Health workshop recommended that the term *idiopathic pneumonia syndrome* (IPS) should be used to avoid histopathologic terms and to define the inherent heterogeneity of this disorder.[72] IPS accounts for more than 40% of deaths related to bone marrow transplantation.[72] Suggested causes of IPS include radiation or chemotherapy regimens prior to transplantation, graft-versus-host disease, unrecognized infections, and other inflammation-related lung injuries.[73,74] IPS is characterized by dyspnea, hypoxemia, nonproductive cough, diffuse alveolar damage, and interstitial pneumonitis in the absence of lower respiratory infection. IPS has been reported early and late, up to 24 months after bone marrow transplantation.[74]

The lung damage following ingestion of the contact herbicide paraquat classically resembles hyperoxic lung damage. Hyperoxia accelerates the lung damage induced by paraquat. Lung toxicity from paraquat occurs following oral administration in humans and aerosol administration and inhalation in experimental animals.[71] The pulmonary specificity of paraquat results in part from its active uptake into lung tissue. Paraquat readily accepts an electron from reduced nicotinamide-adenine dinucleotide phosphate and then is reoxidized rapidly, forming superoxide and other oxygen radicals.[71] The toxicity may be a result of nicotinamide-adenine dinucleotide phosphate depletion (see Fig. 31–1) and/or excess oxygen free radical generation with lipid peroxidation. Treatment with exogenous superoxide dismutase has had limited and conflicting results.[71]

A number of furans have been shown to produce oxidant injury to lungs.[71] Occasionally, patients with acute nitrofurantoin lung toxicity will progress to a chronic reaction leading to fibrosis, and rarely, a patient may develop chronic toxicity without an antecedent acute reaction. Like paraquat, nitrofurantoin undergoes cyclic reduction and reoxidation that may produce superoxide radicals or deplete nicotinamide-adenine dinucleotide phosphate. In addition, nitrofurantoin inhibits glutathione reductase, an enzyme involved in the glutathione antioxidant system (see Fig. 31–1). Table 31–7 lists possible nondrug causes of pulmonary fibrosis.

TABLE 31-6 Drugs That Induce Pneumonitis and/or Fibrosis

Drug	Relative Frequency of Reactions	Drug	Relative Frequency of Reactions
Oxygen	F	Chlorambucil	R
Radiation	F	Melphalan	R
Bleomycin	F	Lomustine and semustine	R
Busulfan	F	Zinostatin	R
Carmustine	F	Procarbazine	R
Hexamethonium	F	Teniposide	R
Paraquat	F	Sulfasalazine	R
Amiodarone	F	Phenytoin	R
Mecamylamine	I	Gold salts	R
Pentolinium	I	Pindolol	R
Cyclophosphamide	I	Imipramine	R
Practolol	I	Penicillamine	R
Methotrexate	I	Phenylbutazone	R
Mitomycin	I	Chlorphentermine	R
Nitrofurantoin	I	Fenfluramine	R
Methysergide	I	Leflunomide	R
Sirolimus	I	Mefloquine	R
Azathioprine, 6-mercaptopurine	R	Pergolide	R

F, frequent; I, infrequent; R, rare.

TABLE 31-7 Possible Causes of Pulmonary Fibrosis

Idiopathic pulmonary fibrosis (fibrosing alveolitis)
Pneumoconiosis (asbestosis, silicosis, coal dust, talc berylliosis)
Hypersensitivity pneumonitis (molds, bacteria, animal proteins, toluene diisocyanate, epoxy resins)
Smoking
Sarcoidosis
Tuberculosis
Lipoid pneumonia
Systemic lupus erythematosus
Rheumatoid arthritis
Systemic sclerosis
Polymyositis/dermatomyositis
Sjögren syndrome
Polyarteritis nodosa
Wegener granuloma
Byssinosis (cotton workers)
Siderosis (arc welders' lung)
Radiation
Oxygen
Chemicals (thioureas, trialkylphosphorothioates, furans)
Drugs (see Tables 31-5, 31-6, and 31-8)

DRUGS ASSOCIATED WITH PULMONARY FIBROSIS

ANTINEOPLASTICS

A number of cancer chemotherapeutic agents produce pulmonary fibrosis. In an excellent review,[70] six predisposing factors for the development of cytotoxic drug–induced pulmonary disease were described: (a) cumulative dose, (b) increased age, (c) concurrent or previous radiotherapy, (d) oxygen therapy, (e) other cytotoxic drug therapy, and (f) preexisting pulmonary disease. Drugs that are directly toxic to the lung would be expected to show a dose–response relationship. Dose–response relationships have been established for bleomycin, busulfan, and carmustine (BCNU).[70] Bleomycin and busulfan exhibit threshold cumulative doses below which a very small percentage of patients exhibit toxicity, but carmustine shows a more linear relationship.[71] Older patients appear to be more susceptible, possibly as a result of a decrease in the antioxidant defense system.

Excessive irradiation produces a pneumonitis and fibrosis thought to be caused by oxygen free radical formation.[70] Evidence for synergistic toxicity with radiation exists for bleomycin, busulfan, and mitomycin.[70] Hyperoxia has shown synergistic toxicity with bleomycin, cyclophosphamide, and mitomycin.[70] Carmustine, mitomycin, cyclophosphamide, bleomycin, and methotrexate all appear to show increased lung toxicity when they are part of multiple-drug regimens.

NITROSOUREAS

BCNU is associated with the highest incidence of pulmonary toxicity (20% to 30%).[70] The lung pathology generally resembles that produced by bleomycin and busulfan. Unique to BCNU is the finding of fibrosis in the absence of inflammatory infiltrates. BCNU preferentially inhibits glutathione reductase, the enzyme required to regenerate glutathione, thus reducing glutathione tissue stores.[70,71] The patients present with dyspnea, tachypnea, and nonproductive cough that may begin within a month of initiation of therapy but may not develop for as long as 3 years.[70] Most patients receiving BCNU develop fibrosis that may remain asymptomatic or become symptomatic any time up to 17 years after therapy.[75] The cumulative dose has ranged from 580 to 2,100 mg/m^2.[71] The disease is usually slowly progressive with a mortality rate from 15% to greater than 90% depending on the study and period of followup. In a retrospective study, the risk factors for development of IPS and prognostic factors for outcomes were evaluated in 94 patients with relapsed Hodgkin disease treated with BCNU containing high-dose chemotherapy and hematopoietic support. The risk factors for pulmonary fibrosis and mortality were female sex and dose of BCNU, with all deaths reported in those who received BCNU at doses of more than 475 mg/m^2.[76] Rapid progression and death within a few days occur in a small percentage of patients.[70] Corticosteroids do not appear to be effective in reducing damage.[70] Other nitrosoureas, lomustine, and semustine also have been reported to produce lung damage in patients receiving unusually high doses.[70]

BLEOMYCIN

Bleomycin is the best-studied cytotoxic pulmonary toxin. Because of its lack of bone marrow suppression, pulmonary toxicity is the dose-limiting toxicity of bleomycin therapy. The incidence of bleomycin lung toxicity is approximately 4%, which may be affected by the following risk factors: bleomycin cumulative dose, age, high concentration of inspired oxygen, radiation therapy, and multidrug regimens, particularly those with cyclophosphamide.[63] Age at the time of treatment with bleomycin also may be a risk factor; patients younger than 7 years of age at the time of receiving bleomycin therapy are more likely to develop pulmonary toxicity compared with older subjects.[63] The cumulative dose above which the incidence of toxicity significantly increases is 450 to 500 units.[70] However, rapidly fatal pulmonary toxicity has occurred with doses as low as 100 units.[70]

Experimentally, bleomycin generates superoxide anions, and the lung toxicity is increased by radiation and hyperoxia.[70] Pretreatment with superoxide dismutase and catalase reduces toxicity in experimental animals.[70] Bleomycin also oxidizes arachidonic acid, which may account for the marked inflammation. Bleomycin also may affect collagen deposition by its stimulation of fibroblast growth.[70] Combination of bleomycin with other cytotoxic agents, particularly regimens containing cyclophosphamide, may predispose patients to pulmonary damage.

There are two distinct clinical patterns of bleomycin pulmonary toxicity. Chronic progressive fibrosis is the most common; acute hypersensitivity reactions occur infrequently. Patients present with cough and dyspnea. The first physiologic abnormality seen is a decreased diffusing capacity of carbon monoxide.[70] Chest radiographs show a bibasilar reticular pattern, and gallium scans show marked uptake in the involved lung.[70] Chest radiographic changes lag behind pulmonary function abnormalities. Spirometry tests before each bleomycin dose are not predictive of toxicity. The single-breath diffusing capacity of carbon monoxide is the most sensitive indicator of bleomycin-induced lung disease. Although it is not absolutely predictive, a drop of 20% or greater in the diffusing capacity of carbon monoxide is an indication for using alternative therapies.[70] The prognosis of bleomycin lung toxicity has improved as a consequence of early detection, but the mortality rate is approximately 25%. Mild cases respond to discontinuation of bleomycin therapy.[63] Corticosteroid therapy appears to be helpful in patients with acute pneumonitis, although there have been no controlled trials. Patients with chronic fibrosis are less likely to respond. Although corticosteroids have been used for a number of drug-induced pulmonary problems, a study in mice showing a potential for worsening of lung damage when administered early during the repair stage should sound a word of caution against their indiscriminate use.[77]

MITOMYCIN

Mitomycin is an alkylating antibiotic that produces pulmonary fibrosis at a frequency of 3% to 12%.[70] The mechanism is unknown, but oxygen and radiation therapy appear to enhance the development of toxicity.[70] The clinical presentation and symptoms are the same as for bleomycin. The mortality rate is approximately 50%. Early withdrawal of the drug and administration of corticosteroids appear to improve the outcome significantly.

ALKYLATING AGENTS

A number of alkylating agents are associated with pulmonary fibrosis (see Table 31–5). The incidence of clinical toxicity is around 4%, although subclinical damage is apparent in up to 46% of patients at autopsy. The mechanism of toxicity is unknown; however, epithelial cell damage that triggers the arachidonic acid inflammatory cascade may be the initiating event.[70] The clinical presentation is insidious, with 4 years being the average duration of therapy before the onset of symptoms.[70] Patients present with low-grade fever, weight loss, weakness, dyspnea, cough, and rales.[70] Pulmonary function tests initially show abnormal diffusion capacity followed by a restrictive pattern (low vital capacity). The histopathologic findings are nonspecific. The prognosis is one of slow progression with a mean survival of 5 months following diagnosis.[70] Although there is no direct dose-dependent correlation, patients receiving less than 500 mg of busulfan do not develop the syndrome without concomitant radiation or use of other pulmonary toxic chemotherapeutic agents.[70] There are anecdotal reports of beneficial responses to corticosteroids, but no controlled studies have been done.

Cyclophosphamide infrequently produces pulmonary toxicity. More than 20 well-documented cases have been reported to date. In animal models, cyclophosphamide produces reactive oxygen radicals. High oxygen concentrations produce synergistic toxicity with cyclophosphamide. The duration of therapy before the onset of symptoms is highly variable, and there may be a delay of several months between the onset of symptoms and discontinuation of the drug.[70] Cyclophosphamide may potentiate carmustine lung toxicity.[70] Clinical symptoms usually consist of dyspnea on exertion, cough, and fever. Inspiratory crackles and the bibasilar reticular pattern typical of cytotoxic drug-induced radiographic changes are present. Histopathologic changes are also nonspecific. Approximately 60% of patients recover. Corticosteroid therapy has been reported to be beneficial; however, death despite corticosteroid administration also has been reported.

Chlorambucil, melphalan, and uracil mustard also are associated with pulmonary fibrosis. Of the alkylating agents, only nitrogen mustard and thiotepa have not been reported to cause fibrotic pulmonary toxicity.[70]

ANTIMETABOLITES

Methotrexate was first reported to induce pulmonary toxicity in 1969.[70] The pulmonary toxicity to methotrexate is unique in that discontinuation is not always necessary, and reinstitution of the drug may not produce recurrence of symptoms.[6] Methotrexate pulmonary toxicity most commonly appears to result from hypersensitivity,[65] and it can occur 3 or more years following methotrexate therapy.[78] Age, sex, underlying pulmonary disease, duration of therapy, or smoking is not associated with an increased risk of pneumonitis with methotrexate.[78] Serial pulmonary function tests did not help to identify pneumonitis in patients receiving methotrexate before the onset of clinical symptoms.[78] Reductions in diffusing capacity of carbon monoxide and lung volumes are the most common manifestations of methotrexate lung toxicity.[63] Pulmonary edema and eosinophilia are common, and fibrosis occurs in only 10% of the patients who develop acute pneumonitis.[70] Systemic symptoms of chills, fever, and malaise are common before the onset of dyspnea, cough, and acute pleuritic chest pain. Methotrexate also is associated with granuloma formation.[70]

The prognosis of methotrexate-induced pulmonary toxicity is good, with a 1% or less mortality rate.[65] Pulmonary toxicity has followed intrathecal as well as oral administration and has occurred after single doses as well as long-term daily and intermittent administration.[70] Pneumonitis has been reported to occur up to 4 weeks following discontinuation of therapy.[70] Numerous anecdotal reports have claimed dramatic benefit from corticosteroid therapy. It is unknown whether intermittent (weekly) dosing, as is done for rheumatoid arthritis, decreases the risk of methotrexate-induced pulmonary toxicity because pneumonitis has occurred with this form of dosing.

Rarely, azathioprine and its major metabolite 6-mercaptopurine have been reported to produce an acute restrictive lung disease. Procarbazine, a methylhydrazine associated more commonly with Loeffler syndrome, rarely has been associated with pulmonary fibrosis.[65] The vinca alkaloids vinblastine and vindesine have been reported to produce severe respiratory toxicity in association with mitomycin. The incidence with the combination is 39% and may represent a true synergistic effect between these agents.[70]

NONCYTOTOXIC DRUGS

Pulmonary fibrosis associated with the ganglionic-blocking agent hexamethonium was first reported in 1954 (see Table 31–6).[6] Patients developed extreme dyspnea after several months on the drug. Pathologic findings were consistent with bronchiectasis, bronchiolectasis, and fibrosis.[6] This phenomenon has occurred occasionally with use of the other ganglionic blockers (i.e., mecamylamine and pentolinium).[6]

In 1959, radiographic changes characteristic of diffuse pulmonary fibrosis were reported in 27 (87%) of 31 patients who had taken phenytoin for 2 years or more.[61] Since then, studies have been conflicting. If phenytoin does produce chronic fibrosis, it would appear to be a relatively rare event.

Gold salts (sodium aurothiomalate) used in the treatment of rheumatoid arthritis have produced pulmonary fibrosis with cough, dyspnea, and pleuritic pain 5 to 16 weeks following institution of therapy.[61] Pulmonary function tests show a restrictive defect, and patients generally have an eosinophilia. The reactions improve on discontinuation of the gold therapy and recur promptly on reexposure. The pulmonary deficit may not resolve completely.

AMIODARONE

Amiodarone, a benzofuran derivative, produces pulmonary fibrosis when used for supraventricular and ventricular arrhythmias (see Table 31–6).[79] The duration of amiodarone therapy before the onset of symptoms has ranged from 4 weeks to 6 years.[61,79] The estimated incidence is 1 in 1,000 to 2,000 treated patients per year. The clinical course is variable, ranging from acute onset of dyspnea with rapid progression into severe respiratory failure and death caused by slowly developing exertional dyspnea over a few months. Patients generally improve on discontinuation of the drug.[79] The majority of patients develop reactions while taking maintenance doses greater than 400 mg daily for more than 2 months or smaller doses for more than 2 years. The risk of amiodarone pulmonary toxicity is higher during the first 12 months of therapy even at a low dosage.[80] Other risk factors include cardiopulmonary surgery combined with the administration of high concentrations of oxygen.[80] Routine spirometry does not appear to be predictive of patients at risk.[81] Carbon monoxide diffusing capacity studies are sensitive indicators of amiodarone pulmonary toxicity but have only a 21% positive predictive value.[81] Clinical findings include exertional dyspnea, nonproductive cough, weight loss, and occasionally low-grade fever.[61,81] Radiographic changes are nondiagnostic and consist of diffuse bilateral interstitial changes consistent with a pneumonitis. Pulmonary function abnormalities include hypoxia, restrictive changes, and diffusion abnormalities.

The mechanism of amiodarone-induced pulmonary toxicity is multifactorial. Amiodarone and its metabolite can damage lung tissue directly by a cytotoxic process or indirectly by immunologic reactions.[80] Amiodarone is an amphiphilic molecule that contains both a highly apolar aromatic ring system and a polar side chain with a positively charged nitrogen atom.[79] Amphiphilic drugs characteristically produce a phospholipid storage disorder in the lungs of experimental animals and humans.[71] Chlorphentermine, an anorectic, is the prototype amphiphilic compound. The mechanism is currently believed to be the inhibition of lysosomal phospholipases.[71] The inflammation and fibrosis are thought to be a late finding resulting from nonspecific inflammation following the breakdown of phospholipid-laden macrophages.[79]

In a review of 39 cases, 9 patients died, and the remaining 30 patients had resolution of abnormalities after withdrawal of the drug.[79] Some patients have had resolution with lowering of the dosage, and therapy has been reinstituted at lower doses without problems in others. Of the patients who died, one-half had received corticosteroids. There are reports of a protective effect with prophylactic corticosteroids and other reports of patients developing amiodarone lung toxicity while on corticosteroids.[79] At this time, any benefit of corticosteroids is unclear because most patients improve after stopping the drug.

PULMONARY HYPERTENSION

Pulmonary hypertension is a rare disorder, occurring with an approximate incidence of 1 to 2 cases per 1 million in the general population.[82] With progression of the disease, right ventricular afterload increases, and the ability to increase cardiac output with activity decreases. This progresses to right-sided heart failure and death.[83]

Patients with pulmonary hypertension often complain of exertional dyspnea, chest pain, and syncope. Because of the nonspecific nature of these symptoms and lack of a noninvasive diagnostic test for detecting pulmonary hypertension, there are often delays in the diagnosis of the disease, frequently up to a year after the onset of symptoms.[83]

The factors leading to the development of pulmonary hypertension are unclear, although associations with portal hypertension and pregnancy have been detected. Obesity by itself may double the risk of pulmonary hypertension.[84] Additionally, the use of cocaine or oral contraceptives, infection with the human immunodeficiency virus (HIV), the use of anorexic agents,[85] hepatic cirrhosis, genetic susceptibility, and female sex in the third to fourth decades of life also are implicated as predisposing factors.[84] Exposure of patients to fenfluramine or dexfenfluramine is associated with 20% of all diagnosed cases of pulmonary hypertension.[84]

The first reports of the association between pulmonary hypertension and the use of anorexic agents occurred in the late 1960s and early 1970s in Western Europe when the drug aminorex was used for weight reduction.[86] The incidence of pulmonary hypertension returned to baseline after the drug was removed from the market. In the early 1990s, an association between fenfluramine use and pulmonary hypertension was established.[87] Shortly thereafter, the International Primary Pulmonary Hypertension Study Group investigated the potential role of anorexic agents in causing pulmonary hypertension.[85] Included in this multinational case-control study were 95 patients with pulmonary hypertension and 355 controls from general practices matched for gender and age. The use of anorexic agents, primarily fenfluramine and dexfenfluramine, within the last year was associated with an increased risk of pulmonary hypertension with an odds ratio of 10:1. When anorexic drugs were used for a total of more than 3 months, the odds ratio increased to 23:1.

In a 12-year observational study, 62 patients with fenfluramine-associated pulmonary hypertension were compared with 125 sex-matched patients with pulmonary hypertension unrelated to the use of fenfluramine derivatives. In most of the cases (81%), fenfluramine derivatives were used for at least 3 months. The time frame between the initiation of the therapy and the onset of dyspnea ranged from 27 days to 23 years. Both the fenfluramine-associated pulmonary hypertension group and the control group had similar levels of New York Heart Association functional class and symptoms, as well as an overall survival rate of 50% in 3 years.[88]

The mechanism by which anorexic agents cause pulmonary hypertension is unknown. Studies show that fenfluramine, dexfenfluramine, and aminorex inhibit potassium channels in isolated pulmonary artery smooth muscle cells in rats, which results in vasoconstriction. Potassium channel activity is altered in pulmonary artery smooth muscle cells obtained from patients with pulmonary hypertension, leading to speculation that anorexic agents may cause vasoconstriction followed by vascular growth and remodeling.[83] Another potential mechanism involves serotonin, which has been found in increased levels in patients with pulmonary hypertension.[83] Serotonin can be stored in the platelet when serotonin plasma concentration is high. Serotonin acts as a pulmonary vasoconstrictor when it is released from the platelets.[84]

Patients with pulmonary hypertension associated with anorexic use may experience a considerable improvement in their condition or possibly even remission within 1 to 3 months following discontinuation of the drug.[84,89] Pharmacologic agents used in the treatment of pulmonary hypertension include high dosage of calcium channel blockers and anticoagulants.[82] Epoprostenol, also known as *prostacyclin*, a strong vasodilator of all vascular beds was approved for the long-term therapy of pulmonary hypertension in 1995.[90] Additionally, lung and heart-lung transplantations have played a role in the treatment of pulmonary hypertension. However, the 4-year survival rate is less than 60% in pulmonary hypertension patients receiving any transplant.[90] Bosentan, an endothelin receptor antagonist indicated for primary pulmonary hypertension, also may have a role, but no studies currently exist describing its use.

In September 1997, the FDA requested the manufacturers of fenfluramine and dexfenfluramine to voluntarily withdraw their products from the market. This was done following case reports of valvular heart disease in patients taking either medication as monotherapy or in combination with another anorexic agent, phentermine. Because no association has been found between phentermine alone and valvular heart disease, it is still available. Isolated case reports of pulmonary hypertension and phentermine monotherapy have been reported,[91,92] but present data do not support an association. Although fenfluramine and phentermine were both approved by the FDA to be used as anorectic agents, the combination therapy, "fen-phen," was never approved.

MISCELLANEOUS PULMONARY TOXICITY

Drugs may produce serious pulmonary toxicity as part of a more generalized disorder. The pleural thickening, effusions, and fibrosis that occur as an extension of the retroperitoneal fibrotic reactions of methysergide and practolol or as part of a drug-induced lupus syndrome are the most common examples (Table 31–8).

Methysergide therapy for prophylaxis of poorly controlled migraine headache occasionally results in pulmonary toxicity associated with pleural effusions. The patients develop pleural pain, dyspnea, and fever. Chest radiography reveals a uniform hazy shadowing over the lower lung fields, and a loud pleural rub is heard on auscultation.[6] The mechanism is unknown, and most patients improve with discontinuation of the drug. Pleural and pulmonary fibrosis has been reported in one patient taking pindolol, a β-blocker structurally similar to prac-

TABLE 31-8 Drugs That May Induce Pleural Effusions and Fibrosis

	Relative Frequency of Reactions
Idiopathic	
Methysergide	F
Practolol	F
Pindolol	R
Methotrexate	R
Nitrofurantoin	R
Drug-induced lupus syndrome	
Procainamide	F
Hydralazine	F
Isoniazid	R
Phenytoin	R
Mephenytoin	R
Griseofulvin	R
Trimethadione	R
Sulfonamides	R
Phenylbutazone	R
Streptomycin	R
Ethosuximide	R
Tetracycline	R
Pseudolymphoma syndrome	
Cyclosporine	R
Phenytoin	R

F, frequent; I, infrequent; R, rare.

tolol, an agent known to produce fibrosis.[61] Acute pleuritis with pleural effusions and fibrosis is a prominent manifestation of drug-induced lupus syndrome. Procainamide is associated with the largest number of pulmonary reactions, with 46% of patients with the lupus syndrome developing pulmonary complications.[6] Symptoms include pleuritic pain and fever with muscle and joint pain. Chest radiographs show bilateral pleural effusions and linear atelectasis. Patients have a positive antinuclear antibody test. Symptoms usually resolve within 6 weeks of drug withdrawal.[6]

Hydralazine is the next most common cause of lupus syndrome. Most patients who develop pleuropulmonary manifestations have antecedent symptoms of generalized lupus.[6] Other drugs that produce the lupus syndrome include isoniazid and phenytoin. Phenytoin also can produce hilar lymphadenopathy as part of a generalized pseudolymphoma or lymphadenopathy syndrome.[6]

MONITORING THERAPEUTIC OUTCOMES

Monitoring for drug-induced pulmonary diseases consists primarily of having a high index of suspicion that a particular syndrome may be drug-induced. Most hypersensitivity or allergic reactions (bronchospasm) occur rapidly, within the first 2 weeks of therapy with the offending agent, and reverse rapidly with appropriate therapy (e.g., withdrawal of the offending agent and administration of corticosteroids and bronchodilators). Dyspnea associated with Loeffler syndrome and acute pulmonary edema syndromes also improve rapidly in 1 to 2 days. However, some residual defect in diffusion capacity and the roentgenogram may persist for a few weeks. It is probably unnecessary to do followup spirometry or diffusion capacity determinations in these patients unless there is some concern that the syndrome will progress to pulmonary fibrosis (through the use of bleomycin or nitrofurantoin).

The routine monitoring of patients receiving known pulmonary toxins with dose-dependent toxicity such as amiodarone, bleomycin, or carmustine is still controversial. For chronic fibrosis, the diffusing capacity of carbon monoxide is the most sensitive test and may be useful in patients receiving bleomycin for detecting and preventing further deterioration of lung function with continued administration. Carmustine lung toxicity may be delayed up to 10 years following administration, and routine monitoring has not proved preventive. Monitoring patients receiving amiodarone in doses greater than 400 mg/day every 4 to 6 months may prove useful in detecting early disease that requires lowering the amiodarone or stopping the drug. Because there is no evidence of a cumulative dose effect once it has been established that the patient can tolerate the elevated dose, continued routine monitoring past the first year is unnecessary.

ABBREVIATIONS

ACE: angiotensin-converting enzyme

COPD: chronic obstructive pulmonary disease

EDTA: ethylenediamine tetraacetic acid

FDA: Food and Drug Administration

FEV_1: forced expiratory volume in the first second of expiration

IPS: idiopathic pneumonia syndrome

NSAIDs: nonsteroidal antiinflammatory drugs

REFERENCES

1. Martys CR. Adverse reactions to drugs in general practice. Br Med J 1979;2:1194–1197.
2. Messaad D, Sahla H, Benahmed S, Godard P, et al. Drug provocation tests in patients with a history suggesting an immediate drug hypersensitivity reaction. Ann Intern Med 2004;140:1001–1006.
3. Levy M, Kewitz H, Altwein W, et al. Hospital admissions due to adverse drug reactions: A comparative study from Jerusalem and Berlin. Eur J Clin Pharmacol 1980;17:25–31.
4. Shapiro S, Slone D, Lewis GP, et al. Fatal drug reactions among medical inpatients. JAMA 1971;216:467–472.
5. Porter J, Jick H. Drug-related deaths among medical inpatients. JAMA 1977;237:879–881.
6. Brewis RAL. Respiratory disorders. In: Davies DM, ed. Textbook of Adverse Drug Reactions, 2d ed. New York: Oxford University Press, 1981:154–178.
7. Hansen-Flaschen J, Cowen J, Raps EC. Neuromuscular blockade in the intensive care unit: More than we bargained for. Am Rev Respir Dis 1993;147:234–236.
8. Lieu F, Powers SK, Herb RA, et al. Exercise and glucocorticoid-induced diaphragmatic myopathy. J Appl Physiol 1993;75:763–771.
9. Dekhuijzen PNR, Gayan-Ramirez G, de Bock V, et al. Triamcinolone and prednisolone affect contractile properties and histopathology of rat diaphragm differently. J Clin Invest 1993;92:1534–1542.
10. Decramer M, Lacquet LM, Fagard R, et al. Corticosteroids contribute to muscle weakness in chronic airflow obstruction. Am J Respir Crit Care Med 1994;150:11–16.
11. Fisher HK. Drug-induced asthma syndromes. In: Weiss EB, Segal MS, Stein M, eds. Bronchial Asthma: Mechanisms and Therapeutics, 3d ed. Boston: Little, Brown, 1993:938–949.
12. McKeever TM, Lewis S, Smit HA, et al. The association of acetaminophen, aspirin, and ibuprofen with respiratory disease and lung function. Am J Respir Crit Care Med 2005:171;966–971.
13. Settipane GA. Aspirin and allergic diseases: A review. Am J Med 1983;74(Suppl 6a):102–109.
14. Stevenson DD. Diagnosis, prevention, and treatment of adverse reactions to aspirin and nonsteroidal anti-inflammatory drugs. J Allergy Clin Immunol 1984;74:617–622.
15. Szczeklik A, Gryglewski RJ. Asthma and antiinflammatory drugs: Mechanisms and clinical patterns. Drugs 1983;25:533–543.
16. Matsuse H, Shimoda T, Matsua N, et al. Aspirin-induced asthma as a risk factor for asthma mortality. J Asthma 1997;34:314–317.
17. Szcezklik A, Nizankowaska E. Clinical features and diagnosis of aspirin induced asthma. Thorax 2000;55(Suppl 2):S42–S44.
18. Dahlen B, Melillo G. Inhalation challenge in ASA-induced asthma. Respir Med 1998;92:378–384.
19. Dahlen B, Zetterstrom O. Comparison of bronchial and per oral provocation with aspirin in aspirin-sensitive asthmatics. Eur Respir J 1990;3:527–534.
20. Berges-Gimeno MP, Simon RA, Stevenson DD. Long term treatment with aspirin desensitization in asthmatic patients with aspirin-exacerbated respiratory disease. J Allergy Clin Immunol 2003;111:180–186.
21. Mathison DA, Stevenson DD, Simon RA. Precipitating factors in asthma: Aspirin, sulfites, and other drugs and chemicals. Chest 1985;87(Suppl):50–54.
22. American Academy of Pediatrics, Committee on Drugs. "Inactive" ingredients in pharmaceutical products: Update. Pediatrics 1997;99:268–278.
23. Yoshida S, Ishizaki Y, Onuma K, et al. Selective cyclooxygenase 2 inhibitor in patients with aspirin-induced asthma. J Allergy Clin Immunol 2000;106:1201–1202.
24. Szczeklik A, Niankowska E, Bochenek G, et al. Safety of a specific COX-2 inhibitor in aspirin-induced asthma. Clin Exp Allergy 2001;31:219–225.
25. Dahlen B, Szczeklik A, Murray JJ. Celecoxib in patients with asthma and aspirin intolerance. N Engl J Med 2001;344:142.
26. Stevenson DD, Simon RA. Lack of cross-reactivity between rofecoxib and aspirin-sensitive patients with asthma. J Allergy Clin Immunol 2001;108:47–51.
27. Israel E, Fischer A, Rosenberg M, et al. The pivotal role of 5-lipoxygenase products in the reaction of aspirin-sensitive asthmatics to aspirin. Am Rev Respir Dis 1993;148:1447–1451.
28. Paul JD, Simon RA, Daffern PJ, et al. Lack of effect of the 5-lipoxygenase inhibitor zileuton in blocking oral aspirin challenges in aspirin-sensitive asthmatics. Ann Allergy Asthma Immunol 2000;85:40–45.

29. Stevenson DD, Simon RA, Mathison DA, Christiansen SC. Montelukast is only partially effective in inhibiting aspirin response in aspirin-sensitive asthmatics. Ann Allergy Asthma Immunol 2000;85:477–482.
30. Berges-Gimeno MP, Simon RA, Stevenson DD. The effect of leukotriene-modifier drugs on aspirin-induced asthma and rhinitis reactions. Clin Exp Allergy 2002;32:1491–1496.
31. Menendez R, Venzor J, Ortiz G. Failure of zafirlukast to prevent ibuprofen-induced anaphylaxis. Ann Allergy Asthma Immunol 1998;80:225–226.
32. Robuschi M, Gambaro G, Setini P, et al. Attenuation of aspirin-induced bronchoconstriction by sodium cromoglycate and nedocromil sodium. Am J Respir Crit Care Med 1997;155:1461–1464.
33. Dahlen S, Malmstrom K, Nizankowska E, et al. Improvement of aspirin-intolerant asthma by montelukast, a leukotriene antagonist: A randomized, double-blind, placebo-controlled trial. Am J Respir Crit Care Med 2002;165:9–14.
34. Reiss TF, Chervinsky P, Dockhorn RJ, et al. Montelukast, a once-daily leukotriene receptor antagonist, in the treatment of chronic asthma: A multicenter, randomized, double-blind trial. Arch Intern Med 1998;158:1213–1220.
35. Riddell JG, Shanks RG. Effects of betaxolol, propranolol, and atenolol on isoproterenol-induced β-adrenoceptor responses. Clin Pharmacol Ther 1985;38:554–559.
36. Hauck RW, Schulz CH, Emslander HP, Bohm M. Pharmacological actions of the selective and non-selective β-adrenoreceptor antagonists celiprolol, bisoprolol and propranolol on human bronchi. Br J Pharmacol 1994;113:1043–1049.
37. Fraunfeder FT, Barker AF. Respiratory effects of timolol. N Engl J Med 1984;311:1441.
38. Dunn TL, Gerber MJ, Shen AS, et al. The effect of topical ophthalmic instillation of timolol and betaxolol on lung function in asthmatic subjects. Am Rev Respir Dis 1986;133:264–268.
39. Anonymous. Systemic adverse reactions with betaxolol eye drops. Med J Aust 1995;162:84.
40. Simon RA. Update on sulfite sensitivity. Allergy 1998;53:78–79.
41. Anibarro B, Caballero T, Garcia-Ara C, et al. Asthma with sulfite intolerance in children: A blocking study with cyanocobalamin. J Allergy Clin Immunol 1992;90:103–109.
42. Beasley R, Rafferty P, Holgate ST. Adverse reactions to the nondrug constituents of nebulizer solutions. Br J Clin Pharmacol 1988;25:283–287.
43. Zhang YG, Wright WJ, Tam WK, et al. Effect of inhaled preservatives on asthmatic subjects: II. Benzalkonium chloride. Am Rev Respir Dis 1990;141:1405–1408.
44. Beasley R, Fishwick, D, Miles JF, et al. Preservatives in nebulizer solutions: Risks without benefit. Pharmacotherapy 1998;18:130–139.
45. Asmus MJ, Barros MD, Liang J, et al. Pulmonary function response to EDTA, an additive in nebulized bronchodilators. J Allergy Clin Immunol 2001;107:68–72.
46. Greenberger PA. Contrast media reactions. J Allergy Clin Immunol 1984;74:600–605.
47. Tilles SA. Occupational latex allergy: Controversies in diagnosis and prognosis. Ann Allergy Asthma Immunol 1999;83:640–644.
48. Yunginger JW. Natural rubber latex allergy. In: Middleton E Jr, Reed CE, Ellis EF, et al. eds. Allergy Principles and Practice, 5th ed. St. Louis: CV Mosby, 1998;1073–1078.
49. Poley GE, Slater JE. Latex allergy. J Allergy Clin Immunol 2000;105:1054–1062.
50. Leynadier F, Herman D, Vervolet D, Andre C. Specific immunotherapy with a standardized latex extract versus placebo in allergic healthcare workers. J Allergy Clin Immunol 2000;106;585–590.
51. Sastre J, Fernandez-Nieto M, Rico P, et al. Specific immunotherapy with a standardized latex extract in allergic workers: A double-blind, placebo-controlled study. J Allergy Clin Immunol 2003;111:985–994.
52. Luque CA, Ortiz MV. Treatment of ACE inhibitor-induced cough. Pharmacotherapy 1999;19:804–810.
53. Sebastian JL, McKinney WP, Kaufman J, et al. Angiotensin-converting enzyme inhibitors and cough: Prevalence in an outpatient medical clinic population. Chest 1991;99:36–39.
54. Simon SR, Black HR, Moser M, Berland WE. Cough and ACE inhibitors. Arch Intern Med 1992;152:1698–1700.
55. Israili ZH, Hall WD. Cough and angioneurotic edema associated with angiotensin-converting enzyme inhibitor therapy: A review of the literature and pathophysiology. Ann Intern Med 1992;117:234–242.
56. Kaufman J, Casanova JE, Riendl P, et al. Bronchial hyperreactivity and cough due to angiotensin-converting enzyme inhibitors. Chest 1989;95:544–548.
57. Malini PL, Strocchi E, Zanardi M, et al. Thromboxane antagonism and cough induced by angiotensin-converting enzyme inhibitor. Lancet 1997;350:15–18.
58. Allen TL, Gora-Harper ML. Cromolyn sodium for ACE inhibitor-induced cough. Ann Pharmacother 1997;31:773–775.
59. Dicpinigaitis PV, Thomas SA, Sherman MB, et al. Losartan-induced bronchospasm. J Allergy Clin Immunol 1996;98:1128–1130.
60. Pylypchuk GB. ACE inhibitor- versus angiotensin II blocker-induced cough and angioedema. Ann Pharmacother 1998;32:1060–1066.
61. Cooper JAD, White DA, Matthay RA. Drug-induced pulmonary disease: 2. Noncytotoxic drugs. Am Rev Respir Dis 1986;133:488–505.
62. Henderson CA, Reynolds JE. Acute pulmonary edema in a young male after intravenous nalmefene. Anesth Analg 1997;84:218–219.
63. Copper JA Jr. Drug-induced lung disease. Adv Intern Med 1997;42:231–268.
64. Oshima T, Kasuya Y, Okumura Y, et al. Identification of independent risk factors for fentanyl-induced cough. Can J Anaesth 2006:53;753–758.
65. Obermiller T, Lakshminarayan S. Drug-induced hypersensitivity reactions in the lung. Immunol Allergy Clin North Am 1991;11:575–594.
66. Frank L, Massaro D. Oxygen toxicity. Am J Med 1980;69:117–126.
67. Jackson RM. Pulmonary oxygen toxicity. Chest 1985;88:900–905.
68. Elliott CG, Rasmusson BY, Crapo RO, et al. Prediction of pulmonary function abnormalities after adult respiratory distress syndrome (ARDS). Am Rev Respir Dis 1987;135:634–638.
69. Neff TA, Stocker R, Frey HR, et al. Long-term assessment of lung function in survivors of severe ARDS. Chest 2003;123:845–853.
70. Cooper JAD, White DA, Matthay RA. State of the art: Drug-induced pulmonary disease: 1. Cytotoxic drugs. Am Rev Respir Dis 1986;133:321–340.
71. Kehrer JP, Kacew S. Systematically applied chemicals that damage lung tissue. Toxicology 1985;35:251–293.
72. Clark JG, Hansen JA, Hertz MI, et al. Idiopathic pneumonia syndrome after bone marrow transplantation. Am Rev Respir Dis 1993;147:1601–1606.
73. Wiedemann HP. Toward an understanding of idiopathic pneumonia syndrome after bone marrow transplantation. Crit Care Med 1999;27:2040–2041.
74. Quabeck K. The lung as a critical organ in marrow transplantation. Bone Marrow Transplant 1994;14:S19–S28.
75. O'Driscoll BR, Hasleton PS, Taylor PM, et al. Active lung fibrosis up to 17 years after chemotherapy with carmustine (BCNU) in childhood. N Engl J Med 1990;323:378–382.
76. Rubio C, Hill ME, Milan S, et al. Idiopathic pneumonia syndrome after high-dose chemotherapy for relapsed Hodgkin's disease. Br J Cancer 1997;75:1044–1048.
77. Jantz MA, Sahn SA. Corticosteroids in acute respiratory failure. Am J Respir Crit Care Med 1999;160:1079–1100.
78. Lynch JP, McCune WJ. Immunosuppressive and cytotoxic pharmacotherapy for pulmonary disorders. Am J Crit Care 1997;155:395–420.
79. Rakita L, Sobol SM, Mostow N, et al. Amiodarone pulmonary toxicity. Am Heart J 1983;106:906–914.
80. Jessurun GAJ, Boersma WG, Crijns HJGM. Amiodarone-induced pulmonary toxicity: Predisposing factors, clinical symptoms and treatment. Drug Saf 1998;18:339–344.
81. Gleadhill IC, Wise RA, Schonfeld SA, et al. Serial lung-function testing in patients treated with amiodarone: A prospective study. Am J Med 1989;86:4–10.
82. Rubin LJ. Primary pulmonary hypertension. N Engl J Med 1997;336:111–117.
83. McCann UD, Seiden LS, Rubin LJ, Ricaurte GA. Brain serotonin neurotoxicity and primary pulmonary hypertension from fenfluramine and dexfenfluramine: A systematic review of the evidence. JAMA 1997;278;666–672.
84. Vivero LE, Anderson PO, Clark RF. Pharmacology in emergency medicine: A close look at fenfluramine and dexfenfluramine. J Emerg Med 1998;16:197–295.
85. Abenhaim L, Moride Y, Brenot F, et al. Appetite-suppressant drugs and the risk of primary pulmonary hypertension. N Engl J Med 1996;335:609–616.
86. Gurtner HP. Aminorex and pulmonary hypertension: A review. Cor Vasa 1985;27:160–171.

87. Brenot F, Herve P, Petitpretz P, et al. Primary pulmonary hypertension and fenfluramine use. Br Heart J 1993;70:537–541.
88. Simonneau G, Fartoukh M, Sitbon O, et al. Primary pulmonary hypertension associated with the use of fenfluramine derivatives. Chest 1998;114:195–199S.
89. Nall KC, Rubin LJ, Lipskind S, Sennesh JD. Reversible pulmonary hypertension associated with anorexigen use. Am J Med 1991;91:97–99.
90. Bever KA, Perry PJ. Dexfenfluramine hydrochloride: An anorexigenic agent. Am J Health Syst Pharm 1997;54:2059–2072.
91. Heuer L, Benoit W, Heydrich D. Diagnostic error: Pulmonary hypertension caused by an appetite suppressant (Mirapront). Chir Praxis 1978;23:497–504.
92. Schnabel KF, Schultz V, Busch S, Just H. Drug-induced primary vascular pulmonary hypertension. Med Welt 1976;27:1300–1303.

CHAPTER 32

Cystic Fibrosis

GARY MILAVETZ

KEY CONCEPTS

1. Cystic fibrosis is a disorder of the chloride ion transport in epithelial cells. It especially affects the cells that line the pulmonary and gastrointestinal systems, although the functions of other exocrine glands are altered.
2. The chloride ion transport dysfunction is multifaceted and results in thickened secretions that typically lead to obstruction, infection and inflammation in the affected systems. These in turn lead to the morbidity and mortality associated with cystic fibrosis.
3. Thickened secretions from the pancreas lead to deficiencies of digestive enzymes and bicarbonate, which leads to malabsorption of foodstuffs; malabsorption leads to maldigestion and malnutrition.
4. Treatment of the gastrointestinal component includes pancreatic enzyme and vitamin supplementation aimed at providing adequate nutritional needs.
5. Airway obstruction and pulmonary infection occur as a result of bacterial colonization and infection, thickened secretions and inflammation.
6. Acute antibiotic treatment is aimed at bacterial eradication while prophylactic treatment reduces the progression of the disease. *Pseudomonas aeruginosa* is the most common pathogen found in patients with cystic fibrosis.
7. The progression of pulmonary disease is prevented by a two-pronged approach. Reducing or eradicating inflammation decreases cellular and tissue alterations associated with cystic fibrosis. Reducing the bacterial burden in the pulmonary tree may decrease acute exacerbations and alter the disease course.
8. Gene therapy may be the treatment of the future but current trial results have been disappointing.
9. The goal of cystic fibrosis therapy is to slow or stop the progression of the disease and allow young patients to normally grow and develop and to have as normal of a lifestyle as possible.

Cystic fibrosis is the most common lethal, genetic disease in the white population. The disease mainly involves the exocrine glands and thus affects a number of organ systems (Table 32–1). The more common manifestations of this disease involve the gastrointestinal and pulmonary systems, with premature mortality associated with the latter. Most of the disease process results from a defect in electrolyte transport caused by a loss of functional chloride channels in epithelial cells. The protean nature of this disease dictates that care be multidisciplinary with a wide variety of therapeutic interventions.

Learning objectives, review questions, and other resources can be found at **www.pharmacotherapyonline.com.**

EPIDEMIOLOGY

Cystic fibrosis is primarily inherited through an autosomal (mendelian) recessive mode. Within a couple, with each parent being a carrier (heterozygous for the trait), a child has a 1:4 chance of having the disease, a 1:2 chance of being a carrier, and a 1:4 chance of being normal (having neither the disease nor the trait). The incidence of cystic fibrosis is greatest in the white population; it occurs in about 1 of every 2,000 live births in the United States.[1] Thus, the incidence of the trait (carrier state) in this group is approximately 5%. The frequency of this disease is considerably less in other races, occurring in about 1 in 17,000 blacks and in 1 in 90,000 Asians.[2]

After years of intensive research, the cystic fibrosis gene was identified and cloned in 1989.[3–5] The gene is located on the long arm of chromosome 7 and encodes for a protein called the cystic fibrosis transmembrane regulator (CFTR); this membrane protein functions as a chloride channel involved in the transport of electrolytes and water. In addition to the inherited recessive mutation affecting the CFTR protein, spontaneous mutation also occurs. More than 1,000 cystic fibrosis-associated mutations within the cystic fibrosis gene have been described, but the most common mutation involves a three-base pair deletion that results in the absence of a phenylalanine residue at position 508 of the CFTR protein.[3–5] This common mutation, referred to as the ΔF_{508} allele, is present in approximately 70% of patients in the United States. The mutations have been divided into four classes: I—defective protein production; II—defective protein processing; III—defective channel regulation; and IV—defective channel conductance.[6] Patients homozygous for the ΔF_{508} mutation, which falls primarily into class II, tend to be diagnosed at an earlier age, owing to a greater frequency of pancreatic insufficiency (99% vs. 72% in heterozygotes and 36% in patients with other genotypes).[7,8]

PATHOPHYSIOLOGY

Cystic fibrosis is a disease of epithelia, especially those cells lining the intestinal tract, pancreatic ducts, hepatobiliary tree, vas deferens, sweat ducts, and airway lumen. In the normal state, these epithelial cells can transport chloride through CFTR chloride channels with sodium and water accompanying this ion flux. (1) Chloride transport through CFTR channels is activated by protein kinases in response to an increase in the intracellular second messenger, cyclic adenosine 3′,5′-monophosphate.[9] In cystic fibrosis, a loss of functional CFTR

TABLE 32-1 Organ Involvement in Cystic Fibrosis

Organ System/ Organ	Abnormality	Consequence
Gastrointestinal		
Pancreas	Digestive enzyme deficiency	Maldigestion
		Malnutrition
	Insulin deficiency	Glucose intolerance
Intestines	Viscous secretions	Obstruction
Liver	Biliary cirrhosis/fatty infiltration	Portal hypertension/ esophageal varices
Pulmonary	Viscous secretions	Chronic obstruction
	Infection	Endobronchial infection
Sweat glands	Failure to reabsorb sodium	Hyponatremia
Reproductive	Obstruction of epididymis, vas deferens, and seminal vesicles	Aspermia
	Viscous cervical mucus	Decreased fertility
Hematologic	Chronic disease?	Anemia
Bone and joint	Unknown	Arthritis, osteopenia

chloride channels leads to defective cyclic adenosine 3′,5′-monophosphate-stimulated chloride transport; in most epithelia, this defect results in decreased chloride secretion and increased sodium absorption (Fig. 32–1). ❷ Defective electrolyte transport is thought to alter the volume or composition of the fluid secreted by the pancreas, hepatobiliary tree, reproductive tract, sweat gland, and the airways.

GASTROINTESTINAL TRACT

The gastrointestinal tract may be involved in cystic fibrosis with either intestinal obstruction or deficient secretion of digestive enzymes by the pancreas. In 10% to 16% of cystic fibrosis patients, the first gastrointestinal manifestation of the disease is small bowel obstruction, which is evident shortly after birth and known as *meconium ileus.* In these patients, the basic electrolyte transport defect is thought to cause abnormally tenacious meconium that cannot be evacuated. A similar condition, known as *distal intestinal obstruction syndrome* or *meconium ileus equivalent,* occurs in older cystic fibrosis patients; it is also thought to result from abnormally tenacious gastrointestinal secretions and fecal impaction. Other intestinal complications include intussusception, volvulus, gastroesophageal reflux, atresia, perforation, giant cystic meconium peritonitis, and rectal prolapse.

A relative deficiency of pancreatic digestive enzymes (pancreatic achylia) is present with most genotypes and is clinically apparent in 85% of patients. Pancreatic lesions including fibrosis, fatty replacement, and cyst formation are secondary to obstruction of small pancreatic ducts by thickened secretions and cellular debris. Inspissated eosinophilic material may accumulate in the acini and ductules. As a result, the volume of pancreatic secretions and the concentration of pancreatic enzymes and bicarbonate are reduced. Affected enzyme concentrations include trypsin, chymotrypsin, carboxypeptidase, amylase, and lipase. This leads to a maldigestion of ingested nutrients,

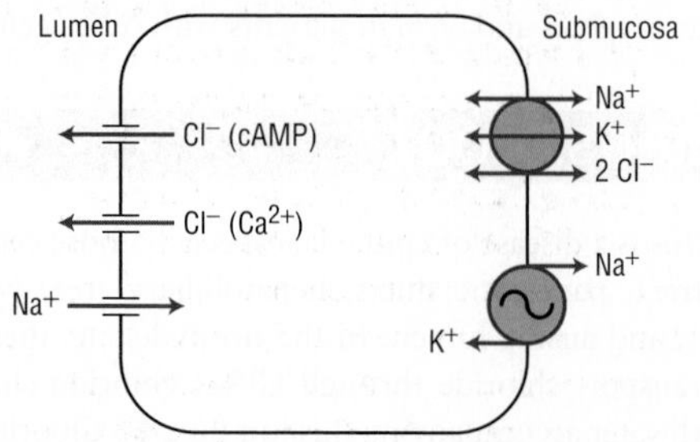

FIGURE 32-1. Electrolyte transport in the airway epithelial cell. The cystic fibrosis transmembrane regulator is the cyclic-3′,5′-AMP (cAMP)-dependent chloride channel.

including fats and protein. Increased fecal losses of bile acids (binding to undigested fecal fat decreases enterohepatic recycling) also may contribute to fat maldigestion. The maldigestion brings added foodstuffs into the colon, reducing transit time and contributing to additional malnutrition. ❸

Because of the lipase deficiency, fat-soluble vitamin (A, D, E, and K) deficiencies may occur. ❹ Whether lipase activity or bile acids (e.g., in micelle formation) are involved in fat-soluble vitamin absorption with steatorrhea is unclear. Vitamin B_{12} and zinc deficiencies also may occur as a result of pancreatic enzyme deficiency. Although pancreatic involvement is predominantly and initially exocrine in nature, insulin deficiency with glucose intolerance also occurs in cystic fibrosis patients, especially as they advance in age. This probably occurs as a result of chronic inflammatory changes causing fibrotic changes to the entire pancreas including the endocrine function. Carbohydrate intolerance is characterized by low insulin concentrations and enhanced peripheral sensitivity to insulin, but not by the presence of islet cell or antiinsulin antibodies. Carbohydrate intolerance in cystic fibrosis is not usually associated with the ketosis as commonly occurs in type 1 diabetes. This complication involves an increase in the number of insulin receptors with decreased affinity for insulin. Despite a concomitant increase in tissue affinity for insulin, 8% of cystic fibrosis children older than 12 years of age require insulin therapy.

The liver can be involved in cystic fibrosis. Biliary cirrhosis secondary to bile duct obstruction occurs in as many as 18% of patients, whereas fatty infiltration occurs in approximately 30% of patients in a pattern unrelated to nutritional status. Bile ducts may be obstructed by inspissated mucus which may lead to focal or multilobar cirrhosis.[10] Such hepatic involvement can occur at any age, but is more common with advancing age and can lead to portal hypertension, esophageal varices and hypersplenism. The most common laboratory abnormality associated with hepatic involvement is elevated serum hepatic isoenzymes (γ-glutamyltranspeptidase, alanine aminotransferase, aspartate aminotransferase, and alkaline phosphatase).

PULMONARY SYSTEM

The pulmonary manifestations of cystic fibrosis result from an incompletely characterized defect in innate host defenses at the airway surface including an exaggerated inflammatory response, defective bactericidal activity, and altered mucus clearance.[11–13] Chronic bacterial endobronchitis is the essential disease process that defines the pulmonary component of cystic fibrosis. ❺ The three factors influencing the endobronchitis are airway infection, inflammation, and obstruction. Together, these culminate in long-term airway destruction. The ongoing controversy of which comes first—inflammation or infection—was studied in an effort to clarify this issue. Children diagnosed with cystic fibrosis detected by newborn screening but lacking signs and symptoms of infection were compared to controls with chronic stridor. In this group of children with cystic fibrosis, inflammation seems to be initiated and sustained by infection.[14] Other pathophysiology aspects of airways disease in cystic fibrosis are the defects found in natural pulmonary defenses and especially mucus clearance.[15] The mucus glands in cystic fibrosis appear to have defective anion-mediated fluid secretion resulting in hyposecretion rather than hyperabsorption of fluid.[16] Regulation of airway surface liquid also is an important part of the normal pulmonary defense system. Patients with cystic fibrosis are only partially able to adjust airway surface liquid volume related to the lack of CFTR.[17] The airway surface liquid in patients with cystic fibrosis also appears to be deficient in the antimicrobial factors that are present in normal airway surface liquid. The understanding of how defective CFTR influences the disease process has improved although a clear comprehension and its implications for disease treatment is still elusive.

The combination of persistent obstruction along with inflammation often leads to air trapping, atelectasis, and, eventually, bronchiectasis that progresses until respiratory insufficiency develops. The lung disease usually progresses from small airway obstruction to more generalized airway obstruction, and, finally, toward a component of restrictive lung disease as individual segments become completely obstructed and nonfunctional. Hyperinflation or dilation of the air spaces is a common finding. Furthermore, persistent obstruction of the small airways with mucus, an excellent culture medium for microorganisms, may facilitate the growth of bacteria within an extracellular matrix or biofilm, making the infection relatively resistant to antibiotics. Although bacterial infections are thought to be a major contributor to cystic fibrosis airway disease, viruses and other nonbacterial pathogens also play an important pathologic role.[13,18,19] Environmental factors, such as exposure to tobacco smoke, may also contribute.[20]

The three most common bacterial pathogens isolated from the respiratory secretions (sputum) of cystic fibrosis patients are *Staphylococcus aureus, Pseudomonas aeruginosa,* and *Haemophilus influenzae,* with *P. aeruginosa* usually predominating throughout life. *Proteus, Klebsiella* species and *Stenotrophomonas maltophilia* are observed less frequently. Mucoid strains (alginate producers) of *P. aeruginosa* commonly observed in cystic fibrosis may be particularly resistant to antibiotics,[21] as are nonmotile forms. The isolation of *Burkholderia cepacia* from the sputum of cystic fibrosis patients has become more common at some cystic fibrosis centers. The significance of this contagious organism varies from one patient to the next. Three fairly distinct syndromes associated with this *B. cepacia* have been described, these being asymptomatic colonization, chronic deterioration with intermittent fever and weight loss, and rapid, usually fatal, deterioration.[22] The nature of the initially cultured oropharyngeal flora in patients younger than 2 years of age has prognostic significance. The finding of *P. aeruginosa* or *P. aeruginosa* plus *S. aureus* in initial cultures appears related to increased morbidity and mortality, respectively.[23]

The presence of the above bacteria contributes to the destructive changes in the airways of cystic fibrosis patients by direct damage from bacterial toxins and the body's immune reaction to these bacteria. For example, *P. aeruginosa* elaborates a number of extracellular toxins, proteases, hemolysins, and exopolysaccharides, which may be responsible for direct airway damage, increased mucin production by the airway epithelium, and the production of immune complexes (immunoglobulins G and M) which may contribute to local damage. Elevated levels of such mediators as granulocyte elastase, tumor necrosis factor-α, interleukins 1 and 2, and related complexes with associated inhibitors are well documented in cystic fibrosis patients. One inflammatory mediator that clearly contributes to pulmonary pathophysiology is neutrophil elastase. Present in excess, it overwhelms and neutralizes native antiproteases (α_1-antitrypsin and secretory leukocyte protease inhibitor), destroys structural fibers, and inhibits complement-mediated phagocytosis and antipseudomonal antibodies. Combined with other inflammatory mediators, a self-sustaining vicious cycle leading to progressive and often permanent tissue damage is established. The neutrophil influx that is part of this cycle results in release of neutrophil-derived DNA, which is thought to contribute to sputum viscosity. The occasional presence of *Aspergillus fumigatus* in the sputum of these patients may also contribute to the pulmonary pathology because it can induce a steroid-responsive allergic reaction.

The consequence of these pulmonary processes is a decrease in gas exchange by the lungs. The challenge of moving air through obstructed airways often requires the use of accessory muscles, resulting in an increased anterior–posterior chest diameter (also referred to as "barrel chest"), a flattened diaphragm, and pulmonary hypertension. The increased work of breathing in these patients produces a relative exercise intolerance and increased resting energy expenditure. Hemoptysis secondary to bronchiectasis occurs but is seldom massive. Other respiratory complications include gastroesophageal reflux, pneumothorax, and right-sided heart failure (cor pulmonale), secondary to the pulmonary hypertension. Although seldom overt clinically, the findings of right ventricular hypertrophy, increased heart weight, and right atrial and right ventricular chamber dilation are usually present at autopsy. Digital clubbing, a common finding in cystic fibrosis as well as in other chronic pulmonary conditions, may be related to chronic hypoxia.

The upper respiratory tract is also commonly involved in cystic fibrosis. Sinusitis and nasal polyposis occur in 90% and 50% of patients, respectively.[24] Sinusitis is chronic in character and acute symptoms are unusual. Although its etiology is not entirely clear, sinusitis may result from obstruction of the sinus ducts, thus preventing drainage. The bacteria generally isolated in these cases include *P. aeruginosa, H. influenzae,* streptococci, and anaerobes. Usually, the same strain of *P. aeruginosa* found in the lungs is present in the upper airways (nasopharynx and sinuses), which may represent a reservoir for the pathogen.

SWEAT GLANDS

Abnormally high concentrations of sodium and chloride are found in the sweat of cystic fibrosis patients as a result of defective chloride absorption across the water-impermeable sweat duct epithelium. This forms the basis for measuring sweat chloride concentration as a diagnostic test for cystic fibrosis. This defect in salt absorption rarely causes clinical symptoms except in warmer environments or during hot weather, when excessive sweating may lead to salt depletion; this clinical problem can be prevented by supplementing the diet with salt. In the sweat coil where salt and water are excreted into the gland lumen, sodium and chloride are not excreted at abnormally high concentrations in cystic fibrosis because chloride is secreted through chloride channels other than the CFTR. However, as sweat progresses through the sweat duct toward the skin surface, chloride absorption across the water-impermeable epithelium is reduced because of a loss of CFTR chloride channels. Similar abnormalities can be seen in the excretions of the salivary glands.

REPRODUCTIVE SYSTEM

Approximately 95% of males with cystic fibrosis are sterile because of obstruction of the epididymis, vas deferens, and seminal vesicles resulting in aspermia. There is late maturation of the reproductive system with delayed onset of puberty in both sexes. Females also have reduced fertility owing to the production of abnormal cervical mucus. Menstrual irregularity and oligomenorrhea are also common. Nonetheless, owing to greater life expectancy in these patients, increasing numbers are becoming mothers. In these individuals, the course and tolerance of pregnancy are related to the pregravid nutritional and pulmonary status.

HEMATOLOGIC SYSTEM

Anemia is observed in some cystic fibrosis patients despite chronic hypoxia. The apparent deficient erythroid response occurs, at least in part, from disturbances in erythropoietin regulation and iron availability (impaired gastrointestinal absorption). Despite chronic hypoxia in some patients with cystic fibrosis, erythropoietin concentrations are normal or low. The condition is characterized by decreased hematocrit and serum ferritin, increased carboxyhemoglobin, and normal or low hemoglobin. Many patients may have iron deficiency as a consequence of decreased dietary intake, malabsorption, or blood loss.

BONES AND JOINTS

Arthritis may occur in cystic fibrosis and can take one of several forms.[25] The arthritis may be either mono- or polyarticular and is usually nondestructive. An episodic form is most common and may be a result of immune complexes formed in response to the chronic pulmonary infections. Hypertrophic osteoarthropathy occurs in cystic fibrosis as it does in association with other pulmonary diseases. The incidence of arthritis may be increasing as median survival age increases. Osteopenia and osteoporosis also occur more frequently in adults with cystic fibrosis. The causes of the resultant bone demineralization are multifactorial and include vitamin D malabsorption, decreased vitamin D conversion (via sunlight), delayed puberty and endocrine development, poor nutrition, limited physical activity, and chronic acidosis.

CLINICAL PRESENTATION

The clinical findings of cystic fibrosis develop as a direct consequence of the pathophysiologic processes described above. Thus, the clinical findings can be conveniently subdivided by organ system.

GASTROINTESTINAL SYSTEM

Intestinal symptoms are usually secondary to either intestinal obstruction or maldigestion of nutrients. Obstruction, manifested as meconium ileus, distal intestinal obstruction syndrome or intussusception, causes abdominal distension, pain, vomiting, or a change in stool output.

More commonly, the gastrointestinal symptoms of cystic fibrosis are caused by maldigestion of food causing steatorrhea and malnutrition. The stools are foul odorous, bulky, greasy, and more frequent in number; rectal prolapse may occur, especially in the presence of excessive weight loss. The stool's high fat content results from a relative lipase deficiency. Perhaps the most significant consequence of maldigestion is malnutrition; that is, cystic fibrosis children characteristically fall below their age-related norms for both weight and height.

PULMONARY SYSTEM

The respiratory symptoms of cystic fibrosis are usually those of obstructive airway disease such as coughing, sputum production, labored breathing, wheezing, retractions, pleurisy, and cyanosis. Digital clubbing is a common finding thought to be associated with bronchiectasis. Increased anterior–posterior chest diameter, a flattened diaphragm, and hyperaeration may be noted on chest roentgenogram.

The respiratory status usually follows a cyclical pattern, from a state of relative well-being to one of acute pulmonary deterioration theoretically paralleling the course of the airway infection. There may be significant declines in pulmonary function referred to as acute respiratory exacerbations and generally associated with symptoms of bacterial endobronchial infection. Common pathogens found in the lungs of a cystic fibrosis patient include *S. aureus, H. influenzae* and *P. aeruginosa*. Less-common pathogen include *S. maltophilia* and *B. cepacia*, which used to be referred to as *Pseudomonas cepacia*. Increased coughing, increased sputum production, changes in sputum character (e.g., thicker and darker in color), tachypnea, dyspnea, increasing oxygen requirement, and a decrease in exercise tolerance are common. Symptoms of chronic sinusitis and nasal polyposis may include nasal obstruction, pain over affected sinuses, and anosmia.

Concomitantly, laboratory testing of peripheral blood may reveal an increased white blood count with increased polymorphonuclear leukocytes and immature forms consistent with an acute infection. Tests of pulmonary function often demonstrate both intermittent and persistent decreases in forced vital capacity, forced expiratory volume at 1 second (FEV_1), and increased residual volume. Tests of small airway function are more markedly affected as the pulmonary disease progresses. Arterial blood gases may reveal hypoxia or hypercapnia as the disease progresses.

OTHER SIGNS AND SYMPTOMS

The relative insulin deficiency observed in older cystic fibrosis patients is often asymptomatic and only detected on laboratory analysis of serum performed for other reasons. However, cystic fibrosis-related diabetes may present as a recent decline in weight without the typical gastrointestinal symptoms of malabsorption. They may also present as untreated cases of diabetes mellitus type 2. Cor pulmonale is not usually clinically evident unless signs of left-sided heart failure ensue, although enlargement in cardiac size may be noted on routine chest roentgenogram prior to that time. Signs and symptoms of anemia and arthritis with cystic fibrosis patients do not differ from those caused by other chronic diseases.

Excessive losses of sodium and chloride in the sweat of cystic fibrosis patients seldom result in symptoms of heat prostration, but this phenomenon may cause a "salty" taste on the skin.

DIAGNOSIS

The diagnosis of cystic fibrosis is usually made on the basis of elevated sweat chloride concentrations (sweat chloride testing)[26] and may be confirmed with CFTR mutational analysis. Another test, recording the potential difference across the nasal epithelium is usually reserved for cases in which the results of sweat testing and mutational analysis are nondiagnostic.[27] For sweat chloride determination, two samples of sweat are collected with the use of pilocarpine iontophoresis and the concentration of chloride in each sample is measured. Duplicate sweat chloride concentrations of 60 mEq/L or more are considered diagnostic of cystic fibrosis. However, a number of disorders, such as adrenal insufficiency, hypothyroidism, protein calorie malnutrition, anorexia nervosa, ectodermal dysplasia, mucopolysaccharidosis, nephrosis with edema, type 1 glycogen storage disease, familial hypoparathyroidism syndrome, fucosidosis, nephrogenic diabetes insipidus, and Mauriac syndrome may be associated with elevated sweat chloride concentrations, but generally these conditions do not present a problem in the differential diagnosis of cystic fibrosis. Ninety-eight percent of cystic fibrosis patients will have a sweat chloride concentration 60 mEq/L or greater. The remaining 2% usually have sweat chloride concentrations between 50 and 60 mEq/L and the test may have to be repeated one or more times to obtain definitive results. Nevertheless, the results of sweat testing alone may not be able to confirm the presence or absence of cystic fibrosis. The presence of chronic obstructive respiratory disease, exocrine pancreatic insufficiency, and/or a positive family history of the disease may also provide additional support for the diagnosis. Genetic (CFTR mutation) analysis and recording of nasal transepithelial potential difference may be helpful in making a diagnosis. Genetic (CFTR mutation) analysis may be used to confirm the diagnosis in utero or to detect heterozygotes (carriers) with obvious implications for genetic counseling. Newborn screening for the disease has been adopted in some states, though the benefits of making a presymptomatic diagnosis on long-term outcome are still being assessed.[28]

COURSE

Cystic fibrosis is a heterogeneous disease in terms of initial presentation, organ involvement, and clinical course. Some children are diagnosed at birth because of meconium ileus, which occurs in approximately 16%

of people with cystic fibrosis. Neonatal screening programs are increasing, but the benefits of presymptomatic diagnosis are still being assessed; prenatal diagnosis is early in its implementation. Most patients are diagnosed by 1 year of age because of a history of steatorrhea and poor weight gain. The median age at diagnosis is 7 months and most patients are diagnosed by 12 years of age.[29]

The course of the disease after diagnosis varies from one patient to another. A patient may have a rapid downhill course from early pulmonary involvement, while another may suffer only from gastrointestinal complaints for many years without significant pulmonary symptoms. Although the expected life span of cystic fibrosis patients has increased to longer than 30 years of age in the last two decades, some patients still die early in life, secondary to a fulminant pulmonary process. Still others, owing to minimal involvement and a mild course, may not be diagnosed until their second decade of life. The increased longevity now realized with early diagnosis and aggressive treatment may have led to an increase in formerly less-common complications such as diabetes and hepatic disease. Two-year mortality rates greater than 50% are associated with an FEV_1 less than 30% of predicted, PaO_2 less than 50 mm Hg, or PCO_2 greater than 50 mm Hg.[30]

TREATMENT

Cystic Fibrosis

■ DESIRED OUTCOME

The desired pharmacotherapeutic outcomes for cystic fibrosis are both long- and short-term. ❾ In the long-term, one obviously tries to halt or delay progression of the disease to allow for normal growth and development. In the short-term, acute problems must be dealt with. The ultimate goal of pharmacotherapy for the gastrointestinal involvement of cystic fibrosis is optimal nutrition. On a day-to-day basis, normal bowel habits, continued weight gain, and normal vitamin levels are desirable. The goal of therapy for the pulmonary component is to reduce the signs and symptoms of airway infection, inflammation, and obstruction. Thus, antibiotic, antiinflammatory, bronchodilator, and mucolytic therapy are geared toward treating the complications that compromise lung function. For an acute pulmonary exacerbation, a return of pulmonary function to the preexacerbation status is the central goal of therapy.

■ GENERAL APPROACH TO TREATMENT

The Cystic Fibrosis Foundation has published clinical guidelines for the diagnosis and care of cystic fibrosis patients, including applicable pharmacotherapy.[31] The following information is generally in agreement with those guidelines, although it may contain more current information. The interested reader is referred to that publication for more detail on the drug treatment of cystic fibrosis and its various complications.

Gastrointestinal System

The treatment of gastrointestinal involvement is ultimately aimed at correcting the nutritional deficit present in many patients.[32] ❹ In addition to the pancreatic enzyme replacement and other drug therapy described below, nutritional supplementation is frequently employed. Nutritional interventions range from behavioral modification to nocturnal feedings via gastrostomies.[33]

Pancreatic Enzyme Supplementation The backbone of gastrointestinal therapy in cystic fibrosis is pancreatic enzyme replacement or supplementation.[34] The preferred products are microencapsulated pancreatic enzymes, although powders are marketed and are useful in patients unable to swallow capsules or to otherwise use the microencapsulated beads they contain. Microencapsulated products protect the contained enzymes from destruction by gastric acid and may be given in much lower doses than their predecessors, which were susceptible to acid breakdown. Most contemporary enzyme replacement products vary mainly in enzyme content per capsule, with lipase content being the chief variable. Table 32–2 lists representative products and their contents are presented. Infants are normally given 2,000 to 4,000 lipase units per 120 mL of formula or breast milk, which provides 450 to 900 lipase units per gram of ingested fat. In general, patients require 500 to 4,000 lipase units per gram of ingested fat, with the average pediatric or adult patient requiring 1,800 units per gram of fat. Enzymes may also be dosed based on weight, with an initial dose of 1,000 lipase units being administered per kilogram of body weight per meal. One-half that amount is administered with snacks.

Before the introduction of microencapsulated enzyme products, various maneuvers were used to circumvent or overcome the problem of acid breakdown. The most obvious of these was to administer large quantities of enzyme product. Enteric-coated (microencapsulated) pancreatic enzymes have largely solved this problem. The occasional patient may yet require large quantities of even the microencapsulated enzyme product. Whether such difficulties are caused by residual acid breakdown or perhaps low pH in the upper small intestine (secondary to deficient bicarbonate excretion by the pancreas) resulting in a failure to dissolve the coating of the microencapsulated beads is unknown. Defective enteric coating on some generic brands has also been described and led to FDA reclassification of these products, requiring bioequivalence data. Histamine H_2-receptor antagonists and proton pump inhibitors have been used to reduce the enzyme dose when residual acid breakdown of enzymes is suspected. Another possible maneuver is

TABLE 32-2 Pancreatic Enzyme Products

Trade Name	Manufacturer	Lipase	Protease	Amylase	Form[a]
Ku-Zyme	Schwarz Pharma	8,000	30,000	30,000	C
Pancrease	McNeil	4,000	25,000	20,000	ECM
Pancrease MT4		4,000	12,000	12,000	ECM
Pancrease MT10		10,000	30,000	30,000	ECM
Pancrease MT16		16,000	48,000	48,000	ECM
Pancrease MT20		20,000	65,000	65,000	C
Pancrelipase	Geneva	4,000	25,000	20,000	ECM
Ultrase		4,500	25,000	20,000	C
Ultrase MT12	Scandipharm	12,000	39,000	39,000	ECM
Ultrase MT20		20,000	65,000	65,000	ECM
Ultrase MT18		24,000	78,000	78,000	ECM
Viokase 8	Robins	8,000	30,000	30,000	T
Viokase		16,800	20,000	70,000	P[b]

[a]Dosage form: C, capsule; ECM, enteric-coated microspheres or beads; T, tablet; P, powder.
[b]Viokase powder, units of enzymes per 700 mg.

to administer both microencapsulated and non–enteric-coated enzyme products (e.g., powder) concomitantly.

For patients who are unable to swallow capsules, the contents may be emptied into applesauce, jelly, or some other nonalkaline vehicle, provided the patient does not chew the microencapsulated beads. Side effects are uncommon with pancreatic enzyme products. Perianal irritation resembling diaper rash may occur in infants fed excess quantities of enzyme powders. Hyperuricosuria has also been reported to occur secondary to pancreatic enzyme use, apparently related to the high purine content of the products. Proximal colonic stricture (fibrosing colonopathy) is a dose-related side effect associated with lipase doses in excess of 24,000 units/kg/day.[35]

Vitamin Supplementation Patients should receive multivitamin tablets daily to provide adequate water-soluble vitamins along with reasonable amounts of vitamins D and K. ❹ Although clinically evident fat-soluble vitamin deficiencies are unusual in those patients who are taking adequate pancreatic enzymes and receiving a balanced diet, obvious vitamin K deficiency, manifested as bleeding diathesis, can occur. Demineralization of bone has also been described and vitamin E deficiency has been related to neurologic dysfunction. In addition, appropriate laboratory tests (serum carotene, vitamin E, and cholecalciferol concentrations) will often help document other deficiencies, leading to recommendations for additional supplementation of these vitamins. Water-miscible vitamin A, 4,000 international units/day, and vitamin E, 100 to 400 international units/day should also be administered either singly or in the form of a water-miscible combination product (containing vitamins A, D, E, and K). Vitamin K, in a dose of 5 mg twice weekly, should be given to those patients with prolonged international normalized ratio. It should also be noted that appropriately adjusted doses of fat-soluble preparations may be more cost-effective than their water-miscible counterparts (e.g., 800 international units fat-soluble vitamin E vs. 200 international units water-miscible vitamin E).[36]

Treating Meconium Ileus and Distal Intestinal Obstruction Syndrome The treatment of meconium ileus or distal intestinal obstruction syndrome can sometimes be limited to the use of enemas with isoosmolar contrast. Unfortunately, surgery (bowel resection and primary anastomosis) is often necessary to treat meconium ileus and prevent its complications. Distal intestinal obstruction syndrome usually responds to management by oral or nasogastric administration of electrolyte lavage solutions. The adequacy of enzyme dosage should also be reassessed in the face of distal intestinal obstruction.

Prevention and Treatment of Cirrhosis Ursodeoxycholic acid, a bile acid with choleretic properties, has been shown to produce morphologic and functional improvement in affected patients. The effects are dose related and 15 to 20 mg/kg/d has been used, sometimes in combination with taurine supplementation.[37] Administering this agent prophylactically to patients at risk for liver disease, if feasible, has been proposed.[38]

Cardiovascular System

Various modalities have been used in attempts to treat pulmonary hypertension and secondary cor pulmonale of cystic fibrosis. These treatments, which include the use of vasodilators, inotropic agents, and diuretics, have all resulted in limited and transient effects. This is most likely due to the fact that none of these modes of therapy address the underlying cause of the cor pulmonale, hypoxia. Likewise, supplemental (often nocturnal) oxygen treatment has also failed to affect mortality rates or disease progression, although it does appear to prevent oxygen desaturation that occurs with exercise as well as that occurring during sleep. Thus, the most beneficial approach may be to attempt to improve oxygenation with aggressive pulmonary therapy.

Pulmonary System

Management of the pulmonary component of cystic fibrosis can be broken down into three general areas: antiobstructive, antiinflammatory, and antiinfective therapy.[39]

Antiobstructive Therapy The cornerstone of pulmonary therapy is percussion and postural drainage, which aids in the clearance of pulmonary mucus and is performed once or twice daily in "healthy" patients and as often as six times daily during acute pulmonary exacerbations. ❼ New flutter devices may also be useful adjuncts in this regard. A flutter device is a hand-held unit that produces vibrations in the airways when exhaled through. These vibrations loosen and facilitate the removal of mucus and secretions from the airways. Percussion is sometimes preceded by nebulizer therapy during which nebulized sterile water or 0.9% sodium chloride solution is breathed to liquefy pulmonary secretions. Bronchodilators may be added to the nebulizer solution to prevent bronchospasm and mucolytic agents (e.g., *N*-acetylcysteine; Mucomyst, Bristol-Myers Squibb Company, Princeton, NJ) may be added to liquefy pulmonary secretions or enhance mucus clearance. Although the effects of bronchodilators administered by inhalation can be demonstrated with pulmonary function testing, the efficacy of mucolytic agents are not readily demonstrated. Moreover, many patients prefer not to use *N*-acetylcysteine because of its unpleasant taste and odor and because it may induce bronchospasm. Normal saline and sodium bicarbonate solution may be administered by aerosol as aids to sputum expectoration, but documentation of efficacy is elusive.

Recombinant human DNAse has been approved for use in cystic fibrosis. When given by inhalation (2.5 mg once or twice daily), Rh DNAse reduces the viscosity of cystic fibrosis sputum and leads to statistically significant, though modest, improvement in pulmonary function.[40] More importantly, the regular use of Rh DNAse may help decrease the incidence of (or lengthen the time between) respiratory exacerbations, thereby improving their quality of life and indirectly decreasing the overall costs of care in patients with mild to moderate disease. Should these outcomes be borne out in additional long-term studies, especially before the onset of clinical symptoms, this therapy may be justified as a way to prevent or delay the progression of pulmonary disease.

Hypertonic saline inhalation recently came to light as an additional therapy to slow the progression of lung damage associated with cystic fibrosis.[41,42] A 7% solution has generally been used, although other concentrations have been used with similar results. Unfortunately, this product is not commercially available, so it must be extemporaneously compounded. Because of the hypertonic nature of the solution, this solution is associated with an increased incidence of local bothersome respiratory symptoms even though it is safe and effective. Preceding hypertonic saline therapy with a bronchodilator may reduce the incidence of these bothersome symptoms. This therapy may be used concurrently with other inhaled treatments, but should not be mixed with other nebulizer solutions, as it will change the osmolarity of the resulting solution. As with other nebulized therapies, to assure appropriate delivery it should only be used with the recommended nebulizer.

Because some cystic fibrosis patients have a component of reactive airway disease that may contribute to their pulmonary disease, systemic bronchodilators such as theophylline and β-agonists may provide some benefit. Recurrent wheezing or dyspnea that improves with bronchodilators represents a legitimate indication for these agents; however, responsiveness to such agents (>15% improvement in FEV_1) should be documented, before a protracted course is begun. Standard antiasthmatic doses of most bronchodilators should be appropriate for cystic fibrosis patients, although theophylline clearance may differ in cystic fibrosis patients and bioavailability of some products may be decreased, sometimes necessitating the use of higher-than-usual doses.[43] Because of the necessity of pharmacokinetic monitoring and its involvement in a number of common drug interactions, theophylline should be considered second-line bronchodilator therapy at most in these patients. Because cystic fibrosis patients are at high risk to develop complications from influenza, the influenza vaccine should be administered on a yearly basis, and amantadine prophylaxis or treatment may be indicated as well. Other interventions that would be appropriate include immunization for influenza, pneumococcal infections and *H. influenzae.*

Antiinflammatory Therapy In an attempt to block the consequences of the inflammatory component of this disease, corticosteroid therapy has been evaluated. ❼ Although results of preliminary trials were encouraging, a large, multicenter, placebo-controlled trial found that alternate-day prednisone treatment at 2 mg/kg to have beneficial effects on pulmonary function, but undesirable effects on linear growth and glucose metabolism.[44] Further analysis of the data from this same study suggested that the benefits of a 1 mg/kg dose might outweigh the risks.[45] Data concerning the efficacy of inhaled corticosteroids are scant. A long-term trial of oral ibuprofen indicates a beneficial effect by slowing the rate of progression of pulmonary disease.[46] Unfortunately, therapeutic drug monitoring (periodic determination of ibuprofen serum concentrations) is required.

Antibiotic Therapy Young children with cystic fibrosis have an extended period of time, perhaps months or years, when they have no evidence of airway infection. Later, they develop a mild airway infection or early bacterial colonization often without associated symptoms. However, bronchoalveolar lavage fluid reveals evidence of infection and inflammation (high neutrophil count with a predominance of proinflammatory cytokines). ❻ Eventually, they develop a chronic airway infection that cannot be fully eradicated, not even with prolonged use of systemic or topical antibiotics. This scenario is best explained by the ability of bacteria such as *P. aeruginosa* to achieve high-density growth within small airways whereby they become organized into a community that grows more slowly and secretes an extracellular matrix that protects the bacteria from local host defenses and/or most antibiotics. This complex growth pattern is referred to as a biofilm community. Acute exacerbations of cystic fibrosis are thought to involve satellite foci of bacterial proliferation that stimulate mucus production in response to bacterial exoproducts, worsening airway obstruction as a consequence of the host's proinflammatory response.

Because of the complexities of bacterial infections in cystic fibrosis, antibiotics are used with three different goals in mind. ❻ First, before an infection develops the primary goal is to detect infections early in their course so that treatment is successful at preventing the bacteria from developing into a biofilm community (bacterial eradication). Second, once biofilm growth has become established, the primary goal is to use antibiotics to prevent rapid bacterial proliferation (bacterial suppression) to avoid excess sputum production, decreased lung function, and the concomitant loss of appetite and weight. Finally, once an acute exacerbation has developed, the primary goal is to eliminate bacterial proliferation, reduce the bacterial load and the degree of sputum production, return lung function to the preexacerbation (target) value, improve nutritional intake and to correct any weight losses (treatment of acute exacerbations).

However, the use of antibiotics in cystic fibrosis is somewhat controversial and certainly challenging. ❻ Controversy exists because innate host defenses in cystic fibrosis may certainly be sufficient to eliminate most pathogens including *P. aeruginosa* from the airways. Without antibiotics, some patients with cystic fibrosis appear to go many years before they develop typical airway infections caused by *P. aeruginosa*. In addition, some cystic fibrosis patients have transiently positive throat and bronchoalveolar lavage cultures for *P. aeruginosa* that resolve without exogenous antibiotics. Thus, it is unclear when antibiotics are actually needed to help eradicate these pathogens. Moreover, once bacterial eradication with antibiotics is accomplished, will some other organism soon initiate another airway infection? In other words, are the early stages of bacterial colonization merely a marker for a decrease in host defenses? Does this decrease in host defense persist suggesting that repeated courses of antibiotics will be required regardless of whether eradication therapy was successful? The answers to these questions remain unknown, thus the use of antibiotics in cystic fibrosis lung disease is controversial.

The chronic use of antibiotics to suppress bacteria in cystic fibrosis is controversial because antibiotic resistance may be induced or enhanced. Suppressive therapy is prescribed with the intention of prolonging the time between acute exacerbations and to slow the rate of progression of lung disease. Although intuitively attractive, this practice is not supported by well-designed clinical trials.[47] Moreover, the practice of routine, quarterly administration of intravenous courses of antibiotics used at some European centers still lacks proof of efficacy.[48]

Antibiotic treatment for acute pulmonary exacerbations usually results in clinical improvement without eliminating bacteria from the sputum. In this case, the antibiotics are thought to lessen the bacterial burden within the airways, and thereby inhibit the quantity of exotoxins produced or the degree of host inflammation against the bacteria or their exoproducts.[49] The failure to eradicate the organism suggests that bacteria may be colonizing the airway surface, rather than penetrating the tissues as a pathogen. The bacteria may remain viable within an environment protected from the antibiotics, such as enclosed within a biofilm community. It also suggests the possibility that antibiotics may not be essential for the treatment of acute exacerbations. One study comparing antibiotic therapy to placebo indicated that antibiotics are not essential for recovery from an acute exacerbation.[50] However, because the study size was small and only included patients with mild to moderate disease, these results may not be applicable to all acute exacerbations. These results are also consistent with the notion that viral infections, air pollutants, irritants, allergens, or some other factors play a role in clinical exacerbations.

Finding known bacterial pathogens at high density in airway secretions, along with the clinical setting of increased cough, increased sputum production that is thicker and darker than baseline, and a significant decrease in lung function, loss of appetite and exercise tolerance, supports the addition of antibiotics to treat this clinical exacerbation. However, deciding to start antibiotic therapy leads to a number of other important, and sometimes perplexing, issues. These include the selection of the best antibiotic(s) for that individual patient, the optimal route of administration, the best dosage and dosage regimen to use, especially in light of altered pharmacokinetics in patients with cystic fibrosis, the potential emergence of antibiotic-resistant bacteria, and the identification of appropriate end points of therapy.

❻ ***Selection of Antibiotic.*** Suppressive therapy may be accomplished with the use of common orally administered antibiotics such as trimethoprim-sulfamethoxazole, amoxicillin-clavulanic acid, or one of the many oral cephalosporins. Specific therapy for acute exacerbations is directed at proven or likely pathogens such as *P. aeruginosa* and *S. aureus* and usually includes an aminoglycoside and an extended-spectrum penicillin. As most *S. aureus* encountered are β-lactamase producers, use of an extended-spectrum penicillin–β-lactamase inhibitor combination (e.g., ticarcillin-clavulanate) will help avoid the necessity of triple-drug therapy. Single-agent therapy with newer antibiotics, especially on an outpatient basis, is frequently employed at some centers where significant resistance to these agents has not yet emerged. Such agents would include ceftazidime, aztreonam, and ciprofloxacin. However, the evidence supporting the clinical superiority of two-drug combinations over single-agent therapy leads many clinicians to only treat with combinations.[51–54] The fact that such combinations are sometimes synergistic in vitro and the possibility that they may act to suppress or delay the emergence of resistance provide attractive rationales for their use. Furthermore, in vitro synergism has been reported to persist even in the face of resistance to one of the single agents in a given combination.[55] Lastly, monodrug therapy has been met with rapid emergence of resistance.[56]

Unlike other cases of lower respiratory tract infection, organism-specific drug treatment may be based on results from sputum cultures in cystic fibrosis patients because good agreement between sputum and thoracotomy cultures has been demonstrated.[57] Typically, such results will lead one to prescribe or recommend aminoglycoside–extended-spectrum penicillin combinations, although other antibiotics, such as ciprofloxacin, and older agents, such as colistin, also may play a role. While the complete eradication of *S. aureus* and *H. influenzae* are practical goals or end points of antibiotic therapy, the total eradication of *Pseudomonas* species is infrequent and transient. Thus, once a patient has been colonized/infected with *P. aeruginosa*, it is prudent to assume that it is always present regardless of culture results. Consistent with these infectious phenomena, the complete resolution of pulmonary signs and symptoms becomes less and less likely as the disease progresses. *B. cepacia* and *S. maltophilia* are generally resistant to most antibiotics. These bacteria may be susceptible to trimethoprim-sulfamethoxazole or chloramphenicol. *B. cepacia* from cystic fibrosis patients is frequently susceptible to ceftazidime, whereas some strains of *S. maltophilia* may be susceptible to other agents such as doxycycline and piperacillin.

Selection of Dose-Altered Pharmacokinetics. Although altered pharmacokinetics in cystic fibrosis are not limited to antibiotics (Table 32–3), this drug class has been the most extensively studied.[58] As is true for theophylline, many cystic fibrosis patients have increased total body clearance for many antibiotics, including the aminoglycosides, some of the β-lactams, and trimethoprim-sulfamethoxazole. Thus higher doses of these agents may be necessary to produce therapeutic concentrations (Table 32–4). Unfortunately, these alterations in pharmacokinetics are neither consistent nor predictable. Why the pharmacokinetics of these antibiotics are different in cystic fibrosis patients is unknown. It appears that for many β-lactam antibiotics, increased total body clearance could be accounted for by increased renal clearance. However, it should be pointed out that renal function, as reflected by glomerular filtration rate and renal blood flow, is not different in cystic fibrosis patients as compared to noncystic fibrosis controls.[59] Moreover, a concomitant increase in renal clearance does not completely explain the increase in total-body clearance of aminoglycosides, leading some to speculate about extra-renal pathways for elimination. In any event, increased total body clearance dictates higher doses in many but not all patients. However, a range of dosage requirements should be expected, consistent with a range in the variation of pharmacokinetics in these patients. For example, experience with netilmicin revealed a dosage requirement range of 7 to 17 mg/kg/d to achieve peak concentrations (one-half hour after the end of a drug infusion) of 8 mcg/mL or greater.[60] The mean dosage requirement in this study was approximately 12 mg/kg/day. Peak concentrations of this magnitude are felt to be necessary to adequately treat pneumonia caused by gram-negative bacteria.[61,62] Variations in hepatic metabolic activity or in phenotypic distribution of metabolic polymorphisms may explain some pharmacokinetic differences in cystic fibrosis.[63,64]

Although alterations in pharmacokinetics of antibiotics may correlate with the severity of pulmonary disease,[65,66] it is not possible to predict changes in antibiotic pharmacokinetics in cystic fibrosis patients based on markers of clinical status or disease progression. Attempts to correlate antibiotic pharmacokinetics with Shwachman score (a gross method for quantitation of disease status) have been unsuccessful.[67,68] Attempts to guide aminoglycoside dosing are often based on measured serum concentrations during a course of therapy. However, this method may also meet with mixed success owing to changing pharmacokinetics of this family of antibiotics during an acute pulmonary exacerbation.[69] This observation should not, however, deter one from attempts to adjust doses to desirable concentrations based on serum concentration determinations and subsequent pharmacokinetic calculations.

TABLE 32-3 Changes in Pharmacokinetics in Cystic Fibrosis

Agent	$\beta t_{1/2}$	V_D	Cl_B	Cl_R
Antibiotics				
Methicillin	NC	I	I	I
Cloxacillin	D	I	I	I
Dicloxacillin	I	NR	NR	I
Azlocillin	D	I	I	NR
Piperacillin	D	I	I	NR
Ticarcillin	D	NC	I	I
Aztreonam	D	I	I	I
Ceftazidime	D	I	I	I
Imipenem	NC	I	I	NR
Trimethoprim-sulfamethoxazole	D/D	NC/NC	I/I	I/NC
Gentamicin	NC	I	I	NR
Tobramycin	NC	I	I	NC
Amikacin	NC	I	I	I
Netilmicin	NC	I	I	NR
Fleroxacin	D	D	I	D
Other				
Theophylline	D	I	I	I
Furosemide	NC	NC	I	NC
Acetaminophen	NC	NR	I	NR

$\beta t_{1/2}$, elimination half-life; Cl_B, total body clearance, Cl_R, renal clearance; D, decreased; I, increased; NC, no change; NR, not reported; V_D, apparent volume of distribution.
Data from Konstan et al. and Lindsay and Bosso.[46,58]

TABLE 32-4 Antibiotic Doses in Cystic Fibrosis

Antibiotic	Dose (mg/kg/d)	Regimen	Adult Maximum Dose (g/d)
Parenteral antibiotics			
Tobramycin,[a] gentamicin,[a] or netilmicin[a]	6–9	q 8 h	NA
Amikacin[a]	20–30	q 8 h	NA
Azlocillin	400	q 4–6 h	24
Aztreonam	200	q 6 h	8
Ceftazidime	150	q 8 h	6
Colistin	2.5–6	q 6–8 h	NA
Imipenem	45–100	q 6 h	4
Nafcillin	100	q 4–6 h	6
Ticarcillin or ticarcillin/clavulanate	400	q 4–6 h	18
Piperacillin	400	q 4–6 h	18
Oral antibiotics			
Amoxicillin	20	q 8 h	
Amoxicillin/clavulanate	20	q 6 h	
Ciprofloxacin[b]	1,500 mg/d	q 12 h	1.5
Cephalexin	50–100	q 6–8 h	6
Dicloxacillin	80–100	q 6 h	6
Trimethoprim-sulfamethoxazole	10–15[c]	q 12 h	0.64[c]
Inhaled antibiotics			
Colistin	150 mg/d	q 6–12 h	NA
Gentamicin or tobramycin	600–1,800 mg/d	q 12 h	NA
Polymyxin B	250 mg/d	q 6–12 h	NA

[a]Starting doses; adjust to desired serum concentrations based on dose–serum concentration relationship.
[b]Adult dose.
[c]Based on trimethoprim.

Alternate Routes of Administration. An additional route of antibiotic administration that is intuitively attractive in patients with cystic fibrosis is by inhalation of aerosolized solution. Theoretically, such a route of administration should deliver the drug to the actual site of infection and perhaps avoid systemic toxicity. Certainly, many classes of antibiotics including β-lactams, aminoglycosides, and polymyxins have been administered to cystic fibrosis patients in this fashion, often in conjunction with systemic antibiotics. However, until recently, no clear effect or advantage had been consistently demonstrated. Early studies suffered from lack of controls, small sample size, and a failure to ensure that the respiratory equipment used would, in fact, guarantee that drug is delivered to the small airways. In a subsequent, placebo-controlled, multicenter trial, 600 mg tobramycin administered by aerosol three times daily was found to produce a small but statistically significant improvement in FEV_1, forced vital capacity, forced expiratory flow 25% to 75%, *P. aeruginosa* density in sputum, and peripheral white blood cell count.[70] This being recognized, appropriate clinical circumstances for this form of therapy (type and condition of patient), length of therapy, and frequency of therapy remain to be clarified. One-half of this dose is apparently also effective and a 300-mg dose is the current norm. If such doses are to be used, preservative-free antibiotic preparations should be used. The efficacy of smaller doses of inhaled aminoglycosides remains unproven.

Bacterial Resistance. As already noted, emergence of antimicrobial resistance seems to follow the introduction and use of a new antibiotic.[56] *P. aeruginosa* can exhibit many resistance mechanisms revealed as resistance to quinolones (altered DNA gyrase target site), β-lactams (production of Bush group 1 β-lactamase), aminoglycosides (decreased permeability and modifying enzymes), and carbapenems (decreased permeability). *B. cepacia* is inherently resistant to most antibiotics. Methicillin-resistant staphylococci are increasingly common in institutional settings and will become a more pervasive problem in cystic fibrosis populations. These phenomena require close attention to susceptibility reports in selecting therapy and the avoidance of unnecessary or unnecessarily protracted courses of antibiotic therapy. Another area of increasing concern is the management of transmission of pathogens from one patient to another.[71]

Recommendations for Antibiotic Therapy. Despite these inherent difficulties, a number of recommendations regarding the use of systemic antibiotics in cystic fibrosis can be made. ❻ The selection of antibiotics should be based on specific culture and susceptibility results. When instituting empiric therapy in the absence of culture results, the clinician can be guided by the most recent laboratory data or institute therapy based on likely pathogens in the patient's age group. Aminoglycosides should be initially dosed at the upper end of the normal dosage range (e.g., 6 to 7.5 mg/kg/d for tobramycin), and serum concentrations should be determined so that dosage can be appropriately adjusted to achieve peak concentrations of at least 8 mcg/mL. It should be kept in mind that aminoglycoside serum half-lives may lengthen during the course of treatment so that a constant relationship between dose and serum concentration may not exist. Consequently, upward adjustments in dosage should be made with some degree of caution and should be followed with further determination of serum concentrations. Once-daily administration of aminoglycosides is gaining popularity as in other settings. Obviously, such a dosing practice would result in much larger peak concentrations than those mentioned above. Comparative efficacy and safety of such dosing regimens in cystic fibrosis patients have not yet been fully elucidated, but this practice is likely to be increasingly employed as cystic fibrosis-specific data are generated.

β-Lactam antibiotics such as extended-spectrum penicillins should be prescribed with aminoglycosides to take advantage of their frequent synergy and prevent the emergence of resistance. These agents should be prescribed in large doses to delay stepwise resistance. Ticarcillin, azlocillin, and piperacillin should be prescribed in a dose of at least 350 mg/kg/day divided into four to six doses. For patients with *P. aeruginosa* and *S. aureus*, the combination of an aminoglycoside and ticarcillin-clavulanate or piperacillin-tazobactam is appropriate. Selection among these agents should be based on local susceptibility patterns and cost considerations. The possible increased incidence of fever and exanthema with the newer penicillins should be kept in mind.[72] Aztreonam would be a safe and effective β-lactam to use in patients experiencing these serum sickness-like reactions to the penicillins.[73] In older patients with *P. aeruginosa* isolates with broad resistance patterns, the clinician should work closely with the microbiology laboratory to identify effective agents or combinations. The potential use of older agents with unique mechanisms of action, such as colistin, should not be overlooked.

Oral antibiotics may be prescribed in symptomatic outpatients with susceptible pathogens in their sputum. Agents with activity against common pathogens such as *S. aureus* and *H. influenzae* are useful in this setting. These typically include such antibiotics as first-generation cephalosporins, trimethoprim-sulfamethoxazole, and amoxicillin-clavulanic acid. The use of such agents on a "prophylactic" basis is discouraged because the data available at present suggest that a beneficial effect does not outweigh the risk of development of resistance among the common bacterial pathogens of cystic fibrosis.[74] The 4-fluoroquinolone antibiotic ciprofloxacin possesses potent activity against most cystic fibrosis pathogens and has been evaluated in adult patients undergoing pulmonary exacerbations. Although not conclusive because of shortcomings in the studies, available data suggest that this oral agent is as effective as standard intravenous therapy.[75] The availability of a potent, oral antipseudomonal agent poses a number of potential uses in the cystic fibrosis population. However, it should be kept in mind that repeated or long-term use will likely lead to resistance and that antibiotics play only a supportive role in the treatment of these patients. Thus oral antibiotic therapy, regardless of efficacy, does not negate the need for other forms of therapy which are often best administered in the hospital setting. It should also be pointed out that although ciprofloxacin appears to be safe in patients younger than 18 years of age with little evidence of joint or cartilage toxicity,[76] this agent should be used with caution in the younger population.

Treatment of Other Pulmonary Complications The drug and nondrug treatments of the most serious of pulmonary complications, including pulmonary hypertension, right-sided heart failure, respiratory failure, pneumothorax, and hemoptysis, are beyond the scope of this chapter. In general, the therapeutic approach does not vary substantively from that caused by other respiratory diseases.

EVALUATION OF THERAPEUTIC OUTCOMES

GASTROINTESTINAL

Normal growth requires adequate nutrition and because of the increased energy needs and possible malabsorption, the nutritional needs of patients with cystic fibrosis cannot be overstated.[77] ❹ The patient's nutritional status should be closely monitored on both short-term and long-term bases. Growth in children and adolescents along with height and weight in all patients should be followed with time; anthropometric measurements give more precise information. The adequacy of pancreatic enzyme replacement can be grossly assessed by following stool patterns with the goal of normal number per day and normal consistency. Any evidence of steatorrhea may indicate suboptimal enzyme therapy. A more precise method would involve assessment of fat quantities in the stool. If a patient does not respond to normal doses of enzyme supplement, other factors that can cause similar symptoms (bloating, abdominal pain, symptomatic steatorrhea) should be considered. These would include lack of adherence with directions for taking the enzymes, outdated enzymes, dietary factors such as excessive fruit juice consumption, high-fat meals, and concomitant gastrointestinal disease (e.g., enteric bacterial or parasitic infection, celiac disease, inflammatory bowel disease). Vitamin status can be assessed though serum monitoring of fat-soluble vitamin concentrations.

PULMONARY

Pulmonary status can be monitored with a combination of clinical observation and examination and a variety of laboratory tests. Over the long run, pulmonary function is usually followed with spirometry, lung volumes and oxygenation. Physical examination should focus on signs and symptoms of upper and lower respiratory tract infection. In addition, exercise tolerance, recent character of sputum production, and oxygen requirements are key to long-term and short-term assessment. With antibiotic and bronchodilator treatment of acute respiratory exacerbations, a return to preexacerbation clinical status, based on physical examination or pulmonary function testing, becomes a practical end point for antimicrobial treatment. Although the goal of bacterial eradication is desirable, other attainable end points may be more reasonable, as discussed earlier. Bacterial density in sputum, sputum DNA and protein content, and C-reactive protein all have proven value as monitoring parameters but may not be available at many centers. Of the objective parameters, pulmonary function tests correlate best with clinical observations and scoring systems.[78] Response to intravenous antibiotics and aggressive chest physiotherapy, as measured by FEV_1 at the end of 1 week of treatment, has been used to predict total length of therapy necessary. In patients whose FEV_1 had recovered more than 40% at the end of 1 week, a total of 2 weeks of therapy was generally sufficient.[79] Little has been done by way of pharmacodynamic studies in treating cystic fibrosis. Therefore, symptomatic improvement is largely relied on to assess the relative success of antibiotic therapy. Oral antibiotic therapy should also be limited in length with specific end points, such as decreased cough and/or improved pulmonary function, identified as treatment commences.

GROWTH AND DEVELOPMENT IN CHILDREN

Realization that early detection and general growth early in life is important for development and general good clinical health status in children with cystic fibrosis, several new areas of investigation have arisen. Early diagnosis and treatment, where appropriate, is recognized as an important contributor to improved health for cystic fibrosis patients. Some states now require newborn screening so as to identify patients early and refer for further followup and education.[80] Another new area has been the use of growth hormone. Administration of growth hormone improves the growth of prepubertal children with cystic fibrosis.[81,82] Furthermore, it improves the general clinical status of the patients.

NEW DIRECTIONS IN THERAPY

❽ Now that the gene and gene product of cystic fibrosis are identified, gene therapy has obvious potential as treatment.[83] Research to date has centered on introduction of the correct gene into affected tissues. Viral vectors, chiefly adenovirus, have been studied in animal models, and human trials are under way. Liposomes may represent another useful delivery mode to introduce the correct gene.

Other novel approaches to therapy are currently being investigated and, for the most part, are directed at the inflammatory component of the disease or the basic cellular defect. Protease inhibitors hold potential in this condition for reasons cited earlier. α_1-Antitrypsin administered by aerosol shows promise, as does secretory leukocyte protease inhibitor and other antiproteases.[84–86] Pentoxifylline, which is known to inhibit tumor necrosis factor-α transcription and its stimulatory effect on polymorphonuclear leukocytes, also shows promise.[87] In an attempt to directly approach the cellular defect in cystic fibrosis, the diuretic amiloride was shown to possess positive activity in improving respiratory secretion rheology and clearance,[88] presumably by blocking excessive sodium reabsorption, but was found to be no more effective than placebo in a large-scale controlled trial. At a similar level, the secretagogues adenosine and uridine triphosphate have been shown to increase chloride excretion in epithelial cells of cystic fibrosis patients.[89] The combination of amiloride and uridine triphosphate (thereby both blocking sodium absorption and stimulating chloride secretion) may also promote clearance of airway secretions.[90] Other experimental therapies interact with the defects in CFTR production or processing. Studies with phenylbutyrate (which increases the amount of functional protein that reaches the cell surface), 8-cyclopentyl-1,3-dipropylxanthine (CPX), milrinone (a phosphodiesterase inhibitor), and genistein (a tyrosine-kinase inhibitor), each of which activate mutant CFTR, and low concentration gentamicin, which suppresses certain premature stop mutations in CFTR, are all active.

It is hoped that some, if not all, of these approaches will provide viable additions to our pharmacologic armamentarium for this disease. For older, more severely affected patients who may not be able to benefit from such advances, organ transplantations (single lung, double lung, heart–lung) are more widely available and reasonably successful.[91]

CONCLUSIONS

Pharmacotherapeutic intervention plays an important role in the management of these patients but is complex. The clinician is, as yet, faced with many unresolved issues in attempting to apply sound therapeutic principles in this population. Although close attention should be paid to pharmacologic treatment, the approach to these patients should be multifaceted and multidisciplinary in character. In addition to the involvement of such pediatric subspecialties as pulmonology, gastroenterology, pharmacology, and infectious diseases, contributions from such areas as nutrition support and social work should be a regular and ongoing part of the management effort.

ABBREVIATIONS

CFTR: cystic fibrosis transmembrane regulator

FEV_1: forced expiratory volume at 1 second

PaO_2: partial pressure of arterial oxygen

$PaCO_2$: partial pressure of arterial carbon dioxide

REFERENCES

1. Steinberg AG, Brown DC. On the incidence of cystic fibrosis of the pancreas. Am J Hum Genet 1960;12:416–424.
2. Wright SE, Morton NE. Genetic studies on cystic fibrosis in Hawaii. Am J Hum Genet 1968;20:157–169.
3. Rommens JM, Iannuzzi MC, Kerem B, et al. Identification of the cystic fibrosis gene: Chromosome walking and jumping. Science 1989;245:1059–1065.
4. Riordan JR, Rommens JM, Kerem B, et al. Identification of the cystic fibrosis gene: Cloning and characterization of complementary DNA. Science 1989;245:1066–1073.

5. Kerem B, Rommens JM, Buchanan JA, et al. Identification of the cystic fibrosis gene: Genetic analysis. Science 1989;245:1073–1080.
6. Welsh MJ, Smith AE. Molecular mechanisms of CFTR chloride channel dysfunction in cystic fibrosis. Cell 1993;73:1251–1254.
7. Kerem E, Corey M, Kerem B, et al. The relationship between genotype and phenotype in cystic fibrosis—Analysis of the most common mutation (ΔF_{508}). N Engl J Med 1991;323:1517–1522.
8. Mohon RT, Wagener JS, Abman SH, et al. Relationship of genotype to early pulmonary function in infants with cystic fibrosis identified through neonatal screening. J Pediatr 1993;122:550–555.
9. Collins FC. Cystic fibrosis: Molecular biology and therapeutic implications. Science 1992;256:774–779.
10. Feigelson J, Anagnostopoulos C, Poquet M, et al. Liver cirrhosis—Therapeutic implications and long-term follow-up. Arch Dis Child 1993;68:653–657.
11. Goldman, MJ, Anderson GM, Stolzenberg ED, et al. Human β-defensin-1 is a salt-sensitive antibiotic in lung that is inactivated in cystic fibrosis. Cell 1997;88:553–560.
12. Pier GB, Grout M, Zaida TS, et al. Role of mutant CFTR in hypersusceptibility of cystic fibrosis patients to lung infections. Science 1996;271:64–67.
13. Wang EEL, Prober CG, Manson B, et al. Association of respiratory viral infections with pulmonary deterioration in patients with cystic fibrosis. N Engl J Med 1984;311:1653–1658.
14. Armstrong DS, Hook SM, Jamsen KM, et al. Lower airway inflammation in infants with cystic fibrosis detected by newborn screening. Pediatr Pulmonol 2005;40:500–510.
15. Knowles MR, Boucher RC. Mucus clearance as a primary innate defense mechanism for mammalian airways. J Clin Invest 2002;109:571–577.
16. Joo NS, Irokawa T, Robbins RC and Wine JJ. Hyposecretion, and not hyperabsorption, is the basic defect of cystic fibrosis airway glands. J Biol Chem 2006;281:7392–7398.
17. Tarran R, Trout L, Donaldson SH, Boucher RC. Soluble mediators, and not cilia, determine airway surface liquid volume in normal and cystic fibrosis superficial airway epithelia. J Gen Physiol 2006;127:591–604.
18. Abman SH, Ogle JW, Butler-Simon N, et al. Role of respiratory syncytial virus in early hospitalizations for respiratory distress of young infants with cystic fibrosis. J Pediatr 1988;113:826–830.
19. Pribble CG, Black PG, Bosso JA, et al. Clinical manifestations of exacerbations of cystic fibrosis associated with nonbacterial infections. J Pediatr 1990;117:200–204.
20. Campbell PW, Parker RA, Roberts BT, et al. Association of poor clinical status and heavy exposure to tobacco smoke in patients with cystic fibrosis who are homozygous for the F_{508} deletion. J Pediatr 1992;120:261–264.
21. May TB, Shinabarger D, Mahara R, et al. Alginate synthesis by *Pseudomonas aeruginosa:* A key pathogenic factor in chronic pulmonary infections of cystic fibrosis patents. Clin Microbiol Rev 1991;4:191–206.
22. Isles A, Maclusky I, Corey M, et al. *Pseudomonas cepacia* infection in cystic fibrosis: An emerging problem. J Pediatr 1984;104:206–210.
23. Hudson VL, Wielinski CL, Regelmann WE. Prognostic implications of initial oropharyngeal bacterial flora in patients with cystic fibrosis diagnosed before the age of two years. J Pediatr 1993;122:854–860.
24. Triglia JM, Belus JF, Dessi P, et al. Rhinonasal manifestations of cystic fibrosis. Ann Otolaryngol Chir Cervicofac 1993;110:98–102.
25. Lawrence JM, Moore TL, Madson KL, et al. Arthropathies of cystic fibrosis: Case reports and review of the literature. J Rheumatol 1993;20(Suppl 38):12–15.
26. LeGrys VA, Yankaskas JR, Quittelli, LN, et al. Diagnostic sweat testing: Cystic Fibrosis Foundation guidelines. J Pediatr 2007;151:85–89.
27. Rosenstein BJ, Cutting GR. The diagnosis of cystic fibrosis: A consensus statement. J Pediatr 1998;132:589–595.
28. Newborn screening for cystic fibrosis: A paradigm for public health genetics policy development. Proceeding of a 1997 workshop. Morbidity and Mortality Weekly Reports 1997;46(RR-16):1–24.
29. FitzSimmons SC. The changing epidemiology of cystic fibrosis. J Pediatr 1993;122:1–9.
30. Kerem E, Reisman J, Corey M, et al. Prediction of mortality in patients with cystic fibrosis. N Engl J Med 1992;326:1187–1191.
31. Clinical Practice Guidelines for Cystic Fibrosis Committee. Clinical practice guidelines for cystic fibrosis. Bethesda, MD: Cystic Fibrosis Foundation, 1997.
32. Riedel BD. Gastrointestinal manifestations of cystic fibrosis. Pediatr Ann 1997;26;235–241.
33. Ramsey BW, Farrell PM, Pencharz P, et al. Nutritional assessment and management in cystic fibrosis. Am J Clin Nutr 1992;55:108–116.
34. Ferrone M, Raimon do M, Solapio JS. Pancreatic enzyme pharmacotherapy. Pharmacotherapy 2007;27:910–920.
35. FitzSimmons SC, Burkhart GA, Borowitz D, et al. High-dose pancreatic-enzyme supplements and fibrosing colonopathy in children with cystic fibrosis. N Engl J Med 1997;336:1283–1289.
36. Nasr SZ, O'Leary MH, Hillerman C. Correction of vitamin E deficiency with fat-soluble versus water-miscible preparations of vitamin E in patients with cystic fibrosis. J Pediatr 1993;122:810–812.
37. Colombo C, Battezzati PM, Podda M, et al. Ursodeoxycholic acid for liver disease associated with cystic fibrosis: A double-blind multicenter trial. Hepatology 1996;23:1484–1490.
38. Columbo C, Grazia M, Ferrari M, et al. Analysis of risk factors for the development of liver disease associated with cystic fibrosis. J Pediatr 1994;124:393–399.
39. Ramsey BW. Management of pulmonary disease in patients with cystic fibrosis. N Engl J Med 1996;335:179–188.
40. Fuchs HJ, Borwitz DS, Christainsen DH, et al. Effect of aerosolized recombinant human DNAse on exacerbations of respiratory symptoms and on pulmonary function in patients with cystic fibrosis. N Engl J Med 1994:331:637–642.
41. Elkins MR, Robinson M, Rose BR, et al. A controlled trial of long-term inhaled hypertonic saline in patients with cystic fibrosis. N Engl J Med 2006;354:229–240.
42. Donaldson SH, Bennett WE, Zeman KL, et al. Mucus clearance and lung function in cyctic fibrosis with hypertonic saline. N Engl J Med 2006;354:241–250.
43. Spino M. Pharmacokinetics of drugs in cystic fibrosis. Clin Rev Allergy 1991;9:169–210.
44. Rosenstein BJ, Eigen H. Risks of alternate-day prednisone in patients with cystic fibrosis. Pediatrics 1991;87:245–246.
45. Eigen H, Rosenstein BJ, FitzSimmons S, et al. A multicenter study of alternate-day prednisone therapy in patients with cystic fibrosis. J Pediatr 1995;126:515–523.
46. Konstan MW, Byard PJ, Hoppel CL, et al. Effect of high-dose ibuprofen in patients with cystic fibrosis. N Engl J Med 1995;332:848–854.
47. Beardsmore CS, Thompson JR, Williams A, et al. Pulmonary function in infants with cystic fibrosis: The effect of antibiotic treatment. Arch Dis Child 1994;71:133–137.
48. Jensen T, Pedersen SS, Høiby N, et al. Use of antibiotics in cystic fibrosis: The Danish approach. Antibiot Chemother 1989;42:237–246.
49. Grimwood K, Semple RA, Rabin HR, et al. Elevated exoenzyme expression by *Pseudomonas aeruginosa* is correlated with exacerbations of lung disease in cystic fibrosis. Pediatr Pulmonol 1993;15:135–139.
50. Gold R, Carpenter S, Heurter H, et al. Randomized trial of ceftazidime versus placebo in the management of acute respiratory exacerbations in patients with cystic fibrosis. J Pediatr 1987;111:907–913.
51. Parry MF, Neu HC, Merlino M, et al. Treatment of pulmonary infections in patients with cystic fibrosis: A comparative study of ticarcillin and gentamicin. J Pediatr 1977;90:144–148.
52. Møller NE, Høiby N. Antibiotic treatment of chronic *Pseudomonas aeruginosa* infection in cystic fibrosis patients. Scand J Infect Dis 1981;24(Suppl):87–91.
53. Friis B. Chemotherapy of chronic infections with mucoid *Pseudomonas aeruginosa* in lower airways of patients with cystic fibrosis. Scand J Infect Dis 1979;11:211–217.
54. Krause PJ, Young LS, Cherry JD, et al. The treatment of exacerbations of pulmonary disease in cystic fibrosis: Netilmicin compared with netilmicin and carbenicillin. Curr Ther Res 1979;25:609–617.
55. Aronoff SC, Klinger JD. In vitro activities of aztreonam, piperacillin and ticarcillin combined with amikacin against amikacin-resistant *Pseudomonas aeruginosa* and *P. cepacia* isolates from children with cystic fibrosis. Antimicrob Agents Chemother 1984;25:279–280.
56. Bosso JA, Allen JE, Matsen JM. Changing susceptibility of *Pseudomonas aeruginosa* isolates from cystic fibrosis patients with the clinical use of newer antibiotics. Antimicrob Agents Chemother 1989;33:526–528.
57. Thomassen MJ, Klinger JD, Badger SJ, et al. Cultures of thoracotomy specimens confirm usefulness of sputum cultures in cystic fibrosis. J Pediatr 1984;104:352–356.
58. Lindsay CA, Bosso JA. Optimization of antibiotic therapy in cystic fibrosis patients. Clin Pharmacokinet 1993;24:496–506.

59. Spino M, Chai RP, Isles AF, et al. Assessment of glomerular filtration rate and effective renal plasma flow in cystic fibrosis. J Pediatr 1985;107:64–70.
60. Bosso JA, Townsend PL, Herbst JJ, et al. Pharmacokinetics and dosage requirements of netilmicin in cystic fibrosis patients. Antimicrob Agents Chemother 1985;28:829–831.
61. Moore RD, Smith CR, Lietman PS. Association of aminoglycoside plasma levels with therapeutic outcome in gram-negative pneumonia. Am J Med 1984;77:657–662.
62. Noone P, Parsons MC, Pattison JR, et al. Experience in monitoring gentamicin therapy during treatment of serious gram negative sepsis. Br J Med 1974;1:477–481.
63. Kearns GL. Hepatic drug metabolism in cystic fibrosis: Recent developments and future directions. Ann Pharmacother 1993;27:74–79.
64. Bosso JA, Liu Q, Evans WE, et al. CYP2D6 *N*-acetylation, and xanthine oxidase activity in cystic fibrosis. Pharmacotherapy 1996;16:749–753.
65. MacDonald NE, Anas NG, Peterson RG, et al. Renal clearance of gentamicin in cystic fibrosis. J Pediatr 1983;103:985–990.
66. Nahata MC, Lubion AH, Visconti JA. Cephalexin pharmacokinetics in patients with cystic fibrosis. Dev Pharmacol Ther 1984;7:221–228.
67. Spino M, Chai RP, Isles AF, et al. Cloxacillin absorption and disposition in cystic fibrosis. J Pediatr 1984;105:829–835.
68. Jacobs RF, Trang JM, Kearns GL, et al. Ticarcillin/clavulanic acid pharmacokinetics in children and young adults with cystic fibrosis. J Pediatr 1985;106:1001–1007.
69. Bosso JA, Relling MV, Townsend PL, et al. Intrapatient variations in aminoglycoside disposition in cystic fibrosis. Clin Pharm 1987;6:54–58.
70. Ramsey BW, Dorkin HL, Eisenberg JD, et al. Efficacy of aerosolized tobramycin in patients with cystic fibrosis. N Engl J Med 1993;328:1740–1746.
71. Saiman L, Siegel J, and the Cystic Fibrosis Foundation Consensus Conference on Infection Control Participants. Infection control recommendations for patients with cystic fibrosis: Microbiology, important pathogens, and infection control practices to prevent patient-to-patient transmission. Infect Control Hosp Epidemiol 2003;37:S6–52.
72. Møller NE, Eriksen KR, Feddersen C, et al. Chemotherapy against *Pseudomonas aeruginosa* in cystic fibrosis. A study of carbenicillin, azlocillin or piperacillin in combination with tobramycin. Eur J Respir Dis 1982;63:130–139.
73. Jensen T, Koch C, Pedersen SS, et al. Aztreonam for cystic fibrosis patients who are hypersensitive to other β-lactams. Lancet 1987;1:1319–1320.
74. Beardsmore CS, Thompson JR, Williams A, et al. Pulmonary function in infants with cystic fibrosis. Arch Dis Child 1994;71:133–137.
75. Bosso JA. Use of ciprofloxacin in cystic fibrosis patients. Am J Med 1989;87(Suppl 5A):123S–127S.
76. Høiby N, Pedersen SS, Jensen T, et al. Fluoroquinolones in the treatment of cystic fibrosis. Drugs 1993;45(Suppl 3):98–101.
77. Borowitz D, Baker RD, Stallings V. Consensus report on nutrition for pediatric patients with cystic fibrosis. J Pediatr Gastroenterol Nutr 200;35:246–259.
78. Bosso JA, Walker KB. Lack of correlation between objective indicators and clinical-response scores during antimicrobial therapy for acute pulmonary exacerbations of cystic fibrosis. Clin Pharm 1988;7:897–901.
79. Rosenberg SM, Schramm CM. Predictive value of pulmonary function testing during pulmonary exacerbations in cystic fibrosis. Pediatr Pulmonol 1993;16:227–235.
80. Farrell PM, Kosorok MR, Rock MJ, et al. Early diagnosis of cystic fibrosis through neonatal screening prevents severe malnutrition and improves long-term growth. J Pediatr 2001;107:1–13.
81. Hardin DS, Ellis KJ, Dyson M, et al. Growth hormone improves clinical status in prepubertal children with cystic fibrosis: Results of a randomized controlled trial. J Pediatr 2001;139:636–642.
83. Hardin DS, Adams-Huet B, Brown D, et al. Growth hormone improves clinical status in prepubertal children with cystic fibrosis: Results of a randomized controlled trial. J Clin Endocrinol Metab 2006;91:4925–4929.
83. Rosenfeld MA, Collins FS. Gene therapy for cystic fibrosis. Chest 1996;109:241–252.
84. McElvaney NG, Hubbard RC, Birrer P, et al. Aerosol α_1-antitrypsin treatment for cystic fibrosis. Lancet 1991;337:392–394.
85. McElvaney NG, Nakamura H, Birrer P, et al. Modulation of airway inflammation in cystic fibrosis: In vivo suppression of interleukin-8 levels on the respiratory epithelial surface by aerosolization of recombinant secretory leukoprotease inhibitor. J Clin Invest 1992;90:296–301.
86. Meyer KC, Kewandeski JR, Zimmerman JJ, et al. Human neutrophil elastase and elastase/alpha$_1$-antiprotease complex in cystic fibrosis. Am Rev Respir Dis 1991;144:580–585.
87. Aronoff SC, Quinn FJ, Carpenter LS, et al. Effects of pentoxifylline on sputum neutrophil elastase and pulmonary function in patients with cystic fibrosis: Preliminary observations. J Pediatr 1994;125:992–997.
88. Knowles MR, Church NL, Waltner WE, et al. A pilot study of aerosolized amiloride for the treatment of lung disease in cystic fibrosis. N Engl J Med 1990;322:1189–1194.
89. Knowles MR, Clarke LL, Boucher RC. Activation by extracellular nucleotides of chloride secretion in the airway epithelia of patients with cystic fibrosis. N Engl J Med 1991;325:533–538.
90. Bennett WD, Olivier KN, Zeman KL, et al. Effect of uridine 5'-triphosphate plus amiloride on mucociliary clearance in adult cystic fibrosis. Am J Respir Crit Care Med 1996;153:1796–1801.
91. Yankaskas JR, Westerman JH, Thompson JT, et al. Improved results of lung transplantation for patients with cystic fibrosis. J Thorac Cardiovasc Surg 1995;109:224–234.

SECTION 4
GASTROINTESTINAL DISORDERS

CHAPTER 33

Evaluation of the Gastrointestinal Tract

KEITH M. OLSEN, MARIE A. CHISHOLM-BURNS, AND MARK W. JACKSON

KEY CONCEPTS

1. The patient history is key to evaluating GI disorders and should include the problem onset, the setting in which it developed, and its presentation. Patient warning signs should be identified that require immediate referral for further evaluation.
2. A complete physical examination should be performed with severity and location of symptoms directing the focus of the examination.
3. Barium sulfate allows evaluation of the hollow organs of the digestive tract for mucosal lesions and stricture.
4. The upper GI series involves radiographic visualization of the esophagus, stomach, and small intestine; whereas the lower GI series involves visualization of the colon and rectum.
5. Enteroclysis is used to evaluate the small bowel by introducing contrast agents by tube through the nose or mouth.
6. GI ultrasonography, computed tomography, and magnetic resonance imaging provide images of the gallbladder, liver, pancreas, and abdominal wall.
7. Radionuclide imaging is useful to visualize the liver, spleen, bile ducts, gallbladder, and gut.
8. The endoscope, an illuminated optical instrument, remains an important tool for the diagnosis and management of GI disorders with common endoscopic studies, including esophagogastroduodenoscopy, colonoscopy, sigmoidoscopy, and endoscopic retrograde cholangiopancreatography.
9. Ambulatory pH-metry is an important diagnostic test for gastroesophageal reflux disease. The traditional method is gradually being replaced by wireless systems.
10. Multichannel intraluminal impedance and pH monitoring combines acid exposure with impedance changes in resistant flow to aide the diagnosis of reflux in patients receiving a proton pump inhibitor.
11. Capsule endoscopy takes pictures of the GI tract in the assessment of the small bowel.

Learning objectives, review questions, and other resources can be found at **www.pharmacotherapyonline.com.**

The gastrointestinal (GI) tract is composed of organs and tissues that have diverse forms and functions. It includes the esophagus, stomach, small intestine, large intestine, colon, rectum, biliary tract, gallbladder, liver, and pancreas. Despite the rapid proliferation of technology for the diagnosis of digestive diseases, the patient history and physical examination remain important for initial assessment, triage, and direction of further diagnostic interventions. When combined with a thorough patient history and physical examination, diagnostic procedures are essential in the evaluation of GI disorders. This chapter describes the most commonly used tools available in clinical practice to evaluate patients with GI diseases.

SYMPTOMS OF GASTROINTESTINAL DYSFUNCTION

A variety of symptoms can arise from GI dysfunction. Common GI symptoms include heartburn, abdominal pain, dyspepsia, nausea, vomiting, diarrhea, constipation, and gastrointestinal bleeding. Signs and symptoms of malabsorption, hepatitis, and GI infection are also commonly seen. All clinicians must recognize warning symptoms that include weight loss, intractable vomiting, anemia, dysphagia, and bleeding, and a patient presenting with any of these symptoms should be immediately referred for further diagnostic interventions. The next sections describe methods that are commonly used to assess patients with GI complaints. For specific details concerning each GI disease state, please consult that particular chapter in this book.

PATIENT HISTORY

A comprehensive patient history is the cornerstone in the evaluation of a patient with digestive complaints. A clear, detailed, chronologic account of the patient's problems should be ascertained. This account

TABLE 33-1 General Questions in a Gastrointestinal History

1. Tell me about the problem that you are experiencing. When did it start?
2. Where is your pain located? Please point to the area where you feel pain. What were you doing when the pain occurred? How rapidly did the pain come on? Is your pain constant or intermittent? What factors exacerbate or alleviate your pain? Does the pain awaken you at night?
3. What medications are you taking to help the pain? How much do you take? Do these medications work?
4. What other medications are you currently taking? Why are you taking them?
5. Have you recently had a change in dietary intake? If so, please describe. Can you draw any correlation between the foods that you eat and your gastrointestinal (GI) complaint?
6. Have you recently had a change in bowel habits? Have you experienced any diarrhea or constipation lately? Do you experience painful bowel movements?
7. Have you experienced any nausea or vomiting lately? If so, please describe conditions centered around this event.
8. Have you experienced any recent change in weight? Was this intentional? How many pounds have you gained or lost and over what time period did this occur? How has your appetite been?
9. Have you passed any blood from your rectum or vomited blood? Have you noticed any dark, tarry stools?
10. Have you had any acid indigestion?
11. Do you have difficulty swallowing?
12. Has anyone in your family experienced similar GI complaints? If so, please describe. Does anyone in your family have a history of GI disorders, including cancer of the GI tract?
13. Describe your past medical history, including illnesses and surgeries.
14. Please describe any past injuries that you have experienced.
15. Have you recently traveled outside of the United States? If so, where? When? How long did you stay? What kind of living conditions did you experience? What foods and drinks did you ingest?

should include the onset of the problem, the setting in which it developed, and its manifestations. The symptoms onset often provides important information that helps to formulate a differential diagnosis. For example, biliary pain, such as that encountered with symptomatic gallstone disease, typically evolves over minutes and lasts for hours, but pain caused by pancreatitis evolves over hours and lasts for days. The setting is always relevant as it provides clues to the possible origin of the disorder. For example, in the patient with complaints of reflux or ulcer disease, when do the symptoms occur, are they alleviated or worsened by food and does the pain diminish when administered acid-suppressive therapy? Is the patient immunosuppressed (opportunistic infection)? Also aiding in the diagnosis is identification of factors that alleviate or exacerbate the principal symptom. For instance, ingesting a meal often relieves the pain of duodenal ulcer, but worsens that of gastric ulcer. The healthcare professional should ask questions that address the potential etiologic possibilities, including motility disorders, structural diseases, malignancies, infections, psychosocial factors, dietary factors, and travel-associated diseases.[1,2] Questions concerning past medical and family history detailing illnesses, surgeries, injuries, foreign travel, living conditions, and habits are valuable (Table 33–1). Because some pharmacologic agents cause GI injury, a medication history is vital (Table 33–2).

PHYSICAL EXAMINATION

Because the organ systems of the body interact and may provide important data needed for diagnosis, it is necessary to perform a thorough physical examination.[3] A comprehensive evaluation of the patient should be performed with notable attention to physical appearances and vital signs as they may suggest clues to the patient's overall condition and stability. Depending on the acuteness and severity of the clinical presentation, careful examination of the abdomen is an essential part of the workup. Examination of the

TABLE 33-2 Drugs That May Cause Gastrointestinal Injury[15–17]

Gastrointestinal mucosal injury
- Aspirin
- Bisphosphonates
- Chemotherapeutic agents
- Corticosteroids
- Ethacrynic acid
- Ethanol
- Iron preparations
- Nonsteroidal antiinflammatory agents
- Pancreatic enzymes
- Potassium chloride
- Reserpine
- Warfarin

Jaundice
- Acetohexamide
- Androgens
- Chlorpropamide
- Corticosteroids
- Erythromycin
- Estrogens
- Ethanol
- Gold salts
- Nitrofurantoin
- Phenothiazines
- Warfarin

Liver damage
- Acetaminophen
- Allopurinol
- Amiodarone
- Aminosalicylic acid
- Dapsone
- Erythromycin
- Ethanol
- Glyburide
- Isoniazid
- Ketoconazole
- Lovastatin
- Methotrexate
- Methyldopa
- Monoamine oxidase inhibitors
- Nevirapine
- Niacin
- Nifedipine
- Nitrofurantoin
- Phenazopyridine
- Phenytoin
- Propylthiouracil
- Rifampin
- Salicylates
- Sulfonamides
- Telithromycin
- Tetracycline
- Valproic acid
- Verapamil
- Warfarin
- Zidovudine

Pancreatitis
- Azathioprine
- Corticosteroids
- Didanosine
- Estrogens
- Ethacrynic acid
- Ethanol
- Furosemide
- Metronidazole
- Opiates
- Pentamidine
- Sulfonamides
- Tetracycline
- Thiazides

abdomen classically includes inspection, auscultation, percussion, and palpation. Inspection of the abdomen may reveal scars, hernias, bulges, or peristalsis. Auscultation is mainly focused on analysis of bowel sounds and identification of bruits. Percussion of the abdomen allows for detection of tympany, measurement of visceral organs, and detection of ascites. Palpation may allow the clinician to identify tenderness, rigidity, masses, and hernias. A digital rectal examination is used to detect masses and tenderness, and to assess muscle tone. Stool on the examiner's glove obtained during rectal examination is often subjected to testing for detection of occult blood.[2,3] Patients presenting with upper gastrointestinal symptoms need more careful questioning to distinguish symptoms of reflux disease versus peptic ulcer disease. Additionally, once cardiovascular disease is eliminated, patients with chest pain may have a gastrointestinal source to their symptoms and further diagnostic workup may be needed.

LABORATORY AND MICROBIOLOGIC TESTS

Laboratory and microbiologic tests may be used to (a) assess organ function, (b) screen for certain GI disorders, and (c) evaluate the effectiveness of therapy. To achieve an accurate diagnosis and provide the best care, it is important to assess the patient's fluid and electrolyte status, nutritional status, and abdominal organ function. A complete blood cell count should be completed early in the evaluation to provide information concerning infection, malignancy, bone marrow suppression, anemia, and blood loss.[4] A serum chemistry panel provides clinicians with valuable information. For example, serum creatinine and blood urea nitrogen are often used as a measure of hydration status, as well as serving as indicators for renal function. Elevations in serum creatinine and blood urea nitrogen may be indicative of renal dysfunction or dehydration, and bleeding from the GI tract may lead to elevations in blood urea nitrogen. Albumin and prealbumin levels can be used to assess the patient's nutritional and hydration status and provide information concerning hepatic and renal function. Specifically, low albumin may be indicative of malnutrition, hepatic dysfunction, nephrotic syndromes, or protein-losing enteropathies such as Crohn's disease and ulcerative colitis. Serum measurements of sodium, chloride, and potassium are useful to determine electrolyte abnormalities associated with diarrheal illnesses.

Specific laboratory blood tests are used as screening tools for certain GI disorders. Measurements of serum aspartate transaminase and alanine transaminase are elevated in most diseases of the liver, and serum alkaline phosphatase and bilirubin are often elevated in hepatobiliary disorders. Prothrombin time and international normalized ratio are related to hepatocyte synthesis of vitamin K-dependent clotting factors and serve as indirect measurements of hepatic function. When evaluating patients with suspected pancreatitis, serum and urine measurements of amylase and lipase are important, because these will be elevated in most patients with acute pancreatitis (see Chap. 41).

Microbiologic and related studies are useful in evaluating patients with unexplained diarrhea, abdominal pain, and suspected GI infections. Examination studies of the stool may be used to detect the presence of bacteria, parasites, or toxins. Pathogens most often responsible for infectious diarrhea and enteritis include bacteria such as *Shigella, Salmonella, Escherichia coli, Yersinia,* and *Clostridium difficile;* viruses such as cytomegalovirus, especially in acquired immune deficiency syndrome (AIDS) patients; and parasites such as *Entamoeba histolytica* and *Giardia lamblia.*[5] Patients presenting with watery, pseudomembranous diarrhea following antibiotic exposure within the previous 1–3 months should have their stool checked for *C. difficile* toxins A and B. Because *Helicobacter pylori* is a significant factor associated with peptic ulcer disease and MALT lymphomas, identification of this organism is critical in patients experiencing upper gastrointestinal symptoms (see Chap. 35).[5]

DIAGNOSIS

The patient's history, physical examination, and routine laboratory tests are valuable in establishing a diagnosis, but frequently more specific studies are required to confirm or disprove a clinical suspicion. The most appropriate diagnostic test depends on the anatomic region involved, the suspected abnormality, reliability of the test (e.g., sensitivity vs. specificity), patient preference, the patient's overall condition, and clinical manifestations of the patient. The next sections outline the most frequently used diagnostic studies and procedures and their roles in evaluating the GI tract.

RADIOLOGY

Radiologic procedures rely on the differential absorption of radiation of adjacent tissues to highlight anatomy and pathology. Radiologic procedures important in evaluating the GI tract include plain radiography, upper GI series, lower GI series, and enteroclysis.[6,7]

Plain Radiography of the GI System

Radiographic evaluation of the GI tract often starts with plain films of the abdomen, which are straightforward, noncontrast radiographs.[7] Specific abdominal structures that may be identified include the kidneys, ureters, and bladder; esophagus; stomach; intestine; stones; and vessels. Plain films are often used to evaluate abdominal pain. Clinicians frequently employ plain radiographic fluoroscopy to guide and position other instruments that are used to evaluate and treat GI disorders; an example is the manipulation of dilation devices to treat esophageal strictures. Bowel obstruction and perforation are especially well identified by this technique.

Contrast Agents

Barium sulfate is the contrast agent of choice for studying the esophagus, stomach, and intestine; but it has largely been replaced to a great extent by direct visualization of the GI tract.[7] Barium sulfate is a metallic material detected by radiography after swallowing the agent; it is termed the *barium swallow*. Barium sulfate is not generally absorbed, and constipation is the most frequent adverse effect reported with its use. Barium sulfate can reveal mucosal lesion defects and lumen size, and is helpful in diagnosing hiatal hernias, strictures along the GI tract, polyps, tumors, and ulcers. The barium esophagram should not serve as a primary diagnostic tool for patients with heartburn.

Upper GI Series

The upper GI series refers to the radiographic visualization of the esophagus, stomach, and small intestine. Patient preparation for an upper GI series usually consists of instructing patients to refrain from eating or drinking 8 to 12 hours prior to testing, which allows the upper GI tract to empty. A contrast agent such as barium sulfate is administered to the patient at the beginning of the study. The observed swallowing of the contrast agent permits visualization and monitoring of esophageal structural and motor functions. As the contrast medium flows into the stomach and small intestine, several regional radiographic films are taken in order to inspect these areas. This tracking of contrast agents through the small intestine is referred to as the *small bowel follow-through.* The upper GI series with small bowel follow-through commonly uncovers gastric cancer, peptic ulcer disease, esophagitis, gastric outlet obstruction, and Crohn's disease (Fig. 33–1). In general, the barium swallow is plagued by low sensitivity and specificity for many GI disorders.

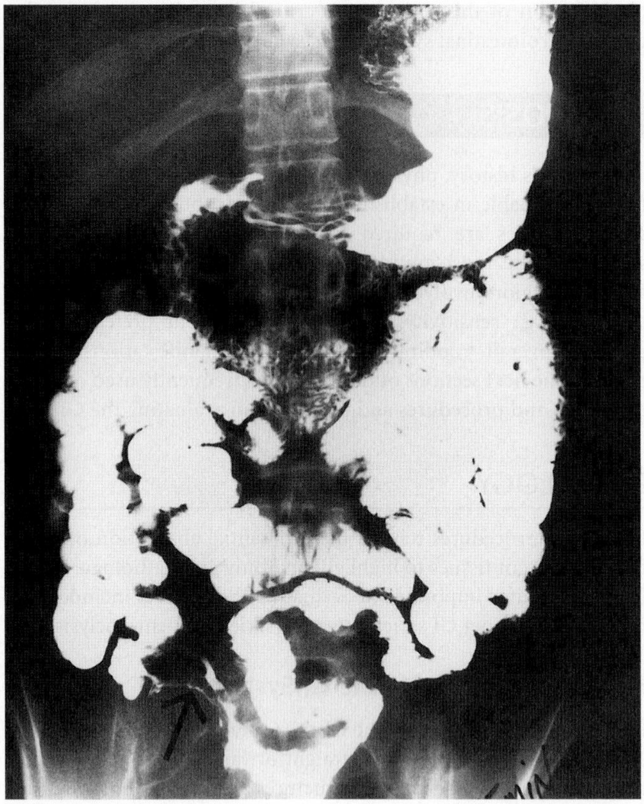

FIGURE 33-1. Upper GI series with small bowel follow-through demonstrating narrowed distal terminal ileum and separation of small bowel loops *(arrow)*. These findings are consistent with Crohn's disease.

Lower GI Series

The lower GI series is used to examine the colon and rectum. Patients complaining of lower abdominal pain, constipation, or diarrhea are often referred for a lower GI series. The colon is prepared for the procedure by instructing the patient to refrain from eating or drinking 8 to 12 hours before the procedure, and by administering bowel-cleansing agents such as bisacodyl, magnesium citrate, magnesium hydroxide, or polyethylene glycol-electrolyte solution. During a lower GI series, a barium sulfate enema is given to contrast the terminal large intestine and rectum. The lower GI series is useful to detect and evaluate enterocolitis, obstructions, volvulus, and mucosal and structural lesions.[7] The lower GI series is commonly used to diagnose Crohn's disease, ulcerative colitis, colon cancers, and diverticulitis.

Small Bowel Enteroclysis

Enteroclysis, or small bowel enema, refers to the technique of direct small bowel introduction of a contrast agent through a tube inserted through the patient's mouth or nose. Intermittent radiographic films are taken of the small bowel as the contrast agent flows distally (Fig. 33–2). Because enteroclysis provides detailed imaging, it is an accurate method for evaluating the small bowel and for detecting small mucosal lesions that may be overlooked on the traditional small bowel follow-through.[9] Methylcellulose is used to enhance the detail of the small intestine in enteroclysis, thereby improving visualization. Patient preparation for this procedure involves instructing patients to refrain from eating or drinking 8 to 12 hours before testing and administering bowel-cleansing agents. The most frequent disorder evaluated by enteroclysis is obscure GI bleeding.

IMAGING STUDIES

By using computer-assisted techniques, it is possible to generate cross-sectional radiographic images of the body. Ultrasonography,

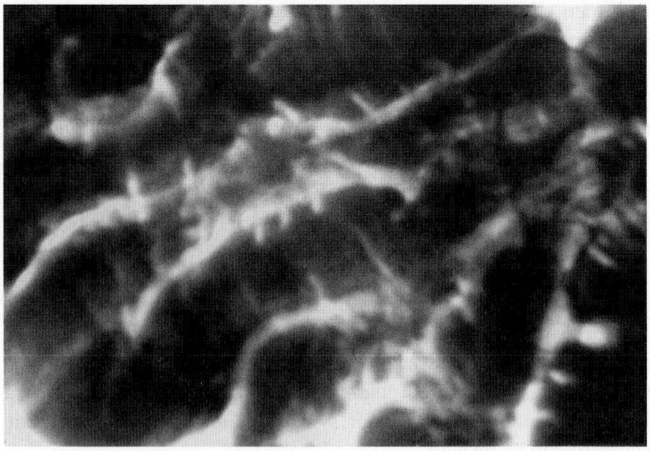

FIGURE 33-2. Normal small bowel enteroclysis. Contrast agents are instilled into the small bowel to highlight tumors, strictures, or other lesions. In this image, one can identify the normal circular folds.

computed tomography, radionuclide scanning, and magnetic resonance imaging are frequently used imaging procedures for evaluating digestive disorders.[6,7]

Ultrasonography

Ultrasonography provides images of deeper structures such as the gallbladder, liver, pancreas, and abdominal wall. The clinician is able to image slices of the GI tract by directing a narrow beam of high-energy sound waves into the body and recording the reflections from the various organs and structures. Because ultrasonography is non-invasive, relatively inexpensive, requires no ionizing radiation, and can be performed at bedside with a portable unit, it is a well-accepted and useful technology. It accurately depicts gallstones and gallbladder, and hepatobiliary and pancreatic diseases (Fig. 33–3). When combined with Doppler technologies, ultrasonography can image GI vascularity. Ultrasonography is limited by the presence of bowel gas and excessive amounts of body fat.[6,7]

Computed Tomography

Computed tomography (CT) or computed axial tomography (CAT) scans provide detailed images of the GI system in which transverse planes of tissue are swept by a radiographic beam and a computer analysis of the variance in absorption produces a precise reconstructed image of that area.[6] Contrast agents may be added in a CT procedure to illuminate specific hollow structures and vascularity of the GI tract. The abdominal CT displays organs from the diaphragm down to the pelvic brim, and is especially valuable for detecting GI diseases of the liver, pancreas, spleen, and colon. Patient preparation for CT includes refraining from eating or drinking for a minimum of 4 hours before the test. The remarkable detail that CT offers in imaging organs and tissues adds to its popularity for evaluation of the GI system. CT is useful in the identification of liver cancer, pancreatitis, pancreatic cancer, intra-abdominal abscesses, and cysts (Fig. 33–4).[6,7] Unlike ultrasonography, patient body size or the presence of gas does not limit the quality of imaging with CT.

Radionuclide Imaging

Radionuclide imaging involves intravenous injections of a radiopharmaceutical imaging agent and the use of a computerized detection camera to gather images. Although the choice of a radiopharmaceutical agent depends on the specific organ or function being studied, the most commonly used agent is technetium (^{99m}Tc) tagged to a carrier molecule. Radiographic imaging is useful to visualize the liver and spleen (liver-spleen scan), bile ducts, gallbladder (HIDA [hepatoimin-

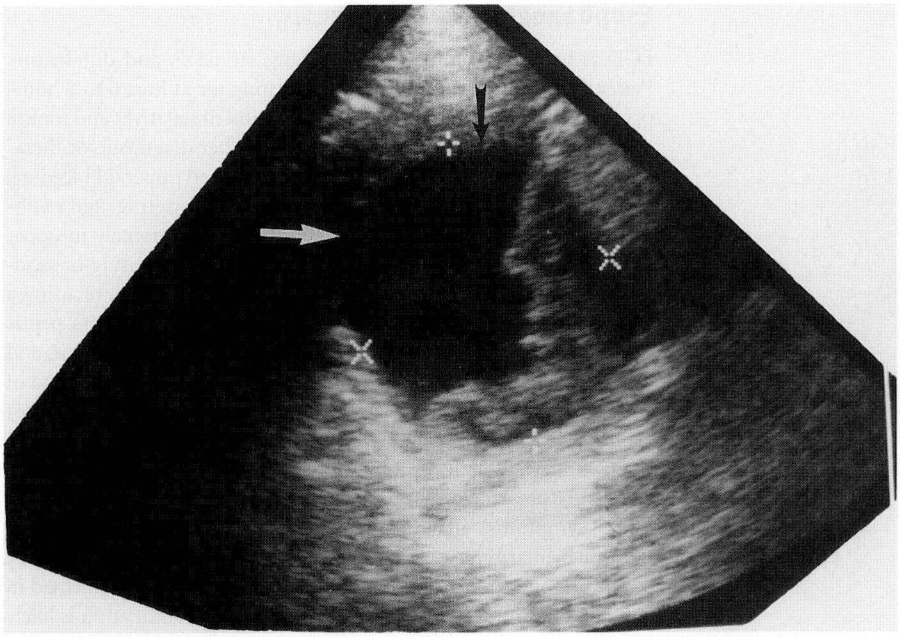

FIGURE 33-3. Abdominal ultrasonogram demonstrating a chronic pancreatic pseudocyst *(arrows)*.

odiacetic acid] scan), and gut (bleeding scan).[6,7] Cysts, abscesses, tumors, and obstructions are detected and displayed as areas of differential uptake of radioactivity (Fig. 33–5).[6] Radionuclide bleeding scans may detect hemorrhages and may assist in localization. Contrast media nephrotoxicity in patients with preexisting renal impairment remains a clinically significant problem. Pretest treatment in high-risk patients with pharmacologic agents has demonstrated mixed results.

Magnetic Resonance Imaging

Magnetic resonance imaging (MRI) places the patient in close proximity to a high-strength magnetic field through which pulses of radiofrequency radiation are projected, thereby exciting the nuclei of hydrogen, phosphorus, oxygen, and other elements. The radiofrequency signals are manipulated and recorded by a computer, and a two-dimensional image representing a section of the patient is produced.[6,7] MRI has greater sensitivity for identifying liver tumors than do ultrasonography, CT, and radionuclide imaging. Significant advances in MRI technology and imaging capabilities often makes this a preferred diagnostic test.[6,7]

Arteriography

Arteriography of the gut depicts the configuration of visceral blood vessels after intravenous administration of a contrast medium. Arteriography may be employed for detecting tumors and bleeding lesions and therapeutic applications, including embolization of bleeding vessels, fistulas, and inoperable tumors.[6,7]

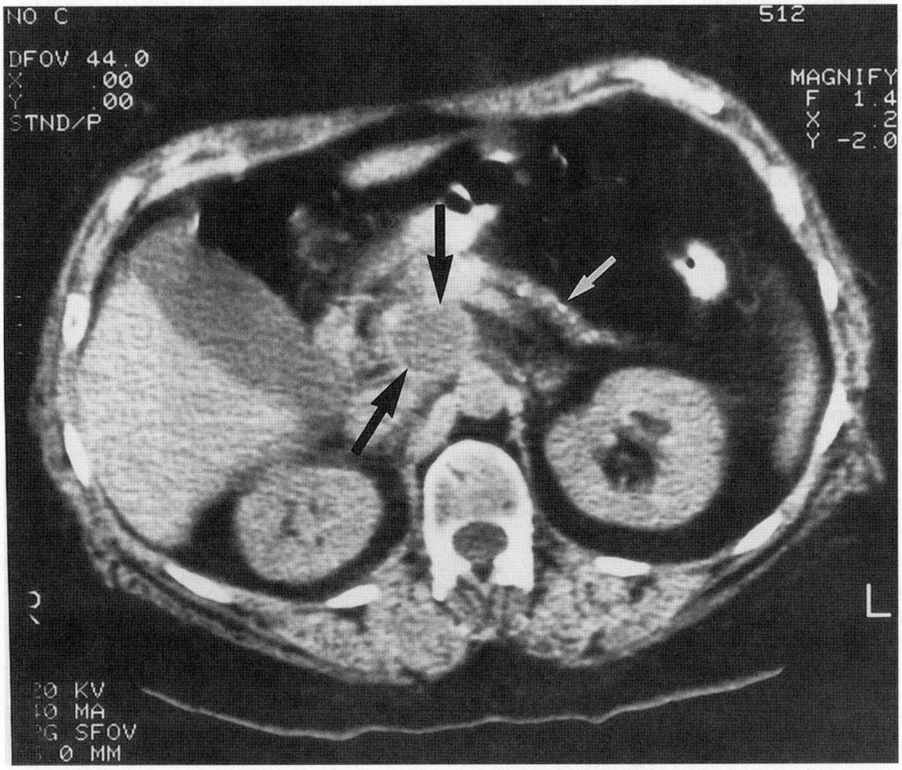

FIGURE 33-4. CT scan of the abdomen showing pancreatitis with calcification *(white arrow)* and pancreatic pseudocyst *(black arrows)*.

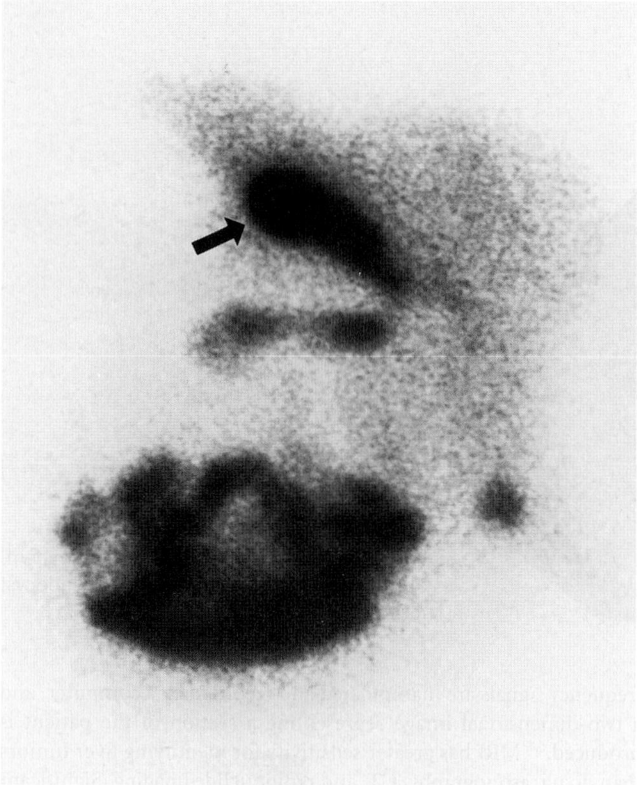

FIGURE 33-5. HIDA scan demonstrating normal gallbladder *(arrow)*.

ENDOSCOPY

Refinement in optical engineering and fiber optics has made possible the development of the endoscope, which revolutionized the management of GI disorders. An endoscope is an illuminated white-light optical instrument designed to inspect the interior of the GI tract. Endoscopes enable the practitioner to inspect intraluminal mucosal lesions and to obtain biopsies and washings for cytology studies. Upper GI tract endoscopy (esophagogastroduodenoscopy [EGD]) is capable of inspecting the esophagus, stomach, and proximal small bowel. Lower GI tract endoscopy of the rectum and colon may be accomplished by colonoscopy or sigmoidoscopy. Endoscopy can also be used to perform many therapeutic procedures.[8]

Preparation for endoscopic examinations includes instructing patients to refrain from eating or drinking for at least 8 to 12 hours prior to the endoscopic procedure. Bowel cleansing is necessary for colonoscopy and sigmoidoscopy. Topical pharyngeal anesthetics, such as viscous lidocaine or benzocaine, usually improve patient acceptance of the upper endoscopic tube. Intravenous sedating agents, such as the benzodiazepines, lorazepam, midazolam, and, more recently, propofol, are among the most common agents used to induce "conscious sedation" prior to the endoscopy. These sedating agents tend to improve patient acceptance and ease of the procedure. The agents should not be used without appropriate monitoring and the availability of flumazenil, a benzodiazepine antagonist. Serious adverse events have occurred with these agents when used for conscious sedation. In addition, antimuscarinic agents such as atropine sulfate are occasionally used for their cardiovascular effects, such as increasing a patient's heart rate, or for their antispasmodic effects, such as reducing duodenal and colonic motility. Because of its effectiveness at reducing bowel motility, glucagon may be used. Endoscopy should be used with caution in patients with severe respiratory or cardiac failure, and for patients with suspected perforated viscera. The most commonly used endoscopic studies are upper endoscopy, colonoscopy, sigmoidoscopy, and endoscopic retrograde cholangiopancreatography.[8]

Esophagogastroduodenoscopy

EGD is used to examine the esophagus, stomach, and duodenum. Patient preparation for EGD includes fasting for at least 6 to 8 hours prior to the procedure and the administration of sedatives and topical anesthetics. Common indications may be either diagnostic or therapeutic in nature, and include evaluating suspected upper GI bleeding, obstructions, upper abdominal pain, persistent vomiting, and radiographic abnormalities.[12] EGD can be used interventionally in upper gastrointestinal bleeding for ligation procedures, sclerosing or vasoconstrictive agent administration at the site of the bleed, or using a heat probe on a bleeding vessel. EGD commonly uncovers peptic ulcers and is the method of choice to diagnose Barrett esophagus and other esophageal erosions (Fig. 33–6). Once viewed as the method of choice to diagnosis gastroesophageal reflux disease, EGD has lost ground to the wide availability of proton pump inhibitors. Because of the favorable side-effect profile of proton pump inhibitors, they are frequently prescribed by primary care physicians for heartburn and other symptoms attributed to gastroesophageal reflux disease. Because primary care physicians usually refer patients only when they fail to respond to therapy, by the time an endoscopy is performed in patients on proton pump inhibitor therapy, the examination is likely to reveal normal-appearing mucosa.[8]

Colonoscopy

Colonoscopy permits direct examination of the large intestine and rectum. To prepare for colonoscopy, the patient should fast for at least 8 to 12 hours prior to the examination, and bowel cleansing should be completed. A benzodiazepine and a short-acting narcotic agent are given to produce conscious sedation. As with upper GI endoscopy, indications for lower GI endoscopy can be either diagnostic or therapeutic in nature, and include evaluation and detection of abnormalities visualized by radiography, as well as GI hemorrhage, colonic lesions, volvulus, ulcerative colitis, Crohn disease, diverticulitis, and excision of colonic polyps.[9]

Sigmoidoscopy

Sigmoidoscopy is used to evaluate the sigmoid colon and rectum (Fig. 33–7). Flexible sigmoidoscopy has virtually replaced rigid sigmoidoscopy because of increased patient comfort and superior performance. The major indication for this examination is to evaluate symptoms related to the colon or rectum, and to conduct screening of asymptomatic patients for colon polyps or cancer. Patient preparation involves instructing patients to abstain from eating or drinking for at least 8 hours prior to the procedure and the administering of bowel-cleansing agents. Anoscopy is especially useful in evaluating the anus.

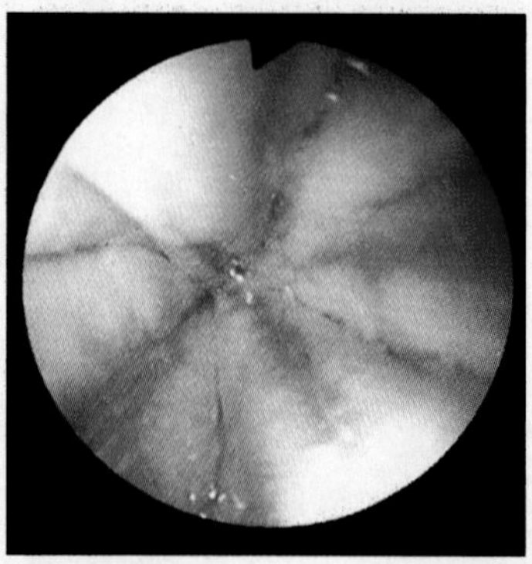

FIGURE 33-6. EGD demonstrating linear red streaks with a central white streak extended up the esophagus in peptic regurgitant esophagitis. *(From Kasper DL, Braunwald E, Hauser S, et al., eds. Harrison's Principles of Internal Medicine, 16th ed. New York: McGraw-Hill, 2005:1731, with permission.)*

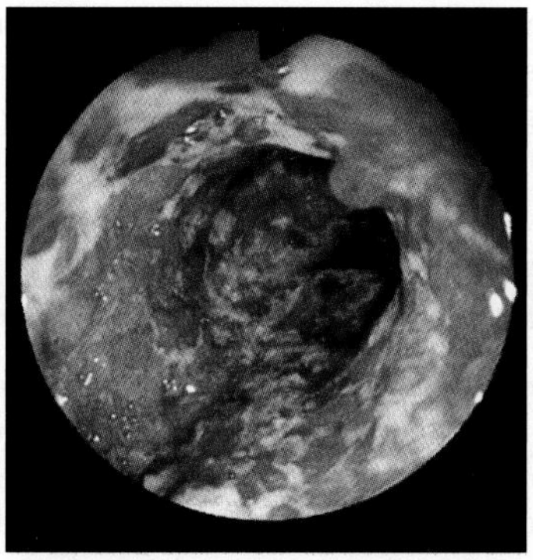

FIGURE 33-7. Sigmoidoscopic photograph demonstrating severe ulcerative colitis with diffuse ulceration, bleeding, and exudation. *(From Kasper DL, Braunwald E, Hauser S, et al., eds. Harrison's Principles of Internal Medicine, 16th ed. New York: McGraw-Hill, 2005:1732, with permission.)*

The major indications for anoscopic examination include symptoms related to the anus and rectum, such as bleeding, protrusions or swelling, pain, and severe itching. Patients undergoing sigmoidoscopy or anoscopy generally do not require sedation.

Endoscopic Retrograde Cholangiopancreatography

Endoscopic retrograde cholangiopancreatography (ERCP) is an important procedure that is used to evaluate and treat diseases of the biliary tree and pancreas. By injecting contrast agents through a catheter placed in the pancreaticobiliary ducts during ERCP, abnormalities such as obstructions, calculi, and strictures can be examined. ERCP also allows for the use of therapeutic techniques such as the removal of ductal stones, stenting of strictures, and sphincterotomy. Preparation for ERCP consists of conscious sedation and glucagon to relax gut motility. Common reasons for ERCP include detection and evaluation of pancreatic malignancy, pancreatitis, biliary obstruction, bile duct stones, jaundice, and patients whose clinical presentation suggests biliary disease (Fig. 33–8).[7,9]

Capsule Endoscopy

Capsule endoscopy allows the visualization of the small intestine, and consists of a vitamin-pill–sized video camera that is swallowed and acts as an endoscope. As the video capsule travels naturally through the digestive tract, images are transmitted to a recording device. Patients return the recording device to the practitioner so that the images can be downloaded to a computer and evaluated. Eventually, the camera is naturally excreted and not retrieved.[10]

MISCELLANEOUS TESTS

Esophageal Manometry

Esophageal manometry is used to evaluate diseases of the esophagus by assessing esophageal motor functions. Common indications for this procedure include dysphagia and obscure chest pain. A special catheter equipped with pressure transducers is placed into the esophagus to measure esophageal pressures and peristalsis. Provocative testing with pharmacologic agents such as edrophonium chloride, a cholinergic muscle stimulant, may be used to precipitate esophageal pain during this procedure. Typical indications for esophageal manometry include evaluating esophageal dysmotility, nonobstructive dysphagia, obscure chest pain, scleroderma, intestinal pseudoobstruction, achalasia, and aiding in positioning instruments such as pH probes.

Ambulatory Esophageal pH Monitoring

Esophageal pH monitoring is considered by many clinicians as the gold standard for studying gastric fluid pH in patients who complain of gastroesophageal reflux. Ambulatory 24-hour pH monitoring is an elegant way to link esophageal acid exposure, as detected by a probe in the esophagus, with patient symptoms. The pH probe is placed approximately 5 cm above the distal esophagus. Because intraesophageal pH is normally higher (pH 6) than that of the stomach (pH approximately 1 to 3), the pH probe will record a decrease in pH if gastroesophageal reflux occurs. The most accepted method to identify gastroesophageal reflux during monitoring is the sudden decrease in pH below 4.0. The ambulatory 24-hour pH study links the patient's symptom to an acid event (Fig. 33–9). Wireless pH monitoring systems have gradually replacing the older methods that required a wire probe placement. A capsule is attached to the distal esophagus by a delivery system. The capsule then transmits measured pH data to a receiver by radiotelemetry technique. Wireless systems offer the advantage of better patient acceptance and extended monitoring of up to 96 hours versus 24 hours of the wire method. There are limitations to ambulatory pH monitoring in patients receiving proton pump inhibitor therapy or in the detection of nonacidic or weakly acidic refluxate.[11]

Multichannel intraluminal impedance monitoring is an emerging technique to study acid and nonacid reflux. The method combines pH measurements with manometry that enables the measurement of

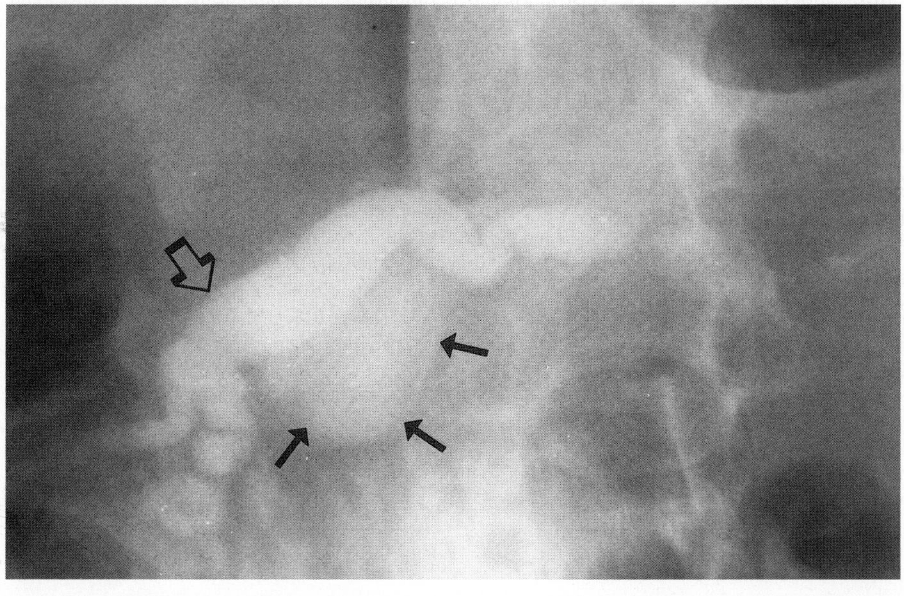

FIGURE 33-8. Endoscopic retrograde cholangiopancreatography (ERCP) demonstrating a dilated, irregular pancreatic duct with areas of stricturing *(large arrow)*. A pancreatic pseudocyst is visible immediately adjacent to the spine *(small arrows)*.

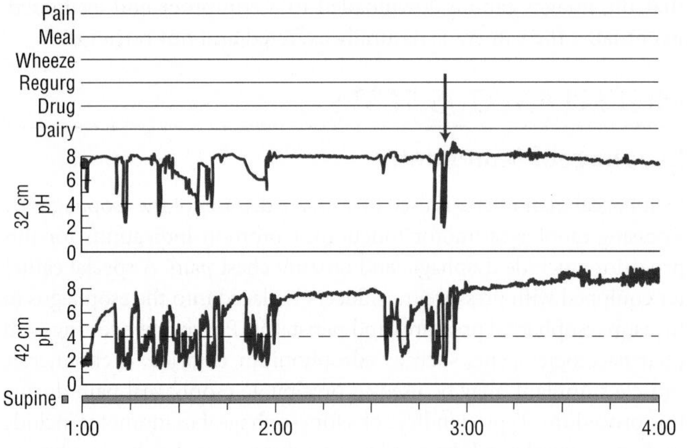

FIGURE 33-9. Ambulatory pH monitoring. The pH recordings from two esophageal probes are plotted over a 3-hour interval. Notice that the patient's symptom of regurgitation correlates with a low pH (<4) event *(arrow)*.

and distinction between swallowing and reflux. In patients who have failed symptomatically to respond to empiric proton pump inhibitor therapy in GERD, the test can separate those in whom symptoms are associated with acid reflux from those in whom symptoms are associated with non-acid reflux. Outcomes studies are required to further evaluate the usefulness of this diagnostic method.[12,13]

The Bernstein test, an older procedure that is used to measure gastric fluid pH, has largely been replaced by ambulatory pH monitoring. The procedure requires inserting a nasogastric tube and administrating alternating dripped solutions of normal saline and 0.1 N hydrochloric acid (HCl) into the esophagus via the nasogastric tube. If patient symptoms are reproduced by the acid perfusion and not the saline, the study is considered abnormal and indicative of acid hypersensitivity.[14]

Endoscopic Ultrasonography

Endoscopic ultrasonography is useful in the diagnosis and staging of gastroenterologic disorders. The instrument itself functions very much like a typical upper endoscope but with the added feature of an ultrasound transducer. The examiner is then able to see the regional anatomy and pathology beneath the mucosa. The major advantage of this procedure is its capability to deliver the ultrasound transducer to close proximity of deep tissues for enhanced image resolution. In clinical practice, endoscopic ultrasonography is highly useful in detecting and defining gastrointestinal and pancreatic malignancies. It also plays a role in the diagnosis of submucosal lesions and small pancreatic malignancies. Endoscopic ultrasonographic guidance of fine-needle biopsy is increasingly performed.

Laparoscopy

Laparoscopy uses a tube-like device with an elaborate optical system that permits distinct visualization of the peritoneal cavity. General anesthesia is often required and a surgical incision is made in the abdomen to allow the passage of the laparoscope. The exterior of the liver, gallbladder, spleen, peritoneum, diaphragm, and pelvic organs may be examined during the laparoscopic examination. Similar to the other endoscopic techniques mentioned, biopsies and therapeutic interventions may be performed during the laparoscopy. Reasons for doing laparoscopy include evaluating patients with ascites, abdominal masses, chronic abdominal pain, abnormalities indicated on liver–spleen scan, liver diseases, obstructive jaundice, and hepatic malignancy.

CONCLUSIONS

Evaluation of the GI tract begins with a careful history and comprehensive physical examination. It then proceeds in a deliberate and thoughtful manner to establish the correct diagnosis and appropriate management. Laboratory and microbiologic tests, radiography, ultrasonography, computed tomography, radionuclide scanning, magnetic resonance imaging, arteriography, endoscopy, esophageal manometry, pH monitoring, endoscopic ultrasonography, and laparoscopy have definite roles in diagnosing and evaluating GI disorders. Clinicians should be aware of warning signs that require immediate referral for further diagnostic studies.

REFERENCES

1. Kearney DJ. Approach to the patient with gastrointestinal disorders. In: Friedman SL, McQuaid KR, et al., eds. Diagnosis & Treatment in Gastroenterology. New York: Lange Medical Books/McGraw-Hill, 2003:1–33.
2. Powell DW. Approach to the patient with gastrointestinal disease. In: Goldman L, Ausiello D, eds. Cecil's Textbook of Medicine. Philadelphia: WB Saunders, 2004:782–785.
3. Bates B. A Guide to Physical Examination. Philadelphia: Lippincott, 2005.
4. Farkas J, Farkas P, Hyde D. Liver and gastroenterology tests. In: Lee M, ed. Interpreting Laboratory Data. Baltimore, MD: ASHP, 2004:323–364.
5. Bouckengooghe AR, DuPont HL. Approach to the patient with diarrhea. In: Gorbach SL, Bartlett JG, Blacklow NR, eds. Infectious Diseases. Philadelphia: Lippincott, 2004:597–603.
6. Novelline RA. Squire's Fundamentals of Radiology. Cambridge, MA: Harvard University Press, 2004.
7. Wittich GR. Diagnostic imaging procedures in gastroenterology. In: Goldman L, Ausiello D, eds. Cecil's Textbook of Medicine. Philadelphia: WB Saunders, 2004:784–789.
8. Tytgat GNJ. Upper gastrointestinal endoscopy. In: Yamada T, Alpers DH, Kaplowitz N, eds., et al. Gastroenterology. Philadelphia: Lippincott, 2003:138:2825–2844.
9. Hay DW, Onion SK. Blackwell's Primary Care Essentials: Gastrointestinal and Liver Disease. Malden, MA: Blackwell Science, 2002:363.
10. News from Mayo Clinic in Jacksonville. Capsule Endoscopy Goes Where Few Endoscopes Have Gone Before. 2002, *http:www.mayoclinic.org/news2002-md32.html.*
11. Lutsi B, Hirano I. Ambulatory pH monitoring: New advances and indications. Gastroenterol Hepatol 2006;2:825–842.
12. Tutuian R, Vela MF, Shay SS, Castell DO. Multichannel intraluminal impedance in esophageal function testing and gastroesophageal reflux monitoring. J Clin Gastroenterol 2003;37:206–215.
13. Sandler RS. Bernstein (acid perfusion) test. In: Drossman DA, ed. Manual of Gastroenterologic Procedures. New York: Raven, 1993:56–60.
14. Nguyen HN, Domingues GRS, Lammert F. Technological insights: Combined impedance manometry for esophageal motility testing—Current results and further implications. World J Gastroenterol 2006;39:6266–6273.
15. Lewis J H, Ahmed M, Shobassy A, Palese C. Drug-induced liver disease. Curr Opin Gastroenterol 2006;22:223–233.
16. Saukkonen JJ, Cohn DL, Jasmer RM, et al. An official ATS statement: Hepatotoxicity of antituberculosis therapy. Am J Respir Crit Care Med 2006;174:935–952.
17. Nathwani RA, Kaplowitz N. Drug hepatotoxicity. Clin Liver Dis 2006;10:207–217.

CHAPTER 34 Gastroesophageal Reflux Disease

DIANNE B. WILLIAMS AND ROBERT R. SCHADE

KEY CONCEPTS

1. Patients should be assessed for symptoms, such as heartburn, and for signs and symptoms of complications (e.g., dysphagia) that require immediate medical attention.

2. Endoscopy is used to evaluate mucosal damage from gastroesophageal reflux disease (GERD) and to assess for the presence of Barrett's esophagus or other complications; ambulatory reflux monitoring is useful for confirming GERD in patients with persistent symptoms without evidence of mucosal damage or in patients with atypical symptoms; manometry is useful in patients who are candidates for antireflux surgery and for ensuring proper placement of pH probes.

3. The goals of GERD treatment are to alleviate symptoms, decrease the frequency of recurrent disease, promote healing of mucosal injury, and prevent complications.

4. GERD treatment is determined by disease severity and includes lifestyle changes and patient-directed therapy, pharmacologic treatment, and interventional approaches (antireflux surgery or endoscopic therapies).

5. Patients with typical GERD symptoms should be treated with lifestyle modifications and a trial of empiric acid-suppression therapy. Those who do not respond to empiric therapy or who present with alarm symptoms should undergo endoscopy.

6. Interventional approaches offer an alternative treatment for selected patients when long-term pharmacologic management is undesirable.

7. Acid suppression is the mainstay of GERD treatment. H_2-receptor antagonists are effective in less-severe GERD. Proton pump inhibitors provide the greatest symptom relief and the highest healing rates, especially in patients with erosive disease or moderate to severe symptoms.

8. Many patients with GERD will relapse if medication is withdrawn, so long-term maintenance treatment may be required. A proton pump inhibitor is the drug of choice for maintenance of patients with moderate to severe GERD.

9. Patient medication profiles should be reviewed for drugs that may aggravate GERD. Patients should be monitored for adverse drug reactions and potential drug–drug interactions.

Learning objectives, review questions, and other resources can be found at **www.pharmacotherapyonline.com.**

Gastroesophageal reflux disease (GERD) is a common medical disorder seen by clinicians from various specialties. GERD refers to symptoms or mucosal damage that results from abnormal reflux of the stomach contents into the esophagus.[1] When the esophagus is repeatedly exposed to refluxed material for prolonged periods of time, inflammation of the esophagus (reflux esophagitis) occurs, and in some cases, it can progress to erosion of the squamous epithelium of the esophagus (erosive esophagitis). Gastroesophageal reflux associated with disease processes in organs other than the esophagus, such as the lungs or larynx, is referred to as atypical (or extraesophageal) GERD. Severe reflux symptoms associated with normal endoscopic findings are referred to as "symptomatic GERD," nonerosive reflux disease (NERD), or endoscopy-negative reflux disease (ENRD). Complications of long-term reflux may include the development of strictures, Barrett's esophagus, or adenocarcinoma of the esophagus.

Many patients suffering from mild GERD do not go on to develop erosive esophagitis and are often managed with lifestyle changes, antacids, and nonprescription histamine-2 (H_2)-receptor antagonists or nonprescription proton pump inhibitors. Those with more severe symptoms (with or without endoscopic findings) predictably follow a course of relapsing disease, requiring more intensive treatment with acid-suppression therapy followed by long-term maintenance therapy. Interventional approaches, including antireflux surgery and endoscopic therapies, offer an alternative for selected patients in whom prolonged medical management is undesirable.

EPIDEMIOLOGY

Gastroesophageal reflux disease occurs in people of all ages but is most common in those older than age 40 years. Although mortality associated with GERD is rare, GERD symptoms may have a significant impact on quality of life. The true prevalence and incidence of GERD is difficult to assess because many patients do not seek medical treatment, symptoms do not always correlate well with the severity of the disease, and there is no standardized definition or universal gold standard method for diagnosing the disease. However, an estimated 10% to 20% of people in Western countries suffer from GERD symptoms on a weekly basis.[2] Heartburn is the hallmark symptom of GERD and is generally described as a substernal sensation of warmth or burning rising up from the abdomen that may radiate to the neck. It may be waxing and waning in character.

The prevalence of GERD varies depending on the geographic region, but appears highest in Western countries.[2] Except during pregnancy and possibly NERD, there does not appear to be a major difference in incidence between men and women. NERD tends to be more common in women and in patients who are approximately a decade younger than patients who develop erosive disease. Although gender does not generally play a major role in the development of GERD, it is an important factor in the development of Barrett's esophagus, a complication of GERD in which the normal squamous epithelium is replaced with specialized columnar epithelium. Barrett's esophagus is most prevalent in white adult males in Western countries. The presence of Barrett's esophagus increases the risk for adenocarcinoma of the esophagus. Other risk factors and comorbidities that may contribute to the development or worsening of GERD symptoms include family history, obesity, smoking, alcohol consumption, certain medications and foods, respiratory diseases, and chest pain.

PATHOPHYSIOLOGY

The key factor in the development of GERD is the abnormal reflux of gastric contents from the stomach into the esophagus.[1] In some cases, gastroesophageal reflux is associated with defective lower esophageal sphincter (LES) pressure or function. Patients may have decreased gastroesophageal sphincter pressures related to (a) spontaneous transient LES relaxations, (b) transient increases in intraabdominal pressure, or (c) an atonic LES, all of which may lead to the development of gastroesophageal reflux. Problems with other normal mucosal defense mechanisms, such as anatomic factors, esophageal clearance, mucosal resistance, gastric emptying, epidermal growth factor, and salivary buffering, may also contribute to the development of GERD. Aggressive factors that may promote esophageal damage upon reflux into the esophagus include gastric acid, pepsin, bile acids, and pancreatic enzymes. Thus the composition and volume of the refluxate, as well as duration of exposure, are important aggressive factors in determining the consequences of gastroesophageal reflux. Rational therapeutic regimens in the treatment of gastroesophageal reflux are designed to maximize normal mucosal defense mechanisms and attenuate the aggressive factors.

LOWER ESOPHAGEAL SPHINCTER PRESSURE

The lower esophageal sphincter is a manometrically defined zone at the distal esophagus with an elevated basal resting pressure. The sphincter is normally in a tonic, contracted state, preventing the reflux of gastric material from the stomach, but relaxes on swallowing to permit the free passage of food into the stomach.

Mechanisms by which defective LES pressure may cause gastroesophageal reflux are threefold. First, and probably most importantly, reflux may occur following spontaneous transient LES relaxations that are not associated with swallowing. Although the exact mechanism is unknown, esophageal distension, vomiting, belching, and retching have all been shown to cause relaxation of the LES. While not thought to contribute significantly to erosive esophagitis, these transient relaxations, which are normal postprandially, may play an important role in intermittent nonerosive reflux. Transient decreases in sphincter pressure are responsible for more than half of the reflux episodes in patients with GERD. The propensity to develop gastroesophageal reflux secondary to transient decreases in LES pressure is probably dependent on numerous factors, including the degree of sphincter relaxation, efficacy of esophageal clearance, patient position (more common in recumbent position), gastric volume, and intragastric pressure. Second, reflux may occur following transient increases in intraabdominal pressure (stress reflux). An increase in intraabdominal pressure such as that occurring during straining, bending over, coughing, eating, or a Valsalva maneuver may overcome a weak LES, and thus may lead to reflux. Third, the LES may be atonic, thus permitting free reflux as seen in patients with scleroderma. Although transient relaxations are more likely to occur when there is normal LES pressure, the latter two mechanisms are more likely to occur when the LES pressure is decreased by such factors as fatty foods, gastric distension, smoking, or certain medications. Table 34–1 lists medications and foods that affect lower esophageal sphincter pressure.[3] Various foods aggravate esophageal reflux by decreasing LES pressure or by precipitating symptomatic reflux by direct mucosal irritation (e.g., spicy foods, orange juice, tomato juice, and coffee).

TABLE 34-1 Foods and Medications That May Worsen GERD Symptoms

Decreased lower-esophageal sphincter pressure	
Foods	
Fatty meal	Garlic
Carminatives (peppermint, spearmint)	Onions
Chocolate	Chili peppers
Coffee, cola, tea	
Medications	
Anticholinergics	Ethanol
Barbiturates	Nicotine (smoking)
Caffeine	Nitrates
Dihydropyridine calcium channel blockers	Progesterone
Dopamine	Tetracycline
Estrogen	Theophylline
Direct irritants to the esophageal mucosa	
Foods	
Spicy foods	Tomato juice
Orange juice	Coffee
Medications	
Alendronate	Iron
Aspirin	Quinidine
Nonsteroidal antiinflammatory drugs	Potassium chloride

Pregnancy is a condition in which reflux is common. There are many postulated reasons for the increased incidence of heartburn during pregnancy, including hormonal effects on esophageal muscle, LES tone, and physical factors (increased intraabdominal pressure) resulting from an enlarging uterus.

A decrease in LES pressure resulting from any of the previously mentioned causes is not always associated with gastroesophageal reflux. Likewise, individuals who experience decreases in sphincter pressures and subsequently reflux, do not always develop GERD. The other natural defense mechanisms (anatomic factors, esophageal clearance, mucosal resistance, and other gastric factors) must be evoked to explain this phenomenon.

ANATOMIC FACTORS

Disruption of the normal anatomic barriers by a hiatal hernia was once thought to be a primary etiology of gastroesophageal reflux and esophagitis. Now it appears that a more important factor related to the presence or absence of symptoms in patients with hiatal hernia is the LES pressure. The size of a hiatal hernia is proportional to the frequency of transient LES relaxations. Patients with hypotensive LES pressures and large hiatal hernias are more likely to experience gastroesophageal reflux following abrupt increases in intraabdominal pressure compared to patients with a hypotensive LES and no hiatal hernia. Although anatomic factors are still considered significant by some, the diagnosis of hiatal hernia is currently considered a separate entity with which gastroesophageal reflux may or may not simultaneously occur.

ESOPHAGEAL CLEARANCE

In many patients with GERD, the problem is not that they produce too much acid, but that the acid produced spends too much time in contact with the esophageal mucosa. This is not surprising, because the symptoms and/or severity of damage produced by gastroesophageal reflux are partially dependent on the duration of contact between the gastric contents and the esophageal mucosa. This contact time is, in turn, dependent on the rate at which the esophagus clears the noxious material, as well as the frequency of reflux. The esophagus is cleared by primary peristalsis in response to swallowing, or by secondary peristalsis in response to esophageal distension and gravitational effects. Swallowing contributes to esophageal clearance by increasing salivary flow. Saliva contains bicarbonate that buffers the residual gastric material on the surface of the esophagus. The production of saliva decreases with increasing age, making it more difficult to maintain a neutral intraesophageal pH. Therefore esophageal damage caused by reflux occurs more often in the elderly, and similarly in patients with Sjögren's syndrome or xerostomia. Swallowing is also decreased during sleep, making nocturnal GERD a problem in many patients.

MUCOSAL RESISTANCE

Within the esophageal mucosa and submucosa there are mucus-secreting glands. The mucus secreted by these glands may contribute to the protection of the esophagus.[4] Bicarbonate moving from the blood to the lumen can neutralize acidic refluxate in the esophagus. When the mucosa is repeatedly exposed to the refluxate in GERD, or if there is a defect in the normal mucosal defenses, hydrogen ions diffuse into the mucosa, leading to the cellular acidification and necrosis that ultimately cause esophagitis. In theory, mucosal resistance may be related not only to esophageal mucus, but also to tight epithelial junctions, epithelial cell turnover, nitrogen balance, mucosal blood flow, tissue prostaglandins, and the acid–base status of the tissue.[4] Saliva is also rich in epidermal growth factor, stimulating cell renewal.

GASTRIC EMPTYING

Delayed gastric emptying can contribute to gastroesophageal reflux. An increase in gastric volume may increase both the frequency of reflux and the amount of gastric fluid available to be refluxed. Gastric volume is related to the volume of material ingested, rate of gastric secretion, rate of gastric emptying, and amount and frequency of duodenal reflux into the stomach. Factors that increase gastric volume and/or decrease gastric emptying, such as smoking and high-fat meals, are often associated with gastroesophageal reflux. This partially explains the prevalence of postprandial gastroesophageal reflux. Fatty foods may increase postprandial gastroesophageal reflux by increasing gastric volume, delaying the gastric emptying rate, and decreasing the LES pressure. Patients with gastroesophageal reflux, particularly infants, may have a defect in antral motility. The delay in emptying may promote regurgitation of feedings, which might, in turn, contribute to two common complications of GERD in infants (e.g., failure to thrive and pulmonary aspiration).[5]

COMPOSITION OF REFLUXATE

The composition, pH, and volume of the refluxate are important aggressive factors in determining the consequences of gastroesophageal reflux. In animals, acid has two primary effects when it refluxes into the esophagus. First, if the pH of the refluxate is less than 2, esophagitis may develop secondary to protein denaturation. In addition, pepsinogen is activated to pepsin at this pH and may also cause esophagitis. Duodenogastric reflux esophagitis, or "alkaline esophagitis," refers to esophagitis induced by the reflux of bilious and pancreatic fluid. The term *alkaline esophagitis* may be a misnomer in that the refluxate may be either weakly alkaline or acidic in nature. An increase in gastric bile concentrations may be caused by duodenogastric reflux as a result of a generalized motility disorder, slower clearance of the refluxate, or after surgery.[6]

Although bile acids have both a direct irritant effect on the esophageal mucosa and an indirect effect of increasing hydrogen ion permeability of the mucosa, symptoms are more often related to acid reflux than to bile reflux. Specifically, the percentage of time that the esophageal pH is below 4 is greater for patients with severe disease as compared to those with mild disease. Esophageal pH monitoring in conjunction with 24-hour bile monitoring has shown a higher incidence of Barrett's esophagus in patients who have both acid and alkaline reflux.[6] More study is needed to substantiate this finding. Nevertheless, the combination of acid, pepsin, and/or bile is a potent refluxate in producing esophageal damage.

COMPLICATIONS

Several complications may occur with gastroesophageal reflux, including esophageal strictures, Barrett's esophagus, and adenocarcinoma of the esophagus. Strictures are common in the distal esophagus and are generally 1 to 2 cm in length. The use of nonsteroidal antiinflammatory drugs or aspirin has been implicated as an additional risk factor that may contribute to the development or worsening of GERD complications.[2] Although GERD may lead to esophageal bleeding, the blood loss is usually chronic and low grade in nature, but anemia may occur. In some patients, the reparative process leads to the replacement of the squamous epithelial lining of the esophagus by specialized columnar-type epithelium. This condition, known as Barrett's esophagus, is more likely to occur in those patients with a long history (years) of symptomatic reflux.[7] Patients with Barrett's esophagus have a greater than 30% incidence of esophageal stricture formation. The stricture is often the presenting finding, as once Barrett's esophagus is found, the patient gets treatment. Additionally, the risk of esophageal adenocarcinoma is 30 to 60 times higher in patients with Barrett's esophagus as compared to the general population.[8]

The pathophysiology of gastroesophageal reflux is a complex cyclic process. It is difficult, if not impossible, to determine which occurs first: gastroesophageal reflux leading to defective peristalsis with delayed clearing, or an incompetent LES pressure leading to gastroesophageal reflux. Understanding the factors associated with the development of GERD provides insight into the treatment modalities currently used to manage patients suffering from this disease.

CLINICAL PRESENTATION

❶ Patients with GERD may display symptoms described as (a) typical, (b) atypical, or (c) alarm. Table 34–2 summarizes each of these clinical presentations of GERD. The severity of the symptoms of gastroesophageal reflux does not always correlate with the degree of esophagitis, but it does correlate with the duration of reflux. Patients with nonerosive disease may have symptoms as severe as those with endoscopic findings.

It is important to distinguish GERD symptoms from those of other diseases, especially when chest pain or pulmonary symptoms are present. Interestingly, close to half of patients presenting with chest pain who have a normal electrocardiogram have GERD.[9] Similarly, approximately half of patients with asthma have GERD.[9] Patients presenting with asthma (especially nocturnal asthma) that is poorly responsive to standard medical therapies should be evaluated to determine if GERD contributes to their symptoms. Pulmonary symptoms result from either direct irritation of the vagus nerve when refluxed acid comes in contact with the esophageal mucosa, causing bronchospasm (the reflex theory) or, less commonly, from aspiration of the refluxate into the lungs, causing chemical irritation that manifests as pneumonia or pulmonary fibrosis (the reflux theory).

As previously mentioned, patients who are inadequately treated for GERD may go on to develop complications from long-term acid exposure. Long-term, recurrent reflux symptoms that are not ade-

TABLE 34-2 Clinical Presentation of GERD

Typical symptoms: May be aggravated by activities that worsen gastroesophageal reflux such as recumbent position, bending over, or eating a meal high in fat.
- Heartburn
- Water brash (hypersalivation)
- Belching
- Regurgitation

Atypical symptoms: In some cases, these extraesophageal symptoms may be the only symptoms present, making it more difficult to recognize GERD as the cause, especially when endoscopic studies are normal.
- Nonallergic asthma
- Chronic cough
- Hoarseness
- Pharyngitis
- Chest pain
- Dental erosions

Alarm symptoms: These symptoms may be indicative of complications of GERD such as Barrett's esophagus, esophageal strictures, or esophageal cancer.
- Continual pain
- Dysphagia
- Odynophagia
- Unexplained weight loss
- Choking

quately treated may lead to the development of Barrett's esophagus and may be an independent risk factor for the development of esophageal adenocarcinoma.[8] Esophageal strictures may be present in patients presenting with dysphagia. However, these symptoms may occur in other esophageal disorders such as esophageal diverticulum, achalasia, obstruction, esophageal spasm, esophageal infections, scleroderma, and malignancy. The presence of alarm symptoms should be further investigated to differentiate other diseases as the cause.

The most useful tool in the diagnosis of gastroesophageal reflux is the clinical history, including both presenting symptoms and associated risk factors. Patients presenting with mild, typical symptoms of reflux (heartburn and regurgitation) do not usually require invasive esophageal evaluation. These patients generally benefit from an initial empiric trial of acid-suppression therapy. A clinical diagnosis of GERD can be assumed in patients who respond to appropriate therapy.[1] Further diagnostic evaluation should be performed in those patients do not respond to therapy, for those who present with alarm symptoms (e.g., dysphagia, weight loss), and in those with long-standing GERD symptoms. Alarm symptoms may indicate more complicated disease and long-standing GERD symptoms increase the risk for Barrett's esophagus.

❷ Useful tests in diagnosing GERD include endoscopy, ambulatory reflux monitoring, and manometry. Endoscopy is the preferred technique for assessing the mucosa for esophagitis, identifying Barrett's esophagus and diagnosing complications.[1] It enables visualization and biopsy of the esophageal mucosa. Although endoscopy is a highly specific test, it is not extremely sensitive. In mild cases of GERD, the esophageal mucosa may appear relatively normal. In addition, noninflammatory GERD and major motor disorders may be missed by endoscopy. A camera-containing capsule swallowed by the patient offers the newest technology for visualizing the esophageal mucosa. The PillCam ESO is less invasive and takes less than 15 minutes to perform in the clinician's office. Images of the esophagus are downloaded through sensors placed on the patient's chest that are connected to a data collector. The camera-containing capsule is passed in the stool.

Although less expensive than endoscopy, barium radiography lacks the sensitivity and specificity needed to accurately determine the presence of mucosal injury or to distinguish between Barrett's esophagus and esophagitis. For these reasons, barium radiography has limited use in the routine diagnosis of GERD. Unfortunately, the presence or absence of mucosal damage does not prove the patient's symptoms are reflux related; for that, ambulatory reflux monitoring is useful.

Ambulatory pH testing identifies patients with excessive esophageal acid exposure and helps determine if symptoms, both typical and atypical, are acid related. However, pH monitoring may be less reliable in confirming laryngopharyngeal reflux.[10] Interestingly, patients may have severe symptoms, including esophagitis, even when total acid exposure is considered normal.[1] Ambulatory pH testing may also be useful in patients who are on what is considered adequate therapy, but whose symptoms are not improving. However, GERD that is truly refractory to medical therapy is uncommon. Ambulatory pH testing can be performed by passing a small pH probe transnasally and placing it approximately 5 cm above the LES.[11,12] Patients are asked to keep a diary of symptoms that later are correlated with the pH measurement corresponding to the time the symptom was reported. In addition to correlating symptoms to abnormal esophageal acid exposure, ambulatory pH testing also documents the percentage of time the intraesophageal pH is below 4 and determines the frequency and severity of reflux. Two recent developments related to ambulatory reflux monitoring include (a) the use of combined impedance and acid testing and (b) the use of a tubeless method of acid monitoring.[1] Whereas ambulatory pH testing only measures acid reflux, combined impedance and acid testing measures both acid and nonacid reflux. This may be useful when evaluating patients on acid suppression therapy. The second method involves the attachment of a radiotelemetry capsule to the esophageal mucosa. The advantages of this method are that a longer period of monitoring is possible (48 hours) and it is more comfortable for the patient because a nasogastric tube is unnecessary.

The empiric use of standard- or even double-dose proton pump inhibitor (specifically omeprazole) as a therapeutic trial for diagnosing the presence of GERD may be useful in patients with atypical symptoms. This approach is less expensive, more convenient, and more readily available than ambulatory reflux monitoring. Problems with using a proton pump inhibitor as a diagnostic tool include lack of a standardized dosing regimen and duration of the diagnostic trial.

Esophageal manometry may be used to ensure the proper placement of esophageal pH probes and to evaluate esophageal peristalsis and motility prior to antireflux surgery. To perform manometry, a multilumen pressure sensing tube is passed into the stomach and the pressures are measured as the tube is pulled back across the lower esophageal sphincter, esophagus, and pharynx. The recent advancement of the tubeless pH monitoring system using endoscopic landmarks for placement may negate the need for manometry for ensuring proper placement of esophageal pH probes.[1]

TREATMENT

■ DESIRED OUTCOMES

❸ Therapeutic modalities used in the treatment of gastroesophageal reflux are targeted at reversing the various pathophysiologic abnormalities. The goals of treatment are to (a) alleviate or eliminate the patient's symptoms; (b) decrease the frequency or recurrence and duration of gastroesophageal reflux; (c) promote healing of the injured mucosa; and (d) prevent the development of complications. Therapy is directed at augmenting defense mechanisms that prevent reflux and/or decrease the aggressive factors that worsen reflux or mucosal damage (Fig. 34–1). Specifically, therapy is directed at (a) decreasing the acidity of the refluxate; (b) decreasing the gastric volume available to be refluxed; (c) improving gastric emptying; (d) increasing LES pressure; (e) enhancing esophageal acid clearance; and (f) protecting the esophageal mucosa.

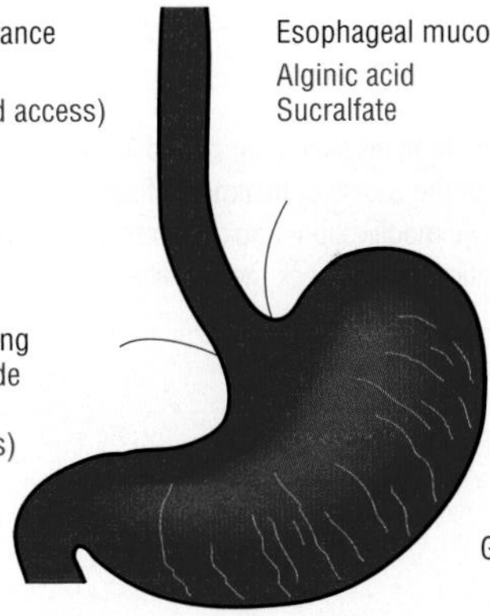

FIGURE 34-1. Therapeutic interventions in the management of gastroesophageal reflux disease. Pharmacologic interventions are targeted at improving defense mechanisms or decreasing aggressive factors. (LES, lower esophageal sphincter.)

■ GENERAL APPROACH TO TREATMENT

❹ The treatment of GERD is categorized into one of the following modalities: (a) lifestyle modifications and patient-directed therapy with antacids, nonprescription H_2-receptor antagonists, and/or nonprescription proton pump inhibitors; (b) pharmacologic intervention with prescription-strength acid suppression therapy; (c) and interventional therapies (antireflux surgery or endoscopic therapies; Table 34–3). The initial therapeutic modality used is in part dependent on the patient's condition (frequency of symptoms, degree of esophagitis, and presence of complications). Historically, a step-up approach was used, starting with noninvasive lifestyle modifications and patient-directed therapy, and progressing to pharmacologic management or interventional approaches (Table 34–4). A step-down approach, starting with a proton pump inhibitor given once or twice daily instead of an H_2-receptor antagonist, and then stepping down to the lowest degree of acid suppression needed to control symptoms, is also effective. Neither the "step-up" nor the "step-down" approach has superior efficacy over the other. The clinician should determine the most appropriate approach for the individual patient. Every attempt should be made to aggressively control symptoms and to prevent relapses early in the course of the patient's disease in order to prevent the complications that are seen with long-standing symptomatic GERD.[13] In patients with moderate to severe GERD, especially those with erosive disease, starting with a proton pump inhibitor as initial therapy is advocated because of its superior efficacy over H_2-receptor antagonists.

Dietary and lifestyle modifications with education about factors that may worsen GERD symptoms is reasonable to discuss with the patient even though they are unlikely to control the patient's symptoms in most cases.[1] Table 34–5 lists many of the lifestyle modifications that can be recommended.[1] Although most patients do not respond to lifestyle changes alone, education about their potential benefits should be stressed on a routine basis. Patients with mild or infrequent symptoms may see improvement with the inexpensive nonprescription H_2-receptor antagonists, proton pump inhibitors, antacids, or alginic acid.

❺ Patients who do not respond to lifestyle modifications and patient-directed therapy after 2 weeks should seek medical attention and are generally started on empiric therapy consisting of an acid-suppression agent. Acid-suppression therapy with proton pump inhibitors or H_2-receptor antagonists is the mainstay of GERD treatment. Patients presenting with moderate to severe symptoms (with or without esophageal erosions) should be started on a proton pump inhibitor as initial therapy because it provides the most rapid symptomatic relief and healing in the highest percentage of patients.[1] H_2-receptor antagonists in divided doses are effective in patients with mild GERD. Standard H_2-receptor antagonist doses may be increased to 2 to 4 times the normal dose in patients who do not respond to standard doses. However, if this is necessary, it is more cost-effective to switch to a proton pump inhibitor.

Promotility agents are not as effective as acid-suppression agents. Combining promotility agents with acid-suppression drugs offers only modest improvements in symptoms over standard doses of H_2-receptor antagonists and should not be routinely recommended. In addition, the availability of a promotility agent that has an acceptable adverse effect profile is lacking. Mucosal protectants, such as sucralfate, have a very limited role in the treatment of GERD.

TABLE 34-3 Evidence-Based Treatment Recommendations for GERD

Recommendations	Level of Evidence[a]
Lifestyle modifications	
Patients may benefit from lifestyle modifications but most will require acid suppression therapy to control symptoms.	IV
Patient-directed therapy	
Over-the-counter antacids, H_2-receptor antagonists, and proton pump inhibitors may be used in patients with mild, infrequent heartburn or regurgitation. Patients experiencing continuous symptoms for longer than 2 weeks should be seen by their clinician. Patients experiencing alarm symptoms should seek medical attention as soon as possible.	IV
Acid-suppression therapy	
Acid-suppression therapy is the preferred treatment for GERD. Proton pump inhibitors provide more rapid relief of symptoms and are more effective at healing the esophageal mucosa compared to H_2-receptor antagonists in patients with moderate to severe GERD.	I
Promotility therapy	
Promotility therapy may be useful in some patients when combined with acid-suppression therapy. They are generally not recommended as monotherapy in patients with GERD.	II
Maintenance therapy	
Most patients with GERD will require continuous therapy to control symptoms and to prevent complications.	I
Surgery	
Antireflux surgery represents a viable maintenance option for patients with an established diagnosis of GERD.	II
Endoscopic therapy	
Symptom control may be achieved with the use of endoscopic therapies in some patients with an established diagnosis of GERD.	III
Refractory GERD	
GERD that is refractory to adequate acid suppression is uncommon. In these cases, the diagnosis should be confirmed through further diagnostic tests, preferably ambulatory pH testing, before antireflux surgery is considered.	IV

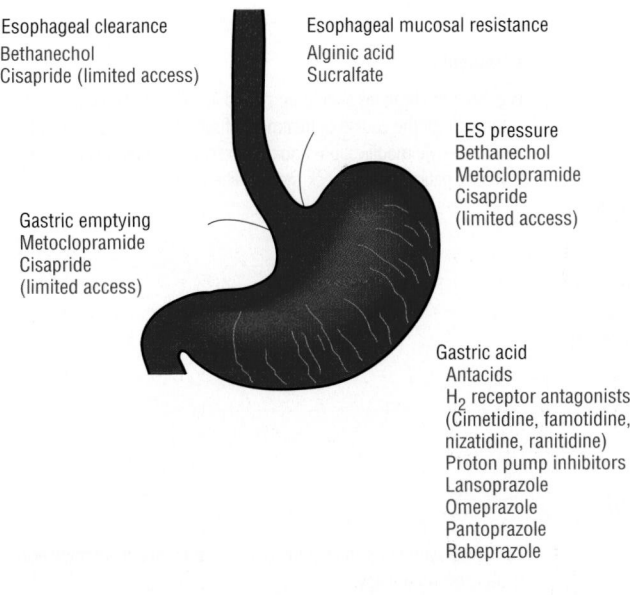

[a]Level of evidence:
I = Strong evidence from at least one published systematic review of multiple, well-designed, randomized, controlled trials.
II = Strong evidence from at least one published, properly designed, randomized, controlled trial of appropriate size and in an appropriate clinical setting.
III = Strong evidence from published, well-designed trials without randomization, single group, pre-post, cohort, time series, or matched case-controlled studies.
IV = Evidence from well-designed nonexperimental studies from more than one center or research group or opinion of respected authorities, based on clinical evidence, descriptive studies, or reports of expert consensus committees.
Data from DeVault KR, Castell DO. Updated guidelines for the diagnosis and treatment of gastroesophageal reflux disease. Am J Gastroenterol 2005;100:190–200.

TABLE 34-4 Therapeutic Approach to GERD in Adults

Patient Presentation	Recommended Treatment Regimen	Comments
Intermittent, mild heartburn	**Lifestyle modifications** **plus** **patient-directed therapy** Antacids • Maalox or Mylanta 30 mL as needed or after meals and at bedtime • Gaviscon 2 tabs after meals and at bedtime • Calcium carbonate 500 mg, 2–4 tablets as needed **and/or** Nonprescription H_2-receptor antagonists (taken up to twice daily) • Cimetidine 200 mg • Famotidine 10 mg • Nizatidine 75 mg • Ranitidine 75 mg **or** Nonprescription proton pump inhibitor (taken once daily) • Omeprazole 20 mg	Lifestyle modifications should be started initially and continued throughout the course of treatment. If symptoms are unrelieved with lifestyle modifications and nonprescription medications after 2 weeks, patient should seek medical attention.
Symptomatic relief of GERD	**Lifestyle modifications** **plus** **prescription-strength acid suppression therapy**	For typical symptoms, treat empirically with prescription-strength acid-suppression therapy. If symptoms recur, consider maintenance therapy (MT). Note: Most patients will require standard doses for MT.
	H_2-receptor antagonists (for 6–12 weeks) • Cimetidine 400 mg twice daily • Famotidine 20 mg twice daily • Nizatidine 150 mg twice daily • Ranitidine 150 mg twice daily **or**	Mild GERD can usually be treated effectively with H_2-receptor antagonists.
	Proton pump inhibitors (for 4–8 weeks); all are given once daily • Esomeprazole 20 mg • Lansoprazole 15 mg • Omeprazole 20 mg • Pantoprazole 40 mg • Rabeprazole 20 mg	Patients with moderate to severe symptoms should receive a proton pump inhibitor as initial therapy.
Healing of erosive esophagitis or treatment of patients presenting with moderate to severe symptoms or complications	**Lifestyle modifications** **plus** Proton pump inhibitors for 4–16 weeks (up to twice daily) • Esomeprazole 20–40 mg daily • Lansoprazole 30 mg daily • Omeprazole 20 mg daily • Rabeprazole 20 mg daily • Pantoprazole 40 mg daily **or**	For atypical or alarm symptoms, obtain endoscopy (if possible) to evaluate mucosa. Give a trial of a proton pump inhibitor. If symptoms are relieved, consider MT. Proton pump inhibitors are the most effective maintenance therapy in patients with atypical symptoms, complications, and erosive disease.
	High-dose H_2-receptor antagonist (for 8–12 weeks) • Cimetidine 400 mg four times daily or 800 mg twice daily • Famotidine 40 mg twice daily • Nizatidine 150 mg four times daily • Ranitidine 150 mg four times daily	Patients not responding to pharmacologic therapy, including those with persistent atypical symptoms, should be evaluated via ambulatory reflux monitoring to confirm the diagnosis of GERD (if possible).
Interventional therapies	Antireflux surgery or endoscopic therapies	

Maintenance therapy is generally necessary to control symptoms and to prevent complications. In patients with more severe symptoms (with or without esophageal erosions), or in patients with other complications, maintenance therapy with a proton pump inhibitor is most effective. Routine use of combination therapy has no role in maintenance therapy of GERD. GERD that is refractory to adequate acid suppression is rare. In these cases, the diagnosis should be confirmed through further diagnostic tests before long-term, high-dose therapy or interventional approaches (antireflux surgery or endoscopic therapies) are considered.[1]

NONPHARMACOLOGIC THERAPY

Nonpharmacologic treatment of GERD includes (a) lifestyle modifications, which should be started initially and continued throughout the treatment course for GERD, and (b) interventional approaches (antireflux surgery or endoscopic therapies), which may be viable maintenance modalities in selected patients.

Lifestyle Modifications

The most common lifestyle modifications that a patient should be educated about include (a) weight loss; (b) elevation of the head of the bed; (c) consumption of smaller meals and not eating 3 hours prior to sleeping; (d) avoidance of foods or medications that exacerbate GERD; (e) smoking cessation; and (f) avoidance of alcohol (see Table 34–5).

Obesity increases the risk of GERD, most likely through increased intraabdominal pressure. Disruption of the esophagogastric junction has also been seen in obese patients.[14] A high-fat meal will decrease LES pressure for 2 hours or more postprandially. In contrast, a high-protein, low-fat meal will elevate LES pressure. Consequently, weight loss and a low-fat diet may help to improve GERD symptoms. Elevating the head of the bed approximately 6 to 8 inches with a foam wedge under the mattress (not just elevating the head with pillows) decreases nocturnal esophageal acid contact time and should be recommended. Many foods may worsen the

TABLE 34-5 Nonpharmacologic Treatment of GERD with Lifestyle Modifications

- Elevate the head of the bed (increases esophageal clearance). Use 6- to 8-inch blocks under the head of the bed. Sleep on a foam wedge.
- Dietary changes
  - Avoid foods that may decrease lower esophageal sphincter pressure (fats, chocolate, alcohol, peppermint, and spearmint)
  - Avoid foods that have a direct irritant effect on the esophageal mucosa. (spicy foods, orange juice, tomato juice, and coffee)
  - Include protein-rich meals in diet (augments lower esophageal sphincter pressure)
  - Eat small meals and avoid eating immediately prior to sleeping (within 3 hours if possible; decreases gastric volume)
  - Weight reduction (reduces symptoms)
- Stop smoking (decreases spontaneous esophageal sphincter relaxation)
- Avoid alcohol (increases amplitude of the lower esophageal sphincter, peristaltic waves, and frequency of contraction)
- Avoid tight-fitting clothes
- Discontinue, if possible, drugs that may promote reflux (calcium channel blockers, β-blockers, nitrates, theophylline)
- Take drugs that have a direct irritant effect on the esophageal mucosa with plenty of liquid if they cannot be avoided (bisphosphonates, tetracyclines, quinidine, and potassium chloride, iron salts, aspirin, nonsteroidal antiinflammatory drugs)

Data from DeVault KR, Castell DO. Updated guidelines for the diagnosis and treatment of gastroesophageal reflux disease. Am J Gastroenterol 2005;100:190–200.

symptoms of GERD. Fats and chocolate can decrease LES pressure, whereas citrus juice, tomato juice, coffee, and pepper may irritate damaged endothelium.

It is important to evaluate patient profiles and to identify potential medications that may exacerbate GERD symptoms. Medications, such as anticholinergics, barbiturates, calcium channel blockers, and theophylline decrease LES pressure. Other medications, including aspirin, iron, nonsteroidal antiinflammatory drugs, quinidine, potassium chloride, and bisphosphonates can act as direct contact irritants to the esophageal mucosa. Patients taking bisphosphonates (e.g., alendronate) should be instructed to drink 6 to 8 ounces of plain tap water and remain upright for at least 30 minutes following administration. Proper patient education can help prevent dysphagia or esophageal ulceration. Patients should be closely monitored for worsening symptoms when any of these medications are started. If symptoms worsen, alternative therapies may be warranted. The clinician must weigh the risks and benefits of continuing a drug known to worsen GERD and esophagitis.

Smoking can cause aerophagia, which leads to increased belching and regurgitation. However, data are lacking to show that symptoms improve in patients who quit smoking. Nevertheless, patients with GERD should be encouraged to quit smoking. Alcohol, although not thought to play a role in severe disease, decreases LES pressure and may exacerbate symptoms such as heartburn.

Many patients are noncompliant with lifestyle modifications, and even those who do comply generally continue to have symptoms that require acid-suppression therapy. Nonetheless, it is important to regularly stress the potential benefits of lifestyle modifications.

Interventional Approaches

Interventional approaches include antireflux surgery and endoscopic therapies.

Antireflux Surgery ❻ Surgical intervention is a viable maintenance alternative for selected patients with well-documented GERD.[1] The goal of antireflux surgery is to reestablish the antireflux barrier, to position the lower esophageal sphincter within the abdomen where it is under positive (intraabdominal) pressure, and to close any associated hiatal defect.[15] Antireflux surgery should be considered in patients (a) who fail to respond to pharmacologic treatment; (b) who opt for surgery despite successful treatment because of lifestyle considerations, including age, time, or expense of medications; (c) who have complications of GERD (e.g., Barrett's esophagus, strictures); or (d) who have atypical symptoms and reflux documented with ambulatory reflux monitoring.[15]

The antireflux surgical procedure chosen depends on the surgeon's expertise and preference, as well as on anatomic considerations.[15] In general, 90% of patients have symptom resolution following successful open Nissen's fundoplication. Because of the diminished surgical complications with the newer laparoscopic surgical procedures (Nissen's fundoplication being one of the most commonly performed procedures), the role of surgery in the long-term management of GERD has become more appealing. The major complications with antireflux surgery include gas bloat syndrome (inability to belch or vomit), dysphagia, vagal denervation, splenic trauma, and, very rarely, death. In contrast, death has not occurred as a consequence of pharmacologic treatment with a proton pump inhibitor.

Antireflux surgery is superior to medical management with an H_2-receptor antagonist or a promotility agent. However, omeprazole doses of 40 to 60 mg were equally efficacious to antireflux surgery. Long-term effectiveness of antireflux surgery is uncertain. Patients younger than 50 years old and those with typical symptoms that are responsive to medical therapy have the best outcomes with surgery.[1]

Endoscopic Therapies Several new endoscopic approaches for the management of GERD include endoscopic sewing devices and endoluminal application of radiofrequency heat energy resulting in tissue injury or nerve ablation (the Stretta procedure).[16] These techniques are FDA-approved, but their exact role in the management of GERD has yet to be determined.

An endoscopic sewing device (EndoCinch) and full-thickness plication devices (NDO Surgical) significantly reduce symptoms of heartburn and regurgitation, and improve the quality-of-life scores. Use of acid suppression therapy may be reduced by as much as 70% at 12-month followup.[17]

The Stretta device delivers radiofrequency energy through specialized needles placed into the submucosal tissue of the esophagus while monitoring esophageal mucosal surface temperatures, resulting in an increase in the LES reflux barrier. The primary outcome has been reduction in symptomatic heartburn and improvement in quality of life. Because of the paucity of sufficient data, it is unclear what the role of this device will be in the management of GERD.

CLINICAL CONTROVERSY

Some clinicians believe that patients should be offered the newer endoscopic therapies instead of proton pump inhibitors for long-term maintenance of GERD. Although the newer endoscopic therapies provide good results and less recovery time than surgery, the long-term effects are still unknown. Conversely, many patients prefer not to have to take medication indefinitely, and in some cases still complain of symptoms despite drug therapy.

■ PHARMACOLOGIC THERAPY

Pharmacologic treatment consists of (a) patient-directed therapy with nonprescription antacids, H_2-receptor antagonists, or proton pump inhibitors and (b) prescription-strength acid suppression therapy or promotility medications.

Patient-Directed Therapy

Patient-directed therapy is appropriate for mild, intermittent symptoms. Patients with continuous symptoms lasting longer than 2 weeks should seek medical attention.

Antacids and Antacid-Alginic Acid Products

Patients should be educated that antacids are an appropriate component of treating mild GERD, even though documentation of their efficacy in placebo-controlled clinical trials is lacking.[1] Although the literature is somewhat controversial on the superiority of antacids to placebo, clinicians and patients clearly consider antacids to be effective for immediate symptomatic relief, and antacids are often used concurrently with other acid-suppression therapies. Maintaining the intragastric pH >4 decreases the activation of pepsinogen to pepsin, a proteolytic enzyme. Also, neutralization of gastric fluid leads to increased LES pressure. Patients who require frequent use of antacids for chronic symptoms should be treated with prescription-strength acid suppression therapy because their illness is considered more significant.

An antacid product combined with alginic acid is not a potent neutralizing agent and does not enhance LES pressure; however, it does form a highly viscous solution that floats on the surface of the gastric contents. This viscous solution is thought to serve as a protective barrier for the esophagus against reflux of gastric contents. It also reduces the frequency of the reflux episodes. The combination product may be superior to antacids alone in relieving the symptoms of GERD.[1] Efficacy data indicating endoscopic healing are lacking.

Antacid or antacid combination products may cause gastrointestinal adverse effects (diarrhea or constipation, depending on the product), alterations in mineral metabolism, and acid–base disturbances. Aluminum-containing antacids may bind to phosphate in the gut and lead to bone demineralization. In addition, antacids interact with a variety of medications by altering gastric pH, increasing urinary pH, adsorbing medications to their surfaces, providing a physical barrier to absorption, or forming insoluble complexes with other medications. Antacids have clinically significant drug interactions with tetracycline, ferrous sulfate, isoniazid, quinidine, sulfonylureas, and quinolone antibiotics. Antacid–drug interactions are influenced by composition, dose, dosage schedule, and formulation of the antacid.

Dosage recommendations for antacids in the management of GERD are somewhat difficult to derive from the literature. Doses range from hourly to an as-needed basis (see Table 34–4). In general, antacids have a short duration of action, which necessitates frequent administration throughout the day to provide continuous neutralization of acid. Taking antacids after meals can increase the duration of action from about 1 hour to 3 hours; however, nighttime acid suppression cannot be maintained with bedtime doses.

Nonprescription H_2-Receptor Antagonists and Proton Pump Inhibitors

Nonprescription H_2-receptor antagonists (cimetidine, famotidine, nizatidine, and ranitidine) are effective in lowering gastric acid when taken prior to meals and decrease GERD symptoms associated with exercise. Antacids may have a slightly faster onset of action, while the H_2-receptor antagonists have a much longer duration of action compared with antacids.

The proton-pump inhibitor omeprazole is available over-the-counter. A dose of 20 mg per day is indicated for short-term (14 days) treatment of heartburn. Patients who do not respond to lifestyle modifications and patient-directed therapy after 2 weeks should be seen by their clinician.

Acid-Suppression Therapy

❼ Acid-suppression therapy with prescription-strength H_2-receptor antagonists and proton pump inhibitors are the mainstay of GERD treatment.

H_2-Receptor Antagonists (Cimetidine, Famotidine, Nizatidine, and Ranitidine) H_2-receptor antagonists in divided doses are effective in treating patients with mild to moderate GERD.[1] The majority of the trials assessing the efficacy of standard doses of H_2-receptor antagonists indicate that symptomatic improvement is achieved in an average of 60% of patients after 12 weeks of therapy.[1] However, endoscopic healing rates tend to be lower, an average of 50%.[1]

The efficacy of H_2-receptor antagonists in the management of GERD is extremely variable and is frequently lower than desired. Response to the H_2-receptor antagonists is dependent on the (a) severity of disease, (b) dosage regimen used, and (c) duration of therapy. These factors are important to keep in mind when comparing various clinical trials and/or assessing a patient's response to therapy. The severity of esophagitis at baseline has a profound impact on the patient's response to H_2-receptor antagonists. For symptomatic relief of mild GERD, low-dose, nonprescription H_2-receptor antagonists or standard doses given twice daily may be beneficial. Patients who do not respond to standard doses may be hypersecreters of gastric acid and will require higher doses. Although higher doses of H_2-receptor antagonists may provide higher symptomatic and endoscopic healing rates, limited information exists regarding the safety of these regimens, and they can be less effective and more costly than once-daily proton pump inhibitors. Unlike duodenal ulcer disease, in which the duration of therapy is relatively short (e.g., 4 to 6 weeks), prolonged courses of H_2-receptor antagonists are frequently required in the treatment of GERD.

Because all of the H_2-receptor antagonists have similar efficacy, selection of the specific agent to use in the management of GERD should be based on factors such as differences in pharmacokinetics, safety profile, and cost. In general, the H_2-receptor antagonists are well tolerated. The most common adverse effects are headache, somnolence, fatigue, dizziness, and either constipation or diarrhea. Patients should be monitored for the presence of adverse effects as well as potential drug interactions, especially when on cimetidine. Cimetidine may inhibit the metabolism of theophylline, warfarin, phenytoin, nifedipine, and propranolol, among others. An alternate H_2-receptor antagonist should be selected if the patient is on any of these medications.

Proton Pump Inhibitors (Esomeprazole, Lansoprazole, Omeprazole, Pantoprazole, and Rabeprazole) Proton pump inhibitors are superior to H_2-receptor antagonists in treating patients with moderate to severe GERD. This includes not only those patients with erosive esophagitis or complications (e.g., Barrett's esophagus, strictures), but also those patients with nonerosive GERD who have moderate to severe symptoms. FDA-approved doses (per day) of proton pump inhibitors are omeprazole 20 mg, esomeprazole 20 mg, lansoprazole 30 mg, rabeprazole 20 mg, and pantoprazole 40 mg. Symptomatic relief is seen in approximately 83% of patients after 8 weeks treated with a proton pump inhibitor, whereas the endoscopic healing rate at 8 weeks is 78%.[1]

Proton pump inhibitors block gastric acid secretion by inhibiting gastric H^+/K^+-adenosine triphosphatase in gastric parietal cells.[18] This produces a profound, long-lasting antisecretory effect capable of maintaining the gastric pH above 4, even during postprandial acid surges. A correlation appears to exist between the percentage of time the gastric pH remains above 4 during the 24-hour period and healing erosive esophagitis.

A few trials have compared proton pump inhibitors to each other. In general, healing rates at 4 weeks and 8 weeks are similar; lansoprazole and rabeprazole, however, may relieve symptoms faster after the first dose when compared to omeprazole. Healing rates at 4 weeks and 8 weeks were similar. Whether proton pump inhibitors have a role in the management of Barrett's esophagus remains a topic for debate. The use of high-dose omeprazole (40 mg twice daily) caused partial regression of Barrett's esophagus, but no change was noted in patients receiving ranitidine 150 mg twice daily.[19] Others propose that these islands of normal squamous cells that appear in patients with Barrett's esophagus after high-dose proton pump inhibitors may be covering Barrett's esophagus epithelium and may mask the development of cancerous changes in the mucosa.[20] It is unknown whether regression of Barrett's esophagus reduces the risk of adenocarcinoma in someone who already has Barrett's esophagus, but aggressive therapy aimed at adequate suppression of acid reflux early in the course of a patient's disease may help to prevent the development of this GERD complication. No drug has FDA approval for treating Barrett's esophagus. However, drugs can be used to manage reflux in patients with Barrett's esophagus as it is known that reflux is very common in this patient population.

The proton pump inhibitors are usually well tolerated; however, potential adverse effects include headache, dizziness, somnolence, diarrhea, constipation, nausea, and vitamin B_{12} deficiency. The frequency of adverse events appears to be similar to that seen with the H_2-receptor antagonists.

Drug interactions with the proton pump inhibitors vary with each agent. All proton pump inhibitors can decrease the absorption of drugs such as ketoconazole or itraconazole, which require an acidic environment to be absorbed. All proton pump inhibitors are metabolized by the cytochrome P450 system to some extent, specifically by the CYP2C19 and CYP3A4 enzymes. However, no interactions with lansoprazole, pantoprazole, or rabeprazole have been seen with CYP2C19 substrates such as diazepam, warfarin, and phenytoin.[13] Esomeprazole does not appear to interact with warfarin or phenytoin, and an interaction with diazepam is generally not considered clinically relevant. Pantoprazole is also metabolized by a cytosolic sulfotransferase and is therefore less likely to have significant drug interactions compared with the other proton pump inhibitors. Although generally not causing major concern, omeprazole has the potential to inhibit the metabolism of warfarin, diazepam, and phenytoin, and lansoprazole may decrease theophylline concentrations. Patients taking warfarin should be monitored for potential bleeding.

Drug interactions with omeprazole are of particular concern in patients who are considered "slow metabolizers," which is more common in the Asian population, but also found in approximately 3% of the caucasian population. Unfortunately, it is unclear which patients have the polymorphic gene variation that makes them slow metabolizers. Like omeprazole, the metabolism of esomeprazole may also be altered in patients with this polymorphic gene variation. Patients on potentially interacting drugs, such as warfarin, should be monitored closely for potential problems. In general, all of these agents are safe and effective and the choice of a particular agent will most likely be based on cost.

The proton pump inhibitors degrade in acidic environments and are therefore formulated in a delayed-release capsule or tablet formulation. Lansoprazole, esomeprazole, and omeprazole contain enteric-coated (pH-sensitive) granules in a capsule form. For patients who are unable to swallow the capsule, or for pediatric patients, the contents of the delayed-release capsule can be mixed in applesauce or placed in orange juice. If a patient has a nasogastric tube, the contents of an omeprazole capsule can be mixed in 8.4% sodium bicarbonate solution. Esomeprazole granules can be dispersed in water. Lansoprazole comes in a packet for oral suspension and a delayed-release, orally disintegrating tablet. Although these dosage forms are beneficial for those who cannot swallow the capsule, such as elderly or pediatric patients, the packet for oral suspension should not be placed through a nasogastric tube. Patients taking pantoprazole or rabeprazole should be instructed not to crush, chew, or split the delayed-release tablets. Lansoprazole, esomeprazole, and pantoprazole are available in an intravenous formulation, which offers an alternative route of administration for patients who are unable to take an oral proton pump inhibitor. Importantly, the intravenous product is not more efficacious than oral proton pump inhibitors and is significantly more expensive. Careful patient selection is necessary to avoid the increased cost from the use of the intravenous product.

The newest dosage form is omeprazole in a nonprescription delayed-release tablet and a combination product with sodium bicarbonate in an immediate-release capsule and oral suspension (Zegerid). It is the first immediate-release proton pump inhibitor and should be taken on an empty stomach at least 1 hour before a meal. Zegerid offers an alternative to the delayed-release capsules or the intravenous formulation in adult patients with a nasogastric tube.

Patients should be instructed to take their proton pump inhibitor in the morning, 15 to 30 minutes before breakfast, to maximize efficacy, because these agents inhibit only actively secreting proton pumps. Patients with nocturnal symptoms may benefit from taking their proton pump inhibitor prior to the evening meal. If dosed twice daily, the second dose should be administered approximately 10 to 12 hours after the morning dose and prior to a meal or snack.[13] Twice daily dosing may also be appropriate during a diagnostic trial for noncardiac chest pain, in patients with atypical or complicated symptoms, and in those with breakthrough symptoms.[1]

Promotility Agents

Promotility agents may be useful as an adjunct to acid suppression therapy in patients with a known motility defect (e.g., LES incompetence, decreased esophageal clearance, delayed gastric emptying). Unfortunately, all available promotility agents are fraught with undesirable side effects and are not generally as effective as acid-suppression therapy. Extrapyramidal effects, sedation, and irritability are common with bethanechol and metoclopramide.

Cisapride Cisapride has comparable efficacy to H_2-receptor antagonists in treating patients with mild esophagitis. Unfortunately, cisapride is no longer available for routine use because of life-threatening cardiac arrhythmias when it is combined with certain medications and other disease states. It is currently available only through a limited access program from the manufacturer.

Metoclopramide Metoclopramide, a dopamine antagonist, increases LES pressure in a dose-related manner, and accelerates gastric emptying in gastroesophageal reflux patients. Unlike cisapride, however, metoclopramide does not improve esophageal clearance. Metoclopramide provides symptomatic improvement for some patients with gastroesophageal reflux disease; however, substantial data indicating that metoclopramide provides endoscopic healing are lacking. In addition, metoclopramide's side effect profile and the incidence of tachyphylaxis with continued use limits its usefulness in treating many patients with GERD. The risk of adverse effects is much greater in elderly patients and in patients with renal dysfunction because the drug is primarily eliminated by the kidneys. Contraindications include Parkinson's disease, mechanical obstruction, concomitant use of other dopamine antagonists or anticholinergic agents, and pheochromocytoma.

Bethanechol Bethanechol, a promotility drug, has very limited value in the treatment of GERD because of unwanted side effects. Bethanechol is not routinely recommended for the treatment of GERD.

Other Promotility Drugs Under Investigation Other promotility drugs under investigation include domperidone, a dopamine antagonist, itopride, and baclofen. Because domperidone does not cross the blood–brain barrier, it does not cause the central nervous system effects seen with metoclopramide. However, it is not currently available in the United States. Baclofen, an aminobutyric acid (GABA) receptor type B agonist, may decrease esophageal acid exposure and the number of reflux episodes by decreasing the number of transient relaxations of the LES. However, this agent has many side effects, limiting its usefulness in GERD.

Mucosal Protectants

Sucralfate, a nonabsorbable aluminum salt of sucrose octasulfate, has very limited value in the treatment of GERD. Sucralfate is not routinely recommended for use in the treatment of GERD.

Combination Therapy

Combination therapy with an acid suppression agent and a promotility agent or a mucosal protectant agent would seem logical given the multifactorial nature of the disease, particularly in light of the disappointing results seen with many monotherapy regimens. However, sufficient data to support combination therapy are limited, and this approach should not be routinely recommended unless a patient has GERD plus motor dysfunction occurring. The addition of an H_2-receptor antagonist at bedtime to proton pump inhibitor therapy for the treatment of nocturnal symptoms has been evaluated. The effectiveness of this strategy may decrease over time.[21]

Maintenance Therapy

8 Although healing and/or symptomatic improvement may be achieved via many different therapeutic modalities, a large percentage of patients with gastroesophageal reflux will relapse following discontinuation of therapy, especially those with more severe disease. Patients who have symptomatic relapse following discontinuation of therapy or lowering of dose, including patients with complications such as Barrett's esophagus, strictures, or hemorrhage, should be considered for long-term maintenance therapy to prevent complications or worsening of esophageal function.[1] The goal of maintenance therapy is to improve quality of life by controlling the patient's symptoms and preventing complications. These goals cannot generally be achieved by decreasing the dose of the therapeutic modality used for initial healing or switching to a less potent acid suppression agent. Most patients will require standard doses to prevent relapses. Patients should be counseled on the importance of complying with lifestyle changes and long-term maintenance therapy in order to prevent recurrence or worsening of disease.[1]

H_2-receptor antagonists may be effective maintenance therapy for patients with mild disease.[1] The proton pump inhibitors are the drugs of choice for maintenance treatment of moderate to severe esophagitis or symptoms. Lower doses of a proton pump inhibitor or alternate-day dosing may be effective in some patients with less-severe disease, thereby allowing titration in some cases. "On-demand" maintenance therapy, by which patients take their proton pump inhibitor only when they have symptoms, may be effective for patients with endoscopy-negative GERD.[1] Although not well studied, many patients with only mild to moderate symptoms may decide on their own to take their medication this way for the financial benefit. However, patients with more-severe disease and/or complications should be maintained on standard doses of proton pump inhibitors.

Long-term chronic use of higher doses of proton pump inhibitors is not indicated unless the patient has complicated symptoms, has erosive esophagitis per endoscopy, or has had further diagnostic evaluation to determine the level of acid exposure. Metoclopramide is not approved for maintenance therapy and use is limited by adverse effect profile. Antireflux surgery and endoscopic therapies may also be considered a viable alternative to long-term drug therapy for maintenance of healing in patients who are candidates.

Maintenance Therapy with Proton Pump Inhibitors Long-term use of the proton pump inhibitors are safe, with no evidence of carcinoid tumors directly linked to their use. Prolonged hypergastrinemia leading to the development of colonic polyps, and potentially adenocarcinoma, was also a concern that has proven unfounded with long-term use.[22] However, the role of *Helicobacter pylori* status in patients with GERD has been questioned. As a consequence of the controversy surrounding *H. pylori* and GERD, specific guidelines on how to handle these patients are lacking. Most clinicians would probably opt to eradicate *H. pylori* infections once detected. Further studies are needed to determine the role of *H. pylori* in patients with GERD.

CLINICAL CONTROVERSY

The role of *Helicobacter pylori* infection in GERD patients remains unclear. One study suggested that long-term proton pump inhibitor use in the presence of *H. pylori* may increase the risk of atrophic gastritis with subsequent increase in risk for gastric cancer.[23] Conversely, the presence of *H. pylori* infection may actually have a protective effect on GERD and clearing the symptoms may worsen GERD symptoms.[24]

Maintenance Therapy with H_2-Receptor Antagonists The studies evaluating the efficacy of the H_2-receptor antagonists in maintaining GERD patients in remission have been disappointing. Currently, ranitidine 150 mg twice daily is the only H_2-receptor antagonist regimen that is FDA approved for maintenance of healing of erosive esophagitis.

SPECIAL POPULATIONS

There are several special populations that should be considered when discussing GERD, such as patients with atypical symptoms, patients with nonerosive symptoms, pediatric patients, elderly patients, and patients with refractory symptoms.

PATIENTS WITH ATYPICAL GERD SYMPTOMS

Patients presenting with atypical symptoms may require higher doses and longer treatment courses as compared with patients with typical symptoms. These patients are best diagnosed with ambulatory reflux monitoring.[25] In patients who present with noncardiac chest pain, a short course (1 to 8 weeks) of omeprazole 20 mg twice daily has been advocated.[25] In patients with asthma, antireflux medications improve asthma symptoms and even decrease antiasthma medication use, but have little or no effect on lung function.[26] A trial of 3 months has been advocated using twice-daily proton pump inhibitor therapy for both asthma and laryngeal symptoms thought to be associated with GERD. Omeprazole doses as high as 60 mg daily have been used.[25] In patients with chronic cough, ambulatory reflux monitoring, when available, is the preferred approach for evaluation of GERD.[27] Maintenance therapy is generally indicated in patients who respond to the therapeutic trial or have endoscopic evidence of reflux. Antireflux surgery or endoscopic therapies may be an option in selected patients.

PATIENTS WITH ENDOSCOPY-NEGATIVE REFLUX DISEASE

Although the integrity of the esophageal mucosa is best evaluated with endoscopy, endoscopy does not confirm whether or not the patient's symptoms are related to GERD.[1] In some cases, patients with typical symptoms and increased acid exposure have no evidence of esophageal damage. Many patients with persistent severe symptoms but normal endoscopy will require therapy similar to those with positive endoscopic findings. Patients who present with normal esophageal mucosa on endoscopy should undergo ambulatory reflux monitoring to further confirm the diagnosis of GERD.

PEDIATRIC PATIENTS WITH GERD

Gastroesophageal reflux occurs in approximately 18% of the infant population. Most have physiologic reflux with no clinical consequence.[28] Complications, although rare, include distal esophagitis, failure to thrive, esophageal peptic strictures, Barrett's esophagus, and pulmonary disease.[29] Chronic vomiting associated with gastroesophageal reflux must be distinguished from other causes, such as neurologic, metabolic, eating, and rumination disorders. Developmental immaturity of the LES is one suspected cause of gastroesophageal reflux in infants.[29] Like adults, transient LES relaxations seem to be the most common cause of gastroesophageal reflux in children. Other causes include impaired luminal clearance of gastric acid, neurologic impairment, and type of infant formula. Uncomplicated gastroesophageal reflux usually resolves without incident by 12 to 18 months of life, and usually responds to supportive therapy, including dietary adjustments, postural management, and reassurance for the parents.[29] Thickened feedings may be useful in milder cases. Smaller, more frequent feedings may also be beneficial. If there is no improvement, medical therapy might be indicated. Combined use of a promotility agent and an acid suppression agent seems to work the fastest.[29] Unfortunately, with the removal of cisapride, there is no longer a readily available promotility agent without major side effects. Metoclopramide is used as a promotility agent in pediatric patients. Ranitidine is commonly used at a dose of 2 mg/kg twice daily.[29]

The use of proton pump inhibitors is becoming more common in pediatrics. Lansoprazole is indicated for treating symptomatic and erosive GERD in pediatric patients older than age 1 year. A dose of 15 mg once daily is recommended for children who weigh 30 kg or less, and a dose of 30 mg once daily is recommended for those who weigh more than 30 kg. Although not FDA approved for use in children, there is evidence supporting the effectiveness of omeprazole in treating children with GERD. A common dose for treating esophagitis is 1 mg/kg per day (divided once or twice daily).[30] Even though no major adverse events have been noted in children receiving proton pump inhibitors for up to 7 years, the relative safety of prolonged proton pump inhibitor use in children remains unknown.[30] There are no data involving the other proton pump inhibitors in the treatment of GERD in pediatric patients.

ELDERLY PATIENTS WITH GERD

Many elderly patients have decreased host defense mechanisms, such as saliva production. More aggressive therapy with a proton pump inhibitor may be warranted in patients older than 60 years of age with symptomatic GERD. Often these patients do not seek medical attention because they feel their symptoms are part of the normal aging process. They may present with atypical symptoms such as chest pain, asthma, hoarseness, coughing, wheezing, poor dentition, or jaw pain. Decreased GI motility is a common problem in elderly patients. Unfortunately, there are no good promotility agents available to these patients. Cisapride is not available for general use and elderly patients are especially sensitive to the central nervous system effects of metoclopramide. They may also be sensitive to the central nervous system effects of H_2-receptor antagonists. Proton pump inhibitors appear to be the most useful treatment modality because they have superior efficacy and are dosed once daily, which is beneficial in all patients, but is especially beneficial in the elderly.

PATIENTS WITH REFRACTORY GERD

GERD refractory to medical management is rare. Other causes for the patient's symptoms should be evaluated. The majority of patients with refractory symptoms experience nocturnal acid breakthrough. Other reasons for refractory symptoms may be related to timing of proton pump inhibitor and drug metabolism differences in certain patients. Because of this, switching to another proton pump inhibitor may be effective for refractory symptoms in some patients. Ambulatory reflux monitoring is useful in patients who are not responding to therapy. Adding an H_2-receptor antagonist at bedtime for nocturnal symptoms has been suggested; however, the effect may be short-lived.[21] Antireflux surgery and endoscopic therapies may also be considered in this patient population.

PHARMACOECONOMIC CONSIDERATIONS

In addition to the traditional clinical end points that demonstrate that a certain therapy is effective, the cost-effectiveness of the therapy in relation to predicted outcomes and its effects on quality of life must be evaluated. For GERD, one must consider the primary goals of treatment: to relieve symptoms, to heal injury, to prevent recurrence, and to prevent complications. These factors must be evaluated separately, because different costs are associated with achieving each end point. For example, patients with complications associated with GERD, such as strictures, would be more likely to use medical resources as a consequence of revisits and diagnostic tests. Although effects on quality of life may be difficult to evaluate when your goal is preventing recurrence, untreated GERD has a more negative impact on psychological well being than untreated hypertension, mild heart failure, angina pectoris, or menopause. Improving a patient's quality of life is a measure of treatment success and may help decide which therapy a patient receives.

The proton pump inhibitors are generally more expensive than the H_2-receptor antagonists or promotility agents. Omeprazole's generic and over-the-counter availability makes this less of an issue. However, the most expensive therapy is the one that is ineffective. If the H_2-receptor antagonist does not accomplish the treatment goals, then it costs more because the patient must be retreated.

Patient compliance is another factor that affects the outcome of drug therapy. Drug regimens that are easily managed improve compliance, and thus improve outcome for the patient. This especially can be a problem in patients who require high-dose therapy with H_2-receptor antagonists. Not only is the patient required to take the drug more often in higher doses, but there is also increased expense associated with such regimens. The patient may be unable to afford the drug. Choosing a drug that is least expensive and provides the greatest benefit related to dosing interval and number of tablets taken is the optimal regimen. Studies comparing various treatment strategies for GERD show that proton pump inhibitors are more cost-effective than H_2-receptor antagonists, especially in patients with moderate to severe disease.

Decision analysis has been used to evaluate the cost-effectiveness of lifestyle modifications and/or patient-directed therapy alone or combined with omeprazole 20 mg daily or ranitidine 150 mg twice daily for patients with persistent symptomatic GERD. A complex model that evaluated the influence of empiric versus definitive therapy, compliance, and efficacy of the three treatment regimens was employed. Although the retail cost of omeprazole was highest among the treatments evaluated, it was the most cost-effective strategy and was associated with the lowest overall cost. Studies also show that proton pump inhibitors improve quality-of-life measures in symptomatic patients with erosive esophagitis.[31] Additional studies are needed to evaluate the impact of various treatment regimens on quality-of-life issues and cost, and to compare long-term medical management with antireflux surgery and endoscopic therapies. At least one study showed that proton pump inhibitors were as effective as antireflux surgery and slightly more cost effective at 5 years. However, the costs were similar after 10 years.[32]

EVALUATION OF THERAPEUTIC OUTCOMES

⑨ The long-term benefits of treatment are difficult to assess because of the limited information known about the epidemiology and natural history of GERD. Consequently, successful outcomes are generally measured in terms of three separate end points: (a) relieving symptoms, (b) healing the injured mucosa, and (c) preventing complications.

The short-term goal of therapy is to relieve symptoms such as heartburn and regurgitation to the point at which they do not impair the patient's quality of life. Patients should be educated regarding lifestyle modifications that should be adhered to throughout the course of therapy, including smoking cessation, weight loss, raising the head of the bed, eating smaller meals, and avoiding eating prior to bedtime. Patients should also be instructed to avoid or limit foods that aggravate GERD symptoms, such as fat and chocolate. In addition, the patient's drug profile should be reviewed to identify medications that may contribute to GERD symptoms. These agents should be avoided if possible. Table 34–6 has recommendations for providing pharmaceutical care to patients with GERD.

The clinician should take an active role in educating the patient about potential adverse effects and drug interactions that may occur with drug therapy. The frequency and severity of symptoms should be monitored and patients should be counseled on symptoms that suggest the presence of complications requiring immediate medical attention, such as dysphagia or odynophagia. Patients with persistent symptoms should be evaluated for the presence of strictures or other complications. Patients should also be monitored for the presence of atypical symptoms such as cough, nonallergic asthma, or chest pain. These symptoms require further diagnostic evaluation. Long-term maintenance treatment is indicated in patients who have strictures because the strictures commonly recur if reflux esophagitis is not treated.

The second goal is to heal the injured mucosa. Again, lifestyle modifications and the importance of complying with the therapeutic regimen chosen to heal the mucosa should be stressed. Patients should be educated about the risk of relapse and the need for long-term maintenance therapy to prevent recurrence or complications.

TABLE 34-6 Recommendations for Providing Pharmaceutical Care to Patients with GERD

1. Assess the patient's symptoms to determine if patient-directed therapy is appropriate or whether patient should be evaluated by a clinician. Determine the type of symptoms, frequency, and exacerbating factors. Refer any patient with alarm or atypical symptoms to a clinician for further diagnostic workup.
2. Obtain a thorough history of prescription, nonprescription, and natural drug product use.
3. Counsel the patient on lifestyle modifications that will improve symptoms.
4. Recommend appropriate drug therapy based on patient presentation.
5. Develop a plan to assess effectiveness of acid suppression therapy after an appropriate amount of time (8 to 16 weeks). Recommend alternative therapy if necessary.
6. Assess improvement in quality-of-life measures such as physical, psychological, and social functioning and well-being.
7. Evaluate the patient for the presence of adverse drug reactions, drug allergies, and drug interactions.
8. Stress the importance of compliance with the therapeutic regimen, including lifestyle modifications. Recommend a therapeutic regimen that is easy for the patient to accomplish.
9. Provide patient education with regard to disease state, lifestyle modifications, and drug therapy. Patients should be counseled on:
   - What causes GERD and what things to avoid
   - When to take their medications
   - What potential adverse effects may occur
   - Which drugs may interact with their therapy
   - What alarm signs they should report to their clinician

The final, more long-term goal of therapy is to decrease the risk of complications (esophagitis, strictures, and Barrett's esophagus). A small subset of patients may continue to fail treatment despite therapy with high doses of H_2-receptor antagonists or a proton pump inhibitor. Patients should be monitored for the presence of continual pain, dysphagia, or odynophagia.

CONCLUSIONS

Gastroesophageal reflux disease is a common disease that classically presents as heartburn. The pathophysiology of reflux is complex, involving both aggressive factors (acid, pepsin, bile acids, pancreatic enzymes, and prostaglandins) and defense mechanisms (anatomic factors, LES pressure, esophageal clearance, and gastric emptying). Therapeutic modalities are designed to minimize the aggressive factors and/or augment the defense mechanisms.

ABBREVIATIONS

ENRD: endoscopy-negative reflux disease

GERD: gastroesophageal reflux disease

GI: gastrointestinal

H_2: histamine type-2

LES: lower esophageal sphincter

NERD: nonerosive reflux disease

REFERENCES

1. DeVault KR, Castell DO. Updated guidelines for the diagnosis and treatment of gastroesophageal reflux disease. Am J Gastroenterol 2005;100:190–200.
2. Dent J, El-Serag HB, Wallander MA, Johansson S. Epidemiology of gastro-oesophageal reflux disease: a systematic review. Gut 2005;54:710–717.
3. DeVault KR. Review article: The role of acid suppression in patients with non-erosive reflux disease or functional heartburn. Aliment Pharmacol Ther 2006;23(Suppl 1):33–39.
4. Goldstein JL, Schlesinger PK, Mozwecz HL, et al. Esophageal mucosal resistance: A factor in esophagitis. Gastroenterol Clin North Am 1990;19:565–585.
5. Rudolph CD, Mazur LJ, Liptak GS, et al. Guidelines for evaluation and treatment of gastroesophageal reflux in infants and children: Recommendations of the North American Society for Pediatric Gastroenterology and Nutrition. J Pediatr Gastroenterol Nutr 2001;32(Suppl 2):1–31.
6. Hirano I. Review article: Modern technology in the diagnosis of gastro-oesophageal reflux disease—Bilitec, intraluminal impedance and Bravo capsule pH monitoring. Aliment Pharmacol Ther 2006;23(Suppl 1):12–24.
7. Spechler SJ. Barrett's Esophagus. N Engl J Med 2002;346(11):836–842.
8. Lagergren J, Bergstrom R, Lindgren A, Nyren O. Symptomatic gastroesophageal reflux as a risk factor for esophageal adenocarcinoma. N Engl J Med 1999;340:825–831.
9. Liu JJ, Carr-Lock DL, Osterman MT, et al. Endoscopic treatment for atypical manifestations of gastroesophageal reflux disease. Am J Gastroenterol 2006;101:440–445.
10. Postma GN. Ambulatory pH monitoring methodology. Ann Otol Rhinol Laryngol Suppl 2000;184:10–14.
11. Pandolfino JE, Kahrilas PJ. Prolonged pH monitoring: Bravo capsule. Gastrointest Endosc Clin N Am 2005;15:307–318.
12. Pandolfino JE, Schreiner MA, Lee TJ, et al. Comparison of the Bravo wireless and Digitrapper catheter-based pH monitoring systems for measuring esophageal acid exposure. Am J Gastroenterol 2005;100:1466–1476.
13. Welage LS, Berardi RR. Evaluation of omeprazole, lansoprazole, pantoprazole, and rabeprazole in the treatment of acid-related disorders. J Am Pharm Assoc 2000;40:52–62.

14. Pandolfino JE, El-Serag HB, Zhang Q, et al. Obesity: A challenge to esophagogastric junction integrity. Gastroenterology 2006;130:639–649.
15. Anonymous. Guideline for the surgical treatment of gastroesophageal reflux disease (GERD). Surg Endosc 1998;12:186–188.
16. Johnson DA. Endoscopic therapy for GERD—baking, sewing, or stuffing: An evidence-based perspective. Rev Gastroenterol Disord 2003;3:142–149.
17. Pleskow D, Rothstein R, Lo S, et al. Endoscopic full-thickness plication for the treatment of GERD: 12-month follow-up for the North American open-label trial. Gastrointest Endosc 2005;61:643–649.
18. Horn J. The proton-pump inhibitors: Similarities and differences. Clin Ther 2000;22:266–280.
19. Peters FT, Ganesh S, Kuipers EJ, et al. Endoscopic regression of Barrett's oesophagus during omeprazole treatment: A randomised double blind study. Gut 1999;45:489–494.
20. Sampliner RE, Camargo E. Normalization of esophageal pH with high-dose proton pump inhibitor therapy does not result in regression of Barrett's esophagus. Am J Gastroenterol 1997;92:582–585.
21. Fackler WK, Ours TM, Vaezi MF, et al. Long-term effect of H2RA therapy on nocturnal gastric acid breakthrough. Gastroenterology 2002;122:625–632.
22. Garrett WR. Considerations for long-term use of proton-pump inhibitors. AJHP 1998;55:2268–2279.
23. Kuipers EJ, Lundell L, Klinkenberg-Knol EC, et al. Atrophic gastritis and *Helicobacter pylori* infection in patients with reflux esophagitis treated with omeprazole or fundoplication. N Engl J Med 1996;334:1018–1022.
24. O'Connor HJ. *Helicobacter pylori* and gastro-oesophageal reflux disease—Clinical implications and management. Aliment Pharmacol Ther 1999;13:117–127.
25. DeVault KR. Overview of therapy for extraesophageal manifestations of gastroesophageal reflux disease. Am J Gastroenterol 2000;95:S39–S44.
26. Field SK, Sutherland LR. Does medical antireflux therapy improve asthma in asthmatics with gastroesophageal reflux? A critical review of the literature. Chest 1998;114:275–283.
27. Irwin RS, Boulet LP, Cloutier MM, et al. Managing cough as a defense mechanism and a symptom: A consensus panel report of the American College of Chest Physicians. Chest 1998;114(Suppl):133S–181S.
28. Vandenplas Y, Belli D, Benhamou P-H, et al. Current concepts and issues in the management of regurgitation in infants: A reappraisal. Management guidelines from a working party. Acta Paediatr 1996;85:531–534.
29. Faubion WA, Zein NN. Gastroesophageal reflux in infants and children. Mayo Clin Proc 1998;73:166–173.
30. Patel AS, Pohl JF, Easley DJ. Proton pump inhibitors in pediatrics. Pediatr Rev 2003;24:12–15.
31. Revicki D, Wood M, Maton PM, et al. The impact of gastroesophageal reflux disease on health-related quality of life. Am J Med 1998;104:252–258.
32. Heudebert GR, Marks R, Wilcox CM, et al. Choice of long-term strategy for the management of patients with severe esophagitis: A cost-utility analysis. Gastroenterology 1997;112:1078–1086.

CHAPTER 35

Peptic Ulcer Disease

ROSEMARY R. BERARDI AND LYNDA S. WELAGE

KEY CONCEPTS

1. Patients with peptic ulcer disease should reduce psychological stress, cigarette smoking, and nonsteroidal antiinflammatory drug (NSAID) use, and should avoid foods and beverages that exacerbate ulcer symptoms.

2. Eradication is recommended for all *Helicobacter pylori*-positive patients with an active ulcer, a documented history of a prior ulcer, or a history of ulcer-related complications.

3. Treatment with a conventional antiulcer drug (H_2-receptor antagonist, proton pump inhibitor, or sucralfate) may be an alternative to *H. pylori* eradication, but is discouraged because of the high rate of ulcer recurrence and ulcer-related complications. Combining conventional antiulcer drugs adds to treatment costs without enhancing efficacy.

4. Maintenance therapy with a low-dose H_2-receptor antagonist or proton pump inhibitor may be indicated for high-risk patients who fail *H. pylori* eradication, patients with severe complications, heavy smokers, or those with *H. pylori*-negative ulcers.

5. The selection of an *H. pylori* eradication regimen should be based on efficacy, safety, antibiotic resistance, cost, and the likelihood of medication adherence. Treatment should be initiated with a proton pump inhibitor-based three-drug regimen. If a second course of *H. pylori* therapy is required, the regimen should contain different antibiotics.

6. Proton pump inhibitor cotherapy reduces the risk of NSAID-related gastric and duodenal ulcers and is at least as effective as recommended dosages of misoprostol and superior to the H_2-receptor antagonists.

7. Standard dosages of a proton pump inhibitor and a nonselective NSAID are as effective as a selective cyclooxygenase-2 (COX-2) inhibitor in reducing the risk of NSAID-induced ulcers and upper GI complications.

8. The eradication of *H. pylori* improves clinical outcomes and decreases the use of healthcare resources when compared to conventional antisecretory therapy. Misoprostol or proton pump inhibitor cotherapy, or switching to a selective COX-2 inhibitor is cost-effective in patients with the highest risk for NSAID-related ulcers and upper GI complications.

9. Patients with peptic ulcer disease, especially those receiving *H. pylori* eradication or misoprostol cotherapy, require patient education regarding their disease and drug treatment to successfully achieve a positive therapeutic outcome.

Learning objectives, review questions, and other resources can be found at **www.pharmacotherapyonline.com.**

Acid-related diseases (gastritis, erosions, and peptic ulcer) of the upper gastrointestinal (GI) tract require gastric acid for their formation.[1–4] Peptic ulcer disease (PUD) differs from gastritis and erosions in that ulcers typically extend deeper into the muscularis mucosa.[1] There are three common forms of peptic ulcers: *Helicobacter pylori* (*H. pylori*)-associated, nonsteroidal antiinflammatory drug (NSAID)-induced, and stress ulcers (Table 35–1). The term "stress-related mucosal damage" (SRMD) is preferred to stress ulcer or stress gastritis, because the mucosal lesions range from superficial gastritis and erosions to deep ulcers.

Chronic peptic ulcers vary in etiology, clinical presentation, and tendency to recur (see Table 35–1). *H. pylori*-associated and NSAID-induced ulcers develop most often in the stomach and duodenum of ambulatory patients (Fig. 35–1). Occasionally, ulcers develop in the esophagus, jejunum, ileum, or colon. Peptic ulcers are also associated with Zollinger-Ellison's syndrome (ZES), radiation, chemotherapy, and vascular insufficiency (Table 35–2).[1,4] In contrast, acute ulcers (stress-related mucosal damage [SRMD]) occur primarily in the stomach in critically ill hospitalized patients (see Table 35–1). This chapter focuses on chronic PUD associated with *H. pylori* and NSAIDs. A brief discussion of ZES and upper GI bleeding related to PUD and SRMD is included.

The natural course of chronic PUD is characterized by frequent ulcer recurrence. Approximately 60% to 100% of ulcers recur within 1 year of initial ulcer healing with conventional antiulcer regimens.[1] The most important factors that influence ulcer recurrence are *H. pylori* infection and NSAID use. Other factors include gastric acid hypersecretion, cigarette smoking, alcohol use, a long duration of PUD, ulcer-related complications, and patient noncompliance. The cause of ulcer recurrence is most likely multifactorial.

EPIDEMIOLOGY

Approximately 10% of Americans develop chronic PUD during their lifetime.[1] The incidence varies with ulcer type, age, gender, and geographic location. Race, occupation, genetic predisposition, and societal factors may play a minor role in ulcer pathogenesis, but are attenuated by the importance of *H. pylori* infection and NSAID use. The prevalence of PUD in the United States has shifted from predominance in men to nearly comparable prevalence in men and women. Recent trends suggest a declining rate for younger men and an increasing rate for older women.[1] Factors influencing these trends include the declining smoking rates in younger men and the increased use of NSAIDs in older adults.

TABLE 35-1 Comparison of Common Forms of Peptic Ulcer

Characteristic	*H. pylori* Induced	NSAID Induced	SRMD
Condition	Chronic	Chronic	Acute
Site of damage	Duodenum > stomach	Stomach > duodenum	Stomach > duodenum
Intragastric pH	More dependent	Less dependent	Less dependent
Symptoms	Usually epigastric pain	Often asymptomatic	Asymptomatic
Ulcer depth	Superficial	Deep	Most superficial
GI bleeding	Less severe, single vessel	More severe, single vessel	More severe, superficial mucosal capillaries

H. pylori, Helicobacter pylori; NSAID, nonsteroidal antiinflammatory drug; SRMD, stress-related mucosal damage.

Since 1960, ulcer-related physician visits, hospitalizations, operations, and deaths have declined in the United States by more than 50%, primarily because of decreased rates of PUD among men.[1] The decline in hospitalizations has resulted from a reduction in hospital admissions for uncomplicated duodenal ulcer. However, hospitalizations of older adults for ulcer-related complications (bleeding and perforation) have increased.[1] Although the overall mortality from PUD has decreased, death rates have increased in patients older than 75 years of age, most likely a result of increased consumption of NSAIDs and an aging population. Patients with gastric ulcer have a higher mortality rate than do patients with duodenal ulcer because gastric ulcer is more prevalent in older individuals. Despite these trends, PUD remains one of the most common GI diseases, resulting in impaired quality of life, work loss, and high-cost medical care.

ETIOLOGY AND RISK FACTORS

Most peptic ulcers occur in the presence of acid and pepsin when *H. pylori*, NSAIDs, or other factors (see Table 35–2) disrupt normal mucosal defense and healing mechanisms.[1] Hypersecretion of acid is the primary pathogenic mechanism in hypersecretory states such as ZES.[4] Ulcer location is related to a number of etiologic factors. Benign gastric ulcers can occur anywhere in the stomach, although most are located on the lesser curvature, just distal to the junction of the antral and acid-secreting mucosa (see Fig. 35–1). Most duodenal ulcers occur in the first part of the duodenum (duodenal bulb).

HELICOBACTER PYLORI

H. pylori infection causes chronic gastritis in all infected individuals and is causally linked to PUD, gastric cancer, and mucosa-associated lymphoid tissue (MALT) lymphoma (Fig. 35–2).[1,5–7] However, only a small number of infected individuals will develop symptomatic PUD (approximately 20%) or gastric cancer (less than 1%).[1,7] Serologic studies confirm an association between *H. pylori* and gastric cancer.[1] Evidence for PUD is based on the fact that most non-NSAID ulcers are infected with *H. pylori*, and that *H. pylori* eradication markedly decreases ulcer recurrence.[1,5] Host-specific cofactors and *H. pylori* strain variability play an important role in the pathogenesis of PUD and gastric cancer.[5–7] Although an association between *H. pylori* and PUD bleeding is less clear, eradication of *H. pylori* decreases recurrent bleeding.[8] No specific link has been established between *H. pylori* and dyspepsia, nonulcer dyspepsia (NUD), or gastroesophageal reflux disease (GERD).[9,10] There is insufficient data to support a link between *H. pylori* and extragastric manifestations, for example, cardiovascular disease.[11]

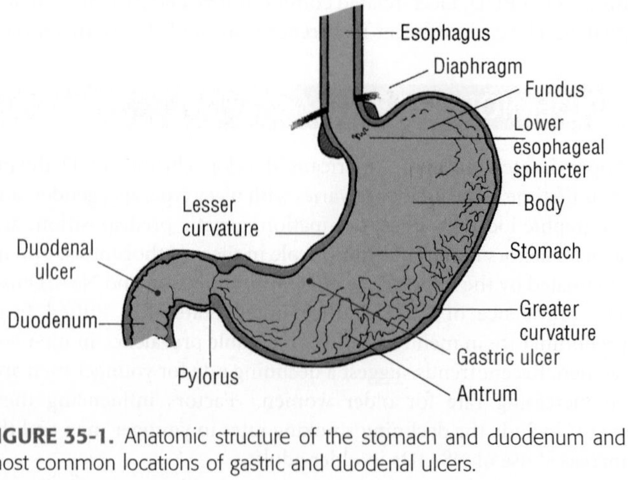

FIGURE 35-1. Anatomic structure of the stomach and duodenum and most common locations of gastric and duodenal ulcers.

The prevalence of *H. pylori* varies by geographic location, socioeconomic conditions, ethnicity, and age. In developing countries, *H. pylori* prevalence exceeds 80% in adults and correlates with lower socioeconomic conditions.[5] In industrialized countries, the prevalence of *H. pylori* in adults is between 20% and 50%.[5] The prevalence of *H. pylori* in the United States is 30% to 40%, but remains higher in ethnic groups such as African and Latin Americans. During the last few years, the incidence of *H. pylori* has declined dramatically in developed countries, most likely as a consequence of improved living standards and socioeconomic conditions.[6] There is an increased *H. pylori* prevalence with age, but this mainly reflects acquisition during infancy and early childhood.[1] Infection rates do not differ with gender or smoking status.

H. pylori is transmitted person-to-person by three possible pathways; fecal–oral, oral–oral, and gastro–oral.[1,6] Transmission of the organism most likely is by the fecal–oral route, either directly from an infected person, or indirectly from fecal-contaminated water or food.[1] Members of the same household are likely to become infected when someone in the same household is infected.[1,6] Risk factors include crowded living conditions, a large number of children, unclean water, and consumption of raw vegetables. Transmission by the oral–oral route has been postulated, but this is an unlikely route of transmission. *H. pylori* could be transmitted by the gastro–oral route by vomiting or iatrogenically with the use of inadequately sterilized endoscopes.[1]

NONSTEROIDAL ANTIINFLAMMATORY DRUGS

NSAIDs are one of the most widely prescribed classes of medications in the United States, particularly in individuals 60 years of age and older.[1] There is overwhelming evidence linking chronic nonselective

TABLE 35-2 Potential Causes of Peptic Ulcer

Common causes
Helicobacter pylori infection
Nonsteroidal antiinflammatory drugs
Critical illness (stress-related mucosal damage)
Uncommon causes
Hypersecretion of gastric acid (e.g., Zollinger-Ellison's syndrome)
Viral infections (e.g., cytomegalovirus)
Vascular insufficiency (crack cocaine associated)
Radiation
Chemotherapy (e.g., hepatic artery infusions)
Rare genetic subtypes
Idiopathic

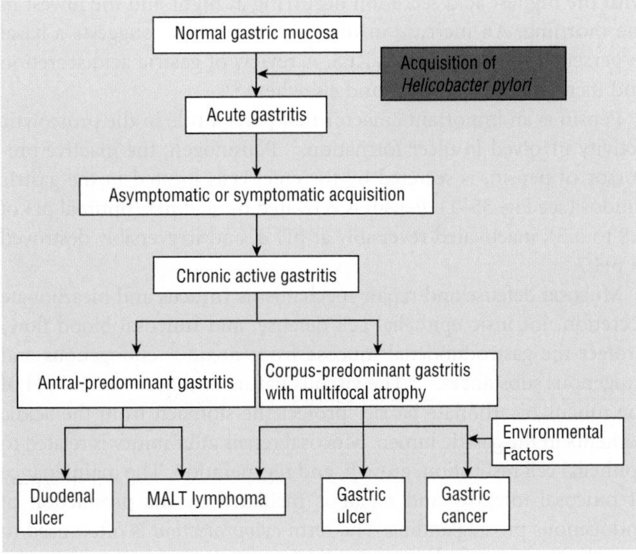

FIGURE 35-2. The natural history of *Helicobacter pylori* infection in the pathogenesis of gastric ulcer and duodenal ulcer, mucosa-associated lymphoid tissue (MALT) lymphoma, and gastric cancer.

NSAID (including aspirin) use to a variety of GI tract injuries (Table 35–3).[1,12–14] Subepithelial gastric hemorrhages occur within 15 to 30 minutes of ingestion, and progress to gastric erosions with continued ingestion.[1,12] These lesions heal within a few days with continued NSAID use and do not lead to GI complications. Gastroduodenal ulcers occur in 15% to 30% of regular NSAID users and may develop within a week or with continued treatment (6 months or longer).[12] Gastric ulcers are most common, occur primarily in the antrum (see Fig. 35–1), and are of greater concern than erosions because of their potential to bleed or perforate (see Table 35–1). NSAID-induced ulcers occur less frequently in the esophagus and colon.[1,15] Each year, nonselective NSAIDs account for at least 16,500 deaths and 107,000 hospitalizations in the United States.[1] Clinically important upper GI events occur in 3% to 4.5% of arthritis patients who are taking NSAIDs, and about 1.5% of patients taking NSAIDs have a serious upper GI complication.[12]

Table 35–4 lists the risk factors for NSAID-induced ulcers and GI-related complications. Combinations of factors confer an additive risk. The risk of NSAID complications is increased as much as 14-fold in patients with a previous history of an ulcer or ulcer-related complication.[1] Advanced age is an independent risk factor and increases linearly with the age of the patient.[1] The high incidence of ulcer complications in older individuals may be explained by age-related changes in gastric mucosal defense. The risk for NSAID-induced ulcers and complications is dose related, but can occur with low dosages of nonprescription NSAIDs or low cardioprotective dosages of aspirin (81 to 325 mg/day).[1,12–16] Adverse GI events may occur at any time, during treatment. The use of low-dose aspirin in combination with another NSAID increases the risk of upper GI complications to a greater extent than the use of either drug alone.[1] NSAID-related dyspepsia that is not relieved by antiulcer medications may suggest an ulcer or ulcer complication, but dyspepsia does not correlate directly with mucosal injury or clinical events.

TABLE 35-3 Selected Nonsteroidal Antiinflammatory Drugs (NSAIDs) and Cyclooxygenase-2(COX-2) Inhibitors

Nonsalicylates[a]
Nonselective (traditional) NSAIDs: indomethacin, piroxicam, ibuprofen, naproxen, sulindac, ketoprofen, ketorolac, flurbiprofen
Partially selective NSAIDs: etodolac, nabumetone, meloxicam, celocoxib, diclofenac
Selective COX-2 inhibitors: rofecoxib,[b] valdecoxib[b]
Salicylates
Acetylated: aspirin
Nonacetylated: salsalate, trisalicylate

[a]Based on COX-1/COX-2 selectivity ratio.
[b]Withdrawn from U.S. market.

TABLE 35-4 Risk Factors for Nonsteroidal Antiinflammatory Drug (NSAID)-Induced Ulcers and Upper Gastrointestinal Complications[a]

Established risk factors
Older than 60 years of age
Previous peptic ulcer
Previous ulcer-related upper GI complication
Concomitant use of corticosteroid
High-dose NSAIDs
Multiple NSAID use or NSAID plus aspirin use
Choice of NSAID
Aspirin (including cardioprotective dosages)
Concomitant use of anticoagulant or coagulopathy
Concomitant use of antiplatelet drug such as clopidogrel
Concomitant use of oral bisphosphonates
Concomitant use of selective serotonin reuptake inhibitor
Chronic illness (e.g., cardiovascular disease)
Possible risk factors
NSAID-related dyspepsia
Helicobacter pylori infection
Rheumatoid arthritis (extent of disability)
Alcohol consumption
Questionable risk factors
Cigarette smoking

[a]Combinations of risk factors are additive.
From Del Valle et al.,[1] Suerbaum and Michetti,[5] Laine,[12] Naesdal and Brown,[13] Lanas et al.,[15] and Tata et al.[17]

Corticosteroids, when used alone, do not increase the risk of ulcer or complications, but ulcer risk is increased twofold in corticosteroid users who are also taking concurrent NSAIDs.[1] The risk of GI bleeding markedly increases when NSAIDs are taken concurrently with anticoagulants,[1] and may increase with concurrent use of serotonin reuptake inhibitors.[17] Whether *H. pylori* infection is a risk factor for NSAID-induced ulcers remains controversial.[13,18] However, *H. pylori* and NSAIDs act independently to increase ulcer risk and ulcer-related bleeding and appear to have additive effects.[14] The incidence of peptic ulcer is reported to be higher in *H. pylori*-positive NSAID users when the two factors are combined.[19,20]

There is little evidence to support clinically important differences in ulcer frequency and upper GI complications among most available nonaspirin, nonselective NSAIDs (see Table 35–3) when used in equipotent antiinflammatory dosages.[1] However, the nonacetylated salicylates (e.g., salsalate) and the partially selective NSAIDs (e.g., etodolac, nabumetone, meloxicam, diclofenac, and celecoxib) may be associated with a decreased incidence of GI toxicity.[1,13,21,22] NSAIDs that selectively inhibit cyclooxygenase-2 (COX-2) decrease the incidence of gastroduodenal ulcers and related GI complications when compared to the nonselective NSAIDs.[13,21] The use of buffered or enteric-coated aspirin confers no added protection from ulcer or GI complications.[13,22]

CIGARETTE SMOKING

Epidemiologic evidence links cigarette smoking to PUD, but it is uncertain whether smoking causes peptic ulcers.[1] The risk is proportional to the number of cigarettes smoked and is modest when fewer than 10 cigarettes are smoked per day. Death rates are higher among patients who smoke than among nonsmoking patients, although it is not known whether the increase in mortality reflects PUD or the cardiac and pulmonary sequelae of smoking. The exact mechanism by which cigarette smoking contributes to PUD remains unclear. Possible mechanisms include delayed gastric emptying of solids and liquids, inhibition of pancreatic bicarbonate secretion, promotion of duodenogastric reflux, and reduction in mucosal prostaglandin (PG) production. Smoking increases gastric acid secretion, but this effect is inconsistent. Whether nicotine or other components of smoke are responsible for these physiologic alterations is unknown. Cigarette smoking may provide a favorable milieu for *H. pylori* infection.

PSYCHOLOGICAL STRESS

The importance of psychological factors in the pathogenesis of PUD remains controversial.[1] Clinical observation suggests that ulcer patients are adversely affected by stressful life events. However, results from controlled trials are conflicting and have failed to document a cause-and-effect relationship.[1] Emotional stress may induce behavioral risks such as smoking and the use of NSAIDs, or alter the inflammatory response or resistance to *H. pylori* infection. The role of stress and how it affects PUD is complex and probably multifactorial.

DIETARY FACTORS

The role of diet and nutrition in PUD is uncertain, but may explain regional variations.[1] Coffee, tea, cola beverages, beer, milk, and spices may cause dyspepsia, but do not increase the risk for PUD. Beverage restrictions and bland diets do not alter the frequency of ulcer recurrence. Although caffeine is a gastric acid stimulant, constituents in decaffeinated coffee or tea, caffeine-free carbonated beverages, beer, and wine may also increase gastric acid secretion. In high concentrations, alcohol ingestion is associated with acute gastric mucosal damage and upper GI bleeding; however, there is insufficient evidence to confirm that alcohol causes ulcers.[1]

DISEASE ASSOCIATED WITH PEPTIC ULCERS

There is epidemiologic evidence linking duodenal ulcers with certain chronic diseases, but the pathophysiologic mechanisms of these associations are unclear.[1] A strong association exists with systemic mastocytosis, multiple endocrine neoplasia type 1, chronic pulmonary diseases, chronic renal failure, kidney stones, hepatic cirrhosis, and α_1-antitrypsin deficiency. An association may exist with cystic fibrosis, chronic pancreatitis, Crohn's disease, coronary artery disease, polycythemia vera, and hyperparathyroidism.

PATHOPHYSIOLOGY

A physiologic imbalance between aggressive factors (gastric acid and pepsin) and protective factors (mucosal defense and repair) remain important issues in the pathophysiology of gastric and duodenal ulcers. Gastric acid is secreted by the parietal cells, which contain receptors for histamine, gastrin, and acetylcholine. Acid (as well as *H. pylori* infection and NSAID use) is an independent factor that contributes to the disruption of mucosal integrity. Increased acid secretion has been observed in patients with duodenal ulcers and may be a consequence of *H. pylori* infection.[23,24] Patients with ZES (described later in the chapter; see Zollinger-Ellison's Syndrome) have profound gastric acid hypersecretion resulting from a gastrin-producing tumor.[4] Patients with gastric ulcer usually have normal or reduced rates of acid secretion (hypochlorhydria).

Acid secretion is expressed as the amount of acid secreted under basal or fasting conditions, basal acid output (BAO); after maximal stimulation, maximal acid output (MAO); or in response to a meal.[23] Basal, maximal, and meal-stimulated acid secretion varies according to time of day and the individual's psychological state, age, gender, and health status. The BAO follows a circadian rhythm, with the highest acid secretion occurring at night and the lowest in the morning. An increase in the BAO:MAO ratio suggests a basal hypersecretory state such as ZES. A review of gastric acid secretion and its regulation can be found elsewhere.[23]

Pepsin is an important cofactor that plays a role in the proteolytic activity involved in ulcer formation.[23] Pepsinogen, the inactive precursor of pepsin, is secreted by the chief cells located in the gastric fundus (see Fig. 35–1). Pepsin is activated by acid pH (optimal pH of 1.8 to 3.5), inactivated reversibly at pH 4, and irreversibly destroyed at pH 7.

Mucosal defense and repair mechanisms (mucus and bicarbonate secretion, intrinsic epithelial cell defense, and mucosal blood flow) protect the gastroduodenal mucosa from noxious endogenous and exogenous substances.[1,24] The viscous nature and near-neutral pH of the mucus-bicarbonate barrier protect the stomach from the acidic contents in the gastric lumen. Mucosal repair after injury is related to epithelial cell restitution, growth, and regeneration. The maintenance of mucosal integrity and repair is mediated by the production of endogenous prostaglandins. The term *cytoprotection* is often used to describe this process, but *mucosal defense* and *mucosal protection* are more accurate terms, as prostaglandins prevent deep mucosal injury and not superficial damage to individual cells. Gastric hyperemia and increased prostaglandin synthesis characterize adaptive cytoprotection, the short-term adaptation of mucosal cells to mild topical irritants. This phenomenon enables the stomach to initially withstand the damaging effects of irritants. Alterations in mucosal defense that are induced by *H. pylori* or NSAIDs are the most important cofactors in the formation of peptic ulcers.

HELICOBACTER PYLORI

H. pylori is a spiral-shaped, pH-sensitive, gram-negative, microaerophilic bacterium that resides between the mucus layer and surface epithelial cells in the stomach, or any location where gastric-type epithelium is found.[1,5] The combination of its spiral shape and flagellum permits it to move from the lumen of the stomach, where the pH is low, to the mucus layer, where the local pH is neutral. The acute infection is accompanied by transient hypochlorhydria, which permits the organism to survive in the acidic gastric juice.[24] The exact method by which *H. pylori* initially induces hypochlorhydria is unclear. One theory is that *H. pylori* produces large amounts of urease, which hydrolyzes urea in the gastric juice and converts it to ammonia and carbon dioxide.[5] The local buffering effect of ammonia creates a neutral microenvironment within and surrounding the bacterium, which protects it from the lethal effect of acid. *H. pylori* also produces acid-inhibitory proteins, which allows it to adapt to the low-pH environment of the stomach.[24] *H. pylori* attaches to gastric-type epithelium by adherence pedestals, which prevent the organism from being shed during cell turnover and mucus secretion. Antral organisms colonize gastric metaplastic tissue (which is thought to arise secondary to changes in acid or bicarbonate secretion, products of *H. pylori*, or host inflammatory responses) in the duodenal bulb, leading to duodenal ulcer (see Fig. 35–2).[1] Colonization of the corpus (body) of the stomach is associated with gastric ulcer.

Bacterial and host factors contribute to the ability of *H. pylori* to cause gastroduodenal mucosal injury. Pathogenic mechanisms include (a) direct mucosal damage, (b) alterations in the host immune/inflammatory response, and (c) hypergastrinemia leading to increased acid secretion.[1,5] In addition, *H. pylori* enhances the carcinogenic conversion of susceptible gastric epithelial cells.[7,25,26]

Direct mucosal damage is produced by virulence factors (vacuolating cytotoxin, cytotoxin-associated gene protein, and growth-inhibitory factor), elaborating bacterial enzymes (lipases, proteases, and urease), and adherence.[1,5,26] Approximately 50% of *H. pylori* strains produce vacuolating cytotoxin (Vac A) that leads to cell death and is important in the development of gastric cancer.[1,26] Strains with cytotoxin-associated gene (cagA) protein are associated with duodenal ulcer, atrophic gastritis, and gastric cancer.[1,5,7,25] Lipases and proteases degrade gastric mucus, ammonia produced by urease may be toxic to gastric epithelial cells, and bacterial adherence enhances the uptake of toxins into gastric epithelial cells. *H. pylori* infection alters the host inflammatory response and damages epithelial cells directly by cell-mediated immune mechanisms, or indirectly by activated neutrophils or macrophages attempting to phagocytose bacteria or bacterial products.[1,5] Host polymorphisms are important markers of disease susceptibility and may identify high-risk patients.[26] Polymorphisms of interleukin-1 and its receptor antagonist may be associated with either increased gastric acid secretion and duodenal ulcer or decreased acid output, atrophic gastritis, and gastric cancer.[1,7]

NONSTEROIDAL ANTIINFLAMMATORY DRUGS

Nonselective NSAIDs, including aspirin (see Table 35–3), cause gastric mucosal damage by two important mechanisms: (a) direct or topical irritation of the gastric epithelium and (b) systemic inhibition of endogenous mucosal prostaglandin synthesis.[1,13,14] Although the initial injury is initiated topically by the acidic properties of many of the NSAIDs, systemic inhibition of the protective prostaglandins plays the predominant role in the development of gastric ulcer.[1,13,14] Cyclooxygenase (COX) is the rate-limiting enzyme in the conversion of arachidonic acid to prostaglandins and is inhibited by NSAIDs (Fig. 35–3).

Two similar COX isoforms have been identified: cyclooxygenase-1 (COX-1) is found in most body tissue, including the stomach, kidney, intestine, and platelets; cyclooxygenase-2 (COX-2) is undetectable in most tissues under normal physiologic conditions, but its expression can be induced during acute inflammation and arthritis (Fig. 35–4).[1,13] COX-1 produces protective prostaglandins that regulate physiologic processes such as GI mucosal integrity, platelet homeostasis, and renal function. COX-2 is induced (unregulated) by inflammatory stimuli such as cytokines, and produces prostaglandins involved with inflammation, fever, and pain. COX-2 is also constitutionally expressed in organs such as the brain, kidney, and reproductive tract. Adverse effects (e.g., GI or renal toxicity) of NSAIDs are primarily associated with the inhibition of COX-1, whereas antiinflammatory actions result primarily from NSAID inhibition of COX-2.[1,13] Nonselective NSAIDs, including aspirin (see Table 35–3), inhibit both COX-1 and COX-2 to varying degrees.[1,13] The COX-1–to–COX-2 inhibitory ratio determines the relative GI toxicity of a specific NSAID. In addition, aspirin and nonaspirin NSAIDs irreversibly inhibit platelet COX-1, resulting in decreased platelet aggregation and prolonged bleeding times, thereby increasing the potential for upper and lower GI bleeding.[1]

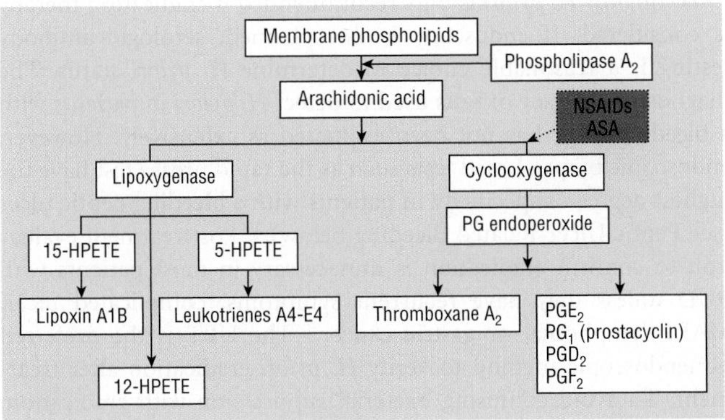

FIGURE 35-3. Metabolism of arachidonic acid after its release from membrane phospholipids. *Broken arrow* indicates inhibitory effects. (ASA, aspirin; HPETE, hydroperoxyeicosatetraenoic acid; NSAIDs, nonsteroidal antiinflammatory drugs; PG, prostaglandin.)

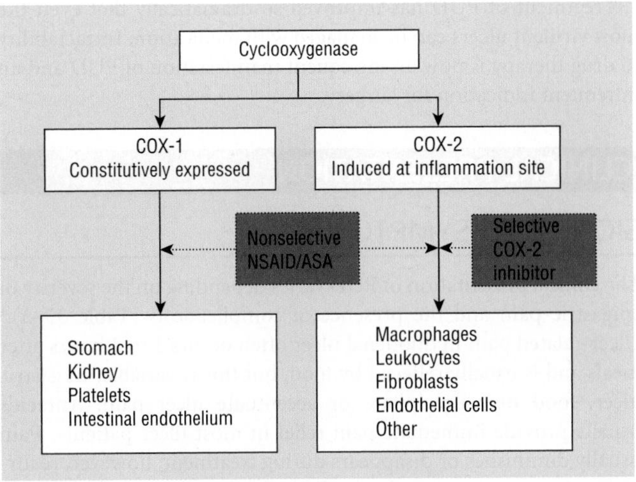

FIGURE 35-4. Tissue distribution and actions of cyclooxygenase (COX) isoenzymes. Nonselective nonsteroidal antiinflammatory drugs (NSAIDs) including aspirin (ASA) inhibit COX-1 and COX-2 to varying degrees; COX-2 inhibitors inhibit only COX-2. *Broken arrow* indicates inhibitory effects.

Other mechanisms may also contribute to the development of NSAID-related mucosal injury.[1]

Topical irritant properties are predominantly associated with acidic NSAIDs (e.g., aspirin) and their ability to decrease the hydrophobicity of the mucous gel layer in the gastric mucosa.[1] Most nonaspirin NSAIDs have topical irritant effects, but aspirin is the most damaging. Although NSAID prodrugs, enteric-coated aspirin tablets, salicylate derivatives, and parenteral or rectal preparations are associated with less-acute topical gastric mucosal injury, they can cause ulcers and related GI complications as a result of their systemic inhibition of endogenous PGs.

COMPLICATIONS

Upper GI bleeding, perforation, and obstruction occur with *H. pylori*-associated and NSAID-induced ulcers and constitute the most serious, life-threatening complications of chronic PUD.[1,2] Bleeding is caused by the erosion of an ulcer into an artery and occurs in approximately 10% to 15% of patients.[1,2] The bleeding may be occult (hidden) and insidious, or may present as melena (black-colored stools) or hematemesis (vomiting of blood). The use of NSAIDs (especially in older adults) is the most important risk factor for upper GI bleeding. Deaths occur primarily in patients who continue to bleed, or in those patients who rebleed after the initial bleeding has stopped (see Upper Gastrointestinal Bleeding).

Ulcer-related perforation into the peritoneal cavity occurs in approximately 7% of patients with PUD.[1] The incidence of perforation is increasing with the increased use of NSAIDs. Mortality is usually higher for perforated gastric ulcer than duodenal ulcer. The pain of perforation is usually sudden, sharp, and severe, beginning first in the epigastrium, but quickly spreading over the entire abdomen. Most patients experience ulcer symptoms prior to perforation. However, older patients who experience perforation in association with NSAID use may be asymptomatic. Penetration occurs when an ulcer burrows into an adjacent structure (pancreas, biliary tract, or liver) rather than opening freely into a cavity.

Gastric outlet obstruction occurs in approximately 2% of patients with peptic ulcers.[1] Mechanical obstruction is caused by scarring or edema of the duodenal bulb or pyloric channel and can lead to gastric retention. Symptoms usually occur over several months and include early satiety, bloating, anorexia, nausea, vomiting, and weight loss. Perforation, penetration, and gastric outlet obstruction occur most often in patients with long-standing PUD.

Treatment of PUD has improved so dramatically that even the most virulent ulcers can be managed with medication. Intractability to drug therapy is now an infrequent manifestation of PUD and an infrequent indication for surgery.

CLINICAL PRESENTATION

SIGNS AND SYMPTOMS

The clinical presentation of PUD varies depending on the severity of epigastric pain and the presence of complications (Table 35–5).[1] Ulcer-related pain in duodenal ulcer often occurs 1 to 3 hours after meals and is usually relieved by food, but this is variable. In gastric ulcer, food may precipitate or accentuate ulcer pain. Antacids usually provide immediate pain relief in most ulcer patients. Pain usually diminishes or disappears during treatment; however, recurrence of epigastric pain after healing often suggests an unhealed or recurrent ulcer.

Epigastric pain does not define an ulcer.[1,14] The absence of pain does not preclude the diagnosis especially in the elderly who may present with "silent" ulcer complications. The reasons for this are unclear, but may relate to differences in the way the elderly perceive pain or the analgesic effect of NSAIDs. Dyspepsia in itself is of little clinical value when assessing subsets of patients who are most likely to have an ulcer. Patients taking NSAIDs often report dyspepsia, but dyspeptic symptoms do not directly correlate with an ulcer. Patients with dyspeptic symptoms may have either uninvestigated (no upper endoscopy) or investigated (underwent upper endoscopy) dyspepsia. If an ulcer is not confirmed in a patient with ulcer-like symptoms at the time of endoscopy, the disorder is referred to as *nonulcer dyspepsia*.[3] Ulcer-like symptoms may occur in the absence of peptic ulceration in association with *H. pylori* gastritis or duodenitis. There is no one sign or symptom that differentiates between *H. pylori*-associated and NSAID-induced ulcer.

TABLE 35-5 Presentation of Peptic Ulcer Disease

General
- Mild epigastric pain or acute life-threatening upper gastrointestinal complications

Symptoms
- Abdominal pain that is often epigastric and described as burning, but may present as vague discomfort, abdominal fullness, or cramping
- A typical nocturnal pain that awakens the patient from sleep (especially between 12 AM and 3 AM)
- The severity of ulcer pain varies from patient to patient, and may be seasonal, occurring more frequently in the spring or fall; episodes of discomfort usually occur in clusters, lasting up to a few weeks and followed by a pain-free period or remission lasting from weeks to years
- Changes in the character of the pain may suggest the presence of complications
- Heartburn, belching, and bloating often accompany the pain
- Nausea, vomiting, and anorexia, are more common in patients with gastric ulcer than with duodenal ulcer, but may also be signs of an ulcer-related complication

Signs
- Weight loss associated with nausea, vomiting, and anorexia
- Complications, including ulcer bleeding, perforation, penetration, or obstruction

Laboratory tests
- Gastric acid secretory studies
- Fasting serum gastrin concentrations are only recommended for patients who are unresponsive to therapy, or for those in whom hypersecretory diseases are suspected
- The hematocrit and hemoglobin are low with bleeding, and stool hemoccult tests are positive
- Tests for *Helicobacter pylori* (see Table 35–6)

Other diagnostic tests
- Fiberoptic upper endoscopy (esophagogastroduodenoscopy) detects more than 90% of peptic ulcers and permits direct inspection, biopsy, visualization of superficial erosions, and sites of active bleeding
- Routine single-barium contrast techniques detect 30% of peptic ulcers; optimal double-contrast radiography detects 60% to 80% of ulcers

From Del Valle et al.[1] and Yuan et al.[14]

DIAGNOSIS

Routine laboratory tests are not helpful in establishing the diagnosis of uncomplicated PUD (see Table 35–5).[1]

TESTS FOR *HELICOBACTER PYLORI*

The diagnosis of *H. pylori* infection can be made using endoscopic or nonendoscopic tests (Table 35–6).[1,5,27] The tests that require upper endoscopy are invasive, more expensive, and usually require a mucosal biopsy for histology, culture, or detection of urease activity. At least three tissue samples are taken from specific areas of the stomach, as patchy distribution of *H. pylori* infection can lead to false-negative results. Because certain medications may decrease the sensitivity of these tests, antibiotics and bismuth salts should be withheld for 4 weeks and proton pump inhibitors (PPIs) for 1 to 2 weeks prior to endoscopic testing. A new method permits the in vivo observation of *H. pylori* in their natural niche during endoscopy.[28]

Two types of nonendoscopic tests are available: tests that identify active infection and tests that detect antibodies (see Table 35–6). Antibody tests do not differentiate between active infection and previously eradicated *H. pylori*. The nonendoscopic tests are noninvasive, more convenient, and less expensive than the endoscopic tests and include the urea breath test (UBT), serologic antibody detection tests, and the stool antigen test.[1,5,27] The UBT is the most accurate noninvasive test and is based on *H. pylori* urease activity.[27] The ^{13}carbon (nonradioactive isotope) and ^{14}carbon (radioactive isotope) tests require that the patient ingest radiolabeled urea, which is then hydrolyzed by *H. pylori* (if present in the stomach) to ammonia and radiolabeled bicarbonate. The radiolabeled bicarbonate is absorbed in the blood and excreted in the breath. A mass spectrometer is used to detect ^{13}carbon, whereas ^{14}carbon is measured using a scintillation counter. Serologic tests are a cost-effective alternative for the initial diagnosis of *H. pylori* infection in the untreated patient. However, serology should not be used to confirm *H. pylori* eradication and is unreliable in young children.[1,5,27] Office-based tests provide rapid results but are less accurate than laboratory-based enzyme-linked immunosorbent assay (ELISA) tests. The stool antigen test is less expensive and easier to perform than the UBT, and may be useful in children. Although comparable to the UBT in the initial detection of *H. pylori*, the stool antigen test is less accurate when used to confirm *H. pylori* eradication posttreatment. Salivary and urine antibody tests are under investigation.[1,27]

Testing for *H. pylori* is only recommended if eradication therapy is considered. If endoscopy is not planned, serologic antibody testing is a reasonable choice to determine *H. pylori* status. The diagnostic accuracy of tests used to detect *H. pylori* in patients with a bleeding ulcer has not been evaluated as extensively. However, endoscopic biopsy-based tests such as the rapid urease test have the highest degree of specificity in patients with a bleeding peptic ulcer (see Peptic Ulcer-Related Bleeding below).[29] Posttreatment evaluation to confirm eradication is unnecessary in most patients with PUD unless they have recurrent symptoms, complicated ulcer, MALT lymphoma, or gastric cancer.[1] The UBT is the preferred nonendoscopic method to verify *H. pylori* eradication after treatment. To avoid confusing bacterial suppression with eradication, the UBT must be delayed at least 4 weeks after the completion of treatment. The term *eradication* or *cure* is used when posttreatment tests conducted 4 weeks after the end of treatment do not detect the organism. Quantitative antibody tests are considered impractical

TABLE 35-6 Tests for Detection of *Helicobacter pylori*

Test	Description	Comments
Endoscopic tests		
Histology	Microbiologic examination using various stains	Gold standard; >95% sensitive and specific; permits classification of gastritis; results are not immediate; not recommended for initial diagnosis; tests for active *H. pylori* infection
Culture	Culture of biopsy	Enables sensitivity testing to determine appropriate treatment or antibiotic resistance; 100% specific; results are not immediate; not recommended for initial diagnosis; used after failure of second-line treatment; tests for active *H. pylori* infection
Biopsy (rapid) urease	*H. pylori* urease generates ammonia, which causes a color change	Test of choice at endoscopy; >90% sensitive and specific; easily performed; rapid results (usually within 24 hours); tests for active *H. pylori* infection
Nonendoscopic tests		
Antibody detection (laboratory based)	Detects antibodies to *H. pylori* in serum; in the U.S., only FDA-approved anti-*H. pylori* IgG antibody should be used	Quantitative; less sensitive and specific than endoscopic tests; more accurate than in-office; unable to determine if antibody is related to active or cured infection; antibody titers vary markedly between individuals and take 6 months to 1 year to return to the uninfected range; not affected by PPIs or bismuth; antibiotics given for unrelated indications may cure the infection but antibody test will remain positive
Antibody detection (can be performed in office or near patient)	Detects IgG antibodies to *H. pylori* in whole blood or fingerstick	Qualitative; quick (within 15 minutes); unable to determine if antibody is related to active or cured infection; most patients remain seropositive for at least 6 months to 1 year after *H. pylori* eradication; not affected by PPIs, bismuth, or antibiotics
Urea breath test	*H. pylori* urease breaks down ingested labeled C-urea, patient exhales labeled CO_2	Tests for active *H. pylori* infection; 95% sensitive and specific; results take about 2 days; antibiotics, bismuth, PPIs, and H_2RAs may cause false-negative results; withhold PPIs or H_2RAs (1–2 weeks) and bismuth or antibiotics (4 weeks) prior to testing; may be used posttreatment to confirm eradication
Stool antigen	Identifies *H. pylori* antigen in stool, leading to color change that can be detected visually or by spectrophotometer	Tests for active *H. pylori* infection; sensitivity and specificity comparable to urea breath test when used for initial diagnosis; antibiotics, bismuth, and PPIs may cause false-negative results, but to a lesser extent than with the urea breath test; may be used posttreatment to confirm eradication

H_2RA, H_2-receptor antagonist; PPI, proton pump inhibitor.

for posttreatment eradication as antibody titers remain elevated for long periods of time.

IMAGING AND ENDOSCOPY

The diagnosis of PUD depends on visualizing the ulcer crater either by upper GI radiography or upper endoscopy (see Table 35–5).[1] Because of its lower cost, greater availability, and greater safety, radiography is often the initial diagnostic procedure in patients with suspected uncomplicated PUD. If complications are thought to exist, or if an accurate diagnosis is warranted, upper endoscopy is the diagnostic procedure of choice. If a gastric ulcer is found on radiography, malignancy should be excluded by direct endoscopic visualization and histology.

CLINICAL COURSE AND PROGNOSIS

The natural history of PUD is characterized by periods of exacerbations and remissions.[1] Ulcer pain is usually recognizable and episodic, but symptoms are variable, especially in older adults and in patients taking NSAIDs. Antiulcer medications, including the histamine-2 receptor antagonists (H_2RAs), PPIs, and sucralfate, relieve symptoms, accelerate ulcer healing, and reduce the risk of ulcer recurrence, but they do not cure the disease. Both duodenal ulcers and gastric ulcers recur unless the underlying cause (*H. pylori* or NSAID) is removed. Successful *H. pylori* eradication markedly decreases ulcer recurrence and complications. Prophylactic cotherapy or a COX-2 inhibitor dramatically decreases the risk for ulcers and related complications in high-risk patients who are taking NSAIDs. Approximately 20% of patients with chronic PUD experience upper GI bleeding, perforation, or obstruction. Mortality in patients with gastric ulcer is slightly higher than in duodenal ulcer and the general population. The development of adenocarcinoma in *H. pylori*-infected patients is a slow process that occurs over 20 to 40 years and is associated with a lifetime risk of less than 1%.[1,7]

TREATMENT

DESIRED OUTCOME

The treatment of chronic PUD varies depending on the etiology of the ulcer (*H. pylori* or NSAID), whether the ulcer is initial or recurrent, and whether complications have occurred (Fig. 35–5). Overall treatment is aimed at relieving ulcer pain, healing the ulcer, preventing ulcer recurrence, and reducing ulcer-related complications. The goal of therapy in *H. pylori*-positive patients with an active ulcer, a previously documented ulcer, or a history of an ulcer-related complication, is to eradicate *H. pylori*, heal the ulcer, and cure the disease. Successful eradication heals ulcers and reduces the risk of recurrence to less than 10% at 1 year.[1] The goal of therapy in a patient with a NSAID-induced ulcer is to heal the ulcer as rapidly as possible. Patients who are at high risk of developing NSAID ulcers should receive prophylactic cotherapy or be switched to a COX-2 inhibitor (if available) to reduce ulcer risk and related complications. When possible, the most cost-effective drug regimen should be used.

GENERAL APPROACH TO TREATMENT

The treatment of PUD centers on healing the ulcer and reducing the risk of ulcer recurrence and related complications. Drug regimens containing antimicrobials such as clarithromycin, metronidazole, amoxicillin, and bismuth salts and antisecretory drugs (PPIs or H_2RAs) relieve ulcer symptoms, heal the ulcer, and eradicate *H. pylori* infection. Successful eradication will alter the natural history of PUD and cure the disease. PPIs are preferred to H_2RAs or sucralfate for healing *H. pylori*-negative NSAID ulcers because they accelerate ulcer healing and provide more effective relief of symptoms. Treatment with a PPI should be extended to 8 to 12 weeks if the NSAID must be continued. A PPI-based *H. pylori* eradication regimen is recommended in *H. pylori*-positive patients with an active ulcer who are also taking an NSAID. Prophylactic cotherapy with either a PPI or miso-

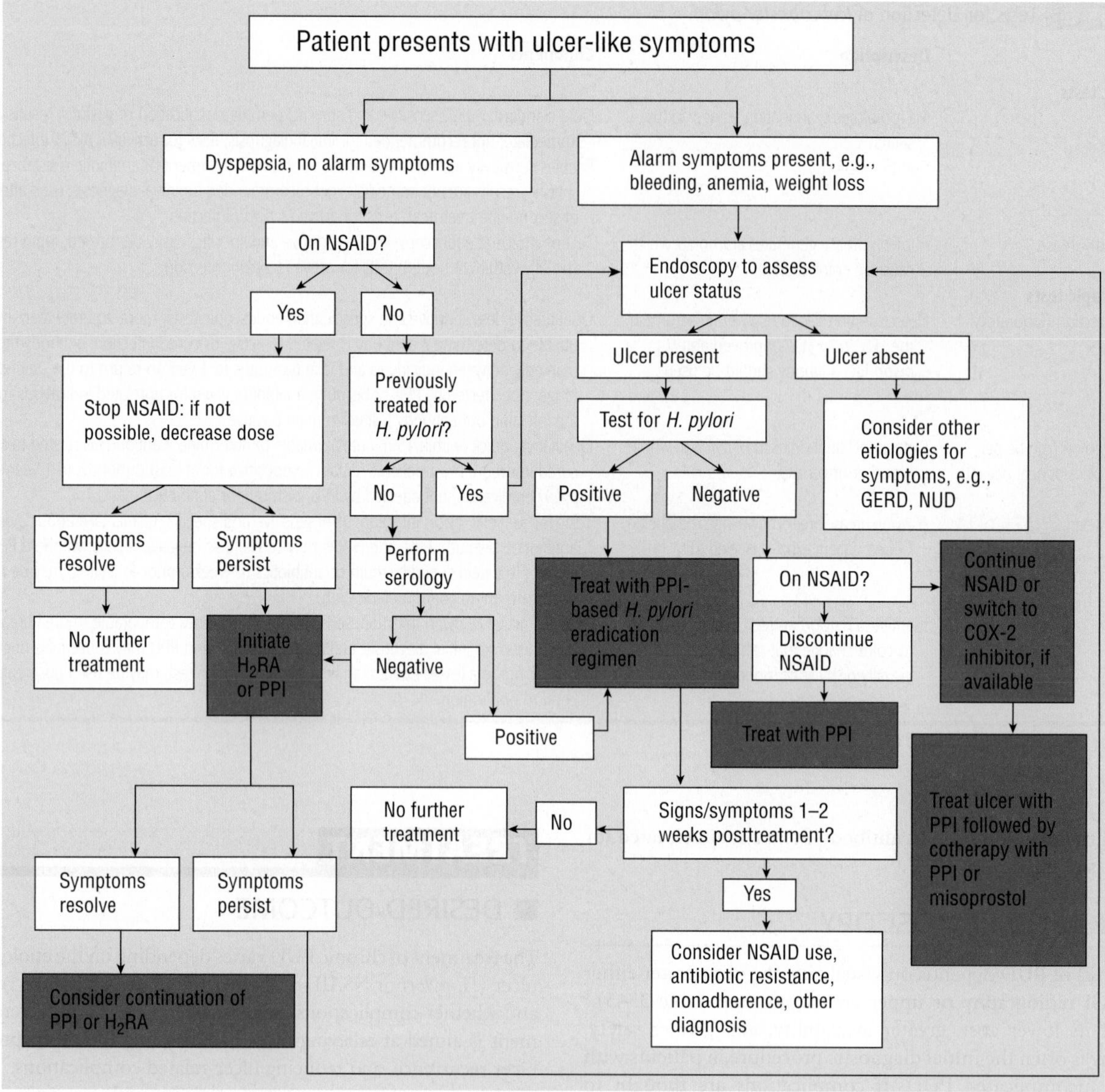

FIGURE 35-5. Algorithm. Guidelines for the evaluation and management of a patient who presents with dyspeptic or ulcer-like symptoms. (COX-2, cyclooxygenase-2; GERD, gastroesophageal reflux disease; *H. pylori*, *Helicobacter pylori*; H_2RA, H_2-receptor antagonist; PPI, proton pump inhibitor; NSAID, nonsteroidal antiinflammatory drug; NUD, nonulcer dyspepsia.)

prostol decreases ulcer risk and upper GI complications in patients taking nonselective NSAIDs. A COX-2 inhibitor may be used as an alternative to a nonselective NSAID, but the risk of adverse cardiovascular effects must be weighted against the gastroprotective benefits in each patient. The optimal therapeutic strategy for patients at very high risk of NSAID-related GI events is not known, but selected patients may benefit from the use of a COX-2 inhibitor and a PPI.

Dietary modifications are important for patients who are unable to tolerate certain foods and beverages. Lifestyle modifications such as reducing stress and decreasing or stopping cigarette smoking is encouraged. Some patients may require radiographic or endoscopic procedures for a definitive diagnosis or for complications such as bleeding. Surgery may be necessary in patients with ulcer-related complications.

■ NONPHARMACOLOGIC THERAPY

❶ Patients with PUD should eliminate or reduce psychological stress, cigarette smoking, and the use of nonselective NSAIDs (including aspirin). Although there is no "antiulcer diet," the patient should avoid foods and beverages (e.g., spicy foods, caffeine, and alcohol) that cause dyspepsia or that exacerbate ulcer symptoms. If possible, alternative agents such as acetaminophen, nonacetylated salicylate (e.g., salsalate), or COX-2 inhibitors should be used for relief of pain.

Elective surgery for PUD is rarely performed today because of highly effective medical management such as the eradication of *H. pylori* and the use of potent acid inhibitors.[30] A subset of patients, however, may require emergency surgery for bleeding, perforation, or obstruction. In the past, surgical procedures were performed for medical treatment failures and included vagotomy with pyloroplasty or vagotomy with antrectomy.[30] Vagotomy (truncal, selective, or parietal cell) inhibits vagal stimulation of gastric acid. A truncal or selective vagotomy frequently results in postoperative gastric dysfunction and requires a pyloroplasty or antrectomy to facilitate gastric drainage. When an antrectomy is performed, the remaining stomach is anastomosed with the duodenum (Billroth I) or with the jejunum (Billroth II). A vagotomy is unnecessary when an antrectomy is performed for gastric ulcer. The postoperative consequences associated with these procedures include postvagotomy diarrhea, dumping syndrome, anemia, and recurrent ulceration.

TABLE 35-7 Guidelines for the Eradication of *Helicobacter pylori* Infection

Strongly recommended

- Gastric and duodenal ulcer (active or inactive), including complicated ulcers, and following gastric surgery for peptic ulcer
- Mucosa-associated lymphoid tissue (MALT) lymphoma
- Atrophic changes in the gastric mucosa (atrophic gastritis)
- Following resection of gastric cancer
- Infected patients who are first-degree relatives of patients with gastric cancer
- Infected patients who are aware and concerned about the risks of infection

Controversial

- Use of nonsteroidal antiinflammatory drugs (*H. pylori* infection and the use of nonsteroidal antiinflammatory drugs or aspirin are independent risk factors for peptic ulcer disease)
- Nonulcer dyspepsia
- Patients with gastroesophageal reflux disease receiving long-term proton pump inhibitor therapy

From Malfertheiner et al.[35] and Chex and Wong.[36]

PHARMACOLOGIC THERAPY

Recommendations

❷ Table 35–7 presents guidelines for the eradication of infection in *H. pylori*-positive individuals. Table 35–8 lists the recommended *H. pylori* eradication regimens. First-line therapy should be initiated with a PPI-based three-drug regimen for a minimum of 7 days, but preferably for 10 to 14 days. If a second course of treatment is required, the PPI-based three-drug regimen should contain different antibiotics or a four-drug regimen with bismuth subsalicylate, metronidazole, tetracycline, and a PPI should be used.

❸ Treatment with a conventional antiulcer drug, such as a PPI, an H_2RA, or sucralfate alone (Table 35–9), is an alternative to *H. pylori* eradication, but is discouraged because of the high rate of ulcer recurrence and ulcer-related complications associated with these regimens. Concomitant therapy (e.g., an H_2RA and sucralfate or an H_2RA and a PPI) is not recommended because it adds to drug costs without enhancing efficacy. Maintenance therapy with a PPI or H_2RA is recommended for high-risk patients with ulcer complications, patients who fail eradication, and those with *H. pylori*-negative ulcers.

❹ Patients with NSAID-induced ulcers should be tested to determine their *H. pylori* status. If *H. pylori*-positive, treatment should be initiated with a PPI-based three-drug eradication regimen. If *H. pylori*-negative, the NSAID should be discontinued and the patient treated with either a PPI, H_2RA, or sucralfate. If the NSAID must be continued, treatment should be initiated with a PPI (if *H. pylori*-negative) or with a PPI-based three-drug eradication regimen (if *H. pylori*-positive). Prophylactic cotherapy with a PPI or misoprostol or switching to a selective COX-2 inhibitor (if available) is recommended for patients at risk of developing ulcer-related upper GI complications (Table 35–10).

Treatment of *Helicobacter pylori*-Associated Ulcers

The following discussion focuses on the eradication of *H. pylori* in adults. Guidelines for the treatment of *H. pylori* infection in the elderly,[31,32] children,[33] and patients with chronic renal insufficiency[34] are found elsewhere.

❺ The goal of *H. pylori* drug therapy is eradication of the organism. Treatment should be effective, well-tolerated, easy to comply with, and cost-effective. *H. pylori* regimens should have eradication (cure) rates of at least 80% based on intention-to-treat analysis, or at least 90% based on per-protocol analysis, and should minimize the potential for antimicrobial resistance.[1,5,36–37] The use of a single antibiotic, bismuth salt, or antiulcer drug does not achieve this goal.[1,5] However, clarithromycin is the single most effective antibiotic.[1] Two-drug regimens that combine a PPI and either amoxicillin or clarithromycin have yielded marginal and variable eradication rates in the United States and are not recommended.[1,5] In addition, the use of only one antibiotic is associated with a higher rate of antimicrobial resistance.[1]

Eradication regimens (see Table 35–8) that combine two antibiotics and one antisecretory drug (triple therapy) or a bismuth salt, two antibiotics, and an antisecretory drug (quadruple therapy) increase eradication rates to an acceptable level and reduce the risk of antimicrobial resistance.[35–38] When selecting a first-line eradication regimen, an antibiotic combination should be used that permits second-line treatment (if necessary) with different antibiotics. The antibiotics that have been most extensively studied and found to be effective in various combinations include clarithromycin, amoxicillin, metronidazole, and tetracycline.[1,5] Although other antibiotics may be effective, they should not be used as part of the initial *H. pylori* regimen. Because of insufficient data, ampicillin should not be substituted for amoxicillin, doxycycline should not be substituted for tetracycline, and azithromycin or erythromycin should not be substi-

TABLE 35-8 Drug Regimens to Eradicate *Helicobater pylori*[a]

Drug #1	Drug #2	Drug #3	Drug #4
Proton pump inhibitor-based 3-drug regimens			
Omeprazole 20 mg twice daily *or* lansoprazole 30 mg twice daily *or* pantoprazole 40 mg twice daily *or* esomeprazole 40 mg daily *or* rabeprazole 20 mg daily	Clarithromycin 500 mg twice daily	Amoxicillin 1 g twice daily *or* metronidazole 500 mg twice daily	
Bismuth-based 4-drug regimens[b]			
Omeprazole 40 mg twice daily *or* lansoprazole 30 mg twice daily *or* pantoprazole 40 mg twice daily *or* esomeprazole 40 mg daily *or* rabeprazole 20 mg daily *or* standard ulcer-healing dosages of an H_2-receptor antagonist taken for 4–6 weeks (see Table 35–9)	Bismuth subsalicylate 525 mg four times daily	Metronidazole 250–500 mg four times daily	Tetracycline 500 mg four times daily *or* amoxicillin 500 mg four times daily, or, clarithromycin 250–500 mg four times daily

[a]Although treatment is minimally effective if used for 7 days, 10–14 days of treatment is recommended. The antisecretory drug may be continued beyond antimicrobial treatment in patients with a history of a complicated ulcer, e.g., bleeding or in heavy smokers.

[b]In the setting of an active ulcer, acid suppression is added to hasten pain relief.

TABLE 35-9 Oral Drug Regimens Used to Heal Peptic Ulcers or Maintain Ulcer Healing

Drug	Duodenal or Gastric Ulcer Healing (mg/dose)	Maintenance of Duodenal or Gastric Ulcer Healing (mg/dose)
Proton pump inhibitors		
Omeprazole	20–40 daily	20–40 daily
Lansoprazole	15–30 daily	15–30 daily
Rabeprazole	20 daily	20 daily
Pantoprazole	40 daily	40 daily
Esomeprazole	20–40 daily	20–40 daily
H_2-receptor antagonists		
Cimetidine	300 four times daily 400 twice daily 800 at bedtime	400–800 at bedtime
Famotidine	20 twice daily 40 at bedtime	20–40 at bedtime
Nizatidine	150 twice daily 300 at bedtime	150–300 at bedtime
Ranitidine	150 twice daily 300 at bedtime	150–300 at bedtime
Promote mucosal defense		
Sucralfate	1 g four times daily 2 g twice daily	1–2 g twice daily 1 g four times daily

tuted for clarithromycin. Amoxicillin should not be used in penicillin-allergic patients and metronidazole should be avoided if alcohol is consumed.[36] Bismuth salts have a topical antimicrobial effect.[1] Explanations as to why antisecretory drugs enhance the efficacy of antibiotics include increased activity or stability of the antibiotic at a higher intragastric pH and enhanced topical antibiotic concentration resulting from decreased intragastric volume.

Proton Pump Inhibitor-Based Three-Drug Regimens

Proton pump inhibitor-based three-drug regimens with two antibiotics (see Table 35–8) constitute first-line therapy for eradication of *H. pylori*.[1,5,35,36] There is now consensus that PPI-based regimens that combine either clarithromycin and amoxicillin or clarithromycin and metronidazole provide successful efficacy[1,35,36] and that the amoxicillin–metronidazole combination may be less effective.[1] In most cases, increasing the antibiotic dosage dose not improve eradication rates. Amoxicillin is preferred over clarithromycin for initial eradication because bacterial resistance is almost absent and it has fewer adverse effects.[14] It also leaves metronidazole as a backup agent for second-line therapy. The PPI–clarithromycin–metronidazole regimen should be used as first-line treatment in penicillin-allergic patients (see Table 35–8).[36]

An initial 7-day course of therapy provides minimally acceptable eradication rates and has been approved by the FDA and is recommended in Europe.[1,5,35,36] The duration of therapy, however, remains controversial in the United States, as longer treatment periods (10- and 14-day) favor higher eradication rates and are less likely to be associated with antimicrobial resistance.[1,5,36] A number of other antibiotics and antibiotic combinations have been evaluated as part of the PPI-based three-drug regimen with varying degrees of success.[1,5,36,39]

The PPI is an integral part of the three-drug regimen and should be taken 30 to 60 minutes before a meal along with the two antibiotics (see Table 35–8). Prolonged PPI treatment beyond 2 weeks after eradication is not necessary for ulcer healing.[40] A single daily dose of a PPI may be less effective than a double dose when used as part of a triple-therapy *H. pylori* eradication regimen.[41] Substitution of one PPI for another is acceptable and does not appear to enhance or diminish *H. pylori* eradication.[42] An H_2RA should not be substituted for a PPI, because more effective eradication rates have been demonstrated with a PPI.[43] Pretreatment with a PPI does not influence *H. pylori* eradication.[44]

Sequential therapy with a PPI and amoxicillin for 5 days followed by a PPI, clarithromycin, and metronidazole for an additional 5 days has achieved eradication rates which are superior to the traditional PPI-based three-drug regimens.[36,45] The rationale for sequential eradication therapy is to initially treat the patient with antibiotics that rarely promote resistance (e.g., amoxicillin) to reduce the bacterial load and preexisting resistant organisms and then to follow with different antibiotics (e.g., clarithromycin and metronidazole) to kill the remaining organisms. Sequential drug regimens must be validated in the United States before they can be recommended as first-line eradication therapy.

CLINICAL CONTROVERSY

Some clinicians favor an initial 7-day *H. pylori* regimen, whereas others favor a 10- or 14-day treatment course. The optimal duration of therapy is uncertain, as shorter periods may enhance compliance, but longer treatment periods in compliant patients favor higher eradication rates and are less likely to be associated with antimicrobial resistance. Patients receiving a second course of therapy after an unsuccessful eradication should receive treatment for 14 days.

Bismuth-Based Four-Drug Regimens

The bismuth-based four-drug regimens presented in Table 35–8 are used as first-line therapy to eradicate *H. pylori*. Eradication rates for a 14-day regimen containing bismuth, metronidazole, tetracycline,

TABLE 35-10 Risk Assessment and Suggested Guidelines for Reducing Gastrointestinal Risk in Patients Receiving Chronic NSAID Therapy

Risk Assessment (see Table 35–4)	Definition	Suggested Guidelines
Low	No risk factors or age <65 years and no aspirin, no prior ulcer, no history of ulcer-related GI complication	Nonselective NSAID or partially selective NSAID (see Table 35–3)
Moderate	1–2 risk factors (e.g., age >65 years, low-dose aspirin, high-dose NSAID)	Nonselective NSAID or partially selective NSAID plus PPI or misoprostol cotherapy; selective COX-2 inhibitor (if available)
High	≥3 risk factors or concomitant use of low-dose aspirin and either corticosteroids, warfarin, or clopidogrel	Nonselective or partially selective NSAID plus PPI or misoprostol cotherapy; COX-2 inhibitor if available plus PPI or misoprostol cotherapy
Very high	Prior ulcer or ulcer-related complication plus additional risk factors (e.g., age >65 years, concomitant use of low-dose aspirin, corticosteroids, warfarin, or clopidogrel)	Nonselective or partially selective NSAID plus PPI or misoprostol cotherapy; COX-2 inhibitor if available plus PPI or misoprostol cotherapy; consider NSAID or COX-2 inhibitor if available plus PPI and misoprostol cotherapy

COX-2, cycloxygenase-2 inhibitor; NSAID, nonsteroidal antiinflammatory drug; PPI, proton pump inhibitor.
From Del Valle et al.,[1] Elta,[2] Naesdal and Brown,[13] Dubois et al.,[51] and Chan and Graham.[52]

and an H_2-receptor antagonist are similar to those achieved with PPI-based triple therapy.[1,5,36,46] Increasing the duration of treatment to 1 month does not substantially increase eradication. Substitution of amoxicillin for tetracycline lowers the eradication rate and is usually not recommended.[1,46] Substitution of clarithromycin 250 to 500 mg four times a day for tetracycline yields similar results, but increases adverse effects. The antisecretory drug is used to hasten pain relief in patients with an active ulcer. Although the original bismuth-based four-drug regimen is effective and inexpensive, it is associated with frequent adverse effects and poor compliance. Comparable eradication rates occur when bismuth subcitrate potassium (biskalcitrate) is used in place of bismuth subsalicylate.

First-line treatment with quadruple therapy using a PPI (with bismuth, metronidazole, and tetracycline) in place of the H_2RA achieves similar eradication rates as those of PPI-based triple therapy and permits a shorter treatment duration (7 days).[1,46] Although evidence supports the efficacy of bismuth-based quadruple therapy as first-line treatment, it is often recommended as second-line treatment when a clarithromycin-amoxicillin regimen is used initially (see section on eradication regimens after initial treatment failure). All medications except the PPI should be taken with meals and at bedtime.

Eradication Regimens after Initial Treatment Failure

H. pylori eradication is often more difficult after initial treatment fails and successful eradication is extremely variable.[5,36,37] Because there are limited data on second attempts to eradicate *H. pylori*, treatment failures should be handled on a case-by-case basis. Patients who fail first-line regimens should be referred to a gastroenterologist for further diagnostic evaluation.

Second-line treatment should (a) use antibiotics that were not previously used during initial therapy; (b) use antibiotics that do not have resistance problems; (c) use a drug that has a topical effect such as bismuth; and the duration of treatment should be extended to 14 days.[47] Thus after unsuccessful initial treatment with a PPI–amoxicillin–clarithromycin regimen, second-line therapy should be instituted with bismuth subsalicylate, metronidazole, tetracycline, and a PPI for 14 days (see Table 35–8).[5,47] Other second-line regimens are discussed elsewhere.[36,47,48]

Factors That Contribute to Unsuccessful Eradication

Factors that contribute to unsuccessful eradication include poor medication adherence, resistant organisms, low intragastric pH, and a high bacterial load.[37,47,49] Medication adherence decreases with multiple medications, increased frequency of administration, increased length of treatment, intolerable adverse effects, and costly drug regimens. Although longer treatment duration may contribute to nonadherence, missed doses in a 7-day regimen may also lead to failed eradication.[47] Tolerability varies with different regimens. Metronidazole-containing regimens increase the frequency of adverse effects (especially when the dose is >1 g/day). Other common adverse effects include taste disturbances (metronidazole and clarithromycin), nausea, vomiting, abdominal pain, and diarrhea. Antibiotic-associated colitis, a serious complication, occurs occasionally. Oral thrush and vaginal candidiasis may also occur.

An important determinant of successful *H. pylori* eradication is the presence of preexisting antimicrobial resistance.[1,26,37,47] Metronidazole resistance is most common (10% to 60%), but varies depending on prior antibiotic exposure and geographic region.[1,26,37] The clinical importance of metronidazole resistance in eradicating *H. pylori* remains uncertain, as the synergistic effect of combining metronidazole with other antibiotics appears to render resistance to metronidazole less important. Primary resistance to clarithromycin is lower (10% to 15%) than with metronidazole, but it is more likely to affect the clinical outcome.[1,47] Secondary resistance occurs in up to two-thirds of treatment failures. Resistance to tetracycline and amoxicillin is uncommon.[1] Resistance to bismuth has not been reported. The role of antibiotic sensitivity testing before initiating *H. pylori* treatment has not been established.

Probiotics

Probiotics (e.g., strains of *Lactobacillus* and *Bifidobacterium*) and foodstuffs (e.g., cranberry juice and some milk proteins) with bioactive components have been used to proactively control *H. pylori* colonization in at-risk individuals and may have a possible role in decreasing mucosal inflammation and healing gastric ulcer in the *H. pylori*-infected patient.[50] Thus, regular intake of probiotics may eventually constitute a low-cost alternative for individuals who are at-risk for *H. pylori* colonization and, in combination with antibiotics, may increase eradication rates. A review of this subject is found elsewhere.[50]

Treatment of NSAID-Induced Ulcers

Nonselective NSAIDs should be discontinued (when possible) if an active ulcer is confirmed. If the NSAID is stopped, most uncomplicated ulcers will heal with standard regimens of an H_2-receptor antagonist, PPI, or sucralfate (see Table 35–9).[1,12,14] PPIs are usually preferred because they provide more rapid relief of symptoms and ulcer healing than H_2RAs or sucralfate. If the NSAID must be continued despite ulceration, consideration should be given to reducing the NSAID dose, or switching to acetaminophen, a nonacetylated salicylate, a partially selective COX-2 inhibitor, or a selective COX-2 inhibitor (see Table 35–3). The PPIs are the drugs of choice when the NSAID must be continued, as potent acid suppression is required to accelerate ulcer healing.[1,12,14] H_2RAs and sucralfate are less effective in the presence of continued NSAID use. If *H. pylori* is present, eradication should be initiated with a regimen that contains a PPI.[1,12–14]

Strategies to Reduce the Risk of NSAID-Induced Ulcers and Upper GI Complications There are three therapeutic approaches to reducing the risk of nonselective NSAID-related ulcers and serious upper GI complications (see Table 35–10). Medical cotherapy with either a PPI or misoprostol decreases ulcer risk and GI complications in high-risk patients.[1,12–14,21,51,52] The use of a selective COX-2 inhibitor instead of a nonselective NSAID also decreases risk of ulcers and serious GI events.[1,12–14,21,51,52] Unfortunately, these strategies, when used alone, do not completely eliminate ulcer recurrence and complications in patients at the "highest risk." Strategies aimed at reducing the topical irritant effects of nonselective NSAIDs—prodrugs, slow-release formulations, and enteric-coated products—do not prevent ulcers or GI complications.

Misoprostol Cotherapy Misoprostol, 200 mcg orally four times per day, reduces the risk of NSAID-induced gastric and duodenal ulcer, and ulcer-related GI complications, but diarrhea and abdominal cramping limit its use.[12–14,21] Because a dosage of 200 mcg three times per day is comparable in efficacy to 800 mcg/day, the lower dosage should be considered in patients unable to tolerate the higher dose.[1,12–14] Reducing the misoprostol dosage to 400 mcg per day or less to minimize diarrhea compromises its beneficial effects. A fixed combination of misoprostol 200 mcg and diclofenac (50 mg or 75 mg) is available and may enhance compliance, but the flexibility to individualize drug dosage is lost. A large clinical trial in rheumatoid arthritis patients provides the most compelling evidence that misoprostol reduces the risk of serious upper GI complications in high-risk patients.[53]

Proton Pump Inhibitor Cotherapy ❻ Proton pump inhibitor cotherapy reduces the risk of nonselective NSAID-related gastric and duodenal ulcer[1,12–14,21] and is superior to the H_2RAs.[1,13,52] All

PPIs, when used in standard PPI dosages (see Table 35–9) are effective. When lansoprazole (15 or 30 mg/day) was compared to misoprostol 800 mcg/day or placebo, both dosages of lansoprazole and misoprostol effectively reduced the risk of ulcer recurrence, although the PPI was better tolerated.[54] A greater proportion of those in the misoprostol group reported treatment-related adverse events and withdrew early from the study. Two small studies report a reduction in serious upper GI complications in patients with a history of upper GI bleeding receiving PPI cotherapy.[55,56]

H_2-Receptor Antagonist Cotherapy Standard H_2-receptor antagonist dosages (e.g., famotidine 40 mg/day) are effective in reducing the risk of NSAID-induced duodenal ulcer, but not gastric ulcer (the most frequent type of ulcer associated with NSAIDs).[1,12–14,21] Higher dosages (e.g., famotidine 40 mg twice daily, ranitidine 300 mg twice daily) may reduce the risk of gastric and duodenal ulcer, but results from clinical trials are variable.[1,13,21] It is unknown whether H_2RAs reduce the risk of ulcer-related upper GI complications. Therefore, the H_2RAs are not recommended as prophylactic cotherapy. However, the H_2RAs may be used when necessary to relieve NSAID-related dyspepsia.

Selective COX-2 Inhibitors Two large, multicenter, clinical trials with selective COX-2 inhibitors have reported a reduction in the risk of symptomatic ulcers and upper GI complications by 50% to 60% when compared to nonselective NSAIDs.[57,58] Patients in the Celecoxib Long-term Arthritis Safety Study (CLASS) trial who were taking celecoxib and required cardioprotection (antiplatelet effects of aspirin), were permitted to also take low-dose aspirin.[57] The initial 6-month analysis of the CLASS trial found a higher rate of ulcer complications in those treated with nonselective NSAIDs compared to celecoxib, but longer-term data presented at the FDA Advisory Meeting found the rate of ulcer complications to be nearly identical in both groups.[59] The most likely explanation for these results is that celecoxib is not a highly selective COX-2 inhibitor as was originally anticipated. Today, celecoxib is no longer considered a selective COX-2 inhibitor (Table 35–3) because its improved GI safety when compared to nonselective NSAIDs has not been established. A post hoc analysis confirmed that patients who were taking aspirin had a nearly identical event incidence rate with those who were taking nonselective NSAIDs, and that the only benefit of celecoxib was in patients who were not taking aspirin. Thus the gastroprotective benefits of celecoxib were negated in aspirin users. Similar effects have been observed with rofecoxib.

The Vioxx Gastrointestinal Outcomes Research (VIGOR) trial excluded aspirin users and found that ulcers and ulcer-related complications were lower with rofecoxib than with naproxen.[58] However, there was an increased number of nonfatal myocardial infarctions observed in the rofecoxib group compared to those taking naproxen. It was initially suggested that the lack of antiplatelet effects from rofecoxib, in contrast to the platelet inhibition associated with naproxen, was responsible for the increased thrombotic events observed in the rofecoxib group. Rofecoxib was later withdrawn from the market following an interim analysis of a study to prevent colorectal adenomas that revealed an increased risk of myocardial infarction and thrombotic stoke with rofecoxib when compared to placebo.[60] Subsequently, valdecoxib was withdrawn from the market amid concerns about cardiovascular risk.

Cardiovascular safety was also evaluated in the CLASS trial, but serious cardiovascular thromboembolic events were no different between celecoxib and the comparative nonselective NSAIDS. Increased risk appears to be dependent on a number of factors including increased COX-2 selectivity, higher dosages, and a longer duration of treatment.[61] Although celecoxib remains on the market in the United States (at the time of writing), individual patient risk factors for cardiovascular disease must be considered when determining treatment and the lowest effective dose should be used for the shortest duration of time. Patients should be counseled about the signs and symptoms of cardiovascular disease and what they should do if they occur. It remains unclear as to whether cardiovascular effects are limited to the selective COX-2 inhibitors or also apply to other NSAIDs, for example, ibuprofen, diclofenac, meloxicam. Although retrospective trials suggest an association, causality has not been prospectively demonstrated.[62] Dyspepsia and abdominal pain, fluid retention, hypertension, and renal toxicity are associated with both nonselective NSAIDs and the COX-2 inhibitors.[21] New classes of COX-2 inhibitors (e.g., nitric oxide donors, 5-lipoxygenase inhibitors) are under investigation.

❼ Two small, non–placebo-controlled trials in *H. pylori*-negative patients at high risk for NSAID-related complications, found that the use of a PPI and a nonselective NSAID was equivalent to the use of a selective COX-2 inhibitor with regard to incidence of ulcer complications.[63,64] In one trial,[63] patients were randomized to receive celecoxib or naproxen plus lansoprazole, and in the other,[64] celecoxib was compared to diclofenac plus omeprazole. A substantial number of patients in both trials had recurrent bleeding after 6 months of treatment. Cotherapy using a PPI and a COX-2 inhibitor in high-risk patients should be considered, but this regimen is likely to have a very modest benefit when compared to a PPI plus a nonselective NSAID.[65]

CLINICAL CONTROVERSY

Some clinicians favor the concomitant use of an NSAID and low-dose aspirin in a high-risk patient, whereas others favor the use of a selective COX-2 inhibitor and low-dose aspirin. Ulcer risk is increased when a nonselective NSAID and aspirin are used concomitantly, but the benefit of the COX-2 inhibitor may be reduced in a patient taking low-dose aspirin. The comparative risks and benefits of these two methods to reduce ulcer complications has not been studied and remains controversial.

Conventional Treatment of Active Ulcers and Long-Term Maintenance of Ulcer Healing

Conventional treatment with standard dosages of H_2-receptor antagonist or sucralfate relieves ulcer symptoms and heals the majority of gastric and duodenal ulcers in 6 to 8 weeks (see Table 35–9).[1] Proton pump inhibitors provide comparable ulcer healing rates over a shorter treatment period (4 weeks).[1] A higher daily dose or a longer treatment duration is sometimes needed to heal larger gastric ulcers. Antacids are not used as single agents to heal ulcers because of the high volume and frequent doses required.[1] When conventional antiulcer therapy is discontinued after ulcer healing, most patients develop a recurrent ulcer within 1 year.[1,5]

Continuous antiulcer therapy (see Table 35–9) is aimed at the long-term maintenance of ulcer healing and at preventing ulcer-related complications. Because *H. pylori* eradication dramatically decreases ulcer recurrence (<10% at 1 year), continuous maintenance therapy has become largely obsolete.[1] However, maintenance therapy may be indicated for patients who have previous ulcer-related complications, failed *H. pylori* eradication therapy, or who are heavy smokers or NSAID users.

Treatment of Refractory Ulcers

Ulcers are considered refractory to therapy when symptoms, ulcers, or both persist beyond 8 weeks (duodenal ulcer) or 12 weeks (gastric ulcer) despite conventional treatment, or when several courses of *H. pylori* eradication fail.[1] Poor patient compliance, antimicrobial resistance, cigarette smoking, NSAID use, gastric acid hypersecretion, or tolerance to the antisecretory effects of an H_2RA (see Antiulcer

Agents below) may contribute to refractory PUD. Patients with refractory ulcers should undergo upper endoscopy to confirm a nonhealing ulcer, exclude malignancy, and assess *H. pylori* status. *H. pylori*-positive patients should receive eradication therapy (see Treatment of *Helicobacter pylori*-Associated Ulcers). In *H. pylori*-negative patients, higher PPI dosages (e.g., omeprazole 40 mg/day) heal the majority of ulcers.[1] Continuous treatment with a PPI is often necessary to maintain healing, as refractory ulcers typically recur when therapy is discontinued or the dose is reduced. Switching from one PPI to another is not beneficial. Patients with refractory gastric ulcer may require surgery because of the fear of malignancy.

Antiulcer Agents

A comprehensive review of the pharmacology, pharmacokinetics, pharmacodynamics, efficacy, drug interactions, and tolerability of the antiulcer agents is found elsewhere.[1,66–69]

Proton Pump Inhibitors The PPIs (omeprazole, esomeprazole, lansoprazole, rabeprazole, and pantoprazole) dose-dependently inhibit basal and stimulated gastric acid secretion.[1,66,68] When PPI therapy is initiated, the degree of acid suppression increases over the first 3 to 4 days of therapy, as more and more proton pumps are inhibited.[66,68] Because PPIs inhibit only those proton pumps that are actively secreting acid, they are most effective when taken 30 to 60 minutes before meals.[66,68] The duration of acid suppression is a function of binding to the H^+/K^+-adenosine triphosphatase (ATPase) enzyme and is substantially longer that beyond that predicted based on the short half-lives of the agents.[66]

The PPIs are formulated in delayed-release enteric-coated dosage forms, including pH-sensitive granules contained in gelatin capsules (omeprazole, esomeprazole, and lansoprazole), rapidly disintegrating tablets (lansoprazole), and delayed release enteric-coated tablets (rabeprazole, pantoprazole, and nonprescription omeprazole). The pH-sensitive enteric coating prevents degradation and premature protonation of the drug in stomach acid. The enteric coating dissolves in the duodenum at pH values above approximately 6 and then the drug is systemically absorbed.[66,68] Omeprazole is also available in immediate release formulations that contain sodium bicarbonate (oral suspension, oral capsule) or sodium bicarbonate and magnesium hydroxide (oral tablet).[69–71] In this case, sodium bicarbonate and magnesium hydroxide serve as antacids to raise gastric pH and protect the immediate release omeprazole from premature protonation.[69] Intravenous products available in the U.S. include pantoprazole, lansoprazole, and esomeprazole.[66] The various formulations provide numerous options for administering proton pump inhibitors (Table 35–11).

All five PPIs provide similar ulcer-healing rates, maintenance of ulcer-healing rates, and relief of ulcer symptoms when used in recommended dosages (see Tables 35–8 and 35–9).[1,67,72] When higher dosages are indicated, the daily dose should be divided in order to obtain better 24-hour pH control.[66,68] A dosage reduction is unnecessary in patients with renal impairment or in older adults, but should be considered in severe hepatic disease.[1,73]

The short-term adverse effects of the PPIs are similar to those observed with the H_2RAs and include headache, nausea, and abdominal pain.[1,67] Because the immediate-release formulations contain sodium bicarbonate, these formulations are contraindicated in patients with metabolic alkalosis and hypocalemia.[69,70] In addition, the sodium content in the immediate-release formulations should be taken into consideration in patients who are on sodium-restricted diets.[67] Because all PPIs increase intragastric pH, they may alter the bioavailability of some orally administered drugs, such as ketoconazole (weak bases) and digoxin, or in pH-dependent dosage forms.[1,67,68] Omeprazole and esomeprazole selectively inhibit hepatic cytochrome P450 (CYP450) isoenzyme 2C19 and decrease the elimination of phenytoin, and diazepam.[1,67,68] Lansoprazole produces a slight increase in the metabolism of theophylline, presumably by inducing CYP1A.[1,67,68] A review of the FDA database for the years 1997 to 2001 revealed that drug interactions with PPIs are rare and usually do not constitute a major clinical risk.[74]

Consequences of Prolonged Hypochlorhydria. All PPIs dose-dependently increase serum gastrin concentrations approximately two- to fourfold as a function of their potent acid-inhibitory effect.[1,75] Fasting gastrin elevations are usually within the normal range and return to baseline within 1 month of discontinuing the drug. In humans, use of PPIs may lead to enterochromaffin-like (ECL) hyperplasia as a result of the hypergastrinemia; however, there has been no evidence that these changes result in dysplasia, carcinoid tumors, or gastric adenocarcinoma.[1,75] Long-term PPI

TABLE 35-11 Proton Pump Inhibitor Formulations and Options for Administration

	Omeprazole	Esomeprazole	Lansoprazole	Pantoprazole	Rabeprazole
Commercially available oral formulations					
Capsule	X[a]	X	X		
Tablet	X[b]			X	X
Oral disintegrating tablet			X		
Packet for oral suspension	X[c]	X[c]			
Extemporaneous oral preparations					
Pellets from capsule in water		X			
Pellets from capsule in applesauce	X		X		
Pellets from capsule in juice	X	X[d]	X		
Extemporaneous preparation of delayed release PPI in bicarbonate	X		X	X	
Parenteral formulations					
Intravenous	Not available in U.S.	X		X	

X, product is available.

[a]Omeprazole available as delayed-release enteric-coated pellets in a capsule or as immediate-release formulation that contains 20 or 40 mg of omeprazole with 1100 mg sodium bicarbonate. Because 20- and 40-mg dosages contain the same amount of bicarbonate, two 20- mg tablets should not be substituted for the 40-mg immediate-release omeprazole–bicarbonate capsule

[b]Omeprazole oral tablets are available as 20-mg delayed-release tablets over-the-counter, as well as in an immediate-release formulation containing 20 or 40 mg of omeprazole, 600 mg sodium bicarbonate, and 700 mg magnesium hydroxide. Because 20- and 40-mg dosages contain the same amount of bicarbonate, two 20-mg tablets should not be substituted for the 40-mg immediate-release omeprazole–bicarbonate–magnesium hydroxide tablet.

[c]Omeprazole oral suspension is available as 20 or 40 mg omeprazole with 1680 mg sodium bicarbonate. Because 20- and 40-mg dosages contain the same amount of bicarbonate, two 20-mg tablets should not be substituted for the 40-mg immediate-release omeprazole–bicarbonate packet.

[d]No published data; information extrapolated from omeprazole.

From Devlin et al.,[66] Welage,[68] Castell,[69] reference 70, and Waknine.[71]

therapy in *H. pylori*-positive patients is associated with progressive atrophic gastritis of the gastric body.[75] At this time there is inadequate evidence to link the long-term use of PPIs with gastric cancer in *H. pylori*-positive patients or to support an association between PPIs, colonic polyps, and colorectal cancer.[1] Although bacterial overgrowth occurs in the stomach as a consequence of hypochlorhydria which may lead to carcinogenic *N*-nitroso compounds in animals, it is unlikely to result in significant gastric nitrosation in humans.[1,75,76] PPI therapy is associated with an increased risk of enteric infections (*Salmonella, Campylobacter, Clostridium difficile*); however, data suggesting that PPI therapy predisposes patients to infections outside of the gastrointestinal tract remains controversial.[76] A decrease in vitamin B_{12} has been reported in some patients received long-term PPI therapy, but it is not a major concern.[75]

H_2-Receptor Antagonists Ulcer healing is comparable among H_2RAs (cimetidine, famotidine, nizatidine, and ranitidine) with equipotent multiple daily doses or a single full dose given after dinner or at bedtime (see Table 35–9), but tolerance to their antisecretory effect occurs.[1] Twice-daily administration suppresses daytime acid and benefits patients with daytime ulcer pain. Cigarette smokers may require higher doses or a longer duration of treatment. H_2-receptor antagonists are eliminated renally and therefore a dosage reduction is recommended in patients with moderate to severe renal failure.[1]

The short- and long-term safety of all four H_2RAs is similar.[1] Thrombocytopenia, the most common hematologic effect, is reversible and occurs with all four H_2RAs. However, the propensity for H_2RAs to cause thrombocytopenia is likely overestimated.[1,77] Cimetidine inhibits several CYP450 isoenzymes, resulting in numerous drug interactions (e.g., theophylline, lidocaine, phenytoin, and warfarin).[1,78] Ranitidine binds less avidly to hepatic CYP450 isoenzymes than does cimetidine, and has less potential for drug interactions. Famotidine and nizatidine do not interact with drugs metabolized by hepatic CYP450 isoenzymes. Because the H_2RAs decrease acid secretion they may alter the bioavailability of some orally administered drugs, similar to that seen with the PPIs.[78]

Sucralfate Sucralfate should be taken on an empty stomach to prevent binding to dietary protein and phosphate. Deterrents to its use include multiple doses per day, large tablet size, and the need to separate the drug from meals and potentially interacting medications. Constipation is most common and develops in approximately 3% of patients.[1] Seizures may occur in dialysis patients who are also receiving aluminum-containing antacids. Hypophosphatemia may develop with long-term treatment. Gastric bezoar formation has been reported. The concomitant use of sucralfate with oral fluoroquinolones, phenytoin, digoxin, theophylline, quinidine, amitriptyline, warfarin, and ketoconazole may reduce their bioavailability.[1,78] The interaction is often minimized by giving the interacting drug at least 2 hours before sucralfate. Alternative antiulcer therapy may be warranted in patients taking oral fluoroquinolones.

Prostaglandins Misoprostol, a synthetic prostaglandin E_1 analog, moderately inhibits acid secretion and enhances mucosal defense.[1,79] Antisecretory effects are dose-dependent over the range of 50 to 200 mcg; cytoprotective effects occur in humans at doses of greater than 200 mcg. Because protective effects occur at higher doses, it is difficult to establish the protective effect independent of the antisecretory action. Although not recommended in the United States, a dose of 200 mcg four times daily or 400 mcg twice daily heals duodenal ulcers and gastric ulcers comparable to standard H_2RA or sucralfate regimens.[1]

Diarrhea, the most troublesome adverse effect, is dose dependent and develops in 10% to 30% of patients.[1,79] Abdominal cramping, nausea, flatulence, and headache typically accompany the diarrhea. Taking the drug with or after meals and at bedtime may minimize the diarrhea. Because misoprostol is uterotropic and produces uterine contractions that may endanger pregnancy, it is contraindicated for use by pregnant women to reduce the risk of NSAID-induced ulcers.[79] If misoprostol is prescribed to women in their childbearing years, use of adequate contraceptive measures must be confirmed and a negative serum pregnancy test should be documented within 2 weeks of initiating treatment. Patients should be counseled about the GI effects and the need to avoid magnesium antacids, as they may increase the propensity for GI adverse effects.

Bismuth Preparations Bismuth subsalicylate and bismuth subcitrate potassium (biskalcitrate) are currently the only available bismuth salt in the United States.[1] Possible ulcer-healing mechanisms include an antibacterial effect, a local gastroprotective effect, and stimulation of endogenous prostaglandins. Bismuth salts do not inhibit or neutralize acid. Bismuth subsalicylate is regarded as safe and has few adverse effects when taken in recommended dosages. Because renal insufficiency may decrease bismuth elimination, bismuth salts should be used with caution in older patients and in renal failure. Bismuth subsalicylate may cause salicylate sensitivity or bleeding disorders, and should be used with caution in patients receiving concurrent salicylate therapy. Patients should be advised that bismuth salts may impart a black color to the stool and possibly the tongue (liquid preparations).

Antacids Antacids neutralize gastric acid, inactivate pepsin, and bind bile salts. Aluminum-containing antacids also suppress *H. pylori* and enhance mucosal defense.[1,80,81] GI adverse effects are most common with antacids and are dose dependent.[1,81] Magnesium salts cause an osmotic diarrhea, whereas aluminum salts cause constipation. Diarrhea usually predominates with magnesium/aluminum preparations. Aluminum-containing antacids (except aluminum phosphate) form insoluble salts with dietary phosphorus and interfere with phosphorus absorption.[1] Hypophosphatemia occurs most often in patients with low dietary phosphate intake (e.g., malnutrition or alcoholism). Combined treatment with sucralfate may amplify the hypophosphatemia and the potential for aluminum toxicity.

Magnesium-containing antacids should not be used in patients with a creatinine clearance of less than 30 mL/min because magnesium excretion is impaired which may lead to toxicity.[81] Hypercalcemia may occur in patients with normal renal function taking more than 20 g/day of calcium carbonate, and in patients with renal failure who are taking more than 4 g/day. The milk-alkali syndrome (hypercalcemia, alkalosis, renal stones, increased blood urea nitrogen, and increased serum creatinine concentration) occurs with high calcium intake in patients with systemic alkalosis produced by either ingestion of absorbable antacids (sodium bicarbonate) or prolonged vomiting. Antacids may alter the absorption and excretion of drugs when administered concomitantly.[1,78,81] Important interactions may occur when antacids are administered with iron supplements, tetracycline, warfarin, digoxin, quinidine, isoniazid, ketoconazole, or the fluoroquinolones. Most interactions can be avoided by separating the antacid from the oral drug by at least 2 hours.

Pharmacoeconomic Considerations

❽ The eradication of *H. pylori* improves clinical outcomes and decreases the use of healthcare resources when compared to conventional antisecretory therapy.[82] Thus the costs of continued treatment and recurrence far outweigh the cost of *H. pylori* drug regimens. The cost-effectiveness of misoprostol cotherapy is greatest in patients with the highest risk for NSAID-related GI complications.[83] The use of a PPI with a nonselective NSAID or switching to a selective COX-2 inhibitor (if available) is also cost-effective in high-risk patients.[84]

EVALUATION OF THERAPEUTIC OUTCOMES

❾ Table 35–12 lists the recommendations for treating and monitoring patients with PUD. Relief of epigastric pain should be monitored

TABLE 35-12 Recommendations for Treating and Monitoring Patients with *Helicobacter pylori*-Associated and Nonsteroidal Antiinflammatory Drug (NSAID)-Induced Ulcers

Helicobacter pylori-associated ulcer

1. Recommend drug treatment as presented in the chapter text.
2. Assess patient allergies to determine if allergic to penicillin (or other antibiotics) so that drug regimens that contain penicillin (or other antibiotics) can be avoided. Avoid regimens that contain tetracycline in children.
3. Assess patient use of alcohol or alcohol-containing products with metronidazole and oral birth control medications with antibiotics and counsel appropriately.
4. Assess likelihood of nonadherence to the drug regimen as a cause of treatment failure.
5. Recommend a different antibiotic combination if *H. pylori* eradication fails and a second treatment is planned.
6. Inform the patient of change in stool color when bismuth salicylate is included in an *H. pylori* eradication regimen.
7. Assess and monitor patients for potential adverse effects, especially those associated with metronidazole, clarithromycin, and amoxicillin.
8. Assess and monitor patients for potential drug interactions, especially those receiving metronidazole, clarithromycin, or cimetidine.
9. Monitor patients for salicylate toxicity, especially patients receiving cotherapy with other salicylates, anticoagulants, and patients with renal failure.
10. Monitor patients for persistent or recurrent symptoms within 14 days after completion of a course of *H. pylori* eradication therapy.
11. Provide patient education to patients who are receiving *H. pylori* eradication therapy, including why antibiotic and antiulcer combinations are used; when and how to take medications; adverse effects; alarm symptoms; the importance of adherence to the entire course of drug treatment; and to contact their healthcare provider if alarm symptoms develop (e.g., blood in the stools, black tarry stools, vomiting, severe abdominal pain), or if symptoms persist or return after *H. pylori* eradication.

NSAID-induced ulcer

1. Recommend drug treatment as presented in the chapter text.
2. Assess risk factors for NSAID-induced ulcers and ulcer-related complications, and when indicated recommend appropriate strategies for reducing ulcer risk (see Table 35–10).
3. Recommend eradication treatment for *H. pylori*-positive patients taking NSAIDs.
4. Monitor patients for signs and symptoms of NSAID-related upper GI complications.
5. Assess and monitor patients for potential drug interactions and adverse effects (especially misoprostol).
6. Provide patient education to patients who are at risk of NSAID-induced ulcers or GI-related complications, including why cotherapy is used with nonselective NSAIDs; when and how to take medications; adverse effects; alarm symptoms; when to contact their healthcare provider; and the importance of adherence to drug treatment.

throughout the course of treatment in patients with either *H. pylori*- or NSAID-related ulcers. Ulcer pain typically resolves in a few days when NSAIDs are discontinued, and within 7 days upon initiation of antiulcer therapy. Most patients with uncomplicated PUD will be symptom free after treatment with any one of the recommended antiulcer regimens. The persistence, or recurrence, of symptoms within 14 days after the end of treatment suggests failure of ulcer healing or *H. pylori* eradication, or an alternative diagnosis such as GERD. The majority of patients with uncomplicated *H. pylori*-positive ulcers do not require confirmation of ulcer healing or *H. pylori* eradication. However, eradication should be confirmed after treatment in individuals who are at high-risk for complications, for example, individuals who had a prior bleeding ulcer. When endoscopy is not indicated, the UBT is the preferred test to confirm *H. pylori* eradication. Medication adherence should be assessed in patients who fail therapy.

High-risk patients on NSAIDs should be closely monitored for signs or symptoms of bleeding, obstruction, penetration, or perforation. Patients who remain symptomatic, have recurrent attacks, or who have ulcer-related complications should be referred to a gastroenterologist. Follow-up endoscopy can be justified in patients with frequent symptomatic recurrence, refractory disease, complications, or suspected hypersecretory states.

ZOLLINGER-ELLISON'S SYNDROME (ZES)

ZES is characterized by gastric acid hypersecretion and recurrent peptic ulcers that result from a gastrin-producing tumor (gastrinoma).[4,67,85,86] In the United States, ZES accounts for 0.1% to 1% of patients with duodenal ulcer; however, this may be an underestimation of the true incidence because of the heterogeneity of clinical manifestations.[86] Gastrinomas are classified as those associated with multiple endocrine neoplasia type 1 (MEN 1) or sporadic tumors, which have a greater tendency to behave as malignant tumors. In more than 80% of cases, gastrinomas are localized in an area referred to as the "triangle of gastrinomas," which includes the convergence of the cystic duct and the common bile duct, the junction of the second and third portion of the duodenum, and the junction of the head and body of the pancreas.[85] Malignant gastrinomas occur in up to 65% of patients, with metastases to regional lymph nodes, liver, and bone.[85]

A diagnosis of ZES should be considered in patients with multiple ulcers and recurrent or refractory PUD, often accompanied by esophagitis or ulcer complications.[4,85,86] Ulcers occur most often in the duodenum, but may involve the stomach or jejunum. Diarrhea occurs in approximately 50% of patients and results from high concentrations of acid that overwhelm the duodenum's buffering capacity and damage the mucosa.[4,85] Intraluminal acid also causes steatorrhea by inactivating pancreatic lipase and precipitating bile acids. Vitamin B_{12} malabsorption may result from reduced intrinsic factor activity. The diagnosis is established when the serum gastrin is higher than 1,000 pg/mL and the BAO is greater than 15 mEq/h in patients with an intact stomach (BAO >5 mEq/h in patients with previous gastric surgery) or when the hypergastrinemia is associated with a gastric pH value of <2.[4,86] In situations in which the serum gastrin is between 100 and 1,000 pg/mL and gastric pH is <2, a secretin or calcium proactive test is used to aid the diagnosis.[86] Identification of the location of the tumor with imaging techniques is essential, as early surgical resection prior to liver metastases is often curative.[4,85] Unfortunately, effective medical therapy may delay the recognition of the disease and adversely influence outcome. The widespread use of PPIs, although effective in reducing symptoms, may mask the clinical presentation and complicate the diagnosis.[4,85] In addition, PPIs can cause hypergastrinemia, which may further complicate the diagnosis of ZES.[75,85,87]

Treatment is based on the presence or absence of peptic ulcers, esophagitis, diarrhea, and a gastrinoma, which may be malignant. The PPIs are the oral drugs of choice for managing gastric acid hypersecretion. Treatment should be instituted with omeprazole 60 mg/day (or an equivalent dose of esomeprazole, lansoprazole, rabeprazole, or pantoprazole) and should be adjusted based on individual patient response.[4,85,86] Dividing the daily dose and giving the PPI every 8 to 12 hours is most effective in controlling acid output and relieving symptoms. Although doses as high as 360 mg/day of omeprazole have been administered, an average dose of 60 to 100 mg/day reduces basal acid output to target levels.[85,86] The goal of therapy for uncomplicated patients is to maintain BAO between 1 and 10 mEq/h, in the hour preceding the next dose of the PPI.[86] In complicated cases, such as patients with MEN 1, GERD, or those who are undergoing partial gastrectomy, the BAO should be maintained below 5 mEq/h. A gradual reduction in PPI dose is recommended after the initial dose required for adequate control of gastric acid hypersecretion is achieved.[4,86] Intravenous PPIs are used to suppress gastric acid secretion in patients who are unable to take oral PPIs.[67,85]

Octreotide directly inhibits gastric acid secretion and the release of gastrin.[4] Although a subcutaneous dose of 100 to 250 mcg three times a day substantially reduces gastric acid secretion, octreotide is not considered first-line therapy. The long-acting repeatable octreotide formulation is efficacious in patients with gastrointestinal neuroendocrine tumors and has been shown to stabilize tumor growth in between 37% and 80% of patients.[85] However, it is important to demonstrate that the patient tolerates octreotide prior to converting to the long-acting product. Usually an initial dose of octreotide long-acting repeatable depot 20 mg is given intragluteally once every 4 weeks and is subsequently titrated based on response. The most common side effects of somatostatin analogs like octreotide include abdominal pain, diarrhea, gallstones, and pain at the injection site.[4,85] Patients with metastatic gastrinoma require tumor resection or treatment with chemotherapeutic agents.

UPPER GASTROINTESTINAL BLEEDING

There are approximately 170 cases of upper GI bleeding per 100,000 adults annually.[88] Despite a decreased incidence of PUD and improvements in the management of upper GI bleeding, the mortality rate associated with acute hemorrhage remains approximately 7%.[2,88] Upper GI bleeding can be broadly categorized as variceal or nonvariceal bleeding. Two common types of nonvariceal bleeding are bleeding from chronic peptic ulcers and bleeding from SRMD (stress gastritis, stress ulcer, or stress erosions), both of which are acid–peptic complications.[2,67,88,89] The presentation and pathophysiology of these two conditions are different, as bleeding associated with chronic PUD usually precedes hospital admission, whereas bleeding associated with SRMD develops in severely ill patients during hospitalization.[1,2,89]

The underlying pathophysiology of bleeding from a peptic ulcer or from SRMD is similar in that impaired mucosal defense in the presence of gastric acid and pepsin leads to mucosal damage. In chronic PUD, *H. pylori* infection and NSAID use are the most important etiologic factors, whereas the primary pathogenic factor in SRMD is thought to be mucosal ischemia resulting from reduced gastric blood flow.[1,89,90] In contrast to chronic PUD, stress-related mucosal lesions are characteristically asymptomatic, multiple, located in the proximal stomach, and are unlikely to perforate.[90] Bleeding from SRMD occurs from superficial mucosal capillaries, whereas bleeding associated with chronic PUD usually results from a single vessel. The mortality rate associated with clinical significant stress-related mucosal bleeding (SRMB) approximates 50% and is related to the underlying severity in the patient population.[67,89,90] In contrast, the mortality associated with chronic PUD-related bleeding is approximately 12%, but can increase dramatically in selected patient populations.[88,91–93] Although the initial management of acute upper GI bleeding focuses on aggressive resuscitative measures and ensuring hemodynamic stability, and is the same for both PUD-related bleeding and SRMB, the medical management of each condition is distinctly different.[88,90]

PEPTIC ULCER-RELATED BLEEDING

The degree of risk must be assessed to determine how aggressively to treat the patient with chronic PUD-related bleeding.[88,91] Patients older than 60 years of age who have comorbid conditions, high transfusion requirements, ongoing blood loss, presence of shock, prolonged prothrombin time (or increased international normalized ratio [INR]), and erratic mental status generally have poorer prognoses and usually require more aggressive intervention including admission to an intensive care unit (ICU).[88,92] Diagnostic endoscopy is usually performed to identify the source of the bleeding, assess the potential risk for rebleeding, and if appropriate, therapeutic interventions are employed to promote hemostasis.[2,92] Several endoscopic treatment approaches (e.g., thermocoagulation, laser therapy, injection sclerotherapy, hemoclipping, and ligation) can be used; however, to maximize the likelihood of positive outcomes, patients are usually treated with a combination of thermocoagulation and injection with epinephrine.[92] The appearance of the ulcer at the time of endoscopy is a prognostic indicator for the risk of rebleeding.[88,92] Clean-based ulcers are most commonly seen and are associated with a low risk of rebleeding.[92] In most cases, these patients can be immediately discharged after endoscopy on antiulcer therapy. Patients with an adherent clot overlying the ulcer base are at intermediate risk of rebleeding, and controversy exists as to the appropriate management of these patients.[92,93] It has been recommended that adherent clots be removed and then the lesion be reclassified based on what is observed following clot removal.[93] Patients with a visible vessel or active bleeding are at high risk of rebleeding, and must be carefully managed, as rebleeding increases the mortality rate 10-fold.[92,93]

Antisecretory therapy is often used as adjuvant therapy to prevent PUD rebleeding in high-risk patients because acid impairs clot stability.[67,92,93] H_2-receptor antagonists are ineffective in preventing PUD rebleeding because they do not achieve an intragastric pH of 6 (which is needed to promote clot stability), and tolerance to their antisecretory effect develops rapidly.[67,88,91–93] In contrast, PPI therapy significantly reduces the incidence of rebleeding, and need for surgery, but has no significant impact on mortality.[67,88,91–95] A post hoc analysis, however, of the Cochrane Collaboration review assessing PPI therapy for ulcer bleeding, revealed a significant decrease in all-cause mortality when data from Asian randomized, controlled trials were pooled and compared to other trials.[96] The greater reduction in rebleeding rates, need for surgery, and significant reduction in mortality rate in Asian studies may be a result of several factors, including lower parietal cell mass, increased prevalence of *H. pylori* infection, and a higher prevalence of the CYP2C19 slow metabolizer phenotype leading to higher plasma PPI concentrations in Asian patients.

Both the precise route (oral or intravenous) and the dose of PPI remain controversial with no significant differences emerging in a recent meta-analysis.[91] Based on the theoretical goal of maintaining gastric pH values >6, and data from randomized, controlled trials, practice guidelines recommend that high-dose continuous infusion PPI (equivalent to omeprazole 80 mg given intravenously as a loading dose, followed by 8 mg/h continuous infusion for 3 days) be used to reduce the risk of rebleeding in high-risk patients who have undergone endoscopy hemostasis.[67,88,91–95] Administration of high-dose continuous-infusion PPI therapy given prior to endoscopy hastened resolution of bleeding stigmata.[94] However, PPI therapy is not a replacement for interventional endoscopy in patients who are at high risk of rebleeding, as data demonstrate that the combination of a high-dose PPI continuous intravenous infusion with therapeutic endoscopy is superior to either strategy alone.[95] High-dose oral PPI therapy (omeprazole 80 mg/day for 5 days) is also effective; however, concerns exist whether critically ill patients will absorb the medication.[67,91,92] The risk of rebleeding is greatest within the first 72 hours (especially the first 24 hours) and it is during this time that antisecretory therapy to prevent rebleeding in high-risk patients should be employed.[88,92] Subsequently, the patient's underlying PUD should be evaluated and treated.

Patients with upper GI bleeding should be tested for *H. pylori* at the time of endoscopy (see Tests for *Helicobacter pylori* above). However, tests are associated with an increased rate of false-negatives when obtained during acute bleeding episodes.[29] If the initial results of the rapid urease test and/or histology are negative, a confirmatory test (^{14}C-urea breath test or serology) should be performed following the acute bleeding episode. There is no rationale for using intravenous therapy to eradicate *H. pylori*. Ulcer treatment, including *H. pylori* eradication, if appropriate, should be initiated after the acute bleeding episode (see Treatment of *Helicobacter pylori*-Associated Ulcers and Treatment of NSAID-Induced Ulcers above).

STRESS-RELATED MUCOSAL BLEEDING

More than 75% of critically ill patients develop SRMD within 24 hours of admission to an ICU, but the incidence of clinically significant SRMB is considered to be in the range of 1.2% to 6%.[89,90] Clinically significant bleeding increases the length of ICU stay by approximately 4 to 8 days, results in excessive healthcare costs, and is associated with an increased mortality rate.[67,90] Thus attempts to prevent SRMB are warranted in high-risk patients. Prophylactic therapy to prevent bleeding is most effective if initiated early in the patient's course.

Patients who are at risk for SRMB include those with respiratory failure (need for mechanical ventilation for longer than 48 hours), coagulopathy, hypotension, sepsis, hepatic failure, acute renal failure, multiple trauma, severe burns (>35% of body surface area), head injury, traumatic spinal cord injury, major surgery, or history of GI bleeding.[67,89,90,97] Although the relative importance of the various risk factors remains controversial, most clinicians concur that patients with respiratory failure (mechanical ventilation for longer than 48 hours) or coagulopathy should receive prophylaxis, as these two factors have been shown to be independent risk factors.[67] In the absence of these two risk factors, some clinicians only administer prophylaxis to patients who have two of the aforementioned risk factors.[89] Although exactly who should receive prophylaxis remains controversial, not all patients in a hospital or ICU are at increased risk of SRMB. A cost-effective approach is to target prophylactic therapy at high-risk patients.

Prevention of SRMB includes resuscitative measures that restore mucosal blood.[89,90] Although the benefits of enteral nutrition to patient outcome (e.g., improved nutritional status enhances mucosal integrity) are of overall clinical importance, its precise role as a sole modality to prevent SRMB remains controversial.[90] Therapeutic options for the prevention of SRMB include antacids (which are of historical interest, as they are no longer used because of cumbersome dosage schedules and side effects), antisecretory drugs (H_2RAs and PPIs), and sucralfate, a mucosal protectant.[67,89,90,97–100] Cimetidine, given as a continuous intravenous infusion, is FDA-labeled for the prevention of SRMB; however, intermittent intravenous H_2RAs are more commonly used in clinical practice.[67,90]

Immediate-release omeprazole sodium bicarbonate suspension (40 mg × 2 doses, then 40 mg/day) was more effective than continuous infusion cimetidine in maintaining intragastric pH >4 in critically ill patients; however, there was no difference in the incidence of clinically important SRMD between the two groups.[98] Based on meeting the prespecified criteria for noninferiority criteria, immediate-release omeprazole gained FDA labeling for the prevention of SRMB.[69,98]

Antisecretory therapy is generally preferred for SRMB prophylaxis for several reasons. First, a large landmark study demonstrated that intravenous ranitidine was superior to oral sucralfate in preventing SRMB.[99] Second, ranitidine did not increase the risk for nosocomial pneumonia, as the incidence of pneumonia was not different between the two treatment groups.[99] Finally, sucralfate therapy is cumbersome, requiring multiple daily dosage administration which may clog nasogastric tubes, cause constipation, and/or interact with several medications.[90] Although controversy exists as to which antisecretory agent should be used to prevent SRMB, data published in 2004 indicated that H_2RAs were the most commonly prescribed agents.[100] Extensive studies and years of experience support the use of H_2RAs.[89,90,100] However, PPIs are more potent than H_2RAs in inhibiting acid secretion and unlike H_2RAs tolerance does not develop to PPIs.[67,90,97] Although limited data exists assessing the efficacy of PPIs for the prevention of SRMB, based on data from Conrad and others, one would conclude oral PPI suspensions may be used as alternatives to H_2RAs or sucralfate for preventing SRMB.[97,98] However numerous question remain unanswered regarding the use of PPIs for the prevention of SRMB. What is the efficacy and optimal dosage of intravenous PPIs for the prevention of SRMB? What is the role of the various enteral PPI formulations (see Table 35–11)? What is the preferred route of administration for this indication?[67]

Improvement in the patient's overall medical condition (discharge from the ICU, extubation, and oral intake) suggests that prophylactic therapy can be discontinued. If a patient develops clinically important bleeding, endoscopic evaluation of the GI tract is indicated along with aggressive antisecretory therapy.

CONCLUSIONS

H. pylori eradication and antisecretory drugs are the mainstay of today's treatment strategies for PUD. Although *H. pylori* can be successfully treated with available regimens, there is a need for new therapies that will simplify treatment while improving eradication rates. In the future, new classes of COX-2 inhibitors may reduce cardiovascular concerns by maintaining antiplatelet effects while decreasing GI damage. Identification of genetic markers linked to PUD may eventually help identify patients who are at high risk of developing gastric and duodenal ulcers. In the interim, this common disease will continue to impact quality of life and the cost of healthcare.

ABBREVIATIONS

BAO: basal acid output

COX-1: cyclooxygenase-1

COX-2: cyclooxygenase-2

CYP450: cytochrome P450

ECL: enterochromaffin-like

ELISA: enzyme-linked immunosorbent assay

GERD: gastroesophageal reflux disease

H. pylori: *Helicobacter pylori*

H_2RA: histamine-2 receptor antagonist

ICU: intensive care unit

MALT: mucosa-associated lymphoid tissue

MAO: maximal acid output

MEN: multiple endocrine neoplasia

NSAID: nonsteroidal antiinflammatory drug

NUD: nonulcer dyspepsia

PG: prostaglandin

PPI: proton pump inhibitor

PUD: peptic ulcer disease

SRMB: stress-related mucosal bleeding

SRMD: stress-related mucosal damage

UBT: urea breath test

ZES: Zollinger-Ellison's syndrome

REFERENCES

1. Del Valle J, Chey WD, Scheiman JM, et al. Acid peptic disorders. In: Yamada T, Aplers DH, Kaplowitz N, et al., eds. Textbook of Gastroenterology, 4th ed. Philadelphia: Lippincott Williams & Wilkins, 2003:1321–1376.
2. Elta GH. Approach to the patient with gross gastrointestinal bleeding. In: Yamada T, Aplers DH, Kaplowitz N, et al., eds. Textbook of Gastroenterology, 4th ed. Philadelphia: Lippincott Williams & Wilkins, 2003:698–723.
3. American Gastroenterologic Association. Medical position statement: Evaluation of dyspepsia. Gastroenterol 2005;129:1753–1755.

4. Del Valle J, Scheiman JM. Zollinger-Ellison's syndrome. In: Yamada T, Aplers DH, Kaplowitz N, et al., eds. Textbook of Gastroenterology, 4th ed. Philadelphia: Lippincott Williams & Wilkins, 2003:1377–1394.
5. Suerbaum S, Michetti P. *Helicobacter pylori* infection. N Engl J Med 2002;347:1175–1186.
6. Queiroz DMM, Luzza F. Epidemiology of *Helicobacter pylori* infection. Helicobacter 2006;2005;11(Suppl 1):1–5.
7. Starzynska T, Malfertheiner P. *Helicobacter* and digestive malignancies. Helicobacter 2006;11(Suppl 1):32–35.
8. Gisbert JP, Khorrami S, Carballo F, et al. Meta-analysis: *Helicobacter pylori* eradication therapy vs. antisecretory noneradication therapy for the prevention of recurrent bleeding from peptic ulcer. Aliment Pharmacol Ther 2004;19:617–629.
9. Matysiak-Budnik T, Laszewicz W, Lamarque D, Chaussade S. *Helicobacter pylori* and non-malignant diseases. Helicobacter 2006;11(Suppl 1):27–31.
10. Delaney B, McColl K. Review article: *Helicobacter pylori* and gastro-oesophageal reflux disease. Aliment Pharmacol Ther 2005;22(Suppl 1):32–40.
11. Solnick JV, Franceschi F, Roccarina D, Gasbarrini A. Extragastric manifestations of *Helicobacter pylori* infection—Other *Helicobacter* species. Helicobacter 2006;11(Suppl 1):46–51.
12. Laine L. Approaches to nonsteroidal anti-inflammatory drug use in the high-risk patient. Gastroenterology 2001;120:594–606.
13. Naesdal J, Brown K. NSAID-associated adverse effects and acid control aids to prevent them: A review of current treatment options. Drug Safety 2006;29:119–132.
14. Yuan Y, Padol IT, Hunt RH. Peptic ulcer disease today. Nat Clin Pract Gastroenterol Hepatol 2006;3:80–89.
15. Lanas A, Perez-Aisa MA, Feu F, et al. A nationwide study of mortality associated with hospital admission due to severe gastrointestinal events and those associated with nonsteroidal antiinflammatory drug use. Am J Gastroenterol 2005;100:1685–1693.
16. Thomas J, Straus WL, Bloom BS. Over-the-counter nonsteroidal anti-inflammatory drugs and risk of gastrointestinal symptoms. Am J Gastroenterol 2002;97:2215–2219.
17. Tata LJ, Fortun PJ, Hubbard RB, et al. Does concurrent prescription of selective serotonin reuptake inhibitors and non-steroidal anti-inflammatory drugs substantially increase the risk of upper gastrointestinal bleeding? Aliment Pharmacol Ther 2005;22:175–181.
18. Laine L. Review article: The effect of *Helicobacter pylori* infection on nonsteroidal anti-inflammatory drug-induced upper gastrointestinal tract injury. Aliment Phamacol Ther 2002;16(Suppl 1):34–39.
19. Huang JQ, Sridhar S, Hunt RH. Role of *Helicobacter pylori* infection and nonsteroidal anti-inflammatory drugs in peptic ulcer disease: A meta-analysis. Lancet 2002;369:14–22.
20. Lanas A, Fuentes J, Benito R, et al. *Helicobacter pylori* increases the risk of upper gastrointestinal bleeding in patients taking low-dose aspirin. Aliment Phamacol Ther 2002;16:779–786.
21. Micklewright R, Lane S, Linley W, et al. Review article: NSAIDs, gastroprotection and cyclo-oxygenase-II–selective inhibitors. Aliment Pharmacol Ther 2003;17:321–332.
22. Garcia Rodriguez LA, Harnandez-Diaz S, de Abajo FJ. Association between aspirin and upper gastrointestinal complications: Systematic review of epidemiologic studies. Br J Clin Pharmacol 2001;52:563–571.
23. Del Valle J, Todisco A. Gastric secretion. In: Yamada T, Aplers DH, Kaplowitz N, et al., eds. Textbook of Gastroenterology, 4th ed. Philadelphia: Lippincott Williams & Wilkins, 2003:266–307.
24. Sachs G, Shin M, Munson K, et al. The control of gastric acid and *Helicobacter pylori* eradication. Aliment Pharmacol Ther 2000;14:1383–1401.
25. Hatakeyama M, Brzozowski T. Pathogenesis of *Helicobacter pylori* infection. Helicobacter 2006;11(Suppl 1):14–20.
26. Basset C, Holton J, Gatta L, et al. *Helicobacter pylori* infection: Anything new should we know? Aliment Pharmacol Ther 2004;20(Suppl 2):31–41.
27. Dzierzanowska-Fangrat K, Lehours P, Megraud F, et al. Diagnosis of *Helicobacter pylori* infection. Helicobacter 2006;11(Suppl 1):6–13.
28. Kiesslich R, Goetz M, Burg J, et al. Diagnosing *Helicobacter pylori* in vivo by confocal laser endoscopy. Gastroenterology 2005;128:2119–2123.
29. Gisbert JP, Abraiira V. Accuracy of *Helicobacter pylori* diagnostic tests in patients with bleeding peptic ulcer: a systematic review and meta-analysis. Am J Gastroenterol 2006;101:848–863.
30. Seymour NE, Andersen DK. Surgery for peptic ulcer disease and postgastrectomy syndromes. In: Yamada T, Aplers DH, Kaplowitz N, et al., eds. Textbook of Gastroenterology, 4th ed. Philadelphia: Lippincott Williams & Wilkins, 2003:1441–1454.
31. Pilotto A, Malfertheiner P. Review article: An approach to *Helicobacter pylori* infection in the elderly. Aliment Pharmacol Ther 2002;16:683–691.
32. Anderson J, Gonzalez J. *H. pylori* infection: Review of the guidelines for diagnosis and treatment. Geriatrics 2000;55:44–49.
33. Mourad-Baars P, Chong S. *Helicobacter pylori* infection in pediatrics. Helicobacter 2006;11(Suppl 1):40–45.
34. Sheu BS, Huang JJ, Yang HB, et al. The selection of triple therapy for *Helicobacter pylori* eradication in chronic renal insufficiency. Aliment Pharmacol Ther 2003;17:1283–1290.
35. Malfertheiner P, Megraud F, O'Morain C, et al. Current concepts in the management of *Helicobacter pylori* infection—The Maastricht Maastrict III Consensus Report Gut 2007;56:772–781.
36. Chex WD, Wong BCY, Another Practice Parameters Committee of American College of Gastroenterology, American College of Gastroenterology. Guidelines on the Management of *Helicobacter pylori* infection. Am J Gastroenterol 2007;102:1808–1825.
36. Qasim A, O'Morain CA. Review article: Treatment of *Helicobacter pylori* infection and factors influencing eradication. Aliment Pharmacol Ther 2002;16(Suppl 1):24–30.
37. Cavallaro LG, Egan B, O'Morain C, et al. Treatment of *Helicobacter pylori* infection. Helicobacter 2006;11:(Suppl 1):36–39.
39. Sullivan B, Coyle W, Nemec R, et al. comparison of azithromycin and clarithromycin in triple therapy regimens for the eradication of *Helicobacter pylori*. Am J Gastroenterol 2002;97:2536–2539.
40. Gisbert JP, Pajares JM. Systematic review and meta-analysis: Is 1-week proton pump inhibitor-based triple therapy sufficient to heal peptic ulcer? Aliment Pharmacol Ther 2005;21:795–804.
41. Vallve M, Vergara M, Gisbert JP, et al. Single vs. double dose of a proton pump inhibitor in triple therapy for *Helicobacter pylori* eradication: A meta-analysis. Aliment Pharmacol Ther 2002;16:1149–1156.
42. Vergara M, Vallve M, Gisbert JP, et al. Meta-analysis: Comparative efficacy of different proton-pump inhibitors in triple therapy for *Helicobacter pylori* eradication. Aliment Pharmacol Ther 2003;18:647–654.
43. Gisbert JP, Khorrami S, Calvet X, et al. Meta-analysis: Proton pump inhibitors vs. H_2-receptor antagonists—Their efficacy with antibiotics in *Helicobacter pylori* eradication. Aliment Pharmacol Ther 2003;18:757–766.
44. Janssen MJR, Laheij RJF, Boer WA, et al. Meta-analysis: the influence of pre-treatment with a proton pump inhibitor on *Helicobacter pylori* eradication. Aliment Pharmacol Ther 2005;21:341–345.
45. Varia D, Zullo N, Vakil N, et al. Sequential therapy versus standard triple-drug therpay for *Heliobacter pylori* eradication. Ann Intern Med 2007;146:556–563.
46. Gene E, Calvet X, Azagra R, et al. Triple vs quadruple therapy for treating *Helicobacter pylori* infection: A meta-analysis. Aliment Pharmacol Ther 2003;17:1137–1143.
47. Megraud F, Lamouliatte H. Review article: The treatment of refractory *Helicobacter pylori* infection. Aliment Pharmacol Ther 2003;17:1333–1343.
48. Saad RJ, Schoenfeld P, Kim HM, et al. Levofloxacin-based triple therapy versus bismuth-based quadruple therapy for persistant *Helicobacter pylori* infection: A meta-analysis. Am J Gastroenterol. 2006;101:488–496.
49. Lee M, Kemp JA, Canning A, et al. A randomized controlled trial of an enhanced patient compliance program for *Helicobacter pylori* therapy. Arch Intern Med 1999;159:2312–2316.
50. Gotteland M, Brunser O, Cruchet S. Systematic review: are probiotics useful in controlling gastric colonization by *Helicobacter pylori*. Aliment Pharmacol Ther 2006;23:1077–1086.
51. Dubois RW, Melmed GY, Henning JM, et al. Guidelines for the appropriate use of non-steroidal anti-inflammatory drugs, cyclo-oxygenase-2-specific inhibitors and proton pump inhibitors in patients requiring chronic anti-inflammatory therapy. Aliment Pharmacol Ther 2004;19:197–208.
52. Chan FKL, Graham DY. Review article: Prevention of non-steroidal anti-inflammatory drug gastrointestinal complications—Review and recommendations based on risk assessment. Aliment Pharmacol Ther 2004;19:1051–1061.
53. Silverstein FE, Graham DY, Senior JR, et al. Misoprostol reduces serious gastrointestinal complications in patients with rheumatoid arthritis receiving nonsteroidal anti-inflammatory drugs: A randomized, double-blind, placebo-controlled trial. Ann Intern Med 1995; 123:241–249.

54. Graham DY, Agrawal NM, Campbell DR, et al. Ulcer prevention in long-term users of nonsteroidal anti-inflammatory drugs: Results of a double-blind, randomized, multicenter, active- and placebo-controlled study of misoprostol vs lansoprazole. Arch Intern Med 2002;152:169–175.
55. Chan FK, Chung SC, Suen BY, et al. Preventing recurrence of upper gastrointestinal bleeding in patients with *Helicobacter pylori* infection who are taking low-dose aspirin or naproxen. N Engl J Med 2001;344:967–973.
56. Lai KC, Lam SK, Chu KM, et al. Lansoprazole for the prevention of recurrences of upper gastrointestinal complications from long-term low-dose aspirin use. N Engl J Med 2002;346:2033–2038.
57. Silverstein F, Faich G, Goldstein JL, et al. Gastrointestinal toxicity with celecoxib vs nonsteroidal antiinflammatory drugs for osteoarthritis and rheumatoid arthritis. The CLASS study: A randomized controlled trial. JAMA 2000;284:1247–1255.
58. Bombardier C, Laine L, Reicin A, et al. Comparison of upper intestinal toxicity of rofecoxib and naproxen in patients with rheumatoid arthritis. VIGOR Study Group. N Engl J Med 2000;343:1520–1528.
59. US Food and Drug Administration Advisory Committee. CLASS. Celecoxib Long-term Arthritis Safety Study Agenda. FDA. Gaithersburg, MD. Meeting February 7, 2001, *http://www.fda.gov/ohrms/dockets/ac/01/slides/3677S_01__sponsor.pdf.*
60. Bresalier RS, Sandler RS, Quan H, et al. Cardiovascular events associated with rofecoxib in colorectal adenoma chemoprevention trial. N Engl J Med 2005:352:1092–1102.
61. White WB. Cardiovascular effects of the cyclooxygenase inhibitors. Hypertension 2007;49:408–418.
62. Kearney PM, Baigent C, Godwin J, et al. Do selective cyclooxygenase-2 inhibitors and traditional non-steroidal antiinflammatory drugs increase the risk of atherothrombosis? Meta-analysis of randomized trials. BMJ 2006;322:1302–1308.
63. Chan FD, Huang LC, Suen BY, et al. Celecoxib versus diclofenac and omeprazole in reducing the risk of recurrent ulcer bleeding in patients with arthritis. N Engl J Med 2002;347:2104–2111.
64. Lai KC, Chu KM, Hui WM, et al. COX-2 inhibitor compared with proton pump inhibitor in the prevention of recurrent ulcer complications in high-risk patients taking NSAIDs [abstract]. Gastroenterology 2001;120:A104.
65. Scheiman JM, Yeomans ND, Talley NJ, et al. Prevention of ulcers by esomeprazole in at-risk patients using nonselective NSAIDs and COX-2 inhibitors. Am J Gastroenterol 2006;101:701–710.
66. Devlin JW, Welage LS, Olsen KM. Proton pump inhibitor formulary considerations in the acutely ill part 1: Pharmacology, pharmacodynamics and available formulations. Ann Pharmacother 2005;39:1667–1677.
67. Devlin JW, Welage LS, Olsen KM. Proton pump inhibitor formulary considerations in the acutely ill—Part 2: Clinical efficacy, safety, and economics. Ann Pharmacother 2005;39:1844–1851.
68. Welage L. Pharmacologic properties of proton pump inhibitors. Pharmacotherapy 2003;23(10 Pt 2):74S–80S.
69. Castell D. Review of immediate-release omeprazole for the treatment of gastric acid-related disorders. Expert Opin Pharmacother 2005;6:2501–2510.
70. Package insert. Zegerid (omeprazole/sodium bicarbonate). San Diego, CA. Santarus, Inc. *http://www.zegerid.com/assets/pdfs/prescribing_information.pdf.*
71. Waknine Y. FDA approvals: Zegerid chewable, OsmoPrep, Tasmar. Medscape Gastroenterology Medical News [Internet]. March 2006, *http://www.medscape.com/viewarticle/528790.* (Registration required for access.)
72. Gisbert JP. Potent gastric acid inhibition in *Helicobacter pylori* eradication. Drugs 2005;65(Suppl 1):83–96.
73. Stedman CA, Barclay ML. Review article: Comparison of the pharmacokinetics, acid suppression and efficacy of proton pump inhibitors. Aliment Pharmacol Ther 2000;14:963–978.
74. Labenz J, Petersen KU, Rosch W, Koelz HR. A summary of Food and Drug Administration-reported adverse events and drug interactions occurring during therapy with omeprazole, lansoprazole, and pantoprazole. Aliment Pharmacol Ther 2003;17:1015–1019.
75. Laine L, Ahnen D, McClain C, et al. Review article: Potential gastrointestinal effects of long-term acid suppression with proton pump inhibitors. Aliment Pharmacol Ther 2000;14:651–668.
76. Williams C, McColl KE. Review article: Proton pump inhibitors and bacterial overgrowth. Aliment Pharmacol Ther 2006;23:3–10.
77. Wade EE, Rebuck JA, Healey MA, Rogers FB. H_2 antagonist-induced thrombocytopenia: Is this a real phenomenon? Intensive Care Med 2002;28:459–465.
78. Welage LS, Berardi RR. Drug interactions with antiulcer agents: Considerations in the treatment of acid-peptic disease. J Pharm Pract 1994;VII:177–195.
79. Chong YS, Su LL, Arulkumaran S. Misoprostol: A quarter century of use, abuse and creative misuse. Obstet Gynecol Surg 2004;59:128–140.
80. Kamiya S, Yamaguchi H, Osaki T, et al. Effect of an aluminum hydroxide-magnesium hydroxide combination drug on adhesion, IL-8 inducibility, and expression of HSP60 by *Helicobacter pylori*. Scand J Gastroenterol 1999;34:663–670.
81. Maton PN, Burton ME. Antacids revisited: A review of their clinical pharmacology and recommended therapeutic use. Drugs 1999;57:855–870.
82. Sonnenberg A, Schwartz JS, Cutler AF, et al. Cost savings in duodenal ulcer therapy through *Helicobacter pylori* eradication compared with conventional therapies: Results of a randomized, double-blind, multicenter trial. Arch Intern Med 1998;158:852–860.
83. Maetzel A, Ferraz MB, Bombardier C. The cost-effectiveness of misoprostol in preventing serious gastrointestinal events associated with the use of nonsteroidal anti-inflammatory drugs. Arthritis Rheum 1998;41:16–25.
84. El-Serag HP, Graham DY, Richardson P, et al. Prevention of complicated ulcer disease among chronic users of nonsteroidal antiinflammatory drugs: The use of a nomogram in cost-effectiveness analysis. Arch Intern Med 2002;162:2105–2110.
85. Tomassetti P, Campana D, Piscitelli L, et al. Treatment of Zollinger Ellison's syndrome. World J Gastroenterol 2005;11:5423–5432.
86. Campana D, Piscitelli L, Mazzotta E, et al. Zollinger-Ellison's syndrome. Minerva Med 2005;96:187–206.
87. Corleto VD, Annibale B, Gibril F, et al. Does the widespread use of proton pump inhibitors mask, complicate and/or delay the diagnosis of Zollinger-Ellison's syndrome? Aliment Pharmacol Ther 2001;15:1555–1561.
88. Barkun AN, Barbou M, Marshall JK. Consensus recommendations for managing patients with nonvariceal upper gastrointestinal bleeding. Ann Intern Med 2003;139:843–857.
89. American Society of Health-System Pharmacists Therapeutic Guidelines on Stress Ulcer Prophylaxis. Am J Health Syst Pharm 1999;56:347–379.
90. Stollman N, Metz DC. Pathophysiology and prophylaxis of stress ulcer in intensive care unit patients. J Crit Care 2005;20:35–45.
91. Leontiadis GI, Sharma VK, Howden CW. Proton pump inhibitor treatment for acute peptic ulcer bleeding [review]. Cochrane Database Syst Rev 2006;(1):CD002094.
92. Sung JJ. The role of acid suppression in the management and prevention of gastrointestinal hemorrhage associated with gastroduodenal ulcers. Gastroenterol Clin N Am 2003;32:S11–S23.
93. McCarthy DM. Management of bleeding peptic ulcer: Current status of intravenous proton pump inhibitors. Best Prac Res Clin Gastroenterol 2004;18(5):7–12.
94. Lau JY, Leung WK, Wu JC, et al. Early Administration of High-Dose Intravenous Omeprazole Prior to Endoscopy in Patients with Upper Gastrointestinal Bleeding: A Double-Blind, Placebo-Controlled, Randomized Trail (abstract 347). Presented at: 2005 Digestive Disease Week Meeting. Chicago, IL, May 15–18, 2005.
95. Sung JJ, Chan FK, Lau JY. The effect of endoscopic therapy in patients receiving omeprazole for bleeding ulcers with nonbleeding visible vessels or adherent clots. Ann Intern Med 2003;139:237–243.
96. Leontiadis GI, Sharma VK, Howden CW. Systematic review and meta-analysis: Enhanced efficacy of proton pump inhibitor therapy for peptic ulcer bleeding in Asia—A post hoc analysis from the Cochrane Collaboration. Aliment Pharmacol Ther 2005;21(9):1055–1061.
97. Jung R, MacLaren R. Proton-pump inhibitors for stress ulcer prophylaxis in critically ill patients. Ann Pharmacother 2002;36:1929–1937.
98. Conrad SA, Gabrielli A, Margolis B, et al. Randomized, double-blind comparison of immediate-release omeprazole oral suspension versus intravenous cimetidine for the prevention of upper gastrointestinal bleeding in critically ill patients. Crit Care Med 2005;33:760–765.
99. Cook D, Guyatt G, Marshall J, et al. A comparison of sucralfate and ranitidine for the prevention of upper gastrointestinal bleeding in patients requiring mechanical ventilation. N Engl J Med 1998;338:791–797.
100. Daley RJ, Rebuck JA, Welage LS, Rogers FB. Prevention of stress ulceration: Current trends in critical care. Crit Care Med 2004;32:2008–2013.

CHAPTER 36

Inflammatory Bowel Disease

BRIAN A. HEMSTREET AND JOSEPH T. DIPIRO

KEY CONCEPTS

1. The exact cause of inflammatory bowel disease (IBD) is unknown, although there are components that appear to be infectious and other components that suggest immune dysregulation. Genetic variations explain some of the increased risk of disease occurrence.

2. Ulcerative colitis is confined to the rectum and colon, causes continuous lesions, and affects primarily the mucosa and the submucosa. Crohn's disease can involve any part of the GI tract, often causes discontinuous (skip) lesions, and is a transmural process that can result in fistulas, perforations, or strictures.

3. Common gastrointestinal complications of IBD include rectal fissures, fistulas (Crohn's disease), perirectal abscess (ulcerative colitis), and colon cancer; possible extraintestinal manifestations include hepatobiliary complications, arthritis, uveitis, skin lesions (including erythema nodosum and pyoderma gangrenosum), and aphthous ulcerations of the mouth.

4. The severity of ulcerative colitis may be assessed by factors such as stool frequency, presence of blood in stool, fever, pulse, hemoglobin, erythrocyte sedimentation rate, C-reactive protein, abdominal tenderness, and radiologic or endoscopic findings. The severity of Crohn's disease can be assessed using similar parameters, in addition to the Crohn's disease activity index, which includes stool frequency, presence of blood in stool, endoscopic appearance, and physician's global assessment.

5. The goals of treatment of IBD are resolution of acute inflammation and complications, alleviation of systemic manifestations, maintenance of remission, and in some patients, surgical palliation or cure.

6. The first-line treatment for mild to moderate ulcerative colitis or Crohn's colitis consists of oral aminosalicylates, such as sulfasalazine or mesalamine; mesalamine or steroid enemas or suppositories may be used for rectosigmoid disease. Delayed-release oral formulations of mesalamine may be used for Crohn's ileitis.

7. Corticosteroids are often required for acute ulcerative colitis or Crohn's disease. The duration of steroid use should be minimized and the dose tapered gradually over 3 to 4 weeks. Infliximab is an option for patients with moderate to severe active ulcerative colitis, and for those patients with ulcerative colitis who are depend on corticosteroids.

8. Intravenous continuous infusion of cyclosporine is effective in treating severe colitis that is refractory to steroids.

9. Sulfasalazine and mesalamine derivatives can prevent recurrence of acute disease in many patients, while steroids are ineffective for this purpose.

10. Other drugs that are useful for treatment of Crohn's disease include metronidazole (for perineal disease), azathioprine or mercaptopurine (for inadequate response or to reduce steroid dosage), cyclosporine (for refractory disease), and infliximab for refractory or fistulizing disease.

Learning objectives, review questions, and other resources can be found at **www.pharmacotherapyonline.com.**

There are two forms of idiopathic inflammatory bowel disease (IBD): (a) ulcerative colitis, a mucosal inflammatory condition confined to the rectum and colon; and (b) Crohn's disease, a transmural inflammation of the gastrointestinal tract that can affect any part, from the mouth to the anus. The etiologies of both conditions are unknown, but they may have some common pathogenic mechanisms.

EPIDEMIOLOGY

Inflammatory bowel disease is most prevalent in western countries and in areas of northern latitude.[1] The reported rates of IBD are highest in Scandinavia, Great Britain, and North America.[2] Crohn's disease has a reported incidence of 3.6 to 8.8 per 100,000 persons in the United States and a prevalence of 20 to 40 per 100,000 people.[3] The incidence of Crohn's disease varies considerably among studies, but has clearly increased dramatically over the last three or four decades.[3] Ulcerative colitis incidence ranges from 3 to 15 cases per 100,000 persons per year among the white population, with a prevalence of 80 to 120 per 100,000 persons.[3] The incidence of ulcerative colitis has remained relatively constant over many years.[2] Although most epidemiologic studies combine ulcerative proctitis with ulcerative colitis, from 17% to 49% of cases are proctitis.

Both sexes are affected equally with inflammatory bowel disease, although some studies show slightly greater numbers of women with Crohn's disease and males with ulcerative colitis.[2] Ulcerative colitis and Crohn's disease have bimodal distributions in age of initial presentation. The peak incidence occurs in the second or third decades of life, with a second peak occurring between 60 and 80 years of age.[1,2] A significantly increased incidence of ulcerative colitis (four to five times normal) has been observed in Ashkenazi Jews, whereas blacks and Asians have a relatively low incidence of occurrence.[2,4,5]

ETIOLOGY

1 Although the exact etiology of ulcerative colitis and Crohn's disease is unknown, similar factors are believed responsible for both

TABLE 36-1 Proposed Etiologies for Inflammatory Bowel Disease

Infectious agents
Viruses (e.g., measles)
L-Forms of bacteria
Mycobacteria
Chlamydia
Genetics
Metabolic defects
Connective tissue disorders
Environmental factors
Diet
Smoking (Crohn's disease)
Immune defects
Altered host susceptibility
Immune-mediated mucosal damage
Psychological factors
Stress
Emotional or physical trauma
Occupation

conditions (Table 36–1). The major theories of the cause of IBD involve a combination of infectious, genetic, and immunologic factors.[6] The inflammatory response with IBD may indicate abnormal regulation of the normal immune response or an autoimmune reaction to self-antigens. The microflora of the gastrointestinal tract may provide an environmental trigger to activate inflammation.[7] Crohn's disease has been described as a disorder mediated by T lymphocytes that arises in genetically susceptible individuals as a result of a breakdown in the regulatory constraints on mucosal immune responses to enteric bacteria."[8]

INFECTIOUS FACTORS

Microorganisms are a likely factor in the initiation of inflammation in IBD.[7] However, no definitive infectious cause of IBD has been found, even though the presentation is similar to that caused by some invasive microbial pathogens. Patients with IBDs have increased numbers of surface-adherent and intracellular bacteria.[9] IBD may involve a loss of tolerance toward normal bacterial flora.[10] Other supporting evidence for an infectious etiology is that colitis does not appear to occur in genetically altered germ-free animals, intestinal lesions in IBD typically predominate in areas of highest bacterial exposure, and observed differences in the existing makeup of the resident luminal and mucosal bacterial flora in healthy subjects versus those with IBD.[7]

Suspect infectious agents include the measles virus, protozoans, mycobacteria, such as *Mycobacterium paratuberculosis*, and other bacteria such as *Listeria monocytogenes*, *Chlamydia trachomatis*, and *Escherichia coli*.[11] Also, certain strains of bacteria produce toxins (necrotoxins, hemolysins, and enterotoxins) that cause mucosal damage. Bacteria elaborate peptides (e.g., formyl-methionyl-leucyl-phenylalanine) that have chemotactic properties and that cause an influx of inflammatory cells with subsequent release of inflammatory mediators and tissue destruction. Microbes may elaborate superantigens, which are capable of global T-lymphocyte stimulation and subsequent inflammatory response.[12] As many as 60% of patients with Crohn's disease have circulating antibody to *Saccharomyces cerevisiae*, but this may not represent a disease mechanism.[8]

GENETIC FACTORS

Genetic factors predispose patients to IBDs, particularly Crohn's disease. In studies of monozygotic twins, there has been a high concordance rate, with both individuals of the pair having an IBD (particularly Crohn's disease).[8] Also, first-degree relatives of patients with IBD may have up to a 20-fold increase in the risk of disease.[9] Several genetic markers have been identified that occur more frequently in patients with IBD. The CARD15 gene on chromosome 16, formerly referred to as NOD2, is thought to account for 20% of the genetic predisposition to Crohn's disease. Human leukocyte antigen (HLA) DR2 has been associated with ulcerative colitis in Japanese subjects, while HLA-DR3 has been associated with ulcerative colitis in European subjects.[11,13] Additionally the multidrug-resistance gene 1 (ABCB/MDR 1) on chromosome 7 is a potential susceptibility gene for ulcerative colitis.[14] Multiple other genes have been associated with IBD, including DLG5, OCTN1, and CARD4; however, the nature of these gene products has not been established.[11,13]

IMMUNOLOGIC MECHANISMS

The immune system is known to play a critical role in the underlying pathogenesis of IBD. In Crohn's disease, the bowel wall is infiltrated with lymphocytes, plasma cells, mast cells, macrophages, and neutrophils. Similar infiltration has been observed in the mucosal layer of the colon in patients with ulcerative colitis. Inflammation in IBD is maintained by an influx of leukocytes from the vascular system into sites of active disease. This influx is promoted by expression of adhesion molecules (such as α_4-integrins) on the surface of endothelial cells in the microvasculature in the area of inflammation.[10,15] Many of the systemic manifestations of IBD have an immunologic etiology (e.g., arthritis or uveitis). Finally, IBD is typically responsive to immunosuppressive drugs (e.g., corticosteroids and azathioprine).

The immune theory of IBD assumes that IBD is caused by an inappropriate reaction of the immune system. Potential immunologic mechanisms include both autoimmune and nonautoimmune phenomena.[9] Autoimmunity may be directed against mucosal epithelial cells or against neutrophil cytoplasmic elements. Some patients with IBD have abnormal structural features for colonic epithelial cells even in the absence of active disease. Autoantibodies to these structures have been reported. Also, antineutrophil cytoplasmic antibodies are found in a high percentage of patients with ulcerative colitis (70%) and much less frequently with Crohn's disease.[9] Presence of antineutrophil cytoplasmic antibodies in left-sided ulcerative colitis is associated with resistance to medical therapy.[16] Dysregulation of cytokines is a component of IBD. Specifically, T-helper type 1 (TH_1) cytokine activity (which enhances cell-mediated immunity and suppresses humoral immunity) is excessive with Crohn's disease, whereas T-helper type 2 (TH_2) cytokine activity (which inhibits cell-mediated immunity and enhances humoral immunity) is excessive with ulcerative colitis.[17] The result is that patients have inappropriate T-cell responses to antigens from their own intestinal microflora.[17] Expression of interferon γ (a TH_1 cytokine) in intestinal mucosa of diseased patients is increased, whereas interleukin-4 (a TH_2 cytokine) is reduced.[6,18]

Tumor necrosis factor-α (TNF-α) is a pivotal proinflammatory cytokine in Crohn's disease. TNF-α can recruit inflammatory cells to inflamed tissues, activate coagulation, and promote the formation of granulomas. Production of TNF-α is increased in the mucosa and intestinal lumen of patients with Crohn's disease.[6,9,18] Eicosanoids such as leukotriene B_4 are increased in rectal dialysates and tissues of IBD patients and are related to disease activity. Leukotriene B_4 enhances neutrophil adherence to vascular endothelium and acts as a neutrophil chemoattractant. These findings have led to the consideration of leukotriene inhibitor strategies for therapy.

PSYCHOLOGICAL FACTORS

Mental health changes appear to correlate with remissions and exacerbations, especially of ulcerative colitis, but psychological factors overall are not thought to be an etiologic factor. There is a weak association between the number of stressful events experienced and the time to relapse of ulcerative colitis.[19]

DIET, SMOKING, AND NONSTEROIDAL ANTIINFLAMMATORY DRUG USE

Changes in diet by people in industrialized countries where Crohn's disease is more common have not been consistently associated with the disease. Studies of increased intake of refined sugars or chemical food additives and reduced fiber intake have provided conflicting results regarding risk for Crohn's disease. Smoking plays an important but contrasting role in ulcerative colitis and Crohn's disease.

Smoking is protective for ulcerative colitis.[9] The risk of developing ulcerative colitis in smokers is approximately 40% of that in nonsmokers.[2] Clinical relapses are associated with smoking cessation, and nicotine transdermal administration has been effective in improving symptoms in patients with ulcerative colitis.[20,21] In contrast, smoking is associated with a twofold increased frequency of Crohn's disease.[2] Crohn's disease patients who stop smoking have a more benign course than patients who continue smoking.[22] The mechanisms of these differing effects have not been identified.

Use of nonsteroidal antiinflammatory drugs (NSAIDs) can trigger disease occurrence or lead to disease flares.[9,23] The effect of NSAIDs to inhibit prostaglandin production through cyclooxygenase inhibition may impair mucosal barrier protective mechanisms. The increased risk seems to be present for cyclooxygenase-2 inhibitors as well as cyclooxygenase-1 inhibitors, however it is unclear whether cyclooxygenase-2 inhibitors may be somewhat safer in select patients with IBD.[24,25]

PATHOPHYSIOLOGY

Ulcerative colitis and Crohn's disease differ in two general respects: anatomic sites and depth of involvement within the bowel wall. There is, however, overlap between the two conditions, with a small fraction of patients showing features of both diseases. Confusion can occur, particularly when the inflammatory process is limited to the colon. Table 36–2 compares pathologic and clinical findings of the two diseases.

TABLE 36-2 Comparison of the Clinical and Pathologic Features of Crohn's Disease and Ulcerative Colitis

Feature	Crohn's Disease	Ulcerative Colitis
Clinical		
Malaise, fever	Common	Uncommon
Rectal bleeding	Common	Common
Abdominal tenderness	Common	May be present
Abdominal mass	Common	Absent
Abdominal pain	Common	Unusual
Abdominal wall and internal fistulas	Common	Absent
Distribution	Discontinuous	Continuous
Aphthous or linear ulcers	Common	Rare
Pathologic		
Rectal involvement	Rare	Common
Ileal involvement	Very common	Rare
Strictures	Common	Rare
Fistulas	Common	Rare
Transmural involvement	Common	Rare
Crypt abscesses	Rare	Very common
Granulomas	Common	Rare
Linear clefts	Common	Rare
Cobblestone appearance	Common	Absent

ULCERATIVE COLITIS

❷ Ulcerative colitis is confined to the rectum and colon, and affects the mucosa and the submucosa. In some instances, a short segment of terminal ileum may be inflamed; this is referred to as *backwash ileitis*. Unlike Crohn's disease, the deeper longitudinal muscular layers, serosa, and regional lymph nodes are not usually involved.[1,9,10] Fistulas, perforation, or obstruction are uncommon because inflammation is usually confined to the mucosa and submucosa.

The primary lesion of ulcerative colitis occurs in the crypts of the mucosa (crypts of Lieberkühn) in the form of a crypt abscess. Here, frank necrosis of the epithelium occurs; it is usually visible only with microscopy, but may be seen grossly when coalescence of ulcers occurs. Extension and coalescence ulcers may surround areas of uninvolved mucosa. These islands of mucosa are called *pseudopolyps*. Other typical ulceration patterns include a "collar-button ulcer," which results from extensive submucosal undermining at the ulcer edge.[9,26,27] The extensive mucosal damage seen in ulcerative colitis can result in significant diarrhea and bleeding, although a small percentage of patients experience constipation.

❸ Ulcerative colitis can be accompanied by complications that may be local (involving the colon or rectum) or systemic (not directly associated with the colon). With either type the complications may be mild, serious, or even life-threatening. Local complications occur in the majority of ulcerative colitis patients. Relatively minor complications include hemorrhoids, anal fissures, or perirectal abscesses, and are more likely to be present during active colitis. Enteroenteric fistulas are rare.

A major complication is toxic megacolon, which is a segmental or total colonic distension of >6 cm with acute colitis and signs of systemic toxicity.[28] It is a severe condition that occurs in up to 7.9% of ulcerative colitis patients admitted to hospitals and results in death rates up to 50%. With toxic megacolon, ulceration extends below the submucosa, sometimes even reaching the serosa. Vasculitis, swelling of the vascular endothelium, and thrombosis of small arteries occurs; involvement of the muscularis propria causes loss of colonic tone, which leads to dilation and potential perforation. The patient with toxic megacolon usually has a high fever, tachycardia, distended abdomen, and elevated white blood cell count, and a dilated colon is observed on radiography.[6,28] Colonic perforation, however, may occur with or without toxic megacolon and is a greater risk with the first attack. Another infrequent major local complication is massive colonic hemorrhage. Colonic stricture, sometimes with clinical obstruction, may also complicate long-standing ulcerative colitis.

The risk of colonic carcinoma is much greater in patients with ulcerative colitis as compared to the general population. The risk of colon cancer begins to increase 10 to 15 years after the diagnosis of ulcerative colitis. The absolute risk may be as high as 30% 35 years after diagnosis, and as high as 49% for patients who have a long history of disease and who were younger than 15 years of age at the time of diagnosis.

The inflammatory response seen in IBD has also been blamed for the systemic complications seen in both Crohn's disease and ulcerative colitis. The next section summarizes the systemic extraintestinal complications of ulcerative colitis.

Hepatobiliary Complications

Approximately 11% of patients with ulcerative colitis are reported to have hepatobiliary complications, with frequencies ranging from 5% to 95% in IBD patients overall.[29–32] Hepatic complications include fatty liver, pericholangitis, chronic active hepatitis, and cirrhosis. Biliary complications include sclerosing cholangitis, cholangiocarcinoma, and gallstones.

Fatty infiltration of the liver may be a result of malabsorption, protein-losing enteropathy, or concomitant steroid use. The most common hepatic complication is pericholangitis (acute inflammation surrounding the intrahepatic portal venules, bile ducts, and lymphatics), which occurs in up to one-third of ulcerative colitis patients. This is associated with progressive fibrosis of intrahepatic and extrahepatic bile ducts in a small percentage of ulcerative colitis patients, and is referred to as primary sclerosing cholangitis. Cirrhosis may be a sequela of cholangitis or of chronic active hepatitis. Often the severity of hepatic disease does not correlate with gastrointestinal disease activity.

Gallstones occur commonly in patients with Crohn's disease (particularly with terminal ileal disease) and may be related to bile salt malabsorption. Also, cholangiocarcinoma occurs 10 to 20 times more frequently in IBD patients as compared to the general population.[29]

Joint Complications

Arthritis commonly occurs in IBD patients and is typically asymmetric (unlike rheumatoid arthritis) and migratory, involving one or a few, usually large, joints.[29,31,32] The joints most often affected, in decreasing frequency, are the knees, hips, ankles, wrists, and elbows. Sacroiliitis also occurs commonly. Arthritis associated with ulcerative colitis is generally related to the severity of colonic disease, and resolution without recurrence is seen with proctocolectomy. Also, arthritis in this setting is different from rheumatoid arthritis in that rheumatoid factors are generally not detected. It is nondeforming and nondestructive, even after multiple episodes.

Another potential joint complication is ankylosing spondylitis, which is often unresponsive to treatment. The incidence of ankylosing spondylitis in patients with ulcerative colitis is 30 times that of the general population and occurs most commonly in patients with the HLA-B27 phenotype.

Ocular Complications

Ocular complications, including iritis, uveitis, episcleritis, and conjunctivitis, occur in up to 10% of patients with IBD.[29,31,32] The most commonly reported symptoms with iritis and uveitis include blurred vision, eye pain, and photophobia. Episcleritis is associated with scleral injection, burning, and increased secretions. These complications may parallel the severity of intestinal disease, and recurrence after colectomy with ulcerative colitis is uncommon.

Dermatologic and Mucosal Complications

Skin and mucosal lesions associated with IBD include erythema nodosum, pyoderma gangrenosum, and aphthous ulceration. Five to 10% of IBD patients experience dermatologic or mucosal complications.[1,31,32]

Raised, red, tender nodules, which vary in size from 1 cm to several centimeters, are manifestations of erythema nodosum. They are typically found on the tibial surfaces of the legs and arms. These lesions are more commonly observed in Crohn's disease patients and are noted to correlate with disease severity.

Pyoderma gangrenosum occurs more commonly in patients with ulcerative colitis (1% to 5% incidence) and is characterized by discrete skin ulcerations that have a necrotic center and a violaceous color of the surrounding skin.[31] They can be seen on any part of the body but are more commonly found on the lower extremities.

Oral lesions are found in 6% to 20% of patients with Crohn's disease and 8% of patients with ulcerative colitis.[31] The most common lesion is aphthous stomatitis, seen with Crohn's disease. The severity of these lesions tends to parallel GI disease.

CROHN'S DISEASE

❷ Crohn's disease is best characterized as a transmural inflammatory process. The terminal ileum is the most common site of the disorder, but it may occur in any part of the GI tract from mouth to anus. About two-thirds of patients have some colonic involvement, and 15% to 25% of patients have only colonic disease.[9,12] Patients often have normal bowel separating segments of diseased bowel; that is, the disease is discontinuous.

Regardless of the site, bowel wall injury is extensive and the intestinal lumen is often narrowed. The mesentery first becomes thickened and edematous and then fibrotic. Ulcers tend to be deep and elongated and extend along the longitudinal axis of the bowel, at least into the submucosa. The "cobblestone" appearance of the bowel wall results from deep mucosal ulceration intermingled with nodular submucosal thickening.

❸ Complications of Crohn's disease may involve the intestinal tract or organs unrelated to it. Small-bowel stricture and subsequent obstruction is a complication that may require surgery. Fistula formation is common and occurs much more frequently than with ulcerative colitis.[12] Fistulae often occur in the areas of worst inflammation, where loops of bowel have become matted together by fibrous adhesions. Fistulae may connect a segment of the GI tract to skin (enterocutaneous fistula), two segments of the GI tract (enteroenteric fistula), or the intestinal tract with the bladder (enterovesicular fistula) or vagina. Crohn's disease fistulae or abscesses associated with them frequently require surgical treatment.

Bleeding with Crohn's disease is usually not as severe as with ulcerative colitis, although patients with Crohn's disease may have hypochromic anemia. Also, as with ulcerative colitis, the risk of carcinoma is increased but not as greatly as with ulcerative colitis.

Systemic complications of Crohn's disease are common, and similar to those found with ulcerative colitis. Arthritis, iritis, skin lesions, and liver disease often accompany Crohn's disease. Renal stones occur in up to 10% of patients with Crohn's disease (less frequently with ulcerative colitis) and are caused by fat malabsorption, which allows for greater oxalate absorption and formation of calcium oxalate stones. Gallstones also occur with greater frequency in patients with ileitis, possibly because of bile acid malabsorption at the terminal ileum.

Nutritional deficiencies are common with Crohn's disease.[33,34] Reported frequencies of various nutritional parameters are weight loss, 40% to 80%; growth failure in children, 15% to 88%; iron-deficiency anemia, 25% to 50%; vitamin B_{12} deficiency, 20% to 37%; folate deficiency, 13% to 37%; hypoalbuminemia, 25% to 76%; hypokalemia, 33%; and osteomalacia, 36%. There are usually decreased fat stores and lean tissue. Growth failure in children may be associated with hypozincemia.

CLINICAL PRESENTATION

The patterns of clinical presentation of IBD can vary widely. Patients may have a single acute episode that resolves and does not recur, but most patients experience acute exacerbations after periods of remission. With more severe disease, prolonged illness may occur.

ULCERATIVE COLITIS

Although a typical clinical picture of ulcerative colitis can be described, there is a wide range of presentation, from mild abdominal cramping with frequent small-volume bowel movements to profuse diarrhea (Table 36–3). Most patients with ulcerative colitis experience intermittent bouts of illness after varying intervals with no symptoms. Only a small percentage of patients have continuous unremitting symptoms or have a single acute attack with no subsequent symptoms.

❹ Complex disease classifications are generally not used in clinical practice for ulcerative colitis. The arbitrarily determined distinctions of mild, moderate, and severe disease activity are generally used, and these are determined largely by clinical signs and symptoms.[35,36]

TABLE 36-3 Clinical Presentation of Ulcerative Colitis

Signs and symptoms
- Abdominal cramping
- Frequent bowel movements, often with blood in the stool
- Weight loss
- Fever and tachycardia in severe disease
- Blurred vision, eye pain, and photophobia with ocular involvement
- Arthritis
- Raised, red, tender nodules that vary in size from 1 cm to several centimeters

Physical examination
- Hemorrhoids, anal fissures, or perirectal abscesses may be present
- Iritis, uveitis, episcleritis, and conjunctivitis with ocular involvement
- Dermatologic findings with erythema nodosum, pyoderma gangrenosum

Laboratory tests
- Decreased hematocrit/hemoglobin
- Increased erythrocyte sedimentation rate
- Leukocytosis and hypoalbuminemia with severe disease

Mild—Fewer than 4 stools daily, with or without blood, with no systemic disturbance and a normal erythrocyte sedimentation rate.

Moderate—More than 4 stools per day but with minimal systemic disturbance.

Severe—More than 6 stools per day with blood, with evidence of systemic disturbance as shown by fever, tachycardia, anemia, or erythrocyte sedimentation rate of >30.

It is also important to determine disease extent; that is, which part of the colon is involved—rectum, descending colon only, or the entire colon. Patients with "distal" disease have inflammation limited to areas below the splenic flexure (also referred to as *left-sided* disease), whereas those with "extensive disease" have inflammation extending proximal to the splenic flexure.[35,36] Likewise, inflammation confined to the rectal area is referred to as *proctitis*, whereas disease involving the rectum and sigmoid colon is referred to as *proctosigmoiditis*.[26] Inflammation of the majority of the colon is deemed *pancolitis*.

Two-thirds of patients with ulcerative colitis have mild disease, which almost always starts in the rectum. Occasionally, the mild form may progress to severe disease, which may be called "fulminant" if it occurs acutely. Systemic signs and symptoms of the disease (e.g., arthritis, uveitis, or pyoderma gangrenosum) may be present in these patients, and in fact may be the reason the patient seeks medical attention. Patients with mild disease are believed to be at lower risk of colon cancer. Moderate disease is observed in one-fourth of patients.

With severe disease, the patient is usually found to be in acute distress, has profuse bloody diarrhea, and often has a high fever with leukocytosis and hypoalbuminemia. Often, the patient is dehydrated, and therefore may be tachycardic and hypotensive. This presentation may have a sudden onset with rapid progression.

The diagnosis of ulcerative colitis is made on clinical suspicion and confirmed by biopsy, stool examinations, sigmoidoscopy or colonoscopy, or barium radiographic contrast studies. The presence of extracolonic manifestations such as arthritis, uveitis, and pyoderma gangrenosum may also aid in establishing the diagnosis.[35]

CROHN'S DISEASE

As with ulcerative colitis, the presentation of Crohn's disease is highly variable. A single episode may not be followed by further episodes, or the patient may experience continuous, unremitting disease. The time between the onset of complaints and the initial diagnosis may be as long as 3 years. The patient typically presents with diarrhea and abdominal pain. Hematochezia occurs in about one-half of the patients with colonic involvement and much less frequently when there is no colonic involvement. Commonly, a patient first presents with a perirectal or perianal lesion (Table 36–4). The diagnosis should also be suspected in children with growth retardation, especially with abdominal complaints.

TABLE 36-4 Clinical Presentation of Crohn's Disease

Signs and symptoms
- Malaise and fever
- Abdominal pain
- Frequent bowel movements
- Hematochezia
- Fistula
- Weight loss
- Arthritis

Physical examination
- Abdominal mass and tenderness
- Perianal fissure or fistula

Laboratory tests
- Increased white blood cell count and erythrocyte sedimentation rate

Much like ulcerative colitis, guidelines classify the severity of active Crohn's disease by the presence of several signs and symptoms.[37] Patients with mild to moderate Crohn's disease are typically ambulatory and have no evidence of dehydration, systemic toxicity, loss of body weight, or abdominal tenderness, mass, or obstruction. Crohn's disease is considered moderate to severe in patients who fail to respond to treatment for mild to moderate disease, and in those with fever, weight loss, abdominal pain or tenderness, vomiting, intestinal obstruction, or significant anemia. Severe to fulminant Crohn's disease is classified as the presence of persistent symptoms or evidence of systemic toxicity despite outpatient corticosteroid treatment, or presence of cachexia, rebound tenderness, intestinal obstruction, or abscess.

The course of Crohn's disease is characterized by periods of remission and exacerbation. Some patients may be free of symptoms for years, whereas others experience chronic problems in spite of medical therapy. As with ulcerative colitis, the diagnosis of Crohn's disease involves a thorough evaluation using laboratory, endoscopic, and radiologic testing to detect the extent and characteristic features of the disease. Because of similarities that may exist between ulcerative colitis and Crohn's disease confined to the colon, a definitive diagnosis cannot be made in up to 15% of cases, even with pathologic specimens in hand. Small-bowel involvement and strictures detected on radiographs are characteristic of Crohn's disease.

TREATMENT

Inflammatory Bowel Disease

■ DESIRED OUTCOME

❺ To treat IBD properly, the clinician must have a clear concept of realistic therapeutic goals for each patient. These goals may relate to resolution of acute inflammatory processes, resolution of attendant complications (e.g., fistulas and abscesses), alleviation of systemic manifestations (e.g., arthritis), maintenance of remission from acute inflammation, or surgical palliation or cure. The approach to the therapeutic regimen differs considerably with varying goals, as well as with the two diseases, ulcerative colitis and Crohn's disease.

When determining goals of therapy and selecting therapeutic regimens it is important to understand the natural history of IBD.[38] Some cases of acute ulcerative colitis are self-limited. With mild to moderate acute colitis without systemic symptoms, 20% of patients may experience spontaneous improvement in their disease within a few weeks; however, a small percentage of patients may go on to experience more serious disease. With severe colitis, improvement without treatment cannot be expected. For instance, the response to medical management of toxic megacolon is variable and emergent colectomy may be required. When remission of ulcerative colitis is achieved, it is likely to last at least 1 year with medical therapy. In the absence of medical therapy, one-half to two-thirds of patients are likely to relapse within 9 months.[37] In some reports, remission rates with placebo have approached those found with active treatment.

A considerable number of patients with active Crohn's disease may achieve at least temporary remission without drug therapy. In two large trials, 26% and 42% of ambulatory patients on placebo achieved remission.[39,40] Once remission is achieved, two-thirds to three-fourths of patients remain in remission up to 2 years without drug therapy.[40] The implication of these data is that up to 40% of patients with active Crohn's disease improve in 3 to 4 months with observation alone, and that most patients remain in remission for prolonged periods without medical intervention. These observations apply more to mild or moderate disease than to severe disease.

■ GENERAL APPROACH TO TREATMENT

❻ Treatment of IBD centers on agents used to relieve the inflammatory process. Salicylates, corticosteroids, antimicrobials, and immunosuppressive agents such as azathioprine, mercaptopurine, and methotrexate are commonly used to treat active disease and, for some agents, to lengthen the time of disease remission. Information regarding the extent and distribution of the disease should be taken into account, as this often dictates the route and formulation of drug therapy that are most effective.

In addition to the use of drugs, surgical procedures are sometimes performed when active disease is inadequately controlled or when the required drug dosages pose an unacceptable risk of adverse effects. For most patients with IBD, nutritional considerations are also important, because these patients are often malnourished. Finally, a variety of therapies may be used to address complications or symptoms of IBD. For example, antidiarrheals may be used in some patients, although these are generally to be avoided in severe ulcerative colitis because they may contribute to the development of toxic colonic dilation. Antimicrobial agents may be used in conjunction with surgical drainage when abscesses are present. Iron may be required, particularly with ulcerative colitis, where blood loss from the colon can be significant.

■ NONPHARMACOLOGIC THERAPY

Nutritional Support

Proper nutritional support is an important aspect of the treatment of patients with IBD, not because specific types of diets are useful in alleviating the inflammatory conditions, but because patients with moderate to severe disease are often malnourished either because the inflammatory process results in significant malabsorption or maldigestion, or because of the catabolic effects of the disease process. Elevated levels of interleukin-6 and TNF-α are known to increase protein turnover, resulting in protein loss and muscle wasting.[34] Malabsorption may occur in the patient with Crohn's disease with inflammatory involvement of the small bowel, where many nutrients are absorbed, as well as in patients who have undergone multiple small-bowel resections with subsequent reduction in absorptive surface ("short gut"). Maldigestion with accompanying diarrhea can occur if there is a bile salt deficiency in the gut.

Many specific diets have been tried to improve the condition of patients with IBD, but none has gained widespread acceptance. With each individual it is helpful to eliminate specific foods that exacerbate symptoms. This elimination process must be conducted cautiously, as patients have been known to exclude a wide range of nutritious products without adequate justification. Some patients with IBD, although not the majority, have lactase deficiency; consequently, diarrhea may be associated with milk intake. In these patients, avoidance of milk or supplementation with lactase generally improves the patient's symptoms. Patients with small-bowel strictures as a consequence of Crohn's disease should avoid excessive high-residue foods, such as citrus fruits and nuts.[1]

The nutritional needs of the majority of patients can be adequately addressed with enteral supplementation.[41] In severe acute ulcerative colitis, enteral nutrition resulted in a significantly greater increase in serum albumin, fewer adverse effects related to the nutritional regimen, and fewer postoperative infections, as compared to isocaloric, isonitrogenous parenteral nutrition.[42] The regimens were similar with regard to remission rate and the need for colectomy. Consideration should be given to lipid administration for its caloric value, as well as in recognition of depleted peripheral fat stores in many IBD patients and the greater potential for fatty acid deficiency. The use of enteral nutrition in patients with Crohn's disease is preferable, as favorable effects on modulation of proinflammatory cytokine production may lead to enhanced maintenance of nutritional stores and increased growth rates in children.[43,44] Likewise, use of enteral nutrition may facilitate induction of remission in up to 60% of patients with active Crohn's disease.[43,45]

Parenteral nutrition is an important component of the treatment of severe Crohn's disease or ulcerative colitis. The use of parenteral nutrition allows complete bowel rest in patients with severe ulcerative colitis, which may alter the need for proctocolectomy. Parenteral nutrition has also been valuable in Crohn's disease, because remission may be achieved with parenteral nutrition in about 50% of patients.[46] In some patients, the disease may worsen when parenteral nutrition is stopped. Patients who have severe Crohn's disease may require a course of parenteral nutrition to attain a reasonable nutritional status or in preparation for surgery, as poor perioperative nutritional status is associated with an increased incidence of postoperative complications.[34] Patients with enterocutaneous fistulas of various etiologies benefit from parenteral nutrition.[46] Parenteral nutrition may also be valuable in children or adolescents with growth retardation associated with Crohn's disease, but surgery is often necessary with severe disease. Finally, when possible, home parenteral nutrition should be used for patients requiring long-term therapy, particularly those with "short gut" as a consequence of surgical resection.

There is a growing interest in using probiotic approaches for IBD. Probiotics involves the reestablishment of normal bacterial flora within the gut by oral administration of live bacteria such as nonpathogenic *E. coli*, bifidobacteria, lactobacilli, or *Streptococcus thermophilus*. Probiotic formulations have been effective in maintaining remission in ulcerative colitis.[47,48]

Surgery

Even with medical therapy 30% to 40% of patients with ulcerative colitis and 70% to 80% of patients with Crohn's disease require surgical intervention at some point in their life.[49] Although surgery (proctocolectomy) is curative for ulcerative colitis, this is not the case for Crohn's disease. Surgical procedures involve resection of segments of intestine that are affected, as well as correction of complications (e.g., fistulas) or drainage of abscesses.

For ulcerative colitis, colectomy may be necessary when the patient has disease uncontrolled by maximum medical therapy or when there are complications of the disease such as colonic perforation, toxic dilation (megacolon), uncontrolled colonic hemorrhage, or colonic strictures. Colectomy may be indicated in patients with long-standing disease (longer than 8 years), as a prophylactic measure against the development of cancer, and in patients with premalignant changes (severe dysplasia) on surveillance mucosal biopsies. The most common surgical procedures include proctocolectomy, after which the patient is left with a permanent ileostomy, and abdominal colectomy, with removal of the mucosa of the rectum and anastomosis of an ileal pouch to the anus (ileal pouch–anal anastomosis).[49] The risk from

TABLE 36-5 Mesalamine Derivatives for Treatment of Inflammatory Bowel Disease

Product	Trade Name(s)	Formulation	Dose/Day	Site of Action
Sulfasalazine	Azulfidine Azulfidine EN-tabs	Immediate-release or enteric-coated tablets	4–6 g	Colon
Mesalamine	Rowasa, Salofalk	Enema	1–4 g	Rectum, distal colon
	Asacol	Mesalamine tablet coated with Eudragit-S (delayed-release acrylic resin)	2.4–4.8 g	Distal ileum and colon
	Pentasa	Mesalamine capsules encapsulated in ethylcellulose microgranules	2–4 g	Small bowel and colon
	Lialda	Mesalamine tablet formulated with MMX delayed release technology (pH-dependent outer coat with polymeric matrix core); allows for once-daily dosing	2.4–4.8g	Colon
	Canasa	Mesalamine suppository	500–1,000 mg	Rectum
Olsalazine	Dipentum	Dimer of 5-aminosalicylic acid oral capsule	1.5–3 g	Colon
Balsalazide	Colazal	Capsule	6.75 g	Colon

surgery in these patients is relatively low if the operations are performed on a nonemergent basis.

The indications for surgery with Crohn's disease are not as well established as for ulcerative colitis, and surgery is usually reserved for the complications of the disease. A recognized problem with intestinal resection for Crohn's disease is the high recurrence rate. Surgery may be appropriate in well-selected patients who have severe or incapacitating disease or obstruction in spite of aggressive medical management. The surgical procedures performed include resections of the major intestinal areas of involvement. In some patients with severe rectal or perianal disease, particularly abscesses, diversion of the fecal stream is performed with a colostomy. Other indications for surgery include strictures, resection of colon cancer or an inflammatory mass, or management of intestinal perforations or fistulae.

PHARMACOLOGIC THERAPY

Drug therapy plays an integral part in the overall treatment of IBD. None of the drugs used for IBD are curative; at best they serve to control the disease process. Therefore a reasonable goal of drug therapy is resolution of disease symptoms such that the patient can carry on normal daily functions. The major types of drug therapy used in IBD include aminosalicylates, corticosteroids, immunosuppressive agents (azathioprine, mercaptopurine, cyclosporine, and methotrexate), antimicrobials (metronidazole and ciprofloxacin), and agents to inhibit TNF-α (anti–TNF-α antibodies) (Table 36–5).

Sulfasalazine, an agent that combines a sulfonamide (sulfapyridine) antibiotic and mesalamine (5-aminosalicylic acid) in the same molecule, has been used for many years to treat IBD but was originally intended to treat arthritis. Sulfasalazine is cleaved by gut bacteria in the colon to sulfapyridine (which is mostly absorbed and excreted in the urine) and mesalamine (which mostly remains in the colon and is excreted in stool).[45,50,51]

The active component of sulfasalazine is mesalamine.[45,50,51] The mechanism of action of mesalamine is not well understood. Cyclooxygenase or lipoxygenase inhibition alone does not entirely account for the agent's effects. Aminosalicylates may block production of prostaglandins and leukotrienes, inhibit bacterial peptide-induced neutrophil chemotaxis and adenosine-induced secretion, scavenge reactive oxygen metabolites, and inhibit activation of the nuclear regulatory factor nuclear factor kappa B.[9]

Because the mechanism of action of sulfasalazine is not related to the sulfapyridine component, and because sulfapyridine is believed to be responsible for many of the adverse reactions to sulfasalazine, mesalamine alone can be used. Mesalamine can be used topically as an enema or suppository for the treatment of proctitis, or given orally in slow-release formulations that deliver mesalamine to the small intestine and colon (Table 36–6 and Fig. 36–1). Slow-release oral formulations of mesalamine, such as Pentasa®, release mesalamine from the duodenum to the ileum, with up to 59% of the drug passing into the colon.[50] Lialda® is a newly available tablet formulation of mesalamine that uses a pH-dependent coating in combination with a polymeric matrix core, which releases the drug evenly throughout the colon and allows for once-daily dosing.[51] Olsalazine is a dimer of two 5-aminosalicylate molecules linked by an azo bond. Mesalamine is released in the colon after colonic bacteria cleave olsalazine. Balsalazide is a mesalamine prodrug that is enzymatically cleaved in the colon to produce mesalamine. The recommended daily doses of the oral mesalamine derivatives are intended to approximate the molar equivalent of mesalamine present in 4 g of sulfasalazine. At present, sulfasalazine is often used versus oral mesalamine derivatives, mainly because it costs much less. However, it is not tolerated as well as the mesalamine alternatives. Because the oral mesalamine formulations are coated tablets or granules, they should not be crushed or chewed. Unlike sulfasalazine, all of these agents are safe to use in patients with sulfonamide allergies.

Corticosteroids and adrenocorticotropic hormone have been widely used for the treatment of ulcerative colitis and Crohn's disease, given parenterally, orally, or rectally.[52] Corticosteroids are believed to modulate the immune system and inhibit production of cytokines and mediators. It is not clear whether the most important steroid effects are systemic or local (mucosal). Budesonide is a corticosteroid that is administered orally in a controlled-release formulation designed to release in the terminal ileum. The drug undergoes extensive first-pass metabolism, so systemic exposure is thought to be minimized.[53] Immunosuppressive agents such as azathioprine, mercaptopurine (a metabolite of azathioprine), methotrexate, or cyclosporine are sometimes used for the treatment of IBD.

Azathioprine and mercaptopurine are effective for long-term treatment of Crohn's disease and ulcerative colitis.[45,54] These agents are generally reserved for patients who are refractory to steroids, and they may be associated with serious adverse effects such as lymphomas, pancreatitis, or nephrotoxicity. They are usually used in conjunction with mesalamine derivatives and/or steroids, and must be used for long periods of time (from a few weeks up to 6 months) before benefits may be observed.[54] Remission can be prolonged by azathioprine in steroid-dependent patients with ulcerative colitis. Cyclosporine has also been of short-term benefit in treatment of acute, severe ulcerative colitis when used in a continuous intravenous infusion. Lower-dose continuous infusions (2 mg/kg vs. 4 mg/kg daily), or oral daily doses of 5 to 6 mg/kg may in conjunction with steroids may be an effective option for those with fulminant disease.[55] The agent poses a risk of nephrotoxicity and neurotoxicity. Some studies evaluating tacrolimus for the treatment of IBD suggest a potential role for its use in patients with fistulizing Crohn's disease, in patients unresponsive to steroids or infliximab, and in management of some extraintestinal manifestations.[56] Methotrexate given 15 to 25 mg intramuscularly once weekly is useful for treatment and maintenance of Crohn's disease but not ulcerative colitis.[57,58]

Antimicrobial agents, particularly metronidazole, are frequently used in attempts to control Crohn's disease but are not useful in ulcerative colitis.[37,59] Metronidazole is of value in some patients with

TABLE 36-6 Levels of Evidence for Therapeutic Interventions in Inflammatory Bowel Disease

Interventions	Evidence Grades
Ulcerative colitis	
Mild-moderate active distal disease may be treated with oral aminosalicylates, topical mesalamine, or topical steroids	A
Combined oral and topical aminosalicylates are more effective than either alone for mild-moderate active distal disease	A
Oral prednisone in doses of 40–60 mg/day or 1 mg/kg/day may be used in patients with mild-moderate distal disease unresponsive to oral or topical aminosalicylates	B
Sulfasalazine in doses of 4–6 g/day or an alternate aminosalicylate in doses of up to 4.8 g/g of the active 5-aminosalicylate moiety are effective for induction of mild-moderate extensive colitis	A
Infliximab is effective for moderate to severe disease in those patients not responding to corticosteroids or an immunosuppressive agent	A
Systemic corticosteroids are effective in moderate to severe active disease	A
Hospitalization for parenteral steroids is indicated for patients with severe disease or those failing to respond to oral steroids	A
Failure to demonstrate improvement following 7–10 days of parenteral steroids in patients with severe disease is an indication for cyclosporine or colectomy	B
Mesalamine suppositories (proctitis) and enemas (distal colitis) are effective in maintenance of remission when dosed as infrequently as every third night	A
Sulfasalazine, mesalamine, or balsalazide are effective in maintenance of remission of distal disease; combining oral and topical mesalamine is more effective than either alone	A
Sulfasalazine, olsalazine, mesalamine, and balsalazide are effective in preventing relapses in patients with mild to moderate extensive disease	A
Corticosteroids are ineffective as maintenance treatment	A
Azathioprine, mercaptopurine, or infliximab are effective in lowering or eliminating corticosteroid use in corticosteroid-dependent patients	A
Azathioprine, mercaptopurine, or infliximab may be effective in patients with severe disease flares or those requiring retreatment with corticosteroids within 1 year	C
Oral cyclosporine is effective in patients with corticosteroid refractory disease but requires concomitant administration of azathioprine or mercaptopurine	C
Infliximab therapy is effective for maintenance if there is an initial response	A
Crohn's disease	
Oral aminosalicylates are effective for mild-moderate ileal, ilealocolonic, or colonic active disease	D
Metronidazole may be effective in patients not responding to sulfasalazine	D
Ileal-release budesonide is effective for mild-moderate ileal or right-sided colonic disease	A
Topical hydrocortisone is effective for distal colonic inflammation	A
Systemic corticosteroids are effective in moderate to severe active disease	A
Systemic corticosteroids are not effective in patients with perianal fistulas	C
Hospitalization for parenteral steroids is indicated for patients with severe disease or those failing to respond to oral steroids	A
Parental methotrexate is effective for induction of remission in patients with active disease, and to reduce corticosteroid dependency	B
Infliximab is effective for moderate to severe disease in those patients not responding to corticosteroids or an immunosuppressive agent	A
Infliximab is effective for those patients with fistulas who have not responded to antibiotics, immunosuppressive agents, or surgical drainage	A
High-dose oral cyclosporine (7.6 mg/kg) has short-term efficacy in patients with active disease	B
Intravenous cyclosporine is effective for the treatment of fistulizing disease	B
Corticosteroids are ineffective as maintenance treatment	A
Budesonide is effective as short-term maintenance therapy (3 months) but not as long-term therapy	A
Azathioprine, 6-mercaptopurine, or infliximab is effective in lowering or eliminating corticosteroid use in corticosteroid-dependent patients.	A
Azathioprine, 6-mercaptopurine, or infliximab may be effective in patients with severe disease flares or those requiring retreatment with corticosteroids within 1 year	A
Azathioprine or 6-mercaptopurine are effective for maintenance of remission regardless of disease distribution	A
Azathioprine or 6-mercaptopurine may be effective for treating perianal or enteric fistulae	C
Methotrexate maintenance therapy (15–25 mg IM weekly) is effective for patients whose active disease has responded to IM methotrexate	A
Methotrexate IM 25 mg IM weekly for up to 16 weeks followed by 15 mg IM weekly is effective for patients with chronic active disease	A
Infliximab therapy is effective for maintenance if there is an initial response	A

Grade A: Homogenous evidence from multiple well-designed, randomized (therapeutic) or cohort (descriptive) controlled trials, each involving a number of participants so as to be of sufficient statistical power.
Grade B: Evidence from at least one large, well-designed clinical trial with or without randomization from cohort or case control analytic studies or well-designed meta-analysis.
Grade C: Evidence based on clinical experience, descriptive studies, or reports of expert committees.
Grade D: Not rated.
Compiled from Kornbluth and Sachar,[36] Hanauer et al.,[69] and Simms and Steinhart.[97]

active Crohn's disease, particularly involving the perineal area or fistulas.[59] The mechanism of metronidazole's effect on Crohn's disease has not been determined but is theorized to relate to interruption of a bacterial role in the inflammatory process. Ciprofloxacin has also been used for treatment of IBD. Rifaximin, a new nonabsorbable antibiotic, has also shown some efficacy in treatment of both ulcerative colitis and Crohn's disease.[59]

Infliximab is an immunoglobulin G_1 chimeric monoclonal antibody that binds TNF-α and inhibits its inflammatory effect in the gut. The agent is useful for moderate to severe active disease and steroid-dependent or fistulizing disease, but the cost far exceeds that of other regimens.[60]

Adalimumab is also an IgG1 antibody to TNF-α, however this agent, unlike infliximab is fully humanized and contains no murine sequences. Theoretically, the lack of a murine component in adalimumab avoids the problem of antibody development seen with use of infliximab. This agent can be given subcutaneously, unlike infliximab,

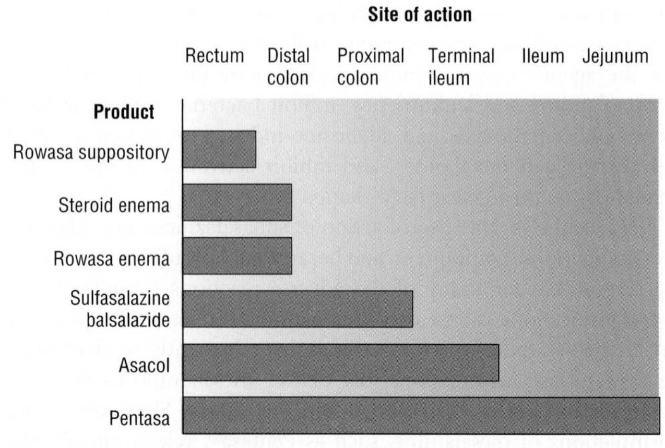

FIGURE 36-1. Site of activity of various agents used to treat inflammatory bowel disease.

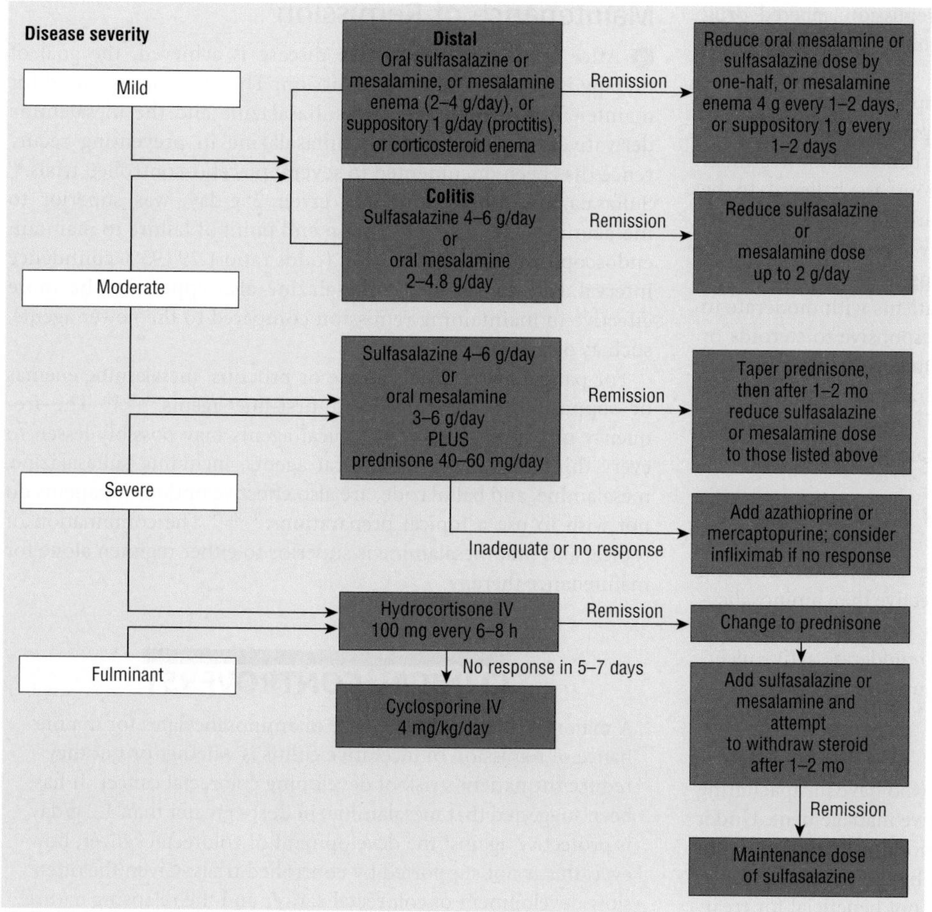

FIGURE 36-2. Treatment approaches for ulcerative colitis.

which is given intravenously. Adalimumab is a treatment option for patients with moderate to severe active Crohn's disease previously treated with infliximab who have lost response.[61,62,63]

Ulcerative Colitis

Mild to Moderate Disease Most patients with active ulcerative colitis have mild to moderate disease and do not require parenteral medications (Fig. 36–2). The first line of drug therapy for patients with extensive disease is oral sulfasalazine or an oral mesalamine derivative.[36] Topical mesalamine is more effective than oral mesalamine or topical steroids for distal disease.[36] The combination of oral and topical mesalamine is more effective than either alone for active distal disease.[26,36,64,65] When given orally, usually 4 to 6 g/day, and possibly up to 8 g/day, of sulfasalazine is required to attain control of active inflammation. There does not appear to be an increased rate of response with increased dosage over 6 g/day, although side effects increase. Even with the use of adequate doses, patient improvement usually takes 4 weeks, and sometimes longer.[36] The dosage of sulfasalazine that can be given is usually limited by the patient's tolerance of the agent; most adverse effects of sulfasalazine are dose related (GI disturbances, headache, and arthralgia).[35] Sulfasalazine therapy should be instituted at 500 mg/day and increased every few days up to 4 g/day or the maximum tolerated. It should not be used in patients with allergy to sulfonamide containing drugs.

Oral mesalamine derivatives (such as those listed in Table 36–5) are reasonable alternatives to sulfasalazine for treatment of ulcerative colitis. Oral mesalamine products are used for patients with extensive disease, while topical agents, such as enemas and suppositories, are used for distal disease. Mesalamine is clearly more effective than placebo but no more effective than sulfasalazine for extensive disease.[66,67] Mesalamine preparations are typically better tolerated, and the majority of patients intolerant to sulfasalazine or topical steroids should tolerate one of the other oral mesalamine derivatives.[35,36] Dose-related effects do exist and when used orally for active extensive disease, the equivalent of 4.8 g of the active 5-aminosalicylic acid moiety should be administered when possible.[36,66,67] Studies comparing daily doses of 2.4 g versus 4.8 g of mesalamine (Asacol formulation) in patients with moderate active ulcerative colitis demonstrated greater efficacy at 6 weeks of therapy (58% vs. 72%, $P < 0.05$).[64,68,69] Although the dosage range for Pentasa is 2 to 4 g/day, 4 g/day appears to be more effective.[66] Olsalazine (a dimer of 5-aminosalicylic acid that is given orally) is effective for treatment of mild to moderate ulcerative colitis. However, of patients taking olsalazine, 15% to 25% experience severe diarrhea, often necessitating discontinuation of the drug. This results from a direct osmotic effect of the drug to induce small-bowel fluid secretion. For this reason it is not the drug of first choice.[36] Balsalazide is another viable agent that couples mesalamine with the inert carrier molecule 4-aminobenzoyl-B-alanine, and is effective for treatment of mild to moderate ulcerative colitis.[70,71] When used topically, mesalamine suppositories will only reach to approximately 10 to 20 cm and thus should be reserved for patients with proctitis. Because enema formulations reach to the splenic flexure, they can be used for distal disease.[26,36]

❼ Steroids have a place in the treatment of moderate to severe active ulcerative colitis regardless of disease location, or in those patients who are unresponsive to maximal doses of oral and/or topical mesalamine derivatives.[36,71] Oral steroids (usually up to 1 mg/kg per day of prednisone equivalent or 40 to 60 mg daily) may be used for patients who do not have an adequate response to sulfasalazine or mesalamine.[36] Overall, steroids and sulfasalazine appear to be equally efficacious; however, the response to steroids may be evident sooner. Oral steroids should not be used as initial therapy for mild to moderate ulcerative colitis, mainly because of the known risks of steroid use. If steroids are used to attain remission, tapered drug withdrawal should be accomplished to minimize long-term steroid exposure.

Rectally administered steroids given as suppositories, enemas, or foams can be used as initial therapy for patients with ulcerative proctitis or distal colitis. Rectal agents are also beneficial for treatment of tenesmus. With these agents, local actions are believed to be responsible for drug effects. Rectal steroids are effective in the treatment of active, distal ulcerative colitis. However, rectal mesalamine is more effective than rectal steroids for inducing remission.[26,36,64,65,72]

Infliximab is another viable option for patients with moderate to severe active ulcerative colitis who are unresponsive to steroids or other immunosuppressive agents.[60,64,72,73] Outpatients with moderately active ulcerative colitis have response rates of up to 69% at 8 weeks following initial doses of 5 mg/kg.[74] Hospitalized patients have mixed results, with some demonstrating reduced rates of colectomy for patients receiving infliximab.[73,75,76]

Nicotine has been proposed as a treatment for ulcerative colitis (but not as a treatment for Crohn's disease) based on the observation of the onset of a flare of ulcerative colitis after smoking cessation in some individuals. While less effective than aminosalicylates, transdermal nicotine in daily doses of 15 to 25 mg may improve symptoms in patients with mild to moderate active ulcerative colitis and can be considered as an adjunctive therapy.[36,77]

Severe or Intractable Disease

Patients with uncontrolled severe colitis or who have incapacitating symptoms require hospitalization for effective management. Under these conditions, patients generally receive nothing by mouth to put the bowel at rest. Most medication is given by the parenteral route. Sulfasalazine or mesalamine derivatives are not beneficial for treatment of severe colitis because of rapid elimination of these agents from the colon with diarrhea, thereby not allowing sufficient time for gut bacteria to cleave the molecules. Overall it is difficult to evaluate drugs in this setting, because patients with severe disease almost always receive additional medications including steroids.

Steroids have been valuable in the treatment of severe disease because the use of these agents may allow some patients to avoid colectomy. Intravenous hydrocortisone 300 to 400 mg daily in three divided doses or methylprednisolone 48 to 60 mg once daily are considered first-line agents.[36,72] Methylprednisolone is typically preferred because of its lesser mineralocorticoid effects. A trial of steroids is warranted in most patients before proceeding to colectomy, unless the condition is grave or rapidly deteriorating. The length of the medical trial before consideration of surgery is open to debate. Steroids increase surgical risk, particularly infectious risk, if an operation is required later. After a colectomy is performed, steroids should no longer be required for the disease; however, they must be withdrawn gradually (usually over 3 to 4 weeks) to avoid hypoadrenal crisis because of adrenal suppression.

❽ Patients who are unresponsive to parenteral corticosteroids after 7 to 10 days should receive cyclosporine by intravenous infusion. Seventy to 80% of hospitalized patients who are unresponsive to corticosteroids will respond to cyclosporine.[55] Continuous intravenous infusion of cyclosporine (4 mg/kg per day) is typically effective in steroid-resistant acute severe ulcerative colitis and may reduce the need for emergent colectomy.[55,78] Intravenous cyclosporine has also been recommended as an alternative to steroids in patients with severe attacks of ulcerative colitis (fulminant colitis).[79] Patients who are controlled on intravenous cyclosporine can then be switched to an oral cyclosporine taper regimen with subsequent transition to azathioprine or 6-mercaptopurine.[72] As mentioned earlier, infliximab is also an alternative to cyclosporine, and may also deter the need for colectomy in patients with severe disease not responsive to steroids.[72,73–75]

Maintenance of Remission

❾ After remission from active disease is achieved, the goal of therapy is to then maintain remission. The major agents used for maintenance of remission are sulfasalazine and the mesalamine derivatives.[66,80] The value of sulfasalazine in preventing recurrences has been documented in several placebo-controlled trials.[80] Sulfasalazine, most commonly given 2 g/day, was superior to mesalamine when using the main end point of failure to maintain endoscopic or clinical remission (odds ratio 1.29 [95% confidence interval 1.05 to 1.57]).[80] Sulfasalazine also appears to be more effective in maintaining remission compared to the newer agents, such as olsalazine.

For patients with distal disease or proctitis, mesalamine enemas or suppositories are considered first-line agents.[26,36,65] The frequency of administration of topical agents may possibly lessen to every third night over time. Oral agents, including sulfasalazine, mesalamine, and balsalazide, are also effective options if patients do not wish to use a topical preparations.[26,36,65] The combination of topical and oral mesalamine is superior to either regimen alone for maintenance therapy.

CLINICAL CONTROVERSY

A major question about the use of aminosalicylates for maintenance of remission of ulcerative colitis is whether or not they reduce the patient's risk of developing colorectal cancer. It has been suggested that mesalamine, in doses greater than 1.2 g/day, is protective against the development of colorectal cancer; however, this is not supported by controlled trials. Given the often slow development of colorectal cancer and the relapsing nature of ulcerative colitis, these significantly limit the ability to conduct long-term surveillance studies in patients in remission.

Steroids do not have a role in the maintenance of remission with ulcerative colitis because they are ineffective.[36] Steroids should be gradually withdrawn after remission is induced (over 3 to 4 weeks). If they are continued, the patient will be at risk for steroid induced adverse effects without likelihood of benefits. For patients who require chronic steroid use (steroid dependency), there is a strong justification for alternative therapies or colectomy. Azathioprine is effective in preventing relapse of ulcerative colitis for periods exceeding 4 years.[54,69,72,81] However, 3 to 6 months may be required before beneficial effects are noted. For patients who initially respond to infliximab, continued dosing of 5 mg/kg as maintenance therapy every 8 weeks is another alternative for corticosteroid dependent patients, or those failing immunosuppressive therapy.[60,72,73]

■ CROHN'S DISEASE

Management of Crohn's disease often proves more difficult than management of ulcerative colitis, partly because of the greater complexity of presentation with Crohn's disease (Fig. 36–3). The disease may involve any segment of the GI tract, from mouth to anus, and may involve other visceral structures and soft tissues through fistulization. There is a greater reliance on drug therapy with Crohn's disease, because resection of all involved intestine may not be possible. Unfortunately, recurrence of Crohn's disease is common following surgery with reported rates of up to 64% recurrence following surgical resection of affected areas of bowel.[49]

Active Crohn's Disease

The goal of treatment for active Crohn's disease is to achieve remission; however, in many patients, reduction of symptoms so the patient may carry out normal activities, or reduction of the steroid dose

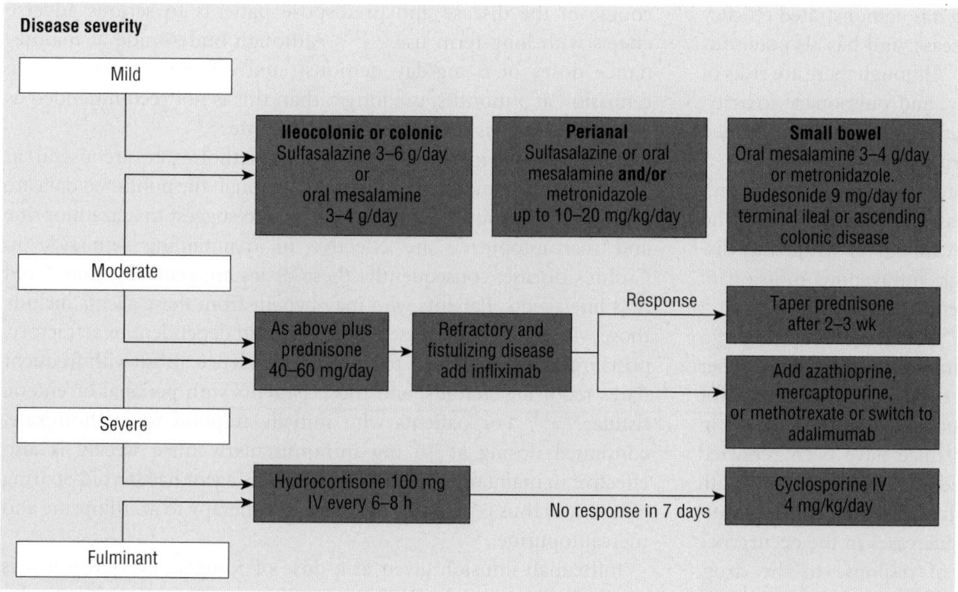

FIGURE 36-3. Treatment approaches for Crohn's disease.

required for control, is a significant accomplishment. In the majority of patients, active Crohn's disease is treated with sulfasalazine, mesalamine derivatives, or steroids, although azathioprine, mercaptopurine, methotrexate, infliximab, and metronidazole are frequently used.

The role of sulfasalazine in the treatment of active Crohn's disease is not as well established as its role in the treatment of ulcerative colitis. Sulfasalazine is superior to placebo, but is more effective when Crohn's disease involves the colon.[37] In these circumstances, sulfasalazine is as effective as prednisone.[36,82,83] Mesalamine formulations such as Pentasa or Asacol have the ability to release mesalamine in the small bowel, thus targeting ileal disease, yet have demonstrated variable results in patients with active Crohn's disease.[82,83] Only a few small trials using Asacol at 3.8 g/day or Pentasa at 4 g/day have demonstrated superiority to placebo for treatment of active Crohn's disease.[82,83] Despite variable effectiveness, the mesalamine derivatives may be better tolerated than sulfasalazine, particularly at higher doses. Thus, a trial of sulfasalazine or an oral mesalamine derivative is reasonable as initial therapy in patients with mild to moderate active Crohn's disease with ileal, ileocolonic, or colonic involvement.[36]

❼ Steroids are frequently used for the treatment of active Crohn's disease, particularly with more moderate to severe presentations, or in those patients unresponsive to aminosalicylates. Budesonide (Entocort) is a viable first-line option for patients with mild to moderate ileal or right-sided (ascending colonic) disease.[53,72,84] This agent is superior to placebo and has demonstrated superiority to mesalamine in some trials.[81] Budesonide is inferior to traditional systemic steroids for severe disease, although it carries a lower risk of adverse effects, and does not reach areas distal to the ascending colon. Oral systemic steroids are effective in inducing remission in up to 70% of patients and should be reserved for patients with moderate to severe disease who have failed aminosalicylates or budesonide.[72,82] Hospitalized patients with severe or fulminant disease, or those who are unable to tolerate oral therapy, are candidates for administration of parenteral steroids.[53,72] Systemic steroids do not appear to be effective for treatment of perianal fistulas.[72]

❿ Metronidazole (given orally up to 20 mg/kg per day in divided doses) has demonstrated variable efficacy, but may possibly be useful in some patients with Crohn's disease, particularly in patients with colonic or ileocolonic involvement, or in those patients with perineal disease.[59,82,83,85] For most patients with colonic or perineal disease, metronidazole is added to a mesalamine product or steroids as adjunctive therapy, where satisfactory control of Crohn's disease is not gained with first-line agents, or in attempts to reduce steroid dosage.[73] Ciprofloxacin has gained attention as an alternative to metronidazole, and has demonstrated some efficacy in small trials only.[82,83] The combination of metronidazole and ciprofloxacin appears to be efficacious in some patients with perianal disease.[59,85]

The immunosuppressive agents (azathioprine and its metabolite mercaptopurine) are effective, but are generally limited to use in patients who are not achieving adequate response to standard medical therapy, or to reduce steroid doses when high steroid doses are required.[54,72,82,86] Azathioprine and mercaptopurine have both demonstrated long-term benefits in patients with Crohn's disease.[54,81] The usual dose of azathioprine is 2 to 3 mg/kg per day; the usual dose of mercaptopurine is 1 to 1.5 mg/kg per day.[72] Starting doses are typically 50 mg/day and increased at 2-week intervals; complete blood counts with differential should be monitored every 2 weeks while doses are being titrated.[72] The onset of therapeutic effects is delayed with both azathioprine and mercaptopurine, and a minimum of 3 to 4 months is often required to see clinical benefits.[72,82]

Clinical response to mercaptopurine is related to whole-blood concentrations of the metabolite 6-thioguanine (6-TGN), while toxicity is correlated with concentrations of another metabolite, 6-methylmercaptopurine (6-MMPR).[13,54,87] Metabolic inactivation of azathioprine and mercaptopurine occurs mainly by the enzyme thiopurine S-methyltransferase (TPMT), which exhibits genetic polymorphism. Enzyme-deficient patients are at greater risk of bone marrow suppression from these agents.[14,54] Determination of TPMT activity is possible, and may be necessary to determine which patients require lower doses of these agents.[14,54] Alternatively, a newer strategy for evaluating a patient's risk for toxicity is to perform a TPMT genotype or phenotype.[54,72] This is recommended prior to therapy with subsequent dose adjustments based on the patient's genotypic profile.[72]

CLINICAL CONTROVERSY

Although thiopurines, such as azathioprine and mercaptopurine, are effective for maintenance of remission of Crohn's disease, it is debated how long treatment should be continued once remission is achieved. Evidence has demonstrated efficacy of these agents in maintaining remission for longer than 4 years; however, some authors argue that long-term exposure to these potentially toxic agents outweighs the benefit.

Although mostly used in the setting of maintenance therapy, methotrexate is another option for use as induction therapy.[82] Use of a weekly intramuscular injection of 25 mg has demonstrated efficacy for induction of remission in Crohn's disease, and has also demonstrated corticosteroid-sparing effects.[72,82,88] Although there are risks of bone marrow suppression, hepatotoxicity, and pulmonary toxicity, use of low-dose methotrexate appears relatively safe when continued as maintenance therapy if proper monitoring is implemented.

Infliximab is used for treating moderate to severe active Crohn's disease in patients failing immunosuppressive therapy, in those who are corticosteroid dependent, and for treatment of fistulizing disease.[60,72,89] In large trials, a 5-mg/kg single intravenous infusion of infliximab resulted in clinical improvement in 58% of patients at 2 weeks and in 65% of patients at 8 weeks.[60,89] Continued dosing of 5 mg/kg at 2 and 6 weeks following the initial dose leads to higher response rates, and is recommended as the regimen of choice for induction therapy in active disease.[72] Response rates of up to 62% in the reduction of number of draining fistulae have been reported following induction therapy and continued maintenance dosing with infliximab.[60,89,90] Patients who receive infliximab often develop antibodies to infliximab, which can result in increases in the occurrence of serious infusion reactions and loss of response to the drug. Strategies to reduce formation of antibodies to infliximab include administration of a second dose within 8 weeks of the first dose, concurrent administration of steroids (hydrocortisone 200 mg intravenously on the day of the infusion or oral prednisone the day prior), and use of concomitant immunosuppressive agents.[60,72,89] Induction of tolerance using a dose escalation technique was also effective in administering infliximab to patients with previous severe infusion reactions.[91]

Cyclosporine is typically not recommended for treatment of Crohn's disease except for acute management of patients with severe fistulizing disease.[72,90,92] Up to 83% of patients with refractory fistulas responded to intravenous cyclosporine (4 mg/kg per day) within a mean of 7.9 days.[82] The dose of cyclosporine is important in determining efficacy. An oral dose of 5 mg/kg per day is ineffective, whereas 7.6 mg/kg per day has demonstrated effectiveness in some trials.[72,92] However, toxic effects limit the routine use of this higher dosage. At present, the therapeutic blood or plasma concentration range for cyclosporine has not been established for Crohn's disease, but whole-blood trough concentrations of 300 to 500 ng/mL for intravenous therapy or 200 to 400 ng/mL for oral therapy are reasonable goals.[72,82] When using cyclosporine clinicians should recognize the accompanying long-term risk of renal toxicity and infection, as well as the potential for drug interactions.

Trials evaluating treatment with adalimumab in patients with moderately to severe active Crohn's disease who have lost response to infliximab have demonstrated up to a 54% complete response in some instances.[61,62,63] Doses used are typically 160 mg subcutaneously initially, followed by 80 mg subcutaneously at week two, with subsequent doses of 40 mg subcutaneously every over week thereafter.

Maintenance of Remission

❾ Prevention of recurrence of disease is clearly more difficult with Crohn's disease than with ulcerative colitis. There is minimal evidence to support sulfasalazine and oral mesalamine derivatives' effectiveness for maintenance of Crohn's disease following medically induced remission.[82,93,94] Despite these findings, an attempt to maintain remission with sulfasalazine and oral mesalamine following a medically induced remission is reasonable given the favorable side-effect profile of these drugs compared to that of the immunosuppressive agents and infliximab.[79] Mesalamine does appear to have some efficacy in preventing postsurgical relapse following resection, with absolute risk reductions of 10% to 15% for relapse reported in some studies.[94,95]

Systemic steroids have no place in the prevention of recurrence of Crohn's disease. These agents do not appear to alter the long-term course of the disease and predispose patients to serious adverse effects with long-term use.[37,72,96] Although budesonide at maintenance doses of 6 mg/day demonstrated efficacy in maintaining remission at 3 months, use longer than this is not recommended as a loss of efficacy is seen after this timeframe.[72,97]

Azathioprine, mercaptopurine, and methotrexate are useful in some patients to maintain remission. Although the published data are somewhat inconsistent, there is evidence to suggest that azathioprine and mercaptopurine are effective in maintaining remission in Crohn's disease; consequently, these drugs are generally considered first-line agents. Patients who may benefit from these agents include those with quiescent disease who are steroid dependent or refractory, postsurgical patients so as to prevent recurrence, those with frequent flares requiring steroids, and those patients with perianal or enteric fistulae.[54,72,82] For patients who initially respond to methotrexate, continued dosing at 15 mg intramuscularly once weekly is also effective in maintaining remission.[72,82] This agent has steroid-sparing effects, and thus represents an alternative therapy to azathioprine and mercaptopurine.

Infliximab infusion given at a dose of 5 mg/kg every 8 weeks is more effective than placebo in maintaining remission in patients who initially respond to infliximab for active Crohn's disease.[60,64,72,74,89] An increase in the dose to 10 mg/kg is acceptable if loss of efficacy over time is evident. Additionally, infliximab is the most effective maintenance therapy for fistulizing disease; however, given the high cost of this agent, some have questioned whether this approach is the most cost-effective.[90]

Adalimumab is also a treatment option for maintenance therapy of Crohn's disease. Following induction therapy, dose of 40 mg subcutaneously every other week have resulted in clinical remission rates of 36–46% adter 56 weeks of therapy.[98,99] Again this agent should be reserved for those patients unresponsive to conventional therapies, including infliximab.

CLINICAL CONTROVERSY

Given the delayed onset of azathioprine some have advocated using infliximab as a "bridge" therapy, using three induction doses to treat active Crohn's disease in steroid-dependent patients while waiting for the therapeutic effects of azathioprine to become evident. Although one recent study has demonstrated this to be effective, some argue that this regimen only delays relapse and does not prevent it, while adding significant expense.[100,101]

SELECTED COMPLICATIONS

TOXIC MEGACOLON

The treatment required for toxic megacolon includes general supportive measures to maintain vital functions, consideration for early surgical intervention, and use of various drugs (steroids, cyclosporine, and antimicrobials).[28,36] Aggressive fluid and electrolyte management is required for dehydration. Fluids and electrolytes may be lost through vomiting, diarrhea, and nasogastric intubation, as well as through fluid accumulation in the bowel. When the patient has lost significant amounts of blood (through the rectum), blood replacement may be necessary. Opiates and medications with anticholinergic properties should be discontinued because these agents enhance colonic dilatation, thereby increasing the risk of bowel perforation. Broad-spectrum antimicrobials that include coverage for gram-negative bacilli and intestinal anaerobes should be used as preemptive therapy in the event that perforation occurs.[28] Fortunately perforation occurs in only 2% to 3% of cases.[36] The duration of the antimicrobial regimen (often 2 to 3 weeks) should be determined with consideration that there may be significant intraabdominal contamination with signs and symptoms hidden by steroid effects.

If the patient is not on steroids, then high-dose intravenous therapy should be administered to reduce acute inflammation. Recommended regimens include hydrocortisone 100 mg every 8 hours, methylprednisolone 15 mg every 6 hours, or corticotropin 40 units every 8 hours.[28] Although the duration of steroid administration is uncertain, most clinicians continue the high-dose steroids for up to 2 weeks after improvement is observed, and then reduce the dosage (approximately 0.5 to 1 mg/kg per day) for a few additional weeks.

Emergent surgical intervention, mainly an abdominal colectomy with formation of an ileostomy, is an important consideration in patients with toxic megacolon and prevents death in some patients.[28,36,49] Surgical resection is usually reserved for patients failing maximal medical therapy, however the timing of surgery following initiation of medical therapy is somewhat controversial. Some authors advocate 24 to 72 hours of observation following initiation of medical treatment before performing a colectomy,[36,49] whereas others advocate waiting up to 7 days as long as the patient is stable.[28]

SYSTEMIC MANIFESTATIONS

The common systemic manifestations of IBD include arthritis, anemia, skin manifestations such as erythema nodosum and pyoderma gangrenosum, uveitis, and liver disease. These problems may be related to the inflammatory process. For some of these manifestations specific therapies can be instituted, whereas for others the treatment that is used for the GI inflammatory process also addresses the systemic manifestations.

Anemia occurs when there is significant blood loss from the GI tract. If the patient can consume oral medication, ferrous sulfate should be administered. If the patient is unable to take oral medication and the patient's hematocrit is sufficiently low, blood transfusions or intravenous iron infusions may be required.[31,32] Anemia may also be related to malabsorption of vitamin B_{12} or folic acid, particularly in patients who have had ileal resection, so these may also be required. Patients with IBD are also at high risk for bone loss, osteoporosis, and fractures.[32,102] Screening for osteoporosis via digital X-ray absorptiometry is recommended for patients using steroids for longer than 3 months, in postmenopausal females, males older than age 50 years, and those who have sustained a low-stress fracture.[32,102] If the patient is deemed at high risk for osteoporosis, vitamin D and calcium should be instituted. If osteoporosis is present, then calcium, vitamin D, and a bisphosphonate are recommended.[32,102] Corticosteroid use should be limited and weight-bearing exercise initiated.

There are no consistently recommended therapies for aphthous ulcers, liver disease, episcleritis, or uveitis associated with IBD. Some reports suggest that these manifestations are worse during exacerbations of the intestinal disease and that measures improving intestinal disease will improve these systemic manifestations. Unfortunately, this association has not been demonstrated consistently. For arthritis associated with IBD, aspirin or another NSAID may be beneficial, as might be steroids. However NSAID use may exacerbate the underlying IBD. Liver transplantation is being used more frequently for definitive treatment of primary sclerosing cholangitis. Infliximab has demonstrated efficacy in treatment of some arthritic and skin manifestations such as ankylosing spondylitis, erythema nodosum, and pyoderma gangrenosum.[32,103]

SPECIAL CONSIDERATIONS

PREGNANCY

Either the occurrence or consideration of pregnancy may cause significant concerns in the patient with IBD. Patients with IBD have similar infertility rates as the general female population, thus the rate of normal childbirth is similar to that for healthy populations.[104] Some studies have noted a greater risk of spontaneous abortions in patients with IBD. Also, there is a greater incidence of low birth weight infants in mothers with chronic idiopathic ulcerative colitis.[104] Pregnancy has minimal effects on the course of IBD.[104,105] Likewise, IBD appears to have little effect on the course of pregnancy, particularly if the IBD is quiescent at the time of conception.[104,105] Patients who are pregnant experience IBD recurrence rates similar to those of nonpregnant females. Also, there is no justification for therapeutic abortion with IBD because termination of the pregnancy has not been observed to improve the disease. There is also unfounded concern that the drugs required to treat IBD may be teratogenic.

Steroids and sulfasalazine my be administered during pregnancy with the same guidelines that would be applied to the nonpregnant patient.[104,105] Steroids given systemically do not appear to be detrimental to the fetus. Sulfasalazine is generally well tolerated; however it does interfere with folate absorption, so supplementation with folic acid 1 mg twice daily should be used during the pregnancy.[104] Interestingly, sulfasalazine has also been reported to cause decreased sperm counts and reduced fertility in males.[104] This effect is reversible on discontinuation of the drug, and it is not reported with mesalamine. Immunosuppressive drugs (azathioprine and mercaptopurine) may be associated with fetal deformities in humans; however, they have been used without detriment in some patients.[104,105] Infliximab also appears to be safe for use in pregnant patients.[104] Metronidazole may be used for short courses for treatment of trichomoniasis, but prolonged use should be avoided due to potential mutagenic effects.[104] Methotrexate should not be used during pregnancy, as it is a known abortifacient (category X).[72,104]

Overall, drug therapy for IBD is not a contraindication for pregnancy, and most pregnancies are well managed in patients with these diseases. The indications for medical and surgical treatment are similar to those in the nonpregnant patient. If a patient has an initial bout of IBD during pregnancy, a standard approach to treatment should be initiated. Recommendations for the use of drugs in nursing mothers vary. Although prednisone and prednisolone can be detected in breast milk, breast-feeding is believed to be safe for the infant when low doses of prednisone are used.[105] Sulfasalazine does not pose a risk of kernicterus, as levels of sulfapyridine in breast milk are low or undetectable. Metronidazole should not be given to nursing mothers because it is excreted into breast milk.[105]

ADVERSE DRUG EFFECTS

Drug intolerance often limits the usefulness of agents used to treat IBD. Many patients receiving sulfasalazine, mesalamine, corticosteroids, metronidazole, azathioprine, mercaptopurine, methotrexate, or infliximab experience undesired effects. In some cases, these adverse effects can be significant and require discontinuation of the therapy. Knowledge of the common or important adverse reactions will assist in avoiding or minimizing their effects.

Sulfasalazine is often associated with adverse drug effects and these effects may be classified as either dose related or idiosyncratic.[106,107] The sulfapyridine portion of the sulfasalazine molecule is believed to be responsible for much of the sulfasalazine toxicity.[106] Dose-related side effects usually include GI disturbances such as nausea, vomiting, diarrhea, or anorexia, but may also include headache and arthralgia. These adverse reactions tend to occur more commonly on initiation of therapy and decrease in frequency as therapy is continued. Approaches to the management of these adverse effects include discontinue the agent for a short period and then reinstitute therapy at a reduced dosage with subsequent slower dose escalation, administration with food, or substitution of another enteric-coated mesalamine product.[106,107] Folic acid absorption is impaired by sulfasalazine, which may lead to anemia. Patients receiving sulfasalazine should receive oral folic acid supplementation.

Adverse effects that are idiosyncratic are not dose related and most commonly include rash, fever, or hepatotoxicity, as well as relatively uncommon but serious reactions such as bone marrow suppression, thrombocytopenia, pancreatitis, pneumonitis, interstitial nephritis, and hepatitis. For most patients with idiosyncratic reactions, sulfasalazine must be discontinued. In some patients who have experienced allergic reactions to sulfasalazine, a desensitization procedure can be instituted. By gradually increasing sulfasalazine dosage over weeks to months, patient tolerance has been improved.[107]

Oral mesalamine derivatives may impose a lower frequency of adverse effects as compared to sulfasalazine.[52] Up to 90% of patients who are intolerant to sulfasalazine will tolerate oral mesalamine derivatives.[106] However, olsalazine, may cause watery diarrhea in up to 25% of patients, often requiring drug discontinuation.[106]

Adverse reactions to corticosteroids are well recognized and may occur when corticosteroids are used for any indication. However, there is a greater potential for adverse effects when corticosteroids are used for the treatment of IBD because high doses must often be used for extended periods. In the National Cooperative Crohn's Disease Study, half of patients receiving high-dose steroid therapy experienced side effects, as did one-third of the patients on the lower-dose regimens for maintenance.[39] The well-appreciated adverse effects of corticosteroids include hyperglycemia, hypertension, osteoporosis, acne, fluid retention, electrolyte disturbances, myopathies, muscle wasting, increased appetite, psychosis, and reduced resistance to infection. In addition, corticosteroid use may cause adrenocortical suppression. To minimize corticosteroid effects, clinicians have used alternate-day steroid therapy; however, some patients do not do well clinically on the days when no steroid is given. For most patients a single daily corticosteroid dose suffices, and divided daily doses are unnecessary. Another problem with corticosteroids is adrenal insufficiency after abrupt steroid withdrawal. This necessitates gradual tapering of steroid therapy for patients using these agents daily for more than 2 to 3 weeks.[106]

Immunosuppressants such as azathioprine and mercaptopurine have a significant potential for adverse reactions and have resulted in withdrawal rates in clinical trials of up to 20%.[54] Adverse events to thiopurines are typically divided into two groups, type A and type B.[54] Type A are dose related and include malaise, nausea, infectious complications, hepatitis, and myelosuppression. As mentioned earlier, the myelosuppression from azathioprine and mercaptopurine is related to a deficiency of TPMT with subsequent accumulation of toxic metabolites. Type B reactions are considered idiosyncratic and include fever, rash, arthralgia, and pancreatitis (3% to 15% of patients).[54,106] Mercaptopurine causes adverse reactions similarly to azathioprine; however, there are fewer reports of lymphomas with this agent. In one cohort of IBD patients, adverse effects from mercaptopurine were as follows: pancreatitis, 1.2%; allergic reactions, 3.9%, significant leukopenia, 11.5%; and infectious complications, 14%.[108] Allopurinol inhibits the metabolism of mercaptopurine, and a dosage reduction of the latter is required when the two are used in combination.

Most patients receiving metronidazole for Crohn's disease tolerate the agent fairly well; however, mild adverse effects occur frequently. They commonly include nauseas, metallic taste, urticaria, and glossitis.[59,106] More serious effects that occur with long-term use include development of paresthesia and reversible peripheral neuropathy.[59,106] Other effects include a disulfiram-like reaction if alcohol is ingested in conjunction.

Infliximab has been related to adverse effects such as infusion reactions, serum sickness, and increases in serious infections such as sepsis and reactivation of latent tuberculosis.[60,89] Infusion reactions and serum sickness relate to the immune response to foreign protein. Patients often develop antiinfliximab antibodies with multiple infusions. Serum sickness has occurred in patients who received infliximab doses separated by a long period of time.[60] Sepsis and tuberculosis may occur because of the inhibition of TNF-protective mechanisms. Patients should receive a tuberculin skin test (purified protein derivative) and a chest radiograph prior to initiating therapy to rule out undiagnosed tuberculosis.[60] Patients with clinically significant active infections should not receive infliximab. Lastly, infliximab may worsen existing heart failure and should be avoided in patients with severe or decompensated disease. Despite the potential for adverse effects, the reported rate of nonadherence to infliximab is low.[109]

Adalimumab carries similar risks to infliximab, and therefore the same screening and monitoring that is used for infliximab should also be implemented for adalimumab.

EVALUATION OF THERAPEUTIC OUTCOMES

The success of therapeutic regimens to treat IBD can be measured by patient-reported complaints, signs, and symptoms; by direct clinician examination (including endoscopy); by history and physical examination; by selected laboratory tests; and by quality-of-life measures. Evaluation of IBD severity is difficult because much of the assessment is subjective.[110] To create more objective measures, disease rating scales or indices have been created. The Crohn's Disease Activity Index is a commonly used scale, particularly for evaluation of patients during clinical trials.[111] The scale incorporates eight elements: (a) number of stools in the past 7 days; (b) sum of abdominal pain ratings from the past 7 days; (c) rating of general well-being in the past 7 days; (d) use of antidiarrheals; (e) body weight; (f) hematocrit; (g) finding of abdominal mass; and (h) a sum of extraintestinal symptoms present in the past week. Elements of this index provide a guide for those measures that may be useful in assessing the effectiveness of treatment regimens. A subsequent scale was developed specifically for perianal Crohn's disease, known as the Perianal Crohn's Disease Activity Index.[110] The Perianal Crohn's Disease Activity Index includes five items: (a) presence of discharge; (b) pain; (c) restriction of sexual activity; (d) type of perianal disease; and (e) degree of induration.

Standardized assessment tools have also been constructed for ulcerative colitis.[112] Elements in these scales include (a) stool frequency; (b) presence of blood in the stool; (c) mucosal appearance (from endoscopy); and (d) physician's global assessment based on physical examination, endoscopy, and laboratory data.

Additional studies that are often useful include direct endoscopic examination of affected areas and radiocontrast studies. For patients with acute disease, assessment of fluid and electrolyte status is important, because these may be lost during diarrheal episodes. Other laboratory tests, such as serum albumin, transferrin, or other markers of visceral protein status, as well as markers of inflammation (erythrocyte sedimentation rate), may be used.

Assessment of the IBD patient must include consideration of adverse drug effects. Because many of the agents used have a relatively high probability of causing adverse effects, particularly corticosteroids and other immunosuppressive agents, patient assessment should include collection of history and physical and laboratory data that are necessary to prevent or recognize adverse drug effects.

Finally, a patient quality-of-life assessment should be performed regularly.[110] Agents that appear clinically equivalent may differ substantially in resulting quality of life. Inquiry should be made regarding general well-being, emotional function, and social function. Social function may include assessment of the ability to perform routine daily functions, maintain occupational activities, sexual function, and recreation. The most common tool used to assess quality of life is the Inflammatory Bowel Disease Questionnaire, a 32-item questionnaire that covers four disease dimensions: bowel function, emotional status, systemic symptoms, and social function.[110] The Inflammatory Bowel Disease Questionnaire has shown good correlation with the Crohn's Disease Activity Index.[110] A shortened version has also been developed for use in the community practice setting.[113] A less-frequently used tool is the Rating Form of Inflammatory Bowel Disease Patient Concerns.[110]

Quality-of-life studies have been conducted with infliximab. To balance the exceptionally high cost of this therapy, Crohn's disease patients who receive infliximab have improved quality of life, fewer emergency room visits, a reduced requirement for surgery, and are more likely to be employed.[114,115]

ABBREVIATIONS

HLA: human leukocyte antigen

IBD: inflammatory bowel disease

NSAIDs: nonsteroidal antiinflammatory drugs

TPMT: thiopurine S-methyltransferase

TNF-α: tumor necrosis factor-α

REFERENCES

1. Langmead L, Rampton D. A GP guide to inflammatory bowel disease. Practitioner 2001;245:224–229.
2. Sandler RS, Eisen GM. Epidemiology of inflammatory bowel disease. In: Kirsner JB, ed. Inflammatory Bowel Diseases. Philadelphia: WB Saunders, 2000:89–112.
3. Feldman M. Sleisenger and Fordtran's Gastrointestinal and Liver Disease, 7th ed. New York: Elsevier, 2002.
4. Cross RK, Jung C, Wasan S, et al. Racial differences in disease phenotypes in patients with Crohn's disease. Inflamm Bowel Dis 2006;12:192–198.
5. Straus WL, Eisen Gm, Sandler RS, et al. Crohn's disease: Does race matter? Am J Gastroenterol 2000;95(2):479–483.
6. Viscido A, Aratari A, Maccioni F, et al. Inflammatory bowel diseases: Clinical update of practical guidelines. Nucl Med Commun 2005;26:649–655.
7. Seksik P, Sokol H, Lepage P, et al. Review article: The role of bacteria in onset and perpetuation of inflammatory bowel disease. Aliment Pharmacol Ther 2006;24(Suppl 3):11–18.
8. Shanahan F. Crohn's disease. Lancet 2003;359:62–69.
9. Podolsky DK. Inflammatory bowel disease. N Engl J Med 2002;347:417–429.
10. Farrell RJ, Peppercorn MA. Ulcerative colitis. Lancet 2002;359:331–340.
11. Lakatos PL, Fischer S, Lakatos L, et al. Current concept on the pathogenesis of inflammatory bowel disease-crosstalk between genetic and microbial factors: Pathogenic bacteria and altered bacterial sensing or changes in mucosal integrity take "toll." World J Gastroenterol 2006;12(12):1829–1841.
12. Shanahan F. Pathogenesis of ulcerative colitis. Lancet 1993;342:407–411.
13. Vermeire S. Review article: Genetic susceptibility and application of genetic testing in clinical management of inflammatory bowel disease. Aliment Pharmacol Ther 2006;24(Suppl 3):2–10.
14. Herrlinger KR, Jewell DP. Review article: Interactions between genotype and response to therapy in inflammatory bowel diseases. Aliment Pharmacol Ther 2006;24:1403–1412.
15. Lanzaratto F, Carpani M, Chaudhary R, Ghosh S. Novel treatment options for inflammatory bowel disease: Targeting α_4 integrin. Drugs 2006;66:1179–1189.
16. Sandborn WJ, Landers CJ, Tremaine WJ, Targan BR. Association of antineutrophil cytoplasmic antibodies with resistance to treatment of left-sided ulcerative colitis: Results of a pilot study. Mayo Clin Proc 1996;71:431–436.
17. Blumberg RS, Strober W. Prospects for research in inflammatory bowel disease. JAMA 2001;285:643–647.
18. MacDonald TT, DiSabatino A, Gordon JN. Immunopathogenesis of Crohn's disease. JPEN J Parenter Enteral Nutr 2005;29(4):S118–S125.
19. Bitton A, Sewitch MJ, Peppercorn MA, et al. Psychosocial determinants of relapse in ulcerative colitis: A longitudinal study. Am J Gastroenterol 2003;98:2112–2115.
20. Pullan RD, Rhodes J, Ganesh S, et al. Transdermal nicotine for active ulcerative colitis. N Engl J Med 1994;330:811–815.
21. Sandborn WJ, Tremaine WJ, Offord KP, et al. Transdermal nicotine for mildly to moderately active ulcerative colitis. Ann Intern Med 1997;126:364–371.
22. Cosnes J, Beaugerie L, Carbonnel F, Gendre JP. Smoking cessation and the course of Crohn's disease: An intervention study. Gastroenterology 2001;120:1093–1099.
23. Cipolla G, Crema F, Sacco S, et al. Nonsteroidal anti-inflammatory drugs and inflammatory bowel disease: Current perspectives. Pharmacol Res 2002;46:1–6.
24. Mahadevan U, Loftus EV, Tremaine WJ, Sandborn WJ. Safety of selective cyclooxygenase inhibitors in inflammatory bowel disease. Am J Gastroenterol 2002;97:910–914.
25. Bonner GF. Using COX-2 inhibitors in IBD. Anti-inflammatories inflame a controversy [editorial]. Am J Gastroenterol 2002;97783–97785.
26. Regueiro MD. Diagnosis and treatment of ulcerative proctitis. J Clin Gastroenterol 2004;38:733–740.
27. Geboes K. Review article: What are the important endoscopic lesions for detection of dysplasia in inflammatory bowel disease? Aliment Pharmacol Ther 2006;24(Suppl 3):50–55.
28. Gan SI, Beck PL. A new look at toxic megacolon: An update and review of incidence, etiology, pathogenesis, and management. Am J Gastroenterol 2003;98:2363–2371.
29. Monsen V, Sorstad J, Hellers G, et al. Extracolonic diagnosis in ulcerative colitis: An epidemiologic study. Am J Gastroenterol 1990;85:711–716.
30. Harmatz A. Hepatobiliary manifestations of inflammatory bowel disease. Med Clin North Am 1994;78:1387–1398.
31. Rankin GB. Extraintestinal and systemic manifestations of inflammatory bowel disease. Med Clin North Am 1990;74:39–50.
32. Kethu SR. Extraintestinal manifestations of inflammatory bowel diseases. J Clin Gastroenterol 2006;40:467–475.
33. O'Keefe SJD, Rosser BG. Nutrition and inflammatory bowel disease. In: Targan SR, Shanahan F, eds. Inflammatory Bowel Disease: From Bench to Bedside. Baltimore: Williams & Wilkins, 1994:461–477.
34. Filippi J, Al-Jaouni R, Wiroth JB, et al. Nutritional deficiencies in patients with Crohn's disease in remission. Inflam Bowel Dis 2006;12:185–191.
35. Collins P, Rhodes J. Ulcerative colitis: Diagnosis and management. BMJ 2006;333:340–343.
36. Kornbluth A, Sachar DB. Ulcerative practice guidelines in adults (update): American College of Gastroenterology, Practice Parameters Committee. Am J Gastroenterol 2004;99:1371–1385.
37. Hanauer SB, Sandborn W. Management of Crohn's disease in adults. Am J Gastroenterol 2001;96:635–643.
38. Janowicz HD. The "natural history" of inflammatory bowel disease and therapeutic decisions. Am J Gastroenterol 1987;82:498–503.
39. Summers RW, Switz DM, Sessions JT, et al. National Cooperative Crohn's Disease Study: Results of drug treatment. Gastroenterology 1979;77:847–869.
40. Malchow H, Ewe K, Brandes JW, et al. European Cooperative Crohn's Disease Study (ECCDS): Results of drug treatment. Gastroenterology 1984;86:249–266.
41. Wu S, Craig RM. Intense nutritional support in inflammatory bowel disease. Dig Dis Sci 1995;40:843–852.
42. Gonzalez-Huix F, Fernandez-Banares F, Esteve-Comas M, et al. Enteral versus parenteral nutrition as adjunct therapy in acute ulcerative colitis. Am J Gastroenterol 1993;88:227–232.
43. Griffiths AM. Enteral nutrition in the management of Crohn's Disease. JPEN J Parenter Enteral Nutr 2005;29:S108–S117.
44. Sanderson IR, Croft NM. The anti-inflammatory effects of enteral nutrition. JPEN J Parenter Enteral Nutr 2005;29:S134–S140.
45. Buning C, Lochs H. Conventional therapy for Crohn's disease. World J Gastroenterol 2006;12(30):4794–4806.
46. Lewis JD, Fisher RL. Nutritional support in inflammatory bowel disease. Med Clin North Am 1994;78:1443–1456.

47. Gassull MA. Review article: The intestinal lumen as a therapeutic target in inflammatory bowel disease. Aliment Pharmacol Ther 2006;24(Suppl 3):90–95.
48. Sullivan A, Nord CE. Probiotics and gastrointestinal diseases. J Intern Med 2005;257:78–92.
49. Hancock L, Windsor AC, Mortensen. Inflammatory bowel disease: The view of the surgeon. Colorectal Dis 2006;8(Suppl 1):10–14.
50. Sandborn WJ, Hanauer SB. Systematic review: The pharmacokinetic profiles of oral mesalazine formulations and mesalazine pro-drugs used in the management of ulcerative colitis. Aliment Pharmacol Ther 2003;17:29–42.
51. Hanauer SB. New lessons: Classic treatments, expanding options in ulcerative colitis. Colorectal Dis 2006;8(Suppl 1):20–24.
52. Friend Dr. Review article: Issues in oral administration of locally acting glucocorticoids for the treatment of inflammatory bowel disease. Aliment Pharmacol Ther 1998;12:591–603.
53. Hofer KN. Oral budesonide in the management of Crohn's disease. Ann Pharmacother 2003;37;1457–1464.
54. Derijks LJJ, Gilissen LPL, Hooymans PM, Hommes DW. Review article: Thiopurines in inflammatory bowel disease. Aliment Pharmcol Ther 2006;24:715–729.
55. Durai D. Hawthorne AB. Review article: How and when to use ciclosporin in ulcerative colitis. Aliment Pharmacol Ther 2005;22:907–916.
56. Gonzalez-Lama Y, Gisbert JP, Mate J. The role of tacrolimus in inflammatory bowel disease: A systematic review. Dig Dis Sci 2006;51:1833–1840.
57. Schroder O, Stein J. Low dose methotrexate in inflammatory bowel disease: Current status and future directions. Am J Gastroenterol 2003;98:530–537.
58. Vandell AG, DiPiro JT. Low-dose methotrexate for treatment and maintenance of remission in patients with inflammatory bowel disease. Pharmacotherapy 2002;22:613–620.
59. Guslandi M. Antibiotics for inflammatory bowel disease: Do they work? Eur J Gastroenterol Hepatol 2005:17;145–147.
60. Rutgeerts P, Van Assche G, Vermeire S. Review article: Infliximab for inflammatory bowel disease—Seven years on. Aliment Pharmacol Ther 2006;23:451–463.
61. Konstantinos AP, Shaye OA, Vasiliaukas EA, et al. Safety and efficacy of adalimumab (D2E7) in Crohn's disease patients with an attenuated response to infliximab. Am J Gastrenterol 2005;100:75–79.
62. Sandborn WJ, Rutgeert P, Enns R, et al. Adalimumab induction therapy for Crohn's disease previously treated with infliximab. Ann Intern Med 2007;146:829–838.
63. Hanauer SB, Sanborn WJ, Rutgeerts P, et al. Human anti-tumor necrosis factor monocolonal antibody (adalimumab) in Crohn's disease: The C1ASSIC-I trial. Gastroenterology 2006;130:323–333.
64. Sandborn WJ. What's new: Innovative concepts in inflammatory bowel disease. Colorectal Dis 2006;8(Suppl 1):3–9.
65. Gionchetto P, Rizzello F, Morselli C, et al. Review article: Aminosalicylates for distal colitis. Aliment Pharmacol Ther 2006;24(Suppl 3):41–44.
66. Hanauer SB. Review article: High dose aminosalicylates to induce and maintain remission in ulcerative colitis. Aliment Pharmacol Ther 2006;24(Suppl 3):37–40.
67. Sutherland L, MacDonald JK. Oral 5-aminosalicylic acid for induction of remission in ulcerative colitis. Cochrane Database Syst Rev 2006;(2):CD000543.
68. Hanauer SB, Sandborn WJ, Kornbluth A, et al. Delayed-release oral mesalamine 4.8 g/day (800 mg tablet) versus 2.4 g/day (400 mg tablet) for treatment of moderately active ulcerative colitis: Combined analysis of two randomized, double blind, controlled trials. Gastroenterology 2005;128:A75.
69. Hanauer SB, Sandborn WJ, Kornbluth A, et al. Delayed-release oral mesalamine 4.8 g/day (800 mg tablet) for treatment of moderately active ulcerative colitis. The ASCEND II Trial. Am J Gastroenterol 2005;100:2478–2485.
70. Sandborn WJ. Rational selection of oral 5-aminosalicylate formulations and prodrugs for the treatment of ulcerative colitis [editorial]. Am J Gastroenterol 2002;97(12):2939–2941.
71. Pruitt R, Hanson J, Safdi M, et al. Balsalazide is superior to mesalamine in the time to improvement of signs and symptoms of acute mild-to-moderate ulcerative colitis. Am J Gastroenterol 2002;97:3078–3086.
72. American Gastroenterological Association Institute technical review on corticosteroids, immunomodulators, and infliximab in inflammatory bowel disease. Gastroenterology 2006;130;940–987.
73. Lawson MM, Thomas AG, Akobeng AK. Tumour necrosis factor alpha blocking agents for induction of remission in ulcerative colitis. Cochrane Database Syst Rev 2006;(3):CD005112.
74. Rutgeerts P, Sandborn WJ, Feagan BG, et al. Infliximab for induction and maintenance therapy for ulcerative colitis. N Engl J Med 2005;353;2462–2476.
75. Janerot G, Hertervig E, Friis-Liby I, et al. Infliximab as rescue therapy in severe to moderately severe ulcerative colitis: A randomized, placebo controlled study. Gastroenterology 2005;128:1805–1811.
76. Regueiro M, Curtis J, Plevy S. Infliximab for hospitalized patients with severe ulcerative colitis. J Clin Gastroenterol 2006;40:476–481.
77. McGrath J,McDonald JWD, MacDonald JK. Transdermal nicotine for induction of remission in ulcerative colitis. Cochrane Database Syst Rev 2004;(4):CD004722.
78. Shibolet O, Regushevskaya E, Brezis M, Soares-Weiser K. Cyclosporine A for induction of remission in severe ulcerative colitis. Cochrane Database Syst Rev 2005;(1):CD004277.
79. D'Haens G, Lemmens L, Geboes K, et al. Intravenous cyclosporine versus corticosteroids as single therapy for severe attacks of ulcerative colitis. Gastroenterology 2001;120:1323–1329.
80. Sutherland L, MacDonald JK. Oral 5-aminosalicylic acid for maintenance of remission in ulcerative colitis. Cochrane Database Syst Rev 2006;(2):CD000544.
81. Holtmann MH, Krummenauer F, Claas C, et al. Long-term effectiveness of azathioprine in IBD beyond 4 years: A European multicenter study in 1176 patients. Dig Dis Sci 2006;51:1516–1524.
82. Gionchetti P. Conventional therapy for Crohn's disease. World J Gastroenterol 2006;12:4794–4806.
83. Sandborn WJ. Evidenced based treatment algorithm for mild to moderate Crohn's disease. Am J Gastroenterol 2003;98:S1–S5.
84. Otley A, Steinhart AH. Budesonide for induction of remission in Crohn's disease. Cochrane Database Syst Rev 2005;(4):CD000296.
85. AGA Technical review on perianal Crohn's Disease. Gastroenterology 2003;125:1508–1530.
86. Sandborn W, Sutherland L, Pearson D, May G, Modigliani R, Prantera C. Azathioprine or 6-mercaptopurine for induction of remission in Crohn's disease. Cochrane Database Syst Rev 2000;(3):CD000545.
87. Dubinsky MC, Lamothe S, Yang HY, et al. Pharmacogenomics and metabolite measurement for 6-mercaptopurine therapy in inflammatory bowel disease. Gastroenterology 2000;18:705–713.
88. Alfadhli AAF, McDonald JWD, Feagan BG. Methotrexate for induction of remission in refractory Crohn's disease. Cochrane Database Syst Rev 2004;(4):CD003459.
89. Kamm MA. Review article: Biological drugs in Crohn's disease. Aliment Pharmacol Ther 2006;24(Suppl 3):80–89.
90. Bressler B, Sands BE. Review article: Medical therapy for fistulizing Crohn's disease. Aliment Pharmacol Ther 2006;24:1283–1293.
91. Duburque C, Lelong J, Iacob R, et al. Successful induction of tolerance to infliximab in patients with Crohn's disease and prior severe infusion reactions. Aliment Pharmacol Ther 2006;24:851–858.
92. McDonald JWD, Feagan BG, Jewell D, Brynskov J, Stange EF, MacDonald JK. Cyclosporine for induction of remission in Crohn's disease. Cochrane Database Syst Rev 2005;(2):CD000297.
93. Akobeng AK, Gardener E. Oral 5-aminosalicylic acid for maintenance of medically-induced remission in Crohn's disease. Cochrane Database Syst Rev 2005;(1):CD003715.
94. Feagan BG. Maintenance therapy for inflammatory bowel disease. Am J Gastroenterol 2003;98:S6–S17.
95. Lemann M. Review article: Can post-operative recurrence in Crohn's disease be prevented? Aliment Pharm Ther 2006;24(Suppl 3):22–28.
96. Steinhart AH, Ewe K, Griffiths AM, Modigliani R, Thomsen OO. Corticosteroids for maintenance of remission in Crohn's disease. Cochrane Database Syst Rev 2003;(4):CD000301.
97. Simms L, Steinhart AH. Budesonide for maintenance of remission in Crohn's disease. Cochrane Database Syst Rev 2001;(1):CD002913.
98. Hanauer SB, Sandborn WJ, Rutgeerts P, et al. Adalimumab for maintenance treatment of Crohn's disease: Results of the C1ASSIC-II trial. Gut 2007;56:1232–1239.

99. Colombel J, Sanborn WJ, Rutgeerts P, et al. Adalimumab for maintenance of clinical response and remission in patients with Crohn's disease: The CHARM trial. Gastroenterology 2007;132:52–65.
100. Lemann M, Mary J-Y, Duclos B, et al. Infliximab plus azathioprine for steroid dependent Crohn's disease patients. Gastroenterology 2006; 130:1054–1061.
101. Travis S. Infliximab and azathioprine: Bridge or parachute? [editorial]. Gastroenterology 2006;130(4):1354–1357.
102. American Gastroenterological Association medical position statement: Guidelines on osteoporosis in gastrointestinal diseases. Gastroenterology 2003;124:791–794.
103. Padovan M, Castellino G, Govoni M, Trotta F. The treat of the rheumatological manifestations of the inflammatory bowel diseases. Rheumatol Int 2006;26:953–958.
104. Steinlauf AF, Present DH. Medical management of the pregnant patient with inflammatory bowel disease. Gastroenterol Clin North Am 2004;33:361–385.
105. Ferrero S, Ragni N. Inflammatory bowel disease: Management issues during pregnancy. Arch Gynecol Obstet 2004;270:79–85.
106. Navarro F, Hanauer SB. Treatment of inflammatory bowel disease: Safety and tolerability issues. Am J Gastroenterol 2003;98(Suppl 12):S18–S23.
107. Kung SJ, Choudhary C, McGeady SJ, Cohn JR. Lack of cross-reactivity between 5-aminosalicylic acid-based drugs: A case report and review of the literature. Ann All Asthma Immunol 2006;97:284–287.
108. Warman JI, Korelitz BI, Fleisher MR, Janardhanam R. Cumulative experience with short- and long-term toxicity to 6-mercaptopurine in the treatment of Crohn's disease and ulcerative colitis. J Clin Gastroenterol 2003;37:220–225.
109. Kane S, Dixon L. Adherence rates with infliximab therapy in Crohn's disease. Aliment Pharmcol Ther 2006;24:1099–1103.
110. Sostegni R, Daperno M, Scaglione N. Review article: Crohn's disease: Monitoring disease activity. Aliment Pharmacol Ther 2006;17(Suppl 2):11–17.
111. Best WR, Becktel JM, Singleton JW, et al. Development of a Crohn's disease activity index. Gastroenterology 1976;70:439–444.
112. Sanborn WJ, Tremaine WJ, Schroeder KW, et al. Cyclosporine enemas for treatment-resistant, mildly to moderately active, left-sided ulcerative colitis. Am J Gastroenterol 1993;88:640–645.
113. Irvine EJ, Zhou Q, Thompson AK. The short inflammatory bowel disease questionnaire: A quality of life instrument for community physicians managing inflammatory bowel disease. CERPT investigators. Canadian Crohn's Relapse Prevention Trial. Am J Gastroenterol 1996;91:1571–1578.
114. Lichtenstein GR, Yan S, Balla M, Hanauer S. Remission in patients with Crohn's disease is associated with improvement in employment and quality of life and a decrease in hospitalizations and surgeries. Am J Gastroenterol 2004;99:91–96.
115. Rubenstein JH, Chong RY, Cohen RD. Infliximab decreases resource use among patients with Crohn's disease. J Clin Gastroenterol 2002;35:151–156.

CHAPTER 37

Nausea and Vomiting

CECILY V. DIPIRO

KEY CONCEPTS

1. Nausea and/or vomiting may be a part of the symptom complex for a variety of gastrointestinal, cardiovascular, infectious, neurologic, metabolic, or psychogenic processes.
2. Nausea or vomiting may be caused by a variety of medications or other noxious agents.
3. The overall goal of treatment should be to prevent or eliminate nausea and vomiting regardless of etiology.
4. Treatment options for nausea and vomiting include drug and nondrug modalities such as relaxation, biofeedback, and self-hypnosis.
5. The primary goal with chemotherapy-induced nausea and vomiting (CINV) is to *prevent* nausea and/or vomiting. Optimal control of acute nausea and vomiting positively impacts the incidence and control of delayed and anticipatory nausea and vomiting.
6. The emetic risk of the chemotherapeutic regimen is the primary factor to consider when selecting prophylactic antiemetics for CINV.
7. Patients at high risk of vomiting should receive prophylactic antiemetics for postoperative nausea and vomiting (PONV).
8. Patients receiving single-exposure, high-dose radiation therapy to the upper abdomen or receiving total or hemibody irradiation, should receive prophylactic antiemetics for radiation-induced nausea and vomiting (RINV).

Nausea and vomiting are common complaints among many individuals with gastrointestinal (GI) disorders. However, because of the variable etiologies of these problems, management can be quite simple or detailed and complex, essentially innocuous or associated with therapy-induced adverse reactions. This chapter provides an overview of nausea and vomiting, two multifaceted problems.

Nausea is usually defined as the inclination to vomit or as a feeling in the throat or epigastric region alerting an individual that vomiting is imminent. Vomiting is defined as the ejection or expulsion of gastric contents through the mouth and is often a forceful event. Either condition may occur transiently with no other associated signs or symptoms; however, these conditions also may be only part of a more complex clinical presentation.

Learning objectives, review questions, and other resources can be found at **www.pharmacotherapyonline.com.**

ETIOLOGY

1 Nausea and vomiting may be associated with a variety of clinical presentations. In addition to GI diseases, either or both may accompany cardiovascular, infectious, neurologic, or metabolic disease processes. Nausea and vomiting may be a feature of such conditions as pregnancy, or may follow operative procedures or administration of certain medications, such as those used in cancer chemotherapy. Psychogenic etiologies of these symptoms may be present, especially in young women with an underlying emotional disturbance. Anticipatory etiologies may be involved, such as in patients who have previously received cytotoxic chemotherapy. Table 37–1 lists specific etiologies associated with nausea and vomiting.[1]

In addition to identifying conditions associated with nausea and vomiting, it is important to address the specific causative medical problems. For example, nausea and vomiting may occur in as many as 70% of patients with inferior myocardial infarction or diabetic ketoacidosis. Eighty percent to 90% of patients with an Addisonian crisis, acute pancreatitis, or acute appendicitis may present with nausea and vomiting.

The etiology of nausea and vomiting may vary with the age of the patient. For example, vomiting in the newborn during the first day of life suggests upper digestive tract obstruction or an increase in intracranial pressure. Other illnesses associated with vomiting in children include pyloric stenosis, duodenal ulcer, stress ulcer, adrenal insufficiency, septicemia, and diseases of the pancreas, liver, or biliary tree. Also, the hepatocellular failure seen in Reye syndrome may lead to profound cerebral edema followed by persistent emesis. A common etiology of vomiting in children is viral gastroenteritis caused by rotavirus. Vomiting in infants may be associated with something as simple as overfeeding, rapid feeding, inadequate burping, or lying down too soon after feeding. These types of vomiting are usually indicative of minor problems and may be altered by changing the approach to feeding.

2 Drug-induced nausea and vomiting are of particular concern, especially with the increasing number of patients receiving cytotoxic treatment. A four-level classification system defines the risk for emesis with specific cytotoxic agents (Table 37–2).[2] Although some agents may have greater emetic risk than others, combinations of agents, high doses, clinical settings, psychological conditions, prior treatment experiences, and unusual stimulus of sight, smell, or taste may alter a patient's response to drug treatment. In this setting, nausea and vomiting may be unavoidable and some patients experience these problems so intensely that chemotherapy is postponed or discontinued. In addition to the emetic risk of various cytotoxic regimens, a variety of other common etiologies have been proposed for the development of nausea and vomiting in cancer patients (Table 37–3).[3,4]

TABLE 37-1 Specific Etiologies of Nausea and Vomiting

Gastrointestinal mechanisms
Mechanical obstruction
Gastric outlet obstruction
Small bowel obstruction
Functional gastrointestinal disorders
Gastroparesis
Nonulcer dyspepsia
Chronic intestinal pseudoobstruction
Irritable bowel syndrome
Organic gastrointestinal disorders
Peptic ulcer disease
Pancreatitis
Pyelonephritis
Cholecystitis
Cholangitis
Hepatitis
Acute gastroenteritis
Viral
Bacterial
Cardiovascular diseases
Acute myocardial infarction
Congestive heart failure
Radiofrequency ablation
Neurologic processes
Increased intracranial pressure
Migraine headache
Vestibular disorders
Metabolic disorders
Diabetes mellitus (diabetic ketoacidosis)
Addison disease
Renal disease (uremia)
Psychiatric causes
Psychogenic vomiting
Anxiety disorders
Anorexia nervosa
Therapy-induced causes
Cytotoxic chemotherapy
Radiation therapy
Theophylline preparations
Anticonvulsant preparations
Digitalis preparations
Opiates
Antibiotics
Drug withdrawal
Opiates
Benzodiazepines
Miscellaneous causes
Pregnancy
Noxious odors
Operative procedures

Reprinted and adapted from Hasler WL, Chey WD. Gastroenterology, 2003, Vol. 25, 1860–1867.

TABLE 37-2 Emetic Risk of Intravenous Cytotoxic Agents

Emetic Risk (If No Prophylactic Medication is Administered)	Cytotoxic Agent (in Alphabetical Order)
High (>90%)	Carmustine
	Cisplatin
	Cyclophosphamide ≥1,500 mg/m^2
	Dacarbazine
	Dactinomycin
	Mechlorethamine
	Streptozotocin
Moderate (30% to 90%)	Carboplatin
	Cytarabine >1 g/m^2
	Cyclophosphamide <1,500 mg/m^2
	Daunorubicin
	Doxorubicin
	Epirubicin
	Idarubicin
	Ifosfamide
	Irinotecan
	Oxaliplatin
Low (10% to 30%)	Bortezomib
	Cetuximab
	Cytarabine ≤1 g/m^2
	Docetaxel
	Etoposide
	Fluorouracil
	Gemcitabine
	Methotrexate
	Mitomycin
	Mitoxantrone
	Paclitaxel
	Pemetrexed
	Topotecan
	Trastuzumab
Minimal (<10%)	Bevacizumab
	Bleomycin
	Busulfan
	2-Chlorodeoxyadenosine
	Fludarabine
	Rituximab
	Vinblastine
	Vincristine
	Vinorelbine

Adapted from Results of the 2004 Perugia International Antiemetic Consensus Conference.[2]

PATHOPHYSIOLOGY

The three consecutive phases of emesis include nausea, retching, and vomiting. Nausea, the imminent need to vomit, is associated with gastric stasis and may be considered a separate and singular symptom. Retching is the labored movement of abdominal and thoracic muscles before vomiting. The final phase of emesis is vomiting, the forceful expulsion of gastric contents caused by GI retroperistalsis. The act of vomiting requires the coordinated contractions of the abdominal muscles, pylorus, and antrum, a raised gastric cardia, diminished lower esophageal sphincter pressure, and esophageal dilatation.[5] Vomiting should not be confused with regurgitation, an act in which the gastric or esophageal contents rise to the pharynx because of pressure differences caused by, for example, an incompetent lower esophageal sphincter. Accompanying autonomic symptoms of pallor, tachycardia, and diaphoresis account for many of the distressing feelings associated with emesis.

Vomiting is triggered by afferent impulses to the vomiting center, a nucleus of cells in the medulla. Impulses are received from sensory centers, such as the chemoreceptor trigger zone (CTZ), cerebral cortex, and visceral afferents from the pharynx and GI tract. When excited, afferent impulses are integrated by the vomiting center, resulting in efferent impulses to the salivation center, respiratory center, and the pharyngeal, GI, and abdominal muscles, leading to vomiting.

The CTZ, located in the area postrema of the fourth ventricle of the brain, is a major chemosensory organ for emesis and is usually associated with chemically induced vomiting. Because of its location, bloodborne and cerebrospinal fluid toxins have easy access to the CTZ. Therefore, cytotoxic agents primarily stimulate this area rather than the cerebral cortex and visceral afferents. Similarly, pregnancy-associated vomiting probably occurs through stimulation of the CTZ.

Numerous neurotransmitter receptors are located in the vomiting center, CTZ, and GI tract, including cholinergic, histaminic, dopaminergic, opiate, serotonergic, neurokinin, and benzodiazepine receptors. Chemotherapeutic agents, their metabolites, or other emetic compounds theoretically trigger the process of emesis through stimulation of one or more of these receptors. Effective antiemetics are able to antagonize or block the emetogenic receptors.

TABLE 37-3 Nonchemotherapy Etiologies of Nausea and Vomiting in Cancer Patients

Fluid and electrolyte abnormalities
Hypercalcemia
Volume depletion
Water intoxication
Adrenocortical insufficiency
Drug induced
Opiates
Antibiotics
Antifungals
Gastrointestinal obstruction
Increased intracranial pressure
Peritonitis
Metastases
Brain
Meninges
Hepatic
Uremia
Infections (septicemia, local)
Radiation therapy

From Stephenson and Davies,[3] and American Society of Health-System.[4]

CLINICAL PRESENTATION

Because it is impossible to discuss all clinical settings in which the presence of nausea and vomiting might be a pertinent finding, these processes are presented in Table 37–4 as they might occur together, and also as *simple* or *complex* in presentation.

TREATMENT

Nausea and Vomiting

DESIRED OUTCOME

❸ The overall goal of antiemetic therapy is to prevent or eliminate nausea and vomiting. This should be accomplished without adverse effects or with clinically acceptable adverse effects. Although this goal may be accomplished easily in patients with simple nausea and vomiting, patients with more complex problems require greater assistance. In addition to these clinical goals, appropriate cost issues should be considered, particularly in the management of chemotherapy-induced and postoperative nausea and vomiting.

TABLE 37-4 Presentation of Nausea and Vomiting

General
Depending on severity of symptoms, patients may present in mild to severe distress
Symptoms
Simple: Self-limiting, resolves spontaneously and requires only symptomatic therapy
Complex: Not relieved after administration of antiemetics; progressive deterioration of patient secondary to fluid–electrolyte imbalances; usually associated with noxious agents or psychogenic events
Signs
Simple: Patient complaint of queasiness or discomfort
Complex: Weight loss; fever; abdominal pain
Laboratory tests
Simple: None
Complex: Serum electrolyte concentrations; upper/lower GI evaluation
Other information
Fluid input and output
Medication history
Recent history of behavioral or visual changes, headache, pain, or stress
Family history positive for psychogenic vomiting

GENERAL APPROACH TO TREATMENT

❹ Treatment options for nausea and vomiting include drug and nondrug modalities. The treatment of nausea and vomiting is quite varied depending on the associated medical situation. Even though a number of potentially effective measures are available, most patients receive a medication at some point in their care. For simple nausea and vomiting, patients may choose to do nothing or to select from a variety of nonprescription drugs. As symptoms become worse or are associated with more serious medical problems, patients are more likely to benefit from prescription antiemetic drugs. When prescribed according to reliable clinical information, these agents often provide acceptable relief; however, some patients will never be totally free of symptoms. This lack of relief is most disabling when it is associated with an unresolved medical problem or when the necessary therapy for this condition is the cause of the nausea or vomiting, as in the case of patients who are receiving chemotherapy of moderate or high emetic risk.

NONPHARMACOLOGIC MANAGEMENT

Nonpharmacologic management of nausea and vomiting may include a variety of dietary, physical, or psychological changes consistent with the etiology of symptoms. For patients with simple complaints, perhaps resulting from excessive or disagreeable food or beverage consumption, avoidance or moderation in dietary intake may be preferable. Patients suffering symptoms of systemic illness may improve dramatically as their underlying condition resolves. Finally, patients in whom these symptoms result from labyrinthine changes produced by motion may benefit quickly by assuming a stable physical position.

Cancer patients who are undergoing chemotherapy may experience nausea and/or vomiting despite receiving prophylactic antiemetics. Anticipatory nausea or vomiting rarely occurs unless the patient has previously experienced posttreatment nausea or vomiting, suggesting that the mechanism for anticipatory nausea and vomiting is a learned process involving elements of classic conditioning.[6] This conditioning model may also be important in understanding the development of pregnancy-related nausea. Nonpharmacologic interventions are classified as behavioral interventions and include relaxation, biofeedback, self-hypnosis, cognitive distraction, guided imagery, and systematic desensitization.[7,8]

The management of psychogenic vomiting is greatly dependent on psychological intervention. However, because the underlying problems are so complex and intertwined in personal relationships, psychological therapy may require lengthy, in-depth treatment. Pharmacologic therapy offers only minimal benefit in these patients. Surgery, such as gastroenterostomy, is of no value.

PHARMACOLOGIC THERAPY

❹ Although many approaches to the treatment of nausea and vomiting have been suggested, antiemetic drugs (nonprescription and prescription) are most often recommended. These agents represent a variety of pharmacologic and chemical classes, as well as dosage regimens and routes of administration. With so many treatment possibilities available, factors that enable the clinician to discriminate among various choices include (a) the suspected etiology of the symptoms; (b) the frequency, duration, and severity of the episodes; (c) the ability of the patient to use oral, rectal, injectable, or transdermal medications; and (d) the success of previous antiemetic medications. Table 37–5 gives information concerning commonly available antiemetic preparations.

The treatment of simple nausea and vomiting usually requires minimal therapy. For these symptoms, patients may choose from a lengthy list of nonprescription products. Both nonprescription and

TABLE 37-5 Common Antiemetic Preparations and Adult Dosage Regimens

Drug	Adult Dosage Regimen	Dosage Form/Route	Availability
Antacids			
Antacids (various)	15–30 mL every 2–4 h prn	Liquid	OTC
Histamine (H_2) antagonists			
Cimetidine (Tagamet HB)	200 mg twice daily prn	Tab	OTC
Famotidine (Pepcid AC)	10 mg twice daily prn	Tab	OTC
Nizatidine (Axid AR)	75 mg twice daily prn	Tab	OTC
Ranitidine (Zantac 75)	75 mg twice daily prn	Tab	OTC
Antihistaminic–anticholinergic agents			
Cyclizine (Marezine)	50 mg before departure; may repeat in 4–6 h prn	Tab	OTC
Dimenhydrinate (Dramamine)	50–100 mg every 4–6 h prn	Tab, chew tab, cap	OTC
Diphenhydramine (Benadryl)	25–50 mg every 4–6 h prn	Tab, cap, liquid	Rx/OTC
	10–50 mg every 2 to 4 h prn	IM, IV	
Hydroxyzine (Vistaril, Atarax)	25–100 mg every 4–6 h prn	IM (unlabeled use)	Rx
Meclizine (Bonine, Antivert)	12.5–25 mg 1 h before travel; repeat every 12–24 h prn	Tab, chew tab	Rx/OTC
Scopolamine (Transderm Scop)	1.5 mg every 72 h	Transdermal patch	Rx
Trimethobenzamide (Tigan)	300 mg three to four times daily	Cap	Rx
	200 mg three to four times daily	IM, supp	
Phenothiazines			
Chlorpromazine (Thorazine)	10–25 mg every 4–6 h prn	Tab, liquid	Rx
	25–50 mg every 4–6 h prn	IM, IV	
Prochlorperazine (Compazine)	5–10 mg three to four times daily prn	Tab, liquid	
	5–10 mg every 3 to 4 h prn	IM	Rx
	2.5–10 mg every 3 to 4 h prn	IV	Rx
	25 mg twice daily prn	Supp	Rx
Promethazine (Phenergan)	12.5–25 mg every 4–6 h prn	Tab, liquid, IM, IV, supp	Rx
Thiethylperazine (Torecan)	10 mg one to six times daily prn	Tab, IM, IV	Rx
Cannabinoids			
Dronabinol (Marinol)	5–15 mg/m^2 every 2–4 h prn	Cap	Rx (C-III)
Nabilone (Cesamet)	1–2 mg twice daily	Cap	Rx (C-II)
Butyrophenones			
Haloperidol (Haldol)	1–5 mg every 12 h prn	Tab, liquid, IM, IV	Rx
Droperidol (Inapsine)[a]	2.5 mg; additional 1.25 mg may be given	IM, IV	Rx
Benzodiazepines			
Alprazolam (Xanax)	0.5–2 mg three times per day prior to chemotherapy	Tab	Rx (C-IV)
Lorazepam (Ativan)	0.5–2 mg on night before and morning of chemotherapy	Tab	Rx (C-IV)
Miscellaneous agents			
Metoclopramide (Reglan), for delayed CINV	20–40 mg three to four times daily	Tab	Rx

C-II, C-III, C-IV, controlled substance schedule 2, 3, and 4, respectively; cap, capsule; chew tab, chewable tablet; CINV, chemotherapy-induced nausea and vomiting; liquid, oral syrup, concentrate, or suspension; OTC, nonprescription; Rx, prescription; supp, rectal suppository; tab, tablet.

[a]See text for current warnings.

prescription drugs useful in the treatment of simple nausea and vomiting are usually effective in small, infrequently administered doses. Side effects and toxic effects in these settings are also usually minimal. Although suitable for occasional simple nausea and vomiting, nonprescription agents are often abandoned by the patient as symptoms continue or become progressively worse. As the patient's condition warrants, prescription medications may be chosen, either as single-agent therapy or in combination.

The management of complex nausea and vomiting, for example, in patients who are receiving cytotoxic chemotherapy, may require combination therapy. In combination regimens, the goal is to achieve symptomatic control through administration of agents with different pharmacologic mechanisms of action.

■ ANTACIDS

Patients who are experiencing simple nausea and vomiting may use various antacids. In this setting, single or combination nonprescription antacid products, especially those containing magnesium hydroxide, aluminum hydroxide, and/or calcium carbonate, may provide sufficient relief, primarily through gastric acid neutralization.

Common antacid regimens for the relief of acute or intermittent nausea and vomiting include one or more 15 to 30 mL doses of single- or multiple-agent products. Potential adverse effects from antacids are usually related to the presence of magnesium, aluminum, or calcium salts. Specifically, osmotic diarrhea from magnesium and constipation from aluminum or calcium salts may be of concern to patients, particularly those self-medicating with high or frequently administered antacid doses. Generally, however, when used occasionally for acute episodic relief of nausea and vomiting, antacids do not produce serious toxicities.

■ H_2-RECEPTOR ANTAGONISTS

Patients may use histamine$_2$-receptor antagonists in low doses to manage simple nausea and vomiting associated with heartburn or gastroesophageal reflux. Individual dosages of cimetidine 200 mg, famotidine 10 mg, nizatidine 75 mg, or ranitidine 75 mg may be used for brief periods. Except for potential drug interactions with cimetidine, these agents cause few side effects when used for episodic relief.

■ ANTIHISTAMINE–ANTICHOLINERGIC DRUGS

Antiemetic drugs from the antihistaminic–anticholinergic category appear to interrupt various visceral afferent pathways that stimulate nausea and vomiting and may be appropriate in the treatment of simple nausea and vomiting. Adverse reactions associated with the use of the antihistaminic–anticholinergic agents primarily include drowsiness, confusion, blurred vision, dry mouth, and urinary retention, and possibly tachycardia, particularly in elderly patients. Also, as doses are increased or are more frequently administered, patients with narrow-angle glaucoma, prostatic hyperplasia, or asthma are at greater risk of complications from the anticholinergic effects of these drugs.

■ PHENOTHIAZINES

Phenothiazines have been the most widely prescribed antiemetic agents and appear to block dopamine receptors, most likely in the CTZ. Phenothiazines are marketed in an array of dosage forms, none of which appears to be more efficacious than another. These agents may be most practical for long-term treatment and are inexpensive in comparison with newer drugs. Rectal administration is a reasonable alternative in patients in whom oral or parenteral administration is not feasible.

Phenothiazines are most useful in adult patients with simple nausea and vomiting. Intravenous prochlorperazine provides quicker and more complete relief with less drowsiness than intravenous promethazine in adult patients treated in an emergency department for nausea and vomiting associated with uncomplicated gastritis or gastroenteritis.[9] There are numerous potential side effects with these medications, including extrapyramidal reactions, hypersensitivity reactions with possible liver dysfunction, bone marrow aplasia, and excessive sedation.

■ BUTYROPHENONES

Two butyrophenone compounds that have antiemetic activity are haloperidol and its congener droperidol; both block dopaminergic stimulation of the CTZ. Although each agent is effective in relieving nausea and vomiting, haloperidol is not considered first-line therapy for uncomplicated nausea and vomiting but has been used in palliative care situations.[10] The current labeling of droperidol recommends that all patients should undergo a 12-lead electrocardiogram prior to administration, followed by cardiac monitoring for 2 to 3 hours after administration because of the possibility of the development of potentially fatal QT prolongation and/or torsade de pointes.[11] The clinical use of droperidol has effectively ceased outside of clinical trials in anesthesia.

■ CORTICOSTEROIDS

Corticosteroids have demonstrated antiemetic efficacy since the initial recognition that patients who received prednisone as part of their Hodgkin disease protocol appeared to develop less nausea and vomiting than did those patients who were treated with protocols that excluded this agent. Methylprednisolone has also been used as a component of an antiemetic regimen, but the majority of trials have included dexamethasone.

Dexamethasone has been used successfully in the management of chemotherapy-induced and postoperative nausea and vomiting, either as a single agent or in combination with selective serotonin reuptake inhibitors (SSRIs). For chemotherapy-induced nausea and vomiting (CINV), dexamethasone is effective in the prevention of both cisplatin-induced acute emesis and when used alone or in combination for the prevention of delayed nausea and vomiting associated with CINV.[12–15] For patients with simple nausea and vomiting, steroids are not indicated and may be associated with unacceptable risks.

■ METOCLOPRAMIDE

Metoclopramide, procainamide's congener, provides significant antiemetic effects by blocking the dopaminergic receptors centrally in the CTZ. Metoclopramide increases lower esophageal sphincter tone, aids gastric emptying, and accelerates transit through the small bowel, possibly through the release of acetylcholine. Metoclopramide is used for its antiemetic properties in patients with diabetic gastroparesis and with dexamethasone for prophylaxis of delayed nausea and vomiting associated with chemotherapy administration. Its use as prophylaxis for acute chemotherapy-induced nausea and vomiting was supplanted by the introduction of the SSRIs in the early 1990s. These agents have greater efficacy and decreased toxicity compared with metoclopramide in patients who are receiving cisplatin-based regimens.[16,17]

■ CANNABINOIDS

Thirty randomized, controlled trials from 1975 to 1996 were analyzed to quantify the antiemetic efficacy and adverse effects of cannabis when given to 1,366 patients who received chemotherapy.[18] Oral nabilone, oral dronabinol, and intramuscular levonantradol were compared with conventional antiemetics (prochlorperazine, metoclopramide, chlorpromazine, thiethylperazine, haloperidol, domperidone, and alizapride) or placebo. Across all trials, cannabinoids were slightly more effective than active comparators and placebo when the chemotherapy regimen was of moderate emetogenic potential, and patients preferred them. No dose–response relationships were evident to the authors. The cannabinoids were also more toxic; side effects included euphoria, drowsiness, sedation, somnolence, dysphoria, depression, hallucinations, and paranoia. The efficacy of cannabinoids as compared to SSRIs has not been studied. Use of these agents should be considered when other regimens do not provide desired efficacy.

■ SUBSTANCE P/NEUROKININ 1 RECEPTOR ANTAGONISTS

Substance P is a peptide neurotransmitter in the neurokinin (NK) family whose preferred receptor is the NK_1 receptor.[19] The acute phase of CINV is believed to be mediated by both serotonin and substance P, whereas substance P is believed to be the primary mediator of the delayed phase. Aprepitant is the first substance P/NK_1 receptor antagonist in clinical use; others are in development. The efficacy of aprepitant was demonstrated in patients receiving high-dose cisplatin-based chemotherapy[14,15] and in patients receiving doxorubicin and cycophosphamide,[20] a regimen of moderate emetic risk. The three-drug regimen of aprepitant, dexamethasone, and ondansetron provided improved protection from vomiting for the 5 days after chemotherapy administration as compared with the combination of dexamethasone and ondansetron.

Aprepitant has the potential for numerous drug interactions because it is a substrate, moderate inhibitor, and an inducer of cytochrome isoenzyme CYP3A4 and an inducer of CYP2C9. Aprepitant can increase serum concentrations of many drugs metabolized by CYP3A4, including docetaxel, paclitaxel, etoposide, irinotecan, ifosfamide, imatinib, vinorelbine, vincristine, and vinblastine. In clinical studies, aprepitant was concomitantly administered with etoposide, vinorelbine, or paclitaxel, with no adjustment in the doses of these agents to account for potential drug interactions. The efficacy of oral contraceptives may be reduced when given with aprepitant. Concomitant administration with warfarin may result in a clinically significant decrease in the international normalized ratio.[21] The dose of oral dexamethasone should be reduced 50% when coadministered with aprepitant, because of the 2.2-fold increase in observed area under the plasma-concentration-versus-time curve.[22] Aprepitant is not approved for use in children.

■ SELECTIVE SEROTONIN REUPTAKE INHIBITORS

SSRIs block presynaptic serotonin receptors on sensory vagal fibers in the gut wall, effectively blocking the acute phase of CINV. These agents do not completely block the acute phase of CINV and are less efficacious in preventing the delayed phase, but they are the standard of care in the management of chemotherapy-induced, radiation-induced, and postoperative nausea and vomiting. Issues involved in the use of dolasetron, granisetron, ondansetron, and palonosetron are reviewed in detail in the sections that follow. The most common side effects associated with these agents are constipation, headache, and asthenia. Safety and efficacy in children younger than 2 years old have not been established.

CHEMOTHERAPY-INDUCED NAUSEA AND VOMITING

5 Nausea and vomiting that occurs within 24 hours of chemotherapy administration is defined as acute, whereas when it starts more than 24 hours after chemotherapy administration, it is defined as delayed. The primary goal with CINV is to *prevent* nausea and/or vomiting. Optimal control of acute nausea and vomiting positively impacts the incidence and control of delayed and anticipatory nausea and vomiting. Clinical practice guidelines for the use of antiemetics in CINV have been published.[2,23,24] Despite the availability of these practice guidelines, product availability and recommended doses are institution-specific and may vary considerably from the doses listed in Table 37–6.

Factors to consider when selecting an antiemetic for CINV include the following:

- The emetic risk of the chemotherapy agent or regimen (see Table 37–2).
- Patient-specific factors.
- Patterns of emesis after administration of specific chemotherapy agents or regimens.

Prophylaxis of CINV

6 The emetic risk of the chemotherapeutic agent (see Table 37–2) is the primary factor to consider when deciding whether to administer prophylactic agents and which antiemetic(s) to select. Tables 37–6 and 37–7 summarize recommendations from the updated American Society of Clinical Oncology (ASCO) antiemetic guidelines.[23] Antiemetic guidelines published by other groups are in overall agreement with the ASCO guidelines. Minor differences reflect the volume of literature published and the varying doses studied.

Patients receiving chemotherapy that is classified as being of high emetic risk should receive a combination antiemetic regimen containing three drugs on the day of chemotherapy administration (day 1)—a SSRI (e.g., dolasetron, granisetron, ondansetron, or palonosetron) + dexamethasone + NK_1 inhibitor (e.g., aprepitant). Patients receiving regimens that are classified as being of moderate emetic risk should receive a combination antiemetic regimen containing a SSRI + dexamethasone on day 1. The exception to this is patients who are receiving an anthracycline plus cyclophosphamide; these patients should receive the triple-drug combination described for regimens of high emetic risk. Dexamethasone alone is recommended for prophylaxis prior to regimens of low emetic risk.

SSRIs are considered to be of equivalent efficacy and safety when equivalent doses are used for the prevention of acute emesis. When available in both oral and intravenous dosage forms, oral products are equally effective as intravenous products. The decision as to which SSRI to use should be based on patient-specific factors and cost.

TABLE 37-6 Recommendations for the Use of Antiemetics in Patients Receiving Chemotherapy

Emetic Risk	Prophylaxis of Acute Phase of CINV on Day of Chemotherapy Administration (Day 1)	Prophylaxis of Delayed Phase of CINV
High	SSRI + dexamethasone + aprepitant	Days 2 and 3 after chemotherapy: dexamethasone + aprepitant
Moderate	**Anthracycline + cyclophosphamide:**	
	SSRI + dexamethasone + aprepitant	Days 2 and 3 after chemotherapy: aprepitant
	All other regimens of moderate emetic risk:	Days 2–4 after chemotherapy: dexamethasone or SSRI
	SSRI + dexamethasone	
Low	Dexamethasone	None
Minimal	None	None

CINV, chemotherapy-induced nausea and vomiting; SSRI, selective serotonin reuptake inhibitor.

TABLE 37-7 Dosage Recommendations for CINV

Emetic Risk	Prophylaxis of Acute Phase of CINV (one dose administered prior to chemotherapy)	Prophylaxis of Delayed Phase of CINV
High	SSRI:	
	Dolasetron 100 mg PO or 100 mg IV or 1.8 mg/kg IV	
	Granisetron 2 mg PO or 1 mg IV or 0.01 mg/kg IV	
	Ondansetron 24 mg PO or 8 mg IV or 0.15 mg/kg IV	
	Palonosetron 0.25 mg IV	
	and Dexamethasone 12 mg PO (with aprepitant) or 20 mg PO	Dexamethasone 8 mg PO days 2 and 3 after chemotherapy
	and Aprepitant 125 mg PO	Aprepitant 80 mg PO days 2 and 3 after chemotherapy
Moderate	Anthracycline + cyclophosphamide:	
	SSRI: (as above)	
	and Dexamethasone 12 mg PO (with aprepitant)	
	and Aprepitant 125 mg PO	Aprepitant 80 mg PO days 2 and 3 after chemotherapy
	All other regimens of moderate emetic risk:	
	SSRI:	
	Dolasetron 100 mg PO or 100 mg IV or 1.8 mg/kg IV	SSRI: Dolasetron 100 mg PO daily[a]
	Granisetron 2 mg PO or 1 mg IV or 0.01 mg/kg IV	Granisetron 1 mg PO daily[a]
	Ondansetron 16 mg PO or 8 mg IV or 0.15 mg/kg IV	Ondansetron 8 mg PO daily or twice daily[a]
	Palonosetron 0.25 mg IV	
	and Dexamethasone 8 mg IV	or Dexamethasone 8 mg PO daily[a]
Low	Dexamethasone 8 mg PO	None
Minimal	None	None

CINV, chemotherapy-induced nausea and vomiting; SSRI, selective serotonin reuptake inhibitor.
[a]For 2–4 days following chemotherapy.
Doses included in the above table reflect the recommendations from published guidelines (refs. 3, 28, 29). These doses may differ from manufacturer labeling; they reflect the consensus of the guideline participants.

Treatment of CINV

Some patients who are receiving chemotherapy experience nausea and/or vomiting despite the use of multiagent prophylaxis. All patients receiving chemotherapy should have antiemetics available for rescue of breakthrough nausea and vomiting. Chlorpromazine, prochlorperazine, promethazine, methylprednisolone, lorazepam, metoclopramide, dexamethasone, and dronabinol can be used for adult patients. Around-the-clock dosing should be considered

TABLE 37-8 Risk Factors for Postoperative Nausea and Vomiting

Patient-specific factors
Female gender
Nonsmoking status
History of motion sickness/postoperative nausea and vomiting
Anesthetic risk factors
Use of volatile anesthetics
Nitrous oxide
Use of opioids (intraoperative or postoperative)
Surgical risk factors
Duration of surgery
Operative procedure (intraabdominal, ear-nose-throat, major gynecologic, orthopedic, or laparoscopic)

From Gan et al.[29]

rather than as-needed administration. The choice of agent should be based on patient-specific factors, including potential adverse drug reactions, and cost. Granisetron, dolasetron, and ondansetron are effective in the treatment of breakthrough nausea and vomiting, but they are not superior to the less expensive antiemetics listed above. Chlorpromazine, lorazepam, and methylprednisolone (or dexamethasone) are recommended for pediatric patients.

Prophylaxis of Delayed CINV

The best strategy to prevent delayed CINV—nausea and/or vomiting occurring 24 or more hours after chemotherapy—is to control acute CINV.[24] Aprepitant, dexamethasone and metoclopramide have demonstrated efficacy in preventing delayed CINV, whereas the results with SSRIs are inconsistent.[23]

Patients receiving cisplatin and other agents are at highest risk to experience delayed CINV. The addition of aprepitant in the recommended three-drug combination on the day of cisplatin administration and additional doses of aprepitant and dexamethasone on the 2 days after cisplatin administration improved the control of vomiting as compared with patients who received the dexamethasone alone postchemotherapy, the standard of care prior to the availability of aprepitant.[14,15] Current practice guidelines recommend administration of aprepitant and dexamethasone on the 2 days following the administration of chemotherapy of high emetic risk.[2,23]

The incidence of delayed CINV following chemotherapy agents of moderate emetic risk is less-well defined. The current recommendation is to give single-agent dexamethasone or an SSRI to patients in this group, except to patients who are receiving an anthracycline and cyclophosphamide for whom single-agent aprepitant is recommended for the 2 days following chemotherapy.[23] Other practice guidelines offer alternate recommendations for the prophylaxis of delayed CINV after regimens of moderate emetic risk.[2,24]

Management of delayed CINV has challenged practitioners. With the addition of aprepitant, the number of patients not experiencing delayed emesis after cisplatin chemotherapy increased from 51% to 72% as compared with dexamethasone,[14,15] and from 49% to 55% in patients receiving an anthracycline plus cyclophosphamide, as compared with twice-daily ondansetron,[20] but the problem has not been eliminated. The availability of palonosetron, an injectable SSRI with a prolonged serum half-life and higher receptor binding affinity, may offer another option for prophylaxis of delayed nausea and vomiting. Given once every 7 days,[25] palonosetron was found to protect more patients from delayed emesis than either ondansetron or dolasetron in adult patients receiving chemotherapy of moderate emetic risk,[26,27] but the studies were not designed to determine superiority.

CLINICAL CONTROVERSY

Is one SSRI more efficacious than another in preventing CINV associated with chemotherapy regimens of high emetic risk? Current practice guidelines[23] state that SSRIs have equivalent safety and efficacy and are interchangeable based on current literature. Triple-drug therapy that includes dexamethasone and aprepitant is the current standard of care, but head-to-head trials of palonosetron versus dolasetron or granisetron or ondansetron, in combination with dexamethasone and aprepitant, have not been reported.

POSTOPERATIVE NAUSEA AND VOMITING

Postoperative nausea and vomiting (PONV) complicates surgical procedures for approximately 25% to 30% of patients undergoing anesthesia.[28] Factors to be considered for PONV prophylaxis and treatment include risk factors, potential morbidity, potential adverse events associated with antiemetics, antiemetic efficacy, and costs. Most patients undergoing an operative procedure do not require preoperative prophylactic antiemetic therapy and universal PONV prophylaxis is not cost-effective. Table 37–8 summarizes the risk factors for PONV. Prophylaxis and treatment of PONV should adhere to consensus guidelines.[29] Other strategies to reduce baseline PONV risk factors among patients at highest risk, in addition to prophylactic antiemetics, include use of regional anesthesia, propofol, supplemental oxygen, and hydration, as well as avoiding nitrous oxide, volatile anesthetics, and opioids. Total intravenous anesthesia reduced the risk of PONV similar to the prophylactic administration of a single antiemetic.[30]

Prophylaxis of PONV

❼ Although the optimal management of PONV is not known, patients at highest risk of vomiting should receive prophylactic antiemetics. Patients at low risk for PONV are unlikely to benefit from prophylaxis and may potentially experience adverse reactions from the medications. Cyclizine, dexamethasone, dolasetron, droperidol, granisetron, metoclopramide, ondansetron, and tropisetron are effective as compared with placebo for the prophylaxis of PONV.[31] Table 37–9 summarizes the doses for prophylactic antiemetics from the consensus guidelines.[29] Patients at moderate risk for PONV should receive one prophylactic antiemetic, whereas those at high risk should receive two prophylactic antiemetic agents from different classes.[29,30] Optimal dosing of agents used in combination has not been determined.

TABLE 37-9 Recommended Prophylactic Doses of Antiemetics for Postoperative Nausea and Vomiting

Drug	Adult Dose (IV)	Pediatric Dose (IV)	Timing of Dose[a]
Dolasetron	12.5 mg	350 mcg/kg up to 12.5 mg	At end of surgery
Granisetron	0.35–1 mg		At end of surgery
Ondansetron	4–8 mg	50–100 mcg/kg up to 4 mg	At end of surgery
Tropisetron	5 mg		At end of surgery
Dexamethasone	5–10 mg	150 mcg/kg up to 8 mg	At induction
Droperidol	0.625–1.25 mg	50–70 mcg/kg up to 1.25 mg	At end of surgery

[a]Based on recommendations from consensus guidelines; may differ from manufacturer's recommendations.

From Gan et al.[29]

Dexamethasone is an effective, inexpensive prophylactic agent when administered either alone or in combination with other antiemetic drugs before the induction of anesthesia.[30–32] Droperidol is one of the most effective agents for PONV prophylaxis, but concerns about the development of torsade de pointes severely limit its use.[33] With equivalent efficacy and safety profiles, acquisition cost was the primary factor that differentiated the SSRIs from each other.[29] SSRIs are most effective when given at the end of surgery.

Aprepitant was recently approved for the prevention of PONV at a dose of 40 mg given orally within 3 hours prior to induction of anesthesia.[21] Whether it will be used as monotherapy or in combination with other prophylactic agents is yet to be determined.

Treatment of PONV

Most patients given a drug to prevent PONV will not benefit from it and 1 to 5 of every 100 patients given PONV prophylaxis may experience a mild adverse reaction such as headache, sedation, or dry mouth.[31] If a patient develops nausea and/or vomiting despite prophylaxis, treatment options are limited. Use of the same drug for treatment is ineffective when it was used for prophylaxis.[34]

SSRIs in doses of dolasetron 12.5 mg, granisetron 0.1 mg, ondansetron 1 mg or tropisetron 0.5 mg are recommended in patients who experience PONV despite prophylactic dexamethasone or when no prophylactic agent was used.[29] Treatment doses of SSRIs, when an SSRI was used as prophylaxis, are not recommended until 6 hours after surgery.[34] Patients who experience PONV after receiving prophylactic treatment with a SSRI plus dexamethasone should receive a rescue dose from a different drug class such as a phenothiazine or droperidol.[35]

■ RADIATION-INDUCED NAUSEA AND VOMITING (RINV)

Nausea and vomiting associated with radiation therapy is not well understood. It is neither as predictable nor as severe as CINV, and many patients receiving radiation therapy will not experience nausea or vomiting. Risk factors associated with the development of RINV include the site of radiation, the dose, dose rate, and area of the body to be irradiated.

❽ Patients receiving single-exposure, high-dose radiation therapy to the upper abdomen, or total- or hemibody irradiation, should receive prophylactic antiemetics for RINV.

Prophylaxis of RINV

Four radiotherapy-induced emesis risk groups have been defined by the Antiemetic Subcommittee of the Multinational Association of Supportive Care in Cancer (MASCC) and the ASCO antiemetic practice guidelines.[2,23] Both groups recommend preventive therapy with a SSRI and dexamethasone in patients who are receiving total-body irradiation (high emetic risk). The efficacy of oral granisetron 2 mg and ondansetron 8 mg was demonstrated in 34 patients who underwent hyperfractionated total-body irradiation.[36] Patients undergoing radiation therapy procedures with moderate to low emetic risk should receive a SSRI prior to each fraction.

■ DISORDERS OF BALANCE

A variety of clinical conditions may be associated with vertigo and dizziness. The etiology of these complaints may include diseases that are infectious, postinfectious, demyelinative, vascular, neoplastic, degenerative, traumatic, toxic, psychogenic, or idiopathic. Symptoms of imbalance perceived by the patient present a particular clinical challenge. Whether associated with a minor or complex disorder, motion sickness may be associated with nausea and vomiting.

Although much progress has been made in the management of other illnesses associated with emesis, motion sickness represents an area in which newer agents have provided little benefit. Beneficial therapy for patients in this setting can most reliably be found among the antihistaminic–anticholinergic agents. However, the precise mechanisms of action of these agents are currently unknown. Neither the antihistaminic nor the anticholinergic potency appears to correlate well with the ability of these agents to prevent or treat the nausea and vomiting associated with motion sickness. When used for their depressant effects on labyrinth excitability, these agents produce variable efficacy and safety profiles. Oral regimens of antihistaminic–anticholinergic agents given one to several times each day may be effective, especially when the first dose is administered prior to motion.

Scopolamine is commonly used to prevent nausea or vomiting caused by motion. The usefulness of scopolamine in preventing motion sickness was enhanced with the development of the transdermal system (patch) that increased patient satisfaction and decreased untoward side effects. A review of 12 randomized, controlled studies showed that scopolamine provided better protection from motion-induced sickness than did placebo, but was not superior to antihistamines and combinations of scopolamine and ephedrine.[37]

■ ANTIEMETIC USE DURING PREGNANCY

As many as 75% of pregnant women experience nausea and vomiting to some degree during the first trimester of pregnancy. The severity of the symptoms varies considerably, from mild nausea to incapacitating nausea and vomiting. The etiology of nausea and vomiting of pregnancy (NVP) is not well understood. For the majority of women, these symptoms are self-limited, although approximately 1% to 3% develop hyperemesis gravidarum, a serious condition marked by severe physical symptoms and/or medical complications requiring hospitalization. In its most severe state, hyperemesis gravidarum may result in volume contraction, starvation, and electrolyte abnormalities.

Initial management of NVP often involves dietary changes and/or lifestyle modifications. Nonpharmacologic interventions for NVP include ginger[38] and acupressure, although efficacy trials for acupressure are lacking. Persistent nausea and/or vomiting leads to the consideration of drug therapy at a time when teratogenic potential of each agent must be considered.

Table 37–10 summarizes the NVP treatment recommendations from the American College of Obstetricians and Gynecologists (ACOG).[39] A comprehensive review of treatment options for NVP was published.[40] Pyridoxine (10 to 25 mg 1 to 4 times daily), with or without doxylamine (12.5 to 20 mg 1 to 4 times daily), is recommended as first-line therapy. If symptoms persist, addition of an histamine$_1$-receptor antagonist such as dimenhydrinate (50 to 100 mg orally or rectally every 4 to 6 hours as needed), diphenhydramine (25 to 50 mg orally or 10 to 50 mg intravenously [IV] every 4 to 6 hours as needed), or meclizine (25 mg orally every 4 to 6 hours as needed) is recommended. Dopamine antagonists can also be added if symptoms continue (metoclopramide 5 to 10 mg IV every 8 hours as needed; promethazine 12.5 to 25 mg IV every 4 hours as needed; prochlorperazine 5 to 10 mg orally every 6 hours as needed).

Patients with persistent NVP or who show signs of dehydration should receive intravenous fluid replacement with thiamine. Ondansetron 2 to 8 mg orally/IV every 8 hours as needed may alleviate NVP, but the only randomized, controlled trial of intravenous ondansetron showed it to be no more effective than promethazine for treatment of severe NVP.[41] Corticosteroids should be reserved for patients with refractory NVP or hyperemesis gravidarum; methylprednisolone 16 mg orally/IV every 8 hours for 3 days followed by a 2-week taper is recommended. This regimen may

TABLE 37-10 Treatment Recommendations for the Management of Nausea and Vomiting of Pregnancy

Recommendations	Recommendation Grades[a]
The severity of nausea and vomiting of pregnancy (NVP) may be decreased by taking a multiple vitamin at the time of conception.	A
First-line pharmacotherapy for the treatment of NVP should consist of pyridoxine (vitamin B_6) or pyridoxine + doxylamine.	A
Treatment of NVP with ginger has shown beneficial effects and can be considered as a nonpharmacologic option.	B
Antihistamine H_1-receptor blockers, phenothiazines, and benzamides have been shown to be safe and efficacious in cases of refractory NVP.	B
Early treatment of NVP is recommended to prevent progression to hyperemesis gravidarum.	B
Treatment of severe NVP or hyperemesis gravidarum with methylprednisolone may be efficacious in refractory cases; however, the risk profile of methylprednisolone suggests it should be a treatment of last resort.	B
Intravenous hydration should be used for the patient who cannot tolerate oral liquids for a prolonged period or if clinical signs of dehydration are present.	C
Correction of ketosis and vitamin deficiency should be strongly considered.	C
Dextrose and vitamins, especially thiamine, should be included in the therapy when prolonged vomiting is present.	C
Enteral or parenteral nutrition should be initiated for any patient who cannot maintain weight because of vomiting.	C

[a]Strength of recommendations: A = good and consistent scientific evidence. B = limited or inconsistent scientific evidence. C = consensus and expert opinion.

Used with permission. Nausea and vomiting of pregnancy. ACOG Practice Bulletin No. 52. American College of Obstetricians and Gynecologists. Obstet Gynecol 2004;103(4):803–815.

be repeated if necessary, but treatment should not exceed a total of 6 weeks.

■ ANTIEMETIC USE IN CHILDREN

Practice guidelines recommend that a corticosteroid plus SSRI should be administered to children receiving chemotherapy of high or moderate emetic risk.[23] The best doses or dosing strategies for children (by age, weight, or body surface area) have not been clearly established. Standard adult doses of SSRIs may not provide consistent antiemetic protection in children due to wider interpatient variations in metabolism and clearance.[42]

For nausea and vomiting associated with pediatric gastroenteritis, emphasis should be placed on rehydration measures rather than on pharmacologic intervention. Promethazine suppositories were the most commonly prescribed antiemetic for pediatric gastroenteritis in a survey of physicians, despite the lack of prospective trials for this agent.[43] In 2004, the Food and Drug Administration reviewed all cases (125) of serious adverse events that involved children (age range: birth to 16 years) who had received any formulation of promethazine. Serious outcomes, including death, occurred with all routes of administration (oral, rectal, and parenteral) at doses ranging from 0.45 to 6.4 mg/kg. Subsequently, a black box warning was added to the promethazine labeling that included a contraindication for use of any product containing promethazine in children younger than age 2 years and a strengthened warning with regard to use in children 2 years of age or older.[44]

■ PHARMACOECONOMIC CONSIDERATIONS

There are many important variables to consider when attempting to document the overall costs of using a medication in a particular medical situation. Medication costs alone cannot begin to explain the true pharmacoeconomic outcome associated with the use of antiemetic drugs. For example, the costs associated with an unexpected hospital admission because of vomiting after an outpatient surgical procedure quickly offset the savings related to the selection of an inexpensive antiemetic drug. In this and other similar situations, it is economically and clinically important to develop antiemetic protocols based on appropriate decision analysis and clinical outcomes in order to optimize drug product selection. The clinical practice guidelines that have been previously described are valuable tools when developing institution-specific antiemetic protocols. The availability of new, more expensive agents will only increase the costs associated with the prophylaxis of CINV and PONV. The need to control antiemetic costs for health systems is universal and formulary management strategies have been described.[45]

EVALUATION OF THERAPEUTIC OUTCOMES

In accordance with the information presented concerning age and clinical condition, individualized therapy is possible through drug selection and dosage adjustment. Monitoring criteria for drug therapy should include the subjective assessment of the patient's severity of nausea, as well as objective parameters, such as changes in patient weight, the number of vomiting episodes each day, the volume of vomitus lost, and evaluation of fluid, acid–base balance, and electrolyte status, with particular attention to serum sodium, potassium, and chloride concentrations. In addition, evaluation of renal function may become important, particularly in patients with volume contraction and progressive electrolyte disturbances. Specific parameters include daily urine volume, urine specific gravity, and urine electrolyte concentrations. Physical assessment of patients should include evaluation of mucous membranes and skin turgor, because dryness of these tissues may be indicative of significant volume loss.

ABBREVIATIONS

ASCO: American Society of Clinical Oncology

CINV: chemotherapy-induced nausea and vomiting

CTZ: chemoreceptor trigger zone

NK_1: $neurokinin_1$

NVP: nausea and vomiting of pregnancy

PONV: postoperative nausea and vomiting

RINV: radiation-induced nausea and vomiting

SSRI: selective serotonin reuptake inhibitor

REFERENCES

1. Hasler WL, Chey WD. Nausea and vomiting. Gastroenterology 2003;125:1860–1867.
2. Prevention of chemotherapy- and radiotherapy-induced emesis. Results of the 2004 Perugia International Antiemetic Consensus Conference. Ann Oncol 2006;17:20–28.
3. Stephenson J, Davies A. An assessment of etiology-based guidelines for the management of nausea and vomiting in patients with advanced cancer. Support Care Cancer 2006;14:348–353.
4. American Society of Health-System (ASHP) therapeutic guidelines on the pharmacologic management of nausea and vomiting in adult and pediatric patients receiving chemotherapy or radiation therapy or undergoing surgery. Am J Health-Syst Pharm 1999;56:729–764.
5. Lee M. Nausea and vomiting. In: Feldman M, ed. Sleisenger and Fordtran's Gastrointestinal and Liver Disease: Pathophysiology/Diagnosis/Management. St. Louis: Elsevier, 2006:119–130.

6. Montgomery GH, Bovbjerg DH. The development of anticipatory nausea in patients receiving adjuvant chemotherapy for breast cancer. Physiol Behav 1997;61:737–741.
7. King CR. Nonpharmacologic management of chemotherapy-induced nausea and vomiting. Oncol Nurs Forum 1997;24:S41–S48.
8. Matteson S, Roscoe J, Hickok J, Morrow GR. The role of behavioral conditioning in the development of nausea. Am J Obstet Gynecol 2002;186:S239–S243.
9. Ernst A, Weiss SJ, Park S, et al. Prochlorperazine versus promethazine for uncomplicated nausea and vomiting in the emergency department: A randomized, double-blind clinical trial. Ann Emerg Med 2000;36:89–94.
10. Critchley P, Plach N, Grantham M, et al. Efficacy of haloperidol in the treatment of nausea and vomiting in the palliative patient: A systematic review. J Pain Symptom Manage 2001;22:631–634.
11. Inapsine (droperidol). *www.fda.gov/medwatch/SAFETY/2001/inapsine.htm.*
12. Italian Group for Antiemetic Research. Double-blind, dose-finding study of four intravenous doses of dexamethasone in the prevention of cisplatin-induced acute emesis. J Clin Oncol 1998;16:2937–2942.
13. Ioannidis JT, Hesketh PJ, Lau J. Contribution of dexamethasone to control of chemotherapy-induced nausea and vomiting: A meta-analysis of randomized evidence. J Clin Oncol 2000;18:3409–3422.
14. Poli-Bigelli S, Rodrigues-Pereira J, Carides AD, et al. Addition of the neurokinin 1 receptor antagonist aprepitant to standard antiemetic therapy improves control of chemotherapy-induced nausea and vomiting. Results from a randomized, double-blind, placebo-controlled trial in Latin America. Cancer 2003;97:3090–3098.
15. Hesketh PJ, Grunbert SM, Gralla RJ, et al. The oral neurokinin-1 antagonist aprepitant for the prevention of chemotherapy-induced nausea and vomiting: A multinational, randomized, double-blind, placebo-controlled trial in patients receiving high-dose cisplatin—The Aprepitant Protocol 052 Study Group. J Clin Oncol 2003;21:4112–4119.
16. De Mulder PH, Seynaeve C, Vermorken JB, et al. Ondansetron compared with high-dose metoclopramide in prophylaxis of acute and delayed cisplatin-induced nausea and vomiting: A multicenter, randomized, double-blind, crossover study. Ann Intern Med 1990;113:834–840.
17. Heron JF, Goedhals L, Jordaan JP, et al. Oral granisetron alone and in combination with dexamethasone: A double-blind randomized comparison against high-dose metoclopramide plus dexamethasone in prevention of cisplatin-induced emesis. Ann Oncol 1994;5:579–584.
18. Tramer MR, Carroll D, Campbell FA, et al. Cannabinoids for control of chemotherapy induced nausea and vomiting: Quantitative systematic review. BMJ 2001;323:1–8.
19. Stahl SM. The ups and downs of novel antiemetic drugs, Part 1: Substance P, 5-HT, and the neuropharmacology of vomiting. J Clin Psychol 2003;64:498–499.
20. Warr DG, Hesketh PJ, Gralla RJ, et al. Efficacy and tolerability of aprepitant for the prevention of chemotherapy-induced nausea and vomiting in patients with breast cancer after moderately emetogenic chemotherapy. J Clin Oncol 2005;23:2822–2830.
21. Emend [package insert]. Whitehouse Station, NJ: Merck & Co, June 2006.
22. McCrea JB, Majumdar AK, Goldberg MR, et al. Effects of the neurokinin-1 receptor antagonist aprepitant on the pharmacokinetics of dexamethasone and methylprednisolone. Clin Pharmacol Ther 2003;74:17–24.
23. Kris MG, Hesketh PJ, Somerfield MR, et al. American Society of Clinical Oncology guideline for antiemetics in oncology: Update 2006. J Clin Oncol 2006;24:2932–2947.
24. National Comprehensive Cancer Network. Clinical Practice Guidelines in Oncology. Antiemesis Version 1.2007. 2006, *http://www.nccn.org/professionals/physician_gls/PDF/antiemesis.pdf.*
25. Aloxi [package insert]. Bloomington, MI: MGI PHARMA Inc., January 2006.
26. Eisenberg P, Figueroa-Vadillo J, Zamora R, et al. Improved prevention of moderately emetogenic chemotherapy-induced nausea and vomiting with palonosetron, a pharmacologically novel 5-HT_3 receptor antagonist: Results of a phase III, single-dose trial versus dolasetron. Cancer 2003;98:2473–2482.
27. Gralla R, Lichinitser M, Van Der Vegt S, et al. Palonosetron improves prevention of chemotherapy-induced nausea and vomiting following moderately emetogenic chemotherapy: Results of a double-blind randomized phase III trial comparing single doses of palonosetron with ondansetron. Ann Oncol 2003;14:1570–1577.
28. Kovac AL. Prevention and treatment of postoperative nausea and vomiting. Drugs 2000;59:213–243.
29. Gan TJ, Meyer T, Apfel CC, et al. Consensus guidelines for managing postoperative nausea and vomiting. Anesth Analg 2003;97:62–71.
30. Apfel CA, Korttila K, Abdalla M, et al. A factorial trial of six interventions for the prevention of postoperative nausea and vomiting. N Engl J Med 2004;350:2441–2451.
31. Carlisle JB, Stevenson CA. Drugs for preventing postoperative nausea and vomiting. Cochrane Database Syst Rev 2006;3:CD004125.
32. Wang JJ, Ho ST, Tzeng JI, Tang CS. The effect of timing of dexamethasone administration on its efficacy as a prophylactic antiemetic for postoperative nausea and vomiting. Anesth Analg 2000;91:136–139.
33. Hill RP, Lubarsky DA, Phillips-Bute B, et al. Cost-effectiveness of prophylactic antiemetic therapy with ondansetron, droperidol or placebo. Anesthesiology 2000;92:958–967.
34. Kovac AL, O'Connor TA, Pearman MH, et al. Efficacy of repeat intravenous dosing of ondansetron in controlling postoperative nausea and vomiting: A randomized, double-blind, placebo-controlled multicenter trial. J Clin Anesth 1999;11:453–459.
35. Kreisler NS, Spiekermann BF, Ascari CM, et al. Small-dose droperidol effectively reduces nausea in a general surgical adult patient population. Anesth Analg 2000;91:1256–1261.
36. Spitzer TR, Friedman CJ, Bushnell W, et al. Double-blind, randomized, parallel-group study on the efficacy and safety of oral granisetron and oral ondansetron in the prophylaxis of nausea and vomiting in patients receiving hyperfractionated total body irradiation. Bone Marrow Transplant 2000;26:203–210.
37. Spinks AB, Wasiak J, Villaneuva EV, Bernath V. Scopolamine for preventing and treating motion sickness. Cochrane Database Syst Rev 2004;3:CD002851.
38. Portnoi G, Chng LA, Karimi-Tabesh L, et al. Prospective comparative study of the safety and effectiveness of ginger for the treatment of nausea and vomiting in pregnancy. Am J Obstet Gynecol 2003;189:1374–1377.
39. Nausea and vomiting of pregnancy. ACOG Practice Bulletin No. 52. American College of Obstetricians and Gynecologists. Obstet Gynecol 2004;103:803–815.
40. Badell ML, Ramin SM, Smith JA. Treatment options for nausea and vomiting during pregnancy. Pharmacotherapy 2006;26:1273–1287.
41. Sullivan CA, Johnson CA, Roach H, Martin RW, et al. A pilot study of intravenous ondansetron for hyperemesis gravidarum. Am J Obstet Gynecol 1996;174:1565–1568.
42. Wade I, Takeda T, Sato M, et al. Pharmacokinetics of granisetron in adults and children with malignant diseases. Biol Pharm Bull 2001;24:432–435.
43. Kwon KT, Rudkin SE, Langdorf MI. Antiemetic use in pediatric gastroenteritis: A national survey of emergency physicians, pediatricians, and pediatric emergency physicians. Clin Pediatr 2002;41:641–652.
44. Starke PR, Weaver J, Chowdhury BA. Boxed warning added to promethazine labeling for pediatric use. N Engl J Med 2005;352:2653.
45. Lucarelli CD. Formulary management strategies for type 3 serotonin receptor antagonists. Am J Health Syst Pharm 2003;60:S4–S11.

CHAPTER 38

Diarrhea, Constipation, and Irritable Bowel Syndrome

WILLIAM J. SPRUILL AND WILLIAM E. WADE

KEY CONCEPTS

1. Diarrhea is caused by many viral and bacterial organisms. It is most often a minor discomfort, not life-threatening, and it is usually self-limited.
2. The four pathophysiologic mechanisms of diarrhea have been linked to the four broad diarrheal groups, which are secretory, osmotic, exudative, and altered intestinal transit. The three mechanisms by which absorption occurs from the intestines are active transport, diffusion, and solvent drag.
3. Management of diarrhea focuses on preventing excessive water and electrolyte losses, dietary care, relieving symptoms, treating curable causes, and treating secondary disorders.
4. Bismuth subsalicylate is marketed for indigestion, relieving abdominal cramps, and controlling diarrhea, including traveler's diarrhea, but may cause interactions with several components if given excessively.
5. Underlying causes of constipation should be identified when possible and corrective measures taken (e.g., alteration of diet or treatment of diseases such as hypothyroidism).
6. The foundation of treatment of constipation is dietary fiber or bulk-forming laxatives that provide 10 to 15 g/day of raw fiber.
7. Irritable bowel syndrome (IBS) is one of the most common gastrointestinal disorders. It is characterized by lower abdominal pain, disturbed defecation, and bloating. Many nongastrointestinal manifestations also exist with IBS. Recent studies have found that visceral hypersensitivity is a major culprit in the pathophysiology of the disease.
8. Diarrhea-predominant IBS should be managed by dietary modification and when diet changes alone are insufficient to promote control of symptoms, by drugs such as loperamide.
9. Several drug classes are involved in the treatment of the pain associated with IBS, including tricyclic compounds and the gut-selective calcium channel blockers.

DIARRHEA

Diarrhea is a troublesome discomfort that affects most individuals in the United States at some point in their lives and can be thought of as both a symptom and a sign. Usually diarrheal episodes begin abruptly and subside within 1 or 2 days without treatment. This chapter focuses primarily on noninfectious diarrhea, with only minor reference to infectious diarrhea (see Chap. 117 for a discussion of gastrointestinal infections). Diarrhea is often a symptom of a systemic disease and not all possible causes of diarrhea are discussed in this chapter. Acute diarrhea is commonly defined as <14 days' duration, persistent diarrhea as more than 14 days' duration, and chronic diarrhea as more than 30 days' duration.

To understand diarrhea, one must have a reasonable definition of the condition; unfortunately, the literature is extremely variable on this. Simply put, diarrhea is an increased frequency and decreased consistency of fecal discharge as compared to an individual's normal bowel pattern. Frequency and consistency are variable within and between individuals. For example, some individuals defecate as often as three times per day, whereas others defecate only two or three times per week. A Western diet usually produces a daily stool weighing between 100 and 300 g, depending on the amount of nonabsorbable materials (mainly carbohydrates) consumed. Patients with serious diarrhea may have a daily stool weight in excess of 300 g; however, a subset of patients experience frequent small, watery passages. Additionally, vegetable fiber-rich diets, such as those consumed in some Eastern cultures, such as those in Africa, produce stools weighing more than 300 g/day.

Diarrhea may be associated with a specific disease of the intestines or secondary to a disease outside the intestines. For instance, bacillary dysentery directly affects the gut, whereas diabetes mellitus causes neuropathic diarrheal episodes. Furthermore, diarrhea can be considered as acute or chronic disease. Infectious diarrhea is often acute; diabetic diarrhea is chronic. Congenital disorders in gastrointestinal ion-transport mechanisms are another cause of chronic diarrhea.[1] Whether acute or chronic, diarrhea has the same pathophysiologic causes that help identification of specific treatments.

EPIDEMIOLOGY

The epidemiology of diarrhea varies in developed versus developing countries.[2,3] In the United States, diarrheal illnesses are usually not reported to the Centers for Disease Control and Prevention (CDC) unless associated with an outbreak or an unusual organism or condition. For example, the acquired immune deficiency syndrome (AIDS) has been identified with protracted diarrheal illness. Diarrhea is a major problem in daycare centers and nursing homes, probably because early childhood and senescence plus environmental conditions are risk factors. Although an exact epidemiologic profile in the United States is not available through the CDC or published literature, chronic diarrhea affects approximately 5% of the adult population and ranges from 3% to 20% in children worldwide.[4] In developing countries, diarrhea is a leading cause of illness and death in children, creating a tremendous economic strain on healthcare costs.

❶ Most cases of acute diarrhea are caused by infections with viruses, bacteria, or protozoa and are generally self-limited.[5] Although viruses are more commonly associated with acute gastroenteritis, bacteria are responsible for more cases of acute diarrhea.[6]

Evaluation of a noninfectious cause is considered if diarrhea persists and no infectious organism can be identified, or if the patient falls into a high-risk category for metabolic complications with persistent diarrhea. Common causative bacterial organisms include *Shigella*, *Salmonella*, *Campylobacter*, *Staphylococcus*, and *Escherichia coli*. Food-borne bacterial infection is a major concern, as several major food poisoning episodes have occurred that were traced to poor sanitary conditions in meat-processing plants. Acute viral infections are attributed mostly to the Norwalk and rotavirus groups.

PHYSIOLOGY

In the fasting state, 9 L of fluid enters the proximal small intestine each day. Of this fluid, 2 L are ingested through diet, while the remainder consists of internal secretions. Because of meal content, duodenal chyme is usually hypertonic. When chyme reaches the ileum, the osmolality adjusts to that of plasma, with most dietary fat, carbohydrate, and protein being absorbed. The volume of ileal chyme decreases to about 1 L/day upon entering the colon, which is further reduced by colonic absorption to 100 mL daily. If the small intestine water absorption capacity is exceeded, chyme overloads the colon, resulting in diarrhea. In humans, the colon absorptive capacity is about 5 L daily. Colonic fluid transport is critical to water and electrolyte balance.

Absorption from the intestines back into the blood occurs by three mechanisms: active transport, diffusion, and solvent drag. Active transport and diffusion are the mechanisms of sodium transport. Because of the high luminal sodium concentration (142 mEq/L), sodium diffuses from the sodium-rich gut into epithelial cells, where it is actively pumped into the blood and exchanged with chloride to maintain an isoelectric condition across the epithelial membrane.

Hydrogen ions are transported by an indirect mechanism in the upper small intestine. As sodium is absorbed, hydrogen ions are secreted into the gut. Hydrogen ions then combine with bicarbonate ions to form carbonic acid, which then dissociates into carbon dioxide and water. Carbon dioxide readily diffuses into the blood for expiration through the lung. The water remains in the chyme.

Paracellular pathways are major routes of ion movement. As ions, monosaccharides, and amino acids are actively transported, an osmotic pressure is created, drawing water and electrolytes across the intestinal wall. This pathway accounts for significant amounts of ion transport, especially sodium. Sodium plays an important role in stimulating glucose absorption. Glucose and amino acids are actively transported into the blood via a sodium dependent cotransport mechanism. Cotransport absorption mechanisms of glucose-sodium and amino acid-sodium are extremely important for treating diarrhea.

Gut motility influences absorption and secretion. The amount of time in which luminal content is in contact with the epithelium is under neural and hormonal control. Neurohormonal substances, such as angiotensin, vasopressin, glucocorticoid, aldosterone, and neurotransmitters also regulate ion transport.

PATHOPHYSIOLOGY

❷ Four general pathophysiologic mechanisms disrupt water and electrolyte balance, leading to diarrhea, and are the basis of diagnosis and therapy. These are (a) a change in active ion transport by either decreased sodium absorption or increased chloride secretion; (b) change in intestinal motility; (c) increase in luminal osmolarity; and (d) increase in tissue hydrostatic pressure. These mechanisms have been related to four broad clinical diarrheal groups: secretory, osmotic, exudative, and altered intestinal transit.

Secretory diarrhea occurs when a stimulating substance either increases secretion or decreases absorption of large amounts of water and electrolytes. Substances that cause excess secretion include vasoactive intestinal peptide (VIP) from a pancreatic tumor, unabsorbed dietary fat in steatorrhea, laxatives, hormones (such as secretion), bacterial toxins, and excessive bile salts. Many of these agents stimulate intracellular cyclic adenosine monophosphate and inhibit Na^+/K^+-adenosine triphosphatase (ATPase), leading to increased secretion. Also, many of these mediators inhibit ion absorption simultaneously. Clinically, secretory diarrhea is recognized by large stool volumes (>1 L/day) with normal ionic contents and osmolality approximately equal to plasma. Fasting does not alter the stool volume in these patients.

Poorly absorbed substances retain intestinal fluids, resulting in osmotic diarrhea. This process occurs with malabsorption syndromes, lactose intolerance, administration of divalent ions (e.g., magnesium-containing antacids), or consumption of poorly soluble carbohydrate (e.g., lactulose). As a poorly soluble solute is transported, the gut adjusts the osmolality to that of plasma; in so doing, water and electrolytes flux into the lumen. Clinically, osmotic diarrhea is distinguishable from other types, as it ceases if the patient resorts to a fasting state.

Inflammatory diseases of the gastrointestinal tract discharge mucus, serum proteins, and blood into the gut. Sometimes bowel movements consist only of mucus, exudate, and blood. Exudative diarrhea affects other absorptive, secretory, or motility functions to account for the large stool volume associated with this disorder.

Altered intestinal motility produces diarrhea by three mechanisms: reduction of contact time in the small intestine, premature emptying of the colon, and bacterial overgrowth. Chyme must be exposed to intestinal epithelium for a sufficient time period to enable normal absorption and secretion processes to occur. If this contact time decreases, diarrhea results. Intestinal resection or bypass surgery and drugs (such as metoclopramide) cause this type of diarrhea. On the other hand, an increased time of exposure allows fecal bacteria overgrowth. A characteristic small intestine diarrheal pattern is rapid, small, coupling bursts of waves. These waves are inefficient, do not allow absorption, and rapidly dump chyme into the colon. Once in the colon, chyme exceeds the colonic capability to absorb water.

Etiologic Examination of the Stool

Stool characteristics are important in assessing the etiology of diarrhea. A description of the frequency, volume, consistency, and color provides diagnostic clues. For instance, diarrhea starting in the small intestine produces a copious, watery or fatty (greasy), and foul-smelling stool; contains undigested food particles; and is usually free from gross blood. Colonic diarrhea appears as small, pasty, and sometimes bloody or mucoid movements. Rectal tenesmus with flatus accompanies large intestinal diarrhea.

CLINICAL PRESENTATION

Table 38–1 outlines the clinical presentation of diarrhea and Table 38–2 shows common drug-induced causes of diarrhea. A medication history is extremely important in identifying drug-induced diarrhea. Many agents, including antibiotics and other drugs, cause diarrhea or, less commonly, pseudomembranous colitis. Self-inflicted laxative abuse for weight loss is popular.

Most acute diarrhea is self-limiting, subsiding within 72 hours. However, infants, young children, the elderly, and debilitated persons are at risk for morbid and mortal events in prolonged or voluminous diarrhea. These groups are at risk for water, electrolyte, and acid–base disturbances, and potentially cardiovascular collapse and death. The prognosis for chronic diarrhea depends on

TABLE 38-1 Clinical Presentation of Diarrhea

General
- Usually, acute diarrheal episodes subside within 72 hours of onset, whereas chronic diarrhea involves frequent attacks over extended time periods.

Signs and symptoms
- Abrupt onset of nausea, vomiting, abdominal pain, headache, fever, chills, and malaise.
- Bowel movements are frequent and never bloody, and diarrhea lasts 12 to 60 hours.
- Intermittent periumbilical or lower right quadrant pain with cramps and audible bowel sounds is characteristic of small intestinal disease.
- When pain is present in large intestinal diarrhea, it is a gripping, aching sensation with tenesmus (straining, ineffective, and painful stooling). Pain localizes to the hypogastric region, right or left lower quadrant, or sacral region.
- In chronic diarrhea, a history of previous bouts, weight loss, anorexia, and chronic weakness are important findings.

Physical examination
- Typically demonstrates hyperperistalsis with borborygmi and generalized or local tenderness.

Laboratory tests
- Stool analysis studies include examination for microorganisms, blood, mucus, fat, osmolality, pH, electrolyte and mineral concentration, and cultures.
- Stool test kits are useful for detecting gastrointestinal viruses, particularly rotavirus.
- Antibody serologic testing shows rising titers over a 3- to 6-day period, but this test is not practical and is nonspecific.
- Occasionally, total daily stool volume is also determined.
- Direct endoscopic visualization and biopsy of the colon may be undertaken to assess for the presence of conditions such as colitis or cancer.
- Radiographic studies are helpful in neoplastic and inflammatory conditions.

TABLE 38-2 Drugs Causing Diarrhea

Laxatives
Antacids containing magnesium
Antineoplastics
Auranofin (gold salt)
Antibiotics
- Clindamycin
- Tetracyclines
- Sulfonamides
- Any broad-spectrum antibiotic

Antihypertensives
- Reserpine
- Guanethidine
- Methyldopa
- Guanabenz
- Guanadrel
- Angiotensin-converting enzyme inhibitors

Cholinergics
- Bethanechol
- Neostigmine

Cardiac agents
- Quinidine
- Digitalis
- Digoxin

Nonsteroidal antiinflammatory drugs
Misoprostol
Colchicine
Proton pump inhibitors
H_2-receptor blockers

the cause; for example, diarrhea secondary to diabetes mellitus waxes and wanes throughout life.

TREATMENT

Diarrhea

PREVENTION

Acute viral diarrheal illness often occurs in daycare centers and nursing homes. As person-to-person contact is the mechanism by which viral disease spreads, isolation techniques must be initiated, For bacterial, parasite, and protozoal infections, strict food handling, sanitation, water, and other environmental hygiene practices can prevent transmission. If diarrhea is secondary to another illness, controlling the primary condition is necessary. Antibiotics and bismuth subsalicylate are advocated to prevent traveler's diarrhea, in conjunction with treatment of drinking water and caution with consumption of fresh vegetables.

DESIRED OUTCOME

❸ If prevention is unsuccessful and diarrhea occurs, therapeutic goals are to (a) manage the diet; (b) prevent excessive water, electrolyte, and acid–base disturbances; (c) provide symptomatic relief; (d) treat curable causes; and (e) manage secondary disorders causing diarrhea (Figs. 38–1 and 38–2).

Clinicians must clearly understand that diarrhea, like a cough, may be a body defense mechanism for ridding itself of harmful substances or pathogens. The correct therapeutic response is not necessarily to stop diarrhea at all costs.

NONPHARMACOLOGIC MANAGEMENT

Dietary management is a first priority in the treatment of diarrhea. Most clinicians recommend discontinuing consumption of solid foods and dairy products for 24 hours. However, fasting is of questionable value, as this treatment modality has not been extensively studied. In osmotic diarrhea, these maneuvers control the problem. If the mechanism is secretory, diarrhea persists. For patients who are experiencing nausea and/or vomiting, a mild, digestible, low-residue diet should be administered for 24 hours. If vomiting is present and uncontrollable with antiemetics (see Chap. 37), nothing is taken by mouth. As bowel movements decrease, a bland diet is begun.

Feeding should continue in children with acute bacterial diarrhea. Fed children have less morbidity and mortality, whether or not they receive oral rehydration fluids. Studies are not available in the elderly or in other high-risk groups to determine the value of continued feeding in bacterial diarrhea.

Water and Electrolytes

Rehydration and maintenance of water and electrolytes are primary treatment goals until the diarrheal episode ends. If the patient is volume depleted, rehydration should be directed at replacing water and electrolytes to normal body composition. Then water and electrolyte composition are maintained by replacing losses. Many patients will not develop volume depletion and therefore will only require maintenance fluid and electrolyte therapy. Parenteral and enteral routes may be used for supplying water and electrolytes. If vomiting and dehydration are not severe, enteral feeding is the less costly and preferred method. In the United States, many commercial oral rehydration preparations are available (Table 38–3).

Because of concerns about hypernatremia, physicians continue to hospitalize patients and intravenously correct fluid and electrolyte deficits in severe dehydration. Oral solutions are strongly recommended.[7,8] In developing countries, the World Health Organization Oral Rehydration Solution (WHO-ORS) saves the lives of millions of children annually.

During diarrhea, the small intestine retains its ability to actively transport monosaccharides such as glucose. Glucose actively carries sodium with water and other electrolytes. Because the WHO-ORS has a high sodium concentration, physicians have been reluctant to

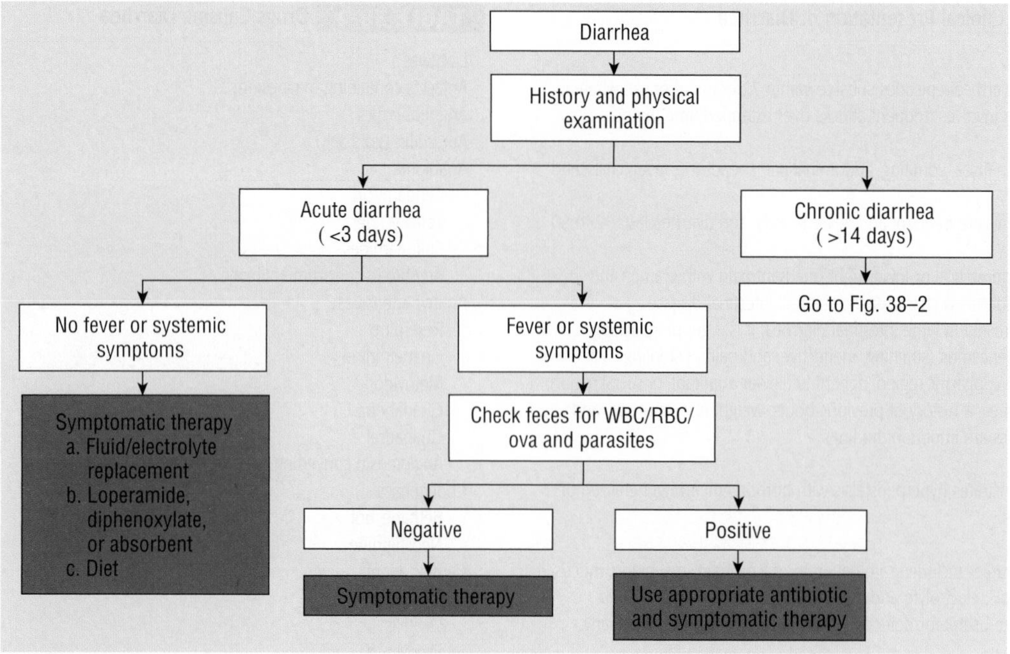

FIGURE 38-1. Recommendations for treating acute diarrhea. Follow these steps: (a) Perform a complete history and physical examination. (b) Is the diarrhea acute or chronic? If chronic diarrhea, go to Fig. 38–2. (c) If acute diarrhea, check for fever and/or systemic signs and symptoms (i.e., toxic patient). If systemic illness (fever, anorexia, or volume depletion), check for an infectious source. If positive for infectious diarrhea, use appropriate antibiotic/anthelmintic drug and symptomatic therapy. If negative for infectious cause, use only symptomatic treatment. (d) If no systemic findings, then use symptomatic therapy based on severity of volume depletion, oral or parenteral fluid/electrolytes, antidiarrheal agents (see Table 38–4), and diet. (RBC, red blood cells; WBC, white blood cells.)

use it in well-nourished children. Yet controlled comparative studies describe more favorable results with the WHO-ORS than with parenteral fluids.[9] The recommended WHO-ORS (see Table 38–3) has now been reformulated to have a lower osmolarity, sodium content, and glucose load. Rice-based oral solution is also a hyposmotically active substrate that elutes glucose without increasing stool or urine outflows. Rehydration of infants with acute diarrhea using a rice-based solution is effective.[9] Decreased stool output and greater absorption and retention of fluid and electrolytes also results. In summary, oral rehydration solution is a lifesaving treatment for millions afflicted in developing countries. Acceptance in developed countries is less enthusiastic; however, the advantage of this product in reducing hospitalizations may prove its use as a cost-effective alternative, saving millions of dollars in healthcare expenditures.

■ PHARMACOLOGIC THERAPY

Various drugs have been used to treat diarrheal attacks (Table 38–4). These drugs are grouped into several categories: antimotility, adsorbents, antisecretory compounds, antibiotics, enzymes, and intestinal microflora. Usually these drugs are not curative but palliative.

Opiates and Their Derivatives

Opiates and opioid derivatives (a) delay the transit of intraluminal contents or (b) increase gut capacity, prolonging contact and absorption. Enkephalins, which are endogenous opioid substances, regulate fluid movement across the mucosa by stimulating absorptive processes. Limitations to the use of opiates include an addiction potential (a real concern with long-term use) and worsening of diarrhea in selected infectious diarrhea.

Most opiates act through peripheral and central mechanisms with the exception of loperamide, which acts only peripherally. Loperamide is antisecretory; it inhibits the calcium-binding protein calmodulin, controlling chloride secretion. Loperamide, available as 2-mg capsules or 1 mg/5 mL solution (both are nonprescription products), is suggested for managing acute and chronic diarrhea. The usual adult dose is initially 4 mg orally, followed by 2 mg after each loose stool, up to 16 mg/day. Used correctly, this agent has rare side effects, such as dizziness and constipation. If the diarrhea is concurrent with a high fever or bloody stool, the patient should be referred to a physician. Also, diarrhea lasting 48 hours beyond initiating loperamide warrants medical attention. Loperamide can also be used in traveler's diarrhea. It is comparable to bismuth subsalicylate for treatment of this disorder.[10]

Diphenoxylate is available as a 2.5-mg tablet and as a 2.5 mg/5mL solution. A small amount of atropine (0.025 mg) is included in the product to discourage abuse. In adults, when taken as 2.5 to 5 mg three or four times daily, not to exceed a 20-mg total daily dose, diphenoxylate is rarely toxic. Some patients may complain of atropinism (blurred vision, dry mouth, and urinary hesitancy). Like loperamide, it should not be used in patients who are at risk of bacterial enteritis with *E. coli*, *Shigella*, or *Salmonella*.

Difenoxin, a diphenoxylate derivative also chemically related to meperidine, is also combined with atropine and has the same uses, precautions, and side effects. Marketed as a 1-mg tablet, the adult dosage is 2 mg initially, followed by 1 mg after each loose stool, not to exceed 8 mg/day.

Paregoric, tincture of opium, is marketed as a 2 mg/5 mL solution and is indicated for managing both acute and chronic diarrhea. It is not widely prescribed today because of its abuse potential.

Adsorbents

Adsorbents are used for symptomatic relief. These products, many not requiring a prescription, are nontoxic, but their effectiveness remains unproven. Adsorbents are nonspecific in their action; they adsorb nutrients, toxins, drugs, and digestive juices. Polycarbophil absorbs 60 times its weight in water and can be used to treat both diarrhea and constipation. It is a nonprescription product and is

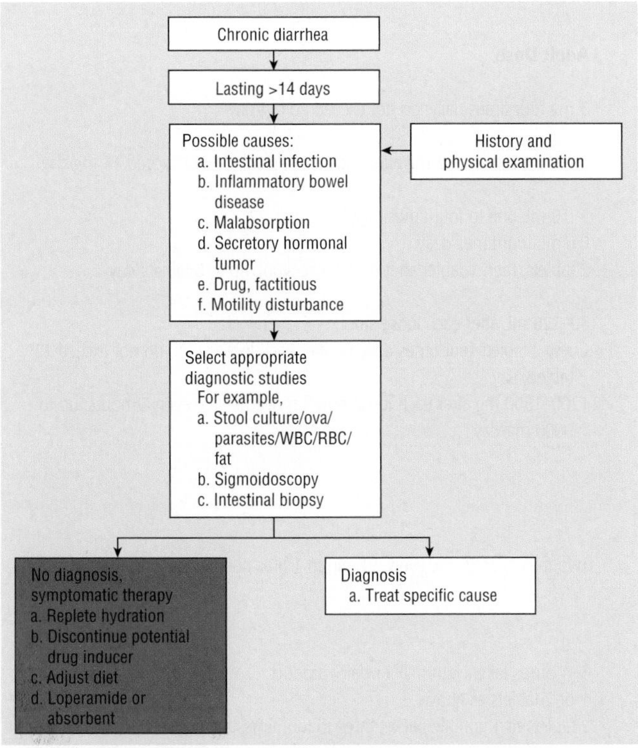

FIGURE 38-2. Recommendations for treating chronic diarrhea. Follow these steps: (a) Perform a careful history and physical examination. (b) The possible causes of chronic diarrhea are many. These can be classified into intestinal infections (bacterial or protozoal), inflammatory disease (Crohn's disease or ulcerative colitis), malabsorption (lactose intolerance), secretory hormonal tumor (intestinal carcinoid tumor or vasoactive intestinal peptide-secreting tumor [VIPoma]), drug (antacid), factitious (laxative abuse), or motility disturbance (diabetes mellitus, irritable bowel syndrome, or hyperthyroidism). (c) If the diagnosis is uncertain, selected appropriate diagnostic studies should be ordered. (d) Once diagnosed, treatment is planned for the underlying cause with symptomatic antidiarrheal therapy. (e) If no specific cause can be identified, symptomatic therapy is prescribed. (RBC, red blood cells; WBC, white blood cells.)

sold as a 500-mg chewable tablet. This hydrophilic nonabsorbable product is safe and may be taken four times daily, up to 6 g/day in adults. See Table 38–4 for selected antidiarrheal preparations.

Antisecretory Agents

Bismuth subsalicylate appears to have antisecretory, antiinflammatory, and antibacterial effects. As a nonprescription product, it is marketed for indigestion, relieving abdominal cramps, and controlling diarrhea, including traveler's diarrhea. Bismuth subsalicylate dosage strengths are a 262-mg chewable tablet, 262 mg/5 mL liquid, and 524 mg/15 mL liquid. The usual adult dose is 2 tablets or 30 mL every 30 minutes to 1 hour up to 8 doses per day.

❹ Bismuth subsalicylate contains multiple components that might be toxic if given excessively to prevent or treat diarrhea. For instance, an active ingredient is salicylate, which may interact with anticoagulants or may produce salicylism (tinnitus, nausea, and vomiting). Bismuth reduces tetracycline absorption and may interfere with select gastrointestinal radiographic studies. Patients may complain of a darkening of the tongue and stools with repeat administration. Salicylate can induce gout attacks in susceptible individuals.

Bismuth subsalicylate suspension has been evaluated in the treatment of secretory diarrhea of infectious etiology as well. In a dose of 30 mL every 30 minutes for 8 doses, unformed stools decrease in the first 24 hours. Bismuth subsalicylate may also be effective in preventing traveler's diarrhea.

Octreotide, a synthetic octapeptide analog of endogenous somatostatin, is proven effective for the symptomatic treatment of carcinoid tumors and other peptide-secreting tumors, dumping syndrome, and chemotherapy-induced diarrhea.[11] It has had limited success in patients with AIDS-associated diarrhea and short-bowel syndrome, does not appear to have an advantage over various opiate derivatives in the treatment of chronic idiopathic diarrhea, and has the disadvantage of being administered by injection.[12] Metastatic intestinal carcinoid tumors secrete excessive amounts of vasoactive substances, including histamine, bradykinin, serotonin, and prostaglandins. Primary carcinoid tumors occur throughout the gastrointestinal tract, with most in the ileum. Predominant signs and symptoms experienced by patients with these tumors are attributable to excessive concentrations of 5-hydroxytryptophan and serotonin. The totality of their clinical effects is termed the carcinoid syndrome. Paroxysmal vasomotor attacks characterize carcinoid syndrome, most notably sudden red to purple flushing of the face and neck. These attacks are often caused by emotional outbursts or by ingestion of food or alcohol. Some patients have a violent, watery diarrhea with abdominal cramping. Initially, diarrhea might be managed with various agents such as codeine, diphenoxylate, cyproheptadine, methysergide, phenoxybenzamine, or methyldopa. But octreotide has more recently been considered first-line therapy.

Octreotide blocks the release of serotonin and many other active peptides, and has been effective in controlling diarrhea and flushing. It is reported to have direct inhibitory effects on intestinal secretion and stimulatory effects on intestinal absorption. Non–gastrin-secreting adenomas of the pancreas are tumors associated with profuse watery diarrhea. This condition has been referred to as Verner-Morrison's

TABLE 38-3 Oral Rehydration Solutions

	WHO-ORS[a]	Pedialyte[b] (Ross)	Rehydralyte[b] (Ross)	Infalyte (Mead Johnson)	Resol[b] (Wyeth)
Osmolality (mOsm/L)	311	249	304	200	269
Carbohydrates[b] (g/L)	13.5	25	25	30[c]	20
Calories (cal/L)	65	100	100	126	80
Electrolytes (mEq/L)					
Sodium	75	45	75	50	50
Potassium	20	20	20	25	20
Chloride	65	35	65	45	50
Citrate	–	30	30	34	34
Bicarbonate	30	–	–	–	–
Calcium	–	–	–	–	4
Magnesium	–	–	–	–	4
Sulfate	–	–	–	–	–
Phosphate	–	–	–	–	5

[a]World Health Organization reduced osmolarity Oral Rehydration Solution.
[b]Carbohydrate is glucose.
[c]Rice syrup solids are carbohydrate source.

TABLE 38-4 Selected Antidiarrheal Preparation

	Dose Form	Adult Dose
Antimotility		
Diphenoxylate	2.5 mg/tablet 2.5 mg/5 mL	5 mg four times daily; do not exceed 20 mg/day
Loperamide	2 mg/capsule 1 mg/5 mL	Initially 4 mg, then 2 mg after each loose stool; do not exceed 16 mg/day
Paregoric	2 mg/5 mL (morphine)	5–10 mL one to four times daily
Opium tincture	5 mg/mL (morphine)	0.6 mL four times daily
Difenoxin	1 mg/tablet	2 tablets, then 1 tablet after each loose stool; up to 8 tablets/day
Adsorbents		
Kaolin–pectin mixture	5.7 g kaolin + 130.2 mg pectin/30 mL	30–120 mL after each loose stool
Polycarbophil	500 mg/tablet	Chew 2 tablets four times daily or after each loose stool; do not exceed 12 tablets/day
Attapulgite	750 mg/15 mL 300 mg/7.5 mL 750 mg/tablet 600 mg/tablet 300 mg/tablet	1200–1500 mg after each loose bowel movement or every 2 hours; up to 9000 mg/day
Antisecretory		
Bismuth subsalicylate	1050 mg/30 mL 262 mg/15 mL 524 mg/15 mL 262 mg/tablet	Two tablets or 30 mL every 30 min to 1 h as needed up to 8 doses/day
Enzymes (lactase)	1,250 neutral lactase units/4 drops 3,300 FCC lactase units per tablet	3–4 drops taken with milk or dairy product 1 or 2 tablets as above
Bacterial replacement (*Lactobacillus acidophilus, Lactobacillus bulgaricus*)		2 tablets or 1 granule packet three to four times daily; give with milk, juice, or water
Octreotide	0.05 mg/mL 0.1 mg/mL 0.5 mg/mL	Initial: 50 mcg subcutaneously One to two times per day and titrate dose based on indication up to 600 mcg/day in two to four divided doses

syndrome, WDHA (watery diarrhea, hypokalemia, and achlorhydria) syndrome, pancreatic cholera, watery diarrhea syndrome, and vasoactive intestinal peptide-secreting tumor (VIPoma). Excessive secretion of VIP from a retroperitoneal or pancreatic tumor produces most of the clinical features. Excessive VIP is isolated in about half of patients, along with numerous other peptide hormones (peptide histidine methionine [PHM], serotonin, somatostatin, gastrin, and glucagon). Surgical tumor dissection is the treatment of choice. In nonsurgical candidates, the profuse watery diarrhea and other symptoms commonly encountered are managed with octreotide.

The dose of octreotide varies with the indication, disease severity and patient response.[11] For managing diarrhea and flushing associated with carcinoid tumors in adults, the initial dosage range is 100 to 600 mcg/day in two to four divided doses subcutaneously for 2 weeks. For controlling secretory diarrhea of VIPomas, the dosage range is 200 to 300 mcg/day in two to four divided doses for 2 weeks. Some patients may require higher doses for symptomatic control. Patients responding to these initial doses may be switched to Sandostatin LAR Depot, a long-acting octreotide formulation. This product consists of microspheres containing the drug. Initial doses consist of 20 mg given intramuscularly intragluteally at 4-week intervals for 2 months. It is recommended that during the first 2 weeks of therapy the short-acting formulation also be administered subcutaneously. At the end of 2 months, patients with good symptom control may have the dose reduced to 10 mg every 4 weeks, while those without sufficient symptom control may have the dose increased to 30 mg every 4 weeks. For patients experiencing recurrence of symptoms on the 10-mg dose, dosage adjustment to 20 mg should be made. It is not uncommon for patients with carcinoid tumors or VIPomas to experience periodic exacerbation of symptoms. Subcutaneous octreotide for several days should be reinstituted in these individuals. In so-called carcinoid crisis, octreotide is given as an intravenous infusion at 50 mcg/h for 8 to 24 hours.

Because octreotide inhibits many other gastrointestinal hormones, it has a variety of intestinal side effects. With prolonged use, gallbladder and biliary tract complications such as cholelithiasis have been reported. Approximately 5% to 10% of patients complain of nausea, diarrhea, and abdominal pain. Local injection pain occurs with about an 8% incidence. With high doses, octreotide may reduce dietary fat absorption, leading to steatorrhea.

Two other somatostatin analogs, lanreotide and vapreotide, have been studied.[13] Lanreotide, not currently available in the United States but available in Europe, is indicated for patients with carcinoid tumors in a dose of 30 mg intramuscularly (as a depot) every 14 days. If necessary the dose can be increased to 30 mg intramuscular every 7 to 10 days. Vapreotide is an orphan drug that is indicated for pancreatic and gastrointestinal fistulas as well as esophageal variceal bleeding.

Miscellaneous Products

Lactobacillus preparations such as Lactinex granules are considered probiotics agents that contain bacteria or yeast, such as lactic acid bacteria are dietary supplements that have been used for many years in hopes of replacing colonic microflora. This supposedly restores normal intestinal function and suppresses the growth of pathogenic microorganisms. However, a dairy product diet containing 200 to 400 g of lactose or dextrin is equally effective in producing recolonization of normal flora. The dosage of lactobacillus preparations varies depending on the brand used and lactobacillus preparations should be administered with milk, juice, water, or cereal. Intestinal flatus is the primary patient complaint experienced with this modality.

Anticholinergic drugs such as atropine block vagal tone and prolong gut transit time. Drugs with anticholinergic properties are present in many nonprescription products. Their value in controlling diarrhea is questionable and limited because of side effects. Angle-closure glaucoma, selected heart diseases, and obstructive uropathies are relative contraindications to the use of anticholinergic agents.

Lactase enzyme products are helpful for patients who are experiencing diarrhea secondary to lactose intolerance. Lactase is required for carbohydrate digestion. When a patient lacks this enzyme, eating dairy products causes an osmotic diarrhea. Several products are available for use each time a dairy product, especially milk or ice cream, is consumed.

CLINICAL CONTROVERSY

Long-term use of oral opiates is not routinely recommended for several pharmacologic reasons. Some opioids such as morphine and codeine have the tendency to cause constipation by slowing down the peristaltic action of the bowels, which can also result in a functional ileus. This effect can be minimized by administering laxatives and/or stool softeners in patients who require long-term opiate therapy. Prokinetic agents may also be helpful in treating opiate-related constipation.

Investigational Drugs

Several new classes of compounds are undergoing clinical trials for efficacy in acute diarrhea.[14] Enkephalins are endogenous opiate compounds in the gut that have antisecretory and proabsorptive activity in the small intestine. They promote sodium and chloride reabsorption via stimulation of a nonadrenergic, noncholinergic neurotransmitter. Enkephalinase inhibitors, compounds that slow down the enzymatic (i.e., enkephalinase) breakdown of endogenous enkephalins found in the small intestines. They exert an antisecretory effect without affecting GI motility or CNS-related effects/side effects. One specific compound, originally called acetorphan but now referred to as racecadotril, has been extensively tested in humans and found to be equal to other opiate anti-diarrheals such as loperamide, while causing less GI motility side effects such as abdominal bloating, pain, and constipation.[15,16] Racecadotril is currently licensed only in France and a few other developing countries with a high incidence of childhood diarrhea, but it is expected to be approved by other countries as well in the near future.

Vaccines are a new therapeutic frontier in controlling infectious diarrheas, especially in developing countries.[17,18] An oral vaccine for cholera is licensed and available in other countries (Dukoral from SBL Vaccines) appears to provide somewhat better immunity and have fewer adverse effects than the previously available parenteral vaccine. However, the CDC does not recommend cholera vaccines for most travelers, nor is the vaccine available in the United States.

Oral *Shigella* vaccine, although effective under field conditions, requires 5 weekly oral doses and repeat booster doses, thereby limiting its practicality for use in developing nations. With about 1,500 serotypes for *Salmonella*, a vaccine is not currently available for humans. There are two newer typhoid vaccine formulations, one a parenteral inactivated whole-cell vaccine and the other an oral live-attenuated (Ty21a) vaccine that is administered in 4 doses on days 1, 3, 5, and 7, to be completed at least l week before exposure. Rotavirus vaccine is effective in infants and children; and is administered as a three-oral-dose sequence. A rotavirus vaccine program has been formed to reduce child morbidity and mortality from diarrheal disease by accelerating the availability of rotavirus vaccines appropriate for use in developing countries.

■ EVALUATION OF THERAPEUTIC OUTCOMES

General Outcomes Measures

Therapeutic outcomes are directed toward key symptoms, signs, and laboratory studies. Constitutional symptoms usually improve within 24 to 72 hours. Monitoring for changes in the frequency and character of bowel movements on a daily basis in conjunction with vital signs and improvement in appetite are of utmost importance. Also, the clinician needs to monitor body weight, serum osmolality, serum electrolytes, complete blood cell counts, urinalysis, and culture results (if appropriate).

Acute Diarrhea

Most patients with acute diarrhea experience mild to moderate distress. In the absence of moderate to severe dehydration, high fever, and blood or mucus in the stool, this illness is usually self-limiting within 3 to 7 days. Mild to moderate acute diarrhea is usually managed on an outpatient basis with oral rehydration, symptomatic treatment, and diet. Elderly persons with chronic illness and infants may require hospitalization for parenteral rehydration and close monitoring.

Severe Diarrhea

In the urgent/emergent situation, restoration of the patient's volume status is the most important outcome. Toxic patients (fever dehydration, hematochezia, or hypotension) require hospitalization, intravenous fluids and electrolyte administration, and empiric antibiotic therapy while awaiting culture and sensitivity results. With timely management, these patients usually recover within a few days.

CONSTIPATION

Constipation is a commonly encountered medical condition in the United States for which many patients initiate self-treatment. One reason constipation continues to be a frequent problem in this country is lack of adequate dietary fiber. Another unfortunate problem is that many people have misconceptions about normal bowel function, and think that daily bowel movements are required for health and well being. Others believe that the lack of a daily bowel movement contributes to the accumulation of toxic substances or is associated with various somatic complaints. These misconceptions often lead to the inappropriate use of laxatives by the general public.

Constipation does not have a single, generally agreed upon definition. When using the term, the lay public or healthcare professional may be referring to several difficult-to-quantify variables: bowel movement frequency, stool size or consistency, and such symptoms as the sensation of incomplete defecation. Stool frequency is most often used to describe constipation; however, the frequency of bowel movements used to define constipation is not well established.

Normal people pass at least 3 stools per week. Some of the definitions of constipation used in clinical studies include (a) less than 3 stools per week for women and 5 stools per week for men despite a high-residue diet, or a period of more than 3 days without a bowel movement; (b) straining at stool greater than 25% of the time and/or 2 or fewer stools per week; or (c) straining at defecation and less than 1 stool daily with minimal effort. These varying definitions demonstrate the difficulty in characterizing this problem. An international committee defined and classified constipation on the basis of stool frequency, consistency, and difficulty of defecation.[19,20]

Functional constipation is defined as two or more of the following complaints present for at least 12 months in the absence of laxative use: (a) straining at least 25% of the time; (b) lumpy or hard stools at least 25% of the time; (c) a feeling of incomplete evacuation at least 25% of the time; or (d) two or fewer bowel movements in a week. Rectal outlet delay is defined as anal blockage more than 25% of the time and prolonged defecation or manual disimpaction when necessary.

EPIDEMIOLOGY

A systematic review of the epidemiology of constipation in North America reported a prevalence range for constipation of 1.9% to 27%, with the most reported estimates ranging from 12% to 19%. Prevalence estimates by gender were female-to-male ratio of 2.2:1.[21] Results from 42,375 participants of the National Health Interview Survey on Digestive Disorders demonstrated that there is not an age-related increased incidence of infrequent bowel movements; however, there is an age-related increased incidence of laxative use.[22] The frequency of subjects reporting two or fewer bowel movements per week was 5.9% for those younger than 40 years of age; 3.8% for subjects 60 to 69 years of age; and 6.3% for subjects older than 80 years of age. In a prospective study of 3,166 people older than 65 years of age in a Florida community,[23] 26% of women and 15.8% of men reported recurrent constipation. Factors found to correlate with self-reported constipation were age, sex (higher frequency in females), total number of drugs taken, abdominal pain, and hemorrhoids.

PATHOPHYSIOLOGY

❺ Constipation is not a disease, but a symptom of an underlying disease or problem. Approaches to the treatment of constipation should begin with attempts to determine its cause. Disorders of the GI tract (irritable bowel syndrome or diverticulitis), metabolic disorders (diabetes), or endocrine disorders (hypothyroidism) may be involved. Constipation commonly results from a diet low in fiber or from use of constipating drugs such as opiates. Finally, constipation may sometimes be psychogenic in origin.[24] Each of these causes is discussed in the following sections.

Constipation is a frequently reported problem in the elderly, probably the result of improper diets (low in fiber and liquids), diminished abdominal wall muscular strength, and possibly diminished physical activity. However, as previously stated, the frequency of bowel movements is not decreased with normal aging. In addition, diseases that may cause constipation, such as colon cancer and diverticulitis, are more common with increasing age. Table 38–5 lists common causes of constipation in specific disease states.

Drug-Induced Constipation

Use of drugs that inhibit the neurologic or muscular function of the GI tract, particularly the colon, may result in constipation (Table 38–6).

The majority of cases of drug-induced constipation are caused by opiates, various agents with anticholinergic properties, and antacids containing aluminum or calcium. With most of the agents listed in Table 38–6, the inhibitory effects on bowel function are dose dependent, with larger doses clearly causing constipation more frequently.

Opiates have effects on all segments of the bowel, but effects are most pronounced on the colon. The major mechanism by which opiates produce constipation has been proposed to be prolongation of intestinal transit time by causing spastic, nonpropulsive contractions. An additional contributory mechanism may be an increase in electrolyte absorption.

All opiate derivatives are associated with constipation, but the degree of intestinal inhibitory effects seems to differ between agents. Orally administered opiates appear to have greater inhibitory effects than parenterally administered products. Orally administered enkephalins (endogenous opiate-like polypeptides) are recognized to have antimotility properties.

TABLE 38-5 Possible Causes of Constipation

Conditions	Possible Causes
GI disorders	Irritable bowel syndrome
	Diverticulitis
	Upper GI tract diseases
	Anal and rectal diseases
	Hemorrhoids
	Anal fissures
	Ulcerative proctitis
	Tumors
	Hernia
	Volvulus of the bowel
	Syphilis
	Tuberculosis
	Helminthic infections
	Lymphogranuloma venereum
	Hirschsprung's disease
Metabolic and endocrine disorders	Diabetes mellitus with neuropathy
	Hypothyroidism
	Panhypopituitarism
	Pheochromocytoma
	Hypercalcemia
	Enteric glucagon excess
Pregnancy	Depressed gut motility
	Increased fluid absorption from colon
	Decreased physical activity
	Dietary changes
	Inadequate fluid intake
	Low dietary fiber
	Use of iron salts
Neurogenic causes	CNS diseases
	Trauma to the brain (particularly the medulla)
	Spinal cord injury
	CNS tumors
	Cerebrovascular accidents
	Parkinson's disease
Psychogenic causes	Ignoring or postponing urge to defecate
	Psychiatric diseases
Drug induced	See Table 38–6

CLINICAL PRESENTATION

Table 38–7 shows the general clinical presentation of constipation.

TABLE 38-6 Drugs Causing Constipation

- Analgesics
  - Inhibitors of prostaglandin synthesis
  - Opiates
- Anticholinergics
  - Antihistamines
  - AntiParkinsonian agents (e.g., benztropine or trihexyphenidyl)
  - Phenothiazines
  - Tricyclic antidepressants
- Antacids containing calcium carbonate or aluminum hydroxide
- Barium sulfate
- Calcium channel blockers
- Clonidine
- Diuretics (non–potassium-sparing)
- Ganglionic blockers
- Iron preparations
- Muscle blockers (D-tubocurarine, succinylcholine)
- Nonsteroidal antiinflammatory agents
- Polystyrene sodium sulfonate

TABLE 38-7 Clinical Presentation of Constipation

Signs and symptoms
- It is important to ascertain whether the patient perceives the problem as infrequent bowel movements, stools of insufficient size, a feeling of fullness, or difficulty and pain on passing stool.
- Signs and symptoms include hard, small, or dry stools, bloated stomach, cramping abdominal pain and discomfort, straining or grunting, sensation of blockade, fatigue, headache, and nausea and vomiting.

Laboratory tests
- A series of examinations, including proctoscopy, sigmoidoscopy, colonoscopy, and barium enema, may be necessary to determine the presence of colorectal pathology.
- Thyroid function studies may be performed to determine the presence of metabolic and endocrine disorders.

TREATMENT

Constipation

■ GENERAL APPROACH TO TREATMENT

The patient should be asked about the frequency of bowel movements and the chronicity of constipation. Constipation occurring recently in an adult may indicate significant colon pathology such as malignancy; constipation present since early infancy may be indicative of neurologic disorders. The patient also should be carefully questioned about usual diet and laxative regimens. Does the patient have a diet consistently deficient in high-fiber items and containing mainly highly refined foods? What laxatives or cathartics has the patient used to attempt relief of constipation? The patient should be questioned about other concurrent medications, with interest focused on agents that might cause constipation.

For most patients who complain of constipation, a thorough physical examination is not required after it is established that constipation (a) is not a chronic problem, (b) is not accompanied by signs of significant GI disease (e.g., rectal bleeding or anemia), and (c) does not cause severe discomfort. In these circumstances, the patient may be referred directly to the first-line therapies for constipation described in the next section (mainly bulk-forming laxatives and dietary fiber with occasional use of saline or stimulant laxatives). Table 38–8 presents a general treatment algorithm for the management of constipation.

❻ The proper management of constipation requires a number of different modalities; however, the basis for therapy should be dietary modification. The major dietary change should be an increase in the amount of fiber consumed daily. In addition to dietary management, patients should be encouraged to alter other aspects of their lifestyles if necessary. Important considerations are to encourage patients to exercise (achieved even by brisk walking after dinner) and to adjust bowel habits so that a regular and adequate time is made to respond to the urge to defecate. Another general measure is to increase fluid intake. This is generally recommended and believed beneficial, although there is little objective evidence to support this measure.

If an underlying disease is recognized as the cause of constipation, attempts should be made to correct it. GI malignancies may be removed via surgical resection. Endocrine and metabolic derangements should be corrected by the appropriate methods. For example, when hypothyroidism is the cause of constipation, cautious institution of thyroid-replacement therapy is the most important treatment measure.

As discussed earlier, many drug substances may cause constipation. If a patient is consuming medications well known to cause constipation, consideration should be given to alternative agents. For some medications (e.g., antacids), nonconstipating alternatives exist. If no reasonable alternatives exist to the medication thought to be responsible for constipation, consideration should be given to lowering the dose. If a patient must remain on constipating medications, then more attention must be given to general measures for prevention of constipation, as discussed in the next section.

TABLE 38-8 Constipation Treatment Algorithm

History
- Stool frequency
- Stool consistency
- Difficulty of defecation

Possible causes
- Diet deficient in high-fiber items and consisting mainly of highly refined foods
- GI disorders
- Metabolic and endocrine disorders
- Pregnancy
- Neurogenic
- Psychogenic
- Drug induced
- Laxative abusers

Symptoms seen with chronic constipation
- Fluid and electrolyte imbalances (hypokalemia)
- Protein-losing gastroenteropathy with hypoalbuminemia
- Syndromes resembling colitis

Select appropriate diagnostic studies
- Proctoscopy
- Sigmoidoscopy
- Colonoscopy
- Barium enema

Diagnosis
1. Treat specific cause
2. No diagnosis, symptomatic therapy
   A. Bulk-forming agents
   B. Dietary modification
   C. Alter lifestyle (exercise)
   D. Increase fluid intake
   E. Discontinue potential drug inducer

■ NONPHARMACOLOGIC THERAPY

Dietary Modification and Bulk-Forming Agents

The most important aspect of therapy for constipation for the majority of patients is dietary modification to increase the amount of fiber consumed. Fiber, the portion of vegetable matter not digested in the human GI tract, increases stool bulk, retention of stool water, and rate of transit of stool through the intestine. The result of fiber therapy is an increased frequency of defecation. Also, fiber decreases intraluminal pressures in the colon and rectum, which is thought to be beneficial for diverticular disease and for irritable bowel syndrome. The specific physiologic effects of fiber are not well understood. Patients should be advised to include at least 10 g of crude fiber in their daily diets.[26] Fruits, vegetables, and cereals have the highest fiber content. Bran, a by-product of milling of wheat, is often added to foods to increase fiber content and contains a high amount of soluble fiber, which may be extremely constipating in larger doses. Raw bran is generally 40% fiber. Medicinal products, often called "bulk-forming agents," such as psyllium hydrophilic colloids, methylcellulose, or polycarbophil, have properties similar to those of dietary fiber and may be taken as tablets, powders, or granules (Table 38–9).

A trial of dietary modification with high-fiber content should be continued for at least 1 month before effects on bowel function are determined. Most patients begin to notice effects on bowel function 3 to 5 days after beginning a high-fiber diet, but some patients may require a considerably longer period of time. Patients should be cautioned that abdominal distension and flatus may be particularly

TABLE 38-9 Dosage Recommendations for Laxatives and Cathartics

Agent	Recommended Dose
Agents that cause softening of feces in 1–3 days	
Bulk-forming agents/osmotic laxatives	
Methylcellulose	4–6 g/day
Polycarbophil	4–6 g/day
Psyllium	Varies with product
Polyethylene glycol 3350	
Emollients	
Docusate sodium	50–360 mg/day
Docusate calcium	50–360 mg/day
Docusate potassium	100–300 mg/day
Lactulose	15–30 mL orally
Sorbitol	30–50 g/day orally
Mineral oil	15–30 mL orally
Agents that result in soft or semifluid stool in 6–12 h	
Bisacodyl (oral)	5–15 mg orally
Senna	Dose varies with formulation
Magnesium sulfate (low dose)	<10 g orally
Agents that cause watery evacuation in 1–6 h	
Magnesium citrate	18 g 300 mL water
Magnesium hydroxide	2.4–4.8 g orally
Magnesium sulfate (high dose)	10–30 g orally
Sodium phosphates	Varies with salt used
Bisacodyl	10 mg rectally
Polyethylene glycol-electrolyte preparations	4 L

troublesome in the first few weeks of fiber therapy, particularly with high bran consumption. In most cases these problems resolve with continued use.

Bulk-forming laxatives have few adverse effects. The only major caution in the use of bulk-forming laxatives is that obstruction of the esophagus, stomach, small intestine, and colon has been reported when the agents have been consumed without sufficient fluid and in patients with intestinal stenosis.

Surgery

In a small percentage of patients who present with complaints of constipation, surgical procedures are necessary because of the presence of colonic malignancies or GI obstruction from a number of other causes. In each case, the involved segment of intestine may be resected or revised. Surgery may be required in some endocrine disorders that cause constipation, such as pheochromocytoma, which requires removal of a tumor.

Biofeedback

The majority of patients with constipation related to pelvic floor dysfunction can benefit from electromyogram-guided biofeedback therapy.[25] The value of biofeedback in children with chronic constipation has not been well demonstrated.[26]

■ PHARMACOLOGIC THERAPY

Drug Regimens of Choice

Treatment and prevention of constipation should consist of bulk-forming agents in addition to dietary modifications that increase dietary fiber.[27] A variety of products are available that provide adequate bulk. Whichever agent is chosen, it should be used daily and continued indefinitely in most patients, particularly those with chronic constipation.

For most persons with acute constipation, infrequent use (less than every few weeks) of laxative products is acceptable. Acute constipation may be relieved by the use of a tap-water enema or a glycerin suppository; if neither is effective, the use of oral sorbitol, low doses of bisacodyl or senna, or saline laxatives (e.g., milk of magnesia) may provide relief. If laxative treatment is required for longer than 1 week, the person should be advised to consult a physician to determine if there is an underlying cause of constipation that requires treatment with other modalities.

For some bedridden or geriatric patients, or others with chronic constipation, bulk-forming laxatives remain the first line of treatment, but the use of more potent laxatives may be required relatively frequently. Fiber should be avoided in bedridden patients who are cognitively impaired.[25] When other than bulk-forming laxatives are used, they should be administered in the lowest effective dose and as infrequently as possible to maintain regular bowel function (more than 3 stools per week). Agents that may be used in these situations include bisacodyl, senna, milk of magnesia, and sorbitol or lactulose. Mineral oil should be avoided, particularly in bedridden patients, because of the risk of aspiration and lipoid pneumonia. Some patients with chronic constipation may present with fecal impactions. Before vigorous oral laxatives can be used, the impaction needs to be removed using mechanical methods, including tap-water or saline enemas and digital extraction.

In the hospitalized patient without GI disease, constipation may be related to the use of general anesthesia and/or opiate substances. Most orally or rectally administered laxatives may be used in these situations. For prompt initiation of bowel evacuation, either a tap-water enema, glycerin suppository, or oral milk of magnesia are recommended.

With infants and children, constipation may occur commonly. In patients with persistent problems, the underlying etiology may be neurologic, metabolic, or secondary to anatomic abnormalities. Management of constipation in this age group should consist of dietary modification with an emphasis on high-fiber foods.

For acute constipation in most age groups, a tap-water enema or glycerin suppository may be helpful. Occasional use of milk of magnesia or an anthraquinone laxative in low doses is justified as well.

Drug Classes

The traditional classification system for laxatives and cathartics by suspected mode of action is not very useful, as this is not clearly understood for many agents. In general, most of these products induce bowel evacuation by one or more of the mechanisms associated with the etiology of diarrhea, including active electrolyte secretion, decreased water and electrolyte absorption, increased intraluminal osmolarity, and increased hydrostatic pressure in the gut. Laxatives convert the intestine from primarily an organ that absorbs water and electrolytes to an organ that secretes these substances.

The various classes of laxatives are discussed in this section. These agents are divided into three general classifications: (a) those causing softening of feces in 1 to 3 days (bulk-forming laxatives, docusates, and lactulose); (b) those that result in soft or semifluid stool in 6 to 12 hours (diphenylmethane derivatives and anthraquinone derivatives); and (c) those causing water evacuation in 1 to 6 hours (saline cathartics, castor oil, and polyethylene glycol-electrolyte lavage solution).

Emollient Laxatives

Emollient laxatives are surfactant agents, docusate in its various salts, which work by facilitating mixing of aqueous and fatty materials within the intestinal tract. They may increase water and electrolyte secretion in the small and large bowel. These products are generally given orally, although docusate potassium has also been used rectally. These products result in a softening of stools within 1 to 3 days of therapy.

Emollient laxatives are ineffective in treating constipation, but are used mainly to prevent this condition. They may be helpful in situations in which straining at stool should be avoided, such as after recovery from myocardial infarction, with acute perianal disease, or after rectal surgery. It is unlikely that these agents would be effective in preventing constipation if major causative factors (e.g., heavy opiate use, uncorrected pathology, or inadequate dietary fiber) are not concurrently addressed.

Although docusates are generally safe, a few adverse effects have been noted. They may increase the intestinal absorption of agents administered concurrently and alter toxic potential.

Lubricants

Mineral oil is the only lubricant laxative in routine use. This agent, obtained from petroleum refining, acts by coating stool and allowing for easier passage. It inhibits colonic absorption of water, thereby increasing stool weight and decreasing stool transit time. Mineral oil may be given orally or rectally in a dose of 15 to 45 mL. Generally, the effect on bowel function is noted after 2 or 3 days of use.

Mineral oil is helpful in situations similar to those suggested for docusates: to maintain a soft stool and to avoid straining for relatively short periods of time (a few days to 2 weeks); however, it possesses a much greater potential for adverse effects and its routine use should be discouraged. Mineral oil may be absorbed systemically and can cause a foreign-body reaction in lymphoid tissue. Also, in debilitated or recumbent patients, mineral oil may be aspirated, causing lipoid pneumonia.[28] Mineral oil may decrease the absorption of fat-soluble vitamins (A, D, E, and K) with chronic use by causing retention in the GI tract. Finally, even when given orally, mineral oil may leak from the anal sphincter, causing pruritus and soiling of clothing.

Lactulose and Sorbitol

Lactulose is a disaccharide that is used orally or rectally. It is metabolized by colonic bacteria to low-molecular-weight acids, resulting in an osmotic effect whereby fluid is retained in the colon.[29] The fluid retained in the colon lowers the pH and increases colonic peristalsis. Lactulose is generally not recommended as a first-line agent for the treatment of constipation because it is costly and not necessarily more effective than such agents as sorbitol or milk of magnesia. It may be justified as an alternative for acute constipation, and has been particularly useful in elderly patients. Occasionally, the use of lactulose may result in flatulence, cramps, diarrhea, and electrolyte imbalances.[30] Sorbitol, a monosaccharide, exerts its effect by osmotic action and has been recommended as a primary agent in the treatment of functional constipation in cognitively intact patients.[25] It is as effective as lactulose and much less expensive.

Diphenylmethane and Anthraquinone Derivatives

Bisacodyl, the only remaining diphenylmethane derivative with the withdrawal of phenolphthalein, exerts its therapeutic effect by stimulating the mucosal nerve plexus of the colon. Bisacodyl exhibits significant interpatient variability in effective dose, with doses that cause no effect in one patient resulting in excessive cramping and fluid evacuation in others. Bisacodyl is not recommended for regular daily use but can be used intermittently (every few weeks) to treat constipation or as a bowel preparation before diagnostic procedures in which cleansing of the colon is necessary. Bisacodyl may sometimes cause severe abdominal cramping as well as significant fluid and electrolyte imbalances with chronic use.

Senna or sennosoids are the only remaining anthraquinone derivatives after removal of cascara sagrada and casanthrone (cascara extracts). Laxative effects are limited to the colon, and stimulation of the Auerbach plexus may be involved. As with bisacodyl, senna is only recommended for intermittent use and daily use should be strongly discouraged.

Saline Cathartics

Saline cathartics are composed of relatively poorly absorbed ions such as magnesium, sulfate, phosphate, and citrate, which produce their effects primarily by osmotic action in retaining fluid in the GI tract. Magnesium stimulates the secretion of cholecystokinin, a hormone that causes stimulation of bowel motility and fluid secretion. These agents may be given orally or rectally. A bowel movement may result within a few hours after oral doses and in 1 hour or less after rectal administration.

These agents should be used primarily for acute evacuation of the bowel, which may be necessary before diagnostic examinations, after poisonings, and in conjunction with some anthelmintics to eliminate parasites. Such agents as milk of magnesia (an 8% suspension of magnesium hydroxide) may be used occasionally (every few weeks) to treat constipation in otherwise healthy adults. Saline cathartics should not be used on a routine basis. The enema formulations of these agents may be useful in fecal impactions.

As with most laxatives, these agents may cause fluid and electrolyte depletion. Also, magnesium or sodium accumulation may occur when magnesium-containing cathartics are used in patients with renal dysfunction or when sodium phosphate is used in patients with congestive heart failure.

Castor Oil

Castor oil is metabolized in the GI tract to an active compound, ricinoleic acid, which stimulates secretory processes, decreases glucose absorption, and promotes intestinal motility, primarily in the small intestine. Castor oil usually results in a bowel movement within 1 to 3 hours of administration. Because the agent has such a strong purgative action, it should not be used for the routine treatment of constipation.

Glycerin

Glycerin is usually administered as a 3-g suppository and exerts its effect by osmotic action in the rectum. As with most agents given as suppositories, the onset of action is usually less than 30 minutes. Glycerin is considered a very safe laxative, although it may occasionally cause rectal irritation. Its use is acceptable on an intermittent basis for constipation, particularly in children.

Polyethylene Glycol-Electrolyte Lavage Solution

Whole-bowel irrigation with polyethylene glycol-electrolyte lavage solution (PEG-ELS) has become popular for colon cleansing before diagnostic procedures or colorectal operations.

Four liters of this solution is administered over 3 hours to obtain complete evacuation of the GI tract. The solution is not recommended the routine treatment of constipation and its use should be avoided in patients with intestinal obstruction.

Lubiprostone

The FDA recently approved the first new drug in a class called "chloride channel activators," which are designed to act locally in the gut to open chloride channels on the GI luminal epithelium, which, in turn, stimulates chloride-rich intestinal fluid secretion and accelerates GI transit time and delays gastric emptying.[31] Lubiprostone (Amitiza), is approved for "chronic idiopathic constipation in adults" at a recommended dose of one 24-mg capsule twice daily with food. Clinical trials have shown a significant increase in spontaneous bowel movements versus placebo.[32] Common adverse effects include headache (13%), diarrhea, and nausea, as a result of delayed gastric emptying, which were more prominent with twice-daily dosing.

Other Agents

Tap-water enemas may be used to treat simple constipation. The administration of 200 mL of tap water by enema to an adult often results in a bowel movement within 30 minutes. Soap-suds enemas are no longer recommended as their use may result in proctitis or colitis.

Prevention

For certain groups of patients, such as those recovering from myocardial infarction or rectal surgery, straining at defecation is to be avoided. The basis of preventive therapy in these patients should be bulk-forming laxatives. Additionally, the use of docusate is popular, although its effectiveness is debated. In pregnant patients, constipation may result because of alterations in anatomy or iron supplementation. As described earlier, bulk-forming laxatives and docusates should be the first line of prevention.

LAXATIVE ABUSE SYNDROME

Misconceptions about normal bowel patterns and the effect of laxatives have contributed to a syndrome of laxative abuse that is relatively common in the United States. The availability of laxatives as chocolates or gums conveys to the public that the use of these agents is without adverse consequences. Abuse of laxatives has occurred traditionally in persons trying to maintain daily bowel function, but more recently has extended to others who use laxatives for the purpose of controlling weight. In either case, the consistent abuse of strong laxatives and cathartics may lead to serious illness.

Laxative abuse for the purpose of maintaining daily bowel function begins with misconceptions about the frequency, quantity, or consistency of stools. With the use of strong purgatives, the colon may be so thoroughly cleansed that a bowel movement may not occur normally until a few days later. This delay reinforces the need for more purgatives and the cycle of laxative dependence is begun. Eventually the patient may require daily laxatives to maintain bowel function. A variation of laxative abuse is seen in persons who use them as a means of weight loss.

The laxative abuser may present with contradictory findings of diarrhea and weight loss. In addition, long-term abusers of laxatives lend to have vomiting, abdominal pain, lassitude, weakness, thirst, edema, and bone pain (caused by osteomalacia). With prolonged use of laxatives a number of serious illnesses may arise, including fluid and electrolyte imbalances (including acid–base imbalances and hypokalemia), protein-losing gastroenteropathy with hypoalbuminemia, and syndromes resembling colitis.

The determination of laxative abuse syndrome can be difficult because many laxative abusers vigorously deny laxative use. Middle-aged women tend to be the most common laxative abusers. The chronic laxative abuse problem should be addressed by a combination of measures, including psychiatric evaluation, dietary modification with reliance on bulk-forming laxatives, and specific guidelines to the patient for the withdrawal of stimulant laxatives.

EVALUATION OF THERAPEUTIC OUTCOMES

The ultimate goal of treatment for constipation is alteration of lifestyle (particularly diet) to prevent further episodes of constipation. Short-term goals include alleviation of acute constipation with relief from symptoms. For patients with chronic constipation, the goals are more long-term and include use of proper diet and decreased reliance on laxatives. Effective treatment of constipation requires the patient to become more knowledgeable about the causes of constipation, proper diet, and appropriate use of laxatives.

IRRITABLE BOWEL SYNDROME

Irritable bowel syndrome (IBS) is a gastrointestinal syndrome characterized by chronic abdominal pain and altered bowel habits in the absence of any organic cause. It is the most commonly diagnosed gastrointestinal condition.

EPIDEMIOLOGY

The prevalence of IBS is approximately 10% to 15% based on North American and European population-based studies; however, there is a wide variation in prevalence by individual country.[33–36] IBS affects men and women, young patients, and the elderly. However, younger patients and women are more likely to be diagnosed with IBS. A systematic review estimated that there is an overall 2:1 female predominance in North America.[34] Although only 15% of those affected actually seek medical attention, IBS is the cause of between 25% and 50% of all referrals to gastroenterologists.[37]

PATHOPHYSIOLOGY

Although the exact pathophysiologic abnormalities with IBS are still being actively investigated, it is currently thought that IBS results from altered somatovisceral and motor dysfunction of the intestine from a variety of causes. Abnormal central nervous system processing of afferent signals may lead to visceral hypersensitivity, with the specific nerve pathway affected determining the exact symptomatology expressed. This visceral hypersensitivity is a neuroenteric phenomenon that is independent of motility and psychological disturbances.[27] Factors known to contribute to these alterations include genetics, motility factors, inflammation, colonic infections, mechanical irritation to local nerves, stress, and other psychological factors.

Serotonin-Type Receptors

The enteric nervous system contains a significant percentage of the body's 5-hydroxytryptamine (serotonin, 5-HT).[38] Two types of serotonin exists within the gut: serotonin type 3 (HT_3) and serotonin type 4 (HT_4), which are responsible for secretion, sensitization, and motility.[39] Previous studies show that there is an increase in the postprandial levels of 5-HT in those who suffer from diarrhea predominant IBS when compared with nonsufferers.[38] Therefore, stimulation and antagonism of these serotonin receptors has become a focused area for research on new drug therapies for both diarrhea- and constipation-predominant disease.

CLINICAL PRESENTATION

❼ Irritable bowel syndrome presents as either diarrhea-predominant or constipation-predominant disease and can be defined as lower abdominal pain, disturbed defecation (constipation, diarrhea, or an alternating pattern of both), and bloating in the absence of structural or biochemical factors that might explain these symptoms (Table 38–10). Because IBS can consist of a variable number of signs and symptoms, two diagnostic criteria "check lists" are commonly used to aid in the workup of a patient suspected of having IBS. The Manning criteria was first proposed in 1978, whereas the Rome criteria was initially proposed in 1999 and revised as recently as 2006 by an international working group in an effort to help standardize the diagnostic criteria used in clinical research protocols. Table 38–11 shows the symptom criteria for both of the Manning[40] and Rome III[41] symptom-based criteria.

Additional diagnostic steps that can be taken include sigmoidoscopy or colonoscopy; examination of the stool for occult blood and ova and parasites; complete blood cell count; erythrocyte sedimen-

TABLE 38-10 Clinical Presentation of Irritable Bowel Syndrome

Signs and symptoms
• Lower abdominal pain
• Abdominal bloating and distension
• Diarrhea symptoms, >3 stools/day
• Extreme urgency
• Mucus passage
• Constipation symptoms, <3 stools/wk, straining, incomplete evacuation
• Psychological symptoms such as depression and anxiety
Nongastrointestinal symptoms
• Urinary symptoms
• Fatigue
• Dyspareunia
Other concurrent conditions
• Fibromyalgia
• Functional dyspepsia
• Chronic fatigue syndrome
Reduced health-related quality of life

tation rate; and serum electrolytes. In some cases, radiographic imaging studies, such as computed tomography scans or barium swallows or enemas, may also be necessary if the findings of the above assessment are not typical for IBS.[42]

TREATMENT

Irritable Bowel Syndrome

■ GENERAL APPROACH TO TREATMENT

The treatment approach to IBS is based upon the predominant symptoms and their severity (Fig. 38–3). Milder, less frequent episodes can be managed with dietary restrictions and a higher-fiber diet, with addition of bulk-forming laxatives, if necessary. More persistent disease may require as-needed uses of various antispasmodic or antidiarrheal agents such as loperamide. Lastly, the most-severe forms of this disease may call for pharmacologic agents directed specifically at the underlying neurohormonal imbalance, such as the 5-HT_4 agonists, such as tegaserod, or the 5-HT_3 receptor antagonists, such as alosetron.

CLINICAL CONTROVERSY

The newer serotonin receptor agonists and antagonists tegaserod and alosetron act on GI-specific serotonin receptors to treat constipation-predominant and diarrhea predominant IBS, respectively. However, both drugs are currently only indicated for women. Efficacy and safety in men has not been established because the initial manufacturer's sponsored clinical trials contained insufficient numbers of men with IBS to provide the necessary statistical power to prove efficacy and safety. Ongoing studies should determine if these drugs are indicated in men.

Alosetron, a 5-HT_3 receptor antagonist, was withdrawn from the U.S. market in 2000 as a result of serious adverse effects, including severe constipation and ischemic colitis that did not appear in the initial clinical trials. It was reintroduced in 2002 and is now limited to an FDA-approved restricted-use program in lower initial doses, and requires extensive postmarketing surveillance. Results of these trials are necessary to definitively determine alosetron's true safety profile, especially with regard to its association with or causation of fatal ischemic colitis.

TABLE 38-11 Symptom-Based Criteria for Irritable Bowel Syndrome

The Manning criteria[40]
Chronic or recurrent abdominal pain for at least 6 months and two or more of the following:
1. Abdominal pain relieved with defecation
2. Abdominal pain associated with more frequent stools
3. Abdominal pain associated with looser stools
4. Abdominal distension
5. Feeling of incomplete evacuation after defecation
6. Mucus in stools
Rome III diagnostic criteria for irritable bowel syndrome[41]
Recurrent abdominal pain or discomfort at least 3 days per month in the last 3 months associated with 2 or more of the following:
1. Relieved with defecation
2. Onset associated with a change in frequency of stool
3. Onset associated with a change in form (appearance) of stool

■ CONSTIPATION-PREDOMINANT DISEASE

In the constipation-predominant patient, dietary fiber may be beneficial. Patients should be instructed to begin with 1 tablespoonful of fiber with 1 meal daily and gradually increase the dose to include fiber with 2 and 3 meals a day until the desired outcome is achieved. End points that the patient should aim for include bulkier and more easily passed stools. For patients unable to tolerate dietary

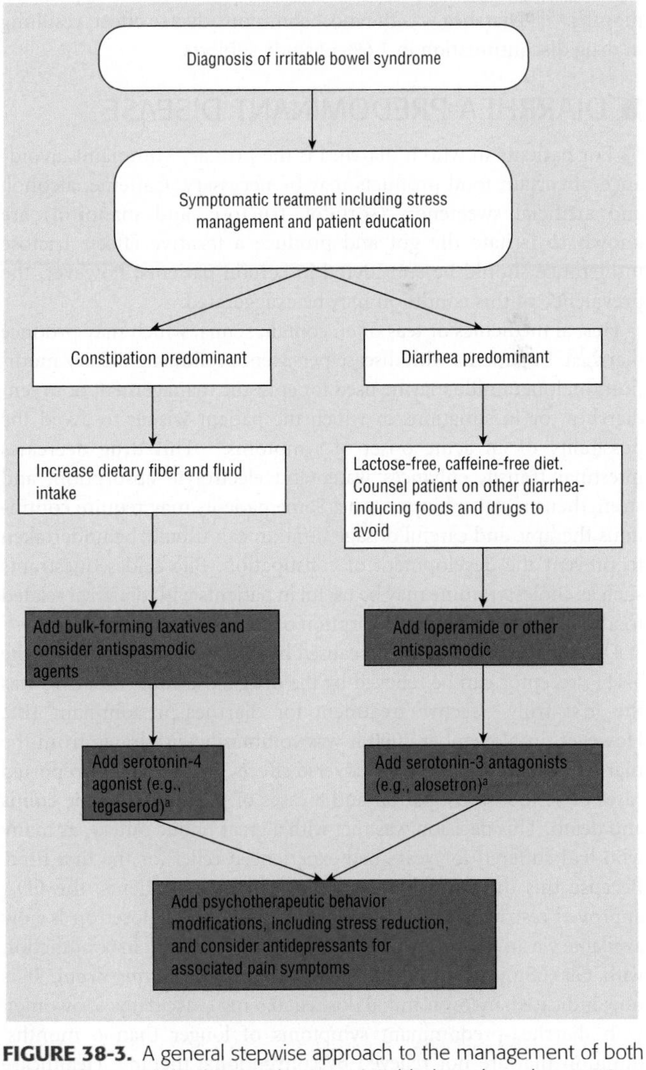

FIGURE 38-3. A general stepwise approach to the management of both constipation- and diarrhea-predominant irritable bowel syndrome. [a]Consider manufacturer sponsored patient access program.

bran, bulking agents such as psyllium may be substituted.[30] Laxative use is not encouraged in these patients, and it should only be used in the smallest dose for the least amount of time in cases of severe constipation.

The 5-HT_4 partial agonist tegaserod was the first therapy approved by the FDA specifically for short-term, intermittent treatment of constipation-predominant IBS.[42] Tegaseride was suspended from marketing in early 2007 at the request of the FDA due to an analysis of clinical trial data showing a small, yet significant, increase in ischemia events (MI < CVA, and unstable angina) in patients with pre-existing cardiovascular disease and/or cardiovascular risk factors. In July 2007, the drug's manufacturer, Novartis, began tegaseride (Zelnorm®) restricted access program to patients in the United States via either a manufacturer sponsored FDA-approved investigational new drug (IND) protocol or through the FDA via an emergency INID protocol. Tegaserod is a serotonin derivative that activates 5-HT_4 receptors on the neurons in the gastrointestinal tract, increasing GI motility and decreasing visceral sensations. It is approved as 2-mg or 6-mg doses given twice daily 30 minutes prior to a meal with water for up to 12 weeks.[43] Stimulation of the 5-HT_4 receptors by tegaserod increases gastric secretions and promotes motility, with improvement in symptoms generally occurring within the first week of therapy. Currently this therapy is only approved for use in women, as efficacy and safety in men has not been established because of inadequate numbers of men enrolled in clinical trials to date.[44] In addition, length of effective therapy has only been approved for 12 weeks[45]; however, tegaserod may provide safe and effective therapy for up to 12 months.[44,46] Diarrhea was the most common adverse effect, resulting in drug discontinuation in 1.6% of study subjects.

■ DIARRHEA-PREDOMINANT DISEASE

❽ For patients in whom diarrhea is the primary complaint, avoidance of certain food products may be necessary. Caffeine, alcohol, and artificial sweeteners (sorbitol, fructose, and mannitol) are known to irritate the gut and produce a laxative effect. Lactose intolerance should be considered in certain patients; however, the prevalence of this condition may be exaggerated.

Herbal medicines or teas often contain senna, which may produce diarrhea. In patients with disease persistence following dietary modification, loperamide may be used for episodic management of urgent diarrhea, or in situations in which the patient wishes to avoid the possibility of an acute onset of symptoms.[43] This drug decreases intestinal transit, enhances water and electrolyte absorption, and strengthens rectal sphincter tone. Some patients may require continuous therapy, and careful dosage titration can usually be undertaken to prevent the development of constipation. Bile acid sequestrants such as cholestyramine may be useful in patients with diarrhea related to idiopathic bile acid malabsorption or following cholecystectomy.[42]

Diarrhea-predominant IBS caused by excessive stimulation of the 5-HT_3 receptor can be relieved by the drug alosetron. Alosetron was the first truly effective treatment for diarrhea-predominant IBS. However, in November 2000 it was voluntarily withdrawn from the market because of severe GI adverse effects, including 113 reported cases of serious constipation and 8 cases of possible ischemic colitis and death. This decision was met with a great public outcry, as many who had suffered for years had experienced relief for the first time. Because this drug was highly effective in many patients, the FDA approved restricted use of alosetron in June 2002. Alosetron is now available via an FDA-approved restricted-use program in conjunction with GlaxoSmithKline as detailed at *http://www.lotronex.com*. It is now indicated, in lower initial doses of 0.5 mg twice daily, for women with diarrhea-predominant symptoms of longer than 6 months' duration that are not relieved by conventional therapy. Healthcare providers must use extreme caution in therapy with this drug, and must follow strict FDA-mandated guidelines.

Use of Antidepressants in IBS

Tricyclic antidepressants have shown some benefit in treatment of diarrhea-predominant IBS associated with moderate to severe abdominal pain, by modulating perception of visceral pain, altering GI transit time, and treating underlying comorbidities.[47,48] Selective serotonin reuptake inhibitors are less-well studied, with only one report with paroxetine showing some improvement in stool passage and "well being" but no decrease in abdominal pain.[49]

Figure 38–3 shows a general stepwise approach to the management of both constipation and diarrhea-predominant irritable bowel syndrome.

■ PAIN IN IBS

❾ Select patients with IBS suffer significant pain associated with their disease. Data supporting the use of antispasmodic agents in these patients are conflicting.[50,51] In these cases, a trial of low-dose antidepressant therapy is indicated, especially if pain is associated with eating. Both tricyclic antidepressants and serotonin reuptake inhibitors produce analgesia, and may relieve depressive symptoms if present. Preprandial doses of drugs containing anticholinergic properties may suppress pain (and/or diarrhea) associated with an overactive postprandial gastrocolonic response. Tricyclic antidepressants should be avoided in patients with pain and constipation. In addition, psychotherapy, including cognitive behavioral therapy, relaxation therapy, and hypnotherapy, has been shown to decrease IBS symptoms.[52]

■ DRUG CLASSES CURRENTLY UNDER INVESTIGATION FOR THE TREATMENT OF IBS

Probiotics (see Diarrhea above) such as *Lactobacillus* and *Bifidobacterium* reduced IBS symptoms in several investigation trials.[53,54] Another 5-HT_3 antagonist, cilansetron, has demonstrated similar efficacy to that of alosetron in phase II trials and enrolled enough male patients to show benefit in males as well. This drug is currently in phase III trials. In addition, other compounds being evaluated include neurokinin$_1$ (NK1) and neurokinin$_3$ (NK3) receptor antagonists, gut-selective calcium channel blockers, cholecystokinin receptor antagonists, and agents capable of stimulating motilin receptors (motilin mimetics).[55]

■ EVALUATION OF THERAPEUTIC OUTCOMES

IBS is usually classified as constipation-predominant, diarrhea-predominant, or IBS with abdominal pain and bloating. Therapeutic goals in IBS should focus on the patient's primary complaint. Dietary and drug therapy goals should focus on end-organ treatment to relieve abdominal pain (antispasmodic drugs) or disturbed bowel habits (antidiarrheals and bulk-forming agents). Additionally, severe symptoms from central nervous system dysregulation should be treated with antidepressants, psychotherapy, relaxation/stress management, cognitive behavior treatment, and/or hypnosis aimed at specific affective disorders.[55] Lastly, the serotonin receptor agonists and antagonists can be used in carefully selected patients whose symptoms are not adequately controlled with other agents. The American Gastroenterology Association recommends that patients with severe IBS consider psychological treatments such as psychotherapy, relaxation/stress management, and/or cognitive behavior treatment.

ABBREVIATIONS

5-HT: serotonin

IBS: irritable bowel syndrome

ORS: oral rehydration solution

PEG-ELS: polyethylene glycol-electrolyte lavage solution

PHM: peptide histidine methionine

VIP: vasoactive intestinal peptide

REFERENCES

1. Binder HJ. Causes of chronic diarrhea. N Engl J Med 2006;355(3):236–239.
2. Dupont HL. Diarrheal diseases in the developing world. Infect Dis Clin North Am 1995;9(2):313–324.
3. Feldman RA, Banatvala N. The frequency of culturing stools from adults with diarrhea in Great Britain. Epidemiol Infect 1994;113 (1):41–44.
4. Sandler RS, Stewart WF, Liberman JN, Ricci JA, Zorich NL. Abdominal pain, bloating, and diarrhea in the United States: Prevalence and impact. Dig Dis Sci 2000;45(6):1166–1171.
5. Musher DM, Musher BL. Contagious acute gastrointestinal infections. N Engl J Med 2004;351(23):2417–2427.
6. Jones TF, Bulens SN, Gettner S, et al. Use of stool collection kits delivered to patients can improve confirmation of etiology in foodborne disease outbreaks. Clin Infect Dis 2004;39(10):1454–1459.
7. Fine KD, Schiller LR. AGA technical review on the evaluation and management of chronic diarrhea. Gastroenterology 1999;116(6):1464–1486.
8. Mahalanabis D. Current status: Of oral rehydration as a strategy for the control of diarrhoeal diseases. Indian J Med Res 1996;104:115–124.
9. Pizarro D, Posada G, Sandi L, Moran JR. Rice-based oral electrolyte solutions for the management of infantile diarrhea. N Engl J Med 1991;324(8):517–521.
10. Ansdell VE, Ericsson CD. Prevention and empiric treatment of traveler's diarrhea. Med Clin North Am 1999;83(4):945–973.
11. Harris AG, Odorisio TM, Woltering EA, et al. Consensus statement—Octreotide dose titration in secretory diarrhea. Diarrhea Management Consensus Development Panel. Dig Dis Sci 1995;40(7): 1464–1473.
12. Schiller LR. Review article: Anti-diarrhoeal pharmacology and therapeutics. Aliment Pharmacol Ther 1995;9(2):87–106.
13. Ruszniewski P, Ducreux M, Chayvialle JA, et al. Treatment of the carcinoid syndrome with the long-acting somatostatin analogue lanreotide: A prospective study in 39 patients. Gut 1996;39(2):279–283.
14. Farthing MJ. Antisecretory drugs for diarrheal disease. Dig Dis 2006;24(1–2):47–58.
15. Prado D. A multinational comparison of racecadotril and loperamide in the treatment of acute watery diarrhoea in adults. Scand J Gastroenterol 2002;37(6):656–661.
16. Lecomte JM. An overview of clinical studies with racecadotril in adults. Int J Antimicrob Agents 2000;14(1):81–87.
17. Thompson RF, Bass DM, Hoffman SL. Travel vaccines. Infect Dis Clin North Am 1999;13(1):149–167.
18. Tacket CO, Kotloff KL, Losonsky G, et al. Volunteer studies investigating the safety and efficacy of live oral El Tor Vibrio cholerae 01, vaccine strain CVD 111. Am J Trop Med Hygiene 1997;56(5):533–537.
19. Koch A, Voderholzer WA, Klauser AG, Müller-Lissner S. Symptoms in chronic constipation. Dis Colon Rect 1997;40(8):902–906.
20. Romero Y, Evans JM, Fleming KC, Phillips SF. Constipation and fecal incontinence in the elderly population. Mayo Clin Proc 1996;71(1):81–92.
21. Higgins PD, Johanson JF. Epidemiology of constipation in North America: A systematic review. Am J Gastroenterol 2004;99(4):750–759.
22. Harari D, Gurwitz JH, Avorn J, Bohn R, Minaker KL. Bowel habit in relation to age and gender. Findings from the National Health Interview Survey and clinical implications. Arch Intern Med 1996;156 (3):315–320.
23. Stewart RB, Moore MT, Stat M, Marks RG, Hale WE. Correlates of constipation in an ambulatory elderly population. Am J Gastroenterol 1992;87(7):859–864.
24. Browning SM. Constipation, diarrhea, and irritable bowel syndrome. Primary Care 1999;26(1):113–136.
25. Ko CY, Tong J, Lehman RE, Shelton AA, Schrock TR, Welton ML. Biofeedback is effective therapy for fecal incontinence and constipation. Arch Surg 1997;132(8):829–833.
26. van der Plas RN, Benninga MA, Büller HA, et al. Biofeedback training in treatment of childhood constipation: A randomised controlled study. Lancet 1996;348(9030):776–780.
27. Drossman DA. Review article: An integrated approach to the irritable bowel syndrome. Aliment Pharmaco Ther 1999;13:3–14.
28. Gattuso JM, Kamm MA. Adverse effects of drugs used in the management of constipation and diarrhea. Drug Safety 1994;10(1):47–65.
29. Clausen MR, Mortensen PB. Lactulose, disaccharides and colonic flora—Clinical consequences. Drugs 1997;53(6):930–942.
30. Thompson WG. Irritable bowel syndrome: A management strategy. Baillieres Best Pract Res Clin Gastroenterol 1999;13(3):453–460.
31. Cuppoletti J, Malinowska DH, Tewari KP, et al. SPI-0211, activates T84, cell chloride transport and recombinant human ClC-2 chloride currents. Am J Physiol Cell Physiol 2004;287(5):C1173–C1183.
32. Winpenny JP. Lubiprostone. Drugs 2005;8(5):416–422.
33. Hungin AP, Chang L, Locke GR, Dennis EH, Barghout V. Irritable bowel syndrome in the United States: Prevalence, symptom patterns and impact. Aliment Pharmacol Ther 2005;21(11):1365–1375.
34. Brandt LJ, Bjorkman D, Fennerty MB, et al. Systematic review on the management of irritable bowel syndrome in North America. Am J Gastroenterol 2002;97(11 Suppl):S7–S26.
35. Thompson WG, Irvine EJ, Pare P, Ferrazzi S, Rance L. Functional gastrointestinal disorders in Canada: First population-based survey using Rome II criteria with suggestions for improving the questionnaire. Dig Dis Sci 2002;47(1):225–235.
36. Hungin AP, Whorwell PJ, Tack J, Mearin F. The prevalence, patterns and impact of irritable bowel syndrome: An international survey of 40,000 subjects. Aliment Pharmacol Ther 2003;17(5):643–650.
37. Everhart JE, Renault PF. Irritable bowel syndrome in office-based practice in the United States. Gastroenterology 1991;100(4):998–1005.
38. Bearcroft CP, Perrett D, Farthing MJG. Postprandial plasma 5-hydroxytryptamine in diarrhoea predominant irritable bowel syndrome: A pilot study. Gut 1998;42(1):42–46.
39. Chey WD. Tegaserod and other serotonergic agents: What is the evidence? Rev Gastroenterol Disord 2003;3 Suppl 2:S35–S40.
40. Manning AP, Thompson WG, Heaton KW, Morris AF. Towards positive diagnosis of the irritable bowel. Br Med J 1978;2(6138):653–654.
41. Longstreth GF, Thompson WG, Chey WD, Houghton LA, Mearin F, Spiller RC. Functional bowel disorders. Gastroenterology 2006;130(5):1480–1491.
42. Camilleri M. Review article: Tegaserod. Aliment Pharmacol Ther 2001;15(3):277–289.
43. Tougas G, Snape WJ, Otten MH, et al. Long-term safety of tegaserod in patients with constipation-predominant irritable bowel syndrome. Aliment Pharmacol Ther 2002;16(10):1701–1708.
44. Muller-Lissner SA, Fumagalli I, Bardhan KD, et al. Tegaserod, a 5-HT_4 receptor partial agonist, relieves symptoms in irritable bowel syndrome patients with abdominal pain, bloating and constipation. Aliment Pharmacol Ther 2001;15(10):1655–1666.
45. Kim HJ, Camilleri M, McKinzie S, et al. A randomized controlled trial of a probiotic, VSL#3, on gut transit and symptoms in diarrhoea-predominant irritable bowel syndrome. Aliment Pharmacol Ther 2003;17(7):895–904.
46. Layer P, Keller J, Mueller-Lissner S, Ruegg P, Loeffler H. Tegaserod: Long-term treatment for irritable bowel syndrome patients with constipation in primary care. Digestion 2005;71(4):238–244.
47. Jackson JL, O'Malley PG, Tomkins G, Balden E, Santoro J, Kroenke K. Treatment of functional gastrointestinal disorders with antidepressant medications: A meta-analysis. Am J Med 2000;108(1):65–72.
48. Drossman DA, Toner BB, Whitehead WE, et al. Cognitive-behavioral therapy versus education and desipramine versus placebo for moderate to severe functional bowel disorders. Gastroenterology 2003;125(1):19–31.
49. Tabas G, Beaves M, Wang J, Friday P, Mardini H, Arnold G. Paroxetine to treat irritable bowel syndrome not responding to high-fiber diet: A double-blind, placebo-controlled trial. Am J Gastroenterol 2004;99 (5):914–920.

50. Scarpignato C, Pelosini I. Management of irritable bowel syndrome: Novel approaches to the pharmacology of gut motility. Can J Gastroenterol 1999;13 Suppl A:50A–65A.
51. Jailwala J, Imperiale TF, Kroenke K. Pharmacologic treatment of the irritable bowel syndrome: A systematic review of randomized, controlled trials. Ann Intern Med 2000;133(2):136–147.
52. Heymann-Monnikes I, Arnold R, Florin I, Herda C, Melfsen S, Monnikes H. The combination of medical treatment plus multicomponent behavioral therapy is superior to medical treatment alone in the therapy of irritable bowel syndrome. Am J Gastroenterol 2000;95(4):981–994.
53. Verdu EF, Collins SM. Irritable bowel syndrome and probiotics: From rationale to clinical use. Curr Opin Gastroenterol 2005;21(6): 697–701.
54. Kajander K, Hatakka K, Poussa T, Farkkila M, Korpela R. A probiotic mixture alleviates symptoms in irritable bowel syndrome patients: A controlled 6-month intervention. Aliment Pharmacol Ther 2005;22(5):387–394.
55. Drossman DA, Whitehead WE, Camilleri M. Irritable bowel syndrome: A technical review for practice guideline development. Gastroenterology 1997;112(6):2120–2137.

CHAPTER 39 Portal Hypertension and Cirrhosis

JULIE M. SEASE, EDWARD G. TIMM, AND JAMES J. STRAGAND

KEY CONCEPTS

1. Cirrhosis is a severe, chronic, irreversible disease associated with significant morbidity and mortality. However, the progression of cirrhosis secondary to alcohol abuse can be interrupted by abstinence. Consequently, it is imperative for the clinician to educate and support abstinence from alcohol as part of the overall treatment strategy of the underlying liver disease.
2. Patients with cirrhosis and portal hypertension should be considered for endoscopic screening and patients with varices should receive primary prophylaxis with β-adrenergic blockade therapy.
3. When nonselective β-adrenergic blocker therapy is used to prevent rebleeding, it is essential that the dose be titrated to achieve a heart rate goal of 60 beats per minute (beats/min) or a heart rate that is 25% lower than the baseline heart rate.
4. Octreotide is the preferred vasoactive agent employed in the medical management of variceal bleeding. Endoscopy employing endoscopic band ligation is the primary therapeutic tool in the management of acute variceal bleeding.
5. The combination of spironolactone and furosemide is the recommended initial diuretic therapy for patients with ascites.
6. All patients who have survived an episode of spontaneous bacterial peritonitis should receive long-term antibiotic prophylaxis.
7. The mainstay of therapy of hepatic encephalopathy involves therapy to lower blood ammonia concentrations, and includes diet therapy, lactulose, and antibiotics alone or in combination with lactulose.

Chronic liver disease and exposure to hepatotoxic substances causes damage to normal liver tissue resulting in an inflammatory response and abnormal collagen secretion. The initial result of this inflammation and collagen secretion is hepatic fibrosis.[1] Fibrosis, defined as the excessive accumulation of proteins, such as collagen, in the liver's extracellular matrix, is currently considered a wound-healing response to chronic liver injury. If fibrotic liver disease advances, collagen bands progress to bridging fibrosis and eventually frank hepatic cirrhosis.[2] The word *cirrhosis* is derived from the Greek *kirrhos,* meaning orange-colored, and refers to the yellow-orange hue of the cirrhotic liver seen by the pathologist or surgeon. Cirrhosis is defined histologically based on three criteria: diffuse disease, presence of fibrosis, and replacement of normal liver architecture by abnormal nodules.[3] As fibrotic tissue replaces normal hepatic parenchyma, resistance to blood flow results in the clinical problems of portal hypertension and the development of varices and ascites. Hepatocyte loss and intrahepatic shunting of blood result in diminished metabolic and synthetic function which leads to hepatic encephalopathy and coagulopathy.

❶ While cirrhosis has many causes (Table 39–1), in the United States, excessive alcohol intake and hepatitis B and C are the most common causes.[1,3] This chapter elucidates the pathophysiology of cirrhosis and the resultant effects on human anatomy and physiology. Treatment strategies for managing the most commonly encountered clinical complications of cirrhosis are discussed.

Learning objectives, review questions, and other resources can be found at **www.pharmacotherapyonline.com.**

EPIDEMIOLOGY

The exact prevalence of cirrhosis is unknown, with nearly 30% to 40% of diagnoses being made on autopsy.[3] Cirrhosis is responsible for more than 26,000 deaths each year in America and chronic liver disease is currently ranked twelfth among the leading causes of death in the United States.[4] Acute variceal bleeding and spontaneous bacterial peritonitis are among the immediately life-threatening complications of cirrhosis. Associated conditions causing significant morbidity include ascites and hepatic encephalopathy. Approximately 50% of patients with cirrhosis develop ascites during 10 years of observation and half of the cirrhotic patients who develop ascites will die within 2 years of diagnosis.[5]

PATHOPHYSIOLOGY OF CIRRHOSIS

Any discussion of cirrhosis must be based on a firm understanding of hepatic anatomy and vascular supply. Conceptually, the liver can be thought of as an elaborate blood filtration system receiving blood from the hepatic artery and the portal vein (Fig. 39–1) with portal blood originating from the mesenteric, gastric, splenic, and pancreatic veins. Blood enters the liver via the portal triad which contains branches of the portal vein and hepatic artery, bile ducts, and lymphatic and nerve tissue. It then drains through the sinusoidal spaces of the hepatic lobule (Fig. 39–2), which are lined by the workhorses of the liver, the hepatocytes. Individual hepatocytes are arranged in plates 1 cell thick, expanding from the portal veins to the terminal hepatic venules. The six or more surfaces of each individual hepatocyte either make contact with adjacent hepatocytes, border the bile canaliculi, or are exposed to the sinusoidal space. Filtered blood travels into the terminal hepatic venules, also called central veins, and then empties into larger hepatic veins and eventually into the inferior vena cava. The hepatic lobule can be subdivided into three functional zones based on relative oxygen supply. The hepatic artery supplies oxygen-rich blood to the portal triad. Hepatocytes at

TABLE 39-1 Etiology of Cirrhosis

Chronic alcohol consumption
Chronic viral hepatitis (types B, C, and D)
Metabolic liver disease
Hemochromatosis
Wilson disease
α_1-Antitrypsin deficiency
Nonalcoholic steatohepatitis ("fatty liver")
Cholestatic liver diseases
Primary biliary cirrhosis
Secondary biliary cirrhosis (possible causes: gallstones, strictures, parasitic infection)
Primary sclerosing cholangitis (associated with ulcerative colitis and cholangiocarcinoma)
Budd-Chiari syndrome
Severe congestive heart failure and constrictive pericarditis
Drugs and herbals
Isoniazid, methyldopa, amiodarone, methotrexate, phenothiazine, estrogen, anabolic steroids, black cohosh, Jamaican bush tea

the periphery therefore receive a higher level of oxygen than the cells near the terminal hepatic venules.[6]

In areas of hepatocellular injury, regardless of the nature of the inciting agent, hepatic stellate cells undergo an abnormal transformation. Stellate cells normally reside in the sinusoidal space and are involved in the storage of retinoids like vitamin A. However, when hepatic injury occurs, stellate cells in the affected areas begin to resemble fibroblasts, express contractile proteins, and become a major source of collagen and other matrix proteins that proliferate

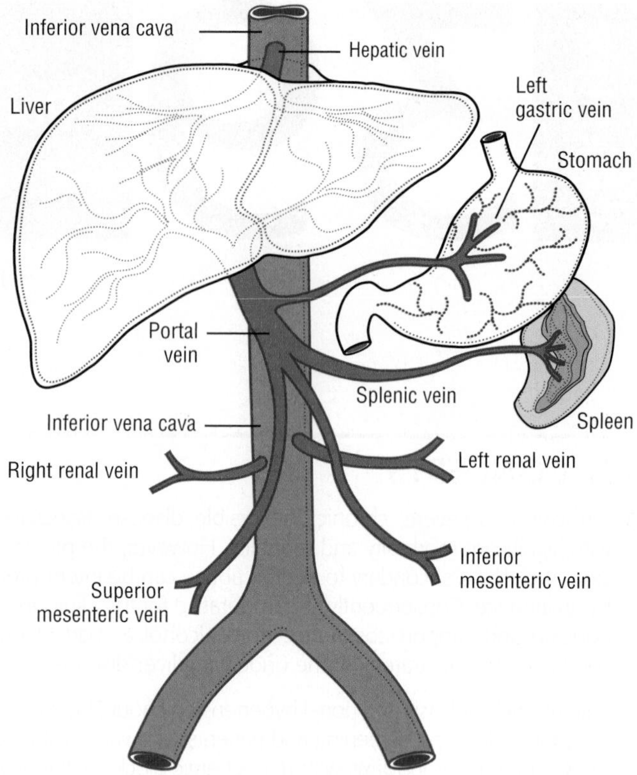

FIGURE 39-1. The portal venous system.

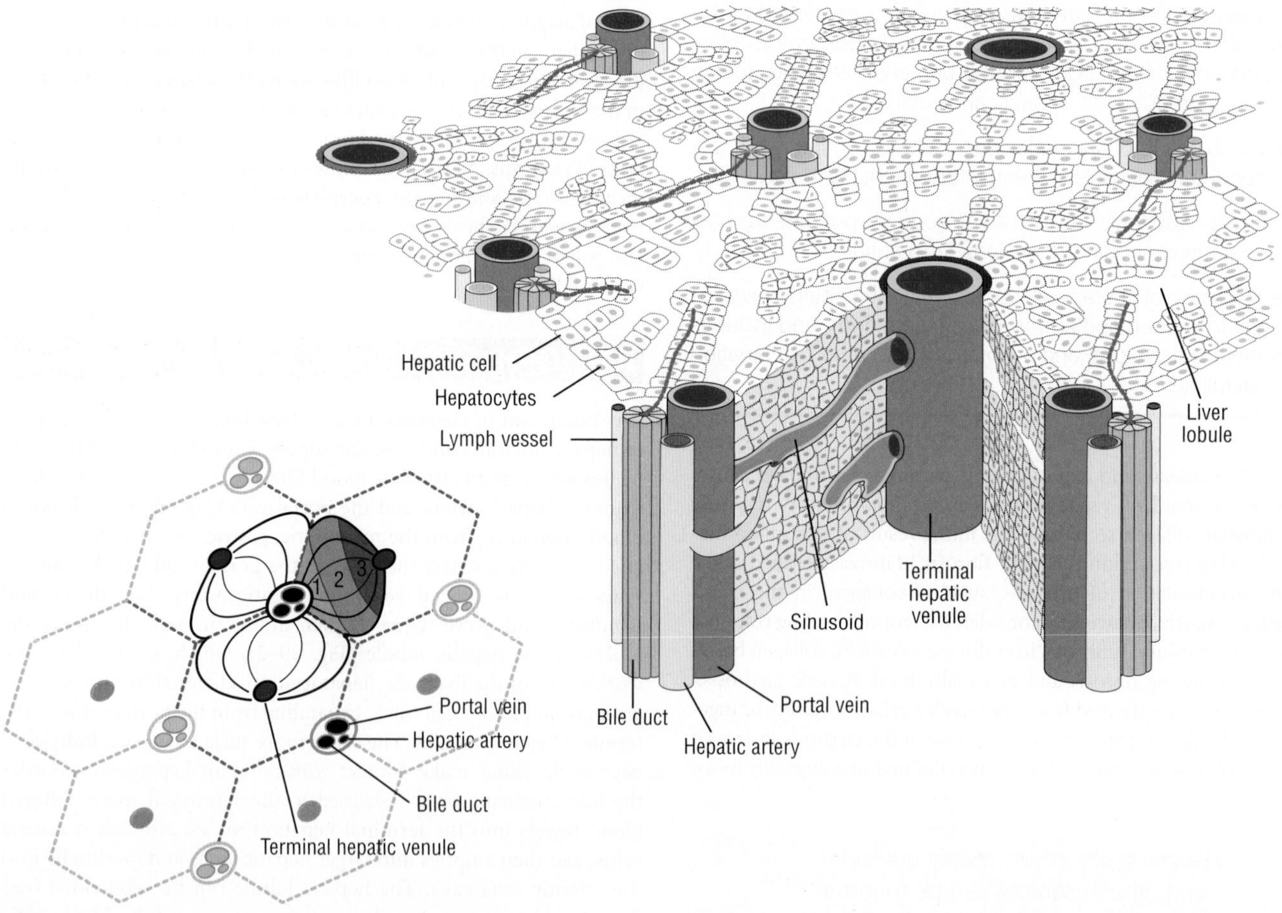

FIGURE 39-2. The hepatic lobule. 1, 2, and 3 indicate thte three functional zones based on relative oxygen supply (1 being the highest).

during fibrosis, eventually causing the permanent hepatic scarring characteristic of cirrhosis.[1] The progressive deposition of fibrous material within the sinusoids disrupts the normal blood flow through the hepatic lobule. Resistance to portal blood flow increases as fibrous tissue accumulates resulting in persistent and progressive elevations in portal blood pressures or portal hypertension.

Changes occur in cirrhosis to the vasodilatory and vasoconstricting mediators that regulate the hepatic sinusoidal blood flow. A decrease in the production of nitric oxide, which acts as a vasodilator, and an increase in the levels of endogenous vasoconstrictors, such as endothelin, combine to increase the resistance to blood flow through the sinusoidal space. Concurrently, there also appears to be an increase in the blood flow to the splanchnic vasculature through a nitric oxide-mediated effect on the splanchnic arteriole.[7,8] These pathophysiologic changes mark the current and past targets of pharmacologic therapy for the treatment of portal hypertension and prevention of variceal bleeding.

In summary, cirrhosis results in elevation of portal blood pressure because of fibrotic changes within the hepatic sinusoids, changes in the levels of vasodilatory and vasoconstrictor mediators, and an increase in blood flow to the splanchnic vasculature.

ANATOMIC AND PHYSIOLOGIC EFFECTS OF CIRRHOSIS

Cirrhosis and the pathophysiologic abnormalities that cause it result in the commonly encountered problems of ascites, portal hypertension, esophageal varices, hepatic encephalopathy, and coagulation disorders. Other, less commonly seen problems in patients with cirrhosis include hepatorenal syndrome, hepatopulmonary syndrome, and endocrine dysfunction.

ASCITES

Ascites, from the Greek *askos,* meaning water bag or wineskin, is the pathologic accumulation of lymph fluid within the peritoneal cavity. It is one of the earliest and most common presentations of cirrhosis.[9] More than 50% of cirrhotic patients develop ascites within 10 years of diagnosis.[5] The mechanism for the development of ascites is multifactorial. Recent theory states that severe portal hypertension and hepatic insufficiency lead to splanchnic arterial vasodilation and decreased peripheral resistance. The resulting systemic hypotension causes increased activity of the sympathetic nervous system and renin–angiotensin–aldosterone system, which causes increased sodium and water retention and vasoconstrictor production (Fig. 39–3). Although vascular resistance is increased in most major vascular territories (kidney, brain, skin, and muscle) by this increase in vasoconstrictor release, the splanchnic vasculature does not seem to have the same response. Instead, splanchnic arterial dilation occurs and causes a rapid inflow of arterial blood into the liver and other splanchnic organs. Hydrostatic pressure increases leading to excessive splanchnic lymph production and leakage. The leaked fluid accumulates in the abdominal cavity, forming ascites, which is continuously perpetuated by ongoing sodium and water retention by the kidneys.[10]

PORTAL HYPERTENSION AND VARICES

The most important clinical sequelae of portal hypertension are the development of varices or alternative routes of blood flow from the portal to the systemic circulation, bypassing the liver (see Fig. 39–1). Varices decompress the portal venous system and return blood to the systemic circulation. Varices can occur at any level of the gastrointestinal tract; however, the route with the most clinical significance is through the left gastric vein with the development of esophageal varices. Patients with cirrhosis are at risk for variceal bleeding when

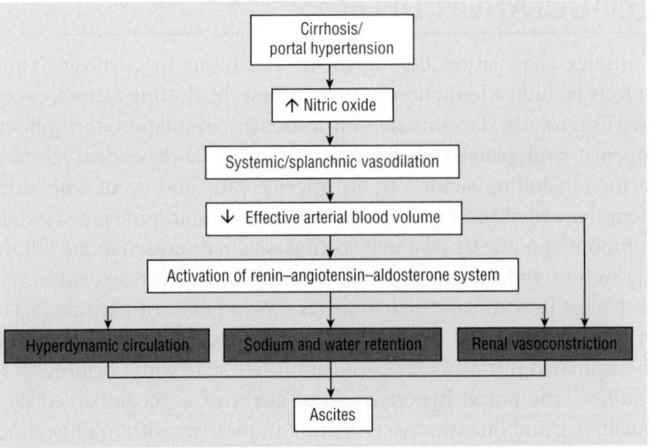

FIGURE 39-3. Pathogenesis of ascites.

portal venous pressure is 12 mm Hg greater than vena cava pressure.[7] Hemorrhage from varices occurs in 25% to 40% of patients with cirrhosis, and each episode of bleeding carries a 25% to 30% risk of death.[11] Rebleeding is common following initial hemorrhage, especially within the first 72 hours. More than 50% of recurrent bleeding episodes occur within the first 10 days of the initial bleed and risk returns to baseline after 6 weeks.[11] The risk of bleeding from esophageal varices is related to the tension on the variceal wall, which, in turn, is related to portal vein pressure and, ultimately, to the degree of cirrhosis.[7] It should be apparent from this understanding that the primary strategy for the treatment of esophageal varices is the reduction of portal hypertension by pharmacologic and surgical approaches.

HEPATIC ENCEPHALOPATHY

Hepatic encephalopathy (HE) can be defined as a central nervous system disturbance with a wide range of neuropsychiatric symptoms, and which is associated with hepatic insufficiency and liver failure.[12,13] Symptoms of HE are thought to result from an accumulation of gut-derived nitrogenous substances in the systemic circulation as a consequence of decreased hepatic functioning and shunting through portosystemic collaterals bypassing the liver. Once these substances enter the central nervous system, they cause alterations of neurotransmission that affect consciousness and behavior.[12] Ammonia is the most commonly cited culprit in the pathogenesis of HE, but glutamate, benzodiazepine receptor agonists, and manganese have also been recognized as potential causes.[12,13] Arterial ammonia levels are increased commonly in both acute and chronic liver disease, but an established correlation between blood ammonia levels and mental status does not exist.[12] Despite this, interventions to lower blood ammonia levels remain the mainstay of treatment for HE.

HE is now categorized as type A, B, or C, based on nomenclature developed by the 11th World Congress of Gastroenterology. Type A is HE induced by acute liver failure; type B is a result of portal–systemic bypass without associated intrinsic liver disease; and type C is HE that occurs in patients with cirrhosis. The duration and characteristics of HE are classified as episodic, persistent, and minimal. Episodic HE occurs spontaneously or is precipitated by a clinical factor, such as gastrointestinal bleeding. Recurrent HE is defined by two episodes of spontaneous or precipitated HE occurring within 1 year, and the hallmark of persistent HE is chronic cognitive deficits that decrease a patient's quality of life. Minimal HE refers to cirrhotic patients who do not suffer clinically overt cognitive dysfunction, but who are found to have cognitive impairment on psychological studies.[13] HE associated with chronic liver failure has a gradual onset, is commonly associated with known precipitating factors, and has a poor prognosis with the need for long-term treatment of the underlying liver disease.[12]

COAGULATION DEFECTS

Complex coagulation derangements can occur in cirrhosis. These defects include a reduction in the synthesis of clotting factors, excessive fibrinolysis, disseminated intravascular coagulation, thrombocytopenia, and platelet dysfunction. Vitamin K-dependent clotting factors, including factor VII, are affected early and occur with sufficient frequency and rapidity that the prothrombin time is a standard component of the Child-Pugh scoring system discussed in the following section. In fact, a reduction in clotting factor VII is so common in end-stage liver disease that it affects 75% to 85% of patients.[14] The presence of activated clotting factors in cirrhosis creates a low-grade disseminated intravascular coagulation-like state with fibrinolysis. In addition, the portal hypertension of cirrhosis is accompanied by a qualitative and quantitative reduction in platelets with mild to moderate thrombocytopenia occurring in 49% to 64% of patients with end-stage liver disease.[14] The net effect of these events is the development of bleeding diathesis.

CLINICAL PRESENTATION

Cirrhotic patients may present in a variety of ways, from asymptomatic patients with abnormal laboratory tests noted on routine blood tests to acute life-threatening hemorrhage in an emergency room. The approach to a patient with suspected liver disease begins with a thorough history and physical examination. Table 39–2 describes some of the typical presenting characteristics of patients with cirrhosis.[3,15] Clinical jaundice is often a late manifestation of cirrhosis and its absence does not exclude the diagnosis.

A thorough history of alcohol or drug use, with the input of family and friends is important, as the patient often underestimates the amount of alcohol consumed. Family history can also provide clues regarding problems such as hemochromatosis. The social history provides information regarding potential occupational exposures to toxic agents. A history of acute pain and fever may indicate an obstructive process caused by gallstones, or an inflammatory condition such as viral or alcoholic hepatitis.

The classic clinical signs of cirrhosis, such as palmar erythema, spider angiomata, and gynecomastia, are neither sensitive nor specific for this disease.[15,16] Only a combination of physical and laboratory findings provides a reasonable indicator of liver disease. A decreased albumin level was the most common finding in patients with cirrhosis, but was nonspecific and occurred in a variety of conditions. An elevated prothrombin time was the single most reliable manifestation of cirrhosis. The combination of thrombocytopenia, encephalopathy, and ascites was found in just over half of cirrhotics, but had the highest predictive value.[12]

TABLE 39-2 Clinical Presentation of Cirrhosis

Signs and symptoms
Asymptomatic
Hepatomegaly, splenomegaly
Pruritus, jaundice, palmar erythema, spider angiomata, hyperpigmentation
Gynecomastia, reduced libido
Ascites, edema, pleural effusion, and respiratory difficulties
Malaise, anorexia, and weight loss
Encephalopathy
Laboratory tests
Hypoalbuminemia
Elevated prothrombin time
Thrombocytopenia
Elevated alkaline phosphatase
Elevated aspartate transaminase (AST), alanine transaminase (ALT), and γ-glutamyl transpeptidase (GGT)

LABORATORY ABNORMALITIES

There are no laboratory or radiographic tests of hepatic function despite the commonly ordered *liver function tests*. These commonly measured markers are substances produced by the liver and released into the bloodstream during hepatocellular injury, and are more correctly termed *liver dysfunction tests*. True liver function tests that assess the ability of the liver to eliminate substances that undergo hepatic metabolism, such as the ^{14}C-aminopyrine breath test, are limited by complexity and availability.

Routine liver tests include alkaline phosphatase, bilirubin, aspartate transaminase (AST), alanine transaminase (ALT), and γ-glutamyl transpeptidase (GGT). Additional markers of hepatic synthetic activity include albumin and prothrombin time. Liver function tests are often the first step in the evaluation of patients who present with symptoms or signs suggestive of cirrhosis. Liver function tests are typically elevated in chronic inflammatory liver disease such as hepatitis C, but may be normal in patients with a previous toxic exposure or resolved infectious process such as hepatitis B.

The use of liver function tests in the diagnosis and management of cirrhosis is discussed in the following sections. It is useful to group the tests into two broad categories: markers of hepatocyte damage, such as the transaminases, and markers of hepatocellular synthetic function, such as prothrombin time and albumin.

Aminotransferases

The aminotransferases, AST and ALT, are enzymes located in the cytoplasm of hepatocytes and their levels are elevated with hepatocellular injury. The degree of elevation and rate of rise in aminotransferase serum levels is helpful in suggesting possible etiologies. The highest levels are typically seen in acute viral, ischemic, or toxic liver injury.[17] In contrast, alcoholic liver disease resulted in AST elevations of only 6 to 7 times the upper limit of normal in 98% of patients in a landmark study by Cohen and Kaplan.[18]

The ratio of AST to ALT also provides information in patients with suspected alcoholic liver disease. Seventy percent of patients with alcoholic liver disease had ratios greater than 2 compared to only 4% of patients with viral hepatitis.[18]

Alkaline Phosphatase and γ-Glutamyl Transpeptidase

Elevated serum levels of alkaline phosphatase and GGT occur as a result of the bile flow obstruction that accompanies conditions such as primary biliary cirrhosis, primary sclerosing cholangitis, drug-induced cholestasis, gallstone disease, and autoimmune cholestatic liver disease. Neither alkaline phosphatase nor GGT are found solely in the liver, and elevations in either of these biomarkers can occur in a variety of disease states, affecting other bodily tissues. However, the combination of an elevation in alkaline phosphatase level with a concomitant elevation in GGT level is considered to be both a sensitive and specific marker of cholestatic liver disease.[17]

Child-Pugh Classification and Mayo End-Stage Liver Disease Score

The Child-Pugh classification system has gained widespread acceptance as a means of quantifying the myriad effects of the cirrhotic process on the laboratory and clinical manifestations of this disease.[19] Recommended drug-dosing adjustments for patients in liver failure, when available, are normally based upon the Child-Pugh score. The newer Mayo End-Stage Liver Disease (MELD) scoring system is now the accepted classification scheme used by the United Network for Organ Sharing (UNOS) in the allocation livers for transplantation.[20] The Child-Pugh classification system employs a combination of physical and laboratory findings (Table 39–3),

TABLE 39-3 Criteria and Scoring for the Child-Pugh Grading of Chronic Liver Disease

Score	1	2	3
Bilirubin (mg/dL)	1–2	2–3	>3
Albumin (mg/dL)	>3.5	2.8–3.5	<2.8
Ascites	None	Mild	Moderate
Encephalopathy (grade)	None	1 and 2	3 and 4
Prothrombin time (seconds prolonged)	1–4	4–6	>6

Grade A, <7 points; grade B, 7–9 points; grade C, 10–15 points.

whereas the MELD score calculation takes into account a patient's serum creatinine, bilirubin, international normalized ratio (INR), and etiology of liver disease, omitting the more subjective reports of ascites and encephalopathy used in the Child-Pugh system. The MELD scoring calculation is as follows[21]:

$$\text{MELD score} = 0.957 \times \text{Log}_e(\text{creatinine mg/dL}) + 0.378 \times \text{Log}_e(\text{bilirubin mg/dL}) + 1.120 \times \text{Log}_e(\text{INR}) + 0.643$$

These classification systems are important because they are used to assess and define the severity of the cirrhosis, and as a predictor for patient survival, surgical outcome, and risk of variceal bleeding.

CLINICAL CONTROVERSY

The Child-Pugh classification system has been used for decades to quantify liver impairment in patients with cirrhosis. A problem with this system is that it relies on subjective scoring components related to ascites and encephalopathy, leading to the possibility of interpretation differences and scoring disparities. UNOS now employs the MELD scoring system, which relies solely on objective laboratory measurements, to stratify the severity of a patient's liver dysfunction and assist with transplant allocation. Controversy surrounds whether or not the Child-Pugh scoring system should be abandoned for the more objective MELD scoring system to describe the severity of a patient's liver dysfunction, assist with clinical decision making, and eventually guide drug dosing.

Bilirubin

Bilirubin is a breakdown product of hemoglobin derived from senescent red blood cells. Elevations of the serum bilirubin are common in end-stage liver disease and obstruction of the common bile duct caused by gallstones or malignancy; however, there are other causes of an elevated bilirubin (Table 39–4).

TABLE 39-4 Etiology of Hyperbilirubinemia

Etiology	Diagnosis
Unconjugated bilirubin	
Excessive production	Hemolysis
Immature enzyme systems	Jaundice of newborn
	Jaundice of prematurity
Inherited defects	Gilbert syndrome
	Crigler-Najjar syndrome
Drug effects	
Conjugated bilirubin	
Impaired intrahepatic excretion	
Hepatocellular disease	Hepatitis, cirrhosis, drugs
Intrahepatic cholestasis	Drugs, pregnancy
Congenital	Dubin-Johnson syndrome
	Rotor syndrome
Obstruction	
Extrahepatic	Calculus, stricture, neoplasm
Intrahepatic	Sclerosing cholangitis, cirrhosis, neoplasm

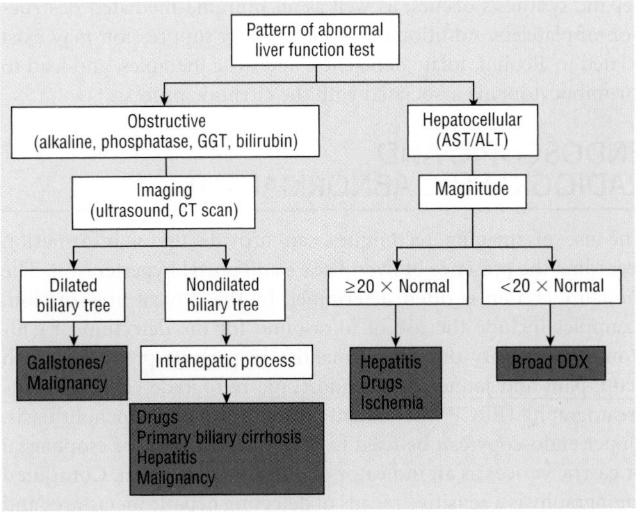

FIGURE 39-4. Interpretation of liver function tests. (CT, computed tomography; DDX, differential diagnosis.)

When cirrhosis has been established, the degree of bilirubin elevation has prognostic significance and is used as a component of the Child-Pugh and MELD scoring systems for quantifying the degree of cirrhosis.

Figure 39–4 describes a general algorithm for the interpretation of liver function tests. The algorithm first separates the tests into two categories based on the underlying pathology (pattern of elevations): obstructive (alkaline phosphatase, GGT, and bilirubin) versus hepatocellular (AST and ALT). If a hepatocellular pattern predominates, the magnitude of elevation provides diagnostic assistance. If the degree of elevation is ≥20 times normal, the etiology is likely a result of drugs or other toxins, ischemia, or acute viral hepatitis. Elevations <20 times normal have a broad differential. Unfortunately, most liver enzyme abnormalities will fall into a mixed pattern, providing limited diagnostic assistance.

Albumin and Coagulation Factors

Albumin and coagulation proteins are markers of hepatic synthetic activity and are therefore used to estimate the level of functioning hepatocytes in cirrhosis. They are both used in the Child-Pugh system for liver disease and the INR is used in the MELD scoring system as a marker of coagulation. Albumin levels can be affected by a number of factors, including the patient's nutritional status, acute illnesses, which result in redistribution of albumin, and protein losses from renal and intestinal sources.

Coagulation factors I, II, V, VII, VIII, IX, X, XI, XII, and XIII are synthesized in the liver and, when circulating levels of factors I, V, VII, IX, and X are sufficiently reduced, the prothrombin time (PT) becomes prolonged. PT prolongation is related to the severity of liver disease and decreased synthetic activity in the liver. The PT is used as one of the prognostic factors found in the Child-Pugh scoring system. Likewise, the INR, which is calculated based upon the PT, is used in the MELD system.[22] The PT has also been used in acute liver disease as an outcome measurement in acetaminophen overdose and acute alcoholic hepatitis.[23]

Thrombocytopenia

Thrombocytopenia (generally defined as a platelet count less than 150,000) is a common feature of chronic liver disease found in 30% to 64% of cirrhotic patients. The etiology of thrombocytopenia in liver disease is multifactorial involving primarily splenomegaly caused by portal hypertension with pooling of platelets in the spleen. A decrease in thrombopoietin as a consequence of decreased hepatic synthesis occurs, as well as an immune-mediated destruction of platelets. Additionally, bone marrow suppression may exist related to alcohol, folate deficiency, and drug therapies, and lead to thrombocytopenia associated with the cirrhotic process.[22]

ENDOSCOPIC AND RADIOGRAPHIC ABNORMALITIES

The use of imaging techniques can provide useful information regarding the presence of liver disease and portal hypertension. The modality chosen is often determined by the clinical presentation. Examples include the use of ultrasound for the detection of gallstones and biliary duct abnormalities in patients presenting with acute pain and jaundice, or endoscopic retrograde cholangiopancreatography (ERCP) for patients with known choledocholithiasis. Upper endoscopy can be used to detect the presence of esophageal or gastric varices as an indicator of portal hypertension. Computed tomography is a sensitive means of detecting hepatic metastases and is used for directing liver biopsy.

LIVER BIOPSY

Liver biopsy plays a central role in the diagnosis and staging of liver disease. However, for the diagnosis of cirrhosis, percutaneous liver biopsy has a significant false-negative rate because of the presence of regenerating nodules within the liver.

TREATMENT

Cirrhosis

GENERAL APPROACHES TO TREATMENT

The clinical manifestations of cirrhosis are protean and it is difficult to provide overall management guidelines. General approaches to therapy should include:

1. Identifying and eliminating, where possible, the causes of cirrhosis (e.g., alcohol abuse).
2. Assessing the risk for variceal bleeding and beginning pharmacologic prophylaxis when indicated. Reserve prophylactic endoscopic therapy for patients with contraindications or intolerance to β-adrenergic blockers. Endoscopic therapy is also appropriate for patients suffering acute bleeding episodes. Variceal obliteration with endoscopic techniques is the recommended treatment of choice in patients with acute bleeding.
3. Evaluating the patient for clinical signs of ascites and managing with pharmacologic therapy (e.g., diuretics and paracentesis). Careful monitoring for spontaneous bacterial peritonitis should be used in patients with ascites who undergo acute deterioration.
4. Monitoring for hepatic encephalopathy, which is a common complication of cirrhosis that requires clinical vigilance and treatment with dietary restriction, elimination of central nervous system depressants, and therapy to lower ammonia levels.
5. Monitoring frequently for signs of hepatorenal syndrome, pulmonary insufficiency, and endocrine dysfunction is necessary.

DESIRED OUTCOMES

The desired therapeutic outcomes can be viewed in two categories: *resolution of acute complications*, such as tamponade of bleeding and resolution of hemodynamic instability for an episode of acute variceal hemorrhage; and *prevention of complications*, through lowering of portal pressure with medical therapy using β-adrenergic blocker therapy, or supporting abstinence from alcohol. Treatment end points and desired therapeutic outcomes are presented for each of the recommended therapies discussed.

PORTAL HYPERTENSION AND VARICEAL BLEEDING

Portal hypertension is characterized by an increased gradient between the portal venous and central venous pressures which leads to esophageal and gastric varices. Once the gradient increases above 12 mm Hg, variceal bleeding can occur causing a potentially life-threatening complication of cirrhosis.[11] Mortality from the first incidence of variceal bleeding is approximately 50%.[24] In one study, varices arose in 5% of cirrhotic patients within 1 year and in 28% within 3 years. The 2-year risk of variceal bleeding was 12% and the 30-day mortality of variceal bleeding ranged from 20% to 29%. Progression was predicted by the Child-Pugh scoring system.[25]

MANAGEMENT OF PORTAL HYPERTENSION AND VARICEAL BLEEDING

The management of varices involves three strategies: (a) primary prophylaxis (prevention of the first bleeding episode); (b) treatment of acute variceal hemorrhage; and (c) secondary prophylaxis, prevention of rebleeding in patients who have previously bled.[8]

Primary Prophylaxis

β-Adrenergic Blockade The mainstay of primary prophylaxis is the use of nonselective β-adrenergic blocking agents such as propranolol or nadolol.[11] These agents reduce portal pressure by reducing portal venous inflow via two mechanisms: a decrease in cardiac output through β_1-adrenergic blockade and a decrease in splanchnic blood flow through β_2-adrenergic blockade.[26]

Meta-analysis of 12 trials assessing the effectiveness of the β-adrenergic blockers propranolol and nadolol demonstrated the effectiveness of these agents in the prevention of bleeding over a median follow up of 2 years and a trend toward a reduction in mortality. The average reduction in the incidence of initial bleeding achieved by nonselective β-adrenergic blockade is approximately 25%. Benefit was proven irrespective of variceal size or the presence of ascites.[27] Nadolol reduces the rate of growth of small esophageal varices in patients with cirrhosis.[28] However, β-adrenergic blocker therapy does not prevent the formation of first varices and prophylactic therapy is not recommended until an assessment of esophageal varices is made.[7,26] Once started, β-adrenergic blocker therapy should be continued for life unless it is not tolerated.[29]

Treatment Recommendations: Variceal Bleeding—Primary Prophylaxis

❷ All patients with cirrhosis should be screened for varices upon diagnosis and all patients found to have varices, regardless of variceal size, should receive prophylaxis therapy with a ❸ nonselective β-adrenergic blocker.[7] Initiate therapy with oral propranolol 10 mg three times daily or nadolol 20 mg once daily and titrate to a reduction in the resting heart rate of 20% to 25%, an absolute heart rate of 55 to 60 beats/min, or the development of adverse effects. Patients with contraindications or intolerance to β-adrenergic blockers should be considered for alternative prophylactic therapy.[30] Endoscopic band ligation (EBL) is superior to both β-adrenergic blockers and nitrates for preventing first bleeding.[31–36] Because EBL does not improve survival and long-term benefits are still uncertain, use of EBL for primary prophylaxis should be reserved for patients with contraindications or intolerance to β-adrenergic blockers.[7] Nitrates are no longer recommended as alternative therapy for primary prophylaxis against variceal bleeding in patients with intolerance to β-adrenergic blockers.[7] Additionally, there is insufficient evidence to recommend use of nitrates in addition to β-adrenergic blockers in an attempt to further lower portal pressure.[7,37] At this time, there is also insufficient evidence to support the use of other agents which decrease hepatic resistance and blood flow such as carvedilol, prazosin, irbesartan, or losartan in the management of portal hypertension.[8] Nonselective β-adrenergic blocker therapy remains the mainstay of therapy in portal hypertension patients with known varices to avoid first variceal bleeding.

■ ACUTE VARICEAL HEMORRHAGE

Variceal hemorrhage typically presents with hematemesis or melena. Important risk factors include active alcohol abuse, use of nonsteroidal antiinflammatory agents or aspirin, or previous variceal hemorrhage.[30] It is important to note, however, that variceal bleeding secondary to portal hypertension can occur in patients without signs of liver disease; for example, in patients with portal vein thrombosis. The initial assessment should determine the severity of the bleeding, severity of other organ dysfunction, and the severity of the liver disease.[30]

Management of Acute Variceal Hemorrhage

Initial treatment goals include (a) adequate fluid resuscitation; (b) correction of coagulopathy and thrombocytopenia; (c) control of bleeding; (d) prevention of rebleeding; and (e) preservation of liver function. Prompt stabilization and aggressive fluid resuscitation of patients with active bleeding is followed by endoscopic examination. General resuscitation measures should be applied in the initial management of variceal hemorrhage. Airway management is critical in patients with variceal hemorrhage because of depressed reflexes and/or combative behavior associated with drug and alcohol use. The endoscopic approach to bleeding also requires a quiet and cooperative patient, and elective intubation for airway control and adequate sedation is often necessary. Clinical practice guidelines approved by the American College of Gastroenterology recommend esophagogastroduodenoscopy (EGD) employing endoscopic injection sclerotherapy (EIS) or endoscopic band ligation (EBL) of varices as the primary diagnostic and treatment strategy for upper GI tract hemorrhage secondary to portal hypertension and varices.[38]

Fluid resuscitation involves colloids initially and subsequent blood products after blood bank matching procedures are completed. Packed red blood cells, fresh-frozen plasma, and platelets may be employed both as volume expanders and corrective therapy for underlying clotting abnormalities. Vasoactive drug therapy (somatostatin, octreotide, or terlipressin) to stop or slow bleeding is routinely used early in patient management to allow stabilization of the patient and to permit endoscopy to proceed under more favorable conditions. Antibiotic therapy to prevent sepsis should also be implemented early, especially for patients with signs of infection or ascites. Figure 39–5 presents an algorithm for the management of variceal hemorrhage.

Drug Therapy

Drugs employed to manage acute variceal bleeding include octreotide or somatostatin, vasopressin, and terlipressin (triglycyl-lysine vasopressin). These agents work as splanchnic vasoconstrictors thus decreasing portal blood flow and pressure.[39,40]

Somatostatin and Octreotide Somatostatin is a naturally occurring 14-amino-acid peptide with a half-life of 1 minute, necessitating continuous intravenous infusion; octreotide is its more potent synthetic octapeptide analog with a half-life of 10 to 22 minutes, which can be dosed via intravenous infusion or subcutaneous injection. Somatostatin and octreotide decrease splanchnic arterial blood flow with a subsequent decrease in portal inflow through inhibition of vasodilatory gastrointestinal peptides including glucagon, vasoactive intestinal peptide, calcitonin gene-related peptide, and substance P. Somatostatin and octreotide are associated with few side effects.[41] Unlike vasopressin, systemic vasoconstriction and elevations in blood

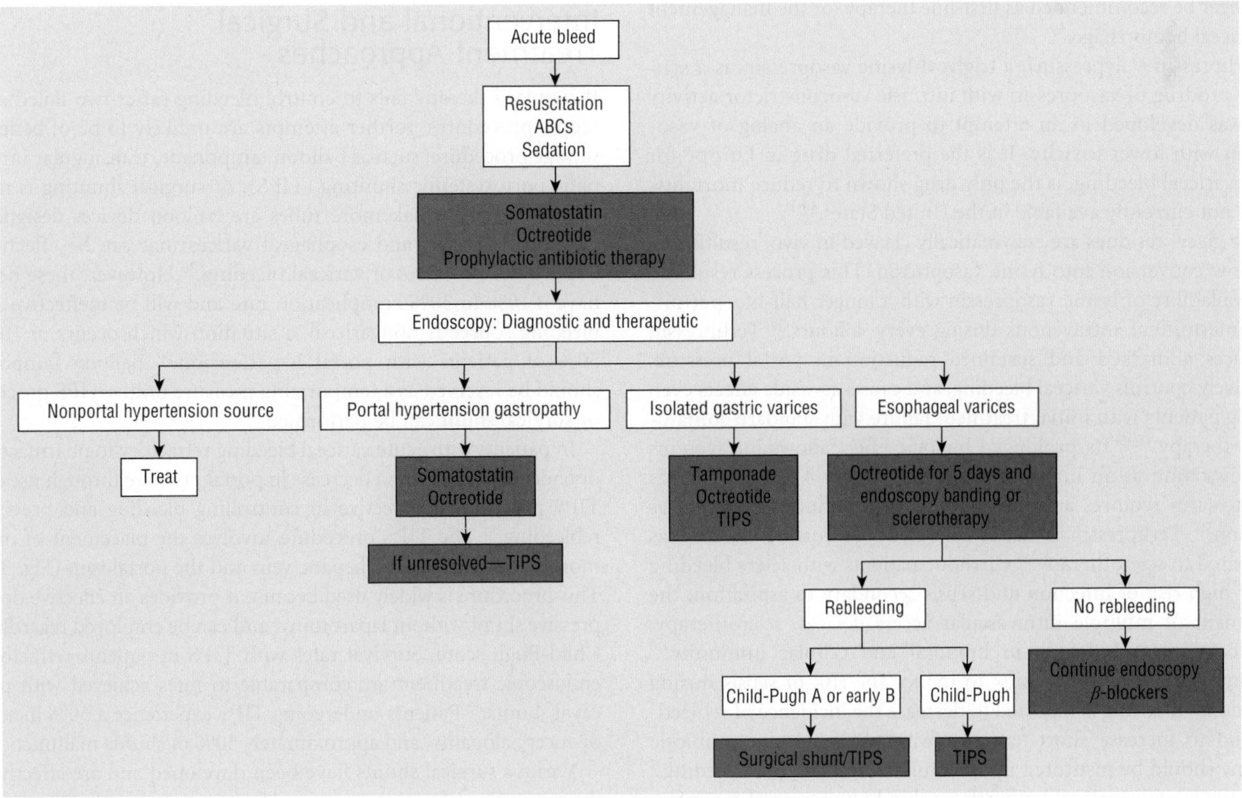

FIGURE 39-5. Management of acute variceal hemorrhage. (TIPS, transjugular intrahepatic portosystemic shunt.)

pressure are not seen because the vasoconstriction that occurs with somatostatin and octreotide is selective for the mesenteric circulation. Clinical trial data with somatostatin and octreotide are somewhat conflicting. For somatostatin, meta-analysis of clinical trials has been performed for studies comparing the drug with both placebo and vasopressin. Somatostatin controlled bleeding better than vasopressin, and had a superior side effect profile, but, oddly, was not found to control bleeding better when trials comparing the drug to placebo were analyzed.[42,43] A meta-analysis of 13 studies comparing octreotide with terlipressin, vasopressin, or placebo found improved control of bleeding with octreotide over each of the other three therapeutic options. Efficacy was similar to sclerotherapy with fewer side effects than terlipressin or vasopressin.[44]

Vasopressin (also known as antidiuretic hormone) is a potent, nonselective vasoconstrictor that has been recommended for many years for the management of acute variceal bleeding. Vasopressin reduces portal pressure by causing splanchnic vasoconstriction, which reduces splanchnic blood flow. Unfortunately, the vasoconstrictive effects of vasopressin are nonselective—the vasoconstriction produced is not restricted to the splanchnic vascular bed. Potent systemic vasoconstriction occurs in the coronary and mesenteric circulation as well, resulting in hypertension, severe headaches, coronary ischemia, myocardial infarction, and arrhythmias. A meta-analysis of 15 randomized controlled clinical trials of vasopressin for variceal hemorrhage demonstrated that vasopressin was significantly more effective than no treatment; however, control of hemorrhage was achieved in only 50% of the bleeding episodes.[42] Adverse effects were reported in 45% of patients, and vasopressin was discontinued in 25% of patients secondary to adverse effects. To minimize adverse effects associated with the peripheral vasoconstriction secondary to vasopressin, and to further lower portal pressure, the combination of vasopressin and intravenous nitroglycerin has been evaluated.[9] The combination trended toward improved control of hemorrhage with reduced side effects when compared to vasopressin alone. However, with the recent addition of safer and equally effective treatment alternatives, vasopressin, alone or combined with nitroglycerin, can no longer be recommended as first-line therapy for the management of variceal hemorrhage.[30]

Terlipressin (Glypressin), a triglycyl-lysine vasopressin, is a synthetic prodrug of vasopressin with intrinsic vasoconstrictor activity that was developed in an attempt to provide an analog of vasopressin with lower toxicity. It is the preferred drug in Europe for acute variceal bleeding, is the only drug shown to reduce mortality, but is not currently available in the United States.[30]

The glycyl residues are enzymatically cleaved in vivo, resulting in the slow conversion into lysine vasopressin. This process results in the availability of lysine vasopressin with a longer half-life, permitting intermittent intravenous dosing every 4 hours.[30] Terlipressin produces a marked and sustained reduction in portal pressure, effectively controls variceal bleeding, and causes few side effects even among patients with initial treatment failure with standard somatostatin therapy.[45,46] Its prolonged biologic effect allows intravenous administration as an intermittent infusion every 4 hours, whereas somatostatin requires administration as a continuous intravenous infusion.[47] Terlipressin is better tolerated and equally effective as compared to sclerotherapy.[45] Cirrhotic patients with active bleeding are at high risk of infection and sepsis secondary to aspiration, the placement of multiple intravascular access devices, sclerotherapy, translocation, and defects in humoral and cellular immunity.[30] Prophylactic antibiotic therapy to reduce the risk of sepsis during episodes of bleeding is reported to decrease the incidence of rebleeding and to increase short-term survival.[48] Prophylactic antibiotic therapy should be instituted upon admission for variceal bleeding.[7] All patients with variceal hemorrhage should be screened for infection and pan cultured. Patients should be evaluated at admission and observed throughout therapy for signs and symptoms of spontaneous bacterial peritonitis.[49]

Endoscopic Interventions: Sclerotherapy and Band Ligation

❹ The American College of Gastroenterology published clinical practice guidelines in 1997 recommending EGD employing EIS or EBL of varices as the primary diagnostic and treatment strategy for upper GI tract hemorrhage secondary to portal hypertension and varices.[38] Since that time, the Baveno IV Consensus Report was published stating that EBL is the recommended form of endoscopic therapy for acute variceal bleeding, although EIS may be employed if ligation is technically difficult.[7] EIS involves injection of 1 to 4 mL of a sclerosing agent into the lumen of the varices to tamponade blood flow. EBL consists of placement of rubber bands around the varix through a clear plastic channel attached to the end of the endoscope. After the rubber bands are in place, the varix will slough off after 48 to 72 hours. Endoscopic approaches can successfully stop bleeding in up to 95% of cases, but rebleeding may occur in 50% of cases.[30]

Various clinical trials have been completed comparing the effectiveness of EBL, EIS, and drug therapy to control variceal bleeding. In a meta-analysis of 15 trials comparing EIS with vasoactive drug therapy, the rates of treatment failure and mortality were found to be similar between treatment strategies, while EIS was related to significantly more adverse effects as compared to somatostatin.[50] In a trial comparing EBL and somatostatin, EBL was found superior at controlling bleeding and adverse effects were similar.[51] A meta-analysis of 13 randomized controlled trials comparing EBL, EIS, and vasoactive drug therapy found EBL to be the most effective treatment option with EIS and drug therapy being equally effective, but significantly less effective than EBL.[52] Endoscopic injection of the tissue adhesive *n*-butyl 2-cyanoacrylate has been found to control active bleeding as well as EBL, and was associated with a lower rate of rebleeding in one trial.[53]

Interventional and Surgical Treatment Approaches

If standard therapy fails to control bleeding (after two failed endoscopic procedures, further attempts are unlikely to be of benefit) a salvage procedure, such as balloon tamponade, transjugular intrahepatic portosystemic shunting (TIPS), or surgical shunting is necessary. Sengstaken-Blakemore tubes are balloon devices designed to tamponade gastric and esophageal varices that can be effective in 70% to 90% of cases of variceal bleeding.[30] However, these devices have a 10% to 30% complication rate and will be ineffective if the bleeding source is nonvariceal, a situation which occurs in 10% to 50% of patients with portal hypertension.[30] Balloon tamponade should be reserved as a temporizing measure until a TIPS procedure or surgical shunt can be performed.[49]

In patients with acute variceal bleeding refractory to pharmacologic or endoscopic therapy, a decrease in portal pressure through use of the TIPS procedure is effective in controlling bleeding and preventing rebleeding.[54] The TIPS procedure involves the placement of one or more stents between the hepatic vein and the portal vein (Fig. 39–6). This procedure is widely used because it provides an effective decompressive shunt without laparotomy, and can be employed regardless of Child-Pugh score. Survival rates with TIPS in patients refractory to endoscopic treatment are comparable to rates achieved with portacaval shunts.[30] Patients undergoing TIPS experience a 30% incidence of encephalopathy, and approximately 50% of shunts malfunction.[49]

Various surgical shunts have been developed and are effective for the prevention of recurrent variceal hemorrhage in patients refractory to β-adrenergic blockade and endoscopy.[49]

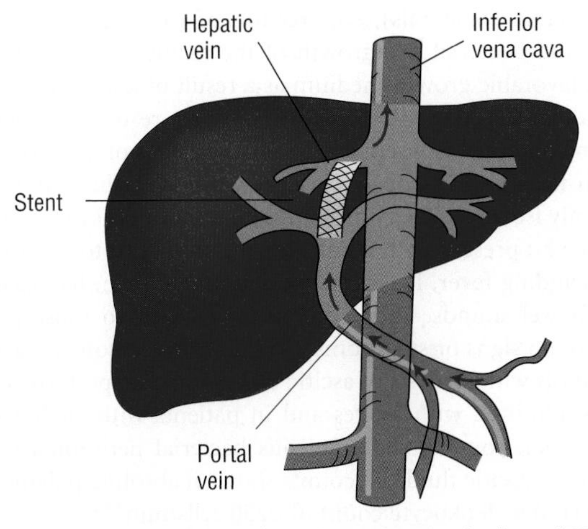

FIGURE 39-6. Transjugular intrahepatic portosystemic shunt (TIPS).

Treatment Recommendations: Variceal Hemorrhage

Patients require prompt resuscitation with colloids and blood products to correct intravascular losses and to reverse existing coagulopathies. ❹ Drug therapy with octreotide or somatostatin should be initiated early to control bleeding and facilitate diagnostic and therapeutic endoscopy. Based on availability, octreotide is preferred. Therapy is initiated with an IV bolus of 50 to 100 mcg and is followed by a continuous infusion of 25 mcg/h, up to a maximum rate of 50 mcg/h. Monitor patients for hypo- or hyperglycemia, especially patients with diabetes, and assess for cardiac conduction abnormalities. Vasopressin is no longer recommended for control of variceal bleeding. Endoscopy is recommended in any patient with upper gastrointestinal bleeding caused by ruptured varices. EBL is the recommended form of endoscopic therapy but EIS may also be employed and an additional endoscopic therapy option is injection of the tissue adhesive *n*-butyl 2-cyanoacrylate.[7] Antibiotic prophylaxis is recommended if ascites is present and EIS is planned. Appropriate choices include a third-generation cephalosporin (e.g., ceftazidime or ceftriaxone), a penicillin/β-lactamase inhibitor combination (e.g., piperacillin-tazobactam), or a fluoroquinolone (e.g., ofloxacin). Surgical shunts and TIPS are employed as salvage therapy in patients who have failed repeated endoscopy and vasoactive drug therapy.

Secondary Prophylaxis: Prevention of Rebleeding Because the risk of rebleeding after initial control of variceal hemorrhage can approach 80%, and rebleeding significantly increases the risk of death, it is inappropriate to simply observe patients for evidence of further bleeding. Traditionally, pharmacologic therapy using β-adrenergic blockers was recommended as the initial approach for prevention of rebleeding. Combination therapy with β-adrenergic blockers and chronic EBL to eradicate varices has been recognized as the likely best treatment option for secondary prophylaxis of variceal bleeding.[7] Alternatives for the secondary prevention of rebleeding include surgical or interventional shunting.

Drug Therapy. Drug therapy of variceal hemorrhage is less expensive, offers fewer serious complications, and is usually preferred by patients. In patients without contraindications, β-adrenergic blocking agents should be the initial step in secondary prophylaxis, along with EBL.[7,30] A meta-analysis of 11 randomized controlled clinical trials demonstrated a significant 21% reduction in rebleeding with β-blockers as compared to untreated controls, and a 5.4% improvement in the 2-year overall survival rate.[55] Secondary prophylaxis with β-adrenergic blockade therapy also resulted in a significant 7.4% reduction in death as a consequence of rebleeding. Propranolol was used in 10 trials; nadolol was used in one trial. Patients treated with β-adrenergic blocking agents experienced significantly more adverse events, 22% versus 9% compared to untreated controls,[55] with 5.7% requiring discontinuation of β-adrenergic blockade therapy.

When considering the benefits associated with β-adrenergic blockers, it is important to appreciate that at least 30% of cirrhotic patients will not achieve a reduction in portal pressures sufficient to prevent bleeding even with adequate β-adrenergic blockade.[31] Use of a long-acting β-blocker (such as nadolol) is usually recommended to improve compliance, and gradual, individualized dose escalation may help to minimize side effects. Ideally, portal pressure monitoring can help to assess the response to β-adrenergic blocker therapy and identify nonresponders earlier in the treatment course. A decrease in hepatic venous pressure gradient (HVPG) to <12 mm Hg or a reduction of more than 20% from baseline are considered therapeutic targets.[8]

CLINICAL CONTROVERSY

The procedure for measuring portal pressures is invasive, expensive, and not available in most facilities. Additionally, the cost-effectiveness of this approach (baseline and posttherapy) has not been compared with simply monitoring heart rate reduction with β-blockers.[56] However, for patients who fail to achieve sufficient reductions in portal pressure with β-blocker therapy alone, combination therapy with nitrates may more effectively lower portal pressure potentially reducing bleeding rates.[57] Controversy currently surrounds whether or not routine HVPG monitoring should be employed in secondary prophylaxis patients so as to better identify those with insufficient portal pressure lowering on standard β-adrenergic blocker therapy who may potentially benefit from the addition of nitrate therapy.

Comparisons of β-adrenergic blocker therapy alone with EIS suggest that less variceal rebleeding is seen with EIS, but this benefit is offset by an increase in complications.[58] However, β-adrenergic blocker therapy in combination with nitrates is more effective than EIS at lower risk of rebleeding with fewer side effects.[59] Several studies have been conducted comparing EIS with EBL at preventing rebleeding. EBL is safer and more effective at decreasing the rate of recurrent bleeding. EBL requires fewer sessions to obliterate varices and improves survival as compared to EIS.[60–62] Combined drug therapy with nadolol plus isosorbide mononitrate was more effective than EBL at preventing rebleeding than EBL with a lower rate of major complications.[57] More studies are required to make combination therapy with a β-adrenergic blocker and a nitrate the definitive choice over EBL for prevention of rebleeding. Current guidelines suggest that a combination of drug therapy and EBL is likely the best therapeutic choice for secondary prophylaxis at this time.

Shunting. When drug therapy and endoscopy fail, alternatives include TIPS placement or shunt surgery. Regular documentation of patency and the requirement of repeat procedures make it an unsuitable long-term solution. In patients with well-compensated hepatic function (Child-Pugh grade A or B) surgical shunting is an excellent option.

Treatment Recommendations: Secondary Prophylaxis The preferred initial approach to secondary prophylaxis is currently unsettled with both pharmacotherapy and interventional procedures being accepted means. Endoscopic therapy using either EIS or EBL and pharmacologic therapy are both effective in reducing the risk of rebleeding. As a consequence of decreased complications, bleeding, and possibly mortality, EBL has emerged as the endoscopic treatment of choice.[60–62] ❹ Either EBL alone or the combination of EBL with pharmacologic therapy can be considered appropriate initial therapy. Pharmacologic therapy should be initiated with a nonselective β-blocker such as propranolol 20 mg three times a day, or nadolol at a dose of 20

TABLE 39-5 Evidence-Based Table of Selected Treatment Recommendations: Variceal Bleeding in Portal Hypertension

Recommendation	Grade
Prevention of variceal bleeding	
Nonselective β-blockers should be initiated in patients with medium or large esophageal varices	1A
EBL should be offered to patients who have contraindications or intolerance to nonselective β-blockers	5D
Treatment of variceal bleeding	
Antibiotic prophylaxis should be instituted on admission	1A
Vasoactive drugs should be started as soon as possible, prior to endoscopy, and maintained for 2–5 days	1A
EBL is the recommended form of endoscopic therapy for acute esophageal variceal bleeding and should be used in conjunction with vasoactive drug therapy	1A
Secondary prophylaxis of variceal bleeding	
Nonselective β-blockers, EBL, or both should be used for prevention of recurrent variceal bleeding	1A

EBL, endoscopic band ligation.
Recommendation Grading: Level of Evidence 1 = highest; 5 = lowest and Grade of Recommendation: 1 = strongest; D = weakest.
Data from DeFranchis R. Updating consensus in portal hypertension. Report of the Baveno III consensus workshop on definitions, methodology and therapeutic strategies in portal hypertension. J Hepatol 2000;33:846–852.

to 40 mg once daily, and titrated weekly to achieve a goal heart rate of 55 to 60 beats/min or a heart rate that is 25% lower than the baseline heart rate. Assessment of portal pressures can identify nonresponders for whom combination therapy with β-blockers and nitrates may be attempted to achieve portal pressure gradients <12 mm Hg. Monitor patients for evidence of heart failure, bronchospasm, and glucose intolerance, particularly hypoglycemia in patients with insulin-dependent diabetes. Table 39–5 summarizes the evidence-based treatment recommendations regarding portal hypertension and variceal bleeding.

■ ASCITES AND SPONTANEOUS BACTERIAL PERITONITIS

Patients with cirrhosis fail to maintain normal extracellular fluid volumes secondary to abnormal sodium and fluid retention and an impaired capacity to eliminate water.[9] The classic physical examination findings of ascites are a distended abdomen with a fluid thrill or shifting dullness. The development of ascites in patients with cirrhosis is an indication of advanced liver disease and is a poor prognostic sign. The principal therapeutic goal for patients with ascites is to improve the patient's sense of well-being and quality of life by minimizing respiratory difficulties, loss of appetite, and discomfort from abdominal distension or leg swelling. Treatment of ascites is expected to have little effect on survival, however.[63] Pleural effusions are common, and in some cases can be the primary manifestation of the fluid retention. Workup includes a history and physical examination, laboratory tests to assess liver function, abdominal ultrasound to rule out hepatocellular carcinoma, endoscopy to evaluate esophageal and gastric varices, abdominal paracentesis with analysis of ascitic fluid, and a complete evaluation of circulatory and renal function. Treatment of ascites has risks. Depending on the treatment approach and the goals selected, significant adverse reactions can occur, including electrolyte disturbances, acid–base abnormalities, hepatic encephalopathy, hypovolemia, and renal insufficiency.

Spontaneous bacterial peritonitis (SBP), infection of preexisting ascitic fluid, in the absence of any evidence of a primary intraabdominal source of infection, is a common complication in patients with ascites, developing in 10% to 25% of patients followed prospectively for at least 1 year.[9] The pathogenesis of SBP is unknown, but presumably results from altered gut permeability (cirrhosis permits enteric organisms direct access to the bloodstream via the portosystemic collaterals), suppression of the reticuloendothelial system, and bacterial overgrowth of the ascitic fluid. Ascitic fluid offers a favorable growth medium as a result of leukocyte dysfunction and decreased ascitic fluid defenses as a result of a decreased albumin content.[64] Consequently, most episodes of SBP are caused by gram-negative Enterobacteriaceae, with *Escherichia coli* the most commonly isolated. The clinical presentation of SBP can vary from patients who present with all of the signs and symptoms of peritonitis, including fever, leukocytosis, abdominal pain, hypoactive or absent bowel sounds, and rebound tenderness, to those patients who have no signs or symptoms at all. For this reason, a diagnostic paracentesis with analysis of ascitic fluid should be performed in all patients admitted with ascites and in patients with cirrhosis who suddenly deteriorate.[5,9] Spontaneous bacterial peritonitis is diagnosed when ascitic fluid cell counts show an absolute polymorphonuclear (PMN) leukocyte count of ≥250 cells/mm^3.[64]

Management of Ascites and Spontaneous Bacterial Peritonitis

The following treatment guidelines for the management of adult patients with ascites and spontaneous bacterial peritonitis were developed and approved by the Practice Guidelines Committee of the American Association for the Study of Liver Diseases (AASLD).[5]

Ascites In adult patients with new-onset ascites as determined by physical examination or radiographic studies, abdominal paracentesis should be performed and ascitic fluid analysis should include a cell count with differential and a serum-ascites albumin gradient (SAG). If infection is suspected, ascitic fluid cultures should be obtained at the time of the paracentesis. The SAG can accurately determine whether ascites is a result of portal hypertension or another process. If the SAG is >1.1 g/dL, portal hypertension is present with 97% accuracy.[5] If the SAG is <1.1 g/dL, with similar certainty, the patient does not have portal hypertension. This is important because patients without portal hypertension will not respond to salt restriction and diuretics. The treatment of ascites secondary to portal hypertension is relatively straightforward and includes abstinence from alcohol, sodium restriction, and diuretics. This strategy is effective in approximately 90% of patients. Fifteen percent of patients will respond to dietary sodium restriction alone, and an additional 75% of patients will respond to the addition of diuretics.[65]

❹ Abstinence from alcohol is an essential element of the overall treatment strategy. Abstinence from alcohol can result in improvement of the reversible component of alcoholic liver disease and normalize portal pressures in some patients.[5] Even in those patients with cirrhosis from another cause (e.g., autoimmune hepatitis) abstinence from alcohol can reverse alcohol-related effects and result in substantial improvement of the underlying liver disease. Patients with cirrhosis not caused by alcohol have less reversible liver disease, and by the time ascites is present, given the poor prognosis, these patients may be best managed with liver transplantation rather than protracted medical therapy.[5]

Beyond avoidance of alcohol, the primary treatment of ascites caused by portal hypertension and cirrhosis is salt restriction and oral diuretic therapy.[5] Fluid loss and weight change depend directly on sodium balance in these patients. To monitor them appropriately, evaluation of urinary sodium excretion, using a 24-hour urine collection, is recommended.[5] However, severe hyponatremia, serum sodium <120 mEq/L, does warrant fluid restriction; rapid correction of asymptomatic hyponatremia (patients with cirrhosis usually are not symptomatic until their serum sodium concentrations are <110 mEq/L) is not recommended.

Diuretic Therapy ❺ The AASLD practice guidelines recommend that diuretic therapy be initiated with the combination of spironolactone and furosemide. At one time, spironolactone was commonly recommended for initial therapy as a single agent. However, because of the likelihood for development of drug-induced hyperkalemia with spironolactone when used as monotherapy, the drug is now only recommended for use as a lone diuretic agent in patients with minimal fluid overload.[5] If tense ascites is present, paracentesis should be performed prior to institution of diuretic therapy and salt restriction.[5] For patients who respond to diuretic therapy, this approach is preferred over the use of serial paracenteses.[5] In patients with refractory ascites, serial paracenteses may be employed. Albumin infusion postparacentesis is controversial, but reasonable for extraction volumes exceeding 5 L.[5] Laboratory tests for renal function and electrolytes need to be monitored during therapy. Liver transplantation should be considered in patients with refractory ascites. For patients who are not transplant candidates and who fail repeated paracentesis because of loculated ascites, TIPS or peritoneal venous shunts may be considered. Both of these procedures have significant complication rates and are not recommended for the routine treatment of ascites.[5]

Spontaneous Bacterial Peritonitis Relatively broad-spectrum antibiotic therapy that adequately covers the three most commonly encountered pathogens (*E. coli, Klebsiella pneumoniae,* and *Streptococcus pneumoniae)* is warranted in patients with documented or suspected SBP.[5] Delaying antibiotic therapy while awaiting evidence of a positive ascitic fluid culture is not recommended and can result in overwhelming infection and death.[5] In some patients, signs and symptoms of infection are present such as fever, abdominal pain, and encephalopathy at the bacterascites stage (i.e., signs and symptoms are present before the PMN count in the ascitic fluid is elevated). In these patients, signs and symptoms of infection justify empiric antibiotic therapy until culture results are known, regardless of the PMN count in the ascitic fluid.[5]

Cefotaxime, or a similar third-generation cephalosporin, is considered the drug of choice for SBP.[5] Cefotaxime is more effective than aztreonam or the combination of ampicillin and tobramycin.[9] A 5-day course of antibiotic therapy was as efficacious as 10 days of therapy in a randomized trial involving 100 patients with SBP.[66] Fluoroquinolone antibiotics provide good activity against the usual pathogens encountered in SBP, excellent oral bioavailability, and high penetration into ascitic fluid. Ofloxacin 400 mg every 12 hours administered orally is equivalent to intravenous cefotaxime for treatment of SBP in patients without vomiting, shock, significant hepatic encephalopathy, or serum creatinine over 3 mg/dL.[67] For many patients, oral ofloxacin therapy offers a simple, cost-effective alternative to intravenous therapy with third-generation cephalosporins.

Secondary bacterial peritonitis, ascitic fluid infection caused by a treatable intraabdominal source, can masquerade as SBP and should be considered when multiple or atypical organisms are cultured, a very high ascitic fluid PMN count is seen, or in patients who fail to respond to appropriate antibiotic therapy. A dramatic clinical response is typical of uncomplicated SBP once treatment is initiated. A followup paracentesis revealing a PMN count that continues to rise despite antibiotic therapy can be helpful in detecting secondary peritonitis.[5]

❻ Antibiotic therapy for the *prevention* of SBP should be considered in all patients who are at high risk for this complication, including those who have experienced a prior episode of SBP or variceal hemorrhage, and those with low-protein ascites (<1 g/dL). Patients with gastrointestinal hemorrhage should receive short-term (7 days) norfloxacin twice daily or trimethoprim-sulfamethoxazole to prevent SBP. An intravenous quinolone can be used for patients actively bleeding.[5] Patients who survive an episode of SBP should receive long-term prophylaxis with norfloxacin or trimethoprim-sulfamethoxazole.[5] It may also be appropriate to provide antibiotic prophylaxis (either short-term or long-term) to those patients with ascites and no gastrointestinal bleeding, a total ascitic protein <1 g/dL, and a serum bilirubin >2.5 mg/dL.[5] Antibiotic prophylaxis should be limited only to patients in one of the above high-risk groups as selective intestinal decontamination does promote the growth of resistant gut flora. Additionally, prophylaxis regimens should be continued long-term only in patients who have survived an episode of SBP or possibly in those with ascites whose total ascitic protein is <1 g/dL and serum bilirubin is >2.5 mg/dL.[5]

Treatment Recommendations: Ascites and Spontaneous Bacterial Peritonitis

Adult patients admitted to the hospital with new-onset ascites should have an abdominal paracentesis performed to establish the serum-ascites albumin gradient, the ascitic fluid PMN count, and to obtain ascitic fluid cultures. Patients who drink alcohol should be strongly discouraged from further alcohol use. ❺ Sodium restriction to 2,000 mg/day, together with spironolactone and furosemide, is the mainstay of therapy. Diuretic therapy should be initiated with single morning doses of spironolactone 100 mg and furosemide 40 mg administered orally with the goal of a 0.5-kg maximum daily weight loss. Titrate diuretic therapy using the 100-mg:40-mg ratio, to a maximum daily dose of 400 mg spironolactone and 160 mg furosemide. This combination ratio is used because it usually maintains normokalemia. Fluid restriction, unless the serum sodium is <120 mEq/L, and bedrest are not recommended. Monitor urinary sodium excretion using a 24-hour urine collection, and monitor serum potassium and renal function frequently. Avoid rapid correction of asymptomatic hyponatremia in patients with cirrhosis. If tense ascites is present, a 4- to 6-L paracentesis should be performed prior to institution of diuretic therapy and salt restriction. For patients who respond to diuretic therapy, this approach is preferred over the use of serial paracenteses. Discontinue diuretic therapy in patients who experience encephalopathy, severe hyponatremia (serum sodium <120 mEq/L) despite fluid restriction, or renal insufficiency (serum creatinine >2 mg/dL). Serial paracenteses may be considered for patients with refractory ascites with albumin infusion postparacentesis when volumes exceeding 5 L are removed.

Patients with documented SBP, positive ascitic fluid cultures, or ascitic fluid PMN count ≥250 cells/mm^3, regardless of symptoms, should receive broad-spectrum empiric antibiotic therapy with cefotaxime 2 g every 8 hours, or a similar third-generation cephalosporin, plus albumin 1.5 g/kg within 6 hours of admission and 1 g/kg on day 3. Patients with ascitic fluid PMN counts <250 cells/mm^3, but with signs and symptoms of infection (abdominal pain, tenderness, fever, encephalopathy, renal failure, acidosis, or peripheral leukocytosis), should also receive empiric antibiotic treatment with cefotaxime 2 g every 8 hours, or a similar third-generation cephalosporin. Short-term prophylaxis should be considered for the prevention of SBP in patients with low-protein ascites (<1 g/dL) and in patients with variceal hemorrhage.[5]

❻ All patients who have survived an episode of SBP should receive long-term antibiotic prophylaxis.[5] Table 39–6 summarizes the evidence-based treatment recommendations regarding ascites and SBP.

■ HEPATIC ENCEPHALOPATHY

The clinical manifestations of HE vary widely.[68] Patients with minimal HE often experience only minor motor and attentional deficits and compensate on their own without the need for therapy. Those with persistent HE who have more significant deficits that impact activities of daily living can benefit from intervention.[12]

The prevalence of HE among cirrhotics is variable but may be found in up to 70% of patients.[13] To determine the severity of HE, a grading system that relates neurologic and neuromuscular signs can

TABLE 39-6 Evidence-Based Table of Selected Treatment Recommendations: Ascites and Spontaneous Bacterial Peritonitis

Recommendation	Grade
Ascites	
Initial therapeutic paracentesis should be performed in patients with tense ascites	II-3
Sodium restriction of 2,000 mg/day should be instituted, as well as oral diuretic therapy with spironolactone and furosemide	I
Diuretic-sensitive patients should be treated with sodium restriction and diuretics rather than serial paracentesis	III
Refractory ascites	
Serial therapeutic paracenteses may be performed	III
Postparacenteses albumin infusion of 8–10 g/L of fluid removed can be considered if more than 4–5 L are removed during paracenteses	II-2
Treatment of SBP	
If ascitic fluid PMN counts are greater than 250 cells/mm^3, empiric antibiotic therapy should be instituted (cefotaxime 2 g every 8 hours)	I
If ascitic fluid PMN counts are less than 250 cells/mm^3, but signs or symptoms of infection exist, empiric antibiotic therapy should be initiated while awaiting culture results	II-3
Ofloxacin 400 mg twice daily may be substituted for cefotaxime in patients without vomiting, shock, grade II or higher encephalopathy, or serum creatinine greater than 3 mg/dL	I
If ascitic fluid PMN counts are greater than 250 cells/mm^3 and clinical suspicion of SBP is present, 1.5 g/kg albumin should be infused within 6 hours of detection and 1 g/kg albumin infusion should also be given on day 3	I
Prophylaxis against SBP	
Twice-daily norfloxacin or trimethoprim-sulfamethoxazole should be used for 7 days to prevent SBP in cirrhosis patients with gastrointestinal hemorrhage; intravenous quinolone therapy may be used in active bleeding	I
Patients who survive an episode of SBP should receive long-term prophylaxis with either daily norfloxacin or trimethoprim-sulfamethoxazole	I
Short-term or long-term prophylaxis may be justified in patients with ascites whose ascitic total protein is less than 1g/dL or whose serum bilirubin is greater than 2.5 mg/dL	I

PMN, polymorphonuclear leukocyte; SBP, spontaneous bacterial peritonitis.
Recommendation Grading: I = randomized controlled trials; II-1 = controlled trials without randomization; II-2 = cohort or case-control analytic studies; II-3 = multiple time series, dramatic uncontrolled experiments; III = opinions of authorities, descriptive epidemiology.
Data from Runyon BA. Management of adult patients with ascites due to cirrhosis. Hepatology 2004;39(3):841–856.

be used (Table 39–7). Presently, the primary substances thought to be involved in the development of HE are ammonia, manganese, and the γ-aminobutyric acid (GABA)–benzodiazepine receptors.[12,68]

Management of Hepatic Encephalopathy

Episodic HE usually develops in a clinically stable cirrhotic patient as the result of an acute precipitating event.[12] Table 39–8 lists the most commonly encountered precipitating factors and suggests general treatment alternatives.[12,13,68] Table 39–9 describes the treatment goals for patients with HE and contrasts the differences between episodic and persistent HE. The general approach to the management of HE is to first identify and treat any precipitating factors, which often results in prompt resolution of the encephalopathy. The development of mental status changes in cirrhosis is associated with increased morbidity and mortality.[12] However, universal treatment of patients with subclinical HE is not recommended because the consequences of motor and attention deficits are considered minor, and prevention of progression to more severe HE has not been studied.[12]

Treatment approaches for episodic and persistent HE include (a) reducing ammonia blood concentrations by dietary restrictions and drug therapy aimed at inhibiting ammonia production or enhancing its removal and (b) inhibition of the GABA–benzodiazepine receptors. Additionally, treatment for persistent HE should include avoidance and prevention of precipitating factors in an effort to avoid acute decompensation.[12]

Hyperammonemia ❼ Despite criticisms of the ammonia hypothesis, treatment interventions to reduce ammonia blood concentrations are beneficial in patients with HE.[12] Decreasing ammonia blood concentrations by limiting its availability and production, or by enhancing its metabolism, remains a mainstay of therapy for patients with both episodic and persistent HE.[12]

Decreasing ammonia blood concentrations can be attempted by reducing ammonia production or by decreasing the availability of ammonia in the colon. Limiting dietary protein acutely usually results in a lowering of ammonia concentrations and improvement in HE.

Guidelines for nutritional support of patients with liver disease have been published by the European Society for Parenteral and Enteral Nutrition.[69] Protein withdrawal is a cornerstone of treatment for patients during acute episodes of HE. However, prolonged restriction can lead to malnutrition and poorer prognosis among HE patients.[12,70] Therefore, once successful reversal of HE symptoms is achieved, protein is added back to the diet initially with 0.5 to 0.6 g/kg per day and advanced by 0.25 to 0.5 g/kg per day every 3 to 5 days until either a target of 1 to 1.5 g/kg per day is reached or progression of HE occurs.[69] Vegetable-source protein may be preferable to animal-source protein because it contains fewer aromatic amino acids (phenylalanine, tryptophan, and tyrosine) and methionine which, when elevated in the serum, can worsen the symptoms of HE.[12,69,70] Also, the higher fiber content of vegetable protein increases colonic transit time and lowers colonic pH secondary to its fermentation by colonic bacteria.[12,69] Most patients will tolerate at least 1 g/kg per day of standard proteins without becoming encephalopathic.[70] Branched-chain amino acid formulations may provide a better tolerated source of protein in those patients with protein intolerance.[12] Bowel cleansing using cathartics or lactulose enemas (see below) results in rapid removal of ammonia substrate from the colon and may be combined with dietary intervention to help patient eliminate ammonia and tolerate dietary protein.

TABLE 39-7 Grading System for Hepatic Encephalopathies

Grade	Level of Consciousness	Personality/Intellect	Neurologic Abnormalities	Electroencephalogram Abnormalities
0	Normal	Normal	None	None
Minimal	Normal	Normal	Psychological only	None
1	Inverted sleep patterns/restless	Forgetful, mild confusion, agitation, irritable	Tremor, apraxia, incoordination, impaired handwriting	Triphasic waves
2	Lethargic, slow responses	Disorientation for time, amnesia, decreased inhibitions, inappropriate behavior	Asterixis, dysarthria, ataxia, hypoactive reflexes	Triphasic waves
3	Somnolent but arousable, confused	Disorientation for place, aggressive	Asterixis, hyperactive reflexes, Babinski sign, muscle rigidity	Triphasic waves
4	Coma/unarousable	None	Decerebrate	Delta activity

TABLE 39-8 Portosystemic Encephalopathy: Precipitating Factors and Therapy

Factor	Therapy Alternatives
Gastrointestinal bleeding	
Variceal	Band ligation/sclerotherapy
	Octreotide
Nonvariceal	Endoscopic therapy
	Proton pump inhibitors
Infection/sepsis	Antibiotics
	Paracentesis
Electrolyte abnormalities	Discontinue diuretics
	Fluid and electrolyte replacement
Sedative ingestion	Discontinue sedatives/tranquilizers
	Consider reversal (flumazenil/naloxone)
Dietary excesses	Limit daily protein
	Lactulose
Constipation	Cathartics
	Bowel cleansing/enema
Renal insufficiency	Discontinue diuretics
	Discontinue nonsteroidal antiinflammatory drugs, nephrotoxic antibiotics
	Fluid resuscitation

The use of lactulose, a nonabsorbable disaccharide (and Lactinol, which is not available in the United States), is standard therapy for both acute and chronic HE.[12] Lactulose, when administered orally, passes through the gastrointestinal tract and reaches the colon unchanged.[12,71] For patients unable to take lactulose orally or via tube administration, it may be administered as an enema.[12] Lactulose increases osmotic pressure in the colon and also undergoes fermentation by gut flora resulting in production of organic acids which lower colonic pH. Together, these actions increase peristalsis and exert a cathartic effect.[71]

Acidification of the colon through lactulose administration lowers ammonia levels in the blood in several ways: (a) it supplies carbohydrate to the gut thereby decreasing amino acid breakdown; (b) it changes bacterial flora metabolism in the gut reducing protein degradation; (c) it supplies energy for the growth of the bacterial mass in the gut (nitrogen-containing compounds are used in this growth process and therefore expended); and (d) it decreases bacterial urea degradation.[71] Lactulose also enhances the net movement of ammonia from the blood into the bowel.[12] More than 30 clinical trials have demonstrated the efficacy of lactulose in the management of acute HE, and more than 20 studies support its use in chronic HE.[15] Clinical improvement is noted in approximately 86% of patients with acute HE, and in approximately 77% of patients with chronic HE.

Inhibiting the activity of urease-producing bacteria by using neomycin or metronidazole can decrease production of ammonia.[72,73] Neomycin at doses of 3 to 6 g daily can be given for 1 to 2 weeks during an acute episode of HE.[12] For persistent HE, a dose of 1 to 2 g daily could be used with periodic renal and annual auditory monitoring.[12] Despite poor absorption, chronic use of neomycin can lead to irreversible ototoxicity, nephrotoxicity, and the possibility of staphylococcal superinfection. As such, neomycin should not be considered first-line therapy for HE. In patients with an inadequate response to lactulose alone, combination therapy with neomycin may be tried.[12] Metronidazole 250 mg twice daily may also produce a favorable clinical response in HE.[12] However, neurotoxicity caused by impaired hepatic clearance of the drug may be problematic.[12]

TABLE 39-9 Treatment Goals: Episodic and Persistent Hepatic Encephalopathy (HE)

Episodic HE	Persistent HE
Control precipitating factor	Reverse encephalopathy
Reverse encephalopathy	Avoid recurrence
Hospital/inpatient therapy	Home/outpatient therapy
Maintain fluid and hemodynamic support	Manage persistent neuropsychiatric abnormalities
	Manage chronic liver disease
Expect normal mentation after recovery	High prevalence of abnormal mentation after recovery

It has been speculated that ammonia generated by *Helicobacter pylori* in the stomach is associated with precipitating or worsening HE in patients with cirrhosis.[74] However, a prospective clinical trial showed no significant improvement in mental status or serum ammonia levels in patients with HE who underwent *H. pylori* eradication.[75] Consequently, routine eradication of *H. pylori* is not recommended.[12]

Enhancing ammonia removal by stimulating its detoxification by supporting alternative metabolic pathways can reduce blood ammonia concentrations. L-Ornithine L-aspartate stimulates residual hepatic urea cycle activity and promotes peripheral glutamine synthesis.[76] The effectiveness of intravenous L-ornithine L-aspartate at reducing blood ammonia and improving the clinical symptoms of hepatic encephalopathy in cirrhosis patients has been studied and proven to be effective in patients with grade 1 and grade 2 HE with clinical response rates similar to those of lactulose.[77] Oral L-ornithine L-aspartate is effective at reducing blood ammonia and improving clinical symptoms in patients with grade 2 HE.[78]

Zinc is a cofactor of urea cycle enzymes and can be deficient in cirrhotic patients, especially in cases of malnourishment. Both supportive and nonsupportive studies evaluating the efficacy of zinc replacement at decreasing ammonia levels and improving symptoms of HE have been published.[12] In a controlled trial in cirrhotic patients with mild HE, the administration of zinc sulfate 600 mg/day for 3 months resulted in increased urea formation and lower ammonia levels, along with improvement in psychological test scores.[79] Zinc supplementation is recommended for long-term management in patients with cirrhosis who are zinc deficient.[12]

Inhibition of GABA–Benzodiazepine Receptors The GABA-receptor complex is the primary inhibitory neural network within the central nervous system. An enhanced GABAergic tone and an increased amount of endogenous benzodiazepines have been postulated to contribute to HE.[12] Based on evidence of an increase in benzodiazepine receptor ligands in patients with hepatic encephalopathy, flumazenil has been evaluated for the treatment of HE. Among five prospective, placebo-controlled trials, three reported benefit with flumazenil, whereas two found no difference when compared to placebo. With dosages of 0.2 to 15 mg IV, response rates were variable, ranging from 17% to 78%; improvements, however, were often transient.[80] Flumazenil, which is only available in an intravenous dosage form, may be considered for short-term therapy in refractory patients with suspected benzodiazepine intake, but cannot be recommended for routine clinical use.

Treatment Recommendations: Hepatic Encephalopathy

Treatment recommendations depend on the type of HE being managed, episodic HE, persistent HE, or minimal HE. The general approach to the management of HE is to first identify patients with acute episodic HE and then to provide aggressive management of any precipitating events (see Table 39–8). When the precipitating event has been discovered and appropriate therapy initiated, steps to rapidly reverse the encephalopathy should be implemented. Remember that the altered sensorium associated with HE itself is associated with increased morbidity and mortality.

❼ The mainstay of therapy of HE involves measures to lower blood ammonia concentrations, and includes diet therapy, lactulose, and antibiotics, alone or in combination with lactulose. Other adjunctive therapies include zinc replacement in patients with zinc deficiency.

In patients with episodic HE, protein is withheld or limited to 10 to 20 g/day while maintaining the total caloric intake, until the clinical situation improves. Titrate protein based on tolerance, increasing intake in increments of 10 to 20 g/day every 3 to 5 days to a total of 1 to 1.5 g/kg per day. In patients with persistent HE, restrict protein to 40 g/day. Consider the addition of dietary fiber to animal-source protein diets.

In episodic HE, lactulose is initiated at a dose of 45 mL orally every hour (or by retention enema, 300 mL lactulose syrup in 1 L water, held for 60 minutes) until catharsis begins. The dose is then decreased to 15 to 45 mL orally every 8 to 12 hours (enemas every 6 to 8 hours) and titrated to produce two to three soft, acidic stools per day. Patients are maintained on this regimen to prevent recurrence of episodic HE. Monitor electrolytes periodically, follow patients for changes in mental status, and titrate to the number of stools as above.

Antibiotic therapy with either metronidazole or neomycin is reserved for patients who have not responded to diet and lactulose therapy, where the combination may provide additive effects and improved clinical response. Zinc acetate supplementation at a dose of 220 mg twice daily is recommended for long-term management in patients with cirrhosis who are zinc deficient.

Other adjunctive therapies that may be considered for patients refractory to standard therapy include L-ornithine L-aspartate or flumazenil 0.2 mg up to 15 mg IV. Universal treatment of patients with minimal HE is not recommended; however, therapy to improve performance of daily activities, or in patients with more significant deficits, may be considered with close monitoring for adverse effects. Finally, supportive measures to manage the underlying liver failure need to be implemented.

■ SYSTEMIC COMPLICATIONS

In addition to the more common complications of chronic liver disease discussed above, a number of other complications can occur, including hepatorenal syndrome, hepatopulmonary syndrome, coagulation disorders, and endocrine dysfunction.

Hepatorenal syndrome, functional renal failure in the setting of cirrhosis in the absence of intrinsic renal disease, occurs in patients with cirrhosis as a result of intense vasoconstriction within the renal cortical vasculature. It is common and develops in approximately 40% of patients with cirrhosis and ascites within 5 years.[81] The resultant reduction in blood supply to the kidneys causes avid sodium retention and oliguria. The pathophysiologic mechanism responsible for these effects is unknown, but is linked to both the increased vasoconstrictor and decreased vasodilator factors acting on the renal circulation. The three predominant factors involved in this process include the hemodynamic changes that decrease renal perfusion pressure, a stimulated renal sympathetic nervous system, and an increased synthesis of humoral and renal vasoactive mediators.[81]

Management of hepatorenal syndrome consists of excluding all other potential nephrotoxins, such as nonsteroidal antiinflammatory agents and aminoglycosides, and assessment for prerenal azotemia secondary to overaggressive diuretic use. Withholding diuretic therapy and administering a fluid challenge of up to 1.5 L is recommended for early diagnosis and therapy.[81] Other therapies studied in the management of hepatorenal syndrome include low (subpressor)-dose dopamine, ornipressin, terlipressin, and midodrine in combination with octreotide, misoprostol, *n*-acetylcysteine, and dialysis.[81] Liver transplantation, which if successful results in full recovery of renal function, remains the treatment of choice for refractory hepatorenal syndrome.

Hepatopulmonary syndrome affects somewhere between 10% and 70% of patients with cirrhosis.[82] This abnormality is caused by alterations in lung mechanics caused by edema and tense ascites, an abnormal ventilation-to-perfusion ratio, the presence of arterial venous shunts, and changes in the alveolar–arterial membrane.[82] These patients present with dyspnea, and arterial oxygenation is often impaired. In the absence of intrinsic cardiopulmonary disease, cirrhotic patients with these findings should be evaluated for hepatopulmonary syndrome which is diagnosed based upon the presence of arterial hypoxemia, an increased alveolar–arterial oxygen gradient, and intrapulmonary vasodilation.[82] Long-term management requires control of ascites (see Management of Ascites and Spontaneous Bacterial Peritonitis above), supportive therapy with supplemental oxygen, and optimizing fluid status. The prognosis for these patients is poor. Ultimately, liver transplantation offers the best chance for long-term recovery.

Coagulation disorders are common in patients with chronic liver disease. These disorders increase the risk of bleeding and tend to become more profound as the liver failure becomes more severe. Correction of the coagulopathy is essential for patients actively bleeding (see Management of Acute Variceal Hemorrhage above), but is not required for patients who present with only minor symptoms such as bruising or nose bleeds and who are not actively bleeding. The pathophysiology of the coagulopathy is complex and involves impaired synthesis of clotting factors, excessive fibrinolysis, disseminated intravascular coagulation, thrombocytopenia, and platelet dysfunction.[14] Acute therapy involves platelet transfusions for thrombocytopenia, and fresh-frozen plasma for prolongation of the prothrombin time because of clotting factor deficiencies. Long-term management of cirrhotic patients with identified coagulopathies is supportive for the management of the underlying cause of cirrhosis; for example, encouraging abstinence from alcohol.

The presence of cirrhosis can produce abnormal regulation and function of multiple endocrine systems.[83] Most common are feminization and hypogonadism, and hypothyroidism. Cirrhosis perturbs the hypothalamic–pituitary axis, which is required for normal regulation of sex and thyroid hormones. In men with cirrhosis, testosterone levels are depressed, while estrogen levels are increased. The clinical manifestations of these changes include loss of libido, muscle wasting, and gynecomastia. These clinical findings are commonly seen and have been reported to occur in up to 60% of cirrhotic patients.[83] In women, feminization changes are less-well studied. Alcohol use complicates and can worsen sex hormone abnormalities.

Both central and peripheral defects in thyroid secretion are noted in patients with cirrhosis. Alcohol plays a major role with direct toxic effects on the thyroid gland. Management includes thyroid hormone replacement for hypothyroidism with the usual doses (levothyroxine 50 to 100 mcg/day) and oral testosterone replacement (testosterone 200 mg three times daily) may be attempted to decrease prevalence of gynecomastia. Routine hormone replacement has not been shown to impact survival or disease progression.[83]

■ LIVER TRANSPLANTATION

The complications seen in patients with chronic liver disease are essentially functional as a secondary effect of the circulatory and metabolic changes that accompany liver failure. Consequently, liver transplantation is the only treatment that can offer a cure for complications of end-stage cirrhosis. However, patient selection, evaluation, and pre- and postsurgical management are beyond the scope of this review.

PHARMACOKINETIC AND PHARAMACODYNAMIC CHANGES IN LIVER FAILURE

Cirrhosis modulates the behavior of drugs in the body by inducing kinetic alterations in drug absorption, distribution, and clearance. Additionally, patients with cirrhosis may exhibit pharmacodynamic changes with increased sensitivity to the effects of certain drugs, namely opiates, benzodiazepines, and nonsteroidal antiinflammatory drugs (NSAIDs). These pharmacodynamic changes are separate and distinct from the enhancement of drug effects seen in cirrhosis patients as a result of pharmacokinetic changes.[84] Hepatic drug clearance is primarily dependent upon protein binding, hepatic blood flow, and metabolic enzyme activity.[85] The pathophysiologic changes that occur in patients with cirrhosis, including reduced liver blood flow, altered microcirculatory distribution of blood flow within the liver, diminished metabolic and synthetic function, and changes in the endothelial lining of the sinusoids, can have a significant impact on each of these factors. The consequence of these changes is a reduction in intrinsic metabolic activity, a reduction in the delivery of blood to the liver that decreases clearance and prolongs half-life, and a reduction in the degree of protein binding that increases the fraction of unbound drug in the serum. Finally, patients with cirrhosis frequently accumulate large amounts of interstitial fluid resulting in substantial changes in the volume of distribution, which also prolongs drug half-life. These changes occur most commonly in combination in patients with cirrhosis and are dynamic throughout the disease course. The effect that these changes will have depends on the drug and the type of biotransformation that the drug undergoes.

Drugs with a high extraction ratio (high-extraction drugs) are dependent on blood flow for metabolism and the rate of metabolism is sensitive to changes in blood flow. Drugs with a low extraction ratio (low-extraction drugs) are dependent on intrinsic metabolic activity for metabolism and the rate of metabolism reflects changes in intrinsic clearance and protein binding.[84,85] Furthermore, hepatic biotransformation involves two types of metabolic processes: phase I reactions and phase II reactions. Phase I reactions involve the cytochrome P450 system and include hydrolysis, oxidation, dealkylation, and reduction reactions. Phase II reactions involve conjugation of the drug with an endogenous molecule such as sulfate or an amino acid, rendering it more water soluble and enhancing its elimination. Drugs metabolized by phase I reactions, especially oxidation, tend to be significantly impaired in patients with cirrhosis, whereas drugs eliminated by conjugation are relatively unaffected.[86]

The variability and complexity of the interaction between the extent and severity of liver disease and individual characteristics of the drug makes it very difficult to predict the degree of pharmacokinetic perturbation in an individual patient. Unfortunately, there are no sensitive and specific clinical or biochemical markers that allow us to quantify the extent of liver insufficiency or the degree of metabolic activity. In addition, renal insufficiency and alterations that commonly accompany cirrhosis further complicate empiric dosing recommendations in these patients.[84] Dosing recommendations are most commonly nonspecific, with recommendations labeled for patients with mild to moderate liver impairment. Dosing information for patients with more severe liver impairment is not available. As a result, when patients with cirrhosis require therapy with drugs that undergo hepatic metabolism (e.g., benzodiazepines), monitoring response to therapy and anticipating drug accumulation and enhanced effects is essential. In the case of benzodiazepines, selection of an agent such as lorazepam, an intermediate-acting agent that is metabolized via conjugation and has no active metabolites, is easier to monitor than a drug such as diazepam, a long-acting benzodiazepine that is oxidized in the liver and has an active metabolite with a long half-life of its own. Up-to-date drug dosing recommendation information for patients with liver disease has been published.[87]

PHARMACOECONOMIC CONSIDERATIONS

A number of issues related to the drug therapy and monitoring of cirrhosis have been studied over the years. Two such studies, both related to the prevention of variceal bleeding and published recently, are mentioned here. A recent analysis provides evidence that HVPG monitoring is not cost-effective for use in patients with varices and no history of variceal bleeding as compared to treatment with standard β-blocker therapy without invasive monitoring.[88] A cost-utility evaluation of secondary prophylaxis therapies concluded that patients are best served by treatment with either EBL or EBL plus medical management as compared to TIPS placement.[89] Because treatment approaches for patients with cirrhosis can range from supportive medical therapy, to repeated endoscopic procedures with serious complications, to liver transplantation, the need for application of economic analysis is obvious. Of critical importance is the question of when, in the course of chronic liver disease, are the various treatment interventions employed and should liver transplantation be attempted earlier, thereby avoiding most of the complications associated with chronic liver disease.

EVALUATION OF THERAPEUTIC OUTCOMES

Table 39–10 summarizes the management approach for patients with cirrhosis, including monitoring parameters and therapeutic out-

TABLE 39-10 Management Approach and Outcome Assessments

Complication	Treatment Approach	Monitoring Parameter	Outcome Assessment
Ascites	Diet, diuretics, paracentesis, TIPS	Daily assessment of weight	Prevent or eliminate ascites and its secondary complications
Spontaneous bacterial peritonitis	Antibiotic therapy, prophylaxis if undergoing paracentesis	Evidence of clinical deterioration (e.g., abdominal pain, fever, anorexia, malaise, fatigue)	Prevent/treat infection to decrease mortality
Variceal bleeding	Pharmacologic prophylaxis	Child-Pugh score, endoscopy, CBC	Appropriate reduction in heart rate and portal pressure
	Endoscopy, vasoactive drug therapy (octreotide), ligation or sclerotherapy, volume resuscitation, pharmacologic prophylaxis	CBC, evidence of overt bleeding	Acute: control acute bleed Chronic: variceal obliteration, reduce portal pressures
Coagulation disorders	Blood products (PPF, platelets), vitamin K	CBC, prothrombin time, platelet count	Normalize PT time, maintain/improve hemostasis
Hepatic encephalopathy	Ammonia reduction (lactulose, cathartics), elimination of drugs causing CNS depression, limit excess protein in diet	Grade of encephalopathy, EEG, psychological testing, mental status changes, concurrent drug therapy	Maintain functional capacity, prevent hospitalization for encephalopathy, decrease ammonia levels, provide adequate nutrition
Hepatorenal syndrome	Eliminate concurrent nephrotoxins (NSAIDs), decrease or discontinue diuretics, volume resuscitation, liver transplantation	Serum and urine electrolytes, concurrent drug therapy	Prevent progressive renal injury by preventing dehydration and avoiding other nephrotoxins Liver transplantation for refractory hepatorenal syndrome
Hepatopulmonary syndrome	Paracentesis, O_2 therapy	Dyspnea, presence of ascites	Acute: relief of dyspnea and hypoxia Chronic: manage ascites as above

CBC, complete blood cell count; CNS, central nervous system; EEG, electroencephalogram; PT, prothrombin time; NSAID, nonsteroidal antiinflammatory drug; PPF, plasma protein fraction; TIPS, transjugular intrahepatic portosystemic shunt.

comes. Cirrhosis is generally a chronic progressive disease that requires aggressive medical management to prevent or delay common complications. Table 39–10 also lists monitoring criteria that need to be carefully followed in order to achieve the maximum benefit from the medical therapies employed and prevent adverse effects. A therapeutic plan including therapeutic end points for each medical and diet therapy needs to be developed and discussed with the patient.

ABBREVIATIONS

AASLD: American Association for the Study of Liver Diseases
ALT: alanine transaminase
AST: aspartate transaminase
EBL: endoscopic band ligation
EGD: esophagogastroduodenoscopy
EIS: endoscopic injection sclerotherapy
ERCP: endoscopic retrograde cholangiopancreatography
GABA: γ-aminobutyric acid
GGT: γ-glutamyl transpeptidase
HE: hepatic encephalopathy
HVPG: hepatic venous pressure gradient
MELD: Mayo End-Stage Liver Disease
NSAIDs: nonsteroidal antiinflammatory drugs
PMN: polymorphonuclear
SAG: serum-ascites albumin gradient
SBP: spontaneous bacterial peritonitis
TIPS: transjugular intrahepatic portosystemic shunt
UNOS: United Network for Organ Sharing

REFERENCES

1. Iredale JP. Cirrhosis: New research provides a basis for rational and targeted treatments. BMJ 2003;327:143–147.
2. Bataller R, Brenner DA. Liver fibrosis. J Clin Invest 2005;115(2):209–218.
3. Anand BS. Cirrhosis of liver. West J Med 1999;171:110–115.
4. Minino AR, Heron MP, Smith BL. Deaths: Preliminary data for 2004. Natl Vital Stat Rep 2006;54(19):1–49.
5. Runyon BA. Management of adult patients with ascites due to cirrhosis. Hepatology 2004;39(3):841–856.
6. Malarkey DE, Johnson K, Ryan L, et al. New insights into functional aspects of liver morphology. Toxicol Pathol 2005;33:27–34.
7. DeFranchis R. Evolving concensus in portal hypertension. Report of the Baveno IV Consensus Workshop on methodology of diagnosis and therapy in portal hypertension. J Hepatol 2005;43:167–176.
8. Abraldes JG, Angermayr B, Bosch J. The management of portal hypertension. Clin Liv Dis 2005;9:685–713.
9. Cadenas A, Bataller R, Qarroyo V. Mechanisms of ascites formation. Clin Liver Dis 2000;4:447–465.
10. Arroyo V. Pathophysiology, diagnosis and treatment of ascites in cirrhosis. Ann Hepatol 2002;1(2):72–79.
11. Wright AS, Rikkers LF. Current management of portal hypertension. J Gastrointest Surg 2005;9(7):992–1005.
12. Blei AT, Cordoba J. Hepatic encephalopathy. Am J Gastroenterol 2001;96:1968–1976.
13. Stewart CA, Cerhan J. Hepatic encephalopathy: A dynamic or static condition. Metab Brain Dis 2005;20(3):193–204.
14. Kujovich JL. Hemostatic defects in end stage liver disease. Crit Care Clin 2005;21:563–587.
15. Talwalkar JA, Lindor KD. Primary biliary cirrhosis. Lancet 2003;362:53–61.
16. DeFranchis R, Primigrani M. Natural history of portal hypertension in patients with cirrhosis. Clin Liver Dis 2001;5:645–663.
17. Giannini EG, Testa R, Savarino V. Liver enzyme alteration: A guide for clinicians. CMAJ 2005;172(3):367–379.
18. Cohen JA, Kaplan MM. The SGOT/SGPT ratio—An indicator of alcoholic disease. Dig Dis Sci 1979;24:835–838.
19. Pugh RNH, Murray-Lyon IM, Dawson JL, et al. Transection of the oesophagus for bleeding oesophagus varices. Br J Surg 1973;60:646–649.
20. Malinchoc M, Kamath PS, Gordon FD, et al. A model to predict poor survival in patients undergoing transjugular intrahepatic portosystemic shunts. Hepatology 2000;31:864–871.
21. MELD/PELD calculator documentation. October 20, 2006, *http://www.unos.org/waitlist/includes_local/ pdfs/meld_peld_calculator.pdf.*
22. Amitrano L, Guardascione MA, Brancaccio V, Baizano A. Coagulation disorders in liver disease. Semin Liver Dis 2002;22(1):83–96.
23. O'Grady JG, Alexander GJM, Hayllat KM, et al. Early indicators of prognosis in fulminant hepatic failure. Gastroenterology 1989;97:439–445.
24. Gow PJ, Chapman RW. Modern management of oesophageal varices. Postgrad Med J 2001;77:75–81.
25. El Serag HB, Everhart JE. Improved survival after variceal hemorrhage over an 11-year period in the Department of Veterans Affairs. Am J Gastroenterol 2000;95:3566–3573.
26. Groszmann RJ, Guadalupe G, Bosch J, et al. Beta-blockers to prevent gastroesophageal varices in patients with cirrhosis. N Engl J Med 2005;353:2254–2261.
27. D'Amico G, Pagliaro L, Bosch J. Pharmacologic treatment of portal hypertension: An evidence-based approach. Semin Liver Dis 1999;19:475–505.
28. Merkel C, Marin R, Angeli P, et al. A placebo-controlled clinical trial of nadolol in the prophylaxis of growth of small esophageal varices in cirrhosis. Gastroenterology 2004;127:476–484.
29. Abraczinskas DR, Ookubo R, Grace ND, et al. Propranolol for the prevention of first esophageal variceal hemorrhage: A lifetime commitment? Hepatology 2001;34:1096–1102.
30. Patch D, Burroughs AK. Variceal hemorrhage. In: Cohen S, Davis GL, Gianella RA, et al., eds. Therapy of Digestive Disorders: A Companion to Sleisenger and Fordtran's Gastrointestinal and Liver Disease. Philadelphia: WB Saunders, 2000:355–372.
31. Lui HF, Stanley AJ, Forrest EH, et al. Primary prophylaxis of variceal hemorrhage: A randomized controlled trial comparing band ligation, propranolol, and isosorbide mononitrate. Gastroenterology 2002;123:735–744.
32. Jutabha R, Jensen DM, Martin P, et al. Randomized study comparing banding and propranolol to prevent initial variceal hemorrhage in cirrhotics with high-risk esophageal varices. Gastroenterology 2005;128:870–881.
33. Psilopoulos D, Galanis P, Goulas S, et al. Endoscopic variceal ligation vs. propranolol for prevention of first variceal bleeding: A randomized controlled trial. Eur J Gastroenterol Hepatol 2005;17:1111–1117.
34. Sarin SK, Wadhawan M, Agarwal SR, et al. Endoscopic variceal ligation plus propranolol versus endoscopic variceal ligation alone in primary prophylaxis of variceal bleeding. Am J Gastroenterol 2005;100:797–804.
35. Schepke M, Kleber G, Nurnberg D, et al. Ligation versus propranolol for the primary prophylaxis of variceal bleeding in cirrhosis. Hepatology 2004;40(1):65–72.
36. Lay CS, Tsai YT, Lee FY, et al. Endoscopic variceal ligation versus propranolol in prophylaxis of first variceal bleeding in patients with cirrhosis. J Gastroenterol Hepatol 2006;21(2):413–419.
37. Garcia-Pagan JC, Morillas R, Banares R, et al. Propranolol plus placebo versus propranolol plus isosorbide-5-mononitrate in the prevention of a first variceal bleed: A double-blind RCT. Hepatology 2003;37:1260–1266.
38. Grace ND. Diagnosis and treatment of gastrointestinal bleeding secondary to portal hypertension [practice guidelines]. Am J Gastroenterol 1997;92:1082–1091.
39. Volk ML and Marrero JA. Advances in critical care hepatology. Minerva Anestesiol 2006;72:269–281.
40. Baik SK, Jeong PH, Ji SW, et al. Acute hemodynamic effects of octreotide and terlipressin in patients with cirrhosis: A randomized comparison. Am J Gastroenterol 2005;100:631–635.
41. Wolf DC. The management of variceal bleeding: Past, present, and future. Mt Sinai J Med 1999;66:1–13.
42. Imperiale TF, Teran JC, McCullough AJ. A meta-analysis of somatostatin vs vasopressin in the treatment of acute esophageal variceal hemorrhage. Gastroenterology 1995;109:1289–1294.
43. Gotzsche PC, Gjorup I, Bonnen H, et al. Somatostatin vs placebo in bleeding oesophageal varices: Randomized trial and meta-analysis. BMJ 1995;310:1495–1498.

44. Corley D, Cello J, Adkisson W, et al. Octreotide for acute esophageal variceal bleeding: A meta-analysis. Gastroenterology 2001;120:946–954.
45. Escorsell A, Del Arbol LR, Planas R, et al. Multicenter randomized controlled trial of terlipressin versus sclerotherapy in the treatment of acute variceal bleeding: The TEST study. Hepatology 2000;32:471–476.
46. Villanueva C, Planella M, Aracil C, et al. Hemodynamic effects of terlipressin and high somatostatin dose during acute variceal bleeding in nonresponders to the usual somatostatin dose. Am J Gastroenterol 2005;100:624–630.
47. Feu F, Del Arbol LR, Banares R, et al. Double-blind randomized controlled trial comparing terlipressin and somatostatin for acute variceal hemorrhage. Gastroenterology 1996;111:1291–1299.
48. Goulis J, Armonis A, Patch D, et al. Bacterial infection is independently associated with failure to control bleeding and early rebleeding in cirrhotic patients with gastrointestinal hemorrhage. Hepatology 1998;27:1207–1212.
49. Shahara AJ, Rockey OC. Gastrointestinal variceal hemorrhage. N Engl J Med 2001;345:669–681.
50. D'Amico G, Pietrosi G, Tarantino I, Pagliaro L. Emergency sclerotherapy versus vasoactive drugs for variceal bleeding in cirrhosis: A Cochrane meta-analysis. Gastroenterology 2003;124(5):1277–1291.
51. Chen WC, Lo GH, Tsai WL, et al. Emergency endoscopic variceal ligation versus somatostatin for acute esophageal variceal bleeding. J Chin Med Assoc 2006;69:60–67.
52. Gross M, Schiemann U, Muhlhofer A, Zoller WG. Meta-analysis: Efficacy of therapeutic regimens in ongoing variceal bleeding. Endoscopy 2001;33:737–746.
53. Tan P, Hou M, Lin H, et al. A randomized trial of endoscopic treatment of acute gastric variceal hemorrhage; *n*-butyl-2-cyanoacrylate injection versus band ligation. Hepatology 2006;43:690–697.
54. Wong F. The use of TIPS in chronic liver disease. Ann Hepatol 2006;5:5–15.
55. Bernard B, LeBrec D, Mathurin P, et al. Beta-adrenergic antagonists in the prevention of gastrointestinal rebleeding in patients with cirrhosis: A meta-analysis. Hepatology 1997;25:63–70.
56. Patch D, Sabin CA, Gerunda G, et al. A randomized controlled trial of medical therapy versus endoscopic ligation for the prevention of variceal rebleeding in patients with cirrhosis. Gastroenterology 2002;123:1013–1019.
57. Villanueva C, Minana J, Ortiz J, et al. Endoscopic ligation compared with combined treatment with nadolol and isosorbide mononitrate to prevent recurrent variceal bleeding. N Engl J Med 2001;345(9):647–655.
58. D'Amico G, Pagliaro, L, Bosch J. The treatment of portal hypertension. A meta-analytic review. Hepatology 1995;22:332–354.
59. Villanueva C, Balanzo J, Vonella MT, et al. Nadolol plus isosorbide mononitrate compared with sclerotherapy for the prevention of variceal rebleeding. N Engl J Med 1996;334:1624–1629.
60. Stiegman GV, Goff JS, Michaletz-Onody PA, et al. Endoscopic sclerotherapy as compared with endoscopic ligation for bleeding esophageal varices. N Engl J Med 1992;326:1527–1532.
61. Gimson AES, Ramage JK, Panos MZ, et al. Randomized trial of varices banding ligation versus injection sclerotherapy for bleeding oesophageal varices. Lancet 1993;342:391–394.
62. Laine L, el-Newihi HM, Migikovscky B, et al. Endoscopic ligation compared with sclerotherapy for the treatment of bleeding esophageal varices. Ann Intern Med 1993;119:1–7.
63. Krige JEJ, Beckingham IJ. ABC of diseases of liver, pancreas, and biliary system: Portal hypertension—2. Ascites, encephalopathy, and other conditions. BMJ 2001;322:416–418.
64. Parsi MA, Atreja A, Zein NN. Spontaneous bacterial peritonitis: Recent data on incidence and treatment. Cleve Clin J Med 2004;71:569–576.
65. Zervos EE, Rosemurgy AS. Management of medically refractory ascites. Am J Surg 2001;181:256–264.
66. Runyon BA, McHutchison JG, Antillon MR, et al. Short-course vs long-course antibiotic treatment of spontaneous bacterial peritonitis: A randomized controlled trial of 100 patients. Gastroenterology 1991;100:1737–1742.
67. Navasa M, Follo A, Llovet JM, et al. Randomized, comparative study of oral ofloxacin versus intravenous cefotaxime in spontaneous bacterial peritonitis. Gastroenterology 1996;111:1011–1017.
68. Mas A. Hepatic encephalopathy: From pathophysiology to treatment. Digestion 2006;73(Suppl 1):86–93.
69. Plauth M, Merli M, Kondrug J, et al. ESPEN guidelines for nutrition in liver disease and transplantation. Clin Nutr 1997;16(2):43–55.
70. Charlton M. Branched-chain amino acid enriched supplements as therapy for liver disease. J Nutr 2006;136:295S–298S.
71. Schumann C. Medical, nutritional and technological properties of lactulose. An update. Eur J Nutr 2002;41(Suppl 1):I17–I25.
72. Hawkins RA, Jessy J, Mans AM, et al. Neomycin reduces the intestinal production of ammonia from glutamine. Adv Exp Med Biol 1994;368:125–134.
73. Morgan MH, Read AE, Speller DC. Treatment of hepatic encephalopathy with metronidazole. Gut 1982;23:1–7.
74. Gubbins GP, Moritz TE, Marsano LS, et al. *Helicobacter pylori* is a risk factor for hepatic encephalopathy in acute alcoholic hepatitis: The ammonia hypothesis revisited. The Veterans Administration Cooperative Study Group no. 275. Am J Gastroenterol 1993;88:1906–1910.
75. Vasconez C, Elizalde JI, Llach J, et al. *Helicobacter pylori*, hyperammonemia and subclinical portosystemic encephalopathy: Effects of eradication. J Hepatol 1999;30:260–264.
76. Butterworth RF. Pathophysiology of hepatic encephalopathy: A new look at ammonia. Metab Brain Dis 2002;17:221–227.
77. Kircheis G, Nilium R, Held C, et al. Therapeutic efficacy of L-ornithine–L-aspartate infusions in patients with cirrhosis and hepatic encephalopathy: Results of a placebo-controlled, double-blind study. Hepatology 1997;25:1351–1360.
78. Stauch S, Kircheis G, Adler G, et al. Oral L-ornithine–L-aspartate therapy of chronic hepatic encephalopathy. Results of a placebo-controlled double-blind study. J Hepatol 1998;28:856–864.
79. Marchesini G, Fabbri A, Bianchi G, et al. Zinc supplementation and amino acid–nitrogen metabolism in patients with advanced cirrhosis. Hepatology 1996;23:1084–1092.
80. Als-Nielson B, Kjaergard LL, Glaudd C. Benzodiazepine receptor antagonists for acute and chronic hepatic encephalopathy. Cochrane Database Syst Rev 2001;4:CD002798.
81. Dagher L, Moore K. The hepatorenal syndrome. Gut 2001;49:729–737.
82. Moller S, Henriksen JH. Cardiopulmonary complications in chronic liver disease. World J Gastroenterol 2006;12:526–538.
83. Fitz JG. Hepatic encephalopathy, hepatopulmonary syndrome, hepatorenal syndrome, coagulopathy, and endocrine complications of liver disease. In: Feldman M, Tschumy WO, Friedman LS, Sleisenger MH, eds. Sleisinger and Fordtran's Gastrointestinal and Liver Disease: Pathophysiology/Diagnosis/Management, 7th ed. Philadelphia: WB Saunders, 2002:1543–1565.
84. Fabiola D, Tchambaz L, Schlienger R, et al. Dose adjustments in patients with liver disease. Drug Safety 2005;28:529–545.
85. DePaepe P, Belpaire FM, Buylert WA. Pharmacokinetic and pharmacodynamic considerations when treating patients with sepsis and septic shock. Clin Pharmacokinet 2002;41:1135–1151.
86. Kashuba ADM, Joohyun JP, Persk AM, Brouwer LR. Drug metabolism, transport, and the influence of hepatic disease. In: Burton ME, Shaw LM, Schentag JJ, et al., eds. Applied Pharmacokinetics and Pharmacodynamics: Principles of Therapeutic Drug Monitoring, 4th ed. Baltimore: Lippincott, Williams & Wilkins, 2006:121–164.
87. Elbekai RH, Korashy HM, El-Kadi AOS. The effect of liver cirrhosis on the regulation and expression of drug metabolizing enzymes. Curr Drug Metab 2004;5:157–167.
88. Hicken BL, Sharara AI, Abrams GA, et al. Hepatic venous pressure gradient measurements to assess response to primary prophylaxis in patients with cirrhosis: A decision analytical study. Aliment Pharmacol Ther 2003;17:145–153.
89. Rubenstein JH, Eisen GM, Inadomi JM. A cost-utility analysis of secondary prophylaxis for variceal hemorrhage. Am J Gastroenterol 2004;99:1274–1288.

CHAPTER 40 Drug-Induced Liver Disease

WILLIAM R. KIRCHAIN AND RONDALL E. ALLEN

KEY CONCEPTS

1. Drug-induced liver disease occurs as several different clinical presentations: idiosyncratic reactions, allergic hepatitis, toxic hepatitis, chronic active toxic hepatitis, toxic cirrhosis, and liver vascular disorders.
2. The mechanisms of drug-induced liver disease are diverse, representing many phases of biotransformation, and are susceptible to genetic polymorphism.
3. The assessment of a possible liver injury caused by drugs should include what is known in the literature, the timing involved, the clinical course, and, always, an exploration for preexisting conditions that may have encouraged the lesion's development.
4. Liver enzyme assays can help to determine if a particular type of liver damage is present.
5. Monitoring for drug-induced liver disease must be tailored to the drug and the patient's potential risk factors.

The number of drugs associated with adverse reactions involving the liver is extensive.[1] One of the more common reasons for the withdrawal of a drug from the marketplace is an elevation of serum concentrations of liver enzymes.[2] Its impact on the pharmaceutical industry has led regulatory agencies to withdraw drugs from the market, restrict the use of certain medications, and issue black box warnings.[3] Alcohol-induced liver disease is the most common type of drug-induced liver disease. All other drugs together account for less than 10% of patients hospitalized for elevated liver enzymes.[4] Overall, the reported incidence of drug-induced liver disease is around 1 in 10,000 to 1 in 100,000 patients.[1]

In approximately 75% of these cases liver transplantation is ultimately required for patient survival.[2] The liver's function affects almost every other organ system in the body, but there are no specific diagnostic tests for drug-induced liver disease or a means to single out an implicated drug. Therefore it is important to know the patterns of drug-related pathology in order to assess adverse reactions when they occur. It is also important to understand how and when to monitor for these reactions.

PATTERNS OF DRUG-INDUCED LIVER DISEASE

HEPATOCELLULAR INJURY

Hepatocellular injury is characterized by significant elevations in the aminotransferases in serum which usually precede elevations in total bilirubin levels and alkaline phosphatase levels.[5] Most injuries occur within 1 year of initiating the offending agent. Hepatocellular injury can lead to fulminant hepatitis with a corresponding 20% survival rate with supportive care.[6] For those patients who present with the combination of hepatocellular injury and jaundice, there is a 10% mortality rate.[7] Acarbose, allopurinol, fluoxetine, and losartan are capable of causing hepatocellular injury.[5]

Hepatocellular injuries can be further subdivided by specific histologic patterns and clinical presentations. Centrolobular necrosis, steatohepatitis (steatonecrosis), phospholipidosis, and generalized hepatocellular necrosis are each identifiable by particular biopsy results and subtle differences in clinical presentation.

CENTROLOBULAR NECROSIS

Centrolobular necrosis is often a dose-related, predictable reaction secondary to drugs such as acetaminophen; however, it also can be associated with idiosyncratic reactions, such as those caused by the anesthetic halothane. Also called direct or metabolite-related hepatotoxicity, centrolobular necrosis is usually the result of the production of a toxic metabolite (Fig. 40–1). The damage spreads outward from the middle of a lobe of the liver.

Patients suffering from centrolobular necrosis tend to present in one of two ways, depending on the extent of necrosis. Mild drug reactions, involving only small amounts of parenchymal liver tissue, may be detected as asymptomatic elevations in the serum aminotransferases. If the reaction is diagnosed at this stage, most of these patients will recover with minimal cirrhosis and thus minimal chronic liver impairment. More severe forms of centrolobular necrosis are accompanied by nausea, vomiting, upper abdominal pain, and jaundice.[8,9]

These reactions are predictable, often dose-related effects in the liver caused by specific agents. When taken in overdose, acetaminophen becomes bioactivated to a toxic intermediate known as *N*-acetyl-*p*-benzoquinone imine (NAPQI). NAPQI is very reactive, with a high affinity for sulfhydryl groups. The amino acid glutathione provides a ready source of available sulfhydryl groups within the hepatocyte. When the liver's glutathione stores are depleted and there are no longer sulfhydryl groups available to detoxify this metabolite, it begins to react directly with the hepatocyte (see Fig. 40–1). Replenishing the liver's sulfhydryl capacity through the administration of *N*-acetylcysteine early after ingestion of the overdose halts this pro-

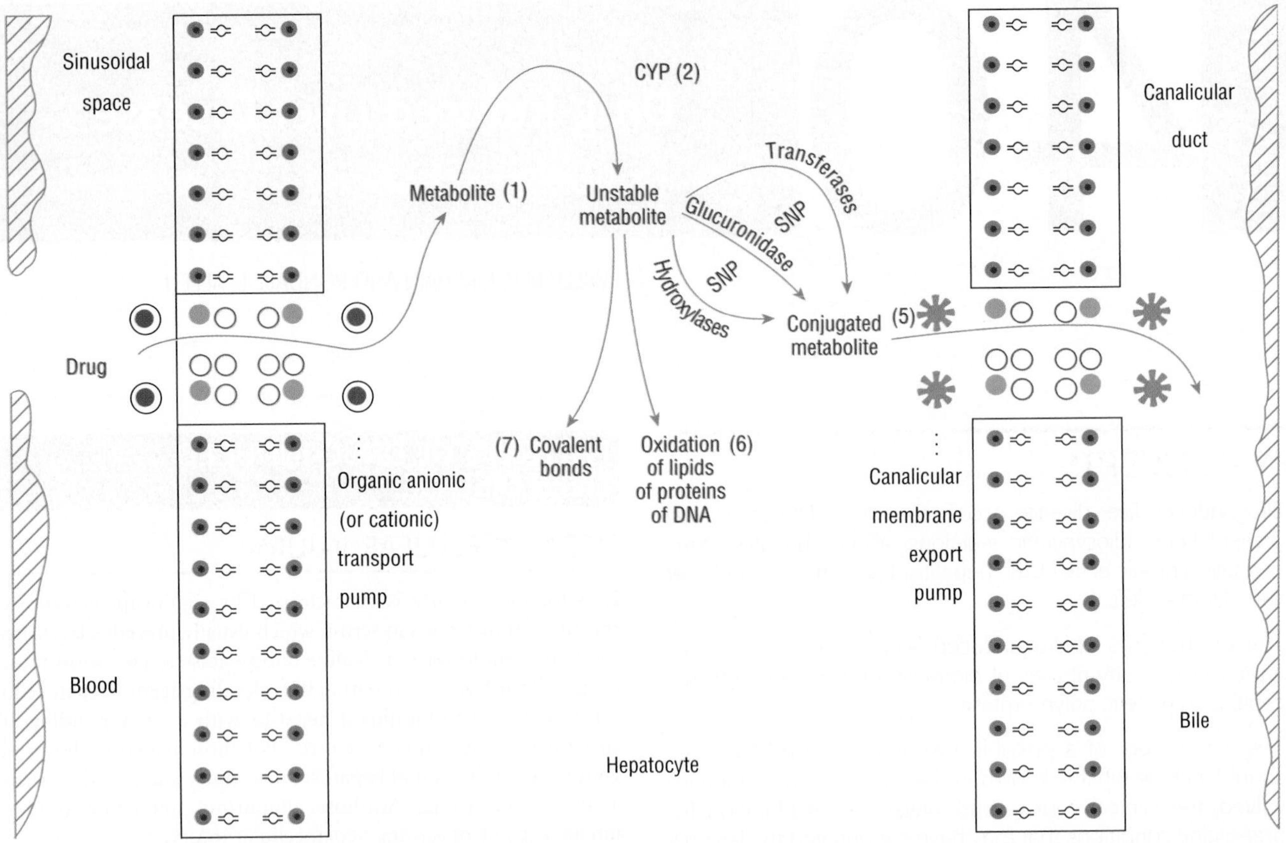

FIGURE 40-1. A general diagram of biotransformation. (*1*) The drug is actively transported into the hepatocyte by the organic anion transport pump, a transmembrane protein. (*2*) The metabolite (drug) interacts with one of a number of enzymes, the most common being CYP2C9, 2C19, 2D6, and 3A4. This family of enzymes is regulated by the complementary DNA xenobiotic receptor. The xenobiotic receptor is in turn upregulated by other drugs, changes in cholesterol catabolism, and bile acids. (*3*) The immediate result of the action of these phase I enzymes is the production of an unstable metabolite. (*4*) The unstable metabolite then reacts with glucuronidase, various transferases, or hydroxylases to form a conjugated metabolite. The efficacy of these enzymes is affected by the patient's nutritional state and genetic polymorphism, leading to variations in individual risk for toxicity. (*5*) The conjugated metabolite is removed from the hepatocyte by the canalicular membrane export pump, one of a large family of membrane proteins (other members of this family pump conjugated metabolites back into the blood for excretion by the kidney). These proteins are subject to genetic polymorphism as well, again leading to some patients having an increased risk for toxicity. (*6*) If unable to form a conjugate, the unstable metabolite can participate in oxidative reactions that damage lipids, proteins, or even DNA. (*7*) Alternatively the unstable metabolite may form damaging covalent bonds with available anions or cations. (SNP, indicates points in this process that are influenced by an individual's single nucleotide polymorphisms.)

cess.[10,11] During the first hours after ingestion, some patients report mild symptoms of nausea and vomiting, but no elevations of the commonly measured liver enzymes are seen. Not for 40 to 50 hours after ingestion do serum elevations in the liver enzymes begin.[11]

Reye's syndrome is an aggressive form of toxic hepatitis often associated with aspirin use in children. Valproate toxicity can also present in this pattern. Early in the process of Reye's syndrome, mitochondrial dysfunction leads to the depletion of acyl-coenzyme A and carnitine. Fatty acids accumulate and gluconeogenesis is impaired, resulting in hypoglycemia. A concurrent disruption of the urea cycle occurs, leading to a decrease in the removal of ammonia and a slowing of protein use. A threefold rise in the blood ammonia level and an increase in the prothrombin time are common findings. In advanced stages of Reye's syndrome, many patients develop intracranial hypertension that can be life-threatening and refractory to therapy.[12,13]

STEATOHEPATITIS

Steatohepatitis (also known as steatonecrosis) is a specialized type of acute necrosis resulting from the accumulation of fatty acids in the hepatocyte. Drugs or their metabolites that cause steatonecrosis do so by affecting fatty-acid oxidation within the mitochondria of the hepatocyte (see Fig. 40–1). Hepatic vesicles become engorged with fatty acids, eventually disrupting the homeostasis of the hepatocyte. The liver biopsy is marked by a massive infiltration by polymorphonuclear leukocytes, degeneration of the hepatocytes, and the presence of Mallory bodies.[4]

Alcohol is the drug that most commonly produces steatonecrotic changes in the liver. When alcohol is converted into acetaldehyde, the synthesis of fatty acids is increased.[14,15] When the hepatocyte has become completely engorged with microvesicular fat, it often breaks open, spilling into the blood. If enough hepatocytes break open, an inflammatory response begins. If the offending agent is withdrawn before significant numbers of hepatocytes become necrotic, the process is completely reversible without long-term sequelae. In nonalcoholic steatohepatitis, the same end point is often achieved through oxidation of lipid peroxidases.[16]

Tetracycline produces steatohepatitis and steatosis.[17] The lesions are characterized by large vesicles of fat found diffused throughout the liver. The development of this reaction is related to the high concentrations achieved when tetracycline is given intravenously and in doses greater than 1.5 g/day. The mortality of tetracycline steatohepatitis is high (70% to 80%), and those who do survive often develop cirrhosis. Sodium valproate also can produce steatonecrosis through the process of bioactivation. Cytochrome P450 converts valproate to *delta*-4-valproic acid, a potent inducer of microvesicular fat accumulation.[18]

Patients experiencing steatohepatitis may present with abdominal fullness or pain as their only complaint. Patients with more severe steatonecrosis will present with all the symptoms characteristic of alcoholic hepatitis such as nausea, vomiting, steatorrhea, abdominal pain, pruritus, and fatigue.

PHOSPHOLIPIDOSIS

Phospholipidosis is the accumulation of phospholipids instead of fatty acids. The phospholipids usually engorge the lysosomal bodies of the hepatocyte.[19] Amiodarone is associated with this reaction. Patients treated with amiodarone who develop overt hepatic disease tend to have received higher doses of the drug. These patients also have higher amiodarone–to–N-desethyl-amiodarone ratios, indicating a greater accumulation of the parent compound. Amiodarone and its major metabolite *N*-desethyl-amiodarone remain in the liver of all patients for several months after therapy is stopped. Usually the phospholipidosis develops in patients treated for more than 1 year. The patient can present with either elevated aminotransferases or hepatomegaly; jaundice is rare.[4,20]

GENERALIZED HEPATOCELLULAR NECROSIS

Generalized hepatocellular necrosis mimics the changes associated with the more common viral hepatitis. The onset of symptoms is usually delayed as much as a week or more after exposure to toxin. Bioactivation is often important for toxic hepatitis to develop, but may not be the immediate cause of damage. Many drugs that are associated with toxic hepatitis produce metabolites that are not inherently toxic to the liver. Instead, they act as haptens, binding to specific cell proteins and inducing an autoimmune reaction (see Fig. 40–1).[21]

The rate of bioactivation can vary between males and females and between individuals of the same sex.[22,23] The cytochrome P450 (CYP450) system tends to metabolize lipophilic substrates that are actively pumped into the hepatocyte by an organic anion (or cation) transporting protein. The CYP450 subspecies 2C, 2D, 3A, and 4A are regulated by the highly inducible xenobiotic receptor on complementary DNA. The receptor is found in the liver, and to a lesser extent in the cells lining the intestinal tract, and is responsible for cholesterol catabolism and bile acid homeostasis. The activity of this receptor is subject to genetic polymorphism as well. This results in a wide variation in the sensitivity of the population to generalized hepatocellular necrosis and other forms of hepatic damage.[16,24]

The long-term administration of isoniazid can lead to hepatic dysfunction in 10% to 20% of those receiving the drug. Yet severe toxic hepatitis develops in only 1% or less of this population.[25] The *N*-acetyltransferase 2 (NAT2) genotype appears to play a role in determining a patient's relative risk. In one study, patients with the slow-type NAT2 genotype had a 28-fold greater risk of developing serum aminotransferase elevations than did patients with the fast-type NAT2 genotype.[26] Isoniazid is metabolized by several pathways, acetylation being the major pathway. It is acetylated to acetylisoniazid, which, in turn, is hydrolyzed to acetylhydrazine.[27] The acetylhydrazine, and to a lesser extent the acetylisoniazid, are directly toxic to the cellular proteins in the hepatocyte, but rapid acetylators also detoxify acetylhydrazine very rapidly, converting it to diacetylhydrazine (a nontoxic metabolite).

Isoniazid simultaneously is an example of the potential predictability of drug-induced liver disease based on single nucleotide polymorphism and a lesson in the limitations of our current understanding. There are definite links to NAT2 genotype and toxicity.[28] The risk for this reaction is also influenced heavily by the age of the patient, with older patients having a much higher risk than younger patients. In fact, age may be more important than genotype.[25,26,28]

Ketoconazole produces generalized hepatocellular necrosis or milder forms of hepatic dysfunction in 1% to 2% of patients treated for fungal infections. This reaction is fatal in high numbers of patients who are infected with the human immunodeficiency virus. The onset is usually early in therapy, although it can be delayed until several months into therapy. In immune-compromised patients in whom ketoconazole is used for long periods of time, special care should be taken to watch for changes in liver function.[29]

TOXIC CIRRHOSIS

The scarring effect of hepatitis in the liver leads to the development of cirrhosis. Some drugs tend to cause such a mild case of hepatitis that it may not be detected. Mild hepatitis can be easily mistaken for a more routine generalized viral infection. If the offending drug or agent is not discontinued, this damage will continue to progress. The patient eventually presents not with hepatitis, but with cirrhosis. Methotrexate causes periportal fibrosis in most patients who experience hepatotoxicity.

The lesion results from the action of a bioactivated metabolite produced by CYP450.[30] This process occurs most commonly in patients treated for psoriasis and arthritis. The extent of damage can be reduced or controlled by increasing the dosage interval to once weekly or by routine use of folic acid supplements.[31] Vitamin A is normally stored in liver cells, and causes significant hypertrophy and fibrosis when taken for long periods in high doses. Hepatomegaly is a common finding, along with ascites and portal hypertension. In patients with vitamin A toxicity, gingivitis and dry skin are also very common. This is accelerated by ethanol, which competes with retinol for aldehyde dehydrogenase.[14]

CHOLESTATIC INJURY

A second pattern of hepatic damage is an injury that primarily involves the bile canalicular system and is know as cholestatic injury. In cholestatic disease, disturbance of the subcellular actin filaments around the canaliculi prevents the movement of bile through the canalicular system.[31] The inability of the liver to remove bile causes intrahepatic accumulation of toxic bile acids and excretion products.[32] Although rare, some patients develop progressive destruction of the cholangiocytes leading to the vanishing bile duct syndrome.

Drug-induced cholestasis can occur as an acute disorder (e.g., cholestasis with or without hepatitis and cholestasis with bile duct injury) or as a chronic disorder (e.g., vanishing bile duct syndrome, sclerosing cholangitis, and cholelithiasis).[33] However, the most common form of drug-induced cholestasis is cholestasis with hepatitis. Most patients with this acute disorder present with nausea, malaise, jaundice, and pruritus.[5] Elevations in serum alkaline phosphatase levels are more prominent and usually precede the elevations of other liver enzymes in serum.[5] On histologic examination, portal inflammation and hepatocyte necrosis are noted.[34] Although the antipsychotic drug chlorpromazine appears to be the prototype drug for this disorder, other medications are associated with other forms of cholestatic injury, such as erythromycin estolate, amoxicillin-clavulanic acid, and carbamazepine.[6]

Cholestatic injury, also known as cholestatic jaundice or cholestasis, can be classified by the area of the bile canalicular or ductal system that is impaired. Canalicular cholestasis is often associated with long-term high-dose estrogen therapy. Clinically, these patients are often asymptomatic and present with mild to moderate elevations of serum bilirubin.[35] An intravenous form of vitamin E, α-tocopherol acetate, causes cholestatic jaundice, primarily involving the canalicular duct in premature infants. The incidence of this reaction in those receiving this formulation was high (>10%) and the mortality even higher (>50%).[36]

The administration of total parenteral nutrition for periods greater than 1 week induces cholestatic changes and nonspecific enzyme elevations in some patients. Patients with low serum albumin concentrations may be at greater risk than patients with normal serum albumin concentrations.[4] This reaction also has been reported to occur rarely with sulfonamides, sulfonylureas, erythromycin estolate and ethylsuccinate, captopril, lisinopril, and other phenothiazines.[37]

MIXED HEPATOCELLULAR AND CHOLESTATIC INJURY

The final pattern of hepatic damage is a combining of the previous two patterns. This presentation can be the result of three different processes. In some patients, an injury may begin as hepatocellular (or cholestatic) and simply spread so rapidly that by the time the patient presents for diagnosis and treatment, all areas of the liver are affected. In other patients, the underlying mechanism of damage is such that cells are injured regardless of their anatomical location or primary metabolic role.

LIVER VASCULAR DISORDERS

Focal lesions in hepatic venules, sinusoids, and portal veins occur with various drugs. The most commonly associated drugs are the cytotoxic agents used to treat cancer, the pyrrolizidine alkaloids, and the sex hormones. A centralized necrosis often follows and can result in cirrhosis. Azathioprine and herbal teas that contain comfrey (a source of pyrrolizidine alkaloids) are associated with the development of venoocclusive disease. The exact incidence is rare and may be dose related.[4] Peliosis hepatitis is a rare type of hepatic vascular lesion that can be seen as both an acute and a chronic disease. The liver develops large, blood-filled lacunae (space or cavity) within the parenchyma. Rupture of the lacunae can lead to severe peritoneal hemorrhage. Peliosis hepatitis is associated with exposure of the liver to androgens, estrogens, tamoxifen, azathioprine, and danazol. Androgens with a methyl alkylation at the 17-carbon position of the testosterone structure are the most frequently reported agents that cause peliosis hepatitis, usually after at least 6 months of therapy.[38]

MECHANISMS OF DRUG-INDUCED LIVER DISEASE

STIMULATION OF AUTOIMMUNITY

Autoimmune injuries involve antibody mediated cytotoxicity or direct cellular toxicity.[34,39] This type of injury occurs when enzyme-drug adducts migrate to the cell surface and form neoantigens. The neoantigens serve as targets for cytolytic attack by T cells.[5] The injury may be exacerbated by the recruitment of inflammatory cells. Halothane, sulfamethoxazole, carbamazepine, and nevirapine are associated with autoimmune injuries.[32] Stimulation of autoimmunity is often associated with some stage of all fulminant presentations. It is the primary cause of injury in idiosyncratic reactions.

Dantrolene, isoniazid, phenytoin, nitrofurantoin, and trazodone are associated with a type of autoimmune-mediated disease in the liver called *chronic active hepatitis*.[8,40] Patients experience periods of symptomatic hepatitis followed by periods of convalescence, only to repeat the experience months later. It is a progressive disease with a high mortality rate and is more common in females than males. Antinuclear antibodies appear in most patients. These drugs appear to form antiorganelle antibodies.[21] The exact identification of a causative agent is sometimes difficult as diagnosis requires multiple episodes occurring long after exposure to the offending drug.

IDIOSYNCRATIC REACTIONS

Idiosyncratic drug-related hepatotoxicity is rare and usually occurs in a small proportion of individuals. These adverse reactions are often categorized into allergic and nonallergic reactions. The allergic reactions are characterized by fever, rash, and eosinophilia. They are usually dose-related and have a short latency period (<1 month). Upon reexposure to the offending agent, the patient will experience rapid recurrence of hepatotoxicity. Studies show that minocycline, nitrofurantoin, and phenytoin can cause allergic reactions.[3]

Unlike the allergic reactions, the nonallergic idiosyncratic reactions are devoid of the hypersensitivity features and usually have a long latency period (several months). These patients often have normal liver function tests for 6 months or longer and then suddenly develop hepatotoxicity. Dependent on the medication, the incident can be independent of dose or dose-related. Amiodarone, isoniazid, and ketoconazole are associated with nonallergic drug-related hepatotoxicity.[3]

DISRUPTION OF CALCIUM HOMEOSTASIS AND CELL MEMBRANE INJURY

Drug-induced damage to the cellular proteins that are involved with calcium homeostasis can lead to an influx of intracellular calcium that causes a decline in adenosine triphosphate levels and disruption of the actin fibril assembly. The resulting impact on the cell is blebbing of the cell membrane, rupture, and cell lysis.[32] Lovastatin, venlafaxine, and phalloidin, which is the active component of mushrooms, impair calcium homeostasis.[32,39]

METABOLIC ACTIVATION OF THE CYTOCHROME P450 ENZYMES

Most hepatocellular injuries involve the production of high-energy reactive metabolites by the CYP450 system. ❷ These reactive metabolites are capable of forming covalent bonds with cellular proteins (enzymes) and nucleic acids that lead to adduct formation. In the case of acute toxicity, the enzyme-drug adduct can cause cell injury or cell lysis. Adducts that form with DNA can cause long-term consequences such as neoplasia. Acetaminophen, furosemide, and diclofenac are examples of this mechanism of liver injury.[41] Individual genetic differences can play a role in the significance of this process. Patients with a single nucleotide polymorphism (SNP) that codes for slow-reacting variants of CYP450 will react differently from those with a SNP that codes for very-fast-reacting variants.

STIMULATION OF APOPTOSIS

Apoptosis represents a distinct pattern of cell lysis that is characterized by cell shrinkage and fragmentation of nuclear chromatin. Apoptotic pathways are triggered by interactions between death ligands (tumor necrosis factor and Fas ligand) and death receptors (tumor necrosis factor receptor-1 and Fas). These interactions activate caspases which cleave cellular proteins and eventually lead to cell death.[42] Cumulative doses of acetaminophen cause apoptosis.[39]

MITOCHONDRIAL INJURY

Drugs that impair mitochondrial structure, function, or DNA synthesis can disrupt β-oxidation of lipids and oxidative energy production within the hepatocyte.[31] In acute disease, prolonged interruption of β-oxidation leads to microvesicular steatosis, whereas, in chronic disease, macrovesicular disease is present.[6] Severe damage to the mitochondria eventually leads to hepatic failure and death. Aspirin, valproic acid, and tetracycline cause mitochondrial injury by inhibiting β-oxidation and amiodarone via disruption of oxidative phosphorylation.[32]

LIVER NEOPLASTIC DISEASE

A large body of the current literature on adverse reactions and the liver addresses the development of neoplasms following drug therapy. Both carcinoma- and sarcoma-like lesions have been identified. Fortunately, hepatic tumors associated with drug therapy are usually benign and remit when drug therapy is discontinued. Except in rare instances, these lesions are associated with long-term exposure to the offending agent.[43] Androgens, estrogens, and other hormonal-related agents are the most frequently associated causes of neoplastic disease. The model for drug-induced hepatic cancer is polyvinyl chloride exposure. Used in the production of many types of plastic products, polyvinyl chloride induces angiosarcoma in exposed workers after as few as 3 years of exposure.[44]

ASSESSMENT

The best and most important technique for assessing and monitoring drug-induced liver disease is the patient's history. ❸ Questions addressing the patient's drug use along with a thorough review of systems are essential. The use of a protocol, such as that proposed by Danan and Benichou, can significantly improve the accuracy of the assessment (Table 40–1).[45] The use of drugs for recreational purposes must not be overlooked. Cocaine has been directly linked to liver disease.[46] Ecstasy, the street name of methylenedioxymethamphetamine, has induced fulminant hepatitis, which has led to death in some cases.[47] The more pervasive impact of street drugs on the incidence of hepatic disease is the concomitant injection or ingestion of adulterants. Many of these adulterants are either directly toxic or serve to enhance the toxicity of the drug.

It is also important to determine nondrug hepatic disease risk. Arsenic, for example, is known to induce both acute and chronic hepatic reactions. Arsenic in low concentrations is found in insect-resistant lumber.[47] Following Occupational Safety and Health Administration guidelines should decrease the danger of using these products, but will not eliminate it. Even if exposure to an environmental toxin in and of itself does not produce a hepatic reaction, it may predispose a patient to a hepatic reaction when a drug is added. Table 40–2 lists some of the more common hepatic toxins found in occupational or environmental exposures that can add to a patient's risk for developing a hepatic lesion.[48]

A person's use of alternative medicine must be solicited. Many herbal remedies were once wisely abandoned because of their common adverse reactions. Comfrey tea is a common cause of hepatocellular damage. As in the case of the Chinese remedy *jin bu huan*, or as in the case of the more elegantly presented chaparral capsules containing grease wood leaves, the end of therapy with these types of agents is occasionally severe disability or death from fulminant hepatic failure.[49] Pennyroyal oil, margosa oil, and clove oil cause a dose-related hepatotoxicity.[49]

The nutritional status of a patient can be as important to the development of a drug-induced liver disease as the hepatotoxin itself.[47] Patients who are malnourished because of illness or long-term alcohol abuse make up the most troublesome group.[50] Low serum levels of vitamins E and C, along with lutein and the α- and β-carotenes are associated with asymptomatic elevations in transaminases. Conversely, high serum iron, transferrin, and selenium levels are also associated with asymptomatic elevations of transaminases.[51]

All potential drug reactions should be judged as to the timing of the reaction versus drug administration, pharmacokinetic considerations, the information in the literature records about previous reactions, the inclusion of alternative nondrug causes, and close clinical observation when the drug in question is stopped. It is also important to keep in mind that most elevations in liver enzymes will not be associated with a drug. In a study of all patients admitted to a hospital in the United Kingdom with elevated liver aminotransferases, only 9% of cases involved a drug other than alcohol as the possible cause.[3] In all cases, titers of serum antibodies to hepatitis A, B, and C should be drawn. Even in cases in which the drug is absolutely targeted as the cause, viral hepatitis may be a complication.

TABLE 40-1 An Approach to Evaluating a Suspected Hepatotoxic Reaction Using a Clinical Diagnostic Scale

Patient Presents with Elevated Liver Enzymes	Score	Component Subscore
Literature		
Literature supports this drug (drug combination) and pattern of liver enzyme elevation	+2	
No literature supports this, but the drug has been on the market less than 5 years	+0	—
No literature supports this and the drug has been on the market for 5 years or more	−3	
Alternative causes		
Alternative causes (e.g., viral, alcohol) are completely ruled out	+3	
Alternative causes are partially ruled out	+0	—
Alternative causes cannot be ruled out and are possible or even probable	−1	
Presentation		
The presentation includes 4 or more extrahepatic (fever, malaise, etc.) symptoms	+3	
The presentation includes 2–3 extrahepatic symptoms	+2	—
The presentation includes only 1 identifiable extrahepatic symptom	+1	
The presentation is essentially a laboratory abnormality, with no extrahepatic symptoms	+0	
Temporality		
Initiation of drug therapy to onset is 4–56 days	+3	
Initiation of drug therapy to onset is <4 or >56 days	+1	
Discontinuance of therapy to onset is 0–7 days	+3	—
Discontinuance of therapy to onset is 8–15 days	+0	
Discontinuance of therapy to onset is >15 days	−1	
Rechallenge		
Rechallenge was positive	+3	—
Rechallenge was negative or not attempted	+0	
Total Score		—

The likelihood that this presentation is an adverse reaction in the liver increases linearly with an increasing score. The maximum score is 14, and scores below 7 are associated with an ever-decreasing likelihood that the drug or drug combination in question caused the problem. This approach is not designed for the assessment of hepatic cancers or cirrhotic conditions.

Reprinted from J Clin Epidemiol, Vol 46, Danan G, Benichou C. Causality assessment of adverse reactions to drugs–I. A novel method based on the conclusions of international consensus meetings: Application to drug-induced liver injuries: pages 1323–1330, Copyright 1993, with permission from Elsevier.

TABLE 40-2 Environmental Hepatotoxins and Associated Occupations at Risk for Exposure

Hepatotoxin	Associated Occupations at Risk for Exposure
Arsenic	Chemical plant, construction, agricultural workers
Carbon tetrachloride	Chemical plant workers, laboratory technicians
Copper	Plumbers, outdoor sculpture artists, copper foundry workers
Dimethylformamide	Chemical plant workers, laboratory technicians
2,4-Dichlorophenoxyacetic acid	Horticulturists
Fluorine	Chemical plant workers, laboratory technicians
Toluene	Chemical plant, agricultural workers, laboratory technicians
Trichloroethylene	Printers, dye workers, cleaners, laboratory technicians
Vinyl chloride	Plastics plant workers; also found as a river pollutant

TABLE 40-3 Relative Patterns of Hepatic Enzyme Elevation versus Type of Hepatic Lesion

Enzyme	Abbreviations	Necrotic	Cholestatic	Chronic
Alkaline phosphatase	Alk Phos, AP	↑	↑↑↑	↑
5'-Nucleotidase	5-NC, 5NC	↑	↑↑↑	↑
γ-Glutamyltransferase	GGT, GGTP	↑	↑↑↑	↑↑
Aspartate aminotransferase	AST, SGOT	↑↑↑	↑	↑↑
Alanine aminotransferase	ALT, SGPT	↑↑↑	↑	↑↑
Lactate dehydrogenase	LDH	↑↑↑	↑	↑

↑, <100% of normal; ↑↑, >100% of normal; ↑↑↑, >200% of normal.

Often there is no good clinical test available to determine the exact type of hepatic lesion, short of liver biopsy. ❹ There are certain patterns of enzyme elevation that have been identified and can be helpful (Table 40–3).[52,53] The specificity of any serum enzyme depends on the distribution of that enzyme in the body. Alkaline phosphatase is found in the bile duct epithelium, bone, and intestinal and kidney cells. 5'-Nucleotidase is more specific for hepatic disease than alkaline phosphatase, because most of the body's store of 5'-nucleotidase is in the liver. Glutamate dehydrogenase is a good indicator of centrolobular necrosis because it is found primarily in centrolobular mitochondria. Most hepatic cells have extremely high concentrations of transaminases. Aspartate aminotransferase (AST) and alanine aminotransferase (ALT) are commonly measured in serum. Because of their high concentrations and easy liberation from the hepatocyte cytoplasm, AST and ALT are sensitive indicators of necrotic lesions within the liver. After an acute hepatic lesion is established, it may take weeks for these concentrations to return to normal.[53]

Serum bilirubin concentration is a sensitive indicator of most hepatic lesions and has significant prognostic value. High peak bilirubin concentrations are associated with poor survival. Other important findings that indicate poor survival are a peak prothrombin time greater than 40 seconds, elevated serum creatinine, and low arterial pH. The presence of encephalopathy or prolonged jaundice are not good signs for the survival of the patient and are strong indicators for transplantation.[54]

Bilirubin concentrations and serum enzyme elevations give a static picture of the liver's condition and are not good indicators of hepatic function. Clinically available tests to predict hepatic function include measurement of serum proteins (albumin or transferrin). As a hepatic function decreases, serum protein concentrations in the body decrease at a rate determined by each protein's own elimination rate. Overhydration and starvation can also decrease serum protein concentrations. Changes in the prothrombin time often occur earlier than the changes in albumin or transferrin. The response of the prothrombin time to the administration of 10 mg of parenteral vitamin K is often used to differentiate between hepatic and extrahepatic disease.

MEASUREMENT OF LIVER FUNCTION

A good compound for a liver function test would theoretically be (a) nontoxic and lacking any pharmacologic effect; (b) either rapidly and completely absorbed orally or easily administered via a peripheral vein; (c) eliminated only by the liver; and (d) easily measured (drug and its metabolite) in blood, saliva, or urine.[55]

Several tests are used in research settings and in liver transplant patients to indicate liver function. Tests such as sulfobromophthalein, indocyanine green, or sorbitol measure qualities of hepatic clearance. There are also a few drugs that have been used to test liver function. The advantage of sorbitol over indocyanine green is a much lower incidence of allergic reactions. It is partially cleared by the kidney, and urine levels must also be determined during the test.[56] A good estimate of hepatic clearance can be obtained by serial blood levels of a variety of hepatically eliminated drugs if an assay is locally available. Ultrasound and computed tomographic imaging can be used on a periodic basis to monitor for the development of fibrosis or vascular lesions in the liver and for hepatocellular carcinomas.[57]

If a liver biopsy has been performed, the injury should be classified by the histologic findings. In cases in which there is no biopsy, the pattern of liver enzyme elevation can estimate the type of injury. Hepatocellular injuries are marked by elevations in transaminase that are at least two times normal. If the alkaline phosphatase is also elevated, a hepatocellular lesion is still suspected when the elevation of ALT is notably higher than the elevation of alkaline phosphatase. If the magnitude of elevation is nearly equal between ALT and alkaline phosphatase, the lesion is likely cholestatic.

A liver injury is acute if it lasts less than 3 months; it is considered chronic after 3 months of consistent symptoms or enzyme elevation. A liver injury is severe if the patient has marked jaundice, if the prothrombin time does not improve by more than 50% after the

TABLE 40-4 An Approach to Determining a Drug-Monitoring Plan to Detect Hepatotoxicity

The patient is to be started on a drug that may cause a hepatotoxic reaction

↓

Is the patient pregnant?
Is the patient older than age 60 years?
Is the patient exposed to an environmental hepatotoxin at work or at home?
Is the patient drinking more than one alcoholic beverage per day or bingeing on weekends?
Is the patient using any injected recreational drug?
Is the patient using herbal remedies or tisanes that are associated with hepatic damage?
Is the patient's diet deficient in magnesium, vitamin E, vitamin C, or α- or β-carotenes?
Is the patient's diet excessive in vitamin A, iron, or selenium?
Does the patient have hypertriglyceridemia or type 2 diabetes mellitus?
Does the patient have juvenile arthritis or systemic lupus erythematosus?
Is the patient HIV-positive, have AIDS, or on reverse transcriptase inhibitors?
Does the patient have chronic or chronic remitting viral hepatitis (hepatitis B or C)?

↓

Draw a baseline set of blood samples for liver enzymes, bilirubin, albumin, and transferrin before beginning the drug

↓

Does the patient have more than two risk factors?
Is the drug identified as one that may cause a predictable hepatotoxic reaction?[a]

↓Yes	↓No
Redraw liver enzymes every 60–90 days depending on the drug, for the first year	Redraw liver enzymes if other signs or symptoms manifest

If no toxicity is manifested during the first year of therapy, then redraw liver enzymes every 6–12 months; assess liver for cirrhosis every 1–2 years by ultrasound and every 4–6 years by CT or MRI scan; biopsy as directed by other findings

AIDS, acquired immunodeficiency syndrome; CT, computer tomography; HIV, human immunodeficiency virus; MRI, magnetic resonance imaging.

[a]A drug can become a predictable risk if it is administered concurrently with another drug or food that is known to induce or inhibit its metabolism.

administration of vitamin K, or if encephalopathy is detectable. If an acute liver injury progresses from normal to severe in a matter of a few days or weeks, it is considered fulminant.[58,59]

MONITORING

The serum transaminases AST and ALT are the most commonly used transaminases in the clinical setting. There are often no set rules available for a particular drug. ❺ The general guidelines found in Table 40–4 can help in determining a monitoring schedule for drugs where no prior recommendations are published. Concentrations of these enzymes should be obtained approximately every 4 weeks, depending on the reported characteristics of the reaction in question. Methotrexate should be monitored every 4 weeks, because toxicity usually develops over a period of several weeks to months.[57] In addition, some recommend that sulfobromophthalein or indocyanine-green excretion studies be performed on a regular basis and that patients treated for very long periods of time should have a liver biopsy performed every 12 months.[60]

ABBREVIATIONS

ALT: alanine aminotransferase

AST: aspartate aminotransferase

CYP450: cytochrome P450 liver enzyme system

NAPQI: *N*-acetyl-*p*-benzoquinone imine

NAT2: *N*-acetyltransferase 2 genotype

SNP: single nucleotide polymorphism

REFERENCES

1. Biour M, Jaillon PJ. [Drug-induced hepatic diseases]. Pathol Biol (Paris) 1999;47:928–937.
2. Lee W. Drug-induced hepatotoxicity. N Engl J Med 2003;349:474–485.
3. Kaplowitz N. Idiosyncratic drug hepatotoxicity. Nat Rev Drug Discov 2005;4:489–499.
4. Lewis J. Drug-induced liver disease. Med Clin North Am 2000;84:1275–1311.
5. Navarro V, Senior J. Drug-related hepatotoxicity. N Engl J Med 2006;354:731–739.
6. Watkins P, Seeff L. Drug-induced liver injury: Summary of a single topic clinical research conference. Hepatology 2006;43:618–631.
7. Bjornsson E. Drug-induced liver injury: Hy's rule revisited. Clin Pharmacol Ther 2006;79:521–528.
8. Fernandes NF, Martin RR, Schenker S. Trazodone-induced hepatotoxicity: A case report with comments on drug-induced hepatotoxicity. Am J Gastroenterol 2000;95:532–535.
9. Fontana RJ, McCashland TM, Benner KG, et al. Acute liver failure associated with prolonged use of bromfenac leading to liver transplantation. The Acute Liver Failure Study Group. Liver Transpl Surg 1999;5:480–484.
10. Buckley NA, Whyte IM, O'Connell DL, Dawson AHJ. Oral or intravenous *N*-acetylcysteine: Which is the treatment of choice for acetaminophen (paracetamol) poisoning? J Toxicol Clin Toxicol 1999;37:759–767.
11. Black M. Acetaminophen hepatotoxicity. Gastroenterology 1980;78:382–392.
12. Belay ED, Bresee JS, Holman RC, et al. Reye's syndrome in the United States from 1981 through 1997 [see comments]. N Engl J Med 1999;340:1377–1382.
13. Monto AS. The disappearance of Reye's syndrome—A public health triumph [editorial; comment] [see comments]. N Engl J Med 1999;340:1423–1424.
14. Leo MA, Lieber CSJ. Alcohol, vitamin A, and beta-carotene: Adverse interactions, including hepatotoxicity and carcinogenicity. Am J Clin Nutr 1999;69:1071–1085.
15. Agarwal DP, Goedde HW. Human aldehyde dehydrogenases: Their role in alcoholism. Alcohol 1989;6:517–523.
16. Bohan A, Boyer J. Mechanisms of hepatic transport of drugs: Implications for cholestatic drug reactions. Semin Liver Dis 2002;22:123–136.
17. Lee WM. Acute hepatic failure. N Engl J Med 1993;329:1862–1872.
18. Konig SA, Schenk M, Sick C, et al. Fatal liver failure associated with valproate therapy in a patient with Friedreich's disease: Review of valproate hepatotoxicity in adults. Epilepsia 1999;40:1036–1040.
19. Lullman H, Lullman R, Wasserman O. Drug-induced phospholipidosis, II. Tissue distribution of the amphiphilic drug chlorphentermine. CRC Crit Drug Rev Toxicol 1975;4:185–218.
20. Chang CC, Petrelli M, Tomashefski JF Jr, McCullough AJJ. Severe intrahepatic cholestasis caused by amiodarone toxicity after withdrawal of the drug: A case report and review of the literature. Arch Pathol Lab Med 1999;123:251–256.
21. Beane PH, Bourdi M. Autoantibodies against cytochrome P450 in drug-induced autoimmune hepatitis. Ann NY Acad Sci 1993;685:641–645.
22. Evans WE, Relling MV. Pharmacogenomics: Translating functional genomics into rational therapeutics. Science 1999;286:487–491.
23. Hunt CM, Westerkam WR, Stave GM. Effect of age and gender on the activity of human hepatic CYP3A. Biochem Pharmacol 1992;44:275–283.
24. Liddle C, Goodwin B. Regulation of hepatic drug metabolism: Role of nuclear receptors PXR and CAR. Semin Liver Dis 2002;22:115–122.
25. Tsagaropoou-Stinga H, Mataki-Emmanouilidon R, Karida-Kavalioti S, et al. Hepatotoxic reactions in children with severe tuberculosis treated with isoniazid-rifampin. Pediatr Infect Dis 1985;4:270–273.
26. Ohno M, Yamaguchi I, Yamamoto I, et al. Slow *N*-acetyltransferase 2 genotype affects the incidence of isoniazid and rifampicin-induced hepatotoxicity. Int J Tuberc Lung Dis 2000;4:256–261.
27. Kergueris MF, Bourin M, Larousse C. Pharmacokinetics of isoniazid: Influence of age. Eur J Clin Pharm 1986;30:335–340.
28. Vuilleumier N, Rossier MF, Chiappe A, et al. CYP2E1 genotype and isoniazid-induced hepatotoxicity in patients treated for latent tuberculosis. Eur J Clin Pharmacol 2006;62:423–429.
29. Van Puijenbroek EP, Metselaar HJ, Berghuis PH, et al. [Acute hepatocytic necrosis during ketoconazole therapy for treatment of onychomycosis. National Foundation for Registry and Evaluation of Adverse Effects.] Ned Tijdschr Geneeskd 1998;142:2416–2418.
30. Hashkes PJ, Balistreri WF, Bove KE, et al. The relationship of hepatotoxic risk factors and liver histology in methotrexate therapy for juvenile rheumatoid arthritis. J Pediatr 1999;134:47–52.
31. Leonard PA, Clegg DO, Carson CC, et al. Low dose pulse methotrexate in rheumatoid arthritis: An 8-year experience with hepatotoxicity. Clin Rheumatol 1987;6:575–582.
32. Cullen P. Mechanistic classification of liver injury. Toxicol Pathol 2005;33:6–8.
33. Jaeschke H, Gores G, Cederbaum A, et al. Mechanisms of hepatotoxicity. Toxicol Sci 2002;65:166–176.
34. Levy C, Lindor K. Drug-induced cholestasis. Clin Liver Dis 2003;7:311–330.
35. Foitl DR, Hyman G, Leftowitch JH. Jaundice and intrahepatic cholestasis following high-dose megestrol acetate for breast cancer. Cancer 1989;63:438–439.
36. Lorch V, Murphy D, Hoersten L, et al. Unusual syndrome among premature infants: Associated with a new intravenous vitamin E product. Pediatrics 1985;75:598–601.
37. Olsson R, Wiholm BE, Sand C, et al. Liver damage from flucloxacillin, cloxacillin and dicloxacillin. J Hepatol 1992;15:154–161.
38. Soe KL, Soe M, Gluud CN. [Liver pathology associated with anabolic androgenic steroids]. Ugeskr Laeger 1994;156:2585–2588.
39. Lee W. Drug-induced hepatotoxicity. N Engl J Med 2003;349:474–485.
40. Lee WM. Drug-induced hepatotoxicity. N Engl J Med 1995;333:1118–1127.
41. Park B, Kitteringham N, Maggs J, et al. The role of metabolic action in drug-induced hepatotoxicity. Annu Rev Pharmacol Toxicol 2005;45:177–202.
42. Malhi H, Gores G, Lemasters J. Apoptosis and necrosis in the liver: A tale of two deaths? Hepatology 2006;43:S31–S44.
43. Lee FI, Smith PM, Bennett B, Williams DMJ. Occupationally related angiosarcoma of the liver in the United Kingdom 1972–1994. Gut 1996;39:312–318.
44. Anonymous. Epidemiologic notes and reports: Angiosarcoma of the liver among polyvinyl chloride workers—Kentucky. MMWR Morb Mortal Wkly Rep 1997;46:99–101.

45. Danan G, Benichou C. Causality assessment of adverse reactions to drugs—I. A novel method based on the conclusions of international consensus meetings: Application to drug-induced liver injuries. J Clin Epidemiol 1993;46:1323–1330.
46. Van Thiel DH, Perper JA. Hepatotoxicity associated with cocaine abuse. Recent Dev Alcohol 1992;10:335–341.
47. Jones AL, Simpson KJJ. Review article: Mechanisms and management of hepatotoxicity in ecstasy (MDMA) and amphetamine intoxications. Aliment Pharmacol Ther 1999;13:129–133.
48. Wang JS, Groopman JD. Toxic liver disorders. In: Rom WN, ed. Environmental and Occupational Medicine, 3rd ed. Philadelphia: Lippincott-Raven, 1998:831–840.
49. Steadman C. Herbal hepatotoxicity. Semin Liver Dis 2002;22:195–206.
50. Seef LB, Cuccherin BA, Zimmerman HJ, et al. Acetaminophen hepatotoxicity in alcoholics: A therapeutic misadventure. Ann Intern Med 1986;104:399–404.
51. Ruhl CE, Everhart JE. Relation of elevated serum alanine aminotransferase activity with iron and antioxidant levels in the United States. Gastroenterology 2003;124:1821–1829.
52. Whitehead MW, Haukes ND, Hainesworth I, Kingham JGC. A prospective study of causes of notably raised aspartate aminotransferase of liver origin. Gut 1999;45:129–133.
53. Choppa S, Griffin PH. Laboratory tests and diagnostic procedures in evaluation of liver disease. Am J Med 1985;79:221–230.
54. O'Grady JG, Alexander GJM, Hayllar KM, Williams R. Early indicators of prognosis in fulminant hepatic failure. Gastroenterology 1989;97:439–445.
55. Barstow L, Smith RE. Liver function assessment by drug metabolism. Pharmacotherapy 1990;10:280–288.
56. Zech J, Lange H, Bosch J, et al. Steady-state extrarenal sorbitol clearance as a measure of hepatic plasma flow. Gastroenterology 1988;95:749–759.
57. Mathieu D, Kobeiter H, Maison P, et al. Oral contraceptive use and focal nodular hyperplasia of the liver. Gastroenterology 2000;118:560–564.
58. Anonymous. Standardization of definitions and criteria of causality assessment of adverse drug reactions, drug-induced liver disorders: Report of an international consensus meeting. Int J Clin Pharmacol Ther Toxicol 1990;28:317–322.
59. Newman M, Auerbach R, Feiner H, et al. The role of liver biopsies in psoriatic patients receiving long-term methotrexate treatment: Improvement in liver abnormalities after cessation of treatment. Arch Dermatol 1989;125:1218–1224.
60. O'Connor GT, Olmstead EM, Sug K, et al. Detection of hepatotoxicity associated with methotrexate therapy for psoriasis. Arch Dermatol 1989;125:1209–1217.

CHAPTER 41

Pancreatitis

ROSEMARY R. BERARDI AND PATRICIA A. MONTGOMERY

KEY CONCEPTS

ACUTE PANCREATITIS

1. Patients with severe acute pancreatitis require early and aggressive intravenous fluid resuscitation.
2. Treatment requires that if at all possible, medications that potentially cause pancreatitis be discontinued.
3. Use parenteral narcotic analgesics to control abdominal pain. Meperidine is not recommended as a first-line agent because of dosing limitations and the risk for seizures in patients with renal failure.
4. Octreotide may be used in severe acute pancreatitis, but its efficacy in decreasing complications and mortality remains uncertain.
5. Antibiotics should not be used in the absence of signs of infection except in patients with severe acute pancreatitis when pancreatic necrosis is present.

CHRONIC PANCREATITIS

6. Abstinence from alcohol is an important factor in preventing abdominal pain in the early stages of alcohol-induced chronic pancreatitis.
7. Initiate pain control with nonnarcotic analgesics such as acetaminophen or a nonsteroidal antiinflammatory agent. The dose and frequency of administration should be increased before the patient is switched to a narcotic. Parenteral narcotics should be reserved for patients with severe pain that is unresponsive to oral agents. Patients with frequent or constant pain should receive the lowest effective analgesic dose scheduled around the clock.
8. A trial of non–enteric-coated pancreatic enzymes with either an H_2-receptor antagonist or a proton pump inhibitor should be considered for pain control in patients with mild to moderate disease.
9. Pancreatic enzyme supplementation and a reduction of dietary fat are used to treat malabsorption and steatorrhea. An initial lipase dose of about 30,000 international units should be given with each meal.
10. Symptomatic patients whose steatorrhea is not corrected by pancreatic enzyme supplementation and a reduction in dietary fat may benefit from the addition of an H_2-receptor antagonist or a proton pump inhibitor.

Learning objectives, review questions, and other resources can be found at **www.pharmacotherapyonline.com.**

Pancreatitis is inflammation of the pancreas with variable involvement of regional tissues or remote organ systems.[1] Acute pancreatitis (AP) is characterized by severe pain in the upper abdomen and elevations of pancreatic enzymes in the blood.[2] In the majority of patients, AP is a mild, self-limiting disease that resolves spontaneously without complications. Approximately 20% of adults have a severe course, and 10% to 30% of those with severe AP die.[3,4] Although exocrine and endocrine pancreatic function may remain impaired for variable periods after an attack, AP seldom progresses to chronic pancreatitis.[2]

Chronic pancreatitis (CP) is characterized by permanent damage to pancreatic structure and function because of progressive inflammation and long-standing pancreatic injury.[1,5–7] In the early stages of the disease, recurrent, acute, symptomatic exacerbations resemble attacks of AP and may not be distinguishable from AP. Most patients have periods of intractable upper abdominal pain, which is the dominant feature. Progressive pancreatic exocrine and endocrine insufficiency leads to maldigestion and diabetes mellitus. CP patients are at an increased risk of developing pancreatic cancer.[5,7] Patients with AP and CP suffer from many of the same complications.

EPIDEMIOLOGY

The prevalence of pancreatitis varies widely with geographic, etiologic (e.g., alcohol consumption), environmental, and genetic factors. The reported prevalence of AP among men and women in the United States is less than 1%, whereas the prevalence of CP is 0.05% in males and 0.01% in females, but the true spectrum of these diseases is probably underestimated.[7] Hospitalizations for AP have increased in the United States, most likely related to an increase in gallstones in association with obesity.[8] The incidence of gallstone-related AP is increased among white women older than age 60 years.[3] Alcoholic CP is more common in men and has a peak incidence between 35 and 45 years of age.[7] Blacks are more likely than whites to be hospitalized for CP than for alcoholic cirrhosis, but an underlying genetic factor remains elusive.[7]

PHYSIOLOGY OF EXOCRINE PANCREATIC SECRETION

The pancreas possesses both endocrine and exocrine functions. The islets of Langerhans, which contain the cells of the endocrine pancreas, secrete insulin, glucagon, somatostatin, and other polypeptide hormones. The exocrine pancreas is composed of acini that secrete about 1 to 2 L/day of isotonic fluid that contains water, electrolytes,

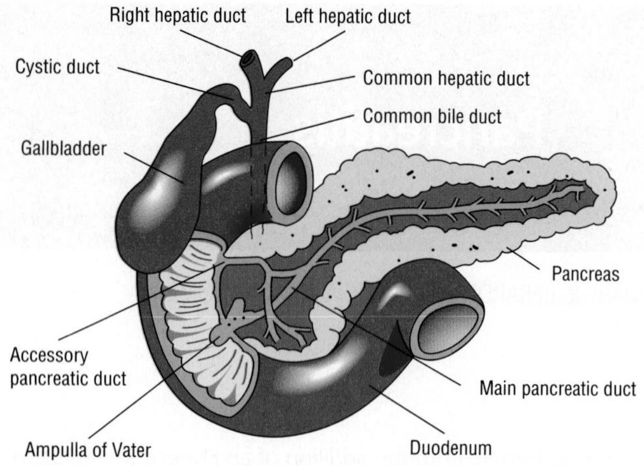

FIGURE 41-1. Anatomic structure of the pancreas and biliary tract.

and pancreatic enzymes necessary for digestion. Bicarbonate is secreted primarily by the centroacinar (ductular) cells and is the principal ion of physiologic importance. Pancreatic juice is delivered to the duodenum via the pancreatic ducts (Fig. 41–1) where the alkaline secretion (pH approximately 8.3) neutralizes gastric acid and provides an appropriate pH for maintaining the activity of pancreatic enzymes.[9]

The major pancreatic exocrine enzyme groups are:

- *Proteolytic:* trypsinogen, chymotrypsinogen, procarboxypeptidase, and proelastase
- *Amylolytic:* amylase
- *Lipolytic:* lipase, procolipase, prophospholipase A_2, and carboxylesterase lipase
- *Nucleolytic:* ribonuclease, deoxyribonuclease
- *Other:* trypsin inhibitor

The proteolytic enzymes are synthesized within the acinar cells and secreted as zymogens (inactive enzymes), which are activated in the lumen of the duodenum. Enterokinase secreted by the duodenal mucosa converts trypsinogen to trypsin, which then activates all other proteolytic zymogens. Two important mechanisms protect the pancreas from the potential degradative action of its own digestive enzymes. The synthesis of proteolytic enzymes as zymogens requires extrapancreatic trigger enzymes for activation. In addition, pancreatic juice contains a low concentration of trypsin inhibitor, which inactivates trypsin and partially inhibits chymotrypsin. Proteolytic activity in the intestinal lumen is not inhibited because the concentration is minimal. Lipase, amylase, ribonuclease, and deoxyribonuclease are secreted by the acinar cells in their active form. Colipase facilitates the action of lipase by binding to the bile salt-lipid surface and lowering the optimum pH of lipase from 8.5 to 6.5, the normal luminal pH in the duodenum.[9]

The regulation of exocrine pancreatic secretion is complex and depends on stimulatory and inhibitory factors exerted through hormonal and neuronal mechanisms. Two hormones, secretin (SC) and cholecystokinin (CCK), play an important role in mediating postprandial pancreatic secretion and have synergistic effects: SC stimulates ductular cells to increase water and bicarbonate; CCK stimulates acinar cells to secrete a juice that is low in volume and bicarbonate, but rich in enzyme content. The release of SC from the intestinal mucosa is pH dependent and occurs when the duodenal pH is approximately 4.5. Below this pH, titratable acid in the duodenum governs pancreatic bicarbonate output. Although the postprandial release of SC is small, nonacid factors such as products of fat digestion and bile can also stimulate SC release. The release of CCK from the small intestine depends on the presence of fatty acids and amino acids in the duodenum. Vasoactive intestinal polypeptide is structurally similar to SC and exhibits weak secretin-like effects on exocrine pancreatic secretion. Gastrointestinal peptides such as somatostatin inhibit enzyme secretion by modulating cholinergic transmission. Intestinal serotonin (5-hydroxytryptamine) is released in response to a number of stimuli, including duodenal acidification, and may play a role in postprandial pancreatic secretion.[9]

There are three phases of pancreatic exocrine secretion: cephalic, gastric, and intestinal. In the fasted state, basal secretion occurs at a low rate; output fluctuates in cycles with the interdigestive migrating motor complex (IMMC), so that peak secretions occur during phase III of the IMMC.[9] The cephalic phase is stimulated by the sight and smell of food and is mediated by vagal pathways. Gastric distension and the rate of gastric emptying stimulate an increase in enzyme-rich pancreatic fluid. In the intestinal phase, chyme and acid stimulate pancreatic secretion through the release of SC and CCK. A more in-depth discussion of pancreatic physiology is found elsewhere.[9]

ACUTE PANCREATITIS

AP varies from mild to severe disease, in which the severity of the attack correlates with the degree of pancreatic involvement and complications. The morphologic appearance of the pancreas and surrounding tissue ranges from interstitial edema and inflammatory cells (interstitial pancreatitis) to pancreatic and extrapancreatic necrosis (necrotizing pancreatitis), which has a higher risk of infection, organ failure, and mortality.[2] The rupture of blood vessels within or around the pancreas may lead to a collection of blood in the retroperitoneal spaces.

ETIOLOGY

Table 41–1 lists the etiologic risk factors associated with AP. Gallstones and alcohol abuse together account for 70% to 80% of all cases of AP.[8] Approximately 20% of adult cases are idiopathic (a cause cannot be determined).[3,10] AP occurs in 5% to 15% of all patients who have undergone endoscopic retrograde cholangiopancreatography (ERCP), and in 30% to 40% of high-risk patients.[8,11] End-stage renal disease increases the risk of AP, with patients who are receiving chronic peritoneal dialysis being at higher risk than those receiving hemodialysis.[12] Cigarette smoking appears to increase the risk of pancreatitis, especially in alcohol-related disease.[13] Pregnancy is not

TABLE 41-1 Etiologic Risk Factors Associated with Acute Pancreatitis

Structural	Gallstone disease, sphincter of Oddi dysfunction, pancreas divisum, pancreatic tumors
Toxins	Alcohol (ethanol) consumption, scorpion bite, organophosphate insecticides
Infectious	Bacterial, viral (including AIDS), parasitic
Metabolic	Genetic hypertriglyceridemia, chronic hypercalcemia
Genetic	Cystic fibrosis, α_1-antitrypsin deficiency, hereditary (trypsinogen gene mutations)
Medications	See Table 41–2 for specific drugs
Iatrogenic	Abdominal surgery, ERCP
Renal disease	Chronic renal failure, dialysis related
Trauma	Blunt trauma to the abdomen
Vascular	Vasculitis, atherosclerosis, cholesterol emboli, coronary bypass surgery
Other etiologies	Congenital, Crohn's disease, autoimmune, tropical, solid-organ transplantation (liver, kidney, heart), refeeding
Idiopathic	Undetermined cause

AIDS, acquired immune deficiency syndrome; ERCP, endoscopic retrograde cholangiopancreatography.
From references 1, 2, 8, 10, 12.

TABLE 41-2 Medications Associated with Acute Pancreatitis

Class I Definite Association	Class II Probable Association	Class III Possible Association	
5-Aminosalicylic acid	Acetaminophen	Aldesleukin	Indomethacin
Asparaginase	Carbamazepine	Amiodarone	Infliximab
Azathioprine	Cisplatin	Asparaginase	Ketoprofen
Corticosteroids	Enalapril	Calcium	Ketorolac
Cytarabine	Erythromycin	Celecoxib	Lipid emulsion
Didanosine	Hydrochlorothiazide	Clozapine	Lisinopril
Estrogens	Interferon α_{2b}	Cholestyramine	Mefenamic acid
Furosemide	Lamivudine	Cimetidine	Metformin
Mercaptopurine	Octreotide	Ciprofloxacin	Methyldopa
Opiates		Clarithromycin	Metolazone
Pentamidine		Clonidine	Metronidazole
Pentavalent antimonials		Cyclosporine	Nitrofurantoin
Sulfasalazine		Danazol	Omeprazole
Sulfamethoxazole and trimethoprim		Diazoxide	Ondansetron
Sulindac		Etanercept	Oxyphenbutazone
Tetracycline		Ethacrynic acid	Paclitaxel
Valproic acid/salts		Famciclovir	Pravastatin
		Glyburide	Propofol
		Gold therapy	Propoxyphene
		Granisetron	Rifampin
		Ibuprofen	Sertraline
		Indinavir	Zalcitabine

From references 14–24.

considered a cause of AP as pregnant women develop pancreatitis as a result of a coincident process, most commonly cholelithiasis.

Medications

The incidence of drug-induced AP ranges from 2% in the general population to as high as 40% in human immunodeficiency virus (HIV)-positive patients.[14] It is not clear how drugs cause AP, but once the process is initiated, disease severity is determined by the propagation of proinflammatory mediators. Numerous drugs are believed to cause AP, but ethical and practical considerations prevent rechallenge with the suspected agent.[14,15] In the past, drugs were divided based on a definite, probable, or possible association with AP.[15] Recently, a new, updated classification was devised that improves the strength of evidence implicating a drug as a cause of AP (Table 41–2).[14] Class I (definite association) implies a temporal relationship of drug administration to abdominal pain and hyperamylasemia in at least 20 reported cases with at least 1 positive response to rechallenge with the offending agent. Class II medications are implicated in more than 10 (but less than 20) reported cases of AP and suggest a probable association. Class III medications include all drugs implicated in AP (including classes I and II), as well as numerous others with a possible association (10 or fewer reported cases or unpublished reports in pharmaceutical or U.S. Food and Drug Administration files). Table 41–2 lists medications according to this updated classification but only includes selected class III medications. A comprehensive list of class III drugs (including references) is found elsewhere.[14]

Most information on drug-induced AP is obtained from case reports.[16–24] Proton pump inhibitors and histamine$_2$-receptor antagonists may be initiated in response to early symptoms of unrecognized pancreatitis and may confound the association between the drug and the disease. A retrospective cohort study, however, does not support an association between AP and proton pump inhibitors or histamine$_2$-receptor antagonists.[16] Medications such as propofol and tamoxifen are associated with hyperlipidemia and pancreatitis.[17,18] Metformin is associated with AP in toxic levels.[19] The clinician should be especially suspicious of drug-induced AP in high-risk patients, such as those receiving multiple medications or immunomodulating drugs, and in geriatric, HIV-positive, and cancer patients.[14] AP is an infrequent complication of drug therapy, but it is prudent to withdraw medication when an association is suspected. Allergic reactions (e.g., urticaria) usually do not accompany drug-induced AP.

PATHOPHYSIOLOGY

The pathophysiology of AP is based on events that initiate the injury and secondary events that establish and perpetuate the injury (Fig. 41–2). The premature activation of trypsinogen to trypsin leads to activation of other digestive enzymes and autodigestion of the gland.[1,2] Genetic abnormalities in pathways that protect the pancreas from autodigestion also play a pathophysiologic role.[1] The release of activated pancreatic enzymes into the pancreas and surrounding tissues produces tissue damage and necrosis to the pancreas, the surrounding fat, and adjacent structures. Lipase damages the fat cells, producing noxious substances that cause further pancreatic and peripancreatic injury. The release of cytokines by the acinar cell directly injures the acinar cell and enhances the inflammatory response.[25–27] Injured acinar cells liberate chemoattractants that attract neutrophils, macrophages, and other cells to the area of inflammation. Vascular damage and ischemia causes the release of kinins, which makes capillary walls

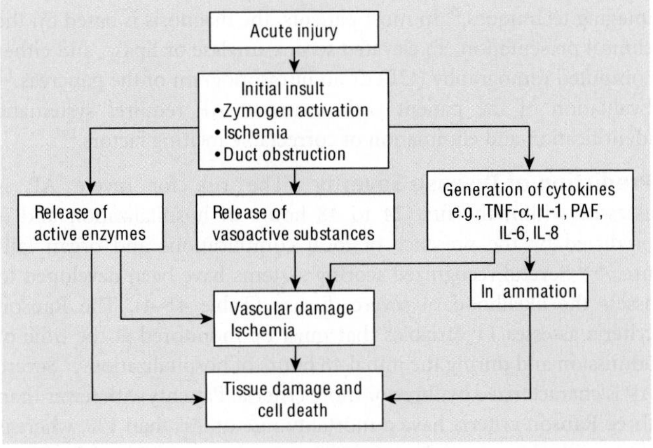

FIGURE 41-2. Pathophysiology of acute pancreatitis: initiating and secondary events. (IL-1β, interleukin-1β; IL-6, interleukin-6; IL-8, interleukin-8; PAF, platelet-activating factor; TNF-α, tumor necrosis factor-α.)

permeable and promotes tissue edema. The release of damaging oxygen-free radicals appears to correlate with the severity of pancreatic injury.[2] Pancreatic infection may result from increased intestinal permeability and translocation of colonic bacteria. The release of activated pancreatic enzymes into the systemic circulation may progress to distant organ damage, multiorgan failure, and death.[2–4]

COMPLICATIONS

Local complications—including acute fluid collection, pancreatic necrosis, infection, abscess (collection of pus in or adjacent to the pancreas), and pseudocyst (collection of pancreatic juice and tissue debris enclosed by a wall of fibrous or granulation tissue)—develop approximately 3 to 4 weeks after the initial attack. Pancreatic infections occur in 15% to 30% of those with pancreatic necrosis and are usually secondary infections of necrotic tissue.[8] Most deaths result from infected necrosis, pancreatic abscess, and sepsis.[2] Pancreatic ascites occurs when pancreatic secretions spread throughout the peritoneal cavity. Systemic complications include cardiovascular, renal, pulmonary, metabolic, hemorrhagic, and central nervous system abnormalities.[2] Of the early complications, shock is the main cause of death. Hypotension results from hypovolemia, hypoalbuminemia, the release of kinins, and sepsis. Renal complications are usually caused by hypovolemia. Pulmonary complications develop when fluid accumulates within the pleural space and compresses the lung and the acute respiratory distress syndrome (ARDS) restricts gas exchange. The most common cause of hypoxemia in patients with AP is ARDS. Pleural effusions occur in 4% to 17% of patients, and occur more frequently on the left.[2] Gastrointestinal bleeding occurs secondary to numerous causes including rupture of a pseudocyst. Severe AP is associated with confusion and coma.

CLINICAL PRESENTATION

Signs and Symptoms

The clinical presentation of AP varies depending on the severity of the inflammatory process and whether damage is confined to the pancreas or involves local and systemic complications (Table 41–3).[2,3,8]

Diagnosis

The definitive diagnosis of AP is surgical examination of the pancreas or pancreatic histology. In the absence of these procedures, the diagnosis depends on the recognition of an etiologic factor, the clinical signs and symptoms, abnormal laboratory tests, and imaging techniques that predict the severity of the disease (see Table 41–3). ERCP is usually reserved for abnormalities found by less-invasive imaging techniques.[28] In most patients, the diagnosis is based on the clinical presentation, an elevated serum amylase or lipase, and either computed tomography (CT) or an ultrasonogram of the pancreas.[1,2] Evaluation of the patient with recurrent AP requires systematic identification and elimination of correctable inciting factors.[29]

Prediction of Disease Severity The risk for severe AP is assessed within the first 24 to 48 hours of hospitalization and is predicted by the presence of local complications and organ failure.[2,4,30] Several recognized scoring systems have been developed to assess the likelihood of severe disease (Table 41–4). The Ranson criteria assesses 11 variables that must be monitored at the time of admission and during the initial 48 hours of hospitalization.[2,3] Severe AP is characterized by three or more criteria. Patients with fewer than three Ranson criteria have a mortality rate of less than 1%, whereas those with six or more have a 100% mortality rate.[2] Some modifications of the Ranson criteria have dropped the base deficit and fluid requirements, whereas others have added obesity as an independent risk factor.[2] The Acute Physiology and Chronic Health Evaluation (APACHE II) system uses 12 indicators of physiologic and biochemical function, age, and previous health status with a score of ≥8 points considered as the threshold for severe AP.[2,3,8] The APACHE II score is calculated within the first 24 hours and is considered among the best predictors of severity on admission. The Atlanta scoring system

TABLE 41-3 Presentation of Acute Pancreatitis

General
• The patient may have acute mild symptoms or present with a severe acute attack with life-threatening complications.
Symptoms
• The patient may present initially with moderate abdominal discomfort to excruciating pain, nausea, shock, and respiratory distress.
• Abdominal pain occurs in 95% of patients. The pain is usually epigastric and radiates to either of the upper quadrants or the back in two-thirds of patients. In gallstone pancreatitis, the pain is typically sudden and quite severe and the intensity is often described as "knife-like" or "boring." The pain usually reaches its maximum intensity within 30 minutes and may persist for hours or days. Repositioning the patient relieves very little of the pain. In alcohol abuse and other cases, the onset of pain may be less abrupt and poorly localized. Pain may not be the dominant symptom if it is masked by multiorgan failure.
• Nausea and vomiting occur in 85% of patients and usually follows the onset of abdominal pain. Vomiting does not provide relief of the abdominal pain.
Signs
• Marked epigastric or diffuse tenderness on palpation with rebound tenderness and guarding in severe cases. The abdomen is often distended and tympanic, with bowel sounds decreased or absent in severe disease.
• Vital signs may be normal, but hypotension, tachycardia, and low-grade fever are observed, especially with widespread pancreatic inflammation and necrosis.
• Dyspnea and tachypnea are often signs of acute respiratory complications. Jaundice and altered mental status may be present and have multiple causes. Other signs of alcoholic liver disease may be present in patients with alcoholic pancreatitis.
Laboratory tests
• Leukocytosis is frequently present; hyperglycemia or hypoalbuminemia may be present. Liver transaminases, alkaline phosphatase, and bilirubin are usually elevated in gallstone pancreatitis and in patients with intrinsic liver disease.
• The hematocrit may be normal, but hemoconcentration results from multiple factors, e.g., vomiting. In patients with third-space fluid loss, hemoconcentration is present and a reasonably accurate marker of severe disease.
• The total serum calcium is usually normal initially, but hypocalcemia disproportionate to the hypoalbuminemia may develop. Marked hypocalcemia is an indication of severe necrosis and a poor prognostic sign.
• The serum amylase concentration usually rises within 4 to 8 hours of the initial attack, peaks at 24 hours, and returns to normal over the next 8 to 14 days. Serum amylase concentrations greater than three times the upper limit of normal are highly suggestive of acute pancreatitis. Persistent elevations suggest extensive pancreatic necrosis and related complications. Normal concentrations may be observed if testing is delayed (amylase may have returned to normal) or in patients with hyperlipidemic pancreatitis (marked triglyceride elevations may interfere with amylase assay).
• Serum lipase is specific to the pancreas and concentrations are elevated and parallel the elevations in serum amylase. Levels remain elevated with pancreatic inflammation and return to normal when the inflammatory process resolves. Because of its longer half-life, elevations of serum lipase can be detected after the serum amylase has returned to normal.
• C-reactive protein is elevated by 48 hours after the onset of symptoms and may be useful in differentiating between mild and severe pancreatitis.
• Thrombocytopenia and an increase in the international normalized ratio are seen in some patients with severe acute pancreatitis.
Abdominal imaging
• Contrast-enhanced computed tomography (CT) is used to identify the cause of pancreatitis and confirm the diagnosis. It is less accurate for evaluating the gallbladder and biliary ducts. The test distinguishes interstitial from necrotizing pancreatitis, but does not distinguish between fat necrosis and acute fluid collection.
• Magnetic resonance imaging is used to grade the severity of acute pancreatitis, identify biliary duct problems that are not seen on CT, or if there are contraindications to contrast-enhanced CT.
• Ultrasonography of the abdomen is useful to determine pancreatic enlargement and peripancreatic fluid collections. It is also sensitive for detecting dilated biliary ducts and stones in the gallbladder.

From Topazian and Gorelick,[2] Whitcomb,[3] Draganov and Forsmark,[8] and Yadav et al.[32]

TABLE 41-4 Prognostic Indicators for Severe Acute Pancreatitis

Prognostic Factor	Criterion
Ranson criteria	
On admission	
Age (y)	>55
White cell count/mm^3	>16,000
Glucose (mg/dL)	>200
Lactic dehydrogenase (international units/L)	>350
Aspartate aminotransferase (units/L)	>250
Within 48 hours	
Decrease in hematocrit (% points)	>10
Increase in blood urea nitrogen (mg/dL)	>5
Calcium (mg/dL)	<8
Partial pressure of oxygen (mm Hg)	<60
Base deficit (mmol/L)	>4
Estimated fluid deficit (L)	>6
Atlanta criteria	
Unfavorable prognostic signs	
Ranson criteria	≥3
APACHE II score	≥8
Organ failure (shock)	
Systolic blood pressure (mm Hg)	<90
Pulmonary insufficiency (PAO_2 mm Hg)	<60
Renal failure after hydration [creatinine (mg/dL)]	>2
Gastrointestinal tract bleeding (mL in 24 h)	>500
Systemic complications	
Disseminated intravascular coagulation	
Platelets (mm^3)	≤100,000
Fibrinogen (g/L)	<1
Fibrin-split products (m/mL)	>80
Metabolic disturbance	
Calcium (mg/dL)	≤7.5
Local complications	
Pseudocyst	Present
Necrosis	Present
Abscess	Present

APACHE, Acute Physiology and Chronic Health Evaluation; PAO_2, partial pressure arterial oxygen.
From Topazian and Gorelick,[2] Whitcomb,[3] and Draganov and Forsmark.[8]

consolidates clinical indicators, organ failure, and local complications and provides an ongoing assessment of disease severity.[3,8,31]

Laboratory Tests Laboratory test results vary depending on the severity of the inflammatory process, whether damage is confined to the pancreas or involves contiguous organs, and the time course from the onset of the acute attack (see Table 41–3).[8,32] C-reactive protein greater than 150 mg/L can be used to identify severe pancreatitis. Serum amylase and lipase are the most widely used for detecting elevations of pancreatic enzymes in AP, but elevations do not necessarily correlate with either the etiology or severity of the disease. In addition, many nonpancreatic diseases may be associated with hyperamylasemia, including salivary, renal, hepatobiliary, metabolic, female reproductive tract, and neoplastic diseases.[2,8,32] Pancreatic isoamylase studies assist in determining the origin of elevated serum amylase concentrations, but are not useful for the diagnosis of AP because the diseases that simulate pancreatitis cause pancreatic rather than nonpancreatic amylase levels to rise. Serum concentrations of proinflammatory cytokines such as tumor necrosis factor-α and interleukin-6 are markers of disease severity, but elevations are not specific for pancreatitis and the tests are not widely available.[25,26,32] Newer markers (e.g., urinary trypsinogen activation peptide) provide both diagnostic and prognostic information, but are not routinely used in practice. Other tests have been used to detect pancreatic enzymes in the serum (e.g., elastase) and urine (e.g., amylase), but most are not useful in the diagnosis of AP.[1,2,32]

Abdominal Imaging A number of radiologic imaging techniques reveal pancreatic abnormalities during the disease course (see Table 41–3). Although no single imaging technique provides a positive diagnosis for AP, CT is usually considered the gold standard.

CLINICAL COURSE AND PROGNOSIS

The clinical course of AP varies from a mild transitory disorder to a severe necrotizing disease. Mild AP is self-limiting and subsides spontaneously within 3 to 5 days. Mortality increases with unfavorable early prognostic signs, local complications, and organ failure. The mortality of pancreatic necrosis is 10%, but increases to 30% to 40% in infected pancreatic necrosis.[2] Mortality is influenced by etiology, as idiopathic or postoperative AP have higher rates than gallstone- or alcoholic-induced disease. Mortality is higher during the first or second attacks than during recurrent acute episodes. Death during the first few days results from systemic complications. When death occurs after this period, it is associated with local complications.

TREATMENT

Acute Pancreatitis

■ DESIRED OUTCOME

Treatment of AP is aimed at relieving abdominal pain and nausea, replacing fluids, minimizing systemic complications, and preventing pancreatic necrosis and infection. Management varies depending on the severity of the attack (Fig. 41–3). Patients with mild AP respond very well to the initiation of supportive care and the reduction of pancreatic secretions. Patients with severe AP follow a more fulminant course and should be treated aggressively and monitored closely.

■ GENERAL APPROACH TO TREATMENT

All patients with AP should receive supportive care, including intravenous fluid resuscitation, adequate nutrition, and effective relief of pain and nausea. The use of nasogastric aspiration offers no clear advantage in patients with mild AP, but is beneficial in patients with profound pain, severe disease, paralytic ileus, and intractable vomiting.[2] Patients predicted to follow a severe course will require treatment of cardiovascular, respiratory, renal, and metabolic complications. ❶ Aggressive fluid resuscitation is essential to correct intravascular volume. The prognosis of the patient often depends on the rapidity and adequacy of volume restoration, as large quantities of fluid are sequestered within the peritoneal and retroperitoneal spaces. Vasodilation from the antiinflammatory response, vomiting, and nasogastric suction contribute to hypovolemia and fluid and electrolyte losses. Intravenous colloids may be required to maintain intravascular volume and blood pressure because fluid losses are rich in protein. Patients with pancreatitis and systemic inflammatory response syndrome may benefit from treatment with drotrecogin alfa. Intravenous potassium, calcium, and magnesium are used to correct deficiency states. Insulin is used to treat hyperglycemia. Local complications resolve as the inflammatory process subsides; however, patients with necrotizing pancreatitis may require antibiotics and surgical intervention. ❷ Medications listed in Table 41–2 should be discontinued, if possible.

■ NONPHARMACOLOGIC THERAPY

Nonpharmacologic therapy includes ERCP for removal of an underlying biliary tract gallstone, surgery, and nutritional support. Surgery is indicated in patients with pseudocyst, pancreatic abscess, or to drain the pancreatic bed if hemorrhagic or necrotic material is present.

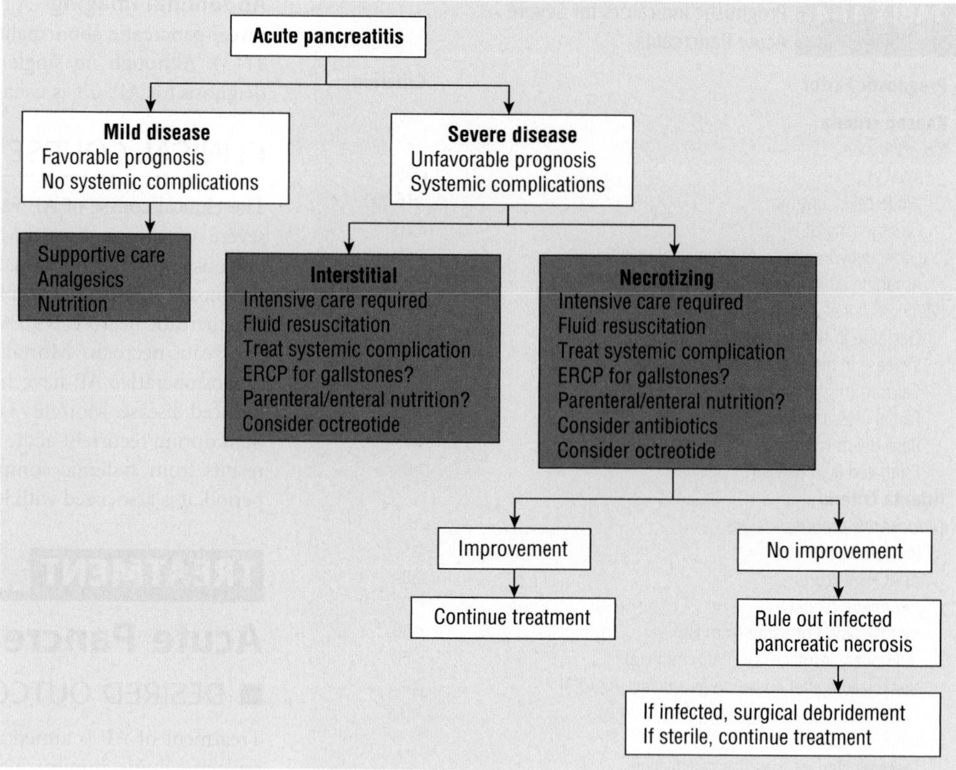

FIGURE 41-3. Algorithm of guidelines for evaluation and treatment of acute pancreatitis. (ERCP, endoscopic retrograde cholangiopancreatography.)

Nutrition and Probiotics

Nutritional support plays an important role in the management of patients with mild or severe disease as AP creates a catabolic state that promotes nutritional depletion, which can impair recovery, increase the risk of complications, and prolong hospititalization.[33–35] Patients with mild AP can begin oral feeding when bowel sounds have returned and pain has resolved.[8] In severe or complicated disease, nutritional deficits develop rapidly and are complicated by tissue necrosis, organ failure, and surgery. Enteral or parenteral nutrition should be initiated if it is anticipated that oral nutrition will be withheld for more than 1 week, but the optimal means of providing nutrition is controversial.[35–37] In the past, there was concern that enteral feeding stimulated pancreatic enzyme secretion and exacerbated the underlying disease. Today, there is consensus among studies in patients with severe AP that enteral feeding is the preferred route of administration because it is as safe and as effective as parenteral nutrition, attenuates the acute inflammatory response, and improves disease severity.[34–37] Although nasojejunal administration has been used, the nasogastric route also appears to be safe and effective.[33,38] If enteral feeding is not possible or if the patient is unable to obtain sufficient nutrients, total parenteral nutrition should be implemented before protein and calorie depletion becomes advanced. Intravenous lipids should not be withheld unless the serum triglyceride concentration is greater than 500 mg/dL.[2] Preliminary data suggest that the early nasojejunal administration of probiotics (such as lactobacillus) to enteral nutrition may reduce bacterial translocation and possibly decrease pancreatic necrosis and abscess.[39–42]

■ PHARMACOLOGIC THERAPY

Recommendations

Patients with mild AP respond well to supportive care, intravenous fluid resuscitation, nutrition, and relief of pain and nausea. Pain and nausea can be treated with moderate dosages of intravenous analgesics and antiemetics. Antibiotics are not indicated in mild disease. Patients with severe AP require intensive care, vigorous fluid resuscitation, nutritional support, and analgesia. Antisecretory drugs may be used to prevent stress-related mucosal bleeding. Octreotide may be tried in severe AP, but its efficacy remains uncertain (see Fig. 41–3). The use of prophylactic antibiotics is controversial in the absence of signs of infection except in patients with biliary tract gallstones, or in severe AP when pancreatic necrosis or abscess is likely.

Relief of Abdominal Pain

Analgesics are administered to reduce the severity of abdominal pain. The most important factors to consider in selecting an analgesic are efficacy and safety. Although the administration of some narcotics is associated with mild and transient increases in serum amylase and lipase, these effects are not deleterious to the patient. Traditionally, treatment was usually initiated with parenteral meperidine (50 to 100 mg every 3 to 4 hours) because it did not cause pancreatitis or significantly alter the function of the sphincter of Oddi, thereby worsening the pancreatitis.[43,44] ❸ Today many hospitals have either restricted or eliminated the use of meperidine because, unlike other narcotics, there is a ceiling on the dose and it is contraindicated in patients with renal failure. Active metabolites of meperidine accumulate in renal impairment and may cause seizures or psychosis. The maximum recommended parenteral dose of meperidine is 600 mg/day in patients with normal renal function, but it should not be used in patients with renal failure.

Parenteral morphine is often recommended for pain control because it provides a longer duration of pain relief than meperidine with less risk of seizures. However, its use in AP is sometimes avoided because it is thought to cause spasm of the sphincter of Oddi, increases in serum amylase, and, rarely, pancreatitis.[2] Although morphine increases biliary pressure, there is no evidence to indicate that it is contraindicated for use in AP as no studies have compared clinical outcomes of AP using various analgesics.[44] Hydromorphone may be used because it also has a longer half-life than meperidine. Patient-controlled analgesia should be considered in patients who require frequent narcotic dosing (e.g., every 2 to 3 hours) and usually achieves adequate pain control. Dosing should be monitored carefully and adjusted daily. There is no evidence that antisecretory drugs (such as H_2-receptor antagonists or proton pump inhibitors) prevent an exacerbation of abdominal pain.[45]

Limitation of Systemic Complications and Prevention of Pancreatic Necrosis

Aggressive fluid resuscitation and support of respiratory, renal, cardiovascular, and hepatobiliary function may limit systemic complications.[2,30,46,47] However, there is no proven method to prevent these complications.[45] Although hemoconcentration (decreased intravascular volume) is strongly associated with pancreatic necrosis, it is not clear whether vigorous fluid resuscitation alone during the first 24 hours can prevent pancreatic necrosis.[48] Procedures such as ERCP, hypothermia, nasogastric suction, pancreatic irradiation, peritoneal lavage, and thoracic duct drainage remain unproven.[2,45]

A number of agents have been investigated to limit disease progression by either directly or indirectly reducing pancreatic secretion, inhibiting the action of circulating inflammatory mediators, or increasing pancreatic microcirculation.[30,46,47,49–51] The use of parenteral H_2-receptor antagonists or proton pump inhibitors does not improve the overall outcome of patients with AP.[8] Corticosteroids are not helpful in limiting systemic complications and altering the course of the disease.[47] Clinical studies with protease inhibitors such as aprotinin and gabexate fail to reduce mortality in AP.[8,46–48,50] Conflicting or inconclusive data exists regarding the efficacy of atropine, lexipafant, low-molecular weight dextran, antioxidants such as *N*-acetylcysteine, indomethacin, interleukin-10, and infliximab.[47,49,51]

Somatostatin and its synthetic analog octreotide are potent inhibitors of pancreatic enzyme secretion and have been used to interrupt the inflammatory process. Several studies and a meta-analysis that evaluated the efficacy of somatostatin and octreotide suggest a slight trend toward benefit.[52–54] A randomized, open-label trial in severe AP indicates that octreotide 0.1 mg subcutaneously every 8 hours decreased mortality, sepsis, and length of hospital stay.[53] In a study using higher dosages (0.5 mcg/kg per hour given by continuous intravenous infusion), octreotide provided a decrease in serum amylase, greater improvement in pancreatic edema, and earlier return to oral intake than controls.[54] These studies are confounded by the lack of a reliable scoring system for severe AP, had small numbers of patients, were not placebo-controlled, and included patients with mild disease.[46]

❹ There is insufficient data to support the routine use of somatostatin or octreotide in the treatment of AP.

CLINICAL CONTROVERSY

Some clinicians believe that octreotide should be used routinely to decrease pancreatic secretions in patients with AP, whereas others believe it is unnecessary. Octreotide can be used in selected patients with severe AP, but its efficacy in decreasing mortality remains uncertain.

Prevention of Infection

❺ Patients with severe AP complicated by necrosis should receive antibiotic prophylaxis with a broad-spectrum antibiotic (Fig. 41–4).[1–3,45,55] The use of antibiotic prophylaxis in those without CT-proven necrosis is controversial.[3,8,55] Prophylactic antibiotics do not offer any benefit in cases of mild AP or when there is no necrosis.

Antibiotic prophylaxis in early clinical trials showed no benefit, but the studies were flawed, as they included all degrees of disease severity and did not have a sufficient number of patients with severe necrotiz-

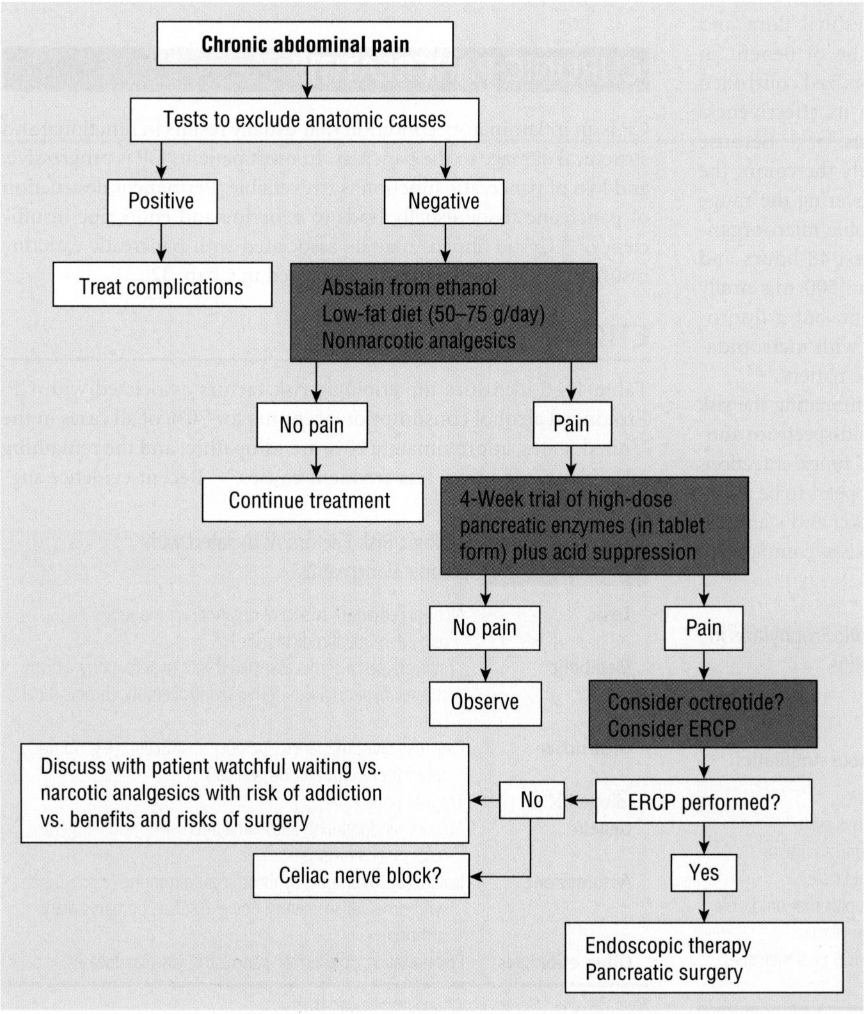

FIGURE 41-4. Algorithm of guidelines for the treatment of chronic abdominal pain in chronic pancreatitis. (ERCP, endoscopic retrograde cholangiopancreatography.)

ing AP.[1,47] In addition, the studies used ampicillin, which does not penetrate well into pancreatic tissue.[47] Imipenem-cilastatin, metronidazole, cefotaxime, piperacillin, mezlocillin, ofloxacin, and ciprofloxacin all achieve satisfactory bactericidal tissue concentrations, whereas aminoglycosides have poor penetration.[46,47,55] However, the importance of antibiotic penetration into pancreatic tissue has been debated, as it is the peripancreatic retroperitoneal necrotic fat and debris, not the pancreas itself, that becomes infected.

At present, there is sufficient evidence to recommend that patients with severe acute necrotizing pancreatitis receive antibiotic prophylaxis as soon as possible after diagnosis. Several randomized clinical trials have compared antibiotic prophylaxis with no antibiotics in patients with acute necrotizing pancreatitis, with varying results (Table 41–5).[56–61] In one study, prophylaxis with cefuroxime 4 to 5 g/day lowered mortality, length of hospital stay, and the overall infection rate, but a decrease in the total number of infections was attributed to fewer urinary tract infections in the antibiotic group.[56] In contrast, other antibiotic regimens decreased the incidence of sepsis, but had no effect on mortality.[57–59] Another study with imipenem-cilastatin found a reduction in the need for surgery, but no effect on mortality or sepsis.[60] Studies that included severe AP without CT demonstration of necrosis failed to show a beneficial effect on mortality.[58,61] Despite differences among the studies, two meta-analyses and a Cochrane review concluded that prophylaxis with broad-spectrum antibiotics decreases sepsis and mortality in patients with severe AP and necrosis.[62–64] Generally, treatment is initiated with imipenem-cilastin or a fluoroquinolone plus metronidazole and continued for 10 to 14 days.[8,55] Early antibiotic treatment may improve the prognosis of necrotizing AP,[65] but benefits must be weighed against inappropriate antibiotic prophylaxis and increasing microbial resistance.

Selective gut decontamination with oral nonabsorbable antibiotics is aimed at eradicating bacteria in the intestinal flora and reducing translocation.[55,66] This alternative may be of benefit in reducing the risk of pancreatic infection, but randomized controlled trials in patients with AP are needed to confirm its effectiveness when compared to parenteral antibiotic prophylaxis.[1,2,47,55] Because the source of bacterial contamination is most likely the colon, the choice of antibiotic should be broad-spectrum, covering the range of enteric aerobic gram-negative bacilli and anaerobic microorganisms. Treatment should be initiated within the first 48 hours and continued for 2 to 3 weeks. Imipenem-cilastatin (500 mg orally every 8 hours) is probably the most effective agent, but a fluoroquinolone (such as ciprofloxacin or levofloxacin) with metronidazole should be considered for the penicillin-allergic patient.[1,47]

Antibiotic prophylaxis is not always effective in eliminating the risk of infected pancreatic necrosis. Patients receiving broad-spectrum antibiotics are at increased risk for resistant bacterial and fungal infections leading to a worsening of the disease course. There appears to be a shift toward gram-positive infections (primarily enterococci and staphylococci) in AP patients who receive antibiotic prophylaxis as compared to earlier studies when patients did not receive antibiotic prophylaxis.[67] The use of prophylactic antibiotics may also alter the bacteriology of infected necrosis and is associated with an increase in the incidence of fungal and β-lactam–resistant gram-positive organisms.[68] The rise in fungal infections has led some clinicians to consider the addition of an antifungal agent to the prophylactic regimen.[69] Although agents such as fluconazole penetrate pancreatic tissue,[70] the effectiveness of prophylactic antifungal agents remains unproven and there are no definitive recommendations for use. Once infection develops in the patient with necrotic AP, surgical debridement is required.

TABLE 41-5 Clinical Trials of Intravenous Antibiotic Prophylaxis in Patients with Severe Acute Pancreatitis

Investigators	Patients (n)	Cause of Acute Pancreatitis	Intravenous Antibiotics
Sainio et al.[56]	30	Alcohol	Cefuroxime
Pederzoli et al.[57]	74	Biliary	Imipenem-cilastin
Delcenserie et al.[58]	23	Alcohol	Ceftazidime, amikacin, metronidazole
Schwartz et al.[59]	26	Biliary	Ofloxacin plus metronidazole
Nordback et al.[60]	58	Alcohol	Imipenem-cilastin
Isenmann et al.[61]	114	Alcohol	Ciprofloxacin plus metronidazole

CLINICAL CONTROVERSY

Some clinicians believe that antibiotic prophylaxis is necessary in patients with severe AP so as to prevent pancreatic infection, whereas others believe that this practice is unnecessary. Antibiotic use in AP remains controversial especially in patients without definite proof of pancreatic necrosis. Patients with severe AP complicated by necrosis should receive prophylactic treatment with a broad-spectrum antibiotic.

POST-ERCP PANCREATITIS

The clinical characteristics of post-ERCP pancreatitis are similar to those of AP from other causes. In most cases, the pancreatitis is mild and resolves in several days. Pretreatment with octreotide, corticosteroids, calcium channel blockers, natural β-carotene, and aprotinin has been disappointing,[1,11,71,72] but somatostatin, diclofenac suppositories, and gabexate have shown some benefit.[1,73–75] To date, there have not been any studies to evaluate the cost-effectiveness of prophylactic therapy.

CHRONIC PANCREATITIS

CP is an inflammatory condition that usually results in functional and structural damage to the pancreas. In most patients CP is progressive, and loss of pancreatic function is irreversible. Permanent destruction of pancreatic tissue usually leads to exocrine and endocrine insufficiency.[5–8] Cystic fibrosis may be associated with pancreatic exocrine insufficiency in children and is discussed in Chap. 32.

ETIOLOGY

Table 41–6 identifies the etiologic risk factors associated with CP. Prolonged alcohol consumption accounts for 70% of all cases in the United States, approximately 20% are idiopathic, and the remaining 10% constitute other, less-frequent causes.[5–8] Recent evidence sug-

TABLE 41-6 Etiologic Risk Factors Associated with Chronic Pancreatitis

Toxic	Alcohol (ethanol), tobacco, organotin compounds (e.g., di-*n*-butyltin dichloride)
Metabolic	Chronic hypercalcemia associated with hyperparathyroidism, chronic hypertriglyceridemia (controversial), chronic renal failure
Obstructive	Pancreas divisum, pancreatic duct obstruction (e.g., tumor), sphincter of Oddi (controversial)
Idiopathic	Tropical pancreatitis
Genetic	Autosomal dominant, autosomal recessive/modifier genes (e.g., cystic fibrosis)
Autoimmune	Isolated autoimmune, syndromic autoimmune (e.g., Sjögren syndrome, inflammatory bowel disease, primary biliary cirrhosis)
Other etiologies	Postirradiation, postnecrotic pancreatitis, vascular diseases

From Owyang,[5] Stevens et al.,[6] and Etemad and Whitcomb.[7]

gests that there is a strong association between cigarette smoking and CP.[5,6] Autoimmune pancreatitis may be isolated or occur in association with immune-mediated disorders.[76] Although cholelithiasis may coexist with CP, gallstones rarely lead to chronic disease.

PATHOPHYSIOLOGY

The exact mechanism by which alcohol causes CP is uncertain. One major theory is that alcohol-induced pancreatitis progresses from inflammation to cellular necrosis, and that fibrosis occurs over time. Chronic alcoholism results in a number of changes in pancreatic fluid that creates an environment for the formation of intraductal protein plugs that block small ductules.[5] Blockage of the ductules produces progressive structural damage in the ducts and the acinar tissue. Calcium complexes to the protein plugs, first in the small ductules and then in the main pancreatic duct (see Fig. 41–1), eventually resulting in injury and destruction of pancreatic tissue. Newer theories have been hypothesized, all of which lead to pancreatic destruction and insufficiency.[6,77]

The pathogenesis of the abdominal pain associated with CP is multifactorial and related in part to increased intraductal pressure secondary to continued pancreatic secretion, pancreatic inflammation, and abnormalities involving pancreatic nerves. Malabsorption of protein and fat occurs when the capacity for enzyme secretion is reduced by 90%.[5] Lipase secretion decreases more rapidly than the proteolytic enzymes. Bicarbonate secretion may be decreased, leading to a duodenal pH of less than 4.[5] A minority of patients develop complications, including pancreatic pseudocyst, abscess, and ascites or common bile duct obstruction, leading to cholangitis or secondary biliary cirrhosis. Bleeding is associated with a variety of causes.

CLINICAL PRESENTATION

Signs and Symptoms

The clinical presentation of CP varies depending on the etiology of the disease, the severity of the inflammatory process, and the extent of irreversible damage to the pancreas (Table 41–7).[5–8] The classic features are abdominal pain, malabsorption, weight loss, and diabetes. Most alcoholic patients have chronic pain; others have intermittent attacks or painless pancreatitis. Abstinence from ethanol may relieve pain, but does not prevent exocrine dysfunction.[5] The course of pain is unpredictable, but may lessen as pancreatic insufficiency progresses.[78]

TABLE 41-7 Presentation of Chronic Pancreatitis

General

- The patient may appear well-nourished or have coexistent signs of malnutrition and chronic alcoholic liver disease. During the acute attack, the patient may be thought to have acute pancreatitis until the diagnosis of chronic pancreatitis is established.

Symptoms

- Dull epigastric or abdominal pain that radiates to the back is seen. Pain is the most prominent clinical feature and tends to be episodic initially, but becomes more consistent as the disease progresses. A minority of patients will have no pain.
- Characteristically the pain is deep-seated, positional, frequently nocturnal, and unresponsive to medication. The intensity of the pain varies from mild to severe, and does not usually correlate directly with the inflammatory process or other physical findings. Severe attacks last from several days to several weeks and may be aggravated by eating.
- Nausea and vomiting often accompany the pain.

Signs

- Steatorrhea (excessive loss of fat in the feces) and azotorrhea (excessive loss of protein in the feces) are seen in most patients. Steatorrhea is often associated with diarrhea and bloating.
- Weight loss may be seen.
- Approximately 50% of patients with advanced pancreatic insufficiency present with vitamin B_{12} malabsorption.
- Jaundice occurs in approximately 10% of patients.
- Pancreatic diabetes is usually a late manifestation that is commonly associated with pancreatic calcification. Ketoacidosis, vascular complications, and nephropathy are uncommon with this form of diabetes.
- Neuropathy is sometimes seen.
- Complications, including pancreatic pseudocysts, pleural effusions, and ascites, may be detected on physical examination.

Laboratory tests

- The white blood cell count, fluids, and electrolytes usually remain normal unless fluids and electrolytes are lost as a result of vomiting and diarrhea.
- Serum amylase and lipase concentrations usually remain normal unless the pancreatic duct is blocked or a pseudocyst is present.

Other diagnostic tests

- Malabsorption of fat can be detected by Sudan staining of the feces or by a 72-hour quantitative measurement of fecal fat.
- Ultrasonography is the simplest and least expensive of the imaging techniques. Abdominal computed tomography is often used in patients who have a negative or unsatisfactory ultrasonogram examination.
- Endoscopic retrograde cholangiopancreatography is the most sensitive and specific test for the diagnosis of chronic pancreatitis. However, because it is associated with complications, it is reserved for patients for whom the diagnosis cannot be established by imaging techniques.

From Owyang,[5] Etemad and Whitcomb,[7] and Draganov and Forsmark.[8]

DIAGNOSIS

Most patients with CP have a history of heavy alcohol use and attacks of recurrent upper abdominal pain. The diagnosis is suspected in those with suggestive signs and symptoms and confirmed by the classic triad of calcification of the pancreas, steatorrhea, and diabetes, but surgical biopsy of the pancreas through laparoscopy or laparotomy is the gold standard.[5] In the absence of histologic samples, imaging techniques (see Table 41–7) are helpful in detecting pancreatic calcification, other causes of pain (ductal obstruction secondary to stones, strictures, or pseudocysts), and in differentiating CP from pancreatic cancer. Direct tests of pancreatic exocrine function involve the collection of pancreatic fluid after stimulation with exogenous hormones such as secretin or cholecystokinin. The functional tests are not diagnostic, but serve as a sign of CP and a measure of the severity of injury.[79] Because these tests are complicated and require intubation and special collection techniques, they are not routinely performed.

CLINICAL COURSE AND PROGNOSIS

Patients with alcoholic CP usually present with an initial acute attack followed by successive attacks that are slower to resolve. Continued alcohol use leads to chronic abdominal pain and progressive exocrine and endocrine insufficiency.[8] In approximately 50% of patients, the pain diminishes 5 to 10 years after the onset of symptoms.[80] Steatorrhea, calcification, and diabetes usually develop after 10 to 20 years of heavy ethanol ingestion. Most patients present with varying degrees of pain, malnutrition, and glucose intolerance. The 10-year survival rate is approximately 70%, whereas the 20-year survival rate is 45%.[8] Approximately 15% to 20% of patients with alcohol-related CP die of complications associated with acute attacks. Most deaths occur as a consequence of malnutrition, infection, or ethanol, narcotic, and tobacco use. CP is a risk factor for pancreatic adenocarcinoma, which contributes to the high mortality.[5,7] The clinical course of idiopathic CP is more favorable than that of alcoholic pancreatitis.[5,10]

TREATMENT

Chronic Pancreatitis

■ DESIRED OUTCOME

The treatment of uncomplicated CP is aimed primarily at the control of chronic abdominal pain (see Fig. 41–4) and the correc-

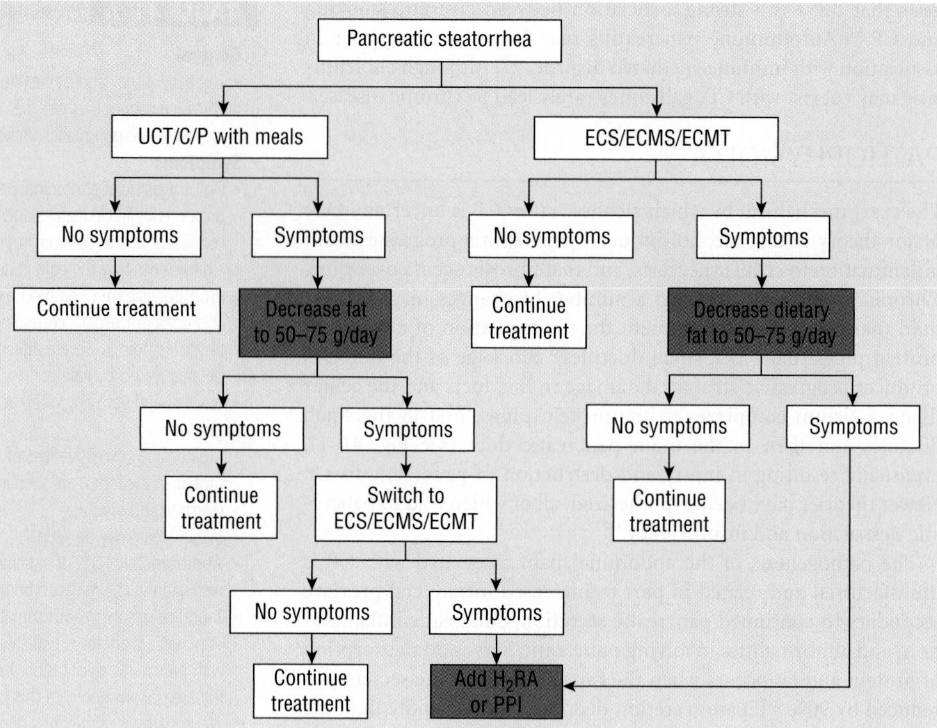

FIGURE 41-5. Algorithm of guidelines for the treatment of pancreatic steatorrhea in chronic pancreatitis. (C, capsule; ECMS, enteric-coated microsphere; ECS, enteric-coated sphere; ECMT, enteric-coated microtablet; H_2RA, H_2-receptor antagonist; P, powder; PPI, proton pump inhibitor; UCT, uncoated tablet.)

tion of malabsorption with pancreatic enzymes (Fig. 41–5). Diabetes associated with CP may require exogenous insulin.

■ GENERAL APPROACH TO TREATMENT

The majority of patients with alcohol-related CP require pain control and pancreatic enzyme supplementation.[5,8,80–83] Avoidance of alcohol usually decreases pain, but oral analgesics remain the cornerstone of therapy. Nonnarcotic analgesics such as acetaminophen, nonsteroidal antiinflammatory drugs (NSAIDs), or tramadol should be tried initially. The dose and frequency of administration is usually increased before the patient is switched to a narcotic. Patients unresponsive to nonnarcotic analgesics should be given a trial of non–enteric-coated pancreatic enzymes prior to using narcotics. Narcotics are required for patients with severe pain. Specific endoscopic or surgical procedures may be necessary in patients refractory to drug therapy. Patients with malabsorption require pancreatic enzymes to reduce steatorrhea and azotorrhea. Most patients achieve satisfactory results with standard-dosage regimens of either the non–enteric-coated or microencapsulated enteric-coated dosage forms. In patients who remain symptomatic, dietary fat should be reduced. An antisecretory drug should be added to the regimen when enzymes alone provide an inadequate reduction in steatorrhea or when low duodenal pH is documented.

■ NONPHARMACOLOGIC THERAPY

❻ Abstinence from alcohol is the most important factor in preventing abdominal pain in the early stages of alcoholic CP, although reports of the effect of abstinence from alcohol have varied.[5,80] Small and frequent meals (6 meals per day) and a diet restricted in fat (50 to 75 g/day) are recommended to minimize postprandial pancreatic secretion and resulting pain.[83] Enteral nutrition (elemental diets) may be necessary if oral calorie intake is insufficient or if the patient is chronically debilitated.[33] Parenteral nutrition should be instituted when an enteral tube cannot be placed, gastric decompression is required, or a complicated fistula is present.[33]

In some patients, pain may be associated with pseudocysts, peptic ulcer, cholelithiasis, biliary or duodenal obstruction, or pancreatic cancer, and if detected may be amenable to other forms of treatment (see Fig. 41–4), including endoscopic procedures such as sphincterotomy, pancreatic duct stenting, and lithotriptic destruction of pancreatic calculi.[5,8,80,84] The most common indication for surgery is abdominal pain that is refractory to medical therapy. Surgical procedures that alleviate pain include a subtotal pancreatectomy, decompression of the main pancreatic duct, or interruption of the splanchnic nerves.[5,8,80,84] Although the pain may diminish as the gland deteriorates, it is unreasonable to wait years for spontaneous relief. A percutaneous injection of a corticosteroid or endoscopic ultrasonography-guided injection of a local anesthetic into the celiac ganglion (celiac plexus block) may be attempted. Pain relief obtained by these procedures lasts only a few months and repeated treatments are not as effective.[80,84,85]

■ PHARMACOLOGIC THERAPY

Recommendations

Pain management should begin with nonnarcotic analgesics such as acetaminophen or NSAIDs (see Fig. 41–4). If pain persists, the response to exogenous non–enteric-coated pancreatic enzymes should be evaluated in patients with mild to moderate CP. If these measures fail, an oral narcotic should be added to the drug regimen. Parenteral narcotics should be reserved for patients with severe pain that is unresponsive to oral analgesics. Nonnarcotic modulators of chronic pain should be considered in patients with difficult-to-manage pain.

Most patients with malabsorption will require pancreatic enzyme supplementation and a reduction in dietary fat so as to achieve satisfactory nutritional status and become relatively asymptomatic. An initial prandial dose of 30,000 international units of lipase (uncoated tablet, capsule, or powder) is recommended to be given with each meal (see Fig. 41–5). Unlike the treatment of pain, the use of the microencapsulated enteric-coated pancreatic enzyme dosage forms are often selected to treat steatorrhea because of their higher potency and the need to take fewer tablets or capsules. The total daily lipase dose should be titrated to reduce steatorrhea. In some patients, a reduction in dietary fat may be necessary. An antisecretory drug should be added to the regimen when there is an inadequate response to enzyme therapy alone (see Fig. 41–5). If these measures are ineffective, documentation of the diagnosis and exclusion of other diseases should be undertaken.

Relief of Chronic Abdominal Pain

Analgesics ❼ Nonnarcotic analgesics such as acetaminophen or NSAIDs should be given before meals to prevent postprandial exacerbation of pain (Table 41–8).[5,80–84] Treatment should be individualized and should begin with the lowest effective dose. The dosage regimen should usually be maximized before switching to narcotic alternatives. Analgesics should be scheduled around the clock, because they may be more effective and the total amount of medication required over 24 hours may be less. If the nonnarcotic analgesic is ineffective, consideration should be given to using tramadol or adding a low-dose narcotic to the regimen (e.g., acetaminophen plus codeine). Severe pain relief necessitates the use of opiate analgesics. Narcotics should not be withheld because of the risk of inducing addiction. Oral agents should be used before parenteral narcotics are administered. Nonnarcotic modulators of chronic pain such as selective serotonin reuptake inhibitors (e.g., paroxetine) or tricyclic antidepressants should be considered in difficult-to-manage patients.[1,81,84] Tricyclic antidepressants are useful adjuncts, as they not only treat depression, but have a direct effect on pain and potentiate the effect of opioid narcotics.[84] Referral to a dedicated pain clinic should be considered when available.

Pancreatic Enzymes ❽ The use of orally administered pancreatic enzymes to relieve abdominal pain remains controversial, although a consensus review has advocated their use (see Table 41–8).[80] Results from clinical trials are conflicting, especially when non–enteric-coated preparations were compared to enteric-coated enzyme products.[5,81–84,86,87] Only those studies that used a non–enteric-coated dosage form plus a gastric acid suppressant demonstrated a reduction in pain.[8] The administration of non–enteric-coated pancreatic enzymes may afford pain relief by suppressing pancreatic enzyme secretion through a negative feedback mechanism involving proteases present in the duodenum.[88] Effective enzyme therapy reduces pancreatic stimulation, diminishes intraductal pressure, and should decrease pain. Enteric-coated enzyme preparations deliver proteases too far distally to achieve a negative-feedback effect. Possible reasons for failure of enzymes to relieve abdominal pain include insufficient concentrations of trypsin in the pancreatic enzyme preparation and gastric acid inactivation or proteolytic destruction of trypsin.[5,84,86,87] The addition of an antisecretory drug to the non–enteric-coated enzyme preparation is recommended, as it reduces the degradation of proteases in the stomach.[5,81] A trial of non–enteric-coated enzymes may be beneficial in a subset of individuals, primarily those with mild to moderate disease and in patients with a nonalcoholic etiology.[5,80,84]

CLINICAL CONTROVERSY

Some clinicians believe that pancreatic enzyme supplementation should be used to relieve mild to moderate abdominal pain, whereas others believe that these agents are ineffective. A trial of non–enteric-coated pancreatic enzyme supplementation and an antisecretory drug should be given to patients with mild to moderate disease when nonnarcotic medications have failed and before initiating treatment with narcotics.

Other Agents A number of other agents, including octreotide, allopurinol, and antioxidant therapy (e.g., organic selenium, vitamin E, vitamin C, or β-carotene), have been investigated for the purposes of relieving pain in chronic pancreatitis.[5,80] There is insufficient evidence to support the use of these agents.

TABLE 41-8 Guidelines for the Pharmacologic Treatment of Chronic Pancreatitis

Treatment of chronic pain (oral drug regimens)
Nonnarcotic
• Acetaminophen: Dosage should be limited to 500 mg four times a day if patient drinks more than two alcoholic beverages per day; increased risk of hepatotoxicity, especially in chronic heavy alcohol use
• Nonsteroidal antiinflammatory drugs (NSAIDs): Standard dosage regimens of aspirin or traditional NSAIDs (e.g., ibuprofen). Use with caution in patients at risk for upper GI bleeding and in renal insufficiency
• Tramadol: 50–100 mg every 4–6 h not to exceed 400 mg/day; has narcotic-like effect; contraindicated in alcohol or hypnotic intoxication; drug interactions; expensive
• Consider use of selective serotonin reuptake inhibitors (e.g., paroxetine) or tricyclic antidepressants in difficult-to-manage patients
Narcotics
• Codeine 30–60 mg every 6 h; hydrocodone 5–10 mg every 4–6 h; oxycodone 5–10 mg every 6 h; fentanyl patch 25–100 mcg/h; pentazocine 25–50 mg every 4–6 h; propoxyphene 65 mg every 4–6 h not to exceed 390 mg/day; methadone 2.5–10 mg every 4–6 h; morphine sulfate (extended-release) 30–60 mg every 8–12 h; hydromorphone 2–4 mg every 4–6 h
• Risk of potentiation with alcohol; impaired respiration; constipation; hypotension
• Dosing is usually based on providing continuous pain relief; consider combining narcotic with acetaminophen or NSAIDs; narcotic dependence is common; narcotic abuse is a concern in alcoholics; tolerance to narcotics may develop
Pancreatic enzymes
• Requires that high doses of proteases be delivered to the duodenum for relief of pain; non–enteric-coated pancreatic enzymes are recommended and should be taken with each meal and at night if needed; recommend name brands with proven efficacy and safety, as generic products have been associated with treatment failure; add H_2-receptor antagonist or proton pump inhibitor
• Viokase-8 tablets or Ku-Zyme HP capsules: 6–8 with each meal (see Table 41–9) plus either an H_2-receptor antagonist or proton pump inhibitor
• May cause nausea, cramping, hyperuricemia; hypersensitivity to pork protein
Treatment of maldigestion and steatorrhea
Non–enteric-coated pancreatic enzymes
• Viokase-8 tablets or Ku-Zyme HP capsules, 6–8 with each meal and at bedtime if needed (see Table 41–9)
• Addition of antisecretory drug (H_2-receptor antagonist or proton pump inhibitor) may increase efficacy, but also increases cost
• May cause nausea, cramping, hyperuricemia; hypersensitivity to pork protein
Enteric-coated pancreatic enzymes
• Enteric-coated spheres, microspheres, and microtablets are available (see Table 41–9)
• Usually requires fewer capsules or tablets per meal than non–enteric-coated enzymes; may enhance compliance
• Does not usually require additional antisecretory agents; may be less expensive than non–enteric-coated plus H_2-receptor antagonist or proton pump inhibitor
• May cause nausea, cramping, hyperuricemia; hypersensitivity to pork protein
• Fibrosing colonopathy has occurred in children using preparations that contain the methacrylic acid copolymer coating
Antisecretory drugs
• May improve enzyme treatment of steatorrhea

From references 5, 81–84, 86, 87, 89–91.

Treatment of Malabsorption

Malabsorption requires treatment when steatorrhea is documented (>7 g of fat in the feces per 24 hours while on a diet of 100 g/day of fat) and persistent weight loss occurs despite efforts to correct it. The combination of pancreatic enzymes (lipase, amylase, and protease) and a reduction in dietary fat (to <25 g/meal) enhances the patient's nutritional status and reduces (but does not totally correct) steatorrhea. ❾ The success of a pancreatic enzyme preparation requires that it contain a high concentration of lipase and proteases, be enteric-coated to avoid destruction by gastric acid, and be the appropriate size to permit efficient delivery of the enzymes to the small intestine.[5,89–92] A critical amount of enzymes must be delivered to the duodenum in sufficient concentrations for digestion to occur. The maximal delivery of endogenous pancreatic lipase following a meal is approximately 140,000 international units per hour for 4 hours.[5] Malabsorption is minimized if the concentration of enzymes delivered to the duodenum is at least 5% of normal maximal enzyme output. This requires that approximately 30,000 international units of lipase and 10,000 international units of trypsin be delivered during the 4-hour postprandial period.[5,89] In many cases, the lipase dose will need to be increased (up to a maximum of 75,000 international units) because of insufficient lipolytic activity.[90] Most exogenous lipase is rapidly and irreversibly destroyed at an intragastric pH below 4.[5,89–92] Enteric coating is an effective way to protect the acid-labile enzymes, but the enzymes must be emptied from the stomach at the same rate as the ingested food and released in the duodenum. The polymer used to coat the enzyme is pH-dependent and dissolves in the duodenum at a pH of >5, where the enzymes are released.[5,89] If an intragastric pH of <4 prevails, the enteric coating will remain intact and the enzymes will be released in the upper portion of the small intestine. A duodenal pH of <4 may prolong dissolution of the enteric coating and release of the enzymes. The size of the enteric-coated enzyme preparation influences the timing of enzyme delivery to the duodenum.[5,89,93,94] Microencapsulated enteric-coated preparations with a microcapsular diameter of about 1.4 mm empty from the stomach in synchrony with food and mix effectively with intestinal chyme.[5,89] Large enteric-coated tablets and some microspheres (microcapsular diameter >2 mm) do not empty at the same rate as stomach contents, and thus are not as effective in treating steatorrhea.

Pancreatic Enzyme Supplements Oral pancreatic enzyme supplements are available as a powder, uncoated or coated tablet, capsule, enteric-coated sphere (ECS) and microsphere (ECMS), or enteric-coated microtablet (ECMT) encased in a cellulose or gelatin capsule (Table 41–9). Recommended dosages of microencapsulated enteric-coated products are not necessarily more effective than recommended dosages of the non–enteric-coated enzyme preparations.[5,89] This is because a lesser quantity of lipase is usually administered at each meal with the enteric-coated preparations. Thus the most important determinant in reducing steatorrhea is the total amount of active lipase that reaches the duodenum and empties with the meal. Generic pancreatic enzyme preparations have been associated with treatment failures when substituted for brand-name products.[95]

Pancreatic enzyme supplements differ in enzyme content and activity, bioavailability, clinical efficacy, patient acceptance, and cost. Compliance is often a problem because of the number of tablets or capsules required per dose, the need to take them with each meal or snack, and the cost of pancreatic enzyme therapy. The efficacy of enzyme supplements may be optimized by administration during or after meals.[96] Consideration should be given to selecting a product that contains higher lipase activity (see Table 41–9) so that fewer tablets or capsules are required. However, reports of colonic strictures and intestinal obstruction in cystic fibrosis patients taking high-dose pancreatic enzymes (>20,000 international units lipase per capsule) have led to their withdrawal from the market in the United States.[5,97] Pancreatic enzymes contain nucleic acids, and when given in high therapeutic doses, they have been associated with hyperuricosuria, hyperuricemia, and kidney stones.[5,82] Impaired folic acid absorption by oral pancreatic enzymes may lead to folic acid deficiency. Gastrointestinal side effects appear to be dose-related, but occur less frequently with the enteric-coated products. Sensitization and allergic reactions are uncommon but may occur in patients taking the powder.

TABLE 41-9 Frequently Used Pancreatic Enzyme Preparations

Product	Dosage Form	Enzyme Content (Units)[a] Lipase	Amylase	Protease
Creon-10	ECMS	10,000	33,200	37,500
Creon-20	ECMS	20,000	66,400	75,000
Ku-Zyme HP	C	8,000	30,000	30,000
Lipram-CR10	ECMS	10,000	33,200	37,500
Lipram-PN16	ECMS	16,000	48,000	48,000
Lipram-CR20	ECMS	20,000	66,400	75,000
Lipram-PN20	ECMS	20,000	56,000	44,000
Lipram-UL12	ECMS	12,000	39,000	39,000
Lipram-PN10	ECMS	10,000	30,000	30,000
Lipram-UL18	ECMS	18,000	58,500	58,500
Lipram-UL20	ECMS	20,000	65,000	65,000
Pancrease	ECMS	4,500	20,000	25,000
Pancrease MT-4	ECMT	4,000	12,000	12,000
Pancrease MT-10	ECMT	10,000	30,000	30,000
Pancrease MT-16	ECMT	16,000	48,000	48,000
Pancrease MT-20	ECMT	20,000	56,000	44,000
Ultrase MT 12	ECMT	12,000	39,000	39,000
Ultrase MT 18	ECMT	18,000	58,500	58,500
Ultrase MT 20	ECMT	20,000	65,000	65,000
Viokase[b]	P	16,800	70,000	70,000
Viokase 8	UCT	8,000	30,000	30,000
Viokase 16	UCT	16,000	60,000	60,000

C, powder encased in a cellulose capsule; ECS, enteric-coated sphere encased in a cellulose capsule; ECMS, enteric-coated microspheres encased in a cellulose or gelatin capsule; ECMT, enteric-coated microtablets encased in a cellulose capsule; P, powder; UCT, uncoated tablet.

[a]All listed products contain pancrelipase. Pancrelipase contains not less than 24 USP units of lipase activity, not less than 100 USP units of amylase activity, and not less than 100 USP units of protease activity per milligram.

[b]Units of 0.7 g of powder.

Adjuncts to Enzyme Therapy The use of antisecretory drugs as adjuncts to enzyme therapy may improve the efficacy of pancreatic enzyme supplementation.[5,89,98] The beneficial effects of an H_2-receptor antagonist or proton pump inhibitor result from both an increase in pH and a decrease in intragastric volume.[5,98] These agents should maintain luminal gastric and duodenal pH above 4 and enhance lipase activity. Increased duodenal pH also prevents bile acid precipitation, increasing fatty acid solubility. Antacids appear to have little or no added effect in reducing steatorrhea.[5]

⑩ Symptomatic patients whose steatorrhea is not corrected by enzyme replacement therapy and a reduction in dietary fat may benefit from the addition of an H_2-receptor antagonist. A proton pump inhibitor should be considered in patients who fail to benefit from the addition of an H_2-receptor antagonist. The additional cost of antisecretory therapy and the potential for adverse effects and drug interactions should be considered.

PHARMACOECONOMIC CONSIDERATIONS

The pharmacoeconomic issues associated with the medical treatment of AP and CP have not been extensively examined. Aggressive medical and surgical care decreases mortality in AP, but the overall cost-effectiveness of a specific treatment is unknown. The relief of abdominal pain in AP and CP, as well as pancreatic enzyme supplementation in patients with CP, improves quality of life and nutritional status.[99] Although the efficacy of octreotide in AP remains uncertain, its use in severe AP is reasonable and potentially cost-effective. Antibiotic prophylaxis of targeted patients may reduce mortality and length of hospital stay, but pharmacoeconomic studies have not confirmed this suspicion. However, a reduction in the length of stay could offset the cost of antibiotic therapy.

In some cases, medications that cost more may be more cost-effective. This is particularly true with pancreatic enzymes and the microencapsulated enteric-coated dosage forms. These latter products may cost more per unit, but they offer greater patient acceptance and compliance when compared to uncoated tablets. In addition, when cost is based on the total number of tablets or capsules per day, rather than the cost of a single tablet or capsule, the high-potency preparations are usually similar in price to the uncoated products. The addition of an H_2-receptor antagonist or proton pump inhibitor may actually be cost-effective for patients who are inadequately controlled on maximal enzyme therapy.

EVALUATION OF THERAPEUTIC OUTCOMES

ACUTE PANCREATITIS

Pain control, fluid and electrolyte status, and nutrition should be assessed periodically in patients with mild AP, depending on the degree of abdominal pain and fluid loss. Patients with severe AP should receive intensive care and close monitoring of vital signs, fluid and electrolyte status, white blood cell count, blood glucose, lactic dehydrogenase, aspartate aminotransferase, serum albumin, hematocrit, blood urea nitrogen, serum creatinine, and international normalized ratio. Continuous hemodynamic and arterial blood gas monitoring is essential. Serum lipase, amylase, and bilirubin require less-frequent monitoring. The patient should be monitored for signs of infection, relief of abdominal pain, and adequate nutritional status. Therapeutic outcome depends on the severity of the acute attack, medical management (which is primarily supportive), and prevention or treatment of infection. Despite appropriate supportive therapy, deterioration of respiratory, renal, and cardiovascular function may lead to death.

CHRONIC PANCREATITIS

The severity and frequency of abdominal pain should be assessed periodically so as to determine the efficacy of the patient's pain control regimen. Most patients with abdominal pain can be adequately controlled with acetaminophen or NSAIDs. A trial of non–enteric-coated pancreatic enzymes and either an H_2-receptor antagonist or proton pump inhibitor may relieve pain in patients with mild to moderate disease. Patients with severe pain will require narcotics. In these patients, pain should be monitored daily and medications adjusted accordingly. Some patients will require endoscopic therapy or pancreatic surgery.

The effectiveness of pancreatic enzyme supplementation in treating malabsorption is measured by improvement in body weight and stool consistency or frequency. The 72-hour stool test for fecal fat may be used when there is concern regarding the adequacy of treatment. Serum uric acid and folic acid concentrations should be monitored yearly in patients prone to hyperuricemia or folic acid deficiency. Blood glucose must be closely monitored in the diabetic patient. Therapeutic outcome depends in part on the ability of the patient to discontinue alcohol and tobacco use and to maintain adequate nutrition. Pain control and pancreatic enzyme supplementation are important therapeutic measures that contribute to the patient's quality of life. A small number of patients die from complications associated with an acute attack.

CONCLUSIONS

Important advances have been made regarding our understanding of acute and chronic pancreatitis, especially as it relates to genetics, pathogenesis, and the natural history of the diseases. Although there has been a reduction in the mortality of patients with severe AP, controversy remains regarding the use of antibiotic prophylaxis. Patients with CP benefit from improved strategies for managing pain and malabsorption. New and improved diagnostic techniques and medical treatments will replace many of the procedures and drugs we use today.

ABBREVIATIONS

AP: acute pancreatitis

ARDS: acute respiratory distress syndrome

CT: computed tomography

CCK: cholecystokinin

CP: chronic pancreatitis

ERCP: endoscopic retrograde cholangiopancreatography

IMMC: interdigestive migrating motor complex

NSAID: nonsteroidal antiinflammatory drug

SC: secretin

REFERENCES

1. Mitchell RMS, Byrne MF, Baillie J. Pancreatitis. Lancet 2003;361:1447–1455.
2. Topazian M, Gorelick FS. Acute pancreatitis. In: Yamada T, Aplers DH, Kaplowitz N, et al., eds. Textbook of Gastroenterology, 4th ed. Philadelphia: Lippincott Williams & Wilkins, 2003:2026–2061.
3. Whitcomb DC. Acute pancreatitis. N Engl J Med 2006;354:2142–2150.
4. Swaroop VS, Chari ST, Clain JE. Severe acute pancreatitis. JAMA 2004;291:2865–2868.
5. Owyang C. Chronic pancreatitis. In: Yamada T, Aplers DH, Kaplowitz N, et al., eds. Textbook of Gastroenterology, 4th ed. Philadelphia: Lippincott Williams & Wilkins, 2003:2061–2090.
6. Stevens T, Conwell DL, Zuccaro G. Pathogenesis of chronic pancreatitis: An evidence-based review of past theories and recent developments. Am J Gastroenterol 2004;99:2256–2270.
7. Etemad B, Whitcomb DC. Chronic pancreatitis: Diagnosis, classification and new genetic developments. Gastroenterology 2001;120:682–707.
8. Draganov P, Forsmark, CE. Diseases of the Pancreas. February 2006, *http://www.acpmedicine.com/sample/med0405.pdf.*
9. Owyang C, Williams JA. Pancreatic secretion. In: Yamada T, Aplers DH, Kaplowitz N, et al., eds. Textbook of Gastroenterology, 4th ed. Philadelphia: Lippincott Williams & Wilkins, 2003:340–366.
10. Draganov P, Forsmark CE. "Idiopathic" pancreatitis. Gastroenterology 2005;128;756–763.
11. Cheng C-L, Sherman S, Watkins JL, et al. Risk factors for post-ERCP pancreatitis: A prospective multicenter study. Am J Gastroenterol 2006;101:139–147.
12. Quraishi ER, Goel S, Gupta M, et al. Acute pancreatitis in patients on chronic peritoneal dialysis: An increased risk? Am J Gastroenterol 2005;100:2288–2293.
13. Morton C, Klatsky AL, Udaltosova N. Smoking, coffee, and pancreatitis. Am J Gastroenterol 2004;99:731–738.
14. Trivedi CD, Ptichumoni CS. Drug-induced pancreatitis. J Clin Gastroenterol 2005;39:709–716.
15. Eland IA, van Puijenbroek EP, Sturkenboom MJCM, et al. Drug-associated acute pancreatitis: Twenty-one years of spontaneous reporting in the Netherlands. Am J Gastroenterol 1999;94:2417–2422.
16. Eland A, Alvarez H, Stricker BH, Rodriguez AG. The risk of acute pancreatitis associated with acid-suppressing drugs. Br J Clin Pharmacol 2000;49:473–478.
17. Devlin JW, Lau AD, Tanios MA. Propofol-associated hypertriglyceridemia and pancreatitis in the intensive care unit: An analysis of frequency and risk factors. Pharmacotherapy 2005;25:1348–1352.
18. Lin H-H, Hsu C-H, Chao Y-C. Tamoxifen-induced severe acute pancreatitis: A case report. Dig Dis Sci 2004:49:997–999.
19. Mallick S. Metformin induced acute pancreatitis precipitated by renal failure. Postgrad Med J 2004;80:239–240.
20. McDornald KB, Garbor BG, Perreault MM. Pancreatitis associated with simvastatin plus fenofibrate. Ann Pharmacother 2002;36:275–279.
21. Fisher AA, Bassett ML. Acute pancreatitis associated with angiotensin II receptor antagonists. Ann Pharmacother 2002;36:1883–1886.
22. Blomgren KB, Sundstrom A, Steineck G, et al. Obesity and treatment of diabetes with glyburide may both be risk factors for acute pancreatitis. Diabetes Care 2002;25:298–302.
23. Spigwet O, Hagg S, Bate A. Hepatic injury and pancreatitis during treatment with serotonin reuptake inhibitors: Data from the World Health Organization (WHO) database of adverse drug reactions. Int Clin Psychopharmacol 2003;18:157–161.

24. Blomgren KB, Sündstrom A, Steineck G, et al. A Swedish case-control network for studies of drug-induced morbidity—Acute pancreatitis. Eur J Clin Pharmacol 2002;58:275–283.
25. Mayer J, Rau B, Gansauge F, et al. Inflammatory mediators in human acute pancreatitis: Clinical and pathophysiological implications. Gut 2000;47:546–552.
26. Riche FD, Cholley BO, Laisne MJC, et al. Inflammatory cytokines, C reactive protein, and procalcitonin as early predictors of necrosis infection in acute necrotizing pancreatitis. Surgery 2003;133:257–262.
27. Nagar AB, Gorelick FS. Acute Pancreatitis. Curr Opin Gastroenterol 2004;20:439–443.
28. Adler DG, Baron TH, Egan J, et al. ASGE guideline: The role of ERCP in diseases of the biliary tract and the pancreas. Gastrointest Endosc 2005;62:1–8.
29. Somogyi L, Martin SP, Venkatesan T, et al. Recurrent acute pancreatitis: An algorithmic approach to identification and elimination of inciting factors. Gastroenterology 2001;120:708–717.
30. Tenner S. Initial management of acute pancreatitis: Critical issues during the first 72 hours. Am J Gastroenterol 2004;99:2489–2494.
31. Venkatesan T, Moulton JS, Ulrich CD, Martin SP. Prevalence and predictors of severity as defined by Atlanta criteria among patients presenting with acute pancreatitis. Pancreas 2003;26:107–110.
32. Yadav D, Agarwal N, Pitchumoni S. A critical evaluation of laboratory tests in acute pancreatitis. Am J Gastroenterol 2002;97:1309–1318.
33. Meier R, Beglinger C. Nutrition in pancreatic diseases. Best Pract Res Clin Gastroenterol 2006;20:507–529.
34. McClave SA, Chang WK, Dhaliwal R, Heyland DK. Nutrition support in acute pancreatitis: A systematic review of the literature. J Parent Ent Nutr 2006;30:143–156.
35. Mayerle J, Hlouschek V, Lerch MM. Current management of acute pancreatitis. Nat Clin Pract Gastroenterol Hepatol 2005;2:473–483.
36. Al-Omran M, Groof A, Wilke D. Enteral versus parenteral nutrition for acute pancreatitis. Cochrane Database Syst Rev 2003;1:CC002837.
37. Marik PE, Zaloga GP. Meta-analysis of parenteral nutrition versus enteral nutrition in patients with acute pancreatitis. BMJ 2004;328:1407.
38. Eatock FC, Brombacher GD, Steven A, et al. Nasogastric feeding in severe acute pancreatitis may be practical and safe. Int J Pancreatol 2000;28:23–29.
39. Penner R, Fedorak RN, Madsen KL. Probiotics and nutraceuticals: Non-medicinal treatments of gastrointestinal diseases. Curr Opin Pharmacol 2005;5:596–603.
40. Oláh A, Issekutz A, Gamal ME, et al. Randomized clinical trial of specific lactobacillus and fiber supplement to early enteral nutrition in patients with acute pancreatitis. Br J Surg 2002;89:1103–1107.
41. Kecskes G, Belagyi T, Olah A. Early jejunal nutrition with combined pre- and probiotics in acute pancreatitis—Prospective, randomized, double-blind investigations. Magy Seb 2003;563–568.
42. Bengmark S. Bio-ecological control of acute pancreatitis: The role of enteral nutrition, pro- and synbiotics. Curr Opin Clin Nutr Metab Care 2005:8:447–561.
43. Isenhower HL, Mueller BA. Selection of narcotic analgesics for pain associated with pancreatitis. Am J Health Syst Pharm 1998;55:480–486.
44. Thompson DR. Narcotic analgesic effects on the sphincter of Oddi: A review of the data and therapeutic implications in treating pancreatitis. Am J Gastroenterol 2001;96:1266–1272.
45. Banks PA. Practice guidelines in acute pancreatitis. Am J Gastroenterol 1997;92:377–386.
46. Yousaf M, McCallion K, Daimond T. Management of severe acute pancreatitis. Br J Surg 2003;90:407–420.
47. Norton ID, Clain JE. Optimizing outcomes in acute pancreatitis. Drugs 2001;61:1581–1591.
48. Brown A, Baillargeon JD, Hughes MD, et al. Can fluid resuscitation prevent pancreatic necrosis in severe acute pancreatitis? Pancreatology 2002;2:104–107.
49. Fantini L, Tomassetti P, Pezzilli R. Management of acute pancreatitis: Current knowledge and future perspectives. World J Emer Surg 2006;1–6.
50. Singh VP, Chan ST. Protease inhibitors in acute pancreatic: Lessons from the bench and failed clinical trials. Gastroenterology 2005;126:2172–2174.
51. Holtz HG, Schmidt J, Ryschich EW, et al. Isovolemic hemodilution with dextran prevents contrast medium-induced impairment of pancreatic microcirculation in necrotizing pancreatitis of the rat. Am J Surg 1995;169:161–166.
52. Andriulli A, Leandro G, Clemente R, et al. Meta-analysis of somatostatin, octreotide and gabexate mesylate in the therapy of acute pancreatitis. Aliment Pharmacol Ther 1998;12:237–245.
53. Paran H, Mayo A, Paran D. Octreotide treatment in patients with severe acute pancreatitis. Dig Dis Sci 2000;45:2247–2251.
54. Karakoyunlar O, Sivrel E, Tanir N, et al. High-dose octreotide in the management of acute pancreatitis. Hepatogastroenterology 1999;46:1968–1971.
55. Lankisch PG, Lerch MM. The role of amitotic prophylaxis in the treatment of acute pancreatitis. J Clin Gastroenterol 2006;40:149–155.
56. Sainio V, Kemppainen P, Poulallainen P, et al. Early antibiotic treatment in acute necrotizing pancreatitis. Lancet 1995;346:663–667.
57. Pederzoli P, Bassi C, Vesentini S, et al. A randomized multicenter clinical trial of antibiotic prophylaxis with imipenem. Surg Gynecol Obstet 1993;176:480–483.
58. Delcenserie R, Yzet T, Ducroix JP. Prophylactic antibiotics in treatment of severe acute alcoholic pancreatitis. Pancreas 1996;13:198–201.
59. Schwartz M, Isenmann R, Meyer H, Berger HG. Antibiotic use in necrotizing pancreatitis. Results of a controlled study. (English Abstract) Dtsch Med Wschr 1997;122:356–361.
60. Nordback I, Sand J, Saaristo R, Paajanen H. Early treatment with antibiotics reduces the need for surgery in acute necrotizing pancreatitis—A single-center randomized study. J Gastrointest Surg 2001;5:113–118; discussion 118–120.
61. Isenmann R, Runzi M, Kron M, et al. Prophylactic antibiotic treatment in patients with predicted severe acute pancreatitis: A placebo-controlled double-blind trial. Gastroenterology 2004;126:997–1004.
62. Golub R, Siddiai F, Pohl D. Role of antibiotics in acute pancreatitis: A meta-analysis. J Gastrointest Surg 1998;2:496–503.
63. Sharma VK, Howden CW. Prophylactic antibiotic administration reduces sepsis and mortality in acute necrotizing pancreatitis: A meta-analysis. Pancreas 2001;22:1–4.
64. Villatoro E, Larvin M, Bassi C. Antibiotic therapy for prophylaxis against infection of pancreatic necrosis in acute pancreatitis. Cochrane Database Syst Rev 2006;(4):CD002941.
65. Manes G, Uomo I, Menchise A, et al. Timing of antibiotic prophylaxis in acute pancreatitis: A controlled randomized study with meropenem. Am J Gastroenterol 2006;101:1348–1353.
66. Luiten EJ, Bruining HA. Antimicrobial prophylaxis in acute pancreatitis: Selective decontamination versus antibiotics. Baillieres Best Pract Res Clin Gastroenterol 1999;13:317–330.
67. Gloor B, Muller CA, Worni M, et al. Pancreatic infection in severe pancreatitis: The role of fungus and multiresistant organisms. Arch Surg 2001;136:592–596.
68. Howard TJ, Temple MB. Prophylactic antibiotics alter the bacteriology of infected necrosis in severe acute pancreatitis. J Am Coll Surg 2002:195:759–767.
69. De Waele JJ, Vogelaers D, Blot S, Colardyn F. Fungal infections in patients with severe acute pancreatitis and the use of prophylactic antibiotics. Clin Infect Dis 2003;37:208–213.
70. Shrikhande S, Friess H, Issenegger C. Fluconazole penetration into the pancreas. Antimicrob Agents Chemother 2000;44:2569–2571.
71. Poon RT, Fan ST. Antisecretory agents for prevention of post-ERCP pancreatitis: Rationale for use and clinical results. JOP 2003;4:33–40.
72. Lavy A, Karban A, Suissa A, Yassin K, Hermesh I, Ben-Amotz A. Natural β-carotene for the prevention of post-ERCP pancreatitis. Pancreas 2004;29:45–50.
73. Murray B, Carter R, Imrie C, Evans S, O'Suilleabhain C. Diclofenac reduces the incidence of acute pancreatitis after endoscopic retrograde cholangiopancreatography. Gastroenterology 2003;124:1786–1791.
74. Arvanitidies D, Anagnostopoulous GI, Giannopoulous D, et al. Can somatostatin prevent post-ERCP pancreatitis? Results of a randomized controlled trial. J Gastroenterol Hepatol 2004;19:278–282.
75. Hoogerwerf WA. Pharmacological management of pancreatitis. Curr Opin Pharmacol 2005;5:578–582.
76. Kim K-P, Kim M-H, Song MH, et al. Autoimmune chronic pancreatitis. Am J Gastroenterol 2004;99:1605–1616.
77. Lerch MM, Albrecht E, Ruthenburger M, et al. Pathophysiology of alcohol-induced pancreatitis. Pancreas 2003;27:291–296.
78. Ammann RW, Muelihaupt B, Zurich Pancreatitis Study Group. The natural history of pain in alcoholic chronic pancreatitis. Gastroenterology 1999;116:1132–1140.

79. Chowdhury RS, Forsmark CE. Review article: Pancreatic function testing. Aliment Pharmacol Ther 2003;17:733–750.
80. Warshaw A, Banks PA, Fernandez-del C. American Gastroenterological Association Technical Review: Treatment of pain in chronic pancreatitis. Gastroenterology 1998;115:765–776.
81. Andren-Sandberg A, Hoem D, Gislason H. Pain management in chronic pancreatitis. Eur J Gastroenterol 2002;14:957–970.
82. Whitcomb D, Pfutzer RH, Slivka A. Alcoholic chronic pancreatitis. Curr Treat Option Gastroenterol 1999;2:273–282.
83. American Gastroenterological Association Medical Position Statement: Treatment of pain in chronic pancreatitis. Gastroenterology 1998;115:763–764.
84. Conwell DL, Zuccaro G. Pain management in chronic pancreatitis. Curr Treat Option Gastroenterol 1999;2:295–304.
85. Bhutani MS, Pasricha PJ. Neurolytic approaches for the treatment of pain in patients with chronic pancreatitis. Curr Treat Option Gastroenterol 2003;6:375–379.
86. Brown A, Hughes M, Tenner S, et al. Does pancreatic enzyme supplementation reduce pain in patients with chronic pancreatitis: A meta-analysis. Am J Gastroenterol 1997;92:2032–2035.
87. Mossner J. Palliation of pain in chronic pancreatitis: Use of enzymes. Surg Clin North Am 1999;79:861–872.
88. Walkowiak J, Witmanowski H, Strzykala K, et al. Inhibition of endogenous pancreatic enzyme secretion by oral pancreatic enzyme treatment. Eur J Gastroenterol 2003;33:65–69.
89. Greenberger NJ. Enzymatic therapy in patients with chronic pancreatitis. Gastroenterol Clin North Am 1999;28:687–693.
90. Keller J, Layer P. Pancreatic enzyme supplementation therapy. Curr Treat Option Gastroenterol 2003;6:369–374.
91. Layer P, Keller J, Lankich PG. Pancreatic enzyme replacement therapy. Curr Gastroenterol Rep 2001;3:101–108.
92. Apte MN, Keogh GW, Wilson JS. Chronic pancreatitis: Complications and management. J Clin Gastroenterol 1999;29:225–240.
93. Bruno MJ, Borm JJ, Hock FJ, et al. Gastric transit and pharmacodynamics of a two-millimeter enteric-coated pancreatin microsphere preparation in patients with chronic pancreatitis. Dig Dis Sci 1998;43:203– 213.
94. Halm U, Loser C, Lohr M, et al. A double-blind randomized, multicentre, crossover study to prove equivalence of pancreatin minimicrospheres versus microspheres in exocrine pancreatic insufficiency. Aliment Pharmacol Ther 1999;13:951–957.
95. Hendeles L, Hochhaus G, Kazerounian S. Generic and alternative brand-name pharmaceutical equivalent: Select with caution. Am J Hosp Pharm 1993;50:323–329.
96. Dominguez-Munoz JE, Iglesias-Garcia J, Iglesias-Rev M, et al. Effect of the administration schedule on the therapeutic efficacy of oral pancreatic supplements in patients with exocrine pancreatic insufficiency: A randomized, three-way crossover study. Aliment Pharmacol Ther 2005;21:993–1000.
97. Littlewood JM. Update on intestinal strictures. J R Soc Med 1999;92(Suppl 37):41–49.
98. DiMagno EP. Gastric acid suppression and treatment of severe exocrine pancreatic insufficiency. Best Pract Res Clin Gastroenterol 2001:15:477–486.
99. Wehler M, Nichterlein R, Fischer B, et al. Factors associated with health-related quality of life in chronic pancreatitis. Am J Gastroenterol 2003;98:138–146.

CHAPTER 42 Viral Hepatitis

PAULINA DEMING, RENEE-CLAUDE MERCIER, AND MANJUNATH P. PAI

KEY CONCEPTS

1. Hepatitis A is transmitted via the fecal–oral route. Transmission is most likely to occur through travel to countries with high rates of hepatitis A, poor sanitation and hygiene, and overcrowded areas.
2. Hepatitis A causes an acute, self-limiting illness and does not lead to chronic infection. There are three stages of infection: incubation, acute hepatitis, and convalescence. Rarely the infection progresses to liver failure.
3. Treatment of hepatitis A consists of supportive care. There is no role for antiviral agents in treatment.
4. Hepatitis B causes both acute and chronic infection. Infants and children are at high risk for chronic infection.
5. Several therapies are available for hepatitis B, including lamivudine, interferon α_{2b}, pegylated interferon α_{2a}, entecavir, adefovir, and telbivudine. Patient status, extent of disease, viral load, and viral resistance are all considered when deciding on treatment.
6. Chronic hepatitis B patients may require long-term therapy. Long-term therapy poses a challenge because of the potential for developing resistance. Resistance to lamivudine is most common, although resistance mutations to telbivudine, adefovir, and entecavir have also been seen. Optimal treatment of resistant strains is unknown.
7. Prevention of hepatitis B infections focuses on immunization of all children and at-risk adults.
8. Hepatitis C is an insidious, blood-borne infection. Injection drug use is the major mode of transmission in the United States.
9. Combination pegylated interferon and ribavirin therapy is the treatment of choice for hepatitis C. Treatment duration for hepatitis C infections is 48 weeks for viral genotype 1, and 24 weeks for genotypes 2 and 3. However, therapy may be optimized based on infecting genotype and virologic response. Viral genotype 1 is most difficult to treat.
10. Side effects of hepatitis C therapy pose a significant obstacle to completion of therapy and chance for cure. Adjunct pharmacologic therapy and dose reductions may be necessary to prevent premature cessation of treatment.

Learning objectives, review questions, and other resources can be found at **www.pharmacotherapyonline.com.**

The major hepatotrophic viruses responsible for viral hepatitis are hepatitis A, hepatitis B, hepatitis C, delta hepatitis, and hepatitis E. All share clinical, biochemical, immunoserologic, and histologic findings. Both hepatitides A and E are spread through fecal–oral contamination; whereas hepatitides B, C, and delta are transmitted parenterally. Infection with delta hepatitis requires coinfection with hepatitis B. Although the rates of acute infection have declined, viral hepatitis remains a major cause of morbidity and mortality with a significant impact on healthcare costs in the United States. Significant therapeutic advances have occurred with hepatitis B with the approval of new agents and updated guidelines for care. For hepatitis C, the challenge remains of increasing successful outcomes while minimizing side effects of therapy. This chapter focuses on hepatitides A, B, and C.

HEPATITIS A

Hepatitis A virus (HAV), or infectious hepatitis, is often a self-limiting and acute viral infection of the liver posing a health risk worldwide. The infection is rarely fatal. According to the Centers for Disease Control and Prevention (CDC), the 4,488 reported cases of acute clinical hepatitis A infection in the United States in 2005 were the lowest in recorded history.[1] Although vaccine preventable, HAV continues to be one of the most commonly reported infections.

EPIDEMIOLOGY

Various patient groups are at increased risk for infection with HAV. Children pose a particular problem with the spread of the disease because they often remain clinically asymptomatic and are infectious for longer periods of time than adults. Traditionally, the most likely patient group to be affected is household or close personal contacts of an infected person. (1) Infection primarily occurs through the fecal–oral route, by person-to-person, or by ingestion of contaminated food or water. Incidentally, HAV's prevalence is linked to regions with low socioeconomic status and specifically to those with poor sanitary conditions and overcrowding. Rarely, the virus can be spread through blood or blood products. Despite being detectable in saliva, there are no data to suggest transmission through this mode of contact.[2] International travel and immigration also mitigate potential exposure to the virus.

Analysis of the 5,683 cases reported in the United States in 2004 revealed a change in risk factors for infectivity.[3] Although rates have declined as a result of successful vaccination programs to a record low of 1.9 cases per 100,000 people in 2004, HAV rates have increased among international travelers, injection-drug users (IDUs), and men who have sex with men (MSM).[3] Travel to HAV endemic areas now represents the largest proportion of acute HAV cases.[1,3] Additional patient groups that are at risk include patients with chronic liver disease and persons working with nonhuman primates. In pregnant women, acute HAV infection may be associated with maternal complications and preterm labor.[4] Food-borne outbreaks also occur; a 2003 outbreak in Pennsylvania was associated with more than 500 persons infected and 3 deaths, and was linked to green onions imported from Mexico.[5]

HAV infections acquired through international travel create significant HAV-associated costs in terms of loss of work time and healthcare costs. Despite low endemic rates and successful vaccinations of at-risk populations in the United States, unvaccinated children acquiring HAV infections abroad can serve as reservoirs of the virus upon return to the United States, even while remaining clinically asymptomatic themselves. Nearly 40% of children younger than age 15 years with HAV had international travel as a risk factor in 2004.[3] According to the CDC, the majority of travel-related cases correspond to travel to Central and South America and Mexico.[3] Most Americans traveling to Mexico do not consider that country to be a risk in part because of Mexico's proximity to the United States. Moreover, most tourists falsely believe that higher-end resorts imply safety and that short visits to foreign countries are not associated with a risk for infection. In fact, frequent, short visits will have a cumulative risk for infection that should not be ignored.[6]

TABLE 42-1 Clinical Presentation of Acute Hepatitis A

Signs and symptoms
• The preicteric phase brings nonspecific influenza-like symptoms consisting of anorexia, nausea, fatigue, and malaise
• Abrupt onset of anorexia, nausea, vomiting, malaise, fever, headache, and right upper quadrant abdominal pain with acute illness
• Icteric hepatitis is generally accompanied by dark urine, acholic (light-colored) stools, and worsening of systemic symptoms
• Pruritus is often a major complaint of icteric patients
Physical examination
• Icteric sclera, skin, and secretions
• Mild weight loss of 2 to 5 kg
• Hepatomegaly
Laboratory tests
• Positive serum immunoglobulin M anti-hepatitis A virus
• Mild elevations of serum bilirubin, γ-globulin, and hepatic transaminase (alanine transaminase and aspartate transaminase) values to about twice normal in acute anicteric disease
• Elevations of alkaline phosphatase, γ-glutamyl transferase, and total bilirubin in patients with cholestatic illness

ETIOLOGY

Hepatitis A is a RNA virus belonging to the genus *Hepatovirus* of the Picornaviridae family. Humans are the only known reservoir for the virus and transmission occurs primarily through the fecal–oral route.[7] The virus is stable in the environment for at least a month and requires heating foods to a minimum of 85°C (185°F) for 1 minute or disinfecting with a 1:100 dilution of sodium hypochlorite (bleach) in tap water for inactivation.[2,8]

Multiple genotypes of the virus exist and although the clinical implications of infection by particular type are unknown, types I and III are the most commonly identified in human outbreaks.[7]

PATHOPHYSIOLOGY

HAV infection is usually acute, self-limiting, and confers lifelong immunity. HAV's life cycle in the human host classically begins with ingestion of the virus. Absorption in the stomach or small intestine allows entry into the circulation and uptake by the liver. Replication of the virus occurs within hepatocytes and gastrointestinal epithelial cells. New virus particles are released into the blood and secreted into bile by the liver. The virus is then either reabsorbed to continue its cycle or excreted in the stool. The enterohepatic cycle will continue until interrupted by antibody neutralization.[7] The exact mechanism of replication and secretion is unknown; however, the initial viral expansion does not seem to be associated with hepatic injury as peak viral fecal excretion precedes clinical signs and symptoms of infection.[2]

On biopsy, acute hepatitis is marked by hepatocellular degeneration, inflammatory infiltrate, and hepatocyte regeneration. Hepatocellular degeneration occurs as a result of immune-mediated injury and not as a direct cytopathic effect of the virus.[9] Clinical symptoms of HAV typically identify the onset of the immune response. Cytolytic T cells mediate hepatocyte lysis to eradicate the virus and mark the cellular immune response with rising hepatic enzyme levels.[7]

CLINICAL PRESENTATION

❷ The incubation period of HAV is approximately 28 days, with a range of 15 to 50 days. Viremia occurs within 1 to 2 weeks of exposure as patients begin to shed the virus.[2] Table 42–1 summarizes the clinical features of acute hepatitis A. Peak fecal shedding of the virus precedes the onset of clinical symptoms and elevated liver enzymes. Acute hepatitis follows, beginning with the preicteric or prodromal period. The phase is marked by an abrupt onset of nonspecific symptoms, some very mild.[2] Other, more unusual symptoms include chills, myalgia, arthralgia, cough, constipation, diarrhea, pruritus, and urticaria. The phase generally lasts 2 months. There are no specific symptoms unique to HAV. Liver enzyme levels rise within the first weeks of infection, peaking approximately in the fourth week and normalizing by the eighth week. Conjugated bilirubinemia, or dark urine, precedes the onset of the icteric period. The concentration of virus declines at this point and patients are generally considered noninfectious approximately 1 week after the onset of jaundice.[10] Gastrointestinal (GI) symptoms may persist or subside during this time and some patients may have hepatomegaly. Duration of the icteric period varies and corresponds to disease duration. It averages between 7 and 30 days.[7]

Symptoms and severity of HAV vary according to age. Children younger than 6 years of age typically are asymptomatic. Symptoms, if they do occur, do not include jaundice. In older children and adults, the majority of patients present with symptoms that last less than 2 months and 70% of adults experience jaundice. Peak viral shedding precedes the onset of GI symptoms in adults. In young children, shedding can occur for months following diagnosis.[2] Because children are often asymptomatic and will shed the virus for long periods of time they can serve as a reservoir for the spread of HAV.

HAV RNA is detectable in the serum for an average of 17 days before peak alanine aminotransferase (ALT) levels and can persist for an average of 79 days after the onset of symptoms. In some patients, serum HAV is detectable for more than a year.[11] Immunoglobulin (Ig) M antibody to HAV (anti-HAV) is required for a diagnosis of acute infection. It becomes detectable 5 to 10 days before the onset of symptoms and can persist for months after. IgG anti-HAV replaces IgM and indicates host immunity following the acute phase of the infection. Serologic tests exist but should be interpreted with caution.[8] FDA-approved assays for serologic testing detect IgM and total anti-HAV (IgG and IgM). Patients who have detectable total anti-HAV and a negative IgM have resolved their infection. Although patients who are successfully immunized will have IgG, assays are not sensitive enough to detect anti-HAV in most patients. Similarly, patients who receive intramuscular (IM) Ig will also have anti-HAV but concentrations are below the level of detection of most assays.[2,8] Concentrations of antibody often fall to 10 to 100 times lower than what would be expected after a natural course of infection. Although a positive anti-HAV result confirms protection, undetectable concentration of anti-HAV may not necessarily imply that protective levels were not achieved.[8]

HAV does not lead to chronic infections. Some patients may experience symptoms for up to 9 months. Rarely, patients experience complications from HAV including relapsing hepatitis, cholestatic hepatitis, and fulminant hepatitis. Fatalities from HAV are generally rare though more likely in patients older than age 50 years and in persons with preexisting liver disease.[8] Fulminant hepatitis occurs mostly in young children and adults with chronic liver disease. Although occurring in 0.01% of clinical infections, fulminant hepatitis has a high fatality rate and therapy consists of supportive care.[9]

Diagnosis

A diagnosis of HAV is based on clinical criteria of an acute onset of fatigue, abdominal pain, loss of appetite, intermittent nausea and vomiting, jaundice or elevated serum aminotransferase levels, and serologic testing for IgM anti-HAV. Serologic testing is necessary to differentiate the diagnosis from other types of hepatitis.

TREATMENT

Hepatitis A Virus

■ DESIRED OUTCOME

❸ The majority of people infected with HAV can be expected to fully recover without clinical sequelae.[7] Nearly all individuals will have clinical resolution within 6 months of the infection, and a majority will have done so by 2 months. Rarely, symptoms persist for longer or patients relapse. The ultimate goal of therapy is complete clinical resolution. Other goals include reducing complications from the infection, normalization of liver function, and reducing infectivity and transmission.

■ GENERAL APPROACH TO TREATMENT

No specific treatment options exist for HAV infections. Instead, patients should receive general supportive care. In patients who develop liver failure, transplant is the only option. Although hepatocellular damage occurs through immune-mediated responses, steroid use is not recommended.[12] Prevention and prophylaxis are key to managing the virus. The importance of good hand hygiene cannot be overemphasized in preventing disease transmission. Immunoglobulin is used for pre- and postexposure prophylaxis, and offers passive immunity. Active immunity is achieved through vaccination. Vaccines were approved for use in 1995 and implemented in the routine vaccination of children, as well as at-risk adults, to reduce the overall incidence of HAV.[8]

Prevaccination serologic testing to determine susceptibility is generally not recommended. In some cases, testing may be cost-effective if the cost of the test is less than that of the vaccine and if the person is from a moderate to high endemic area and likely to have prior immunity. Prevaccination serologic testing of children is not recommended. Similarly, because of high vaccine response, postvaccine serologic testing is not recommended.[8]

PREVENTION OF HEPATITIS A

HAV is easily preventable with vaccination. Because children often serve as reservoirs of the disease, vaccine programs have targeted children as the most effective means to control HAV. Two vaccines for HAV are available and are incorporated into the routine childhood vaccination schedule. In October 2005, the FDA reduced the minimum age for the vaccines to 12 months of age. In response, the Advisory Committee on Immunization Practices recommended expanding vaccine coverage to all children, including catch-up programs for children living in areas without existing vaccination programs. The new recommendations were enacted in the attempt to further reduce HAV incidence rates and possibly to eradicate the virus.[13] Adult vaccination recommendations also exist (Table 42–2).

TABLE 42-2 Recommendations for Hepatitis A Virus (HAV) Vaccination

All children at 1 year of age
In areas without existing hepatitis A vaccination programs, catch-up vaccination of children ages 2–18 years can be considered
Persons traveling to or working in countries that have high or intermediate endemicity of infection[a]
Men who have sex with men
Illegal-drug users
Persons with occupational risk for infection (e.g., persons who work with HAV-infected primates or with HAV in a research laboratory)
Persons who have clotting factor disorders
Persons with chronic liver disease

[a]Travelers to Canada, Western Europe, Japan, Australia, or New Zealand are at no greater risk for infection than they are in the United States. All other travelers should be assessed for HAV risk.
From Centers for Disease Control and Prevention.[8,13]

Routine prevention of HAV transmission includes regular hand washing with soap and water after using the bathroom, changing a diaper, and before food preparation. For travelers to countries with high endemic rates of HAV, even short-term stays in urban and upscale resorts are not risk-free.[8] In particular, contaminated water and ice, fresh produce, and any uncooked foods pose a risk.[7]

Vaccines to Prevent Hepatitis A

Two inactivated virus vaccines are currently licensed in the United States: Havrix and Vaqta. Both vaccines are inactivated virus and are available for pediatric and adult use. The differences in the two vaccines are in the use of a preservative and in expression of antigen content. Vaqta is formulated without a preservative and uses units of HAV antigen to express potency. Havrix uses 2-phenoxyphenol as a preservative and antigen content is expressed as enzyme-linked immunosorbent assay units. Pediatric dosing is indicated for children 12 months of age through 18 years of age, and adult dosing is for patients ages 19 years and older (Table 42–3).[8] Although high seroconversion rates of ≥94% are achieved with the first dose, both vaccines recommend a booster shot to achieve the highest possible antibody titers. There are insufficient data to suggest the vaccines offer sufficient postexposure protection in outbreak settings. Both vaccines may be given concomitantly with immunoglobulin and the two brands are interchangeable for booster shots.[8]

Vaccine efficacy may be reduced in certain patient populations. In HIV (human immunodeficiency virus)-infected patients, greater immunogenic response may correlate with higher baseline CD4 cell counts. Response to the HAV vaccine as determined by detection of anti-HAV after vaccination found that among HIV patients, females and patients with CD4 counts >200 cells/mm^3 at vaccination had a higher response rate.[15]

The most common side effects of the vaccines include soreness and warmth at the injection site, headache, malaise, and pain.

TABLE 42-3 Recommended Dosing of Havrix and Vaqta

Vaccine	Age (y)	Dose	No. of Doses	Schedule (mo)
Havrix	1–18	720 ELISA units	2	0, 6–12
	≥19	1,440 ELISA units	2	0, 6–12
Vaqta	1–18	25 units	2	0, 6–18
	≥19	50 units	2	0, 6–18

ELISA, enzyme-linked immunoabsorbent assay.
From Centers for Disease Control and Prevention.[13]

Reported serious adverse events include anaphylaxis, Guillain-Barré syndrome, brachial plexus neuropathy, transverse myelitis, multiple sclerosis, encephalopathy, and erythema multiforme. However, causality of these reported events has not been established. Furthermore, incidence of serious adverse events in the vaccinated population did not differ from the incidence in nonvaccinated populations. It is important to note that more than 65 million doses of the vaccine have been administered and despite routine monitoring for adverse events, there are no data to suggest a greater incidence of serious adverse events among vaccinated people compared to nonvaccinated. The vaccine is considered safe.[8]

Twinrix is a bivalent vaccine for hepatitides A and B that was approved by the FDA in 2001. The vaccine is approved for people ages 18 and older and is given at 0, 1, and 6 months. Although seroconversion exceeds 90% for HAV after the first dose, the full three-dose series is required for maximal hepatitis B virus (HBV) seroconversion. The combined vaccine offers the advantage of immunization against both types of hepatitis in a single vaccine.

Immunoglobulin

Ig is used when pre- or postexposure prophylaxis against HAV infection is needed. A sterile preparation of concentrated antibodies against HAV, Ig provides protection by passive transfer of antibody. Ig is most effective if given in the incubation period of the infection. Receipt of Ig within the first 2 weeks of infection will reduce infectivity and moderate the infection in 85% of patients. Patients who received at least 1 dose of the HAV vaccine at least 1 month earlier do not need pre- or postexposure prophylaxis with Ig.[8] Ig is available both as an intravenous (IV) and IM injection but for HAV exposure, only the IM is used. If given to infants or pregnant women, the thimerosal-free formulation should be used.

International travelers are the major patient population receiving preexposure prophylaxis with Ig. HAV vaccination or prophylaxis with Ig is recommended for travelers to countries with high endemic rates of HAV. Serious adverse events are rare. Anaphylaxis has been reported in patients with Ig A deficiency. Patients who had an anaphylaxis reaction to Ig should not receive it. There is no contraindication for use in pregnancy or lactation.

Dosing of Ig is the same for adults and children. For postexposure prophylaxis and for short-term preexposure coverage of <3 months, a single dose of 0.02 mL/kg is given intramuscularly. For long-term preexposure prophylaxis of ≤5 months, a single dose of 0.06 mL/kg is used. Either the deltoid or gluteal muscle may be used. In children younger than 24 months of age, Ig can be given in the anterolateral thigh muscle.[8]

For people who were recently exposed to HAV and who had not been previously vaccinated, Ig is indicated in the following situations: (a) when in close personal contact with an HAV-infected person; (b) all staff and attendees of daycare centers when HAV is documented; (c) if they were involved in a common source exposure; for example, in a food-borne outbreak with an HAV-infected food handler, other food handlers at the location should receive Ig; if the case person handled food and had poor hygiene or diarrhea, patrons of the location should also receive Ig if they can be identified and located within the 2 weeks of the exposure; (d) classroom contacts of an index case patient; and (e) schools, hospitals, and work settings where close personal contact occurred with the case patient.[8]

Ig can be given concomitantly with the HAV vaccine. Although the antibody titer will be lower than if the vaccine were administered alone, the response is still protective. However, Ig can interfere with the response of other vaccines and should be delayed. The measles, mumps, and rubella (MMR) vaccine should be delayed for a minimum of 3 months after receipt of Ig. The varicella vaccine must be delayed for 5 months. Conversely, Ig should not be given to patients who received the MMR within 2 weeks or the varicella vaccine within 3 weeks. In situations where the benefits of Ig outweigh the benefits of the other vaccines, revaccination can be performed after Ig administration. For the MMR, revaccination should be at least 3 months later, and for the varicella vaccine, at least 5 months later.[8] In general, Ig does not interfere with inactivated vaccines and may be administered safely with other vaccines traditionally given to travelers to some developing countries, such as the oral poliovirus or yellow fever vaccine.[8]

PHARMACOECONOMIC CONSIDERATIONS

Although the costs of an HAV outbreak are significant, routine vaccination of all individuals is not cost-effective. Rather, by targeting at-risk populations, the majority of cases can be prevented. Children play a pivotal role in disease persistence. The use of the HAV vaccine is cost-effective in children and offers the most benefit to the personal contacts of children, reflecting the role of children as a reservoir for the disease.[15] The use of the combined HAV-HBV vaccine is effective in reducing costs associated with HAV among persons who are at increased risk for infection. Among 100,000 healthcare workers in high endemic states, the vaccine was anticipated to reduce the number of related work loss days from 34,463 to 4,667 days, an estimated savings of $6.1 million.[15] Nearly $2 million in savings could be seen in costs associated with HAV treatment. In a sexually transmitted diseases clinic serving 1 million patients, the combined vaccine was expected to prevent 2,263 occult infections and cost $13,397 per quality-adjusted life-year (QALY).[16] Both studies predicted between $2 and $2.5 million in savings associated with HAV treatment, realized mostly in reduced hospitalizations. The risk of HAV from food transmission in the United States is low and can be avoided in many cases by adherence to basic hygiene practices.

HEPATITIS B

Although a vaccine was made available in 1981, HBV has acutely infected more than 2 billion people globally, leading to chronic infection in more than 350 million people.[17] Chronic infection with HBV is a major public health issue as it serves as a reservoir for continued HBV transmission and poses a significant risk of death resulting from liver disease. More than 1 million people per year die as a result of liver cirrhosis and hepatocellular carcinoma (HCC).

EPIDEMIOLOGY

According to the CDC, only 12% of the global population lives in an area of low prevalence for hepatitis B, defined as an area where <2% of the population is HB_sAg (hepatitis B surface antigen)-positive.[17] Prevalence can vary regionally; however, areas commonly associated with high infectivity rates include sub-Saharan Africa, most of Asia, as well as the Amazon and southern parts of Eastern and Central Europe.[17] Areas of high prevalence, approximately 45% of the global population, are of special concern because most infections are of infants and children and >90% of cases lead to a chronic carrier state. Although less than 1% of people have chronic infection in both Western Europe and North America,[17] in the United States, HBV is the second most common type of acute viral hepatitis and the third most reported preventable disease, second only to HAV.[18] There are approximately 1.25 million chronically infected HBV people in the United States. In 2005, an estimated 51,000 people developed new infections. Annually, an estimated 3,000 to 5,000 people die from chronic liver disease attributable to HBV.[1]

HBV is transmitted sexually, parenterally, and perinatally. In areas of high HBV prevalence, perinatal transmission from mother to infant is most common, whereas in areas of intermediate prevalence, horizontal transmission from child to child is most common. Sexual contact, both homosexual and heterosexual, and injection-drug use are the predominant forms of transmission in low-endemic countries such as the United States.[19] Concentration of HBV is high in blood, serum, and wound exudates of infected persons. The virus is detectable in moderate quantities in semen, vaginal fluid, and saliva, and is present in low concentrations in urine, feces, sweat, tears, and breast milk.[18,20] Transmission can occur through contact with infected body fluids in the absence of blood, as the virus may be stable in the environment for a number of days.[20,21] In the United States in 2004, no risk factor could be identified for the majority of acute infections with HBV. International travel was the most prevalent identifiable risk factor, followed by injection drug use and sexual or household contact with a hepatitis B-infected person. Among children younger than 15 years of age, the largest overall risk factor in 2004 was international travel.[3] No cases were documented for patients receiving transfusions or on hemodialysis.[17] Among racial and ethnic groups, HBV is highest among non-Hispanic blacks. Asians/Pacific Islanders and non-Hispanic whites have similar rates, while Hispanics have the lowest HBV rates.[3]

The mode of transmission has clinical implications because chronic infections are associated with infection acquired in younger patients, especially those infected perinatally and in early childhood.[20]

ETIOLOGY

The HBV is a DNA virus of the family Hepadnaviridae. It is a partially double-stranded, circular DNA with 3,200 base pairs that typically infects liver cells, although it has been found in kidney, pancreas, and mononuclear cells.[22,23] Seven HBV genotypes exist (A to H) with distinct geographic distribution (Table 42–4). It is possible that genotype prevalence may be dependent on mode of transmission as types B and C are found in areas where vertical transmission is the primary mode of infection.[24] Correlations between clinical outcomes and HBV genotypes have been suggested, with genotype C associated with more severe liver injury, including liver cirrhosis and progression to HCC.[24] A noted limitation of studies is frequently small sample sizes and a predominance of research from Asia, primarily comparing genotypes B and C.[24] Nonetheless, a study of a diverse patient immigrant population infected with genotypes A, B, C, D, and E, confirmed that more severe liver fibrosis was significantly higher in HBV genotypes A, C, and D-infected patients. Genotype B may be more benign because it is associated with faster seroconversion.[25] Resistance mutations may contribute to genotype virulence and hence impact severity of liver disease in infection.[26]

PATHOPHYSIOLOGY

Upon infection, replication of the virus begins by attachment of the virion to the hepatocyte cell surface receptors. The particles are transported to the nucleus where the DNA is converted into closed, circular DNA that serves as a template for pregenomic RNA. Viral RNA is then transcribed and transported back to the cytoplasm where it can alternatively serve as a reservoir for future viral templates or bud into the intracellular membrane with the viral envelope proteins and infect other cells.[22,27] The viral genome has four reading frames coding for various proteins and enzymes required for viral replication and spread. Several of these proteins are used diagnostically (Table 42–5). The HB_sAg is the most abundant of the three surface antigens and is detectable at the onset of clinical symptoms. Its persistence past 6 months after initial detection corresponds to chronic infection and poses an increased risk for cirrhosis, hepatic decompensation, and HCC. Development of antibody to HB_sAg (anti-HB_sAg) confers immunity to the virus and clearance of HB_sAg is associated with favorable outcomes.[23,28] The precore polypeptide encodes for the secretory protein hepatitis B_e antigen (HB_eAg) and the hepatitis B core antigen (HB_cAg) proteins. Although HB_eAg's role in infection is nebulous, it is present in an acute infection and is replaced by antibodies (anti-HB_eAg) once an infection is resolved. HB_eAg was assumed to be a marker of viral replication and infectivity; however, it is now known that some viral mutants exist that are unable to have or have downregulated expression of HB_eAg, although their ability to replicate is not affected.[29] HB_eAg-negative mutants pose a particular clinical challenge because they are refractory to treatment. The HB_cAg is a nucleocapsid protein that, when expressed on hepatocytes, promotes immune-mediated cell death. High levels of antibodies (IgM anti-HB_cAg) are detectable during acute infections. The detection of IgM anti-HB_cAg is also a reliable assay for diagnosing fulminant acute hepatitis where HB_sAg and HBV DNA are often undetectable.[22,30] Patients who respond to vaccine will have anti-HB_sAg only.[8]

HBV itself does not seem to be pathogenic to cells; rather, it is thought that the immune response to the virus is cytotoxic to hepatocytes. Antigen nonspecific inflammatory responses triggered by T cells may be responsible for most hepatic injury, with progression to cirrhosis and HCC.[20,22] The immune response includes major histocompatibility complex (MHC) class I CD8 cytotoxic T cells and MHC class II CD4 T-helper cells. In both an acute and chronic

TABLE 42-4 Worldwide Distribution of Hepatitis B Virus Genotypes

Genotype	Geographic Distribution
A	Northern/central Europe, North America, sub-Saharan Africa
B, C	Southeast Asia, Japan
D	Mediterranean region, Middle East, India
F	Central and South America, North American Indians, Polynesia
G	France, North America
H	Central America

Data from Ganne-Carrie N, Williams V, Kaddouri H, et al. Significance of hepatitis B virus genotypes A to E in a cohort of patients with chronic hepatitis B in the Seine Saint Denis district of Paris (France). J Med Virol 2006;78:335–340.

TABLE 42-5 Interpretation of Serologic Tests in Hepatitis B Virus

Tests	Result	Interpretation
HB_sAg	(–)	
Anti-HB_c	(–)	Susceptible
Anti-HB_s	(–)	
HB_sAg	(–)	
Anti-HB_c	(+)	Immune because of natural infection
Anti-HB_s	(+)	
HB_sAg	(–)	Immune because of vaccination (valid only if test performed 1–2 months after third vaccine dose)
Anti-HB_c	(–)	
Anti-HB_s	(+)	
HB_sAg	(+)	
Anti-HB_c	(+)	Acute infection
IgM anti-HB_c	(+)	
HB_sAg	(+)	
Anti-HB_c	(+)	Chronic infection
IgM anti-HB_c	(–)	
Anti-HB_s	(–)	
HB_sA	(–)	Four interpretations possible:
Anti-HB_c	(+)	1. Recovery from acute infection
Anti-HB_s	(–)	2. Distant immunity and test not sensitive enough to detect low level of HB_s in serum
		3. Susceptible with false-positive anti-HB_c
		4. May have undetectable level of HB_sAg in serum and be chronically infected

HB_c, hepatitis B core; HB_s, hepatitis B surface; HB_sA, hepatitis B surface associated; HB_sAg, hepatitis B surface antigen; IgM, immunoglobulin M.

From Centers for Disease Control and Prevention: Hepatitis B Serology, http://www.cdc.gov/ncidod/diseases/hepatitis/b/Bserology.htm.

infection, the antibody response is strong. In an acute infection, however, the cytotoxic T-cell response is critical to viral clearance. If the response is weak, chronic infection is likely.[22] Moreover, liver injury is likely caused by secondary, nonspecific inflammation activated by the initial cytotoxic lymphocyte response and as an attempt by the immune system to clear the virus by destroying HBV antigen presenting hepatocytes. Destruction of hepatocytes results in release of circulating, and hence increased, ALT levels.

Cirrhosis

Cirrhosis results as the liver attempts to regenerate while in an environment of persistent inflammation. Like in other viral hepatitis-induced cirrhoses, continued alcohol consumption exacerbates hepatocellular damage. Most patients with compensated cirrhosis are either asymptomatic or have mild symptoms of epigastric pain and dyspepsia.[25] During cirrhosis, the liver enters a cycle of ongoing liver damage, fibrosis, and attempts at regeneration. The classical appearance of a small and knobby liver reflects the irreversible effect of nodules of regenerating cells integrated with infiltrates of inflammatory induced fibrous tissue. Both viral and clinical factors affect the outcome of cirrhosis (Table 42–6). The development of cirrhosis is mostly insidious and patients can remain stable for years before disease progression. An estimated 20% of all chronic hepatitis B patients develop complications of hepatic insufficiency and portal hypertension as their compensated cirrhosis progresses to decompensated cirrhosis within a 5-year period.[27] Typically, the initial clinical findings of decompensated cirrhosis are ascites, jaundice, variceal bleed, encephalopathy, or a combination of symptoms.[25] Damage is irreversible. Treatment is supportive care and patients are candidates for liver transplantation.

Hepatocellular Carcinoma

HBV is a known risk factor for the development of HCC and in areas of high HBV endemicity, a major complication of the infection.[20,22] The development of HCC can be insidious, occurring in the absence of cirrhosis or in the presence of clinically silent, compensated cirrhosis. Many patients with HCC have no signs of decompensated cirrhosis.[25] The virus itself is not likely the causative agent of the cancer. In most cases, HCC develops after years of inflammatory processes provoked by ongoing HBV infection. Compared to hepatitis C virus (HCV), however, HBV does seem to provoke a more direct carcinogenic effect as evidenced by its presence in less-severe liver disease, and among patients with advanced HCC, HBV infection is associated with a worse survival rate.[31] Several factors influence the development of HCC, as well as predict survival (see Table 42–6). HCC is more prevalent in males; in older patients; in patients coinfected with HCV or delta hepatitis; and in patients with serologic markings of past or present HBV infection, preexisting cirrhosis, or continued alcohol ingestion. Risks for death and decompensation increase with underlying liver disease. Other host-specific or environmental factors may impact the course of liver disease. In Asian patients, HCC tumors are commonly seen in otherwise healthy patients, whereas HCC is typically seen in white patients with chronic liver disease.[32] Persistently elevated HBV DNA levels (≥10,000 copies/mL) predict HCC development, even after adjusting for sex, age, cigarette smoking, alcohol consumption, HB_eAg status, ALT level, and liver cirrhosis.[33] HB_eAg status is not a risk factor. In otherwise healthy patients without coinfection or who do not have HCC or decompensation at the time of seroclearance, HB_sAg seroclearance does predict a favorable long-term outcome.[28] Additional predictors of survival include younger age and maintenance of liver function as evidenced by laboratory findings.[25]

TABLE 42-6 Factors Associated with Hepatitis B Virus (HBV) Cirrhosis and Disease Progression

Persistence of HBV serum DNA
Infection with genotype C
Coinfection with HCV, delta hepatitis, or HIV
Age at diagnosis
Severity of liver disease at diagnosis
Male sex
Frequency of severe hepatic flares
Alcohol use
Laboratory/physical findings of abnormal liver function

HCV, hepatitis C virus; HIV, human immunodeficiency virus.
Compiled from Fattovich,[25] Lok et al.,[27] and Wright.[34]

CLINICAL PRESENTATION

❹ The clinical symptoms and course of an HBV infection are indistinguishable from other types of viral hepatitis. Three phases of an HBV infection exist. During the initial or acute phase of a HBV infection in adults and older children, the HBV enters a 4- to 10-week incubation period, during which antibodies toward the HBV core are produced and the virus replicates profusely. Active viral replication results in high serum HBV DNA levels and HB_eAg secretion.[22] ALT levels may rise slightly, but most patients will remain asymptomatic. Symptoms, if they do occur, include fever, anorexia, nausea, vomiting, jaundice, dark urine, clay-colored or pale stools, and abdominal pain. Most neonates and children are anicteric and have no clinical symptoms, whereas up to half of adult patients are icteric.[25] HB_sAg does not become detectable until after significant viremia. The initial phase is considered immunotolerant because no hepatic injury is sustained, as evidenced by generally normal ALT levels. Patients are highly infectious during this time.[24] In perinatally acquired infections, and in young children, the phase can last for decades—until adulthood.[23] Infected children pose a particular risk because they are often asymptomatic, undiagnosed, and highly infectious.

The immunoactive phase marks a decrease in HBV DNA levels with ongoing secretion of HB_eAg. Patients are symptomatic with intermittent flares of hepatitis and marked increases in ALT levels. More frequent flares are associated with disease progression.[34] The phase can last a few weeks in acute disease, and for years in patients with chronic disease. As the host immune system attempts to gain control of the infection by stopping active viral replication, serum HBV DNA levels drop to undetectable, ALT levels normalize, and liver necroinflammation resolves.[25]

If the infection is self-limiting, HBV DNA quickly subsides, HB_eAg disappears within weeks, and HB_sAg usually resolves within 4 months. The final phase is seroconversion and is defined by the replacement of HB_eAg with anti-HB_eAg. Factors favoring seroconversion include female sex, older age, biochemical activity, and genotype. Flares of hepatitis with ALT levels >5 times the upper limits of normal, compared to <5 times the upper limits of normal, correspond to increased immune system activity and precede seroconversion. The B genotype is associated with earlier seroconversion than genotype C.[25]

Chronic HBV

❹ Patients who continue to have detectable HB_sAg and HB_eAg and a high serum titer of HBV DNA for more than 6 months have chronic HBV.[25] Table 42–7 lists the clinical features of chronic hepatitis B. The most predictive factor for developing a chronic infection is age. Perinatal infections almost always result in chronic infections because of immune tolerance to the virus.[35] Risks of chronicity declines to a rate of 30% in infants and to less than 5% of acute adult infections.[23]

Chronic infections can be controlled in many cases, but cure is not possible because the HBV template is integrated into the host

TABLE 42-7 Clinical Presentation of Chronic Hepatitis B[a]

Signs and symptoms
• Easy fatigability, anxiety, anorexia, and malaise
• Ascites, jaundice, variceal bleeding, and hepatic encephalopathy can manifest with liver decompensation
• Hepatic encephalopathy is associated with hyperexcitability, impaired mentation, confusion, obtundation, and eventually coma
• Vomiting and seizures
Physical examination
• Icteric sclera, skin, and secretions
• Decreased bowel sounds, increased abdominal girth, and detectable fluid wave
• Asterixis
• Spider angiomata
Laboratory tests
• Presence of hepatitis B surface antigen for at least 6 months
• Intermittent elevations of hepatic transaminase (alanine transaminase and aspartate transaminase) and hepatitis B virus DNA greater than 10^5 copies/mL
• Liver biopsies for pathologic classification as chronic persistent hepatitis, chronic active hepatitis, or cirrhosis

[a]Chronic hepatitis B can be present even without all the signs, symptoms, and physical examination findings listed being apparent.

TABLE 42-8 Recommendations for Hepatitis B Virus (HBV) Vaccination

Infants
Adolescents including all previously unvaccinated children <19 years old
All unvaccinated adults at risk for infection
All unvaccinated adults seeking vaccination (specific risk factor not required)
Men and women with a history of other sexually transmitted diseases and persons with a history of multiple sex partners (>1 partner/6 months)
Men who have sex with men
Injection-drug users
Household contacts and sex partners of persons with chronic hepatitis B infection and healthcare and public safety workers with exposure to blood in the workplace
Clients and staff of institutions for the developmentally disabled
International travelers who plan to spend >6 months in countries with high rates of HBV infection and who will have close contact with the local population
Recipients of clotting-factor concentrates
Sexually transmitted disease clinic patients
HIV patient/HIV-testing patients
Drug-abuse treatment and prevention clinic patients
Correctional facilities inmates
Chronic dialysis/ESRD patients

ESRD, end-stage renal disease; HIV, human immunodeficiency virus.
From Centers for Disease Control.[21]

genome. In patients with recurring cycles of viral expression and host immune response, progressive liver damage ensues.[35] Patients can be divided into two types of chronic hepatitis B: those who are HB_eAg-positive and those who are HB_eAg-negative. The ability to express HB_eAg by the virus differentiates the two types of chronic infection. Patients who are HB_eAg-negative can be further subdivided into the active or inactive carrier. HB_eAg-negative chronic HBV patients who are active carriers have high serum HBV DNA, elevated ALT levels, and liver necroinflammation.[25] The clinical course tends to be worse with a very low rate of spontaneous remission. Patients may have long periods of disease remission but recurring flares of hepatitis with increased frequency and severity can progress to cirrhosis and HCC. HB_eAg-negative chronic HBV patients who are inactive carriers have detectable HB_sAg and anti-HB_eAg and have normal ALTs. This patient population usually experiences a more benign course of disease, with the possibility of long-term remission, even seroconversion, although reactivation is possible with the progression to cirrhosis and HCC. Rarely, patients will resolve their infection. Patients with undetectable HB_sAg but with anti-HB_sAg and anti-HB_cAg represent a small portion of patients who are not likely to experience reinfection or reactivation unless immunosuppressed.[25]

HBV MUTATIONS

❺ Among the DNA viruses, HBV is notable for its significantly higher mutation rate.[29] One of the most common mutations consists of a nucleotide substitution either preventing or causing downregulation of the production of HB_eAg. This mutation results in a chronic infection that may have a poorer long-term prognosis. Typically the mutation emerges during the infection and not as an infection by a mutant form of the virus.[29] The selective pressures of the L-nucleoside analog antivirals, including lamivudine, cause the YMDD mutation. The mutation is associated with the active site of the DNA polymerase and causes an altered active site. The incidence of lamivudine resistance increases with each subsequent year of therapy and may be associated with a more severe disease progression.[29] Cross-resistance of lamivudine-resistant YMDD mutants to telbivudine has been demonstrated and patients treated with both lamivudine and telbivudine showed resistance mutations to both drugs. Telbivudine-specific resistance can also occur at rates lower than that seen in lamivudine.[36] Other mutations include resistance to adefovir and entecavir. The addition of lamivudine in adefovir resistance may overcome resistance although the optimal management of either adefovir or entecavir resistant strains is not clear.[29,37]

PREVENTION OF HEPATITIS B

Despite the introduction of the HBV vaccine in 1981 and recommendations on vaccination in 1982, rates of HBV did not decline in the early 1980s. Initial declines in incidence were likely attributable to behavioral changes among high risk groups as a result of the acquired immune deficiency syndrome (AIDS) epidemic. A 94% decline in rates between 1990 and 2004 was seen in children and adolescents, which began with the initiation of screening of pregnant women and subsequent immunizations of infants and recommendations set forth in the 1990s to immunize adolescents. Regulations enacted by Occupational Safety and Health Administration (OSHA) further reduced overall U.S. rates by 75%.[18,21]

❼ Prophylaxis against HBV can be achieved by vaccination or by passive immunity in postexposure cases with hepatitis B immunoglobulin. Vaccination is the most effective strategy to prevent infection and a comprehensive vaccination strategy has been implemented in the United States (Table 42–8). Vaccines use HB_sAg for the antigen via recombinant DNA technology using yeast to prompt active immunity. More than 60 million adolescents and more than 40 million infants and children have received a HBV vaccine in the United States since 1982. The vaccine is considered safe. Since 2000, vaccines licensed in the United States either contain none or trace amounts of thimerosal as a preservative. Available vaccines include two single-antigen products and three combination products. The two single-antigen products are Recombivax HB and Engerix-B. Twinrix is a combination vaccine for HAV and HBV in adults. Comvax and Pediarix are used for children and are used for HBV along with other scheduled vaccines.

Passive immunity in the form of anti-HB_sAg offers temporary protection against HBV and is used in conjunction with the hepatitis B vaccine for postexposure prophylaxis.[21]

TREATMENT

Hepatitis B Virus

■ DESIRED OUTCOME

HBV infections are not curable; rather, the goals of therapy are to increase the chances for seroclearance, prevent disease progression to cirrhosis and HCC, and to minimize further injury in patients with ongoing liver damage.

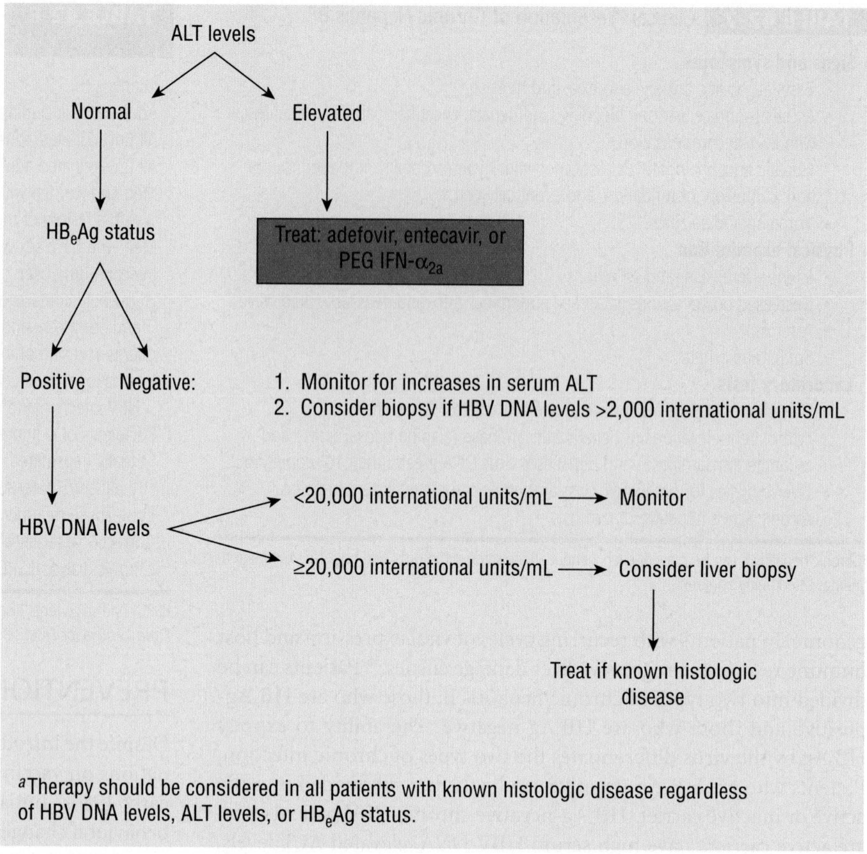

FIGURE 42-1. Suggested treatment algorithm for chronic hepatitis B virus infection based on the recommendations of the American Gastroenterological Association. (ALT, alanine transaminases; HB$_e$Ag, hepatitis B e antigen; PEG INF, pegylated interferon.) *(Adapted from reference 29.)*

■ GENERAL APPROACH TO TREATMENT

❺ Response to therapy is monitored by biochemical (normalization of ALT levels), histologic examination of liver cells from biopsy (a minimum 2-point decrease in histology activity compared to baseline biopsy), and virologic response (undetectable serum HBV DNA levels and loss of HB$_e$Ag in HB$_e$Ag-positive patients).[27] Maintenance of viral suppression is defined as durability of response. In HB$_e$Ag-positive patients, successful therapy includes loss of HB$_e$Ag status and seroconversion to anti-HB$_e$Ag. Other serologic markers are typically not evaluated in clinical trials. Recommendations for treatment consider the patient's age, serum HBV DNA and ALT levels, as well as histologic evidence and clinical progression of disease (Figs. 42–1 and 42–2). Not all chronic HBV patients are candidates for treatment. Some patients may be best managed with periodic monitoring for disease progression because the chances for therapeutic response are unlikely and do not outweigh the risks and costs associated with treatment. Various guidelines have been published and updates made as more drugs are indicated for use in HBV.[27,29,38]

■ NONPHARMACOLOGIC THERAPY

All chronic HBV patients should be counseled on preventing disease transmission. Sexual and household contacts should be vaccinated. To minimize further liver damage, all chronic HBV patients should avoid alcohol and be immunized against HAV. No level of alcohol use has been established as safe.[29] Moreover, patients are encouraged to consult their medical provider before using any new medications, including herbals and nonprescription drugs.[21]

Herbal medicines are an intriguing option to many patients. Four common preparations include *Phyllanthus*, milk thistle, glycyrrhizin (licorice root extract), and a mixture of herbs known as Liv 52. Although some of the products may have some benefits, the methodologic qualities of the trials evaluating the herbs are poor. Randomized, placebo-controlled studies and long-term followup data are lacking. Meta-analysis of existing studies demonstrated that milk thistle and Liv 52 do not affect the course of liver disease. Herbal treatment is not recommended for patients with chronic hepatitis B.[39]

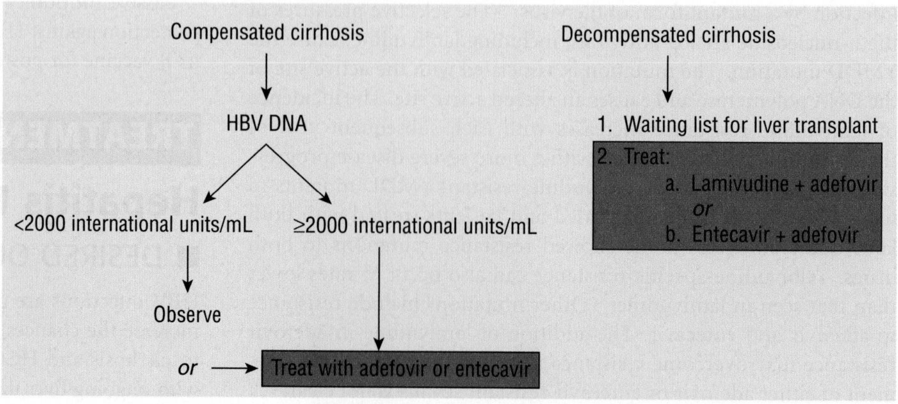

FIGURE 42-2. Suggested treatment algorithm based on the recommendations of the American Gastroenterological Association for chronic hepatitis B virus-infected patients with cirrhosis. *(Adapted from reference 29.)*

■ PHARMACOLOGIC THERAPY

❺ Because hepatic damage is sustained by ongoing viral replication, drug therapy aims to suppress viral replication by either immune mediating or antiviral agents. In the United States, interferon (IFN)-α_{2b}, lamivudine, telbivudine, adefovir, entecavir, and pegylated IFN-α_{2a} are all approved as first-line therapy options for chronic HBV.[29]

Interferon

IFN-α_{2b} therapy was the first approved therapy for treatment of HBV and improves long-term outcomes and survival.[20] Acting as a host cytokine, it has antiviral, antiproliferative, and immunomodulatory effects in chronic HBV.[40] Several factors correlate with improved response to IFN therapy, including increased ALT and HBV DNA levels, high histologic activity score at biopsy, and being non-Asian. Asian patients tend to have more normal ALT levels in chronic infection, confounding the actual impact of ethnicity on infection.[40]

Patients who respond to IFN therapy tend to have a more durable response than that seen with lamivudine, likely as a consequence of IFN's stimulation of the immune response for seroconversion. Seroconversion rates range from 30% to 40% and are often permanent, although relapse is more likely in HB_eAg-negative patients.[35,41] The duration of therapy is finite, although the optimal duration of treatment is unclear. Treatment for a minimum of 12 months is associated with greater sustained virologic response rates than treatment for 4 to 6 months. Seroconversion can occur during or after therapy is complete. An extended treatment duration of 24 months may benefit the difficult-to-treat HB_eAg-negative patient.[35] Conventional IFN therapy is plagued with numerous problems, including the inconvenience of thrice-weekly injections; however, standard interferon therapy has virtually been replaced by the use of pegylated IFN (PEG-IFN) because of the benefits in ease of administration, decreased side effect profile, and improvements in efficacy. Compared to conventional IFN, PEG-IFN has a longer half-life enabling once-weekly injections. For HBV treatment, the approved PEG-IFN formulation is PEG-IFN-α_{2a}. Studies comparing PEG-IFN-α_{2a} monotherapy with PEG-IFN-α_{2a}–lamivudine combination therapies suggest that combination therapy caused greater HBV DNA suppression than PEG-IFN-α_{2a} monotherapy, PEG-IFN-α_{2a} monotherapy better achieved HB_eAg seroconversion than lamivudine monotherapy with no difference in combination therapy, and combination therapy resulted in less lamivudine resistance than lamivudine monotherapy. Interferon-based therapies are still limited by multiple adverse effects (Table 42–9). The high risk of infection precludes use of IFN in decompensated cirrhotic patients.[29] In patients with compensated cirrhosis, IFN appears to be safe and effective, although it can provoke hepatic flares and precipitate hepatic decompensation.[29,35]

Lamivudine

Lamivudine, a nucleoside analog, has antiviral activity against both HIV and HBV. It is dosed at 100 mg daily; the optimal duration of treatment is unknown. In both HB_eAg-positive and -negative patients, lamivudine demonstrates profound viral suppression. HBV DNA serum levels are undetectable in 90% of lamivudine-treated patients after 4 weeks.[35] Normalization of ALT levels occurs gradually over 3 to 6 months in most patients. Additionally, fibrotic changes are reduced and may be reversed in some cases. Response to lamivudine is dependent on baseline ALT levels, with higher levels corresponding to greater likelihood of seroconversion. Seroconversion rates increase with duration of therapy and are at 50% by the fifth year of therapy.[29] The advantages of lamivudine-based therapy include its safety profile and patient tolerability and the convenience of an oral tablet. Moreover, lamivudine can safely be used in immunosuppressed and cirrhotic patients.[41] However, lamivudine therapy is not without problems. There is no clear duration of treatment and HB_eAg-negative patients have a less than 20% viral suppression rate after 12 months of therapy. Serum HBV DNA levels return to baseline upon cessation of therapy.[42] Seroconversion rates are less than 20% after 1 year of therapy and will relapse in up to 58% of patients. Relapse rates are highest among Asian patients.[41] Resistance is inevitable and can undermine the value of treatment. The emergence of YMDD mutants increases with each subsequent year of therapy, with rates approaching 70% after 4 years of therapy, and is associated with returns of serum HBV DNA and elevated ALT levels.[20,22] Although seroconversion can occur even after the appearance of resistant mutants,[22] the prognosis is poor for most patients who develop resistance.[35] In HB_eAg-negative chronic hepatitis B, where therapy is long-term and the exact duration of therapy unknown, resistance is an especially daunting problem.[43]

TABLE 42-9	Common Side Effects Associated with Peginterferon Therapy (Experienced by >20% of Patients)
Fatigue	Arthralgia
Fever	Musculoskeletal pain
Headache	Insomnia
Nausea	Depression
Anorexia	Anxiety/emotional lability
Rigors	Alopecia
Myalgia	Injection site reactions

Adefovir

Adefovir dipivoxil is an acyclic nucleoside analog of adenosine monophosphate. The drug acts by inhibiting HBV DNA polymerase. It is dosed at 10 mg daily for 1 year, although the optimal duration of therapy is unknown.[29] A 48-week course of treatment is effective in improving histologic findings, reducing serum HBV DNA and ALT levels, and increasing HB_eAg seroconversion in both HB_eAg-negative and -positive patients.[44,45] Further suppression of HBV DNA and ALT levels occurred in long-term therapy over 4 to 5 years with improved histologic findings.[37] In HB_eAg-negative patients treated for 48 weeks, the benefits of therapy were lost within 4 weeks of stopping adefovir. In contrast, patients treated for 144 weeks maintained benefits throughout the treatment duration and saw continued improvement in fibrosis as the therapy continued. However, rates of seroconversion were low.[37] Historically, increases in serum creatinine limited treatment to doses of 30 mg/day or less. In patients treated chronically at a dose of 10 mg daily, the incidence of nephrotoxicity was the same as placebo. In patients treated with 10 mg/day for a subsequent 48 weeks, the incidence of serum creatinine abnormalities did not change from the first year of therapy.[37] Resistance to adefovir has not been seen within the first year of therapy. Resistant mutants have been identified and do respond to lamivudine therapy, although the full impact on clinical outcomes is not known.[29] In patients with developing lamivudine resistance as demonstrated by rising HBV DNA levels, the addition of adefovir was more effective if done while ALT levels were still normal.[46]

Entecavir

Entecavir is a guanosine nucleoside analog that acts by inhibiting HBV polymerase. An oral agent, it is more potent than lamivudine in suppressing serum HBV DNA levels and is effective in lamivudine-resistant HBV.[29,47] The drug is dosed at 0.5 mg daily in treatment-naive or non–lamivudine-resistant infections and at 1 mg daily in lamivudine-refractory patients. In a 48-week trial comparing it to lamivudine, entecavir resulted in significantly higher rates of histologic improvement, HBV DNA reduction and undetectability, and ALT normalization. No difference in HB_eAg loss or seroconversion was observed in HB_eAg-positive patients.[48] Among all patients, no differences in fibrosis improvement were seen and resistance to entecavir was not detected after 2 years of therapy.[48,49] However, treatment response in lamivudine-resistant patients is lower overall and entecavir-resistant mutants can develop during the course of treatment.[29] Resistance is most likely to occur in patients with preexisting lamivudine resistance.[47] In terms of safety, entecavir is comparable to lamivudine. Patients switched from lamivudine to entecavir are at risk for hepatic flares, although severe flares are unlikely.[47]

Telbivudine

The most recently approved drug for HBV treatment is telbivudine, a HBV-specific nucleoside analog. Telbivudine acts as a competitive inhibitor of viral reverse transcriptase and DNA polymerase. The drug inhibits HBV DNA synthesis with no activity against other viruses or human polymerases.[36] Compared to lamivudine, telbivudine is a more potent suppressor of HBV DNA with greater median HBV DNA log reductions and more patients achieving undetectable viral loads.[36,47] More patients also experienced a normalization of ALT levels. Although more telbivudine-treated patients experienced seroconversion, the difference was not significant. Compared to adefovir, telbivudine significantly reduced HBV DNA levels, although no difference was seen for HB_eAg loss or ALT normalization.[50] Resistance may limit telbivudine's efficacy, although long-term data are needed.[47] During a 1-year study, 5% of patients developed resistance and data suggest telbivudine should not be used in patients with resistance to lamivudine.[36] Varying degrees of hepatic impairment do not alter the kinetics of the drug, nor does the coadministration of lamivudine or adefovir.[51,52] Combination therapy of telbivudine and lamivudine did demonstrate greater seroconversion rates but the difference was not statistically different from monotherapy.[55] The most commonly associated adverse event with telbivudine is upper respiratory tract infection.[50]

ALTERNATIVE DRUG TREATMENTS

Emtricitabine is a cytosine analog approved for use in HIV and with activity against HBV. It is currently not approved for HBV. In a comparative study with placebo, emtricitabine showed a significant decrease in viral load to undetectable in 54% of patients, normalization of ALT levels in 65% of patients, and improvement in necroinflammatory score. However, seroconversion to anti-HB_eAg and HB_eAg loss did not differ between placebo and emtricitabine. Emtricitabine safety was comparable to placebo. At the end of the 48-week treatment, 20 emtricitabine-treated patients had YMDD or YMDD-related resistance mutations.[53]

Tenofovir is a nucleotide analog approved for use in HIV and with activity against HBV. Compared to adefovir in lamivudine-resistant chronic hepatitis B, it showed an earlier and greater suppression of HBV DNA. Toxicity is minimal compared to adefovir. Resistance has not been seen.[41]

Combination therapy has been proposed to counter the issues of resistance. YMDD mutants remain susceptible to adefovir.[46] Adding adefovir to patients on lamivudine when HBV DNA levels began to increase better maintained normal ALT levels and suppressed HBV DNA than waiting to add adefovir until after ALT levels increased.[46] Combination therapy with interferon and lamivudine creates less resistance than lamivudine monotherapy, but the combination did not change the posttherapy response in chronic HB_eAg-negative patients. The American Gastroenterology Association recommends combination therapy with lamivudine or entecavir plus adefovir for decompensated cirrhotic patients with chronic HBV regardless of HBV DNA levels or HB_eAg status.[29]

SPECIAL POPULATIONS

The decision to treat cirrhotic patients depends on disease progression. Patients with decompensated cirrhosis require referral for liver transplant. Most recently updated guidelines suggest lamivudine, adefovir, and entecavir are possible agents for use in cirrhotic patients (see Fig. 42–2).[29] In patients coinfected with HCV, the more dominant form of the virus is targeted for treatment. The current recommendation is to treat HCV according to published guidelines and consider the addition of entecavir or adefovir if HBV DNA levels remain stable or rise.[29]

In HIV coinfected patients, therapy should be tailored specifically to the patient. If the patient is being treated for HIV, certain regimens may be optimized to include drugs with efficacy against HBV, including tenofovir or lamivudine. If patients are on a stable regimen that does not include HBV-active drugs, adefovir may be added.[29]

Although the majority of chronic HBV patients are adults, children may be treated. Lamivudine is indicated for children ages 2 years and older and interferon is approved for use in children ages 1 year and older. Entecavir is approved for adolescents ages 16 years and older, whereas pegylated interferon and adefovir do not have indications for pediatric dosing.

PHARMACOECONOMIC CONSIDERATIONS

Cost considerations in HBV include the cost-effectiveness of the HBV vaccine and available antiviral treatments. The use of a combined HAV/HBV vaccine is cost-effective.[16] Routine use of the HBV vaccine in HIV counseling and testing sites, including sexually transmitted disease clinics, showed it to be an effective and cost-effective measure in preventing HBV among high-risk groups. The model, which considered four different strategies in vaccination, including no vaccination, found that routine vaccination would cost $4,400 per QALY and per life-year saved. When costs of HBV treatment and transplants were included, the cost decreased to $2,200 per QALY, further supporting routine vaccination as a cost-effective measure.[55]

The cost-effectiveness of therapy for chronic HBV patients must address the approval of new agents for treatment. For noncirrhotic chronic HBV patients with elevated ALT levels, the most cost-effective therapy consisted of initiating treatment with lamivudine and switching to adefovir with the development of lamivudine resistance. The salvage strategy cost $8,447 per QALY. Pegylated interferon was not compared.[56] In chronic HBV patients with cirrhosis, entecavir was the most effective, yet more expensive, option. Entecavir cost $25,626 per QALY as compared to adefovir's $19,731 per QALY. Salvage therapy was not found to be cost-effective in this patient population.[57] Pegylated interferon was not compared for initial treatment because of its relative novelty in HBV treatment; because interferon is not considered a treatment option for cirrhosis, it was not included in the analysis of cirrhotic patients.

CLINICAL CONTROVERSY

Although previously published guidelines do not support the use of IFN in cirrhosis because of the potential for an IFN-induced hepatic flare progressing to decompensation, some experts suggest PEG-IFN-α_{2a} may be an option for some patients with compensated cirrhosis. Moreover, some experts argue that lamivudine, although indicated for use in cirrhosis, may cause clinical decompensation because of the drug's high risk for resistance and hence, viral rebound triggering decompensation.

HEPATITIS C

HCV is approximately five times as common as HIV and is responsible for an estimated 10,000 chronic liver disease-associated deaths per year.[1] More than 190,000 deaths from HCV-related disease are expected between 2010 and 2019, with projected costs exceeding $10 billion.[58] Most acute infections are asymptomatic and the course of the infection is insidious. As a result, many patients are not diagnosed until significant disease progression.

EPIDEMIOLOGY

❽ HCV is the most common blood-borne pathogen. In the United States, approximately 3.2 million people are chronically infected with HCV.[1] An estimated 20,000 new HCV infections occurred in 2005; however, because of the clinically silent nature of acute infections and the 20- to 30-year disease progression to cirrhosis, it is the 200,000 patients infected per year in the late 1980s who contribute to today's HCV burden.[58] Considering that HCV infection is prevalent in high-risk populations such as prisoners, IDUs, and the homeless, and that this population is generally excluded from most surveys, it is estimated that the actual number of chronically infected people is significantly higher. Nearly 75% of infected people may not be identified.[58] The single largest risk factor for infection is injection drug use. Some experts also consider other illicit drug use, for example intranasal cocaine, as a risk factor because of the possible contamination of drug paraphernalia not limited to syringes and needles.[3] Historically, blood transfusion posed a major risk for infection. Patients who received blood transfusions or transplants before 1992, clotting factors before 1987, or were ever on chronic hemodialysis represent a majority of chronic HCV infections.[59] Improved screening of blood in 1992 decreased the risk of transfusion-related HCV.[60] Currently hemodialysis and transfusions both represent less than 1% of risk factors in known HCV exposures.[3] Although sexual transmission is an often-identified risk factor, the actual risk is very low and may be confounded by other behaviors. Studies of monogamous couples in long-term relationships do not support the use of barrier methods for preventing transmission. Testing of sexual partners in a monogamous relationship is mainly recommended for ease of mind.[61] Although sexual contact is considered an inefficient means of HCV transmission, multiple sexual partners and coinfection with sexually transmitted diseases, including HIV, increase the risk for HCV sexual transmission.[62]

Screening

Although acute HCV infections are often not recognized and many progress to chronic infections, routine screening for infection is not recommended. Various guidelines and position papers for the screening and treatment of chronic HCV infection exist.[59,61] Screening is warranted in patients who are at high risk for infection (Table 42–10).

TABLE 42-10 Recommendations for Hepatitis C Virus (HCV) Screening

Current or past use of injection drug use
Coinfection with HIV
Received blood transfusions or organ transplantations before 1992
Received clotting factors before 1987
Ever on chronic hemodialysis
Patients with unexplained elevated ALT levels or evidence of liver disease
Healthcare and public safety workers after an occupational exposure
Children born to HCV-positive mothers
Immigrants from countries with a high prevalence of HCV infection

ALT, alanine transaminase; HIV, human immunodeficiency virus.
Data from Hoofnagle.[63]

Although the risk of HCV in monogamous relationships is very low and barrier methods are not recommended, sexual partners may be tested for the sake of reassurance.[59] The risk of infection from other needle-borne exposures, such as acupuncture, tattooing, and body piercing, is unclear and at this time not an indication for routine screening for HCV.[61]

ETIOLOGY

HCV is a single-stranded RNA virus of the family Flaviviridae notable for lacking a proofreading polymerase and enabling frequent viral mutations.[58,63] The virus replicates within hepatocytes and like hepatitis B, is not directly cytopathic. HCV replicates copiously with an estimated serum half-life of 2 to 3 hours. The result is a proliferate, persistently mutating virus posing an immense challenge for immune-mediated control.[63]

HCV is differentiated into six major genotypes, numbered 1 to 6, and varying in nucleotide sequence by 30% to 50%. Genotypes are further classified into subtypes (a, b, c, etc.), which differ by 10% to 30% in nucleotide sequence. The most widely distributed genotypes are 1 and 2, with genotype 1 the most common (Table 42–11). In the United States, the majority of infections are caused by genotypes 1a and 1b, followed by genotypes 2 and 3. Although infection caused by any of the genotypes can lead to cirrhosis, end-stage liver disease (ESLD), or HCC, the significance of the infecting genotype is related to therapeutic response. Genotypes 2 and 3 are at least twice as likely to respond to therapy as genotype 1. Genotypes 4, 5, and 6 are not well understood but are expected to respond with rates similar to genotype 1.[63]

PATHOPHYSIOLOGY

In the vast majority of cases, an acute HCV infection leads to chronic infection. The immune response in an acute HCV infection is mostly insufficient to eradicate the virus. During the early phases of infection, natural killer cells are activated as HCV RNA levels rapidly rise. A combined effort of HCV specific CD4 and CD8 T lymphocytes and interferon coexpression decrease viral replication. The eradication of HCV by cytotoxic T lymphocytes may occur either as a result of induced apoptosis by infected hepatocytes or by the release of interferon to stifle viral replication. The extent of hepatocyte apoptosis may correlate with the course of the disease. Liver damage and HCC are associated with high levels of hepatocyte apoptosis. Low levels of apoptosis are associated with viral persistence. Moreover, CD4 T-helper cells are unlikely to mediate liver injury, but rather may promote an environment conducive for other immune responses damaging to the liver. Bystander killing may also play a role in hepatic damage. Although HCV infects less than 10% of hepatocytes, up to 20% of cells are activated for apoptosis.[64]

HCV poses a daunting challenge for immune control because of its rapid viral diversification. HCV genomic mutations are detectable within 1 year of infection. Resolved cases of HCV are defined by a vigorous T-cell response with highly active CD8 and persistent

TABLE 42-11 Worldwide Hepatitis C Virus Genotype Distribution

Genotype	Region
1	Worldwide, especially United States, Northern Europe
2	Worldwide, especially Northern Europe, Japan
3	India
4	Middle East, Africa
5	South Africa
6	Hong Kong, Southeast Asia

From Hoofnagle.[63]

CD4 cell response. It is hypothesized that the CD8 activity mediates protective immunity but requires the aid of CD4 cells to maintain the response during viral mutations.[64]

CLINICAL PRESENTATION

In an acute HCV infection, most patients are asymptomatic and undiagnosed. HCV RNA is detectable within 1 to 2 weeks of exposure and levels rise quickly during the initial weeks. The HCV RNA levels plateau at 10^5 to 10^7 international units/mL and precede a peak in ALT levels and the onset of symptoms. Rising ALT levels indicate hepatic injury and cell necrosis. It is not unusual for levels to exceed values 10 times the upper limits of normal.[63] Although HCV RNA serum levels can show interpatient variability, the levels tend to be stable for the individual patient.[65] Typically, symptoms occur 7 weeks after the infection, with a range of 3 to 12 weeks. Approximately one-third of adults will experience some mild and nonspecific symptoms, including fatigue, anorexia, weakness, jaundice, abdominal pain, or dark urine.[58,63] Acute infections rarely progress to fulminant hepatitis, although the course can be severe and prolonged. If the infection is self-limiting, symptoms last several weeks as ALT and HCV RNA levels subside. Almost all patients, including immunosuppressed patients, will develop antibodies to HCV. Typically, antibodies are not detectable until either at the time of or shortly after the development of symptoms and are not used diagnostically in an acute infection because a third of infected patients may test negative at the onset of symptoms despite infection.[63]

Up to 85% of acutely infected patients will go on to develop a chronic HCV infection, defined as persistently detectable HCV RNA for 6 months or more. HCV RNA levels and ALT levels can fluctuate and even have periods of undetectable HCV RNA and normal ALTs. Most patients will have few, if any symptoms. The most common symptom is persistent fatigue. Additional symptoms include right upper quadrant pain, nausea, or poor appetite. On physical examination, hepatomegaly is usually present. With advanced disease, stigmata of liver disease is evident, such as spider nevi, splenomegaly, palmar erythema, testicular atrophy, and caput medusae. However, almost all patients with chronic HCV will have some degree of necroinflammatory disease on liver biopsy. The extent of structural damage varies considerably.[63] Chronic inflammation of the liver from chronic HCV infection may result in fibrosis. Fibrosis is defined by altered hepatic perfusion creating a distorted structure and affecting normal function.[66] The speed of fibrosis progression can vary and is not necessarily predicative of cirrhosis development. An estimated 20% of chronic HCV patients will develop cirrhosis and half of those patients will progress to either decompensated cirrhosis or HCC. Historically, one-third of untreated patients may expect to develop cirrhosis within 20 years, while another third of patients may delay the onset of cirrhosis for 50 years or never develop it.

It is currently not possible to definitively identify patients at risk for disease progression.[66] Several factors may correlate with a decreased risk for chronicity. Being younger than 40 years old, female, nonblack, not immunosuppressed, and with a symptomatic acute HCV infection decreases the risk of developing a chronic infection. Being older than age 20 years at infection triples the risk for chronic HCV. Blacks, especially black men, are more likely to develop chronic infection and have lower treatment responses.[67] Becoming symptomatic and having jaundice is associated with a lower likelihood of chronic infection, perhaps correlating to a stronger immune response to the acute infection. Finally, immunosuppressed patients, such as those with HIV, are more prone to chronic infection although they are not inherently unable to clear the infection.[63] Similarly, disease progression is associated with increased age, male sex, continued alcohol intake, and HIV coinfection. Diabetes, as well as steatosis and obesity, may also potentiate fibrosis progression. Viral load and genotypes other than genotype 3 are not factors. Genotype 3 may be associated with fibrosis progression.[66] The development of HCV cirrhosis poses a 30% risk over 10 years for the development of ESLD, as well as a 1% to 2% risk per year of developing HCC.[61] Progression to cirrhosis is the primary concern in patients infected with HCV for 2 decades or longer. Unfortunately, because acute infections are typically not recognized, the diagnosis of HCV is often not made until disease progression.

HCV is also rarely associated with extrahepatic manifestations. The most common is cryoglobulinemia, a local deposition of immune complexes that cause vasculitis. Typical manifestations involve the skin and internal organ damage, predominantly affecting the kidneys. Symptoms of cryoglobulinemia include fatigue, skin rash, purpura, arthralgias, renal disease, and neuropathy.[63] Other, more rare symptoms include B-cell non-Hodgkin's lymphoma, Sjögren syndrome, glomerulonephritis, arthritis, corneal ulcers, thyroid disease, neuropathies, and porphyria cutanea tarda.[68]

DIAGNOSIS

For many patients, a diagnosis of hepatitis C is incidental. Some patients are diagnosed after persistently abnormal transaminases. Unfortunately, those patients who present with symptoms typically have advanced disease. A diagnosis of chronic HCV is confirmed with a reactive enzyme immunoassay for anti-HCV. Testing for anti-HCV is not routinely recommended because of the low prevalence of HCV in the general population and the nonspecificity of the test. Although many professional associations advocate testing for both symptomatic and asymptomatic persons with risk factors for HCV, the U.S. Preventative Task Force does not recommend routine screening of high-risk individuals.[69]

TREATMENT

Hepatitis C Virus

■ DESIRED OUTCOME

The primary goal of therapy is to eradicate HCV infection. Resolving the infection prevents the development of chronic HCV infection sequelae. Even patients who are unable to achieve cure may see histological improvements with therapy.[59]

■ GENERAL APPROACH TO TREATMENT

Treatment for HCV is necessary because nearly 85% of acutely infected patients develop chronic infections and are at risk of developing cirrhosis, ESLD, and HCC. Moreover, HCV infection is the most common indication for liver transplant. Treatment is indicated for patients previously untreated who have chronic HCV, circulating HCV RNA, increased ALT levels, evidence on biopsy of moderate to severe hepatic grade and stage, and compensated liver disease.[59] According to the American Association for the Study of Liver Diseases, among chronic HCV patients, symptomatic cryoglobulinemia is an indication for HCV antiviral therapy irrespective of the stage of liver disease.[61] Therapy is not without risk, and in some cases may not be recommended, such as in patients with decompensated liver disease, a history of severe uncontrolled psychiatric disorder, and in patients with severe hematologic cytopenias.[59] Table 42–12 lists the contraindications to therapy.

Before therapy is initiated, quantitative HCV testing, genotyping, and a liver biopsy are performed. Quantitative amplification assays for HCV RNA are performed in patients who are candidates for therapy to obtain baseline information on the viral load. A baseline HCV RNA level serves as a prognostic indicator for response and is

TABLE 42-12 Contraindications to Hepatitis C Virus Combination Therapy

Autoimmune hepatitis
Decompensated liver disease
Women who are pregnant or patients whose female partners are pregnant
Patients with hemoglobinopathies
Patients with creatinine clearance <50 mL/min
Patients on hemodialysis
Patients with ischemic cardiovascular or cerebrovascular disease

used to monitor virologic response once therapy is initiated. Genotyping is also necessary for treatment candidates because response to therapy and duration of therapy vary depending on the infecting genotype. Liver biopsy is used to determine histologic grade and stage and to guide therapy.[61] Because most chronic HCV patients are not diagnosed for years, a biopsy can provide clinical information on the extent of hepatic damage incurred since infection and offer baseline data to assess disease progression.[59] In some patients, liver biopsy may support a decision to delay treatment.

Overall, the greatest predictor of treatment response is infection with nongenotype 1. Adherence to therapy is a crucial component in response, especially among genotype 1-infected patients. Patients who take at least 80% of their medications for at least 80% of the treatment time are more likely to successfully respond to therapy.[74] Treatment response is monitored according to the following terminology:

Early virologic response (EVR): patient who experiences at least a 2-log reduction in viral load by the 12th week of treatment

End-of-treatment response (ETR): patient with no detectable viral load at the end of treatment

Sustained virologic response (SVR): patient with no detectable viral load at the conclusion of therapy and 6 months later

Relapser: patient who responds to therapy but whose viral load becomes detectable at the conclusion of therapy

Nonresponder: patient with a stable viral load during the course of therapy

Partial responder: patient with at least a 2-log reduction in viral load but who never has undetectable viral levels

Patients who experience an EVR are more likely to also have an SVR. Less than 3% of patients who fail to have an EVR can be expected to achieve an SVR.[59,61] If the goal of therapy is viral eradication and an EVR is not achieved, therapy may be discontinued. In some patients, however, histologic benefits can occur without an EVR and histologic improvements alone may warrant continuation of therapy.[59]

NONPHARMACOLOGIC THERAPY

All chronic HCV patients should be vaccinated against hepatitides A and B. Lifestyle changes are an important factor in reducing health consequences in hepatitis C. Continued alcohol use is a known risk factor for disease progression and severity. There is no established lower limit of alcohol consumption at which disease progression is not seen. Obesity is also a factor and patients should be encouraged to eat a balanced diet and exercise regularly to maintain a normal weight. Smoking may contribute to disease progression. Patients should be encouraged to maintain good overall health, stop smoking, and avoid alcohol and illicit drugs.[61,71] The use of herbal therapy is ineffective.[39]

PHARMACOLOGIC THERAPY

❾ The current standard of care for chronic HCV patients is a combination therapy of a once-weekly injection of PEG-IFN and a daily oral dose of ribavirin. Overall response rates are greatest with combination therapy at an SVR rate of 54% to 56%.[59] Therapy is optimized based on genotype, patient weight, and response to therapy. Table 42–13 lists current therapeutic regimens. For genotype 1, evaluation for an EVR at 12 weeks is recommended as an indicator of the probability of achieving an SVR. Because therapy is not without a significant side-effect profile and because failure to achieve EVR is so strongly correlated with treatment failure, some clinicians will terminate therapy early in genotype 1 patients (Fig. 42–3). Conversely, because genotypes 2 and 3 respond so well to therapy, there are data to support early treatment termination in patients who show an EVR at 4 weeks (Fig. 42–3).[72]

TABLE 42-13 Recommended Hepatitis C Virus Treatment Dosing

Genotype	Peg-IFN Dose	Ribavirin Dose		Duration[a]
1	Peginterferon α_{2a} 180 mcg/wk *or*	<75 kg[b]	1,000 mg	48 weeks
	Peginterferon α_{2b} 1.5 mcg/wk	≥75 kg	1,200 mg	
2, 3	Peginterferon α_{2a} 180 mcg/wk *or* Peginterferon α_{2b} 1.5 mcg/wk		800 mg	24 weeks

[a]Actual treatment duration may be reduced depending on early virologic response.
[b]Patient weight.

Interferon

Historically, treatment of HCV involved the use of IFN-α. Although IFN monotherapy resulted in an SVR in less than 10% of patients, the

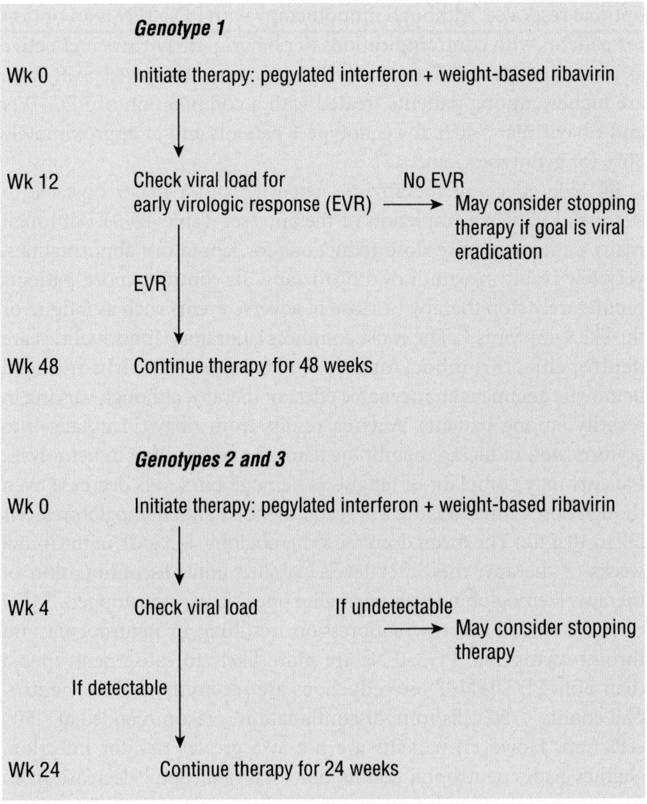

FIGURE 42-3. Suggested response-optimized chronic hepatitis C virus infection treatment regimens based on the recommendations of the American Gastroenterological Association. *(Adapted from reference 59.)*

TABLE 42-14 Pegylated Interferon Comparison

	Pegasys	PEG-Intron
Interferon	Alpha-2a	Alpha-2b
Indications	HBV, HCV	HCV
PEG moiety (weight)	Branched (40 kDa)	Linear (12 kDa)
Distribution	8–12 L; highest concentration in liver, spleen, kidneys	Body-weight dependent: 1 L/kg; distributes throughout body
Metabolism	Liver	Liver
Excretion	Renal	Renal
Dosing	Fixed: 180 mcg/wk subcutaneously	Weight dependent: 1.5 mcg/kg/wk subcutaneously

HBV, hepatitis B virus; HCV, hepatitis C virus.

response was durable. The addition of a pegylated moiety to IFN improved the pharmacokinetic profile of the drug to reduce injection frequency from three times to once a week, and doubled SVR rates. Even among cirrhotic patients, PEG-IFN was safe and effective.[59] Two PEG-IFNs are available, PEG-IFN-α_{2a} (Pegasys) and PEG-IFN-α_{2b} (PEG-Intron). Table 42–14 lists the differences between the two drugs. It is unclear which therapy is superior. A comparison trial on the antiviral effects of the two therapies found that PEG-IFN-α_{2b} had a greater decrease in HCV RNA during the first 4 weeks of monotherapy than PEG-IFN-α_{2a}.[73] Achievement of SVR may be more likely in patients with an early and intense viral suppression. Nonetheless, head-to-head trials are lacking and the true clinical difference between therapies remains unknown.

Ribavirin

Ribavirin, a synthetic guanosine analog, is ineffective as a monotherapy for HCV and its exact mechanism of action is unknown. When added to IFN, ribavirin significantly increases SVR rates, especially among genotypes 2 and 3. Ribavirin is dosed based on weight for optimal response. Although monotherapy with PEG-IFN is an option for patients with contraindications to ribavirin, ribavirin is ineffective as monotherapy and should not be used alone. However, SVR rates are highest among patients treated with a combination of PEG-IFN and ribavirin at >40% for genotype 1 patients and at approximately 80% for genotypes 2 and 3.[59]

⑩ Side effects of therapy are extensive and a major obstacle to successful patient completion of therapy (see Table 42–9). Although many patients require dose reductions for laboratory abnormalities, very few result in withdrawal of therapy. In contrast, more patients prematurely stop therapy because of adverse events such as fatigue or flu-like symptoms.[74] The most common laboratory abnormalities are neutropenia, thrombocytopenia, and anemia. Ribavirin-induced hemolytic anemia is an inevitable effect of therapy, although varying in severity among patients. Anemia results from ribavirin uptake into erythrocytes, inducing membrane damage and resulting in hemolysis. Patients may complain of fatigue as hemoglobin levels decrease even though dose reductions are not recommended until hemoglobin levels fall to 10 g/dL. The mean decrease in hemoglobin is 3 g/dL in the initial weeks of therapy; thereafter levels stabilize until discontinuation of therapy. Hemoglobin levels normalize once ribavirin is stopped.[74] IFN can cause bone marrow suppression, resulting in neutropenia and thrombocytopenia. PEG-IFNs are more likely to cause neutropenia than non–PEG-IFN. Dose reductions are recommended for neutrophil counts <750 cells/mm; discontinuation is recommended at <500 cells/mm. However, patients are not at a greater risk for infection. Neither nadir neutrophil counts nor total neutrophil decrease from baseline are related to infection. One study examined the risk for total, viral, fungal, and bacterial infections and concluded that neither dose reductions of interferon nor the addition of granulocyte-stimulating factor in HCV-treatment–induced neutropenia is warranted.[75]

Up to one-third of patients are expected to experience some degree of depression during treatment partly because of interferon's interference with the serotonin pathways.[54] Although many patients can be managed with selective serotonin reuptake inhibitors, various degrees of counseling and psychiatric consultations may be necessary. Severe depression and suicidal behaviors are rare but not undocumented. More common side effects include flu-like symptoms, which can be managed by acetaminophen or nonsteroidal inflammatory drugs.[59]

Alternative Treatments

Currently investigated drug treatments for chronic HCV include VX-950 and valopcitabine (NM283). VX-950 is a reversible, selective, and specific inhibitor of HCV replication. It is an oral drug and current data suggest optimal dosing to be three times per day. Although VX-950 demonstrated great viral load reduction even among previous interferon nonresponders, when taken alone it demonstrated viral breakthrough within 2 weeks of initiation.[76] Valopcitabine, or NM283, is a ribonucleoside analog inhibiting viral replication. Studies in treatment-naive and treatment-refractory patients are ongoing.

Special Populations

Clinical trials are conducted with a patient population that generally does not reflect the patient spectrum encountered in clinical practice. There are no contraindications to the treatment of intravenous-drug users, prisoners, persons with substance abuse issues, or persons with psychiatric disorders. However, barriers exist that can prevent access to care. A multidisciplinary approach to HCV treatment that includes mental health and substance abuse professionals should be considered in providing care to special populations.[77]

Published recommendations for treatment in various special populations are as follows.[59,61]

Patients with Normal ALTs The decision to treat patients with normal ALTs is somewhat controversial and made on individual patient basis. Clinicians should consider the risks and benefits of therapy, including histologic data, genotype, likelihood for response, and other factors, such as patient willingness to undergo therapy. Successful treatment significantly improves patient quality of life and reduce fatigue.[78]

Patients with Decompensated Cirrhosis Patients with evidence of decompensation are candidates for liver transplantation. Therapy is not recommended.

Relapsed Patients The decision to re-treat should consider the previous therapeutic regimen. Patients with prior treatment with IFN monotherapy or IFN and ribavirin should be considered for retreatment with PEG-IFN and ribavirin. The likelihood for SVR is lower, but may be as high as 50%.

Nonresponders Retreatment with PEG-IFN and ribavirin can increase SVR rates in patients previously treated with IFN monotherapy or IFN and ribavirin. Previous adherence, treatment tolerance, severity of underlying liver disease, as well as factors affecting treatment response, such as genotype, should be considered before deciding to retreat.

Accidental Needle-Stick Exposures Prophylactic treatment immediately following an accidental needle-stick exposure is not recommended for multiple reasons. Risk of transmission is considered low and among those infected, a percentage will successfully seroconvert and not require treatment. Because an initial delay in therapy does not increase the risk for developing a chronic infection, most experts wait 2 to 3 months before initiating treatment. Treatment is continued for a minimum of 24 weeks.

Intravenous-Drug Users Injection drug use is a major factor in the cycle of HCV transmission. There are no recommendations against treatment for active IDUs although ongoing drug abuse can create many complications and expert opinion dictates that the decision to treat be made on a case-by-case basis. Treatment is recommended for recovering drug users, including those in drug treatment programs. Reinfection rates are low among intravenous drug users who achieve SVR.[79]

Alcoholism Because continued alcohol use affects disease progression and severity and thus response to therapy, the cessation of alcohol use during therapy is recommended. Moreover, a period of abstinence before initiation of therapy is also recommended.

End-Stage Renal Disease The role of chronic HCV treatment is not defined for patients with end-stage renal disease. Hemodialysis is a contraindication for ribavirin use. Monotherapy with IFN is an option in patients with renal insufficiency or with end-stage renal disease. PEG-IFN can pose toxicity problems and requires careful monitoring.

HIV Coinfection A large portion of HIV-infected patients who acquired the virus via intravenous drug use will be coinfected with HCV. Treatment poses additional problems because of hepatotoxicity issues associated with highly active antiretroviral treatment, hepatic complications from HIV-associated diseases, as well as flares in hepatitis as CD4 counts recover. The American Gastroenterological Association recommends a 48-week course of therapy regardless of genotype. The prognosis for an SVR is worse than in patients infected with HCV only. In general, treatment is recommended and both HIV and HCV therapies can be coadministered with the exception of ribavirin and didanosine. Other potential ribavirin drug interactions include zidovudine and stavudine.[80]

Children Currently therapy is indicated for children ages 3 years and older and consists of IFN-α_{2b} monotherapy or in combination with ribavirin. PEG-IFN is not yet indicated for pediatric use. IFN is dosed at 3 million international units/m^2 (this is the dose used in the majority of pediatric studies) and ribavirin is available in a liquid formulation. Pediatric patients tend to better tolerate therapy than adults.

PREVENTION

No vaccine is available for HCV. It is unlikely that a vaccine will be developed in the near future because of the mutagenesis of the virus. Patients infected with HCV should be counseled on not being blood, organ, or semen donors. Although the likelihood of household transmission is small, patients should minimize risks by avoiding possible blood or mucus exposure, such as not sharing razors or toothbrushes and covering open wounds. Patients who continue to use illegal drugs should avoid sharing all drug paraphernalia, as risk of transmission is not limited to needles and syringes.

PHARMACOECONOMIC CONSIDERATIONS

The progression of HCV-induced liver disease is highly variable and identifying which patients will progress remains a clinical challenge. Because not all patients will develop clinical sequelae, therapy may not be necessary in all patients. Given the relative unreliability of treatment to achieve an SVR, the costs associated with therapy, and the side-effect profile of the drugs, the cost-effectiveness of therapy may be questioned. Several studies have assessed the economic values of treating chronically infected HCV patients.

Issues of cost-effectiveness must weigh the public health impact of HCV against the costs of therapy. Despite the decreased incidence of acute HCV infections, epidemiologic data suggest the greatest disease burden will occur in 2015, reflecting the slow progression of disease in patients infected in the late 1970s and early 1980s. At the same time, HCV-related mortality is expected to triple.[81] A projected 720,000 patient-years will be lost as a result of decompensated cirrhosis and HCC. Predicted costs exceed $21 billion from the development of clinical sequelae. In patients who are younger than age 65 years, the costs associated with premature death are even higher—an expected $54 billion.[58] Although not all patients will develop HCV-related liver disease, it is not currently possible to identify which patients will have disease progression. Moreover, HCV-infected patients are prone to high levels of fatigue and neuropsychiatric and cognitive impairment, further contributing to decreased patient quality of life.[81]

Treatment with PEG-IFN therapy compared to traditional IFN is a cost-effective approach among noncirrhotic patients who are infected with any of the genotypes, especially in patients who are infected with nongenotype 1.[82] A review of studies published on the cost-effectiveness of therapies for HCV found that HCV therapy is cost-effective most of the time. Reduced cost-effectiveness was seen in patients treated with normal transaminases and healthy biopsies. However, most clinicians would opt not to treat such patients. Moreover, evaluating virologic response by week 12 and terminating therapy if no response is evident substantially lowers treatment costs by more than $15,000. Overall, various studies found that HCV treatment falls within the accepted cost-effectiveness margin, defined as less than $50,000 per QALY. The studies concluded that antiviral therapy costs offset costs associated with disease sequelae.[81]

CLINICAL CONTROVERSIES

In patients with advanced disease, a biopsy may be risky and offer no additional clinical information whether to treat or not. Some clinicians believe that if therapy is to be initiated regardless, the liver biopsy offers no additional information. In patients with genotype 2 or 3, because response to therapy is so high and most clinicians treat despite biopsy results, there may not be a reason for biopsy.

Histologic improvement is not limited to patients who experience an SVR. Some clinicians believe IFN-based antiviral therapies, regardless of response, can decrease the incidence of HCC development.

ABBREVIATIONS

ALT: alanine transaminase

Anti-HAV: antibody to hepatitis A virus

CDC: Centers for Disease Control and Prevention

ESLD: end-stage liver disease

ETR: end-of-treatment response

EVR: early virologic response

FDA: Food and Drug Administration

GI: gastrointestinal

HAV: hepatitis A virus

HB_cAg: hepatitis B core antigen

HB_eAg: hepatitis B e antigen

HB_sAg: hepatitis B surface antigen

HBV: hepatitis B virus

HCC: hepatocellular carcinoma

HCV: hepatitis C virus

HIV: human immunodeficiency virus
IDU: injection-drug user
IFN: interferon
Ig: immunoglobulin
MMR: measles, mumps, rubella
MSM: men who have sex with men
QALY: quality-adjusted life-year(s)
SVR: sustained virologic response

REFERENCES

1. Centers for Disease Control and Prevention. U.S. Disease Burden Data 1980–2005: Disease Burden from Hepatitis A, B, and C in the United States (2006). 2006, *http//www.cdc.gov/Ncidod/diseases/hepatitis/resource/dz_burden.htm.*
2. Nainan OV, Xia G, Vaughan G, Margolis HA. Diagnosis of hepatitis A virus infection: A molecular approach. Clin Microbiol Rev 2006;19:63–79.
3. Centers for Disease Control and Prevention. Hepatitis Surveillance Report No. 61. Atlanta, GA: U.S. Department of Health and Human Services, Centers for Disease Control and Prevention, 2006.
4. Elinav E, Ben-Dov IZ, Shapira Y, et al. Acute hepatitis A infection in pregnancy is associated with high rates of gestational complications and preterm labor. Gastroenterol 2006;130:1129–1134.
5. Centers for Disease Control and Prevention. Hepatitis A outbreak associated with green onions at a restaurant—Monaca, Pennsylvania, 2003. MMWR Morb Mortal Wkly Rep 2003;2002;52(47):1155–1157.
6. Steffen R. Changing travel-related global epidemiology of hepatitis A. Am J Med 2005;118(Suppl 10A):46s–49s.
7. Cuthbert JA. Hepatitis A. Old and new. Clin Microbiol Rev 2001;14:38–58.
8. Centers for Disease Control and Prevention. Prevention of hepatitis A through active or passive immunizations: Recommendations of the Advisory Committee on Immunization Practices (ACIP). MMWR Morb Mortal Wkly Rep 1999;48(RR-12):1–37.
9. World Health Organization position paper: Hepatitis A vaccines. Wkly Epidemiol Rec 2000;5:37–44.
10. Leach CT. Hepatitis A in the United States. Pediatr Infect Dis J 2004;23:551–552.
11. Bower WA, Nainan OV, Han X, Margolis HS. Duration of viremia in hepatitis A virus infection. J Infect Dis 2000;182:12–17.
12. Rawls RA, Vega KJ. Viral hepatitis in minority America. J Clin Gastroenterol 2005;39:144–151.
13. Centers for Disease Control and Prevention. Prevention of hepatitis A through active or passive immunizations: Recommendations of the Advisory Committee on Immunization Practices (ACIP). MMWR Morb Mortal Wkly Rep 2006;55(RR-7):1–23.
14. Weissman S, Feucht C, Moore BA. Response to hepatitis A vaccine in HIV-positive patients. J Viral Hepat 2006;13:81–86.
15. Jacobs RJ, Gibson GA, Meyerhoff AS. Cost-effectiveness of hepatitis A/B vaccine versus hepatitis B vaccine for healthcare and public safety workers in the western United States. Infect Control Hosp Epidemiol 2004;25:563–569.
16. Jacobs RD, Meyerhoff AS. Cost-effectiveness of hepatitis A/B vaccine versus hepatitis B vaccine in public sexually transmitted disease clinics. Sex Transm Dis 2003;30:859–865.
17. World Health Organization. Hepatitis B. Fact Sheet No. 204 (2000). 2000, *http//www.who.int/mediacentre/factsheets/fs204/en.*
18. Centers for Disease Control and Prevention. Hepatitis B Slide Kit. Division of Viral Hepatitis (2003). 2003, *http//www.cdc.gov/ncidod/diseases/hepatitis/slides/index.htm.*
19. Lok ASF. Chronic hepatitis B. N Engl J Med 2002;346:1682–1683.
20. Lavanchy D. Hepatitis B virus epidemiology, disease burden, treatment, and current and emerging prevention and control measures. J Viral Hepat 2004;11:97–107.
21. Centers for Disease Control. A comprehensive immunization strategy to eliminate transmission of hepatitis B virus infection in the United States: Recommendations of the Advisory Committee on Immunization Practices (ACIP) Part 1: Immunization of infants, children, and adolescents. MMWR Morb Mortal Wkly Rep 2005;54(RR-16):1–31.
22. Ganem D, Prince AM. Hepatitis B virus infection—Natural history and clinical consequences. N Engl J Med 2004;350:1118–1129.
23. Lee WM. Hepatitis B virus infection. N Engl J Med 1997;337:1733–1745.
24. Kao JH. Hepatitis B viral genotypes: Clinical relevance and molecular characteristics. J Gastroenterol Hepatol 2002;17:643–650.
25. Fattovich G. Natural history of hepatitis B. J Hepatol 2003;39:s50–s58.
26. Ganne-Carrie N, Williams V, Kaddouri H, et al. Significance of hepatitis B virus genotypes A to E in a cohort of patients with chronic hepatitis B in the Seine Saint Denis district of Paris (France). J Med Virol 2006;78:335–340.
27. Lok ASF, McMahon BJ. AASLD practice guidelines: Chronic hepatitis B. Hepatology 2001;34:1225–1241.
28. Arase Y, Ikeda K, Suzuki F, et al. Long-term outcome after hepatitis B surface antigen seroclearance in patients with chronic hepatitis B. Am J Med 2006;119:71.e9–71e.16.
29. Keeffe EB, Dieterich DT, Han SB, et al. A treatment algorithm for the management of chronic hepatitis B virus infection in the United States: An update. Clin Gastroenterol Hepatol 2006;4:936–962.
30. Raimondo G, Pollicino T, Squadrito G. Clinical virology of hepatitis B virus infection. J Hepatol 2003;39(Suppl 1):s26–s30.
31. Cantarini MC, Trevisani F, Morselli-Labate AM, et al. Effect of the etiology of viral cirrhosis on the survival of patients with hepatocellular carcinoma. Am J Gastroenterology 2006;101:91–98.
32. Bruxi J, Llovet JM. Hepatitis B virus and hepatocellular carcinoma. J Hepatol 2003;39(Suppl 1):s59–s63.
33. Chen CJ, Yang HI, Su J, et al. Risk of hepatocellular carcinoma across a biological gradient of serum hepatitis B virus DNA level. JAMA 2006;295:65–73.
34. Wright TL. Introduction to chronic hepatitis B infection. Am J Gastroenterol 2006;101(Suppl 1):s1–s6.
35. Farrell GC, Teoh NC. Management of chronic hepatitis B virus infection: A new era of disease control. Intern Med J 2006;36:100–113.
36. Kim JW, Park SH, Louie SG. Telbivudine: A novel nucleoside analog for chronic hepatitis B. Ann Pharmacother 2006;40:472–478.
37. Hadziyannis SJ, Tassopoulos NC, Heathcote EJ, et al. Long-term therapy with adefovir dipivoxil for HB_eAg-negative chronic hepatitis B. N Engl J Med 2005;352:2673–2681.
38. Lok ASF, McMahon BJ. Chronic hepatitis B. Update of recommendations. Hepatology 2004;39:1–5.
39. Dhiman RK, Chawla YK. Herbal medicines for liver diseases. Dig Dis Sci 2005;50:1807–1812.
40. Asmuth DM, Nguyen HH, Melcher GP, et al. Treatments for hepatitis B. Clin Infect Dis 2004;39:1353–1362.
41. Craxi A, Antonucci G, Camma C. Treatment options in HBV. J Hepatol 2006;44 (Suppl 1):s77–s83.
42. Jacobson IM. Therapeutic options for chronic hepatitis B. considerations and controversies. Am J Gastroenterol 2006;101(Suppl 1):s13–s18.
43. Wong SN, Lok ASF. Update on viral hepatitis: 2005. Curr Opin Gastroenterol 2006;22:241–247.
44. Marcellin P, Chang TT, Lim SG, et al. Adefovir dipivoxil for the treatment of hepatitis B e antigen-positive chronic hepatitis B. N Engl J Med 2003;348:808–816.
45. Hadziyannis SJ, Tassopoulos NC, Heathcote EJ, et al. Adefovir dipivoxil for the treatment of hepatitis B e antigen-negative chronic hepatitis B. N Engl J Med 2003;348:800–807.
46. Lampertico P, Vigano M, Manenti E, et al. Adefovir rapidly suppresses hepatitis B in HB_eAg-negative patients developing genotypic resistance to lamivudine. Hepatology 2005;42:1414–1419.
47. Dienstag JL. Looking to the future: New agents for chronic hepatitis B. Am J Gastroenterology 2006;101(Suppl 1):s19–s25.
48. Chang TT, Gish RG, de Man R, et al. A comparison trial of entecavir and lamivudine for HB_eAg-positive chronic hepatitis B. N Engl J Med 2006;354:1001–1010.
49. Lai CL, Shouval D, Lok AS, et al. Entecavir versus lamivudine for patients with HB_eAg-negative chronic hepatitis B. N Engl J Med 2006;354:1011–1020.
50. Jones R, Nelson M. Novel anti-hepatitis B agents: A focus on telbivudine. Int J Clin Pract 2006;60:1295–1299.
51. Zhou XJ, Marbury TC, Alcorn HW, et al. Pharmacokinetics of telbivudine in subjects with various degrees of hepatic impairment. Antimicrob Agents Chemother 2006;50:1721–1726.

52. Zhou XJ, Fielman BA, Lloyd DM, et al. Antimicrob Agents Chemother 2006;50:2309–2315.
53. Lim SG, Ng TM, Kung N, et al. A double-blind placebo-controlled study of emtricitabine in chronic hepatitis B. Arch Intern Med 2006;166:49–56.
54. Marcellin P, Lau GKK, Bonino F, et al. Peginterferon alfa-2a alone, lamivudine alone, and the two in combination in patients with HB_eAg-negative chronic hepatitis B. N Engl J Med 2004;351:1206–1217.
55. Kim SY, Billah K, Lieu TA, et al. Cost effectiveness of hepatitis B vaccination at HIV counseling and testing sites. Am J Prev Med 2006;30:498–506.
56. Kanwal F, Gralnek IM, Martin P, et al. Treatment alternatives for chronic hepatitis B virus infection: A cost-effectiveness analysis. Ann Intern Med 2005;142:821–831.
57. Kanwal F, Farid M, Martin P, et al. Treatment alternatives for hepatitis B cirrhosis: A cost-effectiveness analysis. Am J Gastroenterol 2006;101:2076–2089.
58. McHutchison JG, Bacon BR. Chronic hepatitis C: An age wave of disease burden. Am J Manag Care 2005;11(Suppl 10):s286–s295.
59. Dienstag JL, McHutchison JG. American Gastroenterological Association technical review of the management of hepatitis C. Gastroenterology 2006;130:231–264.
60. Lauer GM, Walker BD. Hepatitis C virus infection. N Engl J Med 2001;345:41–52.
61. Strader DB, Wright T, Thomas DL, Seeff LB. American Association for the Study of Liver Diseases: Diagnosis, management, and treatment of hepatitis C. Hepatology 2004;39:1147–1171.
62. Terrault NA. Sexual activity as a risk factor for hepatitis C. Hepatology 2002;36(5 Suppl 1):s99–s105.
63. Hoofnagle JH. Course and outcome of hepatitis C. Hepatology 2002;36(5 Suppl 1):s21–s29.
64. Kanto T, Hayashi N. Immunopathogenesis of hepatitis C virus infection: Multifaceted strategies subverting innate and adaptive immunity. Intern Med 2006;45:183–191.
65. National Institutes of Health Consensus Development Conference Statement: Management of hepatitis C. 2002–June 10–12. Hepatology 2002;36(Suppl 1):s3–s20.
66. Massard J, Ratziu V, Thabut D, et al. Natural history and predictors of disease severity in chronic hepatitis C. J Hepatol 2006;44:s19–s24.
67. Muir AJ, Bornstein JD, Killenberg PG, Peginterferon alfa-2b and ribavirin for the treatment of chronic hepatitis C in blacks and non-Hispanic whites. N Engl J Med 2004;350:2265–2271.
68. Mayo, MJ. Extrahepatic manifestations of hepatitis C infection. Am J Med Sci 2002;325:135–148.
69. U.S. Preventive Services Task Force. Screening for hepatitis C virus infection in adults: Recommendation statement. Ann Intern Med 2004;140:462–464.
70. McHutchison JG, Manns M, Patel K, et al. Adherence to combination therapy enhances sustained response in genotype-1 infected patients with chronic hepatitis C. Gastroenterology 2002;123:1061–1069.
71. Seeff LB. Natural history of chronic hepatitis C. Hepatology 2002;36(Suppl 1):s35–s46.
72. Mangia A, Santoro R, Minerva N, et al. Peginterferon alfa-2b and ribavirin for 12 vs. 24 weeks in HCV genotype 2 or 3. N Engl J Med 2005;352:2609–2617.
73. Silva M, Poo J, Wagner F, et al. A randomized trial to compare the pharmacokinetic, pharmacodynamic, and antiviral effects of peginterferon alfa-2b and peginterferon alfa-2a in patients with chronic hepatitis C (COMPARE). J Hepatol 2006;45:204–213.
74. Fried MW. Side effects of therapy of hepatitis C and their management. Hepatology 2002;36(Suppl 1):s237–s244.
75. Cooper CL, Al-Bedwawi S, Lee C, Garber G. Rate of infectious complications during interferon-based therapy for hepatitis C is not related to neutropenia. Clin Infect Dis 20063;42:1674–1678.
76. Reesink HW, Zeuzem S, Weegink CJ, et al. Rapid decline of viral RNA in hepatitis C patients treated with VX-950: A phase 1b, placebo-controlled, randomized study. Gastroenterology 2006;131:997–1002.
77. Geppert CMA, Arora S, Ethical issues in the treatment of hepatitis C. Clin Gastroenterol Hepatol 2005;3:937–944.
78. Arora S, O'Brien C, Zeuzem S, et al. Treatment of chronic hepatitis C patients with persistently normal alanine aminotransferase levels with the combination of peginterferon alpha-2a (40 kDa) plus ribavirin: Impact on health-related quality of life. J Gastroenterol Hepatol 2006;21:406–412.
79. Grebely J, Conway B, Raffa JD, et al. Hepatitis C virus reinfection in injection drug users. Hepatology 2006;44:1139–1145.
80. Swan T. Care and Treatment for Hepatitis C and HIV Coinfection. U.S. Department of Health and Human Services Health Resources and Services Administration HIV/AIDS Bureau, April 2006. Available at *http://hab.hrsa.gov/tools/coninfection/index.html*
81. Wong JB. Hepatitis C: Cost of illness and considerations for the economic evaluation of antiviral therapies. Pharmacoeconomics 2006;24:661–672.
82. Sullivan SD, Craxi A, Alberti A, et al. Cost-effectiveness of peginterferon alpha-2a plus ribavirin versus interferon alpha-2b plus ribavirin as initial therapy for treatment-naïve chronic hepatitis C. Pharmacoeconomics 2004;22:257–265.
83. Centers for Disease Control and Prevention. Recommendations for prevention and control of hepatitis C virus (HCV) infection and HCV-related chronic disease. MMWR Morb Mortal Wkly Rep 1998;47:1–39.

CHAPTER 43 Drug Therapy Individualization in Patients with Hepatic Disease or Genetic Alterations in Drug Metabolizing Activity

Y. W. FRANCIS LAM

KEY CONCEPTS

1. Hepatic elimination of drugs is primarily dependent on three variables: activity of metabolizing enzymes, plasma protein binding, and liver blood flow, each of which could be altered significantly in patients with liver diseases.
2. Hepatic extraction ratio represents a conceptual measure of the efficiency of extraction of drug from the blood by the liver, and is not a measure of the metabolic capacity of the liver per se.
3. Increased systemic bioavailability is primarily a concern for orally administered drugs that have a high hepatic extraction ratio.
4. Evaluation of patient's liver function for assessment of need of dosage adjustment is difficult, with most clinicians opting to use the Child-Pugh classification system.
5. Genetic polymorphisms affecting the drug metabolizing enzymes represent an additional patient-specific factor to consider in optimization of drug therapy.
6. Both phase I and phase II enzymes are associated with altered drug exposure.
7. Currently, there are few examples of how metabolic genotypes or phenotypes can be used to determine dosage of individual drugs.
8. An increasing number of attempts have been made to incorporate pharmacogenetics in clinical studies during drug development and in regulatory review.

Although there are many patient-related variables that can change the pharmacokinetics of drugs and potentially necessitate dosage regimen modification, the most common dosing changes are due to alterations in elimination capacity of the two primary eliminating organs—the liver and the kidneys. This chapter focuses on the changes in drug pharmacokinetics and pharmacodynamics resulting from altered hepatic drug metabolism in patients with hepatic dysfunction, and the implications for dosing. In addition, genetic changes in metabolic capacity of individuals also affect drug elimination from the liver, and examples of how pharmacogenetic information can impact drug dosage regimen modification and labeling are discussed.

Learning objectives, review questions, and other resources can be found at **www.pharmacotherapyonline.com.**

DRUG ELIMINATION BY THE LIVER

1 Drugs are primarily eliminated from the body by metabolism and excretion. Of these two biologic processes, the liver plays a pivotal role in the metabolism of parent drugs and formation of metabolites prior to their excretion by the kidneys. The overall capacity of the liver to carry out its metabolic role is primarily dependent on three factors: activity of the metabolizing enzymes within the smooth endoplasmic reticulum and the cytosol of the hepatocyte; the degree of protein binding in the blood, which affects the amount of unbound drugs available for uptake into the hepatocyte; and liver blood flow, which delivers drugs to the hepatocyte via the portal vein for orally administered drugs and via the systemic circulation for all administered drugs. As such, any patient-specific factors that affect enzymatic activity, protein binding, or liver blood flow would potentially result in significant alteration in drug disposition and therapeutic response. An understanding of the pharmacokinetic basis of hepatic drug elimination is helpful to conceptualize and quantify altered drug disposition in patients with liver dysfunction, and is the focus of the next section.

PHARMACOKINETIC BASIS OF HEPATIC DRUG ELIMINATION

Within a healthy liver, only the unbound drugs can be transported from the vasculature to the hepatocyte, where biotransformation occurs via the activity of the metabolic enzymes. Consequently, blood flow to the liver, the degree of plasma protein binding, and the intrinsic metabolic activity all affect the efficiency of the liver to eliminate a specific drug. The intrinsic metabolic activity measures the ability of the hepatocyte to eliminate drug in the absence of drug supply limitations such as plasma protein binding and blood flow. Thus, in essence, it reflects the inherent activity of the drug metabolizing enzymes within the hepatocyte, and is quantified as intrinsic clearance (Cl_{int}) in the literature. The hepatic clearance (Cl_H), or elimination of a drug, is related to the three physiologic determinants by the following mathematical relationship:

$$Cl_H = \frac{Q_H \times fu_B \times Cl_{int}}{Q_H + fu_B \times Cl_{int}}$$

where Q_H is hepatic blood flow, fu_B is unbound drug fraction in the blood, and Cl_{int} is intrinsic clearance.

Based on this mathematical relationship, when enzyme activity (Cl_{int}) and fu_B are very low relative to hepatic blood flow, they will become the primary determinants and rate-limiting process for hepatic clearance, as Cl_H approximates $fu_B \times Cl_{int}$. On the other hand, when enzyme activity and fu_B are very high in relation to blood flow, Cl_H would approximate Q_H and blood flow carrying drug to the liver is the rate-limiting process for hepatic elimination. A more detailed review of the complex mathematical relationship between hepatic clearance and the three physiologic determinants, as well as the different pharmacokinetic models used to explain the physiologic approaches to hepatic drug clearance, are provided by Wilkinson et al.[1,2]

❷ The hepatic clearance for any drug can also be conceptualized as the product of blood flow across the liver and the hepatic extraction ratio (ER_H) for that drug. The ER_H is a semiquantitative measure of the efficiency of extraction of drug from the blood by the liver, with a numerical value that ranges from zero to one. In general, the liver effectively "removes" high extraction ratio drugs (usually defined as $ER_H \geq 0.7$) from the blood as soon as they are presented via the blood supply. As such, the elimination of these drugs is more sensitive to changes in, and rate limited by, hepatic blood flow. Examples of drugs with this flow-dependent elimination characteristic are metoprolol, nitroglycerin, and verapamil (Table 43–1). Conversely, the liver does not exhibit a large metabolic capacity for drugs with a low extraction ratio (usually defined as $ER_H \leq 0.3$). The elimination of these drugs is more sensitive to changes in the degree of plasma protein binding and/or intrinsic metabolic activity, and rate limited by these two factors rather than by hepatic blood flow (flow-independent elimination). Warfarin, diazepam, erythromycin, phenytoin, theophylline, and valproic acid are representative examples of low-extraction ratio drugs.

Although it seems confusing that extensively metabolized drugs such as warfarin, phenytoin, and theophylline are classified as "low extraction" drugs, it is important to remember that the ER_H does not measure metabolic capacity per se; rather, it is a conceptual semiquantitative measure to help define the ease of extraction of a drug by the liver as the drug is delivered to the hepatocyte via the blood flow across the liver. Based on the degree of plasma protein binding, drugs with a low extraction ratio are sometimes further subgrouped as binding sensitive (e.g., phenytoin) and binding insensitive (e.g., theophylline). As such, the mathematical relationship discussed in the preceding paragraph would dictate that hepatic clearance of a highly protein-bound, low-extraction-ratio drug would depend on both intrinsic clearance and the degree of plasma protein binding, whereas the intrinsic clearance of unbound drug is the primary factor affecting hepatic clearance for a low-extraction-ratio drug with a low degree of plasma protein binding.

ALTERED HEPATIC DRUG ELIMINATION IN LIVER DISEASES

Patients with liver diseases can have altered drug elimination either at the level of hepatic blood flow, plasma protein binding, or intrinsic metabolic activity. Although there are different types of liver diseases that can result in reduced functional capacity, most disease states, such as hepatitis, liver cancer, and hepatosplenic schistosomiasis, are usually not associated with significant or prolonged alteration in drug metabolism unless cirrhosis is present, where there is irreversible hepatic damage. Jorga et al.[3] showed that there was no difference in the unbound clearance of tolcapone in patients with moderate chronic hepatitis compared to that in healthy volunteers. In contrast, patients with cirrhosis showed a significant decrease in unbound clearance of tolcapone. In fact, most literature studies that investigated the effect of liver diseases on drug disposition were primarily conducted in patients with cirrhosis.

CHANGES IN HEPATIC BLOOD FLOW

❸ Perfusion of the liver is provided by blood supply from the hepatic artery, which carries oxygenated blood from the aorta, and the portal vein, which carries nutrient-rich blood from the gastrointestinal tract. The terminal branches of the hepatic artery and the portal vein merge into the hepatic sinusoids, the vascular capillaries of the hepatocyte. The hepatic vein allows blood to exit from the liver into the inferior vena cava and then the systemic circulation. The portal vein provides approximately 75% of the liver's total blood supply of about 1.5 L/min in healthy adults. Consequently, the liver is the first site of elimination for orally administered drugs before they reach the systemic circulation (Fig. 43–1). This "first-pass effect" primarily affects high extraction ratio drugs and the extent of drug elimination can be significant, resulting in low systemic bioavailability (see Table 43–1). Simply put, under the assumptions of complete drug dissolution, absence of drug degradation in the gastrointestinal tract, and absence of gut wall metabolism, a drug with $ER_H \geq 70\%$, will have a bioavailability of $\leq 30\%$. Although the extent of drug loss can be circumvented by oral administration of a larger dose compared to that for intravenous administration, the oral bioavailability of some drugs could be very low and variable, necessitating administration by alternative routes such as sublingual for nitroglycerin.

In patients with chronic liver diseases such as cirrhosis, blood flow across the liver is usually decreased.[4] In addition, cirrhosis also causes alteration of vasculature within the liver, resulting in intra- and extrahepatic portosystemic shunting. Shunt formation allows up to 80% of blood supply to bypass the hepatocytes.[5] These changes in normal blood supply to the liver prevent a significant amount of drug from entering the site of metabolic inactivation. Furthermore, the permanent loss of hepatocyte function in patients with cirrhosis also results in reduced metabolic capacity. These two pathologic processes together decrease hepatic clearance significantly for orally administered, high extraction ratio drugs, and the reduced first-pass effect results in dramatic increase in systemic bioavailability (see Table 43–1).[6–11] Pentikainen et al.[12] reported that in patients without cirrhosis, the oral bioavailability of clomethiazole, a sedative commonly used in Europe, is 10 ± 7%. In patients with cirrhosis, the bioavailabil-

TABLE 43-1 Examples of High Extraction Drugs with Corresponding Reported Percent Increase in Bioavailability in the Presence of Cirrhosis

High Extraction Ratio (≥0.7) Flow Dependent	Reported Increases in Bioavailability in Presence of Cirrhosis
Labetalol	91%
Midazolam	100%
Morphine	115%
Nifedipine	78%
Propranolol	67%
Verapamil	60%

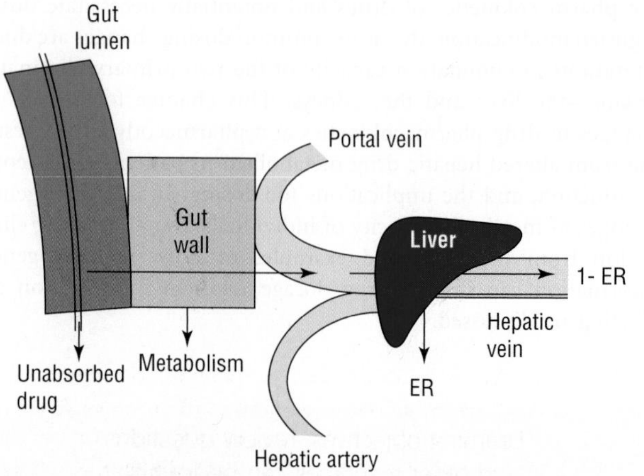

FIGURE 43-1. Schematic representation of the liver integrating the concept of hepatic extraction and first-pass effect. (ER, extraction ratio.)

TABLE 43-2 Example of Drugs with Documented Changes in Phase 2 Metabolic Capacity in Patients with Liver Diseases

Drug	Types or Severity of Liver Disease	Changes in Pharmacokinetic Parameters	Recommended Dosing Modification	References
Diflunisal	Histologically proven cirrhosis	36% reduction in clearance of unbound diflunisal 38% reduction in formation of phenolic and acyl glucuronides	None	23
Oxazepam	Biopsy-proven cirrhosis	54% reduction in oral clearance	None	24
Tolcapone	Child-Pugh class B	44% reduction in unbound clearance	50% dose reduction	3
Zidovudine	Child-Pugh class B or C	73% reduction in oral clearance	50% dose reduction	26

Data from Kirchheiner J, Brosen K, Dahl M, et al. CYP2D6 and CYP2C19 genotype-based dose recommendations for antidepressants: a first step towards subpopulation-specific dosages. Acta Psychiatr Scand Suppl 2001;104:173–192.

ity is 116 ± 25%, representing a greater than 10-fold increase. This can have significant impact on occurrence of adverse drug reaction and dosage adjustment for patients with liver diseases, and is discussed in subsequent sections. In contrast, low extraction ratio drugs have minimal first-pass effect and therefore exhibit high bioavailability after oral administration, as long as bioavailability is not reduced by additional biologic processes other than hepatic first-pass metabolism.

CHANGES IN METABOLIC CAPACITY

In addition to altering the liver vasculature, cirrhosis also causes irreversible hepatic damage and cell death. Although it is anticipated that extensive hepatic damage is associated with reduced drug metabolism with resultant decreased Cl_{int} and impaired hepatic drug elimination, the extent of impairment is variable among patients, as well as among different metabolic reactions.

In general, phase I oxidative metabolism mediated by the cytochrome P450 (CYP) enzyme system is more sensitive to the effect of cirrhosis than phase II conjugation reactions such as glucuronidation. For example, among the benzodiazepines, the clearances of diazepam[13] and midazolam,[7] but not of oxazepam[14] and temazepam,[15] are reduced in patients with cirrhosis. This differential effect between phase I oxidation and phase II conjugation reactions may be related to impaired uptake of oxygen caused by sinusoidal capillarization associated with cirrhosis,[16,17] as hypoxia has an important role in suppressing CYP-mediated drug metabolism in both animal[18–20] and human[21] studies. Froomes et al.[22] showed that oxygen supplementation in cirrhotic patients resulted in normalization of clearance of the phase I substrate theophylline but not of acetaminophen, a phase II substrate. Despite the general belief of "sparing" of phase II conjugation reactions in patients with cirrhosis, it is important to note that more recent studies have shown conjugation reactions can be reduced in patients with liver dysfunction, especially those with severe liver cirrhosis (Table 43–2).[3,23–26] The conflicting result between the study of Sonne et al.[24] and that of Shull et al.[14] might be related to the difference in severity of liver diseases in the two study populations.

Given the presence of multiple isoforms of human CYP enzymes, different studies have investigated whether there are selective differences in expression and activity of individual isoenzymes. George et al.[27,28] showed that compared to livers obtained from 20 healthy controls, the total CYP amount in the livers obtained from 50 patients with different types of end-stage chronic liver disease was reduced. Based on the Child-Pugh classification, 4 of the 50 patients have class A, 17 have class B, and 29 have class C cirrhosis. In addition, 18 patients also have cholestasis.

Selective alteration in amount, catalytic activities, and messenger ribonucleic acid (mRNA) level among CYP1A2, CYP2C8/10, CYP2E1, and CYP3A were reported in these 50 patients, and the presence or absence of cholestasis also have an effect on the observed changes. CYP1A2 amount and catalytic activity were significantly reduced with a corresponding decrease in mRNA level in patients with both cholestatic and noncholestatic cirrhosis. CYP3A4 amount, catalytic activity, and mRNA were significantly reduced only in patients without cholestasis. The amount and catalytic activity of CYP2E1 were decreased only in cirrhotic patients with cholestasis, whereas the CYP2E1 mRNA level was lower in both types of cirrhosis. In contrast, CYP2C amount and catalytic activity were not reduced in either type of cirrhosis. Although the corresponding level of mRNA was shown to be decreased in both cirrhosis types, the use of a nonspecific polyclonal antibody to identify CYP2C8/10 might have recognized other 2C isoenzymes and produced erroneous results. In summary, although it is clear that based on in vitro studies at the protein level[27,28] the extent of hepatic dysfunction-induced impairment in drug metabolism is dependent on both severity and type of disease, as well as the specific isoenzyme affected, the exact mechanism for this differential effect remains to be elucidated. In addition, the ability to extrapolate these results to the *in vivo* setting and possible dosage recommendation would likely require incorporation of the effect of additional patient-specific variables such as concurrent medications and disease states.

An additional complicating factor occurs for low-extraction, binding-sensitive drugs. In patients with cirrhosis, production of drug-binding proteins such as albumin and α_1-acid glycoprotein decrease, resulting in an increase in the unbound concentration of acidic and basic drugs, respectively. This not only would lead to increased toxicity, but also increased hepatic elimination as the unbound fraction increases. The magnitude and duration of the elevated unbound concentration are difficult to predict.

ADDITIONAL EFFECTS OF LIVER DISEASES ON DRUG DISPOSITION AND EFFECTS

EFFECT ON DRUG ABSORPTION

Delayed gastric emptying possibly related to altered action of gastrointestinal hormones occurs in patients with cirrhosis.[29,30] Although this will delay the rate of absorption, the extent of drug absorption is generally not reduced. Even though the liver has no functional role in affecting the absorption of drug from the gastrointestinal tract per se, its unique anatomical positioning within the circulating system makes it a primary site of loss for orally administered drug prior to its entry into the systemic circulation. As discussed in previous sections, drugs with a high extraction ratio will undergo significant "presystemic metabolism" or first-pass effect, resulting in low systemic bioavailability. In patients who have cirrhosis with associated portosystemic shunting and/or reduction in metabolic capacity, oral administration of these drugs could result in a significant increase in their systemic bioavailability and hence pharmacodynamic effect. In contrast, drugs with a low extraction ratio generally have a negligible first-pass effect and, hence, only minimal changes in systemic bioavailability is expected in the presence of cirrhosis.

EFFECT ON DRUG EXCRETION

Reduced glomerular filtration rate and renal plasma flow have been observed in patients with liver cirrhosis,[31,32] potentially accounting for reported decreased renal elimination of several drugs, including fluconazole,[33] lithium,[34] and ofloxacin.[35] In addition, in individual patients, advanced liver disease can be complicated by the presence of hepatorenal syndrome with renal failure. In these patients, dosage reduction would need to be considered even for drugs that are primarily excreted unchanged by the kidney.

EFFECT ON DRUG PHARMACODYNAMICS

Changes in therapeutic response to a drug can occur in patients with liver disease even in the absence of any changes in pharmacokinetics. The increased drug sensitivity can occur as a result of altered affinity of the drug to its target, altered binding to the target, alteration in the target itself, altered permeability of the blood-brain barrier, or increases in γ-aminobutyric acid (GABA) receptors or GABA-ergic activity. Altered pharmacodynamic responses have been reported in the literature with analgesics,[36] benzodiazepines,[37] loop diuretics, and β-blockers.

Bakti et al.[38] reported that with similar unbound triazolam concentration at 2.25 hours after drug administration, cirrhotic patients experienced on average a 30% greater impairment in psychometric performance tests, including the digit symbol substitution test, flicker sensitivity, and pursuit rotor, when compared to healthy control subjects. Test performance was similar in both groups prior to administration of triazolam. The study results suggest that the increased sensitivity is not a result of altered pharmacokinetic profile, and might explain why clinically some cirrhotic patients develop encephalopathy and other CNS effects even when administered standard doses of benzodiazepines, cimetidine,[39] and quinolones.[40]

Conversely, resistance to the pharmacodynamic effect of loop diuretics in patients with cirrhosis has been reported for bumetamide,[41] furosemide,[42,43] torasemide,[43,44] and triamterene.[45] For these drugs, the sigmoidal curve that describes the relationship between drug concentration and pharmacologic response is shifted to the right in patients with cirrhosis, indicating a reduced response compared to healthy individuals. Downregulation of β_2-adrenoreceptors in patients with cirrhosis[46] has been suggested as a possible mechanism of lower therapeutic response observed with metipranolol[47] in patients with cirrhosis.

ADDITIONAL VARIABLES AFFECTING DRUG DISPOSITION

Drugs and metabolites that are excreted into the bile reach the small intestine via the biliary tract. Within the small intestine, these metabolites, especially the glucuronides, can be converted back to the parent compound, resulting in reabsorption of both parent and metabolites and thus complete the enterohepatic circulation. Consequently, interruption of this enterohepatic circulation could reduce systemic drug exposure. There is little information on the role of biliary excretion to the overall drug elimination and the effect of how biliary excretion of drugs could be affected by liver diseases.

Finally, it is important to note that it is only recently that the role of hepatic transport proteins, such as the organic anion transporting polypeptides and P-glycoprotein, was recognized. Research in elucidating the clinical significance of the different hepatic transport proteins in drug disposition will be forthcoming, but currently there is little information regarding how liver disease affects the function of these proteins and therefore drug uptake into the hepatocyte.

LIVER FUNCTION ASSESSMENT

In contrast to renal impairment, accurate quantification of liver function in patients with hepatic impairment is difficult to perform, especially for the purpose of dosage adjustment. The severity of liver function impairment is usually assessed clinically with the Pugh modification of the Child-Turcotte classification.[48] Based on the clinical evidence of ascites and encephalopathy and laboratory parameters that measure the liver's synthetic and excretory functions, patients are assigned different scores in accordance to the level of impairment in these parameters (Table 43–3). The classification is easy to use and useful for following the clinical course of an individual patient or comparing groups of patient among studies. However, despite the expected correlation between decline in liver function such as synthesis of albumin or clotting factors and the corresponding changes in their respective laboratory parameters, the presence of patient-specific variables, such as nutritional status and vitamin K intake, would complicate the usefulness of these parameters. In addition, in contrast to renal impairment, none of the clinically used liver function tests, including those used in the Child-Pugh classification, correlate well with drug pharmacokinetic parameters. This not only is a result of their inability to quantify the primary physiologic determinants of hepatic clearance, including intrinsic clearance and hepatic blood flow, but also a reflection of the complex and multiple physiologic processes not being accurately accounted for by any individual laboratory test.

TABLE 43-3 Severity of Liver Disease Based on the Child-Pugh Classification

Clinical or Laboratory Parameters	1 Point	2 Points	3 Points
Ascites	absent	mild	moderate
Encephalopathy (grade)	absent	grade 1 or 2	grade 3 or 4
Serum albumin (g/dL)	>3.5	2.8–3.5	<2.8
Serum bilirubin (mg/dL)	1–2	2–3	>3
Prothrombin time (seconds >control)	1–4	4–10	>10

Note: A value of 5 suggests absence of liver impairment, whereas 15 would indicate severe liver failure. The original Child-Turcotte classification consisted of grades A, B, and C, with grade C being the most severe liver disease. Similar to the Pugh modification, the Child-Turcotte classification includes albumin, bilirubin, and ascites, plus assessment of nutrition and neurologic disorder.

The inability of endogenous markers to provide a quantitative measurement of the liver capacity to metabolize drug has led to the administration of exogenous model substrates and calculation of their clearances as quantitative liver function measurements. Based on the physiologic determinants of hepatic clearance discussed previously, these exogenously administered model substrates can be generally categorized into flow-dependent, for example, indocyanine green,[49] lidocaine,[50] and sorbitol;[51] and flow-independent, for example, aminopyrine,[52] antipyrine,[53] caffeine,[54] and erythromycin.[55] However, none of these markers have been shown to be better than the Child-Pugh classification for assessing liver function in patients. The time and invasive procedure for performing these tests also limit their clinical usefulness. Indeed, to date, they have not gained widespread acceptance for predicting drug kinetics and aiding dosage adjustment in patients with liver dysfunction.

Furthermore, studies showed that administration of a flow-dependent and flow-independent model substrate in the same subjects did not result in an independent measure of the physiologic determinants of hepatic clearance. Rather, a correlation between the two test measures was unexpectedly obtained.[56,57] Because cirrhosis causes both irreversible hepatic cell damage and altered vasculature via portosystemic shunting, the pharmacokinetic profile of a drug can be affected by changes in hepatic blood flow and drug-metabolizing enzyme activity. However, it is not known to what extent reduced hepatocyte function would impact elimination of flow-dependent drugs. Nevertheless, the "intact hepatocyte hypothesis," which suggests the presence of intrahepatic shunts in chronic liver disease, has been proposed as a possible explanation for the reduced extraction of flow-dependent drugs, accounting for the observed positive correlation between the clearances of both flow-dependent and flow-independent drugs.[56,57] In addition, given the complexity of the CYP enzyme system, simultaneous administration of several model substrates for different metabolic enzymes as advocated by various cocktail approaches[58–60] would be necessary to characterize the changes in metabolic capacities in patients with liver dysfunction.

DRUG DOSING IN PATIENTS WITH LIVER IMPAIRMENT

Similar to dosing considerations in patients with kidney dysfunction, dosing adjustment in patients with liver diseases can, in general, be accomplished by either a dose reduction or an extended dosing interval, or by a combination of both strategies. However, the lack of a clinical laboratory test that correlates well with the metabolic capacity of the liver hampers the development of dosing guidelines or algorithms similar to that for patients with kidney dysfunction.

Nevertheless, based on an understanding of the pharmacokinetic basis of hepatic drug metabolism, knowledge of the likely etiology of liver dysfunction (reduced liver blood flow, portosystemic shunting, or hepatic failure), and characteristics of the drug in question (flow-dependent or flow-independent, extent of plasma protein binding), a conceptual framework for rational dosing can be made. For drugs with a high ER_H and administered orally, the initial and maintenance doses in patients with cirrhosis need to be reduced because of the significant decrease in first-pass effect caused by portosystemic shunting and decreased hepatic blood flow across the liver. The challenge for adopting this conceptual framework to clinical practice is our ability to predict the magnitude of dose reduction needed. Given the data of Pentikainen[12] and the ranges of reported percent increase in bioavailability for some commonly used drugs (see Table 43–1), one prudent approach is to assume 100% bioavailability unless there is specific bioavailability data or specific dosage adjustment guidelines, and estimate the reduced maintenance dose proportionally by the following mathematical expression:

$$D_H/D_N = F/100$$

where F is the known bioavailability of the drug available from the literature or the manufacturer, and D_H and D_N are the doses used in patients with liver dysfunction and normal liver function, respectively. If drugs with a high ER_H were administered intravenously, then only the maintenance dose would need to be reduced as a result of reduced hepatic blood flow. For drugs with a low ER_H, change in bioavailability is minimal after oral administration and the initial dose for both oral and intravenous routes could be the same as patients with normal liver function. Conversely, the maintenance dose for both administration routes would need to be reduced in patients with cirrhosis according to the reduction in metabolic capacity.

Based on this concept, the oral dose of theophylline can be reduced by up to 50%, which would be in line with the clearance of 0.042 L/kg/h in patients with cirrhosis, as compared to 0.062 L/kg/h in patients with normal liver function.[61] Similarly, the dosage of tolcapone could also be reduced by 50% given the difference in pharmacokinetic profiles in patients with Child-Pugh class B cirrhosis.[3] Obviously, this dose modification serves only as a starting point, consideration of the therapeutic index of the drug in question and good clinical judgment with close monitoring of other factors that can further change the metabolic capacity (e.g., in the case of theophylline, viral illness, smoking, drug–drug interaction, congestive heart failure) would greatly enhance the ability of a clinician to optimize drug therapy in patients with liver dysfunction.

❹ Since there is no equivalent of serum creatinine or creatinine clearance for assisting dosage adjustment in patients with liver dysfunction, the Child-Pugh classification, despite its limitation, is still used primarily by clinicians to assess the extent of liver dysfunction and dose adjustment if needed.[62] As a total Child-Pugh score of 5 and 15 represent, respectively, normal liver function and severe hepatic impairment, it is reasonable to reduce the maintenance dose by 25% for a drug that is primarily dependent on the liver for elimination (≥65% to 70%) in a patient with a score of 8 to 9. A dose reduction of 50% would be prudent for a patient with a score of ≥10. Likewise, Child-Turcotte grades B and C classifications[63] could result in similar 50% and 75% reduction, respectively, of the daily maintenance dose. For both classification systems, depending on the severity of the liver dysfunction and clinical judgment, extension of the dosing interval should also be considered.

In addition, the Food and Drug Administration, through official guidance, also recommend the use of the Child-Pugh classification to categorize the extent of hepatic impairment in patients.[64] As a result, even though the recommendation is not binding, the classification has been employed during drug development in most studies designed to provide dosage recommendation for patients with liver diseases. As an example, a two- to four-fold increases, respectively, in the area under the curve of atomoxetine in patients with Child-Pugh B and C classifications, has led to the labeling recommendations of 50% and 75% reduction of the normal dose used in patients with normal liver function.[65] A summary of such dosage recommendations for 23 recently approved drugs was recently published and is the most quantatative resource currently available.[66]

PHARMACOGENETIC ALTERATION IN DRUG METABOLIZING ENZYME ACTIVITIES

❺ Although many factors, including age, gender, smoking, and diet, can influence drug disposition and therapeutic response in individual patients, recent research emphasis has focused on the effect of pharmacogenetics on drug pharmacokinetics and pharmacodynamics. Chapter 6 provides a more in-depth discussion of the concept of pharmacogenetics and how drug disposition and response are related to specific genotypes and/or phenotypes. The focus of the subsequent sections is to provide information on how pharmacogenetic testing has been reported in the literature for dosing individualization or labeling changes for specific drugs that rely on polymorphic enzymes for their metabolism.

Pharmacogenetic testing for presence of altered metabolic activity can be achieved by phenotyping, genotyping, or both methods. In general, a genotype is a trait marker of an individual's metabolic activity for a specific polymorphic enzyme, and is independent of time and external factors such as concurrent medications, smoking status, or diet. Currently, most laboratory genotyping tests only analyze the more common alleles of a specific polymorphic gene, for example, **2* and **3* for *CYP2C9* and *CYP2C19*, **3*, **4*, **5*, **6*, **2xN* for *CYP2D6*, **28* for *UGT1A1*. Consequently, ethnicity would be important patient-specific information for CYP genotyping if ethnic-specific alleles, such as **5* and **6* for *CYP2C9*, **10*, **17*, and **21* for *CYP2D6*, are to be determined.

Phenotype, on the other hand, represents the metabolic activity at a specific time, which could be susceptible to changes in the presence of concurrent drug therapy. However, in patients receiving concurrent therapy, this usually conceived disadvantage of phenotype might be more useful than genotype in assessing metabolic capacity and hence dosing consideration. For example, in the presence of a potent CYP2D6 inhibitor, the CYP2D6 metabolic capacity of a genotypic extensive metabolizer could be significantly decreased to a level similar to that of a poor metabolizer.[67] In such a scenario, the metabolic capacity would be more reflected by the phenotype, and the dose of a CYP2D6 substrate in a genotypic extensive metabolizer might needed to be adjusted lower, so long as the patient is receiving the CYP2D6 inhibitor concurrently.

DOSING IN PATIENTS WITH GENETICALLY ALTERED METABOLIC CAPACITIES

❻ ALTERATION IN PHASE 1 ENZYMES

CYP2C9

Metabolism of the pharmacologically active *S*-warfarin is mediated by the polymorphic CYP2C9, with the **3* allele having a greater influence on its disposition than the **2* allele. The racemic warfarin doses in patients carrying either of these two allelic variants were in general 15% to 30% lower than those with the wild-type **1* allele.[68] Japanese patients with the *CYP2C9*1/*3* and *CYP2C9*3/*3* genotypes had median dosage requirements that were 48% (0.031 mg/kg/day) and 88% (0.007 mg/kg/day) lower, respectively, than the maintenance dose of 0.06 mg/kg/day in patients with the *CYP2C9*1/*1* genotype.[69] Aithal et al.[68] and Margaglione et al.[70] both reported higher incidence of bleeding complications in patients with the **2* or the **3* allele compared to patients with the **1* allele. Although these and other results[71–74] demonstrate a role for the CYP2C9 polymorphism in determining warfarin dose requirement and minimizing toxicity, the presence of polymorphisms in other target genes, including those affecting the activities of vitamin K 2,3-epoxide reductase complex, subunit 1,[75–78] γ-glutamyl carboxylase,[77,79] epoxide hydrolase,[80] and calumenin,[81] as well as the uptake of vitamin K,[82–84] suggest that we still need to develop a better dosing algorithm or model for widespread genotype-based warfarin dosing in clinical practice.[85] The FDA recently accepted the recommendation of its advisory committee to test for genetic variations in patients receiving warfarin therapy and thus the labeling of warfarin has been updated. Even though it might be difficult and expensive to conduct a randomized genotype-guided warfarin dosing trial, in April 2007 the National Institute of Health issued a Request for Proposal for a Clinical Trial Coordinating Center to conduct a large, multicenter, double-blind randomized trial to compare different approaches to guiding warfarin therapy initiation. The clinical trial primarily aims to evaluate whether using a genotype-enhanced dosing algorithm based on clinical information and knowledge of genetic variants known to affect warfarin metabolism to initiate warfarin treatment will improve anticoagulation status when compared to dosing algorithm using only clinical information.

CYP2C19

The polymorphic CYP2C19 is the primary isoenzyme responsible for the metabolism for proton pump inhibitors. Although there are up to 10-fold differences in systemic exposure between carriers of the *CYP2C19*1* allele versus **2* and **3* alleles, patients possessing one or two of these variant alleles did not experience higher incidence of concentration-related toxicity, likely a reflection of the wide margin of safety for this group of drugs. Rather, the clinical relevance of the CYP2C19 polymorphism lies with the efficacy, with a gene-dose effect in disease cure rate demonstrated for 30 mg of lansoprazole,[86] 20 mg of omeprazole,[87] and 10 mg of rabeprazole,[88] but not for a higher 40 mg dose of omeprazole.

Furata et al.[89] reported the results of pharmacogenomics-based tailored lansoprazole regimens designed to achieve sufficient acid inhibition for eradication of *Helicobacter pylori.* Based on 24-hour intragastric pH monitoring, lansoprazole dosage regimens that achieved intragastric pH ≥5.0 were documented to be 30 mg three times daily for homozygous carriers of the **1* allele, 15 mg three times daily for heterozygous carriers of the **1* allele, and 15 mg twice daily for homozygous carriers of the **2* or **3* alleles. For achieving intragastric pH ≥5.8, the corresponding dosage regimens in the three *CYP2C19* genotypes groups were 30 mg four times daily, 15 mg four times daily, and 15 mg twice daily, respectively. Three hundred *H. pylori*-positive patients were then randomly assigned to receive either the standard regimen consisting of lansoprazole 30 mg, clarithromycin 400 mg, and amoxicillin 750 mg, all given twice daily, or the pharmacogenomics-based regimen consisting of lansoprazole dosed according to patient's *CYP2C19* genotype and antibiotic regimen according to genetic testing of bacterial susceptibility to clarithromycin. The eradication rate for the pharmacogenomics-based regimen was 96% (144 of 150 patients), significantly higher than the 70% (105 of 150 patients) achieved with the standard regimen (P <0.001). In addition, the per-patient cost required for successful eradication for the genotype-based regimen ($669) was similar to that of the standard regimen ($657), lending support not only to the clinical usefulness, but also the cost-effectiveness of pharmacogenomic-based therapeutic approach.

CYP2D6

The report of a female patient found to be resistant to normal doses of nortriptyline[90] represented some of the earliest evidence of how altered metabolic capacity can impact drug dosing and response. The clinical observation and subsequent metabolic phenotyping and genotyping identified three extra copies of the *CYP2D6* gene in the patient,[91] thereby accounting for her extremely high dose requirement of 500 mg/day for nortriptyline. This and other patients with similar high CYP2D6 activity were subsequently categorized as ultrarapid metabolizers.

Since these clinical observations and molecular discoveries, there has been a dramatic increase in the identification, cloning, and investigation of the functional significance of numerous additional *CYP2D6* alleles. To date, it is probably safe to label CYP2D6 as the most studied, yet most variable gene, with significant differences in activity among patients. The presence of multiple alleles with significant interindividual (20% to 96%) and intraindividual (12% to 140%) variabilities in enzyme activity[92,93] may be partially responsible for the time gap between the nortriptyline case report and subsequent attempts to use metabolic genotyping or phenotyping for antidepressant dose recommendation.[94] The investigators compared the pharmacokinetic profiles of 32 CYP2D6- and CYP2C19-dependent antidepressants in subjects with different *CYP2D6* and *CYP2C19* genotypes, took into consideration of the contribution of the polymorphic isoenzymes to the overall elimination of each antidepressant, and provided dose recommendation for 14 of the 32 antidepressants in extensive metabolizers, intermediate metabolizers, and poor metabolizers of CYP2D6 (Fig. 43–2) or CYP2C19. In general, poor metabolizers need approximately 50% of the normal dose of tricyclic antidepressants whereas the dose reduction was smaller for the selective serotonin reuptake inhibitors.

Using the approach proposed by Kirchheiner et al.,[94] nortriptyline maintenance dose requirements for attainment of comparable systemic exposure or therapeutic plasma concentrations could be estimated to be 50% and up to 230% of the average dose, respectively, in poor metabolizers and ultrarapid metabolizers. In contrast, the dose requirements would be 70% to 90% of the average dose in intermediate metabolizers and 100% to 140% of the average dose in extensive metabolizers. Unfortunately, even though there are multiple literature reports of increased adverse effects in poor metabolizers of CYP2D6, there were no other documented reports of therapeutic failure for CYP-dependent antidepressants in ultrarapid metabolizers. Kirchheiner et al.[94] acknowledged the lack of data preclude any dose recommendation in ultrarapid metabolizers for most antidepressants, with the exception being nortriptyline, desipramine, and mianserin, and the dose recommendations are based on data from very few patients. They further noted that only 5 of 54 reviewed studies included evaluation of efficacy in relation to genotypes, and only the study of Mihara et al.[95] showed a significant relationship (P

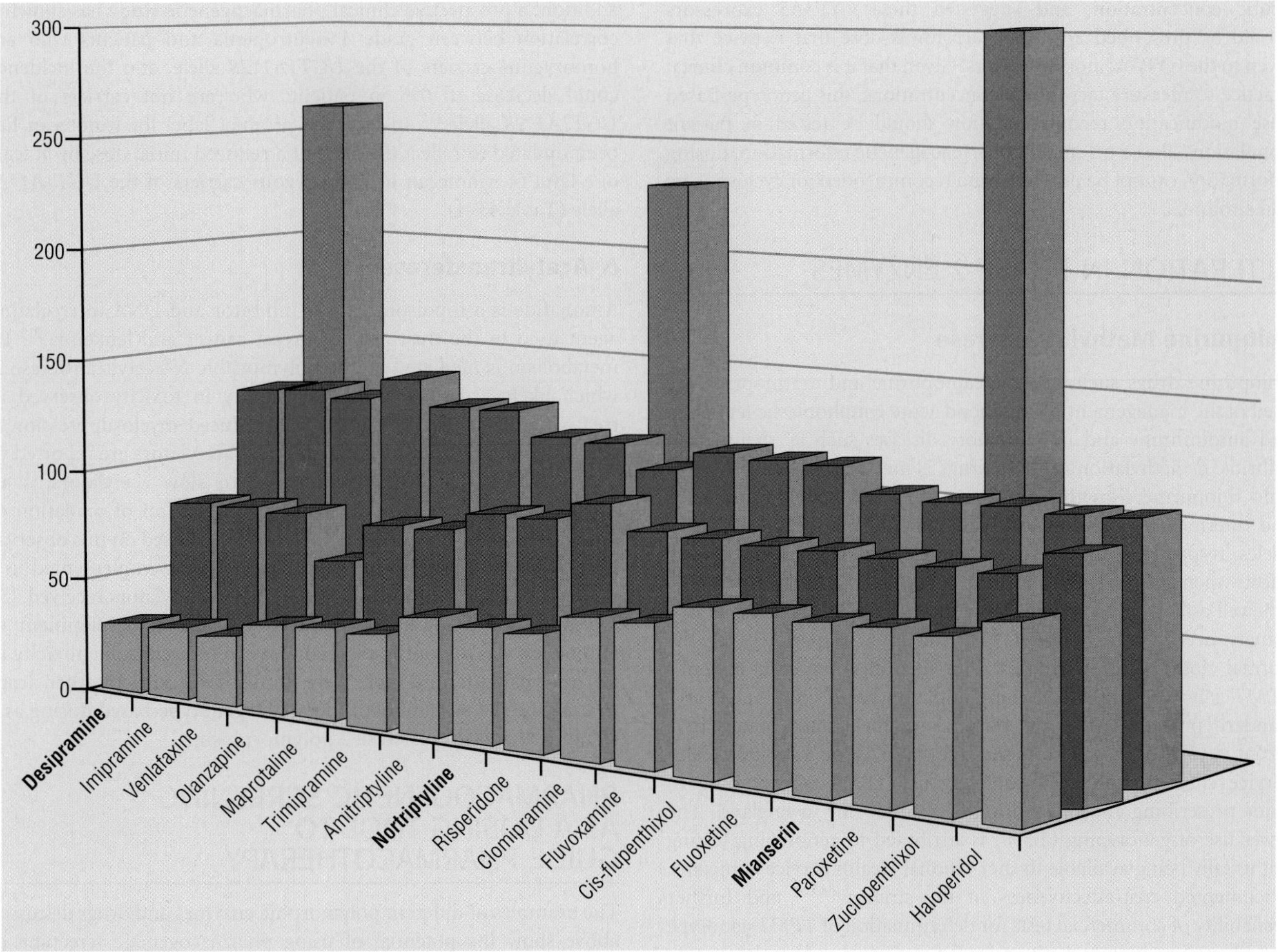

FIGURE 43-2. Schematic representation of dosage adjustment (percent of normal dose) of selected antidepressants and antipsychotics based on CYP2D6 genotypes (starting from the foreground: poor metabolizer, intermediate metabolizer, extensive metabolizer, and ultrarapid metabolizer). *(Data from Kirchheiner J, Brosen K, Dahl M, et al. Acta Psychiatr Scand Suppl 2001;104:173–192.)*

= 0.023). More recently, Brockmoller et al.[96] reported that the clearance of *S*-mirtazapine in ultrarapid metabolizers is 12.6-fold higher than in poor metabolizers, and suggested that poor response might occur in ultrarapid metabolizers as a result of lesser degree of presynaptic α_2-antagonism and lower norepinephrine and serotoninergic activities. Despite implying that a higher dosage for this metabolic group was appropriate, there was no specific recommendation.

❼ Although significant relationship between *CYP2D6* genotype and steady-state antipsychotic pharmacokinetic parameters or drug concentrations have been reported for haloperidol,[97] perphenazine,[98] risperidone,[99] and zuclopenthixol,[98] there were few studies that evaluated or documented how genetic polymorphism could impact clinical outcome,[100] with most of the data showing a higher incidence of concentration-dependent toxicity in poor metabolizers. The study of Brockmoller et al.[97] suggested a nonsignificant trend toward better response to haloperidol in poor metabolizers and lesser response in ultrarapid metabolizers, possibly reflecting the difficulty of relating rating-scale-based changes in psychotic symptoms to specific metabolic genotypes. There is no study that evaluates use of genotyping or phenotyping for dose recommendation of antipsychotics.

The formation of the active metabolite *O*-desmethyltramadol from tramadol is dependent on CYP2D6, and similar to the report with codeine, analgesic relief from tramadol is reported to be lower in poor metabolizers.[101] Although tramadol also possesses other opioid and nonopioid-dependent mechanisms for its analgesic effect, Stamer et al.[102] showed in a prospective study with 300 patients recovering from abdominal surgery, that there is a significant difference in the percentage of nonresponders (based on need for rescue pain medication and patient's satisfaction upon interview) between *CYP2D6* poor metabolizers (46.7%) and extensive metabolizers (21.6%) (P = 0.005). More importantly, they reported a difference in the loading dose of tramadol between the two groups: 144.7 ± 22.6 mg and 108.2 ± 56.9 mg, respectively (P <0.001). 43.3% of genotypic poor metabolizers, compared to 21.6% of genotypic extensive metabolizers, required rescue medication in the recovery room. The authors concluded that poor metabolizers have a higher analgesic consumption. Even though there are likely other significant pharmacogenetic variables affecting opioid analgesic response, the difference in dosing requirement shown in this study suggest that 30% dose increase might be necessary in poor metabolizers of CYP2D6.

CYP3A

Despite the existence of significant interindividual variability in activity, study evaluations of the role of *CYP3A* genes (*CYP3A4*, *CYP3A5*, and *CYP3A7*) in mediating disposition and response so far have not been conclusively clarified. The most convincing evidence showing a genetic influence is *CYP3A5*3* allele affecting tacrolimus pharmacokinetics. Homozygous carriers of the **3* allele were shown to have a higher plasma tacrolimus concentration than patients with the *CYP3A5*1* allele, although considerable overlap exists between the *CYP3A5* genotypes and achievable concentration/dose.[103,104] MacPhee et al.[105] showed that homozygous and heterozygous carriers of the *CYP3A5*1* allele required a longer time to achieve therapeutic concentration, and suggested these CYP3A5 expressors should be prescribed an initial tacrolimus dose that is twice that given to the CYP3A5 nonexpressors. Given that it is common clinical practice to measure tacrolimus concentrations, this genotype-based dose modification recommendation should be tested in patient populations. Based on current pharmacogenetic information, dosing information cannot be predicted and recommended for cyclosporine and sirolimus.

ALTERATION IN PHASE 2 ENZYMES

Thiopurine Methyltransferase

Thiopurine drugs such as 6-mercaptopurine and azathioprine are used in the management of childhood acute lymphoblastic leukemia and autoimmune and inflammatory diseases such as rheumatoid arthritis. *S*-methylation of these drugs is mediated by the polymorphic thiopurine *S*-methyltransferase (TPMT). Poor metabolizers and intermediate metabolizers with two and one deficient *TPMT* alleles, respectively, are prone to significant hematopoietic adverse effects when given standard doses as normal metabolizers. Currently, it is well established that patients with low and intermediate TPMT activity need a maximum of 10% and 50%, respectively, of the normal dose of thiopurines,[106] and identification of a patient's *TPMT* genotype prior to therapy initiation has been adopted as a standard procedure in some hospitals in the United States. In a recent study, Fargher et al.[107] showed that 67% of National Health Service clinicians surveyed routinely use TPMT phenotyping to guide prescribing and monitoring of azathioprine in England. The lower use of genotyping (5.3%) is attributed to genotyping testing not usually being available to the National Health Service clinicians. Documented cost-effectiveness of the strategy[108,109] and further availability of commercial tests for determination of *TPMT* genotype and phenotype may make it easier for justifying and implementing genotype-based thiopurine dosing in other medical centers and clinics.

Uridine Diphosphate Glucuronosyltransferase

The polymorphic uridine diphosphate glucuronosyltransferase 1A1 (UGT1A1) is important for the glucuronidation of several anticancer drugs including irinotecan. Irinotecan is a prodrug and the pharmacologically active moiety, SN-38, is inactivated by UGT1A1. Poor metabolizers of UGT1A1 have reduced SN-38 inactivation[110] and a higher incidence of dose-limiting toxicities such as diarrhea.[111] In addition, a prospective clinical pharmacogenetic study has shown a correlation between grade 4 neutropenia and patients who are homozygous carriers of the *UGT1A1*28* allele, and the incidence could decrease to 0% in patients who are not carriers of the *UGT1A1*28* allele.[112] In fact, the product label for irinotecan has been updated to reflect the need of a reduced initial dose by at least one level of irinotecan in homozygous carriers of the *UGT1A1*28* allele (Table 43–4).

N-Acetyltransferase

Amonafide is a topoisomerase II inhibitor and DNA intercalating agent used in the treatment of breast cancer and leukemia.[113] Its metabolism is mediated by the polymorphic *N*-acetyltransferase 2, which likely accounts for the variability in toxicity observed in treated patients. The extent of drug-induced myelosuppression is correlated to acetylation extent, and fast acetylators are reported to experience greater toxicity compared to slow acetylators,[114] an unexpected phenomenon attributed to inhibition of oxidation of amonafide by the *N*-acetylated metabolite.[115] Based on this observation, genotype-based dosing modifications were implemented in a phase I clinical trial, in which fast and slow acetylators received 250 mg/m^2 and 375 mg/m^2, respectively.[116] Clinical development of amonafide was discontinued secondary to unpredictable toxicity in different patients, and there were no further studies of other drugs to examine the possibility of metabolic genotype-based dosing as a result of *N*-acetyltransferase 2 polymorphism.

PHARMACOGENETIC SCREENING AS A DOSING TOOL TO GUIDE PHARMACOTHERAPY

The examples of different polymorphic enzymes and drugs discussed above show the potential of using pharmacogenetic screening of patients for dosing and optimizing therapy. The value of early detection of patients with deficient metabolic genotype and/or phenotype is clearly demonstrated with the thiopurines and irinotecan, whereas clinical experience with specific tricyclic agents showed that optimal therapeutic response can be achieved earlier with detection of duplicated or amplified *CYP2D6*2* allele. Although there is no documented report of an association between metabolic polymorphisms and selective serotonin reuptake inhibitor efficacy, poor metabolizers do have significant side effects with venlafaxine[117] and paroxetine.[118] Given the high incidence of nonadherence to antidepressants,[119,120] one can also make a case that genotype-based dose reduction in poor

TABLE 43-4 Examples of Label Changes Incorporating Pharmacokinetic Data or Therapeutic Response in Patients with Liver Diseases or Genetic Alteration in Metabolic Capacity

Drug	Relevant Pharmacokinetic Data or Therapeutic Response as a Result of Patient-Specific Alteration in Disposition	Label Information Incorporating Study Data
Atomoxetine	4-fold and 2-fold increases in AUC in patients with Child-Pugh grades C and B classification, respectively	Reduce normal dose by 75% and 50%, respectively, in the two groups of patients.
6-Mercaptopurine (6-MP)	6-MP is inactivated via TPMT to the inactive metabolite methyl-6-MP; TPMT activity is controlled by a genetic polymorphism, with a defined correlation between deficiency in TPMT activity and myelotoxicity	Patients with intermediate TPMT activity may be at increased risk of myelotoxicity if receiving conventional doses of 6-MP. Patients with low or absent TPMT activity are at an increased risk of developing severe, life-threatening myelotoxicity if receiving conventional doses of 6-MP. TPMT genotyping or phenotyping (red blood cell TPMT activity) can help identify patients who are at an increased risk for developing 6-MP toxicity. The optimal starting dose for homozygous-deficient patients has not been established.
Irinotecan	Irinotecan is converted to the active metabolite SN-38, which is subsequently inactivated by UGT1A1; irinotecan toxicity is related to SN-38 exposure	Individuals homozygous for the *UGT1A1*28 allele* are at increased risk for neutropenia after irinotecan administration. A reduction in the starting dose by at least 1 level of irinotecan should be considered for patients known to be homozygous for the *UGT1A1*28 allele*. The appropriate dose reduction in this patient population is unknown.

AUC, area under the curve; TPMT, thiopurine *S*-methyltransferase.

metabolizers might improve therapeutic outcome through a lower incidence of side effects and better adherence to the medication regimen.

Unfortunately, despite the evidence of benefit, the pace of pharmacogenetic-guided individualized therapy is slow.[121] Currently, pharmacogenetic screening of deficiency in TPMT remains one of the few examples of how pharmacogenetics can guide dosing and individualize drug therapy of thiopurines in clinical practice.[107] Even the updated label of irinotecan is lacking specific information of how much the dose reduction should be for homozygous carriers of the *UGT1A1*28* allele. Additionally, genotype-based dosing information is not available for many other drugs. Given the extensive literature on genotype-related differences in drug pharmacokinetics, the lack of dosing information is unfortunate. As an example, clearance of tolbutamide in homozygous carriers of *CYP2C9*3* is 84% lower than in patients with the *CYP2C9*1/*1* genotype, whereas heterozygous carriers of the **2* allele have an approximately 50% lower clearance.[122] Based on these results, dose reductions of approximately 90% and 50% would seem to be an appropriate recommendation in these patients for controlled clinical trials to evaluate whether the goal of genotype-based therapy could be achieved in clinical practice. However, no such prospective trial has been performed. Since efficacy of the oral sulfonylureas can be evaluated easily in clinical practice, implementation of these dose recommendations in clinics or physician offices in lieu of expensive and time-consuming clinical trials might be the first step to take in achieving pharmacogenetic-based dosing and therapy individualization.

Yet it is clear that not all drugs are candidates for genotype-based dose recommendation. The drug in question not only has to be primarily metabolized by a polymorphic enzyme, it also needs to have a narrow therapeutic index. In the study by Brockmoller et al.,[97] although there was a trend toward lower efficacy with increasing number of active *CYP2D6* genes and higher efficacy in the poor metabolizers, there was significant overlap in the haloperidol daily doses among the four metabolic groups, with 14 ± 10 mg in ultrarapid metabolizers versus 13 ± 9 mg in the poor metabolizers. This could be a result of the complex metabolic disposition of haloperidol that includes CYP2D6- and CYP3A4-mediated oxidation, glucuronidation, and interconversion with reduced haloperidol. The clinical usefulness of *CYP2D6* genotyping is further minimized by significant interethnic variabilities in metabolic disposition.[123] In addition, as demonstrated with risperidone, the presence of an active metabolite would also make it difficult to demonstrate the clinical relevance of genotype-based dose recommendation for the parent compound.

❽ Nevertheless, it is encouraging to find that pharmaceutical companies have chosen to include pharmacogenetic screening to identify special populations for evaluation of pharmacokinetics, pharmacodynamics, and clinical outcomes.[124] As an example, *CYP2D6* genotype was one of the patient-related variables included in the evaluation of differences in systemic exposure of atomoxetine in specific populations. Although no specific dose recommendation arose from the results, the information was incorporated into the drug labeling, acknowledging the higher incidence of some adverse drug effect being related to the *CYP2D6* poor metabolizer genotype.[65]

As additional data regarding the clinical relevance of pharmacogenetic screening testing for dosing and therapy individualization become available, the information can be incorporated for drug development as well as for approved drugs. It is noteworthy that over the last few years, the FDA has updated the labeling of 6-mercaptopurine, azathioprine, and irinotecan[125–127] to reflect the risk of toxicity and the need of dosage adjustment in poor metabolizers and intermediate metabolizers of these two polymorphisms. Within the same time period, the FDA has also approved AmpliChip CYP genotyping test for screening of common *CYP2C19* and *CYP2D6* alleles, and the UGT1A1 Molecular Assay for genotyping *UGT1A1* alleles.[128,129] Given that the revised label information does not specifically address the precise dose reduction for patients receiving either 6-mercaptopurine, azathioprine, or irinotecan (see Table 43–4) because of lack of study data using patients' individualized *TPMT* or *UGT1A1* genotypes, it is clear much work, similar to the study of Furuta et al.,[89] needs to be done through additional clinical trials before pharmacogenetics-guided dosing can be achieved in clinical practice.

ABBREVIATIONS

Cl_H: hepatic clearance

Cl_{int}: intrinsic clearance

CYP: cytochrome P450

ER_H: hepatic extraction ratio

fu_B: unbound drug fraction in the blood

Q_H: hepatic blood flow

TPMT: thiopurine *S*-methyltransferase

REFERENCES

1. Wilkinson GR, Shan DG. Commentary: A physiological approach to hepatic drug clearance. Clin Pharmacol Ther 1975;18:377–390.
2. Wilkinson GR. Clearance approaches in pharmacology. Pharmacol Rev 1987;39:1–47.
3. Jorga KM, Crossman JM, Fettler B, et al. Effect of liver impairment on the pharmacokinetics of tolcapone and its metabolites. Clin Pharmacol Ther 1998;63:646–654.
4. Miyajima H, Nomura M, Muguruma N, et al. Relationship among gastric motility, autonomic activity, and portal hemodynamics in patients with liver cirrhosis. J Gastroenterol Hepatol 2001;16:647–650.
5. Grozman R, Kotelanski B, Cohn JN, Khatri IM. Quantification of portosystemic shunting from the splenic and mesenteric beds in alcoholic liver disease. Am J Med 1972;53:715–722.
6. Homeida M, Jackson L, Roberts CJC. Decreased first pass metabolism of labetalol in chronic liver disease. Br Med J 1978;2:1048–1050.
7. Pentikainen PJ, Valisalmi L, Himberg JJ, et al. Pharmacokinetics of midazolam following intravenous and oral administration in patients with chronic liver disease and in healthy subjects. J Clin Pharmacol 1989;29:272–277.
8. Hasselstrom J, Eriksson S, Persson A, et al. The metabolism and bioavailability of morphine in patients with severe liver cirrhosis. Br J Clin Pharmacol 1990;29:289–297.
9. Kleinbloesem CH, van Harten J, Wilson JP, et al. Nifedipine kinetics and hemodynamic effects in patients with liver cirrhosis after intravenous and oral administration. Clin Pharmacol Ther 1986;40:21–28.
10. Rocher I, Decourt S, Leneveu A, et al. Hemodynamic and pharmacokinetic study of propranolol and atenolol in cirrhosis patients. Int J Clin Pharmacol Ther Toxicol 1985;23:406–410.
11. Somogyi A, Albrecht M, Kliems G, et al. Pharmacokinetics, bioavailability, and ECG response of verapamil in patients with liver cirrhosis. Br J Clin Pharmacol 1981;12:51–60.
12. Pentikainen PI, Neuvonen PJ, Jostell KG. Pharmacokinetics of clomethiazole in healthy volunteers and patients with cirrhosis of the liver. Eur J Clin Pharmacol 1980;17:275–284.
13. Andreasen PB, Hendel J, Greisen G, Hvidberg EF. Pharmacokinetics of diazepam in disordered liver function. Eur J Clin Pharmacol 1976;10:115–120.
14. Shull HJ, Wilkinson GR, Johnson R, Schenker S. Normal disposition of oxazepam in acute viral hepatitis and cirrhosis. Ann Intern Med 1976;84:420–425.
15. Ghabrial H, Desmond PV, Watson KJ, et al. The effects of age and chronic liver disease on the elimination of temazepam. Eur J Clin Pharmacol 1986;30:93–97.
16. Morgan DJ, McLean AJ. Therapeutic implications of impaired hepatic oxygen diffusion in chronic liver disease. Hepatology 1991;14:1280–1282.

17. Martinez-Hernandez A, Martinez J. The role of capillarization in hepatic failure: Studies in carbon tetrachloride-induced cirrhosis. Hepatology 1991;14:864–874.
18. Hickey PL, Angus PW, McLean AJ, Morgan DJ. Oxygen supplementation restores theophylline clearance to normal in cirrhotic rats. Gastroenterol 1995;108:1504–1509.
19. Hickey PL, McLean AJ, Angus PW, et al. Increased sensitivity of propranolol clearance to reduced oxygen delivery in the isolated perfused cirrhotic rat liver. Gastroenterology 1996;111:1039–1048.
20. Proulx M, Du Sovich P. Acute moderate hypoxia in conscious rabbits: Effect on hepatic cytochrome P450 and on reactive oxygen species. J Pharm Pharmacol 1995;47:392–397.
21. Richer M, Lam YWF. Hypoxia, arterial pH and theophylline disposition. Clin Pharmacokinet 1993;25:283–299.
22. Froomes PR, Morgan DJ, Smallwood RA, Angus PW. Comparative effects of oxygen supplementation on theophylline and acetaminophen clearance in human cirrhosis. Gastroenterology 1999;116:915–920.
23. Macdonald JI, Wallace SM, Mahachai V, Verbeeck RK. Both phenolic and acyl glucuronidation pathways of diflunisal are impaired in liver cirrhosis. Eur J Clin Pharmacol 1992;42:471–474.
24. Sonne J, Anderson PB, Loft S, et al. Glucuronidation of oxazepam is not spared in patients with hepatic encephalopathy. Hepatology 1990;11:951–956.
25. Furlan V, Demirdjian S, Bourdon O, et al. Glucuronidation of drugs by hepatic microsomes derived from healthy and cirrhotic human livers. J Pharmacol Exp Ther 1999;289:1169–1175.
26. Taburet AM, Naveau S, Zorza G, et al. Pharmacokinetics of zidovudine in patients with liver disease. Clin Pharmacol Ther 1990;47:731–739.
27. George J, Murray M, Byth K, Farrell GG. Differential alterations of cytochrome P450 proteins in livers from patients with severe chronic liver disease. Hepatology 1995;21:120–128.
28. George J, Liddle C, Murray M, et al. Pre-translational regulation of cytochrome P450 genes is responsible for disease-specific changes of individual P450 enzymes among patients with cirrhosis. Biochem Pharmacol 1995;49:873–881.
29. Ishizu H, Shiomi S, Kawamura E, et al. Gastric emptying in patients with chronic liver diseases. Ann Nucl Med 2002;16:177–182.
30. Usami A, Mizukami Y, Onji M. Abnormal gastric motility in liver cirrhosis: Role of secretin. Dig Dis Sci 1998;43:2392–2397.
31. Rodriguez A, Martin A, Oterino JA, et al. Renal function in compensated hepatic cirrhosis: Effects of an amino acid infusion and relationship with nitric acid. Dig Dis 1999;17:235–240.
32. Woitas RP, Heller J, Stoffel-Wagner B, et al. Renal functional reserve and nitric oxide in patients with compromised liver cirrhosis. Hepatology 1997;26:858–864.
33. Ruhnke M, Yeates RA, Pfaff G, et al. Single-dose pharmacokinetics of fluconazole in patients with liver cirrhosis. J Antimicrob Chemother 1995;35:641–647.
34. Diez J, Simon MA, Anton F, et al. Tubular sodium handling in cirrhotic patients with ascites as analyzed by the renal lithium clearance method. Eur J Clin Invest 1990;20:266–271.
35. Orlando R, Sawadogo A, Miglioli PA, et al. Oral disposition kinetics of ofloxacin in patients with compromised liver cirrhosis. Chemotherapy 1992;38:1–6.
36. Laidlaw J, Read AE, Sherlock S. Morphine tolerance in hepatic cirrhosis. Gastroenterology 1961;40:389–396.
37. Ochs HR, Greenblatt DJ, Eckardt B, et al. Repeated diazepam dosing in cirrhotic patients: Cumulation and sedation. Clin Pharmacol Ther 1983;33:471–476.
38. Bakti G, Fisch HU, Karlaganis G, et al. Mechanism of the excessive sedative response of cirrhotics to benzodiazepines: Model experiments with triazolam. Hepatology 1987;7:629–638.
39. Kimelblatt BJ, Cerra FB, Calleri G, et al. Dose and serum concentration relationships in cimetidine-associated mental confusion. Gastroenterology 1980;78:791–795.
40. Chapuis L, Cadranel JF, Nordmann P, et al. Grand mal seizures as a complication of treatment with pefloxacin in patients with cirrhosis: A report of three cases. J Hepatol 1993;19:383–384.
41. Marcantonio LA, Auld WHR, Murdoch WR, et al. The pharmacokinetics and pharmacodynamics of the diuretic bumetanide in hepatic and renal disease. Br J Clin Pharmacol 1983;15:245–252.
42. Villeneuve JP, Verbeeck RK, Wilkinson GR, Branch RA. Furosemide kinetics and dynamics in cirrhosis. Clin Pharmacol Ther 1986;40:14–20.
43. Gentilni P, La Villa G, Marra F, et al. Pharmacokinetics and pharmacodynamics of torasemide and furosemide in patients with diuretic resistant ascites. J Hepatol 1996;25:481–490.
44. Schwartz S, Brater DC, Pound D, et al. Bioavailability, pharmacokinetics, and pharmacodynamics of torasemide in patients with cirrhosis. Clin Pharmacol Ther 1993;54:90–97.
45. Dao MT, Villeneuve JP. Kinetics and dynamics of triamterene at steady-state in patients with cirrhosis. Clin Invest Med 1988;11:6–9.
46. Gerbes AL, Remien J, Jungst D, et al. Evidence for down-regulation of β_2-adrenoreceptors in cirrhosis patients with severe cirrhosis. Lancet 1986;1:1409–1411.
47. Janku I, Perlik F, Tkaczykova M, et al. Disposition kinetics and concentration-effect relationship of metipranolol in patients with cirrhosis and healthy subjects. Eur J Clin Pharmacol 1992;42:337–340.
48. Pugh RN, Murray-Lyon IM, Dawson JL, et al. Transection of the oesophagus for bleeding oesophageal varices. Br J Surg 1973;60:646–649.
49. Soons PA, De Boer A, Cohen AF, Breimer DD. Assessment of hepatic blood flow in healthy subjects by continuous infusion of indocyanine green. Br J Clin Pharmacol 1991;32:697–704.
50. Oellerich M, Burdelski M, Lautz HU, et al. Lidocaine metabolite formation as a measure of liver function in patients with cirrhosis. Ther Drug Monit 1990;12:219–226.
51. Zeeh J, Lange H, Bosch J, et al. Steady-state extrarenal sorbitol clearance as a measure of hepatic plasma flow. Gastroenterology 1988;95:749–759.
52. Villeneuve JP, Infante-Rivard C, Ampelas M, et al. Prognostic value of the aminopyrine breath test in cirrhotic patients. Hepatology 1986;6:928–931.
53. Fabre D, Bressolle F, Comeni R, et al. Identification of patients with impaired hepatic drug metabolism using a limited sampling procedure for estimation of phenazone (antipyrine) pharmacokinetic parameters. Clin Pharmacokinet 1993;24:333–343.
54. Renner E, Wietholtz H, Huguenin P, et al. Caffeine: A model compound for measuring liver function. Hepatology 1984;4:38–46.
55. Watkins PB, Hamilton TA, Annesley TM, et al. The erythromycin breath test as a predictor of cyclosporine blood levels. Clin Pharmacol Ther 1990;48:120–129.
56. Colli A, Buccino G, Cocciolo M, et al. Disposition of a flow-limited drug (lidocaine) and a metabolic capacity limited drug (theophylline) in liver cirrhosis. Clin Pharmacol Ther 1988;44:642–649.
57. Forrest JA, Finlayson ND, Adjepon-Yomoah KK, Prescott LF. Antipyrine, paracetamol, and lignocaine elimination in chronic liver disease. Br Med J 1977;1(6073):1384–1387.
58. Frye RF, Matzke GR, Adedoyin A, et al. Validation of the five-drug "Pittsburgh Cocktail" approach for assessment of selective regulation of drug metabolizing enzymes. Clin Pharmacol Ther 1997;62:365–376.
59. Chainuvati S, Nafziger AN, Leeder JS, et al. Combined phenotypic assessment of cytochrome p450 1A2, 2C9, 2C19, 2D6 and 3A, *N*-acetyltransferase-2 and xanthine oxidase activities with the "Cooperstown 5+1 cocktail." Clin Pharmacol Ther 2003;74:437–447.
60. Jerdi MC, Daali Y, Oestreicher MK, et al. A simplified analytical method for a phenotyping cocktail of major CYP450 biotransformation routes. J Pharm Biomed Anal 2004;35:1203–1212.
61. Piafsky KM, Sitar DS, Rangno RE, Ogilvie RI. Theophylline disposition in patients with hepatic cirrhosis. N Engl J Med 1977;296:1495–1497.
62. Lucena MI, Andrade RJ, Tognoni G, et al. Drugs use for non-hepatic associated conditions in patients with liver cirrhosis. Eur J Clin Pharmacol 2003;59:71–76.
63. Child CI, Turcotte JG. Surgery and portal hypertension. In Child CI, ed. the Liver and Portal Hypertension. Philadelphia: WB Sanders, 1964:1–85.
64. Food and Drug Administration. Guidance for industry: Pharmacokinetics in patients with impaired hepatic function: Study design, data analysis, and impact on dosing and labeling. May 2003, *http://www.fda.gov/cder/guidance/3625fnl.pdf*.
65. Food and Drug Administration. Labeling Information. 2002, *http://www.accessdata.fda.gov/scripts/cder/drugsatfda*.
66. Spray JW, Willett K, Chase D, et al. Dosage recommendation for hepatic dysfunction based on Child-Pugh scores. Am J Health Syst Pharm 2007;64:690–693.
67. Alfaro C, Lam YWF, Simpson J, Ereshefsky L. CYP2D6 status of extensive metabolizers following multiple dose administration of flu-

voxamine, fluoxetine, sertraline, or paroxetine. J Clin Psychopharmacol 1999;19:155–163.

68. Aithal GP, Day CP, Kesteven PJ, Daly AK. Association of polymorphisms in cytochrome P450 CYP2C9 with warfarin dose requirement and risk of bleeding complications. Lancet 1999;353(9154):717–719.
69. Takahashi H, Wilkinson GR, Caraco Y, et al. Population differences in *S*-warfarin metabolism between CYP2C9 genotype-matched Caucasian and Japanese patients. Clin Pharmacol Ther 2003;73:253–263.
70. Margaglione M, Colaizzo D, D'Andrea G, et al. Genetic modulation of oral anticoagulation with warfarin. Thromb Haemost 2000;84:775–778.
71. Higashi MK, Veenstra DL, Kondo LM, et al. Association between CYP2C9 genetic variants and anticoagulation-related outcomes during warfarin therapy. JAMA 2002;287:1690–1698.
72. Hill MA, Wilke RA, Caldwell MD, et al. Relevant impact of covariates in prescribing warfarin according to CYP2C9 genotype. Pharmacogenetics 2004;4:539–547.
73. Peyvandi F, Spreafico M, Siboni SM, et al. CYP2C9 genotypes and dose requirements during the induction phase of oral anticoagulant therapy. Clin Pharmacol Ther 2004;75:198–203.
74. Hillman MA, Wilke RA, Yale SH, et al. A prospective, randomized pilot trial of model-based warfarin dose initiation using CYP2C9 genotype and clinical data. Clin Med Res 2005;3:137–145.
75. D'Andrea G, D'Ambroiso RL, Di Perna P, et al. A polymorphism in the VKORC1 gene is associated with an inter-individual variability in the dose-anticoagulant effect of warfarin. Blood 2005;105:645–649.
76. Rieder MJ, Reiner AP, Gage BF, et al. Effect of VKORC1 haplotypes on transcriptional regulation and warfarin dose. N Engl J Med 2005;352:2285–2293.
77. Wadelius M, Chen LY, Downes K, et al. Common VKORC1 and GGCX polymorphisms associated with warfarin dose. Pharmacogenomics J 2005;5:262–270.
78. Schelleman H, Chen Z, Kealey C, et al. Warfarin response and vitamin K epoxide reductase complex 1 in African Americans and Caucasians. Clin Pharmacol Ther 2007;81:742–747.
79. Shikata E, Ieiri I, Ishiguro S, et al. Association of pharmacokinetic (CYP2C9) and pharmacodynamic (factors II, VII, IX, and X; proteins S and C; and γ-glutamyl carboxylase) gene variants with warfarin sensitivity. Blood 2004;103:2630–2635.
80. Loebstein R, Vecsler M, Kurnik D, et al. Common genetic variants of microsomal epoxide hydrolase affect warfarin dose requirements beyond the effect of cytochrome P4502C9. Clin Pharmacol Ther 2005;77:365–372.
81. Vecsler M, Loebstein R, Almog S, et al. Combined genetic profiles of components and regulators of the vitamin K-dependent γ-carboxylase system affect individual sensitivity to warfarin. Thromb Haemost 2006;95:205–211.
82. Kohnke H, Sorlin K, Granath G, Wadelius M. Warfarin dose related to apolipoprotein E (APOE) genotype. Eur J Clin Pharmacol 2005;61:381–388.
83. Kohnke H, Seordo MG, Pengo V, et al. Apolipoprotein E (APOE) and warfarin dosing in an Italian population. Eur J Clin Pharmacol 2005;61:781–783.
84. Visser LE, Trienekens PH, De Smet PA, et al. Patients with an ApoE epsilon4 allele require lower doses of coumarin anticoagulants. Pharmacogenet Genomics 2005;15:69–74.
85. Gage BF, Eby C, Milligan PE, et al. Use of pharmacogenetics and clinical factors to predict the maintenance dose of warfarin. Thromb Haemost 2004;91:87–94.
86. Furata T, Shirai N, Watanabe F, et al. Effect of cytochrome P4502C19 genotypic differences on cure rates for gastroesophageal reflux disease by lansoprazole. Clin Pharmacol Ther 2002;72:453–460.
87. Furata T, Ohashi K, Kamata T, et al. Effect of genetic differences in omeprazole metabolism on cure rates for *Helicobacter pylori* infection and peptic ulcer. Ann Intern Med 1998;129:1027–1030.
88. Furata T, Shirai N, Takashima M, et al. Effects of genotypic differences in CYP2C19 status on cure rates for *Helicobacter pylori* infection by dual therapy with rabeprazole plus amoxicillin. Pharmacogenetics 2001;11:341–348.
89. Furata T, Shirai N, Kodaira M, et al. Pharmacogenomic-based tailored versus standard therapeutic regimen for eradication of *H. pylori*. Clin Pharmacol Ther 2007;81:521–528.
90. Bertilsson L, Aberg-Wistedt A, Gustaffson LL. Extremely rapid hydroxylation of debrisoquine: A case report with implication for treatment with nortriptyline and other tricyclic antidepressants. Ther Drug Monit 1985;7:478–480.
91. Bertilsson L, Dahl ML, Sioqvist F, et al. Molecular basis for rational megaprescribing in ultrarapid hydroxylators of debrisoquine [letter]. Lancet 1993;341:63.
92. Kashuba AD, Nafziger AN, Kearns G, et al. Quantification of intraindividual variability and the influence of menstrual cycle phase on CYP2D6 activity as measured by dextromethorphan phenotyping. Pharmacogenetics 1998;8:403–410.
93. Labbe L, Sirois C, Pilote S, et al. Effect of gender, sex hormones, time variables and physiological urinary pH on apparent CYP2D6 activity as assessed by metabolic ratios of marker substrates. Pharmacogenetics 2000;10:425–438.
94. Kirchheiner J, Brosen K, Dahl M, et al. CYP2D6 and CYP2C19 genotype-based dose recommendations for antidepressants: A first step towards subpopulation-specific dosages. Acta Psychiatr Scand Suppl 2001;104:173–192.
95. Mihara K, Otani K, Tybring G, et al. The CYP2D6 genotype and plasma concentrations of mianserin enantiomers in relation to therapeutic response to mianserin in depressed Japanese patients. J Clin Psychopharmacol 1997;17:467–471.
96. Brockmoller J, Meineke I, Kirchheiner J. Pharmacokinetics of mirtazapine: Enantioselective effects of the CYP2D6 ultra rapid metabolizer genotype and correlation with adverse effects. Clin Pharmacol Ther 2007;81:699–707.
97. Brockmoller J, Kirchheiner J, Schmider J, et al. The impact of the *CYP2D6* polymorphism on haloperidol pharmacokinetics and on the outcome of haloperidol treatment. Clin Pharmacol Ther 2002;72:438–452.
98. Jerling M, Dahl ML, Aberg-Wistedt A, et al. The CYP2D6 genotype predicts the oral clearance of the neuroleptic agents perphenazine and zuclopenthixol. Clin Pharmacol Ther 1996;59:423–428.
99. Scordo MG, Soina E, Facciola G, et al. Cytochrome P450 2D6 genotype and steady state plasma levels of risperidone and 9-hydroxyrisperidone. Psychopharmacology (Berl) 1999;147:300–305.
100. Schillevoort I, de Boer A, van der Weider J, et al. Antipsychotic-induced extrapyramidal syndromes and cytochrome P450 2D6 genotype: A case-control study. Pharmacogenetics 2002;12:235–240.
101. Poulsen L, Arendt-Nielsen L, Brosen K, Sindrup SH. The hypoanalgesic effect of tramadol in relation to CYP2D6. Clin Pharmacol Ther 1996;60:636–644.
102. Stamer UM, Lehnen K, Hothker F, et al. Impact of CYP2D6 genotype on postoperative tramadol analgesia. Pain 2003;105:231–238.
103. Haufroid V, Mourad M, Van Kerckhove V, et al. The effect of CYP3A5 and MDR1 (ABCB1) polymorphisms on cyclosporine and tacrolimus dose requirements and trough blood levels in stable renal transplant patients. Pharmacogenetics 2004;14:147–154.
104. Zheng H, Zeevi A, Schuetz E, et al. Tacrolimus dosing in adult lung transplant patients is related to cytochrome P4503A5 gene polymorphism. J Clin Pharmacol 2004;44:135–140.
105. MacPhee IA, Fredericks S, Tai T, et al. The influence of pharmacogenetics on the time to achieve target tacrolimus concentrations after kidney transplantation. Am J Transplant 2004;4:914–919.
106. Evans WE, Hon YY, Bomgaars L, et al. Preponderance of thiopurine *S*-methyltransferase deficiency and heterozygosity among patients intolerant to mercaptopurine or azathioprine. J Clin Oncol 2001;19:2293–2301.
107. Fargher EA, Tricker K, Newman W, et al. Current use of pharmacogenetic testing: A national survey of thiopurine methyltransferase testing prior to azathioprine prescription. J Clin Pharm Therap 2007;32:187–195.
108. Tavadia SM, Mydlarski PR, Reis MD, et al. Screening for azathiopurine toxicity: A pharmacoeconomic analysis based on a target case. J Am Acad Dermatol 2000;42:628–632.
109. Oh KT, Anis AH, Bae SC. Pharmacoeconomic analysis of thiopurine methyltransferase polymorphism screening by polymerase chain reaction for treatment with azathioprine in Korea. Rheumatology 2004;43:156–163.
110. Rouits E, Boisdron-Celle M, Dumont A, et al. Relevance of different UGT1A1 polymorphisms in irinotecan-induced toxicity: A molecular and clinical study of 75 patients. Clin Cancer Res 2004;10:5151–5159.

111. Gupta E, Lestingi TM, Mick R, et al. Metabolic fate of irinotecan in humans: Correlation of glucuronidation with diarrhea. Cancer Res 1994;54:3723–3725.
112. Innocenti F, Undevia SD, Iyer L, et al. Genetic variants in the UDP-glucuronosyltransferase 1A1 gene predict the risk of severe neutropenia of irinotecan. J Clin Oncol 2004;22:1382–1388.
113. Costanza ME, Berry D, Henderson IC, et al. Amonafide: An active agent in the treatment of previously untreated advanced breast cancer—A cancer and leukemia group B study (CALGB 8642). Clin Cancer Res 1995;1:699–704.
114. Ratain MJ, Mick R, Berezin F, et al. Paradoxical relationship between acetylator phenotype and amonafide toxicity. Clin Pharmacol Ther 1991;50:573–579.
115. Ratain MJ, Rosner G, Allen SL, et al. Population pharmacodynamic study of amonafide: A Cancer and Leukemia Group B study. J Clin Oncol 1995;13:741–747.
116. Ratain MJ, Mick R, Berezin F, et al. Phase 1 study of amonafide dosing based on acetylator phenotype. Cancer Res 1993;53:2304–2308.
117. Lessard E, Yessine MA, Hamelin BA, et al. Influence of CYP2D6 activity on the disposition and cardiovascular toxicity of the antidepressant agent venlafaxine in humans. Pharmacogenetics 1999;9:435–443.
118. Murphy GM Jr., Kremer C, Rodriguez HE, Schatzberg AF. Pharmacogenetics of antidepressant medication intolerance. Am J Psychiatry 2003;160:1830–1835.
119. Kaplan EM. Antidepressants noncompliance as a factor in the discontinuance syndrome. J Clin Psychiatry 1997;58:31–36.
120. Thompson C, Peveler RC, Stephenson D, McKendrick J. Compliance with antidepressant medication in the treatment of major depressive disorder in primary care: A randomized comparison of fluoxetine and a tricyclic antidepressant. Am J Psychiatry 2000;157:338–343.
121. Zineh I, Pebanco GD, Aquilante CL, et al. Discordance between availability of pharmacogenetic studies and pharmacogenetics-based prescribing information for the top 200 drugs. Ann Pharmacother 2006;40:639–644.
122. Kirchheiner J, Bauer S, Meineke I, et al. Impact of CYP2C9 and CYP2C19 polymorphisms on tolbutamide kinetics and on the insulin and glucose response in healthy volunteers. Pharmacogenetics 2002; 12:101–109.
123. Lam YWF, Jann MW, Chang WH, et al. Intra- and interethnic variability in reduced haloperidol to haloperidol ratios. J Clin Pharmacol 1995;35:128–136.
124. Chou M, Huang SM, Sahajwalla C, Lesko LJ. An informal survey of pharmacogenetics/pharmacogenomics (PGTX) in a sample of INDs and NDAs [abstract]. Clin Pharmacol Ther 2003;73:P33.
125. Purinethol product label, Gate Pharmaceuticals, North Wales, PA, July 2004.
126. Imuran product label, Prometheus Laboratories, Inc., San Diego, CA, July 2005.
127. Camptosar product label, Pfizer, New York, NY, July 2005.
128. Food and Drug Administration, Department of Health and Human Services. Medical devices, clinical chemistry and clinical toxicology devices: Drug metabolizing enzyme genotyping system. Final rule. Fed Regist 2005;70:865–867.
129. Hasegawa Y, Sarashina T, Ando M, et al. Rapid detection of UGT1A1 gene polymorphisms by newly developed Invader assay. Clin Chem 2004;50:1479–1480.

SECTION 5
RENAL DISORDERS

CHAPTER 44

Quantification of Renal Function

THOMAS C. DOWLING

KEY CONCEPTS

1. The stage of chronic kidney disease (CKD) should be determined for all individuals based on the level of kidney function, independent of etiology, according to the National Kidney Foundation (NKF) Kidney Disease/Dialysis Outcome Quality Initiative (K/DOQI) CKD classification system.

2. Persistent proteinuria indicates the presence of chronic kidney disease.

3. Quantitation of urine protein excretion, such as the measurement of a spot urine albumin-to-creatinine ratio, is recommended for determining the severity of CKD and monitoring the rate of disease progression.

4. The glomerular filtration rate (GFR) is the single best indicator of kidney function.

5. Measurement of the GFR is most accurate when performed following the exogenous administration of inulin, iothalamate, or radioisotopes such as technetium-99m diethylenetriamine pentaacetic acid (^{99m}Tc-DPTA).

6. Measurement of creatinine clearance is not routinely recommended; however, pretreatment with cimetidine improves the accuracy of this "measure" of GFR.

7. Equations to estimate creatinine clearance or GFR are commonly used in ambulatory and inpatient settings, and incorporate patient laboratory and demographic variables such as serum creatinine, age, gender, weight, and ethnicity.

8. Longitudinal assessment of GFR and proteinuria is important for monitoring the efficacy of therapeutic interventions, such as angiotensin-converting enzyme inhibitors and angiotensin receptor blockers, which are used to slow or halt the progression of kidney disease.

9. The measurement of a serum creatinine concentration (S_{cr}), evaluation of a plot of the reciprocal of S_{cr} versus time and serum cystatin C concentration should be used with caution to estimate the rate of decline in renal function in CKD patients, as these indices do not consider patient age, lean body mass, gender, diet, concomitant diseases and drug therapy, circadian rhythm, stability of kidney function, or tubular secretion of creatinine.

10. Other assessments of the kidney, such as radiography, computed tomography, magnetic resonance imaging, sonography, and biopsy, are predominantly used for determining the diagnosis of a given condition as they provide evidence of the functional and structural changes associated with kidney disease.

Learning objectives, review questions, and other resources can be found at **www.pharmacotherapyonline.com.**

Kidney disease is a worldwide health problem. It is estimated that 11% of the U.S. population has impaired renal function, with many cases being undiagnosed. Evaluation of renal function using both qualitative and quantitative methods is an important part of the evaluation of patients and an essential characterization of individuals who participate in clinical research investigations. Estimation of creatinine clearance has been considered the clinical standard for assessment of renal function for more than 40 years. Other tests, such as urinalysis, radiographic procedures, and biopsy, are also valuable tools in the assessment of kidney disease, and these qualitative assessments are useful for determining the pathology and etiology of kidney disease. Urinalysis, for example, may give clues to the primary location, such as glomerular or tubular, of the renal disease. Followup studies, such as imaging procedures or kidney biopsy, may then further differentiate the specific cause, thereby guiding the selection of the optimal therapeutic intervention.

1 Quantitative indices, such as the assessment or estimation of glomerular filtration rate (GFR), is now considered the most useful diagnostic tool for the identification of the presence of chronic kidney disease (CKD).[1,2] This index, as well as creatinine clearance, can also be used to quantify changes in function that may occur as a result of disease progression, therapeutic intervention, or a toxic insult.[3] The measurement or estimation of creatinine clearance, however, remains the most commonly used index for individualizing medication dosage regimens for patients with acute or chronic kidney disease.

TABLE 44-1 Markers of Renal Function

Renal plasma/blood flow	*p*-Aminohippurate (PAH)
	^{131}I-Orthoiodohippurate (^{131}I-OIH)
	^{99m}Tc-mercaptoacetyltriglycine (^{99m}Tc-MAG3)
Glomerular filtration rate	Inulin, sinistrin
	Iothalamate
	Iohexol
	^{99m}Tc-diethylenetriaminepentaacetic acid (^{99m}Tc-DTPA)
	^{125}I-Iothalamate
	Creatinine
	Cystatin C
Tubular function	*p*-Aminohippurate (PAH)
	N^1-Methylnicotinamide (NMN)
	Tetraethylammonium (TEA)
	β_2-Microglobulin
	Retinol-binding protein (RBP)
	Protein HC (α_1-microglobulin)
	N-Acetylglucosaminidase (NAG)
	Alanine aminopeptidase (AAP)
	Adenosine binding protein (ABP)

Renal "function" includes the processes of filtration, secretion, and reabsorption, as well as endocrine and metabolic functions. Alterations of all five renal functions, whether declining or improving, are associated primarily with GFR. This chapter critically evaluates the various methods that can be used for the quantitative assessment of kidney function in individuals with normal renal function, as well as in those with chronic kidney disease and acute renal failure (Table 44–1). Where appropriate, discussion regarding the qualitative assessment of the renal function is also presented, including specialized tests such as kidney biopsy.

EXCRETORY FUNCTION

The most important contribution of the kidney to overall maintenance of body homeostasis is the urinary excretion of water, electrolytes, endogenous substances such as urea, and environmental toxins. Through the combined processes of glomerular filtration, tubular secretion, and reabsorption, the nephron, as the functional unit of the kidney, regulates the output of water, electrolytes and solutes from the body, and is the key organ responsible for maintenance of homeostasis despite fluctuations in the dietary ingestion.

FILTRATION

Glomerular filtration is a passive process by which water and small-molecular-weight ions (<5 to 10 kDa) and molecules diffuse across the glomerular–capillary membrane into the Bowman capsule and then enter the proximal tubule (Fig. 44–1). Because most proteins are too large (>60 kDa) to be substantially filtered, or their filtration is impeded by the electronegative charge on the epithelial surface of the glomerulus, compounds presented to the glomerulus in the protein-bound state are not filtered and thus remain in the peritubular circulation.

SECRETION

Secretion is an active process that predominantly takes place in the proximal tubule and facilitates the elimination of compounds from the renal circulation into the tubular lumen. Several highly efficient anionic and cationic transport systems for a wide range of endogenous and exogenous substances have been identified and the renal clearance of these actively secreted entities can greatly exceed GFR; for example, their clearance may be in the range of 600 to 1,000 mL/min.

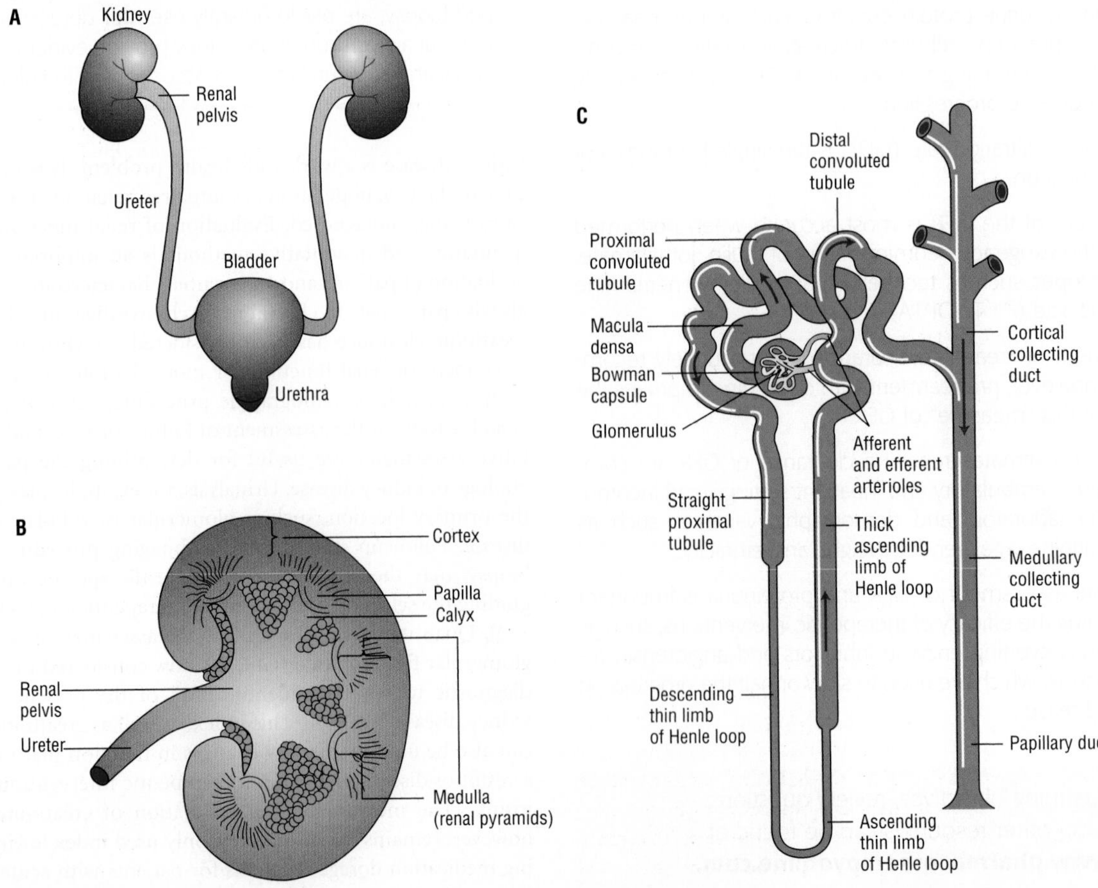

FIGURE 44-1. Structures of the *(A)* urinary system, *(B)* kidney, and *(C)* nephron, the functional unit of the kidney.

Probenecid, *p*-aminohippurate (PAH), and penicillin are examples of anionic substances, whereas creatinine, cimetidine, and procainamide are well-characterized cations.[4] These transport systems are not mutually exclusive, as probenecid has been observed to compete with the tubular secretion of cimetidine.[5] Other transport pathways, such as P-glycoprotein and multidrug resistance protein, are also present in several tissues, including the kidney, liver, jejunum, colon, and brain. These efflux proteins are now recognized as important contributors to the renal elimination of many drugs.[6] For example, P-glycoprotein, which is located on the apical membrane of the proximal tubule, plays an important role in the renal elimination of a wide range of drugs, such as cimetidine, digoxin, and procainamide. Blockade of P-glycoprotein could result in decreased renal elimination of such compounds, leading to an increased drug exposure. Verapamil and cyclosporine are the two most widely studied agents that reduce the activity of this tubular transport mechanism.[5] Further investigations into the exact role of the P-glycoprotein and multidrug resistance protein efflux pathways on drug elimination are presently underway.

REABSORPTION

Reabsorption of water and solutes occurs throughout the nephron, whereas the reabsorption of most medications occurs predominantly along the distal tubule and collecting duct. Urine flow rate and physicochemical characteristics of the molecule influence these processes: highly ionized compounds are not reabsorbed unless pH changes within the urine increase the fraction unionized, so that reabsorption may be facilitated.

INTACT NEPHRON HYPOTHESIS

The "intact nephron hypothesis" described by Bricker,[8] which was published more than 40 years ago, proposes that "kidney function" of patients with renal disease is the net result of a reduced number of appropriately functioning nephrons. As the number of nephrons is reduced from the initial complement of 2 million, those which are unaffected compensate; that is, they hyperfunction. The cornerstone of this hypothesis is that glomerulotubular balance is maintained, such that those nephrons capable of functioning will continue to perform in an appropriate fashion. Extensive studies have indeed shown that single-nephron glomerular filtration rate increases in the unaffected nephrons, thus the whole-kidney GFR which represents the sum of the single-nephron glomerular filtration rates of the remaining functional nephrons may remain close to normal until there is extensive injury. Based on this, one would presume that a measure of one component of nephron function could be used as an estimate of all renal functions. This, indeed, has been and remains our clinical approach.

FILTRATION CAPACITY

GFR is dependent on numerous factors, one of which is protein load. Bosch[9] suggested that an appropriate comprehensive evaluation of renal function should include the measurement of "filtration capacity" of the kidney. This is similar in context to a cardiac stress test. The patient may have no hypoxic symptoms, for example, angina while resting, but it may become quite evident when the patient begins to exercise. Subjects with normal renal function administered an oral or intravenous protein load prior to measurement of GFR have been noted to increase their GFR by as much as 50%.[9] As renal function declines, the kidneys usually compensate by increasing the single-nephron glomerular filtration rate. The renal reserve, the maximal degree by which GFR can be increased will be reduced in those individuals whose kidneys are already functioning at higher-than-normal levels because of preexisting renal injury. Thus this may be a complementary, insightful index of renal function reserve for many individuals with as yet unidentified CKD.

Quantification of renal function is not only an important component of a diagnostic evaluation, but it also serves as an important parameter for monitoring therapy directed at the etiology of the diminished function itself, thereby allowing for objective measurement of the success or failure of treatment. Measurement of renal function also serves as a useful indicator of the ability of the kidneys to eliminate drugs from the body. Furthermore, alterations of drug distribution and metabolism have been associated with the degree of renal function. A discussion of pharmacokinetic changes in renal disease is extensively reviewed in Chap. 51. Although several indices have been used for the quantification of filtration capacity or GFR in the research setting, estimation of creatinine clearance and GFR are the primary ones used in the clinical arena.

ENDOCRINE FUNCTION

The kidney synthesizes and secretes many hormones involved in maintaining fluid and electrolyte homeostasis. Secretion of renin by the cells of the juxtaglomerular apparatus and production and metabolism of prostaglandins and kinins are among the kidney's endocrine functions. In addition in response to decreased oxygen tension in the blood which is sensed by the kidney, erythropoietin is produced and secreted by peritubular fibroblasts. Because these functions are related to renal mass, decreased endocrine activity is associated with the loss of viable kidney cells. In the presence of stages 3 to 5 chronic kidney disease and moderate to severe acute renal injuries, secretion of erythropoietin is impaired leading to reduced red blood cell formation; normocytic anemia and symptoms of reduced oxygen delivery to tissues such as fatigue, dyspnea, and angina (see Chaps. 46 and 47). Renal anemia is clearly associated with many comorbidities, such as left ventricular hypertrophy, which is present in more than 40% of CKD patients.[10] Indeed, anemia-induced renal hypoxia results indirectly in erythropoietin gene activation, tubular necrosis, and apoptosis, thereby contributing to further renal cell injury.[11] This cyclic relationship between kidney disease, suppression of erythropoietin secretion, and cardiovascular disease is also referred to as the cardiorenal anemia syndrome.

METABOLIC FUNCTION

The kidneys perform a wide variety of metabolic functions, including the activation of vitamin D_3, gluconeogenesis, and metabolism of endogenous compounds such as insulin, steroids, and xenobiotics. Impaired renal function results in decreased formation of activated vitamin D_3 and decreased insulin metabolism. It is common for patients with diabetes and chronic renal failure to have reduced requirements for exogenous insulin,[12] and supplemental therapy with activated vitamin D_3 (calcitriol) or other vitamin D analogs (paricalcitol, doxercalciferol) is often necessary to avert the bone loss and pain associated with renal osteodystrophy.[13] Cytochrome P450, *N*-acetyltransferase, glutathione transferase, renal peptidases, and other enzymes responsible for the degradation and activation of selected endogenous and exogenous substances have been identified in the kidney. The cytochrome P450 (CYP) system in the kidneys is as active as that in the liver, when corrected for organ mass. In vitro studies have demonstrated impaired function of CYP3A4 and CYP2C9, whereas CYP1A2, CYP2C19, and CYP2D6 are not affected. This data is supported by recent clinical trials in end-stage renal disease patients receiving hemodialysis, where hepatic CYP3A activity was reported to be reduced by 28% from values observed in age-matched controls; partial correction was

TABLE 44-2 Presentation of Chronic Kidney Disease (CKD)

	Early CKD (Stages 1–2)	Late CKD (Stages 3–4)
General	The patient may not appear in distress	Patient may have edema
Symptoms	Not likely present	The patient may have fatigue, malaise, pruritus, nausea
Signs	Not likely present	May present with fluid retention, anemia, dyspnea, reduced urine output
Laboratory tests	Microalbuminuria Mildly-elevated serum creatine and blood urea nitrogen	Persistent proteinuria Reduced glomerular filtration rate or creatine clearance rate Abnormal urinalysis
Other diagnostic tests		Renal ultrasound shows reduced kidney mass

noted following the hemodialysis procedure.[14,15] See Chap. 51 for a more detailed discussion.

QUALITATIVE AND SEMIQUANTITATIVE INDICES OF KIDNEY FUNCTION

Patients who develop CKD remain relatively asymptomatic until impairment has progressed to the point that systemic manifestations and/or secondary complications become evident (Table 44–2).

As renal function declines, patients may develop de novo or experience an exacerbation of hypertension, edema, electrolyte abnormalities, anemia, or other complications (see Chaps. 46 and 47). The National Kidney Foundation (NKF) currently recommends that all patients with CKD, and those at increased risk for CKD, undergo at least yearly a comprehensive laboratory assessment comprised of (a) serum creatinine to estimate GFR; (b) albumin-to-creatinine ratio in a spot urine specimen; (c) examination of urine sediment for red blood cell and white blood cell counts; (d) renal ultrasonography; (e) serum electrolytes, including sodium, potassium, chloride, and bicarbonate; (f) urine pH; and (g) urine specific gravity.[16] The role of each of these indices in the identification and monitoring of CKD are discussed in detail below.

LABORATORY PROCEDURES TO DETECT THE PRESENCE OF KIDNEY DISEASE

Urinalysis is an important tool for detecting and differentiating various aspects of kidney disease, which often goes unnoticed as the result of its asymptomatic presentation. Urinalysis can be used to detect and monitor the progression of diseases such as diabetes mellitus, glomerulonephritis, and chronic urinary tract infections.[16–18] A typical urinalysis provides information about physical and chemical composition, most of which can be completed quickly and inexpensively by visual observation (volume and color) and dipstick testing. Microscopic urinalysis requires use of a light microscope to determine cellular content as described below.

Chemical Analysis of Urine

pH The normal urine pH typically ranges from 4.5 to 7.8, and an elevation above this may suggest the presence of urea-splitting bacteria. In patients with renal tubular acidosis, urine pH is usually >5.5 because of impaired hydrogen ion secretion in the distal tubule or collecting duct.

Glucose Glucose is usually not present in the urine because the kidney normally completely reabsorbs all the glucose filtered at the glomerulus. When a patient's blood glucose concentration exceeds the maximum threshold for glucose reabsorption in the kidney (~180 mg/dL), glucosuria will be present. Routine assessment of glucosuria has been replaced by newer methods of direct blood glucose measurements. Urine glucose testing is now predominantly used as a screening tool for the detection of diabetes.

Ketones Acetoacetate and acetone are not normally found in the urine; they are however excreted in patients with diabetic ketoacidosis. They are also present under conditions of fasting or starvation. Typically, values of acetone excretion are reported as small (<20 mg/dL), moderate (30 to 40 mg/dL), and large (>80 mg/dL).

Nitrite Nitrite is not usually present in urine. The presence of nitrite is most commonly the result of conversion from urinary nitrate by bacteria present in the urine. The presence of nitrite thus suggests that the patient has a urinary tract infection, commonly caused by gram-negative rods such as *Escherichia coli*. Although false-positive results are very rare, false-negative results are more common and may be caused by lack of dietary nitrate, reduced urine nitrate concentration as a consequence of diuresis, or infections caused by bacteria such as enterococci and *Acinetobacter*, which do not reduce nitrate, and pseudomonads, which convert nitrate to nitrogen gas.

Leukocyte Esterase Leukocyte esterase is released from lysed granulocytes in the urine; its presence is suggestive of urinary tract infection. False-positive tests can result from delayed processing of the urine sample, contamination of the sample with vaginal secretions (such as blood or heavy mucus discharge), or by *Trichomonas* infection (such as trichomoniasis). False-negative tests can be produced by the presence of high levels of protein or ascorbic acid.

Heme The heme test indicates the presence of hemoglobin or myoglobin in the urine. A positive test without the presence of red blood cells suggests either red cell hemolysis or rhabdomyolysis.

Protein or Albumin Persistent proteinuria or albuminuria, that is, observation of its presence on at least three occasions over a period of 3 to 6 months, is now considered the principal marker of kidney damage.[16,17] ❷ Evaluation of urinary protein or albumin is now a standard tool used to characterize the severity of CKD and to monitor the rate of disease progression or regression. Under normal conditions, plasma proteins remain in the glomerular capillaries as blood perfuses the kidney and thus do not cross the glomerular basement membrane or enter the urinary space. Some of these proteins, such as albumin and globulins are not filtered by the glomerulus as a result of charge and size selectivity (>40 kDa). Smaller proteins (<20 kDa) pass across the glomerular basement membrane but are readily reabsorbed in the proximal tubule. Most healthy individuals excrete between 30 and 150 mg/day of total protein consisting of approximately 30 mg/day of albumin. The remainder of the protein in the urine is secreted by the tubules (Tamm-Horsfall, immunoglobulin A, and urokinase) or comprised of smaller proteins such as β_2-microglobulin, apoproteins, enzymes, and peptide hormones. Increased excretion of these low-molecular-weight proteins in the urine is considered a sensitive marker of tubulointerstitial disease.

Historically, the sulfosalicylic acid test was used as a crude measure of proteinuria. This test is performed by adding sulfosalicylic acid to urine and then visually comparing this admixture with a tube of untreated urine; the presence of turbidity indicates the qualitative presence of proteinuria. Dipstick tests are now the most common means to determine in a semiquantitative fashion a patient's daily urine protein or albumin excretion. False-positive results can occur in the presence of alkaline urine (pH more than 7.5), when the dipstick is immersed too long, in those with highly concentrated urine, in the presence of drugs such as penicillin, sulfonamides, or tolbutamide, as well as blood, pus, semen, or vaginal secretions. False-negative results occur with dilute urine (specific gravity <1.015) and when proteinuria is caused by nonalbumin or low-molecular-weight proteins such as heavy or light chains or Bence Jones proteins. The results of these dipstick tests are graded as negative (<10 mg/dL), trace (10 to 20 mg/dL), 1+ (30 mg/dL), 2+ (100 mg/dL), 3+ (300 mg/dL), or 4+ (>1,000 mg/dL). Portable desktop analyzers such as the Chemstrip 101 Urine Analyzer (Roche Diagnostics) and Clinitek 50 Urine Chemistry Analyzer (Bayer Corporation) can also be used as an alternative to visual urinalysis test-strip evaluation.

❸ Because most dipstick methods are not specific for albumin, test strips that are specific for low levels of albuminuria (30 to 300 mg/day) should be employed. Microalbuminuria test strips, such as the Chemstrip Micral-Test II (Roche Diagnostics), when dipped into a urine sample assume a color ranging from white (0 mg/L) to red (100 mg/L), depending on the amount of albumin present in the sample. In patients with a positive protein or albumin dipstick test, a 24-hour urine collection with measurement of albumin excretion can be used to further define the degree of albuminuria. However, this method requires a high degree of patient compliance and is being replaced by a similarly accurate but less cumbersome technique: calculation of the ratio of protein or albumin (in milligrams) to creatinine (in grams) obtained from an untimed (spot) urine specimen. The normal ratio is <30 mg albumin or <200 mg protein per gram of creatinine in the urine, with values between 30 and 300 mg of albumin per gram of creatinine considered to be in the microalbuminuria range.[16] Positive test results should be repeated, particularly in patients without an underlying cause for renal disease, such as diabetes or hypertension. Monitoring of the degree of glomerular injury in CKD patients should use the albumin-to-creatinine ratio, whereas for patients with clinical proteinuria, that is, excretion of >500 mg per day or an albumin-to-creatinine ratio >500 mg/g, the protein-to-creatinine ratio can be used.

CLINICAL CONTROVERSY

In the past, measurement of urinary protein excretion rate was accomplished using a 24-hour urine collection in patients who were at risk for CKD. However, many now advocate the use of an untimed "spot" urine sample with either an albumin-specific dipstick or measurement of the albumin-to-creatinine ratio.

Specific Gravity Specific gravity is a measure of urine weight relative to water (1.00) that is performed using a refractometer. Thus, specific gravity is dependent on water intake and urine-concentrating ability. Normal values range from 1.003 to 1.030. Osmolality, which is a measure of the number of solute particles in the urine, is a more accurate measure of the kidney's ability to make a concentrated urine. Generally the two values correlate; however, when large quantities of heavier molecules, such as glucose, are in the urine, the specific gravity may be elevated relative to the osmolality. These tests are used in the assessment of urine-concentrating ability and are most informative when interpreted along with the hydration status of the patient and plasma osmolality.

Microscopic Analysis of Urine Formed elements that may be detected in the urine include erythrocytes and leukocytes, casts, and crystals. An important consideration in the assessment of hematuria is whether the cells are of renal origin. More than 2 cells per high-power field is abnormal, and the presence of dysmorphic cells suggest renal parenchymal origin either because of damage as they pass through the glomerulus or during exposure to the varying osmotic environments of the tubular lumen. White blood cells may be present in the urine in association with infection or inflammatory conditions, such as interstitial nephritis. More than 1 cell per high-power field is usually considered abnormal. Contamination of the sample should also be considered when there are many cells and may be a result of the presence of menses or of inadequate sample collection. Casts are cylindrical forms composed of protein, with or without cells that take the shape of the collecting tubules, where they are formed. Casts without cells are labeled *hyaline casts* and consist of the Tamm-Horsfall mucoprotein, secreted by the renal tubules. They are nonspecific and may appear in concentrated urine. In the presence of red or white blood cells, casts may be formed that include the cells, indicating that the cells were of renal origin. Solubility of the Tamm-Horsfall protein is increased as urine pH rises; therefore, sample collection for casts should occur with the first morning void when the urine is most acidic. Otherwise, casts may dissolve and elude detection.

A variety of crystals may be present in the urine, including uric acid, calcium oxalate, calcium phosphate, calcium magnesium ammonium pyrophosphate, and cystine. Many of these have a unique crystalline form, which permits them to be identified with microscopy.

Serum or Blood Urea Nitrogen

Amino acids metabolized to ammonia are subsequently converted in the liver to urea, the production of which is dependent on protein availability (diet) and hepatic function. Urea undergoes glomerular filtration followed by reabsorption of up to 50% of the filtered load in the proximal tubule. The reabsorption rate of urea is predominantly dependent on the reabsorption of water. The excretion of urea may, therefore, be decreased under conditions which necessitate water conservation such as dehydration although the GFR may be normal or only slightly reduced. This condition is evident when a patient exhibits prerenal azotemia, or an increase of the blood urea nitrogen to a greater extent than the serum creatinine. The normal blood urea nitrogen-to-creatinine ratio is 10 to 15:1, and an elevated ratio is suggestive of a decreased effective circulating volume, which stimulates increased water, and hence, urea reabsorption. Creatinine is not reabsorbed to any significant extent by the kidneys. Despite these limitations, the blood urea nitrogen is usually used in combination with the serum creatinine concentration as a simple screening test for the detection of renal dysfunction.

Serum Creatinine

Creatinine is the standard laboratory marker for the detection of kidney disease. The third National Health and Nutrition Examination Survey (NHANES III) revealed a mean serum creatinine of 0.96 mg/dL in women, and 1.16 mg/dL in men in the United States.[19] Values were lower among Mexican Americans, and higher among non-Hispanic blacks. For all groups, the serum creatinine increased with age. The report also noted that among community-dwelling adults, 10.9 million have a serum creatinine greater than 1.5 mg/dL; 3.0 million have a serum creatinine greater than 1.7 mg/dL; and 0.8 million have a serum creatinine greater than 2.0 mg/dL. Although the serum creatinine concentration alone is not an optimal measure of kidney function, it is often used as a marker for referral to a nephrologist. There is presently no accepted single standard for an "abnormal" serum creatinine, as it is gender, race, and age-dependent.

The concentration of creatinine in serum is a function of creatinine production and renal excretion. Creatinine is a product of creatine metabolism from muscle; therefore, its production is directly dependent on muscle mass. At steady state, the "normal" serum creatinine concentration range is 0.5 to 1.5 mg/dL for males and females. Creatinine is eliminated primarily by glomerular filtration, and as GFR declines, the serum creatinine concentration rises (Fig. 44–2).

Several methods are used for the determination of the serum creatinine concentration, most of which use the nonspecific Jaffe reaction, a colorimetric method based on the reaction of creatinine

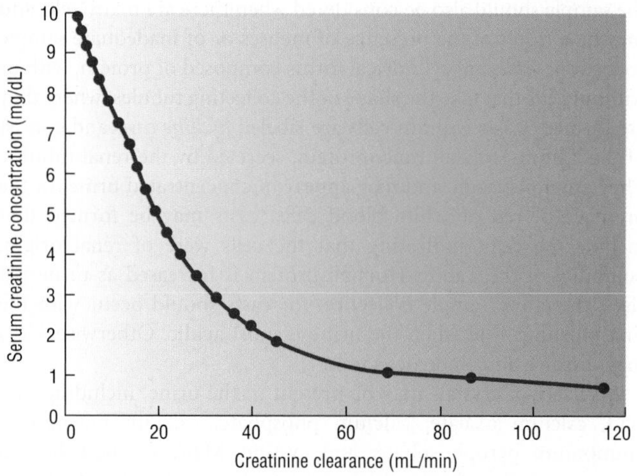

FIGURE 44-2. Relationship between serum creatinine and creatinine clearance.

with alkaline picrate. This nonspecific method also reacts with noncreatinine chromogens in the serum, which may result in a falsely increased serum creatinine concentration.[17] The noncreatinine chromogens are not present in the urine in sufficient quantities to interfere with the urinary creatinine measurement, because the concentration of creatinine in urine is several-fold greater than the serum concentration. The impact of this interference is seen with the creatinine clearance (CL_{cr}) calculation:

$$CL_{cr} = (U_{cr} \times V) / S_{cr} \times t)$$

where U_{cr} = urine creatinine concentration, V = urine volume, S_{cr} = serum creatinine concentration, and t = duration of the urine collection.

This "normal" interference results in an increase in the serum creatinine concentration of approximately 10% and thereby the measured creatinine clearance would underestimate the true GFR by 10%. In subjects with normal renal function, this tends to counterbalance the effect of the contribution of tubular secretion of creatinine, which increases urine creatinine by nearly 10%. Thus, CL_{cr} has been proposed to serve as a good measure of GFR in subjects with normal renal function. However, this false increase in serum creatinine becomes less noticeable as the true creatinine concentration rises, due to the increasing contribution of tubular secretion to the renal clearance of creatinine.[20] This becomes of major importance when kidney function is reduced to less than 50% of normal.

Diabetic ketoacidosis may produce increased concentrations of acetoacetate, which serves as a chromophore in the Jaffe reaction, thereby increasing the serum creatinine concentration. Other substances that also react with this procedure in the serum include glucose, protein, pyruvate, fructose, uric acid, and ascorbic acid (Table 44–3). In addition, some cephalosporin antibiotics are associated with a false increase in the serum creatinine concentration, including cephalothin, cefazolin, cephalexin, cefoxitin, cefaclor, and cephradine,[21] whereas other antibiotics, such as the fluoroquinolones (ciprofloxacin, fleroxacin, lomefloxacin, ofloxacin, levofloxacin, sparfloxacin, and temafloxacin), do not produce a false elevation in serum creatinine.[22] The degree of interference is dependent on the serum concentration of the antibiotic, so blood samples for creatinine should be obtained when the antibiotic concentration is lowest (at the end of a dosing interval). These interferences are not observed when the serum creatinine is measured using an enzymatic technique. The antifungal agent 5-flucytosine causes an increase in the serum creatinine when measured using the Ektachem enzymatic system, but does not interact with the Jaffé method.[23] Daly et al.[24] reported a false-negative effect of dobutamine and dopamine on the serum creatinine value when measured using the Ektachem system.

TABLE 44-3 Factors That May Alter Creatinine Clearance Determinations

Analytical	Physiologic
Acetoacetate	Age, weight, gender
Ascorbic acid	Diet
Cephalosporins (cephalothin, cefazolin, cephalexin, cefoxitin, cefaclor, cephradine)	Diurnal variation
	Cimetidine
Dobutamine	Trimethoprim
Dopamine	Probenecid
5-Flucytosine	Exercise
Fructose	
Glucose	
Protein	
Pyruvate	
Uric acid	

The interference is concentration dependent and results in a 10% to 100% decrease of the serum creatinine concentration. The authors hypothesized that both drugs compete with the chromogenic dye for oxidation by hydrogen peroxide in a concentration-dependent manner. The problem is most evident when blood samples are contaminated with residual IV solution containing the interfering drug. These differences emphasize the need to standardize a method within the clinic setting and require the clinician to be aware of the methods employed in the laboratory for the determination of creatinine concentrations.

Other compounds are known to interfere with the serum creatinine concentration by inhibition of the active tubular secretion of creatinine. Among these are cimetidine and trimethoprim, which compete for creatinine secretion at the cationic transport system in a dose-dependent fashion. Cimetidine, given as a single 400-mg dose can result in a reduction of the CL_{cr}-to-inulin clearance ratio from 1.30 to 1.03, without a change in inulin clearance. Ranitidine, an H_2-receptor antagonist similar to cimetidine, however, does not have a similar effect on creatinine secretion following single doses of 300 to 1,200 mg.[25]

The serum creatinine concentration is dependent on the "input" function, or formation rate, and "output" function, or elimination rate. Its formation rate depends on the zero-order production from creatine metabolism, as well as input from other sources, such as dietary intake. Creatine metabolism is directly proportional to muscle mass; therefore, individuals with more muscle mass have a higher serum creatinine concentration at any given degree of kidney function than those with less muscle mass. Strenuous exercise is associated with an increase of approximately 10% in the serum creatinine concentration. In contrast, cachectic patients, as the result of minimal muscle mass, will have very low serum creatinine concentrations, as do those with spinal cord injuries.[26] Elderly patients and those with poor nutrition may also have low serum creatinine concentrations (<1.0 mg/dL) secondary to decreased muscle mass. Other factors that influence the serum creatinine concentration include the dietary intake of creatine. During the cooking of meat, some creatine is converted to creatinine, which is rapidly absorbed following ingestion.

Serum creatinine concentrations may rise as much as 50% within 2 hours of a meat meal and remain elevated for as long as 8 to 24 hours.[27] Ingestion of creatine as an ergogenic dietary supplement is currently popular. There are conflicting reports as to the effect of creatine ingestion on the serum creatinine concentration. Poortsmans et al.[28] evaluated a short-term regimen of 20 g creatine per day for 5 days in healthy subjects, and reported no significant change in the serum creatinine, creatinine excretion rate, or creatinine clearance. Robinson et al.,[29] however, reported a 25% to 40% increase in the serum creatinine concentration after ingestion of 20 g creatine per day for either 5 days or 8 weeks. The renal excretion rate of creatinine was not measured. The issue of whether creatine ingestion adversely affects kidney function was studied by Edmonds et al.[30] They noted that creatine supplementation led to an increase in renal disease progression in a rat model for renal cystic disease, suggesting that creatine supplementation may be a risk factor in patients with preexisting renal disease. These conditions present a problem only when a single serum creatinine concentration is used to represent the entire 24-hour collection period, which is usually the case. An alternative is to obtain multiple samples and calculate the area under the serum concentration time curve and divide this by the collection time interval to obtain the average plasma creatinine concentration. This is rarely done in clinical practice, but points out the need to question patients regarding dietary intake for the 24 hours preceding the measurement of CL_{cr}.

Diurnal variation in serum creatinine concentration may also affect the accuracy of the CL_{cr} determination. Although the fluctuation is minimal, the observed peak plasma creatinine concentration generally occurs at approximately 7:00 PM, whereas the nadir is in the morning. To minimize this effect, the CL_{cr} is usually performed over a 24-hour period with the plasma creatinine obtained in the morning, as long as the patient has stable kidney function. Collection of urine remains a limiting factor in the 24-hour CL_{cr} because of incomplete collections, and interconversion between creatinine and creatine that can occur if the urine is not maintained at a pH <6.

Cystatin C

Cystatin C is a 132-amino-acid (13.3-kDa) cysteine protease inhibitor produced by all nucleated cells of the body that is being investigated as a potential biomarker of renal function. It is freely filtered at the glomerulus and undergoes some reabsorption and catabolism in the proximal tubule. However, it has been shown that serum cystatin C concentrations can be altered by many factors other than kidney function, such as age, nutritional status, gender, weight, height, cigarette smoking, serum C-reactive protein levels, steroid therapy, and rheumatoid arthritis.[31–33] Originally introduced in Europe, it has been recommended as a test of kidney function because of findings that serum concentrations significantly correlated with GFR as well as serum creatinine. The recent development of an automated immunoassay technique has resulted in the development of suggested reference ranges of 0.70 to 1.38 mg/L in children older than 1 year of age, and 0.54 to 1.21 mg/L in adults. Its sensitivity as an indicator of renal function relative to other markers such as serum creatinine is yet to be fully defined. Early evidence suggests that it may be a more sensitive index of kidney disease; comparison of ^{125}I-iothalamate with serum creatinine and cystatin C showed that the serum creatinine began to increase when the GFR was 75 mL/min/1.73 m^2 as compared to 88 mL/min/1.73 m^2 for cystatin C.[31] However, Keevil et al.[34] reported that serum cystatin C had greater intraindividual variability than serum creatinine in healthy individuals, which may limit its use in longitudinal evaluations of renal function.

Several recent studies suggest that there is still much to discover before we know whether this test will be a replacement for creatinine or a confounding ancillary test. In a 4-year longitudinal study in 30 Pima Indians without CKD, the reciprocal cystatin C index (100/cystatin C) was shown to be a better predictor of declining GFR than was reciprocal serum creatinine, estimated GFR, or CL_{cr}.[35] However in patients being treated for malignant disease, Page et al.[36] reported increased cystatin C concentrations that were independent of CL_{cr}. Cystatin C concentrations were also noted to be independent of GFR and weakly associated with measured creatinine clearance, in pediatric and adult renal transplant recipients, possibly due to the formation of cystatin–immunoglobulin complexes or reduced tubular catabolism.[37,38] Two additional studies have shown a strong association between serum cystatin C and cardiovascular disease in elderly and non-CKD patients, suggesting that it may provide useful prognostic information in some populations.[39,40] It appears that cystatin C is a nonspecific marker of GFR that likely is a more sensitive index than serum creatinine of early changes in GFR. Further longitudinal evaluations will be necessary to clarify its usefulness as a prognostic index of trends in renal function and/or cardiovascular outcomes.

MEASUREMENT OF KIDNEY FUNCTION

The gold standard quantitative index of kidney function is a measured GFR. A variety of methods may be used to measure and estimate kidney function in the acute care and ambulatory settings. Estimation of GFR is important for early recognition and monitoring of patients with chronic kidney disease. Estimation of CL_{cr} is important as a guide for drug dose adjustment in the presence of renal impairment.

It is important to recognize conditions that may alter renal function independent of underlying renal pathology. For example, protein intake, such as oral protein loading or an infusion of amino acid solution, may increase GFR.[9] As a result, inter- and intrasubject variability must be considered when it is used as a longitudinal marker of renal function. Dietary protein intake has been demonstrated to correlate with GFR in healthy subjects. Brändle et al.[41] evaluated renal function in four groups of healthy volunteers, each ingesting a diet controlled for protein over a 4-month period. The GFR was nonlinearly related to the urine nitrogen excretion, with an observed maximum of 181.7 mL/min at a urinary nitrogen excretion rate of 20 g/day, or 125 g/day protein intake. Subjects who are vegetarian have a lower GFR than individuals who consume a similar caloric but normal-protein-content diet because of their reduced dietary protein intake. When challenged with a protein load, the vegetarian subjects are able to increase their GFR to the "normal" range.[9] Findings from the Nurses' Health Study[42] indicate that longitudinal changes in GFR are independent of the source of protein (nondairy animal, dairy, or vegetable) in women with normal renal function. However, women with mild renal insufficiency (GFR 71 ± 7 mL/min) who consumed the highest amount of protein (93 g/day) had a threefold greater risk of a ≥5-mL/min decline in GFR compared to the lowest protein group (60 g/day); rates of decline were highest in those consuming nondairy animal protein. The increased GFR following a protein load is the result of renal vasodilation accompanied by an increased renal plasma flow. The exact mechanism of the renal response to protein is unknown, but may be related to extrarenal factors such as glucagon, prostaglandins, and angiotensin II, or intrarenal mechanisms, such as tubular transport and tubuloglomerular feedback.[43,44] Despite the evidence of a "renal reserve," standardized evaluation techniques have not been developed. Therefore, assessment of the standard GFR measurement technique must consider the dietary protein status of the patient at the time of the study.

CLINICAL CONTROVERSY

Estimation of creatinine clearance in vegetarians is controversial. Some clinicians advocate use of the 24-hour creatinine clearance in these patients since this method is based on the renal clearance of creatinine. The six-variable Modification of Diet in Renal Disease Study equation, which incorporates nutritional parameters such as blood urea nitrogen and albumin, has yet to be evaluated in this non-CKD population.

MEASUREMENT OF GLOMERULAR FILTRATION RATE

4 A measured GFR remains the single best index of functioning renal mass. As renal mass declines in the presence of age-related loss

of nephrons or coexisting disease states such as hypertension or diabetes, there is a progressive decline in GFR. The rate of decline in GFR can be used to predict the time to onset of stage 5 CKD, as well as the risk of complications of CKD. Accurate measurement of GFR in clinical practice is a critical variable for the individualization of the dosage regimens of renally excreted medications so as to maximize their therapeutic efficacy and avoid potential toxicity.

The GFR is expressed as the volume of plasma filtered across the glomerulus per unit time, based on total renal blood flow and capillary hemodynamics. The normal values for GFR are 127 ± 20 mL/min/1.73 m^2 and 118 ± 20 mL/min/1.73 m^2 in healthy men and women, respectively. For example, if the normal renal blood flow were approximately 1.0 L/min/1.73 m^2, plasma volume was 60% of blood volume, and filtration fraction across the glomerulus was 20%, then the normal GFR would be approximately 120 mL/min/1.73 m^2.

Because GFR cannot be measured directly in humans, clearance methods that use substances that are freely filtered without additional clearance because of tubular secretion or reduction as the result of reabsorption are required. Additionally, the substance should not be susceptible to metabolism within renal tissues and should not alter renal function. Given these conditions, the GFR is equivalent to the renal clearance of the solute marker:

$$\text{GFR} = \text{renal CL} = (A_e) / \text{AUC}_{0\text{–}t}$$

where renal CL is renal clearance of the marker, A_e is the amount of marker excreted in the urine in a specified period of time, t, and $\text{AUC}_{0\text{-}t}$ is the area under the plasma-concentration-versus-time curve of the marker.

Under steady-state conditions, for example during a continuous infusion of the marker, the expression simplifies to

$$\text{GFR} = \text{renal CL} = (A_e) / [C_{ss}) \times \text{t}]$$

where C_{ss} is the steady-state plasma concentration of the marker achieved during continuous infusion. The continuous infusion method can also be employed without urine collection, where plasma clearance is calculated as CL = infusion rate/C_{ss}. Requirements of this method include steady-state plasma concentrations and accurate measurement of infusate concentrations. Plasma clearance can also be determined following a single-dose intravenous injection with multiple sampling of blood to estimate area under the curve ($\text{AUC}_{0\text{-}\infty}$). Here, clearance is calculated as CL = dose/AUC. These plasma clearance methods commonly yield clearance values 10% to 15% higher than urine collection methods.[45,46]

The GFR marker is most often administered as a combination of IV loading dose and continuous infusion, designed to achieve the desired target plasma concentration. Following an equilibration period, sequential measurements of GFR are made over three or more 30 to 60 minute time periods. Urine is collected, and blood samples are collected at the beginning and end of each urine collection period. It is necessary to maintain adequate hydration during the test because GFR is dependent on renal blood flow and it assures adequate urine output during the procedure. A relatively constant urine flow will decrease the variability among repeated measurements and should be within the range of 1 to 5 mL/min. Carefully timed renal clearance studies should ensure adequate bladder emptying and accurate measurement of urine volume. In patients with impaired bladder emptying, such as those with benign prostatic hypertrophy or neurogenic bladder, urinary catheterization may be required.

❺ Several markers have been used for the measurement of GFR and include both exogenous and endogenous compounds. Those administered as exogenous agents, such as inulin, iothalamate, iohexol, and radioisotopes, require specialized administration techniques and detection methods for the quantification of function, but generally provide a more accurate measure of GFR. Methods that employ endogenous compounds, such as creatinine, require less-technical expertise, but produce results with greater variability. The marker of choice depends on the purpose and cost of the test (e.g., ^{125}I-iothalamate costs $2,000 per vial [Glofil-125, QOL Medical]); research protocols will generally use a more accurate test than one used in the clinical setting (Table 44–4).

TABLE 44-4 Sensitivity and Clinical Utility of Renal Function Tests

	Accuracy	Clinical Utility	Cost
Inulin clearance	++++	+	$$$$
Radiolabeled markers	+++	+	$$$
Nonisotopic contrast agents	+++	++	$$$
Creatinine clearance	++	+++	$$
Serum creatinine	+	++++	$

+, least acceptable; ++, adequate; +++, better; ++++, best.

Inulin Clearance

Inulin is a relatively large fructose polysaccharide (5,200 daltons), obtained from plant tubers of the Jerusalem artichoke, dahlia, and chicory plants. It is not bound to plasma proteins, is freely filtered at the glomerulus, is not secreted or reabsorbed, and is not metabolized by the kidney. The volume of distribution of inulin approximates extracellular volume, or 20% of ideal body weight. Because it is eliminated by glomerular filtration, its elimination half-life is dependent on renal function and is approximately 1.3 hours in subjects with normal renal function. Measurement of plasma and urine inulin concentrations can be performed using high-performance liquid chromatography.[47] Sinistrin, another polyfructosan, has similar characteristics to inulin; it is filtered at the glomerulus and not secreted or reabsorbed to any significant extent. It is a naturally occurring substance derived from the root of the North African vegetable red squill, *Urginea maritime* that has a much higher degree of water solubility than inulin. Assay methods for sinistrin have been described using enzymatic procedures, as well as high-performance liquid chromatography with electrochemical detection.[48]

Iothalamate Clearance

Alternatives have been sought for inulin as a marker for GFR because of the problems of availability, high cost, sample preparation, and assay variability. Iothalamate is an iodine-containing radiocontrast agent that is available in both radiolabeled (^{125}I) and nonradiolabeled forms. This agent is handled in a manner similar to that of inulin; it is freely filtered at the glomerulus and does not undergo substantial tubular secretion or reabsorption. The nonradiolabeled form is most widely used to measure GFR in ambulatory and research settings, and can safely be administered by IV bolus, continuous infusion, or subcutaneous injection.[49] Plasma and urine iothalamate concentrations can be measured using high-performance liquid chromatography.[50] Plasma iothalamate clearance methods that do not require urine collections have been shown to be highly correlated with iothalamate renal clearance. The observed positive bias of approximately 10 mL/min suggests that there is some degree of nonrenal clearance of this agent. If one "corrects" the plasma clearance value by subtracting the population mean nonrenal clearance, the resultant estimate of GFR is well-suited for longitudinal evaluations of renal function.[45]

Iohexol

Iohexol, a nonionic, low osmolar, iodinated contrast agent, has also been used for the determination of GFR. It is eliminated almost entirely by glomerular filtration, and plasma and renal clearance values are similar to observations with other marker agents: strong correlations of 0.90 or greater and significant relationships such as $\text{CL}_{\text{iohexol}} = 0.90\ \text{CL}_{\text{iothalamate}} + 6.8$ mL/min have been reported.[51–53]

These data support iohexol as a suitable alternative marker for the measurement of GFR. One key advantage of this agent is that a single plasma sample can be used to quantify iohexol, clearance provided sufficient time has elapsed since injection. For patients with a reduced GFR more time must be allotted—more than 24 hours if the estimated GFR is less than 20 mL/min.[51]

Radiolabeled Markers

The GFR has also been quantified using radiolabeled markers, such as ^{125}I-iothalamate (614 daltons, radioactive half-life of 60 days), ^{99m}Tc-diethylenetriamine pentaacetic acid (^{99m}Tc-DPTA; 393 daltons, radioactive half-life of 6.03 hours), and ^{51}Cr-ethylenediaminetetraacetic acid (^{51}Cr-EDTA; 292 daltons, radioactive half-life of 27 days).[54] These relatively small molecules are minimally bound to plasma proteins and do not undergo tubular secretion or reabsorption to any significant degree. ^{125}I-iothalamate and ^{99m}Tc-DPTA are used in the United States, whereas ^{51}Cr-EDTA is used extensively in Europe. The use of radiolabeled markers allows one to determine the individual contribution of each kidney to total renal function.[55] Various protocols exist for the administration of these markers and subsequent determination of GFR using either plasma or renal clearance calculation methods. The nonrenal clearance of these agents appears to be low (3 to 8 mL/min), suggesting that plasma clearance is an acceptable technique except in patients with severe renal insufficiency (GFR <30 mL/min). Indeed, highly significant correlations between renal clearance among radiolabeled markers has been demonstrated.[56] Although total radioactive exposure to patients is usually minimal, use of one of these agents does require compliance with radiation safety committees and appropriate biohazard waste disposal.

Estimation of GFR

A series of equations proposed by Levey and colleagues[2,57–59] have gained widespread support for the estimation of GFR in many patient populations. These equations were derived from multiple regression analysis of data obtained from the 1,628 patients enrolled in the Modification of Diet in Renal Disease Study (MDRD). The initial regression model yielded the following six-variable Modification of Diet in Renal Disease Study (MDRD6) equation:

$$\text{GFR} = 170 \times (P_{cr})^{-0.999} \times [\text{Age}]^{-0.176} \times [0.762 \text{ if patient is female}] \times [1.180 \text{ if patient is black}] \times [\text{SUN}]^{-0.170} \times [\text{Alb}]^{0.318}$$

where P_{cr} = plasma creatinine, SUN = serum nitrogen concentration, and Alb = serum albumin concentration. Comparison of various prediction equations showed that the new equation (r^2 = 90.2%) provided a more precise estimate of GFR than measured CL_{cr} (r^2 = 86.6%) or CL_{cr} estimated by the Cockcroft-Gault equation (r^2 = 84.2%) in the MDRD population. More recently,[16] a modified, four-variable version of the original MDRD equation (MDRD4) has been shown to provide a similar estimate of GFR results compared to its six-variable predecessor:

$$\text{GFR} = 186^{*}\ (\text{Pcr})^{-1.154} \times (\text{Age})^{-0.203} \times (0.742 \text{ if patient is female}) \times (1.210 \text{ if patient is black})$$

This equation, based on plasma creatinine, age, sex, and race, was validated in the MDRD study sample and is now recommended by the NKF and the National Kidney Disease Education Program (NKDEP) for calculating the estimated GFR (eGFR) in patients with a history of CKD risk factors and a GFR <60 mL/min/1.73 m^2. The performance of MDRD6, and more recently the MDRD4, has been assessed in a variety of patient populations. In renal transplant patients with severe renal insufficiency (CL_{cr} <30 mL/min/1.73 m^2), the MDRD6 equation was highly correlated with mean CL_{cr} and urea clearances, less biased, and more precise than the Cockcroft-Gault equation.[58] However, this equation was less accurate than the Cockcroft-Gault equation in healthy subjects, diabetic patients with normal GFR (88 to 182 mL/min/1.73 m^2), and healthy potential kidney donors.[59,60] In cirrhotic patients being evaluated for liver transplant (GFR 58 ± 5.1 mL/min/1.73 m^2) the MDRD4, MDRD6, and Cockcroft-Gault equations significantly overestimated GFR by 30% to 50%, and were imprecise estimates of GFR before and after liver transplantation.[61,62] In a small study of elderly subjects (age >68 years) with mild/moderate CKD (GFR 53 ± 18 mL/min/1.73 m^2) the MDRD6 equation was slightly positively biased compared to the Cockcroft-Gault equation (8% vs. 10%), but precision was similar between methods relative to measured GFR.[63] Beddhu et al. reported that the MDRD6 equation, like the Cockcroft-Gault equation, is dependent on creatinine production and is susceptible to bias in malnourished patients with end-stage renal disease.[64] The MDRD equations should not be used in ill, hospitalized patients,[65] nor in individuals with normal renal function,[60] and should be used with caution in children, the elderly, and those with extremes in muscle mass (cachectic and obese) until further performance data is available. The MDRD equations also should not be used for renal drug dose adjustment until further studies evaluating the relationship between eGFR and drug clearance/elimination are conducted. Several online resources are available to assist clinicians with eGFR calculations, such as the NKDEP.[66]

CLINICAL CONTROVERSY

Some practitioners are advocating the use of the MDRD4 equation in patients without CKD, although it appears to have a weaker correlation with GFR than the Cockcroft-Gault equation. However, recent evidence suggests that the MDRD4 equation should be reserved for patients with a GFR <60 mL/min. The use of standardized isotope dilution mass spectrometry traceable creatinine assays may improve the performance of the MDRD4 equation in patients with GFR >60 mL/min.

A recent approach to standardize and reduce analytical errors associated with serum creatinine assays, and thereby improve the accuracy of eGFR results, has been proposed for implementation in clinical laboratories.[59] This assay calibration, called isotope dilution-mass spectrometry, will likely reduce the inter-laboratory variability in serum creatinine values. In settings using the isotope dilution-mass spectrometry assay, a revised MDRD eGFR equation is recommended, which accounts for an approximate 5% reduction in creatinine values. The NKDEP also recommends reporting serum creatinine values in mg/dL to two decimal places (e.g., 0.93 mg/dL), and values in μmol/L to the nearest whole number (e.g., 84 μmol/L). This practice will likely reduce rounding errors that in the past contributed to bias between creatinine-based GFR or CL_{cr} estimates. However the impact of this approach on the accuracy of eGFR results or renal drug dose adjustments remains to be determined.

CLINICAL CONTROVERSY

Drug-dose individualization is often required in patients with CKD. Approved drug labeling typically includes a dose-adjustment table based on the patient's estimated CL_{cr} using the Cockcroft-Gault method. With many hospital laboratories now reporting MDRD eGFR values, the usefulness of this measure as a guide for drug-dose adjustments needs to be clarified.

Measured Creatinine Clearance

❻ Despite the common use of a measured (24-hour) CL_{cr} as an index of renal function, its use is now more controversial then ever. Short-duration witnessed CL_{cr} correlates with iothalamate clearance performed using the single-injection technique. In a multicenter study[67] of 136 patients with type I diabetic nephropathy, the correlations of simultaneous CL_{cr}, Cockcroft-Gault CL_{cr}, and 24-hour CL_{cr} (compared to $CL_{iothalamate}$) were 0.81, 0.67, and 0.49, respectively, indicating increased variability with the 24-hour clearance determination. In a selected group of 110 patients, measurement of a 4-hour CL_{cr} during water diuresis provided the best estimate of the GFR as determined by the $CL_{iothalamate}$. Furthermore, the ratio of CL_{cr} to $CL_{iothalamate}$ did not appear to increase as the GFR decreased. These data suggest that a short collection period with a water diuresis may be the best method for estimation of GFR by creatinine clearance.

A limitation of using creatinine as a filtration marker is that it undergoes varying degrees of tubular secretion. Tubular secretion augments the filtered creatinine by approximately 10% in subjects with normal kidney function. If the nonspecific Jaffe reaction is used, which overestimates the serum creatinine concentration by approximately 10% because of the noncreatinine chromogens, then the creatinine clearance is a very good measure of GFR in patients with normal kidney function. Tubular secretion, however, increases to as much as 100% in patients with renal insufficiency.[20] As renal impairment develops, the remaining nephrons hypertrophy, and the degree of tubular secretion decreases less than the decrease in filtration. The result is an overestimation of creatinine clearance as a function of GFR assessed by inulin or iothalamate clearance. For example, Bauer et al.[20] reported that the CL_{cr}-to-CL_{inulin} ratio in subjects with mild impairment was 1.20; for moderate impairment, it was 1.87; and for severe impairment, it was 2.32. Thus, creatinine clearance is a poor indicator of GFR in patients with moderate to severe renal insufficiency.

Because cimetidine blocks the tubular secretion of creatinine the potential role of several oral cimetidine regimens to improve the accuracy and precision of creatinine clearance as an indicator of GFR has been evaluated. The CL_{cr}-to-CL_{DPTA} ratio declined from 1.33 with placebo to 1.07 when 400 mg of cimetidine was administered four times a day for 2 days prior to and during the clearance determination.[68] Similar results were observed when a single 800-mg dose of cimetidine was given 1 hour prior to the simultaneous determination of CL_{cr} and $CL_{iothalamate}$; the ratio of CL_{cr} to $CL_{iothalamate}$ was reduced from a mean of 1.53 to 1.12.[69] Thus a single oral dose of cimetidine 800 mg should provide adequate blockade of creatinine secretion to improve the accuracy of a creatinine clearance measurement as an estimate GFR in patients with stages 3 to 5 CKD.

Estimation of Creatinine Clearance

❼ Many equations describing the mathematical relationships between various patient factors and CL_{cr} have been reported over the past 3 decades. Most equations incorporate factors such as age, gender, weight, and serum creatinine concentration, without the need for urine collection. The most widely used of these estimators is the Cockcroft-Gault equation,[70] which identified age and body mass as factors which significantly contribute to the estimate of CL_{cr}. This relationship was based on observations from 249 male patients with stable kidney function in whom the creatinine production rates were estimated.

For obese individuals, that is those weighing more than 30% above their ideal body weight (IBW), it is recommended that IBW be used in place of actual body weight (ABW)[71] in the Cockcroft-Gault equation, where:

$$\text{IBW(kg, males)} = 50 + 2.3 \text{ (Height in inches} >60)$$

$$\text{IBW (kg, females)} = 45 + 2.3 \text{ (Height in inches} >60)$$

An alternative approach for estimating CL_{cr} (mL/min) in obese patients is the Salazar-Corcoran equation which has been shown to be unbiased and superior to the Cockcroft-Gault equation in this population.[71,72]

Luke et al.[73] evaluated the ability of the Cockcroft-Gault method and four other methods to predict CL_{cr}, with inulin clearance being considered the standard measure of GFR. The simultaneously determined inulin and creatinine clearances correlated best, $r^2 = 0.85$, and the CL_{cr} overestimated CL_{inulin} by approximately 15% due to tubular secretion of creatinine. For the five calculated clearances, Cockcroft-Gault and Mawer et al.[74] correlated the best with inulin clearance. The Cockcroft-Gault method showed a linear relationship with CL_{inulin} equal to 1.121 of CL_{cr} plus 20.6 mL/min ($r^2 = 0.66$), whereas for Mawer et al. the relationship was CL_{inulin} equal to 1.051 of CL_{cr} plus 18.3 mL/min ($r^2 = 0.66$). Other methods, such as Jelliffe[75] and Hull et al.,[76] consistently underestimated the CL_{cr}. As kidney function declined, there was an increase in the fraction of creatinine eliminated by secretion as measured by the CL_{cr}-to-CL_{inulin} ratio, consistent with earlier reports. This limitation should be taken into consideration when attempting to use CL_{cr} for the estimation of renal function and the individualization of drug dosage regimens. Gault et al.[77] also evaluated the performance of the Cockcroft-Gault estimator of renal function compared with inulin and ^{99m}Tc-DPTA. Except for conditions of unstable kidney function, it performed similar to the 24-hour creatinine clearance method (Table 44–5).

Patients undergoing screening for participation in the African American Study of Kidney Disease (AASK) were evaluated for kidney function based on an estimated CL_{cr} compared with the simultaneous CL_{cr} and ^{125}I-iothalamate, and 24-hour CL_{cr}.[78] The simultaneous CL_{cr} provided the best estimate of GFR. The Cockcroft-Gault method was the preferred method for estimation of GFR, based on performance and ease of use. This method was noted to underestimate the GFR by 9%, perhaps because of the increased excretion rate of creatinine by black patients.[78,79]

Administration of cimetidine has also resulted in improved performance of the Cockcroft-Gault equation to predict GFR. Ixkes et al.[80] gave patients three 800-mg doses of cimetidine in 24 hours, and measured creatinine plasma levels from 3 to 7 hours following the final dose. During this 4-hour period, the $CL_{iothalamate}$ was determined as the measure of GFR. The Cockcroft-Gault calculations were performed with the plasma creatinine measurement 3 hours after the last dose of cimetidine. The ratio of the Cockcroft-Gault estimated CL_{cr}-to-$CL_{iothalamate}$ decreased from 1.28 ± 0.21 to 0.98 ± 0.11 in the presence of cimetidine. This cimetidine dosing schedule also improved the accuracy of Cockcroft-Gault estimates relative to GFR in renal transplant patients with GFR values ranging from 20 to 80 mL/min/1.73m^2.[81,82]

TABLE 44-5 Equations for the Estimation of Creatinine Clearance in Adults with Stable Renal Function

Cockroft and Gault[80]	Men: $CL_{cr} = (140 - \text{age})\ \text{ABW}/(S_{cr} \times 72)$ Women: $CL_{cr} \times 0.85$
Jelliffe[89]	Men: $CL_{cr} = (100/S_{cr}) - 12$ Women: $CL_{cr} = (80/S_{cr}) - 7$
Jelliffe[90]	Men: $CL_{cr} = 98 - [0.8\ (\text{age} - 20)]/S_{cr}$ Women: $CL_{cr} \times 0.9$
Mawer et al.[88]	Men: $\text{IBW}\ [29.3 - (0.203 \times \text{age})]\ [1 - (0.03 \times S_{cr}]/(14.4 \times S_{cr})$ Women: $\text{IBW}\ [25.3 - (0.175 \times \text{age})]\ [1 - (0.03 \times S_{cr})]/(14.4 \times S_{cr})$
Hull et al.[91]	Men: $CL_{cr} = [(145 - \text{age})/S_{cr}] - 3$ Women: $Cl_{cr} \times 0.85$
Levey et al. (MDRD6)[72]	$\text{GFR} = 170 \times (S_{cr})^{-0.999} \times [\text{age}]^{-0.176} \times [0.762 \text{ if patient is female}] \times [1.180 \text{ if patient is black}] \times [\text{SUN}]^{-0.170} \times [\text{Alb}]^{0.318}$
Levey et al. (MDRD4)[24]	$\text{GFR} = 186 \times (S_{cr})^{-1.154} \times (\text{Age})^{-0.203} \times (0.742 \text{ if patient is female}) \times (1.210 \text{ if patient is black})$

Alb, serum albumin concentration (g/dL); CL_{cr}, creatinine clearance in mL/min; IBW, ideal body weight (kg); S_{cr}, serum or plasma creatinine (mg/dL); SU, serum urea nitrogen concentration (mg/dL).

Liver Disease

The prediction of CL_{cr} or eGFR is particularly problematic in patients with preexisting liver disease and renal impairment. Lower-than-expected serum creatinine values may result from reduced muscle mass, protein-poor diet, diminished hepatic synthesis of creatine (a precursor of creatinine), and fluid administration can lead to significant overestimation of creatinine clearance. Orlando et al.[83] evaluated 10 healthy subjects, 10 patients with mild liver disease, and 10 with severe liver disease, and observed a measured CL_{cr}-to-CL_{inulin} ratio of 1.05, 1.03, and 1.04 for each group, respectively. When the CL_{cr} of patients with severe liver disease was estimated using the Cockcroft-Gault equation, the resultant ratio (CL_{cr} Cockcroft-Gault-to-CL_{inulin}) was 1.23. Lam et al.[84] likewise noted an overprediction by Cockcroft-Gault of the measured CL_{cr} in patients with severe disease, by 40% to 100%.

Studies of renal function in patients with severe hepatic disease confirm the earlier observations of Hull et al.[76] and Caregaro et al.[85] who reported that measured CL_{cr} overestimated GFR by 50% in hepatic patients with a GFR of 56 ± 19 mL/min/1.73 m^2 because of increased tubular secretion of creatinine. The effect of cimetidine administration on measured CL_{cr} was recently evaluated in a small study by Sansoe et al.[86] In 12 patients with compensated cirrhosis, serum creatinine values increased from 0.68 ± 0.11 to 0.94 ± 0.14 mg/dL during coadministration of cimetidine (1,000 mg given as 400 mg × 1 then 200 mg every 3 hours) during a 9-hour clearance period. The CL_{cr} was reduced from 138 ± 20 to 89 ± 13 mL/min, with no change in measured GFR.

CLINICAL CONTROVERSY

In patients with liver disease, falsely low serum creatinine values frequently occur as a result of malnourishment, muscle wasting, and tubular secretion of creatinine. Preliminary data suggests that the use of cimetidine may improve the accuracy of measured creatinine clearance compared to measured GFR in patients with cirrhosis. However, the effect of this approach on methods to estimate CL_{cr} or GFR is unknown.

DeSanto et al.[87] studied 19 patients with mild liver disease whose inulin and creatinine clearances were 90 ± 4.4 and 122 ± 7 mL/min/1.73 m^2, respectively. The degree of overestimation of GFR by creatinine clearance was inversely correlated with GFR ($r = 0.452$, $P < 0.04$). Thus, measurement of renal function in patients with hepatic disease should be performed by using a method specific for glomerular filtration, and estimation of creatinine clearance should be avoided.

Other Special Populations

Davis and Chandler[88] confirmed the accuracy of the Cockcroft-Gault equation to predict CL_{cr} in trauma patients with stable kidney function, and Thakur et al.[26] demonstrated its successful use in 42 paraplegic subjects. Renal transplant recipients are frequently monitored for renal function, as numerous complications may occur during the life of the allograft. Goerdt et al.[89] assessed the bias and precision with which several nomographic methods predicted GFR (iohexol clearance) in 127 patients with stable kidney function. The Cockcroft-Gault method performed poorly, overestimating iohexol clearance. This is expected, as iohexol clearance provides a true measure of GFR, whereas the Cockcroft-Gault CL_{cr} estimate is falsely high because of the tubular secretion of creatinine. Huang et al.[90] reported the inability of several CL_{cr} equations to predict renal function in hospitalized patients with advanced human immunodeficiency virus (HIV) disease. All of the prediction methods overestimated the measured 24-hour CL_{cr}. The reasons for the poor predictability of these methods are unclear, although 24-hour collection methods result in increased variability, often because of inadequate collection of urine.

Renal function assessment during pregnancy is usually performed using a 24-hour creatinine clearance determination. Quadri et al.[91] evaluated the Cockcroft-Gault method during each trimester in 34 pregnant women and compared these estimates with the measured 24-hour CL_{cr}. Prepregnancy weights were used throughout the study for the Cockcroft-Gault method, and results correlated well with the measured clearances ($r^2 = 0.76$). The maximal CL_{cr} occurred during the second trimester for both methods.

Unstable Renal Function

Patients with unstable kidney function present a unique situation because serum creatinine values are changing, and steady state cannot be assumed when estimating CL_{cr}. It can take several days for serum creatinine values to reach steady state in early acute renal failure, but this time can be reduced when renal function is improving. In patients with previously normal renal function, a change in the serum creatinine concentration of more than 50% over a period of 1 day is suggestive of unstable renal function. In patients with preexisting CKD (S_{cr} >2.0 mg/dL) an increase in serum creatinine by 30% or more than 1.0 mg/dL over a 24- to 48-hour period indicates the presence of acute renal failure. Methods to measure GFR in this population, such as ^{125}I-iothalamate clearance, are cumbersome and costly especially in the acute care setting. Table 44–6 lists several equations for estimating renal function under these conditions.[92–94] Although these equations are commonly used to estimate CL_{cr} in patients with acute renal failure, a rigorous evaluation of the accuracy and precision of each of these proposed methods is lacking. Also lacking is a method to estimate GFR, an equivalent to the MDRD equation for patients with CKD, for patients with acute renal failure.

The equation proposed by Jelliffe is a revised dynamic model of creatinine kinetics based on theoretical estimates of creatinine production and adjusted for age and changes in serum creatinine; however, its ability to predict changes in drug clearance (and dose adjustments) has not been evaluated.[92] In the acute setting, factors previously discussed that may alter the serum creatinine concentration must be evaluated to avoid misinterpretation. The inappropriate use of the Cockcroft-Gault equation in those with acute renal failure can significantly overestimate the value of CL_{cr} when compared to equations that are designed to account for changes in serum creatinine in patients with unstable renal function. It is thus, ultimately, most important to recognize that renal function in patients with acute renal failure is generally markedly lower than one would estimate using steady-state methods, and dose adjustments should be made if necessary to avoid drug toxicity (see Chap. 45 and Tables 44–7 and 44–8).

CLINICAL CONTROVERSY

Serum creatinine values can fluctuate widely in patients with unstable renal function. Although some practitioners advocate use of the Cockroft-Gault equation using the highest of the two serum creatinine values, most recommend calculation of CL_{cr} using either the Brater or Jelliffe equations.

Kidney Function in Children

Kidney function in the neonate is difficult to assess because of difficulty in urine and blood collection, the frequent presence of a non–steady-state serum creatinine, and apparent disparity between development of glomerular and tubular function. Preterm infants demonstrate significantly reduced GFR prior to 34 weeks, which

TABLE 44-6 Equations for the Estimation of Creatine Clearance in Adults with Unstable Renal Function

Reference	Units	Equations: *Males*	Equations: *Females*
Jelliffe[92]	mL/min per 1.73 m²	$E^{ss} = wt^a[29.3 - 0.203\ (age)]$ $E^{ss}_{corr} = E^{ss}[1.035 - 0.0337\ (S_{cr})]$ $E = E^{ss}_{corr} - \frac{[4wt^a(S_{cr_2} - S_{cr_1})]}{\Delta t\ day}$ $CL_{cr} = \frac{E}{14.4(S_{cr})}$	$E^{ss} = wt^a[25.1 - 0.175\ (age)]$ $E^{ss}_{corr} = E_{ss}\ [1.035 - 0.0337\ (S_{cr})]$ $E = E^{ss}_{corr} - \frac{[4wt^a(S_{cr_2} - S_{cr_1})]}{\Delta t day}$ $CL_{cr} = \frac{E}{14.4(S_{cr})}$
Chiou et al.[93]	mL/min	$V_d = 0.6\ L\ (wt^a)$ $CL_{cr} = \frac{2[28 - 0.2\ (age)]}{14.4(S_{cr_1} + S_{cr_2})} + \frac{2[V_d(S_{cr_1} - S_{cr_2})]}{(S_{cr_1} + S_{cr_2})\ \Delta t\ min} - [CrCl^{NR} \times wt^a]$	$V_d = 0.6\ L\ (wt^a)$ $CL_{cr} = \frac{2wt^a[22.4 - 0.16\ (age)]}{14.4(S_{cr_1} + S_{cr_2})} + \frac{2[V_d(S_{cr_1} - S_{cr_2})]}{(S_{cr_1} + S_{cr_2})\ \Delta t\ min} - [CrCl^{NR} \times wt^a]$
Brater[94]	mL/min per 70 kg	$CL_{cr} = \frac{[293 - 2.03\ (age) \times [1.035 - 0.01685\ (S_{cr_1} + S_{cr_2})]}{(S_{cr_1} + S_{cr_2})} + \frac{49(S_{cr_1} - S_{cr_2})}{(S_{cr_1} + S_{cr_2})\ \Delta t\ day}$	CL_{cr} = Male value × 0.86

CL_{cr}, creatinine clearance; $CrCl^{NR}$, nonrenal clearance of creatinine = 0.048 mL/min per kg; E, creatinine excretion; E^{ss}, steady-state creatinine excretion; E^{ss}_{corr}, corrected steady-state creatinine excretion; Δt day, time in days between S_{cr_1} and S_{cr_2}; Δt min, time in minutes between S_{cr_1}, and S_{cr_2}; S_{cr_1}, first serum creatinine value; S_{cr_2}, second serum creatinine value; S_{cr}, average of S_{cr_1} and S_{cr_2}; V_d, volume distribution of creatinine.
[a]Use ideal body weight (IBW) if weight >30% above IBW.

rapidly increases and becomes similar to term infants within the first week of life.[95] Evaluation of GFR in preterm infants on day 3 of life, using an inulin infusion, failed to identify a relationship between patient weight and GFR. Gestational age, which ranged from 23.4 to 36.9 weeks (mean: 30.2 weeks), however, correlated with both GFR and reciprocal of serum creatinine. The inulin clearance increased from 0.67 to 0.85 mL/min in those with gestational age <28 weeks versus those of 32 to 37 weeks of age, while S_{cr} decreased from 1.05 to 0.73 mg/dL, respectively. Creatinine was measured using a specific enzymatic method to avoid interference from bilirubin or drugs.[96] Creatinine clearance has also been evaluated in infants younger than 1 week of age, and values of 17.8 mL/min/1.73 m² on day 1 increased to 36.4 mL/min/1.73 m² by day 6.[97] In light of these rapid changes in GFR, estimation of GFR is not recommended for infants younger than 1 week of age. Kidney function expressed as GFR standardized to body surface area increases with age and stabilizes at approximately 1 year. In older children, GFR is best assessed using standard measurement techniques for GFR. Subcutaneous administration of ^{125}I-iothalamate has been effectively used to measure GFR in children ranging in age from 1 to 20 years.[98]

Estimation of CL_{cr} as described by Schwartz et al.[99] is dependent on the child's age and length:

$$GFR = [length\ (cm) \times k]\ /\ S_{cr}$$

where k is defined by age group: infant (1 to 52 weeks) = 0.45; child (1 to 13 years) = 0.55; adolescent male = 0.7; and adolescent female = 0.55.

Subsequent studies verified these relationships in children with normal renal function or mild renal impairment. However, variability increases at clearance values <50 mL/min. Al-Harbi and Lireman[100] reported a good correlation of the predicted CL_{cr} with measured 4-hour CL_{cr} and ^{99m}Tc-DPTA ($r = 0.75$) in 48 pediatric renal allograft recipients 3 to 19 years of age. However, predictive performance measures of bias and precision were not reported. Fong et al.[101] evaluated the method in critically ill children (mean age: 5.6 years; range: 0.1 to 20.8 years) and concluded that the method significantly overestimated the measured CL_{cr} (bias = 45%). Peirrat et al. recently compared the MDRD, Schwartz, and Cockcroft-Gault equations in

TABLE 44-7 Scenario A (Worsening Renal Function)

J.R. is a 50-year-old male (weight: 70 kg; body surface area: 1.73m²), admitted to the intensive care unit following an automobile accident. His renal function was normal prior to admission; however his serum creatinine has increased from 0.6 mg/dL to 3.0 mg/dL in the past 24 hours.

Equation	Cl_{cr}	Assumptions
Jelliffe[105]	21.9 mL/min/1.73 m²	E^{ss} = 1341.2 mg/day E^{ss}_{corr} = 1241 mg/day S_{cr} = 1.8 mg/dL $S_{cr}1$ = 0.6 mg/dL $S_{cr}2$ = 3.0 mg/dL Δt = 1 day Wt = 70 kg
Brater[107]	19.1 mL/min	$S_{cr}1$ = 0.6 mg/dL $S_{cr}2$ = 3.0 mg/dL Δt = 1 day
Cockcroft-Gault[80]	29.2 mL/min	S_{cr2} = 3.0 mg/dL Wt = 70 kg

Cl_{cr}, creatinine clearance rate; Δt, time between $S_{cr}1$ and $S_{cr}2$; E^{ss}, steady-state creatinine excretion; E^{ss}_{corr}, steady-state creatinine excretion corrected, S_{cr}, average serum creatinine; $S_{cr}1$, first serum creatinine value; $S_{cr}2$, second serum creatinine value; Wt, weight.

TABLE 44-8 Scenario B (Improving Renal Function)

J.R. has been in the intensive care unit for 1 week, and his status is improving. His serum creatinine has decreased from 3.0 mg/dL to 1.0 mg/dL in the past 24 hours.

Approach	Cl_{cr}	Assumptions
Jelliffe[105]	64.5 mL/min/1.73 m²	E^{ss} = 1341.2 mg/day E^{ss}_{corr} = 1297.7 mg/day S_{cr} = 2.0 mg/dL $S_{cr}1$ = 3.0 mg/dL $S_{cr}2$ = 1.0 mg/dL Δt = 1 day Wt = 70 kg
Brater[107]	78.7 mL/min	$S_{cr}1$ = 3.0 mg/dL $S_{cr}2$ = 1.0 mg/dL Δt = 1 day
Cockcroft-Gault[80]	87.5 mL/min	S_{cr} = 1.0 mg/dL Wt = 70 kg

Cl_{cr}, creatinine clearance rate; Δt, time between $S_{cr}1$ and $S_{cr}2$; E^{ss}, steady-state creatinine excretion; E^{ss}_{corr}, steady-state creatinine excretion corrected; S_{cr}, serum creatinine, $S_{cr}1$, first serum creatinine value; $S_{cr}2$, second serum creatinine value; Wt, weight.

children 3 to 19 years of age.[102] In children <12 years, the Schwartz and MDRD equations were significantly more biased than Cockcroft-Gault, and Cockcroft-Gault provided the best prediction of GFR in children >12 years. Because the MDRD equation was developed in the adult population, the results of these investigations suggest that further studies will be needed to clarify the value of any of these predictive methods in children. Dose adjustments and other therapeutic decisions based on kidney function warrant appropriate measures of renal status to avoid incorrect decisions.

Kidney Function in the Elderly

Cross-sectional studies demonstrate decreased GFR as a function of age when GFR is measured as inulin, iothalamate, or creatinine clearance.[70,103] The Baltimore Longitudinal Study on Aging,[104] an evaluation of 254 normal healthy subjects, revealed that creatinine clearance decreases at the rate of approximately 0.75 mL/min/1.73 m^2/y beginning at the fourth decade of life. These subjects were evaluated prospectively for up to 23 years. Interestingly, approximately one-third of the subjects showed no change in renal function from their baseline value, and a small number showed an increased clearance. These changes may be a result of normal physiologic changes or of subclinical insults to the kidneys initiating the events leading to chronic progressive loss of renal function. Fliser et al.[105] studied renal functional reserve in healthy young (23 to 32 years) and elderly (61 to 82 years) volunteers using an amino acid infusion technique. Inulin clearance was used as the measure of GFR, which increased 16% in young and 17% in elderly subjects following the infusion. Renal functional reserve thus appears to be maintained in healthy elderly individuals.

Interpretation of the serum creatinine concentration alone is difficult in the elderly patient primarily because of the decreased muscle mass and resultant lower production rate of creatinine. Thus, the serum creatinine often remains within the normal range despite a reduction in the number of functional nephrons. As renal function declines, the kidneys excrete a larger fraction of creatinine. This perpetuates the "normal" serum creatinine. Recent recommendations such as the adoption of standardized creatinine assays by clinical laboratories and reporting of serum creatinine values to two decimal places, will likely improve the accuracy of renal function estimation in the elderly population.[59]

The Cockcroft-Gault formula[70] can be used to estimate the CL_{cr} of elderly patients. Smythe et al.[106] estimated CL_{cr} in 23 patients >60 years of age using seven different methods, and compared the results to a measured 24-hour CL_{cr} determination. Estimations were performed with the actual serum creatinine concentration and also with the serum creatinine rounded up to 1.0 mg/dL if the actual value was <1.0 mg/dL. Rounding the serum creatinine to 1.0 mg/dL resulted in a significantly lower (bias = 28.8 mL/min) estimate of GFR, as compared with the actual clearance, than when the unadjusted serum creatinine (bias = 2.3 mL/min) was used. These data strongly suggest that one should not arbitrarily fix the serum creatinine concentration in elderly patients at 1.0 mg/dL. An alternative to the estimation of GFR or a 24-hour clearance determination is a 4-hour clearance performed during water diuresis.[67] This correlated with the inulin clearance as well as with an inpatient 24-hour CL_{cr}. However, one must be aware of the potential risk of hyponatremia in the geriatric patient who is unable to tolerate an oral water load, as well as the need for complete bladder emptying to ensure accurate results. O'Connell et al.[107] assessed the accuracy of 2- and 8-hour urine collections compared with 24-hour creatinine clearance determinations in 45 hospitalized patients >65 years old with indwelling urethral catheters. Single, timed urine collections for CL_{cr} showed minimal bias with the 8-hour collection as compared with the 24-hour value, whereas the 2-hour determination was both biased and imprecise.

Assessment of Progression

Chronic kidney disease (see Chap. 46) will eventually lead to end-stage renal disease (see Chap. 47), necessitating dialysis or transplantation for survival (see Chaps. 48 and 92). The rate of progression can be slowed and in some cases halted through dietary modification, strict blood pressure control, initiation of angiotensin-converting enzyme inhibitor or angiotensin receptor blocker therapy to reduce urinary protein excretion, and improved glucose control in patients with diabetes mellitus (see Chap. 46). The efficacy of these interventions is optimally assessed with the sequential measurement of an accurate and sensitive index of GFR such as iohexol, iothalamate, or radioisotope clearance.[108]

❽ Alternatively, use of newer methods to estimate GFR, such as the MDRD4 equation, or traditional methods, such as the linear decline in the reciprocal of the serum creatinine concentration as a function of time, are simple clinical tools that can be used to evaluate the rate of progression of renal disease and to predict the time when dialysis will be needed.[2,19] It is known that serum creatinine concentration is a function of input from the breakdown of creatine or the ingestion of dietary sources and elimination occurs predominantly through glomerular filtration and tubular secretion. Under steady-state conditions, the formation rate of creatinine equals the elimination rate (R), and CL_{cr} is inversely related to S_{cr} as:

$$S_{cr} = R/CL_{cr}$$

The reciprocal relationship between S_{cr} and CL_{cr} is then expressed as:

$$1/S_{cr} = 1/R \times CL_{cr}$$

❾ Figure 44–3A depicts the reciprocal relationship between S_{cr} and CL_{cr}. As renal function declines, the reciprocal of the serum creatinine concentration decreases as a linear function of the CL_{cr}, and the slope of the relationship is the reciprocal of the elimination rate of creatinine. Clinicians can use the reciprocal serum creatinine plotted as a function of time as a prognostic tool, to predict when dialysis may be needed (when $1/S_{cr}$ ~0.1) or as a marker for evaluating the success of therapeutic interventions to alter the rate of decline in renal function (Fig. 44–3B). Several factors, such as changes in dietary intake of creatinine and decreased muscle mass, which are associated with a reduction in the production of creatinine, may alter the utility of the relationship. Furthermore, if tubular secretion increases in response to nephron hypertrophy disproportionately to filtration, or if nonrenal routes of elimination of creatinine, such as metabolism by intestinal bacteria, become more important, then changes in the slope of the reciprocal creatinine versus time relationship may be altered. It is most important to be aware of the limitations of serum creatinine measurement and to realize that it is not an adequate test to detect early chronic renal disease or to precisely estimate the rate of progression.

Microalbuminuria has been identified as an early marker of renal disease in patients with diabetic nephropathy[109] and numerous other conditions, such as hypertension and obesity.[110,111] Albuminuria is a more sensitive marker than total protein for monitoring CKD progression, as well as a modifiable risk factor for renal disease progression and cardiovascular disease.[39] Thus patients with microalbuminuria (30 to 300 mg/day) on at least two or three occasions or overt albuminuria (>300 mg/day) should begin to receive pharmacotherapy. For children, microalbuminuria is considered present if albumin excretion exceeds 0.36 mg/kg/day, and overt albuminuria has been defined as an excretion rate that exceeds 4 mg/kg/day. The urinary albumin-to-creatinine ratio is also an accurate predictor of 24-hour proteinuria, a marker of renal disease. Guidelines for monitoring indicate that a urine albumin to creatinine ratio of >30 mg/g places the patient at increased risk of developing diabetic

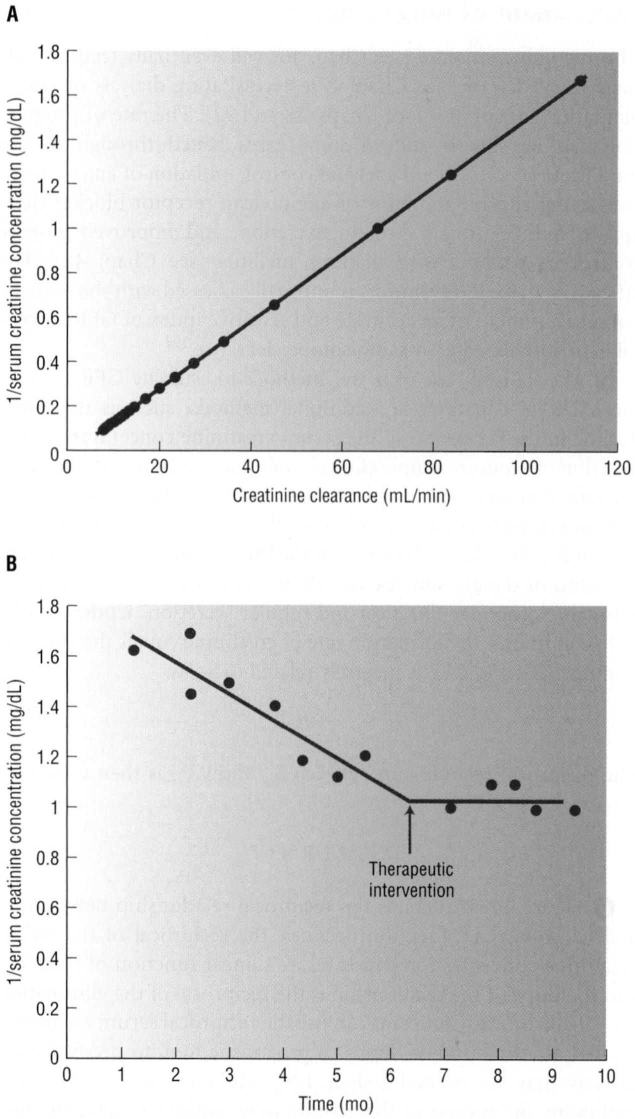

FIGURE 44-3. Linear relationship between 1/serum creatinine concentration and creatinine clearance *(A)* and 1/serum creatinine concentration as a function of time in a hypothetical patient with progressive renal impairment *(B)*. The *arrow* indicates a change in the rate of progression, which may be related to a therapeutic intervention.

nephropathy and is an indication for the initiation of pharmacotherapeutic intervention.[18] Microalbuminuria has also been suggested as a risk factor for renal dysfunction among patients with essential hypertension.[112]

Measurement of Renal Plasma and Blood Flow

Measurement of renal plasma and blood flow is rarely if ever determined in the clinical setting; rather, it is reserved for research settings to evaluate hemodynamic changes related to disease or drug therapy. The kidneys receive approximately 20% of cardiac output and representative values of renal blood flow in men and women of about 1,200 ± 250 and 1,000 ± 180 mL/min/1.73 m^2 have been reported, respectively.[113] Renal plasma flow (RPF) is estimated to be 60% of blood flow if it is assumed that the average hematocrit is 40% and that it can be measured by the use of model compounds that are eliminated from the plasma compartment on a single pass through the kidneys. Because only 20% of the plasma is filtered at the glomerulus, the compound must undergo active tubular secretion and minimal to no reabsorption to be completely eliminated. To accurately reflect RPF, the extraction through the kidney must be nearly 100%. PAH is an organic anion that has been used extensively for the quantification of renal plasma flow. PAH is approximately 17% bound to plasma proteins and is eliminated extensively by active tubular secretion. Because PAH elimination is active, saturation of the transport processes should be anticipated, and concentrations of PAH in plasma should not exceed 10 to 20 mg/L. Dowling et al.[114] used a sequential infusion technique and observed concentration-dependent renal clearance of PAH at concentrations above 100 mg/dL. Furthermore, PAH is also metabolized, possibly within the kidney, to *N*-acetyl-PAH, and it is important for the analytical method to differentiate the parent compound and metabolite.[50] Prescott et al.[115] noted that the renal clearance of PAH decreases at low plasma concentrations, while the clearance of the acetyl metabolite increases. Further studies are necessary to evaluate the mechanisms and significance of these findings. The extraction ratio (ER) for PAH is 70% to 90% at plasma concentrations of 10 to 20 mg/L, hence the term "effective" renal plasma flow (ERPF) has been used when the clearance of PAH is not corrected for the extraction ratio or if it is assumed to be 1.[4] Normal values are about 650 ± 160 mL/min for men and 600 ± 150 mL/min for women.[113] Children will reach normalized adult values by 3 years of age, and ERPF will begin to decline as a function of age after 30 years, reaching about one-half of its peak value by 90 years of age. The method for calculation of ERPF is based on the relationship between organ clearance, ER, and flow:

$$\text{ERPF} = \text{renal PAH CL} = \text{RPF} \times \text{ER}$$

Effective renal blood flow (ERBF) can be estimated from ERPF by assuming the extraction ratio is 1 and correcting for the red blood cell volume of the blood (hematocrit [HCT]):

$$\text{ERBF} = \text{ERPF}/(1 - \text{HCT})$$

ERPF can also be measured using the radioisotopes ^{131}I-orthoiodohippurate (^{131}I-OIH) or ^{99m}Tc-mercaptoacetyltriglycine (^{99m}Tc-MAG3).[116] One important advantage of this method is its ability to measure ERPF in total or for each kidney independently, as well as its ability to produce renal images. Russell and Dubovsky,[117] using a single-injection technique, compared clearance methods with and without urine collection and showed similar results with each method.

QUANTITATIVE ASSESSMENT OF TUBULAR FUNCTION

Although GFR is the best overall indicator of renal function, it may not provide an accurate measure of tubular function, either secretory capacity or cellular function, suitable for use in the research environment.[118] Tubular secretory function can be assessed by measuring PAH transport as the prototype marker of the organic anion secretory system. N^1-methylnicotinamide (NMN) and tetraethylammonium are prototype compounds secreted by the cationic transport system and may be used as markers of cationic secretory capacity.[4,118] Edwards et al.[119] demonstrated delayed recovery of NMN clearance among patients with psoriasis treated with low-dose cyclosporine, as compared with the recovery of GFR and renal blood flow. Earlier studies with NMN suggested its use to assess the effects of selected renal diseases on drug handling by the kidneys.[120] Dowling et al.[114] explored the usefulness of famotidine as a marker for cationic transport, but was unable to demonstrate saturation, perhaps due to the contribution from other secretory pathways such as P-glycoprotein.

Furthermore, Karyekar et al.[121] demonstrated that itraconazole, a P-glycoprotein inhibitor, significantly reduced the renal tubular secretion of cimetidine in healthy individuals, suggesting that cimetidine may be used as an in vivo probe of renal P-glycoprotein function. It should also be recognized that these transport systems are not necessarily mutually exclusive. Indeed, probenecid, which is secreted by the anionic pathway, inhibits the secretion of cationic compounds. Quantitative measures of tubular transport capacity are currently limited primarily to the research setting.

Other measures of tubular function are less specific and are regarded primarily as indices of damage within the nephron. Schentag and Plaut[122] demonstrated a delay in the increase of serum creatinine following aminoglycoside toxicity when compared to markers for tubular damage such as the low-molecular-weight protein β_2-microglobulin (11.8 kDa) and urinary enzymes. The rise in β_2-microglobulin is related to an early functional defect in the proximal tubular cell. This is followed by a rise in the excretion of enzymes released as a result of structural damage of the cells, and, finally, by the formation and excretion of cellular casts. Other low-molecular-weight proteins used as markers of tubular function include retinol-binding protein (21 kDa) and protein HC (also known as α_1-microglobulin, 27 kDa).[123] These proteins are normally freely filtered at the glomerulus and then completely reabsorbed by the proximal tubule. Increases in their excretion are thus suggestive of tubular dysfunction but are not diagnostic, as an increased production rate or GFR of less than 30 mL/min may lead to increased excretion. In both cases, the maximal reabsorptive capacity may be exceeded, leading to net excretion of the protein. Retinol-binding protein and protein HC are elevated with tubular damage and may be more appropriate markers than β_2-microglobulin.

Numerous urinary enzymes such as *N*-acetylglucosaminidase, alanine aminopeptidase, alkaline phosphatase, γ-glutamyltransferase, pyruvate kinase, glutathione transferase, lysozyme, and pancreatic ribonuclease have been used as diagnostic markers for renal disease. Jung et al.[124] compared the ability of five enzymes (*N*-acetylglucosaminidase, alanine aminopeptidase, alkaline phosphatase, γ-glutamyltransferase, and lysozyme) to detect early rejection episodes in kidney transplant patients. Only *N*-acetylglucosaminidase and alanine aminopeptidase were early predictors of rejection. *N*-acetylglucosaminidase is an enzyme contained within the lysosome of the tubular cell and is released when the lysosome is damaged, whereas alanine aminopeptidase is an enzyme of the brush border. Both markers were increased approximately 2 days earlier than serum creatinine in patients with transplant rejection.

QUALITATIVE DIAGNOSTIC PROCEDURES

Radiologic Studies

⑩ The etiology of kidney disease can be evaluated using several qualitative diagnostic techniques, including radiography, ultrasonography, magnetic resonance imaging, and biopsy. The standard radiograph of the kidneys, ureters, and bladder provides a gross estimate of kidney size and identifies the presence of calcifications.[54] Although an easy test to perform, the value of the information is minimal, and more detailed evaluations are often necessary. The intravenous urogram (formerly known as intravenous pyelogram) involves the administration of a contrast agent to facilitate visualization of the urinary collecting system. It is primarily used in the assessment of structural changes that may be associated with hematuria, pyuria, or flank pain, resulting from recurrent urinary tract infections, obstruction, or stone formation. For patients with low GFRs, retrograde administration of dye into the ureters may be performed to facilitate visualization of the collecting system. Contrast agents are also employed during renal angiography for the assessment of renovascular disease. As a test for the diagnosis of renovascular hypertension, the captopril (angiotensin-converting enzyme inhibitor) test is a useful adjunct. Under conditions of unilateral renal artery stenosis, the affected kidney produces large quantities of angiotensin II, which constricts the efferent arteriole to maintain GFR. The administration of an angiotensin-converting enzyme inhibitor results in reduced uptake of the contrast agent because the efferent arteriole is dilated, thereby decreasing the perfusion pressure of the affected kidney. For patients with bilateral disease, a decrease in uptake is observed in both kidneys.[125] Computed tomography is a cross-sectional anatomic imaging procedure based on x-ray data. The procedure is frequently performed with contrast to enhance imaging. Spiral, or helical, computed tomography, a more recent technique, provides for three-dimensional reconstruction of tissues. Computed tomography is performed as a test for the evaluation of obstructive uropathy, malignancy, and infections of the kidney.

Renal Ultrasonography

Ultrasonography uses sound waves to generate a two-dimensional image. The echogenicity of the kidney is compared with that of an adjacent organ—liver on the right and spleen on the left—with an increased echogenicity indicating an abnormal finding. Ultrasonography can distinguish the renal pyramids, medulla, and cortex, and abnormalities in structure, such as occurs with obstruction. Renal ultrasonography is also used as a guide for site localization during percutaneous kidney biopsy.

Magnetic Resonance Imaging

Magnetic resonance imaging is based on aligning hydrogen nuclei in the body with the use of a powerful magnet and applying radiofrequency pulses. The signals emitted by the hydrogen nuclei during realignment on repeated pulses allows for generation of the tissue image. Realignment times can also be altered with the use of contrast agents (gadolinium, gadopentetate), leading to increased signal intensity and improved imaging. Magnetic resonance imaging is useful for the assessment of obstruction, malignancy, and renovascular lesions. The relative advantages and limitations of these procedures are discussed in more detail in recent reviews.[54,126]

Biopsy

Renal biopsy is used in several conditions to facilitate diagnosis when clinical, laboratory, and imaging findings prove inconclusive. Proteinuria and hematuria are both associated with renal parenchymal disease. When less-invasive studies are unsuccessful in differentiating the cause and the possible causes have different therapeutic approaches, biopsy may be indicated. Functional status of the kidney is not assessed with biopsy, and severity of disease and progression is best measured using quantitative tests discussed above. Contraindications to renal biopsy include a solitary kidney, severe hypertension, bleeding disorder, severe anemia, cystic kidney, and hydronephrosis, among others. Complications resulting from biopsy primarily include hematuria, which may last for several days, and perirenal hematoma.[18]

CONCLUSIONS

The prevalence of kidney disease has increased dramatically over the past two decades, indicating a need for early identification, risk classification and monitoring of renal function in CKD patients. Comprehensive approaches to evaluating renal function in CKD patients in the clinical setting include the Cockcroft-Gault equation for estimating creatinine clearance and drug dosing, the MDRD4 equation to estimate GFR, and measurement of urinary protein excretion or albumin-to-creatinine ratio as a marker of the integrity of the glomerular basement membrane. Accurate measurement of GFR using exogenous administration of inulin, iothalamate, or radioisotope techniques such as ^{99m}Tc-DPTA is typically reserved for research settings to assess drug therapy outcomes and progression of disease. Use of qualitative assessments of renal function, such as radiography, computed tomography, magnetic resonance imaging, sonography, and biopsy, can help to determine the underlying cause of kidney disease.

ABBREVIATIONS

AUC: area under the plasma concentration vs. time curve

CKD: chronic kidney disease

CL: clearance

CL_{cr}: creatinine clearance

C_{ss}: concentration of a substance in plasma under steady-state conditions

CT: computerized tomography

ER: extraction ratio

ERBF: effective renal blood flow

ERPF: effective renal plasma flow

GFR: glomerular filtration rate

HCT: hematocrit

IBW: ideal body weight

MDRD: Modification of Diet in Renal Disease study

NKF: National Kidney Foundation

PAH: para-aminohippuric acid

S_{cr}: serum creatinine

U_{cr}: urine creatinine concentration

REFERENCES

1. Levey AS, Eckardt KU, Tsukamoto Y, et al. Definition and classification of chronic kidney disease: A position statement from Kidney Disease: Improving Global Outcomes (KDIGO). Kidney Int 2005;67(6):2089–2100.
2. Stevens LA, Coresh J, Greene T, Levey AS. Assessing kidney function—Measured and estimated glomerular filtration rate. N Engl J Med 2006;354(23):2473–2483.
3. Campens D, Buntinx F. Selecting the best renal function tests. Int J Technol Assess Health Care 1997;13:343–356.
4. Sica DA, Schoolwerth AC. Renal handling of organic anions and cations: Excretion of uric acid. In: Brenner BM, ed. Brenner and Rector's The Kidney, 6th ed. Philadelphia: WB Saunders, 2000:680–700.
5. Hsyu PH, Gisclon LG, Hui AC, Giacomini KM. Interactions of organic anions with the organic cation transporter in renal BBMV. Am J Physiol 1988;254:F56–F61.
6. Bendayan R. Renal drug transport: A review. Pharmacotherapy 1996;16:971–985.
7. Sikic BI. Pharmacologic approaches to reversing multidrug resistance. Semin Hematol 1997;34:40–47.
8. Bricker NS. On the meaning of the intact nephron hypothesis. Am J Med 1969;46:1–11.
9. Bosch JP. Renal reserve. A functional view of glomerular filtration rate. Semin Nephrol 1995;15:381–385.
10. Levin A, Singer J, Thompson CR, Ross H, Lewis M. Prevalent left ventricular hypertrophy in the predialysis population: Identifying opportunities for intervention. Am J Kidney Dis 1996;27:347–354.
11. Lacombe C, Mayeux P. The molecular biology of erythropoietin. Nephrol Dial Transplant 1999;1994;14(Suppl 2):22–28.
12. Alvestrand A. Carbohydrate and insulin metabolism in renal failure. Kidney Int Suppl 1997;62:S48–S52.
13. Martin KJ, Olgaard K, Coburn JW, et al. Diagnosis, assessment, and treatment of bone turnover abnormalities in renal osteodystrophy. Am J Kidney Dis 2004;43(3):558–565.
14. Dowling TC, Briglia AE, Fink JC, et al. Characterization of hepatic cytochrome P4503A (CYP3A) activity in ESRD patients. Clin Pharmacol Ther 2003;73(5):427–434.
15. Nolin TD, Appiah K, Kendrick SA, Le P, McMonagle E, Himmelfarb J. Hemodialysis acutely improves hepatic CYP3A4, metabolic activity. J Am Soc Nephrol 2006;17(9):2363–2367.
16. Keane WF, Eknoyan G. Proteinuria, albuminuria, risk, assessment, detection, elimination (PARADE): A position paper of the National Kidney Foundation. Am J Kidney Dis 1999;33:1004–1010.
17. Kasiske BL, Keane WF. Laboratory assessment of renal disease: Clearance, urinalysis, and renal biopsy. In: Brenner BM, ed. Brenner and Rector's The Kidney, 6th ed. Philadelphia: WB Saunders, 2000:1129–1170.
18. Rose BD, Renneke HG. Renal Pathophysiology—The Essentials. Baltimore: Williams & Wilkins.
19. Jones CA, McQuillan GM, Kusek JW, et al. Serum creatinine levels in the US population: Third National Health and Nutrition Examination Survey. Am J Kidney Dis 1998;32:992–999.
20. Bauer JH, Brooks CS, Burch RN. Clinical appraisal of creatinine clearance as a measurement of glomerular filtration rate. Am J Kidney Dis 1982;2:337–346.
21. Green AJE, Halloran SP, Mould GP, et al. Interference by newer cephalosporins in current methods for measuring creatinine. Clin Chem 1990;36:2139–2140.
22. Massoomi F, Matthews HG III, Destache CJ. Effect of seven fluoroquinolones on the determination of serum creatinine by the picric acid and enzymatic methods. Ann Pharmacother 1993;27:586–588.
23. Young DS, ed. Effects of Drugs on Clinical Laboratory Tests, 4th ed. Washington, DC: AACC Press, 1995:3.190–3.211.
24. Daly TM, Kempe KC, Scott MG, et al. "Bouncing" creatinine levels [letter]. N Engl J Med 1996;334:1749–1750.
25. Van den Berg, Koopman MG, Arisz L. Ranitidine has no influence on tubular creatinine secretion. Nephron 1996;74:705–708.
26. Thakur V, Reisin E, Solomonow M, et al. Accuracy of formula-derived creatinine clearance in paraplegic subjects. Clin Nephrol 1997;47:237–242.
27. Mayersohn M, Conrad KA, Achari R. The influence of a cooked meat meal on creatinine plasma concentration and creatinine clearance. Br J Clin Pharmacol 1983;15:227–230.
28. Poortsmans JR, Francaux M. Long-term oral creatine supplementation does not impair renal function in healthy athletes. Med Sci Sports Exerc 1999;31:1108–1110.
29. Robinson TM, Sewell DA, Casey A, et al. Dietary creatine supplementation does not affect some haematological indices, or indices of muscle damage and renal function. Br J Sports Med 2000;34:284–288.
30. Edmunds JW, Jayapalan S, DiMarco NM, et al. Creatine supplementation increases renal disease progression in Han:SPRD-cy Rats. Am J Kidney Dis 2001;37:73–78.
31. Coll E, Botey A, Alvarez L, et al. Serum cystatin C as a new marker for noninvasive estimation of glomerular filtration rate and as a marker for early renal impairment. Am J Kidney Dis 2000;36:29–34.
32. Knight EL, Verhave JC, Spiegelman D, et al. Factors influencing serum cystatin C levels other than renal function and the impact on renal function measurement. Kidney Int 2004;65:1416–1421.
33. Levin A. Cystatin C, serum creatinine, and estimates of kidney function: Searching for better measures of kidney function and cardiovascular risk. Ann Intern Med 2005;142:586–588.
34. Keevil BG, Kilpatrick ES, Nichols SP, Maylor PW. Biological variation of cystatin C. Implications for the assessment of glomerular filtration rate. Clin Chem 1998;44(7):1535–1539.
35. Perkins BA, Nelson RG, Ostrander BE, et al. Detection of renal function decline in patients with diabetes and normal or elevated GFR by serial measurements of serum cystatin C concentration: Results of a 4-year follow-up study. J Am Soc Nephrol 2005;16:1404–1412.
36. Page MK, Bükki B, Luppa P, Neumeier D. Clinical value of cystatin C determination. Clin Chim Acta 2000;297:67–72.
37. Bokenkamp A, Domanetzki M, Zinck R, et al. Cystatin C serum concentrations underestimate glomerular filtration rate in renal transplant recipients. Clin Chem 1999;45:1866–1868.
38. Akbas SH, Yavuz A, Tuncer M, et al. Serum cystatin C as an index of renal function in kidney transplant patients. Transplant Proc 2004;36(1):99–101.
39. Brosius FC, Hostetter TH, Kelepouris E, et al. Detection of chronic kidney disease in patients with or at increased risk of cardiovascular

disease: A science advisory from the American Heart Association Kidney and Cardiovascular Disease Council; the Councils on High Blood Pressure Research, Cardiovascular Disease in the Young, and Epidemiology and Prevention; and the Quality of Care and Outcomes Research Interdisciplinary Working Group: Developed in collaboration with the National Kidney Foundation. Circulation 2006;114(10):1083–1087.
40. Shlipak MG, Katz R, Sarnak MJ, et al. Cystatin C and prognosis for cardiovascular and kidney outcomes in elderly persons without chronic kidney disease. Ann Intern Med 2006;145(4):237–246.
41. Brändle E, Sieberth HG, Hautman RE. Effect of chronic dietary protein intake on the renal function in healthy subjects. Eur J Clin Nutr 1996;50:734–740.
42. Knight EL, Stampfer MJ, Hankinson SE, Spiegelman D, Curhan GC. The impact of protein intake on renal function decline in women with normal renal function or mild renal insufficiency. Ann Intern Med 2003;138(6):460–467.
43. Brenner BM, Lawler EV, Mackenzie HS. The hyperfiltration theory: A paradigm shift in nephrology. Kidney Int 1996;49:1774–1777.
44. Woods LL. Intrarenal mechanisms of renal reserve. Semin Nephrol 1995;15:386–395.
45. Dowling TC, Frye RF, Fraley DS, Matzke GR. Comparison of iothalamate clearance methods for measuring GFR. Pharmacotherapy 1999;19(8):943–950.
46. Florijn KW, Barendregt JNM, Lentjes EGWM, et al. Glomerular filtration rate measurement by "single-shot" injection of inulin. Kidney Int 1994;46:252–259.
47. Dall'Amico R, Montini G, Pisanello L, et al. Determination of inulin in plasma and urine by reverse-phase high-performance liquid chromatography. J Chromatogr B Biomed Appl 1995;672:155–159.
48. Soper CPR, Bending MR, Barron JL. An automated enzymatic inulin assay, capable of full sinistrin hydrolysis. Eur J Clin Chem Clin Biochem 1995;33:497–501.
49. Agarwal R. Ambulatory GFR measurement with cold iothalamate in adults with chronic kidney disease. Am J Kidney Dis 2003;41(4):752–759.
50. Dowling TC, Frye RF, Zemaitis MA. Simultaneous determination of *p*-aminohippuric acid, acetyl-*p*-aminohippuric acid and iothalamate in human plasma and urine by high-performance liquid chromatography. J Chromatogr B Biomed Sci Appl 1998;716(1–2):305–313.
51. Frennby B, Sterner G, Almén T, et al. The use of iohexol clearance to determine GFR in patients with severe chronic renal failure—A comparison between different clearance techniques. Clin Nephrol 1995;43:35–46.
52. Rocco MV, Buckalew VM Jr, Moore LC, Shihabi ZK. Measurement of glomerular filtration rate using nonradioactive iohexol: Comparison of two one-compartment models. Am J Nephrol 1996;16:138–143.
53. Lundqvist S, Hietala SO, Groth S, Sjödin JG. Evaluation of single sample clearance calculations in 902 patients. A comparison of multiple and single sample techniques. Acta Radiol 1997;38(1):68–72.
54. Hricak H, Meux M, Reddy GP. Radiologic assessment of the kidney. In: Brenner BM, ed. Brenner and Rector's The Kidney, 6th ed. Philadelphia: WB Saunders, 2000:1171–1200.
55. Frennby B, Almén T, Lilja B, et al. Determination of the relative glomerular filtration rate of each kidney in man. Acta Radiol 1995;36:410–417.
56. Morton K, Pisani DE, Whiting JH Jr, et al. Determination of glomerular filtration rate using technitium-99m-DTPA with differing degrees of renal function. J Nucl Med Technol 1997;25:110–114.
57. Levey AS, Bosch JP, Lewis JB, et al. A more accurate method to estimate glomerular filtration rate from serum creatinine: A new prediction equation. Ann Intern Med 1999;130:461–470.
58. Levey AS, Greene T, Kusek J, Beck G. A simplified equation to predict glomerular filtration rate from serum creatinine. J Am Soc Nephrol 2000;11:155A.
59. Myers GL, Miller WG, Coresh J, et al. Recommendations for improving serum creatinine measurement: A report from the Laboratory Working Group of the National Kidney Disease Education Program. Clin Chem 2006;52:5–18.
60. Rule AD, Gussak HM, Pond GR, et al. Measured and estimated GFR in healthy potential kidney donors. Am J Kidney Dis 2004;43(1):112–119.
61. Skluzacek PA, Szewc RG, Nolan CR, et al. Prediction of GFR in liver transplant candidates. Am J Kidney Dis 2003;42(6):1169–1176.
62. Gonwa TA, Jennings L, Mai ML, et al. Estimation of glomerular filtration rates before and after orthotopic liver transplantation: Evaluation of current equations. Liver Transpl 2004;10(2):301–309.
63. Lamb EJ, Webb MC, Simpson DE, Coakley AJ, Newman DJ, O'Riordan SE. Estimation of glomerular filtration rate in older patients with chronic renal insufficiency: Is the modification of diet in renal disease formula an improvement? J Am Geriatr Soc 2003;51(7):1012–1017.
64. Beddhu S, Samore MH, Roberts MS, et al. Creatinine production, nutrition, and glomerular filtration rate estimation. J Am Soc Nephrol 2003;14(4):1000–1005.
65. Poggio ED, Nef PC, Wang X, et al. Performance of the Cockcroft-Gault and modification of diet in renal disease equations in estimating GFR in ill hospitalized patients. Am J Kidney Dis 2005;46(2):242–252.
66. National Kidney Disease Education Program. 2007, *http://www.nkdep.nih.gov.*
67. Lemann J, Bidani AK, Bain RP, et al. Use of the serum creatinine to estimate glomerular filtration rate in health and early diabetic nephropathy. Am J Kidney Dis 1990;16:236–243.
68. Roubenoff R, Drew H, Moyer M, et al. Oral cimetidine improves the accuracy and precision of creatinine clearance in lupus nephritis. Ann Intern Med 1990;113:501–506.
69. Zaltzman JS, Whiteside C, Cattran D, et al. Accurate measurement of impaired glomerular filtration using single-dose oral cimetidine. Am J Kidney Dis 1996;27:504–511.
70. Cockroft DW, Gault MH. Prediction of creatinine clearance from serum creatinine. Nephron 1976;16:31–41.
71. Spinler SA, Nawarskas JJ, Boyce EG, et al. Predictive performance of ten equations for estimating creatinine clearance in cardiac patients. Iohexol Cooperative Study Group. Ann Pharmacother 1998;32(12):1275–1283.
72. Salazar DE, Corcoran GB. Predicting creatinine clearance and renal drug clearance in obese patients from estimated fat-free body mass. Am J Med 1988;84(6):1053–1060.
73. Luke DR, Halstenson CE, Opsahl JA, et al. Validity of creatinine clearance estimates in the assessment of renal function. Clin Pharmacol Ther 1990;48:503–508.
74. Mawer CE, Knowles BR, Lucas SB, et al. Computer-assisted prescribing of kanamycin for patients with renal insufficiency. Lancet 1972;1:12–15.
75. Jelliffe RW. Creatinine clearance: Bedside estimate. Ann Intern Med 1973;79:604–605.
76. Hull JH, Hak LJ, Koch GC, et al. Influence of range of renal function and liver disease on predictability of creatinine clearance. Clin Pharmacol Ther 1981;29:516–521.
77. Gault MH, Longerich LL, Harnett JD, et al. Predicting glomerular function from adjusted serum creatinine. Nephron 1992;62:249–256.
78. Coresh J, Toto RD, Kirk KA, et al. Creatinine clearance as a measure of GFR in screens for the African-American study of kidney disease. Am J Kidney Dis 1998;32:32–42.
79. Goldwasser P, Aboul-Magd A, Maru M. Race and creatinine excretion in chronic renal insufficiency. Am J Kidney Dis 1997;30:16–22.
80. Ixkes MCJ, Koopman MG, van Acker BAC, et al. Cimetidine improves GFR-estimation by the Cockcroft-Gault formula. Clin Nephrol 1997;47:229–236.
81. Schiff J, Paraskevas S, Keith D, et al. Prediction of the glomerular filtration rate using equations in kidney-pancreas transplant patients receiving cimetidine. Transplantation 2006;81(3):469–472.
82. Kemperman FA, Surachno J, Krediet RT, Arisz L. Cimetidine improves prediction of the glomerular filtration rate by the Cockcroft-Gault formula in renal transplant recipients. Transplantation 2002;73(5):770–774.
83. Orlando R, Floreani M, Padrini R, Palatini P. Evaluation of measured and calculated creatinine clearances as glomerular filtration markers in different stages of liver cirrhosis. Clin Nephrol 1999;51:341–347.
84. Lam NP, Sperelakis R, Kuk J, et al. Rapid estimation of creatinine clearances in patients with liver dysfunction. Dig Dis Sci 1999;44:1222–1227.
85. Caregaro L, Menon F, Angeli P, et al. Limitations of serum creatinine level and creatinine clearance as filtration markers in cirrhosis. Arch Intern Med 1994;154:201–205.
86. Sansoe G, Ferrari A, Castellana CN, Bonardi L, Villa E, Manenti F. Cimetidine administration and tubular creatinine secretion in patients with compensated cirrhosis. Clin Sci 2002;102(1):91–98.
87. DeSanto NG, Anastasio P, Loguercio C, et al. Creatinine clearance: An inadequate marker of renal filtration in patients with early posthepa-

titic cirrhosis (Child A) without fluid retention and muscle wasting. Nephron 1995;70:421–424.
88. Davis GA, Chandler MHH. Comparison of creatinine clearance estimation methods in patients with trauma. Am J Health Syst Pharm 1996;53:1028–1032.
89. Goerdt PJ, Heim-Duthoy KL, Macres M, Swan SK. Predictive performance of renal function equations in renal allografts. Br J Clin Pharmacol 1997;44:261–265.
90. Huang E, Hewitt R, Shelton M, Morse GD. Comparison of measured and estimated creatinine clearance in patients with advanced HIV disease. Pharmacotherapy 1996;16:222–229.
91. Quadri KH, Bernardini J, Greenberg A, et al. Assessment of renal function during pregnancy using a random urine protein to creatinine ratio and Cockcroft-Gault formula. Am J Kidney Dis 1994(3);24: 416–420.
92. Jelliffe RW. Estimation of creatinine clearance in patients with unstable renal function, without a urine specimen. Am J Nephrol 2002;22(4):320–324.
93. Chiou WL, Hsu FH. A new simple rapid method to monitor renal function based on pharmacokinetic considerations of endogenous creatinine. Res Commun Chem Pathol Pharmacol 1975;10:315–330.
94. Brater DC. Drug Use in Renal Disease. Balgowlah, Australia: ADIS Health Science Press, 1983:22–56.
95. Arant BS Jr. Developmental patterns of renal functional maturation compared in the human neonate. J Pediatr 1978;92:705–712.
96. van den Anker, de Groot R, Broerse HM, et al. Assessment of glomerular filtration rate in preterm infants by serum creatinine: Comparison with inulin clearance. Pediatrics 1995;96:1156–1158.
97. Sertel H, Scopes J. Rates of creatinine clearance in babies less than one week of age. Arch Dis Child 1973;48:717–720.
98. Bajaj G, Alexander SR, Browne R, et al. ^{125}Iodine-iothalamate clearance in children. A simple method to measure glomerular filtration. Pediatr Nephrol 1996;10:25–28.
99. Schwartz GJ, Brion LP, Spitzer A. The use of plasma creatinine concentration for estimating glomerular filtration rate in infants, children, and adolescents. Pediatr Clin North Am 1987;34:571–590.
100. Al-Harbi N, Lireman D. Comparison of three different methods of estimating the glomerular filtration rate in children after renal transplantation. Am J Nephrol 1997;17:68–71.
101. Fong J, Johnston S, Valentino T, Notterman D. Length/serum creatinine ratio does not predict measured creatinine clearance in critically ill children. Clin Pharmacol Ther 1995;58:192–197.
102. Pierrat A, Gravier E, Saunders C, et al. Predicting GFR in children and adults: A comparison of the Cockcroft-Gault, Schwartz, and modification of diet in renal disease formulas. Kidney Int 2003;64(4):1425–1436.
103. Lindeman RD, Tobin J, Shrock NW. Longitudinal studies on the rate of decline in renal function with age. J Am Geriatr Soc 1985;33:278–281.
104. Lindeman RD. Assessment of renal function in the old: Special considerations. Clin Lab Med 1993;13:269–277.
105. Fliser D, Ritz E, Franek E. Renal reserve in the elderly. Semin Nephrol 1995;15:463–467.
106. Smythe M, Hoffman J, Kizy K, et al. Estimating creatinine clearance in elderly patients with low serum creatinine concentrations. Am J Hosp Pharm 1994;51:198–204.
107. O'Connell MB, Wong MO, Bannick-Mohrland SD, et al. Accuracy of 2- and 8-hour urine collections for measuring creatinine clearance in the hospitalized elderly. Pharmacotherapy 1993;13:135–142.
108. Agodoa L, Eknoyan G, Ingelfinger J, et al. Assessment of structure and function in progressive renal disease. Kidney Int Suppl 1997;63:S144–S150.
109. Rossing P, Astrup AS, Smidt UM, et al. Monitoring kidney function in diabetic nephropathy. Diabetologia 1994;37:708–712.
110. Valensi P, Assayag M, Busby M, et al. Microalbuminuria in obese patients with or without hypertension. Int J Obes Relat Metab Disord 1996;20:574–579.
111. Berrut G, Bouhanick B, Fabbri P, et al. Microalbuminuria as a predictor of a drop in glomerular filtration rate in subjects with non-insulin-dependent diabetes mellitus and hypertension. Clin Nephrol 1997;48:92–97.
112. Mimran A, Ribstein J, DuCailar G. Is microalbuminuria a marker of early intrarenal vascular dysfunction in essential hypertension? Hypertension 1994;23:1018–1021.
113. Dworkin LD, Sun AM, Brenner BM. The renal circulations. In: Brenner BM, ed. Brenner and Rector's The Kidney, 6th ed. Philadelphia: WB Saunders, 2000:277–318.
114. Dowling TC, Frye RF, Fraley DS, Matzke GR. Characterization of tubular functional capacity in humans using para-aminohippurate and famotidine. Kidney Int 2001;59:295–303.
115. Prescott LF, Freestone S, McAuslane JAN. The concentration-dependent disposition of intravenous *p*-aminohippurate in subjects with normal and impaired renal function. Br J Clin Pharmacol 1993;35:20–29.
116. Taylor A, Manatunga A, Morton K, et al. Multicenter trial validation of a camera-based method to measure Tc-99m mercaptoacetyltriglycine, or Tc-99m MAG_3, clearance. Radiology 1997;204:47–54.
117. Russell CD, Dubovsky EV. Comparison of single-injection multisample renal clearance methods with and without urine collection. J Nucl Med 1995;36:603–606.
118. Nassseri K, Daley-Yates PT. A comparison of *N*-1-methylnicotinamide clearance with 5 other markers of renal function in models of acute and chronic renal failure. Toxicol Lett 1990;53:243–245.
119. Edwards BD, Maiza A, Daley-Yates PT, et al. Altered clearance of *N*-1-methylnicotinamide associated with the use of low doses of cyclosporine. Am J Kidney Dis 1994;23:23–30.
120. Maiza A, Daley-Yates PT. Estimation of the renal clearance of drugs using endogenous *N*-1-methylnicotinamide. Toxicol Lett 1990;53:231–235.
121. Karyekar CS, Eddington ND, Briglia AE, Gubbins PO, Dowling TC. Renal interaction between itraconazole and cimetidine. J Clin Pharmacol 2004;44:919–927.
122. Schentag JJ, Plaut ME. Patterns of urinary β_2-microglobulin excretion by patients treated with aminoglycosides. Kidney Int 1980;17:654–661.
123. Jung K, Diego J, Strobelt V, et al. Diagnostic significance of some urinary enzymes for detecting acute rejection crises in renal transplant recipients: Alanine aminopeptidase, alkaline phosphatase, γ-glutamyl transferase, *N*-acetyl-β-glucosaminidase, and lysozyme. Clin Chem 1986;32:1807–1811.
124. Jung K. Urinary enzymes and low-molecular-weight proteins as markers of tubular dysfunction. Kidney Int Suppl 1994;47:S29–S33.
125. Taylor A, Nally JV. Clinical applications of renal scintigraphy. AJR Am J Roentgenol 1995;164:31–41.
126. Higgins TJ, Mindell HJ, Fairbank JT. Kidney imaging techniques. In: Greenberg A, ed. Primer on Kidney Diseases, 4th ed. Philadelphia: Elsevier Saunders, 2005:47–55.

CHAPTER 45

Acute Renal Failure

WILLIAM DAGER AND ANNE SPENCER

KEY CONCEPTS

1. Acute renal failure (ARF) is a common complication in the hospitalized patient and is associated with a high mortality rate.
2. ARF is predominantly categorized based on the anatomic area of injury or malfunction: (a) prerenal—decreased renal blood flow, (b) intrinsic—a structure within the kidney is damaged, and (c) postrenal—an obstruction is present within the urine collection system.
3. Risk factors for ARF include advanced age, acute infection, preexisting chronic respiratory or cardiovascular disease, dehydration, and chronic kidney disease.
4. ARF lacks a specific and sensitive sign to herald its onset. Hence, a thorough patient history, including medications, recent procedures and illnesses, physical examination, and laboratory assessment of serum and urine are necessary components of an ARF evaluation after an elevated serum creatinine (S_{cr}) is noted.
5. Prevention is key; there are very few therapeutic options for the therapeutic management of established ARF.
6. Supportive management remains the primary approach to prevent or reduce the complications associated with ARF. Supportive therapies include: renal replacement therapies (RRTs), nutritional support, avoidance of nephrotoxins, and blood pressure and fluid management.
7. For those patients with prolonged or severe ARF, RRTs are the cornerstone of support and facilitate an aggressive approach to fluid, electrolyte and waste management.
8. Diuretic resistance is a common phenomenon in the patient with ARF and can be addressed with aggressive sodium restriction, combination diuretic therapy, or a continuous infusion of a loop diuretic.
9. Drug-dosing regimens for ARF patients receiving intermittent hemodialysis (IHD) are predominantly extrapolated from data derived from patients with chronic kidney disease (CKD); however, important pharmacokinetic differences exist in patients with ARF that should be considered.
10. Drug dosing guidelines for ARF patients receiving continuous renal replacement therapies (CRRTs) are poorly characterized and individualized doses may need to be determined by estimating the clearance of medications associated with a high risk of toxicity by the patient and the CRRT procedure.

Learning objectives, review questions, and other resources can be found at **www.pharmacotherapyonline.com.**

The development of acute renal failure (ARF) presents a difficult challenge to the clinician because there are many possible causes and the onset is often asymptomatic. In the ambulatory setting, patients may not notice ARF symptoms for days to weeks. Changes in clinical and laboratory markers of its presence can be subtle and are often overlooked. Despite its often insidious presentation, the consequences of ARF can be serious, especially in hospitalized patients, among whom mortality rates of up to 60% have been reported.[1,2]

Supportive therapy is the focus of management for those with established ARF, as there is no therapy that directly reverses the injury associated with the numerous causes of ARF. Management goals include maintenance of blood pressure, fluid, and electrolyte homeostasis, all of which may be dramatically altered in the presence of ARF. Additional therapies designed to eliminate or minimize the insult that precipitated ARF include discontinuation of the offending drug (i.e., the nephrotoxin), cardiac support of the failing heart, removal of the obstruction from the urinary collection system, corticosteroids to minimize any intrinsic inflammatory process, antibiotic therapy to treat any infection, or other specific maneuvers to limit or reverse the kidney injury. Because of the poor clinical outcomes and lack of specific therapies, the importance of preventing ARF cannot be overemphasized. Individuals at highest risk, such as those with chronic kidney disease (CKD) and the elderly with chronic medical conditions, need to be identified and their exposure to harmful diagnostic or therapeutic procedures or medications minimized.

Renal replacement therapies (RRTs) such as hemodialysis and peritoneal dialysis have been available for decades, but have not resulted in dramatic improvements in the outcomes of patients with ARF. However, newer RRT modalities including an array of continuous renal replacement therapies (CRRTs) appear to offer some benefits, although available resources may limit their use and drug dosing is handicapped by a paucity of data. Careful patient monitoring for response to these therapies and attention to pharmacokinetic alterations make it possible to develop rational drug-dosing regimens for these complex patients. Despite the supportive care that CRRTs offer, development of ARF is frequently a catastrophic event. In this chapter, the epidemiology and multiple etiologies of ARF, as well as the clinical features associated with the most common types of ARF, are presented. Methods to recognize and identify the extent of functional loss are also discussed. Finally preventative strategies and management approaches for those with established ARF are reviewed.

DEFINITION OF ACUTE RENAL FAILURE

ARF is broadly defined as a decrease in glomerular filtration rate (GFR), generally occurring over hours to days, sometimes over weeks, that is associated with an accumulation of waste products, including urea and creatinine. This relatively abrupt decline in renal function is in contrast to CKD, which is defined by the presence of proteinuria/albuminuria for at least 3 months, in combination with a GFR of <90 mL/min/1.73 m^2.[3] A decrease in urine output is often observed, but is not required for ARF to be present.[4] Compared to a normal urine output of ≥1,200 mL/day, patients with ARF are often categorized as being anuric (urine output <50 mL/day), oliguric (urine output <500 mL/day), or nonoliguric (urine output >500 mL/day).

Currently, there is no universally accepted definition of ARF in clinical practice: in fact, more than 30 definitions for ARF are reported in the medical literature.[5] Many of these definitions incorporate selective aspects of ARF observed in different patient populations. Comparisons between studies that describe incidences, treatment effects, and patient outcomes can thus be difficult, if not impossible to interpret. Although a serum creatinine (S_{cr}) or calculated creatinine clearance (Cl_{cr}) may not provide a reliable characterization of renal function in all ARF situations, clinicians frequently use some combination of the absolute S_{cr} value, change in S_{cr} value over time, and/or urine output as the primary criteria for diagnosing the presence of ARF.[4,6] The commonly used and highly variable definitions for ARF are nonspecific and open to various interpretations. On a patient-by-patient basis, the semantics of the ARF definition are relatively meaningless. However, to move the prevention and treatment of ARF forward, consistent definitions must be employed. Without them, clinicians will be unable to accurately use any data generated because the nonspecific classification of ARF will be an insurmountable barrier to the identification of who was studied, and hence, to whom the data apply. A means to standardize the various aspects of the clinical presentation is necessary to allow integration of the literature observations to bedside management. A new consensus-derived definition and classification system for ARF was recently proposed, and is currently being validated (Fig. 45–1).[7,8] This three-tiered classification uses both GFR and urine output, plus two clinical outcomes that may occur subsequent to an episode of ARF as components of the paradigm. Definitions of risk of dysfunction (R), injury to the kidney (I), and failure of the kidney (F) are outlined. The clinical outcomes of loss of function (L), and end-stage renal disease (E) complete the RIFLE acronym. Thus far, validation studies have confirmed the value of these criteria in predicting hospital mortality, although further assessment is still necessary.[9,10]

EPIDEMIOLOGY

ARF is an uncommon condition in the community-dwelling, generally healthy population, with an annual incidence of approximately 0.02% (Table 45–1).[11] In individuals with preexisting CKD, however, the incidence may be as high as 13%. In nonhospitalized patients, dehydration, exposure to selected pharmacologic agents such as contrast media, and the presence of heart failure are associated with an increased risk of ARF. Additionally, trauma, rhabdomyolysis, vessel thrombosis, and drugs are common culprits in the development of ARF.[11] The pharmacologic agents commonly associated with ARF, including contrast media, chemotherapeutic agents, nonsteroidal antiinflammatory drugs (NSAIDs), angiotensin-converting enzyme inhibitors, angiotensin receptor blockers, and antiviral medications are discussed in detail in Chap. 49.[11,12]

❶ The hospitalized individual is at high risk of developing ARF; the reported incidence is 7%.[13] The incidence of ARF is markedly higher in critically ill patients, ranging from 6% to 23%.[6] The high mortality rate related to ARF, which is reported to range from 35% to 80%, is a significant clinical concern that has been relatively unresponsive to therapeutic intervention over the last four decades. Although the relative contribution of ARF to mortality rates of the underlying disease states is unclear given that current illness and ARF cannot be reliably quantified, it is certain that the presence of ARF will independently contribute significantly to overall mortality.[6] For survivors of ARF, subsequent morbidity or development of some degree of CKD is also a consideration. Although 90% of individuals recover enough renal function to live normal lives, approximately half of these are left with subclinical deficits. Five percent will not regain

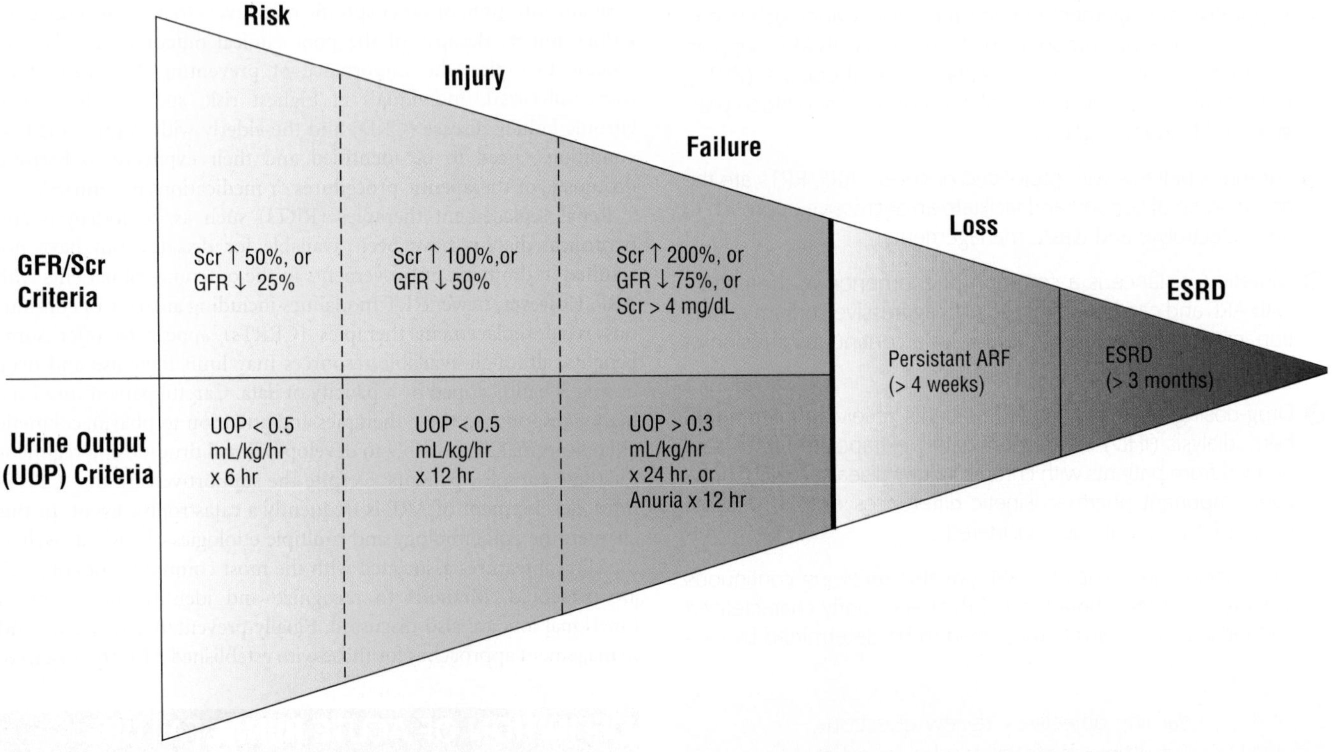

FIGURE 45-1. RIFLE classification for acute renal failure (ARF). (ESRD, end-stage renal disease; GFR, glomerular filtration rate; S_{cr}, serum creatinine). *(Reprinted and adapted from Crit Care Clin, Vol. 21, Bellomo R. Defining, quantifying, and classifying acute renal failure, pages 223-237, Copyright © 2005, with permission from Elsevier.)*

TABLE 45-1 Incidence and Outcomes of Acute Renal Failure Relative to Where It Occurs

	Community-Acquired	Hospital-Acquired	ICU-Acquired
Incidence	Low (<1%)	Moderate (2%–5%)	High (6%–23%)
Cause	Single	Single or multiple	Multifactorial
Overall survival rate	70%–95%	30%–50%	10%–30%
Worsened outcome if:	RRT required Poor preadmission health Other failed organ systems	RRT required Poor preadmission health Ischemic ARF cause Other failed organ systems	Intrinsic renal disease Ischemic ARF cause Septic RRT required Poor preadmission health Other failed organ systems
Better outcome if:	Nonoliguric	Nonoliguric Nephrotoxic cause	Prerenal cause Postrenal cause Nonoliguric Nephrotoxic cause Hyperglycemia prevented

ARF, acute renal failure; RRT, renal replacement therapy.

sufficient renal function to live independently and thus require long-term peritoneal or hemodialysis or transplantation. An additional 5% will suffer from a progressive deterioration in kidney function after initial recovery, likely as a consequence of hyperfiltration and sclerosis of the remaining glomeruli.[14]

ETIOLOGY

❷ The etiology of ARF can be divided into broad categories based on the anatomic location of the injury associated with the precipitating factor(s). The management of patients presenting with this disorder is largely predicated on identification of the specific etiology responsible for the patient's current acute kidney injury (Table 45–2). Traditionally, the causes of ARF have been categorized as (a) prerenal, which results from decreased renal perfusion in the setting of undamaged parenchymal tissue, (b) intrinsic, the result of structural damage to the kidney, most commonly the tubule from a ischemic or toxic insult, and (c) postrenal, caused by obstruction of urine flow downstream from the kidney (Fig. 45–2).

❸ The most common cause of hospital-acquired ARF is prerenal ischemia as the result of reduced renal perfusion secondary to sepsis, reduced cardiac output, and/or surgery. Drug-induced ARF may account for 18% to 33% of in-hospital occurrences. Other risk factors for developing ARF while hospitalized include advanced age (>60 years of age), male gender, acute infection, and preexisting chronic diseases of the respiratory or cardiovascular systems.[6]

PATHOPHYSIOLOGY

PSEUDORENAL AND FUNCTIONAL ACUTE RENAL FAILURE

In selected situations their can be a rise in either the blood urea nitrogen (BUN) or the S_{cr}, suggesting presence of renal dysfunction when in fact GFR is not diminished. This could be the result of cross-reactivity with the assay used to measure the BUN or S_{cr}, or selective inhibition of the secretion of creatinine into the proximal tubular lumen (see Chap. 44). The initiation or discontinuation of such agents should be considered in the assessment for acute changes in renal function, and should be looked for as part of the work up in any patient who is suspected to have ARF.

In functional ARF, a decline in GFR secondary to a reduced glomerular hydrostatic pressure, which is the driving force for the formation of ultrafiltrate, can occur without damage to the kidney itself. The decline in glomerular hydrostatic pressure may be a direct consequence of changes in glomerular afferent (vasoconstriction) and efferent (vasodilation) arteriolar circumference. These clinical conditions are most commonly seen in individuals who have reduced effective blood volume (e.g., heart failure, cirrhosis, severe pulmonary disease, or hypoalbuminemia) or renovascular disease (e.g., renal artery stenosis) and who cannot compensate for changes in afferent or efferent arteriolar tone. A decrease in efferent arteriolar resistance as the result of initiation of angiotensin-converting enzyme inhibitor or angiotensin receptor blocker therapy is a common cause of this syndrome. The hepatorenal syndrome is also included in this classification because the kidney itself may be damaged, and there is intense afferent arteriolar vasoconstriction leading to a decline in glomerular hydrostatic pressure. In all the above conditions, the urinalysis is no different from its baseline state and the urinary indices suggest prerenal azotemia.

Functional ARF is very common in individuals with heart failure who receive an angiotensin converting enzyme inhibitor or an angiotensin receptor blocker in an attempt to improve their left ventricular function. Because the decline in efferent arteriolar resistance resulting from the inhibition of angiotensin II occurs within days, if the dose of the angiotensin-converting enzyme inhibitor is increased too rapidly, a decline in GFR with a concomitant rise in the serum creatinine will be noticeable. If the increase in the serum creatinine is mild to moderate (an increase of less than 30% from baseline) the medication can be continued.

PRERENAL ACUTE RENAL FAILURE

Prerenal ARF results from hypoperfusion of the renal parenchyma, with or without systemic arterial hypotension. Renal hypoperfusion with systemic arterial hypotension may be caused by a decline in intravascular or effective blood volume that can occur in those with acute blood loss (hemorrhage), dehydration, hypoalbuminemia, or diuretic therapy. Renal hypoperfusion without systemic hypotension is most commonly associated with bilateral renal artery occlusion, or unilateral occlusion in a patient with a single functioning kidney. The initial physiologic responses to a reduction in effective blood volume by the body includes activation of the sympathetic nervous and the renin–angiotensin–aldosterone systems, and release of antidiuretic hormone if hypotension is present. These responses work together to directly maintain blood pressure via vasoconstriction and stimulation of thirst to increase fluid intake and the promotion of sodium and water retention. Additionally, GFR may be maintained by afferent arteriole dilation and efferent arteriole constriction. In concert, these homeostatic mechanisms are often able to maintain arterial pressure and renal perfusion, potentially averting the progression to ARF.[15] If, however, the decreased renal perfusion is severe or prolonged, these compensatory mechanisms may be overwhelmed and ARF will then

TABLE 45-2 Classification of Acute Renal Failure

Category	Abnormality Causing Acute Renal Failure	Possible Causes
Prerenal	Intravascular volume depletion resulting in arterial hypotension	Dehydration Inadequate fluid intake Excessive vomiting, diarrhea or gastric suctioning Increased insensible losses (e.g., fever, burns) Diabetes insipidus High serum glucose (glucosuria) Overdiuresis Hemorrhage Decreased cardiac output Hypoalbuminemia Liver disease Nephrotic syndrome
	Arterial hypotension (regard less of volume status)	Anaphylaxis Sepsis Excessive antihypertensive use
	Decreased cardiac output	Heart failure Sepsis Pulmonary hypertension Aortic stenosis (and other valvular abnormalities) Anesthetics
	Isolated renal hypoperfusion	Bilateral renal artery stenosis (unilateral renal artery stenosis in solitary kidney) Emboli Cholesterol Thrombotic Medications Cyclosporine Angiotensin-converting enzyme inhibitors Nonsteroidal antiinflammatory drugs Radiocontrast media Hypercalcemia Hepatorenal syndrome
Intrinsic	Vascular damage	Vasculitis Polyarteritis nodosa Hemolytic uremic syndrome-thrombotic thrombocytopenic purpura Emboli Atherosclerotic Thrombotic Accelerated hypertension
	Glomerular damage	Systemic lupus erythematosus Poststreptococcal glomerulonephritis Antiglomerular basement membrane disease
	Acute tubular necrosis	Ischemic Hypotension Vasoconstriction Exogenous toxins Contrast dye Heavy metals Drugs (amphotericin B, aminoglycosides, etc.) Endogenous toxins Myoglobin Hemoglobin
	Acute interstitial nephritis	Drugs Penicillins Ciprofloxacin Sulfonamides Infection Viral Bacterial
Postrenal	Bladder outlet obstruction	Prostatic hypertrophy, infection, cancer Improperly placed bladder catheter Anticholinergic medication
	Ureteral	Cancer with abdominal mass Retroperitoneal fibrosis Nephrolithiasis
	Renal pelvis or tubules	Nephrolithiasis Oxalate Indinavir Sulfonamides Acyclovir Uric acid

be clinically evident. If renal artery stenosis is present, narrowing bilaterally (both kidneys) or unilaterally (one functional kidney) of the artery responsible for blood flow to the kidney can lead to reduced renal function. The most common cause is atherosclerosis, with severe abrupt occlusion sometimes occurring as the result of an embolism.[16]

INTRINSIC ACUTE RENAL FAILURE

Acute intrinsic renal failure results from damage to the kidney itself. Conceptually, acute intrinsic renal failure can be categorized on the basis of the structures within the kidney that are injured: the renal vasculature, glomeruli, tubules, and the interstitium. Many diverse mechanisms have been associated with the development of intrinsic ARF, many of which are categorized in Table 45–2.

Renal Vasculature Damage

Occlusion of the larger renal vessels resulting in ARF is not common, but can occur if large atheroemboli or thromboemboli occlude the bilateral renal arteries, or one vessel of the patient with a single kidney. Atheroemboli most commonly develop during vascular procedures that cause atheroma dislodgement, such as angioplasty or aortic manipulations. Thromboemboli may arise from dislodgement of a mural thrombus in the left ventricle of a patient with severe heart failure, or from the atria of a patient with atrial fibrillation. Renal artery thrombosis may occur in a similar fashion to coronary thrombosis, in which a thrombus forms in conjunction with an atherosclerotic plaque.

Although smaller vessels can also be obstructed by atheroemboli or thromboemboli, the damage is limited to the vessels involved, and the development of significant ARF is unlikely. However, these small vessels are susceptible to inflammatory processes that lead to microvascular damage and vessel dysfunction when the renal capillaries are affected. Neutrophils invade the vessel wall, causing damage that can include thrombus formation, tissue infarction, and collagen deposition within the vessel structure. Diffuse renal vasculitis can be mild or severe, with severe forms promoting concomitant ischemic acute tubular necrosis (ATN). The S_{cr} is usually elevated as the lesions are diffuse, and thus the area of damage is large. Accelerated hypertension that is not treated may also compromise renal microvascular blood flow, and thus cause diffuse renal capillary damage.

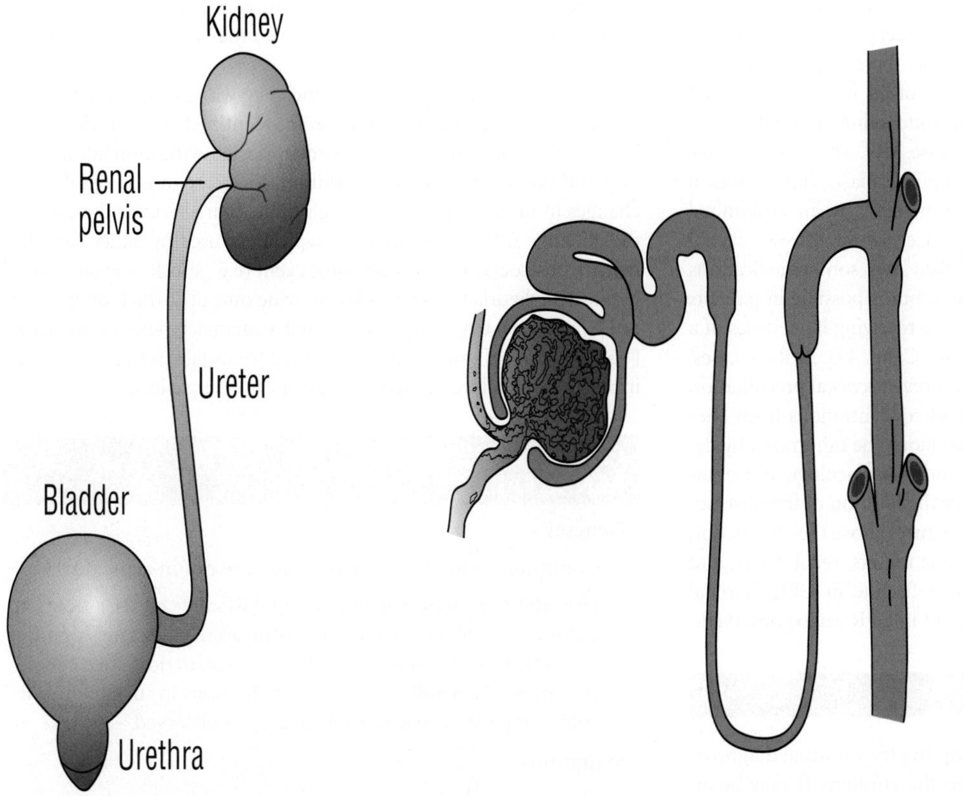

FIGURE 45-2. Physiologic classification of ARF. Blood flows through the afferent arteriole, to the glomerulus and exits through the efferent arteriole. The formation of glomerular ultrafiltrate is dependent on the surface area of the capillaries within the glomerular region, their permeability, and the net hydrostatic pressure across the capillary wall. A decrease in blood flow and renal perfusion can lead to a prerenal reduction in renal function. Under conditions in which renal blood flow is diminished, the kidney maintains glomerular ultrafiltration by vasodilating the afferent and vasoconstricting the efferent arterioles. Medications that may interfere with these processes might result in an abrupt decline in glomerular filtration. Damage to the glomerular or tubular regions leads to intrinsic ARF. Obstruction of urine flow once in the collecting tubule, ureter, bladder, or urethra is termed postrenal failure.

Glomerular Damage

Only 5% of the cases of intrinsic ARF are of glomerular origin. The glomerulus is one of two capillary beds in the kidney, and serves to filter fluid and solute into the tubules while retaining proteins and other large blood components in the intravascular space. Because it's a capillary system, glomerular damage can occur by the same mechanisms described for the renal vasculature, and one additional mechanism, that is, severe inflammatory processes specific to the glomerulus. The pathophysiology and specific therapeutic approaches used to combat the inflammatory processes are described in detail in Chap. 50.

Tubule Damage

Approximately 85% of all cases of intrinsic ARF are caused by ATN, of which 50% are a result of renal ischemia, often arising from an extended prerenal state. The remaining 35% are the result of exposure to direct tubule toxins, which can be endogenous (myoglobin, hemoglobin, or uric acid) or exogenous (contrast agents, heavy metals, or aminoglycoside antibiotics). The tubules located within the medulla of the kidney are particularly at risk from ischemic injury, as this portion of the kidney is metabolically active and thus has high oxygen requirements, yet even in the best of situations, receives relatively low oxygen delivery (as compared to the cortex). Thus, ischemic conditions caused by severe hypotension or exposure to vasoconstrictive drugs preferentially affect the tubules more than any other portion of the kidney.

The clinical evolution of ATN is characterized by the initial injury causing tubule epithelial cell necrosis or apoptosis, followed by an extension phase with continued hypoxia and an inflammatory response involving the nearby interstitium.[17] The onset of ATN can occur over days to weeks, and rarely longer than that depending on the factors responsible for the damage to the tubular epithelial cells.[18] Once tubular cells die, they slough off into the tubular lumen. The debris causes increased tubular pressure and reduces glomerular filtration.[19] Additionally, the loss of epithelial cells leaves only the basement membrane between the filtrate and the interstitium, which results in dysregulation of fluid and electrolyte transfer across the tubular epithelium. Regardless of the etiology, tubular injury leads to a loss in the ability to concentrate urine, to defective distal sodium reabsorption, and, ultimately, to a reduction in the GFR.[20] Continued kidney hypoxia or toxin exposure after the original insult kills more cells, and propagates the inflammatory response and can extend the injury and delay the recovery process. With prolonged ischemia, the tubular epithelial cells in the corticomedullary junction are damaged and die. When the toxin or ischemia is removed, a maintenance phase ensues (typically 2 to 3 weeks), followed by a recovery phase (2 to 3 weeks) during which new tubule cells are regenerated. The recovery phase is associated with a notable diuresis, which requires attention to fluid balance to ensure that a secondary prerenal injury does not occur. However, if the ischemia or injury is extremely severe or prolonged, cortical necrosis may occur, preventing any tubule cell regrowth in the affected areas.

Interstitial Damage

The interstitium of the kidney is rarely the primary cause of end-stage renal disease (ESRD), but it can become severely inflamed and lead to ARF. Acute interstitial nephritis is most commonly caused by medications (see Chap. 49), or bacterial or viral infections.[21] Up to 30% of cases have no identifiable cause.[22] Whatever the inciting event, interstitial nephritis is characterized by lesions comprised of monocytes, macrophages, B cells, or T cells, clearly identifying an immunologic response as the injurious process affecting the interstitium.[23] Because of the interwoven nature of the interstitium and the tubules, the widespread inflammation and edema affect the function of the tubules, and may cause fibrosis if the administration of the nephrotoxin is not discontinued and inflammation quickly controlled.[24]

POSTRENAL ACUTE RENAL FAILURE

Postrenal ARF may develop as the result of obstruction at any level within the urinary collection system from the renal tubule to urethra (see Table 45–2). However, if the obstructing process is above the bladder, it must involve both kidneys (one kidney in a patient with a single functioning kidney) to cause significant ARF. Bladder outlet obstruction, the most common cause of obstructive uropathy, is often caused by a prostatic process (hypertrophy, cancer or infection) causing a physical impingement on the urethra and thereby preventing the passage of urine. It may also be the result of an improperly placed urinary catheter. Neurogenic bladder or anticholinergic medications may also prevent bladder emptying and cause ARF. The blockage may occur at the ureter level, secondary to nephrolithiasis, blood clots, a sloughed renal papillae, or physical compression by an abdominal process such as retroperitoneal fibrosis, cancer, or an abscess. Crystal deposition within the tubules from oxalate and some medications severe enough to cause ARF is uncommon, but is possible in patients with severe volume contraction and in those receiving large doses of a drug with relatively low urine solubility (see Chap. 49). In these cases, patients have insufficient urine volume to prevent crystal precipitation in the urine.[25] Extremely elevated uric acid concentrations from chemotherapy-induced tumor lysis syndrome should be minimized by the initiation of an aggressive fluid regimen and pharmacologic preventative therapies in at-risk patients. Wherever the location of the obstruction, urine will accumulate in the renal structures above the obstruction and cause increased pressure upstream. The ureters, renal pelvis, and calyces all expand, and the net result is a decline in GFR. If renal vasoconstriction ensues, a further decrement in GFR will be observed.

CLINICAL PRESENTATION

❹ The initiating sign or symptom prompting the eventual diagnosis of ARF is highly variable, depending on the etiology. It may be an elevated S_{cr}, decreased urine output, blood in the urine, pain during voiding, or severe abdominal or flank pain. The first step is to determine if the renal complication is acute, chronic, or the result of an acute change in a patient with known CKD. BUN, potassium, phosphorous, and, potentially, magnesium concentrations in serum will likely become elevated and should be promptly evaluated. For those presenting in the outpatient environment it may be difficult to determine when the onset was as the initial presentation of ARF may have been asymptomatic. The onset of ARF may, in fact, trigger independently symptoms of a concurrent medical condition or excessive drug response from a renally eliminated agent.

PATIENT ASSESSMENT

A past medical history for renal disease-related chronic conditions, such as poorly controlled hypertension or diabetes mellitus, previous laboratory data documenting the presence of proteinuria or an elevated S_{cr}, and the finding of bilateral small kidneys on renal ultrasonography suggests the presence of CKD. A thorough medical history and a review of past medical records, if available, that includes recent procedures and illnesses, should be done as soon as possible. The medication and recent procedure history may suggest causes for acute interstitial nephritis or other nephrotoxic effects. An exhaustive review of their recent prescription, as well as nonprescription, complementary, and alternative medications, should be completed. Special attention should be focused on diuretics, NSAIDs, antihypertensives, recent contrast dye exposure and any other recent additions or changes in the patient's medications. Patients may have noticed an acute change in their voiding habits with an increase in urinary frequency or nocturia, both suggesting a urinary concentrating defect. A decrease in the force of the urinary stream may suggest an obstruction. The presence of cola-colored urine also often stimulates people to seek medical care and its presence is indicative of blood in the urine, a finding commonly associated with acute glomerulonephritis. The onset of flank pain is suggestive of a urinary stone; however, if bilateral, it may suggest swelling of the kidneys secondary to acute glomerulonephritis or acute interstitial nephritis. Complaints of severe headaches may suggest the presence of severe hypertension as a result of ARF. A recent increase in the patient's weight or complaints of tight-fitting rings secondary to salt and water retention also may be helpful in defining the time of onset of renal failure.

Patients who develop renal insufficiency while hospitalized usually have an acute initiating event that can be identified from a review of the laboratory data, urine output record, and the medication administration and procedure records. In addition to its prognostic significance, changes in urine output may be helpful in characterizing the cause of the patient's ARF. Acute anuria is typically caused by either complete urinary obstruction or a catastrophic event (e.g., shock or acute cortical necrosis). Oliguria (<500 mL/day of urine output), which often develops over several days, suggests prerenal azotemia, whereas nonoliguric (>500 mL/day of urine output) renal failure usually results from acute intrinsic renal failure or incomplete urinary obstruction.

CLINICAL PRESENTATION OF ACUTE RENAL FAILURE

General

- Community-dwelling patients often are not in acute distress.
- Hospitalized patients may develop ARF after either a notable reduction in blood pressure or intravascular volume, significant insult to the kidney, or sudden obstruction after catheterization. Generally, an acute reduction in urine output coinciding with a rise in BUN and S_{cr} is observed.

Symptoms

- *Outpatient:* Change in urinary habits, sudden weight gain, or flank pain.
- *Inpatient:* Typically, ARF is recognized by clinicians before the patient, who may not experience any obvious symptoms.

Signs

- Patient may have edema; urine may be colored or foamy; orthostatic hypotension in volume-depleted patients, hypertension in the fluid-overloaded patient or in the presence of acute or chronic hypertensive kidney disease.

Laboratory Tests

- Elevations in the serum potassium, BUN, creatinine, and phosphorous, or a reduction in calcium and the pH (acidosis), may be present. The clinical findings are different based on the cause of the ARF.
- An increased serum white blood cell count may be present in those with sepsis-associated ARF, and eosinophilia suggests acute interstitial nephritis.
- Urine microscopy can reveal cells, casts, or crystals that help distinguish among the possible etiologies and/or severities of ARF.
- An elevated urine specific gravity suggests prerenal ARF, as the tubules are concentrating the urine. Urine chemistry also indicates the presence of protein, which suggests glomerular injury, and blood, which can result from damage to virtually any kidney structure.

Other Diagnostic Tests

- Renal ultrasonography or cystoscopy may be needed to rule out obstruction; renal biopsy is rarely used, and is reserved for difficult diagnoses.

A physical examination, including assessment of the patient's volume and hemodynamic status, is an important step in evaluating individuals with ARF. Table 45–3 lists common physical findings in patients with ARF. The physical exam should be thorough, as clues regarding the etiology of the patient's ARF can be evident from the patient's head (eye exam) to toe (evidence of dependent edema).

TABLE 45-3 Physical Examination Findings in Acute Renal Failure

Physical Examination Finding	Possible Diagnosis	Category of Acute Renal Failure
Vital signs		
Orthostatic hypotension	Volume depletion	Prerenal
Febrile	Sepsis	Intrinsic–tubule necrosis
Skin		
Tenting	Volume depletion	Prerenal
Rash	Hypersensitivity reaction	Intrinsic–interstitial nephritis
Petechiae	Thrombotic thrombocytopenic purpura	Intrinsic–vasculitis
	Hemolytic uremic syndrome	
	Sepsis	Intrinsic–tubule necrosis
Splinter hemorrhages	Endocarditis	Intrinsic–glomerulonephritis
Janeway lesions		
Osler nodes		
Edema	Total-body volume overload	Intrinsic or prerenal because of heart failure Other types of prerenal unlikely
HEENT		
Hollenhorst plaque	Cholesterol emboli	Intrinsic–vascular
Roth spots	Endocarditis	Intrinsic–glomerulonephritis
Elevated jugular venous pressure	Heart failure Pulmonary hypertension	Prerenal
Heart		
S_3 heart sound	Heart failure	Prerenal
New or increased murmur	Endocarditis	Intrinsic–glomerulonephritis
Lung		
Rales	Heart failure	Prerenal
Abdomen		
Renal artery bruit	Renal artery stenosis	Prerenal
Ascites	Liver failure or right-heart failure	Prerenal Hepatorenal syndrome
Bladder distension	Bladder outlet obstruction	Postrenal
Genitourinary		
Prostatic enlargement	Prostatic hypertrophy or cancer	Postrenal
Gynecologic		
Abnormal bimanual examination	Possible bilateral ureteral obstruction or cervical cancer	Postrenal

HEENT, head, eyes, ears, nose, and throat.

Observations will either support or refute the cause as prerenal, intrinsic or postrenal. In those with prerenal ARF, low effective arterial blood volume may be evidenced by the presence of postural hypotension and decreased jugular venous pressure (JVP). Fluid overload as a consequence of ATN on the other hand is often reflected by rales in the lower lung fields and/or the presence of peripheral edema. If ascites or pulmonary edema is present, the effective arterial blood volume perceived by the kidneys may be low and thus suggest the diagnosis of functional ARF.

When the interstitium of the kidney is damaged (e.g., acute allergic interstitial nephritis), the concentrating gradient within the kidney may be attenuated and ammonia handling disrupted, resulting in a very dilute-appearing urine. Consequently, patients presenting with acute interstitial nephritis frequently are unable to concentrate the urinary solutes. Blood pressure should be evaluated for elevations that may accompany intrinsic renal damage. Any recent history of an infection may suggest postinfective glomerulonephritis. Although uncommon, thromboembolism occurring in the renal artery or vein can potentially result in ischemic damage, and should be a component of the physical assessment. Physical examination may detect possible postrenal obstruction, such as the presence of a urinary catheter, an enlarged prostate in males or cervical/uterine abnormalities in females. Renal artery stenosis can be identified via Doppler ultrasound by measuring changes in flow distal to the narrowing if visible, or by computed tomography (CT) angiography, which can describe the anatomy of the renal vessels.

TABLE 45-4 Diagnostic Parameters for Differentiating Causes of Acute Renal Failure

Laboratory Test	Prerenal Azotemia	Acute Intrinsic Renal Failure	Postrenal Obstruction
Urine sediment	Normal	Casts, cellular debris	Cellular debris
Urinary RBC	None	2–4+	Variable
Urinary WBC	None	2–4+	1+
Urine sodium	<20	>40	>40
FE_{Na} (%)	<1	>2	Variable
Urine/serum osmolality	>1.5	<1.3	<1.5
Urine/S_{cr}	>40:1	<20:1	<20:1
BUN/S_{cr}	>20	~15	~15

ARF, acute renal failure; BUN, blood urea nitrogen; FE_{Na}, fractional excretion of sodium; S_{cr}, serum creatinine; RBC, red blood cell; WBC, white blood cell.

Common laboratory tests are used to classify the cause of ARF. Functional ARF, which is not included in this table, would have laboratory values similar to those seen in prerenal azotemia. However, the urine osmolality-to-plasma osmolality ratios may not exceed 1.5, depending on the circulating levels of antidiuretic hormone. The laboratory results listed under acute intrinsic renal failure are those seen in acute tubular necrosis, the most common cause of acute intrinsic renal failure.

LABORATORY TESTS AND INTERPRETATION

The commonly available laboratory tests used to evaluate the patient with renal insufficiency are described in Chap. 44, and those of particular value in the assessment of renal function in patients with ARF are highlighted in Table 45–4. There is currently no consensus on the degree and time frame of changes in S_{cr} values that clearly defines the presence of ARF. The difficulty of using S_{cr} as a diagnostic laboratory test for patients with ARF is its lack of sensitivity to rapid changes in GFR. An abrupt cessation in glomerular filtration will not yield an immediate measurable change in S_{cr}. The reasons for this are: creatinine generation and accumulation is relatively slow, there is a lag time between test and clinical event, lab tests may not be very sensitive to small changes in GFR, and fluid retention that commonly accompanies ARF dilutes the retained creatinine.[26] Additionally, when decreased filtration of creatinine occurs, functional tubules can increase the secretion of creatinine into the urine, further complicating the interpretation of S_{cr}.

An example of this phenomenon is illustrated by an acute renal artery thrombus that results in abrupt cessation of GFR in one kidney as a consequence of the complete obstruction of blood flow to that kidney (Fig. 45–3). Although 5 minutes following the event GFR is decreased 50% (assuming the other kidney is functioning and unaffected), the serum creatinine remains unchanged. Assuming a standard daily creatinine production of approximately 20 mg/kg of lean body weight, one can expect approximately 1.4 g of creatinine production in a 24-hour period in a 70-kg individual. In pharmacokinetic terms, daily creatinine production is analogous to a continuous infusion, and GFR determines the elimination rate of creatinine. In the patient with normal renal function (GFR of 120 mL/min), the half-life of creatinine is 3.5 hours with 95% of steady state achieved in approximately 14 hours. If GFR declines to 60, 30, or 12 mL/min, the half-life of creatinine increases, resulting in prolongation of the time to reach 95% of steady state, specifically taking 1, 2, and 4 days, respectively.[27]

Other biomarkers for acute renal injury and failure are being explored. One such marker, serum cystatin C (see Chap. 44) has been explored as a more sensitive and rapid means to detect renal dysfunction and injury.[28] Although an elevation in serum creatinine or

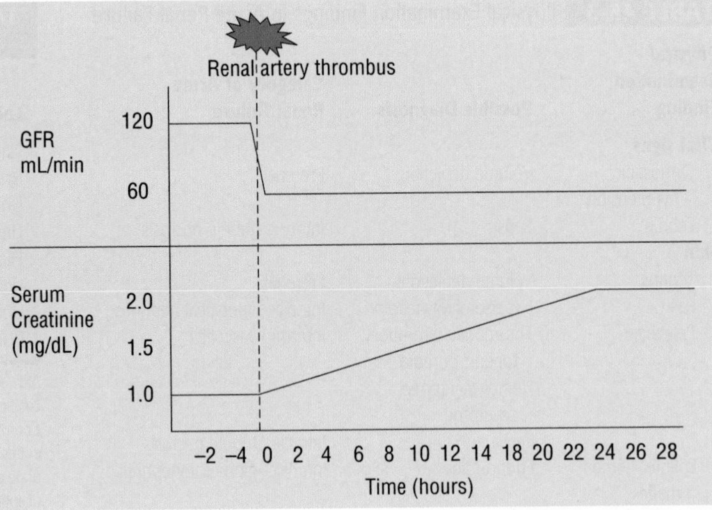

FIGURE 45-3. Glomerular filtration rate (GFR; mL/min) and serum creatinine (S_{cr}; g/dL) versus time following acute renal injury. Prior to time 0, a GFR of 120 mL/min and a S_{cr} of 1.0 g/dL exist. At time 0, an abrupt renal artery thrombus forms, depriving one kidney of renal blood flow. Composite GFR immediately declines by 50% to approximately 60 mL/min. However, S_{cr} does not increase immediately, as it is dependent on creatinine production and attainment of steady-state serum concentrations.

cystatin C may be clearly indicative of a reduction in renal function, these are not quantitative indices that allow one to ascertain the degree of remaining function the patient has. Although several methods, such as the Cockcroft-Gault or one of the Modification of Diet in Renal Disease equations (see Table 44–4), have been extensively used to estimate GFR in patients with CKD, they are not applicable for ARF patients with changing S_{cr} values because by the nature of the condition, renal function is unstable. In ARF, these equations can overestimate GFR when the ARF is worsening, and underestimate it when the ARF is resolving. To avoid missing changes in renal function when relying on equations to predict renal function, consider looking at the sequence of S_{cr} values to determine if renal function is potentially improving (values declining) or worsening (values rising). The most recent S_{cr} value reflects the time-averaged kidney function over the preceding time period. Assessment of urine output can assist in verifying observed serum laboratory values, as well as providing an up-to-the-moment means of identifying any changes in the kidney function. While dependent on several factors such as hydration status and medications, urine output measured over a finite period of time (e.g., 4 hours) is a useful short-term assessment of kidney function. An abrupt decline or increase compared to previous values is highly suggestive of a change in functional status. Because of the shortcomings associated with serum creatinine, urine output is an extremely useful parameter in the assessment of the patient with ARF. Anuria, defined as <50 mL/day of urine, suggests complete kidney failure. Conversely, oliguria (<17 mL/h urine output) certainly indicates kidney damage; however, some function is present. In the setting of ARF, any urine production >17 mL/h indicates the presence of nonoliguric ARF. Despite reasonable urine output, the quality of the urine being produced is not reliably composed of the expected waste products and solutes. Damaged tubules may allow substantial urine to be produced; however, the electrolyte, protein, and acid–base functions of the kidney may be severely compromised. For these reasons, urine output alone is an unreliable marker of kidney function.

Instead of using fixed numbers to determine renal function, changes in the value, even if it remains within the normal range, may indicate marked impairment of renal function. For example, patients with reduced creatinine production, such as those with low muscle mass either because of being bedridden for long periods of time or a concurrent emaciated state, may have very low baseline S_{cr} values (<0.6 mg/dL) and thus the presence of a gradual S_{cr} rise to normal values (0.8 to 1.2 mg/dL) may actually indicate reduced GFR. When coupled with a decline in urine output, this might suggest the presence of ARF. However, in the presence of improved nutrition and an expanding muscle mass, it may be a true representation of the person's current renal status. In contrast, a high S_{cr} value may be present if drawn prior to removal of a postrenal obstruction, such as a nonfunctional Foley catheter, with liters of urine now being voided over a relatively short period of time (hours). S_{cr} and BUN are extensively removed during acute hemodialysis treatments, so when assessing any change in these parameters in the ARF patient, one must pay close attention to when the lab specimens were collected relative to the dialysis procedure.

Several mathematical approaches to estimate GFR in patients with unstable S_{cr} that incorporate the principles of creatinine accumulation and elimination have been proposed[29–31] and are discussed in detail in Chap. 44. These methods have not been extensively validated in the setting of acute alterations in renal function and their value for adjusting medication dosing is questionable. Additionally, these equations are complex, rendering bedside implementation difficult and highly likely to be complicated by calculation errors.

Another approach to measuring renal function when S_{cr} values alone are not reflective of function is to directly measure urine Cl_{cr} over a short period of time, such as 4 to 12 hours.[32] Although potentially precise and fairly simple to do, accuracy is questionable because the urine output is generally low and if the collection is incomplete, the lost urine can have a dramatic impact on the clearance determination.

To facilitate its diagnosis and management, ARF can be classified into several broad categories based on precipitating factors (see Table 45–2). Traditionally this includes prerenal (resulting from decreased renal perfusion), acute intrinsic (resulting from structural damage to the kidney), and postrenal failure (obstruction of urine from removal). A fourth category, functional acute renal failure, is characterized by hemodynamic changes at the glomerulus independent of decreased perfusion or structural damage. Identifying the cause of ARF, which strongly influences potential outcomes and therapies, is of paramount importance.

Selected blood tests in addition to BUN and S_{cr} can be quite valuable in differentiating the cause of ARF and also contribute to optimal patient management. For example, infectious causes of ARF can be assessed using a complete blood cell count with differential. Serum electrolyte values are likely to be abnormal because of the acute decline of the kidney's ability to regulate electrolyte excretion, and particular attention should be paid to serum potassium and phosphorus values, which can be markedly elevated and cause life-threatening complications.

In individuals with normal renal function, the ratio between the BUN and S_{cr} is usually less than 15:1. In the presence of prerenal ARF, reabsorption of BUN exceeds that of creatinine and thus one often sees a ratio greater than 20:1. Given the limited usefulness of solely using S_{cr} or BUN concentrations to differentiate the etiology of ARF, urinary electrolytes and osmolality should be determined, and both a micro-

TABLE 45-5 Urine Analysis Findings as a Guide to the Etiology of Acute Renal Failure

Presence of	Suggestive of
Leukocyte esterase	Pyelonephritis
Nitrite	Pyelonephritis
Protein	
Mild	Tubular damage
Moderate	Glomerulonephritis, pyelonephritis, tubular damage
Large	Lupus nephritis
Hemoglobin	Glomerulonephritis, pyelonephritis, renal infarction, papillary necrosis, renal tumors, kidney stones, tubular necrosis from rhabdomyolysis
Specific gravity	
Low	Tubular necrosis
High	Prerenal
Myoglobin	Rhabdomyolysis-associated tubular necrosis
Urobilinogen	Hemolysis-associated tubular necrosis

TABLE 45-6 Differential Diagnosis of Acute Renal Failure on the Basis of Urine Microscopic Examination Findings

Urine Sediment	Suggestive of
Cells	
Microorganisms	Pyelonephritis
Red blood cells	Glomerulonephritis, pyelonephritis, renal infarction, papillary necrosis, renal tumors, kidney stones
White blood cells	Pyelonephritis, interstitial nephritis
Eosinophils	Drug-induced allergic interstitial nephritis, renal transplant rejection
Epithelial cells	Tubular necrosis
Casts	
Granular casts	Tubular necrosis
White blood cell casts	Pyelonephritis, interstitial nephritis
Red blood cell casts	Glomerulonephritis, renal infarct, lupus nephritis, vasculitis
Crystals	
Urate	Postrenal obstruction
Phosphate	Alkaline urine, possibly secondary to *Proteus* sp. infection, postrenal obstruction

scopic and chemical analysis of the urine should be performed (Table 45–5). The finding of a high urinary specific gravity, in the absence of glucosuria or mannitol administration, suggests an intact urinary concentrating mechanism, and that the cause of the patient's ARF is likely prerenal azotemia. The presence of urinary protein is often difficult to interpret, especially in the setting of acute on chronic renal failure. A patient with CKD may have a baseline proteinuria, thus clouding the clinical presentation, unless this is known at the time of ARF assessment. Classically, proteinuria is a hallmark of glomerular damage. However, tubular damage can also result in proteinuria, as the tubules are responsible for reabsorbing small proteins that are normally filtered by all glomeruli. The presence of blood also results in a positive urine protein test, so this confounder must always be assessed for when a positive urine protein is obtained. Hematuria suggests acute intrinsic ARF secondary to glomerular or injury to other kidney tissue. On microscopic examination, the key findings are cells, casts, and crystals, and the presence of one or more of these suggests specific etiologies of the ARF (Table 45–6). The presence of crystals may suggest nephrolithiasis and a postrenal obstruction. If red blood cells or red blood cell casts are present, one should consider the presence of a physical injury to the glomerulus, renal parenchyma or vascular beds. The finding of white blood cells or white blood cell casts suggests interstitial inflammation (i.e., interstitial nephritis), which can be secondary to an allergic, granulomatous, or infectious process.

Simultaneous measurement of urine and serum electrolytes is also helpful in the setting of ARF (see Table 45–4). From these values a fractional excretion of sodium can be calculated. The equation for the calculation of the fractional excretion of sodium (FeNa) is:

$$\text{FeNa} = (\text{excreted Na/filtered Na}) \cdot 100 = (U_{vol} \cdot U_{Na})/(\text{GFR} \cdot S_{Na}) \cdot 100$$

where

$$\text{GFR} = (U_{vol} \cdot U_{cr})/(S_{cr} \cdot t)$$

Thus

$$\text{FeNa} = (U_{Na} \cdot S_{cr} \cdot 100)/(U_{cr} \cdot S_{Na})$$

where U_{vol} is urine volume; U_{cr} is urine creatinine concentration; U_{Na} is urine sodium; S_{cr} is serum creatinine concentration; S_{Na} is serum sodium concentration, which usually does not vary much; GFR is the glomerular filtration rate; and t is the time period over which the urine is collected.

The fractional excretion of sodium is one of the better diagnostic parameters to differentiate the cause of ARF. A low urinary sodium concentration (<20 mEq/L) and low fractional excretion of sodium (<1%) in a patient with oliguria suggest that there is stimulation of the sodium-retentive mechanisms in the kidney and that tubular function is intact. These findings are most characteristic of prerenal azotemia. Unfortunately, diuretic use in the preceding days limits the usefulness of the fractional excretion of sodium calculation by increasing natriuresis, even in hypovolemic patients. The fractional excretion of urea (FeUrea), which can be calculated similarly to the FeNa, is sometimes used as an alternative means to assess tubule function.

The inability to concentrate urine results in a high fractional excretion of sodium (>2%), suggesting tubular damage is the primary cause of the intrinsic ARF. Diagnosing the type of ARF using fractional excretion of sodium is not absolute, as there are some intrinsic causes that can be associated with a low fractional excretion of sodium (e.g., contrast nephropathy, myoglobinuria, and interstitial nephritis). Highly concentrated urine (>500 mOsm/L) suggests stimulation of antidiuretic hormone and intact tubular function. These findings are consistent with prerenal azotemia.

DIAGNOSTIC PROCEDURES

When the source of renal failure is unclear after a history, physical examination, and assessment of laboratory values, then imaging techniques such as abdominal radiography (kidneys, ureters, and bladder), CT, or ultrasonography may be helpful. These may reveal small, shrunken kidneys indicative of CKD, and postrenal obstruction can often be identified with a renal ultrasonogram and/or CT scan. Renal ultrasonography is a useful means to detect obstruction or hydronephrosis. Nephrolithiases as small as 5 nm, or narrowing of the ureteral tract can be detected by ultrasonography. No contrast dye is required, and it is noninvasive, simple, portable, and rapid to accomplish. In selected conditions under the guidance of a nephrologist, more invasive procedures, such as cystoscopy or biopsy, may be considered to detect the presence of malignancy, prostate hypertrophy, uterine fibroids, nephrolithiases or ureterolithiases.

If insertion of a urinary catheter into the patient's bladder after the patient has voided or attempted to void does not yield a large volume of urine (>500 mL), then one can usually exclude postrenal obstruction distal to the bladder as the cause of ARF. Cystoscopy with retrograde pyelography may be helpful if the possibility of obstruction exists, and the insertion of a catheter did not result in a significant volume of urine.

In cases in which the cause of ARF is not evident, renal biopsies are useful in determining the cause in the majority of patients.[33] Because of the associated risk of bleeding, a renal biopsy is rarely undertaken and should only be performed in those rare circumstances when a definitive diagnosis is needed to guide therapy, such as the precise etiology of glomerulonephritis (see Chap. 50).

PREVENTION AND TREATMENT

Acute Renal Failure

■ DESIRED OUTCOME

❺ Given the dismal outcome of established ARF, prevention is critical. In some cases, the risk of developing ARF may be predictable, such as decreased perfusion secondary to abdominal surgery, coronary bypass surgery, acute blood loss in trauma, and uric acid nephropathy, where preventative strategies can be effective. When patients with risk factors for developing ARF are scheduled for surgery, the clinician should be aware that the likelihood of the patient developing ARF is high and consider preventative measures, including discontinuation of medications that may enhance the likelihood of renal damage (e.g., NSAIDs, angiotensin-converting enzyme inhibitors). Consequently the goals are (a) to prevent ARF, (b) avoid or minimize further renal insults that would worsen the existing injury or delay recovery, and (c) provide supportive measures until kidney function returns.

■ GENERAL APPROACH TO PREVENTION

The general approach to the prevention of ARF is dependent on the setting the patient is in. To prevent the development of ARF, healthcare professionals should educate the patient on preventative measures. The patient should receive guidance regarding their optimal daily fluid intake (approximately 2 L/day) to avoid dehydration, and if they are to receive any treatment that can pose a risk for insult to the kidney (e.g., chemotherapy or uric acid nephropathy). The patient's fluid balance can be evaluated by measuring acute changes in weight, as other typical sources for weight changes in an adult occur over more prolonged periods, and blood pressure changes. If the patient has a history of nephrolithiasis, they may benefit from dietary restrictions, depending on the type of stones that were present in the past. If a patient has a Foley catheter in place, proper care and monitoring needs to be performed to ensure that postobstructive ARF does not develop. Selected strategies to prevent drug-related ARF are discussed briefly below and in detail in Chap. 49.

■ NONPHARMACOLOGIC THERAPIES

There are many situations in which administration of a nephrotoxin cannot be avoided, such as when radiocontrast dye is to be administered. In these settings, one of several nonpharmacologic therapies can be employed in an attempt to prevent the development of ARF. Adequate hydration and sodium loading prior to radiocontrast dye administration have been shown to be beneficial therapies. A trial comparing infusions of 0.9% NaCl or 5% dextrose with 0.45% NaCl administered prior to radiocontrast dye infusion conclusively demonstrated that normal saline was superior in preventing ARF.[34] The intravenous solution infusion rate used in this study was 1 mL/kg per hour beginning the morning that the radiocontrast dye was going to be given, and all subjects were encouraged to drink fluids liberally as well. The benefits of 0.9% NaCl infusions have been found in similar studies,[35] suggesting this regimen should be used in all at-risk patients who can tolerate the sodium and fluid load. In addition to the correction of dehydration, saline administration may result in dilution of contrast media, prevention of renal vasoconstriction leading to ischemia, and avoidance of tubular obstruction. The results of one recent study suggest that hydration with sodium bicarbonate provides more protection than saline, perhaps by reducing the formation of pH-dependent oxygen free radicals.[36]

In some cases, when nephrotoxic agent use cannot be avoided, there may be ways to administer them in a manner that reduces their nephrotoxic potential. A good example of this is the use of amphotericin B to treat fungal infections. Amphotericin is a highly nephrotoxic agent, causing ARF in approcimately 30% of patients who receive it.[37] However, there are many infections for which no good alternative treatment exists. The nephrotoxic potential of amphotericin B deoxycholate can be reduced significantly simply by slowing the infusion rate from a standard 4-hour infusion to a slower 24-hour infusion of the same dose.[38] In a patient with risk factors for the development of ARF, liposomal forms of amphotericin B can be used. These liposomal formulations are more expensive, but have been associated with a lower incidence of kidney damage.[39]

Preventive Dialysis

A novel approach to reducing the incidence of nephrotoxicity associated with radiocontrast dye administration is to provide RRT prophylactically to patients who are at high risk of ARF. Hemofiltration initiated prior to and continued for 24 hours after dye administration has resulted in a significant reduction in mortality and a reduced need for dialysis.[40] In contrast, the use of hemodialysis within 1 hour of contrast dye infusion did not yield an improvement in nephrotoxicity rates, possibly because the toxicity caused by dye occurs within minutes of its administration.[41] Overall, evidence to date does not support any consistent significant benefit with the routine use of extracorporeal blood purification to prevent radiocontrast dye–induced nephropathy over standard medical therapy.[42]

■ PHARMACOLOGIC THERAPIES

Dopamine and Diuretics

Given the dismal outcome of established ARF, many drugs have been investigated for its prevention. Almost all of these approaches have been shown to be of little to no value. Low doses of dopamine (≤2 mcg/kg/min) increase renal blood flow and might be expected to increase GFR. Theoretically, this could be considered beneficial, as an enhanced GFR might flush nephrotoxins from the tubules, minimizing their toxicity. Furthermore, loop diuretics may decrease tubular oxygen consumption by reducing solute reabsorption.[43] Despite these theoretical suggestions, controlled studies have not supported these theories. Dopamine (2 mcg/kg/min) worsened renal perfusion indices compared to saline in a crossover study in patients with ARF.[44] A blinded and randomized trial conducted in patients who were undergoing cardiac surgery compared dopamine at 2 mcg/kg/min, furosemide at 0.5 mcg/kg/min, and a 0.9% NaCl given at initiation of surgery to determine whether any of the these interventions is beneficial.[45] Postoperative increases in S_{cr} occurred significantly more often in the furosemide-treated patients than in the other two groups. Dopamine afforded no benefit compared to the 0.9% NaCl infusion, and thus also should not be used routinely in this manner.

CLINICAL CONTROVERSIES

Despite most studies not showing improved patient outcomes with its use, low-dose dopamine continues to be commonly used. The risks associated with dopamine use (extravasation and the potential for significant dosing errors) suggest that its use should be avoided whenever possible.

Giving low-dose dopamine infusions (≤2 mcg/kg/min) for the prevention of ARF is a surprisingly common practice given the paucity of data to support its use. Although most studies do report an increase in urine output when low-dose dopamine is administered, almost none report that this practice yields a benefit to the patient. A meta-analysis of all low-dose dopamine studies conducted from 1966 to 2000 concluded that low-dose dopamine does not prevent ARF and its use cannot be justified.[46]

The use of diuretics to prevent nephrotoxicity may actually result in intravascular volume depletion and thereby increase the risk of ARF. A trial of forced diuresis, in which mannitol, furosemide, and/or dopamine were given, and the resultant urinary losses were replaced with intravenous solutions, found that diuretic use resulted in little benefit compared to the administration of IV solutions alone.[47] Interestingly, these investigators noted that patients who were unable to increase their urine output after diuretic administration were more likely to develop ARF than were patients who did respond to diuretics. While this unresponsiveness to diuretics might simply be an indication of preexisting kidney damage, similar reports have linked diuretic unresponsiveness to increased mortality rates in critically ill patients with ARF.[48]

Fenoldopam

Fenoldopam mesylate is a selective dopamine A-1 receptor agonist that increases blood flow to the renal cortex that has been investigated for its ability to prevent the development of ARF in many settings including contrast dye induced nephropathy (CIN). Originally approved for use as an intravenous antihypertensive agent, several small studies suggested that fenoldopam had salutary properties for the prevention of drug-induced nephrotoxicity. The largest, multicenter, randomized, placebo-controlled trial of fenoldopam conducted to date in patients with CKD found that fenoldopam use did not reduce the risk of CIN.[49] Indeed, the CIN Consensus Working Panel stated that, fenoldopam along with dopamine, calcium channel blockers, atrial natriuretic peptide, and 1-arginine, were not effective preventative therapeies to reduce the incidence of CIN.[50] However, a recent systematic review of randomized controlled trials of critically ill patients or those undergoing major surgery, revealed that fenoldopam significantly reduced the risk of acute kidney injury and the need for renal replacement therapy. This analysis suggests that fenoldopam may be a viable entity to prevent the development of ARF in some clinical settings.[51] A prospective, appropriately powered trial will need to be performed to validate this observation.

Acetylcysteine

N-acetylcysteine is a thiol-containing antioxidant that may effectively reduce the risk of developing CIN in patients with pre-existing kidney disease, although a therapeutic benefit has not been consistently demonstrated.[52,53] The mechanism for *N*-acetylcysteine's ability to reduce the incidence of contrast dye induced nephrotoxicity is not clear, but likely is due to its antioxidant effects. Given the consistent findings of its efficacy and its relatively low cost, *N*-acetylcysteine should be given to all patients at risk for CIN.[52,54–57] The recommended *N*-acetylcysteine dosing regimen for prevention of CIN is 600 mg orally every 12 hours for 4 doses with the first dose administered prior to contrast exposure. Several other drugs have been investigated for the prevention of ARF with varying degrees of success.[42,52,53]

Theophylline may reduce the incidence of CIN with an efficacy that is perhaps comparable to that reported in studies of *N*-acetylcysteine. However, findings are inconsistent across studies.[58] A large, well-designed trial that incorporates the evaluation of clinically relevant outcomes is required to more adequately assess the role of theophylline in CIN prevention.

Glycemic Control

Perhaps the most promising agent for the prevention of hospital-acquired ARF is a very old drug, but its use in the prevention of ARF is new. Van den Berghe et al. randomized patients in a surgical intensive care unit to receive either standard control (<200 mg/dL) or intensive glucose control measures (goal blood glucose concentrations of 80 to 110 mg/dL).[59] Tight blood glucose resulted in significant improvements in mortality and a 41% reduction in the development of ARF. While it appears that blood glucose control was the key factor associated with the mortality benefit, the reduction in ARF may have been a consequence of the total dose of insulin used to treat the patient, suggesting a direct protective effect of insulin.[60] Strict glycemic control is recognized as an important goal for outpatient diabetics[61]; however, intensive insulin therapy may now also become the standard of care for all critically ill patients to prevent ARF and improve mortality.

MANAGEMENT

Established Acute Renal Failure

■ DESIRED OUTCOMES

Short-term goals include minimizing the degree of insult to the kidney, reducing extrarenal complications, and expediting the patient's recovery of renal function. The ultimate goal is to have the patient's renal function restored to their pre-ARF baseline.

■ GENERAL APPROACH TO TREATMENT

Prerenal sources of ARF should be managed with hemodynamic support and volume replacement. If the cause is immune related, as may be the case with interstitial nephritis or glomerulonephritis, appropriate immunosuppressive therapy must be promptly initiated. Postrenal therapy focuses on removing the cause of the obstruction. It is important to approach the treatment of established ARF with an understanding of the patient's comorbidities and baseline renal function. Loss of kidney function combined with other clinical conditions, such as cardiac and liver failure, are associated with higher mortality than that associated with the development of ARF alone.[62] At times, the most efficacious remedy for ARF is management of the comorbid precipitating event. Appreciation of the baseline renal function is also important at the outset of ARF management, because the presence of CKD indicates the highest degree of renal function that can be attained after ARF resolution. Finally, the presence of CKD indicates that the kidneys have less reserve, and thus there is a greater likelihood that the individual may not fully recover from the current insult.

❻ Once acute renal failure is established, the cause is known, and any specific therapy implemented, supportive care is the mainstay of ARF management regardless of etiology. RRT may be necessary to maintain fluid and electrolyte balance while removing accumulating waste products. The slow process of renal recovery cannot begin until there are no further insults to the kidney. In the case of ATN, the recovery process typically occurs within 10 to 14 days after resolution of the last insult. The recovery period will be prolonged if the kidney is exposed to repeated insults.

■ NONPHARMACOLOGIC

Initial modalities to reverse or minimize prerenal ARF include removal of medications associated with diminished renal blood flow or the physical removal of a prerenal obstruction. If dehydration is evident, then appropriate fluid replacement therapy, as described below, should be initiated. Moderately volume-depleted patients can be given oral rehydration fluids; however, if intravenous fluid is required, isotonic normal saline is the replacement fluid of choice, and large volumes may be necessary to provide adequate fluid resuscitation. Typically, IV fluid challenges are initiated with 250 to 500 mL of normal saline over 15 to 30 minutes with an assessment after each challenge of the patient's volume status. Unless profound dehydration is present, as may be seen in diabetic ketoacidosis or hyperosmolar hyperglycemic states, 1 to 2 L is usually adequate. Patients with diabetic ketoacidosis or a hyperosmolar hyperglycemic state often have a 10% to 15% total-body water deficit, and more aggressive fluid replacement is necessary. The patient should be monitored for pulmonary edema, peripheral edema, adequate blood pressure (diastolic blood pressure >60 mm Hg), normoglycemia and electrolyte balance. Urine output may not be promptly observed, as the kidney continues to retain sodium and water until rehydration is achieved. Up to 10 L may be required in the septic patient during the first 24 hours, because of the profound increase in vascular capacitance and fluid leakage into the extravascular, interstitial space.[63]

Patients with ARF on top of preexisting CKD should not be expected to produce urine beyond their preexisting baseline. In patients with anuria or oliguria, slower rehydration, such as 250-mL boluses or 100 mL/h infusions of normal saline, should be considered to reduce the risk for pulmonary edema, especially if heart failure or pulmonary insufficiency exists. Other replacement fluids may be considered if the dehydration is accompanied by a severe electrolyte imbalance amenable to large and relatively rapid infusions. For example, dehydration resulting from severe diarrhea is often accompanied by metabolic acidosis caused by bicarbonate losses. A reasonable IV rehydration fluid in this situation is 5% dextrose with 0.45% NaCl plus 50 mEq of sodium bicarbonate per liter, administered as boluses as described above, followed by a brisk continuous infusion (200 mL/h) until rehydration is complete, acidosis corrected, and diarrhea resolved. This fluid will remain mostly in the intravascular space, providing the necessary perfusion pressure to the kidneys, and also provide a substantial amount of bicarbonate to correct the acidosis.

If the prerenal ARF is a result of blood loss, or complicated by symptomatic anemia, red blood cell transfusion to a hematocrit no higher than 30% is the treatment of choice.[64] Although albumin is sometimes used as a resuscitative agent, its use should be limited to individuals with severe hypoalbuminemia (e.g., liver disease, nephritic syndrome) who are resistant to crystalloid therapy. These patients have severe hypoalbuminemia-associated third spacing that complicates fluid management, and albumin may be useful in this setting.

The most common interventions that must be made when treating patients with intrinsic or postobstructive ARF involve fluid and electrolyte management. Most patients with these types of ARF, as well as those with a prerenal cause who are excessively fluid resuscitated ultimately become fluid overloaded. This means drug infusions and nutrition solutions must be maximally concentrated. So-called keep vein open or maintenance intravenous infusions should be minimized unless the patient is euvolemic or is receiving RRT to maintain fluid balance. Supportive care goals for the hospitalized patient with any type of ARF include maintenance of adequate cardiac output and blood pressure to allow adequate tissue perfusion. However, a fine balance must be maintained in anuric and oliguric patients unless the patient is hypovolemic or is able to achieve fluid balance via RRT. If fluid intake is not minimized, edema may rapidly develop, especially in hypoalbuminemic patients. In contrast, vasopressors, like dopamine at doses of ≥2 mcg/kg/min or norepinephrine when used to maintain adequate tissue perfusion, may also induce kidney hypoxia as the result of a reduction in renal blood flow. Consequently, Swan-Ganz monitoring may be necessary for critically ill patients (see Chap. 25).

❼ Because there is no current definitive therapy for ARF, supportive management remains the primary approach to prevent or reduce associated complications or death. In the presence of severe ARF, RRTs are commonly prescribed to manage uremia, metabolic acidosis, hyperkalemia and complications of excess fluid retention, such as pulmonary edema or accumulation of renally cleared medications. Although precise indications for starting RRT are unclear, some general guidelines for therapy have been proposed (Table 45–7).

Renal Replacement Therapies

RRTs can be administered either intermittently or continuously. The optimal mode for hemodialysis is unclear, and varies depending on the clinical presentation of the patient. It is unclear in many situations if dialysis can improve survival in ARF. Some recent data suggest that more aggressive approaches using RRTs in a more liberal fashion may improve survival in critically ill ARF patients.[65] The choice of whether continuous therapies or intermittent RRTs are used is a matter of debate and is usually determined by physician preference and the resources available at the hospital.

TABLE 45-7 The AEIOUs That Describe the Indications for Renal Replacement Therapy

Indication for Renal Replacement Therapy	Clinical Setting
A Acid–base abnormalities	Metabolic acidosis resulting from the accumulation of organic and inorganic acids
E Electrolyte imbalance	Hyperkalemia, hypermagnesemia
I Intoxications	Salicylates, lithium, methanol, ethylene glycol, theophylline, phenobarbital
O fluid Overload	Postoperative fluid gain
U Uremia	High catabolism of acute renal failure

Intermittent Hemodialysis

Intermittent hemodialysis (IHD) is the most frequently used RRT and has several advantages. IHD machines are readily available in most acute care facilities and healthcare workers are familiar with their use. Hemodialysis treatments usually last 3 to 4 hours with blood flow rates to the dialyzer typically ranging from 200 to 400 mL/min. Advantages of IHD include rapid removal of volume and solute, and rapid correction of most of the electrolyte abnormalities associated with ARF. IHD can be scheduled at times to maximize staffing availability and treatments per day per machine, while minimizing inconvenience to the patient. The primary disadvantage is hypotension, typically caused by rapid removal of intravascular volume over a short period of time. Venous access for dialysis can be difficult in hypotensive patients and can limit the effectiveness of IHD, leading to ineffective solute clearance, lack of acidosis correction, continued volume overload, and delayed recovery because of further renal ischemia insults. If hemodialysis is carefully monitored and hypotension avoided, better patient outcomes can be achieved.[66] Patients with stage 5 CKD generally achieve adequate solute and volume control with thrice-weekly dialysis, but hypercatabolic, fluid-overloaded patients with ARF may require daily hemodialysis treatments.[67] The use of daily versus thrice-weekly IHD in the setting of ARF patients is associated with a reduction in dialysis-related hypotension and a shorter period of time to full recovery of kidney function.[68] Chapter 48 provides a more detailed explanation of the principles and processes of hemodialysis.

Continuous Renal Replacement Therapies

In contrast to IHD, CRRTs that were developed over the past 15 years have proven to be a viable management approach for hemodynamically unstable patients with ARF.[69] Several CRRT variants have been developed, including continuous venovenous hemofiltration (CVVH), continuous venovenous hemodialysis (CVVHD), and continuous venovenous hemodiafiltration (CVVHDF). They differ in the degree of solute and fluid clearance that can be clinically achieved as a result of the use of diffusion, convection, or a combination of both. Although solute removal is slower, a greater amount can be removed over a 24-hour period compared to IHD, which is associated with improved outcomes in critically ill patients with ARF.[70]

In CVVH, solute and fluid clearance is primarily a result of convection where passive diffusion of fluids containing solutes is removed while volume absent of the solutes is replaced to the patient (Fig. 45–4). Continuous venovenous hemodialysis (CVVHD) provides extensive solute removal primarily by diffusion, where solute molecules at a higher concentration (plasma) pass through the dialysis membrane to a lower concentration (dialysate) and some fluid is removed as a

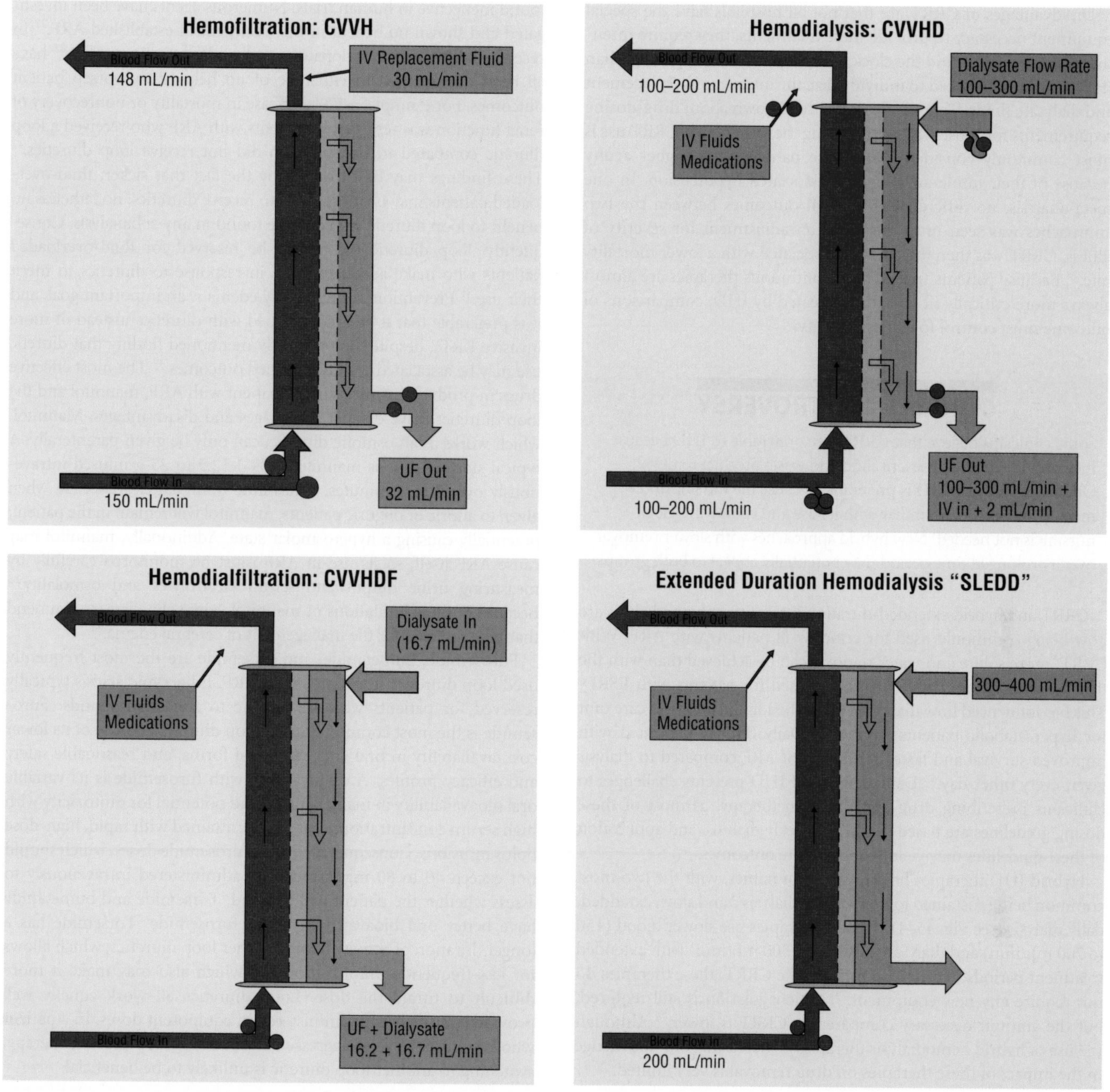

FIGURE 45-4. Several RRTs are commonly utilized in ARF patients including one of the three primary CRRT variants: (a) continuous veno-venous hemofiltration (CVVH), (b) continuous veno-venous hemodialysis (CVVHD), (c) continuous veno-venous hemodiafiltration (CVVHDF), and the hybrid intermittent hemodialysis therapy (d) slow extended daily dialysis (SLEDD). The blood circuit in each diagram is represented in red, while the hemofilter/dialyzer membrane is yellow and the ultrafiltration/dialysate compartment is depicted in brown. Excess body water and accumulated endogenous waste products are removed solely by convection when CVVH is employed. With CVVHD, waste products are predominantly removed as the result of passive diffusion from the blood where they are in high concentration to the dialysate. The degree of fluid removal which is accomplished by convection is usually minimal. CVVHDF utilizes convection to a degree similar to that employed during CVVH as well as diffusion, and thus is often associated with the highest clearance of drugs and waste products. Finally, SLEDD employs lower blood and dialysate flow rates that IHD, but due to its extended duration it is a gentler means of achieving adequate waste product and fluid removal.

function of the ultrafiltration coefficient of the dialyzer. Because the dialysate flows in a countercurrent direction to the plasma flow on the other side of the membrane, the concentration gradient is maximized. This procedure is associated with a lower incidence of clotting than CVVH because of reduced hemoconcentration as there is less fluid removal during the process. CVVHDF combines both hemofiltration and hemodialysis, achieving even higher solute and fluid removal rates (Fig. 45–4). The ultrafiltration rate is an important determinant of the effectiveness of all three forms of CRRT: achievement of a removal rate of 35 mL/kg/h is associated with improved survival.[70]

Because of the reduced blood flow rates relative to IHD, thrombosis is a significant concern with CRRT, and thus some form of anticoagulation is generally necessary for almost all patients. Typical anticoagulation is achieved by the administration of unfractionated heparin, or in some cases, a low-molecular-weight heparin, a direct thrombin inhibitor, or citrate solution.[71] Replacement fluids can be infused either just before or after the dialyzer/hemofilter. Infusing fluids after the hemofilter can result in hemoconcentration within the filter, a factor associated with an increased risk of thrombosis of the dialyzer. Replacing fluids before the filter reduces thrombosis risk, but also reduces solute clearance.

Disadvantages of CRRT are that not all hospitals have the special equipment necessary to provide these treatments, they require intensive nursing care around the clock, and they are more expensive than IHD because of the need to individualize the intravenous replacement and dialysate fluids. There is also very little known about drug-dosing requirements for those who are receiving these therapies. CRRT use is most commonly considered for those patients with higher acuity because of their intolerance of IHD-associated hypotension. In one meta-analysis, no difference in clinical outcomes between the two approaches was seen until there was an adjustment for severity of illness. CRRT was then found to be associated with a lower mortality rate.[72] Because patients treated with continuous therapies are almost always more critically ill than those treated by IHD, comparisons of outcome must control for illness severity.

CLINICAL CONTROVERSY

Some clinicians believe that CRRTs are preferable to IHD because they provide more consistent fluid and waste product removal. Others suggest that IHD is preferable because the nursing and medical staff is more familiar with its use and round-the-clock nursing is not needed. New hybrid approaches with slower removal over a prolonged time period may potentially appeal to both groups.

CRRT and hybrid extended-duration intermittent hemodialysis are now being commonly used for critically ill patients with ARF. With CRRT, more solute and water removal can be achieved than with the thrice-weekly hemodialysis treatments used for patients with ESRD. This has influenced how dialysis is prescribed in the intensive care unit for hypercatabolic patients with ARF. Daily IHD is associated with improved survival and faster resolution of ARF compared to dialysis given every other day.[62] Daily delivery of IHD presents challenges to clinicians prescribing drug and nutrition therapy, as most of these dosing guidelines are based on thrice-weekly dialysis, and application of these guidelines may yield inappropriate outcomes.

Hybrid IHD therapies have a variety of names, with the two most common being sustained low-efficiency dialysis[73] and slow, extended, daily dialysis (see Fig. 45–4).[74] These therapies use slower blood (150 to 200 mL/min) and dialysate flow rates (300 mL/min) with extended treatment periods of 6 to 12 hours. Unlike CRRT, these therapies do not require any new equipment.[74] Anticoagulation is still required, but the amount necessary compared to CRRT is lower.[74] Although the use of hybrid hemodialysis therapies is increasing, our knowledge of the impact of these therapies on drug removal is very limited.[75,76]

■ PHARMACOLOGIC

Once the kidney has been damaged by an acute insult (e.g., reduced perfusion or exposure to exogenous or endogenous nephrotoxins), initial therapies should be directed to prevent further insults to the kidney, thereby minimizing extension of the injury.[20] If sepsis is present, antibiotic therapy regimens should be adjusted for decreased renal elimination, the potential for increased elimination if the agent is removed by hemodialysis, and the ability to treat the infection to prevent further damage to the kidney. The time to recovery from ARF is determined from the most recent insult to the kidney, not the first insult. Hospitalized patients with ARF are at high risk for repeated episodes of kidney injury as the result of repeated exposures to nephrotoxic agents and hypotensive episodes, among other problems. These increased risks, coupled with the fact that no drugs have been found to accelerate ARF recovery, dictate the way clinicians approach the ARF patient.

To date, no pharmacologic approach to reverse the decline or accelerate the recovery of renal function has been proven to be clinically useful. Many agents have looked promising in animal trials, only to be found ineffective in human trials. Numerous agents have been investigated and shown no benefit in the treatment of established ARF.[77] In recent years thyroxine,[78] dopamine,[79,80] and loop diuretics[47,81,82] have all been documented to either be of no help or to worsen patient outcomes. For example, a 77% increase in mortality or nonrecovery of renal function was reported in patients with ARF who received a loop diuretic compared to patients who did not receive loop diuretics.[47] These findings may be explained by the fact that sicker, fluid-overloaded patients may be more likely to receive diuretics, nonetheless no benefit to loop diuretic use could be found in any subanalysis. Consequently, loop diuretic use should be reserved for fluid-overloaded patients who make adequate urine in response to diuretics to merit their use.[81] Prevention of pulmonary edema is an important goal, and it is preferable that it be accomplished with diuretics instead of more invasive RRTs, despite the previously mentioned finding that diuretic use may be associated with diminished outcomes.[47] The most effective drugs in producing diuresis in the patient with ARF, mannitol and the loop diuretics, have distinct advantages and disadvantages. Mannitol, which works as an osmotic diuretic, can only be given parenterally. A typical starting dose is mannitol (20%) 12.5 to 25 g infused intravenously over 3 to 5 minutes. It has little nonrenal clearance, so when given to anuric or oliguric patients, mannitol will remain in the patient, potentially causing a hyperosmolar state. Additionally, mannitol may cause ARF itself, so its use in ARF must be monitored carefully by measuring urine output and serum electrolytes and osmolality.[83] Because of these limitations of mannitol, some clinicians recommend that it be reserved for the management of cerebral edema.[84]

Furosemide, bumetanide, and torsemide are the most frequently used loop diuretics in patients with ARF. Ethacrynic acid is typically reserved for patients who are allergic to sulfa compounds. Furosemide is the most commonly used loop diuretic because of its lower cost, availability in oral and parenteral forms, and reasonable safety and efficacy profiles. A disadvantage with furosemide is its variable oral bioavailability in many patients and potential for ototoxicity with high serum concentrations that may be attained with rapid, high-dose bolus infusions. Consequently, initial furosemide doses, which should not exceed 40 to 80 mg, are usually administered intravenously to assess whether the patient will respond. Torsemide and bumetanide have better oral bioavailability than furosemide. Torsemide has a longer duration of activity than the other loop diuretics, which allows for less-frequent administration but which also may make it more difficult to titrate the dose. Loop diuretics all work equally well provided that they are administered in equipotent doses. In a patient who is unresponsive to aggressive intravenous loop diuretic therapy, switching to another loop diuretic is unlikely to be beneficial.

Diuretic Resistance

8 Inability to respond to administered diuretics is common in ARF and is associated with a poor patient outcome (Table 45–8).[47] An effective technique to overcome diuretic resistance is to administer loop diuretics via continuous infusions instead of intermittent boluses. Less natriuresis occurs when equal doses of loop diuretics are given as a bolus instead of as a continuous infusion. Furthermore, adverse reactions from loop diuretics (myalgia and hearing loss) occur less frequently in patients receiving continuous infusion compared to those receiving intermittent boluses, ostensibly because higher serum concentrations are avoided. However, these adverse effects still may occur with continuous infusion of loop diuretics and should be monitored.[85] The finding that the continuous infusions of loop diuretics have efficacy that is at least as good as intermittent bolus dosing, with fewer adverse effects, appears to be consistent for all agents, including furosemide,[86] bumetanide,[87] and torsemide.[88] When a continuous loop diuretic infusion is used, an initial loading dose is given (equivalent to furosemide 40 to 80 mg) prior to the initiation of a continuous infusion at 10 to 20 mg/h of furosemide or its equivalent. Patients with low

TABLE 45-8 Common Causes of Diuretic Resistance in Patients with Acute Renal Failure

Causes of Diuretic Resistance	Potential Therapeutic Solutions
Excessive sodium intake (sources may be dietary, IV fluids, and drugs)	Remove sodium from nutritional sources and medications
Inadequate diuretic dose or inappropriate regimen	Increase dose, use continuous infusion or combination therapy
Reduced oral bioavailability (usually furosemide)	Use parenteral therapy; switch to oral torsemide or bumetanide
Nephrotic syndrome (loop diuretic protein binding in tubule lumen)	Increase dose, switch diuretics, use combination therapy
Reduced renal blood flow	
Drugs (NSAIDs ACEIs, vasodilators)	Discontinue these drugs if possible
Hypotension	Intravascular volume expansion and/or vasopressors
Intravascular depletion	Intravascular volume expansion
Increased sodium resorption	
Nephron adaptation to chronic diuretic therapy	Combination diuretic therapy, sodium restriction
NSAID use	Discontinue NSAID
Heart failure	Treat the heart failure, increase diuretic dose, switch to better-absorbed loop diuretic
Cirrhosis	High-volume paracentesis
Acute tubular necrosis	Higher dose of diuretic, diuretic combination therapy, add low-dose dopamine

ACEIs, angiotensin-converting enzyme inhibitors; NSAIDs, nonsteroidal antiinflammatory drugs.

creatinine clearances may have much lower rates of diuretic secretion into the tubular fluid; consequently, higher doses are generally used in patients with renal insufficiency.[84] Diuretic resistance may occur simply because excessive sodium intake overrides the ability of the diuretics to eliminate sodium. However, other reasons for diuretic resistance often exist in this population. Patients with ATN have a reduced number of functioning nephrons on which the diuretic may exert its action. Other clinical states, like glomerulonephritis, are associated with heavy proteinuria. Intraluminal loop diuretics cannot exert their effect in the loop of Henle because they are extensively bound to proteins present in the urine. Still other patients may have greatly reduced bioavailability of oral furosemide because of intestinal edema, often associated with high preload states, which further reduces oral furosemide absorption. Table 45–8 includes possible therapeutic options to counteract each form of diuretic resistance. Combination therapy of loop diuretics plus a diuretic from a different pharmacologic class may be an alternative approach in the setting of ARF.[89] Loop diuretics increase the delivery of sodium chloride to the distal convoluted tubule and collecting duct. With time, these areas of the nephron compensate for the activity of the loop diuretic and increase sodium and chloride resorption. Diuretics that work at the distal convoluted tubule (chlorothiazide and metolazone) or the collecting duct (amiloride, triamterene, and spironolactone) may have a synergistic effect when administered with loop diuretics by blocking the compensatory increase in sodium and chloride resorption. The combination of loop diuretics and usual doses of thiazide diuretics may be effective in renal disease despite the accumulation of endogenous organic acids in renal disease that blocks the transport of loop diuretics into the lumen. If oral thiazides cannot be given to the patient, chlorothiazide 500 mg can be administered parenterally.

Several drug combinations with loop diuretics have been investigated, including the addition of one or more of the following: theophylline, acetazolamide, spironolactone, thiazides, or metolazone.[83] Of these combinations, oral metolazone is used most frequently with furosemide. Metolazone, unlike other thiazides, produces effective diuresis at a GFR below 20 mL/min. This combination of metolazone and a loop diuretic has been used successfully in the management of fluid overload in patients with heart failure, cirrhosis, and nephrotic syndrome. Despite a lack of supporting evidence, oral metolazone at a dose of 5 mg is commonly administered 30 minutes prior to an intravenous loop diuretic to allow time for absorption. Additionally, this combination has been found to be efficacious in pediatric patients in addition to adults.[90] The combination of mannitol plus intravenous loop diuretics is used by some practitioners,[51] but no convincing evidence of the superiority of this combination regimen to conventional dosing of either diuretic alone exists.

■ ELECTROLYTE MANAGEMENT

Hypernatremia and fluid retention are frequent complications of ARF, and thus sodium restriction is a necessary intervention. In general, patients should receive no more than 3 g of sodium per day from all sources, including intravenous fluids, drugs, and enteral intake. Clinicians should be vigilant about sources of sodium. Excessive sodium intake is a common reason diuretic therapy fails. Commonly administered intravenous antibiotics, as well as other medications, may contain significant amounts of sodium; for example, 1 L of 0.9% NaCl yields 154 mEq (3.5 g) of sodium. At usual doses, intravenous metronidazole provides 1.3 g of sodium per day, ampicillin up to 800 mg, piperacillin approximately 700 mg, and fluconazole 500 mg. The cumulative effect of a few sodium-containing medications and fluids can be significant.

In continuous and intermittent RRTs there usually is less concern about hyponatremia developing because these therapies often incorporate isonatremic (135 to 140 mEq/L of sodium) solutions as the dialysate or ultrafiltrate replacement solutions. Serum sodium concentrations should be monitored daily. Hyperkalemia, hyperphosphatemia, and, to a lesser extent, hypermagnesemia are electrolyte disorders that are frequently seen in patients with ARF. This is generally not a serious concern in those who are receiving RRT, but electrolytes should be monitored closely in all patients with ARF.

The most common electrolyte disorder encountered in ARF patients is hyperkalemia, as more than 90% of potassium is renally eliminated. Life-threatening cardiac arrhythmias may occur when the serum potassium is over 6 mmol/L, so potassium restriction is essential. All patients with ARF should have serum potassium monitored at least daily, and twice daily for those who are seriously ill. This frequency is a consequence of the seriousness of the potential arrhythmias, the dynamic nature of potassium serum concentrations in the acutely ill patient, the potential for metabolic acidosis leading to increased extracellular potassium concentrations, and potassium's ubiquitous presence in foods and some medications. Commonly encountered medications that contain substantial amounts of potassium include oral phosphorous replacement powders (e.g., Neutra-Phos and Neutra-Phos-K) and alkalinizers (Polycitra). Many foods are high in potassium, including potatoes, beans, and various fruits. Some medications may promote potassium retention by the kidneys, and should also be avoided or closely monitored (see Chap. 54). Typically no potassium should be added to parenteral solutions unless hypokalemia is documented. Patients receiving enteral nutrition should be limited to a 3-g potassium diet. Patients receiving RRT should also have their serum potassium concentration measured at least daily. Some centers add no potassium to their CRRT solutions and hypokalemia can result unless one is prospectively monitoring for its development. Chapter 54 discusses the treatment of hyperkalemia in detail.

Other electrolytes that require monitoring include phosphorous and magnesium. Both are eliminated by the kidneys and are not removed efficiently by dialysis. In the early stages of ARF, hyperphosphatemia might be more common than hypophosphatemia. Patients who have significant tissue destruction (e.g., trauma, rhabdomyolysis, tumor lysis syndrome) may have significant phosphorus released from the destroyed tissue. Treatment of the hyperphosphatemic state can include CRRT. Calcium-containing antacids should be avoided to prevent precipitation of calcium phosphate in the soft tissues. Typically, the dietary intake of phosphorous and magnesium is restricted, but in patients receiving prolonged renal replacement, deficiency states can occur, particularly in pediatric patients because of their reduced body stores. In contrast to the patient with CKD, calcium balance is usually not an important issue for the ARF patient because of the limited duration of the illness. One exception to this is in patients who are receiving CRRT with citrate as the anticoagulant. Citrate binds to serum calcium and without an adequate concentration of calcium, blood cannot form a clot. Citrate is thus typically infused before the dialyzer/hemofilter to maintain the dialyzer circuit calcium levels between 0.35 and 0.50 mmol/L. Calcium chloride (10 g of CaCl diluted in 500 mL normal saline), or gluconate (20 g of calcium gluconate to 500 mL normal saline) is then administered prior to returning the blood to the patient to maintain systemic ionized calcium levels between 1.11 to 1.31 mmol/L.[92] The citrate that reaches the systemic circulation is subsequently metabolized by the liver. Severe hypocalcemia can result in arrhythmias, and even death, so frequent monitoring of unbound serum calcium concentrations is essential.

■ NUTRITIONAL INTERVENTIONS

Baseline nutritional status is a strong predictor of outcomes in patients with ARF.[93] The provision of enteral nutrition to patients with ARF in intensive care units is associated with an improvement in outcomes.[94] Parenteral nutrition, however, has not demonstrated the same benefit and some have questioned whether it should be used in this population.[95] (see Chapter 147 for a detailed discussion.)

Because fluid intake often must be restricted in severely volume-overloaded ARF patients, the design and provision of adequate parenteral or enteral nutrition are problematic (see Chap. 147). Septic patients with ARF usually are hypercatabolic and normalized protein catabolic rates of up to 1.75 g/kg/day have been reported, but this value varies widely among patients.[96] Most patients with ARF have difficulty tolerating the amount of intravenous fluid required to replace catabolized protein unless they are receiving CRRT or daily hemodialysis.

Although patients with ARF typically experience elevated levels of potassium, magnesium, and phosphorus, which often necessitate restriction of these from nutrition formulas, it is not uncommon for deficiency states to occur in patients receiving CRRT, despite incorporation of these electrolytes into the replacement fluid solutions. The effect of CRRT on the delivery and removal of macro- and micronutrients must also be taken into account. The dextrose contained in CRRT replacement solutions may contribute a significant amount of calories to the patient's regimen. The removal of protein during dialysis, especially during peritoneal dialysis, may necessitate an increase of the protein intake up to 2.5 g/kg/day in some patients (see Chap. 147).

Another nutritional consideration for patients receiving CRRT is the heat losses as a consequence of the cooling of the patient's blood as it traverses the extracorporeal circuit and as a result of the use of room-temperature intravenous ultrafiltrate replacement solutions.[97] The energy loss for patients who are receiving continuous hemofiltration is estimated to be as high as 800 kcal/day.[98] Most of this heat loss can be attenuated by warming the intravenous ultrafiltrate replacement solution.[98] However, many hospitals are unable to heat intravenous solutions as they are infused, so recognition of this large source of energy loss is necessary so that the clinician can design an adequate nutritional prescription.

■ DRUG-DOSING CONSIDERATIONS

❾ Optimization of drug therapy for patients with ARF is often quite challenging. The multiple variables influencing responses to the drug regimen include the patient's residual drug clearance, the accumulation of fluids, which can markedly alter a drug's volume of distribution, and delivery of CRRT or IHD, which can increase drug clearance and impact the patient's fluid status to further complicate the clinician's projection of the optimal dosage regime. For renally eliminated drugs (>30% excreted unchanged in the urine), particularly for agents with a narrow therapeutic range, serum drug concentration measurements and assessment of pharmacodynamic responses are likely to be necessary. If hepatic function is intact, choosing an agent eliminated primarily by the liver may be preferred. However, any renally eliminated active metabolites may accumulate to a point where they can elicit an undesired pharmacologic effect. Renal failure can also independently impair drug metabolism.[99] Clinical experiences and pharmacokinetic studies in patients with established ARF are fairly limited. The use of dosing guidelines based on data derived from patients with stable CKD, however, may not reflect the clearance and volume of distribution in critically ill ARF patients (see Chap. 51).[100]

Edema, which is common in ARF, can significantly increase the volume of distribution of many drugs, particularly water-soluble ones with relatively small volumes of distribution. Increased fluid distribution into the tissues (i.e., sepsis, anasarca in heart failure) can also contribute to a larger volume of distribution for many drugs and thereby reduce the proportion of drug in the plasma that is available to be removed by CRRT or IHD. ARF frequently occurs in critically ill patients and thus multisystem organ failure must often be contended with. Reductions in cardiac output or liver function in addition to volume overload can significantly alter the pharmacokinetic profile of many drugs such as vancomycin, aminoglycosides, and low-molecular-weight heparins.[101,102]

In almost all cases where rapid onset of activity is desired, a loading dose may be necessary to promptly achieve desired serum concentrations because the expanded volume of distribution and the prolonged elimination half-life result in an extended time (3.5 times the half-life) until steady-state concentrations are achieved. Maintenance dosing regimens should be reassessed frequently and be based on the patient's current renal function. A dose that provides the desired serum concentration on one day may be inappropriate only a few days later if the patient's fluid status or renal function has changed dramatically.

CLINICAL CONTROVERSY

In the volume-depleted patient requiring a renally eliminated medication, dosing regimens based on the initial S_{cr} prior to fluid therapy have the potential to underestimate renal function and drug elimination, resulting in subtherapeutic serum concentrations. Although not accepted as a standard practice, an initial 24-hour dosing regimen with a bolus might be optimal for many patients.

Drug therapy individualization for the ARF patient who is receiving any form of renal replacement therapy is complicated by the fact that patients with ARF may have a higher residual nonrenal clearance than CKD patients who have a similar CL_{cr}. This has been reported with some drugs, such as ceftriaxone, imipenem, and vancomycin.[103–106] Alterations in the activity of some, but not all, cytochrome P450 enzymes have been demonstrated in patients with CKD.[99] The nonrenal clearance of imipenem in patients with ARF (91 mL/min) is between the values observed in stage 5 CKD patients (50 mL/min) and those with normal renal function (130 mL/min).[106] This may be the result of less accumulation of uremic waste products that may alter hepatic function. A nonrenal clearance value in a patient with ARF that is higher than anticipated based on data from individuals with CKD would result in lower-than-expected, possibly subtherapeutic, serum concentrations. For example, to maintain comparable serum concentrations, the imipenem dose requirement in patients with ARF would be 2,000 mg/24 hours as compared to the recommended dosage for patients with ESRD of 1,000 mg/24 hours.[106] As ARF persists, the nonrenal clearance values appear to approach those observed in patients with CKD.[107,108] Finally, the clearance of aminoglycosides has been reported to be higher and the elimination half-life shorter in those with severe ARF compared to ESRD patients requiring hemodialysis.[100] Thus, application of dosing regimens derived from studies in patients with CKD and ESRD may result in underdosing of these agents and thereby contribute to less than optimal clinical outcomes.

IHD Compared to CRRT

In addition to patient-specific differences, there are marked differences between IHD and the three primary types of CRRT—CVVH, CVVHD, and CVVHDF—with regard to drug removal.[109–111]

CRRT During CVVH, drug removal primarily occurs via convection/ultrafiltration (the passive transport of drug molecules at the concentration at which they exist in plasma water into the ultrafiltrate). Convective removal is most efficient for smaller agents, typically less than 15,000 daltons in size, and those that are primarily unbound in the plasma. The clearance of a drug by either of these methods is thus a function of the membrane permeability for the drug, which is called the sieving coefficient (SC) and the rate of ultrafiltrate formation (UFR). Alteration in the pore size of the filter and surface charge relative to the molecule being removed may vary between different dialyzers. If diffusion of the drug is not dependent on the filter pore size, then the SC can be calculated as follows:

$$SC = (2 \times C_{UF})/[(C_a) + (C_v)]$$

where C_a and C_v are the concentrations of the drug in the plasma going into and returning from the dialyzer/hemofilter, respectively, and C_{UF} is the concentration in the ultrafiltrate. The SC is often approximated by the fraction unbound (f_u) because this information may be more readily available. Thus the clearance by CVVH can be calculated as:

$$Cl_{CVVH} = UFR \times SC$$

or approximated as:

$$Cl_{CVVH} = UFR \times f_u$$

In CVVHDF, clearance is a combination of both diffusion and convection. The Cl_{CVVHDF} can be mathematically approximated providing the blood flow rate is greater than 100 mL/min and the dialysate flow rate (DFR) is between 8 and 33 mL/min as:

$$Cl_{CVVHDF} = (UFR \times f_u) + Cl_{diffusion}$$

where $Cl_{diffusion}$ is the clearance via diffusion from plasma water to the dialysate. In the clinical setting, it is not possible to separate these two components (UFR and DFR) of Cl_{CVVHDF}. In essence the Cl_{CVVHDF} is calculated as the product of the combined ultrafiltrate and dialysate volume (V_{df}) and the concentration of the drug in this fluid (C_{df}) divided by the plasma concentration (C_p^{mid}) at the midpoint of the V_{df} collection period.

⑩ Individualization of therapy for a patient receiving CRRT therapy is dependent on the patient's residual renal function and the clearance of the drug by the mode of CRRT the patient is receiving. There are differences in the rate of drug removal, not only between the three primary modes of CRRT, but also within each mode.[105,109–112] This is a result of differences in the filter membrane composition, variable degrees of drug binding to the membrane, and the permeability characteristics of the membrane.[113–116] The primary factors that influence drug clearance during CRRT are thus ultrafiltration rate, blood flow rate, and dialysate flow rate. For example, clearance in CVVH is directly proportional to the ultrafiltration rate, whereas clearance during CVVHDF, which depends on both the ultrafiltration rate and the dialysate flow rate, increases as either flow rate increases. An increase in ultrafiltration flow rate (5 to 45 mL/min) and dialysate flow rate (8.3 to 33.3 mL/min), however, can have dramatic effects on clearance of

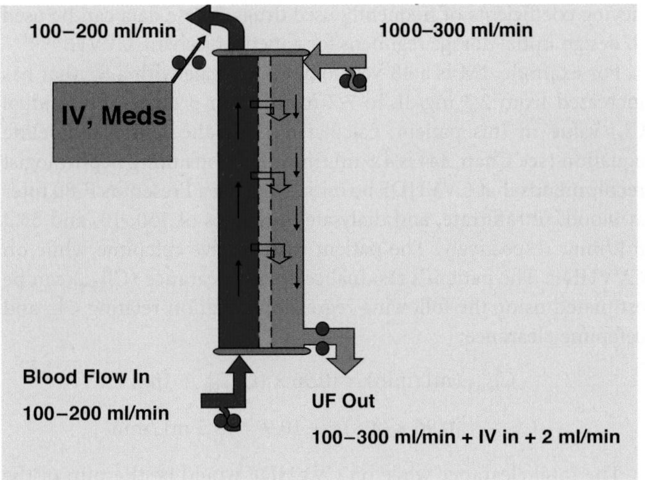

FIGURE 45-5. The effect of increasing ultrafiltration rate (UFR in milliliters per minute) and dialysate flow rate (DFR in milliliters per minute) on the clearance of ceftazidime. *(Adapted from reference 116.)*

agents such as ceftazidime during CVVH and CVVHD, respectively (Fig. 45–5).[116]

Another readily apparent factor that changes drug dosing is the type of RRT used in the patient. CRRT can rapidly remove excess fluid from edematous patients, thereby changing the volume of distribution (V_D) of drugs with limited distribution (low V_D suggesting a greater proportion in the plasma or extracellular fluid) fairly rapidly. Drug clearances attained by IHD, CRRTs, and hybrid RRTs all differ from each other and must be added to any endogenous drug clearance that the patient generates.[105] An algorithmic approach for drug dosage adjustment in patients undergoing CRRT has been proposed.[110] In CRRT, the clearance of a given agent may be ascertained from published reports.[110,117,118] Table 45–9 summarizes the

TABLE 45-9 Predicted and Measured Sieving Coefficients of Selected Drugs

Drug	Predicted	Measured
Amikacin	0.95	0.88
Amphotericin	0.01	0.32–0.4
Ampicillin	0.80	0.6–0.69
Cefepime	0.97	0.47-0.97
Cefoperazone	0.10	0.27–0.69
Cefotaxime	0.62	0.55–1.1
Cefoxitin	0.30	0.32
Ceftazidime	0.90	0.38–0.78
Ceftriaxone	0.10	0.71–0.82
Clindamycin	0.25	0.49–0.98
Digoxin	0.75	0.96
Erythromycin	0.25	0.37
5-Fluorocytosine	0.96	0.98
Gentamicin	0.95	0.81–0.75
Imipenem	0.80	0.78
Metronidazole	0.80	0.80
Mezlocillin	0.68	0.68
N-acetylprocainamide	0.80	0.92
Nafcillin	0.20	0.47
Netilmicin	–	0.85
Oxacillin	0.05	0.02
Phenobarbital	0.60	0.86
Phenytoin	0.10	0.45
Procainamide	0.80	0.86
Theophylline	0.47	0.85
Tobramycin	0.95	0.78–0.86
Vancomycin	0.90	0.5–0.8

Adapted from references 109–112, 117 and 118.

sieving coefficients of frequently used drugs. These data can be used to design initial dosage regimens for patients receiving CVVH.[109,112]

For example, IM is a 48-year-old, 60-kg male with a S_{cr} that has increased from 2.3 mg/dL to 7.2 mg/dL over 3 days. The residual Cl_{cr} value in this patient, calculated using the Jeliffe and Jeliffe equation (see Chap. 44) is 4.8 mL/min. The consulting nephrologist recommends that CVVHDF be initiated using a Fresenius F-80 filter at blood, ultrafiltrate, and dialysate flow rates of 150, 15, and 33.3 mL/min, respectively. The patient is to receive cefepime while on CVVHDF. The patient's residual cefepime clearance (Cl_{RES}) can be estimated using the following regression equation relating Cl_{cr} and cefepime clearance:

$$Cl_{RES}\ (\text{mL/min}) = [0.96 \times (Cl_{cr})]\ + 10.9$$

$$Cl_{RES} = [0.96 \times (4.8)]\ + 10.9 = 15.5\ \text{mL/min}$$

The total clearance while on CVVHDF would be the sum of the patient's residual clearance and the cefepime clearance associated with CVVHDF (which can be approximated as described above) as follows:

$$Cl_{CVVHDF} = [(UFR + DFR) \times f_u)]$$

$$Cl_{CVVHDF} = [(15 + 33) \times 0.97]$$

$$Cl_T = CL_{RES} + CL_{CVVHDF}$$

$$Cl_T = 15.5\ \text{mL/min} + 47\ \text{mL/min} = 62.1\ \text{mL/min}$$

This patient's clearance value can be used to adjust the cefepime dose as described below. The cefepime clearance in a patient with normal renal function would be calculated as:

$$Cl_{norm}\ (\text{mL/min}) = [0.96 \times (Cl_{cr})]\ + 10.9$$

$$Cl_{norm} = [0.96 \times 120]\ + 10.9$$

$$Cl_{norm} = 126.1$$

The dosage adjustment factor would then be:

$$Q = Cl_T/Cl_{norm}$$

$$Q = 62.1 \div 126 = 0.49$$

For this patient's situation, the normal regimen of cefepime would be 2,000 mg (D_n) every 12 hours (τ_n). If one wanted to maintain D_n and extend the dosing interval, then τ_f would be calculated as:

$$\tau_f = \tau_n/Q$$

$$\tau_f = 12\ \text{hours}/0.49$$

$$\tau_f \approx 24\ \text{hours}$$

This approach suggests the patient should receive cefepime 2,000 mg every 24 hours. If the additional clearance associated with CVVHDF (40.2 mL/min) was not considered, the calculated dosing interval would have been considerably longer. Several variables can impact the outcome of these calculations, including the multiple variables within the dialysis therapy—for example, UFR, blood flow rate, and DFR—and interpatient variability in nonrenal and renal drug clearance, to name just two.

Intermittent Hemodialysis Limitations of IHD-based dosing charts include variability in the patients' individual pharmacokinetic parameters, differences in the dialysis prescription, such as dialyzer blood flow or duration, and the use of new IHD dialyzers. The approach to hemodialysis may also change on a daily basis, especially in unstable individuals with ARF. This could include, for example, the dialyzer/filter used, the duration, the degree of hemofiltration compared to convection, and blood flow rate. Individualization of a dosing regimen may require daily assessment of the clinical status of the patient and any planned or recently administered hemodialysis.

CLINICAL CONTROVERSY

Some clinicians use a standard ESRD dosage regimen despite the fact that renal function can fluctuate such that the patient may be in one dosing range one day and in another the next. Others believe, however, that the patient's clinical need for the drug and any change in the volume of distribution or the RRT therapy should be considered if one has any chance of achieving the target serum concentrations.

Overall, there are a tremendously large number of potential pharmacokinetic and pharmacodynamic alterations to be aware of in the patient with ARF. Unfortunately, there is a dearth of data to quantify these changes, and even less evidence to prove that if one incorporates these considerations into patient care that the associated outcomes will be improved.

EVALUATION OF THERAPEUTIC OUTCOMES

Vigilant monitoring of patients with ARF is essential, particularly in those who are critically ill (Table 45–10). Once the laboratory-based tests (e.g., urinalysis, fractional excretion of sodium calculations) have been conducted to diagnose the cause of ARF, they usually do not have to be repeated. In established ARF, daily measurements of urine output, fluid intake, and weight should be performed. Vital signs should be monitored at least daily, more often if patient acuity of illness is high. Daily blood tests for electrolytes, BUN, and a complete blood cell count should be considered routine for hospitalized patients.

Therapeutic drug monitoring should be performed for drugs that have a narrow therapeutic window that can be measured by the hospital laboratory. If results from these serum drug concentrations cannot be obtained in a timely fashion (<24 hours) to the patient's care team, then their value is limited. When considering approaches to measuring serum concentrations, consensus is limited. Measuring a serum drug concentration prior to hemodialysis has the advantage of allowing time for the result to be reported and redosing done shortly

TABLE 45-10 Key Monitoring Parameters for Patients with Established Acute Renal Failure

Parameter	Frequency
Fluid ins/outs	Every shift
Patient weight	Daily
Hemodynamics (blood pressure, heart rate, mean arterial pressure, etc.)	Every shift
Blood chemistries	
Sodium, potassium, chloride, bicarbonate, calcium, phosphate, magnesium	Daily
Blood urea nitrogen/serum creatinine	Daily
Drugs and their dosing regimens	Daily
Nutritional regimen	Daily
Blood glucose	Daily (minimum)
Serum concentration data for drugs	After regimen changes and after renal replacement therapy has been instituted
Times of administered doses	Daily
Doses relative to administration of renal replacement therapy	Daily
Urinalysis	
Calculate measured creatinine clearance	Every time measured urine collection performed
Calculate fractional excretion of sodium	Every time measured urine collection performed
Plans for renal replacement	Daily

after dialysis with minimal delay. This is especially important if the desired pharmacologic effects are lost during or after hemodialysis is complete because the serum concentrations have become subtherapeutic. Knowledge based on previous observations of how a particular agent is removed for a given dialysis approach and any prehemodialysis serum concentration of the agent can assist in estimating the amount removed and predicting any necessary postdialysis dose. Serum concentrations drawn after hemodialysis may reflect plasma concentrations that are transiently depressed until the drug can reequilibrate from the tissues (plasma rebound effect). The advantage with an after-dialysis level is the greater accuracy in determining how much drug was cleared during hemodialysis, but may delay reestablishing target effects. Greater therapeutic drug monitoring may be necessary in patients with ARF than what is done routinely for other patients because of the potential changes in dynamic status (changing volume status, changing renal function, and RRTs) of ARF patients.

PHARMACOECONOMIC CONSIDERATIONS

ARF is a large financial burden on the healthcare system. Much of this cost is because many of these patients are in intensive care units where daily costs are high. It is estimated that the average total hospital cost of a patient with ARF who requires RRT is approximately $50,000.[119] Most patients who survive ARF regain life-sustaining renal function, but the 5% who do not regain renal function[14] continue to incur the economic and personal costs of dialysis or kidney transplantation. The financial burden is estimated to be $50,000 per year greater than the non–dialysis-dependent patient whose kidneys recovered from ARF. Nonetheless, patients who required RRT for their ARF generally have a good quality of life after recovery.[119]

Medical intervention costs can be normalized to assess total costs using quality-adjusted life-years (QALYs) gained by the intervention. The use of a QALY approach to treatment of critically ill patients with ARF indicates that treating these patients is very expensive relative to other common medical interventions.[120] For example, in 2001, the treatment of critically ill ARF patient cost per QALY was $168,711, compared to treatment of acute myocardial infarction cost per QALY of $45,000, and the routine treatment of hypertension cost per QALY of $31,321.[6] A typical cost per QALY of <$100,000 is considered cost-effective. Although nobody is suggesting that serious ARF not be treated, it is clear that research needs to be done to improve the ARF survival rate to reduce this cost per QALY. Furthermore, it underscores the need to prevent the occurrence of ARF in the first place.

CONCLUSIONS

The unique characteristics of ARF compared to CKD can lead to notable differences in how renal function is measured and how treatment regimens are developed. Most management approaches currently involve prevention and support of the patient once ARF is established, so as to minimize the potential for additional harm to either the patient or kidney. Understanding the constantly changing status inherent to ARF, and how to adjust management regimens is a key component to optimizing therapy.

ACKNOWLEDGMENT

We gratefully acknowledge Bruce Mueller, PharmD, FCCP, BCPS, for his contributions to the prior editions of this chapter.

ABBREVIATIONS

ARF: acute renal failure

ATN: acute tubular necrosis

BUN: blood urea nitrogen

CKD: chronic kidney disease

CL_{cr}: creatinine clearance

CRRT: continuous renal replacement therapy

CT: computed tomography

CVVH: continuous venovenous hemofiltration

CVVHD: continuous venovenous hemodialysis

CVVHDF: continuous venovenous hemodiafiltration

FE_{Na}: fractional excretion of sodium

GFR: glomerular filtration rate

IHD: intermittent hemodialysis

NSAID: nonsteroidal antiinflammatory drug

QALY: quality-adjusted life-year

RRT: renal replacement therapy

S_{cr}: serum creatinine

REFERENCES

1. Uchino S, Kellum JA, Bellomo R, et al. Acute renal failure in critically ill patients: A multinational, multicenter study. JAMA 2005;294:813–818.
2. Ympa YP, Sakr Y, Reinhart K, Vincent JL. Has mortality from acute renal failure decreased? A systematic review of the literature. Am J Med 2005;118:827–832.
3. National Kidney Foundation. K/DOQI clinical practice guidelines for chronic kidney disease: Evaluation, classification, and stratification. Am J Kidney Dis 2002;39:S1-S266.
4. Lameire N, Hoste E. Reflections in the definition, classification, and diagnostic evaluation of ARF. Curr Opin Crit Care 2004;10:468–475.
5. Kellum J, Levin N, Bouman C, Lameire N. Developing a consensus classification system for ARF. Curr Opin Crit Care 2002;8:509–514.
6. Pruchnicki MC, Dasta JF. Acute renal failure in hospitalized patients: Part I. Ann Pharmacother 2002;36:1261–1267.
7. Bellomo R. Defining, quantifying, and classifying acute renal failure. Crit Care Clin 2005;21:223–237.
8. Kellum J, Ronco C, Mehta R, Bellomo R. Consensus development in acute renal failure: The Acute Dialysis Quality Initiative. Curr Opin Crit Care 2005;11:527–532.
9. Hoste EA, Kellum JA. RIFLE criteria provide robust assessment of kidney dysfunction and correlate with hospital mortality. Crit Care Med 2006;34:2016–2017.
10. Uchino S, Bellomo R, Goldsmith D, et al. An assessment of the RIFLE criteria for acute renal failure in hospitalized patients Crit Care Med 2006;34:1913–1917.
11. Lameire N, Van Biesen WV, Vanholder R. The changing epidemiology of ARF. Nat Clin Prac Nephrol 2006;2:364–377.
12. Kalra PA, Kumwenda M, MacDowell P, Roland MO. Questionnaire study and audit of use of angiotensin converting enzyme inhibitors and monitoring in general practice: The need for guidelines to prevent renal failure. BMJ 1999;318:234–237.
13. Nash K, Hafeez A, Hou S. Hospital-acquired renal insufficiency. Am J Kidney Dis 2002;39:930–936.
14. Brady HR, Clarkson MR, Lieberthal W. Acute Renal Failure. In: Brenner B, ed. The Kidney, 7th ed. Philadelphia: WB Saunders, 2004:1215–1292.
15. Badr KF, Ichikawwa I. Prerenal failure: A deleterious shift from renal compensation to decompensation. N Engl J Med 1988;319:623–629.
16. Khati NJ, Hill MC, Kimmel PL. The role of ultrasound in renal insufficiency: The essentials. Ultrasound Q 2005;21:227–244.
17. Lameire N. The pathophysiology of acute renal failure Crit Care Clin 2005;21:197–210.
18. Tillyard A, Keays R, Soni N. The diagnosis of acute renal failure in intensive care: Mongrel or pedigree? Anaesthesia 2005;60:903–914.
19. Kelly KJ, Molitoris BA. ARF in the new millennium: Time to consider combination therapy. Semin Nephrol 2000;20:4–19.

20. Sutton TA, Fisher CJ, Molitoris BA. Microvascular endothelial injury and dysfunction during ischemic ARF. Kidney Int 2002;62:1539–1549.
21. Kelly CJ, Neilson EG. Tubulointerstitial Diseases. In: Brenner B, ed. The Kidney, 7th ed. Philadelphia: WB Saunders, 2004:1483–1511.
22. Laberke HG, Bohle A. Acute interstitial nephritis: Correlations between clinical and morphological findings. Clin Nephrol 1980;14:263–273.
23. Meyers CM. New insights into the pathogenesis of interstitial nephritis. Curr Opin Nephrol Hypertens 1999;8:287–292.
24. Olsen TS, Wassef NF, Olsen HS, Hansen HE. Ultrastructure of the kidney in acute interstitial nephritis Ultrastruct Pathol 1986;10:1–16.
25. Perazella MA. Crystal-induced ARF. Am J Med 1999;106:459–465.
26. Mehta RL, McDonald B, Gabbai F, et al. Nephrology consultation in ARF. does timing matter? Am J Med 2002;113:456–461.
27. Comstock TJ, Whitley KV. The kidneys. In: Lee M, ed. Basic Skills in Interpreting Laboratory Data, 3rd ed. Bethesda, MD: American Society of Health-System Pharmacists, 2004:233–262.
28. Westhuyzen J. Cystatin C. A promising marker and predictor of impaired renal function. Ann Clin Lab Sci 2006;36:387–394.
29. Brater DC. Drug Use in Renal Disease. Balgowlah, Australia: ADIS Health Science Press, 1983:22–56.
30. Chiou WL, Hsu FH. A new simple and rapid method to monitor the renal function based on pharmacokinetic consideration of endogenous creatinine. Res Commun Chem Pathol Pharmacol 1975;10:315–330.
31. Jelliffe RW, Jelliffe SM. A computer program for estimation of creatinine clearance from unstable concentration. Math Biosci 1972;14:17–24.
32. Baumann TJ, Staddon JE, Horst HM, Bivins BA. Minimum urine collection periods for accurate determination of creatinine clearance in critically ill patients. Clin Pharm 1987;6:393–398.
33. Haas M, Spargo BH, Wit EJC, Meehan SM. Etiologies and outcome of acute renal insufficiency in older adults: A renal biopsy study of 259 cases. Am J Kidney Dis 2000 2000;35:433–447.
34. Mueller C, Buerkle G, Buettner HJ. Prevention of contrast media-associated nephropathy. Arch Intern Med 2002;162:329–336.
35. Solomon R, Werner C, Mann D, et al. Effects of saline, mannitol, and furosemide to prevent acute decreases in renal function induced by radiocontrast agents. N Engl J Med 1994;331:1416–1420.
36. Merten GJ, Burgess WP, Gray LV, et al. Prevention of contrast-induced nephropathy with sodium bicarbonate: A randomized controlled trial. JAMA 2004;291:2328–2334.
37. Bates DW, Su L, Yu DT, et al. Mortality and costs of ARF associated with amphotericin B therapy. Clin Infect Dis 2001;32:686–693.
38. Eriksson U, Seifert B, Schaffner A. Comparison of effects of amphotericin B deoxycholate infused over 4 or 24 hours: Randomized controlled trial. BMJ 2001;322:1–6.
39. Walsh TJ, Finberg RW, Arndt C, et al. Liposomal amphotericin B for empirical therapy in patients with persistent fever and neutropenia. N Engl J Med 1999;340:764–771.
40. Marenzi G, Marana I, Lauri G, et al. The prevention of radiocontrast-agent-induced nephropathy by hemofiltration. N Engl J Med 2003;349:1333–1340.
41. Huber W, Jeschke B, Kreymann B, et al. Haemodialysis for the prevention of contrast-induced nephropathy. Invest Radiol 2002;37:471–481.
42. Cruz DN, Perazella MA, Bellomo R, et al. Extracorporeal blood purification therapies for prevention of radiocontrast-induced nephropathy: A systematic review. Am J Kidney Dis 2006;48:361–371.
43. Ronco C, Bellomo R. Prevention of ARF in the critically ill. Nephron Clin Pract 2003;93:c13-c20.
44. Lauschke A, Teichgraber UKM, Frei U, Eckardt KU. "Low-dose" dopamine worsens renal perfusion in patients with acute renal failure. Kidney Int 2006;69:1669–1674.
45. Lassnigg A, Donner E, Grubhofer G, et al. Lack of renoprotective effects of dopamine and furosemide during cardiac surgery. J Am Soc Nephrol 2000;11:97–104.
46. Kellum J, Decker J. Use of dopamine in ARF. A meta-analysis. Crit Care Med 2001;29:1526–1531.
47. Stevens MA, McCullough PA, Tobin KJ, et al. A prospective randomized trial of prevention measures in patients at high risk for contrast nephropathy. J Am Coll Cardiol 1999;33:403–411.
48. Mehta R, Pascual M, Soronko S, Chertow G. Diuretics, mortality, and nonrecovery in ARF. JAMA 2002;288:2547–2553.
49. Stone GW, McCollough PA, Tumlin JA, et al. Fenoldopam mesylate for the prevention of contrast-induced nephropathy. JAMA 2003;290:2284–2292.
50. Stacul F, Adams A, Becker CR, et al. Strategies to reduce the risk of contrast-induced nephropathy. Am J Cardiol 2006 Sep 18;98(6A):59K–77K.
51. Landoni G, Biondi-Zoccal GG, Tumlin JA, et al. Beneficial impact of fenoldopam in critically ill patients with or at risk for acute renal failure: A meta analysis of randomized trials. Am J Kidney Dis 2007 Jan;49(1):56–68.
52. Rudnick MR, Kesselheim A, Goldfard S. Contrast-induced nephropathy: How it develops, how to prevent it. Cleve Clin J Med 2006;73:75–77.
53. Marenzi G, Assanelli E, Marana I, et al. *N*-acetylcysteine and contrast-induced nephropathy in primary angioplasty. N Engl J Med 2006;354:2773–2782.
54. Maeder M, Klein M, Fehr T, Rickli H. Contrast nephropathy: Review focusing on prevention. J Am Coll Cardiol 2004;44:1763–1771.
55. Bagshaw SM, MacAlister FA, Manns BJ, Ghali WA. Acetylcysteine in the prevention of contrast-induced nephropathy: A case study of the pitfalls in the evolution of evidence. Arch Intern Med 2006;166:161–166.
56. Asif A, Epstein M. Prevention of radiocontrast-induced nephropathy. Am J Kideny Dis 2004;44:12–24.
57. Briguori C, Airoldi F, D'Andrea D, et al. Renal Insufficiency Following Contrast Media Administration Trial (REMEDIAL): A randomized comparison of 3 preventive strategies. Circulation 2007;115:1211–1217.
58. Bagshaw SM, Ghali WA. Theophylline for prevention of contrast-induced nephropathy: A systematic review and meta-analysis. Arch Intern Med. 2005;165(10):1087–1093.
59. Van den Berghe G, Wouters P, Weekers F, et al. Intensive insulin therapy in critically ill patients. N Engl J Med 2001;345:1359–1367.
60. Van den Berghe G, Wouters PJ, Bouillon R, et al. Outcome benefit of intensive insulin therapy in the critically ill: Insulin dose versus glycemic control. Crit Car Med 2003;31:359–366.
61. ASHP Commission on Therapeutics. ASHP therapeutic position statement on strict glycemic control in patients with diabetes. Am J Health Syst Pharm 2003;60:2357–2362.
62. McAlister FA, Ezekowitz J, Tonelli M, Armstrong PW. Renal insufficiency and heart failure: Prognostic and therapeutic implications from a prospective cohort study. Circulation 2004;109:1004–1009.
63. Ognibene FP. Hemodynamic support during sepsis. Clin Chest Med 1996;17:279–287.
64. Hébert PC, Wells G, Blajchman MA, et al. A multicenter, randomized, controlled clinical trial of transfusion requirements in critical care. N Engl J Med 1999;340:409–417.
65. Saudan P, Niederberger M, Seigneux SD, et al. Adding a dialysis dose to continuous hemofiltration increases survival in patients with acute renal failure. Kidney Int 2006;70:1312–1317.
66. Schortgen F, Soubrier N, Delclauz C, et al. Hemodynamic tolerance of intermittent hemodialysis in critically ill patients. Am J Respir Crit Care Med 2000;162:197–202.
67. Clark WR, Mueller BA, Kraus MA, Macias WL. Extracorporeal therapy requirements for patients with ARF. J Am Soc Nephrol 1997;8:804–812.
68. Schiffl H, Lang SM, Fischer R. Daily hemodialysis and the outcome of ARF. N Engl J Med 2002;346:305–310.
69. Ronco C, Bellomo R, Kellum JA. Continuous renal replacement therapy: Opinions and evidence. Adv Ren Replace Ther 2002;9:229–244.
70. Ronco C, Bellomo R, Homel P, et al. Effects of different doses in continuous veno-venous hemofiltration on outcomes of ARF. A prospective, randomized trial. Lancet 2000;356:26–30.
71. Oudemans-van Straaten HM, Wester JPJ, de Ponte ACJM, Schetz MRC. Anticoagulation strategies in continuous renal replacement therapy: Can the choice be evidence based? Intensive Care Med 2006;32:188–202.
72. Kellum JA, Angus DC, Johnson JP, et al. Continuous versus intermittent renal replacement therapy: A meta-analysis. Intensive Care Med 2002;28:29–37.
73. Marshall MR, Golper TA, Shaver MJ, et al. Urea kinetics during sustained low-efficiency dialysis in critically ill patients requiring renal replacement therapy. Am J Kidney Dis 2002;39:556–570.
74. Kumar VA, Craig M, Depner TA, Yeun JY. Extended daily dialysis: A new approach to renal replacement for ARF in the intensive care unit. Am J Kidney Dis 2000;36:294–300.
75. Dager WE. Filtering out important considerations for developing drug-dosing regimens in extended daily dialysis. Crit Care Med 2006;34:240–241.
76. Manley HJ, Bailie GR, McClaran ML, Bender WL. Gentamicin pharmacokinetics during slow daily home hemodialysis. Kidney Int 2003;63:1072–1078.

77. Pruchnicki MC, Dasta JF. Acute renal failure in hospitalized patients: Part II. Ann Pharmacother 2002;36:1430–1442.
78. Acker CG, Singh AR, Flick RP. A trial of thyroxine in ARF. Kidney Int 2000;57:293–298.
79. ANZICS Clinical Trials Group. Low-dose dopamine in patients with early renal dysfunction: A placebo-controlled randomised trial. Lancet 2000;356:2139–2143.
80. Schrier RW, Wang W. Acute renal failure and sepsis. N Engl J Med 2004;351:159–169.
81. Bagshaw SM, Delaney A, Haase M, et al. Loop diuretics in the management of acute renal failure: A systematic review and meta analysis. Crit Care Resusc 2007;9:60–68.
82. Davis A, Gooch I. The use of loop diuretics in renal failure in critically ill patients to reduce mortality, maintain renal function, or avoid requirements for renal support. Emerg Med 2006;23:569–570.
83. Better OS, Rubinstein I, Winaver JM, Knochel JP. Mannitol therapy revisited. Kidney Int 1997;51:886–894.
84. Brater DC. Diuretic therapy. N Engl J Med 1998;339:387–395.
85. Howard PA, Dunn MI. Severe musculoskeletal symptoms during continuous infusion of bumetanide. Chest 1997;111:359–364.
86. Schuller D, Lynch JP, Fine D. Protocol-guided diuretic management: Comparison of furosemide by continuous infusion and intermittent bolus. Crit Care Med 1997;25:1969–1975.
87. Rudy DW, Voelker JR, Greene PK, et al. Loop diuretics for chronic renal insufficiency: A continuous is more efficacious than bolus therapy. Ann Intern Med 1991;115:360–366.
88. Kramer WG, Smith WB, Ferguson J, et al. Pharmacodynamics of torsemide administered as an intravenous injection and as a continuous infusion to patients with congestive heart failure. J Clin Pharmacol 1996;36:265–270.
89. Ellison DH. Diuretic resistance: Physiology and therapeutics. Semin Nephrol 1999;19:581–597.
90. Segar JL, Chemtob S, Bell EF. Changes in body water compartments with diuretic therapy in infants with chronic lung disease. Early Hum Dev 1997;48:99–107.
91. Sirivella S, Gielchinsky I, Parsonnet V. Mannitol, furosemide, and dopamine infusion in postoperative renal failure complicating cardiac surgery. Ann Thorac Surg 2000;69:501–506.
92. Amanzadeh J, Reilly RF. Anticoagulation and continuous renal replacement therapy. Semin Dial 2006;19:311–316.
93. Fiaccadori E, Lombardi M, Leonardi S, et al. Prevalence and clinical outcome associated with preexisting malnutrition in ARF. A prospective cohort study. J Am Soc Nephrol 1999;10:581–591.
94. Metnitz PGH, Krenn CG, Steitzer H, et al. Effect of ARF requiring renal replacement therapy on outcome in critically ill patients. Crit Care Med 2002;30:2051–2058.
95. Koretz RL. Does nutritional intervention in protein-energy malnutrition improve morbidity or mortality? J Ren Nutr 1999;9:119–121.
96. Leblanc M, Garred LJ, Cardinal J, et al. Catabolism in critical illness: Estimation from urea nitrogen appearance and creatinine production during continuous renal replacement therapy. Am J Kidney Dis 1998;32:444–453.
97. Yagi N, Leblanc M, Sakai K, et al. Cooling effect of continuous renal replacement therapy in critically ill patients. Am J Kidney Dis 1998;32:1023–1030.
98. Manns M, Maurer E, Steinbach B, Evering HG. Thermal energy balance during in vitro continuous veno-venous hemofiltration. ASAIO J 1998;44:M601-M605.
99. Nolin TD, Frye RF, Matzke GR. Hepatic drug metabolism and transport in patients with kidney disease. Am J Kidney Dis 2003;42:906–925.
100. Dager W, King J. Aminoglycosides in intermittent hemodialysis: Pharmacokinetics with individual dosing. Ann Pharmacother 2006;40:9–14.
101. Haas CE, Nelsen JL, Raghavendran K, et al. Pharmacokinetics and pharmacodynamics of enoxaparin in multiple trauma patients. J Trauma 2005;59:1336–1344.
102. Kane-Gill SL, Feng Y, Bobek MB, et al. Administration of enoxaparin by continuous infusion in a naturalistic setting: Analysis of renal function and safety. J Clin Pharm Ther 2005;30:207–213.
103. Heinemeyer G, Link J, Weber W, et al. Clearance of ceftriaxone in critical care patients with ARF. Intensive Care Med 1990;16:448–453.
104. Macias WL, Mueller BA, Scarim SK. Vancomycin pharmacokinetics in ARF. Preservation of non-renal clearance. Clin Pharmacol Ther 1991;50:688–694.
105. Mueller BA, Pasko DA, Sowinski KM. Higher renal replacement therapy dose delivery influences on drug therapy. Artif Organs 2003;27:808–814.
106. Tegeder I, Bremer F, Oelkers R, et al. Pharmacokinetics of imipenem-cilastatin in critically ill patients undergoing continuous venovenous hemofiltration. Antimicrob Agents Chemother 1997;41:2640–2645.
107. Macias W, Mueller B, Scarim S, et al. Continuous venovenous hemofiltration: An alternative to continuous arteriovenous hemofiltration and hemodiafiltration in acute renal failure. Am J Kidney Dis 1991;18:451–458.
108. Mueller B, Scarim S, Macias W. Comparison of imipenem pharmacokinetics in patients with acute or chronic renal failure treated with continuous hemofiltration. Am J Kidney Dis 1993;21:172–179.
109. Bugge JF. Pharmacokinetics and drug dosing adjustments during continuous venovenous hemofiltration or hemodiafiltration in critically ill patients. Acta Anaesthesiol Scand 2001;45:929–934.
110. Joy MS, Matzke GR, Armstrong DK, et al. A primer on continuous renal replacement therapy for critically ill patients. Ann Pharmacother 1998;32:362–375.
111. Veltri MA, Neu AM, Fivush BA, et al. Drug dosing during intermittent hemodialysis and continuous renal replacement therapy: Special considerations in pediatric patients. Paediatr Drugs 2004;6:45–65.
112. Bohler J, Donauer J, Keller F. Pharmacokinetic principles during continuous renal replacement therapy: Drugs and dosage. Kidney Int Suppl 1999;72:S24-S28.
113. Joy MS, Matzke GR, Frye RF, Palevsky PM. Determinants of vancomycin clearance by CVVH and CVVHD. Am J Kidney Dis 1998;31:1019–1027.
114. Kronfol NO, Lau AH, Barakat MM. Aminoglycoside binding to polyacrylonitrile hemofilter membranes during continuous hemofiltration. ASAIO Trans 1987;33:300–303.
115. Lau AH, Kronfol NO. Determinants of drug removal by continuous hemofiltration. Int J Artif Organs 1994;17:373–378.
116. Matzke GR, Frye RF, Joy MS, Palevsky PM. Determinants of ceftazidime clearance by continuous venovenous hemofiltration and continuous venovenous hemodialysis. Antimicrob Agents Chemother 2000;44:1639–1644.
117. Bressolle F, Kinowski JM, de la Coussaye JE, et al. Clinical pharmacokinetics during continuous hemofiltration. Clin Pharmacokinet 1994;26:457–471.
118. Reetze-Bonorden P, Bohler J, Keller E. Drug dosage in patients during continuous renal replacement therapy. Clin Pharmacokinet 1993;24:362–379.
119. Korkeila M, Ruokonen E, Takala J. Costs of care, long-term prognosis and quality of life in patients requiring renal replacement therapy during intensive care. Intensive Care Med 2000;26:1824–1831.
120. Hamel MB, Phillips RS, Davis RB, et al. Outcomes and cost-effectiveness of initiating dialysis and continuing aggressive care in seriously ill hospitalized adults. Ann Intern Med 1997;127;195–202.

CHAPTER 46 Chronic Kidney Disease: Progression-Modifying Therapies

MELANIE S. JOY, ABHIJIT KSHIRSAGAR, AND NORA FRANCESCHINI

KEY CONCEPTS

1. The prevalence of chronic kidney disease (CKD) is estimated at nearly 19 million people in the United States.
2. Because the development of CKD is a complex phenomenon, the Kidney Disease Outcomes Quality Initiative (K/DOQI) has recommended categorizing risk factors associated with CKD as susceptibility, initiation, and progression factors.
3. Reduction of kidney mass, development of glomerular hypertension, and intratubular proteinuria are key mechanisms responsible for the progression of chronic kidney disease.
4. CKD is classified into five stages based on the presence of kidney structural damage (e.g., proteinuria) and/or kidney function (glomerular filtration rate), Stage1 is indicative of mild structural changes with "normal" kidney function while Stage 5 is analogous to end stage renal disease for which dialysis or kidney transplantation may be necessary.
5. Serum creatinine is not a reliable marker of kidney function among the elderly, the malnourished, and children. Therefore, it is important to estimate the glomerular filtration rate rather than just measuring the serum creatinine, especially in these three populations.
6. Stage 5 CKD manifests as asterixis, pruritus, dysgeusia, nausea, vomiting, anorexia, weight loss and susceptibility to bleeding. These signs and symptoms of uremia are foundational to the decision to implement kidney replacement therapy.
7. The progression of CKD can be limited by optimal control of hyperglycemia and hypertension.
8. Diabetic patients with or without hypertension who demonstrate persistent microalbuminuria despite intensive insulin therapy should have their ACEI or ARB dose titrated to achieve maximal suppression of urinary albumin excretion to halt or slow CKD progression.
9. Angiotensin-converting enzyme inhibitors (ACEIs) and angiotensin receptor blockers (ARBs) are key pharmacologic treatments of chronic kidney disease because of their hemodynamic and blood pressure reduction effects, which help to limit kidney disease progression.
10. Supportive therapies that may help to slow the rate of CKD progression include dietary protein restriction, lipid-lowering medications, smoking cessation, and anemia management.

Learning objectives, review questions, and other resources can be found at **www.pharmacotherapyonline.com.**

Under normal conditions each of the two million nephrons of the kidneys work in an organized fashion to filter, reabsorb, and excrete various solutes and water. The kidney is a primary regulator of sodium and water balance, as well as of acid–base homeostasis. The kidney also produces hormones necessary for red blood cell synthesis and calcium homeostasis. Impairment of kidney function is often referred to as CKD. Based on the time course of development, CKD is divided into two broad categories. Acute renal failure refers to the rapid loss of kidney function over days to weeks. Chronic kidney disease, also called chronic renal insufficiency or progressive kidney disease by some, is defined as a progressive loss of function occurring over several months to years, and is characterized by the gradual replacement of normal kidney architecture with interstitial fibrosis.

The working group of the National Kidney Foundation's (NKF) Kidney Dialysis Outcomes and Quality Initiative (K/DOQI) has developed a CKD classification system based on the presence of structural kidney damage and/or functional changes in glomerular filtration rate (GFR) present for a period of 3 months or more.[1] CKD is categorized by the level of kidney function (as defined by GFR) into stages 1 through 5, with each increasing number indicating a more advanced stage of the disease (Table 46–1).[1] The use of GFR versus serum creatinine to define the stages of CKD was chosen because the serum creatinine is an inaccurate index of GFR, and there is marked variability in GFR between subjects with similar serum creatinine values (see Chap. 44). Although the stages are defined functionally by the GFR, the classification system also accounts for structural evidence of kidney damage. Normal kidney function in adults is approximately 120 mL/min/1.73 m^2 of GFR. Even though a GFR of >90 mL/min/1.73 m^2 is considered normal kidney function, a patient can be diagnosed with CKD if the patient has proteinuria, hematuria, or evidence of structural damage from a kidney biopsy. Stage 5 CKD was previously referred to as end-stage renal disease (ESRD) or end-stage kidney disease.

EPIDEMIOLOGY OF CKD

The epidemiology of stage 5 CKD has been well documented through the efforts of the United States Renal Data System (USRDS), a national data system that collects, analyzes, and distributes information about U.S. patients on hemodialysis and peritoneal dialysis, as well as kidney transplant recipients.[2] Information on the epidemiology of the earlier stages of CKD is less-well characterized. In the United States alone, there are several major epidemiologic studies currently in progress or in development to elucidate the natural history of CKD, its progression, and concurrent morbid-

TABLE 46-1 Definition and Prevalence of the Stages of Chronic Kidney Disease

Stage	Glomerular Filtration Rate[a]	Prevalence[c]
1	≥90[b]	10,500,000
2	60–89	7,100,000
3	30–59	7,600,000
4	15–29	400,000
5	<15 (includes patients on dialysis)	300,000

[a]Glomerular filtration rate in mL/min per 1.73 m^2 body surface area.
[b]Chronic kidney disease can be present with a normal or near normal GFR if other markers of kidney disease are present, such as proteinuria, hematuria, biopsy results showing kidney damage, or anatomic abnormalities (e.g., cysts).
[c]Based on measurement of an elevated albumin-to-creatinine ratio.

TABLE 46-2 Risk Factors Associated with Chronic Kidney Disease

Risk Factor	Key Studies
Susceptibility	
Advanced age	Lindeman et al.,[17] Goetz et al.[75]
Reduced kidney mass and low birth weight	Lackland et al.[24]
Racial/ethnic minority	Tierney et al.,[21] Rostand et al.,[22] Perry et al.[23]
Family history	Freedman et al.,[25] FIND Research Group[26]
Low income or education	Byrne et al.,[19] Perneger et al.[20]
Systemic inflammation	Kshirsagar et al.,[27] Erlinger et al.[28]
Dyslipidemia	Muntner et al.,[29] Schaeffner et al.[30]
Initiation	
Diabetes mellitus	Hasslacher et al.,[32] Brancati et al.[34]
Hypertension	Coresh et al.,[39] Perneger et al.,[40] Klag et al.
Glomerulonephritis	Massy et al.[46]
Progression	
Glycemia (among diabetic patients)	Reichard et al.,[62] DCCT Research Group[63]
Hypertension	Klahr et al.,[51] Jafar et al.,[52] Bakris,[57] UKPDS Group,[58] UKPDS Group,[59] Bakris[60]
Proteinuria	Keane et al.,[50] Klahr,[51] Jafar et al.[52]
Smoking	Orth et al.,[66] Orth et al.[76]
Obesity	Hsu et al.,[82] Iseki et al.,[83] Ejerblad et al.[84]

ities. One study targets individuals with polycystic kidney disease,[3] while another study targets African Americans with hypertensive nephrosclerosis.[4] The CKD Cohort study, funded by the National Institutes of Health,[5] and an Amgen Inc. and Fresenius cosponsored study (Stride Registry)[6] are investigating progressive CKD and its relationship with comorbid cardiovascular disease. The National Kidney Foundation has recognized the importance of early detection and has initiated the Kidney Early Evaluation Program[7] to identify, educate, and provide free screening for people at increased risk of developing kidney disease. Furthermore, U.S. governmental agencies have targeted CKD as one of 28 major focus areas for improvement by the year 2010, as set forth in the Healthy People 2010 document.[8] Over the next decade, as a result of these initiatives, our understanding of the epidemiology, pathophysiology, and management of mild (stage 1) to moderate (stage 4) CKD will undoubtedly increase.

❶ CKD has been described as a silent epidemic[9] and is a worldwide public health problem.[10] Three different national surveys have estimated that CKD affects 5% of the adult U.S. population when CKD is defined by a serum creatinine concentration greater than 1.2 to 1.5 mg/dL.[11–13] The Third National Health and Nutritional Examination Survey (NHANES III), a nationally representative sample of the U.S. adult population, projected that at least 10.9 million people had reduced kidney function as evidenced by serum creatinine concentrations equal or higher than 1.5 mg/dL.[11] When data on the presence of microalbuminuria and proteinuria was included, the estimated prevalence of CKD is 10.9% of U.S. population age 20 years or older, or 19 million individuals.[1] The prevalence of CKD is thus similar to that of other chronic conditions such as hypertension, diabetes mellitus, and cardiovascular disease.

Incidence estimates of stage 5 CKD are obtained from the USRDS.[2] During the two decades spanning 1980 to 2000, the number of patients entering stage 5 (and requiring renal replacement therapy) increased by 5% to 10% per year. However, beginning in 2003 and continuing to the present, the rate of increase has declined to less than 1%.[14] The main factor attributed to this decline has been the implementation of angiotensin-converting enzyme inhibitor (ACEI) and angiotensin receptor blocker (ARB) therapy as a standard of care for those with early stage CKD.[14] The role and impact of ACEI and ARB therapy for patients with hypertension- and diabetes mellitus-associated renal disease is discussed in detail later in this chapter. The four most common causes of incident (new cases of) stage 5 CKD in the United States are diabetes mellitus, hypertension, glomerulonephritis, and polycystic kidney disease. The causes and incidence rates include diabetic nephropathy (150 cases/million), hypertensive nephropathy (80 cases/million), glomerulonephritis (22 cases/million), and polycystic kidney disease (5 cases/million).[2] Individuals over 65 years of age and black race are at higher risk of CKD.[2] For example, the rate of stage 5 CKD is fourfold higher for blacks as compared to whites.[2]

It is often assumed that all early stages of CKD progress continuously toward stage 5. Thus, information on risk factors obtained from USRDS data is assumed to be generalizable to all stages of CKD. The validity of this approach to projecting future incidence data has not been tested. Further complicating these issues is the fact that the development and progression of the early stages of CKD is a complex phenomenon.[15] The risk factors associated with CKD are numerous and varied and many of these are not those one would traditionally consider as having a direct influence on the causal pathway. The working group of K/DOQI has recommended categorizing CKD risk factors as susceptibility factors, initiation factors, or progression factors to help clinicians stratify the overall risks of individual patients (Table 46–2).[10]

The focus of the current chapter is on the initiation and progression of CKD. Because diabetes mellitus and hypertension are the two most prevalent etiologies for CKD, a considerable amount of attention is given to discussing the course and treatments designed to slow the progressive kidney function decline that is commonly observed in patients with either of these two diseases. This chapter focuses on the early CKD stages, that is, stages 1, 2, and 3, which are the critical battleground if one hopes to minimize the number of patients who ultimately require renal replacement therapy. CKD is a continuous and progressive disease state that often results in the appearance of several concomitant complications that commence at various stages in the disease. Chapter 47 will address the pathophysiology and consequences and complications of CKD that tend to become evident in those with stage 4 or 5 CKD. The treatment options for these conditions and monitoring parameters are also discussed.

ETIOLOGY

SUSCEPTIBILITY FACTORS

Susceptibility factors to CKD are advanced age,[16–18] low income or education,[19,20] and racial/ethnic minority status,[21–23] as well as reduced kidney mass, low birth weight,[24] and family history of CKD.[25,26] These factors have not been proven to directly cause kidney damage. Novel proposed susceptibility factors are systemic inflammation[27,28] and dyslipidemia.[29,30] Although most of these susceptibility factors may not be amenable to pharmacologic or lifestyle interventions, they may be useful for identifying populations that are at high risk of CKD.

INITIATION FACTORS

❸ Initiation factors are conditions that directly result in kidney damage, and are modifiable by pharmacologic therapy. Diabetes mellitus, hypertension, autoimmune diseases, polycystic kidney disease, systemic infections, urinary tract infections, urinary stones, lower urinary tract obstructions, and drug toxicity are all considered initiation factors. Because diabetes mellitus, hypertension, and glomerular diseases are, respectively, the three most common causes of CKD in the United States, the following discussion focuses on these conditions.

Diabetes Mellitus

Individuals with type 1 diabetes mellitus have a 40% lifetime risk of developing CKD of any stage,[31] whereas individuals with type 2 diabetes mellitus have a 50% lifetime risk.[32] Given the greater prevalence of type 2 diabetes mellitus as compared to type 1—generally a 10:1 ratio exists in most countries[33]—the majority of CKD from diabetes would be among individuals with type 2 disease. Although not all individuals with diabetic nephropathy progress to stage 5 CKD, the lifetime risk is considerable. A prospective study of over 300,000 individuals screened from the Multiple Risk Factor Intervention Trial estimated that approximately 3% of individuals with diabetes mellitus will develop stage 5 CKD during their lifetime.[34] Thus diabetic subjects have a 12-fold greater relative risk of developing stage 5 CKD than does someone without diabetes. Subjects with diabetes also have an increased risk of nondiabetic causes of CKD, suggesting an underlying genetic susceptibility to kidney diseases.[35]

Hypertension

Hypertension also increases the risk of CKD although the exact role as a cause or consequence is often debated as the kidney has a role in the development and modulation of high blood pressure.[36–38] Therefore, the interpretation of epidemiologic studies regarding the presence of high blood pressure and the risk of progressive kidney disease may be limited by reverse causation. Hypertension generally develops concomitantly with progressive kidney disease. For example, hypertension is present in 40% of individuals with a GFR of 90 mL/min per 1.73 m^2; in 55% of those with a GFR of 60 mL/min per 1.73 m^2; and 75% of individuals with a GFR of 30 mL/min per 1.73 m.[21] Furthermore, in the NHANES III survey, a serum creatinine of 1.6 mg/dL or higher for men and 1.4 mg/dL or higher for women was more common in persons with hypertension (9.1%) than in persons without hypertension (1.1%).[39]

Conversely, prospective studies have shown that elevated blood pressure increases the risk for the development of CKD among subjects without initial kidney disease.[40,41] A recent prospective study of 316,675 adult managed care patients showed increased odds of incident ESRD (stage 5 CKD) in those with increased baseline blood pressure. The odds of CKD development were 2.0 (95% confidence interval [CI] 1.6 to 2.5) for blood pressure ranges of 120 to 129 mm Hg systolic over 80 to 84 mm Hg diastolic, and 4.3 (95% CI 2.6 to 6.9) for blood pressure higher than 210/120 mm Hg as compared to blood pressure lower than 120/80 mm Hg. Patients were devoid of baseline kidney disease in this study.[41]

In the Multiple Risk Factor Intervention Trial, a primary prevention trial to test the effect of an intervention program on mortality from coronary heart disease, the overall lifetime risk of developing stage 5 CKD for individuals with hypertension was 5.6%.[42] The risk varied dramatically by level of blood pressure, from 0.33% at stage 1 hypertension (systolic blood pressure 140 to 150 mm Hg and/or diastolic blood pressure 90 to 100 mm Hg) to 4.5% for systolic blood pressure levels greater than 180 mm Hg or diastolic blood pressure levels greater than 110 mm Hg over a followup period of approximately 16 years.[42]

Glomerulonephritis

Glomerular diseases are also considered initiation factors of CKD. The epidemiology and pathophysiology of glomerular diseases are variable and thus all diseases should not justifiably be lumped into one disease category. Some conditions, such as Goodpasture's disease or Wegener's granulomatosus, may progress rapidly to stage 5 CKD, and thus may best be categorized as causes of acute renal failure. Other conditions, such as immunoglobulin (Ig) A nephropathy, membranous nephropathy, focal segmental glomerulosclerosis, lupus nephritis, and others, are more indolent diseases, and are considered causes of CKD (see Chap. 50). The chronic glomerular diseases progress at variable rates, with the loss of GFR ranging from 1.4 to 9.5 mL/min per year.[43–46]

PROGRESSION FACTORS

❹ Progression risk factors are those associated with further kidney damage. This is generally evident as an increase in the rate of decline in kidney function in those who already have damaged kidneys. The most important predictors of progressive CKD are the persistence of underlying initiation factors (e.g., diabetes mellitus, hypertension, glomerulonephritis, and polycystic kidney disease), and the progression factors of proteinuria, elevated blood pressure, and smoking.

Proteinuria

Numerous studies have documented the importance of proteinuria in the progression of both diabetic[47–50] and nondiabetic[51,52] kidney disease. Most of these findings are from secondary analyses of intervention trials. In diabetic kidney disease (types 1 and 2), an albumin excretion rate higher than 30 mg per 24 hours (microalbuminuria) strongly predicted the development of overt nephropathy (proteinuria) and subsequent loss of kidney function.[47–49,53] In nondiabetic kidney disease, the Modification of Diet in Renal Disease Study (MDRD), a randomized clinical trial examining the effects of oral protein restriction and blood pressure control on the progression of CKD among individuals with preexisting CKD, demonstrated that a patient's baseline level of proteinuria strongly predicted future loss of GFR.[51] Furthermore, individuals with the highest levels of baseline proteinuria benefited the most from pharmacologic reduction of blood pressure. A recent study of more than 1,800 individuals with varying stages of CKD demonstrated a strong, graded risk of CKD based on the level of proteinuria; a fivefold increased risk of progression was observed for each 1.0 g/day increase in proteinuria.[52]

The joint role of blood pressure and proteinuria in the progression of CKD was investigated by Jafar et al. using data from 11 randomized, controlled trials that compared the efficacy of antihypertensive regimens for patients with predominantly nondiabetic kidney disease.[54] The increased risk for CKD progression at higher systolic blood pressure levels was greater in patients with urine protein excretion greater than 1.0 g/day (P <0.006).[54]

Hypertension

The early treatment of hypertension and the achievement of aggressive target values has been demonstrated to slow the rate of progression of CKD.[51,52,55–59] Bakris et al. demonstrated a direct correlation between the level of achieved blood pressure and preservation of kidney function in diabetic patients.[60] The analysis included 10 studies in which diabetic patients were treated with various antihypertensive agents. The change in GFR was measured during each study. An inverse linear relationship between the average attained blood pressure at study completion and average GFR was observed; and the lower final mean arterial blood pressure resulted in a lower average decline in GFR. For example, a systolic blood pressure of 180 mm Hg was associated with a 14 mL/min per year decline in GFR, whereas patients with a systolic blood pressure of 135 mm Hg had only a 2 mL/min per year decline in GFR.[60]

A recent extended followup analysis of the MDRD original cohort showed that patients assigned to lower blood pressure target (mean arterial pressure: <92 mm Hg) were 32% less likely to develop stage 5 CKD than those in the usual target blood pressure (mean arterial pressure: <107 mm Hg).[61] Therefore, low blood pressure slowed the progression of nondiabetic kidney disease in patients with an existing moderately to severely decreased GFR.

Diabetes Mellitus

Hyperglycemia is an initiation and progression risk factor for CKD. Two large prospective studies performed in the early 1990s showed the benefits of blood glucose control in both the development and progression of microvascular complications.[62,63] These findings were confirmed by two additional British studies.[55,56] The largest of these studies, the Diabetes Control and Complications Trial (DCCT) enrolled 1,441 patients with type 1 diabetes mellitus who were randomized to conventional blood glucose control or to intensive glucose control.[63] Conventional control consisted of up to two insulin injections per day guided by blood glucose levels. Intensive control consisted of administration of insulin three or more times daily by injection or by external pump to achieve a hemoglobin A_{1c} ≤6.0%. The main outcome measure of efficacy was retinopathy, a marker of microvascular disease that is usually associated with diabetic nephropathy among individuals with type 1 diabetes mellitus. Roughly half of the patients had mild retinopathy. Primary prevention was defined as a reduction in new occurrence of retinopathy among patients with no baseline retinopathy, and secondary prevention was defined as a reduction in the rate of progression of retinopathy among individuals with baseline retinopathy. A primary risk reduction of retinopathy of 76% and secondary risk reduction of 54% were noted with intensive control. The intensive therapy was associated with a 39% reduction in the risk for the development of "microalbuminuria" (urinary albumin excretion ≥40 mg/day), and a 54% reduction in the development of "frank albuminuria" (urinary albumin excretion ≥300 mg/day) compared to conventional therapy. The beneficial effect of intensive therapy on the development of proteinuria remained after completion of the randomized phase of the DCCT.[64] Individuals initially randomized to the intensive therapy had a 59% reduction in the development of new microalbuminuria, and 84% reduction in the development of albuminuria compared to the conventional group 7 to 8 years after completion of the DCCT.

Smoking

Recent studies suggest that smoking may promote initiation and progression of CKD in subjects with type 1 and type 2 diabetes.[65–68] Smoking increased the rate of CKD progression in diabetes by approximately twofold in one study.[69] The "cigarette pack years" was an independent predictive factor for CKD progression among diabetic subjects.[70] In addition, smoking has also been associated with CKD in hypertension,[71] especially among hypertensive black subjects.[72] Some studies have demonstrated an association between smoking and microalbuminuria and the development of stage 5 CKD.[73–75] Smoking has also been identified as a risk factor for progression in patients with IgA nephropathy, polycystic kidney disease, and systemic lupus erythematosus.[76,77]

Hyperlipidemia

Dyslipidemia may be associated with kidney disease. Three epidemiologic studies[29,30,78] demonstrated that dyslipidemia predicts incident CKD among individuals considered at low risk for CKD.[79] CKD with or without nephrotic syndrome is frequently accompanied by abnormalities in lipoprotein metabolism. The prevalence of hyperlipidemia appears to increase as kidney function declines and hyperlipidemia is a characteristic of the nephrotic syndrome.[80] In 85% to 90% of patients with decreased kidney function and proteinuria greater than 3 g/day, elevated plasma total and low-density lipoprotein cholesterol occurs. Approximately 50% of these patients have low levels (<35 mg/dL) of high-density lipoprotein cholesterol, and 60% have triglyceride concentrations greater than 200 mg/dL.[80] Lipid-lowering agents can decrease the extent of glomerular injury in animal models with hyperlipidemia and kidney disease.[81] Therefore, treatment of lipid abnormalities in patients with CKD may have a beneficial effect on slowing the rate of progression of the kidney disease.

Obesity

Recent studies show an association of obesity with development of stage 5 CKD.[82,83] Iseki et al. examined the relationship between body mass index (BMI) and the development of ESRD among 47,504 men and 53,249 women using data from a 1983 community-based screening in Okinawa, Japan.[83] BMI was associated with an increased risk of the development of ESRD in men (odds ratio [OR] 1.3; 95% CI 1.1 to 1.4) but not in women. Another large population study using data from Kaiser Permanente revealed an increased risk of ESRD in overweight (relative risk [RR] 1.9; 95% CI 1.6 to 2.1 for BMI 25 to 29.9 kg/m^2) and obese subjects (RR 3.6 [95% CI 3.1 to 4.2] for those with a BMI of 30 to 34.9 kg/m^2; RR 6.1 [95% CI 5.0 to 7.5] for those with a BMI of 35 to 39.9 kg/m^2; and RR 7.1 [95% CI 5.4 to 9.3] for those with a BMI greater than 40 kg/m^2). Higher baseline BMI remained an independent predictor for ESRD after adjustments for baseline blood pressure level as well as presence of diabetes mellitus.[82]

A recent population-based study showed that a BMI ≥25 kg/m^2 at age 20 years is associated with a threefold increase in risk of CKD compared to a BMI lower than 25 kg/m^2. Obesity (BMI ≥30) among men and morbid obesity (BMI ≥35) among women was associated with three- to fourfold increases in risk.[84]

Other Factors

Other identified risk factors for progression are lead exposure[85] and illicit drug use.[86] A recent population-based study suggested that apolipoprotein E genetic variants are also associated with progression of CKD in both whites and blacks.[87]

PATHOPHYSIOLOGY

Kidney damage can result from heterogeneous causes. For example, diabetic nephropathy is characterized by glomerular mesangial expansion; in hypertensive nephrosclerosis, the kidney's arterioles have arteriolar hyalinosis; and renal cysts are present in polycystic kidney disease. Therefore, the initial structural damage may depend on the primary disease affecting the kidney. However, the majority of progressive nephropathies share a final common pathway to irreversible renal parenchymal damage and ESRD (Fig. 46–1).[88,89] The key elements of this pathway are: (a) loss of nephron mass; (b) glomerular capillary hypertension; and (c) proteinuria.

The exposure to any of the initiation risk factors can result in loss of nephron mass. The remaining nephrons hypertrophy to compensate for the loss of renal function and nephron mass.[90] Initially, this compensatory hypertrophy may be adaptive. Over time, the hyper-

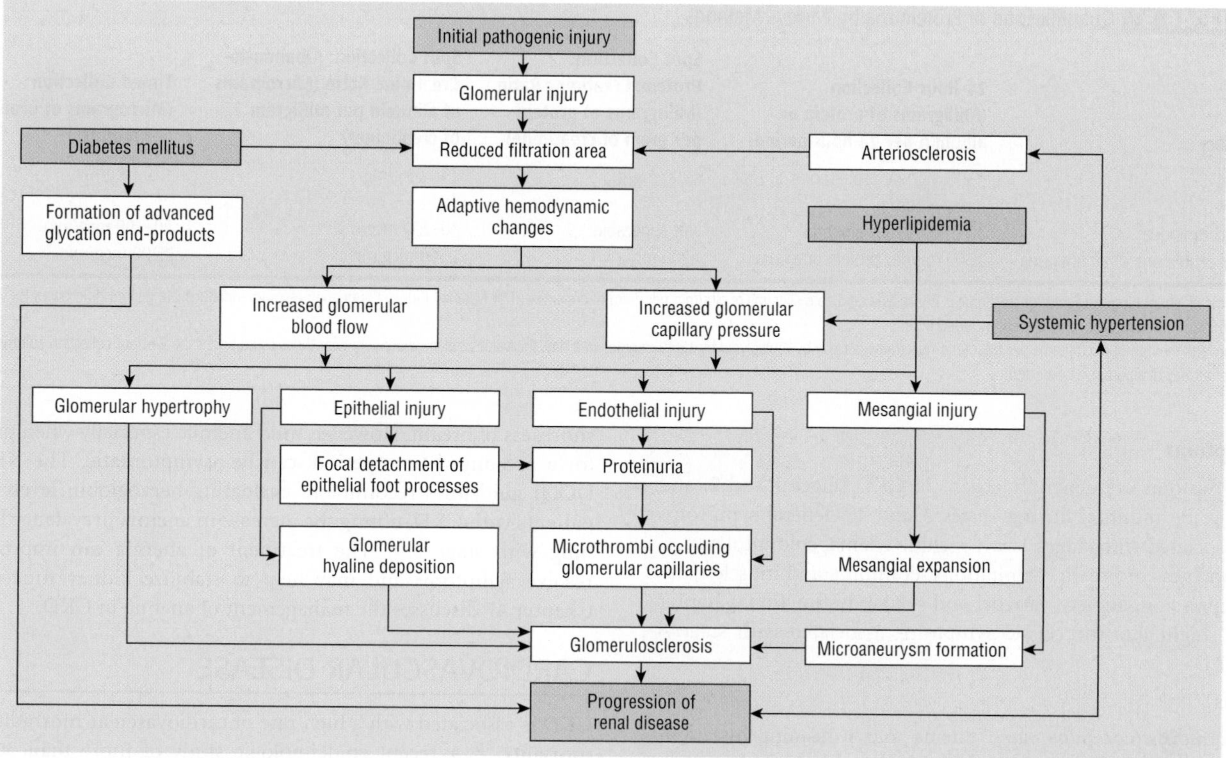

FIGURE 46-1. Proposed mechanisms for progression of renal disease.

trophy can lead to the development of intraglomerular hypertension, possibly mediated by angiotensin II.[91,92] Angiotensin II is a potent vasoconstrictor of both the afferent and efferent arterioles, but preferentially affects the efferent arterioles, leading to increased pressure within the glomerular capillaries and consequent increased filtration fraction. The development of intraglomerular hypertension usually correlates with the development of systemic arterial hypertension. Animal studies have demonstrated that high intraglomerular capillary pressure impairs the size-selective function of the glomerular permeability barrier, resulting in increased urinary excretion of albumin and frank proteinuria.[93,94] Angiotensin II may also mediate renal disease progression through nonhemodynamic effects.[95]

Proteinuria alone may promote progressive loss of nephrons as a result of direct cellular damage.[88,95] Filtered proteins such as albumin, transferrin, complement factors, immunoglobulins, cytokines, and angiotensin II are toxic to kidney tubular cells. Numerous studies have demonstrated that the presence of these proteins in the renal tubule activates tubular cells which leads to the upregulated production of inflammatory and vasoactive cytokines, such as endothelin, monocyte chemoattractant protein (MCP-1), and RANTES (regulated upon activation, normal T-cell expressed and secreted).[88,96–99] Proteinuria is also associated with the activation of complement components on the apical membrane of proximal tubules.[100] Accumulating evidence now suggests that intratubular complement activation may be the key mechanism of damage in the progressive proteinuric nephropathies.[101–103] These events ultimately lead to scarring of the interstitium, progressive loss of structural nephron units, and reduction in GFR.

CLINICAL PRESENTATION

CKD is often asymptomatic, and should be suspected in individuals with conditions such as diabetes, hypertension, genitourinary abnormalities, and autoimmune diseases. In addition, individuals of older age and those with a family history of kidney disease should be considered for CKD screening. Recommended screening studies include serum creatinine and GFR measurement, urinalysis, and/or imaging studies of the kidneys. Abnormal elevations of serum creatinine, reflecting decreases in GFR, or presence of urinary or imaging study abnormalities are indications for a full evaluation of CKD.[1]

❺ The rate of GFR loss can vary in CKD because of differences in the underlying disease process and extent of kidney damage, treatment responsiveness, and compliance with therapies. The NKF K/DOQI developed a classification system that divides CKD into five stages, with each increasing number indicating a more advanced stage of the disease, as defined by GFR[1] (see Table 46–1). These stages are based on kidney function and evidence of kidney damage. Therefore, one can have CKD with a normal GFR (>90 mL/min per 1.73 m^2) if there is evidence of structural damage to the kidneys (e.g., presence of proteinuria). The GFR rather than serum creatinine was used to define kidney function in this official classification system because the serum creatinine is an inadequate measure of kidney function (see Chap. 44).

The NKF K/DOQI defines kidney damage as the presence of clinical proteinuria. Table 46–3 summarizes the methods available to detect and interpret proteinuria and albuminuria. In addition, Chap. 44 provides a detailed discussion of the relative merits of the various methods currently available for the detection of urinary protein.

CLINICAL PRESENTATION OF CKD STAGES 1 TO 4

General

- CKD development and progression may be insidious in onset, often without noticeable symptoms. The diagnosis of CKD requires measurement of serum creatinine, estimation of GFR, and assessment of the urine (urinalysis) for protein and/or albumin excretion. CKD stages 3, 4, and 5 require further workup for CKD complications of anemia, cardiovascular disease, metabolic bone disease, malnutrition, and disorders of fluids and electrolytes.

TABLE 46-3 Quantification of Proteinuria by Various Methods

Category	24-Hour Collection (Milligrams of protein or albumin per 24-hour period)	Spot Collection: Protein: Creatinine Ratio (Milligrams of protein per gram of creatinine)	Spot Collection: Albumin-to-Creatinine Ratio (Micrograms of albumin per milligram of creatinine[a])	Timed Collection (Micrograms of protein per minute[b])
Normal	<300 mg/day protein or <30 mg/day albumin	<200 mg/g	<30 mcg/mg	<20 mcg/min
Microalbuminuria	30–300 mg/day albumin	Not applicable	30–299 mcg/mg	20–199 mcg/min
Clinical proteinuria or albuminuria	≥300 mg/day protein or albumin	>200 mg/g	≥300 mcg/mg	≥200 mcg/min

[a]Micrograms of albumin per milligram of creatinine is equal, as a ratio, to milligrams of albumin per gram of creatinine. The National Kidney Foundation recommendations cite gender differences for values of spot albumin-to-creatinine ratios that are not included here.
[b]If one converts the rate of micrograms per minute to milligrams per day by multiplying by 1,440 minutes in a day, the values obtained are very near those listed under the 24-hour collection column of milligrams per day of albumin, as expected.

Symptoms

- Symptoms are generally absent in CKD stages 1 and 2, and may be minimal during stages 3 and 4. General symptoms associated with stages 1 to 4 include edema, cold intolerance, shortness of breath, palpitations, cramping and muscle pain, depression, anxiety, fatigue, and sexual dysfunction. Chapter 47 highlights the classic symptoms associated with stage 5 CKD.

Signs

- *Cardiovascular–pulmonary:* Edema and worsening hypertension, electrocardiographic evidence of left ventricular hypertrophy, arrhythmias, hyperhomocysteinemia, and dyslipidemia
- *Gastrointestinal:* Gastroesophageal reflux disease, weight loss
- *Endocrine:* Secondary hyperparathyroidism, decreased vitamin D activation, β_2-microglobulin deposition, and gout
- *Hematologic:* Anemia of CKD, iron deficiency, and bleeding
- *Fluid/electrolytes:* Hyper- or hyponatremia, hyperkalemia, and metabolic acidosis

Patients with stage 1 or 2 CKD disease usually do not have any symptoms or metabolic derangements such as acidosis, anemia, and bone disease. In addition, the most common measure of impairment of kidney function, serum creatinine, may be only slightly elevated in these early CKD stages. Consequently, estimation of the GFR is imperative for recognition of early stages of CKD.

❻ Because the early stages of CKD are often undetected, the diagnosis requires a high level of suspicion in patients with chronic conditions such as hypertension and diabetes. Signs and symptoms associated with CKD become more prevalent in stages 3, 4, and 5. Anemia, abnormalities of calcium and phosphorus metabolism (secondary hyperparathyroidism), malnutrition, and fluid and electrolyte abnormalities become more common as kidney function deteriorates (see Chap. 47).

ANEMIA

Because the kidneys secrete 90% of the endogenous hormone erythropoietin, an endogenous hormone necessary for erythropoiesis, declining kidney function can lead to erythropoietin deficiency and anemia. The prevalence of anemia at specific stages of CKD is difficult to ascertain because of limited available data and use of various definitions.[1] Estimates of anemia (hemoglobin of less than 12 g/dL) prevalence in patients with a GFR greater than 80 mL/min per 1.73 m^2 are between 1% and 30%.[104] The true prevalence rate estimation is unclear as other factors, such as ethnicity, age, and gender, can also contribute to anemia. The prevalence of a hemoglobin less than 13 g/dL increases considerably in stages 3 to 5 CKD.[1] Anemia can lead to symptoms of fatigue, weakness, and shortness of breath. However, mild anemia, especially when present for a prolonged time period, can be asymptomatic. The NKF K/DOQI guidelines recommend evaluating hemoglobin levels in all patients with CKD, noting the increase in anemia prevalence beginning with stage 3.[105] The treatment of anemia can improve or resolve symptoms and may help to stabilize kidney function.[106] Chapter 47 discusses the management of anemia in CKD.

CARDIOVASCULAR DISEASE

CKD is associated with a high rate of cardiovascular morbidity and mortality.[107] A recent epidemiologic study of more than 300,000 individuals demonstrated a strong relationship between GFR and cardiovascular disease: the lower the level of GFR, the higher the incidence of cardiovascular events.[108] In fact, individuals with stages 2 to 4 CKD were more likely to die from cardiovascular disease complications than to survive to the initiation of renal-replacement therapy;[109] consequently, monitoring for the presence or development of cardiovascular disease in patients with CKD is an important aspect of their care. It is established that patients with CKD have 16% to 37% of the life expectancy of a matched population without kidney disease.[110] Appropriate traditional and nontraditional cardiovascular risk factor assessments are necessary in the evaluation of the patient with CKD. Guidelines for the evaluation, monitoring, and treatment of cardiovascular diseases in patients with CKD have been published and a detailed discussion can be found in the cited reference.[107]

DISORDERS OF CALCIUM AND PHOSPHORUS HOMEOSTASIS

Abnormalities in calcium and phosphorus metabolism typically occur in stages 3 to 5 CKD. Secondary hyperparathyroidism, however, can develop earlier despite normal serum calcium and phosphorus levels, at a GFR of 80 mL/min per 1.73 m^2 or below.[111] Thus, to detect secondary hyperparathyroidism and limit the bone complications, it is recommended that parathyroid hormone concentration, vitamin D levels, and calcium and phosphorus be monitored beginning in stage 3 CKD.[112] Additional systemic benefits of correcting abnormalities in calcium, phosphorus, and parathyroid hormone may include cardiovascular risk reduction. Chapter 47 discusses the management of bone disease caused by CKD.

MALNUTRITION

Anorexia and malnutrition are complications of CKD. Although there are limited data defining at exactly which stage malnutrition develops, the NKF K/DOQI guidelines recommend evaluating for signs of malnutrition when the GFR is lower than 60 mL/min per 1.73 m^2 (stages 3, 4, and 5).[113] An investigation for malnutrition should include a dietary assessment for protein and calorie intake, serum albumin, and/or assessment of protein appearance in the urine (as a marker of protein intake). Chapter 143 discusses the interpretation of these tests and Chap. 147 discusses nutritional recommendations for patients with CKD.

TREATMENT

Chronic Kidney Disease

■ GOAL OF THERAPY

The goal of therapy is to delay the progression of CKD, thereby minimizing the development or severity of associated complications including cardiovascular disease. Nonpharmacologic and pharmacologic interventions are available to slow the rate of CKD progression and they may also decrease the incidence and prevalence of ESRD.

❼ Usually the patient with CKD will benefit from modest dietary protein restriction (as a nondrug therapy) as well as pharmacologic therapy. The pharmacologic therapy's main purpose is to control the underlying conditions, such as diabetes mellitus and hypertension, that have precipitated the kidney damage so as to prevent further declines in function. Patients generally require a multimodality treatment approach irrespective of the cause of their kidney disease. Therapy with ACEIs and/or ARBs is a key therapeutic component for almost all patients.

■ NONPHARMACOLOGIC THERAPY

Dietary Protein Restriction

Experimental studies of kidney disease in animals suggest that dietary protein restriction delays the rate of progression of kidney function decline.[114] This hypothesis was tested in humans in the MDRD study, a randomized controlled trial that evaluated the benefits of dietary protein restriction and blood pressure reduction on the rate of CKD progression.[51,115] Most enrolled subjects had nondiabetic kidney disease and 24% of them had a diagnosis of polycystic kidney disease. Subjects with moderate CKD (GFR of 25 to 55 mL/min per 1.73 m^2) were randomized by dietary protein intake groups (1.3 g/kg per day or 0.58 g/kg per day), in addition to blood pressure grouping (usual mean arterial pressure [MAP] [107 mm Hg] or low MAP [92 mm Hg]), for a total of four groups. Subjects with advanced CKD (GFR 13 to 24 mL/min per 1.73 m^2) were randomized to a low-protein diet (0.58/kg/day) or a very-low-protein diet (0.28 g/kg/day) with a ketoamine acid supplement, in addition to the usual and low MAP as defined above for a total of four groups. After a mean followup of 2.2 years, protein restriction failed to show a statistical benefit in slowing the progression of CKD in any of the study groups. However, a secondary analysis of the MDRD study was conducted and revealed that in those patients with a GFR of less than 25 mL/min per 1.73 m^2, a protein intake of 0.6 g/kg per day was significantly associated with a decreased rate of progressive renal disease.[115] In addition, this analysis showed that the rate of progression to ESRD was significantly reduced by 41% for each 0.2 g/kg per day reduction in dietary protein intake. The discrepancy in results between the primary and secondary analyses can be explained by the different statistical methods used in each of the two analyses, in that the later analysis evaluated participants who were actually compliant with their dietary prescription.

Because of concerns of inadequate power of individual studies, meta-analyses have been performed to determine effect of protein restriction on the progression of CKD. Two notable meta-analyses, using almost the same individual studies have come to somewhat varying conclusions.[116,117] The first, by Pedrini et al., used only randomized, controlled trials of protein restriction, and demonstrated 33% risk reduction in the development of renal failure or death among nondiabetic patients, and a 44% risk reduction in the progression of proteinuria or CKD among diabetic individuals.[116] The second meta-analysis demonstrated a statistically beneficial effect of protein restriction on the progression of CKD; yet the authors concluded that the absolute effect, a reduction in the rate of decline of GFR by 0.53 mL/min per year after the addition of a low-protein diet does not compare well to other strategies.[117]

Thus, the available data suggests only a relatively small benefit from dietary protein restriction in CKD patients. Because low protein diets may lead to malnutrition in patients with advanced CKD and those with nephrotic-range proteinuria, the NKF K/DOQI has advocated a dietary protein intake of 0.6 g/kg per day in patients with a GFR <25 mL/min per 1.73 m^2.[113] Titration of protein intake up to 0.75 g/kg per day is suggested for patients who cannot achieve or maintain adequate nutritional status with the lower-protein (0.6 g/kg per day) diet.[113]

■ PHARMACOLOGIC THERAPY

Guidelines for CKD treatment usually recognize the differences in pathogenesis and course of diabetic and nondiabetic CKD. Consequently, pharmacologic interventions are discussed separately for these conditions within this chapter. The major focus of this chapter is on the impact of ACEI and ARB therapies on progressive CKD. Pharmacologic therapies specific for glomerulonephritis are discussed in Chap. 50, while therapies for the treatment of complications of kidney disease are covered in Chap. 47.

Diabetic Chronic Kidney Disease

■ INTENSIVE INSULIN THERAPY

The DCCT was the first study to show the long-term benefits of intensive insulin therapy (IIT) on kidney and other diabetes-related outcomes.[63] IIT was achieved by administration of three or more times daily insulin injections or by insulin pump infusion so as to attain preprandial and postprandial blood glucose levels of 70 to 120 mg/dL and <180 mg/dL, respectively. IIT effectively reduced the incidence of microalbuminuria as compared to standard therapy in both the primary prevention and secondary prevention groups, as described previously.[63] However, IIT was associated with at least one episode of hypoglycemia in 65% of patients as compared to 35% in the standard treatment group.[63] Other studies confirm the beneficial effects of IIT in prevention and progression of diabetic complications.[118,119] A meta-analysis of 16 clinical studies showed a benefit in reducing the frequency and severity of diabetic complications, and delaying the development and progression of diabetic nephropathy with intensive blood glucose control in type 1 diabetes.[118] A 4-year followup study of the DCCT participants, the Epidemiology of Diabetes Interventions and Complications study, showed a continued benefit of IIT on the risk of diabetic nephropathy with a 53% reduction in microalbuminuria.[119]

The United Kingdom Prospective Diabetes Study's Intensive Glucose Control Study also presented data on prevention of microvascular complications among individuals with type 2 diabetes mellitus.[55] Individuals newly diagnosed with type 2 diabetes mellitus (n = 3,867) were randomized to intensive therapy (goal fasting plasma glucose of <6 mmol/L) or conventional therapy (goal fasting plasma glucose of <15 mmol/L) after a 3-month period of dietary counseling. Individuals in either group could use oral sulfonylureas or insulin. After 10 years of followup, the intensive group was associated with an 11% reduction in median hemoglobin A_{1c}, and a 12% reduction in any diabetes-related end point compared to the conventional group. Most of the observed benefit was in a reduction in microvascular end points, primarily proliferative retinopathy.[55]

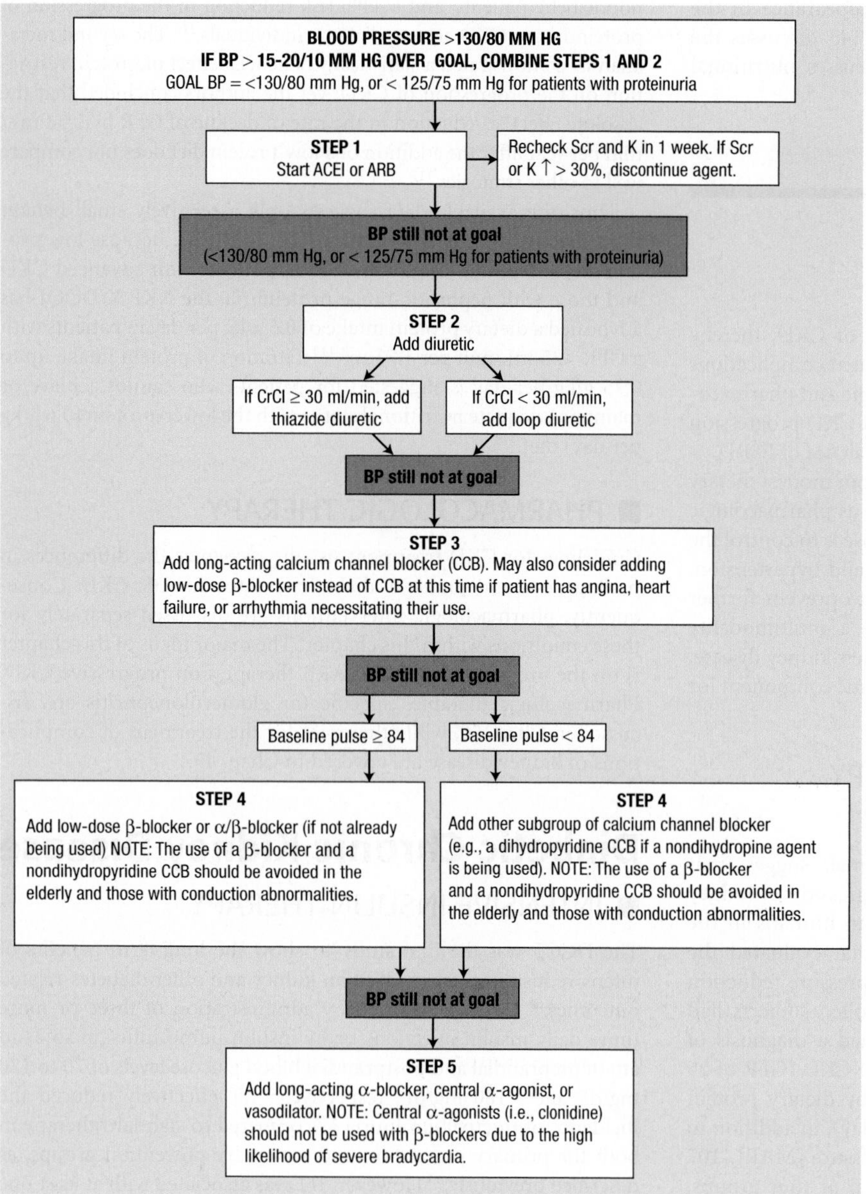

FIGURE 46-2. Hypertension management algorithm for patients with CKD. Dosage adjustments should be made every 2 to 4 weeks as needed. The dose of one agent should be maximized before another is added. (ACEI, angiotensin-converting enzyme inhibitor; ARB, angiotensin receptor blocker; BP, blood pressure; CAD, coronary artery disease; CCB, calcium channel blocker; CHF, congestive heart failure; MI, myocardial infarction; UP:Cr, urinary protein-to-creatinine ratio.) *(Adapted from reference 136 with permission.)*

The data from the DCCT, meta-analyses, and United Kingdom Prospective Diabetes Study provide levels of support for reducing microvascular complications, including nephropathy, by instituting intensive therapy for patients with type 1 and type 2 diabetes mellitus. Intensive therapy can include insulin or oral drugs, but employ the testing of blood sugar at least three times daily. Furthermore, the goals of therapy include an A_{1c} of <7%, and preprandial plasma and peak postprandial blood glucose of 92 to 130 mg/dL and <180 mg/dL, respectively.[120] The clinician is encouraged to review Chap. 77 for a thorough review of dosing, monitoring, and goals of therapies to treat diabetes mellitus.

■ OPTIMAL HYPERTENSION CONTROL

Reduction of blood pressure in type 1 and type 2 diabetic patients has been associated with lower rates of CKD progression.[58,59,121–130] The United Kingdom Prospective Diabetes Study[59] was a randomized trial of captopril or atenolol among 1,148 hypertensive type 2 diabetic patients designed to evaluate the effect of blood pressure reduction to a level of <150/85 mm Hg versus <180/105 mm Hg on macrovascular and microvascular outcomes. Reductions of 24% in diabetes-related end points, 32% in deaths related to diabetes, 44% in strokes, and 37% in microvascular end points were observed after a median follow up of 8.4 years. [59] The benefit of blood pressure control has been confirmed in subsequent studies of type 2 diabetic subjects with microalbuminuria.[121,122,127,131–134] These studies used either ACEI (Table 46–4) or ARB (Table 46–5) classes of drugs, which likely have nonhemodynamic beneficial effects on CKD progression, as discussed below, as well as blood-pressure-lowering effects. In type 1 diabetes with nephropathy, a rigorous blood pressure goal (MAP of ≤92 mm Hg) leads to decreased proteinuria.[129]

The Seventh Joint National Committee on Prevention, Detection, Evaluation, and Treatment of High Blood Pressure recommends a goal blood pressure of <130/80 mm Hg for patients with CKD.[135] Elevated blood pressure is often more difficult to control in patients with CKD than in those with normal kidney function. Therefore, to achieve adequate blood pressure goals, three or more different blood pressure medications are usually required.[136] Figure 46–2 depicts the proposed algorithm for the management of hypertension in people with CKD and diabetes. The selection of individual classes of drugs for limiting progression of CKD is presented in the following sections.

TABLE 46-4 Summary of Angiotensin-Converting Enzyme Inhibitor Studies in Diabetic Patients

Drug, Dose, and Study Design	Baseline Renal Characteristics	Number of Subjects and Disease	Study Duration	Outcome	Reference and Study Name
Captopril 25 mg three times a day; randomized, placebo-controlled trial	UPE ≥500 mg/day, S_{cr} ≤2.5 mg/dL	409 Type 1 DM	3 years	Risk reduction of doubling S_{cr} was 48% with captopril treatment; subanalysis showed a larger risk reduction with more elevated S_{cr} (76% when the S_{cr} was 2 g/dL)	Lewis et al.[123]
Enalapril once daily; randomized, placebo-controlled trial	Normotensive, UAE 20–200 mcg/min	103 Type 2 DM	5 years	Risk reduction of 66.7% for progression to clinical albuminuria with enalapril	Ahmad et al.[124]
Enalapril 10 mg once daily; randomized, placebo-controlled trial	Normotensive, UAE ≤30 mg/day	156 Type 2 DM	6 years	Risk reduction of 12.5% for microalbuminuria with enalapril treatment; GFR reductions were two times greater in the placebo-treated patients at 6 years	Ravid et al.[125]
Lisinopril 10 mg once daily with titration to BP; placebo-controlled trial	Normotensive patients with either normoalbuminuria or microalbuminuria	530 Type 1 DM	2 years	18.8% lower UPE with lisinopril treatment; greater treatment effect in those with baseline microalbuminuria (34.2 mcg/min vs. 1 mcg/min)	EUCLID Study Group[126]
Ramipril 10 mg once daily; randomized, placebo-controlled trial	Normoalbuminuria or microalbuminuria	3,577 Type 2 DM	4.5 years	Ramipril lowered risk of overt nephropathy with and without baseline microalbuminuria (relative risk of 0.8); lower UP:Cr at 1 and 4.5 years with ramipril treatment	HOPE and MICROHOPE[127]
Captopril 50 mg twice a day; randomized, placebo-controlled trial	Normotensive patients with microalbuminuria	143 Type 1 DM	2 years	Risk reduction of 67.8% for clinical proteinuria with captopril treatment; GFR reductions of 7.9 mL/min per 1.73 m^2 per year in placebo group while stable in captopril group	North American Microalbuminuria Study Group[128]
Enalapril 5 mg once daily, titrated to BP; placebo-controlled trial	Hypertensive, GFR of 30–100 mL/min per 1.73 m^2	121 Type 2 DM	3 years	Clinical albuminuria progression in 7% of enalapril vs. 21% of placebo group; enalapril therapy preserved GFR, whereas placebo treatment resulted in a loss of 0.33 mL/min per 1.73 m^2 per month	Lebovitz et al.[130]

BP, blood pressure; DM, diabetes mellitus; GFR, glomerular filtration rate; S_{cr}, serum creatinine; UAE, urinary albumin excretion; UP:Cr, urinary protein-to-creatinine ratio; UPE, urinary protein excretion.

Patients diagnosed with both hypertension and diabetes mellitus have been estimated to have up to a sixfold higher risk of developing ESRD than do those patients with diabetes mellitus alone.[136] Adequate blood pressure control can reduce the rate of decline in GFR and the degree of albuminuria in hypertensive type 1 and type 2 diabetic patients.[136] Although interventions that reduce blood pressure have historically shown reductions in urinary albumin and protein excretion, the ACEIs were the first agents shown to reduce glomerular capillary pressure and volume, which, in animal models and human studies, have resulted in preservation of renal function.[137–139] Table 46–6 summarizes the documented effects of the other various available antihypertensive agents on renal blood flow and GFR.[140,141]

TABLE 46-5 Summary of Angiotensin Receptor Blocker Studies in Diabetic Patients

Drug, Dose, and Study Design	Baseline Characteristics	Number of Subjects and Disease	Duration	Outcomes	Reference and Study Name
Irbesartan 300 mg once daily; amlodipine 10 mg once daily, randomized, placebo-controlled trial	Hypertensive, UPE ≥900 mg/day	1,715 Type 2 DM	2.6 years	Irbesartan therapy resulted in a 20% (for placebo) and 23% (for amlodipine) risk reduction in primary composite end point of doubling of S_{cr}, development of ESRD, or death	Lewis et al.[134]
Irbesartan 150 mg once daily; irbesartan 300 mg once daily; randomized, placebo-controlled trial	Hypertensive, AER of 20–200 mcg/min	590 Type 2 DM	2 years	Irbesartan 150 mg resulted in a 24% reduction in UAE; irbesartan 300 mg resulted in a 38% reduction in UAE; placebo resulted in a 2% decrease; hazard ratio for diabetic nephropathy was 0.56 and 0.32 in the 150-mg and 300-mg irbesartan groups, respectively	Parving et al.[133]
Losartan 50–100 mg once daily; randomized placebo-controlled trial	Hypertensive, UA:U_{cr} of at least 300 and S_{cr} 1.3–3 mg/dL	1,513 Type 2 DM	3.4 years	Losartan therapy resulted in a 16% risk reduction of primary composite end point of doubling of S_{cr}, ESRD, or death; level of proteinuria declined by 35% with losartan therapy	Brenner et al.[132]
Irbesartan 150 mg twice a day; randomized, placebo-controlled trial, crossover study	Hypertensive and normotensive, microalbuminuria	128 Type 2 DM	120 days	Irbesartan had a beneficial effect on reducing AER in both hypertensive and normotensive patients with type 2 diabetes	Sasso et al.[131]

AER, albumin excretion rate; DM, diabetes mellitus; ESRD, end-stage renal disease; S_{cr}, serum creatinine; UA:U_{cr}, urinary albumin-to-urinary creatinine ratio; UAE, urinary albumin excretion; UPE, urinary protein excretion.

TABLE 46-6 Effects of Antihypertensive Agents on Renal Blood Flow (RBF) and Glomerular Filtration Rate (GFR)

Antihypertensive Agent	Mechanism of Action	Effects on Renal Hemodynamics
Diuretics	Sodium and volume depletion	↓ GFR and RBF
	↑ Vasodilatory prostaglandin levels (IV loop diuretics)	↑ RBF
	Renal vasoconstriction (IV thiazide diuretics)	↓ GFR and RBF
β-Adrenergic blockers	↓ Cardiac output	↓ GFR and RBF
	↑ Renal vascular resistance (nonselective agents)	↓ GFR and RBF
	↑ Renal vascular resistance (β_1-selective agents)	No change in GFR and RBF
Centrally acting antiadrenergic drugs	↓ Renal vascular resistance (methyldopa)	No change in GFR and RBF
	↓ Renal perfusion pressure (clonidine, α_2-adrenergic agonist)	↓ GFR and RBF
Peripherally acting antiadrenergic drugs	Direct vasodilation (postsynaptic α_1-adrenoreceptor blocking agents)	No change in GFR and RBF
Direct vasodilator agents	↓ Renal vascular resistance (hydralazine, minoxidil)	↑ RBF and no effect on GFR
	Arterial vasodilation plus dilatation of venous capacitance vessels (nitroprusside)	↓ GFR and RBF (acute effect)
Calcium channel blockers	↓ Renal vascular resistance by vasodilation of afferent arterioles (hypertensive patients)	↑ RBF and no change in GFR

↓, decrease; ↑, increase.

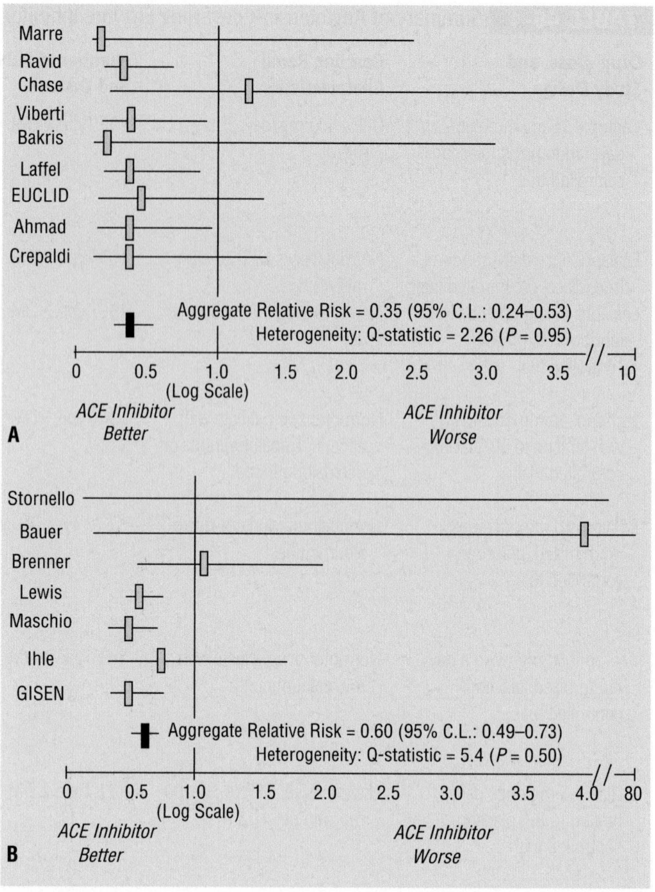

FIGURE 46-3. *A.* Relative risk for developing microalbuminuria with 95% confidence intervals (CIs) in each study, and the aggregate relative risk with 95% CIs for all studies (N = 642 with diabetes). *B.* Relative risk for doubling serum creatinine concentration or development of ESRD with 95% CIs in each study, and aggregate relative risk with 95% CIs for all studies (N = 1,277; 479 with diabetes). (ACE, angiotensin-converting enzyme.) (*From reference 143 with permission.*)

Antihypertensive Drug Choice

❽ Several studies have confirmed the beneficial effects of ACEIs on renal function in patients with and without diabetes. Table 46–4 shows the results of the key studies that evaluated more than 100 diabetic subjects followed over 2 to 6 years.[123–125,127,128,130,142] These studies show that the benefit of ACEI use in CKD is seen in both type 1 and 2 diabetic subjects, across different degrees of kidney damage (normoalbuminuria, microalbuminuria, frank proteinuria, and reduction in GFR), and are drug-class specific. These findings consistently support the role of ACEI therapy in the management of CKD. It is customary to begin at low doses and increase the dose at 4-week intervals to control the level of proteinuria. The dose is usually increased until proteinuria is reduced by 30% to 50% or the development of side effects such as elevations in serum creatinine or potassium occurs.

A meta-analysis that pooled several of the small and large randomized, controlled studies showed beneficial effects of ACEI therapy on diabetic nephropathy.[143] Progression to proteinuria was reduced by 65% in patients with diabetes mellitus and microalbuminuria, and progression of nephropathy (doubling of serum creatinine) was reduced by 40% in patients with overt proteinuria (comprised of 30% diabetics and 70% nondiabetics; Fig. 46–3).[143] However, a recent meta-analysis of 127 studies with more than 30,000 subjects suggests that the benefit of ACEIs and ARBs over other pharmacologic agents is related to blood pressure attained during the study rather than to special properties of the ACEI or ARB (e.g., antiproteinuric effects).[144]

Some of the discrepancy in these results may be due to aldosterone escape in renin–angiotensin–aldosterone system blockade. Type 2 diabetic subjects with nephropathy who had increased aldosterone plasma levels during a mean 35-month treatment with losartan had a faster decline in the rate of GFR compared to those without aldosterone escape.[145] Combination therapy of ACEI and ARBs or addition of an aldosterone inhibitor to ACEI or ARB was recently suggested to improve suppression of the renin–angiotensin–aldosterone system.[146] Another study exploring the addition of an aldosterone receptor blocker to ACEI or ARB for renoprotection in type 1 diabetes was recently published.[147] This study, conducted in 20 patients with proteinuria, showed a reduction in albuminuria by 30% with a significant daytime reduction of blood pressure in patients treated with spironolactone 25 mg once daily. The results are intriguing and need to be confirmed with larger numbers of patients with close monitoring for complications such as hyperkalemia.

The ARBs have also been shown to slow the progression of diabetic kidney disease.[131–134] Table 46–5 summarizes data from several studies (with at least 100 patients) evaluating ARB efficacy in type 2 diabetes. All patients in these trials had at least a level of proteinuria consistent with microalbuminuria and all were hypertensive. With the exception of one, the studies were of a sufficiently long duration to determine the beneficial effects of ARBs on nephropathy. Of note, the beneficial effect of delaying the onset of diabetic nephropathy was significant in type 2 diabetic patients who received irbesartan 300 mg daily for up to 2 years.[133] A similar trend (although not statistically significant) was observed in those subjects who received a lower dose of irbesartan (150 mg daily). The Evaluation of Losartan in the Elderly (ELITE) study, which assessed losartan versus captopril in diabetics and nondiabetics, showed comparable renal benefits of both ARBs and ACEIs in a population of heart failure patients.[148] Currently, the data show efficacy of both ACEIs and ARBs in type 2 diabetes, whereas only ACEIs have been adequately evaluated in patients with type 1 diabetes. Thus, until head-to-head trials with these agents are assessed, they should not be considered interchangeable in all forms of diabetes.[149]

Because ACEIs and ARBs have demonstrated efficacy in patients with diabetes, the possibility of using both agents in type 2 diabetics has been investigated.[150] A short-term (12 to 24 week) study evaluated lisinopril (20 mg once daily) and candesartan (16 mg once daily) versus the combination in 199 patients. The reduction of urinary albumin-to-creatinine ratios was greater with combination therapy (50%) than with either lisinopril (39%) or candesartan (24%) alone. However, blood pressure reduction was also significantly greater in the combination therapy patients, making it unclear if the combination produced an enhanced antiproteinuric effect or if the reduction in the albumin-to-creatinine ratio could be attributable to the greater reduction in blood pressure.[150]

Studies suggest that no individual ACEI drug is superior to any other ACEI.[143] In patients with hypertension, the primary goal is to optimally treat the blood pressure to target, and the secondary goal is to control proteinuria. For normotensive patients with microalbuminuria, one should titrate the ACEI to reduce the degree of microalbuminuria. The antihypertensive ceiling effect noted for ACEI dosage titration has not been confirmed for lowering urinary protein excretion. However, patients with hypertension and proteinuria can still exhibit side effects associated with blood pressure lowering, and hence dosages should be titrated to the maximal level of proteinuria reduction without reducing the blood pressure to a level associated with adverse events including renal function compromise. Patients should be initiated on the lowest possible dose of ACEI and titrated to blood pressure control and proteinuria reduction. A specific recommendation regarding the dose to initiate therapy with a specific ACEI has not been established; consequently, the lowest recommended dose for the management of hypertension may be appropriate until such information is available. The clinician needs to evaluate the insurance coverage of specific agents in specific patients. In addition, one needs to consider the presence of other concomitant diseases and past history of treatment, as well as any side effects demonstrated with particular agents. Generally, ACEIs are more cost-effective than ARBs because of the availability of generic formulations. If and when patients exhibit adverse effects such as cough and/or hyperkalemia, a switch to an ARB is appropriate.

Because the clearance of all ACEIs (with the exception of fosinopril) is reduced in CKD, it is prudent to commence therapy at lower initial doses and subsequently titrate to achieve the optimal therapeutic effects and minimize potential toxicity.[151] The antiproteinuric effects of ACEIs are not necessarily attained at the same doses as the antihypertensive effects. Thus patients who have reached their blood pressure goals may require further dosage adjustments to achieve maximal reductions in urinary protein excretion. Serum potassium needs to be monitored when initiating therapy with ACEIs, especially when patients are concurrently receiving drugs that may increase the risk of hyperkalemia, such as nonsteroidal antiinflammatory agents. Chapter 15 has a thorough discussion of dose, dose titration, monitoring, and adverse effects of ACEIs and ARBs.

Some calcium channel blockers (CCBs) decrease glomerular injury without negatively changing renal hemodynamics.[138] The postulated mechanisms for this decrease in renal injury include suppression of glomerular hypertrophy, inhibition of platelet aggregation, and decreased salt accumulation.[138] Although the data regarding dihydropyridine calcium channel blockers do not suggest any beneficial effects beyond those attributable to reducing blood pressure, there is some suggestion that the nondihydropyridine agents (diltiazem and verapamil) may have beneficial effects on proteinuria that are similar to those of ACEIs.[152–154] A few studies suggest that the efficacy of combination therapy with ACEIs and nondihydropyridine CCBs may be superior in terms of proteinuria reduction than the use of either agent alone.[155] Most clinicians, however, tend to use the combination of ACEI plus ARBs instead of either of the former agents plus a nondihydropyridine CCB. In general, nondihydropyridine CCBs are used as second-line antiproteinuric drugs when ACEIs or ARBs are not tolerated.

CLINICAL CONTROVERSY

Some clinicians believe that combinations of ACEI and ARB medications or ACEI and nondihydropyridine calcium channel blockers are additive in terms of reductions in proteinuria reduction over single therapy, whereas others believe that single-agent therapy with ACEI or ARB is adequate.

Nondiabetic Chronic Kidney Disease

■ ANTIHYPERTENSIVE AGENTS

❾ Reduction of blood pressure is key to decreasing cardiovascular and renal sequelae. However, all antihypertensive agents are not equal in their ability to preserve kidney function despite similar efficacy in terms of blood pressure reduction. Among the different antihypertensives available, ACEIs and ARBs are currently considered the first choice in patients with CKD because they reduce intraglomerular pressure. Several short- and long-term clinical trials have assessed the effect of ACEIs on renal function in patients without diabetes; Table 46–7 summarizes these trials.[142,156–159] These studies vary in length from 12 weeks to 7 years, and several enrolled a small number of subjects. Most patients had nephropathy associated with proteinuria and advanced CKD. Significant reductions in the risk of doubling serum creatinine, requirement for dialysis, and/or proteinuria were demonstrated for patients receiving the ACEIs. In one study, ramipril (1.25 to 5 mg daily) reduced proteinuria and the rate of GFR decline to a greater extent than that expected from blood pressure reduction alone.[142] The proteinuria reduction was greatest in those patients with the highest baseline levels of proteinuria. A limitation of this study was that the additional antihypertensive agents that were administered to study participants were not specified. A subsequent study in patients with mean proteinuria of 3 g/day showed that the relative risk of developing ESRD was 2.3 times higher in the conventional therapy plus placebo arm as compared to the conventional therapy plus ramipril arm.[159] These studies and the summary results of a meta-analysis revealed that ACEIs conferred a 40% reduction in the risk of developing ESRD or doubling of serum creatinine in patients with overt proteinuria (>300 mg protein/24 hours) and renal disease of various etiologies; see Fig. 46–3).[143] However, a recent meta-analysis failed to show a significant benefit of ACEI and/or ARBs over other antihypertensive agents in CKD progression.[144] A post hoc analysis of the African American Study of Kidney Disease and Hypertension (AASK), which evaluated two different blood pressure targets and three different treatment regimens in subjects with a GFR between 20 and 65 mL/min per 1.73 m^2, showed that the change in the level of proteinuria over 6 months of treatment predicted the progression of hypertensive CKD.[160] In addition, a post hoc analysis of the Antihypertensive and Lipid-Lowering Treatment to Prevent Heart Attack Trial (ALLHAT), where hypertensive subjects were randomized to chlorthalidone, amlodipine, or lisinopril for a mean of 4.9 years, revealed similar incident rates of ESRD in the three treatment groups irrespective of the cause of renal disease.[161] Therefore, although the drug class versus absolute blood pressure reduction is an evolving area of investigation, current treatment guidelines recommend use of ACEI or ARBs in subjects with CKD.

The ARBs, although evaluated to a lesser extent than ACEIs, appear to have similar efficacy in terms of kidney protection in patients with

TABLE 46-7 Summary of Studies with Angiotensin-Converting Enzyme Inhibitors in Patients without Diabetes

Drug, Dose, and Study Design	Baseline Characteristics	Number of Subjects and Disease	Duration	Outcomes	Reference and Study Name
Benazepril 10 mg once daily; randomized, placebo-controlled trial	Mild (46–60 mL/min GFR) and moderate (30–45 mL/min GFR) renal insufficiency	583 Patients with various renal disorders including diabetes mellitus	3 years	Benazepril afforded a 53% risk reduction in primary end point of doubling of S_{cr} or requirement for dialysis; 71% and 46% risk reductions in the mild and moderate renal insufficiency groups, respectively	Maschio et al.[156]
Ramipril 2.5 mg once daily and titrated to BP; randomized, placebo-controlled trial	GFR 20–70 mL/min per 1.73 m^2 UPE ≥1 g/day	352 Proteinuric patients	5 years	Rate of loss of GFR was 0.89 mL/min per month in placebo group versus 0.39 mL/min per month in ramipril group; twice the numbers of patients receiving placebo vs. ramipril reached primary composite end point of doubling of S_{cr} or ESRD	The GISEN Group[142]
Enalapril 20 mg once daily vs. losartan 50 mg once daily; randomized trial	Proteinuria	93 Hypertensives	12 weeks	UP:Cr was reduced by 43% in losartan group vs. 23% in enalapril group ($P = 0.05$)	Nielsen et al.[157]
Enalapril 5–40 mg daily vs. other antihypertensive agents; randomized, controlled trial	UPE ≥0.5 g/day S_{cr} ≥1.5 mg/dL	44 IgAN patients	7 years	Renal survival was significantly better in the enalapril group (100%) versus the other antihypertensive group (70%) after 4 years, and 92% vs. 55% respectively, after 7 years; proteinuria significantly decreased in the enalapril group, whereas it tended to increase in the control group	Praga et al.[158]
Ramipril 1.25–5 mg daily vs. conventional therapy; randomized controlled trial	Proteinuria 1–3 g/day	186 Chronic nephropathies	31 months	Progression to use ESRD was half as common in the ramipril group; patients with GFR ≤45 mL/min per 1.73 m^2 and proteinuria ≥1.5 g/24 hours had the greatest benefit from ramipril therapy	Ruggenenti et al.[159]

ESRD, end-stage renal disease; GFR, glomerular filtration rate; IgAN, immunoglobulin A nephropathy; S_{cr}, serum creatinine; UP:Cr, urinary protein-to-creatinine ratio; UPE, urinary protein excretion.

several forms of glomerulonephritis (Table 46–8).[162,163] Proteinuria reduction on the order of 25% to 47% was shown with ARB therapy. However, these studies employed small numbers of patients with short followup time frames as compared to studies in diabetic patients. Despite these limitations, most clinicians use either ACEI or ARB therapy as the standard of care in patients with nondiabetic CKD and proteinuria. The combination use of ARBs with ACEIs has been proposed and preliminary data suggest that this approach is safe and results in a greater decrease in proteinuria than that seen with either agent alone.[164] A recent study prospectively evaluated the use of losartan 100 mg daily alone, trandolapril 3 mg daily alone, or the combination of the two in 336 patients with nondiabetic kidney diseases. The primary end point, time to doubling of serum creatinine or ESRD, was observed in 11% of combination therapy patients and in 23% of each of the single-agent treatment groups.[165] The selection of ACEIs versus ARBs in the control of proteinuria in nondiabetic kidney disease is essentially predicated on cost of therapy, patient tolerance, and clinician preference.

The CCBs are also effective treatments for hypertension in patients with nondiabetic CKD. However, as was mentioned previously, only the nondihydropyridine CCBs have been studied and shown to reduce the rate of decline of kidney function.[152,166] There are currently no data to suggest that higher doses of nondihydropyridine CCBs are needed to elicit a reduction in proteinuria as compared to a reduction in blood pressure.

Although diuretics are commonly used to treat fluid overload and hypertension in patients with CKD, there are no compelling data to suggest any renal protection in terms of proteinuria regression or a reduction in the rate of progression. Chapter 52 addresses the use of diuretics for managing volume overload. Other available antihypertensive agents are used to control blood pressure in patients with kidney disease. Additional central and peripherally acting antihy-

TABLE 46-8 Summary of Studies with Angiotensin Receptor Blockers in Patients without Diabetes

Drug, Dose, and Study Design	Baseline Characteristics	Number of Subjects and Disease	Duration	Outcomes	Reference
Losartan 50 mg once daily vs. control	Normotensive, proteinuria	23 FSGS patients	1 year	Proteinuria decreased 47% in the losartan group at 1 year, while there was a significant increase in proteinuria in the control group; total serum protein and albumin concentrations also increased in the losartan group; cholesterol levels of the losartan group were significantly reduced	Usta et al.[162]
Losartan 25 mg once daily vs. enalapril 10 mg once daily; randomized, controlled trial	GFR 36–93 mL/min	34 Primary glomerulonephritis	3 months	Proteinuria reduced 25% vs. 45% in losartan and enalapril groups, respectively; significant decline in GFR in enalapril group and no change in losartan group	Tylicki et al.[163]

FSGS, focal segmental glomerulosclerosis; GFR, glomerular filtration rate; UPE, urinary protein excretion.

pertensive agents can be used in patients with CKD. One must consider the need for dosage reductions caused by reductions in GFR for drugs that are excreted by the kidneys and/or supplemental doses as a consequence of dialysis removal of hydrophilic β-blockers such as nadolol, acebutolol, and atenolol.

Regardless of the treatment regimen, hypertension should be treated to the currently accepted targets in patients with CKD. If proteinuria is present, the use of ACEIs, ARBs, and possibly nondihydropyridine CCBs may be superior to conventional agents in decreasing proteinuria and glomerular hypertension.

As precipitous reductions in blood pressure may be deleterious to kidney function in patients with underlying CKD, blood pressure targets in these patients should be achieved over several weeks to allow the kidney to adapt to reduced perfusion pressures.[135] Typically there is an acute but sustained reduction in GFR of approximately 25% to 30% within 3 to 7 days after initiation of ACEI therapy as a result of a reduction in intraglomerular pressure.[167] If a sustained increase in the serum creatinine by more than 30% after ACEI therapy initiation is observed, ACEI therapy discontinuation should be strongly considered (see Chap 49). It is necessary to realize that although ACEI therapy may be effective in reducing the rate of nephropathy progression, one needs to consider their propensity for hyperkalemia and potential for acute GFR reduction especially in patients who already have compromised GFR.

CLINICAL CONTROVERSY

Some clinicians fail to prescribe ACEI or ARB medications when the GFR is less than 20 to 30 mL/min per 1.73 m^2 because of fear of the patient developing a further elevation in serum creatinine, whereas other clinicians prescribe these medications and just evaluate serum creatinine closely after therapy initiation and dosage increases.

OTHER INTERVENTIONS TO LIMIT DISEASE PROGRESSION

⑩ Other interventions such as lipid-lowering regimens, smoking cessation, and anemia management may also slow the progression of CKD.

HYPERLIPIDEMIA TREATMENT

Although several drugs are available for lipid lowering, the β-hydroxy-β-methylglutaryl coenzyme A (HMG-CoA) reductase inhibitors and gemfibrozil have been most often used in dyslipidemic patients with CKD with and without proteinuria.[80] The primary goal of treatment is to adequately treat hyperlipidemia so as to decrease the risk for progressive atherosclerotic cardiovascular disease. However, a meta-analysis of 13 studies of lipid-lowering agents showed a reduction in the rate of CKD progression by only 0.156-mL/min per month.[168] The mechanisms for this effect are unknown, but HMG-CoA may reduce monocyte infiltration, mesangial cell proliferation, mesangial matrix expansion, and tubulointerstitial inflammation and fibrosis.[169] Consequently, a secondary goal of lipid-lowering treatment is to reduce proteinuria and renal function decline. Additional therapies that show favorable benefits on lipids are carnitine, fish oil, low-molecular-weight heparins, and exercise.[170] The National Cholesterol Education Program III and NKF K/DOQI guidelines should be consulted for a thorough review of lipid reduction and cardiovascular disease in patients with CKD.[112,171]

SMOKING CESSATION

Although the adverse cardiovascular disease health risks of smoking are well documented, only recently have the adverse effects of smoking on the progression of CKD been recognized. Smoking is associated with an acute reduction in GFR, and increased heart rate and blood pressure, likely secondary to nicotine exposure. [172] Nicotine has also been associated with an increase in urinary albumin excretion.[69,172] Although the effectiveness of smoking cessation on limiting progressive CKD has not been prospectively evaluated, one study suggested that smoking cessation resulted in a protective effect against proteinuria and reduced GFR.[173] This later study showed that although current smokers had a significantly higher albumin excretion (and reduced GFR) versus nonsmokers, those patients who quit smoking had a statistical association with only microalbuminuria.[173] Based on the evolving data concerning the detrimental effects of smoking on the kidney, it is prudent to educate patients regarding this risk, and institute appropriate therapeutic options for smoking cessation as discussed in Chap. 69.

ANEMIA TREATMENT

Prolonged anemia is associated with left ventricular hypertrophy and heart failure. It has been suggested that anemia may increase the rate of CKD progression.[174] Researchers have coined the phrase "cardiorenal anemia syndrome" to describe the interrelationship between anemia, heart failure, and CKD.[174] It has been hypothesized that the treatment of heart failure and anemia may reduce the progression of both heart failure and CKD.[175,176]

A study in renal transplant recipients showed an absence of renal function decline in newly anemic patients who had erythropoietin therapy initiated and a reduction in the loss of further renal function in patients who had ongoing anemia for a short time period and subsequently received therapy with erythropoietin.[177] Longer renal graft survival in erythropoietin-treated patients was also reported. These data support further study of the potential role of anemia management in reducing CKD progression. Tissue hypoxia associated with anemia may be a stimulus for continued renal injury in those with stages 3 to 5 CKD. In addition, anemia-related alterations of renal sympathetic nerve activity and related increases in oxidative stress have been reported.[178] Chapter 47 discusses anemia as a complication of CKD.

PHARMACOECONOMIC CONSIDERATIONS

The financial and societal costs of the care of individuals with CKD are high, especially the care of those with ESRD—this population of beneficiaries comprises only 0.5% of the total Medicare population, yet accounts for 5% of all Medicare expenditures.[179] Annualized expenditures per beneficiary ranged from $36,000 for those 24 years of age and younger to $51,000 for those 75 years of age and older.[179] These costs for the care of advanced CKD are estimated to increase dramatically over the next decade, reaching an estimated $28 billion dollars by the year 2010 for Medicare alone.[180]

There have been a few evaluations of the potential pharmacoeconomic impact of screening for microalbuminuria and the subsequent initiation of various pharmacotherapeutic regimens in type 1 diabetic patients.[181,182] According to one study, the historical standard approach to proteinuria reduction was considered to be treatment with hydrochlorothiazide at the time of hypertension diagnosis, while the newer treatment approach assumed three different screening and treatment strategies with ACEIs. The results from this evaluation suggested that with early screening and treatment of persistent microalbuminuria with ACEIs, it is possible to realize a cost-effectiveness of $7,900 to $16,500 per year of life saved. This amount is similar to the cost-effectiveness associated with treating hypertension in the general population. A similar cost-effectiveness analysis using different strategies but the same basic model was also performed[182] and projected that treating all patients with an ACEI 5 years after the diagnosis of diabetes was as cost-

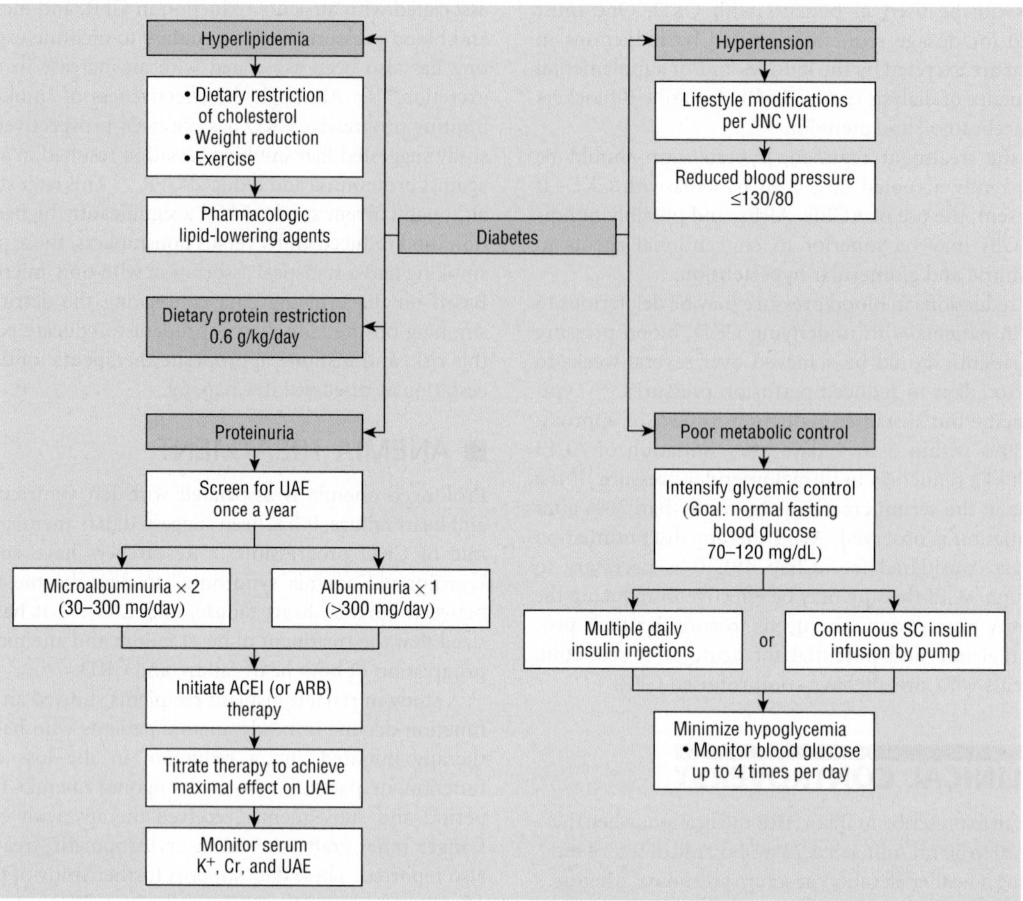

FIGURE 46-4. Therapeutic strategies to prevent progression of renal disease in diabetic individuals. (ACEI, angiotensin-converting enzyme inhibitor; ARB, angiotensin receptor blocker; JNC VII, the seventh report of the Joint National Committee on Prevention, Detection, Evaluation, and Treatment of High Blood Pressure; SC, subcutaneous; UAE, urinary albumin excretion.)

effective as annual screening for microalbuminuria beginning 5 years after diagnosis, with the initiation of an ACEI when and if persistent microalbuminuria was detected. The DCCT Research Group evaluated the cost-effectiveness of intensive insulin therapy as compared with conventional diabetes treatment.[183] The analysis demonstrated that implementing intensive insulin therapy would result in an incremental cost per year of life gained of $28,661, which represents a good value to the healthcare system. Overall, it appears that aggressive insulin therapy, as well as treatment with ACEIs when persistent microalbuminuria is identified, reduces complications and ultimately increases length of life at reasonable costs to society. The results of these simulated analyses remain to be prospectively confirmed.

The United Kingdom Prospective Diabetes Study also included a cost-effectiveness study that compared tight blood pressure control (ACEI and β-blocker therapy) with less-optimized control. The main outcomes included use of healthcare resources and the time free from diabetes-related end points. The investigators concluded that tight blood pressure control in patients with type 2 diabetes and hypertension produced a positive cost-effectiveness ratio as a result of reducing the cost of complications and increasing the interval without complications.[184] Another study concluded that all middle-aged patients with newly diagnosed type 2 diabetes should be treated with an ACEI rather than be screened for microalbuminuria and then treated.[185] That study determined that this treatment method would provide additional benefit with only a modest increase in cost.

CONCLUSIONS

DIABETICS

Based on the available clinical and experimental data, pharmacologic interventions can help to limit the progression of CKD in diabetic patients. Figure 46–4 summarizes these interventions. All patients with type 1 diabetes of more than 5 years' duration and all type 2 diabetics should be screened yearly for microalbuminuria (urinary albumin excretion or urinary albumin-to-creatinine ratio).[120] Blood glucose should be maintained within or close to the normal range by frequent insulin doses or by using a continuous subcutaneous insulin infusion, while minimizing the risk of hypoglycemia by frequent blood glucose monitoring.[120] ACEI therapy should be initiated in normotensive and hypertensive type 1 or type 2 diabetic patients with persistent microalbuminuria (30 to 300 mg/day) or overt albuminuria (>300 mg/day). ACEIs should be titrated every 1 to 3 months to achieve a maximal reduction in urinary albumin excretion. Within 1 week of initiating or increasing the dose of an ACEI, serum creatinine and potassium should be evaluated to detect abrupt reductions in GFR or development of hyperkalemia. ARBs should be considered as another first-line therapy in type 2 diabetic patients for the reduction of persistent proteinuria or albuminuria. A nondihydropyridine CCB may be an effective secondary alternative agent in patients who are unable to tolerate either an ACEI or an ARB. A combination of an ACEI with

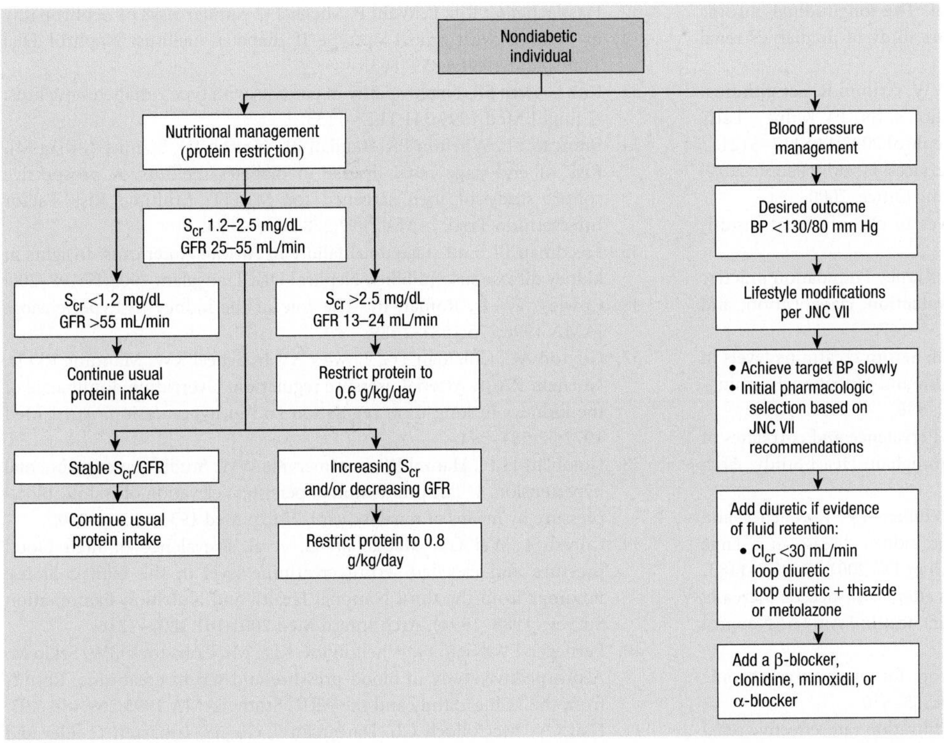

FIGURE 46-5. Therapeutic strategies to prevent progression of renal disease in nondiabetic individuals. ACEI, angiotensin-converting enzyme inhibitor; ARB, angiotensin receptor blocker; BP, blood pressure; GFR, glomerular filtration rate; CL_{cr}, creatinine clearance; MAP, mean arterial pressure; S_{cr}, serum creatinine.

an ARB may result in a greater reduction in proteinuria or albuminuria than either agent alone, and thus may be a therapeutic alternative in patients who are not maximally responding to single-agent therapy. Addition of an aldosterone receptor blocker may be considered in subjects with documented aldosterone escape.

NONDIABETIC PATIENTS

Figure 46–5 summarizes therapeutic interventions for nondiabetic patients with CKD. Nutritional management should be monitored frequently, regardless of the amount of protein intake prescribed, to avoid malnutrition. Based on the results of the MDRD study, a low-protein diet is of variable benefit in patients with moderate kidney dysfunction (GFR 25 to 55 mL/min per 1.73 m^2). Thus it is probably reasonable to prescribe a standard-protein diet unless the patient develops rapid progression of their kidney disease.[186] For patients with severe kidney dysfunction, as defined by the MDRD study as a GFR of 13 to 24 mL/min per 1.73 m^2, a low-protein diet of 0.6 g/kg per day may reduce the rate of decline in kidney function, time to reach end-stage kidney disease, and onset of uremic symptoms.[115]

Blood pressure control should target normotensive levels of <130/80 mm Hg in patients with CKD.[120,187] In patients with proteinuria above 3 g/day and CKD, an ACEI or ARB is still considered to be first-line therapy. Hyperlipidemia should also be treated to decrease cardiovascular risks and the suggested association between lipid abnormalities and CKD progression.

As kidney function decreases and subjects approach CKD stage 4, the patient should begin to get prepared for renal-replacement therapy. Hemodialysis, peritoneal dialysis, and renal transplantation need to be discussed (see Chaps. 48 and 92). Early referral to a nephrologist or other clinician specializing in the care of patients with progressive CKD may allow the proper dialysis vascular access placement, evaluation for uremia symptoms, and may allow for identification and treatment of the complications including anemia, and metabolic abnormalities.[188]

ABBREVIATIONS

ACEI: angiotensin-converting enzyme inhibitor

ARB: angiotensin receptor blocker

CCB: calcium channel blocker

CKD: chronic kidney disease

DCCT: Diabetes Control and Complications Trial

ESRD: end-stage renal disease

GFR: glomerular filtration rate

HMG-CoA: β-hydroxy-β-methylglutaryl coenzyme A (reductase)

IIT: intensive insulin therapy

K/DOQI: Kidney Dialysis Outcomes and Quality Initiative

MAP: mean arterial blood pressure

MDRD: Modification of Diet in Renal Disease

NHANES III: Third National Health and Nutritional Examination Survey

USRDS: United States Renal Data System

REFERENCES

1. K/DOQI clinical practice guidelines for chronic kidney disease: Evaluation, classification, and stratification. Kidney Disease Outcome Quality Initiative. Am J Kidney Dis 2002;39:S1–S246.
2. USRDS. USRDS 2007 Annual Data Report. Bethesda, MD: National Institutes of Health, National Institute of Diabetes and Digestive and Kidney Disease, 2007.
3. 2003, *http://www.nih.gov/news/pr/jav2006/niddk-24.htm.*
4. Gassman JJ, Greene T, Wright JT, Jr, et al. Design and statistical aspects of the African American Study of Kidney Disease and Hypertension (AASK). J Am Soc Nephrol 2003;14:S154–S165.
5. Feldman HI, Appel LJ, Chertow GM, et al. The Chronic Renal Insufficiency Cohort (CRIC) Study: Design and methods. J Am Soc Nephrol 2003;14:S148–S153.

6. Perlman RL, Kiser M, Finkelstein F, et al. The longitudinal chronic kidney disease study: A prospective cohort study of predialysis renal failure. Semin Dial 2003;16:418–423.
7. Ohmit SE, Flack JM, Peters RM, Brown WW, Grimm R. Longitudinal Study of the National Kidney Foundation's (NKF) Kidney Early Evaluation Program (KEEP). J Am Soc Nephrol 2003;14:S117–S121.
8. U.S. Department of Health and Human Services. Healthy People 2010. Washington, DC: U.S. Government Printing Office, 2000.
9. Pereira BJ. Introduction: New perspectives in chronic renal insufficiency. Am J Kidney Dis 2000;36:S1–S3.
10. Levey AS, Coresh J, Balk E, et al. National Kidney Foundation practice guidelines for chronic kidney disease: Evaluation, classification, and stratification. Ann Intern Med 2003;139:137–147.
11. Jones CA, McQuillan GM, Kusek JW, et al. Serum creatinine levels in the U.S. population: Third National Health and Nutrition Examination Survey. Am J Kidney Dis 1998;32:992–999.
12. Culleton BF, Larson MG, Evans JC, et al. Prevalence and correlates of elevated serum creatinine levels: The Framingham Heart Study. Arch Intern Med 1999;159:1785–1790.
13. Nissenson AR, Pereira BJ, Collins AJ, Steinberg EP. Prevalence and characteristics of individuals with chronic kidney disease in a large health maintenance organization. Am J Kidney Dis 2001;37:1177–1183.
14. Ruggenenti P RG. Kidney failure stabilizes after a two-decade increase: Impact on global (renal and cardiovascular) health. J Am Soc Nephrol 2007;2:146–150.
15. McClellan WM, Flanders WD. Risk factors for progressive chronic kidney disease. J Am Soc Nephrol 2003;14:S65–S70.
16. Davies DR SN. Age changes in glomerular filtration rate, effective renal plasma flow, and tubular excretory capacity in adult males. J Clin Invest 1950;29:496–507.
17. Lindeman RD, Tobin J, Shock NW. Longitudinal studies on the rate of decline in renal function with age. J Am Geriatr Soc 1985;33:278–285.
18. Rowe JW, Andres R, Tobin JD, Norris AH, Shock NW. The effect of age on creatinine clearance in men: A cross-sectional and longitudinal study. J Gerontol 1976;31:155–163.
19. Byrne C, Nedelman J, Luke RG. Race, socioeconomic status, and the development of end-stage renal disease. Am J Kidney Dis 1994;23:16–22.
20. Perneger TV, Whelton PK, Klag MJ. Race and end-stage renal disease. Socioeconomic status and access to health care as mediating factors. Arch Intern Med 1995;155:1201–1208.
21. Tierney WM, Harris LE, Copley JB, Luft FC. Effect of hypertension and type II diabetes on renal function in an urban population. Am J Hypertens 1990;3:69–75.
22. Rostand SG. US minority groups and end-stage renal disease: A disproportionate share. Am J Kidney Dis 1992;19:411–413.
23. Perry HM Jr, Miller JP, Fornoff JR, et al. Early predictors of 15-year end-stage renal disease in hypertensive patients. Hypertension 1995;25:587–594.
24. Lackland DT, Bendall HE, Osmond C, Egan BM, Barker DJ. Low birth weights contribute to high rates of early-onset chronic renal failure in the Southeastern United States. Arch Intern Med 2000;160:1472–1476.
25. Freedman BI, Bowden DW, Rich SS, Appel RG. Genetic initiation of hypertensive and diabetic nephropathy. Am J Hypertens 1998;11:251–257.
26. Genetic determinants of diabetic nephropathy: The family investigation of nephropathy and diabetes (FIND). J Am Soc Nephrol 2003;14:S202–S204.
27. Kshirsagar AV, Elter J., Beck J, Offenbacher S, Coresh J, Falk R. Periodontal disease is associated with moderate renal insufficiency in a general population sample [abstract]. J Am Soc Nephrol 2001;12:218.
28. Erlinger TP, Tarver-Carr ME, Powe NR, et al. Leukocytosis, hypoalbuminemia, and the risk for chronic kidney disease in U.S. adults. Am J Kidney Dis 2003;42:256–263.
29. Muntner P, Coresh J, Smith JC, Eckfeldt J, Klag MJ. Plasma lipids and risk of developing renal dysfunction: The atherosclerosis risk in communities study. Kidney Int 2000;58:293–301.
30. Schaeffner ES, Kurth T, Curhan GC, et al. Cholesterol and the risk of renal dysfunction in apparently healthy men. J Am Soc Nephrol 2003;14:2084–2091.
31. Favre L, Glasson P, Vallotton MB. Reversible acute renal failure from combined triamterene and indomethacin: A study in healthy subjects. Ann Intern Med 1982;96:317–320.
32. Hasslacher C, Ritz E, Wahl P, Michael C. Similar risks of nephropathy in patients with type I or type II diabetes mellitus. Nephrol Dial Transplant 1989;4:859–863.
33. Ritz E, Orth SR. Nephropathy in patients with type 2 diabetes mellitus. N Engl J Med 1999;341:1127–1133.
34. Brancati FL, Whelton PK, Randall BL, Neaton JD, Stamler J, Klag MJ. Risk of end-stage renal disease in diabetes mellitus: A prospective cohort study of men screened for MRFIT. Multiple Risk Factor Intervention Trial. JAMA 1997;278:2069–2074.
35. Freedman BI. End-stage renal failure in African Americans: Insights in kidney disease susceptibility. Nephrol Dial Transplant 2002;17:198–200.
36. Cowley AW Jr, Roman RJ. The role of the kidney in hypertension. JAMA 1996;275:1581–1589.
37. Guyton AC, Coleman TG, Cowley AV Jr, Scheel KW, Manning RD Jr, Norman RA Jr. Arterial pressure regulation. Overriding dominance of the kidneys in long-term regulation and in hypertension. Am J Med 1972;52:584–594.
38. Goldblatt H LJ, Hanzal RF, Summerville WW. Studies on experimental hypertension. 1. The production of persistent elevation of systolic blood pressure by means of renal ischemia. J Exp Med 1934;59:347–379.
39. Coresh J, Wei GL, McQuillan G, et al. Prevalence of high blood pressure and elevated serum creatinine level in the United States: Findings from the third National Health and Nutrition Examination Survey (1988–1994). Arch Intern Med 2001;161:1207–1216.
40. Perneger TV, Nieto FJ, Whelton PK, Klag MJ, Comstock GW, Szklo M. A prospective study of blood pressure and serum creatinine. Results from the "Clue" Study and the ARIC Study. JAMA 1993;269:488–493.
41. Hsu CY, McCulloch CE, Darbinian J, Go AS, Iribarren C. Elevated blood pressure and risk of end-stage renal disease in subjects without baseline kidney disease. Arch Intern Med 2005;165:923–928.
42. Klag MJ, Whelton PK, Randall BL, et al. Blood pressure and end-stage renal disease in men. N Engl J Med 1996;334:13–18.
43. Rekola S, Bergstrand A, Bucht H. Deterioration of GFR in IgA nephropathy as measured by ^{51}Cr-EDTA clearance. Kidney Int 1991;40:1050–1054.
44. Pei Y, Cattran D, Greenwood C. Predicting chronic renal insufficiency in idiopathic membranous glomerulonephritis. Kidney Int 1992;42:960–966.
45. Hannedouche T, Chauveau P, Kalou F, Albouze G, Lacour B, Jungers P. Factors affecting progression in advanced chronic renal failure. Clin Nephrol 1993;39:312–320.
46. Massy ZA, Khoa TN, Lacour B, Descamps-Latscha B, Man NK, Jungers P. Dyslipidaemia and the progression of renal disease in chronic renal failure patients. Nephrol Dial Transplant 1999;14:2392–2397.
47. Viberti GC, Hill RD, Jarrett RJ, Argyropoulos A, Mahmud U, Keen H. Microalbuminuria as a predictor of clinical nephropathy in insulin-dependent diabetes mellitus. Lancet 1982;1:1430–1432.
48. Mogensen CE, Christensen CK. Predicting diabetic nephropathy in insulin-dependent patients. N Engl J Med 1984;311:89–93.
49. Wirta O, Pasternack A, Mustonen J, Oksa H, Koivula T, Helin H. Albumin excretion rate and its relation to kidney disease in non-insulin-dependent diabetes mellitus. J Intern Med 1995;237:367–373.
50. Keane WF, Brenner BM, de Zeeuw D, et al. The risk of developing end-stage renal disease in patients with type 2 diabetes and nephropathy: The RENAAL study. Kidney Int 2003;63:1499–1507.
51. Klahr S, Levey AS, Beck GJ, et al. The effects of dietary protein restriction and blood-pressure control on the progression of chronic renal disease. Modification of Diet in Renal Disease Study Group. N Engl J Med 1994;330:877–884.
52. Jafar TH, Stark PC, Schmid CH, et al. Proteinuria as a modifiable risk factor for the progression of non-diabetic renal disease. Kidney Int 2001;60:1131–1140.
53. Keane WF. Proteinuria: Its clinical importance and role in progressive renal disease. Am J Kidney Dis 2000;35:S97–S105.
54. Jafar TH, Stark PC, Schmid CH, et al. Progression of chronic kidney disease: The role of blood pressure control, proteinuria, and angiotensin-converting enzyme inhibition: A patient-level meta-analysis. Ann Intern Med 2003;139:244–252.
55. Intensive blood-glucose control with sulphonylureas or insulin compared with conventional treatment and risk of complications in patients with type 2 diabetes (UKPDS 33). UK Prospective Diabetes Study (UKPDS) Group. Lancet 1998;352:837–853.

56. Effect of intensive blood-glucose control with metformin on complications in overweight patients with type 2 diabetes (UKPDS 34). UK Prospective Diabetes Study (UKPDS) Group. Lancet 1998;352:854–865.
57. Bakris GL. Treatment of stage I hypertension and development of renal dysfunction. J Hum Hypertens 2001;15:81–84.
58. Tight blood pressure control and risk of macrovascular and microvascular complications in type 2 diabetes: UKPDS 38. UK Prospective Diabetes Study Group. BMJ 1998;317:703–713.
59. Efficacy of atenolol and captopril in reducing risk of macrovascular and microvascular complications in type 2 diabetes: UKPDS 39. UK Prospective Diabetes Study Group. BMJ 1998;317:713–720.
60. Bakris GL. A practical approach to achieving recommended blood pressure goals in diabetic patients. Arch Intern Med 2001;161:2661–2667.
61. Sarnak MJ, Greene T, Wang X, et al. The effect of a lower target blood pressure on the progression of kidney disease: Long-term follow-up of the modification of diet in renal disease study. Ann Intern Med 2005;142:342–351.
62. Reichard P, Nilsson BY, Rosenqvist U. The effect of long-term intensified insulin treatment on the development of microvascular complications of diabetes mellitus. N Engl J Med 1993;329:304–309.
63. The effect of intensive treatment of diabetes on the development and progression of long-term complications in insulin-dependent diabetes mellitus. The Diabetes Control and Complications Trial Research Group. N Engl J Med 1993;329:977–986.
64. Sustained effect of intensive treatment of type 1 diabetes mellitus on development and progression of diabetic nephropathy: The Epidemiology of Diabetes Interventions and Complications (EDIC) study. JAMA 2003;290:2159–2167.
65. Muhlhauser I, Bender R, Bott U, et al. Cigarette smoking and progression of retinopathy and nephropathy in type 1 diabetes. Diabet Med 1996;13:536–543.
66. Orth SR, Ritz E, Schrier RW. The renal risks of smoking. Kidney Int 1997;51:1669–1677.
67. Holl RW, Grabert M, Heinze E, Debatin KM. Objective assessment of smoking habits by urinary cotinine measurement in adolescents and young adults with type 1 diabetes. Reliability of reported cigarette consumption and relationship to urinary albumin excretion. Diabetes Care 1998;21:787–791.
68. Ejerblad E, Fored CM, Lindblad P, et al. Association between smoking and chronic renal failure in a nationwide population-based case-control study. J Am Soc Nephrol 2004;15:2178–2185.
69. Ritz E, Benck U, Franek E, Keller C, Seyfarth M, Clorius J. Effects of smoking on renal hemodynamics in healthy volunteers and in patients with glomerular disease. J Am Soc Nephrol 1998;9:1798–1804.
70. Sawicki PT, Didjurgeit U, Muhlhauser I, Bender R, Heinemann L, Berger M. Smoking is associated with progression of diabetic nephropathy. Diabetes Care 1994;17:126–131.
71. Regalado M, Yang S, Wesson DE. Cigarette smoking is associated with augmented progression of renal insufficiency in severe essential hypertension. Am J Kidney Dis 2000;35:687–694.
72. Bakris G, Rahman M, Lea J, Ward H, Massry S, Wang S, and the AASK Study Group. Associations between cardiovascular risk factors and glomerular filtration rate at baseline in the African American Study of Kidney Disease (AASK) trial. J Am Soc Nephrol 1998;10:A0717.
73. Whelton PK. The evolving epidemic of cardiovascular and renal diseases: A worldwide challenge. Curr Opin Nephrol Hypertens 1995;4:215–217.
74. Haroun MK, Jaar BG, Hoffman SC, Comstock GW, Klag MJ, Coresh J. Risk factors for chronic kidney disease: A prospective study of 23,534 men and women in Washington County, Maryland. J Am Soc Nephrol 2003;14:2934–2941.
75. Goetz FC, Jacobs DR Jr, Chavers B, Roel J, Yelle M, Sprafka JM. Risk factors for kidney damage in the adult population of Wadena, Minnesota. A prospective study. Am J Epidemiol 1997;145:91–102.
76. Orth SR, Stockmann A, Conradt C, et al. Smoking as a risk factor for end-stage renal failure in men with primary renal disease. Kidney Int 1998;54:926–931.
77. Chapman AB, Johnson AM, Gabow PA, Schrier RW. Overt proteinuria and microalbuminuria in autosomal dominant polycystic kidney disease. J Am Soc Nephrol 1994;5:1349–1354.
78. Fox CS, Larson MG, Leip EP, Culleton B, Wilson PW, Levy D. Predictors of new-onset kidney disease in a community-based population. JAMA 2004;291:844–850.
79. Cases A, Coll E. Dyslipidemia and the progression of renal disease in chronic renal failure patients. Kidney Int Suppl 2005:S87–S93.
80. Kasiske BL. Hyperlipidemia in patients with chronic renal disease. Am J Kidney Dis 1998;32:S142–S156.
81. Walker WG. Relation of lipid abnormalities to progression of renal damage in essential hypertension, insulin-dependent and non insulin-dependent diabetes mellitus. Miner Electrolyte Metab 1993;19:137–143.
82. Hsu CY, McCulloch CE, Iribarren C, Darbinian J, Go AS. Body mass index and risk for end-stage renal disease. Ann Intern Med 2006;144:21–28.
83. Iseki K, Ikemiya Y, Kinjo K, Inoue T, Iseki C, Takishita S. Body mass index and the risk of development of end-stage renal disease in a screened cohort. Kidney Int 2004;65:1870–1876.
84. Ejerblad E, Fored CM, Lindblad P, Fryzek J, McLaughlin JK, Nyren O. Obesity and risk for chronic renal failure. J Am Soc Nephrol 2006;17:1695–1702.
85. Lin JL, Lin-Tan DT, Hsu KH, Yu CC. Environmental lead exposure and progression of chronic renal diseases in patients without diabetes. N Engl J Med 2003;348:277–286.
86. Vupputuri S, Batuman V, Muntner P, et al. The risk for mild kidney function decline associated with illicit drug use among hypertensive men. Am J Kidney Dis 2004;43:629–635.
87. Hsu CC, Kao WH, Coresh J, et al. Apolipoprotein E and progression of chronic kidney disease. JAMA 2005;293:2892–2899.
88. Remuzzi G, Bertani T. Pathophysiology of progressive nephropathies. N Engl J Med 1998;339:1448–1456.
89. Remuzzi G, Ruggenenti P, Perico N. Chronic renal diseases: Renoprotective benefits of renin-angiotensin system inhibition. Ann Intern Med 2002;136:604–615.
90. Platt R. Structural and functional adaptation in renal failure. Br Med J 1952;1:1372–1377.
91. Hostetter TH, Olson JL, Rennke HG, Venkatachalam MA, Brenner BM. Hyperfiltration in remnant nephrons: A potentially adverse response to renal ablation. Am J Physiol 1981;241:F85–F93.
92. Brenner BM, Meyer TW, Hostetter TH. Dietary protein intake and the progressive nature of kidney disease: The role of hemodynamically mediated glomerular injury in the pathogenesis of progressive glomerular sclerosis in aging, renal ablation, and intrinsic renal disease. N Engl J Med 1982;307:652–659.
93. Yoshioka T, Mitarai T, Kon V, Deen WM, Rennke HG, Ichikawa I. Role for angiotensin II in an overt functional proteinuria. Kidney Int 1986;30:538–545.
94. Yoshioka T, Rennke HG, Salant DJ, Deen WM, Ichikawa I. Role of abnormally high transmural pressure in the permselectivity defect of glomerular capillary wall: A study in early passive Heymann nephritis. Circ Res 1987;61:531–538.
95. Aros C, Remuzzi G. The renin-angiotensin system in progression, remission and regression of chronic nephropathies. J Hypertens Suppl 2002;20:S45–S53.
96. Park CH, Maack T. Albumin absorption and catabolism by isolated perfused proximal convoluted tubules of the rabbit. J Clin Invest 1984;73:767–777.
97. Zoja C, Morigi M, Figliuzzi M, et al. Proximal tubular cell synthesis and secretion of endothelin-1 on challenge with albumin and other proteins. Am J Kidney Dis 1995;26:934–941.
98. Wang Y, Chen J, Chen L, Tay YC, Rangan GK, Harris DC. Induction of monocyte chemoattractant protein-1 in proximal tubule cells by urinary protein. J Am Soc Nephrol 1997;8:1537–1545.
99. Zoja C, Donadelli R, Colleoni S, et al. Protein overload stimulates RANTES production by proximal tubular cells depending on NF-kappa B activation. Kidney Int 1998;53:1608–1615.
100. Nath KA, Hostetter MK, Hostetter TH. Pathophysiology of chronic tubulo-interstitial disease in rats. Interactions of dietary acid load, ammonia, and complement component C3. J Clin Invest 1985;76:667–675.
101. Morita Y, Nomura A, Yuzawa Y, et al. The role of complement in the pathogenesis of tubulointerstitial lesions in rat mesangial proliferative glomerulonephritis. J Am Soc Nephrol 1997;8:1363–1372.
102. Nangaku M, Pippin J, Couser WG. Complement membrane attack complex (C5b-9) mediates interstitial disease in experimental nephrotic syndrome. J Am Soc Nephrol 1999;10:2323–2331.
103. Morita Y, Ikeguchi H, Nakamura J, Hotta N, Yuzawa Y, Matsuo S. Complement activation products in the urine from proteinuric patients. J Am Soc Nephrol 2000;11:700–707.

104. Hsu CY, McCulloch CE, Curhan GC. Epidemiology of anemia associated with chronic renal insufficiency among adults in the United States: Results from the Third National Health and Nutrition Examination Survey. J Am Soc Nephrol 2002;13:504–510.
105. KDOQI Clinical Practice Guidelines and Clinical Practice Recommendations for Anemia in Chronic Kidney Disease. Am J Kidney Dis 2006;47:S11–S145.
106. Jungers P, Choukroun G, Oualim Z, Robino C, Nguyen AT, Man NK. Beneficial influence of recombinant human erythropoietin therapy on the rate of progression of chronic renal failure in predialysis patients. Nephrol Dial Transplant 2001;16:307–312.
107. K/DOQI clinical practice guidelines for cardiovascular disease in dialysis patients. Am J Kidney Dis 2005;45:S1–S153.
108. Go AS, Chertow GM, Fan D, McCulloch CE, Hsu CY. Chronic kidney disease and the risks of death, cardiovascular events, and hospitalization. N Engl J Med 2004;351:1296–1305.
109. Keith DS, Nichols GA, Gullion CM, Brown JB, Smith DH. Longitudinal follow-up and outcomes among a population with chronic kidney disease in a large managed care organization. Arch Intern Med 2004;164:659–663.
110. Obrador GT, Ruthazer R, Arora P, Kausz AT, Pereira BJ. Prevalence of and factors associated with suboptimal care before initiation of dialysis in the United States. J Am Soc Nephrol 1999;10:1793–1800.
111. Martinez I, Saracho R, Montenegro J, Llach F. The importance of dietary calcium and phosphorous in the secondary hyperparathyroidism of patients with early renal failure. Am J Kidney Dis 1997;29:496–502.
112. National Kidney Foundation. K/DOQI clinical practice guidelines for managing dyslipidemias in chronic kidney disease. Am J Kidney Dis 2003;41:S1–S92.
113. Kopple JD. National kidney foundation K/DOQI clinical practice guidelines for nutrition in chronic renal failure. Am J Kidney Dis 2001;37:S66–S70.
114. Brenner BM. Hemodynamically mediated glomerular injury and the progressive nature of kidney disease. Kidney Int 1983;23:647–655.
115. Levey AS, Adler S, Caggiula AW, et al. Effects of dietary protein restriction on the progression of advanced renal disease in the Modification of Diet in Renal Disease Study. Am J Kidney Dis 1996;27:652–663.
116. Pedrini MT, Levey AS, Lau J, Chalmers TC, Wang PH. The effect of dietary protein restriction on the progression of diabetic and nondiabetic renal diseases: A meta-analysis. Ann Intern Med 1996;124:627–632.
117. Kasiske BL, Lakatua JD, Ma JZ, Louis TA. A meta-analysis of the effects of dietary protein restriction on the rate of decline in renal function. Am J Kidney Dis 1998;31:954–961.
118. Wang PH, Lau J, Chalmers TC. Meta-analysis of effects of intensive blood-glucose control on late complications of type I diabetes. Lancet 1993;341:1306–1309.
119. Retinopathy and nephropathy in patients with type 1 diabetes four years after a trial of intensive therapy. The Diabetes Control and Complications Trial/Epidemiology of Diabetes Interventions and Complications Research Group. N Engl J Med 2000;342:381–389.
120. Standards of medical care in diabetes—2007. Diabetes Care 2007;2001;30(Suppl 1):S4–S41.
121. Savage S, Johnson Nagel N, Estacio RO, et al. The ABCD (Appropriate Blood Pressure Control in Diabetes) trial. Rationale and design of a trial of hypertension control (moderate or intensive) in type II diabetes. Online J Curr Clin Trials 1993; Doc No 104.
122. Viberti G, Wheeldon NM. Microalbuminuria reduction with valsartan in patients with type 2 diabetes mellitus: A blood pressure-independent effect. Circulation 2002;106:672–678.
123. Lewis EJ, Hunsicker LG, Bain RP, Rohde RD. The effect of angiotensin-converting-enzyme inhibition on diabetic nephropathy. The Collaborative Study Group. N Engl J Med 1993;329:1456–1462.
124. Ahmad J, Siddiqui MA, Ahmad H. Effective postponement of diabetic nephropathy with enalapril in normotensive type 2 diabetic patients with microalbuminuria. Diabetes Care 1997;20:1576–1581.
125. Ravid M, Brosh D, Levi Z, Bar-Dayan Y, Ravid D, Rachmani R. Use of enalapril to attenuate decline in renal function in normotensive, normoalbuminuric patients with type 2 diabetes mellitus. A randomized, controlled trial. Ann Intern Med 1998;128:982–988.
126. Randomised placebo-controlled trial of lisinopril in normotensive patients with insulin-dependent diabetes and normoalbuminuria or microalbuminuria. The EUCLID Study Group. Lancet 1997;349:1787–1792.
127. Effects of ramipril on cardiovascular and microvascular outcomes in people with diabetes mellitus: Results of the HOPE study and MICRO-HOPE substudy. Heart Outcomes Prevention Evaluation Study Investigators. Lancet 2000;355:253–259.
128. Laffel LM, McGill JB, Gans DJ. The beneficial effect of angiotensin-converting enzyme inhibition with captopril on diabetic nephropathy in normotensive IDDM patients with microalbuminuria. North American Microalbuminuria Study Group. Am J Med 1995;99:497–504.
129. Lewis JB, Berl T, Bain RP, Rohde RD, Lewis EJ. Effect of intensive blood pressure control on the course of type 1 diabetic nephropathy. Collaborative Study Group. Am J Kidney Dis 1999;34:809–817.
130. Lebovitz HE, Wiegmann TB, Cnaan A, et al. Renal protective effects of enalapril in hypertensive NIDDM. role of baseline albuminuria. Kidney Int Suppl 1994;45:S150–S155.
131. Sasso FC, Carbonara O, Persico M, et al. Irbesartan reduces the albumin excretion rate in microalbuminuric type 2 diabetic patients independently of hypertension: A randomized double-blind placebo-controlled crossover study. Diabetes Care 2002;25:1909–1913.
132. Brenner BM, Cooper ME, de Zeeuw D, et al. Effects of losartan on renal and cardiovascular outcomes in patients with type 2 diabetes and nephropathy. N Engl J Med 2001;345:861–869.
133. Parving HH, Lehnert H, Brochner-Mortensen J, Gomis R, Andersen S, Arner P. The effect of irbesartan on the development of diabetic nephropathy in patients with type 2 diabetes. N Engl J Med 2001;345:870–878.
134. Lewis EJ, Hunsicker LG, Clarke WR, et al. Renoprotective effect of the angiotensin-receptor antagonist irbesartan in patients with nephropathy due to type 2 diabetes. N Engl J Med 2001;345:851–860.
135. Chobanian AV, Bakris GL, Black HR, et al. Seventh report of the Joint National Committee on Prevention, Detection, Evaluation, and Treatment of High Blood Pressure. Hypertension 2003;42:1206–1252.
136. Bakris GL, Williams M, Dworkin L, et al. Preserving renal function in adults with hypertension and diabetes: A consensus approach. National Kidney Foundation Hypertension and Diabetes Executive Committees Working Group. Am J Kidney Dis 2000;36:646–661.
137. Parving HH. Impact of blood pressure and antihypertensive treatment on incipient and overt nephropathy, retinopathy, and endothelial permeability in diabetes mellitus. Diabetes Care 1991;14:260–269.
138. Dworkin LD, Benstein JA, Parker M, Tolbert E, Feiner HD. Calcium antagonists and converting enzyme inhibitors reduce renal injury by different mechanisms. Kidney Int 1993;43:808–814.
139. Kasiske BL, Kalil RS, Ma JZ, Liao M, Keane WF. Effect of antihypertensive therapy on the kidney in patients with diabetes: A meta-regression analysis. Ann Intern Med 1993;118:129–138.
140. Schlueter WA, Batlle DC. Renal effects of antihypertensive drugs. Drugs 1989;37:900–925.
141. Risler T, Kramer B, Muller GA. The efficacy of diuretics in acute and chronic renal failure. Focus on torsemide. Drugs 1991;41 Suppl 3:69–79.
142. Randomised placebo-controlled trial of effect of ramipril on decline in glomerular filtration rate and risk of terminal renal failure in proteinuric, non-diabetic nephropathy. The GISEN Group (Gruppo Italiano di Studi Epidemiologici in Nefrologia). Lancet 1997;349:1857–1863.
143. Kshirsagar AV, Joy MS, Hogan SL, Falk RJ, Colindres RE. Effect of ACE inhibitors in diabetic and nondiabetic chronic renal disease: A systematic overview of randomized placebo-controlled trials. Am J Kidney Dis 2000;35:695–707.
144. Casas JP, Chua W, Loukogeorgakis S, et al. Effect of inhibitors of the renin-angiotensin system and other antihypertensive drugs on renal outcomes: Systematic review and meta-analysis. Lancet 2005;366:2026–2033.
145. Schjoedt KJ, Andersen S, Rossing P, Tarnow L, Parving HH. Aldosterone escape during blockade of the renin-angiotensin-aldosterone system in diabetic nephropathy is associated with enhanced decline in glomerular filtration rate. Diabetologia 2004;47:1936–1939.
146. Rossing K, Schjoedt KJ, Smidt UM, Boomsma F, Parving HH. Beneficial effects of adding spironolactone to recommended antihypertensive treatment in diabetic nephropathy: A randomized, double-masked, cross-over study. Diabetes Care 2005;28:2106–2112.
147. Schjoedt KJ, Rossing K, Juhl TR, et al. Beneficial impact of spironolactone on nephrotic range albuminuria in diabetic nephropathy. Kidney Int 2006;70:536–542.

148. Pitt B, Segal R, Martinez FA, et al. Randomised trial of losartan versus captopril in patients over 65 with heart failure (Evaluation of Losartan in the Elderly Study, ELITE). Lancet 1997;349:747–752.
149. Hostetter TH. Prevention of end-stage renal disease due to type 2 diabetes. N Engl J Med 2001;345:910–912.
150. Mogensen CE, Neldam S, Tikkanen I, et al. Randomised controlled trial of dual blockade of renin-angiotensin system in patients with hypertension, microalbuminuria, and non-insulin dependent diabetes: The Candesartan and Lisinopril Microalbuminuria (CALM) study. BMJ 2000;321:1440–1444.
151. Sica DA, Gehr T.W. The pharmacokinetics of angiotensin-converting enzyme inhibitors in end-stage renal disease. Semin Dialysis 1994;7:205–213.
152. Maki DD, Ma JZ, Louis TA, Kasiske BL. Long-term effects of antihypertensive agents on proteinuria and renal function. Arch Intern Med 1995;155:1073–1080.
153. Weidmann P, Schneider M, Bohlen L. Therapeutic efficacy of different antihypertensive drugs in human diabetic nephropathy: An updated meta-analysis. Nephrol Dial Transplant 1995;10 Suppl 9:39–45.
154. Bakris GL, Copley JB, Vicknair N, Sadler R, Leurgans S. Calcium channel blockers versus other antihypertensive therapies on progression of NIDDM associated nephropathy. Kidney Int 1996;50:1641–1650.
155. Epstein M. Effects of ACE inhibitors and calcium antagonists on progression of chronic renal disease. Blood Press Suppl 1995;2:108–112.
156. Maschio G, Alberti D, Janin G, et al. Effect of the angiotensin-converting-enzyme inhibitor benazepril on the progression of chronic renal insufficiency. The Angiotensin-Converting-Enzyme Inhibition in Progressive Renal Insufficiency Study Group. N Engl J Med 1996;334:939–945.
157. Nielsen S, Dollerup J, Nielsen B, Jensen HA, Mogensen CE. Losartan reduces albuminuria in patients with essential hypertension. An enalapril controlled 3 months study. Nephrol Dial Transplant 1997;12 Suppl 2:19–23.
158. Praga M, Gutierrez E, Gonzalez E, Morales E, Hernandez E. Treatment of IgA nephropathy with ACE inhibitors: A randomized and controlled trial. J Am Soc Nephrol 2003;14:1578–1583.
159. Ruggenenti P, Perna A, Gherardi G, et al. Renoprotective properties of ACE-inhibition in non-diabetic nephropathies with non-nephrotic proteinuria. Lancet 1999;354:359–364.
160. Lea J, Greene T, Hebert L, et al. The relationship between magnitude of proteinuria reduction and risk of end-stage renal disease: Results of the African American study of kidney disease and hypertension. Arch Intern Med 2005;165:947–953.
161. Rahman M, Pressel S, Davis BR, et al. Renal outcomes in high-risk hypertensive patients treated with an angiotensin-converting enzyme inhibitor or a calcium channel blocker vs a diuretic: A report from the Antihypertensive and Lipid-Lowering Treatment to Prevent Heart Attack Trial (ALLHAT). Arch Intern Med 2005;165:936–946.
162. Usta M, Ersoy A, Dilek K, et al. Efficacy of losartan in patients with primary focal segmental glomerulosclerosis resistant to immunosuppressive treatment. J Intern Med 2003;253:329–334.
163. Tylicki L, Rutkowski P, Renke M, Rutkowski B. Renoprotective effect of small doses of losartan and enalapril in patients with primary glomerulonephritis. Short-term observation. Am J Nephrol 2002;22:356–362.
164. Ruilope LM. Is it wise to combine an ACE inhibitor and an angiotensin receptor antagonist? Nephrol Dial Transplant 1999;14:2855–2856.
165. Nakao N, Yoshimura A, Morita H, Takada M, Kayano T, Ideura T. Combination treatment of angiotensin-II receptor blocker and angiotensin-converting-enzyme inhibitor in non-diabetic renal disease (COOPERATE): A randomised controlled trial. Lancet 2003;361:117–124.
166. Tarif N, Bakris GL. Preservation of renal function: The spectrum of effects by calcium-channel blockers. Nephrol Dial Transplant 1997;12:2244–2250.
167. Apperloo AJ, de Zeeuw D, de Jong PE. A short-term antihypertensive treatment-induced fall in glomerular filtration rate predicts long-term stability of renal function. Kidney Int 1997;51:793–797.
168. Fried LF, Orchard TJ, Kasiske BL. Effect of lipid reduction on the progression of renal disease: A meta-analysis. Kidney Int 2001;59:260–269.
169. Oda H, Keane WF. Recent advances in statins and the kidney. Kidney Int Suppl 1999;71:S2–S5.
170. Massy ZA, Ma JZ, Louis TA, Kasiske BL. Lipid-lowering therapy in patients with renal disease. Kidney Int 1995;48:188–198.
171. Executive Summary of the third report of The National Cholesterol Education Program (NCEP) Expert Panel on Detection, Evaluation, and Treatment of High Blood Cholesterol in Adults (Adult Treatment Panel III). JAMA 2001;285:2486–2497.
172. Halimi JM, Mimran A. Renal effects of smoking: Potential mechanisms and perspectives. Nephrol Dial Transplant 2000;15:938–940.
173. Pinto-Sietsma SJ, Mulder J, Janssen WM, Hillege HL, de Zeeuw D, de Jong PE. Smoking is related to albuminuria and abnormal renal function in nondiabetic persons. Ann Intern Med 2000;133:585–591.
174. Silverberg D, Wexler D, Blum M, Wollman Y, Iaina A. The cardiorenal anaemia syndrome: Does it exist? Nephrol Dial Transplant 2003;18 Suppl 8:viii7–12.
175. Silverberg DS, Wexler D, Blum M, et al. The correction of anemia in severe resistant heart failure with erythropoietin and intravenous iron prevents the progression of both the heart and the renal failure and markedly reduces hospitalization. Clin Nephrol 2002;58 Suppl 1:S37–S45.
176. Silverberg DS, Wexler D, Blum M, et al. Effect of correction of anemia with erythropoietin and intravenous iron in resistant heart failure in octogenarians. Isr Med Assoc J 2003;5:337–339.
177. Becker BN, Becker YT, Leverson GE, Heisey DM. Erythropoietin therapy may retard progression in chronic renal transplant dysfunction. Nephrol Dial Transplant 2002;17:1667–1673.
178. Deicher R, Horl WH. Anaemia as a risk factor for the progression of chronic kidney disease. Curr Opin Nephrol Hypertens 2003;12:139–143.
179. Rettig RA. The social contract and the treatment of permanent kidney failure. JAMA 1996;275:1123–1126.
180. USRDS. USRDS 2001 Annual Data Report. Bethesda, MD: National Institutes of Health, National Institute of Diabetes and Digestive and Kidney Disease, 2001.
181. Siegel JE, Krolewski AS, Warram JH, Weinstein MC. Cost-effectiveness of screening and early treatment of nephropathy in patients with insulin-dependent diabetes mellitus. J Am Soc Nephrol 1992;3:S111–S119.
182. Kiberd BA, Jindal KK. Routine treatment of insulin-dependent diabetic patients with ACE inhibitors to prevent renal failure: An economic evaluation. Am J Kidney Dis 1998;31:49–54.
183. Lifetime benefits and costs of intensive therapy as practiced in the diabetes control and complications trial. The Diabetes Control and Complications Trial Research Group. JAMA 1996;276:1409–1415.
184. Cost effectiveness analysis of improved blood pressure control in hypertensive patients with type 2 diabetes: UKPDS 40. UK Prospective Diabetes Study Group. BMJ 1998;317:720–726.
185. Golan L, Birkmeyer JD, Welch HG. The cost-effectiveness of treating all patients with type 2 diabetes with angiotensin-converting enzyme inhibitors. Ann Intern Med 1999;131:660–667.
186. Jacobson HR, Striker GE. Report on a workshop to develop management recommendations for the prevention of progression in chronic renal disease. Am J Kidney Dis 1995;25:103–106.
187. The sixth report of the Joint National Committee on prevention, detection, evaluation, and treatment of high blood pressure. Arch Intern Med 1997;157:2413–2446.
188. Eknoyan G, Levin N. NKF-K/DOQI Clinical Practice Guidelines: Update 2000. Foreword. Am J Kidney Dis 2001;37:S5–S6.

CHAPTER 47

Chronic Kidney Disease: Management of Complications

JOANNA Q. HUDSON

KEY CONCEPTS

1. The number of patients with chronic kidney disease (CKD) is increasing, and it is expectated that the number of patients with end-stage renal disease (ESRD) will double by 2020.
2. Common complications of stages 4 and 5 CKD include anemia, hyperphosphatemia, secondary hyperparathyroidism, fluid and electrolyte abnormalities, metabolic acidosis, and malnutrition.
3. Cardiovascular complications are prevalent in the CKD population and are the leading cause of mortality in patients with ESRD. For this reason, all ESRD patients at the initiation of dialysis should be assessed for cardiovascular disease, which includes assessment for coronary artery disease, cardiomyopathy, valvular heart disease, cerebrovascular disease, and peripheral vascular disease in addition to screening for both traditional and nontraditional cardiovascular risk factors.
4. The management of CKD and the associated secondary complications should be initiated prior to development of ESRD.
5. Guidelines by the National Kidney Foundation Kidney Disease/Dialysis Outcomes Quality Initiative (NKF-K/DOQI) should be used as a basis for the workup of CKD and the design of appropriate therapy for associated complications.
6. Patient education plays a critical role in the appropriate management of patients with stage 4 or 5 CKD and related complications. A multidisciplinary team structure is a rational approach to provide this education and effectively design and implement the extensive nonpharmacologic and pharmacologic interventions required.
7. Anemia of CKD, which is primarily caused by a deficiency in the production of endogenous erythropoietin by the kidney, is a common complication observed in patients with stages 4 and 5 CKD and contributes to cardiovascular disease.
8. Management of anemia includes administration of erythropoietic-stimulating agents (ESAs) (epoetin alfa and darbepoetin alfa) and regular iron supplementation (oral or intravenous administration) to achieve a target hemoglobin of at least 11 g/dL and to potentially prevent the development of left ventricular hypertrophy if therapy is initiated early. The target upper limit of hemoglobin is not clearly defined, but evidence does not support exceeding a hemoglobin of 12 g/dL.
9. Hyperphosphatemia, changes in calcium homeostasis, and secondary hyperparathyroidism are common in patients with CKD and contribute to extravascular calcifications and an increased risk of cardiovascular mortality.
10. Management of hyperphosphatemia, calcium balance, and secondary hyperparathyroidism includes dietary phosphorus restriction, prudent use of phosphate binding agents, vitamin D, and calcimimetic therapy.

Learning objectives, review questions, and other resources can be found at **www.pharmacotherapyonline.com.**

The clinical syndrome that develops insidiously as kidney function declines to the most severe stages, stages 4 and 5 chronic kidney disease (CKD), begins with nonspecific symptoms such as nausea and vomiting, which become progressively worse as the glomerular filtration rate (GFR) drops below 15 mL/min. It is at this stage that renal replacement therapy, either dialysis (see Chap. 48) or transplantation (see Chap. 92), is indicated to remove uremic toxins and to maintain hemodynamic stability. The patient with stage 5 CKD requiring chronic dialysis or renal transplantation for relief of uremic symptoms is said to have end-stage renal disease (ESRD). In this chapter, ESRD refers specifically to patients who are receiving chronic dialysis.

The staging system for CKD is designed not only to trigger implementation of appropriate interventions to delay progression of CKD, as discussed in Chap. 46, but also as an index of when to consider initiating management of the complications of CKD. The most frequent complications of CKD discussed here include fluid and electrolyte abnormalities, anemia, secondary hyperparathyroidism and renal osteodystrophy, hypertension and hyperlipidemia, metabolic acidosis, and miscellaneous complications resulting from the effects of CKD on other organ systems, including malnutrition, pruritus, and uremic bleeding (Table 47–1 lists other complications of CKD). Diagnostic and therapeutic approaches to the management of fluid and electrolyte abnormalities, hypertension, hyperlipidemia, and metabolic acidosis in patients without CKD are presented elsewhere in this text. Cardiovascular disease as a common complication in patients with CKD also requires early and aggressive intervention.[1] Often complications of CKD are unrecognized or are inappropriately managed, and for many patients lead to significant morbidity, premature mortality, or a poor prognosis by the time they reach ESRD.[2] This chapter discusses the epidemiology of ESRD and the pathophysiology and pharmacotherapeutic management of the complications and comorbidities that occur frequently in patients with stages 4 and 5 CKD (including ESRD).

EPIDEMIOLOGY

1 In 2000, approximately 19 million people in the United States were estimated to have CKD: 8 million of this total had an estimated GFR less than 60 mL/min per 1.73 m^2 (stage 3, 4, or 5 CKD), the

TABLE 47-1 Other Complications of Chronic Kidney Disease

Organ System or Complication	Effects
Amyloidosis	Accumulation of β_2-microglobulin Manifests as carpal tunnel syndrome
Bleeding	Potentially result of platelet abnormalities
Endocrine	Thyroid function – symptoms of hypothyroidism Hypothermia Glycemic control – ↑ in hypoglycemic episodes as kidney disease progresses (result of ↓ degradation of insulin by the kidney)
Gastrointestinal	Nausea, vomiting, diarrhea, anorexia, GI bleeding
Immune system	Imparied cell-mediated immunity Lymphopenia
Neurologic	Peripheral neuropathies Restless leg syndrome Uremic encephalopathy

point at which secondary complications are more prevalent.[3] In 2005, the latest year for which data are available, a total of more than 106,000 new cases of ESRD were reported and the prevalence as of the end of the year was 484,693, including 341,000 patients on dialysis and 143,693 with a functioning kidney after transplantation.[2] Incidence rates are higher in blacks (fourfold higher), Native Americans (twofold higher), and Hispanics (twofold higher) compared to whites, a trend that has persisted over the last decade.[2] The incidence has also increased dramatically in patients 65 years of age and older. Although the overall number of patients with ESRD is substantial now, it is projected that by the year 2020 the number will exceed 780,000 patients, the majority of cases attributable to diabetes.

ESRD patients have a mortality rate up to four times higher than comparable patients age 65 years or older without kidney disease.[2] Associated predictors of mortality at the start of dialysis include a lower estimated GFR, decreased serum albumin, and the presence of comorbidities, such as diabetes and cardiovascular disease.[4] Lower hemoglobin levels and body mass index are also associated with increased mortality. The association of mortality with these factors highlights the need to address complications as soon as they are detected and ideally prior to the time of consideration for renal replacement therapy.

ETIOLOGY

Many clinical conditions and diseases lead to progressive kidney damage and ESRD (see Chap. 46). Diabetes mellitus continues to be the leading cause of CKD and, ultimately, of ESRD in the United States.[2] The incidence rate of ESRD attributed to diabetes has doubled, while the prevalence has more than tripled, in the last 10 years, although the incidence rate has remained fairly stable since 2001. Diabetes is particularly common in Native Americans. Approximately 80% of Native Americans diagnosed with ESRD have diabetes, classified as either a primary cause of ESRD or a comorbid condition.[2]

Hypertension, the second leading cause of ESRD in the United States, was also associated with an almost 50% increase in incident rate in the last decade, with the greatest increase being in the black population.[2] Glomerulonephritis which includes a wide variety of glomerular lesions caused by immunologic, vascular, and other idiopathic diseases (see Chap. 50) is the third leading cause of ESRD in the United States. Other diseases and conditions, such as cystic kidney disease, Wegener granulomatosis, vascular diseases, and acquired immunodeficiency syndrome (AIDS) nephropathy account for relatively few cases of ESRD compared to diabetes and hypertension.[2] The increase in the incidence of AIDS nephropathy was most dramatic between 1991 and 1995, but has since stabilized.

PATHOPHYSIOLOGY

Progression of CKD to ESRD occurs over years to decades in the majority of cases, with the precise mechanism of kidney damage dependent on the etiology of the disease (see Chaps. 46 and 50); however, the consequences and complications of marked reductions in kidney function are fairly uniform irrespective of the underlying etiology. The mechanisms of progression of CKD and measures to delay progression are essential elements for primary care clinicians to consider as they design intervention strategies for their patients. Those clinicians who care for patients with ESRD or stages 4 and 5 CKD must also have a clear understanding of the pathogenesis, clinical presentation, and management strategies for secondary complications and comorbidities to improve quality of care and outcomes.

No single toxin is responsible for all of the signs and symptoms of uremia observed in patients with stage 4 or 5 CKD. Accumulation of one or several of these known and potential toxins may be the result of increased secretion, as with the biologically active substances such as parathyroid hormone (PTH) and atrial natriuretic peptide; decreased clearance because of reduced metabolism within the kidney for compounds such as PTH, gastrin, growth hormone, glucagon, somatostatin, prolactin, calcitonin, and insulin; and/or decreased renal clearance of metabolic by-products of protein metabolism. The buildup of these uremic toxins ultimately results in altered organ and immune function, and leads to a myriad of secondary complications.

❷ Altered fluid and electrolyte homeostasis, metabolic acidosis, anemia of CKD, secondary hyperparathyroidism and renal osteodystrophy, and cardiovascular disease are among the common complications associated with a substantial decline in GFR. The pathophysiology of these complications is described here.

FLUID AND ELECTROLYTE ABNORMALITIES

Sodium and Water

In persons with normal kidney function, sodium balance is maintained at a sodium intake of 120 to 150 mEq/day. The fractional excretion of sodium (FeNa) is approximately 1% to 3%. Water balance is also maintained, with a normal range of urinary osmolality of 50 to 1,200 mOsm/kg (average range 500 to 800 mOsm/kg). An osmotic diuresis occurs with an increase in FeNa leading to obligatory water losses and impairment in the kidney's ability to dilute or concentrate urine (urinary osmolality is often fixed at that of plasma or approximately 300 mOsm/L). Nocturia is present relatively early in the course of CKD (stage 3) secondary to the defect in urinary concentrating ability. In patients with severe CKD (stages 4 and 5), serum sodium concentration is generally maintained as the result of an increase in FeNa by as much as 30%, but results in a volume-expanded state.[5] Total renal sodium excretion decreases despite an increase in sodium excretion by remaining nephrons. Volume overload with pulmonary edema can result, but the most common manifestation of increased intravascular volume is systemic hypertension.

Potassium Homeostasis

Serum potassium is freely filtered at the glomerulus, reabsorbed in the proximal tubule and loop of Henle, and actively secreted into the urine at the cortical collecting duct. The kidneys normally excrete 90% to 95% of the daily potassium dietary load. The fractional excretion of potassium (FE_K) is approximately 25%. Normally only 5% to 10% of ingested potassium is excreted through the gut. Potassium homeostasis is also maintained by shifting extracellular potassium intracellularly immediately following ingestion of a potassium load. In patients with CKD, potassium balance is maintained by an increase in distal tubular potassium secretion in which aldosterone plays an important role; FE_K can increase to as high as five times normal.[5] Thus the serum potassium concentration is usually maintained in the normal range until the GFR is less than 20 mL/min per 1.73 m^2 body surface area, at which point mild hyperkalemia is likely to develop. A significant increase in potassium secretion by the colon also contributes to the maintenance of potassium balance, but this adaptation cannot compensate fully for the decrease in renal potassium excretion.

METABOLIC ACIDOSIS

Individuals with normal kidney function generate enough hydrogen ion to reclaim all filtered bicarbonate and to secrete approximately 1 mEq/kg per day of hydrogen ions, which are generated from the metabolism of dietary proteins (see Chap. 55). As a result, they maintain a constant body fluid pH through the buffering of hydrogen ion by proteins, hemoglobin, phosphate, and bicarbonate. Renal ammoniagenesis and phosphate excretion buffer the urine and facilitate acid excretion. In severe CKD, all filtered bicarbonate is reclaimed, but the ability of the kidneys to synthesize ammonia is impaired. This decrease in urinary buffer results in decreased net acid excretion and continuous positive hydrogen ion balance; consequently, metabolic acidosis develops. A clinically significant metabolic acidosis is commonly seen when the GFR drops below 20 to 30 mL/min (stage 4 CKD). In these patients, the plasma bicarbonate concentration tends to stabilize at 15 to 20 mEq/L.

ANEMIA OF CHRONIC KIDNEY DISEASE

❼ The primary cause of anemia in CKD patients is a decrease in production of the hormone erythropoietin by the progenitor cells of the kidney, where 90% of production typically occurs. Plasma concentrations of erythropoietin increase exponentially in individuals with normal kidney function as hemoglobin/hematocrit decline (i.e., in response to decreased oxygenation). In contrast, there is no correlation between the degree of anemia and erythropoietin concentrations in anemic ESRD patients. The result is a normochromic, normocytic anemia, unless the individual has concomitant iron deficiency, which can result in a microcytic anemia, or a folate or B_{12} deficiency, which can result in a macrocytic anemia. Additional factors contributing to the development of anemia of CKD are the decreased red cell life span in the presence of uremia (from the normal of 120 days to approximately 60 days in ESRD), iron deficiency, blood loss from regular laboratory testing, and blood loss with hemodialysis for patients requiring this modality of renal replacement therapy. Iron deficiency is the primary cause of resistance to therapy with erythropoietic-stimulating agents (ESAs; i.e., epoetin alfa or darbepoetin alfa).

SECONDARY HYPERPARATHYROIDISM AND RENAL OSTEODYSTROPHY

❾ Calcium and phosphorus balance is mediated through the complex interplay of hormones and their effects on bone, the GI tract, kidney, and parathyroid gland. What begins as relatively minor imbalances in phosphorus and calcium homeostasis leads to secondary hyperparathyroidism (sHPT) in the short-term and ultimately renal osteodystrophy (ROD) if these metabolic abnormalities are not corrected (Fig. 47–1). ROD progresses insidiously for several years before patients become symptomatic. When symptoms such as bone pain and skeletal fractures occur, the disease is not easily amenable to treatment.

As kidney function declines there is a decrease in phosphorus elimination, which results in hyperphosphatemia and when severe a reciprocal decrease in serum calcium concentration. Hypocalcemia is the primary stimulus for release of PTH by the parathyroid glands, the effects of which are mediated by the interaction of ionized calcium with the calcium-sensing receptor on the chief cells of the parathyroid gland. Hyperphosphatemia also increases PTH synthesis and release through its direct effects on the parathyroid gland and production of prepro-PTH messenger RNA.[6] In an attempt to normalize ionized calcium, PTH decreases phosphorus reabsorption and increases calcium reabsorption by the proximal tubules of the kidney (at least until the GFR falls to less than approximately 30 mL/min), and also increases calcium mobilization from bone. The result is a correction in calcium and phosphorus, at least in the early stages of CKD; however, this occurs at the expense of an elevated PTH ("the trade-off hypothesis"). The increase in PTH is most notable when GFR is less than 60 mL/min per 1.73 m^2 (stage 3 CKD) and worsens as kidney function further declines.[7]

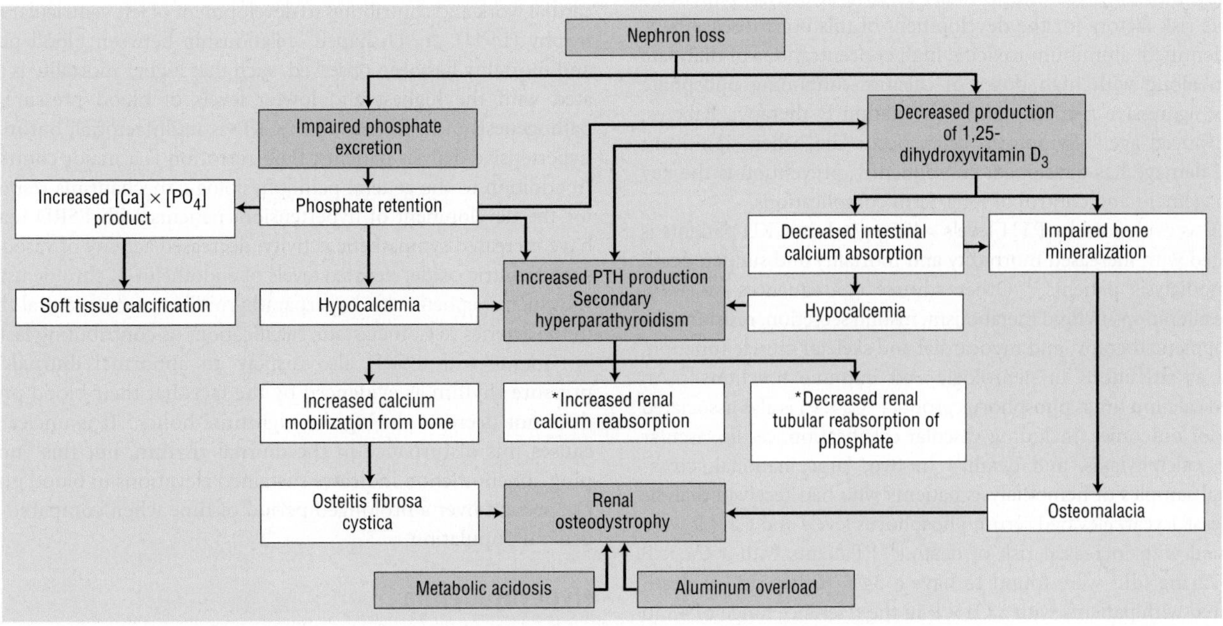

FIGURE 47-1. Pathogenesis of secondary hyperparathyroidism and renal osteodystrophy in patients with chronic kidney disease. (*These adaptations are lost as kidney disease progresses.) PTH, parathyroid hormone.

Active vitamin D (1,25-dihydroxyvitamin D_3 or calcitriol) promotes increased intestinal absorption of calcium, which helps to normalize ionized calcium. Calcitriol also works directly on the parathyroid gland to suppress PTH production. The enzyme 1α-hydroxylase is responsible for the final hydroxylation and conversion of the vitamin D precursor, 25-hydroxyvitamin D, to the active form in the kidney. As kidney disease progresses this conversion is impaired and vitamin D deficiency results. Calcitriol levels decrease significantly before there is a perceptible rise in PTH in CKD patients.[7] Other differences in vitamin D metabolism observed in patients with CKD that lead to deficiencies in the 25-hydroxyvitamin D precursor include decreased dermal synthesis of vitamin D, decreased exposure to sunlight, and reduced dietary intake of vitamin D.[8] In patients with stage 3 or 4 CKD, 25-hydroxyvitamin D levels of <30 ng/mL are associated with increased PTH.[8] As a result of such findings, evaluation of 25-hydroxyvitamin D levels and supplementation in patients with observed deficiencies are recommended for stages 3 and 4 CKD.[8]

A multiplicity of metabolic disorders in patients with CKD contributes to worsening sHPT and the associated consequences (see Fig. 47–1). The continuous production of PTH by the parathyroid glands leads to parathyroid hyperplasia (nodular or diffuse). Nodular tissue demonstrates more rapid growth potential and appears to be associated with fewer vitamin D and calcium-sensing receptors, resulting in resistance to the effects of calcium and vitamin D therapy and subsequent development of ROD.[6] Bone loss can be detected in patients with early stages of kidney disease and multiple types of bone lesions have been identified from bone biopsies of patients on dialysis.[9] The skeletal complications associated with ROD include osteitis fibrosa cystica (high bone turnover disease), osteomalacia (low bone turnover disease), and adynamic bone disease. Osteitis fibrosa cystica is characterized by areas of peritrabecular fibrosis. Dynamic measurements show a high bone formation rate, which results from high circulating concentrations of PTH. Bone marrow fibrosis and decreased erythropoiesis are also consequences of severe osteitis fibrosa cystica. Osteomalacia was historically caused by aluminum toxicity in hemodialysis patients, a finding less common today with decreased use of aluminum-containing phosphate binders and changes in the processing of dialysate solutions to decrease aluminum absorption. Adynamic lesions are characterized by low amounts of fibrosis or osteoid tissue and low bone formation rates. The incidence of adynamic lesions has increased over the last 10 years and may be present in as many as 50% of dialysis patients.[10] Multiple risk factors for the development of this bone disease have been identified: aluminum toxicity; high concentrations of dialysate calcium along with high doses of calcium-containing phosphate binders; aggressive management with vitamin D therapy; diabetes; and advanced age.[10] Symptoms often occur late, when significant skeletal damage has developed; consequently, prevention is the key to management and control of long-term complications.

sHPT as evidenced by PTH levels >495 pg/mL in CKD patients is associated with increased morbidity and mortality and sudden death in hemodialysis patients.[11] Other adverse consequences of sHPT include alterations in lipid metabolism, insulin secretion, resistance to erythropoietic therapy, and myocardial and skeletal muscle function, as well as alterations in neurologic and immune functions.[12] An elevated calcium times phosphorus product (Ca × P) is also associated with poor outcomes, including vascular calcification, cardiovascular disease, calciphylaxis, and death.[13] In two, large, national, cross-sectional samples of hemodialysis patients who had received dialysis for at least 1 year, elevated serum phosphorus levels and Ca × P were associated with increased risk of death.[13,14] Patients with a Ca × P above 72 mg^2/dL^2 were found to have a 34% higher risk of death compared with patients with a Ca × P in the reference range of 43 to 52 mg^2/dL^2.[13] Calcium scores, as measured by electron-beam computed tomography, were significantly higher in hemodialysis patients than in patients without kidney disease who had proven coronary artery disease. Intake of calcium from calcium-based binders also appears to be a significant contributor to coronary artery calcification, even in young dialysis patients.[15] These data underscore the need to consider all the consequences of elevated PTH and Ca × P, not only their consequences on bone.

CARDIOVASCULAR DISEASE

❸ Patients with CKD are at increased risk of cardiovascular disease, independent of the etiology of their kidney disease. Although a clearly unique pathogenesis of cardiovascular disease specific to CKD has not been identified, it is known that manifestations of kidney disease are contributory.[16] In addition, uremic toxins can induce pericarditis, a potentially fatal complication. Currently, screening of this high-risk population for cardiovascular risk factors is not routinely considered.[16,17]

Mortality secondary to cardiovascular disease is 10 to 30 times greater in dialysis patients than in the general population.[16] In addition to traditional cardiac risk factors such as hypertension and hyperlipidemia, diabetes, tobacco use, and physical inactivity, patients with kidney disease have other unique risk factors. Among these are hyperhomocysteinemia, elevated levels of C-reactive protein, increased oxidant stress, and hemodynamic overload.[1] Complications such as anemia and metabolic disorders (i.e., abnormalities in Ca, P, and PTH) of CKD are also contributory. In particular, arterial vascular disease (e.g., atherosclerosis) and cardiomyopathy are the primary types of cardiovascular disorders present in the CKD population.[1,16] These disorders lead to development of ischemic heart disease and its manifestations including myocardial infarction. As a predominant comorbidity, cardiovascular disorders and their sequela are the leading cause of death in the ESRD population.[1,2]

Hypertension

As a primary cause or consequence of progressive loss of kidney function, hypertension is prevalent in the majority of patients with CKD (see Chap. 46). Approximately 50% to 60% of dialysis patients are hypertensive, defined as a predialysis blood pressure greater than 150/90 mm Hg, and only a small percentage of dialysis patients do not require antihypertensive therapy.[1] Hypertension induced by volume expansion and increased systemic vascular resistance increases myocardial work and contributes to development of left ventricular hypertrophy (LVH). A "U-shaped" relationship between blood pressure and mortality has been observed, such that higher mortality is associated with the highest and lowest levels of blood pressure.[1] The pathogenesis of hypertension in CKD is multifactorial, but in many hypertensive dialysis patients, fluid retention is a major contributor. In addition to the general pathophysiologic mechanisms responsible for the development of hypertension, patients with ESRD may also have increased sympathetic activity, decreased activity of vasodilators such as nitric oxide, elevated levels of endothelin-1, chronic use of an ESA such as epoetin alfa, hyperparathyroidism, and structural changes in the arteries (e.g., metastatic calcification) as contributing factors.[1]

Patients with ESRD also display an abnormal diurnal blood pressure rhythm as evidenced by the fact that their blood pressure does not decrease during the nighttime hours.[1] It is unclear what causes this disturbance in the diurnal rhythm, but this "nondipping" phenomenon indicates sustained elevations in blood pressure are present over a prolonged period of time when compared to the general population.

Hyperlipidemia

CKD with or without nephrotic syndrome is frequently accompanied by abnormalities in lipoprotein metabolism. It is well established that dyslipidemias cause atherosclerotic cardiovascular disease and there are many compelling reasons to aggressively treat these disorders.[18] A clear association between hypercholesterolemia, hypertriglyceridemia, or other lipoprotein changes in patients with CKD and the high incidence of cardiovascular disease has not been demonstrated in large prospective studies. However, it is likely that the same lipoprotein abnormalities that confer increased risk of cardiovascular disease in the general population would also be harmful to patients with kidney disease. A low or declining serum cholesterol in patients with ESRD also is associated with higher mortality, a paradoxical effect.[1,19] These findings beg the question of whether aggressive lipid lowering is warranted in this population. Further analysis, however, shows that low cholesterol levels were observed in conjunction with inflammation and malnutrition, factors that increase mortality. In the absence of these confounding factors, it is the higher cholesterol levels, not lower levels, that were associated with increased mortality, thus supporting treatment of hypercholesterolemia in ESRD patients.[1]

The lipid panel generally observed in patients with CKD without nephrotic syndrome is a normal total and low-density lipoprotein (LDL) cholesterol, low high-density lipoprotein (HDL), and high triglycerides (plasma concentrations >200 mg/dL).[20] Although the concentrations of LDL are not uniformly increased in patients with kidney disease, these patients appear to produce small, dense LDL particles that are more susceptible to oxidation and more atherogenic than larger LDL subfractions. Other lipoprotein abnormalities include changes in apoprotein content of lipoprotein molecules and increased very-low-density and intermediate-density lipoproteins. For patients with CKD and a urinary protein excretion greater than 3 g/day, the major lipid abnormalities are elevation of plasma total and LDL cholesterol, with or without low HDL cholesterol (<35 mg/dL) and elevated triglycerides. Treatment of proteinuria resolves the hyperlipidemia in most patients with nephrotic syndrome.

CLINICAL PRESENTATION

Damage to the kidney has detrimental consequences on many other organ systems, particularly once patients develop ESRD. The subjective and objective findings of CKD that may be present in an individual are dependent on the severity of disease (i.e., stage of CKD). At the time of referral to a nephrologist patients may present with some, but rarely all, of the signs and symptoms associated with uremia and secondary complications of CKD, unless they are in the more advanced stages of the disease (stage 4 or 5 CKD). It is apparent that management of CKD requires treatment of multiple secondary complications.

CLINICAL PRESENTATION OF STAGE 4 OR 5 CHRONIC KIDNEY DISEASE

Symptoms

- Uremic symptoms (fatigue, weakness, shortness of breath, mental confusion, nausea and vomiting, bleeding, and loss of appetite), as well as itching, cold intolerance, weight gain, and peripheral neuropathies are common in patients with stage 5 disease.

Signs

- Edema, changes in urine output (volume and consistency), "foaming" of urine (indicative of proteinuria), and abdominal distension.

Laboratory Tests[a]

- *Decreased:* creatinine clearance, bicarbonate (metabolic acidosis), hemoglobin/hematocrit (anemia), iron stores (iron deficiency), vitamin D levels, albumin (malnutrition), glucose (may result from decreased degradation of insulin with impaired kidney function or poor oral intake), calcium (in early stages of CKD), HDL.
- *Increased:* serum creatinine, blood urea nitrogen, potassium, phosphorus, PTH, blood pressure (hypertension is a common cause and result of CKD), glucose (uncontrolled diabetes is a cause of CKD), low-density lipoprotein and triglycerides, T_4 levels (hypothyroidism), calcium (in ESRD)
- *Other:* May be Hemoccult-positive if GI bleeding occurs secondary to uremia.

Other Diagnostic Tests

- Left ventricular hypertrophy may be observed, as well as increased homocysteine levels and increased C-reactive protein.

[a]Indicative of common secondary complications of CKD.

Recommendations for the evaluation and workup of several of the most common secondary complications of CKD are described in detail in the remainder of this chapter.

ANEMIA OF CHRONIC KIDNEY DISEASE

All patients with CKD should have their hemoglobin (Hb) measured at least annually. Testing should be conducted more frequently in individuals with more severe CKD, as well as in those at any stage who are diagnosed with anemia. If the Hb is less than 12 g/dL in adult females or less than 13.5 g/dL in adult males, a complete workup for anemia of CKD should be done.[21] This includes evaluation of other causes of anemia such as bleeding, deficiencies in vitamin B_{12} or folate, or other disease states that contribute to anemia, including human immunodeficiency virus infection and malignancies. As the primary cause of resistance to therapy for anemia of CKD, iron status must be evaluated. Red blood cell indices and iron indices should be measured, including the red blood cell indices (mean corpuscular hemoglobin, mean corpuscular volume, mean corpuscular hemoglobin concentration), white blood cell count, differential and platelet count, absolute reticulocyte count, transferrin saturation (TSat) or content of hemoglobin in the reticulocytes, and serum ferritin. A stool guaiac test should also be performed to rule out GI bleeding.

Iron deficiency manifests as a microcytic anemia and is accompanied by a low mean corpuscular volume, whereas deficiencies in vitamin B_{12} and folate present as a macrocytic anemia with an increase in mean corpuscular volume. The TSat is calculated as ([serum iron/TIBC] × 100), where TIBC is the total iron-binding capacity. If the TSat and serum ferritin values are below the desired threshold (see Table 47–2), iron supplementation is warranted prior to starting ESA therapy. If all other causes of anemia are ruled out and the anemia persists despite iron supplementation, patients should be treated with either epoetin alfa or darbepoetin alfa.

Iron supplementation is required by most patients with ESRD because of the increased iron demand that results from stimulation of red blood cell production with ESAs. As CKD worsens, a progressive decline in Hb despite ESA therapy may be observed. Consequently, regular followup of Hb and iron status is warranted to ensure the desired outcomes are met and to make necessary dose adjustments in ESAs and iron therapy (see Treatment of Anemia of Chronic Kidney Disease below).

The effects of anemia and decreased oxygen delivery on other comorbid conditions, including LVH, must also be considered given the burden of cardiovascular complications in this population.[22] The negative effects of anemia on quality of life are also important from a patient perspective and a compelling reason for early and aggressive treatment.[23]

SECONDARY HYPERPARATHYROIDISM AND RENAL OSTEODYSTROPHY

Disorders of calcium and phosphorus homeostasis including sHPT are prevalent in the CKD population. A recent evaluation of a cohort of outpatients found elevated PTH levels in approximately 21% of patients with an estimated GFR between 60 and 69 mL/min/1.73 m^2 and in 56% of patients with stage 3, 4, or 5 CKD (estimated GFR less than 60 mL/min/1.73 m^2).[7] Calcitriol deficiency was observed at all levels of GFR, but was more prevalent (greater than 60%) in the group with an estimated GFR of less than 30 mL/min/1.73 m.[2] These percentages are even higher in the ESRD population.[8,14] Consequently, preventative measures should be initiated in patients in the early stages of CKD.

The workup for sHPT and the associated metabolic abnormalities includes evaluation of serum phosphorus, calcium, Ca × P product, and PTH. These labs should be assessed at least every 3 months in the patient with stage 4 CKD. For the ESRD population, PTH should be evaluated at least every 3 months and the calcium and phosphorus assessed at least monthly. Many dialysis facilities have developed protocols that call for evaluation of all these parameters on a monthly basis. Measurement of the active vitamin D precursor, 25-hydroxyvitamin D, is recommended in patients with stage 4 CKD who have elevated PTH levels to determine the appropriate form of vitamin D supplementation required (see Treatment of Secondary Hypoparathyroidism below).

Bone mineral density and serum calcium and calcitriol concentrations decrease progressively, whereas serum PTH, osteocalcin, bone-specific alkaline phosphatase, and phosphorus concentrations increase as GFR declines.[7,9] Evaluation of bone histology may be warranted in patients with severe sHPT or in symptomatic stage 4 or 5 CKD patients. Bone disease can be diagnosed using iliac crest bone biopsy and bone histomorphometric analysis. Bone mineral densitometry studies may also be used to detect bone loss in patients with CKD and are useful to monitor response to therapeutic interventions. Coronary artery calcification can be evaluated by noninvasive means using electron-beam computed tomography. Invasive procedures such as coronary angiography can also be used to ascertain the degree of damage if the newer technology is not available.

Monitoring of serum aluminum levels should be done at least annually and as frequently as every 3 months in patients receiving aluminum-containing phosphate binders or other aluminum-based medications, although regular use of these agents is not recommended in patients with CKD.[8] If aluminum concentrations are elevated (60 to 200 mcg/L) a deferoxamine test should be done. The deferoxamine infusion test is based on the concept that the amount of aluminum mobilized following a single dose of deferoxamine is representative of the total-body burden of aluminum. A dose of 5 mg/kg of deferoxamine is administered, generally over the last hour of dialysis for hemodialysis patients. The serum aluminum level predose and 2 days postdose are compared. A change in serum aluminum concentration of ≥50 mcg/L is considered a positive test. A change of this magnitude in conjunction with an intact parathyroid hormone (iPTH) of <150 pg/mL is indicative of aluminum bone disease, which should then be confirmed by bone biopsy.[8]

PTH is secreted from the parathyroid gland as intact PTH, an 84-amino-acid peptide chain (1–84 PTH) that is biologically active, and as smaller carboxy-terminal PTH fragments.[24] Circulating levels of these fragments (e.g., 7–84 PTH) may increase substantially in patients with CKD and actively antagonize the effects to 1–84 PTH. Available immunoradiometric and immunochemiluminescent assays for measurement of intact PTH, such as the Nichols Institute Allegro immunoradiometric assay (IRMA), measure not only the intact molecule, but also fragments, which may lead to overestimation of biologically active PTH. The goal iPTH based on this assay method in ESRD patients is three to five times the upper limits of normal (approximately 200 to 300 pg/mL). Clinicians involved in the care of patients with CKD should become familiar with available assays used in their facilities so as to provide optimal care for their patients.

METABOLIC ACIDOSIS

Serum electrolytes should be measured routinely in patients with stage 4 and 5 CKD. If the results suggest the presence of an acidotic state, arterial blood gases should be measured. These patients should also have a complete medical history and review of medications to determine if there are other potential causes of acid–base disturbances (e.g., diabetic ketoacidosis, ingestion of toxins, or GI disorders). The anion gap, indicating the differences in unmeasured anions and cations, should also be calculated (see Chap. 55). An elevated anion gap (>17 mEq/L) is often present in patients with stage 4 or 5 CKD because of the accumulation of organic anions, phosphates, and sulfates. Treatment of metabolic acidosis in patients with CKD generally includes administration of bicarbonate to correct acidemia, the time course of which depends on the severity of the acidosis. Asymptomatic patients with mild acidosis (bicarbonate of 12 to 20 mEq/L; pH of 7.2 to 7.4) generally do not require emergent therapy and gradual correction over days to weeks is appropriate.

CARDIOVASCULAR DISEASE

The Kidney Disease/Dialysis Outcomes Quality Initiative (K/DOQI) guidelines on cardiovascular disease in dialysis patients recommend that all patients starting dialysis be assessed for cardiovascular disease (including coronary artery disease, cardiomyopathy, valvular heart disease, cerebrovascular disease, and peripheral vascular disease) and be screened for traditional (e.g., hypertension and hyperlipidemia) and nontraditional cardiovascular risk factors.[1]

Hypertension

Patients with stages 4 and 5 CKD should have their blood pressure evaluated at every clinic visit and at home, if appropriate. Patients with ESRD should have blood pressure monitored at every scheduled clinic visit (or hemodialysis session) and they should be encouraged to learn how to monitor their blood pressure while at home. Patients who have required extensive surgeries in both arms to establish vascular accesses should have blood pressure measured in the thighs or legs. Blood pressure monitoring with an appropriate-size cuff should be measured prior to insertion of the needles for hemodialysis.

Hyperlipidemia

A complete fasting lipid profile including total cholesterol, LDL, HDL, and triglycerides should be done in all CKD patients. Lipoprotein levels may be influenced by several factors, including GFR and proteinuria. It is recommended that CKD patients have their lipid profile assessed more frequently than the general population to identify abnormalities and treat them early. In patients on hemodialysis the lipid profile should be done prior to dialysis or on nondialysis days.[25] Patients should also be evaluated for other conditions that are known to cause dyslipidemias (e.g., liver disease).

TREATMENT

Chronic Kidney Disease

Once a patient is diagnosed with CKD, implementation of therapy to address the primary cause (e.g., diabetes, hypertension, or glomerulonephritis) and potentially delay progression is a priority. Chapter 46 discusses the key concepts involved in the management of these critical issues in detail. When patients reach stage 4, progression to ESRD is almost inevitable, although the process may be delayed if appropriate therapy is initiated. It is during stage 4 CKD that plans for renal replacement therapy (hemodialysis or peritoneal dialysis) need to be made, and patients educated about dialysis modalities and options for transplantation if they are candidates.

❹ Regardless of the stage of CKD at which the patient presents, the management of secondary complications (e.g., anemia and secondary hyperparathyroidism) and comorbid conditions, if they are present, is critical to maximize the length and optimize the quality of the patient's life. Historically, these conditions have not been appropriately managed.[26] Laboratory data to diagnose such complications (e.g., iron studies and PTH levels) are often not evaluated until the patient has reached ESRD. According to data from the 2007 United States Renal Data System report, the likelihood of a CKD patient receiving calcium and phosphorus testing (1.0 being ideal) was 0.29 and the probability of lipid monitoring was 0.64 for those with Medicare coverage.[2] Medicare patients with both diabetes and hypertension were more likely to be tested. With regard to anemia of CKD, based on claims data to evaluate care of CKD patients, it was determined that in the year prior to initiation of dialysis only 10.5% of patients had received an ESA and 6.8% a prescription iron product, despite more than 40% having been diagnosed with anemia.[27] Lack of attention to the disorder, problems with payment for drug therapy by third-party payers, and the logistics of maintaining the regular followup necessary for therapy with ESAs contribute to this poor management. Late referral to a nephrologist may in part account for this poor management; however, even in ideal clinical environments such as nephrology clinics, these secondary complications may be overlooked.

DESIRED OUTCOME

The overall goal of therapy is to optimize the patient's duration and quality of life. Patients who reach CKD stage 4 almost inevitably experience progression to ESRD and thus require dialysis to sustain their life. Chapter 48 discusses the considerations involved in selecting from among the dialysis options available for the management of ESRD. The following discussion thus focuses on minimizing the risks associated with the development of the consequences and complications of ESRD and their management.

GENERAL APPROACH TO PATIENT CARE

To delay the development of the consequences and secondary complications of ESRD frequent medication reviews are paramount to reduce the risk of drug-related problems and exposure of these patients to nephrotoxic agents (see Chap. 49). Drug-dosing guidelines based on the degree of kidney function should be followed, and a complete medication history of prescription and nonprescription medications, as well as herbals and nutritional supplements, should be obtained and routinely updated. Chronic use of nonsteroidal antiinflammatory drugs and cyclooxygenase-2 inhibitors should be avoided when possible. Patients should be instructed on all brand and generic names of these classes of medications to reduce the risk of exposure. Appropriate measures should also be taken for hospitalized patients to decrease the risk of nephrotoxicity from radiocontrast agents (for procedures requiring such dyes), and antibiotics such as aminoglycosides, as well as from nonsteroidal antiinflammatory drugs and angiotensin-converting enzyme inhibitors (ACEIs) (see Chaps. 45 and 49).

Continued patient education, initiated prior to development of ESRD, is essential to help patients become active participants in their own care and knowledgeable about medications, which they often require on a chronic basis. Pharmacists involved with the dialysis population have identified many specific drug-related problems (e.g., inappropriate dose or indication for a medication, adverse drug reactions) that commonly occur in the ESRD population and have demonstrated that the provision of clinical pharmacy services reduce such problems and contributes to improvements in patient quality of life.[28–30]

❺ When a patient with stage 4 or 5 CKD is initially evaluated, one of the most important steps is an early evaluation for the presence of secondary complications, as outlined in the Clinical Presentation above. Prompt initiation of management based on available consensus guidelines and the best clinical practices such as those developed by the National Kidney Foundation (K/DOQI) offer the most likely avenue for a successful patient outcome. The guidelines and recommendations were developed based on evidence, when available and the opinion of the expert group of individuals when the evidence was sparse. This process, although a standard approach to developing a consensus on patient care, is subject to criticism, especially those recommendations based solely or primarily on opinion. The K/DOQI guidelines should not replace clinical judgment, but rather provide a basis upon which treatment decisions can be made in the context of both evidence and opinion. The secondary complications that are addressed in the currently available clinical practice guidelines include anemia of CKD, bone metabolism and disease, cardiovascular disease in dialysis patients, dyslipidemias, hypertension, and nutrition.

❻ Appropriate management of secondary complications of CKD usually involves a multidisciplinary approach to manage the nonpharmacologic and pharmacologic interventions, dietary education, and social/financial concerns. The typical team includes physicians (primary care physicians and nephrologists), nurses, dietitians, and social workers in outpatient dialysis facilities. In some outpatient dialysis centers pharmacists are also active members of the care team, although this is more common in institutionalized environments. A strong emphasis on patient education by all clinicians cannot be overemphasized.[28–30]

FLUID AND ELECTROLYTE ABNORMALITIES

Maintenance of fluid volume, osmolarity, electrolyte balance, and acid–base status are all regulated in large part by the kidney, and their homeostasis is altered in patients with impaired kidney function. Chapters 52, 53, and 54 provide a comprehensive discussion of fluid and electrolyte disorders and treatment options. The unique aspects of treatment of sodium, water, and potassium disorders in stage 4 CKD and dialysis patients are highlighted here.

Desired Outcomes

Sodium and Water Homeostasis The goal is to maintain a normal serum sodium concentration (135 to 145 mEq/L) while maintaining euvolemia. By achieving these goals, the risk of developing or worsening hypertension secondary to volume overload is reduced.

Potassium Homeostasis The focus is on prevention of the acute adverse consequences, particularly cardiac effects, while maintaining potassium concentrations of approximately 4 to 5.5 mEq/L. This is often achieved through dietary restriction of potassium, minimizing exposure to medications that may increase serum potassium, and use of sodium–potassium exchange resins when indicated. If hyperkalemia develops, management options are based on the degree to which potassium is elevated (see Chap. 54).

Nonpharmacologic Therapy

Sodium and Water Balance The ability of the kidney to adjust to abrupt changes in sodium intake is greatly diminished in patients with severe CKD. Sodium restriction beyond a no-added-salt diet should not be recommended except in the face of hypertension or edema. The kidney maintains the ability to lower urinary sodium content to essentially zero, but this can only be accomplished by very gradual sodium restriction over a period of several days. Hospitalized patients should not routinely be sodium restricted because they have adapted to their outpatient intake. Negative sodium balance and its resultant volume contraction can result in decreased perfusion to the kidney and a subsequent further acute decline in GFR.

Fluid restriction is generally unnecessary for all but those patients with stage 5 CKD provided sodium intake is controlled. An intact thirst mechanism maintains total-body water and effective plasma osmolality near normal. Large amounts of free water administered orally or as IV fluid may induce hyponatremia and volume overload. Sodium retention and volume expansion also contribute to hypertension in many patients with severe CKD, and diuretic therapy may be necessary to control edema or blood pressure. When the patient develops ESRD, dialysis (specifically ultrafiltration) or a kidney transplant becomes necessary to maintain normovolemia.

Potassium Homeostasis Hyperkalemia is more common in patients with stage 5 CKD and in those who require dialysis. The majority of patients can be managed with a dietary potassium restriction of 50 to 80 mEq/day and a reduction in dialysate potassium concentrations for patients receiving hemodialysis or peritoneal dialysis (see Chap. 48). Hyperkalemia is less common, however, in the peritoneal dialysis population because of the more extensive removal of potassium by the peritoneal dialysis procedure and, in general, these patients are allowed more liberal dietary potassium intake.

Pharmacologic Therapy

Sodium and Water Balance Diuretic therapy is often necessary to prevent edema and the associated symptoms from volume overload. Loop diuretics increase urine volume and renal sodium excretion even in those with stage 4 CKD. A combination of a loop diuretic with a thiazide diuretic (such as hydrochlorothiazide or metolazone) can result in a profound excretion of sodium and water. Saline-containing IV solutions should be used cautiously in patients with CKD because the kidney's ability to excrete a salt load is impaired and thus they are prone to volume overload.

Potassium Homeostasis The definitive treatment of severe hyperkalemia for an ESRD patient is hemodialysis. In reality, there is often a delay between diagnosis of hyperkalemia and institution of dialysis, which necessitates the use of other temporizing measures, such as IV calcium gluconate, insulin and glucose, nebulized β_2-adrenergic agonists (albuterol), and sodium polystyrene sulfonate (see Chap. 54). Unfortunately, shifting potassium into the intracellular fluid compartment with insulin and glucose or with albuterol makes removal of potassium via dialysis more difficult. Multiple dialysis sessions may be necessary following potassium redistribution to the extracellular space. Sodium polystyrene sulfonate (with sorbitol), a potassium–sodium exchange resin, can be given orally in doses of 25 to 50 g to increase potassium excretion via the ileum and colon. Lastly, sodium bicarbonate therapy is no longer advocated in the treatment of ESRD hyperkalemia unless severe metabolic acidosis is also present, because the potassium-lowering effect is unreliable. Loop diuretics, a standard pharmacologic treatment option for hyperkalemia, are ineffective in patients with ESRD.

A review of medications to identify those that increase serum potassium should also be done regularly. This includes potassium-sparing diuretics, β-blockers, which interfere with the extrarenal translocation of potassium into cells, and ACEIs, which may cause hyperkalemia by reducing aldosterone production. Polycitra, used for the treatment of metabolic acidosis, contains potassium citrate and should not be prescribed for patients with severe CKD. The contribution of dialysis modalities to potassium homeostasis in patients with ESRD must also be considered (see Chap. 48). Constipation in patients with CKD can interfere with colonic potassium excretion; therefore a good bowel regimen is also important.

CLINICAL CONTROVERSY

Spironolactone and eplerenone decrease cardiovascular mortality in patients with severe heart failure. However, because data on use of these agents in patients with ESRD are very limited, and because these agents contribute to hyperkalemia, they should be used with great caution in patients with ESRD. It may be prudent to avoid prescribing these agents until additional studies are reported supporting their safety in the ESRD population.

Evaluation of Therapeutic Outcomes

Monitoring of volume status and serum electrolyte levels should be done at each followup visit in patients with stages 4 and 5 CKD, particularly given the risk and detrimental consequences of volume overload and extracellular fluid volume expansion (e.g., hypertension and pulmonary edema) and hyperkalemia (e.g., arrhythmias). Clinicians should evaluate patients for signs and symptoms of volume overload (e.g., pitting edema, rales, ascites, shortness of breath, and increased weight). Blood pressure monitoring in the clinic setting and at home, if feasible, to monitor the efficacy of the antihypertensive regimen is also warranted. As kidney disease progresses dietary intervention and diuretic therapy (based on the degree of kidney function) will likely become necessary. Laboratory evaluation of serum potassium is warranted to identify hyperkalemia. The patient should also be instructed about how to do a self-evaluation for signs and symptoms of edema and about nonpharmacologic interventions to prevent volume overload and hyperkalemia.

Patients with stage 5 CKD on hemodialysis are seen in the dialysis facilities much more frequently (three times per week) than patients with early stage CKD and peritoneal dialysis patients. Assessment of electrolytes is generally done once per month, although this is evaluated more frequently if necessary. Other pertinent observations in this population include a rise in the predialysis weight over a relative short period of time and shortness of breath, both indicative of volume overload. In these situations, the dialysis prescription may be altered acutely to remove more volume during the dialysis procedure (see Chap. 48) and the patient will require counseling on appropriate dietary intake of sodium and water.

■ ANEMIA OF CHRONIC KIDNEY DISEASE

Desired Outcome

The desired outcomes of anemia management are to increase oxygen-carrying capacity, thereby decreasing dyspnea, orthopnea, and fatigue, and to prevent long-term consequences such as LVH and cardiovascular mortality. To achieve these goals one must have adequate iron, folate, and B_{12}, and sufficient levels of ESAs. Other factors that contribute to worsening of anemia, such as blood loss and other causes of resistance to ESA therapy, should also be identified and corrected if possible. Specific targets for hemoglobin and iron indices, recommendations for appropriate use of ESAs and iron preparations, and recommendations on adjuvant therapy for anemia management based on the K/DOQI guidelines and clinical practice recommendations are discussed in the following sections. Table 47–2 lists the target hemoglobin and iron indices.

Target Hemoglobin The Hb is the preferred monitoring parameter for anemia because hematocrit (HCT) fluctuates with volume

TABLE 47-2 Target Parameters for Anemia Management in Chronic Kidney Disease

Parameter	Stage 4 CKD and Peritoneal Dialysis Patients	Hemodialysis Patients
Hb	11–12 g/dL	11–12 g/dL
TSat[a]	>20%	>20%
CHr	–	>29 pg/cell
Serum ferritin[a]	>100 ng/mL	>200 ng/mL

CHr, content of hemoglobin in reticulocytes; CKD, chronic kidney disease; Hb, hemoglobin; TSat, transferrin saturation.

[a]No upper limit defined; be aware of the risk of iron overload.

Data from KDOQI Clinical Practice Guidelines and Clinical Practice Recommendations for Anemia in Chronic Kidney Disease. Am J Kidney Dis 2006;47:S11–145.

status and may be falsely elevated if the blood sample has been stored for a prolonged period of time. The lower end of the target hemoglobin concentration (Hb) range in patients treated for anemia of CKD prior to March 2007 had been greater than 11 g/dL (corresponding HCT 33%), a value lower than that accepted in patients without CKD. However, no absolute ceiling Hb was recommended; rather, there was a statement in the guidelines that there is insufficient evidence to recommend maintaining Hb levels at 13.0 g/dL or greater.

A higher mortality rate for ESRD patients with Hb/HCT values above the target ranges has been reported, particularly in patients with cardiac disorders;[31] however, beneficial effects of increasing the HCT up to 39% have also been observed, including improvements in cardiac function, cognitive ability, and quality of life.[32] Hence, the target Hb range in CKD patients continues to be debated. Two recently published randomized clinical trials have provided more information, yet stimulated more debate, on the target Hb in early stage CKD. In the Correction of Hemoglobin and Outcomes in Renal Insufficiency (CHOIR) trial, patients with an estimated GFR of 15 to 50 mL/min/1.73 m^2 were treated with human erythropoietin (epoetin alfa) to achieve a high Hb (13.5 g/dL) or a lower Hb (11.3 g/dL) to evaluate differences in risk of complications from cardiovascular causes and death; primary end points were time to the composite of death, myocardial infarction, hospitalization for congestive heart failure (excluding renal replacement therapy), or stroke.[33] After 16 months there were 125 events in the high Hb group (n = 715), achieved Hb was12.6 g/dL, and 97 events in the low Hb group (n = 717), achieved Hb was 11.3 g/dL, indicating a higher risk of adverse events with a higher Hb (hazard ratio: 1.34; 95% confidence interval: 1.03 to 1.74; $P = 0.03$). Those who reached the target Hb in the higher Hb group received larger doses of epoetin alfa (10,694 units) compared to those who achieved the target Hb in the lower Hb group (6,057 units). In the Cardiovascular Risk Reduction by Early Anemia Treatment with Epoetin Beta (CREATE) trial, the effect of complete anemia correction (Hb 13.0 to 15.0 g/dL) versus partial anemia correction (Hb 10.5 to 11.5 g/dL) on cardiovascular outcomes (time to first cardiovascular event) in patients with an estimated GFR of 15 to 35 mL/min/1.73 m^2 was evaluated.[34] After 3 years of treatment there was no significant difference in the risk of a first cardiovascular event between the complete correction (n = 301) and partial correction (n = 302) groups (hazard ratio: 0.78; 95% confidence interval: 0.53 to 1.14; $P = 0.20$).

Based on these data and more recent observations, the FDA and the manufacturer of these products agreed, in March 2007, on revised product labeling that includes updated warnings, a new boxed warning, and modifications to the dosing instructions. The new boxed warning advises health care providers to monitor Hb and to adjust the ESA dose to maintain the lowest hemoglobin level needed to avoid blood transfusions. Health care providers and patients should carefully weigh the risks of ESAs against risks of transfusion. Other recently completed studies describe an increased risk of death, blood clots, strokes, and heart attacks in patients with chronic kidney failure when ESAs were given at higher than recommended doses. Based on the most currently available, albeit controversial, information, the target upper limit for Hb in patients treated for anemia of CKD should be individualized based on the patient's condition and dosage regimen adjusted to avoid Hb values greater than 12 g/dL until further evidence is available.

Additional information about treatment of anemia with ESAs will likely be available in the near future. The Trial to Reduce Cardiovascular Events with Aranesp Therapy (TREAT) is currently ongoing, with a planned enrollment of 4,000 patients. This is a randomized, placebo-controlled study in patients with type 2 diabetes and an estimated GFR of less than 60 mL/min/1.73 m^2 to evaluate differences in the composite primary end point of cardiovascular death, heart failure, myocardial infarction, stroke, and hospitalization for unstable angina treatment for patients who receive darbepoetin alfa (Aranesp) to achieve a target Hb of 13 g/dL versus a target Hb greater than 9 g/dL. Patients in the latter group will receive darbepoetin if the Hb falls to less than 9 g/dL, but otherwise will receive placebo. This trial may provide information to answer questions regarding treatment of anemia in a population at high risk of cardiovascular events.

Iron Status Iron indices that should be monitored include the TSat, an indicator of iron immediately available for delivery to the bone marrow, and serum ferritin, an indirect measure of storage iron. Transferrin is the carrier protein for iron and, as a protein, may be affected by nutritional status. Serum ferritin is an acute-phase reactant, meaning it may be elevated under certain inflammatory conditions and give a false indication of storage iron. The content of hemoglobin in reticulocytes also is reliable in assessing iron status in hemodialysis patients and is recommended in the K/DOQI guidelines as an alternative to TSat to assess iron deficiency in this population.[21,35] Table 47–2 lists the recommended target iron indices to achieve prior to initiation of ESA therapy and to maintain during therapy.[21] The higher acceptable level for serum ferritin of greater than 200 ng/mL in hemodialysis patients is based on the information showing improved outcomes (lower ESA doses and improved response to iron) at this level of ferritin. The current K/DOQI anemia guidelines differ from the previous guidelines which had recommended an upper level for TSat of 50% and serum ferritin of 800 ng/mL to reduce the risk of iron overload. No upper level for these iron indices has been clearly established in the current recommendations based on available safety information; however, the risk of iron overload always needs to be considered with IV iron supplementation. According to the K/DOQI recommendations there is insufficient evidence to recommend routine administration of IV iron if the patient's serum ferritin level is greater than 500 ng/mL.[21] Since ferritin can be elevated by many conditions the intepretations of singular values is challenging. The decision of whether or not to give IV iron is thus primarily based on clinical judgements.

Nonpharmacologic Therapy

Nonpharmacologic therapy for anemia of CKD includes maintaining adequate dietary intake of iron. A relatively small amount of dietary iron, approximately 1 to 2 mg (or approximately 10%), is absorbed each day, primarily in the duodenum. Although there is some debate as to whether GI absorption of iron is significantly altered in patients with severe CKD, it is clear that oral intake from dietary sources alone is generally insufficient to meet the increased iron requirements that are necessitated by the initiation of erythropoietic therapy.[21]

Pharmacologic Therapy

8 Pharmacologic therapy for anemia of CKD includes chronic therapy with an ESA to correct erythropoietin deficiency and iron supplementation to correct and prevent iron deficiency caused by ongoing blood loss and increased iron demands associated with the initiation of erythropoietic therapy (Figs. 47–2 and 47–3). Iron

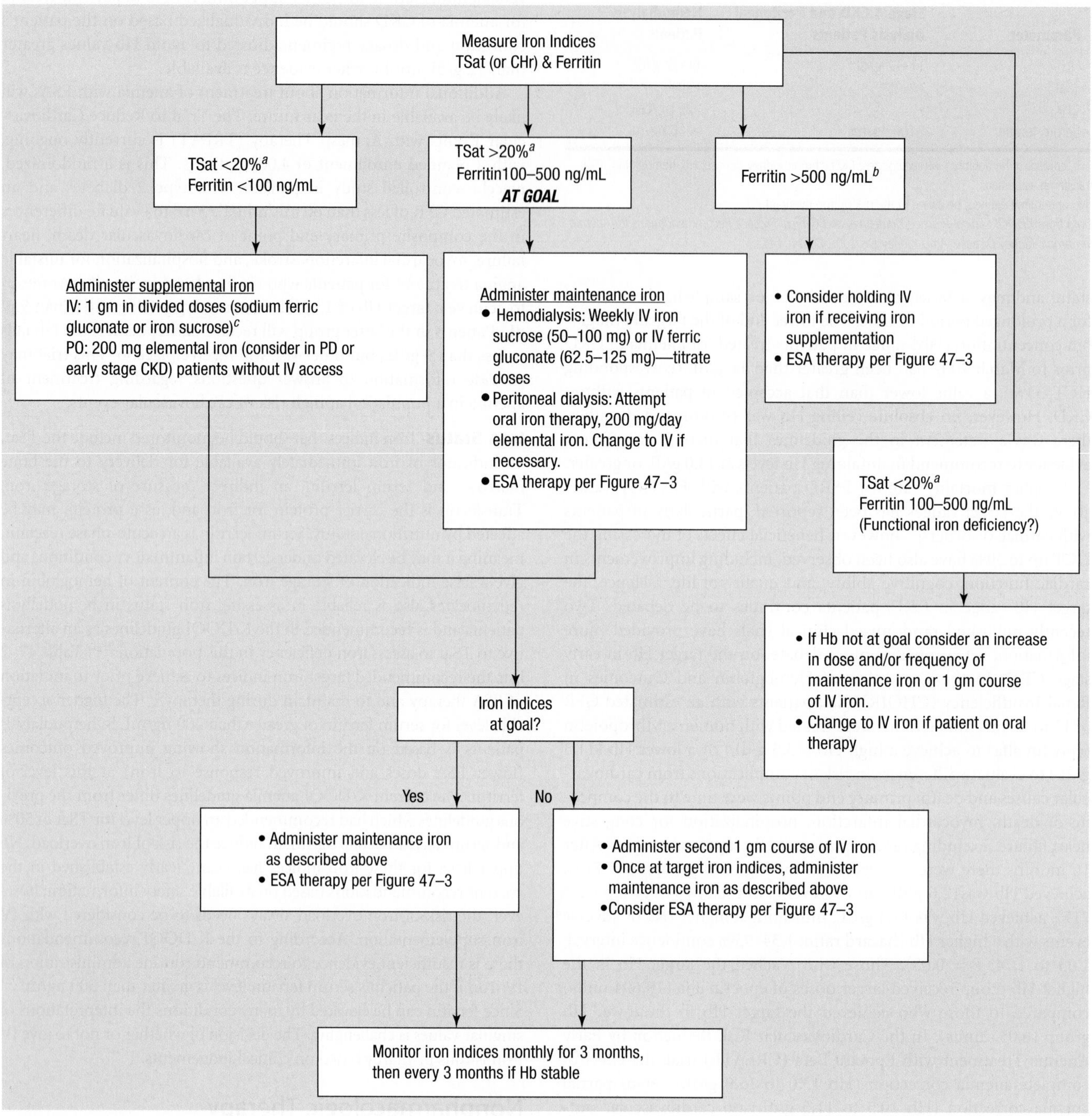

[a] Or CHr <29 pg/cell in hemodialysis patients
[b] Clinical judgement should be used to determine if iron supplementation should be continued when ferritin >500 ng/mL
[c] IV iron regimen may be divided over 8–10 HD sessions (depending on product used) or given in larger doses over a prolonged administration time (e.g. up to 400 mg iron sucrose over 2.5 hrs) for patients on PD

FIGURE 47-2. Guidelines for iron therapy in the management of the anemia of chronic kidney disease. (CHr, content of hemoglobin in the reticulocytes; ESA, erythropoietic-stimulating agent; Hb, hemoglobin; TSat, transferrin saturation.)

therapy is first-line therapy for anemia of CKD if iron deficiency is diagnosed, and for some patients the target Hb may be achieved without concomitant ESA therapy. Coadministration of iron and an ESA is often required to effectively stimulate erythropoiesis and prevent microcytic anemia that occurs with iron deficiency.

Iron Supplementation If TSat (or content of hemoglobin in the reticulocytes) and serum ferritin are below goal indices, iron supplementation is recommended. Options for iron supplementation include oral and IV therapy (Tables 47–3 and 47–4). Available oral iron preparations differ in their content of elemental iron. Products available for oral therapy include ferrous salts (ferrous sulfate, ferrous fumarate, and ferrous gluconate), polysaccharide iron complex, and, most recently, a heme iron polypeptide formulation. Four IV iron products are currently available in the United States (Table 47–4): two composed of iron dextran (INFeD, molecular weight [MW] 96,000; and Dexferrum, MW 267,000), sodium ferric gluconate (Ferrlecit, MW 350,000), and iron sucrose (Venofer, MW 43,000).

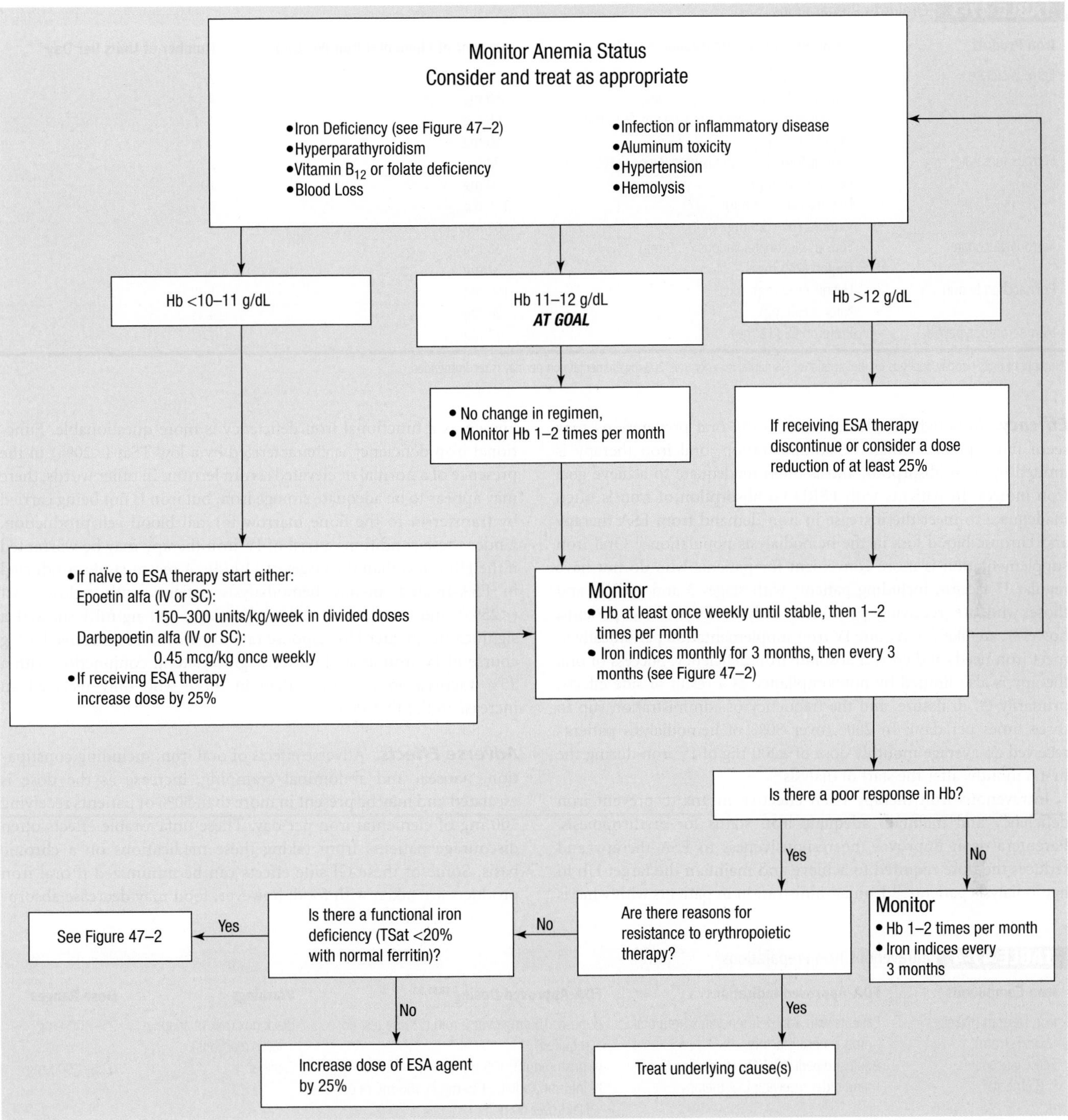

FIGURE 47-3. Guidelines for erythropoietic stimulating agent therapy in the management of the anemia of chronic kidney disease. (ESA, erythropoietic-stimulating agent; Hb, hemoglobin; SC, subcutaneous; TSat, transferrin saturation.)

Pharmacology and Mechanism of Action. Iron supplements provide the elemental iron required for production of hemoglobin and its subsequent incorporation in red blood cells, the net result of which is an increase in the transportation of oxygen to tissues. Supplementation of iron is necessary to replete iron stores and maintain adequate iron for transport to the bone marrow.

Pharmacokinetics. Approximately 10% of orally administered iron is absorbed in the duodenum and upper jejunum. Absorption of iron is decreased by food and achlorhydria. The heme form of oral iron binds to a different receptor in the GI tract than nonheme iron, is absorbed to a greater extent, and may be better tolerated.[36] Some oral iron formulations also include ascorbic acid to enhance iron absorption. Although there is an association between ascorbic acid intake and oxalate formation, this association is generally not observed at doses of ascorbic acid contained in these iron formulations.

Intravenous iron preparations differ in the composition of the complex to which elemental iron is bound. These differences affect the rate of dissociation of iron from the complex to the reticuloendothelial system and subsequent storage as ferritin. The half-life of these formulations also differ: ferric gluconate (1 hour), iron sucrose (6 hours), and iron dextran (40 to 60 hours). However, there is minimal to no correlation between the pharmacokinetics of these formulations and their pharmacodynamic effects.[37]

TABLE 47-3 Oral Iron Preparations

Iron Product	Common Agents and Available Units	Amount of Elemental Iron Per Unit	Number of Units Per Day[a]
Ferrous sulfate	Fer-In-Sol (75 mg/0.6 mL)	75 mg	2–3
	Feosol (200 mg)	50 mg	4
	Ferrous sulfate, various preparations (325 mg)	65 mg	3–4
	Slow FE (160 mg)	50 mg	4
Ferrous fumarate	Ferrous fumarate, various preparations (300 mg)	99 mg	2
	Femiron (20 mg)	20 mg	10
	Nephro-Fer (350 mg)	115 mg	2
	Vitron-C (65–125 mg)	65 mg	3
Ferrous gluconate	Ferrous gluconate, various (325 mg)	36 mg	6
	Fergon (240 mg)	27 mg	6
Polysaccharide iron	Hytinic (150 mg)	150 mg	1–2
	Niferex (50 mg)	50 mg	4
Heme iron polypeptide	Proferrin-ES (12 mg)	12 mg	17

[a]Number of units per day depends on the amount of elemental iron per unit; 200 mg elemental iron per day is recommended.

Efficacy. Although supplementation using oral preparations may seem more practical than IV administration, oral iron therapy is limited by poor absorption and is often inadequate to achieve goal iron indices. In patients with ESRD GI absorption of iron is often inadequate to meet the increase in iron demand from ESA therapy and chronic blood loss in the hemodialysis population.[21] Oral iron supplementation is more convenient for patients who do not have regular IV access, including patients with stages 3 and 4 CKD and those who are receiving peritoneal dialysis. Even these patients, however, are likely to require IV iron supplementation periodically to meet iron needs and correct absolute iron deficiency. Success of oral therapy is also limited by noncompliance as a result of side effects, primarily GI in nature, and the frequency of administration (up to three times per day). In 2005, over 80% of hemodialysis patients received an average monthly dose of ≥200 mg of IV iron during the first 6 months after the start of dialysis.[2]

Intravenous iron therapy is an effective means to prevent iron deficiency and maintain adequate iron status for erythropoiesis. Parenteral iron improves the responsiveness to ESA therapy and reduces the dose required to achieve and maintain the target Hb in hemodialysis patients.[21] Iron administration in patients with what is known as a functional iron deficiency is more questionable. Functional iron deficiency is characterized by a low TSat (<20%) in the presence of a normal or elevated serum ferritin. In other words, there may appear to be adequate storage iron, but iron is not being carried by transferrin to the bone marrow for red blood cell production. Under these conditions a trial of IV iron therapy may be warranted if the Hb is less than the target of 11 g/dL. A recent study conducted in ESA-treated anemic hemodialysis patients with a low TSat (<25%) and an elevated serum ferritin (>500 ng/mL) showed a significantly greater Hb response rate in patients who received a 1-g course of IV iron as sodium ferric gluconate in conjunction with a 25% increase in ESA dose than in those who only received an increase in the ESA dose.[38]

Adverse Effects. Adverse effects of oral iron, including constipation, nausea, and abdominal cramping, increase as the dose is escalated and may be present in more than 50% of patients receiving 200 mg of elemental iron per day. These unfavorable effects often discourage patients from taking these medications on a chronic basis. Some of these GI side effects can be minimized if oral iron products are taken with food; however, food may decrease absorp-

TABLE 47-4 Intravenous Iron Preparations[a]

Iron Compounds	FDA-Approved Indications	FDA-Approved Dosing[48,51,52]	Warnings	Dose Ranges[b]
Iron Dextran (INFeD, DexFerrum)[c]	Patients with iron deficiency in whom oral iron is unsatisfactory	IV push: 100 mg over 2 min (25-mg test dose required)	Black box (risk of anaphylactic reactions)	25–1,000 mg
Ferric gluconate (Ferrlecit)[d]	Adult and pediatric HD patients age 6 years and older receiving ESA therapy	IV push (adult): 125 mg over 10 min IV infusion (adult): 125 mg in 100 mL of 0.9% NaCl over 60 min IV infusion (pediatric): 1.5 mg/kg in 25 mL of 0.9% of NaCl over 60 min; maximum dose 125 mg	General	62.5–1,000 mg
Iron sucrose (Venofer)[e]	HD patients with CKD receiving ESA therapy	IV push: 100 mg over 2–5 min IV infusion: 100 mg in maximum of 100 mL of 0.9% NaCl over 15 min	General	25–1,000 mg
	Nondialysis-CKD patients receiving or not receiving ESA therapy	IV push: 200 mg over 2–5 min on 5 different occasions within 14-day period		
	PD patients receiving ESA therapy	IV infusion: 2 infusions, 14 days apart, of 300 mg in maximum 250 mL of 0.9% NaCl over 1.5 h, followed by 1 infusion, 14 days later, of 400 mg in maximum 250 mL of 0.9% NaCl over 2.5 h		

CKD, chronic kidney disease; ESA, erythropoietin-stimulating agent; HD, hemodialysis; PD, peritoneal dialysis.
[a]All products may be administered IV push (small doses only).
[b]Small dosing ranges (e.g., 25–150 mg per week) generally used for maintenance regimens. Larger doses (e.g. 1 gram) should be administered in divided doses.
[c]Supplied in 2-mL single dose vials containing 50 mg of elemental iron per mL.
[d]Available in colorless glass ampules containing 62.5 mg elemental iron (12.5 mg/mL).
[e]Supplied in 5-mL single-dose vials containing 100 mg elemental iron (20 mg/mL).

tion of oral iron. Patients should initially be instructed to take oral iron on an empty stomach; however, if side effects lead to intolerance and noncompliance these agents can be administered with food or an alternative agent may be prescribed.

Adverse effects of IV iron include allergic reactions, hypotension, dizziness, dyspnea, headaches, lower back pain, arthralgia, syncope, and arthritis. Some of these reactions, in particular hypotension, can be minimized by decreasing the dose or rate of infusion of iron. The most concerning potential consequence of IV iron administration is anaphylaxis. Anaphylactoid reactions to iron dextran have been reported in up to 1.8% of patients, with serious reactions including respiratory complications and cardiovascular collapse occurring in approximately 0.6%.[39] Such reactions are believed to be partly a response to antibody formation to the dextran component. Adverse reactions have been reported more frequently in those receiving Dexferrum compared to INFeD; a two- to eightfold increase in the incidence was noted with Dexferrum.[40] Such differences were particularly influential in product selection prior to the availability of sodium ferric gluconate and iron sucrose. These IV iron formulations have a better safety record than either of the iron dextran products, based on their history of use in Europe over the last four decades and recent data in the United States since these products were approved.[41,42] Sodium ferric gluconate and iron sucrose do not require a test dose prior to administration of the full dose, unlike iron dextran, which requires a 25-mg test dose to evaluate the risk of anaphylactic reactions. As a precaution with all IV preparations, patients should be observed during and immediately following administration for any adverse reactions.

Administration of IV iron also introduces a risk of iron overload. Deposition of excess iron may affect several organ systems, leading to hepatic, pancreatic, and cardiac dysfunction. Bone marrow biopsy provides the most definitive diagnosis of iron overload, but because it is an extremely invasive procedure, it is not widely employed in most clinical settings. Maintaining serum ferritin and TSat values that demonstrate efficacy in preventing iron deficiency yet are safe is the most reasonable approach to minimize the risk of iron toxicity. The challenge is in defining these upper limits, particularly for serum ferritin, which may be elevated in inflammatory conditions and not reflective of true iron stores in such situations. If symptomatic overload does occur, deferoxamine (Desferal) or phlebotomy may be necessary.

The safety and efficacy of high-dose IV iron regimens have been evaluated to determine the most cost-effective and efficacious dosing strategies. Iron dextran has been safely administered to dialysis patients in total-dose infusions ranging from 400 mg to 2 g.[43] Similar high-dose regimens of 500 mg have also been safely administered to patients with stages 3 and 4 CKD.[44] Although such iron dextran regimens have been safely administered, it is important to consider that with the information available today on the safety profile of sodium ferric gluconate and iron sucrose, many clinicians would consider these newer agents as first-line therapy. Sodium ferric gluconate has been safely administered at doses of 250 mg infused over 1 hour (4.2 mg/min).[45] In this same evaluation, 19 doses greater than 250 mg were administered; 1 dose of 312.5 mg, 14 doses of 375 mg, and 4 doses of 500 mg, with infusion rates varying from 1.22 mg/min to 25 mg/min. No serious adverse events were reported, although nonserious events, such as pruritus, did occur in 4 of the 144 patients who received the 250-mg dose. Doses in these higher ranges should not be adopted as standard of care until further safety data become available. If doses higher than those currently approved are used in practice, they should be administered over a prolonged time period (at least 2 hours). Iron sucrose at doses of up to 500 mg administered over 3 hours on consecutive days has been successful in maintaining iron stores without causing serious adverse events.[46] When administered over a shorter time period this same dose was associated with dizziness, hypotension, and nausea.[47] In this same evaluation the administration of lower doses of 200 to 300 mg given over 2 hours resulted in fewer adverse events. Higher dose regimens for iron sucrose have been approved in patients with early stage CKD and peritoneal dialysis patients (see Table 47–4), populations in whom administration of higher doses are more convenient as these patients are seen less frequently by healthcare providers than the hemodialysis population.[48]

Although there are conflicting reports, most clinicians believe that exposure to iron may contribute to the risk of bacterial infection because iron is used by microorganisms for metabolic functions.[49] The association of IV iron with oxidative stress, acceleration of atherosclerosis, and other cardiovascular conditions has also been suggested.[50] These potential long-term risks of IV iron therapy are not clearly defined and there are no data that unequivocally confirm that aggressive use of IV iron in CKD patients treated with ESA therapy increases patient morbidity or mortality.

Drug–Drug and Drug–Food Interactions. Drugs commonly used in the CKD population that may decrease absorption of oral iron include calcium preparations and antacids. Oral iron may also decrease the absorption of quinolone antibiotics. Medications that increase gastric pH, such as H_2-antagonists and proton pump inhibitors, may also decrease iron absorption as iron absorption in the duodenum is maximized at an acidic pH.

Dosing and Administration. Correction of absolute iron deficiency (TSat less than 20%, serum ferritin less than 100 ng/mL [less than 200 ng/mL in hemodialysis patients]) requires administration of iron. The route of administration may be oral or IV in the stage 4 CKD and peritoneal dialysis patients. If oral therapy is initiated, the recommended dose is 200 mg of elemental iron per day (see Table 47–3). The IV route of administration is preferred in hemodialysis patients. For the hemodialysis population typical repletion dosing regimens are 100 mg as iron sucrose or iron dextran over 10 dialysis sessions, or 125 mg of sodium ferric gluconate over 8 dialysis sessions (see Table 47–4).[48,51,52] These regimens are FDA-approved and reduce the risk of adverse reactions to IV iron therapy.

Administration of 1 g of IV iron is also reasonable to initially replete hemodialysis patients with an absolute iron deficiency; however, without ongoing iron supplementation, many patients quickly become iron deficient. There is sufficient evidence to support use of maintenance doses of IV iron in hemodialysis patients (e.g., iron sucrose or iron dextran 25 to 100 mg/wk; sodium ferric gluconate 62.5 to 125 mg/wk).[53]

Erythropoietic-Stimulating Agent Therapy

Pharmacology and Mechanism of Action. ESAs are required to stimulate differentiation of erythroid progenitor stem cells and induce the release of reticulocytes from the bone marrow to the bloodstream where they mature into erythrocytes (red blood cells). Available ESAs include epoetin alfa (distributed as Epogen by Amgen, Inc., Thousand Oaks, CA; and Procrit by Ortho Biotech, Johnson & Johnson, Raritan, NJ) and darbepoetin alfa (Aranesp by Amgen, Inc.). Epoetin beta is available from several different sources outside the United States. These agents are glycoproteins manufactured by recombinant DNA technology that have the same biologic activity as endogenous erythropoietin. Although the amino acid sequence of epoetin alfa is identical to the endogenous protein, the carbohydrate structure differs. Since 1989, epoetin alfa has been the mainstay of therapy for anemia of CKD and substantially reduced the percentage of patients dependent on transfusions for management of anemia. Darbepoetin alfa was approved for treatment of anemia of CKD in September 2001. Darbepoetin alfa differs from epoetin alfa by the addition of two N-linked carbohydrate side chains, which increases the sialic acid content of darbepoetin compared with epoetin alfa, resulting in a higher molecular weight (~38,000 daltons for darbepoetin compared with 30,400 daltons for epoetin alfa).[54]

Pharmacokinetics and Pharmacodynamics. Epoetin alfa may be administered by either the IV or subcutaneous (SC) routes. Although bioavailability with SC administration is poor (approximately 20%), the low peak serum concentrations and the prolonged half-life (approximately 24 hours as compared to 8.5 hours IV)[55] yield a Hb response that is at least as good or better than that attained with IV administration.[56] This enhanced efficacy is presumed to be caused by a more prolonged physiologic stimulation of erythroid precursors. The SC doses required to achieve and maintain the target Hb have been reported as 15% to 50% lower than doses required with IV administration.[53] Darbepoetin alfa has a longer half-life and extended biologic activity than does epoetin alfa (darbepoetin alfa 25.3 hours IV, 48.8 hours SC) as a consequence of the increased sialic acid content.[57] The prolonged half-life of darbepoetin offers the advantage of less-frequent dosing, starting at once-a-week or once-every-other-week dosing when given IV or SC.[58] This is of particular benefit in nondialysis CKD patients and in the peritoneal dialysis population, who are not seen by healthcare providers in the clinic as often. Prolonged dosing intervals, as infrequent as once every 4 weeks, have also been effective in maintaining target Hb in many CKD patients, including nondialysis CKD and ESRD patients.[59,60]

The pharmacodynamics of epoetin and darbepoetin are important to consider when evaluating response to therapy. With initiation of ESA therapy or a change in dose, the Hb may begin to rise as the result of demargination of reticulocytes; however, it takes approximately 10 days before erythrocyte progenitor cells mature and are released into the circulation. The Hb continues to increase until the life span of the cells stimulated by epoetin or darbepoetin is reached (mean 2 months; range 1 to 4 months in patients with ESRD). At this point a new steady state is achieved (i.e. the rate at which red blood cells are being produced equals the rate at which they are leaving the circulation). For this reason it is important to evaluate the Hb response over several weeks as opposed to making changes in the dosing regimen prematurely.

Efficacy. Efficacy of ESA therapy is determined by the change in Hb after initiation of therapy or following a dose adjustment, with the ultimate goal of achieving the target Hb of 11 to 12 g/dL. Patients will generally respond to ESA therapy in a dose-related fashion unless there are factors present that may cause resistance to therapy. The K/DOQI guidelines define failure to respond to therapy when there has been a significant increase in the ESA dose required to maintain a target Hb or a significant decrease in Hb at a constant ESA dose, or when the Hb fails to increase to greater than 11 g/dL despite an ESA dose equivalent to epoetin greater than 500 international units/kg/wk.[21] A number of factors and conditions may cause resistance to ESA therapy, including iron deficiency, hospitalization, catheter insertion, hypoalbuminemia, elevated C-reactive protein, chronic bleeding, aluminum toxicity, malnutrition, hyperparathyroidism, cancer and chemotherapy, AIDS, inflammation, and infection.[21]

As the most common cause of resistance, iron deficiency must be routinely evaluated for and treatment begun prior to initiation of ESAs. Inflammation (localized or systemic infection, active inflammatory disease, or surgical trauma) is associated with defective iron utilization known as *reticuloendothelial block.* Reticuloendothelial block is characterized by a reduction in iron delivery from body stores to the bone marrow, and is generally refractory to iron therapy. Erythropoietic therapy may be continued in the infected or postoperative patient, even though increased doses are often required to maintain or slow the rate of decline in Hb. Deficiencies in folate and vitamin B_{12} should also be considered as potential causes of resistance to ESA therapy, as both are essential for optimal erythropoiesis. Patients on hemodialysis or peritoneal dialysis should be routinely supplemented with water-soluble vitamins (including B_{12} and folate) as these vitamins are often depleted with dialysis therapy. There is also some evidence to suggest that patients receiving ACEIs may be relatively resistant to erythropoietic therapy, although these findings have not been consistently demonstrated.[61] An increase in the dosage of ESAs may be necessary in patients receiving ACEIs who do not maintain a stable Hb.

Studies have demonstrated reduced morbidity, increased exercise capacity and tolerance, and enhanced quality of life when ESA therapy was initiated, iron stores maintained, and target Hb attained.[21,32] Data also suggest a stabilization or regression of LVH in patients with early kidney disease and in those with ESRD when anemia is successfully treated.[62] Whether there is an optimal Hb target to prevent development of LVH remains to be determined. In a 2-year study, no difference in left ventricular mass index was observed between patients with stages 3 or 4 CKD maintained at a Hb of 9 to 10 g/dL versus 12 to 13 g/dL.[63] Given these observations and the recent concerns regarding the target Hb level additional prospective studies addressing this question will be needed to resolve the controversy.

Adverse Effects. Epoetin alfa and darbepoetin alfa are generally well tolerated; hypertension is the most common adverse event reported.[21] Protocols established in some clinical settings, primarily in outpatient dialysis clinics, sometimes recommend withholding ESA therapy if blood pressure is above a defined threshold. K/DOQI guidelines for anemia do not recommend withholding ESA therapy for elevated blood pressure, but advocate more judicious use of antihypertensive agents and dialysis to control blood pressure.[21] However, FDA approved product labeling advise that ESAs not be used in those with uncontrolled blood pressure. Although seizures have occurred in patients treated with epoetin, the incidence does not appear to be increased over the baseline levels seen in placebo control groups. Vascular access thrombosis may be more frequent during epoetin therapy, but this finding has not been supported to the extent necessary to advocate increased monitoring for this effect. The K/DOQI guidelines specifically state that vascular access occlusion, inadequate dialysis, history of seizures, or compromised nutritional status are not contraindications to ESA therapy.[21]

Neutralizing antibodies to ESAs and endogenous erythropoietin have been identified in a small number of patients treated with ESAs.[64] These patients develop antibody-mediated pure red cell aplasia (PRCA), which results in an absolute resistance to ESA therapy and intermittent blood transfusions as the primary therapeutic option. Case reports increased dramatically between 1998 and 2002 and occurred in parallel with the increase in SC administration primarily with one epoetin alfa product manufactured outside the United States, Eprex (Johnson & Johnson, Manati, Puerto Rico). Differences in this formulation that were noted at the time of the increase in PRCA cases were the substitution of human albumin with polysorbate 80 and use of uncoated rubber stoppers in the single-dose syringes, factors that in combination may increase release of organic compounds and increase immunogenicity of SC-administered epoetin alfa.[21] Changes in packaging of these syringes with fluororesin-coated stoppers and prohibiting SC administration practices in both Europe and Canada have led to a decrease in PRCA case reports. No case of antibody-associated PRCA has been documented in patients receiving only IV administration of ESAs and few cases have been reported with other ESAs.[65]

Although the case reports of antibody-associated PRCA are relatively few in number and the primary problem with the formulation addressed, clinicians should be aware of this rare phenomenon in patients resistant to ESA therapy. Further evaluation for antibody-mediated PRCA should be considered for patients receiving ESA therapy for more than 4 weeks who develop a sudden rapid decrease in Hb level (rate of 0.5 to 1.0 g/dL/wk) or require 1 to 2 red blood cell transfusions per week and who have a normal platelet and white blood cell count with an absolute reticulocyte count of less than 10,000/μL.[21] Discontinuation of ESA therapy is recommended in antibody-mediated PRCA because antibodies are cross-reactive and continued exposure may lead to anaphylactic reactions. Immunosuppressive therapy has been effective for some patients, although is still considered investigative. The question remains as to whether patients who develop antierythropoietin antibodies should receive other ESAs. Although switching to another ESA has been successful in at least one case report, this practice cannot be recommended without further evidence of safety.[66]

Drug–Drug Interactions. No significant drug interactions have been reported with the available ESAs.

Dosing and Administration. Recommended starting doses of epoetin alfa are 50 to 100 units/kg IV or SC three times per week for hemodialysis patients.[67] Less-frequent dosing is preferred in stage 4 CKD patients and with early stage CKD and peritoneal dialysis patients since these patients are seen in the outpatient clinic setting on a relatively infrequent basis. Studies have been done to evaluate extended dosing intervals for SC administration of epoetin alfa in early stage CKD patients.[68–70] Improved erythropoiesis and reduced transfusion requirements were observed in patients with anemia (Hb <10 g/dL) who received once weekly SC doses of 10,000 units of epoetin alfa.[70] Monthly dosing intervals for epoetin alfa SC have also been effective in maintaining target Hb values in this population.[69]

The starting dose of darbepoetin alfa in patients not previously receiving ESA therapy is 0.45 mcg/kg IV or SC administered once weekly.[71] A conversion table for patients who are to be switched from epoetin alfa (units per week) to darbepoetin alfa (micrograms per week) is available in the package insert for darbepoetin.[71] Frequency of dosing of darbepoetin is weekly for patients previously receiving epoetin two to three times per week and every other week for patients receiving epoetin once weekly. Extended dosing intervals of darbepoetin as infrequent as every 4 weeks have been successful in maintaining Hb levels in early stage CKD and dialysis patients.[72,73] This extended-dosing regimen is most beneficial for stage 4 CKD patients.

The IV route of administration is preferred for most hemodialysis patients based, in part, on the risk for PRCA associated with SC administration (see Adverse Effects above) and convenient IV access for these patients during the hemodialysis procedure.[21] Subcutaneous administration of ESAs is preferable for chronic ambulatory peritoneal dialysis patients and the nondialysis CKD population because these patients do not usually have regular IV access.

Figures 47–2 and 47–3 provide an algorithmic approach to management of anemia using ESAs and iron therapy in patients with ESRD.

Transfusions and Adjunct Therapies Red blood cell transfusions are currently a third-line treatment option for anemia of CKD. Red blood cell transfusions carry many risks and therefore should only be used in select situations, such as acute management of symptomatic anemia, following significant acute blood loss, and prior to surgical procedures that carry a high risk of blood loss, with the goal of preventing inadequate tissue oxygenation or cardiac failure. Androgen therapy was used extensively before the availability of ESAs; today, however, there is insufficient evidence to support use of androgens.[21] The risks of liver toxicity, malignancy, virilization in females, and hypertriglyceridemia outweigh the benefits of androgen therapy. L-Carnitine supplementation and vitamin C were previously suggested as adjunctive treatments of anemia associated with kidney disease, but are no longer recommended because of the lack of evidence supporting improved anemia management with these therapies.

Investigational Agents

Iron. Investigational agents for iron supplementation include ferumoxytol, a polysaccharide-coated iron oxide administered IV; iron oligosaccharide, elemental iron complexed with glucose; and ferric pyrophosphate, a water-soluble form of iron that may be administered via the dialysate solution used for hemodialysis and peritoneal dialysis.[74]

Erythropoietic-Stimulating Agents. Continuous erythropoietin receptor activator is a new ESA that is undergoing review by the FDA and may provide another option for treatment of anemia of CKD. This agent interacts with the erythropoietin receptors to cause stimulation of erythropoiesis, but has receptor-binding characteristics that differ from native erythropoietin. The half-life of this agent is notably longer than other available ESAs, approximately 70 to 122 hours after IV and 102 to 147 hours after SC administration which translates into a longer duration of action and thus potentially less frequent dosing for CKD.[74,75]

Hypoxia-inducible factor is a transcription factor found in erythropoietin-producing cells that activates erythropoietin during hypoxic conditions and regulates iron absorption. In conditions causing destabilization of this transcription factor erythropoietin production does not occur. An oral agent known as an hypoxia-inducible factor-stabilizing agent that prevents destabilization of hypoxia-inducible factor is being investigated and may be promising for patients with CKD.[74]

A synthetic peptide-based ESA known as Hematide that has the same biologic properties as endogenous erythropoietin, but a completely different amino acid sequence has been developed for treatment of anemia associated with CKD and cancer and is currently undergoing phase II studies.[74]

Pharmacoeconomic Considerations

Pharmacoeconomic considerations in the management of anemia of CKD relate primarily to the costs associated with ESAs and the increased use of IV iron to sustain erythropoiesis. Over the last decade there has been a steady rise in cost associated with the provision of ESA and IV iron for the dialysis population: the cost to Medicare has stabilized at just over $1 billion per year during the last 2 to 3 years.[2] Cost advantages can be realized, however, from the benefits associated with appropriate management of anemia, including fewer days of hospitalization, decreased mortality, and increased transplant success.[2,32] Implementation of maintenance IV iron therapy, as well as SC administration of ESAs, also has the potential to reduce Medicare cost for anemia management. Current Medicare reimbursement rates for epoetin and IV iron produce profits of 12% and 45%, respectively for most dialysis programs, and thus there is little incentive to minimize the use of either agent. In the case of iron therapy, IV iron is reimbursable by Medicare, whereas oral iron must either be paid for by the patient out-of-pocket or by secondary insurers (usually with a copayment). Capitation of payments for medications such as ESAs and IV iron therapy may force the dialysis community to change their clinical practices and thereby optimize their use. Considerations are a bit different in patients with early stage CKD as Medicare does not cover medication costs for this population. The lack of payment is a deterrent to timely implementation of therapy and likely contributes to the development of secondary complications such as anemia.

Other factors that affect the pharmacoeconomics of using ESAs include drug acquisition costs, frequency of administration, and the treatment environment (inpatient or outpatient setting).[76] Less-frequent dosing of ESAs may be beneficial from a pharmacoeconomic perspective because cost associated with administration may be reduced. Given that both epoetin alfa and darbepoetin alfa are effective at treating anemia, cost has become the primary decision factor for drug selection. Pharmaceutical companies that distribute these products have bundled these agents with their other products and thus complicated the pharmacoeconomic evaluation picture.

CLINICAL CONTROVERSY

There is limited evidence to support routine administration of IV iron if the serum ferritin is greater than 500 ng/mL. This presents a clinical challenge in deciding if iron supplementation is warranted in anemic dialysis patients with a TSat of less than 20% (or content of hemoglobin in the reticulocytes <29 pg/cell) and an elevated serum ferritin (>500 ng/mL). The clinical judgement that must be made is whether the elevated ferritin is indicative of iron overload or a result of inflammation or reticuloendothelial iron blockade (in which case a trial of iron therapy may be rational).

Evaluation of Therapeutic Outcomes

Figures 47–2 and 47–3 depict algorithmic approaches to the evaluation of patient outcomes. Iron status should be assessed every month during initial ESA treatment, and every 3 months for those receiving a stable ESA regimen or for those hemodialysis patients not treated with an ESA.[21] For all ESAs, the dose and subsequent adjustments of ESAs should be determined by the patient's Hb level relative to the target Hb level, and the most recent observed rate of increase in Hb level.[21] Hemoglobin should be monitored at least monthly in patients receiving ESA therapy, although more frequent monitoring (e.g., every 2 weeks) is warranted after initiation of an ESA or following a dose change until the Hb is stable. The response to ESA therapy should be evaluated at least over 2 to 4 weeks before a change in the dose of epoetin alfa or darbepoetin alfa is made. If the change in Hb is <1 g/dL over a 4-week time period, the dose of the ESA should be increased by 25%. If the change in Hgb is >1 g/dL over a 2-week time period, the dose of epoetin alfa or darbepoetin alfa should be reduced by 25%.[71,77] New FDA and CMS recommendations now advise health care providers to withhold ESA therapy if the Hb is >12 g/dl; some clinicians, however, may institute a dosage reduction of ≥25% to prevent drastic shifts in Hb levels. An inadequate response to ESA therapy justifies a complete evaluation for causes of resistance (see Efficacy section above).

SECONDARY HYPERPARATHYROIDISM AND RENAL OSTEODYSTROPHY

Desired Outcome

The overall goal of therapy is to prevent sHPT, hyperphosphatemia, and ROD, and the detrimental consequences of these disorders, including cardiovascular and extravascular calcifications. Although clinicians are becoming more aware of such consequences, efforts to improve evaluation and management in patients prior to development of more severe disease are needed.

K/DOQI guidelines for the diagnosis and management of bone disease in CKD proposed criteria for calcium, phosphorus, Ca × P, and iPTH based on the stage of CKD (Table 47–5).[8] The recommended corrected serum calcium for patients with stage 3 or 4 CKD is within the normal range, whereas the proposed range for patients with stage 5 CKD is slightly lower than what is considered a normal total calcium. This is based on the observation of an increased risk of soft tissue and vascular calcifications in this population and the exposure to dialysate calcium for the ESRD population. It is important to note that these are calcium concentrations corrected for the degree of protein binding (i.e., corrected based on serum albumin concentration). The corrected calcium value should also used to determine the Ca × P product. Recommended serum phosphorus concentrations are 2.7 to 4.6 mg/dL, with higher concentrations acceptable in stage 5 CKD. The proposed Ca × P of 55 mg^2/dL^2 is much lower than the previous recommendation of 65 to 70 mg^2/dL^2, which is still cited in some references. The iPTH recommended for patients with stage 4 or 5 CKD is above the normal range so as to prevent oversuppression of PTH and reduce the risk of adynamic bone disease. Serum aluminum levels should also be maintained below 20 mcg/L to minimize the risk of developing aluminum toxicity, a contributing factor to bone disease.[8]

TABLE 47-5 Kidney Disease/Dialysis Outcomes Quality Initiative (K/DOQI) Guidelines for Calcium, Phosphorus, Calcium Phosphorus Product, and Intact Parathyroid Hormone

	Chronic Kidney Disease		
Parameter	***Stage 3***	***Stage 4***	***Stage 5***
Corrected calcium (mg/dL)	"Normal"	"Normal"	8.4–9.5
Phosphorus (mg/dL)	2.7–4.6	2.7–4.6	3.5–5.5
Ca × P (mg^2/dL^2)	<55	<55	<55
Intact parathyroid hormone (pg/mL)	35–70	70–110	150–300

From Eknoyan G et al. [8]

⑩ Management of PTH, phosphorus, and calcium balance, and minimization of patient exposure to aluminum are important in preventing the development of sHPT and slowing or preventing the progression of sHPT, ROD, and cardiovascular and extravascular calcifications. Patients with ESRD usually require a combination of phosphate-binding medication, vitamin D, and calcimimetic therapy to achieve these goals. Control of serum phosphorus is paramount because hyperphosphatemia is an initiating event in the development of other metabolic disturbances. Unfortunately, hyperphosphatemia is difficult to control and hypercalcemia may develop as a result of treatment with calcium-containing phosphate binders.[15] There are different considerations in management of sHPT based on the stage of CKD. Hyperphosphatemia and sHPT in patients with stage 3 or 4 CKD are often overlooked. If these patients are not evaluated early in the course of the disease, they have a higher likelihood of developing metabolic abnormalities that contribute to poor outcomes by the time they reach stage 5 CKD or ESRD. Many patients with CKD are receiving suboptimal management of their disorders of calcium, phosphorus, and PTH homeostasis.

Nonpharmacologic Therapy

Dietary Phosphorus Restriction Dietary phosphorus restriction should be a first-line intervention for management of hyperphosphatemia in patients with CKD and should be initiated for most patients with stage 3, 4, or 5 CKD. The K/DOQI guidelines recommend phosphorus restriction to 800 to 1,000 mg/day when the upper levels of phosphorus are reached (see Table 47–5).[8] This recommendation also holds true for patients with iPTH levels above the recommended range, given the evidence that lowering phosphorus ingestion directly decreases PTH synthesis and secretion.[78] The challenge with dietary restriction of phosphorus is providing enough protein to prevent malnutrition, a common problem in the CKD population, because foods high in phosphorus are generally high in protein. Examples of foods or beverages that contain high amounts of phosphorus include meats, dairy products, dried beans, nuts, colas, peanut butter, and beer. Nutritional goals must be evaluated on an individual basis, preferably by a dietitian specializing in the care of CKD patients. Dialysis patients require a higher protein intake (1.2 to 1.3 g/kg per day) making restriction of phosphorus even more challenging. Removal of phosphorus does occur with peritoneal dialysis and hemodialysis (approximately 2 to 3 g/wk, dependent on the dialysis prescription); however, dialysis alone usually does not adequately control hyperphosphatemia.

One of the most common obstacles to the success of dietary phosphorus restriction is patient noncompliance because of the poor palatability and inconvenience. Regular counseling by a dietitian is essential to improve patient compliance.

Parathyroidectomy Parathyroidectomy is the last therapeutic option for patients with sHPT. The K/DOQI guidelines for bone metabolism and disease recommend surgery only for those patients with persistently elevated iPTH (iPTH >800 pg/mL) associated with hypercalcemia and/or hyperphosphatemia that are refractory to medical therapy.[8] Surgical approaches include either subtotal parathyroidectomy or total parathyroidectomy with autotransplantation of parathyroid tissue to an accessible site, such as the forearm. Postoperative hypocalcemia, hypophosphatemia, and hypomagnesemia may occur because of a marked increase in bone production in relation to bone absorption ("hungry bone syndrome"). Following surgery frequent monitoring of ionized calcium is required (every 4 to 6 hours for the first 48 to 72 hours after surgery). Ionized calcium should be maintained above 3.6 mg/dL (0.9 mmol/L), using calcium gluconate infusions if necessary. The recommended dose of calcium gluconate is 1 to 2 mg of elemental calcium per kilogram per hour, adjusted to maintain ionized calcium at 4.6 to 5.4 mg/dL (1.15 to 1.36 mmol/L). Once the ionized calcium is stable, oral therapy may be initiated with 1 to 2 g of calcium carbonate in conjunction with calcitriol in doses of up to 2 mcg per day. Adjustments in phosphate binders will also be necessary to maintain target phosphorus levels (see section on pharmacologic therapy).[8] Treatment with supplemental calcium and vitamin D may be required for weeks or months.

Pharmacologic Therapy

As kidney function declines, dietary restriction of phosphorus alone is usually inadequate to control serum phosphorus, and phosphate-binding agents are necessary, along with vitamin D therapy and/or calcimimetic therapy, to prevent sHPT.

Phosphate-Binding Agents

Pharmacology and Mechanism of Action. Drugs that bind dietary phosphorous in the GI tract form insoluble aluminum, calcium, or magnesium phosphate which is excreted in feces, thus reducing phosphorus absorption and serum phosphorus concentrations. A variety of phosphate-binding agents are available, including calcium-, lanthanum-, aluminum-, and magnesium-containing compounds, and the nonelemental agent sevelamer hydrochloride (Table 47–6). Patients must be instructed to take these agents with meals to minimize absorption of phosphorus from dietary sources.

Efficacy. Oral calcium compounds are well established as first-line agents for control of both serum phosphorus and calcium concentrations, at least in the early stages of CKD when hypocalcemia is more common. Calcium carbonate and calcium acetate are the primary preparations used; calcium citrate is also available, but is not recommended since the citrate component increases aluminum absorption. The chloride salt is also not recommended because it is very astringent and unpalatable, and absorbed chloride may contribute to systemic acidosis. Calcium carbonate is marketed in a variety of dosage forms (see Table 47–6) and is relatively inexpensive. Unfortunately, many calcium carbonate products are considered food supplements and thus are not required by law to meet United States Pharmacopeia (USP) disintegration and dissolution requirements. In general, nationally advertised brands meet USP quality standards for disintegration and dissolution, but it is difficult to determine whether private label or house brands conform to these standards. Variability in gastric pH may also affect disintegration or dissolution, and thus phosphate-binding efficacy. Calcium carbonate is more soluble in an acidic medium, and therefore should be administered prior to meals when stomach acidity is highest. In addition, acid-suppressing agents such as ranitidine and proton pump inhibitors may reduce the phosphate-binding activity of calcium carbonate by increasing gastric pH. Calcium acetate binds approximately twice as much phosphorus as calcium carbonate at comparable doses of elemental calcium.[8] Increased binding potency limits GI calcium absorption; however, calcium acetate is more soluble, and therefore better absorbed than calcium carbonate in an alkaline pH, which may explain the similar incidence of hypercalcemia. Patients with a corrected calcium of less than 8.4 mg/dL should receive calcium carbonate or calcium acetate as a calcium supplement (with or without vitamin D therapy).

Although calcium-containing phosphate-binding agents continue to be used as first-line therapy, their chronic use may increase the risk for vascular and tissue calcification.[15] The K/DOQI guidelines now recommend that the total dose of elemental calcium provided by calcium-containing binders not exceed 1,500 mg per day and the total daily intake from all sources not exceed 2,000 mg.[8] This presents clinicians with a challenge for patients in whom maximum doses do not achieve the goal phosphorus. In such situations, a non–calcium-based binder alone or in combination with a calcium product may be needed. Calcium-containing binders are not recommended in dialysis patients when on two consecutive measurements the serum calcium is >10.2 mg/dL or the iPTH is <150 pg/mL.[8]

Sevelamer hydrochloride is a nonabsorbable hydrogel phosphate-binding agent that does not contain aluminum, calcium, or magnesium. The dosage needed to control serum phosphorus concentrations may be as high as 6.3 g/day.[79] Sevelamer also significantly lowers LDL cholesterol and increases HDL by a mean of 30% and 18%, respectively. This is an added beneficial effect in a population at risk for cardiovascular events. Recent evidence has shown a decreased rate of vascular calcification in hemodialysis patients receiving this agent relative to those prescribed calcium-containing binders.[80] Sevelamer is now recommended as primary therapy in dialysis patients with severe vascular or soft tissue calcifications, and may also be used as a first-line phosphate-binding agent in patients with stage 5 CKD.[8] Sevelamer carbonate received FDA approval in October 2007 and is expected to be available in early 2008. This agent contains a carbonate buffer which may help maintain bicarbonate levels in the recommended range and reduce the potential for GI side effects.

Lanthanum carbonate is a phosphate binder recently approved for patients with ESRD.[81] Short-term (6 to 28 weeks) and long-term (2 to 3 years) therapy with lanthanum has demonstrated efficacy in controlling phosphorus and maintaining PTH in the target range with less risk of hypercalcemia than calcium-containing binders.[82,83] Initial daily doses are in the range of 750 to 1,500 mg (administered in divided doses with meals) with doses of 1,500 to 3,000 mg often being required to maintain target phosphorus in ESRD patients. The poor GI absorption, which limits systemic effects, and high binding capacity with phosphorus makes this an attractive phosphate-binding agent, particularly when options other than calcium-containing binders are needed. Lanthanum is available as a chewable tablet, which may be appealing for some patients.

Aluminum salts were widely used in the 1980s as phosphate-binding agents because of their high binding potency. They should be considered as third-line agents now and be reserved for acute treatment of severe hyperphosphatemia or used at low doses in combination with either calcium-containing binding agents or sevelamer hydrochloride in cases of hyperphosphatemia that is not responding to therapy with a single agent. The duration of aluminum therapy should be limited to 4 weeks.[8] Magnesium-containing antacids are also effective phosphate binders and may decrease the amount of

TABLE 47-6 Phosphate-Binding Agents Used in the Treatment of Hyperphosphatemia in CKD Patients

Compound	Trade Name	Compound Content (mg)	Dose Titration[b]	Starting Doses	Comments
Calcium carbonate[a] (40% elemental calcium)	Tums	500, 750, 1,000, 1,250	Increase or decrease by 500 mg per meal (200 mg elemental calcium)	0.5–1 g (elemental calcium) three times a day with meals	First-line agent; dissolution characteristics and phosphate binding affect may vary from product to product; try to limit daily intake of elemental calcium to 1,500 mg/day Approximately 39 mg phosphorus bound per 1 g calcium carbonate
	Oscal-500	1,250			
	Caltrate 600	1,500			
	Nephro-Calci	1,500			
	LiquiCal	1,200			
	CalciChew	1,250			
Calcium acetate (25% elemental calcium)	PhosLo	667	Increase or decrease by 667 mg per meal (168 mg elemental calcium)	0.5–1 g (elemental calcium) three times a day with meals	First-line agent; comparable efficacy to calcium carbonate with half the dose of elemental calcium; do not exceed 1.5 gms of elemental calcium per day Approximately 45 mg phosphorus bound per 1 g calcium acetate By prescription only
Sevelamer hydrochloride	Renagel	400, 800	Increase or decrease by 800 mg per meal	800–1,600 mg three times a day with meals	First-line agent; lowers low-density lipoprotein cholesterol More expensive than calcium products; preferred in patients at risk for extraskeletal calcification
Sevelamer carbonate	Renvela	800	Same as HCL salt	Same as HCL salt	Same as HCL; associated with a lower risk of GI adverse events than Renagel.
Lanthanum carbonate	Fosrenol	250, 500, 750, 1,000	Increase or decrease by 250–500 mg per meal	250–500 mg three times a day with meals	First line agent Available as chewable tablets
Aluminum hydroxide	Alterna GEL	600 mg/5 mL	–	300–600 mg three times a day with meals	Third-line agents; do not use concurrently with citrate-containing products Reserve for short-term use (4 weeks) in patients with hyperphosphatemia not responding to other binders
	Amphojel	300, 600 (tablet); 320 mg/5 mL (suspension)			
	Alu-Cap	400			
Aluminum carbonate	Basaljel	500 (tablet, capsule); 400 mg/5 mL (suspension)	–	450–500 mg three times a day with meals	Same as for aluminum hydroxide
Magnesium carbonate	Mag-Carb	70 capsule	–	70 mg three times a day with meals	Third-line agent; diarrhea common; monitor serum magnesium
Magnesium hydroxide	Milk of magnesia	300, 600 (tablet); 400 mg/5 mL, 800 mg/5 mL (suspension)	–	300–400 mg three times a day with meals	Same as for magnesium carbonate
Magnesium carbonate/calcium carbonate	MagneBind 200	200	160	200 mg three times a day with meals (based on magnesium content)	Same as for calcium carbonate and magnesium carbonate

[a]Multiple preparations available which are not listed.
[b]Based on phosphorus levels, titrate every 2 to 3 weeks until phosphorus goal reached.

calcium-containing binders necessary for control of phosphorus; however, their use may be limited by the frequent occurrence of GI side effects and the potential for magnesium accumulation.

Adverse Effects. Adverse effects of calcium-containing phosphate binders, as well as of sevelamer and lanthanum, are generally limited to GI side effects, including constipation, diarrhea, nausea, vomiting, and abdominal pain. The risk of hypercalcemia is also a concern and may necessitate restriction of calcium intake from the combination of calcium-containing binders and dietary intake. Aluminum binders can no longer be recommended as first-line therapy because of the CNS toxicity and the worsening of anemia associated with aluminum accumulation. Although an effective phosphate binder, use of magnesium is often limited by side effects that include diarrhea, abdominal cramps, hypermagnesemia, and hyperkalemia.

Drug–Drug and Drug–Food Interactions. Calcium-containing phosphate-binding agents interfere with the absorption of several other oral medications that are commonly prescribed for CKD patients, including oral iron, zinc, and quinolone antibiotics. Data regarding drug interactions with sevelamer are limited; however, in recent evaluations, no drug interactions with digoxin, warfarin, metoprolol, enalapril, or oral iron were observed.[84–86] Coadministration with ciprofloxacin did, however, result in a 50% decrease in bioavailability of the antibiotic.[84] There is also some information to suggest a potential interaction between sevelamer and cyclosporine (decreased bioavailability of cyclosporine) and altered phosphorus binding in the presence of agents that increase gastric pH (e.g., omeprazole).[87,88] Consequently, it is prudent to monitor for changes in phosphorus levels following initiation of concomitant therapy with agents known to alter gastric pH. Drug interaction studies with lanthanum, although limited, have shown that coadministration with warfarin, digoxin, and metoprolol did not affect the bioavailability of those agents.[81] In general, it is rational to separate the administration time of oral medications for which a reduction in bioavailability has a clinically significant effect (e.g., quinolones) from phosphate binders by at least 1 hour before or 3 hours after administration of the phosphate binder. This is a key patient-counseling recommendation as patients are often switched from one phosphate binder to another and it is easier for them to remember this general concept regarding phosphate binders and other medications. Many phosphate binders are marketed as antacids or calcium supplements and often CKD patients do not know why they have been prescribed these agents.

Regular patient counseling is essential to enhance compliance and minimize the potential for drug interactions.

Dosing and Administration. Table 47–6 lists starting doses of phosphate-binding agents and suggested dose titrations. Doses should be titrated to achieve the recommended serum phosphorus concentrations based on stage of CKD, yet avoid complications such as hypercalcemia. The daily dose of elemental calcium should not exceed 1,500 mg (2,000 mg from phosphate binders and dietary intake).[8]

Vitamin D Therapy Vitamin D compounds include ergocalciferol (vitamin D_2) and cholecalciferol (vitamin D_3) that must be converted to the active form in the kidney. Calcitriol (1,25-dihydroxyvitamin D_3) is the most active form of vitamin D and is available as an oral formulation (Rocaltrol) as well as an IV formulation (Calcijex). The currently available vitamin D analogs include paricalcitol (19-*nor*-1,25-dihydroxyvitamin D_2; Zemplar) and doxercalciferol (1α-hydroxyvitamin D_2; Hectorol). Calcitriol or one of the vitamin D analogs is required for patients with severe kidney disease because these agents do not require conversion by the kidney to the biologically active form.

Pharmacology and Mechanism of Action. Active vitamin D suppresses PTH secretion by stimulating absorption of serum calcium by intestinal cells and through direct activity on the parathyroid gland to decrease PTH synthesis. As a result, the serum calcium concentration is raised and the parathyroid glands decrease the rate of secretion and formation of PTH. The set point for calcium (i.e., the calcium concentration at which PTH secretion is decreased by 50%), which is generally raised in sHPT, is lowered when active vitamin D therapy is initiated. This indicates that a lower ionized calcium concentration is effective at suppressing secretion of PTH. All of these actions are mediated by the interaction of vitamin D with vitamin D receptors, which are located in many organs, including the parathyroid gland, GI tract, and kidney.[89] Calcitriol also upregulates vitamin D receptors, which ultimately may reduce parathyroid hyperplasia. Unfortunately, the enhanced GI absorption of calcium and phosphorus with calcitriol therapy frequently leads to hypercalcemia and hyperphosphatemia. There is also evidence that hyperphosphatemia results in resistance to the PTH-suppressing effects of vitamin D analogs and directly stimulates PTH release. These actions contribute to the increase in the Ca × P product, which can lead to soft-tissue and vascular calcification.[14,15] Consequently, reasonable control of calcium and phosphorus must be achieved before initiation and during continued vitamin D therapy. Although this does not mean that vitamin D therapy should be withheld or discontinued in patients with a Ca × P product greater than 55 mg^2/dL^2, interventions, including use of agents with less risk of hypercalcemia and hyperphosphatemia, and more prudent use of phosphate binders to lower the calcium and phosphorus are necessary in such patients.

The unique interactions of vitamin D with the vitamin D receptors have been a focus of research and have led to the development of vitamin D analogs, which vary in their affinity for these receptors and thus may result in less hypercalcemia, while retaining the positive physiologic actions on bone and parathyroid tissue. Paricalcitol and doxercalciferol are D_2 compounds that effectively lower PTH in dialysis patients.[90,91] Paricalcitol differs from calcitriol by the absence of the exocyclic carbon 19 and the fact that it is a vitamin D_2 derivative. This agent is available as an IV formulation for use in patients with stage 5 CKD and an oral form which is approved for use in those with stage 3 and 4 CKD. Doxercalciferol, in contrast to calcitriol and paricalcitol, is a prohormone that needs to be hydroxylated in the liver to its active 1,25-dihydroxyvitamin D_2 product. Doxercalciferol is also available for both IV and oral administration.

Pharmacokinetics. Calcitriol can be administered orally as well as by IV injection. Oral absorption occurs rapidly; therefore oral and IV therapies are both reasonable options for treatment of sHPT. Although historically a topic of controversy, a review of the available literature leads to the conclusion that intermittent IV administration of calcitriol is more effective than daily oral calcitriol for sHPT.[8] When paricalcitol is administered IV, its half-life is similar to that of calcitriol (up to 30 hours). The half-life in for oral administration of paricalcitol is 17 to 20 hours in patients with stages 3 and 4 CKD.[92] Doxercalciferol as a prodrug has a slightly prolonged half-life of 45 hours, although this difference in half-life compared to other agents is not of clinical significance.

Efficacy. Administration of calcitriol by either the oral or IV route may be based on conventional dosing (usually 0.25 to 0.5 mcg/day) or pulse dosing (0.5 to 2 mcg two to three times per week). Logistically, IV dosing is more practical in hemodialysis patients, whereas oral therapy is more practical for those with stage 3 or 4 CKD and peritoneal dialysis patients. Conventional daily oral doses of calcitriol (0.25 mcg) may be more frequently associated with hypercalcemia and hyperphosphatemia, because vitamin D receptors are located in intestinal mucosa where direct stimulation can occur.

Although hypercalcemia is less likely with the newer analogs, elevated calcium concentrations have been observed with these agents in patients with ESRD. However, some of these cases were associated with excessive dosing of these agents and oversuppression of PTH, a condition more likely to promote hypercalcemia. When administered at doses 10 times that of calcitriol and at a dose equivalent to doxercalciferol, paricalcitol has been less frequently associated with hypercalcemia in animal studies and in human trials.[93,94] Doxercalciferol and paricalcitol have also been evaluated in patients with stages 3 and 4 CKD. They are effective in reducing PTH to target levels; however, differences in the magnitude of elevations of calcium and phosphorus have not been directly compared in this population.[95,96]

Although comparisons between vitamin D analogs are relatively limited there is some information comparing clinical indicators in ESRD patients receiving these agents. In one study, fewer cases of hyperphosphatemia were reported with paricalcitol than with calcitriol when administered at high doses to hemodialysis patients.[93] A more rapid suppression of PTH was also observed in paricalcitol-treated patients than with calcitriol, although the more clinically significant finding from this study was the decrease in incidence of hypercalcemia and elevated Ca × P in the paricalcitol-treated patients.[97] Nontraditional effects of vitamin D, including a potential survival benefit, have also been reported.[98–100] An improvement in 3-year survival in a large dialysis population receiving paricalcitol was observed compared with a historic cohort that received calcitriol.[98] This survival advantage was also observed for hemodialysis patients who received vitamin D (either calcitriol or paricalcitol) compared to no vitamin D and was independent of calcium, phosphorus, and PTH.[99] The relationship between all available vitamin D agents (calcitriol, doxercalciferol, and paricalcitol) and mortality was further evaluated in a retrospective analysis of more than 7,700 hemodialysis patients.[101] After a median followup of 37 weeks, mortality (all-cause and atherosclerotic cardiovascular mortality) was similar for doxercalciferol- and paricalcitol-treated patients and similar to the calcitriol-treated patients when adjusted for laboratory values (e.g., calcium, PTH, albumin, phosphorus) and standardized mortality for the dialysis clinics included in this study. Vitamin D therapy, regardless of agent, was associated with lower mortality. Antiproteinuric effects of paricalcitol have also been reported in patients with stages 3 and 4 CKD.[100] These findings are of interest when considering other potential effects of vitamin D beyond suppression of PTH.

Adverse Effects. Although all agents are effective in suppressing PTH levels, they differ in the degree to which they cause other metabolic abnormalities. Adverse effects of note with vitamin D therapy in patients treated for sHPT include hypercalcemia and hyperphosphatemia. Differences in calcitriol and vitamin D analogs have been demonstrated in animal studies and in clinical trials evaluating the effect on reduction of PTH while minimizing the risk of these adverse consequences.[93,94]

Drug–Drug and Drug–Food Interactions. Cholestyramine may reduce the absorption of orally administered calcitriol and doxercalciferol. In vitro data suggest that paricalcitol is metabolized by the hepatic enzyme CYP3A4 and has the potential to interact with other agents that are metabolized by this enzyme.[92] When ketoconazole, a CYP3A4 inhibitor, was given concomitantly, paricalcitol serum concentrations doubled. Caution is also advised when CYP3A4 inhibitors are given to those receiving doxercalciferol. No other significant interactions have been reported.

Dosing and Administration. Recommendations for vitamin D therapy differ based on the stage of CKD.[8] Because changes in vitamin D metabolism can lead to deficiencies in vitamin D precursors in patients with stage 3 or 4 CKD, 25-hydroxyvitamin D levels should be measured in patients with PTH values above the upper recommended ranges of 70 pg/mL or 110 pg/mL for stages 3 and 4 CKD, respectively (see Table 47–5). If the 25-hydryoxyvitamin D level is less than 30 ng/mL, a vitamin D precursor (e.g., ergocalciferol) is recommended (Table 47–7).[8] To prevent vitamin D insufficiency, doses of 600 to 800 units per day of ergocalciferol are recommended. According to the guidelines, active vitamin D or an analog should be administered orally (e.g., as oral calcitriol, doxercalciferol, or paricalcitol) when PTH remains elevated despite adequate 25-hydroxyvitamin D levels.

Active vitamin D therapy should be initiated, when warranted, in patients with stage 3 or 4 CKD as an oral daily dose of 0.25 mcg calcitriol, 1 mcg doxercalciferol, or 1 mcg paricalcitol.[102] For paricalcitol the recommended daily dose is 2 mcg if the PTH is greater than 500 pg/mL. If these agents are administered intermittently (generally three times per week), the recommended initial dose is twice the daily dose.[102] Higher starting doses may be required based on the severity of sHPT. Prior to starting therapy the serum calcium and phosphorus should be well controlled (serum calcium <9.5 mg/dL and phosphorus <4.6 mg/dL) to minimize the risk of hypercalcemia and an elevated Ca × P. In patients with ESRD there is a clearly defined role for treatment with active vitamin D or a vitamin D analog because the conversion of precursors to active vitamin D is impaired. Table 47–8 lists dosing recommendations based on PTH. Serum calcium and Ca × P should be monitored regularly while the patient is receiving therapy.[8] Dose adjustments should be made every 2 to 4 weeks based on PTH concentrations. For patients who need to be converted from calcitriol to paricalcitol, a dosing conversion ratio of 1:4 of IV calcitriol to paricalcitol has been proposed; however, some clinicians suggest a ratio of 1:3 to avoid oversuppression of PTH.[8]

TABLE 47-7 Dosing Recommendations for Vitamin D in Patients with Stages 3 and 4 Chronic Kidney Disease

Definition	Serum 25(OH)D (ng/mL)	Dose of Ergocalciferol[a]
Severe vitamin D deficiency	<5	50,000 international units/wk orally × 12 weeks, then monthly × 6 months or 500,000 international units as a single intramuscular dose
Mild vitamin D deficiency	5–15	50,000 international units/wk orally × 4 weeks, then monthly × 6 months
Vitamin D insufficiency	16–30	50,000 international units/month orally 6 months

25(OH)D, 25 hydroxyvitamin D.
[a]25(OH)D levels should be measured following the 6-month course of therapy for patients with mild and severe vitamin D deficiency.
From Eknoyan G et al. [8]

TABLE 47-8 Dosing Recommendations for Vitamin D in Patients with Stage 5 Chronic Kidney Disease and Those on Hemodialysis[a]

PTH (pg/mL)	IV and Oral Calcitriol Dose per HD	IV Paricalcitol Dose per HD	Oral and IV Doxercalciferol Dose per HD
300–600[b]	0.5–1.5 mcg oral or IV	2.5–5 mcg	5 mcg oral, 2 mcg IV
600–1,000[b]	1–4 mcg oral 1–3 mcg IV	6–10 mcg	5–10 mcg oral, 2–4 mcg IV
>1,000[c]	3–7 mcg oral 3–5 mcg IV	10–15 mcg	10–20 mcg oral, 4–8 mcg IV

HD, hemodialysis; PTH, parathyroid hormone.
[a]Peritoneal dialysis patients may be treated with oral doses of calcitriol (0.5–1.0 mcg) or doxercalciferol (2.5–5 mcg) two or three times weekly. May also use oral calcitriol at 0.25 mcg daily.
[b]If serum calcium <9.5 mg/dL, phosphorus <5.5 mg/dL, and Ca P <55 mg^2/dL^2.
[c]If serum calcium <10 mg/dL, phosphorus <5.5 mg/dL, and Ca × P <55 mg^2/dL^2.
From Eknoyan G et al. [8]

Calcimimetics

Pharmacology and Mechanism of Action. Cinacalcet hydrochloride (Sensipar) is a calcimimetic agent approved for treatment of sHPT in ESRD patients and for treatment of hypercalcemia in patients with parathyroid carcinoma. Cinacalcet is the first agent in this class to receive FDA approval. This compound acts on the calcium-sensing receptor on the surface of the chief cell of the parathyroid gland to mimic the effect of extracellular ionized calcium and increase the sensitivity of the calcium-sensing receptor to calcium, subsequently reducing PTH secretion.

Pharmacokinetics. The maximum plasma concentration of cinacalcet is achieved in approximately 2 to 6 hours following oral administration. The half-life is approximately 30 to 40 hours. Cinacalcet has a large volume of distribution (approximately 1,000 L), and is 93% to 97% bound to plasma proteins, both characteristics indicating that removal by dialysis is negligible. Cinacalcet is metabolized by the liver, specifically by the cytochrome P450 isoenzymes CYP3A4, CYP2D6, and CYP1A2.[103]

Efficacy. In placebo-controlled clinical trials conducted in dialysis patients (predominantly those receiving hemodialysis) cinacalcet significantly decreased PTH and the Ca × P product within the 6-month study period, regardless of the severity of sHPT.[104] The starting dose of 30 mg per day was titrated every 3 or 4 weeks to a maximum dose of 180 mg per day to achieve the target PTH of ≤250 pg/mL and avoid hypocalcemia. Approximately 66% and 93% of patients in the clinical trials were receiving concurrent vitamin D and phosphate binders, respectively. If a patient experienced symptoms of hypocalcemia or had a serum calcium <8.4 mg/dL, calcium supplements and/or calcium-based phosphate binders could be increased. If ineffective, the vitamin D dose could be increased. The median dose required to achieve the desired PTH by the end of the study period was 90 mg. Cinacalcet has also been studied in patients with Stage 3 and 4 CKD with sHPT and was effective in lowering PTH while maintaining the Ca and P within the target ranges.[105] This drug is however not approved for use in those with stage 2 CKD because of the risk of hypocalcemia. Because cinacalcet was approved after the K/DOQI guidelines on bone disease became available, the challenge to clinicians is in deciding how to most effectively use cinacalcet in conjunction with other therapies to manage hyperphosphatemia and sHPT.

Adverse Effects. The most frequently reported adverse events with cinacalcet were nausea and vomiting. Although nausea and vomiting occurred more frequently with cinacalcet, these events were generally transient, mild to moderate in nature, and infrequently led to withdrawal from clinical trials.[103]

Because cinacalcet lowers serum calcium and may cause hypocalcemia, this agent should not be started if the serum calcium is less than the lower limit of normal, approximately 8.4 mg/dL. Serum calcium should be measured within 1 week after initiation or dose adjustment of cinacalcet. Once the maintenance dose is established, serum calcium should be measured approximately monthly. Potential manifestations of hypocalcemia include paresthesia, myalgia, cramping, tetany, and convulsions.

Drug–Drug and Drug–Food Interactions. Because cinacalcet is metabolized by multiple hepatic enzymes there is potential for drug interactions. Cinacalcet is also a potent inhibitor of the enzyme CYP2D6. As a result, dose adjustments of concomitant medications that are predominantly metabolized by this enzyme and have a narrow therapeutic index, such as flecainide, thioridazine, vinblastine, and most tricyclic antidepressants (i.e., amitriptyline), may be required.[100,103]

Several agents commonly used in the CKD population have been evaluated for interactions with cinacalcet.[103] Coadministration of calcium carbonate or sevelamer did not affect the pharmacokinetics of cinacalcet. Pantoprazole did not alter the pharmacokinetics of cinacalcet HCl, an important finding since pantoprazole alters gastric pH, and the solubility of cinacalcet decreases as the gastric pH rises over 5.5. Coadministration of cinacalcet with warfarin also did not affect the pharmacokinetics of warfarin. Coadministration of cinacalcet and ketoconazole, a strong inhibitor of cytochrome P450 (CYP) 3A4, resulted in an increase in the area under the curve and maximum concentration of 2.3 and 2.2 times, respectively. Concurrent administration of cinacalcet with amitriptyline increased amitriptyline exposure and nortriptyline (active metabolite) exposure by approximately 20% in CYP2D6-extensive metabolizers.

Food has been shown to increase absorption of cinacalcet by up to 81% compared to fasting; therefore this medication should be taken with meals to achieve the maximal effect.

Dosing and Administration. The recommended starting oral dose of cinacalcet is 30 mg once daily. The dose should be titrated every 2 to 4 weeks to a maximum dose of 180 mg once daily to achieve the desired PTH levels and to maintain near-normal serum calcium concentrations. Patients with hepatic disease may require lower doses, as studies have shown a decrease in metabolism of cinacalcet in this patient population. Cinacalcet is available as a film-coated tablet containing 30, 60, or 90 mg.

Pharmacoeconomic Considerations

Pharmacoeconomic considerations in the management of sHPT and ROD include medication costs, the cost associated with laboratory procedures (e.g., monitoring of 25-hydroxyvitamin D and more frequent evaluation of iPTH in patients with stage 3 or 4 CKD), and the medical expenditures associated with the management of cardiovascular disease and bone fractures. The pattern of vitamin D product use in U.S. dialysis units has been strongly influenced by Medicare reimbursement. Currently, IV vitamin D products are separately reimbursable expenses for dialysis programs. In fact, dialysis programs often generate significant profit from the IV administration of these agents. In contrast, oral administration of vitamin D is more convenient for patients with stage 3 or 4 CKD and the peritoneal dialysis population; however, these agents are not separately reimbursable, and because they must be purchased by the patient, compliance becomes an issue.

The cost-to-benefit ratio associated with more aggressive management of metabolic disorders (e.g., hyperphosphatemia and hypercalcemia) and sHPT has not been formally evaluated. If the associated complications such as vascular and soft-tissue calcifications that may increase morbidity and hospitalizations can be significantly reduced, the additional medication costs may ultimately be of minimal consequence.

CLINICAL CONTROVERSY

Although the National Kidney Foundation's K/DOQI guidelines recommend supplementation with ergocalciferol in stage 3 and 4 CKD patients with 25-hydryoxyvitamin D deficiency, there is little evidence to support this recommendation. Indeed some clinicians begin active vitamin D therapy in this clinical setting.

Evaluation of Therapeutic Outcomes

The goals for treatment with dietary phosphate restriction, phosphate-binding agents, vitamin D therapy, and/or calcimimetic therapy are to prevent sHPT and subsequent ROD without inducing adynamic bone disease from oversuppression of PTH or vascular or extravascular calcifications. Regular monitoring of serum calcium, phosphorus, Ca × P, iPTH, and vitamin D status to achieve and maintain target goals is currently the most practical and effective means of achieving these outcomes.

The serum calcium, phosphorus, and iPTH levels should be measured in all patients with a GFR of less than 60 mL/min.[8] Patients with stage 3 CKD should have followup measurements done at least every 12 months; those with stage 4 CKD should have follow up done every 3 months. More frequent monitoring is required for ESRD patients: monitor iPTH every 3 months and calcium and phosphorus every month. More frequent monitoring (monthly for iPTH and every 2 weeks for calcium and phosphorus) may be warranted following any change in the therapeutic interventions to correct these abnormalities.

■ CHRONIC METABOLIC ACIDOSIS

Desired Outcome

The goals of therapy for patients with CKD are to normalize the pH of the blood (pH of approximately 7.35 to 7.45) and maintain the serum bicarbonate within the normal range (22 to 26 mEq/L). In patients on hemodialysis, the goal of therapy is to maintain a predialysis or stabilized bicarbonate concentration at or above 22 mEq/L.[19] Metabolic acidosis appears to stimulate protein catabolism, which can contribute to a negative nitrogen balance and lower albumin concentrations, as well as cause growth retardation in children. Lower serum bicarbonate levels in peritoneal dialysis patients have also been associated with a higher hospitalization rate and longer hospital stays.[19] Severe acidemia (blood pH <7.1 to 7.2) suppresses myocardial contractility, predisposes patients to cardiac arrhythmias, and may lead to a decrease in total peripheral vascular resistance and blood pressure, reduced hepatic blood flow, and impaired oxygen delivery.[107] The prevention and treatment of severe metabolic acidosis in patients with kidney disease is also important to prevent the development of renal bone disease.

Nonpharmacologic Therapy

Therapy for metabolic acidosis requires pharmacologic intervention to correct the acidemia. Treatment of other underlying disorders that may be contributory is also warranted.

Pharmacologic Therapy

In patients with stage 4 or 5 CKD, the use of alkalinizing salts, such as sodium bicarbonate or citrate/citric acid preparations, is useful to replenish depleted body bicarbonate stores. Sodium bicarbonate tablets are manufactured in 325- and 650-mg strengths (a 650-mg tablet contains 7.6 mEq sodium and 7.6 mEq bicarbonate). Shohl's solution and Bicitra contain 1 mEq/mL of sodium and the equivalent of 1 mEq/mL of bicarbonate as sodium citrate/citric acid. Citrate is metabolized in the liver to bicarbonate, and citric acid is metabolized to CO_2 and water. Polycitra, which contains potassium citrate, (1 mEq/mL of sodium, 1 mEq/mL of potassium, and 2 mEq/mL of bicarbonate) should not be used in patients with severe CKD as hyperkalemia may result.

The replacement dose of alkali (base) needed to restore the serum bicarbonate concentration to normal (24 mEq/L) can be approximated by multiplying the volume of distribution of bicarbonate (0.5 L/kg) by the patient's body weight (in kilograms) and the patient's base deficit (difference between the patient's serum bicarbonate value and the normal value of 24 mEq/L). The calculated amount of bicarbonate replacement therapy (in milliequivalents) should be administered over several days to prevent volume overload from excessive sodium intake. After the serum bicarbonate has normalized, a maintenance regimen of bicarbonate to neutralize daily acid production may be all that is necessary (12 to 20 mEq/day in divided doses). Doses are subsequently titrated to maintain normal plasma bicarbonate concentrations. Patients with renal tubular acidosis may require higher doses of alkalinizing agents (see Chap. 55). Fluid balance should be monitored carefully because of the sodium content of these agents. Citrate-containing solutions should not be used in combination with aluminum-containing compounds because they can enhance aluminum absorption and increase the risk of aluminum intoxication. Excessive doses of alkalinizing agents may cause metabolic alkalosis, as well as lethargy or cardiac depression secondary to a decrease in ionized serum calcium concentration. Gastrointestinal distress characterized by gastric distension and flatulence is relatively common with high doses of oral sodium bicarbonate. Patients with severe acidosis (serum bicarbonate <8 mEq/L; pH <7.2) may require IV therapy (see Chap. 55).

Metabolic acidosis in both adult and pediatric patients undergoing dialysis can often be managed with the use of higher concentrations of bicarbonate or acetate in the dialysate (>38 mEq/L bicarbonate is safe and effective). Administration of oral bicarbonate salts as described above may also be necessary for some dialysis patients.

Evaluation of Therapeutic Outcomes

Regular monitoring of arterial blood gases and serum electrolytes, particularly potassium, are necessary to determine the effectiveness of therapy. A gradual correction is appropriate to avoid overcorrection and subsequent complications such as alkalosis and other electrolyte abnormalities (see Chap. 55). Laboratory measurement of serum bicarbonate is associated with several technical problems. Blood collection techniques, transportation, and assay methodology can affect the measured concentrations. Blood samples should not have contact with air; process delays should be avoided; and consistent analytical methods should be used with serial measurements to improve accuracy.[19]

■ TREATMENT OF CARDIOVASCULAR DISEASE IN CHRONIC KIDNEY DISEASE

Specific recommendations regarding the management of cardiovascular disease in the ESRD population are included in K/DOQI guidelines. Two common risk factors for cardiovascular disease—hypertension and hyperlipidemia—are further discussed in this section.

Desired Outcome

Hypertension The goal blood pressure for cardiovascular risk reduction, in patients with early stage CKD is less than 130/80 mm Hg.[107] The target blood pressure in patients with ESRD is not well defined; however, the K/DOQI guidelines propose a predialysis blood pressure of less than 140/90 mm Hg and a postdialysis blood pressure of less than 130/80 mm Hg, although this recommendation is not based on data from prospective controlled studies.[1] The targets may need to be individualized for patients who experience intradialytic hypotension. These goals can rarely be achieved using lifestyle modifications alone in CKD patients. Thus aggressive antihypertensive therapy is often required.

Hyperlipidemia Based on strong evidence of risk reduction and the benefits of lipid-lowering therapy in the general population, and the high prevalence of atherosclerotic cardiovascular disease in patients with CKD, the consensus is that CKD patients are among the highest-risk group for cardiovascular conditions (i.e., equivalent to that of patients with known coronary heart disease) and should be treated aggressively for dyslipidemia to an LDL cholesterol goal below 100 mg/dL.[18,25] The decision to lower LDL cholesterol to less than 70 mg/dL based on more recent data in high-risk populations is a therapeutic option that is not supported by strong evidence from clinical trials. Table 47–9 lists the goals for patients with stage 5 CKD based on lipid abnormality, as well as the appropriate course of therapy.

Nonpharmacologic Therapy

Hypertension A primary intervention for management of hypertension in patients with ESRD is sodium restriction to approximately 2 to 3 g/day. Fluid intake should be restricted in patients with volume overload, particularly in patients on hemodialysis who are at risk for substantial fluid accumulation between dialysis sessions. Regular dietary counseling becomes critical to the success of nonpharmacologic interventions, given the large number of lifestyle changes typically required by CKD patients. Other lifestyle modifications, including regular exercise, weight loss, and smoking cessation, are also recommended, but difficult to implement.

In hemodialysis patients, achievement of an individual's "dry weight" is necessary to control blood pressure and may be done through dietary intervention, increased ultrafiltration, and longer dialysis sessions (see Chap. 48). Aggressive ultrafiltration in hemodialysis patients has shown beneficial effects of lowering blood pressure and decreasing left ventricular mass index. Prolonged hemodialysis also better maintains normal blood pressure, improves survival, and reduces the need for antihypertensive medications; however, the majority of hemodialysis programs in the United States use shorter dialysis sessions (3- to 4-hour sessions three times per week).[1]

Hyperlipidemia In patients with elevated triglyceride levels (≥500 mg/dL) and/or LDL between 100 and 129 mg/dL, lifestyle changes

TABLE 47-9 Management of Dyslipidemia in Patients with Chronic Kidney Disease

Dyslipidemia	Goal	Initial Therapy	Modification in Therapy[a]	Alternative[a]
TG ≥500 mg/dL	TG <500 mg/dL	TLC	TLC + fibrate or niacin	Fibrate or niacin
LDL 100–129 mg/dL	LDL <100 mg/dL	TLC	TLC + low-dose statin	Bile acid sequestrant or niacin
LDL ≥130 mg/dL	LDL <100 mg/dL	TLC + low-dose statin	TLC + maximum-dose statin	Bile acid sequestrant or niacin
TG ≥200 mg/dL and non-HDL ≥130 mg/dL	Non-HDL <130 mg/dL	TLC + low-dose statin	TLC + maximum-dose statin	Fibrate or niacin

HDL, high-density lipoprotein; LDL, low-density lipoprotein; Non-HDL, total cholesterol minus HDL cholesterol; TG, triglycerides; TLC, therapeutic lifestyle changes.

[a]Dosing of selected agents by class: fibrate (gemfibrozil 600 mg twice a day); niacin (1.5–3 g/day of immediate-release product); statin (simvastatin 10–40 mg/day if glomerular filtration rate [GFR] <30 mL/min, 20–80 mg/day if GFR >30 mL/min); bile acid sequestrant (cholestyramine 4–16 g/day). See Chap. 23 for more complete dosing information.

From reference 25.

without pharmacologic therapy are recommended as initial therapy (see Chap. 21). Unfortunately, most patients with CKD have already been advised to adhere to difficult dietary regimens, which may include protein, phosphorus, sodium, potassium, and fluid restrictions. Thus, although diet therapy is a reasonable first-step approach, it may not be successful in many patients with CKD because of noncompliance. A dietitian who is well versed in the management of kidney disease should be consulted.

Pharmacologic Therapy

Hypertension Most patients with hypertension and CKD require drug regimens that include three or more antihypertensive agents to achieve target blood pressure. Blood pressure reductions can be achieved with agents in all antihypertensive classes, although there is a preference for agents that inhibit the renin–angiotensin system, and choice should be guided by the individual patient's concomitant disease states.

Diuretic therapy is beneficial for management of blood pressure in patients with early CKD; however, thiazide diuretics are not generally effective in patients with a GFR of <30 mL/min. Loop diuretics can be used throughout all stages of CKD; however, patients with ESRD who have minimal to no residual kidney function will often not respond to these agents.

ACEIs or angiotensin receptor blockers are the preferred agents for patients with progressive CKD and proteinuria. They are also preferred in patients with ESRD because of their potential benefits, including regression of LVH, reduction in sympathetic nerve activity and pulse-wave velocity, improvement in endothelial function, and reduced oxidative stress.[1] Lower initial doses of these agents may be necessary because the elimination half-lives of the parent compound (captopril and lisinopril) or active metabolite (enalapril, benazepril, and ramipril) are prolonged in ESRD patients. Available angiotensin receptor blockers do not require dosage adjustment for decreased kidney function and they are not effectively removed by hemodialysis.

Calcium channel blockers that selectively lower systemic vascular resistance also appear to be effective in the treatment of hypertension in patients with ESRD and are associated with decreased total and cardiovascular mortality.[1] β-Blockers may be particularly useful in hypertensive CKD patients given the beneficial effects after myocardial infarction. Agents such as esmolol, timolol, pindolol, metoprolol, or labetalol, which are metabolized and not significantly removed by dialysis, may be easier to dose titrate than agents that are both dialyzable and extensively eliminated unchanged by the kidney (e.g., acebutolol, atenolol, bisoprolol, and nadolol). Agents requiring less-frequent dosing may be used to improve patient compliance.

Use of other antihypertensive agents in the patient with CKD should be based on recommendations in the general population (see Chap. 15). In the ESRD population, agents that act on the sympathetic nervous system, such as prazosin, terazosin, doxazosin, clonidine, guanabenz, and guanfacine, may be required in patients who are unresponsive to ACEIs, calcium channel blockers, or β-blocker therapy, and used in conjunction with adequate dialysis. Central α_2-agonists such as clonidine appear to be the safest of these agents; however, adverse effects, such as dry mouth, may lead to extra fluid consumption in some patients. Postsynaptic α-blockers (e.g., prazosin) are associated with postural hypotension following hemodialysis. Guanethidine and methyldopa should be avoided because of potential complications, including severe postural hypotension, severe dialysis-related hypotension, and impotence. The addition of vasodilators such as minoxidil may prove useful in patients resistant to combinations of the previously mentioned agents.

Hyperlipidemia Management of dyslipidemia in patients with CKD should be based on the report from the National Cholesterol Education Program and the K/DOQI guidelines for dyslipidemia in patients with CKD.[18,25] If lifestyle changes are not effective in achieving goal triglyceride and LDL levels after a few months, drug therapy is warranted (see Table 47–9). Drug therapy is also recommended for those with more extreme elevations in LDL (≥130 mg/dL).

Drug classes that may prove useful in treatment of lipid disorders include: 3-hydroxy-3-methylglutaryl coenzyme A (HMG-CoA) reductase inhibitors (statins); the bile acid sequestrants; nicotinic acid; and fibric acids (gemfibrozil and clofibrate). Statins are the most effective drugs for lowering LDL and total cholesterol in patients with kidney disease (with or without nephrotic syndrome) and generally should be regarded as the drugs of first choice. Drug therapy for hypertriglyceridemia includes a fibrate or nicotinic acid; in general, fibrates are better tolerated. Studies evaluating statins have shown cholesterol-lowering benefits in addition to reduction in risk of nonfatal myocardial infarction and cardiac death in a relatively limited number of patients with early stage CKD.[1] In contrast results from a 4-year study evaluating the effect of atorvastatin therapy on morality caused by cardiac events, nonfatal myocardial infarction and stroke in more than 1,200 hemodialysis patients with type 2 diabetes (a group at high risk for cardiovascular events), showed no significant benefit in the composite end point compared to the placebo group.[108] When evaluated individually there was a significantly greater relative risk of fatal stroke in the atorvastatin treated patients. These findings do not support initiation of statin therapy in ESRD patients with type 2 diabetes, but rather initiation at an earlier time point. It is not yet known how these results would compare with findings from a nondiabetic ESRD population.

Several potential drug interactions and/or side effects have been observed in those CKD patients receiving antilipemic therapy. The nonselective binding activity of bile acid sequestrants may reduce absorption of corticosteroids, digoxin, thiazide diuretics, warfarin, and other commonly used medications. Myositis and myalgia, along with increased serum creatine phosphokinase (CPK), may occur in ESRD patients who use clofibrate. Determining the optimal dose of clofibrate in this patient population is difficult, as plasma protein-binding changes markedly affect free concentrations of the active metabolite, clofibric acid, which has a prolonged half-life in patients with stage 5 CKD. Gemfibrozil may be a safer alternative, as the half-life is not altered with kidney dysfunction. Lower doses of 300 mg twice a day with close monitoring of CPK is recommended by some clinicians, based on an association of standard dose therapy with increases in CPK concentrations in dialysis patients.

Although HMG-CoA reductase inhibitors are remarkably free of adverse effects in otherwise healthy subjects, one should be cognizant of the potential myotoxic effects of these drugs, especially when administered with interacting agents including, but not limited to, azole antibiotics, cyclosporine, gemfibrozil, niacin, and in the presence of hepatic disease.[25] Patients receiving sevelamer as a phosphate binder may reap the benefits of its cholesterol-lowering effects.

Pharmacoeconomic Considerations

Hypertension Compliance and economic factors must be considered in the selection of antihypertensive therapy for CKD patients. Patients with ESRD are prescribed an average of 9 to 12 medications. Choosing agents that can be administered once or twice daily may improve patient compliance. In addition, there are now many options within some antihypertensive classes, such as calcium channel blockers, ACEIs, angiotensin receptor blockers, and β-blockers, which allow for less-frequent dosing. In most cases, no clear therapeutic advantage has been demonstrated with any particular agent within a class. Therefore, selecting the least costly agent that can be administered once or twice daily is reasonable.

As more information becomes available from studies evaluating the effects of long-term therapy of hypertension on cardiovascular events in patients with ESRD, cost benefits from potentially decreasing the occurrence of such events and their comorbidities may be quantified.

Hyperlipidemia Statin therapy for treatment of dyslipidemias has been shown to be cost-effective in patients at high risk for coronary heart disease. Although this has not specifically been evaluated in patients with CKD, this population is considered in the highest-risk group for coronary heart disease and cardiovascular events. It may be reasonable at least in theory to extrapolate this information on the cost benefits of therapy to the CKD population, although findings from the atorvasatin trial in ESRD patients contradict this rationale.

CLINICAL CONTROVERSY

Currently, there is no strong consensus on whether the predialysis or postdialysis blood pressure (or an average of the two) should be used to guide therapy and assess cardiovascular risk in the hemodialysis population. This issue, along with the question of the target blood pressure in this population, mean many decisions about pharmacologic therapy are based more on clinical judgement than evidence.

Evaluation of Therapeutic Outcomes

Hypertension Blood pressure monitoring to determine the effectiveness of therapy should be done at each visit for patients with ESRD, particularly following initiation of therapy (nonpharmacologic or pharmacologic) and at home when feasible. Patients on hemodialysis should have blood pressure measured before, during, and after dialysis to determine the effect of changes in their volume status on blood pressure. Some hemodialysis patients experience a paradoxical rise in blood pressure during dialysis. In these cases, the effect of dialysis on removal of antihypertensive agents and the dosing times relative to the dialysis procedure need to be evaluated. Similarly, patients may need to adjust the time of administration of antihypertensive therapy relative to the dialysis session if intradialytic hypotension occurs. Such decisions should be based on the pharmacokinetic profile of the antihypertensive agent in patients with ESRD. In cases when antihypertensive agents need to be discontinued, they should be withdrawn slowly. Chapter 15 discusses other aspects of monitoring blood pressure and associated complications.

Hyperlipidemia Patients should have their lipid profile reassessed 2 to 3 months following a change in treatment and at least annually thereafter.[25] Periodic evaluations of cardiovascular performance, as described in Chapters 13 and 23, are also warranted.

■ OTHER COMPLICATIONS OF CHRONIC KIDNEY DISEASE

Pruritus

Despite advances in dialysis treatment, pruritus (itching) remains a problem for 60% to 90% of ESRD patients.[109] The pathogenesis of uremic pruritus is poorly understood, but has been attributed to multiple factors such as inadequate dialysis, skin dryness, secondary hyperparathyroidism, increased vitamin A and histamine plasma concentrations, and increased sensitivity to histamine. In hemodialysis patients who experienced pruritus based on responses to a questionnaire (completed by a total of 453 of 1,773 patients) more than 70% also reported difficulties with sleep during a 24-month followup period.[110] Other factors associated with pruritus were male gender, high blood urea nitrogen and β_2-microglobulin levels, hypercalcemia, and hyperphosphatemia. Treatment options for pruritus, beyond control of metabolic abnormalities and delivery of adequate dialysis, have been fairly limited, but include antihistamines, 5-HT_3 receptor blockers such as ondansetron, and gabapentin.[110–112]

Nutritional Status

Protein-energy malnutrition is very common among patients with advanced CKD (stages 4 and 5) (see Chap. 147).[19] Causes of malnutrition in these patients include inadequate food intake secondary to anorexia, altered taste sensation, and the unpalatability of prescribed diets. Other factors in the ESRD population, such as the effect of the dialysis procedure on removal of nutrients, hypercatabolism induced by other inflammatory conditions, and blood loss are also contributory. Protein restriction as an intervention to potentially delay progression of kidney disease in patients with stage 3 or 4 CKD may also lead to protein malnutrition by the time a patient reaches ESRD; therefore the risks versus the benefits of this intervention must be considered on an individual basis (see Chap. 46) as hypoalbuminemia and malnutrition have a strong association with mortality in chronic dialysis patients.

Patients with ESRD have increased nutritional needs relative to the general population, based on the effect of the disease state and the dialysis procedure on nutritional status. The recommended dietary protein intake in chronic hemodialysis patients is 1.2 g/kg body weight per day.[19] The recommended intake for chronic peritoneal dialysis patients is at least 1.2 to 1.3 g/kg body weight per day, based on the increased protein loss that occurs with this dialysis modality. Protein requirements are higher in patients who are acutely ill (see Chap. 147). The recommended total daily energy intake in both hemodialysis and peritoneal dialysis patients is 35 kcal/kg body weight per day.[19] For peritoneal dialysis patients, this includes intake from both diet and that obtained from the glucose absorbed from peritoneal dialysate. For patients older than 60 years of age this criterion differs, because increasing age is generally associated with reduced physical activity and lean body mass. Daily energy intake for these patients is 30 to 35 kcal/kg body weight per day. Nutritional support should be considered for those patients who cannot achieve these goals with oral intake alone. Another option for nutritional supplementation in patients on hemodialysis includes interdialytic parenteral nutrition (see Chap. 147).

Vitamin requirements for ESRD patients receiving dialysis differ from those of a healthy person because of dietary modifications, kidney dysfunction, and dialysis therapy. The plasma concentrations of vitamins A and E are elevated in ESRD, whereas those of the water-soluble vitamins (B_1, B_2, B_6, B_{12}, niacin, pantothenic acid, folic acid, biotin, and vitamin C) tend to be low in this population, in large part because many are dialyzable. The goal for vitamin supplementation in this population should be to prevent subclinical and frank deficiency and to avoid pathology from overdosage. Special vitamin supplements have been formulated for the dialysis population, which primarily include B vitamins with C and folic acid.

Supplementation with L-carnitine has been advocated for its potential benefits in patients with ESRD including management of hypertriglyceridemia, hypercholesterolemia, and anemia.[113] Although some of these benefits have been demonstrated, the evidence does not strongly support routine supplementation with L-carnitine in patients with ESRD. Cost and the addition of yet another medication to the already complex regimen prescribed for many of these patients also mitigates against the routine use of this agent.

Uremic Bleeding

Bleeding complications in patients with CKD are usually mild, but can result in major hemorrhagic events. The primary mechanisms underlying the hemostatic problem are platelet biochemical abnormalities and alterations in platelet–vessel wall interactions. Decreased platelet aggregation and adhesiveness have been shown in a number of studies in ESRD patients.[114] Additionally, there is a decreased plasma concentration and defective binding of the large multimer of von Willebrand factor (vWF), which results in abnormal platelet–

blood vessel wall interactions. Patients on hemodialysis are at even greater risk of bleeding, not only because of the hemodialysis process itself, but from administration of other medications. Heparin is frequently administered during dialysis procedures to prevent clotting during dialysis. Patients who are at high risk for bleeding may require alternative anticoagulation procedures rather than traditional hemodialysis with systemic heparinization. In addition, dialysis patients often receive systemic anticoagulation (warfarin) or antiplatelet therapy (aspirin or clopidogrel) for prevention of access clotting or other cardiovascular disorders.

There are several nondialytic adjunctive therapies that may temporarily shorten the increased bleeding time observed in patients with kidney disease. Cryoprecipitate is rich in factor VIII, fibrinogen, and fibronectin, and shortens bleeding time. Desmopressin (1-deamino-8-D-arginine vasopressin) has minimal vasoconstrictive effects as compared to vasopressin, but effectively releases autologous factor VIII (vWF) from the endothelial lining of vessel walls. A consistent lowering of bleeding time has been observed with intravenous, subcutaneous, and intranasal routes of administration. A drawback to the use of desmopressin is tachyphylaxis with repeated doses; response may return after 3 to 4 days. This effect is felt to be caused by depletion of vWF stores following the first dose.

Administration of estrogens is also effective as an intervention to reduce bleeding time in uremic patients, a strategy based on the observation that women with von Willebrand disease improved during pregnancy.[114] Oral conjugated estrogens and low-dose transdermal patches are also effective. Side effects, which are uncommon and usually mild, include hot flashes, nausea, vomiting, hypertension, gynecomastia, and loss of libido. An increased risk of thromboembolism may result from estrogen therapy, especially with chronic use.

CONCLUSIONS

The number of patients with and at risk for CKD is increasing, with a substantial rise in the population with stage 5 CKD expected in the next decade. Although efforts to delay progression of CKD are paramount, measures to diagnose and manage the associated secondary complications and comorbid conditions early in the course of the disease are also essential. Common complications of stages 4 and 5 CKD include anemia, secondary hyperparathyroidism, fluid and electrolyte abnormalities, metabolic acidosis, and malnutrition. Cardiovascular complications are also prevalent in the population with CKD being the leading cause of mortality in patients with stage 5 disease. Patient education plays a critical role in the appropriate management of CKD and related complications. A multidisciplinary team structure is a rationale approach to provide this education and effectively design and implement the extensive nonpharmacologic and pharmacologic interventions required.

ABBREVIATIONS

ACEI: angiotensin-converting enzyme inhibitor

AIDS: acquired immunodeficiency syndrome

Ca × P: calcium phosphorus product; serum calcium multiplied by serum phosphorus

CKD: chronic kidney disease

CPK: creatine phosphokinase

ESAs: erythropoietic stimulating agents

ESRD: end-stage renal disease

FE_K: fractional excretion of potassium

FeNa: fractional excretion of sodium

GFR: glomerular filtration rate

Hb: hemoglobin

HCT: hematocrit

HDL: high-density lipoprotein

HMG-CoA: 3-hydroxy-3-methylglutaryl coenzyme A (reductase)

iPTH: intact parathyroid hormone

LDL: low-density lipoprotein

LVH: left ventricular hypertrophy

K/DOQI: Kidney Disease Outcomes Quality Initiative

PTH: parathyroid hormone

ROD: renal osteodystrophy

sHPT: secondary hyperparathyroidism

TSat: transferrin saturation

vWF: von Willebrand factor

REFERENCES

1. K/DOQI clinical practice guidelines for cardiovascular disease in dialysis patients. Am J Kidney Dis 2005;45:16–153.
2. U.S. Renal Data System. USRDS 2007 Annual Data Report: Atlas of Chronic Kidney Disease and End-Stage Renal Disease in the United States, National Institutes of Health, National Institute of Diabetes and Digestive and Kidney Diseases, Bethesda, MD, 2007.
3. K/DOQI clinical practice guidelines for chronic kidney disease: Evaluation, classification, and stratification. Am J Kidney Dis 2002;39:S1–S266.
4. Pereira BJ. Overcoming barriers to the early detection and treatment of chronic kidney disease and improving outcomes for end-stage renal disease. Am J Manag Care 2002;8:S122–S135; quiz S136–S139.
5. Brenner RM, Brenner BM. Adaptation to renal injury. In: Kasper DL, Braunwald E, Fauci AS, Hauser SL, Longo DL, Jameson JL, eds. Harrison's Principles of Internal Medicine, 16th ed. New York: McGraw-Hill, 2005:1639–1644.
6. Fukagawa M, Nakanishi S, Kazama JJ. Basic and clinical aspects of parathyroid hyperplasia in chronic kidney disease. Kidney Int Suppl 2006;102:S3–S7.
7. Levin A, Bakris GL, Molitch M, et al. Prevalence of abnormal serum vitamin D, PTH, calcium, and phosphorus in patients with chronic kidney disease: Results of the study to evaluate early kidney disease. Kidney Int 2007;71:31–38.
8. Eknoyan G, Levin A, Levin NW. Bone metabolism and disease in chronic kidney disease. Am J Kidney Dis 2003;42:1–201.
9. Lobao R, Carvalho AB, Cuppari L, et al. High prevalence of low bone mineral density in pre-dialysis chronic kidney disease patients: Bone histomorphometric analysis. Clin Nephrol 2004;62:432–439.
10. Coen G. Adynamic bone disease: An update and overview. J Nephrol 2005;18:117–122.
11. Ganesh SK, Stack AG, Levin NW, Hulbert-Shearon T, Port FK. Association of elevated serum PO(4), Ca PO(4) product, and parathyroid hormone with cardiac mortality risk in chronic hemodialysis patients. J Am Soc Nephrol 2001;12:2131–2138.
12. Bro S, Olgaard K. Effects of excess PTH on nonclassical target organs. Am J Kidney Dis 1997;30:606–620.
13. Block GA, Hulbert-Shearon TE, Levin NW, Port FK. Association of serum phosphorus and calcium x phosphate product with mortality risk in chronic hemodialysis patients: A national study. Am J Kidney Dis 1998;31:607–617.
14. Block GA, Port FK. Re-evaluation of risks associated with hyperphosphatemia and hyperparathyroidism in dialysis patients: Recommendations for a change in management. Am J Kidney Dis 2000;35:1226–1237.
15. Goodman WG, Goldin J, Kuizon BD, et al. Coronary-artery calcification in young adults with end-stage renal disease who are undergoing dialysis. N Engl J Med 2000;342:1478–1483.
16. Sarnak MJ, Levey AS, Schoolwerth AC, et al. Kidney disease as a risk factor for development of cardiovascular disease: A statement from the American Heart Association Councils on Kidney in Cardiovascular

Disease, High Blood Pressure Research, Clinical Cardiology, and Epidemiology and Prevention. Hypertension 2003;42:1050–1065.
17. Collins AJ, Li S, Gilbertson DT, Liu J, Chen SC, Herzog CA. Chronic kidney disease and cardiovascular disease in the Medicare population. Kidney Int Suppl 2003:S24–S31.
18. Executive Summary of The Third Report of The National Cholesterol Education Program (NCEP) Expert Panel on Detection, Evaluation, and Treatment of High Blood Cholesterol in Adults (Adult Treatment Panel III). JAMA 2001;285:2486–2497.
19. Clinical practice guidelines for nutrition in chronic renal failure. K/DOQI, National Kidney Foundation. Am J Kidney Dis 2000;35:S1–140.
20. Ritz E, Wanner C. Lipid changes and statins in chronic renal insufficiency. J Am Soc Nephrol 2006;17:S226–S230.
21. KDOQI clinical practice guidelines and clinical practice recommendations for anemia in chronic kidney disease. Am J Kidney Dis 2006;47:S11–145.
22. Levin A. Clinical epidemiology of cardiovascular disease in chronic kidney disease prior to dialysis. Semin Dial 2003;16:101–105.
23. Walters BA, Hays RD, Spritzer KL, Fridman M, Carter WB. Health-related quality of life, depressive symptoms, anemia, and malnutrition at hemodialysis initiation. Am J Kidney Dis 2002;40:1185–1194.
24. Herberth J, Fahrleitner-Pammer A, Obermayer-Pietsch B, et al. Changes in total parathyroid hormone (PTH), PTH-(1–84) and large C-PTH fragments in different stages of chronic kidney disease. Clin Nephrol 2006;65:328–334.
25. K/DOQI Clinical Practice Guidelines for managing dyslipidemias in patients with chronic kidney disease. Am J Kidney Dis 2003;41:S1–S91.
26. Owen WF, Jr. Patterns of care for patients with chronic kidney disease in the United States: Dying for improvement. J Am Soc Nephrol 2003;14:S76–S80.
27. London R, Solis A, Goldberg GA, Wade S, Chan WW. Examination of resource use and clinical interventions associated with chronic kidney disease in a managed care population. J Manag Care Pharm 2003;9:248–255.
28. Manley HJ, Carroll CA. The clinical and economic impact of pharmaceutical care in end-stage renal disease patients. Semin Dial 2002;15:45–49.
29. Joy MS, DeHart RM, Gilmartin C, et al. Clinical pharmacists as multidisciplinary health care providers in the management of CKD. A joint opinion by the Nephrology and Ambulatory Care Practice and Research Networks of the American College of Clinical Pharmacy. Am J Kidney Dis 2005;45:1105–1118.
30. Zillich AJ, Saseen JJ, Dehart RM, et al. Caring for patients with chronic kidney disease: A joint opinion of the ambulatory care and the nephrology practice and research networks of the American College of Clinical Pharmacy. Pharmacotherapy 2005;25:123–143.
31. Besarab A, Bolton WK, Browne JK, et al. The effects of normal as compared with low hematocrit values in patients with cardiac disease who are receiving hemodialysis and epoetin. N Engl J Med 1998;339:584–590.
32. Collins AJ. Influence of target hemoglobin in dialysis patients on morbidity and mortality. Kidney Int Suppl 2002:44–48.
33. Singh Ak, Szczech L, Tang KL, et al. Correction of anemia with epoetin alfa in chronic kidney disease. N Engl J Med 2006;355:2085–2098.
34. Drueke TB, Locatelli F, Clyne N, et al. Normalization of hemoglobin level in patients with chronic kidney disease and anemia. N Engl J Med 2006;355:2071–2084.
35. Tsuchiya K, Okano H, Teramura M, et al. Content of reticulocyte hemoglobin is a reliable tool for determining iron deficiency in dialysis patients. Clin Nephrol 2003;59:115–123.
36. Nissenson AR, Berns JS, Sakiewicz P, et al. Clinical evaluation of heme iron polypeptide: Sustaining a response to rHuEPO in hemodialysis patients. Am J Kidney Dis 2003;42:325–330.
37. Seligman P, NV D, J S, et al. Single-dose pharmacokinetics of sodium ferric gluconate complex in iron-deficient subjects. Pharmacotherapy 2004;24:564–573.
38. Coyne DW, Kapoian T, Suki W, et al. Ferric gluconate is highly efficacious in anemic hemodialysis patients with high serum ferritin and low transferrin saturation: Results of the Dialysis Patients' Response to IV Iron with Elevated Ferritin (DRIVE) Study. J Am Soc Nephrol 2007;18:975–984.
39. Fishbane S. Safety in iron management. Am J Kidney Dis 2003;41:18–26.
40. Fletes R, Lazarus JM, Gage J, Chertow GM. Suspected iron dextran-related adverse drug events in hemodialysis patients. Am J Kidney Dis 2001;37:743–749.
41. Charytan C, Levin N, Al-Saloum M, Hafeez T, Gagnon S, Van Wyck DB. Efficacy and safety of iron sucrose for iron deficiency in patients with dialysis-associated anemia: North American clinical trial. Am J Kidney Dis 2001;37:300–307.
42. Michael B, Coyne DW, Fishbane S, et al. Sodium ferric gluconate complex in hemodialysis patients: Adverse reactions compared to placebo and iron dextran. Kidney Int 2002;61:1830–1839.
43. Auerbach M, Winchester J, Wahab A, et al. A randomized trial of three iron dextran infusion methods for anemia in EPO-treated dialysis patients. Am J Kidney Dis 1998;31:81–86.
44. Dahdah K, Patrie JT, Bolton WK. Intravenous iron dextran treatment in predialysis patients with chronic renal failure. Am J Kidney Dis 2000;36:775–782.
45. Folkert VW, Michael B, Agarwal R, et al. Chronic use of sodium ferric gluconate complex in hemodialysis patients: Safety of higher-dose (> or = 250 mg) administration. Am J Kidney Dis 2003;41:651–657.
46. Blaustein DA, Schwenk MH, Chattopadhyay J, et al. The safety and efficacy of an accelerated iron sucrose dosing regimen in patients with chronic kidney disease. Kidney Int Suppl 2003:S72–S77.
47. Chandler G, Harchowal J, Macdougall IC. Intravenous iron sucrose: Establishing a safe dose. Am J Kidney Dis 2001;38:988–991.
48. Venofer. Package insert. Shirley, NY: American Regent Laboratories, February 2007.
49. Brewster UC, Perazella MA. Intravenous iron and the risk of infection in end-stage renal disease patients. Semin Dial 2004;17:57–60.
50. Afzali B, Goldsmith DJ. Intravenous iron therapy in renal failure: Friend and foe? J Nephrol 2004;17:487–495.
51. INFeD. Package insert. Florham Park, NJ: Watson Pharma, March 2006.
52. Ferrlecit. Package insert. Corona, CA: Watson Pharma, September 2006.
53. NKF-K/DOQI clinical practice guidelines for anemia of chronic kidney disease: Update 2000. Am J Kidney Dis 2001;37:S182–S238.
54. Egrie JC, Browne JK. Development and characterization of novel erythropoiesis stimulating protein (NESP). Nephrol Dial Transplant 2001;16(Suppl 3):3–13.
55. Ateshkadi A, Johnson CA, Oxton LL, Hammond TG, Bohenek WS, Zimmerman SW. Pharmacokinetics of intraperitoneal, intravenous, and subcutaneous recombinant human erythropoietin in patients on continuous ambulatory peritoneal dialysis. Am J Kidney Dis 1993;21:635–642.
56. McClellan WM, Frankenfield DL, Wish JB, Rocco MV, Johnson CA, Owen WF Jr. Subcutaneous erythropoietin results in lower dose and equivalent hematocrit levels among adult hemodialysis patients: Results from the 1998 End-Stage Renal Disease Core Indicators Project. Am J Kidney Dis 2001;37:E36.
57. Macdougall IC, Gray SJ, Elston O, et al. Pharmacokinetics of novel erythropoiesis stimulating protein compared with epoetin alfa in dialysis patients. J Am Soc Nephrol 1999;10:2392–2395.
58. Vanrenterghem Y, Barany P, Mann JF, et al. Randomized trial of darbepoetin alfa for treatment of renal anemia at a reduced dose frequency compared with rHuEPO in dialysis patients. Kidney Int 2002;62:2167–2175.
59. Agarwal AK, Silver MR, Reed JE, et al. An open-label study of darbepoetin alfa administered once monthly for the maintenance of haemoglobin concentrations in patients with chronic kidney disease not receiving dialysis. J Intern Med 2006;260:577–585.
60. Theodoridis M, Passadakis P, Kriki P, et al. Efficient monthly subcutaneous administration of darbepoetin in stable CAPD patients. Perit Dial Int 2005;25:564–569.
61. Abu-Alfa AK, Cruz D, Perazella MA, Mahnensmith RL, Simon D, Bia MJ. ACE inhibitors do not induce recombinant human erythropoietin resistance in hemodialysis patients. Am J Kidney Dis 2000;35:1076–1082.
62. Silverberg D. Outcomes of anaemia management in renal insufficiency and cardiac disease. Nephrol Dial Transplant 2003;18 Suppl 2:ii7–ii12.
63. Roger SD, McMahon LP, Clarkson A, et al. Effects of early and late intervention with epoetin alpha on left ventricular mass among patients with chronic kidney disease (stage 3 or 4): Results of a randomized clinical trial. J Am Soc Nephrol 2004;15:148–156.
64. Macdougall IC. Antibody-mediated pure red cell aplasia (PRCA): Epidemiology, immunogenicity and risks. Nephrol Dial Transplant 2005;20 Suppl 4:iv9–iv15.
65. Bennett CL, Luminari S, Nissenson AR, et al. Pure red-cell aplasia and epoetin therapy. N Engl J Med 2004;351:1403–1408.

66. Asari A, Gokal R. Pure red cell aplasia secondary to epoetin alpha responding to Darbepoetin alpha in a patient on peritoneal dialysis. J Am Soc Nephrol 2004;15:2204–2207.
67. Epogen. Package insert. Thousand Oaks, CA: Amgen, March 2007.
68. Provenzano R, Bhaduri S, Singh AK. Extended epoetin alfa dosing as maintenance treatment for the anemia of chronic kidney disease: The PROMPT study. Clin Nephrol 2005;64:113–123.
69. Germain M, Ram CV, Bhaduri S, Tang KL, Klausner M, Curzi M. Extended epoetin alfa dosing in chronic kidney disease patients: A retrospective review. Nephrol Dial Transplant 2005;20:2146–2152.
70. Provenzano R, Garcia-Mayol L, Suchinda P, et al. Once-weekly epoetin alfa for treating the anemia of chronic kidney disease. Clin Nephrol 2004;61:392–405.
71. Aranesp. Package insert. Thousand Oaks, CA: Amgen, April 2007.
72. Ling B, Walczyk M, Agarwal A, Carroll W, Liu W, Brenner R. Darbepoetin alfa administered once monthly maintains hemoglobin concentrations in patients with chronic kidney disease. Clin Nephrol 2005;63:327–334.
73. Jadoul M, Vanrenterghem Y, Foret M, Walker R, Gray SJ. Darbepoetin alfa administered once monthly maintains haemoglobin levels in stable dialysis patients. Nephrol Dial Transplant 2004;19:898–903.
74. Rastogi A, Nissenson AR. New approaches to the management of anemia of chronic kidney disease: Beyond Epogen and INFeD. Kidney Int Suppl 2006:S14–S16.
75. Macdougall IC. CERA (Continuous Erythropoietin Receptor Activator): A new erythropoiesis-stimulating agent for the treatment of anemia. Curr Hematol Rep 2005;4:436–440.
76. Brophy DF, Ripley EB, Holdford DA. Pharmacoeconomic considerations in the health system management of anaemia in patients with chronic kidney disease and end stage renal disease. Expert Opin Pharmacother 2003;4:1461–1469.
77. Procrit. Package insert. Raritan, NJ: Ortho Biotech, March 2007.
78. Moe SM, Drueke TB. Management of secondary hyperparathyroidism: The importance and the challenge of controlling parathyroid hormone levels without elevating calcium, phosphorus, and calcium-phosphorus product. Am J Nephrol 2003;23:369–379.
79. Chertow GM, Burke SK, Dillon MA, Slatopolsky E. Long-term effects of sevelamer hydrochloride on the calcium phosphate product and lipid profile of haemodialysis patients. Nephrol Dial Transplant 2000;15:559.
80. Block GA, Spiegel DM, Ehrlich J, et al. Effects of sevelamer and calcium on coronary artery calcification in patients new to hemodialysis. Kidney Int 2005;68:1815–1824.
81. Fosrenol. Package insert. Wayne, PA: Shire U.S., July 2007.
82. Joy MS, Kshirsagar A, Candiani C, Brooks T, Hudson JQ. Lanthanum carbonate. Ann Pharmacother 2006;40:234–240.
83. Hutchison AJ, Maes B, Vanwalleghem J, et al. Long-term efficacy and tolerability of lanthanum carbonate: Results from a 3-year study. Nephron Clin Pract 2006;102:c61–c71.
84. Renagel. Package insert. Cambridge, MA: Genzyme, April 2007.
85. Burke S, Amin N, Incerti C, Plone M, Watson N. Sevelamer hydrochloride (Renagel), a nonabsorbed phosphate-binding polymer, does not interfere with digoxin or warfarin pharmacokinetics. J Clin Pharmacol 2001;41:193–198.
86. Burke SK, Amin NS, Incerti C, Plone MA, Lee JW. Sevelamer hydrochloride (Renagel), a phosphate-binding polymer, does not alter the pharmacokinetics of two commonly used antihypertensives in healthy volunteers. J Clin Pharmacol 2001;41:199–205.
87. Capitanini A, Lupi A, Osteri F, et al. Gastric pH, sevelamer hydrochloride and omeprazole. Clin Nephrol 2005;64:320–322.
88. Guillen-Anaya MA, Jadoul M. Drug interaction between sevelamer and cyclosporin. Nephrol Dial Transplant 2004;19:515.
89. Slatopolsky E, Finch J, Brown A. New vitamin D analogs. Kidney Int Suppl 2003:S83–7.
90. Maung HM, Elangovan L, Frazao JM, et al. Efficacy and side effects of intermittent intravenous and oral doxercalciferol (1-alpha-hydroxyvitamin D(2)) in dialysis patients with secondary hyperparathyroidism: A sequential comparison. Am J Kidney Dis 2001;37:532–543.
91. Lindberg J, Martin KJ, Gonzalez EA, Acchiardo SR, Valdin JR, Soltanek C. A long-term, multicenter study of the efficacy and safety of paricalcitol in end-stage renal disease. Clin Nephrol 2001;56:315–323.
92. Zemplar Capsules. Package insert. Abbott Park, IL: Abbott Laboratories, 2005.
93. Joist HE, Ahya SN, Giles K, Norwood K, Slatopolsky E, Coyne DW. Differential effects of very high doses of doxercalciferol and paricalcitol on serum phosphorus in hemodialysis patients. Clin Nephrol 2006;65:335–341.
94. Brown AJ, Finch J, Slatopolsky E. Differential effects of 19-nor-1,25-dihydroxyvitamin D(2) and 1,25-dihydroxyvitamin D(3) on intestinal calcium and phosphate transport. J Lab Clin Med 2002;139:279–284.
95. Coburn JW, Maung HM, Elangovan L, et al. Doxercalciferol safely suppresses PTH levels in patients with secondary hyperparathyroidism associated with chronic kidney disease stages 3 and 4. Am J Kidney Dis 2004;43:877–890.
96. Coyne D, Acharya M, Qiu P, et al. Paricalcitol capsule for the treatment of secondary hyperparathyroidism in stages 3 and 4 CKD. Am J Kidney Dis 2006;47:263–276.
97. Sprague SM, Lerma E, McCormmick D, Abraham M, Batlle D. Suppression of parathyroid hormone secretion in hemodialysis patients: Comparison of paricalcitol with calcitriol. Am J Kidney Dis 2001;38:S51–6.
98. Teng M, Wolf M, Lowrie E, Ofsthun N, Lazarus JM, Thadhani R. Survival of patients undergoing hemodialysis with paricalcitol or calcitriol therapy. N Engl J Med 2003;349:446–456.
99. Teng M, Wolf M, Ofsthun MN, et al. Activated injectable vitamin D and hemodialysis survival: A historical cohort study. J Am Soc Nephrol 2005;16:1115–1125.
100. Agarwal R, Acharya M, Tian J, et al. Antiproteinuric effect of oral paricalcitol in chronic kidney disease. Kidney Int 2005;68:2823–2828.
101. Tentori F, Hunt WC, Stidley CA, et al. Mortality risk among hemodialysis patients receiving different vitamin D analogs. Kidney Int 2006;70:1858–1865.
102. Hudson JQ. Secondary hyperparathyroidism in chronic kidney disease: Focus on clinical consequences and vitamin D therapies. Ann Pharmacother 2006;40:1584–1593.
103. Sensipar (cinacalcet HCl) Tablets Package Insert. Amgen Inc., Thousand Oaks, CA. October 2007.
104. Quarles LD. Cinacalcet HCl: A novel treatment for secondary hyperparathyroidism in stage 5 chronic kidney disease. Kidney Int Suppl 2005:S24–8.
105. Charytan C, Coburn JW, Chonchol M, et al. Cinacalcet hydrochloride is an effective treatment for secondary hyperparathyroidism in patients with CKD not receiving dialysis. Am J Kidney Dis 2005;46:58–67.
106. Kraut JA, Kurtz I. Use of base in the treatment of severe acidemic states. Am J Kidney Dis 2001;38:703–727.
107. Abosaif NY, Arije A, Atray NK, et al. K/DOQI clinical practice guidelines on hypertension and antihypertensive agents in chronic kidney disease. Am J Kidney Dis 2004;43:S1–290.
108. Wanner C, Krane V, Marz W, et al. Atorvastatin in patients with type 2 diabetes mellitus undergoing hemodialysis. N Engl J Med 2005;353:238–248.
109. Zucker I, Yosipovitch G, David M, Gafter U, Boner G. Prevalence and characterization of uremic pruritus in patients undergoing hemodialysis: Uremic pruritus is still a major problem for patients with end-stage renal disease. J Am Acad Dermatol 2003;49:842–846.
110. Narita I, Alchi B, Omori K, et al. Etiology and prognostic significance of severe uremic pruritus in chronic hemodialysis patients. Kidney Int 2006;69:1626–1632.
111. Weisshaar E, Dunker N, Rohl FW, Gollnick H. Antipruritic effects of two different 5-HT3 receptor antagonists and an antihistamine in haemodialysis patients. Exp Dermatol 2004;13:298–304.
112. Manenti L, Vaglio A, Costantino E, et al. Gabapentin in the treatment of uremic itch: An index case and a pilot evaluation. J Nephrol 2005;18:86–91.
113. Matera M, Bellinghieri G, Costantino G, Santoro D, Calvani M, Savica V. History of L-carnitine: Implications for renal disease. J Ren Nutr 2003;13:2–14.
114. Kaw D, Malhotra D. Platelet dysfunction and end-stage renal disease. Semin Dial 2006;19:317–322.

CHAPTER 48

Hemodialysis and Peritoneal Dialysis

EDWARD F. FOOTE AND HAROLD J. MANLEY

KEY CONCEPTS

1. The hemodialysis procedure involves the perfusion of blood and dialysate on opposite sides of a semipermeable membrane. Substances are removed from the blood by diffusion and convection. Excess plasma water is removed via ultrafiltration.

2. The native arteriovenous fistula is the preferred access for hemodialysis because of fewer complications and a longer survival rate. Venous catheters are plagued by complications such as infection and thrombosis and often deliver relatively poor blood flow rates.

3. Adequacy of hemodialysis can be assessed by the *Kt/V* and urea reduction ratio (URR). The National Kidney Foundation's Kidney Disease Outcomes Quality Initiative has set the minimum goal *Kt/V* at greater than 1.2 per treatment and the URR at greater than 65%. In practice, most patients on hemodialysis exceed this goal.

4. During hemodialysis, patients commonly experience hypotension and cramps. Other more serious complications include infection and thrombosis of the vascular access.

5. The peritoneal dialysis procedure involves the instillation of dialysate into the peritoneal cavity via a permanent peritoneal catheter. The peritoneal membrane lines the highly vascularized abdominal viscera and acts as the semipermeable membrane across which diffusion and ultrafiltration occur. Substances are removed from the blood across the peritoneum via diffusion and ultrafiltration. Excess plasma water is removed via ultrafiltration created by osmotic pressure generated by various dextrose or icodextrin concentrations.

6. Patients on peritoneal dialysis are required to instill and drain, manually or via automated systems, several liters of fresh dialysate each day. The more exchanges a patient completes each day results in greater solute removal.

7. Peritonitis is a common complication of peritoneal dialysis. Initial empiric therapy for peritonitis should include intraperitoneal antibiotics that are effective against both gram-positive and gram-negative organisms.

8. Nasal carriage of *Staphylococcus aureus* is associated with an increased risk of catheter-related infections and peritonitis. Prophylaxis with intranasal mupirocin (twice a day for 5 days every month) or mupirocin (daily) at the exit site can effectively reduce *S. aureus* infections.

The complete chapter, learning objectives, and other resources can be found at **www.pharmacotherapyonline.com.**

The three primary treatment options for patients with end-stage renal disease (ESRD) are hemodialysis (HD), peritoneal dialysis (PD), and kidney transplantation. The United States Renal Data System is the national system that "collects, analyzes, and distributes" data relating to the United States ESRD program.[1] According to the United States Renal Data System, at the end of 2005 (the most recent data available), there were 483,750 patients in the United States with ESRD. Of these, 314,162 and 25,895 patients were being treated with HD and PD, respectively, and 143,693 had a functioning kidney transplant. The vast majority of incident (new) dialysis patients are treated with HD. Since mid-1990, the number of prevalent PD patients has decreased. Although the number of patients who have received a kidney transplant has risen steadily, transplantation has not kept pace with the growing prevalence of ESRD in the United States.

Since 1972, the treatment of ESRD (both dialysis and kidney transplantation) has been covered by Medicare. Total spending for ESRD in 2005 was $32 billion; approximately one-third of this was from non-Medicare payers. ESRD patients consume a disproportionate amount of healthcare dollars. Approximately 1% of the patients in the Medicare program have ESRD, yet 8.2% of the budget is consumed by the ESRD program. Although total spending for ESRD treatment continues to climb, per-patient spending (after adjusting for inflation) was fairly flat between 2004 and 2005.

There are some positive signs as it relates to public health and ESRD. Although the total number of dialysis patients is increasing in the United States, the incident rate (number of new dialysis patients per total population) has stabilized or slightly decreased from the highest value observed in 1997. The prevalent population of ESRD continues to climb, reflective of reduced mortality and enhanced patient care. The primary diagnosis for incident patients with ESRD is diabetes.[1] Chapter 46 provides a thorough discussion on the epidemiology of chronic kidney disease.

This chapter serves as a primer on the principles and practice of dialysis. The chapter focuses on HD and PD as the dialysis modalities most commonly employed for the management of ESRD (see Chap. 45 for a discussion of the role of dialysis in the management of acute renal failure). The pertinent factors which should be considered before the initiation of dialysis are described. The morbidity and mortality associated with HD and PD are compared, as these considerations may influence the dialysis method chosen by patients and clinicians. Because dialysis by either method is not a generic procedure, the variants of HD and PD are detailed. The multiple types of vascular and peritoneal access used to provide HD and PD, including various catheters and surgical techniques, are illustrated. The concept of dialysis adequacy for each modality is briefly reviewed. Finally, the clinical presentation of the common complications of both dialytic therapies is presented, along with pertinent nonpharmacologic and pharmacologic therapeutic approaches.

CHAPTER 49

Drug-Induced Kidney Disease

THOMAS D. NOLIN AND JONATHAN HIMMELFARB

KEY CONCEPTS

1. The initial diagnosis of drug-induced kidney disease typically involves detection of elevated serum creatinine and blood urea nitrogen, for which there is a temporal relationship between the toxicity and use of a potentially nephrotoxic drug.
2. Drug-induced kidney disease is best prevented by avoiding the use of potentially nephrotoxic agents in patients at increased risk for toxicity. However, when exposure to these drugs cannot be avoided, recognition of risk factors and specific techniques, such as hydration, may be used to reduce potential nephrotoxicity.
3. Acute tubular necrosis is the most common presentation of drug-induced kidney disease in hospitalized patients. The primary agents implicated are aminoglycosides, radiocontrast media, cisplatin, amphotericin B, foscarnet, and osmotically active agents.
4. Angiotensin-converting enzyme inhibitors and nonsteroidal antiinflammatory drugs are associated with hemodynamically mediated kidney injury, the pathogenesis of which is a decrease in glomerular capillary hydrostatic pressure.
5. Acute allergic interstitial nephritis is the underlying cause for up to 3% of all cases of acute kidney injury. Clinical manifestations of allergic interstitial nephritis typically present approximately 14 days after initiation of therapy and include fever, maculopapular rash, eosinophilia, pyuria, hematuria, proteinuria, and oliguria.

Drug-induced kidney disease or nephrotoxicity (DIN) is a relatively common complication of several diagnostic and therapeutic agents. It is seen in both inpatient and outpatient settings with variable presentations depending on the drug and clinical setting. Manifestations of DIN include acid–base abnormalities, electrolyte imbalances, urine sediment abnormalities, proteinuria, pyuria, and/or hematuria.[1] However, the most common manifestation of DIN is a decline in the glomerular filtration rate (GFR), which results in a rise in the serum creatinine (S_{cr}) and blood urea nitrogen (BUN). Initial diagnosis of DIN is often delayed as it typically involves detection of elevated S_{cr} and BUN, for which there is a temporal relationship between the toxicity and use of a potentially nephrotoxic drug. This is consistent with the classic qualitative definition of acute renal failure (ARF) i.e., an "abrupt and sustained decrease in glomerular filtration, urine output, or both."[2] Unfortunately, numerous definitions of ARF and nephrotoxicity based on various quantitative changes in the serum creatinine concentration and other clinical end points have been published.[2,3] Consequently, it is extraordinarily difficult to ascertain the true incidence of ARF and/or DIN because broad ranges have been reported for the same agent. This may be alleviated if the recently developed new diagnostic criteria based on physiologic measurements (e.g., S_{cr} and urine output) are broadly accepted, and if the new term *acute kidney injury* (AKI) supplants the use of ARF (see Chap. 45).[4–6]

DIN is often reversible on discontinuation of the offending agent, but may also lead to acute kidney injury and/or end-stage renal disease (ESRD). Currently, many different mechanisms are responsible for the pathogenesis of DIN and the introduction of new drugs with novel mechanisms of action provides the potential for the identification of new presentations of AKI and chronic kidney disease (CKD). This chapter reviews the epidemiology, pathophysiology, risk factors, and basic principles of prevention of DIN. Detailed discussions of these issues plus management strategies are presented for widely used agents that have been associated with a moderate to high likelihood of DIN.

EPIDEMIOLOGY

The incidence and characteristics of outpatient or community-acquired DIN are not well understood as mild toxicity is often unrecognized in this setting. However, the pharmacoepidemiology of these effects has become more important as care increasingly shifts to the outpatient setting. Up to 20% of hospital admissions, as a result of AKI, have been attributed specifically to community-acquired DIN.[7] Conversely, DIN has been studied for years in the acute care hospital setting where it has been implicated in 8% to 60% of all cases of in-hospital AKI and as such is a recognized source of significant morbidity and mortality.[8] In-hospital drug use may contribute to 35% of all cases of acute tubular necrosis, most cases of allergic interstitial nephritis (AIN), as well as nephrotoxicity due to alterations in renal hemodynamics and postrenal obstruction.[9] The incidence of antibiotic-induced nephrotoxicity alone may be as high as 36%.[1] Aminoglycoside antibiotics, radiocontrast media, conventional nonselective nonsteroidal antiinflammatory drugs (NSAIDs) and selective cyclooxygenase-2 (COX-2) inhibitors, amphotericin B, and angiotensin-converting enzyme inhibitors (ACEIs) have also been frequently implicated.[10–12] Computer-guided medication dosing for hospital inpatients may improve the safety of some of these potentially harmful drugs and minimize the occurrence of DIN in this setting.[13]

CLINICAL PRESENTATION

1 Because the most common manifestation of DIN is a decline in GFR leading to a rise in S_{cr} and BUN, the onset of toxicity in hospitalized, acutely ill patients is most often recognized by routine laboratory monitoring of these two chemistries. Decreased urine output may also be an early sign of toxicity, particularly with radiographic contrast media, NSAIDs, and ACEIs. In the outpatient setting, nephrotoxicity is often recognized by symptoms such as malaise, anorexia, vomiting, volume overload (shortness of breath or edema), and hypertension. S_{cr} or BUN concentrations and urine collection for creatinine clearance may subsequently be measured to quantify the degree of loss of glomerular filtration. Marked intrasubject between-day variability of S_{cr} values has been noted (±20% for values within the normal range; see Chap. 44). Furthermore, they may be altered as the result of dietary changes and initiation of drug therapy, which may interfere with the assay procedure. Thus a change in S_{cr} of at least 0.5 mg/dL for subjects with a baseline S_{cr} <2 mg/dL and an increase of approximately 30% for those with S_{cr} >2 mg/dL, when correlated temporally with the initiation of drug therapy, is a common threshold for the identification of DIN.

CLINICAL PRESENTATION OF DRUG-INDUCED KIDNEY DISEASE

General

- The most common manifestation is a decline in GFR leading to a rise in S_{cr} and BUN.

Symptoms

- Malaise, anorexia, vomiting, shortness of breath, or edema.

Signs

- Decreased urine output may be an early sign of toxicity, particularly with radiographic contrast media, NSAIDs, and ACEIs, with progression to volume overload and hypertension.
- *Proximal tubular injury:* metabolic acidosis with bicarbonaturia; glycosuria in the absence of hyperglycemia; and reductions in serum phosphate, uric acid, potassium, and magnesium as a result of increased urinary losses.
- *Distal tubular injury:* polyuria from failure to maximally concentrate urine, metabolic acidosis from impaired urinary acidification, and hyperkalemia from impaired potassium excretion.

Laboratory Tests

- A change in S_{cr} of at least 0.5 mg/dL for subjects with a baseline S_{cr} <2 mg/dL and an increase of >30% for those with S_{cr} >2 mg/dL, when correlated temporally with the initiation of drug therapy is commonly observed.[3,10]

Other Diagnostic Tests

- Urinary excretion of *N*-acetyl-*β*-D-glucosaminidase, *γ*-glutamyl transpeptidase, glutathione *S*-transferase, and interleukin-18 are markers of proximal tubular injury and have been used for the early detection of AKI in critically ill patients.[14,15]
- Kidney injury molecule-1 (KIM-1) is expressed in the proximal tubule and is upregulated in patients with ischemic acute tubular necrosis, appearing in the urine within 12 hours after the ischemic insult.[15]
- Neutrophil gelatinase-associated lipocalin (NGAL) protein may be detected in the urine within 3 hours of ischemic injury.[15]

TABLE 49-1 Drug-Induced Renal Structural–Functional Alterations

Tubular epithelial cell damage	
Acute tubular necrosis	• Pentamidine
• Adefovir, cidofovir, tenofovir	• Radiographic contrast media
• Aminoglycoside antibiotics	• Zoledronate
• Amphotericin B	Osmotic nephrosis
• Cisplatin, carboplatin	• Dextran
• Cyclosporine, tacrolimus	• Intravenous immunoglobulin
• Foscarnet	• Mannitol
Hemodynamically mediated kidney injury	
• Angiotensin-converting enzyme inhibitors	• Cyclosporine, tacrolimus
	• Nonsteroidal antiinflammatory drugs
• Angiotensin II receptor blockers	• OKT3
Obstructive nephropathy	
Intratubular obstruction	Nephrolithiasis
• Acyclovir	• Indinavir
• Foscarnet	• Sulfonamides
• Indinavir	• Triamterene
• Methotrexate	
• Sulfonamides	
Glomerular disease	
• Gold	• Nonsteroidal antiinflammatory drugs, cyclooxygenase-2 inhibitors
• Lithium	• Pamidronate
Tubulointerstitial disease	
Acute allergic interstitial nephritis	Nephrocalcinosis
• Ciprofloxacin	• Oral sodium phosphate solution
• Loop diuretics	Papillary necrosis
• Nonsteroidal antiinflammatory drugs, cyclooxygenase-2 inhibitors	• Nonsteroidal antiinflammatory drugs, combined phenacetin, aspirin, and caffeine analgesics
• Penicillins	
• Proton pump inhibitors	
Chronic interstitial nephritis	
• Cyclosporine	
• Lithium	
• Aristolochic acid	
Renal vasculitis, thrombosis, and cholesterol emboli	
Vasculitis and thrombosis	• Mitomycin C
• Hydralazine	• Methamphetamines
• Propylthiouracil	• Cyclosporine, tacrolimus
• Allopurinol	Cholesterol emboli
• Penicillamine	• Warfarin
• Gemcitabine	• Thrombolytic agents

Nephrotoxicity may be evidenced by alterations in renal tubular function without loss of glomerular filtration (Table 49–1). Indicators of proximal tubular injury include metabolic acidosis with bicarbonaturia; glycosuria in the absence of hyperglycemia; and reductions in serum phosphate, uric acid, potassium, and magnesium as a result of increased urinary losses. Indicators of distal tubular injury include polyuria from failure to maximally concentrate urine, metabolic acidosis from impaired urinary acidification, and hyperkalemia from impaired potassium excretion. Urinary enzymes and low-molecular-weight proteins are also used as early markers of nephrotoxicity. For example, urinary excretion of *N*-acetyl-*β*-D-glucosaminidase, *γ*-glutamyl transpeptidase, glutathione *S*-transferase, and interleukin-18 are markers of proximal tubular injury and have been used for the early detection of acute kidney damage in critically ill patients. The transmembrane protein KIM-1 is expressed in the proximal tubule and is upregulated in patients with ischemic acute tubular necrosis, appearing in the urine within 12 hours after the ischemic insult. Similarly, NGAL protein is detected in the urine within 3 hours of ischemic injury in rodent models of kidney disease. In the future, novel urinary biomarkers such as interleukin-18, KIM-1, and NGAL may facilitate the earlier diagnosis of nephrotoxicity and minimize the long-term consequences of this common drug-induced disorder.

PRINCIPLES FOR PREVENTION OF DRUG-INDUCED NEPHROPATHY

❷ The primary principle for prevention of DIN is to avoid the use of potentially nephrotoxic agents in patients at increased risk for toxicity. However, because exposure to these drugs often cannot be avoided, several interventions have been proposed to reduce the potential for the development of nephrotoxicity, for example, careful and adequate hydration to establish high renal tubular urine flow rates.[8] However, other strategies to reduce drug toxicity are still theoretical and/or investigational and relate directly to the specific nephrotoxic mechanisms of the drug. For example, adefovir is a nucleotide antiviral that is actively transported by OAT1.[16] Inhibition of OAT1-mediated transport with NSAIDs minimizes accumulation of adefovir in renal proximal tubule cells and results in a reduction in DIN.[17]

Table 49–1 lists the several specific drug-induced renal structural–functional alterations that are responsible for the vast majority of cases of DIN. This chapter discusses the pathophysiologic mechanisms responsible for the development of DIN with these agents in detail, along with clinical presentation, prevention strategies, therapeutic management approaches, and relevant monitoring plans.

TUBULAR EPITHELIAL CELL DAMAGE

❸ Renal tubular epithelial cell damage may be caused by either direct toxic or ischemic effects of drugs. Damage is most often localized in the proximal and distal tubular epithelia, and when observed as cellular degeneration and sloughing from proximal and distal tubular basement membranes is termed acute tubular necrosis.[18] Swelling and vacuolization of proximal tubular cells may also be noted in those with osmotic nephrosis.[12] Acute tubular necrosis is the most common presentation of DIN in the inpatient setting. The primary agents implicated in renal tubular epithelial cell damage are aminoglycosides, radiocontrast media, cisplatin, amphotericin B, foscarnet, and osmotically active agents such as immunoglobulins, dextrans, and mannitol.[1,12]

ACUTE TUBULAR NECROSIS

Aminoglycoside Nephrotoxicity

Incidence Although nephrotoxicity has been reported in up to 58% of patients who are receiving aminoglycoside therapy, most recent reviews suggest rates of 5% to 15%.[19,20] The large variance is in part a result of the use of different definitions of toxicity, variability between agents in the class, and the risk factors present in the study population.

Clinical Presentation A gradual progressive rise in the serum creatinine concentration and decrease in creatinine clearance after 6 to 10 days of therapy are the initial clinical manifestations of toxicity. Patients typically present with nonoliguria, maintaining urine volumes greater than 500 mL/day. Although renal magnesium wasting can occur, that is, daily excretion of more than 10 to 30 mg, the risk of hypomagnesemia is generally low. Severe kidney injury does not usually develop if aminoglycoside therapy is stopped promptly upon notation of a signficant rise in serum creatinine, but occasionally it may, and for these individuals dialysis therapy may be required (see Chap. 48). Aminoglycoside-associated nephropathy must be evaluated carefully because not all AKI during a course of therapy is caused by the aminoglycoside. Dehydration, sepsis, ischemia, and other nephrotoxic drugs frequently contribute to and complicate the identification of the causative agent or condition.

Pathogenesis The reduction of GFR in patients receiving aminoglycosides is predominantly the result of proximal tubular epithelial cell damage leading to obstruction of the tubular lumen and back leakage of the glomerular filtrate across the damaged tubular epithelium.[21] Toxicity may be related to cationic charge, which facilitates binding of filtered aminoglycosides to renal tubular epithelial cell luminal membranes, followed by intracellular transport and concentration in lysosomes.[1,21,22] Cellular dysfunction and death may result from release of lysosomal enzymes into the cytosol, generation of reactive oxygen species, altered cellular metabolism, and alterations in cell membrane fluidity, leading to reduced activity of membrane-bound enzymes, including Na^+-K^+-adenosine triphosphatase, dipeptidyl peptidase IV, and neutral aminopeptidase.

Risk Factors Multiple risk factors for aminoglycoside nephrotoxicity have been identified. These relate to the aggressiveness of aminoglycoside dosing, synergistic toxicity as the result of combination drug therapy, and preexisting clinical conditions of the patient (Table 49–2).[21]

Prevention Aminoglycoside-induced nephrotoxicity may be prevented by more discriminating selection of patients in whom the drugs are used. Moreover, alternative antibiotics should be used whenever possible and as soon as microbial sensitivities are known. Commonly used alternatives include fluoroquinolones (e.g., ciprofloxacin or levofloxacin) and third- or fourth-generation cephalosporins (e.g., ceftazidime or cefepime). When aminoglycosides are necessary, the specific drug used does not appear to significantly affect the risk of nephrotoxicity, and therapy should be selected to optimize antimicrobial efficacy. Furthermore, it is imperative to avoid volume depletion, limit the total aminoglycoside dose administered, and avoid concomitant therapy with other nephrotoxic drugs. Future therapeutic alternatives may include nonnephrotoxic aminoglycoside congeners, which are in development, that retain the desired bactericidal activity and yet are devoid of nephrotoxicity.[23]

Prospective, individualized pharmacokinetic monitoring has been used for more than 25 years. Although many have reported a decrease in the incidence of aminoglycoside-induced nephrotoxicity, the studies are often small and statistically underpowered. High intermittent dosing of aminoglycosides, termed *once-daily dosing*, used in combina-

TABLE 49-2 Risk Factors for Aminoglycoside Nephrotoxicity

A. Related to aminoglycoside dosing:
Large total cumulative dose
Prolonged therapy
Trough concentration exceeding 2 mg/L
Recent previous aminoglycoside therapy
B. Related to synergistic nephrotoxicity. Aminoglycosides in combination with:
Amphotericin B
Cyclosporine
Diuretics
Vancomycin
C. Related to predisposing conditions in the patient:
Dehydration
Gram-negative bacteremia
Hypoalbuminemia
Increased age
Liver disease
Obstructive jaundice
Preexisting kidney disease
Poor nutrition
Potassium or magnesium deficiencies
Shock

tion with other antibiotics, has been intensively investigated as a practical cost-effective method to maintain antimicrobial efficacy while reducing nephro-, vestibular, and ototoxicity.[24,25] Nephrotoxicity may be reduced because proximal tubular aminoglycoside uptake appears to be limited during the transient, high-peak serum concentrations, and because low aminoglycoside concentrations for a greater proportion of the dosing interval facilitate excretion of the aminoglycoside. Although greater clinical efficacy and reduced nephrotoxicity may be realized with once-daily compared to standard dosing, seriously ill, immunocompromised, and elderly patients, as well as patients with preexisting kidney disease, are not ideal candidates for this approach because of altered aminoglycoside clearance in these patients.[25]

Management Serum creatinine concentrations should be measured frequently (every 2 to 4 days) during therapy. Aminoglycoside use should be discontinued or the dosage regimen revised if a S_{cr} increase of 0.5 mg/dL or more is noted that is not attributable to another cause. Other nephrotoxic drugs should be discontinued if possible, and the patient should be maintained adequately hydrated and hemodynamically stable. Short-term dialysis may be necessary, but ESRD has rarely been reported to be solely the result of aminoglycoside toxicity.

Radiographic Contrast Media Nephrotoxicity

Incidence Nephrotoxicity associated with radiographic contrast media administration is the third leading cause of hospital-acquired AKI.[26,27] The incidence rises from <2% in patients with a low risk of AKI to 40% to 50% in patients with a high risk, such as those with CKD or diabetes mellitus.[26,28,29] The risk of contrast-induced nephrotoxicity increases as the number of risk factors increases, and diabetic patients with CKD have the greatest risk.[28,30]

Clinical Presentation Contrast nephrotoxicity presents most commonly as nonoliguric, transient tubular enzymuria. However, irreversible oliguric (urine volume <500 mL/day) kidney injury requiring dialysis has been reported in high-risk patients. Kidney injury typically manifests within the first 12 to 24 hours after the administration of contrast. The serum creatinine concentration usually peaks between 2 and 5 days after exposure, with recovery after 4 to 10 days. Urinalysis typically reveals only hyaline and granular casts, but may also be completely bland.[30] The urine sodium concentration and fractional excretion of sodium are frequently low. Although toxicity has generally been considered to be mild and reversible, an in-hospital mortality rate of 35% has been reported in patients with severe contrast media-induced AKI requiring dialysis, compared to 7% in those with contrast nephrotoxicity not requiring dialysis.[28]

Pathogenesis Contrast nephrotoxicity appears to be caused by direct tubular toxicity and/or renal ischemia.[28,29] Direct tubular toxicity is suggested by the frequent presence of renal tubular enzymuria and biopsy findings of proximal tubular epithelial cell vacuolization and acute tubular necrosis. In contrast to these findings, the frequent finding of a low urine sodium concentration and low fractional excretion of sodium suggests that renal tubular function is preserved. Renal ischemia may result from systemic hypotension associated with contrast injection, as well as renal vasoconstriction mediated by an imbalance of humoral agents, including prostaglandins, adenosine, atrial natriuretic peptide, nitric oxide, and endothelin.[28,30] Renal ischemia may also result from dehydration as the result of osmotic diuresis associated with the use of hyperosmolar agents (900 to 1,780 mOsm/kg) and increased blood viscosity caused by red blood cell crenation and aggregation.[28]

Risk Factors Preexisting kidney disease, particularly in diabetic patients, is the major risk factor.[28,30] Conditions associated with decreased renal blood flow, including congestive heart failure and dehydration, also confer risk. The presence of multiple myeloma has been considered a relative contraindication for contrast use, but the risk appears to be associated with concomitant dehydration, kidney disease, or hypercalcemia rather than the diagnosis itself. Both larger doses of contrast and use of hyperosmolar contrast agents have been associated with an increased risk in susceptible patients.[28]

Prevention Because contrast nephrotoxicity can be anticipated in the majority of patients who are at risk, the use of preventative procedures is justified for most patients. Table 49–3 lists the recommended interventions for prevention of contrast nephrotoxicity. All patients scheduled to receive radiocontrast media should be assessed for risk factors, and the risk-to-benefit ratio should be considered.[27–32] High-risk patients can be identified by evaluating medical history and indication for the contrast study, along with their most recent serum creatinine concentrations. Nephrotoxicity is best prevented in high-risk patients by using alternative imaging procedures (e.g., ultrasound, magnetic resonance imaging, and nuclear medicine scans). However, if contrast media must be used, the smallest adequate dose should be administered. Dose reduction proportional to the level of kidney function may be protective, but may limit the adequacy of imaging.[33]

Low-osmolality nonionic (iohexol and iopamidol) and ionic (ioxaglate) contrast agents may be used to prevent nephrotoxicity. Standard contrast media are not reabsorbed in the kidney and cause osmotic diuresis, which contributes to the renal toxicity observed with these agents. The second generation of contrast agents have half the osmolality of standard agents and are associated with less toxicity, especially when used in patients with preexisting kidney disease.[30] The incidence of contrast nephrotoxicity in nondiabetic

TABLE 49-3 Recommended Interventions for Prevention of Contrast Nephrotoxicity

Intervention	Recommendation	Recommendation Grade[a]
Contrast	• Minimize contrast volume/dose	A-1
	• Use noniodinated contrast studies	A-2
	• Use low- or isoosmolar contrast agents	A-2
Medications	• Avoid concurrent use of potentially nephrotoxic drugs (e.g., nonsteroidal antiinflammatory drugs, aminoglycosides)	A-2
Normal (0.9%) saline	• Initiate infusion at least 3 hours prior to contrast exposure and continue 8–24 hours postexposure • Infuse at 1 mL/kg/hr up to 150 mL/h, adjusting postexposure as clinically indicated	A-1
Sodium bicarbonate 154 mEq/L	• Initiate infusion at 3 mL/kg/h, beginning 1 hour prior to contrast exposure, then continue at 1 mL/kg/h for 6 hours postexposure	B-2
N-acetylcysteine	• Administer 600 mg orally, every 12 hours × 4 doses beginning prior to contrast exposure (i.e., one dose prior to exposure and 3 doses postexposure)	B-1

[a]Strength of recommendations: A, B, C, good, moderate, and poor evidence to support recommendation, respectively. Quality of evidence: 1, Evidence from more than one properly randomized, controlled trial. 2, Evidence from more than one well-designed clinical trial with randomization, from cohort or case-controlled analytic studies or multiple time series; or dramatic results from uncontrolled experiments. 3, Evidence from opinions of respected authorities, based on clinical experience, descriptive studies, or reports of expert communities.

Derived from data in references 27, 28, 31, 32.

patients with underlying kidney disease is more than twofold higher in those receiving standard contrast agents than in those receiving low-osmolar agents.[26] However, use of low-osmolar agents does not preclude the development of nephrotoxicity and preventive measures should be considered.

CLINICAL CONTROVERSY

Some clinicians believe that low-osmolar contrast agents should be used in virtually all patients who are at risk for toxicity. Others believe that the cost-to-benefit ratio of using low-osmolar contrast agents to prevent nephrotoxicity is questionable except in patients at high risk, because low-osmolar agents are considerably (three to five times) more expensive than standard higher osmolar ionic agents.

Dehydration should be corrected before contrast administration, other nephrotoxic drugs discontinued if possible, and subsequent contrast studies appropriately timed to minimize cumulative toxicity.[27,28] Hydration with isotonic saline before and after contrast administration reduces the incidence of toxicity, particularly in high-risk patients, and is currently the most widely accepted preventative intervention.[28] In addition to the correction of dehydration, saline administration may result in dilution of contrast media, prevention of renal vasoconstriction leading to ischemia, and avoidance of tubular obstruction. The results of one recent study suggest that hydration with sodium bicarbonate provides more protection than saline, perhaps by reducing the formation of pH-dependent oxygen free radicals.[34] *N*-acetylcysteine is a thiol-containing antioxidant that may effectively reduce the risk of developing contrast nephrotoxicity in patients with preexisting kidney disease, although a therapeutic benefit has not been consistently demonstrated.[28,35] Nevertheless, its use should be considered, along with hydration, in all patients who are at risk of toxicity.[28,29,31,35–37] The recommended *N*-acetylcysteine dosing regimen for prevention of contrast nephrotoxicity is 600 mg orally every 12 hours × 4 doses, with the first dose administered prior to contrast exposure (see Table 49–3).

CLINICAL CONTROVERSY

Some clinicians believe that insufficient evidence exists to justify use of acetylcysteine for the prevention of contrast nephrotoxicity, whereas others feel that its safety profile, ease of use, low cost, and potential for benefit are adequate justification for use in all patients.

Continuous venovenous hemofiltration may also be an effective means of preventing contrast nephrotoxicity and was associated with improved outcomes in one study of patients with CKD.[38] However, because of the logistical issues (e.g., technical difficulty) and high cost of hemofiltration, this approach is not widely used.[28,36] Use of mannitol and furosemide to prevent toxicity remains controversial,[29] and recent evidence indicates that the dopamine$_1$-receptor agonist fenoldopam may not prevent contrast-induced nephropathy in CKD patients.[27,36] Consequently, these approaches are generally not recommended for the prevention of contrast nephrotoxicity.

Management Currently there is no specific therapy available for managing established contrast nephrotoxicity. Care is supportive as described in Chap. 45. Renal function (e.g., S_{cr}, urine output) and volume status should be closely monitored, and dialysis used as needed in patients with the most severe kidney injury.

Cisplatin and Carboplatin Nephrotoxicity

Incidence Platin-containing compounds are important chemotherapeutic agents that frequently cause renal tubular damage.[39–41] The incidence of cisplatin nephrotoxicity was 50% to 100% in the 1980s. Subsequently, the incidence of toxicity has decreased to 6% to 13%, primarily as the result of limiting the total drug dose and reducing the rate of administration. However, when used in combination with other nephrotoxins, high-dose cisplatin continues to contribute to DIN. A 20% to 40% decline in GFR is frequently observed in patients treated with cisplatin.[39] Carboplatin, a second-generation platinum analog, is associated with a much lower incidence of nephrotoxicity than cisplatin and thus is the preferred agent in high-risk patients.[40]

Clinical Presentation Peak serum creatinine concentrations occur approximately 10 to 12 days after initiation of therapy, with recovery by 21 days. However, kidney damage is dose related and cumulative with subsequent cycles of therapy, so the serum creatinine concentration may continue to rise. Irreversible kidney injury may result. Renal magnesium wasting is common and can be accompanied by hypocalcemia and hypokalemia. Hypomagnesemia may be severe, and associated with seizures, neuromuscular irritability, or personality changes, and persist long after chemotherapy has ended. Hypomagnesemia results primarily from increased urinary losses as a result of renal tubular damage as well as saline hydration and diuretic therapy to prevent toxicity. Anorexia and diarrhea also contribute, because of decreased intake and increased loss of magnesium, respectively.

Pathogenesis Proximal tubular damage appears acutely after administration of platin-containing compounds, as the result of impairment of cell energy production, possibly by binding to proximal tubular cellular proteins and sulfhydryl groups with disruption of cell enzyme activity and uncoupling of oxidative phosphorylation.[41] The initial proximal tubular damage is followed by a progressive loss of glomerular filtration and impaired distal tubular function.[39] Renal biopsies generally show sparing of glomeruli with necrosis of proximal and distal tubules and collecting ducts.

Risk Factors Risk factors include increased age, dehydration, renal irradiation, concurrent use of aminoglycoside antibiotics, and alcohol abuse.[39]

Prevention Toxicity is best prevented by prospective dose reduction and decreased frequency of administration, which usually requires using the platin compounds in combination with other chemotherapeutic agents, and avoiding concurrent use of other nephrotoxic drugs. Vigorous hydration with isotonic saline is important and should be used in all patients with a goal of maintaining at least 100 mL/h of urine output during and after cisplatin treatment. Hydration is initiated up to 24 hours prior to, and continued during and for 4 to 8 hours after, cisplatin administration; saline doses range from a total of 1 to 4 L administered at rates as high as 250 mL/h immediately prior to cisplatin treatment, to as high as 3 L/m^2 for high-dose carboplatin.[39] Hydration is continued during and after cisplatin administration at rates of 150 to 250 mL/h as tolerated. Although protective roles for furosemide or mannitol-induced diuresis are less clear,[28] their use is often necessary to maintain volume homeostasis, particularly when saline infusion rates of 250 mL/h are used. Furosemide 20 mg to 40 mg is commonly administered 30 minutes prior to cisplatin, or mannitol 12.5 g up to 50 g is administered with cisplatin to maintain ≥100 mL/h of urine output.

Amifostine, an organic thiophosphate that is converted to an active metabolite, chelates cisplatin in normal cells and reduces the nephrotoxicity, neurotoxicity, ototoxicity, and myelosuppression associated with cisplatin and carboplatin therapy.[42] The renoprotective effect of amifostine administration has been demonstrated in patients receiving cisplatin/ifosfamide-based chemotherapy.[43] Amifostine fully preserved GFR in patients with solid tumors after administration of two cycles of chemotherapy compared to a 30% reduction in GFR in controls. In addition, although hypomagnesemia and tubular damage were still observed in the amifostine group they were markedly less severe. Pretreatment with amifostine should be considered in patients who are at risk for kidney injury, particularly patients who are elderly, volume depleted, have CKD, or are receiving other nephrotoxic drugs concurrently.

Promising investigational techniques include the use of hypertonic saline (e.g., administration of each dose in 250 mL of 3% saline) to reduce tubular cisplatin uptake,[44] *N*-acetylcysteine to reduce oxidative damage by acting as a sulfhydryl donor, and disulfiram metabolite diethyldithiocarbamate to reduce cytochrome P450 2E1-mediated generation of hydroxyl radicals.[39,45] Recently, the protective effect of melatonin,[46] and the ability of cisplatin-incorporated polymeric micelles to maintain antitumor activity while reducing nephrotoxicity were demonstrated.[47] Finally, reduced renal exposure can be achieved with the use of localized intraperitoneal administration in conjunction with systemic administration of sodium thiosulfate for those with peritoneal tumors.

Management Acute kidney injury caused by cisplatin therapy is usually partially reversible with time and supportive care, including dialysis. Renal function indices should be closely followed, with S_{cr} and BUN concentrations checked daily. Serum magnesium, potassium, and calcium concentrations should be monitored daily and corrected as needed. Hypocalcemia and hypokalemia may be difficult to reverse until hypomagnesemia is corrected. Progressive kidney disease caused by cumulative nephrotoxicity may be irreversible and in some cases may require chronic dialysis support.

Amphotericin B Nephrotoxicity

Incidence Amphotericin B toxicity may be seen with cumulative doses as low as 300 to 400 mg, and reaches an incidence of 80% when cumulative doses approach 4 g.[48,49] Although numerous studies demonstrate lower rates of nephrotoxicity with liposomal formulations compared to conventional amphotericin B, it is difficult to compare rates of toxicity between products and studies because of the variability in the study populations, doses administered, and inconsistent definitions of nephrotoxicity and methods of assessment.[50]

Clinical Presentation Toxicity relates to cumulative dosage and usually manifests after administration of 2 to 3 g as renal tubular potassium, sodium, and magnesium wasting, impaired urine concentrating ability, and distal renal tubular acidosis as a consequence of a leak of hydrogen ions out of the tubular lumen.[49] Renal blood flow and GFR decreases are common, resulting in a rise in S_{cr} and BUN concentrations, and potassium and magnesium replacement may be necessary.[48] Consequently, renal function indices should be closely followed, with S_{cr} and BUN concentrations checked daily, and serum magnesium, potassium, and calcium concentrations monitored every other day and corrected as needed.

Pathogenesis The mechanisms of kidney injury include direct tubular epithelial cell toxicity with increased tubular permeability and necrosis, as well as arterial vasoconstriction and ischemic injury.[48] Overall, the combined effects of increased cell energy and oxygen requirements because of greater cell membrane permeability, and reduced cellular oxygen delivery because of renal vasoconstriction, result in renal medullary tubular epithelial cell necrosis and kidney injury.

Risk Factors Risk factors include CKD, higher average daily doses, volume depletion, and concomitant administration of diuretics and other nephrotoxins (cyclosporine in particular).[49,51] Rapid infusions of amphotericin B have the potential to increase toxicity. A recent comparison of 24-hour continuous infusions with conventional 4-hour infusions revealed a significant reduction of toxicity, attributed to decreased "pretubular" effects (e.g., effects on renal blood flow and GFR).[52]

Prevention Several liposomal amphotericin B formulations are now available and should be used in most high-risk patients as they have been reported to reduce nephrotoxicity by enhancing drug delivery to sites of infection, thereby reducing exposure of mammalian cell membranes.[49,51,53] Nephrotoxicity can also be minimized by limiting the cumulative dose and avoiding concomitant administration of other nephrotoxins, particularly cyclosporine.[54] Additionally, providing hydration with 1 L intravenous 0.9% sodium chloride daily during the course of therapy appears to reduce toxicity. Mannitol infusion to induce an osmotic diuresis, however, has not been shown to be protective.[51]

CLINICAL CONTROVERSY

Many clinicians recommend using liposomal formulations of amphotericin B in all patients with CKD and those at risk for developing nephrotoxicity, whereas others maintain that the safety and efficacy of liposomal formulations are not yet established enough to warrant their use in all patients.

Management Amphotericin nephrotoxicity is best treated by discontinuation of therapy and substitution of alternative antifungal therapy, if possible. Renal tubular dysfunction and glomerular filtration will improve gradually to some degree in most patients, but damage may be irreversible. Renal function indices should be closely followed, with S_{cr} and BUN concentrations checked daily, and serum magnesium, potassium, and calcium concentrations should be monitored daily and corrected as needed.

OSMOTIC NEPHROSIS

Several drugs, including mannitol, low-molecular-weight dextran, and radiographic contrast media, or drug vehicles, such as sucrose and propylene glycol, are associated with vacuolization, swelling, and, ultimately, necrosis of proximal tubular epithelial cells with a decline in renal function.[12] The decline in renal function may be a result of the hypertonic and osmotically active nature of these agents. Intravenous immunoglobulin solutions contain hyperosmolar sucrose and may cause osmotic nephrosis and acute kidney injury, which is usually reversible shortly after discontinuing therapy.[55] Toxicity may be prevented by diluting the solution and reducing the rate of infusion. Hydroxyethyl starch, used as a plasma volume expander, has also been implicated in the development of osmotic nephrosis.[12]

Mannitol may rarely cause oligoanuric kidney injury with proximal tubular cell vacuolization on biopsy.[1] It can also cause direct renal vasoconstriction or induce an osmotic diuresis with increased solute delivery to the macula densa and subsequent tubuloglomerular feedback, leading to vasoconstriction of the glomerular afferent arteriole and decreased renal blood flow. Risk factors for mannitol toxicity include excessive doses, preexisting kidney disease, and concomitant diuretic or cyclosporine therapy. Nephrotoxicity may be prevented by limiting the dose and avoiding dehydration and concomitant diuretic therapy. Patients usually recover normal renal function when elevated mannitol concentrations decrease following drug withdrawal or hemodialysis.

HEMODYNAMICALLY MEDIATED KIDNEY INJURY

❹ The kidneys constitute only 0.4% of body weight, but receive approximately 25% of resting cardiac output.[1] This enhances the kidney's exposure to circulating drugs. Within each nephron, blood flow and pressure are regulated by glomerular afferent and efferent arterioles to maintain intraglomerular capillary hydrostatic pressure, glomerular filtration, and urine output. Afferent and efferent arteriolar vasoconstriction are primarily mediated by angiotensin II, whereas afferent vasodilation is primarily mediated by prostaglandins (Fig. 49–1). This specialized blood flow is precisely regulated by interrelations between arachidonic acid metabolites, natriuretic factors, nitric oxide, the sympathetic nervous system, the renin–angiotensin system, and the macula densa response to distal tubular solute delivery. Hemodynamically mediated kidney injury results from a decrease in intraglomerular pressure. Mechanisms commonly include a decrease in renal blood flow, vasoconstriction of glomerular afferent arterioles, and vasodilation of glomerular efferent arterioles.

ANGIOTENSIN-CONVERTING ENZYME INHIBITORS AND ANGIOTENSIN II RECEPTOR BLOCKERS

Incidence

The incidence of ACEI- or angiotensin II receptor blocker (ARB)-mediated kidney injury has not been established. However, hospitalized patients with congestive heart failure, and those with CKD, including diabetic nephropathy, are most likely to experience a significant decline in renal function when therapy with one of these agents is initiated. Although ACEI-induced AKI has accounted for 9% of all cases of AKI requiring hospitalization,[56] reductions in GFR have been reported primarily in patients with severe atherosclerotic renal artery stenosis.[57] The rise is often minimal in renovascular disease if only one renal artery is stenotic, but is more apparent in patients with a single kidney, congestive heart failure, volume depletion, or bilateral renal small vessel disease. Up to one-third of patients with bilateral renal artery stenosis demonstrate a rise in serum creatinine >30% after starting ACEI therapy.[56]

Clinical Presentation

Therapy with ACEIs and ARBs will acutely reduce GFR, so a moderate rise in serum creatinine of 0.1 to 0.3 mg/dL should be anticipated.[58] Importantly, a distinction must be made between a potentially detrimental reduction in GFR and a normal, predictable rise in serum creatinine. A rise in S_{cr} of 0.5 mg/dL or more in the course of 1 to 2 weeks may necessitate discontinuance of the offending drug. Dose-related elevations in serum creatinine should be anticipated in most patients prescribed ACEIs, based on their pathophysiologic effects.[59] An increase in serum creatinine of up to 30% within 2 to 5 days of initiating therapy is an indication that the drug has begun to exert its desired pharmacologic effect. The increase in creatinine usually stabilizes within 2 to 3 weeks and is usually reversible upon stopping the drug. Furthermore, an association exists between acute increases in serum creatinine of ≤30% from baseline that stabilize within the first 2 months of initiating therapy and preservation of renal function.

Pathogenesis

The kidney normally attempts to maintain GFR by dilating the afferent arteriole and constricting the efferent arteriole in response to a decrease in renal blood flow. During states of reduced blood flow, the juxtaglomerular apparatus increases renin secretion. Plasma renin converts angiotensinogen to angiotensin I, and ultimately angiotensin II by angiotensin-converting enzyme. Angiotensin II constricts the afferent and efferent arterioles resulting in a net increase in intraglomerular pressure. Additionally, renal prostaglandins, prostaglandin E_2 in particular, are released and induce a net dilation of the afferent arteriole, thereby improving blood flow into the glomerulus. Together these processes maintain GFR and urine output (Fig. 49–2).

ACEI- or ARB-mediated kidney injury is the result of a decrease in glomerular capillary hydrostatic pressure sufficient to reduce glomerular ultrafiltration.[12] When ACEI therapy (e.g., enalapril or ramipril) is initiated, the synthesis of angiotensin II is decreased, thereby preferentially dilating the efferent arteriole. This reduces outflow resistance from the glomerulus and decreases hydrostatic pressure in the glomerular capillaries, which alters Starling forces across the glomerular capillaries to decrease intraglomerular pres-

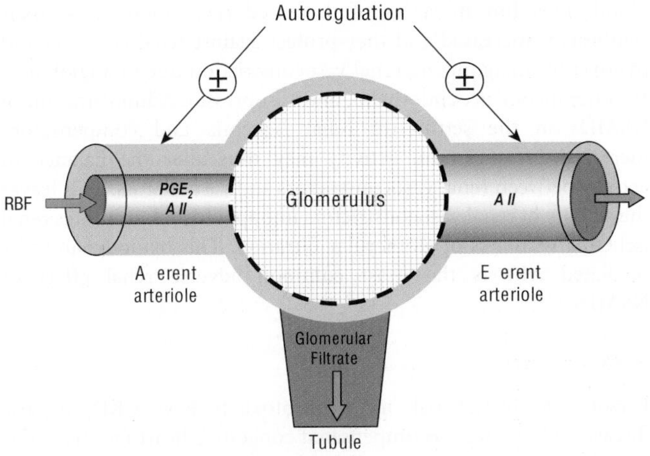

FIGURE 49-1. Normal glomerular autoregulation serves to maintain intraglomerular capillary hydrostatic pressure, glomerular filtration rate (GFR), and, ultimately, urine output. (A II, angiotensin II; PGE_2, prostaglandin E_2; RBF, renal blood flow.)

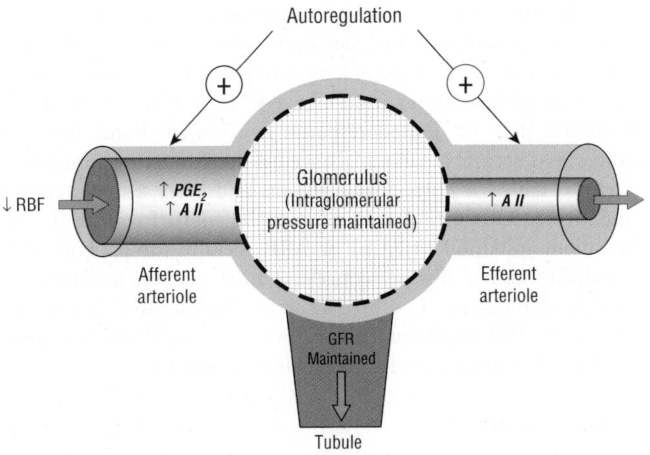

FIGURE 49-2. Glomerular autoregulation during "prerenal" states (i.e., reduced blood flow). (A II, angiotensin II; GFR, glomerular filtration rate; PGE_2, prostaglandin E_2; RBF, renal blood flow.)

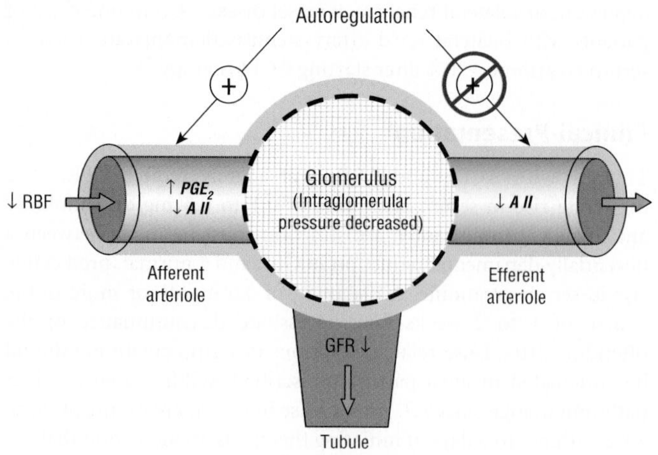

FIGURE 49-3. Pathogenesis of angiotensin-converting enzyme inhibitor (ACEI) nephropathy. (A II, angiotensin II; GFR, glomerular filtration rate; PGE_2, prostaglandin E_2; RBF, renal blood flow.)

sure, GFR, and then often leads to nephrotoxicity, particularly in the setting of reduced renal blood flow or effective arterial blood volume (Fig. 49–3), that is, "prerenal" settings in which glomerular afferent arteriolar blood flow is reduced and the efferent arteriole is vasoconstricted to maintain sufficient glomerular capillary hydrostatic pressure for ultrafiltration.

Risk Factors

Patients at greatest risk are those dependent on angiotensin II to maintain blood pressure and renal efferent arteriolar constriction. These include patients with hemodynamically significant renal artery stenosis, particularly bilateral stenosis, and those with decreased effective arterial blood volume (i.e., prerenal states), especially those with congestive heart failure, volume depletion from excess diuresis or gastrointestinal fluid loss, hepatic cirrhosis with ascites, and the nephrotic syndrome.[12,58]

Prevention

Hemodynamically mediated AKI caused by ACEIs or ARBs is frequently preventable by recognizing the presence of preexisting kidney disease or decreased effective renal blood flow as a result of volume depletion, heart failure, or liver disease.[58] A common strategy for at-risk patients is to initiate therapy with very low doses of a short-acting ACEI (e.g., captopril 6.25 mg to 12.5 mg), then gradually titrate the dose upward and convert to a longer-acting agent after patient tolerance has been demonstrated. Outpatients may be started on low doses of long-acting ACEIs (e.g., enalapril 2.5 mg) with gradual dose titration every 2 to 4 weeks until the maximum dose or desired response is achieved. Renal function indices and serum potassium concentrations must be monitored carefully, daily for hospitalized patients and every 2 to 3 days for outpatients. Monitoring may need to be more frequent during outpatient initiation of ACEI or ARB therapy for patients with preexisting kidney disease, congestive heart failure, or suspected renovascular disease. Use of concurrent hypotensive agents and other drugs that affect renal hemodynamics (e.g., NSAIDs, diuretics) should be discouraged and dehydration avoided.

Management

Acute decreases in renal function and the development of hyperkalemia usually resolve over several days after ACEI or ARB therapy is discontinued. Occasionally patients will require management of severe hyperkalemia, usually with sodium polystyrene sulfonate suspension (see Chap. 54). ACEI or ARB therapy may frequently be reinitiated, particularly for patients with congestive heart failure, after intravascular volume depletion has been corrected or diuretic doses reduced. Slight reductions in renal function (maintenance of a serum creatinine concentration of 2 to 3 mg/dL) may be an acceptable trade-off for hemodynamic improvement in certain patients with severe congestive heart failure or renovascular disease not amenable to revascularization.[57]

NONSTEROIDAL ANTIINFLAMMATORY DRUGS AND SELECTIVE CYCLOOXYGENASE-2 INHIBITORS

Incidence

NSAIDs have an overall favorable safety profile resulting in nonprescription availability in the United States of ibuprofen, naproxen, and ketoprofen for short-term therapy. Although potential adverse renal effects from nonprescription NSAIDs have been a concern, conventional nonselective NSAIDs and selective COX-2 inhibitors are unlikely to impair renal function in the absence of renal ischemia or excess renal vasoconstrictor activity. Nevertheless, given the fact that 50 million U.S. citizens report NSAID use, it has been estimated that 500,000 to 2.5 million people will develop NSAID nephrotoxicity in the United States annually.[60]

Clinical Presentation

Kidney injury can occur within days of initiating therapy, particularly with a short-acting NSAID such as ibuprofen.[60] Patients typically present with complaints of diminished urine output, weight gain, and/or edema. Urine volume and sodium concentration are usually low, and BUN, S_{cr}, and potassium are typically elevated. The urine sediment is usually unchanged from baseline, but may show granular casts. Hemodynamically mediated kidney injury associated with COX-2 inhibitors presents similarly.[12]

Pathogenesis

NSAIDs inhibit COX-catalyzed prostaglandin production and impair renal function by decreasing synthesis of vasodilatory prostaglandins from arachidonic acid.[60] Renal prostaglandins are synthesized in the renal cortex and medulla by vascular endothelial and glomerular mesangial cells. Their effects are primarily local and result in renal vasodilation (particularly prostacyclin and prostaglandin E_2). They have limited activity in states of normal renal blood flow, but in states of decreased renal blood flow their synthesis is increased and they protect against renal ischemia and hypoxia by antagonizing renal vasoconstriction due to angiotensin II, norepinephrine, endothelin, and vasopressin. Administration of NSAIDs in the setting of renal ischemia and compensatory increased prostaglandin activity may thus alter the balance of activity between renal vasoconstrictors and vasodilators. This leaves the activity of renal vasoconstrictors unopposed and promotes renal ischemia with loss of glomerular filtration. This hemodynamically mediated AKI is the most common adverse renal effect of NSAIDs.[1,12]

Risk Factors

Persons at greatest risk for nephrotoxicity have CKD, hepatic disease with ascites, decompensated congestive heart failure, intravascular volume depletion, or systemic lupus erythematosus.[12] Additional risk factors include atherosclerotic cardiovascular disease and concurrent diuretic therapy. The elderly are also at higher risk because of interaction of prevalent medical problems, multiple-drug therapies, and reduced renal hemodynamics. NSAID use in patients older than 65 years of age may increase the risk of AKI by up to 58%.[61] Combined NSAID or COX-2 inhibitor and ACEI or ARB therapy is also a concern and should be avoided in high-risk patients.

Prevention

NSAID- and COX-2 inhibitor-induced AKI can be prevented by recognizing high-risk patients and using analgesics with less prostaglandin inhibition, such as acetaminophen, nonacetylated salicylates, aspirin, and possibly nabumetone. Nonnarcotic analgesics (e.g., tramadol) may also be useful, but do not provide antiinflammatory activity.[60] When NSAID therapy is essential for high-risk patients, the minimal effective dose should be used for the shortest duration possible, along with optimal management of predisposing medical problems and frequent renal function monitoring. Moreover, use of concurrent hypotensive agents and other drugs which affect renal hemodynamics (e.g., ACEIs, ARBs, diuretics) should be discouraged in high-risk patients and dehydration avoided.

Traditional, nonselective NSAIDs inhibit COX-1 and COX-2, whereas the selective drugs meloxicam, celecoxib, and valdecoxib preferentially inhibit COX-2. COX-2 inhibitors were anticipated to be beneficial in high-risk patients. However, recent data indicate that they affect renal function similarly to nonselective NSAIDs and thus caution is warranted with their use, particularly in high-risk patients.[12,62]

Management

NSAID-induced AKI is treated by discontinuation of therapy and supportive care. Kidney injury is rarely severe and recovery is usually rapid. Occasionally, the hemodynamic insult is sufficiently severe to cause frank tubular necrosis, which can prolong injury.[12] The differential diagnosis of NSAID hemodynamically mediated AKI must also include NSAID-induced acute interstitial nephritis, with or without the nephrotic syndrome, because steroid therapy may benefit this type of renal injury.

CYCLOSPORINE AND TACROLIMUS

The calcineurin inhibitors cyclosporine and tacrolimus have dramatically enhanced the success of solid-organ transplantation. Nephrotoxicity, however, remains a major dose-limiting adverse effect of both drugs.[63] Although delayed chronic interstitial nephritis has been reported, acute hemodynamically mediated kidney injury is the primary mechanism of nephrotoxicity.[8,12]

Incidence

Historically, reversible AKI occurred frequently in transplant recipients during the first 6 months of cyclosporine therapy. Recent data indicate that the 5-year risk of CKD after transplantation of a nonrenal organ ranges from 7% to 21%, depending on the type of organ transplanted.[63] In addition, the occurrence of CKD in these patients is associated with more than a fourfold increase in the risk of death.

Clinical Presentation

The clinical presentation of acute hemodynamically mediated kidney injury secondary to cyclosporine and tacrolimus is quite different than the presentation of chronic nephrotoxicity (see Chronic Interstitial Nephritis below for a discussion of the presentation). AKI may occur within days of initiating therapy. S_{cr} concentration rises and creatinine clearance decreases. Hypertension, hyperkalemia, sodium retention, and hypomagnesemia may occur. No urine sediment abnormalities are seen. Renal biopsy usually reveals thickening of arterioles, mild focal glomerular sclerosis, proximal tubular epithelial cell vacuolization and atrophy, and interstitial fibrosis. Biopsy is useful to distinguish acute cyclosporine nephrotoxicity from renal allograft rejection, the latter being evidenced by cellular infiltration.[64]

Pathogenesis

A dose-related hemodynamic mechanism is likely during the initial months of therapy because renal function improves rapidly following dose reduction. Reversible vasoconstriction and injury to glomerular afferent arterioles occurs, possibly as a result of increased activity of thromboxane A_2, endothelin, and the sympathetic nervous system, or diminished activity of nitric oxide or prostacyclin.[65,66] Vasoconstriction caused by increased renin–angiotensin system activity may also contribute. In contrast, renal arteriolar hyalinization and chronic renal ischemia, as well as increased extracellular matrix synthesis, appear to be the primary mechanisms that contribute to cyclosporine-induced CKD.[65,66]

Risk Factors

Risk factors include age over 65 and higher initial cyclosporine dose, as well as renal graft rejection, hypotension, infection, and concomitant therapy with nephrotoxic drugs such as aminoglycosides, amphotericin B, acyclovir, NSAIDs, and radiocontrast agents, as well as drugs that inhibit cyclosporine hepatic metabolism.[64] The incidence of AKI with potential progression to chronic nephropathy has decreased since the introduction of lower-dose-therapy regimens. Unfortunately, there has been no apparent reduction in the incidence of the slow, dose-dependent decline in glomerular filtration.[66]

Prevention

Because acute hemodynamically mediated kidney injury secondary to cyclosporine and tacrolimus appears to be concentration related, pharmacokinetic and pharmacodynamic monitoring is an important means of preventing toxicity. However, the persistent presence of therapeutic or low cyclosporine concentrations does not totally preclude the development of nephrotoxicity. Calcium channel blockers may antagonize the vasoconstrictor effect of cyclosporine by dilating glomerular afferent arterioles and preventing acute decreases in renal blood flow and glomerular filtration.[64] Lastly, decreased doses of cyclosporine or tacrolimus, primarily when used in combination with other nonnephrotoxic immunosuppressants, may minimize the risk of toxicity, but this may increase the risk of chronic rejection.

Management

AKI usually improves with dose reduction, and treatment of contributing illness or the discontinuation of interacting drugs. CKD is usually irreversible, but progressive toxicity may be limited by discontinuation of cyclosporine (or tacrolimus) therapy or dose reduction, with the continuation of other immunosuppressants. S_{cr} and BUN should be closely monitored (daily if possible), as should cyclosporine or tacrolimus concentrations, to ensure that serum concentrations are within the narrow therapeutic range.

OBSTRUCTIVE NEPHROPATHY

Obstructive nephropathy is the result of mechanical obstruction to urine flow following glomerular filtration, and is most commonly caused by intratubular obstruction or postrenal obstruction secondary to nephrolithiasis or prostatic hypertrophy.[12,67]

INTRATUBULAR OBSTRUCTION

Drug-induced acute renal tubular obstruction can be caused by intratubular precipitation of tissue-degradation products or drugs and/or their metabolites. Acute uric acid nephropathy following tumor-tissue degradation as the result of chemotherapy (i.e., tumor lysis syndrome) is the most common cause of this type of kidney injury. Acute oliguric or anuric kidney injury develops rapidly. The diagnosis is supported by a urine uric acid-to-creatinine ratio greater than 1. Uric acid precipitation can be prevented by pretreatment hydration with normal saline to maintain urine output of >2.5 L/day, administration of allopurinol 300 to 600 mg daily started 2 to 3 days prior to chemotherapy, and urinary alkalinization to pH 7.0.

Drug-induced rhabdomyolysis can lead to intratubular precipitation of myoglobin, and if severe, AKI. The most common cause of drug-induced rhabdomyolysis is direct myotoxicity from β-hydroxy-β-methylglutaryl-coenzyme A reductase inhibitors, including lovastatin and simvastatin.[68] The risk of rhabdomyolysis is increased when this class of drugs is administered concurrently with gemfibrozil, niacin, or inhibitors of the CYP3A4 metabolic pathway (e.g., erythromycin and itraconazole). Rhabdomyolysis may also result from pressure necrosis as the result of stupor or coma following ingestion of CNS depressants (e.g., alcohol and narcotics), or extreme neuromuscular agitation associated with abuse of central nervous system stimulants (e.g., amphetamines, cocaine, ecstasy, and phencyclidine).[68]

Intratubular precipitation of drugs or their metabolites can also cause AKI.[12,69] Urine pH decreases to approximately 4.5 during maximal stimulation of renal tubular hydrogen ion secretion. Certain solutes can precipitate and obstruct the tubular lumen at this acid pH, particularly when urine is concentrated, such as in patients with volume depletion. For example, acyclovir is relatively insoluble at physiologic urine pH and is associated with intratubular precipitation in dehydrated oliguric patients.[12,16,67] Sulfadiazine when used at high doses, and methotrexate may also precipitate in acidic urine and can cause oligo-anuric kidney injury. Massive administration of ascorbic acid can also result in obstruction of renal tubules with calcium oxalate crystals. Oxalate, a poorly soluble ascorbic acid metabolite, can also precipitate and worsen renal function when ascorbic acid is administered to patients with AKI or the congenital nephrotic syndrome. Low-molecular-weight dextran therapy for volume expansion and rheologic effects has also caused kidney injury, possibly by intratubular precipitation of filtered dextran. Triamterene may also precipitate in renal tubules and cause kidney injury.[69] Foscarnet complexation with ionized calcium may result in precipitation of calcium-foscarnet salt crystals in renal glomeruli, causing primarily a crystalline glomerulonephritis. The salt crystals may then secondarily precipitate in the renal tubules causing tubular necrosis.[70] The protease inhibitor indinavir has been associated with crystalluria, crystal nephropathy, dysuria, urinary frequency, back and flank pain, or nephrolithiasis in approximately 8% of treated patients.[12] Intratubular indinavir crystal precipitation is prevented in nearly 75% of treated patients via consumption of 2 to 3 L of fluid per day.[12]

Kidney injury caused by intratubular precipitation of most tissue-degradation products or drugs and their metabolites can be largely prevented and possibly treated by administering the drug after vigorously prehydrating the patient, maintaining a high urine volume, and urinary alkalinization.[8]

NEPHROLITHIASIS

Nephrolithiasis (formation of renal calculi or kidney stones) does not present as classic nephrotoxicity as GFR is usually not decreased. Drug-induced nephrolithiasis can be the result of abnormal crystal precipitation in the renal collecting system, potentially causing pain, hematuria, infection, or, occasionally, urinary tract obstruction with kidney injury. The overall prevalence of drug-induced nephrolithiasis is estimated to be 1%.[67]

Renal stone formation, possibly also accompanied by intratubular precipitation of crystalline material, has been a rare complication of drug therapy. Until the acquired immune deficiency syndrome (AIDS) era, triamterene had been the drug most frequently associated with renal stone formation, with a prevalence of 0.4%.[67] However, it has been unclear whether triamterene or its metabolites actually initiated stone formation, or are passively absorbed onto the organic matrix of preexisting calculi. Sulfadiazine is a poorly soluble sulfonamide that has caused symptomatic acetylsulfadiazine crystalluria with stone formation and flank or back pain, hematuria, or kidney injury in up to 29% of patients treated with the drug.[58] A high urine volume and urinary alkalinization to pH >7.15 may be protective. AKI caused by intratubular precipitation of indinavir and collecting system obstruction from nephrolithiasis have occurred.[67] Because indinavir is more water soluble at acidic pH, urine acidification could be protective but is impractical. Maintaining a high urine volume may be most protective.[67] Numerous other drugs have been implicated in the development of nephrolithiasis, including the antiviral drugs nelfinavir and foscarnet, the antibacterial agents ciprofloxacin, amoxicillin, and nitrofurantoin, and various products containing ephedrine, norephedrine, and pseudoephedrine.[67]

GLOMERULAR DISEASE

Proteinuria with or without a decline in the GFR is a hallmark sign of glomerular injury (see Chap. 50). Several different glomerular lesions may occur, mostly by immune mechanisms rather than direct cellular toxicity. Although drug-induced glomerular disease is uncommon, a variety of agents have been implicated.[71]

Minimal change glomerular injury with nephrotic range proteinuria (i.e., >3.5 g/day) caused by drugs is frequently accompanied by interstitial nephritis and is most common during NSAID therapy.[60,71] Ampicillin, rifampin, phenytoin, and lithium have also been implicated. The pathogenesis is unknown, but nephrotic-range proteinuria as a consequence of NSAID therapy is frequently associated with a T-lymphocytic interstitial infiltrate, suggesting disordered cell-mediated immunity. Proteinuria usually resolves rapidly after discontinuation of the offending drug, and a 3- to 4-week course of corticosteroids may help resolve the lesion.[72]

Focal segmental glomerulosclerosis (FSGS) is characterized by patchy areas of glomerular sclerosis with interstitial inflammation and fibrosis (see Chap. 50). FSGS has been described in the setting of chronic heroin abuse (heroin nephropathy).[73,74] The pathogenesis is unknown but may include direct toxicity by heroin or adulterants and injury from bacterial or viral infections accompanying intravenous drug use. FSGS is also the predominant renal lesion in AIDS patients and may result from human immunodeficiency virus (HIV) infection or heroin abuse. Glomerulosclerosis caused by HIV infection may be distinguished from heroin nephropathy by tubuloreticular structures in endothelial cells on electron microscopy and the more rapid course and poorer prognosis. The bisphosphonate pamidronate, commonly used to treat malignancy-associated hypercalcemia, has also been associated with the development of collapsing FSGS. Patients receiving either high doses or prolonged therapy are at highest risk.[75,76]

Membranous nephropathy is characterized by immune complex formation along glomerular capillary loops, and although rarely seen, has classically been associated with gold therapy, penicillamine, and NSAID use.[12,71] The pathogenesis may involve damage to proximal tubule epithelium with antigen release, antibody formation, and glomerular immune complex deposition.

TUBULOINTERSTITIAL DISEASE

Tubulointerstitial diseases involve the renal tubules and the surrounding interstitial tissue.[18] The presentation may be acute and reversible with interstitial inflammatory cell infiltrates, rapid loss of renal function, and systemic symptoms. A chronic and irreversible presentation associated with interstitial fibrosis, and minimal to no systemic symptoms have also been observed.

ACUTE ALLERGIC INTERSTITIAL NEPHRITIS

Incidence

❺ AIN is the underlying cause for up to 3% of all cases of AKI.[72] Multiple drugs have been implicated (Table 49–4). AIN usually manifests 2 weeks after exposure to a drug but may occur sooner if the patient was previously sensitized.[11]

TABLE 49-4 Drugs Associated with Allergic Interstitial Nephritis

Antimicrobials	
Acyclovir	Indinavir
Aminoglycosides	Rifampin
Amphotericin B	Sulfonamides
β-Lactams	Tetracyclines
Erythromycin	Trimethoprim-sulfamethoxazole
Ethambutol	Vancomycin
Diuretics	
Acetazolamide	Loop diuretics
Amiloride	Triamterene
Chlorthalidone	Thiazide diuretics
Neuropsychiatric	
Carbamazepine	Phenytoin
Lithium	Valproic acid
Phenobarbital	
Nonsteroidal antiinflammatory drugs	
Aspirin	Ketoprofen
Cyclooxygenase-2 inhibitors	Naproxen
Diclofenac	Phenylbutazone
Diflunisal	Piroxicam
Ibuprofen	Zomepirac
Indomethacin	
Miscellaneous	
Acetaminophen	Lansoprazole
Allopurinol	Methyldopa
Aspirin	Omeprazole
Azathioprine	*P*-aminosalicylic acid
Captopril	Phenylpropanolamine
Cimetidine	Propylthiouracil
Clofibrate	Radiographic contrast media
Cyclosporine	Ranitidine
Glyburide	Sulfinpyrazone
Gold	Warfarin
Interferon-alfa	

β-Lactams

Clinical Presentation Although methicillin-induced allergic interstitial nephritis is the prototype for AIN, it is now recognized that AIN is associated with all β-lactam antobiotics.[72] Clinical signs present approximately 14 days after initiation of therapy and include (with their approximate incidence) fever (80%), maculopapular rash (25%), eosinophilia (80%), pyuria and hematuria (90%), low-level proteinuria (90%), and oliguria (20%). Systemic hypersensitivity findings of fever, rash, eosinophilia, and eosinophiluria suggest the diagnosis, but this constellation of findings is not consistently reliable as one or more are frequently absent. Eosinophiluria, an important marker of drug-induced AIN, is frequently absent, possibly because of fragility of eosinophils in urine and inadequate laboratory methodology. Anemia, leukocytosis, and elevated immunoglobulin E levels may occur. Tubular dysfunction may be manifested by acidosis, hyperkalemia, salt wasting, and concentrating defects.[11,18,72]

NSAIDs

Clinical Presentation NSAID-induced AIN has a different clinical presentation than that seen with most other drugs.[12,72] Patients are typically older than age 50 years (reflecting NSAID use for degenerative joint disease), the onset is delayed a mean of 6 months from initiation of therapy compared to 2 weeks with β-lactams, and there is a much lower incidence of fever, rash, and eosinophilia. These extrarenal symptoms are observed in only 10% of patients.[12,72] Concomitant nephrotic syndrome (proteinuria >3.5 g/day) occurs in more than 70% of patients. Fenoprofen-allergic interstitial nephritis is considered the prototype for NSAID-induced AIN because it accounts for nearly 50% of cases.[72] Prompt diagnosis of allergic interstitial nephritis is important as discontinuation of the offending drug may prevent irreversible renal damage.[18] Renal biopsy is the most specific method for diagnosis but is usually not possible in acutely ill patients.

Pathogenesis AIN is characterized as a diffuse or focal interstitial infiltrate of lymphocytes, plasma cells, eosinophils, and occasional polymorphonuclear neutrophils.[18,72] Granulomas and tubular epithelial cell necrosis are relatively common with drug-induced AIN. The pathogenesis is an allergic hypersensitivity response. Occasionally a humoral antibody-mediated mechanism is implicated by the presence of circulating antibody to a drug hapten–tubular basement membrane complex, low serum complement levels, and deposition of immunoglobulin G and complement in the tubular basement membrane. More commonly, a cell-mediated immune mechanism is suggested by the absence of these findings and the presence of a predominantly T-lymphocyte infiltrate with an increased helper-to-suppressor cell ratio. In particular, NSAID interstitial nephritis involves T lymphocytes, possibly in response to altered prostaglandin synthesis.[11,18]

Risk Factors No specific risk factors have been identified because these are idiosyncratic hypersensitivity reactions. Individuals with other drug allergies may have increased risk and warrant close monitoring.

Prevention No specific preventive measures are known because of the idiosyncratic nature of these reactions. Patients must be monitored carefully to recognize the signs and symptoms, because promptly discontinuing the offending drug often leads to full recovery.[18]

Management Prednisone therapy has been beneficial, particularly in patients whose renal function does not improve within 1 week after stopping the offending drug, but no prospective treatment trials have been reported to date.[18,72] Various dosage regimens have been used, but an initial dose of 1 mg/kg/day for a week, which is then tapered over 3 weeks to discontinuation, has been recommended.[72,77] Typical renal function indices (e.g., S_{cr}, BUN) and signs and symptoms of AIN should be monitored closely for improvement.

CHRONIC INTERSTITIAL NEPHRITIS

Lithium, cyclosporine, aristolochic acid, and only a few other drugs have been reported to cause chronic interstitial nephritis, which is usually a progressive and irreversible lesion.[1,18]

Lithium

Incidence Several renal tubular lesions are associated with lithium therapy; an impaired ability to concentrate urine (nephrogenic diabetes insipidus) has been seen in up to 87% of patients.[78] Acute tubular necrosis and chronic tubulointerstitial nephritis are less-frequently noted, and incomplete distal renal tubular acidosis is observed in up to 50% of patients.[79] Historically, the most important question regarding lithium use was whether long-term therapy, with lithium concentrations maintained in the therapeutic range, caused chronic tubulointerstitial nephritis. It is now established that long-term lithium therapy is associated with nephrotoxicity in the absence of episodes of acute intoxication, and that the duration of therapy and the cumulative dose are the major determinants of toxicity.[80]

Clinical Presentation Polydipsia (excessive thirst) and polyuria (excessive urination) are observed in 40% and 20%, respectively, of patients with nephrogenic diabetes insipidus (see Chap. 52).[79] They adapt well to their urinary-concentrating defect and these concerns are usually minimal. Acute tubular necrosis is sometimes observed in the setting of acute lithium toxicity. Urinalysis may show moderate proteinuria, a few red and white blood cells, and granular casts. Renal function usually returns to baseline values after lithium concentrations are reduced to the therapeutic range. Nephrotoxicity may develop insidiously and only be recognized by rising BUN or creatinine concentrations or the onset of hypertension.

Pathogenesis Impaired ability to concentrate urine is a result of a dose-related decrease in collecting duct response to antidiuretic hormone. This results from impaired formation of cellular cyclic adenosine monophosphate in response to antidiuretic hormone. Lithium-induced AKI occurs predominantly during episodes of acute lithium intoxication. The pathogenesis includes dehydration secondary to nephrogenic diabetes insipidus, as well as direct proximal and distal tubular cell toxicity. Chronic tubulointerstitial nephritis attributed to lithium is evidenced most commonly by biopsy findings of interstitial fibrosis, tubular atrophy, and glomerular sclerosis.[18,80] The pathogenesis may involve cumulative direct lithium toxicity as duration of therapy correlates with the decline in the GFR. Finally, some patients may have increased susceptibility to lithium toxicity. Although the reason for this is unknown, this could explain the difficulty in characterizing the nephrotoxic effects of chronic lithium therapy.

Risk Factors The major risk factor for AKI is an elevated lithium concentration, particularly in association with dehydration. Concomitant therapy with neuroleptic agents may contribute. Chronic nephrotoxicity may result from cumulative damage caused by repeated episodes of acute renal injury.

Prevention Prevention of acute and chronic toxicity includes maintaining lithium concentrations as low as therapeutically possible, avoiding dehydration, and monitoring renal function. It is unknown whether progression to chronic kidney disease can be prevented by stopping lithium use when mild kidney injury is first recognized. This poses a dilemma as lithium is highly effective for affective disorders and the risks and potential benefits of discontinuing such a beneficial drug need to be carefully considered.[80] However, if lithium therapy is continued, renal function must be monitored and therapy discontinued if it continues to decline.

Management Symptomatic polyuria and polydipsia can be reversed by discontinuation of lithium therapy or ameliorated with amiloride 10 mg daily during continued lithium therapy (see Chap. 52).[79] If polyuria does not resolve within 7 to 10 days of therapy, then the amiloride dose should be increased to 20 mg daily.[81] AKI is usually reversible with supportive care, including dialysis to reduce toxic blood lithium concentrations. Progressive chronic interstitial nephritis is treated by discontinuation of lithium therapy, adequate hydration, and avoidance of other nephrotoxic agents. Lithium serum concentrations, as well as renal function indices, including urine output, BUN, and S_{cr} should be monitored closely for resolution of signs and symptoms of toxicity.

Cyclosporine

Delayed chronic interstitial nephritis has been reported after 6 to 12 months of therapy and can result in irreversible kidney disease. Toxicity usually manifests as a slowly rising S_{cr} concentration and decreased creatinine clearance that may not reflect the severity of histopathologic changes. Typical biopsy findings include arteriolar hyalinosis, glomerular sclerosis, and a striped pattern of tubulointerstitial fibrosis.[64–66,79] The pathogenesis appears to involve sustained renal arteriolar endothelial cell injury which ultimately results in chronic renal ischemia because of increased release of endothelin-1, decreased production of nitric acid, and increased expression of transforming growth factor-β.[82] Nephrotoxicity has been dose dependent in some, but not all analyses, and occurs even during low-dose therapy.[65]

Aristolochic Acid (Chinese Herb Nephropathy)

Incidence In the early 1990s, a cluster of young women with rapidly progressive kidney disease leading to ESRD were reported in Brussels, Belgium.[83] The patients had strikingly similar pathologic findings of interstitial fibrosis with tubular atrophy on renal biopsy. Further investigation revealed that all the women were patients of the same weight-loss clinic and had received a weight-loss treatment containing Chinese herbs. Subsequent analysis of the herb-based treatment demonstrated significant amounts of *Aristolochia fangchi* (Guang fang ji), known to contain aristolochic acid, the major alkaloid of the botanical species *Aristolochia*.[83] The term *Chinese herb nephropathy* was established and associated with aristolochic acid exposure after confirmatory renal biopsies were obtained from additional Belgian kidney disease patients with prior exposure to the same Chinese herb-based treatment. Approximately 3% to 5% of patients who received the weight-loss regimen developed disease, and numerous additional cases of nephropathy and ESRD associated with the use of *Aristolochia* species have been reported from around the globe.[83]

Clinical Presentation Patients with Chinese herb nephropathy typically present with mild to moderate hypertension, mild proteinuria, glucosuria, and moderately elevated S_{cr} concentrations.[83] Anemia and shrunken kidneys are also common on initial presentation. The overwhelming majority of cases reported to date have been in women. The main pathologic lesions observed in the kidneys are interstitial fibrosis with atrophy and destruction of tubules throughout the renal cortex; in general, the glomeruli are not affected. Perhaps the most remarkable feature of Chinese herb nephropathy is the rate at which it progresses. In most individuals, ESRD requiring dialysis or transplantation develops within 6 to 24 months of exposure. An alarming high prevalence (approximately 40%) of urothelial transitional cell carcinoma has been observed in Belgian patients who underwent renal transplantation.[83,84]

Pathogenesis Although the precise mechanism of aristolochic acid-induced nephropathy and urothelial carcinoma is yet to be characterized, recent data indicate direct DNA damage may be the cause. The major components of aristolochic acid are metabolized to mutagenic compounds called aristolactam I and aristolactam II, respectively, which have been demonstrated to form DNA adducts in humans.[83]

Prevention The primary means of preventing Chinese herb nephropathy appears to be the limitation of exposure to compounds containing aristolochic acids. Several countries, including the United Kingdom, Canada, Australia, and Germany, have banned the use of *Aristolochia*-containing herbs.[82]

NEPHROCALCINOSIS

Nephrocalcinosis is a clinical–pathologic condition characterized by extensive tubulointerstitial precipitation and deposition of calcium phosphate leading to marked tubular calcification.[85,86] Typical risk factors for developing nephrocalcinosis include clinical conditions associated with hypercalcemia, including hyperparathyroidism, increased bone turnover, hypercalcemia of malignancy, and increased intake of calcium or vitamin D. Recently, however, several documented cases of nephrocalcinosis in patients without hypercalcemia have pointed to oral sodium phosphate solution (OSPS) used for bowel cleansing as the causative agent.[85,86] The term acute phosphate nephropathy was coined specifically to describe OSPS-induced nephrocalcinosis, as its pathogenesis is the result of increased phosphate intake rather than hypercalcemia.[85] The incidence of acute phosphate nephropathy is unknown but rare. Patients usually present with AKI several days to months after exposure to OSPS. Patients in one cohort of 21 cases of acute phosphate nephropathy presented with AKI and a mean serum creatinine of 3.9 mg/dL at a median of 1 month after colonoscopy.[85] Low-grade proteinuria (<1.0 g/day), normocalcemia, and a bland urinary sediment are usually observed. Extensive deposition of calcium phosphate in the distal tubules and collecting ducts without glomerular or vascular injury is the hallmark of OSPS-induced nephrocalcinosis.[85,86] Risk factors include bowel conditions associated with prolonged intestinal transit, and high sodium phosphate dosage, along with concomitant volume depletion and diuretic, NSAID, ACEI, or ARB therapy. Advanced age may also be a risk factor as most reported cases are in the elderly. OSPS should be avoided in patients with CKD.

PAPILLARY NECROSIS

Papillary necrosis is a form of chronic tubulointerstitial nephritis characterized by necrosis of the renal papillae, the regions of the kidney where the collecting ducts enter the renal pelvis.[18] Analgesic use is the most common cause of papillary necrosis, accounting for a third of all cases.[87]

Analgesic Nephropathy

Incidence "Classic" analgesic nephropathy is characterized by chronic tubulointerstitial nephritis with papillary necrosis.[18] Chronic excessive consumption of combination analgesics, particularly those containing phenacetin, was believed to be the major cause and led to the removal of phenacetin and phenacetin mixtures from most world markets. However, contemporary analgesics, particularly aspirin, acetaminophen, and NSAIDs, alone or in combination, are also associated with the development of analgesic nephropathy. A recent review suggests that currently there is insufficient evidence to definitively associate these non–phenacetin-containing analgesics with nephropathy.[88] Analgesic nephropathy is reported as the primary cause of ESRD by as many as 9% of dialysis patients.[89]

Clinical Presentation Analgesic nephropathy evolves insidiously over years. It is difficult to recognize and may be underdiagnosed as a cause of ESRD. The most sensitive and specific diagnostic criteria include (a) a history of chronic daily habitual analgesic ingestion (classically this equated to daily use for at least 5 years); (b) intravenous pyelography, renal ultrasound, or renal computed tomography imaging, which reveals decreased renal mass and bumpy renal contours; and (c) papillary calcifications.[89] Frequently, however, imaging only demonstrates chronic pyelonephritis and small kidneys with thin renal cortices and blunted calyces. Hypertension and atherosclerotic cardiovascular disease are common. Early renal manifestations include impaired maximal urinary concentration, sterile pyuria, microscopic hematuria, and low levels of proteinuria. Urinary tract infection is common. Renal biopsy reveals nonspecific chronic interstitial inflammation and scarring.[18]

Pathogenesis Mechanisms of analgesic nephropathy remain unclear. The renal lesion begins in the papillary tip as a result of accumulated toxic metabolites, decreased blood flow, and impaired cellular energy production. The metabolism of phenacetin to acetaminophen, which is then oxidized to toxic free radicals that are concentrated in the papilla, appears to be the initiating factor that causes toxicity by mechanisms analogous to acetaminophen hepatotoxicity. Toxicity is prevented by availability of reduced glutathione. However, salicylates deplete renal glutathione and thereby facilitate phenacetin and acetaminophen toxicity.[18,79]

Risk Factors The epidemiology of analgesic use and analgesic nephropathy continues to evolve.[88,90] The classic concept persists that risk for ESRD increases with cumulative consumption of combination analgesics, phenacetin, or acetaminophen and aspirin or NSAIDs. Caffeine contained in combination analgesics may increase risk, but the role is not clear.[89] Chronic use of therapeutic doses of NSAIDs alone, but not aspirin or salicylates alone, can cause analgesic nephropathy. Case-control studies associate high-dose acetaminophen use alone with an increased risk for ESRD. However, these associations remain inconclusive as a consequence of study design flaws, as acetaminophen has been the preferentially prescribed analgesic for patients with chronic kidney disease.[88]

Prevention Prevention has depended primarily on public health efforts to restrict the sale of phenacetin and combination analgesics. This has effectively reduced analgesic nephropathy in Australia and Europe. However, risk continues with continued availability of nonprescription combination analgesics containing aspirin, acetaminophen, and caffeine in the United States and throughout the world.

Individuals requiring chronic analgesic therapy may reduce risk by limiting the total dose, avoiding combined use of two or more analgesics, and maintaining good hydration to prevent renal ischemia and decrease the papillary concentration of toxic substances. Acetaminophen remains the preferred nonopiate analgesic for patients with preexisting kidney disease.

Management Treatment of established nephrotoxicity requires cessation of analgesic consumption. This can prevent progression and may improve renal function. Renal function indices, including urine output, BUN, and S_{cr}, should be monitored every several months. Patients should also be monitored for the development of transitional cell carcinoma of the renal pelvis, calyces, ureters, and bladder, which may present years after analgesic nephropathy is diagnosed.

RENAL VASCULITIS, THROMBOSIS, AND CHOLESTEROL EMBOLI

Numerous drugs are associated with the development of vasculitis.[91,92] For example, propylthiouracil is associated with cutaneous, renal, and pulmonary vasculitis; allopurinol is associated with cutaneous, renal, and hepatic vasculitis; hydralazine is associated with cutaneous, renal, and pulmonary vasculitis; and isotretinoin is associated with cutaneous, renal, pulmonary, and gastrointestinal vasculitis.[91,92] Systemic polyarteritis nodosa, a vasculitis with involvement of small- and medium-size renal arteries, has been described following minocycline use.[92] Patients may present with hematuria, proteinuria, reduced renal function, and hypertension. Hydralazine, propylthiouracil, allopurinol, and penicillamine have been implicated in the development of antineutrophil cytoplasmic antibody-positive vasculitis.[93] Patients exposed to these drugs who subsequently develop antineutrophil cytoplasmic antibody-positive vasculitis appear to exhibit high titers of antimyeloperoxidase antibodies. Treatment of vasculitis typically consists of withdrawing the offending drug and a tapering course of prednisone, and usually leads to resolution of symptoms within weeks to months.[91]

Numerous medications, including mitomycin C, oral contraceptive agents, cyclosporine, tacrolimus, muromonab-CD3, antineoplastic agents, interferon, ticlopidine, clopidogrel, and quinine can cause a thrombotic microangiopathy (hemolytic uremic syndrome or thrombotic thrombocytopenic purpura) manifested by endothelial proliferation and thrombus formation in the renal and central nervous system vasculature.[94,95] The association with mitomycin C is notable because the pathogenesis appears to be a direct, dose-related toxic effect, rarely occurring in patients who receive doses <30 mg/m^2. Nephrotoxicity has occurred following chemotherapy with mitomycin C alone or with 5-fluorouracil, cisplatin, bleomycin, a vinca alkaloid, and tamoxifen. Microangiopathic hemolytic anemia and thrombocytopenia are usually present. Systemic endothelial damage with multisystem organ failure has occurred. Kidney injury can be severe and irreversible, although corticosteroids, antiplatelet agents, vincristine, plasma exchange, plasmapheresis, and high-dose intravenous immunoglobulin G have each induced clinical improvement. Gemcitabine is a pyrimidine analog used for the treatment of various solid tumors which was recently associated with the development of hemolytic uremic syndrome, with an estimated incidence of 0.015%.[12,39]

Anticoagulants and thrombolytics, particularly warfarin, can systemically embolize cholesterol particles from aortic atherosclerotic plaques to small arteries and arterioles, including renal arterioles. These agents remove or prevent thrombus formation over ulcerative plaques, causing emboli.[1] Cholesterol emboli induce an inflammatory obliterative vascular response, causing renal ischemia. Purple discoloration of the toes and mottled skin over the legs are important clinical clues.

COSTS OF DRUG-INDUCED KIDNEY DISEASE

The pharmacoeconomics of drug-induced kidney disease are not well defined. An analysis of aminoglycoside therapy in the acute care environment for 1984 to 1985 revealed 7.3% of patients experienced nephrotoxicity. The mean additional cost for each episode of toxicity (in 1984 dollars) was $2,501,[96] and more than $4,500 per case in the late 1990s.[20] Individualized pharmacokinetic monitoring efforts were recently reported to decrease costs associated with aminoglycoside nephrotoxicity by more than $900 per patient.[19] Outpatient care costs of NSAID toxicity have also been evaluated. Costs for hospital care for NSAID-induced acute hemodynamically-mediated kidney injury and interstitial nephritis combined have been estimated at $990 million per year.[97] The risk of ESRD stemming from immunosuppressant-induced nephrotoxicity contributes substantially to the cost of heart transplantation.[64] The estimated cost per transplantation patient was $6,700 within 5 years, increasing to $14,200 within 8 years after transplantation. Finally, patients who develop ESRD require dialysis, which typically costs more than $50,000 per year.

ABBREVIATIONS

ACEI: angiotensin-converting enzyme inhibitor

AIDS: acquired immune deficiency syndrome

AIN: allergic interstitial nephritis

AKI: acute kidney injury

ARB: angiotensin II receptor blocker

ARF: acute renal failure

BUN: blood urea nitrogen

CKD: chronic kidney disease

COX: cyclooxygenase

CYP: cytochrome P450

DIN: drug-induced nephrotoxicity

ESRD: end-stage renal disease

FSGS: focal segmental glomerulosclerosis

GFR: glomerular filtration rate

HIV: human immunodeficiency virus

KIM-1: kidney injury molecule-1

NGAL: neutrophil gelatinase-associated lipocalin

NSAID: nonsteroidal antiinflammatory drug

S_{cr}: serum creatinine

REFERENCES

1. Choudhury D, Ahmed Z. Drug-associated renal dysfunction and injury. Nat Clin Pract Nephrol 2006;2:80–91.
2. Kellum JA, Levin N, Bouman C, Lameire N. Developing a consensus classification system for acute renal failure. Curr Opin Crit Care 2002;8:509–514.
3. Mehta RL, Chertow GM. Acute renal failure definitions and classification: Time for change? J Am Soc Nephrol 2003;14:2178–2187.
4. Warnock DG. Towards a definition and classification of acute kidney injury. J Am Soc Nephrol 2005;16:3149–3150.
5. Hoste EA, Clermont G, Kersten A, et al. RIFLE criteria for acute kidney injury are associated with hospital mortality in critically ill patients: A cohort analysis. Crit Care 2006;10:R73.
6. Hoste EA, Kellum JA. Acute kidney injury: Epidemiology and diagnostic criteria. Curr Opin Crit Care 2006;12:531–537.
7. Elasy TA, Anderson RJ. Changing demography of acute renal failure. Semin Dial 1996;9:438–443.
8. Schetz M, Dasta J, Goldstein S, Golper T. Drug-induced acute kidney injury. Curr Opin Crit Care 2005;11:555–565.
9. Thadhani R, Pascual M, Bonventre JV. Acute renal failure. N Engl J Med 1996;334:1448–1460.
10. Nash K, Hafeez A, Hou S. Hospital-acquired renal insufficiency. Am J Kidney Dis 2002;39:930–936.
11. Markowitz GS, Perazella MA. Drug-induced renal failure: A focus on tubulointerstitial disease. Clin Chim Acta 2005;351:31–47.
12. Perazella MA. Drug-induced nephropathy: An update. Expert Opin Drug Saf 2005;4:689–706.
13. Chertow GM, Lee J, Kuperman GJ, et al. Guided medication dosing for inpatients with renal insufficiency. JAMA 2001;286:2839–2844.
14. D'Amico G, Bazzi C. Urinary protein and enzyme excretion as markers of tubular damage. Curr Opin Nephrol Hypertens 2003;12:639–643.
15. Han WK, Bonventre JV. Biologic markers for the early detection of acute kidney injury. Curr Opin Crit Care 2004;10:476–482.
16. Izzedine H, Launay-Vacher V, Deray G. Antiviral drug-induced nephrotoxicity. Am J Kidney Dis 2005;45:804–817.
17. Mulato AS, Ho ES, Cihlar T. Nonsteroidal anti-inflammatory drugs efficiently reduce the transport and cytotoxicity of adefovir mediated by the human renal organic anion transporter 1. J Pharmacol Exp Ther 2000;295:10–15.
18. Silva FG. Chemical-induced nephropathy: A review of the renal tubulointerstitial lesions in humans. Toxicol Pathol 2004;32 Suppl 2:71–84.
19. Streetman DS, Nafziger AN, Destache CJ, Bertino AS Jr. Individualized pharmacokinetic monitoring results in less aminoglycoside-associated

nephrotoxicity and fewer associated costs. Pharmacotherapy 2001;21:443–451.

20. Slaughter RL, Cappelletty DM. Economic impact of aminoglycoside toxicity and its prevention through therapeutic drug monitoring. Pharmacoeconomics 1998;14:385–394.
21. Mingeot-Leclercq MP, Tulkens PM. Aminoglycosides: Nephrotoxicity. Antimicrob Agents Chemother 1999;43:1003–1012.
22. Nagai J, Takano M. Molecular aspects of renal handling of aminoglycosides and strategies for preventing the nephrotoxicity. Drug Metab Pharmacokinet 2004;19:159–170.
23. Sandoval RM, Reilly JP, Running W, et al. A non-nephrotoxic gentamicin congener that retains antimicrobial efficacy. J Am Soc Nephrol 2006;17:2697–2705.
24. Maglio D, Nightingale CH, Nicolau DP. Extended interval aminoglycoside dosing: From concept to clinic. Int J Antimicrob Agents 2002;19:341–348.
25. Olsen KM, Rudis MI, Rebuck JA, et al. Effect of once-daily dosing vs. multiple daily dosing of tobramycin on enzyme markers of nephrotoxicity. Crit Care Med 2004;32:1678–1682.
26. Waybill MM, Waybill PN. Contrast media-induced nephrotoxicity: Identification of patients at risk and algorithms for prevention. J Vasc Interv Radiol 2001;12:3–9.
27. Barrett BJ, Parfrey PS. Clinical practice. Preventing nephropathy induced by contrast medium. N Engl J Med 2006;354:379–386.
28. Rudnick MR, Kesselheim A, Goldfarb S. Contrast-induced nephropathy: How it develops, how to prevent it. Cleve Clin J Med 2006;73:75–77.
29. Maeder M, Klein M, Fehr T, Rickli H. Contrast nephropathy: Review focusing on prevention. J Am Coll Cardiol 2004;44:1763–1771.
30. Murphy SW, Barrett BJ, Parfrey PS. Contrast nephropathy. J Am Soc Nephrol 2000;11:177–182.
31. Bagshaw SM, McAlister FA, Manns BJ, Ghali WA. Acetylcysteine in the prevention of contrast-induced nephropathy: A case study of the pitfalls in the evolution of evidence. Arch Intern Med 2006;166:161–166.
32. Schweiger MJ, Chambers CE, Davidson CJ, et al. Prevention of contrast induced nephropathy: Recommendations for the high risk patient undergoing cardiovascular procedures. Catheter Cardiovasc Interv 2006;69:135–140.
33. Gerlach AT, Pickworth KK. Contrast medium-induced nephrotoxicity: Pathophysiology and prevention. Pharmacotherapy 2000;20:540–548.
34. Merten GJ, Burgess WP, Gray LV, et al. Prevention of contrast-induced nephropathy with sodium bicarbonate: A randomized controlled trial. JAMA 2004;291:2328–2334.
35. Marenzi G, Assanelli E, Marana I, et al. *N*-acetylcysteine and contrast-induced nephropathy in primary angioplasty. N Engl J Med 2006;354:2773–2782.
36. Asif A, Epstein M. Prevention of radiocontrast-induced nephropathy. Am J Kidney Dis 2004;44:12–24.
37. Briguori C, Airoldi F, D'Andrea D, et al. Renal Insufficiency Following Contrast Media Administration Trial (REMEDIAL): A randomized comparison of 3 preventive strategies. Circulation 2007;115:1211–1217.
38. Marenzi G, Marana I, Lauri G, et al. The prevention of radiocontrast-agent-induced nephropathy by hemofiltration. N Engl J Med 2003;349:1333–1340.
39. Kintzel PE. Anticancer drug-induced kidney disorders. Drug Saf 2001;24:19–38.
40. Hartmann JT, Lipp HP. Toxicity of platinum compounds. Expert Opin Pharmacother 2003;4:889–901.
41. Taguchi T, Nazneen A, Abid MR, Razzaque MS. Cisplatin-associated nephrotoxicity and pathological events. Contrib Nephrol 2005;148:107–121.
42. Koukourakis MI. Amifostine in clinical oncology: Current use and future applications. Anticancer Drugs 2002;13:181–209.
43. Hartmann JT, Knop S, Fels LM, et al. The use of reduced doses of amifostine to ameliorate nephrotoxicity of cisplatin/ifosfamide-based chemotherapy in patients with solid tumors. Anticancer Drugs 2000; 11:1–6.
44. de Jongh FE, van Veen RN, Veltman SJ, et al. Weekly high-dose cisplatin is a feasible treatment option: Analysis on prognostic factors for toxicity in 400 patients. Br J Cancer 2003;88:1199–1206.
45. Al Ghamdi SS, Chatterjee PK, Raftery MJ, et al. Role of cytochrome P4502E1 activation in proximal tubular cell injury induced by hydrogen peroxide. Ren Fail 2004;26:103–110.
46. Sener G, Satiroglu H, Kabasakal L, et al. The protective effect of melatonin on cisplatin nephrotoxicity. Fundam Clin Pharmacol 2000;14:553–560.
47. Mizumura Y, Matsumura Y, Hamaguchi T, et al. Cisplatin-incorporated polymeric micelles eliminate nephrotoxicity, while maintaining antitumor activity. Jpn J Cancer Res 2001;92:328–336.
48. Fanos V, Cataldi L. Amphotericin B-induced nephrotoxicity: A review. J Chemother 2000;12:463–470.
49. Costa S, Nucci M. Can we decrease amphotericin nephrotoxicity? Curr Opin Crit Care 2001;7:379–383.
50. Wingard JR, White MH, Anaissie E, et al. A randomized, double-blind comparative trial evaluating the safety of liposomal amphotericin B versus amphotericin B lipid complex in the empirical treatment of febrile neutropenia. L Amph/ABLC Collaborative Study Group. Clin Infect Dis 2000;31:1155–1163.
51. Deray G. Amphotericin B nephrotoxicity. J Antimicrob Chemother 2002;49 Suppl 1:37–41.
52. Eriksson U, Seifert B, Schaffner A. Comparison of effects of amphotericin B deoxycholate infused over 4 or 24 hours: Randomised controlled trial. BMJ 2001;322:579–582.
53. Carrigan HC, Hanf-Kristufek L. Comparison of nephrotoxicity of amphotericin B products. Clin Infect Dis 2001;32:990–991.
54. Bates DW, Su L, Yu DT, et al. Correlates of acute renal failure in patients receiving parenteral amphotericin B. Kidney Int 2001;60:1452–1459.
55. Orbach H, Tishler M, Shoenfeld Y. Intravenous immunoglobulin and the kidney—A two-edged sword. Semin Arthritis Rheum 2004;34:593–601.
56. Wynckel A, Ebikili B, Melin JP, et al. Long-term follow-up of acute renal failure caused by angiotensin converting enzyme inhibitors. Am J Hypertens 1998;11:1080–1086.
57. Epstein BJ. Elevations in serum creatinine concentration: Concerning or reassuring? Pharmacotherapy 2004;24:697–702.
58. Perazella MA. Drug-induced renal failure: Update on new medications and unique mechanisms of nephrotoxicity. Am J Med Sci 2003;325:349–362.
59. Bakris GL, Weir MR. Angiotensin-converting enzyme inhibitor-associated elevations in serum creatinine: Is this a cause for concern? Arch Intern Med 2000;160:685–693.
60. Whelton A. Nephrotoxicity of nonsteroidal anti-inflammatory drugs: Physiologic foundations and clinical implications. Am J Med 1999;106:13S–24S.
61. Griffin MR, Yared A, Ray WA. Nonsteroidal antiinflammatory drugs and acute renal failure in elderly persons. Am J Epidemiol 2000;151:488–496.
62. Szeto CC, Chow KM. Nephrotoxicity related to new therapeutic compounds. Ren Fail 2005;27:329–333.
63. Ojo AO, Held PJ, Port FK, et al. Chronic renal failure after transplantation of a nonrenal organ. N Engl J Med 2003;349:931–940.
64. de Mattos AM, Olyaei AJ, Bennett WM. Nephrotoxicity of immunosuppressive drugs: Long-term consequences and challenges for the future. Am J Kidney Dis 2000;35:333–346.
65. Burdmann EA, Andoh TF, Yu L, Bennett WM. Cyclosporine nephrotoxicity. Semin Nephrol 2003;23:465–476.
66. Liptak P, Ivanyi B. Primer: Histopathology of calcineurin-inhibitor toxicity in renal allografts. Nat Clin Pract Nephrol 2006;2:398–404.
67. Daudon M, Jungers P. Drug-induced renal calculi: Epidemiology, prevention and management. Drugs 2004;64:245–275.
68. Vanholder R, Sever MS, Erek E, Lameire N. Rhabdomyolysis. J Am Soc Nephrol 2000;11:1553–1561.
69. Perazella MA. Crystal-induced acute renal failure. Am J Med 1999;106:459–465.
70. Maurice-Estepa L, Daudon M, Katlama C, et al. Identification of crystals in kidneys of AIDS patients treated with foscarnet. Am J Kidney Dis 1998;32:392–400.
71. Izzedine H, Launay-Vacher V, Bourry E, et al. Drug-induced glomerulopathies. Expert Opin Drug Saf 2006;5:95–106.
72. Rossert J. Drug-induced acute interstitial nephritis. Kidney Int 2001;60:804–817.

73. D'agati V. Pathologic classification of focal segmental glomerulosclerosis. Semin Nephrol 2003;23:117–134.
74. Jaffe JA, Kimmel PL. Chronic nephropathies of cocaine and heroin abuse: A critical review. Clin J Am Soc Nephrol 2006;1:655–667.
75. Markowitz GS, Appel GB, Fine PL, et al. Collapsing focal segmental glomerulosclerosis following treatment with high-dose pamidronate. J Am Soc Nephrol 2001;12:1164–1172.
76. Albaqumi M, Soos TJ, Barisoni L, Nelson PJ. Collapsing glomerulopathy. J Am Soc Nephrol 2006;17:2854–2863.
77. Alexopoulos E. Drug-induced acute interstitial nephritis. Ren Fail 1998;20:809–819.
78. Markowitz GS, Radhakrishnan J, Kambham N, et al. Lithium nephrotoxicity: A progressive combined glomerular and tubulointerstitial nephropathy. J Am Soc Nephrol 2000;11:1439–1448.
79. Braden GL, O'Shea MH, Mulhern JG. Tubulointerstitial diseases. Am J Kidney Dis 2005;46:560–572.
80. Presne C, Fakhouri F, Noel LH, et al. Lithium-induced nephropathy: Rate of progression and prognostic factors. Kidney Int 2003;64:585–592.
81. Finch CK, Kelley KW, Williams RB. Treatment of lithium-induced diabetes insipidus with amiloride. Pharmacotherapy 2003;23:546–550.
82. Olyaei AJ, de Mattos AM, Bennett WM. Nephrotoxicity of immunosuppressive drugs: New insight and preventive strategies. Curr Opin Crit Care 2001;7:384–389.
83. Cosyns JP. Aristolochic acid and "Chinese herbs nephropathy": A review of the evidence to date. Drug Saf 2003;26:33–48.
84. Nortier JL, Martinez MC, Schmeiser HH, et al. Urothelial carcinoma associated with the use of a Chinese herb (*Aristolochia fangchi*). N Engl J Med 2000;342:1686–1692.
85. Markowitz GS, Stokes MB, Radhakrishnan J, D'Agati VD. Acute phosphate nephropathy following oral sodium phosphate bowel purgative: An underrecognized cause of chronic renal failure. J Am Soc Nephrol 2005;16:3389–3396.
86. Gonlusen G, Akgun H, Ertan A, et al. Renal failure and nephrocalcinosis associated with oral sodium phosphate bowel cleansing: Clinical patterns and renal biopsy findings. Arch Pathol Lab Med 2006;130:101–106.
87. Brix AE. Renal papillary necrosis. Toxicol Pathol 2002;30:672–674.
88. Feinstein AR, Heinemann LA, Curhan GC, et al. Relationship between nonphenacetin combined analgesics and nephropathy: A review. Ad Hoc Committee of the International Study Group on Analgesics and Nephropathy. Kidney Int 2000;58:2259–2264.
89. De Broe ME, Elseviers MM. Analgesic nephropathy. N Engl J Med 1998;338:446–452.
90. Michielsen P, de Schepper P. Trends of analgesic nephropathy in two high-endemic regions with different legislation. J Am Soc Nephrol 2001;12:550–556.
91. ten Holder SM, Joy MS, Falk RJ. Cutaneous and systemic manifestations of drug-induced vasculitis. Ann Pharmacother 2002;36:130–147.
92. Cuellar ML. Drug-induced vasculitis. Curr Rheumatol Rep 2002;4:55–59.
93. Choi HK, Merkel PA, Walker AM, Niles JL. Drug-associated antineutrophil cytoplasmic antibody-positive vasculitis: Prevalence among patients with high titers of antimyeloperoxidase antibodies. Arthritis Rheum 2000;43:405–413.
94. Pisoni R, Ruggenenti P, Remuzzi G. Drug-induced thrombotic microangiopathy: Incidence, prevention and management. Drug Saf 2001;24:491–501.
95. Dlott JS, Danielson CF, Blue-Hnidy DE, McCarthy LJ. Drug-induced thrombotic thrombocytopenic purpura/hemolytic uremic syndrome: A concise review. Ther Apher Dial 2004;8:102–111.
96. Eisenberg JM, Koffer H, Glick HA, et al. What is the cost of nephrotoxicity associated with aminoglycosides? Ann Intern Med 1987;107:900–909.
97. McGoldrick MD, Bailie GR. Nonnarcotic analgesics: Prevalence and estimated economic impact of toxicities. Ann Pharmacother 1997;31:221–227.

CHAPTER 50

Glomerulonephritis

ALAN H. LAU

KEY CONCEPTS

1. Glomerulonephritis is a collection of glomerular diseases mediated by different immunologic pathogenic mechanisms, resulting in varied clinical presentation and therapeutic outcomes.
2. The signs and symptoms associated with glomerulonephritis can be nephritic in nature, characterized by inflammatory injury, or nephrotic in nature, characterized by proteinuria.
3. In the absence of specific and effective therapy for many types of glomerulonephritis, supportive treatments for edema, hypertension, hyperlipidemia, and intravascular thrombosis play important roles in reducing the complications associated with the disease.
4. To maximize therapeutic benefits and minimize drug-induced complications, patients have to be monitored closely to assess their therapeutic responses as well as the development of any treatment-induced toxicities.
5. Among all the types of glomerulonephritis, minimal-change nephropathy is most responsive to treatment. Steroids can induce good responses in most patients during initial treatment as well as relapse.
6. Because of the lack of consistently effective treatment for primary focal segmental glomerular sclerosis, angiotensin-converting enzyme inhibitors or angiotensin receptor blockers are commonly used for patients with mild disease to control symptoms. Steroids and immunosuppressive agents are reserved for patients with severe disease.
7. The optimal treatment for lupus nephritis depends on the underlying lesion and disease activity, as well as the severity and duration of the clinical presentation.
8. The treatment of poststreptococcal glomerulonephritis is mainly supportive and symptomatic. Antibiotic therapy does not prevent subsequent diseases but may reduce the severity.

Despite the recent advances in cell and molecular biology, the precise pathogenetic mechanisms of many glomerular diseases remain unknown and the available therapeutic regimens are still far from optimal. This chapter provides an overview of the primary causes of glomerulonephritis with a focus on their etiology, the pathophysiologic mechanisms responsible for glomerular injury, and the clinical presentation of the eight predominant types of glomerulonephritis. Treatment options and monitoring approaches for each of these common forms of glomerulonephritis are also discussed. Although diabetes mellitus and amyloidosis are important secondary causes of glomerular diseases, a thorough discussion of the pathophysiology and management of these entities is beyond the scope of this chapter.

Learning objectives, review questions, and other resources can be found at **www.pharmacotherapyonline.com.**

NORMAL GLOMERULAR ANATOMY AND FUNCTION

The glomerulus, which is enclosed within the Bowman capsule, consists of two important components: the filtration barrier and the mesangium (Fig. 50–1). The capillary wall, which serves as a filtration barrier, consists of three well-defined layers: fenestrated endothelium, glomerular basement membrane (GBM), and epithelial cells. The epithelial cells, also known as podocytes, have specialized foot processes embedded in the outer layer of the GBM. It is across this barrier that fluid flows and ultimately forms ultrafiltrate. Under normal conditions, the GBM appears to function as a compact hydrated gel of matrix proteins with a pore-like structure. The mesangium provides support for the glomerular capillaries and also modulates blood flow through the capillaries. It consists of mesangial cells embedded in an extracellular matrix.

The unique capillary bed of the glomerulus allows small nonprotein plasma constituents up to the size of inulin, which has a molecular weight of 5,200 daltons, to pass freely while excluding macromolecules equal to or larger than albumin, which has a molecular weight of 69,000 daltons. Both the size and charge of the molecules affect the ease of passage through the glomerular membrane. Fixed, negatively charged sites are found within the glomeruli in all three layers of the capillary wall: the endothelium, the epithelium, and the GBM. The movement of negatively charged molecules is thus restricted more than that of neutral or positively charged molecules. Different glomerular diseases affect this size- and charge-selective barrier to different extents; consequently, glomerulopathies present with varied clinical features and solute-excretion patterns.

Some of the glomerular cells, such as the epithelial cells, have phagocytic function that can remove macromolecules trapped within the filtration barrier. They are also capable of synthesizing the GBM. In contrast, the mesangial cells regulate glomerular hemodynamics by responding to angiotensin II and producing prostaglandins. They also synthesize and respond to various cytokines and thus play a key role in immune-mediated glomerular diseases. There are also resident phagocytes in the mesangium, removing macromolecules trapped in the basement membrane into the urinary space. These phagocytes are involved in the development of both immune and nonimmune glomerular injury.

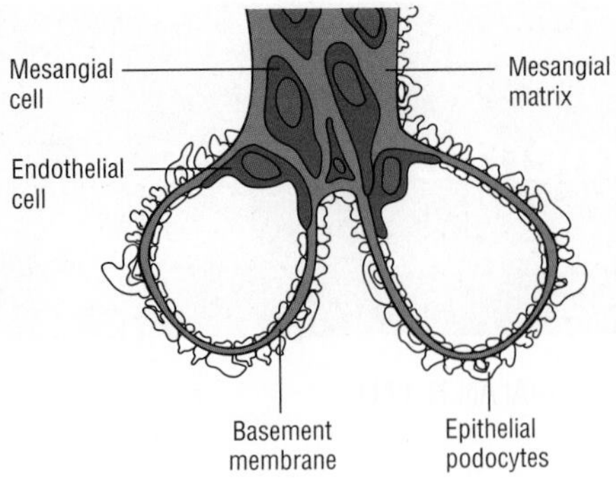

FIGURE 50-1. Microanatomy of the glomerulus.

EPIDEMIOLOGY AND ETIOLOGY

In the United States in 2004, glomerulonephritis was the third most common cause of end-stage renal disease (ESRD), accounting for approximately 16% of all the living ESRD patients. About 8,500 patients (8.1% of all patients) develop ESRD because of glomerulonephritis each year.[1]

Humoral and cellular immunologic mechanisms participate in the pathogenesis of most glomerulonephritis. Abnormalities in coagulation and metabolism, as well as hereditary and vascular diseases, also contribute to glomerular damage. The histopathologic manifestations vary substantially among the different types of glomerulonephritis. An overview of the primary pathogenetic mechanisms is presented in this section, and specific abnormalities for each of the primary types of glomerulonephritis are presented in subsequent sections.

PATHOPHYSIOLOGY

❶ The glomerular lesion may be diffuse (involving all glomeruli), focal (involving some but not all glomeruli), or segmental, also known as local (involving part of the individual glomerulus). The pathologic manifestations may also be described as proliferative (overgrowth of epithelium, endothelium, or mesangium), membranous (thickening of GBM), and/or sclerotic.

The glomerular capillary wall is particularly susceptible to immune-mediated injury. Antigen and antibody tend to localize in the glomerulus, probably because of its high blood flow and capillary hydrostatic pressure. Parenchymal damage can be induced as a result of humoral- and cell-mediated immune reactions (Table 50–1). Antibodies and sensitized T lymphocytes are the primary mediators of glomerular injury.[2,3]

Production of antibodies to endogenous or exogenous antigens that are recognized as foreign by the host is the first step in humoral immunologic damage to the glomerulus. Endogenous antigens may be intrinsic glomerular antigens, such as Heymann antigen on the epithelial cell or Goodpasture's antigen on the GBM, or previously sequestered antigens, such as DNA or thyroglobulin. Exogenous antigens are most often viral, bacterial, parasitic, or fungal in origin. Antineutrophil cytoplasmic autoantibodies (ANCAs), autoantibodies that react to the cytoplasmic components of neutrophils and monocytes, are found in patients with idiopathic crescentic glomerulonephritis and also in the accompanying vasculitis.

TABLE 50-1 Immunologic Mechanisms of Glomerular Injury

Circulating immune complexes
In situ antigen–antibody interaction
Intrinsic glomerular antigen; e.g., glomerular basement membrane antigens
Exogenous planted antigens
Cell-mediated mechanism

Complexes of antigens and antibodies may be formed in the circulation and then passively entrapped in the glomerular capillary or mesangium. Alternately, experimental antibodies may combine with endogenous glomerular antigens or exogenous antigens entrapped in the glomerulus to form complexes locally, or in situ.[3] The type and extent of glomerular damage are dependent on the location of the immune complex formation and the rate at which it is removed. Impaired removal facilitates the growth of the complex and thus increases the likelihood of glomerular damage.

Subsequent to antigen–antibody formation, a series of biologic events is triggered that ultimately leads to glomerular injury. Noninflammatory lesions can result from the binding of noncomplement-fixing antibody to the glomerular epithelial cell (mechanism 1), or the activation of the complement system to form the C5b-9 membrane attack complex (mechanism 2).[3] Both mechanisms can damage the glomerular epithelial cell and result in capillary wall injury and proteinuria. Inflammatory lesions are induced by glomerular infiltration of circulating inflammatory cells such as neutrophils, monocytes/macrophages, and platelets (mechanism 3), or proliferation of resident glomerular mesangial cells (mechanism 4), resulting in GBM damage.[3] The migration of neutrophils and monocytes to the glomerular tufts is promoted by chemoattractants such as complement fragments (C3a and C5a), platelet-activating factor, interleukin-8, and monocyte chemotactic protein-1.[4] Various cytokines, chemokines, and growth factors are then released to participate in the inflammatory process.[2]

T cells sensitized to glomerular antigen, macrophages, and resident mesangial cells are important participants in cell-mediated injury. Sensitized T cells can cause glomerular hypercellularity in the absence of antibody deposition.[2–4] Cytotoxic T cells may bind with the target cells and destroy them. Alternatively, a delayed-type hypersensitivity reaction may be initiated by activated T cells through the release of lymphokines, to attract, activate, and transform monocytes into macrophages.[3] These humoral and cellular mediators, in conjunction with a host of toxic molecular entities including reactive oxygen species, proteinases, eicosanoids, and procoagulants, which are secreted by neutrophils, macrophages, platelets, and resident glomerular cells can alter the permeability, blood flow, and function of the glomeruli. Vascular constriction and occlusion follow and result in the eventual destruction of the glomeruli.

Acute forms of glomerular injury may frequently lead to chronic and persistent renal dysfunction, even though the original immune factors that induce glomerular injury have resolved. Progression to ESRD may be inevitable. Experimental and clinical investigations suggest that a variety of factors may participate in the progression of renal injury. These factors include systemic and glomerular hypertension; high dietary protein intake; proteinuria; glomerular hypertrophy; hyperlipidemia; activation of the coagulation system; abnormalities of calcium and phosphorus balance; and tubulointerstitial injury. Tubulointerstitial injury is an important factor in the progression of glomerular disease. Much interest has been focused on the role of proteinuria in causing glomerular and tubulointerstitial damage. The degree of proteinuria not only is an index of the severity of glomerular disease, but also provides a measure of the rate of progression of renal injury. Heavy proteinuria is an indicator of poor prognosis in various glomerular diseases.

Proteinuria is also accompanied by an increased flux of macromolecules across the mesangium. The mesangial overload may then lead to structural damage. The passage of serum components, such as complement, across the GBM may have a pathophysiologic effect on the glomerular epithelial cells and alter the integrity of the glomerular filtration barrier. The damaging effects of macromolecules other than albumin, such as immunoglobulins, lipoproteins, transferrin, and complement, remain to be characterized.

TABLE 50-2 Tendencies of Glomerular Diseases to Manifest Nephrotic and Nephritic Features

	Nephrotic Features	Nephritic Features
Minimal-change nephropathy	++++	–
Membranous nephropathy	++++	+
Diabetic glomerulosclerosis	++++	+
Amyloidosis	++++	+
Focal segmental glomerulosclerosis	+++	++
Mesangioproliferative glomerulonephritis	++	++
Membranoproliferative glomerulonephritis	++	+++
Proliferative glomerulonephritis	++	+++
Acute poststreptococcal glomerulonephritis	+	++++
Crescentic glomerulonephritis[a]	+	++++

[a]Can be immune complex-mediated, antiglomerular basement membrane antibody-mediated, or associated with antineutrophil cytoplasmic autoantibodies.

CLINICAL PRESENTATION

❷ Although patients with glomerular disease may present with an array of signs and symptoms, they are often categorized into one of two broad classifications: nephritic or a nephrotic syndrome (Table 50–2). The unique clinical presentation characteristics of the predominant glomerulopathies are described in the individual disease sections, presented later in the chapter.

Nephritic syndrome reflects glomerular inflammation and frequently results in hematuria. White cells and cellular and granular casts are commonly found in the urine. In contrast, nephrotic syndrome reflects noninflammatory injury to the glomerular structures, and results in few cells or cellular casts in the urine. Initially, there may be limited or no reduction in renal excretory function.

Hematuria occurs when red blood cells leak through the openings of the GBM. The presence of red cell casts is highly indicative of glomerulonephritis or vasculitis. The presence of dysmorphic red blood cells in the urine is suggestive of glomerular disease. The red blood cells are damaged as they pass through the openings in the GBM or the cells may sustain osmotic injury as they travel through the different osmotic environments within the lumen of the kidney tubules.

The presence of proteinuria indicates a defect of the size- and/or charge-selective barriers within the GBM. Normal urinary protein excretion is between 40 and 80 mg/day, with a maximum of 150 mg. Fewer than 20 mg of the excreted proteins are albumin. Most of the albumin that enters the glomerular filtrate is either reabsorbed or catabolized by the tubular epithelium. The dipsticks that are commonly used to identify proteinuria detect only albumin; they become positive when protein excretion is more than 300 to 500 mg/day. They are therefore unable to detect the early stages of renal injury secondary to diabetes mellitus or hypertension, which often result in microalbuminuria with urinary albumin excretion ranges between 30 and 300 mg/day. Chemstrip Micral-Test II (Roche Diagnostics, Indianapolis, IN), a simple immunoassay on a dipstick, permits specific and semiquantitative determination of urinary albumin concentrations at five levels: 0, 10, 20, 50, and 100 mg/L. Another qualitative test, Micro-Bumintest (Bayer Diabetes Care, Mishawaka, IN), registers a positive reading when the urine albumin concentration is greater than 40 mg/L.

Hypertension is common in patients with glomerular diseases, as a result of renal salt retention causing plasma volume expansion. In contrast, increased activity of vasoconstrictors such as angiotensin II is often the cause in patients with chronic glomerular diseases. Scarring of the glomerulus resulting in regional ischemia is thought to be responsible for the hypertension. Activation of the sympathetic nervous system and the release of vasoconstrictor substances may also contribute.

NEPHRITIC SYNDROME

Glomerular bleeding resulting in hematuria is typical in nephritic syndrome. Dysmorphic red cells, especially acanthocytes, are a sensitive and specific marker of glomerular bleeding. The presence of pus and cellular and granular casts in the urine is common. The extent of proteinuria is variable. Patients with severe nephritic glomerular injury have renal function impairment because of the reduced glomerular surface area available for filtration, as a result of constriction of the capillary lumen by proliferating mesangial cells or inflammatory cells.

CLINICAL PRESENTATIONS OF NEPHRITIC AND NEPHROTIC SYNDROMES

General

- The patients are generally not in acute distress

Symptoms

- The patients may not experience any major symptoms

Nephritic Signs

- Hematuria
- Hypertension and edema as renal function declines

Nephrotic Signs

- Edema
- Weight gain
- Fatigue

Laboratory Tests

Nephritic:

- Proteinuria (up to 3 g/day or more
- Pus, cellular and granular casts in urine is common
- Hypoproteinemia
- Hypercoagulable state in some patients

Nephrotic:

- Proteinuria, >3.5 g/day/1.73 m^2
- Hyperlipidemia
- Lipiduria

NEPHROTIC SYNDROME

Nephrotic syndrome is characterized by proteinuria greater than 3.5 g/day per 1.73 m^2, hypoproteinemia, edema, and hyperlipidemia. A hypercoagulable state may also be present in some patients. The syndrome may be the result of primary diseases of the glomerulus, or be associated with systemic diseases such as diabetes mellitus, lupus, amyloidosis, and preeclampsia. Hypoproteinemia, especially hypoalbuminemia, results from increased urinary loss of albumin and an increased rate of catabolism of filtered albumin by proximal tubular cells. The compensatory increase in hepatic synthesis of albumin is insufficient to replenish the protein loss, probably because of malnutrition.

Edema formation in patients with nephrotic syndrome was traditionally thought to be driven by the reduced plasma oncotic pressure secondary to hypoalbuminemia. If the oncotic pressure is low, the movement of fluid from the vascular space to the interstitial compartment results in a reduction of the plasma volume, which can trigger compensatory renal sodium and water retention through the activation of the renin–angiotensin–aldosterone axis, vasopressin, and the sympathetic nervous system (the "underfill" mechanism). However, experimental data reveal that the plasma volume is actually normal or elevated. Hypoalbuminemia may not cause edema until the serum albumin concentration is less than 2 g/dL. In addition, the transcapillary oncotic pressure gradient is not as high as previously thought because increased lymphatic flow reduces the interstitial oncotic pressure by removing protein and fluid from the interstitium, thereby reducing the transcapillary oncotic pressure gradient.[5] Instead, fluid retention is likely mediated by a primary increase in sodium reabsorption at the distal nephron, which is probably caused by tubular resistance to the action of atrial natriuretic peptide (the "overflow" mechanism).[6] It is likely that both mechanisms may contribute to nephrotic edema in different patients.[6]

Albuminuria greater than 3 g daily is associated with a significant increase in serum cholesterol concentrations in patients with primary glomerular disease.[7] Hyperlipidemia in nephrotic syndrome is characterized by elevated serum total cholesterol and triglyceride concentrations, with increased very-low-density lipoprotein (VLDL) and low-density lipoprotein (LDL) cholesterol concentrations. Lipoprotein (a) levels may also be increased The reduced plasma oncotic pressure as a result of hypoalbuminemia may stimulate hepatic synthesis of lipids and lipoproteins. The increased VLDL production and increased liver cholesterol synthesis, along with a decrease in LDL receptor activity, can then lead to an increase in LDL cholesterol concentrations. In addition, reduced serum albumin or the loss of a liporegulatory substance may result in reduced VLDL clearance.[8] Nephrotic patients with hyperlipidemia, especially those with concomitant hypertension, are presumed to have an increased risk for atherosclerotic vascular disease. Hyperlipidemia also promotes the progression of glomerular injury, as evidenced by glomerulosclerosis, mesangial expansion, and hyalinosis.[8,9]

Many patients with nephrotic syndrome have a hypercoagulable state caused by defects of several control proteins in the coagulation cascade. The concentration of the coagulation inhibitor antithrombin III is reduced because of increased loss in the urine. A reduced amount of the coagulation inhibitors proteins C and S, along with increased concentrations of factors V and VIII, increased fibrinogen concentrations, and abnormal platelet function, may also contribute to the hypercoagulable state. The net result of these alterations in coagulation is an increased risk for arterial and venous thrombosis, especially in the deep veins and renal veins. As many as 25% of patients with membranous nephropathy may have renal vein thrombosis.

DIAGNOSIS

Patients with suspected glomerular disease should have an extensive medical history obtained to identify potential systemic causes (Table 50–3). Medication, environmental, and occupational histories may also help identify possible exposure to potentially nephrotoxic agents. A carefully conducted physical examination and laboratory evaluation may reveal the presence of systemic diseases that may contribute to the development of glomerular disease (Fig. 50–2). In addition, the patient's age, gender, and ethnic background may be helpful in

TABLE 50-3 Evaluation of Patients Suspected of Having Glomerular Disease

Medical history

To identify symptoms of medical conditions that may cause glomerular disease
- Diabetes mellitus
- Amyloidosis
- Systemic lupus erythematosus
- Other familial conditions associated with renal disease

To identify symptoms suggestive of nephrotic syndrome
- Reduced appetite
- Fatigue
- Weight gain
- Edema

Medication, environmental, and occupational histories

To identify possible exposure to potentially nephrotoxic drugs, toxins, or chemicals

Physical examination

To identify signs and symptoms associated with systemic diseases
- Hypertension
- Rash
- Arthritis
- Retinopathy
- Neuropathy
- Lymphadenopathy
- Hepatomegaly
- Malignancy

Laboratory evaluation

Urinalysis
- To determine nephrotic nature of glomerular disease
  - Proteinuria, >3 g/day
  - Lipiduria
- To determine nephritic nature of glomerular disease
  - Hematuria
  - Pyuria
  - Cellular, granular casts

Glomerular filtration rate
- To determine extent of glomerular damage

Other tests
- To identify type and etiology of glomerular disease
  - Serum complement concentration
  - Antinuclear and anti-DNA antibodies
  - Antistreptolysin antibodies
  - Circulating antiglomerular basement membrane antibodies
  - Cryoglobulins

Percutaneous renal biopsy
- To provide definitive diagnosis of glomerular disease

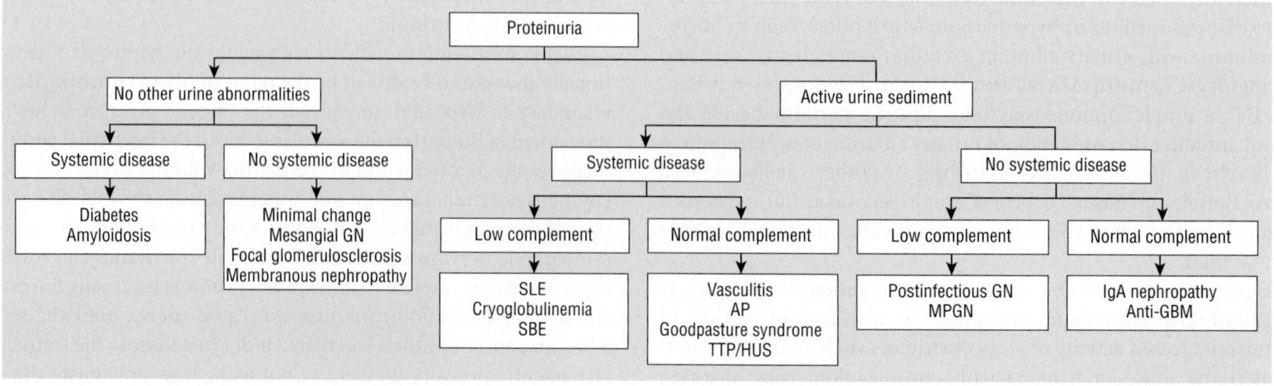

FIGURE 50-2. Clinical presentations of glomerulonephritis. (AP, anaphylactoid purpura; GBM, glomerular basement membrane; GN, glomerulonephritis; HUS, hemolytic uremic syndrome; IgA, immunoglobulin A; MPGN, membranoproliferative glomerulonephritis; SBE, subacute bacterial endocarditis; SLE, systemic lupus erythematosus; TTP, thrombotic thrombocytopenic purpura.)

pinpointing the specific type of glomerular disease. Many of the conditions are more prevalent in certain age groups, although they may occur at any age. For example, proliferative glomerulonephritis is more common in those younger than 40 years of age, whereas the incidence of membranous glomerulonephritis is dramatically higher in those older than 50 years of age.

Laboratory evaluation such as urinalysis can help differentiate the nephrotic or nephritic nature of the disease. The glomerular filtration rate (GFR) may be used to determine the extent of glomerular damage. In the early stages of the disease, the GFR may remain normal. Initial injury to the glomerulus primarily lowers the permeability coefficient (K_f) of the GBM, by reducing the surface area available for filtration and/or the unit permeability of the membrane. The reduced permeability is compensated by an elevation in the glomerular capillary hydrostatic pressure through afferent arteriolar dilation and efferent arteriolar constriction. Extensive glomerular damage may therefore be present before a substantial reduction of total GFR is evident.

Although the cause of glomerular disease may be established from clinical and laboratory evaluation, sometimes percutaneous renal biopsy may be needed to provide a definitive diagnosis.

TREATMENT

Glomerulonephritis

■ GENERAL APPROACH TO TREATMENT

The management of patients with glomerulonephritis involves specific pharmacologic therapy for the glomerular disease, and supportive measures to prevent and/or treat the pathophysiologic sequelae, namely hypertension, edema, and progression of renal disease. In patients with nephrotic syndrome, supportive therapy should also address the management of extrarenal complications of heavy proteinuria, namely hypoalbuminemia, hyperlipidemia, and thromboembolism. Because patients with significant proteinuria tend to have more rapid decline of renal function, reduction of proteinuria thus becomes critical in delaying the rate of progression toward end-stage renal disease.

Immunosuppressive agents, alone or in combination, are commonly used to alter the immune processes that are responsible for the glomerulonephritides. Corticosteroids, in addition to their immunosuppressive effect, also possess antiinflammatory activities. They reduce the production and/or release of many substances that mediate the inflammatory process, such as prostaglandins, leukotrienes, platelet-activating factors, tumor necrosis factors, and interleukin (IL)-1. Movement of leukocytes and macrophages to the site of inflammation is also inhibited. The immunosuppressive effects of corticosteroids are mediated through the inhibition of the release of IL-1 and tumor necrosis factor by activated macrophages, and IL-2 by activated T cells. In addition, the actions of migration-inhibiting factor and γ-interferon are inhibited. Processing of antigens is thus affected by the presence of corticosteroids. Cytotoxic agents, such as cyclophosphamide, chlorambucil, or azathioprine, are commonly used to treat glomerular diseases. Cyclosporine can reduce lymphokine production by activated T lymphocytes and it may decrease proteinuria by improving the permselectivity of the GBM. Mycophenolate mofetil is useful in different glomerulonephritides because of its effects on T and B cell lymphocytes.

Because many immune factors are implicated in the pathogenesis of glomerulonephritis, plasmapheresis may be used to remove these mediators. During the procedure, whole blood is removed from the body and centrifugation is used to separate the cellular elements from the plasma. The cells are then infused back to the patient after resuspension in saline or plasma substitute. The plasma proteins, presumably including the pathogenic immune factors, are thereby removed from the patient.

Recently, many novel targets were identified and new agents are being evaluated for their usefulness to control the disease, preserve renal function, and improve patient outcome. To stay abreast of the expanding availability of treatment options, one can routinely consult one of the clinical trial registries, such as *www.clinicaltrials.gov*.[10]

■ SUPPORTIVE THERAPY

❸ In patients with nephrotic syndrome, dietary measures involve restriction of sodium intake to 50 to 100 mEq/day,[11] protein intake of 0.8 to 1 g/day,[11,12] and a low-lipid diet of less than 200 mg cholesterol. Total fat should account for less than 30% of daily total calories.[11] Sodium restriction is important not only in the control of edema, but also in the control of hypertension and proteinuria. Similarly, protein restriction not only helps to reduce proteinuria, but also has a potential role in retarding the progression of renal disease. Patients should also stop smoking because a dose-dependent increase in risk for developing ESRD was observed in men with primary inflammatory (immunoglobulin A glomerulonephritis) or noninflammatory (polycystic kidney disease) renal diseases.[13]

Edema

Management of nephrotic edema involves salt restriction, bedrest, and use of support stockings and diuretics. However, severe salt restriction is difficult to achieve and prolonged bedrest could predispose nephrotic patients to thromboembolism. Hence the use of a loop diuretic such as furosemide is frequently required. Although the delivery of diuretic to the kidney tubules is normal, the presence of large amounts of protein in the urine promotes drug binding, and thereby reduces the availability of the diuretic to the luminal receptor sites. In addition, reduced sodium delivery to the distal tubule secondary to decreased glomerular perfusion may also alter diuretic effectiveness. Large doses of the loop diuretic, such as 160 to 480 mg of furosemide, may be needed for patients with moderate edema (see Chap. 52). In some instances, a thiazide diuretic or metolazone may be added to enhance natriuresis.[11,14] Alternatively, continuous intravenous infusion of a loop diuretic, such as furosemide 160 to 480 mg/day, may be employed.[15] In patients with morbid edema, albumin infusion may be used to expand plasma volume and to increase diuretic delivery to the renal tubules, thus enhancing diuretic effect. However, it may precipitate congestive heart failure and may also reduce therapeutic response to steroid in minimal-change nephropathy. In patients with significant edema, the goal of treatment should be a daily loss of 1 to 2 lb of fluid until the patient's desired weight has been obtained.

Hypertension

Optimal control of hypertension in patients with glomerular disease is important in reducing both the progression of renal disease and the risk for cardiovascular disease[12] (see Chaps. 15 and 46). The target blood pressure to be 130/80 mm Hg in patients with chronic renal insufficiency defined by GFR <60 mL/min or albuminuria >300 mg/day is 130/80 mm Hg.[16] Angiotensin-converting enzyme inhibitors (ACEIs) and angiotensin II receptor blockers (ARBs) delay the loss of renal function in patients with diabetic and nondiabetic (primarily glomerulonephritis) renal diseases.[17] Nondihydropyridine calcium channel blockers (e.g., diltiazem, verapamil) reduce proteinuria and preserve renal function, and could be used as an additional agent. In contrast, the dihydropyridine calcium channel blockers (e.g., nifedipine, amlodipine, or nisoldipine) are effective in lowering blood pressure, but without the benefit of proteinuria reduction.[18]

Proteinuria

Dietary protein restriction reduces proteinuria and may retard renal function deterioration. Secondary analysis of the Modification of Diet in Renal Disease Study in patients with moderate renal insufficiency (GFR of 25 to 55 mL/min/1.73 m^2) revealed that reduced protein intake (0.66 g/kg/day) delayed the rate of GFR deterioration in patients with severe renal insufficiency (GFR of 13 to 24 mL/min/1.73 m^2).[19] Consequently, modest protein restriction of 0.8 g/kg/day is reasonable for patients with moderate renal insufficiency. Decreasing dietary protein also reduces the intake of phosphorus and potassium. In many instances, the potential benefits of protein restriction have to be balanced against the need for protein intake to overcome nutritional deficiencies. For nondialyzed patients who have GFRs of less than 25 mL/min/1.73 m^2, dietary protein intake should be reduced to 0.6 g/kg/day.[12]

It is now recognized that proteinuria is an independent risk factor for renal function decline and cardiovascular disease.[20] Reducing proteinuria can retard renal function loss and delay the progression to ESRD.[21] The antiproteinuric effect of ACEIs is associated with a fall in filtration fraction, suggesting a reduction in intraglomerular pressure. Recent studies show that ACEIs and ARBs may also have direct effects on podocytes, resulting in reduction of proteinuria and glomerular scarring. [22] In addition, angiotensin-converting enzyme (ACE) inhibition may also reduce the effect of angiotensin II on renal cell proliferation, thereby reducing sclerosis. These beneficial effects on proteinuria are beyond what can be attributed by the drug's antihypertensive effects (see Chap. 46).[23,24]

The combined use of an ACEI and an ARB reduces the rate of renal function decline more than either treatment alone.[17,25] Such combination maximizes blockade of the renin–angiotensin system by counteracting the effects of angiotensin II produced by non-ACE pathways. In addition, with the blockade of the angiotensin II type 1 receptor, the angiotensin II produced by the non-ACE pathways may still act on the angiotensin II type 2 receptors, further facilitating vasodilation.[26] An angiotensin II receptor antagonist should therefore be added to the regimen for those patients who do not attain full and persistent remission of proteinuria with an ACEI alone.

Nonsteroidal antiinflammatory drugs (NSAIDs) probably reduce proteinuria through prostaglandin E_2 inhibition, resulting in a reduction of intraglomerular pressure, a decrease in GFR, and restoration of the barrier size-selectivity of the GBM.[11] Indomethacin and meclofenamate are the two most-evaluated NSAIDs. Their antiproteinuric effect is comparable to that attained with ACEIs, and combined treatment with an ACEI results in additional proteinuria reduction.[27] However, adherence to a low-sodium diet or concurrent use of a diuretic is needed to maximize the antiproteinuric effect. Because of their potential for nephrotoxicity, especially in patients with poor renal function, long-term use of an NSAID for renoprotection is not preferred.[23]

Hyperlipidemia

An abnormal lipoprotein profile increases the risk of atherosclerosis and coronary heart disease in patients with nephrotic syndrome. It is therefore important to treat patients with persistent nephrotic syndrome and sustained dyslipidemia, especially those with high VLDL and LDL cholesterol levels in the presence of a normal or low high-density lipoprotein cholesterol level (see Chaps. 23 and 47). Therapy is especially needed for those with concurrent atherosclerotic cardiovascular disease, or with additional risk factors for atherosclerosis, such as smoking and hypertension.[8]

A low-fat diet is usually not sufficient to correct hyperlipoproteinemia.[11] β-Hydroxy-β-methylglutaryl-coenzyme A (HMG-CoA) reductase inhibitors, also known as the statins such as lovastatin, pravastatin, simvastatin, and fluvastatin, are considered the treatment of choice.[11] They reduce total plasma cholesterol concentration, LDL cholesterol, and total plasma triglyceride concentrations.[8] Aside from the lipid-lowering effects, statins may confer renoprotection through different mechanisms, including reduction of cell proliferation and mesangial matrix accumulation and antiinflammatory and immunomodulatory effects.[28] Recent clinical studies show that they can reduce proteinuria and delay renal function loss.[29,30] The combined use of an ACEI with a statin may offer additional benefits in controlling nephrotic hyperlipidemia.[19]

Anticoagulation

Renal vein thrombosis, pulmonary emboli, or other thromboembolic events, are serious and common complications of nephrotic syndrome, and are frequently seen in those with membranous nephropathy. Although patients who have documented thromboembolic episodes should be anticoagulated with warfarin until remission of nephrotic syndrome, the use of prophylactic anticoagulation is controversial. A decision analysis study suggested that prophylactic anticoagulation is beneficial in patients with membranous nephropathy.[31] Anticoagulation should also be considered for those patients at high risk for thrombosis; e.g., those who require prolonged bedrest, those receiving high-dose intravenous steroids, post surgical patients, as well as those who are dehydrated.[11]

■ DISEASE PROGRESSION AND TREATMENT CONSIDERATIONS

The course and prognosis of the different glomerular diseases are extremely variable and depend on the underlying etiology. In glomerular diseases with a secondary cause, such as poststreptococcal glomerulonephritis, after the initiating factor is removed, the prognosis of the renal disease is often good. In contrast, the rates of renal function deterioration among the primary glomerulonephritides vary according to the form of glomerulonephritis. The majority of patients with minimal-change disease, IgA nephropathy, and membranous nephropathy have a fairly good prognosis. However, those with focal segmental glomerulosclerosis who are resistant to therapy, as well as those with rapidly progressive glomerulonephritis who are untreated, are likely to experience rapid loss of renal function. In some instances, half of the renal function may be lost within a 3-month period. Certain glomerulonephritides, such as minimal-change nephropathy, are very responsive to treatment. In contrast, for some other types of glomerulonephritis, such as membranous proliferative glomerulonephritis, consistently effective therapy has yet to be found.

Because of the variable courses exhibited by the different glomerulonephritides, specific treatment approaches have been developed for each disease. The natural history of the glomerulonephritis has to be well delineated before a promising regimen can be evaluated, from both therapeutic and economic perspectives. Otherwise patients will be exposed to unnecessary treatment-related toxicities if they have a type of glomerulonephritis that is likely to undergo spontaneous remission. The potential therapeutic benefits of treatment regimens should always be weighed against the risks to which the patients are being exposed. It is therefore imperative to identify patients who are most likely to benefit from treatment, especially those who have other risk factors that may contribute to the deterioration of their renal function. In those instances in which satisfactory regimens are not available to treat the primary disease, appropriate supportive measures should be employed. Optimization of systemic and glomerular pressure, reducing proteinuria, and possibly controlling hyperlipidemia may all improve the long-term outcome as well as the quality of life of these patients.

Evaluation of Therapeutic Outcomes

❹ Patients should be monitored closely for therapeutic response as well as the development of treatment-related toxicities. Although the rate of renal function deterioration is an important indicator of the long-term success of treatment, resolution of nephrotic and nephritic signs and symptoms associated with the glomerulopathies is an important short-term therapeutic target.

Serum creatinine concentration as well as creatinine clearance should be evaluated prior to and during treatment; 24-hour urine outflow should be collected to determine the extent of proteinuria. Alternatively, the daily urine protein excretion may be estimated by the urinary total protein-to-creatinine concentration ratio. After establishing the correlation between the 24-hour urinary protein excretion and the protein-to-creatinine ratio, single, random urine specimens may be used in place of a 24-hour urine collection. Blood pressure should be monitored periodically to assess the need for, and the adequacy of, antihypertensive therapy. The pressures should also be evaluated in conjunction with clinical signs and symptoms of edema and fluid overload to gauge the need for volume control as well as diuretic use. For patients with nephrotic syndrome, serum lipid concentrations should be monitored. If the patient has hematuria, urinalysis and a complete blood count should be obtained. The clinician should also be aware of the patient's appetite and energy level, because these are indicators of the patient's overall state of well-being. At times, renal biopsy is needed to assess response to treatment and disease progression, to determine future treatment strategy, and to confirm the initial diagnosis.

Patients receiving cytotoxic drug treatment should be evaluated for drug-related toxicities every week during the initial treatment period. After 1 month of treatment, the frequency of monitoring may be reduced. When the patient is on long-term steroid treatment, monthly visits are often required for assessment of both efficacy and toxicities. If a favorable response is obtained after a course of treatment, the patient may be evaluated every 3 to 4 months. The patient's renal function, proteinuria, urinalysis, blood pressure, lipid profile, and the overall state of health should be assessed during these regular followup visits.

INDIVIDUAL GLOMERULOPATHIES

MINIMAL-CHANGE NEPHROPATHY

Epidemiology and Etiology

Minimal-change nephropathy (also termed *minimal-change disease*) is commonly found in children, accounting for more than 90% of all cases of nephrotic syndrome in children between 1 and 4 years of age. The percentage drops gradually to less than 50% after age 10 years, and accounts for less than 20% of all cases of idiopathic nephrotic syndrome in adults. Secondary causes of minimal-change nephropathy include NSAIDs, lupus, and various T-cell–related disorders, such as Hodgkin disease and leukemias.

Pathophysiology

Minimal-change disease is also known as "nil" disease, primarily because of the absence of definitive pathologic changes observed under light and immunofluorescence microscopy. The characteristic lesion in patients with minimal-change disease, as visualized under electron microscopy, is the spreading and fusion of the foot processes of epithelial cells over an unchanged GBM. *Lipoid nephrosis* is another term that has been used to describe this type of glomerular disease because lipids, as well as renal tubular cells, are found in the urine. The pathogenesis of minimal-change disease is unknown. Altered cell-mediated immunologic response, specifically T-cell dysfunction or changes in the T-cell subpopulations, may be responsible. The activated lymphocytes are thought to secrete lymphokines that reduce the production of anions in the GBM. The permeability of the GBM to plasma albumin is increased through a reduction of electrostatic repulsion. The loss of anionic charges also results in fusion of the epithelial cell foot processes. Other vascular permeability factors, such as hemopexin, IL-4, and vascular endothelial growth factor, also have been suggested to be responsible.

Clinical Presentation

Most patients present initially with edema, frequently acute in onset, following a nonspecific upper respiratory tract infection, allergic reaction, or vaccinations, which might have activated the T lymphocytes. Nephrotic syndrome with massive proteinuria (substantially more than 40 mg/m^2 per hour for children and 3 g/day for adults), edema, hypoalbuminemia, and hyperlipidemia is common. The patient's weight may increase dramatically because of sodium and fluid retention. Nephrotic features, such as gross hematuria, are uncommon. Hypertension and decreased renal function are uncommon in children but are more common in older adults.[32] In some patients, volume depletion may result in mild to moderate azotemia.

TREATMENT

Minimal-Change Nephropathy

■ PHARMACOLOGIC THERAPY

Steroids

❺ Minimal-change disease is most responsive to initial treatment with corticosteroids. In children, steroid therapy is expected to reduce proteinuria in approximately 90% of the patients, with >95% 10-year renal survival.[33] Because of the excellent response to initial therapy with steroids and the prevalence of this glomerular disease in children, reduction of proteinuria secondary to steroid treatment is considered diagnostic for minimal-change disease without the need for biopsy. Prednisone is commonly administered at 60 mg/m^2 per day initially for 4 to 6 weeks. The dose is then reduced to 40 mg/m^2 per day every other day for another 4 to 6 weeks, with or without tapering afterwards (Fig. 50–3).[34] Proteinuria will disappear in 50% of patients after 1 week and in 90% of patients after 4 weeks of treatment. Different versions of the steroid regimen are available as there is no consensus on the optimal dose and duration. Studies are being conducted to identify to best strategy to induce remission, reduce disease recurrence, and minimize adverse effects of the therapy. Commonly, the initial episode is treated with an extended course (months) of therapy, followed by shorter treatment (weeks) for relapses.[35]

Initial therapy For adults, prednisone 1 mg/kg per day is given initially for 4 weeks with a reduction to 0.75 mg/kg every other day for the next 4 weeks. Proteinuria will disappear in 50% to 60% of patients after 8 weeks of treatment, and complete remission will be attained in 80% of patients after 28 weeks of therapy.[32]

Relapse As many as 85% of the patients who respond to initial steroid therapy (steroid sensitive) will experience a relapse of proteinuria, mostly within 6 to 12 months after disease onset. The risk of relapse is affected by the duration of initial steroid therapy.[11,34] Children who were asymptomatic with proteinuria diagnosed during routine urine screening tend to have less-frequent relapses and a more favorable clinical course. In those who relapse, 50% to 65% may have steroid-responsive relapse episodes over the subsequent 3- to 5-year period. The dose and duration of steroid treatment for the relapse do not influence the subsequent rate of relapse.[11,34] Commonly, 60 mg/m^2 per day of prednisone is given until the urine is free of protein for 3 days, to be followed by 4 weeks of alternate-day prednisone at 40 mg/m^2 per dose.[34]

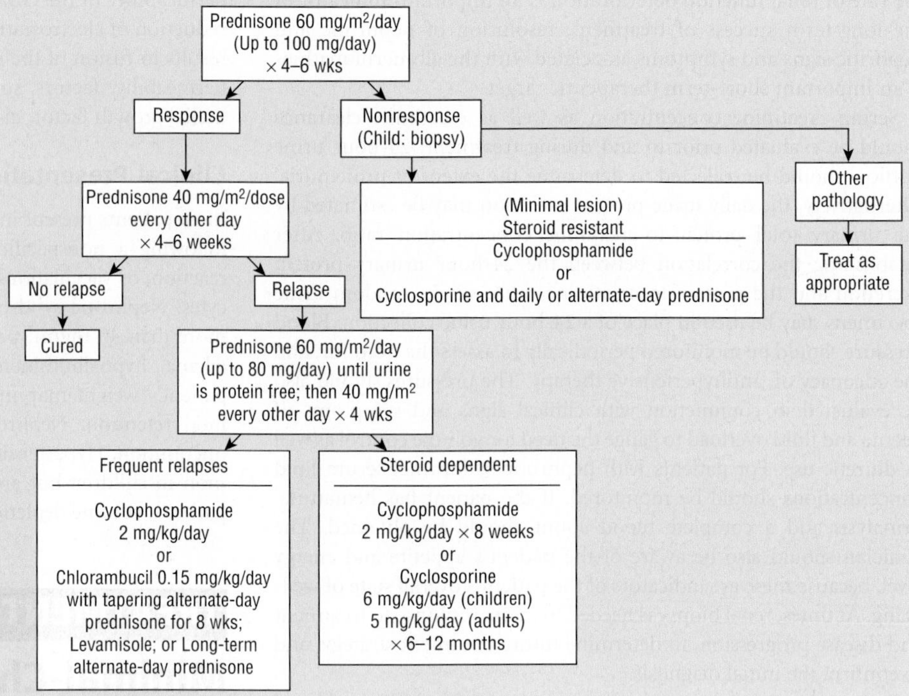

FIGURE 50-3. Treatment algorithm for minimal-change nephropathy. *(Modified from reference 34.)*

Frequent Relapse Approximately 10% to 20% of children will experience three or four relapses that are responsive to steroid. Half of them will then relapse frequently and become steroid dependent, requiring continuous low-dose alternate-day prednisone to maintain an extended relapse-free period.[34] A small number of patients eventually develop resistance to steroids, and a biopsy done at that time often reveals another pathology such as focal segmental glomerulosclerosis. It is controversial whether minimal-change disease progresses into focal segmental glomerulosclerosis or whether the glomerulosclerosis that was present at the time of initial diagnosis was inadvertently diagnosed as minimal-change nephropathy because of tissue-sampling error during the renal biopsy.

Cytotoxic Agents

Cytotoxic agents are often considered for patients who are steroid resistant, as well as for those who require large doses of steroids to sustain remission (steroid dependent). These agents are also beneficial for pediatric patients who experience growth inhibition secondary to chronic use of steroid.[11] Cytotoxic agents are effective in inducing remission and the duration of remission tends to be longer than that induced by steroid. In those patients who relapse after cytotoxic therapy, they may respond to steroid better than before.

Cyclophosphamide at 2 mg/kg per day for 10 to 12 weeks given alone or with prednisone (50 to 75 mg/m^2) is very effective in inducing remission and restoring steroid responsiveness in patients who were previously steroid dependent and then became steroid resistant. Alternatively, chlorambucil at 0.1 to 0.2 mg/kg per day may be used. This agent, however, is associated with more adverse effects than cyclophosphamide. Azathioprine has also been used; however, treatment for 6 to 12 months is often needed before any favorable response is apparent.

The immunosuppressive effect of cytotoxic agents, with or without the concurrent use of steroids, can result in serious infections, which are the primary cause of death in patients with minimal-change nephropathy. Other toxicities associated with cyclophosphamide include gonadal fibrosis, which results in sterility, hemorrhagic cystitis, alopecia, and a potential to develop malignancy in those on long-term treatment.

Cyclosporine

Cyclosporine decreases lymphokine production by activated T lymphocytes and thereby reduces proteinuria by reversing the lymphokine-induced alterations in the anionic charge and permeability of the GBM to albumin. In patients with steroid-sensitive or steroid-dependent disease, cyclosporine induces remission in 80% to 85% of patients. However, the disease-free period is not often sustained, and relapse, which is usually not as responsive to cyclosporine retreatment, may occur as soon as the drug is tapered or discontinued.[36] The steriod-sparing effect of cyclosporine is also useful for steroid-dependent patients, especially those who have experienced significant adverse effects.

The usual starting dose of cyclosporine for remission induction is 5 mg/kg per day for adults and 100 to 150 mg/m^2 per day for children. Similar dosages are used to maintain remission long-term. The optimal cyclosporine blood concentrations, as well as the need to monitor them, are controversial. No correlation has been found between the severity of the cyclosporine-induced tubulointerstitial lesions and the mean dose or trough drug concentration. However, monitoring of the area under the serum concentration-time curve has been suggested and target exposures have been proposed. Testing the in vitro sensitivity of peripheral blood lymphocytes to cyclosporine in the presence of a T-cell mitogen may offer a novel method to predict response and individualize therapy.[37]

Because of the risk of toxicities associated with long-term therapy, cyclosporine should not be given for more than 4 months in the absence of any beneficial effect.[36] Consequently, it is indicated for patients (a) who relapse frequently or are steroid dependent, after failing to respond to a course of cyclophosphamide; (b) for whom cyclophosphamide is contraindicated or when gonadal toxicity is a concern; (c) who are steroid dependent when a "steroid holiday" is needed for catch-up growth and puberty; or (d) who have steroid-resistant disease.[34]

Levamisole

Levamisole, an immunostimulant, can promote the maturation of young T cells and restore the function of T cells and phagocytes when the immune system is depressed. It may also inhibit the production of an immunosuppressive lymphokine. Levamisole was found to have a steroid-sparing effect and was capable of maintaining remission in children who had frequent relapse steroid-dependent nephrotic syndrome.[38] In addition, it is as effective as cyclophosphamide in reducing relapse rate and steroid dosages.[39] The most serious adverse effect of levamisole is neutropenia, which is generally reversible. At present the drug is no longer available in the United States; however, it is still used elsewhere in the world for selected steroid-dependent patients.

Mycophenolate Mofetil

Mycophenolate mofetil is an immunosuppressant that can suppress T- and B-cell lymphocyte proliferation, B-lymphocyte antibody production, and expression of adhesion molecules. It is reported to have steroid-sparing effects and to be useful in steroid-dependent patients, as well as in those who fail cytotoxic thereapy.[40,41]

Therapeutic Outcomes

The long-term prognosis of most patients with minimal-change disease is good. The majority of pediatric patients will not experience any relapse of the disease 10 years after the initial onset, and most will be free of the proteinuria after puberty. In adults, an 85% to 90% survival rate is seen 10 years after disease onset. Although this condition may spontaneously remit in up to 70% of untreated adults, life-threatening complications may be associated with untreated nephrotic syndrome. Significant deterioration in renal function is uncommon in both adult and pediatric patients and is observed only in those who are steroid resistant or steroid dependent. Because of the overall favorable outcome of the disease and the relatively uncommon progression into chronic renal failure, aggressive use of cytotoxic agents is not indicated even in most patients with frequent relapses. Toxicities associated with aggressive therapy do not justify the need to induce remission in those patients who fail to respond to steroids and the nonaggressive use of cytotoxic agents. Symptomatic therapy with diuretics to control edema, in conjunction with a low-salt diet and albumin infusion as needed for acute development of anasarca, is often a more rewarding therapeutic approach. NSAIDs and ACEIs may also be used to reduce the proteinuria.

FOCAL SEGMENTAL GLOMERULOSCLEROSIS

Etiology and Epidemiology

Focal segmental glomerulosclerosis (FSGS) is a clinicopathologic condition that can be idiopathic (primary) or secondary to a variety of causes. FSGS accounts for less than 15% of the cases of idiopathic nephrotic syndrome in children, and approximately 15% to 20% in adults; however, it may account for 36% to 80% of the cases in African Americans.[42] The incidence of FSGS has been rapidly increasing, so that it now is the most common glomerular disease causing ESRD. Conditions such as sickle cell disease, cyanotic congenital heart disease, and morbid obesity can induce hemodynamic stress on an initially normal nephron population and result in FSGS. Severe glomerular injury can also be seen in patients with nephropathy associated with heroin abuse, human immunodeficiency virus (HIV) infection, and genetic mutations involving the podocin and WT1 genes.[42] The primary and secondary sclerotic lesions may be morphologically similar, but they represent diseases with different courses and responses to therapy.

Pathophysiology

Sclerotic lesions are characteristically found in some of the glomeruli (focal) and usually involve only a portion of the glomeruli (segmental).[43] Similar to minimal-change disease, fusion of foot processes is commonly seen in those glomeruli that are not sclerotic. It is thought that both minimal-change disease and FSGS share similar pathogenetic mechanisms, with FSGS resulting in severe injury to the glomerular epithelial cells. During the early stage of FSGS, only a small number of glomeruli may have the segmental sclerotic lesion and the disease may be confined to the juxtamedullary region. If an inadequate number of glomeruli are sampled during renal biopsy, the diagnosis of FSGS may be missed, or the patient may be thought to have minimal-change disease. Resistance to steroid therapy may thus be one of the first clues that the patient, indeed, has FSGS rather than minimal-change disease. Alternatively, a patient may have the steroid-sensitive minimal-change disease initially, which subsequently progresses to steroid-resistant FSGS.

Clinical Presentation

Almost all the patients present with proteinuria, and many of them have all the features of nephrotic syndrome. The proteinuria is nonselective, containing albumin and other higher-molecular-weight proteins, and is usually less severe when compared to patients who have minimal-change disease. Hypertension, microscopic hematuria, and renal dysfunction may be seen in up to half of the patients. Reduced renal function becomes more prevalent as the disease progresses.

The presenting clinical features in nephrotic adults with minimal-change nephropathy can be indistinguishable from that of FSGS, and renal biopsy is therefore critical in the treatment of adults with nephrotic syndrome. African Americans have a four-time higher risk of developing FSGS than white or Asian patients. They tend to develop the disease earlier and present with nephrotic range proteinuria more often. They are less responsive to steroids and are more likely to experience a rapid decline in renal function, resulting in ESRD.

TREATMENT

Focal Segmental Glomerulosclerosis

■ PHARMACOLOGIC THERAPY

Steroids

❻ The treatment of FSGS is controversial because of the lack of data from randomized, prospective, controlled trials. A course of prednisone (1 to 2 mg/kg per day) with tapering after 3 to 4 months of treatment is first used for nephrotic patients.[42,43] Urinary protein excretion and serum albumin concentration should be monitored to assess efficacy. The median time to induce complete remission is 3 to 4 months, although 5 to 9 months may be needed in some patients.[42] In general, 30% to 40% of all patients can be expected to attain complete remission; for those who are not responding, treatment should be continued for 6 months before they are considered steroid resistant.[44]

If the patient develops a relapse after an adequate response to the initial treatment, a second course of steroids is generally sufficient.[42] However, if relapse occurs frequently, cytotoxic agents or cyclosporine would be indicated.

For patients who are not nephrotic, their relatively favorable prognosis does not support using steroids or other immunosuppressive agents. However, close followup and good blood pressure control with ACEIs are necessary to minimize disease progression.[43]

Most of the studies conducted thus far include mostly white patients. In a recent retrospective review of 72 patients that included 65 African American patients, steroid use was not found to associate with renal survival or the induction of proteinuria remission.[45] The initial creatinine level, blood pressure, and severity of renal lesion are significant factors for renal survival. About one third of the patients who received steroids developed complications such as diabetes and significant weight gain.

Cytotoxic Agents

When used with steroids during initial therapy, cytotoxic agents were not found to offer any additional beneficial effect.[42] In those patients who are not responding to steroids during initial therapy, cytotoxic agents such as cyclophosphamide (2 mg/kg/day) and chlorambucil (0.1 to 0.2 mg/kg/day) have been used with pulse methylprednisolone to induce remission. Response rates as high as 66% have been reported in uncontrolled trials, although such favorable responses have not been universally observed.[42]

Cyclosporine

In steroid-resistant patients, cyclosporine therapy has produced a complete or partial remission in 70% of patients, with a relapse rate of 47%.[46] Encouraging results have also been reported with the concurrent use of cyclosporine and steroid.[42] Adverse effects of cyclosporine commonly include gingival hyperplasia, hypertrichosis, hypertension, and renal insufficiency. In an attempt to minimize the long-term side effects, a regimen that included periodic cyclosporine dose reduction when given with steroid, cyclophosphamide, and mycophenolate mofetil was developed and favorable effects were observed.[47]

Mycophenolate Mofetil

Mycophenolate mofetil has been reported by several small studies to have favorable effects in patients who were steroid resistant, many of whom had failed to respond to other cytotoxic agents and cyclosporine.[48] Forty-four percent of the patients had reduced proteinuria and the improvement was sustained in 50% for up to 1 year. Deterioration of renal function was not observed. Other investigators have reported similar experiences. Further studies are needed to define the role of this agent among the various treatment options.

Symptomatic Therapy

Because of the lack of a consistently effective regimen for primary FSGS, many patients with mild disease are treated conservatively. ACEIs and ARBs are effective in reducing proteinuria and in stabilizing renal function in many patients with primary or secondary FSGS.[42] For patients who have nephrotic range proteinuria, elevated serum creatinine concentration and interstitial scarring on biopsy, corticosteroids with or without immunosuppressive agents are often used.

THERAPEUTIC OUTCOMES

ESRD develops within 10 years in 10% or less of the 30% to 50% of adults and children who had attained complete remission.[46,49] For those patients who are resistant to therapy, the rate of renal function deterioration to ESRD may be rapid, within 1 year, or slow, over as long as 10 to 20 years; approximately 50% develop ESRD within 10 years.[49] Those patients with severe proteinuria (>10 to 15 g/day), high serum creatinine concentration at diagnosis, initial steroid resistance, or interstitial fibrosis on renal biopsy are likely to have a more rapid decline in renal function.[43] African American patients may also have a higher risk. Kidney transplantation is often indicated for those patients who develop ESRD; however, FSGS has recurred in 20% to 50% of the renal allografts soon after transplantation. Children and those with severe disease or rapid progression to ESRD prior to transplantation are more likely to experience a recurrence. The proteinuria may reappear within hours after transplantation and graft failure may occur in one third to one half of the patients. The median time to recurrence was reported to be 14 days in one study. Although cyclosporine is ineffective in preventing the recurrence of nephrotic syndrome after transplantation, a high dose of the agent (up to 35 mg/kg per day) induces a remission of the recurrent disease. ACEIs and plasmapheresis are also used to prolong graft survival. The effectiveness of these therapies and the rapid recurrence of the disease in the transplanted kidney substantiate the possibility that a circulating humoral mediator is responsible for the nephropathy.

MEMBRANOUS NEPHROPATHY

Etiology and Epidemiology

Membranous nephropathy is the most common disorder responsible for idiopathic nephrotic syndrome in adults, accounting for about 20% to 25% of cases. It is also a frequent cause of renal failure secondary to glomerulonephritis. The hallmark histologic features of membranous nephropathy are glomerular capillary wall thickening with subepithelial deposits under light and electron microscopy. Most cases are idiopathic, but approximately 25% of adults and 80% of children have secondary causes.[50,51] In the United States, the most common etiologies are autoimmune diseases (e.g., lupus), infection (e.g., hepatitis B and C), syphilis, neoplasm (e.g., carcinoma of the lung, breast, gastrointestinal tract, or kidney), and medications (e.g., gold, penicillamine, or captopril). Malaria and schistosomiasis are common causes in other parts of the world. De novo membranous nephropathy can also occur in the allografts of renal transplant patients. Because the response to therapy as well as the prognosis for idiopathic and secondary membranous nephropathy are different, it is important to identify any potential underlying causes for the nephropathy prior to treatment. Although this glomerular disease can occur at any age, the peak incidence is between ages 30 and 50 years and is especially likely in patients older than age 50 years who present with nephrotic syndrome.[50]

Pathophysiology

Examination of kidney tissue under light microscopy reveals normal mesangium and normocellularity. The glomerular capillary wall may be thickened in well-developed lesions. In the advanced stage, the capillary wall is markedly thickened and intramembranous deposits are found. Progressive changes in capillary lumen patency parallel those in the GBM, resulting in glomerulosclerosis with capillary collapse and tubular atrophy in end-stage membranous nephropathy. Immunofluorescence microscopy shows strong capillary wall staining of IgG and C3 on the epithelial side of the basement membrane. Antibody-mediated immune injury appears to be the main pathogenetic mechanism. The immune complex can be formed in situ or deposited from circulating immune complexes.

Clinical Presentation

Most patients with membranous nephropathy present with heavy proteinuria (exceeding 3.5 g/day). Those patients excreting large amounts of IgG and α_1-microglobulin, indicating more significant tubulointerstitial damage, have a lower remission rate and are more likely to progress toward renal failure.[50]

The signs and symptoms are usually insidious in onset and may consist of anorexia, malaise, edema, anasarca, or ascites, and pericardial and pleural effusions may also be present. As a result of a hypercoagulable state, pulmonary embolism may develop, but rarely results in death. The incidence of renal vein thrombosis varies from 5% to 62%,[51] and membranous nephropathy should be suspected when there is a sudden onset of hematuria; loin pain; pulmonary embolus; fluctuating or worsening proteinuria or glomerular filtration rate; renal tubular acidosis; or an increase in leg edema. Hypertension is found in approximately 30% of patients and is more common with renal insufficiency or in advanced disease.

In addition to heavy proteinuria, urinalysis often reveals lipiduria and oval fat bodies. Microhematuria is seen in fewer than 25% of patients, and gross hematuria and red cell casts are rare. In idiopathic membranous nephropathy, the serum complement concentrations are normal. Low levels of complement should alert one to search for secondary causes, such as lupus, hepatitis B infection, or an alternative diagnosis. Similarly, antinuclear antibodies, anti-DNA antibodies, rheumatoid factor, hepatitis B serologies, and serum cryoglobulins are generally negative in idiopathic membranous nephropathy. Occult malignancy has been found in as many as 10% of elderly patients with membranous nephropathy.

The natural course of idiopathic membranous nephropathy is variable. Up to 30% of the patients experience spontaneous remission, commonly within 2 years of disease onset. Half of the remaining patients have persistent proteinuria with long-term preservation of renal function, while the other half has gradual loss of renal function.[50] Heavy proteinuria (>10 g/day); male gender; elevated serum creatinine concentration at the time of presentation; poorly controlled hypertension; advanced age at onset of disease; non-Asian race; certain human leukocyte antigen phenotypes; and tubulointerstitial fibrosis on initial renal biopsy are associated with progressive renal disease.[50,51] A predictive algorithm, incorporating the level of proteinuria, initial creatinine clearance, as well as the slope of renal function decline over 6 month, has been developed to determine the risk for disease progression.[50]

In general, patients with idiopathic membranous nephropathy have a relatively benign course with mean 10-year survival of approximately 70%. Those who present with persistent nonnephrotic proteinuria seldom develop renal insufficiency and have a normal life expectancy. Fewer than 10% of patients develop a remitting and relapsing course.[51] The prognosis for secondary membranous nephropathy depends on the underlying cause. Remission occurs when the infection resolves or when the causative medication is withdrawn.

TREATMENT

Membranous Nephropathy

The treatment of idiopathic membranous nephropathy is controversial and ranges from supportive therapy to immunosuppression. Conservative management of patients with mild disease includes edema control with salt restriction and diuretics[5] and reduction of proteinuria with protein restriction and ACEIs (Fig. 50–4).[51] Management of hypertension and hyperlipidemia is required for most patients, whereas prophylactic anticoagulation, despite having benefits shown to outweigh the risks, is usually given only for patients with renal vein thrombosis or documented pulmonary embolus.[31,51]

■ PHARMACOLOGIC THERAPY

Steroids

Remission of proteinuria, whether spontaneously or treatment related, may confer a good prognosis. Corticosteroids alone were ineffective in improving proteinuria remission rate in all controlled trials and in preventing progression in all but one study.[51] The result of a meta-analysis also confirmed the lack of efficacy of steroids when used alone.

Cytotoxic Agents

Cytotoxic agents, when used in conjunction with corticosteroids, are effective in increasing the remission rate of proteinuria and preserving renal function. Ponticelli and colleagues devised such a regimen by combining intravenous methylprednisolone (1 g) for 3 days followed by oral methylprednisolone (0.4 mg/kg) for the subsequent 27 days of months 1, 3, and 5. Oral chlorambucil (0.2 mg/kg) is to be given daily in months 2, 4, and 6.[52] The 10-year renal survival was increased to 92% when compared with 60% in the control group. They later substituted cyclophosphamide (2.5 mg/kg per day) for chlorambucil, which resulted in similar rates of proteinuria remission and relapse, but with fewer serious side effects in those who received cyclophosphamide.[53]

Results from a recent meta-analysis of randomized, controlled trials affirmed that cytotoxic agents, but not steroids, are effective in reducing nephrotic-range proteinuria, with cyclophosphamide having fewer adverse effects than chlorambucil.[54]

Cyclosporine

A controlled trial found that cyclosporine, given at a dose of 3 to 4 mg/kg/day for 6 months, was effective in patients with medium risk for disease progression.[50] For patients with severe nephrotic syndrome and deteriorating renal function who do not respond to cytotoxic therapy, cyclosporine may offer some benefits; however, the risk for cyclosporine nephrotoxicity is of concern, especially

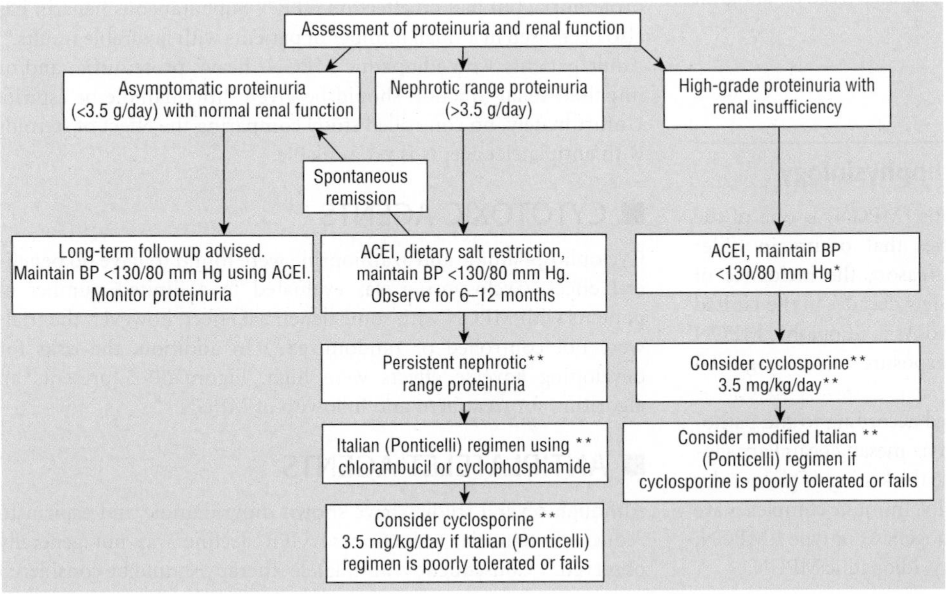

FIGURE 50-4. Treatment algorithm for idiopathic membranous nephropathy. Patients may change from one category to another during the course of followup. *, Supported by evidence from controlled trials; **, introduction of risk reduction strategies for both secondary effects of disease and adverse effects of immunotherapy; (ACEI, angiotensin-converting enzyme inhibitor; BP, blood pressure.) *(Modified from reference 51.)*

during long-term therapy. A 12-month course of cyclosporine (mean dose: 3.8 mg/kg/day) was found to reduce proteinuria as well as the rate of renal deterioration.[55] In a recent study of 41 patients who received cyclosporine, many with concurrent steroid and ACE inhibitor therapy, the median treatment time to complete remission was 225 days among the 34% of patients who attained complete remission.[56] During such long-term treatment, hypertension may be exacerbated and the serum creatinine concentration may be increased because of nephrotoxicity. When the renal function declines, the dose of cyclosporine should be reduced.

Alternative Therapeutic Options

Because spontaneous remission is common and only approximately 25% of patients with new-onset idiopathic membranous nephropathy ultimately develop ESRD in 20 to 30 years, it is prudent not to aggressively treat all patients at the onset of the disease. Patients who have a low risk for renal disease progression can be managed with observation and symptomatic therapy. Normalizing the blood pressure and reducing proteinuria with ACEIs and/or ARBs are important as both hypertension and proteinuria are independent risk factors for the progression of renal failure.[50] Patients with low risk for renal disease progression include children 2 to 16 years of age, adult males with proteinuria less than 2 g/day, or adult females with proteinuria less than 5 g/day and normal renal function. In contrast, patients who have a high risk of developing renal failure, including those with proteinuria greater than 10 g/day with or without impaired renal function, and patients with symptomatic nephrotic syndrome with a plasma albumin of less than 2 g/dL, should be aggressively treated to induce remission. An alkylating agent such as cyclophosphamide or chlorambucil, combined with steroids, should be given to induce remission. Recently, mycophenolate mofetil, rituximab, and eculizumab were shown separately to be effective in treating a small number of patients.[57–59] A synthetic analog of adrenocorticotropic hormone, tetracosactide, has also been shown in small studies to offer results superior to the cytotoxic–steroid combination regimen.[60]

The cytoxic–steroid combination regimen may be effective in inducing remission in the 30% to 40% of the medium-risk patients who relapse within 2 years after treatment discontinuation. Alternately, cyclosporine may be used with similar effectiveness.[50] The cyclophosphamide–steroid combination should also be used for relapse in high-risk patients.

In patients with a transplanted kidney, both de novo and recurrent membranous nephropathy may occur. Patients with primary membranous nephropathy are more at risk. Recurrence is typically associated with nephrotic syndrome and a high risk of allograft failure from disease and/or rejection.

MEMBRANOPROLIFERATIVE GLOMERULONEPHRITIS

Etiology, Epidemiology, and Pathophysiology

Membranoproliferative glomerulonephritis (MPGN) is one of the least-common renal morphologic entities that occurs in older children and adults. For some unclear reason, the incidence of MPGN has been decreasing over the past few decades in the United States and Europe. However, in Africa and Asia, idiopathic MPGN is still common, perhaps secondary to exposure to unrecognized infectious and parasitic agents.

The several types of MPGN are classified according to the pathologic features. Type I MPGN, also known as mesangiocapillary glomerulonephritis, is characterized by diffuse thickening of glomerular capillary walls and mesangial hypercellularity. Immune complexes are presumed to have a major role in the pathogenesis of type I MPGN, which is the most common type of primary, idiopathic MPGN.

Type II MPGN is also known as dense-deposit disease because of the presence of dense deposits of C3 within the glomerular basement membrane, which gives rise to a ribbon-like appearance. Other variants of the disease include type III MPGN, which is seen rarely and consists of subendothelial and subepithelial deposits with lamination and disruption of the lamina densa of the GBM.

Type I MPGN is a slowly progressive disease that accounts for 80% of all MPGN, but only 5% to 15% of all cases of nephrotic syndrome seen in pediatric and adult patients. It occurs most frequently in patients between 5 and 30 years of age, and because remissions are rare, many patients eventually develop ESRD. The renal survival is 60% to 65% at 10 years, and the presence of nephrotic syndrome, interstitial disease, and hypertension are poor prognostic indicators.[61] Type II MPGN is a more aggressive disease that constitutes approximately 15% of all patients with MPGN. Only 20% of patients remain stable for more than a few years and the median time before the development of ESRD is 7 years.

Clinical Presentation

Nephrotic syndrome is the most common presenting condition although some patients may also have a nephritic component (hematuria), hypertension, and renal insufficiency. Hypocomplementemia is commonly seen.

TREATMENT

Membranoproliferative Glomerulonephritis

■ STEROIDS

The efficacy of corticosteroids, cyclophosphamide, antiplatelet drugs, and anticoagulants has been evaluated for the treatment of MPGN. In children, prednisone 40 mg/m^2 given on alternate days is effective, when compared with placebo, in reducing the decline in GFR.[62] This observation was confirmed by other uncontrolled studies.[61] Consequently, prednisone should be given for 6 to 12 months to children with MPGN, proteinuria (more than 3 g/day), and/or impaired renal function.[61] Other studies suggest that this regimen may also be beneficial in children with mild proteinuria.

Although the effect of steroids has not been proven in adults, antiplatelet drugs, such as dipyridamole and aspirin, as well as warfarin, were found in randomized controlled trials to reduce proteinuria, but had no effect on GFR.[61] Subcutaneous heparin has also been used in a small number of patients with favorable results.[63] Adult patients with idiopathic MPGN, heavy proteinuria, and/or impaired renal function should be given dipyridamole or aspirin. Unfortunately, no controlled study comparing the effect of steroids with antiplatelet agents is yet available.

■ CYTOTOXIC AGENTS

Cyclophosphamide and azathioprine were found to have no beneficial effect. Cyclosporine was evaluated in a limited number of patients with MPGN with some beneficial effect; however, the trials were not controlled or randomized.[64] In addition, the risks for developing adverse effects were high. Figure 50–5 presents an algorithm for treatment and followup of MPGN.

■ ANTIPLATELET AGENTS

Although several studies have shown dipyridamole and aspirin to reduce proteinuria, reduction of GFR decline was not generally observed.[61] Consequently, antiplatelet therapy should be considered

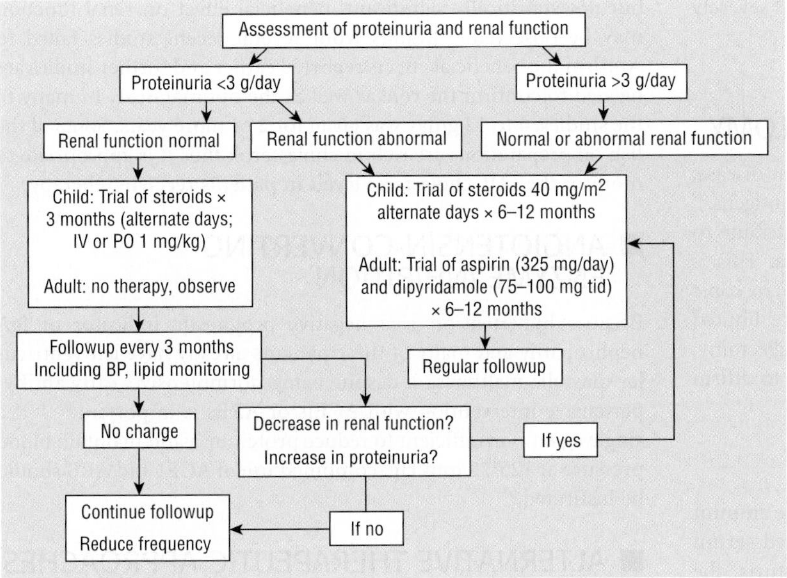

FIGURE 50-5. Treatment algorithm for membranoproliferative glomerulonephritis. (BP, blood pressure.) *(Modified from reference 61.)*

as a viable option only for those patients with significant proteinuria. There should be periodic followup of patients to assess proteinuria and renal function.

It is difficult to conduct large-scale controlled trials for MPGN because of the low incidence of the disease. Based on the available studies, many of the drugs evaluated do not have any consistent, beneficial effect on renal function and proteinuria. Renal transplantation is an alternative; however, the recurrence rate is close to 100% for type II MPGN and is approximately 20% to 30% for type I MPGN. Half of the allografts ultimately fail.[63]

IMMUNOGLOBULIN A NEPHROPATHY

Etiology and Epidemiology

IgA nephropathy, also known as Berger disease, was first described in France in 1968. It now is the most common primary glomerulonephritis in the world, and accounts for 10% of patients with ESRD in many countries. The prevalence among patients with glomerulonephritis or patients who had kidney biopsy varies from as high as 50% in Japan and East Asia to 10% to 30% in Europe. In the United States, the overall prevalence is approximately 10% to 15%, but is as high as 35% among Native Americans living in New Mexico.[65] These differences in prevalence may reflect variations in genetic predisposition, as well as the criteria used for urinary screening and kidney biopsy.

IgA nephropathy is more frequently seen in younger adults and is two to six times more common in males than in females. It is uncommon in blacks, both in the United States and in Africa.[65] IgA nephropathy was once thought to be a benign disease presenting with asymptomatic hematuria; however, its ability to present with any clinical syndrome associated with glomerular disease is now recognized. Some patients will develop ESRD over variable periods of time.

Pathophysiology

Primary IgA nephropathy is an immune-complex–mediated disease in which IgA deposits and other pathologic lesions are found in kidney tissues. In contrast, Henoch-Schönlein purpura, a systemic disease that is believed to be closely linked to IgA nephropathy, shares similar immunohistologic findings in the kidneys. Both typically have vasculitis affecting the joints, skin, and gastrointestinal tract, which may result from the same pathologic process of IgA nephropathy. The diagnosis of IgA nephropathy is established by the presence of mesangial IgA deposits upon immunofluorescence examination of the kidney biopsy. The IgA immune complex, composed of IgA antibody bound with an environmental antigen, such as a virus, bacteria, or food substances, is presumed to be deposited from the systemic circulation. Alternately, the complex may be formed in situ, with the IgA antibody bound with an endogenous antigen in the mesangium. In the mesangium, IgA can bind with receptors on the mesangial cells to induce proliferation and cytokine production. In addition, it can activate complement through the alternate pathway to induce glomerular damage.[66] The extent of the injury depends on the characteristics of the IgA that favor mesangial deposition, the susceptibility of the mesangium toward deposition, the ability to mount an inflammatory response to the deposits, and the response of the kidney to the injury in a way that favors progressive renal damage.[67]

Clinical Presentation

IgA nephropathy commonly presents in the second and third decades of life, but it can occur at any age. Many patients have microscopic hematuria and proteinuria for years, persistently or intermittently, during the early stages of the disease. About half of the patients present with gross hematuria concurrent with an infection, commonly in the upper respiratory tract.[65] The hematuria may occur 1 to 2 days after the onset of infection symptoms, which is different from the 10- to 14-day delay seen after the pharyngitis in poststreptococcal glomerulonephritis. Proteinuria is common and nephrotic range often indicates advanced disease. Hypertension and edema are infrequent but are common in poststreptococcal glomerulonephritis.

Renal dysfunction is uncommon at the initial presentation; however, approximately 10% to 20% of the patients develop ESRD within 10 years, and 30% develop it after 20 years.[68] Hypertension, severe proteinuria, renal function impairment, old age, and the severity of histologic lesions are all predictive factors for poor long-term outcome.[66–68]

TREATMENT

Immunoglobulin A Nephropathy

Spontaneous remission is seen in only 10% to 25% of children and 5% to 7.5% of adults. Unfortunately, no therapy is known to be consistently effective for the treatment of IgA nephropathy. Because of the slow progression of the disease to ESRD, it is very difficult to conduct trials to evaluate the long-term effectiveness of specific treatments. The lack of understanding of the pathogenetic mechanisms and the unavailability of appropriate animal models severely limit the development of rational treatment regimens.

NONPHARMACOLOGIC THERAPY: LOW-GLUTEN DIET AND TONSILLECTOMY

Restriction of dietary gluten is effective in patients with celiac disease, but not in patients with no identifiable nephritogenic antigens.[69] Removal of the tonsils, which produce IgA_1 and may contribute to IgA nephropathy, may reduce proteinuria and hematuria. This is especially helpful in patients who developed recurrent macroscopic hematuria as provoked by bacterial tonsillitis. There are limited studies to show the long-term renoprotective effects of tonsillectomy; however, larger studies with longer followup are needed to affirm such beneficial effect.[67]

PHENYTOIN

Phenytoin was evaluated because of its ability to reduce the amount of polymeric IgA in the circulation.[69] Although it reduced serum IgA concentrations and frequency of macroscopic hematuria, the glomerular lesions deteriorated in some of the patients and the drug is not generally used nowadays.

CORTICOSTEROIDS

Corticosteroids with or without immunosuppressive agents have been used to treat IgA nephropathy for many years. A recent meta-analysis of available trials showed that steroid therapy is associated with reduction in proteinuria, risk for progression to ESRD, as well as the rate of renal function deterioration.[70] Low-dose, short-term (<3 months) steroid therapy is not expected to yield favorable results. In contrast, larger doses of steroids (IV methylprednisolone 1g/day for 3 days at months 1, 3, and 5, and oral prednisone 0.5 mg/kg every other day for 6 months) were able to reduce proteinuria and renal function deterioration.[71] However, the dose of the steroids and the risk for toxicity might be considered high by many.[67] Patients with nephrotic range proteinuria and impaired renal function are likely candidates for steroid therapy; however, the responses to such treatment are not favorable.

CYTOTOXIC AGENTS

Several studies have evaluated the efficacy of azathioprine and cyclophosphamide. In some of the studies, cyclophosphamide was used in conjunction with dipyridamole, heparin and warfarin. It is difficult to assess which of these agents contributed to the limited favorable effects observed. In addition, in many of these studies, blood pressure control and ACE inhibition were not always optimal. At present, there is no clear evidence to support the use of these cytotoxic agents for IgA nephropathy, except perhaps for those patients with advanced rapidly progressive disease.[67]

FISH OIL

The third approach is to reduce glomerular inflammation and glomerulosclerosis induced by IgA deposits. Antiinflammatory agents, antiplatelet drugs, and anticoagulants have been tried without success to decrease the production or action of mediators responsible for IgA immune complex-induced glomerular damage. However, the *n*-3 fatty acids in fish oil reduce the production or action of prostaglandins and leukotrienes, thus limiting the renal damage caused by inflammation, platelet aggregation, and vasoconstriction.[24] In a controlled trial on patients with heavy proteinuria and mildly impaired renal function, daily use of fish oil delayed the progression of renal failure with modest reduction in proteinuria.[72] A meta-analysis of five controlled studies indicated that a minor, but not statistically significant, beneficial effect on renal function may be observed.[73] Results from several recent studies failed to confirm the beneficial effects reported earlier and further studies are needed to confirm the role as well as the optimal dose. In many of the studies, 4 to 12 g/day was given for 2 or more years. Some of the fish oil preparations are rich in cholesterol; thus it is appropriate to monitor the LDL cholesterol levels in patients receiving therapy.

ANGIOTENSIN-CONVERTING ENZYME INHIBITION

Because hypertension is a negative prognostic indicator of IgA nephropathy and many of these patients already have left ventricular diastolic malfunction despite being normotensive, early antihypertensive intervention with ACEIs or ARBs is important.[65,66] If a single agent is insufficient to reduce proteinuria and maintain blood pressure at 125/75 mm Hg, combined use of ACEI and ARB should be instituted.[67]

ALTERNATIVE THERAPEUTIC APPROACHES

Patients with IgA nephropathy have abnormal production of IgA and several different immunoglobulins. Immunoglobulins, administered intravenously initially and then intramuscularly, may have beneficial effects through immunomodulation, increased catabolism of autoantibodies, and blockade of receptors.[74] The doses in this experimental trial, which has not been independently replicated, were very high: 1 g/kg/day × 2 days IV every month × 3, then 0.35 mL/kg IM every 15 days × 6 months. Plasmapheresis with albumin replacement was performed before the 2- to 12-hour IV infusions to avoid serum sickness. Reduction in proteinuria, hematuria, GFR decline, and histologic activity index were observed in 11 patients with a progressive course of the disease. Renal survival was prolonged in eight of these patients who were followed for 3 to 10 years.[75] Larger, randomized, controlled trials are needed before one can recommend this regimen with confidence.

Urokinase, danazol, dapsone, sodium cromoglycate, and plasma exchange have also been evaluated, but none is consistently effective nor shown to affect renal function.[68,74] Cyclosporine treatment was found in a limited number of studies to reduce proteinuria; however, renal function decreased during treatment. Consequently, its use is limited by the potential for nephrotoxicity.[24,74]

The HMG-CoA reductase inhibitor fluvastatin was reported to reduce urinary protein excretion in moderately proteinuric (0.6 to 1.6 g/day) patients who had IgA nephropathy with normal renal function.[76] Creatinine clearance remained stable during the 6-month study. Although longer-term evaluation in a larger patient population is needed to confirm this beneficial effect, statin use is an obvious choice for hyperlipidemic patients with IgA.

Antiplatelet agents are commonly used in Japan and rarely outside of Asia for IgA nephropathy.[77] A recent meta-analysis of seven trials (four in Japan and three in Hong Kong) revealed that these agents reduced proteinuria and stabilized renal function.[78] Mycophenolate mofetil and several new strategies are being evaluated as experimental treatments for IgA nephropathy on the premise that they may reduce IgA synthesis and mesangial uptake and/or suppress the effects of proinflammatory or profibrogenic mediators.[78]

TREATMENT ALGORITHM

Normotensive patients with normal renal function, isolated microhematuria, and proteinuria less than 1 g/day should be observed closely without specific treatment.[66] It has been suggested that patients with minimal proteinuria of 0.5 to 1 g/day receive fish oil and an ACE inhibitor (ACEI) or ARB (Fig. 50–6).[24] Because corticosteroids reduce proteinuria, a course of alternate-day prednisone

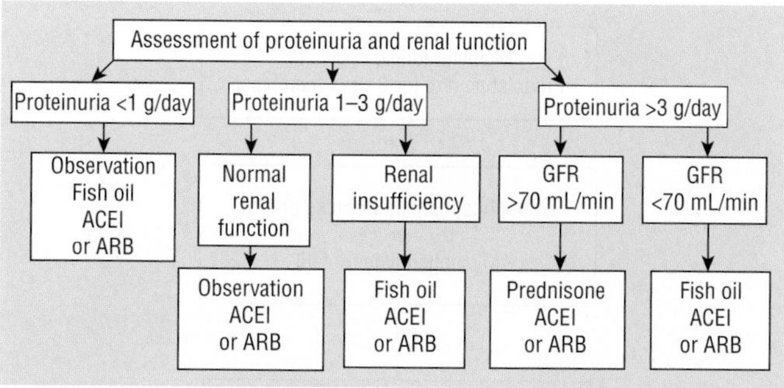

FIGURE 50-6. Treatment algorithm for biopsy-proven IgA nephropathy. (ACE, angiotensin-converting enzyme; GFR, glomerular filtration rate.) *(Modified from reference 68.)*

(1 mg/kg/day) with subsequent tapering is indicated for patients with proteinuria greater than 3 g/day who have good renal function (>70 mL/min).[68] A more aggressive IV or oral steroid regimen may be considered, even though its efficacy has not been definitively established. For patients with a slow progressive decline in creatinine clearance (<70 mL/min), fish oil should be given. Azathioprine, cyclophosphamide, mycophenolate mofetil, or dipyridamole/warfarin therapy may also be used, although the efficacy of these agents has not been established. If the patient experiences rapid GFR decline of more than 2 mL/min per month, immunoglobulin therapy may be considered despite the fact that only limited data are available. Other therapies that may be considered for these patients include pulse steroids, a cyclophosphamide–steroid combination, mycophenolate mofetil, and plasmapheresis.[24,66,68,79]

■ THERAPEUTIC OUTCOMES

Urinary protein excretion and the mean arterial blood pressure at followup correlate well with the progression of disease. The risk of developing ESRD is proportional to the amount of proteinuria, under the influence of ACEI and ARB therapy, after 1 year of followup.[80] For those patients who develop end-stage renal failure, transplantation is appropriate, especially for young adults. Recurrence of IgA mesangial deposits in the renal allograft may occur in up to 50% of patients in 5 years and be universally present at 10 years or more posttransplant, but the recurrence of clinical disease is only approximately 10% to 15%.[65,66] There is also no correlation between the aggressiveness of the primary disease and the rate of recurrence.[65] Immunosuppression using corticosteroids, azathioprine, and/or cyclosporine is not expected to prevent the recurrent nephropathy.

LUPUS NEPHRITIS

Etiology and Epidemiology

Glomerulonephritis is one of the most serious complications of systemic lupus erythematosus (SLE) and accounts for much of the morbidity and mortality of patients afflicted with the disease. SLE predominantly affects young women between 15 and 40 years of age, with an incidence of 1 in 2,000 women in the United States. African Americans are more susceptible; they develop the disease at a younger age, have nephritis earlier in the course and are more likely to progress to end-stage kidney disease.

The renal manifestations of lupus nephritis are variable and encompass a wide spectrum of histopathologic lesions.[81] The underlying histopathology is associated with different prognoses and responses to therapy, which cannot be predicted solely based on clinical manifestations. Thus, a renal biopsy is required to assess the severity of the disease and to predict the short-term and long-term outcomes associated with therapy. Drugs, such as hydralazine and procainamide, are known to precipitate a lupus syndrome; however, they are unlikely to cause disease that affects the kidney.

Pathophysiology

Immune complex deposits, whether formed in the circulation or in situ, can be found in various regions of the glomerulus, as well as the peritubular interstitium and vasculature outside the glomerulus. Based on light, immunofluorescence, and electron microscopy findings, lupus nephritis can be categorized into six World Health Organization (WHO) classes: I—normal; II—mesangial; III—focal proliferative; IV—diffuse proliferative; V—membranous; and VI—advanced sclerosing.[82] In an attempt to enhance the predictive values of the histologic findings, semiquantitative assessments of active lesions and sclerotic changes are used to determine activity index and chronicity index, respectively. In 2003, the ISN/RPS (International Society of Nephrology/Renal Pathology Society) classification was developed to reduce interobserver reproducibility and provide a practical and standardized approach to biopsy interpretation so that outcome data can be compared worldwide.[83]

The hallmark feature in the pathogenesis of SLE is B-cell hyperactivity and the dysregulated production of autoantibodies against multiple antigens in the body, including DNA and various ribonucleoproteins.[81,84] The size and location of the immune complexes in the glomerulus correlate with the nature and severity of renal injury. Deposition of small numbers of stable immune complexes of intermediate size in the mesangium tends to produce less-severe inflammation in the glomerulus. The sequestration of the immune complexes in the mesangium prevents them from activating inflammatory mediators. Hence, the lesion is noninflammatory in nature. In contrast, large numbers of intermediate-sized or large immune complexes result in infiltration of inflammatory cells and release of necrotizing enzymes.

Clinical Presentation

Females have a higher risk for developing lupus, especially in the adult years. Nephritis is commonly seen within the first 4 years of diagnosis of SLE, but may also be the first manifestation of the disease. The clinical presentation ranges from minimal hematuria and proteinuria to severe, rapidly progressive diffuse glomerulonephritis. Proteinuria is very common and nephrotic syndrome is seen in most patients with membranous lesions. Microscopic hematuria is almost always present, whereas macroscopic hematuria, which commonly indicates severe renal involvement, is rare.[82] Active urinary sediments (red cell casts, dysmorphic red cells, and hematuria) are suggestive of the diffuse proliferative lesion.[81] Hypertension is present in 25% to 45% of patients, and is associated with a worse prognosis. Other conditions found to be associated with poor prognosis include elevated serum creatinine concentration, heavy proteinuria, anemia (hematocrit <26%), black race, and disease onset during childhood or in those >60 years of age. Most patients have hypocomplementemia and increased antibody titers for anti–double-stranded DNA, particularly those with focal or diffuse proliferative lesions. Serum creatinine concentration at the time of diagnosis is most predictive of short-term outcome.

TREATMENT

Lupus Nephritis

❼ The choice of therapy depends on the underlying lesion and the activity, as well as the chronicity indices. Acute life-threatening disease involving multiple organs requires induction treatment that can suppress the disease promptly. In contrast, long-term management of chronic indolent disease requires therapy with more acceptable side-effect profiles. Corticosteroids are the cornerstone of therapy. However, for severe lupus nephritis, primarily the diffuse proliferative type, alkylating agents may be needed to reduce or prevent the progression to ESRD. Newer alternatives with fewer side effects are now available.

Optimal blood pressure control is important. ACE inhibitor or ARB has been shown to reduce proteinuria. Patients with normal renal function and less than 2 g of proteinuria usually do not require therapy, except for the management of extrarenal lupus manifestations. The prognosis of these patients is generally good and renal biopsy can be delayed. However, close followup of renal function and urinalysis is required.

■ ACUTE INDUCTION TREATMENT

Steroids and Cytotoxic Agents

Patients with more than 2 g of proteinuria, deteriorating renal function, and/or active urinary sediments require a renal biopsy to define the underlying lesion and determine the activity and chronicity of disease. Patients with proliferative lesions, class IV and class III with subendothelial deposits and signs of severe disease activity, should be treated with pulse intravenous methylprednisolone followed by low-dose oral steroids. Cyclophosphamide is used concurrently because it is a powerful B-cell inhibitor and can suppress the resynthesis of autoantibodies to normal levels.[82] Combined use of intravenous cyclophosphamide and methylprednisolone is more effective than either agent alone in inducing remission.[84,85] Cyclophosphamide is given orally in some of the regimens.[86] Azathioprine has also been used in conjunction with cyclophosphamide. The risk for adverse events, such as infection, gonadal damage, amenorrhea, and cervical dysplasia, and malignancy is increased with the cytotoxic regimens.[84] Studies show that cyclophosphamide toxicities may be related to the cumulative doses rather than the route of administration.[86] Because oral doses of cyclophosphamide tend to accrue easily, it is prudent to use it only for those who are high risk and had failed other therapies.

Mycophenolate Mofetil

Several trials have found that mycophenolate mofetil with concurrent steroid therapy is an effective agent for induction therapy. It was as effective as cyclophosphamide in inducing remission but with fewer side effects. Many of these trials were conducted in Asia and may not reflect the American patient population. However, two recent trials that included African Americans, who are at risk for poorer prognosis, also show that mycophenolate mofetil was more efficacious than intravenous cyclophosphamide and resulted in fewer adverse effects.[84,87] Based on the recently available data, mycophenolate mofetil seems to be a viable alternative to cyclophosphamide; however, the duration of followup in these trials was not as long as the trials that were conducted to establish the efficacy of cyclophosphamide-based regimens. The ability of mycophenolate mofetil to sustain the remission long-term is still unclear (Fig. 50–7).

■ CHRONIC MAINTENANCE TREATMENT

Steroids and Cytotoxic Agents

Oral steroid is most frequently used for maintenance treatment (prednisolone 5 to 15 mg/day or equivalent).[82] Alternate-day regimens, although not evaluated, are often used in children to minimize growth retardation. Monthly pulse IV steroids in conjunction with cyclophosphamide resulted in more sustained remission, fewer relapses, and no significant increase in side effects.[88] Meta-analysis shows this combination to be more beneficial than steroid or cyclophosphamide alone. Cyclophosphamide, because of its bladder and gonadal toxicity, has been given as monthly and then bimonthly

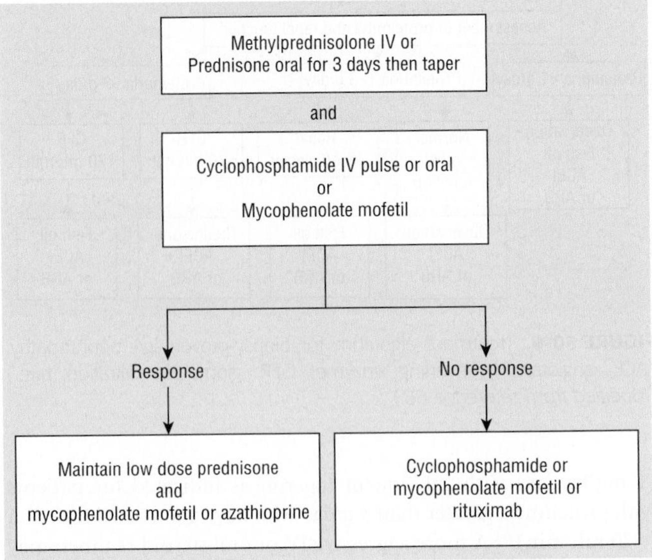

FIGURE 50-7. Treatment algorithm for proliferative lupus nephritis.

intravenous injection, instead of daily administration, for 2 or more years. However, toxicity is still a concern. A study conducted in Europe showed that after initial lower pulse doses of IV cyclophosphamide, oral azathioprine was able to attain remission rates similar to those of higher initial pulse doses of cyclophosphamide with quarterly followup doses.[89] Recently, daily doses of mycophenolate mofetil or azathioprine for 2 years have been shown to be more effective than intravenous pulses of cyclophosphamide in reducing relapse while being less toxic.[90]

Cyclosporine

Cyclosporine may reduce proteinuria and lupus activity, stabilize renal function, and improve kidney morphology. However, flares of disease activity may occur when the drug is discontinued or the dosage tapered. Nephrotoxicity is also a concern after prolonged use.

■ ALTERNATIVE THERAPEUTIC AGENTS

Many new agents have been developed to target the various pathways, costimulatory molecules, and immune mediators responsible for the pathologic autoantibody production.

LJP-394 (Riquent, abetimus sodium), composed of four double-stranded oligodeoxynucleotides, render specific B lymphocytes unresponsive to immunogen by cross-linking with the surface immunoglobulin receptors, thereby reducing anti-DNA antibody production. It may reduce renal and systemic SLE flares in a subgroup of patients whose anti-DNA antibodies are bound avidly to the compound.[91] However, a subsequent study did not reveal such a beneficial effect when compared with placebo.[84]

Rituximab is a monoclonal antibody directed against CD20, which is a membrane-associated glycoprotein on B lymphocytes. It causes B-lymphocyte depletion without affecting plasma cells, which do not have CD20. In patients, the B-cell depletion correlates with clinical response. However, the studies available are uncontrolled and different regimens were used in heterogenous groups of patients.[84] Results from ongoing randomized trials are needed to confirm its efficacy. Studies are also underway to evaluate epratuzumab (anti-CD22).

Disruption of communication between B and T cells can result in reduced autoimmune response. Different anti-CD40 ligand monoclonal antibodies, such as BG9588 (ruplizumab) and IDEC-131, have been evaluated; however, they were not found to be useful because of life-threatening thromboembolic complications.[92]

TREATMENT OUTCOME

The prognosis of patients with class II disease is generally good and often no specific treatment is needed. In patients with class V disease, steroids alone commonly induce partial or complete remission. Immunosuppressive agents can be used for those who are not responsive to steroids. The survival of patients with classes III and IV disease has improved during the last two to three decades to approximately 74% to 80% at 10 years.[81] With the recent use of mycophenolate mofetil, better understanding of the optimal cytotoxic regimens, the use of lower steroid dosages, and better management of complications such as hypertension, infections, hyperlipidemia, and other metabolic complications of the disease, the long-term outcome has became more favorable. Lupus patients with end-stage kidney disease on dialysis fare as well as those with non–lupus-related renal disease. In those patients who received a renal transplant, the allograft outcome of patients with lupus nephritis is favorable. Recurrence of lupus in the renal allograft can occur, but is usually of minor clinical importance.

RAPIDLY PROGRESSIVE GLOMERULONEPHRITIS

Etiology and Epidemiology

Rapidly progressive glomerulonephritis (RPGN) describes a clinicopathologic syndrome of rapid loss of renal function—usually a greater than 50% decrement of the glomerular filtration rate within 3 months. The predominant histologic finding of RPGN is extensive crescent formation, usually in more than 50% of the glomeruli. Hence, it is also known as crescentic glomerulonephritis. RPGN accounts for 2% to 7% of all renal biopsy findings, and is responsible for up to 5% of patients with end-stage kidney disease. The age ranges of susceptible patients vary with the type of RPGN. For example, types I and II RPGN are more common in younger patients, whereas type III is seen more frequently in older individuals.

RPGN is not a single disease entity. A variety of glomerulonephritides with or without systemic diseases may present as RPGN, including anti-GBM glomerulonephritis, Goodpasture's syndrome, lupus nephritis, poststreptococcal glomerulonephritis, membranoproliferative glomerulonephritis, IgA nephropathy, polyarteritis nodosa, Wegener's granulomatosis, and idiopathic crescentic glomerulonephritis.

Primary RPGN is categorized according to the immunofluorescence microscopic findings, indicating different immunopathogenesis, therapeutic approaches, and clinical outcome. Type I is characterized by the linear localization of immunoglobulins, mainly IgG, along the GBM, signifying anti-GBM antibody-induced injury. Type II is defined by the coarse granular deposition of immunoglobulins and complement within the capillary walls and mesangium, indicating immune-complex–mediated injury. Type III is characterized by scanty or complete lack of immune complex deposits; consequently, it is also known as pauci-immune RPGN. Circulating ANCAs are often detected in type III RPGN.

Pathophysiology

Different etiologic factors are implicated as the cause of RPGN: toxins, drugs, viral and bacterial infections, neoplasms, autoimmune mechanisms, and various immunogenetic factors.[93] Regardless of the etiology and type of RPGN, damage in the glomerular capillary wall by both humoral and cellular pathways of inflammation is common. Activation of the terminal C5b-9 (membrane-attacking complex) of the complement system produces severe capillary wall injury. Proteinases and reactive oxygen species released by neutrophils and macrophages may result in severe glomerular injury. Platelets and the coagulation system are activated and result in capillary thrombosis. The ruptured capillaries release fibrinogen and procoagulants which may come into contact with thrombogenic tissue debris and lead to fibrinoid changes. In anti-GBM glomerulonephritis, the direct attack of the anti-GBM antibody on the GBM is responsible for the capillary wall injury.[93] In patients with ANCA-associated disease, the interaction of ANCAs with neutrophils and monocytes, which have been primed by concurrent infections or inflammatory processes, can lead to activation of these leukocytes and release of toxic oxygen species and lytic enzymes, resulting in vascular injury.

The disruption of the capillary wall allows movement of macrophages and other plasma constituents into Bowman's space and stimulates the formation of crescents, which are composed mainly of parietal epithelial cells, as well as macrophages and fibroblasts. Crescent formation indicates the severity of the glomerular capillary disease but not its pathogenesis.

Clinical Presentation

Among the crescentic glomerulonephritides, the pauci-immune RPGN (type III) is the most frequent, accounting for more than 50% of cases, whereas the anti-GBM antibody-mediated RPGN (type I) is the least frequent, occurring in roughly 10% to 20% of patients. Of patients with type I RPGN, 60% to 70% may have concurrent pulmonary hemorrhage and Goodpasture's syndrome, which is caused by antibodies directed against the pulmonary alveolar basement membrane. Most patients with immune-complex–mediated RPGN (type II) have collagen vascular disease, systemic infections, or a severe form of primary glomerular disease. Approximately 70% of patients with type III RPGN also present with evidence of systemic vasculitis, such as Wegener's granulomatosis and polyarteritis nodosa. Some patients have only renal manifestations, and are said to have idiopathic crescentic glomerulonephritis or renal vasculitis.

The clinical presentation is dominated by progressive renal insufficiency with complaints of tea-colored urine, malaise, anorexia, low-grade fever, and migratory polyarthropathy. Type I RPGN is more common in younger patients, whereas patients with ANCA-mediated disease tend to be older.[96] Urinalysis commonly shows nephritic sediments with hematuria, erythrocyte casts, and proteinuria. However, overt nephrotic syndrome is rare.

Serologic analysis is very useful in distinguishing the different types of RPGN. The detection of serum anti-GBM antibodies with the appropriate clinical presentation confirms the diagnosis of anti-GBM glomerulonephritis. More than 80% of patients with pauci-immune or idiopathic crescentic glomerulonephritis have circulating ANCAs. ANCAs are autoantibodies specific for the cytoplasmic constituents of neutrophil granules and monocyte lysosomes. Patients with ANCA-associated disease limited to renal involvement often have P-ANCA (perinuclear staining), whereas patients with Wegener's granulomatosis tend to have C-ANCA (cytoplasmic staining). Both the anti-GBM antibody and the ANCAs are absent in patients with type II RPGN. Measurements of circulating immune complexes are not useful for making a specific diagnosis, but detection of specific serum antibodies known to mediate immune complex–associated nephritis is helpful, using anti-DNA antibody as a marker for lupus nephritis and elevated antistreptolysin O titers for poststreptococcal glomerulonephritis.

TREATMENT

Rapidly Progressive Glomerulonephritis

Early aggressive therapy has improved the renal prognosis of patients with crescentic glomerulonephritis. The rapid deterioration of renal function and the paucity of a large number of patients make randomized controlled studies very difficult to conduct. Based on the available data, immunosuppressive therapy alone appears to be ineffective for type I RPGN, while types II and III RPGN respond well to high-dose steroid therapy.[93,94] Regardless of the type of RPGN, poor response to therapy and an ominous renal survival are expected if the patient presents with oliguria, has a serum creatinine concentration greater than 6 or 7 mg/dL, is dialysis dependent, or has a renal biopsy showing advanced chronic parenchymal disease.[95] Because of the differences in response, the therapeutic approaches for each type of RPGN are presented separately below:

■ ANTIGLOMERULAR BASEMENT MEMBRANE GLOMERULONEPHRITIS (TYPE I)

Steroids and cyclophosphamide, in conjunction with plasma exchange, have been used effectively to control the disease. Plasma exchanges remove the pathogenic anti-GBM antibodies in circulation and are conducted for 2 weeks or until the antibodies disappear. Steroids (prednisolone 1 mg/kg/day, tapered over 6 months) and cyclophosphamide (2 to 3 mg/kg/day for 3 months) are then given to prevent new antibody production.[94,96] Patients with mild disease generally respond well to plasma exchange alone or immunosuppression (steroid and/or cytotoxic agents). In patients with severe disease (poor renal function and extensive crescent formation), most are expected to respond to the combination of plasma exchange and steroid/cytotoxic drug therapy. Pulse intravenous administration of corticosteroids (methylprednisolone 30 mg/kg/day for 3 days) has been used successfully to alleviate pulmonary hemorrhage, but the results are not as convincing for glomerulonephritis.[93,94] Because of the rapid decline in renal function, diagnosis should be established early so that therapy can proceed without delay. When the serum creatinine concentration is 6 mg/dL or above, or the patient is oliguric or requires dialysis, the response to therapy is usually poor and the patient should be treated conservatively.[94,96] Poor response should also be expected when crescents are found in more than 85% of the glomeruli.

■ IMMUNE-COMPLEX–MEDIATED GLOMERULONEPHRITIS (TYPE II)

Patients with postinfectious RPGN generally have a favorable prognosis even without treatment. Complete spontaneous recovery occurs in 50% of cases, whereas chronic renal failure develops in 32%.[93] Pulse doses of methylprednisolone (30 mg/kg/day, every other day × 3), followed by oral prednisone (1 mg/kd/day, tapered over several months) and then tapering, are beneficial in type II RPGN, with a response rate of 85% in patients with acute disease and 70% in those with more chronic disease.[93,94] Plasmapheresis does not appear to provide any additional benefit.[94]

■ ANTINEUTROPHIL CYTOPLASMIC AUTOANTIBODY-ASSOCIATED GLOMERULONEPHRITIS (TYPE III)

Combined use of high-dose corticosteroids and cyclophosphamide induces remission in more than 90% of patients.[95] Cyclophosphamide, if given intravenously, is associated with fewer infectious complications while being as effective as the oral route in inducing remission; however, the risk of relapse may be higher.[97] Because approximately 30% of the patients may relapse, cyclophosphamide also has been used for maintenance therapy. Mycophenolate mofetil and methotrexate are now being used and they have been shown in limited studies to be effective.[95,97] Plasmapheresis is not expected to have any additional benefits for patients with mild to moderate disease who are receiving immunosuppressive therapy. However, as an adjunct to immunosuppressive therapy, it may be beneficial for patients with severe disease presenting with acute renal failure, especially those with pulmonary hemorrhage.[97]

■ RENAL TRANSPLANTATION

Anti-GBM nephritis may recur in up to 55% of patients who received a renal transplant. However, only 25% of these patients showed clinical disease activity, with rare allograft failure. Because the frequency of recurrence and its severity are related to the presence of circulating anti-GBM antibody, it is recommended that transplantation should not be performed until the anti-GBM antibody is undetectable for at least 6 to 12 months. The recurrence rate of ANCA-associated nephritis is 17%, with the average time to relapse from transplantation of 31 months.[98]

POSTSTREPTOCOCCAL GLOMERULONEPHRITIS

Etiology and Epidemiology

Poststreptococcal glomerulonephritis (PSGN) and glomerulonephritis caused by other infectious agents, such as bacteria, viruses, and parasites, were once common. Improved sanitation, personal hygiene, medical care, and public health measures helped to decrease the incidence of group A streptococcal infection both in the United States and in other developed countries, resulting in a decline of PSGN. In contrast, glomerulonephritis secondary to other infectious agents, such as hepatitis C and HIV, is seen with increasing frequency.

PSGN is now the most common form of glomerulonephritis in children, but is less common than the other types of glomerulonephritis in adults. PSGN is seen mostly in children aged between 5 and 15 years and is uncommon in children younger than 2 years of age and in adults older than 50 years of age. It normally follows pharyngeal or skin infection caused by the nephritogenic strains of group A streptococci; however, other strains of streptococci, such as groups C and G, have also been reported to cause PSGN. Streptococcal pharyngitis is more common in winter and early spring, whereas skin infection is frequently found in the summer. The risk for developing acute glomerulonephritis secondary to the nephritogenic strains of bacteria is approximately 10% to 15% in infected patients. However, three to four times more patients may experience a subclinical form of the disease.

Pathophysiology

Streptococcal antigens may induce changes in the glomerular components rendering them immunogenic or autologous IgG may be altered to become antigenic. Alternately, the streptococcal antigens may induce antibodies that react with glomerular antigens. In situ immune complexes are then formed and result in a complement-mediated inflammatory response. The kinin and coagulation cascades are activated and chemotactic factors are released to recruit neutrophils and monocytes, resulting in acute glomerular lesions.

Examination of the acute PSGN kidneys reveals hypercellular glomeruli with proliferation of mesangial and endothelial cells. Infiltration of neutrophils, monocytes, and eosinophils is apparent within the capillary lumen and also in the mesangial areas. Crescent formation may be seen in patients with severe disease, and if found in more than 30% of the glomeruli, RPGN may be present concurrently.[99] The prognosis is generally poor for these patients and complete recovery is unlikely. Immunofluorescence examination reveals diffuse granular deposits of IgG and C3 along the glomerular basement membrane and also in the mesangium.

Clinical Presentation

The nephritis is preceded by a latent period following a streptococcal infection. The latent period is commonly 7 to 14 days for pharyngitis and 14 to 28 days for skin infection. An acute nephritic syndrome then develops, commonly with hematuria and edema.

Gross hematuria is seen in 70% of patients, and microscopic hematuria can be found in all patients. Hypertension is usually mild to moderate and results from sodium and water retention. Many patients have signs and symptoms associated with volume overload, which include dyspnea, orthopnea, and cough. Urinalysis of patients with PSGN reveals hematuria, dysmorphic red blood cells, and red cell casts. Proteinuria is common, but often not in the nephrotic range. Renal function is frequently mildly impaired.

Throat or skin culture may be positive for group A streptococci, despite the latent period following the initial infection. However, antibiotic therapy may render the culture result negative. Serologic measurements of antibodies to different streptococcal antigens can confirm recent exposure to the infection. Titers that can be measured include antistreptolysin O (ASO), antistreptokinase, antihyaluronidase (AHase), antideoxyribonuclease B (ADNase B), and antinicotyladenine dinucleotidase (NADase).[100] In most patients with streptococcal pharyngitis, the ASO titers begin to rise about 10 to 14 days later, peak at 3 to 4 weeks, and persist for several months before decreasing. The rise in ASO titers can be reduced by antibiotic treatment and may not be seen in patients with streptococcal skin infection in whom the streptolysin may be bound to skin lipids. ADNase B and AHase titers should be used instead because they are specific and are positive in the majority of patients. The streptozyme test is a combined assay for ASO, ADNase B, NADase, and AHase. Antibodies to other antigens such as zymogen, streptococcal cationic proteinase exotoxin B (SPEB), and plasmin receptor (Plr), were evaluated recently.[101]

Serum complement levels are often decreased in patients with PSGN. If the C3 level is depressed for more than 6 to 8 weeks, MPGN, lupus nephritis, or glomerulonephritis related to endocarditis or occult visceral abscess should be suspected. Renal biopsy is not normally indicated unless the patient has prolonged hematuria, proteinuria, or depressed C3 level. Renal biopsy is needed to detect other types of glomerulonephritis such as lupus, RPGN, or MPGN.

TREATMENT

Poststreptococcal Glomerulonephritis

8 The treatment of PSGN is mainly supportive and symptomatic. Early antibiotic therapy does not prevent subsequent PSGN, but it may reduce the severity of the disease. It can, however, prevent the spread of the streptococcal infection to other family members. Antibiotic prophylaxis is not recommended because infected patients will develop long-lasting, often lifelong immunity against the strain of streptococci. Exposure to another nephritogenic strain of streptococci is possible, but unlikely.

Supportive measures, as discussed earlier in this chapter, should be used to control fluid volume and blood pressure. Because the hypertension is of the low-renin type, ACEIs and β-blockers are not expected to be useful. If the patient has crescentic disease, use of pulse steroids and/or immunosuppressive agents can be considered; however, the efficacy and safety of these agents have not been established for this condition.

The acute manifestations of PSGN are normally self-limited, and for more than 95% of patients renal function has returned to baseline within 3 to 6 weeks. Diuresis usually begins 7 to 10 days after onset of the acute episode, whereas hypertension and azotemia resolve in 1 to 2 weeks. Gross hematuria lasts for 1 to 2 weeks and proteinuria usually resolves within 6 months in more than 90% of children. However, microscopic hematuria may persist for up to 2 years. In general, children have more rapid recovery than adults. Prognosis is often better when PSGN occurs during an epidemic than in cases found sporadically. Most of the children will recover fully and be free from chronic complications of PSGN if they have no preexisting renal disorder, heavy proteinuria, or crescentic glomerular lesions, or did not require hospitalization during the acute episode. In contrast, adult patients have a less-favorable long-term outcome. As many as 50% of the patients may develop persistent proteinuria, hypertension, and renal insufficiency, with some resulting in end-stage renal failure.

PHARMACOECONOMIC CONSIDERATIONS

Prospective, randomized, controlled comparative trials need to be conducted in a sizable patient population before the efficacy and economic implications of a new regimen can be established. This type of large-scale study is potentially feasible for the more common forms of glomerulonephritis, such as minimal-change disease, IgA nephropathy, and membranous nephropathy. In contrast, prospective controlled trials are difficult to conduct for the relatively uncommon glomerulonephritides such as membranous proliferative glomerulonephritis. After defining the natural history and the optimal drug regimen for each glomerulonephritis, in conjunction with the incidence of drug-induced complications, the economic implications of the individual treatment approach can be assessed. However, the optimal approaches for treating most types of glomerulonephritis have not been identified and the economic implications of the individual treatment regimens thus remain to be established.

CONCLUSIONS

A better understanding of the pathogenetic mechanisms leading to glomerular injury has improved the treatment of glomerulonephritis. However, the glomerulopathies are a heterogeneous group of immune disorders with different clinical courses, prognoses, and responses to current immunologic and nonimmunologic therapies. The clinician should understand the natural history and prognosis of each subgroup of glomerulonephritis, the efficacy of different immunomodulating regimens in inducing disease remission and preserving renal function, and the characteristics of at-risk patients who warrant aggressive therapy. Judicious use of immunosuppressive agents with careful monitoring of their adverse effects cannot be overemphasized. In addition, treatment of the disease complications and control of factors that lead to progression of renal disease are important in reducing the morbidity and mortality of patients with glomerulonephritis.

ABBREVIATIONS

ACE: angiotensin-converting enzyme

ADNase B: antideoxyribonuclease B

AHase: antihyaluronidase

ANCA: antineutrophil cytoplasmic autoantibody

ARB: angiotensin II receptor blocker

ASO: antistreptolysin O

ESRD: end-stage renal disease

GBM: glomerular basement membrane

GFR: glomerular filtration rate

FSGS: focal segmental glomerulosclerosis

HIV: human immunodeficiency virus

HMG-CoA: hydroxymethylglutaryl coenzyme A (reductase)

IL: interleukin

LDL: low-density lipoprotein (cholesterol)

MPGN: membranoproliferative glomerulonephritis

NADase: antinicotyladenine dinucleotidase
PSGN: poststreptococcal glomerulonephritis
RPGN: rapidly progressive glomerulonephritis
SLE: systemic lupus erythematosus
VLDL: very-low-density lipoprotein (cholesterol)
WHO: World Health Organization

REFERENCES

1. U.S. Renal Data System 2006 Annual Data Report. Minneapolis, MN: USRDS Coordinating Center. 2006, *http://www.usrds.org*.
2. Schena FP, Gesualdo L, Grandaliano G, Montinaro V. Progression of renal damage in human glomerulonephritides: Is there sleight of hand in winning the game? Kidney Int 1997;52:1439–1457.
3. Couser WG. Mediation of immune glomerular injury. J Am Soc Nephrol 1990;1:13–29.
4. Remuzzi G, Zoja C, Perico N. Proinflammatory mediators of glomerular injury and mechanisms of activation of autoreactive T cells. Kidney Int Suppl 1994;44:S8–S16.
5. Humphreys MH. Mechanisms and management of nephrotic edema. Kidney Int 1994;45:266–281.
6. Schrier RW, Fassett RG. A critique of the overfill hypothesis of sodium and water retention in the nephrotic syndrome. Kidney Int 1998;53:1111–1117.
7. Warwick GL, Fox JG, Boulton-Jones JM. The relationship between urinary albumin excretion rate and serum cholesterol in primary glomerular disease. Clin Nephrol 1994;41:135–137.
8. Wheeler DC, Bernard DB. Lipid abnormalities in the nephrotic syndrome: Causes, consequences, and treatment. Am J Kidney Dis 1994;23:331–346.
9. Kaysen GA, De Sain-van der Verlden M. New insights into lipid metabolism in the nephrotic syndrome. Kidney Int Suppl 1999;71:S18–S21.
10. Nachman PH, Martin J. Developments in the immunotherapy of glomerular disease. J Pharm Prac 2002;15:472–489.
11. Ponticelli C, Passerini P. Treatment of the nephrotic syndrome associated with primary glomerulonephritis. Kidney Int 1994;46:595–604.
12. Klahr S, Levey A, Beck G, et al. The effects of dietary protein restriction and blood pressure control on the progression of chronic renal disease. N Engl J Med 1994;330:877–884.
13. Orth SR, Stockmann A, Conradt C, et al. Smoking as a risk factor for end-stage renal failure in men with primary renal disease. Kidney Int 1998;54:926–931.
14. Fliser D, Schroter M, Neubeck M. Coadministration of thiazides increases the efficacy of loop diuretics even in patients with advanced renal failure. Kidney Int 1994;46:482–488.
15. Rudy DW, Voelker JR, Greene PK, et al. Loop diuretics for chronic renal insufficiency: A continuous infusion is more efficacious than bolus therapy. Ann Intern Med 1991;115:360–366.
16. Chobanian AV, Bakris GL, Black HR, et al. The seventh report of the joint national committee on prevention, detection, evaluation and treatment of high blood pressure: The JNC 7 report. JAMA 2003;289:2560–2572.
17. Ruggenenti P, Remuzzi G. Is therapy with combined ACE inhibitor and angiotensin receptor antagonist the new gold standard of treatment for nondiabetic, chronic proteinuric nephropathies? NephSAP 2003;2:235–237.
18. Gashti CN, Bakris GL. The role of calcium antagonists in chronic kidney disease. Curr Opin Nephrol Hypertens 2004;18:155–161.
19. Levey AS, Adler S, Caggiula AW, et al. Effects of dietary protein restriction on the progression of advanced renal disease in the Modification of Diet in Renal Disease Study. Am J Kidney Dis 1996;27:652–663.
20. Toto R. Proteinuria reduction: Mandatory consideration or option when selecting an antihypertensive agent? Curr Hypertens Rep 2005;7:374–378.
21. The GISEN group (Gruppo Italiano di Studi Epidemiologici in Nefrologia). Randomized placebo-controlled trial effect of ramipril on decline in glomerular filtration rate and risk of terminal renal failure in proteinuric, non-diabetic nephropathy. Lancet 1997;349:1857–1863.
22. Jefferson JA, Shank SJ. Glomerular disease: The podocyte is ready for prime time and may already be center stage. NephSAP 2006;331–338.
23. Vogt L, Navis G, de Zeeuw D. Renoprotection: A matter of blood pressure reduction or agent-characteristics? J Am Soc Nephrol 2002;13(Suppl 3):S202–S207.
24. Alexopoulos E. Treatment of primary IgA nephropathy. Kidney Int 2004;65:341–355.
25. Combination treatment of angiotensin-II receptor blocker and angiotensin-converting-enzyme inhibitor in non-diabetic renal disease (COOPERATE): A randomized controlled trial. Lancet 2003;361:117–124.
26. Taal MV, Brenner BM. Combination ACEI and ARB therapy: Additional benefit in renoprotection? Curr Opin Nephrol Hypertens 2002;11:377–381.
27. Perico N, Remuzzi A, Sangalli F, et al. The antiproteinuric antagonism in human IgA nephropathy is potentiated by indomethacin. J Am Soc Nephrol 1998;9:2308–2317.
28. Oda H, Keane WF. Recent advances in statins and the kidney. Kidney Int Suppl 1999;71:S2–S5.
29. Tonelli M, Moyé L, Sacks FM. Effect of pravastatin on loss of renal function in people with moderate chronic renal insufficiency and cardiovascular disease. J Am Soc Nephrol 2003;14:1605–1613.
30. Agarwal R. Effects of statins on renal function. Am J Cardiol 2006;97:748–755.
31. Sarasin FP, Schifferli JA. Prophylactic oral anticoagulation in nephrotic patients with idiopathic membranous nephropathy. Kidney Int 1994;45:578–585.
32. Nolasco F, Cameron JS, Heywood EF, et al. Adult-onset minimal-change nephrotic syndrome: A long-term follow-up. Kidney Int 1986;29:1215–1223.
33. Jennette JC, Mandal AK. The nephrotic syndrome. In: Mandal AK, Jennette JC, eds. Diagnosis and Management of Renal Disease and Hypertension, 2nd ed. Durham, NC: Carolina Academic Press, 1994:235–272.
34. Bargman JM. Management of minimal lesion glomerulonephritis: Evidence-based recommendations. Kidney Int Suppl 1999;70:S3–S16.
35. Tune BM, Mendoza SA. Treatment of the idiopathic nephrotic syndrome: Regimens and outcomes in children and adults. J Am Soc Nephrol 1997;8:824–832.
36. Niaudel P, Habib R. Cyclosporine in the treatment of idiopathic nephrosis. J Am Soc Nephrol 1994;5:1049–1056.
37. Yoshida M, Yoshikawa N, Akashi M, et al. Lymphocyte drug sensitivity is useful for prediction of the antiproteinuric effect and relapse rate in cyclosporine treatment for frequent-relapse minimal change nephrotic syndrome. Kidney Blood Press Res 2005;28:226–229.
38. Fu LS, Shien CY, Chi CS. Levamisole in steroid-sensitive nephrotic syndrome children with frequent relapses and/or steroid dependency: Comparison of daily and every-other-day usage. Nephron Clin Pract 2004;97:c137–c141.
39. Alsaran K, Grisaru S, Stephens D, et al. Levamisole vs. cyclophosphamide for frequently-relapsing steroid-dependent nephrotic syndrome. Clin Nephrol 2001;56:289–294.
40. Novak I, Frank R, Vento S, et al. Efficacy of mycophenolate mofetil in pediatric patients with steroid-dependent nephrotic syndrome. Pediatr Nephrol 2005;20:1265–1268.
41. Day CJ, Cockwell P, Lipkin GW, et al. Mycophenolate mofetil in the treatment of resistant idiopathic nephrotic syndrome. Nephrol Dial Transplant 2002;17:2011–2013.
42. Korbet SM. Treatment of primary focal segmental glomerulosclerosis. Kidney Int 2002;62:2301–2310.
43. Korbet SM. Primary focal segmental glomerulosclerosis. J Am Soc Nephrol 1998;9:1333–1340.
44. Burgess E. Management of focal segmental glomerulosclerosis: Evidence-based recommendations. Kidney Int Suppl 1999;70:S26–S32.
45. Crook ED, Habeeb D, Gowdy O, et al. Effects of steroids in focal segmental glomerulosclerosis in a predominantly African-American population. Am J Med Sci 2005;330:19–24..
46. Frassinetti Castelo Branco Camurça Fernandes P, Bezerra Da Silva G Jr, De Sousa Barros FA, et al. Treatment of steroid-resistant nephrotic syndrome with cyclosporine: Study of 17 cases and a literature review. J Nephrol 2005;18:711–720.
47. El-Reshaid K, El-Reshaid W, Madda J. Combination of immunosuppressive agents in treatment of steroid-resistant minimal change disease and primary focal segmental glomerulosclerosis. Ren Fail 2005;27:523–530.
48. Cattran DC, Wang GG, Appel GB, et al. Mycophenolate mofetil in the treatment of focal segmental glomerulosclerosis. Clin Nephrol 2004; 62:405–411.

49. Chishti AS, Sorof JM, Brewer ED, et al. Long-term treatment of focal segmental glomerulosclerosis in children with cyclosporine given as a single daily dose. Am J Kidney Dis 2001;38:754–760.
50. Cattran D. Management of membranous nephropathy: When and what for treatment.. J Am Soc Nephrol 2005;16:1188–1194.
51. Geddes CC, Cattran DC. The treatment of idiopathic membranous nephropathy. Semin Nephrol 2000;20:299–308.
52. Ponticelli C, Zucchelli P, Passerini P, et al. A 10-year follow-up of a randomized study with methylprednisolone and chlorambucil in membranous nephropathy. Kidney Int 1995;48:1600–1604.
53. Ponticelli C, Altieri P, Scolari F, et al. A randomized study comparing methylprednisolone plus chlorambucil versus methylprednisolone plus cyclophosphamide in idiopathic membranous nephropathy. J Am Soc Nephrol 1998;9:444–450.
54. Perna A, Schieppati A, Zamora J, et al. Immunosuppressive treatment for idiopathic membranous nephropathy: A systematic review. Am J Kidney Dis 2004;44:385–401.
55. Cattran DC, Greenwood C, Ritchie S, et al. A controlled trial of cyclosporine in patients with progressive membranous nephropathy. Kidney Int 1995;47:1130–1135.
56. Fritsche L, Budde K, Farber L, et al. Treatment of membranous glomerulopathy with cyclosporin A: How much patience is required? Nephrol Dial Transplant 1999;14:1036–1038.
57. Choi MJ, Eustace JA, Gimenez LF. Mycophenolate mofetil treatment for primary glomerular diseases. Kidney Int 2002, 61:1098–1114.
58. Ruggenenti P, Chiurchiu C, Brusegan V, et al. Rituximab in idiopathic membranous nephropathy: A one-year prospective study. J Am Soc Nephrol 2003;14:1851–1857.
59. Appel G, Nachman P, Hogan S, et al. Eculizumab (C5 complement inhibitor) in the treatment of idiopathic membranous nephropathy [abstract]. J Am Soc Nephrol 2002;13:668A.
60. Ponticelli C, Passerini P, Salvadori M, et al. A randomized pilot trial comparing methylprednisolone plus a cytotoxic agent versus synthetic adrenocorticotropic hormone in idiopathic membranous nephropathy. Am J Kidney Dis 2006;47:233–240.
61. Levin A. Management of membranoproliferative glomerulonephritis: Evidence-based recommendations. Kidney Int Suppl 1999;70:S41–S46.
62. Tarshish P, Bernstein J, Tobin JN, et al. Treatment of mesangiocapillary glomerulonephritis with alternate-day prednisone—A report of the International Study of Kidney Disease in Children. Pediatr Nephrol 1992;6:123–130.
63. Appel GB, Cook HT, Hageman G, et al. Membranoproliferative glomerulonephritis type II (dense deposit disease): An update. J Am Soc Nephrol 2005;16:1392–1404.
64. Klein M, Radhakrishnan J, Appel G. Cyclosporine treatment of glomerular diseases. Annu Rev Med 1999;50:1–15.
65. Donadio JV, Grande JP. Immunoglobulin A nephropathy. N Engl J Med 2002;347:738–748.
66. Floege J, Feehally J. IgA nephropathy: Recent developments. J Am Soc Nephrol 2000;11:2395–2403.
67. Barratt J, Feehally J. IgA nephropathy. J Am Soc Nephrol 2005;16:2088–1097.
68. Nolin L, Courteau M. Management of IgA nephropathy: Evidence-based recommendations. Kidney Int Suppl 1999;70:S56–S62.
69. Glassock RJ. The treatment of IgA nephropathy at the end of the millennium. J Nephrol 1999;12:288–296.
70. Samuels JA, Strippoli GF, Craig JC, et al. Immunosuppressive treatments for immunoglobulin A nephropathy: A meta-analysis of randomized controlled trials. Nephrology (Carlton) 2004;9:177–185.
71. Pozzi C, Andrulli S, Del Vecchio L, et al. Corticosteroids effectiveness in IgA nephropathy: Long-term results of a randomized, controlled trial. J Am Soc Nephrol 2004;15:157–163.
72. Donadio JV, Jr., Grande JP, Bergstralh EJ, et al. The long-term outcome of patients with IgA nephropathy treated with fish oil in a controlled trial. Mayo Nephrology Collaborative Group. J Am Soc Nephrol 1999;10:1772–1777.
73. Dillon JJ. Fish oil therapy for IgA nephropathy: Efficacy and interstudy variability. J Am Soc Nephrol 1997;8:1739–1744.
74. Glassock GJ. The treatment of IgA nephropathy: Status at the end of the millennium. J Nephrol 1999;12:288–296.
75. Rasche FM, Keller E, Lepper PM, et al. High-dose intravenous immunoglobulin pulse therapy in patients with progressive immunoglobulin A nephropathy: A long-term follow-up. Clin Exp Immunol 2006;146:47–53.
76. Buemi M, Allegra A, Corica F, et al. Effect of fluvastatin on proteinuria in patients with immunoglobulin A nephropathy. Clin Pharmacol Ther 2000;67:427–431.
77. Taji Y, Kuwahara T, Shikata S, et al. Meta-analysis of antiplatelet therapy for IgA nephropathy. Clin Exp Nephrol 2006;10:268–273.
78. Lai KN. Future directions in the treatment of IgA nephropathy. Nephron 2002;92:263–270.
79. Sanz-Guajardo D. Plasmapheresis in the treatment of glomerulonephritis: Indications and complications. Am J Kidney Dis 2000;36:liv–lvi.
80. Donadio JV, Bergstralh EJ, Grande JP, et al. Proteinuria patterns and their association with subsequent end-stage renal disease in IgA nephropathy. Nephrol Dial Transplant 2002;17:1197–1203.
81. Contreras G, Roth D, Pardo V, et al. Lupus nephritis: A clinical review for practicing nephrologists. Clin Nephrol 2002;57:95–107.
82. Cameron JS. Lupus nephritis. J Am Soc Nephrol 1999;10:413–424.
83. Weening JJ, D'Agati VD, Schwartz MM, et al. The classification of glomerulonephritis in systemic lupus erythematosus revisited. Kidney Int 2004;65:521–530.
84. Waldman M, Appel GB. Update on the treatment of lupus nephritis. Kidney Int 2006;70:1403–1412.
85. Gourley MF, Austin HA, Scott D, et al. Methylprednisolone and cyclophosphamide, alone or in combination, in patients with lupus nephritis. A randomized, controlled trial. Ann Intern Med 1996;125:549–557.
86. Lai KN, Tang SCW, Mok CC. Treatment for lupus nephritis: A revisit. Nephrology (Carlton) 2005;10:180–188.
87. Ginzler EM, Dooley MA, Aranow C, et al. Mycophenolate mofetil or intravenous cyclophosphamide for lupus nephritis. N Engl J Med 2005;353;2219–2228.
88. Illei GG, Austin HA, Crane M, et al. Combination therapy with pulse cyclophosphamide plus pulse methylprednisolone improves long-term renal outcome without adding toxicity in patients with lupus nephritis. Ann Intern Med 2001;135:248–257.
89. Houssiau FA, Vasconcelos C, D'Cruz D, et al. Immunosuppressive therapy in lupus nephritis: The Euro-Lupus Nephritis Trial, a randomized trial of low-dose versus high-dose intravenous cyclophosphamide. Arthritis Rheum 2002;46:2121–2131.
90. Contreras G, Pardo V, Leclercq B, et al. Sequential therapies for proliferative lupus nephritis. N Engl J Med 2004;350:971–980.
91. Alarcon-Segovia D, Tumlin JA, Furie RA, et al. LJP 394 for the prevention of renal flare in patients with systemic lupus erythematosus: Results from a randomized, double-blind, placebo-controlled study. Arthritis Rheum 2003;48:442–454.
92. Boumpas DT, Furie R, Manzi S, et al. A short course of BG9588 (anti-CD40 ligand antibody) improves serologic activity and decreases hematuria in patients with proliferative lupus glomerulonephritis. Arthritis Rheum 2003;48:719–727.
93. Couser WG. Rapidly progressive glomerulonephritis: Classification, pathogenetic mechanisms, and therapy. Am J Kidney Dis 1988;11:449–464.
94. Bolton WK. Treatment of glomerular disease: ANCA-negative RPGN. Semin Nephrol 2000;20:244–255.
95. Jennette JC. Rapidly progressive crescentic glomerulonephritis. Kidney Int 2003;63:1164–1177.
96. Little MA, Pusey CD. Rapidly progressive glomerulonephritis: Current and evolving treatment strategies. J Nephrol 2004;17:10–19.
97. de Groot K, Adu D, Savage CO. The value of pulse cyclophosphamide in ANCA-associated vasculitis: Meta-analysis and critical review. Nephrol Dial Transplant 2001;16:2018–2027.
98. Nachman PH, Segelmark M, Westman K, et al. Recurrent ANCA-associated small-vessel vasculitis after transplantation: A pooled analysis. Kidney Int 1999;56:1544–1550.
99. Couser WG, Johnson RJ. Postinfective glomerulonephritis. In: Neilson EG, Couser WG, eds. Immunologic Renal Diseases, 2nd ed. Philadelphia: Lippincott-Raven, 2001:899–929.
100. Rodriguez-Iturbe B, Parra G. Glomerulonephritis associated with infection: Poststreptococcal glomerulonephritis. In: Massry SG, Glassock RJ, ed. Massry & Glassock's Textbook of Nephrology, 4th ed. Philadelphia: Lippincott Williams & Wilkins, 2001:667–671.
101. Rodriguez-Iturbe B. Nephritis-associated streptococcal antigens: Where are we now? J Am Soc Nephrol 2004;15:1961–1962.

CHAPTER 51

Drug Therapy Individualization for Patients with Renal Insufficiency

GARY R. MATZKE AND REGINALD F. FRYE

KEY CONCEPTS

1. Chronic kidney disease has been demonstrated to result in minimal alterations in the absorption or bioavailability of only a few drugs.
2. The volume of distribution of many drugs is increased in the presence of acute and chronic kidney disease as a consequence of volume expansion and reduced protein binding.
3. In addition to the expected decrement in renal clearance, nonrenal clearance (i.e., gastrointestinal and hepatic drug metabolism) of several drugs is also reduced in patients with chronic kidney disease.
4. Individualization of a drug dosage regimen for a patient with reduced kidney function (RKF) is based on the pharmacodynamic/pharmacokinetic characteristics of the drug and the patient's degree of residual renal function.
5. The drug dosing guidelines for patients with RKF in many drug information resources is highly variable and thus many are ill suited for clinical use.
6. The effect of hemodialysis or peritoneal dialysis on drug elimination is dependent on the characteristics of the drug and the dialysis prescription.
7. The application of dialysis clearance data to guide drug dosage regimen design for hemodialysis patients is limited and prospective monitoring of serum concentrations is warranted.

Patients with chronic kidney disease (CKD) are commonly encountered in clinical practice. Indeed, it is estimated that nearly 15 million people in the United States have serum creatinine values of 1.5 mg/dL or greater.[1] In children, renal function does not mature to reach adult values until one year of age.[2] In older adults, age-related declines in renal function combine with an increased use of medications to make this patient group particularly susceptible to adverse effects secondary to the lack of appropriate pharmacotherapy individualization.[3,4] The presence of reduced kidney function (RKF) in any patient necessitates that the clinician know how and why drug disposition is altered in the presence of CKD and the appropriate methods to individualize drug therapy to maximize therapeutic outcomes.

Learning objectives, review questions, and other resources can be found at **www.pharmacotherapyonline.com.**

CKD is often accompanied by the development of anemia, hyperparathyroidism, bleeding abnormalities, hyperlipidemia, hypertension, and changes in gastrointestinal tract integrity (see Chaps. 46 and 47). Thus CKD patients are often prescribed an extensive array of medications. There are now many reports that document changes in the disposition of some drugs in patients with CKD as the result of changes in bioavailability,[5,6] distribution volume,[7,8] and metabolic activity.[9] Thus some degree of drug therapy individualization is warranted for most patients with CKD. In the simplest situation, a drug that is almost entirely renally eliminated unchanged, a dosage regimen adjustment may be calculated on the basis of the patient's residual creatinine clearance.[10] However, for medications that are extensively metabolized or for which dramatic changes in protein binding and/or distribution volume have been noted, a more complex adjustment strategy may need to be employed.[8,11] Furthermore, because of the physiologic and biochemical changes associated with progressive CKD, patients may respond to a given dose or serum concentration of a drug differently than patients with normal renal function.[5]

Knowledge of basic pharmacokinetic principles combined with the drug disposition properties of a particular compound and the degree and type of pathophysiologic alterations associated with RKF makes it possible for the clinician to design individualized therapeutic regimens to optimize therapeutic outcomes and minimize adverse events. This chapter describes the influence of CKD on drug absorption, distribution, metabolism, and elimination. The array of drug information resources for the adjustment of the dosage regimens for patients with RKF is critiqued. A practical framework for drug dosage individualization for patients with RKF based on continuous versus categorical classifications is presented and the influences of peritoneal dialysis and hemodialysis on drug disposition are discussed. Finally drug administration strategies for those receiving hemodialysis are presented. Chapter 45 discusses drug-dosage-regimen adjustment strategies for patients with acute renal failure, including those who are receiving continuous renal replacement therapy.

EFFECT ON DRUG ABSORPTION

(1) There is little quantitative information regarding the influence of CKD on drug absorption and bioavailability. Changes in gastrointestinal transit time and gastric pH, edema of the gastrointestinal tract, vomiting and diarrhea (frequent complications of severe renal insufficiency), and antacid administration have all been proposed as a rationale for alterations in the bioavailability of drugs in CKD patients. Evaluations of bioavailability are generally conducted in those with severe stable renal insufficiency, that is, stage 5 CKD, which is also called end-stage renal disease (ESRD). The assessment of bioavailability in this patient population is, however, complicated, because most of these patients are prescribed multiple medications (often in excess of 10 to 12 different agents), many of which cannot be discontinued during the course of a bioavailability study.

Some of the drug absorption "bioavailability" studies in ESRD patients were not designed to provide an assessment of absolute bioavailability (i.e., they did not include intravenous administration of the drug). Rather, the principal outcomes were the documentation of alterations in the peak concentration (C_{max}), time at which the peak concentration was attained (t_{max}), or in the fractional amount of drug recovered in the urine in a finite time period. Unfortunately, this limited information has been extrapolated by some into a general conclusion that drug absorption is slowed and/or that the extent of absorption is reduced as the result of the development of CKD.[6]

In fact the absolute bioavailability of only a few drug compounds is affected by ESRD.[5,8] An increase in bioavailability as the result of a decrease in metabolism during the drug's first pass through the gastrointestinal tract and liver has been noted for some β-blockers (i.e., bufuralol, oxprenolol, propranolol, and tolamolol), dextropropoxyphene, and dihydrocodeine.[5,8] Although the bioavailability of these compounds is increased, clinical consequences (development of excessive or unexpected adverse effects) have only been demonstrated with dextropropoxyphene and dihydrocodeine. The lack of association between the altered serum concentration time profile and clinical consequences of the β-blockers may result from an alteration in the responsiveness of patients with renal disease to these agents, as has been reported with propranolol in the elderly.[3]

EFFECT ON DRUG DISTRIBUTION

The volume of distribution of many drugs is increased in patients with moderate to severe CKD as well as those with preexisting CKD who develop acute renal failure (Table 51–1).[8,12,13] An increase in distribution volume may result from decreased protein binding, increased tissue binding, or pathophysiologic alterations in body composition (e.g., the fractional contribution of total-body water to total-body weight).

Generally, the plasma protein binding of acidic drugs (e.g., warfarin and phenytoin) is decreased in those with ESRD,[7,14] whereas the binding of basic drugs (e.g., quinidine and lidocaine) is usually normal or only slightly decreased or increased (Table 51–2).[7,15,16] The decrease in binding of acidic drugs has been attributed to qualitative changes in the binding sites, accumulation of endogenous inhibitors of binding, and decreased concentrations of albumin. The first two of these mechanisms appear to account for most of the observed changes in binding. In addition, the high concentrations of metabolites of some compounds that accumulate in patients with ESRD may interfere with the protein binding of the parent compound.

❷ As a result of the decrease in protein binding, the unbound fraction of many acidic drugs increases in CKD patients. A new equilibrium is ultimately established as a result of increased drug elimination/distribution, such that the unbound concentrations remain comparable despite the fact that total concentrations are reduced. Thus the net effect of changes in protein binding is an alteration in the relationship between total drug concentration and pharmacodynamic effect. This can be illustrated with the anticonvulsant phenytoin. The protein binding of this acidic drug, which binds to albumin, is significantly reduced as a result of endogenous substances that accumulate in patients with renal failure and compete for binding, as well as by conformational changes in albumin in CKD patients.[17] This change in protein binding alters the relationship between total phenytoin concentration and effect or toxicity. The resulting increase in unbound fraction, from the normal of 10% to ~20% or more, results in increased hepatic clearance and decreased total concentrations. Thus in patients with CKD, the therapeutic range based on total phenytoin concentration is shifted downward from normal values of 10 to 20 mg/L as the degree of residual renal

TABLE 51-1 Volume of Distribution of Selected Drugs in Patients with End-Stage Renal Disease

Drug	Normal (L/kg)	ESRD (L/kg)	Change from Normal (%)
Increased			
Amikacin	0.20	0.29	45
Azlocillin	0.21	0.28	33
Cefazolin	0.13	0.17	31
Cefoxitin	0.16	0.26	63
Cefuroxime	0.20	0.26	30
Clofibrate	0.14	0.24	71
Dicloxacillin	0.08	0.18	125
Erythromycin	0.57	1.09	91
Furosemide	0.11	0.18	64
Gentamicin	0.20	0.32	60
Isoniazid	0.6	0.8	33
Minoxidil	2.6	4.9	88
Nalmefene	7.9	14.7	86
Phenytoin	0.64	1.4	119
Trimethoprim	1.36	1.83	35
Vancomycin	0.64	0.85	33
Decreased			
Chloramphenicol	0.87	0.60	−31
Digoxin	7.3	4.0	−45
Ethambutol	3.7	1.6	−57
Pipemidic acid	2.0	0.84	−58

TABLE 51-2 Unbound Fraction of Selected Drugs in Patients with Normal Renal Function and End-Stage Renal Disease

Acidic Drugs	Normal	ESRD	Change from Normal (%)
Abecarnil	4	15	275
Azlocillin	62.5	75	20
Cefazolin	16	29	81
Cefoxitin	27	59	119
Ceftriaxone	10	20	100
Clofibrate	3	9	200
Dicloxacillin	3	9	200
Diflunisal	12	44	267
Doxycycline	12	28	133
Furosemide	4	6	50
Methotrexate	57.2	63.8	12
Metolazone	5	10	100
Moxalactam	48	64	33
Pentobarbital	34	41	21
Phenytoin	10	21.5	115
Salicylate	8	20	150
Sulfamethoxazole	34	58	71
Valproic acid	8	23	188
Warfarin	1	2	100
Basic Drugs	**Normal**	**ESRD**	**Change from Normal (%)**
Decreased			
Bepridil	0.3	0.1	−67
Clonidine	55.6	47.6	−14
Disopyramide	32	28	−13
Propafenone	3.4	2.4	−29
Increased			
Amphotericin B	3.5	4.1	17
Chloramphenicol	45	64	42
Clonazepam	13.9	16	15
Diazepam	2	8	300
Fluoxetine	5.5	6.5	18
Ketoconazole	1	1.5	50
Prazosin	6	10.1	68
Rosiglitazone	0.16	0.22	38
Triamterene	19	43	126

function declines. However, the unbound concentration therapeutic range is unchanged in the presence of RKF. Unbound concentration measurements thus provide the best means for individualizing phenytoin therapy in patients with RKF and should be used whenever they are available. Several equations have been proposed to approximate the equivalent "total" phenytoin concentration in an ESRD patient relative to an individual with normal renal function.[17] Although these approaches have not been rigorously evaluated, they may be useful in some clinical settings to predict dosage requirements via a standard nonlinear approach. The principal binding protein for several basic drug compounds is α_1-acid glycoprotein, an acute-phase reactant protein whose plasma concentrations are increased in renal transplant and hemodialysis patients.[8] As a result of this increase, the unbound fraction of those drugs may be significantly decreased in ESRD patients.

Altered tissue binding may also affect the apparent volume of distribution of a drug. For example, the distribution volume of digoxin has been reported to be reduced by 30% to 50% from normal values in patients with stage 5 CKD, as well as in hemodialysis patients.[18] This reduction in the distribution volume may be secondary to a decrease in tissue binding as a result of competitive inhibition by endogenous or exogenous substances. Multiple methods have been proposed to estimate the degree of reduction in digoxin's distribution volume.[18] Acidosis or the presence of digoxin-like immunoreactive substances that bind to and inhibit membrane adenosine triphosphatase may also contribute to this phenomenon.[19] In this situation, the absolute amount of digoxin bound to the receptor is reduced and the resultant serum digoxin concentration is higher than anticipated.

Knowledge of protein and tissue binding changes in patients with renal insufficiency is critically important in the interpretation of serum drug concentrations, as the unbound concentration of several drugs in plasma correlates more closely with the concentration of drug at the receptor site and, therefore, with the pharmacologic effect, than does the total concentration of drug in plasma.[20] Because an alteration in plasma protein or tissue binding of a drug will likely alter the total drug concentration, the usual expected relationship between total drug concentration and pharmacologic response will be perturbed, but the relationship to unbound drug should not be affected.

Thus in patients with renal insufficiency, particularly in those with ESRD, a "normal" total drug concentration may be associated with either an adverse reaction secondary to elevated unbound drug concentrations, or a subtherapeutic response because of an altered plasma-to-tissue drug concentration ratio. The monitoring of unbound drug concentrations in this patient population is warranted for those drugs that have a narrow therapeutic range, are highly protein bound (free fraction of <20%), and for which marked variability in the free fraction has been reported (e.g., phenytoin and disopyramide).

Finally, the method used to calculate the volume of distribution may be influenced by renal insufficiency. The three most commonly used volume of distribution terms are: volume of the central compartment (V_c), volume of the terminal phase (V and V_{area}), and volume of distribution at steady state (V_{ss}). The V_c for many drugs approximates extracellular fluid volume and thus may be increased or decreased by acute changes. Oliguric acute renal failure, is often accompanied by fluid overload and a resultant increased V_c for many drugs. The V_{area} or V_β represents the proportionality constant between plasma concentrations in the terminal elimination phase and the amount of drug remaining in the body. V_β is affected by both distribution characteristics, as well as by the terminal elimination rate constant. V_β and V_{ss} will often be similar in magnitude, with V_β being slightly larger. Because V_{ss} has the advantage of being independent of drug elimination, it is the most appropriate volume term to use when one desires to compare drug distribution volumes between patients with renal insufficiency and those with normal renal function.[21]

EFFECT ON METABOLISM

❸ A decrease in the renal clearance of drugs in patients with RKF is well appreciated. However, there is now good preclinical evidence that CKD may lead to alterations in nonrenal clearance in some cases as the result of changes in cytochrome P450 (CYP)-mediated metabolism in the liver and other organs.[9,22,23] The observed clinical reductions in nonrenal clearance in CKD patients have been generally proportional to the reductions in glomerular filtration rate (GFR) (Table 51–3).[8] However, the effect(s) of RKF on nonrenal drug clearance also appear to depend on whether the renal failure is acute or chronic in nature. The degree of reduction in those with acute renal failure does not appear to be as great as that observed in ESRD patients.[12]

In general, these studies should be interpreted with caution because concurrent drug intake, age, smoking status, and alcohol intake were often not controlled. Furthermore, the possibility of pharmacogenetic variation in drug-metabolizing enzymes (e.g., CYP enzymes) must be considered. Prediction of the effect of renal insufficiency on the metabolism of a particular drug is thus difficult and there is currently no quantitative strategy to factor these changes into an individualized treatment regimen. However, some qualitative insight can be gained if one knows what enzyme is involved in the metabolism of the drug of interest and how the enzyme(s) is affected by the presence of renal insufficiency.

Investigations of the effect of chronic renal failure on hepatic enzyme activity in animals have demonstrated reductions in some, but not all, pathways of drug metabolism.[9,22,23] The mechanism(s) by which RKF affects hepatic drug metabolism is not clearly known, but may relate to accumulation of endogenous inhibitors (e.g., uremic toxins) or to the fact that CKD patients exist in a chronic inflammatory state and have increased levels of oxidative stress,[24] and other factors known to downregulate CYP enzymes.[25] In rat models of chronic renal failure, protein expression of several CYP enzymes, including CYP3A1 and CYP3A2 (corresponding to human CYP3A4), is reduced in the liver by as much as 75%. The mechanism of this decrease in protein content and messenger ribonucleic acid expression, suggests transcriptionally mediated downregulation.[22] The in vivo relevance of these findings was demonstrated in rats with chronic renal failure using enzyme-selective breath tests; the results showed

TABLE 51-3 Effect of End-Stage Renal Disease on Nonrenal Clearance of Selected Drugs

Decreased			
Acyclovir	Aztreonam	Bufuralol	Captopril
Cefmenoxime	Cefmetazole	Cefonicid	Cefotaxime
Cefotiam	Cefsulodin	Ceftizoxime	Cilastatin
Cimetidine	Ciprofloxacin	Cortisol	Encainide
Erythromycin	Imipenem	Isoniazid	Methylprednisolone
Metoclopramide	Moxalactam	Nicardipine	Nimodipine
Nitrendipine	Procainamide	Quinapril	Repaglinide
Verapamil	Zidovudine		
Unchanged			
Acetaminophen	Chloramphenicol	Clonidine	Codeine
Diflunisal	Indomethacin	Insulin	Isradipine
Lidocaine	Morphine	Metoprolol	Nisoldipine
Nortriptyline	Pentobarbital	Propafenone	Quinidine
Theophylline	Tocainide	Tolbutamide	
Increased			
Bumetanide	Cefpiramide	Fosinopril	Nifedipine
Phenytoin	Rosiglitazone	Sulfadimidine	

that CYP2C11 and CYP3A2 activity was significantly reduced (by up to 35%), while CYP1A2 activity was no different from that in control animals.[23] Consistent with these observations in animals, CYP3A activity as measured by the erythromycin breath test is 28% lower in ESRD patients as compared to healthy controls.[26] Although baseline CYP3A activity was lower in these patients, the increase in CYP3A activity observed following enzyme induction with rifampin was similar.[26] Collectively, these data indicate that CKD has a detrimental effect on some important pathways of hepatic drug metabolism in animals and man.

In addition to changes in hepatic metabolism, chronic renal failure has also been shown in animals to affect the expression and activity of CYP enzymes in the intestine.[27] CYP1A1 and CYP3A2 enzyme content was reduced by 43% and 71%, respectively, and corresponding messenger ribonucleic acid levels were decreased by 32% and 36%, respectively. Although this has not been evaluated in humans, it may become clinically relevant for those drugs for which intestinal metabolism is known to be important (e.g., CYP3A substrates with low bioavailability).

Thus, current data suggest a differential effect on the individual CYP enzymes with the activity of some enzymes (e.g., CYP3A4 and CYP2C9) being reduced,[26,28] while others (e.g., CYP2E1) are not affected.[29] This differential effect on individual enzymes may help to explain some of the conflicting reports of whether drug metabolism is altered in the presence of RKF.

EFFECT OF RENAL INSUFFICIENCY ON METABOLITE ELIMINATION

Patients with severe renal insufficiency who are receiving chronic treatment with some agents may experience accumulation of metabolite(s) as well as parent compound. Metabolites of several drugs have been reported to have significant pharmacologic and/or toxicologic activity. However, the pharmacokinetics and pharmacology of metabolites are not often fully elucidated in humans. In a sense, the patient with severe renal impairment is being exposed to a new pharmacologic entity if the serum concentrations of the metabolite exceed those reported in patients with normal renal function.

The metabolite may have pharmacologic activity similar to that of the parent drug and thus contribute significantly to clinical response; that is true, for example, of oxypurinol. Alternatively, the metabolite may have qualitatively dissimilar pharmacologic action; for example, normeperidine has central nervous system (CNS) stimulatory activity that reportedly produces seizures, whereas meperidine has CNS depressant actions.[30] Because of the multiplicity of potential interactions of compounds that are primarily metabolized, the practical consequences of metabolite accumulation are difficult to predict and are most often identified in those patients at risk by trial and error.

EFFECT OF RENAL INSUFFICIENCY ON RENAL EXCRETION

Renal clearance (CL_R) of a drug is the composite of GFR, tubular secretion, and reabsorption ($CL_R = (GFR \times f_u) + CL_{secretion} - CL_{reabsorption}$), where f_u is the fraction of the drug unbound to plasma proteins. Drug elimination by filtration occurs by a diffusion process, while tubular secretion and reabsorption are bidirectional processes that involve carrier-mediated renal transport systems.[31] Renal transport systems have been broadly classified on the basis of substrate selectivity into the anionic and cationic renal transport systems, which are responsible for the transport of a number of organic acidic and basic drugs, respectively. Renal organic anion transport is mediated by transporters, transporting polypeptides, and multidrug resistance-associated protein transporters.[31] Several drugs, including β-lactam antibiotics, diuretics, and nonsteroidal antiinflammatory drugs, are actively secreted by one or more of these transporter families which also have an essential role in the elimination of glucuronide metabolites. Organic cation transport systems mediate the reabsorption and excretion of endogenous cationic compounds and drugs (e.g., cimetidine, famotidine, and quinidine). The P-glycoprotein transport system in the kidney is also involved in the secretion of cationic and hydrophobic drugs (e.g., digoxin and vinca alkaloids).[31] Other important renal transport systems include the peptide transporters, which are involved in the uptake of peptide-like drugs including β-lactam antibiotics and angiotensin-converting enzyme inhibitors, while nucleoside transporter proteins are involved in uptake of nucleosides and nucleoside analogs (e.g., zidovudine and dideoxyinosine).

Alterations in filtration, secretion, or reabsorption, secondary to CKD may have a dramatic effect on drug disposition: for drugs that are primarily filtered, a reduction in glomerular filtration rate will result in a proportional decrease in renal drug clearance. However, for drugs that are extensively renally secreted (CL_R >300 mL/min), the loss of filtration clearance (up to 120 mL/min) will have less of an impact. In the absence of data delineating the contribution of tubular function to renal clearance, the clinical measurement or estimation of creatinine clearance remains the guiding factor for drug-dosage regimen design.[8,10] Although several methods have been proposed to estimate GFR from routinely available clinical data (see Chap. 44) the usefulness of a calculated GFR to guide drug dosing has not been extensively evaluated.[32,33]

The importance of an alteration in renal function on drug elimination depends on two factors: the fraction of drug normally eliminated by the kidney unchanged and the degree of renal insufficiency. Quantitation of the patient's renal function can be accomplished by measurement of creatinine clearance or estimation based on the stable serum creatinine concentration (see Chap. 44). Because of the time delay involved and problems in obtaining complete urine collections, measured creatinine clearance values are infrequently used for initial drug-dosage regimen design. Therefore the calculation of initial drug dosage regimens relies on the estimation of creatinine clearance (CL_{cr}) in adults and children from such routinely available clinical data as age, gender, height, weight, and serum creatinine. These relationships are most accurate for individuals of average muscle mass for their age, weight, and height. The creatinine clearance of emaciated and obese adult patients is difficult to predict, and incorrect estimates have been obtained with most methods.

Several methods are also available for estimating creatinine clearance in adults with acute renal failure using age, height, weight, serum creatinine, and time data (see Chap. 44). These methods have not been independently validated and their usefulness for approximating renal function in complex patient situations is not currently recommended.

DRUG-DOSAGE REGIMEN DESIGN FOR CHRONIC KIDNEY DISEASE PATIENTS

❹ Table 51–4 lists the typical steps involved in designing a dosage regimen for a patient with CKD. The design of the optimal dosage regimen for patients with RKF is dependent on the availability of an accurate characterization of the relationship between the pharmacokinetic parameters of the drug and renal function, and an accurate assessment of the patient's renal function, CL_{cr}. Prior to 1998 there was no consensus regarding the explicit criteria for characterization of the relationship between the pharmacokinetics and pharmacodynamics of a drug and renal function. The United States Food and Drug Administration (FDA) industry guidance issued in May 1998 provided a framework to help companies decide when

TABLE 51-4 A Stepwise Approach to Adjust Drug Dosages for Patients with Renal Insufficiency

Step 1	Obtain history and relevant demographic/clinical information	Record demographic information, obtain past medical history including history of renal disease, and record current laboratory information (e.g., serum creatinine)
Step 2	Estimate creatinine clearance	Use Cockcroft-Gault equation to estimate creatinine clearance, or calculate creatinine clearance from timed urine collection
Step 3	Review current medications	Identify drugs for which individualization of the treatment regimen will be necessary
Step 4	Calculate individualized treatment regimen	Determine treatment goals (see text); calculate dosage regimen based on pharmacokinetic characteristics of the drug and the patient's renal function
Step 5	Monitor	Monitor parameters of drug response and toxicity; monitor drug levels if available/applicable
Step 6	Revise regimen	Adjust regimen based on drug response or change in patient status (including renal function) as warranted

TABLE 51-5 Relationship Between Creatinine Clearance and Total-Body Clearance and Terminal Elimination Rate Constant of Selected Drugs

Drug	Elimination Rate Constant	Total Body Clearance
Acyclovir		$CL = 3.37 (CL_{cr}) + 0.41$
Amikacin	$k = (0.0024 \times CL_{cr}) + 0.01$	$CL = 0.6 (CL_{cr}) + 9.6$
Ceftazidime	$k = (0.004 \times CL_{cr}) + 0.004$	$CL = 1.15 (CL_{cr}) + 10.6$
Ciprofloxacin		$CL = 2.83 (CL_{cr}) + 363$
Digoxin		$CL = 0.88 (CL_{cr}) + 23$
Gentamicin	$k = (0.0029 \times CL_{cr}) + 0.015$	$CL = 0.983 (CL_{cr})$
Lithium		$CL = 0.20 (CL_{cr})$
Ofloxacin		$CL = 1.04 (CL_{cr}) + 38.7$
Piperacillin	$k = (0.0049 \times CL_{cr}) + 0.21$	$CL = 1.36 (CL_{cr}) + 1.50$
Tobramycin	$k = (0.0029 \times CL_{cr}) + 0.01$	$CL = 0.801 (CL_{cr})$
Vancomycin	$k = (0.00083 \times CL_{cr}) + 0.0044$	$CL = 0.69 (CL_{cr}) + 3.7$

CL, total-body clearance; CL_{cr}, creatinine clearance.

they should conduct such a "characterization" study and proposed explicit recommendations for study design, data analysis, and assessment of the impact of the study results on drug dosing.[34] Thus the quality of data available to clinicians has improved dramatically in the last 10 years.

Most dosage-adjustment guidelines have proposed the use of a fixed dose or interval for patients with broad ranges of renal function.[11,13,35–39] Indeed, normal renal function has often been ascribed to anyone who has a CL_{cr} >90 mL/min even though there are many individuals who have CL_{cr} values in the range of 120 to 180 mL/min. Mild renal insufficiency encompasses the range of 60 to 89 mL/min, moderate renal insufficiency encompasses the CL_{cr} range of 30 to 59 mL/min, and severe renal insufficiency and ESRD often are defined as a creatinine clearance of 15 to 29 mL/min, and <15 mL/min, respectively. Each of these categories encompasses at least a twofold range in renal function, and thus the calculated drug regimen may not be optimal for all patients whose renal function lies within the given range.

❺ Secondary references, such as the American Hospital Formulary Service Drug Information Service,[35] the British National Formulary,[36] *Drug Prescribing in Renal Failure*,[37] and *Martindale: The Complete Drug Reference*,[38] are generally touted as excellent sources of information about a drug's pharmacokinetic characteristics in subjects with normal and impaired renal function. A recent systematic comparison of these four sources strongly suggests a need for a more consistent quantitative approach to drug dosage regimen individualization for those with CKD.[40] The authors concluded that the remarkable variation in recommendations along with the paucity of details of the methods used to generate the dosing advice, as well as the lack of reference to primary literature made these sources of drug information ill suited for clinical use. None of these sources consistently provide the explicit relationships of the kinetic parameters of interest (total body clearance, elimination rate constant, and distribution volume) with a continuous index of renal function, such as CL_{cr}. To find this information, one may need to identify the original research study that assessed the drug's disposition or a comprehensive review article on the class of drugs of interest. For many drugs one may be able to identify several of these relationships—some derived from rigorous premarketing evaluations of new drugs conducted in adequately sized studies and others from population analysis of already marketed drugs. The relationship of the most clinical value will be dependent on the similarities between the population of subjects/patients who were studied and the patient's given clinical situation. Ideally, one should be able to identify a relationship between total body clearance (CL) or elimination rate constant (k) with CL_{cr}, such as those depicted in Table 51–5. This information, along with the patient's CL_{cr}, will enable prediction of the patient's disposition parameters and then formulation of a therapeutic regimen to attain the desired therapeutic outcome.

If specific literature recommendations and/or the relationship of kinetic parameters to CL_{cr} are not available, then one can estimate the CL or k of the patient with the method of Rowland and Tozer,[10] provided the fraction of the drug that is eliminated renally unchanged (f_e) in subjects with normal renal function is known.[13] This approach assumes that the change in CL and k are proportional to CL_{cr}, that renal disease does not alter the drug's metabolism, that the metabolites, if formed, are inactive and nontoxic, that the drug obeys first-order (linear) kinetic principles, and that it is adequately described by a one-compartment model. If these assumptions are true, then the kinetic parameter/dosage adjustment factor (Q) can be calculated as:

$$Q = 1 - [f_e(1 - KF)]$$

where KF is the ratio of the patient's CL_{cr} to the assumed normal value of 120 mL/min. Thus for a drug that is 85% eliminated renally unchanged in a patient who has a CL_{cr} of 10 mL/min, the Q factor would be:

$$\begin{aligned} Q &= 1 - [0.85(1 - (10/120))] \\ &= 1 - [0.85(0.92)] \\ &= 1 - 0.78 \\ &= 0.22 \end{aligned}$$

The estimated total body clearance for this patient can then be calculated as $CL_{PT} = CL_{norm} \times Q$, where CL_{norm} is the mean value in patients with normal renal function as reported in the literature.

After the kinetic parameters for the patient are estimated, the best method for dosage-regimen adjustment should be selected. Specifically, one must determine whether the desired goal is the maintenance of a similar peak, trough, or average steady-state drug concentration. If there is a significant relationship between peak concentration and clinical response[41] (e.g., aminoglycosides) or toxicity[42] (e.g., quinidine, phenobarbital, and phenytoin), then attainment of the specific target values is critical. If, however, no specific target values for peak or trough concentrations have been reported (e.g., antihypertensive agents, benzodiazepines, and cephalosporins), then a regimen goal of attaining the same average steady-state concentration may be appropriate.

Although several methods have been proposed to attain the desired average steady-state concentration profile, the principal choices are to decrease the dose or prolong the dosing interval. If the size of the dose is reduced while the dosing interval remains unchanged, the desired average steady-state concentration will be

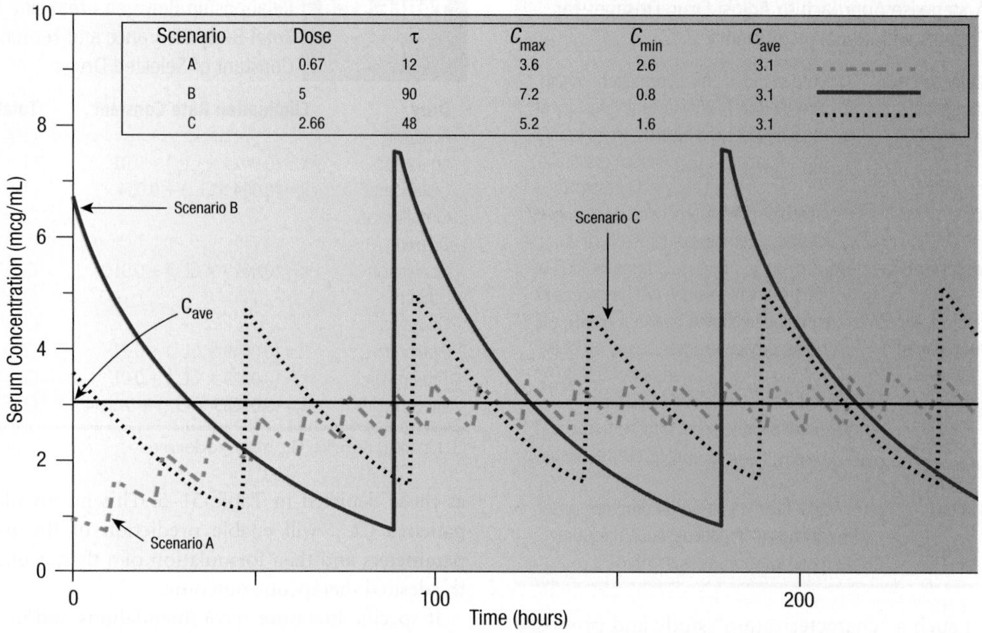

FIGURE 51-1. Although the average steady-state concentrations *(C_{ave})* are identical regardless of which dosage adjustment strategy one decides to implement, the concentration–time profile will be markedly different if one changes the dose and maintains the dosing interval (τ) constant *(Scenario A)*, versus changing the dosing interval and maintaining the dose constant *(Scenario B)* or changing both *(Scenario C)*.

similar; however, the peak will be lower and the trough higher (Fig. 51–1). Alternatively, if the dosing interval is increased and the dose size remains unchanged, the peak and trough concentrations in the patient with reduced renal function will be similar to those in the patient with normal renal function. This dosage adjustment method is often recommended because it is likely to yield significant cost savings as a result of a reduction in nursing and pharmacy time, as well as a reduction in the supplies associated with frequent drug administration. Finally, the dose and dosing interval may both need to be changed to allow the administration of a clinically feasible dose (500 mg vs. a calculated value of 487 mg) or a practical dosing interval, for example, 12 hours instead of 17 hours.

The first step in the process, if the relationship between the pharmacokinetic parameters of the drug and renal function are known, is to estimate the drug disposition parameters in the patient with renal insufficiency. The ratio (*Q*) of the estimated elimination rate constant or total body clearance of the patient relative to subjects with normal renal function (CL_{cr} = 120 mL/min) may then be calculated. This parameter may be used to determine the dose or dosing interval alterations necessary for the patient.

For example, the following relationship between total clearance (CL) and creatinine clearance has been reported for ganciclovir[43]:

$$CL(mL/min/1.8\ m^2) = 1.25(CL_{cr}) + 8.57$$

Thus CL for a subject with normal renal function (CL_{norm}) would be calculated as:

$$CL_{norm} = [1.25(120)] + 8.57$$

$$CL_{norm} = 158.6\ mL/min\ per\ 1.8\ m^2$$

Clearance (CL_{fail}) for a patient with a creatinine clearance of 10 mL/min would be:

$$CL_{fail} = [1.25(10)] + 8.57$$

$$CL_{fail} = 21.1\ mL/min\ per\ 1.8\ m^2$$

Ganciclovir is commonly used in solid-organ transplantation patients as prophylaxis against or treatment for cytomegalovirus infection.[44] The inhibitory concentration of 50% (IC_{50}) of ganciclovir against most clinical isolates of cytomegalovirus is between 0.1 and 2.8 mcg/mL (approximately 0.4 to 11 μmol/L).[43] Consequently, trough concentrations should be maintained within this range, but caution is warranted as neutropenia is associated with the attainment of ganciclovir trough concentrations exceeding 2.6 mcg/mL (10 μmol/L).[45] If a patient with ESRD received the typical ganciclovir dose for a patient with normal renal function, the predicted trough concentrations would approach 20 μmol/L. Consequently, a dosage modification in this patient is necessary to avoid potential toxicity. The dosing regimen can be modified using the ratio of the predicted clearance values. The quotient or *Q* for this patient is calculated as:

$$Q = CL_{fail}/CL_{norm}$$

$$Q = 21.1/158.6$$

$$Q = 0.133$$

where CL_{norm} is the clearance in a patient with normal renal function and CL_{fail} is the clearance of the patient with impaired renal function.

The maintenance dose (D_f) for the patient or the adjusted dosing interval (τ_f) may then be calculated from the following relationships, where D_n is the normal dose and τ_n is the normal dosing interval:

$$D_f = D_n \times Q$$

$$\tau_f = \tau_n/Q$$

For this patient situation, the normal dose and dosing interval of ganciclovir would be 5 mg/kg and 12 hours, respectively. If we wanted to maintain the dosing interval at 12 hours, then D_f would be calculated as:

$$D_f = (5\ mg/kg) \times (0.133) = 0.67\ mg/kg$$

This regimen would result in decreased peak and trough concentrations compared to a patient with this degree of renal insufficiency who received a normal dosage regimen (Fig. 51–1, Scenario A). However, the peak concentrations would be lower and the trough concentrations higher than those observed when a patient with normal renal function received a standard regimen.

If we want to maintain D_n and extend the dosing interval, τ_f would be calculated as:

$$\tau_f = \tau_n/Q = 12/0.133 = 90 \text{ hours}$$

This regimen would yield similar peak and trough concentrations in the renally impaired patient as in the patient with normal renal function, but there is a risk of missed doses with such an unorthodox interval (Fig. 51–1, Scenario B). In addition, the prolonged period below the steady-state drug concentration (C_{ss}) average concentration may be less than optimal.

Finally, a practical dosing interval (τ_p) may be selected and then a dose based on that interval can be calculated. If a dosage interval τ_f of 24 hours were selected, because in many institutions there is an increased risk of missed doses with longer dosing intervals, then the D_f would be calculated as follows:

$$D_f = [D_n \times Q \times \tau_f]/\tau_p$$

$$= [(5 \text{ mg/kg}) \times (0.133) \times (24)]/12$$

$$= 1.33 \text{ mg/kg}$$

This method would likely be most appropriate in this case, as prolonged subtherapeutic concentrations are avoided and troughs are reduced from the first method (Fig. 51–1, Scenario C). The selection of which dosage adjustment method to use to calculate an optimal regimen depends on the drug characteristics and the patient care situation. This dosage adjustment method assumes that the protein binding and volume of distribution of the drug are not significantly altered by renal insufficiency. Thus this approach cannot be used with accuracy for those drugs with demonstrated differences in these pharmacokinetic parameters.

If the volume of distribution (V_D) of a drug is significantly altered in patients with renal insufficiency or in whom one desires to attain a specific maximum or minimum concentration, the estimation of a dosage regimen becomes more complex. If the relationship between V_D and creatinine clearance has been characterized, then V_D may be estimated. If one assumes that a one-compartment linear model can describe the drug, the predicted V_D may then be used with the predicted elimination rate constant (k) of the drug to yield an adjusted dosing interval and intravenous or oral dose. For orally administered drugs, the τ_f can be calculated and the dose can then be approximated as:

$$\tau_f = [(-1/k_f)(\ln[C_{min}/C_{max}])] + t_{peak}$$

$$\text{Dose}_{po} = [FC^t_p\, V_D\, (k_a - k)]/[k_a\, (e^{-kt}/1 - e^{-k\tau})\, (e^{-kat}/1 - e^{-ka\tau})]$$

where, F equals bioavailability, C^t_p equals the desired plasma concentration at time t, and k_a is the absorption rate constant. This approach allows for the individualization of an oral dosage regimen for attainment of specific peak and trough serum concentrations. If the drug is absorbed extremely rapidly, one can approximate the τ_f and the dose using equations original proposed for IV dosing as:

$$\tau_f = (-1/k_f)(\ln\, [C_{min}/C_{max}])$$

$$\text{Dose}_{po} = V_D \times (C_{max} - C_{min})$$

Digoxin is a frequently used oral medication for which the V_D is decreased in patients with renal insufficiency, and for which one usually desires to closely control the plasma concentration time profile. The V_D and CL_{fail} of digoxin can be estimated for a 70-kg patient with a CL_{cr} of 12 mL/min per 1.73 m^2 as summarized by Job[18]:

$$V_D = 226 + [(298(CL_{cr}))/(29.1 + CL_{cr})]$$

$$= 226 + [(298(12))/(29.1 + 12)]$$

$$= 226 + 87.0$$

$$= 313 \text{ L}$$

$$CL_{fail} = (0.88 \times CL_{cr}) + 23 \text{ mL/min}$$

$$= 10.6 + 23$$

$$= 33.6 \text{ mL/min}$$

$$k_f = CL_{fail}/V_D$$

$$= (33.6 \text{ mL/min} \times 1440 \text{ min/d})/313 \text{ L}$$

$$= (48.3 \text{ L/d})/313 \text{ L}$$

$$= 0.154 \text{ day}^{-1}$$

The t_{peak} is generally at 2 hours, and the k_a from the literature is about 0.76 hour^{-1} or 18 day^{-1}.[13] Thus one now has all the information needed to calculate the τ_f and dose for this patient:

$$\tau_f = [(-1/k_f)(\ln[C_{min}/C_{max}])] + t_{peak}$$

$$= [(-1/0.154)(\ln[0.8/1.4])] + 2 \text{ hours}$$

$$= [(-6.49)(-0.56)] + 2 \text{ hours}$$

$$= 3.6 \text{ days} + 2 \text{ hours}$$

$$\approx 4 \text{ days}$$

$$\text{Dose}_{po} = [(1)(1.4)(313)(18 - 0.154)]/[18(e^{-0.154(0.083)}/1 - e^{-0.154(4)}) - (e^{-18(0.083)}/1 - e^{-18(4)})]$$

$$= 0.226 \text{ mg or one 0.25 mg oral capsule every 4 days}$$

Alternatively, the predicted volume of distribution and elimination rate constant or the total body clearance may be used to calculate a dose regimen that will maintain the desired average C_{ss} of the drug:

$$\text{Dose (mg/h)} = C_{ss}\, [(k_f \times V_D) \text{ or } (CL_f)]$$

Depending on how much variance above and below the average steady state one desires, the dosing interval may range from hourly to as infrequently as every 48 hours or longer. For example, if the calculated dose were 10 mg/h, the desired average steady-state concentration would be maintained with a dosing interval of 60 mg every 6 hours or 480 mg every 48 hours.

PATIENTS RECEIVING CONTINUOUS RENAL REPLACEMENT THERAPY

Continuous renal replacement therapies are used for the management of fluid overload and the removal of uremic toxins in patients with acute renal failure and other conditions.[46] The several forms of continuous renal replacement therapy in clinical use today are extensively described in Chap. 45. Which of these therapies will be optimal for a given patient is dependent on several factors, including bleeding risk, degree of hypercatabolism, acid–base balance, and experience of the healthcare provider. Chapter 45 discusses drug therapy individualization for the patient receiving any one of the most popular continuous renal replacement therapy variants.

PATIENTS RECEIVING CHRONIC PERITONEAL DIALYSIS

Although the majority of patients with ESRD receive treatment with hemodialysis, as of 2004 approximately 25,765 receive one of the multiple variants of chronic peritoneal dialysis.[47] Peritoneal dialysis, like other dialysis modalities, has the potential to affect drug disposition; however, drug therapy individualization is often less complicated in these patients as a result of the limited drug clearances achieved with the procedures (see Chap. 48).

Many of the factors that are important in determining drug dialyzability for other treatment modalities pertain to peritoneal dialysis as well.[48,49] Peritoneal dialysis involves the instillation of 1 to 3 L of dialysis solution into the peritoneal cavity. Waste products and other substances, including drugs, move from the blood and surrounding tissues into the dialysis solution by means of diffusion and ultrafiltration. Factors that influence drug dialyzability in peritoneal dialysis include drug-specific characteristics such as molecular weight, solubility, degree of ionization, protein binding, and volume of distribution. The intrinsic properties of the peritoneal membrane that affect drug removal include blood flow, pore size, and peritoneal membrane surface area, which is approximately equal to the body surface area. There is an inverse relationship between peritoneal drug clearance and molecular weight, protein binding, and volume of distribution. Also, drug compounds that are ionized at physiologic pH will diffuse across the membrane more slowly than unionized compounds. In general, hemodialysis is more effective in removing drug substances than peritoneal dialysis such that if a drug is not removed by hemodialysis, it is unlikely to be removed by peritoneal dialysis. Detailed reviews of the disposition of other drugs in chronic peritoneal dialysis patients are reported elsewhere.[48,50] Antiinfective agents are the most commonly studied drugs because of their primary role in the treatment of peritonitis.[49,51] (See Chap. 48.) Most other drugs can generally be dosed based on the residual renal function of the patient because the additional clearance by peritoneal dialysis is so small.

PATIENTS RECEIVING CHRONIC HEMODIALYSIS

The number of patients with ESRD who receive chronic hemodialysis has steadily increased since the early 1970s; currently, more than 309,269 patients are being treated with this life-sustaining therapy.[47] Although many new hemodialyzers have been introduced in the past 20 years and more than 100 different ones were available in the United States in 2007, the effect of hemodialysis on drug disposition is rarely reevaluated after it is initially reported. Thus most of the literature probably represents an underestimation of the impact of hemodialysis on drug disposition.

❻ The impact of hemodialysis on a patient's drug therapy is dependent on several factors, including the characteristics of each drug, the dialysis conditions, and the clinical situation for which dialysis is performed. Drug-related factors that affect dialyzability include the molecular weight or size, degree of protein binding, and distribution volume.[8] Prior to the mid-1980s these were the primary factors that needed to be known to assess the degree of dialyzability of a given drug, because the vast majority of dialysis filters were composed of cellulose, cellulose acetate, or regenerated cellulose (cuprophane; see Chap. 48), which were generally impermeable to drugs with a molecular weight greater than 1,000 daltons, and the clearance by hemodialysis tended to decline dramatically (by up to 60%) as molecular weight increased from 100 to 500 daltons. Drugs that are small but highly protein bound also are not well dialyzed because both of the principal binding proteins, α_1-acid glycoprotein and albumin, have a very high molecular weight. Finally, those drugs that are widely distributed throughout the body are poorly removed by hemodialysis.

The dialysis prescription for the patient can also dramatically affect the dialysis clearance. The primary factors that can vary between patients are the composition of the dialysis filter, the filter surface area, the blood and dialysate flow rates, and whether or not the dialysis unit reuses the dialysis filter. Dialysis membranes are composed of cellulose-based, semisynthetic, or synthetic materials (e.g., polysulfone, polymethylmethacrylate, or acrylonitrile). The synthetic filters are available for low-, medium-, and high-flux modes of dialysis (see Chap. 48), with the principal difference between modes being the degree of water transport which is expressed as the ultrafiltration coefficient in mL of water removal per mm Hg pressure in the dialysate circuit (see Chap. 48). High-flux dialysis membranes have the largest pore sizes and more closely mimic the filtration characteristics of the human kidney than the filters used to deliver conventional hemodialysis. This allows the passage of most solutes, including drugs, that have a molecular weight of 20,000 daltons or less.[52] Thus high-molecular-weight drugs such as vancomycin are extensively cleared by this mode of dialysis, although their clearance by conventional dialysis is minimal. An increase in removal has also been reported with several other drugs that have lower molecular weights (Table 51–6).[53] Figure 51–2 shows the plasma concentration–time profile of gentamicin in a patient receiving dialysis with a low-flux conventional (cellulose acetate [CA170]) or a high-flux (polysulfone [F80]) dialyzer. Because the clearance of gentamicin with the high-flux dialysis procedure is significantly greater than with the low-flux conventional procedure, the patient receiving high-flux dialysis will require larger doses relative to the patient receiving low-flux dialysis to maintain a similar plasma concentration–time profile.

The impact of hemodialysis on drug therapy should thus not be viewed as a generic procedure such that a certain percentage of drug

TABLE 51-6 Drug Disposition during Dialysis Depends on Dialyzer Characteristics

	Hemodialysis Clearance (mL/min)		Half-Life during Dialysis (h)	
Drug	***Conventional***	***High Flux***	***Conventional***	***High Flux***
Ceftazidime	55–60	155[a]	3.3	1.2[a]
Cefuroxime	NR	103[b]	3.8	1.6[b]
Foscarnet	183	253[b]	NR	NR
Gentamicin	58.2	116[b]	3.0	4.3[b]
Netilmicin	46	87–109	5.0–5.2	2.9–3.4
Ranitidine	43.1	67.2[b]	5.1	2.9[b]
Vancomycin	9–21	31–60[c]	35–38	12.0[c]
		40–150[b]		4.5–11.8[b]
		72–116[d]		NR[d]

NR, not reported.
[a]Polyamide filter.
[b]Polysulfone filter.
[c]Polyacrylonitrile filter.
[d]Polymethylmethacrylate.
Data from Matzke GR, J Pharmacy Practice, Vol. 15, pp. 405–418, Copyright 2002 by Sage Publications, Inc. Reprinted by Permission of Sage Publications, Inc.

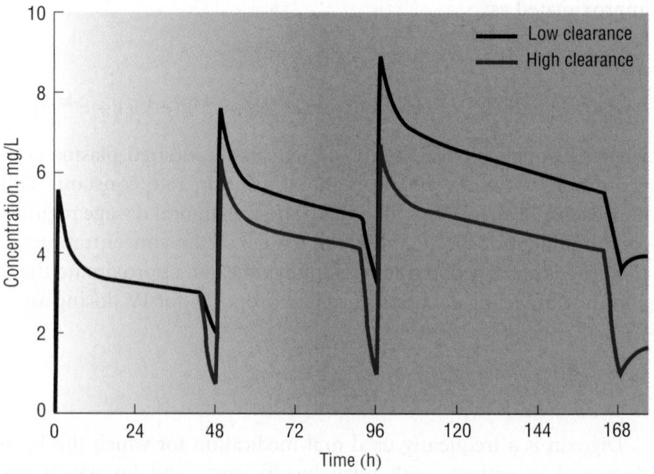

FIGURE 51-2. Clearance of gentamicin by low- and high-clearance dialyzers in a patient given the same gentamicin dose after each dialysis treatment. Concentrations in the patient receiving dialysis with a low-clearance dialyzer will experience a steady rise in the serum concentrations, whereas concentrations in the patient receiving dialysis with the high-clearance dialyzer will be maintained at the same peak and predialysis concentrations observed after the third dose.

in the body is removed with each dialysis session; neither should simple "yes–no" answers on the dialyzability of drug compounds be considered sufficient information to make therapeutic decisions. Reference materials that indicate "yes–no" status regarding the dialyzability of drug compounds provide no quantification of the impact of hemodialysis, and are thus of little value to the clinician who needs to design a dosing regimen for a patient. Compounds considered nondialyzable with low-flux dialyzers in fact may be significantly removed by high-flux hemodialyzers. Characteristics of the dialysis procedure that was studied, such as membrane composition and surface area, and blood and dialysis flow rates, are thus critical data that should be known before one uses the hemodialysis clearance data to prospectively design a drug-dosing regimen for a hemodialysis patient.

The quantitative impact of hemodialysis on drug disposition can be calculated in several ways.[8] The determination of the half-life during dialysis ($t_{1/2,\text{onHD}}$), has frequently been used as an index of drug removal by dialysis. Unfortunately, the $t_{1/2,\text{onHD}}$ may not be interpretable because declining plasma drug concentrations during dialysis represent elimination by the body as well as by dialysis. Furthermore, if significant rebound in drug concentrations after dialysis has been reported, the half-life of drug during dialysis procedure may be artificially low.[54–58] An alternative and more accurate means of assessing the effect of hemodialysis is to calculate the dialyzer clearance (CL_D) of the drug.[8] The CL_D can be calculated by several approaches. The CL^b_D from blood can be calculated as $CL^b_D = Q_b\ [(A_b - V_b)/A_b]$, where Q_b is blood flow through the dialyzer, A_b is the concentration of drug in blood going into the dialyzer, and V_b is the blood concentration of drug leaving the dialyzer. This equation is valid only if the drug concentrations are measured in whole blood and if the drug rapidly and completely distributes into red blood cells. Because drug concentrations are generally determined in plasma, the previous equation is usually modified to $CL^p_D = Q_p[(A_p - V_p)/A_p]$ where p represents plasma and Q_p is plasma flow, which equals Q_b (1 – hematocrit). This clearance calculation most accurately reflects dialysis drug clearance as most drugs do not significantly penetrate red blood cells or bind to formed blood elements. However, one must keep in mind that venous plasma concentrations may be artificially high and CL^p_D will be low if plasma water is removed from the blood at a faster rate than drug. This tends to occur when extensive ultrafiltration is performed simultaneously with diffusion during dialysis.

The recovery clearance approach, the benchmark for the determination of dialyzer clearance, can be calculated as[8]:

$$CL^r_D = R/AUC_{0-t}$$

where R is the total amount of drug recovered unchanged in the dialysate and AUC_{0-t} is the area under the predialyzer plasma concentration–time curve during the period of time that the dialysate was collected. To determine the AUC_{0-t}, at least two, and preferably three to four, plasma concentrations should be obtained during dialysis.

The hemodialysis clearance values reported in the literature may vary significantly depending on which of these methods were used to calculate CL_D. The principal reason for this is that for most medications we do not know the degree and rapidity with which the drug crosses the red blood cell membrane. Because the CL^r_D method incorporates no assumption of the degree of red blood cell permeability, it can be reliably used as the benchmark value. The primary limitation of this calculation is that the concentrations of the drug in the dialysate may be below the sensitivity limits of the assay.

The following principles may be used to generate a drug-dosage regimen recommendation for hemodialysis patients by using a value of CL_D that is reported in the literature.[8,53] Because clearance terms are additive, the total clearance during dialysis can be calculated as the sum of the patient's residual renal and nonrenal clearance during the interdialytic period (CL_{RES}) and dialyzer clearance (CL_D):

$$CL_T = CL_{RES} + CL_D$$

The half-life during the period between dialysis treatments and during dialysis can then be calculated from the following relationships using an estimate of the drug's distribution volume (V_D), which can be obtained from the literature[13]:

$$t_{1/2,\text{offHD}} = 0.693\ [V_D/CL_{RES}]$$

$$t_{1/2,\text{onHD}} = 0.693\ [V_D/(CL_{RES} + CL_D)]$$

Once the key pharmacokinetic parameters have been estimated/calculated, they may be used to simulate the plasma concentration–time profile of the drug for the individual patient and then one can ascertain how much drug to administer and when. This approach to drug therapy individualization can be accomplished in a stepwise fashion assuming first-order elimination of the drug and a one-compartment model.

For example, a 34-year-old male with ESRD was admitted to a hospital from the outpatient hemodialysis unit, where he experienced shaking and chills and had a temperature of 40°C (104°F). He weighed 70 kg and was 69 inches tall, had a residual CL_{cr} of 3 mL/min, and received high-flux dialysis for 3 hours three times a week on an F80 polysulfone dialyzer. He received 140 mg of gentamicin at the end of his most recent hemodialysis treatment, which ended less than an hour prior to admission to the hospital.

The first step is to estimate this patient's pharmacokinetic parameters of gentamicin on the basis of published population data.[13] The volume of distribution in this patient is 23.1 L (0.33 L/kg × 70 kg), and his residual total body clearance (CL_{RES}) estimated from the relationship between CL and creatinine clearance [$CL_{RES} = CL_{cr} \times 0.98$] is 3 mL/min or 0.176 L/h. The elimination rate constant can be approximated as:

$$k = CL_{RES} \div V_D$$

$$= 0.176\ \text{L/h} \div 23.1\ \text{L}$$

$$= 0.0076\ \text{hr}^{-1}$$

The hemodialysis clearance of gentamicin is dependent on the dialyzer, and a value of 116 mL/min was recently reported by Amin et al.[59]

One now can predict what the plasma concentrations of gentamicin will be over the next 24 to 48 hours, assuming the infusion time for the drug (t') was 30 minutes. The concentration at the end of the 30-minute infusion (C_{max}) would be:

$$C_{max} = \frac{(\text{Dose}/t')1 - e^{-kt'}}{CL_{RES}}$$

$$C_{max} = \frac{(280\ \text{mg/h})1 - e^{-(0.0076)0.5}}{0.176\ \text{L/H}}$$

$$C_{max} = (1{,}944\ \text{mg/L})\ (0.003) = 6.0\ \text{mg/L}$$

The plasma concentration prior to the next dialysis session (C_{bD}), which is 44 hours away, and the concentration after dialysis (C_{aD}) can be calculated as:

$$C_{bD} = C_{max} \times e^{-(CL_{RES}/VD) \times t}$$

$$= 6.0 \times e^{-0.0076 \times 44}$$

$$= 4.3\ \text{mg/L}$$

$$C_{aD} = C_{bD} \times e^{-((CL_{RES} + CLD)/VD) \times t}$$

$$= 4.3 \times e^{-((0.176 + 6.96)/23.1) \times 4}$$

$$= 4.3 \times e^{-0.309 \times 4}$$

$$= 1.25 \text{ mg/L}$$

On the basis of these data, a second dose will likely be required at the end of the next dialysis session as one generally desires to have gentamicin concentrations fall below 2 mg/L before administering another dose.

During this interdialytic interval, however, several blood samples were collected to characterize this patient's residual gentamicin clearance, distribution volume, and the clearance of gentamicin during dialysis. Blood samples were therefore collected at the following times after the first dose:

DAY 1:	7 PM (2 hours after dose)	6.5 mg/L
DAY 2:	8 AM (39 hours after dose; just before dialysis)	4.1 mg/L
DAY 3:	12 noon (immediately after dialysis)	2.0 mg/L

The C_{max} can be calculated by back-extrapolation to the end of the infusion as described in Chap. 5. The elimination rate during the interdialytic period (k_{ID}) and during dialysis (k_{DD}), and the V_D can be calculated as:

$$V_D = \frac{Dose/t'}{k_{ID}} \quad \frac{1 - e^{-kIDt'}}{(C_{max} - C_{min}e^{-kIDt'})}$$

$$V_D = \frac{140/0.5}{0.0125} \quad \frac{1 - e^{-(0.0125)0.5}}{(6.7 - 0.0e^{-(0.0125)0.5})}$$

$$V_D = \frac{134.4}{6.7} = 20 \text{ L}$$

$$k_{ID} = (\ln C_1/C_2)/\Delta t$$

$$k_{ID} = (\ln 6.5/4.1)/37 = 0.0125/\text{h}$$

$$k_{DD} = (\ln C_2/C_3)/\Delta t$$

$$k_{DD} = (\ln 4.1/2.0)/4 = 0.179/\text{h}$$

where Δt is the time in hours between the two measured concentrations and C_{min} is the gentamicin concentration in plasma prior to the administration of this dose.

The patient's residual clearance (CL_{RES}) of gentamicin can then be calculated as:

$$CL_{RES} = V_D \times k_{ID}$$

$$CL_{RES} = 20.0 \text{ L} \times 0.0125 = 0.25 \text{ L/h or } 4.2 \text{ mL/min}$$

The dialyzer clearance (CL_D) can be calculated as follows because one knows the total clearance during dialysis (CL_T) and CL_{RES}:

$$CL_D = CL_T - CL_{RES}$$

$$CL_D = (k_{DD} \times V_D) - 4.2 \text{ mL/min}$$

$$CL_D = (0.179/\text{h} \times 20.0 \text{ L}) - 4.2 \text{ mL/min}$$

$$CL_D = (3.6 \text{ L/h or } 59.6 \text{ mL/min}) - 4.2 \text{ mL/min}$$

$$CL_D = 55.4 \text{ mL/min}$$

This case illustrates the need for individualizing drug therapy for hemodialysis patients as this patient's V_D was 13% smaller, CL_{RES} was 42% greater, and CL_D was more than 50% less than the estimates based on population parameters.

The ultimate reason for measuring the plasma concentrations of aminoglycosides and several other agents is to individualize the patient's dosage regimen to achieve a bacteriologic cure while preserving residual renal function. Thus there remains one important step in our evaluation: the calculation of the dose this patient should receive next. The two factors that enter into this decision are the desired peak and trough concentrations and the degree of rebound in drug concentrations, after the end of dialysis. Because gentamicin concentrations have been noted to increase by approximately 25% within 1.5 to 2 hours after the end of hemodialysis, the trough concentration of this patient can be considered to be 2.5 mg/L (2.0 mg/L × 1.25). Although this value is higher than one might like to maintain in an individual with normal renal function, a prolonged period of almost 24 hours would be required just to have the concentration drop below 2.0 mg/L. It is frequently necessary in critically ill individuals with ESRD to redose the patient even though the postdialysis trough serum concentration is between 2 and 3 mg/L. Assuming the desired peak concentration was 7.0 mg/L, the postdialysis dose this patient would need can then be calculated using the simplified approach below, because the elimination half-life is extremely prolonged relative to the infusion time, and thus minimal drug is eliminated during the infusion period:

$$\text{Dose} = V_D \times (C_{max} - C_{min})$$

$$= 20.0 \text{ L} \times (7.0 - 2.5) = 90 \text{ mg}$$

❼ It is common practice in most hemodialysis units to administer drugs after the patient has received dialysis on the premise that it is desirable to minimize the loss of drug that would result from the additional clearance during hemodialysis. Certainly, administration of antihypertensive agents and vasoactive drugs should be avoided in the hours prior to a hemodialysis session to minimize the likelihood of hypotension. However, emerging pharmacokinetic and pharmacodynamic considerations suggest that this may not be the optimal approach for several other agents, such as aminoglycosides and vancomycin.[60–63] Two evaluations of predialysis and one of intradialytic dosing of aminoglycosides indicate that similar peak concentrations, a prime indicator of efficacy, can be obtained in these scenarios relative to those observed with postdialysis dosing.[60,62,63] The area under the concentration–time curve during the dosing interval and the subsequent predialysis concentrations were noted to be significantly reduced and thus the risk of ototoxicity and further renal injury may be minimized. The best dosing schedule, a dose roughly twice that traditionally employed for postdialysis administration, in the 26 patients evaluated by Teigen et al., resulted in the achievement of the desired peak and area under the concentration–time curve in approximately 90% of patients.[62] The administration of traditional doses of tobramycin (1.5 mg/kg) or vancomycin (1,000 mg) during dialysis has been associated with markedly lower areas under the concentration–time curve than those observed when the same dose was administered postdialysis; consequently, higher dosage regimens are necessary to compensate for the additional loss of drug during the dialysis procedure.[61,63] Although these observations are intriguing, the doses proposed by Teigen et al. are only starting conditions and it is highly recommended that aminoglycoside concentrations be measured after the first dose and individualized accordingly using Bayesian methodology.

CONCLUSIONS

Subtherapeutic or supratherapeutic responses to drugs in patients with renal insufficiency are often misinterpreted and not recognized as such. The adverse outcomes associated with inappropriate drug use and dosing have not been quantified but do warrant future investigations. Sound pharmacokinetic principles, used in concert with reliable population pharmacokinetic estimates, should ultimately yield the optimal approach to drug dosage regimen design for patients with renal insufficiency. Individualization of therapy should be undertaken whenever clinical therapeutic monitoring tools are available.

The key action step is to use the knowledge we have to improve patient outcomes. The recent study of van Dijk et al. is an unfortunate reminder of how far we still have to go.[64] They observed that although dosage adjustments based on renal function were warranted in 24% of the prescriptions of the patients with CL_{cr} less than 51 mL/min, such adjustments were only performed in 59% of cases.

ABBREVIATIONS

A_b: concentration of drug in blood going into the dialyzer (arterial side)

A_p: concentration of drug in plasma going into the dialyzer (arterial side)

AUC_{0-t}: the area under the predialyzer plasma concentration–time curve during hemodialysis

C_a: concentration of the drug in the plasma going into a filter

C_{aD}: plasma concentration after dialysis

C_{ave}: average plasma concentration

C_{bD}: plasma concentration prior to the next dialysis session

C_{df}: concentration of drug in the dialysis fluid

C_{ss}: average steady-state plasma concentration

CL: total-body clearance

$CL^b{}_D$: dialyzer clearance from blood

CL_{cr}: creatinine clearance

CL_D: dialyzer clearance

CL_{fail}: clearance of a drug in a patient with impaired renal function

CL_{norm}: clearance of a drug in patients with normal renal function

$CL^p{}_D$: dialyzer clearance from plasma

CL_{PT}: estimated total body clearance for a given patient

CL_R: net renal excretion

$CL_{reabsorption}$: tubular reabsorption

CL_{RES}: residual drug clearance in a dialysis patient

$CL_{secretion}$: tubular secretion

C_{max}: peak drug concentration

CNS: central nervous system

$C^t{}_p$: desired plasma concentration at time t

CYP: cytochrome P450 enzymes

D_f: maintenance dose for a patient with renal insufficiency

D_n: dose for a patient with normal renal function

ESRD: end-stage renal disease

f_e: fraction of drug eliminated unchanged in the urine

f_u: fraction of drug unbound to plasma proteins

GFR: glomerular filtration rate

IC_{50}: inhibitory concentration of 50%

k_a: absorption rate constant

k: elimination rate constant

k_{DD}: elimination rate constant during dialysis

KF: ratio of the patient's creatinine clearance to the assumed normal value of 120 mL/min

k_{ID}: elimination rate constant between dialysis sessions (interdialytic)

Q: kinetic parameter/dosage adjustment factor

Q_b: blood flow through the dialyzer

Q_p: plasma flow through the dialyzer = Q_b (1 HCT)

R: the total amount of drug recovered unchanged in the dialysate

τ_f: dosing interval in a patient with renal failure

τ_p: practical dosing interval for a patient with renal failure

τ_n: dosing interval in a patient with normal renal function

t_{max}: time to peak drug concentration

$t_{1/2}$: half-life

$t_{1/2,onHD}$: half-life during dialysis

$t_{1/2,offHD}$: half-life off dialysis

V_{area}: volume of distribution area

V_β: volume of distribution

V_c: volume of the central compartment

V_D: volume of distribution

V_{ss}: volume of distribution at steady state

REFERENCES

1. Jones CA, McQuillan GM, Kusek JW, et al. Serum creatinine levels in the U.S. population: Third National Health and Nutrition Examination Survey. Am J Kidney Dis 1998;32:992–999.
2. Kearns GL, Abdel-Rahman SM, Alander SW, et al. Developmental pharmacology—Drug disposition, action, and therapy in infants and children. N Engl J Med 2003;349:1157–1167.
3. Mangoni AA, Jackson SH. Age-related changes in pharmacokinetics and pharmacodynamics: Basic principles and practical applications. Br J Clin Pharmacol 2004;57:6–14.
4. Hammerlein A, Derendorf H, Lowenthal DT. Pharmacokinetic and pharmacodynamic changes in the elderly. Clinical implications. Clin Pharmacokinet 1998;35:49–64.
5. Matzke GR, Frye RF. Drug administration in patients with renal insufficiency: Minimising renal and extrarenal toxicity. Drug Saf 1997;16:205–231.
6. Cusack BJ. Pharmacokinetics in older persons. Am J Geriatr Pharmacother 2004;2(4):274–302.
7. Grandison MK, Boudinot FD. Age-related changes in protein binding of drugs: Implications for therapy. Clin Pharmacokinet 2000;38:271–290.
8. Matzke GR, Comstock TJ. Influence of renal disease and dialysis on pharmacokinetics. In: Evans WE, Schentag JJ, Burton ME, eds. Applied Pharmacokinetics: Principles of Therapeutic Drug Monitoring, 4th ed. Baltimore: Lippincott Williams & Wilkins, 2005:187–212.
9. Nolin TD, Frye RF, Matzke GR. Hepatic drug metabolism and transport in patients with kidney disease. Am J Kidney Dis 2003;42:906–925.
10. Rowland M, Tozer TN. Clinical Pharmacokinetics: Concepts and Applications, 3rd ed. Philadelphia: Lea and Febiger, 1995:156–183.
11. Matzke GR, Dowling TD. Dosing concepts in renal dysfunction. In: Murphy JE, ed. Clinical Pharmacokinetics Pocket Reference, 4th ed. Bethesda, MD: American Society of Health-System Pharmacists, 2008:427–443.
12. Matzke GR, Clermont G. Clinical pharmacology and therapeutics. In: Murray PT, Brady HR, Hall JB, eds. Intensive Care in Nephrology. Boca Raton, FL: Taylor and Francis, 2006:245–265.
13. Thummel KE, Shen DD, Isoherranen N, Smith HE. Design and optimization of dosage regimens: Pharmacokinetic data. In: Hardman JG, Limbird LE, Goodman GA, eds. Goodman & Gilman's The Pharmacological Basis of Therapeutics, 11th ed. New York: McGraw-Hill, 2006:1787–1888.
14. Vanholder R, Van Landsehoot N, De Smet R, et al. Drug protein binding in chronic renal failure: Evaluation of nine drugs. Kidney Int 1988;33:996–1004.
15. Chan GL, Axelson JE, Price JD, et al. In vitro protein binding of propafenone in normal and uraemic human sera. Eur J Clin Pharmacol 1989;36:495–499.
16. Pritchard JF, Matzke GR, Opsahl JA, et al. Effects of hemodialysis on plasma protein binding of bepridil. J Clin Pharmacol 1995;35:137–141.

17. Winter ME. Phenytoin and Fosphenytoin. In: Murphy JE, ed. Clinical Pharmacokinetics Pocket Reference, 4th ed. Bethesda, MD: American Society of Health-System Pharmacists, 2008:247–259.
18. Job ML. Digoxin. In: Murphy JE, ed. Clinical Pharmacokinetics Pocket Reference, 4th ed. Bethesda, MD: American Society of Health-System Pharmacists, 2008:139–147.
19. Malini PL, Strocchi E, Feliciangeli G, et al. Digitalis receptors and digoxin sensitivity in renal failure. Clin Exp Pharmacol Physiol 1985;12:115–120.
20. Lam YW, Banerji S, Hatfield C, Talbert RL. Principles of drug administration in renal insufficiency. Clin Pharmacokinet 1997;32:30–57.
21. Koup J. Disease states and drug pharmacokinetics. J Clin Pharmacol 1989;29:674–679.
22. Leblond F, Guevin C, Demers C, et al. Downregulation of hepatic cytochrome P450 in chronic renal failure. J Am Soc Nephrol 2001;12:326–332.
23. Leblond FA, Giroux L, Villeneuve JP, Pichette V. Decreased in vivo metabolism of drugs in chronic renal failure. Drug Metab Dispos 2000;28:1317–1320.
24. Himmelfarb J, Stenvinkel P, Ikizler TA, Hakim RM. The elephant in uremia: Oxidant stress as a unifying concept of cardiovascular disease in uremia. Kidney Int 2002;62:1524–1538.
25. Morgan ET, Li-Masters T, Cheng PY. Mechanisms of cytochrome P450 regulation by inflammatory mediators. Toxicology 2002;181–182:207–210.
26. Dowling TC, Briglia AE, Fink JC, et al. Characterization of hepatic cytochrome P4503A activity in patients with end-stage renal disease. Clin Pharmacol Ther 2003;73:427–434.
27. Leblond FA, Petrucci M, Dube P, et al. Downregulation of intestinal cytochrome p450 in chronic renal failure. J Am Soc Nephrol 2002;13:1579–1585.
28. Dreisbach AW, Japa S, Gebrekal AB, et al. Cytochrome P4502C9 activity in end-stage renal disease. Clin Pharmacol Ther 2003;73:475–477.
29. Nolin TD, Gastonguay MR, Bies RR, et al. Impaired 6-hydroxychlorzoxazone elimination in patients with kidney disease: Implication for cytochrome P450 2E1 pharmacogenetic studies. Clin Pharmacol Ther 2003;74:555–568.
30. Murphy EJ. Acute pain management for the patient with concurrent renal or hepatic disease. Anaesth Intensive Care 2005;33(3):311–322.
31. Lee W, Kim RB. Transporters and renal drug elimination. Annu Rev Pharmacol Toxicol 2004;44:137–166.
32. Wargo KA, Eiland EH, Hamm W, English TM, Phillippe HM. Comparison of the Modification of Diet in Renal Disease and Cockroft-Gault equations for antimicrobial dosage adjustments. Ann Pharmacother 2006;40:1248–1253.
33. Spruill WJ, Wade WE, Cobb HH. Estimating glomerular filtration rate with a Modification of Diet in Renal disease equation: Implications for pharmacy. Am J Health Syst Pharm 2007;64:652–660.
34. Anonymous. Characterization of the relationship between the pharmacokinetics and pharmacodynamics of a drug and renal function. U.S. Department of Health and Human Services (*http://www.fda.gov/cber/guidelines.htm*), FDA Guidance, May 1998.
35. McEvoy GK, Litvak K, Welsh OH, et al. American Hospital Formulary Service, Drug Information. Bethesda, MD: American Society of Hospital Pharmacists, 2001.
36 Joint formulary committee. British National Formulary, 48th ed. London: British Medical Association and Royal Pharmaceutical Society of Great Britain, 2004. (*http://www.bnf.org/bnf/.*)
37. Aronoff GR, Berns JS, Brier ME, et al. Drug Prescribing in Renal Failure: Dosing Guidelines for Adults, 4th ed. Philadelphia: American College of Physicians-American Society of Internal Medicine, 1999.
38. Sweetman SC, ed. Martindale: The Complete Drug Reference. London: Pharmaceutical Press, 2004.
39. Munar MY, Singh H. Drug dosing adjustments in patients with chronic kidney disease. Am Fam Physician 2007;75:1487–1496.
40. Vidal L, Shavit M, Fraser A, Paul M, Leibovici L. Systematic comparison of four sources of drug information regarding adjustment of dose for renal function. BMJ 2005;331:263–266.
41. Craig WA. Pharmacokinetic/pharmacodynamic parameters: Rationale for antibacterial dosing of mice and men. Clin Infect Dis 1998;26:1–12.
42. Murphy JE. Clinical Pharmacokinetics Pocket Reference, 4th ed. Bethesda, MD: American Society of Health-System Pharmacists, 2008.
43. Scott JC, Partovi N, Ensom MH. Ganciclovir in solid organ transplant recipients: Is there a role for clinical pharmacokinetic monitoring? Ther Drug Monit 2004;26:68–77.
44. Pescovitz MD, Pruett TL, Gonwa T, et al. Oral ganciclovir dosing in transplant recipients and dialysis patients based on renal function. Transplantation 1998;66:1104–1107.
45. Balfour HH. Management of cytomegalovirus disease with antiviral drugs. Rev Infect Dis 1990;12:S849–S860.
46. Joy MS, Matzke GR, Armstrong DK, et al. A primer on continuous renal replacement therapy for critically ill patients. Ann Pharmacother 1998;32:362–375.
47. U.S. Renal Data Systems. USRDS 2006 Annual Data Report. Bethesda, MD: The National Institutes of Health, Institute of Diabetes and Digestive and Kidney Diseases, 2006.
48. Taylor CA, Abdel-Rahman E, Zimmerman SW, Johnson CA. Clinical pharmacokinetics during continuous ambulatory peritoneal dialysis. Clin Pharmacokinet 1996;31:293–308.
49. Manley HJ, Bailie GR. Treatment of peritonitis in APD. pharmacokinetic principles. Semin Dial 2002;15:418–421.
50. Veltri MA, Neu AM, Fivush BA, et al. Drug dosing during intermittent hemodialysis and continuous renal replacement therapy: Special considerations in pediatric patients. Paediatr Drugs 2004;6:45–65.
51. Piraino B, Bailie GR, Bernardini J, et al. Peritoneal dialysis related infections: 2005 update. Perit Dial Int 2005;25(2):107–131.
52. Cheung AK. Hemodialysis and Hemofiltration. In: Greenberg A, Cheung AK, Coffman TM, Falk RJ, Jennette JC, eds. Primer on Kidney Disease, 4th ed. Philadelphia: WB Saunders, 2005:464–475.
53. Matzke GR. Status of hemodialysis of drugs in 2002. J Pharm Pract 2002;15:405–418.
54. Barbhaiya RH, Knupp CA, Forgue ST, et al. Pharmacokinetics of cefepime in subjects with renal insufficiency. Clin Pharmacol Ther 1990;48:268–276.
55. Halstenson CE, Guay DR, Opsahl JA, et al. Disposition of cefmetazole in healthy volunteers and patients with impaired renal function. Antimicrob Agents Chemother 1990;34:519–523.
56. Matzke GR, O'Connell ME, Collins AJ, Keshaviah PR. Disposition of vancomycin during hemofiltration. Clin Pharmacol Ther 1986;40:425–430.
57. Kelloway JS, Awni WM, Lin CC, et al. Pharmacokinetics of ceftibuten-cis and its trans metabolite in healthy volunteers and in patients with chronic renal insufficiency. Antimicrob Agents Chemother 1991;35:2267–2274.
58. Halstenson CE, Berkseth RO, Mann HJ, Matzke GR. Aminoglycoside redistribution phenomenon after hemodialysis: Netilmicin and tobramycin. Int J Clin Pharmacol Ther Toxicol 1987;25:48–55.
59. Amin NB, Padhi ID, Touchette MA, et al. Characterization of gentamicin pharmacokinetics in patients hemodialyzed with high-flux polysulfone membranes. Am J Kidney Dis 1999;34:222–227.
60. Matsuo H, Hayashi J, Ono K, et al. Administration of aminoglycosides to hemodialysis patients immediately before dialysis: A new dosing modality. Antimicrob Agents Chemother 1997;41:2597–2601.
61. Scott Mk, Macias WL, Kraus MA, et al. Effects of dialysis membrane on intradialytic vancomycin administration. Pharmacotherapy 1997;17(2):256–262.
62. Teigen MMB, Duffull S, Dang L, Johnson DW. Dosing of gentamicin in patients with end-stage renal disease receiving hemodialysis. J Clin Pharmacol 2006;46:1259–1267.
63. Mohamed OHK, Wahba IM, Watnick S, et al. Administration of tobramycin in the beginning of the hemodialysis session: A novel intradialytic dosing regimen. Clin J Am Soc Nephrol 2007;2:694–699.
64. van Dijk EA, Drabbe NRG, Kruijtbosch M, De Smet PAGM. Drug dosage adjustments according to renal function at hospital discharge. Ann Pharmacother 2006;40:1254–1260.

CHAPTER 52 Disorders of Sodium and Water Homeostasis

JAMES D. COYLE AND MELANIE S. JOY

KEY CONCEPTS

1. Hypovolemic, hypotonic, hyponatremia is relatively common in patients taking thiazide diuretics. Thiazide-induced hyponatremia is usually mild and relatively asymptomatic, but it can be severe and symptomatic. Hyponatremia rarely if ever occurs with loop diuretics.

2. The syndrome of inappropriate secretion of antidiuretic hormone causes euvolemic, hypotonic, hyponatremia. Common causes of this syndrome include lung cancer, CNS disorders, pulmonary disorders, and a variety of drugs.

3. Symptoms of hyponatremia are usually neurologic in nature and symptom severity depends both on the magnitude of the decrease in serum sodium concentration and the rate at which it developed. Treatment of hyponatremia is associated with a risk of osmotic demyelination syndrome, a severe neurologic complication that can develop if the rate of serum sodium correction exceeds 8 to 12 mEq/L within 24 hours.

4. Asymptomatic or mildly symptomatic hyponatremic patients should generally be managed conservatively with treatment directed at the underlying cause. A 0.9% sodium chloride infusion can be cautiously used to correct the serum sodium in patients with hypovolemic, hypotonic, hyponatremia and moderate to severe symptoms. A 3% sodium chloride infusion can be cautiously used in patients with euvolemic or hypervolemic, hypotonic, hyponatremia and moderate to severe symptoms.

5. Hypernatremia most commonly occurs when increased water or hypotonic fluid losses are not offset by increased water intake or administration. For example, patients with diabetes insipidus excrete large volumes of dilute urine, but usually develop hypernatremia only if their water intake does not increase to offset the increased water losses.

6. Symptoms of hypernatremia are usually neurologic in nature, and range in severity from weakness, lethargy, restlessness, irritability, and confusion to twitching, seizures, coma, and death. The severity of symptoms depends on both the magnitude of the increase in serum sodium and the rate at which it developed.

7. The treatment goals in patients with hypernatremia include cautious correction of the serum sodium concentration and, when appropriate, restoration of a normal extracellular fluid volume. Too rapid correction of the serum sodium can result in cerebral edema, seizures, neurologic damage, and possibly death. To minimize the risk of these complications, the serum sodium concentration should be corrected at a maximum rate of 0.5 to 1 mEq/L per hour, depending on the rate of hypernatremia development, and be limited to no more than 10 mEq/L per day.

8. Patients with central diabetes insipidus should be treated with intranasal desmopressin acetate, with goals of decreasing urine volume to less than 2 L per day while maintaining the serum sodium concentration between 137 and 142 mEq/L. Patients with nephrogenic diabetes insipidus should be treated by correcting the underlying cause when possible, and sodium chloride restriction in conjunction with a thiazide diuretic to decrease the extracellular fluid volume by approximately 1 to 1.5 L.

9. Edema can develop as a primary defect in renal sodium handling or as a response to a decreased effective circulating volume. It is usually first detected in the feet or pretibial areas of ambulatory patients. Pulmonary edema, evidenced by auscultatory crackles, can be life-threatening.

10. Diuretics are the primary pharmacologic means for achieving the desired therapeutic outcomes of minimization of edema and improving organ function. Diuretic resistance can be overcome by using an increased dose or by using a combination of a loop diuretic and a thiazide or thiazide-like diuretic.

Learning objectives, review questions, and other resources can be found at **www.pharmacotherapyonline.com.**

The human body tightly regulates blood volume and plasma osmolality as both are essential for normal cellular function. Blood volume is important because it is a determinant of tissue perfusion, and effective tissue perfusion is required to deliver oxygen and nutrients to and remove metabolic waste products from tissues. Plasma osmolality is an important determinant of intracellular volume. Maintenance of normal intracellular volume is particularly critical in the brain, where alterations can result in significant neural dysfunction and potentially death.

The homeostatic mechanisms for regulating blood volume and plasma osmolality involve control of sodium and water balance.[1] Interestingly, the homeostatic mechanisms for controlling blood volume are focused on controlling sodium balance. In contrast, the homeostatic mechanisms for controlling plasma osmolality, which is largely determined by serum sodium concentration, are focused on controlling water balance. Thus, sodium and water balance are closely related and are frequently considered together. Disorders of sodium and water homeostasis are common and potentially serious. They usually result in either hypo- or hypernatremia, depending on the disorder. It is important for clinicians to understand these disorders because they can both be caused by and treated with medications. This chapter reviews the etiology, classification, clinical presentation, and therapy for disorders of sodium and water homeostasis.

TABLE 52-1 Composition of Intravenous Replacement Solutions

Solution	Dextrose (g/dL)	[Na⁺] (mEq/L)	[Cl⁻] (mEq/L)	Tonicity	Distribution		Free Water/L
					% ECF	*% ICF*	
D_5W	5	0	0	Hypotonic	40	60	1,000 mL
0.45% sodium chloride	0	77	77	Hypotonic	73	37	500 mL
0.9% sodium chloride	0	154	154	Isotonic	100	0	0 mL
3% sodium chloride[a]	0	513	513	Hypertonic	100	0	−2,331 mL

Cl^-, chloride; D_5W, 5% dextrose in water; ECF, extracellular fluid; ICF, intracellular fluid; Na^+, sodium.
[a]This solution will result in osmotic removal of water from the intracellular space.

SODIUM AND WATER HOMEOSTASIS

Hypo- and hypernatremia are syndromes of altered plasma tonicity and cell volume that reflect a change in the ratio of total exchangeable body sodium to total body water. Many factors affect tonicity and water balance and a sound understanding of the pathogenesis and evaluation approaches are of utmost importance if one is to successfully prevent and manage these syndromes.

Sixty percent of total body water is located intracellularly whereas 40% is contained in the extracellular space.[1] Sodium and its accompanying anions, chloride and bicarbonate, comprise more than 90% of the total osmolality of the extracellular fluid (ECF), whereas intracellular osmolality is primarily dependent on the concentration of potassium and its accompanying anions (mostly organic and inorganic phosphates). The differential concentrations of sodium and potassium in the intra- and extracellular fluid are maintained by the sodium-potassium-adenosine triphosphatase (Na^+-K^+-ATPase) pump.[1,2] Most cell membranes are freely permeable to water, and thus the osmolality of intra- and extracellular body fluids is the same.

Solutes that cannot freely cross cell membranes, such as sodium, are referred to as effective osmoles. The concentration of effective osmoles in the ECF determines the tonicity of the ECF, which directly affects the distribution of water between the extra- and intracellular compartments.[1] Addition of an isotonic solution to the ECF will result in no change in intracellular volume because there will be no change in the effective osmolality of the ECF. Addition of a hypertonic solution to the ECF, however, will result in a decrease in cell volume, whereas addition of a hypotonic solution to the ECF will result in an increase in cell volume. Table 52–1 summarizes the composition of commonly used intravenous solutions and their respective distribution into extracellular and intracellular compartments following infusion.

The serum sodium concentration is tightly regulated, and usually varies by no more than 2% to 3%. Regulation of serum sodium concentration occurs indirectly via mechanisms that control its determinants, plasma osmolality, and blood volume.[1] The kidney regulates water excretion through a feedback mechanism with the hypothalamus, such that the serum osmolality remains relatively constant (275 to 290 mOsm/kg) despite day-to-day variations in water intake. Plasma osmolality is largely determined by the concentrations of sodium and the accompanying anions chloride and bicarbonate, and can be estimated as:

$$\text{Sosm} = (2 \times S_{Na}) + (B_{glucose}/18) + (BUN/2.8)$$

where Sosm = serum osmolality in milliosmoles per kilogram; S_{Na} = serum sodium concentration in mEq/L; $B_{glucose}$ = glucose concentration in mg/dL; and BUN = blood urea nitrogen concentration in mg/dL.[1,3]

Arginine vasopressin (AVP), commonly known as antidiuretic hormone (ADH), is released from the posterior pituitary when the plasma osmolality increases by 1% to 2% or more.[1] AVP binds to the vasopressin-2 (V2) receptors on the basolateral surface of renal tubular epithelial cells, resulting in the insertion of water channels (aquaporin-2) into the apical tubular lumen surface of the cell.[4] Water can then pass through the cell into the peritubular capillary space where it is then reabsorbed into the systemic circulation. An increase in serum osmolality sensed in the hypothalamus results not only in AVP release, but also in stimulation of thirst. The combination of an increase in water intake and a decrease in water excretion results in a decrease in the serum osmolality and inhibition of AVP secretion once the plasma osmolality is restored to normal.

Nonosmotic release of AVP occurs when a decrease in a person's effective circulating volume results in a decrease in systemic blood pressure.[1] The effective circulating volume is that part of the ECF that is located in the arterial system and is responsible for organ perfusion.[1] A decrease in the effective circulating volume (more accurately, the pressure associated with that volume) activates arterial baroreceptors in the carotid sinus and glomerular afferent arterioles, resulting in stimulation of the renin-angiotensin system and increased synthesis of angiotensin II. Angiotensin II stimulates both nonosmotic release of AVP and thirst. This volume stimulus overrides osmotic inhibition of AVP release, and conservation of water fosters restoration of effective circulating volume and blood pressure at the expense of hypo-osmolality.

Proper assessment of a patient with an abnormal serum sodium concentration requires knowledge of the fact that changes in the serum sodium concentration do not necessarily correlate with changes in ECF volume or sodium content as the sodium concentration is determined by the ratio of the ECF sodium content and ECF volume.[1] Although hyponatremia and hypernatremia can be associated with conditions of high, low, or normal ECF sodium and volume, both conditions are most commonly the result of abnormalities of water metabolism.[1]

HYPONATREMIA

EPIDEMIOLOGY AND ETIOLOGY

Hyponatremia (serum sodium <135 mEq/L) is the most common electrolyte abnormality encountered in clinical practice.[5,6] Although its prevalence is not well-established and varies with the patient population studied, it has been estimated to be as high as 28% in patients admitted to an acute care hospital, 14% in patients seen in ambulatory hospital clinics, and 7% in community clinics.[7] Increasing age (>40 years) is clearly a risk factor for hyponatremia.[7]

Recognition of the high prevalence of hyponatremia is important because this condition is associated with significant morbidity and mortality.[8] Transient or permanent brain dysfunction can result from either the acute effects of hypo-osmolality or from too rapid correction of hypo-osmolality in patients with symptomatic hyponatremia. Hyponatremia is predominantly the result of an excess of extracellular water relative to sodium because of impaired water excretion. The kidney normally has the capacity to excrete large volumes of dilute urine after ingestion of a water load. Nonosmotic release of AVP, however, can lead to retention of water and to a drop in serum sodium concentration, despite a fall in both serum

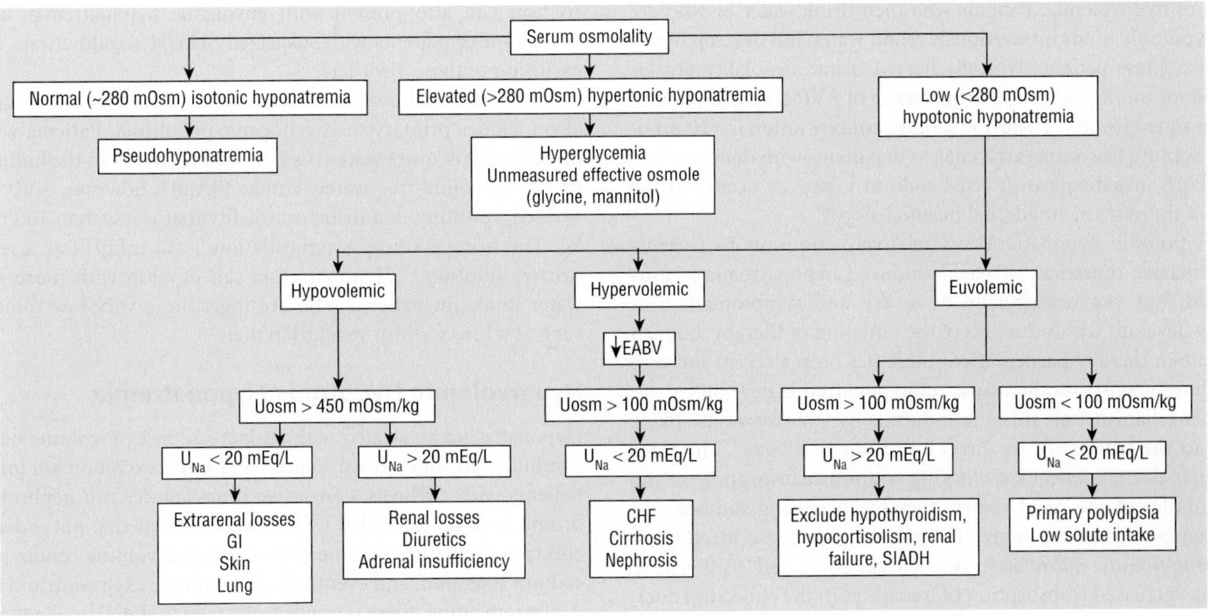

FIGURE 52-1. Diagnostic algorithm for the evaluation of hyponatremia. (CHF, congestive heart failure; SIADH, syndrome of inappropriate secretion of antidiuretic hormone; U_{Na}, urine sodium concentration; Uosm, urine osmolality.)

and intracellular osmolality. The causes of nonosmotic release of AVP include hypovolemia; decreased effective circulating volume as seen in patients with chronic heart failure (CHF), nephrosis, and cirrhosis; and the syndrome of inappropriate antidiuretic hormone secretion (SIADH). The pathophysiology, clinical features, and management of hyponatremia are detailed below.

PATHOPHYSIOLOGY

Hyponatremia can be associated with normal, increased, or decreased plasma osmolality, depending on its cause (Fig. 52–1).[1,3] Hyponatremia in patients with normal serum osmolality can be caused by hyperlipidemia or hyperproteinemia. Historically this form of hyponatremia, termed *pseudohyponatremia*, was an artifact of the method of serum sodium concentration measurement. This laboratory artifact is uncommon today and has been overcome with the use of ion-specific electrodes to measure the serum sodium concentration. If the sodium concentration in a laboratory is still measured by flame photometry, the volume of serum is overestimated because the elevated lipids or proteins account for a greater proportion of the total volume of the sample (Fig. 52–2). Because the sodium is distributed in only the water component of serum, the measured serum sodium concentration is falsely decreased. The measurement of serum osmolality, however, is not significantly affected, leading to a discrepancy between the calculated and measured serum osmolality.

Hyponatremia associated with increased serum osmolality, termed *hypertonic hyponatremia*, suggests the presence of excess, nonsodium effective osmoles in the ECF.[1,3] This is most frequently encountered in patients with hyperglycemia. Elevated concentrations of glucose provide effective plasma osmoles, resulting in diffusion of water from the cells into the extracellular compartment thereby expanding the ECF, which results in decrease in the serum sodium concentration. For every 100 mg/dL increase in the serum glucose concentration, the serum sodium level decreases by 1.7 mEq/L, and the serum osmolality increases by 2 mOsm/kg.[3] It should be noted that this correction is only a rough estimate because the increase in serum sodium varies substantially with the degree of hyperglycemia.[9] Other substances such as mannitol, glycine, and sorbitol that do not cross cellular membranes provide effective osmoles and can also cause hypertonic hyponatremia. The presence of these unmeasured osmoles should be suspected in patients with hypertonic hyponatremia if there is a significant osmolal gap, the difference between the measured and calculated plasma osmolality.[1]

Hyponatremia associated with decreased plasma osmolality, termed *hypotonic hyponatremia*, is the most common form of hyponatremia and has many potential causes (see Fig. 52–1).[1,3] An important step in the diagnostic evaluation of patients with hypotonic hyponatremia is clinical assessment of the patient's extracellular fluid volume.[3] Categorization of these patients into one of three groups (decreased, increased, or clinically normal ECF volume) is very helpful in identifying the pathophysiologic mechanisms responsible for the hyponatremia and an appropriate treatment regimen.

Hypovolemic Hypotonic Hyponatremia

Most patients with ECF volume contraction lose fluids that are hypotonic relative to plasma and thus can be transiently hypernatremic. This includes patients with fluid losses caused by diarrhea, excessive sweating, and diuretics. This transient hypernatremic hyperosmolality results in osmotic release of AVP and stimulation of thirst. If sodium and water losses continue, more AVP is released as

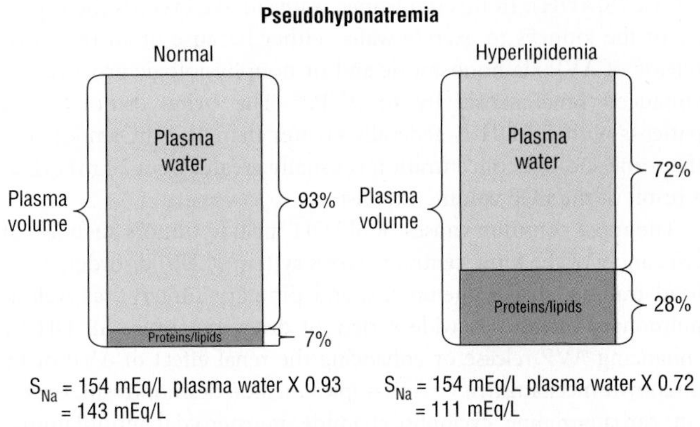

FIGURE 52-2. Elevated lipids or proteins result in a larger discrepancy between the volume of the sample and plasma water, leading to a falsely low measurement of the serum sodium concentration when using the method of flame photometry.

a result of hypovolemia. Patients who then drink water or who are given hypotonic fluids intravenously retain water and develop hyponatremia. These patients typically have a urine osmolality greater than 450 mOsm/kg, reflecting the presence of AVP and formation of a concentrated urine.[10] The urine sodium concentration is <20 mEq/L when sodium losses are extrarenal, as in patients with diarrhea, and >20 mEq/L in patients with renal sodium losses, as occurs in the setting of diuretic use or adrenal insufficiency.[10]

❶ Hypotonic hyponatremia is relatively common in patients taking thiazide diuretics.[11] Thiazide-induced hyponatremia is usually mild, but can occasionally be severe and symptomatic.[12] It typically develops within 2 weeks of the initiation of therapy, but can occur late in therapy particularly if there has been a recent increase in the diuretic dose or other causes of hyponatremia develop.[1,12]

The mechanism of thiazide-induced hyponatremia is likely related to the balance of its direct and indirect effects.[1] Thiazides exert their diuretic effect by blocking sodium reabsorption in the distal tubules of the renal cortex, thereby increasing sodium and water removal from the body. The resulting decrease in effective circulating volume stimulates AVP release. Increased AVP release results in increased reabsorption of free water in the collecting duct, as well as increased water intake because of stimulation of thirst. Hyponatremia results because the net result of these effects is the loss of more sodium than water.

Interestingly, hyponatremia occurs infrequently with loop diuretics.[1] This difference between thiazide and loop diuretics likely relates to their different sites of action. Loop diuretics exert their diuretic effect by blocking sodium reabsorption in the ascending limbs of the loop of Henle, many of which are located in the renal medulla. This action decreases medullary osmolality. Thus, when the loop diuretics decrease effective circulating volume and stimulate AVP release, less water reabsorption occurs in the collecting ducts than would occur if the osmolality of the renal medulla were normal. Thiazide diuretics do not alter medullary osmolality as their site of action is located in the renal cortex rather than in the medulla. In addition, most loop diuretics have a shorter half-life than the thiazides, and patients can therefore replete the urinary sodium and water losses prior to taking the next dose, thereby minimizing AVP stimulation.

Euvolemic Hypotonic Hyponatremia

❷ Euvolemic hypotonic hyponatremia is associated with a normal or slightly decreased ECF sodium content and increased total body water and ECF volume. The increase in ECF volume is usually not sufficient to cause peripheral or pulmonary edema, and thus patients appear clinically euvolemic. Euvolemic hyponatremia is most commonly the result of the syndrome of inappropriate ADH release (SIADH). In this syndrome, water intake exceeds the capacity of the kidneys to excrete water, either because of an increased release of AVP via nonosmotic and/or nonphysiologic processes or enhanced renal sensitivity to AVP.[13] The urine osmolality in patients with SIADH is generally greater than 100 mOsm/kg, and the urine sodium concentration is usually greater than 20 mEq/L as a result of the ECF volume expansion.

The most common causes of SIADH include tumors such as oat cell cancer of the lung, central nervous system (CNS) disorders (e.g., head trauma, stroke, meningitis, and pituitary surgery), as well as pulmonary disease.[3] A wide variety of drugs can cause SIADH by enhancing AVP release or enhancing the renal effect of AVP or by unknown mechanisms.[3,10,14] Examples include desmopressin, oxytocin, carbamazepine, cyclophosphamide, nonsteroidal antiinflammatory drugs (NSAIDs), selective serotonin reuptake inhibitors, tricyclic antidepressants, phenothiazines, opiates, and methylenedioxymethamphetamine, a drug of abuse commonly known as "ecstasy."[3,10,14] Patients with renal insufficiency, adrenal insufficiency, and hypothyroidism can also present with euvolemic hyponatremia, and the evaluation of patients with suspected SIADH should always include exclusion of these disorders.

The differential diagnosis of euvolemic hypotonic hyponatremia also includes primary or psychogenic polydipsia. Patients with this disorder drink more water (usually >20 L/day) than the kidneys can excrete as solute-free water. Unlike SIADH, however, AVP is suppressed, resulting in a urine osmolality that is less than 100 mOsm/kg. The urine sodium is typically low (<15 mEq/L) as a result of urinary dilution.[15] Hyponatremia can develop with more modest water intake in patients who are ingesting a very-low-solute diet, such as a low-sodium vegetarian diet.

Hypervolemic Hypotonic Hyponatremia

Hyponatremia associated with an increase in ECF volume occurs in conditions in which renal sodium and water excretion are impaired. Patients with cirrhosis, congestive heart failure, and nephrotic syndrome have an expanded ECF volume and edema, but a decreased effective circulating volume. This decreased volume results in renal sodium retention, and eventually ECF volume expansion and edema. At the same time, there is nonosmotic release of AVP and retention of water in excess of sodium, thus perpetuating the hyponatremia.

CLINICAL PRESENTATION

❸ Patients with chronic, mild hyponatremia (serum sodium concentration greater than 125 to130 mEq/L) are usually asymptomatic, with hyponatremia being discovered incidentally when serum electrolytes are measured for other purposes.[1,3,16] However, recent data from a small number of carefully evaluated patients suggest that it might be more accurate to say that symptoms of mild hyponatremia are frequently unnoticed by both physician and patient.[17] These data suggest that chronic, mild hyponatremia is associated with impairment of attention, posture, and gait, all of which contribute to a substantially increased risk of falls.

Patients with moderate (serum sodium concentration of 115 to 125 mEq/L) to severe (serum sodium concentration less than 110 to 115 mEq/L) or rapidly developing hypotonic hyponatremia often present with a range of neurologic symptoms resulting from hypoosmolality-induced volume expansion of brain cells.[1,3,16] Classic symptoms include nausea and malaise, headache, lethargy, restlessness, and disorientation, and in some seizures, coma, permanent brain damage, respiratory arrest, brainstem herniation, and death.

The presence of these symptoms and their severity depend on both the magnitude of the hyponatremia and the rate at which the hyponatremia developed.[1,3,16] The magnitude of the hyponatremia is important because serum osmolality decreases in direct proportion to the serum sodium concentration, and water movement into brain cells increases as serum osmolality decreases. The rate of osmolality change is an important factor because brain cells are able to adjust their intracellular osmolality to minimize cellular volume changes in response to volume changes, but time is required for this adaptation to occur.[1,18] When a decline in plasma osmolality causes movement of water into brain cells, sodium, potassium, and *organic osmolytes* move out of the cells to decrease intracellular osmolality and minimize intracellular water movement. Organic osmolytes, primarily myoinositol in humans, are osmotically active substances that contribute substantially to controlling intracellular osmolality without directly altering cellular function.[18] The various components of this adaptive mechanism occur over different time frames, with sodium and potassium efflux occurring over minutes to several hours and organic osmolyte efflux occurring over hours to days.[18] Maximal compensation for a decrease in plasma osmolality typically requires up to 48 hours. Thus, acute changes in plasma osmolality are not compensated for instantaneously and are more likely to be associated with symptoms. Recent studies suggest that patients with concurrent respiratory failure and hypoxemia are at greater risk for adverse neurologic outcomes because hypoxemia diminishes the capacity of the brain to actively transport solute out of cells, leading to a higher incidence of cerebral edema.[19]

In addition to neurologic symptoms, patients with hypovolemic hyponatremia can present with signs and symptoms of hypovolemia including dry mucous membranes, decreased skin turgor, tachycardia, decreased jugular venous pressure, and orthostatic hypotension. These findings are helpful in identifying the type of hyponatremia.

The brain's adaption to changes in plasma osmolality is also relevant to symptoms that can develop if hyponatremia is corrected too rapidly (i.e., >12 mEq/L per day). These patients might experience an acute decrease in brain cell volume, which contributes to the pathogenesis of *osmotic demyelination syndrome*.[20,21] Patients with this complication might develop para- or quadriparesis, pseudobulbar palsy, and locked-in syndrome 5 to 7 days after treatment because of demyelination lesions in the pons.[21,22] Patients who have a significant degree of cerebral adaptation to hypotonic hyponatremia are at higher risk of experiencing this syndrome.[21] This is presumably because these patients have lower intracellular osmolalities at the initiation of therapy, which results in greater decreases in intracellular volume when the plasma osmolality is raised rapidly. Brain adaptation to increases in plasma osmolality requires time, just as was true for its initial adaptation to decreases in serum sodium concentration.

CLINICAL PRESENTATION OF HYPONATREMIA

General

- Hyponatremia is asymptomatic in most patients. Symptoms directly attributable to hyponatremia include neurologic dysfunction associated with cerebral edema.

Symptoms

- The presence and severity of symptoms are related both to the magnitude and rapidity of onset of the hyponatremia. Nausea and malaise are the earliest findings, followed by headache, lethargy, restlessness, and disorientation, and eventually seizures, coma, permanent brain damage, respiratory arrest, brainstem herniation, and death if hyponatremia is severe or develops rapidly. Other symptoms that can be seen with hyponatremia are those attributable to its underlying cause, such as volume depletion in patients with hypovolemic hypotonic hypo-osmolality or volume excess in patients with hypervolemic hypotonic hyponatremia.

Signs

- General: Dry mucous membranes, decreased skin turgor, tachycardia, decreased jugular venous pressure, and postural hypotension can be present in hypovolemic patients.
- Pulmonary: Noncardiogenic pulmonary edema has been described.
- Neurologic: Depressed reflexes. Rapid correction of hyponatremia can result in an acute decrease in brain cell volume resulting in demyelinating brain injury.

Laboratory Tests

- Serum sodium values lower than 135 mEq/L are present. Plasma osmolality and urine sodium concentration can be helpful in diagnosing the cause. Tests including but not limited to serum glucose and lipids and tests to assess kidney and thyroid function should be conducted to identify or rule out potential causes.

TREATMENT

Hyponatremia

DESIRED OUTCOME

❹ The goal of treating patients with hypovolemic hypotonic hyponatremia is to resolve the underlying cause of the sodium and ECF volume deficits, and safely correct the hyponatremia. The treatment goals for hypervolemic and euvolemic hypotonic patients depend on the underlying cause of the hyponatremia and the severity of the patient's symptoms. Patients with an acute onset of hyponatremia or severe symptoms require more aggressive therapy to correct the hypotonicity. The initial goal for these patients is to increase plasma tonicity enough to control the severe symptoms; this typically requires a relatively small increase in serum sodium concentration of ~5%.[3] Once control of the severe symptoms is achieved, full correction of the serum sodium concentration should be achieved at a controlled rate. Asymptomatic patients and patients with mild to moderate symptoms do not require rapid correction of the serum sodium, and the treatment is dictated by the underlying etiology. In all cases the goal is to avoid an increase in the serum sodium concentration greater than 12 mEq/L in 24 hours.[1,3,23] Some recommend that the maximal rate of correction not exceed 8 mEq/L in 24 hours.[16]

GENERAL APPROACH TO TREATMENT

The following principles serve as general guidelines for the treatment of patients with hyponatremia[1,3,10,16,23]: (1) It is important for both the short- and long-term management of the patient to treat the underlying cause of hyponatremia. (2) Appropriate treatment of patients with hypotonic hyponatremia requires balancing the risks of the hyponatremia versus the risk of osmotic demyelination syndrome. In general, patients who acutely developed moderate to severe hyponatremia and/or patients who have severe symptoms are at greatest risk and potentially benefit most from more rapid correction of their hyponatremia. (3) Active correction of hypovolemic hypotonic hyponatremia is usually best accomplished with 0.9% sodium chloride solution as these patients have both sodium and water deficits, and 100% of the water stays in the ECF compartment. (4) Active correction of euvolemic and hypervolemic hypotonic hyponatremia in patients who do not require rapid correction is usually best accomplished by water restriction. Demeclocycline, vasopressin V2 receptor antagonists, or sodium chloride plus a loop diuretic, can be used if the initial response is not adequate. In patients with severe symptoms, 3% sodium chloride solution (possibly combined with furosemide) should initially be used to more rapidly correct the hyponatremia. Furosemide can be administered concurrently to enhance the serum sodium correction by increasing the excretion of water. (5) Long-term management is required for patients in whom the underlying cause of hyponatremia cannot be corrected. This can include water restriction, increasing sodium intake, and/or the use of an AVP antagonist. Application of these principles to the treatment of patients with various forms of hypotonic hyponatremia is discussed in the following sections.

ACUTE OR SEVERELY SYMPTOMATIC HYPOTONIC HYPONATREMIA

A patient who has or is at high risk of experiencing severe symptoms caused by hyponatremia should receive either 3% or 0.9% sodium chloride solution until severe symptoms resolve.[1,3,10,16,23] Resolution of severe symptoms frequently requires only a small, 5% increase in serum sodium, although some suggest that the initial target should be to increase serum sodium to approximately 120 mEq/L.[3,24] Choice of infusion solution's sodium chloride concentration depends on the cause of hyponatremia. The relative concentrations of urine sodium and potassium (osmotically effective urine cations) must be compared with those of the infusate in planning a treatment regimen for patients with hypotonic hyponatremia. For the serum sodium to increase after infusion of a solution of sodium chloride, the concentration of sodium in the infusate must exceed the sum of the sodium and potassium concentration in the urine to effect net-free water excretion.

Patients with SIADH often have urinary concentrations of osmotically effective urine cations that exceed the sodium concentration of 0.9% sodium chloride (154 mEq/L), and thus these patients should be preferentially treated with 3% sodium chloride (513 mEq/L). In this case use of isotonic sodium chloride carries the potential hazard of actually worsening hyponatremia.[1,24] The relatively high concentration of urinary sodium in patients with SIADH stems from the fact that the ECF is expanded, thus minimizing reabsorption of sodium along the nephron. When the urine osmolality exceeds 300 mOsm/kg, it is generally advisable to add an intravenous loop diuretic, not only to increase the excretion of solute-free water, but also to prevent volume overload, which can result from infusion of hypertonic sodium chloride. Intravenous furosemide, initially at a dose of 40 mg every 6 hours, is generally sufficient to prevent volume overload and to decrease the concentration of osmotically active urine cations to less than 150 mEq/L.

Patients with hypovolemic hypotonic hyponatremia, conversely, can be treated with 0.9% sodium chloride solution. In contrast to patients with SIADH, patients with this condition avidly reabsorb sodium throughout the nephron when the effective circulating blood volume is decreased. Thus the urine osmolality is primarily comprised of urea, and the concentration of urine sodium is often less than 20 mEq/L, which is substantially less than the sodium concentration in 0.9% sodium chloride solution. Use of 3% sodium chloride solution will also effectively correct hyponatremia in these patients, but its use should be reserved for situations requiring very rapid correction of the hyponatremia.

Hypervolemic hypotonic hyponatremic patients are particularly problematic to manage acutely because the sodium and volume required to minimize the risk of cerebral edema or seizures can worsen their already compensated hepatic, cardiac, or renal function. It is generally agreed that these patients should be treated with hypertonic sodium chloride and prompt initiation of fluid restriction. Loop diuretic therapy will also likely be required to facilitate urinary excretion of free water.

■ DETERMINATION OF SODIUM CHLORIDE INFUSION REGIMEN

Several methods for determining the correct sodium chloride solution infusion regimen for a hyponatremic patient have been proposed.[1,3,25–29] It is important to recognize that usual approaches provide only a rough estimate of the correct infusion regimen as their use involves known but yet incorrect assumptions. More accurate equations have recently been derived, but the benefits of this more complex approach relative to the approach outlined below remains to be determined.[26,27]

One commonly used approach is based on estimation of the change in plasma sodium resulting from the infusion of one liter of 3% or 0.9% sodium chloride solution as follows[3,25]:

$$\text{Change in } S_{Na} \text{ with 1 liter of infusate}$$

$$= [IV_{Na} - S^1_{Na}] \div (BW + IV_{vol})$$

where S^1_{Na} = initial patient serum sodium concentration; IV_{Na} = sodium concentration of infusate (154 mEq/L for 0.9% sodium chloride or 513 mEq/L for 3% sodium chloride); IV_{vol} = 1 L of infusate; and BW = total body water (in liters), which can be estimated as a fraction of body weight (kilograms) as follows[30]:

$$0.6 \times \text{body weight for children and men} < 70 \text{ years old}$$

$$0.5 \times \text{body weight for men} \geq 70 \text{ years old and females} < 70 \text{ years old}$$

$$0.45 \times \text{body weight for women} \geq 70 \text{ years old}$$

The appropriate infusion volume for a given patient can then be estimated based on the proportion of the estimated change that would result from a 1-liter infusion that is actually desired in that patient. Finally, an appropriate infusion rate can be calculated for this infusion volume to control the rate of increase in the serum sodium concentration.

For example, consider the case of a 170 centimeter (5 feet 7 inch), 60 kilogram (132 pound), 66-year-old woman who presents with nausea, vertigo, and disorientation that have developed over the past several days. She was started on carbamazepine 10 days ago for the treatment of trigeminal neuralgia. Her serum sodium is currently 108 mEq/L. Assuming this woman has carbamazepine-induced SIADH, an initial approach to treatment might include discontinuing her carbamazepine and partially correcting her hyponatremia by raising her serum sodium to approximately 120 mEq/L over the first 24 hours of hospitalization. This should be an adequate response to alleviate her current symptoms, decrease the risk of more severe symptoms, and minimize the risk of osmotic demyelination syndrome. Assuming that use of 3% sodium chloride solution is appropriate, the infusion regimen required to increase her serum sodium to 120 mEq/L over the next 24 hours can be calculated as follows:

$$\text{Change in } S^1_{Na} \text{ with 1 L of infusate} =$$
$$(513 \text{ mEq/L} - 108 \text{ mEq/L}) \div [(0.5 \text{ L/kg} \times 60 \text{ kg}) + 1.0 \text{ L}]$$

$$= 13.1 \text{ mEq/L or } 1.31 \text{ mEq/100 mL}$$

Because infusion of 1 L of 3% sodium chloride solution would produce a 13.1 mEq/L rise in the serum sodium, and we desire only a 12 mEq/L increase, the appropriate infusion volume is 916 mL [(12 mEq/L ÷ 13.1 mEq/L) × 1,000 mL]. In the presence of symptoms, the serum sodium should be increased by approximately 1.5 mEq/L per hour over the first 2 to 4 hours (for a total of 3 to 6 mEq/L) or until the symptoms have resolved. Thus an initial infusion rate of 114 mL/h [1.5 mEq/L per hour ÷ 1.31 mEq/L per 100 mL] for the first 2 to 4 hours, followed by an infusion rate of approximately 23 to 31 mL/h for the next 20 to 22 hours, respectively, would be a reasonable initial treatment plan. The approach to this calculation would be similar if 0.9% sodium chloride solution were used, except that the expected increase in serum sodium concentration would be only 1.5 mEq/L per liter infused, and an infusion volume of approximately 8 liters would be required to achieve the targeted serum sodium concentration.

CLINICAL CONTROVERSY

Clinicians often disagree whether or not to administer 3% sodium chloride to patients with symptomatic hypotonicity. Advantages of 3% sodium chloride include more rapid correction of serum sodium concentration and smaller infusion volumes. In addition, 3% sodium chloride solution is required in conditions characterized by high urine osmolality caused by high sodium and potassium content (e.g., SIADH). The disadvantage of 3% sodium chloride is a higher risk of exceeding maximum recommended rates of correction and causing osmotic demyelination syndrome. The clinician must carefully consider the cause of the patient's hyponatremia as well as the relative risk of slower correction of the hyponatremia versus the development of osmotic demyelination syndrome.

■ EVALUATION OF THERAPEUTIC OUTCOMES

Patients with severely symptomatic hypotonic hyponatremia should be admitted to the intensive care unit or to a highly monitored setting for close monitoring of neurologic and volume status. Serial physical examinations of the heart, lungs, and neurologic status should be performed several times over the initial 12 hours of hospitalization. The serum sodium concentration should be measured every 2 to 4 hours, and the urine osmolality, sodium, and potassium should be measured every 4 to 6 hours over the first day of therapy. The rate of administration of the infusate should then be adjusted to avoid exceeding a rise in the serum sodium greater than 12 mEq/L per day.

NONEMERGENT HYPOVOLEMIC HYPOTONIC HYPONATREMIA

Most patients with hypovolemic hypotonic hyponatremia do not require rapid correction of their hyponatremia because they are either asymptomatic or have only mild-to-moderate symptoms. Many of these patients are at higher risk of developing osmotic demyelination syndrome if serum sodium correction occurs too rapidly because they have chronic hyponatremia that has been maximally compensated for by the brain's osmotic adaptation. The combination of the adaptive decrease in intracellular osmolality and rapid increase in serum osmolality results in excessive movement of water out of the brain cells, intracellular volume depletion, and thereby increased risk of osmotic demyelination syndrome. Treatment of these patients should include correction of the underlying condition, if possible. When direct treatment of the hyponatremia is justified, a 0.9% solution of sodium chloride should be used.[1] This solution effectively replaces both the sodium and water deficits that characterize these patients and presents a lower risk of an excessive rate of correction than 3% sodium chloride solution.

A patient's ECF volume deficit (ECFVd) can be estimated based on sex, change in body weight, and age. For example, consider the case of a 56-year-old woman who was started on hydrochlorothiazide 10 days ago for the treatment of hypertension. She is 172.7 centimeters (5 feet 8 inches) tall and weighed 62 kilograms (136.7 pounds) at that time. Today she presents with complaints of mild nausea and "feeling dizzy" when she stands up. Her weight is 55.3 kilograms (122 pounds). Physical examination reveals dry mucous membranes and orthostatic hypotension. Her serum sodium is 125 mEq/L. The patient's ECFVd could be estimated as follows[31]:

$$\text{ECFVd} = \text{ECFV}_{\text{norm}} - \text{ECFV}_{\text{current}}$$

$$\text{ECFVd} = [\text{TBW}_{\text{norm}} \times 0.5\ \text{L/kg} \times 0.33] - [\text{TBW}_{\text{current}} \times 0.5\ \text{L/kg} \times 0.33]$$

$$\text{ECFVd} = [62\ \text{kg} \times 0.5\ \text{L/kg} \times 0.33] - [55.3\ \text{kg} \times 0.5\ \text{L/kg} \times 0.33]$$

$$\text{ECFVd} = 1.1\ \text{L}$$

If the patient's previous weight were not known, it could be roughly estimated based on clinical signs and symptoms. The presence of hyponatremia suggests an ECFVd of 5% or more, whereas the presence of orthostatic hypotension suggests an ECFVd of at least 10% to 15%. A 0.9% solution of sodium chloride is considered to be isotonic and thus is optimal to correct the volume deficit because it will remain in the ECF space (see Table 52–1).

The expected increase in the serum sodium concentration following infusion of 1 liter 0.9% sodium chloride (154 mEq/L) can be estimated as:

$$\text{Change in } S_{\text{Na}} \text{ with 1 liter of infusate} = [\text{IV}_{\text{Na}} - S^{1}_{\text{Na}}] \div (\text{BW} + \text{IV}_{\text{vol}})$$

$$= [154\ \text{mEq/L} - 125\ \text{mEq/L}] \div [(0.5\ \text{L/kg} \times 55.3\ \text{kg}) + 1.0\ \text{L}]$$

$$= 1.0\ \text{mEq/L}$$

Thus the infusion of 1.1 L of 0.9% sodium chloride will result in an increase of serum sodium of 1.1 mEq/L (1.1 L × 1.0 mEq/L). The patient's sodium serum concentration can thus be predicted to be 126 mEq/L (125 mEq/L + 1.1 mEq/L) following the infusion.

Because the overriding initial treatment goal is to restore effective circulating volume, it might be necessary to infuse 0.9% sodium chloride at 200 to 400 mL/h until symptoms of hypovolemia moderate. The infusion rate can then be decreased to 100 to 150 mL/h so the serum sodium level increases no more than 12 mEq/L over the initial 24 hours. Infusion of 0.9% sodium chloride at rates greater than 250 mL/h should be used cautiously in patients with a history of left ventricular dysfunction or renal insufficiency. It is important to recognize that the rate of increase in the serum sodium concentration can substantially increase once hypovolemia has been corrected if infusion rates are not decreased.[1] Once the ECF volume is restored, AVP secretion will cease, and a rapid water diuresis can ensue, which can potentially result in an increase in the serum sodium at a rate greater than 12 mEq/L per day. Ideally, the potential for this increase in correction rate is recognized prospectively, and infusion rates are appropriately adjusted. Estimation of the patient's ECFVd at the initiation of therapy can help in this regard. If the serum sodium is observed to be increasing at a rate greater than 12 mEq/L per day the infusate should be changed to 0.45% sodium chloride, and the infusion rate set to one that approximates urine output (approximately 1.5 to 2 mL/kg per hour is a reasonable initial rate), to slow the rate of increase in the serum sodium concentration.[3]

■ EVALUATION OF THERAPEUTIC OUTCOMES

Patients presenting with evidence of volume depletion should be reexamined frequently during the initial few hours of therapy. The serum sodium concentration should be measured every 2 to 4 hours to allow timely adjustment of the rate and composition of intravenous fluids to avoid an increase in the serum sodium greater than 12 mEq/L per day. Intravenous 0.9% sodium chloride should be administered judiciously in patients with a history of congestive heart failure or renal insufficiency, with frequent assessments of the cardiopulmonary examination so the infusion rate can be appropriately decreased at the earliest sign of pulmonary congestion.

NONEMERGENT EUVOLEMIC HYPOTONIC HYPONATREMIA

The treatment of SIADH always involves water restriction and correction of the underlying cause, if possible. Drugs that could be contributing should be identified and discontinued. The goal is to induce negative water balance by restricting water intake to less than 1,000 to 1,200 mL/day, such that water losses from insensible sources (skin and lung) and from obligate urine and fecal losses exceed intake. Daily insensible water losses via skin and lungs are approximately 900 mL/day, whereas approximately 200 mL and a minimum of 500 mL/day is lost in stool and in urine output, respectively. Because approximately 850 mL of water per day is ingested in food, and an additional 350 mL are generated from oxidative processes, the water intake reduction should result in a negative water balance of several hundred milliliters per day.[1] Other goals include maintenance of the serum sodium level above 125 mEq/L to prevent symptoms of hypotonicity, and avoidance of iatrogenic hypo- or hypervolemia.

Patients with chronic SIADH who are unable to restrict water sufficiently to maintain the serum sodium greater than 120 to 125 mEq/L can be treated by increasing solute intake with sodium chloride and/or loop diuretics.[3] Sodium chloride or urea tablets increase the obligatory daily solute excretion, which augments the capacity for renal water excretion. The goal is to increase the daily solute intake and excretion to approximately 900 mOsm per day. Because an average diet contains approximately 600 mOsm, 9 grams of sodium chloride would be required to increase the osmolar excretion to 900 mOsm/day (each 1-gram sodium chloride tablet contains 17 mmol of sodium and 17 mmol of chloride). Because extracellular volume expansion is an expected adverse effect, a loop diuretic should be administered concurrently to avoid pulmonary congestion and peripheral edema. Loop diuretics also enhance water excretion by limiting the formation of the medullary concentration gradient.[32]

Demeclocycline is another treatment option for patients who are not adequately controlled by fluid restriction alone. Demeclocycline inhibits tubular AVP activity, resulting in increased water excretion.[1,33] The usual dose of demeclocycline is 300 mg two to four times daily. Because of its delayed onset of action (3 to 6 days), this agent has no role in the acute management of severe hyponatremia, and dosage changes should be made no more frequently than every 3 to 4 days during its use.[1,33] Demeclocycline should not be used in patients with liver disease or compromised fluid intake, who are at high risk for demeclocycline-induced renal tubular toxicity and acute renal failure, or in children because it can interfere with bone development.[1,34]

There is substantial interest in the use of a new class of drugs called vasopressin receptor antagonists to treat SIADH, as well as other causes of euvolemic and hypervolemic hypotonic hyponatremia.[35–37] These agents competitively bind to the vasopressin V2 receptor on the basolateral surface of epithelial cells in the collecting duct. Blockade of AVP binding to the V2 receptor prevents aquaporin-2 water channel transport to the apical surface, thereby decreasing AVP-dependent water reabsorption in the collecting duct. These agents have been called "aquaretics" because they increase the excretion of water without significantly increasing the excretion of electrolytes.[35] Several V2 antagonists are under investigation and show promise for the treatment of chronic hypo-osmolal syndromes such as chronic SIADH.[35,36] One agent, conivaptan, has been recently approved by the FDA for treatment of euvolemic hyponatremia in hospitalized patients. Unlike the other vasopressin receptor antagonists being developed, conivaptan is a mixed vasopressin V1a and V2 receptor antagonist. Because it is available only for administration by intravenous infusion, its use for treatment of chronic SIADH is not practical. Other vasopressin receptor antagonists currently under development are oral medications that can play a substantial role in the management of chronic SIADH in the future.[37] The use of intravenous conivaptan in the management of SIADH in hospitalized patients is appealing, but its role relative to 3% sodium chloride solution remains to be established. It is important to recognize that vasopressin receptor antagonists are contraindicated in hypovolemic patients as their use would worsen the hypovolemia.

■ EVALUATION OF THERAPEUTIC OUTCOMES

The serum sodium level should be measured every 24 to 48 hours after the water restriction is initiated until it stabilizes at a concentration of greater than 125 mEq/L. A continued decline in the serum sodium level would indicate either nonadherence to the prescribed restriction or the need for a more stringent restriction. Once the serum sodium level has stabilized above 125 mEq/L, patients should then be seen every 2 to 4 weeks to assess neurologic status and to obtain serum and urine for sodium, potassium, and osmolality. Again, attention should be given to volume status (i.e., blood pressure, mucous membranes, skin turgor, and heart and lung examination), particularly in patients who are being treated with sodium chloride tablets and loop diuretics.

NONEMERGENT HYPERVOLEMIC HYPOTONIC HYPONATREMIA

The initial treatment goals for patients with asymptomatic or minimally symptomatic hypotonic hyponatremia and an expanded ECF volume include achieving a negative water balance while minimizing rapid changes in cell volume until the serum sodium is greater than 125 mEq/L. This entails correction of the underlying cause when possible, as well as restriction of water intake to a volume less than 1,000 to 1,200 mL/day. Dietary intake of sodium should be restricted to 1,000 to 2,000 mg/day, depending on the degree of ECF volume expansion and edema.

Patients with hypervolemic hypotonic hyponatremia caused by congestive heart failure should be treated with measures that can potentially improve cardiac contractility and improve the effective circulating volume, thereby limiting the nonosmotic release of AVP. Therapeutic options include digitalis or afterload reduction with angiotensin-converting enzyme inhibitors (ACEIs) or angiotensin II receptor blockers (ARBs). Of these, only ACEIs have been shown in clinical trials to be of benefit in partially correcting hyponatremia in patients with congestive heart failure.[38] No specific ACE inhibitor offers any particular advantage for this indication, and the dose should be titrated to keep the systolic blood pressure in the 110 to 130 mm Hg range. Dose-limiting adverse effects include hyperkalemia (serum potassium >5.5 mEq/L), as well as a decline in renal function. The benefits and risks of continuing ACE inhibition must be weighed carefully in each case, but a decrease in glomerular filtration rate (GFR) of less than 30% that stabilizes within 2 months of therapy initiation generally does not require dosage reduction or discontinuation of the ACE inhibitor.[39]

CLINICAL CONTROVERSY

Some clinicians regard any increase in serum creatinine in patients on ACEIs as a reason to decrease dosage or discontinue the medication. ACEIs selectively dilate the afferent arteriole, causing a decrease in intraglomerular pressure and reduced GFR. Although this might be viewed negatively, many experts suggest that the decrease in pressure is likely renoprotective, and that one does not need to reduce the dosage or discontinue therapy unless the resulting decrease in GFR is greater than 30% and does not stabilize within 2 months.

Other potentially treatable causes of asymptomatic hyponatremia associated with an expanded ECF volume include nephrotic syndrome and cirrhosis. ACEIs can be used to decrease proteinuria in patients with nephrotic syndrome, leading to partial correction of hypoalbuminemia and to a decrease in nonosmotic AVP release. Patients with advanced cirrhosis can benefit from placement of a transjugular intrahepatic portosystemic shunt, which can increase the effective circulating volume and thus reduce the nonosmotic release of AVP. This procedure can potentially exacerbate or precipitate hepatic encephalopathy, and should be avoided in patients with a history of encephalopathy. V2 receptor antagonists also show promise for treating hyponatremia in the setting of cirrhosis.[40]

Vasopressin receptor antagonists have also been proposed for the treatment of hypervolemic hypotonic hyponatremia in patients with congestive heart failure and cirrhosis.[35–37] The role of these agents in the management of these conditions, particularly congestive heart failure, is currently under intense investigation with promising early results.[37,41–43] Vasopressin receptor antagonists are expected to play a major role in the acute and chronic management of hyponatremia in these patients in the future.

EVALUATION OF TREATMENT OUTCOMES

Patients should initially be evaluated on a daily basis for lung congestion, ascites, peripheral edema, and signs or symptoms of hyponatremia. The serum sodium concentration should be measured daily until it stabilizes above 125 mEq/L following initiation of water restriction. Patients should then be assessed 1 week following discharge, and then every 2 to 4 weeks to assess compliance with the water restriction and other treatment measures, volume status, and hyponatremia-related symptoms.

HYPERNATREMIA

EPIDEMIOLOGY AND ETIOLOGY

5 Hypernatremia (serum sodium >145 mEq/L) is always associated with hypertonicity and results from a deficit of water relative to ECF sodium content.[1] Hyperosmolar states are a potent stimulus for thirst, and therefore hypernatremia is most commonly observed in patients with an impaired thirst response or in those without access to water. Infants and comatose patients, as well as elderly or disabled patients with an impaired sensorium or functional status are therefore at highest risk for this disorder.[44] The incidence of hypernatremia in general medical-surgical hospital patients and intensive care unit patients has been estimated to be at least 1% and 7.9% respectively.[45,46] Outcome generally depends on the rapidity with which the hypernatremia developed. Mortality from acute hypernatremia in children, which develops in less than 72 hours, ranges from 10% to 70%. In contrast, chronic hypernatremia in children, defined as that which develops over 3 or more days, has a mortality rate of 10%.[47] An acute increase in serum sodium in adults to greater than 160 mEq/L is associated with a 75% mortality rate.[28] Adults in whom the hypernatremia developed at a slower rate have a lower but still high mortality rate of approximately 60%. Hypernatremia in adults is often associated with a serious underlying illness, which likely contributes to the high mortality rate.

PATHOPHYSIOLOGY

Hypernatremia can result from either loss of water or hypotonic fluids, or less commonly from administration of hypertonic fluids or ingestion of sodium. Patients develop hypovolemic, hypervolemic, or isovolemic hypernatremia depending on the relative magnitude of sodium and water loss or gain caused by the underlying condition (Fig. 52–3).

Water loss commonly occurs as a result of insensible losses (evaporative losses of water through the skin and lungs) in patients deprived of water. Hospitalized patients who are febrile or receiving mechanical ventilation are often treated with intravenous fluids containing insufficient free water to replace insensible losses. Hypernatremia can be observed in patients with hypotonic gastrointestinal losses (diarrhea or vomiting) or in patients who have been exposed to high temperatures who suffer large water losses from both sweat and insensible losses.

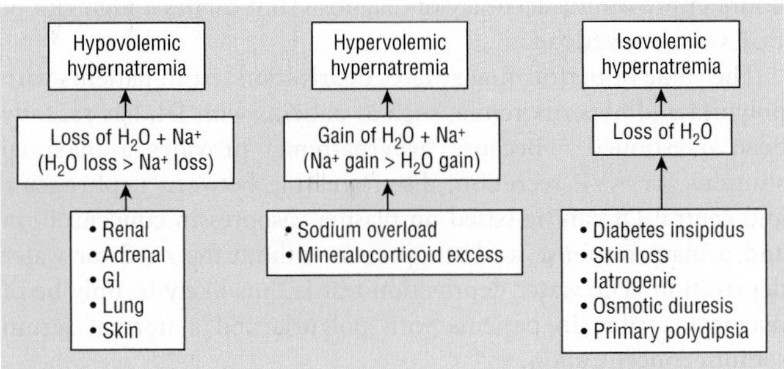

FIGURE 52-3. Common etiologies of hypernatremia. (H_2O, water; Na^+, sodium.)

TABLE 52-2 Causes of Diabetes Insipidus

Central DI	Nephrogenic DI
Idiopathic	Lithium toxicity
Familial	Hypercalcemia
Neurosurgery	Hypokalemia
Head trauma	Cidofovir
CNS malignancy	Foscarnet
Hypoxic encephalopathy	Inherited aquaporin-2 defect
Sheehan syndrome	Inherited vasopressin V2 receptor defect
	Demeclocycline

CNS, central nervous system; DI, diabetes insipidus.

Diabetes insipidus (DI) is a condition characterized by decreased AVP secretion or decreased renal response to AVP.[1,48,49] Patients excrete large volumes (3 to 20 L/day) of dilute urine, resulting in large urinary losses of water. DI is classified as either central (decreased AVP secretion) or nephrogenic (decreased renal response to AVP). Table 52–2 summarizes the causes of DI. Patients with central DI often present with sudden onset of polyuria, whereas patients with nephrogenic DI develop polyuria more gradually.

Administration of hypertonic sodium chloride can result in hypernatremia and an expanded ECF volume. This is typically iatrogenic, and can follow administration of sodium bicarbonate, use of hypertonic sodium chloride enemas, or intrauterine injection of hypertonic sodium chloride. Rarely, patients with hyperaldosteronism spontaneously present with an expanded ECF and mild hypernatremia.[44]

CLINICAL PRESENTATION

6 The symptoms of hypernatremia are primarily caused by a decrease in neuronal cell volume and can include weakness, lethargy, restlessness, irritability, and confusion.[1,44] Symptoms of more severe or rapidly developing hypernatremia include twitching, seizures, coma, and death. Hypernatremia results in movement of water from the intracellular space to the extracellular fluid. As discussed above, neurons can adapt to ECF tonicity changes by adjusting intracellular osmolality, including decreasing or increasing the concentration of organic osmolytes. In the case of hypernatremia, ECF hypertonicity results in generation of intracellular organic osmolytes within 24 hours of onset. This increase in intracellular fluid tonicity then draws water into the neurons, thus limiting the decrease in cell volume. Patients with chronic hypernatremia are therefore less likely to present with symptoms caused by this cerebral adaptation than patients with acute hypernatremia.

Hypernatremia is often associated with serious underlying illness, and signs and symptoms related to that illness can also be present. Patients with a history of severe diarrhea or vomiting can present with ECF volume depletion. Elderly patients deprived of water after sustaining a stroke or hip fracture often present with mental status changes and signs of ECF volume depletion. Clinically detectable extracellular fluid volume depletion, however, might not be evident until the serum sodium concentration exceeds 160 mEq/L, because these patients primarily have water loss, two-thirds of which is derived from the intracellular space. The urine is concentrated, osmolality often exceeds 450 mOsm/kg, as a result of both osmotic and nonosmotic release of AVP. The first step in evaluating patients with hypernatremia is the clinical assessment of the ECF volume, urine volume, and urine osmolality (Fig. 52–4).

Patients with a contracted ECF volume and a low urine output include those who have sustained insensible water losses that exceed intake, as well as those with extrarenal losses of hypotonic fluids. On physical examination, one should search for postural hypotension,

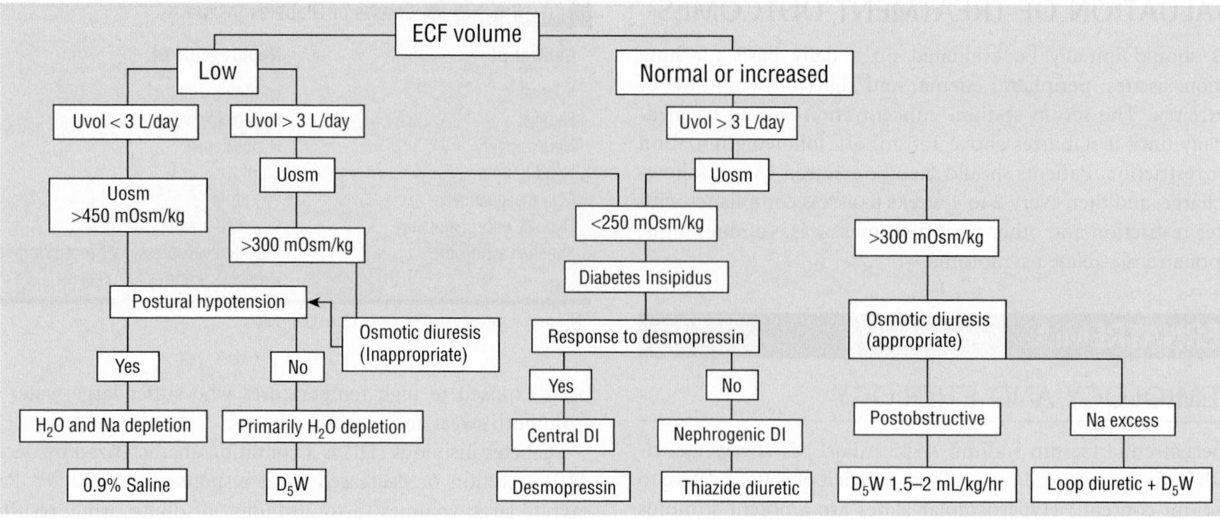

FIGURE 52-4. Diagnostic and treatment algorithm for hypernatremia. (D_5W, 5% dextrose in water; ECF, extracellular fluid; H_2O, water; Na, sodium; Uosm, urine osmolality; Uvol, daily urine volume.) See text for guidelines regarding calculations of infusion rates for intravenous solutions.

diminished skin turgor, and delayed capillary refill. The daily urine output is typically less than 1 liter.

A recent multicenter, case-control study examined the clinical presentation of hypernatremia in 150 elderly patients in geriatric care facilities.[50] Low blood pressure, tachycardia, dry oral mucosa, decreased skin turgor, and recent changes in consciousness were all more common in hypernatremic patients than in controls. Perhaps not surprisingly in this mixed patient population, the presence of signs of dehydration was variable, with orthostatic hypotension and decreased subclavicular and forearm skin turgor present in at least 60% of patients. Abnormal subclavicular and thigh skin turgor, dry oral mucosa, and recent change in consciousness were significantly and independently associated with hypernatremia.

CLINICAL PRESENTATION OF HYPERNATREMIA

General

- The rise in the plasma sodium concentration and osmolality causes acute water movement from the intracellular to the extracellular fluid. In the brain this decrease in volume can cause rupture of the cerebral veins, leading to focal intracerebral and subarachnoid hemorrhages and possible irreversible neurologic damage.

Symptoms

- The clinical manifestations of this disorder begin with lethargy, weakness, confusion, restlessness, and irritability, and can progress to twitching, seizures, coma, and death. Severe symptoms usually require an acute elevation in the plasma sodium concentration to above 160 mEq/L. Values above 180 mEq/L are associated with a high mortality rate.

Signs

- Signs of hypernatremia can include postural hypotension, tachycardia, dry oral mucosa, diminished skin turgor, and reduced or increased output of dilute or concentrated urine, depending on cause.
- Signs associated with chronic hypernatremia are often difficult to detect because most affected adults have underlying neurologic disease.

Laboratory Tests

- Serum sodium levels are generally higher than 145 mEq/L. Measurement of urine volume and osmolality may be helpful in diagnosing the cause.

Osmotic Diuresis Patients undergoing an osmotic diuresis generally have urine volumes greater than 3 L/day. Excessive urinary excretion of glucose, sodium, urea, or an exogenously administered solute such as mannitol, are identified either by history or by direct measurement of serum and urinary concentrations of the suspected solute. Patients with postobstructive diuresis, such as those with bladder outlet obstruction caused by prostatic hypertrophy, are usually volume expanded as a result of retained excess solute because of a decline in the GFR.[1] The osmotic diuresis that follows alleviation of the obstruction is appropriate in that it promotes excretion of the excess retained solute. Patients with severe hyperglycemia, conversely, present with signs of volume depletion, and the diuresis is therefore inappropriate, further exacerbating the degree of ECF volume contraction.

Diabetes Insipidus Patients with DI tend to maintain a normal ECF volume as long as they are conscious and have free access to water. Patients typically have only a slight elevation in the serum sodium concentration (usually in the 141 to 145 mEq/L range), and a daily urine volume greater than 3 liters.[51] A water deprivation test is sometimes recommended to aid in the differential diagnosis between central and nephrogenic DI.[23] This consists of depriving patients of water for 8 to 12 hours. Urine osmolality, urine volume, and body weight, are then measured before and after subcutaneous administration of 5 mcg of desmopressin acetate. Patients with central DI will show a prompt increase in urine osmolality to approximately 600 mOsm/kg and a decrease in urine volume after desmopressin administration. Those with nephrogenic DI will be unable to increase the urine osmolality above 300 mOsm/kg.[1] The direct measurement of vasopressin levels after infusion of 5% sodium chloride at a rate of 0.05 mL/kg/min for no more than 2 hours improves the accuracy of diagnosis, but carries a high risk of ECF volume overload.[52]

The value of performing a water deprivation test in patients with polyuria and hypernatremia, such as patients with DI, has recently been questioned.[53] Because hypernatremia provides a maximal stimulus for AVP secretion, discriminating between nephrogenic and central DI can be based on plasma vasopressin concentration and urinary response to desmopressin without the need for water deprivation. The water deprivation test is thus likely to only be of diagnostic value in patients with polyuria and a normal serum sodium concentration.

Sodium Overload Patients who have ingested large amounts of sodium (>4 tablespoons [1,400 mEq Na^+] of sodium chloride) or who have received greater than 5 liters of hypertonic fluids are volume expanded, although this may not always be clinically evident as edema. This results in an osmotic diuresis, polyuria, and a urine osmolality greater than 300 mOsm/kg. The excess sodium will be excreted in the urine in patients with normal renal function.

TREATMENT

Hypernatremia

DESIRED OUTCOME

7 The desired goals for patients with hypernatremia include correction of the serum sodium concentration at a rate that restores and maintains cell volume as close to normal as possible, as well as normalizing the ECF volume in states of ECF volume depletion or expansion. Adequate treatment should result in the resolution of symptoms associated with hypovolemia. Careful titration of fluids and medications should minimize the adverse effects from too rapid correction. Rapid correction can result in movement of excessive water into the brain cells, resulting in cerebral edema, seizures, neurologic damage, and potentially death.[1] Modulation of dietary sodium intake and sodium replacement can be necessary to prevent recurrence of hypernatremia.

PHARMACOLOGIC THERAPY

Hypovolemic Hypernatremia

Hypovolemic hypernatremia (postural hypotension, tachycardia, and decreased skin turgor) should initially be treated with 0.9% sodium chloride until hemodynamic stability is restored. An initial infusion rate of 200 to 300 mL/h will likely be appropriate for many patients. Once intravascular volume is restored, 0.45% sodium chloride or 5% dextrose in water (D5W) can then be infused to correct the water deficit,[31] the volume of which can be estimated as:

$$\text{Water Deficit} = \text{Present TBW} \times [(S^1_{Na} / 140) - 1]$$

where TBW = total body water; S^1_{Na} = initial patient serum sodium concentration (in mEq/L); and 140 = normal or goal S_{Na} (in mEq/L).

The rate of correction depends on the rapidity with which the hypernatremia developed. Hypernatremia that has developed over a few hours can be corrected at a rate of approximately 1 mEq/L per hour, whereas a rate of 0.5 mEq/L per hour should be used when it has developed more slowly.[16,44] The rate of correction should generally be limited to no more than 10 mEq/L per day.[23,44]

Treatment of hyperglycemia-induced osmotic diuresis consists of correcting the hyperglycemia with insulin, as well as administering 0.9% sodium chloride until signs of ECF volume depletion resolve. Once hemodynamic stability is restored, the water deficit should be corrected in a manner analogous to that described for patients with hypovolemic hypernatremia above. The corrected serum sodium level should be calculated by adding 1.7 mEq/L for every 100-mg/dL increase in the serum glucose concentration before estimating the water deficit.[3]

Hypernatremia in patients undergoing a postobstructive diuresis should be treated with infusion of hypotonic fluids such as 0.45% sodium chloride at maintenance rates of approximately 1.5 mL/kg per hour. It is important to avoid the temptation to administer fluids to replace urine output on a 1:1 volume basis, because this tends to perpetuate the diuresis.

The serum sodium concentration and fluid status should be monitored every 2 to 3 hours over the first 24 hours of admission in patients with symptomatic hypernatremia to permit appropriate adjustment in the rate of infusion of hypotonic fluids. After symptoms resolve and the serum sodium is less than 148 mEq/L, serum sodium determinations every 6 to 12 hours and fluid status assessment every 8 to 24 hours are generally sufficient to follow the course of therapy.

Central Diabetes Insipidus

8 Patients with central DI should generally receive AVP replacement therapy with desmopressin, an AVP analog.[1,16] Because of variable absorption of oral desmopressin, DI is best treated with the intranasal formulation 1-desamino-8-D-arginine vasopressin (DDAVP); however, oral tablets are available and can be useful in some patients. The beginning intranasal dose should be 10 mcg once daily. Ultimately the dose may need to be titrated up to 10 mcg twice daily for most adults. Each insufflation of intranasal DDAVP delivers 10 mcg of desmopressin acetate at a concentration of 100 mcg/mL. Several medications with antidiuretic properties have been used successfully in the management of central and nephrogenic DI (Table 52–3). They can be used as an alternative to DDAVP or adjunctively.

The desmopressin dose should be adjusted to achieve adequate urinary concentration during sleep to prevent nocturia, to result in a daily urine volume of approximately 1.5 to 2 L, and to maintain the serum sodium concentration in the 137 to 142 mEq/L range. The serum sodium concentration should be measured every 3 to 4 days during the initial dose titration period, and then every 2 to 4 months. Administration of desmopressin results in nonsuppressible AVP activity and presents a risk of water intoxication caused by excess water retention.[1] Patients using desmopressin should therefore be monitored for signs and symptoms of hyponatremia and hypervolemia. It has been suggested that patients using desmopressin who experience water intoxication can minimize the risk of a second episode by delaying a dose of desmopressin each week until polyuria and thirst develop, thus demonstrating the need for additional desmopressin doses.[16]

Nephrogenic Diabetes Insipidus

Hypercalcemia and hypokalemia should be corrected, and medications that contribute to the pathogenesis should be discontinued. One key goal in treating nephrogenic DI is to induce a mild ECFVd (1 to 1.5 L) with a thiazide diuretic and dietary sodium restriction (85 mEq Na^+ or 2,000 mg sodium chloride per day), which often can decrease urine volume by as much as 50% (see Table 52–3). This will increase proximal water reabsorption, decrease the volume of filtrate delivered to the distal nephron, and decrease urine volume. NSAIDs such as indomethacin at a dose of 50 mg three times a day can potentiate the activity of AVP and can be used as adjunctive therapy.[1,54] Patients with lithium-induced nephrogenic DI can derive particular benefit from amiloride at a dose of 5 to 10 mg

TABLE 52-3 Drugs Used to Manage Central and Nephrogenic Diabetes Insipidus

Drug	Indication	Dose
Desmopressin acetate	Central and nephrogenic	5–20 mcg intranasally every 12–24 hours
Chlorpropamide	Central	125–250 mg orally daily
Carbamazepine	Central	100–300 mg orally twice a day
Clofibrate	Central	500 mg orally four times a day
Hydrochlorothiazide	Central and nephrogenic	25 mg orally every 12–24 hours
Amiloride	Lithium-related nephrogenic	5–10 mg orally daily
Indomethacin	Central and nephrogenic	50 mg orally every 8–12 hours

daily; amiloride directly inhibits uptake of lithium from the tubular lumen into principal cells in the cortical collecting duct.[1,55]

CLINICAL CONTROVERSY

The relative merits of the various drug treatment options, including NSAIDs and amiloride, for nephrogenic DI have not been well studied. Choice of agents is therefore subject to clinician variability. It is unclear if there is a significant difference among these agents in the risk of clinically important decreases in GFR when they are used to produce mild ECF volume decreases.

■ EVALUATION OF TREATMENT OUTCOMES

Physical examination with attention to volume status and measurement of serum and urine sodium concentration and osmolality should be assessed every 2 to 3 months during chronic therapy. A 24-hour urine collection to measure urine volume and sodium excretion will help guide therapy with diuretics and determine adherence to sodium restriction.

Sodium Overload

Treatment of sodium overload consists of administration of loop diuretics to facilitate excretion of the excess sodium, as well as intravenous D_5W. The latter should be infused at a rate that will decrease the serum sodium at approximately 0.5 mEq/L per hour, or 1 mEq/L per hour in cases in which the hypernatremia developed rapidly over several hours.[44] The volume of infusate may be estimated as described previously. Furosemide should be administered at a dose of 20 to 40 mg intravenously every 6 hours.

The serum sodium should initially be measured every 2 to 4 hours, and the diuretic continued until signs of ECF volume overload (pulmonary congestion and edema) resolve. The serum sodium concentration can be determined every 6 to 12 hours once the serum sodium level is less than 148 mEq/L and symptoms of hypertonicity resolve.

EDEMA

The body closely monitors blood volume to help ensure adequate tissue perfusion. A decline in the effective circulating volume (actually the blood pressure resulting from that volume) results in decreased sodium and water excretion by the kidney.[1] Under these conditions, the kidneys retain all of the water and sodium ingested until the effective circulating volume is restored to normal. An increase in dietary sodium is accompanied by an increase in water intake caused by the initial increase in serum osmolality and stimulation of thirst. The resultant increase in ECF volume augments renal perfusion, effecting a transient increase in GFR which leads to enhanced sodium filtration and excretion.[56] These homeostatic mechanisms are crucial in maintaining sodium balance, as retention of just a few milliequivalents of sodium per day can eventually lead to an expanded ECF volume and edema formation.

PATHOPHYSIOLOGY

❾ Edema may be defined as a clinically detectable increase in interstitial fluid volume. Clinical detectability in adults generally requires an interstitial volume increase of at least 2.5 to 3 L.[1] Edema develops when excess sodium is retained either as a primary defect in renal sodium excretion, or as a response to a decrease in the effective circulating volume despite an already normal or expanded ECF volume. An increase in the capillary hydrostatic pressure because of an expansion of the ECF volume, or an increase in central venous pressure may lead to edema formation. Edema may also occur when there is an alteration in Starling forces within the capillary.[57] The Starling equation denotes the relationship between factors affecting the movement of fluid between the capillary and interstitium and is discussed in detail in Chap. 26.

Edema may develop rapidly as in the setting of acute decompensation in myocardial contractility which leads to an elevation in pulmonary venous pressure that is transmitted back to the pulmonary capillaries resulting in acute pulmonary edema. Edema may also develop insidiously as in the case of renal sodium and water retention due to diminished effective circulating volume which leads to a rise in the ECF volume and edema formation in both peripheral and pulmonary interstitial tissues.

Edema formation in patients with nephrotic syndrome is primarily related to renal sodium and water retention. A decrease in capillary oncotic pressure does not appear to play a major role until the serum albumin concentration falls to less than 2 g/dL. This is explained by the fact that both capillary and interstitial oncotic pressure decrease proportionately above a serum albumin concentration of 2 g/dL, and thus the transcapillary oncotic gradient is not significantly altered.[58]

Patients with cirrhosis initially develop ascites as a result of an increase in the pressure in the portal circulation proximal to the diseased liver. Sequestration of fluid in the abdominal cavity (ascites) and peripheral vasodilation as a consequence of increased levels of circulating cytokines, result in a decrease in the effective circulating volume, activation of the sympathetic nervous system, and secondary hyperaldosteronism. Therefore, renal sodium retention leads to worsened ascites and edema.

CLINICAL PRESENTATION

Edema is usually first detected in the feet or pretibial area of ambulatory patients and in the presacral area of bed-bound individuals. Edema is described as "pitting" when a depression created by exerting pressure for several seconds over a bony prominence such as the tibia does not rapidly refill. The severity of the edema should be rated on a semi-quantitative scale of 1+ to 4+ depending on the depth of the pit (1+ = 2 mm, 2+ = 4 mm, 3+ = 6 mm, and 4+ = 8 mm).

The extent of the edema should also be quantified according to the area of involvement. Pretibial edema, for example, should be quantified according to how far it extends up the lower leg (e.g., one-third up the lower leg). Pulmonary edema, an increase in lung interstitial and alveolar water, is often evidenced by crackles (also called rales) upon auscultation. It should be quantified according to how far the crackles extend from the dependent portion of the lung(s). So, for example, edema limited to the ankles and feet would indicate less severe edema than edema that extends halfway up the lower legs, and crackles limited to the base of both lungs in an upright person would indicate less severe pulmonary edema than crackles throughout both lung fields.

TREATMENT

Edema

■ GENERAL APPROACH TO TREATMENT

❿ The goals of diuretic therapy are to minimize tissue edema and thus improve organ function, as well as to relieve symptoms of edema such as dyspnea in patients with congestive heart failure (CHF) or abdominal distention in patients with ascites. It is important to emphasize that the presence of edema does not always dictate the need for instituting pharmacologic (diuretic) therapy. Only pulmo-

TABLE 52-4 Maximal Effective Dose and Dosing Interval for Edema Management with Loop Diuretics

Diuretic	Dosing Interval	Normal	Cirrhosis	CHF	Nephrotic Syndrome	GFR (10–50 mL/min)	GFR (<10 mL/min)
Furosemide							
IV	6–8 hours	10–40 mg	40 mg	40–80 mg	120 mg	80 mg	200 mg
Oral	6–8 hours	20–80 mg	80 mg	80–160 mg	240 mg	160 mg	320–400 mg
Bumetanide							
IV/Oral	6–8 hours	1 mg	1 mg	2–3 mg	3 mg	2–3 mg	8–10 mg
Torsemide							
IV/Oral	24 hours	15–20 mg	10–20 mg	20–50 mg	50 mg	20–50 mg	50–100 mg

CHF, congestive heart failure; GFR, glomerular filtration rate.

nary edema requires immediate pharmacologic treatment because it is life-threatening. Other forms of edema may be treated gradually, with a comprehensive approach that includes not only diuretics, but also sodium restriction and treatment of the underlying disease state. Sodium intake should generally be restricted to 1,000 to 2,000 mg/day. A slow, more judicious approach in non–life-threatening situations will help to minimize complications of diuretic therapy and excessive fluid removal. These may include impaired vital organ perfusion, azotemia, and impaired cardiac output due to a fall in the left ventricular end-diastolic filling pressure.

PHARMACOLOGIC THERAPY

Diuretics are the primary pharmacologic therapy for the management of edema. Patients with expanded ECF volume and edema often require therapy with diuretics when treatment of the underlying disease and daily sodium restriction are insufficient to relieve the edema. Diuretics can be categorized according to the site in the nephron where sodium reabsorption is inhibited. Loop diuretics inhibit the sodium-potassium-chloride (Na^+-K^+-$2Cl^-$) carrier in the loop of Henle. Thiazide diuretics inhibit the Na^+-Cl^- carrier in the distal tubule. Finally, potassium-sparing diuretics inhibit the sodium channel in the cortical collecting duct either directly (triamterene and amiloride), or by interfering with aldosterone activity (spironolactone and eplerenone). The efficacy of a diuretic depends on the presence of several factors, including the amount of filtered solute normally reabsorbed at the site of action, the amount of solute reabsorbed distal to the site of action, and adequate delivery of drug to the site of action in the nephron.

Loop diuretics are the most potent diuretics, as evidenced by the fact that they increase peak fractional excretion of sodium (FeNa) to 20% to 25%. Thiazide- and potassium-sparing diuretics are less potent and increase peak FeNa to 3% to 5% and 1% to 2%, respectively.[1] Although a large portion of the filtered sodium is reabsorbed in the proximal nephron, the efficacy of proximal-acting diuretics such as acetazolamide is limited by reabsorption of the excess fluid and sodium in the loop of Henle.

The effectiveness of thiazide and loop diuretics is dependent on the concentration of the drug in the tubular lumen. These diuretics are delivered to the tubular lumen of the kidney by active transport by the proximal tubular cells. Osmotic diuretics, conversely, are freely filtered into the tubular lumen in the proximal tubule, whereas spironolactone gains access to mineralocorticoid receptors in the cortical collecting duct through diffusion from the systemic circulation.

A threshold concentration of loop or thiazide diuretic must be delivered to the active site (e.g., loop of Henle or distal tubule) to achieve a natriuresis.[1,59] Once this concentration is achieved, further increases in diuretic dose will not elicit an increase in diuretic response. Thus a ceiling dose of diuretic is recognized. Administration of 40 mg of intravenous furosemide to a normal subject will result in excretion of 200 to 250 mEq of sodium in 3 to 4 liters of urine over a 3- to 4-hour period.[59] Table 52–4 summarizes the maximal effective doses and dosing intervals for loop diuretics in patients with cirrhosis, CHF, nephrotic syndrome, as well as those with reduced renal function. Patients with renal insufficiency often require larger doses of diuretics to achieve adequate concentrations of the drug at the active site. The natriuretic response is decreased in patients with renal insufficiency because the filtered load of sodium falls proportionately as GFR declines. This can be partially overcome by dosing diuretics more frequently, as well as by using continuous infusions in critically ill hospitalized patients.[1,60,61] The latter will maintain more consistent levels of the diuretic above the threshold concentration. Patients who are diuretic resistant should be treated with both a loop and a thiazide-type diuretic. Patients with CHF and a normal GFR have impaired oral absorption of furosemide. An adequate diuresis is most readily sustained by increasing the frequency of diuretic administration (Fig. 52–5).

Diuretic resistance can be caused by increased uptake of sodium in the distal tubule, impaired delivery of diuretics to the site of action, or decreased intrinsic diuretic activity. Animal studies have demonstrated binding of furosemide to albumin in the tubular lumen, which decreases the availability of the drug to the active site.[62] Human studies, however, have demonstrated that when albumin binding is inhibited by concurrent administration of sulfasoxazole, diuretic resistance persists, suggesting a decrease in intrinsic tubular sensitivity to loop diuretics.[63] This impaired natriuretic response can be overcome by using higher diuretic doses to increase the delivery of free drug to the secretory site in the nephron.[60,61] Combinations of loop diuretics with distally-acting diuretics are generally necessary to promote a natriuresis that exceeds tubular sodium reabsorption (Fig. 52–6).

CLINICAL CONTROVERSY

Some clinicians advocate using combinations of diuretics in cases of diuretic resistance associated with nephrotic syndrome, while others prefer to use larger-than-average doses of single agents to overcome enhanced protein binding in the tubular lumen associated with proteinuria.

Secondary hyperaldosteronism plays a major role in the pathogenesis of edema in patients with cirrhosis. Therefore, these patients

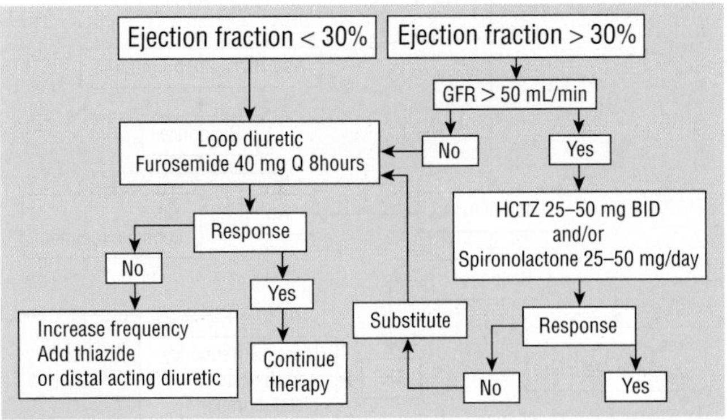

FIGURE 52-5. Therapeutic algorithm for diuretic use in patients with congestive heart failure. (GFR, glomerular filtration rate; HCTZ, hydrochlorothiazide.)

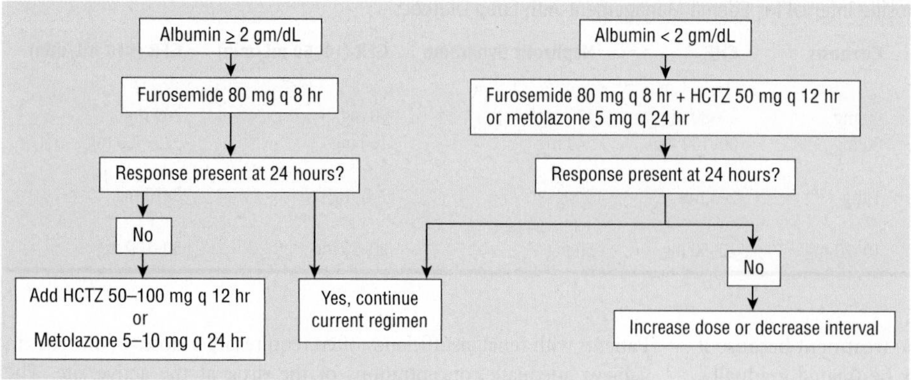

FIGURE 52-6. Therapeutic algorithm for diuretic therapy in patients with nephrotic syndrome. (HCTZ, hydrochlorothiazide.)

should initially be treated with spironolactone in the absence of impaired GFR and hyperkalemia. Thiazides can then be added for patients with a creatinine clearance >50 mL/min. For those patients who remain diuretic resistant, a loop diuretic can replace the thiazide. Patients with impaired GFR (creatinine clearance of <40 mL/min) can require a loop diuretic, with addition of a thiazide in those who do not achieve adequate diuresis.[61] Care should be taken to avoid hypokalemia, which can precipitate hepatic encephalopathy by increasing ammoniagenesis (Fig. 52–7).[64]

Complications of loop and thiazide diuretic therapy include hypokalemia, excess depletion of ECF volume, hyponatremia, hypomagnesemia, metabolic alkalosis, and hyperuricemia. Thiazides can also cause hypercalcemia, particularly in patients with mild subclinical hyperparathyroidism. Chronic therapy with potassium-sparing diuretics, including triamterene, amiloride, and spironolactone, can cause a mild metabolic acidosis and can precipitate hyperkalemia. Patients with moderate to severe kidney dysfunction or those receiving NSAIDs, ACEIs, or ARBs are at highest risk for this complication. In addition, spironolactone can cause reversible gynecomastia in patients receiving therapy for more than several weeks. This side effect, however, has not been associated with eplerenone, a newly available aldosterone antagonist.[65]

EVALUATION OF THERAPEUTIC OUTCOMES

Patients should be monitored by careful history and intermittent physical examinations to detect signs and symptoms of edema as well as adverse effects of treatment. Physical examination should include measurement of blood pressure and pulse in either supine or seated positions and after standing for 2 to 3 minutes. ECF volume can be estimated based on the height of the jugular venous pressure, extent of edema, auscultation of the heart and lungs, and skin mobility. Followup monitoring (10 to 14 days after initiation of therapy) should include determinations of serum sodium, potassium, chloride, bicarbonate, magnesium, calcium, BUN, serum creatinine, and uric acid. A new steady state will have developed over that time period and further fluctuations in ECF volume and electrolyte balance should not occur in the absence of a change in clinical status, diuretic dose, or dietary intake. Repeated blood tests are not necessary at every visit unless there is a change in the patient's clinical status.

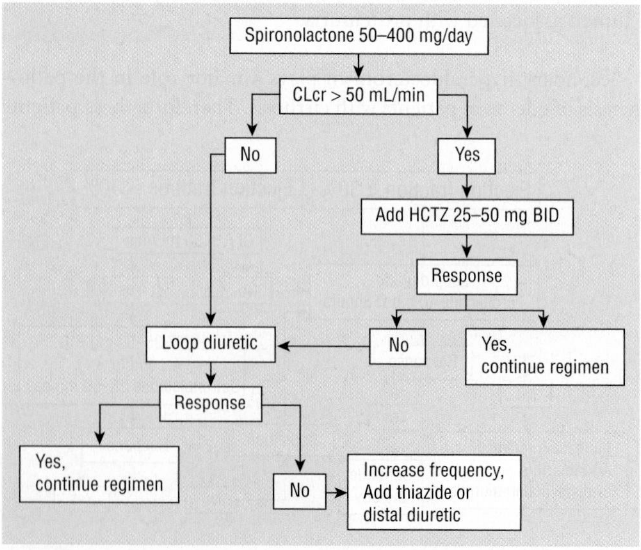

FIGURE 52-7. Therapeutic algorithm for diuretic use in patients with cirrhosis. (CL_{cr}, creatinine clearance; HCTZ, hydrochlorothiazide.)

ABBREVIATIONS

ACEI: angiotensin-converting enzyme inhibitor

AVP: arginine vasopressin, also known as antidiuretic hormone or ADH

ATPase: adenosine triphosphatase

BUN: blood urea nitrogen

CHF: congestive heart failure

CNS: central nervous system

DDAVP: 1-desamino-8-D-arginine vasopressin

D5W: 5% dextrose in water

DI: diabetes insipidus

ECF: extracellular fluid

ECFVd: extracellular fluid volume deficit

$ECFV_{current}$: current extracellular fluid volume

$ECFV_{norm}$: normal extracellular fluid volume

FeNa: fractional excretion of sodium

GFR: glomerular filtration rate

IV_{Na}: sodium concentration of infusate

IV_{vol}: volume of infusate

NSAID: nonsteroidal antiinflammatory drug

S^1_{Na}: initial patient serum sodium concentration

SIADH: syndrome of inappropriate secretion of antidiuretic hormone

TBW: total body water

$TBW_{current}$: current total body water

TBW_{norm}: normal total body water

V2: vasopressin-2

REFERENCES

1. Rose DR, Post TW. Clinical Physiology of Acid-Base and Electrolyte Disorders, 5th ed. New York: McGraw-Hill, 2001.
2. Andreoli TE. Water: Normal balance, hyponatremia, and hypernatremia. Ren Fail 2000;2:711–735.
3. Androgué HJ, Madias NE. Hyponatremia. N Engl J Med 2000;342:1581–1589.
4. Deen PM, Verdijk MA, Knoers NV, et al. Requirement of human renal water channel aquaphorin-2 for vasopressin-dependent concentration of urine. Science 1994;264:92–95.
5. Upadhyay A, Jaber BL, Madias NE. Incidence and prevalence of hyponatremia. Am J Med 2006;119(7A):S30–S35.
6. Anderson RJ. Hospital-associated hyponatremia. Kidney Int 1986;29:1237–1247.
7. Hawkins RC. Age and gender as risk factors for hyponatremia and hypernatremia. Clin Chim Acta 2003;337:169–172.
8. Nzerue CM, Baffoe-Bonnie H, You W, et al. Predictors of outcome in hospitalized patients with severe hyponatremia. J Natl Med Assoc 2003;95:335–343.
9. Kurtz I, Nguyen MK. Evolving concepts in the quantitative analysis of the determinants of the plasma water sodium concentration and the pathophysiology and treatment of dysnatremias. Kidney Int 2005;68:1982–1993.
10. Reynolds RM, Seckl JR. Hyponatremia for the clinical endocrinologist. Clin Endocrinol 2005;63:366–374.
11. Chow KM, Szeto CC, Wong,TY-H, et al. Risk factors for thiazide-induced hyponatremia. Q J Med 2003;96:911–917.
12. Sonnenblick M, Friedlander Y, Rosin AJ. Diuretic-induced severe hyponatremia: Review and analysis of 129 reported patients. Chest 1993;103:601–606.
13. Smith DM, McKenna K, Thompson CJ. Hyponatremia. Clin Endocrinol 2000;52:667–678.
14. Jacob S, Spinler SA. Hyponatremia associated with selective serotonin-reuptake inhibitors in older adults. Ann Pharmacother 2006;40:1618–1622.
15. Hairprasad MK, Eisinger RP, Nadler IM, et al. Hyponatremia in psychogenic polydipsia. Arch Intern Med 1980;140:1639–1642.
16. Reynolds RM, Padfield PL, Seckl JR. Disorders of sodium balance. BMJ 2006;332:702–705.
17. Decaux G. Is asymptomatic hyponatremia really asymptomatic? Am J Med 2006;119(7A):S79–S82.
18. Sterns RH, Silver SM. Brain volume regulation in response to hypo-osmolality and its correction. Am J Med 2006;119(7A):S12–S16.
19. Ayus JC, Arrief AI. Chronic hyponatremic encephalopathy in post-menopausal women—Association of therapies with morbidity and mortality. JAMA 1999;281:2299–2304.
20. Sterns RH. Severe symptomatic hyponatremia: Treatment and outcome: A study of 64 cases. Ann Intern Med 1987;107:656–664.
21. Murase TM, Sugimura Y, Takefuji S, et al. Mechanisms and therapy of osmotic demyelination. Am J Med 2006;119(7A):S69–S73.
22. Sterns RH, Riggs JE, Schochet SS Jr. Osmotic demyelination syndrome following correction of hyponatremia. N Engl J Med 1986;314:1535–1542.
23. Ellison DH. Core curriculum in nephrology: Disorders of sodium and water. Am J Kidney Dis 2005;46:356–361.
24. Decaux G, Soupart A. Treatment of symptomatic hyponatremia. Am J Med Sci 2003;326:25–30.
25. Androgue HJ, Madias NE. Aiding fluid prescription for dysnatremias. Intensive Care Med 1997;23:309–316.
26. Nguyen MK, Kurtz I. A new quantitative approach to the treatment of the dysnatremias. Clin Exp Nephrol 2003;7:125–137.
27. Kurtz I, Nguyen MK. Evolving concepts in the quantitative analysis of the determinants of the plasma water sodium concentration and the pathophysiology and treatment of the dysnatremias. Kidney Int 2005;68:1982–1993.
28. Kraft MD, Btaiche IF, Sacks GS, Kudsk KA. Treatment of electrolyte disorders in adult patients in the intensive care unit. Am J Health Syst Pharm 2005;62:1663–1682.
29. Liamis G, Kalogirou M, Saugos V, Moses E. Therapeutic approach in patients with dysnatremias. Nephrol Dial Transplant 2006;21:1564–1569.
30. Fanestil DD, Moore FD. Compartmentation of body water. In: Narins RG, ed. Maxwell and Kleeman's Fluid and Electrolyte Metabolism, 5th ed. New York: McGraw-Hill, 1994:1–20.
31. Mange K, Matsuura D, Cizman B, et al. Language guiding therapy: The case of dehydration versus volume depletion. Ann Intern Med 1997;127:848–853.
32. Decaux G, Waterlot Y, Genette F, Mockel J. Treatment of the syndrome of inappropriate secretion of antidiuretic hormone with furosemide. N Engl J Med 1981;304:329–330.
33. Verbalis JG. Hyponatremia and hyposmolar disorders. In: Greenberg A, ed. Primer on Kidney Diseases, 4th ed. Philadelphia: WB Saunders, 2005:58–65.
34. Curtis NJ, van Heyningen C, Turner JJ. Irreversible nephrotoxicity from demeclocycline in the treatment of hyponatremia. Age Ageing 2002;31:151–152.
35. Greenberg A, Verbalis JG. Vasopressin receptor antagonists. Kidney Int 2006;69:2124–2130.
36. Palm CP, Pistrosch F, Herbrig K, Gross P. Vasopressin antagonists as aquaretic agents for the treatment of hyponatremia. Am J Med 2006;119(7A):S87–S92.
37. Schrier RW, Gross P, Gheorghiade M, et al. Tolvaptan, a selective oral vasopressin V_2-receptor antagonist, for hyponatremia. N Engl J Med 2006;355:2099–2112.
38. Elisaf M, Theodorou J, Pappas C, Siamopoulos K. Successful treatment of hyponatremia with angiotensin-converting enzyme inhibitors in patients with congestive heart failure. Cardiology 1995;86:477–480.
39. Bakris GL, Weir MR. Angiotensin-converting enzyme inhibitor-associated elevation of creatinine: Is this a cause for concern? Arch Intern Med 2000;160:685–693.
40. Gerbes AL, Gulberg V, Gines P, et al. Therapy of hyponatremia in cirrhosis with a vasopressin receptor antagonist: A randomized double-blind multicenter trial. Gastroenterology 2003;124:933–939.
41. Goldsmith SR. Vasopressin receptor antagonists: Mechanisms of action and potential effects of heart failure. Cleve Clin J Med 2006;73(Suppl 2):S20–S23.
42. Gheorghiade M. The clinical effects of vasopressin receptor antagonists in heart failure. Cleve Clin J Med 2006;73(Suppl 2):S24–S29.
43. Sanghi P, Uretsky BF, Schwarz ER. Vasopressin antagonism: A future treatment option in heart failure. Eur Heart J 2005;26:538–543.
44. Androgué HJ, Madias NE. Hypernatremia. N Engl J Med 2000;342:1493–1499.
45. Palevsky PM, Bhagrath R, Greenberg A. Hypernatremia in hospitalized patients. Ann Intern Med 1996;124:197–203.
46. Aiyagari V, Deibert E, Diringer MN. Hypernatremia in the neurologic intensive care unit: How high is too high? J Crit Care 2006;21:163–172.
47. Moritz ML, Ayus JC. The changing pattern of hypernatremia in hospitalized children. Pediatrics 1999;104:435–439.
48. Sands JM, Bichet DG. Nephrogenic diabetes insipidus. Ann Intern Med 2006;144:186–194.
49. Garofeanu CG, Weir M, Rosas-Arellano P, et al. Causes of reversible nephrogenic diabetes insipidus: A systematic review. Am J Kidney Dis 2005;45:626–637.
50. Chassagne P, Druesne L, Capet C, Menard JF, Bercoff E. Clinical presentation of hypernatremia in elderly patients: A case control study. J Am Geriatr Soc 2006;54:1225–1230.
51. Andreoli TE. The polyuric syndromes. Nephrol Dial Transplant 2001;16(Suppl 6):10–12.
52. Zerbe RL, Robertson GL. A comparison of plasma vasopressin measurements with a standard indirect test in the differential diagnosis of polyuria. N Engl J Med 1981;304:1539–1546.
53. Moritz ML. A water deprivation test is not indicated in the evaluation of hypernatremia [letter]. Am J Kidney Dis 2005;46:1150–1151.
54. Monnens L, Jonkman A, Thomas C. Response to indomethacin and hydrochlorothiazide in nephrogenic diabetes insipidus. Clin Sci 1984;66:709–715.
55. Battle DC, Von Riotte AB, Gaviria M, Grupp M. Amelioration of polyuria by amiloride in patients receiving long-term lithium therapy. N Engl J Med 1985;312:408–414.
56. Bonventre JV, Leaf A. Sodium homeostasis: Steady states without a setpoint. Kidney Int 1982;21:880–883.
57. Taylor AE. Capillary fluid filtration: Starling forces and lymph flow. Circ Res 1981;49:557–575.

58. Schrier RW. Pathogenesis of sodium and water retention in high-output and low-output cardiac failure, nephrotic syndrome, cirrhosis, and pregnancy. N Engl J Med 1988;319:1127–1134.
59. Brater DC. Diuretic therapy. N Engl J Med 1998;339:387–395.
60. Rudy DW, Voelker JR, Greene PK, et al. Loop diuretics for chronic renal insufficiency: A continuous infusion is more efficacious than bolus therapy. Ann Intern Med 1991;115:360–366.
61. Ellison DH. Edema and the clinical use of diuretics. In: Greenberg A, ed. Primer on Kidney Diseases, 4th ed. Philadelphia: Saunders, 2005:136–148.
62. Kirchner KA, Voelker JR, Brater DC. Intratubular albumin blunts the response to furosemide—A mechanism for diuretic resistance in the nephrotic syndrome. J Pharmacol Exp Ther 1990;252:1097–1101.
63. Agarwal R, Gorski JC, Sundblad K, Brater DC. Urinary protein binding does not affect response to furosemide in patients with nephrotic syndrome. J Am Soc Nephrol 2000;11:1100–1105.
64. Weiner ID, Wingo CS. Hypokalemia—Consequences, causes, and correction. J Am Soc Nephrol 1997;8:1179–1188.
65. Liew D, Martin J, Krum H. Eplerenone. Pharmacia. Curr Opin Investig Drugs 2003;4:316–322.

CHAPTER 53

Disorders of Calcium and Phosphorus Homeostasis

AMY BARTON PAI, MARK ROHRSCHEIB, AND MELANIE S. JOY

KEY CONCEPTS

1. Severe acute hypercalcemia can result in cardiac arrhythmias, whereas chronic hypercalcemia can lead to calcium deposition in soft tissues including blood vessels and the kidney.
2. The correction of hypercalcemia can include multiple pharmacotherapeutic modalities such as hydration, diuretics, bisphosphonates, and steroids, depending on the etiology and acuity of the hypercalcemia
3. Hypocalcemia is typically associated with an insidious onset, however, some drugs such as cinacalcet are associated with rapid decreases in serum calcium.
4. Acute treatment of hypocalcemia requires calcium supplementation whereas chronic management may require other therapies such as vitamin D to maintain serum calcium values.
5. Hyperphosphatemia occurs most frequently in patients with chronic kidney disease.
6. Treatment of nonemergent hyperphosphatemia includes the use of phosphate binders to decrease absorption of phosphorus from the gastrointestinal tract.
7. Hypophosphatemia is a relatively common complication among critically ill patients.
8. Treatment of acute hypophosphatemia usually requires intravenous supplementation of phosphorous salts.

Homeostasis of fluid and electrolytes is necessary for the body's normal physiologic functions. Disorders of calcium and phosphorus are common complications of multiple acute and chronic diseases. These disorders are frequently seen in the acute care setting; however, they are also often present in ambulatory patients albeit in a less severe state. The consequences of electrolyte disorders can range from asymptomatic to life-threatening requiring hospitalization and emergent treatment. The maintenance of fluid and electrolyte homeostasis requires adequate functioning of feedback mechanisms, hormones, and multiple organ systems.

Many common drug therapies can disturb the normal homeostatic mechanisms that maintain calcium and phosphorous balance. In addition, with some drug therapies, toxicity is enhanced when underlying electrolyte disorders are present. Drug-induced disorders respond well to discontinuation of the offending agent(s); however, additional therapies are sometimes required to correct the disorder. This chapter reviews the etiology, classification, clinical presentation, and therapy for the most common disorders of calcium and phosphorus homeostasis.

Learning objectives, review questions, and other resources can be found at **www.pharmacotherapyonline.com.**

DISORDERS OF CALCIUM HOMEOSTASIS

The maintenance of physiologic calcium concentrations in the intracellular and extracellular spaces is vital for the preservation and function of cell membranes; propagation of neuromuscular activity; regulation of endocrine and exocrine secretory functions; blood coagulation cascade; platelet adhesion process; bone metabolism; muscle cell excitation/contraction coupling; and mediation of the electrophysiologic slow-channel response in cardiac and smooth-muscle tissue.

The disorders of calcium homeostasis are related to the calcium content of the extracellular fluid, which contains less than 0.5% of the total body stores of calcium. Skeletal bone contains more than 99% of total body stores of calcium.[1] Extracellular fluid (ECF) calcium is moderately bound to plasma proteins (46%), primarily albumin.[2] Unbound or ionized calcium is the physiologically active form and is the fraction that is homeostatically regulated.[3] Extracellular calcium, however, is most commonly measured as the total serum calcium level, which includes both bound and unbound calcium.[2] The normal total calcium serum concentration range is 8.5 to 10.5 mg/dL.[3]

Proper assessment of total serum calcium concentrations includes measurement of the patient's serum albumin concentration. Hypoalbuminemia, which can be associated with many chronic disease states, is probably the most common cause of "laboratory hypocalcemia." Patients remain asymptomatic because the unbound or ionized fraction of serum calcium remains normal (normal range 4.4 to 5.4 mg/dL). A corrected total serum calcium (S_{ca}) concentration can be calculated based on the measured total serum calcium and the difference between a patient's measured albumin concentration and the normative value of 4 g/dL by the following equation:

$$\text{Corrected } S_{ca}\ (\text{mg/dL}) = \text{measured } S_{ca}\ (\text{mg/dL}) + [0.8 \times (4.0\ \text{g/dL} - \text{measured albumin (g/dL)})].$$

The concentration of ionized calcium is closely regulated by the interactions of parathyroid hormone (PTH), phosphorus, vitamin D, and calcitonin (Fig. 53–1). PTH increases serum calcium concentrations by stimulating calcium release from bone, reducing renal calcium excretion, and enhancing absorption in the gastrointestinal tract secondary to increased renal production of 1,25-dihydroxyvitamin D_3. Vitamin D directly increases serum calcium, as well as phosphorus concentrations, by increasing gastrointestinal absorption. Indirectly, it can also lead to calcium release from bone and reduced renal excretion. Calcitonin inhibits osteoclastic bone resorption. Its plasma concentrations are increased when ionized calcium concentrations

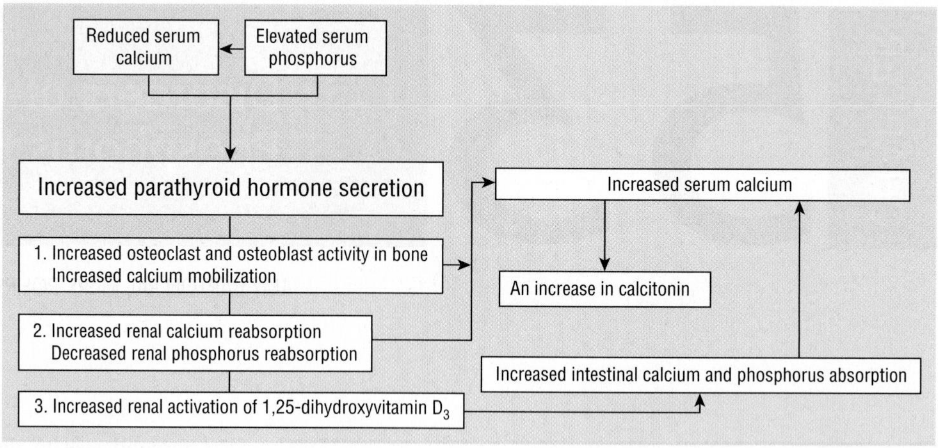

FIGURE 53-1. Homeostatic mechanisms to maintain serum calcium concentrations.

are high as the body attempts to return the calcium level to the normal range. Disruption of these homeostatic mechanisms results in the clinical manifestations of hypercalcemia or hypocalcemia.

Any factor that alters the concentration of albumin or its binding of calcium can be expected to change the unbound fraction of total serum calcium. The most significant cause of changes in calcium binding to albumin is a change in extracellular fluid pH. In the presence of metabolic alkalosis the fraction of calcium bound to albumin is increased, thus reducing the plasma concentration of ionized calcium. This can result in symptomatic hypocalcemia; that is, paresthesia, muscle cramping and spasms, memory loss, and seizures.[1] Conversely, metabolic acidosis decreases calcium binding to albumin and results in increased ionized calcium. Hypoalbuminemic states are probably the most common cause of "laboratory hypocalcemia." When the albumin level is decreased, the ionized calcium concentration can be normal although total concentration is reduced. Each 1 g/dL drop in the serum albumin concentration below 4 g/dL will result in a decrease of total serum calcium concentration by 0.8 mg/dL.[1,2] This approach of calculating an albumin-adjusted calcium concentration has been found to overestimate the degree of hypercalcemia and usually fails to identify hypocalcemia in critically ill patients, therefore ionized calcium values should be used to assess calcium status in these patients.[4,5]

HYPERCALCEMIA

Hypercalcemia (total serum calcium >10.5 mg/dL) has been associated with a multitude of causes (Table 53–1). The most common causes of hypercalcemia are cancer and primary hyperparathyroidism. The reported incidence of primary hyperparathyroidism in the United States ranges from 10 to 30 cases per 100,000 people.[6] Hypercalcemia of cancer occurs in approximately 20% to 40% of cancer patients at some time during the course of their disease.[7] Cancer-associated hypercalcemia is predominantly encountered in hospitalized patients, whereas primary hyperparathyroidism accounts for the vast majority of cases in the outpatient setting.[8,9]

PATHOPHYSIOLOGY

Hypercalcemia is the result of one of three primary mechanisms: increased bone resorption, increased gastrointestinal absorption, or decreased elimination by the kidneys (see Fig. 53–1). Many tumors secrete PTH–related protein, which binds to the PTH receptors in bone and renal tissues, leading to increased bone resorption and renal tubular reabsorption.[10] Tumors can also secrete substances such as vitamin D, transforming growth factor, interleukins, prostaglandins, interferon, tumor necrosis factor, and granulocyte-macrophage colony stimulating factor, which are associated with the development of hypercalcemia.[7] Hypercalcemia of malignancy is a common complication of squamous cell carcinomas of the lung, head, and neck, hematologic malignancies such as multiple myeloma and T-cell lymphomas, and carcinomas of ovary, kidney, bladder, and breast. The most frequent types of malignancy associated with hypercalcemia are carcinomas of the lung and breast.[9] Furthermore, up to 40% of patients with multiple myeloma can develop hypercalcemia.[9] Primary hyperparathyroidism is the most common cause of hypercalcemia in the general population. Benign parathyroid adenomas account for 80% to 85% of these cases of hyperparathyroidism, parathyroid hyperplasia accounts for 15%, and parathyroid carcinoma is the cause in less than 1% of cases.[7,8]

Other causes of hypercalcemia include medications, endocrine and granulomatous disorders, immobilization, high bone-turnover states (adolescence and Paget's disease), and rhabdomyolysis. Increased gastrointestinal absorption can be the result of excessive ingestion of vitamin D analogs, calcium supplements, and lithium. Lithium and vitamin A therapy can increase bone resorption, whereas increased renal tubular reabsorption of calcium can occur with thiazide and lithium therapy. Aluminum antacids prevent calcium deposition in the bone; thereby increasing serum concentrations.[11] Addison's disease, acromegaly, and thyrotoxicosis are endocrine disorders that can lead to hypercalcemia because of increased renal tubular reabsorption and increased bone resorption. Finally, the granulomatous disorders (sarcoidosis, tuberculosis, histoplasmosis, and leprosy) are

TABLE 53-1 Etiologies of Hypercalcemia

Neoplasms	**Medications**
Bone metastasis	Thiazides
Breast	Lithium
Multiple myeloma	Vitamin D
Lymphoma	Vitamin A
Leukemia	Calcium
Humoral induced	Aluminum/magnesium antacids
Ovary	Theophylline
Kidney	Tamoxifen
Pheochromocytoma	Ganciclovir
Multiple endocrine neoplasia	**Granulomatous disease**
Lung	Sarcoidosis
Head and neck	Tuberculosis
Esophagus	Cryptococcus
Cervix	Berylliosis
Lymphoproliferative disease	Histoplasmosis
Hyperparathyroidism	Coccidioidomycosis
Primary	Leprosy
Tertiary	**Endocrine disease**
Miscellaneous	Adrenal insufficiency
Immobilization	Hyperthyroidism
Paget's disease	Acromegaly
Familial hypocalciuric hypercalcemia	
Adolescence	
Rhabdomyolysis	

associated with hypercalcemia caused by an increase in gastrointestinal absorption.[12] Milk-alkali syndrome is the term applied to those situations where an individual develops hypercalcemia following the ingestion of calcium and absorbable alkali (e.g., calcium carbonate) and is an important cause of hypercalcemia in patients who are not on dialysis.[13,14]

CLINICAL PRESENTATION

Patients with mild to moderate hypercalcemia, that is, total serum calcium concentrations of less than 13 mg/dL, can often be asymptomatic. This is usually the case in drug-induced hypercalcemia and the vast majority of patients with primary hyperparathyroidism.[8,15,16] In fact, one study noted normocalcemia in approximately 20% of patients with a diagnosis of primary hyperparathyroidism, suggesting target tissue resistance to PTH.[16] The signs and symptoms of severe hypercalcemia that are usually present if the total serum calcium concentration is >13 mg/dL may differ depending on the acuity of onset.[2] Hypercalcemia of malignancy usually develops quickly and is accompanied by a classic symptom complex of anorexia, nausea and vomiting, constipation, polyuria, polydipsia, and nocturia.[15] Polyuria and nocturia secondary to a urinary-concentrating defect constitute some of the most frequent renal effects of hypercalcemia.[15] Hypercalcemic crisis is characterized by an acute elevation of total serum calcium to a value >15 mg/dL, acute renal insufficiency, and obtundation (inability to arouse).[15] If untreated, hypercalcemic crisis can progress to oliguric renal failure, coma, and life-threatening ventricular arrhythmias.[15] The primary complications associated with chronic hypercalcemia (hyperparathyroidism) include metastatic calcification, nephrolithiasis, and chronic renal insufficiency.[15]

CLINICAL PRESENTATION OF HYPERCALCEMIA

General

- The signs and symptoms of hypercalcemia depend on severity and on the rapidity of onset.

Symptoms

- Symptoms include fatigue, weakness, anorexia, depression, anxiety, cognitive dysfunction, vague abdominal pain, and constipation. Renal symptoms can include polyuria, polydipsia, and nocturia. Rarely, severe hypercalcemia leads to acute pancreatitis

Signs

- Renal: The most important renal manifestations which are generally the result of chronic hypercalcemia are nephrolithiasis; renal tubular dysfunction, particularly decreased concentrating ability; and acute and chronic renal insufficiency.
- Cardiovascular: Long-standing hypercalcemia can lead to the deposition of calcium in heart valves, coronary arteries, and myocardial fibers. Hypercalcemia also directly shortens the myocardial action potential, which is reflected in a shortened QT interval and coving of the ST-T wave. Spontaneous ventricular tachyarrhythmias and elevations in blood pressure have also been reported.
- Musculoskeletal: A number of rheumatologic complaints have been described in hyperparathyroidism, including gout, pseudogout, and chondrocalcinosis. The relative roles of hypercalcemia and PTH excess in these problems are not known.
- Other signs: Band keratopathy, a reflection of subepithelial calcium phosphate deposits in the cornea, is a very rare finding associated with hypercalcemia. It extends as a horizontal band across the cornea in the area that is exposed between the eyelids.

Laboratory Tests

- Serum calcium concentrations of more than 10.5 mg/dL are considered to represent hypercalcemia. Patients with values up to 13 mg/dL are generally considered to have mild or moderate hypercalcemia, whereas those with values greater than this indicate the presence of severe hypercalcemia.

Calcium and/or calcium-phosphorus complex deposition in blood vessels and multiple organs is a complication of chronic hypercalcemia and/or concomitant hyperphosphatemia and hyperparathyroidism (see Chap. 47). Calcium deposits in atherosclerotic lesions contribute to cardiac disease.[17] Intracardiac and arterial calcifications have been found in patients with Paget's disease who have normal renal function. It is hypothesized that similar calcification processes occur in both bone and vascular tissue, leading to cardiovascular diseases including heart failure, systolic hypertension, and ischemic heart disease.[18]

The electrocardiographic changes associated with hypercalcemia include shortening of the QT interval and coving of the ST-T wave.[15] Very high serum calcium concentrations can cause T-wave widening, indicating a repolarization defect that may be associated with spontaneous ventricular tachyarrhythmias.[15] Hypertension and arrhythmias have occurred in the setting of hypercalcemia. The effects of digoxin on cardiac conduction including lowering of the excitation threshold, shortening of the effective refractory period and increased atrioventricular refractoriness, can be potentiated by hypercalcemia.[19]

Nephrolithiasis (kidney stones) and nephrocalcinosis (calcium deposits in the kidney) are the primary renal complications arising from long-standing hypercalcemia, as the result of primary hyperparathyroidism. Stone formation is dependent on a favorable milieu within the kidney or urinary tract: such as oversaturation of the urine and/or reduced concentrations of endogenous inhibitors of crystal formation (e.g., citrate or pyrophosphate). It is estimated that hyperparathyroidism accounts for 2% to 8% of all patients with calcium stones.[20,21] Of note, in those patients with low glomerular filtration rates (GFRs), the 24-hour urinary calcium will actually diminish secondary to the reduced urine flow. However, the fractional excretion of calcium might increase.[21] Sarcoidosis is the other hypercalcemic condition frequently associated with calcium stones.[21] Other causes of nephrolithiasis with calcium-containing stones include hypocitraturia, renal tubular acidosis, hyperoxaluria, and hyperuricosuria.[22,23] Stone formers who have primary hyperparathyroidism are more likely to be female, older than 50 years of age, and have a family history of multiple endocrine disorders.[20] High dietary sodium intake can also raise urinary calcium concentrations, perhaps due to a reduction in calcium reabsorption in the kidney, thus predisposing patients to calcium stones. Although chronic renal failure can be the ultimate result of persistent stones, it is the primary cause of renal disease in <2% of the end-stage renal disease population.

TREATMENT

Hypercalcemia

■ DESIRED OUTCOME

The indications for the treatment of acute hypercalcemia are dependent on the severity of hypercalcemia, acuity of its development, and presence or absence of symptoms requiring emergent treatment (e.g., necrotizing pancreatitis). Treatment should include interventions that reverse signs and symptoms, restore normocalcemia, treat the underlying cause of hypercalcemia, and prevent long-term consequences.

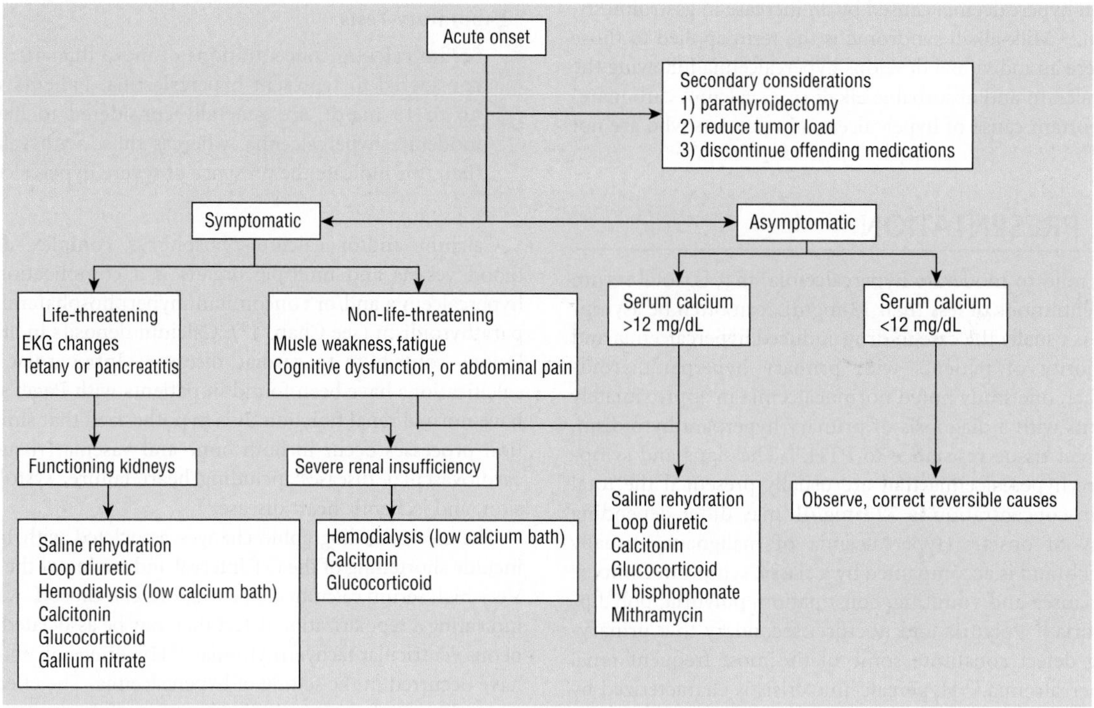

FIGURE 53-2. Pharmacotherapeutic options for the acutely hypercalcemic patient.

Chronic hypercalcemia is usually caused by an underlying medical condition or prescribed therapies. The treatment of malignancies can help mitigate acute hypercalcemic episodes. Treatment of hyperparathyroidism should reduce serum calcium concentrations as well as reduce the development of long-term complications such as vascular complications, chronic kidney disease (CKD), and kidney stones.

NONPHARMACOLOGIC THERAPY

Hypercalcemic crisis and acute symptomatic severe hypercalcemia should be considered medical emergencies and treated immediately (Fig. 53–2). These patients can require immediate-acting interventions to promptly reduce the serum calcium concentration if they are experiencing ECG changes, neurologic manifestations, or pancreatitis. Pharmacologic therapy consisting of volume expansion and enhancement of urinary calcium excretion with loop diuretics is usually the initial management strategy. Hemodialysis against a zero- or low-calcium dialysate solution should be considered for patients with severely impaired renal function (CKD stage 4 or 5) who cannot tolerate large fluid loads and in whom diuretics have limited efficacy.[11] Effective treatment of moderate to severe hypercalcemia in the absence of life-threatening symptoms begins with attention to the underlying disorder and correction of associated fluid and electrolyte abnormalities. Patients with primary hyperparathyroidism might ultimately need surgery, particularly if they have systemic manifestations. Patients with malignancy often require surgical reduction of tumor load to control the exogenous supply of cytokines and hormones that cause the hypercalcemia. In contrast, patients with drug-induced hypercalcemia generally respond to discontinuation of the offending agent.

CLINICAL CONTROVERSY

Although dialysis is the best method for rapidly reducing highly elevated serum calcium in patients with CKD, many clinicians choose a pharmacologic approach as the initial therapy.

PHARMACOLOGIC THERAPY

❷ For those patients with normal to moderately impaired renal function (CKD stage 3 and 4), the cornerstone of initial treatment of severe hypercalcemia or hypercalcemic crisis is volume expansion to increase urinary calcium excretion (see Table 53–3). Patients with symptomatic hypercalcemia are often dehydrated secondary to vomiting and polyuria; thus rehydration with saline-containing fluids is necessary to interrupt the stimulus for sodium and calcium reabsorption in the renal tubule.[24] Rehydration can be accomplished by the infusion of normal saline at rates of 200 to 300 mL/h, until the patient is fluid resuscitated and serum calcium approaches the upper limit of the normal range. The precise rate depends on concomitant conditions (primarily cardiovascular and renal) and extent of hypercalcemia. The saline infusion rate can be decreased to a rate that approximates the patient's intake of oral or intravenous fluids. (See Chap. 52 for a thorough discussion of the concepts and calculations of water deficit.) Adequacy of hydration is assessed by measuring fluid intake and output or by central venous pressure monitoring.[9,10] Loop diuretics such as furosemide (40 to 80 mg IV every 1 to 4 hours) or ethacrynic acid (for patients with sulfa allergies) can also be instituted to increase urinary calcium excretion and to minimize the development of volume overload from the administration of saline[9] (Fig 53–2 and Table 53–2). Loop diuretics such as furosemide block calcium (and sodium) reabsorption in the thick ascending limb of the loop of Henle and augment the calciuric effect of saline alone. The importance of rehydration prior to loop diuretic use is critical because if dehydration persists or becomes worse the serum calcium can actually increase because of enhanced proximal tubule calcium reabsorption.[2] Potassium chloride, 10 to 20 mEq/L, should be added to the saline solution after rehydration is accomplished to maintain normokalemia in the presence of diuretic therapy. Serum magnesium levels should also be monitored, and magnesium replacement instituted if magnesium levels fall below 1.8 mg/dL. Rehydration with saline and administration of furosemide can result in a decrease of 2 to 3 mg/dL in total serum calcium within 24 to 48 hours.[9]

TABLE 53-2 Drug Therapy Used to Treat Acute Hypercalcemia

Drug	Starting Dosage	Time Frame to Initial Response	Contraindications	Adverse Effects
0.9% saline ± electrolytes	200–300 mL/h	24–48 hours	Renal insufficiency; congestive heart failure	Electrolyte abnormalities; fluid overload
Loop diuretics	40–80 mg IV every 1–4 hours	N/A	Allergy to sulfas (use ethacrynic acid)	Electrolyte abnormalities
Calcitonin	4 units/kg every 12 hours SQ/IM 10–12 units/h IV	1–2 hours	Allergy to calcitonin	Facial flushing, nausea/vomiting, allergic reaction
Pamidronate	30–90 mg IV over 2–24 hours	2 days	Renal insufficiency	Fever
Etidronate	7.5 mg/kg per day IV over 2 hours	2 days	Renal insufficiency	Fever
Zoledronate	4–8 mg IV over 15 minutes	1–2 days	Renal insufficiency	Fever, fatigue, skeletal pain
Ibandronate	2–6 mg IV bolus	2 days	Renal insufficiency	Fever, musculoskeletal pain
Gallium nitrate	200 mg/m^2 per day	?	Severe renal insufficiency	Nephrotoxicity; hypophosphatemia; nausea/vomiting/diarrhea; metallic taste
Mithramycin	25 mcg/kg IV over 4–6 hours	12 hours	Decreased liver function; renal insufficiency; thrombocytopenia	Nausea/vomiting; stomatitis; thrombocytopenia; nephrotoxicity; hepatotoxicity
Glucocorticoids	40–60 mg oral prednisone equivalents	?	Serious infections; hypersensitivity	Diabetes; osteoporosis; infection

SQ, subcutaneous.

In those patients in whom saline hydration therapy is contraindicated (e.g., those with severe chronic heart failure [CHF] or moderate to severe renal dysfunction), short-term therapy with calcitonin is a viable alternative agent to initiate reduction of serum calcium levels; within 24 to 48 hours. Calcitonin has a rapid onset of action (within 1 to 2 hours); however, the degree and extent of serum calcium level reduction are often unpredictable.[2] Calcitonin decreases serum calcium concentrations, primarily by inhibiting bone resorption. It can also reduce renal tubular reabsorption of calcium, thus promoting calciuresis. Calcitonin from salmon sources is most commonly administered subcutaneously or intramuscularly (for larger volumes) in a starting dose of 4 units/kg every 12 hours. The side effects from intravenously administered calcitonin (facial flushing, nausea, and vomiting) limit patient acceptability. Allergic reactions, although rare, do occur; therefore a test dose (intradermal injection of 0.1 mL of a 10-units/mL solution) is recommended prior to starting therapy. If marked erythema and/or wheal formation does not occur within 15 minutes after administration, therapy can begin. Salmon calcitonin therapy is associated with tachyphylaxis caused by antibody formation to foreign proteins or molecules resembling the calcitonin polypeptide.[25] Tachyphylaxis has been primarily documented in patients receiving therapy for more than 4 months and thus might not be clinically significant in the acute care setting. The addition of corticosteroid therapy or conversion to human calcitonin increases effectiveness.[2] Finally, intravenous phosphate has been used to rapidly reduce ionized calcium concentrations through the formation of insoluble calcium-phosphate salts. However, intravenous phosphate is extremely hazardous because extraskeletal precipitation of calcium-phosphate can result in metastatic calcification, hypotension, acute renal failure, or death and thus it currently does not have a role in the management of acute hypercalcemia.[2]

Bisphosphonates block bone resorption very efficiently, render the hydroxyapatite crystal of bone mineral resistant to hydrolysis by phosphatases, and also inhibit osteoclast precursors from attaching to the mineralized matrix, thus blocking their transformation into mature functioning osteoclasts.[9,15,26] The antiresorptive properties of this class of agents can provide long term control of serum calcium and are the first-line therapy for cancer-associated hypercalcemia. Pamidronate is very effective in controlling hypercalcemia associated with malignancy and slightly more effective than etidronate.[7] The usual dose of pamidronate is 30 to 90 mg as an IV infusion given over 2 to 24 hours. Pamidronate also has the advantage of single-day therapy.[9] Etidronate, when administered in doses of 7.5 mg/kg per day by slow intravenous infusion over at least 2 hours for 3 days, is effective in the therapy of hypercalcemia of malignancy.[9] Zoledronate and ibandronate are the newest high-potency bisphosphonates with demonstrated effectiveness in the treatment of hypercalcemia of malignancy. Complete response has been reported in 88.4% to 86.7% of zoledronate-versus 69.7% of pamidronate-treated patients.[27,28] Zoledronate intravenous doses of 4 to 8 mg given over 5 minutes have resulted in normalization of serum calcium concentrations.[28] Intravenous infusions of 0.02 or 0.04 mg/kg diluted in 5% dextrose (given over 20 to 50 minutes) have also been effective.[29] A similar hypocalcemic response has been noted with ibandronate in comparison to pamidronate (76.5% versus 75.8%); however, the time period to a relapse of hypercalcemia was longer with ibandronate (14 days versus 4 days), suggesting a therapeutic advantage.[30] In contrast to other bisphosphonates, ibandronate can be administered by bolus injection. Single doses of 4 to 6 mg when administered every 3 to 4 weeks have been effective in managing hypercalcemia of malignancy.[31] The onset of serum calcium concentration decline is slower with bisphosphonate therapy (concentrations begin to decline in 2 days and reach a nadir in 7 days); thus calcitonin therapy can be necessary if rapid serum level reduction is required.[9,31] Duration of normocalcemia varies, but usually does not exceed 2 to 3 weeks. It appears to be dependant on the severity and treatment response of the underlying malignancy.[2] The duration of response has been suggested to be longer with zoledronate (4 to 5 weeks), although the data is sparse.[29] Fever is a common side effect of intravenous bisphosphonate therapy. Although oral bisphosphonates are useful for the treatment of bone turnover in Paget's disease, there are insufficient data to suggest their use for the initial treatment of hypercalcemia. The use of oral bisphosphonates for maintenance therapy in patients predisposed to hypercalcemia (malignancy) has been successful in some cases.[32] The safety of continuous bisphosphonate therapy in patients with moderate to severe renal insufficiency is currently unknown. Renal function monitoring (serum creatinine) is advised with the use of bisphosphonates, as cases of acute tubular necrosis have been reported.[33,34] Although there are no published guidelines for frequency of serum creatinine monitoring, it is advisable to evaluate serum creatinine within a week after the infusion and just prior to the next scheduled dose.

CLINICAL CONTROVERSY

Bisphosphonates are renally eliminated and prescribing information advises caution in patients with GFR <30 to 35 mL/min, however, emerging evidence suggests that these agents may slow the rate of cardiovascular calcification in patients with kidney disease.

Gallium nitrate is indicated for the treatment of symptomatic hypercalcemia of malignancy not responsive to hydration therapy.[35] However, because of its adverse side-effect profile, it is generally reserved for those who fail to respond to less toxic agents. Gallium nitrate inhibits bone resorption, and may be superior to calcitonin in inducing normocalcemia. It can provide a longer duration of normocalcemia as compared to etidronate. The initial dose is usually a continuous IV infusion of 200 mg/m^2 per day for 5 consecutive days. Gallium nitrate can be more effective in achieving normocalcemia in patients with epidermoid (squamous) cancers.[36] Because gallium nitrate is nephrotoxic, the initial dose should be conservative and the patient's renal function closely monitored if it is coadministered with other nephrotoxic drugs, including some chemotherapeutic agents, nonsteroidal antiinflammatory drugs (NSAIDs), and antibiotics (e.g., gentamicin). Other common adverse effects include hypophosphatemia, nausea, vomiting, diarrhea, hypocalcemia, and metallic taste.

Mithramycin (plicamycin) is a potent cytotoxic antibiotic that inhibits osteoclast-mediated bone resorption and thereby reduces hypercalcemia. Mithramycin can be administered at a dose of 25 mcg/kg via intravenous infusion over 4 to 6 hours in saline or 5% dextrose solutions. This therapy can be repeated daily for 3 to 4 days or on alternating days for 3 to 8 doses.[9,37] Serum calcium levels begin to fall within 12 hours of a mithramycin dose, with the peak effect generally occurring over 48 to 96 hours.[2,9] Single doses are usually well tolerated.[37] Common dose-related adverse effects of mithramycin include nausea, vomiting, stomatitis, thrombocytopenia, inhibition of platelet function, and renal and hepatotoxicity can be avoided by limiting the number of doses administered to less than four.[2] Mithramycin is usually limited to short-term therapy (typically one to two doses) in patients who have not responded to alternative therapies. Complete blood count, liver function, and renal function should be monitored within 1 to 2 days after administration. Mithramycin should be avoided in patients with thrombocytopenia and liver and renal insufficiency (creatinine clearance <30 mL/min).[9]

Prednisone or an equivalent agent in the corticosteroid class is usually effective in the treatment of hypercalcemia resulting from multiple myeloma, leukemia, lymphoma, sarcoidosis, and hypervitaminoses A and D.[2,26,37] These agents are effective because they reduce gastrointestinal calcium absorption, increase urinary calcium excretion, and decrease bone resorption and osteoblast proliferation.[8] Daily doses of 40 to 60 mg of prednisone or the equivalent are effective at reducing serum calcium within 3 to 5 days followed by a reduction in urinary calcium excretion within 7 to 10 days. The disadvantages of corticosteroid therapy are its relatively slow onset of action and the potential for diabetes mellitus, osteoporosis, and increased susceptibility to infection.[6,25]

CHRONIC HYPERCALCEMIA

Chronic, asymptomatic hypercalcemia can be treated with subcutaneous administration of salmon calcitonin; 50 to 100 international units daily or three times weekly for patients with Paget's disease. The intranasal formulation of calcitonin has been used in doses of 200 to 400 international units daily; unfortunately this has resulted in only mild decreases in serum calcium. The lack of significant efficacy of the synthetic intranasal formulation is the result of the lower potency and shorter duration of action as compared to salmon calcitonin.

Asymptomatic patients with mild hypercalcemia may be carefully observed, especially if treatment for the underlying condition (malignancy) is initiated. The calcimimetic agent cinacalcet HCl was recently approved for its calcium-lowering effect in the management of parathyroid carcinoma.[40,41] These agents bind to the calcium-sensing receptor, albeit at a different location than calcium, and increase the sensitivity for receptor activation by extracellular calcium. This results in reduced PTH and serum calcium concentrations.[40,41] Cinacalcet HCl administered at a starting dose of 30 mg orally twice daily has been used for the treatment of parathyroid carcinoma. The dosage is titrated every 2 to 4 weeks in 30-mg increments until the desired serum calcium level is achieved. The maximum approved dosage is 90 mg three to four times daily. Patients should have serum calcium measured within 1 week after starting or increasing the dose of this agent.[42,43] Patients who develop nephrolithiasis from hypercalciuria are most often treated with sodium citrate to enhance stone dissolution, thiazide diuretics to decrease urinary calcium excretion, or shock wave lithotripsy (Table 53–3).

TABLE 53-3 Treatment of Nephrolithiasis Associated with Chronic Hypercalcemia and Hypercalciuria

Intervention	Indications	Comments
Extracorporeal shock wave lithotripsy		
Uses sound waves to break up stones which then can pass spontaneously	Obstruction of the urinary tract especially with stones >5 mm.	Consider adjunctive use of potassium citrate to inhibit aggregation of residual fragments.
Enhancement of stone dissolution		
Alkalinizing agents	Treatment for non emergent active stones. Can also be used for prevention.	Potassium citrate preferred over sodium citrate as it decreases urinary calcium, inhibits calcium oxalate precipitation, and increases urinary citrate more
Potassium citrate 20 mEq twice daily		
Sodium citrate 20 to 30 mEq twice daily		
Decrease urinary calcium excretion		
Thiazide diuretics	Prevention	Drug of choice in patients with low bone density
Hydrochlorothiazide 50 mg everyday		
Indapamide 25 mg everyday		
Chlorthalidone 25 mg everyday		
Binding intestinal calcium		
Cellulose sodium phosphate (Calcibind)	Prevention for those with absorptive hypercalciuria	Alternative to thiazides if intolerant or ineffective, monitor bone density
Calcium binding ion-exchange resin that decreases gastrointestinal absorption of calcium: 5 g PO twice daily with oxalate restriction		
Inhibition of crystal formation		
Phyllanthus nituri plant extract	Prevention, after shock wave lithotripsy	Commercial preparations with *P. nituri as* the sole ingredient can be difficult to obtain
Inhibits calcium oxalate stone formation by incorporating glycosaminoglycans into the calculi: 2 grams daily		
Low calcium diet		
<400 mg per day	Prevention	Monitor bone density prior to and periodically during treatment, limit oxalate restriction, can increase hyperoxaluria, data suggest high calcium intake may actually be more beneficial

HYPOCALCEMIA

The incidence of hypocalcemia in intensive care unit patients ranges from 70% to 90% based on total serum calcium values of less than 8.5 mg/dL, to 15% to 50% based on the observation of ionized calcium concentrations of less than 4.4 mg/dL.[3] Emergent treatment of hypocalcemia is rarely warranted unless life-threatening symptoms are present (e.g., frank tetany or seizures). Hypocalcemia occurs infrequently in the outpatient setting and is most common in elderly, malnourished patients and those who have received sodium phosphate as a bowel preparation agent.

PATHOPHYSIOLOGY

Hypocalcemia is the result of alterations in the effect of PTH and vitamin D on the bone, gut, and kidney (see Fig. 53–1). The primary causes of hypocalcemia are postoperative hypoparathyroidism and vitamin D deficiency. Other causes include magnesium deficiency, thyroid surgery, medications, hypoalbuminemia, blood transfusions, peripheral blood progenitor cell harvesting, tumor lysis syndrome, and mutations in the calcium-sensing receptor.[44–49] PTH concentrations are elevated in conditions of hypocalcemia, with the exception of hypoparathyroidism and hypomagnesemia.[50]

An acute, symptomatic rapid fall in total serum calcium concentrations (to values <7 mg/dL) is common in patients who have had a parathyroidectomy or thyroidectomy. Hypocalcemia in these postsurgical patients is generally transient in nature.[51] The "hungry bone syndrome" is a condition of profound hypocalcemia whereby the bone avidly incorporates calcium and phosphorus from the blood in an attempt to recalcify bone. This is common after surgical parathyroidectomy in patients who have had a prolonged state of hyperparathyroidism and/or hyperthyroidism. Serum calcium concentrations should be monitored every 6 hours during the 24 to 48 hours following such surgeries, and pharmacologic doses of calcium can be necessary to prevent or minimize the drop in serum calcium. Additionally, mild to moderate hypocalcemia can be a long-term consequence of parathyroidectomy in hemodialysis patients.[51]

Vitamin D and its metabolites play an important role in the maintenance of extracellular calcium concentrations and in normal skeletal structure and mineralization. Vitamin D is necessary for the optimal absorption of calcium and phosphorus. On a worldwide basis, the most common cause of chronic hypocalcemia is nutritional vitamin D deficiency. In malnourished populations, manifestations include rickets and osteomalacia. Nutritional vitamin D deficiency is uncommon in Western societies because of the fortification of milk with ergocalciferol.[51] The most common cause of vitamin D deficiency in Western societies is gastrointestinal disease.[15] Gastric surgery, chronic pancreatitis, small-bowel disease, intestinal resection, and bypass surgery are associated with decreased concentrations of vitamin D and its metabolites.[15] Vitamin D replacement therapy might need to be administered by the intravenous route if poor oral bioavailability is noted. Decreased production of 1,25-dihydroxyvitamin D_3 can occur as a result of a hereditary defect resulting in vitamin D–dependent rickets. Recently, polymorphisms of the vitamin D receptor have been identified, and these genetic variations can contribute to increased risk of rickets associated with vitamin D and calcium deficient diets, especially in certain African and East Asian populations.[52] It also can occur secondary to chronic renal insufficiency if there is insufficient production of the 1-α-hydroxylase enzyme for the production of the most active metabolite, 1,25-dihydroxyvitamin D_3.[53] Treatment of hypocalcemia associated with CKD is reviewed in Chap. 47.

Hypomagnesemia of any cause can be associated with severe symptomatic hypocalcemia that is unresponsive to calcium replacement therapy (see Chap. 54). Reduced serum magnesium concentrations can impair PTH secretion and induce resistance of target organs to the actions of PTH.[43] Normalization of serum calcium concentrations in these patients is thus dependent on appropriate replacement of magnesium.

Drug-induced hypocalcemia has been reported in patients receiving furosemide, calcitonin, bisphosphonates, gallium nitrate, mithramycin, cinacalcet, fluoride, ketoconazole, and pentamidine.[43,54] Oral phosphorus therapy, commonly used to treat patients with malabsorption syndromes caused by gastrointestinal diseases, can also result in hypocalcemia. The anticonvulsants phenobarbital and phenytoin cause hypocalcemia by increasing catabolism of vitamin D and thereby impairing calcium release from bone and reducing intestinal calcium absorption.[43] Drugs that cause hypomagnesemia (aminoglycosides, amphotericin B, cyclosporine, diuretics, foscarnet, and cisplatin) are also associated with an increased risk of hypocalcemia. Chelating agents in blood (citrate) and in radiographic contrast media (ethylenediamine tetraacetate) can also cause transient hypocalcemia.[44,45,55] Concentrated citrate is increasingly being used in hemodialysis catheter locks and to anticoagulate the dialysis circuit during continuous renal replacement therapy. Symptomatic hypocalcemia (ionized calcium <2.4 mg/dL) has been reported in patients exposed to citrate solutions, which appears to be related to the concentration of the citrate solution.[56] Injection of citrate solutions greater than the volume of the dead space of the catheter lumen or accidental injection of citrate catheter lock solutions that are not intended for systemic administration have been associated with serious cardiovascular problems such as hypotension or cardiac arrest.[57]

CLINICAL PRESENTATION

The clinical manifestations of hypocalcemia are quite variable. The more acute the drop in ionized calcium concentration, the more likely the patient will develop symptoms.[50] Increases in plasma pH enhances the binding of calcium to albumin thus alkalosis can result in rapid decreases in ionized calcium. Concomitant hypomagnesemia, hypokalemia, hyponatremia, and additive side effects from prescribed medications also increase the likelihood of symptomatic presentation.

Hypocalcemia can manifest as neuromuscular, CNS, dermatologic, and cardiac sequelae.[15] Acute hypocalcemia is more likely to manifest as neuromuscular (paresthesia, muscle cramps, tetany, and laryngeal spasm) and cardiovascular symptoms, whereas chronic hypocalcemia often presents as CNS (depression, anxiety, memory loss, confusion, hallucinations, and tonic-clonic seizures) and dermatologic symptoms (hair loss, grooved and brittle nails, and eczema).[43] The hallmark sign of acute hypocalcemia is tetany caused by enhanced peripheral neuromuscular irritability.[15] Tetany manifests as paresthesia around the mouth and in the extremities, muscle spasms and cramps, carpopedal (hands and feet) spasms, and rarely as laryngospasm and bronchospasm.[15] Chvostek's and/or Trousseau's sign can be elicited during physical examination.[43] Chvostek's sign is elicited as twitching of facial muscles when the facial nerve is tapped anterior to the ear. Trousseau's sign is elicited by carpal spasm when a blood pressure cuff is inflated above systolic blood pressure for 3 minutes.

The cardiovascular manifestations of hypocalcemia result in electrocardiographic changes characterized by a prolonged QT interval and symptoms of decreased myocardial contractility often associated with congestive heart failure.[43] Both acute and chronic hypocalcemia can result in a reversible syndrome characterized by acute myocardial failure or refractory congestive heart failure.

Other cardiovascular manifestations include arrhythmias, bradycardia, and hypotension that is unresponsive to fluid and pressor administration.[43]

CLINICAL PRESENTATION OF HYPOCALCEMIA

General

- Hypocalcemia is caused in part by disorders of vitamin D or PTH. Acute causes of hypocalcemia result in rapid decreases in serum ionized calcium and can be associated with sepsis, alkalosis, or drugs. Parathyroidectomy or thyroidectomy are also associated with a rapid reduction in serum calcium. Malnutrition associated with vitamin D deficiency should not be overlooked as an etiology of chronic hypocalcemia.

Symptoms

- The symptoms of hypocalcemia, usually associated with an acute decrease in serum calcium, include tetany, paresthesia, muscle cramps, and laryngeal spasms. Chronic hypocalcemia is usually associated with the symptoms of depression, anxiety, memory loss, and confusion.

Signs

- Neurologic: The hallmark of acute hypocalcemia is tetany, which is characterized by neuromuscular irritability including seizure potential. Extrapyramidal disorders, mainly parkinsonism but also dystonia, hemiballismus, choreoathetosis, and oculogyric crises, occur in 5% to 10% of patients with idiopathic hypoparathyroidism. Chvostek's and/or Trousseau's signs can be elicited during physical examination.
- Dermatologic: The skin can be dry, puffy, and coarse. Other dermatologic manifestations can include hyperpigmentation, dermatitis and eczema, and psoriasis. Hair and skin signs including coarse, brittle, and sparse hair with patchy alopecia and brittle nails can also appear.
- Ophthalmologic: Cataract development has been reported to occur with hypocalcemia.
- Dental manifestations: These are usually associated with the presence of chronic hypocalcemia in early development. Signs include dental hypoplasia, failure of tooth eruption, defective enamel and root formation, and abraded carious teeth.
- Cardiovascular: Hypotension, decreased myocardial performance, and congestive heart failure have been reported. A prolonged QT interval, arrhythmias, and bradycardia can also occur but are more common with acute or very severe hypocalcemia.
- Gastrointestinal: Steatorrhea can be associated with chronic hypocalcemia.
- Musculoskeletal: Although patients with chronic hypocalcemic disorders have skeletal abnormalities, such findings do not appear to be direct consequences of hypocalcemia. Some patients with hypocalcemia have myopathy.
- Endocrine: Hypocalcemia alone can impair insulin release. In addition, idiopathic hypoparathyroidism can be associated with polyglandular autoimmune syndromes.

Laboratory Tests

- Serum calcium levels of less than 8.5 mg/dL are considered to represent hypocalcemia. Ionized calcium values less than 4.4 mg/dL (<1.1 mmol/L), which are often measured in critically ill patients, are also indicative of hypocalcemia.

TREATMENT

Hypocalcemia

DESIRED OUTCOME

The goals of therapy for patients with normal renal function are the resolution of signs and symptoms of hypocalcemia, restoration of normocalcemia, management of associated electrolyte abnormalities, and treatment of the underlying cause of hypocalcemia. The goals for patients with chronic renal insufficiency are different and are discussed in detail in Chap. 47. Asymptomatic hypocalcemia associated with hypoalbuminemia requires no treatment because ionized (physiologically active) plasma calcium concentrations are normal. Treatment of hypocalcemia is dependent on identification of the pathogenesis of the underlying disorder, acuteness of onset, and presence and severity of symptoms. Acute symptomatic hypocalcemia requires parenteral administration of soluble calcium salts (Fig 53–3).

PHARMACOLOGIC THERAPY

The initial therapeutic intervention for patients with acute symptomatic hypocalcemia is to administer 100 to 300 mg of elemental calcium intravenously over 5 to 10 minutes.[58] This can be accomplished by the administration of 1 g of calcium chloride (27% elemental calcium) or 2 to 3 g of calcium gluconate (9% elemental calcium). Calcium gluconate is generally preferred over calcium chloride for peripheral venous administration because calcium gluconate is less irritating to veins. The use of calcium gluconate provides a less predictable and slightly smaller increase in plasma ionic calcium compared with calcium chloride. Calcium should not be infused at a rate greater than 60 mg of elemental calcium per minute because severe cardiac dysfunction, including ventricular fibrillation, can result.[58] Intravenous calcium administration should be used with caution in patients receiving digitalis glycosides because of the possibility of bradycardia or atrioventricular (A-V) block.[3] The bolus dose of calcium is only effective for 1 to 2 hours and should be followed by a continuous infusion of elemental calcium at a rate of 0.5 to 2 mg/kg per hour.[3] The calcium concentrations should be monitored every 4 to 6 hours during the intravenous infusions. The ionized calcium concentration usually normalizes within 4 hours, and the maintenance infusion rate of elemental calcium can then be decreased to 0.3 to 0.5 mg/kg per hour to maintain the desired calcium concentration.[2] Calcium should not be added to bicarbonate- or phosphate-containing solutions because of the possibility of precipitation.

Once acute hypocalcemia is corrected by parenteral administration, further treatment modalities should be individualized according to the cause of hypocalcemia. If hypomagnesemia is present, magnesium supplementation is indicated (see Chap. 54). Hypocalcemia secondary to hungry bone syndrome following parathyroidectomy has been attenuated by pretreatment with bisphosphonates.[59] Asymptomatic and chronic hypocalcemia associated with hypoparathyroidism and vitamin D–deficient states can be managed by oral calcium and vitamin D supplementation (see Tables 47–6 and 47–7). Therapy is begun with 1 to 3 g/day of elemental calcium.[1] Average maintenance doses range from 2 to 8 g of elemental calcium per day in divided doses. If serum calcium does not normalize, a vitamin D preparation might need to be added.

Treatment of hypocalcemia associated with vitamin D–deficient states should be individualized. In patients with malabsorption, vitamin D requirements vary markedly, and large doses can be required. In contrast, vitamin D deficiency associated with anticonvulsant medication can be corrected with smaller doses of vitamin D. Oral doses of 1,25-dihydroxyvitamin D_3 usually range from 0.5 to

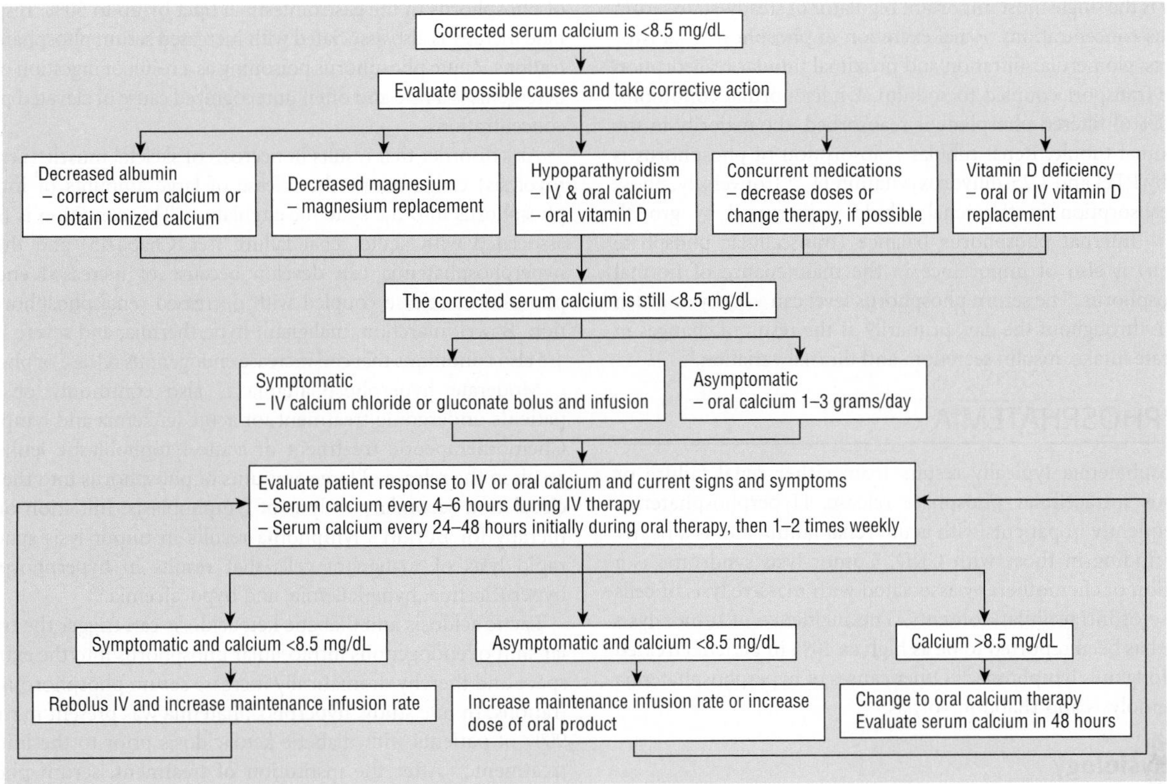

FIGURE 53-3. Hypocalcemia diagnostic and treatment algorithm.

3 mcg daily. The usual initial oral dose of ergocalciferol is 50,000 international units daily.[58] Vitamin D doses are usually adjusted approximately every 4 weeks. Vitamin D deficiency is highly prevalent especially in areas of low sun exposure and limited dietary sources of vitamin D.[60] New data suggest that current dietary recommendations are not sufficient to maintain 25-hydroxyvitamin D_3 concentrations at or above 32 mcg/L.[60] The treatment of vitamin D deficiency associated with CKD generally requires the administration of 1,25-dihydroxyvitamin D_3 or another synthetic vitamin D_2 analog, such as paricalcitol or doxercalciferol. Patients who have reduced 25-hydroxylase activity (e.g., hepatic disease) can also require treatment with calcitriol (1,25-dihydroxyvitamin D_3). The newer vitamin D_2 analogs (paricalcitol and doxercalciferol) were developed to preferentially suppress PTH secretion with less effect on serum calcium concentration and thus their efficacy for the management of hypocalcemia may be minimal. In selected cases, increasing calcium ingestion can be required if vitamin D replacement alone is ineffective in returning calcium concentrations to normal.

Adverse effects of oral calcium and vitamin D supplementation include hypercalcemia and hypercalciuria, especially in the hypoparathyroid patient, in whom the renal calcium-sparing effect of PTH is absent. Hypercalciuria can increase the risk of calcium stone formation and nephrolithiasis in susceptible patients. One maneuver to help prevent calcium stones is to maintain the urine calcium excretion below 300 mg per day. Intermittently monitoring 24-hour urine collections for total calcium excretion can help to minimize the occurrence of hypercalciuria. The addition of thiazide diuretics for patients at risk for stone formation can result in a reduction of both urinary calcium excretion and vitamin D requirements.[58]

DISORDERS OF PHOSPHORUS HOMEOSTASIS

Phosphorus is an essential element in phospholipid cell membranes, nucleic acids, and phosphoproteins, which are required for mitochondrial function.[61] Phosphorus regulates the intermediary metabolism of carbohydrates, fats, and proteins. Phosphorus also regulates enzymatic reactions including glycolysis, ammoniagenesis, and the 1-hydroxylation of 25-hydroxyvitamin D_3.[61] In addition, phosphorus is required for the generation of 2,3-diphosphoglycerate (2,3-DPG) in red blood cells, which is required for normal oxygen-hemoglobin dissociation and delivery of oxygen to the tissues.[62] Phosphorus is the source of the high-energy bonds of adenosine triphosphate (ATP), thus fueling a wide variety of physiologic processes, including muscle contractility, electrolyte transport, neurologic function, and other important biochemical reactions.[61] Considering its diverse biologic importance, it is not difficult to appreciate the clinical implications of disorders of phosphorus homeostasis.

Phosphorus, the major intracellular anion, is present in living organisms mainly as organic phosphate esters such as 2,3-DPG, adenosine, guanosine triphosphate, and fructose 1,6-diphosphate.[61] Only a small fraction of intracellular phosphorus exists as inorganic phosphate; however, this fraction is critical because it is the source from which ATP is resynthesized.[61] The majority of inorganic phosphate is located in the extracellular space where it is the prime determinant of intracellular phosphate; thus small increments in the organic phosphate levels can profoundly alter both the extracellular and intracellular phosphate levels. Metabolic disturbances (acidosis, alkalosis, and ketoacidosis), hydrogen ion shifts, and hormones (PTH, calcitonin, cortisol, and vitamin D) all can cause transcellular shifts in phosphorus concentrations. Because of these phenomena, the serum phosphorus level does not accurately reflect total body stores.[62]

The typical Western diet provides a daily intake of 800 to 1,600 mg of phosphorus. Approximately 60% to 80% of this is absorbed in the gastrointestinal tract by passive and active transport (vitamin D mediated). PTH, 1,25-dihydroxyvitamin D_3, and low-phosphate diets mediate increased absorption. Decreased absorption occurs under conditions of increased dietary intake of phosphorus and magnesium, glucocorticoid therapy, and hypothyroidism. The normal serum phosphorus concentration in adults is 2.5 to 4.5 mg/dL and for children younger than 12 years old it is 4 to 5.6 mg/dL. Excretion by the kidney is the single most important regulator of steady-state serum phosphorus concentrations. Renal excretion of phosphorus is a two-step process: glomerular filtration and proximal tubular reabsorption by passive transport coupled to sodium. Under normal conditions, 85% to 90% of filtered phosphate is reabsorbed, the majority in the early proximal tubule. Renal tubular reabsorption of phosphorus is inhibited by PTH and 1,25-dihydroxyvitamin D_3.[61] Conversely, phosphorus reabsorption in the renal tubule is increased by growth hormone.[61] Internal phosphorus balance (transcellular phosphate distribution) is also of importance in the maintenance of normal serum phosphorus. The serum phosphorus level can vary by as much as 2 mg/dL throughout the day, primarily as the result of changes in carbohydrate intake, insulin secretion, and diurnal variation.[61]

HYPERPHOSPHATEMIA

Hyperphosphatemia typically results from either renal failure or endogenous intracellular phosphate release. Hyperphosphatemia occurs frequently in patients with acute renal failure and is a nearly universal finding in those with CKD. Tumor lysis syndrome is a complication of chemotherapy associated with massive lysis of cells and release of intracellular contents. The incidence of tumor lysis syndrome has been reported to be as high as 40% in patients treated for non-Hodgkin's lymphoma.[61] Other causes of hyperphosphatemia include hemolysis and rhabdomyolysis.

Pathophysiology

The most common cause of hyperphosphatemia is a decrease in urinary phosphorus excretion secondary to decreased GFR.[63] Retention of phosphorus decreases vitamin D synthesis and induces hypocalcemia, which leads to an increase in PTH; a finding that can be seen in those with stage 2 to 3 CKD. This physiologic response inhibits further tubular reabsorption of phosphorus as the kidney attempts to correct hyperphosphatemia and normalize serum calcium concentrations. Patients with excessive exogenous phosphorus administration or who experience massive tissue breakdown or cell lysis in the setting of acute renal failure can rapidly develop moderate to severe hyperphosphatemia (serum phosphorus >6.5 mg/dL).[61] Severe hyperphosphatemia (serum phosphorus >7.0 mg/dL) is commonly encountered in patients with CKD, especially those with GFRs less than 15 mL/min per 1.73 m^2 (see Chap. 47).

Hyperphosphatemia caused by an increase in renal tubular reabsorption associated with hypoparathyroidism is usually less severe than that observed in patients with severe renal failure or excessive exogenous or endogenous introduction of phosphorus into the ECF. Acromegaly and thyrotoxicosis can also cause hyperphosphatemia by reducing urinary phosphorus excretion.

Iatrogenic causes of hyperphosphatemia have been widely reported, and clinicians should be aware of the phosphorus content of intravenous, oral, and rectally administered products. Large doses of phosphorus administered intravenously to treat hypercalcemia can ultimately result in severe life-threatening hyperphosphatemia. Although less-well recognized, oral and rectal administration of phosphate-containing solutions such as sodium phosphate (Fleet Phospho-Soda) can also result in severe and life-threatening hyperphosphatemia, especially in patients with moderate and severe renal insufficiency.[63,64] The risk of mortality is dependent on the amount of phosphorus absorbed from the administered product, however, fatalities have occurred at lower phosphorus concentrations.[63] Acute phosphate nephropathy and renal failure have also been reported with the use of oral sodium phosphate bowel preparations. Recently the FDA issued a safety warning regarding the use of these products in patients at risk (the elderly, those with CKD) or on medications known to effect renal hemodynamics (e.g., diuretics, NSAIDs or renin-angiotensin aldosterone system inhibitors).[65] Intravenous or oral vitamin D therapy can increase absorption of phosphorus in the gastrointestinal tract by up to 50%. Bisphosphonate therapy is also associated with increased serum phosphate concentrations. Acute phosphorus poisoning as a result of ingestion of laundry detergents is a rare and often unrecognized cause of elevated phosphate concentrations.

Any disorder that results in necrosis of skeletal muscle (i.e., rhabdomyolysis) can generate the release of large amounts of intracellular phosphorus into the systemic circulation. This condition is frequently associated with acute renal failure (see Chap. 45) and thus severe hyperphosphatemia can develop because of increased endogenous phosphorus release coupled with decreased renal phosphorus excretion. Bowel infarction, malignant hyperthermia, and severe hemolysis are also conditions that can increase endogenous release of phosphorus.

Moderate hyperphosphatemia is also commonly observed in patients undergoing treatment for acute leukemia and lymphomas.[66] Chemotherapeutic treatment of acute lymphoblastic leukemia can result in the release of large amounts of phosphorus into the systemic circulation secondary to lysis of lymphoblasts. Initiation of chemotherapy for Burkitt's lymphoma results in tumor lysis syndrome, a rapid lysis of malignant cells that results in hyperphosphatemia, hyperuricemia, hyperkalemia, and hypocalcemia.[66]

Lactic acidosis and diabetic ketoacidosis can trigger the transcellular shift of endogenous intracellular phosphorus into the extracellular space and thereby dramatically increase serum phosphorous concentrations. In one study, hyperphosphatemia was present in more than 90% of patients with diabetic ketoacidosis prior to the initiation of treatment.[67] After the institution of treatment, serum phosphorus levels should be checked hourly as they can decrease rapidly, and patients can ultimately develop hypophosphatemia.

Clinical Presentation

The severe acute onset of hyperphosphatemia can result in calcium and phosphorus complexation and lead to the precipitation of calcium phosphate into soft tissues, intrarenal calcification, nephrolithiasis, or obstructive uropathy. Other symptoms associated with moderate to severe hyperphosphatemia include nausea, vomiting, diarrhea, lethargy, and seizures. The major effects of long-term hyperphosphatemia are related to the development of hypocalcemia (caused by phosphate inhibition of renal 1-α-hydroxylase) and its related consequences, as well as vascular and organ damage resulting from the deposition of calcium-phosphate crystals. Extravascular calcification can result in band keratopathy, "red eye," pruritus, and periarticular calcification, especially in CKD patients. In addition, soft-tissue calcifications in the conjunctiva, skin, heart, cornea, lung, gastric mucosa, and kidney have been observed, primarily in CKD patients with chronic disordered mineral metabolism.[61] Hyperphosphatemia associated with CKD can result in renal osteodystrophy because of overproduction of PTH. This condition is discussed in detail in Chap. 47.

CLINICAL PRESENTATION OF HYPERPHOSPHATEMIA

General

- As the serum phosphate concentration is primarily determined by the ability of the kidneys to excrete dietary phosphate, hyperphosphatemia is uncommon in patients with normal kidney function.

Symptoms

- Acute symptoms include GI disturbances, lethargy, obstruction of the urinary tract, and rarely seizures. Symptoms associated with chronic hyperphosphatemia are associated with deposition of calcium-phosphate crystals and include "red eye" and pruritus.

Signs

- The elevated calcium-phosphate product results in precipitation in arteries, joints, soft tissues, and the viscera. This can result in tissue ischemia, termed *calciphylaxis*.

Laboratory Tests

- Serum phosphate levels higher than 4.5 mg/dL represent hyperphosphatemia.

TREATMENT

Hyperphosphatemia

DESIRED OUTCOME

Management of patients with acutely elevated serum phosphorus should be directed at avoiding gastrointestinal and neurologic symptoms and preventing deposition in the urinary tract to avoid the development of acute renal failure. The treatment of hyperphosphatemia is focused on returning serum phosphate concentrations to the normal or near normal (for those with CKD) range, with the hope that one can minimize the long-term cardiovascular consequences of calcium-phosphorus crystal deposition in the vasculature. Calcium-phosphate crystals are likely to form in vivo when the product of the serum calcium and phosphate concentrations exceeds 50 to 60 mg^2/dL^2.[38] The recently published National Kidney Foundation's Dialysis Outcomes Quality Initiative guidelines for bone metabolism and disease defines the goal calcium-phosphorus product as less than 55 mg^2/dL^2.[68] Furthermore, serum phosphorus concentrations greater than 6.5 mg/dL, have been independently associated with increased morbidity and mortality. Serum phosphorus concentrations should be maintained in the 2.7 to 4.6 mg/dL range for those with stage 3 and 4 CKD, whereas for patients in stage 5 CKD the goal is to maintain values between 3.5 and 5.5 mg/dL.[68]

PHARMACOLOGIC THERAPY

Severe symptomatic hyperphosphatemia manifesting as hypocalcemia and tetany should be treated by the intravenous administration of calcium salts. Although this can seem counterintuitive in a patient with a phosphorus of 16 mg/dL and a calcium of 7 mg/dL (the calcium-phosphorus product is 112 mg^2/dL^2), correction of severe hypocalcemia is of primary importance because of the critical nature of this disorder. If calcium concentrations are not critically low, the initial management strategy should include limitation of all exogenous sources of phosphorus and efforts to block further absorption should be initiated. Dialysis can be initiated if the patient remains symptomatic despite these interventions.

In general, the most effective way to treat asymptomatic chronic hyperphosphatemia is to decrease phosphate absorption from the GI tract by the use of phosphate-binding agents.[61] Antacids containing divalent and trivalent cations (calcium, lanthanum, magnesium, and aluminum), or sevelamer are the agents most frequently used in the prevention and treatment of hyperphosphatemia (see Table 47–6).[69,70] Long-term treatment with aluminum hydroxide and aluminum carbonate should be discouraged because the use of these agents has been associated with anemia, CNS disorders, and bone disease.[71] Short-term therapy with these agents is effective and safe. Aluminum and calcium are available in oral suspension formulations, which can aid administration in acutely ill patients with G-tubes. The most frequent adverse effect from phosphate-binding agents (especially calcium) is constipation (see Table 47–6). Calcium salts are the preferred phosphate-binding agents except when there is concomitant hypercalcemia. Therapy with the polymer agent (sevelamer) or lanthanum carbonate might avoid the detrimental effects associated with aluminum, magnesium, or calcium therapy.[11]

CLINICAL CONTROVERSY

Emerging data suggest that noncalcium, nonaluminum phosphate binders (e.g., sevelamer) can slow progression of cardiac calcification in chronic hemodialysis patients, however there are no data to suggest that there are any benefits to using sevelamer for the management of those with normal renal function who develop acute hyperphosphatemia.

HYPOPHOSPHATEMIA

Mild to moderate hypophosphatemia is defined as a serum phosphorus concentration of 1 to 2 mg/dL, whereas severe hypophosphatemia is defined as a serum phosphorus concentration of less than 1 mg/dL.[72] Hypophosphatemia has been observed in approximately 1% to 3% of the laboratory screening panels of patients who have been admitted to a hospital.[62] The incidence in hospitalized critically ill patients is 18% to 28%.[72] Unlike its severe form, mild or moderate hypophosphatemia seldom causes recognizable signs and symptoms.[66]

PATHOPHYSIOLOGY

Hypophosphatemia can be the result of decreased gastrointestinal absorption, increased urinary excretion, or extracellular to intracellular redistribution.[61] Although mild to moderate hypophosphatemia is common and can occur in inpatients and outpatients, severe hypophosphatemia is predominantly encountered in the acute care setting and can be associated with life-threatening symptoms, including seizures, coma, and rhabdomyolysis (Table 53–4).

Phosphate-binding substances such as sucralfate, calcium carbonate, sevelamer, lanthanum carbonate, and aluminum- or magnesium-containing antacids have the potential to bind large amounts of phosphorus in the gut, thereby preventing absorption. If phosphate-binding agents are ingested on a chronic basis in conjunction with a dietary phosphorus deficiency, hypophosphatemia can result.[66] Patients who are receiving long-term phosphate-binding agents, those with peptic ulcer disease or CKD, and those who may be predisposed to moderate hypophosphatemia (alcoholics) are at highest risk for the development of severe hypophosphatemia. Hyperparathyroidism can cause hypophosphatemia as a result of decreased gastrointestinal absorption of dietary phosphorus.

Increased renal losses of phosphorus can occur in hyperparathyroid (primary and secondary) patients with normal renal function and those with vitamin D deficiency. Elevated PTH levels lead to an increase in serum calcium concentrations and decreased serum phosphorus concentrations. Serum phosphorus is decreased as the result of a reduction in renal tubular reabsorption.[72] Recovery from extensive third-degree burns is associated with development of an anabolic state as stress levels decrease and nutritional therapies take effect as well as a marked diuretic phase associated with an impressive renal loss of phosphate.[66] Because phosphorus is rapidly incorporated into the new cells, this can contribute to the severity of the hypophosphatemia. Drugs that cause increased renal elimination of phosphorus include diuretics (acetazolamide and osmotic diuretics), glucocorticoids, and sodium bicarbonate.

Rapid refeeding of malnourished patients with high-carbohydrate, high-calorie diets with inadequate amounts of supplemental phosphorus can result in severe symptomatic hypophosphatemia. This phenomenon is especially prevalent in patients with other underlying risk factors for the development of hypophosphatemia, such as alcoholism.[73] The etiology of severe hypophosphatemia associated with hyperalimentation and nutritional recovery can be separated into two phases: acute, rapid hypophosphatemia secondary to intracellular shifts of phosphorus resulting from glucose-induced insulin secretion;

TABLE 53-4 Conditions Associated with the Development of Hypophosphatemia

Decreased gastrointestinal absorption
Phosphate-binding drugs
Sucralfate
Calcium carbonate
Aluminum/magnesium antacids
Sevelamer
Lanthanum carbonate
Decreased dietary phosphorus intake
Glucocorticoids
Vitamin D deficiency/resistance
Hypoparathyroidism
Chronic diarrhea
Steatorrhea
Increased urinary excretion
Hyperparathyroidism (primary and secondary)
Recovery from burns
Rickets
Malignant neoplasms
Fanconi syndrome
Acute volume expansion
Metabolic acidosis
Renal transplantation
Vitamin D deficiency and/or resistance
Diuretics
Acetazolamide
Osmotic agents
Glucocorticoids
Sodium bicarbonate
Internal redistribution
Refeeding syndrome
Parenteral nutrition
Parathyroidectomy (hungry bone syndrome)
Alcoholism
Respiratory alkalosis
Diabetic ketoacidosis (correction)
Dextrose solutions
Insulin
Catecholamines
Anabolic steroids
Glucagon
Calcitonin
Erythropoietin

and the gradual decrease in serum phosphorus concentration over 5 to 10 days secondary to tissue repair in the presence of phosphorus deprivation.[74] The development of severe hypophosphatemia secondary to hyperalimentation can be prevented by the administration of 12 to 15 mmol of phosphorus per liter of hyperalimentation solution or 15 mmol per 1,000 calories of dextrose.[75] Transcellular shifts in phosphorus also occur after parathyroidectomy, causing severe hypocalcemia and hypophosphatemia because of hungry bone syndrome (deposition of phosphorus and calcium in the bone).

Severe and prolonged respiratory alkalosis (a result of hyperventilation, pain, anxiety, and sepsis) can cause hypophosphatemia.[62] Respiratory alkalosis is thought to contribute significantly to the hypophosphatemia observed during alcohol withdrawal.[62] Although patients with diabetic ketoacidosis may present with hyperphosphatemia, the institution of therapy to correct it can cause serum phosphorus concentrations to decrease rapidly as phosphorus shifts back into the intracellular compartment. In addition, the acidosis associated with the diabetic ketoacidotic state can cause a decomposition of organic compounds inside the cell and a release of inorganic phosphorus into the plasma and subsequently into the urine.[61] The combination of intracellular phosphorus breakdown and the shift of phosphorus into cells on initiation of treatment can lead to severe hypophosphatemia. Drugs associated with transcellular shifts in phosphorus include dextrose solutions, glucagon, insulin, catecholamines, calcitonin, erythropoietic agents, and anabolic steroids.

Chronic ethanol abusers are prone to a variety of serum electrolyte disorders including hypocalcemia, hypomagnesemia, hypokalemia, and hypophosphatemia. The etiology of hypophosphatemia in the alcoholic patient is multifactorial. Malnutrition, poor dietary intake, diarrhea, vomiting, and the use of phosphate-binding antacids can all contribute to the hypophosphatemia of alcoholism.[61] In addition, serum phosphorus concentrations may decrease after hospitalization in the alcoholic patient with the institution of dextrose-containing intravenous fluids, as a result of an intracellular shift of phosphorus.[61,74] Hyperventilation associated with the alcohol withdrawal syndrome can also contribute to the development of hypophosphatemia.[66] Alcoholic patients are particularly susceptible to the complications of hypophosphatemia such as rhabdomyolysis, which is often seen during withdrawal or refeeding.[66,74] Thus serum phosphorus concentrations should be routinely monitored in alcoholic patients.

CLINICAL PRESENTATION

The clinical manifestations of severe hypophosphatemia are diverse and can affect many organ systems. It is likely that two primary biochemical abnormalities are responsible for most of the clinical manifestations of severe hypophosphatemia.[61] First, intracellular energy stores may be decreased secondary to depletion of intracellular ATP, which is dependent on inorganic intracellular phosphate. This can result in disruptions in cellular function. Second, reduced red blood cell 2,3-DPG concentrations are associated with a shift to the left of the oxyhemoglobin saturation curve. This shift is associated with a decrease in the release of oxygen to peripheral tissues (increased oxygen affinity for hemoglobin) and may result in tissue hypoxia.[61] These metabolic disorders can be seen in a wide variety of organ systems.

Neurologic (CNS) manifestations of severe hypophosphatemia result in a metabolic encephalopathy syndrome. This progressive syndrome of irritability, apprehension, weakness, numbness, paresthesia, dysarthria, confusion, obtundation, seizures, and coma has been described in patients with severe hypophosphatemia.[66,73] Neuropsychiatric disturbances include apathy, delirium, hallucinations, and paranoia. Peripheral neuropathy and symptoms resembling Guillain-Barré syndrome have also been reported.[73]

Severe hypophosphatemia can result in significant dysfunction of skeletal muscle ranging from myalgia, bone pain, and weakness, with chronic hypophosphatemia, to potentially fatal rhabdomyolysis with severe acute hypophosphatemia.[73] Laboratory evaluations can help to distinguish between chronic and acute on chronic hypophosphatemia. Elevated alkaline phosphatase, normal creatine phosphokinase, and normal to low phosphorus and calcium are present in cases of chronic hypophosphatemia. In contrast, hyperkalemia, hyperuricemia, elevated blood urea nitrogen (BUN) and creatinine, hypercalcemia, and myoglobinuria are present in cases in which rhabdomyolysis complicates the acute or chronic hypophosphatemia.[73] Hypophosphatemia can result in acute respiratory failure secondary to respiratory muscle weakness and diaphragmatic contractile dysfunction. Thus frequent assessment of serum phosphorus concentration is indicated in patients at risk for respiratory failure. Likewise, adequate treatment of hypophosphatemia in respiratory failure can aid in successful weaning from the ventilator.[62] Dysphagia and ileus have also been attributed to hypophosphatemia.[62]

Cardiac muscle function has been reported to be impaired in the setting of hypophosphatemia and has resulted in congestive cardiomyopathy. This has been reported in alcoholics, and postoperative and intensive care patients. A depletion in cardiac ATP stores has been hypothesized as the cause of this syndrome.[73] Arrhythmias have also been reported in patients with hypophosphatemia. Because hypophosphatemia is a potentially reversible cause of heart failure, it should be considered in patients who experience an acute deterioration in ventricular function.

Hematologic manifestations of hypophosphatemia include decreased levels of 2,3-DPG, decreased red blood cell ATP, and membrane rigidity.[61] When red blood cell ATP decreases to below 15% of normal, cells become spherocytic and rigid, and are trapped and destroyed in the spleen.[61] Therefore hemolysis can be a manifestation of severe hypophosphatemia. Reduction in ATP content of white blood cells can result in mobility, chemotaxis, phagocytosis, and bactericidal dysfunction.[66] These changes can contribute to an increased risk of infection in hypophosphatemic patients. Animal studies also demonstrate platelet abnormalities in the setting of hypophosphatemia.[73] The implications of hypophosphatemia for human platelet function, however, have not been determined.

Finally, prolonged hypophosphatemia may result in osteopenia and osteomalacia because of enhanced osteoclastic resorption of bone. Glucose intolerance from hypophosphatemia caused by tissue insensitivity to insulin has also been described.

CLINICAL PRESENTATION OF HYPOPHOSPHATEMIA

General

- The manifestations of hypophosphatemia depend on the chronicity and severity of the phosphate depletion. The major conditions associated with symptomatic hypophosphatemia are chronic alcoholism, intravenous hyperalimentation without adequate phosphate supplementation, and the chronic ingestion of antacids. Severe hypophosphatemia can also be seen during treatment of diabetic ketoacidosis and with prolonged hyperventilation.

Symptoms

- Except for the effects on mineral metabolism, the symptoms of hypophosphatemia are caused by two consequences (reduction of red cell 2,3-DPG and reduction of intracellular ATP levels), and can impact virtually all organ systems. The symptoms are predominantly neurological and can include irritability, apprehension, weakness, numbness, paresthesia, and confusion. Severe acute development of hypophosphatemia can result in seizures or coma.

Signs

- The initial response of bone to hypophosphatemia contributes to hypercalcemia and hypercalciuria. Prolonged hypophosphatemia can also result in rickets and osteomalacia.
- Neurologic: Severe hypophosphatemia can lead to a metabolic encephalopathy.
- Cardiopulmonary: Impaired myocardial contractility, respiratory failure secondary to ATP depletion, congestive heart failure, new onset or worsening of an existing condition.
- Musculoskeletal: Proximal myopathy, dysphagia, and ileus have been reported. Acute hypophosphatemia superimposed on preexisting severe phosphate depletion can lead to rhabdomyolysis.
- Hematologic: Alterations in the hematopoietic system can also occur, resulting in hemolysis, reduction in phagocytotic and granulocyte chemotactic ability, as well as defective clot retraction and thrombocytopenia.

Laboratory Tests

- Serum phosphate levels below 2.4 mg/dL are indicative of hypophosphatemia.

TREATMENT

Hypophosphatemia

DESIRED OUTCOME

The goals of therapy are the reversal of signs and symptoms of hypophosphatemia, normalization of serum phosphorus concentrations, and management of underlying conditions. Awareness of the clinical situations in which hypophosphatemia is anticipated (alcoholism, diabetic ketoacidosis, and parenteral nutrition) is of vital importance in preventing iatrogenic hypophosphatemia. The routine addition of phosphorus in concentrations of 12 to 15 mmol/L to intravenous hyperalimentation solutions is of utmost importance for the prevention of severe hypophosphatemia in hospitalized patients.

PHARMACOLOGIC THERAPY

Severe (<1 mg/dL) or symptomatic hypophosphatemia should be treated with parenteral phosphorus replacement. Oral phosphorus supplementation is usually reserved for patients who are asymptomatic or who exhibit mild to moderate hypophosphatemia. Estimation of total body phosphorus deficit is difficult because phosphorus is an intracellular electrolyte. Dosage and infusion recommendations, as well as response to parenteral phosphorus replacement, are highly variable.[72] The infusion of 15 mmol of phosphorus in 250 mL 5% dextrose or 0.9% sodium chloride over 3 hours is a safe and effective treatment for severe hypophosphatemia.[72] Mean increases in serum phosphate of 0.5 to 0.8 mg/dL have been reported. Doses of 15 to 30 mmol of phosphorus can be given over 1 to 3 hours in patients without hypercalcemia (serum calcium >10.5 mg/dL).[72,75] Other authors recommend a wider dosage range of 0.08 to 0.64 mmol/kg body weight (5 to 45 mmol in a 70-kg patient) given over 4 to 12 hours.[65,76] Intravenous phosphate therapy produces the desired increase in serum phosphorus at 24 hours in 20% to 80% of patients. Response is dependent on the degree of phosphate depletion and replacement dose administered.[61] Furthermore, the initial success is often followed in 48 to 72 hours by recurrent hypophosphatemia, necessitating close monitoring of serum phosphorus and repeated administration of phosphorus products as warranted.

CLINICAL CONTROVERSY

The recommended initial dosage of intravenous phosphorus in conditions of severe hypophosphatemia is not well established and can range from 5 to 45 mmol of phosphorus.

Parenteral phosphorus supplementation is associated with risks of hyperphosphatemia, metastatic soft tissue deposition of calcium-phosphate product, hypomagnesemia, hypocalcemia, and hyperkalemia or hypernatremia (caused by intravenous phosphorus salt) (Table 53–5). Inappropriate administration of large doses of parenteral phosphorus over relatively short time periods has resulted in symptomatic hypocalcemia and soft-tissue calcification.[61] The rate of infusion and choice of initial dosage should therefore be based on severity of hypophosphatemia, presence of symptoms, and coexistent medical conditions. Patients should be closely monitored with frequent (every 6 hours) serum phosphorus determinations for 48 to 72 hours after starting intravenous therapy. It can be necessary to continue administration of intravenous phosphorus for several days in some patients, although other patients may be able to tolerate an oral maintenance regimen. Monitoring should also include assessment of serum potassium, calcium, and magnesium concentrations. Hypomagnesemia secondary to intracellular shifts occurs frequently (27% to 80%) in severely hypophosphatemic patients.[72] Therapy with parenteral phos-

TABLE 53-5 Phosphorus Replacement Therapy

Product (Salt)	Phosphate Content	Initial Dosing Based on Serum K
Oral therapy (potassium phosphate + sodium phosphate)		
Neutra-Phos (7 mEq/packet each of Na and K)	250 mg (8 mmol)/packet	1 packet three times daily[a]
Neutra-Phos-K (14.25 mEq/packet of K)	250 mg (8 mmol)/packet	Serum K >5.5 mEq/L Not recommended
K-Phos Neutral (13 mEq/tablet Na and 1.1 mEq/tablet K)	250 mg (8 mmol)/tablet	Serum K >5.5 mEq/L 1 tablet three times daily
Uro-KP-Neutral (10.9 mEq/tablet Na and 1.27 mEq/tablet K)	250 mg (8 mmol)/tablet	Serum K >5.5 mEq/L 1 tablet three times daily
Fleets Phospho-soda (Sodium phosphate solution)	4 mmol/mL	Serum K >5.5 mEq/L 2 mL three times daily
Intravenous therapy		
Sodium PO_4 (4.0 mEq/mL Na)	3 mmol/mL	Serum K >3.5 mEq/L 15–30 mmol IVPB
Potassium PO_4 (4.4 mEq/mL K)	3 mmol/mL	Serum K < 3.5 mEq/L 15–30 mmol IVPB

IVPB, intravenous piggyback; K, potassium; Na, sodium; PO_4, phosphate.
[a]Monitor serum K closely + intravenous piggy back.

phorus should be undertaken with great caution and at reduced dosage for patients with hypercalcemia or renal dysfunction.[66,74]

Mild to moderate or asymptomatic hypophosphatemia can be treated by the administration of oral phosphorus salts in doses of 1.5 to 2 g (50 to 60 mmol) daily in divided doses (see Table 53–5). Phosphorus concentrations should be monitored daily, with the goal of correcting the reduced phosphorus concentration in approximately 7 to 10 days. The primary dose-limiting adverse effect associated with oral phosphorus replacement is the development of osmotic diarrhea. Patients with mild to moderate hypophosphatemia and moderate to severe renal insufficiency should receive reduced daily oral doses (i.e., 1 g or approximately 30 mmol of phosphorus) with careful monitoring of serum phosphorus concentration because they are predisposed to phosphorus retention. In addition to phosphorus supplementation for hypophosphatemia, dipyridamole can decrease renal phosphate leaking and increase serum phosphorus. Doses of 75 mg four times daily have resulted in increases in serum 1,25-dihydroxyvitamin D_3 and decreases in serum calcium and urolithiasis events.[77]

CONCLUSIONS

Clinicians play an integral part in the management of fluid and electrolyte abnormalities; initially they should review the patient's medication history to determine if any of the patient's current drug therapy contributed to the existing abnormalities. They should also carefully evaluate all drug therapy options to reduce the risk of developing new electrolyte problems and to optimize the outcome of the current management plan. This proactive interventional approach will facilitate the management of mild disorders in the community and can reduce the need for hospitalization.

ABBREVIATIONS

ATP: adenosine triphosphate
BUN: blood urea nitrogen
CHF: congestive heart failure
CKD: chronic kidney disease
CNS: central nervous system
2,3-DPG: 2,3-diphosphoglycerate
NSAID: nonsteroidal antiinflammatory drug
PTH: parathyroid hormone
S_{ca}: serum calcium

REFERENCES

1. Reber PM, Heath H III. Hypocalcemic emergencies. Med Clin North Am 1995;79:93–106.
2. Nussbaum SR. Pathophysiology and management of severe hypercalcemia. Endocrinol Metab Clin North Am 1993;22:343–362.
3. Zaloga GP. Hypocalcemia in critically ill patients. Crit Care Med 1992;20:251–262.
4. Slomp J, van der Voort PH, Gerritsen RT, et al. Albumin-adjusted calcium is not suitable for diagnosis of hyper- and hypocalcemia in the critically ill. Crit Care Med 2003;31:1389–1393.
5. Byrnes MC, Huynh K, Helmer SD, et al. A comparison of corrected serum calcium levels to ionized calcium levels among critically ill surgical patients. Am J Surg 2005;189(3):310–314.
6. Levine MA. Primary hyperparathyroidism: 7,000 years of progress. Cleve Clin J Med 2005;72:1084–1097.
7. Zojer N, Keck AV, Pecherstorfer M. Comparative tolerability of drug therapies for hypercalcemia of malignancy. Drug Saf 1999;21:389–406.
8. Rude RK. Hyperparathyroidism. Otolaryngol Clin North Am 1996;29:663–679.
9. Chisholm MA, Mulloy AL, Taylor AT. Acute management of cancer-related hypercalcemia. Ann Pharmacother 1996;30:507–513.
10. Strewler GJ. The physiology of parathyroid hormone-related protein. N Engl J Med 2000;342:177–185.
11. Ralston SH, Coleman R, Fraser WD, et al. Medical management of hypercalcemia. Calcif Tissue Int 2004;74:1–11.
12. Schmidt-Gayk H, Haerdt H. Differential diagnosis of hypercalcemia: Laboratory assessment. Recent Results Cancer Res 1994;137:122–137.
13. Picolis MK, Lavis VR, Orlander PR. Milk-alkali is a major cause of hypercalcemia. Clin Endocrinol (Oxf) 2005;63:566–576.
14. Beall DP, Henslee HB, Webb HR, et al. Milk-alkali syndrome: A historical review and description of the modern version of the syndrome. Am J Med Sci 2006;331:233–242.
15. Agus ZS, Wasserstein A, Goldfarb S. Disorders of calcium and magnesium homeostasis. Am J Med 1982;72:473–488.
16. Maruani G, Hertig A, Paillard M, Houillier P. Normocalcemic primary hyperparathyroidism: Evidence for a generalized target-tissue resistance to parathyroid hormone. J Clin Endocrinol Metab 2003;88:4641–4648.
17. Abedin M, Tintut Y, Demer LL. Vascular calcification: Mechanisms and clinical ramifications. Arterioscler Thromb Vasc Biol 2004;24:1161–1170.
18. Bevilacqua M, Dominguez LJ, Rosini S, Barbagallo M. Bisphosphonates and atherosclerosis: Why? Lupus 2005;14:773–779.
19. Vella A, Gerber TC, Hayes DL, et al. Digoxin, hypercalcemia and cardiac conduction. Postgrad Med 1999;75:554–556.
20. Rodman JS, Mahler RJ. Kidney stones as a manifestation of hypercalcemic disorders. Hyperparathyroidism and sarcoidosis. Urol Clin North Am 2000;27:275–285.

21. Yamashita H, Noguchi S, Uchino S, et al. Influence of renal function on clinico-pathological features of primary hyperparathyroidism. Eur J Endocrinol 2003;148:597–602.
22. Dretler SP. The physiologic approach to the medical management of stone disease. Urol Clin North Am 1998;25:613–623.
23. Coe FL, Evan A, Worcester E. Kidney stone disease. J Clin Invest 2005;115:2598–2608.
24. Mundy GR, Guise TA. Hypercalcemia of malignancy. Am J Med 1997;103:134–145.
25. Grauer A, Ziegler R, Raue F. Clinical significance of antibodies against calcitonin. Exp Clin Endocrinol Diabetes 1995;103:345–351.
26. Stewart AF. Hypercalcemia associated with cancer. N Engl J Med 2005;352:373–379.
27. Wellington K, Goa KL. Zoledronic acid: A review of its use in the management of bone metastases and hypercalcemia of malignancy. Drugs 2003;63:417–437.
28. Major P, Lortholary A, Hon J, et al. Zoledronic acid is superior to pamidronate in the treatment of hypercalcemia of malignancy: A pooled analysis of two randomized, controlled clinical trials. J Clin Oncol 2001;19:558–567.
29. Body JJ, Lortholary A, Romieu G, et al. A dose-finding study of zoledronate in hypercalcemic cancer patients. J Bone Miner Res 1999;14:1557–1561.
30. Pecherstorfer M, Steinhauer EU, Rizzoli R, et al. Efficacy and safety of ibandronate in the treatment of hypercalcemia of malignancy: A randomized multicenter comparison to pamidronate. Support Care Cancer 2003;11:539–547.
31. Guay DR. Ibandronate, an experimental intravenous bisphosphonate for osteoporosis, bone metastases and hypercalcemia of malignancy. Pharmacother 2006;26:655–673.
32. Rastad J, Benson L, Johansson H, et al. Clodronate treatment in patients with malignancy-associated hypercalcemia. Acta Med Scand 1987;221:489–494.
33. Banerjee D, Asif A, Striker L, et al. Short-term, high-dose pamidronate-induced acute tubular necrosis: The postulated mechanisms of bisphosphonate nephrotoxicity. Am J Kidney Dis 2003;41:E18.
34. Markowitz GS, Fine PL, Stack JI, et al. Toxic acute tubular necrosis following treatment with zoledronate (Zometa). Kidney Int 2003;64:281–289.
35. Leyland-Jones B. Treatment of cancer-related hypercalcemia: The role of gallium nitrate. Semin Oncol 2003;30(2 Suppl 5):13–19.
36. Cvitkovic F, Armand JP, Tubiana-Hulin M, et al. Randomized, double-blind, phase II trial of gallium nitrate compared with pamidronate for acute control of cancer-related hypercalcemia. Cancer J 2006;12:47–52.
37. Edelson GW, Kleerekoper M. Hypercalcemic crisis. Med Clin North Am 1995;79:79–92.
38. Manolagas SC, Weinstein RS. New developments in the pathogenesis and treatment of steroid-induced osteoporosis. J Bone Miner Res 1999;14:1061–1066.
39. Block GA, Klassen PS, Lazarus JM, et al. Mineral metabolism, mortality and morbidity in maintenance hemodialysis. 2004;15:2208–2218.
40. Collins MT, Skarulis MC, Bilezikian JP, et al. Treatment of hypercalcemia secondary to parathyroid carcinoma with a novel calcimimetic agent. J Clin Endocrinol Metab 1998;83:1083–1088.
41. Franceschini N, Joy MS, Kshirsagar A. Cincacet HCl: A calcimimetic agent for the management of primary and secondary hyperparathyroidism. Expert Opin Investig Drugs 2003;12:1413–1421.
42. Sensipar (cinacalcet HCl) [package insert]. Thousand Oaks, CA: Amgen, Inc; 2004.
43. Cinacalcet: New drug. Secondary hyperparathyroidism: Where are the clinical data? Prescrire Int 2006;15:90–93.
44. Guise TA, Mundy GR. Evaluation of hypocalcemia in children and adults. J Clin Endocrinol Metab 1995;80:1473–1478.
45. Jawan B, de Villa V, Luk HN, et al. Ionized calcium changes during living-donor liver transplantation in patients with and without administration of blood-bank products. Transpl Int 2003;16:510–514.
46. Kishimoto M, Ohto H, Shikama Y, et al. Treatment for the decline of ionized calcium levels during peripheral blood progenitor cell harvesting. Transfusion 2002;42:1340–1347.
47. Yarpuzlu AA. A review of clinical and laboratory findings and treatment of tumor lysis syndrome. Clin Chim Acta 2003;333:13–18.
48. Alvarez-Hernandez D, Santamaria I, Rodriguez-Garcia M, et al. A novel mutation in the calcium-sensing receptor responsible for autosomal dominant hypocalcemia in a family with two uncommon parathyroid hormone polymorphisms. J Mol Endocrinol 2003;31:255–262.
49. Hu J, Mora S, Colussi G, et al. Autosomal dominant hypocalcemia caused by a novel mutation in the loop 2 region of the human calcium receptor extracellular domain. J Bone Miner Res 2002;17:1461–1469.
50. Singer FR. Medical management of nonparathyroid hypercalcemia and hypocalcemia. Otolaryngol Clin North Am 1996;29:701–710.
51. Ariyan CE, Sosa JA. Assessment and management of patients with abnormal calcium. Crit Care Med 2004;32:S146-S154.
52. Fischer PR, Thacher TD, Pettifor JM, et al. Vitamin D polymorphisms and nutritional rickets in Nigerian children. J Bone Miner Res 2000;15:2206–2210.
53. Fouser L. Disorders of calcium, phosphorus and magnesium. Pediatr Ann 1995;24:38, 41–46.
54. Maalouf NM, Heller HJ, Odvina CV, et al. Bisphosphonate-induced hypocalcemia: Report of 3 cases and review of the literature. Endocr Pract 2006;12:48–53.
55. Choyke PL, Knopp MV. Pseudohypocalcemia with MR imaging contrast agents: A cautionary tale. Radiology 2003;227:639–646.
56. Uhl L, Maillet S, King S, Kruskall MS. Unexpected citrate toxicity and severe hypocalcemia during apheresis. Transfusion 1997;37:1063–1065.
57. Polaschegg HD, Sodemann K. Risks related to catheter locking solutions containing concentrated citrate. Nephrol Dial Transplant 2003;18:2688–2689.
58. Tohme JF, Bilezikian JP. Hypocalcemic emergencies. Endocrinol Metab Clin North Am 1993;22:363–375.
59. Lee I, Sheu WH, Tu ST, et al. Bisphosphonate pretreatment attenuates hungry bone syndrome postoperatively in subjects with primary hyperparathyroidism. J Bone Miner Metab 2006;24:255–258.
60. Hollis BW. Circulating 25-hydroxyvitamin D levels indicative of vitamin D sufficiency: Implications for establishing a new effective dietary intake recommendation for vitamin D. J Nutr 2005;135:317–322.
61. Hruska K, Gupta A. Disorders of phosphate homeostasis. In: Avioli LV, Krane SM, eds. Metabolic Bone Disease and Clinically Related Disorders, 3rd ed. New York: Academic Press, 1998:207–236.
62. Weisinger JR, Bellorin-Font E. Magnesium and phosphorus. Lancet 1998;352:391–396.
63. Fine A, Patterson J. Severe hyperphosphatemia following phosphate administration for bowel preparation in patients with renal failure: Two cases and a review of the literature. Am J Kidney Dis 1997;29:103–105.
64. Aydogan T, Kanbay M, Uz B, et al. Fatal hyperphosphatemia secondary to a phosphosoda bowel preparation in a geriatric patient with normal renal function. J Clin Gastroenterol 2006;40:177.
65. U.S. Food and Drug Administration. Oral Sodium Phosphate (OSP) Products for Bowel Cleansing. FDA Alert. 2006, *http://www.fda.gov/cder/drug/infopage/osp_solution/default.htm*.
66. Amanzadeh J, Reilly RF. Hypophosphatemia: An evidence-based approach to its clinical consequences and management. Nat Clin Pract Nephrol 2006;2:136–148.
67. Kelsler R, McDonald RD, Cadnapaphornchai P. Dynamic changes in serum phosphorus levels in diabetic ketoacidosis. Am J Med 1985;79:571–576.
68. Eknoyan G, Levin A, Levin NW. K/DOQI clinical practice guidelines for bone metabolism and disease in chronic kidney disease. Am J Kidney Dis 2003;42(Suppl 3):S1–201.
69. Joy MS, Finn WF. Randomized, double-blind, placebo-controlled, dose-titration, Phase III study assessing the efficacy and tolerability of lanthanum carbonate: A new phosphate binder for the treatment of hyperphosphatemia. Am J Kidney Dis 2003;42:96–107.
70. D'Haese PC, Spasovski GB, Sikole A, et al. A multicenter study on the effects of lanthanum carbonate (Fosrenol) and calcium carbonate on renal bone disease in dialysis patients. Kidney Int 2003;85:S73–S78.
71. Coladonato JA. Control of hyperphosphatemia among patients with ESRD. J Am Soc Nephrol 2005;16: S107–114.
72. Perreault MM, Ostrop NJ, Tierney MG. Efficacy and safety of intravenous phosphate replacement in critically ill patients. Ann Pharmacother 1997;31:683–688.
73. Subramanian R, Khardori R. Severe hypophosphatemia. Pathophysiologic implications, clinical presentation, and treatment. Medicine (Baltimore) 2000;79:1–78.
74. Hoggson SF, Hurley DL. Acquired hypophosphatemia. Endocrinol Metab Clin North Am 1993;22:397–409.

75. Charron T, Bernard F, Skrobik Y, et al. Intravenous phosphate in the intensive care unit: More aggressive repletion regimens for moderate and severe hypophosphatemia. Intensive Care Med 2003;29:1273–1278.
76. Clark CL, Sacks GS, Dickerson RN, et al. Treatment of hypophosphatemia in patients receiving specialized nutrition support using a graduated dosing scheme: Results from a prospective clinical trial. Crit Care Med 1995;23:1504–1511.
77. Prie D, Blanchet FB, Essig M, et al. Dipyridamole decreases renal phosphate leak and augments serum phosphorus in patients with low renal phosphate threshold. J Am Soc Nephrol 1998;9:1264–1269.

CHAPTER 54 Disorders of Potassium and Magnesium Homeostasis

DONALD F. BROPHY AND TODD W. B. GEHR

KEY CONCEPTS

1. Potassium is the primary intracellular ion in the human body.
2. The normal serum potassium concentration range is 3.5 to 5 mEq/L (3.5 to 5 mmol/L).
3. Potassium regulates many biochemical processes in the body and is a key ion for electrical action potentials across cellular membranes.
4. Potassium chloride is the preferred potassium supplement for the most common causes of hypokalemia.
5. In patients with concomitant hypokalemia and hypomagnesemia, it is imperative to correct the hypomagnesemia before the hypokalemia.
6. Hyperkalemia is a common occurrence in patients with acute or chronic kidney disease.
7. Magnesium is an important cofactor for many cellular functions.
8. The normal serum magnesium concentration range is 1.4 to 1.8 mEq/L (0.85 to 1.15 mmol/L).
9. Hypomagnesemia is commonly caused by excessive gastrointestinal or renal magnesium wasting.
10. Hypermagnesemia is commonly observed in patients with acute or chronic kidney disease.

Potassium and magnesium are electrolytes that are responsible for numerous metabolic activities. Disorders of these electrolytes are frequently seen in both the acute care and community ambulatory care settings. Clinicians should have a firm understanding of the etiology, pathophysiology, symptoms, pharmacotherapy, and monitoring of these disorders. This chapter describes the homeostatic mechanisms that are responsible for the maintenance of normal potassium and magnesium serum concentrations. The clinical disorders responsible for the development of hyperkalemia, hypermagnesemia, hypokalemia, and hypomagnesemia are also reviewed.

POTASSIUM

❶ Potassium is the most abundant cation in the body, with estimated total body stores of 3,000 to 4,000 mEq.[1] Ninety-eight percent of this amount is contained within the intracellular compartment, and the remaining 2% is distributed within the extracellular compartment. The sodium potassium adenosine triphosphatase (Na^+-K^+-ATPase) pump located in the cell membrane is responsible for the compartmentalization of potassium. This pump is an active transport system that maintains increased intracellular stores of potassium by transporting sodium out of the cell and potassium into the cell at a ratio of 3:2. Consequently, the pump maintains a higher concentration of potassium inside the cell.

❷ The normal serum concentration range for potassium is 3.5 to 5.0 mEq/L, whereas the intracellular potassium concentration is usually approximately 150 mEq/L.[2] Approximately 75% of the intracellular potassium is located in skeletal muscle; the remaining 25% is located in the liver and red blood cells. Extracellular potassium is distributed throughout the serum and interstitial space. Potassium is dynamic in that it is constantly moving between the intracellular and extracellular compartments according to the body's needs. Thus the serum potassium concentration alone does not accurately reflect the total body potassium content.

❸ Potassium has many physiologic functions within cells, including protein and glycogen synthesis and cellular metabolism and growth. It is also a determinant of the electrical action potential across the cell membrane.[1] The ratio of the intracellular to extracellular potassium concentration is the major determinant of the resting membrane potential across the cell membrane. Thus the resting membrane potential is greatly affected by variations in extracellular potassium concentration. Serum potassium concentrations outside the normal range can have disastrous effects on neuromuscular activity, in particular cardiac conduction. Hypo- and hyperkalemia are both associated with potentially fatal cardiac arrhythmias, along with other neuromuscular disturbances.

CONTROL OF POTASSIUM HOMEOSTASIS

Potassium homeostasis, the maintenance of serum potassium within the normal range, is affected by dietary intake, gastrointestinal and urinary excretion, hormones, acid–base balance, and body fluid tonicity.[3]

The recommended daily allowance for dietary potassium intake is approximately 50 mEq/day.[1] Potassium is found in abundance in fruits, vegetables, and meats. The typical American ingests approximately 50 to 150 mEq of potassium daily.[3] Nearly all of this is absorbed, with only 10 to 20 mEq/day eliminated in feces. The amount eliminated in the feces increases, however, in patients with diarrhea, and in those with underlying chronic kidney disease (CKD).[4]

The kidney is the primary route of potassium elimination. Potassium is freely filtered but almost all of it is reabsorbed passively in the proximal tubule and the thick ascending limb of the loop of Henle.[5] Therefore urinary potassium excretion is primarily determined by potassium secretion from the luminal cells of the distal tubule and collecting duct. Although the amount of potassium filtered by the

Learning objectives, review questions, and other resources can be found at **www.pharmacotherapyonline.com.**

glomerulus approaches 700 mEq per day, only approximately 10% to 20% is actually excreted in the urine.[1] However, this amount can vary based on dietary intake, serum potassium concentration, and aldosterone activity. For example, more potassium is renally excreted in conditions that result in high aldosterone activity (e.g., dehydration) when the body is attempting to conserve sodium or when there is an increase in dietary potassium intake.

Hormones such as insulin, catecholamines, and aldosterone dramatically affect potassium homeostasis. Insulin is the most important hormonal mediator of potassium balance because it stimulates the cellular Na^+-K^+-ATPase pump to increase transport of potassium into liver, muscle, and adipose tissue.[3] There is a complex negative feedback loop in which insulin secretion tightly regulates serum potassium concentrations: an increase of only a few tenths of a milliequivalent stimulates pancreatic insulin secretion in an attempt to prevent hyperkalemia from developing.[1] If hyperkalemia does occur, glucagon is released from the liver to protect against insulin-induced hypoglycemia. Conversely, hypokalemia inhibits insulin secretion, a finding that explains why some patients receiving diuretics develop hyperglycemia.

An elevation in circulating catecholamines such as epinephrine usually results in the intracellular movement of potassium by two mechanisms.[6] They stimulate the β-receptor, which directly activates the Na^+-K^+-ATPase pump. Second, they stimulate glycogenolysis, which raises blood glucose concentrations, thereby increasing insulin secretion. This dual mechanism is often used therapeutically in patients with hyperkalemia to normalize serum potassium concentrations.

Aldosterone, a mineralocorticoid that is secreted from the adrenal glands in response to high serum potassium concentrations, promotes urinary potassium excretion. Aldosterone works in the distal tubule and collecting duct to promote the reabsorption of sodium and water in exchange for potassium. Aldosterone may also have extrarenal activity by stimulating cellular Na^+-K^+-ATPase pump activity.[6]

Changes in acid–base status significantly affect the serum potassium concentration. For example, the infusion of metabolic inorganic acids, such as hydrochloric acid, results in an increase in serum potassium. The body compensates for excessive hydrogen ions by moving them from the serum into the cell, in exchange for intracellular potassium, to maintain electroneutrality. The process by which this occurs is complex, and a cellular H^+-K^+-ATPase pump has been identified. The efflux of potassium into the serum can result in hyperkalemia. A commonly quoted approximation of the pH effect is that for every 0.1 unit decrease in pH, there is a corresponding increase in serum potassium of 0.6 to 0.8 mEq/L (with a wide range of 0.2 to 1.7).[5] This is often referred to as *false hyperkalemia* because there is not a true excess of total body potassium. Metabolic acidosis associated with lactic acidosis and ketoacidosis, does not result in hyperkalemia, because both cations and anions enter the cell, thus maintaining electroneutrality.[1] Respiratory acidosis also does not significantly affect the serum potassium concentration.[6]

Conversely, metabolic alkalosis has been associated with hypokalemia. As a result of a net loss of hydrogen ion from the serum, intracellular hydrogen ions enter the serum to increase the acidity of the blood. To maintain electroneutrality extracellular potassium ions are shifted intracellularly. This creates a relative deficiency of potassium in the serum. Serum potassium decreases approximately 0.6 mEq/L for each 0.1 unit increase in blood pH. This is frequently termed *false hypokalemia* because there is not a true deficiency in total body potassium.

Finally, hyperosmolality can result in enhanced movement of potassium from the cell into the extracellular fluid. This occurs most likely because of the associated cell shrinkage and water loss, which increases the intracellular-to-extracellular potassium gradient.[3] This is seen most commonly in conditions such as diabetic ketoacidosis. Conversely, hypo-osmolality does not seem to affect potassium distribution.

HYPOKALEMIA

Epidemiology

Hypokalemia (defined as a serum potassium concentration <3.5 mEq/L) is one of the most commonly encountered electrolyte abnormalities in clinical practice.[7,8] Hypokalemia can be categorized as mild (serum potassium 3 to 3.5 mEq/L), moderate (serum potassium 2.5 to 3 mEq/L), or severe (<2.5 mEq/L). When hypokalemia is detected, a diagnostic workup that evaluates the patient's comorbid disease states and concomitant medications should be initiated. Hypokalemia is virtually nonexistent in healthy adults. This is due in part to the relatively high potassium content in the typical Western diet as well as the body's effective potassium-sparing mechanisms, which tightly regulate the serum potassium concentration. However it has been estimated that as many as 50% of patients who receive thiazide or loop diuretics have serum potassium concentrations less than 3.5 mEq/L.[8]

Etiology and Pathophysiology

Hypokalemia results when there is a total body potassium deficit, or when serum potassium is shifted into the intracellular compartment. Total body deficits occur in the setting of poor dietary intake of potassium, or when there are excessive renal and gastrointestinal losses of potassium.

Maintaining a consistent dietary intake of potassium is important because the body has no effective method for storing potassium. At steady state, potassium excretion matches potassium intake; approximately 90% of ingested potassium is renally excreted, whereas 10% is excreted in feces.[9] This underscores the importance of eating a well-balanced diet. Elderly patients with chronic diseases and those undergoing surgery are at increased risk for developing hypokalemia because of insufficient intake or losses resulting from surgery.

Many drugs can cause hypokalemia by a variety of mechanisms including intracellular potassium shifting and increased renal or stool losses (Table 54–1). The most common cause of drug-induced hypokalemia is loop and thiazide diuretic administration as these agents inhibit renal sodium reabsorption, which results in increased sodium delivery to the distal tubule. Consequently, hypokalemia develops because the distal tubule selectively reabsorbs sodium, and excretes potassium down its concentration gradient. Second, because

TABLE 54-1 Mechanism of Drug-Induced Hypokalemia

Transcellular Shift	Enhanced Renal Excretion	Enhanced Fecal Elimination
β_2-Receptor agonists	**Diuretics**	**Sodium polystyrene sulfonate**
Epinephrine	Acetazolamide	**Phenolphthalein**
Albuterol	Thiazides	**Sorbitol**
Terbutaline	Indapamide	
Pirbuterol	Metolazone	
Salmeterol	Furosemide	
Isoproterenol	Torsemide	
Ephedrine	Bumetanide	
Pseudoephedrine	Ethacrynic acid	
Tocolytic agents	**High-dose penicillins**	
Ritodrine	Nafcillin	
Nylidrin	Ampicillin	
Theophylline	Penicillin	
Caffeine	**Mineralocorticoids**	
Insulin overdose	**Miscellaneous**	
	Aminoglycosides	
	Amphotericin B	
	Cisplatin	

diuretics result in volume contraction, aldosterone is secreted which further promotes the renal excretion of potassium. If concomitant potassium supplements are not provided to patients receiving loop and thiazide diuretics, mild to moderate hypokalemia is inevitable.

The second most common etiology of hypokalemia is excessive loss of potassium-rich GI fluid as a result of diarrhea and/or vomiting. The typical potassium loss in feces is approximately 10 mEq per day.[7] In diarrheal states, this amount increases proportionally with the volume of stool output. Vomiting also accounts for substantial potassium losses, which have been estimated to be as high as 30 to 50 mEq per liter of vomitus.[8] Metabolic alkalosis can also occur in cases of severe diarrhea and vomiting as a result of loss of these bicarbonate-rich fluids. This causes an intracellular shifting of potassium, which lowers the serum concentration of potassium even further. Prolonged diarrhea and vomiting can significantly affect children and elderly patients because their kidneys are unable to effectively maintain adequate fluid status.

Hypomagnesemia can also contribute to the development of hypokalemia because it reduces the intracellular potassium concentration and promotes renal potassium wasting.[10] The intracellular potassium concentration decreases because hypomagnesemia impairs the function of the Na^+-K^+-ATPase pump. The precise mechanism of the accelerated renal loss of potassium is unknown. It is unclear whether hypomagnesemia directly causes hypokalemia, because the two are often found together as a result of drugs (diuretic administration) or disease states (diarrhea). When concomitant hypokalemia and hypomagnesemia occur, the magnesium deficiency should be corrected first, otherwise full repletion of the potassium deficit is difficult.

CLINICAL PRESENTATION OF HYPOKALEMIA

General

- The signs and symptoms of hypokalemia are usually nonspecific and highly variable between patients.

Symptoms

- Symptoms are highly dependent on the degree of hypokalemia and its rapidity of onset.
- Mild hypokalemia is often asymptomatic.
- Moderate hypokalemia is associated with cramping, weakness, malaise, and myalgias.

Signs

- Cardiovascular: In severe hypokalemia, electrocardiogram (ECG) changes often include ST-segment depression or flattening, T-wave inversion, and U-wave elevation. Clinical arrhythmias include heart block, atrial flutter, paroxysmal atrial tachycardia, ventricular fibrillation, and digitalis-induced arrhythmias.
- Musculoskeletal: Cramping and impaired muscle contraction.

Laboratory Tests

- Serum potassium concentration less than 3.5 mEq/L is diagnostic. Hypomagnesemia (serum magnesium concentration <1.7 mg/dL) can also be present.

TREATMENT

Hypokalemia

■ DESIRED OUTCOME

The goals of hypokalemia management are to prevent the development of and to treat if present serious life-threatening complications, to normalize the serum potassium concentration, to identify and correct the underlying cause of hypokalemia, and to prevent overcorrection of the serum potassium concentration.

■ GENERAL APPROACH TO THERAPY

The general approach to therapy depends on the degree and rapidity with which hypokalemia developed and the presence of symptoms. Serum potassium concentrations between 3.5 and 4 mEq/L are a sign of early potassium depletion. No pharmacologic therapy is recommended at this point; however, these patients should be encouraged to increase their dietary intake of potassium-rich foods. When the serum potassium concentration is between 3 and 3.5 mEq/L, it is debatable whether pharmacologic therapy should be initiated. Oral potassium supplementation should be initiated in patients with underlying cardiac conditions that predispose them to cardiac arrhythmias.[11] This includes patients receiving concomitant digoxin therapy. Patients with serum potassium concentrations below 3 mEq/L should always be treated to achieve values between 4 and 4.5 mEq/L. In asymptomatic patients, oral therapy is the preferred route of administration. Intravenous potassium can be necessary in symptomatic patients with severe depletion, or in patients who are intolerant to oral supplementation. In patients with concomitant moderate to severe hypomagnesemia, the magnesium deficit should be corrected before potassium supplementation, to prevent refractory hypokalemia.[10,12]

■ NONPHARMACOLOGIC THERAPY

Various nonpharmacologic therapies have been used to prevent and treat hypokalemia. The best and most abundant source of potassium supplementation comes from dietary sources, in particular, fresh fruits and vegetables, fruit juices, and meats.[12] Table 54–2 lists foods that are excellent sources of potassium. Salt substitutes that contain potassium chloride are another effective, inexpensive source of potas-

TABLE 54-2 Foods That Are High in Potassium

Highest content (>1,000 mg/100 g)
Dried figs
Molasses
Very high content (>500 mg/100 g)
Dried fruits (dates, prunes)
Nuts
Avocados
Bran cereals
Lima beans
High content (>250 mg/100 g)
Vegetables
Spinach
Tomatoes
Broccoli
Squash
Beets
Cauliflower
Carrots
Potatoes
Fruits
Bananas
Cantaloupe
Kiwi
Oranges
Mangos
Meats
Ground beef
Steak
Pork
Lamb
Veal

sium. Increased dietary intake of foods with high potassium content is not recommended long-term for many patients because it can add unwanted calories to the patient's diet. Moreover, dietary potassium is almost entirely coupled with phosphate, rather than chloride, so it is not as effective in correcting potassium loss associated with hypochloremic conditions such as vomiting, nasogastric suctioning, and diuretic therapy.[12]

PHARMACOLOGIC THERAPY

Guidelines for potassium supplementation were last published by the National Council on Potassium in Clinical Practice in 2000 (Table 54–3).[12] These guidelines provide a comprehensive framework for potassium prophylaxis and replacement in many distinct patient populations. When deciding on appropriate pharmacotherapy to replete potassium, five factors must be considered: (1) the patient's normal baseline potassium concentration; (2) underlying medical conditions that can affect potassium balance; (3) concomitant medications that can affect potassium balance; (4) the patient's dietary and salt intake; and (5) the patient's ability to comply with the therapeutic regimen.[12]

A general rule for potassium replacement is that for every 1-mEq/L decrease of potassium below 3.5 mEq/L, there is a corresponding total body potassium deficit of 100 to 400 mEq. Because of the wide variance in projected deficits, each patient's therapy must be individualized and adjustments made on the basis of the patients signs, symptoms, and frequent measurements of serum potassium. In patients receiving chronic loop or thiazide diuretic therapy, 40 to 100 mEq of potassium can correct mild to moderate potassium deficits. Doses up to 120 mEq can be required in more severe deficiencies. When providing oral potassium supplementation, the total daily dose should be divided into three to four doses to minimize the developement of GI side effects. Patients receiving diuretics can become chronically hypokalemic and can benefit from combination potassium-sparing diuretic therapy.

TABLE 54-3 General Consensus Guidelines for Potassium Replacement

Guideline	Comment
Potassium replacement therapy should accompany dietary consumption of potassium-rich foods.	Potassium-rich foods often cannot completely replace potassium associated with chloride losses (vomiting, diuretics, or nasogastric suction) because it is almost entirely coupled to phosphate. Furthermore, increasing dietary intake of these foods can lead to unwanted weight gain.
Potassium replacement is recommended for patients who are sodium sensitive, and hypertensive patients.	A high-sodium diet often results in excessive urinary potassium excretion.
Potassium replacement is recommended in patients who are subject to vomiting, diarrhea, or diuretic/laxative abuse.	These conditions promote excessive renal and GI potassium loss.
Potassium supplementation is best administered orally in divided doses over several days to achieve full repletion.	
Laboratory measurement of serum potassium is convenient but not always accurate.	Clinicians should be aware of the factors that result in transcellular potassium shifts. Monitoring 24-hour urinary potassium excretion can be necessary in high-risk patients.
Patient adherence to potassium replacement can be increased with compliance-enhancing regimens.	Microencapsulated products have no bitter smell or aftertaste and have much better GI tolerance. Regimens should be made as simple as possible to follow.
A potassium dosage of 20 mEq/day is usually sufficient to prevent hypokalemia from occurring. Doses of 40–100 mEq are usually sufficient to treat hypokalemia.	

CLINICAL CONTROVERSY

The replacement of potassium intravenously can be accomplished by IV piggyback or Buretrol administration. A pharmacist usually prepares the potassium IV piggyback, double checks the concentration and fluid, and then dispenses the final product to the medical unit. However, with Buretrol administration, essentially any clinician (e.g., nurse or physician) can prepare the solution on the medical unit, and infuse the potassium solution into the patient. The Joint Commission and the United States Pharmacopeia 797 Standards now advocate that all parenteral products be compounded in a sterile, laminar flow environment, and be double-checked by a pharmacist to assure patient safety. Many hospitals to date have not adapted these recommendations, which were developed to improve patient safety.

❹ Whenever possible, potassium supplementation should be administered by mouth. Three salts are available for oral potassium supplementation: chloride, phosphate, and bicarbonate. Potassium phosphate should be used when patients are both hypokalemic and hypophosphatemic; potassium bicarbonate is most commonly used when potassium depletion occurs in the setting of metabolic acidosis. Potassium chloride, however, is the primary salt form used because it is the most effective treatment for the most common causes of potassium depletion (i.e., diuretic-induced and diarrhea-induced) as these conditions are associated with potassium and chloride losses.

Potassium chloride can be administered in either tablet or liquid formulations (Table 54–4). The liquid forms are generally less expensive; however, patient compliance can be low because of their strong, unpleasant taste.[12] Two sustained-release solid dosage forms are currently available in the United States: a wax-matrix formulation, and a microencapsulated formulation. The microencapsulated tablet is generally preferred because it disintegrates better in the stomach and is associated with less GI irritation.[7,12]

Intravenous potassium use should be limited to: (1) severe cases of hypokalemia (serum concentration <2.5 mEq/L); (2) patients exhibiting signs and symptoms of hypokalemia such as ECG changes or muscle spasms; or (3) patients unable to tolerate oral therapy. Intravenous supplementation is more dangerous than oral therapy because it is more likely to result in hyperkalemia, phlebitis, and pain at the site of infusion.

The vehicle in which IV potassium is administered is important. Whenever possible, potassium should be prepared in saline-containing solutions (e.g., 0.9% or 0.45% sodium chloride [NaCl]). Dextrose-containing solutions stimulate insulin secretion, which can

TABLE 54-4 Differentiation of Available Potassium Supplements

Supplement	Comment
Controlled-release microencapsulated tablet	Disintegrates better in GI tract; fewer GI erosions as compared to wax-matrix tablets
Encapsulated controlled-release microencapsulated particles	Fewer erosions as compared to wax-matrix tablets
Potassium chloride elixir	Inexpensive, poor taste, poor compliance, immediate effect
Potassium chloride effervescent tablets for solution	More expensive than elixir, convenient
Wax-matrix extended-release tablets	Easier to swallow; more GI erosions as compared to other therapies

cause intracellular shifting of potassium worsening the patient's hypokalemia, and should be avoided whenever possible.[13] Generally, 10 to 20 mEq of potassium is diluted in 100 mL 0.9% NaCl for intravenous administration. These concentrations are safe when administered through a peripheral vein over 1 hour. When infusion rates exceed 10 mEq/h, ECG monitoring should be performed to detect cardiac changes. The serum potassium concentration should be evaluated following the infusion of each 30 to 40 mEq, to direct further potassium replacement requirements. Multiple doses of potassium can be repeated as needed until the serum potassium concentration normalizes. To allow adequate time for the potassium to equilibrate between the intra- and extracellular spaces, the clinician should wait at least 30 minutes from the end of each infusion before obtaining a serum concentration. Care should be taken to avoid sampling from the same line in which the potassium was infused, as this can result in a spuriously high potassium concentration.

In cases of severe potassium depletion, patients can require as much as 300 to 400 mEq/day. In this instance, it is common practice to dilute 40 to 60 mEq in 1,000 mL 0.45% NaCl and infuse at a rate not exceeding 40 mEq/h. When possible, this should be performed in an intensive care unit under continuous ECG monitoring. Because of the high potassium concentration, and the risk for burning pain and peripheral venous sclerosis, the infusion should be through a central intravenous line into a large vein (e.g., superior vena cava). Given the volume required to infuse this dose of potassium, this infusion strategy might be impractical in certain clinical situations (e.g., patients requiring fluid restriction). A reasonable alternative is to split the potassium dose between the oral and intravenous routes. For example, if a symptomatic patient requires 120 mEq of potassium, the clinician can give 60 mEq as the immediate-release potassium liquid, and the other 60 mEq can be given via the intravenous route (20 mEq/100 mL/h in three doses). When giving large potassium doses, serum monitoring should be performed following the administration of half the dose to guide the clinician as to the need for additional potassium. This can also help avoid the development of hyperkalemia.

■ ALTERNATIVE THERAPIES

Potassium-sparing diuretics are an alternative to chronic exogenous potassium supplementation, especially when patients are concomitantly receiving drugs that are known to deplete potassium (e.g., diuretics or amphotericin B). Spironolactone inhibits the effect of aldosterone in the distal convoluted tubule, thereby decreasing potassium elimination in the urine. Spironolactone is especially effective as a potassium-sparing agent in patients with primary or secondary hyperaldosteronism. Amiloride and triamterene act by an aldosterone-independent mechanism; however, the precise mechanism of their potassium sparing is unknown.

Spironolactone is available as 25-mg, 50-mg, and 100-mg tablets. The usual starting dose is 25 to 50 mg daily, and can be titrated to a maximum dose of 400 mg/day. The potassium-retaining effects generally take approximately 48 hours to occur. Important side effects include hyperkalemia, gynecomastia, breast tenderness, and impotence in men.

Triamterene is available as 50-mg and 100-mg capsules. The usual starting dose is 50 mg twice daily, which can be titrated to 100 mg twice daily. Triamterene 50 mg is available as a combination product with hydrochlorothiazide 25 mg and is commonly used for the treatment of hypertension. Common side effects include hyperkalemia, sodium depletion, and metabolic acidosis.

Amiloride is available as a 5-mg tablet. The usual starting dose is 5 mg daily; however, 10 mg can be given in those with severe hypokalemia. This is also available as a combination product with hydrochlorothiazide 50 mg. The most common side effects are hyperkalemia and metabolic acidosis.

Generally, concomitant use of potassium supplementation with potassium-sparing diuretics is not necessary. There is a significant risk of hyperkalemia during combination therapy, especially in patients with underlying renal insufficiency or diabetes mellitus.

To date, there have been no pharmacoeconomic evaluations of the different pharmacotherapeutic alternatives to manage hypokalemia. The most economical source of chronic potassium supplementation is to increase the amount in the diet. Thus patients receiving diuretic therapy should be instructed to increase their dietary intake of potassium-rich foods. By doing so, they can often avert the need for exogenous potassium therapy.

■ EVALUATION OF THERAPEUTIC OUTCOMES

❺ Serum potassium concentrations should be monitored regularly while the patient is receiving potassium supplementation. For patients receiving prophylactic potassium supplementation during diuretic therapy, the serum potassium and magnesium concentrations, as well as renal function should be monitored every 1 to 2 months in stable patients. In hospitalized patients receiving oral therapy for mild hypokalemia, the potassium concentration should be monitored every 2 to 3 days. Generally, the potassium concentration begins to increase within 72 hours. If it does not increase by at least 1 mEq/L within 96 hours, the clinician should suspect concomitant magnesium depletion. If present, correcting the magnesium deficit generally results in normalization of potassium. Patients receiving IV potassium supplementation require close ECG monitoring if the infusion rate is greater than 20 mEq/h. Doses greater than this should be administered only in the presence of continuous ECG monitoring. Additionally, the patient should have potassium concentrations obtained halfway through, and 30 minutes following completion of the total potassium dose to guide further potassium dosing. Finally, the patient should be assessed for adverse effects such as burning pain at the infusion site or phlebitis.

HYPERKALEMIA

Hyperkalemia, defined as a serum potassium concentration greater than 5.5 mEq/L, can be further classified according to its severity: mild hyperkalemia (serum potassium 5.5 to 6 mEq/L), moderate hyperkalemia (6.1 to 6.9 mEq/L), and severe hyperkalemia (>7 mEq/L).[14]

Epidemiology

Hyperkalemia is much less common than hypokalemia. In fact, if all patients with acute and chronic kidney disease were excluded, the true prevalence of hyperkalemia would be insignificant.[14] Indeed, the incidence of hyperkalemia in hospitalized patients is highly variable, and reports have ranged from 1.4% to 10%.[15] Most cases of hyperkalemia are the result of overcorrection of hypokalemia with intravenous potassium supplements. Severe hyperkalemia occurs more commonly in elderly patients with renal insufficiency who receive chronic oral potassium supplementation.[15,16]

Etiology and Pathophysiology

Hyperkalemia develops when potassium intake exceeds excretion (true hyperkalemia) (i.e., elevated total body stores), or when the transcellular distribution of potassium is disturbed (i.e., normal total body stores). The four primary causes of hyperkalemia—(1) increased potassium intake, (2) decreased potassium excretion, (3) tubular unresponsiveness to aldosterone, and (4) redistribution of potassium into the extracellular space—are discussed below.

Hyperkalemia Associated with Increased Potassium Intake

Hyperkalemia in this setting is almost always associated with renal insufficiency. Patients with stage 4 or 5 CKD and dialysis patients who are noncompliant with dietary potassium restrictions often present with life-threatening hyperkalemia. Many of these patients do not realize that fresh fruits and vegetables contain large amounts of potassium. Anecdotally, in many dialysis centers the incidence of hyperkalemia peaks during the summer months, when fresh garden produce is available. Another common dietary source associated with the development of hyperkalemia is potassium chloride salt substitutes. Many dialysis patients are instructed to use salt substitutes to avoid excessive sodium intake in an attempt to control volume overload. These patients unwittingly become hyperkalemic because these products contain approximately 10 to 15 mEq potassium per gram, or 200 mEq per tablespoon. Finally, many over-the-counter herbal and alternative medicine products may contain significant concentrations of potassium.[17] Indeed, noni juice, a product touted for its many health benefits, has been implicated as a cause of hyperkalemia in patients with renal dysfunction.[18]

It is essential for patients with CKD to receive education regarding dietary sources of potassium as well as information on the potassium content of herbal products because the ingestion of these can lead to hyperkalemia.

Hyperkalemia Associated with Decreased Renal Potassium Excretion ❻ The kidneys excrete 80% of the daily potassium intake. Therefore when the kidney is unable to excrete potassium appropriately, as in acute renal failure (ARF) and stage 4 to 5 CKD, potassium is retained and often results in hyperkalemia. Finally, many drugs can inhibit the kidney's ability to excrete potassium by inhibiting aldosterone and thus contribute to an increase in serum potassium concentrations.

Severe hyperkalemia is more common in ARF than in CKD because patients are often hypercatabolic and can have underlying disorders, such as rhabdomyolysis or tumor lysis syndrome, which result in release of potassium from injured or lysed cells.[19] Severe hyperkalemia is rare in stable CKD patients, perhaps because of enhanced GI and renal potassium excretion.[20] Data suggest that hyperkalemia actually directly stimulates renal K^+ excretion through an effect that is independent of, and additive to, that of aldosterone.[20] Renal excretion of potassium is also inhibited by various endocrinologic disorders, including adrenal insufficiency, Addison's disease, and selective hypoaldosteronism. All of these disorders involve a decreased production of aldosterone, which results in the retention of potassium.

Several drugs have profound effects on the kidney's ability to regulate potassium.[21] Four drug classes in particular have specific effects on the kidney: angiotensin-converting enzyme inhibitors (ACEIs), angiotensin-II receptor blockers (ARBs), potassium-sparing diuretics, and prostaglandin inhibitors such as nonsteroidal antiinflammatory drugs (NSAIDs). Although hyperkalemia with these drugs is typically dose-dependent, the rates of hyperkalemia have been reported to range from 5% to 10% in most clinical trials. Other commonly used drugs that can cause hyperkalemia are digoxin, cyclosporine, tacrolimus, trimethoprim-sulfamethoxazole, heparin, and pentamidine.[21]

Tubular Unresponsiveness to Aldosterone Certain medical conditions, such as sickle cell anemia, systemic lupus erythematosus, and amyloidosis, can produce a defect in tubular potassium secretion, possibly as the result of an alteration in the aldosterone-binding site. The exact mechanism of the tubular unresponsiveness is unknown.

Redistribution of Potassium into the Extracellular Space The efflux of potassium from within the cell into the extracellular fluid, which is associated with no change in total body potassium stores, is to be expected in the presence of metabolic acidosis, diabetes mellitus, chronic renal failure, or lactic acidosis. β-Blockers can also result in a transcellular potassium shift.[21]

The serum potassium concentration can also be falsely elevated in some conditions, and not reflect the actual in vivo potassium concentration. This is termed *pseudohyperkalemia*. Pseudohyperkalemia occurs most commonly in the setting of extravascular hemolysis of red blood cells.[14] When a blood specimen is not processed promptly and cellular destruction occurs, intracellular potassium is released into the serum. Pseudohyperkalemia can also occur in conditions of thrombocytosis or leukocytosis. If severe hyperkalemia is found in a patient who is asymptomatic with an otherwise normal laboratory report, the hyperkalemia is most likely pseudohyperkalemia, and a repeat blood sample should be evaluated. Truly elevated potassium concentrations are normally associated with other laboratory abnormalities, such as low carbon dioxide (acidosis) or elevated blood urea nitrogen and creatinine concentrations (indicating renal insufficiency).

CLINICAL PRESENTATION OF HYPERKALEMIA

General

- Related to the effects of excessive potassium on neuromuscular, cardiac, and smooth muscle cell function.

Symptoms

- Frequently asymptomatic.
- The patient might complain of heart palpitations or skipped heartbeats.

Signs

- ECG changes (see Fig. 54–1 for description).

Laboratory Tests

- Serum potassium concentration >5.5 mEq/L.

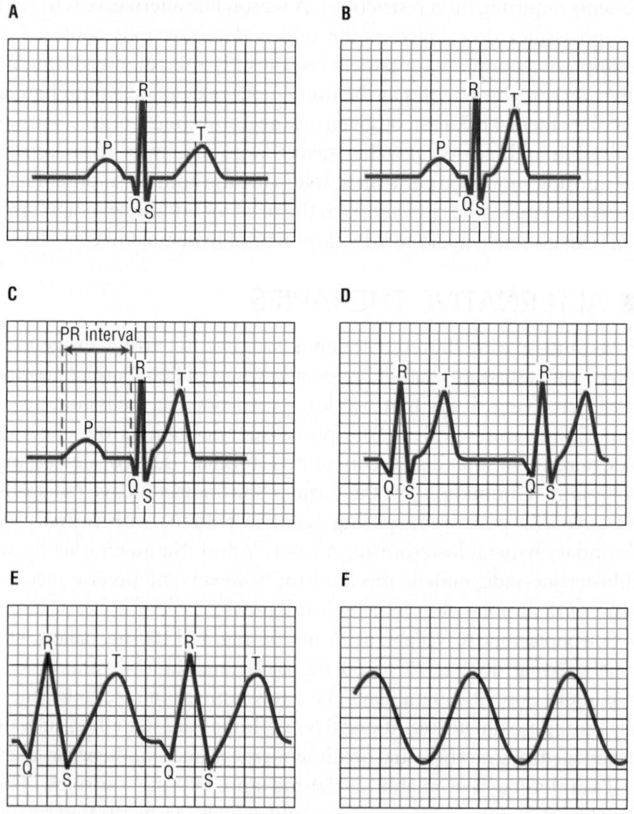

FIGURE 54-1. The earliest electrocardiographic manifestation of hyperkalemia is an increase in the rate of ventricular repolarization, which results in a peaking of the T wave at serum potassium concentrations of ~5.5 to 6 mEq/L *(B)*, relative to the normal ECG presentation *(A)*. Further increases in the serum potassium concentration above 6 mEq/L result in conduction delays through the His-Purkinje system, the atrial myocardium, and the ventricular myocardium. The ECG manifestations of these conduction delays and the sequence in which they occur are a widening of the PR interval *(C)*, delay through the His-Purkinje system, a loss of the P wave *(D)*, delay through the atrial myocardium, a widening of the QRS complex *(E)*, and delay through the ventricular myocardium. Finally, there is a merging of the QRS complex with the T wave *(F)*, which results in a sine-wave appearance.

TREATMENT

Hyperkalemia

■ DESIRED OUTCOME

The goals of therapy for the treatment of hyperkalemia are to antagonize adverse cardiac effects, reverse any symptoms that are present, and return the serum and total body stores of potassium to normal. Asymptomatic patients with mild hyperkalemia usually require no specific therapy other than the tincture of time, dietary education to control intake, and monitoring of serum potassium daily if an inpatient or weekly if an outpatient to assure resolution. Severe hyperkalemia (>7 mEq/L) or moderate hyperkalemia (6.1 to 6.9 mEq/L), when associated with clinical symptoms or ECG changes, requires immediate treatment. Initial treatment of severe and moderate symptomatic hyperkalemia is focused on antagonism of the cardiac membrane actions of hyperkalemia (e.g., with calcium). Secondarily, one should attempt to decrease extracellular potassium concentration by promoting its intracellular movement (e.g., with glucose, insulin, β_2-receptor agonists, or sodium bicarbonate) or enhance its removal from the body by hemodialysis and/or the oral administration of cation-exchange resins. In any case, the underlying cause of hyperkalemia should be identified and reversed, and exogenous potassium must be withheld.

■ GENERAL APPROACH TO TREATMENT

The general treatment approach for patients with hyperkalemia is outlined in Fig. 54–2. In patients who have acute ECG changes, calcium should be administered to prevent or treat any cardiac manifestations of hyperkalemia. Once the patient is hemodynamically stabilized, the serum potassium concentration should be rapidly decreased to <5.5 mEq/L within minutes by administering drugs that cause an intracellular shift. If the patient is asymptomatic, rapid correction is not necessary. The clinician can administer an ion exchange resin (e.g., sodium polystyrene sulfonate [SPS]) that results in removal of potassium from the body over several hours to days.

■ NONPHARMACOLOGIC THERAPY

Hemodialysis patients who present with severe hyperkalemia, or with cardiac manifestations of hyperkalemia, should undergo an additional hemodialysis treatment as soon as possible. Because even in emergent situations it takes a while to arrange for a dialysis treatment, bicarbonate, epinephrine, or insulin plus glucose therapy are often administered while the patient is waiting for or in transit to the dialysis unit. Other forms of dialysis can be performed (e.g., peritoneal dialysis or continuous renal replacement therapy), although they are less effective means to acutely lower an elevated serum potassium.[22]

■ PHARMACOLOGIC THERAPY

Various drug therapies have been used to lower the serum potassium concentration. The optimal regimen for a given patient is dependent on the rapidity and degree of lowering that is necessary. Table 54–5 provides an overview of the available therapies, and their respective onset and the degree of change one can expect.

In asymptomatic patients with mild to moderate hyperkalemia (serum concentration 5.5 to 6.9 mEq/L), aggressive therapy is usually not indicated. However, the clinician should have a low threshold for giving intravenous calcium in asymptomatic patients with known cardiac histories. In patients with normal renal function, or those with stage 3 or 4 CKD, loop diuretics can be administered in the short term to promote urinary potassium excretion. Furosemide 20 to 40 mg orally is a common starting dose, and this can be titrated to

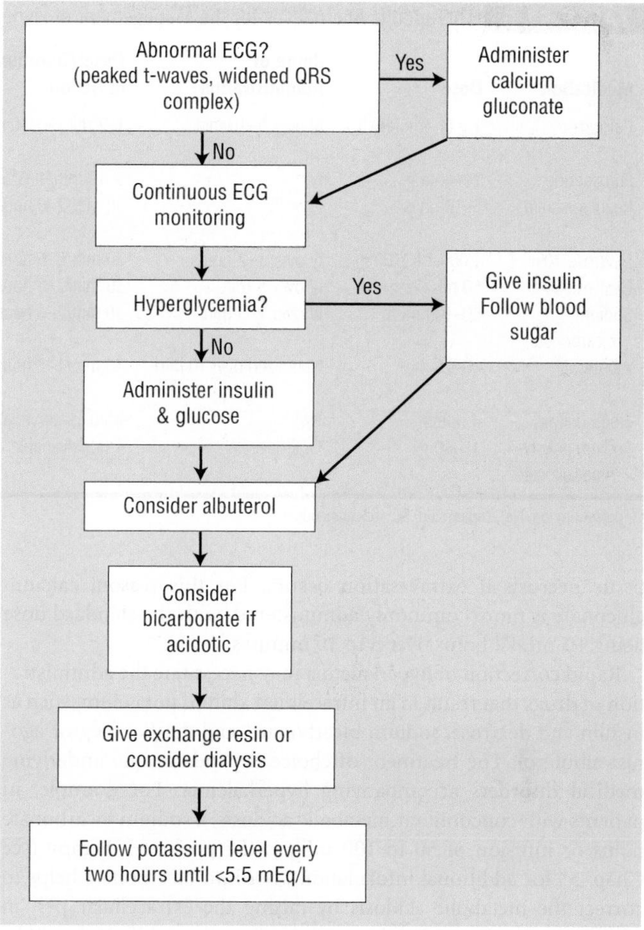

FIGURE 54-2. Treatment approach for hyperkalemia.

response. Its onset of activity is within minutes, and its duration of activity is approximately 4 to 6 hours. Close monitoring of the patient's volume status and other electrolyte concentrations is required while the patient is receiving loop diuretic therapy. Alternatively, SPS (Kayexalate), a cation-exchange resin, can be administered orally or rectally by enema. SPS is available in powder form or prepackaged as a 70% sorbitol suspension. The oral route is more effective than the enema and is better tolerated by the patient. As the resin passes through the intestines, each gram of SPS exchanges 1 mEq of sodium for 1 mEq of potassium ions, which are in a relatively higher concentration in the large intestine. The onset of action of SPS is within 1 hour, and it can be repeated every 4 hours as needed. The sorbitol component of the suspension promotes the excretion of the cationically modified potassium exchange resin by inducing diarrhea. The usual oral dose of SPS is 15 to 60 g in the 70% sorbitol suspension. A retention enema prepared by mixing 60 to 100 g SPS in 100 to 200 mL of a 30% sorbitol or 10% dextrose suspension warmed to body temperature will usually remove 0.5 mEq of potassium per gram of SPS.[23] The enema may be retained in the rectum for several hours as tolerated by the patient.

In symptomatic patients, or in those with severe hyperkalemia (serum potassium >7 mEq/L), emergency care is indicated. Initial therapy in this setting is the administration of intravenous calcium to protect the heart from life-threatening arrhythmias.[19,22] Calcium antagonizes the cardiac membrane effect of hyperkalemia and reverses ECG changes within minutes. Its duration of action is 30 to 60 minutes, and it can be repeated as needed based on ECG findings. Intravenous calcium can be given as either the chloride or gluconate salt; each is available as a 10% solution by weight. Calcium chloride provides approximately three times more calcium than equal volumes of the gluconate salt; however, it can cause

TABLE 54-5 Therapeutic Alternatives for the Management of Hyperkalemia

Medication	Dose	Route of Administration	Onset/Duration of Action	Acuity	Mechanism of Action	Expected Result
Calcium	1 g (1 ampule)	IV over 5–10 min	1–2 min/10–30 min	Acute	Raises cardiac threshold potential	Reverses electrocardiographic effects
Furosemide	20–40 mg	IV	5–15 min/4–6 hours	Acute	Inhibits renal Na^+ reabsorption	Increased urinary K^+ loss
Regular insulin	5–10 units	IV or SC	30 min/2–6 hours	Acute	Stimulates intracellular K^+ uptake	Intracellular K^+ redistribution
Dextrose 10%	1,000 mL (100 g)	IV over 1–2 hours	30 min/2–6 hours	Acute	Stimulates insulin release	Intracellular K^+ redistribution
Dextrose 50%	50 mL (25 g)	IV over 5 min	30 min/2–6 hours	Acute	Stimulates insulin release	Intracellular K^+ redistribution
Sodium bicarbonate	50–100 mEq	IV over 2–5 min	30 min/2–6 hours	Acute	Raises serum pH	Intracellular K^+ redistribution
Albuterol	10–20 mg	Nebulized over 10 min	30 min/1–2 hours	Acute	Stimulates intracellular K^+ uptake	Intracellular K^+ redistribution
Hemodialysis	4 hours	N/A	Immediate/variable	Acute	Removal from serum	Increased K^+ elimination
Sodium polystyrene sulfonate	15–60 g	Oral or rectal	1 hour/variable	Nonacute	Resin exchanges Na^+ for K^+	Increased K^+ elimination

K^+, potassium ion; Na^+, sodium ion; SC, subcutaneous.

tissue necrosis if extravasation occurs. For this reason, calcium gluconate is more commonly administered, with the standard dose being 10-mL IV bolus over 5 to 10 minutes.

Rapid correction of hyperkalemia may necessitate the administration of drugs that result in an intracellular shift of potassium, such as insulin and dextrose, sodium bicarbonate, and the β_2-receptor agonist albuterol. The treatment of choice depends on the underlying medical disorders accompanying hyperkalemia. For example, in patients with concomitant metabolic acidosis, a sodium bicarbonate bolus or infusion of 50 to 100 mEq is the preferred therapy (see Chap. 55 for additional information). Sodium bicarbonate helps to correct the metabolic acidosis by raising the extracellular pH, in addition to causing a rapid intracellular potassium shift. It should be noted that sodium bicarbonate is much less effective when hyperkalemia is not related to metabolic acidosis.[19] Sodium bicarbonate is also less effective in patients with end-stage renal disease (ESRD), in whom a decrease in serum potassium may not be seen for as long as 4 hours.[23] Sodium bicarbonate can also lead to sodium and volume overload in patients with stage 4 or 5 CKD. Administration of insulin (5 to 10 units IV) and dextrose (10% or 50%) is an effective method of reducing potassium. Insulin increases the activity of the Na^+-K^+-ATPase pump, thereby intracellularly shifting potassium. Glucose should be given with insulin unless the serum glucose is greater than 250 mg/dL because hypoglycemia can develop with unopposed insulin therapy. β_2-Adrenergic agonists, such as albuterol, have a dual mechanism for lowering serum potassium. First, they stimulate the Na^+-K^+-ATPase pump to promote intracellular potassium uptake. Second, they stimulate pancreatic β-receptors to increase insulin secretion. Albuterol can be administered intravenously (0.5 mg given over 15 minutes) or via nebulizer (10 to 20 mg nebulized over 10 minutes); however, it should be noted that injectable albuterol is not available in the United States. There are important limitations with albuterol therapy, most notably variable bioavailability via the inhaled route (leading to potential over- or underdosing and unpredictability of response) and second, cardiac side effects such as tachycardia can be undesirable in patients who already have abnormal ECGs.

A recent Cochrane review evaluated the emergency treatment of hyperkalemia.[24] Many of the reviewed studies were small, and not all intervention groups had sufficient data for meta-analysis to be performed. However, given these limitations, inhaled and nebulized β-agonists, and IV insulin-and-glucose were all deemed effective. The combination of nebulized β-agonists with IV insulin-and-glucose appeared to be more effective than either agent alone. The meta-analysis results were equivocal for IV bicarbonate, and notably, SPS was not effective by 4 hours.

A major problem with drawing conclusions from this meta-analysis is the heterogeneity of the study population. Most of the data were from nonrandomized, noncontrolled observational studies and case reports. Doses of the drugs were not standardized and followup was often lacking. Therefore, the clinician should exercise caution when extrapolating these findings to their clinical practice. For example, SPS has been used clinically with good results for many years. However, the Cochrane database found few data to support its use. This underscores the need for clinicians to be able to interpret the limitations of the published literature. Nonetheless, the Cochrane database review corroborates the approach detailed in Fig. 54–2.

EVALUATION OF THERAPEUTIC OUTCOMES

The evaluation of therapeutic outcomes differs based on the severity of hyperkalemia. For example, mild or moderate asymptomatic hyperkalemia is observed much more frequently compared to symptomatic, severe hyperkalemia. Many drugs such as ACEIs, ARBs, and spironolactone result in asymptomatic hyperkalemia. In patients with normal renal function, once these drugs are initiated and the dose titrated, clinicians should check the potassium concentration at least monthly. For those patients with renal dysfunction, monitoring can be more frequent, such as biweekly until the dose is stabilized. In the case where the patient has been on a stable dose for a long period of time and hyperkalemia develops, the clinician should attempt to downward titrate the dose or switch to another medication without hyperkalemia as a side effect (e.g., calcium channel blocker).

In patients who have acute symptomatic hyperkalemia (e.g., ECG changes), frequent potassium concentration and ECG monitoring is warranted. The patient should receive continuous ECG telemetry monitoring until the serum potassium concentration decreases below 5 mEq/L, and the ECG abnormalities resolve. Similarly, while the patient is receiving emergent therapy, serial serum potassium concentrations should be obtained every hour until the potassium concentration decreases below 5 mEq/L. For patients who receive insulin and dextrose therapy for hyperkalemia, blood glucose monitoring should be performed hourly, or more frequently if patients demonstrate signs and symptoms of hypoglycemia. For patients who receive large doses of sodium bicarbonate therapy for hyperkalemia, an arterial blood gas or serum chemistry profile should be obtained to assess their acid–base status. Furthermore, the patient should be evaluated for signs of fluid overload secondary to the high sodium load. Patients receiving albuterol therapy should be questioned regularly regarding the development of palpitations and tachycardia. In asymptomatic patients receiving SPS, serum potassium concentrations can be obtained within 4 hours, and the dose repeated as necessary. The patient's medication records should be reviewed to assure the patient is not receiving drug therapy that increases the serum potassium concentration. Furthermore, the patient should be questioned regarding the occurrence of diarrheal stool output.

DISORDERS OF MAGNESIUM HOMEOSTASIS

7 Magnesium plays a central role in cellular function and is an important cofactor in more than 300 biochemical reactions in the body, especially those systems that are dependent on adenosine triphosphate.[25] Mitochondrial function, protein synthesis, cell membrane function, and parathyroid hormone (PTH) secretion are just a few important functions affected by magnesium. It is the fourth most abundant extracellular cation and second most abundant intracellular cation. Disorders of magnesium homeostasis are commonly encountered in clinical situations and most frequently are manifested as alterations in cardiovascular and neuromuscular function. Life-threatening conditions such as paralysis and cardiac arrhythmias can occur, making the proper recognition and treatment of these problems of paramount importance.

8 Magnesium is principally distributed in bone (67%) and muscle (20%). Because of its predominantly intracellular distribution, measurement of magnesium in the extracellular compartment may not accurately reflect the total body magnesium content. The majority of magnesium in the extracellular fluid is in the ionized form as only 20% is bound to serum proteins. The normal range for serum magnesium is 1.4 to 1.8 mEq/L, which is equivalent to 1.7 to 2.3 mg/dL or 0.85 to 1.15 mmol/L.

The maintenance of magnesium homeostasis depends on the balance between intake and output. Thirty to forty percent of ingested magnesium is absorbed in the small bowel. A small amount is present in intestinal secretions and reabsorbed in the sigmoid colon. The kidneys play a major role in maintaining magnesium balance. Renal magnesium handling is unique in that approximately 20% of the filtered magnesium is reabsorbed in the proximal tubule; the majority of reabsorption occurs in the thick ascending limb of the loop of Henle.[1] This explains why loop diuretics often cause profound urinary magnesium wasting. Unlike most other important electrolytes, there is no hormonal regulation of the distribution of magnesium between bone and circulating or intracellular magnesium pools. Because of this, both hypomagnesemia and hypermagnesemia commonly occur.

HYPOMAGNESEMIA

Epidemiology

Hypomagnesemia is a common problem in both ambulatory and hospitalized patients. Although the exact prevalence is difficult to estimate, it has been reported that up to 65% of intensive care unit patients are magnesium deficient.[26] Although serum magnesium concentrations are not a reliable index of total body magnesium content, they remain the primary diagnostic tool to evaluate body stores.

Etiology and Pathophysiology

9 Hypomagnesemia is usually associated with disorders of the intestinal tract or kidney. Drugs or conditions that interfere with intestinal absorption or increase renal excretion of magnesium can result in hypomagnesemia (Table 54–6). Decreased intestinal absorption as a result of small bowel disease is the most common cause of hypomagnesemia worldwide. These disorders include regional enteritis; radiation enteritis; ulcerative colitis; acute and chronic diarrhea; pancreatic insufficiency and other malabsorptive syndromes; small-bowel bypass surgery; and chronic laxative abuse.[27] Hypomagnesemia is commonly associated with alcoholism. The etiology is often multifactorial, including reduced intake, pancreatic insufficiency, chronic vomiting and diarrhea, and urinary magnesium wasting. In addition, patients who are hospitalized for acute alcohol withdrawal often receive IV glucose and can experience even greater reductions in their serum magnesium concentration. Because hypomagnesemia can contribute to the development of delirium tremens associated with alcohol withdrawal, aggressive magnesium replacement is indicated for these patients, especially those with tachyarrhythmias, hypocalcemia, or hypokalemia.

Primary renal magnesium wasting can be caused by a defect in renal tubular magnesium reabsorption, or inhibition of sodium reabsorption in those segments in which magnesium transport follows passively. The former condition is associated with hypercalciuria, nephrolithiasis, and progressive renal disease. The latter is associated with Gitelman and Bartter syndromes.[28] Much more common than these is renal magnesium wasting secondary to thia-

TABLE 54-6 Causes of Hypomagnesemia

Gastrointestinal
Reduced intake
Protein-calorie malnutrition
Prolonged parenteral fluid administration without magnesium
Alcoholism
Reduced absorption
Primary hypomagnesemia
Malabsorption syndromes (e.g., tropical sprue, celiac disease, radiation enteritis, or intestinal lymphectasia)
Short-bowel syndrome (e.g., small-bowel resection or ileal bypass)
Pancreatic insufficiency
Increased loss
Excessive vomiting
Prolonged nasogastric suction
Excessive laxative use
Intestinal and biliary fistulas
Prolonged diarrhea (ulcerative colitis, Crohn's disease, or cancer of the colon)
Renal
Primary tubular disorders
Primary renal magnesium wasting
Bartter syndrome
Renal tubular acidosis
Diuretic phase of acute tubular necrosis
Postobstructive diuresis
Postrenal transplant diuresis
Glomerulonephritis
Pyelonephritis
Drug-induced renal losses
Aminoglycosides
Amphotericin B
Cyclosporine
Diuretics
Digitalis
Cisplatin
Hormone-induced renal losses
Primary hyperparathyroidism
Hyperthyroidism
Aldosteronism
"Hungry bone syndrome" after parathyroidectomy
Internal redistribution
Diabetic ketoacidosis
Glucose, amino acid, or insulin administration
Massive blood transfusion (citrate)
Pancreatitis with lipidemia (magnesium soap)
Other
Excessive sweating and lactation
Hypercalcemia and hypercalciuria
Phosphate depletion
Chronic alcoholism
Extracellular fluid volume expansion

zide and loop diuretics.[27] Other commonly used drugs that can cause renal magnesium wasting include aminoglycosides, amphotericin B, cyclosporine, tacrolimus, cisplatin, pentamidine, and foscarnet.[26]

Clinical Presentation

Hypomagnesemia is typically an asymptomatic condition.[27] However, because hypomagnesemia is often associated with a variety of other electrolyte abnormalities such as hypokalemia and hypocalcemia, it is difficult to ascribe specific clinical manifestations solely to magnesium deficiency. Hypocalcemia is one of the most prominent symptoms of hypomagnesemia. The etiology of hypocalcemia is not entirely clear, but it is probably caused by decreased secretion of PTH, low 1,25-$(OH)_2$ vitamin D concentrations, and skeletal resistance to PTH.[28] As with hypokalemia, hypocalcemia accompanied by hypomagnesemia is most effectively treated with magnesium administration.

CLINICAL PRESENTATION OF HYPOMAGNESEMIA

General

- The dominant organ systems affected by hypomagnesemia are the neuromuscular and cardiovascular systems.

Symptoms

- Neuromuscular symptoms such as tetany, twitching, and generalized convulsions are common.
- Cardiac symptoms include heart palpitations.

Signs

- Neuromuscular: Presence of Chvostek sign, Trousseau sign, tremor, and tetany.
- Cardiovascular: Cardiac arrhythmias (ventricular fibrillation, torsade de pointes, or digoxin-induced arrhythmias), sudden cardiac death, and hypertension can be present. ECG abnormalities include widened QRS complex and peaked T waves with mild hypomagnesemia; and prolonged PR interval, progressive widening of QRS complex, and flattened T waves with moderate to severe hypomagnesemia.

Laboratory Tests

- Serum magnesium concentration less than 1.4 mEq/L. Serum potassium and calcium concentrations can also be low.

TREATMENT

Hypomagnesemia

■ DESIRED OUTCOME

The treatment goals in the management of hypomagnesemia are (1) resolution of the corresponding signs and symptoms, (2) restoration of normal magnesium concentrations, (3) correction of concomitant electrolyte abnormalities, and (4) identification and correction of the underlying cause of magnesium depletion.

■ GENERAL APPROACH TO TREATMENT

Nearly all of the data regarding magnesium replacement therapy have been derived from reports in acutely ill, hospitalized patients. Magnesium supplementation can be given by the oral, IM, or IV route. Table 54–7 outlines one approach to the hypomagnesemic patient. The severity of the magnesium depletion and the presence of severe signs and symptoms should dictate the route of administration. Because IM administration is painful, it should be reserved for those patients with severe hypomagnesemia and limited venous access. IV bolus

TABLE 54-7 Guidelines for Treatment of Magnesium Deficiency in Adults

1. Serum magnesium <1 mEq/L (1.2 mg/dL) with life-threatening symptoms (seizure or arrhythmia)
Day 1
2 g magnesium sulfate (1 g magnesium sulfate = 8.1 mEq Mg^{2+}) mixed with 6 mL 0.9% NaCl in 10-mL syringe and administer IV push over 1 minute
Follow with 1.0 mEq Mg^{2+}/kg lean body weight IV infusion over 24 hours
Days 2–5
0.5 mEq Mg^{2+}/kg lean body weight per day divided in maintenance IV fluids
2. Serum magnesium <1 mEq/L (1.2 mg/dL) without life-threatening symptoms
Day 1
Total of 1 mEq Mg^{2+}/kg lean body weight per day as continuous IV infusion, or divided and given IM every 4 hours for five doses
Days 2–5
0.5 mEq Mg^{2+}/kg lean body weight IV infusion per day as continuous IV infusion or divided and given IM every 6–8 hours
3. Serum magnesium >1 mEq/L (1.2 mg/dL) and <1.5 mEq/L (1.8 mg/dL) without symptoms
As in no. 2, above, or
Milk of magnesia 5 mL four times daily as tolerated, or
Magnesium-containing antacid 15 mL three times daily as tolerated, or
Magnesium oxide tablets 400 mg four times daily; increase to two tablets four times daily as tolerated

Mg^{2+}, magnesium ion; NaCl, sodium chloride.

administration is associated with flushing, sweating, and a sensation of warmth; thus bolus administration should be avoided if possible. There have been no clinical trials assessing the optimal regimen for magnesium replacement, however, most clinicians agree that 8 to 12 g of magnesium sulfate in the first 24 hours followed by 4 to 6 g per day for 3 to 5 days is adequate to replete body stores.[27] Even if severe magnesium depletion is present, approximately 50% of the administered dose is excreted in the urine. Consequently, magnesium replacement should be performed over 3 to 5 days, and continued supplementation should be provided for patients unable to eat and for those patients with continued magnesium wasting.

■ PHARMACOLOGIC THERAPY

Asymptomatic patients, or those patients with serum magnesium concentrations greater than 1 mEq/L (1.2 mg/dL), can be treated with oral supplements, such as magnesium-containing antacids or laxatives, or magnesium oxide tablets or capsules. The typical dose of magnesium oxide is 400 to 800 mg given three or four times daily until repleted. However, as expected, diarrhea is the most common dose-limiting side effect of oral therapy, which can greatly reduce patient compliance. Moreover many oral products contain very little magnesium, which necessitates frequent dosing.

In cases of severe magnesium depletion (serum concentrations <1 mEq/L), or if signs and symptoms are present regardless of the serum concentration, IV magnesium should be administered. A 50% solution of magnesium sulfate is available for injection in 2-mL or 10-mL ampules (4 mEq/mL). The 50% solution should be diluted to 20% before injection to prevent venous sclerosis and pain. Therapy should be continued until the signs and symptoms have completely resolved. In patients with renal insufficiency, the dose should be reduced by 50%.

■ EVALUATION OF THERAPEUTIC ENDPOINTS

In patients with acute, asymptomatic mild to moderate hypomagnesemia receiving therapy, serum magnesium concentrations should be obtained at least daily during their hospitalization. Patients receiving oral magnesium therapy should be questioned regarding GI

TABLE 54-8 Causes of Hypermagnesemia

Decreased renal excretion	
Acute renal failure	
Chronic kidney disease with exogenous intake	
Excessive intake	
Treatment of toxemia of pregnancy	
Ureteral irrigants (hemiacidrin)	
Cathartics	
Other	
Lithium therapy	
Hypothyroidism	
Milk-alkali syndrome	
Addison's disease	
Viral hepatitis	
Acute diabetic ketoacidosis	

tolerance and the occurrence of diarrhea. Patients being treated for symptomatic severe hypomagnesemia should have their serum magnesium concentration monitored hourly until the serum concentration reaches 1.5 mEq/L and the symptoms resolve. At that point the serum magnesium concentration can be monitored every 6 to 12 hours for the next 24 hours while receiving magnesium supplementation. Once the magnesium concentration is stable in the normal range, a concentration can be obtained daily. It should be reiterated that it typically takes 3 to 5 days to fully replete total body magnesium stores.

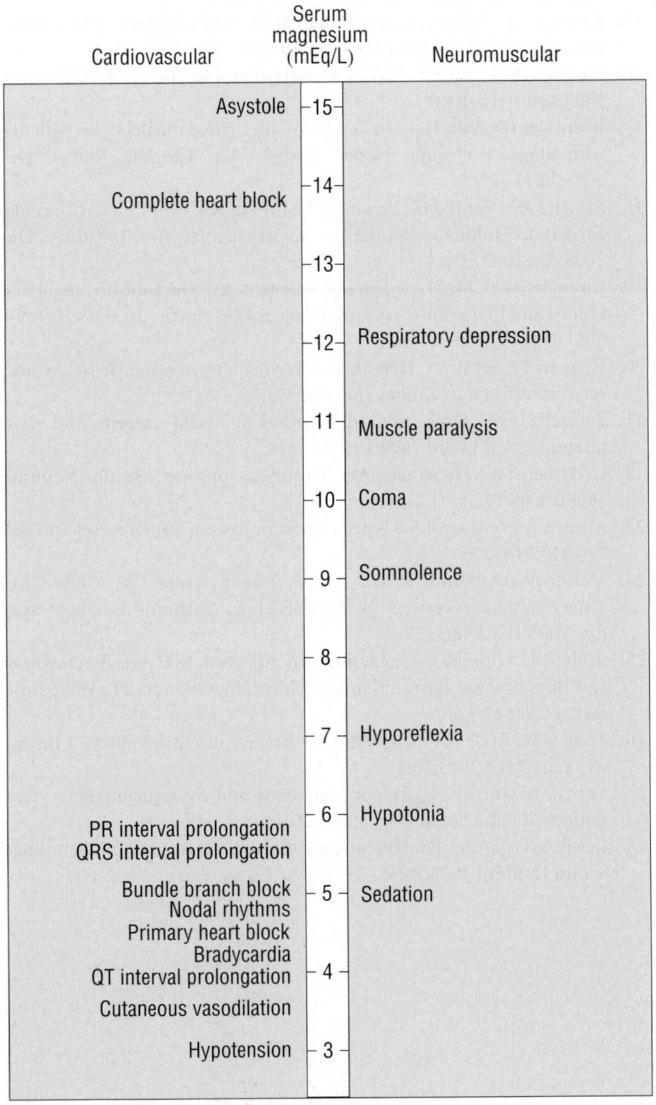

FIGURE 54-3. Clinical findings associated with hypermagnesemia.

Patients receiving oral magnesium-containing antacids or supplements should be asked regularly about the occurrence of diarrhea.

HYPERMAGNESEMIA

Epidemiology

⑩ Hypermagnesemia (serum magnesium >2 mEq/L) is a rare occurrence that is generally seen in patients with stage 4 or 5 CKD when magnesium intake exceeds the excretory capacity of the kidneys. Elderly patients are prone to hypermagnesemia because of their reduced glomerular filtration rate (GFR) and because of their tendency to consume magnesium-containing antacids and vitamins.

Etiology and Pathophysiology

Because absolute magnesium excretion decreases as GFR declines, serum magnesium concentrations tend to increase in patients with moderate to severe CKD. Indeed, magnesium concentrations steadily increase as the GFR decreases below 30 mL/min/1.73m^2. As long as the patient maintains a normal diet, the serum magnesium concentration typically stabilizes at approximately 2.5 mEq/L. If patients with stage 4 or 5 CKD are taking concomitant magnesium-containing antacids, the serum concentration can approach 6 mEq/L, a value associated with signs and symptoms of toxicity. Critically ill patients with multiorgan system failure receiving enteral or parenteral nutrition are also prone to develop hypermagnesemia. Finally, the parenteral treatment of eclampsia with magnesium sulfate can lead to hypermagnesemia. Table 54–8 lists other causes of hypermagnesemia.

Clinical Presentation

The signs and symptoms of hypermagnesemia reflect magnesium's action on the neuromuscular and cardiovascular systems.[27] Symptoms are rare when the serum concentration is less than 4 mEq/L (Fig. 54–3).

TREATMENT

Hypermagnesemia

■ DESIRED OUTCOME

The goals of therapy are to (1) reverse the neuromuscular and cardiovascular manifestations of hypermagnesemia, (2) decrease the magnesium concentration toward normal values, and (3) identify and treat the underlying cause of hypermagnesemia.

■ PHARMACOLOGIC THERAPY

There are three primary means of treating hypermagnesemia: (1) reduce magnesium intake, (2) enhance elimination of magnesium, and (3) antagonize the physiologic effects of magnesemia. The optimal treatment regimen for the management of hypermagnesemia depends on the presence of signs and symptoms and the degree of serum concentration elevation. Intravenous calcium in doses of 100 to 200 mg of elemental calcium directly antagonizes the neuromuscular and cardiovascular effects of hypermagnesemia. Oral calcium is not used because of its relatively poor bioavailability and lack of immediate onset. The clinical effect of calcium is immediate, but the effect is transient; hence repeated intravenous doses of 100 to 200 mg of elemental calcium might need to be administered hourly until the symptoms abate and the magnesium concentration is normalized. Supportive care with cardiac pacing, vasopressors, and mechanical ventilation can be necessary in life-threatening situations. In patients with normal renal function, or those with stage 1, 2, or 3 CKD, forced diuresis with saline and loop diuretics can promote magnesium elimination. An initial loop diuretic intravenous bolus of furosemide 40 mg or a similar equivalent can be used. Subsequent dosing can be determined based on the patient's clinical response. Patients with CKD can require long-term loop diuretic therapy to maintain adequate fluid and electrolyte balance. In dialysis patients, their hemodialysis prescription should be changed to employ magnesium-free dialysate.

■ EVALUATION OF THERAPEUTIC ENDPOINTS

Patients who are receiving intravenous calcium salts for the treatment of severe, symptomatic hypermagnesemia should have their serum magnesium concentration evaluated hourly until symptoms abate and the magnesium concentration decreases below 4 mg/dL. Furthermore the patient should be continuously monitored to detect ECG changes. In CKD patients who can produce urine, forced diuresis with saline and furosemide should reduce the serum magnesium concentration within 6 to 12 hours. Close monitoring of the urine output and physical examination for signs of volume overload are important. Emergency hemodialysis will usually correct the hypermagnesemia within 4 hours and is a reasonable option for those who are currently receiving hemodialysis. To prevent further episodes of hypermagnesemia, the patient should receive dietary education regarding foods and beverages that contain large quantities of magnesium.

In conclusion, disorders of potassium and magnesium are frequently encountered in both the acute care and community ambulatory care settings. If severe, these disorders can have catastrophic results. Clinicians should be able to identify patients at risk for these common electrolyte disorders and quickly design appropriate pharmacotherapy and monitoring regimens to optimize patient outcomes.

ABBREVIATIONS

ACEI: angiotensin-converting enzyme inhibitor

ARB: angiotensin-II receptor blocker

ARF: acute renal failure

CKD: chronic kidney disease

ECG: electrocardiogram

ESRD: end-stage renal disease

GI: gastrointestinal

NSAID: nonsteroidal antiinflammatory drug

PTH: parathyroid hormone

SPS: sodium polystyrene sulfonate

REFERENCES

1. Peterson LN, Levi M. Disorders of potassium metabolism. In: Schrier RW, ed. Renal and Electrolyte Disorders, 6th ed. Philadelphia: Lippincott Williams & Wilkins, 2003:171–215.
2. Schaefer TJ, Wolford RW. Disorders of potassium. Emerg Med Clin North Am 2005;23:723–747.
3. Sharma K, Cox M. Potassium homeostasis. In: Szerlip HM, Goldfarb S, eds. Workshops in Fluid and Electrolyte Disorders. New York: Churchill Livingstone, 1993:71–96.
4. Agarwal R, Afzalpurkar R, Fordtran JS. Pathophysiology of potassium absorption and secretion by the human intestine. Gastroenterology 1994;107:548–571.
5. Rose BD, Rennke HG. Renal Pathophysiology—The Essentials. Baltimore: Williams & Wilkins, 1994:169–190.
6. Wingo CS, Weiner ID. Disorders of potassium balance. In: Brenner BM, ed. The Kidney, 6th ed. Philadelphia: WB Saunders, 2000:998–1036.
7. Gennari FJ. Hypokalemia. N Engl J Med 1998;339:451–458.
8. Weiner ID, Wingo CS. Hypokalemia—Consequences, causes, and correction. J Am Soc Nephrol 1997;8:1179–1188.
9. Gennari FJ. Disorders of potassium homeostasis: Hypokalemia and hyperkalemia. Crit Care Clin 2002;18:273–288.
10. Ryan MP. Interrelationships of magnesium and potassium homeostasis. Miner Electrolyte Metab 1993;19:290–295.
11. Sica DA, Struthers AD, Cushman WC, et al. Importance of potassium in cardiovascular disease. J Clin Hypertens 2002;4:198–206.
12. Cohn JN, Kowey PR, Whelton PK, Prisant LM. New guidelines for potassium replacement in clinical practice: A contemporary review by the National Council on Potassium in Clinical Practice. Arch Intern Med 2000;160:2429–2436.
13. Agarwal A, Wingo CS. Treatment of hypokalemia. N Engl J Med 1999;340:154–155. Letter.
14. Weiner ID, Wingo CS. Hyperkalemia: A potential silent killer. J Am Soc Nephrol 1998;9:1535–1543.
15. Rastegar A, Soleimani M, Rastergar A. Hypokalemia and hyperkaliemia. Postgrad Med J 2001;77:759–764.
16. Luckey AE, Parsa CJ. Fluid and electrolytes in the aged. Arch Surg 2003;138:1055–1060.
17. Burrowes JD, Van Houten G. Use of alternative medicine by patients with stage 5 chronic kidney disease. Adv Chronic Kidney Dis 2005;12:312–325.
18. Mueller BA, Scott MK, Sowinski KM, Prag KA. Noni juice (*Morinda citrifolia*): Hidden potential for hyperkalemia? Am J Kidney Dis 2000;35:310–312.
19. Chmielewski CM. Hyperkalemic emergencies: Mechanisms, manifestations and management. Crit Care Nurs Clin North Am 1998;10:449–458.
20. Gennari FJ, Segal AS. Hyperkalemia: An adaptive response in chronic renal insufficiency. Kidney Int 2002;62:1–9.
21. Perazella MA. Drug-induced hyperkalemia: Old culprits and new offenders. Am J Med 2000;109:307–314.
22. Greenberg A. Hyperkalemia: Treatment options. Semin Nephrol 1998;18:46–57.
23. Ahmed J, Weisberg LS. Hyperkalemia in dialysis patients. Semin Dial 2001;15:348–356.
24. Mahoney BA, Smith WAD, Lo DS, Tsoi K, Tonelli M, Clase CM. Emergency interventions for hyperkalemia. Cochrane Database Syst Rev 2005;18:CD003235.
25. Rude RK. Minerals—Magnesium. In: Stipanuk MH, ed. Biochemical and Physiological Basis of Human Nutrition. Orlando, FL: WB Saunders, 2000:671–685.
26. Tong GM, Rude RK. Magnesium deficiency in critical illness. J Intensive Care Med 2005;20:3–17.
27. Topf JM, Murray PT. Hypomagnesemia and hypermagnesemia. Rev Endocr Metab Disord 2003;4:195–206.
28. Kelepouris E, Agus ZS. Hypomagnesemia: Renal magnesium handling. Semin Nephrol 1998;18:58–73.

CHAPTER 55

Acid–Base Disorders

JOHN W. DEVLIN, GARY R. MATZKE, AND PAUL M. PALEVSKY

KEY CONCEPTS

1. The kidney plays a central role in the regulation of acid–base homeostasis through the excretion or reabsorption of filtered bicarbonate (HCO_3^-), the excretion of metabolic fixed acids and generation of new HCO_3^-.
2. Arterial blood gases, along with serum electrolytes, physical findings, medical and medication history, and the clinical condition of the patient, are the primary tools to determine the cause of an acid–base disorder and to design and monitor a course of therapy.
3. Metabolic acidosis and metabolic alkalosis are generated by a primary change in the serum bicarbonate concentration. In metabolic acidosis, bicarbonate is lost or a nonvolatile acid is gained, whereas metabolic alkalosis is characterized by a gain in bicarbonate or a loss of nonvolatile acid.
4. Renal tubular acidosis refers to a group of disorders characterized by impaired tubular renal acid handling despite normal or near-normal glomerular filtration rates. These patients often present with hyperchloremic metabolic acidosis.
5. Respiratory compensation for a primary metabolic acidosis begins rapidly (within 15 to 30 minutes) but does not reach a steady state for 12 to 24 hours after the onset of metabolic acidosis.
6. Primary therapy of most acid–base disorders must include treatment or elimination of the underlying cause, not just correction of the pH and electrolyte disturbances.
7. Potassium supplementation is always necessary for patients with chronic metabolic acidosis, as the bicarbonaturia resulting from alkali therapy increases the renal potassium wasting.
8. Effective treatment of the underlying cause of some organic acidoses (e.g., ketoacidosis) can result in the regeneration of bicarbonate within hours, thus mitigating the need for alkali therapy.
9. Loss of gastric acid from vomiting or nasogastric suctioning is often responsible for the development of a metabolic alkalosis, characterized by hypochloremia and hyperbicarbonatemia.
10. Aggressive diuretic therapy can produce a metabolic alkalosis, and the accompanying hypokalemia can be serious.
11. The patient's response to volume replacement can be predicted by the urine chloride concentration and permits the differential diagnosis of metabolic alkalosis.
12. Management of these disorders usually consists of treatment of the underlying cause of mineralocorticoid excess. In patients in whom the mineralocorticoid excess cannot be corrected, chronic pharmacologic therapy can be required.
13. In most cases of acute metabolic acidosis, such as following cardiopulmonary arrest, sodium bicarbonate therapy is not indicated and can be detrimental. Blood gas analysis should guide therapy.

Learning objectives, review questions, and other resources can be found at **www.pharmacotherapyonline.com.**

Acid–base disorders are common, and often serious, disturbances that can result in significant morbidity and mortality. This chapter reviews the mechanisms responsible for the maintenance of acid–base balance and the laboratory analyses that aid clinicians in their assessment of acid–base disorders. The pathophysiology of the four primary acid–base disturbances is presented, the therapeutic options are critiqued, and guidelines for the achievement of the desired therapeutic outcomes are presented. Because many drugs affect acid–base homeostasis and many acid–base abnormalities are potentially preventable, clinicians must anticipate drug-related problems to avoid or minimize the clinical consequences, and when necessary, design appropriate treatment regimens.

ACID–BASE CHEMISTRY

An acid (in this equation, hydrochloric acid [HCl]) is a substance that can *donate* protons (hydrogen ion [H^+]):

$$\text{(acid) HCl} \rightarrow H^+ + \text{chloride ion } (Cl^-)$$

A base (in this equation, ammonia [NH_3]) is a substance that can *accept* protons (hydrogen ion [H^+]):

$$\text{Ammonia } (NH_3) + H^+ \rightarrow NH^+_4 \text{ (base)}$$

The acid–base pairs commonly encountered in clinical practice are listed in Table 55–1.

The acidity of body fluids is quantified in terms of the hydrogen ion concentration. By convention, the degree of acidity is expressed as pH, or the negative logarithm (base 10) of the hydrogen ion concentration. Thus hydrogen ion concentration and pH are inversely related. Normally, the pH of blood is maintained at 7.40 ([H^+] of 4×10^{-8} M) with a range of 7.35 to 7.45. A pH of less than 6.7 ([H^+] of 2×10^{-7} M), representing a fivefold increase in hydrogen ion concentration, or greater than 7.7 ([H^+] of 2×10^{-8} M), representing a 50% decrease in hydrogen ion concentration, are considered incompatible with life.

TABLE 55-1 Acid–Base Pairs

Carbonic acid/bicarbonate	H_2CO_3/HCO_3^-
Monobasic/dibasic phosphate	H_2PO_4/HPO_4^-
Ammonium/ammonia	NH_4^+/NH_3
Lactic acid/lactate	$H_6C_3O_2/H_5C_3O_2^-$

The hydrogen ion concentration in blood may not be indicative of that in other body compartments. For example, the pH within cells, within the cerebrospinal fluid, or on the surface of bone can all be altered without causing an alteration in blood pH.[1] Recognizing this caveat, the acid–base status of the body is usually analyzed based on measurement of blood pH. Alterations in blood pH serve as the basis for the diagnosis of acid–base disorders.

Because the dissociation of acid–base pairs is an equilibrium reaction, the relationship between hydrogen ion concentration or pH and the relative concentrations of the acid and base can be described mathematically in terms of the dissociation constant for the acid–base buffer pair. When expressed as a logarithmic relationship, where p*K* is the negative logarithm of the dissociation constant *K*, this is known as the Henderson-Hasselbalch equation:

$$pH = pK + \log([base]/[acid])$$

BUFFERS

The ability of a weak acid and its corresponding anion (base) to resist change in the pH of a solution on the addition of a strong acid or base is referred to as *buffering*. An acid–base pair is most efficient in functioning as a buffer at a pH close to its p*K*. The principal extracellular buffer is the carbonic acid/bicarbonate (H_2CO_3/HCO_3^-) system. Other physiologic buffers include plasma proteins, hemoglobin, and phosphates. Because the isohydric principle requires that all buffer systems remain in chemical equilibrium, the complex buffering of biologic fluids can be analyzed based on a single buffer pair.

The carbonic acid/bicarbonate buffer system plays a unique role in acid–base homeostasis. In addition to being the most abundant extracellular buffer, the components of this buffer pair are under dynamic regulation by the body. In the presence of carbonic anhydrase, carbonic acid, $[H_2CO_3]$ is in equilibrium with carbon dioxide (CO_2) gas. Changes in ventilation that alter the partial pressure of CO_2 (P_{CO_2}) in the blood regulates the carbonic acid level in the blood. The bicarbonate concentration is independently regulated by the kidney. Because the p*K* for the carbonic acid/bicarbonate system is 6.1, the relationship between pH, carbonic acid, and bicarbonate concentrations can be described by the Henderson-Hasselbalch equation. The concentration of carbonic acid is directly proportional to the amount of CO_2 dissolved in blood, which is equal to the product of P_{CO_2} and its solubility in physiologic fluids, ($P_{CO_2} \times 0.03$). This term can therefore be substituted into the equation below in place of $[H_2CO_3]$.

$$pH = 6.1 + ([HCO_3^-]/[H_2CO_3])$$

$$pH = 6.1 + \log([HCO_3^-]/(P_{CO_2} \times 0.03))$$

Thus, hydrogen ion concentration and pH are determined not by the absolute amounts of bicarbonate and P_{CO_2}, but by their ratio.[1] Under normal physiologic conditions, the kidneys maintain the serum bicarbonate at approximately 24 mEq/L (24 mmol/L), whereas the lungs maintain the P_{CO_2} at approximately 40 mm Hg. The normal physiologic pH is thus 7.4:

$$pH = 6.1 + \log[24/(0.03 \times 40)]$$

$$pH = 6.1 + 1.3 = 7.4$$

If, in response to an acid load, the serum bicarbonate concentration were to decrease to 12 mEq/L [12 mmol/L], the predicted pH would be:

$$[HCO_3^-] = 12 \text{ mEq/L } (12 \text{ mmol/L})$$

$$P_{CO_2} = 40 \text{ mm Hg}$$

$$pH = 6.1 + \log[12/(0.03 \times 40)]$$

$$pH = 6.1 + 1.0 = 7.1$$

However, the normal respiratory response to an acid load is hyperventilation. As a result, if the P_{CO_2} decreased to approximately 26 mm Hg, the change in pH would be less:

$$[HCO_3^-] = 12 \text{ mEq/L } (12 \text{ mmol/L})$$

$$P_{CO_2} = 26 \text{ mm Hg}$$

$$pH = 6.1 + \log[12/(0.03 \times 26)]$$

$$pH = 6.1 + 1.19 = 7.29$$

Thus, the physiologic regulation of both P_{CO_2} and $[HCO_3^-]$ permit the carbonic acid/bicarbonate system to provide more effective buffering of the extracellular fluids than could be achieved on the basis of chemical buffering alone.

REGULATION OF ACID–BASE HOMEOSTASIS

Cellular metabolism results in the production of large quantities of hydrogen that need to be excreted to maintain acid–base balance. In addition, small amounts of acid and alkali are also presented to the body through the diet. The bulk of acid production is in the form of CO_2, with the average adult producing approximately 15,000 mmol of CO_2 each day from the catabolism of carbohydrate, protein, and fat.[2] When respiratory function is normal, the amount of CO_2 produced metabolically is equal to the amount lost by respiration, and the blood CO_2 concentration remains constant.

Digestion of dietary substances and tissue metabolism also results in the production of nonvolatile acids. These acids are derived primarily from the sulfur-containing amino acids cysteine and methionine, as well as from ingested sulfur. In addition, phosphates are generated from the metabolism of proteins and phospholipids. Neutral substances such as glucose can also be incompletely metabolized to intermediates, such as lactic and pyruvic acid, and fatty acids can be incompletely metabolized to acetoacetic acid and β-hydroxybutyric acid. These dietary and metabolic fixed acids are excreted, primarily by the kidney, to maintain acid–base homeostasis. On average, daily fixed acid excretion is approximately 0.8 mEq/kg per day.[3]

Three mechanisms, each of which vary in their onset, collectively maintain acid–base balance: extracellular buffering, ventilatory regulation of carbon dioxide elimination, and renal regulation of hydrogen ion and bicarbonate excretion. Extracellular buffering occurs rapidly and is the body's first defense against a sudden increase in hydrogen ion concentration. Hyperventilation will then result in a decrease in P_{CO_2}, returning blood pH toward normal. Finally, the kidney will excrete the excess hydrogen ion, with the resultant return of acid–base balance to normal over a period of day(s).

EXTRACELLULAR BUFFERING

The body's buffering system can be divided into three components: bicarbonate/carbonic acid, proteins, and phosphates. The bicarbonate buffer is the most important of the body's buffers, because (1) there is more bicarbonate present in the extracellular fluid (ECF) than any other buffer component; (2) the supply of carbon dioxide is unlimited; and (3) the acidity of ECF can be regulated by controlling either the bicarbonate concentration or the P_{CO_2}.

Carbonic acid represents the respiratory component of the buffer pair because its concentration is directly proportional to the P_{CO_2}, which is determined by ventilation. Bicarbonate represents the metabolic component because the kidney may alter its concentration by reabsorption, generating new bicarbonate, or altering elimination.[4] The bicarbonate buffer system easily adapts to changes in acid–base status by alterations in ventilatory elimination of acid (P_{CO_2}) and/or renal elimination of base (HCO_3^-).

The phosphate buffer system consists of serum inorganic phosphate (3.5 to 5 mg/dL[1.2 to 1.6 mmol/L]), intracellular organic phosphate, and calcium phosphate in bone. Extracellular phosphate is present only in low concentrations, so its usefulness as a buffer is limited; however, as an intracellular buffer, phsosphate is more useful. Calcium phosphate in bone is relatively inaccessible as a buffer, but prolonged metabolic acidosis will result in the release of phosphate from bone.

Intracellular and extracellular proteins also act as buffering systems. The charged side chains of amino acids provide the buffering action. Because the concentration of protein is much greater intracellularly than extracellularly, protein is much more important as an intracellular buffer.

RESPIRATORY REGULATION

The second mechanism for maintenance of acid–base homeostasis is control of ventilation. Both the rate and depth of ventilation can be varied to allow for excretion of CO_2 generated by diet and tissue metabolism. Medullary chemoreceptors in the brainstem sense changes in P_{CO_2} and in pH and modulate the control of breathing. Increasing minute ventilation (the total amount of air exhaled over a 1-minute period), by increasing respiratory rate and/or tidal volume (the amount of air exhaled in one breath), will increase CO_2 excretion and decrease the blood P_{CO_2}. Conversely, decreasing minute ventilation decreases CO_2 excretion and increases blood P_{CO_2}. This system rapidly adjusts, within minutes, to changes in acid–base balance.[2]

RENAL REGULATION

❶ Because bicarbonate is a small ion, it is freely filtered at the glomerulus. The bicarbonate load delivered to the nephron is approximately 4,500 mEq/day. To maintain acid–base balance, this entire filtered load must be reabsorbed. Bicarbonate reabsorption occurs primarily in the proximal tubule (Fig. 55–1). In the tubular lumen, filtered bicarbonate combines with hydrogen ion secreted by the apical sodium ion (Na^+)-H^+–exchanger to form carbonic acid. The carbonic acid is rapidly broken down to CO_2 and water by carbonic anhydrase located on the luminal surface of the brush border membrane. The CO_2 then diffuses into the proximal tubular cell, where it reforms carbonic acid in the presence of intracellular carbonic anhydrase. The carbonic acid dissociates to form hydrogen ion, that can again be secreted into the tubular lumen, and bicarbonate that exits the cell across the basolateral membrane and enters the peritubular capillary.

Excretion of metabolic fixed acids and generation of new HCO_3^- is achieved through renal ammoniagenesis and distal tubular hydrogen ion secretion. Ammoniagenesis plays a critical role in acid–base homeostasis, with ammonium (NH^+_4) excretion comprising approximately 50% of renal net acid excretion. Ammonium is generated from the deamination of glutamine in the proximal tubule. For each ammonium ion excreted in the urine, one bicarbonate ion is regenerated and returned to the circulation.[5]

Distal tubular hydrogen ion secretion accounts for the remaining 50% of net acid excretion (Fig. 55–2). In the distal tubular cell, CO_2 combines with water in the presence of intracellular carbonic anhydrase to form carbonic acid, which dissociates to H^+ and HCO_3^-. The H^+ is actively transported into the tubular lumen by a H^+- adenosine triphosphatase (ATPase). The bicarbonate exits the cell across the basolateral membrane and enters the circulation.[5]

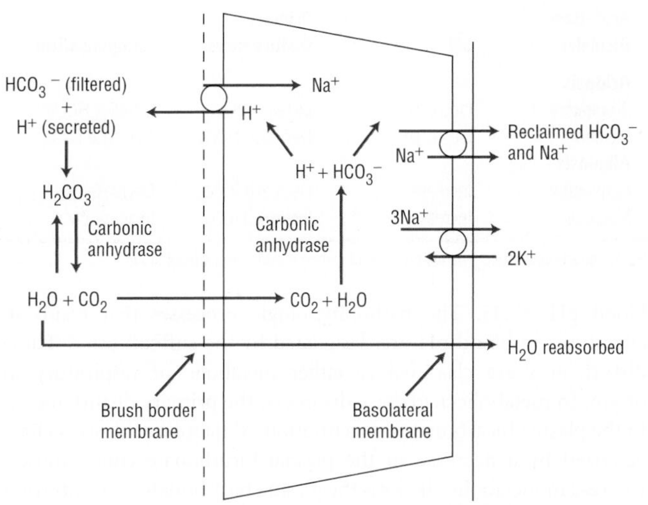

FIGURE 55-1. Proximal tubular bicarbonate reabsorption. In the tubular lumen, filtered bicarbonate (HCO_3^-) combines with hydrogen ion (H^+) secreted by an apical sodium ion (Na^+)-H^+ exchanger to form carbonic acid (H_2CO_3). The carbonic acid is rapidly broken down to carbon dioxide (CO_2) and water by carbonic anhydrase located on the luminal surface of the brush border membrane. The CO_2 then diffuses into the proximal tubular cell, where it reforms carbonic acid in the presence of intracellular carbonic anhydrase. The carbonic acid dissociates to form hydrogen ion, that can again be secreted into the tubular lumen, and bicarbonate that exits the cell across the basolateral membrane and enters the peritubular capillary.

ACID–BASE DISTURBANCES

Alterations in blood pH are designated by the suffix "-emia"; *acidemia* is an arterial blood pH <7.35 and *alkalemia* is an arterial

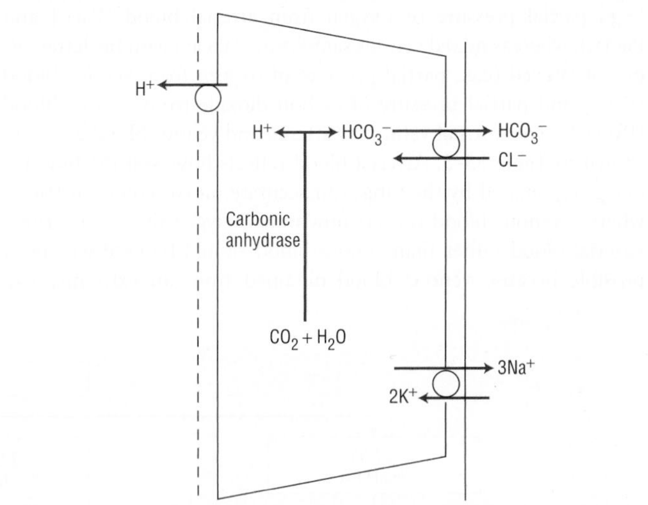

FIGURE 55-2. Collecting duct acid excretion. Hydrogen ion (H^+) and bicarbonate (HCO_3^-) are generated intracellularly from carbon dioxide (CO_2) and water, in the presence of intracellular carbonic anhydrase. The hydrogen ion is actively secreted into the tubular lumen by H^+-adenosine triphosphatase (ATPase) located in the apical (luminal) membrane. Bicarbonate exits the cell across the basolateral membrane and enters the peritubular capillary. (CL^-, chloride ion; Na^+, sodium ion.)

TABLE 55-2 Interpretation of Simple Acid–Base Disorders

Acid–Base Disorder	pH	Primary Disturbances	Compensation
Acidosis			
Respiratory	Decrease	Increase $Paco_2$	Increase HCO_3^-
Metabolic	Decrease	Decrease HCO_3^-	Decrease $Paco_2$
Alkalosis			
Respiratory	Increase	Decrease $Paco_2$	Decrease HCO_3^-
Metabolic	Increase	Increase HCO_3^-	Increase $Paco_2$

HCO_3^-, bicarbonate; $Paco_2$, partial pressure of carbon dioxide from arterial blood.

TABLE 55-3 Normal Blood Gas Values

	Arterial Blood	Mixed Venous Blood
pH	7.40 (7.35–7.45)	7.38 (7.33–7.43)
Po_2	80–100 mm Hg	35–40 mm Hg
Sao_2	95%	70%–75%
Pco_2	35–45 mm Hg	45–51 mm Hg
HCO_3^-	22–26 mEq/L (22–26 mmol/L)	24–28 mEq/L (24–28 mmol/L)

HCO_3^-, bicarbonate; Pco_2, partial pressure of carbon dioxide; Po_2, partial pressure of oxygen; Sao_2, saturation of arterial oxygen.

blood pH >7.45. The pathophysiologic processes that result in alterations in blood pH are designated by the suffix "-osis." These disturbances are classified as either metabolic or respiratory in origin. In metabolic acid–base disorders, the primary disturbance is in the plasma bicarbonate concentration. Metabolic acidosis is characterized by a decrease in the plasma bicarbonate concentration whereas in metabolic alkalosis the plasma bicarbonate concentration is increased. Respiratory acid–base disorders are caused by alterations in alveolar ventilation that produce corresponding changes in the partial pressure of carbon dioxide from arterial blood ($Paco_2$). In respiratory acidosis, the $Paco_2$ is elevated; in respiratory alkalosis it is decreased. Each disturbance has a compensatory (secondary) response that attempts to correct the $[HCO_3^-]:Paco_2$ ratio toward normal and mitigate the change in pH (Table 55–2). Although the time course of the respiratory compensatory responses to metabolic disturbances is rapid, the metabolic compensation for respiratory disturbances is slow. As a result, respiratory disturbances are characterized as acute (minutes to hours in duration), indicating that there has not been sufficient time for metabolic compensation, or chronic (days), indicating sufficient time for metabolic compensation has elapsed.

CLINICAL ASSESSMENT OF ACID–BASE STATUS

❷ Blood gases are measured to determine the patient's oxygenation and acid–base status. Under normal circumstances, there is no clinically significant difference in pH between arterial and mixed venous blood. Arterial samples are designated with the letter "a" (e.g., partial pressure of oxygen from arterial blood [Pao_2] and $Paco_2$), whereas mixed venous samples are labeled with the letter "v" or not labeled (e.g., partial pressure of oxygen from venous blood [Pvo_2] and partial pressure of carbon dioxide from venous blood [$Pvco_2$]). The normal values for arterial and venous blood gases are shown in Table 55–3. Arterial blood reflects how well the blood is being oxygenated by the lungs (an accurate measurement of Pao_2), whereas venous blood reflects how much oxygen tissues are using. Arterial blood rather than venous blood should be used whenever possible because venous blood obtained from an extremity can provide misleading information. If metabolism in the extremity is altered by hypoperfusion, exercise, infection, or some other cause, the difference in the amount of dissolved oxygen between arterial and venous blood can be dramatic. The venous pH and Pco_2 during cardiopulmonary resuscitation, might be significantly lower and higher, respectively, than the arterial pH and arterial Pco_2. This indicates a severe tissue acidosis from CO_2 accumulation caused by hypoperfusion.

ANALYSIS OF ARTERIAL BLOOD GAS DATA

Arterial blood gases provide an assessment of the patient's acid–base status. Low pH values (<7.35) indicate an acidemia, whereas high pH values (>7.45) indicate an alkalemia (Fig. 55–3). In a metabolic acidosis, the pH is decreased in association with a decreased serum bicarbonate concentration and a compensatory decrease in $Paco_2$. In a respiratory acidosis, the pH is decreased; the $Paco_2$, however, is elevated. The serum bicarbonate concentration is variable, depending on whether it is an acute disturbance (minimal increase in serum bicarbonate) or a chronic respiratory acidosis (substantial increase in serum bicarbonate). In a metabolic alkalosis, the pH is elevated in association with an increased bicarbonate concentration and a compensatory increase in $Paco_2$. In respiratory alkalosis, the pH is also elevated; the $Paco_2$, however, is decreased. As with respiratory acidosis, the metabolic compensation is variable, with a minimal decrease in serum bicarbonate in acute respiratory alkalosis and a larger decrease in $[HCO_3^-]$ in chronic respiratory alkalosis. Although each measurement has a normal range (see Table 55–3), it is often easiest to consider the midpoint of each range as the normal value. This would correlate to a pH of 7.4, $Paco_2$ of 40 mm Hg and HCO_3^-, of 24 mEq/L (24 mmol/L). Steps in acid–base interpretation are described in Table 55–4.

When arterial blood gases differ significantly from those expected on the basis of the patient's clinical condition and previous laboratory determinations, additional venous blood samples should be drawn to assess plasma electrolyte concentrations. The bicarbonate calculated from the patient's $Paco_2$ and pH of the blood gas should be compared with the measured total CO_2 content (the amount of CO_2 gas extractable from plasma, consisting of HCO_3^-, H_2CO_3, and Pco_2). Ordinarily, the blood gas bicarbonate value is approximately

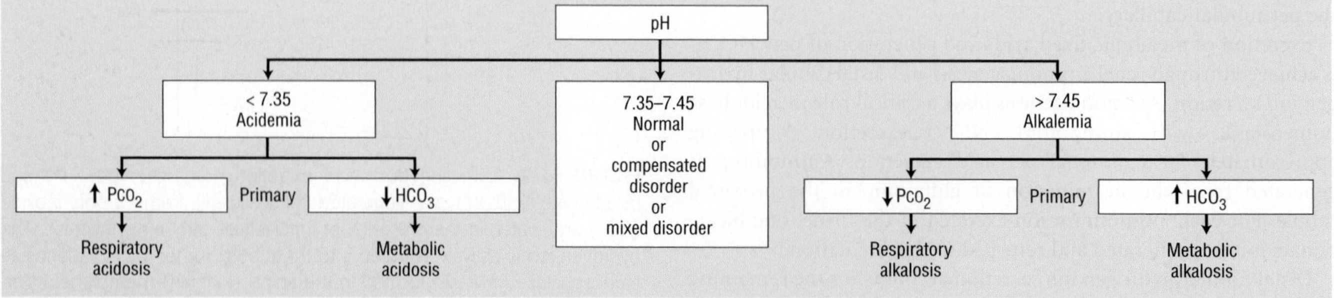

FIGURE 55-3. Analysis of arterial blood gases. (HCO_3^-, bicarbonate; Pco_2, partial pressure of carbon dioxide.)

TABLE 55-4 Steps in Acid–Base Diagnosis

1. Obtain arterial blood gases (ABGs) and electrolytes simultaneously.
2. Compare [HCO_3^-] on ABG and electrolytes to verify accuracy.
3. Calculate anion gap (AG).
4. Is acidemia (pH <7.35) or alkalemia (pH >7.45) present?
5. Is the primary abnormality respiratory (alteration in $Paco_2$) or metabolic (alteration in HCO_3)?
6. Estimate compensatory response (Table 55–7)
7. Compare change in [Cl^-] with change in [Na^+]

[Cl^-], chloride ion; [HCO_3^-], bicarbonate; [Na^+], sodium ion; $Paco_2$, partial pressure of carbon dioxide from arterial blood.

1 to 2 mEq/L (1 to 2 mmol/L) less than total CO_2 content.[3] If these values do not correspond, the results should be interpreted with caution because the difference can reflect an error in the blood collection or storage of the sample, or in the calibration of the blood gas analyzer.

METABOLIC ACID–BASE DISORDERS

METABOLIC ACIDOSIS

Pathophysiology

❸ Metabolic acidosis is characterized by a decrease in pH as the result of a primary decrease in serum bicarbonate concentration. This can result from the buffering (consumption of HCO_3^-) of an exogenous acid, an organic acid accumulating because of a metabolic disturbance (e.g., lactic acid or ketoacids), or the progressive accumulation of endogenous acids secondary to impaired renal function (e.g., phosphates and sulfates).[6] The serum HCO_3^- can also be decreased as the result of a loss of bicarbonate-rich body fluids (e.g., diarrhea, biliary drainage, or pancreatic fistula) or occur secondary to the rapid administration of non–alkali-containing intravenous fluids (dilutional acidosis).

The serum anion gap (SAG), as defined below, can be used to infer whether an organic or mineral acidosis is present.

$$SAG = [Na^+] - [Cl^-] - [HCO_3^-]$$

To maintain electroneutrality, the total concentration of cations in the serum must equal the total concentration of anions.

$$[Na^+] + [UCs] = ([Cl^-] + [HCO_3^-]) + [UAs]$$

The cation concentration is equal to the sodium concentration plus that of "unmeasured" cations (UCs), predominantly magnesium, calcium, and potassium. The anion concentration is equal to the concentrations of chloride, bicarbonate, and "unmeasured" anions (UAs), including proteins, sulfates, phosphates, and organic anions. Therefore, as the result of the combination of the two equations above, the SAG can be expressed as:

$$SAG = [UAs] - [UCs]$$

The normal SAG is approximately 9 mEq/L (9 mmol/L), with a range of 3 to 11 mEq/L (3 to 11 mmol/L). This value is lower than the value of 12 mEq/L (12 mmol/L) cited in the literature in the past because of changes in the instrumentation for measurement of serum electrolytes.[7] Increases in the anion gap to values in excess of 17 to 20 mEq/L (17 to 20 mmol/L) are indicative of the accumulation of unmeasured anions in ECF.

These unmeasured anions are generated as the result of the consumption of HCO_3^- by endogenous organic acids such as lactic acid, acetoacetic acid, or β-hydroxybutyric acid or from the ingestion of toxins such as methanol or ethylene glycol. The degree of elevation in the SAG is dependent on the clearance of the anion, as well as the multiple factors that influence HCO_3^- concentrations. Thus the SAG is a relative rather than an absolute indication of the cause of metabolic acidosis. The SAG can also be elevated in the metabolic acidosis because of renal failure, as the result of the accumulation of various organic anions, phosphates, and sulfates.

In hyperchloremic metabolic acidosis, bicarbonate losses from the ECF are replaced by chloride, and the SAG remains normal. This decrease in bicarbonate results from losses from the gastrointestinal tract, dilution of bicarbonate in the ECF space by the addition of sodium chloride solutions, or the addition of chloride-containing acids to the ECF. Common causes of metabolic acidosis with an increased or a normal SAG are listed in Table 55–5.

Hyperchloremic Metabolic Acidosis

Hyperchloremic metabolic acidosis can result from increased gastrointestinal bicarbonate loss, renal bicarbonate wasting, impaired renal acid excretion, or exogenous acid gain. Gastrointestinal disorders such as diarrhea, biliary or pancreatic drainage through either a surgical drain or fistula can result in the loss of large volumes of bicarbonate-containing fluids. Severe diarrhea, the most common cause of hypochloremic metabolic acidosis, can lead to a daily loss of 5 to 10 L of fluid containing 100 to 140 mEq/L (100 to 140 mmol/L) of sodium, 20 to 40 mEq/L (20 to 40 mmol/L) of potassium, 80 to 100 mEq/L (80 to 100 mmol/L) of chloride, and 30 to 50 mEq/L (30 to 50 mmol/L) of bicarbonate.[4] Patients who have undergone ureteral diversion into the sigmoid colon or isolated ileal loop can also develop a hyperchloremic metabolic acidosis. In these patients, chloride is reabsorbed, and the bicarbonate secreted by the gas-

TABLE 55-5 Common Causes of Metabolic Acidosis

Increased Serum Anion Gap	Normal Serum Anion Gap/ Hyperchloremic States
Lactic acidosis	**Gastrointestinal bicarbonate loss**
Diabetic ketoacidosis	Diarrhea
Lactic acidosis (see Table 55–6)	External pancreatic or small bowel drainage (fistula)
	Ureterosigmoidostomy, ileostomy
Renal failure (acute or chronic)	**Drugs**
	Cholestyramine (bile acid diarrhea)
Methanol ingestion	Magnesium sulfate (diarrhea)
Ethylene glycol ingestion	Calcium chloride (acidifying agent
Salicylate overdosage	**Renal tubular acidosis**
Starvation	Hypokalemia
	Proximal renal tubular acidosis (type II)
	Distal renal tubular acidosis (type I)
	Carbonic anhydrase inhibitors (e.g., acetazolamide)
	Hyperkalemia
	Generalized distal nephron dysfunction (type IV)
	Mineralocorticoid deficiency or resistance
	Tubulointerstitial disease
	Drug-induced hyperkalemia
	Potassium-sparing diuretics (amiloride, spironolactone, triamterene)
	Trimethoprim
	Pentamidine
	Heparin
	Angiotensin-converting enzyme (ACE) inhibitors and receptor blockers
	Nonsteroidal antiinflammatory drugs (NSAIDs)
	Cyclosporin A
	Other
	Acid ingestion (ammonium chloride, hydrochloric acid, hyperalimentation)
	Expansion acidosis (rapid saline administration)

trointestinal epithelial cells while urine retained in the colon or bowel loop results in a net loss of bicarbonate.

Hyperchloremic metabolic acidosis caused by renal bicarbonate wasting is the defining disturbance in proximal renal tubular acidosis and is a complication of therapy with carbonic anhydrase inhibitors. During the treatment of diabetic ketoacidosis, renal loss of β-hydroxybutyrate and acetoacetate, which would otherwise be metabolized to yield bicarbonate, can contribute to the development of hyperchloremic metabolic acidosis. Impaired renal acid excretion that occurs as a result of distal tubular dysfunction in patients with distal renal tubular acidoses can also occur in patients with moderate to severe renal insufficiency from other causes. The metabolic acidosis of renal insufficiency is initially hyperchloremic but can progress to an anion-gap acidosis as the renal insufficiency worsens and sulfates, phosphates, and other anions accumulate. Hyperchloremic metabolic acidosis can also result from the exogenous administration of acid (hydrochloric acid, ammonium chloride) or the unbuffered administration of acid salts from the amino acids in total parenteral nutrition fluids.

Renal Tubular Acidosis

❹ Renal tubular disorders can involve the proximal tubule, with a resultant failure to reabsorb filtered bicarbonate, or affect acid excretion in the distal tubule. The distal renal tubular acidoses (RTAs) are the most common, and are all characterized by impaired net acid excretion. The distal RTAs are subdivided into those that are associated with hypokalemia (type I) and those associated with hyperkalemia (type IV). Patients with classic distal (type I) RTA have impaired hydrogen ion secretion and are unable to excrete the daily acid load necessary to maintain acid–base balance.[4] These patients are unable to maximally acidify their urine (i.e., attain urine pH of <5.5), even in the face of an acid challenge. Type I RTA may be the result of a primary tubular defect or develop secondary to a wide variety of disorders including hypercalcemia, multiple myeloma, systemic lupus erythematosus, Sjögren syndrome, sickle-cell disease, and renal transplant rejection, or following the administration of amphotericin B or ingestion of toluene. The primary form of this disorder usually occurs in children and can result in severe acidosis, slowed growth, nephrocalcinosis, and kidney stones.[7,8] In adults, clinical complications include osteomalacia, nephrocalcinosis, and recurrent kidney stones. The hypokalemia associated with classic distal (type I) RTA results from secondary hypoaldosteronism associated with volume depletion. The renal potassium wasting decreases considerably if bicarbonate therapy is administered.

The hyperkalemic distal (type IV) RTAs are a heterogeneous group of disorders characterized by hypoaldosteronism or generalized distal tubule defects. The most common form of type IV RTA is hyporeninemic hypoaldosteronism. This syndrome is most commonly associated with mild renal insufficiency caused by diabetic nephropathy, but can also be seen in a variety of other disorders, including chronic interstitial nephritis, sickle-cell disease, human immunodeficiency virus (HIV) nephropathy, and obstructive uropathy. The clinical presentation of this syndrome is often exacerbated by pharmacologic therapy with agents that can interfere with the renin-angiotensin-aldosterone axis, such as β-adrenergic blockers, angiotensin-converting enzyme inhibitors, angiotensin receptor blockers, and nonsteroidal antiinflammatory drugs. Heparin can induce the syndrome by inhibiting adrenal aldosterone biosynthesis. Patients with this form of RTA are able to maximally acidify their urine (urine pH <5.5).[7] The primary defect in acid excretion is impaired ammoniagenesis caused by mild renal insufficiency. Hyperaldosteronism predisposes to the development of hyperkalemia, which results in further impairment of ammoniagenesis. Treatment to control the hyperkalemia is usually sufficient to reverse the metabolic acidosis, and mineralocorticoid replacement is frequently unnecessary.

Hyperkalemic distal (type IV) RTA resulting from generalized distal tubule defects is less common than hyporeninemic hypoaldosteronism but is more common than classic distal (type I) RTA. Patients with this defect have impaired tubular potassium secretion in addition to impaired urinary acidification (urine pH >5.5 despite acidemia or acid loading). Urinary obstruction is the most frequent cause of this disorder, which can also be associated with sickle-cell nephropathy, systemic lupus erythematosus, HIV nephropathy, analgesic abuse nephropathy, amyloidosis, renal transplant rejection, and chronic cyclosporine nephrotoxicity.

Proximal (type II) RTA is characterized by defects in proximal tubular reabsorption of bicarbonate. Normally, more than 85% of filtered bicarbonate is reabsorbed in the proximal tubule. Defects in proximal tubular bicarbonate reabsorption result in increased delivery of bicarbonate to the distal nephron, which has a limited capacity for bicarbonate reabsorption. As a result, at a normal serum bicarbonate concentration, the filtered bicarbonate load is incompletely reabsorbed, and is lost in the urine. As the serum bicarbonate concentration decreases, the filtered load of bicarbonate is proportionately decreased. A new equilibrium is established in which the kidney is able to reabsorb the filtered bicarbonate load, albeit at a reduced serum bicarbonate concentration. Thus patients with proximal RTA present with a chronic, nonprogressive hyperchloremic metabolic acidosis. These patients are able to acidify their urine in response to an acid load, but develop bicarbonaturia at a reduced serum bicarbonate concentration following bicarbonate loading. The impaired bicarbonate reabsorption results in salt wasting and secondary hyperaldosteronism. Hypokalemia, which can be severe, usually develops as a result of the hyperaldosteronism and bicarbonaturia.[4,7] Unlike patients with classic distal (type I) RTA, the hyperkalemia if present in proximal RTA is exacerbated by alkali replacement. Proximal RTA can develop as an isolated defect, or it can be associated with generalized proximal tubular dysfunction (Fanconi syndrome), with impaired proximal tubular glucose, phosphate, and amino acid reabsorption. Proximal RTA usually presents as an acquired disorder, secondary to a variety of diseases (amyloidosis, multiple myeloma, or nephrotic syndrome) or exposure to toxins (lead, cadmium, mercury, or outdated tetracyclines). Pharmacologic therapy with carbonic anhydrase inhibitors produces an iatrogenic form of proximal RTA.

Elevated Anion Gap Metabolic Acidosis

Metabolic acidosis with an increased SAG commonly results from increased endogenous organic acid production. In lactic acidosis, lactic acid accumulates as a by-product of anaerobic metabolism. Accumulation of the ketoacids β-hydroxybutyric acid and acetoacetic acid defines the ketoacidosis of uncontrolled diabetes mellitus, alcohol intoxication, and starvation (see Table 55–5). In advanced renal failure, accumulation of phosphate, sulfate, and organic anions is responsible for the increased SAG, which is usually less than 24 mEq/L.[9] The severe metabolic acidosis seen in myoglobinuric acute renal failure caused by rhabdomyolysis may be caused by the metabolism of large amounts of sulfur-containing amino acids released from myoglobin.

The presence of mild elevations in the SAG cannot be automatically attributed to the presence of a high SAG metabolic acidosis. Elevations in the SAG are commonly seen in hospitalized patients, especially those who are critically ill.[10] A variety of factors can contribute to this nonspecific elevation in the SAG, including the presence of alkalemia, which increases the anionic charge of albumin and other plasma proteins. The usefulness of the SAG as a marker of acid–base status is dependent on proper interpretation of a patient's clinical status.[8,9] Despite these limitations, when the SAG exceeds 20 to 25 mEq/L a significant organic acidosis is likely to be present.

High anion gap metabolic acidosis can develop in many clinical settings, including uncontrolled diabetes mellitus (see Chap. 77), alcohol intoxication (see Chaps. 39 and 69), and starvation (see Chap. 66). Toxic ingestions of methanol and ethylene glycol, are also associated with high anion gap metabolic acidosis and can be differentiated from other causes of SAG because of the presence of an elevated osmolar gap (see Chap. 10). The mechanisms responsible for the development of acidosis in these settings are diverse.

Lactic Acidosis Lactic acidosis is one of the most common causes of high SAG metabolic acidosis and can impact approximately 1% of hospitalized patients. Lactic acid is the end product of anaerobic metabolism of glucose (glycolysis). In normal individuals, lactic acid derived from pyruvate enters the circulation in small amounts and is promptly removed by the liver. In the liver, and to a lesser extent in the kidney, lactic acid is reoxidized to pyruvic acid, which is then metabolized to CO_2 and H_2O. The normal plasma lactate concentration in healthy subjects is approximately 1 mEq/L.[6,11] The diagnosis of lactic acidosis should be considered in all patients with metabolic acidosis associated with an increased SAG. Lactic acidosis is considered to be present when lactate concentrations exceed 4 to 5 mEq/L in an acidemic patient.

Classically, lactic acidosis has been differentiated into disorders associated with tissue hypoxia (type A lactic acidosis) and disorders associated with deranged oxidative metabolism (type B lactic acidosis), although the distinction between them is blurred (Table 55–6). The etiologies of lactic acidosis can also be categorized on the basis of changes in lactate production and/or utilization.[4,12] Metabolic disturbances can result in increased tissue pyruvate production or impaired utilization, with proportional increases in lactate concentrations. Increased lactate production is more commonly associated with alterations in tissue redox state, resulting in preferential conversion of pyruvate to lactate. During anaerobic metabolism, reduced nicotinamide adenine dinucleotide accumulates, driving the conversion of pyruvate to lactate and increasing the lactate:pyruvate ratio. States of enhanced metabolic activity (e.g., grand mal seizures, strenuous exercise, or hyperthermia), decreased tissue oxygen delivery (e.g., severe anemia, hypoxia, circulatory shock, or carbon monoxide poisoning) or impaired oxygen utilization (e.g., cyanide toxicity) all are associated with lactic acidosis. Impaired hepatic clearance of lactate, as seen in hypoperfusion states, liver failure, and alcohol intoxication, can also result in lactic acidosis.

Cardiovascular and septic shock, with resultant tissue hypoperfusion, are the most common causes of lactic acidosis. Poor tissue perfusion and hypoxia influence enzymatic pyruvate and lactate metabolism to stimulate anaerobic glycolysis and to decrease lactate utilization. This leads to hyperlactatemia and lactic acidosis. The mortality rate of this type of lactic acidosis can be as high as 80% and correlates with the degree of hyperlactatemia.

Lactic acidosis associated with liver disease, toxins, and congenital enzyme deficiency can be caused by deranged oxidative metabolism or impaired lactate clearance.[4,12] The exact role of diabetes mellitus in the induction of lactic acidosis is not clear. It may involve a decrease in pyruvate dehydrogenase activity, the enzyme responsible for pyruvate metabolism. Lactic acidosis in neoplastic disease is uncommon and reported mostly in patients with myeloproliferative disorders. Leukocytes and neoplastic cells in general have high rates of glycolysis. In the case of a large tumor or tightly packed bone marrow, oxygenation can be decreased, favoring the accumulation of lactate. Lactic acidosis has been reported in patients with massive liver tumors, and it has been postulated that the liver uptake of lactate is decreased in these patients. Lactic acidosis associated with seizures is usually transient and occurs because of excessive muscle activity.[6]

A number of medications can cause lactic acidosis.[13–15] Two of the most common medications associated with the development of lactic acidosis are nucleoside-analog reverse transcriptase inhibitors (NRTIs) (3.9 cases per 1,000 person years) and metformin (0.03 cases per 1,000 person years).[13,14] The proposed mechanism of NRTI-induced lactic acidosis is the inhibition of the enzyme DNA polymerase gamma that is responsible for mitochondrial DNA synthesis.[13] Disruption of this enzyme can inhibit the transport of lactate into the mitochondria, leading to an accumulation in the cytoplasm. Stavudine is the NRTI most frequently associated with lactic acidosis, however the combination of stavudine and didanosine confers the highest risk.

The exact mechanism for metformin-induced lactic acidosis is not completely understood and may occur through a number of pathways including a decrease in hepatic intracellular pH, decreasing cardiac output, increasing gut production of lactate, and increased renal loss of bicarbonate.[14] Risk factors for metformin-induced lactic acidosis include the presence of cardiovascular, pulmonary, renal, and hepatic disorders. Metformin should be discontinued during periods of tissue hypoxia (e.g., myocardial infarction, sepsis), for 3 days after contrast media has been administered or 2 days before general anesthesia administration. In the latter two cases, metformin should only be reinstituted when the patient's renal function is stable.

Propylene glycol is commonly used as a solubilizing agent in intravenous drug preparations (e.g., lorazepam) and is predominantly metabolized to lactic acid via the hepatic enzyme alcohol dehydrogenase. The administration of large doses of propylene glycol, particularly to patients with renal or liver insufficiency, can lead to a lactic acidosis with an osmolar gap and thus serial measurement of the osmolar gap can be used to detect propylene glycol accumulation.[15]

TABLE 55-6 Causes of Lactic Acidosis

Primary decrease in tissue oxygenation
Shock
Severe anemia
Congestive heart failure
Asphyxia
Carbon monoxide poisoning
Deranged oxidative metabolism
Medications
Catecholamines
Linezolid
Metformin
Nalidixic acid
Nucleoside-analog reverse transcriptase inhibitors (didanosine, stavudine, zidovudine)
Overdose (iron, isoniazid, salicylates, theophylline)
Propofol infusion syndrome
Propylene glycol toxicity (IV lorazepam)
Sodium nitroprusside (secondary to cyanide toxicity)
Streptozocin
Diabetes mellitus
Malignancy
Seizures
Methanol, ethanol, or ethylene glycol
Disorders associated with inborn errors of metabolism

CLINICAL PRESENTATION

Chronic metabolic acidosis is usually not associated with severe acidemia and is relatively asymptomatic. The major manifestations are in the bones, where chronic acidemia causes bone demineralization with the development of rickets in children and osteomalacia and osteopenia in adults. In infants and children, chronic metabolic acidosis is associated with growth failure and short stature and can be associated with nonspecific symptoms including anorexia, nausea, weight loss, and muscle weakness.

CLINICAL PRESENTATION OF METABOLIC ACIDOSIS

General

- The patient is usually relatively asymptomatic if the acidosis is acute and mild. In those with severe acidemia (pH <7.15 to 7.20) the cardiovascular, respiratory, and central nervous systems can be affected.

Symptoms

- The patient may complain of loss of appetite, nausea, and vomiting.

Signs

- Cardiac: Flushing, a rapid heart rate, wide pulse pressure, and an increase in cardiac output can be seen initially. This can be followed by a reduction in cardiac output, blood pressure, and liver and kidney blood flow.
- Cerebral: Obtundation or coma.
- Metabolic: Insulin resistance; increased protein degradation; increased metabolic demands.
- Gastrointestinal: Nausea, vomiting, loss of appetite.
- Respiratory: Dyspnea, hyperventilation with deep, rapid respirations is seen in those with severe acidosis.
- Chronic acidemia causes bone demineralization with the development of rickets in children and osteomalacia and osteopenia in adults.

Laboratory Tests

- Serum CO_2 is low. Hyperglycemia and hyperkalemia are common. Patients with a pH <7.2 are deemed to have a severe acidosis.

Severe metabolic acidosis is usually associated with acute processes. The manifestations of severe acidemia (pH <7.20) involve the cardiovascular, respiratory, and central nervous systems. Hyperventilation is often the first sign of metabolic acidosis. At a pH of 7.2, pulmonary ventilation increases approximately fourfold, and an eightfold increase has been noted at a pH of 7.[16] Respiratory compensation can occur as Kussmaul respirations—the deep, rapid respirations seen commonly in patients with diabetic ketoacidosis. In extremely severe acidosis (pH <6.8), CNS function is disrupted to such a degree that the respiratory center is depressed.

CNS depression correlates more closely with spinal fluid pH than with blood pH. For this reason, neurologic symptoms tend to occur more frequently and to a greater degree in patients with respiratory acidosis because the CO_2 accumulated in the respiratory form readily crosses the blood-brain barrier to cause acidosis in the CNS.[1] Because of the slow penetration of administered bicarbonate into the CNS, the CNS pH fails to normalize as rapidly as blood pH. Therefore patients continue to hyperventilate because of sustained CNS acidity, and severe respiratory alkalosis can occur. Sustained lowering of the $Pa{CO_2}$ within 12 to 36 hours is to be anticipated during the correction of any metabolic acidosis.[1]

Systemic acidosis can cause peripheral arteriolar dilatation, characterized by flushing, a rapid heart rate, and wide pulse pressure. Initially, cardiac output can be increased, but as acidosis becomes more severe, myocardial contractility becomes impaired, and cardiac output decreases. The effects of vagal stimulation are also enhanced at pH levels lower than 7.1, probably as a consequence of

TABLE 55-7 Guidelines for Initial Interpretation of Acid–Base Disorders

Acidosis	
Metabolic	$Pa{CO_2}$ (in mm Hg) should decrease by 1.3 times the fall in plasma $[HCO_3^-]$ (in mEq/L)
Acute respiratory	The plasma $[HCO_3^-]$ should increase by 0.1 times the increase in $Pa{CO_2}$ ± 3
Chronic respiratory	The plasma $[HCO_3^-]$ should increase by 0.35 times the increase in $Pa{CO_2}$ ± 4
Alkalosis	
Metabolic	$Pa{CO_2}$ (in mm Hg) should increase by 0.4–0.6 times the rise in plasma $[HCO_3^-]$ (in mEq/L)
Acute respiratory	The plasma $[HCO_3^-]$ should decrease by 0.2 times the decrease in $Pa{CO_2}$ but usually not to less than 18 mEq/L
Chronic respiratory	The plasma $[HCO_3^-]$ should fall by 0.35 times the decrease in $Pa{CO_2}$ but usually not to less than 14 mEq/L

HCO_3^-, bicarbonate; $Pa{CO_2}$, partial pressure of carbon dioxide from arterial blood.
Adapted from Shapiro and Kaehny.[4]

inhibition of acetylcholinesterase. This increases the danger of vagally mediated bradycardia and heart block during acidosis.

Gastrointestinal symptoms of metabolic acidosis include loss of appetite, nausea, and vomiting. Severe acidosis (pH <7.1) interferes with carbohydrate metabolism and insulin utilization, and results in hyperglycemia. Metabolic acidosis alters potassium homeostasis and contributes to the development of hyperkalemia. The magnitude of the effect on serum potassium depends on the type of acidosis: Acidosis caused by mineral acids (e.g., hydrochloric acid) are associated with a greater change in potassium levels than acidosis caused by organic acids (e.g., lactic acidosis), in which the increase in potassium attributable to the acidosis per se is minimal.

COMPENSATION

❺ The patient's primary means to compensate for metabolic acidosis is to increase carbon dioxide excretion by increasing respiratory rate. This results in a decrease in $Pa{CO_2}$. This ventilatory compensation results from stimulation of the respiratory center by changes in cerebral bicarbonate concentration and pH.[1] For every 1-mEq/L (1 mmol/L) decrease in bicarbonate concentration below the average of 24, the $Pa{CO_2}$ decreases by approximately 1 to 1.5 mm Hg from the normal value of 40 (Table 55–7).

The anticipated $Pa{CO_2}$ associated with a given bicarbonate concentration for patients with uncomplicated metabolic acidosis can be calculated as[17]:

$$Pa{CO_2} = (1.5 \times [HCO_3^-]) + 8] \pm 2$$

For example, 95% of patients with a plasma bicarbonate of 16 mEq/L (16 mmol/L) should have an arterial $P{CO_2}$ of 30 to 34 mm Hg. An observed arterial $P{CO_2}$ within this range is consistent with physiologic respiratory compensation for a metabolic acidosis and suggests that there is no respiratory disturbance. In contrast, if the $P{CO_2}$ is less than 30 mm Hg, a superimposed respiratory alkalosis can be present, whereas if the $P{CO_2}$ is greater than 34 mm Hg, a superimposed respiratory acidosis is likely present.

TREATMENT

Metabolic Acidosis

CHRONIC METABOLIC ACIDOSIS

❻ Asymptomatic patients with mild to moderate degrees of acidemia (plasma bicarbonate of 12 to 20 mEq/L ([12 to 20 mmol/L]; pH

TABLE 55-8 Therapeutic Alternatives for Oral Alkali Replacement

Generic Name	Trade Name(s)	Milliequivalents of Alkali	Dosage Form (s)	Comment
Shohl solution Sodium citrate/citric acid	Bicitra (Willen)	1 mEq Na/mL; equivalent to 1 mEq bicarbonate	Solution (500 mg Na citrate, 334 mg citric acid/5 mL)	Citrate preparations increase absorption of aluminum
Sodium bicarbonate	Various (e.g., Sodamint)	3.9 mEq bicarbonate/tablet (325 mg)	325 mg tablet	Bicarbonate preparations can cause bloating because of CO_2 production
		7.8 mEq bicarbonate/tablet (650 mg)	650 mg tablet	
	Baking soda (various)	60 mEq bicarbonate/tsp (5 g/tsp)	Powder	
Potassium citrate	Urocit-K (Mission)	5 mEq citrate/tablet	5 mEq tablet	See above
Potassium bicarbonate/potassium citrate	K-Lyte (Bristol)	25 mEq bicarbonate/tablet	25 mEq tablet (effervescent)	
	K-Lyte DS (Bristol)	50 mEq bicarbonate/tablet (double strength)	50 mEq tablet (effervescent)	See above
Potassium citrate/citric acid	Polycitra-K (Willen)	2 mEq K/mL; equivalent to 2 mEq bicarbonate	Solution (1100 mg K citrate, 334 mg citric acid/5 mL)	See above
		30 mEq bicarbonate/unit dose packet	Crystals for reconstitution (3300 mg K citrate, 1002 mg citric acid/unit dose packet)	
Sodium citrate/potassium citrate/citric acid	Polycitra (Willen) Polycitra-LC (Willen)	1 mEq K, 1 mEq Na/mL; equivalent to 2 mEq bicarbonate	Syrup (Polycitra) solution (Polycitra-LC) (Both contain 550 mg K citrate, 500 mg Na citrate, 334 mg citric acid/5 mL)	See above

of 7.2 to 7.4) do not require emergent therapy. They can usually be managed with gradual correction of the acidemia, over a period of days to weeks, using oral sodium bicarbonate or other alkali preparations (Table 55–8). In all forms of chronic metabolic acidosis, primary therapy should be directed at treating the underlying disease state. Gastrointestinal pathology should be treated to reduce ongoing bicarbonate losses, and factors that exacerbate RTA should be treated. If acidemia persists, alkali therapy should be instituted with the goal of normalization of blood pH. The loading dose (LD) of alkali to initially correct the acidemia can be calculated as follows where V_D is the volume of distribution of bicarbonate[18]:

$$LD(mEq) = (V_D HCO3^- \times \text{body weight [BW]}) \times (\text{desired } [HCO_3^-] - \text{current } [HCO_3^-])$$

For a 60-kg patient with a serum bicarbonate of 15 mEq/L (24 mmol/L to 15 mmol/L), the loading dose is calculated thusly:

$$LD(mEq) = (0.5\ L/kg \times 60\ kg) \times (24\ mEq/L - 15\ mEq/L)$$
$$= 30\ L \times 9\ mEq/L$$
$$= 270\ mEq/L$$

The calculated loading dose of alkali should be administered over several days to avoid volume overload from the accompanying sodium load. For this scenario, a regimen of 60 to 70 mEq (60 to 70 mmol) three times a day for 3 to 5 days should result in an increase in HCO_3^- levels toward normal. In addition to the calculated loading dose, supplemental alkali must also be provided to replace ongoing losses, which can be approximated to be 2 mEq/kg (2 mmol/kg) per day or 40 mEq (40 mmol) three times a day. In patients with associated volume depletion, bicarbonate replacement can be provided simultaneous with volume resuscitation by substituting bicarbonate for chloride in intravenous crystalloid solutions.

In patients with chronic metabolic acidosis because of gastrointestinal bicarbonate losses, maintenance therapy should provide sufficient alkali to replace ongoing bicarbonate losses. The magnitude of this replacement is variable and can be substantial (>10 mEq/kg [10 mmol/kg] per day). In addition, associated losses of other electrolytes, such as potassium and magnesium, may need to be replaced (see Chap. 54).

Proximal (type II) RTA is a bicarbonate-wasting disorder that requires the administration of large maintenance doses of alkali (10 to 15 mEq/kg [10 to 15 mmol/kg] per day). As alkali replacement raises the serum bicarbonate concentration toward normal, the proximal tubule's capacity to reabsorb bicarbonate is overwhelmed, and renal bicarbonate wasting increases. In children, aggressive therapy of proximal RTA is necessary to avoid growth retardation and osteopenia. Because this is generally a mild, nonprogressive acidosis in adults, the benefit of alkali therapy is frequently outweighed by the risks of increased potassium wasting. In patients with classic distal (type I) RTA, maintenance therapy usually requires only enough alkali to buffer the amount of acid generated from dietary intake and metabolism. This usually approximates 1 to 3 mEq/kg per day (1 to 3 mmol/kg).

❼ After initial potassium deficits are replaced, ongoing potassium supplementation may not be required, as renal potassium losses decrease following initiation of appropriate alkali therapy. The use of potassium alkali salts can, however, be desirable in patients with associated nephrolithiasis, because sodium salts can increase urinary calcium excretion.

The metabolic acidosis associated with hyperkalemic distal (type IV) RTA with hyporeninemic-hypoaldosteronemia that is often seen in patients with diabetes mellitus can be corrected by the treatment of hyperkalemia alone (see Chap. 54). The use of supplemental alkali (1 to 2 mEq/kg [1 to 2 mmol/kg] per day) to increase sodium intake and stimulate distal tubular potassium secretion can be beneficial. A minority of patients require the administration of pharmacologic amounts of fludrocortisone.[4] Type IV RTA resulting from a generalized distal tubular disorder often responds to low doses of alkali (1.5 to 2.0 mEq/kg [1.5 to 2.0 mmol/kg] per day).[19] Corrections of the acidosis along with modest dietary potassium restriction (to 1 mEq/kg per day) will often result in the maintenance of serum potassium levels of 5 mEq/L (5 mmol/L) or less.

■ ACUTE SEVERE METABOLIC ACIDOSIS

❽ The management of patients with life-threatening acute metabolic acidosis (plasma bicarbonate of 8 mEq/L [8 mmol/L] and pH <7.20) is dependent on the underlying cause and the patient's cardiovascular status. In some cases patients will require emergent hemodialysis therapy (see Chap. 48). Patients with hyperchloremic acidosis (e.g., diarrhea-induced) are unable to regenerate bicarbonate, and the generation of new bicarbonate by the kidneys can require several days before one can observe a meaningful change in their status.[11] Thus intravenous alkali therapy is often required for these patients.

CLINICAL CONTROVERSY

The role of alkali therapy in patients with severe lactic acidosis is controversial. Treatment should be directed at the underlying causes as serial bicarbonate administration is often not effective and in some settings can be deleterious.

Although conventional wisdom recommends the use of alkali replacement in patients with severe acidemia caused by the deleterious effects of acidemia on circulatory function,[6,11,12] studies have not demonstrated improved outcome with alkali replacement.[20–23]

There are several therapeutic alternatives available for the acute correction of severe metabolic acidosis. Sodium acetate, sodium citrate, and sodium lactate are unreliable sources of alkali because their alkalinizing effect is dependent on their oxidative conversion to bicarbonate. This process is often impaired in critically ill patients, especially those with liver disease or circulatory failure. Although sodium bicarbonate is the most widely used intravenous alkalotic agent,[11] several studies suggest that it is frequently ineffective and can actually be deleterious, especially in patients with lactic acidosis.[20–23] Two of the three remaining alternatives (Carbicarb and dichloroacetate) are investigational and not available in most clinical settings. Tromethamine, or THAM, is a carbon dioxide–consuming, commercially available solution that buffers respiratory as well as metabolic acids.

■ SODIUM BICARBONATE

In theory, sodium bicarbonate administration provides fluid and electrolyte replacement and increases arterial pH, thereby improving cardiac function, perfusion and oxygenation of peripheral tissues, and intracellular pH, and should therefore decrease lactate production and increase clearance. However, sodium bicarbonate administration can actually have paradoxical adverse effects on intracellular pH. When bicarbonate is given by IV infusion, the carbon dioxide generated diffuses more readily than bicarbonate across cell membranes and into cerebrospinal fluid. Therefore the intracellular pH can actually be decreased by administration of bicarbonate.[4]

CLINICAL CONTROVERSY

Although it has been recommended that sodium bicarbonate be administered to raise the arterial pH to approximately 7.20, there are no controlled clinical trials demonstrating that sodium bicarbonate administration is significantly better than general supportive care in reducing morbidity and mortality in these patients.[4,11,20–23]

Excessive sodium bicarbonate administration can result in (1) a shift of the oxyhemoglobin saturation curve to the left thereby impairing oxygen release from hemoglobin to tissues; (2) sodium and water overload, with subsequent pulmonary congestion and hypernatremia; (3) paradoxical tissue acidosis as a result of the production of CO_2 that freely diffuses into myocardial and cerebral cells;[24] and (4) decreased ionized calcium with a resultant decrease in myocardial contractility. If there is an endogenous source of bicarbonate, such as can occur in the case of ketoacidosis or lactic acidosis, a bicarbonate "overshoot" can develop because the ketoacids (acetoacetic acid and β-hydroxybutyric acid) or lactic acid are converted in the liver to bicarbonate once the underlying cause of acidosis is corrected.[10,11,25] Alkalosis can also result if too much sodium bicarbonate is administered too quickly.

If intravenous sodium bicarbonate is used, one must be mindful that the goals are to increase, not normalize, pH (to approximately 7.20) and plasma bicarbonate (to 8 to 10 mEq/L [8 to 10 mmol/L]). There is no calculative method that will assure attainment of these goals with a given dose of sodium bicarbonate because of the multiplicity of competing processes that can affect acid–base status (e.g., vomiting, potential increases in endogenous acid production, and renal failure) and the marked variability in the volume of distribution of bicarbonate (50% of body weight in patients with mild acidosis to approximately 100% in those with severe acidosis).[18] Adrogue and Madias[11] recommended that the dose of sodium bicarbonate be calculated using a distribution volume of 50% of body weight for all patients to avoid overtreatment. The total dose calculated as described previously in the RTA section should be administered as an infusion over one-half to several hours. Followup monitoring of arterial blood gases, beginning no sooner than 30 minutes after the end of the infusion, should be used to guide further therapeutic decisions.

Bicarbonate therapy is generally not necessary in the routine patient with cardiac arrest, even if the initial arrest was unmonitored. The standards and guidelines from the National Conference on Cardiopulmonary and Emergency Cardiac Care state that sodium bicarbonate is most useful in cardiac life support when combined with ventilation in an attempt to maintain near-normal arterial pH during an arrest.[26] During a cardiac arrest, sodium bicarbonate (initial dose 1 mEq/kg [1 mmol/kg]) can be administered by rapid, direct intravenous injection. It should be used only after more proven interventions such as defibrillation, cardiac compression, support of ventilation including intubation, and drug therapies such as epinephrine and antiarrhythmic agents have been employed. Subsequent doses of sodium bicarbonate should be based on measurements of arterial blood pH and $Pa{CO_2}$.

■ TROMETHAMINE

THAM, available as a 0.3 N solution, is a highly alkaline, sodium-free organic amine that acts as a proton acceptor to prevent or correct acidosis.[27] THAM combines with hydrogen ions from carbonic acid to form bicarbonate and a cationic buffer. THAM also acts as an osmotic diuretic to increase urine flow, urine pH, and the excretion of fixed acids, CO_2, and electrolytes. At pH 7.4, 30% of THAM is not ionized and therefore can penetrate into cells and neutralize acidic anions of the intracellular fluid. Intracellular pH increases have been noted within 1 hour after the infusion of THAM. There is, however, no clinical or physiologic evidence that this action is beneficial, or that THAM is more efficacious than sodium bicarbonate.[11,28]

When THAM is used, it must be administered slowly, with careful monitoring to avoid alkalosis. The usual empiric dosage range for tromethamine is 1 to 5 mmol/kg administered intravenously over 1 hour, but doses up to 1.25 mmol/kg can be given over 5 to 15 minutes in acute situations. The dose of THAM can be individualized using the following equation[27]:

$$\text{Dose of THAM (in mL)} = 1.1 \times \text{BW (in kilograms)} \times \text{base deficit}$$

where base deficit = normal $[HCO_3^-]$ minus current $[HCO_3^-]$.

The need for additional THAM is determined by serial measurements of the serum bicarbonate concentration and calculation of the base deficit. Large doses can cause respiratory depression as a result of an increase in blood pH and a decrease in $Pa{CO_2}$ concentration.[28] THAM solution is highly alkaline and can cause severe inflammation, vascular spasm, or tissue damage (necrosis, sloughing, pain, chemical phlebitis, or thrombosis) if infiltration occurs.

Hyperkalemia, hypoglycemia, hypocalcemia, and impaired coagulation have also been reported.[28,29] This agent should only be used with extreme caution in patients with severe liver or kidney failure.

CARBICARB

Carbicarb is an equimolar mixture of sodium carbonate (Na_2CO_3) and sodium bicarbonate ($NaHCO_3$).[30,31] It is no longer commercially available in Canada, and its use in the United States remains investigational. Given that the carbonate ion is a stronger base than bicarbonate, Carbicarb preferentially buffers hydrogen ions resulting in the formation of bicarbonate rather than CO_2. Thus Carbicarb limits, but does not eliminate, the generation of CO_2. Unlike bicarbonate, which can produce a paradoxical intracellular acidosis and thereby impair cardiac function, Carbicarb appears to correct intracellular acidosis if present.[32,33] The risk of hypervolemia and hypertonicity after Carbicarb administration is similar to that of bicarbonate. The small number of trials reporting the clinical utility of this agent and its continued investigational status in most of the world limits its use and availability for the foreseeable future.

DICHLOROACETATE

Dichloroacetate (DCA), another investigational agent, facilitates aerobic lactate metabolism by stimulating the activity of lactate dehydrogenase, thus reversing hyperlactatemia and elevating blood pH.[34,35] DCA, when compared to conventional management in controlled studies, however, has not been shown to improve outcome.[34,36,37] DCA can cause mild drowsiness and peripheral neuropathy, that can be ameliorated or prevented with thiamine supplementation.[35] The future role of DCA in the management of metabolic acidosis, particularly lactic acidosis, remains to be clarified.

METABOLIC ALKALOSIS

Pathophysiology

Metabolic alkalosis is a simple acid–base disorder that presents as alkalemia (increased arterial pH) with an increase in plasma bicarbonate. It is an extremely common entity in hospitalized patients with acid–base disturbances. Under normal circumstances, the kidney is readily able to excrete an alkali load. Thus evaluation of patients with metabolic alkalosis must consider two separate issues: (1) the initial process that generates the metabolic alkalosis; and (2) alterations in renal function that maintain the alkalemic state.[38,39]

Generation ⑨ The generation of metabolic alkalosis can also result from excessive losses of hydrogen ion from the kidneys or stomach or from a gain secondary to the ingestion or administration of bicarbonate-rich fluids. Gastric juice, rich in chloride and hydrogen ion, is secreted at a rate of less than 50 mL/h in the basal state, but can increase up to fivefold with stimulation. In the gastric parietal cells, hydrogen ion and bicarbonate are generated from CO_2 and water.[39] The hydrogen ion is secreted into gastric fluid, and the bicarbonate is retained in the ECF. Normally, an amount of bicarbonate equal to the bicarbonate generated in the stomach is eliminated in the alkaline pancreatic and small-bowel secretions, maintaining hydrogen ion balance. With vomiting and nasogastric suctioning, hydrogen ion is lost externally and metabolic alkalosis results. Diarrhea, as seen with secretory villous adenomas and other secretory diarrheas, often results in excessive gastrointestinal losses of chloride-rich, bicarbonate-poor fluid and thus leads to the generation of metabolic alkalosis.

⑩ Diuretic agents acting on the thick ascending limb of the loop of Henle (e.g., furosemide, bumetanide, and torsemide) and distal convoluted tubule (e.g., thiazides), have most commonly been associated with the generation of metabolic alkalosis.[40] These agents promote the excretion of sodium and potassium almost exclusively in association with chloride, without a proportionate increase in bicarbonate excretion. Collecting duct hydrogen ion secretion is stimulated directly by the increased luminal flow rate and sodium delivery, and indirectly by intravascular volume contraction, which results in secondary hyperaldosteronism. Renal ammoniagenesis can also be stimulated by concomitant hypokalemia, further augmenting net acid excretion.

Increased renal acid excretion can also be the result of excess mineralocorticoid activity. Elevated mineralocorticoid levels directly stimulate collecting duct hydrogen ion secretion and indirectly increase ammoniagenesis by causing hypokalemia.[16] Increased mineralocorticoid activity can result from Cushing's syndrome, primary hyperaldosteronism, or hyperaldosteronism secondary to increased renin activity (e.g., malignant hypertension). In Bartter's and Gitelman's syndromes, defects in sodium transport in the loop of Henle (Bartter's) or distal convoluted tubule (Gitelman's) lead to hypokalemia, secondary hyperaldosteronism, and metabolic alkalosis.[39] In Liddle's syndrome, enhanced sodium reabsorption by the cortical collecting duct epithelial sodium channel results in a syndrome of pseudohyperaldosteronism.[38] Administration of high doses of penicillins (e.g., ticarcillin) can produce metabolic alkalosis because they act as nonreabsorbable anions. High concentrations of poorly reabsorbable anions in the distal renal tubule increase luminal flow rate and luminal electronegativity, which enhances the secretion of potassium and hydrogen ion and results in hypokalemia and metabolic alkalosis.

Metabolic alkalosis can also be generated by the gain of exogenous alkali. This can be seen as a result of bicarbonate administration or from the infusion of organic anions that are metabolized to bicarbonate, such as acetate, lactate, and citrate. The milk-alkali syndrome was historically a common cause of metabolic alkalosis in patients with peptic ulcer disease secondary to the ingestion of large quantities of milk products and antacids. With the advent of alternative therapies for dyspeptic syndromes that are far more effective than milk, this syndrome is now rarely seen.

Maintenance Metabolic alkalosis is predominantly maintained because of an abnormality in renal function. Normally, the kidneys are capable of excreting all of the excess bicarbonate presented to them, even during periods of increased bicarbonate loads.[4] As the serum bicarbonate concentration increases, the filtered bicarbonate load exceeds the maximal rate for bicarbonate reabsorption, and the excess bicarbonate is excreted in the urine. Under normal circumstances, the excess bicarbonate is rapidly excreted, and metabolic alkalosis does not occur or is corrected in a matter of hours.[39]

⑪ Several mechanisms can impair renal bicarbonate excretion and contribute to the maintenance phase of metabolic alkalosis.[38] In general, these mechanisms can be divided into volume-mediated processes (sodium chloride–responsive) and volume-independent processes (sodium chloride–resistant) that are predominantly associated with excess mineralocorticoid activity and hypokalemia (Table 55–9). Intravascular volume depletion maintains metabolic alkalosis through a number of mechanisms. Decreases in the glomerular filtration rate reduce the filtered load of bicarbonate at any given serum concentration, thereby decreasing the kidney's ability to excrete a bicarbonate load. Although this can play a role in patients with chronic kidney disease, it is also an important factor in patients in whom intravascular volume contraction accompanies metabolic alkalosis. Decreased effective arterial blood volume also enhances proximal and distal tubular sodium reabsorption. Sodium reabsorption must be coupled with reabsorption of an anion, such as chloride or bicarbonate, or exchange with a cation, such as potassium or hydrogen, to maintain charge neutrality. In the proximal tubule, increased sodium reabsorption stimulates bicarbonate reabsorption. In the distal nephron, enhanced sodium reabsorption, particularly in the setting of hypokalemia, stimulates hydrogen ion secretion.

TABLE 55-9 Causes of Metabolic Alkalosis Differentiated on the Basis of Their Responsiveness to Sodium Chloride

Sodium chloride–responsive (urinary chloride concentration <10 mEq/L)
Gastrointestinal disorders
Vomiting
Gastric drainage
Villous adenoma of the colon
Chloride diarrhea
Diuretic therapy
Correction of chronic hypercapnia
Cystic fibrosis
Excessive bicarbonate therapy of an organic acidosis
Mild/moderate potassium deficiency
Sodium chloride–resistant (urinary chloride concentration >20 mEq/L)
Excess mineralocorticoid activity
Hyperaldosteronism
Cushing's syndrome
Bartter's syndrome
Gitelman's syndrome
Excessive black licorice intake
Profound potassium depletion
Magnesium deficiency
Liddle's syndrome
Estrogen therapy
Unclassified
Alkali administration
Milk-alkali syndrome
Massive blood or plasma protein fraction transfusion
Nonparathyroid hypercalcemia
Carbohydrate refeeding after starvation
Large doses of penicillin

Mineralocorticoid excess also plays a significant role in the maintenance of metabolic alkalosis. In patients with volume-responsive metabolic alkalosis, intravascular volume depletion stimulates aldosterone secretion. As discussed earlier, excess mineralocorticoid activity can also underlie the generation of metabolic alkalosis. In either situation, the increased mineralocorticoid effect stimulates collecting duct hydrogen ion secretion. Metabolic alkalosis can also be maintained by persistent hypokalemia, enhancing proximal tubular bicarbonate reabsorption, stimulating ammoniagenesis and increasing distal tubular hydrogen ion secretion.[39]

Clinical Presentation

There are no unique signs or symptoms associated with mild to moderate metabolic alkalosis, but patients may complain of symptoms related to the underlying cause of the disorder (e.g., muscle weakness with hypokalemia or postural dizziness with volume depletion). They may have a history of vomiting, gastric drainage, or diuretic use, all of which contribute to the development of metabolic alkalosis. Severe alkalemia (blood pH >7.60) has been associated with cardiac arrhythmias, particularly in patients with heart disease, hyperventilation, and hypoxemia.[41] Neuromuscular irritability can be present, with signs of tetany or hyperactive reflexes, possibly caused by the decreased ionized calcium concentration that occurs secondary to the increase in pH. This decrease in ionized calcium may be caused by a conformational change in the albumin molecules to which the calcium is bound, resulting in increased binding, or by decreased competition from hydrogen ions for binding sites on the albumin molecule. Mental confusion, muscle cramping, and paresthesia can also occur. Lastly, patients will be more difficult to liberate from mechanical ventilation.

Compensation

The respiratory response to metabolic alkalosis is hypoventilation, which results in an increased $Pa{CO_2}$. Respiratory compensation is initiated within hours when the central and peripheral chemoreceptors sense an increase in pH. The $Pa{CO_2}$ increases 6 to 7 mm Hg for each 10-mEq/L (10 mmol/L) increase in bicarbonate, up to a $Pa{CO_2}$ of approximately 50 to 60 mm Hg (see Table 55–7) before hypoxia sensors react to prevent further hypoventilation. If the $Pa{CO_2}$ is normal or less than normal, one should consider the presence of a superimposed respiratory alkalosis, which can be secondary to fever, gram-negative sepsis, or pain.

TREATMENT

Metabolic Alkalosis

Because the body tolerates alkalemia far less well than acidemia, treatment of metabolic alkalosis is nearly always required and should be aimed at correcting the factor(s) responsible for the maintenance of the alkalosis.[38,39,41] For example, vomiting should be treated with antiemetics, gastric losses of hydrogen ion during nasogastric suction can be modulated by giving histamine blockers such as ranitidine or proton pump inhibitors such as omeprazole, and reducing or discontinuing diuretic therapy.[42,43] Metabolic alkalosis will persist until the renal mechanism responsible for maintaining the disorder is corrected, despite the fact that the original cause of the elevated plasma bicarbonate may have resolved. For example, hypovolemia should be treated with sodium chloride (i.e., diuretic abuse or nasogastric suction) to allow excretion of bicarbonate by the kidney. However, patients with severely compromised cardiovascular function may not be able to tolerate this therapeutic approach. In situations such as this and/or the presence of life-threatening alkalosis, some have advocated reduction in pH by control of ventilation.[4] Although controlled hypoventilation, sometimes using inspired CO_2 with supplemental oxygen to prevent hypoxia can be life-saving,[4] this approach is not universally accepted.[39,41] Therapy for metabolic alkalosis can be conceptualized on the basis of the sodium chloride responsiveness of the disorders as shown in Fig. 55–4.

SODIUM CHLORIDE–RESPONSIVE DISORDERS

Sodium chloride–responsive disorders usually result from volume depletion and chloride loss, which can accompany severe vomiting, prolonged nasogastric suction, and diuretic therapy. Initially therapy is directed at expanding intravascular volume and replenishing chloride stores. Sodium and potassium chloride–containing solutions should be administered to patients who can tolerate the volume load.[39,41] Patients with metabolic alkalosis who are volume overloaded or intolerant to volume administration because of congestive heart failure can benefit from the carbonic anhydrase inhibitor acetazolamide. This agent inhibits the action of carbonic anhydrase, thereby inhibiting renal bicarbonate reabsorption. Unfortunately, it also increases the renal losses of potassium and phosphate. Administration of acetazolamide (250 to 375 mg once or twice daily) can promote a sufficient bicarbonate diuresis and return the pH toward normal. However, because the clinical effectiveness of the drug declines as the HCO_3^- concentration decreases, only rarely will this approach fully correct the alkalosis.[38]

Acidifying agents including hydrochloric acid, ammonium chloride, and arginine monohydrochloride can be used to treat severe (pH >7.6) symptomatic metabolic alkalosis. In general, this man-

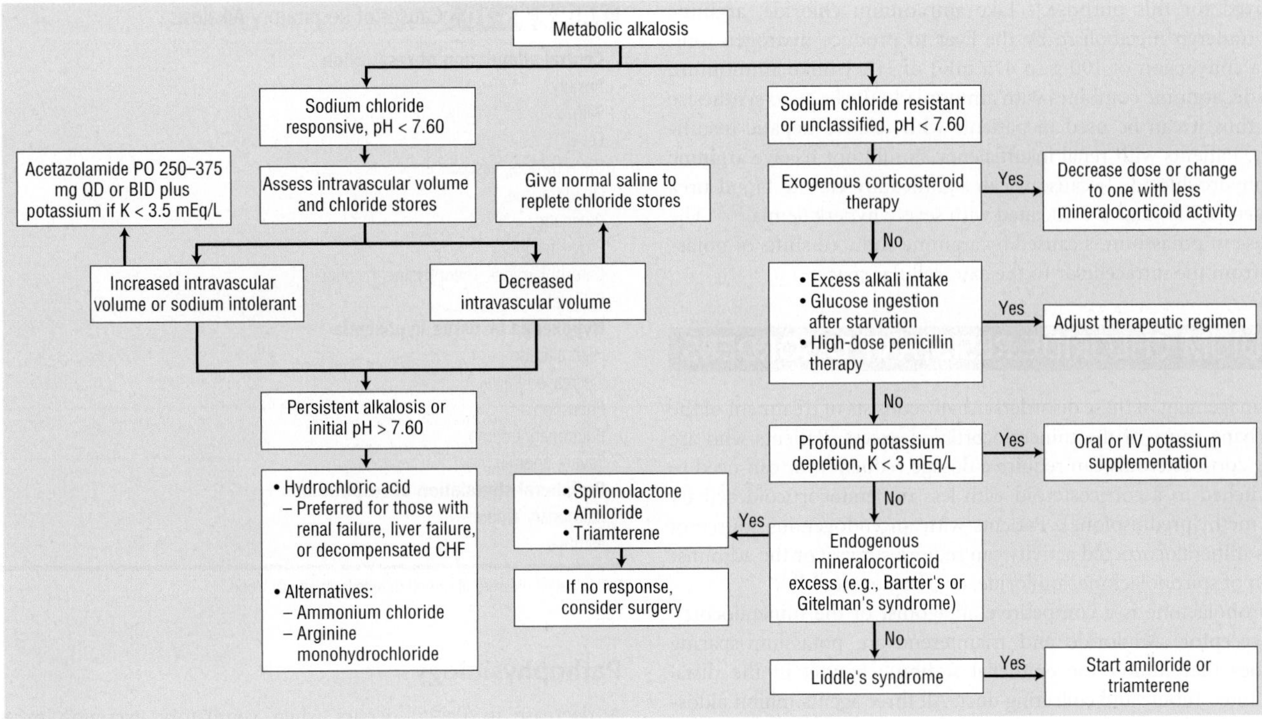

FIGURE 55-4. Treatment algorithm for patients with primary metabolic alkalosis. (BID, twice daily; CHF, chronic heart failure; K, potassium; PO, orally; QD, every day.)

agement is reserved for patients who are unresponsive to conventional fluid and electrolyte management or who are unable to tolerate the requisite volume load because of decompensated congestive heart failure or advanced renal failure.[38,41] Alternatively, hemodialysis using a low-bicarbonate dialysate can be used for the rapid correction of metabolic alkalosis.

HYDROCHLORIC ACID

Hydrochloric acid is usually infused intravenously via a large central vein as a 0.1 to 0.25 N HCl solution in either 5% dextrose or normal saline, although sterile water has also been used. Extemporaneously prepared solutions can be made by adding 100 to 250 mEq (100 to 250 mEq) of HCl through a 0.22-mm filter into a glass container of saline or dextrose. Hydrochloric acid can also be added to parenteral nutrient solutions and administered via a central line without serious degradation of proteins.[44] The rate of infusion should be 100 to 125 mL/h (10 to 25 mEq/h [10 to 25 mEq/h]), with frequent monitoring of arterial blood gases. To prevent overcorrection, the infusion should be stopped when the arterial pH decreases to 7.50.[39]

The dose of hydrochloric acid can be based on an estimate of the total body chloride deficit[27]:

$$\text{Dose HCl (in mEq)} = [0.2\ \text{L/kg} \times \text{BW (in kilograms)}] \times [103 - \text{observed serum chloride}]$$

where the estimated chloride space is 0.2 times the body weight, and the average serum chloride is 103 mEq/L. Alternatively, the dose can be calculated based on the estimated base deficit[41]:

$$\text{Dose HCl (in mEq)} = [0.5\ \text{L/kg} \times \text{BW (in kilograms)}] \times (\text{desired } [HCO_3^-] - \text{observed } [HCO_3^-])$$

CLINICAL CONTROVERSY

At present, there are no comparative data that address the relative accuracy of these two formulas for determining the dose of hydrochloric acid.

The dose of hydrochloric acid is usually infused intravenously over 12 to 24 hours.[45] A severe transient respiratory acidosis can occur if the hydrochloric acid is infused too quickly because of a slower reduction of the elevated bicarbonate concentration in the cerebrospinal fluid than in the extracellular fluid. Improvement is usually seen within 24 hours of initiating therapy. Arterial blood gases and serum electrolytes should be drawn every 4 to 8 hours to evaluate and adjust therapy.

AMMONIUM CHLORIDE

Ammonium chloride has a limited role in the treatment of metabolic alkalosis. The liver converts ammonium chloride (NH_4Cl) to urea and free hydrochloric acid[27]:

$$2NH_4Cl + 2HCO_3^- \rightarrow CO(NH_2)_2 + CO_2 + 3H_2O + 2Cl^-$$

The dose of ammonium chloride can be calculated on the basis of the chloride deficit using the same method as for HCl and assuming that 20 g ammonium chloride will provide 374 mEq (mmol) of H^+. However, only one-half of the calculated dose of ammonium chloride should be administered so as to avoid ammonia toxicity. Ammonium chloride is available as a 26.75% solution containing 100 mEq of H^+ in 20 mL, which should be further diluted prior to administration. A dilute solution can be prepared by adding 20 mL of ammonium chloride to 500 mL of normal saline and infusing the solution at a rate of no more than 1 mEq/min. Improvement in metabolic status is usually seen within 24 hours. CNS toxicity, marked by confusion, irritability, seizures, and coma, has been associated with more rapid rates of administration. Ammonium chloride must be administered cautiously to patients with renal or hepatic impairment. In patients with hepatic dysfunction, impaired conversion of ammonia to urea can result in increased ammonia levels and worsened encephalopathy. In patients with renal failure, the increased urea synthesis can exacerbate uremic symptoms.[27]

ARGININE MONOHYDROCHLORIDE

Arginine monohydrochloride at a dose of 10 g/h given intravenously has been used to treat metabolic alkalosis, although it was never FDA approved for this purpose.[27] Like ammonium chloride, arginine must undergo metabolism by the liver to produce hydrogen ions, with a conversion of 100 g to 475 mEq of H^+. Unlike ammonium chloride, arginine combines with ammonia in the body to synthesize urea; thus it can be used in patients with relative hepatic insufficiency. Patients with renal insufficiency should not receive arginine monohydrochloride because it can significantly elevate blood urea nitrogen (BUN) and is associated with severe hyperkalemia.[27,29] The increase in potassium is caused by arginine-induced shifts of potassium from the intracellular to the extracellular space.

SODIUM CHLORIDE-RESISTANT DISORDERS

⓬ Management of these disorders usually consists of treatment of the underlying cause of the mineralocorticoid excess. Patients who are taking corticosteroids can require a dosage reduction or can need to be switched to a corticosteroid with less mineralocorticoid activity (e.g., methylprednisolone). Patients with an endogenous source of excess mineralocorticoid activity can require surgery or the administration of spironolactone, amiloride, or triamterene.[38,41,46]

Spironolactone is a competitive antagonist of the mineralocorticoid receptor. Amiloride and triamterene are potassium-sparing diuretics that inhibit the epithelial sodium channel in the distal convoluted tubule and collecting duct. All three agents inhibit aldosterone-stimulated sodium reabsorption in the collecting duct. In addition, spironolactone directly inhibits aldosterone-stimulation of the hydrogen ion secretory pump. Thus most patients with mineralocorticoid excess, including Bartter's and Gitelman's syndromes, respond to therapy with these agents.[38,39,46] Liddle's syndrome, which is a form of pseudohypoaldosteronism caused by overactivity of the epithelial sodium channel, is not responsive to spironolactone but can be treated with either amiloride or triamterene. Although experience is limited, some patients with Bartter's and Gitelman's syndromes may respond to nonsteroidal antiinflammatory agents or angiotensin-converting enzyme inhibitors.[47,48] Finally, aggressive potassium repletion can correct the alkalosis in those who have not responded to the approaches outlined above.

RESPIRATORY ACID–BASE DISORDERS

As with the metabolic acid–base disturbances, there are two cardinal respiratory acid–base disturbances: respiratory acidosis and respiratory alkalosis. These disorders are generated by a primary alteration in carbon dioxide excretion, which changes the concentration of carbon dioxide, and therefore the carbonic acid concentration in body fluids. A primary reduction in Pa_{CO_2} causes an increase in pH (respiratory alkalosis), and a primary increase in Pa_{CO_2} causes a decrease in pH (respiratory acidosis). Unlike the metabolic disturbances, for which respiratory compensation is rapid, metabolic compensation for the respiratory disturbances is slow. Hence these disturbances can be further divided into acute disorders, with a duration of minutes to hours, and where metabolic compensation has yet to occur, and chronic disorders that have been present long enough for metabolic compensation to be complete.

RESPIRATORY ALKALOSIS

Respiratory alkalosis is characterized by a primary decrease in Pa_{CO_2} that leads to an elevation in pH. The Pa_{CO_2} decreases when the excretion of CO_2 by the lungs exceeds the metabolic production of CO_2. It is the most frequently encountered acid–base disorder, occurring physiologically in normal pregnancy and in persons living at high altitudes.[45] Respiratory alkalosis also occurs frequently among hospitalized patients (Table 55–10).

TABLE 55-10 Causes of Respiratory Alkalosis

Central stimulation of respiration
Anxiety
Pain
Fever
Brain tumors, vascular accidents
Head trauma
Pregnancy
Progesterone
Catecholamines, theophylline, nicotine
Salicylates
Hypoxemia or tissue hypoxemia
High altitude
Decreased Pa_{CO_2}
Pneumonia
Pulmonary edema
Severe anemia
Peripheral stimulation of respiration
Pulmonary emboli
Asthma

Pa_{CO_2}, partial pressure of carbon dioxide from arterial blood.

Pathophysiology

A decrease in Pa_{CO_2} occurs when ventilatory excretion exceeds metabolic production. Because endogenous production of CO_2 is relatively constant, negative CO_2 balance is primarily caused by an increase in ventilatory excretion of CO_2 (hyperventilation). The metabolic production of CO_2, however, can be increased during periods of stress or with excess carbohydrate administration (e.g., parenteral nutrition). Hyperventilation can develop from an increase in neurochemical stimulation via either central or peripheral mechanisms, or be the result of voluntary or mechanical (iatrogenic) hyperventilation.

A decrease in Pa_{CO_2} can occur in patients with cardiogenic, hypovolemic, or septic shock because oxygen delivery to the carotid and aortic chemoreceptors is reduced. This relative deficit in Pa_{O_2} stimulates an increase in ventilation. The hyperventilation in sepsis is also mediated via a central mechanism. Hyperventilation-induced respiratory alkalosis with an elevation in cardiac index and hypotension without peripheral vasoconstriction can therefore be an early sign of sepsis.

Clinical Presentation

Although most patients are asymptomatic, respiratory alkalosis can cause adverse neuromuscular, cardiovascular, and gastrointestinal effects.[45] During periods of decreased Pa_{CO_2}, there is a decrease in cerebral blood flow, which can be responsible for symptoms of light-headedness, confusion, decreased intellectual functioning, syncope, and seizures. Nausea and vomiting can occur, probably as a result of cerebral hypoxia. In severe respiratory alkalosis, cardiac arrhythmias can occur because of sensitization of the myocardium to the arrhythmogenic effects of circulating catecholamines.[2] Acute respiratory alkalosis has no effect on blood pressure or cardiac output in awake individuals. Anesthetized patients, however, can experience a decrease in both cardiac output and blood pressure, possibly owing to the lack of a tachycardic response.[49]

CLINICAL PRESENTATION OF RESPIRATORY ALKALOSIS

General

- The patient is usually asymptomatic if the condition is chronic and mild.

Symptoms

- The patient may complain of light-headedness, confusion, muscle cramps and tetany, and decreased intellectual functioning.
- Nausea and vomiting can occur, probably as a result of cerebral hypoxia.

Signs

- In severe respiratory alkalosis pH >7.60
- Syncope and seizures
- Cardiac arrhythmias
- Hyperventilation

Laboratory Tests

- Serum chloride concentration is usually slightly increased. Serum ionized calcium, potassium, and phosphorus concentration can be decreased.

The concentration of serum electrolytes can also be altered secondary to the development of respiratory alkalosis. The serum chloride concentration is usually slightly increased, and serum potassium concentration can be slightly decreased. Clinically significant hypokalemia can be a consequence of extreme respiratory alkalosis, although the effect is usually very small or negligible.[2,49] Serum phosphorus concentration can decrease by as much as 1.5 to 2.0 mg/dL (0.5 to 0.6 mmol/L) because of the shift of inorganic phosphate into cells. Reductions in the blood ionized calcium concentration can be partially responsible for symptoms such as muscle cramps and tetany. Approximately 50% of calcium is bound to albumin, and an increase in pH results in an increase in binding.[45]

Compensation

The initial response of the body to acute respiratory alkalosis is chemical buffering: hydrogen ions are released from the body's buffers—intracellular proteins, phosphates, and hemoglobin—and titrate down the serum bicarbonate concentration. This process occurs within minutes. Acutely, the bicarbonate concentration can be decreased by a maximum of 3 mEq/L (3 mmol/L) for each 10–mm Hg decrease in $Paco_2$[16] (see Table 55–7). When only physicochemical buffering has occurred, the disturbance is referred to as acute respiratory alkalosis.

Metabolic compensation occurs when respiratory alkalosis persists for more than 6 to 12 hours. In response to the alkalemia, proximal tubular bicarbonate reabsorption is inhibited, and the serum bicarbonate concentration decreases. Renal compensation is usually complete within 1 to 2 days. The renal bicarbonaturia, as well as decreased NH_4^+ and titratable acid excretion, are direct effects of the reduced $Paco_2$ and pH on renal reabsorption of chloride and bicarbonate.[2] The acuity of the respiratory alkalosis can be assessed on the basis of the degree of renal compensation (see Table 55–7). In fully compensated respiratory alkalosis, the bicarbonate concentration decreases by 4 mEq/L (4 mmol/L) below 24 for each 10–mm Hg drop in $Paco_2$. For example, a sustained decrease in $Paco_2$ of 20 mm Hg will lower serum bicarbonate from 24 to 14 mEq/L (24 to 14 mmol/L) with a resultant pH of 7.46. Bicarbonate concentrations differing from those anticipated using the preceding guidelines suggest a mixed acid–base disorder.

TREATMENT

Respiratory Alkalosis

Because most patients with respiratory alkalosis, especially chronic cases, have few or no symptoms and pH alterations are usually mild (pH not exceeding 7.50), treatment is often not required.[41] The first consideration in the treatment of acute respiratory alkalosis with pH >7.50 is the identification and correction of the underlying cause. Relief of pain, correction of hypovolemia with intravenous fluids, treatment of fever or infection, treatment of salicylate overdose, and other direct measures can prove effective. A rebreathing device, such as a paper bag, can be useful in controlling hyperventilation in patients with the anxiety/hyperventilation syndrome.[45] Oxygen therapy should be initiated in patients with severe hypoxemia. Patients with life-threatening alkalosis (pH >7.60), particularly if it is a mixed respiratory and metabolic condition and they have complications such as arrhythmia or seizures can require mechanical ventilation with sedation and/or paralysis to control hyperventilation.

Respiratory alkalosis in patients receiving mechanical ventilation is usually iatrogenic. It can often be corrected by decreasing either the set respiratory rate or tidal volume although other measures can also be employed. The use of a capnograph and spirometer in the breathing circuit enables a more precise adjustment of the ventilator settings. Another method of treating respiratory alkalosis is to increase the amount of dead space in the ventilator circuit by placing a known length of tubing between the artificial airway and the "Y" piece of the ventilator. This results in "rebreathing" of expired gas, and therefore an increase in the inspired carbon dioxide concentration, which should increase the carbon dioxide tension of the patient, correcting the respiratory alkalosis. In patients breathing more rapidly than the ventilator settings, sedation with or without paralysis can be employed.

RESPIRATORY ACIDOSIS

Pathophysiology

Respiratory acidosis occurs when the lungs fail to excrete carbon dioxide resulting in a lower pH. This can be the result of conditions that centrally inhibit the respiratory center, diseases that interfere with pulmonary perfusion or neuromuscular function, and intrinsic airway or parenchymal pulmonary disease (Table 55–11). Acute respiratory acidosis with hypoxemia, hypercarbia, and acidosis is life-threatening. Those disorders that produce an increase in $Paco_2$ and hypoxemia to a degree compatible with life (e.g., chronic obstructive pulmonary disease), with or without oxygen therapy, can result in chronic respiratory acidosis (Table 55–12). These patients can function normally without noticeable neurologic defects with $Paco_2$ concentrations in the range of 90 to 100 mm Hg (normal, 40 mm Hg), provided adequate oxygenation is maintained.[49]

Clinical Presentation

Respiratory acidosis can produce neurologic symptoms, including altered mental status, abnormal behavior, seizures, stupor, and coma. Hypercapnia can mimic stroke or CNS tumors by producing headache, papilledema, focal paresis, and abnormal reflexes. These CNS symptoms are attributable to the vasodilator effects of CO_2 in the brain that result in an increase in cerebral blood flow.[2] The CNS response to hypercapnia is extremely variable between patients and is most influenced by the acuity of presentation. Given that chronic hypercapnia blunts the usual respiratory stimulus of an elevated $Paco_2$, hypoxemia rather than hypercapnia provides the primary ventilatory stimulus in patients with severe chronic respiratory acidosis.[49]

The degree to which cardiac contractility and heart rate are altered depends on the severity of the acidosis and the rapidity with which it develops. Modest acute hypercapnia ($Paco_2$ of 50 to 55 mm Hg) stimulates a stress-like response, with elevated catecholamines and corticosteroid hormone levels, and can result in increased cardiac output and pulmonary artery pressure.[50] As the severity

TABLE 55-11 Causes of Acute Respiratory Acidosis

Central
Drugs (anesthetics, opioids, sedatives)
Stroke
Head injury
Infection
Status epilepticus
Perfusion abnormalities
Massive pulmonary embolism
Cardiac arrest
Airway and pulmonary abnormalities
Airway obstruction: foreign body, laryngeal edema
Aspiration of vomitus
Asthma
Chronic pulmonary obstructive disease (COPD)
Severe pulmonary edema
Severe pneumonia
Adult respiratory distress syndrome (ARDS)
Smoke inhalation
Pneumothorax
Neuromuscular abnormalities
Brainstem or cervical cord injury
Guillan-Barré syndrome
Myasthenia gravis
Mechanical ventilator
Ventilator malfunction
Inadequate frequency or tidal volume settings
Large dead space
Total parenteral nutrition (increased CO_2 production)

increases, cardiac output declines and vascular resistance decreases leading to refractory hypotension in some patients.[2]

In respiratory acidosis, the serum potassium concentration increases modestly secondary to cellular shifts. The increases are less than those seen with inorganic metabolic acidosis and are difficult to predict for individual patients (see Chap. 54).

CLINICAL PRESENTATION OF RESPIRATORY ACIDOSIS

General

- The patient is usually symptomatic.

Symptoms

- The patient may complain of confusion or difficulty thinking and headache.

Signs

- In severe respiratory acidosis:
- Cardiac: Increased cardiac output if moderate that decreases if severe. Refractory hypotension can be present in some patients.
- CNS: Abnormal behavior, seizures, stupor, and coma. Papilledema, focal paresis, and abnormal reflexes can also be present.

Laboratory Tests

- Serum potassium concentration can be modestly increased. Hypercapnia can be moderate ($Paco_2$ of 50 to 55 mm Hg) to severe ($Paco_2$ of >80 mm Hg). Hypoxia (Pao_2 is <70 mm Hg) is often present.

Compensation

The body responds to acute respiratory acidosis with chemical buffering. The increase in $Paco_2$ results in increased carbonic acid levels. The carbonic acid dissociates, releasing hydrogen ions, which are buffered by nonbicarbonate buffers (i.e., proteins, phosphate, and hemoglobin) and bicarbonate. Thus on the basis of physicochemical factors, increases in $Paco_2$ raise the serum bicarbonate concentration. In general, in acute respiratory acidosis, the bicarbonate concentration increases by 1 mEq/L (1 mmol/L) above 24 for each 10–mm Hg increase in $Paco_2$ above 40 (see Table 55–7).

Metabolic compensation occurs when respiratory acidosis is prolonged beyond 12 to 24 hours. In response to hypercapnia and acidemia, proximal tubular bicarbonate reabsorption, ammoniagenesis, and distal tubular hydrogen secretion are enhanced, resulting in an increase in the serum bicarbonate concentration that raises the pH toward normal. Renal compensation for chronic hypercapnia generally results in the plasma bicarbonate concentration increasing by 4 mEq/L (4 mmol/L) above 24 for each 10–mm Hg increase in $Paco_2$ above 40 (see Table 55–7). The new steady state in acid–base values is generally achieved within 5 days of the onset of hypercapnia in dogs; the time interval necessary for compensation in humans has not been established.

TABLE 55-12 Causes of Chronic Respiratory Acidosis

Neuromuscular abnormalities
Brainstem infarct
Obesity-hypoventilation (Pickwickian) syndrome
Tumors
Poliomyelitis
Multiple sclerosis
Diaphragmatic paralysis
Pulmonary abnormalities
Chronic obstructive pulmonary disease
Kyphoscoliosis
Interstitial pulmonary disease
Overzealous parenteral feeding

TREATMENT

Respiratory Acidosis

The treatment of respiratory acidosis is dependent on the chronicity of the patient's condition. Respiratory decompensation in patients with chronic elevations in $Paco_2$ are frequently seen in those with acute infections and those recently started on narcotic analgesics or oxygen therapy.[41] Aggressive treatment of these conditions can offer considerable benefit and should be initiated. Furthermore, tranquilizers and sedatives should be avoided and supplemental oxygen, if used, should be minimized.

■ ACUTE RESPIRATORY ACIDOSIS

⓭ When carbon dioxide excretion is severely impaired ($Paco_2$ >80 mm Hg) and/or life-threatening, hypoxia is present (Pao_2 <40 mm Hg); the immediate therapeutic goal is to provide adequate oxygenation. Under these circumstances, hypoxia, not acidemia, is the principal threat to life. A patent airway needs to be established, which can necessitate intubation. Excessive secretions must be cleared from the airway and oxygen administered to restore adequate oxygenation. Mechanical ventilation is usually required.

The underlying cause of the acidosis should be treated aggressively (e.g., bronchodilators for treatment of severe bronchospasm; narcotic or benzodiazepine antagonists to reverse the deleterious effects of these agents on the respiratory center). Bicarbonate administration is rarely necessary in the treatment of respiratory acidosis. Furthermore, rapid correction of acidosis with bicarbonate can eliminate the patient's respiratory drive or precipitate metabolic alkalosis. Cautious use of alkali (bicarbonate or THAM) can restore the responsiveness of bronchial muscles to β-adrenergic agonists and thus can be beneficial for those patients with severe bronchospasm.[50] Arterial blood gases should be monitored closely to ensure that the respiratory acidosis is resolving without creating a metabolic alkalosis as the result of compensatory elevation in HCO_3^- and decrease in Pa_{CO_2}. Arterial blood gases should be obtained every 2 to 4 hours during the acute phase and less frequently (every 12 to 24 hours) as the acidosis improves.

ACUTE RESPIRATORY ACIDOSIS IN A COMPENSATED CHRONIC RESPIRATORY ACIDOTIC PATIENT

Patients with a history of chronic respiratory acidosis (e.g., those with chronic obstructive pulmonary disease) can experience an acute worsening of their respiratory acidosis. This can result in severe life-threatening hypoxemia. As with acute respiratory acidosis, the goals of therapy are maintenance of a patent airway and adequate oxygenation. Individuals with chronic respiratory acidosis are routinely able to tolerate a low Pa_{O_2} and an elevated Pa_{CO_2} because of compensation (increased number of red blood cells, hemoglobin content, and 2,3-diphosphoglycerate). The drive to breathe in these patients is dependent on hypoxemia rather than hypercarbia. Administration of oxygen to a patient with chronic respiratory acidosis can eliminate this drive to breathe and result in the syndrome of carbon dioxide narcosis. In this case, if the Pa_{O_2} is 50 mm Hg, no oxygen treatment is necessary. If the Pa_{O_2} is <50 mm Hg, oxygen therapy should be initiated carefully using a controlled flow of oxygen.[2]

Arterial blood gases should be checked periodically to ensure adequate oxygenation. If the Pa_{CO_2} increases during oxygen therapy, it can be a sign of impending carbon dioxide narcosis and oxygen therapy may need to be discontinued. The underlying cause of the acute exacerbation should be aggressively managed. Pulmonary infections should be treated with the appropriate antibiotics and bronchodilators administered as necessary. Excess secretions should be cleared from the airway to allow proper gas exchange. This can involve increasing oral fluid intake to decrease the viscosity of secretions, deep breathing, and postural drainage, suction, or bronchoscopy.

MIXED ACID–BASE DISORDERS

DIAGNOSIS

The diagnosis of a mixed disorder depends on an understanding of the appropriate quantitative response of the compensatory mechanisms for each of the simple acid–base disturbances. To diagnose mixed disorders, one must know how each of the four simple disorders alters pH, Pa_{CO_2}, and $[HCO_3^-]$ (see Table 55–7). If a given set of blood gases does not decrease within the range of expected responses for a simple acid–base disturbance, a mixed disorder should be suspected. In addition to laboratory information, a thorough history and physical examination of the patient will often lead to the diagnosis, even before the laboratory data are available. Examples of common mixed disturbances follow.

Mixed Respiratory Acidosis and Metabolic Acidosis

In mixed respiratory and metabolic acidosis, there is a failure of compensation. The respiratory disorder prevents the compensatory decrease in Pa_{CO_2} expected in the defense against metabolic acidosis. The metabolic disorder prevents the buffering and renal mechanisms from raising the bicarbonate concentration as expected in the defense against respiratory acidosis. In the absence of these compensatory mechanisms the pH decreases markedly.

Mixed respiratory and metabolic acidosis may develop in patients with cardiorespiratory arrest, in those with chronic lung disease who are in shock, and in metabolic acidosis patients who develop respiratory failure when treating this mixed disorder, clinicians need to respond to both the respiratory and metabolic acidosis. Improved oxygen delivery must be initiated to improve hypercarbia and hypoxia. Mechanical ventilation may be needed to reduce Pa_{CO_2}. During the initial stage of therapy, appropriate amounts of alkali should be given to reverse the metabolic acidosis (see Treatment, Metabolic Acidosis, above).

Mixed Respiratory Alkalosis and Metabolic Alkalosis

The combination of respiratory and metabolic alkalosis is the most common mixed acid–base disorder. This mixed disorder occurs frequently in critically ill surgical patients with respiratory alkalosis caused by mechanical ventilation, hypoxia, sepsis, hypotension, neurologic damage, pain, or drugs, and with metabolic alkalosis caused by vomiting or nasogastric suctioning and massive blood transfusions. It can also occur in patients with hepatic cirrhosis who hyperventilate, receive diuretics, or vomit, as well as in patients with chronic respiratory acidosis and an elevated plasma bicarbonate concentration who are placed on mechanical ventilation and undergo a rapid decrease in Pa_{CO_2}.

The renal excretion of bicarbonate that usually occurs as compensation for the respiratory alkalosis is prevented by the complicating metabolic alkalosis. Likewise, the retention of Pa_{CO_2} expected to compensate for metabolic alkalosis is prevented by the primary respiratory alkalosis. The failure of compensation that occurs with mixed respiratory and metabolic alkalosis can result in a severe alkalemia.

Administration of sodium chloride and potassium chloride solutions will help correct the metabolic component of this disorder, and adjustment of the ventilator and/or treatment of an underlying disorder that is causing hyperventilation can correct or ameliorate the respiratory component of this mixed disorder.

Mixed Metabolic Acidosis and Respiratory Alkalosis

This mixed disorder is often seen in patients with advanced liver disease, salicylate intoxication, and pulmonary-renal syndromes. The respiratory alkalosis will decrease the Pa_{CO_2} beyond the appropriate range for the respiratory compensation usually seen with metabolic acidosis. The plasma bicarbonate concentration also decreases below the level expected in compensation for a simple respiratory alkalosis. In a sense, the defense of pH for either disorder alone is enhanced; thus the pH can be normal or close to normal, with a low Pa_{CO_2} and a low $[HCO_3^-]$. Treatment of this disorder should be directed at the underlying cause. Because of the enhanced compensation, the pH is usually closer to normal than in either of the two simple disorders.

Mixed Metabolic Alkalosis and Respiratory Acidosis

This mixed disorder often occurs in patients with chronic obstructive pulmonary disease and chronic respiratory acidosis who are treated with salt restriction, diuretics, and possibly glucocorticoids. When diuretics are initiated, the plasma bicarbonate may increase because of increased renal bicarbonate generation and reabsorption, providing mechanisms for both generating and maintaining metabolic alkalosis. The elevated pH diminishes respiratory drive and may therefore worsen the respiratory acidosis.

Although the pH may not deviate significantly from normal, treatment may need to be initiated to maintain Pa_{O_2} and Pa_{CO_2} at acceptable levels. Because it is often difficult to correctly identify this mixed disorder, it is helpful to observe the patient's response to discontinuation of diuretics and administration of sodium and potassium chloride.[2] If the patient has a simple metabolic alkalosis, the Pa_{CO_2} will normalize, but it will only minimally affect the Pa_{CO_2} if it is a mixed disorder. Treatment should be aimed at decreasing the plasma bicarbonate with sodium and potassium chloride therapy, thereby allowing the renal excretion of retained bicarbonate from the diuretic-induced metabolic alkalosis. This therapy should be used cautiously to avoid exacerbating any underlying congestive heart failure.

EVALUATION OF THERAPEUTIC OUTCOMES

Because acid–base disorders are such a common and widespread problem, pharmacists can play a key role in identifying, preventing, and properly treating acid–base abnormalities. Acid–base disorders do not occur only in the intensive care unit setting. Patients in ambulatory and extended care settings have many chronic conditions and drug therapies that commonly affect acid–base balance. Thus pharmacists in all practice settings should use their knowledge to identify patients at high risk for developing drug-related problems which affect acid–base balance and to undertake appropriate prevention and treatment measures to improve the quality of life of the patients they care for.

ABBREVIATIONS

BW: body weight

CNS: central nervous system

DCA: dichloroacetate

ECF: extracellular fluid

H^+: hydrogen ion

HCO_3^-: bicarbonate

H_2CO_3: carbonic acid

HIV: human immunodeficiency virus

$NH4^+$: ammonium

$Paco_2$: partial pressure of carbon dioxide from arterial blood

Pao_2: partial pressure of oxygen from arterial blood

pH: the negative logarithm (base 10) of the hydrogen ion concentration

p*K*: the negative logarithm of the dissociation constant

$Pvco_2$: partial pressure of carbon dioxide from venous blood

Pvo_2: partial pressure of oxygen from venous blood

RTA: renal tubular acidosis

SAG: serum anion gap

THAM: tromethamine (*Tris*[hydroxymethyl]-aminomethane)

UCs: unmeasured cations

UAs: unmeasured anions

REFERENCES

1. Narins RG. Acid–base disorders: Definitions and introductory concepts. In: Narins RG, ed. Maxwell & Kleeman's Clinical Disorders of Fluid and Electrolyte Metabolism, 5th ed. New York: McGraw-Hill, 1994:765–768.
2. Kaehny WD. Pathogenesis and management of respiratory and mixed acid–base disorders. In: Schrier RW, ed. Renal and Electrolyte Disorders, 5th ed. Philadelphia: Lippincott Williams & Wilkins, 1997:172–191.
3. Adrogue HE, Adrogue HJ. Acid–base physiology. Respir Care 2001;46:328–341.
4. Shapiro JI, Kaehny WD. Pathogenesis and management of metabolic acidosis and alkalosis. In: Schrier RW, ed. Renal and Electrolyte Disorders, 5th ed. Philadelphia: Lippincott Williams & Wilkins, 1997:130–171.
5. Halperin ML, Jungas RL, Cheema-Dhadli S, Brosnan JT. Disposal of the daily acid load: An integrated function of the liver, lungs and kidneys. Trends Biochem Sci 1987;12:197–199.
6. Narins RG, Krishna GG, Yee J, et al. The metabolic acidoses. In: Narins RG, ed. Maxwell & Kleeman's Clinical Disorders of Fluid and Electrolyte Metabolism, 5th ed. New York: McGraw-Hill, 1994:769–826.
7. Halperin ML, Carlisle EJ, Donnelly S, et al. Renal tubular acidosis. In: Narins RG, ed. Maxwell & Kleeman's Clinical Disorders of Fluid and Electrolyte Metabolism, 5th ed. New York: McGraw-Hill, 1994:875–910.
8. Roth KS, Chan JC. Renal tubular acidosis: A new look at an old problem. Clin Pediatr 2001;40:533–543.
9. Salem MM, Mujais SK. Gaps in the anion gap. Arch Intern Med 1992;152:1625–1629.
10. Gauthier PM, Szerlip HM. Metabolic acidosis in the intensive care unit. Crit Care Clin 2002;18:289–308.
11. Adrogue HJ, Madias NE. Management of life-threatening acid–base disorders I. N Engl J Med 1998;338:26–34.
12. Kraut JA, Madias NE. Lactic acidosis. In: Adrogue HJ, ed. Contemporary Management in Critical Care, Vol. 1. Baltimore: Williams & Wilkins, 1995:449–457.
13. Calza L, Manfredi R, Chiodo F. Hyperlactataemia and lactic acidosis in HIV-infected patients receiving antiretroviral therapy. Clin Nutr 2005;24:5–15.
14. Saltpeter SR, Greyber E, Pasternak GA, Salpeter EE. Risk of fatal and nonfatal lactic acidosis with metformin use in type 2 diabetes mellitus: Systemic review and meta-analysis. Arch Intern Med 2003;163:2594–2602.
15. Barnes BJ, Gerst C, Smith JR, et al. Osmolal gap as a surrogate marker for serum propylene glycol concentrations in patients receiving lorazepam for sedation. Pharmacotherapy 2006;26:23–33.
16. Narins RG, Emmett M. Simple and mixed acid–base disorders: A practical approach. Medicine (Baltimore) 1980;59:161–187.
17. Albert MS, Dell RB, Winters RW. Quantitative displacement of acid–base equilibrium in metabolic acidosis. Ann Intern Med 1964;66:312–322.
18. Kraut JA. The role of metabolic acidosis in the pathogenesis of renal osteodystrophy. Adv Ren Replace Ther 1995;2:40–51.
19. Morris RC, Ives HE. Inherited disorders of the renal tubule. In: Brenner BM, ed. Brenner and Rector's the Kidney, Vol. II, 7th ed. Philadelphia: WB Saunders, 2004:1884–1937.
20. Sing RF, Branas CA, Sing RF. Bicarbonate therapy in the treatment of lactic acidosis: Medicine or toxin? J Am Osteopath Assoc 1995;95:52–57.
21. Cooper DJ, Walley KR, Wiggs BR, Russell JA. Bicarbonate does not improve hemodynamics in critically ill patients who have lactic acidosis: A prospective controlled clinical study. Ann Intern Med 1990;112:492–498.
22. Kaplan LJ, Frangos S. Clinical review: Acid–base abnormalities in the intensive care unit-part II. Crit Care 2005;9:198–203.
23. Forsythe SM, Schmidt GA. Sodium bicarbonate for the treatment of lactic acidosis. Chest 2000;117:260–267.
24. Adrogue HJ, Rashad MN, Gorin AB, et al. Assessing acid–base status in circulatory failure: Differences between arterial and central venous blood. N Engl J Med 1989;320:1312–1316.
25. Faber MD, Kupin WL, Heiling CW, Narins RG. Common fluid-electrolyte and acid–base problems in the intensive care unit: Selected issues. Semin Nephrol 1994;14:8–22.
26. Emergency Cardiac Care Committee and Subcommittees, American Heart Association. Guidelines for cardiopulmonary resuscitation and emergency cardiovascular care. Circulation 2005;112: IV-1–IV-211.
27. McEvoy GK, Litvak K, Welsh OH, et al. American Hospital Formulary Service, Drug Information. Bethesda, MD: American Society of Hospital Pharmacists, 2006.
28. Moon PF, Gabor L, Gleed RD, Erb HN. acid–base, metabolic, and hemodynamic effects of sodium bicarbonate or tromethamine administration in anesthetized dogs with experimentally induced metabolic acidosis. Am J Vet Res 1997;58:771–776.
29. Marmarou A, Holdaway R, Ward JD, et al. Traumatic brain tissue acidosis: Experimental and clinical studies. Acta Neurochir 1993;57:160–164.
30. Leung JM, Landow L, Franks M, et al. Safety and efficacy of intravenous Carbicarb in patients undergoing surgery: Comparison with

sodium bicarbonate in the treatment of mild metabolic acidosis. Crit Care Med 1994;22:1540–1549.

31. Shapiro JI. Functional and metabolic responses of the isolated heart during acidosis: Effects of sodium bicarbonate and Carbicarb. Am J Physiol 1990;258:H1835–H1839.
32. Shapiro JI. Pathogenesis of cardiac dysfunction during metabolic acidosis: Therapeutic implications. Kidney Int 1997;51:47–51.
33. Bersin RM, Arieff AI. Improved hemodynamic function during hypoxia with Carbicarb, a new agent for the management of acidosis. Circulation 1988;77:227–233.
34. Stacpoole PW, Wright EC, Baumgartner TG, et al. A controlled clinical trial of dichloroacetate for treatment of lactic acidosis. N Engl J Med 1992;327:1564–1569.
35. Stacpoole PW, Nagaraja NV, Hutson AD. Efficacy of dichloroacetate as a lactate-lowering drug. J Clin Pharmacol 2003;43:683–691.
36. Shangraw RE, Winter R, Hromco J, et al. Amelioration of lactic acidosis with dichloroacetate during liver transplantation in humans. Anesthesiology 1994;81:1127–1138.
37. Vary TC, Siegel JH, Zechnich A, et al. Pharmacologic reversal of abnormal glucose regulation, BCAA utilization, and muscle catabolism in sepsis by dichloroacetate. J Trauma 1988;28:1301–1311.
38. Palmer BF, Alpern RJ. Metabolic alkalosis. J Am Soc Nephrol 1997;8:1462–1469.
39. Khanna A, Kurtzman NA. Metabolic alkalosis. Respir Care 2001;46:354–365.
40. Miltiadous G, Mikhailidis DP, Elisaf M. Acid–base and electrolyte abnormalities observed in patients receiving cardiovascular drugs. J Cardiovasc Pharmacol Ther 2003;8:267–276.
41. Adrogue HJ, Madias NE. Management of life-threatening acid–base disorders II. N Engl J Med 1998;338:107–111.
42. Rowlands BJ, Tindall SF, Elliot DJ. The use of dilute hydrochloric acid and cimetidine to reverse severe metabolic alkalosis. Postgrad Med J 1978;54:118–123.
43. Barton CH, Vaziri ND, Ness RL, et al. Cimetidine in the management of metabolic alkalosis induced by nasogastric drainage. Arch Surg 1979;1:70–74.
44. Mirtallo JM, Rogers KR, Johnson JA, et al. Stability of amino acids and the availability of acid in total parenteral nutrition solutions containing hydrochloric acid. Am J Hosp Pharm 1981;38:1729–1731.
45. Foster GT, Vaziri ND, Sassoon CS. Respiratory alkalosis. Respir Care 2001;46:384–391.
46. Colussi G, Rombola G, De Ferrari ME, et al. Correction of hypokalemia with antialdosterone therapy in Gitelman's syndrome. Am J Nephrol 1994;14:127–135.
47. Hene RJ, Koomans HA, Dorhout Mees EJ, et al. Correction of hypokalemia in Bartter's syndrome by enalapril. Am J Kidney Dis 1987;9:200–205.
48. Vinci JM, Gill JR Jr, Bowden RE, et al. The kallikrein-kinin system in Bartter's syndrome and its response to prostaglandin synthetase inhibition. J Clin Invest 1987;61:1671–1682.
49. Gennari FJ. Respiratory acidosis and alkalosis. In: Narins RG, ed. Maxwell & Kleeman's Clinical Disorders of Fluid and Electrolyte Metabolism, 5th ed. New York: McGraw-Hill, 1994:957–990.
50. Respiratory pump failure: Primary hypercapnia (respiratory acidosis). In: Adrogue HJ, Tobin MJ, eds. Respiratory Failure. Cambridge, MA: Blackwell Science, 1997:125–134.

SECTION 6
NEUROLOGIC DISORDERS

CHAPTER 56

Evaluation of Neurologic Illness

SUSAN C. FAGAN AND FENWICK T. NICHOLS

KEY CONCEPTS

1. The clinical neurologic history and examination are the cornerstones of the neurologic diagnosis and management.
2. Through the patient's history one can determine the main symptoms, the mode of onset (gradual or sudden), progression over time (maximal at onset or steadily gaining intensity), and associated illnesses/risk factors.
3. The neurologic examination is directed at localization of the disease process so that evaluation and management may be planned appropriately.
4. The neurologic examination of a specific patient may be adapted to the patient's specific deficit. For example, a patient with double vision may warrant an extensive cranial nerve examination but a less-extensive assessment of finger strength.

To contribute most effectively to the care of patients with neurologic illness, one must understand the tools used in the diagnosis and management of these patients. In addition, clinicians must be able to gather their own data through a targeted neurologic examination and history taking to ensure optimal pharmacotherapy in neurologic patients. Despite technologic advances that have led to the development of sensitive diagnostic tests in neuroscience, the clinical neurologic history and examination are still the cornerstones of the neurologic diagnosis and management.[1]

SIGNS AND SYMPTOMS

❶ As in all of medicine, obtaining an accurate and complete history is of utmost importance in the evaluation of neurologic diseases. In many instances, the diagnosis can be made on the basis of the history, and the neurologic examination can be tailored to optimally evaluate the patient and confirm the diagnosis. The clinician depends on the patient or family for the details of the illness. Care must be taken to avoid "leading" the patient. Obtaining an accurate history may be difficult because a number of neurologic diseases may affect patients' speech and memory. ❷ Through the patient's history one can determine the main symptoms, the mode of onset (gradual or sudden), progression over time (maximal at onset or steadily gaining intensity), and associated illnesses/risk factors (recent head injury from a motor vehicle accident). The physical examination is important because it can reveal evidence of systemic disease that may have affected the nervous system secondarily (e.g., a seizure in a patient with elevated temperature and stiff neck may suggest meningitis). The neurologic examination is only one component of a complete general physical examination.

Learning objectives, review questions, and other resources can be found at **www.pharmacotherapyonline.com.**

THE NEUROLOGIC EXAMINATION

❸ An assessment of patient effort is necessary to interpret the results of the neurologic examination. It can identify any abnormalities, particularly asymmetry of function, and help to localize the lesion within the nervous system (central versus peripheral and specific location within the central nervous system [CNS] or the peripheral nervous system). The neurologic examination consists of six main components: higher cortical function (mental status), cranial nerves, motor function, reflexes, sensory function, and gait. Table 56–1 describes the common approaches to assessing each of the six domains and includes examples of the diseases in which abnormal findings are common. ❹ A targeted neurologic examination can be performed when a specific deficit is suspected. Table 56–2 describes the cranial nerve examination in more detail. The reader is encouraged to consult other references to better understand the intricacies of the neurologic examination. The clinician must synthesize the results of the history and physical examination to arrive at an anatomic localization of the lesion and create a differential diagnosis.

PROCEDURES USED IN THE DIAGNOSIS

In addition to the neurologic examination, certain imaging techniques and procedures may be essential in the diagnosis of neurologic disorders. Lumbar puncture is used to obtain cerebrospinal fluid (CSF). It is used most often as an evaluation of CNS infections such as meningitis and encephalitis, but it is also useful in subarachnoid

TABLE 56-1 The Neurologic Examination

Domain	Tests Performed	Diseases
Mental status	While obtaining the history: general mental and emotional status, speech, memory, alertness, abstract reasoning, ability to follow commands (motor integration), ability to communicate	Dementias, stroke, metabolic encephalopathies
Cranial nerves	Visual acuity, visual fields, eye movements, jaw strength, corneal reflex, facial symmetry, auditory acuity, gag reflex, shoulder and neck strength	Myasthenia gravis, Parkinson's disease, stroke, amyotrophic lateral sclerosis (ALS)
Motor function	Motor strength with and without resistance, coordination (rapid alternating movements, finger-to-nose), tremors, atrophy, fasciculations	Stroke, myasthenia gravis, Parkinson's disease, ALS
Reflexes	Biceps, triceps, tendon reflexes, plantar response (Babinski sign is an upgoing toe and is abnormal), superficial cutaneous reflexes (abdominal)	Stroke, spinal cord lesions, endocrine diseases (e.g., diabetes, hypothyroidism), peripheral neuropathy
Sensory function	Asymmetry to pinprick, vibration, temperature	Stroke, peripheral neuropathy, migraine aura, diabetes, spinal cord lesions
Gait	Walking, standing (Romberg test = eyes closed, which will accentuate disequilibrium)	Stroke, Parkinson's disease, spinal cord lesions

TABLE 56-2 Cranial Nerve Function and Examples of Testing

I. Olfactory nerve. Smell: identify odors (coffee, cinnamon, lemon; test each nostril separately).
II. Optic nerve. Visual acuity: eye chart. Visual fields: peripheral vision and blind spot; funduscopic exam; pupil size and reaction; color vision (rarely done).
III. Oculomotor (cranial nerves III, IV, and VI have similar functions and are tested as a unit). Eye movements: patient is asked to watch a light as it moved up, down, and on both sides, while eye movements are observed.
IV. Trochlear. See III.
V. Trigeminal nerve. Motor: tests power of jaw opening and sideways deviation against the resistance of a hand placed against the jaw. Sensory: test corneal reflex by touching cornea (also nasal mucosa) with a wisp of cotton.
VI. Abducens. See III.
VII. Facial nerve. Observe asymmetry of face at rest or on speaking, baring teeth, raising eyebrows, or wrinkling forehead. Reflex eye closure to a threatening movement. Glabellar tap: repetitive tapping over bridge of nose—initial blinking should cease after the first few taps.
VIII. Auditory nerve. Vestibular division: observe for nystagmus, positional testing. Auditory division: test acuity with light sound; watch, whisper, rubbing of fingers close to ear.
IX. Glossopharyngeal nerve. Test for gag reflex by touching back of throat with tongue depressor; test swallowing and coughing and note any drooling or pooling of saliva. Test symmetry of palate movement on vocalizing "ah."
X. Vagus nerve. Test gag reflex as in IX.
XI. Spinal accessory nerve. Trapezius and sternomastoid muscles: test power of shrugging shoulders and turning the head to one side against resistance.
XII. Hypoglossal nerve. Motor function of tongue. Look for wasting and abnormal movements.

hemorrhage, multiple sclerosis, and dementia. Opening pressure, cell count and differential, glucose concentration, total protein concentration, and culture and sensitivity are obtained routinely. A space-occupying lesion in the brain with mass effect is a relative contraindication to lumbar puncture because herniation could result. Prior to performing a lumbar puncture, the patient should be checked for papilledema, which may indicate increased intracranial pressure. The opening CSF pressure usually is less than 180 mm H_2O. Normal CSF is clear and colorless and should not contain any red blood cells or polymorphonuclear cells. The presence of up to five mononuclear cells is considered normal. Total protein in the CSF usually is 45 mg/dL or less. Protein may increase with infection, breakdown of the blood–brain barrier (e.g., tumors, stroke, and trauma), and diabetes.

Electroencephalography (EEG) records the electrical activity of the brain. The record is interpreted by observing the basic rhythms and waveforms, the symmetry of the recording, and abnormal electrical discharges. It also may be used to assess the response to photic stimulation or hyperventilation. It is used primarily in the diagnosis of seizures and may be helpful in the evaluation of patients with altered mental status. EEG also may be used to measure evoked potentials. The evoked potentials are the EEG response to repetitive stimuli (visual, auditory, or tactile) and provide information about the presence of abnormalities and disturbances (but not the cause) in the specific pathways tested.

Electromyography (EMG) and nerve conduction velocities (NCVs) are used to assess the function of the peripheral nerves, neuromuscular junction, and muscles. NCVs are measured by stimulating the nerve and recording the speed of conduction of the impulse. NCVs can be used to detect the presence of localized peripheral nerve injuries (e.g., carpal tunnel) or diffuse symmetric neuropathies (which may be inherited or acquired). EMG assesses muscle dysfunction as a result of primary muscle disease or secondary to nerve injury. This test is used to diagnose peripheral neuropathies (inherited and acquired), Guillain-Barré syndrome, myasthenia gravis, amyotrophic lateral sclerosis, radiculopathies, and muscle diseases.

The cerebral circulatory system can be imaged or evaluated in a number of different ways depending on the type and location of the abnormality suspected. Imaging techniques can be used to identify local arterial stenosis, aneurysms, or arteriovenous malformations. Atherosclerosis of the extracranial arteries, a frequent cause of stroke, can be evaluated using ultrasound (referred to as *duplex sonography, carotid Doppler,* or *color-flow Doppler*), magnetic resonance angiography (MRA), spiral computed tomographic angiography (CTA), or intraarterial angiography. The intracranial arterial circulation can be evaluated using transcranial Doppler, MRA, CTA, or intraarterial angiography. Each technique has its own advantages and disadvantages. Intraarterial angiography provides the best imaging of the smaller arteries of the cerebral circulation but is more invasive than the other measures.

Computed tomography (CT) uses x-rays to produce images of "slices" of the brain that are 1 to 10 mm in thickness. CT revolutionized the practice of neurology by allowing direct imaging of the brain anatomy. CT is currently available in most communities and is used to evaluate patients with intracranial disease. CT scans are used to identify tumors, hemorrhages, infarctions, hydrocephalus, and atrophy. Intravenous contrast agents (a contrast-enhanced scan) can be administered to enhance the image of blood vessels and areas of blood–brain barrier damage that may be caused by abscesses, other inflammatory conditions, tumors, or stroke.

Magnetic resonance imaging (MRI) uses the magnetic properties of the hydrogen atom nucleus and proton to produce computer-processed scans that provide improved anatomic detail when compared with CT scans. MRI offers the advantages of better differentiating between white and gray matter and delineating lesions close to bone (brainstem and cerebellum) and has no radiation risk; however, it is not as readily available as CT and is more expensive. MRI has a proven advantage over CT in evaluating lesions in the posterior fossa and in detecting lesions in the white matter, such as plaques in multiple sclerosis. MRI is also useful in the diagnosis of tumors and very early ischemic stroke (diffusion-weighted imaging). Imaging of the spinal canal and its contents can be accomplished either by MRI myelography or CT myelography.

Other imaging techniques such as positron emission tomography (PET) and single-photon emission computed tomography (SPECT) are considered tests of brain function. These tests are being studied extensively in epilepsy as well as in cerebrovascular disorders, cerebral tumors, movement disorders, and dementia. PET scans use a positron-emitting isotope to display chemical activity and the rates of biologic processes within the brain. This method can assess regional metabolic changes in the brain. The expense, technical complexity (a cyclotron is needed), and limited availability of this technique limit its clinical usefulness.

SPECT scans measure radiotracer uptake by tissues and provide cross-sectional images of the brain. This technique has been used extensively to assess cerebral blood flow. Although the resolution of SPECT is not as good as PET, the availability has led to wide clinical use in disorders such as stroke, dementia, and epilepsy.

CONCLUSION

Assessment of the patient with neurologic disease is challenging. The patient by virtue of the neurologic deficit, may or may not be able to provide reliable information regarding medication history or extent of illness. The clinician must develop alternate strategies to obtain a complete data set and develop a pharmacotherapy plan. Ability to interpret and synthesize the results of the neurologic examination and other diagnostic tests will help a great deal in this quest.

ABBREVIATIONS

CNS: central nervous system
CSF: cerebrospinal fluid
CT: computed tomography
CTA: computed tomography angiography
EEG: electroencephalogram
EMG: electromyography
MRA: magnetic resonance angiography
MRI: magnetic resonance imaging
NCVs: nerve conduction velocities
PET: positron-emission tomography
SPECT: single-photon-emission computed tomography

REFERENCE

1. Campbell WW. DeJong's The Neurologic Examination, 6th ed. Philadelphia: Lippincott Williams & Wilkins, 2005.

CHAPTER 57

Multiple Sclerosis

JACQUELYN L. BAINBRIDGE AND JOHN R. CORBOY

KEY CONCEPTS

1. The etiology of multiple sclerosis (MS) is unknown, and currently there is no cure.
2. Multiple sclerosis appears to be an immunologic disorder that is characterized by central nervous system (CNS) demyelination and axonal damage.
3. Multiple sclerosis is classified by the nature of progression over time into several categories, which have different clinical presentations and responses to therapy.
4. Diagnosis of MS requires dissemination of lesions over time in multiple parts of the CNS, and is made primarily on the basis of clinical symptoms and examination. More recent diagnostic criteria also allow for the use of magnetic resonance imaging (MRI), spinal fluid, and evoked potentials to aid in the diagnosis.
5. Acute exacerbations or relapses usually are treated with high-dose glucocorticoids, such as methylprednisolone, and onset of a clinical response to steroid treatment is expected within 3 to 5 days.
6. Treatment with interferon β (Avonex, Rebif, or Betaseron), glatiramer acetate (Copaxone), natalizumab (Tysabri), or mitoxantrone (Novantrone) can reduce annual relapse rate, slow progression of disability, slow cognitive decline, and slow changes seen on brain MRIs in relapsing-remitting MS (RRMS).
7. The only treatment approved for secondary-progressive MS (SPMS) is mitoxantrone, and, if the patient continues to have superimposed relapses, interferon β_{1b}. There are no proven therapies for primary-progressive MS (PPMS).
8. In most cases, treatment with immunomodulating interferon β or glatiramer acetate should begin promptly after the diagnosis of relapsing MS is made and after a single attack if the MRI is suggestive of high risk of further attacks. In RRMS, natalizumab and mitoxantrone should be reserved for those patients who have failed or are intolerant of interferon or glatiramer acetate therapy.
9. The definition of treatment inadequacy is unclear. Thus, therapy after interferon β_{1a} (Avonex or Rebif), interferon β_{1b} (Betaseron), or glatiramer acetate (Copaxone) "treatment failure" in RRMS should be individualized. These therapies are collectively referred to as ABC-R therapy. Options include alternating ABC-R therapy, combining with other agents, using natalizumab or mitoxantrone, or using non–FDA-approved approaches.
10. Patients suffering from MS frequently will have symptoms such as spasticity, bladder dysfunction, fatigue, pain, and depression that can require treatment. Patients must be counseled that therapies such as interferon β and glatiramer acetate will not relieve these symptoms. Depression is common in MS and can pose the risk of suicide.

Learning objectives, review questions, and other resources can be found at **www.pharmacotherapyonline.com.**

MS is an inflammatory disease of the CNS that affects between 250,000 and 350,000 persons in the United States.[1] The term *multiple sclerosis* refers to two characteristics of the disease: the numerous affected areas of the brain and spinal cord producing multiple neurologic symptoms that accrue over time, and the characteristic plaques or sclerosed areas that are the hallmark of the disease.

(1) Although MS was first described almost 140 years ago, the cause remains a mystery, and a cure is still unavailable. Nevertheless, many advances have been made in treating and managing the complications of the disease and improving the quality of life of individuals affected by MS.

EPIDEMIOLOGY

Epidemiologic aspects of MS have been reviewed in a variety of publications.[2–5] MS usually is diagnosed in patients between the ages of 15 and 45 years, and the peak incidence occurs in the fourth decade of life. There are approximately 10,000 new cases diagnosed per year in the United States. Women are afflicted more than men by a ratio of approximately 2:1. Men usually develop the first signs of MS at a later age than women and are also more likely to develop the progressive form of the disease. The most important factors in the determination of risk for developing the disease are geography, age, environmental influences, and genetics. In general, disease prevalence is higher the greater the distance from the equator. Within the United States, the prevalence of MS is higher in states above the 37th parallel. Multiple sclerosis occurs more frequently in whites of Scandinavian ancestry than in other ethnic groups.

ETIOLOGY

It is thought that genetically susceptible individuals between the ages of 10 and 15 years who have lived in a high-risk area for at least 2 years exposed to a crucial environmental agent are at risk for developing MS. Interestingly, an individual who migrates from a low- to a high-risk area prior to the age of 15 years acquires the same chance of developing MS as those who live in a high-risk area all their lives.[6] If the move is made from a high- to a low-risk area, the individual retains the high risk if the move is made after the age of

15 years but acquires the lower risk if the move is made prior to this age.[6] Smoking cigarettes has been associated with both an increased risk of acquiring MS and with more severe progression.[5]

Viral or bacterial infections may be an important environmental cause of MS. Although no clear association has been identified, there are several ways in which a virus or bacteria could play a role in the pathogenesis of MS.[7] These infections might cause either a direct attack on myelin and the oligodendrocyte, or stimulation of an autoimmune response leading to demyelination. Evidence to support a viral etiology includes increased immunoglobulin G (IgG) synthesis in the CNS, increased antibody titers to certain viruses, and epidemiologic studies that indicate a childhood exposure factor, suggesting that "viral" infections may precipitate exacerbations. Immunoglobulin patterns in the cerebrospinal fluid (CSF) are similar in subacute sclerosing panencephalitis (SSPE) and MS. SSPE is a chronic measles infection of the CNS known to be associated with the production of oligoclonal bands in the CSF.[8] In addition, viruses have been shown to cause diseases with prolonged incubation periods, myelin destruction, and a relapsing-remitting course in both humans and experimental animal models.[9]

The most compelling evidence against a microbial etiology is the fact that no single infectious agent has been identified as the cause of MS. Many possible agents have been implicated, including mycoplasma, *Chlamydia pneumoniae,* spirochetes, rabies virus, herpes simplex virus, canine distemper virus, coronavirus, human T-cell leukemia virus type I (HTLV-I), MS-associated retrovirus, measles, and most recently, human herpes virus type 6 (HHV-6)[10,11] and Epstein-Barr virus.[12,13] However, to date, no causal relationship has been established.[9]

The familial recurrence rate of MS is approximately 5%, with siblings being the most commonly reported relationship.[4] Concordance data show a higher prevalence of MS between monozygotic than between dizygotic twins, and a recent study has confirmed the overall concordance among monozygotic twins at approximately 25%, with a risk among females of 34% and males just 5%, similar to that seen in dizygotic twins.[14] This is consistent with the idea that an environmental agent is important in the etiology of MS but also suggests a role for one or more genes. Genetic studies have determined an association between MS and the major histocompatibility complex (MHC) and, in particular, with the human leukocyte antigen (HLA) region on the sixth chromosome that is associated with the genetic control of immune mechanisms.[4,15,16] In African Americans, a locus on chromosome one may be associated with increased susceptibility.[17] In addition, a number of genes have been identified that may alter the speed of progression of the illness, such as apolipoprotein E $\varepsilon 4$ homozygosity,[18] although more recent analysis argues against this.[19] Although African Americans are significantly less likely to be diagnosed with MS compared to whites, there is emerging evidence that African Americans are more likely to have a severe disease course[20] and respond less well to interferon therapy than whites.[21]

PATHOPHYSIOLOGY

❷ The basic physiologic derangement in MS is the stripping of the myelin sheath surrounding CNS axons. This is associated with an inflammatory, perivenular infiltrate consisting of variable numbers and amounts of T and B lymphocytes, macrophages, antibodies, and complement. The lesions are referred to as plaques. Initially, axons, although stripped bare of their myelin sheath, usually are well preserved.[22] Recent studies, however, have shown that damage to axons can be significant, even early in the course of the illness.[23] Axonal damage may be seen as a hypointense lesion, or T_1 hole, on MRI, and these correlate with disability.[24]

It is now well-accepted that MS lesions are heterogeneous, but it remains unclear as to whether this represents differences in the stage of evolution of the lesions over time, differences in underlying immunopathogenesis, or a combination of the two. As reviewed by Frohman and colleagues,[25] acute lesions show demyelination and axonal destruction with lymphocytic hypercellularity, extensive macrophages, loss of oligodendrocytes, but an indistinct margin with little astrocytic proliferation. In contrast, more chronic lesions display less inflammatory lymphocytes but ongoing macrophage deposition with hypertrophic astrocytes and oligodendrocytes with active remyelination.

Acute MS lesions can be divided into four immunopathologic subtypes, with variable degrees of sharpness of borders, loss of specific myelin proteins, and variable numbers of immune cells or immunoglobulins present in the plaques. Types I and II are more consistent with the traditional view of MS as an encephalomyelitis, with type II displaying significant deposition of immunoglobulin and complement. Types III and IV, conversely, appear more consistent with an oligodendrogliopathy. All type IV patients studied so far have PPMS, but otherwise, there is no obvious association of immunopathology and clinical type.[26] These studies have also suggested each patient has only a single pathologic subtype within their nervous system, but multiple pathologies have been seen within a single brain by other investigators.[27] Thus, the true extent and nature of MS pathology within and between patients, and over time, remains unclear.

Just as the full dimensions of the neuropathology are uncertain, so is the pathogenesis of the MS plaque. There is substantial evidence, however, to suggest it is an autoimmune process directed against myelin and oligodendrocytes, the cells that make CNS myelin[25] (Fig. 57–1). The actual mediator of myelin and axonal destruction has not been established, but may reflect a combination of macrophages, destructive cytokines, and reactive oxygen intermediates. The exact trigger for the activation of the T cells in the periphery remains unclear, but the T cells recognize myelin basic protein (MBP), proteolipid protein, myelin oligodendrocyte glycoprotein, and myelin-associated glycoprotein in the blood of patients with MS. A reduction in T-suppressor cells, or suppressor activity, has been reported during active MS and in patients with progressive disease; however, a relative increase in the T-helper–to-suppressor ratio is not found consistently and does not always correlate with disease activity. In patients with stable or mild disease, increased numbers of cells are found that express messenger RNA (mRNA) for transforming growth factor-β (TGF-β) and interleukin-10 (IL-10) compared with patients with severe disease. The complex interplay of the variable cells and cytokines remains to be elucidated.

CLINICAL PRESENTATION OF MULTIPLE SCLEROSIS

General

- Most patients with multiple sclerosis present with nonspecific complaints. Many have problems with their vision or paresthesias.

Primary Symptoms/Signs

- Visual complaints/optic neuritis
- Gait problems
- Paresthesias
- Pain
- Spasticity
- Weakness
- Ataxia
- Speech difficulty
- Psychological changes
- Cognitive changes
- Fatigue

- Bowel/bladder dysfunction
- Sexual dysfunction
- Tremor

Laboratory Tests

- MS is a diagnosis of exclusion
- Magnetic resonance imaging
- Cerebrospinal fluid studies
- Evoked potentials

Secondary Symptoms

- Recurrent urinary tract infections
- Urinary calculi
- Decubiti
- Muscle contractures
- Respiratory infections
- Poor nutrition
- Depression

Tertiary Symptoms

- Financial problems
- Personal/social problems
- Vocational problems
- Emotional problems

CLINICAL PRESENTATION

❸ The clinical presentation of MS is extremely variable among patients and typically varies over time in a given patient. The signs and symptoms of MS can be divided into three categories. Primary symptoms are a direct consequence of conduction disturbances produced by demyelination and axonal damage and reflect the area of the brain or spinal cord that is damaged. Secondary symptoms are complications resulting from primary symptoms. For example, urinary retention, a primary symptom, can lead to frequent urinary tract infections, a secondary symptom. Tertiary symptoms relate to the effect of the disease on the patient's everyday life.[28]

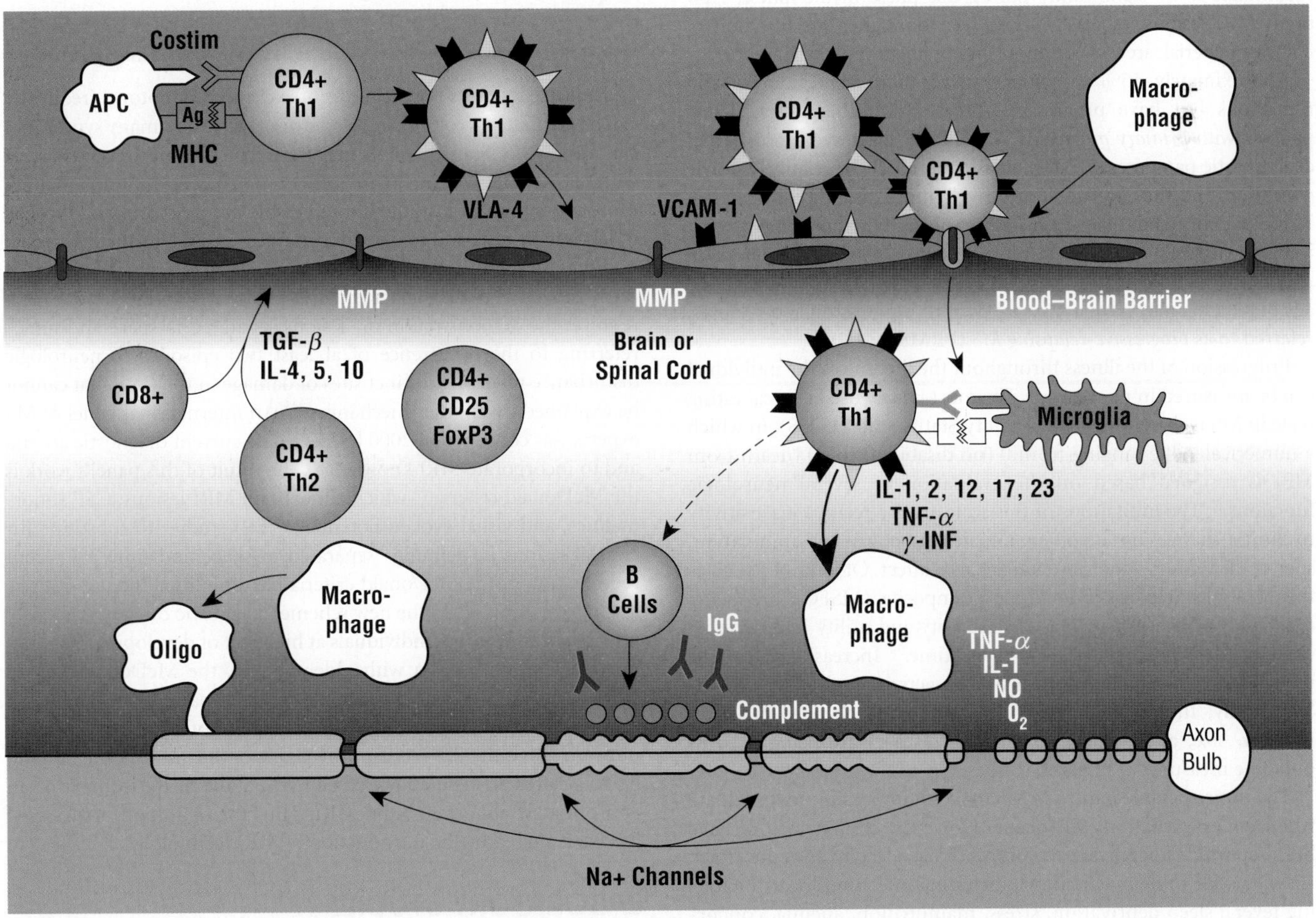

FIGURE 57-1. Autoimmune theory of the pathogenesis of multiple sclerosis (MS). T-helper cells (CD4+) appear to be key initiators of myelin destruction in MS. These autoreactive CD4+ cells, especially of the T-helper cell type 1 (Th1) subtype, are activated in the periphery, perhaps following a viral infection, and express adhesion molecules on their surfaces that allow them to attach and roll along the endothelial cells that constitute the blood-brain barrier. These activated T cells also produce matrix metalloproteinases that help to create openings in the blood-brain barrier, allowing entry of the activated T cells past the blood-brain barrier and into the CNS. Once inside the CNS, the T cells produce pro-inflammatory cytokines, especially interleukins (ILs) 1, 2, 12, 17, and 23, tumor necrosis factor-α (TNF-α), and interferon γ (INF-γ), which further create openings in the blood-brain barrier, allowing entry of B cells, complement, macrophages, and antibodies. The T cells also interact within the CNS with the resident microglia, astrocytes, and macrophages, further enhancing production of proinflammatory cytokines and other potential mediators of CNS damage, including reactive oxygen intermediates and nitric oxide. The role of modulating, or downregulating, cytokines such as IL-4, IL-5, IL-10, and transforming growth factor-β (TGF-β) also has been described. These cytokines are the products of CD4+, CD8+, CD25+, Th1, and FOX P3 regulatory cells. (Ag, antigens; APC, antigen presenting cell; IgG, immunoglobulin G; NA^+, sodium ion; MHC, major histocompatibility complex; VLA, very-late antigen; VCAM, vascular cell adhesion molecule.)

The clinical course of MS is classified into four categories.[29] At the onset of symptoms, about 85% of patients have attacks—new symptoms lasting at least 24 hours and separated from other new symptoms by at least 30 days—followed by remissions (complete or incomplete). Attacks frequently are referred to as *relapses* or *exacerbations,* and the first attack is called a *clinically isolated syndrome* (CIS). This course is called *relapsing-remitting MS* (RRMS). During the RRMS phase, there is a correlation between new brain MRI lesions and clinical attacks, but typically there are many more new MRI lesions than new clinical symptoms. In RRMS patients, attack frequency tends to decrease over time and becomes independent of the development of progressive disabilities.[30] Neurologic recovery following an acute exacerbation is usually quite good early in the disease course, but following repeated relapses, recovery tends to be less complete. Given these features, interpretation and evaluation of potential therapeutic interventions must be done quite cautiously, and control groups are essential in the design of clinical studies.

Up to 10% to 20% of RRMS patients have a benign course, characterized by few relapses, often sensory, with minimal disability accruing over time. Most RRMS patients eventually enter a progressive phase in which attacks and remissions generally are difficult to identify. This is referred to as *secondary-progressive MS* (SPMS). Disability tends to accumulate more significantly during this phase of the illness. New brain MRI lesions, especially those seen only after the injection of contrast material, are less common, and brain atrophy increases.[31]

Approximately 15% of patients never have acute attacks and remissions but have progressive disease from the outset. These patients with *primary progressive MS* (PPMS) have symptoms, especially spastic paraparesis, that may worsen rapidly or relatively slowly over time, and they accrue progressively more disability. In general, PPMS patients tend to have a worse prognosis than those who present initially with RRMS, although more recent data suggest progression may not be as rapid as previously thought.[32] Finally, a small percentage of patients may have a mixture of both progression and relapses, referred to as *progressive-relapsing MS* (PRMS).

Progression of the illness throughout the lifetime of the individual can be measured in many ways. The most widely used clinical rating scale in MS is the Expanded Disability Status Scale (EDSS), in which a numerical value ranging from 0 (no disability) to 10 (death from MS) is assigned based on the evaluation of several neurologic functions.[33] The limitations of this scale are the relative insensitivity to clinical changes not involving impairment of gait and ambulation, such as changes in cognition, fatigue, and affect. Other tools, such as the Multiple Sclerosis Functional Composite (MSFC), are being evaluated for possible increased sensitivity and utility in describing changes in MS-related disability over time.[34] Increasingly, MRI is being used as an index of both disease activity and progression.[35] Specifically, the appearance of new lesions or changes in lesion number, size, and volume (burden of disease) are being used as outcome measures in research studies.

The unpredictable nature of MS makes it impossible to anticipate when an exacerbation will occur. However, certain factors have been reported to aggravate symptoms or even lead to an acute attack (new episode of demyelination), including infections, heat (including fever), sleep deprivation, stress, malnutrition, anemia, concurrent organ dysfunction, exertion, and childbirth.[36] Interestingly, many patients experience a significant reduction in acute relapses during the third trimester of pregnancy, followed by a relative increase postpartum.[36] There are no significant epidemiologic data that support an association between physical trauma and the development or worsening of MS, but this may reflect inadequacy of the studies published to date.[37]

Multiple sclerosis usually does not directly diminish life expectancy. The development of secondary complications such as pneumonia or septicemia (secondary to aspiration of mouth contents with swallowing difficulties, decubitus ulcers, or urinary tract infections) or rapid progression of primary lesions affecting respiratory function can lead to a shorter than expected life span. Most of this decrease in life span is seen in patients with rapidly progressive disease. Suicide rates as high as seven times that expected in the general population have been reported.[38] Clinical and demographic factors that have been used to predict prognosis of MS are listed in Table 57–1.[5,39] Several MRI features also have been shown to correlate with progression of disease (see below).[40–44]

TABLE 57-1 Prognostic Indicators in Multiple Sclerosis

Indicator	Favorable Prognosis	Unfavorable Prognosis
Age at onset	<40 years	>40 years
Gender	Female	Male
Initial symptoms	Optic neuritis or sensory symptoms	Motor or cerebellar symptoms
Attack frequency in early disease	Low	High
Course of disease	Relapsing/remitting	Progressive

Data from Kantarci and Wingerchuk,[5] Swanson,[39] McDonald et al.,[43] and Polman et al.[44]

DIAGNOSIS

❹ Multiple sclerosis is a diagnosis of exclusion; symptoms frequently can be attributed to other neurologic diseases, just as many syndromes can mimic MS. Some patients may have typical symptoms consistent with classic CIS, whereas many others may have symptoms that are more vague. In the past, the unpredictable nature of MS and the lack of laboratory tests and imaging techniques specific for the disease led to difficulties in making this diagnosis, especially in the early stages of the disease. The diagnosis remains primarily a clinical one that requires the demonstration of "lesions separated in space and time," referring to the occurrence of at least two episodes of neurologic disturbance reflecting distinct sites of damage in the CNS that cannot be explained by another mechanism.[43] An international panel of MS experts was convened in 2000 to reevaluate current diagnostic criteria and to incorporate MRI knowledge. The result of this panel's work is the McDonald criteria,[43] which allow brain MRI lesions, CSF abnormalities, and visual evoked potential (VEP) studies to substitute for clinical lesions in defining "separated in space and time." A recent reevaluation of the McDonald criteria has simplified the use of these laboratory studies.[44] In the new scheme, diagnostic categories are MS, possible MS (for those individuals at high risk of developing MS), and not MS. In comparison with older criteria, the McDonald criteria allow for earlier diagnosis.[45] A new consensus panel of the American Association of Neurology endorses the utility of MRI for diagnostic purpose,[46] and the FDA has approved one of the immunotherapies to be used after a single attack of demyelination in the context of an appropriately abnormal brain MRI. Thus the definition of MS itself has been altered by the introduction of MRI technology.

LABORATORY STUDIES

To date, there are no tests specific for MS. Tests that are used frequently include MRI of the brain and spine, CSF evaluation, and evoked potentials. Evidence provided by these studies, used in conjunction with the physical examination and history, aids in establishing the diagnosis of MS.

Imaging Studies

MRI produces images of the brain and spine that reflect damage in the CNS that is characteristic of MS plaques in multiple forms, for instance in the periventricular white matter areas of the brain, as well as more generalized abnormalities such as brain atrophy. MRI is much more sensitive than computed tomography (CT) scans in the detection of MS lesions[47] and is considered the preferred imaging technique. It is extremely helpful for diagnosis and useful for prognosis. Patients with a single, typical attack of demyelination (possible MS or CIS, e.g., optic neuritis) and three or more T_2-weighted lesions on the brain MRI have an almost 90% likelihood of developing a second attack (clinically definite MS) over 15 years.[41] Optic neuritis is a common first symptom of MS and is indicative of a lesion or lesions localizing on the optic nerve. In contrast, similar individuals with normal brain MRIs have only a 19% likelihood of developing MS over 15 years.[41] Total volume of T_2-weighted lesions (called *T_2 burden of disease*) at the onset of CIS also appears to correlate with the development of disability.[47] Lesions that enhance after injection of the contrast material gadolinium indicate new lesions and disruption of the blood-brain barrier and are associated with early conversion to MS in CIS/possible MS patients[48] but do not correlate well over time with progression of disability. Brain atrophy, even early in the course of the illness, probably correlates better with progression of disability.[42]

CSF Evaluation

In MS patients, CNS synthesis of IgG is increased, whereas serum IgG levels are normal. Electrophoretic studies of the CSF show that the IgG separates into a small number of discrete bands, which, when similar bands are not seen in the serum samples taken at the same time, are called *oligoclonal bands* (OCBs).[49] Oligoclonal banding (the presence of two or more oligoclonal bands) of IgG is present in 90% to 95% of patients with clinically definite, established MS but also may be seen in lower percentages of diseases that mimic MS or are quite different clinically.[49] Increasingly, with advances in MRI, CSF analysis is reserved only for patients with atypical clinical scenarios or individuals with possible MS in whom a CSF positive for OCBs may help to define a more definite diagnosis of MS. Although white blood cell counts are often slightly elevated in the CSF of MS patients, the presence of greater than 50×10^6/mL mononuclear cells in the CSF usually indicates a diagnosis other than MS.[49]

Evoked Potentials

Evoked potentials may be helpful in establishing areas of demyelination that are clinically silent. Slowed conduction of visual, brainstem, and somatosensory potentials can be identified, although the sensitivity and specificity of these tests seem to be somewhat less than that seen with MRI or CSF evaluation. Newer diagnostic criteria allow only for the use of VEPs to aid in formal diagnosis.[43,44]

Blood Studies

A recent report has suggested that in CIS patients with abnormal brain MRIs and abnormal CSF consistent with MS, presence or absence of antimyelin antibodies in serum may be helpful in defining prognosis for further events consistent with clinically definite MS.[50] The utility of this test, if any, remains to be defined.

DIFFERENTIAL DIAGNOSIS

A number of disorders can mimic MS. Thus most patients are screened with blood tests for rheumatologic, collagen-vascular, infectious, and sometimes inherited metabolic diseases. MRI may rule out tumors and cervical spondylosis. The use of MRI has led to evaluations for MS in many patients with little or no clinical history consistent with MS; however, almost none of these patients ultimately are diagnosed with MS.[51] There are many causes of nonspecific lesions seen in the subcortical white matter on a brain MRI, and use of established criteria for distinguishing MS lesions from other etiologies (e.g., migraine, hypertension, age older than 50 years, and others) enhances diagnostic accuracy. Electromyography may help in diagnosing amyotrophic lateral sclerosis and neuropathies.

TREATMENT

Multiple Sclerosis

Treatment of MS falls into three broad categories: symptomatic therapy, treatment of acute attacks, and disease-modifying therapies to alter the natural course of the disease. Symptomatic management of the disease is of utmost importance to maintain the patient's quality of life. Treatment of acute attacks will shorten the duration and possibly decrease the severity of the attack. Disease-modifying therapies that alter the course of the illness are most important to diminish progressive disability over time.

A number of different treatment modalities have been studied in the last 30 years, but many older trials had flawed designs. There are no universally accepted treatment algorithms, and treatments vary among clinicians and centers. Perhaps more important, treatment decisions frequently are based on the wishes and goals of individual patients. One potential algorithm for the immunotherapy of RRMS is shown in Fig. 57–2.

CLINICAL CONTROVERSY

When patients initially show signs of RRMS, many practitioners begin treatment with interferon β or glatiramer acetate (ABC-R medications). However, it is controversial which medication to use, and when to start. The role of natalizumab remains unclear. Most practitioners assist patients in making the decision of which medication best fits their lifestyle and offers the maximum efficacy. In patients with severe depression, interferon therapy is contraindicated, and patients are encouraged to use glatiramer acetate. None of the therapies should be used during pregnancy, while attempting to get pregnant, or while breastfeeding.

■ TREATMENT OF ACUTE EXACERBATIONS

❺ Mild acute exacerbations that do not produce functional decline may not require treatment. When functional ability is affected, although treatment suggestions may vary among clinicians, the standard intervention is intravenous injection of high-dose corticosteroids. Results from a large trial of optic neuritis suggest,[52,53] and the American Academy of Neurology recommends,[54] that if treatment with steroids is warranted, it is best to use intravenous methylprednisolone. The mechanism of action for corticosteroids in MS is unknown, but it is speculated that steroids improve recovery by decreasing edema in the area of demyelination. Intravenous methylprednisolone has been shown to shorten the duration of acute exacerbations,[53] and it may delay repeat attacks for up to 2 years after optic neuritis,[54] although it has not been shown definitively to affect the progression of disease.[55] More recently, many practitioners are using high doses of oral methylprednisolone, especially mixing the lyophilized powder in flavored drinks such as smoothies, but there are no comparative data to define this as an equivalent way to deliver the medication.

Methylprednisolone doses can range from 500 to 1,000 mg/day, given intravenously. The duration of therapy is variable and can range from 3 to (rarely) 10 days depending on clinical response. If improvement occurs, it usually begins to be seen after 3 to 5 days. Short-term use of this nature is often accompanied by sleep disturbance, a metallic taste, and rarely gastrointestinal upset. Patients with diabetes mellitus or a predilection to diabetes mellitus may have significant

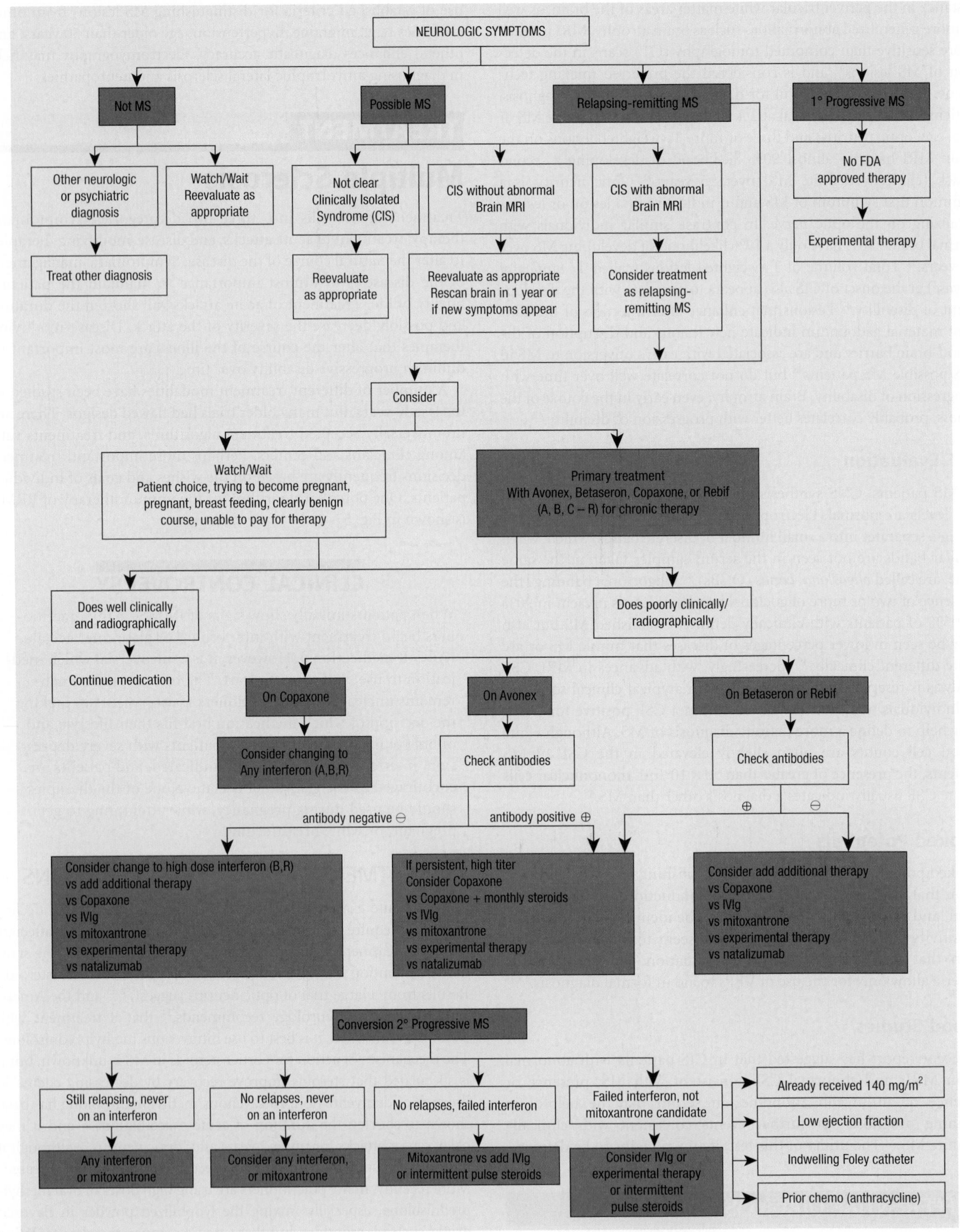

FIGURE 57-2. An algorithm for management of relapsing-remitting multiple sclerosis. (ABC-R, interferon β_{1a} [Avonex], interferon β_{1b} [Betaseron], glatiramer acetate [Copaxone], and interferon β_{1a} [Rebif]; IVIg, intravenous immunoglobulin.)

elevations of blood sugars requiring the use of insulin. Longer durations of intravenous methylprednisolone therapy are associated with acne and fungal infections, mood alteration and rarely, gastrointestinal hemorrhage (especially if used in hospitalized patients or those taking aspirin concurrently).

A very small number of patients have very severe attacks, manifested by hemiplegia, paraplegia, or quadriplegia. If these patients fail to improve with aggressive steroid therapy, plasma exchange every other day for seven treatments can be beneficial for approximately 40% of patients.[56]

CLINICAL CONTROVERSY

If a patient taking interferon decompensates and has high levels of neutralizing antibodies in the blood, most practitioners will stop the medication. In this situation it is controversial whether to rechallenge the patient at a later date with interferon therapy. Many clinicians will only rechallenge with interferon therapy if the patient does not do well on other therapies.

■ DISEASE-MODIFYING THERAPY

Interferon β_{1b} and Interferon β_{1a}

6 Interferon β_{1b} (Betaseron) was the first agent proven to favorably alter the natural history of the illness.[57] In Table 57–2 this agent as well as other disease modifying therapies (DMTs) are listed with evidence-based recommendations from the American Academy of Neurology.[57] Interferon β_{1b} is a nonglycosylated synthetic analog of recombinant interferon β and is produced in *Escherichia coli.* Although the exact mechanism of action is unknown, its effect in MS may be caused by its immunomodulating properties, including the ability to augment suppressor cell function and reduce interferon-γ secretion by activated lymphocytes, its macrophage-activating effect, and its ability to downregulate the expression of interferon-γ–induced class II MHC gene products on antigen-presenting glial cells.[57] Interferon β_{1b} also suppresses T-cell proliferation and may decrease blood-brain barrier permeability.[57] In general, all interferons exert these actions in the periphery and at the blood-brain barrier level. Interferons work at the blood-brain barrier level by decreasing matrix metalloproteinases.

TABLE 57-2 Evidenced-Based Recommendations for Disease Modifying Treatment of Multiple Sclerosis

Recommendations	Recommendation Grades[a]
Interferon β	
• Interferon β has been shown to reduce attack rates in patients with MS or those with CIS who are at high risk of developing MS	A-I
• It is appropriate to consider interferon β for any patient with clinically definite MS or who already has RRMS or SPMS and is still experiencing relapses	A-I
• The effectiveness of interferon β in patients with SPMS but without relapses is uncertain	U-I
• Route of administration of interferon β products is probably not clinically important with regards to efficacy; however, the side effect profile does differ	B-II
• Rate of production of neutralizing antibodies is probably less with interferon β_{1a} than with interferon β_{1b}	B-I
• Presence of neutralizing antibodies may be associated with a reduction in the clinical effectiveness of interferon β treatment	C-I
Glatiramer acetate	
• Glatiramer acetate has been shown to reduce the attack rate in patients with RRMS	A-I
• Treatment with glatiramer acetate may slow sustained disability progression in RRMS	C-I
Mitoxantrone	
• Mitoxantrone probably reduces the attack rate in patients with relapsing forms of MS	B-II, III
• Mitoxantrone may have a beneficial effect on disease progression in MS	C-II, III

CIS, Clinically isolated syndrome; RCT, randomized controlled trial; RRMS, relapsing-remitting MS; SPMS, secondary-progressive MS.

[a]Strength of recommendations: A: established. B: probable. C: possible. U: inadequate data to support recommendation.

Quality of evidence: Class I, evidence from one or more prospective, randomized, controlled clinical trial; Class II, evidence from cohort or RCT not meeting criteria for class I; Class III, evidence from other controlled trials; Class IV, Evidence from uncontrolled studies, case reports, case series or expert opinion.

Reprinted with permission from Goodin et al.[57]

Interferon β_{1b} is administered subcutaneously every other day at a dose of 8 million international units. Clinical trials have demonstrated that at these doses, interferon β_{1b} significantly reduces annual relapse rate and MRI burden of disease compared with placebo. With respect to clinical disability, however, no significant differences were noted between the interferon- and placebo-treated groups.[57] Betaseron is packaged in partially premixed syringes (0.3 mg in 15 prefilled blister units) with a new formulation that does not require refrigeration, and can be used with an autoinjector. Betaseron costs approximately $19,632 per year.

Interferon β_{1a} (Avonex and Rebif) is a natural-sequence glycosylated interferon produced in Chinese hamster ovary cells. Avonex is given as 30 mcg (6 million international units) intramuscularly (IM) once weekly. The prefilled syringes (33 mcg/0.5 mL, 4 per package) should be refrigerated but can be kept at room temperature for 30 days. Avonex costs approximately $18,360 per year. Rebif is made in a very similar fashion as Avonex but given as either 22 or 44 mcg (0.5 mL) subcutaneously three times weekly. It is supplied in a 0.5-mL prefilled syringe with an autoinjector and costs approximately $21,163 per year. Rebif also should be kept refrigerated, but it is stable at room temperature for 30 days.

When given 30 mcg intramuscularly once weekly for two years,[57] patients receiving interferon β_{1a} (Avonex) demonstrated, compared with patients receiving placebo, statistically significant reductions in annual relapse rate (by approximately one-third) as well as disease progression, which was defined as a confirmed decrease of one point on the EDSS. Disease progression also was assessed by MRI studies, and patients receiving active drug had significantly fewer new enhancing lesions compared with placebo-treated patients. Similar results were seen with higher dose (44 mcg), more frequent administration (three times weekly), and subcutaneous injection of interferon β_{1a} (Rebif).[58] Other studies reveal significant effects on slowing brain atrophy[59] and the progression of cognitive decline[60] in patients treated with Avonex. Taken together, these observations show that interferon β possesses significant disease-modifying activity.

Side effects are similar with all the interferons. Baseline complete blood counts, platelet determinations, and liver function tests should be documented before starting therapy, at 1 month, then every 3 months for one year, and every 6 months thereafter. Small percentages of patients develop depressed cell counts and liver enzyme elevations that are usually transient and respond to discontinuation of therapy. Rare patients have developed true liver failure requiring liver transplant, and the package inserts for interferon-β products have been altered, reflecting this risk. The most common adverse effects include injection-site redness, swelling, and rarely necrosis, as well as flu-like symptoms (e.g., fever, chills, myalgias). These symptoms can be mild or severe and are seen in most patients. The flu-like side effects typically occur for up to 24 hours after injection and abate within 1 to 3 months after starting the injections, but they persist in some patients. Injection-site reactions probably are worse with interferon β_{1b}, can occur at any time, and can be lessened by using appropriate injection technique, including site rotation (thighs and buttocks), hydrocortisone cream, applying ice before and after the injection, or use of an autoinjector. Injecting the medications at body temperature (place under armpits) will decrease injection-site pain. Nonsteroidal antiinflammatory agents or acetaminophen taken before and at regular intervals for 24 hours after administration may alleviate the flu-like symptoms. Initiation of one-quarter or one-half the standard dose, and then increasing to full dosage over 1 to 2 months, also may be beneficial in reducing flu-like side effects.[61] Some authors suggest that because of the transient immune activation that can occur following the introduction of interferon β, a short burst of oral prednisone can alleviate some adverse effects.[61]

Less commonly reported side effects include shortness of breath, tachycardia, thyroid dysfunction, and depression. Clinicians must monitor patients carefully for signs of depression and treat accordingly. Although depression is a common finding in MS patients, all the interferons, especially interferon β_{1b}, can produce depressive symptoms. Patients who develop depression should be monitored closely because there can be a risk for suicide. The other side effects usually are transient. Most patients will not feel better or have improvement in symptoms when taking interferons, and many will experience side effects; thus compliance can become a major issue. Finally, safety data on interferon β in pregnancy and lactation are lacking. Abortifacient activity in primates has been noted, however. Until adequate safety data are available, women should be counseled as to appropriate contraception while using these products.

Although the adverse-effect profile of interferon β_{1a} resembles that of interferon β_{1b}, intramuscular interferon β_{1a} (Avonex) may hold several advantages, including markedly fewer local injection-site reactions and once-weekly administration versus subcutaneous injection every other day (or 3 days per week with Rebif).

Glatiramer Acetate (Copaxone)

Glatiramer acetate (Copaxone, formerly known as copolymer-1) is a synthetic polypeptide consisting of L-alanine, L-glutamic acid, L-lysine, and L-tyrosine. Although the precise mechanism of action of this compound is unknown, glatiramer acetate appears to mimic the antigenic properties of MBP.[62] This agent also may act by directly binding to MHC class II receptors and inhibiting binding of MBP peptides to T-cell receptor complexes.[62] Recently, glatiramer acetate has demonstrated that it induces Th2 (anti-inflammatory) lymphocytes in experimental allergic encephalomyelitis (EAE).[62] This is thought to contribute to "bystander" suppression at the site of the MS lesion and thereby reduce inflammation, demyelination, and axonal damage.[63] Glatiramer acetate also may suppress T-cell activation, and recent studies suggest it may be associated with a neuroprotective effect by inducing brain-derived neurotrophic factor.[64]

Given as a daily 20-mg subcutaneous dose, glatiramer acetate appears to have a relatively mild adverse effect profile. Mild pain and pruritus at the injection site are the most frequent patient complaints. Approximately 10% of patients will experience a one-time transient reaction consisting of chest tightness, flushing, and dyspnea beginning several minutes after injection and lasting usually no longer than 20 minutes. If patients have no history or evidence of coronary artery disease, they may be assured these reactions are almost always self-limited and benign. Several adverse effects that have been associated with the interferons, including flu-like symptoms and depression, do not appear to be provoked by glatiramer acetate. Multicenter trials with glatiramer acetate have demonstrated significant reductions in mean annual relapse rate (approximately 29%) that are comparable with the interferons.[57] An extension trial, completed after the original, pivotal 2-year study, suggests that glatiramer acetate may slow the progression of disability in patients with RRMS.[63] Glatiramer acetate also slows development of T_1 holes on brain MRIs,[65] and long-term uncontrolled data show that it remains safe and effective for individuals who continue to take it over 10 years.[66] The annual cost of glatiramer acetate is approximately $19,749 (20 mg/mL in 30 prefilled syringes). The product is stored in the refrigerator but can be kept at room temperature for up to 1 week.

CLINICAL CONTROVERSY

Because of the potential for progressive multifocal leukoencephalopathy (PML), controversy surrounds the proper selection of patients for natalizumab therapy. With the enhanced efficacy of natalizumab over other disease modifying therapies, some clinicians might be tempted to use this drug in patients with early disease and frequent relapses or progressive MS. The limitations imposed by the Tysabri Outreach: Unified Commitment to Health (TOUCH) program make the medication unavailable for these patients.

Natalizumab (Tysabri)

Natalizumab is a partially humanized monoclonal antibody directed at the cell surface adhesion molecule $\alpha_4\beta$-integrin (also known as very-late antigen 1, VLA-1). Natalizumab works by attaching to VLA-1 and blocking its interaction with its ligand on CNS endothelium vascular cell adhesion molecule (VCAM)-1. Thus, activated lymphocytes are denied entry past the blood-brain barrier. In a phase II study, compared to placebo, natalizumab significantly reduced the number of new gadolinium-enhancing lesions by more than 90%, and diminished relapses as well.[67] In a 2-year phase III trial (Atrial Fibrillation Follow-Up Investigation of Rhythm Management [AFFIRM]), compared to placebo, annual relapse rate was reduced by more than 60%, gadolinium-enhancing lesions were lessened by more than 90%, and progression of disability was significantly delayed.[68] In a separate, 2-year, phase III trial (The Safety and Efficacy of Natalizumab in Combination with Interferon Beta-1a in Patients with Relapsing Remitting Multiple Sclerosis [SENTINEL]) in patients already taking interferon β_{1a} (Avonex), those who had natalizumab added to interferon β_{1a} had a relapse rate reduction of more than 50% and gadolinium-enhancing lesion reduction of 84% compared to patients who continued with interferon β_{1a} alone.[69] In these trials natalizumab was injected intravenously every 4 weeks and was relatively well tolerated, although approximately 1% of patients developed infusion reactions, and 6% developed neutralizing antibodies that diminished the efficacy of the drug.

On November 23, 2004, the FDA approved natalizumab, with the stipulation that the studies would continue, for use in relapsing MS in patients with inadequate response or intolerance to other MS therapies. In February 2005, Biogen and Elan voluntarily removed natalizumab from the market after receiving reports of two patients (one patient from the SENTINEL trial, and one patient in a Crohn disease study), who both died after developing PML, a rare brain infection most commonly seen in patients infected with human immunodeficiency virus (HIV).[70–72] One other patient who developed PML in the SENTINEL trial survived.[70–72] Further safety analysis did not identify other cases, and on March 9, 2006, an FDA panel reviewing the data suggested reapproval of natalizumab for use in relapsing patients, who would be required to be placed in an ongoing safety registry (TOUCH). On June 5, 2006, the FDA reapproved use of natalizumab in the United States, and infusions began shortly thereafter.

Natalizumab is indicated as monotherapy, 300 mg every 4 weeks as an infusion. It is indicated for the relapsing forms of MS to delay the accumulation of physical disability and decrease the number of relapses in patients who have a documented inadequate response or intolerance to traditional MS therapies. The wholesale cost of natalizumab is approximately $2,600 per infusion or $31,200 annually (300 mg per 15 mL), which does not include nursing and other fees.[73]

CLINICAL CONTROVERSY

Lifetime exposure to mitoxantrone cannot exceed 140 mg/m^2. This poses a problem when deciding which patients should receive the therapy, as well as when in the disease course they should receive it. Many clinicians feel that treatment should be initiated as soon as the patient meets criteria, whereas others believe therapy should be delayed to not exceed to maximum lifetime dose.

Mitoxantrone

7 Mitoxantrone (Novantrone), a member of the anthracenedione family, is approved by the FDA for reducing neurologic disability and the frequency of clinical relapses in patients with SPMS (chronic), PRMS, or worsening RRMS.[74] The MRI outcomes, however, were not as robust as those typically seen in the trials of relapsing patients alone.[75] Mitoxantrone is administered as a brief (5- to 15-minute) intravenous infusion dosed at 12 mg/m^2 every 3 months. An evaluation

of left ventricular ejection fraction is required prior to administration of each dose and if signs or symptoms of congestive heart failure develop. The maximum allowable lifetime cumulative dose of mitoxantrone is 140 mg/m^2. Other potential side effects noted with this agent are nausea, alopecia, menstrual disorder, amenorrhea, upper respiratory tract infection, urinary tract infection, and leukopenia. The role mitoxantrone will play in the treatment of MS remains unclear because potential cardiac toxicity appears to limit its long-term use. In addition, although patients with SPMS were included in the mitoxantrone in MS (MIMS—Effect of Mitoxantrone on MRI in Progressive MS) trial, resulting in FDA approval for use in SPMS, there was no substudy documenting slowing of progression specifically in this subgroup of patients.[74,75] Thus, support for use of mitoxantrone in this context is less strong.[57] The average wholesale cost of mitoxantrone is approximately $1,982 (average male) or $1,586 (average female) per infusion and will vary based on the patient's body surface area. Nursing, pharmacy, and technical fees must also be added to this estimate.

■ REMAINING QUESTIONS FOR DMT

(8) Despite encouraging results from well-conducted clinical trials, several relevant issues remain. The most important question in the use of the DMTs is when to begin therapy. The Medical Advisory Board of the National Multiple Sclerosis Society has adopted recommendations regarding the use of the current MS DMTs, these are summarized in Table 57–3.[76]

Decisions about the use of any medication rest on determination of the severity of the illness, the efficacy of the medication, and the side effects and costs related to the therapy. Clearly, these drugs slow the course of the illness but do not suppress it completely, and in some individuals, there is no apparent benefit. There is now, however, overwhelming evidence that the vast majority of untreated patients will have progressive disease over time. Pathologic data clearly show that even in acute lesions there is significant axonal damage that is essentially irreversible. MRI data show that 80% to 90% of all new enhancing lesions are asymptomatic, suggesting that a "quiet" clinical course does not necessarily mean there is not ongoing disease activity that ultimately will be reflected in cognitive problems and progressive spastic paraparesis.

TABLE 57-3 Disease Management Consensus Statement

- Initiation of therapy with an interferon β medication (Avonex, Betaseron, Rebif) or glatiramer acetate is advised as soon as possible following a definite diagnosis of MS with active, relapsing disease, and can also be considered for selected patients with a first attack who are at high risk of MS.
- Natalizumab is FDA approved for patients who have had an inadequate response to, or are not able to tolerate other MS therapies.
- Mitoxantrone can be considered for patients with relapsing worsening disease or patients with secondary-progressive MS who are worsening, whether or not relapses are occurring.
- Patients' access to medication should not be limited by the frequency of relapses, age, or level of disability.
- Treatment is not to be stopped during evaluation for continuing treatment.
- Therapy is to be continued indefinitely, unless there is clear lack of benefit, intolerable side effects, new data that reveal other reasons for cessation, or better therapy becomes available.
- Interferon βs (Avonex, Betaseron, Rebif), glatiramer acetate (Copaxone), mitoxantrone (Novantrone), and natalizumab (Tysabri), are all FDA approved for patients with MS and should be included in formularies and covered by third-party payers so that physicians and patients can determine the most appropriate agent on an individual basis.
- Movement from one immunomodulating drug to another should be permitted for medical reasons.
- None of these agents are approved for use in women trying to become pregnant, who are pregnant, or nursing mothers.

Data from Miller et al.[76]

Furthermore, it is now known that very early therapy is effective. In patients with CIS and two or more T_2 lesions on brain MRI (i.e., at high risk for developing clinically definite MS), placebo-controlled studies with all three of the interferon agents have shown significant delay in a second attack and positive outcomes on a variety of MRI measures (BENEFIT = Betaferon in Newly Emerging Multiple Sclerosis for Initial Treatment; CHAMPS = Controlled High Risk Subjects Avonex Multiple Sclerosis Prevention Study; and ETOMS = Early Treatment of Multiple Sclerosis).[77–79] Thus very early therapy is potentially warranted, and interferon β_{1b} and interferon β_{1a} (Avonex) are approved by the FDA after CIS in those with abnormal MRIs consistent with demyelination. The National MS Society recommends that patients with relapsing disease should be placed on Avonex, Betaseron, Copaxone, or Rebif (ABC-R) therapy immediately after the diagnosis.[76]

A second major issue is which drug to use in which patient. There has not been a single, randomized study comparing all four ABC-R drugs with one another in a similar patient population at the same time.[80] The pivotal placebo-controlled trials produced results that were more similar than different when comparing across trials, including a nearly identical one-third reduction in relapse rate for all four drugs over 2 years. There has been speculation for some time, however, that higher dose or more frequent administration of interferon (Rebif or Betaseron) may be more beneficial than the lower dose once-weekly use of interferon (Avonex). To address this issue, two comparative trials of Avonex versus Betaseron (INCOMIN = Independent Comparison of Interferon)[81] and Avonex versus Rebif (EVIDENCE = Evidence of Interferon Dose-Response: European North American Comparative Efficacy)[82] have now been completed. In both cases, Avonex was used in the standard 30 mcg per week intramuscular injection, and the other interferons were used at the usual higher dose, more frequent subcutaneous administration, as in a typical clinical practice. In both studies, there were small but statistically significant differences favoring Betaseron or Rebif in a variety of clinical and MRI measures of efficacy, and it was this short-term (6-month) comparative trial[82] that resulted in FDA approval of Rebif in the United States in 2002. More recently, a randomized, controlled, open-label comparison of interferon β_{1a} at 22 mcg per week versus interferon β_{1b} 250 mcg every other day reported no difference in relapse rate, time to first relapse, or time to sustained progression over a 24 month study.[83] There also have been a variety of other open label comparison trials that were uncontrolled and nonrandomized, and these typically have not shown significant differences in efficacy between the various interferon β products used in the usual manner.

There were many scientific objections to these trials, most important of which was lack of control of dosing versus frequency of administration, absence of blinding of clinical outcomes, and the use of novel primary outcome measures with unclear biologic or clinical significance. In addition, published around the same time was a trial comparing 60 mcg with the standard 30 mcg Avonex in a weekly injection that showed no difference over a 2-year study.[84] Thus, many would conclude there are relatively modest differences between the various interferon preparations, all of which have significant limitations in efficacy, as does glatiramer acetate.

A concern with all three interferon products that further muddies our understanding of the clinical differences between the interferon products is the development of neutralizing antibodies. In clinical trials, 30% to 40% of patients receiving interferon β_{1b} developed antibodies directed against the drug.[85] In these patients, the exacerbation rate was similar to that in placebo-treated patients. In patients on interferon β_{1b} neutralizing antibodies can occur first at 3 to 6 months and up to 18 months. This product tends to be the most antigenic.[85] With interferon β_{1a}, neutralizing antibodies were found in 22% of early trials of Avonex, but later studies reported that only 2% to 5% of treated patients developed antibodies; this decrease was caused by a formulation change of the drug making it the least antigenic.[84,85] Percentages for Rebif are intermediate, therefore moderately antigenic, at approximately 12% and can occur in the first 9 to 15 months of treatment, which is the same time frame for antibody production with Avonex.[58,85,86] The long-term clinical significance of these findings, however, are still not completely clear. Three recent studies, however, have further confirmed the effect of neutralizing antibodies on relapses, MRI lesions, and progression of disability.[86–89] Whether these antibodies are truly cross-reactive between products is unknown, as is the duration during which antibodies can be detected. There are no general consensus guidelines regarding when to test for neutralizing antibodies, which assay to use, or what titer cutoff to apply to patients in clinical settings.[90] An important question is whether production of antibodies might be diminished with treatments such as corticosteroids. Another concern of practitioners is the relationship between active ingredients and varying excipients of interferon therapies and the production of neutralizing antibodies. Significant neutralizing antibodies have not been seen with glatiramer acetate, but neutralizing antibodies are seen in approximately 6% of patients treated with natalizumab, and the antibodies seem to diminish efficacy.[69]

9 We now have experience for more than a decade with MS patients taking DMTs, yet continuing to have more relapses, more lesions on MRI, more disability, and ongoing slippage into SPMS.[91] There is no accepted definition of treatment inadequacy, although the Canadian MS Research Council[92] has suggested a relatively simple approach that incorporates the elements of relapse rate, new MRI lesions, and change on the EDSS. If a patient develops significant and persistent interferon antibodies, movement to a noninterferon (glatiramer acetate, natalizumab, mitoxantrone, or possibly intravenous immunoglobulin) is reasonable. When failing low-dose interferon, options include changing to a higher dose, more frequent administration of interferon, or changing to a noninterferon. A second option is addition of an immunosuppressant agent, such as monthly intravenous methylprednisolone, azathioprine, methotrexate, or mycophenolate. As noted above, the addition of natalizumab to interferon β_{1a} was effective but produced rare cases of PML, and thus this combination will not be used in the future. Small, uncontrolled trials adding mitoxantrone to ABC-R DMT suggest this might be a promising approach for those with ongoing disease activity in spite of DMT. Mitoxantrone or natalizumab will be options for those with relatively severe RRMS, or those who have failed or were intolerant of one or more ABC-R medications.

SYMPTOMATIC MANAGEMENT

10 Many of the symptoms of MS do not require pharmacologic management or do not respond to it. This section covers the primary symptoms in which pharmacologic management may be of benefit (Table 57–4).[28,92–95] See the preceding section (Imaging Studies) on the treatment of acute exacerbations for a discussion on optic neuritis.

Gait Difficulties and Spasticity

Problems with gait can be caused by spasticity, weakness, ataxia, defective proprioception, or a combination of these factors. Spasticity is amenable to pharmacologic intervention, whereas physical therapy may be required in treating gait disturbances owing to any of the other factors. Spasticity is encountered commonly and tends to affect the legs more markedly than the arms. Spasticity can result in falls; however, in the later stages of the disease, the increased muscle tone of a spastic limb often lends strength to patients with underlying weakness. Therefore, when using muscle relaxants, one must be careful not to decrease the tone to an extent that ambulation is actually hindered.[28,93] Baclofen (Lioresal), a γ-aminobutyric acid (GABA) analog, is the preferred agent and usually is started in dosages of 10 mg three times daily and titrated upward to achieve the desired

TABLE 57-4 Treatment of Selected Primary MS Symptoms

Spasticity	Bladder Symptoms	Sensory Symptoms	Fatigue
Baclofen	Propantheline	Carbamazepine	Amantadine
Dantrolene	Oxybutynin	Phenytoin	Antidepressants
Diazepam	Dicyclomine	Amitriptyline or other TCAs	Modafinil
Tizanidine	DDAVP		Methylphenidate
Tiagabine	Self-catheterization	Gabapentin	Dextroamphetamine
Gabapentin	Imipramine or amitriptyline	Lamotrigine	
Pregabalin		Pregabalin	
Botulinum toxin type A	Prazosin		
	Botulinum toxin type A		
	Solifenacin		
	Darifenacin		
	Trospium		
	Hyoscyamine		

DDAVP, desmopressin acetate; TCA, tricyclic antidepressant.
Data from Schapiro,[28] Freedman et al.,[92] Mitchell,[93] Kinn and Larson,[94] and Stenager et al.[95]

response. Most patients achieve a satisfactory response with dosages between 40 and 80 mg/day; however, dosages higher than the recommended daily maximum of 80 mg are required by some patients.[28,93] Continuous intrathecal administration of baclofen may be an option for patients unable to tolerate or unresponsive to oral therapy. Baclofen should not be discontinued abruptly to avoid the possibility of seizures.[93] Small doses of diazepam (Valium) (e.g., 0.5–1 mg) often are added to baclofen in patients in whom optimal response has not been achieved. Tizanidine (Zanaflex) can be added in small dosages to baclofen with sometimes great results and smaller doses of each drug.

Another effective agent, with a different mechanism of action is tizanidine. This short-acting, α-adrenergic agonist acts in the CNS to reduce spasticity by increasing presynaptic inhibition of motor neurons. It appears to have efficacy comparable with that of baclofen.[93] Dosage must be titrated slowly over 2 to 4 weeks, starting with 4 mg at bedtime with adjustments based on clinical response. Effective tolerated dosages have ranged from 2 to 36 mg/day. Sedation, dizziness, and dry mouth are the most commonly reported adverse effects, but hypotension also can occur, as well as a rare but severe hepatotoxicity. In patients who are unable to tolerate baclofen or tizanidine, diazepam (Valium; 2–10 mg/day, clonazepam [Klonopin; 1–3 mg/day]), or dantrolene sodium (Dantrium; 100–400 mg/day), may be considered as alternatives, but they generally are less effective than either baclofen or tizanidine. Mild spasticity also may respond to moderately high doses of gabapentin (Neurontin; 1,800–3,600 mg/day); Tiagabine (Gabitril 8–56 mg/day) may be useful in some patients with spasticity, but side effects can prohibit its use. Pregabalin (Lyrica; 75–300 mg/day) has similar features and mechanism of actions as gabapentin. Although it is approximately three times more potent and does not saturate the L-system transporter system in the gastrointestinal system, it may prove useful in the treatment of spasticity in MS patients.

Botulinum toxin type A (Botox; dose depending on the muscles injected) has been shown to be effective in improving spasticity.[28] The amount of toxin required to exert an effect on spasticity is often too excessive to use safely in the larger muscles; therefore, its use is best limited to smaller areas of focal muscle spasm.

Tremor

Cerebellar symptoms such as tremor can be troubling and difficult to control. Medications that can be helpful include propranolol, primidone, and isoniazid.

Bowel and Bladder Symptoms

Patients commonly complain of incontinence, urgency, frequency, and nocturia, which are indications of a hyperreflexic bladder (i.e., inability to store urine). A number of anticholinergic agents, including oxybutynin chloride (Ditropan; 10–20 mg/day), tolterodine (Detrol; 2–4 mg/day), propantheline bromide (Pro-Banthine; 45–90 mg/day), hyoscyamine (Levsin; 0.75–1.5 mg/day), and dicyclomine hydrochloride (Bentyl; 30–80 mg/day) are used to treat this problem if symptoms are mild. Ditropan is now also available in an extended-release formulation (5 and 10 mg). In addition, tricyclic antidepressants, such as imipramine (Tofranil) and amitriptyline (Elavil), have been used for their anticholinergic properties. With all anticholinergic agents, great care must be used to avoid the problem of constipation, which is worsened by the patient's natural instinct to limit fluid intake (owing to the increasing urge to urinate). Newer medications include antimuscarinic agents such as trospium chloride (Sanctura; 40 mg/day), solifenacin succinate (Vesicare; 5–10 mg/day), and darifenacin hydrobromide (Enablex; 7.5–15 mg/day). As an alternative, the synthetic antidiuretic hormone preparation desmopressin acetate (DDAVP; 0.2–0.6 mg/day) has been reported to be effective in the treatment of urgency and incontinence.[94] Use of DDAVP probably is best limited to bedtime so as to improve sleep and because there can be significant problems with hyponatremia and possible seizures if overused. Patients with significant sphincter dyssynergia may benefit from the oral use of α-adrenergic blockers such as prazosin (Minipress; 10–40 mg/day) or intramuscular use of botulinum toxin type A (Botox; dose depends on the muscles injected).

Intermittent self-catheterization with or without a concomitant anticholinergic agent is recommended in patients with large postvoid urine residual volumes (greater than 100 mL) or when the urinary problem is hyporeflexic in nature (failure to empty). Patients with large postvoid residual volumes are at risk for developing urinary tract infections (UTIs) and often are prescribed urinary acidifiers such as vitamin C or antiseptics such as methenamine mandelate to prevent infections. Antibiotics used for UTI prophylaxis include sulfamethoxazole/trimethoprim, cephalexin, cinoxacin, and nitrofurantoin.

Constipation is the most common bowel complaint. Increases in dietary fiber and hydration may alleviate this problem, but in some instances laxatives or enemas may be necessary.[28]

CLINICAL CONTROVERSY

In a depressed patient with a new diagnosis of MS, it is controversial whether to start interferon therapy because depression is a side effect of the interferon therapies, and the incidence of suicide is higher in this population. Practitioners generally start depressed MS patients on an antidepressant along with the interferon and monitor them closely. Interferon should never be started in a severely depressed patient.

Major Depression

Major depression is common in patients with MS, and the risk of suicide may be increased markedly compared with healthy subjects.[95] Patients should be monitored closely for the development of major depressive symptomatology and treated accordingly (see Chap. 71). Interferon products should be used cautiously in patients with significant depression.

Sensory Symptoms

Numbness and paresthesia are frequent sensory complaints but usually do not require treatment. Some MS patients may develop acute or chronic pain syndromes,[93] such as trigeminal neuralgia and painful dysesthesias, for which treatment is necessary. Carbamazepine (Tegretol; 400–1,200 mg/day) is the preferred agent for the treatment of trigeminal neuralgia, and it is used in the same doses that are used for the treatment of seizure disorders.

Sexual Dysfunction

Sexual dysfunction in both men and women are common in MS, and counseling should be offered to both partners. Sildenafil citrate (Viagra), tadalafil (Cialis), and vardenafil (Levitra) are very effective for men with MS who have erectile dysfunction. Other options for men include alprostadil injection (Caverject) or intraurethral suppositories (MUSE). Viagra is currently being studied in the female population with MS and sexual dysfunction.

Fatigue

Fatigue, one of the most common complaints in MS patients, can be severely disabling, but treatment is often overlooked. Typically present in the late to middle afternoon, it can increase with heat exposure, exertion, intercurrent infection, spasticity, weakness, and depression. Amantadine hydrochloride (100 mg twice daily) is used often and may offer significant relief.[28,92] Pemoline (Cylert), a commonly used therapy, was voluntarily withdrawn from the U.S. market by all manufacturers in late 2005 because of increased risk of liver toxicity. Methylphenidate (Ritalin) and dextroamphetamine (Dexedrine) are used commonly for fatigue in MS. Modafinil (Provigil), at 100 mg twice daily, is helpful for MS-related fatigue.

The aminopyridines, 4-aminopyridine and 3,4-diaminopyridine,[96] are potassium channel blockers that are currently under investigation in the symptomatic treatment of MS. These agents may improve conduction in demyelinated axons and may improve strength and decrease heat sensitivity.

COMPLEMENTARY AND ALTERNATIVE THERAPIES FOR MS

A large percentage of patients with MS use complementary and alternative medicine (CAM) instead of, or in addition to, disease-modifying and symptomatic therapies. Common CAM therapies include diet and dietary supplements, such as vitamins, minerals, and herbs. Antioxidant supplements vitamin A, C, E, α-lipoic acid (ALA), coenzyme Q10 (CoQ_{10}), grape seed, and pine bark extracts have suggestive evidence of benefiting MS patients by making them "feel better overall." However, for patients with MS, there is a theoretical risk involved with taking antioxidant supplements owing to their ability to stimulate the immune system (T cells and macrophages). Stimulating the immune system in patients with MS could be counterproductive, possibly worsening or exacerbating their disease, and may counteract the effects of immunomodulators. Other immune-stimulating supplements that should be used with caution are garlic, ginseng (Asian and Siberian), echinacea, cat's claw, astragalus, alfalfa, and stinging nettle. A few agents that may pose a problem in MS but may have benefit are zinc, melatonin (for insomnia), and dehydroepiandrosterone (DHEA).[97]

In general, there is insufficient data supporting the effectiveness and safety of CAM therapies for MS. However, for patients with MS who are willing to try new approaches with limited evidence, CAM may be a consideration in some cases. Healthcare providers can be a source of objective information regarding the use of CAM for MS and can assist their patients in making the best decision.[97]

PHARMACOECONOMIC CONSIDERATIONS

As with many therapeutic decisions, economic cost, both to the individual and to society, must be considered. Currently, the annual cost of the new potentially disease-modifying therapies is considerable. The Red Book average wholesale price (used for all products in this chapter) of Avonex and each of the currently available interferons is between \$18,000 and \$21,100 per patient per year. Given this expense, it must be remembered that these therapies are not curative and that individual patients may experience variable results. Future investigations evaluating these therapeutic modalities clearly will need to address not only clinical but also economic and humanistic outcomes.

EVALUATION OF THERAPEUTIC OUTCOMES

Response to treatment of acute exacerbations of MS is seen commonly within days. With respect to DMTs, it is important for the clinician to recognize that over the short term (days to weeks), little or no apparent benefit may be noted by either patient or clinician. Evaluation of therapeutic outcomes, such as decreased MS exacerbations and hospitalizations or perhaps slowed disease progression and disability (as measured using scales such as EDSS), must be conducted over a period of months to years. Patients should be provided with realistic goals and expectations of these treatment options and encouraged to participate in the evaluation of therapeutic response. Initially, it may be important to reevaluate patients at relatively short time intervals to monitor for adverse effects.

Safety monitoring of patients on interferon includes regular laboratory monitoring, patient observation, and questioning for adverse effects or changing disability, and regular neurologic examinations. Specific laboratory monitoring for individuals on interferon therapy should include a complete blood count, platelet count, and liver function tests. These should be completed at baseline, every 3 months for 1 year, and every 6 months yearly thereafter. Glatiramer acetate requires no laboratory monitoring. In addition to counseling patients regarding the adverse effects associated with these drugs, pharmacists should actively encourage patients to comply with their prescribed regimens.

CONCLUSIONS

Multiple sclerosis is an inflammatory disease of the CNS that strikes young, genetically susceptible individuals living in high-risk geographic areas. Although the exact etiology of MS is unknown, it is likely that MS is an autoimmune disease triggered by an as yet undetermined environmental agent or agents. There is no cure, but quality of life can be improved through symptomatic management, and the disease course is partially suppressed by presently available DMTs.

ACKNOWLEDGMENT

The authors acknowledge the contributions of Sarah Johnson, PharmD, Leann Nguyen, PharmD, Katherine Hays, PharmD, Christien Paynter, PharmD, Kai Davids, PharmD, Kevin Fanciulli, and Eugene Medley, MS, Khaloud Alsilmi, BS Pharm, and Joan Kaufman, illustrator, for their contributions to this chapter.

ABBREVIATIONS

ABC-R: Avonex, Betaseron, Copaxone, and Rebif
CAM: complementary or alternative medicine
CIS: clinically isolated syndrome
CNS: central nervous system
CSF: cerebrospinal fluid
CT scan: computed tomographic scan
DDAVP: desmopressin
DHEA: dehydroepiandrosterone
DMT: disease modifying therapy
EAE: experimental allergic encephalomyelitis
EDSS: expanded disability status scale
FDA: food and drug administration
GABA: γ-aminobutyric acid
HHV-6: human herpes virus type 6
HIV: human immunodeficiency virus
HLA: human leukocyte antigen
HTLV: human T-cell leukemia virus
IgG: immunoglobulin G
IL-2: interleukin-2
IL-10: interleukin-10
MHC: major histocompatibility complex
MIMS: Effect of Mitoxantrone on MRI in Progressive MS (trial)
MRI: magnetic resonance imaging
MS: multiple sclerosis
MSFC: Multiple Sclerosis Functional Composite
OCBs: oligoclonal bands
PML: progressive multifocal leukoencephalopathy
PPMS: primary-progressive multiple sclerosis
PRMS: primary-relapsing multiple sclerosis
RRMS: relapsing-remitting multiple sclerosis
SPMS: secondary-progressive multiple sclerosis
SSPE: subacute sclerosing panencephalitis
TGF-β: transforming growth factor-β
UTI: urinary tract infection
VEP: visual evoked potential
VLA-1: very late antigen 1

REFERENCES

1. Anderson DW, Ellenberg JH, Leventhal CM, et al. Revised estimate of the prevalence of multiple sclerosis in the United States. Ann Neurol 1992;31:333–336.
2. Sadovnick AD, Ebers GC. Epidemiology of multiple sclerosis: A critical overview. Can J Neurol Sci 1993;20:17–29.
3. Kurtzke JF. Epidemiologic contributions to multiple sclerosis: An overview. Neurology 1980;30(Suppl 2):61–79.
4. Compston A. The epidemiology of multiple sclerosis: Principles, achievements, and recommendations. Ann Neurol 1994;36:S211–S217.
5. Kantarci O, Wingerchuk D. Epidemiology and natural history of multiple sclerosis: New insights. Curr Opin Neurol 2006;19:248–254.
6. Detels R, Visscher BR, Haile RW, et al. Multiple sclerosis and age at migration. Am J Epidemiol 1978;108:386–393.
7. Fujinami RS, von Herrath MG, Christen U, et al. Molecular mimicry, bystander activation, or viral persistence; infections and autoimmune disease. Clin Microbiol Rev 2006;19:80–94.
8. Smith-Jensen T, Burgoon M, Anthony J, et al. Comparison of immunoglobulin G heavy-chain sequences in MS and SSPE brains reveals an antigen-driven response. Neurology 2000;54:1227–1232.
9. Johnson RT. The virology of demyelinating diseases. Ann Neurol 1994;36:S54–S60.
10. Berti R, Soldan SS, Akhyani N, et al. Extended observations on the association of HHV-6 and multiple sclerosis. J Neurovirol 2000;6(Suppl 2):S85–S87.
11. Opsahl ML, Kennedy PG. Early and late HHV-6 gene transcripts in multiple sclerosis lesions and normal appearing white matter. Brain 2005;128:516–527.
12. Buljevac D, van Doornum GJ, Flach HZ, et al. Epstein-Barr virus and disease activity in multiple sclerosis. J Neurol Neurosurg Psychiatry 2005;10:1377–1381.

13. Levin LI, Munger KL, Rubertone MV, et al. Temporal relationship between elevation of Epstein-Barr virus antibody titers and initial onset of neurological symptoms in multiple sclerosis. JAMA 2005;293:2496–2500.
14. Willer CJ, Dyment DA, Risch, et al. Twin concordance and sibling recurrence rates in multiple sclerosis. Proc Natl Acad Sci U S A 2003;100:12877–12882.
15. Hillert J. Human leukocyte antigen studies in multiple sclerosis. Ann Neurol 1994;36:S15–S17.
16. Fierz W. Genetics and immunology. In: Kesselring J, ed. Multiple Sclerosis. Cambridge: Cambridge University Press, 1997:30–48.
17. Reich D, Patterson N, DeJager PL, et al. A whole-genome admixture scan finds a candidate locus for multiple sclerosis susceptibility. Nat Genet 2005;37:1113–1118.
18. Chapman J, Vinokurov S, Achiron A, et al. APOE genotype is a major predictor of long-term progression of disability in MS. Neurology 2001;56:2148–2149.
19. Burwick RM, Ramsay PP, Haines JL, et al. APOE epsilon variation in multiple sclerosis susceptibility and disease severity: Some answers. Neurology 2006;66:1373–1383.
20. Cree BA, Khan O, Bourdette D, et al. Clinical characteristics of African Americans versus Caucasian Americans with multiple sclerosis. Neurology 2004;63:2039–2045.
21. Cree BA, Al-Sabbagh A, Bennett R, et al. Response to interferon beta-1a treatment in African American multiple sclerosis patients. Arch Neurol 2005;62:1681–1683.
22. Sobel RA. The pathology of multiple sclerosis. Neurol Clin 1995;13:1–16.
23. Trapp BD, Peterson J, Ransohoff RM, et al. Axonal transection in the lesions of multiple sclerosis. N Engl J Med 1998;338:278–285.
24. Truyen L, van Wuesberghe JHTM, Barkof F, et al. Accumulation of hypointense lesions ("black holes") on T_1 spin echo MRI correlates with disease progression in multiple sclerosis. Neurology 1996;47:1469–1476.
25. Frohman EM, Racke MK, Raine CS. Multiple sclerosis—The plaque and its pathogenesis. N Engl J Med 2006;354:942–955.
26. Lucchinetti C, Bruck W, Parisi J, et al. Heterogeneity of multiple sclerosis lesions: Implications for the pathogenesis of demyelination. Ann Neurology 2000;47:707–717.
27. Barnett MH, Prineas JW. Relapsing and remitting multiple sclerosis: Pathology of the newly forming lesion. Ann Neurol 2004;55:458–468.
28. Schapiro RT. Managing symptoms of multiple sclerosis. Neurol Clin 2005;23:177–187.
29. Weinshenker BG. Natural history of multiple sclerosis. Ann Neurol 1994;36:S6–S11.
30. Confavreux C, Vukusic S, Moreau T, et al. Relapses and progression of disability in multiple sclerosis. N Engl J Med 2000;343:1430–1438.
31. Zivadinov R, Zorzon M. Is gadolinium enhancement predictive of the development of brain atrophy in multiple sclerosis? A review of the literature. J Neuroimag 2002;12:302–309.
32. Tremlett H, Paty D, Devonshire V. The natural history of primary progressive MS in British Columbia, Canada. Neurology 2005;65:1919–1923.
33. Kurtzke JF. Rating neurologic impairment in multiple sclerosis: An expanded disability status scale (EDSS). Neurology 1983;33:1444–1452.
34. Rudick RA, Cutter G, Reingold S. The multiple sclerosis functional composite: A new clinical outcome measure for multiple sclerosis trials. Mult Scler 2002;8:359–365.
35. Miller DH. Magnetic resonance imaging in monitoring the treatment of multiple sclerosis. Ann Neurol 1994;36:S91–S94.
36. Abramsky O. Pregnancy and multiple sclerosis. Ann Neurol 1994;36:S38–S41.
37. Goodin DS, Ebers GC, Johnson KP, et al. The relationship of MS to physical trauma and psychological stress: Report of the Therapeutics and Technology Assessment Subcommittee of the American Academy of Neurology. Neurology 1999;52:1737–1745.
38. Sadovnick AD, Eisen K, Ebers GC, Paty DW. Cause of death in patients attending multiple sclerosis clinics. Neurology 1991;41:1193–1196.
39. Swanson JW. Multiple sclerosis: Update in diagnosis and review of prognostic factors. Mayo Clin Proc 1989;64:577–586.
40. Filippi M, Paty DW, Kappos L, et al. Correlations between changes in disability and T_2-weighted brain activity in multiple sclerosis: A follow-up study. Neurology 1995;45:255–260.
41. Brex PA, Ciccarelli O, Riordan J, et al. A longitudinal study of abnormalities on MRI and disability from multiple sclerosis. N Engl J Med 2002;346:158–164.
42. Fisher E, Rudick R, Simon J, et al. Eight-year follow-up study of brain atrophy in patients with MS. Neurology 2002;59:1412–1420.
43. McDonald W, Compston A, Edan G, et al. Recommended diagnostic criteria for multiple sclerosis: Guidelines from the international panel on diagnosis of multiple sclerosis. Ann Neurol 2001;50:121–127.
44. Polman CH, Reingold SC, Edan G, et al. Diagnostic criteria for multiple sclerosis: 2005 revisions to the "McDonald Criteria." Ann Neurol 2005;58:840–846.
45. Dalton C, Brex P, Miszkiel K, et al. New T_2 lesions enable an earlier diagnosis of multiple sclerosis in clinically isolated syndromes. Ann Neurol 2003;53:673–676.
46. Frohman EM, Goodin DS, Calabresi PA, et al. The utility of MRI in suspected MS. Report of the Therapeutics and Technology Assessment Subcommittee of the American Academy of Neurology. Neurology 2003;61:1332–1338.
47. O'Riordan JI, Thompson AJ, Kingsley DP, et al. The prognostic value of brain MRI in clinically isolated syndromes of the CNS. A 10-year follow-up. Brain 1998;121:495–503.
48. CHAMPS Study Group. MRI predictors of early conversion to clinically definite MS in the CHAMPS placebo group. Neurology 2002;59:998–1005.
49. Olsson T. Cerebrospinal fluid. Ann Neurol 1994;36:S100–S102.
50. Berger T, Rubner P, Schautzer F, et al. Antimyelin antibodies as a predictor of clinically definite multiple sclerosis after a first demyelinating event. N Engl J Med 2003;349:139–145.
51. Carmosino MJ, Brousseau KM, Arciniegas DB, et al. Initial evaluations for multiple sclerosis in a university multiple sclerosis center: Outcomes and role of magnetic resonance imaging in referral. Arch Neurol 2005;62:585–590.
52. Beck RW, Cleary PA, Anderson MM, et al. A randomized, controlled trial of corticosteroids in the treatment of acute optic neuritis. The Optic Neuritis Study Group. N Engl J Med 1992;326;581–585.
53. Beck RW, Cleary PA, Trobe JD, et al. The effect of corticosteroids for acute optic neuritis on the subsequent development of multiple sclerosis. The Optic Neuritis Study Group. N Engl J Med 1993;329:1764–1769.
54. Kaufman DI, Trobe JD, Eggenberger ER, Whitaker JN. Practice parameter: The role of corticosteroids in the management of acute monosymptomatic optic neuritis. Report of the quality standards subcommittee of the American Academy of Neurology. Neurology 2000;54:2039–2044.
55. Zivadinov R, Rudick RA, De Masi R, et al. Effects of IV methylprednisolone on brain atrophy in relapsing-remitting MS. Neurology 2001;57:1239–1247.
56. Weinshenker BG, O'Brian PC, Petterson TM, et al. A randomized trial of plasma exchange in acute central nervous system inflammatory demyelinating disease. Ann Neurol 1999;46:878–886.
57. Goodin DS, Frohman EM, Garmany GP, et al. Disease-modifying therapies in multiple sclerosis: Report of the therapeutics and technology assessment subcommittee of the American Academy of Neurology and the Multiple Sclerosis Council for Clinical Practice Guidelines. Neurology 2002;58:169–178.
58. PRISMS Study Group and the University of British Columbia MS/MRI Analysis Group. PRISMS-4: Long-term efficacy of interferon-β-1a in relapsing MS. Neurology 2001;56:1628–1636.
59. Simon JH, Jacobs L, Campion M, et al. A longitudinal study of brain atrophy in relapsing MS. Neurology 1999;58:139–145.
60. Fischer JS, Priore RL, Jacobs LD, et al. Neuropsychological effects of interferon-β-la in relapsing multiple sclerosis. Ann Neurol 2000;48:885–892.
61. Frohman E, Phillips T, Kokel K, et al. Disease-modifying therapy in multiple sclerosis: Strategies for optimizing management. Neurology 2002;8:227–236.
62. Aharoni R, Teitelbaum D, Sela M, et al. Copolymer 1 induces T cells of the T helper type 2 that cross-react with myelin basic protein and suppress experimental autoimmune encephalomyelitis. Proc Natl Acad Sci U S A 1997;94:10821–10826.
63. Johnson KP, Brooks BR, Cohen JA, et al. Extended use of glatiramer acetate (Copaxone) is well tolerated and maintains its clinical effect on multiple sclerosis relapse rate and degree of disability. Neurology 1998;50:701–708.

64. Azoulay D, Vachapova V, Shihman B, et al. Lower brain-derived neurotrophic factor in serum of relapsing remitting MS. reversal by glatiramer acetate. J Neuroimmunol 2005;167:215–218.
65. Fillippi M, Rovaris M, Rocca MA, et al. Glatiramer acetate reduces the proportion of new MS lesions evolving into "black holes." Neurology 2001;57:731–733.
66. Ford CC, Johnson KP, Lisak RP, et al. A prospective open-label study of glatiramer acetate: over a decade of continuous use in multiple sclerosis patients. Mult Scler 2006;12:309–320.
67. Miller DH, Khan OA, Sheremata WA, et al. A controlled trial of natalizumab for relapsing multiple sclerosis. N Engl J Med 2003;348:15–23.
68. Polman CH, O'Conor PW, Havrdova E, et al. A randomized, placebo-controlled trial of natalizumab for relapsing multiple sclerosis (AFFIRM). N Engl J Med 2006;354:899–910.
69. Rudick RA, Stuart WH, Calabresi PA, et al. Natalizumab plus interferon beta-1a for relapsing multiple sclerosis (SENTINEL). N Engl J Med 2006;354:911–923.
70. Kleinschmidt-DeMasters BK, Tyler KL Progressive multifocal leukoencephalopathy complicating treatment with natalizumab and interferon beta-1a for multiple-sclerosis. N Engl J Med 2005:353;369–374.
71. Langer-Gould A, Atlas SW, Green AJ, et al. Progressive multifocal leukoencephalopathy in a patient treated with natalizumab. N Engl J Med 2005;353:375–381.
72. Van Assche G, Van Ranst M, Sclot R, et al. Progressive multifocal leukoencephalopathy after natalizumab therapy for Crohn's disease. N Engl J Med 2005;353:362–368.
73. Sweat B. Natalizumab update. Am J Health Syst Pharm 2007;64:705–716.
74. Hartung HP, Gonsette R, Konig N, et al. Mitoxantrone in progressive multiple sclerosis, a placebo-controlled, double-blind, randomized, multicentre trial. Lancet 2002;360:2018–2025.
75. Krapf H, Morrissey SP, Zenker O, et al. Effect of mitoxantrone on MRI in progressive MS. Results of the MIMS trial. Neurology 2005;65:690–695.
76. Miller A, Lisak R, Bohen B, et al. National Multiple Sclerosis Society (NMSS). Disease Management Consensus Statement: Expert Opinion Paper. New York: National MS Society, June 20, 2007:1–8, *http://www.nationalmssociety.org/docs/HOM/Exp_Consensus.pdf*
77. Freedman MS, Kappos L, Polman CH, et al. Betaseron in newly emerging multiple sclerosis for initial treatment (BENEFIT): clinical outcomes. Neurology 2006; June 2006(Suppl 2):A61.
78. Jacobs LD, Beck RW, Simon JH, et al. Intramuscular interferon-β-1a therapy initiated during a first demyelinating event in multiple sclerosis (CHAMPS). N Engl J Med 2000;343:898–904.
79. Comi G, Filippi M, Barkhof F, et al. Effect of early interferon treatment on conversion to definite multiple sclerosis: A randomised study (ETOMS). Lancet 2001;357:1576–1582.
80. Vartanian T. An examination of the results of the EVIDENCE, INCOMIN, and phase III studies of interferon beta products in the treatment of multiple sclerosis. Clin Ther 2003;1:105–118.
81. Durelli L, Verdun E, Bergui M, et al. Every-other-day interferon-β-1b versus once-weekly interferon-β-1a for multiple sclerosis: Results of a 2-year prospective randomized multicentre study (INCOMIN). Lancet 2002;359:1453–1460.
82. Panitch H, Goodin D, Francis G, et al. Randomized, comparative study of interferon-β-1a treatment regimens in MS. The EVIDENCE Trial. Neurology 2002;59:1496–1506.
83. Koch-Henriksen N, Sorensen PS, Christensen T, et al. A randomized study of two interferon-beta treatments in relapsing-remitting multiple sclerosis. Neurology 2006;66:1056–1060.
84. Clanet M, Radue E, Kappos L, et al. A randomized, double-blind, dose-comparison study of weekly interferon-β-1a in relapsing MS. Neurology 2002;59:1507–1517.
85. Namaka M, Pollitt-Smith M, Gupta A, et al. The clinical importance of neutralizing antibodies in relapsing-remitting multiple sclerosis. Curr Med Res Opin 2006;22:223–239.
86. Bertolotto A. Neutralizing antibodies to interferon beta: Implications for the management of multiple sclerosis. Curr Opin Neurol 2004;17:241–246.
87. Francis GS, Rice GP, Alsop JC, et al. Interferon beta 1a in MS. results following development of neutralizing antibodies in PRISMS. Neurology 2005;65:48–55.
88. Kappos L, Clanet M, Sandberg-Wollheim M, et al. Neutralizing antibodies and efficacy of interferon beta-1a: A 4-year controlled study. Neurology 2005;65:40–47.
89. Giovannoni G, Goodman A. Neutralizing anti-IFN-beta antibodies: How much more evidence do we need to use them in practice? Neurology 2005;65:6–8.
90. Goodin DS, Frohman EM, Hurwitz B, et al. Neutralizing antibodies to interferon beta: Assessment of their clinical and radiographic impact: An evidence report. Neurology 2007;67:977–984.
91. Kappos L, Polman C, Pozzilli C, et al. Final analysis of the European multicenter trial on IFNβ-1b in secondary-progressive MS. Neurology 2001;57:1969–1975.
92. Freedman MS, Patry DG, Grand'Maison F, et al. Treatment optimization in multiple sclerosis. Can J Neurol Sci 2004;31:157–168.
93. Mitchell G. Update on multiple sclerosis therapy. Med Clin North Am 1993;77:231–249.
94. Kinn AC, Larsson PO. Desmopressin: A new principle for symptomatic treatment of urgency and incontinence in patients with multiple sclerosis. Scand J Urol Nephrol 1990;24:109–112.
95. Stenager EN, Stenager E, Koch Henriksen N, et al. Suicide and multiple sclerosis: An epidemiological investigation. J Neurol Neurosurg Psychiatry 1992;55:542–545.
96. Beaver CT Jr. The current status of studies of aminopyridine in patients with multiple sclerosis. Ann Neurol 1994;36:S118–S121.
97. Bowling AC. Complementary and alternative medicine in multiple sclerosis, 2nd ed. New York: Demos, 2007.

CHAPTER 58

Epilepsy

SUSAN J. ROGERS AND JOSE E. CAVAZOS

KEY CONCEPTS

1. Patient-specific treatment goals should be identified. Treatment goals can change over time. In general, the goal of treatment should be that the patient be free of seizures and have no adverse effects.
2. Accurate diagnosis and classification of seizure/syndrome type is critical to selection of appropriate pharmacotherapy.
3. Patient characteristics such as age, comorbid conditions, ability to comply with the prescribed regimen, and presence or absence of insurance coverage also can influence the choice of antiepileptic drugs.
4. Pharmacotherapy of epilepsy is highly individualized and requires titration of dose to optimize antiepileptic drug therapy (maximal seizure control with minimal or no side effects). Approximately 50% to 70% of patients can be maintained on one antiepileptic drug.
5. If the therapeutic goal (freedom from seizures and minimal to no adverse effects) is not achieved with monotherapy, a second drug can be added or a switch to an alternative single antiepileptic drug can be made. It is suggested that the second antiepileptic drug should have a different mechanism of action from the first, although there is no evidence in humans to support this.
6. Some patients eventually can discontinue antiepileptic drug therapy. Several factors predict successful withdrawal of antiepileptic drugs.
7. The appropriate use of antiepileptic drugs requires a thorough understanding of their clinical pharmacology, for example, mechanism of action, pharmacokinetics, adverse reaction, dosage forms, and drug interactions.

Epilepsy is a disorder that is best viewed as a symptom of disturbed electrical activity in the brain, which may be caused by a wide variety of etiologies. It is a collection of many different types of seizures that vary widely in severity, appearance, cause, consequence, and management. Seizures that are prolonged or repetitive can be life-threatening. The effect epilepsy has on patients' lives can be significant and extremely frustrating. Indeed, studies have shown that patients with epilepsy who do not experience complete seizure control have lower self-reported quality-of-life scores than patients who are seizure-free. It is also important to recognize that seizures can be just one (albeit the most obvious) symptom of an epileptic disorder. Not uncommonly, patients have other comorbid disorders, including depression, anxiety, and potentially neuroendocrine disturbances. Patients with epilepsy also may display neurodevelopmental delay, memory problems, and/or cognitive impairment. Although, by convention, the focus of drug treatment is on the abolition of seizures, clinicians also need be attentive to addressing these common comorbidities.

Learning objectives, review questions,
and other resources can be found at
www.pharmacotherapyonline.com.

EPIDEMIOLOGY

Each year, 120 per 100,000 people in the United States come to medical attention because of a newly recognized seizure.[1] At least 8% of the general population will have at least one seizure in a lifetime. However, it is common to have a seizure and not have epilepsy. The rate of recurrence of a first unprovoked seizure within 5 years ranges between 23% and 80%. Children with an idiopathic first seizure and a normal electroencephalogram (EEG) have a particularly favorable prognosis. Some seizures occur as single events resulting from withdrawal of central nervous system (CNS) depressants (e.g., alcohol, barbiturates, and other drugs) or during acute neurologic illnesses or systemic toxic conditions (e.g., uremia or eclampsia). Some patients will have seizures only associated with fever. These febrile seizures do not constitute epilepsy.[1]

Epilepsy is a chronic disorder characterized by recurrent unprovoked seizures.[1] The age-adjusted incidence of epilepsy is 44 per 100,000 person-years. Each year, approximately 125,000 new epilepsy cases occur in the United States; only 30% are in people younger than 18 years of age at the time of diagnosis. There is a bimodal distribution in the occurrence of the first seizure, with one peak occurring in newborn and young children and the second peak occurring in patients older than 65 years of age. The relatively high frequency of epilepsy in the elderly is now being recognized.

ETIOLOGY

Seizures occur because a group of cortical neurons discharge abnormally in synchrony. Anything that disrupts the normal homeostasis of neurons and their stability can trigger hyperexcitability and seizures. There are thousands of medical conditions that can cause epilepsy, from genetic mutations to traumatic brain injury. A genetic predisposition to seizures has been observed in many forms of primary generalized epilepsy. Patients with mental retardation, cerebral palsy, head injury, or strokes are at an increased risk for seizures and epilepsy. The more profound the degree of mental retardation as measured by the intelligence quotient (IQ), the greater is the incidence of epilepsy. In the elderly, seizures are primarily of partial onset associated with the focal neuronal injury induced by strokes, neurodegenerative disorders (e.g., Alzheimer disease), and other conditions. In some cases, if an etiology of seizures can be found and corrected, the patient may not require chronic antiepileptic drug (AED) treatment. Patients can also present with unprovoked seizures that do not have an identifiable cause, and thus by definition have idiopathic or cryptogenic epilepsy. *Idiopathic etiology* is the term used for suspected primary generalized seizures, whereas *cryptogenic etiology* is used if no obvious cause is found for partial-onset seizures. The incidence of idiopathic epilepsy is higher in children.[2]

Many factors have been shown to precipitate seizures in susceptible individuals. Hyperventilation can precipitate absence seizures. Sleep, sleep deprivation, sensory stimuli, and emotional stress increase the frequency of seizures. Hormonal changes occurring around the time of menses, puberty, or pregnancy have also been associated with the onset of or an increased frequency of seizures. A careful history should be obtained from patients presenting with seizures because theophylline, alcohol, high-dose phenothiazines, antidepressants (especially maprotiline or bupropion), and street drug use have been associated with provoking seizures. Perinatal injuries and small gestational weight at birth are also risk factors for the development of partial-onset seizures. Immunizations have not been associated with an increased risk of epilepsy.

PATHOPHYSIOLOGY

Seizures result from excessive excitation or in the case of absence seizures from disordered inhibition of a large population of cortical neurons.[3] This is reflected on EEG as a sharp wave or *spike*. Initially, a small number of neurons fire abnormally. Normal membrane conductances and inhibitory synaptic currents break down, and excess excitability spreads, either locally to produce a focal seizure or more widely to produce a generalized seizure. This onset propagates by physiologic pathways to involve adjacent or remote areas. The clinical manifestations depend on the site of the focus, the degree of irritability of the surrounding area of the brain, and the intensity of the impulse.[3]

There are multiple mechanisms that might contribute to synchronous hyperexcitability including: (1) alterations in the distribution, number, type and biophysical properties of ion channels in the neuronal membranes; (2) biochemical modifications of receptors; (3) modulation of second messaging systems and gene expression; (4) changes in extracellular ion concentrations; (5) alterations in neurotransmitter uptake and metabolism in glial cells; and (6) modifications in the ratio and function of inhibitory circuits. In addition local neurotransmitter imbalances could be a potential mechanism for focal epileptogenesis, but human studies on presurgical patients have not shown consistent differences. However, transitory imbalances between the main neurotransmitters, glutamate (excitatory) and γ-aminobutyric-acid (GABA) (inhibitory), and neuromodulators (e.g., acetylcholine, norepinephrine, and serotonin) might play a role in precipitating seizures in susceptible patients.[3]

Control of abnormal neuronal activity with AEDs is accomplished by elevating the threshold of neurons to electrical or chemical stimuli or by limiting the propagation of the seizure discharge from its origin. Raising the threshold most likely involves stabilization of neuronal membranes, whereas limiting the propagation involves depression of synaptic transmission and reduction of nerve conduction.[3]

Prolonged seizures can result in neuronal injury in vulnerable neuronal populations resulting in functional deficits, primarily in memory, and in permanent changes of wiring of the neuronal circuitry. Sprouting and reorganization of neuronal projections might lead to a chronic susceptibility to seizures, neuronal destruction, and brain damage. Also, the continued exposure to glutamate may contribute to neuronal damage. Although individual seizures as such do not cause a significant decrease in intelligence, it has been suggested that patients suffering a large number (greater than 100) of generalized tonic-clonic (GTC) seizures who have multiple episodes of status epilepticus can be at risk for eventual cognitive declines.

CLINICAL PRESENTATION

The International League Against Epilepsy (ILAE) has proposed two major schemes for the classification of seizures and epilepsies: the International Classification of Epileptic Seizures and the International Classification of the Epilepsies and Epilepsy Syndromes.[4,5]

The International Classification of Epileptic Seizures (Table 58–1) combines the clinical description with certain electrophysiologic findings to classify epileptic seizures. Seizures are divided into two main pathophysiologic groups—partial seizures and generalized seizures—by EEG recordings and clinical symptomatology.

Partial (focal) seizures begin in one hemisphere of the brain and—unless they become secondarily generalized—result in an asymmetric motor manifestation. Partial seizures manifest as alterations in motor functions, sensory or somatosensory symptoms, or automatisms. Partial seizures with no loss of consciousness are classified as *simple partial* (SP). In some cases, patients will describe somatosensory symptoms as a "warning" prior to the development of a GTC seizure. These warnings are in fact simple partial seizures and frequently are termed *auras*.

Partial seizures with an alteration of consciousness are described as *complex partial* (CP). With CP seizures, the patient can have automatisms, periods of memory loss, or aberrations of behavior. Some patients with CP epilepsy have been mistakenly diagnosed as having psychotic episodes. CP seizures also can progress to GTC seizures. Patients with CP seizures typically are amnestic to these events.

Generalized seizures have clinical manifestations that indicate involvement of both hemispheres. Motor manifestations are bilateral, and there is a loss of consciousness. Generalized seizures can be further subdivided by EEG and clinical manifestations. A partial seizure that becomes generalized is referred to as a *secondarily generalized seizure*.

Generalized absence seizures are manifested by a sudden onset, interruption of ongoing activities, a blank stare, and possibly a brief upward rotation of the eyes. They generally occur in young children through adolescence. It is important to differentiate absence seizures from complex partial seizures.

TABLE 58-1 International Classification of Epileptic Seizures

- I. Partial seizures (seizures begin locally)
  - A. Simple (without impairment of consciousness)
    - 1. With motor symptoms
    - 2. With special sensory or somatosensory symptoms
    - 3. With psychic symptoms
  - B. Complex (with impairment of consciousness)
    - 1. Simple partial onset followed by impairment of consciousness–with or without automatisms
    - 2. Impaired consciousness at onset–with or without automatisms
  - C. Secondarily generalized (partial onset evolving to generalized tonic-clonic seizures)
- II. Generalized seizures (bilaterally symmetrical and without local onset)
  - A. Absence
  - B. Myoclonic
  - C. Clonic
  - D. Tonic
  - E. Tonic-clonic
  - F. Atonic
  - G. Infantile spasms
- III. Unclassified seizures
- IV. Status epilepticus

Data from Commission on the Classification and Terminology of the International League Against Epilepsy.[4,5]

GTC seizures are what many people think of as epilepsy. The seizure results in a sudden sharp tonic contraction of muscles followed by a period of rigidity and clonic movements. During the seizure, the patient may cry or moan, lose sphincter control, bite the tongue, or develop cyanosis. After the seizure, the patient may have altered consciousness, drowsiness, or confusion for a variable period of time (postictal period) and frequently goes into a deep sleep. Tonic and clonic seizures can occur separately.

Brief shock-like muscular contractions of the face, trunk, and extremities are known as *myoclonic jerks.* They can be isolated events or rapidly repetitive. A sudden loss of muscle tone is known as an *atonic seizure.* This can be described as a head drop, the dropping of a limb, or a slumping to the ground. These patients often wear protective head ware to prevent trauma.

The International Classification of Epilepsies and Epilepsy Syndromes adds components such as age of onset, intellectual development, findings on neurologic examination, and results of neuroimaging studies to define epilepsy syndromes more fully. Syndromes can include one or many different seizure types (e.g., Lennox-Gastaut syndrome). The syndromic approach includes seizure type(s) and possible etiologic classifications (e.g., idiopathic, symptomatic, or unknown). *Idiopathic* describes syndromes that are presumably genetic but also those in which no underlying etiology is documented or suspected. A family history of seizures is commonly present, and neurologic function is essentially normal except for the occurrence of seizures. *Symptomatic* cases involve evidence of brain damage or a known underlying cause. A *cryptogenic* syndrome is assumed to be symptomatic of an underlying condition that cannot be documented. *Unknown* or *undetermined* is used when no cause can be identified. This syndromic classification is more important for prognostic determinations than for a classification based simply on seizure type. The syndrome classification scheme requires more information and, in return, provides a more powerful tool for comprehensive clinical management. A patient's epilepsy is classified based on seizure type (i.e., generalized versus partial) and syndromic type (i.e., idiopathic, symptomatic, or cryptogenic).

CLINICAL PRESENTATION OF EPILEPSY

General

In most cases, the healthcare provider will not be in a position to witness a seizure. Many patients (particularly those with CP or GTC seizures) are amnestic to the actual seizure event. Obtaining an adequate history and description of the ictal event (including time course) from a third party (e.g., significant other, family member, or witness) is critically important. With treatment the typical clinical presentation of the seizure may change.

Symptoms

Symptoms of a specific seizure will depend on seizure type. Although seizures can vary between patients, they tend to be stereotyped within an individual.

- CP seizures can include somatosensory or focal motor features.
- CP seizures are associated with altered consciousness.
- Absence seizures can be almost nondetectable with only very brief (seconds) periods of altered consciousness.
- GTC seizures are major convulsive episodes and are always associated with a loss of consciousness.

Signs

Interictally (between seizure episodes), there are typically no objective or pathognomonic signs.

Laboratory Tests

There are currently no diagnostic laboratory tests for epilepsy. In some cases, particularly following GTC (or perhaps CP) seizures, serum prolactin levels can be transiently elevated. Laboratory tests can be done to rule out treatable causes of seizures (e.g., hypoglycemia, altered electrolyte concentrations, infections, etc.) that do not represent epilepsy.

Other Diagnostic Tests

- EEG is very useful in the diagnosis of various seizure disorders.
- An epileptiform EEG is found in only approximately 50% of the patients who have epilepsy.
- A prolactin serum level obtained within 10 to 20 minutes of a tonic-clonic seizure can be useful in differentiating seizure activity from pseudoseizure activity but not from syncope.[6]
- Although magnetic resonance imaging (MRI) is very useful (especially imaging of the temporal lobes), a computed tomography (CT) scan typically is not helpful except in the initial evaluation for a brain tumor or cerebral bleeding.

TREATMENT

Epilepsy

■ DESIRED OUTCOME

❶ The ultimate goal of treatment for epilepsy is complete elimination of seizures and no side effects with an optimal quality of life. The best quality of life is associated with a seizure-free state.[7] Often, however, a balance between efficacy and side effects must be reached because with the older AEDs used as monotherapy, fewer than 50% of patients become seizure-free.

Because therapy is continued for many years (often a lifetime), chronic side effects must be considered. If the patient is overly sedated or develops other significant side effects, some seizure control may have to be sacrificed to improve functioning. The patient should be involved in deciding what balance between frequency of seizures and the occurrence of side effects is most appropriate. The newer AEDs offer alternatives for balancing seizure frequency and drug side effects.

Providing optimal quality of life goes beyond balancing seizures and side effects. It involves assessing all the concerns of a patient with epilepsy, such as, issues about driving, their future, forming relationships, safety, social isolation, social stigma, and so on. It is also important to recognize that patients with epilepsy can have other neuropsychiatric comorbidities such as depression, anxiety, and sleep disturbances that need treatment.[8,9] Depression is especially important because it has been shown to have a significant impact on quality of life in the patient with treatment-resistant epilepsy.[10]

■ GENERAL APPROACH TO TREATMENT

❷ The general approach to treatment involves identification of goals, assessment of seizure type and frequency, development of a care plan, and a plan for followup evaluation. During the assessment phase, it is critical to establish an accurate diagnosis of the seizure type and classification to help determine the appropriate initial AEDs. Patient-specific treatment goals must be identified, and these can change over time. Despite appropriate AED treatment, approximately 30% to 35% of patients will be refractory to treatment. In this setting, seizure freedom may not be obtained, and more obtainable outcomes should be established (e.g., decrease in the number of seizures and minimized drug adverse effects).

❸ Patient characteristics such as age, medical condition, ability to comply with a prescribed regimen, and insurance coverage also should be explored because these can influence AED choices or help to explain nonadherence to the regimen, a lack of response, or unexpected adverse effects.

Once the assessment is complete, for patients with new-onset seizures, the choice is whether to use drug therapy and, if so, which one. For a patient with long-standing epilepsy, adequacy of the current medication regimen must be evaluated. An AED should not be considered ineffective unless the patient has experienced unacceptable adverse effects with continued seizures.

❹ If a decision is made to start AED therapy, monotherapy is preferred, and approximately 50% to 70% of all patients with epilepsy can be maintained on one drug.[11,12] However, many of these patients are not seizure free. The percentage of patients who are seizure free on one drug varies by seizure type. The prognosis for 12-month seizure freedom is best for those who have only GTC seizures (48% to 55%), worst for those who have only CP seizures (23% to 26%), and intermediate for those with mixed seizure types (25% to 32%).[12] Drugs can be combined in an attempt to help the patient become seizure-free. Combining AEDs with different mechanisms of action can be advantageous, although this approach is as yet unproven. Approximately 65% of patients can be expected to be maintained on one AED and be considered well controlled, although not necessarily seizure-free.

CLINICAL CONTROVERSY

It is believed by some that the upregulation of certain brain efflux transporters such as P-glycoprotein and multidrug-resistant-protein may play a role in drug-resistant epilepsy. The efflux transporters are believed to transport antiepileptic drugs away from the epileptic focus, thus preventing therapeutic concentrations from reaching the site. It is not known if the upregulation is due to genetic or acquired/induced mechanisms or possibly both. P-glycoprotein is encoded in humans by a gene family comprising two genes: MDR1 (ABCB1) and MDR2 (ABCB4). MDR1 appears to be important for the expression of the transporter at the blood–brain barrier. The gene is highly polymorphic with a common polymorphism occurring as C3435T. In one study, C3435T was found to be more prevalent in patients with drug-resistant epilepsy; however, a larger study conducted later was unable to validate these results. A smaller study did partially validate the results.[13]

❺ Of the 35% of patients with unsatisfactory control, 10% will be well controlled with a two-drug treatment. Of the remaining 25%, 20% will continue to have unsatisfactory control despite multiple drug treatment. It has been suggested that there may be a genetic predisposition to epilepsy that is refractory to drug therapy. Some of these patients will become surgical candidates. For some patients, an implantable device such as the vagal nerve stimulator can be an additional nonpharmacologic option.

Once the care plan is established, a prescription is generated for a specific AED. Patient education and assurance of patient understanding of the plan are essential. Detailed directions regarding titration, what to do in the event of a treatment-emergent side effect, and what to do if a seizure occurs must be provided to patients. Documentation of the assessment, care plan, and educational process is essential. Providing the patient with a seizure and side-effect diary will assist in the followup and evaluation phase. At the followup stage of treatment (which can be done in the hospital, clinic, pharmacy, or by phone), the treatment goals must be reviewed. If the goal has been achieved, new goals should be identified. For example, if the GTC seizures are now controlled, the goal may be to control partial seizures. If a patient fails to respond to the first AEDs, trials with other AEDs should be attempted as appropriate. Completion of the evaluation often requires a reassessment of the patient and development of a new care plan taking into account patient compliance, efficacy, and safety of the initial treatment.

Medication noncompliance can be the single most common reason for treatment failure. It is estimated that up to 60% of patients with epilepsy are noncompliant.[14] The rate of noncompliance is increased by the complexity of the drug regimen and by doses taken three and four times a day. Frequent uncontrolled seizures can also predispose a patient to noncompliance secondary to confusion over whether the drug was taken. Noncompliance is not influenced by age, sex, psychomotor development, or seizure type.[14]

Epilepsy is a clinical diagnosis defined by recurrent seizures. Difference of opinion exists as to when the most appropriate time is to initiate AED therapy. Some clinicians start AED treatment after the first seizure, whereas others do not initiate treatment until a second, unprovoked seizure has occurred. Still others initiate prophylactic treatment following a CNS insult thought likely to cause epilepsy eventually (e.g., stroke or head trauma). Appropriate treatment decisions vary depending on individual patient clinical characteristics and circumstances.

Drug treatment may not be indicated in patients whose seizures have minimal impact on their lives or those who have had only a single seizure. If a patient presents after a single isolated seizure, one of three treatment decisions can be made: treat, possibly treat, or do not treat. These decisions are based on the probability of the patient having a second seizure (Table 58–2). For patients with no risk factors, the probability of a second seizure is less than 10% in the first year and approximately 24% by the end of 2 years. If risk factors are present, the recurrence rate can be as high as 80% after 5 years.[15] The decision on whether to start AED therapy often depends on patient-specific factors such as epilepsy syndrome, seizure etiology, presence of a neuroanatomic defect, and the EEG, as well as, the patient's lifestyle and preferences. Patients who have had two or more seizures generally should be started on AEDs.

■ WHEN TO STOP ANTIEPILEPTIC DRUGS

❻ The AEDs used to control seizures may not need to be given for a lifetime. Polypharmacy can be reduced, and some patients can discontinue AEDs altogether. In reducing polypharmacy, the drug considered less appropriate for the seizure type (or the agent deemed most responsible for adverse effects) should be discontin-

TABLE 58-2 Recurrence Risk for Patients Experiencing One Unprovoked Seizure

Type of Patient	First-Year Risk (%)	Fifth-Year Risk (%)
Adults with single unproved seizure		34
No CNS insult	10	29
Influence of family history		
Sibling with seizure	29	46
No sibling with seizures	7	27
EEG patterns		
GSW on EEG	15	58
Normal EEG	9	26
Occurrence of previous seizure	10	39
Caused by an illness or childhood febrile seizure		
Remote symptomatic with Todd paresis	26	48
	41	75
Status epilepticus at onset	37	56
Prior acute seizure	60	80
Idiopathic	10	29

CNS, central nervous system; EEG, electroencephalogram; GSW, generalized spikes and waves.
Data from Leppik[15] and Gross-Tsur et al.[17]

ued first. In some cases, decreasing the number of AEDs a patient is receiving can decrease side effects and increase cognitive abilities. This improvement in cognition may be small, especially if the patient is on a drug that primarily affects psychomotor speed with less effect on higher-order cognitive functioning.

❼ Factors favoring successful withdrawal of AEDs include a seizure-free period of 2 to 4 years, complete seizure control within 1 year of onset, an onset of seizures after age 2 but before age 35, and a normal neurologic examination and EEG. Factors associated with a poor prognosis in discontinuing AEDs, despite a seizure-free interval, include a history of a high frequency of seizures, repeated episodes of status epilepticus, a combination of seizure types, and development of abnormal mental functioning. Children who have irregular generalized spike and wave activity in EEG recordings prior to discontinuation of treatment may have a higher relapse rate (67%) compared with children without epileptiform activity (33%) or children with other types of epileptiform activity (33%) in their last EEG recordings before discontinuation. A 2-year seizure-free period is suggested for absence and rolandic epilepsy, whereas a 4-year seizure-free period is suggested for SP, CP, and absence seizures associated with tonic-clonic convulsions. AED withdrawal generally is not suggested for patients with juvenile myoclonic epilepsy, absence with clonic-tonic-clonic seizures, or clonic-tonic-clonic seizures. The American Academy of Neurology (AAN) has issued guidelines for discontinuing AEDs in seizure-free patients.[16] After assessing the risks and benefits to both the patient and society, AED withdrawal can be considered in a patient meeting the following profile: seizure free for 2 to 5 years, a history of a single type of partial seizure or primary GTC seizures, a normal neurologic exam and normal IQ, and an EEG that has been normalized with treatment. When these factors are present, the relapse rate is expected to be less than 32% for children and 39% for adults.

AED withdrawal should be done gradually, especially in patients with profound developmental disabilities. Some patients will have a recurrence of seizures as the AEDs are withdrawn. Sudden withdrawal is associated with the precipitation of status epilepticus. Withdrawal seizures are of particular concern for agents such as benzodiazepines and barbiturates. Seizure relapse has been reported to be more common if these AEDs are withdrawn over 1 to 3 months than over 6 months.

The risk of seizure relapse has been estimated at 10% to 70%. A meta-analysis determined that the relapse rate was 25% after 1 year and 29% after 2 years. Recurrence of seizures tends to occur early with at least one-half of the recurrences within 6 months of AED withdrawal and 60% to 90% within 1 year. Late reoccurrences are uncommon. Patients who relapse will generally become seizure free and in remission after AEDs are restarted although not necessarily immediately. The underlying epilepsy syndrome appears to determine prognosis for long-term remission.[17]

CLINICAL CONTROVERSY

It is not entirely clear which patients with epilepsy will require lifelong treatment. Although many clinicians feel that AED therapy is lifelong, others would argue that certain patients with idiopathic epilepsy and a normal neurologic examination and EEG are candidates for AED withdrawal following a prolonged period of seizure freedom (e.g., greater than 2 to 3 years). A large amount of the data supporting discontinuing AEDs have been obtained from children. Some adults will be reticent to discontinue AED therapy even if the clinician is in favor of it because of the fear of having a seizure and the consequences (e.g., loss of driver's license) that it would entail. The patient should agree and must be a willing participant in the plan to reduce or withdraw AED therapy.

NONPHARMACOLOGIC THERAPY

Nonpharmacologic therapy for epilepsy includes diet, surgery, and vagus nerve stimulation (VNS). A vagal nerve stimulator is an implanted medical device that is FDA approved for use as an adjunctive therapy in reducing the frequency of seizures in adults and adolescents older than 12 years of age with partial-onset seizures that are refractory to AEDs. It is also used off-label in the treatment of generalized epilepsy.

The mechanisms of antiseizure actions of VNS are unknown in the human, but animal studies have indicated that VNS has multiple activities. Human clinical studies have shown that VNS changes the cerebrospinal fluid (CSF) concentration of inhibitory and stimulatory neurotransmitters and activates specific areas of the brain that generate or regulate cortical seizure activity through increased blood flow. It is believed that the long-term intermittent antiepileptic effects of VNS involve neurotransmitters and or neurochemicals.[18]

The VNS device is relatively safe. The most common side effect associated with stimulation is hoarseness, voice alteration, increased cough, pharyngitis, dyspnea, dyspepsia, and nausea. Serious adverse effects reported include infection, nerve paralysis, hypoesthesia, facial paresis, left vocal cord paralysis, left facial paralysis, left recurrent laryngeal nerve injury, urinary retention, and low-grade fever. Overall, in the VNS studies, the percentage of patients who achieved a 50% or greater reduction in their seizure frequency (responders) ranged from 23% to 50%.

Surgery is the treatment of choice in selected patients with refractory focal epilepsy.[19] The success rate is reported to be between 80% and 90% in properly selected patients. It has been shown that surgery reduces the risk of epilepsy-associated death, and it may also improve depression and anxiety in refractory epilepsy patients.[20,21] A National Institutes of Health Consensus Conference identified three absolute requirements for surgery. They are (1) an absolute diagnosis of epilepsy, (2) failure on an adequate trial of drug therapy, and (3) definition of the electroclinical syndrome. A focus in the temporal lobe has the best chance for a positive outcome; however, extratemporal foci can be excised successfully in more than 75% of patients. The procedure is not without risk. Learning and memory can be impaired postoperatively, and general intellectual abilities are also affected in a small number of patients. Surgery may be particularly useful in children with intractable epilepsy. Patients may need to continue to receive AED therapy for a period of time following successful epilepsy surgery, but they may be able to use a reduced dose of their AEDs.[19,22]

The ketogenic diet was devised in the 1920s. It is high in fat and low in carbohydrates and protein and thus leads to acidosis and ketosis. Protein and calorie intake are set at levels that will meet requirements for growth. Most of the calories are provided in the form of heavy cream and butter, and no sugar is allowed. Vitamins and minerals are supplemented. Medium-chain triglycerides can be substituted for the dietary fats. Fluids are also controlled. It requires strict control and parent compliance. Although some centers find the diet useful for refractory patients, others have found that it is poorly tolerated by patients. Long-term effects have included kidney stones, increased bone fractures, and adverse effects on growth.[23] Recently a modified Atkins diet has been found to be effective in the treatment of intractable pediatric epilepsy.[24]

PHARMACOLOGIC THERAPY

Optimal management of epilepsy, therefore, requires that AED treatment be individualized. Specifically, different patient groups (e.g., children, women of child-bearing potential, and the elderly) may be better suited to receive one AED than another by virtue not only of seizure type but also of susceptibility or relative risk for certain adverse effects. These issues will be highlighted further below.

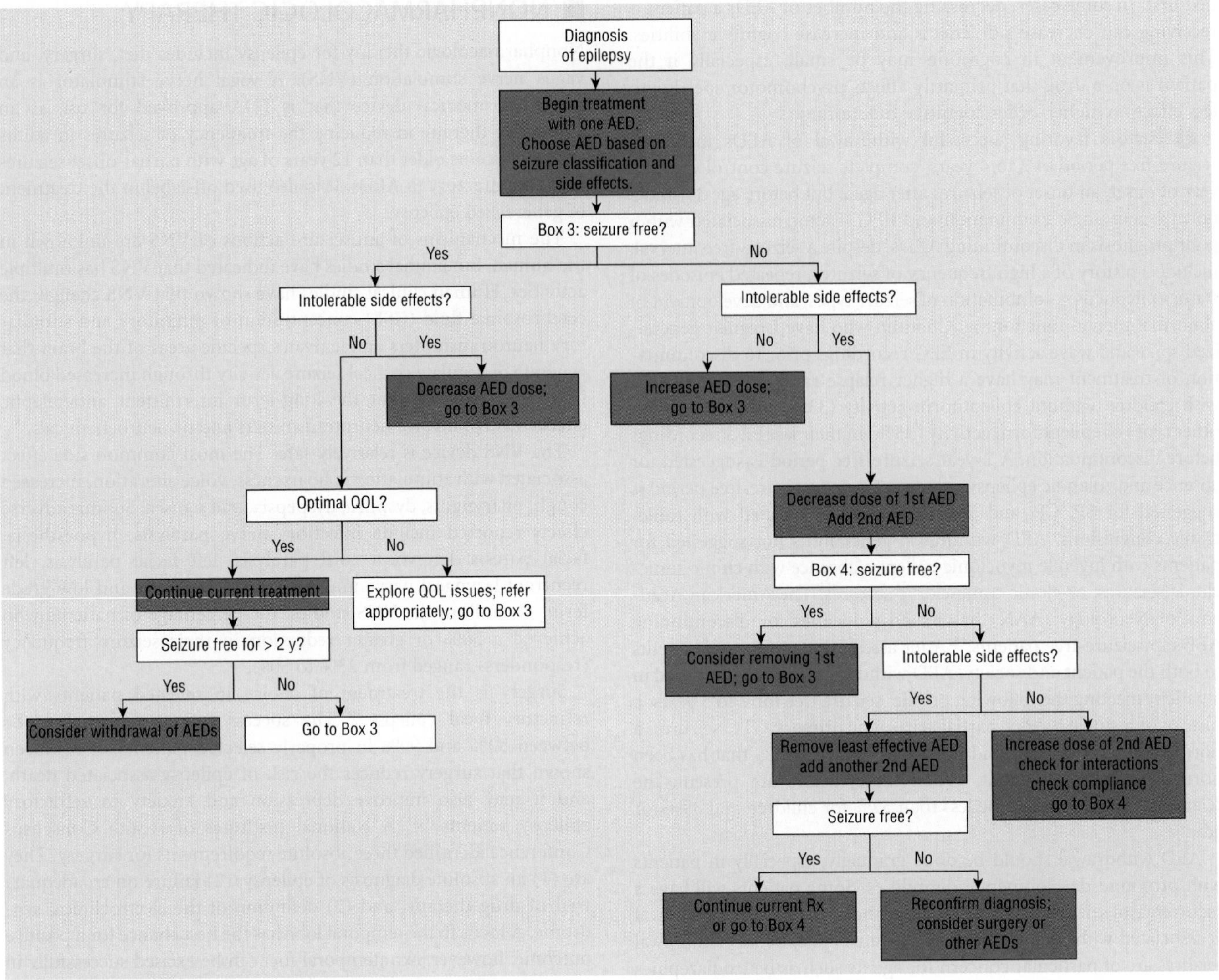

FIGURE 58-1. Algorithm for the treatment of epilepsy. (AED, antiepileptic drug; QOL, quality of life.)

❼ Selection and optimization of AED therapy require not only an understanding of drug mechanism(s) of action and spectrum of clinical activity but also an appreciation of pharmacokinetic variability as well as patterns of drug-related adverse effects. An AED must demonstrate efficacy for the specific seizure type being treated. The drug treatments of first choice depend on the type of epilepsy, as well as on the interface between drug-specific adverse effects and patient preferences. Ultimately, AED effectiveness is the result of the interaction of each of these factors. A suggested algorithm for a general approach to the treatment of epilepsy is shown in Fig. 58–1.

Table 58–3 provides evidenced-based treatment recommendations by three professional/regulatory bodies.[25–29] In addition, recommendations from a U.S. panel of experts, which included more recent drug treatment data compared to the AAN-American Epilepsy Society (AES) recommendations are included.[30]

The mechanism of action of most AEDs can be categorized as either affecting ion channels, augmenting inhibitory neurotransmission, or modulating excitatory neurotransmission. The ion channels affected include the sodium and calcium channels. Augmentation in inhibitory neurotransmission includes increasing CNS concentrations of GABA, whereas efforts to decrease excitatory neurotransmission are primarily focused on decreasing (or antagonizing) glutamate and aspartate neurotransmission. AEDs that are effective against GTC and partial seizures probably reduce sustained repetitive firing of action potentials by delaying recovery of sodium channels from activation. Drugs that reduce corticothalamic T-type calcium currents are effective against generalized absence seizures. Myoclonic seizures respond to drugs that enhance $GABA_A$ receptor inhibition. In addition to mechanism of action, awareness of pharmacokinetic properties (Table 58–4), adverse effects (Table 58–5), AED-AED interactions (Table 58–6), and AED metabolic pathway as well as inducer or inhibitory effects on liver (Table 58–7) can aid in the optimization of AED therapy. Pharmacokinetic interactions are a common complicating factor in AED selection. Interactions can occur in any of the pharmacokinetic processes: absorption, distribution, or elimination. Caution should be used when AEDs are added to or withdrawn from a drug regimen.

Adverse effects of AEDs can be divided into acute and chronic (see Table 58–5). Acute effects can be dose/serum concentration–related or idiosyncratic. Concentration-dependent effects are common and troublesome but not usually life-threatening. Neurotoxic adverse effects are encountered commonly and can include sedation, dizziness, blurred or double vision, difficulty with concentration, and ataxia. In many cases these effects can be alleviated by decreasing drug dose or avoided in some cases by increasing the drug very slowly. Most idiosyncratic reactions owing to an allergic reaction are mild, but they can be more serious if the hypersensitivity involves one or more organ systems. Other idiosyncratic side effects including hepatitis or blood dyscrasias are serious but rare.

Acute organ failure, if it is going to occur, generally occurs within the first 6 months of AED therapy. Unfortunately, screening laboratory evaluations of blood and urine typically are not helpful in

TABLE 58-3 Drugs of Choice for Specific Seizure Disorders

Seizure Type	First-Line Drugs	Alternative Drugs[a]	Comments
Partial seizures (newly diagnosed)			
U.S. guidelines[25,26]	*Adults & adolescents:* Carbamazepine Gabapentin Lamotrigine Oxcarbazepine Phenobarbital Phenytoin Topiramate Valproic acid		*FDA approved:* Carbamazepine Oxcarbazepine Phenobarbital Phenytoin Topiramate Valproic acid
U.K. guidelines[27,28]	Carbamazepine Lamotrigine Oxcarbazepine Topiramate Valproic acid		
ILAE guidelines[29]	*Adults:* Carbamazepine Phenytoin Valproic acid *Children:* Oxcarbazepine *Elderly:* Gabapentin Lamotrigine	*Adults:* Gabapentin Lamotrigine Oxcarbazepine Phenobarbital Topiramate *Children:* Carbamazepine Phenobarbital Phenytoin Topiramate Valproic acid *Elderly:* Carbamazepine	
U.S. Expert Panel 2005[30]	Carbamazepine Lamotrigine Oxcarbazepine	Levetiracetam	
Partial seizures (refractory monotherapy)			
U.S. guidelines[25,26]	Lamotrigine Oxcarbazepine Topiramate		*FDA approved:* Carbamazepine Lamotrigine Oxcarbazepine Phenobarbital Phenytoin Valproic acid
U.K. guidelines[27,28]	Lamotrigine Oxcarbazepine Topiramate		
Partial seizures (refractory adjunct)			
U.S. guidelines[25,26]	*Adults:* Gabapentin Lamotrigine Levetiracetam Oxcarbazepine Tiagabine Topiramate Zonisamide *Children:* Gabapentin Lamotrigine Oxcarbazepine Topiramate		*FDA approved:* Carbamazepine Gabapentin Lamotrigine Levetiracetam Oxcarbazepine Phenobarbital Phenytoin Pregabalin Tiagabine Valproic acid Zonisamide
U.K. guidelines[27,28]	Gabapentin Lamotrigine Levetiracetam Oxcarbazepine Tiagabine Topiramate		
Generalized seizures absence (newly diagnosed)			
U.S. guidelines[25,26]	Lamotrigine		*FDA approved:* Ethosuximide Valproic acid
U.K. guidelines[27,28]	Lamotrigine		
ILAE guidelines[29]	None	Ethosuximide Lamotrigine Valproic acid	
U.S. Expert Panel 2005[30]	Ethosuximide Valproic acid	Lamotrigine	
Primary generalized (tonic-clonic)			
U.S. guidelines[25,26]	Topiramate		*FDA approved:* Lamotrigine Topiramate
U.K. guidelines [27,28]	Lamotrigine Topiramate		
ILAE guidelines[29]	None	*Adults:* Carbamazepine Lamotrigine Oxcarbazepine Phenobarbital Phenytoin Topiramate Valproic acid *Children:* Carbamazepine Phenobarbital Phenytoin Topiramate Valproic acid	
U.S. Expert Panel 2005[30]	Valproic acid	Lamotrigine Topiramate	
Juvenile myoclonic epilepsy			*FDA approved:* Levetiracetam (myoclonic seizures)
ILAE[29]	None	Clonazepam Lamotrigine Levetiracetam Topiramate Valproic acid Zonisamide	
U.S. Expert Panel 2005[30]	Valproic acid	Levetiracetam Topiramate Zonisamide	

[a]Includes possibly effective drugs.

ILAE, International League Against Epilepsy.

Data from French et al.,[25,26] National Institute for Clinical Excellence,[27,28] Glauser et al.,[29] and Karceski et al.[30]

TABLE 58-4 Antiepileptic Drug Pharmacokinetic Data

AED	$t_{1/2}$ (h)	Time to Steady State (days)	Unchanged (%)	V_D (L/kg)	Clinically Important Metabolite	Protein Binding (%)
Carbamazepine	12 M; 5–14 Co	21–28 for completion of auto-induction	<1	1–2	10,11-epoxide	40–90
Ethosuximide	A 60; C 30	6–12	10–20	0.67	No	0
Felbamate	16–22	5–7	50	0.73–0.82	No	~25
Gabapentin[a]	5–40[b]	1–2	100	0.65–1.04	No	0
Lamotrigine	25.4 M	3–15	0	1.28	No	40–50
Levetiracetam	7–10	2		0.7	No	<10
Oxcarbazepine	3–13	2		0.7	10-hydroxy-carbazepine	40
Phenobarbital	A 46–136; C 37–73	14–21	20–40	0.6	No	50
Phenytoin	A 10–34; C 5–14	7–28	<5	0.6–8.0	No	90
Pregabalin	A6-7[b]	1-2	90	0.5	No	0
Primidone	A 3.3–19; C 4.5–11	1–4	40	0.43–1.1	PB	80
Tiagabine	5–13		Negligible		No	95
Topiramate	18–21	4–5	50–70	0.55–0.8 (male); 0.23–0.4 (female)	No	15
Valproic acid	A 8–20; C 7–14	1–3	<5	0.1–0.5	May contribute to toxicity	90–95 binding saturates
Zonisamide	24–60	5–15		0.8–1.6	No	40–60

A, adult; AED, antiepileptic drug; C, child; Co, combination therapy; M, monotherapy; PB, phenobarbital; V_D, volume of distribution.
[a]The bioavailability of gabapentin is dose dependent.
[b]Half-life depends on renal function.
Data from Faught,[31] Leppik,[32] and Bourgeois.[33]

TABLE 58-5 Antiepileptic Drug Side Effects

AED	Acute Side Effects: Concentration Dependent	Acute Side Effects: Idiosyncratic	Chronic Side Effects
Carbamazepine	Diplopia Dizziness Drowsiness Nausea Unsteadiness Lethargy	Blood dyscrasias Rash	Hyponatremia
Ethosuximide	Ataxia Drowsiness GI distress Unsteadiness Hiccoughs	Blood dyscrasias Rash	Behavior changes Headache
Felbamate	Anorexia Nausea Vomiting Insomnia Headache	Aplastic anemia Acute hepatic failure	Not established
Gabapentin	Dizziness Fatigue Somnolence Ataxia	Pedal edema	Weight gain
Lamotrigine	Diplopia Dizziness Unsteadiness Headache	Rash	Not established
Levetiracetam	Sedation Behavioral disturbance	Not established	Not established
Oxcarbazepine	Sedation Dizziness Ataxia Nausea	Rash	Hyponatremia
Phenobarbital	Ataxia Hyperactivity Headache Unsteadiness Sedation Nausea	Blood dyscrasias Rash	Behavior changes Connective tissue disorders Intellectual blunting Metabolic bone disease Mood change Sedation

(continued)

TABLE 58-5 Antiepileptic Drug Side Effects (continued)

	Acute Side Effects		
AED	***Concentration Dependent***	***Idiosyncratic***	**Chronic Side Effects**
Phenytoin	Ataxia Nystagmus Behavior changes Dizziness Headache Incoordination Sedation Lethargy Cognitive impairment Fatigue Visual blurring	Blood dyscrasias Rash Immunologic reaction	Behavior changes Cerebellar syndrome Connective tissue changes Skin thickening Folate deficiency Gingival hyperplasia Hirsutism Coarsening of facial features Acne Cognitive impairment Metabolic bone disease Sedation
Pregabalin	Dizziness Somnolence Blurred vision	Pedal edema Creatine kinase elevation Decrease platelets	Weight gain
Primidone	Behavior changes Headache Nausea Sedation Unsteadiness	Blood dyscrasias Rash	Behavior change Connective tissue disorders Cognitive impairment Sedation
Tiagabine	Dizziness Fatigue Difficulties concentrating Nervousness Tremor Blurred vision Depression Weakness	Spike-wave stupor	Not established
Topiramate	Difficulties concentrating Psychomotor slowing Speech or language problems Somnolence, fatigue Dizziness Headache	Metabolic acidosis Acute angle glaucoma Oligohydrosis	Kidney stones Weight loss
Valproic acid	GI upset Sedation Unsteadiness Tremor Thrombocytopenia	Acute hepatic failure Acute pancreatitis Alopecia	Polycystic ovary–like syndrome Weight gain Hyperammonemia Menstual cycle irregularities
Zonisamide	Sedation Dizziness Cognitive impairment Nausea	Rash Oligohydrosis	Kidney stones Weight loss

AED, antiepileptic drug.
Data from French et al.[25,26] and Leppik.[32]

predicting or detecting the early stage of severe reactions and generally are not recommended in asymptomatic patients. Laboratory assessment including white blood cell counts and liver function tests may be reasonable if the patient reports an unexplained illness (e.g., lethargy, vomiting, fever, or rash).[34] It is important to recognize that adverse effects can occur despite serum concentrations being within the proposed therapeutic range.[35]

Another potential long-term adverse effect of AED treatment is osteomalacia and osteoporosis.[36] The bone disorders associated with AED use consist of a heterogeneous group of disorders. These include findings ranging from asymptomatic high-turnover disease, with findings of normal bone mineral density, to markedly decreased bone mineral density sufficient to warrant the diagnosis of osteoporosis. While the etiology of these osteopathies is still uncertain, it has been hypothesized that certain drugs, including phenytoin, phenobarbital, carbamazepine, oxcarbazepine, and valproic acid, may interfere with vitamin D metabolism. Whether the other AEDs are associated with these effects is as yet unknown. Common laboratory findings in these patients include elevated bone-specific alkaline phosphatase concentration and decreased serum calcium and 25-OH vitamin D concentrations. Patients receiving these drugs should receive supplemental vitamin D and calcium, as well as bone mineral density testing if other risk factors for osteoporosis are present.

The comparative effects of AEDs on cognition have been difficult to evaluate because of differences or inconsistencies in study design, included seizure types, control for serum drug concentrations, and the neuropsychologic tests used. In general, there are not large differences between the older drugs,[37,38] although the barbiturates phenobarbital and primidone appear to cause more cognitive impairment than other commonly used AEDs. Phenytoin, particularly when serum concentrations are above the commonly accepted therapeutic range, may have a greater effect on motor function and speed. Among the older AEDs, valproic acid may cause less impairment of cognition. Improvement in cognition has been reported in patients switched from phen-

TABLE 58-6 Interactions between Antiepileptic Drugs

AED	Added Drug	Effect[a]
Carbamazepine (CBZ)	Felbamate	Incr. 10,11 epoxide Decr. CBZ
	Phenobarbital	Decr. CBZ
	Phenytoin	Decr. CBZ
	Valproic acid	Incr. 10,11 epoxide
Ethosuximide	Carbamazepine	Decr. ethosuximide
	Phenobarbital	Decr. ethosuximide
	Phenytoin	Decr. ethosuximide
Felbamate (FBM)	Carbamazepine	Decr. FBM
	Phenytoin	Decr. FBM
	Valproic acid	Incr. FBM
Gabapentin	No known interactions	
Lamotrigine (LTG)	Carbamazepine	Decr. LTG
	Phenobarbital	Decr. LTG
	Phenytoin	Decr. LTG
	Primidone	Decr. LTG
	Valproic acid	Incr. LTG
Levetiracetam	No known interactions	
Oxcarbazepine	Carbamazepine	Decr. MHD[b]
	Phenobarbital	Decr. MHD[b]
	Phenytoin	Decr. MHD[b]
Phenobarbital (PB)	Felbamate	Incr. PB
	Phenytoin	Incr. or decr. PB
	Valproic acid	Incr. PB
Phenytoin (PHT)	Carbamazepine	Decr. PHT
	Felbamate	Incr. PHT
	Methsuximide	Incr. PHT
	Phenobarbital	Incr. or decr. PHT
	Valproic acid	Decr. Total PHT
	Vigabatrin	Decr. PHT
Pregabalin	No known interactions	
Primidone (PRM)	Carbamazepine	Decr. PRM Incr. PB
	Phenytoin	Decr. PRM Incr. PB
	Valproic acid	Incr. PRM Incr. PB
Tiagabine (TGB)	Carbamazepine	Decr. TGB
	Phenytoin	Decr. TGB
Topiramate (TPM)	Carbamazepine	Decr. TPM
	Phenytoin	Decr. TPM
	Valproic acid	Decr. TPM
Valproic acid (VPA)	Carbamazepine	Decr. VPA
	Felbamate	Incr. VPA
	Lamotrigine	Decr. VPA (slight)
	Phenobarbital	Decr. VPA
	Phenytoin	Decr. VPA
	Primidone	Decr. VPA
	Topiramate	Decr. VPA
Zonisamide	Carbamazepine	Decr. zonisamide
	Phenobarbital	Decr. zonisamide
	Phenytoin	Decr. zonisamide

AED, antiepileptic drug.
[a]Incr. = increased; Decr. = decreased.
[b]MHD = 10-monohydroxymetabolite.
Data from Faught,[31] Leppik,[32] and Bourgeois.[33]

ytoin or phenobarbital to this agent. However, these improvements are subtle and may not be pronounced if patients are in the same relative area of the therapeutic range. Patients changed from polytherapy to monotherapy also may demonstrate improvement in cognition. Some of the newer agents are believed to cause fewer neurobehavioral or cognitive effects. Among the newer AEDs, gabapentin and lamotrigine have been shown in several studies to cause fewer cognitive impairments as compared with older agents, such as carbamazepine.[39,40,41] Conversely, topiramate may cause substantial cognitive impairment, particularly when used at high doses or during rapid dose escalation.[41] In addition, these patients may not be fully aware of their deficits.[42,43] Finally, in some cases, AED treatment itself has been suggested to cause worsening of seizures. This can result from either improper selection of an AED for a specific seizure type or syndrome or can represent a paradoxical toxic effect of the drug.[44]

Because most adult patients have localization-related (partial-onset) seizures, the most widely used AEDs traditionally have been carbamazepine, phenobarbital, phenytoin, and valproic acid. For CP seizures, these AEDs have similar efficacy.[45,46] Of these, carbamazepine and phenytoin are the most commonly prescribed AEDs for use in partial seizures in the United States. In large part, this preference is based on data derived from two landmark trials conducted through the Veterans Administration (VA) Epilepsy Cooperative Study Group. In the first of these trials, patients with new-onset partial or generalized epilepsy were randomized to receive either carbamazepine, phenobarbital, phenytoin, or primidone.[45] At the end of 3 years, patients who received either carbamazepine or phenytoin were equally likely and patients on phenobarbital or primidone were least likely to have remained on their originally assigned treatment. Thus, carbamazepine and phenytoin were considered the drugs of first choice in patients with new-onset partial or generalized seizures. Carbamazepine was associated with fewer side effects. A followup study using almost identical methods compared carbamazepine and valproic acid.[46] Carbamazepine- and valproic acid–treated groups had equal retention rates for tonic-clonic seizures. Carbamazepine was superior to valproic acid for partial seizures. Valproic acid caused slightly more adverse effects.

Based in large part on the earlier VA cooperative trials, carbamazepine traditionally has been recognized as the AED of first choice for partial seizures. Several of the newer-generation AEDs may prove to be reasonable alternatives. The newer antiepileptic drugs were first approved as adjunctive therapy for patients with refractory partial seizures. Monotherapy trials with several of these newer agents including lamotrigine, gabapentin, topiramate, and oxcarbazepine have been completed.[47–49] Comparisons between lamotrigine and older agents including carbamazepine and phenytoin as initial monotherapy in partial seizures have been conducted in Europe, and the results suggest comparable effectiveness and perhaps better tolerability for lamotrigine, particularly in elderly patients. Results from a recently completed VA cooperative trial designed to compare gabapentin, lamotrigine, and carbamazepine in newly diagnosed elderly patients found that gabapentin efficacy is comparable with that of both lamotrigine and carbamazepine, and in fact is better tolerated than carbamazepine and equal to lamotrigine in this population.[50] Clinical data suggest that in newly diagnosed patients, oxcarbazepine is as effective as phenytoin, valproic acid, and immediate-release carbamazepine, with perhaps fewer adverse effects. Interestingly, close examination of the conversion to monotherapy trials suggests that oxcarbazepine demonstrates efficacy even in patients who previously had an inadequate response to carbamazepine, in spite of their structural similarity.

In addition, several monotherapy trials using an active control or pseudoplacebo design also have been performed. Although these study designs do provide evidence of efficacy for the newer drugs, because the comparison is between active drug and placebo in patients who continue to have seizures in spite of current treatment with standard AEDs, it is difficult to compare the efficacy of the newer drugs directly with the older AEDs. A meta-analysis designed to compare some of the newer AEDs found that because of wide and overlapping confidence intervals for both efficacy and tolerability outcome measures, no statistically significant differences between agents could be found.[51] Generally speaking, the newer AEDs appear to have comparable efficacy to the older agents and are perhaps better tolerated.

TABLE 58-7 AED Elimination Pathways and Major Effect on Hepatic Enzymes

AED	Major Hepatic Enzymes	Renal Elimination (%)	Induced	Inhibited
Carbamazepine	CYP3A4; CYP1A2; CYP2C8	<1	CYP1A2; CYP2C; CYP3A; GT	None
Ethosuximide	CYP3A4	12–20	None	None
Felbamate	CYP3A4; CYP2E1; other	50	CYP3A4	CYP2C19; β-oxidation
Gabapentin	None	Almost completely	None	None
Lamotrigine	GT	10	GT	None
Levetiracetam	None (undergoes non-hepatic hydrolysis)	66	None	None
Oxcarbazepine (MHD is active oxcarbazepine metabolite)	Cytosolic system	1 27	CYP3A4; CYP3A5; GT	CYP2C19
Phenobarbital	CYP2C9; other	25	CYP3A; CYP2C; GT	None
Phenytoin	CYP2C9; CYP2C19	5	CYP3A; CYP2C; GT	
Pregabalin	None	100	None	None
Tiagabine	CYP3A4	2	None	None
Topiramate	Not known	70	CYP3A (dose dependent)	CYP2C19
Valproate	GT; β-oxidation	2	None	CYP2C9;GT epoxide hydrolase
Zonisamide	CYP3A4	35	None	None

AED, antiepileptic drug; CYP, cytochrome P450 isoenzyme system; GT, glucuronyltransferase.
Data from Faught[31] and Leppik[32] with permission.

To date, among the newer-generation agents, lamotrigine, oxcarbazepine, and topiramate have received FDA approval for use as monotherapy in patients with partial seizures. Phenobarbital and primidone are also useful in partial seizures, but sedation and cognitive adverse effects limit their utility. Felbamate, which has monotherapy approval, is effective but has been associated with some significant side effects. Interpretation of monotherapy trials with the newer AEDs can be daunting owing to the unique study designs and specific patient populations employed. Although a complete discussion of this topic is beyond the scope of this chapter, several reviews and analyses have been published.[47]

Primarily generalized seizures such as absence seizures may respond differently pharmacologically than other seizure types. Phenytoin, phenobarbital, and carbamazepine, although effective in GTC and partial seizures, are ineffective in treating absence seizures, and in some cases, can precipitate an increase in seizure activity. Absence seizures are best treated with ethosuximide, valproic acid, and perhaps lamotrigine. Levetiracetam, topiramate, or zonisamide also can be effective, although further clinical data are needed to confirm this. Gabapentin and tiagabine do not appear to be effective in treating absence seizures. If the patient has a combination of absence and other generalized or partial seizures, valproic acid is the preferred first choice because it is the only AED effective for absence and other seizure types. If valproic acid is ineffective in treating a mixed seizure disorder that includes absence, ethosuximide should be used in combination with another AED.

The traditional treatment of tonic-clonic seizures is phenytoin or phenobarbital; however, the use of carbamazepine and valproic acid is increasing because these AEDs have a lower incidence of side effects and equal efficacy. Valproic acid generally is considered the drug of first choice for atonic seizures and for juvenile myoclonic epilepsy. Lamotrigine and perhaps topiramate and zonisamide can be alternative agents for these seizure types. Levetiracetam has recently received FDA approval as adjunctive treatment of myoclonic seizures in patients with juvenile myoclonic epilepsy.

In most cases, selection of specific AED will depend on multiple factors, including seizure type, unique patient characteristics, and the expected adverse-effect/pharmacokinetic profile of each AED. An important clinical question remains as to the precise role of the newer-generation drugs. Although several studies would suggest that at least some of the newer agents may have comparable efficacy, as well as improved tolerability compared to the older drugs, definitive comparative studies with all agents are lacking.

Although most of the older AEDs have published therapeutic ranges, the serum concentration should be viewed as a tool with which to optimize therapy for an individual patient, not as a therapeutic end point in and of itself. The serum concentration is a target that should be correlated with clinical outcome. The desired response is the cessation of seizures without side effects. Seizure control can occur before the "minimum" of the published range is achieved, and side effects can appear before the "maximum" of the range is achieved. Some patients may need and tolerate concentrations beyond the maximum. The therapeutic range for AEDs can be different for different seizure types. Serum concentrations may need to be higher to control CP seizures than to control tonic-clonic seizures. Clinicians should define a therapeutic range for an individual patient above which there are side effects and below which the patient experiences seizures. Serum levels can be useful to document lack of efficacy, loss of efficacy, noncompliance, and to determine how much room there is to increase a dose based on expected toxicity. Depending on the AED, they can also be useful in patients with significant renal and/or hepatic disease, patients taking multiple drugs, and women who are pregnant or taking oral contraceptives. To date, therapeutic concentration ranges have not been established conclusively for the newer-generation AEDs.

■ THERAPEUTIC CONSIDERATIONS IN THE ELDERLY AND YOUNG

Use of AEDs in the elderly and young can pose special challenges.[52] Avoidance of AEDs that interact with other medications that the elderly are taking is of upmost importance. Many of the drugs are inducers or inhibitors of the CYP450 system, which can affect the therapeutic drug level of concomitant drugs that can ultimately have a detrimental outcome. Hypoalbuminemia is a common occurrence in the elderly, which can make monitoring and adjustment of serum drug levels of highly albumin-bound AEDs, such as phenytoin, valproic acid, and tiagabine, problematic. The elderly also experience body mass changes such as an increase in fat to lean body mass or decrease in body water, which can affect the volume of distribution of some drugs, and therefore possibly the elimination half-life of the drug. In addition, declining renal and/or hepatic function can occur in the elderly, which can require a lower dose of the AED. Lastly, the pharmacodynamic response to AEDs can change as the patient ages because elderly patients may be more sensitive to various neurocognitive adverse effects of these drugs.

Elderly patients may demonstrate efficacy (e.g., control of seizures) at relatively lower serum concentrations as well.

For neonates and infants, an increase in the total body water to body fat ratio and a decrease in serum albumin and α-acid glycoprotein can result in volume of distribution changes that can affect the elimination half-life of the AEDs. In addition, newborns up to the age of 2 to 3 years display decreased efficiency in renal elimination, with the newborn having the most significant impairment. Hepatic activity is also reduced in this population. However, by age 2 to 3 years, hepatic activity is more robust than that seen in adults. Therefore, children require higher doses of many of the antiepileptics than adults, whereas neonates and infants require lower doses.

■ THERAPEUTIC CONSIDERATIONS IN WOMEN (AND MEN)

Many hormones influence brain electrical excitability, and the steroid hormones estrogen and progesterone may interact in complex ways to alter neuronal excitability and protein synthesis.[53] Estrogen has a seizure-activating effect, whereas progesterone exerts a seizure-protective effect. Estrogen has an inhibitory effect on GABA receptors, potentiates excitatory glutaminergic activity, and can promote the development of kindling. Progesterone has the opposite effect and appears to potentiate GABA receptor activity and reduce neuronal discharge rates. AEDs, especially hepatic metabolizing enzyme inducers, increase the metabolism of steroid hormones and induce the production of sex hormone–binding globulin. This may lead to decreases in the unbound fraction of the hormone. Enzyme-inducing AEDs, including topiramate and oxcarbazepine at higher doses, can cause treatment failures in women taking oral contraceptives owing to induction of the metabolism of both ethinyl estradiol and progestin. A supplemental form of birth control, in addition to oral contraceptives, is advised if breakthrough bleeding occurs. Valproic acid, benzodiazepines, and most of the newer AEDs, such as gabapentin, levetiracetam, tiagabine, and zonisamide, are not enzyme inducers and have not been associated with this effect.

In some women, vulnerability to seizures is highest just before and during the menstrual flow (catamenial seizures) and at the time of ovulation. The risk of catamenial epilepsy is estimated at 12.5%, but it can occur in as many as 50% of women with epilepsy. This pattern of seizure exacerbation can be related to progesterone withdrawal and changes in the estrogen-to-progesterone ratio. Conventional AEDs should be tried first in these women. Intermittent acetazolamide also has been used but with variable and limited success. Hormonal therapy with progestational agents, particularly cyclic natural progesterone therapy, also can be effective. Reproductive endocrine disorders are common in women with epilepsy and include menstrual irregularity, infertility, sexual dysfunction, and possibly an increased risk of polycystic ovary syndrome.[54] Potential mechanisms for these disturbances include disruption of the hypothalamic-pituitary-adrenal (HPA) axis via seizure discharges in limbic structures and/or AEDs.[54] AEDs, particularly the enzyme-inducing agents (e.g., carbamazepine, phenytoin, and phenobarbital), also may affect HPA function by altering the metabolism of the neuroactive sex hormones, including testosterone. Although a definitive causal relationship has not yet been established, an apparent increased incidence of polycystic ovary syndrome has been suggested for women with epilepsy who are receiving valproic acid.[54]

Pregnancy raises several concerns, including the possibility of increased maternal seizures, pregnancy complications, and adverse fetal outcome.[55] Approximately 25% to 30% of women have increased seizures during pregnancy, whereas seizures decrease in a similar number. Increased seizure activity may result from either a direct effect on seizure threshold or a reduction in AED concentration. An increase in clearance has been reported for phenytoin, carbamazepine, phenobarbital, ethosuximide, lamotrigine, oxcarbazepine, and clorazepate. Protein binding also may be altered. The altered disposition of AEDs can begin as early as the first 10 weeks of pregnancy and can take up to 4 weeks postpartum to return to normal. The return to the nonpregnant metabolism and binding requires longer for carbamazepine and phenobarbital than it does for phenytoin.

There is a higher incidence of adverse pregnancy outcomes in women with epilepsy. Although the risk of congenital malformations is 4% to 6% (twice as high as in nonepileptic women), more than 90% of pregnancies in epileptic mothers have satisfactory outcomes. Older data, much of which included AED polytherapy, indicated that barbiturates and phenytoin are associated with congenital heart malformations, orofacial clefts, and other malformations. Valproic acid and carbamazepine are associated with spina bifida (neural tube defect) and hypospadias. From these data the risk of neural tube defect with valproic acid and carbamazepine has been estimated to be 0.5% to 1%, respectively, and appears to be related to drug exposure during gestational days 0 to 28. Other adverse pregnancy outcomes associated with maternal seizures, but not necessarily caused by AEDs, are growth, psychomotor, and mental retardation. Women with epilepsy are also more likely to have miscarriages, and 10% to 20% of infants are born with low birth weight. Guidelines have been developed for counseling and managing pregnant women with epilepsy.

Many of these teratogenic effects can be prevented by adequate folate intake; therefore, prenatal vitamins with folic acid (~0.4–5 mg/day) should be given to any woman of child-bearing potential who is taking AEDs.[55] Higher folate doses should be used in women with a history of a previous pregnancy with a neural tube defect. Higher AED doses and serum concentrations, polytherapy, and a family history of birth defects appear to increase the teratogenic risk. Deciding on the most effective single-drug treatment prior to conception is vitally important. New AEDs are reported to be less teratogenic, and animal reproductive toxicology studies appear to be favorable. At present, clinical data are still limited, and more experience is needed before the true risk (or lack thereof) can be determined. However, multiple registries worldwide are currently collecting prospective data on the outcome of pregnancies in users of newer and older AEDs. To date, results indicate that valproic acid mono- as well as polytherapy appears to cause a significantly higher rate of fetal malformations compared to the other AEDs, especially at doses greater than 1,400 mg/day.[56,57] Some AEDs also can lead to neonatal hemorrhagic disorder, which can be prevented by the administration of vitamin K 10 mg orally, given to the mother daily during the last month of pregnancy.

Although AEDs pass into the breast milk, the concentrations are very low, and the infant receives a subtherapeutic dose. In general, knowledge of the degree of protein binding of a given AED can allow for prediction of breast milk accumulation. Taking AEDs with less protein binding results in more accumulation in breast milk. Treatment with AEDs is not necessarily a reason to discourage breast-feeding. It is advisable that women taking any AED (particularly barbiturates or benzodiazepines) closely observe infants for signs of excess sedation, irritability, or poor feeding.[55]

The perimenopausal period can be associated with worsening of seizures, possibly owing to fluctuations in sex hormones. At menopause, seizures actually can improve, particularly in women who previously presented with a catamenial pattern. The effect of hormone-replacement therapy on seizure control is still unclear, but clinicians should monitor for seizure exacerbation in women receiving supplemental estrogen.

It appears from recent data that men with epilepsy have reduced fertility and that carbamazepine, oxcarbazepine, and valproic acid are associated with sperm abnormalities in these men. In addition,

TABLE 58-8 AED Dosing and Target Serum Concentration Ranges

	Trade Name	Usual Initial Dose	Usual Maximum Daily Dose	Target Serum Concentration Range
Barbiturates				
Mephobarbital	Mebaral	50–100 mg/day	400–600 mg	Not defined
Phenobarbital	Various	1–3 mg/kg/day (10–20 mg/kg LD)	180–300 mg	10–40 mcg/mL
Primidone	Mysoline	100–125 mg/day	750–2,000 mg	5–10 mcg/mL
Benzodiazepines				
Clonazepam	Klonopin	1.5 mg/day	20 mg	20–80 ng/mL
Clorazepate	Tranxene	7.5–22.5 mg/day	90 mg	Not defined
Diazepam	Valium	PO: 4–40 mg IV: 5–10 mg	PO: 4–40 mg IV: 5–30 mg	100–1,000 ng/mL
Lorazepam	Ativan	PO: 2–6 mg IV: 0.05 mg/kg IM: 0.05 mg/kg	PO: 10 mg IV: 0.044 mg/kg	10–30 ng/mL
Hydantoins				
Ethotoin	Peganone	<1,000 mg/day	2,000–4,000 mg with food	15–50 mcg/mL
Mephenytoin	Mesantoin	50–100 mg/day	200–800 mg	25–40 mcg/mL
Phenytoin	Dilantin	PO: 3–5 mg/kg (200–400 mg) (15–20 mg/kg LD)	PO: 500–600 mg	Total: 10–20 mcg/mL Unbound: 0.5–3 mcg/mL
Succinimides				
Ethosuximide	Zarontin	500 mg/day	500–2,000 mg	40–80 mcg/mL
Methsuximide	Celontin	300 mg/day	300–1,200 mg	*N*-desmethyl metabolite 10–40 mcg/mL
Other				
Carbamazepine	Tegretol	400 mg/day	400–2,400 mg	4–14 mcg/mL
Felbamate	Felbatol	1,200 mg/day	3,600 mg	40–100 mcg/mL[a]
Gabapentin	Neurontin	900 mg/day	4,800 mg	4–16 mcg/mL[a]
Lamotrigine	Lamictal	25 mg every other day if on VPA; 25–50 mg/day if not on VPA	100–150 mg if on VPA; 300–500 mg if not on VPA	4–20 mcg/mL[a]
Levetiracetam	Keppra	500–1,000 mg/day	3,000–4,000 mg	5–40 mcg/mL[aa]
Oxcarbazepine	Trileptal	300–600 mg/day	2,400–3,000 mg	12–30 mcg/mL[a] (MHD)
Pregabalin	Lyrica	150 mg/day	600 mg	Not defined
Tiagabine	Gabitril	4–8 mg/day	80 mg	100–300 mcg/mL[a]
Topiramate	Topamax	25–50 mg/day	200–1,000 mg	2–25 mcg/mL
Valproic acid	Depakene Depakote Depacon	15 mg/kg (500–1,000 mg)	60 mg/kg (3,000–5,000 mg)	50–150 mcg/mL[a]
Zonisamide	Zonegran	100–200 mg/day	600 mg	10–40 mcg/mL[a]

AED, antiepileptic drug; IM, intramuscular; LD, loading does; MHD, 10-monohydrate derivative; PO, orally; VPA, valproic acid.
[a]Based on data from clinical trials–no established therapeutic ranges.
Data from Leppik[32] and Bourgeois.[33]

valproic acid seems to cause testicular atrophy resulting in reduced testosterone volume.[58]

■ CLINICAL CONSIDERATIONS WITH SPECIFIC DRUGS

Tables 58–4 through 58–9 list specific data (including pharmacokinetics, adverse effects, AED interactions, metabolism, and dosing) for each of the commonly used AEDs. Below we summarize the relative properties, advantages, and disadvantages, and perspectives as to the place in therapy of each of these agents.

Carbamazepine

Pharmacology and Mechanism of Action The exact mechanism by which carbamazepine suppresses seizure spread is obscure, although it is believed to act primarily through inhibition of voltage-gated sodium channels. In addition, interaction with voltage-gated calcium and potassium channels can also contribute to its activity.[59]

TABLE 58-9 Phenytoin Dosage Forms

Dosage Form	Salt or Acid	Extended or Prompt	Amount of Acid Available
Dilantin capsules	Phenytoin sodium	Extended	
100 mg			92 mg
30 mg			27 mg
Dilantin suspension 125 mg/5 mL	Phenytoin acid	Prompt	125 mg/5 mL
Dilantin Infatabs 50 mg	Phenytoin acid	Prompt	50 mg
Phenytoin injectable 50 mg/mL	Phenytoin sodium	Prompt	46 mg/mL
Fosphenytoin 50 mg PE/mL			50 mg PHT equivalents/mL
Phenytek capsules	Phenytoin sodium	Extended	
200 mg			184 mg
300 mg			276 mg
Phenytoin capsules (generic)	Phenytoin sodium	Prompt	92 mg

PE, phenytoin equivalents; PHT, phenytoin.

Pharmacokinetics The absorption of carbamazepine from immediate-release tablets is slow and erratic because of its low water solubility. There is also a large variability in the peak-to-trough concentrations of up to 40%. There is no first-pass metabolism. Food, especially fat, may enhance the bioavailability of carbamazepine. The suspension dosage form is absorbed faster than the tablets.[60] Controlled-release (Tegretol-XR) and sustained-release (Carbatrol) preparations are also available. These dosage forms are bioequivalent in twice-daily (every 12 hours) dosing to dosing four times daily (every 6 hours) with immediate-release carbamazepine. Compared with immediate-release carbamazepine, both these formulations have lower peaks and higher troughs, which can decrease side effects and improve seizure control. Carbatrol has also been shown to improve quality-of-life measurements compared to the immediate-release product.[61] Patients should be told to take Tegretol-XR with food and that the casing will be excreted in the feces. Tegretol-XR cannot be broken or crushed. Tegretol-XR and Carbatrol appear to be bioequivalent; however, there is less variability in the absorption of Carbatrol.[60]

Carbamazepine is a neutral and highly lipophilic drug that results in high body tissue binding. It binds to α_1-acid glycoprotein and to albumin. The major metabolite is carbamazepine-10,11-epoxide, which has anticonvulsant activity in animals and humans.[60] The formation of the 10,11-epoxide is influenced by concurrent use of other enzyme-inducing or enzyme-inhibiting drugs; thus the 10,11-epoxide concentration may change with the administration of other drugs (e.g., valproate and felbamate) with no change in parent carbamazepine concentration.[60]

Carbamazepine induces its own metabolism (autoinduction) thereby decreasing its half-life after chronic therapy.[60] The presence of enzyme-inducing drugs reduces the half-life even more. The enzyme-induction effect begins within 3 to 5 days of the initiation of therapy and takes 21 to 28 days to complete. Therefore, it is possible to achieve initial concentrations that are within the therapeutic range but have concentrations fall despite continued therapy with good compliance. Some patients who respond well to initial therapy may be labeled refractory or noncompliant if the autoinduction phenomenon is not considered. The autoinduction reverses rapidly if therapy with carbamazepine is discontinued temporarily. Carbamazepine also displays diurnal variation in its serum level with the evening level lower than the morning level.

Adverse Effects Side effects of carbamazepine can fluctuate daily, paralleling the rise and decline of serum concentrations. Neurosensory side effects (e.g., diplopia, blurred vision, nystagmus, ataxia, unsteadiness, dizziness, and headache) are the most common, occurring in 35% to 50% of patients. These side effects are more common during initiation of therapy and can dissipate with continued treatment. Carbamazepine can also cause nausea, which can either be caused by a local effect of the drug on the GI tract, in which case food may help, or caused by an effect on the brainstem, which may ultimately require discontinuation of the drug. Dosage manipulation, including the use of the controlled- or sustained-release preparations, should be tried before the patient is considered to be intolerant of carbamazepine. Carbamazepine can cause hyponatremia, the incidence of which increases with age, however, its occurrence is lower than that seen with oxcarbazepine. Periodic determinations of serum sodium concentration are recommended, especially in the elderly.[60]

Leukopenia is the most common hematologic side effect. An incidence as high as 10% has been reported. Leukopenia usually is transient, even when the drug is continued, and can be caused by a redistribution of white blood cells (WBCs) rather than a decrease in their production. In about 2% of patients, the leukopenia is persistent, but even patients with WBC counts of 3,000/mm^3 or less do not seem to have an increased incidence of infection. A clinical guide is to continue carbamazepine therapy unless the WBC count drops to less than 2,500/mm^3 and the absolute neutrophil count drops to less than 1,000/mm^3.[60]

Drug Interactions Because of concentration-dependent efficacy and side effects, drug interactions with carbamazepine often are very significant. Drugs that inhibit CYP 3A4 potentially may increase carbamazepine serum concentrations. Carbamazepine may interact with other drugs by inducing their metabolism.

Dosing and Administration The variable contributions of the 10,11-epoxide metabolite and free-carbamazepine concentrations have restricted a precise definition of the therapeutic range. Loading doses of carbamazepine are indicated only for critically ill patients. During dosage titration, it should be remembered that carbamazepine clearance increases with time. Doses may be started at one-fourth to one-third the anticipated maintenance dose and increased every 2 to 3 weeks. Because of the auto- and heteroinduction of carbamazepine metabolism, it is necessary to administer the drug two to four times per day. The controlled- and sustained release formulations provide fewer peak-to-trough fluctuations, which can improve adherence, reduce side effects, and improve seizure control. Carbamazepine tablets should not be stored in places where they would be exposed to high heat and high humidity.[60]

Advantages Carbamazepine has been well studied. Oral immediate- and extended-release solid and liquid dosage forms are available. The oral solid dosage form is available as an immediate-release tablet and as a sustained-release capsule and a controlled-release tablet. The sustained- and controlled-release dosage forms allow for twice-daily dosing to reduce the peak-to-trough fluctuations. Compared with other first-generation AEDs, carbamazepine causes minimal cognitive impairment.

Disadvantages Carbamazepine has an active metabolite that can contribute to efficacy and toxicity. Other drugs can alter the concentration of this metabolite without changing the concentration of the parent carbamazepine. It induces its own metabolism, which requires careful dosage titration. It also induces the metabolism of other medications, and other drugs may interact with it and/or the active metabolite. There is no parenteral formulation. There are clinically meaningful CNS side effects including sedation and nausea. One prospective study, however, did find fewer side effects with the sustained release formulation compared to the immediate release formulation.[61] When ingested during the first trimester by pregnant women, carbamazepine has been associated with a 1% risk of spina bifida. Chronic carbamazepine use also has been associated with alterations in bone mineral density in some studies and decreases in 25-hydoxy (OH) vitamin D. The generic formulations of immediate-release tablets have been associated with breakthrough seizures when brands have been switched.

Place in Therapy Carbamazepine should be considered a first-line therapy for patients with newly diagnosed partial seizures and for patients with primary generalized convulsive seizures who are not in an emergent situation.

Ethosuximide

Pharmacology and Mechanism of Action The exact mechanism of action of ethosuximide remains elusive, however, it is believed to exert its main action through inhibition of T-type calcium channels.[59]

Pharmacokinetics Metabolism occurs in the liver by hydroxylation, and the metabolites are believed to be inactive. There is some evidence of a nonlinear metabolic process at higher concentrations.

Adverse Effects The most frequently reported side effects are nausea and vomiting (up to 40%), and these symptoms may be minimized by administration of smaller doses and more frequent dosing.[62]

Drug Interactions Because ethosuximide is not protein bound, displacement interactions do not occur. Valproic acid may inhibit the metabolism of ethosuximide, but only if the metabolism of ethosuximide is near saturation.[63]

Dosing and Administration A loading dose of ethosuximide is not required. Titration over 1 to 2 weeks to maintenance doses of 20 mg/kg per day usually results in therapeutic concentrations. Data suggest that patients can be managed successfully on once-a-day therapy; however, gastrointestinal distress appears to be dose-related, and the total daily dose is usually divided into two equal doses.[60]

Advantages This drug is very effective in the treatment of absence seizures. It is generally well tolerated and has few pharmacokinetic interactions.

Disadvantages Ethosuximide has a very narrow spectrum of activity.

Place in Therapy Ethosuximide is still a first-line treatment for absence seizures.

Felbamate

Pharmacology and Mechanism of Action At therapeutic doses felbamate appears to act by blocking *N*-methyl-D-aspartate (NMDA) synaptic responses and by modulating $GABA_A$ receptors. At higher doses it may modulate sodium channels and inhibit high-voltage activated calcium channels.[59]

Pharmacokinetics Felbamate is rapidly and well absorbed. The absorption is unaffected by food or antacids. Approximately 40% to 50% of a dose of felbamate is metabolized by hydroxylation and conjugation pathways in the liver, with the remainder being excreted unchanged in the urine. Felbamate displays linear pharmacokinetics.[64]

Adverse Effects The most frequently reported side effects with felbamate prior to marketing were anorexia, weight loss, insomnia, nausea, and headache (sometimes severe). Anorexia and weight loss may be especially problematic in children and in patients with diminished caloric intake. After marketing, felbamate was found to be associated with aplastic anemia and acute liver failure. The onset was between 68 and 354 days of therapy. The approximate rate of occurrence of aplastic anemia is 1 in 3,000 and of hepatitis is 1 in 10,000. Data suggest a possible increased risk for aplastic anemia in patients, especially women, with a history of cytopenia, AED allergy or significant toxicity, viral infection, and/or immunologic problems.[25,26,65]

Drug Interactions Depending on the drug, felbamate affects the metabolism of the older AEDs through either inhibition or induction. Interactions with warfarin and felbamate also have been reported.[64]

Dosing and Administration The initial starting dose of felbamate is increased at 2-week intervals.

Advantages Felbamate has a unique mechanism of action. It is approved for treating atonic seizures in patients with the Lennox-Gastaut syndrome and is effective in treating patients with partial seizures.

Disadvantages The use of felbamate is limited by the association with aplastic anemia and hepatotoxicity, as well as multiple drug interactions.

Place in Therapy This agent should be reserved for patients not responding to other AEDs.

Gabapentin

Pharmacology and Mechanism of Action Gabapentin was designed to be a GABA agonist but does not react at the GABA receptor, alter GABA uptake, or interfere with GABA transaminase. Gabapentin appears to bind to an amino acid carrier protein and appears to act at a unique receptor. Gabapentin inhibits high-voltage activated calcium channels.[59] It elevates human brain GABA levels, possibly via alterations in GABA synthesis or reversal of the neuronal GABA transporter, resulting in nonvesicular release of GABA.[66]

Pharmacokinetics Gabapentin is a substrate of the L-amino acid carrier protein in the gut (system L), as well as in the CNS.[67] This amino acid carrier protein transports the drug across the gut membrane by an active process. The binding of gabapentin to this system is saturable, and gabapentin therefore displays dose-dependent bioavailability that appears to vary considerably between individuals.[68] Food, including protein-rich meals, does not appear to interfere with gabapentin oral absorption.[69] Concentrations in human CSF are 5% to 35% of plasma levels, and tissue concentrations are approximately 80% of plasma levels.

Because gabapentin is eliminated exclusively by the kidneys, dosage adjustments are necessary in patients with significantly impaired renal function. In anuric patients, 35% of gabapentin is removed by dialysis.[70]

Adverse Effects Fatigue, somnolence, dizziness, and ataxia are the most frequently reported side effects. Aggressive behavior has been reported in children.[71] The CNS effects of gabapentin are generally less than those of traditional AEDs. A withdrawal reaction characterized by anxiety, insomnia, nausea, sweating, and increased pain has also been reported with abrupt discontinuation in patients taking it for pain.

Drug Interactions Gabapentin does not induce or inhibit liver enzymes; therefore, drug interactions are not likely to occur with gabapentin. There is a 10% reduction in the clearance of gabapentin in patients taking cimetidine and a 20% reduction in the bioavailability if aluminum antacids are taken simultaneously with gabapentin. These interactions are unlikely to be clinically significant.

Dosing and Administration Typical starting doses of gabapentin are 300 mg at bedtime on the first day, increasing to 900 mg/day over 3 days. Faster titration rates (e.g., starting at 300 to 900 mg three times daily) have been well tolerated.[72] Data from a pharmacokinetic study suggest gabapentin should be given at least four times a day when the total daily dose is 3,600 mg or greater.[73] Gabapentin does not appear to be absorbed rectally. Patients with end-stage renal disease maintained on hemodialysis should receive an initial 300- to 400-mg dose with 200 to 300 mg gabapentin given after every 4 hours of hemodialysis.[70]

Advantages Gabapentin has multiple mechanisms of action and is mechanistically different from first-generation AEDs. It is not metabolized and is excreted unchanged by the kidney. Gabapentin has the additional advantages of a broad therapeutic index with minimal CNS adverse effects and no drug interactions. Doses can be escalated rapidly.

Disadvantages Gabapentin is absorbed by an active process that saturates at higher doses. This may require more frequent daily dosing for patients who need doses greater than 3,600 mg/day. Doses exceeding the 3,600 mg/day maximum listed in the package insert may be required in some patients to achieve seizure remission. There is no parenteral formulation.

Place in Therapy Gabapentin is a second-line agent for patients with partial seizures who have failed initial treatment. In addition, although monotherapy trials have no proven efficacy in previously diagnosed refractory patients, there may be a role for this drug in patients with less severe seizure disorders, such as new-onset partial epilepsy, particularly in the elderly patient. Gabapentin also has been shown to be useful in the treatment of chronic pain and other nonepileptic conditions.

Lamotrigine

Pharmacology and Mechanism of Action A primary mechanism of action for lamotrigine appears to be inhibition of voltage-dependent sodium channels, however, the drug also inhibits high voltage-activated calcium channels.[59]

Pharmacokinetics Lamotrigine is completely and rapidly absorbed, with a bioavailability of 98%. Food does not significantly affect drug absorption. Lamotrigine is also absorbed following rectal administration, although the mean area under the curve (AUC) is approximately 50% of that achieved by oral administration. Lamotrigine clearance is higher in children and lower in the elderly compared with young adults. There are only modest differences in the pharmacokinetics of lamotrigine in the elderly versus younger subjects. Hepatic disease, depending on severity, can influence lamotrigine pharmacokinetics. Approximately 17% of a lamotrigine dose can be removed by hemodialysis, with the half-life being reduced to approximately 13 hours. For patients on dialysis, the half-life is much more prolonged between dialyses (57.4 hours) but shorter during dialysis (13 hours).[74] The half-life is prolonged in patients with renal failure.

Adverse Effects The most frequently reported side effects of lamotrigine include diplopia, drowsiness, ataxia, and headache.[75] Adverse effects are more common when lamotrigine is given in combination with other AEDs (e.g., diplopia when given concomitantly with carbamazepine or tremor with valproic acid) as compared with monotherapy, and they can be pharmacodynamic in nature. Lamotrigine can cause rash, which usually appears in the first 3 to 4 weeks of therapy. Patients with a history of developing a rash with another AED are more likely to develop a rash.[76] The rash typically is generalized, erythematous, and morbilliform and frequently is mild to moderate in severity. However, a Stevens-Johnson reaction also has been reported. Some rashes, especially those which develop early, can necessitate the withdrawal of lamotrigine.[77] Risk factors for the emergence of more serious rashes appear to be concomitant use of valproic acid and situations where high initial doses or rapid dosage escalation is used. Data from several European monotherapy trials suggest that when dosed appropriately, the incidence of rash from lamotrigine is similar to that of older agents such as carbamazepine and phenytoin. The incidence is higher in children than in adults.

Drug Interactions Lamotrigine does not inhibit liver enzymes and has a low potential for pharmacokinetic interactions with other drugs. It has been found to decrease the bioavailability of the progesterone component (levonorgestrel) of a combination oral contraceptive by 19%. The clinical relevance of this interaction has not been determined.[78]

Concomitant treatment with oral contraceptives can lead to a reduction in the serum concentrations of lamotrigine because of an induction of lamotrigine glucuronidation by the ethinyl estradiol component of the pill.[79] In addition lamotrigine serum levels can significantly increase during the week off oral contraceptive treatment in some patients on cyclic therapy.[80]

Valproic acid substantially inhibits the metabolism of lamotrigine, with maximal inhibition of lamotrigine metabolism occurring at valproic acid doses and serum concentrations of 500 mg/day and 40 to 50 mcg/mL, respectively.[75] A pharmacodynamic interaction can occur with concurrent carbamazepine therapy, leading to an increase in CNS side effects.

Dosing and Administration In patients who are taking enzyme-inducing drugs, lamotrigine can be started more rapidly than in patients receiving valproic acid. The maintenance doses are also different. These different doses are critical owing to the relationship between rash, concomitant valproic acid treatment, and the dose escalation rate. Removal of inducers from a lamotrigine regimen may necessitate decreases in lamotrigine doses, whereas removal of valproic acid can necessitate an increase in the lamotrigine dose. A dispersible tablet is available for patients who cannot swallow an oral solid dosage form.[25,26,65]

Advantages Lamotrigine is potentially a broad-spectrum AED, having efficacy in partial seizures as well as several types of generalized seizures. A pediatric dosage form is available. It neither induces nor inhibits the metabolism of other AEDs. Lamotrigine has linear pharmacokinetics and is not highly protein bound. Lamotrigine appears to be generally well tolerated in both children and elderly patients and does not cause weight gain.

Disadvantages Lamotrigine is associated with rash, especially in patients who start at a high dose, have rapid dose escalation, and/or are taking concurrent valproic acid. Therefore, the initial doses must be low (lower if the patient is on valproic acid) and escalated slowly in order to maximize patient safety. There is no parenteral dosage form.

Place in Therapy Lamotrigine is useful as both adjunctive treatment in patients with partial seizures and as monotherapy. Lamotrigine appears to have comparable effectiveness with more traditional AEDs such as carbamazepine and phenytoin when used as monotherapy. In addition, lamotrigine may be a useful alternative in patients with primary generalized seizure types such as absence and as adjunctive therapy for patients with primary GTC seizures, the latter of which is an approved indication.

Levetiracetam

Pharmacology and Mechanism of Action Levetiracetam, an *S*-enantiomer pyrrolidone derivative, is chemically unrelated to other available AEDs. Although the precise mechanism of action of levetiracetam has yet to be delineated, it is known that this drug is not active in the classic models used to test antiepileptic drugs. The drug binds in the brain to the synaptic vesicle protein SV2A, which is believed to be important in its activity.[81] This agent may have a unique mechanism of action, including reduction in high-voltage activated calcium ion (Ca^{2+}) currents and delayed-rectifier potassium ion (K^+) currents, as well as a unique action on GABA currents. There is some limited evidence that levetiracetam may have *antiepileptogenic effects,* meaning that this compound may be able to prevent the development of epilepsy under certain circumstances.[82] Clinical confirmation of this animal research is still needed, however.

Pharmacokinetics Levetiracetam is rapidly and completely absorbed following oral administration. The absorption of the drug is not significantly affected by food or enteral nutrition formulas.[83] Renal elimination of unchanged parent drug accounts for the majority of drug clearance (66%), with the remainder being metabolized in blood via nonhepatic enzymatic hydrolysis of an acetamide group to inactive metabolites.[84] This metabolic pathway does not involve either the CYP450 or UGT isozyme systems. Because this drug is eliminated renally, clinicians should anticipate age-related reductions in clearance in elderly patients. Conversely, levetiracetam clearance appears to be approximately 40% higher in children than in adults. In addition patients with severe liver cirrhosis should initially receive one-half the recommended starting dose because of a 57% decrease in clearance of the drug.[85] Currently, data are sparse regarding serum concentration–effect relationships, so the role of therapeutic drug level monitoring remains unclear.

Adverse Effects Adverse effects appear to be modest, with sedation, fatigue, and coordination difficulties being the most common CNS effects. In children and young adults, behavioral disorders including agitation, irritability or somnolence/lethargy are the most frequently reported central nervous side effects.[86] The mechanism underlying these effects is unknown. Formal studies evaluating the cognitive effects of this medication have not yet been conducted.[25,26,65]

Drug Interactions Levetiracetam neither inhibits nor induces the CYP450, UGT, or epoxide hydrolase enzyme systems, and in-vitro data predict a low potential for pharmacokinetic interactions. Levetiracetam does not appear to interact with other AEDs, warfarin, digoxin, or oral contraceptive drugs.[87,88]

Dosing and Administration Levetiracetam is available orally as well as parenterally, the latter for maintenance dosing only. The intravenous (IV) product has not been tested for intramuscular (IM) use, and therefore should not be administered IM. The typical initial dose is given twice daily, with dosage increments every 2 weeks. In order to minimize CNS side effects, clinicians can consider initiating the drug at one-half this rate. The IV formulation should be given at the same frequency and dose as the oral product. Although not FDA approved, the oral dose of levetiracetam has been titrated rapidly up to 3,000 mg in 3 days in some intractable seizure patients with improvement seen in their seizures after day 2.[89]

Advantages Levetiracetam has a novel, although unknown, mechanism of action. It has linear pharmacokinetics and is not metabolized by the cytochrome P450 system. No significant drug interactions, including with oral contraceptives, have been reported. Initial doses can be effective. The drug appears to be well tolerated, with transient sedation being the most troublesome adverse effect in most individuals.

Disadvantages Dose adjustments are needed for patients with decreased renal function, and slower dose escalation may be needed to avoid CNS adverse effects. Behavioral problems can limit therapy in some patients.

Place in Therapy Currently, levetiracetam is indicated for patients with partial seizures who have failed initial therapy. Its role as monotherapy for partial seizures remains to be clarified. The drug was recently approved as adjunctive treatment for myoclonic seizures in patients with juvenile myoclonic epilepsy. Its role as adjunctive treatment in other generalized seizures disorders remains to be defined.

Oxcarbazepine

Pharmacology and Mechanism of Action Oxcarbazepine, which is structurally related to carbamazepine, is a prodrug that is rapidly converted to a 10-monohydrate derivative (MHD), which is the active component. The mechanism of action of oxcarbazepine is similar to that of carbamazepine and perhaps lamotrigine. Oxcarbazepine and MHD block voltage-sensitive sodium channels, modulate the voltage-activated calcium currents, and increase potassium conductance. Interestingly, however, oxcarbazepine can display differing affinities for both sodium channels and Ca^{2+} channels compared with older drugs such as carbamazepine.[90] Whereas carbamazepine may modulate L-type Ca^{2+} channels, oxcarbazepine appears to modulate N- and P-type Ca^{2+} channels.[91] Whether these differences lead to differing patterns of clinical effectiveness is still uncertain. It has no significant interactions with brain neurotransmitters or modulation of receptor sites.

Pharmacokinetics Oxcarbazepine is absorbed completely and is metabolized extensively by noninducible cytosolic ketoreductase to MHD.[92] The MHD is inactivated by glucuronide conjugation and eliminated by the kidneys. Oxcarbazepine and its active metabolite do not undergo autoinduction. The relationship between dose and serum concentration is linear. Children 2 to 6 years of age need larger doses to achieve the same serum concentration, suggesting a more rapid clearance. The maximal drug concentration (C_{max}) and bioavailability of MHD in elderly volunteers were higher than in younger volunteers, and the elimination rate was slower, possibly reflecting decreased renal elimination. Patients with significant renal impairment may require a dosage reduction.

Adverse Effects Oxcarbazepine has been in clinical use worldwide since 1990 and was marketed in more than 50 countries prior to approval in the United States. In U.S. clinical trials the most frequently reported adverse events were dizziness, nausea, headache, diarrhea, vomiting, upper respiratory tract infections, constipation, dyspepsia, ataxia, and nervousness. In comparative trials, oxcarbazepine generally caused fewer side effects than phenytoin, valproic acid, or carbamazepine. Dizziness may be more common in elderly patients than in young adults. CNS adverse effects appear to be far more common at doses greater than 1,200 mg/day. Hyponatremia, defined as a plasma sodium concentration of less than 125 mmol/L, has been reported in up to 25% of patients taking oxcarbazepine and occurs more often in elderly patients. The incidence of hyponatremia with oxcarbazepine is higher than that seen with carbamazepine. Clinicians should be particularly watchful in patients receiving concomitant sodium-depleting drugs such as diuretics. Hyponatremia appears to occur less frequently in children. Clinicians should consider monitoring serum sodium levels following the initiation of oxcarbazepine, and they should instruct patients regarding the symptoms of hyponatremia. Approximately 25% to 30% of patients who develop a rash with carbamazepine will experience a similar reaction with oxcarbazepine.[25,26,65] The tolerability of oxcarbazepine has not been compared with that of extended-release formulations of carbamazepine that have lower peaks and potentially fewer side effects than immediate-release carbamazepine formulations.

Drug Interactions Oxcarbazepine decreases the bioavailability of ethinyl estradiol and levonorgestrel.[93] Women concurrently taking oral contraceptives should be counseled about the potential for contraceptive failure. Unlike carbamazepine, there are no interactions between cimetidine, erythromycin, or warfarin and oxcarbazepine. The administration of oxcarbazepine in doses greater than 1,200 mg with phenytoin has resulted in a 40% increase in the concentration of phenytoin, consistent with inhibition of CYP450 2C19. Oxcarbazepine treatment also may cause modest declines in lamotrigine serum concentrations, suggesting induction of UGT isozymes.[94]

The replacement of carbamazepine with oxcarbazepine may result in a drug interaction because an enzyme-inducing drug is being removed.

Dosing and Administration Doses and titration schedules differ in regards to whether the drug is used for mono- or adjunctive therapy in adults vs children. Although not FDA approved, doses up to 60 mg/kg/day have been used in infants and children younger than 4 years of age to successfully control partial-onset seizures.[95] In patients being converted from carbamazepine, the typical maintenance dose of oxcarbazepine is 1.5 times the carbamazepine dose.

Advantages The efficacy of oxcarbazepine is comparable with that of carbamazepine, phenytoin, and valproic acid. It may be better tolerated than phenytoin as monotherapy and therefore less likely to be discontinued.[96] It has been approved in many countries, and there is broad international experience with this drug.

Disadvantages About 30% of patients who have experienced a rash with carbamazepine have a cross-reaction with oxcarbazepine. There are more reports of hyponatremia with oxcarbazepine, especially in patients at risk. Replacing carbamazepine with oxcarbazepine can result in interactions owing to the removal of carbamazepine. Enzyme-inducing drugs can increase the clearance of MHD. This drug is not likely to be effective in seizure types where carbamazepine is ineffective, such as absence or myoclonic seizures.

Place in Therapy Oxcarbazepine is indicated for use as monotherapy or adjunctive therapy in the treatment of partial seizures in adults and as monotherapy and adjunctive therapy in the treatment of partial seizures in patients as young as 4 years of age with epilepsy. It is also a potential first-line drug for patients with primary generalized convulsive seizures. Oxcarbazepine can also be effective in patients not demonstrating a response to carbamazepine.

Phenobarbital

Pharmacology and Mechanism of Action Phenobarbital may elevate seizure threshold by interacting with GABA receptors to facilitate intrinsic chloride channel function, was well as by blocking high voltage-activated calcium channels. Some of the drug's activity may also be caused by its ability to block α-amino-3-hydroxy-5-methylisoxazole-4-propionic acid (AMPA) and kainate receptors.[59]

Pharmacokinetics Phenobarbital is absorbed rapidly and completely regardless of whether it is given orally, intramuscularly, or rectally.[63] It penetrates the brain at a rate comparable with that of phenytoin, and peak concentrations are achieved 3 to 20 minutes after an IV dose.

Drugs affecting liver enzymes can alter phenobarbital metabolism, but phenobarbital clearance is not affected by liver blood flow. The elimination of phenobarbital is linear. Because tubular reabsorption of phenobarbital is pH dependent, the amount excreted renally can be increased by giving diuretics and urinary alkalinizers.[63] Clearance decreases in the elderly.[97]

Adverse Effects CNS side effects are the primary factors limiting the use of phenobarbital. Tolerance usually develops to initial complaints of fatigue, drowsiness, sedation, and depression. In children, paradoxically, the primary side effect is hyperactivity. Phenobarbital also may cause porphyria and rash, including serious rashes such as Stevens-Johnson.[98]

Drug Interactions Phenobarbital is a potent enzyme inducer and can increase the elimination of any drug metabolized by CYP450- or UGT-mediated metabolism. Cimetidine and chloramphenicol inhibit phenobarbital metabolism, necessitating a decrease in dose. Ethanol increases the metabolism of phenobarbital.[63]

Dosing and Administration In nonacute situations, phenobarbital should be started in low doses and titrated upward. The dose-concentration relationship is linear. Because the half-life of phenobarbital is long, doses can be given once daily, and bedtime dosing may minimize CNS depression.

Advantages Phenobarbital has linear and predictable pharmacokinetics. Multiple dosage forms (e.g., oral solid, oral liquid, IM, and IV) are available, and it is the most inexpensive AED.

Disadvantages Phenobarbital is associated with significant side effects. These include delayed intellectual development and hyperactivity in children and significant cognitive impairment in adults. It is an enzyme inducer and interacts with many other drugs metabolized by the cytochrome P450 system. Phenobarbital has a very long half-life, and dosage adjustments should not be made more often than every 2 to 3 weeks. The parenteral product contains 67% to 75% propylene glycol and 10% alcohol, which can result in significant respiratory depression and hypotension if infused too rapidly.

Place in Therapy Phenobarbital is the drug of choice for neonatal seizures but in other situations is reserved for patients who have failed therapy with other AEDs. It may be useful given intravenously in refractory status epilepticus.

Phenytoin

Pharmacology and Mechanism of Action The primary mechanism of action of phenytoin is believed to be caused by its ability to inhibit voltage-dependent sodium channels.[59]

Pharmacokinetics The pharmacokinetics of phenytoin are complex and fascinating. For a more in-depth understanding, the reader is referred to a more extensive review.[99] The oral absorption of phenytoin is almost complete. Dissolution is the rate-limiting step, and absorption may be saturable at higher doses, such as those used for oral loading doses. Absorption following IM administration of phenytoin is erratic and delayed, and IM injections are painful, however, IM absorption following fosphenytoin is rapid and well tolerated.

Phenytoin enters the brain rapidly and is redistributed to other body tissues, including breast milk and the placenta. Phenytoin competes for albumin sites with other highly protein bound drugs. It is essential to know the patient's serum albumin level in interpreting the serum concentrations of phenytoin.[100] Patients with significant renal dysfunction will have altered phenytoin protein binding. Obesity increases the volume of distribution of phenytoin.

Phenytoin is metabolized in the liver by parahydroxylation. The major isoforms responsible for the metabolism of phenytoin are CYP 2C9 and CYP 2C19; the former displays polymorphism, which may affect the response to phenytoin.[59] Phenytoin displays Michaelis-Menton pharmacokinetics, which means that the metabolism of phenytoin saturates at doses used clinically. The clinical importance of this is that a small change in dose can result in a disproportionally large increase in serum concentrations, potentially leading to toxicity. In some patients the metabolism of phenytoin can saturate even at low serum concentrations within the therapeutic range. The metabolism of phenytoin decreases with age.

Adverse Effects When phenytoin is initiated, the CNS depressant effects can result in lethargy, fatigue, incoordination, blurred vision, higher cortical dysfunction, and drowsiness. These effects usually are transient and can be minimized by slow dosage titration. At very high concentrations greater than 50 mcg/mL, phenytoin can exacerbate seizures.

It is difficult to determine whether the chronic side effects of phenytoin are concentration- or duration-dependent. One of the more common chronic side effects is gingival hyperplasia. Good oral hygiene can minimize gingival hyperplasia and should be encouraged. Other chronic effects include vitamin D deficiency, osteomalacia, carbohydrate intolerance, immunologic disturbances, hypothyroidism, and peripheral neuropathy. Phenytoin is associated with rare hypersensitivity or idiosyncratic reactions resulting in rashes, Stevens-Johnson syndrome, pseudolymphoma, bone marrow suppression, lupus-like reactions, and hepatitis.[101]

Drug Interactions Phenytoin is associated with numerous drug interactions involving altered absorption, metabolism, and protein binding that can enhance or reduce its effects. Phenytoin is an inducer of both CYP450 and UGT isozymes. The absorption of phenytoin can be increased or decreased with the administration of food depending on the composition of the meal. The bioavailability of phenytoin suspension can be decreased in patients receiving continuous enteral nutrient tube feedings. However, a single-dose study of simultaneous administration of enteral feeding found no difference in phenytoin bioavailability, suggesting that the mechanism was something other than physical contact.[99]

Phenytoin decreases folic acid absorption, and folic acid enhances the clearance of phenytoin. Replacement of folic acid can reduce phenytoin concentration and result in loss of efficacy.[99]

Dosing and Administration Four dosage forms are available for oral administration of phenytoin (see Table 58–9), and changing dosage forms can lead to changes in phenytoin serum concentrations. Whether or not a dosage form uses the parent drug or salt form should be considered when changing from one dosage form to another. Phenytoin capsules are designated as immediate-release or extended-release. Only the extended-release capsules should be used in once-a-day dosing. Particle size rather than formulation may determine the rate of absorption. Phenytek has also been marketed in the United States as an extended-release dosage form of phenytoin.

If oral administration is not feasible, IV administration of phenytoin is preferred, as IM administration can cause tissue necrosis. Fosphenytoin is a prodrug for phenytoin and is available as a parenteral dosage form. It is very water-soluble and is converted rapidly to phenytoin systemically. Fosphenytoin can be given rapidly intravenously and intramuscularly with reliable absorption and minimal pain. It is significantly better tolerated than phenytoin.

Because of saturable absorption, an oral loading dose, such as 20 mg/kg, should be divided by four and given at 6-hour intervals. Subsequent dosage adjustments should be done cautiously owing to its nonlinear elimination. One author has suggested that if the serum concentration is less than 7 mcg/mL, the daily dose should be increased by 100 mg; if the serum concentration is between 7 and 12 mcg/mL, the daily dose can be increased by 50 mg; and if the serum concentration is greater than 12 mcg/mL, the daily dose can be increased by 30 mg or less. These increases are reported to result in less than 10% of patients achieving a phenytoin serum concentration greater than 25 mcg/mL.[102]

Advantages Phenytoin has been used for more than 65 years, and its risk-to-benefit ratio is well established. It is available in oral solid, oral liquid, extended-release oral solid, and parenteral (phenytoin and fosphenytoin) dosage forms, allowing flexibility in dosing and use in emergent situations. In some patients the extended release dosage form can be given once a day with good seizure control.

Disadvantages Phenytoin displays Michaels-Menton pharmacokinetics, meaning that the metabolism saturates at doses given clinically. This makes phenytoin a challenging drug to dose. Also, phenytoin is an inducer of cytochrome P450 isozymes, is metabolized by cytochrome P450 enzymes, and is highly protein bound. Therefore, many drug interactions are associated with coadministration of this agent. Phenytoin is associated with multiple significant adverse effects.

Place in Therapy Phenytoin has long been a first-line AED for primary generalized convulsive and partial seizures. Its use in therapy may be reevaluated as more experience is gained with newer AEDs.

Pregabalin

Pharmacology and Mechanism of Action Pregabalin's mechanism of action is unknown, however, it is proposed that the binding of the drug to the subunit of the voltage-gated calcium channel may be responsible for a large part of its activity. This binding results in a decrease in the release of several excitatory neurotransmitters including glutamate, noradrenaline, substance P, and calcitonin gene-related peptide (CGRP).[103]

Pharmacokinetics Pregabalin is a substrate of the L-amino acid carrier protein in the CNS. It does not display dose-dependent bioavailability. Food decreases the rate but not the bioavailability of the drug.[104]

Pregabalin is eliminated from the body primarily by renal excretion as an unchanged drug, and therefore dosage adjustment is required in patients with significantly impaired renal function. In anuric patients, 50% of the dose is removed by hemodialysis.[104]

Adverse Effects Dizziness, somnolence, ataxia, blurred vision, and weight gain are the most frequently reported side effects. It is not known if pregabalin causes aggressive behavior in children. A withdrawal reaction characterized by anxiety, nervousness, and irritability has been noted in patients being treated for generalized anxiety on abrupt discontinuation of the drug. [105]

Drug Interactions Because pregabalin is predominantly excreted unchanged in the urine and undergoes negligible metabolism in humans, drug interactions are unlikely to occur.

Dosing and Administration Starting doses of pregabalin are divided into twice or thrice daily intervals. The manufacturer recommends that patients with end-stage renal disease maintained on hemodialysis should receive a 25 to 75 mg daily dose with 25 to 75 mg given after every 4 hours of hemodialysis.

Advantages Pregabalin is somewhat more potent than gabapentin without the dose-limited gastrointestinal absorption properties. The drug has minimal CNS side effects and no drug interactions.

Disadvantages Pregabalin is a controlled substance class V. Like gabapentin it can cause weight gain and peripheral edema especially as the dose is increased. There is no parenteral formulation available.

Place in therapy Pregabalin is a second-line agent for patients with partial seizures who have failed initial treatment. Pregabalin is also useful in the treatment of chronic neuropathic pain and generalized anxiety disorder.[105]

Tiagabine

Pharmacology and Mechanism of Action Tiagabine is a potent and specific inhibitor of GABA uptake into glial and other neuronal elements. Thus, tiagabine enhances the action of GABA by decreasing its removal from the synaptic space.[106]

Pharmacokinetics Tiagabine is absorbed quickly and nearly completely after oral administration. There is a linear relationship between daily doses and serum concentrations. Children eliminate tiagabine slightly faster than adults. Subjects with hepatic impairment have higher and more prolonged plasma concentrations of total and unbound drug. Renal dysfunction does not change its pharmacokinetics.[106] Tiagabine displays diurnal elimination, i.e., lower evening serum levels compared to morning levels.

Adverse Effects The most frequently reported adverse effects of tiagabine are dizziness, asthenia, nervousness, tremor, diarrhea, and depression. Adverse events usually are mild to moderate in severity and transient, and most were associated with dose titration.[107] CNS side effects can be diminished by taking tiagabine with food, thus slowing the absorption rate. Tiagabine has increased the incidence of nonconvulsive status epilepticus in patients with chronic refractory partial epilepsy.[108] In addition, there have been reports of status epilepticus or new onset seizures occurring in patients without a history of epilepsy, which is noted in the manufacturer's drug labeling.

Drug Interactions Food decreases the rate but not the extent of absorption. Tiagabine is displaced from protein by naproxen, salicylates, and valproate. However, tiagabine does not displace phenytoin, valproic acid, amitriptyline, tolbutamide, or warfarin.[106]

Dosing and Administration A clear dose-response has been demonstrated, and the minimal effective adult dose level is 30 mg/day. The initial dose is increased weekly.

Advantages Tiagabine has a specific, known mechanism of action. It is the first drug marketed in the United States that acts only on GABA reuptake. This drug has linear pharmacokinetics and is not reported to interact with other drugs.

Disadvantages Initially high and rapid dosage escalation is associated with increased CNS side effects. Therefore, the drug must be started at a low dose and titrated gradually to patient response. Lower doses may be needed in patients with liver disease. Tiagabine is metabolized by CYP450 3A4 enzymes, and other drugs may alter its clearance. There is no parenteral formulation.

Place in Therapy Tiagabine is considered a second-line therapy for patients with partial seizures who have failed initial therapy. It does not appear to have a role in primary generalized seizure types.

Topiramate

Pharmacology and Mechanism of Action Topiramate is a sulfamate-substituted monosaccharide that has multiple modes of action involving voltage-dependent sodium channels, GABA receptor subunits, high voltage calcium channels, and kainate/AMPA subunits.[59] The drug also inhibits the enzyme carbonic anhydrase, although this activity does not appear to play a major role in its mechanism of action.[59]

Pharmacokinetics Although generally considered to have linear absorption and elimination pharmacokinetics, a greater than proportional increase in both maximal peak concentration and area under the plasma-concentration-versus-time curve has been observed and probably is explained by saturable binding of the drug to erythrocytes.[109] Approximately 50% of the dose is excreted unchanged renally; however, its metabolism is increased by approximately 50% when topiramate is given with enzyme-inducing AEDs. Renal tubular reabsorption may be involved prominently in the renal handling of topiramate.[110]

Adverse Effects The main adverse events of topiramate are ataxia, impaired concentration, memory difficulties, attentional deficits, confusion, dizziness, fatigue, paresthesia, somnolence, and "thinking abnormally," which rarely has included psychosis. Most of these occurred during rapid titration and at higher doses.[111] Word-finding difficulties can be a problem with topiramate and can occur in a significant number of patients, especially patients with left posterior temporal lobe epilepsy or simple partial seizures.[112] There can be an increased incidence of cognitive dysfunction in patients receiving concomitant therapy with topiramate, valproic acid, or phenobarbital. Nephrolithiasis has occurred in 1.5% of patients receiving topiramate, which is two to four times the incidence in the general population. Patients should be encouraged to maintain adequate fluid intake in order to minimize this problem. Topiramate can cause metabolic acidosis. Risk factors for this condition include patients with renal disease, those with severe respiratory disorders, status epilepticus, diarrhea, surgery, and ketogenic diet. It has been observed at doses as low as 50 mg/day. Metabolic acidosis in part may explain the anorexia and weight loss seen with this drug.[65]

Drug Interactions Oral clearance of digoxin is slightly increased when topiramate is added. Topiramate coadministration can result in increased phenytoin serum concentrations in some patients, an effect consistent with in-vitro studies showing an inhibitory effect of topiramate on the CYP 2C19 isoform. The variable response can be explained by the intersubject variability in the proportion of phenytoin clearance attributed to CYP 2C19 metabolism and whether the patient is a homozygous or heterozygous carrier of the mutant allele responsible for the CYP 2C9 and/or CYP 2C19 "poor metabolizer" phenotype. Topiramate can modestly increase the oral clearance of valproic acid and increase formation of the 4-ene–valproic acid (VPA) metabolite. However, the clinical significance of this interaction is unclear. Topiramate increases the clearance of ethinyl estradiol in a dose-dependant manner. Topiramate doses of less than 200 mg/day are unlikely to alter oral contraceptive pharmacokinetics.[113]

Dosing and Administration Topiramate should be titrated slowly to avoid adverse events with dosage increments every 1 to 2 weeks. For patients on other AEDs, doses of greater than 600 mg/day do not appear to lead to improved efficacy and can cause increased adverse effects; however, higher doses can prove beneficial to individual patients who tolerate them.[114]

Advantages Topiramate has multiple mechanisms of action and is a broad-spectrum AED. The kidney mainly eliminates it, although some liver metabolism occurs, especially if given concomitantly with enzyme inducers. It has liner pharmacokinetics and few drug interactions.

Disadvantages With rapid dosage escalation, topiramate can compromise cognitive functioning, including impaired word finding and short-term memory. Therefore, low initial doses should be used, and the dose must be titrated slowly. Renal stones and weight loss also have been associated with topiramate use. The dose should be decreased in patients with renal failure. There is no parenteral formulation.

Place in Therapy Topiramate is a first-line AED for patients with partial seizures. The drug is also approved for the treatment of tonic-clonic seizures in primary generalized epilepsy.

Valproic Acid/Divalproex Sodium

Pharmacology and Mechanism of Action Initially it was believed that valproic acid increased GABA by inhibiting its degradation or by activating its synthesis. Although this may explain in part the effects of valproic acid, the time course for the increase in GABA compared with the onset of anticonvulsant effects indicates that alterations of the synthesis and degradation of GABA do not fully explain the antiseizure activity of valproic acid. It has been proposed that valproic acid may potentiate postsynaptic GABA responses, may have a direct membrane-stabilizing effect, and may affect potassium channels.[115]

Pharmacokinetics Valproic acid appears to be absorbed completely from available oral dosage forms when administered on an empty stomach.[115] However, the rate of absorption differs among preparations. Peak concentrations occur in 0.5 to 1 hour with the syrup, 1 to 3 hours with the capsule, and 2 to 6 hours with the enteric-coated tablet.[115] The extended-release formulation (Depakote-ER) is FDA approved for use in both patients with migraine headache and epilepsy. It should be noted, however, that the bioavailability of this formulation is approximately 15% less than that of enteric-coated divalproex sodium (Depakote).

Valproic acid is extensively bound to albumin, and this binding is saturable. Accordingly, the valproic acid free fraction will increase as the total serum concentration increases. Because of this saturable binding, measurement of unbound serum concentrations may be a better monitoring parameter than the total valproic acid serum concentration, especially at higher concentrations or in patients with hypoalbuminemia.[63]

The primary route of valproic acid metabolism is β-oxidation, although up to 40% of a dose may be excreted as the glucuronide. At least 10 metabolites of valproic acid have been identified. Some of these may have weak anticonvulsant activity, and at least one metabolite may be responsible for the hepatotoxicity reported with valproic acid. One of the lesser oxidative metabolites, 4-ene-VPA, causes significant hepatotoxicity in rats. The formation of this metabolite is increased when valproic acid is given with enzyme-inducing drugs.[115] Valproic acid displays diurnal elimination with lower evening serum levels occurring than morning levels.

Adverse Effects The most frequently reported side effects are gastrointestinal complaints (up to 20%), including nausea, vomiting, and anorexia, as well as weight gain. Pancreatitis is rare. The gastrointestinal complaints may be minimized but not totally alleviated with the enteric-coated formulation or by giving the drug with food.

Alopecia and hair changes are temporary, and hair growth returns even with continued dosing. Weight gain can be significant for many patients and is associated with an increase in fasting insulin and leptin serum levels.[116] The increase in serum insulin is believed to be caused by the inhibition of metabolism of insulin by the liver.[117] This has led to the development of insulin resistance in obese male and female subjects.[115] Valproic acid causes minimal cognitive impairment.[115]

The most serious side effect reported with valproic acid is hepatotoxicity. Hyperammonemia is common (50%) but does not necessarily imply liver damage; however, fatalities have been attributed to valproic acid hepatotoxicity. Most deaths have occurred in patients who were younger than 2 years of age, mentally retarded, and receiving multiple AEDs. Hepatotoxicity occurred early in the course of therapy. Patients who complain of nausea, vomiting, lethargy, anorexia, and edema in the first 6 to 12 months of therapy should have liver function tests done. Multiple-AED therapy can alter the metabolism of valproic acid, leading to increased formation of the potentially liver-toxic 4-ene-VPA. Valproic acid has been shown to alter carnitine metabolism, and it has been postulated that a deficiency of carnitine alters fatty acid oxidation that could lead to both liver toxicity and hyperammonemia.[118] However, valproic acid hepatotoxicity has occurred in a patient taking supplemental carnitine, and a prospective study demonstrated no effect on well-being when carnitine was added. Although carnitine can ameliorate hyperammonemia in part, it is expensive, and there are only limited data to support routine supplemental use in patients taking valproic acid.[119]

Thrombocytopenia and alterations in platelet aggregation occur in the patients receiving valproic acid, and these phenomena are related to serum concentration. These blood coagulopathies can occur more frequently in children than in adults.[120]

Drug Interactions Because it is highly protein bound, other highly protein-bound drugs can displace valproic acid. Free fatty acids and aspirin can alter valproic acid binding by displacement.

Valproic acid is an enzyme inhibitor that can inhibit specific cytochrome P450 isozymes, epoxide hydrolase, and UGT isozymes. The addition of valproic acid to phenobarbital results in a 30% to 50% decrease in the clearance of phenobarbital and significant toxicity if the dose of phenobarbital is not reduced.

Dosing and Administration Valproic acid in some patients may have a half-life sufficiently long to permit once-daily dosing with enteric-coated divalproex, more frequent dosing is the norm. Based on half-life data, twice-daily dosing is feasible with any valproic acid dosage form; however, children and other patients taking enzyme inducers can require dosing three to four times daily.[63] The serum concentration–dose relationship is curvilinear (e.g., the concentration-dose ratio decreases with increasing dose) probably because of increasing free concentrations and a resulting increase in clearance.[63]

Valproic acid is available as a soft gelatin capsule, an enteric-coated tablet, a syrup, a "sprinkle capsule," an extended-release formulation designed for once-daily dosing, and an IV formulation for replacement of oral therapy or in situations where rapid loading of valproic acid is deemed necessary.[115] This parenteral formulation must not be given intramuscularly because it can cause tissue necrosis. The sprinkle capsule, designed to be opened and mixed with food, has a slower rate of absorption, which results in fewer fluctuations in the peak-to-trough ratio. The syrup is absorbed more rapidly than any solid dosage form. The enteric-coated tablet is not sustained-release; it consists of sodium divalproex, which must be metabolized in the gut to valproic acid. It is enteric coated to reduce the incidence of gastrointestinal distress. The enteric coating does cause delayed absorption, although once the enteric coating dissolves, sodium divalproex has absorption, metabolism, and elimination rates similar to those of the gelatin capsule. If a patient is switched from Depakote to Depakote-ER, the dose should be increased by 14% to 20%. Depakote-ER may be given once daily.

Advantages Valproic acid is available in multiple dosage formulations. The IV formulation is especially well tolerated. It has a wide therapeutic index and can be considered a broad-spectrum AED. It also can be useful in other neurologic or psychiatric disorders, including migraine headache and bipolar disorder.

Disadvantages Some patients report significant weight gain with valproic acid, and this can limit compliance. Valproic acid is also associated with other side effects, such as alopecia, tremor, pancreatitis, polycystic ovary disease, and thrombocytopenia. It has been associated with hepatic necrosis in young children. Valproic acid is an enzyme inhibitor and is involved in multiple drug-drug interactions.

Place in Therapy Valproic acid is first-line therapy for primary generalized seizures such as myoclonic, atonic, and absence seizures. It can be used as both monotherapy and adjunctive therapy for partial seizures, and it can be very useful in patients with mixed seizure disorders.

Zonisamide

Pharmacology and Mechanism of Action Zonisamide, a synthetic 1,2-benzisoxazole derivative classified as a sulfonamide, is chemically different from other AEDs. In animal testing it was demonstrated to be a broad-spectrum AED. It is believed to exert its antiepileptic effect by inhibition of slow sodium channels, by blockade of T-type Ca^{2+} channels, and possibly by inhibition of glutamate release. It also has a weak carbonic anhydrase inhibitory effect.[121]

Pharmacokinetics Zonisamide is well absorbed reaching a maximum peak concentration in 2 to 5 hours. Zonisamide is metabolized by CYP 3A4 and to a much lesser extent by CYP 2C19 and CYP 3A5. Approximately 30% is excreted unchanged in the urine. Zonisamide is distributed to most tissues, but the drug is concentrated in the red blood cells. Zonisamide crosses the placenta. The concentration in breast milk is similar to that in the plasma.[121]

Adverse Effects The most common adverse effects of zonisamide include somnolence, dizziness, anorexia, headache, nausea, agitation, word-finding difficulties, and irritability. Adverse effects may be more common during rapid dose escalation. Because zonisamide is structurally related to sulfonamides, hypersensitivity reactions can occur (0.02% of patients), and zonisamide should be used with caution (if at all) in patients with a confirmed history of allergy to sulfonamide compounds. A 2.6% incidence of symptomatic kidney stones has been reported in patients treated in the United States.[122] Because of reports of modest, reversible declines in renal function in some patients, monitoring of renal function may be advisable for certain patients. Oligohidrosis has been reported. In addition, modest weight loss has been reported with this agent.[25,26,65]

Drug Interactions Zonisamide does not inhibit or induce the cytochrome P450 system.

Dosing and Administration Daily doses should be increased every 2 weeks to response. Zonisamide is stable for 48 hours when mixed with water, apple juice, or pudding for patients who have trouble swallowing oral solid dosage forms.

Advantage Zonisamide has multiple mechanisms of action and may be a broad-spectrum AED. There is broad international experience with this drug. It has a very long half-life, which is suitable for once- or twice-daily dosing. Once-daily dosing is associated with more fluctuations around the mean concentration and perhaps more side effects. Patients may experience modest weight loss with this drug.

Disadvantage The dose of zonisamide should be titrated slowly to patient response. Renal stones and oligohidrosis also have been associated with zonisamide. In addition, cognitive impairment can occur, especially if dosage is escalated rapidly.

Place in Therapy Zonisamide is currently approved for the adjunctive treatment of partial seizures. Thus far, insufficient data exist to support its use as initial monotherapy. Zonisamide is potentially effective in a variety of partial and primary generalized seizure types.

PHARMACOECONOMIC CONSIDERATIONS

CLINICAL CONTROVERSY

The place in therapy of the newer drugs is still being determined. The cost of the newer AEDs generally is much higher that that of the older drugs. Given that, in general, the efficacy of the newer drugs is comparable with that of the older agents, many clinicians (and patients) have been slow to adopt this newer generation of drugs. It is important to recognize that overall effectiveness encompasses both efficacy and tolerability assessments. Generally speaking, the newer generation of AEDs possess fewer adverse effects and seems to be better tolerated than older, far less expensive agents such as the barbiturates. Some may also have less costly long-term adverse effects such as effects on bone metabolism or the fetus, and they may cause fewer drug interactions, which require higher doses of drugs to avoid treatment failures. These differences may well justify the difference in cost, however, this needs to be determined on an individual basis.

The direct costs of epilepsy include the cost of the drug, treatment of adverse events, emergency room visits, drug levels, laboratory tests, physician visits, rehabilitation, and transportation. Indirect costs include the costs associated with time lost from work, the inability to get a job, decreased productivity, and mortality.

It is difficult to assess the entire cost of epilepsy to society. Pashko and coworkers,[123] using a cohort of Pennsylvania Medicaid patients, estimated that the total direct cost of epilepsy is in excess of $10 billion annually, with the majority of the per-patient costs incurred for inpatient hospitalization (uncontrolled seizures or treatment-related toxicity). Another study suggested that the direct costs of epilepsy made up approximately 37% of the total costs, with indirect costs accounting for the remainder.[124] This study also indicated that the costs were much less for a patient who is well controlled than for a patient who is poorly controlled. Drug costs in the Pashko study accounted for approximately 10% of the total costs of epilepsy. In another study, the cost-effectiveness of some of the newer drugs (lamotrigine, vigabatrin, and gabapentin) was estimated for the first year of drug therapy. There was little difference in initial costs, but gabapentin, with fewer adverse effects, resulted in cost savings.[125] The methodology used in this study has been criticized. There have been no pharmacoeconomic studies comparing the older, less expensive AEDs with the newer, more expensive drugs.

Providing the best quality of life possible is a treatment goal for patients with epilepsy, although maintaining a balance between side effects and the number of seizures experienced by patients is very important.[126] Quality of life also takes into account all the concerns of patients with epilepsy, including their social and economic concerns. This can best be assessed by the patient. Complete seizure freedom leads to the best quality of life. In one study, driving was listed as the most important concern by 28% of patients, followed by employment (21%), independence (9%), safety (6%), AED side effects (5%), seizure unpredictability (5%), and seizure avoidance (5%).[127] Assessment of quality of life as a therapeutic outcome ultimately may be more meaningful than measuring blood levels of the AEDs. It is clear that the cheapest drugs in epilepsy (e.g., phenobarbital) are not the best because of the number of side effects. Drug therapy that would control seizures, decrease side effects, improve the quality of life, and reduce the use of other healthcare resources would be cost-effective. Because epilepsy treatment continues to be highly individualized, the drug or combination of drugs that controls seizures with the least number of side effects will be the drug of choice for that patient no matter how expensive the drug acquisition cost.

Because many patients with epilepsy require minimal variation in blood concentrations to prevent seizures and avoid side effects, generic prescribing for epilepsy remains controversial. One study suggested that the money saved by generic prescribing is outweighed by the negative health gain for the person with epilepsy, increased work in general practice, and increased social costs.[128]

EVALUATION OF THERAPEUTIC OUTCOMES

A therapeutic range should be established for each patient. This range should define concentrations that result in minimal side effects and optimal seizure control. This therapeutic plasma concentration range should be used to identify the appropriate patient-specific dose. Patients should be monitored chronically for seizure control, comorbid conditions, social adjustment (including quality-of-life assessments), drug interactions, compliance, and adverse effects. Periodic screening for comorbid neuropsychiatric disorders such as depression and anxiety is also important. Clinical response is more important than the serum drug concentration.

Outcomes can be assessed by prospective clinical monitoring, drug utilization review, and quality-of-life assessments. Clinical monitoring involves identifying the number and type of seizures. Patients should be given a seizure diary, and the severity as well as the frequency of seizures should be monitored. There should be a decrease in the number and/or severity of seizures. Patients should be questioned regularly to determine whether they are seizure-free. It is important to recall that perhaps as many as 30% of patients will be intractable to current pharmacologic treatments. In these patients, if the clinician has determined that AED dosage has been maximized, one should consider either AED combination therapy or, potentially, evaluation for epilepsy surgery or the vagal nerve stimulator.

The treatment of epilepsy begins with a careful identification of the seizure type and selection of the most appropriate AED. Therapy should be initiated slowly, except in life-threatening situations, to avoid acute toxicity. Although most patients can be managed successfully on monotherapy, some patients' seizures remain uncontrolled despite the use of multiple AEDs. Some patients may be genetically refractory to AED therapy. The newer AEDs, as adjunctive therapy or monotherapy, offer additional opportunity to achieve complete seizure control. There is a continuing need for new AEDs and additional research in this area.

ACKNOWLEDGMENTS

The authors acknowledge the contributions of Barry E. Gidal, Pharm.D. and William R. Garnett, Pharm.D., authors of the Epilepsy chapter (Chap. 54) in the 6th edition of *Pharmacotherapy: A Pathophysiologic Approach*.

ABBREVIATIONS

AAN: American Academy of Neurology

AED: antiepileptic drug

AES: American Epilepsy Society

AMPA: α-amino-3-hydroxy-5-methylisoxazole-4-propionic acid

AUC: area under the curve

CGRP: calcitonin gene-related peptide

CP: complex partial

CT: computed tomography

EEG: electroencephalogram

GABA: γ-aminobutyric-acid

GTC: generalized tonic-clonic

HPA: hypothalamic-pituitary-adrenal

IM: intramuscular

ILAE: International League Against Epilepsy

IV: intravenous

IQ: intelligence quotient

MRI: magnetic resonance imaging

NMDA: *N*-methyl-D-aspartate

SP: simple partial

VNS: vagus nerve stimulation

REFERENCES

1. Sander JW. The epidemiology of epilepsy revisited. Curr Opin Neurol 2003;16:165–170.
2. Berg AT. The epidemiologic aspects of epilepsy. In: Wyllie E, ed. The Treatment of Epilepsy, 4th ed. Philadelphia: Lippincott Williams & Wilkins; 2006:109–116.
3. Najm IM, Moddel G, Janigro D. Mechanisms of epileptogenesis and experimental models of seizures. In: Wyllie E, ed. The Treatment of Epilepsy, 4th ed. Philadelphia: Lippincott Williams & Wilkins; 2006:91–102.
4. Commission on Classification and Terminology of the International League Against Epilepsy. Proposal for revised clinical and electroencephalographic classification of epileptic seizures. Epilepsia 1981;22:489–501.
5. Commission on Classification and Terminology of the International League Against Epilepsy. Proposal for revised classification of epilepsies and epileptic syndromes. Epilepsia 1989;30:389–399.
6. Chen DK, So YT, Fisher RS. Use of serum prolactin in diagnosing epileptic seizures. Report of the therapeutic and technology assessment subcommittee of the American Academy of Neurology. Neurology 2005;65:668–675.
7. Vickrey BG, Hays RD, Rausch R, et al. Quality of life of epilepsy surgery patients as compared with outpatients with hypertension, diabetes, heart disease, and/or depressive symptoms. Epilepsia 1994;35:597–607.
8. Schachter SC. Psychiatric comorbidity of epilepsy. In: Wyllie E, ed. The Treatment of Epilepsy, 4th ed. Philadelphia: Lippincott Williams & Wilkins; 2006:1197–1200.
9. Bazil CW. Epilepsy and sleep disturbance. Epilepsy Behav 2003;4:S39–45.
10. Boylan LS, Flint LA, Labovitz DL, et al. Depression but not seizure frequency predicts quality of life in treatment-resistant epilepsy. Neurology 2004;62:258–261.
11. Brodie MJ, French JA. Management of epilepsy in adolescents and adults. Lancet 2000;356:323–328.
12. Mattson RH. Antiepileptic drug monotherapy in adults: Selection and use in new-onset epilepsy. In: Levy RH, Mattson RH, Meldrum BS, eds. Antiepileptic Drugs, 5th ed. Philadelphia: Lippincott Williams & Wilkins, 2002:72–95.
13. Sisodiya SM. Genetics of drug resistance. Epilepsia 2005;46(Suppl 10):33–38.
14. Garnett WR. Antiepileptic drug treatment: Outcomes and adherence. Pharmacotherapy 2000;20:191S–199S.

15 Leppik IE. Contemporary Diagnosis and Management of the Patient with Epilepsy, 6th ed. Newton, PA: Handbooks in Health Care, 2006:66–76.

16. Quality Standards Subcommittee of the American Academy of Neurology. Practice parameter: A guideline for discontinuing antiepileptic drugs in seizure free patients [summary statement]. Neurology 1996;47:600–602.
17. Gross-Tsur V, O'Dell C, Shinnar S. Initiation and discontinuation of antiepileptic drugs. In: Wyllie E, ed. The Treatment of Epilepsy, 4th ed. Philadelphia: Lippincott Williams & Wilkins, 2006:681–694.
18. Wheless J. Vagus nerve stimulation therapy. In: Wyllie E, ed. The Treatment of Epilepsy, 4th ed. Philadelphia: Lippincott Williams & Wilkins, 2006:969–980.
19. Lachhwani DK, Wyllie E. Outcome and complications of epilepsy surgery. In: Wyllie E, ed. The Treatment of Epilepsy, 4th ed. Philadelphia: Lippincott Williams & Wilkins, 2006:1176–1182.
19. Sperling MR, Harris A, Nei M, et al. Mortality after epilepsy surgery. Epilepsia 2005;46(Suppl 11):49–53.
20. Devinsky O, Barr WB, Vickrey BG, et al. Changes in depression and anxiety after resective surgery for epilepsy. Neurology 2005;65:1744–1749.
21. Schiller Y, Casino GD, So EL, Marsh R. Discontinuation of antiepileptic drugs after successful epilepsy surgery. Neurology 2000;54:346–349.
22. Berg AT, Vickrey GB, Langfitt JT, et al. Reduction of AEDs in postsurgical patients who attain remission. Epilepsia 2006;47;64–71.
23. Groesbeck DK, Bluml RM, Kossoff EH. Long-term use of the ketogenic diet: Outcomes of 28 children with over 6 years diet duration. Neurology 2006;66(Suppl 2):A41.
24. Kossoff EH, McGrogan JR, Bluml RM, et al. A modified Atkins diet is effective for the treatment of intractable pediatric epilepsy. Epilepsia 2006;47:421–424.
25. French JA, Kanner AM, Bautista J, et al. Efficacy and tolerability of the new antiepileptic drugs: I. Treatment of new onset epilepsy. Neurology 2004;62:1252–1260.
26. French JA, Kanner AM, Bautista J, et al. Efficacy and tolerability of the new antiepileptic drugs: II. Treatment of refractory epilepsy. Neurology 2004;62:1261–1273.
27. National Institute for Clinical Excellence. Newer Drugs for Epilepsy in Adults. 2006, *http://www.nice.org.uk.*
28. National Institute for Clinical Excellence. Newer Drugs for Epilepsy in Children. 2006, *http://www.nice.org.uk.*
29. Glauser T, Ben-Menachem E, Bourgeois B, et al. ILAE treatment guidelines: Evidenced-based analysis of antiepileptic drug efficacy and effectiveness as initial monotherapy for epileptic seizures and syndromes. Epilepsia 2006;47:1094–1120.
30. Karceski S, Morrell MJ, Carpenter D. Treatment of epilepsy in adults: Expert opinion. Epilepsy Behav 2005;7:S1–S64.
31. Faught E. Pharmacokinetic considerations in prescribing antiepileptic drugs. Epilepsia 2001;42(Suppl 4):19–23.
32. Leppik IE. Contemporary Diagnosis and Management of the Patient with Epilepsy, 6th ed. Newton, PA: Handbooks in Health Care, 2006:92–149.
33. Bourgeois BFD. Pharmacokinetics and pharmacodynamics of antiepileptic drugs. In: Wyllie E. ed. The Treatment of Epilepsy, 4th ed. Philadelphia: Lippincott Williams & Wilkins, 2006:656–669.
34. Harden CL. Therapeutic safety monitoring: What to look for and when to look for it. Epilepsia 2000;41(Suppl 8):S37–44.
35. Perucca E. Is there a role of therapeutic drug monitoring of new anticonvulsants. Clin Pharmacokinet 2000;38:191–204.
36. Pack AM, Olarte LS, Morrell MJ, et al. Bone mineral density in an outpatient population receiving enzyme-inducing antiepileptic drugs. Epilepsy Behav 2003;4:169–174.
37. Meador KJ, Gilliam FG, Kanner AM, Pellock JM. Cognitive and behavioral effects of antiepileptic drugs. Epilepsy Behav 2001;2:S1–17.
38. Vermeulen J, Aldenkamp AP. Cognitive side-effects of chronic antiepileptic drug treatment: A review of 25 years of research. Epilepsy Res 1995;22:65–95.
39. Meador KJ, Loring DW, Ray PG, et al. Differential cognitive effects of carbamazepine and gabapentin. Epilepsia 1999;40:1279–1285.
40. Meador KJ, Loring DW, Ray PG. Differential cognitive effects of carbamazepine and lamotrigine [abstract]. Neurology 2000;54:A84.
41. Martin R, Kuzniecky R, Ho S, et al. Cognitive effects of topiramate, gabapentin and lamotrigine in healthy young adults. Neurology 1999;52:321–327.
42. Fritz N, Glogau S, Hoffman J, et al. Efficacy and cognitive side effects to tiagabine and topiramate in patients with epilepsy. Epilepsy Behav 2005;6:373–381.
43. Salinsky MC, Storzbach D, Spencer DC, et al. Effects of topiramate and gabapentin on cognitive abilities in healthy volunteers. Neurology 2005;64:792–798.
44. Sazgar M, Bourgeois B. Aggravation of epilepsy by antiepileptic drugs. Pediatr Neurol 2005;33:227–234.
45. Mattson RH, Cramer JA, Collins JF, et al. Comparison of carbamazepine, phenobarbital, phenytoin, and primidone in partial and sec-

ondarily generalized tonic-clonic seizures. N Engl J Med 1985;313:145–151.

46. Mattson RH, Cramer JA, Collins JF, et al. A comparison of valproate with carbamazepine for the treatment of complex partial seizures and secondarily generalized tonic-clonic seizures in adults. N Engl J Med 1992;327:765–771.
47. Beydoun A, Kutluay E. Conversion to monotherapy: Clinical trials in patients with refractory partial seizures. Neurology 2003;60(Suppl 4):S13–25.
48. French JA, Kanner AM, Bautista J, et al. Efficacy and tolerability of the new antiepileptic drugs: I. Treatment of new-onset epilepsy. Epilepsia 2004:45;401–409.
49. French JA, Kanner AM, Bautista J, et al. Efficacy and tolerability of the new antiepileptic drugs: II. Treatment of refractory epilepsy. Epilepsia 2004:45;410–423.
50. Rowan AJ, Ramsay ER, Collins JF, et al. New onset geriatric epilepsy: A randomized study of gabapentin, lamotrigine, and carbamazepine. Neurology 2005;64:1868–1873.
51. Marson AG, Kadir ZA, Chadwick DW. New antiepileptic drugs: A systematic review of their efficacy and tolerability. Br Med J 1996;313:1169–1174.
52. Perucca E. Clinical pharmacokinetics of new-generation antiepileptic drugs at the extremes of age. Clin Pharmacokinet 2006;45:351–363.
53. Smith S, Wolley CS. Cellular and molecular effects of steroid hormones and CNS excitability. Cleve Clin J Med 2004;71:S5–10.
54. Morrell MJ, Montouris GD. Reproductive disturbances in patients with epilepsy. Cleve Clin J Med 2004;71:S19–24.
55. Yerby MS, Kaplan P, Tran T. Risks and management of pregnancy in women with epilepsy. Cleve Clin J Med 2004;71:S25–37.
56. Vajda FJE, Eadie MJ. Maternal valproate dosage and foetal malformations. Acta Neurol Scand 2005:112:137–143.
57. Tomson T, Battino D. Teratogenicity of antiepileptic drugs: State of the art. Curr Opin Neurol 2005;18:135–140.
58. Isojaervi JIJ, Loefgren E, Juntunen KST, et al. Effect of epilepsy and antiepileptic drugs on male reproductive health. Neurology 2004;62:247–253.
59. Ferraro TN, Buono RJ. The relationship between the pharmacology of antiepileptic drugs and human gene variation: An overview. Epilepsy Behav 2005;7:18–36.
60. Garnett WR. Carbamazepine. In: Murphy J, ed. Clinical Pharmacokinetics, 2nd ed. Washington, DC: American Society of Health-Systems Pharmacists, 2004.
61. Ficker DM, Privitera M, Krauss G, et al. Improved tolerability and efficacy in epilepsy patients with extended-release carbamazepine. Neurology 2005;65:593–595.
62. Garnett WR. Ethosuximide. In: Murphy J, ed. Clinical Pharmacokinetics. Washington, DC: American Society of Health-Systems Pharmacists, 2004.
63. Garnett WR. Antiepileptics. In: Schumacher GE, ed. Therapeutic Drug Monitoring. Norwalk, CT: Appleton and Lange, 1995:345–395.
64. Pellock JM, Perhach JL, Sofia RD. Felbamate. In: Levy RH, Mattson RH, Meldrum BS, et al., eds. Antiepileptic Drugs, 5th ed. Philadelphia: Lippincott Williams & Wilkins, 2002:301–318.
65. LaRoche SM, Helmers SL. The new antiepileptic drugs: Scientific review. JAMA 2004;291:605–614.
66. Taylor CP, Gee NS, Su TZ, et al. A summary of mechanistic hypothesis of gabapentin pharmacology. Epilepsy Res 1998;29:233–249.
67. Luer MS, Hamani C, Dujovny M, et al. Saturable transport of gabapentin at the blood–brain barrier. Neurol Res 1999;21:559–562.
68. Gidal BE, Radulovic LL, Kruger S, et al. Inter- and intrasubject variability in gabapentin (GBP) absorption and absolute bioavailability. Epilepsy Res 2000;40:123–127.
69. Gidal BE, Maly MM, Kowalski J, et al. Gabapentin absorption: Effect of mixing with foods of varying macronutrient content. Ann Pharmacother 1998;32:405–408.
70. Wong MO, Eldon MA, Keane WF, et al. Disposition of gabapentin in anuric subjects on hemodialysis. J Clin Pharmacol 1995;35:622–626.
71. Lee DO, Steingard RJ, Cesena M, et al. Behavioral side effects of gabapentin in children. Epilepsia 1996;37:87–90.
72. McLean MJ, Gidal BE. Gabapentin in the treatment of epilepsy: A dosing review. Clin Ther 2003;25:1382–1406.
73. Gidal BE, DeCerce J, Bockbrader HR, et al. Gabapentin bioavailability: Effect of dose and frequency of administration in adult patients with epilepsy. Epilepsy Res 1998;31:91–99.
74. Dickins M, Chen C. Lamotrigine: Chemistry, biotransformation, and pharmacokinetics. In: Levy RH, Mattson RH, Meldrum BS, et al., eds. Antiepileptic Drugs, 5th ed. Philadelphia: Lippincott Williams & Wilkins, 2002:369–379.
75. Gilman JT. Lamotrigine: An antiepileptic agent for the treatment of partial seizures. Ann Pharmacother 1995;29:144–151.
76. Hirsch LJ, Weintraub DB, Buchsbaum R, et al. Predictors of lamotrigine-associated rash. Epilepsia 2006;47:318–322.
77. Messenheimer JA. Rash in adult and pediatric patients treated with lamotrigine. Can J Neurol Sci 1998;25:S14–18.
78. Sidhu J, Bulsara S, Job S, Philipson R. A bi-directional pharmacokinetic interaction study of lamotrigine and the combined oral contraceptive pill in healthy subjects [abstract]. Epilepsia 2004;45(Suppl 7):330.
79. Reimers A, Helde G, Brodtkorb E. Ethinyl estradiol, not progestogen, reduces lamotrigine serum concentrations. Epilepsia 2005;46:1414–1417.
80. Contin M, Albani F, Ambrosetto G, et al. Variation in lamotrigine plasma concentrations with hormonal contraceptive monthly cycles in patients with epilepsy. Epilepsia 2006;47:1573–1575.
81. Lynch BA, Lambeng N, Nocka K, et al. The synaptic vesicle protein SV2A in the binding site for the antiepileptic drug levetiracetam. Proc Natl Acad Sci U S A 2004;101:9861–9866.
82. Loscher W, Honack D, Rundfeldt C. Antiepileptogenic effects of the novel anticonvulsant levetiracetam (ucb LO59) in the kindling model of temporal lobe epilepsy. J Pharmacol Exp Ther 1998;284:474–479.
83. Fay MA, Sheth RD, Gidal BE. Oral absorption kinetics of levetiracetam: The effect of mixing with food or enteral nutrition. Clin Ther 2005:27:594–598.
84. Welty TE, Gidal BE, Ficker DM, Privitera MD. Levetiracetam: A different approach to the pharmacotherapy of epilepsy. Ann Pharmacother 2002;36:296–304.
85. Brockmoeller J, Thomsen T, Wittstock M, et al. Pharmacokinetics of levetiracetam in patients with moderate to severe liver cirrhosis (Child-Pugh classes A, B and C): Characterization by dynamic liver function tests. Clin Pharmacol Ther 2005;77:529–541.
86. Coppola G, Mangano S, Tortorella G, et al. Levetiracetam during 1-year follow-up in children, adolescents, and young adults with refractory epilepsy. Epilepsy Res 2004;59:35–42.
87. Perucca E, Gidal BE. Effects of antiepileptic comedication on levetiracetam pharmacokinetics: A pooled analysis of data from randomized adjunctive therapy trials. Epilepsy Res 2003;53:47–56.
88. Gidal BE, Baltes E, Otoul C, Perruca E. Effect of levetiracetam on the pharmacokinetics of adjunctive antiepileptic drugs: A pooled analysis of data from randomized clinic trials. Epilepsy Res 2005;64:1–11.
89. Stefan H, Wang-Tilz Y, Pauli E, et al. Onset of action of levetiracetam: A RCT trial using therapeutic intensive seizure analysis (TISA). Epilepsia 2006;47:516–522.
90. Ambrosio AF, Soares-Da-Silva P, Carvalho CM, Carvalho AP. Mechanisms of action of carbamazepine and its derivatives, oxcarbazepine, BIA 2–093 and BIA 2–024. Neurochem Res 2002;27:121–130.
91. Ambrosio AF, Silva AP, Malva JO, et al. Carbamazepine inhibits L-type Ca^{2+} channels in cultured rat hippocampal neurons stimulated with glutamate receptor agonists. Neuropharmacology 1999;38:1349–1359.
92. Lloyd P, Flesch G, Dieterle W. Clinical pharmacology and pharmacokinetics of oxcarbazepine. Epilepsia 1994;35:10–13.
93. Kalis MM, Huff NA. Oxcarbazepine, an antiepileptic agent. Clin Ther 2001;23:680–700.
94. May TW, Ramback B, Jurgens U. Influence of oxcarbazepine and methsuximide on lamotrigine concentrations in epileptic patients with and without valproic acid comedication: results of a retrospective study. Ther Drug Monit 1999;21:175–181.
95. Pina-Garza JE, Espinoza R, Nordli D, et al. Oxcarbazepine adjunctive therapy in infants and young children with partial seizures. Neurology 2005;65:1370–1375.
96. Muller M, Marson AG, Williamson PR. Oxcarbazepine versus phenytoin monotherapy for epilepsy. Cochrane Database Syst Rev 2006;2:CD003615.
97. Messina S, Battino D, Croci D, et al. Phenobarbital pharmacokinetics in old age: A case-matched evaluation based on therapeutic drug monitoring data. Epilepsia 2005;46:372–377.
98. Baulac M, Cramer JA, Mattson RH. Phenobarbital and other barbiturates: Adverse effects. In: Levy RH, Mattson RH, Meldrum BS, et al., eds. Antiepileptic Drugs, 5th ed. Philadelphia: Lippincott Williams & Wilkins, 2002, 528–540.

99. Tozer TN, Winter ME. Phenytoin. In: Evans WE, Schentag JJ, Jusko WJ, eds. Applied Pharmacokinetics, 3rd ed. Spokane, WA: Applied Therapeutics, 1992:25–1–44.
100. Anderson GD, Pak C, Doane KW, et al. Revised Winter-Tozer equation for normalized phenytoin concentrations in trauma and elderly patients with hypoalbuminemia. Ann Pharmacother 1997;31: 279–284.
101. Bruni J. Phenytoin and other hydantoins: Adverse effects. In: Levy RH, Mattson RH, Meldrum BS, et al., eds. Antiepileptic Drugs, 5th ed. Philadelphia: Lippincott Williams & Wilkins, 2002:605–610.
102. Privitera MD. Clinical rules for phenytoin dosing. Ann Pharmacother 1993;27:1169–1173.
103. Ben-Menachem E. Pregabalin pharmacology and its relevance to clinical practice. Epilepsia 2004;45(Suppl 6):13–18.
104. Bialer M, Johannessen SI, Kupferberg HJ, et al. Progress report on new antiepileptic drugs: A summary of the seventh EILAT conference (EILAT VII). Epilepsy Res 2004;61:1–48.
105. Shneker BF, McAuley JW. Pregablin: A new neuromodulator with broad therapeutic indications. Ann Pharmacother 2005;39:2029–2037.
106. Schachter SC. Tiagabine: Current status and potential clinical applications. Expert Opin Investig Drugs 1996;5:1377–1387.
107. Leppik IE. Tiagabine: The safety landscape. Epilepsia 1995;36:S10–13.
108. Koepp MJ, Edwards M, Collins J, et al. Status epilepticus and tiagabine therapy revisited. Epilepsia 2005;46:1625–1632.
109. Gidal BE, Lensmeyer GL. Therapeutic drug monitoring of topiramate: Evaluation of the saturable distribution between erythrocytes and plasma in whole blood using an optimized HPLC method. Ther Drug Monit 1999;21:567–576.
110. Langtry HD, Gillis JC, Davis R. Topiramate: A review of its pharmacodynamic and pharmacokinetic properties and clinical efficacy in the management of epilepsy. Drugs 1997;54:752–773.
111. Shorvon SD. Safety of topiramate: Adverse events and relationship to dosing. Epilepsia 1996;37(Suppl 2):S18–22.
112. Mula M, Trimble M, Thompson P, et al. Topiramate and word-finding difficulties in patients with epilepsy. Neurology 2003;60:1104–1107.
113. Gidal BE. Topiramate: Drug interactions. In: Levy RH, Mattson RH, Meldrum BS, et al., eds. Antiepileptic Drugs, 5th ed. Philadelphia: Lippincott Williams & Wilkins, 2002:735–739.
114. Privitera M, Fincham R, Penry J, et al. Topiramate placebo-controlled dose-ranging trial in refractory partial epilepsy using 600-, 800-, and 1,000-mg daily dosages. Neurology 1996;46:1678–1683.
115. Davis R, Peters DH, McTavish D. Valproic acid: A reappraisal of its pharmacological properties and clinical efficacy in epilepsy. Drugs 1994;47:332–372.
116. Greco R, Latini G, Chiarelli F, et al. Leptin, ghrelin, and adiponectin in antiepileptic patients treated with valproic acid. Neurology 2005;65;1808–1809.
117. Pylvaenen V, Pakarinen A, Knip M, Isojaervi J. Characterization of insulin secretion in valproate-treated patients with epilepsy. Epilepsia 2006;47:1460–1464.
118. Genton P, Gelissse P. Valproic acid: Adverse effects. In: Levy RH, Mattson RH, Meldrum BS, et al. Antiepileptic Drugs, 5th ed. Philadelphia: Lippincott Williams & Wilkins, 2002:837–851.
119. Gidal BE, Inglese CM, Meyer JM, et al. Diet and valproate mediated transient hyperammonemia: Effect of l-carnitine supplementation in children with epilepsy. Pediatr Neurol 1997;16:301–305.
120. Gerstner T, Teich M, Bell N, et al. Valproate-associated coagulopathies are frequent and variable in children. Epilepsia 2006;47:1136–1143.
121. Welty TE. Zonisamide. In: Wyllie E., ed. The Treatment of Epilepsy, 4th ed. Philadelphia: Lippincott Williams & Wilkins, 2006:891–899.
122. Lee BI. Zonisamide: Adverse effects. In: Levy RH, Mattson RH, Meldrum BS, et al., eds. Antiepileptic Drugs. Philadelphia: Lippincott Williams & Wilkins, 2002;892–898.
123. Pashko S, McCord A, Sena MM. The cost of epilepsy and seizures in a cohort of Pennsylvania Medicaid patients. Med Interface November 1993:84.
124. Begley CE, Annegers JF, Lairson DR, et al. Cost of epilepsy in the United States: A model based on incidence and prognosis. Epilepsia 1994;35:1230–1243.
125. Hughes D, Cockerell OC. A cost minimization study comparing vigabatrin, lamotrigine, and gabapentin for the treatment of intractable partial epilepsy. Seizure 1996;5:89–95.
126. Gilliam F, Carter J, Vahle V. Tolerability of antiseizure medications. Neurology 2004;63(Suppl 4):S9–12.
127. Gilliam F, Kuzniecky R, Faught E, et al. Patient-validated content of epilepsy-specific quality-of-life measurement. Epilepsia 1997;38:233–236.
128. Crawford P, Hall WW, Chappell B, et al. Generic prescribing for epilepsy: Is it safe? Seizure 1996;5:1–5.

CHAPTER 59 Status Epilepticus

STEPHANIE J. PHELPS, COLLIN A. HOVINGA, AND JAMES W. WHELESS

KEY CONCEPTS

1. Status epilepticus (SE) is a neurologic emergency that is associated with significant morbidity and mortality.
2. Generalized convulsive status epilepticus (GCSE) is defined as any recurrent or continuous seizure activity lasting longer than 30 minutes in which the patient does not regain baseline mental status. Any seizure that does not stop within 5 minutes should be treated as impending SE.
3. There are two types of status epilepticus, GCSE and nonconvulsive status epilepticus (NCSE). GCSE is the most common type.
4. Most GCSE develops in patients with no history of epilepsy; however, a patient with preexisting epilepsy may experience GCSE as a result of acute anticonvulsant withdrawal, metabolic disorder, concurrent illness, or progression of neurologic disease.
5. Although the pathophysiology of GCSE is unknown, experimental models have shown that there is a dramatic decrease in γ-aminobutyric acid (GABA)–mediated inhibitory synaptic transmission and that glutamatergic excitatory synaptic transmission sustains the seizures.
6. General treatment includes patient stabilization, adequate oxygenation, preservation of cardiorespiratory function, management of systemic complications, and aggressive assessment of underlying causes.
7. The main purpose of treatment is to prevent or decrease morbidity and mortality of prolonged seizures. Pharmacologic treatment needs to be rapid and aimed at terminating both electrical and clinical seizures. The probability of poorer outcomes increases with increased length of electrographic seizure activity.
8. Lorazepam is the preferred benzodiazepine in treatment of GCSE because of its long duration of action.
9. Currently, the hydantoins (phenytoin and fosphenytoin) are the long-acting anticonvulsants used most frequently. Either phenytoin or fosphenytoin should be given concurrently with benzodiazepines.
10. The maximum rate of infusion for phenytoin and fosphenytoin in adults is 50 mg/min and 150 mg PE/min, respectively.
11. If GCSE is not controlled by two first-line agents (benzodiazepine plus hydantoin or phenobarbital), the GCSE is considered to be refractory. In these cases, newer anticonvulsants and/or pharmacologically induced coma should be used.

INTRODUCTION

❶ Status epilepticus (SE) is a common neurologic emergency that is associated with brain damage and death. ❷ The traditional definition, provided by the International League Against Epilepsy Classification of Epileptic Seizures, defines SE as (1) any seizure lasting longer than 30 minutes whether or not consciousness is impaired or (2) recurrent seizures without an intervening period of consciousness between seizures.[1] Clinically, this definition has limited use particularly in the case of GCSE, as the average seizure is less than 2 minutes; and only 40% of seizures lasting 10 to 29 minutes cease without treatment.[2,3] Pharmacoresistance[4,5] and mortality[3] significantly increase with increased seizure duration. Therefore, aggressive treatment of seizures lasting 5 minutes or more is strongly recommended. ❸ SE can present in several forms (Table 59–1), including GCSE and NCSE.[1]

NCSE occurs in approximately 25% of those with SE and is characterized by a fluctuating or continuous "twilight" state that produces altered consciousness and/or behavior (e.g., lethargy, decreased mental function). An altered electroencephalogram (EEG) is the most important diagnostic and management tool.[6] In most instances, a benzodiazepine and/or valproate remain drugs of choice for NCSE.[6] Although intravenous (IV) hydantoin or phenobarbital can be tried in patients who fail to respond, general anesthesia or barbiturate coma is not appropriate.[6] The reader is referred to several reviews for a more comprehensive discussion of NCSE and its pharmacologic management.[6,7]

GCSE is the most common and severe form of SE and is characterized by repeated primary or secondary generalized seizures that involve both hemispheres of the brain and are associated with a persistent postictal state. This chapter will focus on the epidemiology, pathophysiology, presentation, and management of GCSE.

EPIDEMIOLOGY

It is difficult to determine the incidence of GCSE because most studies fail to consider the patient's age, seizure etiology, and type or duration of the seizure. The worldwide incidence is thought to range between 1.2 and 5 million cases per year, with an annual incidence of 100,000 to 152,000 cases each year in the United States.[8] GCSE has no predilection for gender or socioeconomic status but does occur more frequently in nonwhites across all ages.[9] Most episodes of GCSE occur in individuals with no history of epilepsy; however, approximately 5%

TABLE 59-1 International Classification of Status Epilepticus

Convulsive		Nonconvulsive	
International	***Traditional Terminology***	***International***	***Traditional Terminology***
Primary generalized SE • Tonic-clonic[a,b] • Tonic[c] • Clonic[c] • Myoclonic[b] • Erratic[d]	Grand mal, epilepticus convulsivus	Absence[c]	Petit mal, spike-and-wave stupor, spike-and-slow-wave or 3/s spike-and-wave, epileptic fugue, epilepsia minora continua, epileptic twilight, minor SE
Secondary generalized SE[a,b] • Tonic • Partial seizures with secondary generalization		Partial SE[a,b]	Focal motor, focal sensory, epilepsia partialis continua, adversive SE
		Simple partial Somatomotor Dysphasic Other types	Elementary
		Complex partial	Temporal lobe, psychomotor, epileptic fugue state, prolonged epileptic stupor, prolonged epileptic confusional state, continuous epileptic twilight state

SE, status epilepticus.
[a]Most common in older children.
[b]Most common in adolescents and adults.
[c]Most common in infants and young children.
[d]Most common in neonates.

of adults and 10% to 25% of children with epilepsy will develop GCSE.[7] The incidence of GCSE is highest in the very young (younger than 1 year of age) and the elderly (older than 60 years of age).

ETIOLOGY

Precipitating events for GCSE vary among studies and generally reflect different populations and referral patterns. ❹ Most episodes that occur in known epileptics occur because of acute anticonvulsant withdrawal, a metabolic disorder or concurrent illness, or progression of a preexisting neurologic disease. Common etiologies and mortality rates for pediatric and adult populations are shown in Table 59–2.[9,10] Precipitating events for GCSE are divided into those with and without neurologic structural lesions or those with a precipitating injury or insult. Cases with structural lesions or those with a specific neurologic insult are associated with a poor prognosis.

There are major differences in etiologies for pediatric and adult patients (see Table 59–2). During their first few weeks of life, infants who are born to addicted mothers can develop drug withdrawal seizures. Other neonates can develop GCSE because of a pyridoxine deficiency, which should resolve within hours following treatment with IV pyridoxine (100 mg). Acute encephalopathy and metabolic disorders are the major causes of GCSE in patients younger than 1 year of age. In young children, the cause is frequently a nonspecific illness such as fever and/or a viral illness. Unless accompanied by an underlying neurologic abnormality, fever-induced GCSE is less likely to be associated with sequelae.

The most frequent precipitating events in adults are cerebrovascular disease, withdrawal of anticonvulsants, and low anticonvulsant serum concentrations. Cerebrovascular disease is the leading cause of GCSE in those who have their first seizures after age 60. A number of prescription, over-the-counter, and recreational drugs should be considered in anyone with new-onset GCSE. Elevated anticonvulsant serum concentration or rapid anticonvulsant withdrawal can also precipitate GCSE.

TABLE 59-2 Etiology and Mortality for Pediatric and Adult Cases of Status Epilepticus

Etiology	Number of Cases (% Mortality) *n* = 200 Cases of Pediatric SE	Number of Cases (% Mortality) *n* = 512 Cases of Adult SE
Type I (no structural lesion)		
Infection	55 (5)	6 (35)
CNS infection	11 (0)	2 (20)
Metabolic	20 (5)	12 (36)
Low AED levels	16 (0)	24 (7)
Alcohol	0 (0)	13 (8)
Idiopathic	6 (0)	13 (18)
Type II (structural lesion)		
Anoxia/hypoxia	27 (13)	14 (65)
CNS tumor	3 (50)	5 (22)
CVA	5 (0)	26 (27)
Drug overdose	5 (0)	3 (23)
Hemorrhage	5 (11)	4 (35)
Trauma	13 (0)	3 (23)
Remote causes[a]	33 (5)	7 (13)

AED, antiepileptic drug; CVA, cerebrovascular accident; SE, status epilepticus.
Percentages do not add up to 100% because some patients had multiple etiologies.
[a]More than half of remote causes were congenital malformations and CVA in pediatric and adult patients, respectively.
Data from DeLorenzo et al.[9,10]

MORBIDITY

GCSE is harmful to the brain and is associated with morbidity. However, whether the morbidity results from the underlying etiology or the GCSE itself remains to be determined. Most contend that the GCSE is responsible for the morbidity. Neuronal damage in animal models is evident following 30 to 60 minutes of GCSE regardless of the inducing stimulus, and most animals progress to the development of epilepsy following a prolonged seizure. Interestingly, inhibiting the neuronal damage associated with seizures does not prevent the development of epilepsy, suggesting that the seizures themselves may be harmful. It is difficult to establish a relationship between GCSE and long-term outcomes. This is largely because it is difficult to weigh the effects of seizure type, etiology, duration, concurrent physiologic events, and therapy or lack thereof. However, it has been shown that patients with a history of prolonged febrile seizures who later developed epilepsy share similar histopathologic changes (i.e., hippocampal sclerosis) to those found in animal models of GCSE.[11,12] In these cases the period between the initial GCSE and the first epileptic seizure may be months to decades, suggesting that there may be a link between GCSE and the development of epilepsy. Importantly, studies of GCSE show that the currently available anticonvulsants do not reproducibly prevent the development of epilepsy following prolonged seizures.[11,13]

Patients who develop epilepsy following prolonged GCSE are less likely to experience remission of their seizures and may have decreased cognitive and memory function, mental retardation, or neurologic deficits.[8] Most studies have found that younger children, the elderly, and those with preexisting epilepsy have a higher propensity for sequelae.

MORTALITY

The estimated mortality rate in the United States following GCSE ranges between 22,000 and 42,000 individuals per year.[10] Recent estimates suggest a mortality rate of up to 10% in children,[14] 20% in adults,[8] and 38% in the elderly.[9] When compared with other populations, neonates with seizures have a higher mortality and more neurologic sequelae.

Table 59–2 summarizes the etiology for GCSE and their corresponding mortality rates.[9,11] Interestingly, the mortality associated with many etiologies is significantly greater in adults than in children. Unresponsive patients may die from GCSE, but more frequently they die from the acute illness that precipitated the GCSE. For example, patients with serious central nervous system (CNS) structural changes (e.g., hemorrhage, stroke) have a poor prognosis, whereas those (i.e., 80%–90%) with no structural lesion generally respond to IV phenytoin.

Two variables that affect outcome are the time between onset of GCSE and the initiation of treatment and the duration of the seizure. Mortality significantly increases with increased seizure duration being 2.6% for those with seizures 10 to 29 minutes versus 19% for those with seizures lasting longer than 30 minutes.[2] GCSE lasting longer than 60 minutes have a higher mortality rate (32%) than seizures lasting less than 60 minutes (2.5%).[10] Mortality has decreased over the past decade and probably reflects a recognition of the need to initiate sequenced therapy immediately, and a greater understanding of the pathogenesis of GCSE.

PATHOGENESIS

Seizures occur when the excitatory neurotransmission overcomes inhibitory impulses in one or more brain regions (i.e., neural networks). Most seizures are brief (less than or equal to 5 minutes), largely because the brain's inhibitory mechanisms restore the balance of normal neurotransmission.[14] It is unknown why the mechanisms that control normal brain homeostasis fail. However, when seizures occur in close succession or the magnitude of the proconvulsant stimulus is severe, compensatory mechanisms can be overwhelmed and lead to GCSE.

❺ Although the exact cellular mechanisms responsible for the production of abnormal neural impulses are unknown, it appears that seizure initiation is caused by an imbalance between excitatory (e.g., glutamate, calcium, sodium, substance P, and neurokinin B) and inhibitory neurotransmission (e.g., GABA, adenosine, potassium, neuropeptide Y, opioid peptides, and galanin).[14] Seizure maintenance associated with GCSE is largely caused by glutamate acting on postsynaptic *N*-methyl-D-aspartate (NMDA) and α-amino-3-hydroxy-5-methyl-isoxazole-4-propionate (AMPA)/kainate receptors. Most of what is known about GCSE has focused on gated ion channels, with less known about receptor–second messenger systems (e.g., metabotropic glutamate receptors).[14]

During GCSE, glutamate activation of the NMDA and AMPA receptors causes opening of the gated calcium and sodium channels, respectively. Entry of the respective ions causes neuronal depolarization. Sustained depolarization may maintain GCSE and eventually cause neuronal death through calcium-, free radical-, and kinase-mediated events.[11] Although drugs acting as NMDA and AMPA receptor antagonists seem attractive for the treatment of GCSE, it is likely that glutamate is not the sole mechanism for GCSE and that other mechanisms become increasingly important as the duration of seizures increases.

$GABA_A$ postsynaptic receptors control chloride channels to produce hyperpolarization (inhibition) of the postsynaptic cell membrane. These receptors have binding sites for GABA and select anticonvulsants (e.g., phenobarbital and benzodiazepines) and enhance $GABA_A$-mediated chloride inhibitory currents. It was previously thought that a decrease in presynaptic GABA led to prolonged seizures; however, it is currently held that GABA concentrations increase during the early phases of GCSE and continue to be elevated during late GCSE. Prolonged seizures lead to decreased inhibitory $GABA_A$-receptor density because of postsynaptic receptor endocytosis. Additionally, $GABA_A$ receptors may be modified during SE, such that there is decreased response to both endogenous GABA and GABA agonists.[12] Clinically, this can influence response to both benzodiazepines and phenobarbital in that their relative potencies can be reduced up to tenfold if seizures persist for more than 30 minutes.[12] A similar phenomenon occurs with sodium channel antagonists (phenytoin); however, the magnitude of resistance is believed to be less.[14]

PATHOPHYSIOLOGY

As GCSE continues, there are systemic alterations, progression of motor phenomena, and development of specific EEG findings.[15] Two distinct and predictable phases have been identified. Phase I occurs during the first 30 minutes of seizure activity, and phase II begins 60 minutes later. Although these systemic complications affect the prognosis of GCSE, a prolonged seizure can destroy neurons independent of these systemic events.[11] In fact, the systemic effects of induced seizures in animals can be blocked, but the damage to the neocortex, cerebellum, and hippocampus persists.

During phase I, each seizure produces marked increases in plasma epinephrine, norepinephrine, and steroid concentrations that can cause hypertension, tachycardia, and cardiac arrhythmias.[15] Within minutes, arterial systolic pressures can rise to above 200 mm Hg, and heart rate can increase by 83 beats per minute. Although blood pressure returns to normal within 60 minutes, mean arterial pressure does not fall below 60 mm Hg; hence, cerebral perfusion pressure is not compromised. In animals, cerebral blood flow is also increased, thereby protecting neurons from hypoxic injury.

Seizure-induced increases in sympathetic and parasympathetic stimulation of the heart, in the presence of a hypoxic myocardium, can result in ventricular arrhythmias. Autonomic neuron stimulation can cause a release of insulin and glucagon. Concurrently, circulating catecholamines cause an elevation of hepatic cyclic adenosine monophosphate, producing glycogenolysis. Although the patient can be hyperglycemic initially, serum glucose concentration begins to fall.

Seizure-induced muscular contractions and hypoxia cause lactic acid release, which can produce a severe acidosis that can be accompanied by hypotension and shock. Muscle contractions can be so severe that rhabdomyolysis with secondary hyperkalemia and acute tubular necrosis can occur. The airway can be obstructed, and the patient can become cyanotic or hypoxic at any time. Additionally, an increase in salivation and tracheal and pulmonary secretions can cause aspiration pneumonia. Although transient pleocytosis can develop, it should not be attributed to SE until infectious causes have been eliminated.

Between seizures, the EEG slows, and blood pressure normalizes. Although metabolic demands are increased, the brain is able to adequately compensate. If seizures exceed 60 minutes (phase II), the EEG ictal discharge and clonic motor activity become continuous, and the patient begins to decompensate. Despite elevated levels of catecholamines, the patient can become hypotensive. During the late phase, autoregulation of cerebral blood flow becomes dependent on mean arterial pressure and begins to fail. There continues to be an excessive consumption of oxygen and glucose; however, compensatory mechanisms are no longer able to keep up with demands.

During phase II, the serum glucose concentration may be normal or decreased. Profound hypoglycemia, secondary to hyperinsulinemia, can occur in patients with hepatic dysfunction or in those with reduced glycogen stores. Hyperthermia and respiratory deterioration with hypoxia and ventilatory failure can develop. There also may be metabolic and biochemical complications, including respiratory and metabolic acidosis, hyperkalemia, hyponatremia, and azotemia. There is increased sweating and salivation. This has important clinical ramifications in that a patient's seizures can seem to terminate without treatment or when an ineffective therapy is given.

CLINICAL CONTROVERSY

The choice of long-acting anticonvulsant to give following the initial benzodiazepine is controversial. According to the Working Group on Status Epilepticus, phenytoin should be used in seizures that recur after treatment with a benzodiazepine.[14] Although this has been the practice for decades, no studies have documented the superiority of a hydantoin over other anticonvulsants. Thus, it is questionable if a hydantoin should be administered alone, in larger doses, or at all when seizures recur following benzodiazepine administration.

CLINICAL PRESENTATION AND DIAGNOSIS

Accurate diagnosis requires observation, physical examination, laboratory assessment, EEG, and neurologic imaging. The nature and duration of the seizure should be obtained, and a diagnosis of GCSE should not be made until a clinician has observed at least one seizure. Most patients have an altered consciousness that ranges from obtunded to marked lethargy and somnolence with pronounced eyes-open unresponsiveness and waxy rigidity. Motor features can include muscle contractions, extensor or flexor posturing, and spasms. Over time, the clinical manifestations become less apparent, and the diagnosis requires careful assessment.

In addition to an assessment of language and cognitive abilities, the physical and neurological examinations should assess motor, sensory, and reflex abnormalities, pupillary response, asymmetry, and posturing. The patient should also be examined for secondary injuries (e.g., tongue lacerations, shoulder dislocations, head and facial trauma).

Laboratory tests are essential to the diagnosis of various etiologies. Hypoglycemia, hyponatremia, hypernatremia, hypomagnesemia, hypocalcemia, and renal failure all can cause seizures. A urine drug screen can help eliminate the possibility of illicit drug use or drug overdose. Serum drug concentration(s) should be obtained in those on chronic anticonvulsants, because high concentrations of certain medications can induce seizures, and low concentrations can reflect noncompliance or rapid drug withdrawal. A baseline serum concentration is necessary to determine whether a loading dose of a specific anticonvulsant is required. Assessment of other laboratory parameters (e.g., albumin, renal function, and hepatic function) that affect anticonvulsant dosing also can be useful. An EEG is a valuable diagnostic tool, particularly in those with prolonged GCSE in whom clinically apparent seizures are not always evident, but therapy should not be delayed while awaiting testing or results.

Once seizures have stopped it is important to determine if the patient is febrile or has a systemic or CNS infection. Many physiologic consequences of GCSE (e.g., leukocytosis, pleocytosis, and hyperthermia) produce symptoms that can be confused with other conditions. If a CNS infection is suspected, empiric antibiotics should be started, and a spinal tap should be performed. Computed tomography (CT) or magnetic resonance imaging (MRI) should be obtained to rule out vascular, neoplastic, or infectious etiologies.

CLINICAL PRESENTATION OF GCSE

Symptoms

- Impaired consciousness (e.g., lethargy to coma)
- Disorientation once GCSE is controlled
- Pain associated with injuries (e.g., tongue lacerations, shoulder dislocations, head trauma)

Early Signs

- Generalized convulsions
- Acute injuries or CNS insults that cause extensor or flexor posturing
- Hypothermia or fever suggestive of intercurrent illnesses (e.g., sepsis or meningitis)
- Incontinence
- Normal blood pressure or hypotension and respiratory compromise

Late Signs

- Clinical seizures may or may not be apparent
- Pulmonary edema with respiratory failure
- Cardiac failure (dysrhythmias, arrest, cardiogenic shock)
- Hypotension or hypertension
- Disseminated intravascular coagulation, multisystem organ failure
- Rhabdomyolysis
- Hyperpyremia

Initial Laboratory Tests

- Complete blood count (CBC) with differential
- Serum chemistry profile (e.g., electrolytes, calcium, magnesium, glucose, serum creatinine, alanine aminotransferase [ALT], aspartate aminotransferase [AST])
- Urine drug/alcohol screen
- Blood cultures
- Arterial blood gas to assess for metabolic and respiratory acidosis
- Serum drug concentration if previous anticonvulsant suspected or known

Other Diagnostic Tests

- Spinal tap if CNS infection suspected
- EEG should be obtained on presentation and once clinical seizures are controlled
- CT with and without contrast
- MRI
- Radiograph if indicated to diagnose fractures
- Electrocardiogram (ECG), especially if ingestion confirmed

TREATMENT

Generalized Convulsive Status Epilepticus

DESIRED OUTCOMES

The short-term desired outcomes are (1) immediate termination of all clinical and electrical seizure activity, (2) no clinically significant adverse effects from therapy, and (3) lack of recurrent seizure activity. ❼ The long-term desired outcomes are to minimize or avoid the likelihood of pharmacoresistent epilepsy and/or the development of neurologic sequelae that significantly impact quality of life.

NONPHARMACOLOGIC THERAPY

Vital signs should be assessed, an adequate and protected airway should be established, ventilation should be maintained, and oxygen should be administered. Frequent arterial blood gas determinations should be done to assess for metabolic acidosis, which should be treated with sodium bicarbonate if the pH is less than 7.2. Assisted ventilation should be used to correct respiratory acidosis.

Some patients might continue to have electrical seizures in the absence of clinical motor manifestations. For those who continue to have altered consciousness after clinical control of their seizures, an EEG should be performed. Although hypoglycemia is a rare cause of GCSE, adults should be given 50 mL of a 50% dextrose solution, and children should receive 1 mL/kg of a 25% dextrose solution.[7,8,14] Because Wernicke encephalopathy can develop in alcoholics, adults should receive IV thiamine (100 mg) prior to glucose.[14] Serum glucose concentration should be determined to assess the need for further supplementation.

■ PHARMACOLOGIC THERAPY

When a seizure does not stop automatically within 5 minutes, or when doubt exists regarding the diagnosis, patients should be treated as if they have GCSE. Figure 59–1 provides an algorithm for the treatment of GCSE.

❻ There are four immediate goals in the management of GCSE: (1) patient stabilization, including adequate oxygenation, preservation of cardiorespiratory function, and management of systemic complications; (2) accurate diagnosis of the subtype of GCSE and identification of precipitating factors; (3) termination of clinical and electrical seizures as early as possible; and (4) prevention of seizure recurrence. The three most commonly used classes of anticonvulsants for the initial treatment of GCSE are the benzodiazepines, hydantoins, and barbiturates.

Benzodiazepines

The benzodiazepines are effective initial therapy in most patients with GCSE and should be administered as soon as possible. Generally, one or two IV doses will stop seizures within 2 to 3 minutes.[8] Diazepam, lorazepam, and midazolam are equally effective; therefore the preferred benzodiazepine is determined by differences in the pharmacokinetic and pharmacoeconomic profiles.

Diazepam is an extremely lipophilic moiety with a large volume of distribution (1 to 2 L/kg).[14] Although its initial distribution into the brain occurs within seconds, it rapidly redistributes into fat, causing its CNS half-life to be less than 1 hour and its duration of effect to be less than 30 minutes.[14] If diazepam is the sole anticonvulsant, the rapid decrease in brain concentration can cause seizure recurrence; hence, a longer-acting anticonvulsant (e.g., phenytoin or phenobarbital) should also be given. The initial dose of diazepam (Table 59–3) can be repeated if the patient does not respond within 5 minutes.[14]

❽ Most practitioners consider lorazepam the benzodiazepine of choice.[8,14] It is less lipid soluble than diazepam and takes longer to achieve peak concentrations in the brain; however, its minimal redistribution into fat results in a longer duration of action (i.e., 12 to 24 hours).[8,14] It also has a higher-affinity binding to the benzodiazepine receptor than diazepam.

Initial lorazepam dosing can be found in Table 59–3. This dose can be repeated if the patient does not respond in 5 minutes.[14] Patients chronically on a benzodiazepine (e.g., clonazepam) might have developed tolerance and could require larger doses for response. If successful, lorazepam can provide seizure protection for up to 24 hours. Diazepam and lorazepam cause vein irritation and should be diluted with an equal volume of compatible diluent before administration. Both diazepam and lorazepam contain propylene glycol, which can cause dysrhythmia and hypotension if administered too rapidly.[14] Because of slow and erratic absorption, they should not be given intramuscularly.

Midazolam is water-soluble and diffuses rapidly into the brain. Unfortunately, it has an extremely short half-life and must be given by continuous infusion. Various routes of administration (e.g., buccal, and intramuscular [IM]) have been used successfully to terminate seizures rapidly when IV access cannot be established. Buccal administration is performed easily, and the volume of fluid is small enough (e.g., 2 to 5 mL) that aspiration is unlikely. Because of its increased solubility, IM midazolam has a more reliable absorption than either diazepam or lorazepam. In fact, some practitioners have recommended that IM midazolam be given by emergency personnel as first-line treatment in the out-of-hospital setting.[16]

All benzodiazepines can impair consciousness and interfere with neurologic assessment. Although rare, brief (less than 1 minute) cardiorespiratory depression can occur and can necessitate assisted ventilation or require intubation. This is especially true if a benzodiazepine is used concomitantly with a barbiturate. Hypotension secondary to a reduction in vasomotor tone can occur following large doses.[8]

Phenytoin

❾ A hydantoin is the second-line agent in GCSE that is unresponsive to the benzodiazepines or in seizures that recur after successful treatment with a benzodiazepine.[8] Although it is effective in terminating seizures in 40% to 91% of patients,[14] it can be inferior to lorazepam, phenobarbital, or diazepam plus phenytoin at stopping GCSE within 20 minutes of their infusion.[17,18] Phenytoin has a long half-life (20 to 36 hours) and causes less respiratory depression and sedation than the benzodiazepines or phenobarbital;[14] however, it cannot be delivered rapidly enough to be considered a first-line single agent.

Injectable phenytoin should be diluted to less than or equal to 5 mg/mL in normal saline. Microcrystals will precipitate if it is mixed in a glucose-containing solution. The vehicle (40% propylene glycol) can cause administration-related hypotension and cardiac arrhythmias. These effects are more likely to occur if large loading doses are given to elderly individuals with preexisting cardiac disease or in critically ill patients with marginal blood pressure.[14] Vital signs and an ECG should be obtained during administration. The infusion rate should be slowed if the QT interval widens or if hypotension or arrhythmias develop.[14] ❿ The maximum rate of infusion is 50 mg/min in adults and 3 mg/kg/min in children weighing less than 50 kg (110 lb).[19] The rate should not exceed 25 mg/min in the elderly.

Suggested IV loading doses of phenytoin are provided in Table 59–3.[14] A reduction in the loading dose is recommended for elderly patients,[14] and a larger loading dose is required in obese patients.[20] If the patient has been on phenytoin prior to admission and the serum concentration is known, this should be considered in determining a loading dose. Although some advocate the administration of an additional 5 mg/kg in those with unresponsive GCSE, there is no evidence that this will be beneficial. This practice can cause concentrations to exceed the reference range and produce toxicity. Because phenytoin has poor lipid solubility and enters the brain slowly, it can take up to 60 minutes before the pharmacodynamic effect is apparent. This delay is important when considering administration of a second 5 mg/kg loading dose. Therapeutic serum concentrations, 10 to 20 mg/L, generally do not persist more than 24 hours; hence, maintenance doses (see Table 59–3) should be started within 12 to 24 hours of the loading dose.

Phenytoin has an alkaline pH, which is associated with pain and burning during infusion; phlebitis can occur with chronic infusion, and tissue necrosis is likely on infiltration. IM administration is not recommended because absorption is delayed and erratic, and phenytoin can crystallize in tissue. Oral loading doses have been used in patients not actively seizing; it may take 4 to 12 hours before

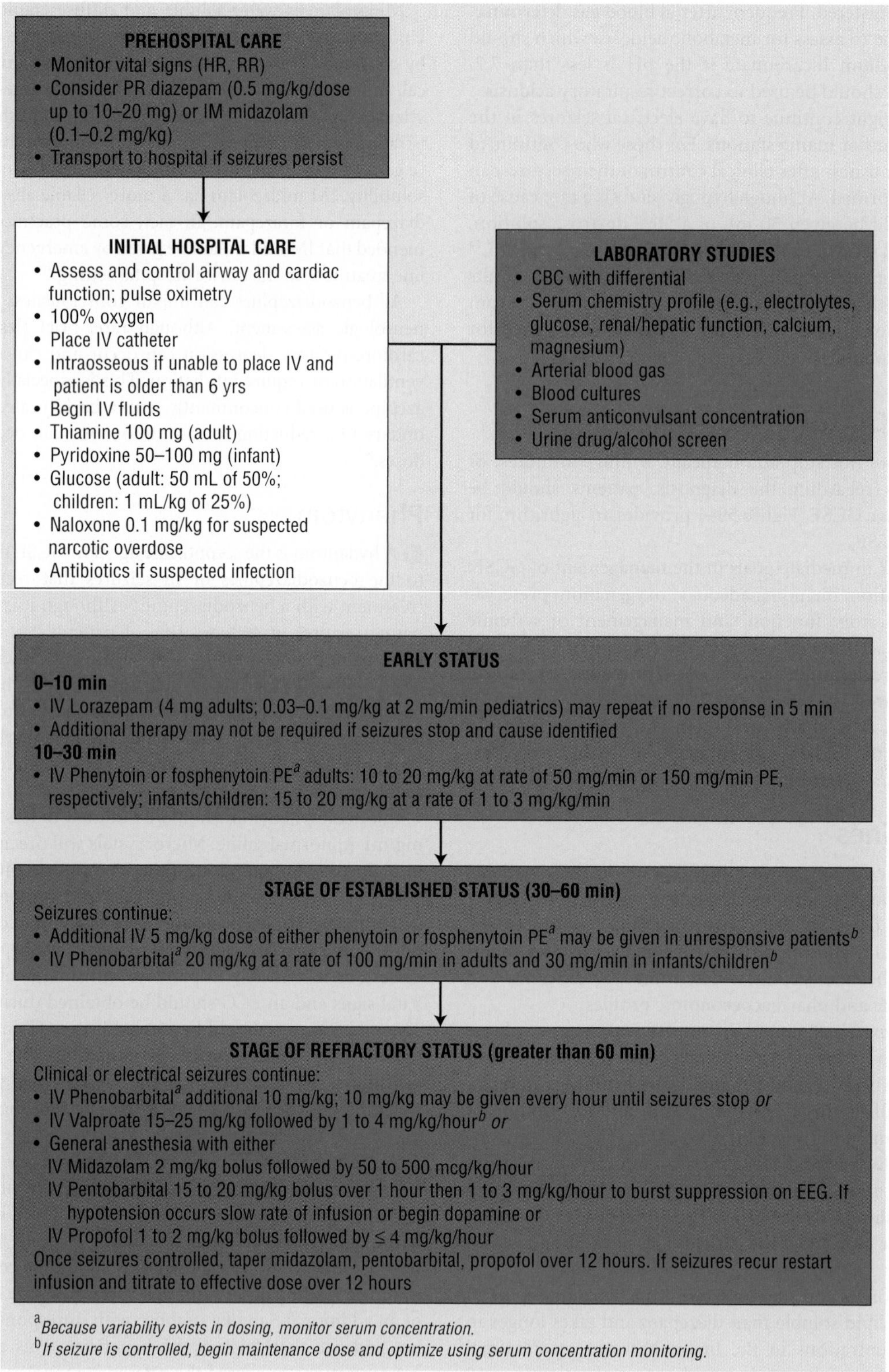

FIGURE 59-1. Algorithm for the treatment of GCSE. (CBC, complete blood count; EEG, electroencephalogram; GCSE, generalized convulsive status epilepticus; HR, heart rate; PR, per rectum; RR, respiratory rate.)

adequate serum concentrations are obtained; therefore, this practice is not recommended.

Fosphenytoin

Fosphenytoin, a water-soluble phosphate ester, has no known pharmacologic activity.[21] It does not contain propylene glycol and is compatible with most common IV fluids. Prior to IV administration it should be diluted in 5% dextrose or normal saline to a concentration of 1.5 to 25 mg phenytoin equivalents/mL.[21] It is converted rapidly (7 to 15 minutes) and completely (100%) to phenytoin by blood and tissue phosphatases after IV and IM dosing.[21] The conversion delay was a concern initially; however, this time is offset by high protein binding, saturable binding at high concentrations, and the rapid rate of infusion.[21]

Nystagmus, dizziness, and ataxia are the most frequent adverse events and are attributed to phenytoin. The frequency of ECG or blood pressure changes is less than that for phenytoin. Nonallergic

TABLE 59-3 Medications Used in the Initial Treatment of GCSE

Anticonvulsant (Route)	Loading Dose (Maximum Dose)		Rate of Infusion		Maintenance Dose	
	Adult	Pediatric	Adult	Pediatric	Adult	Pediatric
Diazepam (IV bolus)	0.25 mg/kg[a,b,c] (40 mg)	0.25–0.5 mg/kg[a,c] (0.75 mg/kg)	<5 mg/min	<5 mg/min	Not used	Not used
Fosphenytoin IV	15–20 mg PE/kg	15–20 mg PE/kg	150 mg PE/min	3 mg PE/kg/min	4–5 mg PE/kg/day	5–10 mg PE/kg/day
Lorazepam (IV bolus)	4 mg[a,b,c] (8 mg)	0.1 mg/kg[a,c] (4 mg)	2 mg/min	2 mg/min	Not used	Not used
Midazolam IV	200 mcg/kg[a,d]	150 mcg/kg[a,d]	0.5–1 mg/min	2–3 min	50–500 mcg/kg/h[e]	60–120 mcg/kg/h[e]
Phenobarbital IV	10–20 mg/kg[e]	15–20 mg/kg[e]	100 mg/min	30 mg/min	1–4 mg/kg/day[e]	3–5 mg/kg/day[e]
Phenytoin IV	10–20 mg/kg[f]	10–20 mg/kg[f]	50 mg/min[g]	1–3 mg/kg/min	4–5 mg/kg/day[e]	5–10 mg/kg/day[e]

GCSE, generalized convulsive status epilepticus; PE, phenytoin equivalents.
[a]Doses can be repeated every 10 to 15 minutes until the maximum dosage is given.
[b]Initial doses in the elderly are 2 to 5 mg.
[c]Larger doses can be required if patients chronically on a benzodiazepine (e.g., clonazepam).
[d]Can be given by the intramuscular, rectal, or buccal routes.
[e]Titrate dose as needed.
[f]Administer additional loading dose based on serum concentration.
[g]The rate should not exceed 25 mg/min in elderly patients and those with known atherosclerotic cardiovascular disease.

paresthesia and pruritus of the face and groin are unique to fosphenytoin and are related to dose and infusion rate, and rarely require discontinuation of fosphenytoin. These side effects typically subside within 5 to 10 minutes after the infusion.[21]

Fosphenytoin should be dosed using PE, thereby obviating the need for interconversion between phenytoin and fosphenytoin. The loading dose and rates of administration of fosphenytoin can be found in Table 59–3. Because of delays in achieving adequate phenytoin serum concentrations, a loading dose should not be given intramuscularly unless IV access is impossible. Continuous ECG, blood pressure, and respiratory status monitoring is recommended for all loading doses of fosphenytoin.

Fosphenytoin serum concentrations are of no clinical value. Serum phenytoin concentrations are the end point for therapeutic drug monitoring, and the desired serum concentration range is the same as that for phenytoin. Fosphenytoin cross-reacts with some phenytoin immunoassays causing an overestimation of phenytoin concentration; hence, blood should not be obtained for at least 2 hours after IV and 4 hours after IM administration.[21]

CLINICAL CONTROVERSY

The debate continues as to which hydantoin is preferred in GCSE. Although phenytoin has been used for decades, it is associated with a variety of problems related to its formulation. Conversely, fosphenytoin is associated with less infusion pain and IV-site complications and fewer hemodynamic effects than phenytoin. Although most practitioners believe that fosphenytoin is clearly a "better" formulation, many struggle with the advantages of fosphenytoin, given its cost.

Phenobarbital

There are three different opinions regarding the use of phenobarbital in GCSE. Because barbiturates cause CNS and respiratory depression, as well as hypotension, most contend that phenobarbital should be the third-line agent when a benzodiazepine plus phenytoin has failed.[8] Others suggest that the barbiturates are as safe and effective as other anticonvulsants and should be the drug of choice after a benzodiazepine has been given. Still others support the continuous-infusion midazolam as the third-line anticonvulsant before the barbiturates.[22]

Although two studies found phenobarbital as effective as diazepam plus phenytoin[17] and lorazepam alone or diazepam plus phenytoin in patients with GCSE,[18] the Working Group on Status Epilepticus recommends that phenobarbital be given after a benzodiazepine plus phenytoin has failed.[14] Currently, most practitioners agree that phenobarbital is the long-acting anticonvulsant of choice in patients with a hypersensitivity to the hydantoins or in those with cardiac conduction abnormalities.

Phenobarbital has biphasic distribution into body organs.[23] During phase I, the drug distributes into highly vascular organs, but it does not distribute into the brain. With the exception of fat, phenobarbital distributes throughout the body during phase II[23]; hence lean body mass should be used in calculating doses in obese patients.[23] Although the highest brain concentrations occur 12 to 60 minutes after an IV dose,[23] seizures are controlled within minutes of the loading dose.[18] The loading and maintenance dose are given in Table 59–3. When necessary, larger loading doses (30 mg/kg) have been used in neonates without adverse effects. If the initial loading dose does not stop the seizures within 20 to 30 minutes, an additional 10 to 20 mg/kg can be given. If seizures continue, a third 10 mg/kg load can be given.[24] Phenobarbital exhibits first-order linear pharmacokinetics, and there is no maximum dose beyond which further doses are likely to be ineffective.[24] Once GCSE is controlled, the maintenance dose should be started within 12 to 24 hours.

Although injectable phenobarbital contains propylene glycol, it can be given more rapidly than phenytoin (see Table 59–3). Phenobarbital can be given IM, but its rate of absorption is too slow to be effective. Phenobarbital can depress consciousness and respiration. The risk of apnea and hypopnea can be more profound in patients treated initially with benzodiazepines.[8,14] If significant hypotension develops, the infusion should be slowed or stopped.[14]

TREATMENT OF REFRACTORY GCSE

⓫ When adequate doses of a benzodiazepine, hydantoin, or barbiturate have failed, the condition is termed *refractory*.[22] Approximately 10% to 15% of patients will develop refractory GCSE, and approximately 30% of patients whose seizures are "clinically" controlled will have persistent electrical manifestations after administration of these anticonvulsants. When a patient develops refractory GCSE, an intense search should be performed for an acute or progressive cause.

It should be remembered that the longer GCSE lasts, the harder it is to treat and that failure to treat aggressively early in the course of disease increases the likelihood of nonresponse.[14] There is no consensus regarding the anticonvulsant of choice, sequencing of therapy, or treatment of refractory GCSE. Regardless of this, the goal is to stop electrical epileptiform activity.

Approaches used include the continuous infusion of a benzodiazepines, medically induced coma, valproate, levetiracetam, topira-

TABLE 59-4 Medications Used to Treat Refractory GCSE

	Loading Dose		Infusion Duration		Maintenance Dose	
Anticonvulsant (Route)	***Adult***	***Pediatric***	***Adult***	***Pediatric***	***Adult***	***Pediatric***
Levetiracetam IV	500–1,000 mg	NA	33–66 mg/min	NA	750–9,000 mg/day	NA
Lidocaine IV	50–100 mg	1 mg/kg (maximum dose = 3–5 mg/kg in first hour)	≤2 minutes	≤2 minutes	1.5–3.5 mg/kg/h	1.2–3 mg/kg/h
Midazolam IV	200 mcg/kg[a]	150 mcg/kg[a]	0.5–1 mg/min	0.5–1 mg/min	50–500 mcg/kg/h[b]	60–120 mcg/kg/h[b]
Pentobarbital IV	10–20 mg/kg	15–20 mg/kg	Over 1–2 hours	Over 1–2 hours	1–5 mg/kg/h[b]	1–5 mg/kg/h[b]
Propofol IV	2 mg/kg	3 mg/kg	Over 10 seconds	Over 20–30 seconds	5–10 mg/kg/h	2–18 mg/kg/h[c]
Topiramate PO	300–1,600 mg	5–10 mg/kg	NA	NA	400–1,600 mg/day	5–10 mg/kg/day
Valproate IV	15–45 mg/kg	20–25 mg/kg	3 mg/kg/min	3 mg/kg/min	1–4 mg/kg/h[b]	1–4 mg/kg/h[b]

GCSE, generalized convulsive status epilepticus; NA, not available; PO, orally.
[a]Doses can be repeated twice every 10 to 15 minutes until the maximum dosage is given.
[b]Titrate dose as needed.
[c]Generally recommended not to exceed a dose of 4 mg/kg/h and a duration of 48 hours.

mate, propofol, paraldehyde, or lidocaine. Doses for these agents can be found in Table 59–4. A meta-analysis compared midazolam, propofol, and pentobarbital in refractory GCSE.[25] Overall response rates were significantly greater in those treated with pentobarbital (92%) compared to midazolam (80%) and propofol (73%). Breakthrough seizures were more commonly observed with midazolam (51%) versus propofol (15%) and pentobarbital (12%). Although pentobarbital had a greater response rate, clinically significant hypotension was more common than with the other agents. Mortality rates were similar for the three drugs.

Benzodiazepines

Some practitioners advocated that midazolam should be the first-line agent in refractory GCSE.[22] Table 59–4 contains the loading and maintenance doses of midazolam. Most patients respond to these doses within an hour, but the continuous-infusion rate should be increased every 15 minutes in those who do not. Because tachyphylaxis can develop, frequent increases in the infusion rate can be necessary, and dosing should be guided by EEG response.[22]

Once GCSE is terminated, dosages can be decreased by 1 mcg/kg/min every 2 hours. Successful discontinuation is enhanced by maintaining the patient's phenytoin and phenobarbital serum concentration(s) above 20 mg/L and 40 mg/L.[22] Because of midazolam's short half-life, patients can return to consciousness more rapidly than those receiving larger doses of more sedating anticonvulsants (e.g., phenytoin, phenobarbital). Generally, continuous-infusion midazolam has been well tolerated, with few cases of hypotension and respiratory depression seen. Hypotension and poikilothermia can occur and can require supportive therapies.

Large-dose continuous-infusion lorazepam and diazepam also have been used successfully in patients unresponsive to phenytoin or phenobarbital.[26] Lorazepam contains propylene glycol, which can accumulate in patients receiving continuous infusions. It has been noted to cause a marked osmolar gap, metabolic acidosis, and renal toxicity, which was attributed to the infusion of propylene glycol.[27–29]

CLINICAL CONTROVERSY

The positioning of midazolam among the medications used to treat GCSE is controversial. Some investigators recommend that midazolam should be the anticonvulsant of first choice and, therefore, should be used in lieu of lorazepam; others argue that it should be used after a hydantoin has failed; still others recommend it only for refractory GCSE.

Medically Induced Coma

If there is an inadequate response to large doses of midazolam, anesthetizing the patient to suppress the cerebral ictal discharge is recommended.[14,25] Although it is likely that the patient is already being mechanically ventilated, intubation and respiratory support are mandatory during barbiturate coma. Because hypotension is a concern, it is essential that vital signs be monitored continuously. A short-acting barbiturate (usually either pentobarbital or thiopental) generally is preferred because it allows a more rapid reversal of coma.

Several sources note that the initial loading dose of pentobarbital is 5 mg/kg.[14] However, this dose is inadequate to produce the serum concentrations (30 to 40 mg/L) necessary to induce an isoelectric EEG. Pentobarbital should be initiated with a loading dose of at least 10 to 20 mg/kg over 1 to 2 hours[25] (see Table 59–4). If hypotension occurs during the loading dose, the rate of administration should be slowed, or dopamine should be administered. The loading dose should be followed immediately by a continuous infusion.[14] Rates are typically begun at 1 mg/kg/h and titrated as needed up to a dose of 5 mg/kg/h. The maintenance infusion should be increased gradually until there is evidence of burst suppression on EEG (i.e., isoelectric EEG) or prohibitive adverse effects occur. Although the duration of barbiturate coma in most studies has been 2 to 3 days, pentobarbital coma has been used safely for 53 days in an 18-year-old patient.[30] To avoid complications (e.g., pneumonia, pulmonary edema), the pentobarbital should be discontinued as soon as possible. Twelve hours after a burst-suppression pattern is obtained, the rate of pentobarbital infusion should be titrated downward every 2 to 4 hours to enable the clinician to determine if the patient's GCSE is in remission. It is important to have other anticonvulsants at therapeutic amounts before pentobarbital is withdrawn so that the risk of seizure recurrence is minimized. Because pentobarbital is a potent hepatic enzyme inducer, doses of most concurrent anticonvulsants will need to be larger than usual maintenance doses. The patient will need to be monitored for side effects as deinduction occurs and anticonvulsant concentrations increase. This can take up to a month after pentobarbital's discontinuation.

Valproate

Limited human data exist regarding the use of valproate in refractory GCSE. Although an IV dosage form has been approved by the FDA, it is not approved for GCSE. A number of loading and continuous-infusion doses (see Table 59–4) have been used to treat GCSE in both adult[31–33] and pediatric patients.[33,34] One study suggested the need to consider the effects of enzyme-inducing anticonvulsants when dosing valproate.[34] This group recommended that the continuous-infusion rate be determined by the presence of concurrent anticonvulsants (no inducers present, 1 mg/kg/h; one or more inducers [e.g., phenytoin, phenobarbital], 2 mg/kg/h; and inducers and pentobarbital coma, 4 mg/kg/h).

Although the manufacturer originally recommended IV valproate be given no faster than 20 mg/min, much faster rates have been studied (2 to 6 mg/kg/min) and are used for administration of the loading dose.[34,35] Currently, the manufacturer recommends that IV valproate be administered at a rate of 3 mg/kg/min. In general, IV valproate has been well tolerated, with no cases of respiratory depression. Hemodynamic instability is extremely rare, but patients' vital signs should be monitored closely during the loading dose.

Propofol

Propofol is extremely lipid soluble, has a large volume of distribution, and has a very rapid onset of action. Its extremely short half-life promotes rapid awakening on drug discontinuation. Propofol has comparative efficacy to midazolam in refractory GCSE.[25,36] Doses can be found in Table 59–4. Although controversial, it has been associated with progressive metabolic acidosis, hemodynamic instability, and bradyarrhythmias that are refractory to aggressive pharmacologic treatments.[37] Finally, a normal adult dose can provide over 1,000 calories per day as lipid at a cost to the patient that may exceed $800 per day.

Other Agents

Oral topiramate has been given in adults (300–1,600 mg/day) and in children (5–10 mg/kg/day most reports, up to 25 mg/kg/day in one) for 2 to 5 days.[38–43] Response tends to be delayed hours to days. Crushing the tablets and dissolving them in small amounts of water is needed in that no parenteral formulation is available. Because topiramate can induce metabolic acidosis and kidney stones, monitoring acid–base status and adequate hydration are recommended. Once seizures are controlled, doses should be tapered to a tolerable maintenance dose.

Oral doses of levetiracetam (750–9,000 mg/day) have been given in case series; however, doses larger than 3,000 mg/day do not add additional efficacy.[44] Levetiracetam is not hepatically metabolized and is minimally protein bound, which makes drug–drug interactions unlikely. Recently, an IV form of levetiracetam was approved.

Lidocaine has been used in refractory GCSE, but its use is not recommended unless other agents have failed.[45] It is administered intravenously and has a rapid onset of action. Table 59–4 gives the recommended initial loading and continuous-infusion doses. Although the reference serum concentration range for the antiarrhythmic effects of lidocaine is 2 to 6 mg/L, the reference range for GCSE has not been established. Serum lidocaine concentrations should be monitored to avoid drug accumulation and toxicity. CNS toxicity (e.g., fasciculations, visual disturbances, and tinnitus) can occur at concentrations between 6 and 8 mg/L; seizures and obtundation can develop when concentrations exceed 8 mg/L.

Halothane, isoflurane, ketamine, and other inhaled anesthetics have been shown to produce EEG suppression; however, these gases are difficult to deliver outside the operating room and require the presence of an anesthesiologist. No proven advantages have been shown over traditional anticonvulsants (e.g., barbiturate coma or continuous-infusion benzodiazepine), and these gases can increase intracranial pressure. If used, dosing is titrated to obtain EEG burst suppression. It is also prudent to validate that the patient does not have a low serum-magnesium concentration, because magnesium deficiency can lower the seizure threshold.

PHARMACOECONOMIC CONSIDERATIONS

The estimated reimbursement of GCSE varies greatly based on the age of the individual and the GCSE etiology. A population study showed that the median and quartile reimbursements for GCSE are $8,417 (25th percentile—$5,592; 75th percentile—$21,155).[46] Median reimbursements were significantly greater for those 17 to 45 years of age ($14,689), those with acute CNS injury ($16,919), and those withdrawing from alcohol or anticonvulsants ($11,239). Lowest median reimbursements were found in those 0 to 16 years of age ($6,140) and those with non-CNS injury ($6,669). For patients with length of stays shorter than 1 week, average reimbursements are $7,000 but increased to $32,907 if the stay was longer than 1 week. For patients staying 1 month or more, reimbursements were more than $60,000. Compared with other acute disorders (myocardial infarction, congestive heart failure, and intracranial hemorrhage), reimbursements for GCSE are 1.6- to 1.9-fold greater.

A number of economic issues can have an impact on formulary considerations. Clearly, there are intra- and interclass differences in medication costs and in ancillary tests or technologies associated with select therapies. For example, if one assumes five treatment options and hypothetically initiates anticonvulsant therapy in a patient weighing 70 kg (154 lb), the following differences in average wholesale prices are noted:

- Diazepam (20 mg) plus generic phenytoin (1 g): $19.33
- Lorazepam alone (8 mg): $8.96
- Midazolam alone (0.25 mg/kg load, 0.1 mg/kg/h): $64.77
- Generic phenytoin (1 g) alone: $14.47
- Diazepam (20 mg) plus fosphenytoin PE (1 g): $158.06
- Phenobarbital (20 mg/kg) alone: $20.89
- IV valproate (25 mg/kg load, 1 mg/kg/h): $106.40

Although many practitioners have heralded the arrival of fosphenytoin as an important therapeutic advancement, it has created a fiscal and ethical dilemma for many institutions. Fosphenytoin is associated with less infusion pain and fewer IV-site complications and hemodynamic adverse effects than phenytoin; however, the cost of this agent ($149/g PE versus $14.47/g phenytoin) has caused many practitioners and administrators to struggle with the practical and ethical importance of the increased safety profile relative to the cost of the product to an institution. When evaluating the difference in cost of these two agents, it is important to remember that phenytoin requires the placement of two IV catheters because of its incompatibility with many solutions and medications that are given concurrently. Additionally, some practitioners are giving fosphenytoin intramuscularly in the emergency room for non-SE indications and thereby avoiding the placement of a catheter and use of an infusion device. Many institutions fail to consider the expense associated with a tissue infiltration of phenytoin. Should an infiltration of phenytoin cause tissue necrosis that necessitates plastic surgery or amputation, the expense of a single multimillion-dollar lawsuit likely will offset the difference between phenytoin and fosphenytoin cost to several institutions.

There is little difference in expense if one advocates phenobarbital over midazolam as third-line therapy, but it might be argued that a patient who experiences phenobarbital-induced respiration depression ultimately may be more expensive to the health system. Finally, a 24-hour infusion of propofol to the same patient will cost in excess of $800.

EVALUATION OF THERAPEUTIC OUTCOMES

Initial success is defined as termination of all clinical and electrical seizure activity, but ultimate success is measured by the patient's quality of life. The morbidity and mortality associated with GCSE are affected by the underlying etiology; however, these can be minimized by the rapid implementation of a rational therapeutic plan. An EEG is an extremely important tool that not only allows practitioners to determine when abnormal electrical activity has been aborted but also can assist in determining which anticonvulsant was effective. Because many of the anticonvulsants affect the cardiorespiratory system, it is imperative that vital signs (e.g., heart rate, respiratory rate, and blood pressure) be monitored during drug infusion. It also may be necessary to monitor the ECG in some patients. Finally, it is imperative that the infusion site be assessed for any evidence of infiltration before and during administration of phenytoin. Information regarding the patient's past medical and drug history and imaging studies (e.g., MRI) also can help to determine if there is a defined etiology for the original episode of GCSE. This information then can be used to guide future medication therapy, as well as help in determining if the patient is at risk for a poor outcome.

CONCLUSION

Our understanding of the cellular basis, physiology, and neuropathology of GCSE continues to evolve. Over the past decade, research into an activated cascade of pathophysiologic changes in neurotransmission, GABAergic inhibition, and NMDA receptor channel–mediated events has enhanced our understanding of this disorder. Although anticonvulsants will continue to be the mainstay of therapy in terminating seizures, specific agents including antagonists of excitatory amino acid neurotransmitters (e.g., glutamate and calcium channel blockers) and agonists of inhibitory neurotransmitters (GABA) may help to block further neuronal damage beyond the epileptogenic focus. Likewise, additional trials investigating the role of newer anticonvulsants in GCSE are warranted.

ABBREVIATIONS

ALT: alanine aminotransferase

AMPA: α-amino-3-hydroxy-5-methyl-isoxazole-4-propionate

AST: aspartate aminotransferase

CBC: complete blood count

CNS: central nervous system

CT: computed tomography

ECG: electrocardiogram

EEG: electroencephalogram, electroencephalography

FDA: Food and Drug Administration

GABA: γ-aminobutyric acid

GCSE: generalized convulsive status epilepticus

MRI: magnetic resonance imaging

NCSE: nonconvulsive status epilepticus

NMDA: *N*-methyl-D-aspartate

SE: status epilepticus

REFERENCES

1. Commission on Classification of Terminology, International League Against Epilepsy. Proposal for revised clinical and electroencephalographic classification of epileptic seizures. Epilepsia 1981;22:489–501.
2. DeLorenzo RJ, Garnett LK, Towne AR, et al. Comparison of status epilepticus with prolonged seizure episodes lasting from 10 to 29 minutes. Epilepsia 1999;40:164–169.
3. Jenssen S, Gracely EJ, Sperling MR. How long do most seizures last? A systematic comparison of seizures recorded in the epilepsy monitoring unit. Epilepsia 2006;47:1499–1503.
4. Lowestein DH, Alldredge BK. Status epilepticus at an urban public hospital in the 1980s. Neurology 1993;43:483–488.
5. Kapur J, MacDonald RL. Rapid seizure-induced reduction of benzodiazepine and Zn^{2+} sensitivity of hippocampal dentate granule cell $GABA_A$ receptors. J Neurosci 1997;17:7532–7540.
6. Walker MC. Diagnosis and treatment of nonconvulsive status epilepticus. CNS Drugs 2001;15:931–939.
7. Shorvon S. The management of status epilepticus. J Neurol Neurosurg Psychiatry 2001;70(Suppl 2):II22–27.
8. Lowenstein DH, Alldredge BK. Status epilepticus. N Engl J Med 1998;338:970–976.
9. DeLorenzo RJ, Pellock JM, Towne AR, Boggs J. Epidemiology of status epilepticus. J Clin Neurophysiol 1995;12:316–325.
10. DeLorenzo RJ, Towne AR, Pellock JM, Ko D. Status epilepticus in children, adults, and the elderly. Epilepsia 1992;33:S15–S25.
11. Pitkanen A. Efficacy of current antiepileptics to prevent neurodegeneration in epilepsy models. Epilepsy Res 2002;50:141–160.
12. Wasterlain CG, Mazarati AM, Naylor D, et al. Short-term plasticity of hippocampal neuropeptides and neuronal circuitry in experimental status epilepticus. Epilepsia 2002;45(Suppl 5):20–29.
13. Temkin NR. Antiepileptogenesis and seizure prevention trials with anti-epileptic drugs: Meta-analysis of controlled trials. Epilepsia 2001;42:515–524.
14. Working Group on Status Epilepticus. Treatment of convulsive status epilepticus: Recommendations of the Epilepsy Foundation of America's Working Group on Status Epilepticus. JAMA 1993;270:854–859.
15. Lothman E. The biochemical basis and pathophysiology of status epilepticus. Neurology 1990;40:13–23.
16. LeDuc TJ, Goellner WE, Sanadi NE. Out-of-hospital midazolam for status epilepticus. Ann Emerg Med 1996;28:377.
17. Shaner DM, McCurdy SA, Herring MO, Gabor AJ. Treatment of status epilepticus: A prospective comparison of diazepam and phenytoin versus phenobarbital and optional phenytoin. Neurology 1988;38:202–207.
18. Treiman DM, Meyers PD, Walton NY, et al. A comparison of four treatments for generalized convulsive status epilepticus. Veterans Affairs Status Epilepticus Cooperative Study Group. N Engl J Med 1998;339:792–798.
19. Appleton R, Sweeney A, Choonara I, et al. Lorazepam versus diazepam in the acute treatment of epileptic seizures and status epilepticus. Dev Med Child Neurol 1995;37:682–688.
20. Abernethy DR, Greenblatt DJ. Phenytoin disposition in obesity: Determination of loading dose. Arch Neurol 1985;42:468–471.
21. Fischer JH, Patel TV, Fischer PA. Fosphenytoin: Clinical pharmacokinetics and comparative advantages in the acute treatment of seizures. Clin Pharmacokinet 2003;42:33–58.
22. Bleck TP. Advances in the management of refractory status epilepticus. Crit Care Med 1993;21:955–957.
23. Dodson WE, Rust RS. Phenobarbital: Absorption, distribution, and excretions. In: Levy R, Mattson R, Meldrum B, eds. Antiepileptic Drugs, 4th ed. New York: Raven Press, 1995:379–387.
24. Crawford TO, Mitchell WG, Fishman LS, Snodgrass SR. Very-high-dose phenobarbital for refractory status epilepticus in children. Neurology 1988;38:1035–1040.
25. Claassen J, Hirsch LJ, Emerson RG, Mayer SA. Treatment of refractory status epilepticus with pentobarbital, propofol, or midazolam: A systematic review. Epilepsia 2002;43:146–153.
26. Labar DR, Ali A, Root J. High-dose IV lorazepam for the treatment of refractory status epilepticus. Neurology 1994;44:1400–1403.
27. Chicella M, Jansen P, Parthiban A, et al. Propylene glycol accumulation associated with continuous infusion of lorazepam in pediatric intensive care patients. Crit Care Med 2002;30:2752–2756.
28. Hayman M, Seidl EC, Ali M, Malik K. Acute tubular necrosis associated with propylene glycol from concomitant administration of IV lorazepam and trimethoprim-sulfamethoxazole. Pharmacotherapy 2003;23:1190–1194.
29. Yaucher NE, Fish JT, Smith HW, Wells JA. Propylene glycol–associated renal toxicity from lorazepam infusion. Pharmacotherapy 2003;23:1094–1099.
30. Mirski MA, Williams MA, Hanlet DF. Prolonged pentobarbital and phenobarbital coma for refractory generalized status epilepticus. Crit Care Med 1995;23:400–404.
31. Giroud M, Gras D, Escousse A, et al. Use of injectable valproic acid in status epilepticus. Drug Invest 1993;5:154–159.

32. Price DJ. Intravenous valproate: Experience in neurosurgery. In: Fourth International Symposium on Sodium Valproate in Epilepsy. London, Royal Society of Medicine International Congress Symposium Series, 1989:197–203.
33. Chez MG, Hammer MS, Loeffel M, et al. Clinical experience of three pediatric patients and one adult case of spike and wave status epilepticus treated with injectable valproic acid. J Child Neurol 1999;14:239–242.
34. Hovinga CA, Chicella MF, Rose DF, et al. Use of IV valproate in three pediatric patients with nonconvulsive or convulsive status epilepticus. Ann Pharmacother 1999;33:579–584.
35. Venkataraman V, Wheless JW. Safety of rapid intravenous infusion of valproate loading doses in epilepsy patients. Epilepsy Res 1999;35:147–153.
36. Brown LA, Levin GM. Role of propofol in refractory status epilepticus. Ann Pharmacother 1998;32:1053–1059.
37. Timpe EM, Eichner SF, Phelps SJ. Propofol-related infusion syndrome in critically ill pediatric patients: Coincidence, association, or causation? J Pediatr Pharmacol Ther 2006;11:17–42.
38. Kahriman M, Minecan D, Kutluay E, et al. Efficacy of topiramate in children with refractory status epilepticus. Epilepsia 2003;44:1353–1356.
39. Reuber M, Evans J, Bamford JM. Topiramate in drug-resistant complex status epilepticus. Eur J Neurol 2002;9:111–112.
40. Towne AR, Garnett LK, Waterhouse EJ, et al. The use of topiramate in refractory status epilepticus. Neurology 2003;60:332–334.
41. Bensalem MK, Fakhoury TA. Topiramate and status epilepticus: Report of three cases. Epilepsy Behav 2003;4:757–760.
42. Blumkin L, Lerman-Sagie T, Houri T, et al. Pediatric refractory partial status epilepticus responsive to topiramate. J Child Neurol 2005;20:239–241.
43. Conway JM, Birnbaum AK, Kriel RL, Cloyd JC. Relative bioavailability of topiramate administered rectally. Epilepsy Res 2003;54:91–96.
44. Rossetti AO, Bromfield EB. Determinants of success in the use of oral levetiracetam in status epilepticus. Epilepsy Behav 2006;8:651–654.
45. Aggarwal P, Wali JP. Lidocaine in refractory status epilepticus: A forgotten drug in the emergency department. Am J Emerg Med 1993;2:243–244.
46. Penberthy LT, Towne A, Garnett LK, Perlin JB. Estimating the economic burden of status epileptic to the health care system. Seizure 2005;14:46–51.

CHAPTER 60

Acute Management of the Brain Injury Patient

BRADLEY A. BOUCHER AND SHELLY D. TIMMONS

KEY CONCEPTS

1. Cerebral ischemia is the key pathophysiologic event triggering secondary neuronal injury following severe traumatic brain injury (TBI). Intracellular accumulation of calcium is postulated to be a central pathophysiologic process in amplifying and perpetuating secondary neuronal injury via inhibition of cellular respiration and enzyme activation.

2. *Guidelines for the Management of Severe Brain Injury,* published by the Brain Trauma Foundation/American Association of Neurological Surgeons, serves as the foundation on which clinical decisions in managing adult neurotrauma patients are based; comparable guidelines for infants, children, and adolescents also have been published.

3. Correcting and preventing early hypotension (systolic blood pressure less than 90 mm Hg) and hypoxemia (PaO_2 less than 60 mm Hg) are primary goals during the initial resuscitative and intensive care of severe TBI patients.

4. The principal monitoring parameter for severe TBI patients within the intensive care environment is intracranial pressure (ICP). Cerebral perfusion pressure (CPP) is also a critical monitoring parameter and should be maintained between 50 and 60 mm Hg (greater than 40 mm Hg in pediatric patients) through the use of fluids, vasopressors, and/or ICP normalization therapy.

5. Nonspecific pharmacologic treatment in the management of intracranial hypertension should include analgesics, sedatives, antipyretics, and paralytics under selected circumstances.

6. Specific pharmacologic treatment in the management of intracranial hypertension includes mannitol, furosemide, and high-dose pentobarbital. Neither routine use of corticosteroids nor aggressive hyperventilation (i.e., $PaCO_2$ less than 25 mm Hg) should be used in the management of intracranial hypertension.

7. Use of phenytoin for the prophylaxis of posttraumatic seizures usually should be discontinued after 7 days if no seizures are observed.

8. Numerous investigational strategies (e.g., calcium antagonists, glutamate antagonists, antioxidants, and free-radical scavengers) targeted at interrupting the pathophysiologic cascade of events occurring following severe TBI have been employed, but no proven therapeutic benefits have been identified.

Learning objectives, review questions, and other resources can be found at **www.pharmacotherapyonline.com.**

Traumatic brain injury (TBI) has been referred to as America's "silent epidemic" and is currently the leading cause of death and disability among children and young adults in the industrialized world.[1,2] Based on an ever-growing understanding of TBI pathophysiology, clinicians and scientists share an optimism that patient outcomes can be improved through the use of evidence-based management guidelines presently and administration of neuroprotective agents in the future. This chapter summarizes TBI epidemiology and pathophysiology and highlights guidelines and systematic reviews of the literature pertaining to the management of severe TBI patients.

EPIDEMIOLOGY

It is estimated that approximately 1.4 million persons sustain a TBI each year in the United States, resulting in 235,000 hospital admissions and 50,000 deaths annually.[2] Importantly, more than 5.3 million Americans currently live with disabilities as a result of their TBI, highlighting the enormous physical and emotional toll of this health-care problem in the United States.[2] The economic effects of acute neurotrauma are also enormous, with estimates of spending on TBI patients requiring hospitalization of $60 billion in the United States in 2000.[3] Economic costs to society from lost productivity are astronomical. While the frequency of TBI remains high, the annual mortality rate following TBI has decreased from nearly 25 per 100,000 to 19.4 per 100,000 population since 1979.[4] Falls are the leading cause of TBI (28%), whereas motor vehicle accidents result in the greatest number of TBI-related hospitalizations and deaths overall.[2] Fall-related TBIs caused the greatest number of deaths in patients 75 years of age and older.[2] Furthermore, TBI-related mortality in males exceeds that in females threefold.[2]

PATHOPHYSIOLOGY

PRIMARY BRAIN INJURY

The neurologic sequelae of brain trauma can occur instantaneously as a consequence of the primary injury or can result from secondary injuries that follow within minutes, hours, or days.[1] Primary injury involves the external transfer of kinetic energy to various structural components of the brain (e.g., neurons, nerve synapses, glial cells, axons, and cerebral blood vessels). The biomechanical forces responsible for primary brain injury can be classified broadly as contact (e.g., blunt-object blow, penetrating-missile injuries) and acceleration/deceleration (e.g., instantaneous brain movements following motor vehicle accidents).[1] Primary injuries are categorized further as focal

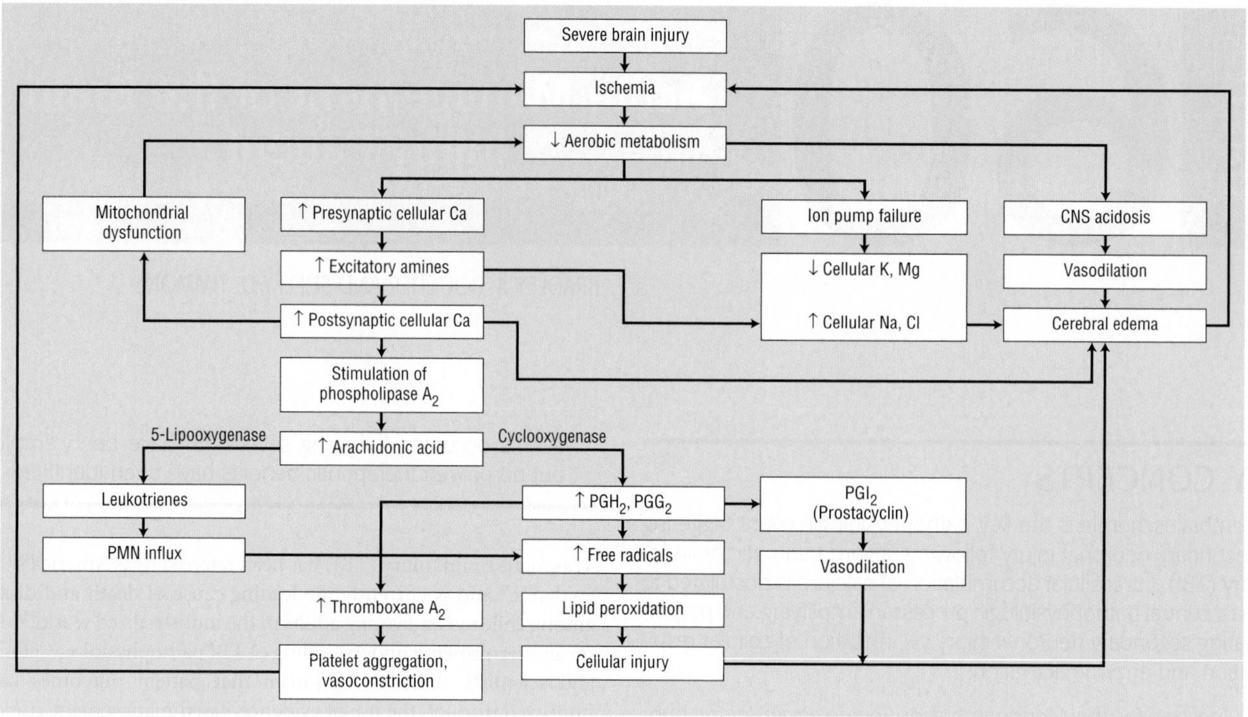

FIGURE 60-1. Schematic illustration of the cascade of biochemical events proposed to occur following severe neurotrauma (secondary brain injury). (Ca, calcium; Cl, chloride; CNS, central nervous system; K, potassium; Mg, magnesium; Na, sodium; PG, prostaglandin; PMN, polymorphonucleocyte.)

(e.g., contusions, hematomas) or diffuse.[5] The latter usually are associated with shearing or stretch forces, which primarily affect axons within the brain (i.e., diffuse axonal injury).[5,6] The type of primary injury (i.e., focal versus diffuse) will be a major factor as to which of the secondary injury mechanisms discussed below will predominate following a TBI; however, many patients, especially those involved in high-speed accidents sustain both types of injury.[7]

SECONDARY BRAIN INJURY

❶ A complex sequence of pathophysiologic events precipitated by primary brain injury may seriously disrupt the normal central nervous system (CNS) balance between oxygen supply and demand.[7] Hypotension during the early posttraumatic period is a major contributor to this imbalance and a primary determinant of outcome.[1,5] The end result of this imbalance may be cerebral ischemia, the key pathophysiologic event triggering secondary injury.[7] Figure 60–1 is a simplified schematic of the processes that constitute secondary brain injury and their various interrelationships. The brain is particularly susceptible to ischemia because of its normally high resting energy requirement and its limited capacity to store oxygen, glucose, and high-energy phosphate compounds (e.g., adenosine triphosphate). Ischemia following brain injury typically occurs in the first 6 to 24 hours following the insult.[8] Thereafter, patients can have hyperemia from days 1 to 3.[8] Vasospasm also can occur.[8] These phenomena can result in imbalances in cerebral oxygen delivery (CDO_2) and consumption ($CMRO_2$), processes that are closely autoregulated under normal circumstances. Factors that can diminish cerebral oxygen supply following brain injury include cerebral edema, expanding mass lesions (e.g., epidural, subdural, and intracerebral hematomas), cerebral vasospasm, and loss of vasoregulatory control. Vasogenic cerebral edema can develop as a consequence of cerebral capillary endothelial damage and disruption of the blood–brain barrier.[7] With cytotoxic and vasogenic edema comes expansion of the intracellular and extracellular fluid spaces, respectively. Elevated intracranial pressure (ICP) is the most detrimental consequence of cerebral edema formation and occurs as the brain tissue volume increases within the nondistensible skull. A significant increase in ICP may further compromise cerebral blood flow (CBF) and extend cytotoxic edema. Hence an increase in ICP can be self-perpetuating unless this cycle is reversed. Hypoxemia can further exacerbate local decreases in cerebral oxygen supply following acute respiratory failure and systemic hypotension. Metabolic demand also can increase following neurotrauma secondary to seizures, agitation, and temperature elevation.

Brain tissue affected by focal ischemia can have a dense core surrounded by a marginally viable region. If adequate CBF is restored, the affected tissue may recover; however, sustained ischemia can result in further loss of cellular integrity and eventual cell death. The loss of ionic homeostasis is postulated to be a key event in fostering secondary brain injury within this ischemic region. Cellular influx of sodium, chloride, and water (i.e., cytotoxic edema) with a corresponding efflux of potassium and magnesium occurs with sodium-potassium-adenosine triphosphatase (Na^+-K^+-ATPase) pump dysfunction.[7] An influx of calcium into the presynaptic terminal ends of damaged neurons is mediated by N-type voltage-sensitive calcium channels. This, in turn, is postulated to stimulate excessive release of the excitatory amines glutamate and aspartate from the affected neurons.[6] The result is ongoing stimulation of postsynaptic cells, which can result in an extension of neurotoxicity and cell death. Influx of calcium and additional sodium is stimulated by activation ionophore receptors including the *N*-methyl-D-aspartate (NMDA) receptor.[7] Calcium influx and its intracellular accumulation initiate a number of events that amplify and perpetuate secondary neuronal injury. High intracellular concentrations of calcium result in mitochondrial dysfunction, which further inhibits cellular respiration, a process already affected by ischemic and/or hypoxic insults.[7] A second major deleterious effect of calcium is to stimulate activation of autodestructive enzymes, including phosphatases, kinases, lipases, and proteases, such as calpain, and caspases.[6,7,9] The effect of phospholipase A_2 stimulation includes formation of several arachidonic acid metabolites derived from membrane lipids: thromboxane A_2, prostaglandins, and leukotrienes.[7] The subsequent effects of these metabolites are lipid peroxidation and the formation of reactive oxygen species.[1,7] Recent data suggest that this event occurs very early after injury (e.g., before hospitalization), which may limit the effectiveness of exogenously administered antioxidants.[10] A common end point with the release of excitatory amines, increases in intracellular calcium, and oxygen free radical generation is apoptosis or programmed cell death and nonprogrammed cellular necrosis.[7,11,12] Cells with a more elaborate dendritic structure (e.g., cortical neurons, hippocampal cells) may be more vulnerable to the effects of apoptosis.[13] Cell-mediated injury involving inflammatory mediators (e.g., cytokines, platelet-activating factor, etc.), nitric oxide, and cell adhesion molecules is yet another possible mechanism involved in secondary neuronal injury.[7] Among the cell lines implicated are polymorphonuclear neutrophils, platelets, endothelial cells, and macrophages. Noteworthy is that limited data suggest that activation of some inflammatory mediators may actually be beneficial such that the relative balance of the mediators versus absolute concentrations may be the most significant pathophysiologic factor following TBI.[14,15] Stimulation of platelet aggregation, vasodilation, and vasoconstriction, intravascularly, also may occur. Lastly, data suggest that there may be a genetic vulnerability to the effects of TBI.[6,16] For example, preliminary evidence indicates that this may be related to faster recovery of aspartate uptake from the cerebrospinal fluid and the cerebrospinal fluid lactate-to-pyruvate ratio in TBI patients in the absence of the apolipoprotein E_4 allele.[17] Noteworthy is that this is the same protein that has been associated with the deleterious effects of various types of Alzheimer disease.[6]

CLINICAL PRESENTATION OF ACUTE BRAIN INJURY

General

- Level of consciousness on admission ranges from awake and alert to completely unresponsive (i.e., GCS 15 to 3, respectively).

Symptoms

- Posttraumatic amnesia (e.g., greater than 1 hour), increasing dizziness, a moderate to severe headache, nausea/vomiting, limb weakness, or paresthesia may indicate more severe injury.

Signs

- CSF otorrhea or rhinorrhea and seizures may indicate more severe injury.
- A rapid deterioration in mental status strongly suggests the presence of an expanding lesion within the skull.
- Severe TBI may be accompanied by significant alterations or instability in vital signs, including abnormal breathing patterns (e.g., apnea, Cheyne-Stokes respirations, tachypnea), hypertension, or bradycardia.

Laboratory Tests

- ABGs indicating hypoxia (i.e., decreased PaO_2) or hypercapnia (i.e., increased $PaCO_2$) may indicate compromised ventilation.
- A positive blood ethanol concentration and/or positive urine drug screen indicates that drug intoxication may be affecting the patient's mental status in addition to the TBI.
- Electrolyte disturbances can cause alterations in mental status, and their effects may interfere with assessment of neurological status relative to brain lesion.

Other Diagnostic Tests

- CT of the head is an important diagnostic tool for detecting the presence of mass lesions.

GCS, Glasgow Coma Scale; CSF, cerebrospinal fluid; TBI, traumatic brain injury; ABG, arterial blood gas; PaO_2, partial pressure of arterial blood oxygen; $PaCO_2$, partial pressure of arterial blood carbon dioxide; CT, computed tomography.

TABLE 60-1 Glasgow Coma Scale

Response	Score
Eyes	
Open spontaneously	4
To verbal command	3
To pain	2
No response	1
Best motor response	
To verbal command	
Obeys	6
To painful stimulus (pressure to nail beds)	
Localizes pain	5
Flexion, withdrawal	4
Flexion, abnormal (decorticate rigidity)	3
Extension (decerebrate rigidity)	2
No response	1
Best verbal response	
(Arouse patient with painful stimulus if necessary)	
Oriented and converses	5
Disoriented and converses	4
Inappropriate words	3
Incomprehensible sounds	2
No response	1
Total	3–15

Data from Teasdale and Jennett.[18]

CLINICAL PRESENTATION

The Glasgow Coma Scale (GCS) is the most widely used system to grade the arousal and functional capacity of the cerebral cortex.[5,18] The GCS defines the level of consciousness according to eye opening, motor response, and verbal response (Table 60–1). A GCS score of 15 corresponds to a normal neurologic examination. GCS scores of 3 to 8, 9 to 12, and 13 to 15 are consistent with severe, moderate, and mild brain injury, respectively.[5] The possibility of ethanol or drug intoxication, hypotension, hypoxia, postictal state, or hypothermia altering the neurologic examination always should be considered. Because narcotics and muscle relaxants affect the neurologic examination, they should not be administered, if at all possible, until the initial examination is complete. Simple, rapidly attainable clinical variables that are predictive of survival include patient age, GCS score (especially the motor score), pupillary reactivity, presence or absence of a hematoma, subarachnoid hemorrhage, midline shift, and appearance of the ventricular cisterns found on a computed tomography (CT) scan of the head.[19]

TREATMENT

Traumatic Brain Injury

❷ In July 1995, the Brain Trauma Foundation (BTF) published an extensive document entitled *Guidelines for the Management of Severe Brain Injury* as a joint initiative with the Guidelines Committee of the American Association of Neurological Surgeons (AANS), the Joint Section on Neurotrauma and Critical Care of the AANS, and the Congress of Neurological Surgeons, with a subsequent revision in 2000 and a third revision pending publication.[20] This landmark publication established for the first time a comprehensive series of evidence-based standards, guidelines, and options for the care of severe TBI patients. A recent survey suggested that significant changes consistent with the BTF/AANS guidelines in the acute management of TBI patients have occurred since 1991, providing indirect evidence as to their overall impact on patient care.[21] Since then guidelines addressing prehospital TBI management,[22] surgical management,[23] and management of penetrating brain injury have been published, and the European Brain Injury Consortium has issued guidelines for the management of severe TBI in adults.[24] Furthermore, TBI management guidelines for infants, children, and adolescents have been developed.[25] In addition, a series of systematic reviews addressing TBI management emanating from The Cochrane Library has been published.[26–31] These reviews have rigorously evaluated the literature for essentially all the major conventional TBI strategies. The recommendations emanating from the published guidelines on TBI management and published systematic reviews are highlighted throughout the remaining portion of this chapter. Until further clinical studies become available, recommendations from the published guidelines should serve as the foundation upon which all clinical decisions in managing severe TBI are based.[6] Nonetheless, it should be noted that the majority of the guidelines are based on class II evidence (primarily prospective clinical trials) and class III evidence (primarily retrospective clinical trials). Few class I evidence studies (i.e., prospective, randomized, controlled trials) are available for traumatic brain injury. Recommendations provided in this chapter pertain to adults and children unless specifically noted to the contrary.

■ DESIRED OUTCOMES

The overall goal in TBI management is not only reduction in morbidity and mortality but also optimization of long-term functional outcome for these patients. This requires careful attention to the following short-term therapeutic goals: (a) establishment of an adequate airway and maintenance of ventilation and circulation during the initial period of resuscitation and evaluation, (b) maintenance of balance between CDO_2 and $CMRO_2$, (c) prevention or attenuation of secondary neuronal injury, and (d) prevention and/or treatment of associated medical complications.

■ INITIAL RESUSCITATION

The first priority in the unconscious patient is the establishment of an airway, which ensures adequate oxygenation and prevents aspiration.[5,32] ❸ Thereafter, restoration of circulating blood volume and maintenance of systolic arterial pressure greater than 90 mm Hg are of utmost importance.[1] In pediatric patients, the systolic arterial pressure goal should be greater than 70 mm Hg + (2 × age in years).[25] Correcting and preventing early hypotension (systolic arterial pressure less than 90 mm Hg) and hypoxia (partial pressure alveolar oxygen [PaO_2] less than 60 mm Hg) are essential because these two factors are among the most powerful predictors of outcome.[20] Isotonic saline (0.9% normal saline) and lactated Ringer solution are generally advocated as initial resuscitation fluids of choice in TBI patients.[20] However, some clinicians believe that hypertonic saline (e.g., 3% or 7.5% saline) is beneficial in the resuscitation of TBI patients.[33] In children, the recommended infusion rate for 3% saline is 0.1 to 1 mL/kg per hour.[25] Clinical studies have yielded equivocal results relative to superiority over isotonic solutions.[1,34,35] Vasopressors and inotropic agents may be needed to maintain an adequate mean arterial pressure (MAP) if hypotension persists after adequate restoration of intravascular volume. Figure 60–2 is an algorithm summarizing treatment priorities in the initial management of acute TBI.

■ POSTRESUSCITATIVE CARE

Following successful resuscitation, priorities shift toward diagnostic evaluation of intracranial and extracranial injuries and emergent surgical intervention as needed. Evacuation of intracranial hematomas (i.e., epidural, subdural, and intracerebral hematomas) is essential to control ICP and improve outcome. Elevation of depressed skull fractures and debridement of penetrating wound tracts are other important emergent surgical procedures in TBI patients. Decompressive craniectomies (i.e., removal of variable amount of skull bone) with or without temporal or frontal lobectomy may be considered in patients with increases in ICP refractory to more conservative measures.[1] The beneficial effects of routine decompressive surgery in adult TBI patients to date are controversial.[36] Nonetheless, improved outcomes with decompressive surgery in pediatric patients have generally yielded more favorable results.[36] Continuous ICP monitoring (e.g., intraventricular catheter, intraparenchymal fiberoptic catheter) is indicated in patients with a GCS score of less than or equal to 8 with an abnormal admission CT scan, in selected patients with abnormal CT scans and higher GCS scores, or in high-risk severe TBI patients with a normal CT scan (i.e., age greater than 40 years, motor posturing, systolic arterial pressure less than 90 mm Hg).[20] Intraventricular catheters have a therapeutic advantage over the other alternatives but are associated with a higher complication rate and can be difficult to place in the setting of the swollen brain. Specifically, cerebrospinal fluid can be drained using this device as a means to lower ICP.[1,5] Continuous ICP monitoring is the only means to objectively evaluate the success of therapies used to decrease ICP. Once the ICP exceeds 20 to 25 mm Hg, therapy should be initiated to decrease ICP below 20 mm Hg.[20,25] Aggressive use of ICP monitors in academic trauma centers across the United States was associated with a reduction in mortality risk as well as a shorter length of stay among survivors.[37] A recent study in Europe, however, demonstrated results at variance with the U.S. study; that is, no improvement in outcome in TBI patients managed with a higher therapeutic intensity level.[38] The use of historical controls in the U.S. study or other differences in patient management could explain the conflicting results from these two studies. Jugular venous oxygen saturation ($SjvO_2$) monitoring is advocated by some practitioners for detection of global cerebral hypoxia (i.e., adequacy of CBF relative to $CMRO_2$), although it is technically difficult to achieve consistent results, and is not currently addressed within the BTF/AANS guidelines.[39] Hence its role remains confined predominantly to use in academic centers and for research.[5,39,40] Cerebral microdialysis techniques have been used successfully as research tools to measure the cerebral extracellular chemistry of TBI patients.[41] Although the widespread use of this methodology by general clinical practices has been slow, the use of brain tissue oxygen monitoring in TBI patients is gaining momentum.[6,42] Recently, the roles of several biochemical markers of TBI (e.g., S-100 protein, neuron-specific enolase) were also reviewed.[43] The usefulness of these or other proteins for the detection of secondary injury in TBI and/or as a treatment-monitoring parameter is yet to be elucidated.

❹ Another important monitoring parameter for severe TBI patients within the intensive care environment is the cerebral perfusion pressure (CPP). The CPP is the difference between MAP and ICP (i.e., CPP = MAP – ICP). Maintenance of an acceptable CPP has been postulated to be critical in reducing cerebral ischemia and secondary injury. The BTF/AANS guidelines originally recommended that CPP be maintained greater than 70 mm Hg based on a number of studies that demonstrated decreased morbidity and mortality in patients whose CPP was actively sustained above 70 to 80 mm Hg.[20] However, in 2003, the BTF/AANS issued an updated recommendation that CPP be maintained at 60 mm Hg or more.[44] In the upcoming guideline revision, maintaining a range of CPP between 50 and 70 mm Hg is suggested as the optimal strategy, tailoring the desired range within those parameters to the individual patient. In children, the recommended CPP goal is greater than 40 mm Hg.[25] Furthermore, the updated recommendation is that aggressive attempts to maintain CPP greater than 70 mm Hg in adults should be avoided in the absence of cerebral ischemia because of the risk of the acute respiratory distress syndrome.[20,45] One recent study challenges the relative importance of CPP in TBI patients, suggesting that the primary focus should be on lowering the ICP to less than 20 mm Hg.[46] In essence, the results of this clinical investigation were that an ICP of 20 mm Hg

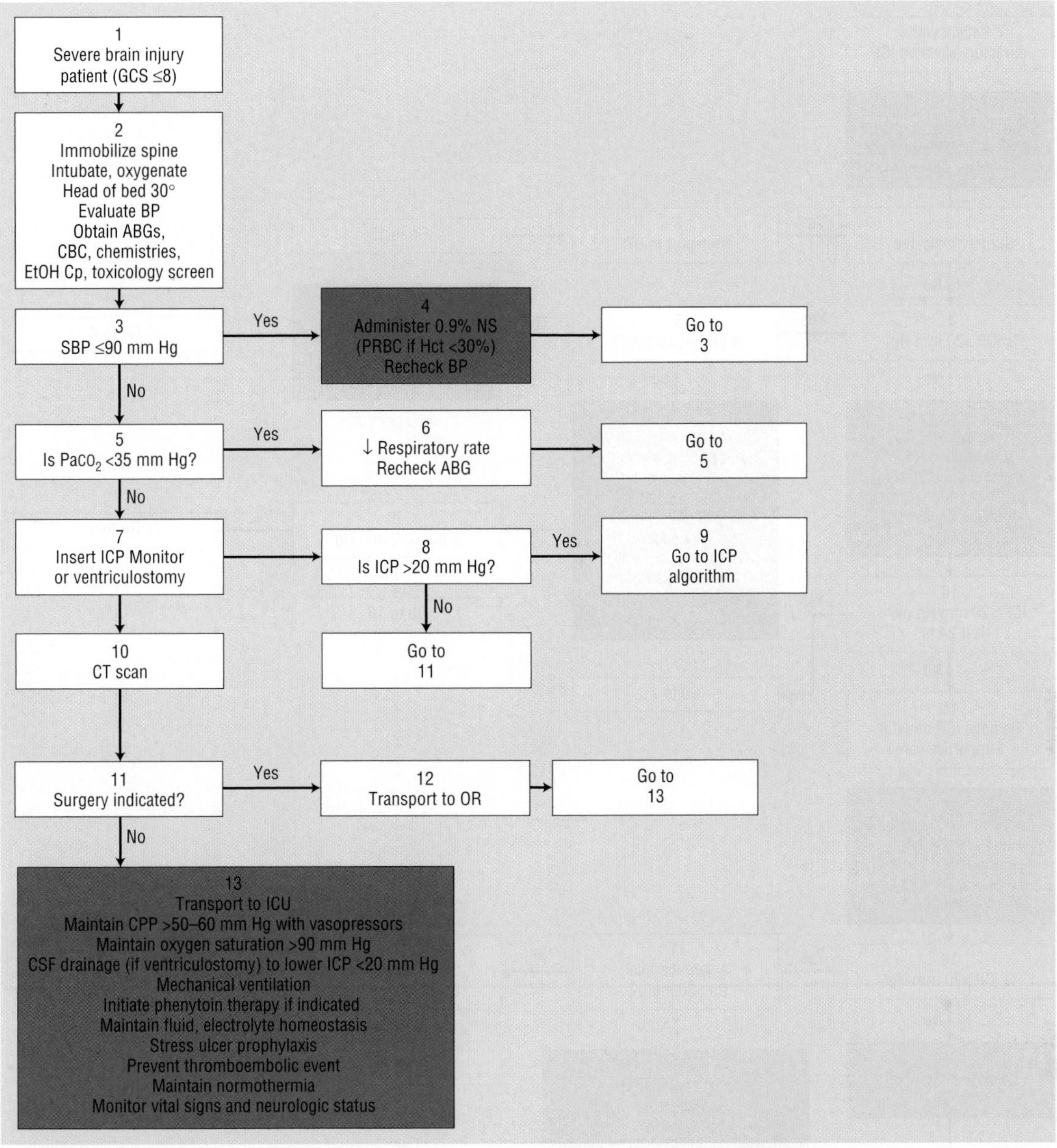

FIGURE 60-2. Algorithm for the acute management of the traumatic brain injury patient. (ABG, arterial blood gas; BP, blood pressure; CBC, complete blood count; CPP, cerebral perfusion pressure; CT, computerized tomography; CSF, cerebrospinal fluid; GCS, Glasgow coma scale; EtOH Cp, ethanol plasma concentration; Hct, hematocrit; ICP, intracranial pressure; ICU, intensive care unit; NS, normal saline; OR, operating room; Pa_{CO_2}, partial pressure of arterial blood carbon dioxide; PRBC, packed red blood cells; SBP, systolic blood pressure.) *(Adapted from Boucher BA. Neurotrauma: Pharmacotherapy Self Assessment Program, 3rd ed., Module 2: Critical Care. Lenexa, KS: American College of Clinical Pharmacy, 1995:215–238. By permission of the American College of Clinical Pharmacy.)*

or more was the most powerful predictor of neurologic deterioration as long as the CPP was maintained above 60 mm Hg.[46]

The goal CPP can be achieved by increasing MAP through the use of fluids and/or vasopressors or by lowering elevated ICP. The goal of volume expansion should be euvolemia as well as avoidance of a hypoosmolar state and negative fluid balance.[25,34,47] If the hematocrit is below 30%, transfusion of packed red blood cells is indicated.[1] Volume status should be targeted to a central venous pressure of 7 to 12 cm H_2O if invasive monitoring is employed.[1] After achievement of euvolemia, the patient's head should be elevated at 30° to promote venous drainage and decrease ICP. If restoration of the intravascular volume is inadequate in elevating MAP to an acceptable level, hypertension should be induced using vasopressors or inotropic support. The drugs employed most commonly to induce hypertension are dopamine, phenylephrine, and norepinephrine.[1] Patients should be monitored for renal dysfunction, lactic acidosis, and signs of peripheral ischemia when these agents are used, especially at large doses.

TREATMENT

Intracranial Hypertension

■ GENERAL PHARMACOLOGIC STRATEGIES

❺ The use of analgesics, sedatives, and paralytics has an important primary role in the management of intracranial hypertension (Fig. 60–3).[48] This is related directly to the association of pain, agitation, excessive muscle movement, and resisting mechanical ventilation with

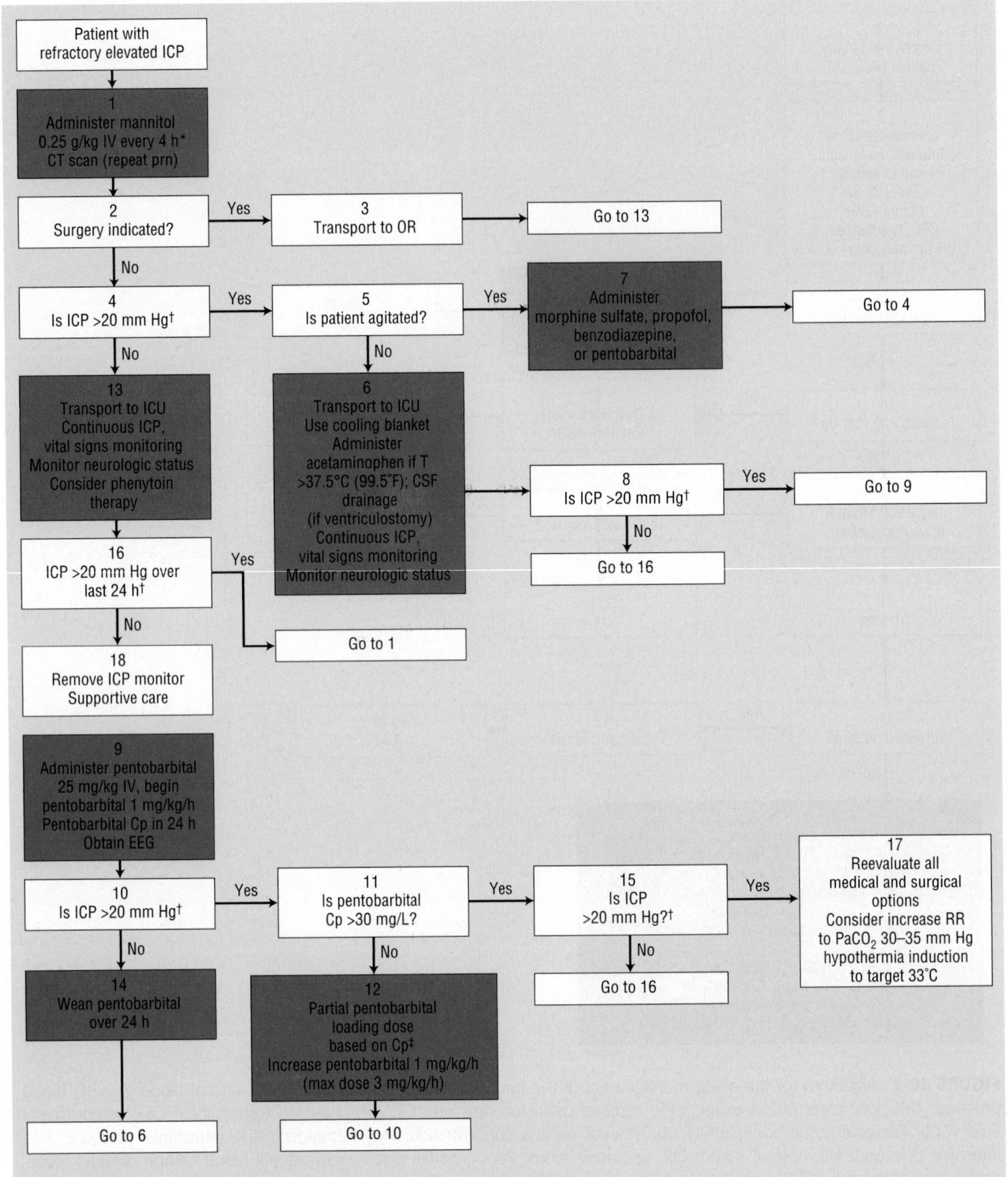

* Alternatively 150 ml 7.5% hypertonic saline. Hold if serum osmolality >320 mOsm/kg

† Treatment thresholds: ICP 20–29 mm Hg for >15 min
ICP 30–39 mm Hg for >2 min
ICP ≥40 mm Hg for >1 min

Note: Transient ICP increases may occur following respiratory procedures (e.g., suctioning, chest physiotherapy, bronchoscopy, intubation).

‡ Partial pentobarbital loading dose (mg) = (30 mg/L – measured Cp) (1 L/kg × wt(kg))

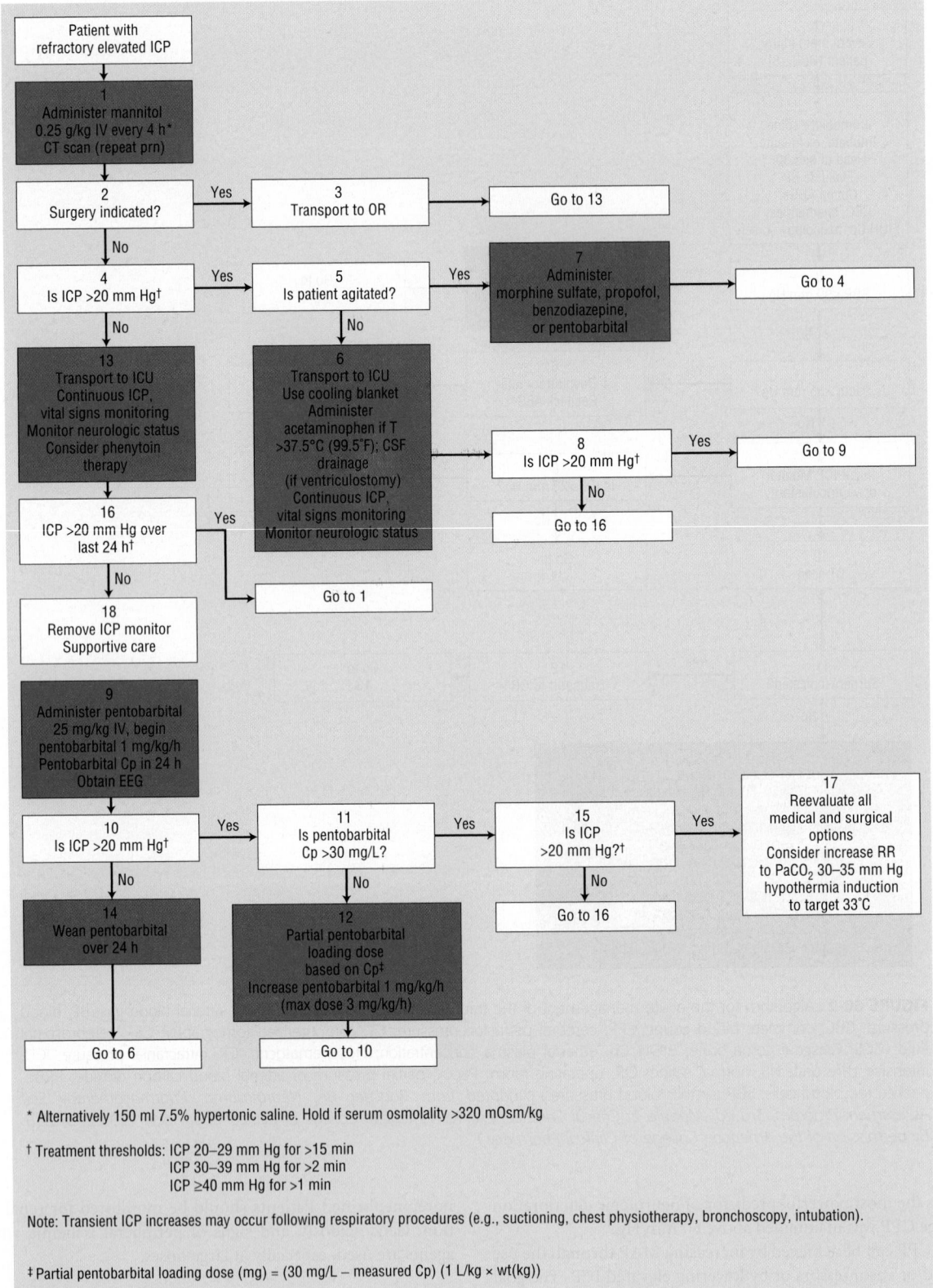

FIGURE 60-3. Algorithm for the management of increased intracranial pressure. (Cp, plasma concentration; CSF, cerebral spinal fluid; CT, computerized tomography; EEG, electroencephalogram; ICP, intracranial pressure; ICU, intensive care unit; OR, operating room; $PaCO_2$, partial pressure of arterial blood carbon dioxide; T, temperature; RR, respiratory rate.) *(Adapted from Boucher BA. Neurotrauma: Pharmacotherapy Self Assessment Program, 3rd ed., Module 2: Critical Care, Lenexa, KS: American College of Clinical Pharmacy, 1995:215–238. By permission of the American College of Clinical Pharmacy.)*

transient increases in ICP. Nonetheless, there have been no studies of the effect of sedation on outcome in patients with severe TBI.[20] Morphine sulfate is the most commonly used analgesic and sedative in this setting.[5] Propofol has become the sedative of choice in TBI patients among many clinicians because of its ease of titration, rapidly reversible effects on discontinuation, and possible neuroprotective effects.[5,49,50] Although it is used for sedation in infants and children who are mechanically ventilated in the ICU setting, the Food and Drug

Administration required that the manufacturer labeling contain specific information that propofol is not approved for sedation of pediatric patients admitted to an intensive care unit (ICU). This is partly a result of the publication of 10 case reports of fatal metabolic acidosis in critically ill children who received propofol.[51] While a direct association between propofol and metabolic acidosis remains unclear, symptoms tend to occur with large doses (greater than 4.8 to 30 mg/kg per hour) and prolonged infusions (longer than 48 to 72 hours). Likewise, long-term infusions in excess of 5 mg/kg per hour should be used cautiously in TBI patients based on a recently published case report series suggesting an association between propofol and cardiac failure.[52] Triglyceride concentrations also should be monitored in patients receiving prolonged propofol infusions and/or high dosages of propofol considering its lipid emulsion formulation and the potential for inducing hypertriglyceridemia under these conditions. Alternative sedatives include etomidate (particularly useful in rapid-induction anesthesia), intermittent low-dose pentobarbital, and short-acting benzodiazepines (e.g., midazolam), especially if there is a reasonable suspicion of alcohol withdrawal as the underlying etiology of the agitation.[5] The potential for these agents to decrease MAP and CPP must be monitored closely. Additionally, the cumulative sedative effects of longer-acting drugs, especially benzodiazepines, must be taken into account. The use of any sedative agent also must be weighed against its potential to obscure the neurologic examination of the patient. Interference with the neurologic examination is also associated with paralytic agents. Prophylactic neuromuscular blockade (i.e., unrelated to ICP control) is not recommended based on evidence indicating increased complications (e.g., pneumonia, prolonged paralysis) and length of stay following use of paralytic agents.[5]

■ HYPERVENTILATION

❻ The practice of prolonged aggressive hyperventilation ($Pa\text{CO}_2$ less than 25 mm Hg) to decrease ICP is no longer recommended.[20] Hyperventilation acutely decreases systemic and cerebral $Pa\text{CO}_2$. The resulting hypocapnia, in turn, induces cerebral vasoconstriction, thereby decreasing CBF and cerebral blood volume.[53] For decades, it was a widely held belief that a reduction in cerebral blood volume and any accompanying decrease in ICP were beneficial. Nonetheless, a systematic review of the literature concluded that data are inadequate to ascertain potential benefit or harm from hyperventilation.[31] Other studies have determined that severe TBI patients with normocapnia, compared to those receiving aggressive hyperventilation, have an improved outcome at 3 and 6 months.[20] Furthermore, recent evidence using microdialysis and local CBF techniques suggests that aggressive hyperventilation may increase extracellular glutamate, a mediator of secondary injury, and lactate concentrations.[54] Despite the decrease in CBF during hyperventilation, no detrimental decrease in $CMR\text{O}_2$ was observed in a recent study.[53] Nonetheless, the potential for decreased CBF to increase the possibility for cerebral ischemia must be weighed. In consideration of the equivocal data relative to the merits of therapeutic hyperventilation in TBI patients, BTF/AANS guidelines recommend that $Pa\text{CO}_2$ be maintained near 35 mm Hg, especially during the first 24 hours.[20] Thereafter, a $Pa\text{CO}_2$ in the range of 30 to 35 mm Hg may be used if ICP control is inadequate.[1,25,50] Aggressive hyperventilation (25 to 30 mm Hg) for brief periods may be considered as second-tier therapy in the setting of refractory intracranial hypertension or in the initial management of patients with signs of cerebral herniation.[20,25] Cerebral tissue oxygen perfusion monitoring may be used to guide the use of this therapeutic intervention.

■ HYPOTHERMIA

Hyperthermia also should be avoided in TBI patients because patients with elevated temperatures have poorer outcomes than normothermic patients.[1,25,55] Hence aggressive maintenance of a core temperature of less than 37.5°C (99.5°F) using acetaminophen, nonsteroidal antiinflammatory drugs, and cooling blankets is indicated for patients following severe TBI. Several experimental cooling techniques, including intravascular cooling for use in TBI patients refractory to conventional management strategies, were discussed in a recent review of this topic.[55]

Although hypothermia has been discussed for nearly 50 years as a cerebral protective maneuver in TBI patients, a resurgence of interest has been fueled by the results of several preliminary studies in the early 1990s demonstrating trends in improvement in mortality and morbidity rates in severe TBI patients randomized to receive mild to moderate hypothermia. However, in the most extensive investigation to date, TBI patients randomized to receive hypothermia (n = 199) within 6 hours of injury (target body temperature 33°C [91.4°F]) and maintained for 48 hours did not have significantly improved outcomes compared with a normothermia group of TBI patients (n = 196) at 6 months.[56] Two meta-analyses confirm these results, concluding that hypothermia is not beneficial in the management of TBI patients.[28,56,57] Regardless, a systematic review of the literature did discern potential benefits in reducing mortality and poor neurologic outcomes based on data combined from 12 trials.[58] Depth and duration of hypothermia, as well as the rate of rewarming after discontinuation of hypothermia, are additional factors that may affect outcomes with this therapeutic maneuver in TBI patients.[58,59] The mechanism underlying a protective effect of hypothermia is likely multifactorial, although a reduction in $CMR\text{O}_2$ is offered most frequently as the basis of any therapeutic benefits. Potential side effects of hypothermia include coagulation disturbances, infectious complications, and cardiac arrhythmias.[57,58] An increase in ICP also may occur secondary to hypothermia-associated shivering that can be prevented with neuromuscular blocking agents. Unfortunately, these agents are also associated with potential adverse events, as discussed previously. Considering these latter risks and equivocal data from clinical trials to date, hypothermia should continue to be considered an investigational treatment.

CLINICAL CONTROVERSY

The optimal initial strategy for acutely lowering increased ICP in TBI patients is equivocal. While the osmotic diuretics have traditionally been used as first-line therapy, use of hypertonic saline solutions is advocated by some clinicians. Not only does hypertonic saline result in plasma volume expansion, but attenuation of immunologic and biochemical events may also be responsible for some of its beneficial effects.

■ OSMOTIC AGENTS

❻ Although a number of osmotic diuretics (e.g., urea, glycerol) can be used to decrease ICP, mannitol is unquestionably the most widely employed.[1] Despite the common practice of administering mannitol to patients with suspected or actual increases in ICP following brain injury, no clinical trial comparing its effects against placebo have been performed.[26] The mechanisms responsible for mannitol's beneficial effects likely relate to (a) an immediate plasma-expanding effect that reduces blood viscosity and increases CBF and (b) establishment of an osmotic concentration gradient across an intact blood–brain barrier that decreases ICP as water diffuses from the brain into the intravascular compartment.[20] If the blood–brain barrier is disrupted as a result of injury, rebound elevations of ICP may occur with prolonged use of the osmotic agent because mannitol accumulates in the brain tissue, resulting in an increase in intracellular brain volume.[51] Recommended doses of mannitol typically range from 0.25 to 1 g/kg intravenously every 4 hours.[20] However, two recent studies using larger bolus doses of mannitol (i.e., approximately 1.4 g/kg) revealed improved clinical outcomes compared with TBI patients with temporal lobe hemorrhages and subdural hematomas treated with conventional dosages.[26,60,61] These two studies not only address the importance of the mannitol dose for this indication, but they also represent the few data substantiating the benefits of mannitol despite its use in managing TBI for over 50 years.[62]

Increased ICP is reduced within minutes following mannitol administration, and the duration of action ranges from 90 minutes to 6 hours, depending on the dose and the clinical conditions that are present.[20] To maximize benefit and minimize adverse events, it is generally recommended that mannitol be administered as a bolus and not as a continuous infusion in this setting.[1,20] However, no clinical trials have directly compared these two administration techniques.[63] Intravenous furosemide (0.5 to 1 mg/kg) may be used in conjunction with mannitol in refractory cases.

Several adverse effects are associated with mannitol. In addition to hypotension resulting from its diuretic effect, a reversible acute renal dysfunction may occur in patients with previously normal renal function after long-term, large-dose administration, especially if the serum osmolality or serum sodium exceeds 320 mOsm/kg and 160 mEq/L, respectively.[1,20] Hence monitoring and maintaining the serum osmolality and sodium, and replacing urinary fluid losses are important to minimize this adverse event. Mannitol should be avoided in patients with renal failure.[5,25] Acute exacerbation of underlying congestive heart failure and pulmonary edema also may occur following rapid intravascular volume expansion. Furosemide is recommended as an alternative diuretic for lowering ICP in these latter patient groups.

Although hypertonic saline solutions have been advocated as a resuscitative fluid following TBI patients as previously mentioned, solutions ranging from concentrations of 3% to 23.4% have been used to acutely lower increased ICP.[32,35] Not only do hypertonic saline solutions create an osmotic gradient in favor of reducing cerebral edema, but recent evidence suggests that they may also have beneficial vasoregulatory, immunologic, and neurochemical effects.[15,64] A recent isovolume head-to-head comparison of 20% mannitol versus 7.5% hypertonic saline in 20 TBI patients refractory to nonspecific therapy (i.e., sedation, analgesia, body positioning) demonstrated significant improvement in the duration and number of elevated ICP episodes per day in those treated with hypertonic saline.[65] No differences in mortality or functional outcome were observed in this study between the two patient groups. Definitive superiority of hypertonic saline therapy compared with osmotic diuretics will require further investigation.

■ BARBITURATES

❻ High-dose barbiturate therapy (i.e., *barbiturate coma*) has been used for decades in the management of increased ICP despite a lack of evidence documenting beneficial effects on patient morbidity and mortality.[30] Nonetheless, based largely on beneficial outcomes observed in a randomized clinical trial published in 1988, BTF/AANS and pediatric guidelines recommend that high-dose barbiturate therapy be considered in hemodynamically stable severe TBI patients refractory to maximal medical ICP-lowering therapy and decompressive surgery.[20,25] Prophylactic use of barbiturates is not advocated in light of insufficient evidence supporting this practice and the potential for adverse events (e.g., hypotension).[20,30] Several mechanisms responsible for the cerebral protective effects of barbiturates have been proposed. These include (a) lowering the regional $CMRO_2$ with a coupled reduction in CBF to these areas, (b) inhibition of lipid peroxidation, and (c) alteration of cerebral vascular tone.[1,48] Prior to inducing a barbiturate coma, the severe TBI patient must be mechanically ventilated with continuous monitoring of arterial blood pressure, electrocardiogram, and ICP. Pentobarbital is the most commonly used barbiturate for this indication, although thiopental also has been used. Pentobarbital should be administered as an intravenous loading infusion totaling 25 mg/kg (i.e., 10 mg/kg over 30 minutes and then 5 mg/kg per hour for 3 hours), followed by a maintenance infusion of 1 to 2 mg/kg per hour.[1,37] If the systolic blood pressure falls during the loading or maintenance infusions, the rate should be slowed temporarily and blood pressure support initiated. The goal of a barbiturate coma is to maintain ICP and CPP at the previously discussed target thresholds in addition to achieving a pentobarbital steady-state concentration of between 30 and 40 mg/L and electroencephalogram burst suppression. Initiation of barbiturate therapy withdrawal can occur when ICP has been controlled satisfactorily for 24 to 48 hours.[20] Barbiturates should be tapered over 24 to 72 hours to prevent ICP spikes.

Side effects associated with high-dose barbiturate therapy involve primarily the cardiovascular system. Hypotension caused by peripheral vasodilation may occur, necessitating decreasing the barbiturate dose or the administration of fluids and vasopressors to maintain blood pressure. A recent systematic review of the literature suggested that one of every four patients receiving barbiturate therapy will develop hypotension.[30] Gastrointestinal (GI) effects of barbiturates include decreased GI muscular tone and decreased amplitude of contraction. On emergence from coma, there may be a period of GI hypermotility. Care should be taken to avoid extravasation of pentobarbital and thiopental solutions because severe tissue damage may occur. Barbiturates should be administered by continuous infusion through a central line dedicated for this purpose. The potential for barbiturates to induce the hepatic drug metabolism of concurrent medications should also be considered. Lastly, the potential for prolonged interference with the proclamation of brain death in TBI patients meeting the locally accepted brain death neurologic criteria must be considered prior to the initiation of high-dose barbiturate therapy.

■ CORTICOSTEROIDS

❻ Although corticosteroids are effective in preventing or reducing cerebral edema in patients with nontraumatic conditions producing vasogenic edema, most studies in TBI patients have not demonstrated that they lower ICP or improve outcome.[20] In addition, use of corticosteroids following TBI is associated with increased complications, including GI bleeding, glucose intolerance, electrolyte abnormalities, and infection. Based on several major randomized trials, the BTF/AANS adult and pediatric guidelines recommend that corticosteroids not be used as the only intervention with evidence supporting a treatment standard put forth in the 2000 version of the guidelines.[24,25] Recent systematic reviews nonetheless have concluded that neither moderate benefits nor moderate harmful effects of corticosteroids in TBI patients can be excluded after review of all clinical trial data collected to date.[66] Noteworthy is that an international investigation known as the CRASH (Corticosteroid Randomization After Significant Head Injury) study was initiated in an attempt to define the merits of corticosteroid therapy in patients with TBI.[67] In this study 10,008 patients with a GCS score less than or equal to 14 were randomized to receive a 48-hour continuous infusion of methylprednisolone or placebo. Results of this study indicate a higher risk of death within 2 weeks of enrollment (relative risk: 1.18) in those patients receiving corticosteroids compared with patients receiving placebo (P <0.001).[67] Thus, corticosteroids should not be used to treat TBI patients regardless of severity.[20,27,67]

TREATMENT AND PROPHYLAXIS

Posttraumatic Seizures

It is generally agreed that patients who have experienced one or more seizures following a moderate to severe TBI should receive anticonvulsant therapy to avoid increases in $CMRO_2$ that occur with the onset of subsequent seizures and to prevent the development of (sometimes subclinical) status epilepticus with associated increase in mortality. Initial therapy in these persons should consist of incremental intravenous doses of diazepam (5 to 40 mg adults; 0.1 to 0.5 mg/kg infants and children) or lorazepam (2 to 8 mg adults; 0.03 to 0.1 mg/kg infants and children) to terminate any active seizure activity followed by intravenous phenytoin to prevent seizure recurrence. Phenytoin dosing regimens for adults and pediatric patients include an intravenous loading dose of 15 to 20 and 10 to 15 mg/kg, respectively, followed by a maintenance dose of 5 mg/kg per day. Alternatively, fosphenytoin, a water-soluble phosphate ester of phenytoin, can be administered intravenously or intramuscularly using the same doses, specified as phenytoin equivalents. The merits of preventive anticonvulsant therapy in patients who have not had a seizure postinjury historically have been more controversial. Risk factors for early posttraumatic seizures (less than 7 days after injury) include a GCS score of less than 10, a cortical contusion, a depressed skull fracture, a subdural hematoma, an epidural hematoma, an intracerebral hematoma, a penetrating head wound, or a seizure within the first 24 hours of injury.[20] In a landmark randomized, placebo-controlled study, the incidence of early posttraumatic seizures in patients receiving placebo was 14.2% compared with 3.6% in patients receiving phenytoin ($P < 0.05$) without a significant increase in drug-related side effects.[68] ❼ A systematic review of the literature corroborated these findings, estimating an improved pooled relative risk for early seizure prevention of 0.34 (95% confidence interval: 0.21 to 0.54) in patients receiving anticonvulsants.[69] Thus it is recommended that phenytoin (or, alternatively, carbamazepine) should be used to prevent seizures in TBI patients who are at high risk for the first 7 days after injury.[20,25,70] Valproate therapy is not recommended based on a trend for higher mortality in a study comparing valproate-treated patients with those receiving phenytoin short-term therapy.[71] The benefits of prophylactic anticonvulsants beyond 7 days have not been demonstrated, and thus their use for this indication is not recommended.[24,69] Unfortunately, despite reducing the incidence of early seizures following brain injury, no beneficial effects have been documented for anticonvulsants on patient mortality or long-term disability.[69]

■ SUPPORTIVE CARE

Although normalizing ICP and maintaining an adequate CPP are the highest priorities in preventing secondary injury following severe TBI, attention also must be given to preventing and/or treating systemic and extracranial complications. This includes careful ongoing fluid and electrolyte management.[35] Common electrolyte disturbances in TBI patients that should be monitored and treated aggressively include hyponatremia, hypomagnesemia, hypokalemia, and hypophosphatemia. Aggressive nutritional support of the TBI patient is another important therapeutic consideration.[20,25] Evidence suggests that early feeding of TBI patients (i.e., by 7 days) may be associated with a trend toward better outcomes in terms of survival and disability.[20,72] Infectious complications commonly encountered in severe TBI patients include nosocomial pneumonia, sepsis, urinary tract infections, and meningitis.[1] Treatment of these potentially devastating infections should be aggressive, with careful attention being paid to antibiotic blood–brain barrier penetration for intracranial infections. Other important therapeutic interventions include correction of any documented coagulopathy,[48] acute gastritis prophylaxis,[5] and prevention of decubitus ulcers and contractures. Prevention of thromboembolic events is also extremely important supportive care in TBI patients.[1] This can be accomplished with the use of intermittent pneumatic compression devices initially with the initiation of systemic therapy (e.g., low-molecular-weight heparin) generally within 2 to 3 days thereafter.[73–75] However, systemic anticoagulation must be used with caution in those patients with intracerebral hemorrhage, or in patients who may need to undergo craniotomy early in their course.

■ CLINICAL PATHWAYS/GUIDELINE IMPLEMENTATION

Use of clinical pathways and formal TBI management guidelines has been demonstrated to improve TBI patient outcomes and reduce institutional resource use. For example, implementation of a severe TBI clinical pathway resulted in a significant reduction in length of stay, ICU stay, and ventilator days among survivors at one institution.[76] Implementation of published TBI guidelines also has been demonstrated to have significant impact on patient outcomes compared with historical controls in three other institutions.[77–79] Few practitioners would dispute the overall importance of integrating current evidence-based management guidelines into clinical practice as a means to optimize care and improve the functional outcome of TBI patients.[80]

■ INVESTIGATIONAL THERAPY

❽ The steady decrease in morbidity and mortality following severe neurotrauma over the last 30 years can be attributed largely to expeditious and aggressive management of events resulting in secondary injury (i.e., ischemia, hypoxia, increased ICP) using conventional treatment strategies.[6] Numerous neuroprotective agents targeting specific pathophysiologic processes that are theorized to occur following severe TBI have been investigated over the last decade in an attempt to further enhance the prospects for a meaningful recovery. Prominent among these strategies have been attempts to modulate calcium influx through the administration of calcium antagonists[29,81] and glutamate antagonists,[6,81–84] and the use of antioxidants/free radical scavengers.[81,85] Inhibitors of inflammatory mediators also are under consideration as neuroprotective agents.[86,87] Unfortunately, none of these agents to date has demonstrated a significant reduction in morbidity or mortality following severe TBI in phase III clinical trials with the exception of nimodipine in a subset of patients.[88] Noteworthy is that a phase II pilot study recently demonstrated a decrease in mortality in 100 TBI patients randomized to receive a 3-day infusion of progesterone compared with placebo.[89] Corroboration of these results is required before this approach can be endorsed. Lastly, various growth factors, including brain-derived neurotrophic factor, nerve growth factor, neurotrophin-3, and erythropoietin,[90] may have a future role in the management of TBI by promoting nerve cell regeneration and differentiation.[86,91] Such neurorestorative strategies can be classified as structural or functional.[6] Importantly, such strategies may be the most fertile targets for genetic manipulation in the future and may have significant implications for post-TBI rehabilitation.[6] Despite generally negative clinical trial findings to date, the search is likely to continue for neuroprotective agents that eventually may improve the long-term outcome in severe TBI patients.

CLINICAL CONTROVERSY

Interest in the use of CNS stimulants, such as methylphenidate and agents that modify the neurochemical balance within the brain, such as Parkinson's disease medications (e.g., amantadine, bromocriptine) and antidepressants following TBI, has existed for years. Relatively small studies using these approaches to improve the cognitive and behavioral outcomes in TBI patients have demonstrated potential benefits. Off-label use of these drugs in TBI patients following the acute phase of their management should be considered investigational until large scale, controlled trials document their utility.

■ OTHER TREATMENT STRATEGIES

The concept of administering commercially available CNS active agents off-label should presently be considered investigative therapy. One example is the use of CNS stimulants in the management and rehabilitation of TBI patients. A comprehensive review of the use of methylphenidate relative to improving cognition in TBI was recently conducted. It was the opinion of the author that the literature does provide a degree of support for improvements in memory, attention, concentration, and mental processing in this patient subset, although results and study designs were highly variable for those investigations included in the analysis.[92] Another example is the use of Parkinson disease medications (e.g., amantadine, bromocriptine, carbidopa/levodopa) in severe TBI patients in an attempt to enhance dopamine release and inhibit reuptake within the injured region of the brain. A review of amantadine following TBI patients indicated that improved cognition and reduced agitation were evident in the majority of patients studied.[93] A recent trial of the rivastigmine used for the treatment of Alzheimer disease demonstrated improved memory in a group of TBI patients with moderate to severe memory loss.[94] Antidepressants represent another class of agents that has been studied in TBI patients. Although intuitively appealing, routine administration of psychostimulants to improve cognitive outcomes in TBI patients or drugs that enhance the biochemical milieu within the CNS following a TBI should be done cautiously until large, well-controlled studies demonstrating beneficial effects are available. Additionally, the timing of administration of these drugs is controversial; the potential for cardiovascular side effects in the face of uncertain benefit would indicate that these drugs should be reserved for the after acute phase of treatment (i.e., weeks to months after injury).

EVALUATION OF THERAPEUTIC OUTCOMES

Table 60–2 summarizes the process for evaluation of therapeutic outcomes. Patients with severe TBI require ICU monitoring initially with the goals of maintaining or reestablishing neurologic and systemic homeostasis as well as readily detecting any neurologic deterioration. This requires frequent evaluation of the patient's neurologic status (e.g., GCS) and measurement of vital signs, urine output, and arterial oxygen saturation (as well as ICP in patients with an ICP monitor in place). Furthermore, careful attention must be paid to the potential for a variety of electrolyte, mineral, and acid–base disturbances, coagulopathies, and infections by obtaining various laboratory tests on a daily basis initially. The intensity of monitoring will be a function of the relative degree of neurologic and hemodynamic stability of the patient in the hours and days following the neurologic insult. Lastly, radiologic tests (e.g., CT scans) are essential not only for the initial diagnostic evaluation of TBI patients but also as a means to evaluate the etiology for any subsequent neurologic deterioration.

TABLE 60-2 Evaluation of Therapeutic Outcomes

General	GCS: record hourly initially, decrease frequency as neurologic status stabilizes
	Vital signs (BP, HR, RR, temperature): record hourly initially, decrease frequency as neurologic status stabilizes
	Urine output: record hourly initially, decrease frequency as neurologic status stabilizes
	Arterial oxygen saturation: continuously while in intensive care unit
Risk of increased ICP	ICP: record hourly, decrease frequency as ICP stabilizes less than 20 mm Hg (usually not until 48–72 hours postinjury at a minimum)[a]
	CPP: record hourly, decrease frequency as CPP stabilizes in the desired range
Laboratory tests	Ethanol concentration and urine drug screen: on admission
	ABGs: daily at a minimum while intubated, repeated as needed based on pulmonary instability requiring ventilator setting changes
	CBC: daily while in intensive care unit
	Serum electrolytes (Na, K, Cl): daily while in intensive care unit; serum sodium and osmolarity may be monitored as frequently as every 6 hours if osmotherapy (mannitol, furosemide, hypertonic saline) is being used
	Minerals (Mg, Ca, P): daily initially until concentrations stable
Radiologic procedures	CT scan: postresuscitation initially with repeat scan(s) as needed based on degree of neurologic instability (e.g., decrease in GCS) or initial CT appearance

ABG, arterial blood gas; BP, blood pressure; Ca, calcium; CBC, complete blood count; Cl, chloride; CPP, cerebral perfusion pressure; CSF, cerebrospinal fluid; CT, computed tomography GCS, Glasgow Coma Scale; HR, heart rate; ICP, intracranial pressure; K, potassium; Mg, magnesium; Na, sodium; P, phosphorus; RR, respiratory rate; TBI, traumatic brain injury.

[a]Continuous monitoring mandated initially if technologically feasible.

ABBREVIATIONS

AANS: American Association of Neurological Surgeons

BTF: Brain Trauma Foundation

CBF: cerebral blood flow

CDO_2: cerebral oxygen delivery

$CMRO_2$: cerebral oxygen consumption

CNS: central nervous system

CPP: cerebral perfusion pressure

CT: computed tomography

GCS: Glasgow Coma Scale

GI: gastrointestinal

ICP: intracranial pressure

MAP: mean arterial pressure

NMDA: *N*-methyl-D-aspartate

$SjVO_2$: jugular venous oxygen saturation

TBI: traumatic brain injury

REFERENCES

1. Cohen SM, Marion DW. Traumatic brain injury. In: Fink MP, Abraham E, Vincent JL, et al., eds. Textbook of Critical Care. Philadelphia: Elsevier Saunders, 2005:377–389.
2. Langlois JA, Rutland-Brown W, Thomas KE. Traumatic brain injury in the United States: Emergency department visits, hospitalizations, and deaths. In: Geberding JL, Arias I, eds. Traumatic Brain Injury in the United States: Emergency Department Visits, Hospitalizations, and Death. Atlanta, GA: Centers for Disease Control and Prevention, National Center for Injury Prevention and Control, 2006:1–55.
3. Finkelstein E, Corso P, Miller T. The Incidence and Economic Burden of Injuries in the United States. New York: Oxford University Press, 2006.
4. Adekoya N, Thurman DJ, White DD, Webb KW. Surveillance for traumatic brain injury deaths—United States, 1989–1998. MMWR Surveill Summ 2002;51:1–14.
5. Marik PE, Varon J, Trask T. Management of head trauma. Chest 2002;122:699–711.
6. Marshall LF. Head injury: Recent past, present, and future. Neurosurgery 2000;47:546–561.
7. Clark RSB, Jenkins L, Lai YC, et al. Biochemical, cellular, and molecular mechanisms of neuronal death and secondary brain injury in critical care. In: Fink MP, Abraham E, Vincent JL, et al., eds. Textbook of Critical Care. Philadelphia: Elsevier Saunders, 2005:263–273.
8. Martin NA, Patwardhan RV, Alexander MJ, et al. Characterization of cerebral hemodynamic phases following severe head trauma: Hypoperfusion, hyperemia, and vasospasm. J Neurosurg 1997;87:9–19.
9. Ray SK, Dixon CE, Banik NL. Molecular mechanisms in the pathogenesis of traumatic brain injury. Histol Histopathol 2002;17:1137–1152.
10. Cristofori L, Tavazzi B, Gambin R, et al. Early onset of lipid peroxidation after human traumatic brain injury: A fatal limitation for the free radical scavenger pharmacological therapy? J Investig Med 2001;49:450–458.
11. Raghupathi R, Graham DI, McIntosh TK. Apoptosis after traumatic brain injury. J Neurotrauma 2000;17:927–938.

12. Ng I, Yeo TT, Tang WY, et al. Apoptosis occurs after cerebral contusions in humans. Neurosurgery 2000;46:949–956.
13. Huang PP, Esquenazi S, Le Roux PD. Cerebral cortical neuron apoptosis after mild excitotoxic injury in vitro: Different roles of mesencephalic and cortical astrocytes. Neurosurgery 1999;45:1413–1422.
14. Singhal A, Baker AJ, Hare GM, et al. Association between cerebrospinal fluid interleukin-6 concentrations and outcome after severe human traumatic brain injury. J Neurotrauma 2002;19:929–937.
15. Dutton RP, McCunn M. Traumatic brain injury. Curr Opin Crit Care 2003;9:503–509.
16. Waters RJ, Nicoll JA. Genetic influences on outcome following acute neurological insults. Curr Opin Crit Care 2005;11:105–110.
17. Kerr ME, Ilyas Kamboh M, Yookyung K, et al. Relationship between apoE4 allele and excitatory amino acid levels after traumatic brain injury. Crit Care Med 2003;31:2371–2379.
18. Teasdale G, Jennett B. Assessment of coma and impaired consciousness. A practical scale. Lancet 1974;2:81–84.
19. Signorini DF, Andrews PJ, Jones PA, et al. Predicting survival using simple clinical variables: A case study in traumatic brain injury. J Neurol Neurosurg Psychiatry 1999;66:20–25.
20. Bullock R, Chesnut RM, Clifton GL, et al. Brain Trauma Foundation, Inc., American Association of Neurological Surgeons. Part 1: Guidelines for the management of severe head injury. New York: Brain Trauma Foundation, 2000:1–165.
21. Marion DW, Spiegel TP. Changes in the management of severe traumatic brain injury: 1991–1997. Crit Care Med 2000;28:16–18.
22. Gabriel EJ, Ghajar J, Jagoda A, et al. Guidelines for prehospital management of traumatic brain injury. J Neurotrauma 2002;19:111–174.
23. Bullock MR, Chesnut R, Ghajar J, et al. Guidelines for the surgical management of traumatic brain injury. Neurosurgery 2006;58(3 Suppl):52–vi.
24. Maas AI, Dearden M, Teasdale GM, et al. EBIC-guidelines for management of severe head injury in adults. European Brain Injury Consortium. Acta Neurochir (Wien) 1997;139:286–294.
25. Adelson PD, Bratton SL, Carney NA, et al. Guidelines for the acute medical management of severe traumatic brain injury in infants, children, and adolescents. Crit Care Med 2003;31:S417-S491.
26. Wakai A, Roberts I, Schierhout G. Mannitol for acute traumatic brain injury. Cochrane Database Syst Rev 2005:CD001049.
27. Alderson P, Roberts I. Corticosteroids for acute traumatic brain injury. Cochrane Database Syst Rev 2005:CD000196.
28. Gadkary CS, Alderson P, Signorini DF. Therapeutic hypothermia for head injury. Cochrane Database Syst Rev 2002;(1):CD001048.
29. Langham J, Goldfrad C, Teasdale G, et al. Calcium channel blockers for acute traumatic brain injury. Cochrane Database Syst Rev 2003;(4): CD000565.
30. Roberts I. Barbiturates for acute traumatic brain injury. Cochrane Database Syst Rev 2000;(2):CD000033.
31. Roberts I, Schierhout G. Hyperventilation therapy for acute traumatic brain injury. Cochrane Database Syst Rev 2000;(2):CD000566.
32. Guha A. Management of traumatic brain injury: Some current evidence and applications. Postgrad Med J 2004;80:650–653.
33. Bhardwaj A, Ulatowski JA. Hypertonic saline solutions in brain injury. Curr Opin Crit Care 2004;10:126–131.
34. Scalea TM. Does it matter how head-injury patients are resuscitated? In: Valadka AB, Andrews BT, eds. Neurotrauma. Evidence-Based Answers to Common Questions. New York: Thieme, 2005:3–7.
35. Rhoney DH, Parker D Jr. Considerations in fluids and electrolytes after traumatic brain injury. Nutr Clin Pract 2006;21:462–478.
36. Sahuquillo J, Arikan F. Decompressive craniectomy for the treatment of refractory high intracranial pressure in traumatic brain injury. Cochrane Database Syst Rev 2006:CD003983.
37. Bulger EM, Nathens AB, Rivara FP, et al. Management of severe head injury: Institutional variations in care and effect on outcome. Crit Care Med 2002;30:1870–1876.
38. Cremer OL, van Dijk GW, van Wensen E, et al. Effect of intracranial pressure monitoring and targeted intensive care on functional outcome after severe head injury. Crit Care Med 2005;33:2207–2213.
39. Stocchetti N. Should I monitor jugular venous oxygen saturation? In: Valadka AB, Andrews BT, eds. Neurotrauma. Evidence-Based Answers to Common Questions. New York: Thieme, 2005:58–67.
40. Latronico N, Beindorf AE, Rasulo FA, et al. Limits of intermittent jugular bulb oxygen saturation monitoring in the management of severe head trauma patients. Neurosurgery 2000;46:1131–1138.
41. Hutchinson PJ. Microdialysis in traumatic brain injury—methodology and pathophysiology. Acta Neurochir Suppl 2005;95:441–445.
42. Kiening KL, Sarrafzadeh AS, Stover JF,Unterberg AW. Should I monitor brain tissue PO_2? In: Valadka AB, Andrews BT, eds. Neurotrauma. Evidence-Based Answers to Common Questions. New York: Thieme, 2005:62–67.
43. Ingebrigtsen T, Romner B. Biochemical serum markers of traumatic brain injury. J Trauma 2002;52:798–808.
44. Cerebral perfusion pressure (update notice). In: Guidelines for the Management of Severe Traumatic Brain Injury. New York: Brain Trauma Foundation; 2003:1–14.
45. Contant CF, Valadka AB, Gopinath SP, et al. Adult respiratory distress syndrome: A complication of induced hypertension after severe head injury. J Neurosurg 2001;95:560–568.
46. Juul N, Morris GF, Marshall SB, Marshall LF. Intracranial hypertension and cerebral perfusion pressure: Influence on neurological deterioration and outcome in severe head injury. The Executive Committee of the International Selfotel Trial. J Neurosurg 2000;92:1–6.
47. Clifton GL, Miller ER, Choi SC, Levin HS. Fluid thresholds and outcome from severe brain injury. Crit Care Med 2002;30:739–745.
48. Maas AIR, Stocchetti N. Intensive care after neurosurgery. In: Fink MP, Abraham E, Vincent JL, et al., eds. Textbook of Critical Care. Philadelphia: Elsevier Saunders, 2005:417–426.
49. Kelly DF, Goodale DB, Williams J, et al. Propofol in the treatment of moderate and severe head injury: A randomized, prospective double-blinded pilot trial. J Neurosurg 1999;90:1042–1052.
50. Bao YP, Williamson G, Tew D, et al. Antioxidant effects of propofol in human hepatic microsomes: Concentration effects and clinical relevance. Br J Anaesth 1998;81:584–589.
51. Mirski M. Anticonvulsants in the intensive care unit. In: Fink MP, Abraham E, Vincent JL, et al., eds. Textbook of Critical Care. Philadelphia: Elsevier Saunders, 2005:1607–1617.
52. Cremer OL, Moons KG, Bouman EA, et al. Long-term propofol infusion and cardiac failure in adult head-injured patients. Lancet 2001;357:117–118.
53. Diringer MN, Yundt K, Videen TO, et al. No reduction in cerebral metabolism as a result of early moderate hyperventilation following severe traumatic brain injury. J Neurosurg 2000;92:7–13.
54. Marion DW, Puccio A, Wisniewski SR, et al. Effect of hyperventilation on extracellular concentrations of glutamate, lactate, pyruvate, and local cerebral blood flow in patients with severe traumatic brain injury. Crit Care Med 2002;30:2619–2625.
55. Thompson HJ, Tkacs NC, Saatman KE, et al. Hyperthermia following traumatic brain injury: A critical evaluation. Neurobiol Dis 2003;12:163–173.
56. Clifton GL, Miller ER, Choi SC, et al. Lack of effect of induction of hypothermia after acute brain injury. N Engl J Med 2001;344:556–563.
57. Harris OA, Colford JM, Jr., Good MC,Matz PG. The role of hypothermia in the management of severe brain injury: A meta-analysis. Arch Neurol 2002;59:1077–1083.
58. McIntyre LA, Fergusson DA, Hebert PC, et al. Prolonged therapeutic hypothermia after traumatic brain injury in adults: A systematic review. JAMA 2003;289:2992–2999.
59. Tokutomi T, Morimoto K, Miyagi T, et al. Optimal temperature for the management of severe traumatic brain injury: Effect of hypothermia on intracranial pressure, systemic and intracranial hemodynamics, and metabolism. Neurosurgery 2003;52:102–111.
60. Cruz J, Minoja G, Okuchi K. Improving clinical outcomes from acute subdural hematomas with the emergency preoperative administration of high doses of mannitol: A randomized trial. Neurosurgery 2001;49:864–871.
61. Cruz J, Minoja G, Okuchi K. Major clinical and physiological benefits of early high doses of mannitol for intraparenchymal temporal lobe hemorrhages with abnormal pupillary widening: A randomized trial. Neurosurgery 2002;51:628–637.
62. Schrot RJ, Muizelaar JP. Mannitol in acute traumatic brain injury. Lancet 2002;359:1633–1634.
63. Roberts I, Schierhout G, Wakai A. Mannitol for acute traumatic brain injury. Cochrane Database Syst Rev 2003:CD001049.

64. Doyle JA, Davis DP, Hoyt DB. The use of hypertonic saline in the treatment of traumatic brain injury. J Trauma 2001;50:367–383.
65. Vialet R, Albanese J, Thomachot L, et al. Isovolume hypertonic solutes (sodium chloride or mannitol) in the treatment of refractory posttraumatic intracranial hypertension: 2 mL/kg 7.5% saline is more effective than 2 mL/kg 20% mannitol. Crit Care Med 2003;31:1683–1687.
66. Alderson P, Roberts I. Corticosteroids for acute traumatic brain injury. Cochrane Database Syst Rev 2005;(1):CD000196.
67. Roberts I, Yates D, Sandercock P, et al. Effect of intravenous corticosteroids on death within 14 days in 10008 adults with clinically significant head injury (MRC CRASH trial): Randomised placebo-controlled trial. Lancet 2004;364:1321–1328.
68. Temkin NR, Dikmen SS, Wilensky AJ, et al. A randomized, double-blind study of phenytoin for the prevention of post-traumatic seizures. N Engl J Med 1990;323:497–502.
69. Schierhout G, Roberts I. Anti-epileptic drugs for preventing seizures following acute traumatic brain injury. Cochrane Database Syst Rev 2001;(4):CD000173.
70. Chang BS, Lowenstein DH. Practice parameter: Antiepileptic drug prophylaxis in severe traumatic brain injury: Report of the Quality Standards Subcommittee of the American Academy of Neurology. Neurology 2003;60:10–16.
71. Temkin NR, Dikmen SS, Anderson GD, et al. Valproate therapy for prevention of posttraumatic seizures: A randomized trial. J Neurosurg 1999;91:593–600.
72. Yanagawa T, Bunn F, Roberts I, et al. Nutritional support for head-injured patients. Cochrane Database Syst Rev 2003:CD001530.
73. Macdonald RL. What is the safest way to prevent deep venous thrombosis and pulmonary embolism after head or spinal cord injury? How soon after surgery or injury can I anticoagulate my patients who develop deep venous thrombosis? In: Valadka AB, Andrews BT, eds. Neurotrauma. Evidence-Based Answers to Common Questions. New York: Thieme, 2005:43–49.
74. Kim J, Gearhart MM, Zurick A, et al. Preliminary report on the safety of heparin for deep venous thrombosis prophylaxis after severe head injury. J Trauma 2002;53:38–42; discussion 43.
75. Norwood SH, McAuley CE, Berne JD, et al. Prospective evaluation of the safety of enoxaparin prophylaxis for venous thromboembolism in patients with intracranial hemorrhagic injuries. Arch Surg 2002;137:696–701.
76. Vitaz TW, McIlvoy L, Raque GH, et al. Development and implementation of a clinical pathway for severe traumatic brain injury. J Trauma 2001;51:369–375.
77. Palmer S, Bader MK, Qureshi A, et al. The impact on outcomes in a community hospital setting of using the AANS traumatic brain injury guidelines. Americans Associations for Neurologic Surgeons. J Trauma 2001;50:657–664.
78. Elf K, Nilsson P, Enblad P. Outcome after traumatic brain injury improved by an organized secondary insult program and standardized neurointensive care. Crit Care Med 2002;30:2129–2134.
79. Patel HC, Menon DK, Tebbs S, et al. Specialist neurocritical care and outcome from head injury. Intensive Care Med 2002;28:547–553.
80. Hartl R, Ghajar J. Does following the recommendations in the Guidelines for the Management of Severe Traumatic Brain Injury make a difference in patient outcome? In: Valadka AB, Andrews BT, eds. Neurotrauma. Evidence-Based Answers to Common Questions. New York: Thieme, 2005:120–123.
81. Farin A, Marshall LF. Why have therapeutic trials in head injury been unable to demonstrate benefits? In: Valadka AB, Andrews BT, eds. Neurotrauma. Evidence-Based Answers to Common Questions. New York: Thieme, 2005:124–131.
82. Knoller N, Levi L, Shoshan I, et al. Dexanabinol (HU-211) in the treatment of severe closed head injury: A randomized, placebo-controlled, phase II clinical trial. Crit Care Med 2002;30:548–554.
83. Merchant RE, Bullock MR, Carmack CA, et al. A double-blind, placebo-controlled study of the safety, tolerability and pharmacokinetics of CP-101,606 in patients with a mild or moderate traumatic brain injury. Ann N Y Acad Sci 1999;890:42–50.
84. Willis C, Lybrand S, Bellamy N. Excitatory amino acid inhibitors for traumatic brain injury. Cochrane Database Syst Rev 2004:CD003986.
85. Maas AI, Steyerberg EW, Murray GD, et al. Why have recent trials of neuroprotective agents in head injury failed to show convincing efficacy? A pragmatic analysis and theoretical considerations. Neurosurgery 1999;44:1286–1298.
86. Doppenberg EM, Choi SC, Bullock R. Clinical trials in traumatic brain injury: Lessons for the future. J Neurosurg Anesthesiol 2004;16:87–94.
87. Sanchez Mejia RO, Ona VO, Li M, Friedlander RM. Minocycline reduces traumatic brain injury-mediated caspase-1 activation, tissue damage, and neurological dysfunction. Neurosurgery 2001;48:1393–1399.
88. Faden AI. Neuroprotection and traumatic brain injury: Theoretical option or realistic proposition. Curr Opin Neurol 2002;15:707–712.
89. Wright DW, Kellermann AL, Hertzberg VS, et al. ProTECT: A randomized clinical trial of progesterone for acute traumatic brain injury. Ann Emerg Med 2006.
90. Buemi M, Cavallaro E, Floccari F, et al. Erythropoietin and the brain: From neurodevelopment to neuroprotection. Clin Sci (Lond) 2002;103:275–282.
91. Teasdale GM, Graham DI. Craniocerebral trauma: Protection and retrieval of the neuronal population after injury. Neurosurgery 1998;43:723–737; discussion 37–38.
92. Siddall OM. Use of methylphenidate in traumatic brain injury. Ann Pharmacother 2005;39:1309–1313.
93. Leone H, Polsonetti BW. Amantadine for traumatic brain injury: Does it improve cognition and reduce agitation? J Clin Pharm Ther 2005;30:101–104.
94. Silver JM, Koumaras B, Chen M, et al. Effects of rivastigmine on cognitive function in patients with traumatic brain injury. Neurology 2006;67:748–755.

CHAPTER 61 Parkinson's Disease

JACK J. CHEN, MERLIN V. NELSON, AND DAVID M. SWOPE

KEY CONCEPTS

1. Thoughtful consideration for selection of initial therapy, management of drug dosing, and use of adjunctive therapies throughout the course of idiopathic Parkinson's disease (IPD) is necessary to optimize long-term therapeutic outcomes and minimize adverse effects.
2. The optimal time to start drug therapy in IPD varies, but in general, treatment is initiated and when the disease begins to interfere with activities of daily living, employment, or quality of life.
3. Anticholinergic medication is useful for mild tremor-predominant IPD but should be used with caution in the elderly and in those with preexisting cognitive difficulties.
4. As monotherapy, amantadine and monoamine oxidase type B (MAO-B) inhibitors provide benefits in early IPD, but the symptomatic effect is less than that of dopamine agonists and carbidopa/levodopa (L-dopa).
5. Carbidopa/L-dopa is the most effective medication for symptomatic treatment and eventually all patients with IPD will require it.
6. Most carbidopa/L-dopa–treated patients will develop motor complications (e.g., fluctuations and dyskinesias).
7. MAO-B inhibitors and catechol-*O*-methyl-transferase inhibitors attenuate motor fluctuations in carbidopa/L-dopa treated patients.
8. Initial monotherapy with a dopamine agonist is effective and, compared to L-dopa, associated with less risk of developing motor complications but is more likely to cause psychiatric symptoms such as hallucinations and impulse control disorders.
9. Surgery is reserved for patients who require additional symptomatic relief or control of motor complications despite receiving medically optimized therapy.

The presence of tremor at rest, rigidity, bradykinesia, and postural instability (instability of balance) are considered the hallmark motor features of idiopathic Parkinson's disease (IPD). These clinical features of IPD were adeptly described in 1817 by James Parkinson.[1]

Learning objectives, review questions, and other resources can be found at **www.pharmacotherapyonline.com.**

EPIDEMIOLOGY

Up to 1 million individuals in the United States have IPD. The approximate annual incidence of IPD (i.e., number of persons diagnosed with IPD per year) is age-dependent and ranges from 10 per 100,000 persons in the sixth decade of life (i.e., 50–59 years of age) to 120 per 100,000 persons in the ninth decade of life (i.e., 80–89 years of age).[2,3] Likewise, the prevalence of IPD also increases with age, affecting 1% of people older than age 65 years and 2.5% of those older than age 80 years. IPD is less frequent in patients younger than age 50 years and the usual age at time of diagnosis ranges between 55 and 65 years. A higher incidence is reported among males, with a male-to-female ratio of up to 2:1.

ETIOLOGY

The true etiology of IPD is unknown, but factors such as genetic constitution and toxin (intrinsic or extrinsic) exposure most likely play a role. In IPD, a key histopathologic feature is degeneration of dopaminergic neurons in the substantia nigra that project to the striatum (i.e., the nigrostriatal pathway).[4] Additionally, neuronal vulnerability in IPD extends beyond the nigrostriatal pathway and includes specific neurons in autonomic ganglia, basal ganglia, spinal cord, and neocortex.[5] In humans, administration of the compound 1-methyl-4-phenyl-1,2,3,6-tetrahydropyridine (MPTP) results in a form of parkinsonism. The MPTP compound is converted by monoamine oxidase (MAO)-B to 1-methyl-4-phenylpyridinium ion (MPP^+), a potent neurotoxin in humans and animals. MPP^+ is toxic to neurons by inhibiting mitochondrial complex 1 of the electron transport chain, which results in the generation of excessive reactive oxygen species and cell death.[6] Several synthetic pesticides have a molecular structure similar to that of MPTP. Although IPD is sporadic in most instances, extensive epidemiologic research associates environmental factors, such as chronic exposure to pesticides and heavy metals (such as iron and manganese), rural living, and drinking well water, with small but demonstrable contributions to the risk for lifetime development of IPD.[7] Interestingly, epidemiologic studies have consistently associated an inverse correlation between cigarette smoking and caffeine consumption for development of IPD.[8,9]

Intrinsically, the substantia nigra pars compacta (SNc) is a region characterized by high levels of oxidative stress because free radicals are generated from dopamine autooxidation mediated by MAO (Fig. 61–1). Several antioxidative molecules (e.g., glutathione) are present in the SNc to limit damage produced by free-radical attack, but in IPD, such protection might be overwhelmed or impaired. Thus cellular damage from oxidant stress is implicated as an etiopathologic component of IPD.[10] The SNc is also rich in iron and copper, essential cofactors in the biosynthesis and metabolism of dopamine. The oxidation–reduction cycle of iron can also generate

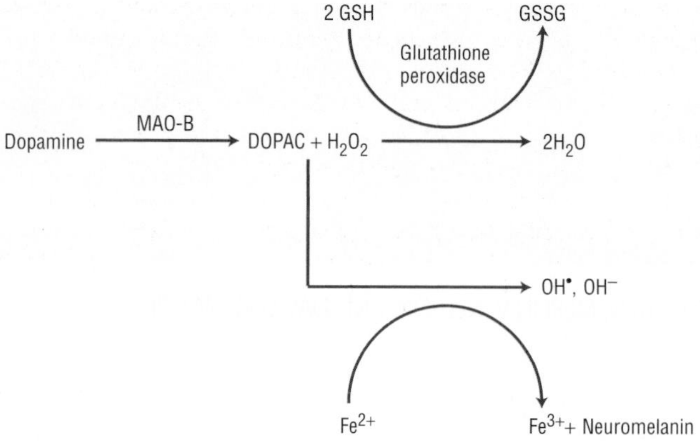

FIGURE 61-1. Dopamine metabolism results in hydrogen peroxide (H_2O_2) formation. If the glutathione system is deficient or excess hydrogen peroxide is present, hydrogen peroxide accepts an electron from ferrous iron (Fe^{2+}), forming ferric iron (Fe^{3+}) and the hydroxyl free radical (OH*). The hydroxyl free radical can cause lipid peroxidation, thereby damaging neuronal cell membranes. (DOPAC, 3,4-dihydroxyphenylacetic acid; GSH, glutathione; GSSG, glutathione disulfide; H_2O, water; OH, the hydroxide ion; MAO-B, monoamine oxidase B.)

free radicals and toxic metabolites (e.g., hydrogen peroxide) (Fig. 61–1). Apoptosis (programmed cell death), excitotoxicity, inflammation, mitochondrial dysfunction, nitric oxide toxicity, proteosomal dysfunction, and autophagic cellular mechanisms are also implicated etiopathologic mechanisms in IPD.

Genetics may play a significant role, particularly if IPD begins before age 50 years.[11,12] More than a dozen gene mutations are associated with forms of parkinsonism. For example, autosomal dominant forms of parkinsonism are associated with mutations of the *α-synuclein* (*PARK1*) and *leucine-rich repeat kinase 2* (*LRRK*) genes. Autosomal recessive forms are associated with mutations of *parkin* and *PINK1* genes. Overall, these forms of genetically linked parkinsonisms constitute only a small percentage of total parkinsonism cases and their pathology and phenotypic aspects differ from that of IPD.

PATHOPHYSIOLOGY

In the SNc, the two hallmark histopathologic features of IPD are depigmentation of dopamine-producing neurons (i.e., loss of SNc neurons) and presence of Lewy bodies (neuronal cytoplasmic filamentous aggregates composed of the presynaptic protein α-synuclein) in the remaining SNc neurons. Lewy bodies appear in degenerating neurons in association with adjacent gliosis. Lewy pathology has been proposed to develop in a predictable anatomic distribution within the parkinsonian brain.[5] In the preclinical (i.e., asymptomatic) stages of IPD, Lewy bodies are initially found in the medulla oblongata, locus coeruleus, raphe nuclei, and olfactory bulb. This may correlate with observations that anxiety, depression, and impaired olfaction is detectable in preclinical stages of IPD. As IPD progresses to clinical stages, Lewy pathology ascends to the midbrain (particularly the SNc) and accounts for development of motor features. In advanced stages, Lewy pathology spreads to the cortex, and this may correlate with behavioral and cognitive changes.

Pathologic findings reveal a correlation between the extent of nigrostriatal dopamine loss and the severity of certain IPD motor features (e.g., bradykinesia). The threshold for onset of clinically detectable IPD appears to be the loss of 70% to 80% of SNc neurons.[13] Functional neuroimaging studies suggest compensatory responses, such as upregulation of dopamine synthesis and downregulation of synaptic dopamine reuptake, occur as adaptive mechanisms in preclinical and very early stages of IPD. These adaptive responses may help to explain why IPD is relatively asymptomatic until profound depletion (70% to 80%) of SNc neurons has occurred.

Dopaminergic projections from the SNc to the striatum (putamen and caudate) synapse on two populations of dopamine receptor-mediated efferent neurons (referred to as the direct and indirect pathways), which, in turn, mediate motor activity via a complex neuronal circuit involving the extrapyramidal system (Fig. 61–2). In IPD, the degeneration of the SNc neurons results in reduced activity within these two efferent pathways. The direct pathway involves activation of striatal D_1 dopamine receptors (which are coupled to adenylate cyclase) and stimulates the inhibitory γ-aminobutyric acid (GABA)/substance P efferents to the globus pallidus interna (GPi) and substantia nigra pars reticulata. The GPi and substantia nigra pars reticulata efferents are inhibitory to the thalamus.[14] In IPD, the reduced activation of D_1 receptors results in greater inhibition of the thalamus. The indirect pathway involves activation of striatal D_2 dopamine receptors (which are coupled to a guanosine triphosphate-binding protein that opens potassium channels to hyperpolarize neurons, thereby reducing the excitability of the neuron).[14] Activation of striatal D_2 dopamine receptors inhibits GABA/enkephalin efferents (medium spiny neurons) to the globus pallidus externa. The globus pallidus externa projects GABA neurons to the subthalamic nucleus. Here, excitatory glutamatergic neurons project to the GPi.

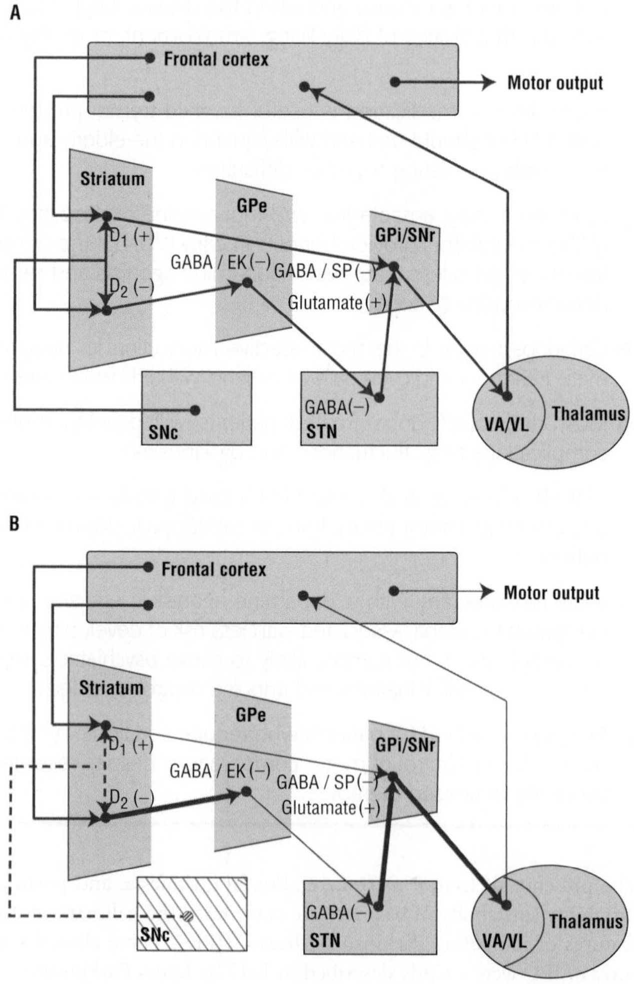

FIGURE 61-2. *A.* The normal balance of the basal ganglia–thalamocortical circuit. *B.* With nigrostriatal degeneration *(dashed line)*, there is loss of inhibition of the GPi by the direct pathway and activation of the GPi via the indirect pathway, resulting in decreased activation of the cortex. See text for details. (GPe, globus pallidus externa; GPi, globus pallidus interna; SNc, substantia nigra pars compacta; SNr, substantia nigra pars reticulata; STN, subthalamic nucleus; VA, ventroanterior nuclei of the thalamus; VL, ventrolateral nuclei of the thalamus.)

TABLE 61-1 Diagnostic Criteria for Idiopathic Parkinson's Disease and Differential Diagnosis

- Idiopathic Parkinson's disease
  - *Clinically possible:* Presence of one of the following: resting tremor, rigidity, or bradykinesia
  - *Clinically probable:* Presence of at least two of the following: resting tremor, rigidity, or bradykinesia
  - *Clinically definite:* Presence of at least two of the following: resting tremor, rigidity, or bradykinesia and a positive response to antiparkinsonian pharmacotherapy
- Essential tremor
- Secondary parkinsonism
  - Pharmacotoxicity (drug-induced)
    - Antiemetics (e.g., metoclopramide, prochlorperazine)
    - Antipsychotics (e.g., phenothiazines, haloperidol, olanzapine, risperidone)
    - Other drugs (α-methyldopa, cinnarizine, flunarizine, tetrabenazine)
  - Environmental toxicity
    - Carbon monoxide poisoning
    - Manganese
    - Methanol
    - MPTP (1-methyl-4-phenyl-1,2,3,6-tetrahydropyridine)
    - Organophosphates
  - Infections
    - Human immunodeficiency virus–associated parkinsonism
    - Postencephalitic parkinsonism
    - Subacute sclerosing panencephalitis
  - Metabolic disorder
    - Hypothyroidism
    - Parathyroid abnormalities
  - Neoplasms, strokes, traumatic lesions involving the nigrostriatal pathways
  - Normal-pressure hydrocephalus
- Parkinsonism with other neuronal system degenerations
  - Alzheimer's with parkinsonism
  - Corticobasal ganglionic degeneration
  - Creutzfeldt-Jakob's disease (CJD)
  - Dementia with Lewy bodies
  - Frontotemporal dementia
  - Progressive supranuclear palsy
  - Multiple-system atrophies
    - Striatonigral degeneration
    - Shy-Drager's syndrome
    - Olivopontocerebellar atrophy
  - Familial (hereditary) parkinsonism
    - Autosomal dominant
      - α-Synuclein gene mutation (PARK1)
      - Frontotemporal dementia parkinsonism (FTDP-17)
      - Levodopa responsive dystonia
      - Leucine-rich repeat kinase 2 (LRRK2) mutation
      - Rapid-onset dystonia parkinsonism (DYT12)
      - Spinocerebellar ataxias (SCA2, SCA3)
    - Autosomal recessive
      - Hallervorden-Spatz disease
      - Neuroacanthocytes
      - Niemann Pick type C
      - Wilson's disease
      - Young-onset parkinsonism (DJ-1, parkin, PINK1)
    - X-linked recessive
      - Fragile X tremor/ataxia syndrome (FXTAS)
      - Lubag (DYT3 or Filipino dystonia parkinsonism)
      - Waisman syndrome (X-linked parkinsonism with mental retardation)

GPi output is inhibitory on the glutamatergic thalamic projections. In IPD, the reduced activation of D_2 receptors translates into greater inhibition of the thalamus. In IPD, restoring activity at the D_2 receptor appears to be of more importance than the D_1 receptor for mediating clinical improvements. Overall, loss of the presynaptic nigrostriatal dopamine neurons in IPD results in inhibition of thalamic activity and reduced activation of the motor cortex. Dopaminergic therapies help to restore motor activity.

In addition to dopamine, the synaptic organization of the basal ganglia also involves a variety of other neurotransmitters and neuromodulators, including acetylcholine, adenosine, enkephalins, GABA, glutamate, serotonin, and substance P. The role for drug modulation of other neurotransmitters and receptor types (e.g., adenosine A_{2A} receptors) is currently being investigated.[15]

Atypical parkinsonian disorders, such as multiple system atrophy and progressive supranuclear palsy are characterized by damage to postsynaptic neurons and dopamine receptors. Therefore, these atypical parkinsonisms are markedly less responsive to dopaminergic therapies.

CLINICAL PRESENTATION

Although IPD is unmistakable in its advanced form, recognizing IPD during the early stages can be challenging. Clinically probable IPD can be diagnosed when at least two of the following are present: limb muscle rigidity, resting tremor (at 3 to 6 Hz and abolished by movement), or bradykinesia (Table 61–1).[16] In early IPD, unilaterality (asymmetry) of features is a conspicuous finding, but as the disease advances, features often become bilateral. For the diagnosis of IPD, other conditions must be reasonably excluded (Table 61–1). Medication-induced parkinsonism can mimic IPD, so it is important to establish if such medications have been used (especially drugs that block D_2 receptors, such as antipsychotics, metoclopramide, or phenothiazine antiemetics). Neurologic conditions that can be mistaken for IPD include atypical parkinsonisms (e.g., corticobasal ganglionic degeneration, multiple system atrophy, progressive supranuclear palsy) and essential tremor. Because the management and prognosis of IPD differs from these other conditions, an accurate diagnosis is important. When the diagnosis is in doubt, referral to a movement disorders specialist is recommended.

PRESENTATION OF IDIOPATHIC PARKINSON'S DISEASE

General Features

- For clinically probable IPD, the patient exhibits at least two of the following: resting tremor, rigidity, or bradykinesia. Asymmetric onset (unilaterality) of these features is usual.
- Postural instability (difficulty with maintaining balance) is more common in advanced IPD.

Motor Symptoms

- The patient experiences decreased manual dexterity, difficulty arising from a seated position, diminished arm swing during ambulation, dysarthria (slurred speech), dysphagia (difficulty with swallowing), festinating gait (tendency to pass from a walking to a running pace), flexed posture (axial, upper/lower extremities), "freezing" at initiation of movement, hypomimia (reduced facial animation), hypophonia (reduced voice volume), and micrographia (diminution of handwritten letters/symbols) (Fig. 61–3).

Autonomic and Sensory Symptoms

- The patient experiences bladder and anal sphincter disturbances, constipation, diaphoresis, fatigue, olfactory disturbance, orthostatic blood pressure changes, pain, paresthesia, paroxysmal vascular flushing, seborrhea, sexual dysfunction, and sialorrhea (drooling).

Mental Status Changes

- The patient experiences anxiety, apathy, bradyphrenia (slowness of thought processes), confusional state, dementia, depression, hallucinosis/psychosis (typically drug-induced), and sleep disorders (excessive daytime sleepiness, insomnia, obstructive sleep apnea, and rapid eye movement sleep behavior disorder).

Laboratory Tests

- No laboratory tests are available to diagnose IPD.

Other Diagnostic Tests

- Genetic testing is not routinely helpful.
- Neuroimaging may be useful for excluding other causes of parkinsonism.
- Medication history should be obtained to rule out drug-induced parkinsonism.

IPD develops insidiously and progressively worsens, although in some patients, clinical symptoms may remain stable for years. Over many years, symptoms may worsen to the point of severe disability, necessitating placement in a skilled nursing facility (especially with the development of dementia or frequent falling).

Tremor of an upper extremity occurring at rest (and occasionally a postural tremor) is often the sole presenting complaint; however, only two-thirds of patients with IPD have tremor on diagnosis, and some never develop this sign. Tremor in IPD is present most commonly in the hands, sometimes with a characteristic pill-rolling motion. Less commonly, tremor may involve the jaw, legs, and toes. Like other motor features of IPD, resting tremor often begins unilaterally and becomes bilateral with disease progression. Stressful or emotional (either negative or positive) situations often increase the tremor amplitude and severity. Usually, volitional movement abolishes resting tremor and it is absent during sleep. Although resting tremor is visibly noticeable in IPD and may cause social embarrassment for the patient, it often is the least physically disabling of the motor features.

Rigidity is the increased muscular resistance to passive range of motion and commonly affects the upper and lower extremities. If tremor is present in the affected extremity, the rigidity is associated with a cogwheel or ratchet-like quality upon examination. Facial muscles also are affected, resulting in hypomimia (masking of facial expressions) that may be erroneously interpreted as apathy, depression, or unfriendliness.

Bradykinesia refers to slowness of movement. Movement in IPD is often slow throughout an intended action, and difficulty with the initiation of movement also occurs. A progressive slowing and decline in dexterity may impair tasks such as finger tapping and handwriting (see Fig. 61–3). Intermittent immobility (*freezing*) is another common characteristic. Freezing is especially likely to occur in situations such as when walking through a narrow doorway or initiating a turn. Patients also may experience a slow shuffling gait with difficulty halting their steps while in motion (festinating gait).

Postural instability, most common in advanced stages of IPD, is one of the most disabling problems of IPD because it increases the fall risk and is least amenable to pharmacotherapy. Testing for impaired postural responses by means of the pull test (in which a patient is unable to recover balance after sudden backward displacement at the shoulders) can help to identify the risk for falling. Many patients with impaired postural responses also have tendencies for propulsive gait (festination) and freezing, which increases the risk of falling.

Although IPD is known predominantly as a disorder of motor capabilities, neuropsychiatric abnormalities also develop. Intellectual deterioration is not inevitable in IPD; however, some patients deteriorate in a manner indistinguishable from Alzheimer's disease and other dementing conditions.[17] IPD patients are also at increased risk for affective disorders such as anxiety and depression.[18] Although the disabilities of IPD may provoke depression in some instances, the biochemical changes in the brain associated with IPD also may predispose for endogenous depression.

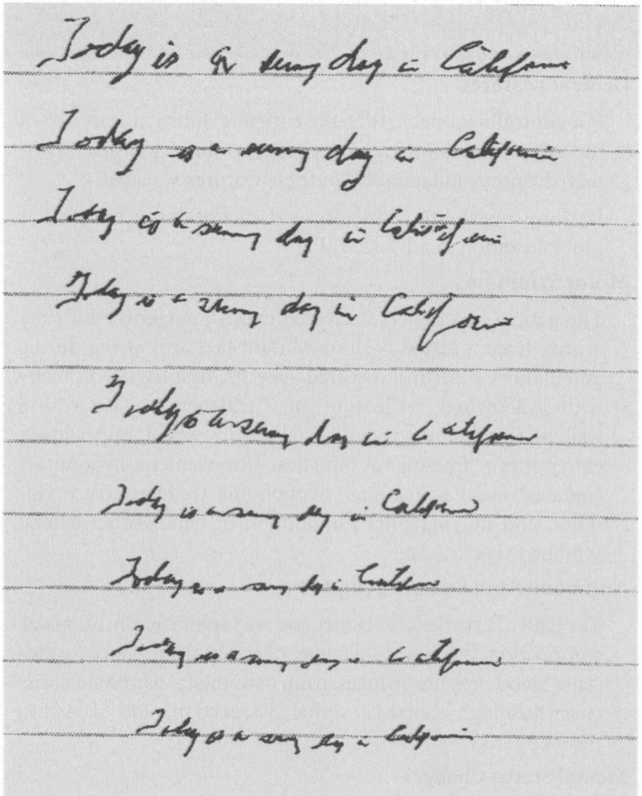

FIGURE 61-3. Example of micrographia in a patient with IPD. As the sentence, "Today is a sunny day in California" is repeatedly handwritten, progressive diminution of letter size occurs (micrographia). The height of each lined row is approximately 5/16 inches (8 mm). *(Courtesy of Jack J. Chen, PharmD, and David M. Swope, MD.)*

TREATMENT

Parkinson's Disease

DESIRED OUTCOMES

The goal in the management of IPD is to improve motor and nonmotor symptoms so that patients are able to maintain the best possible quality of life. Specific objectives to consider when selecting an intervention include preservation of function and ability to perform activities of daily living; improvement of mobility; minimization of adverse effects and treatment complications; and improvement of nonmotor features such as cognitive impairment, depression, fatigue, and sleep disorders. To accomplish some of these objectives, consultation with a specialist is helpful (e.g., movement disorders, physical therapy, psychiatry, sleep medicine).

GENERAL APPROACH TO TREATMENT

❶ Once a correct diagnosis of IPD is made, nonpharmacologic and pharmacologic interventions must be considered. Figure 61–4 illustrates a general treatment approach for early and advanced IPD and Tables 61–2 and 61–3 summarize antiparkinsonian medications and mechanisms of action. Treatment guidelines are updated frequently to keep up with new information and changes in treatment paradigms.[19–23] Clinically proven neuroprotective agents for IPD are not yet available, so the currently available pharmacologic therapies are referred to as symptomatic (i.e., used to improve motor symptoms of IPD).

❷ The definition of functional impairment is highly patient specific. Factors such as employment, lifestyle, and patients' desires must be considered when initiating pharmacotherapy. In general, initial monotherapy begins with a MAO-B inhibitor, or if the patient is "physiologically" young, a dopamine agonist. When additional

TABLE 61-2 Classification of Available Idiopathic Parkinson's Disease Treatments Based on Pharmacologic Mechanism[a]

Anticholinergic
Benztropine
Trihexyphenidyl
Dopamine precursor and augmentation
Levodopa
Inhibit peripheral dopa decarboxylase
Carbidopa
Inhibit catechol-*O*-methyl-transferase
Entacapone
Tolcapone
Inhibit monoamine oxidase type B
Rasagiline
Selegiline
Dopamine receptor agonists
Apomorphine
Bromocriptine
Pramipexole
Ropinirole
Rotigotine
Miscellaneous
Amantadine

[a]Marketed in the United States for idiopathic Parkinson's disease.

TABLE 61-3 Drugs Used in Parkinson's Disease

Generic Name	Trade Name	Dosage Range[a] (mg/day)	Dosage Forms (mg)
Anticholinergic drugs			
Benztropine	Cogentin	0.5–4	0.5, 1, 2
Trihexyphenidyl	Artane	1–6	2, 5
Carbidopa/levodopa products			
Carbidopa/L-dopa	Sinemet	300–1,000[b]	10/100, 25/100, 25/250
Carbidopa/L-dopa ODT	Parcopa	300–1,000[b]	10/100, 25/100, 25/250
Carbidopa/L-dopa CR	Sinemet CR	400–1,000[b]	25/100, 50/200
Carbidopa/L-dopa/entacapone	Stalevo	600–1,600[c]	12.5/50/200, 25/100/200, 37.5/150/200
Carbidopa	Lodosyn	25–75	25
Dopamine agonists			
Apomorphine	Apokyn	3–12	30 per 3 mL
Bromocriptine	Parlodel	15–40	2.5, 5
Pramipexole	Mirapex	1.5–4.5	0.125, 0.25, 0.5, 1, 1.5
Ropinirole	Requip	9–24	0.25, 0.5; 1, 2, 3, 4, 5
Rotigotine	Neupro	2–6	2, 4, 6
COMT inhibitors			
Entacapone	Comtan	200–1,600	200
Tolcapone	Tasmar	300–600	100, 200
MAO-B inhibitors			
Rasagiline	Azilect	0.5–1	0.5, 1
Selegiline	Eldepryl	5–10	5
Selegiline ODT	Zelapar	1.25–2.5	1.25, 2.5
Anticholinergic drugs			
Benztropine	Cogentin	0.5–4	0.5, 1, 2
Trihexyphenidyl	Artane	1–6	2, 5, 2/5 mL
Miscellaneous			
Amantadine	Symmetrel	200–300	100

COMT, catechol-*O*-methyltransferase; CR, controlled release; MAO, monoamine oxidase; ODT, orally disintegrating tablet.
[a]Dosages may vary beyond stated range.
[b]Dosages expressed as L-dopa component.
[c]Dosages expressed as entacapone component.

symptom relief is desired, addition of L-dopa should be considered. With the development of motor fluctuations, addition of a catechol-*O*-methyltransferase (COMT) inhibitor should be considered to extend L-dopa duration of activity, or if the patient is not already on a MAO-B inhibitor or dopamine agonist, addition of either one should be considered. For management of L-dopa induced dyskinesias, the addition of amantadine should be considered. Surgery is considered only in patients who need more symptomatic control or who are experiencing severe motor complications despite pharmacologically optimized therapy.

The treatment plan evolves as the disease progresses and must include consideration of short-term relief and long-term management. Factors that often guide selection of therapies include the "functional" age of the patient, cognitive status, severity of motor features, and response to any previous IPD therapies. Patient education should be communicated with realistic optimism. For example, it should be explained that although there is no cure for IPD, modern medicine has many medications that can provide relief of symptoms. Nonpharmacologic interventions such as exercise should be encouraged, and attention to nonmotor features of IPD should not be neglected.

PHARMACOLOGIC THERAPY

Anticholinergic Medications

❸ Because dopamine tonically inhibits acetylcholine neurons in the striatum, the degeneration of nigrostriatal dopamine neurons also results in a relative increase of striatal cholinergic interneuron activity. This increased cholinergic activity (caused by dopamine depletion) is believed to contribute to the tremor of IPD. The anticholinergic drugs (e.g., benztropine and trihexyphenidyl) are considered effective against tremor but not more so than dopaminergic agents.[19,20] Sometimes dystonic symptoms associated with IPD also will improve. Use of anticholinergic agents is limited because many patients develop intolerable side effects, necessitating dosage reduction or drug discontinuation. Common adverse effects include blurred vision, confusion, constipation, dry mouth, memory difficulty, sedation, and urinary retention. Younger patients are better able to tolerate anticholinergic side effects, whereas patients with preexisting cognitive deficits and advanced age are less tolerant. Anticholinergic drugs can be used alone or in conjunction with L-dopa and other antiparkinson agents.

Amantadine

❹ Amantadine provides modest symptomatic benefit. The precise mechanism of action of amantadine is unknown, but dopaminergic and nondopaminergic mechanisms, such as inhibition of glutamatergic *N*-methyl-D-aspartate (NMDA) receptors are implicated. Amantadine is typically administered 300 mg/day in divided doses. Amantadine is also useful for suppressing L-dopa–induced dyskinesia.[22] The antidyskinetic properties of amantadine are presumed to be mediated by antiglutamate mechanisms. Amantadine is eliminated renally and a reduced dose should be administered when renal dysfunction is present (100 mg/day with creatinine clearances of 30 to 50 mL/min, 100 mg every other day for creatinine clearances of 15 to 29 mL/min, and 200 mg every 7 days for creatinine clearances of less than 15 mL/min and patients on hemodialysis).

Common side effects of amantadine include confusion, dizziness, dry mouth, and hallucinations. The elderly are particularly prone to develop confusion. Not uncommonly, amantadine may cause livedo reticularis, a diffuse mottling of the skin occurs in the upper or lower extremities and often accompanied by lower-extremity edema.

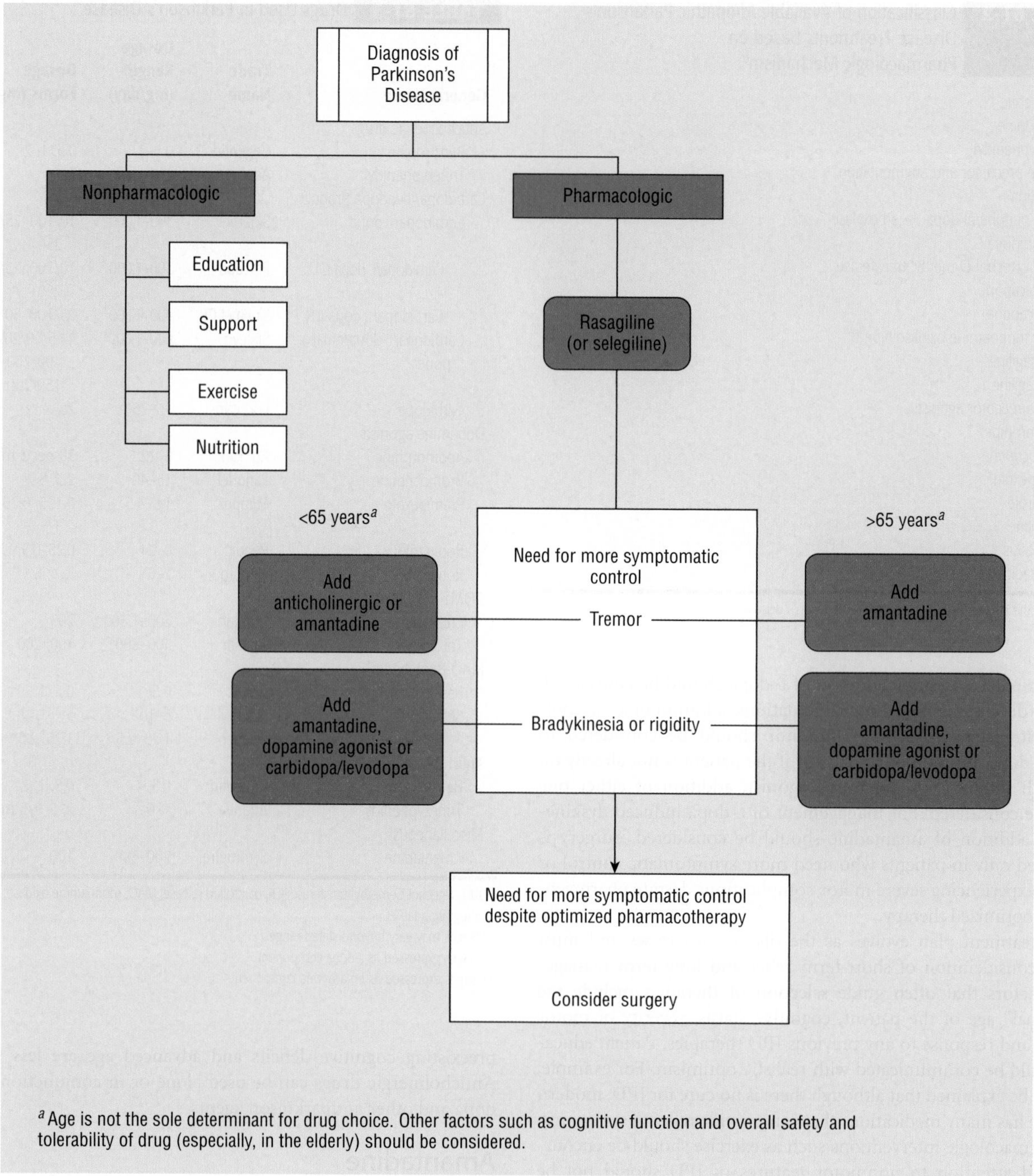

FIGURE 61-4. General approach to the management of early to advanced Parkinson's disease.

Carbidopa/L-Dopa

❺ L-Dopa is the immediate precursor of dopamine and, in combination with a peripherally acting L-amino acid decarboxylase inhibitor (carbidopa or benserazide), remains the most effective drug for the symptomatic treatment of IPD.[19,20] L-Dopa crosses the blood–brain barrier, whereas dopamine, carbidopa, and benserazide do not. The combination of L-dopa with carbidopa or benserazide, reduces the unwanted peripheral conversion of L-dopa to dopamine. As a result, increased amounts of L-dopa are transported into the brain, and peripheral adverse effects of dopamine, such as nausea, are reduced. In the SNc, L-dopa is converted, via decarboxylation, to dopamine by the enzyme L-amino acid decarboxylase (Fig. 61–5). The converted dopamine is stored in the presynaptic SNc neurons until stimulated to be released into the synaptic cleft where upon it binds to the D_1 and D_2 postsynaptic receptors. Dopamine activity is terminated primarily by reuptake back into the presynaptic neuron by means of a dopamine transporter. The enzymes MAO and COMT also inactivate dopamine.

❺ Regardless of what the initial therapeutic agent is, ultimately all patients with IPD will require L-dopa at some point. An initial maintenance L-dopa regimen of 300 mg/day (in divided doses and in combination with carbidopa or benserazide) often is adequate. With regards to carbidopa, about 75 mg/day is required to sufficiently inhibit the peripheral activity of L-amino acid decarboxylase, but some patients require more. Therefore the usual initial maintenance carbidopa/L-dopa regimen is 25/100 mg three times daily. As IPD progresses to more severe symptoms, use of higher dosages is required. There is no maximum allowable total daily L-dopa dose; however, the usual maximal dose needed by patients, even those with severe IPD, is 800 to 1,000 mg/day. Slow buildup of dose (e.g., increments of 100 mg L-dopa per week) can help to minimize treatment emergent side effects such as nausea, postural hypotension, sedation, vivid dreaming, and vomiting.

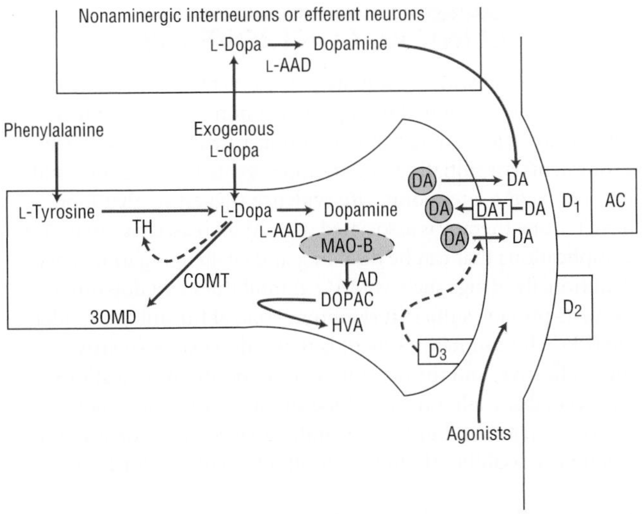

FIGURE 61-5. Dopamine metabolism in presynaptic dopamine neuron. (3OMD, 3-*O*-methyldopa; AC, adenylate cyclase; AD, aldehyde dehydrogenase; COMT, catechol-*O*-methyl transferase; D_1–D_3, dopamine receptors; DA, dopamine; DAT, dopamine transporter; DOPAC, 3,4-dihydroxyphenylacetic acid; HVA, homovanillic acid; L-AAD, L-aromatic amino acid decarboxylase; MAO-B, monoamine oxidase B; TH, tyrosine hydroxylase.)

TABLE 61-4 Common Motor Complications and Possible Treatments

Effect	Possible Treatments
End-of-dose "wearing off" (motor fluctuation)	Increase frequency of carbidopa/L-dopa doses; add either COMT inhibitor or MAO-B inhibitor or dopamine agonist; consider surgery
"Delayed on" or "no on" response	Give carbidopa/L-dopa on empty stomach; use carbidopa/L-dopa ODT; avoid carbidopa/L-dopa CR; use apomorphine subcutaneous; consider surgery
Start hesitation ("freezing")	Increase carbidopa/L-dopa dose; add a dopamine agonist or MAO-B inhibitor; utilize physiotherapy along with assistive walking devices or sensory cues (e.g., rhythmic commands, stepping over objects)
Peak-dose dyskinesia	Provide smaller doses of carbidopa/L-dopa; add amantadine; consider surgery

COMT, catechol-*O*-methyltransferase; CR, controlled release; MAO, monoamine oxidase; ODT, orally disintegrating tablet.

For patients with difficulty swallowing tablets, an orally disintegrating tablet preparation of carbidopa/L-dopa is available. Although this formulation rapidly dissolves on contact with saliva, the carbidopa/L-dopa does not undergo transmucosal absorption and must reach the proximal duodenum for absorption.

Pharmacokinetics There is marked intra- and intersubject variability in the time to peak plasma concentrations after oral L-dopa and this may in part be attributed to differences in gastric emptying. Meals delay gastric emptying, whereas antacids (which decrease gastric acidity) promote gastric emptying. L-Dopa is absorbed primarily in the proximal duodenum by a saturable large neutral amino acid transport system. Competition for this transporter by dietary or supplemental large neutral amino acids (e.g., leucine, phenylalanine) can interfere with L-dopa bioavailability.

L-Dopa is not bound to plasma proteins. Active transport across the blood–brain barrier occurs by the large neutral amino acid transporter system. Because large amounts of dietary large neutral amino acids may compete for transport across the blood–brain barrier and interfere with the clinical response to L-dopa, separation of L-dopa administration with high protein meals has been recommended. However, in patients with early IPD, this interaction is generally not significant. In advanced IPD, special diets involving protein restriction or redistribution may improve L-dopa responsiveness and are sometimes implemented. A metabolite of L-dopa, 3-*O*-methyldopa, also competes for transport, but it is not clear how this affects L-dopa clinical response.

When peripheral decarboxylation of L-dopa is inhibited by carbidopa or benserazide, 3-*O*-methylation (via COMT) becomes the predominant catabolic pathway. The elimination half-life of L-dopa is about 1 hour, and this is extended to about 1.5 hours with the addition of carbidopa or benserazide. With the addition of a COMT inhibitor such as entacapone to carbidopa/L-dopa, the elimination half-life is extended to about 2 to 2.5 hours.

❻ **Motor Complications of L-Dopa** Long-term L-dopa therapy is associated with a variety of motor complications, of which end-of-dose "wearing off" (motor fluctuations) and L-dopa peak-dose dyskinesias are the two most commonly encountered.[24] These motor complications can be disabling and challenging to manage. Approximately 10% of IPD patients will develop involuntary movements ment.[25,26] However, motor complications can occur by as few as 5 to 6 months after starting L-dopa therapy, especially if excessive doses are used initially.[27] Table 61–4 lists the motor complications associated with long-term treatment with carbidopa/L-dopa and suggested management strategies. Initiating therapy with the controlled-release form of carbidopa/L-dopa does not reduce the development of motor complications compared with standard-release carbidopa/L-dopa.[22]

❻ ***End-of-Dose Wearing Off.*** The terms "off" and "on" refer to periods of poor movement (i.e., return of tremor, rigidity, or slowness) and good movement, respectively. End-of-dose wearing off prior to a dose of medication is a common type of response fluctuation. This phenomenon is related to the increasing loss of neuronal storage capability for dopamine as well as the short half-life of L-dopa. Initially, exogenous L-dopa is taken up by the remaining presynaptic (SNc) neurons, converted to dopamine, and stored in synaptic vesicles. With progressive loss of presynaptic neurons, storage capacity, and synthesis of endogenously derived dopamine, patients become more dependent on exogenous L-dopa. Hence the peripheral pharmacokinetic properties of L-dopa increasingly become the determinant of central dopamine synthesis. With advancing IPD, the duration of action of a single carbidopa/L-dopa dose progressively shortens, and in some cases may produce benefits for as little as 1 hour. As a result, carbidopa/L-dopa needs to be given more frequently so as to minimize daytime off episodes and to maximize on time. In addition to administering L-dopa doses more frequently, other options are available (see Table 61–4). In particular, the addition of the COMT inhibitor entacapone or the MAO-B inhibitor rasagiline extends the action of L-dopa and either should be considered.[22]

Alternatively, an oral dopamine agonist also can be added to a carbidopa/L-dopa regimen in an attempt to minimize the occurrence of wearing off. A subcutaneously administered short-acting dopamine agonist, apomorphine, is also available and possesses a rapid onset of effect (within 20 minutes) and may be used, as needed, for relief from off states.[28] A controlled-release (CR) L-dopa product is available that can extend the duration of the carbidopa/L-dopa effect, but it is not considered very effective for management of motor fluctuation.[22] In addition, duodenal/jejunal L-dopa infusions produce constant and smoother stimulation of striatal dopamine receptors and thus stabilize response fluctuations.[29] Although some patients have been maintained on duodenal infusions for long periods of time, this invasive method of administration requires careful planning and is generally not used outside the research setting. If needed, sipping small amounts of carbidopa/L-dopa solution is an easier way to noninvasively titrate drug intake to optimal effect. A solution that is stable for 72 hours at room temperature can be prepared by adding 10 tablets of carbidopa/L-dopa 10/100 (or 25/100) mg and 2 g crystalline ascorbic acid to 1 L of water.[30]

Often, off episodes occur during the night, and patients will awaken in an off state (as a consequence of an overnight decline of drug levels). Bedtime administration of dopamine agonist or a drug formulation that provides sustained drug levels overnight (e.g., carbidopa/L-dopa CR, ropinirole CR, rotigotine transdermal patch) can help reduce nocturnal off episodes and improve functioning upon awakening.

"Delayed-On" and "No-On" Response. "Delayed-on" or "no-on" (drug-resistant off) responses to carbidopa/L-dopa can be a result of delayed gastric emptying or decreased absorption in the duodenum. Chewing a tablet or crushing it and then drinking a full glass of water, or using the orally disintegrating tablet formulation on an empty stomach, decreases gastric disintegration time and facilitates gastric emptying. Additionally, subcutaneously administered apomorphine may be used as rescue therapy from delayed-on or no-on periods. A drug-free period ("drug holiday") has been investigated in an attempt to modify postsynaptic dopamine receptors and thus decrease unpredictable off states. Although not commonly performed because of discomfort (to the patient) and medical risks, when drug holidays are performed, it should be under close medical supervision.

Freezing. "Freezing," or a sudden, episodic inhibition of lower-extremity motor function, may occur and will interfere with ambulation and increase the risk of falls. Patients may report that their "feet are stuck to the floor" and that they have difficulty initiating steps (start hesitation) or turns (turn hesitation). Freezing often is exacerbated by anxiety or when perceived obstacles (e.g., doorways, turnstiles) are encountered. Although changes to the antiparkinson drug regimen may be attempted, improvements are unlikely. Physiotherapy along with various specialized assistive walking devices and sensory cues are helpful.

Dyskinesias. Another complication of L-dopa therapy is "on" period dyskinesias (involuntary choreiform movements involving usually the neck, trunk, and lower/upper extremities). If patients report "shakiness," it is important to clarify if they are referring to tremor or dyskinesias. Dyskinesias usually are associated with peak striatal dopamine levels (peak dose dyskinesia) and, simplistically, can be thought of as too much movement secondary to extension of the pharmacologic effect or too much striatal dopamine receptor stimulation. Less commonly, dyskinesias also can develop during the rise and fall of L-dopa effects (the dyskinesia–improvement–dyskinesia or diphasic pattern of response). In the case of peak-dose dyskinesias, use of lower doses of L-dopa is often beneficial. With the lowering of the L-dopa dose, dyskinesias improve but at the cost of returning parkinsonian features, thereby necessitating an increase in dosage frequency or addition of another agent to counteract the effects of using a lower L-dopa dose. Glutamate overactivity may also be involved as suggested by the antidyskinesia effect of amantadine (NMDA receptor antagonist) and the investigational drug E2007 (α-amino-3-hydroxy-5-methyl-4-isoxazolepropionic acid [AMPA] receptor antagonist). For severe dyskinesias, surgery should be considered.

"Off-Period" Dystonia. In IPD, dystonias (sustained muscle contractions) occur more commonly in a distal lower extremity (e.g., the foot). In fact, clenching of the toes or involuntary turning of the foot can precede the development of IPD. Dystonias often occur in the early morning hours (as a result of waning drug levels) and improve with the first L-dopa dose of the day. Remedies for this problem include bedtime administration of sustained-release products (e.g., carbidopa/L-dopa CR, ropinirole CR, rotigotine transdermal patch), use of baclofen, or selective chemical denervation with injections of botulinum toxin.

CLINICAL CONTROVERSY

The question of when to initiate L-dopa therapy is a matter of debate. Generally, initial therapy with a non–L-dopa agent is often recommended for patients younger than 65 years of age. Proponents for initiating non–L-dopa agents first and then adding L-dopa at a later point, cite evidence suggesting that long-term L-dopa therapy is associated with an increased risk of motor complications that can be disabling and challenging to manage. Additionally, drugs such as MAO-B inhibitors and dopamine agonists provide sufficient symptom control for mild to moderate IPD. The counterargument is that L-dopa is inexpensive, more effective, and the development of motor complications is an acceptable trade-off. Age alone should not be the major deciding factor, and ultimately, individualized considerations of a patient's disability should guide all interventions for IPD.

Monoamine Oxidase B Inhibitors

❹ Two selective MAO-B type B inhibitors, rasagiline and selegiline, are available in the United States for management of IPD. The selective inhibition of MAO-B in the brain interferes with the degradation of dopamine and results in prolonged dopaminergic activity. Both drugs contain a propargylamine moiety, which is essential for conferring irreversible inhibition of MAO-B. At therapeutic doses, these agents preferentially inhibit MAO-B over MAO-A.

The most common concern with use of these agents is regarding interactions with food and other drugs. Practically speaking, at therapeutic doses, these selective MAO-B inhibitors are unlikely to induce a "cheese reaction" (transient hypertension, headache) unless excessive amounts of dietary tyramine (400 mg or greater) are ingested, unlike the nonselective MAO-A/B inhibitors, which require as little as 10 mg or less of dietary tyramine.[31] Additionally, the potential for a hypertensive effect resulting from concomitant administration of sympathomimetic agents (e.g., ephedrine, phenylephrine, pseudoephedrine) that are substrates for MAO-B is unknown, and these medications should be taken concurrently with caution. However, the risk of a severe hypertensive episode associated with occasional administration of nonprescription sympathomimetic agents (e.g., cold products, weight-reducing agents) appears to be minimal.[32]

Concomitant use of MAO-B inhibitors with meperidine and other selected analgesics is contraindicated because of a small risk of serotonin syndrome. Concomitant use of other agents that enhance serotonin levels (e.g., selective serotonin reuptake inhibitors, imipramine, clomipramine, lithium, sibutramine) is not contraindicated.

❹ ❼ Selegiline, also known as L-deprenyl, is marketed for extending L-dopa effects and is typically administered 5 mg twice daily. Selegiline is also available as an orally disintegrating tablet formulation administered 1.25 to 2.5 mg once daily. As monotherapy in early IPD, selegiline provides modest improvements in motor function.[19,20] In more advanced IPD, the adjunctive use of selegiline can provide up to a total of 1 hour of extended on time for patients with wearing off, although the data are inconsistent.[22] This inconsistent effect of conventional selegiline may be explained, in part, by poor and erratic bioavailability of the parent drug.

As an amphetamine pharmacophore, selegiline undergoes first-pass hepatic metabolism (predominantly via cytochrome P450 [CYP] 2B6 and 2C19) to end products of L-methamphetamine and L-amphetamine. Adverse effects of selegiline are minimal but can include insomnia (especially if administered at bedtime), hallucinations, and jitteriness. Selegiline also increases the peak effects of L-dopa and can worsen preexisting dyskinesias or psychiatric symptoms such as delusions. With the selegiline orally disintegrating tablet formulation, first-pass hepatic metabolism is bypassed as a consequence of transmucosal absorption of the drug. Hence, bioavailability characteristics of the parent drug are improved and formation of amphetamine metabolites is reduced. Thus, the selegiline orally disintegrating tablet formulation may provide an improved response relative to conventional selegiline.

❹ ❼ Rasagiline is a second-generation, irreversible, selective MAO-B inhibitor administered at 0.5 or 1 mg once daily. Rasagiline is effective as monotherapy in early IPD and also for managing motor fluctuations in advanced IPD. In a clinical trial, patients initiated on rasagiline monotherapy early in IPD had less functional decline than did patients whose treatment was delayed for 6 months.[33] This suggests that early initiation with rasagiline (perhaps even before the onset of functional impairment) is associated with better long-term outcomes. For the management of patients with motor fluctuations, the efficacy of rasagiline appears similar to that of entacapone, offering approximately 1 hour of extra on time during the day.[34] Consequently, when an adjunctive agent is required for managing motor fluctuations, rasagiline is considered a first-line agent (as is entacapone).[22] Overall, rasagiline is well tolerated and has an incidence of side effects similar to placebo in clinical studies. Rasagiline is metabolized by hepatic CYP1A2 to aminoindan, which is inactive and devoid of amphetamine-like properties.[31]

MAO-B inhibitors with a propargylamine molecular scaffolding have been investigated for neuroprotective properties. These agents inhibit the oxidative deamination of dopamine, which generates hydrogen peroxide and, ultimately, oxyradicals capable of damaging nigrostriatal neurons (see Fig. 61–1). Because MAO-B inhibition diverts dopamine catabolism to an alternate route that does not generate peroxide, MAO-B inhibitor therapy may spare neurons from oxidative stress. Additionally, MAO-B inhibitors have demonstrated antiapoptotic properties in laboratory experiments, further suggesting the possibility of clinical neuroprotection. A placebo-controlled study involving patients with early IPD suggests that rasagiline may provide positive disease-modifying effects when initiated early in the course of IPD, and additional studies are underway to replicate this.[33]

CLINICAL CONTROVERSY

Great interest and considerable controversy surrounds the putative neuroprotective effects of the MAO-B inhibitors. Although preliminary findings suggest that selegiline and rasagiline delay the development of disability in patients with IPD, to date neuroprotective effects have not been clearly shown. Research is underway to address this important question.

COMT Inhibitors

❼ Two COMT inhibitors, entacapone and tolcapone, have been developed to extend the effects from each dose of L-dopa and are indicated for managing wearing off.[22] Both reduce the peripheral conversion of L-dopa to dopamine, thus enhancing central L-dopa bioavailability. Consequently, in the absence of L-dopa, they have no effect on IPD symptoms. For patients with wearing off, these agents can decrease off time significantly by increasing the L-dopa area under the curve by approximately 35%.[35] COMT inhibition is considered more effective than controlled-release carbidopa/L-dopa in providing consistent extension of L-dopa effect.[22] A triple-combination product of carbidopa/ L-dopa/entacapone offers convenience for some patients (i.e., fewer tablets to administer).

Tolcapone inhibits both peripheral and central COMT. Its use is limited by reports of fatal hepatotoxicity, such that strict monitoring of hepatic function, especially during the first 6 months of therapy, is required. Informed consent should also be documented to ensure that patients are aware of this serious but rare adverse effect. Tolcapone is dosed at 100 to 200 mg three times per day. Because of the hepatotoxicity risk, tolcapone is reserved for patients with fluctuations that are not responding to other therapies. Additionally, delayed onset of diarrhea (weeks to months later) can occur in up to 5% of patients.

Entacapone has a shorter half-life than tolcapone, and 200 mg needs to be given with each dose of carbidopa/L-dopa up to a maximum of eight times per day. In clinical trials, both tolcapone and entacapone increased total daily on time by about 1 to 2 hours.[36,37] Dopaminergic adverse effects may occur and generally are manageable by reduction of the carbidopa/L-dopa dosage. Brownish-orange urinary discoloration may occur with both agents. Unlike tolcapone, entacapone is not associated with hepatotoxicity and, if an adjunctive agent is needed for managing motor fluctuations, entacapone is considered one of the first choices.[22]

Dopamine Agonists

Oral dopamine agonists fall into two pharmacologic subtypes: ergot-derived agonists (bromocriptine and pergolide) and the nonergot agonists (pramipexole, ropinirole, rotigotine). The nonergot dopamine agonists are safer than the ergot-derived agonists and are effective as monotherapy in mild-moderate IPD, and also as adjuncts to L-dopa therapy in patients with motor fluctuations.[19,20,22] The dopamine agonists reduce the frequency of off periods and may allow reductions in L-dopa dosage. Use of bromocriptine and pergolide have fallen by the wayside for several reasons. Bromocriptine is not commonly used because of an increased risk of pulmonary fibrosis and reduced efficacy compared to the other agonists.[38] Pergolide use is associated with development of cardiac valve fibrosis and valvular heart disease and is no longer available.[39]

❽ Investigations comparing initial monotherapy with either L-dopa or a dopamine agonists in patients with IPD have revealed a significantly reduced risk of developing motor complications associated with dopamine agonists than with L-dopa.[40,41] These findings have generated divergent opinions as to whether initial treatment of mild IPD should be with an oral dopamine agonist or L-dopa. Younger patients are more likely to develop motor fluctuations; consequently, dopamine agonists are preferred. Older patients are more likely to suffer intolerable side effects (e.g., hallucinations, orthostatic hypotension) from the dopamine agonists; consequently, carbidopa/L-dopa is preferred, particularly if cognitive problems or dementia is present.

Additionally, initial monotherapy with pramipexole or ropinirole is associated with a slower decline in imaging biomarkers of dopaminergic function compared with L-dopa monotherapy, suggesting neuroprotection.[42,43] However, these neuroimaging results are inconclusive because of several issues, including concerns regarding study methodology, accuracy of imaging biomarkers in the presence of dopaminergic agents, and lack of correlation between biomarker and motor function outcomes.

Common adverse effects of dopamine agonists include nausea, confusion, hallucinations, light-headedness, lower-extremity edema, postural hypotension, sedation, and vivid dreaming. Less common but serious adverse effects include compulsive behaviors (e.g., pathologic gambling or shopping), psychosis, and sleep attacks (sudden, unexpected episodes of sleep). Hallucinations and delusion can be managed using a stepwise approach (Table 61–5) that often involves the use of an atypical antipsychotic medication, such as clozapine or quetiapine.[18] The addition of a dopamine agonist to L-dopa therapy also can increase the frequency and severity of L-dopa induced dyskinesias, especially in patients with preexisting dyskinesias.

Initiation of a dopaminergic agonist is best performed by slow titration to minimize side effects. Pramipexole is initiated at a dose of 0.125 mg three times a day and increased every 5 to 7 days, as tolerated, to a maximum of 1.5 mg three times a day. Studies are

TABLE 61-5 Stepwise Approach to Management of Drug-Induced Hallucinosis and Psychosis in Parkinson's Disease

1. General measures such as evaluating for electrolyte disturbance (especially hypercalcemia or hyponatremia), hypoxemia, or infection (especially encephalitis, sepsis, or urinary tract infection).
2. Simplify the antiparkinsonian regimen as much as possible by discontinuing or reducing the dosage of medications with the highest risk-to-benefit ratio first.[a]
   a. Discontinue anticholinergics, including other nonparkinsonian medications with anticholinergic activity such as antihistamines or tricyclic antidepressants.
   b. Taper and discontinue amantadine.
   c. Discontinue monoamine oxidase-B inhibitor.
   d. Taper and discontinue dopamine agonist.
   e. Consider reduction of L-dopa (especially at the end of day) and discontinuation of catechol-*O*-methyltransferase inhibitors.
3. Consider atypical antipsychotic medication if disruptive hallucinosis or psychosis persists.
   a. Quetiapine 12.5–25 mg at bedtime; gradually increase by 25 mg each week if necessary, until hallucinosis or psychosis improved *or*
   b. Clozapine 12.5–50 mg at bedtime; gradually increase by 25 mg each week if necessary until hallucinosis or psychosis improved (requires frequent monitoring for leukopenia).

[a]If dosage reduction or medication discontinuation is either infeasible or undesirable, go to step 3.

underway to investigate the efficacy of twice-daily dosing in early IPD. Ropinirole is initiated at 0.25 mg three times a day and increased by 0.25 mg three times a day on a weekly basis to a maximum of 24 mg/day. A controlled-release ropinirole formulation for once-daily administration may soon be available.[44] Rotigotine is available as a transdermal patch for once-daily administration initiated at 2 mg/day and increased by 2 mg/day on a weekly basis to a maximum of 6 mg for early IPD. The patch formulation provides stable and consistent drug levels over a 24-hour period.

Pramipexole is renally excreted with an 8- to 12-hour half-life. The initial dosage must be adjusted in renal insufficiency (0.125 mg twice daily for creatinine clearances of 35 to 59 mL/min, 0.125 mg once daily for creatinine clearances of 15 to 34 mL/min). Ropinirole has a 6-hour half-life and is metabolized by CYP1A2. Potent inhibitors (e.g., fluoroquinolone antibiotics) and inducers (e.g., cigarette smoking) of this enzyme likely will lead to alterations in ropinirole clearance. Rotigotine is a highly lipophilic agent with a half-life of approximately 5 to 7 hours. The drug has poor oral bioavailability as a consequence of extensive hepatic first-pass metabolism, but is suitable for transdermal delivery. Application sites (e.g., abdomen, hip, shoulder, upper arm, upper thigh) should be rotated to minimize development of patch dermatitis. Because the transdermal delivery system ensures continuous drug delivery and sustained rotigotine levels over a 24-hour period, overnight symptomatic control is improved.[45]

Apomorphine is an injectable nonergot dopamine agonist. It is an aporphine alkaloid originally derived from morphine but lacks narcotic properties. Because of extensive hepatic first-pass metabolism, apomorphine is not suitable for oral administration and is administered subcutaneously. In some countries, apomorphine is also available for continuous subcutaneous injection with minipumps. Apomorphine should not be injected intravenously. For patients with advanced IPD who are experiencing intermittent off episodes despite optimized therapy, administration of subcutaneous apomorphine consistently and effectively triggers an "on" response within 20 minutes.[28] The effective dose ranges from 2 to 6 mg per injection, with most patients requiring approximately 0.06 mg/kg. Sites of injection (abdomen, upper arm, and upper thigh) should be rotated to avoid development of subcutaneous nodules. The route of apomorphine metabolism is unknown. Apomorphine elimination half-life is approximately 40 minutes, and the duration of benefit can be up to 100 minutes. These pharmacokinetic properties make apomorphine a suitable drug for intermittent, as-needed "rescue" administration. Nausea and vomiting are common side effects, and prior to the initiation of apomorphine, patients should be premedicated with the antiemetic trimethobenzamide. Other side effects include dizziness, hallucinations, injection-site irritation, orthostatic hypotension, somnolence, and yawning. As a consequence of reports of severe hypotension and syncope, apomorphine is contraindicated with drugs in the serotonin ($5HT_3$)-receptor blocker class, including dolasetron, granisetron, and ondansetron.

SURGICAL THERAPY

❾ Currently, surgery should be considered as an adjunct to pharmacotherapy when patients are experiencing frequent motor fluctuations or disabling dyskinesia or tremor despite an optimized medical regimen. There are several patient-selection criteria for surgery, including a diagnosis of L-dopa–responsive IPD. Anatomic targets include the thalamus, GPi, and the subthalamic nucleus. Bilateral, chronic, high-frequency electrical stimulation of a target site, also known as deep-brain stimulation (DBS), is the preferred surgical modality.[46]

In DBS surgery, a battery-powered neurostimulator (pacemaker-like device) is implanted subcutaneously below the clavicle and provides constant electrical stimulation, via electrode wires, to the targeted brain structure. Thalamic DBS is very effective for suppressing tremor in the long-term, but it does not significantly improve the other parkinsonian features (bradykinesia, rigidity, motor fluctuations, or dyskinesias). Although debatable, subthalamic nucleus DBS is favored over GPi DBS and is considered a more effective and durable surgical procedure. Subthalamic nucleus DBS is associated with improvements in tremor, rigidity, bradykinesia, motor fluctuations, and dyskinesia, as well as lowering of antiparkinsonian medications.

DBS procedures require adjustment of the electrical stimulation parameters (e.g., voltage, frequency, and pulse width) to achieve optimal control while minimizing side effects. The electrical stimulation parameters (or "electrical dosage") are adjusted via a programmable hand-held device to meet each patient's needs and are performed by trained individuals, including nurse practitioners, physicians, and clinical pharmacists.

Other surgical procedures that have been investigated include grafting or transplantation of human fetal mesencephalon tissue into the striatum.[47,48] This highly experimental procedure is based on the idea that dopaminergic neurons or neuroblasts can be used to replace or "restock" dopaminergic neurons that are lost in patients with IPD.

PHARMACOECONOMIC CONSIDERATIONS

Pharmacoeconomic assessments in IPD are important. IPD places a high economic burden on society.[49] Based on an estimated 1 million cases of IPD in the United States, the direct costs associated with IPD are in the range of $4 to $8 billion per year. If indirect costs, such as lost productivity, are included, the economic burden of IPD significantly increases. Patient-specific factors that influence the cost of IPD include age of symptom onset; level of disability; presence of motor complications, falls, and dementia; and need for skilled nursing. As the severity and level of disability increase, so do the costs associated with IPD. Likewise, the costs of treating patients with motor complications are considerably more than the costs of treating patients without motor complications. A similar trend applies for patients with hallucinations and psychosis who incur greater costs associated with nursing home placement.

Pharmacologic treatments that allow patients to maintain high functioning or reduce the development of motor complications would likely be cost-effective. Similarly, interventions or treatment approaches that slow disease progression (e.g., neuroprotection) are also likely to be cost-effective.

TABLE 61-6 Monitoring Parkinson's Disease Therapy

1. Monitor medication administration times. Educate the patient that immediate-release carbidopa/L-dopa is absorbed best on an empty stomach but is commonly taken with food to minimize nausea. Avoid administration of conventional selegiline in the late afternoon or evening to minimize insomnia.
2. Monitor to ensure that the patient and/or caregivers understand the prescribed medication regimen. For example, catechol-*O*-methyltransferase inhibitors work by enhancing the effect of L-dopa and that the patient should not discontinue medication without notifying the clinician.
3. Monitor and inquire specifically about dose-by-dose effects of medication, including response to doses of medication and the presence of dyskinesias, wearing-off effects, dizziness, nausea, or visual hallucinations. Offer suggestions to help alleviate these or encourage the patient to discuss with their clinician.
4. Monitor and inquire about concerns that caregivers may have about the patient, such as presence of abnormal behaviors, dyskinesias, falls, hallucinations, memory problems, mood changes, and sleep disorders.
5. Monitor for nonadherence and, if present, inquire for possible reasons (e.g., dosing convenience, financial issues, adverse effects) and offer suggestions.
6. Monitor for presence of drugs that can exacerbate idiopathic Parkinson's disease motor features (e.g., D_2 receptor blockers) or if the presence of an anticholinergic agent is causing cognitive impairment.

EVALUATION OF THERAPEUTIC OUTCOMES

Table 61–6 lists the monitoring parameters for Parkinson's disease therapy. It is important to educate patients and caregivers that IPD is a neurodegenerative disease that progresses with time and that some features respond less well to pharmacotherapy (e.g., freezing, postural instability). Patients and caregivers can participate in treatment by recording medication administration times as well as the duration of on and off times that can be reviewed at each visit.

Periodic review of all medications that the patient is taking should be performed to identify use of medications (e.g., D_2-receptor blockers) that can exacerbate IPD motor features. If the patient reports memory problems, the medication profile should be screened for medications with anticholinergic properties and, if present, eliminated when possible. Assessment of the patient's general level of functioning, including activities of daily living, is important to determine when medication adjustments are needed. Screening for anxiety or depressive disorders will help to determine if antidepressant or antianxiety therapy is needed. If falling is a problem, it is important to investigate whether falls are secondary to insufficient motor control or drug side effects such as dizziness and orthostatic hypotension. The former may necessitate an increase in dose of antiparkinson agents, and the latter a reduction in drug dosage. Physical therapy is also helpful for strengthening ambulation and balance skills to minimize falls. The patient should be questioned about any difficulties with their antiparkinson medications, including presence of adverse effects. Recommendations always should be made in view of the patient's perception of the severity of symptoms and effect on quality of life.

CONCLUSIONS

❶ Despite many advances in neuroscience, a universal definitive cause of IPD remains unknown, and the identification of disease-modifying (neuroprotective) therapies remains elusive. The available therapies are symptomatic and include a number of drugs for early and later stages of the disease. Pharmacotherapy can significantly improve a patient's quality of life and functional status. The goal of management remains maintaining acceptable functional control with minimal treatment emergent complications. Thoughtful consideration for choice of initial and adjunctive therapy is critical for optimizing short- and long-term outcomes.

ABBREVIATIONS

COMT: catechol-*O*-methyl-transferase

CR: controlled release

DBS: deep-brain stimulation

GABA: γ-aminobutyric acid

GPi: globus pallidus interna

IPD: idiopathic Parkinson's disease

L-dopa: levodopa

MAO: monoamine oxidase

MPP^+: 1-methyl-4-phenylpyridinium

MPTP: 1-methyl-4-phenyl-1,2,3,6-tetrahydropyridine

NMDA: *N*-methyl-D-aspartate

SNc: substantia nigra pars compacta

REFERENCES

1. Parkinson J. An essay on the shaking palsy. London: Sherwood, Neely, and Jones, 1817:1–66.
2. Van Den Eeden SK, Tanner CM, Bernstein AL, et al. Incidence of Parkinson's disease: Variation by age, gender, and race/ethnicity. Am J Epidemiol 2003;157:1015–1022.
3. Twelves D, Perkins KSM, Counsell C. Systematic review of incidence studies of Parkinson's disease. Mov Disord 2003;18:19–31.
4. Moore DJ, West AB, Dawson VL, et al. Molecular pathophysiology of Parkinson's disease. Annu Rev Neurosci 2005;28:57–87.
5. Braak H, Del Tredici K, Rub U, et al. Staging of brain pathology related to sporadic Parkinson's disease. Neurobiol Aging 2003;24:197–211.
6. Gerlach M, Riederer P, Przuntek H, et al. MPTP mechanisms of neurotoxicity and their implications for Parkinson's disease. Eur J Pharmacol 1991:208:273–286.
7. Gorell JM, Johnston CC, Rybicki BA, et al. Occupational exposures to metals as risk factors for Parkinson's disease. Neurology 1997;48:650–658.
8. Di Monte DA. The environment and Parkinson's disease: Is the nigrostriatal system preferentially targeted by neurotoxins? Lancet Neurol 2003;2:531–533.
9. Logroscino G. The role of early life environmental risk factors in Parkinson disease: What is the evidence? Environ Health Perspect 2005;113(9):1234–1238.
10. Jenner P. Oxidative stress in Parkinson's disease. Ann Neurol 2003;53(Suppl 3):S26–S38.
11. Hofer A, Gasser T. New aspects of genetic contributions to Parkinson's disease. J Mol Neurosci 2004;24:417–424.
12. Hardy J, Cai H, Cookson MR, et al. Genetics of Parkinson's disease and parkinsonism. Ann Neurol 2006;60:389–398.
13. Bernheimer H, Birkmayer W, Hornykiewicz O, et al. Brain dopamine and the syndromes of Parkinson's and Huntington: Clinical, morphological, and neurochemical correlations. J Neurol Sci 1973;20:415–455.
14. Smith Y, Bevan MD, Shink E, Bolam JP. Microcircuitry of the direct and indirect pathways of the basal ganglia. Neuroscience 1998;86:353–387.
15. Schapira AH, Bezard E, Brotchie J, et al. Novel pharmacological targets for the treatment of Parkinson's disease. Nat Rev Drug Discov 2006;5:845–854.
16. Gelb DJ, Oliver E, Gilman S. Diagnostic criteria for Parkinson disease. Arch Neurol 1999;56:33–39.
17. Emre M. Dementia associated with Parkinson's disease. Lancet Neurol 2003;2:229–237.
18. Chen JJ. Anxiety, depression, and psychosis in Parkinson's disease: Unmet needs and treatment challenges. Neurol Clin 2004;22(3 Suppl):S63–S90.
19. Management of Parkinson's disease: An evidence-based review. Mov Disord 2002;17 Suppl 4:S1–S166.
20. Miyasaki JM, Martin W, Suchowersky O, et al. Practice parameter: Initiation of treatment for Parkinson's disease: An evidence based review. Report of the Quality Standards Subcommittee of the American Academy of Neurology. Neurology 2002:58;11–17.

21. Suchowersky O, Gronseth G, Perlmutter J, et al. Quality Standards Subcommittee of the American Academy of Neurology. Practice Parameter: Neuroprotective strategies and alternative therapies for Parkinson disease (an evidence-based review): Report of the Quality Standards Subcommittee of the American Academy of Neurology. Neurology 2006;66:976–982.
22. Pahwa R, Factor SA, Lyons KE, et al. Quality Standards Subcommittee of the American Academy of Neurology. Practice Parameter: Treatment of Parkinson disease with motor fluctuations and dyskinesia (an evidence-based review): Report of the Quality Standards Subcommittee of the American Academy of Neurology. Neurology 2006;66:983–995.
23. Miyasaki JM, Shannon K, Voon V, et al. Quality Standards Subcommittee of the American Academy of Neurology. Practice Parameter: Evaluation and treatment of depression, psychosis, and dementia in Parkinson disease (an evidence-based review): Report of the Quality Standards Subcommittee of the American Academy of Neurology. Neurology 2006;66:996–1002.
24. Hauser RA, McDermott MP, Messing S. Factors associated with the development of motor fluctuations and dyskinesias in Parkinson disease. Arch Neurol 2006;63:1756–1760.
25. Stocchi F. Prevention and treatment of motor complications. Parkinsonism Relat Disord 2003;9(Suppl 2):S73–S81.
26. Pahwa R, Lyons KE. Options in the treatment of motor fluctuations and dyskinesias in Parkinson's disease: A brief review. Neurol Clin 2004;22(3 Suppl):S35–S52.
27. Parkinson Study Group. Levodopa and the progression of Parkinson's disease. N Engl J Med 2004;351:2498–2508.
28. Chen JJ, Obering C. Apomorphine in the management of motor fluctuations associated with Parkinson's disease. Clin Ther 2005;27;1710–1724.
29. Kurth MC. Using liquid levodopa in the treatment of Parkinson's disease. A practical guide. Drugs Aging 1997;10:332–333.
30. Pappert EJ, Buhrfiend C, Lipton JW, et al. Levodopa stability in solution: Time course, environmental effects, and practical recommendations for clinical use. Mov Disord 1996;11:24–26.
31. Chen JJ, Swope D. Clinical pharmacology of rasagiline: A novel, second-generation propargylamine for the treatment of Parkinson disease. J Clin Pharmacol 2005;45:878–894.
32. Jacob JE, Wagner ML, Sage JI. Safety of selegiline with cold medications. Ann Pharmacother 2003;37:438–441.
33. Parkinson Study Group. A controlled, randomized, delayed-start study of rasagiline in early Parkinson disease. Arch Neurol 2004;61:561–566.
34. Rascol O, Brooks DJ, Melamed E, et al. Rasagiline as an adjunct to levodopa in patients with Parkinson's disease and motor fluctuations (LARGO, Lasting effect in Adjunct therapy with Rasagiline Given Once daily, study): A randomised, double-blind, parallel-group trial. Lancet 2005;365:947–954.
35. Ruottinen HM, Rinne UK. COMT inhibition in the treatment of Parkinson's disease. J Neurol 1998;245(suppl 3):25–34.
36. Holm KJ, Spencer CM. Entacapone: A review of its use in Parkinson's disease. Drugs 1999;58:159–177.
37. Keating GM, Lyseng-Williamson KA. Tolcapone. A review of its use in the management of Parkinson's disease. CNS Drugs 2005;19:165–184.
38. McElvaney NG, Wilcox PG, Churg A, et al. Pleuropulmonary disease during bromocriptine treatment of Parkinson's disease. Arch Intern Med 1998;148:2231–2236.
39. Zanettini R, Antonini A, Gatto G, et al. Valvular heart disease and the use of dopamine agonists for Parkinson's disease. N Engl J Med 2007;356:39–46.
40. Rascol O, Brooks DJ, Korczyn AD, et al. A five-year study of the incidence of dyskinesia in patients with early Parkinson's disease who were treated with ropinirole or levodopa. 056 Study Group. N Engl J Med 2000;342:1484–1491.
41. Parkinson Study Group. Pramipexole vs levodopa as initial treatment for Parkinson disease: A 4-year randomized controlled trial. Arch Neurol 2004;61:1044–1053.
42. Parkinson Study Group. Dopamine transporter brain imaging to assess the effects of pramipexole vs levodopa on Parkinson disease progression. JAMA 2002;287:1653–1661.
43. Whone AL, Watts RL, Stoessl AJ. Slower progression in early Parkinson's disease treated with ropinirole vs levodopa: The REAL-PET study. Ann Neurol 2003;54:93–101.
44. Pahwa R, Stacy MA, Factor SA, et al. Ropinirole 24-hour prolonged release: Randomized, controlled study in advanced Parkinson disease. Neurology 2007;68:1108–1115.
45. LeWitt PA, Lyons KE, Pahwa R, et al. Advanced Parkinson disease treated with rotigotine transdermal system: PREFER Study. Neurology 2007;68:1262–1267.
46. Walter BL, Vitek JL. Surgical treatment for Parkinson's disease. Lancet Neurol 2004;3:719–728.
47. Freed CR, Green PE, Breeze RE, et al. Transplantation of embryonic dopamine neurons for severe Parkinson's disease. N Engl J Med 2001;344:710–719.
48. Olanow CW, Goetz CG, Kordower JH, et al. A double-blind controlled trial of bilateral fetal nigral transplantation in Parkinson's disease. Ann Neurol 2003;54:403–414.
49. Dowding CH. Shenton CL, Salek SS. A review of the health-related quality of life and economic impact of Parkinson's disease. Drugs Aging 2006;23:693–721.

CHAPTER 62

Pain Management

TERRY J. BAUMANN AND JENNIFER STRICKLAND

KEY CONCEPTS

1. It is important, whenever possible, to ask patients if they have pain, to identify the source of pain, and to assess the characteristics of the pain.
2. Patients taking analgesics should be monitored for response and side effects, particularly sedation and constipation associated with the opioids.
3. Oral analgesics are preferred over other dosage forms whenever feasible, but it is important to adjust the route of administration to the needs of the patient.
4. Equianalgesic doses are useful as a guide when converting from one agent to another, but further dose titration usually is required to achieve treatment goals.
5. Doses must be individualized for each patient and administered for an adequate duration of time. Around-the-clock regimens should be considered for acute and chronic pain. As-needed regimens should be used for breakthrough pain or when acute pain displays wide variability and/or has subsided greatly.
6. For chronic pain that has a maladaptive inflammatory and/or neuropathic component, anticonvulsants, tricyclic antidepressants, and opioids should be considered.
7. Whenever possible, a multidisciplinary approach and nonpharmacologic strategies should be used.
8. Placebo therapy should not be used as an attempt to diagnose psychogenic pain.

Although the world is full of suffering, it is also full of the overcoming of it.

Helen Keller[1]

Humans have always known and sought relief from pain.[2] The act of relieving pain probably is as old as the medical profession itself. Today, pain's impact on society still is great, and indeed pain complaints remain a primary reason patients seek medical advice.[3]

Regrettably, many healthcare providers do not receive adequate training in this area, and new information is not widely disseminated and/or understood. Clearly, pain management is enhanced when a multidisciplinary approach is applied. Thus, understanding the pathophysiology of pain therapy and maintaining a working knowledge of individual pain regimens are important key factors in addressing pain control.

Learning objectives, review questions, and other resources can be found at **www.pharmacotherapyonline.com.**

DEFINITION

An acceptable definition of pain remains an enigma. Once thought to be a punishment from the gods, the word is derived from the Latin *peone* and the Greek *poine,* meaning "penalty" or "punishment."[2] Aristotle considered pain a feeling and classified it as a passion of the soul, where the heart was the source or processing center of pain.[2] This Aristotelian concept predominated for 2,000 years, although Descartes, Galen, and Vesalius postulated that pain was a sensation in which the brain played an important role. In the 19th century, Mueller, Van Frey, and Goldscheider hypothesized the concepts of neuroreceptors, nociceptors, and sensory input.[2] These theories developed into the current definition of pain: "an unpleasant sensory and emotional experience associated with actual or potential tissue damage or described in terms of such damage."[4] Pain often is so subjective, however, that many clinicians define pain as whatever the patient says it is. The best care is achieved when the patient comes first.[5]

EPIDEMIOLOGY

Fifty million Americans are partially or totally disabled because of pain.[3] The annual cost of pain to U.S. society can be estimated to be in the billions of dollars.[6] In 1 year, an estimated 25 million Americans will experience acute pain due to injury or surgery, and one third of Americans will experience severe chronic pain at some point in their lives.[7] These numbers are expected to rise, as increasingly more Americans work beyond age 60 years and survive into their 80s.[6]

Unfortunately, pain often remains undertreated in hospitals, long-term care facilities, and the community. Seriously ill hospitalized patients have reported a 50% incidence of pain; 15% had extremely or moderately severe pain occurring at least 50% of the time, and 15% were dissatisfied with overall pain control.[8] In a followup report, the authors state that pain control persists as a major problem in hospitalized patients, and some of these patients were still in pain many months after hospitalization and experienced pain even on their deathbeds.[9] In addition, problems with inadequate use of analgesics have been reported in cancer patients residing in nursing homes.[10] In the Michigan pain study, 70% of chronic pain patients claimed to have pain despite treatment, with 22% believing that treatment worsened pain.[6]

PATHOPHYSIOLOGY

The pathophysiology of pain involves a complex array of neural networks in the brain that are acted on by afferent stimuli to produce the experience we know as pain. In acute pain, this modulation is short-lived, but in some situations, the changes may persist, and chronic pain develops.[11,12]

NOCICEPTIVE PAIN

Nociceptive pain typically is classified as either somatic (arising from skin, bone, joint, muscle, or connective tissue) or visceral (arising from internal organs such as the large intestine or pancreas).[13] Whereas somatic pain most often presents as throbbing and well localized, visceral pain can manifest as pain feeling as if it is coming from other structures (referred) or as a well-localized phenomenon.[13] We can think of nociception in terms of stimulation, transmission, perception, modulation,[13] and adaptive inflammation.[12]

Stimulation

The first step leading to the sensation of pain is stimulation of free nerve endings known as *nociceptors.* These receptors are found in both somatic and visceral structures. They distinguish between noxious and innocuous stimuli, and they are activated and sensitized by mechanical, thermal, and chemical impulses.[13] The underlying mechanism of these noxious stimuli (which in and of themselves may sensitize/stimulate the receptor) may be the release of bradykinins, potassium ion (K^+), prostaglandins, histamine, leukotrienes, serotonin, and substance P (among others) that sensitize and/or activate the nociceptors.[14,15] Receptor activation leads to action potentials that are transmitted along afferent nerve fibers to the spinal cord (Fig. 62–1).[13]

Transmission

Nociceptive transmission takes place in Aδ and C-afferent nerve fibers.[13] Stimulation of large-diameter, sparsely myelinated Aδ fibers evokes sharp, well-localized pain, whereas stimulation of unmyelinated, small-diameter C fibers produces dull, aching, poorly localized pain.[13]

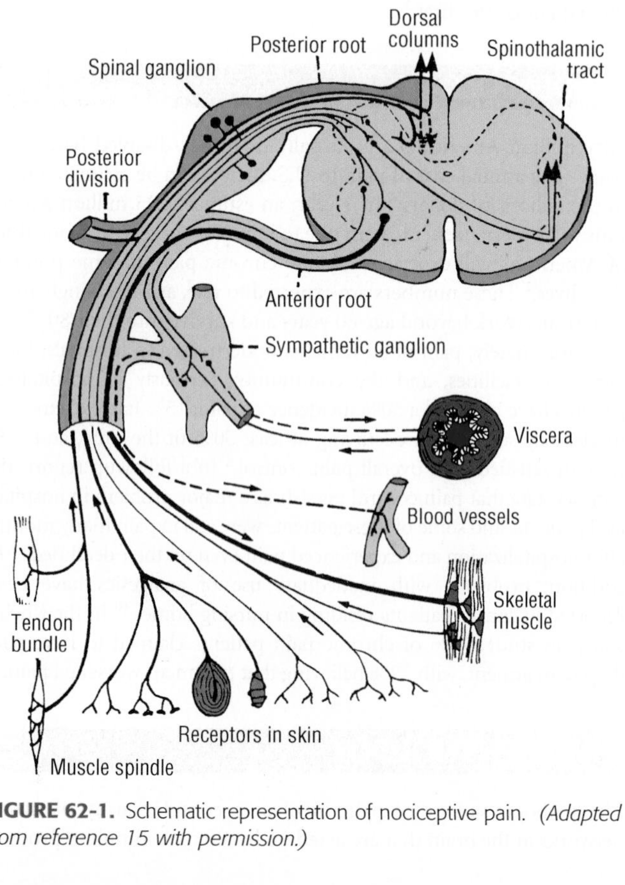

FIGURE 62-1. Schematic representation of nociceptive pain. *(Adapted from reference 15 with permission.)*

These afferent, nociceptive pain fibers synapse in various layers (laminae) of the spinal cord's dorsal horn,[15] releasing a variety of neurotransmitters, including glutamate, substance P, and calcitonin gene–related peptide.[16] The complex array of events that influence pain can be explained in part by the interactions between neuroreceptors and neurotransmitters that take place in this synapse. For example, by stimulating large sensory myelinated fibers (e.g., Aβ) that mutually connect in the dorsal horn with pain fibers, both noxious and nonnoxious stimuli can have an inhibitory effect on pain transmission (Fig. 62–1).[17] Functionally, the importance of the interplay between these different fibers and various neurotransmitters and neuroreceptors is evident in the analgesic response produced by topical irritants or transcutaneous electrical nerve stimulation. These pain-initiated processes reach the brain through a complex array of at least five ascending spinal cord pathways, which include the spinothalamic tract.[18] Information other than pain is also carried along these pathways. Thus, pain is influenced by many factors supplemental to nociception and precludes simple schematic representation. It is postulated that the thalamus acts as a relay station, as these pathways ascend and passs the impulses to central structures where pain can be processed further.[13]

Pain Perception

At this point in transmission, pain is thought to become a conscious experience that takes place in higher cortical structures. The brain may accommodate only a limited number of pain signals, and cognitive and behavioral functions can modify pain. Relaxation, distraction, meditation, and guided mental imagery may decrease pain by limiting the number of processed pain signals.[13] In contrast, a change in our neurobiochemical makeup that results in states such as depression or anxiety may worsen pain.

Modulation

The body modulates pain through a number of complex processes. One, known as the *endogenous opiate system,* consists of neurotransmitters (e.g., enkephalins, dynorphins, and β-endorphins) and receptors (e.g., μ, δ, and κ) that are found throughout the central nervous system (CNS).[18] Like exogenous opioids, endogenous opioids bind to opioid receptor sites and modulate the transmission of pain impulses.[13] Other receptor types also can influence this system. Activation of *N*-methyl-D-aspartate (NMDA) receptors, found in the dorsal horn, can decrease the μ-receptors' responsiveness to opiates.[18]

The CNS also contains a highly organized descending system for control of pain transmission. This system can inhibit synaptic pain transmission at the dorsal horn and originates in the brain.[13] Important neurotransmitters here include endogenous opioids, serotonin, norepinephrine, γ-aminobutyric acid (GABA), and neurotensin.[13]

Adaptive Inflammation

Inflammatory pain can be thought of as the body's shifting from preventing tissue damage to the promotion of healing (e.g., surgical wounds, traumatic injury). As a result of the inflammatory process, the pain threshold is reduced and the injured area becomes more sensitive to pain. This process decreases our contact with and movement of the injured area, thus promoting the progression of healing.[12] When this course of action outlives its functionality or when it is caused by diseases such as arthritis, it can move from an acute to a chronic problem (maladaptive inflammation).[12] "In response to tissue damage and inflammation, a significant alteration occurs in the chemical composition and properties of the neurons that innervate the inflamed tissues. These alterations reflect the nature and levels of the different proteins expressed by the sensory neurons. Altered production of these proteins may modify the phenotypes of the neurons, changing their transduction and transmission properties. Inflammatory pain is also associated with an increase in the excitability or responsiveness of neurons within the CNS, referred to as *central sensitization.* This phenomenon, like peripheral sensitization, is a major cause of hypersensitivity to pain after injury."[19]

NEUROPATHIC PAIN/FUNCTIONAL PAIN

Neuropathic and functional pain is distinctly different from nociceptive pain in that it becomes disengaged from noxious stimuli or healing[12] and often is described in terms of chronic pain. Neuropathic pain is a result of nerve damage, whereas functional pain can be thought of as abnormal operation of the nervous system.[12] A number of neuropathic pain syndromes (e.g., postherpetic neuralgia, diabetic neuropathy) and functional pain syndromes (e.g., fibromyalgia, irritable bowel syndrome, sympathetic induced pain, tension-type headaches, and some noncardiac chest pain)[12] exist. They often are underrecognized and difficult to treat.[13] In addition, the pain reported often is not evident by examining physical findings.[13]

The mechanism responsible for neuropathic and functional pain may be the nervous system's endogenous dynamic nature. Nerve damage or certain disease states may evoke changes seen in inflammatory pain, ectopic excitability, enhanced sensory transmission, nerve structure reorganization, and loss of modulatory pain inhibition.[12,19] Pain circuits rewire themselves both anatomically and biochemically.[16] This produces spontaneous nerve stimulation, autonomic neuronal pain stimulation, and a progressive increase in the discharge of dorsal horn neurons.[13,16]

Clinically, patients present with spontaneous pain transmission (often described as burning, tingling, shock-like, or shooting), exaggerated painful response to normally noxious stimuli (hyperalgesia), and/or painful response to normally nonnoxious stimuli (allodynia).[13,20] This change over time may help to explain why this type of pain often manifests long after the actual nerve-related injury or when no actual injury is identified.

CLASSIFICATION OF PAIN

ACUTE PAIN

Acute pain can be a useful physiologic process warning individuals of disease states and potentially harmful situations. Unfortunately, severe, unremitting, undertreated, acute pain, when it outlives its biologic usefulness, can produce many deleterious effects (e.g., psychological problems). Acute pain usually is nociceptive, although it can be neuropathic in nature, with a relatively strong relationship to levels of pathology.[7] Common causes of acute pain include surgery, acute illness, trauma, labor, and medical procedures.[7]

CHRONIC PAIN

Under normal conditions, acute pain subsides quickly as the healing process decreases the pain-producing stimuli; however, in some instances, pain persists for months to years, leading to a chronic pain state with features quite different from those of acute pain (Table 62–1). This type of pain can be nociceptive, neuropathic/functional, or both.[7] Subtypes include: pain that persists beyond the normal healing time for an acute injury (e.g., complex regional pain syndrome), pain related to a chronic disease (e.g., pain secondary to osteoarthritis), pain without an identifiable organic cause (e.g., fibromyalgia), and a fourth type that many experts believe warrants a discrete classification,[7] pain associated with cancer.[21]

CANCER PAIN

Pain associated with potentially life-threatening conditions is often called malignant pain or simply cancer pain.[7] This type of pain includes both chronic and acute components and often has multiple etiologies. It is pain caused by the disease itself (e.g., tumor invasion, organ obstruction), treatment (e.g., chemotherapy, radiation, surgical incisions), or diagnostic procedures (e.g., biopsy).[7]

TABLE 62-1 Characteristics of Acute and Chronic Pain

Characteristic	Acute Pain	Chronic Pain
Relief of pain	Highly desirable	Highly desirable
Dependence and tolerance to medication	Unusual	Common
Psychological component	Usually not present	Often a major problem
Organic cause	Common	Often not present
Environmental/family issues	Small	Significant
Insomnia	Unusual	Common component
Treatment goal	Cure	Functionality
Depression	Uncommon	Common

Data from Stimmel[2] and Jacobson and Mariano.[68]

CLINICAL PRESENTATION

Clinical presentation of pain is best addressed by proper pain assessment. A patient-oriented approach is essential, and evaluation methods should not differ from those used in other medical conditions.[2] Therefore, a comprehensive history and physical examination are imperative to evaluate underlying diseases and possible ❶ contributing factors.[2] This includes identifying the source of pain when possible.[2] A baseline characterization of pain can be obtained by assessing PQRST characteristics (Table 62–2).[22] Attention also must be given to mental/emotional factors that alter the pain threshold. Anxiety, depression, fatigue, anger, and fear in particular are noted to lower this threshold, whereas rest, mood elevation, sympathy, diversion, and understanding raise the pain threshold.[22]

Clinicians must evaluate all components of the pain experience, e.g., behavioral (part of our reaction to pain is learned),[23] cognitive (thinking processes alter pain experiences),[24] social (pain expression differs in accordance with social environments),[25] and cultural (cultural background may influence pain tolerance).[25] In addition, separating chronic pain from acute pain allows for improved treatment regimens. Acute pain often is localized, well described, and relieved with conventional analgesic therapy (e.g., opioids, acetaminophen, nonsteroidal antiinflammatory drugs [NSAIDs]), whereas chronic pain many times is not well recognized and is not easily treated with conventional analgesics. ❷ Proper patient assessment must include an evaluation of pain management. Pain intensity, pain relief, and medication side effects (e.g., opioid-induced sedation or constipation) must be assessed and reassessed on a regular basis. The timing and regularity of this assessment will depend on the type of pain and the medications administered. Postoperative pain and acute exacerbation of cancer pain may need to be assessed hourly, whereas chronic noncancer pain may require only daily or less frequent assessment. Pain intensity assessment is vital in acute pain,

TABLE 62-2 PQRST Characteristics of Pain

P	Palliative factors	What makes the pain better?
	Provocative factors	What makes the pain worse?
Q	Quality	Describe the pain.
R	Radiation	Where is the pain?
S	Severity/intensity	How does this pain compare with other pain you have experienced?
T	Temporal factors	Does the intensity of the pain change with time?

Data from Twycross.[22]

CLINICAL PRESENTATION OF PAIN

Acute

General

- Often obvious distress (e.g., trauma)

Symptoms

- Can be described as sharp, dull, shock-like, tingling, shooting, radiating, fluctuating in intensity, and varying in location (these occur in a timely relationship with an obvious noxious stimuli)

Signs

- Hypertension, tachycardia, diaphoresis, mydriasis, and pallor, but these signs are *not diagnostic*
- In some cases there are no obvious signs
- Comorbid conditions usually not present
- Outcome of treatment generally predictable

Laboratory Tests

- Pain is always subjective
- There are *no* specific laboratory tests for pain
- Pain is best diagnosed based on patient description and history

Chronic

General

- Can appear to have no noticeable suffering

Symptoms

- Can be described as sharp, dull, shock-like, tingling, shooting, radiating, fluctuating in intensity, and varying in location (these often occur *without* a timely relationship with an obvious noxious stimuli)
- Over time, the pain stimulus may cause symptoms that completely change (e.g., sharp to dull, obvious to vague)

Signs

- Hypertension, tachycardia, diaphoresis, mydriasis, and pallor are seldom present
- In most cases there are NO obvious signs
- Comorbid conditions often present (e.g., sleep problems, depression, relationship problems)
- Outcome of treatment often unpredictable

Laboratory Tests

- Pain is always subjective
- Pain is best diagnosed based on patient description and history
- There are *no* specific laboratory tests for pain; however, history and/or diagnostic proof of past trauma (e.g., computed tomography) or present disease state (e.g., autoantibodies) may be helpful in diagnosing etiology

Data from Twycross[22] and the American Pain Society.[26]

whereas functionality becomes more of an issue in chronic pain. Quality of life must be assessed on a regular basis in all patients.

The clinician must remember, however, that "pain is always subjective. Objective observations of grimacing, limping, or tachycardia may be helpful in assessing patients, but these signs are often absent in patients with chronic pain caused by structural lesions. No neurophysiological or chemical test can measure pain. The clinician must accept the patient's report of pain."[26]

TREATMENT

■ NONPHARMACOLOGIC THERAPY

Stimulation Therapy

Transcutaneous electrical nerve stimulation (TENS) has been used in managing both acute and chronic pain (e.g., surgical, traumatic, low back, arthritis, neuropathy, fibromyalgia, and oral-facial pain).[7,17] However, the studies are contradictory and fail to show any sustained pain relief. As a result, the technique has not gained widespread acceptance.

Psychological Intervention

Even though the cognitive, behavioral, and social aspects of pain are well established, psychological interventions for the treatment of acute pain are not used widely. Simple interventions (e.g., introductory information about sensations to expect after certain procedures) reduce patient distress and greatly reduce postprocedure suffering.[27] Other successful psychological techniques, including relaxation training, imagery, and hypnosis, have proven effective in the management of postprocedure pain and in cancer-related pain.[27,28] Moderate evidence demonstrates that cognitive behavioral therapy and biofeedback also may be useful nonpharmacologic tools in managing chronic pain.[29]

■ PHARMACOLOGIC TREATMENT

Nonopioid Agents

Analgesia should be initiated with the most effective analgesic agent having the fewest side effects. Acetaminophen, acetylsalicylic acid (aspirin), and NSAIDs often are preferred over opiates in the treatment of mild-to-moderate pain (Table 62–3). These drugs (with the exception of acetaminophen) prevent formation of prostaglandins produced in response to noxious stimuli, thereby decreasing the number of pain impulses received by the CNS.[26] Therapeutic outcomes may be less than desired in those who do not expect "mild" analgesics to relieve pain. NSAIDs may be particularly useful in the management of cancer-related bone pain.[28] Studies comparing the efficacy of these agents have been inconsistent. Therefore, the choice of a particular agent often depends on availability, cost, pharmacokinetics, pharmacologic characteristics, and the side-effect profile. Because of the large interpatient variability with NSAIDS, it is considered rational therapy to switch to another member of this drug group after an adequate therapeutic trial of any single agent.

Opioid Agents

Opioids are often the next logical step in the management of acute pain and cancer-related chronic pain. They also are an effective treatment option in the management of chronic noncancer pain; however, this continues to be somewhat controversial. Many times a trial of opioids is warranted, but such a trial should not be done without a complete assessment of the pain complaint.[30]

TABLE 62-3 Adult FDA-Approved Nonopioid Analgesics (Includes Only FDA Approved Agents for Pain)

Class and Generic Name (Brand Name)	Half-Life (h)	Usual Dosage Range (mg)	Maximal Dose (mg/day)
Salicylates			
Acetylsalicylic acid[a]–aspirin (various)	0.25	325–1,000 every 4–6 h	4,000
Magnesium–anhydrous[a] (Doan's, various, various combinations of choline and magnesium are available)	Nd/Nd	304–607 every 4 h 607–934 every 6 h	3,738
Diflunisal (Dolobid, various)	8–12	500–1,000 initial 250–500 every 8–12 h	1,500
para-Aminophenol			
Acetaminophen[a] (Tylenol, various)	2–3	325–1,000 every 4–6 h	4,000[b]
Fenamates			
Meclofenamate (various)	0.8–2.1	50–100 every 4–6 h	400
Mefenamic acid (Ponstel)	2	Initial 500 250 every 6 h (maximum 7 days)	1,000[c]
Pyranocarboxylic acid			
Etodolac (various) (immediate release)	7.3	200–400 every 6–8 h	1,000
Acetic acid			
Diclofenac potassium (Cataflam, various)	1.9	In some patients, initial 100, 50 three times per day	150[d]
Propionic acids			
Ibuprofen[a] (Motrin, various)	2–2.5	200–400 every 4–6 h	3,200[e] 2,400[e] 1,200[f]
Fenoprofen (Nalfon, various)	3	200 every 4–6 h	3,200
Ketoprofen (various)	2	25–50 every 6–8 h	300
Naproxen (Naprosyn, Anaprox, various)	12–17	500 initial 500 every 12 h or 250 every 6–8 h	1,000[c]
Naproxen sodium[a] (Aleve, various)	12–13	In some patients, 440 initial[f] 220 every 8–12 h[f]	660[f]
Pyrrolizine carboxylic acid			
Ketorolac–parenteral (various)	5–6	30–60 (single IM dose only) 15–30 (single IV dose only) 15–30 every 6 h (maximum of 5 days)	30–60 15–30 60–120
Ketorolac–oral, indicated for continuation with parenteral only (various)	5–6	10 every 4–6 h (maximum of 5 days, which includes parenteral doses) In some patients, initial oral dose of 20	40
Cyclooxygenase-2 inhibitors			
Celecoxib (Celebrex)	11	Initial 400 followed by another 200 on first day, then 200 twice daily	400

[a]Available both as an over-the-counter preparation and as a prescription drug.
[b]Some experts believe 4,000 mg may be too high.
[c]Up to 1,250 mg on the first day.
[d]Up to 200 mg on the first day.
[e]Some individuals may respond better to 3,200 mg as opposed to 2,400 mg, although well-controlled trials show no better response; consider risk versus benefits when using 3,200 mg/day.
[f]Over-the-counter dose.
FDA, Food and Drug Administration; Nd, no data.
Data from American Pain Society,[26] Anonymous,[44,45] and Watkins et al.[66]

CLINICAL CONTROVERSY

Many clinicians believe that some chronic painful conditions (e.g., osteoarthritis) never should be treated with opioids, whereas others believe that when other modalities are not effective or seem to pose more of a risk to that particular patient than does conventional therapy (e.g., NSAIDs), then opioids are necessary.

The classification of these agents, their equianalgesic doses, relative histamine-releasing characteristics, pharmacokinetics, and dosing guidelines are outlined in Tables 62–4 and 62–5. The choice of opiate should be based on patient acceptance; analgesic effectiveness; and pharmacokinetic, pharmacodynamic, and side-effect profiles (Tables 62–4 and 62–6).

The pharmacologic activity of opioids depends on their affinity for opiate receptors.[31] Therapeutic activities and side effects range from those exhibited by the opiate agonists (e.g., morphine) to those seen with the opiate antagonists (e.g., naloxone). Partial agonists and antagonists (e.g., pentazocine) compete with agonists for opiate receptor sites and, depending on the inherent agonist and antagonist properties, exhibit mixed agonist–antagonist activity. Mixed agonist–antagonist agents with analgesic activity appear to exhibit selectivity for analgesic receptor sites.[31] This may result in analgesia with fewer undesirable side effects. Efficacy and side effects also may further differ among agents because of receptor subtype variability. Specifically, research has identified multiple

TABLE 62-4 Opioid Analgesics

Class and Generic Name (Brand Name)	Chemical Source	Relative Histamine Release	Route	Equianalgesic Dose in Adults (mg)	Onset (min)/ Half-Life (h)
Phenanthrenes (morphine-like agonists)					
Morphine (various)	Naturally occurring	+++	IM	10	10–20/2
			PO	30	
Hydromorphone (Dilaudid, various)	Semisynthetic	+	IM	1.5	10–20/2–3
			PO	7.5	
Oxymorphone (Numorphan, Opana)	Semisynthetic	+	IM	1	10–20/2–3
			R	5[a]	
			PO	10	
Levorphanol (various)	Semisynthetic	+	IM (acute)	2 (acute)	10–20/12–16
			PO	4 (acute)	
			IM	1 (chronic)	
			PO	1 (chronic)	
Codeine (various)	Naturally occurring	+++	IM	15–30[b]	
			PO	15–30[b]	10–30/3
Hydrocodone (available as combination)	Semisynthetic	N/A	PO	5–10[b]	30–60/4
Oxycodone (various)	Semisynthetic	+	PO	20–30[c]	30–60/2–3
Phenylpiperidines (meperidine-like agonists)					
Meperidine (Demerol, various)	Synthetic	+++	IM	75	10–20/3–4
			PO	50–150[b] This drug is not recommended	
Fentanyl (Sublimaze, Duragesic, various)	Synthetic	+	IM	0.1	7–15/3–4
			Transdermal	25 mcg/h[d]	
			Buccal, transmucosal	Variable[e]	
Diphenylheptanes (methadone-like agonists)					
Methadone (Dolophine, various)	Synthetic	+	IM	Variable[f] (acute)	
			PO	Variable[f] (acute)	30–60/12–190
			IM	Variable[f] (chronic)	
			PO	Variable[f] (chronic)	
Propoxyphene (Darvon, various)	Synthetic	N/A	PO	65[b]	30–60/6–12
Agonist–antagonist derivatives					
Pentazocine (Talwin, various)	Synthetic	N/A	IM	Not recommended	
			PO	50[b]	15–30/2–3
Butorphanol (Stadol, various)	Synthetic	+	IM	2	10–20/3–4
			Intranasal	1[b] (one spray)	
Nalbuphine (Nubain, various)	Semisynthetic	N/A	IM	10	<15/5
Buprenorphine (Buprenex, various)	Semisynthetic	N/A	IM	0.4	10–20/2–3
Antagonists					
Naloxone (Narcan, various)	Synthetic	N/A	IV	0.4–2[g]	1–2 (IV), 2–5 (IM)/ 0.5–1.3
Central analgesic					
Tramadol (Ultram, various)	Synthetic	N/A	PO	50–100[b]	<60/5–7

[a]The American Pain Society[26] considers 5 mg rectal morphine = 5 mg rectal oxymorphone.
[b]Starting dose only (equianalgesia not shown).
[c]Starting doses lower (oxycodone 5–10 mg, meperidine 50–150 mg).
[d]Equivalent PO morphine dose = 45–134 mg/day.
[e]For breakthrough pain only.
[f]The equianalgesic dose of methadone when compared with other opioids will decrease progressively the higher the previous opioid dose has been.
[g]Starting doses to be used in cases of opioid overdose.
IM, intramuscular; IV, intravenous; PO, oral.
Data from references 26, 32, 33, 43, 44, 45, and 67.

subtype μ-receptors with varied expression. This μ-receptor subtype variability may explain why some patients respond differently to certain opioids, specifically μ-receptor agonists.[32]

The effects of the opioid analgesics are relatively selective, and at normal therapeutic concentrations, these agents do not affect other sensory modalities,[33] such as sensitivity to touch, sight, or hearing; however, as the dosage increases, so do the undesirable side effects (Table 62–6). Patients in severe pain may receive very high doses of opioids with no unwanted side effects, but as the pain subsides, patients may not tolerate even very low doses.[34] Frequently, when opioids are administered, pain is not eliminated, but its unpleasantness is decreased.[34] Patients report that although their pain is still present, it no longer bothers them.

Opioids share related pharmacologic attributes and exert a profound effect on the CNS and gastrointestinal tract.[33] Mood changes, sedation, nausea, vomiting, decreased gastrointestinal motility, constipation, respiratory depression, dependence, and tolerance are evident in varying degrees with all agents. Constipation, sedation, and nausea/vomiting are the most common side effects of opioids; respiratory depression is less common.[35] Tolerance to side effects (except to constipation) often develops within the first week of therapy. Consideration of efficacy and side-effect profile assists in selection of the most appropriate agent.

❸ The route of administration depends on individual patient needs. In patients who have oral access, the oral route is preferred. However, the onset of analgesic effects for oral medications is approximately 45 minutes, and the peak effect usually occurs 1 to 2 hours after administration.26 This delay must be a consideration when immediate relief is needed in the management of acute pain. Therefore, in some scenarios, such as acute severe pain (i.e., pain

TABLE 62-5 Dosing Guidelines

Agent(s)	Doses (Titrate Up or Down Based on Patient Response)	Notes
NSAIDs/acetaminophen/aspirin	Dose to maximum before switching to another agent (see Table 62–3)	Used in mild-to-moderate pain May use in conjunction with opioid agents to decrease doses of each Regular alcohol use and high doses of acetaminophen may result in liver toxicity Care must be exercised to avoid overdose when combination products containing these agents are used
Morphine	PO 5–30 mg q 3–4 h[a] IM 5–10 mg q 3–4 h[a] IV 1–2.5 mg q 5 min prn[a] SR 15–30 mg q 12 h (may need to be q 8 h in some patients) Rectal 10–20 mg q 4 h[a]	Drug of choice in severe pain Use immediate-release product with SR product to control "breakthrough" pain in cancer patients Every-24-hour product available
Hydromorphone	PO 2–4 mg q 3–6 h[a] IM 1–4 mg q 3–6 h[a] IV 0.1–0.5 mg q 5 min prn[a] Rectal 3 mg q 6–8 h[a]	Use in severe pain More potent than morphine; otherwise, no advantages
Oxymorphone	IM 1–1.5 mg q 4–6 h[a] IV 0.5 mg initially PO immediate release 5–10 mg q 4–6 h[a] PO extended release 10–20 mg q 12 h[a] Rectal 5 mg q 4–6 h[a]	Use in severe pain No advantages over morphine Use immediate-release product with controlled-release product to control "breakthrough" pain in cancer or chronic pain patients
Levorphanol	PO 2–3 mg q 6–8 h[a] (Levo-Dromoran) PO 2–3 mg q 3–6 h[a] (Levorphanol Tartrate) IM 1–2 mg q 6–8 h[a] IV 1 mg q 3–6 h[a]	Use in severe pain Extended half-life useful in cancer patients In chronic pain, wait 3 days between dosage adjustments
Codeine	PO 15–60 mg q 4–6 h[a] IM 15–60 mg q 4–6 h[a]	Use in moderate pain Weak analgesic; use with NSAIDs, aspirin, or acetaminophen
Hydrocodone	PO 5–10 mg q 4–6 h[a]	Use in moderate/severe pain Most effective when used with NSAIDs, aspirin, or acetaminophen Only available as combination product with other ingredients for pain and/or cough
Oxycodone	PO 5–10 mg q 4–6 h[a] Controlled release 10–20 mg q 12 h	Use in moderate/severe pain Most effective when used with NSAIDs, aspirin, or acetaminophen Use immediate-release product with controlled-release product to control "breakthrough" pain in cancer or chronic pain patients
Meperidine	IM 50–150 mg q 3–4 h[a] IV 5–10 mg q 5 min prn[a]	Use in severe pain Oral not recommended Do not use in renal failure May precipitate tremors, myoclonus, and seizures Monoamine oxidase inhibitors can induce hyperpyrexia and/or seizures or opioid overdose symptoms
Fentanyl	IV 25–50 mcg/h IM 50–100 mcg q 1–2 h[a] Transdermal 25 mcg/h q 72 h Transmucosal (Actiq Lozenge) 200 mcg may repeat × 1, 30 min after first dose is started, then titrate Transmucosal (Fentora Buccal Tablet) 100 mcg, may repeat × 1, 30 min after first dose is started, then titrate Iontophoretic transdermal system 40 mcg per activation	Used in severe pain Do not use transdermal in acute pain Transmucosal for "breakthrough" cancer pain in patients already receiving or tolerant to opioids Iontophoretic transdermal system used for acute pain and can be reactivated every 10 min
Methadone	PO 2.5–10 mg q 3–4 h (acute)[a] IM 2.5–10 mg q 8–12 h (acute)[a] (more frequent dosing may be needed during initial titration) PO 5–20 mg q 6–8 h (chronic)[a]	Effective in severe chronic pain Sedation can be major problem Some chronic pain patients can be dosed every 12 h Equianalgesic dose of methadone when compared with other opioids will decrease progressively the higher the previous opioid dose
Propoxyphene	PO 100 mg q 4 h[a] (napsylate) PO 65 mg q 4 h[a] (HCl) (maximum 600 mg daily of napsylate, 390 mg HCl)	Use in moderate pain Weak analgesic; most effective when used with NSAIDs, aspirin, or acetaminophen This drug is not recommended in the elderly Will cause carbamazepine levels to increase 100 mg of napsylate salt = 65 mg of HCl salt
Pentazocine	PO 50–100 mg q 3–4 h[b] (maximum 600 mg daily)	Third-line agent for moderate-to-severe pain May precipitate withdrawal in opiate-dependent patients Parenteral doses not recommended
Butorphanol	IM 1–4 mg q 3–4 h[b] IV 0.5–2 mg q 3–4 h[b] Intranasal 1 mg (1 spray) q 3–4 h[b] If inadequate relief after initial spray, may repeat in other nostril × 1 in 60–90 min Max 2 sprays (one per nostril) q 3–4 h[b]	Third-line agent for moderate-to-severe pain May precipitate withdrawal in opiate-dependent patients

(continued)

TABLE 62-5 Dosing Guidelines (continued)

Agent(s)	Doses (Titrate Up or Down Based on Patient Response)	Notes
Nalbuphine	IM/IV 10 mg q 3–6 h[b] (maximum 20 mg dose, 160 mg daily)	Second-line agent for moderate-to-severe pain May precipitate withdrawal in opiate-dependent patients
Buprenorphine	IM 0.3 mg q 6 h[b] Slow IV 0.3 mg q 6 h[b] May repeat ×1, 30–60 min after initial dose	Second-line agent for moderate-to-severe pain May precipitate withdrawal in opiate-dependent patients Naloxone may not be effective in reversing respiratory depression
Naloxone	IV 0.4–2 mg	When reversing opiate side effects in patients needing analgesia, dilute and titrate (0.1–0.2 mg q 2–3 min) so as not to reverse analgesia
Tramadol	PO 50–100 mg q 4–6 h[a] If rapid onset not required, start 25 mg/day and titrate over several days Extended release PO 100 mg q 24 h	Maximum dose for nonextended-release, 400 mg/24 h; maximum for extended release, 300 mg/24 h Decrease dose in patient with renal impairment and in the elderly

[a]May start with an around-the-clock regimen and switch to prn if/when the painful signal subsides or is episodic.
[b]May reach a ceiling analgesic effect.
IM, intramuscular; IV, intravenous; NSAID, nonsteroidal antiinflammatory drug; PO, oral; prn, as needed; SR, sustained release.
Data from American Pain Society,[26] Gutstein and Akil,[33] and Anonymous.[44,45]

crisis) or when the patient is unable to take oral medications, alternative routes of therapy (e.g., intravenous) may be preferred. ❹ The opioids differ greatly in equianalgesic dose (Table 62–4), which should be used only as a guide because the nature of pain makes it necessary to individualize pain regimens. True opioid allergies are rare, but Table 62–4 also can be used when treating a patient who is allergic to opiates. Most reactions to opioids, such as itching or rash, are due to the associated histamine release and mast cell degranulation, not to a true allergic or immunoglobulin-E (IgE) response. Although caution is always advised, a decrease in potential cross-sensitivity exists when moving from one opioid structural class to another. The classes are phenanthrenes (morphine-like agonists), phenylpiperidines (meperidine-like agonists), and diphenylheptanes (methadone-like agonists). When considering cross-sensitivity, the mixed agonist–antagonist class acts much like the morphine-like agonists.[36] Reactions due to histamine release may be reduced by choosing agents shown to have less effect on histamine release. Morphine has been associated with the greatest histamine release, whereas agents such as oxycodone and fentanyl typically cause fewer histamine-related reactions (see Table 62–4).

❷ ❺ In the initial stages of acute pain, analgesics should be given around the clock. This should commence after administering a typical starting dose and titrating up or down, depending on the patient's degree of pain and demonstrated side effects (e.g., sedation).[26] As-needed schedules often produce wide swings in analgesic plasma concentrations that create wide swings in pain and sedation. This may initiate a vicious cycle where increasing amounts of pain medications are needed for relief. ❺ As the painful state subsides and the need for medication decreases, as-needed schedules may be appropriate. As-needed schedules also may be useful in patients who present with pain that is intermittent or sporadic in nature (Fig. 62–2). The management of chronic pain is also best accomplished by around-the-clock administration schedules that inhibit serum analgesic concentrations from falling below the point at which a patient experiences the suffering of pain. As-needed schedules are to be used in conjunction with around-the-clock regimens and are used when patients experience breakthrough pain.

TABLE 62-6 Major Adverse Effects of the Opioid Analgesic

Effect	Manifestation
Mood changes	Dysphoria, euphoria
Somnolence	Lethargy, drowsiness, apathy, inability to concentrate
Stimulation of chemoreceptor trigger zone	Nausea, vomiting
Respiratory depression	Decreased respiratory rate
Decreased gastrointestinal motility	Constipation
Increase in sphincter tone	Biliary spasm, urinary retention (varies among agents)
Histamine release	Urticaria, pruritus, rarely exacerbation of asthma (varies among agents)
Tolerance	Larger doses for same effect
Dependence	Withdrawal symptoms upon abrupt discontinuation

Data from Stimmel,[2] Miyoshi and Leckband,[31] and Reisine and Pasternak.[34]

Continuous intravenous and subcutaneous methods of opioid infusion are effective for some postoperative pain, but the probability of unwanted side effects is high.[26] An alternative method is patient-controlled analgesia (PCA). With this technique, patients can self-administer a preset dose of an intravenous opioid via a pump electronically interfaced with a timing device. Compared to traditional as-needed opioid dosing, PCA yields better pain control, improved patient satisfaction, and relatively few differences in side effects.[37]

Administration of opiates directly into the CNS (e.g., epidural and intrathecal/subarachnoid routes) has shown considerable promise in the control of acute, chronic noncancer, and cancer pain (Table 62–7)[13,38,39] and is common in both large and small institutions throughout the United States. Because of reports of marked sedation, respiratory depression, pruritus, nausea, vomiting, urinary retention, and hypotension,[40] these methods of analgesia require careful monitoring and are best used by experienced practitioners. Respiratory depression is of concern and can occur within the first half hour or manifest as late as 12 hours after a single dose of epidural morphine.[40] Naloxone is used to antagonize this effect, but continuous infusion may be required.[40] Analgesia and side effects are evident at lower doses when the opioids are administered intrathecally instead of epidurally. Intrathecally, single morphine doses of 0.1 to 0.3 mg are common, whereas epidurally, doses of 1 to 6 mg are the norm.[38] These intrathecal and epidural opioids often are administered on a continuous-infusion and/or patient-controlled basis, and, when given simultaneously with intrathecal or epidural local anesthetics such as bupivacaine, they have been proven safe and effective.[41] All agents administered directly into the CNS should be preservative-free.

Tolerance, Dependence, Addiction, and Pseudoaddiction

A barrier that consistently causes clinicians to misjudge and mistreat pain is the misunderstanding of opioid tolerance, physical dependence, addiction, and pseudoaddiction. "Tolerance is the diminution of drug effect over time as a consequence of exposure to the drug."[42] It develops at different rates and with tremendous patient variability. However, with stable disease, opioid use often stabilizes, and tolerance does not lead to addiction.[42] "Physical dependence is defined by

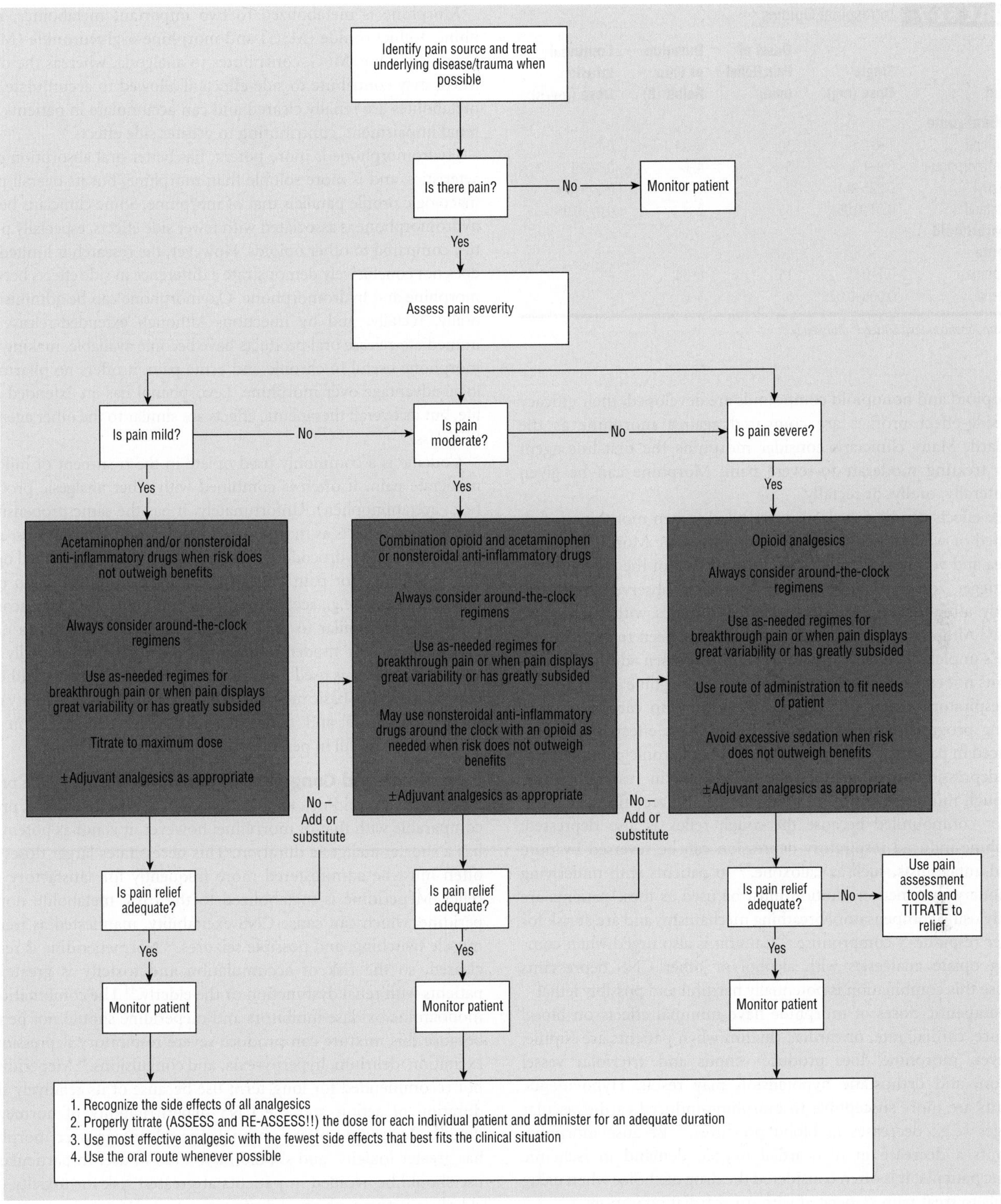

FIGURE 62-2. Algorithm for acute pain. *(Data modified from Omnicare, Inc., Acute Pain Pathway.)*

the occurrence of an abstinence syndrome following administration of an antagonist drug or abrupt dose reduction or discontinuation."[42] Clinicians must understand that physical dependence and tolerance are not equivalent to addiction; however, with chronic opioid use, they are likely to develop.[26] "Addiction is best defined as a behavioral pattern characterized as loss of control over drug use, compulsive drug use, and continued use of a drug despite harm."[42] When opioids are being used, these behaviors must be evaluated continually, but extreme caution is advised when using the term *addiction* because of its many negative connotations, which can lead to a compromised clinician–patient relationship and ineffective pain control.[26,42] In addition, clinicians must be aware that an individual's behaviors may suggest addiction, when in reality the behaviors noted are a reflection of unrelieved pain or pseudoaddiction.[26] The incidence of addiction varies depending on the patient population. In patients with no history of addiction, the risk of addiction is relatively small. "Drug exposure appears to be only one etiologic factor in the development of addiction, and genetics, social, and psychologic factors may be more significant determinants."[7]

Morphine and Congeners Despite the availability of several newer agents, morphine remains the prototype opiate analgesic. As

TABLE 62-7 Intraspinal Opioids

Agent	Single Dose (mg)	Onset of Pain Relief (min)	Duration of Pain Relief (h)	Continual Infusion Dose (mg/h)
Epidural route				
Morphine	1–6	30	6–24	0.1–1
Hydromorphone	0.8–1.5	5–8	4–6	0.1–0.3
Fentanyl	0.025–0.1	5	1–8	0.025–0.1
Sufentanil	0.01–0.06	5	2–4	0.01–0.05
Subarachnoid route				
Morphine	0.1–0.3	15	8–34	–
Fentanyl	0.005–0.025	5	3–6	–

Data from American Pain Society[26] and Ready.[38]

new opioid and nonopioid compounds are developed, their efficacy and side-effect profiles are compared against morphine as the standard. Many clinicians consider morphine the first-line agent when treating moderate-to-severe pain. Morphine can be given parenterally, orally, or rectally.

Side effects can be numerous, particularly when morphine is first initiated or when doses are significantly increased. Morphine causes nausea and vomiting through direct stimulation of the chemoreceptor trigger zone.[33] Opioid-induced nausea is observed most frequently after the initial dose and often subsides with subsequent doses.[43] Although euphoria and dysphoria have been reported, morphine's unpleasant effects are more prominent when administered to patients not experiencing pain.[33] As doses of morphine are increased, the respiratory center becomes less responsive to carbon dioxide, causing progressive respiratory depression. This effect is less pronounced in patients being treated for severe or chronic pain. Respiratory depression often manifests as a decrease in respiratory rate (although minute volume and tidal volume also are affected) and is further compounded because the cough reflex is also depressed. Morphine-induced respiratory depression can be reversed by pure opioid antagonists, such as naloxone.[34] In patients with underlying pulmonary dysfunction, caution must be used as these patients are already using compensatory breathing mechanisms and are at risk for further respiratory compromise.[34] Caution is also urged when combining opiate analgesics with alcohol or other CNS depressants because this combination is potentially harmful and possibly lethal.

Therapeutic doses of morphine have minimal effects on blood pressure, cardiac rate, or cardiac rhythm when patients are supine; however, morphine does produce venous and arteriolar vessel dilation, and orthostatic hypotension may result. Hypovolemic patients are more susceptible to morphine-induced cardiovascular changes (e.g., decreases in blood pressure).[34] Because morphine prompts a decrease in myocardial oxygen demand in ischemic cardiac patients, it is often considered the drug of choice when using opioids to treat pain associated with myocardial infarction.

Morphine decreases the propulsive contractions of the gastrointestinal tract and reduces biliary and pancreatic secretions,[34] resulting in constipation. Morphine-induced spasms of the sphincter of Oddi have been observed.[34] However, the clinical significance of such an occurrence is unclear. Urinary retention is another potential side effect of morphine; tolerance develops to this effect over time.[34] Morphine-induced histamine release often manifests as pruritus, and although not seen often, it may exacerbate bronchospasm in patients with a history of asthma.[34] Therapeutic doses of morphine do not directly affect cerebral circulation, but drug-induced respiratory depression can increase intracranial pressure. Thus, caution is advised in head trauma patients who are not ventilated because morphine may exaggerate this pressure[34] and cloud the neurologic examination results.

Morphine is metabolized to two important metabolites, morphine-3-glucuronide (M3G) and morphine-6-glucuronide (M6G). One metabolite, M6G, contributes to analgesia, whereas the other, M3G, may contribute to side effects if allowed to accumulate. The metabolites are renally cleared and can accumulate in patients with renal impairment, contributing to greater side effects.[33]

Hydromorphone is more potent, has better oral absorption characteristics, and is more soluble than morphine, but its overall pharmacologic profile parallels that of morphine. Some clinicians believe hydromorphone is associated with fewer side effects, especially pruritus, compared to other opioids. However, the research is limited and does not conclusively demonstrate a difference in side effects between morphine and hydromorphone. Oxymorphone can be administered orally, rectally, and by injection. Although extended-release and immediate-release oral products have become available, making oxymorphone useful in chronic and acute pain, it offers no pharmacologic advantage over morphine. Levorphanol has an extended half-life, but its overall therapeutic effects are similar to the other agents in this class.

Codeine is a commonly used opiate in the treatment of mild-to-moderate pain. It often is combined with other analgesic products (e.g., acetaminophen). Unfortunately, it has the same propensity to produce side effects as morphine and may produce more nausea and constipation.[26] Hydrocodone is another commonly prescribed opiate and is available for pain only in combination products with other analgesic agents (e.g., acetaminophen, ibuprofen). Its pharmacologic properties are similar to those of morphine. Oxycodone is a useful oral analgesic for moderate-to-severe pain. This is especially true when the product is used in combination with nonopioids. Although oxycodone shares basic morphine characteristics, the availability of an immediate-release and controlled-release oral dosage form also makes it very useful in persistent pain as well as acute pain.

Meperidine and Congeners (Phenylpiperidines) The prototype phenylpiperidine, meperidine, has a pharmacologic profile comparable with that of morphine; however, it is not as potent and has a shorter analgesic duration. This necessitates larger doses that often must be administered more frequently for satisfactory pain relief. Meperidine is metabolized to the toxic metabolite normeperidine, which can cause CNS excitability, manifested as tremor, muscle twitching, and possible seizures.[33] Normeperidine is renally cleared, so the risk of accumulation and toxicity is greatest in patients with renal dysfunction or the elderly.[44] The combination of monoamine oxidase inhibitors and meperidine should not be used because this mixture can produce severe respiratory depression or excitation, delirium, hyperpyrexia, and convulsions.[34] Meperidine is not recommended for long-term use because of its relatively short duration of action and the CNS hyperirritability of normeperidine.[28] Meperidine offers no analgesic advantage over morphine, has greater toxicity, and should be limited in use. In particular, its use should be avoided in patients at greatest risk for toxicity (e.g., elderly, patients with renal dysfunction).

Fentanyl is a synthetic opioid structurally related to meperidine that is used often in anesthesiology as an adjunct to general anesthesia.[44] This agent is more potent, more lipophilic, and shorter acting than meperidine (Table 62–4). It can be administered parenterally, transmucosally, and transdermally. The fentanyl patch may provide a more convenient dosing alternative in patients on stable regimens. The transdermal patch can provide analgesia for up to 72 hours, but takes 12 to 24 hours for full onset and up to 6 days to reach steady state after dose adjustments. Therefore, the transdermal patch should be limited to patients with chronic pain; it is not appropriate for the management of acute pain.[45] A fentanyl lozenge and a buccal dosage form also are available for treatment of breakthrough cancer pain.[45] Caution should be used when fentanyl is administered to patients who have a very small body habitus, always starting with the smallest expected effective dose and carefully titrating to effect. Most recently an iontophoretic patient controlled transdermal system has been developed for use in acute postoperative pain.[45]

Methadone and Congeners Methadone has gained considerable popularity because of its oral efficacy, extended duration of action, and low cost. Although methadone is effective in acute pain,[45] it has gained particular prominence in treating cancer pain[39] and has increasingly been used in the management of chronic noncancer pain.[46] This despite the fact that, with repeated doses, the analgesic duration of action is prolonged,[45] resulting in an unpredictable half-life, possible excessive sedation, and difficulty in titration. Properties unique to methadone, compared with other opioids, include the D-isomer's ability to antagonize NMDA receptors, agonist effects at κ- and δ-opioid receptors, and blockade of serotonin and norepinephrine reuptake.[46–49] These properties may prove useful in the treatment of neuropathic and chronic pain or in patients with a maladaptive inflammatory component to their pain. The equianalgesic dose of methadone may decrease with higher doses of the previous opioid,[47] complicating conversions from other opioids to methadone.

CLINICAL CONTROVERSY

Some clinicians believe that methadone should be tried before other opioids in many chronic pain conditions where an opioid is warranted because they believe that neuropathic pain is often a component. Other clinicians believe that sustained-released morphine or oxycodone are better first choices.

Propoxyphene usually is used in combination with acetaminophen for treatment of moderate pain. Propoxyphene is metabolized to norpropoxyphene, a potentially toxic metabolite.[26] Elderly patients and those with renal dysfunction are at greatest risk for toxicity; therefore, propoxyphene use is discouraged in these patients.[26,50]

Opioid Agonist–Antagonist Derivatives

Analgesic agents that stimulate the analgesic portion of opioid receptors while blocking or having no effect on the toxicity portion would be considered ideal. The agonist–antagonist derivatives were developed with this in mind. The analgesic class produces analgesia and has a ceiling effect on respiratory depression.[31] These agents also have a lower abuse potential than does morphine, but psychotomimetic responses (e.g., hallucinations and dysphoria, as seen with pentazocine), a ceiling analgesic effect, and a propensity to initiate withdrawal in opioid-dependent populations[31] have diminished their widespread clinical use.

Opioid Antagonists

The pure opioid antagonist naloxone binds competitively to opioid receptors but does not produce an analgesic or opioid side-effect response. Therefore, it is used most often to reverse the toxic effects of agonist- and agonist–antagonist-derived opioids.

Central Analgesic

Tramadol has two basic modes of action: μ-opiate receptor binding and inhibition of norepinephrine and serotonin reuptake. It is indicated for the relief of moderate to moderately severe pain.[51]

Tramadol has a side-effect profile similar to that of the previously mentioned opioid analgesics (e.g., dizziness, euphoria, hallucinations, cognitive dysfunction, and constipation).[44] Tramadol alone may enhance the risk of seizures. In addition, concomitant use with serotonin reuptake inhibitors, opioids, tricyclic antidepressants, monoamine oxidase inhibitors, neuroleptics, or other drugs that can reduce the seizure threshold and use in patients with seizure disorders may increase the risk of seizures.[51] Tramadol may have a place in treating patients with chronic pain, especially neuropathic pain.[52]

Adjuvant Analgesics

Adjuvant analgesics are pharmacologic agents with individual characteristics that make them useful in the management of pain but that typically are not classified as analgesics. Examples of adjuvant analgesics include antidepressants and anticonvulsants. ❻ Chronic pain that has a maladaptive inflammatory (e.g., low back pain) and/or neuropathic component (e.g., diabetic neuropathy) may require such agents (Table 62–8). Anticonvulsants (e.g., gabapentin, which may decrease neuronal excitability), tricyclic antidepressants, serotonin and norepinephrine reuptake inhibitor antidepressants (which block the reuptake of serotonin and norepinephrine, thus enhancing pain inhibition), and topically applied local anesthetics (which decrease nerve stimulation) all have been effective in managing chronic pain.[53,54]

In cancer patients, bone pain can be treated with radiopharmaceuticals. Both strontium 89 and samarium Sm 153 lexidronam have been shown to provide pain relief.[45] Although antihistamines, amphetamines, and steroids have been used as adjuvant pain medications,[28] they have demonstrated only limited success as pain relievers.

Combination Therapy

The combination of opioid and nonopioid analgesics often results in analgesia superior to that produced by either agent alone.[27] This facilitates the use of lower doses and a more favorable side-effect profile, and, when needed, this approach is encouraged.

REGIONAL ANALGESIA

Regional analgesia with properly administered local anesthetics can provide relief of both acute and chronic pain (Table 62–9).[41] These agents can be positioned by injection (e.g., in joints, in the epidural or intrathecal space, along nerve roots, or in a nerve plexus) or topically. Lidocaine in the form of a patch has proven effective in treating focal

TABLE 62-8 Pharmacologic Management of Chronic Noncancer Pain

Type of Pain	Nonopioids	Opioids	Other Medications	Comments
Chronic low back pain	Acetaminophen, NSAIDs	Short-term use for mild-to-moderate flare-ups	TCAs, AEDs	Acetaminophen and NSAIDS first; opioids in selected patients; AEDs or TCAs if neuropathic symptoms
Fibromyalgia	Acetaminophen, NSAIDs	Long-term use not recommended	Tramadol, TCAs; AEDs	Acetaminophen and NSAIDs considered first; tramadol may be better alternative than opioids
Neuropathic pain	Acetaminophen or NSAIDs are rarely effective	Considered first-line therapy but usually are tried after AEDs and/or TCAs, tramadol, lidocaine 5% patch	TCAs, AEDs, SNRIs, tramadol, topical (e.g., 5% lidocaine patch, capsaicin)	Gabapentin, 5% lidocaine patch, tramadol, nortriptyline, desipramine, all considered first-line agents; opioids considered first-line agents but usually are tried after above

AED, antiepileptic drug; NSAIDs, nonsteroidal antiinflammatory drugs; SNRI, serotonin–norepinephrine reuptake inhibitor; TCA, tricyclic antidepressant.
Data from references 7, 19, 53, 54, and 65.

TABLE 62-9 Local Anesthetics[a]

Agent (Brand Name)	Onset (min)	Duration (h)
Esters		
Procaine (Novocain, various)	2–5	0.25–1
Chloroprocaine (Nesacaine)	6–12	0.5
Tetracaine (Pontocaine)	≤15	2–3
Amides		
Mepivacaine (Polocaine, various)	3–5	0.75–1.5
Bupivacaine (Marcaine, various)	5	2–4
Lidocaine (Xylocaine, various)	<2	0.5–1
Prilocaine (Citanest)	<2	≥1
Levobupivacaine[b] (Chirocaine)	≈10	≈8
Articaine with epinephrine[c] (Septodont)	1–6	1
Ropivacaine[d] (Naropin)	11–26	1.7–3.2

[a]Unless otherwise indicated, values are for infiltrative anesthesia.
[b]Epidural administration in cesarean section.
[c]Dental anesthesia.
[d]Epidural administration.
Data from Anonymous.[44,45]

neuropathic pain.[54] Regional anesthetics relieve pain by blocking nociceptive transmission and interrupting sympathetic reflexes.[41] Their lipid solubility, pK_a, percentage of un-ionized drug, drug concentration, vasodilator behavior, and amount of vasoconstrictor (commonly epinephrine) used concomitantly determine the mechanism of action.[41] High plasma concentrations can cause signs of CNS excitation and depression, including dizziness, tinnitus, drowsiness, disorientation, muscle twitching, seizures, and respiratory arrest.[44] Cardiovascular effects include myocardial depression, hypotension, decreased cardiac output, heart block, bradycardia, ventricular arrhythmia, and cardiac arrest.[45] Disadvantages of such methods include the need for skillful technical application, need for frequent administration, and highly specialized followup procedures.

SPECIAL CONSIDERATIONS IN ACUTE PAIN

❶ ❷ ❸ ❺ The World Health Organization (WHO) recommends a three-step ladder approach using the simplest dosage schedules and medications with the least amount of potential harm based on pain intensity ratings from mild to moderate-to-severe.[28] An acute pain algorithm outlining how to use these principles is given in Fig. 62–2. The importance of reassessment and titration during this process cannot be overemphasized.

SPECIAL CONSIDERATIONS IN CANCER PAIN

Managing the pain of cancer encompasses both acute and chronic management techniques. ❼ Thus, pharmacologic treatment and psychological therapies are best combined with surgical methods, anesthetic procedures, and supportive care measures in a multidisciplinary approach to pain relief.[55] The goal is to provide patients with enough pain amelioration to tolerate diagnostic and therapeutic manipulation and permit the patient to function at a level that will allow freedom of movement and choice.[28] Assessment of the factors given in Table 62–2 also applies to cancer patients. Special attention must be given to continual reassessment of the painful state, adverse effects with medications, and aberrant behaviors. ❺ Individualization of therapy is always required.[28] Supportive care, in and outside the hospital, using programs such as hospice, is one of the cancer patient's greatest allies, not only in coping with pain but also in accepting the disease. The positive effect this has on the patient cannot be overstated. Pharmacologic management is the mainstay of therapy, and a typical progression of analgesic use in oncology patients is outlined in Fig. 62–3.

SPECIAL CONSIDERATIONS IN CHRONIC NONCANCER PAIN

❼ The numerous etiologies that produce chronic noncancer pain make treatment complex, and overall management should be multidisciplinary. As pain becomes gradually more chronic, acute symptoms such as hypertension, tachycardia, and diaphoresis become less evident, and symptoms such as depression, sleep disturbances, anxiety, irritability, work problems, and family instability tend to dominate. Patients should not be told that the pain they are feeling is "psychosomatic" or is in their head. In most cases, etiology is not as important as symptomatic relief. Evaluation objectives include establishing an accurate diagnosis, identifying iatrogenic factors, obtaining a comprehensive psychiatric and psychosocial assessment, paying special attention to family and social problems, and obtaining a description of factors that alleviate or exacerbate pain.[2] ❽ Given these objectives, placebos should never be used to diagnose pain.[2]

❼ In all cases of chronic noncancer pain, an integrated systematic approach (such as that often provided by pain clinics), with a strong emphasis on patient–clinician relationships, is essential. The goal is to improve or maintain the patient's level of functioning, decrease the rate of physical deterioration, decrease pain perception, improve the patient's sense of well-being, improve family and social relationships, and decrease dependency on drug therapy.[2] Patients and clinicians must realize that maximum effective treatment may take months or even years.

SPECIAL POPULATIONS

The elderly and the young are at a higher risk for undertreatment because of misunderstandings regarding the pathophysiology of their pain. ❺ In addition, those living with chronic, debilitating, and life-threatening illnesses need specialized pain control and care that is palliative in nature.[56] Although care must be taken in these populations to ensure that proper individualized treatment plans follow accepted guidelines,[56–59] the key concepts in pain management as outlined in this chapter are the guiding tenets in maximizing pain control.

PHARMACOECONOMIC CONSIDERATIONS

The *suffering* component of pain cannot be overemphasized. Most of us know how devastating pain can be to our daily lives. Swift relief from acute and cancer pain and well-planned treatment regimens in chronic nonmalignant pain will allow patients to concentrate on recovery and regaining control of their lives. Although few well-designed pharmacoeconomic studies have been performed,[60–62] most pain clinicians believe that this approach minimizes time in the hospital and time away from work while maximizing quality of life.

EVALUATION OF THERAPEUTIC OUTCOMES

❷ ❺ The key to treating pain effectively is consistent monitoring for effectiveness (pain relief) versus side effects (e.g., sedation) and titrating treatment accordingly. In acute pain, this often must be done several times per day (in the early stages, hourly), whereas in chronic pain this may occur daily or even weekly. The frequency of evaluation also depends on the drug, the administration route, and other therapies being used. When patients cannot be asked about their pain (e.g., coma), monitoring agitation and heart rate is appropriate. Given the subjective nature of pain, the most successful therapies involve not only frequent patient assessment but also a large degree of patient control (as with PCA). With chronic pain, tools such as the Brief Pain Inventory, Initial Pain Assessment

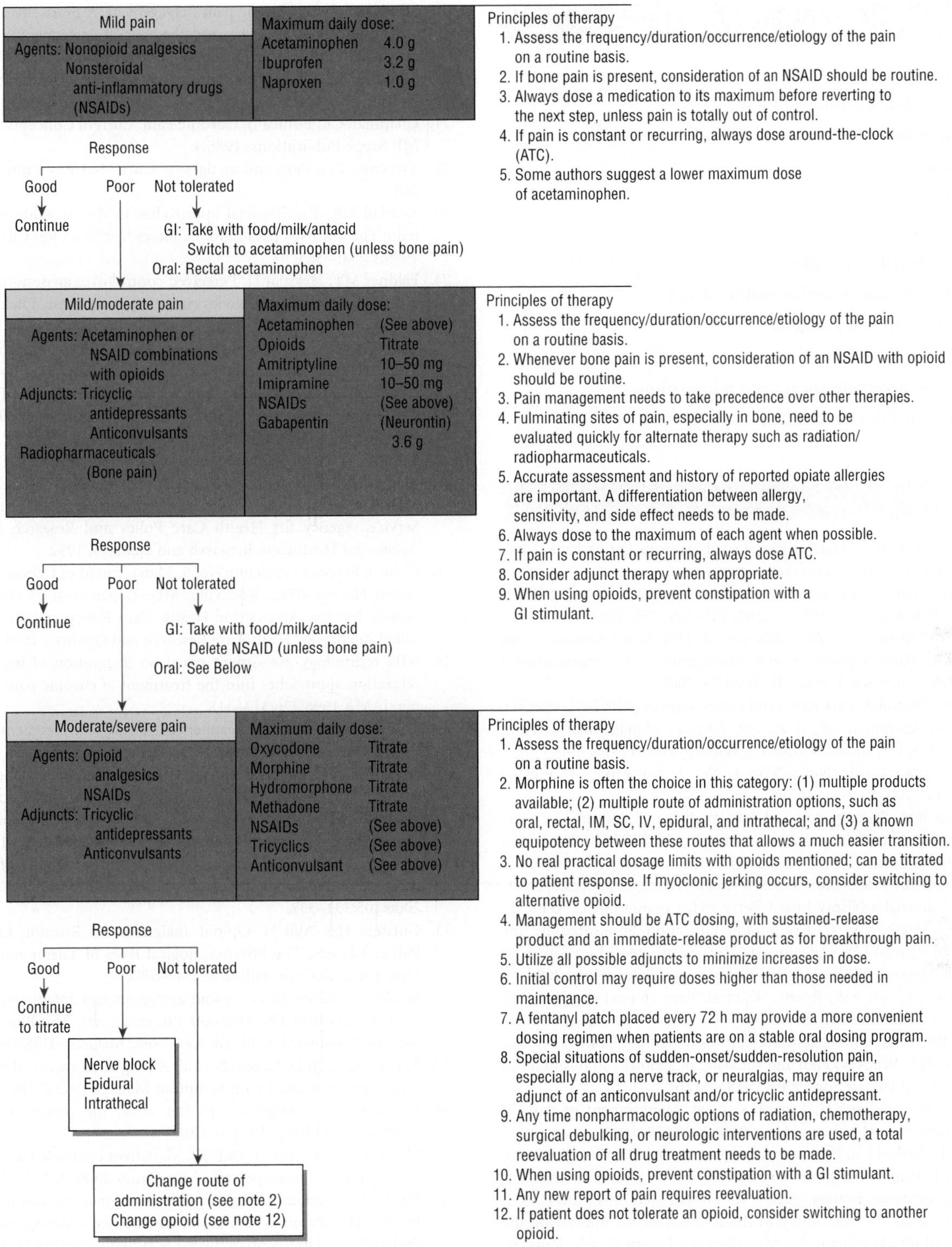
Mild pain
Agents: Nonopioid analgesics
Nonsteroidal anti-inflammatory drugs (NSAIDs)
Maximum daily dose:
Acetaminophen 4.0 g
Ibuprofen 3.2 g
Naproxen 1.0 g
Principles of therapy
1. Assess the frequency/duration/occurrence/etiology of the pain on a routine basis.
2. If bone pain is present, consideration of an NSAID should be routine.
3. Always dose a medication to its maximum before reverting to the next step, unless pain is totally out of control.
4. If pain is constant or recurring, always dose around-the-clock (ATC).
5. Some authors suggest a lower maximum dose of acetaminophen.
Response
Good
Poor
Not tolerated
Continue
GI: Take with food/milk/antacid
Switch to acetaminophen (unless bone pain)
Oral: Rectal acetaminophen
Mild/moderate pain
Agents: Acetaminophen or NSAID combinations with opioids
Adjuncts: Tricyclic antidepressants
Anticonvulsants
Radiopharmaceuticals (Bone pain)
Maximum daily dose:
Acetaminophen (See above)
Opioids Titrate
Amitriptyline 10–50 mg
Imipramine 10–50 mg
NSAIDs (See above)
Gabapentin (Neurontin) 3.6 g
Principles of therapy
1. Assess the frequency/duration/occurrence/etiology of the pain on a routine basis.
2. Whenever bone pain is present, consideration of an NSAID with opioid should be routine.
3. Pain management needs to take precedence over other therapies.
4. Fulminating sites of pain, especially in bone, need to be evaluated quickly for alternate therapy such as radiation/radiopharmaceuticals.
5. Accurate assessment and history of reported opiate allergies are important. A differentiation between allergy, sensitivity, and side effect needs to be made.
6. Always dose to the maximum of each agent when possible.
7. If pain is constant or recurring, always dose ATC.
8. Consider adjunct therapy when appropriate.
9. When using opioids, prevent constipation with a GI stimulant.
Response
Good
Poor
Not tolerated
Continue
GI: Take with food/milk/antacid
Delete NSAID (unless bone pain)
Oral: See Below
Moderate/severe pain
Agents: Opioid analgesics
NSAIDs
Adjuncts: Tricyclic antidepressants
Anticonvulsants
Maximum daily dose:
Oxycodone Titrate
Morphine Titrate
Hydromorphone Titrate
Methadone Titrate
NSAIDs (See above)
Tricyclics (See above)
Anticonvulsant (See above)
Principles of therapy
1. Assess the frequency/duration/occurrence/etiology of the pain on a routine basis.
2. Morphine is often the choice in this category: (1) multiple products available; (2) multiple route of administration options, such as oral, rectal, IM, SC, IV, epidural, and intrathecal; and (3) a known equipotency between these routes that allows a much easier transition.
3. No real practical dosage limits with opioids mentioned; can be titrated to patient response. If myoclonic jerking occurs, consider switching to alternative opioid.
4. Management should be ATC dosing, with sustained-release product and an immediate-release product as for breakthrough pain.
5. Utilize all possible adjuncts to minimize increases in dose.
6. Initial control may require doses higher than those needed in maintenance.
7. A fentanyl patch placed every 72 h may provide a more convenient dosing regimen when patients are on a stable oral dosing program.
8. Special situations of sudden-onset/sudden-resolution pain, especially along a nerve track, or neuralgias, may require an adjunct of an anticonvulsant and/or tricyclic antidepressant.
9. Any time nonpharmacologic options of radiation, chemotherapy, surgical debulking, or neurologic interventions are used, a total reevaluation of all drug treatment needs to be made.
10. When using opioids, prevent constipation with a GI stimulant.
11. Any new report of pain requires reevaluation.
12. If patient does not tolerate an opioid, consider switching to another opioid.
Response
Good
Poor
Not tolerated
Continue to titrate
Nerve block
Epidural
Intrathecal
Change route of administration (see note 2)
Change opioid (see note 12)

FIGURE 62-3. Algorithm for pain management in oncology patients. *(Data modified from the Kaiser Permanente Algorithm for Pain Management in Patients with Advanced Malignant Disease and reference 28.)*

Inventory, McGill Pain Questionnaire, or pain drawings may be helpful.[7]

❷ All opioids can cause constipation. The best management of constipation is prevention. Patients should be counseled on the proper intake of fluids and fiber. A stimulating laxative should be added with chronic opioid use. As noted earlier, CNS depressants (e.g., alcohol, benzodiazepines) amplify CNS depression when used with opioid analgesics, and use of these combinations should be discouraged when possible. When the combinations are used, patients should be monitored closely.

CONCLUSIONS

Poor training of healthcare practitioners in pain assessment and management, improper patient education, and inadequate communication among healthcare professionals are some of the reasons for inadequate pain relief.[63,64] The use of an integrated approach, incorporating the expertise of many disciplines, may well be the most overlooked principle of pain pharmacotherapy. It is the responsibility of all healthcare professionals who deal with pain to work together to ensure proper management.

ABBREVIATIONS

CNS: central nervous system

FDA: Food and Drug Administration

GABA: γ-aminobutyric acid

IM: intramuscular

IV: intravenous

K^+: potassium ion

NMDA: *N*-methyl-D-aspartate

NSAIDs: nonsteroidal antiinflammatory drugs

PCA: patient-controlled analgesia

PO: oral

TENS: transcutaneous electrical nerve stimulation

WHO: World Health Organization

REFERENCES

1. Selected quotes from Helen Keller. David Hawkins Quote Page. 1998, *http://www.river.org/~dhawk/keller-quotes.html.*
2. Stimmel B. Pain, Analgesia and Addiction: The Pharmacology of Pain. New York: Raven Press, 1983:1, 2, 63, 241–245, 259, 266.
3. Joint Commission on Accreditation of Healthcare Organizations (JCAHO). Pain Assessment and Management an Organizational Approach. Oakbrook Terrace, IL: JCAHO, 2000.
4. Turk DC, Okifuji A. Pain terms and taxonomies of pain. In: Loeser JD, Butler SH, Chapman CR, et al., eds. Bonica's Management of Pain. Philadelphia: Lippincott Williams & Wilkins, 2000:17–25.
5. Partners Against Pain News, Vol. 4, No. 3. Norwalk, CT: Purdue Pharma LP, 2000.
6. Gallagher RM. Primary care and pain medicine: A community solution to the public health problem of chronic pain. Med Clin North Am 1999;83:555–583.
7. Pain: Current Understanding of Assessment, Management, and Treatments. Editorial advisory board Berry PH, Covington EC, Dahl JL, Katz JA, Miaskowski C. Continuing Education Sponsored by the American Pain Society and supported by unrestricted education grant from the National Pharmaceutical Council, Inc. Release June 2006.
8. Desbiens NA, Wu AW, Broste SK, et al. Pain and satisfaction with pain control in seriously ill hospitalized adults: Findings from the SUPPORT research investigations. Crit Care Med 1996;24:1953–1961.
9. Desbiens NA, Wu AW. Pain and suffering in seriously ill hospitalized patients. J Am Geriatr Soc 2000;48:S183–S186.
10. Bernabei R, Gambassi G, Lapane K, et al. Management of pain in elderly patients with cancer. JAMA 1998;279:1877–1882.
11. Loeser JD, Melzack R. Pain: An overview. Lancet 1999;353:1607–1609.
12. Woolf CJ. Pain: Moving from symptom control toward mechanism-specific pharmacologic management. Ann Intern Med 2004;140:441–451.
13. Pasero C, Paice JA, McCaffery M. Basic mechanisms underlying the causes and effects of pain. In: McCaffery M, Pasero C, eds. Pain. St. Louis: Mosby, 1999:15–34.
14. Johnson BW. Pain mechanisms: Anatomy, physiology, and neurochemistry. In: Raj PP, Abrams BM, Hahn MB, et al., eds. Practical Management of Pain. St. Louis: Mosby, 2000:117–143.
15. Byers MR, Bonica JJ. Peripheral pain mechanisms and nociceptor plasticity. In: Loeser JD, Butler SH, Chapman CR, et al., eds. Bonica's Management of Pain. Philadelphia: Lippincott Williams & Wilkins, 2000:26–72.
16. Bennett GJ. Neuropathic pain: New insights, new interventions. Hosp Pract 1998;October:95–114.
17. Chabal C. Transcutaneous electrical nerve stimulation. In: Loeser JD, Butler SH, Chapman CR, et al., eds. Bonica's Management of Pain. Philadelphia: Lippincott Williams & Wilkins, 2000:1842–1847.
18. Terman GW, Bonica JJ. Spinal mechanisms and their modulation. In: Loeser JD, Butler SH, Chapman CR, et al., eds. Bonica's Management of Pain. Philadelphia: Lippincott Williams & Wilkins, 2000:73–152.
19. McPherson ML. Chronic pain management: A disease-based approach. In: Chronic Illnesses: A Pharmacotherapy Self-Assessment Program. Kansas City, MO: American College of Clinical Pharmacy, 2005:1–40.
20. Elliott KJ. Taxonomy and mechanisms of neuropathic pain. Semin Neurol 1994;3:195–205.
21. Chapman CR, Bonica JJ. Chronic Pain: Current Concepts. Kalamazoo, MI: Scope Publications, 1985:4.
22. Twycross RG. Pain and analgesics. Curr Med Res Opin 1978;5:497–505.
23. Kendall NA, Psychosocial approaches to the prevention of chronic pain: The low back paradigm. Baillieres Best Pract Res Clin Rheumatol 1999;13:545–554.
24. Feldner MT, Hekmat H. Perceived control over anxiety-related events as a predictor of pain behaviors in a cold pressor task. J Behav Ther Exp Psychiatry 2001;32:191–202.
25. Craig KD. Social modelling influences on pain. In: Sternbach RA, ed. The Psychology of Pain. New York: Raven Press, 1978:73–109.
26. American Pain Society. Principles of Analgesic Use in the Treatment of Acute Pain and Chronic Cancer Pain, 5th ed. Glenview, IL: American Pain Society, 2003.
27. Clinical Practice Guideline. Acute Pain Management: Operative or Medical Procedures and Trauma. Publication No. 92–0032, Rockville, MD: Department of Health and Human Services, Public Health Service, Agency for Health Care Policy and Research (now called Agency for Healthcare Research and Quality), 1992.
28. Clinical Practice Guideline No. 9. Management of Cancer Pain. Publication No. 94–0592, Rockville, MD: Department of Health, Public Health Service, Agency for Health Care Policy and Research (now called Agency for Healthcare Research and Quality), 1994.
29. NIH technology assessment panel on integration of behavioral and relaxation approaches into the treatment of chronic pain and insomnia. JAMA 1996;276:313–318.
30. The use of opioids for the treatment of chronic pain: A consensus statement from the American Academy of Pain Medicine and American Pain Society. Approved 1996, modified September 2003, *www.ampainsoc.org.*
31. Miyoshi HR, Leckband SG. Systemic opioids and analgesics. In: Loeser JD, Butler SH, Chapman CR, et al., eds. Bonica's Management of Pain. Philadelphia: Lippincott Williams & Wilkins, 2000:1682–1709.
32. Landau R. One size does not fit all: Genetic variability of mu-opioid receptor and postoperative morphine consumption. Anesthesiology 2006;105:334–337.
33. Gutstein HB, Akil H. Opioid analgesics. In: Brunton LL, Lazo AS, Parker KL, eds. The Pharmacological Basis of Therapeutics, 11th ed. New York: McGraw-Hill, 2006:547–590.
34. Reisine T, Pasternak G. Opioid analgesics and antagonists. In: Hardman JG, Limbird LE, Molinoff PB, et al., eds. The Pharmacological Basis of Therapeutics, 9th ed. New York: McGraw-Hill, 1995:521–555.
35. Schug SA, Zech D, Grond S, et al. A long term survey of morphine in cancer pain patient. J Pain Symptom Manage 1992;7:259–266.
36. Baumann TJ. Analgesic selection when the patient is allergic to codeine. Clin Pharm 1991;10:658.
37. Momeni M, Crucitti M, DeKock M. Patient controlled analgesia in the management of postoperative pain. Drugs 2006;66:2321–2337.
38. Ready BL. Regional analgesics with intraspinal opioids. In: Loeser JD, Butler SH, Chapman CR, et al., eds. Bonica's Management of Pain. Philadelphia: Lippincott Williams & Wilkins, 2000:1953–1966.
39. Pain (PDQ) Health Professional Version. Modified 2006, *www.cancer.gov.*
40. Littrell RA. Epidural analgesia. Am J Hosp Pharm 1991;48:2460–2474.
41. Buckley PF. Regional anesthesia with local anesthetics. In: Loeser JD, Butler SH, Chapman CR, et al., eds. Bonica's Management of Pain. Philadelphia: Lippincott Williams & Wilkins, 2000:1893–1952.
42. Portenoy RK. Pain specialists and addiction medicine specialists unite to address critical issues. Am Pain Soc Bull 1999;9:2–13.
43. Pasero C, Portenoy RK, McCaffery M. Opioid analgesics. In: McCaffery M, Pasero C, eds. Pain. St. Louis: Mosby, 1999:161–299.
44. Anonymous. American Hospital Formulary Service. In: McVoy GK, ed. Drug Information. Bethesda, MD: American Society of Hospital Pharmacists, 1987, 1991, 1994, 1997, 1999, 2001, 2003, 2004, 2005, 2006, 2007.
45. Anonymous. Facts and Comparisons. Philadelphia: Lippincott, 1986, 1991, 1994, 1997, 2000, 2003, 2004, 2006, 2007.
46. Sandoval JA, Furlan AD, Mailis-Gagnon A. Oral methadone for chronic noncancer pain: A systematic literature review of reasons for administra-

tion, prescription patterns, effectiveness, and side effects. Clin J Pain 2005;21:503–512.
47. Mercadante S, Casuccio A, Fulfaro F, et al. Switching from morphine to methadone to improve analgesia and tolerability in cancer patients: A prospective study. J Clin Oncol 2001;19:2898–2904.
48. Codd EE, Shank RP, Schupsky JJ, Raffa RB. Serotonin and norepinephrine uptake inhibiting activity of centrally acting analgesics: Structural determinants and role in antinociception. J Pharmacol Exp Ther 1995;274:1263–1270.
49. Bennett G, Seratini M, Burchiel K, et al. Evidence-based review of the literature on intrathecal delivery of pain medication. J Pain Symptom Manage 2000;20:512–536.
50. Inturrise CE, Colburn WA, Verbev K, et al. Propoxyphene and norproxyphene kinetics after single and repeated doses of propoxyphene. Clin Pharmcol Ther 1982;31:157–167.
51. Package Insert. Tramadol. Raritan, NJ: Ortho-McNeil, 2004.
52. Sindrup SH, Andersen G, Madsen C, et al. Tramadol relieves pain and allodynia in polyneuropathy: A randomized, double-blind, controlled trial. Pain 1999;83:85–90.
53. Dworkin RH, Backonja M, Fowbotham MC, et al. Advances in neuropathic pain. Arch Neurol 2003;60:1524–1534.
54. Finnerup NB, Otto M, McQuay HJ, et al. Algorithm for neuropathic treatment: An evidenced based proposal. Pain 2005;118:289–305.
55. Foley KM. The treatment of cancer pain. N Engl J Med 1985;313:84–95.
56. Clinical Practice Guidelines for Quality Palliative Care. National Consensus Project for Quality Palliative Care. 2004, *www.nationalconcensusproject.org*.
57. Clinical Practice Guideline, American Geriatrics Society Panel on Persistent Pain in Older Persons. The management of persistent pain in older persons. J Am Geriatr Soc 2002;50:1–20.
58. American Academy of Pediatrics and American Pain Society. The assessment and management of acute pain in infants, children and adolescents. Pediatrics 2001;108:793–797.
59. Consensus statement for the prevention and management of pain in the newborn. Arch Pediatr Adolesc Med. 2001;155:173–180.
60. Thomsen AB, Sorensen J, Sjogren P, Eriksen J. Economic evaluation of multidisciplinary pain management in chronic pain patients: A qualitative systematic review. J Pain Symptom Manage 2001;22:688–698.
61. Ritzwoller DP, Crounse L, Shetterly S, et al. The association of comorbidities, utilization, and costs for patients identified with low back pain. BMC Musculoskelet Disord. 2006;7:72.
62. Lipman AG. Why we need outcomes research and pharmacoeconomics in pain management and palliative care. J Pain Palliat Care Pharmacother 2002;16:1–3.
63. McCaffery M. Pain management problems and progress. In: McCaffery M, Pasero C, eds. Pain. St. Louis: Mosby, 1999:1–14.
64. Bonica JJ, Loeser JD. History of pain concepts and therapies. In: Loeser JD, Butler SH, Chapman CR, et al., eds. Bonica's Management of Pain. Philadelphia: Lippincott Williams & Wilkins, 2000:3–16.
65. Crofford LJ, Robotham MC, Mease PJ, et al. Pregabalin for the treatment of fibromyalgia syndrome. Arthritis Rheum 2005;52:1264–1273.
66. Watkins PB, Kaplowitz N, Slattery TJ, et al. Aminotransferase elevations in healthy adults receiving 4 grams of acetaminophen daily: A randomized controlled trial. JAMA 2006;296:87–93.
67. Nasser SM, Ewan PW. Opiate sensitivity: Clinical characteristics and the role of skin prick testing. Clin Expert Allergy 2001;31:1014–1020.
68. Jacobson L, Mariano AJ. General considerations of chronic pain. In: Loeser JD, Butler SH, Chapman CR, et al., eds. Bonica's Management of Pain. Philadelphia: Lippincott Williams & Wilkins, 2000:241–254.

CHAPTER 63 Headache Disorders

DEBORAH S. MINOR AND MARION R. WOFFORD

KEY CONCEPTS

1. Acute migraine therapies should provide consistent, rapid relief and enable the patient to resume normal activities at home, school, or work.
2. A stratified care approach, in which the selection of initial treatment is based on headache-related disability and symptom severity, is the preferred treatment strategy for the migraineur.
3. Strict adherence to maximum daily and weekly doses of antimigraine medications is essential.
4. Preventive therapy should be considered in the setting of recurring migraines that produce significant disability; frequent attacks requiring symptomatic medication more than twice per week; symptomatic therapies that are ineffective, contraindicated, or produce serious side effects; and uncommon migraine variants that cause profound disruption and/or risk of neurologic injury.
5. The selection of an agent for migraine prophylaxis should be based on individual patient response, tolerability, convenience of the drug formulation, and comorbid conditions.
6. Each prophylactic medication should be given an adequate therapeutic trial (usually 2 to 3 months) to judge its efficacy.
7. A general wellness program and avoidance of migraine triggers should be included in the management plan.
8. After an effective abortive agent and dose have been identified, subsequent treatments should begin with that same regimen.

Headache is one of the most common complaints encountered by healthcare practitioners, accounting for more than 1% of visits to physicians' offices or emergency departments.[1] As one of the top 10 presenting complaints in ambulatory medical care, headache can be symptomatic of a distinct pathologic process or can occur without an underlying cause.[1,2] In 2004, the International Headache Society (IHS) updated its classification system and diagnostic criteria for headache disorders, cranial neuralgias, and facial pain[3] (Table 63–1). Designed to facilitate headache diagnosis in clinical practice and research, the IHS classification provides more precise definitions and standardized nomenclature for both the primary (tension-type, migraine, and cluster headache) and secondary (symptomatic of organic disease) headache disorders. This chapter focuses on the management of the primary headache disorders.

Most recurrent headaches are the result of a benign chronic primary headache disorder.[1] Less often, headaches are symptomatic of a serious underlying medical condition, such as infection, cerebral hemorrhage, or brain mass lesion. The peak prevalence of tension-type and migraine headache, the most common of the primary headache disorders, occurs during the most productive years of life (20 to 55 years of age).[4] Despite the prevalence of these disorders and their associated disability, studies indicate that most migraine and tension-type headache sufferers do not seek medical care for their headaches.[4,5] An improved understanding of the diagnosis and pathophysiologic mechanisms of the primary headache disorders, particularly migraine, has led to the development of specific medications capable of providing rapid relief from moderate to severe attacks. However, a thorough evaluation of the headache history is essential to establish an accurate headache diagnosis and identify patients who can benefit from these newer therapeutic options.

Learning objectives, review questions, and other resources can be found at **www.pharmacotherapyonline.com.**

MIGRAINE HEADACHE

EPIDEMIOLOGY

Results of the American Migraine Study II indicate that 18.2% of women and 6.5% of men in the United States experience one or more migraine headaches per year.[6] The prevalence of migraine varies considerably by age and gender. Before the age of 12 years, migraine is more common in boys than in girls, but prevalence increases more rapidly in girls after puberty.[4] After age 12, females are two to three times more likely than males to suffer from migraine. Gender differences in migraine prevalence have been linked to menstruation, but these differences persist beyond menopause. Prevalence is highest in both men and women between the ages of 25 and 45 years.[7] The usual age of onset is 12 to 17 years of age for females and 5 to 11 years for males, with the incidence of migraine with aura peaking earlier in this range for both.[7] In the American Migraine Study II, 92% of women and 89% of men with migraine reported some headache-related disability, and 53% were severely disabled or needed bed rest during an attack.[6] A number of neurologic and psychiatric disorders, including stroke, epilepsy, major depression, and anxiety disorder, show increased comorbidity with migraine.[4] Whether this relationship is causal or representative of a common pathophysiologic mechanism is unknown. The economic burden of migraine is substantial; however, the direct medical costs associated with migraine treatment are far exceeded by the indirect costs that result from work-related disability.[7]

ETIOLOGY AND PATHOPHYSIOLOGY

The etiologic and pathophysiologic mechanisms of migraine are not completely understood. According to the vascular hypothesis

TABLE 63-1 International Headache Society Classification System: Focus on Migraine Headache

Migraine
Migraine without aura
Migraine with aura
Typical aura with migraine headache (aura lasting less than 1 hour)
Typical aura with nonmigraine headache
Typical aura without headache
Familial hemiplegic migraine
Sporadic hemiplegic migraine
Basilar-type migraine
Childhood periodic syndromes that are commonly precursors of migraine
Cyclical vomiting (self-limiting episodic condition)
Abdominal migraine (episodic midline abdominal pain attacks lasting 1 to 72 hours)
Benign paroxysmal vertigo of childhood (brief episodic vertigo)
Retinal migraine (repeated attacks of monocular visual disturbance)
Complications of migraine
Chronic migraine (occurring on 15 or more days per month for more than 3 months)
Status migrainous (debilitating attack lasting for more than 72 hours)
Persistent aura without infarction (symptoms persisting for more than 1 week)
Migrainous infarction (aura symptoms associated with an ischemic brain lesion)
Migraine-triggered seizure
Probable migraine
Probable migraine without aura
Probable migraine with aura
Probable chronic migraine
Tension-type headache
Cluster headache and other trigeminal autonomic cephalalgias
Other primary headaches
Headache attributed to head and/or neck trauma
Headache attributed to cranial or cervical vascular disorder
Headache attributed to non-vascular intracranial disorder
Headache attributed to a substance or its withdrawal
Headache attributed to infection
Headache attributed to disorder of homeostasis
Headache or facial pain attributed to disorder of cranium, neck, eyes, ears, nose, sinuses, teeth, mouth, or other facial or cranial structures
Headache attributed to psychiatric disorder
Cranial neuralgias and central causes of facial pain
Other headache, cranial neuralgia, central or primary facial pain

Adapted with permission from Headache Classification Committee of the International Headache Society. The international classification of headache disorders, 2nd ed. Cephalalgia 2004;24(Suppl 1):1–151.

proposed by Harold Wolff in 1938, the migraine aura is caused by intracerebral arterial vasoconstriction that is followed by reactive extracranial vasodilation and associated headache.[4] Although studies of regional blood flow in the brain do not support the vascular hypothesis, the aura phase of migraine is associated with a reduction in cerebral blood flow that begins in the occipital region and moves across the cerebral cortex at a rate of 2 to 3 mm/min.[8] However, most clinicians now believe that the positive and negative symptoms of the migraine aura are caused by neuronal dysfunction, not ischemia. The neurologic changes of the aura parallel those that occur during cortical spreading depression, a neuronal event characterized by a wave of depressed electrical activity that advances across the brain cortex at a rate that is consistent with the spread of aura symptoms.[8] Migraine without aura is a neurobiologic disorder.[3] Migraine pain is believed to result from activity within the trigeminovascular system, a network of visceral afferent fibers that arises from the trigeminal ganglia and projects peripherally to innervate the pain-sensitive intracranial extracerebral blood vessels, dura mater, and large venous sinuses[9] (Fig. 63–1). These fibers also project centrally, terminating in the trigeminal nucleus caudalis in the brainstem and upper cervical spinal cord, and thus provide a pathway for nociceptive transmission from meningeal blood vessels into higher centers of the central nervous system (CNS). Activation of trigeminal sensory nerves triggers the release of vasoactive neuropeptides, including calcitonin gene-related peptide (CGRP), neurokinin A, and substance P, from perivascular axons. The released neuropeptides interact with dural blood vessels to promote vasodilation and dural plasma extravasation, resulting in neurogenic inflammation.[8] Orthodromic conduction along trigeminovascular fibers transmits pain impulses to the trigeminal nucleus caudalis, where the information is relayed further to higher cortical pain centers. Continued afferent input can result in sensitization of these central sensory neurons, producing a hyperalgesic state that responds to previously innocuous stimuli and maintains the headache.[8]

Despite recent advances in understanding of the pathophysiology of headache pain, there is still a considerable lack of knowledge regarding the mechanisms involved in the initiation of a migraine attack. Although the exact pathophysiology of migraine needs further elucidation, new imaging techniques have provided insight into mechanisms. Previous vascular and neural theories of migraine development have merged into a combined theory of neurovascular mechanisms through evidence provided by neuroimaging. Activity within the trigeminovascular system may be regulated in part by serotonergic neurons within the brainstem. Thus the pathogenesis of migraine may be related to a defect or dysfunction in the activity of neuronal calcium channels mediating serotonin and excitatory neurotransmitter release in brainstem nuclei that modulate cerebral vascular tone and nociception.[8,9] This dysfunction may result in vasodilation of intracranial extracerebral blood vessels and consequent activation of the trigeminovascular system. Future research might further delineate the role of the brainstem as the "migraine generator."

Genetic factors seem to play an important role in an individual's susceptibility to migraine attacks. Studies in monozygotic twins suggest approximately 50% heritability of migraine with a multifactorial polygenic basis.[10] Although it is possible for any individual to experience a migraine attack, it is the recurrence of attacks in the migraineur that is abnormal. Attack occurrence and frequency are governed by the sensitivity of the CNS to migraine-specific triggers or environmental factors. Migraineurs appear to have a lowered threshold of response to specific environmental circumstances as a result of genetic factors that govern the balance of excitation and inhibition at various levels in the CNS.[10] Thus trigger factors can be viewed as modulators of the genetic set point that predisposes to migraine headache. The hyperresponsiveness of the migrainous brain may be the result of an inherited abnormality in P/Q-type calcium channels that regulate cortical excitability through the release of serotonin and other neurotransmitters.[4] Low levels of magnesium or dopamine, increased levels of excitatory amino acids such as glutamate, and alterations in levels of extracellular potassium also can affect the migraine threshold and initiate and propagate the phenomenon of cortical spreading depression.[11]

Serotonin (5-hydroxytryptamine [5-HT]) has long been implicated as an important mediator of migraine headache. Specific populations of the seven subfamilies of 5-HT receptors (5-HT_1 to 5-HT_7) appear to be involved in the pathophysiology and treatment of migraine headache.[8] Acute antimigraine drugs such as the ergot alkaloids and triptan derivatives are agonists of vascular and neuronal 5-HT_1 receptor subtypes, resulting in vasoconstriction of meningeal blood vessels and inhibition of vasoactive neuropeptide release and pain signal transmission.[8] Drugs used for migraine prophylaxis also modulate neurotransmitter systems. These actions and benefits in migraine management are consistent with the current understanding of migraine pathophysiology and neurovascular disorders.[12]

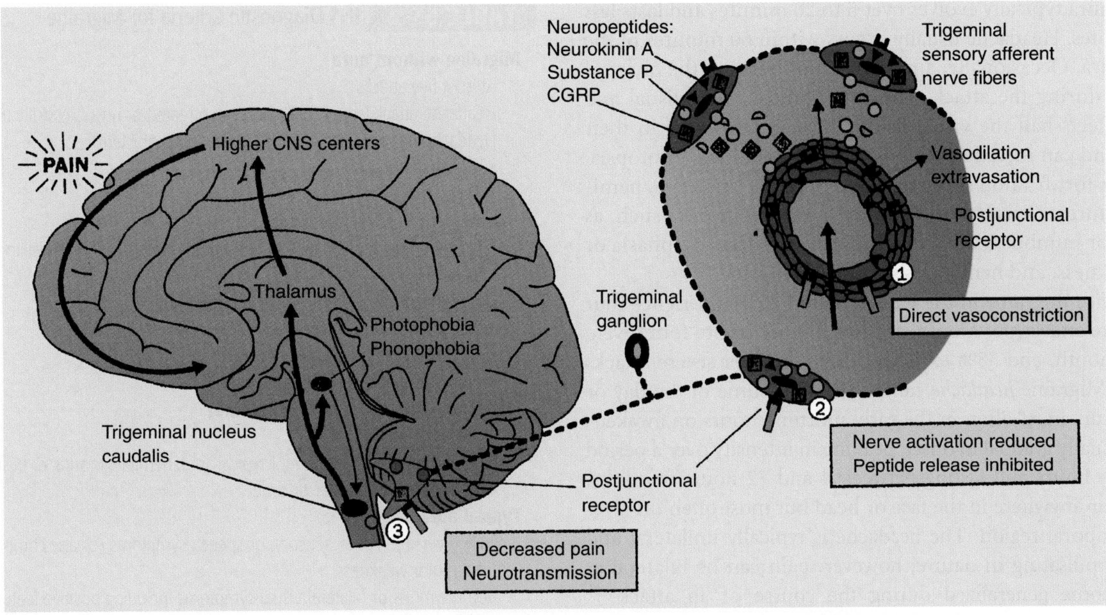

FIGURE 63-1. The pathophysiology of migraine headache. Vasodilation of intracranial extracerebral blood vessels (possibly the result of an imbalance in the brainstem) results in the activation of the perivascular trigeminal nerves that release vasoactive neuropeptides to promote neurogenic inflammation. Central pain transmission may activate other brainstem nuclei, resulting in associated symptoms (nausea, vomiting, photophobia, phonophobia). The antimigraine effects of the $5\text{-HT}_{1B/1D}$ receptor agonists are highlighted at areas 1, 2, and 3. (CGRP, calcitonin gene-related peptide.) *(Adapted with permission from Ferrari MD. Migraine.* Lancet *1998;351:1043–1051. By The Lancet Ltd.)*

CLINICAL PRESENTATION

The migraine attack has been divided into several phases that merit description. *Premonitory symptoms* are experienced by approximately 20% to 60% of migraineurs in the hours or days before the onset of headache.[3,8] The previously popular terms *prodrome* and *warning symptoms* should be avoided because these are often used mistakenly to include aura.[3] Premonitory symptoms vary widely among migraineurs but usually are consistent within an individual. Neurologic symptoms (e.g., phonophobia, photophobia, hyperosmia, and difficulty concentrating) are most common, but psychological (e.g., anxiety, depression, euphoria, irritability, drowsiness, hyperactivity, and restlessness), autonomic (e.g., polyuria, diarrhea, and constipation), and constitutional symptoms (e.g., stiff neck, yawning, thirst, food cravings, and anorexia) also are reported.[4,13]

CLINICAL PRESENTATION OF MIGRAINE HEADACHE

General

- Migraine is a common, recurrent, severe headache that interferes with normal functioning. It is a primary headache disorder divided into two major subtypes, migraine without aura and migraine with aura.

Symptoms

- Migraine is characterized by recurring episodes of throbbing head pain, frequently unilateral, that when untreated can last from 4 to 72 hours. Migraine headaches can be severe and associated with nausea, vomiting, and sensitivity to light, sound, and/or movement. Not all symptoms are present at every attack.
- In the headache evaluation, diagnostic alarms should be identified. These include: acute onset of the "first" or "worst" headache ever, accelerating pattern of headache following subacute onset, onset of headache after age 50 years, headache associated with systemic illness (e.g., fever, nausea, vomiting, stiff neck, and rash), headache with focal neurologic symptoms or papilledema, and new-onset headache in a patient with cancer or human immunodeficiency virus (HIV) infection.

Signs

- A stable pattern, absence of daily headache, positive family history for migraine, normal neurologic examination, presence of food triggers, menstrual association, long-standing history, improvement with sleep, and subacute evolution are all signs of migraine headache. Aura can signal the migraine headache but is not required for diagnosis.

Laboratory Tests

- In selected circumstances and secondary headache presentation, serum chemistries, urine toxicology profiles, thyroid function tests, lyme studies, and other blood tests such as a complete blood count, antinuclear antibody titer, erythrocyte sedimentation rate, and antiphospholipid antibody titer can be considered.

Diagnostic Tests

- Perform a general medical and neurologic physical examination. Check for abnormalities: vital signs (fever, hypertension), funduscopy (papilledema, hemorrhage, and exudates), palpation and auscultation of the head and neck (sinus tenderness, hardened or tender temporal arteries, trigger points, temporomandibular joint tenderness, bruits, nuchal rigidity, and cervical spine tenderness), and neurologic examination (identify abnormalities or deficits in mental status, cranial nerves, deep tendon reflexes, motor strength, coordination, gait, and cerebellar function). Consider neuroimaging studies in patients with abnormal neurologic examination findings of unknown etiology and in those with additional risk factors warranting imaging.

The migraine *aura,* a complex of positive and negative focal neurologic symptoms that precedes or accompanies an attack, is experienced by approximately 31% of migraineurs on some occasions.[14] The aura typically evolves over 5 to 20 minutes and lasts less than 60 minutes. Headache usually occurs within 60 minutes of the end of the aura. Occasionally, aura symptoms begin at the onset of headache or during the attack. The aura is most often visual and frequently affects half the visual field.[3,4] Visual auras vary in their complexity and can include both positive (scintillations, photopsia, teichopsia, or fortification spectrum) and negative (scotoma, hemianopsia) features. Sensory and motor aura symptoms, such as paresthesias or numbness involving the arms and face, dysphasia or aphasia, weakness, and hemiparesis, also are reported.

Of those with migraine in the United States, 25% experience four or more severe attacks per month, 48% experience one to four severe attacks per month, and 38% experience one or fewer severe attacks per month.[6] Migraine *headache* can occur at any time of the day or night but occurs most often in the early morning hours on awakening. Pain is usually gradual in onset, peaking in intensity over a period of minutes to hours and lasting between 4 and 72 hours in adults. Pain can occur anywhere in the face or head but most often involves the frontotemporal region. The headache is typically unilateral and throbbing or pulsating in nature; however, pain can be bilateral at onset or become generalized during the course of an attack.[3,15] Gastrointestinal symptoms almost invariably accompany a migraine headache. During an attack, as many as 90% of migraineurs experience nausea, and emesis occurs in approximately one-third of patients.[8] Other systemic symptoms associated with the headache phase include anorexia, food cravings, constipation, diarrhea, abdominal cramps, nasal stuffiness, blurred vision, diaphoresis, facial pallor, and localized facial, scalp, or periorbital edema. Sensory hyperacuity, manifested as photophobia, phonophobia, or osmophobia, is reported frequently. Because headache pain usually is aggravated by physical activity, most migraineurs seek a dark, quiet room for rest and relief. Impaired concentration, depression, irritability, fatigue, or anxiety often accompany the headache. Once headache pain wanes, patients may experience a *resolution phase* characterized by feeling tired, exhausted, irritable, or listless. Impaired concentration may continue, as well as scalp tenderness or mood changes. Some patients experience depression and malaise, whereas others can feel unusually refreshed or euphoric.[8] The reader is referred to the IHS classification and recent reviews for descriptions of the classic migraine variants and other migraine subtypes[3,4,8,16] (see also Table 63–1).

Although headaches have many potential causes, most are considered to be primary headache disorders. A comprehensive headache history is the most important element in establishing the clinical diagnosis of migraine.[15] A thorough headache history always should be obtained, and information collected should include age at onset, attack frequency and timing, duration of attacks, precipitating or aggravating factors, ameliorating factors, description of neurologic symptoms, characteristics of the headache pain (quality, intensity, location, and radiation), associated signs and symptoms, treatment history, family and social history, and the impact of headaches on daily life.

Secondary headache can be identified or excluded based on the headache history, as well as the results of general medical and neurologic examinations. Diagnostic and laboratory testing also can be warranted in the setting of suspicious headache features or an abnormal examination. The routine use of neuroimaging (computed tomography or magnetic resonance imaging) generally is not indicated in patients with migraine and a normal neurologic examination, but it should be considered in patients with an unexplained abnormal neurologic examination or an atypical headache history.[17] Because migraine headaches usually begin by the second or third decade of life, headaches beginning after age 50 years suggest an organic etiology such as a mass lesion, cerebrovascular disease, or temporal arteritis. Table 63–2 lists the IHS diagnostic criteria for migraine with and without aura.[3]

TABLE 63-2 IHS Diagnostic Criteria for Migraine

Migraine without aura
- At least five attacks
- Headache attack lasts 4 to 72 hours (untreated or unsuccessfully treated)
- Headache has at least two of the following characteristics:
  - Unilateral location
  - Pulsating quality
  - Moderate or severe intensity
- Aggravation by or avoidance of routine physical activity (i.e., walking or climbing stairs)
- During headache at least one of the following:
  - Nausea, vomiting, or both
  - Photophobia and phonophobia
  - Not attributed to another disorder

Migraine with aura (classic migraine)
- At least two attacks
- Migraine aura fulfills criteria for typical aura, hemiplegic aura, or basilar-type aura
- Not attributed to another disorder

Typical aura
- Fully reversible visual, sensory, or speech symptoms (or any combination) but no motor weakness
- Homonymous or bilateral visual symptoms including positive features (e.g., flickering lights, spot, lines) or negative features (e.g., loss of vision) or unilateral sensory symptoms including positive features (e.g., visual loss, pins and needles) or negative features (i.e., numbness), or any combination
- At least one of the following:
  - At least one symptom that develops gradually over a minimum of 5 minutes or different symptoms that occur in succession or both
  - Each symptom lasts for at least 5 minutes and for no longer than 60 minutes
  - Headache that meets criteria for migraine without aura begins during the aura or follows aura within 60 minutes

IHS, International Headache Society.
Adapted with permission from Headache Classification Committee of the International Headache Society. The international classification of headache disorders, 2nd ed. Cephalalgia 2004;24(Suppl 1):1–151.

TREATMENT

Migraines

■ DESIRED OUTCOME

Clinicians who care for migraineurs must appreciate the impact of this painful and debilitating disorder on the life of the patient, the patient's family, and the patient's employer. Treatment strategies must address both immediate and long-term goals. ❶ Acute migraine therapies should provide consistent, rapid relief and enable the patient to resume normal activities at home, school, or work. Recurrence of symptoms and treatment-related adverse effects should be minimal. Ideally, patients should be able to manage their own headaches effectively without a visit to a physician's office or emergency room. In addition, migraineurs should take an active role in the creation of a long-term formal management plan. An individualized approach to treatment can result in a reduction in attack frequency and severity, thus minimizing headache-related disability and emotional distress and improving the patient's quality of life. Goals of long-term and acute treatment of migraine are listed in Table 63–3.

■ GENERAL APPROACH TO TREATMENT

Nonpharmacologic and pharmacologic interventions are available for the management of migraine headache; however, drug therapy remains the mainstay of treatment for most patients. Pharmacotherapeutic management of migraine can be acute (e.g., symptomatic or abortive) or preventive (e.g., prophylactic). When choosing acute or

TABLE 63-3 Goals of Therapy in Migraine Management

Goals of long-term migraine treatment
Reduce migraine frequency, severity, and disability
Reduce reliance on poorly tolerated, ineffective, or unwanted acute pharmacotherapies
Improve quality of life
Prevent headache
Avoid escalation of headache medication use
Educate and enable patients to manage their disease
Reduce headache-related distress and psychological symptoms
Goals for acute migraine treatment
Treat migraine attacks rapidly and consistently without recurrence
Restore the patient's ability to function
Minimize the use of backup and rescue medications[a]
Optimize self-care for overall management
Be cost-effective in overall management
Cause minimal or no adverse effects

[a]Rescue medications are defined as medications used at home when other treatments fail that permit the patient to get relief without a visit to the physician's office or emergency department.

Data from Silberstein[17] and Aukerman et al.[32]

preventive therapies, the clinician should consider the patient's response to specific medications and their tolerability, as well as coexisting illnesses that can limit treatment choices. Abortive or acute therapies can be migraine-specific (e.g., ergots and triptans) or nonspecific (e.g., analgesics, antiemetics, nonsteroidal antiinflammatory drugs [NSAIDs], and corticosteroids) and are most effective at relieving pain and associated symptoms when administered at the onset of migraine[8,18] (Table 63–4). ❷ A stratified care approach in which the selection of initial treatment is based on headache-related disability and symptom severity is the preferred treatment strategy for the migraineur.[17,19] Because attack severity varies in individuals, patients may be advised to use nonspecific agents for mild to moderate headache while reserving migraine-specific medications for more severe attacks. The absorption and efficacy of orally administered drugs can be compromised by the gastric stasis or nausea and vomiting that often accompany migraine.[14] Pretreatment with antiemetic agents or the use of nonoral treatment (e.g., suppositories, nasal sprays, or injections) is advisable when nausea and vomiting are severe.[8]

The frequent or excessive use of acute migraine medications can result in a pattern of increasing headache frequency and drug consumption known as *medication-overuse headache* (or *rebound headache*).[3,19] The syndrome appears to evolve as a self-sustaining headache-medication cycle in which the headache returns as the medication effect wears off, leading to the consumption of more drug for relief. The headache history often reflects the gradual onset of an atypical daily or near-daily headache with superimposed episodic migraine attacks. Medication overuse is one of the most common causes of chronic daily headache.[4] Agents most commonly implicated in this syndrome include simple and combination analgesics, opiates, ergotamine tartrate, and triptans.[3,17] Discontinuation of the offending agent leads to a gradual decrease in headache frequency and severity and a return of the original headache characteristics. Although detoxification usually can be accomplished on an outpatient basis, hospitalization can be necessary for the control of refractory rebound headache and other withdrawal symptoms (e.g., nausea, vomiting, asthenia, restlessness, and agitation). ❸ Regulation of nociceptive systems and renewed responsiveness to therapy may not occur for 3 to 8 weeks following medication withdrawal.[3,4] Most experts recommend limiting use of acute migraine therapies to *2 or 3 days per week* to avoid the development of medication-misuse headache.[8,17]

Preventive migraine therapies are administered on a daily basis to reduce the frequency, severity, and duration of attacks and improve responsiveness to symptomatic migraine therapies[17,20] (Table 63–5). ❹ Preventive therapy should be considered in the setting of recurring migraines that produce significant disability despite acute therapy; frequent attacks requiring symptomatic medication more than twice per week with the risk of developing rebound headache; symptomatic therapies that are ineffective, contraindicated, or produce serious side effects; uncommon migraine variants that cause profound disruption and/or risk of permanent neurologic injury (e.g., hemiplegic migraine, basilar migraine, and migraine with prolonged aura); and patient preference to limit the number of attacks.[17,21] Preventive therapy also may be administered preemptively or intermittently when headaches recur in a predictable pattern (e.g., exercise-induced migraine or menstrual migraine). The efficacy of the various agents used for migraine prophylaxis appears to be similar, but the quality of published data is limited for many commonly used drugs. Only propranolol, timolol, valproate, and topiramate are currently approved by the Food and Drug Administration (FDA) for the indication.[22,23] ❺ Thus the selection of an agent typically is based on its side-effect profile and the patient's comorbid conditions.[21] ❻ A therapeutic trial of 2 to 3 months is necessary to judge the efficacy of each medication, but some reduction in attack frequency can be evident by the first month of therapy.[17,21] Drug therapy should be initiated with low doses and advanced slowly until a therapeutic effect is achieved or side effects become intolerable. Drug doses for migraine prophylaxis are often lower than those necessary for other indications.[4] Overuse of acute headache medications will interfere with the therapeutic effects of preventive treatment.[21] Prophylactic treatment usually is continued for at least 3 to 6 months after the frequency and severity of headaches have diminished and then is tapered gradually and discontinued. Many migraineurs experience fewer and less severe attacks for lengthy periods following discontinuation of prophylactic medications or taper to a lower dose.[21] Figures 63–2 and 63–3 identify treatment and management algorithms for migraine headache.

NONPHARMACOLOGIC THERAPY

Nonpharmacologic therapy of acute migraine headache is limited but can include application of ice to the head and periods of rest or sleep, usually in a dark, quiet environment. Preventive management of migraine should begin with the identification and avoidance of factors that consistently provoke migraine attacks in susceptible individuals[3,24,25] (Table 63–6). Changes in estrogen levels associated with menarche, menstruation, pregnancy, menopause, oral contraceptive use, and other hormone therapies can trigger, intensify, or alleviate migraine.[26] A headache diary that records the frequency, severity, and duration of attacks can facilitate identification of migraine triggers. ❼ Patients also can benefit from adherence to a wellness program that includes regular sleep, exercise, and eating habits, smoking cessation, and limited caffeine intake. Behavioral interventions, such as relaxation therapy, biofeedback (often used in combination with relaxation therapy), and cognitive therapy, are preventive treatment options for patients who prefer nondrug therapy or when symptomatic therapies are poorly tolerated, contraindicated, or ineffective.[17]

CLINICAL CONTROVERSY

Patients are advised to avoid foods and even medications that are identified as migraine triggers. Despite these recommendations, convincing evidence is lacking for many commonly mentioned dietary triggers.[25] Keeping a headache diary can help patients identify risk factors and personal triggers.

TABLE 63-4 Acute Migraine Therapies[a]

Medication	Dosage	Comments
Analgesics		
Acetaminophen	1,000 mg at onset; repeat every 4–6 hours as needed	Maximum daily dose is 4 g
Acetaminophen 250 mg/aspirin 250 mg/caffeine 65 mg	2 tablets at onset and every 6 hours	Available over-the-counter as Excedrin Migraine
Aspirin or acetaminophen with butalbital, caffeine	1–2 tablets every 4–6 hours	Limit dose to 4 tablets/day and usage to 2 days/week
Isometheptene 65 mg/dichloralphenazone 100 mg/acetaminophen 325 mg (Midrin)	2 capsules at onset; repeat 1 capsule every hour as needed	Maximum of 6 capsules/day and 20 capsules/month
Nonsteroidal antiinflammatory drugs		
Aspirin	500–1000 mg every 4–6 hours	Maximum daily dose is 4 g
Ibuprofen	200–800 mg every 6 hours	Avoid doses >2.4 g/day
Naproxen sodium	550–825 mg at onset; can repeat 220 mg in 3–4 hours	Avoid doses >1.375 g/day
Diclofenac potassium	50–100 mg at onset; can repeat 50 mg in 8 hours	Avoid doses >150 mg/day
Ergotamine tartrate		
Oral tablet (1 mg) with caffeine 100 mg	2 mg at onset; then 1–2 mg every 30 minutes as needed	Maximum dose is 6 mg/day or 10 mg/week; consider pretreatment with an antiemetic
Sublingual tablet (2 mg)		
Rectal suppository (2 mg) with caffeine 100 mg	Insert 1/2 to 1 suppository at onset; repeat after 1 hour as needed	Maximum dose is 4 mg/day or 10 mg/week; consider pretreatment with an antiemetic
Dihydroergotamine		
Injection 1 mg/mL	0.25–1 mg at onset IM or subcutaneous; repeat every hour as needed	Maximum dose is 3 mg/day or 6 mg/week
Nasal spray	One spray (0.5 mg) in each nostril at onset; repeat sequence 15 minutes later (total dose is 2 mg or 4 sprays)	Maximum dose is 3 mg/day; prime sprayer 4 times before using; do not tilt head back or inhale through nose while spraying; discard open ampules after 8 hours
Serotonin agonists (triptans)		
Sumatriptan		
Injection	6 mg subcutaneous at onset; can repeat after 1 hour if needed	Maximum daily dose is 12 mg
Oral tablets	25, 50, or 100 mg at onset; can repeat after 2 hours if needed	Optimal dose is 50–100 mg; maximum daily dose is 200 mg
Nasal spray	5, 10, or 20 mg at onset; can repeat after 2 hours if needed	Optimal dose is 20 mg; maximum daily dose is 40 mg; single-dose device delivering 5 or 20 mg; administer one spray in one nostril
Zolmitriptan		
Oral tablets	2.5 or 5 mg at onset as regular or orally disintegrating tablet; can repeat after 2 hours if needed	Optimal dose is 2.5 mg; maximum dose is 10 mg/day Do not divide ODT dosage form
Nasal spray	5 mg (one spray) at onset; can repeat after 2 hours if needed	Maximum daily dose is 10 mg/day
Naratriptan	1 or 2.5 mg at onset; can repeat after 4 hours if needed	Optimal dose is 2.5 mg; maximum daily dose is 5 mg
Rizatriptan	5 or 10 mg at onset as regular or orally disintegrating tablet; can repeat after 2 hours if needed	Optimal dose is 10 mg; maximum daily dose is 30 mg; onset of effect is similar with standard and orally disintegrating tablets; use 5-mg dose (15 mg/day max) in patients receiving propranolol
Almotriptan	6.25 or 12.5 mg at onset; can repeat after 2 hours if needed	Optimal dose is 12.5 mg; maximum daily dose is 25 mg
Frovatriptan	2.5 or 5 mg at onset; can repeat in 2 hours if needed	Optimal dose 2.5–5 mg; maximum daily dose is 7.5 mg (3 tablets)
Eletriptan	20 or 40 mg at onset; can repeat after 2 hours if needed	Maximum single dose is 40 mg; maximum daily dose is 80 mg
Miscellaneous		
Butorphanol nasal spray	1 spray in 1 nostril (1 mg) at onset; repeat in 1 hour if needed	Limit to 4 sprays/day; consider use only when nonopioid therapies are ineffective or not tolerated
Metoclopramide	10 mg IV at onset	Useful for acute relief in the office or emergency department setting
Prochlorperazine	10 mg IV or IM at onset	Useful for acute relief in the office or emergency department setting

ODT, orally disintegrating tablet.

[a]Limit use of symptomatic medications to 2 or 3 days/week when possible to avoid medication-misuse headache.

Data from Ferrari,[9] Silberstein et al.,[18] Matchar et al.,[28] Aukerman et al.,[32] and Tfelt et al.[35]

■ PHARMACOLOGIC MANAGEMENT OF ACUTE MIGRAINE

CLINICAL CONTROVERSY

The availability of many over-the-counter drugs that were formerly prescription medications enables some migraine patients to self-medicate and delay entry into appropriate medical management. Some clinicians feel that over-the-counter products invite patients to take a less effective step-care approach and avoid being treated according to evidence-based guidelines.[27]

Although controversial, some clinicians argue that the efficacy and tolerability of over-the-counter medications for migraine relief are limited because of patient dissatisfaction with the route of administration, the onset of action, the completeness of pain relief, and the length of suffering and prolonged disability.[27]

TABLE 63-5 Prophylactic Migraine Therapies

Medication	Dose
β-Adrenergic antagonists	
Atenolol	25–100 mg/day
Metoprolol[a]	50–300 mg/day in divided doses
Nadolol	80–240 mg/day
Propranolol[a,b]	80–240 mg/day in divided doses
Timolol[b]	20–60 mg/day in divided doses
Antidepressants	
Amitriptyline	25–150 mg at bedtime
Doxepin	10–200 mg at bedtime
Imipramine	10–200 mg at bedtime
Nortriptyline	10–150 mg at bedtime
Protriptyline	5–30 mg at bedtime
Fluoxetine	10–80 mg/day
Phenelzine[c]	15–60 mg/day in divided doses
Gapapentin	900–2,400 mg/day in divided doses
Topiramate[b]	100 mg/day in divided doses
Valproic acid/divalproex sodium[b]	500–1,500 mg/day in divided doses
Verapamil[a]	240–360 mg/day in divided doses
Methysergide[b,c]	2–8 mg/day in divided doses with food
Nonsteroidal antiinflammatory drugs[c]	
Aspirin	1,300 mg/day in divided doses
Ketoprofen[a]	150 mg/day in divided doses
Naproxen sodium[a]	550–1100 mg/day in divided doses
Vitamin B_2	400 mg/day

[a]Sustained-release formulation available.
[b]FDA approved for prevention of migraine.
[c]Daily or prolonged use limited by potential toxicity.
Compiled from Silberstein,[8,17] Silberstein et al.,[18] and Rapopert and Bigal.[22]

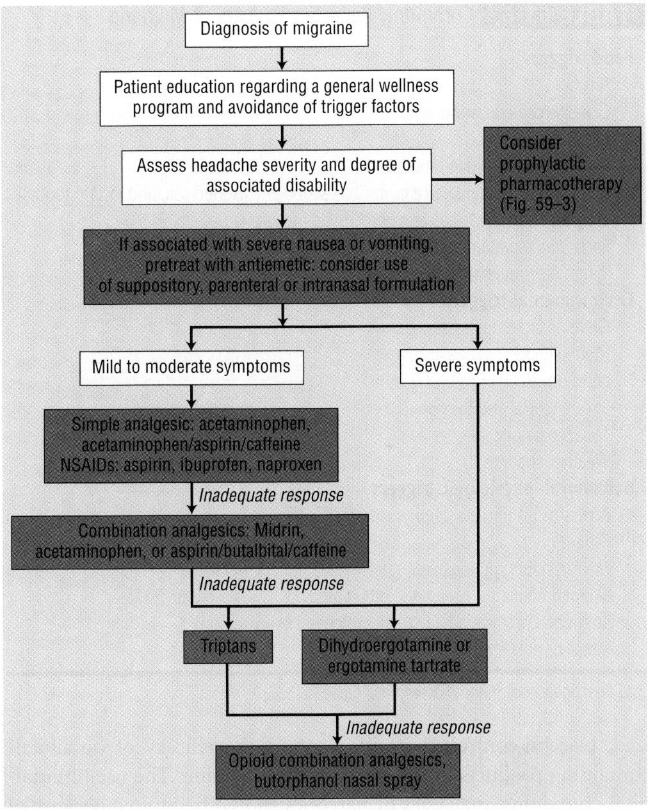

FIGURE 63-2. Treatment algorithm for migraine headaches.

Analgesics and NSAIDs

Simple analgesics and NSAIDs are effective medications for the management of many migraine attacks[6,19,28] (see Table 63–4). They offer a reasonable first-line choice for treatment of mild to moderate migraine attacks or severe attacks that have been responsive in the past to similar NSAIDs or nonopiate analgesics.[17] Of the NSAIDs, aspirin, ibuprofen, naproxen sodium, tolfenamic acid, and the combination of acetaminophen plus aspirin and caffeine have demonstrated the most consistent evidence of efficacy.[24] Evidence for other NSAIDs is either limited (only one study) or inconsistent (some positive and some negative studies).[28] Acetaminophen alone is not generally recommended for migraine because the scientific support is not optimal.[8,17,28] Comparisons with other pharmacotherapeutic classes are limited.

NSAIDs appear to prevent neurogenically mediated inflammation in the trigeminovascular system through the inhibition of prostaglandin synthesis. In general, NSAIDs with a long half-life are preferred as less frequent dosing is needed.[29] Metoclopramide can speed the absorption of analgesics and alleviate migraine-related nausea and vomiting.[25] Suppository analgesic preparations and intramuscular ketorolac are also options when nausea and vomiting are severe.[18] Acute NSAID therapy is associated with gastrointestinal (e.g., dyspepsia, nausea, vomiting, and diarrhea) and CNS side effects (e.g., somnolence, dizziness). NSAIDs should be used cautiously in patients with previous ulcer disease, renal disease, or hypersensitivity to aspirin.[28]

The over-the-counter combination of acetaminophen, aspirin, and caffeine was approved for the treatment of migraine in the United States because of its proven efficacy in relieving migraine pain and associated symptoms.[28] Aspirin and acetaminophen are also available in prescription combination products containing a short-acting barbiturate (butalbital) or narcotic (codeine, propoxyphene). No random-

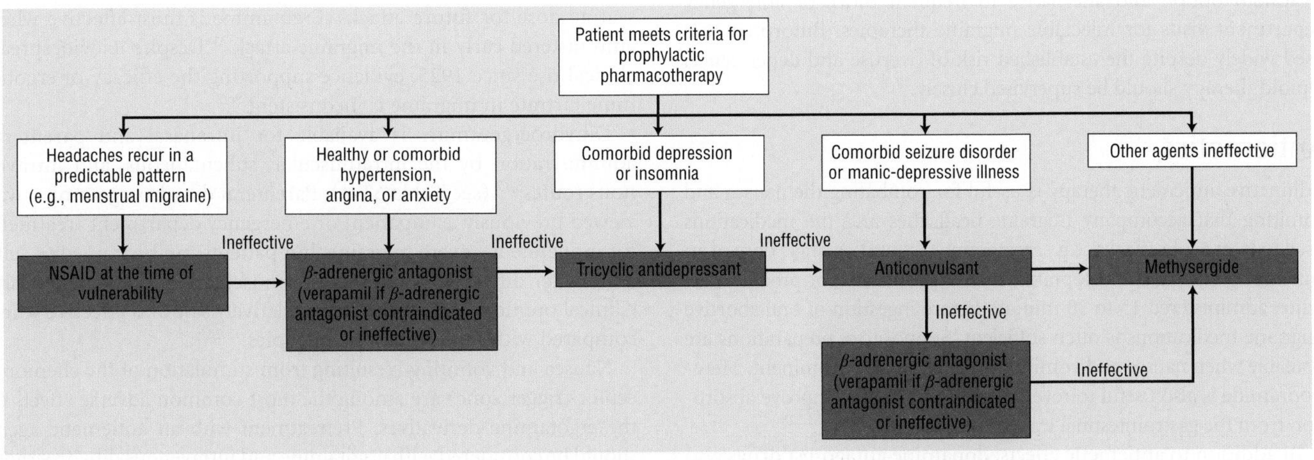

FIGURE 63-3. Treatment algorithm for prophylactic management of migraine headaches. (NSAID, nonsteroidal antiinflammatory drug.)

TABLE 63-6 Commonly Reported Triggers of Migraine

Food triggers
Alcohol
Caffeine/caffeine withdrawal
Chocolate
Fermented and pickled foods
Monosodium glutamate (e.g., in Chinese food, seasoned salt, and instant foods)
Nitrate-containing foods (e.g., processed meats)
Saccharin/aspartame (e.g., diet foods or diet sodas)
Tyramine-containing foods
Environmental triggers
Glare or flickering lights
High altitude
Loud noises
Strong smells and fumes
Tobacco smoke
Weather changes
Behavioral–physiologic triggers
Excess or insufficient sleep
Fatigue
Menstruation, menopause
Skipped meals
Strenuous physical activity (e.g., prolonged overexertion)
Stress or post-stress

Data from Snow et al.,[24] and Diamond and Cady.[25]

ized, placebo-controlled studies support the efficacy of butalbital-containing products in the treatment of migraine. The use of butalbital-containing analgesics or narcotics should be limited because of concerns about overuse, medication-overuse headache, and withdrawal.[8,17,28] Midrin, a combination of acetaminophen, isometheptene mucate (a sympathomimetic amine), and dichloralphenazone (a chloral hydrate derivative), has demonstrated modest benefits in placebo-controlled studies and generally is viewed as an alternative for patients with mild to moderate migraine attacks.[17,28] Although frequent consumption of aspirin or acetaminophen alone can result in medication-overuse headache, combination analgesics appear to pose a greater risk.[8,17]

Opiate Analgesics

Narcotic analgesic drugs (e.g., meperidine, butorphanol, oxycodone, and hydromorphone) are effective but generally should be reserved for patients with moderate to severe infrequent headaches in whom conventional therapies are contraindicated or as "rescue medication" after patients have failed to respond to conventional therapies.[8] Frequent use of narcotic analgesics can lead to the development of dependency and rebound headache.[28] The intranasal formulation of butorphanol, a synthetically derived opioid agonist-antagonist, is a treatment option and alternative to frequent office or emergency department visits for injectable migraine therapies. Butorphanol is used widely despite the established risk of overuse and dependence. Opioid therapy should be supervised closely.[17,28]

Antiemetics

Adjunctive antiemetic therapy is useful for combating the nausea and vomiting that accompany migraine headaches and the medications used to treat acute attacks (e.g., ergotamine tartrate). A single dose of an antiemetic, such as metoclopramide, chlorpromazine, or prochlorperazine, administered 15 to 30 minutes before ingestion of oral abortive migraine medications is often sufficient. Suppository preparations are available when nausea and vomiting are particularly prominent. Metoclopramide is also useful to reverse gastroparesis and improve absorption from the gastrointestinal tract during severe attacks.[17,28]

In addition to antiemetic effects, dopamine antagonist drugs also have been used successfully as monotherapy for the treatment of intractable headache (see Table 63–4). Prochlorperazine administered by the intravenous and intramuscular routes and intravenous metoclopramide provided more effective pain relief than placebo. Chlorpromazine also has provided relief of migraine headache comparable to that provided by intravenous metoclopramide and dihydroergotamine when administered parenterally at doses of 12.5 to 37.5 mg. Domperidone has a possible role for preemptive treatment of migraine. The precise mechanism of action for these agents is unknown. The dopamine antagonists offer an alternative to the narcotic analgesics for the treatment of refractory migraine. Drowsiness and dizziness were reported occasionally with the use of dopamine antagonists in migraineurs. Extrapyramidal side effects were reported infrequently in migraine trials.[28]

Miscellaneous Nonspecific Medications

Corticosteroids can be considered as rescue therapy for status migrainous (a severe, continuous migraine that can last up to 1 week).[17,28] Intravenous dexamethasone at a dose of 6 mg has been tested although there are no high-quality studies supporting the effectiveness of steroids for acute migraine.[28]

Limited studies suggest a role for intranasal lidocaine in the treatment of acute migraine headache.[17,28] Intranasal lidocaine, 1 to 4 drops of a 4% solution, provides rapid pain relief within 15 minutes of administration, but headache recurrence is common. Adverse effects generally are limited to local irritation of the nose or eye, an unpleasant taste, and numbness of the throat.

Preliminary investigations of intramuscular droperidol have yielded favorable results in the treatment of acute migraine headache.[12,30] Future studies might establish a more defined role for this agent in migraine management.

Ergot Alkaloids and Derivatives

Ergotamine tartrate and dihydroergotamine are useful and can be considered for the treatment of moderate to severe migraine attacks.[17] These drugs are nonselective 5-HT_1 receptor agonists that constrict intracranial blood vessels and inhibit the development of neurogenic inflammation in the trigeminovascular system.[8] Central inhibition of the trigeminovascular pathway is also reported. These agents also display activity at α-adrenergic, β-adrenergic, and dopaminergic receptors. Venous and arterial constriction occur with therapeutic doses, but ergotamine tartrate exerts more potent arterial effects than dihydroergotamine.[31]

Ergotamine tartrate is available for oral, sublingual, and rectal administration (see Table 63–4). Oral and rectal preparations contain caffeine to enhance absorption and potentiate analgesia. Some patients respond preferentially to rectal dosing.[8] Dosage requirements should be titrated strictly to establish an effective but subnauseating dose for future attacks. Ergotamine is most effective when administered early in the migraine attack.[31] Despite its widespread clinical use since 1925, evidence supporting the efficacy of ergotamine tartrate in migraine is inconsistent.[8,28]

Dihydroergotamine is available for intranasal and parenteral administration by the intramuscular, subcutaneous, and intravenous routes[8,17] (see Table 63–4). Parenteral dihydroergotamine was viewed previously as inpatient or emergency department treatment for moderate to severe migraine, but patients can be trained to self-administer dihydroergotamine intramuscularly or subcutaneously. Clinical opinion suggests its use is relatively safe and effective when compared with other migraine therapies.[17,28]

Nausea and vomiting (resulting from stimulation of the chemoreceptor trigger zone) are among the most common adverse effects of the ergotamine derivatives. Pretreatment with an antiemetic agent should be considered with ergotamine and intravenous dihydroergotamine therapy. Other common side effects include abdominal pain, weakness, fatigue, paresthesias, muscle pain, diarrhea, and chest tightness. Occasionally, symptoms of severe peripheral ischemia (ergotism), including cold, numb, painful extremities, continuous paresthesias, diminished peripheral pulses, and claudication, can result from the vasoconstrictor effects of the ergot alkaloids. Gangrenous extremities, myocardial infarction, hepatic necrosis, and bowel and brain ischemia have been reported rarely.[4,25,32] Dihydroergotamine is rarely associated with such side effects.[32] Triptans and ergot derivatives should not be used within 24 hours of each other.[32] Recently, reports of severe vasospasm during concomitant therapy with ergotamine and protease inhibitors have appeared in the literature.[33] These cases are attributed to inhibitory effects of the protease inhibitor on the cytochrome P450 3A4 (CYP3A4) isoenzyme and a consequent increase in ergotamine blood levels. Ergotamine derivatives are contraindicated in patients with renal or hepatic failure; coronary, cerebral, or peripheral vascular disease; uncontrolled hypertension; sepsis; and in women who are pregnant or nursing.[4,32] Dihydroergotamine does not appear to cause rebound headache, but dosage restrictions for ergotamine tartrate should be observed strictly to prevent this complication.[4]

Serotonin Receptor Agonists (Triptans)

Introduction of the serotonin receptor agonists, or triptans, represented a significant advance in migraine pharmacotherapy. The first member of this class, sumatriptan, and the second-generation agents zolmitriptan, naratriptan, rizatriptan, almotriptan, frovatriptan, and eletriptan are selective agonists of the 5-HT_{1B} and 5-HT_{1D} receptors. Relief of migraine headache is the result of three key actions: normalization of dilated intracranial arteries through enhanced vasoconstriction, peripheral neuronal inhibition, and inhibition of transmission through second-order neurons of the trigeminocervical complex.[9,14,34] These agents also display varying affinity for 5-HT_{1A}, 5-HT_{1E}, and 5-HT_{1F} receptors. The triptans are appropriate first-line therapy for patients with moderate to severe migraine and are used for rescue therapy when nonspecific medications are ineffective.[17,18]

Sumatriptan, the most extensively studied antimigraine therapy, is available for subcutaneous, oral, and intranasal administration.[34] Subcutaneous sumatriptan is consistently superior to placebo in alleviating migraine headache and associated symptoms, with relief reported in 71% of patients at 1 hour (43% pain-free) and 79% at 2 hours (60% pain-free) in a meta-analysis of placebo-controlled studies.[9,35] In addition to enhanced efficacy, subcutaneous sumatriptan has a more rapid onset of action (10 minutes) when compared with the oral formulation (30 minutes).[18,35] The subcutaneous injection is packaged as an autoinjector device for self-administration by patients. Intranasal sumatriptan provides a faster onset of effect (15 minutes) than the oral formulation and produces similar rates of response (relief in 61% of patients at 2 hours) in placebo-controlled studies.[35] Approximately 30% to 40% of patients who respond to sumatriptan experience headache recurrence within 24 hours.[35] This has been attributed to the drug's short half-life, but recurrence is a problem with most acute migraine therapies.[9,35] A second dose given at the time of recurrence usually is effective.

The second-generation triptans appear to offer an improved pharmacokinetic and pharmacodynamic profile compared with oral sumatriptan.[34–36] These agents have higher oral bioavailability and longer half-lives than oral sumatriptan, which theoretically could improve within-patient treatment consistency and reduce headache recurrence[14,29,34–37] (Table 63–7). Despite the fact that oral absorption can be delayed during migraine attacks, most patients prefer oral formulations, and these account for 80% of all triptan prescriptions.[38]

Results of placebo-controlled studies with each of the second-generation agents reveal somewhat comparable 2-hour response rates. Direct comparative clinical trials are necessary to determine their relative efficacy, but these are available for only a few of the triptans. A recent meta-analysis summarizes the efficacy and tolerability of the different oral triptans across both published and unpublished studies.[38] At all marketed doses, the oral triptans are effective and well tolerated. Across studies for sumatriptan 100 mg, mean results were a 2-hour headache response of 59%, with 29% pain-free at 2 hours, 20% sustained pain-free, and 67% consistency. Compared with sumatriptan 100 mg, rizatriptan 10 mg showed better efficacy and consistency and similar tolerability; eletriptan 80 mg showed better efficacy, similar consistency, but lower tolerability; almotriptan 12.5 mg showed similar efficacy at 2 hours but better other results; naratriptan 2.5 mg and eletriptan 20 mg showed lower efficacy and better tolerability; and zolmitriptan 2.5 and 5 mg, eletriptan 40 mg, and rizatriptan 5 mg all showed similar results. Available data suggest lower efficacy for frovatriptan, although it has the longest half-life of the triptans.[38]

TABLE 63-7 Pharmacokinetic Characteristics of Triptans

Drug	Half-Life (hours)	Time to Maximal Concentration (t_{max})	Bioavailability (%)	Elimination
Almotriptan	3–4	1.4–3.8 hours	70	MAO-A, CYP3A4, CYP2D6
Eletriptan	5	1.4–2.8 hours	50	CYP3A4
Frovatriptan	25	2–4 hours	24–30	CYP1A2
Naratriptan	5–6	2–3 hours	63–74	CYP450 (various isoenzymes)
Rizatriptan	2–3		40–45	MAO-A
Oral tablets		1–1.5 hours		
Disintegrating		1.6–2.5 hours		
Sumatriptan	2			MAO-A
SC injection		12–15 minutes	97	
Oral tablets		2.5 hours	14	
Nasal spray		1–2.5 hours	17	
Zolmitriptan	3		40	CYP1A2, MAO-A
Oral		1.5 hours		
Disintegrating		3 hours		
Nasal		4 hours		

CYP, cytochrome P450; MAO-A, monoamine oxidase type A.
Data from Goadsby et al.,[14] del Rio and Silberstein,[29] Matthew and Loder,[34] Tfelt-Hansen et al.,[35] Deleu and Hanssens,[36] and Pringsheim and Gawel.[37]

Clinical response to the triptans can vary considerably among individual patients. Individual responses cannot be predicted, and if one triptan fails, a patient can be switched successfully to another triptan.[8,38] **8** After an effective agent and dose have been identified, subsequent treatments should begin with that same regimen.

Side effects to the triptans are common but usually mild to moderate in nature and of short duration. Adverse effects are consistent among the class and include paresthesias, fatigue, dizziness, flushing, warm sensations, and somnolence. Local side effects are reported with the subcutaneous (minor injection-site reactions) and intranasal (taste perversion, nasal discomfort) routes. Doses that provide the best ratio of efficacy and safety are considered optimal. Up to 15% of patients receiving a triptan consistently report "chest symptoms," including tightness, pressure, heaviness, or pain in the chest, neck, or throat.[9,18] The mechanism of these symptoms is unknown, but a cardiac source of pain seems unlikely in most patients.[39,40] However, all triptans are partial agonists of human 5-HT coronary artery receptors in vitro, resulting in a small but significant vasoconstrictor response.[14,36] Adverse cardiac events are rare because 5-HT_{2A} receptors mediate most of the effects of serotonin on coronary vessels.[18] Isolated cases of myocardial infarction and coronary vasospasm with ischemia have been reported, but myocardial ischemia is unlikely in patients with normal coronary vasculature.[36] The triptans are contraindicated in patients with a history of ischemic heart disease (e.g., angina pectoris, Prinzmetal's angina, or previous myocardial infarction), uncontrolled hypertension, and cerebrovascular disease. Patients at risk for unrecognized coronary artery disease (e.g., postmenopausal women, men older than 40 years of age, and patients with multiple risk factors) should receive a cardiovascular assessment prior to triptan use and have their initial dose administered under medical supervision. Triptans are also contraindicated in patients with hemiplegic and basilar migraine. The triptans should not be given within 24 hours of the ergotamine derivatives. Administration of sumatriptan, rizatriptan, and zolmitriptan within 2 weeks of therapy with monoamine oxidase inhibitors is not recommended. Concomitant therapy with the selective serotonin reuptake inhibitors (SSRIs) or serotonin-norepinephrine reuptake inhibitors (SNRIs) (e.g., duloxetine, venlafaxine, and sibutramine) can be life-threatening as a result of serotonin syndrome. The potential risk of these combinations should be carefully considered and discussed with the patient.[41] Frequent use of the triptans has been associated with the development of medication-misuse headache.[14,17,28]

■ PROPHYLACTIC PHARMACOLGIC THERAPY

β-Adrenergic Antagonists

β-Adrenergic antagonists are the most widely used drugs for migraine prophylaxis.[21] Propranolol, nadolol, timolol, atenolol, and metoprolol have proven efficacy in controlled clinical trials, reducing the frequency of attacks by 50% in 60% to 80% of patients[21,23] (see Table 63–5). Because the relative efficacy of the individual agents has not been established, selection of a β-blocker can be based on β-selectivity, convenience of the formulation, and tolerability. β-Blockers with intrinsic sympathomimetic activity are ineffective for migraine prophylaxis.[21] Although their precise mechanism of antimigraine action is unknown, they may raise the migraine threshold by modulating adrenergic or serotonergic neurotransmission in cortical or subcortical pathways. β-Blockers are particularly useful in patients with comorbid anxiety, hypertension, or angina. Side effects can include drowsiness, fatigue, sleep disturbances, vivid dreams, memory disturbance, depression, impotence, bradycardia, and hypotension. β-Blockers should be used with caution in patients with congestive heart failure, peripheral vascular disease, atrioventricular conduction disturbances, asthma, depression, and diabetes. Bronchoconstrictive and hyperglycemic effects can be minimized with β_1-selective agents.

Antidepressants

The beneficial effects of antidepressants in migraine are independent of their antidepressant activity and may be related to downregulation of central 5-HT_2 and adrenergic receptors.[21] Amitriptyline, the most widely studied antidepressant for migraine prophylaxis, has demonstrated efficacy in placebo-controlled and comparative studies.[23] Use of other antidepressants is based primarily on clinical and anecdotal experience (see Table 63–5). Other tricyclic antidepressants (TCAs) that have been used successfully for migraine prophylaxis include doxepin, nortriptyline, protriptyline, and imipramine.[17,21] Anticholinergic side effects are common and limit use of these agents in patients with benign prostatic hyperplasia and glaucoma. Evening doses are preferred because of associated sedation. Increased appetite and weight gain can occur. Orthostatic hypotension and cardiac toxicity (slowed atrioventricular conduction) also are reported occasionally. The more favorable side-effect profile of nortriptyline and protriptyline could prove advantageous in patients who are particularly intolerant of the anticholinergic and sedative side effects of amitriptyline.

SSRIs have not been studied extensively for the preventive treatment of migraine headaches, but clinicians have used them nonetheless.[18] Fluoxetine is the most studied SSRI for migraine prevention, but definitive benefit has not been demonstrated in a rigorous clinical study.[21] Prospective data evaluating the other SSRIs (e.g., sertraline, paroxetine, fluvoxamine, and citalopram) are lacking.[17] The SSRIs are considered to be less effective than TCAs for migraine prophylaxis but have gained favor with some clinicians as a result of their more favorable adverse-effect profile.[4] These agents should not be considered as first- or second-line medications for the management of migraine, but they are useful in patients with comorbid depression.[4,21] Preliminary evidence suggests a possible benefit with venlafaxine, an inhibitor of serotonin and norepinephrine reuptake.[42] Again, the potential risk of serotonin syndrome should be considered in patients using SSRIs or SNRIs along with a triptan.[41]

Monoamine oxidase inhibitors (MAOIs), such as phenelzine, have been used in the management of refractory headache, but their complex adverse-effect profile limits their use to experienced prescribers.[42] Strict adherence to a tyramine-free diet is necessary to avoid potentially life-threatening hypertensive crisis. The reader is referred to Chap. 71 for dietary and concurrent medication restrictions for patients taking MAOIs.

Anticonvulsants

Anticonvulsant medications have emerged as an important therapeutic option for the prevention of migraine headaches. The beneficial effects of these agents are likely caused by multiple mechanisms of action, including enhancement of γ-aminobutyric acid (GABA)–mediated inhibition, modulation of the excitatory neurotransmitter glutamate, and inhibition of sodium and calcium ion channel activity.[43] Anticonvulsants, such as divalproex sodium and topiramate, are particularly useful in migraineurs with comorbid seizures, anxiety disorder, or bipolar disorder.[4] The efficacy of valproic acid and divalproex sodium (a 1:1 molar combination of valproate sodium and valproic acid) has been demonstrated in multiple placebo-controlled studies.[21] Nausea and vomiting, the most common early side effects, are self-limited and appear to be less common with divalproex sodium and gradual titration of doses. Alopecia, tremor, asthenia, somnolence, and weight gain are also common complaints.[21,44] The extended-release formulation of divalproex sodium is administered once daily and is better tolerated than the enteric-coated formulation.[44] Hepatotoxicity is the most serious side effect of valproate therapy, but the risk appears to be low in migraineurs (e.g., patients older than 10 years of age who are receiving monotherapy and have no underlying metabolic or neurologic disorder).[21] Baseline liver function tests should be obtained, but routine followup studies are not necessary in asymptomatic adults on monotherapy. Patient evaluation is recommended every 1 to 2 months during the first 6 to 9 months of therapy. Valproate is contraindicated in pregnant women (owing to potential teratogenicity) and patients with a history of pancreatitis or chronic liver disease. Although valproate level determinations can be useful for assessing compliance and toxicity, a recent study suggests that serum levels of less than 50 mcg/mL (346 μmol/L) (usual therapeutic level is 50 to 100 mcg/mL) can provide similar benefit to higher levels.[45]

Topiramate has recently been approved for a migraine prophylaxis indication based on the results of a randomized, double-blind study that demonstrated significantly greater reductions in mean monthly migraine frequency with 100 and 200 mg topiramate daily compared with placebo.[46] Topiramate should be initiated at a low dose, 25 mg, and slowly titrated up to minimize adverse effects. Treatment-emergent adverse events associated with topiramate included paresthesia, fatigue, anorexia, diarrhea, weight loss, difficulty with memory, and nausea. Kidney stones, acute myopia and acute angle-closure glaucoma, and oligohidrosis have been reported infrequently with topiramate use.[47]

A recent study suggests that gabapentin also may be an effective agent for migraine prevention in patients achieving a daily dose of 2400 mg.[21,48] Somnolence, dizziness, and asthenia were the most commonly reported adverse events. Preliminary studies suggest a possible role for other anticonvulsants, including tiagabine, levetiracetam, and zonisamide; however, further clinical studies are needed to confirm their usefulness in migraine prophylaxis.[22,47,49]

Calcium Channel Blockers

The calcium channel blockers generally are considered second- or third-line options for preventive treatment when other drugs with established clinical benefit are ineffective or contraindicated.[18] Verapamil is the most widely used calcium channel blocker for preventive treatment, but it provided only modest benefit in decreasing the frequency of attacks in two placebo-controlled studies.[4] The therapeutic effect of verapamil may not be noted for up to 8 weeks after initiation of therapy.[42] Side effects of verapamil can include constipation, hypotension, bradycardia, atrioventricular block, and exacerbation of congestive heart failure. Evaluations of nifedipine, nimodipine, diltiazem, and nicardipine have yielded equivocal results.[21]

Methysergide

The semisynthetic ergot alkaloid methysergide is a potent 5-HT_2 receptor antagonist that appears to stabilize serotonergic neurotransmission in the trigeminovascular system to block the development of neurogenic inflammation.[28] Although methysergide is an effective preventive medication, its utility is limited by the rare (1 in 5,000 patients) development of retroperitoneal, endocardial, and pulmonary fibrosis during long-term administration.[4] Consequently, a medication-free interval of 4 weeks is recommended following each 6-month treatment period.[28] The dosage should be tapered over a 1-week period to prevent rebound headaches. Monitoring for fibrotic complications should include periodic auscultation of the heart, as well as yearly chest roentgenography, echocardiography, and abdominal magnetic resonance imaging.[21] Methysergide is best tolerated when taken with meals. In addition to gastrointestinal intolerance, muscle aching, leg cramps, claudication, weight gain, and hallucinations are also reported with its use. It is contraindicated in pregnancy, peripheral vascular disorders, coronary artery disease, severe hypertension, thrombophlebitis or cellulitis of the legs, peptic ulcer disease, liver or renal dysfunction, and valvular heart disease.[8] Peripheral vasospasm and severe claudication have been reported occasionally in patients without a prior history of vascular disease. Methysergide is reserved for patients with refractory headaches that do not respond to other preventive therapies.

NSAIDs

NSAIDs are modestly effective for reducing the frequency, severity, and duration of migraine attacks, but potential gastrointestinal and renal toxicity can limit the daily or prolonged use of these agents.[21,23] Consequently, NSAIDs have been used intermittently to prevent headaches that recur in a predictable pattern, such as menstrual migraine. Administration of NSAIDs in the perimenstrual period can be beneficial in women with true menstrual migraine. NSAIDs should be initiated 1 to 2 days prior to the expected onset of headache and continued during the period of vulnerability.[4] Prostaglandin production can be enhanced in women with menstrual migraine, and the preventive mechanism of NSAIDs is thought to involve inhibition of prostaglandin synthesis.[4] If long-term NSAID therapy is initiated, monitoring of renal function and occult blood loss is necessary.

Miscellaneous Prophylactic Agents

A double-blind, placebo-controlled study demonstrated the efficacy of riboflavin (vitamin B_2) 400 mg daily in migraine prophylaxis. Riboflavin was associated with 50% or greater improvement in attack frequency in 59% of patients.[47] More recently, localized injections of botulinum toxin type A have reduced the frequency, severity, and disability associated with migraine headaches significantly in three small double-blind, placebo-controlled trials.[50] The angiotensin-converting enzyme inhibitor lisinopril and the angiotensin II receptor blocker candesartan provided effective migraine prophylaxis in recent double-blind, placebo-controlled, crossover studies of these agents.[51,52] Further research is needed to establish the safety and efficacy of the herbal medication feverfew (*Tanacetum parthenium*) because studies to date have yielded conflicting results.[4] Authors of a recent double-blind, placebo-controlled study concluded that petasites, an extract from the plant *Petasites hybridus*, may be an effective preventive treatment for migraine.[49] Further study is needed to determine the clinical utility and comparative efficacy of these agents for the prophylactic management of migraine.

PHARMACOECONOMIC CONSIDERATIONS

Although migraine is widely recognized as a disease that exacts an enormous toll on the sufferer, the direct and indirect costs associated with migraine headache impose a substantial burden on society as well. The direct medical costs associated with clinic visits for headache and migraine diagnosis and treatment are substantial, exceeding $1 billion per year.[14] Migraine also results in high use of emergency rooms and urgent care centers.[7] Headache accounts for one-third of all over-the-counter analgesic use in the United States, and gross sales from triptans alone total more than $1 billion per year. The indirect costs of the illness related to work absenteeism, decreased productivity, and impairment greatly exceed the direct cost of medical care.[7,53] The estimated indirect cost of migraine-related disability for American employers, the most important determinant of the economic impact of migraine, is approximately $13 billion each year.[7,53]

According to the American Migraine Study II, only 48% of those surveyed with clear symptoms of migraine were diagnosed by a physician.[5,6] Although 96% of severe migraine sufferers take some medication for their headaches, only 41% of those with moderate to severe headache-related disability take prescription medication.[5,6] Because many migraineurs who receive inadequate care experience substantial levels of pain and disability, improvement in migraine diagnosis, care, and treatment potentially could result in lower direct and indirect costs of the disease.

Education of headache patients regarding required behavior changes and effective use of acute and prophylactic pharmacotherapy can be time-consuming, but it is also extremely cost-effective. Oversights can lead to decreased efficacy of medications resulting in repeat dosing and polypharmacy, decreased compliance, increased emergency department use, increased "doctor shopping," and, perhaps, increased use of expensive diagnostic procedures and inpatient services. Recent studies demonstrate that effective migraine treatment can reduce the functional disability and productivity loss associated with a migraine attack.[5,25,34] Patients with stratified care targeted to their needs had higher headache response rates, shorter disability times, less health service utilization, and less loss of productivity.[25]

SUMMARY

Acute and preventive pharmacotherapy for migraine should be individualized based on the individual patient response, tolerability of the available agents, and presence of comorbid conditions. Migraine management should be individualized on the basis of the patient's clinical presentation and medical history. Analgesics and NSAIDs can be considered the drugs of choice for infrequent mild to moderate attacks. The triptans or dihydroergotamine can be used as secondary agents if initial therapies prove ineffective or as first-line therapy in moderate to severe migraine headache. Abortive therapy should be instituted early in the course of the attack to optimize efficacy and minimize migraine-related pain and disability. Preventive therapy should be considered in the setting of recurring migraines that produce significant disability, frequent attacks requiring symptomatic medication more than twice per week, symptomatic therapies that are ineffective, contraindicated, or produce serious side effects, and uncommon migraine variants that cause profound disruption and/or risk of neurologic injury. Efficacy of a prescribed prophylactic regimen should be reassessed periodically. A prolonged headache-free interval could allow for gradual dosage reduction and discontinuation of therapy.

TENSION-TYPE HEADACHE

EPIDEMIOLOGY

Tension-type headache is the most common type of primary headache, with an estimated 1-year prevalence of 63% in men and 86% in women.[2] First onset of tension-type headache typically is early in life (younger than age 20 in 40% of patients), and prevalence peaks between the ages of 20 and 50 years.[2,4] It is more common among women in adulthood, with a female-to-male ratio of 5:4.[2] The mean frequency of attacks is 2.9 days per month, with most sufferers experiencing fewer than one attack per month.[4] The prevalence of chronic tension-type headache (defined as greater than or equal to 180 headache days per year) is estimated at 2% to 3%.[4] Although an estimated 60% of tension-type headache sufferers experience some degree of functional impairment during their attacks, less than 15% of patients seek medical attention for their headaches.[4,2]

PATHOPHYSIOLOGY

Although tension-type headache is the most common type of headache, it is the least studied of the primary headache disorders, and there is limited understanding of key pathophysiologic concepts.[54] Some practitioners theorize that migraine and tension-type headaches represent a continuum of headache severity within the same entity.[55] However, more recently, tension-type headache has been recognized as a distinct disorder. The pain of episodic tension-type headache is thought to originate from myofascial factors and peripheral sensitization of nociceptors. Central mechanisms also are involved.[54] Mental stress, nonphysiologic motor stress, a local myofascial release of irritants or a combination of these may be the initiating stimulus. Following activation of supraspinal pain perception structures, a self-limiting headache results in most individuals owing to central modulation of the incoming peripheral stimuli.[54] Chronic tension-type headache can evolve from episodic tension-type headache in predisposed individuals owing to a disturbance of central nociceptive processing and subsequent sensitization of the CNS.[54] It is likely that other pathophysiologic mechanisms also contribute to the development of tension-type headache.

CLINICAL PRESENTATION

Premonitory symptoms and aura are absent with tension-type headache. The pain usually is mild to moderate in intensity and often is described as a dull, nonpulsatile tightness or pressure.[3,4] Bilateral pain is most common, but the location can vary (frontal and temporal pain are most common; occipital and parietal regions also may be affected).[3] The pain is classically described as having a "hatband" pattern. Associated symptoms generally are absent, but mild photophobia or phonophobia may be reported. The disability associated with tension-type headache typically is minor in comparison with migraine headache, and routine physical activity does not affect headache severity.[3,4] Palpation of the pericranial or cervical muscles can reveal tender spots or localized nodules in some patients.[3] Tension-type headache is classified as either episodic (infrequent or frequent) or chronic based on the frequency and duration of the attacks.[4]

TREATMENT

Tension-Type Headaches

■ GENERAL APPROACH TO TREATMENT

The vast majority of episodic tension-type headache sufferers self-medicate with over-the-counter medications and do not consult a healthcare professional. Although pharmacologic and nonpharmacologic treatments are available, simple analgesics and NSAIDs are the mainstay of acute therapy. Most agents used for tension-type headache have not been studied in controlled clinical trials.[56]

■ NONPHARMACOLOGIC THERAPY

Psychophysiologic therapy and physical therapy have been used in the management of tension-type headache. Psychophysiologic therapy can consist of reassurance and counseling, stress management, relaxation training, and biofeedback. Relaxation training and biofeedback training (alone or in combination) can result in a 50% reduction in headache activity.[4] Evidence supporting physical therapeutic options, such as heat or cold packs, ultrasound, electrical nerve stimulation, stretching, exercise, massage, acupuncture, manipulations, ergonomic instruction, and trigger point injections or occipital nerve blocks, is somewhat inconsistent.[4] However, patients can benefit from selected modalities (e.g., massage) during an acute episode of tension-type headache.

■ PHARMACOLOGIC THERAPY

Simple analgesics (alone or in combination with caffeine) and NSAIDs are effective for the acute treatment of mild to moderate tension-type headache. Acetaminophen, aspirin, ibuprofen, naproxen, ketoprofen, indomethacin, and ketorolac have demonstrated efficacy in placebo-controlled and comparative studies.[4] Failure of over-the-counter agents can warrant therapy with prescription drugs. High-dose NSAIDs and the combination of aspirin or acetaminophen with butalbital or, rarely, codeine are effective options. Use of butalbital and codeine combinations should be avoided when possible owing to the high potential for overuse and dependency. As with migraine headache, acute medication should be taken for episodic tension-type headache no more than 2 days per week to prevent the development of chronic tension-type headache.[4,57] There is no evidence to support the efficacy of muscle relaxants in the management of episodic tension-type headache.[2,4,56] Preventive treatment should be considered if headache frequency (more than two per week), duration (greater than 3–4 hours), or severity results in medication overuse or substantial disability. The principles of preventive treatment for tension-type headache are similar to those for migraine headache. TCAs are prescribed most often for prophylaxis, but other drugs also can be selected after consideration of comorbid medical conditions and respective side-effect profiles.[4] Injection of botulinum toxin into pericranial muscles has demonstrated efficacy in the prophylaxis of chronic tension-type headache in two recently published placebo-controlled studies.[56]

CLUSTER HEADACHE

EPIDEMIOLOGY

Cluster headache, the most severe of the primary headache disorders, is characterized by attacks of severe, unilateral head pain that occur in series lasting for weeks or months (i.e., cluster periods) separated by remission periods usually lasting months or years.[3,4,58] Cluster headaches can be episodic or chronic.[3] Cluster headache is relatively uncommon among the primary headache disorders, but the exact prevalence is uncertain. The prevalence varies from 56 to 401 per 100,000.[58] Men are more likely than women to have cluster headache, and onset generally occurs in those older than 20 years of age.[4,58] Recent genetic epidemiological surveys suggest a predisposition for cluster headache can exist in certain families.[4,58]

PATHOPHYSIOLOGY

The etiologic and pathophysiologic mechanisms of cluster headache are not completely understood. The cyclic nature of attacks implicates a pathogenesis of hypothalamic dysfunction with resulting alterations in circadian rhythms.[4,59] Hypothalamus-regulated changes in cortisol, prolactin, testosterone, growth hormone, leuteinizing hormone, endorphin, and melatonin have been found during periods of cluster headache attack.[59,60] Neuroimaging studies performed during acute cluster headache attacks have demonstrated activation of the ipsilateral hypothalamic gray area, implicating the thalamus as a cluster generator.[59] Significant cranial autonomic activation occurs ipsilateral to the pain, through the same pathways that are activated during migraine.[59]

CLINICAL PRESENTATION

Attacks occur in cluster periods lasting 2 weeks to 3 months in most patients, followed by long pain-free intervals.[3,4] Periods of remission average 2 years in length but have been reported to be from 2 months to 20 years in duration. Approximately 10% of patients have chronic symptoms with attacks recurring for over 1 year without remission or with remission periods of less than 1 month.[3,61] Cluster headache attacks occur commonly at night and appear to be more common in the spring and fall.[61] Attacks occur suddenly, with pain peaking quickly after onset and generally lasting 15 to 180 minutes.[3] Auras are not present with cluster headaches. The pain is excruciating, penetrating, and of a boring intensity in orbital, supraorbital, and temporal unilateral locations.[3,4,61] The headache can be accompanied by conjunctival injection, lacrimation, nasal stuffiness, rhinorrhea, eyelid edema, facial sweating, miosis/ptosis, and restlessness or agitation. During the cluster period, attacks occur from once every other day to eight times per day.[3,4] Whereas migraine patients retreat to a quiet dark room, cluster headache patients generally sit and rock or pace about the room clutching their head.[61] There is a male preponderance in cluster headache, especially in the chronic form, and lifestyle habits such as smoking and consumption of alcohol or coffee are common.[62] Specific diagnostic criteria for cluster headaches are provided within the IHS classification system.[3]

TREATMENT

Cluster Headaches

As in migraine, therapy for cluster headaches involves both abortive and prophylactic therapy. Abortive therapy is directed at managing the acute attack. Prophylactic therapies are started early in the cluster period in an attempt to induce remission and can be transitional using agents not suitable for long-term or chronic use. Patients with chronic cluster headache can require prophylactic medications indefinitely.

■ ABORTIVE THERAPY

Oxygen

The standard acute treatment of cluster headache is inhalation of 100% oxygen by nonbreather facial mask at a rate of 7 to 10 L/min for 15 to 25 minutes.[4,60] Repeat administration can be necessary because of recurrence, as oxygen appears to merely delay, rather than abort, the attack in some patients.[60] No side effects have been reported with the use of oxygen, but caution should be used for those who smoke or have chronic obstructive pulmonary disease.

Ergotamine Derivatives

All forms of ergotamine have been used in cluster headaches, although in general, their role has been supplanted by the triptans. Intravenous dihydroergotamine results in the quickest response, and repeated administration for 3 to 7 days can break the cycle of frequent cluster headache attacks.[60] Ergotamine tartrate also has provided effective relief of cluster headache attacks when administered sublingually or rectally, but the pharmacokinetics of these preparations frequently limit their clinical utility.[60] Dosing guidelines are similar to those for migraine headache therapy.

Triptans

The quick onset of subcutaneous and intranasal triptans make them safe and effective abortive agents for cluster headaches. Subcutaneous sumatriptan (6 mg) is the most effective agent. Nasal sprays are less effective but may be better tolerated in some patients. Adverse events reported in cluster headache patients are similar to those seen in migraineurs. Orally administered triptans have limited use in cluster attacks because of their relatively slow onset of action; oral zolmitriptan (10 mg), however, was beneficial in patients with episodic cluster headache with 60% experiencing mild or no pain at 30 minutes.[37,60]

■ PROPHYLACTIC THERAPY

Verapamil

Verapamil, the preferred calcium channel blocker for the prevention of cluster headaches, is effective in approximately 70% of patients.[4] The beneficial effects of verapamil often appear after 1 week of therapy. A typical suggested dosage range is from 360 mg/day to 720 mg/day.[60]

Lithium

Lithium carbonate is effective for episodic and chronic cluster headache attacks and can be used in combination with verapamil. A positive response is seen in up to 78% of patients with chronic cluster headache, and in up to 63% of patients with episodic cluster headache.[4,60] The usual dose is 600 to 1,200 mg/day, with a suggested starting dose of 300 mg twice daily. Optimal plasma lithium levels for prevention of cluster headache have not been established, but trough values should not be more than 1.0 mEq/L.[4,60]

Initial side effects are mild and include tremor, lethargy, nausea, diarrhea, and abdominal discomfort. Thyroid and renal function must be monitored during lithium therapy. Lithium should be administered with caution to patients with significant renal or cardiovascular disease, dehydration, pregnancy, or concomitant diuretic or NSAID use.[4,60]

Ergotamine

Ergotamine can be an efficacious agent for prophylactic as well as abortive therapy of cluster headaches.[4] A 2-mg bedtime dose is often beneficial for the prevention of nocturnal headache attacks. Daily use of 1 to 2 mg ergotamine alone or in combination with verapamil or lithium can provide effective headache prophylaxis in patients refractory to other agents with little risk of ergotism or rebound headache.[4,60]

Methysergide

In patients unresponsive to other therapies, methysergide 4 to 8 mg/day in divided doses is usually effective in shortening the course of cluster headaches.[60] Response to treatment usually occurs within 1 week of initiation of the drug. Response rates in patients with episodic cluster headache approach 70%, but chronic cluster headache patients receive less benefit.[60] Precautions regarding methysergide use were described earlier in this chapter (see Pharmacologic Management of Acute Migraine above).

Corticosteroids

Corticosteroids are useful for inducing remission.[4,60] Therapy is initiated with 40 to 60 mg/day prednisone and tapered over approximately 3 weeks. Relief appears within 1 to 2 days of initiating therapy. To avoid steroid-induced complications, long-term use is not recommended. Headaches can recur when therapy is tapered or discontinued.

Miscellaneous Agents

Other therapies that have been used in the acute management of cluster headache include intranasal lidocaine, cocaine, capsaicin, and civamide. Limited studies also support the use of divalproex sodium, topiramate, nifedipine, nimodipine, melatonin, and baclofen for cluster prophylaxis. Neurosurgical intervention can be necessary for patients with chronic cluster headache that is resistant to all medical therapies.[4,60]

EVALUATION OF THERAPEUTIC OUTCOMES

Because of the prevalence of headache disorders, clinicians need to be actively involved in patient care issues. Patients should be monitored for frequency, intensity, and duration of headaches, as well as any change in the headache pattern. To this end, migraineurs should be encouraged to keep a headache diary to document the frequency, severity, and duration of migraine attacks, as well as response to medication and potential trigger factors. Careful monitoring is essential to initiate the most appropriate pharmacotherapy, document therapeutic successes and failures, identify medication contraindications, and prevent or minimize adverse events. Patients using acute therapies should be monitored for frequency of use of prescription and over-the-counter medications to identify potential medication-misuse headache. Patient counseling is necessary to allow for proper medication use (e.g., self-injection with sumatriptan), to encourage early use of medications in the headache cycle, and to enhance patient compliance. Strict adherence to dosing guidelines should be stressed to minimize potential toxicity. Patterns of abortive medication use can be documented to establish the need for prophylactic therapy. Prophylactic therapies also should be monitored closely for adverse reactions, abortive therapy needs, adequate dosing, and compliance. Consultation with other health-care practitioners should be encouraged when changes in headache patterns or medication use occur.

CONCLUSIONS

Although headache disorders such as migraine and cluster headaches appear to occur as a result of neuronal dysfunction, the precise etiology and nature of the dysfunction are unknown. Serotonergic neurotransmission and the trigeminovascular system appear to play important roles. A careful patient workup, including patient history, physical examination, and appropriate laboratory tests, should identify most headache patients with major disease. A variety of strategies can be helpful for managing migraine, tension-type, and cluster headaches. Management of primary headache disorders is directed at suppressing acute attacks and preventing recurrences. Continuing research will better define pathophysiologic mechanisms and aid the search for less toxic and more efficacious pharmacologic agents.

ABBREVIATIONS

CGRP: calcitonin gene–related peptide

CNS: central nervous system

GABA: γ-aminobutyric acid

5-HT: serotonin, 5-hydroxytryptamine

FDA: Food and Drug Administration

IHS: International Headache Society

MAOIs: monoamine oxidase inhibitors

NSAIDs: nonsteroidal antiinflammatory drugs

SNRI: serotonin-norepinephrine reuptake inhibitor

SSRI: selective serotonin reuptake inhibitor

TCA: tricyclic antidepressant

REFERENCES

1. Silberstein SD, Lipton RB, Dalessio DJ. Overview, diagnosis, and classification of headache. In: Silberstein SD, Lipton RB, Dalessio DJ, eds. Wolff's Headache and Other Head Pain, 7th ed. New York: Oxford University Press, 2001:6–26.
2. Mueller L. Tension-type, the forgotten headache. Postgrad Med 2002;111:25–50.
3. Headache Classification Committee of the International Headache Society. The international classification of headache disorders, 2nd ed. Cephalalgia 2004;24(Suppl 1):1–151.
4. Silberstein SD, Lipton RB, Goadsby PJ. Headache in Clinical Practice. London: Martin Dunitz, 2002:21–33, 69–128.
5. Lipton RB, Diamond S, Reed M, et al. Migraine diagnosis and treatment: Results from the American Migraine Study II. Headache 2001;41:638–645.
6. Lipton RB, Stewart WF, Diamond S, et al. Prevalence and burden of migraine in the United States: Data from the American Migraine Study II. Headache 2001;41:646–657.
7. Lipton RB, Bigal ME. The epidemiology of migraine. Am J Med 2005;18(Suppl 1):S3–10.
8. Silberstein SD. Migraine. Lancet 2004;363:381–391.
9. Ferrari MD. Migraine. Lancet 1998;351:1043–1051.
10. Gardner KL. Genetics of migraine: An update. Headache 2006;46(Suppl 1):S19–24.
11. Ramadan NM. Targeting therapy for migraine. Neurology 2005;64(Suppl 2):S4–8.
12. Ashkenazi A, Silberstein SD. The evolving management of migraine. Curr Opin Neurol 2003;16:341–345.
13. Kaniecki RG. Diagnostic issues in migraine. Curr Pain Headache Rep 2001;5:183–188.
14. Goadsby PJ, Lipton RB, Ferrari MD. Migraine: Current understanding and treatment. N Engl J Med 2002;346:257–270.
15. Sadovsky R, Dodick DW. Identifying migraine in primary care settings. Am J Med 2005;118(Suppl 1):S11–17.
16. Solomon S. Migraine variants. Curr Pain Headache Rep 2001;5:165–169.
17. Silberstein SD. Practice parameter: Evidence-based guidelines for migraine headache (an evidence-based review). Neurology 2000;55:754–763.
18. Silberstein SD, Goadsby PJ, Lipton RB. Management of migraine: An algorithmic approach. Neurology 2000;55(Suppl 2):S46–52.
19. Lipton RB, Stewart WF, Stone AM, et al. Stratified care vs step care strategies for migraine: The disability in strategies of care study. JAMA 2000;284:2599–2605.
20. Evans RW, Bigal ME, Grosberg B, Lipton RB. Target doses and titration schedules for migraine preventive medications. Headache 2006;46:160–164.
21. Silberstein SD, Goadsby PJ. Migraine: Preventive treatment. Cephalalgia 2002;22:491–512.
22. Rapoport AM, Bigal ME. Preventive migraine therapy: What is new. Neurol Sci 2004;25(Suppl 1):S177–185.

23. Ramadan NM, Silberstein SD, Freitag FG, et al. Evidence-Based Guidelines for Migraine Headache in the Primary Care Setting: Pharmacological Management for Prevention of Migraine. 2000, *www.aan.com/professionals/practice/guidelines*.
24. Snow V, Weiss K, Wall EM, Mottur-Pilson C. Pharmacologic management of acute attacks of migraine and prevention of migraine headache. Ann Intern Med 2002;137:840–849.
25. Diamond M, Cady R. Initiating and optimizing acute therapy for migraine: The role of patient-centered stratified care. Am J Med 2005;118(Suppl 1):S18–27.
26. Kaniecki RG. Migraine and tension-type headache, an assessment of challenges in diagnosis. Neurology 2002;58(Suppl 6):S15–20.
27. Tonore TB, King DS, Noble SL. Do over-the-counter medications for migraine hinder the physician? Curr Pain Headache Rep 2002,6:162–167.
28. Matchar DB, Young WB, Rosenberg JA, et al. Evidence-Based Guidelines for Migraine Headache in the Primary Care Setting: Pharmacological Management of Acute Attacks. The U.S. Headache Consortium. 2000, *www.aan.com/professionals/practice/guidelines.*
29. del Rio MS, Silberstein SD. How to pick optimal acute treatment for migraine headache. Curr Pain Headache Rep 2001;5:170–178.
30. Krusz JC, Scott V, Belanger J. Intravenous propofol: Unique effectiveness in treating intractable migraine. Headache 2000;40:224–230.
31. Diamond S. A fresh look at migraine therapy. Postgrad Med 2001;109(1):49–60.
32. Aukerman G, Knutson D, Miser WF. Management of the acute migraine headache. Am Fam Physician 2002;66:2123–2130, 2140–2141.
33. Eadie MJ. Clinically significant drug interactions with agents specific for migraine attacks. CNS Drugs 2001;15(2):105–118.
34. Matthew NT, Loder EW. Evaluating the triptans. Am J Med 2005;118(Suppl 1):S28–35.
35. Tfelt-Hansen P, DeVries P, Saxena PR. Triptans in migraine: A comparative review of pharmacology, pharmacokinetics, and efficacy. Drugs 2000;60:1259–1287.
36. Deleu D, Hanssens Y. Current and emerging second-generation triptans in acute migraine therapy: A comparative review. J Clin Pharmacol 2000;40:687–700.
37. Pringsheim T, Gawel M. Triptans: Are they all the same? Curr Pain Headache Rep 2002;6:140–146.
38. Ferrari MD, Roon KI, Lipton RB, Goadsby PJ. Oral triptans (serotonin 5-$HT_{1B/1D}$ agonists) in acute migraine treatment: A meta-analysis of 53 trials. Lancet 2001;358:1558–1575.
39. Martin VT, Goldstein JA. Evaluating the safety and tolerability profile of acute treatments for migraine. Am J Med 2005;118(Suppl 1):S36–44.
40. Bigal ME, Lipton RB, Krymchantowski AV. The medical management of migraine. Am J Ther 2004;11(2):130–140.
41. Center for Drug Evaluation and Research. FDA Public Health Advisory: Drug Combination May Result in Serotonin Syndrome. 2006, *www.fda.gov/cder/drug/advisory*.
42. Adelman JU, Adelman, RD. Current options for the prevention and treatment of migraine. Clin Ther 2001;23:772–788.
43. Cutrer FM. Antiepileptic drugs: How they work in headache. Headache 2001;41(Suppl):S3–10.
44. Freitag FG. Divalproex sodium extended-release for the prophylaxis of migraine headache. Expert Opin Pharmacother 2003;4:1573–1578.
45. Kinze S, Clauss M, Reuter U, et al. Valproic acid is effective in migraine prophylaxis at low serum levels: A prospective open-label study. Headache 2001;41:774–778.
46. Brandes JL, Saper JR, Diamond M, et al. Topiramate for migraine prevention: A randomized controlled trial. JAMA 2004;291:965–973.
47. Krymchantowski AV, Bigal ME, Moreira PF. New and emerging prophylactic agents for migraine. CNS Drugs 2002;16:611–634.
48. Mathew NT, Rapoport A, Saper J, et al. Efficacy of gabapentin in migraine prophylaxis. Headache 2001;41:119–128.
49. Bigal ME, Krymchantowski AV, Rapoport AM. New developments in migraine prophylaxis. Expert Opin Pharmacother 2003;4:433–443.
50. Dodick DW. Botulinum neurotoxin for the treatment of migraine and other primary headache disorders: From bench to bedside. Headache 2003;43(Suppl 1):S25–33.
51. Schrader H, Stovner LJ, Helde G, et al. Prophylactic treatment of migraine with angiotensin converting enzyme inhibitor (lisinopril): Randomized, placebo-controlled, crossover study. Br Med J 2001;322:1–5.
52. Tronvik E, Stovner LJ, Helde G, et al. Prophylactic treatment of migraine with an angiotensin II receptor blocker: A randomized, controlled trial. JAMA 2003;289:65–69.
53. Johnson K. Migraine therapy: Balancing efficacy and safety with quality of life and cost. Formulary 2002;37:634–644.
54. Jensen R. Mechanisms of tension-type headache. Cephalalgia 2001:21:786–789.
55. Kaniecki RG. Migraine and tension-type headache: An assessment of challenges in diagnosis. Neurology 2002;58(Suppl 6):S15–20.
56. Jensen R, Olesen J. Tension-type headache: An update on mechanisms and treatment. Curr Opin Neurol 2000;13:285–289.
57. Solomon S, Newman LC. Episodic tension-type headaches. In: Silberstein SD, Lipton RB, Dalessio DJ, eds. Wolff's Headache and Other Head Pain, 7th ed. New York: Oxford University Press, 2001:238–246.
58. Russell MB. Epidemiology and genetics of cluster headache. Lancet Neurol 2004;3:279–83.
59. Schreiber CP. The pathophysiology of primary headache. Prim Care Clin Office Pract 2004;31:261–276.
60. McGeeney, BE. Cluster headache pharmacotherapy. Am J Ther 2005;12(4):351–358.
61. Freitag FG. Cluster headache. Prim Care Clin Office Pract 2004;31:313–329.
62. Favier I, Haan J, Ferrari MD. Chronic cluster headache: A review. J Headache Pain 2005;6:3–9.

SECTION 7
PSYCHIATRIC DISORDERS

CHAPTER 64

Evaluation of Psychiatric Illness

PATRICIA A. MARKEN, MARK E. SCHNEIDERHAN, AND STUART MUNRO

KEY CONCEPTS

1. Patients with psychiatric conditions are treated in all healthcare settings. All clinicians need to develop basic skills in psychiatric assessment to best care for their patients.

2. The *Diagnostic and Statistical Manual of Mental Disorders, 4th Edition, Text Revision* (*DSM-IV-TR*) is the most widely accepted diagnostic reference. It, along with the *American Psychiatric Association Practice Guidelines for the Psychiatric Evaluation of Adults*, provides the clinician a standardized approach for the initial assessment and followup of patients with mental illness.

3. At times, patients suffering from mental illness are challenging to assess, as their condition can prevent them from full cooperation. A range of strategies can be used to gather the needed information while maintaining the safety and comfort of both patient and clinician.

4. A thorough medication history to identify all medications currently taken, as well as those previously taken, is a cornerstone of effective patient management. In addition, it must be determined whether there was an adequate trial (dose and duration) of current and prior medications for psychiatric illnesses.

5. A baseline mental status examination, along with a specific target symptom list, is a critical tool in monitoring response to treatment.

6. Several papers have been published in recent years recommending specific physical assessment and laboratory tests needed for the evaluation of patients with psychiatric conditions. Except for patients taking antipsychotics, no single standard exists, and testing is individualized based on the patient's age, medical history, current physical health, and current medication use and in consideration of the most recent expert opinion. Baseline and followup monitoring for metabolic disturbances should be instituted for all antipsychotic therapies.

Learning objectives, review questions, and other resources can be found at **www.pharmacotherapyonline.com.**

❶ Patients with mental illnesses are treated by all disciplines and in all settings of healthcare and can, in fact, receive the bulk of their care from nonpsychiatrists. Hence the need for good psychiatric assessment skills is not limited to mental health specialists. Along with traditional assessments used across all medical specialties (laboratory tests, medical history, and physical examination), psychiatrists use additional strategies to manage their patients that are perhaps less objective and less familiar to the nonpsychiatrist. This chapter provides a basic overview of appropriate assessment techniques used by clinicians to develop an individualized treatment plan for psychiatric patients. Readers needing greater depth than the materials provided in this chapter are referred to other reference materials.[1–5]

OVERVIEW OF *DIAGNOSTIC AND STATISTICAL MANUAL OF MENTAL DISORDERS*

❷ The *DSM-IV-TR* is the most widely accepted and most important diagnostic reference used in the care of the mentally ill. It provides a common language for practitioners to describe and diagnose psychiatric disorders.[6] Common language is essential because there is considerable overlap of symptoms across many diagnoses. The *Diagnostic and Statistical Manual of Mental Disorders, 1st edition* (*DSM-I*) was introduced in 1952 and was the first manual on mental disorders to contain a description of diagnostic categories. The most recent edition, *DSM-IV-TR*, was released in 2000. The *DSM-IV-TR* uses essentially the same diagnostic criteria sets as *Diagnostic and Statistical Manual of Mental Disorders, 4th edition* (*DSM-IV*).[6] Its purpose is to correct factual errors in *DSM-IV* and update the text sections (e.g., associated features, prevalence, and differential diagnosis) with more contemporary data. A more significant rewriting of diagnostic criteria and introduction of new diagnoses will appear in *Diagnostic and Statistical Manual of Mental Disorders, 5th edition* (*DSM-V*), which probably will not be available until 2011.[6] The *DSM-IV-TR* contains many components that provide a comprehensive understanding of specific mental illnesses and assist in making an accurate diagnosis. For example, the multiaxial patient evaluation ensures that most factors that could contribute to, or complicate, the condition are considered during a patient assessment and throughout treatment planning. Axis I lists the principal psychiatric disorder, developmental disorders, or provisional diagnoses present in the patient. Mental retardation and personality disorders are listed on Axis II. Axis III lists existing physical disorders or conditions. Axis IV lists the severity of psychosocial stressors that might have contributed to a new or recurrent mental disorder or exacerbation of an existing condition. Stressors are rated on a scale of 1 (none) to 6 (catastrophic) and can be acute (lasting less than 6 months) or enduring (lasting longer than 6 months). Examples of stressors include difficulties with interpersonal relationships, parenting, occupation, living circumstances, finances, the legal system, and health. Axis V describes the global assessment of functioning (GAF), rated on a scale from 1 (persistent danger to self or others) to 90 (minimal or absent symptoms). A GAF rating is made based on the current level of functioning and also for the highest level of functioning seen in the previous months to a year prior to the current evaluation. By documenting the baseline level of functioning, the GAF helps evaluate progress toward a patient's therapeutic goals.

DSM-IV-TR provides general information on all mental disorders recognized by the American Psychiatric Association (APA) and includes age of onset, clinical course, complications, predisposing factors, prevalence, and the differential diagnoses. The specific diagnostic criteria for each mental illness and the number of symptoms required to establish a diagnosis are also listed. The *DSM-IV-TR* also includes decision trees for differential diagnosis and a glossary of technical terms. The *Clinical Interview Using DSM-IV* is a companion publication that provides extensive information on interviewing techniques helpful in establishing a specific *DSM-IV* diagnosis.[7]

Additional information besides the *DSM-IV-TR* diagnosis is required before a comprehensive treatment plan can be developed. The *American Psychiatric Association Practice Guidelines for Psychiatric Evaluation of Adults* (2nd edition) includes a full discussion of the domains needed for a thorough clinical evaluation. It also discusses issues of privacy, appropriate setting for assessment, and evaluations in special populations.[5]

In summary, the *DSM-IV-TR* and the APA practice guidelines allow clinicians to evaluate patients in a systematic manner, thereby creating better treatment plans and a more consistent evaluation of response.

THE CLINICAL INTERVIEW

The interview should be conducted in a quiet, nonstimulating, and comfortable area where the patient and the interviewer feel at ease. The setting should be appropriate to the patient's level of acuity and the potential for risk to the patient and clinician. The interviewer should introduce himself or herself and explain what is about to happen to establish a trusting relationship. Generally, open-ended questions come first, followed by questions focused on more specific or personal data. Open-ended questions allow the patient to provide descriptions and other information in his or her own words. Even though more specific questions may then be necessary to fill in the gaps, beginning in this manner minimizes the risk of "leading" the patient. Patients can respond to specific questions and "yes" or "no" questions with answers they think the interviewer wants to hear. The interviewer must be nonjudgmental about the information offered by the patient to develop trust and rapport and to ensure completeness and accuracy of the information. Whether a clinician takes notes or just listens during the interview is an individual decision, with the primary considerations being to make an accurate record of the content of the examination and assuring that the patient is comfortable with the note taking. Table 64–1 provides examples of questions useful for gathering information during the completion of the clinical interview.

TABLE 64-1 Examples of Interview Questions for Assessing Mental Illnesses

Mania
1. Do your thoughts go faster than you can say them?
2. Have you noticed a change in the amount of sleep that you require?
3. Have you spent a lot of money lately, and what did you spend it on?
4. Do you have a lot of extra energy?
(To assess hallucinations and delusions, see Schizophrenia section below.)
Depression
1. Do you cry without any reason?
2. Do you still enjoy the same hobbies/activities that you once did?
3. Has your weight changed recently?
4. Have you had changes in your energy level recently?
5. Do you have any guilty feelings?
6. Do you find it difficult to remember phone numbers, names of friends, appointments, and so on?
(To assess sleep and suicidal potential, see Sleep and Suicide sections below.)
Schizophrenia
Delusions
1. Do you feel that people plot against you?
2. Do you ever feel that you are watched or spied on?
3. Do you have any special abilities?
4. Does anyone ever try to mess with you or bother you?
5. Do others read your thoughts?
Hallucinations
1. Does the TV/radio ever tell you things?
2. Do you hear voices that other people don't hear?
3. What do they say? How many voices?
4. How often do they bother you?
5. Do the voices ever tell you to hurt yourself or someone else?
6. Have you ever heard your name called when there is no one there?
7. Have you ever seen anything strange that you can't explain?
8. Do you ever see things that bother you and no one else?
9. Do you want to act on what the voices say?
Thought broadcasting/insertion
1. If I stood by you could I hear your thoughts?
2. Does your head ever act like a radio?
3. Do you feel that others can put thoughts in your head?
Insight
1. What reasons did your family give you for coming here?
2. What brought you here?
3. Do you consider yourself in need of help?
4. What does your medication do for you?
Sleep
1. Tell me about your sleep.
2. How many hours do you sleep each night at present?
3. How many hours do you usually sleep at night?
4. Do you sleep all through the night?
5. Is there a reason for your waking up?
6. Do you have trouble falling asleep?
7. How do you feel when you wake up?
Suicide potential
1. Do you feel your life is worth living?
2. Do you ever think of hurting yourself?
3. Do you see things improving in the future?
4. Do you think you will try to hurt yourself now?
5. How would you do it?
6. Do you have the means to hurt yourself?

THE CHALLENGING PATIENT

❸ Patient assessment can be challenging when symptoms of the condition prevent effective engagement with the clinician. Patients ramble if their speech patterns are circumstantial or tangential in nature, or they can ruminate as part of a depression. Patients in the manic phases of bipolar disorder may not pause as they speak (pressured speech), making it difficult for the interviewer to interject. In all cases, the interviewer can regain control by politely redirecting the patient back toward the question. Psychotic patients may be paranoid and appear guarded or frightened by the questions. The best approach is to remain calm and respectful; use shorter or close-ended questions; and only seek essential information until the patient is less paranoid. Patients can become agitated and occasionally violent. Often violence is preceded by increased psychomotor agitation as evidenced by pacing, speaking in a loud voice, or gripping the arms of the chair. When there is concern about safety, the interviewer should avoid any behavior that could be misconstrued as threatening, such as touching or unnecessary staring, and interview the patient in the presence of another healthcare provider. Both the patient and interviewer should have equal access to leave the room if either becomes too uncomfortable. If a patient becomes threatening to the interviewer, the interviewer should not hesitate to leave the room and call for help. If a patient describes suicidal thoughts, he or she should be further assessed using the questions outlined in Table 64–1, and depending on the results of further assessment be directed to the appropriate type of care, including hospitalization for patients at immediate risk of harming themselves. A suicidal patient should never be left alone. Asking a patient about suicidal thoughts will not increase the risk. The risk is greater if these questions are never asked or signs of distress are ignored. Before any conclusions are made about a patient interview, the impact of culture on the patient's presentation should be considered. Something that sounds delusional in Western culture can be the norm in others. If a clinician is unclear whether culture of origin accounts for some of the patient's symptoms, he or she should consult with a family member or someone else familiar with the cultural issues for the patient.

PSYCHIATRIC HISTORY

Both the patient's and the patient's family history of mental illness provide important information when formulating a diagnosis and treatment plan. Information should include the current and previous psychiatric diagnoses, the clinical presentation of each illness, time frame between episodes, level of functioning between episodes, length of each episode, total duration of illness, and treatment given during each episode and response to those treatments. Baseline functioning or the highest level of functioning achieved in the past few years is important because it provides a treatment goal. Information on the history of the current episode and reasons for presenting to the clinician also should be gathered. A family history should include a medication history of the immediate relatives because a family member's response to a given medication might predict an individual patient's response to that same medication.

SOCIAL HISTORY

A social history should include educational and occupational background, religion, marital status, substance-use patterns including smoking, and current living situation. By understanding a patient's living environment and social situation, strategies to foster treatment adherence, reduce stress, and increase social support can be developed. To probe this area initially, the clinician can ask patients to describe their social support network. This can be followed by more specific questions such as "To whom are you closest?" or "In whom do you confide?"

MEDICATION HISTORY

❹ A thorough medication history is one of the most important contributions a clinician can make to treatment planning. The history should include medications for both psychiatric and medical conditions. It should list all medications taken by the patient, and report on how each was tolerated and the nature of the response to that drug or combination of drugs. Because most psychiatric medications have a delay in the onset of effect, it is important to determine whether an adequate trial (adequate dose and duration) was provided before the patient was deemed "nonresponsive" to that drug. If a patient has a history of nonadherence, specific causes such as cost, complicated dosing schedules, lack of insight, and adverse effects should be investigated.

MENTAL STATUS EXAMINATION

❺ The mental status examination (MSE) is a key patient assessment tool in psychiatry and is analogous to the physical examination in medicine. The MSE is completed through a direct patient interview and results in a description of current behavior, thoughts, perceptions, and functioning. The MSE provides an objective evaluation used in diagnosis, assessment of the course of the illness, and response to treatment. The MSE is combined with other components of the patient workup (history of present illness, physical examination, appropriate laboratory tests, and medical and psychiatric history) to give a full picture of the presenting problem and factors contributing to the illness. An MSE has several components.[5,7]

Appearance and Attitude Toward Examiner

The appearance of the patient throughout the interview should be noted, including age, dress, grooming and hygiene, use of cosmetics, and facial expressions. A description of appearance also should include unusual physical characteristics and the general state of physical health. The interviewer should note whether the patient is cooperative, mute, hostile, paranoid, guarded, or withdrawn.

Activity

Changes in motor activity include overactivity, underactivity, and catatonia. Overactivity is an increase in purposeful movements or agitation and can include pacing; hand wringing; picking at clothing, skin, or hair; inability to sit still during the interview; and excessive hand gestures. Underactive patients move less than expected. Patients with rigid posture, an absence of movement, and failure to communicate can be catatonic, paranoid, or experiencing medication-induced adverse effects.

Speech and Language

The quantity, flow, and speed of speech and the amount of eye contact should be noted. The appropriateness and degree of eye contact varies significantly between cultures, and before poor eye contact is interpreted, the patient's cultural background should be considered. Speech should be assessed as to whether it proceeds logically in a goal-directed manner or whether the content is vague and poorly organized. Abnormal speech characteristics include blocking, whereby the person suddenly stops speaking without any obvious reason. Thought blocking usually occurs when a hallucination or delusion intrudes into the person's thinking or when upsetting issues are discussed. Circumstantial speech lacks a clear direction because of excess unnecessary information, but the circumstantial patient eventually will make his or her point. In tangential speech, however, the ultimate point is never made. *Perseveration* is repetition of an original answer to subsequent questions. *Flight of ideas* is overproductive, rapid speech during which the patient jumps rapidly from one idea to the next. *Mutism* is identified when the patient does not respond even though he or she is aware of the discussion.

Mood and Affect

Affect describes the patient's current emotional tone, as expressed through facial expression, body posture, and tone of voice, all of which can be objectively observed by the clinician. Mood describes more sustained feelings, which are subjectively reported by the patient. To properly evaluate a patient's mood and affect, his or her appearance and the content of speech must be considered. Change in facial expression and the presence of tears, flushing, sweating, or tremors should be noted. Affect can be described further by its range, appropriateness, intensity, and stability. For example, in schizophrenia or depression, the affect can be flat, whereby no change in expression occurs throughout the interview. In contrast, during a manic episode, the affect is very intense and often labile. *Blunted affect* denotes that the range of emotional expression is reduced, but not absent. An example of *inappropriate affect* is when a patient laughs when he or she is depressed or cries when stating that he or she is happy. A rapidly shifting affect from one extreme to the other is described as *labile.*

Thought and Perceptual Disturbances

A variety of thought disturbances can occur in mental illness. These disturbances generally indicate the presence of psychosis or impaired reality testing. *Delusions* are fixed, false beliefs that are not based in reality or consistent with the patient's religion or culture. Delusions can be paranoid, somatic, or grandiose in nature. Delusions are often unshakable, and although the clinician can challenge the delusional thinking, one should not attempt to talk a patient out of a delusion. *Thought broadcasting* is the belief that one's thoughts are audible to others. *Hallucinations* are false sensory impressions or perceptions that occur in the absence of an external stimulus. Hallucinations can be auditory, visual, olfactory, or gustatory and can be continuous or intermittent. In contrast, *illusions* are visual misperceptions involving a misinterpretation of a real sensory stimulus. For example, a person who initially misperceives a curtain blown by the wind to be an intruder has experienced an illusion. This phenomenon is not indicative of psychiatric illness and can be seen in normal persons. Other thought disturbances are not considered to be psychotic. For example, the couplet of obsessions and compulsions can be indicative of the presence of obsessive-compulsive disorder, which is not considered to be a psychotic disorder. *Obsessions* are unwanted thoughts or ideas that intrude into a person's thinking. *Compulsions* are actions performed in response to the obsessions or to control anxiety associated with the obsession.

Neuropsychiatric Evaluation

A neuropsychiatric evaluation assesses sensorium, attention, concentration, memory, and higher cognitive functions such as orientation and abstraction. Prior to a neuropsychiatric evaluation, the clinician should document whether the patient has received medications with sedative properties, because the outcome of the examination can be altered if central nervous system depressants were recently taken.

Sensorium, or level of consciousness, refers to the alertness of the patient, and if he or she is not fully alert, the amount of stimulation needed to awaken the patient. Attention and concentration can be assessed using serial subtraction by 7s or 3s, or by having a patient spell a five-letter word backward. Language skills are assessed initially by having a patient read something aloud and silently. General intelligence can be assessed loosely by asking factual information about current news items, recent presidents, or popular television shows or sporting events. *Memory* is the ability to recall past experiences and is classified as sensory stores (which lasts seconds), short-term memory (the ability to recall newly acquired information after several minutes), working memory (i.e., immediate application of visual or auditory instructions), and long-term or remote memory (historical facts). Orientation to time, place, person, and situation assesses sensory stores and short-term memory. Asking a patient to recall three objects 5 minutes after they are learned is the definitive test for short-term memory. Patients with depression or anxiety can have deficits in short-term memory. Asking the patient to do a certain task (e.g., pick up a pen with his or her right hand and then fold a piece of paper and pass it to the examiner) can assess the patient's working memory. Patients with cognitive deficits, such as those seen in dementias and schizophrenia, can exhibit deficits in working memory. Remote memory is assessed by asking patients to recall old facts about their lives, such as where they were born or where they went to school. Remote memory usually remains intact the longest in patients with intellectual decline, whereas the ability to create new memories is generally the first sign of a memory deficit. *Abstraction* is the ability to interpret information such as a proverb ("People in glass houses shouldn't throw stones") or identify similarities or differences between words (apple and orange). Abstraction is influenced by education, cultures and linguistic fluency; thus inability to abstract is not always a sign of a psychiatric disorder.

Insight and Judgment

Insight refers to patient awareness that he or she has a mental illness and the consequences of that illness on his or her life. Patients typically demonstrate a lack of insight when they are psychotic. Patients with poor insight are often nonadherent with prescribed medications. *Judgment* is the ability to make decisions appropriate to the situation and can be impaired in a variety of mental illnesses. Judgment can be assessed by asking patients how they would handle either their current or a hypothetical situation. Both insight and judgment can be fluid. For example, intoxicated patients can demonstrate poor insight and judgment only to improve over several hours as their blood alcohol concentration decreases.

PHYSICAL AND LABORATORY ASSESSMENT IN PSYCHIATRY

Patients who present with psychiatric symptoms need a careful medical assessment for many reasons.[1–3]

Both medical illnesses and medications can cause the same psychiatric symptoms. The rapidity of onset of psychiatric symptoms is an important clue that a medical cause is present. Most chronic mental illnesses have a prodromal period, whereas medically-based psychiatric symptoms often have a more rapid onset of symptoms. Patients older than 40 years of age at first presentation are more likely to have a medical cause for their psychiatric symptoms because major psychiatric illnesses such as schizophrenia and bipolar disorder usually first present in adolescence or early adulthood. Family history can provide additional clues. Patients with fluctuating levels of consciousness, disorientation, memory impairment, or visual, tactile, or olfactory hallucinations, substance abuse, and serious medical conditions are more likely to have a medical basis for their presentation.

Patients with psychiatric illnesses, especially depression and anxiety disorders, will often present with only physical complaints, leading to inappropriate care for medical problems that are not present or as serious as they may appear, while the root cause is ignored. Psychotropic medications can cause or exacerbate medical conditions, such as diabetes mellitus, hyperlipidemia, or cardiac arrhythmias, necessitating an understanding of the patient's other risk factors for these conditions before medication is selected. Finally, patients with chronic psychiatric illnesses often receive inadequate healthcare and have poorly controlled medical conditions for many reasons, including their appearance or behavior prohibiting a thorough evaluation, inaccurate information from the patient secondary to impaired memory or perception, and incomplete data to make an appropriate diagnosis and treatment recommendation. A retrospective review found that patients with diabetes or hypertension and diagnoses of schizophrenia, bipolar disorder, or posttraumatic stress disorder were statistically less likely to use medical services than similar patients without these psychiatric conditions.[8]

❻ General laboratory screening is useful for ruling out medical causes of psychiatric illnesses, but extensive testing is usually unnecessary and not cost-effective. Laboratory tests should be individualized to the age, medical/medication history, cooperativeness, and physical health of the patient. Although there is no consensus about specific laboratory tests for diagnosing or evaluating mental illness, antipsychotic therapy warrants patient monitoring for metabolic disturbances.[2,5,9,10] Expert consensus recommends that patients starting on antipsychotic agents should be screened for symptoms of metabolic syndrome including body weight (baseline, weeks 4, 8, and 12, then every 3 months, then annually), waist and hip measurements (baseline and annually), blood pressures (baseline, week 12, and annually), and fasting serum lipids and glucose (if possible at baseline, week 12, and annually). Although a fasting blood glucose determination is preferred over a random measure, this should not be a barrier to adequate monitoring. The clinician can employ random glucose measures or glycosylated hemoglobin A_{1c} if there is difficulty obtaining fasting serum levels. Inadequate lipid monitoring continues to be reported among patients with schizophrenia on second-generation antipsychotics; therefore, lipids should be assessed even if fasting specimens are not available because high-density lipoprotein cholesterol (HDL) levels are a direct measure to identify metabolic abnormalities.[9–12]

A complete physical examination, along with a detailed medical and medication history, vital signs, weight and body mass index, a pregnancy test when indicated, and routine blood chemistry are commonly part of the workup of persons with mental illness. In most cases a physical examination should be chaperoned. Clinicians will want diagnostic tests to evaluate the relative safety of specific medications (e.g., renal status when using lithium or an electrocardiogram when using a tricyclic antidepressant such as amitriptyline or an antipsychotic such as ziprasidone or clozapine) or when baseline information is needed to help document future adverse effects from medications (e.g., lithium-induced hypothyroidism, clozapine-induced leukopenia, antipsychotic-induced diabetes mellitus). Serum concentration monitoring for selected medications (lithium, valproic acid, carbamazepine) is also helpful in increasing probability of response while minimizing adverse effects. Urine drug screens and blood alcohol tests play an important role in identifying the contribution of substances of abuse to the presenting symptoms.

Additional testing can include an electroencephalogram to evaluate for the presence of seizure activity or other neurologic conditions, computed tomography or magnetic resonance imaging to detect structural abnormalities, sedimentation rate and antinuclear antibodies for autoimmune disorders, a human immunodeficiency virus test, thyroid function tests, or vitamin B_{12} and folate concentrations for anemias.[2]

The identification of biologic markers as diagnostic tools and predictors or indicators of drug response is of great interest but currently of little clinical usefulness. The most promising is the dexamethasone suppression test, proposed to be a marker for endogenous melancholic depression. However, its lack of sensitivity and specificity has limited its usefulness as a routine screening tool during a workup for depression.[2]

In summary, a range of assessments aid the clinician in making an accurate diagnosis and identifying underlying or potential drug-related problems. The MSE is the cornerstone of the psychiatric workup, although selective medical tests, a good medical, psychiatric, and medication history, and a thorough physical examination are also important.

PSYCHIATRIC RATING SCALES

Psychiatric rating scales are useful tools to provide an objective way of measuring subjective data (e.g., feelings, thoughts, and perceptions) and to diagnose specific disorders. As there are so many types of scales to choose from, the rater needs training and experience to select and use the most appropriate scale. Rating scales are used in a variety of settings, including research and patient care, and can serve an administrative purpose such as quality control.[4]

Drawbacks to the more frequent use of rating scales include the substantial time commitment for staff to administer the tests and the inability of some patients to tolerate these interviews, especially patients who are severely paranoid or agitated. In addition, repeated ratings are usually necessary to objectively describe longitudinal changes over a defined treatment period as opposed to a snapshot of a complex clinical situation.

Some rating scales are self-administered and do not require a staff member to collect the data; thus they require minimal resources to administer. Patients can be unable to self-administer a questionnaire for a variety of reasons, including literacy and severity of symptoms.

In contrast to symptom-based rating scales (e.g., Brief Psychiatric Rating Scale [BPRS] or Hamilton Depression [HAMD] scale), global rating scales such as the Clinical Global Impression (CGI) scale assess the overall severity of illness based on a rater's clinical experience.[13] In general, these rating scales measure the presence or severity of symptoms and can assist in the diagnostic formulation.

Rating scales are also available to measure adverse side effects from psychiatric medications. Specific adverse side-effect measures can be used for specific categories of medications. Table 64–2 provides a summary of the most common rating scales used to assess and quantify the presence and severity of adverse effects.[14]

Sensitivity, specificity, reliability, and validity are important considerations when selecting a rating scale. *Sensitivity* refers to a test's ability to detect a symptom or illness, given that the symptom or illness is present. *Specificity* refers to a test's ability to determine that a symptom or illness is absent given that the person does not have the illness.

Reliability is the extent to which the score on the scale reflects the hypothetical "true" score and how much interference occurs from outside influences.[15] Reliability is reported by the correlation coefficient, which represents a chance correlation (zero) or perfect correlation (one). Rating scales with reliability correlation coefficients of less than 0.7 are usually considered unreliable for clinical studies. Interrater reliability—agreement in rating scores among clinicians—is important to achieve when multiple clinicians rate the same patient or population. Interrater reliability is established by having all raters independently rate individual patients at the same time to determine the correlation of their scores.

Validity, in contrast, is the ability of a scale to measure what it was designed to measure. Various validity tests are performed on a rating scale to ensure that the scale assesses the appropriate aspects of the illness (content validity), the correlation with diagnoses or clinical change (concurrent validity), and the extent to which the scale measures symptom traits in contrast to a specific symptom (construct validity).

Psychiatric rating scales should not be confused with psychologic tests such as neuropsychologic and intellectual assessments and are best used as only one part of a comprehensive diagnostic plan. Tables 64–3, 64–4, and 64–5 describe commonly used patient-rated and clinician-rated scales for a variety of disease states.[16–21]

SYSTEMATIC MEASUREMENT OF COGNITIVE FUNCTION

Neuropsychiatric rating scales provide specific information such as the rate of change and severity of cognitive decline or improvement. They are useful in situations in which repeated measurements of a patient's mental status are needed because they allow the clinician to determine response to an intervention (e.g., medication) in a more systematic manner. In addition, some cognitive function measures are useful screens for Alzheimer's disease and other causes of cognitive decline. A number of cognitive rating scales are available, the most common being the Mini Mental Status Examination (MMSE).

TABLE 64-2 Adverse Effects Measures

Rating Scale	Type	Scoring	Comments
Systematic Assessment for Treatment of Emergent Events-General Inquiry (SAFTEE-GI)	Structured interview and global assessment	Summary scores of number of events, average severity, and impairment.	5–10 minutes to complete. Baseline and weekly evaluations. Easy to administer. The specific reported information might be more useful than an overall summary score.
MED Watch	Global assessment	No scoring involved.	Minutes to complete. The one-page form requires a narrative description of the problem or adverse reaction. Online submission: *www.fda.gov/medwatch/*.
Abnormal Involuntary Movement Scale (AIMS)	Tardive dyskinesia assessment	12-item, 5-point severity scale. Items 1–4 orofacial movement; 5–7 extremity and truncal movement; 8–10 global severity; 11 and 12 problems with teeth or dentures (yes or no).	5–10 minutes to complete. Commonly used in most clinical settings for dyskinesia assessment. Requires training and clinical experience to make diagnosis. Diagnostic criteria: at least 3 months of antipsychotic treatment. Mild severity score (2) in two discrete areas or moderate severity (3) in one area (i.e., orofacial).
Dyskinesia Identification System: Condensed User Scale (DISCUS)	Tardive dyskinesia assessment	15-item, 5-point severity scale. Items 1, 2 face; 3 eyes; 4, 5 oral; 6–9 lingual; 10, 11 head/neck/trunk; 12, 13 upper limb; 14, 15 lower limb.	10–15 minutes to complete. More descriptive criteria for scoring severity than the AIMS. Scoring based on three dimensions: frequency, detectability, and intensity. A flow chart is provided in the user's manual to assign an item score.
Rating Scale for Extrapyramidal Side Effects (Simpson-Angus EPS Scale)	Drug-induced Parkinson and dystonia assessments	10-item, 5-point anchored severity scale. Mean score is obtained by adding all scores and dividing by 10. A mean score of 0.3 is the upper limit for no EPS.	10 minutes to complete. Item domains include gait, arm dropping, shoulder shaking, elbow rigidity, wrist rigidity, leg pendulousness, head dropping, glabella tap, tremor, and salivation. Requires training and practice to administer.
Barnes Akathisia Scale (BAS)	Drug-induced akathisia	4 items including three 4-point anchored severity scored items and a 5-point global rating score item. Total score of 12 possible.	10 minutes to complete. Items 1–3 (objective akathisia, subjective awareness of restlessness, and subjective distress related to restlessness). Diagnostic criteria: requires both objective and subjective ratings of at least 1 in either two subjective items. Pseudoakathisia is suggested with a positive objective rating, but no subjective score is noted.

EPS, extrapyramidal symptoms.
Data from Schooler and Chengappa[14] and Guy.[13]

The MMSE is a structured interview that globally assesses many cognitive domains including orientation, visuospatial organization, memory, and reasoning to determine an overall score of cognitive function. The maximum score is 30, and a score of 23 or less is indicative of cognitive impairment. The MMSE takes 5 to 10 minutes to administer and is used routinely in the clinical setting.[20] Other examples of cognitive rating scales include the information memory concentration (IMC) test, the dementia rating scale, and the clock drawing and Alzheimer's Disease Assessment Scale.[22–25]

Most of the rating scales involve a structured interview that requires clinician training to ensure accurate administration. Noise and distraction can affect the patient's performance ability; therefore the interview should be conducted in a quiet area with adequate lighting. The interviewer should speak slowly and clearly to the patient when providing instructions or asking questions.

PSYCHOLOGIC TESTING

Although most clinicians do not administer psychologic testing, they can use the results to evaluate the role of medication in relationship to the diagnosis. Psychologic testing alone cannot establish a firm diagnosis but can be a useful diagnostic tool when coupled with clinical judgment. Types of psychologic testing include personality tests (e.g., Rorschach, Minnesota Multiphasic Personality Inventory-2 [MMPI-2]), intelligence tests (e.g., Wechsler Adult Intelligence Scale-Revised, Wechsler Intelligence Scale for Children-Revised), and neuropsychologic tests (e.g., Bender Visual Motor Gestalt Test).[3]

CONCLUSIONS

Patient assessment is the basis from which a pharmaceutical care plan evolves. Problem identification and therapeutic monitoring cannot occur until a thorough assessment is complete. The initial assessment is also the basis for evaluating response to therapy throughout the course of treatment. Psychiatric assessment requires sensitivity and good listening skills on the part of the clinician because it is based primarily on a subjective interview and not objective tests. With careful data collection, clinicians can make substantial contributions to care that improve patient outcomes.

TABLE 64-3 Schizophrenia Rating Scales

Rating Scale	Type	Scoring	Comments
Brief Psychiatric Rating Scale (BPRS)	Clinician-rated	18 items, 7-point severity scale: score ≥38 indicates moderate severity	The anchored BPRS provides descriptions of each severity rating to increase the interrater reliability. The BPRS has four clusters of symptoms: thinking disturbance, anxious depression, withdrawal-retardation, and hostility-suspiciousness.
Scale for Assessment of Negative Symptoms (SANS)	Clinician-rated	30 items, 6-point severity scale: 0 = normal; 5 = severe	Measures degree of affect, alogia, avolition, anhedonia, and attention.
Positive and Negative Syndrome Scale (PANSS)	Clinician-rated	30-item scale, 7-point severity scale	Based on the 18-item brief psychiatric rating scale.
Clinical Global Impression (CGI) Scale	Observational	Severity of illness 7-point rating scale. Global improvement 7-point rating scale. Efficacy index: 1–4 marked improvement; 5–8 moderate; 9–12 minimal; 13–16 unchanged/worse	Observational rating scale to compare severity of illness compared to other similar patients and measures improvement from baseline. The efficacy index measures therapeutic effect and side effects to determine the score.

TABLE 64-4 Depression Rating Scales

Rating Scale	Type	Scoring	Comments
Hamilton Depression Scale (HAMD)	Clinician-rated	17-item scale; <6 = normal mood; 17–25 = mild depression; >25 = severe depression	Used to screen patients for drug studies and to determine severity of symptoms, treatment outcome and is the standard to compare other depression rating scales.
Montgomery-Asberg Depression Rating Scale (MADRS)	Clinician-rated	10-item, 7-point scale. For each item: 0 = no symptoms; 6 = severe symptoms	Differentiates between all the intermediate grades of depression. Decreases bias in patients with other medical illness and increased somatization.
Beck Depression Inventory (BDI)	Patient-rated	21-item scale; 0–9 = normal; 10–15 = mild depression; 16–19 = mild-moderate; 20–29 = moderate-severe; 30–63 = severe depression	The standard for self-rating scales and an objective measure of change in symptoms as a result of treatment.
Zung Self-Rating Depression Scale (ZSDS)	Patient-rated	20-item scale, 4-point severity; <50 normal; 50–59 minimal-mild; 60–69 moderate-marked; ≥70 severe depression	Severity rated by frequency of occurrence of symptoms. May not be as sensitive in measuring changes in severity of symptoms.

TABLE 64-5 Anxiety Rating Scales

Rating Scale	Type	Scoring	Comments
Hamilton Anxiety Scale (HAM-A or HAM-AS or HAMRS)	Clinician-rated	14 items, 5-point scales; scores of ≥18–20 for moderate anxiety	Consists of subscales to measure somatic and psychic anxiety.
Self-Rating Anxiety Scale (Zung SAS)	Patient-rated	20-item scale; 4-point intensity ratings	Correlates to the clinician-rated Anxiety Status Inventory (ASI); however, there is little information on the validity of either test.
Sheehan Panic and Anticipatory Anxiety Scale (SPAAS)	Patient- and clinician-rated	3-part scale	Measures panic attacks, anticipatory anxiety, and limited symptom attacks.
Yale-Brown Obsessive-Compulsive Scale (YBOCS)	Clinician-rated	Semistructured interview	Consists of several clusters of obsessions and compulsions. Used to assess change in treatment studies.

ABBREVIATIONS

APA: American Psychiatric Association

BPRS: Brief Psychiatric Rating Scale

CGI: Clinical Global Impression (scale)

DSM-IV-TR: Diagnostic and Statistical Manual of Mental Disorders, 4th edition, Text Revision

EPS: extrapyramidal symptoms

GAF: global assessment of functioning

HAMD: Hamilton Depression (scale)

IMC: information memory concentration (test)

MMPI-2: Minnesota Multiphasic Personality Inventory-2

MMSE: Mini Mental Status Examination

MSE: mental status examination

REFERENCES

1. Othmer E. Psychiatric interview, history, and mental status examination. In: Sadock BJ, Sadock VA, eds. Comprehensive Textbook of Psychiatry, Vol. 1, 8th ed. Philadelphia: Lippincott Williams & Wilkins, 2005:794–826.
2. Guze BH, Love MJ, Deutsch SI. Medical assessment and laboratory testing in psychiatry. In: Sadock BJ, Sadock VA, eds. Comprehensive Textbook of Psychiatry, Vol. 1, 8th ed. Philadelphia: Lippincott Williams & Wilkins, 2005:916–928.
3. Adams RL, Culbertson JL. Personality assessment: Adults and children. In: Sadock BJ, Sadock VA, eds. Comprehensive Textbook of Psychiatry, Vol. 1, 8th ed. Philadelphia: Lippincott Williams & Wilkins, 2005:874–894.
4. Blacker D. Psychiatric rating scales. In: Sadock BJ, Sadock VA, eds. Comprehensive Textbook of Psychiatry, Vol. 1, 8th ed. Philadelphia: Lippincott Williams & Wilkins, 2005:929–954.
5. McIntyre JS, Charles SC. Psychiatric evaluation of adults second edition. Am J Psychiatry 2006;163(Suppl)1:1–36.
6. American Psychiatric Association. Diagnostic and Statistical Manual of Mental Disorders, 4th ed., text revision (DSM-IV-TR). Washington, DC: American Psychiatric Press, 2000.
7. Othmer E, Othmer SC. The Clinical Interview Using DSM-IV, Vol. 1: Fundamentals. Washington, DC: American Psychiatric Press, 1994.
8. Cradock-O'Leary J, Young AS, Yano EM, et al. Use of general medical services by VA patients with psychiatric disorders. Psychiatr Serv 2002;53:874–878.
9. American Diabetes Association, American Psychiatric Association, American Association of Clinical Endocrinologists, North American Association for the Study of Obesity. Consensus development conference on antipsychotic drugs and obesity and diabetes. Diabetes Care 2004;27:596–601.
10. Cohn TA, Sernyak MJ. Metabolic monitoring for patients treated with antipsychotic medications. Can J Psychiatry 2006;51:492–501.
11. Weissman EM, Zhu CW, Schooler NR, et al. Lipid monitoring in patients with schizophrenia prescribed second-generation antipsychotics. J Clin Psychiatry 2006;67:1323–1326.
12. Ryan MC, Thakore JH. Physical consequences of schizophrenia and its treatment: The metabolic syndrome. Life Sci 2002;71:239–257.
13. Guy W. ECDEU (Early Clinical Drug Evaluation Unit) Assessment Manual for Psychopharmacology, rev. ed. DHEW (Department of Health, Education, and Welfare) Publication (ADM) 76-338. Washington, DC: U.S. Government Printing Office, 1976:158–169.
14. Schooler NR, Chengappa KNR. Adverse effect measures. In: Rush AJ, Pincus HA, First MB, et al., eds. Handbook of Psychiatric Measures, Vol. 11. Washington, DC: American Psychiatric Association, 2000:151–168.
15. Thompson C. Introduction. In: Thompson C, ed. The Instruments of Psychiatric Research. New York: Wiley, 1989:1–16.
16. Fankhauser MP, German ML. Understanding the use of behavioral rating scales in studies evaluating the efficacy of antianxiety and antidepressant drugs. Am J Hosp Pharm 1987;44:2087–2100.

17. Andreasen NC. The scale for assessment of negative symptoms (SANS): Conceptual and theoretical foundations. Br J Psychiatry 1989;155(Suppl 7):49–58.
18. Kay SR, Opler LA, Lindenmayer JP. The positive and negative syndrome scale (PANSS): Rationale and standardization. Br J Psychiatry 1989;155(Suppl 7):59–65.
19. Montgomery SA, Asberg M. A new depression scale designed to be sensitive to change. Br J Psychiatry 1979;134:382–389.
20. Sheehan DV. The Anxiety Disease. New York: Bantam, 1983:114–115.
21. Goodman WK, Price LH, Rasmussen SA, et al. The Yale-Brown Obsessive Compulsive Scale (Y-BOCS): II. Validity. Arch Gen Psychiatry 1989;46:1006–1011.
22. Blessed G, Tomlinson BE, Roth M. The association between quantitative measures of dementia and of senile change in the cerebral grey matter of elderly subjects. Br J Psychiatry 1968;114(512):797–811.
23. Mattis S. Mental status examination for organic mental syndrome in the elderly patient. In: Bellak L, Karasu TB, eds. Geriatric Psychiatry. New York: Grune and Stratton, 1976:77–101.
24. Sunderland T, Hill JL, Mellow AM, et al. Clock drawing in Alzheimer's Disease: A novel measure of dementia severity. Am Geriatric Soc 1989;37:725–729.
25. Rosen WG, Mohs RC, Davis KL. A new rating scale for Alzheimer's Disease. Am J Psychiatry 1984;141:1356–1364.

CHAPTER 65 Childhood Disorders

JULIE ANN DOPHEIDE, JANE TRAN TESORO, AND MICHAEL MALKIN

KEY CONCEPTS

1. Inattention and impulsivity caused by attention-deficit/hyperactivity disorder (ADHD) begins before age 7 years and can continue into adolescence and adulthood, often requiring ongoing drug treatment.
2. Stimulants are first-line treatment for ADHD, atomoxetine and bupropion are second-line, tricyclic antidepressants (TCAs) are third-line, and clonidine or guanfacine are considered fourth-line or as adjuncts to stimulants.
3. Coexisting disorders or symptoms such as anxiety, mood, or behavior dysregulation have an impact on drug selection for ADHD and can necessitate the use of additional agents.
4. Tourette's disorder presents with both motor and vocal tics, which are present during childhood, plateau during adolescence, and can continue during adulthood with a fluctuating course.
5. The decision to medicate patients with Tourette's disorder is based on the degree of concern perceived by the patient, symptom severity, and comorbid disorders.
6. Individuals with Tourette's disorder are particularly sensitive to medication side effects, so medication dosing must be individualized carefully, and close monitoring is essential.
7. Nondrug approaches to enuresis management, such as behavioral interventions or using bed-wetting alarms, are preferred because of lasting cure rates and avoidance of drug side effects.
8. Desmopressin tablets are preferred over TCAs because of better safety and tolerability. Both desmopressin and TCAs have a rapid onset of effect (1–2 weeks), however relapse on drug discontinuation is high.

All neuropsychiatric disorders can first present during childhood.[1] ADHD, Tourette's disorder, and enuresis are the focus of this chapter because, by definition, the onset of symptoms explicitly occurs during childhood.

Treating children with psychotropic drugs requires a very different approach than treating adults. Children undergo neurologic, physiologic, and psychosocial changes throughout development. Age-related pharmacodynamic and pharmacokinetic differences can alter drug disposition and response. Well-defined diagnostic criteria guide drug selection;[1] however, comorbid disorders present treatment challenges.[2,3] Children may not be able to articulate symptom response or adverse effects of a medication. Psychotropic drug treatment of children is intended to control symptoms or behaviors that impair learning and development.[4]

The psychiatric assessment of a child requires obtaining information from the child, parents, caregivers, and teachers.

> Learning objectives, review questions, and other resources can be found at **www.pharmacotherapyonline.com.**

ATTENTION-DEFICIT/HYPERACTIVITY DISORDER

CLINICAL PRESENTATION AND EPIDEMIOLOGY

A diagnosis of ADHD should be considered whenever a child presents with developmentally inappropriate inattention, impulsivity, and or hyperactivity. Symptom presence and severity vary with the situation. It is unusual for a child to display signs of the disorder in all settings or even in the same setting at all times.[1]

1 The onset of ADHD is typically by the age of 3 years and must occur by age 7 years, although the disorder may not require professional attention until the child enters school. ADHD occurs in 3% to 10% of children worldwide and is estimated to be present in 4% of adults.[5,6] In the United States, four boys are diagnosed with ADHD for every girl. This difference is likely because of higher rates of oppositional defiant disorder and conduct disorder in boys, compared with girls, thus referrals for assessment are higher for boys. Symptoms can persist lifelong for both sexes, but hyperactivity is much less prominent in adolescence and adulthood.[4–8]

It is critical to clarify the diagnosis of ADHD in individuals with these symptoms. Inattention and distractibility can be symptoms of an anxiety, mood, or psychotic disorder.[2,3,9] In some cases, other disorders coexist with ADHD; learning deficiencies and conduct or oppositional disorders are common comorbid conditions.[3,7,9] The presence of multiple comorbid conditions, particularly conduct or mood disorder, can increase the likelihood of ADHD chronicity into adulthood.[3,6]

Prescriptions for ADHD medication are increasing in all age groups. As of March 2006, two million prescriptions for ADHD were dispensed monthly for children and adolescents in the United States; this compares to one million ADHD prescriptions dispensed to adults. From January to June 2005, methylphenidate was the most prescribed ADHD medication (47%), amphetamine products were second (33.4%), and atomoxetine was the third (16.4%) most prescribed ADHD agent.[10]

CLINICAL PRESENTATION OF ADHD

General

- Onset of symptoms must be before 7 years of age

Symptoms

- Six or more of the symptoms must be present for 6 months; significant impairment must be seen in two or more settings (e.g., home and school); symptoms must be documented by parent, teacher, and clinician.
- ***Inattention***
  - Often fails to give close attention to details or makes careless mistakes in schoolwork or other activities
  - Often has difficulty sustaining attention in activities
  - Often has difficulty organizing tasks and activities
  - Avoids tasks that require sustained mental effort
  - Often does not seem to listen when spoken to directly
  - Often does not follow through on instructions and fails to finish schoolwork, chores, or duties in the workplace
  - Is easily distracted by extraneous stimuli
  - Is often forgetful in daily activities
  - Loses things necessary for activities
- ***Hyperactivity and Impulsivity***
  - Often fidgets with hands or feet or squirms in seat
  - Often leaves seat when remaining seated is expected
  - Often runs about or climbs excessively at inappropriate times
  - Often has difficulty playing quietly
  - Often interrupts or intrudes on others

Adapted with permission from reference American Psychiatric Association.[1]

ETIOLOGY AND PATHOPHYSIOLOGY

ADHD is a clinical diagnosis with multiple heterogeneous causes.[4,6,9] Both genetic and nongenetic factors are involved. First-degree relatives of an individual with ADHD have a four- to eightfold increased chance of developing ADHD compared to the general population; monozygotic twins have up to a 90% concordance rate for ADHD.[6,9,11] Children with fetal alcohol syndrome, lead poisoning, and meningitis have a higher incidence of ADHD symptomatology.[4,9] ADHD is associated with a variety of environmental risks including obstetric adversity, maternal smoking, and adverse parent-child relationships.[6,11] Dietary causes are unlikely.[4,6]

Although brain studies show no definitive pathophysiologic markers of ADHD, the prefrontal cortex, basal ganglia, and caudate volumes are consistently reported as smaller.[6,12] Individuals with ADHD are twice as likely to display a defective seven-repeat allele of the type 4 dopamine (D_4) receptor gene (DRD4), which has been related to a deficiency in translating the dopaminergic signal to the second messenger system.[6,13,14] Norepinephrine (NE) and epinephrine are agonists at this receptor as well. A genetic variation in the presynaptic dopaminergic transport protein, also known as DAT1, has been linked to ADHD risk and to response to methylphenidate and atomoxetine.[13,14] Clinical implications of these findings are being studied.[6,14]

A prevailing pathophysiologic explanation for ADHD symptoms involves deficits in prefrontal cortex–mediated executive brain function also known as *response inhibition.* Children with ADHD are unable to control their behavior, resist distractions, and develop an awareness of space and time.[2,6] A dysregulation of arousal in front subcortical pathways has also been proposed. Children with ADHD display insufficient alertness during dull and repetitive tasks, alternating with overarousal.[6]

Effective treatments modulate dopamine (DA) and norepinephrine (NE) to improve executive functioning and regulate arousal for improved performance. The clinical response associated with stimulants is not paradoxical and is not diagnostic for ADHD because stimulants can increase attention, decrease motor activity, and improve learning tasks in those with subclinical ADHD or in individuals with such problems from other sources (e.g., fatigue).[4,13]

TREATMENT

Attention-Deficit/Hyperactivity Disorder

STIMULANTS

❷ ❸ Stimulants are considered first-line therapy in most cases of ADHD; however, comorbid conditions have an impact on the drug selection process, calling for a careful, systematic approach. Pharmacotherapy should be considered whenever a thorough diagnostic assessment results in a diagnosis of ADHD. Several studies demonstrate the superiority of stimulants compared with behavioral interventions in alleviating core symptoms of ADHD.[5,15] However, stimulants have not been shown to reliably improve social and academic functioning; therefore multimodal treatment, individualized to the specific needs of the child and family, is crucial for overall positive therapeutic outcome.[4,16–18] Table 65–1 describes behavioral interventions for ADHD. Multimodal treatment includes parent training, family therapy, classroom interventions, and contingency management (e.g., rewards for good behavior).[4,17,18] Figure 65–1 provides an algorithm for drug selection in the treatment of ADHD.

Stimulants (e.g., methylphenidate, dexmethylphenidate, mixed amphetamine salts, and dextroamphetamine) are the most effective drug treatment options, with efficacy ranging from 70% to 96% in trials using wide dosage ranges.[5,16,19]

Despite knowledge of the effects of stimulants on neurotransmitter activity, how these drugs affect the primary symptoms of ADHD is unclear. Methylphenidate and amphetamines block DA and NE reuptake; amphetamines also increase catecholamine release.[13] Both drugs inhibit monoamine oxidase (MAO), amphetamines, more potently

TABLE 65-1 Behavioral Interventions for ADHD

Technique	Description	Example
Positive reinforcement	Providing rewards or privileges contingent on the child's performance	Child completes an assignment and is permitted to play on the computer
Time-out	Removing access to positive reinforcement contingent on performance of unwanted or problem behavior	Child hits sibling impulsively and is required to sit for 5 minutes in the corner of the room
Response cost	Withdrawing rewards or privileges contingent on the performance of unwanted or problem behavior	Child loses free-time privileges for not completing homework
Token economy	Combining positive reinforcement and response cost. The child earns rewards and privileges contingent on performing desired behaviors and loses the rewards and privileges based on undesirable behavior.	Child earns stars for completing assignments and loses stars for getting out of seat. The child cashes in the sum of stars at the end of the week for a prize.

Data from American Academy of Pediatrics[17] with permission.

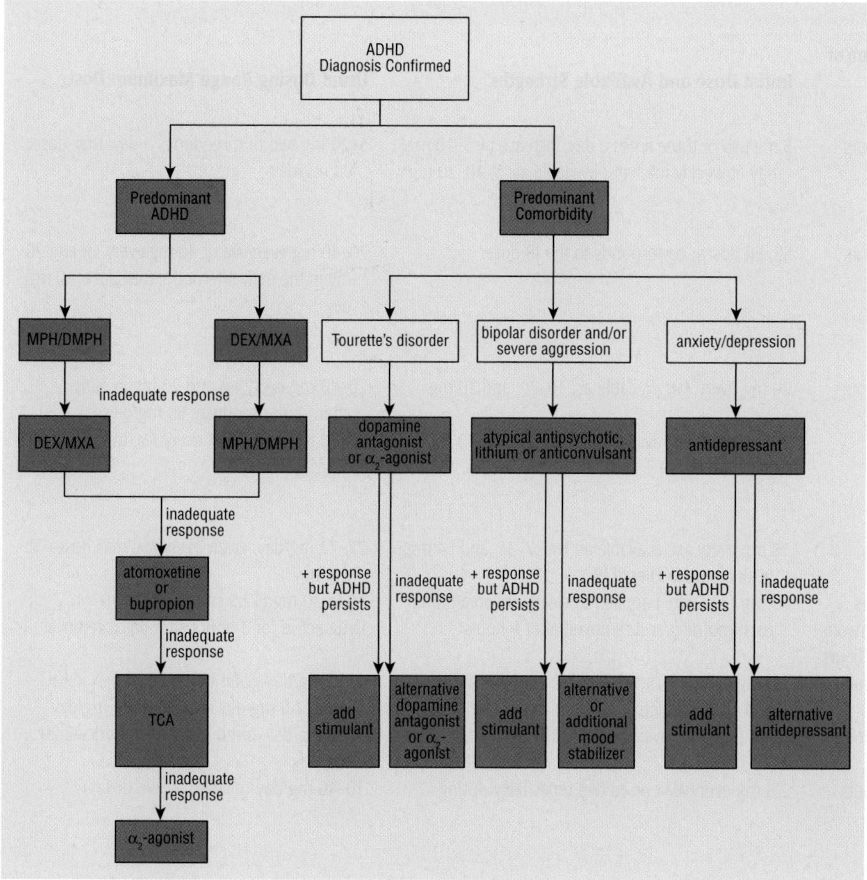

FIGURE 65-1. Algorithm for management of ADHD. Treat predominant disorder first, reassess, and consider alternative or adjunct medications for optimal symptom control. (ADHD, attention-deficit/hyperactivity disorder; DEX, dextroamphetamine; DMPH, dexmethylphenidate; MPH, methylphenidate; MXA, mixed amphetamine salts; TCA, tricyclic antidepressant.) *(Data from Prince,[5] Pliszka et al.,[7] Lopez,[19] Caballerro and Nahata,[30] Kowatch and DelBello,[32] Dopheide,[36] Muller-Vahl,[45] and Jimenez-Jimenez.[46])*

than methylphenidate.[13] Because different stimulants work through slightly different mechanisms, lack of response to one chemical class of stimulant (e.g., methylphenidate or dexmethylphenidate) does not preclude response to another class (e.g., dextroamphetamine or mixed amphetamine salts).[5,7,16]

Stimulant dosing should be titrated for maximum individual efficacy and minimum side effects. Table 65–2 provides initial dose and titration recommendations for stimulants based on manufacturer's recommendations and published guidelines developed by experienced clinicians.[5,16,20]

With immediate-release stimulants, most patients require a two or three times daily dosing schedule because of the short half-lives of these drugs (2 to 4 hours for methylphenidate and dexmethylphenidate and approximately 4 to 6 hours for dextroamphetamine or mixed amphetamine salts).[5,15,19] Drug response is maximal during the absorption phase, is evident in 15 to 30 minutes, and lasts 2 to 6 hours.[5,16,20]

Drug delivery systems of once-daily products (amphetamine aspartate, amphetamine sulfate, dextroamphetamine sulfate, dextroamphetamine saccharate [Adderall XR]; methylphenidate [Concerta]; methylphenidate [Daytrana]; dexmethylphenidate [Focalin XR]; methylphenidate [Metadate CD]; methylphenidate [Ritalin LA]) provide 8 to 12 hours of symptom control.[5,20] Concerta uses an oral osmotic (OROS) controlled-release delivery system, whereas other oral preparations use combinations of immediate-release and extended-release beads containing the drug.[5,19] Concerta is a nondeformable tablet, and it should not be given to children with gastrointestinal narrowing because of the risk of obstruction. Methylphenidate transdermal system provides 12 hours of symptom control when worn for 9 hours.[20] Older wax-matrix sustained-release products (e.g., Ritalin SR) are less effective and infrequently used.[5,16] When choosing between immediate-release or once-daily stimulants, the convenience of once-daily dosing must be weighed against the potential for difficulty falling asleep and risk of increased growth suppression with once-daily or sustained-release products.[5,9,19,21] Adolescents and adults with ADHD are also responsive to stimulants. Methylphenidate is effective in adults in doses up to 1.3 mg/kg per day.[16,22] Lisdexamphetamine is a prodrug conjugated to an amino acid that requires cleavage during metabolism to the active dextroamphetamine. It is available in 30, 50, and 70 mg capsules and is intended to pose less abuse potential.[23]

■ ADVERSE EFFECTS

The most common adverse effects of stimulants and their management strategies are listed in Table 65–3. Uncommon to rare but potentially serious adverse effects are discussed below.

Psychiatric

The FDA has added warnings to the labeling of all stimulants and atomoxetine. Hundreds of post-marketing reports of three broad categories of psychiatric adverse events have been associated with stimulants: (1) psychosis or mania, (2) aggression or violent behavior, (3) severe anxiety or panic attacks. All of these reactions require dose reduction or cessation of stimulant therapy and supportive treatment.[24]

Cardiac

Twenty-five reports of sudden death in children and adults treated with stimulants (17 amphetamine, 8 methylphenidate) were reported to the FDA. Undiscovered structural cardiac defects (thin myocardial wall, valve problems) were found postmortem in 8 of 12 children taking amphetamine and 4 of 7 children taking methylphenidate.[24,25] The risk of sudden unexplained death per 100,000 children exposed to ADHD medication in 2005 is 0.7 for dextroamphetamine/amphetamine, 1.5 with atomoxetine, and 0.2 with methylphenidate.[24] An FDA advisory committee determined the rate was

TABLE 65-2 Stimulant Comparison

Stimulant	Duration of Effect	Initial Dose and Available Strengths	Usual Dosing Range Maximum Dose
Methylphenidate C-II FDA approved for children >6 y old *Short-acting* Immediate release (IR) Ritalin, Methylin, generics	3–5 hours	5 mg two or three times a day; increase by 5–10 mg/day at weekly intervals; available as: 5, 10, 20 mg	5–20 mg two or three times a day; max dose: 60 mg/day
Intermediate-acting Ritalin SR (sustained-release) Methylphenidate SR Metadate ER (extended-release) Methylin ER	3–8 hours	SR, ER doses; corresponds to the IR dose	20–40 mg every AM or 40 mg every AM and 20 mg in the early afternoon; max dose: 60 mg/day
Long-acting Metadate CD 30% IR beads, 70% ER beads	8–12 hours	20 mg every AM; available as: 10, 20, and 30 mg	20–40 mg every AM and 20 mg in early afternoon; max dose: 60 mg/day
Ritalin LA 50% IR, 50% ER beads		20 mg every AM; available as: 20, 30, and 40 mg	20–60 mg/day, given every AM; max dose: 60 mg/day
Concerta (oral osmotic [OROS] controlled-release delivery) ER inner compartments coated with IR methylphenidate		18 mg every AM; available as 18, 27, 36, and 54 mg; 90% bioavailability of IR	27–72 mg/day, given every AM; max dose: 72 mg/day
Daytrana Methylphenidate transdermal system	12 hours when worn for 9 hours	10 mg (12.5 cm^2) applied to clean, dry area on hip each morning and removed after 9 hours	10 to 30 mg (12.5 cm^2–37.5 cm^2) Drug active for 3 hours after patch removal
Dexmethylphenidate (Focalin) C-II FDA approved for children ≥6 y old	3–5 hours	2.5 mg every AM or twice a day; available as: 2.5, 5, and 10 mg tablets	5–10 mg/day given twice a day; max initial dose: 7.5 mg/day max dose: 20 mg/day
Focalin XR 50% IR, 50% ER beads	8–12 hours	5 mg every AM; available as 5, 10, 20 mg capsules	5–20 mg/day, given every AM max dose: 20 mg/day
Mixed Amphetamine Salts C-II FDA approved for children ≥3 y old *Short to intermediate acting* Mixed amphetamine generics Adderall	4–6 hours	2.5 mg every AM one to two times daily dosing	10–40 mg/day (divided in two doses)
Long-acting Adderall XR 50% IR beads, 50% ER beads	8–12 hours	10 mg every AM; available as: 10, 20, and 30 mg	10–30 mg every AM; max dose: 30 mg/day
Dextroamphetamine C-II FDA approved for children ≥3 y old	4–6 hours	2.5 mg every AM to two or three times daily dosing	5–15 mg twice a day
Short-acting Dextroamphetamine generics Dexedrine, Dextrostat	3–5 hours	5 mg every AM; available as: 5 and 10 mg	10–40 mg/day given twice a day
Intermediate-acting Dexedrine Spansule	5–8 hours	Available as: 5-, 10-, and 15-mg spansules	5–30 mg every day or 5–15 mg twice a day; max: 40 mg/day

C-II, schedule II, the Drug Enforcement Administration label that refers to significant abuse potential.
Data from Prince JB,[5] Lopez FA,[19] Anderson VR.[20]

not higher than what would be expected in the general population (0.6–6 cases per 100,000 untreated children), therefore no restriction in use was recommended.[24,25]

Growth

A review of 29 studies examining stimulant effects on growth found a height deficit of approximately 1 cm/y (0.4 in/y) during the first 1 to 3 years of continuous treatment. Dextroamphetamine studies showed more growth attenuation in the first year than methylphenidate studies or studies that combined both stimulants in a single group.[25] A 24-month followup study in 540 children taking methylphenidate showed a 1 cm/y growth deficit, and documented an average loss of 3 kg (6.6 lb) in weight during the first year, with an average 1.2 kg (2.6 lb) decrease in weight during the second year.[26] Proposed mechanisms of stimulant effects on growth include alterations in growth hormone or growth factor, decreased thyroxine secretion, and suppression of appetite leading to reduced caloric intake.[21,27]

In most cases, children should be given a drug-free trial every year. Drug holidays are important because they provide time to reassess treatment.[17] One study showed growth rebound in weight and height occurring over a 3-month period off stimulant, although another study with shorter duration off stimulant (1 month), reported no growth rebound.[26,27] Consideration must be given to the risks of negative effects on learning, socialization, and self-image while off-stimulant therapy when determining the frequency and duration of drug holidays. Drug dosage often varies from year to year, largely because of age-related pharmacokinetic changes. As a child develops, hepatic metabolism slows, and volume of distribution increases.

CLINICAL CONTROVERSY

The use of stimulants to treat ADHD in individuals with substance abuse disorders is controversial. A diagnosis of ADHD confers at least a twofold greater risk of adolescent and adult substance abuse.[2,6,28] The risk is greater if conduct disorder, antisocial personality, or bipolar disorder coexists.[3,28] **PRO:** Stimulant therapy does not increase the risk of substance abuse, and effective treatment of ADHD can facilitate functioning and reduce substance abuse. **CON:** Regardless of the benefits, there is significant misuse or diversion of stimulant medications among older adolescents and young adults, necessitating vigilance among prescribers and careful risk-versus-benefit assessment.[28,29]

TABLE 65-3 Stimulant Adverse Effects and Their Management

Adverse Effect	Recommendation/Management Strategy
Common	
Reduced appetite, weight loss	Give high-calorie meal when stimulant effects are low (at breakfast or at bedtime), or consider cyproheptadine at bedtime
Stomach ache	Administer stimulant on a full stomach, lower dose if possible
Insomnia	Give dose earlier in the day; lower the last dose of the day or give it earlier; consider a sedating medication at bedtime (guanfacine, clonidine, melatonin, or cyproheptadine)
Headache	Divide dose; give with food; or give an analgesic (e.g., acetaminophen or ibuprofen)
Rebound symptoms	Consider longer-acting stimulant trial, atomoxetine or antidepressant
Irritability/jitteriness	Assess for comorbid condition (e.g., bipolar disorder); reduce dosage; consider mood stabilizer or atypical antipsychotic
Uncommon to rare	
Dysphoria	Reduce dosage; reassess diagnosis; consider alternative therapy
Zombie-like state	Reduce dosage or change stimulant medication
Tics or abnormal movements	Reduce dosage; consider alternative medication
Hypertension, pulse fluctuations	Reduce dosage; change medication
Hallucinations	Discontinue stimulant; reassess diagnosis; mood stabilizer and/or antipsychotic may be needed

NONSTIMULANTS

❷ Atomoxetine, a selective norepinephrine reuptake inhibitor, is the first nonstimulant approved by the FDA for the treatment of ADHD. In contrast to the stimulants, it has no abuse potential and is not a controlled substance.[30] Placebo-controlled, short-term trials (6 to 12 weeks) have shown that atomoxetine is effective in reducing ADHD symptoms in children, teens, and adults, and 9-month continuation studies show ongoing benefit for responders. However, available evidence shows lower efficacy rates compared to stimulants.[5,19]

Atomoxetine has a significantly slower onset of therapeutic effect than stimulants (2 to 4 weeks versus 1 hour with an effective stimulant dose). Atomoxetine can be taken once daily by adults or in divided doses in the morning or late afternoon by children.[7,30] Atomoxetine is sometimes combined with a stimulant in partially responsive patients based on case series describing less late-day rebound effects and better sleep when atomoxetine is given in the evening; however, adverse effects are additive.[5,7,19] Table 65–4 provides dosing and titration recommendations for all nonstimulant medications.

Bupropion, a monocyclic antidepressant, is a weak DA and NE reuptake inhibitor with no significant direct effect on serotonin or MAO. Its active metabolites augment noradrenergic and dopaminergic function. Investigations with bupropion in children demonstrated efficacy greater than placebo in two controlled trials and efficacy comparable with methylphenidate (n = 15 children) in another controlled trial.[19] Advantages of bupropion include less toxicity on overdose compared with TCAs and less appetite suppression compared with stimulants. Bupropion also may be effective in adults at antidepressant doses.[5,7,17]

Atomoxetine and bupropion are second-line alternatives to the stimulants for treatment of ADHD in children, teens, and adults. Their potential benefits relative to stimulants include reduced risk of abuse and lower potential for sleep disturbance. TCAs are third-line agents because they are the most dangerous in overdose and pose the greatest risk for cardiovascular side effects.[7,17] Imipramine and desipramine are the most systematically studied TCAs in the treatment of ADHD, although nortriptyline is also effective.[7,17,19] The onset of TCA clinical response occurs within the first 2 to 4 weeks.[7,17]

Variability in dosage requirements for atomoxetine, bupropion, and TCAs can be due to interpatient variability in drug plasma concentration achieved at a given dose. All are metabolized via

TABLE 65-4 Dosing and Adverse Effect Monitoring of Nonstimulant Drugs for ADHD

Drug	Dosing Range and Titration Schedule	Adverse Effect Monitoring
Antidepressants		
Atomoxetine (Strattera)	≤70 kg: start at 0.3 to 0.5 mg/kg every AM or twice a day; max: 1.4 mg/kg per day; ≥70 kg: start at 40 mg every AM or twice a day; max: 100 mg/day	Nausea, anorexia, ↑ blood pressure, ↑ pulse, insomnia, fatigue, sedation, severe liver injury, suicidality
Bupropion (Wellbutrin, SR, XL)	50–300 mg/day; 3 mg/kg per day by end of week one; can increase to 6 mg/kg per day or maximum of 300 mg/day as tolerated	Nausea, insomnia, rash, tics; dose-related risk of seizures
Tricyclic antidepressants: imipramine, desipramine or nortriptyline	50–150 mg/day; start at 0.5–1 mg/kg per day; increase as tolerated to 2–3 mg/kg per day; max: 300 mg/day of desipramine (adults only) or 150 mg/day nortriptyline	Sedation, dizziness, constipation, heart block (check ECG), weight gain, overdose toxicity, rapid heartbeat
Antipsychotics		
Aripiprazole[a] (Abilify)	2–5 mg daily; can titrate weekly as tolerated to response (usual range: 5–20 mg/day)	Nausea, restlessness, insomnia extrapyramidal symptoms, dizziness, sedation
Haloperidol[a] (Haldol)	0.5–1 mg twice daily; can titrate every 3–4 days as tolerated to response (usual range: 0.5–5 mg/day)	Extrapyramidal symptoms, dizziness, ↑ prolactin, sedation
Olanzapine[a] (Zyprexa)	2.5–5 mg every day; can titrate every 3–4 days as tolerated to response (usual range: 7.5–15 mg/day)	Sedation, weight gain, restlessness, extrapyramidal symptoms diabetes, hyperlipidemia
Quetiapine[a] (Seroquel)	25–50 mg twice daily; can titrate every 3–4 days as tolerated to response (usual range: 200–600 mg/day)	Sedation, dizziness, weight gain, diabetes, hyperlipidemia
Risperidone[a] (Risperdal)	0.25–0.5 mg twice daily; can titrate every 3–4 days as tolerated to response, (1–4 mg/day)	Extrapyramidal symptoms, dizziness, ↑ prolactin, hepatotoxicity, weight gain Diabetes, hyperlipidemia
Ziprasidone[a] (Geodon)	10–20 mg twice daily; can titrate every 3–4 days as tolerated to response (usual range: 40–120 mg/day)	Nausea, restlessness, insomnia extrapyramidal symptoms, sedation, QTc prolongation
Other		
Clonidine (Catapres)	0.05 mg two or four times daily; can increase as tolerated to 0.1–0.4 mg/day	Sedation, dizziness, heart block (check ECG), constipation
Guanfacine (Tenex)	0.5 once to twice a day; can increase as tolerated to 1–4 mg/day	Same as above with potentially lower risk of sedation

ADHD, attention-deficit/hyperactivity disorder; ECG, electrocardiogram.
[a]Short-term use (1–4 months) only for severe aggression associated with ADHD.
Data from Shur et al.,[33] Pappadopulus et al.,[34] and Correll et al.[35]

cytochrome P450 (CYP)2D6, and bioavailability and half-life can be 4 to 8 times greater in those taking a CYP2D6 inhibitor (e.g., bupropion, fluoxetine, or paroxetine) or in poor metabolizers. For example, atomoxetine's half-life is 5 hours in extensive metabolizers and 19 hours in poor metabolizers.[7,30] Atomoxetine and bupropion are metabolized faster in prepubertal children and twice daily dosing is optimal (even for bupropion sustained release [SR]).[7] Once daily dosing is possible for most adolescents and adults. If tolerance develops after months of therapy, a dosage adjustment can be necessary to compensate for age-related changes in distribution and metabolism.

❷ Clonidine and guanfacine are less effective alternatives to stimulant, atomoxetine, or bupropion monotherapy. They are prescribed more frequently as adjuncts to reduce disruptive behavior, control aggression, or to improve sleep.[7,19] Clonidine and guanfacine are central α_2-adrenergic agonists, acting both presynaptically to inhibit NE release and post-synaptically to increase blood flow in the prefrontal cortex. Increased blood flow in the prefrontal cortex has been shown to enhance working memory and executive functioning. Both interact with a multitude of neurotransmitter systems including catecholamine, indolamine, cholinergic, α_2-receptors on parasympathetic neurons, opioid, imidazole, and amino acid systems.[13] Guanfacine has a longer elimination half-life (12 to 18 hours) compared with clonidine (2.5 to 4 hours), and its greater selectivity for the α_{2a}-receptor, compared to clonidine, imparts less sedation.[5,31]

❸ Lithium and anticonvulsants are used increasingly to control aggression and explosive behavior in patients with a diagnosis of ADHD. Some patients actually can have childhood-onset bipolar disorder or combined ADHD-bipolar disorder.[7,32] Lithium, valproate, and carbamazepine are effective for explosive behavior, aggression, and impulsivity, but they are not beneficial treatments for a child with the inattentive subtype of ADHD. Dosing starts in low divided doses with titration over 1 to 2 weeks to therapeutic response.[7,32]

Conventional antipsychotics improve symptoms of hyperactivity and impulsivity but can have negative effects on learning and cognitive functioning as well as extrapyramidal side effects (e.g., dystonia and tardive dyskinesia) that limit their usefulness.[7] The atypical antipsychotics: risperidone, olanzapine, quetiapine, ziprasidone, and aripiprazole have been used to control severe aggression in refractory cases of ADHD, particularly if conduct disorder or bipolar disorder coexists. More studies are needed to clarify their place in therapy.[7,33–35]

If multiple drugs are started simultaneously, it is impossible to determine the impact of each drug. The predominance and urgency of symptoms guide the drug-selection process (see Fig. 65–1). For example, if a child presents as severely anxious or depressed with associated attentional problems, then an antidepressant should be initiated first with monitoring to determine if attentional symptoms improve.[7,9,32,36] When a child presents with severe ADHD and associated anxiety or depression, a stimulant should be initiated to treat the more severe ADHD. If ADHD symptoms improve significantly but anxiety or depression persists, then an antidepressant can be added.[7,36] Careful monitoring is needed to detect drug interactions that lead to higher drug plasma levels and increased adverse effects.[7,36] Studies show that stimulants do not routinely make anxiety disorders worse, but they might not improve symptoms either.[7,16,17] In children with epilepsy, methylphenidate is safe and effective; however, the child should be stabilized and seizure-free on an anticonvulsant prior to initiation of the stimulant.[37]

The monoamine oxidase inhibitor (MAOI), tranylcypromine is effective but used infrequently because of the potential for dangerous drug and dietary interactions.[5,13] Selegiline is a MAOI-B selective agent, which has demonstrated comparable efficacy to methylphenidate in small placebo-controlled trials. Dangerous drug and dietary interactions are less likely compared to tranylcypromine. The risks of MAOIs outweigh benefits in children because they are unlikely to remember to adhere to dietary restrictions.[5]

Adverse Effects

Possible atomoxetine adverse effects and their management are similar to those of stimulants including psychiatric and cardiac adverse effects (see Table 65–4). Atomoxetine has been associated with less growth suppression compared to stimulants, 0.44 cm (0.17 in) over 2 years of treatment. It has a greater risk of fatigue, sedation, and dizziness compared to stimulants and bupropion. Unlike stimulants, atomoxetine labeling includes a bolded warning of potential for severe liver injury following reports in two patients. Also, it is the only FDA-approved ADHD medication with a labeled warning for new onset suicidality, 0.4% in atomoxetine treated patients versus 0% in patients receiving placebo.[7,19,24]

Bupropion's adverse effects include nausea, which can resolve over time or with slower dosage titration, and rash, which can require discontinuation of therapy if severe (see Table 65–4). Bupropion should not be used in children with a seizure disorder or eating disorder because of unacceptable risk of seizures in these patients. Bupropion can cause or exacerbate tics.[5,7]

Possible central nervous system (CNS) adverse effects of TCAs include dizziness, aggressiveness, excitement, nightmares, insomnia, forgetfulness, and irritability. Similar to other antidepressants, TCAs carry a warning of the risk of new-onset suicidality in pediatric patients.[35] TCAs should be taken throughout the week and not just on school days. TCA-withdrawal effects are severe in children and include nausea, vomiting, and diarrhea.[36] Signs of CNS toxicity are confusion, impaired concentration, hallucinations, and delusions.

The most common side effects of clonidine and guanfacine are dose-dependent sedation, hypotension, and constipation.[19] Sedation usually subsides after 2 to 3 weeks of therapy.[7,39] Of concern are reports of bradycardia, syncope, rebound hypertension, heart block, and sudden death.[7,40] Four children have died on the combination of methylphenidate and clonidine; however, complicating factors make it impossible to link the drug combination directly with the cause of death.[40] Overdoses, concurrent clonidine and stimulant administration, as well as missed doses of clonidine all add to the risk of adverse cardiovascular events.[39,40] Similar adverse-effect concerns apply to treatment with guanfacine.[19]

PHARMACOECONOMIC CONSIDERATIONS

A study comparing medical care use and costs between persons with and without ADHD over 9 years found that the median cost for a person with ADHD was more than double ($4,306 vs. $1,944; P <0.001) that of someone without ADHD. Increased costs are attributed to accidental injuries, diagnostic assessments, hospital visits, and outpatient visits.[41] The cost-effectiveness of drug treatment has not been assessed. Immediate-release generic methylphenidate, dextroamphetamine, and mixed amphetamine salts appear to provide the most effective and economic therapy because of relatively low drug cost. The cost of once-daily Concerta, Ritalin LA, Metadate CD, Adderall XR, Daytrana, and atomoxetine (Strattera) is approximately 2 to 4 times that of an immediate-release generic stimulant. A retrospective analysis comparing immediate-release methylphenidate use patterns with OROS methylphenidate use patterns in 5,939 patients over 34 months found that OROS methylphenidate use was associated with longer treatment periods, increased patient adherence, and fewer emergency room visits for injury, potentially decreasing overall costs.[42]

Generic bupropion is the least expensive nonstimulant treatment. Imipramine, desipramine, clonidine, and mood stabilizers are relatively inexpensive, but ongoing electrocardiographic and blood-level monitoring can increase costs significantly.[7,41]

EVALUATION OF THERAPEUTIC OUTCOMES

Careful documentation of baseline symptoms and complaints over a 1-month predrug period is essential to the evaluation of therapeutic and adverse outcomes. Investigation regarding family history of psychiatric disorders and cardiac disease is essential to determine risk for related adverse drug reactions and to implement appropriate monitoring.[7] Baseline symptoms can be measured using videotapes, clinician rating scales (e.g., Child Behavioral Checklist or ADHD Rating Scale-IV), or both.[43] In addition, height, weight, and eating and sleeping patterns should be recorded at baseline and every 3 months.[7]

After the initiation and titration of any drug treatment, it is necessary that parents, teachers, and clinicians assess the overall functioning of the child using standardized rating scales to determine if significant therapeutic benefit justifies continuing medication.[7,17,43] Therapeutic effects of the stimulants include decreased motor activity and impulsivity and increased attention span.[13,15,17] This suggests that stimulants are indicated for ADHD symptoms and not for primary learning disorders. The benefits of drug therapy must outweigh the potential for adverse effects.[7,19]

Atomoxetine and bupropion also require monitoring to detect changes in appetite, weight, and sleep patterns, as well as pulse or blood pressure. An adequate trial of atomoxetine or bupropion consists of 6 weeks at maximum tolerated doses unless response occurs at a lower dose.[5,19,30]

When clonidine or guanfacine are given, careful clinical monitoring for fatigue, dizziness, and autonomic changes (e.g., blood pressure and pulse) is recommended.[19] The American Heart Association has stated that electrocardiographic monitoring is not required for clonidine treatment in children, although many clinicians continue to assess for electrocardiogram changes.[40] When discontinuing treatment, clonidine and guanfacine should be withdrawn slowly (0.05 mg clonidine/0.5 mg guanfacine reductions every 3 days) to prevent rebound hypertension or behavioral dyscontrol.[19] A therapeutic trial requires 1 to 2 months to assess therapeutic response, although increased sleep usually occurs immediately.

The effects of TCAs on the electrocardiogram should be monitored carefully. Of more concern are reports of sudden death in children taking desipramine or imipramine.[7,36] Children and adolescents given TCAs should have pretreatment and followup electrocardiograms to assess the effects of TCA therapy on cardiac rate and rhythm.[7,36]

CONCLUSION

The preferred first-line drug therapy for ADHD is either methylphenidate, dexmethylphenidate, mixed amphetamine salts, or dextroamphetamine. Atomoxetine or bupropion are good options for those unresponsive to or unable to tolerate stimulants. TCAs are third-line options, and α_2-agonists are fourth-line or can be used as adjuncts to stimulants. All agents require careful cardiovascular monitoring. Mood stabilizers (e.g., lithium, divalproex, and carbamazepine) and atypical antipsychotics are adjuncts for control of aggression or comorbid bipolar disorder. Other agents require further investigation before their status in the treatment of ADHD can be fully determined.

TOURETTE'S DISORDER

EPIDEMIOLOGY AND CLINICAL PRESENTATION

Once considered rare, Tourette's disorder is present in 0.7% to 1.1% of boys and 0.4% of girls.[44,45] The essential features of this CNS disorder are multiple motor and vocal tics that must be present for more than 1 year before the diagnosis of Tourette's disorder is made. A tic is a sudden, rapid, recurrent, nonrhythmic, stereotyped motor movement or vocalization.[44,45] The clinical presentation can vary from barely noticeable to debilitating, and the type of tic expressed can change over time.[1,44,45] The median age of onset of motor tics is 6 years, with an average delay in diagnosis of 6.8 years.[1,44,45]

❹ Transient tic disorder is diagnosed if motor or vocal tics occur for less than 1 year, with chronic tic disorder diagnosed if motor or vocal tics are present for longer than 1 year.[1,44] Tics are most prominent during childhood and can plateau or attenuate during adolescence. The early 20s frequently bring stabilization of symptoms, although exacerbations occur during adulthood with characteristic fluctuating symptom severity.[1,44,45]

More than 90% of children with Tourette's disorder have coexisting conditions such as ADHD (75%), mood disorders (60%), obsessive-compulsive disorder (40%), other anxiety disorders, or a combination of comorbidities. Tourette's disorder itself does not cause diminished intellectual functioning; however, the severity of tics and associated illnesses can result in significant impairment in school functioning, sometimes necessitating special education classes.[44–46]

CLINICAL PRESENTATION OF TOURETTE'S DISORDER

General

- Onset occurs before 18 years of age

Symptoms

- Multiple motor or one or more vocal tics are present.
- Motor and vocal tics do not need to occur concurrently.
- Tics occur many times a day (usually in bouts) nearly every day or intermittently throughout a period of more than 1 year; during this period there is never a tic-free period of more than 3 consecutive months.
- ***Motor Tics***
  - Eye blinking, lip licking
  - Facial twitching
  - Shoulder shrugging
  - Squatting, twirling
- ***Vocal Tics***
  - Clicks, grunts
  - Barking, yelping
  - Throat clearing, echolalia
  - Coprolalia, palilalia

Data from American Psychiatric Association[1] with permission.

ETIOLOGY AND PATHOPHYSIOLOGY

Tourette's disorder is inherited in a complex polygenic pattern. Symptoms and severity of the disorder vary from one generation to another.[44–46] The neurochemical pathophysiology involves an imbalance in the interaction of dopaminergic, serotonergic, γ-aminobutyric acid (GABA)-ergic, glutamatergic, cholinergic, noradrenergic, and opioid systems in multiple brain regions, most notably the basal ganglia and caudate nucleus. The imbalance can cause a lack of regulation of the brain's inhibitory mechanisms, resulting in tics and associated behavior disorders. This multisystem etiology best explains the success of a variety of treatments.[44–46]

TREATMENT

Tourette's Disorder

5 Whenever symptoms are severe enough to impair the child's ability to function, drug therapy should be initiated. Psychotherapy and behavioral treatment are useful adjuncts.[44–46]

CLINICAL CONTROVERSY

The decision to treat Tourette's disorder with a dopamine type 2 (D_2) receptor antagonist (atypical or conventional) rather than an α_2-agonist is controversial and can be challenging. The choice is usually based on whether high efficacy (D_2 antagonist) or milder adverse effect burden (α_2-agonist) is more desirable in an individual patient.[7,44–46]

Clonidine is the most widely prescribed treatment for Tourette's disorder, according to an international database of 3,500 cases, but its efficacy is not robust, and it is not more effective than DA antagonists.[45,46] In some patients, the response is limited to improvement in attention and behavior with no changes in the frequency of tics. A clonidine trial should be initiated carefully, usually 0.025 to 0.05 mg given in the morning or divided two to three times daily with gradual titration every 4 to 7 days to the usual therapeutic dose of 0.15 to 0.25 mg/day (maximum 0.6 mg/day).[44–46] Doses usually are divided during maintenance therapy for more continuous symptom control and to minimize adverse effects. Case reports describe a positive response from the clonidine patch as well. The onset of therapeutic effects for both tablet and patch is slow, ranging from 2 weeks to a few months.[45,46]

Expert consensus and evidence-based treatment guidelines recommend a trial of atypical antipsychotic before considering the FDA-approved agents, haloperidol or pimozide because of established efficacy (e.g., risperidone) and a lower risk of extrapyramidal side effects.[21,35,46]

Risperidone was significantly more effective than placebo in decreasing motor and vocal tic severity in two controlled trials.[47,48] In parallel comparison trials, risperidone was found to be as effective as pimozide or clonidine. The dose of risperidone in these trials ranged from 0.6–6 mg/day.[47–50] Ziprasidone showed significant efficacy versus placebo in a controlled study at an average dose of 30 mg/day titrated from a starting dose of 5 mg/day.[51,52] An open trial with olanzapine at a mean dose of 10.9 mg/day showed a 50% reduction in global tic severity.[53] One open-label trial and two case reports describe positive therapeutic effects of quetiapine.[54] Aripiprazole has shown modest to robust efficacy in case series and case reports. Clozapine, a 5-hydroxytryptamine 2 ($5\text{-}HT_2$) antagonist with minimal dopamine type 1 (D_1)-blocking and no significant D_2-blocking effects, was found to be ineffective with worsening of symptoms in some Tourette's patients.[45,46]

Therapy with haloperidol or pimozide should be initiated at very low doses of 0.25 to 0.5 mg/day given at bedtime and then increased gradually. Gradual titration over 2 to 3 weeks helps minimize extrapyramidal and sedative effects while permitting careful assessment of response. Symptoms can regress within 48 to 72 hours after an effective dose is reached. Doses less than 5 mg/day are effective in controlling tics for most patients, but occasionally up to 10 or 20 mg/day are required.[45,46] Pimozide is approximately half as potent as haloperidol, and it is considered comparable or possibly superior to haloperidol in efficacy when equivalent doses are used.[44,45]

COMORBIDITY

Pharmacotherapy of Tourette's disorder is challenging because of the common occurrence of coexisting disorders typically requiring medication combinations. Often the behavioral problems precede and are more disturbing than the involuntary movements, making them a treatment priority.

TOURETTE'S AND ADHD

Pharmacotherapy with stimulants increases dopaminergic and noradrenergic activity, which has the potential to aggravate or precipitate tics, although one study in 19 children over 2 years showed no worsening of tics on methylphenidate.[55] A study examined the comparative effects of methylphenidate and dextroamphetamine on tics in children and found the majority experienced improvement in ADHD symptoms with acceptable effects on tics.[45,47] Methylphenidate was better tolerated than dextroamphetamine.

A double-blind, placebo-controlled trial compared methylphenidate or clonidine monotherapy to combination methylphenidate and clonidine in patients with ADHD and Tourette's disorder. Combination therapy demonstrated the greatest benefit in reducing symptoms of ADHD and tics ($P < 0.0001$).[56] Clonidine appeared most helpful for impulsivity and hyperactivity, whereas methylphenidate was most helpful for inattention. All treatments were well tolerated. Patients and caregivers should be aware of the risks of using stimulants in children with Tourette's disorder (see ADHD section); careful monitoring is essential.[45,46,56]

Controlled trials of TCA therapy for comorbid ADHD and chronic tics or Tourette's disorder show significant improvement in inattentive and hyperactive/impulsive symptoms without worsening of tics.[57] In one study, both tics and symptoms of ADHD improved.[57] TCAs offer an alternative to clonidine or combined clonidine/methylphenidate therapy that can be more effective for some patients.

Clonidine or guanfacine alone are less effective alternatives to stimulants in the treatment of children with Tourette's disorder and ADHD. Guanfacine was administered to 34 children (mean age 10.4 years), with ADHD and tic disorder during an 8-week placebo-controlled trial at a dose of 1.5 to 3 mg/day. Tic severity decreased by 31% in the guanfacine group compared to 0% in the placebo group.[31,46] There was a mean improvement of 37% on the teacher-rated ADHD scale compared to 8% improvement with placebo. Because of its similarity to clonidine, guanfacine's cardiovascular effects warrant careful clinical monitoring.[19,40,46]

TOURETTE'S AND ANXIETY OR MOOD DISORDERS

Therapeutic trials (6 to 12 weeks) of an SSRI or clomipramine should be added to tic-specific therapy when obsessive-compulsive, anxiety, or depressive symptoms cause functional impairment in patients with Tourette's disorder.[45,46] Careful monitoring for behavioral activation, disinhibition, and motor restlessness is essential during SSRI or clomipramine therapy, because these symptoms can indicate increased risk for suicidal behavior or a switch to mania requiring drug discontinuation.[36,44,45]

ADJUNCTIVE OR ALTERNATIVE TREATMENTS

For those who are unresponsive, partially responsive, or unable to tolerate DA antagonists or α_2-agonists, there are several adjuncts or alternative treatments available. A small controlled study ($n = 27$) showed metoclopramide (5–40 mg/day) improved symptoms in children and adolescents with tic disorder.[58] Another study demonstrated effectiveness and tolerability of ondansetron (8–24 mg/day) in 30 patients (ages 12 to 46 years) with Tourette's disorder.[59]

Nicotine administration by gum or patch can potentiate the effects of dopamine-blocking agents in relieving tics, according to small controlled trials.[44,45,60] ADHD symptoms can improve as well.[45,60] The long-term adverse effects of nicotine on overall health can limit usefulness.[60] Clonazepam, selegiline, or baclofen appear to offer promise in relieving tics and associated symptoms.[44–46] Opioid agonists or antagonists are not effective. Botulinum toxin requires further study.[44–46] Nonpharmacologic interventions include support groups, "habit-reversal therapy," and even neurosurgery.[44,45,61]

■ ADVERSE EFFECTS

For clonidine and guanfacine, the most common adverse effect is sedation. Fortunately, tolerance usually develops to this effect over days to weeks. The most potentially serious side effects are cardiovascular (see the ADHD section).[19,40] Other α_2-agonist side effects include dry mouth, constipation, headache, mood changes, and even a temporary worsening of tics in approximately 10% of patients.

Atypical antipsychotics (e.g., risperidone, olanzapine, quetiapine, ziprasidone, and aripiprazole) pose similar adverse effect risks in children and adolescents compared to adults (see Table 65–4).[33,35,45,46] Available data show that children and adolescents are at higher risk for experiencing sedation, acute extrapyramidal side effects, hyperprolactinemia, withdrawal dyskinesia, and significant weight gain during treatment compared to adults. Risperidone is associated with more weight gain in youths compared to adults, and ziprasidone and aripiprazole do not seem to be as "weight neutral" in pediatric populations as in adults.[21,35] Children taking quetiapine have shown a decrease in serum total thyroxine (T_4), although thyroid-stimulating hormone (TSH) and T_4 levels are normal suggesting a euthyroid status.[21,35] Ziprasidone carries a risk of QTc prolongation in youth, although torsade de pointes has not been reported, and the clinical significance requires further study.[21,33,35,51]

❻ Adverse effects have been reported with haloperidol doses of 2 mg/day or greater. In one review of 24 patients treated with haloperidol for Tourette's disorder, 66.7% discontinued treatment because of intolerable side effects (e.g., dysphoria, akathisia, nervousness, sedation, dystonia, and cognitive dulling or feeling drugged).[62] Lowering the dose can alleviate side effects. An antiparkinsonian agent such as benztropine (at a starting dose of 0.5 mg orally twice daily) sometimes will reverse extrapyramidal side effects. Whether a patient with Tourette's disorder is developing a new tic or tardive dyskinesia can be difficult to determine. Dosage titration of the medication and careful monitoring will assist in this clinical decision-making process.[45,46]

Pimozide is less likely to cause extrapyramidal side effects compared to haloperidol. Anticholinergic side effects can occur in addition to drowsiness, and occasionally, anxiety will occur. Electrocardiographic changes, including T- and U-wave abnormalities and prolongation of the QTc interval, are found rarely with recommended therapeutic doses for Tourette's disorder; however, drugs that inhibit CYP3A4 (e.g., clarithromycin or fluoxetine) should not be combined with pimozide because of the risk of excessively elevating pimozide blood levels, which can result in lethal QTc prolongation.[7,45,46]

PHARMACOECONOMIC CONSIDERATIONS

No pharmacoeconomic studies have been published on Tourette's disorder. Haloperidol provides the most economic drug therapy because of high efficacy and low drug cost. Pimozide and atypical antipsychotics are more expensive than generic haloperidol. Although generic clonidine is inexpensive, delayed onset of effect and significantly lower efficacy substantially increase total costs of treatment.

EVALUATION OF THERAPEUTIC OUTCOMES

Evaluating therapeutic interventions is challenging, as most patients can suppress their tics voluntarily for minutes to hours.[44,45] Also numerous factors such as stress, concentration, and relaxation can impact tic frequency and severity. The use of regular videotaped assessments in conjunction with standardized rating scales (Yale Global Tic Severity Scale) is helpful in objectively evaluating symptoms, side effects, and overall drug response.[44–46]

❻ Individuals with Tourette's disorder are particularly sensitive to medication side effects, so medication dosing must be individualized with low starting doses and careful weekly titration to response, realizing that it can take 1 to 2 months for an adequate therapeutic trial. Children taking any dopamine-blocking medication should receive monitoring every 3 to 6 months for extrapyramidal effects with a standardized rating scale (e.g., Abnormal Involuntary Movement Scale [AIMS]).[33–35] Patients given pimozide or ziprasidone should receive baseline and followup electrocardiograms.[45,46] Additional monitoring recommendations for individuals receiving atypical antipsychotics include height, weight, body mass index (BMI), level of sedation, appetite, exercise habits, blood pressure, pulse, glucose, and lipids monthly for 3 months and every 3 months, thereafter. Morning prolactin and TSH are recommended annually or if clinical signs and symptoms warrant assessment.[35] Adult patients with Tourette's disorder still can be responsive to drug treatments that were effective during childhood, although the dose and schedule can require adjustment.[44–46]

CONCLUSION

Haloperidol, pimozide, and risperidone have the advantage of greatest efficacy and rapid onset in the treatment of Tourette's disorder. Ziprasidone, olanzapine, quetiapine, and aripiprazole show promise; however, comparison studies with haloperidol, pimozide, or risperidone are needed to determine their relative safety and efficacy. Clonidine and guanfacine have the advantage of no extrapyramidal side effects, but they are significantly less effective and require ongoing cardiovascular monitoring. Drug treatment must be highly individualized, considering comorbid disorders, side-effect sensitivity, and drug interactions.

ENURESIS

ETIOLOGY, PATHOPHYSIOLOGY, AND CLINICAL PRESENTATION

The essential feature of enuresis is repeated involuntary or intentional voiding of urine by day or night that is not caused by a general medical condition.[1] Medical causes of inappropriate voiding (e.g., diabetes mellitus, diabetes insipidus, seizure disorders, or urinary tract infections) should be ruled out. Enuresis can be primary or secondary. Primary enuresis, the most common type, is diagnosed if the child has never established urinary continence. Secondary enuresis follows an established period (3 to 6 months) of urinary continence.

Enuresis occurs in 12% to 25 % of 4 year olds, 7% to 10% of 8 year olds, and 2% to 3% of 12 year olds with 1% to 3% continuing to experience enuresis in late teenage years.[63] After age 5 years, there is a 15% annual rate of spontaneous remission. The ratio of males to females with enuresis is 2:1.[63] Factors that predispose a child to either type of enuresis include a positive family history, institutionalization, low socioeconomic status, reduced functional bladder capacity, delayed or lax toilet training, constipation, psychologic factors, and developmental delay.[63] Some children with nocturnal enuresis lack the normal circadian variation in urine excretion rate, urine osmolality, and antidiuretic hormone (ADH) secretion. Nocturnal enuresis is not associated with a particular sleep stage, although children with enuresis can be more difficult to arouse.[63]

CLINICAL PRESENTATION OF ENURESIS

General

- Patients are 5 years old or older

Symptoms

- Repeatedly voids urine into bed and/or clothes involuntarily or intentionally.
- There is either a frequency of twice weekly for at least 3 consecutive months or the presence of clinically significant distress or impairment in social, academic (occupational), or other area of functioning.

Data from American Psychiatric Association[1] with permission.

TREATMENT

Enuresis

The first step in treating a child with enuresis is to educate the family about the high frequency of the problem, dispel any misconceptions, provide emotional support, and strongly discourage punishment.

❼ Teaching continence skills and various behavioral and conditioning methods remain the primary treatments for enuresis, and drug treatment remains a secondary approach.[63–65] Simple behavioral and physical interventions such as rewarding dry nights, or lifting and waking are often used initially to control nocturnal enuresis and have been shown to work better than no treatment in reducing wet nights without any side effects or safety concerns.[63–65] Complex interventions, such as dry-bed training and full-spectrum home training, in combination with bedwetting alarms can be tried but require time and effort. There is insufficient evidence to support complex interventions without an alarm. After 3 to 4 months of using a bed-wetting alarm, enuresis is cured in two-thirds of children.[63–65]

Alarms are more effective than pharmacotherapy with longer lasting results, although medications work faster, within 2 weeks. Combining medications and alarms has been tried with mixed results.[63–65] Desmopressin tablets are preferred to tricyclic antidepressants (e.g., imipramine) because of lower toxicity risk.[66,67] Oxybutynin or tolterodine may be effective adjuncts to desmopressin in partial responders.[66–69]

■ DESMOPRESSIN

❽ Desmopressin acetate, a synthetic analog of the natural human ADH arginine vasopressin, is currently available in a nasal spray, which is no longer recommended, and a more widely used oral tablet for the treatment of nocturnal enuresis.[63] A rapid dissolve tablet is under study.[70] Desmopressin increases overnight urinary osmotic concentration by increasing water reabsorption and reducing the volume of urine entering the bladder.[67,68] Desmopressin is effective in reducing the number of wet nights in 10% to 65% of children in 1 to 2 weeks, however, up to 80% relapse on discontinuation.[63,66]

In a 6-month, randomized, controlled trial comparing desmopressin (200–400 mcg), imipramine (25 mg), and combination desmopressin (200 mcg) and oxybutynin (5 mg) in 145 enuretic children, (mean age 7.8 years), the combination produced the most rapid results, although the number of wet nights per month at 6 months was similar in the combination desmopressin/oxybutynin group (3.7 ± 5.4) compared to the desmopressin monotherapy group (4.0 ± 4.6). Both treatments were superior to imipramine (9.3 ± 8.3). The mean number of wet nights during the 2-week baseline period in all groups was 13. Tolerability was superior in the desmopressin groups compared to the imipramine group.[68]

Intranasal desmopressin should not be used due to an unacceptable risk of hyponatremia that may cause seizures. Only the tablet form is FDA approved for primary nocturnal enuresis. For children 6 years of age or older, desmopressin tablet can be initiated at 200 mcg at bedtime. Approximately 1% of oral desmopressin is absorbed. Plasma concentrations reach a maximum approximately 45 minutes after administration. Effective dosages range from 200–600 mcg/day of oral desmopressin. The duration of action varies from 10–20 hours, and there is compensatory polyuria the following day when the drug wears off.[63,66]

■ TRICYCLIC ANTIDEPRESSANTS

❽ Imipramine is the most studied TCA, although desipramine, amitriptyline, and nortriptyline are also effective. Imipramine is effective 40% to 60% of the time.[63,71] The mechanism of action of TCAs in treating enuresis is unknown.[63] For children 6 years of age and older, the usual starting dose is 25 mg given 30 minutes before bedtime. Doses can be increased by 25 mg weekly until response is achieved. The usual effective dosing range is 1 to 2.5 mg/kg/night, and doses should not exceed 2.5 mg/kg/night. Most children respond within the first week.[63]

■ ADVERSE EFFECTS

Desmopressin tablets can cause transient headache, chills, dizziness, nausea, and abdominal pain. Rarely, water intoxication, hyponatremia, and subsequent tonic-clonic seizures have been reported.[66] From 1972 to 2005, there were 151 post-marketing reports of hyponatremia in children with nocturnal enuresis, of whom 145 were treated with intranasal desmopressin and 6 received tablets. When desmopressin is administered, evening fluids should be restricted one hour before and for 8 hours after drug administration. Desmopressin tablets should be stopped during acute illnesses that may lead to fluid or electrolyte imbalance. Prompt medical assessment is needed if headache, nausea, or vomiting develops, as these could be signs of hyponatremia. Concomitant medications that may lower sodium (e.g., antidepressants, oxcarbazepine) or illnesses that change hydration status (e.g., the flu) can increase the risk of hyponatremia.[63,66]

TCA adverse effects are dose related and include sedation, dizziness, dry mouth, constipation, weight gain, and the risk of electrocardiographic changes, heart block, and lowering of the seizure threshold.[36]

PHARMACOECONOMIC CONSIDERATIONS

No pharmacoeconomic studies on enuresis are available. The use of a bed-wetting alarm provides the highest overall cure rate, and drugs are a secondary approach. Several types of reusable bed-wetting alarms are available, ranging from $15 to $170 per alarm, compared to $80 to $100 for a 30-day supply of desmopressin.[63,66,72] However, insurance companies commonly reimburse drug therapy, whereas most do not reimburse for alarms. The most inexpensive drug therapy is low-dose TCA; however, electrocardiographic monitoring increases overall costs.[71] Therapy with desmopressin is substantially more expensive than with TCAs because of higher drug cost.

EVALUATION OF THERAPEUTIC OUTCOMES

Before treatment begins, an accurate baseline of bed-wetting frequency must be established. A 50% or greater increase in dry nights is considered a therapeutic response. For example, if baseline dry nights are 2 out of 7 days per week, and drug treatment results in 4 or more dry nights per week, the drug is considered effective. If only one more dry night per week occurs and the drug is at the low end of the dosing range, a dosage increase is needed.[63,66,67]

At least 1 week is needed to evaluate the efficacy of TCAs, and 2 weeks can be needed for evaluation of desmopressin. If drug treatment is ongoing for several months, particularly if enuresis has resolved, attempts to discontinue the drug every 3 to 6 months are recommended to assess for spontaneous remission. Slow tapering of the medication can decrease the frequency of relapse. Unfortunately, therapeutic drug efficacy does not extend beyond drug discontinuation.[63,66,71] Drug plasma level monitoring is not established for desmopressin; and plasma level monitoring for imipramine is inconclusive, and should be recommended only for children who do not respond or poorly tolerate a dose of 2.5 mg/kg/day.[63]

CONCLUSION

Initially, simple interventions such as lift and awaken can be implemented. A bedwetting alarm in combination with complex behavioral interventions provide lasting cures for two-thirds of children. Drug therapy has the advantage of more rapid results, but relapse is high on drug discontinuation.[63,64,66] Desmopressin tablets are preferred over imipramine because of better tolerability and safety.[66,67]

ABBREVIATIONS

ADH: antidiuretic hormone

ADHD: attention-deficit/hyperactivity disorder

AIMS: abnormal involuntary movement scale

BMI: body mass index

CNS: central nervous system

DA: dopamine

DAT1: dopamine transporter protein

D_1, D_2, D_4: dopamine receptors

GABA: γ-Aminobutyric acid

5-HT_2: 5-hydroxytryptamine 2 (serotonin)

MAO: monoamine oxidase

MAOI: monoamine oxidase inhibitor

NE: norepinephrine

SSRI: selective serotonin reuptake inhibitor

TCA: tricyclic antidepressant

REFERENCES

1. American Psychiatric Association. Diagnostic and Statistical Manual of Mental Disorders, 4th ed., Text Revision. Washington, DC: American Psychiatric Press, 2000:39–134.
2. Barkley RA. Major life activity and health outcomes associated with attention-deficit/hyperactivity disorder. J Clin Psychiatry 2002;63(Suppl 12):10–15.
3. Spencer TJ. ADHD and comorbidity in childhood. J Clin Psychiatry 2006;67(Suppl 8):27–31.
4. American Academy of Pediatrics. Clinical practice guideline: Diagnosis and evaluation of the child with attention-deficit/hyperactivity disorder. Pediatrics 2000;105:1158–1170.
5. Prince JB. Pharmacotherapy of ADHD in youth: Update on new stimulant preparations, atomoxetine, novel treatments. Child Adolesc Psychiatr Clin N Am 2006;15:13–50.
6. Biederman J. ADHD: A selective overview. Biol Psychiatry 2005;57:1215–1220.
7. Pliszka SR, Crismon ML, Hughes CW, et al. The Texas children's medication algorithm project: Revision of the algorithm for pharmacotherapy of childhood attention-deficit/hyperactivity disorder. J Am Acad Child Adolesc Psychiatry 2006;45(6):642–657.
8. Weiss MD, Weiss JR. A guide to the treatment of adults with ADHD. J Clin Psychiatry 2004;65(Suppl 3):27–37.
9. Dopheide JA. ASHP therapeutic position statement on the appropriate use of medications in the treatment of ADHD in pediatric patients. Am J Health Syst Pharm 2005;62:1502–1509.
10. Mosholder AD. Use of Drugs for ADHD medications in the United States. 2006, *http://www.fda.gov/ohrms/dockets/ac/06/slides/2006–4210s-index.htm.*
11. Asherson P, Kuntsi J, Taylor E. Unraveling the complexity of ADHD. A behavioural genomic approach. Br J Psychiatry 2005;187:103–105.
12. Castellanos FX, Sharp WS, Gottesman RF, et al. Anatomic brain abnormalities in monozygotic twins discordant for attention deficit hyperactivity disorder. Am J Psychol 2003;160:1693–1696.
13. Wilens TE. Mechanism of agents used for ADHD. J Clin Psychiatry 2006;67(Suppl 8):32–37.
14. Gilbert DL, Wang Z, Sallee FR, et al. Dopamine transporter genotype influences physiologic response to medication in ADHD. Brain 2006;129:2038–2046.
15. National Institutes of Mental Health. Multimodal Treatment Study of ADHD follow-up: 24-Month outcomes of treatment strategies for ADHD. Pediatrics 2004;113(4):754–761.
16. Greenhill LL, Pliszka S, Dulcan MK, et al. Practice parameter for the use of stimulant medications in the treatment of children, adolescents, and adults. J Am Acad Child Adolesc Psychiatry 2002;41(Suppl 2):26S–49S.
17. American Academy of Pediatrics. Clinical practice guideline: Treatment of the school-aged child with ADHD. Pediatrics 2001;108:1033–1044.
18. Pelham WE, Burrows-MacLean L, Gnagy EM, et al. Transdermal methylphenidate, behavioral, and combined treatment for children with ADHD. Exp Clin Psychopharmacol 2005;13(2):111–126.
19. Lopez FA. ADHD: New pharmacological treatments on the horizon. Behavioral and Developmental Pediatrics 2006;27(5):410–416.
20. Anderson VR, Scott LJ. Methylphenidate transdermal system for ADHD in children. Drugs 2006;66(8):1117–1122.
21. Correll CU, Carlson HE. Endocrine and metabolic adverse effects of psychotropic medications in children and adolescents. J Am Acad Child Adolesc Psychiatry 2006;45(7):771–791.
22. Biederman J, Mick E, Surman C, et al. A randomized, placebo-controlled trial of OROS methylphenidate in adults with ADHD. Biol Psychiatry 2006;59:829–835.
23. Biederman J, Krishnan S, Zhang Y, et al. Efficacy and tolerability of lisdexamphetamine in children with ADHD: A phase III multicenter, randomized double-blind forced-dose, parallell-group study. Clin Ther 2007;29:450–463.
24. Cardiovascular and psychiatric risk with drug treatments for ADHD. 2006, *http://www.fda.gov/ohrms/dockets/ac/06/slides/2006–4210s-index.htm.*
25. Wilens TE, Prince JB, Spencer TJ, Biederman J. Stimulants and sudden death: What is a physician to do? Pediatrics 2006;118(3):1215–1219.
26. National Institutes of Mental Health. Multimodal treatment study of ADHD follow-up: Changes in effectiveness and growth at the end of treatment. Pediatrics 2004;113(4):762–769.
27. Poulton A. Growth on stimulant medication. Arch Dis Child 2005;90:801–806.
28. Wilens TE, Faraone SV, Biederman J, et al. Does stimulant therapy of attention-deficit/hyperactivity disorder beget later substance abuse? A meta-analytic review of the literature. Pediatrics 2003;111:179–185.
29. Upadhyaya HP, Rose K, O'Rourke K, et al. ADHD, medication treatment, and substance use patterns among adolescents and young adults. J Child Adolesc Psychopharmacol 2005;15(5):799–809.
30. Caballerro J, Nahata MC. Atomoxetine hydrochloride for the treatment of ADHD. Clin Ther 2003;25:3065–3083.
31. Scahill L, Chappell PB, Kim Young S, et al. A placebo-controlled study of guanfacine in the treatment of children with tic disorders and attention deficit hyperactivity disorder. Am J Psychol 2001;158:1067–1074.
32. Kowatch RA, DelBello MP. Pediatric bipolar disorder: Emerging diagnostic and treatment approaches. Child Adolesc Psych Clin N Am 2006;15:73–108.
33. Schur SB, Sikich L, Fingling RL, et al. Treatment recommendations for the use of antipsychotics for aggressive youth (TRAAY) Part 1: A review. J Am Acad Child Adolesc Psychiatry 2003;42:132–144.
34. Pappadopulos E, Macintyre J, Crismon ML, et al. Treatment recommendations for the use of antipsychotics for aggressive youth (TRAAY) Part 2. J Am Acad Child Adolesc Psychiatry 2003;42:145–161.

35. Correll CU, Penzner JB, Parikh UH, et al. Recognizing and monitoring adverse events of second-generation antipsychotics in children and adolescents. Child Adolesc Psychiatr Clin N Am 2006;15:177–206.
36. Dopheide JA. Recognizing and treating depression in children and adolescents. Am J Health Syst Pharm 2006;63:233–243.
37. Tan M, Appleton R. ADHD, methylphenidate, and epilepsy. Arch Dis Child 2005;90:57–59.
38. Swanson JM, Greenhill LL, Lopez FA, et al. Modafinil film-coated tablets in children and adolescents with ADHD. Results of a randomized, double-blind, placebo-controlled, fixed-dose study followed by abrupt discontinuation. J Clin Psychiatry 2006;67:137–147.
39. Hazell PL, Stuart JE. A randomized controlled trial of clonidine added to psychostimulant medication for hyperactive and aggressive children. J Am Acad Child Adolesc Psychiatry 2003;42:886–894.
40. Klein-Schwartz W. Trends and toxic effects from pediatric clonidine exposures. Arch Pediatr Adolesc Med 2002;156:392–396.
41. Leibson CL, Katusic SK, Barbaresi WJ, et al. Use and costs of medical care for children and adolescents with and without ADHD. JAMA 2001;285:60–66.
42. Kemner JE, Lage MJ. Effect of methylphenidate formulation on treatment patterns and use of emergency room services. Am J Health Syst Pharm 2006;63:317–322.
43. Collett BR, Ohan JL, Myers KM. Ten-year review of rating scales: Scales assessing attention-deficit/hyperactivity disorder. J Am Acad Child Adolesc Psychiatry 2003;42:1015–1037.
44. Jankovic J. Medical progress: Tourette's syndrome. N Engl J Med 2001;345:1184–1192.
45. Muller-Vahl JT. The treatment of Tourette's syndrome: Current opinions. Expert Opin Pharmacother 2002;3:899–914.
46. Jimenez-Jimenez FJ. Pharmacological options for the treatment of Tourette's disorder. Drugs 2001;61:2207–2200.
47. Dion Y, Annable L, Sandor P, et al. Risperidone in the treatment of Tourette syndrome: A double-blind, placebo-controlled trial. J Clin Psychopharmacol 2002;22:31–39.
48. Scahill L, Leckman JF, Schultz RT, et al. A placebo-controlled trial of risperidone in Tourette's syndrome. Neurology 2003;60:1130–1135.
49. Gaffney GR, Perry P, Lund BC, et al. Risperidone versus clonidine in the treatment of children and adolescents with Tourette's syndrome. J Am Acad Child Adolesc Psychiatry 2002;41:330–336.
50. Bruggeman R, van der Linden, Buitelaar JK, et al. Risperidone versus pimozide in Tourette's disorder: A double-blind parallel-group study. J Clin Psychiatry 2001;62:50–56.
51. Sallee FR, Kurlan R, Goetz CG, et al. Ziprasidone treatment of children and adolescents with Tourette's syndrome. J Am Acad Child Adolesc Psychiatry 2000;39:292–299.
52. Sallee FR, Gilbert DL, Vinks AA, et al. Pharmacodynamics of ziprasidone in children and adolescents: Impact on dopamine transmission. J Am Acad Child Adolesc Psychiatry 2003;42:902–907.
53. Budman CL, Gayer A, Lesser M, et al. An open label study of the treatment efficacy of olanzapine for Tourette's disorder. J Clin Psychiatry 2001;62:290–294.
54. Mukaddes NM, Abai O. Quetiapine treatment of children and adolescents with Tourette's disorder. J Child Adolesc Psychopharmacol 2003;13:295–299.
55. Gadow KD, Sverd J. ADHD, chronic tic disorder and methylphenidate. Adv Neurol 2006;99:197–207.
56. Kurlan R and the Tourette's Syndrome Study Group. Treatment of ADHD in children with ties: A randomized controlled trial. Neurology 2002;58:527–536.
57. Spencer T, Biederman J, Coffey B, et al. A double-blind comparison of desipramine and placebo in youth with chronic tic disorder and comorbid ADHD. Arch Gen Psychiatry 2002;59:649–656.
58. Nicolson R, Craven-Thuss MA, Smith J, et al. A randomized, placebo controlled trial of metoclopramide for Tourette's disorder. J Am Acad Child Adolesc Psychiatry 2005;44(7):640–46.
59. Toren P, Weizman A, Ratner S, et al. Ondansetron treatment in Tourette's disorder: A 3-week, randomized, double-blind, placebo-controlled study. J Clin Psychiatry 2005;66:499–503.
60. Silver AA, Shytle D, Philipp MK. Transdermal nicotine and haloperidol in Tourette's disorder: A double-blind placebo-controlled study. J Clin Psychiatry 2001;62:707–714.
61. Wilhelm S, Deckersbach T, Coffey BJ, et al. Habit reversal versus supportive psychotherapy for Tourette's disorder: A randomized controlled trial. Am J Psychiatry 2003;160:1175–1177.
62. Silva RR, Munoz DM, Daniel W, et al. Causes of haloperidol discontinuation in patients with Tourette's disorder: Management and alternatives. J Clin Psychiatry 1996;57:129–135.
63. Fritz G, Rockney R, American Academy of Child and Adolescent Psychiatry Work Group. Practice parameter for the assessment and treatment of children and adolescents with enuresis. J Am Acad Child Adolesc Psychiatry 2004;43(12)1540–1550.
64. Glazener CMA, Evans JHC, Peto RE. Alarm interventions for nocturnal enuresis in children. Cochrane Database Syst Rev 2005;2:CD002911.
65. Glazener CM, Evans JH. Simple behavioral and physical interventions for nocturnal enuresis in children. Cochrane Database Syst Rev 2005;2:CD002561.
66. Glazener CM, Evans JH. Desmopressin for nocturnal enuresis in children. Cochrane Database Syst Rev 2004;3:CD002112.
67. Del Gado R, Donatella DG, Cennamo M, et al. Desmopressin is a safe drug for the treatment of enuresis. Scand J Urol Nephrol 2005;39:308–312.
68. Lee T, Suh HJ, Lee HJ, Lee JE. Comparison of effects of treatment of primary nocturnal enuresis with oxybutynin plus desmopressin alone or imipramine alone: A randomized controlled clinical trial. J Urol 2005;174:1084–1087.
69. Yucel S, Akkaya E, Guntekin E, et al. Should we switch over to tolterodine in every child with incontinence in whom oxybutynin failed? J Urol 2005;65:369–373.
70. Vande Walle JGJ, Bogaert GA, Mattsson S, et al. A new fast-melting oral formulation of desmopressin: A pharmacodynamic study in children with primary nocturnal enuresis. Br J Urol 2006;97:603–609.
71. Glazener CM, Evans JH. Tricyclic and related drugs for nocturnal enuresis in children. Cochrane Database Syst Rev 2003;3:CD002117.
72. Bedwetting alarm prices. 2006, *www.bedwettingstore.com* and *www.drisleeper.com*.

CHAPTER 66 Eating Disorders

STEVEN C. STONER

KEY CONCEPTS

1. The causes of eating disorders are complex, so ongoing multidisciplinary treatment is needed to ensure a positive outcome. Although outpatient treatment is appropriate for the majority of patients, it is important to recognize the factors that indicate a need for inpatient treatment.
2. Careful medical and psychiatric assessments are needed at baseline to determine the severity of illness and comorbid conditions.
3. Nonpharmacologic treatments such as cognitive behavioral therapy, nutritional counseling, family therapy, and interpersonal psychotherapy are the cornerstone of management of anorexia nervosa (AN).
4. In patients with AN, one goal is to achieve and maintain a body weight within 85% of the normal weight for age and height. If the patient is malnourished, oral refeeding with the daily caloric intake starting at 1,000 to 1,600 cal/day and slowly titrating to 2,000 to 3,000 cal/day is preferred. Parenteral refeeding is a treatment of last resort.
5. Antidepressants are considered to be ineffective for the core symptoms of AN and are reserved for patients with mood, anxiety, and obsessional symptoms that persist after weight has improved.
6. Antidepressants can improve both mood and specific target symptoms in bulimia nervosa (BN), but they remain adjunctive to nonpharmacologic treatments.
7. Selective serotonin reuptake inhibitors are first-line agents when medications are indicated for BN. Compared to other antidepressant classes, they are preferred because of improved tolerability and safety, although superior efficacy has not been shown. The dose of fluoxetine in BN is higher (60 mg/day) than the dose usually used in depression.
8. An adequate drug therapy trial in BN is 4 to 8 weeks. If drug treatment fails, consider that the patient might be vomiting or using other purging methods impacting the absorption of the drug.
9. The optimal duration of antidepressant treatment for BN is unknown, but most clinicians continue them for 9 to 12 months in patients who respond and then reevaluate the need for ongoing medication management. The long-term course is variable, but there is the potential for a fatal outcome from cardiac arrest or suicide.
10. Monitoring of patients with BN should include frequency and severity of binge/purge episodes, exercise patterns, use of laxatives or ipecac, mood and anxiety symptoms, eating habits, daily caloric intake, weight, and changes in laboratory abnormalities.

Learning objectives, review questions, and other resources can be found at **www.pharmacotherapyonline.com.**

The eating disorders encompass several complex diseases that share a central pathologic feature of overevaluation of body shape and weight. Eating disorders arise from the interaction between environmental, societal, developmental, psychosocial, genetic, and biologic factors. It is estimated that 5 to 10 million women and 1 million men in the United States have an eating disorder. The urbanization of society, social pressure, and obsession with perfection and being thin have led to an increasing prevalence of eating disorders, with the peak onset being between 16 and 20 years of age.[1–4] AN, BN, and eating disorders not otherwise specified (EDNOS) are the primary disorders that have been identified.[5–9]

Despite an improved understanding of these disabling and potentially fatal disorders, management remains difficult, and pharmacologic intervention is a small part of a comprehensive plan that emphasizes cognitive behavioral therapy and psychotherapy.

EPIDEMIOLOGY

ANOREXIA NERVOSA

AN occurs predominantly in females (90%) and usually presents in late adolescence (median onset 17 years of age) with new cases rarely diagnosed after age 40 years. The estimated prevalence of AN in the general population is 0.3% of females; however, a subthreshold level of symptoms are estimated to affect 0.37% to 1.3% of the population.[2,10–12] Longitudinal management of AN is difficult, even in cases where weight restoration is achieved. Rates of relapse requiring hospitalization within 1 year are estimated to exceed 30%.[13]

The promotion of the virtues of being thin through common electronic media, such as the Internet, is also a potentially negative environmental factor. Many websites inappropriately promote healthy lifestyle aspects of AN and being thin as a means of being in control, successful, and coping with life's pressures.[14]

BULIMIA NERVOSA

BN also occurs predominantly in females (90%) and usually presents in adolescence or early adult life.[5] Between 1% and 4.6% of adolescent and young adult females meet the diagnostic criteria for BN.[3,10,15,16]

EATING DISORDER NOT OTHERWISE SPECIFIED

EDNOS is also described in the American Psychiatric Association's *Diagnostic and Statistical Manual of Mental Disorders,* 4th Edition, Text Revision (DSM-IV-TR).[3,15] Its prevalence is estimated at 1% to 4.7% of the population, with up to 50% of eating disorder patients admitted to tertiary care settings having this condition.[10,17] These individuals present with symptoms characteristic of eating disorders but do not meet specific diagnostic criteria. Two examples of EDNOS are night eating syndrome (NES) and binge eating disorder (BED).

NES is most common in obesity clinic populations, often accompanied by depressive symptoms. The syndrome is defined by early morning anorexia, hyperphagia in the evening, nighttime insomnia, and subsequent early morning awakening with nighttime ingestion of food.[9,18,19] NES impacts an estimated 1.5% of the general population, ranging from 8.9% to 27% in obesity clinics.[20–22] Patients with NES are reported to benefit from antidepressant therapy, most notably sertraline 50 mg to 200 mg daily.[9]

BINGE EATING DISORDER

BED continues to be classified as a research diagnosis. The diagnostic criteria for BED describe recurrent episodes of binge eating without compensatory behaviors (e.g., purging, excessive exercise, or fasting). BED typically presents later in life (older than 40 years of age), and approximately one-fourth of BED patients are male.[17,23]

ETIOLOGY AND PATHOPHYSIOLOGY

❶ The potential etiologic or exacerbating factors for eating disorders represent an array of physiologic, biochemical, developmental, genetic, psychosocial, and psychiatric phenomena. The biologic basis for eating disorders is difficult to delineate because it is unclear if the biologic changes are caused by or are a result of the aberrant eating behavior.

Abnormalities of the hypothalamic-pituitary-gonadal, hypothalamic-pituitary-adrenal, and hypothalamic-pituitary-thyroid axes are described as potential causes of AN. Amenorrhea is found in the majority of females with AN, providing support to the association with gonadotropin.[16] However, symptoms related to these abnormalities do not always correct with weight normalization, suggesting a primary biologic abnormality.[23]

The roles of serotonin, norepinephrine, and dopamine have been studied extensively, as these neurotransmitters have important functions in controlling eating behaviors. Dysfunctions in these systems are thought to be secondary to weight loss. Some aspects of serotonin function do remain abnormal after weight restoration, suggesting that other mechanisms are involved.[24,25] Another molecular genetic target of study is brain-derived neurotrophic factor (BDNF), which is also being studied in disease states such as depression.[26]

Strong genetic influences are present in AN and likely play a role in both BN and BED, independent of the presence of obesity.[27] Twin studies have shown concordance of approximately 55% and 35% in monozygotic twins and 5% and 30% in dizygotic twins for AN and BN, respectively. Genetic mutation studies have focused on polymorphisms of the serotonin 2A receptor, with mixed preliminary results.[23]

Emphasis is also placed on social stress and psychological and developmental issues related to dysfunctional family relationships triggering abnormal eating behavior.[3,16,17,28] Athletes are also at risk for eating disorders, especially female gymnasts, ballet dancers, figure skaters, distance runners, swimmers, male wrestlers, and body builders.[29]

DIAGNOSTIC CRITERIA AND CLINICAL PRESENTATION

❷ AN and BN occur together in approximately 30% to 64% of patients with eating disorders, and may not be distinct diagnostic entities, but rather a continuum of symptoms.[30-32] Many patients initially present with either AN or BN and alternate from one to the other. Figure 66–1 demonstrates similar and unique features of AN and BN.

The use of purging methods is not limited to just BN. Self-induced vomiting is the most common form of purging behavior.[33] Laxative abuse is another form common in both AN and BN, used by an estimated 3% to 70% of patients.[33–35] Although ineffective as a weight-loss strategy, laxative abuse is often used in combination with other behaviors including exercise, diuretics, enemas, and saunas. Within the diagnostic framework of AN, laxative abuse is most common in those identified with the purging subtype.[33] Psychiatric symptoms of depression, anxiety, and borderline personality disorder are also reported in those who abuse laxatives.[33–35]

Depression, schizophrenia, obsessive-compulsive disorder (OCD), and conversion disorders should be included in the differential

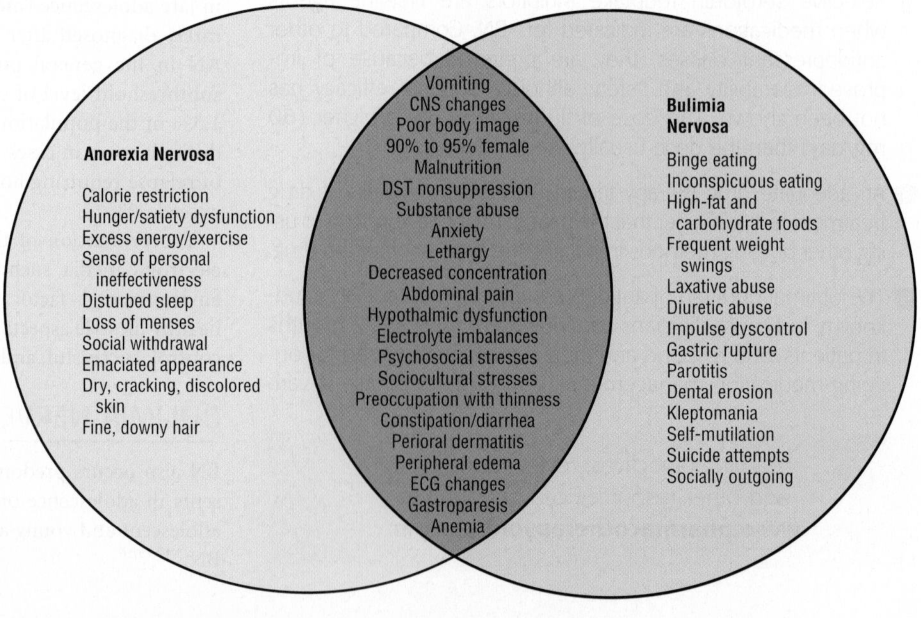

FIGURE 66-1. Signs and symptoms of anorexia nervosa and bulimia nervosa. (DST, dexamethasone suppression test; ECG, electrocardiogram.)

diagnosis of AN and BN because eating abnormalities can be a component of these illnesses. The salient difference is the overriding drive for thinness, disturbed body image, increased energy directed at losing weight, and binge eating episodes which are relatively specific for eating disorders. Most eating disorder patients experience relief of psychiatric symptoms on refeeding.[17]

ANOREXIA NERVOSA

The core features of AN include refusal to maintain a minimal normal body weight (e.g., greater than 85% normal body weight or body mass index greater than 17.5 kg/m^2) or failure to make expected weight gains, intense fear and obsession about weight gain or being "fat," distorted body image, and amenorrhea for at least three consecutive cycles. Patients typically lack an appreciation for the degree of weight loss experienced or are preoccupied with the idea that a part of their body is too large, despite evidence to the contrary. The DSM-IV-TR further classifies AN into restricting type (failure to engage in binge eating or purging behavior) or binge eating/purging type, in which patients regularly participate in bingeing or purging.[15] The AN patient has difficulty sensing when he or she is full (satiety) and commonly complains of feeling bloated after they start eating. Patients also describe not feeling in control of various aspects of their life, particularly caloric intake. AN patients often present with features of major depression, but these symptoms should initially be considered to be secondary to starvation and not a true mood disorder.

CLINICAL PRESENTATION OF ANOREXIA NERVOSA

General

- Patients refuse to maintain body weight and have distorted perceptions about their body.

Symptoms

- Patients have obsessions and fears about eating and gaining weight.
- They complain about feeling full even when they have eaten very little food.
- Denial of symptoms and low self-esteem is the norm. They often feel ineffective and have a lack of self-control.

Signs

- Weakness, lethargy, cachexia, amenorrhea, vomiting, restricted food intake, inappropriate exercise, delayed sexual development, edema, delayed gastric emptying, constipation, bradycardia, hypotension, osteoporosis, dry cracking skin, lanugo, callus on dorsum of hand, perioral dermatitis, and erosion of dental enamel.

Laboratory Abnormalities

- Hypokalemia, hypokalemic alkalosis, hypomagnesemia, leukopenia, QT interval prolongation, ST-segment depression, U waves, hypercholesterolemia, and anemia.

Other Diagnostic Tests

- Nonspecific electroencephalograph (EEG) changes

Psychiatric comorbidity is common, as up to 75% of patients have a primary mood disorder.[36] There is also a link between AN and anxiety disorders, especially social phobia and OCD. The lifetime prevalence of OCD in patients with AN is reported to be as high as 25%, higher than the lifetime prevalence in the general population (2.5%).[36,37] Avoidant and obsessive-compulsive personality disorders are also common in patients with AN.[38,39]

CLINICAL PRESENTATION OF BULIMIA NERVOSA

General

- Patients binge eat and stop when they have abdominal pain or self-induced vomiting or are interrupted by another individual.
- They have a pattern of severe dieting followed by binge-eating episodes.
- They are concerned about their body image but do not have the drive to thinness that is characteristic of AN.

Symptoms

- Patients do not eat regular meals and do not feel satiety at the end of a meal.
- They might use laxatives for weight control.
- They have guilt, depression, and self-disparagement after binges.
- Social isolation can result from frequent bingeing.
- Chaotic and troubled personal relationships and substance abuse are common.

Signs

- Bingeing, vomiting, salivary gland inflammation, erosion of dental enamel, callus on dorsum of hand, perioral dermatitis, dental caries, parotid gland enlargement, abdominal pain, upper end of normal body weight or slightly overweight, frequent weight fluctuations, and diminished masticatory ability.

Laboratory Abnormalities

- Hypokalemia, hypochloremic metabolic acidosis, elevated serum amylase

Other Diagnostic Tests

- None

BULIMIA NERVOSA

The core feature of BN is recurrent episodes of binge eating (an excessive intake of calorie-laden food over a short period of time). Persons with BN are overly sensitive about their weight and have a distorted body image. Most have normal weight, although they might fluctuate between being underweight and overweight. Patients lack control over their eating and participate in recurrent compensatory behavior to prevent weight gain. This can include self-induced vomiting; misuse of laxatives, diuretics, enemas, or other medications; strict dieting or fasting; or excessive exercise. To meet DSM-IV-TR criteria, the binges and compensatory behaviors must occur on average at least twice weekly for 3 months. BN can further be differentiated by purging type (regularly engages in self-induced vomiting or the misuse of laxatives, diuretics, or enemas) or non-purging type (uses other inappropriate compensatory behaviors, such as fasting or excessive exercise, but doesn't engage in purging activities).[15]

Patients typically binge and vomit at least once daily. Caloric intake varies, but patients can consume between 5,000 and 20,000 calories during a single binge. Patients tend to consume foods that are easy to ingest, do not require much chewing or preparation, and are high in carbohydrates or fat. Binge eating is typically secretive and precipitated by a stressful event, followed by post-binge remorse. Binges typically last less than 2 hours but can last for more than 8 hours. To compensate for the excessive caloric intake, many patients fast for prolonged periods, exercise compulsively, purge, or abuse laxatives.

Psychiatric comorbidity includes depression (up to 80%), poor impulse-control, and substance abuse. Approximately 30% to 37% of bulimic patients have a personal history of substance abuse.[40] Kleptomania and borderline and avoidant personality disorders are also frequently observed.[38,39] Patients also commonly steal comfort items such as laxatives, candies, and clothes.[16]

BINGE EATING DISORDER

Patients with binge eating disorder present with recurrent episodes of binging without the compensatory behaviors associated with AN or BN. It is estimated that 5% to 10% of patients seeking treatment for obesity have BED. Comorbid depressive disorder is common, although the self-deprecating focus on body image is less severe than in AN or BN.[21,37] Diagnostic criteria require that episodes of binging occur at least twice per week over a period of 6 months.[15]

MEDICAL COMPLICATIONS OF EATING DISORDERS

The potential medical complications that exist with the presence of eating disorders involve multiple organ systems. The type of medical complication encountered has been shown to be dependent on the type and frequency of the eating disorder behavior. Cardiac complications are of concern and can include wasted cardiac muscle, orthostatic hypotension, decreased cardiac output, arrhythmia, and QTc interval prolongation.[41] During caloric restoration there is a risk for developing a potentially fatal collapse of the cardiovascular system known as *refeeding syndrome*. This risk is reduced by the gradual versus rapid reintroduction of calories.

Metabolic (metabolic acidosis or alkalosis) and electrolyte disturbances (e.g., hypokalemia, hypomagnesemia, hypocalcemia) along with dehydration are often seen. Elevations in bicarbonate levels during periods of hypokalemia can be an indication that the patient is inducing vomiting or using dietary weight-loss medications. Non-anion-gap acidosis has also been reported with the abuse of laxative agents. Additionally, both acute and chronic renal failure has been reported.

Gastrointestinal, oropharyngeal, and dental complications are frequent along with general complaints of lethargy and fatigue.

Hormonal changes related to the hypothalamic-pituitary-gonadal axis resulting from starvation are seen. These abnormalities include effects on estradiol, the gonadotropins (e.g., luteinizing hormone, follicle-stimulating hormone, and gonadotropin-releasing hormone), thyroid function, adrenal function, and growth hormone.[16,41] Specific to female athletes is the *female athlete triad*, defined by the development of irregular menses, osteoporosis, and disordered eating.[41,42] Osteopenia, osteoporosis, and infertility are potential long-term complications of suppressed estrogen. The restoration of weight, specifically in AN, reverses the bone loss, although estrogen supplementation does not appear to be effective. In all cases, the preferred method to address these issues is the normalization of nutrition. The impact on female fertility is not well studied, although the ability to carry a pregnancy to term or to give birth to a child of average birth weight appears reduced.

Chronic starvation can contribute to brain atrophy. Decreases in white matter and cerebrospinal fluid volumes return to normal after a healthy weight is achieved, but gray matter loss can continue to persist.[17,43,44] A thorough physical and laboratory evaluation, as described in Table 66–1, is needed to determine the severity of medical complications.[15,28,45]

TABLE 66-1 Physical and Laboratory Assessment of Eating Disorders

Evaluation	Target Symptoms
Pulse	Bradycardia
Blood pressure	Hypotension, orthostasis
Height/weight	Underweight for size and age/body mass index
Respiratory rate	Rapid if heart failure occurs during refeeding
Temperature	Hypothermia, cold intolerance
Electrocardiogram	ST depression, flat T waves, U waves, increased QT interval, atrioventricular block
Gastrointestinal	Hypoactive bowel sounds, gastritis, abdominal distention
Skin	Dry, scaling, lanugo, hair loss, calluses on fingers and hands
Menses	Amenorrhea
Complete blood count	Leukopenia, anemias, thrombocytopenia
Electrolytes	Hypokalemia, hypomagnesemia, hypo- or hyperphosphatemia
pH	Metabolic alkalosis (acidosis if laxative abuse)
Amylase	Elevated, pancreatitis rare
Liver	Hypoalbuminemia, γ-glutamyl transferase if alcohol abuse
Thyroid	Low to low normal, but not true disease
Cortisol	Elevated with lack of suppression on dexamethasone suppression test
Bone density	Osteoporosis

Data from American Psychiatric Association,[15,17] Halmi,[28] and National Collaborating Center for Mental Health.[53]

TREATMENT

Eating Disorders

DESIRED OUTCOMES

The goals for patients with eating disorders are to reduce distorted body image; restore and maintain healthy body weight; establish normal eating patterns; improve psychologic, psychosocial, and physical problems; resolve contributory family problems; enhance compliance; and prevent relapse.[17] Specific to BED is the additional goal of weight loss.

ANOREXIA NERVOSA

The long-term prognosis of AN patients is not clear, as studies focus only on patients receiving treatment. The course of AN most commonly consists of a single episode with subsequent return to normal weight, although patients can still experience issues with disturbed body image, disordered eating, and other psychiatric problems.[17] Some patients experience an unremitting course leading to death, whereas others suffer episodically. It is estimated that less than 50% of AN patients recover, and 20% remain chronically ill despite weight normalization, return of menses, and improved eating behaviors.[46] The prognosis is more favorable with longer followup care and younger age of onset, whereas a poorer prognosis is associated with chronic illness, lower initial weight, poor family relationships, obsessive-compulsive personality symptoms, and the presence of BN or purging behavior.[23,46–48] Long-term followup shows that more than 5% to 10% of AN patients die, most often the result of cardiac arrest or suicide.[15,46]

BULIMIA NERVOSA

The prognosis of BN, although not well studied, appears to be better than AN patients. Patients with milder presenting symptoms who are treated as outpatients tend to do better, whereas patients with electrolyte imbalances, esophagitis, dental caries, and salivary gland enlargement have a more complicated course.[16] A 6-year followup study of patients who received intensive treatment found that 60% had a "good" response.[47] It is important to note that even in cases in which patients respond, they continue to exhibit symptoms that wax and wane. Total absence of symptoms is an uncommon outcome, and residual symptoms predispose the patient to relapse. The actual definition of recovery varies, as once-a-month binge/purge episodes are considered by some to be recovery if their episodes were previously more frequent, whereas others consider a patient recovered only when complete absence of these behaviors occurs.[48]

GENERAL APPROACH TO TREATMENT

An individualized treatment plan is based on the presence and severity of specific core features of the eating disorder and comorbid medical and psychiatric conditions. Psychiatrists, physician assistants, nurses, nutrition specialists, psychologists, and pharmacists play a role in the care of these complex patients. The absence of an adequate support system of family and friends can be cause for failed treatment. A critical first step is to determine the severity of illness, as that drives both the intensity and the setting for delivery of care. Hospitalization is based on the criteria outlined in Table 66–2 and is limited to only the most severely ill patients.[23,28,29] Medications are rarely indicated as a sole treatment for eating disorders, and many refuse medication, although they remain part of the comprehensive treatment strategy.[49–51] Comparative, double-blind, placebo-controlled trials are sparse with most limited by small sample sizes, ambivalent attitudes toward treatment, medical complications, and high dropout rates.[52]

ANOREXIA NERVOSA

Nonpharmacologic Treatments

❸ Evidence supports that nonpharmacologic treatments have the greatest likelihood of eliciting a response in AN patients.[17,49] This includes cognitive behavioral therapy (CBT), behavioral management, interpersonal psychotherapy, nutritional counseling, and family therapy.[17,28,53] Current guidelines suggest at least 6 months of psychotherapy.[53] CBT helps the patient overcome distorted thinking, including self-worth as measured by body image, feelings of being fat despite evidence to the contrary, and denial. CBT also teaches patients how to use strategies besides eating to cope. Interpersonal psychotherapy focuses on interpersonal relationships and functioning, whereas CBT provides positive reinforcement for weight gain.[36] The benefit of treatment based on an addiction model (12-step program) is not supported by the literature.[17,23] Many psychiatric symptoms in an acutely ill patient, such as depression and anxiety, diminish or disappear with weight restoration. Initial treatment is directed toward restoring a healthy weight (greater than 90% of normal weight for age-matched controls) and treating food phobias.[54] After achieving medical stability and appropriate weight, therapy can be redirected toward addressing ongoing interpersonal problems, weight maintenance, cognitive restructuring, and skill development for relapse prevention.[55] Oral refeeding, initially with liquid formulas if necessary, is the most common approach to weight restoration.

❹ In severe cases, nasogastric refeeding is preferred over intravenous bolus dosing.[17] Total parenteral nutrition is reserved only for the management of severely malnourished patients and if other refeeding methods fail. The decision to administer total parenteral nutrition must be made carefully, because of the potentially devastating psychologic effect on patients who do not wish to gain weight. Current clinical evidence suggests a controlled weight gain of 0.9 to 1.4 kg (2–3 lb) per week in inpatient settings and 0.2 to 0.5 kg (0.5–1 lb) per week in outpatient settings.[15,53,56] Recommendations vary; however, it is considered acceptable for patients to begin refeeding at 1,000 to 1,600 calories per day (30–40 cal/kg per day) with slow titration upwards until they begin to demonstrate sustained weight gain.[17,53,56] This can require the intake of an additional 3,500 to 7,000 extra calories per week.[53] Slow refeeding is important to minimize the risk of medical and psychologic consequences.[23]

Pharmacologic Therapy

Antidepressants Although many studies examine the role of antidepressants in the treatment of AN, they often have small sample sizes and large confidence intervals.[57] Antidepressants currently have no role in the acute treatment of AN, unless there is another clinical indication present.[17,23,49]

TABLE 66-2 Criteria for Hospitalization of Patients with Eating Disorders

- Significant weight loss of 20% or more of normal weight, particularly if weight loss has been recent and rapid, severe starvation symptoms are present, or the patient has been ill for more than 2 years
- Reduced oral intake of food (sudden and persistent)
- Medical complications (e.g., edema) and metabolic abnormalities (e.g., hypoproteinemia) from bingeing, purging, and starvation (e.g., heart rate <40 bpm or > 110 bpm, blood pressure <90/60 mm Hg, glucose <60 mg/dL (3.33 mmol/L), potassium <3 mEq/L (3 mmol/L), or inability to maintain core body temperature
- Co-occurring psychiatric symptoms, notably suicidal ideation, psychotic depression, or substance abuse and dependence
- Nonresponsive to outpatient treatment (after 3–4 months) and poor motivation to recover
- Demoralization or nonfunctional family
- Denial of severity of abnormal eating behaviors
- Continuous supervision required to prevent purging (vomiting or laxative abuse)

Data from American Psychiatric Association,[15,17] Fairburn and Harrison,[23] Halmi,[28] Powers,[29] and National Collaborating Center for Mental Health.[53]

❺ Data suggest that medication is ineffective if a patient weighs less than 85% of their expected weight, thus antidepressants should be initiated only if depression, anxiety, obsessions, or compulsions persist after the target weight is achieved.[23,54,58] The duration of treatment when antidepressants are used in this manner is unclear, but one study showed benefit in treated patients for 1 year and current guidelines suggest 9 to 12 months of therapy.[3,17,53] Antidepressants, along with psychotherapy, have been used to help maintain weight and prevent relapse, but data supporting this are limited.[59] Most clinicians prefer the selective serotonin reuptake inhibitor (SSRI) antidepressants because they are better tolerated and have greater cardiovascular safety than tricyclic antidepressants (TCAs) and monoamine oxidase inhibitors (MAOIs).[17,60] Because these patients are sensitive to anticholinergic and cardiovascular effects, if TCAs or MAOIs are used, low starting doses and a slow titration toward an effective dose is appropriate. The risk of cardiotoxicity in a malnourished population must not be underestimated, and a baseline electrocardiogram (ECG) should be obtained before initiation of these agents.

Fluoxetine continues to be the most widely studied SSRI in AN. Most clinicians initiate at low doses, for example 20 mg/day, and increase to a maximum of 60 mg/day based on response and tolerability.[56,57,59] Some clinical controversy exists regarding when antidepressant therapy should be initiated. During the starvation phases of AN, the majority of clinical trials suggest antidepressants are ineffective, and there is debate as to their effectiveness once weight restoration has occurred. Evidence from a 52-week, randomized, placebo controlled clinical trial of 93 patients with the treatment arm receiving doses from 20 mg/day to 80 mg/day showed no difference between fluoxetine and placebo for time-to-relapse.[61]

Antipsychotics Typical antipsychotics were the first medications used to treat AN because of their potential to reduce obsessive thoughts, paranoid ideation about weight gain, anxiety, and to promote weight gain.[62] However, there was little improvement, and the risks outweighed the benefits. Interest in antipsychotics for acutely ill AN patients has reemerged with the introduction of the atypical agents. Most of the data are from case reports or small trials using risperidone 0.5 to 1.5 mg daily or olanzapine 2.5 to 10 mg daily.[63–68] Improvement has been shown through weight increase and reduction of comorbid anxiety and depressive symptoms, but not all reports are favorable, and these agents require further study. Caution is urged in view of the report of increased QTc in an AN patient taking risperidone.[69] Optimal treatment duration is unknown, as most of the larger studies are less than or equal to 3 months in duration.

Miscellaneous Agents Metoclopramide can be helpful in reducing bloating, early satiety, and abdominal pain commonly found in

AN, but it does not impact weight gain.[17] Low-dose, short-acting benzodiazepines (0.25 mg alprazolam or 0.5 mg lorazepam) given before meals are useful when severe anxiety limits eating.[17] Estrogen replacement has been used, but restoring menses through refeeding is a preferred approach to minimize bone density loss.

CLINICAL CONTROVERSY

Clinicians continue to look for medications that are beneficial during the acute phase of AN. Recent findings from a 52-week study comparing fluoxetine to placebo in patients with anorexia nervosa after successful weight restoration found that fluoxetine did not provide any benefit in preventing relapse. Second generation antipsychotics are being used by some clinicians in acutely ill patients with severe obsessions and paranoia about eating, although the data supporting this approach are limited.

BULIMIA NERVOSA

Nonpharmacologic Therapy

The nondrug strategies used in BN are similar to those used with AN, and they are equally critical to success. CBT has the strongest evidence supporting its benefit in managing BN.[18,24] Current treatment guidelines suggest that CBT should consist of 16 to 20 sessions over a 4- to 5-month period.[53] Interpersonal psychotherapy also plays a role and has a moderate degree of evidence to support its use.[17,23] Nutritional counseling, planned meals, and self-monitoring can help interrupt the binge-purge cycle. Family therapy in BN patients is less critical than with AN, as these patients tend to be older. Programs using self-help and guided self-help manuals based on CBT have shown mixed results; however, when used in combination with fluoxetine, they have improved symptoms.[28,70,71] Data supports the use of 12-step programs, but they should not be used as monotherapy[17,23]

Pharmacologic Therapy

❻ **Antidepressants** Antidepressants are used in the acute and maintenance phase of BN adjunctively with nonpharmacologic approaches. A wide array of antidepressants, including TCAs, MAOIs, trazodone, serotonin-norepinephrine reuptake inhibitors (SNRIs), and SSRIs have been studied. Additionally, several reviews analyzing this body of literature have been published, although there continues to be limited placebo controlled randomized, double-blind clinical studies.[23,49] Antidepressants are reported to reduce depression, anxiety, obsessions, impulsive behaviors such as binge eating and purging, and improve eating habits, although their impact on body dissatisfaction remains unclear. The presence of comorbid mood disorders is not necessary for an antidepressant response.[23,72,73]

The benefit appears to be more robust in the acute phase of the illness, as relapse despite continued antidepressant use is common in patients who are in or near remission.[23,28,51] Antidepressant response usually occurs in 6 to 8 weeks, and reduction in frequency of binge/purge behavior has been as high as 73% and as low as zero.[49] Abstinence rates (elimination of bingeing and purging behaviors) with short-term use range from zero to 68%. More data are needed to determine the long-term benefits of antidepressants for preventing relapse of BN symptoms. One trial evaluating the impact of fluoxetine versus placebo in the maintenance phase showed a better outcome in patients receiving fluoxetine 60 mg/day, although high dropout rates in both groups blurred the overall benefit.[74]

❼ SSRIs are the preferred agents because of their tolerability and because they have been studied in the largest number of patients. Fluoxetine is the only agent to have Food and Drug Administration approval for BN. Tolerability is the primary criterion for selecting an antidepressant in BN because of patients' heightened sensitivity to adverse effects and lack of a clear difference in efficacy between the classes. Even though there is a suggestion that MAOIs produce the most robust effect, the risks of using these medications in impulsive patients limits their use.[51] SNRIs have shown promising results; however, the data supporting their use is limited to case reports.[75] Bupropion is not used in BN patients because of the increased risk of seizures.

Before initiating pharmacologic based therapy, a careful baseline physical examination, ECG, and laboratory workup are essential. Underlying ECG changes secondary to hypokalemia or bradycardia and atrioventricular block from starvation can be present. All antidepressants can cause seizures; thus a careful risk-benefit assessment is warranted if the patient has predisposing factors such as a personal or family history of seizures, cerebrovascular disease, or alcohol or sedative-hypnotic withdrawal.

Doses in BN are in the same range as for patients with depression. Readers are referred to Chap. 71 for antidepressant dosing ranges. For fluoxetine, the higher end of the dosing range, 60 mg/day, can be necessary for response.[76] With other agents, most clinicians initially target the bottom to the middle of the dosing range and increase the dose if there is an inadequate response. Slow titration is needed to allow time to develop tolerance to adverse effects. If TCAs are used, serum concentration monitoring is recommended to ensure that absorption is not compromised by purging.

❽ The time for antidepressant onset of effect in BN is unclear. In the absence of data, the definition of a therapeutic trial from the depression literature (4 to 8 weeks at a therapeutic dose) should be used. As the majority of subjects will not experience a complete remission, and there are few data on predictors of response or whether switching to another class will improve response, a clear and specific target should be stated initially.[17]

❾ Optimal duration of treatment after response is poorly defined, although most clinicians treat for 9 months to 1 year and then reevaluate. The evidence is mixed as to whether any early benefit is sustained, hence the decision to continue treatment should be made based on both initial response and the maintenance of that benefit. If the symptoms return within a few months after antidepressant discontinuation, then the treatment might need to be reinitiated.

Table 66–3 and Fig. 66–2 describe potential guidelines for medication use in BN, but it must be noted that no evidence-based

TABLE 66-3 Guidelines for Medication Use in Bulimia Nervosa

1. Determine baseline frequency of binge and vomiting episodes, laxative abuse, obsessive thoughts, and compulsive behavior. Document weight and patient's subjective feelings of self-image. Describe a baseline level of functioning.
2. Identify comorbid psychiatric conditions (e.g., depression, anxiety disorder, substance abuse, or bipolar disorder).
3. Determine baseline physical status (especially nutritional status, electrocardiogram, and fluid status [dehydration and electrolytes]).
4. Consider whether an antidepressant should be part of a comprehensive treatment plan that includes nonpharmacologic measures, especially cognitive behavioral therapy.
5. If antidepressant is indicated, start at a low dose, and use a selective serotonin reuptake inhibitor unless there is a medical reason not to do so.
6. Monitor carefully for response, adverse effects, and compliance. Response usually is seen after 6 to 12 weeks. Response is determined by change from baseline frequency and severity of target symptoms.
7. If patient responds and response is sustained, continue treatment for 6 to 12 months, then reassess.
8. If response is poor, evaluate compliance and whether patient is vomiting medication. Ensure that the patient is receiving nonpharmacologic therapy.

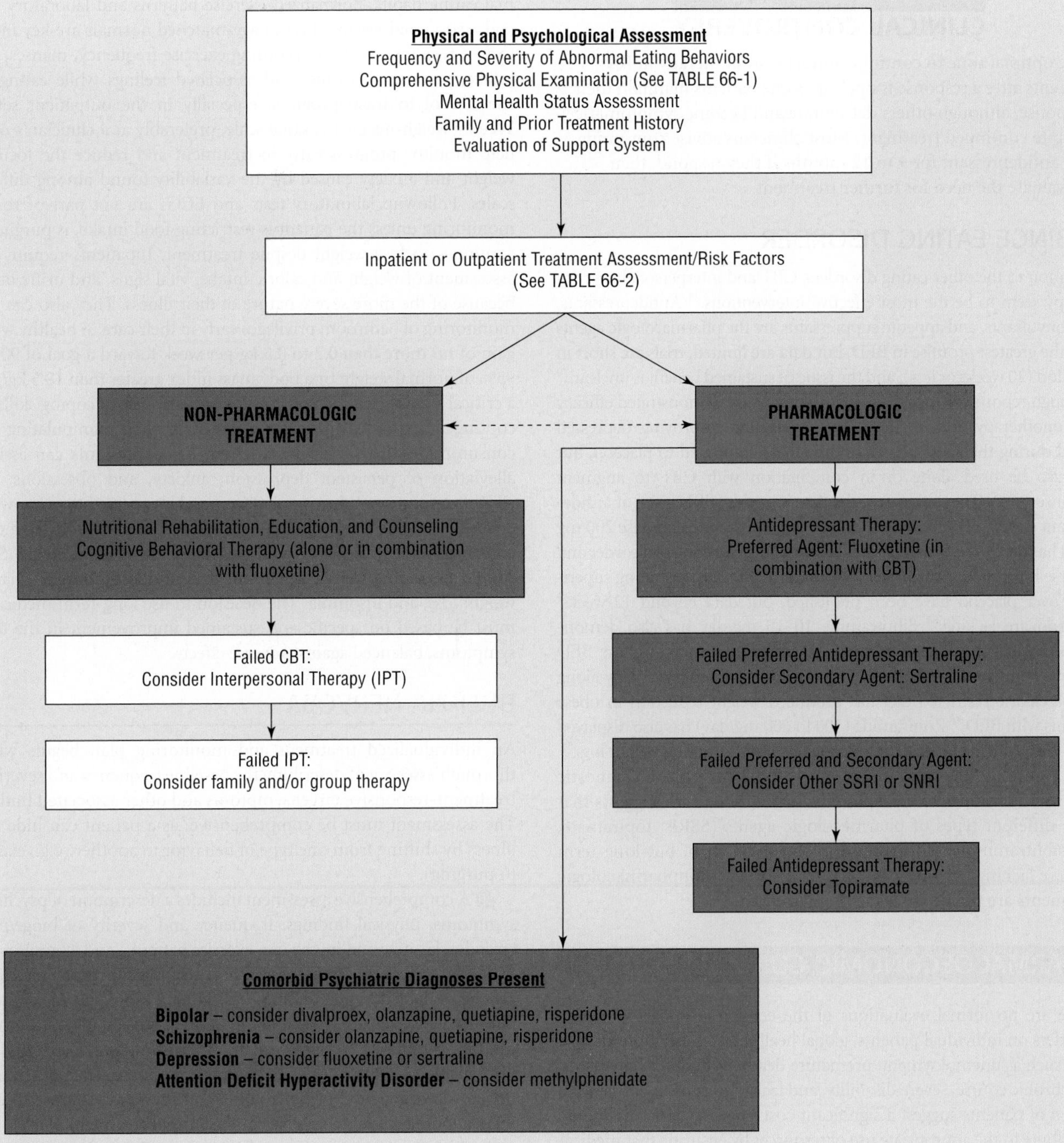

FIGURE 66-2. Bulimia nervosa treatment algorithm. (CBT, cognitive behavioral therapy; IPT, interpersonal pyschotherapy; SNRI, serotonin-norepinephrine reuptake inhibitor; SSRI, selective serotonin reuptake inhibitor.)

consensus for treatment has been endorsed, even with the recent guidelines, meta-analyses, and reviews of the literature.[3,17,23,49,51,53,60]

Mood Stabilizers (Lithium and Anticonvulsants) Because of the lack of evidence demonstrating their benefit, lithium and anticonvulsants are reserved for BN patients with a comorbid bipolar affective disorder.[17,77] Target serum concentrations and doses are similar to those used for patients with seizure or mood disorders. Lithium must be used cautiously, as fluid shifts related to purging and laxative abuse increase the risk of toxicity. The adverse effect of weight gain often makes mood stabilizers and anticonvulsants unacceptable to patients in the long term.

Miscellaneous Agents Low-dose benzodiazepines before meals can help reduce anxiety associated with refeeding, although long-term use is not warranted because of the risk of abuse and dependence. One double-blind trial with ondansetron has shown benefit, but there are insufficient data to recommend a specific role for this agent.[78] Antipsychotics and appetite suppressants do not play a role in managing central BN symptoms.[23]

Nonpharmacologic versus Pharmacologic Approaches

The combination of pharmacologic and nonpharmacologic measures appears to produce the best chance for a positive outcome for patients with BN.[49] Antidepressants, specifically SSRIs, are the class of choice in patients with BN, whereas other medications are reserved for patients with comorbid psychiatric conditions. Only in unusual circumstances should patients be treated with antidepressants alone. Evidence suggests the greatest benefit is during the acute phase of treatment, whereas data are mixed supporting their role in the prevention of relapse.

CLINICAL CONTROVERSY

The optimal time to continue antidepressant therapy in BN patients after a response is unclear. Some patients maintain their response, although others deteriorate and become symptomatic despite continued treatment. Most clinicians advise continuing the antidepressant for 9 to 12 months if they respond, then reevaluate the need for further treatment.

BINGE EATING DISORDER

Common to the other eating disorders, CBT and interpersonal psychotherapy seem to be the most effective interventions.[23] Antidepressants, anticonvulsants, and appetite suppressants are the pharmacologic agents with the greatest promise in BED, but data are limited, trials are short in duration (20 weeks or less), and the issue of sustained benefit is unclear.[79] Although reports are mixed, antidepressants have demonstrated efficacy as monotherapy at reducing binge eating and improving depressed mood during the acute phases of the illness compared to placebo, but can also be used alone or in combination with CBT to augment response.[23,80–83] The majority of the data are with SSRIs given at antidepressant doses.[79] Topiramate 50 to 600 mg daily (a median dose 200 mg daily) has produced benefit in patients with impulse control disorder and because it promotes weight loss. Short-term data demonstrating superiority over placebo have been published, but data beyond 12-weeks' duration are lacking.[84] Sibutramine 10–15 mg/day has also demonstrated benefit in reducing weight and binge frequency in obese BED patients compared to placebo.[85] Orlistat 120 mg three times daily along with a calorie restricted diet has produced weight reduction in obese patients with BED.[86] Zonisamide (100 to 600 mg/day) has also displayed benefit at reducing binge eating frequency and promoting weight loss.[87]

In summary, the question of where BED fits on the diagnostic spectrum continues to be explored. Current literature suggests that three different types of pharmacologic agents (SSRIs, topiramate, and sibutramine) hold promise in the short term, but long-term data are lacking. As with other eating disorders, nonpharmacologic treatments are the key to a successful outcome.

PHARMACOECONOMIC CONSIDERATIONS

There are no formal evaluations of the economic impact of eating disorders on individual patients, global healthcare costs, or on indirect costs such as unemployment, premature death, or disability payments. The chronic course, severe disability, and lack of improvement in up to a third of patients suggest a significant cost impact. Clinicians should contribute to the appropriate use of resources by ensuring that medications are used in situations in which there is evidence demonstrating their benefit and that they are never used as the sole treatment modality. For example, antidepressants are started after normal weight is restored in AN patients and not to treat depressive symptoms in significantly malnourished patients. One study evaluating the relative costs of CBT alone, medication alone, or combination treatment of BN concluded that if overall effectiveness was the prime consideration, then CBT, with medication added if the response was inadequate, was the best approach. If cost-effectiveness was the basis for making treatment decisions, then antidepressants alone as a first step, followed by the addition of CBT when response was inadequate was the preferred.[88]

EVALUATION OF THERAPEUTIC OUTCOMES

ANOREXIA NERVOSA

A combination of subjective and objective measures is used to assess patient response. A reduction in the frequency and severity of abnormal eating habits, normalized exercise patterns and laboratory tests, and a sustained weight close to age-matched normals are key indicators of response. A diary recording exercise frequency, menses, food intake, patterns of eating, and associated feelings while eating is a useful tool to track progress, especially in the outpatient setting. Weekly weigh-ins on the same scale, preferably at a clinician's office, help monitor progress early in treatment and reduce the focus on weight and anxiety caused by the variability found among different scales. Followup laboratory tests and ECGs are not part of routine monitoring unless the patient is restricting food intake, is purging, or continues to lose weight despite treatment. Inpatients require daily assessment of weight and caloric intake, vital signs, and urine output because of the more severe nature of their illness. They also can need monitoring of bathroom privileges early in their care. A healthy weight gain of no more than 0.2 to 0.5 kg per week toward a goal of 90% to 95% of normal weight or a body mass index greater than 18.5 kg/m^2 is a critical sign of treatment success. A patient's use of coping skills and contingencies for dealing with stress other than manipulating food consumption also should be assessed. Antidepressants can assist in alleviation of persistent depression, anxiety, and obsessions, after weight restoration. Improvement in mood is expected to occur within 8 weeks. Patients receiving TCAs should be evaluated for dry mouth, constipation, hypotension, and sedation. Patients receiving SSRIs should be monitored for agitation, drug-induced anorexia, nausea, weight loss, and insomnia. The decision to use long-term medication must be based on specific and sustained improvement in the target symptoms, balanced against adverse effects.

BULIMIA NERVOSA

An individualized treatment and monitoring plan begins with a thorough assessment describing the baseline frequency and severity of treatment-responsive target symptoms and other associated findings. The assessment must be comprehensive, as a patient can hide their illness by shifting from one type of behavior to another (e.g., exercise to purging).

⑩ A comprehensive assessment includes a description of psychiatric symptoms, physical findings, frequency and severity of binge/purge episodes, laxative and ipecac use, exercise patterns, and laboratory and ECG abnormalities. Interpersonal and relationship problems should also be evaluated. Some findings indicating a more chronic course of illness, such as salivary gland inflammation or erosion of dental enamel, can take months to reverse or might never normalize, hence these are not sensitive indicators of early treatment response. Data describing a patient's baseline level of functioning and previous response to treatment should be used to set goals in the current treatment plan.

Antidepressant response usually occurs within 4 to 8 weeks after the onset of treatment. If response does not occur, binge/purge behavior should be considered as a factor potentially contributing to the malabsorption of medication. If this behavior is not present, then every attempt should be made to maximize the dose. Serum concentration monitoring, when appropriate as with TCAs, should be done periodically (every 3 to 6 months if a patient is responding and tolerating the medication, or more frequently if clinically indicated). Evaluation of previously described adverse effects also should be part of the monitoring plan. If the patient responds, they should be followed for 6 to 12 months, then reassess the need for ongoing medication. If the patient relapses on medication discontinuation, then the medication should be restarted.

Ambulatory eating disorder patients present a particular challenge to clinicians. Impulsivity associated with BN can increase the risk for suicide. Prescriptions should be limited to small supplies. In addition, pharmacists should be alert to persons who make large or frequent purchases of laxatives or ipecac syrup, as this is an indicator of possible bulimic behaviors.

CONCLUSIONS

Our understanding of the pathophysiology and symptomatology of eating disorders has improved significantly over the past several years. Medication serves an adjunctive role to a variety of psychosocial therapies in AN, whereas it plays a more central role in BN and BED treatment. By gaining a greater understanding of the underlying physiologic changes and the psychosocial complications associated with eating disorders, treatment plans can be specifically designed for an individual patient with the goal of improving their quality of life.

ACKNOWLEDGMENTS

The author acknowledges the contributions of Patricia A. Marken, PharmD, and Roger W. Sommi, PharmD, authors of the Eating Disorders chapter (Chap. 62) in the 6th edition of *Pharmacotherapy: A Pathophysiologic Approach*.

ABBREVIATIONS

AN: anorexia nervosa

BDNF: brain derived neurotrophic factor

BED: binge eating disorder

BN: bulimia nervosa

CBT: cognitive behavioral therapy

DSM-IV-TR: Diagnostic and Statistical Manual of Mental Disorders, 4th Edition, Text-Revision

ECG: electrocardiogram

EDNOS: eating disorder not otherwise specified

MAOI: monoamine oxidase inhibitor

NES: night eating syndrome

SSRI: selective serotonin reuptake inhibitor

SNRI: serotonin-norepinephrine reuptake inhibitor

TCA: tricyclic antidepressant

REFERENCES

1. Bulik CM, Tozzi FC, Anderson C, et al. The relationship between eating disorders and components of perfectionism. Am J Psychiatry 2003;160:366–368.
2. McKnight Investigators. Risk factors for the onset of eating disorders in adolescent girls: Results of the McKnight longitudinal risk factor study. Am J Psychiatry 2003;160:248–254.
3. Favaro A, Ferrara S, Santonastaso P. The spectrum of eating disorders in young women: A prevalence study in a general population sample. Psychosom Med 2003;65:701–708.
4. Striegel-Moore RH, Dohm FA, Kraemer HC, et al. Eating disorders in white and black women. Am J Psychiatry 2003;160:1326–1331.
5. Gull WW. Anorexia nervosa. Trans Clin Soc (Lond) 1874. In: Kaufman RM, Heifman M, eds. Evolution of Psychosomatic Concepts. Anorexia Nervosa: A Paradigm. New York: International Universities Press, 1964:22–28.
6. Lesegue C. De l'anorexic hysterique. Arch Gen Med 1873. In: Kaufman RM, Heifman M, eds. Evolution of Psychosomatic Concepts. Anorexia Nervosa: A Paradigm. New York: International Universities Press, 1964:385–395.
7. Russel G. Bulimia nervosa: An ominous variant of anorexia nervosa. Psychol Med 1979;9:429–448.
8. Striegel-Moore RH, Franko DL, May A, et al. Should night eating syndrome be included in the DSM? Int J Eat Disord 2006;39:544–549.
9. O'Reardon JP, Allison KC, Martino NS, et al. A randomized, placebo-controlled trial of sertraline in the treatment of night eating syndrome. Am J Psychiatry 2006;163:893–898.
10. Hoek H, van Hoeken D. Review of the prevalence and incidence of eating disorders. Int J Eat Disord 2003;34:383.
11. Bulik CM, Reba L, Siega-Riz AM, Reichborn-Kjennerud T. Anorexia nervosa: Definition, epidemiology, and cycle of risk. Int J Eat Disord 2005;37:52–59.
12. Wittchen HU, Nelson CB, Lachner G. Prevalence of mental disorders and psychosocial impairments in adolescents and young adults. Psychol Med 1998;28:109.
13. Pike KM. Long-term course of anorexia nervosa: Response, relapse, remission, and recovery. Clin Psychol Rev 1998;18:447–475.
14. Norris ML, Boydell KM, Pinhas L, Katzman DK. Ana and the Internet: A review of pro-anorexia websites. Int J Eat Disord 2006;39.
15. American Psychiatric Association. Diagnostic and Statistical Manual of Mental Disorders, 4th ed., Text Revision. Washington, DC: American Psychiatric Press, 2000:583–596.
16. Sadock BJ, Sadock VA, eds. Kaplan and Sadock's Synopsis of Psychiatry. Behavioral Sciences/Clinical Psychiatry, 9th ed. Philadelphia: Lippincott Williams & Wilkins, 2003:739–750.
17. American Psychiatric Association. Treatment of patients with eating disorders, third edition. Am J Psychiatry 2006;163(7 Suppl):4–54.
18. Stunkard A, Grace WJ, Wolff HG. The night eating syndrome: A pattern of food intake in certain obese patients. Am J Med 1955;19:79–86.
19. Birketvedt GS, Florholmen J, Sundsfjord J, et al. Behavioral and neuroendocrine characteristics of the night eating syndrome. JAMA 1999;282:657–663.
20. Gluck ME, Geliebter A, Satov T. Night eating syndrome is associated with depression, low self-esteem, reduced daytime hunger, and less weight loss in obese outpatients. Obes Res 2001;9:264–267.
21. Rand CS, MacGreggor AMC, Stunkard AJ. The night eating syndrome in the general population and among postoperative obesity surgery patients. Int J Eat Disord 1997;22:65–69.
22. Stunkard AJ, Berkowitz R, Wadden T, et al. Binge eating disorder and the night eating syndrome. Int J Obes Relat Metab Disord 1996;20:1–6.
23. Fairburn CG, Harrison PJ. Eating disorders. Lancet 2003;361:407–416.
24. Kaye WH, Frank GK, Meltzer CC, et al. Altered 5-HT2_A receptor activity in women who have recovered from bulimia nervosa. Am J Psychiatry 2001;158:1152–1155.
25. Frank GK, Kaye WH, Meltzer CC, et al. Reduced 5-HT2_A receptor binding after recovery from anorexia nervosa. Biol Psychiatry 2002;52:896–906.
26. Ribases M, Gratacos M, Fernandez-Aranda F, et al. Association of BDNF with anorexia, bulimia, age of onset of weight loss in six European populations. Hum Mol Genet 2004;13(12):1205–1212.
27. Hudson JI, Lalonde JK, Berry JM, et al. Binge-eating disorder as a distinct familial phenotype in obese individuals. Arch Gen Psychiatry 2006;63:313–319.
28. Halmi K. Eating disorders. In: Sadock BJ, Sadock VA, eds. Comprehensive Textbook of Psychiatry, 7th ed. Philadelphia: Lippincott Williams & Wilkins, 2000:1663–1676.
29. Powers PS. Initial assessment and early treatment options for anorexia nervosa and bulimia nervosa. Psychiatr Clin North Am 1996;19:639–655.
30. Casper RC, Hedeker D, McClough JF. Personality dimensions in eating disorders and their relevance for subtyping. J Am Acad Child Adolesc Psychiatry 1992;31:830–840.
31. Eckert ED, Halmi KA, Marchi P, et al. Ten-year follow-up of anorexia nervosa: Clinical course and outcome. Psychol Med 1995;25:143–156.
32. Garner DM, Garfinkel PE, O'Shaughnessy M. Validity of the distinction between bulimia with and without anorexia nervosa. Am J Psychiatry 1985;142:581–587.
33. Tozzi F, Thornton LM, Mitchell J, et al. Features associated with laxative abuse in individuals with eating disorders. Psychosom Med 2006;68:470–477.
34. Garner DM, Garner MV, Rosen LW. Anorexia nervosa "restrictors" who purge: Implications for subtyping anorexia nervosa. Int J Eat Disord 1993;13:171–185.
35. Shroff H, Reba L, Thornton LM, et al. Features associated with excessive exercise in women with eating disorders. Int J Eat Disord 2006;39:454–461.
36. Halmi KA. Eating disorders: Anorexia nervosa, bulimia nervosa, and obesity. In: Hales RE, Yudofsky SC, eds. Essentials of Clinical Psychiatry, 3rd ed. Washington, DC: American Psychiatric Press, 1999:667–685.
37. Braun DL, Sunday SR, Halmi KA. Psychiatric comorbidity in patients with eating disorders. Psychol Med 1994;24:859–867.

38. Skodol AE, Oldham JM, Hyler SE, et al. Comorbidity of DSM-III-R eating disorders and personality disorders. Int J Eat Disord 1993;14:403–416.
39. O'Brien KM, Vincent NK. Psychiatric comorbidity in anorexia and bulimia nervosa: Nature, prevalence, and causal relationships. Clin Psychol Rev 2003;23:53–74.
40. Herzog DB, Keller MB, Sacks NR, et al. Psychiatric comorbidity in treatment seeking anorexics and bulimics. J Am Acad Child Adolesc Psychiatry 1992;31:810–818.
41. Rome ES, Ammerman, S. Medical complications of eating disorders: An update. J Adolesc Health 2003;33:418–426.
42. Birch K. Female athlete triad. Br Med J 2005;330(7485):244–246.
43. Kingston K, Szmukler G, Andrews D, et al. Neuropsychological and structural brain changes in anorexia nervosa before and after refeeding. Psychol Med 1996;26:15–28.
44. Lambe EK, Katzman DK, Mikulis DJ, et al. Cerebral gray matter volume deficits after weight recovery from anorexia nervosa. Arch Gen Psychiatry 1997;54:537–542.
45. Carney CP, Anderson AE. Eating disorders: Guide to medical evaluation and complications. Psychiatr Clin North Am 1996;19:657–679.
46. Steinhausen HC. The outcome of anorexia nervosa in the 20th century. Am J Psychiatry 2002;159(8):1284–1293.
47. Fichter MM, Quadfleig N. Six year course of bulimia nervosa. Int J Eat Disord 1997;22:361–384.
48. Herzog DB, Nussbaum KM, Marmor AK. Comorbidity and outcome in eating disorders. Psychiatr Clin North Am 1996;19:843–859.
49. Mitchell JE, deZwaan M, Roerig JL. Drug therapy for patients with eating disorders. Curr Drug Targets CNS Neurol Disord 2003;2:17–29.
50. Bacaltchuk J, Hay P. Antidepressants versus placebo for people with bulimia nervosa. Cochrane Database Syst Rev 2003;4:CD003391 [updated November 2005].
51. Nakash-Eisikovits O, Dierberger A, Westen D. A multidimensional meta-analysis of pharmacotherapy for bulimia nervosa: Summarizing the range of outcomes in controlled clinical trials. Harv Rev Psychiatry 2002;10:190–211.
52. Halmi KA, Agras WS, Crow S, et al. Predictors of treatment acceptance and completion in anorexia nervosa: Implications for future study designs. Arch Gen Psychiatry 2005;62:776–781.
53. National Collaborating Centre for Mental Health. Eating disorders: Core interventions in the treatment and management of anorexia nervosa, bulimia nervosa and related eating disorders. London: British Psychological Society and Royal College of Psychiatrists, 2004.
54. Zerbe KJ. Multimodal treatment of severe eating disorders. Essent Psychopharmacol 2000;3:1–17.
55. Kleifield EI, Wagner S, Halmi KA. Cognitive-behavioral treatment of anorexia nervosa. Psychiatr Clin North Am 1996;19:715–737.
56. Yager J, Anderson AE. Anorexia nervosa. N Engl J Med 2005;353(14):1481–1488.
57. Gwirtsman HE, Guze BH, Yager J, Gainlsey B. Fluoxetine treatment of anorexia nervosa. An open clinical trial. J Clin Psychiatry 1990;51:378–382.
58. Berg C, Eriksson M, Lindberg G, Sodersten P. Selective serotonin reuptake inhibitors in anorexia. Lancet 1996;348:1459–1450.
59. Kaye WH, Nagata T, Weltzin TE, et al. Double-blind placebo-controlled administration of fluoxetine in restricting- and restricting-purging-type anorexia nervosa. Biol Psychiatry 2001;4:644–652.
60. Jimerson DC, Wolfe BE, Brotman AW, Metzger ED. Medication in the treatment of eating disorders. Psychiatr Clin North Am 1996;19:739–754.
61. Walsh BT, Kaplan AS, Attia E, et al. Fluoxetine after weight restoration in anorexia nervosa: A randomized controlled trial. JAMA 2006;295(22):2605–2612.
62. Dally PJ, Sargant W. A new treatment for anorexia nervosa. Br Med J 1960;1:1770–1773.
63. Carver AE, Miller S, Hagman J, Sigel E. Academy of Eating Disorders Annual Meeting, Boston, April 2002.
64. Powers PS, Santana CA, Bannon YS. Olanzapine in the treatment of anorexia nervosa: An open label trial. Int J Eat Disord 2002;32:146–154.
65. Jensen VS, Mejlhede A. Anorexia nervosa: Treatment with olanzapine. Br J Psychiatry 2000;177:87.
66. Dennis K, LeGrange D, Bremer J. Olanzapine use in adolescent anorexia nervosa. Eat Weight Disord 2006;11(2):53–56.
67. Barbarich N, McConaha C, Gaskill J, et al. An open trial of olanzapine in anorexia nervosa. J Clin Psychiatry 2004;65(11):1480–1482.
68. Malina A, Gaskill J, McConaha C, et al. Olanzapine treatment of anorexia nervosa: A retrospective study. Int J Eat Disord 2003;33:234–237.
69. Newman-Toker JJ. Risperidone in anorexia nervosa. J Am Acad Child Adolesc Psychiatry 2000;39:941–942.
70. Mitchell JE, Fletcher L, Hanson K, et al. The relative efficacy of fluoxetine and manual-based self-help in the treatment of outpatients with bulimia nervosa. J Clin Psychiatry 2001;21:298–304.
71. Walsh BT, Fairburn CG, Mickley D, et al. Treatment of bulimia nervosa in a primary care setting. Am J Psychiatry 2004;161:556–561.
72. Mitchell JE, Groat R. A placebo-controlled, double-blind trial of amitriptyline in bulimia. J Clin Psychopharmacol 1984;4:186–193.
73. Hughes PL, Wells LA, Cunningham CJ, Ilstrup DM. Treating bulimia with desipramine: A double-blind, placebo controlled trial. Arch Gen Psychiatry 1986;43:182–186.
74. Romano SJ, Halmi KA, Sarkar NP, et al. A placebo-controlled study of fluoxetine in continued treatment of bulimia nervosa after successful fluoxetine treatment. Am J Psychiatry 2002;159:96–102.
75. Milano W, Siano C, Putrella C, Capasso A. Treatment of bulimia nervosa with fluvoxamine: a randomized controlled trial. Adv Ther 2005;22(3):278–283.
76. Fluoxetine Bulimia Nervosa Collaborative Study Group. Fluoxetine in the treatment of bulimia nervosa: A multicenter, placebo-controlled, double-blind trial. Arch Gen Psychiatry 1992;49:139–147.
77. McElroy SL, Kotwal R, Hudson JI, et al. Zonisamide in the treatment of binge eating disorder: an open-label, prospective trial. J Clin Psychiatry 2004;65(1):50–56.
78. Faris PL, Kim SW, Meller WH, et al. Effect of decreasing afferent vagal activity with ondansetron on the symptoms of bulimia nervosa: A randomized double-blind trial. Lancet 2000;355:792–797.
79. Carter WP, Hudson JI, Lalonde JK, et al. Pharmacologic treatment of binge eating disorder. Int J Eat Disord 2003;34:S74–S88..
80. Devlin MJ, Goldfein JA, Petkova E, et al. Cognitive behavioral therapy and fluoxetine as adjuncts to group behavioral therapy for binge eating disorder. Obes Res 2005;13(6):1077–1088.
81. Kaplan AS. Academy for Eating Disorders International Conference on Eating Disorders. Expert Opin Investig Drugs 2003;12:1441–1443.
82. McElroy SL, Casuto LS, Nelson EB, et al. Placebo-controlled trial of sertraline in the treatment of binge eating disorder. Am J Psychiatry 2000;157:1004–1006.
83. Hudson J, McElroy SL, Raymond NC, et al. Fluvoxamine in the treatment of binge eating disorder: A multicenter, placebo-controlled, double-blind trial. Am J Psychiatry 1998;155:1756–1762.
84. McElroy SL, Arnold LM, Shapira NA, et al. Topiramate in the treatment of binge eating disorder associated with obesity: A randomized, placebo-controlled trial. Am J Psychiatry 2003;160:255–261.
85. Appolinario JC, Gody-Matos A, Fontanelle LF, et al. An open trial of sibutramine in obese patients with BED. J Clin Psychiatry 2002;63:28–30.
86. Golay A, Laurent-Jaccard A, Habicht F, et al. Effect of orlistat in obese patients with binge eating disorder. Obes Res 2005;13(10):1701–1708.
87. Angras WS, Rossiter EM, Arnow B, et al. One year follow up of psychosocial and pharmacologic treatments for bulimia nervosa. J Clin Psychiatry 1994;55:179–183.

CHAPTER 67 Alzheimer's Disease

PATRICIA W. SLATTUM, RUSSELL H. SWERDLOW, AND ANGELA MASSEY HILL

KEY CONCEPTS

1. Alzheimer's disease (AD) is the most common form of dementing illness, and the prevalence of AD increases with each decade of life.
2. The etiology of AD is unknown, and current pharmacotherapy neither cures nor arrests the pathophysiology.
3. Neuritic plaques and neurofibrillary tangles are the pathologic hallmarks of AD; however, the definitive cause of this disease is yet to be determined.
4. AD affects multiple areas of cognition and is characterized by a gradual onset with a slow, progressive decline.
5. A thorough physical examination (including neurologic examination), as well as laboratory and imaging studies, is required to rule out other disorders and diagnose AD before considering drug therapy.
6. Pharmacotherapy for AD focuses on impacting three domains: cognition, behavioral and psychiatric symptoms, and functional ability.
7. Nondrug therapy and social support for the patient and family are the primary treatment interventions for AD.
8. Cholinesterase inhibitors and memantine are used to treat cognitive symptoms of AD; other medications have been suggested to be beneficial because of their potential preventive or cognitive effects.
9. Appropriate management of vascular disease risk factors may reduce the risk for developing AD and may prevent the worsening of dementia in patients with AD.
10. A thorough behavioral assessment and plan with careful examination of environmental factors should be conducted before initiating drug therapy for behavioral symptoms.
11. Pharmacotherapy may reduce the total cost of treating AD by delaying cognitive decline and time to nursing home placement.

I now begin the journey that will lead me into the sunset of my life.
Ronald Reagan

Learning objectives, review questions, and other resources can be found at **www.pharmacotherapyonline.com.**

Alzheimer's disease (AD), first characterized by Alois Alzheimer in 1907, is a gradually progressive dementia affecting cognition, behavior, and functional status. The exact pathophysiologic mechanisms underlying AD are not entirely known, and no cure exists.[1] Although drugs may reduce AD symptoms for a time, the disease is eventually fatal.

AD profoundly affects the family as well as the patient. The need for supervision and assistance increases until the late stages of the disease, when AD patients become totally dependent on a family member, spouse, or other caregiver for all of their basic needs. These are the all-too-common experiences of the millions of people in the United States who care for someone with AD.

EPIDEMIOLOGY

❶ AD is the most common cause of dementia. AD unassociated with any other pathology accounts for 50% to 60% of cases of late-life cognitive dysfunction. The incidence increases to 80% if AD in conjunction with other pathologic lesions is considered.[2] Table 67–1 lists the most common types of dementia among older adults. Dementia in an individual can result from multiple etiologies. This chapter focuses exclusively on dementia of the Alzheimer's type. However, the reader is encouraged to use the nonpharmacologic approaches and management of behavioral problems outlined in this chapter as a general treatment approach for other types of dementia that may share similar features with AD.

Approximately 4.5 million Americans have AD.[3] By the year 2050, 1 in 5 people will be older than age 65 years, and the number of AD patients is projected to be 13.2 million (Fig. 67–1). Most cases present in persons older than age 65 years, but approximately 5% of cases occur in persons younger than age 65 years. Onset can be as early as age 40 years, resulting in the arbitrary age classifications of early onset (ages 40 to 64 years) and late-onset (ages 65 years and older).[4,5]

Increasing age is the greatest risk factor for AD.[4] The prevalence of AD increases exponentially with age, affecting approximately 7% of individuals ages 65 to 74 years, 53% of those ages 75 to 84, and 40% of persons ages 85 years and older.[3] Genetic inheritance is also a significant risk factor, although other factors may contribute. Factors determining age of onset and rate of progression remain largely undefined.

TABLE 67-1 Common Types of Dementia in Late Life

Alzheimer's disease
Vascular dementia
Lewy body dementia
Frontotemporal dementia including Pick disease
Reversible causes of dementia (e.g., normal-pressure hydrocephalus, thyroid dysfunction, vitamin B_{12} deficiency, depression)

Data from Desai and Grossberg,[2] Rubin,[71] and Chapman et al.[117]

pathways. For example, serotonergic neurons of the raphe nuclei and noradrenergic cells of the locus ceruleus are lost, while monoamine oxidase type B activity is increased. Monoamine oxidase type B is found predominantly in the brain and in platelets, and is responsible for metabolizing dopamine. In addition, abnormalities appear in glutamate pathways of the cortex and limbic structures, where a loss of neurons leads to a focus on excitotoxicity models as possible contributing factors to AD pathology.

Glutamate is the major excitatory neurotransmitter in the cortex and hippocampus. Many neuronal pathways essential to learning and memory use glutamate as a neurotransmitter, including the pyramidal neurons (a layer of neurons with long axons carrying information out of the cortex), hippocampus, and entorhinal cortex. Glutamate and other excitatory amino acid neurotransmitters have been implicated as potential neurotoxins in AD.[42] If glutamate is allowed to remain in the synapse for extended periods of time, it can destroy nerve cells. Toxic effects are thought to be mediated through increased intracellular calcium and accumulation of intracellular free radicals.[42] Dysregulated glutamate activity is thought to be one of the primary mediators of neuronal injury after stroke or acute brain injury. Although intimately involved in cell injury, the role of excitatory amino acids in AD is as yet unclear; however, blockade of *N*-methyl-D-aspartate (NMDA) receptors decreases activity of glutamate in the synapse and may lessen the degree of cellular injury in AD.

BRAIN VASCULAR DISEASE AND HIGH CHOLESTEROL

There is growing evidence of a causal association between cardiovascular disease and its risk factors, with the incidence of AD. Cardiovascular risk factors that are also risk factors for dementia include hypertension, elevated low-density lipoprotein cholesterol, low high-density lipoprotein cholesterol, and, particularly, diabetes.[43] Brain vascular disease may augment the cognitive impairment observed for a given amount of AD pathology in the brain. Dysfunctional blood vessels may impair nutrient delivery to neurons and reduce clearance of βAP from the brain.[1] In addition, vascular disease may accelerate amyloid deposition and increase amyloid toxicity to neurons.[44] Controlling high blood pressure is associated with reduced rate of progression of dementia.[45] Diabetes may increase the risk of dementia through factors related to "metabolic syndrome" (dyslipidemia and hypertension), effects of potentially toxic glucose metabolites on the brain and vasculature, and through insulin itself.[46] Disturbances in insulin-signaling pathways, both in the periphery and the brain, have been linked to AD. Insulin may also regulate the metabolism of βAP and tau protein.[46]

Research has found multiple links between cholesterol and the occurrence of AD. Apo E is a lipoprotein that is synthesized in the liver, central nervous system, and cerebrospinal fluid. It is responsible for transporting cholesterol in the blood through the brain. It is carried by low-density lipoprotein into neurons and binds to NFTs. Apo E4 is associated with increasing deposition of βAP and is thought to act as an accelerating modulator in the course of vascular dementia. The elevated cholesterol levels in brain neurons may alter membrane functioning and result in the cascade leading to plaque formation and AD.

OTHER MECHANISMS

Other hypotheses proposed to explain AD pathogenesis include oxidative stress, mitochondrial dysfunction, and postmenopausal loss of estrogen in women. Each of these mechanisms may contribute to AD pathogenesis, but the extent of the contribution is uncertain. There is a growing body of evidence of a role for oxidative stress and the accumulation of free radicals in the brain of AD patients.[47] Based on epidemiologic studies, vitamin E, and possibly the combination of vitamin E and vitamin C, may prevent AD.[47] Mitochondrial dysfunction may result in disruption of energy metabolism in the neuron.[1] Estrogen is thought to be involved in promoting neuronal growth, and in preventing oxidative damage, which would benefit cells exposed to βAP.[48] Estrogen receptors are present in the brain, and are distributed in a pattern consistent with areas destroyed in AD.[48,49] Estrogen may be important in maintaining normal cholinergic neurotransmission.[49] Estrogen may also increase NMDA receptor numbers in brain areas involved in recording new memories and prevent cell damage by acting as an antioxidant.[48] Additional mechanisms postulated for estrogen's involvement in maintaining memory function are related to the fact that it increases cerebral blood flow and glucose use, reduces plasma levels of Apo E, and blunts stress-related glucocorticoid release. Postmenopausal loss of estrogen may, therefore, impact maintenance of memory functions.

A single common mechanism for producing AD does not exist. Regardless of the source, however, the features remain the same: degeneration of neurons in higher brain areas; accumulation of NFTs and neuritic plaques; profound destruction of cholinergic pathways; and an insidious dementia, slowly progressive until death.

TABLE 67-2 Stages of Alzheimer's Disease

Mild (MMSE score 26–18)	Patient has difficulty remembering recent events. Ability to manage finances, prepare food, and carry out other household activities declines. May get lost while driving. Begins to withdraw from difficult tasks and to give up hobbies. May deny memory problems.
Moderate (MMSE score 17–10)	Patient requires assistance with activities of daily living. Frequently disoriented with regard to time (date, year, season). Recall for recent events is severely impaired. May forget some details of past life and names of family and friends. Functioning may fluctuate from day to day. Patient generally denies problems. May become suspicious or tearful. Loses ability to drive safely. Agitation, paranoia, and delusions are common.
Severe (MMSE score 9–0)	Patient loses ability to speak, walk, and feed self. Incontinent of urine and feces. Requires care 24 hours a day, 7 days a week.

MMSE, Mini Mental Status Examination.
Data from Alzheimer's Association http://www.alz.org,[4] Rubin,[71] Grossberg and Desai.[118]

CLINICAL PRESENTATION OF ALZHEIMER'S DISEASE

❹ The onset of AD is almost imperceptible, without abrupt changes in cognition or function. Deficits occur progressively over time, affecting multiple areas of cognition.[4,50] For treatment and assessment purposes, it is helpful to divide Alzheimer's symptoms into two basic categories: cognitive symptoms and noncognitive (behavioral) symptoms.[50] Cognitive symptoms are present throughout the illness, whereas behavioral symptoms are less predictable.[50] Table 67–2 summarizes the stages of AD.

CLINICAL PRESENTATION OF ALZHEIMER'S DISEASE

General

- The patient may have vague memory complaints initially, or the patient's significant other may report that the patient is "forgetful." Cognitive decline is gradual over the course of illness. Behavioral disturbances may be present in moderate stages. Loss of daily function is common in advanced stages.

Symptoms

Cognitive

- Memory loss (poor recall and losing items)
- Aphasia (circumlocution and anomia)
- Apraxia
- Agnosia
- Disorientation (impaired perception of time and unable to recognize familiar people)
- Impaired executive function

Noncognitive

- Depression, psychotic symptoms (hallucinations and delusions)
- Behavioral disturbances (physical and verbal aggression, motor hyperactivity, uncooperativeness, wandering, repetitive mannerisms and activities, and combativeness)

Functional

- Inability to care for self (dressing, bathing, toileting, and eating)

Laboratory Tests

- Rule out vitamin B_{12} and folate deficiency
- Rule out hypothyroidism with thyroid function tests
- Blood cell counts, serum electrolytes, liver function tests

Other Diagnostic Tests

- CT or MRI scans may aid diagnosis

DIAGNOSIS

A family member often first brings memory complaints to the attention of a primary care clinician. Up to 50% of patients who meet criteria for dementia are not given a diagnosis in the primary care setting, leading some to believe that an appropriate screening tool may be helpful in aiding diagnosis and leading to earlier treatment.[51,52] Despite the phenomenon of underdiagnosis, the United States Preventative Services Task Force concluded that there are insufficient data to recommend for or against cognitive screening for AD, because it could not be determined if the benefits outweigh the risks.[51]

At present the only way to definitively diagnose AD is through direct examination of brain tissue at autopsy or biopsy. Several criteria have been developed for the detection and diagnosis of dementia, including the *Diagnostic and Statistical Manual of Mental Disorders, 4th ed. Text Revision* (DSM-IV-TR) criteria,[53] the Agency for Healthcare Research and Quality (AHRQ) Guidelines,[54] the American Academy of Neurology Guidelines,[55] the National Institute of Neurological Disorders and Stroke (NINDS) criteria,[56] the National Institute of Neurological Communicative Disorders and Stroke (NINCDS), and the Alzheimer's Disease and Related Disorders Association (ADRDA) Criteria.[57]

AD is still primarily a clinical diagnosis.[57] The patient's examination should suggest that cognitive decline from a previously higher baseline has occurred. The history should corroborate this, and further indicate cognitive decline has reached the point where changes in social or occupational functioning are present. It is possible to administer a sophisticated exam that defines cognitive domain strengths and weaknesses, and enables a neuroanatomical localization of the observed deficits. Ideally, evidence of defective retention memory (amnesia) will implicate bimesiotemporal dysfunction. Evidence of parietal cortical dysfunction (visuospatial dysfunction), dorsolateral prefrontal dysfunction (executive dysfunction), or lateral temporal dysfunction (language dysfunction) should also be present. When approached in this way, the exam can indicate a pattern of cognitive decline that is consistent with what would be expected in AD, and assist with rendering a diagnosis that is as much a diagnosis of inclusion as it is of exclusion.

Objectively defining social or occupational dysfunction can prove tricky in the older patient who may be retired, and who may also lead a socially restricted lifestyle for reasons of frailty. For such patients, the minimal requirement is to establish a change in activities of daily living. Early on, this usually involves a change in instrumental activities of daily living (handling finances, organizing medications) rather than basic activities of daily living (hygiene, dressing). Some AD subspecialists use a detailed, standardized, semistructured interview of a nonpatient informant as the most critical piece of the diagnostic evaluation.[58]

Almost any medication can contribute to cognitive impairment in vulnerable individuals, but certain classes of medication are more commonly implicated. Benzodiazepines and other sedative hypnotics, anticholinergics, opioid analgesics, antipsychotics, and anticonvulsants have been associated with cognitive impairment.[59] NSAIDs, histamine H_2 receptor antagonists, digoxin, amiodarone, antihypertensives, and corticosteroids have been implicated in cases of delirium.[59] Because medications are a reversible cause of cognitive symptoms, medication review and management are essential.

❺ For patients who meet criteria for the dementia syndrome (whether the underlying cause is ultimately felt to be AD or not), current recommendations from the American Academy of Neurology include a neuroimaging study (computed tomography or magnetic resonance imaging), as well as a serologic evaluation that includes blood cell counts, serum electrolytes, liver function tests, a test of thyroid function, and a vitamin B_{12} level.[55] Earlier guidelines included a serologic test for syphilis, but this requirement has since been downgraded to optional. When circumstances suggest AD is not the leading entity on the differential diagnosis, other neurologic tests such as spinal fluid analysis or electroencephalogram can occasionally be justified. Neuropsychological testing is also optional, but can prove quite useful for the diagnosis of AD by helping to establish a neuroanatomical localization for the patient's cognitive deficits.

Efforts to define the role of other AD diagnostic tests are ongoing. Positron emission tomography scanning may reveal a pattern of hypometabolism typical of AD (bitemporoparietal hypometabolism), but by itself the diagnostic accuracy of positron emission tomography scanning still lags behind that of the clinical examination and history.[60] Apo E genotyping by itself is also insufficient to make or break a diagnosis of AD, but demonstrating an apo E4 allele in a suspected patient increases the specificity of the diagnosis and can help predict which patients with mild cognitive impairment are most likely to progress to a full-blown diagnosis of AD over the next several years.[61,62] Unless the patient developed dementia prior to age 60 years and also had a parent that developed AD before age 60 years, presenilin 1 genotyping is usually not indicated.

MILD COGNITIVE IMPAIRMENT

It has long been recognized that aging individuals experience changes in cognitive function. Mild cognitive impairment constitutes a syndromic designation that categorizes patients with cognitive complaints insufficient to warrant a syndromic diagnosis of dementia. Persons diagnosed with mild cognitive impairment carry a 10% to 15% chance per year of progressing to an AD diagnosis.[63] A logical extension of this is that what clinicians are actually seeing in most people with mild cognitive impairment is the initial manifestation of a progressive degenerative dementia that will eventually meet AD diagnostic criteria.[64] However, it is important to note that not everyone meeting mild cognitive impairment criteria does or will have AD.

As the mild cognitive impairment designation is increasingly applied, mild cognitive impairment criteria continue to evolve.[65]

TREATMENT

Alzheimer's Disease

DESIRED OUTCOMES

❻ The primary goal of treatment in AD is to symptomatically treat cognitive difficulties and preserve patient function as long as possible. Secondary goals include treating the psychiatric and behavioral sequelae that occur as a result of the disease. Current AD treatments have not been shown to prolong life, cure AD, or halt or reverse the pathophysiologic processes of the disorder.[66]

GENERAL TREATMENT APPROACH

Clinical trials have consistently demonstrated modest benefits of early and continuous treatment with cholinesterase inhibitors.[66] Memantine added in moderate to severe disease may also provide benefit. Following this approach allows for maximum gain and maintenance of cognition and activities of daily living. A symptomatic approach is used to treat behavioral symptoms as they arise.

Provision of education to the patient and family at the time of diagnosis, including discussion of the course of illness, realistic expectations of treatment, and the importance of legal and financial planning, are essential to appropriate treatment. Good communication skills are important to maintain a therapeutic environment and minimize stress throughout the course of illness.

NONPHARMACOLOGIC THERAPY

❼ AD has a profound effect on both the patient and family, so appropriate treatment, both nonpharmacologic and pharmacologic, is needed. Nonmedication interventions are the current primary interventions for management of AD, and medications should be used in the context of multimodal interventions. Behavioral and psychiatric symptoms are among the most challenging and distressing symptoms of the disease and may be the determining factor in a family's decision to seek institutional care. Symptoms such as sleep disturbances, wandering, urinary incontinence, agitation, and aggression in patients with dementia are best managed using behavioral interventions rather than medications whenever possible.[67]

Upon initial diagnosis, the patient and caregiver should be educated on the course of illness, prognosis, available treatments, legal decisions, and quality-of-life issues. Education, including short- and long-term programs, improves caregiver knowledge and confidence, and in some cases, delays time to nursing home placement.[68] Table 67–3 lists basic principles of care for the AD patient.

TABLE 67-3 Basic Principles of Care for the Alzheimer's Patient

- Consider vision, hearing, or other sensory impairments.
- Find optimal level of autonomy and adjust expectations for patient performance over time.
- Avoid confrontation. Remain calm, firm, and supportive if the patient becomes upset.
- Maintain a consistent, structured environment with stimulation level appropriate to the individual patient.
- Provide frequent reminders, explanations, and orientation cues. Employ guiding, demonstration, and reinforcement.
- Reduce choices, keep requests and demands of the patient simple, and avoid complex tasks that lead to frustration.
- Bring sudden declines in function and the emergence of new symptoms to professional attention.

Data from Alzheimer's Association http://www.alz.org,[4] Lyketsos et al.,[44] and Rubin.[71]

Communication between the patient and family members is essential in order to minimize stress on everyone.

The general approach to developing nonmedication strategies for behavioral symptoms is to identify the symptom, identify causative factors, and adapt the caregiving environment to remedy the situation.[4] Environmental triggers may include noise, glare, an insecure space, and too much background distraction, including television. Personal discomfort may also trigger behaviors, so it is important to monitor for pain, hunger, thirst, constipation, full bladder, fatigue, infections and skin irritation, comfortable temperature, fears, and frustrations.[4] Medical comorbidity is a major source of functional and cognitive impairment in patients with AD, so general health maintenance is warranted.[44] Interventions should redirect the patient's attention rather than be confrontational and should specifically address known triggers. Creating a calm environment and removing stressors and triggers is key. Caregivers should be referred to support services such as the Alzheimer's Association for assistance in developing strategies to manage difficult behaviors.

The caregiver must be prepared to face the changes in life that will occur, and acceptance of this does not come easily. Denial on the part of the patient and rationalization on the part of the family are common. The clinician should encourage the family to address legal and financial matters and designate a durable power of attorney for execution of financial and medical decisions once the patient is incompetent. The caregiver will need to address issues such as respite services to provide time for rest, relaxation, and conduct of personal business. Caregiver stress impacts the health and quality of life of the caregiver as well as the patient. Eventually the caregiver will need to face critical questions with respect to institutionalization. This is probably the most difficult decision for the caregiver. Clinician support and referral to social services is vitally important in assisting the caregiver at that moment. The family should also be referred to local resources, such as the Alzheimer's Association, that can provide detailed information regarding support services. Table 67–4 lists some referral sources for caregivers.

Education, communication, and planning are the key nonpharmacologic components of caring for an AD patient. Preparation in the early stages of illness will lessen some of the caregiver stress as the illness progresses.

PHARMACOLOGIC THERAPY

Pharmacotherapy for Cognitive Symptoms

❽ Table 67–5 presents a treatment algorithm for managing cognitive symptoms in AD. Cholinesterase inhibitors and NMDA-receptor

TABLE 67-4 Resources for Caregivers of Persons with Alzheimer's Disease

The following organizations provide educational literature and information on diagnosis, treatment, social support, and ongoing research in Alzheimer's disease:

U.S. Administration on Aging, National Family Caregiver Support Program
http://www.aoa.gov

National Institute on Aging Alzheimer's Disease Education & Referral Center (ADEAR)
http://www.nia.nih.gov/alzheimers

The Alzheimer's Association
http://www.alz.org

The Alzheimer's Research Forum
http://www.alzforum.org

AARP
http://www.aarp.org

National Family Caregivers Association
http://www.thefamilycaregiver.org

ElderCare Online
http://www.ec-online.net

TABLE 67-5 Treatment Options for Cognitive Symptoms in Alzheimer's Disease

- In mild-moderate disease, consider therapy with a cholinesterase inhibitor.
  - Donepezil, or
  - Rivastigmine, or
  - Galantamine
- Titrate to recommended maintenance dose as tolerated.
- In moderate to severe disease, consider adding antiglutamatergic therapy.
  - Memantine
- Titrate to recommended maintenance dose as tolerated.
- Alternatively, consider memantine or cholinesterase inhibitor therapy alone.
- Behavioral symptoms may require additional pharmacologic approaches.

Data from Desai and Grossberg,[2] Lyketsos et al.,[44] and Lleó et al.[47]

antagonists are indicated for treatment of AD. The latest treatment guideline recommends the use of cholinesterase inhibitors for AD, with no preference for a specific agent.[44,69] Donepezil, rivastigmine, and galantamine are indicated in mild to moderate AD, while donepezil is also indicated in severe disease. Memantine is indicated for moderate to severe AD; current evidence does not support its use in earlier stages of the disease.[70] Additional benefit may be achieved when memantine is added to cholinesterase inhibitor therapy in moderate to severe AD.[44,70] There is no evidence supporting combination therapy of more than one cholinesterase inhibitor.

CLINICAL CONTROVERSY

Several cholinesterase inhibitors are now available, raising the question of whether it is appropriate to switch a patient from one to another if the first is not considered effective. Theoretical differences exist in their mechanisms of action, but many clinicians feel that these differences are not clinically meaningful, and therefore that switching is not helpful. Switching is recommended if a patient is not tolerating the initial treatment. Most clinicians probably do switch to another agent, and initial data seem to indicate that some patients do respond to an alternative cholinesterase inhibitor. Usually switching is performed without a washout period and interruptions for longer than 3 weeks are not advised.[47]

Disagreement exists about how to determine effectiveness of treatments for AD. Selection of qualitative versus quantitative assessment may bias a clinician's impression of response. Subtle changes are often detected only by psychometric testing rather than with routine questioning. Because no standard has been suggested to define the effectiveness of these medications, great variation exists between clinicians and the duration of treatment ranges from months to years. Realistic expectations for treatment success may include short-term improvement of symptoms and less decline in behavioral, functional, and cognitive abilities over the longer-term.[66]

Unfortunately, clinical trials have failed to provide answers to key questions in treating AD patients. Information from clinical trials is insufficient to know if a cholinesterase inhibitor dose–response relationship exists, or if additional cognitive improvement may be gained by increasing to the maximum tolerated dose, rather than continuing with the usual recommended daily dosage. Guidance in extrapolating data related to changes in cognition is needed so that a reasonable duration of clinical treatment with cholinesterase inhibitors and NMDA-antagonists can be determined.

In natural disease progression studies, scores on the Alzheimer's Disease Assessment Scale—Cognition (ADAS-cog) have been shown to worsen (increase) by an average of 4 points over 6 months and 7 points over 1 year. Based on these findings, the general consensus is that a 4-point change in the ADAS-cog represents a clinically significant change. Therefore, if a pharmacotherapeutic agent decreases the ADAS-cog by 4 points, one could think of this as having reversed progression of disease symptoms by 6 months. The usefulness of the ADAS-cog in clinical practice is limited because of the time required for administration; it is much more practical to assess changes in disease severity using the Mini Mental Status Examination (MMSE). An untreated patient has an average decline of 2 to 4 points in MMSE score per year. Consequently, successful treatment would reflect a decline of less than 2 points a year. It is reasonable to change to a different cholinesterase inhibitor if the decline in MMSE score is greater than 2 to 4 points after 1 year with the initial agent.

CLINICAL CONTROVERSY

Disagreement exists about the usefulness of current therapies for AD in advanced stages of the disease. Some clinicians believe that patients should be taken off cognitive-enhancing medications once they have reached very severe stages of AD, whereas others believe that these medications may continue to be helpful with managing psychiatric symptoms and maintaining function. Many clinicians discontinue cognitive-enhancing medications once the AD patient is bedridden and unable to perform activities of daily living.

8 Cholinesterase Inhibitors In the early 1980s, researchers began to examine means to enhance cholinergic activity in patients with AD by inhibiting the hydrolysis of acetylcholine through reversible inhibition of cholinesterase. Tacrine was the first such drug to be examined in a systematic fashion. However, tacrine is fraught with significant side effects, including hepatotoxicity, that severely limit its usefulness. For all practical purposes the use of tacrine has been replaced by the use of safer, more tolerable cholinesterase inhibitors. Newer cholinesterase inhibitors donepezil, rivastigmine, and galantamine, show similar efficacy and adverse event profiles to one another and are generally well tolerated. The most frequent adverse events associated with these agents are mild to moderate gastrointestinal symptoms (nausea, vomiting, and diarrhea).[47] Other cholinergic side effects are generally dose-related and include urinary incontinence, dizziness, headache, syncope, bradycardia, muscle weakness, salivation, and sweating. Gradual dose titration over several months can improve tolerability.[69] Abrupt discontinuation can lead to worsening cognition and behavior in some patients.[44] Concurrent use of anticholinergic medications with cholinesterase inhibitors should be avoided.

Table 67–6 summarizes the clinical pharmacology of the cholinesterase inhibitors. The mechanism of action differs slightly between drugs in this class.[71] Donepezil specifically and reversibly inhibits acetylcholinesterase. Rivastigmine inhibits both butyrylcholinesterase and acetylcholinesterase. Galantamine is a selective, competitive, reversible acetylcholinesterase inhibitor and also enhances the action of acetylcholine on nicotinic receptors. The clinical relevance of these differences is unknown. Choice of cholinesterase inhibitor therapy for an individual patient is based on ease of use, patient preference, cost, and safety issues such as potential for drug interactions.[44]

8 Antiglutamatergic Therapy Memantine is the only NMDA-antagonist currently available. Memantine blocks glutamatergic neurotransmission by antagonizing NMDA receptors. Glutamate is an excitatory neurotransmitter in the brain implicated in long-term potentiation, a neuronal mechanism important for learning and memory.[47] By blocking NMDA receptors, excitotoxic reactions, which ultimately lead to cell death, may be prevented, although longer-term studies are needed to assess this hypothesis.[47,70]

Memantine has been studied in patients with moderate and severe AD as monotherapy and in combination with donepezil with

TABLE 67-6 Clinical Pharmacology of the Cholinesterase Inhibitors

	Donepezil	Rivastigmine	Galantamine
Brand name	Aricept	Exelon	Razadyne
Dosage forms	Tablet Orally disintegrating tablet	Capsule Oral solution Patch	Tablet Oral solution Extended-release (ER) capsule
Starting dose	5 mg daily at bedtime	1.5 mg twice a day 4.6 mg/day (patch)	4 mg twice a day (8 mg daily for ER)
Maintenance dose	5–10 mg daily	3–6 mg twice a day 9.5 mg/day (patch)	8–12 mg twice a day (16–24 mg daily for ER)
Meals	No effect of food	Take with food	Take with food
Half-life	70 hours	1.5 hours	7 hours
Protein binding	96%	40%	18%
Metabolism	Substrate (minor) of CYP2D6 and 3A4 Glucuronidation	Cholinesterase-mediated hydrolysis	Substrate (minor) of CYP2D6 and 3A4 Glucuronidation
Renal elimination	Yes	Major pathway	Yes

CYP, Cytochrome P450.
Data from references 72 and 119–122.

modest favorable results on cognition and function.[70] It is currently indicated for use in AD patients with moderate to severe illness. Studies of memantine alone and in combination with cholinesterase inhibitors in mild AD performed to date have provided insufficient evidence to support an indication for mild AD.[4]

Memantine has 100% bioavailability regardless of administration with or without food. Protein binding is low. Memantine is not metabolized by the liver and does not inhibit cytochrome P450. Memantine is primarily excreted unchanged in the urine. The half-life ranges from 60 to 80 hours.[47]

Overall, memantine has been well tolerated in clinical trials. The most common adverse events associated with memantine include constipation, confusion, dizziness, headache, hallucinations, coughing, and hypertension.[73]

Memantine is likely to be used as monotherapy and also in combination with cholinesterase inhibitors in patients with moderate to severe AD. Memantine should be initiated at 5 mg once a day and increased weekly by 5 mg a day to the effective dose of 10 mg twice daily.[73] It may be given with or without food. Dosing of 10 mg daily is recommended in patients with severe renal impairment (creatinine clearance of 5 to 29 mL/min).[73]

Role of Combination Therapy The efficacy of all available AD treatments is limited. Currently, the best possible short-term outcome includes a symptomatic improvement over the pretreatment baseline. Because agents with different mechanisms of action are now available for the treatment of AD, the efficacy of combination therapy has been considered. In the only combination treatment trial published to date, patients receiving donepezil were randomized to receive 20 mg/day of memantine or placebo. During the 6-month course of the trial, those randomized to receive combination therapy performed better on a cognitive scale and an activities of daily living scale than those randomized to donepezil plus placebo.[74] A subsequent report concluded that with donepezil-memantine combination therapy, behavioral benefits were also demonstrable on the Neuropsychiatric Inventory.[75] It is important to note that these studies included subjects with MMSE scores of 5 to 14. Data showing donepezil-memantine combination therapy benefits in AD patients with MMSE scores above 14 are lacking.

Available data suggest treatment strategies currently under investigation will at best slow rather than arrest cognitive decline.[76] It therefore seems reasonable to predict that for the foreseeable future combination therapy will become increasingly common in AD, especially as drugs or treatments with unique mechanisms of action become available, and drugs with neuroprotective modes of action are concomitantly used with symptomatic drugs.

Effect of Current Treatments on Neurodegenerative Processes AD is a progressive disorder. Affected individuals typically experience some degree of cognitive decline and histologic change years (if not decades) before a diagnosis is made. Therefore, the ideal treatment will be one that not only reverses symptoms by enhancing cognitive function (a symptomatic treatment), but also arrests the neurodegeneration-relevant molecular processes that underlie cognitive decline (a disease-modifying treatment).

Clinical trials for AD prompt consideration of whether positive outcomes suggest either a symptomatic or disease-modifying effect. Any rapid performance improvement on cognitive ability, activities of daily living, or behavioral end points is indicative of a symptomatic effect. All cholinesterase inhibitor agents and memantine demonstrate this pattern. On the other hand, arrest of decline or a sustained reduction in the slope of decline would argue the presence of a disease-modifying effect. It has not been possible to unequivocally demonstrate this in trials of the currently approved treatments. Definitive trials evaluating whether cholinesterase inhibitors or memantine have disease-modifying effects are difficult to perform, because doing so requires continuing a placebo arm over an extended period, well beyond demonstration of symptomatic benefit. Also, subject attrition over an extended study would complicate both intent-to-treat and observed cases analyses.

With the currently approved AD drug treatments, placebo-controlled pivotal trials were followed by open-label extension studies. Published studies have lasted as long as 5 years, and as part of these studies, decline in the treatment group was compared to "projected" placebo groups based on the placebo groups followed during the 6-month randomized phase of the efficacy study, as well as natural history cohorts from the precholinesterase inhibitor therapy era. Although analyses of this sort conclude that, for up to at least 5 years, persons receiving treatment exceed their projected nontreatment cognitive performance, no convincing evidence of a disease-modifying effect emerges.[77–80]

Management of Brain Vascular Health

❾ Recent guidelines for the principles of care of patients with AD support the management of vascular brain disease and its associated risk factors as part of the treatment of AD.[44] There is a growing body of evidence that brain vascular disease plays an important role in the progression of dementia. For a given level of Alzheimer's pathology, vascular disease in the brain may add to the degree of cognitive impairment.[44] Brain vascular disease may also accelerate deposition of βAP and increase amyloid toxicity to neurons and the neural synapses.[44] Management of brain vascular disease includes monitoring blood pressure, glucose, cholesterol, and homocysteine and initiation of appropriate interventions.[44] Guidelines recommend initiation of low-dose aspirin therapy in patients with AD with significant brain vascular disease.[44] Elevated homocysteine levels correlate with decreased performance on cognitive tests, but there remains insufficient evidence of a benefit of B vitamin supplementation (B_6, B_{12}, and folic acid) on cognitive function in patients with AD.[81] Reducing the risk for developing brain vascular disease may also be an important strategy in reducing the risk for developing AD. The Alzheimer's Association's Maintain Your Brain campaign is designed to increase awareness of the importance of brain health as a part of healthy aging and recommends staying physically, mentally, and socially active; adopting a low-fat, low-cholesterol diet rich in dark vegetables and fruit; and managing body weight, blood pressure, cholesterol, and blood sugar to reduce the risk of heart disease, stroke, and diabetes.[4] Appropriate management of vascular disease risk factors may reduce the risk for developing AD and may prevent the worsening of dementia in patients with AD.

Other Potential Treatment Approaches

Estrogen Estrogen replacement has been studied extensively for the treatment and prevention for AD. Most, but not all, epidemiologic studies show a lower incidence of AD in women who took estrogen replacement therapy postmenopausally. Results from these epidemiologic surveys prompted researchers to look at the use of estrogen preventively and as a treatment for cognitive decline.

Recent clinical trials have not supported the use of estrogen as a treatment for cognitive decline. Two studies evaluating the potential benefit of conjugated estrogens as a treatment for cognitive decline did not show any benefit;[82,83] behavioral and functional outcomes were not improved either. Conflicting data exist regarding the risk of AD in women who take estrogen replacement therapy. There is clinical evidence that loss of estrogen after menopause is associated with subclinical impairment in some aspects of neuropsychological function. The Women's Health Initiative Memory Study[83] was designed to evaluate the incidence of dementia and mild cognitive impairment in patients taking estrogen plus progestin versus placebo. The number of probable dementia cases in the estrogen plus progestin group was almost double that of the placebo group. The estrogen-alone trial of the Women's Health Initiative was terminated because of an increased risk of stroke and the lack of a significant effect on other cardiovascular disease outcomes. The trial did, however, suggest that estrogen initiated in the late postmenopausal period does not improve global cognitive function and may even adversely affect this outcome. These studies do not support a role for estrogen in treating symptoms of AD.

Antiinflammatory Agents Epidemiologic studies suggest a protective effect against AD in patients who have taken NSAIDs.[84–86] Treatment for less than 2 years is associated with a lower relative risk of AD; however, longer treatment duration lowered this risk further.[85,86]

The benefits of antiinflammatory agents on cognition have been less compelling in clinical studies. Indomethacin, prednisone, and diclofenac/misoprostol administration have had no cognitive benefit in AD patients.[87–89] Tolerability was also problematic.[87,88] Additionally, prednisone treatment was associated with worsening behavioral symptoms,[88] and data from other patient populations suggest that prednisone may be associated with cognitive impairment.[90] Because there is a lack of compelling data and also a significant incidence of adverse effects, particularly gastritis and the possibility of gastrointestinal bleeds, NSAIDs and prednisone are not recommended for general use in the treatment or prevention of AD at the present time.

Recent attention has shifted to the potential benefit of the cyclooxygenase-2 inhibitors in light of their antiinflammatory properties. Rofecoxib has been compared to naproxen and placebo with no demonstrated cognitive benefit after 1 year.[91] Until clinical trials establish benefit of the cyclooxygenase-2 inhibitors, their general use as preventive treatment for AD cannot be recommended. Market withdrawal of rofecoxib and other safety concerns within this class may limit further study in AD.

Lipid-Lowering Agents Interest in the potential protective effects in AD patients of lipid-lowering agents, particularly the 3-hydroxy-3-methylglutaryl-coenzyme A-reductase inhibitors, is growing. Longitudinal epidemiologic studies suggest an association between elevated midlife total cholesterol levels and AD.[92,93] Other studies note that the incidence of AD is lower in patients who have taken either a statin[94,95] or another lipid-lowering agent,[96] but not in patients who were taking other cardiovascular medications.[95] Interestingly, pravastatin and lovastatin, but not simvastatin, were associated with a lower prevalence of AD,[95] suggesting that individual agents rather than a class effect impact AD prevalence. Although these studies have linked cholesterol levels to increased risk of AD, others have yielded conflicting results.[97]

Prospective clinical trials will need to address the cognitive benefit, duration of treatment, class effect versus effectiveness of individual agents, and optimal dosing. Simvastatin has been studied in one clinical trial showing a reduction in βAP in patients with milder AD, but not in those with severe illness.[98] Mixed results were also seen in cognitive outcomes.[98] Atorvastatin is currently being studied in clinical trials. Further studies, including randomized prospective statin trials, are needed to determine cholesterol's role, if any, in the pathogenesis of AD.

Interestingly, cognitive impairment has been recognized as a rare adverse event associated with statin therapy. The extent of cognitive impairment may depend on the lipid solubility of the drug, regulating the amount of drug that is able to cross the blood–brain barrier. As simvastatin and lovastatin have the highest lipophilicity, they may be the most likely candidates to cause memory impairment.[99] More research is needed to understand the complex relationship between cholesterol, statin therapy, and cognitive functioning. For now these agents should be reserved for patients who have other indications for their use.[44]

CLINICAL CONTROVERSY

The antioxidant vitamin E has been proposed as a treatment for AD because of the association of oxygen free radicals with AD, although few studies have documented benefits of treatment. Because of its potential effectiveness, tolerability, and low cost, some clinicians recommend the addition of vitamin E to other therapies for AD. Treatment guidelines from the American Psychiatric Association and the American Academy of Neurology recommend consideration of high-dose vitamin E (e.g., 1,000 international units twice daily) as a treatment option. However, recent findings suggest that vitamin E in high doses is associated with increased mortality in older people.[100] Many clinicians feel that there is insufficient evidence to broadly recommend this as an additive treatment.

Dietary Supplements

Vitamin E Based on pathophysiologic theories involving oxidative stress and the accumulation of free radicals in AD, significant interest has evolved regarding the use of antioxidants in the treatment of AD. Vitamin E is often recommended as adjunctive treatment for AD patients. This recommendation is based on data from the only published clinical trial to date, which evaluated the time to critical end points (i.e., death, institutionalization, loss of ability to perform activities of daily living, or severe dementia) in patients treated with vitamin E, selegiline, the combination, or placebo.[101] Although vitamin E and selegiline were superior to placebo, this study has been criticized because of differences in baseline cognitive severity, calling the validity of the results into question. Nonetheless, vitamin E's potential effectiveness, favorable side effect profile, and low cost have perpetuated its use as adjunctive therapy.

Evidence related to vitamin E's role in prevention of AD is mixed. Epidemiologic studies in individuals without AD have yielded conflicting results, with some studies showing delay in the onset of AD in individuals taking vitamin E supplements, but others failing to find this association.[47] Some studies have also found that dietary intake of vitamin E is associated with reduced risk while others have not.[47] A 3-year study in patients with mild cognitive impairment failed to show that vitamin E had a significant effect on slowing the progression to AD.[47]

Vitamin E treatment may also be associated with risks. Side effects observed with vitamin E administration include impaired hemostasis, fatigue, nausea, diarrhea, and abdominal pain. For example, vitamin E can cause thinning of the blood if it is taken with other medications such as aspirin, ibuprofen, and/or naproxen.[101] A recent meta-analysis found that high dose vitamin E increases mortality in older patients. In light of these findings, doses above 400 international units per day should probably be avoided in patients with AD.[44]

Ginkgo Biloba Ginkgo is one of the most popular dietary supplements used in AD. Hypothesized mechanisms of action in AD include increasing blood flow, decreasing the viscosity of blood, antagonizing platelet activating factor receptors, increasing tolerance to anoxia, inhibiting monoamine oxidase, antiinfective properties, and preventing the damage of membranes caused by free radicals. Ginkgo biloba may also inhibit catecholamine-*O*-methyl transferase. The most important active ingredients include the flavonoids, the ginkgo flavone glycosides, and bioflavonoids. Most studies reporting benefit in patients with AD have studied a standardized extract, EGb 761, in doses of 120 mg per day for at least 4 to 6 weeks. The general recommendations are that if ginkgo biloba is used for dementia it should be used as soon as deterioration of cognitive functioning occurs. Therapeutic response may be noted in 2 to 3 weeks, but 12 weeks of consistent dosing may be needed to get a beneficial effect. It is recommended that doses of 120 to 240 mg of the standard leaf extract twice per day be used.[102,103]

Side effects reported in studies involving EGb 761 are rare and usually mild, and may include nausea, vomiting, diarrhea, headaches, dizziness, palpitations, restlessness, and weakness. Because EGb also has a potent antiplatelet effect, it should not be used in individuals taking anticoagulant or antiplatelet therapies, and should be used cautiously in patients taking NSAIDs.[102,103]

Even if the herbal extract is modestly effective, significant problems exist with its use. The content of herbal products is poorly standardized, and significant variation in purported active ingredient content for some herbals exists from lot to lot and between manufacturers. Until these products are better standardized and their manufacturing and stability better assured, they should be used with caution. Current practice guidelines indicate that, in general, the use of ginkgo is not recommended for AD.[44]

Huperzine A Huperzine A is an alkaloid isolated from the Chinese club moss, *Huperzia serrata.* It reversibly inhibits acetylcholinesterase and is administered orally in doses of 50 to 200 mcg two to four times daily. Clinical studies suggest that huperzine A may be promising for symptomatic treatment of Alzheimer's disease, but more studies are needed to determine its particular place in therapy. In a randomized, placebo-controlled, double-blind study, 58% of patients receiving huperzine A, 200 mcg/day for 8 weeks, had improvements in memory, cognition, and behavioral function compared to 36% who received placebo.[104] No severe side effects were noted. In a randomized, double-blind, placebo-controlled multicenter study in patients with mild to moderate AD, treatment with huperzine A at doses of 400 mcg/day for 12 weeks resulted in improvement in cognition by an average of 4.6 points assessed by ADAS-cog ($P = 0.000$), 2.7 points on the MMSE, and 1.5 points on the Alzheimer's Disease Assessment Scale–noncognition ($P = 0.008$).[104]

Although initial results suggest a potential role for huperzine A in the treatment of AD, it has not been adequately tested for this purpose. Safety issues related to long-term use and lack of careful manufacturing oversight for product purity and consistency remain a concern. Concurrent use with other available cholinesterase inhibitors should be avoided, as there is no evidence for added benefit with increasing cholinesterase inhibitor exposure beyond recommended maintenance doses, but the risk of adverse events increases with dose.

Drugs in Development

Current drug development strategies fall broadly into one of two categories. The first category includes treatments specifically designed to reduce the burden of brain βAP. The second category includes all other strategies.

To reduce brain amyloid levels, approaches to both reducing βAP production and enhancing its removal are undergoing evaluation. βAP is produced through enzymatic processing of APP by two enzyme complexes, the β- and γ-secretases. β-Secretase inhibitors are in phase II human trials. Agents that specifically inhibit γ-secretase could prove problematic from a side-effect perspective, as γ-secretase is also critical for processing Notch3, a protein of developmental importance and perhaps brain maintenance. Certain NSAIDs (ibuprofen and flurbiprofen) influence the γ-secretase but do not inhibit it outright. In general, these NSAIDs alter where γ-secretase cuts the APP protein. An enantiomer of flurbiprofen, R-flurbiprofen, recently completed a phase II human trial and is slated for a phase III efficacy trial.

Immunotherapy approaches have been studied as a way to enhance βAP removal. The most extensive investigation involved AN1792, a βAP-based vaccine. This vaccine first showed efficacy in transgenic mice that produce human βAP. In vaccinated mice, brain βAP loads were reduced, there was preservation of cognitive abilities, and the vaccine was well tolerated.[105] A phase II trial in humans was prematurely halted after a substantial percentage of those mounting a robust immune response to the vaccine experienced encephalitis, a potentially life-threatening brain inflammation. Individuals in this study who were vaccinated, developed a robust immune response, and did not develop encephalitis, as well as those in the trial's placebo group, received ongoing clinical followup. One-year postvaccination neuropsychological data[76] showed that subjects in both of these groups continued to decline, although trends toward lesser decline in the vaccination group were identified. Brain histopathology from vaccinated subjects who subsequently died, demonstrated clear reductions in brain parenchyma βAP.[106–108] In summary, available clinical data are inconclusive but indicate that, over a 1-year period, activating the immune system to remove βAP does not have a robust impact on cognition. The next generation of amyloid clearance therapy is currently under development. This generation includes modifications of the active immunization approach that, hopefully, will not trigger encephalitis. Passive immunization approaches via antibody infusions are also under investigation. The use of unique βAP antibodies is being explored. The usefulness of treating AD subjects with intravenous immunoglobulin preparations, which naturally contain antibodies to βAP, is being evaluated in an open-label study.

The second category of AD treatment development includes efforts not specifically intended to reduce brain βAP levels. Neuroscientists are unraveling intracellular pathways involved in cell information processing, and drugs that can modulate these pathways are under development. Drugs that retard neurofibrillary tangle formation in mice expressing mutant human tau transgenes, such as valproic acid, are being tested in humans. The thiazolidinedione drugs rosiglitazone and pioglitazone, which reduce insulin resistance and which may also have antiinflammatory effects, are undergoing testing in humans with AD. One small open-label trial has involved intracranial implantation of fibroblasts engineered to produce neurotrophic factors.[109]

Obviously, successful development of new AD treatments depends on elucidating AD's true underlying pathophysiology. If AD is a primary amyloidosis, as is postulated by the amyloid cascade hypothesis, then reducing βAP would seem a rational way to proceed with drug development. If AD is not a primary amyloidosis, then the impact antiamyloid therapies have on the disease will be limited at best. Moreover, if AD is not a primary amyloidosis, the usefulness of βAP-overproducing transgenic animals for preclinical drug testing is called into question. Finally, at genetic and epidemiologic levels it is now possible to define several different Alzheimer's "diseases." It is not unreasonable to consider whether treatments useful in one type of AD may not benefit patients with another type.

■ PHARMACOTHERAPY OF NONCOGNITIVE SYMPTOMS

The majority of patients with AD manifest noncognitive symptoms at some point in the illness.[67] These symptoms can be roughly divided into three categories: psychotic symptoms, inappropriate or disruptive behavior, and depression. Effective management of these problems is important because behavioral symptoms are distressing to both the patient and the caregiver, necessitate increased caregiver supervision and patience, and are a leading reason for nursing home placement. In fact, presence of neuropsychiatric symptoms increases caregiver burden more than loss of cognition or self-care.

⑩ Strategies for treatment of psychotic or behavioral symptoms should include environmental interventions first, then pharmacologic interventions if warranted. The need for medications may exist when neuropsychiatric symptoms are of sufficient severity to cause significant distress to the patient or caregiver, interfere with function or cause disability, impede delivery of necessary care, or pose a danger to self or others.[44] The balance between risks of the medication and expected benefits must be acceptable to the patient or surrogate decision maker. Medications should be used cautiously, with adequate monitoring for efficacy and adverse events.

Despite the high prevalence of noncognitive symptoms in AD, little research has been conducted in these patients. Data from clinical trials of antidepressants, cholinesterase inhibitors, and antipsychotics are now emerging, but clearly more research is needed. Because of limited clinical data, treatment is primarily empiric, with side-effect profiles used as a guide in selecting the appropriate treatment. Psychotropic medications with anticholinergic effects should be avoided because they may actually worsen cognition and interfere with cholinesterase inhibitor therapy. Other side effects in the elderly include sedation, medication-induced postural instability, and extrapyramidal side effects, which can decrease the clinical usefulness of traditional psychotropic agents.

General guidelines governing therapy can be summarized as follows: use reduced doses, monitor closely, titrate dosage slowly, and document carefully. Caregivers often have erroneous expectations regarding the effects of psychotropic medications, and the anticipated benefits and risks of therapy should be clearly explained. Disruptive behaviors and delusions wax and wane with disease progression. Attempts to slowly taper and discontinue antipsychotic medication should be undertaken regularly in minimally symptomatic patients, because some patients improve on medication withdrawal.[44] Table 67–7 outlines suggested doses of medications.

TABLE 67-7 Medications Used for Noncognitive Symptoms of Dementia

Drugs	Starting Dose (mg)	Maintenance Dose in Dementia (mg/day)	Target Symptoms
Antipsychotics			Psychosis: hallucinations, delusions, suspiciousness
Haloperidol	0.25	1–3	
Olanzapine	2.5	5–10	Disruptive behaviors: agitation, aggression
Quetiapine	25	100–300	
Risperidone	0.25	0.75–2	
Ziprasidone	20	40–160	
Antidepressants			Depression: poor appetite, insomnia, hopelessness, anhedonia, withdrawal, suicidal thoughts, agitation, anxiety
Citalopram	10	10–20	
Escitalopram	5	20–40	
Fluoxetine	5	10–40	
Paroxetine	10	10–40	
Sertraline	25	75–100	
Venlafaxine	25	75–225	
Trazodone	25	75–150	
Anticonvulsants			Agitation or aggression
Carbamazepine	100	200–600	
Valproic Acid	125	500–1,000	

Data from Lleó et al.,[47] Benoit et al.,[67] and Grossberg and Desai.[118]

CLINICAL CONTROVERSY

Antipsychotic medications have been widely used to treat disruptive behaviors and psychosis in AD patients, although the evidence supporting their modest benefit for some symptoms is limited.[110] Use of antipsychotics to treat severe neuropsychiatric symptoms in AD remains controversial. Recent studies indicate that atypical and typical antipsychotics have been associated with infrequent but serious adverse events, including a small increased risk of death.[44] These findings resulted in a Food and Drug Administration-mandated "black box warning" concerning the use of atypical antipsychotics in the treatment of AD. Careful consideration of risk versus benefit in individual patients is warranted.

Cholinesterase Inhibitors and Memantine

Clinical trials with cholinesterase inhibitors have consistently reported modest benefit in managing neuropsychiatric symptoms, although these are generally not the primary outcomes studied in the trials. In a prospective, randomized, placebo-controlled trial, donepezil significantly improved behavioral symptoms of AD for at least 3 months. Evidence suggests that galantamine and rivastigmine have similar effects.[66] Memantine shows significant behavioral benefits for at least 6 months, either alone or in combination with cholinesterase inhibitors.[66] These treatments can provide modest short-term improvement and possibly slow the development and progression of behavioral symptoms. Cholinesterase inhibitors also have a small beneficial effect on caregiver burden and active time use among caregivers of persons with AD.[111] These benefits should be considered along with cognitive benefits in treatment decisions. Long-term effects on behavior have not been demonstrated to date, and further research is needed. Cholinesterase inhibitors and memantine can be considered as first-line therapy in the early management of behavioral symptoms in AD.[112]

Antipsychotics

Antipsychotics are widely used in the management of neuropsychiatric symptoms in AD. There is modestly convincing evidence that most of the atypical antipsychotics provide some benefit for particular neuropsychiatric symptoms, but these data have been insufficient to gain a Food and Drug Administration approval as an indication for the management of behavioral symptoms in AD. Based on a recent meta-analysis, only 17% to 18% of dementia patients show a treatment response to atypical antipsychotics.[113] In a double-blind, placebo-controlled trial of 421 outpatients with AD and psychosis, aggression, or agitation randomized to receive olanzapine, quetiapine, risperidone, or placebo for up to 36 weeks, there were no significant differences among the treatments in time to discontinuation of treatment or improvement in the Clinical Global Impression of Change scale. The investigators concluded that adverse effects offset advantages in the efficacy of atypical antipsychotic drugs for treatment of psychosis, aggression, or agitation in patients with AD.[113] Adverse events are common with atypical and typical antipsychotics in patients with AD. These adverse events associated with atypical antipsychotics include somnolence, extrapyramidal symptoms, abnormal gait, worsening cognition, cerebrovascular events, and increased risk of death.[110] Typical antipsychotics may also be associated with a small increased risk of death, as well as more severe extrapyramidal effects and hypotension. Chapter 70 has a more detailed discussion of antipsychotic adverse events. Overall, there is a modest expectation of treatment benefit and potential for significant harm associated with antipsychotic use in patients with AD. Individual risk and benefit must be considered when initiating therapy. Diligent monitoring during treatment is essential along with frequent reassessment of continued need.

Antidepressants

Depressive symptoms are common in patients with AD, occurring in as many as 50% of patients.[47] Apathy may be even more frequent, but these symptoms may be difficult to distinguish in patients with dementia. Many trials have studied the efficacy of antidepressants in treating depression in patients with AD, but the results are conflicting. Small sample size, short duration of treatment, and differing measures of therapy outcomes limit comparison across studies and may account in part for conflicting study results.[47] Improvement in patients receiving placebo are also common. In practice, treatment with selective serotonin reuptake inhibitors (SSRIs) is initiated most commonly in patients with AD, based on side-effect profile and evidence of efficacy. Benefit has been shown with sertraline, citalopram, fluoxetine, and paroxetine,[47] although paroxetine causes more anticholinergic effects than other SSRIs. Serotonin/norepinephrine reuptake inhibitors such as venlafaxine may be an alternative.[114] Serotonergic function may also play a role in some of the other behavioral symptoms of AD, and some studies support the use of SSRIs in the management of these behaviors, even in the absence of depression.[71] Tricyclic antidepressants have efficacy similar to the SSRIs, but should generally be avoided because of their anticholinergic activity. There is little evidence for the use of trazodone to manage behavioral or depressive symptoms, but it is commonly recommended to treat insomnia in patients with AD.[71]

Chapter 71 has a more complete discussion of treatment of depression.

Miscellaneous Therapies

Because antipsychotic and antidepressant therapy has shown only modest efficacy and poses a risk of undesirable side effects, medications traditionally used to treat disruptive behaviors and aggression in other psychiatric and neurologic disorders have been suggested as potential alternatives. These alternatives include benzodiazepines, buspirone, selegiline, carbamazepine, and valproic acid.

Benzodiazepines, particularly oxazepam, have been used to treat anxiety, agitation, and aggression, but they generally show inferior efficacy when compared to antipsychotics. Because benzodiazepines impair cognition, can result in disinhibition, and may increase the risk of falls in AD patients, their routine use is not advised.[34] "Mood stabilizer" anticonvulsants such as carbamazepine or valproic acid may be appropriate alternatives, but evidence is conflicting.[112] Clearly, more rigorous placebo-controlled studies are needed to determine the relative efficacy and place in therapy for these medication alternatives.

Noncognitive symptoms are often the most difficult aspect of AD for the caregiver. Selected antipsychotics and antidepressants have been useful for effective management of behavioral, psychotic, and depressive symptoms, thereby easing caregiver burden and allowing the patient to spend additional time at home. Alternative treatments are available in case initial choices are not successful. Adverse events remain an important concern in this population.

PHARMACOECONOMIC CONSIDERATIONS

The economic and social costs of AD are staggering. It is the third most expensive illness in the United States after heart disease and cancer, and the majority of medical and caregiving expenses are left to the patients' families and to government programs (state and federal). The total national cost of AD is estimated at approximately $100 billion annually.[4] In 2005, annual Medicare costs were estimated at $91 billion and Medicaid costs for institutionalized AD patients were estimated at $21 billion.[4] With life expectancy and the number of AD cases increasing, the cost of AD is projected to quadruple over the next 50 years.[4] The potential financial burden of this disease on the healthcare system could reach crisis proportions in the near future unless more effective avenues are developed to provide care for these individuals, to prevent the disease from occurring, or to slow its progression.

Seventy-five percent of care for AD patients is provided by family and friends.[4] Lifetime cost of care for AD is estimated at $174,000.[4] Higher levels of home care have been associated with poorer health and higher rates of emotional stress in caregivers, increasing the likelihood of placing patients in institutionalized care, which is considered the greatest financial cost in treating patients with AD.[4] On average, the cost of yearly nursing home care is $42,000, but exceeds $70,000 per year in some areas of the country.[4] Clearly, the greatest economic burden for the home-living AD patient is the time spent in caring for the patient, whereas in the nursing home the burden is the cost for others to provide care.

Economic data on the cost benefit of medications in AD are growing. Few studies provide prospective cost data from randomized controlled trials, and the data that does exist is for relatively short durations of therapy. Two clinical trials suggest that there is no benefit or disadvantage of donepezil compared to placebo in the cost of healthcare resource use.[69] There are no similar data for galantamine or rivastigmine. One cost analysis trial of memantine found that there was a trade-off between lower costs borne by the caregiver during treatment and higher drug costs borne by the patient.[70] Cost-effectiveness would be established if medications were shown to reduce the cost of care, particularly institutional care, but current randomized controlled trials have not been of sufficient duration to establish this.[69] Most estimates of cost related to AD therapy are based on pharmacoeconomic models involving extrapolation of results from short-term trials, epidemiologic data, and data on resource use in various healthcare delivery models.[115] Each analysis employs different assumptions and incorporates different aspects of cost, making comparisons across analyses difficult. Until long-term data are available, the true cost benefit of various treatment approaches remains unknown.

⓫ Data from current pharmacoeconomic studies in AD suggest that medication therapy may reduce costs of treating this illness;

however, the true cost-effectiveness of these therapies has yet to be established. If AD treatments delay cognitive decline and time to nursing home placement, then they not only have potential economic benefit, but significant effects on the quality of life of patients and caregivers. Future studies, including prospective pharmacoeconomic trials of longer duration and more detailed cost evaluation modeling, are needed to determine the role and benefits of pharmacotherapy on AD.

EVALUATION OF THERAPEUTIC OUTCOMES

An evaluation of therapeutic outcomes in the patient with AD begins with a thorough assessment at baseline and a clear definition of therapeutic goals. Cognitive status, physical status, functional performance, mood, thought processes, and behavior all need to be evaluated before initiation of drug therapy. The clinician should interview both the patient and the caregiver to assess response to drug therapy. Because caregivers often have difficulty giving honest and frank information about their loved one's condition in the loved one's presence, it is often necessary to interview family caregivers separately. In evaluating response to cognitive agents, the clinician should ask questions about the patient's ability to perform daily functional tasks and about mood and behavior, as well as questions about memory and orientation. Objective assessments such as the MMSE for cognition assessment and the Functional Activities Questionnaire for assessment of activities of daily living, should be used to quantify changes in symptoms and function.[54]

Because target symptoms of psychiatric disorders may respond differently in demented patients, a detailed list of symptoms to be treated should be documented in the pharmacotherapy plan to aid in monitoring. These could include, for example, "striking at spouse because patient believes spouse is an impostor," "verbal threats and refusal to allow clothes to be changed," and so on, as opposed to documenting vague symptoms such as "aggression" or "delusions." To make an accurate assessment of depression, multiple symptoms (e.g., sleep, appetite, and activity and interest levels) need to be assessed in addition to the patient's stated mood.

The patient should be observed carefully for potential side effects of drug therapy. The specific side effects to be monitored and the method and frequency of monitoring should be documented. Periodic assessments for drug effectiveness, side effects, compliance, need for dosage adjustment, and change in treatment should occur at least monthly. However, patients need to be treated for an adequate duration to see a therapeutic effect from a given intervention. Because the effects of cognition-enhancing medications are not great, a treatment period of several months to a year may be necessary before it can be determined whether therapy is beneficial. Cognitive effects of the drug are often noticed only as a plateauing during treatment or as deterioration following drug discontinuation. In general, cognitive agents should be continued if the patient is demonstrating no change in clinical status. However, if there is doubt, the medication can be slowly tapered and discontinued, and the patient monitored off the drug for 4 to 6 weeks to determine the need for continued therapy.

ABBREVIATIONS

AD: Alzheimer's disease

ADAS-cog: Alzheimer's Disease Assessment Scale—Cognition

apo E: apolipoprotein E

APP: amyloid precursor protein

βAP: beta-amyloid peptide

MMSE: Mini Mental Status Examination

NFT: neurofibrillary tangle

NMDA: *N*-methyl-D-aspartate

NSAID: nonsteroidal antiinflammatory drug

SSRI: selective serotonin reuptake inhibitor

REFERENCES

1. Blennow K, deLeon MJ, Zetterberg H. Alzheimer's disease. Lancet 2006;368:387–403.
2. Desai AK, Grossberg GT. Diagnosis and treatment of Alzheimer's disease. Neurology 2005;64(Suppl 3):S34–S39.
3. Hebert LE, Scherr PA, Bienias JL, et al. Alzheimer's disease in the U.S. population: Prevalence estimates using the 2000 census. Arch Neurol 2003;60:1119–1122.
4. Alzheimer's Association. *http://www.alz.org/*.
5. Nussbaum RL, Ellis CE. Alzheimer's disease and Parkinson's disease. N Engl J Med 2003;348:1356–1364.
6. Chandra V, Bharucha NE, Schoenberg BS. Conditions associated with Alzheimer's disease at death: Case-control study. Neurology 1986;36:209–211.
7. Goedert M, Spillantini G. A century of Alzheimer's disease. Science 2006;314:777–781.
8. St George-Hyslop PH. Piecing together Alzheimer's. Sci Am 2000;283:76–83.
9. Corder EH, Saunders AM, Risch NJ, et al. Protective effect of apolipoprotein E type 2 allele for late-onset Alzheimer's disease. Nat Genet 1994;7:180–184.
10. Hsiung G, Sadovnick D, Feldman H. Apolipoprotein E4 genotype as a risk factor for cognitive decline and dementia: Data from Canadian Study of Health and Aging. CMAJ 2004;171(8).
11. Rosenberg R. The Molecular and Genetic Basis of AD. The End of the Beginning. The 2000 Wartenberg Lecture. Neurology 2000;54:2045–2054.
12. Martin JB. Molecular Basis of the Neurodegenerative Disorders. N Engl J Med 1999;340(25):1970–1979.
13. Green R, Cupples A, Go R, et al. Risk of dementia among white and African American relatives of patients with Alzheimer's disease. JAMA 2002;287(3):329–336.
14. Skoog I, Kalaria R, Breteler M. Vascular factors and Alzheimer's disease. Alzheimer's Dis Assoc Disord 1999;13(Suppl 3):S106–S114.
15. Elkins J, Douglas V, Johnston SC. Alzheimer's disease risk and genetic variation in ACE. A Meta Analysis. Neurology, 2004;62:363–368.
16. Farrer L, Sherbatich T, Kerynov S, et al. Association between angiotensin-converting enzyme and Alzheimer's disease. Arch Neurol 2000;57:210–214.
17. Jicha GA, Parisi JE, Dickson DW, et al. Alzheimer's and Lewy body pathology in centenarian case series. Neurology 2005;6(Suppl 1):A275.
18. Thomassen R, van Schaick HW, Blansjaar BA. Prevalence of dementia over age 100. Neurology 1998;50:283–286.
19. Blansjaar BA, Thomassen R, Van Schaick HW. Prevalence of dementia in centenarians. Int J Geriatr Psychiatry 2000;15:219–225.
20. Evans DA, Funkenstein HH, Albert MS, et al. Prevalence of Alzheimer's disease in a community population of older persons. Higher than previously reported. JAMA 1989;262:2551–2556.
21. Snowdon DA, Kemper SJ, Mortimer JA, et al. Linguistic ability in early life and cognitive function and Alzheimer's disease in late life. Findings from the Nun Study. JAMA, 1996;275:528–532.
22. Smyth KA, Fritsch T, Cook TB, et al. Worker functions and traits associated with occupations and the development of AD. Neurology 2004;63:498–503.
23. Swerdlow RH. Is aging part of Alzheimer's disease, or is Alzheimer's disease part of aging? Neurobiol Aging 2007;28:1465–1480.
24. Zheng H, Jiang M, Trumbauer ME, et al. β-amyloid precursor protein-deficient mice show reactive gliosis and decreased locomotor activity. Cell 1995;81:525–531.
25. Goate A, Chartier-Harlin MC, Mullan M, et al. Segregation of a missense mutation in the amyloid precursor protein gene with familial Alzheimer's disease. Nature 1991;349:704–706.
26. Hardy J, Allsop D. Amyloid deposition as the central event in the aetiology of Alzheimer's disease. Trends Pharmacol Sci 1991;12:383–388.

27. Hardy JA, Higgins GA. Alzheimer's disease: The amyloid cascade hypothesis. Science 1992;256:184–185.
28. Levy-Lahad E, Wasco W, Poorkaj P, et al. Candidate gene for the chromosome 1 familial Alzheimer's disease locus. Science 1995;269:973–977.
29. Sherrington R, Rogaeva EI, Liang Y, et al. Cloning of a gene bearing missense mutations in early-onset familial Alzheimer's disease. Nature 1995;375:754–760.
30. Wolfe WT, Xia W, Ostaszewski BL, et al. Two transmembrane aspartates in presenilin-1 required for presenilin endoproteolysis and γ-secretase activity. Nature 1999;398:513–517.
31. Kimberly WT, Xia W, Rahmatic J, et al. The transmembrane aspartates in presenilin 1 and 2 are obligatory for γ-secretase activity and amyloid β-protein generation. J Biol Chem 2000;275:3173–3178.
32. Lesne S, Kotilinek L. Amyloid plaques and amyloid-β oligomers: An ongoing debate. J Neurosci 2005;25:9319–9320.
33. Walsh DM, Klyubin I, Shankar GM, et al. The role of cell-derived oligomers of Abeta in Alzheimer's disease and avenues for therapeutic intervention. Biochem Soc Trans 2005;33:1087–1090.
34. Reynolds J, Mintzer J. Alzheimer's disease update: New targets, new options. Drug Benefit Trends 2005:17(2)83–88, 91–95.
35. McGeer PL, Kawamata T, Walker DG, et al. Microglia in degenerative neurological disease. Glia 1993;7:84–92.
36. Sastre M, Klockgether T, Heneka MT. Contribution of inflammatory processes to Alzheimer's disease: Molecular mechanisms. Int J Dev Neurosci 2006;24:167–176.
37. Mrak RE, Griffen WST. Potential inflammatory biomarkers in Alzheimer's disease. J Alzheimers Dis 2005;8:369–375.
38. McGeer PL, Schulzer M, McGeer EG. Arthritis and anti-inflammatory agents as possible protective factors for Alzheimer's disease: A review of 17 epidemiologic studies. Neurology 1996;47:425–432.
39. Rich JB, Rasmusson DX, Folstein MF, et al. Nonsteroidal anti-inflammatory drugs in Alzheimer's disease. Neurology 1995;45:51–55.
40. Aisen PS, Schafer KA, Grundman M, et al. Effects of rofecoxib or naproxen vs placebo on Alzheimer's disease progression: A randomized controlled trial. JAMA 2003;289:2819–2826.
41. Breitner JCS, Zandi PP. Do nonsteroidal anti-inflammatory drugs reduce the risk of Alzheimer's disease? N Engl J Med 2001;345:1567–1568.
42. Wenk GL. Neuropathologic changes in Alzheimer's disease. J Clin Psychiatry 2003;64(Suppl 9):7–10.
43. Stampfer MJ. Cardiovascular disease and Alzheimer's disease: Common links. J Intern Med 2006;260:211–223.
44. Lyketsos CG, Colenda CC, Beck C, et al. Position statement of the American Association for Geriatric Psychiatry regarding principles of care for patients with dementia resulting from Alzheimer's disease. Am J Geriatr Psychiatry 2006;14:561–573.
45. Papademetriou V. Hypertension and cognitive function. Blood pressure regulation and cognitive function: A review of the literature. Geriatrics 2005;60:20–22,24.
46. Biessels GJ, Kappelle LJ. Increased risk of Alzheimer's disease in Type II diabetes: Insulin resistance of the brain or insulin-induced amyloid pathology. Biochem Soc Trans 2005;33:1041–1044.
47. Lleó A, Greenberg SM, Growdon JH. Current pharmacotherapy for Alzheimer's disease. Annu Rev Med 2006;57:513–533.
48. Czlonkowska A, Ciesielska A, Joniec I. Influence of estrogens on neurodegenerative processes. Med Sci Monit 2003;9:RA247–RA256.
49. Simpkins JW, Singh M, Bishop J. The potential role for estrogen replacement therapy in the treatment of the cognitive decline and neurodegeneration associated with Alzheimer's disease. Neurobiol Aging 1994;15:S195–S197.
50. Mohs RC, Haroutunian V. Alzheimer's disease: From earliest symptoms to end stage. In: Davis KL, Charney D, Coyle JT, Nemeroff C, eds. Neuropsychopharmacology: The Fifth Generation of Progress. New York: Lippincott Williams & Wilkins, 2002:1189–1198.
51. Boustani M, Peterson B, Hanson L, et al. Screening for dementia in primary care: A summary of the evidence for the U.S. Preventive Services Task Force. Ann Intern Med 2003;138:927–937.
52. Solomon PR, Murphy CA. Should we screen for Alzheimer's disease? A review of the evidence for and against screening for Alzheimer's disease in primary care practice. Geriatrics 2005;60:26–31.
53. American Psychiatric Association. Diagnostic and Statistical Manual of Mental Disorders, 4th Edition Text Revision. Washington, DC: American Psychiatric Press, 2000.
54. Costa PT Jr, Williams TF, Somerfield M, et al. Early Identification of Alzheimer's Disease and Related Dementias. Clinical Practice Guidelines, Quick Reference Guide for Clinicians, No. 19. Rockville, MD: US Department of Health and Human Services, Public Health Service, Agency for Health Care Policy and Research, 1996.
55. Knopman DS, DeKosky ST, Cummings JL, et al. Practice parameter: Diagnosis of dementia (an evidence-based review): Report of the Quality Standards Subcommittee of the American Academy of Neurology. Neurology 2001;56:1143–1153.
56. Roman GC, Tatemichi TK, Erkinjuntti T, et al. Vascular dementia: Diagnostic criteria for research studies. Report of the NINDS-AIREN international workshop. Neurology 1993;43:250–260.
57. McKhann G, Drachman D, Folstein M, et al. Mental and clinical diagnosis of Alzheimer's disease: Report of the NINCDS-ADRDA Work Group under the auspices of the Department of Health and Human Services Task Force on Alzheimer's disease. Neurology 1984;34:939–944.
58. Fillenbaum GG, Peterson B, Morris JC. Estimating the validity of the Clinical Dementia Rating Scale: The CERAD experience. Consortium to Establish a Registry for Alzheimer's Disease. Aging 1996;8:379–385.
59. Moore AR, O'Keeffe ST. Drug-induced cognitive impairment in the elderly. Drugs Aging 1999;15:15–28.
60. Salmon E, Sadzot B, Maquet P, et al. Differential diagnosis of Alzheimer's disease with PET. J Nucl Med 1994;35:391–398.
61. Petersen RC, Smith GE, Ivnik RJ, et al. Apolipoprotein E status as a predictor of the development of Alzheimer's disease in memory-impaired individuals. JAMA 1995;273:1274–1278.
62. Mayeux R, Saunders AM, Shea S, et al. Utility of the apolipoprotein E genotype in the diagnosis of Alzheimer's disease. Alzheimer's Disease Centers Consortium on Apolipoprotein E and Alzheimer's Disease. N Engl J Med 1998;338:506–511.
63. Petersen RC, Doody R, Kurz A, et al. Current concepts in mild cognitive impairment. Arch Neurol 2001;58:1985–1992.
64. Morris JC. Mild cognitive impairment is early-stage Alzheimer's disease: Time to revise diagnostic criteria. Arch Neurol 2006;63:15–16.
65. Winblad B, Palmer K, Kivipelto M, et al. Mild cognitive impairment—Beyond controversies, towards a consensus: Report of the International Working Group on Mild Cognitive Impairment. J Intern Med 2004;256:240–246.
66. Geldmacher DS, Frolich L, Doody RS, et al. Realistic expectations for treatment success in Alzheimer's disease. J Nutr Health Aging 2006;10:417–429.
67. Benoit M, Arbus C, Blanchard F, et al. Professional consensus on the treatment of agitation, aggressive behaviour, oppositional behaviour and psychotic disturbances in dementia. J Nutr Health Aging 2006;10:410–415.
68. Doody RS, Stevens JC, Beck C, et al. Practice parameter: Management of dementia (an evidence-based review). Neurology 2001;56:1154–1166.
69. Birks J. Cholinesterase inhibitors for Alzheimer's disease. Cochrane Database Syst Rev 2006;1:CD005593.
70. McShane R, Areosa Sastre A, Minakaran N. Memantine for dementia. Cochrane Database Syst Rev 2006;2:CD003154.
71. Rubin CD. The primary care of Alzheimer's disease. Am J Med Sci 2006;332:314–333.
72. Namenda (memantine hydrochloride) package insert. St. Louis, MO: Forest Laboratories, 2005.
73. "Memantine." Geriatric Lexi-Drugs Online. Lexi-Comp. *http://www.crlonline.com/crlonline.*
74. Tariot PN, Farlow MR, Grossberg GT, et al. Memantine treatment in patients with moderate to severe Alzheimer's disease already receiving donepezil: A randomized controlled trial. JAMA 2004;291:317–324.
75. Cummings JL, Schneier E, Tariot PN, et al. Behavioral effects of memantine in Alzheimer's disease patients receiving donepezil treatment. Neurology 2006;67:57–63.
76. Gilman S, Koller M, Black RS, et al. Clinical effects of Abeta immunization (AN1792) in patients with AD in an interrupted trial. Neurology 2005;64:1553–1562.
77. Rogers SL, Doody RS, Pratt RD, Ieni JR. Long-term efficacy and safety of donepezil in the treatment of Alzheimer's disease: Final analysis of a US multicentre open-label study. Eur Neuropsychopharmacol 2000;10(3):195–203.
78. Raskind MA, Peskind ER, Truyen L, et al. The cognitive benefits of galantamine are sustained for at least 36 months: A long-term extension trial. Arch Neurol 2004;61:252–256.

79. Farlow MR, Lilly ML; ENA713 B352 Study Group. Rivastigmine: An open-label, observational study of safety and effectiveness in treating patients with Alzheimer's disease for up to 5 years. BMC Geriatr 2005;5:3.
80. Reisberg B, Doody R, Stoffler A, et al. A 24-week open-label extension study of memantine in moderate to severe Alzheimer's disease. Arch Neurol 2006;63:49–54.
81. Balk EM, Raman G, Tatsioni A, et al. Vitamin B_6 B_{12} and folic acid supplementation and cognitive function. A systematic review of randomized trials. Arch Intern Med 2007;167:21–30.
82. Mulnard RA, Cotman CW, Kawas C, et al. Estrogen replacement therapy for treatment of mild to moderate Alzheimer's disease: A randomized controlled trial. JAMA 2000;283:1007–1015.
83. Writing Group for the Women's Health Initiative Investigators. Risks and benefits of estrogen plus progestin in healthy postmenopausal women. JAMA 2002;288:321–333.
84. McGeer PL, Schulzer M, McGeer EG. Arthritis and anti-inflammatory agents as possible protective factors for Alzheimer's disease: A review of 17 epidemiologic studies. Neurology 1996;47:425–432.
85. Stewart WF, Kawas C, Corrada M. Risk of Alzheimer's disease and duration of NSAID use. Neurology 1997;48:626–632.
86. Etminan M, Gill S, Samii A. Effect of non-steroidal anti-inflammatory drugs on risk of Alzheimer's disease: Systematic review and meta-analysis of observational studies. BMJ 2003;327:128–132.
87. Rogers J, Kirby LC, Hempelman SR, et al. Clinical trial of indomethacin in Alzheimer's disease. Neurology 1993;43:1609–1611.
88. Aisen PS, Davis KL, Berg JD, et al. A randomized controlled trial of prednisone in Alzheimer's disease. Neurology 2000;54:588–593.
89. Scharf S, Mander A, Ugoni A, et al. A double-blind, placebo-controlled trial of diclofenac/misoprostol in Alzheimer's disease. Neurology 1999;53:197–201.
90. Schmidt LA, Fox NA, Goldberg MC. Effects of acute prednisone administration on memory, attention and emotion in healthy human adults. Psychoneuroendocrinology 1999;24:461–483.
91. Aisen PS, Schafer KA, Grundman M, et al. Effects of rofecoxib or naproxen vs placebo on Alzheimer's disease progression. JAMA 2003;289:2819–2826.
92. Notkola IL, Sulkava R, Pekkanen J, et al. Serum total cholesterol, apolipoprotein E4 allele, and Alzheimer's disease. Neuroepidemiology 1998;17:14–20.
93. Kivipelto M, Helkala EL, Laasko MP, et al. Midlife vascular risk factors and Alzheimer's disease in later life: Longitudinal population based study. BMJ 2001;322:1447–1451.
94. Jick H, Zornberg GL, Jick SS, et al. Statins and the risk of dementia. Lancet 2000;356:1627–1631.
95. Wolozin B, Kellman W, Rousseau P, et al. Decreased prevalence of Alzheimer's disease associated with 3-hydroxy-3-methyglutaryl coenzyme A reductase inhibitors. Arch Neurol 2000;57:1439–1443.
96. Rockwood K, Kirkland S, Hogan D, et al. Use of lipid-lowering agents, indication bias, and the risk of dementia in community-dwelling elderly people. Arch Neurol 2002;59:223–227.
97. Tan ZS, Seshadri S, Beiser A, et al. Plasma total cholesterol levels as a risk factor for Alzheimer's disease: The Framingham study. Arch Intern Med 2003;163:1053–1057.
98. Cooper JL. Dietary lipids in the aetiology of Alzheimer's disease. Drugs Aging 2003;20:399–418.
99. Wagstaff L, Mitton M, Mclendon B, et al. Statin-associated memory loss: Analysis of 60 case reports and review of the literature. Pharmacotherapy, 2003;23(7):871–880.
100. Miller ER III, Pastor-Barriuso R, Dalal D, et al. Meta-analysis: High-dosage vitamin E supplementation may increase all-cause mortality. Ann Intern Med 2005;142:37–46.
101. Sano M, Ernesto C, Thomas RG, et al. A controlled trial of selegiline, α-tocopherol, or both as treatment for Alzheimer's disease. N Engl J Med 1997;336:1216–1222.
102. Marcolina S. The use of ginkgo biloba for Alzheimer's dementia. Alternative Medicine Alert 2006;9(6):61–72.
103. Massey A. Effectiveness of ginkgo biloba in memory disorders. J Pharm Prac 1999;12(3):217–224.
104. Diamond BJ, Johnson SK, Torsney K, et al. Complementary and alternative medicines in the treatment of dementia. An evidence-based review. Drugs Aging, 2003;20:981–998.
105. Schenk D, Barbour R, Dunn W, et al. Immunization with amyloid-β attenuates Alzheimer's-disease-like pathology in the PDAPP mouse. Nature 1999;400:173–177.
106. Nicoll JA, Wilkinson D, Holmes C, et al. Neuropathology of human Alzheimer's disease after immunization with amyloid-β peptide: A case report. Nat Med 2003;9:448–452.
107. Ferrer I, Boada Rovira M, Sanchez Guerra ML, et al. Neuropathology and pathogenesis of encephalitis following amyloid-β immunization in Alzheimer's disease. Brain Pathol 2004;14:11–20.
108. Masliah E, Hansen L, Adame A, et al. Abeta vaccination effects on plaque pathology in the absence of encephalitis in Alzheimer's disease. Neurology 2005;64:129–131.
109. Tuszynski MH, Thal L, Pay M, et al. A phase 1 clinical trial of nerve growth factor gene therapy for Alzheimer's disease. Nat Med 2005;11:551–555.
110. Schneider LS, Dagerman K, Insel PS. Efficacy and adverse effects of atypical antipsychotics for dementia: Meta-analysis of randomized, placebo-controlled trials. Am J Geriatr Psychiatry 2006;14:191–210.
111. Lingler JH, Martire LM, Schulz R. Caregiver-specific outcomes in antidementia clinical drug trials: A systematic review and meta-analysis. J Am Geriatr Soc 2005;53:983–990.
112. Beier MT. Treatment strategies for the behavioral symptoms of Alzheimer's disease: Focus on early pharmacologic intervention. Pharmacotherapy 2007;27:399–411.
113. Schneider LS, Tariot PN, Dagerman KS, et al. Effectiveness of atypical antipsychotic drugs in patients with Alzheimer's disease. N Engl J Med 2006;355:1525–1538.
114. Lyketsos CG, Olin J. Depression in Alzheimer's disease: Overview and treatment. Biol Psychiatry 2002;52:243–252.
115. Fillit H, Hill J. Economics of dementia and pharmacoeconomics of dementia therapy. Am J Geriatr Pharmacother 2005;3:39–49.
116. U.S. Census Bureau. 2003,
117. Chapman DP, Williams SM, Strine TW, et al. Dementia and its implications for public health. Prev Chronic Dis [serial online] 2006, *http://www.cdc.gov/pcd/issues/2006/apr/05_0167.htm*.
118. Grossberg GT, Desai AK. Management of Alzheimer's disease. J Gerontol A Biol Sci Med Sci 2003;58A:331–353.
119. Aricept (donepezil hydrochloride) package insert. Teaneck, NJ: Eisai Co, Ltd., 2006.
120. Exelon (rivastigmine tartrate) package insert. East Hanover, NJ: Novartis Pharmaceuticals, 2006.
121. Razadyne (galantamine hydrobromide) package insert. Titusville, NJ: Ortho-McNeil Neurologics, 2006.
122. Exelon (rivastigmine) Patch package insert. East Hanover, N.J.: Novartis Pharmaceutical, 2007.

CHAPTER 68 Substance-Related Disorders: Overview and Depressants, Stimulants, and Hallucinogens

PAUL L. DOERING AND LISA A. BOOTHBY

KEY CONCEPTS

1. Problems related to abuse of chemical substances can occur acutely (e.g., respiratory arrest from using heroin) or after some length of time (e.g., dependence or withdrawal from continued use of an opiate). The treatment approach is distinctly different depending on the type of problem.
2. Withdrawal from certain classes of drugs (e.g., benzodiazepines or barbiturates) can be life-threatening, and steps must be taken to ensure that withdrawal is gradual and that it takes place in closely supervised settings.
3. Although there is much research focusing on drugs to treat the underlying addictive processes, to date the successes have been few. Whereas methadone, *levo-α*-acetylmethadol (LAAM), and now buprenorphine are used for narcotic maintenance, the logical approach at present should center on prevention. Because of their knowledge of pharmacology and the actions of drugs on the body, health professionals can play a key role in education of young people on the dangers of recreational drug use.
4. Pharmacotherapy of substance-related disorders is most often adjunctive to other modes of therapy such as counseling and intense psychotherapy.

Abuse of alcohol, tobacco, and other drugs (ATOD) is the nation's number one health problem, according to a Robert Wood Johnson healthcare report prepared by the Institute for Health Policy, Brandeis University.[1] There are more deaths, illnesses, and disabilities from substance abuse than from any other preventable health condition. The economic cost of substance abuse to the U.S. economy each year is staggering, and it is estimated to be more than $414 billion.[1] A heavy smoker will stay 25% longer when hospitalized than a nonsmoker, and a problem drinker will stay four times as long as a nondrinker.[1] According to the Robert Wood Johnson health report, "Without a reduction in ATOD abuse, healthcare costs cannot be curtailed effectively." Of the more than 2 million deaths each year in the United States, approximately one in four is attributable to alcohol, illicit drug, or tobacco use: 100,000 people die as a result of alcohol, 16,000 die from illicit drug use and deaths related to the acquired immune deficiency syndrome, and 430,700 from tobacco-related illnesses.

In addition, one-half to two-thirds of homicides and serious crimes involve alcohol. Nearly one-half of men arrested for homicide and assault test positive for an illegal drug.[1] ATOD abuse contributes to family problems, with one in four Americans reporting that alcohol has been a cause of trouble in the family, and alcohol abuse plays a part in one of three failed marriages.[1]

Since publication of the last edition of this textbook, a disturbing trend in drug abuse has continued: the use of medicinal drugs for nonmedicinal purposes. Between 1995 and 2002 there was a 163% increase in the number of emergency room visits tied to the abuse of prescription drugs, and these percentages continue to increase.[2] Prescription drugs now are a factor in a quarter of all overdose deaths reported in the United States. Central nervous system (CNS) agents, primarily analgesics (pain relievers), were involved in slightly less than one-half (47%) of all drug-related suicide attempts that presented to emergency departments in 2005, including both prescription and over-the-counter (OTC) formulations. More than 56% of suicide-related emergency department visits included psychotherapeutic agents (e.g., benzodiazepines or antidepressants).[3]

This chapter and the next focus on the problems associated with the abuse of chemical substances and the things clinicians can do to help deal with these problems.

Learning objectives, review questions, and other resources can be found at **www.pharmacotherapyonline.com.**

KEY DEFINITIONS

The lack of a common vocabulary in substance abuse treatment and prevention leads to several problems. Wide arrays of terms are in common use, many without precise meaning. A number of professional disciplines are involved in research, treatment, and education regarding alcohol and other drug-related problems, and each discipline tends to use its own terminology. This lack of universal agreement on language hampers effective communication among professionals and leads to difficulties in formulating public policy and administering third-party reimbursement programs. The Liaison Committee on Pain and Addiction, a collaborative effort of the American Academy of Pain Medicine, the American Pain Society, and the American Society of Addiction Medicine has developed definitions related to the use of medications for the treatment of pain that purport to be consistent with current understanding of relevant neurobiology, pharmacology, and appropriate clinical practice. The ultimate goal of their project was to achieve acceptance and use of uniform definitions by clinicians, regulators, and the public, both nationally and internationally, to promote appropriate treatment of pain throughout the world. The definitions have been approved by each of the three collaborating organizations. The following definitions resulted from this particular consensus development committee.[4]

- *Addiction* is a primary, chronic, neurobiologic disease, with genetic, psychosocial, and environmental factors influencing its development and manifestations. It is characterized by behaviors that include one or more of the following 5Cs:

chronicity, impaired control over drug use, compulsive use, continued use despite harm, and craving.

- *Drug abuse* is a maladaptive pattern of substance use characterized by repeated adverse consequences related to the repeated use of the substance. Examples include failure to fulfill important obligations at work, school, or home; repeated use creating physical danger, such as driving under the influence; legal problems; and social or interpersonal problems such as arguments and fights.
- *Physical dependence* is a state of adaptation that is manifested by a drug class–specific withdrawal syndrome that can be produced by abrupt cessation, rapid dose reduction, decreasing blood level of the drug, and/or administration of an antagonist.
- *Tolerance* is a state of adaptation in which exposure to a drug induces changes that result in a diminution of one or more of the drug's effects over time.

EPIDEMIOLOGY

NATIONAL SURVEY ON DRUG USE & HEALTH

The National Survey on Drug Use and Health (NSDUH) (formerly called the National Household Survey on Drug Abuse)[3] is the primary source of statistical information on the use of illegal drugs by the U.S. population. Conducted by the federal government since 1971, the survey collects data from a representative sample of the population at their place of residence.

In 2005, there were 19.7 million Americans (8.1% of the population ages 12 or older) who used illicit drugs, a rate similar to that observed for the last 4 years. An estimated 22.2 million Americans suffered from substance dependence or abuse because of drugs, alcohol, or both. The 2005 survey found that marijuana is the most commonly used illicit drug, used by 14.6 million Americans. The incidence has remained the same for the last 4 years. The second most popular category of drug use after marijuana is the nonmedical use of prescription drugs. An estimated 6.4 million people, 2.6% of the population 12 years of age or older, were current users of prescription drugs taken nonmedically. Of these, an estimated 4.7 million used narcotic pain relievers, 1.8 million used antianxiety medications, 1.1 million used stimulants, and 272,000 used sedatives.[3]

THE MONITORING THE FUTURE STUDY

Every year the Institute for Social Research of the University of Michigan conducts its Monitoring the Future Study (MTFS), supported under a series of research grants from the National Institute on Drug Abuse.[5] The project has many purposes. Among them is to study changes in the beliefs, attitudes, and behavior of young people in the United States. This study focuses on youth because of their significant involvement in today's social changes, and most importantly because youth in a very literal sense will constitute our future society.[5]

In 2005, 50,000 eighth, tenth, and twelfth grade students in more than 400 public and private secondary schools were surveyed. Use of a number of illicit drugs showed declines in at least one grade; these include 3,4-methylenedioxymethamphetamine (MDMA; "ecstasy"), marijuana, lysergic acid diethylamide (LSD), amphetamines, methamphetamines, steroids, androstenedione, alcohol, and cigarette smoking. Only three drugs of abuse were reported as increased in use among the teenagers surveyed in 2005; these include sedatives, oxycodone extended-release (OxyContin), and inhalants. Among twelfth graders 5% are now current daily marijuana users, down by 1% since 2003. Other interesting trends have emerged for the following drugs[5]:

- *Ecstasy.* Use of this so-called club drug continues to decline from that reported in previous years. Annual prevalence rates in 2005 are down by one-half to two-thirds in eighth, tenth, and twelfth grade compared to 2001 data.
- *Inhalants.* Inhalants, the only class of drug that tends to be more popular among younger teens than older ones, include a wide variety of common household products that youngsters inhale or "huff" in order to get high, such as glues, solvents, butane, gasoline, and aerosols. Some 20.4% of the 2005 eighth graders, 31.7% of the tenth graders, and 40.3% of twelfth graders indicated inhalant use in the prior 12 months, making inhalants the second most widely used class of illicitly used drugs for eighth graders (after marijuana), tenth graders (after alcohol), and twelfth graders (after alcohol). The annual prevalence rate among twelfth-grade students continued to rise in 2005, most likely because of the accessibility of inhalants.
- *Prescription drugs.* Both sedatives and OxyContin abuse continues to rise among twelfth graders. Sedative abuse is at its highest rate among twelfth graders since 1980 at 7.2% in 2005. OxyContin use among twelfth graders continued to increase in 2005 to an annual prevalence of 5.5%. OxyContin use among twelfth graders has increased 40% since 2002.
- *Amphetamine and methamphetamine.* Amphetamine use has continued to decline in all three grades in 2005.

SUBSTANCE ABUSE EMERGENCIES: THE DAWN PROGRAM

Since the early 1970s, the Drug Abuse Warning Network (DAWN),[6] an ongoing national survey of hospital emergency departments, has collected information on patients seeking hospital emergency department treatment related to their use of an illegal drug or the nonmedical use of a legal drug. DAWN serves as an early warning system to the ever-changing patterns of use of illegal drugs. These data allow healthcare professionals to be better prepared to react to medical emergencies arising from illegal drug use and to target prevention and education programs to specific drug-using groups or populations.

DAWN defines a *drug-related episode* as an emergency department visit that was induced by or related to the use of an illegal drug(s) or the nonmedical use of a legal drug for patients aged 6 to 97 years. In 2004, there were 1.3 million drug abuse–related emergency department episodes in the United States.[6] Cocaine-related episodes constituted nearly 30% of all emergency department drug-related episodes in 2004, more than any other illicit substance measured by DAWN. No significant changes from 2004 were evident for the club drugs ecstasy (MDMA) (8,621 mentions in 2004), γ-hydroxybutyrate (GHB) (2,340 mentions), or ketamine (227 mentions). Heroin accounted for 8% (162,137 mentions) in 2004, and amphetamines and methamphetamine combined were involved in 5% of drug abuse–related emergency department episodes. When considered together, narcotic analgesics and combinations comprised 32% of emergency department episodes estimated for the United States in 2004. From 2000 to 2002, the increase for narcotic analgesics was 45% (from 82,373), and over the 8-year period from 1995 to 2002, emergency department episodes related to narcotic analgesics and combinations increased 163% (from 45,254).

ECONOMIC IMPACT OF SUBSTANCE ABUSE

Substance abuse and addiction have an enormous impact on the economy. Over the years, the Center on Addiction and Substance Abuse (CASA) at Columbia University has conducted numerous studies aimed at quantifying the costs to local, state, and federal governments and agencies. CASA reported the results[7] of an intensive

3-year analysis of the impact of substance abuse on state budgets. They discovered that in 1998 states spent $620 billion of their own funds to operate state government and provide public services such as education, Medicaid, child welfare, mental health, and highway safety. Of this amount, a full 13.1%—$81.3 billion—went to dealing with the aftermath of substance abuse and addiction.[7] This figure does not include the financial toll such abuse extracts from federal or local spending or the private costs such as lost productivity or premature death. Each American paid $277 per year in state taxes to deal with the burden of substance abuse and addiction in their social programs and only $10 a year for prevention and treatment. Of every dollar states spend on substance abuse, 95.8 cents goes to pay for the burden of this problem on public programs. For example, untreated substance abuse increases the cost of every state's criminal justice system; elementary and secondary schools; Medicaid; child welfare, juvenile justice and mental heath systems, highways, and state payrolls. These costs totaled $77.9 billion in 1998.[7]

The majority of the substance abuse–related diseases in the Medicaid population are linked to tobacco and illicit drugs, many related to birth complications resulting from cocaine use. More than 60 Medicare ailments are attributable to ATOD abuse. The majority of the substance abuse–related diseases in the Medicare population are associated with tobacco, which accounts for 80% of these diseases. If substance abuse and addiction do not decrease, it will cost the Medicare program alone more than $1 trillion over the next 20 years.[7] Needless to say, reducing the problem of substance abuse and dependence would result in tremendous savings for local, state, and federal governments and would have a net positive impact on the quality of life of our citizens.

ACUTE VERSUS CHRONIC PROBLEMS

❶ Misuse of chemical substances causes problems of two types: those that occur acutely and those that arise after continued use of a drug. Acute problems are usually predictable, given the pharmacology of the drug. Acute drug intoxications usually occur at doses in excess of that normally taken. Chronic abuse of chemical substances can cause a wide array of physical, psychological, and psychiatric ailments. The substance-induced disorders discussed here mainly include intoxication and withdrawal. Psychiatric problems associated with substance abuse, including dementia, psychosis, mood disorders, and anxiety, are discussed elsewhere. Physical illnesses associated with chronic use of chemicals (e.g., alcoholic liver disease) are likewise covered in other chapters.

The essential feature of substance dependence is the continued use of the substance despite adverse substance-related problems. The criteria for substance dependence are the same for each of the drugs or drug classes, varying only to fit the unique pharmacologic properties of each drug. Patients who take prescribed drugs for appropriate medical indications and in correct doses may still show tolerance, physical dependence, and withdrawal symptoms if the drug is stopped abruptly rather than being tapered. Tolerance and physical dependence are inevitable consequences of chronic treatment with opioids and certain other drugs, but by themselves, tolerance and physical dependence do not imply "addiction." To meet *Diagnostic and Statistical Manual of Mental Disorders, 4th edition, Text Revision* (*DSM-IV-TR*) criteria[8] for the diagnosis of substance dependence, at least three of the following must be present at any time in a 12-month period:

1. Tolerance
2. Withdrawal, indicated by the appearance of the characteristic withdrawal syndrome or the use of the same or related drug to relieve or avoid withdrawal symptoms
3. Substance taken in larger amounts or over a longer period of time than was intended
4. Persistent desire or unsuccessful efforts to cut down or control substance use
5. Time spent in activities necessary to obtain the substance, use the substance, or recover from its effects
6. Social, occupational, or recreational activities given up or reduced because of substance use
7. Substance use continued despite knowledge of having a persistent or recurrent physical or psychologic problem caused or exacerbated by the substance

The characteristic feature of *substance abuse* is a maladaptive pattern of substance use indicated by repeated adverse consequences related to the repeated use of the substance. Examples include failure to fulfill important obligations at work, school, or home; repeated use in situations in which it is physically dangerous, such as driving under the influence; legal problems; and social or interpersonal problems such as arguments and fights.[8] *Intoxication* refers to the development of a substance-specific syndrome after recent ingestion and presence in the body of a substance, and it is associated with maladaptive behavior during the waking state caused by the effect of the substance on the central nervous system (CNS). Examples include belligerence, mood lability, impaired judgment, and impaired social or occupational functioning. Evidence for recent intake of the substance can be obtained from the history, physical examination, or laboratory examination. The most common changes involve disturbances in perception, wakefulness, attention, thinking, judgment, motor behavior, and interpersonal behavior.

In addition to the previous definition, *withdrawal* can be further described as the development of a substance-specific syndrome after cessation of or reduction in intake of a substance that was used regularly by the individual to induce a state of intoxication. Withdrawal causes significant distress to the individual and is associated with impairment in social, occupational, or other areas of functioning. Withdrawal is usually associated with substance dependence. Withdrawal generally is also associated with a craving to readminister the drug to relieve the symptoms.

As with most illnesses, the course and prognosis of the disorders of substance use and dependence are variable. Untreated physical withdrawal from the CNS depressants is potentially life-threatening, but withdrawal almost always can be managed successfully with proper medical care. Getting patients who are drug dependent to stop using drugs is very difficult, and many patients return to drug use even after treatment. As many as 75% of treated, substance-dependent patients will relapse at least once. Many patients, however, are able to obtain recovery with treatment and continued care in 12-step programs such as Alcoholics Anonymous (AA) or Narcotics Anonymous (NA). Substance dependence or addiction can be viewed as a chronic illness that can be controlled successfully with treatment but cannot be cured and is associated with a high relapse rate. Without treatment, the course can progress to life-threatening severity, resulting from the effects of the drug, drug contaminants, or medical complications of use.[8] Although an in-depth discussion of the mechanism of drug addiction is beyond the scope of this chapter, the interested reader is directed to a concise review article that presents the current understanding of the biology of drug addiction.[9]

CNS DEPRESSANTS

BENZODIAZEPINES AND OTHER SEDATIVE-HYPNOTICS

The past several years have witnessed a sharp increase in the abuse of prescription drugs. In 2005, an estimated 6.4 million persons were current users of prescription drugs for nonmedical purposes.[3]

Benzodiazepines are among the most popular "party drugs" both on college campuses and in the population at large. DAWN estimates show that from 1995 to 2002, increases were evident for the most frequently mentioned benzodiazepines, alprazolam (62%, from 17,082 to 27,659), clonazepam (33%, from 12,802 to 17,042), and unnamed benzodiazepines (199%, from 11,587 to 34,697).[2] According to DAWN, alprazolam and clonazepam are the most frequent benzodiazepines seen in emergency department visits related to pharmaceutical misuse/abuse (49,842 visits and 26,238 visits, respectively). Benzodiazepines occurring less frequently but still in substantial numbers include diazepam in 15,733 emergency department visits and lorazepam in 16,926 emergency department visits.[6]

In clinical practice, the benzodiazepines largely have replaced the short-acting barbiturates and other nonbarbiturate sedative-hypnotics. Benzodiazepines with faster onset (e.g., diazepam) tend to be preferred by the recreational drug user because they are reinforcing. Flunitrazepam emerged in the mid-1990s as an illegal drug in the United States that was predominantly abused recreationally and associated with sexual assaults.[10] Medically, this benzodiazepine is used in the short-term treatment of insomnia and as a preanesthetic medication. As with other benzodiazepines, flunitrazepam is most commonly ingested orally, frequently in conjunction with alcohol or other drugs. The drug's effects begin within 30 minutes, peak within 2 hours, and can persist for up to 8 hours or more depending on the dosage.[10]

PRESENTATION OF BENZODIAZEPINE INTOXICATION AND WITHDRAWAL

General

- The intoxicated patient may be in acute distress in overdoses or when benzodiazapines are combined with alcohol.
- Patients in withdrawal may also be in acute distress and should be treated with a benzodiazepine taper to prevent seizures.

Symptoms

- The patient may experience memory impairment, drowsiness, visual disturbances, confusion, and gastrointestinal disturbances. Patients may appear intoxicated, with slurred speech, poor coordination, swaying, and bloodshot eyes, with or without the odor of alcohol.[11–14]

Signs

- Hypotension or nystagmus may be observed, and urinary retenion may occur.

Laboratory Tests

- Qualitative testing to confirm presence of benzodiazepines is useful for diagnostic purposes, but quantitative plasma concentrations are usually not clinically useful.

A dramatic drop in cases of flunitrazepam abuse followed the legal reclassification of the drug as a schedule I substance in Florida in February 1997. A recent rise in alprazolam and clonazepam cases coincides with the decreased use of flunitrazepam and represents a new trend in abuse of the benzodiazepines. Alprazolam (Xanax) has become particularly popular and is known on the street by its slang names, Z-Bars, Zandy bars, footballs, and Zannies, among others. Young people will often take alprazolam or other benzodiazepines before going to the bar or dance club, ostensibly to lower the amount of alcoholic beverage needed to attain the desired level of intoxication. Unfortunately, this "pre-partying" is especially popular among women who do not like the taste of beer or find the caloric burden of drinking to be limiting. Sadly, whether taking it intentionally or being given the drug without their knowledge or consent, these women become targets for sexual predators who know that the victim will have diminished recall of the events that take place. When a victim is unable to give precise details of what happened and when it happened, and is unable to identify the perpetrator, the chances of successful prosecution are greatly diminished.

Because all benzodiazepines have abuse and dependence liability, patients cannot be switched from one benzodiazepine to another in hopes of decreasing a pattern of drug abuse or dependence behavior. Zolpidem, a nonbenzodiazepine, nonbarbiturate sedative, has been suggested to have little liability for physical dependence, but tolerance and withdrawal have been reported in association with its use as well.[11] Recent reports in the lay press have linked use of zolpidem to sleep-walking, erratic driving, binge eating, and other similarly bizarre activities.

Benzodiazepines generally do not cause life-threatening respiratory depression, as do the barbiturate-like drugs.[12] Long-term use of even therapeutic doses of benzodiazepines can cause physical dependence and withdrawal symptoms after abrupt discontinuation.[13]

❷ Gradual tapering of dosage is also associated with less withdrawal and rebound anxiety than abrupt discontinuation. Dependence on sedative-hypnotics and benzodiazepines is summarized in Table 68–1.

Occurrence of hallucinations or seizures would indicate severe physical withdrawal. For additional information on benzodiazepine withdrawal, refer to Chap. 73.

γ-HYDROXYBUTYRATE

GHB is a chemical compound structurally similar to the inhibitory brain neurotransmitter γ-aminobutyric acid. Powdered forms of GHB were marketed in health food stores as a nutritional supplement before being removed from the retail market by the Food and Drug Administration (FDA) in 1991. At that time it was used primarily by body builders for its purported ability to increase growth hormone, but it proved to cause serious illness and death when taken in excess doses or in combination with alcohol or other drugs. Primary groups using GHB include party and nightclub attendees. Like flunitrazepam, GHB is also characterized as a date rape drug.[14] Manifestations of acute GHB toxicity include coma, seizures, respiratory depression, and vomiting. Other documented effects of GHB include amnesia and hypotonia (associated with doses of 10 mg/kg of body weight), abnormal sequence of rapid eye movement (REM) and non-REM sleep (doses of 20 to 30 mg/kg), and anesthesia (doses of approximately 50 mg/kg). Doses greater than 50 mg/kg can decrease cardiac output and produce severe respiratory depression, seizure-like activity, and coma[15,16]; coma and respiratory depression can be potentiated by concomitant use of alcohol.[17] There is no antidote for GHB overdose, and treatment is restricted to nonspecific supportive care. Figure 68–1 shows a protocol recommended for treating suspected GHB overdose.

In March 2000, GHB was placed into schedule I of the Controlled Substances Act. Until recently, the majority of GHB sold on the streets was manufactured using inexpensive kits obtained over the Internet. It is mixed largely by nonchemists from recipes that can be flawed or incomplete, and finished products are often of questionable purity, and more important, unknown potency. Improper preparation of GHB can result in a mixture of GHB and sodium hydroxide that can be severely toxic because of the combined effects of the GHB and the direct caustic effects of sodium hydroxide. As there is no way to know the strength of homemade GHB, what might be a safe dose today (e.g., "one capful") could produce a toxic dose tomorrow if a different batch is used. Fortunately, crackdowns in 1997 by the FDA, the Department of Justice, and other enforcement groups has led to decreased availability of ready-made kits on the Internet. Despite the FDA's action, GHB remains available to consumers.

The decreased Internet availability of kits to make GHB has been accompanied by an increased availability of chemical precursors to

TABLE 68-1 Dependence on Sedative-Hypnotics

Generic Name	Common Trade Names	Oral Sedating Dose (mg)	Physical Dependence Daily Dose and Time Needed to Produce Dependence	Time Before Onset of Withdrawal (hours)	Peak Withdrawal Symptoms (days)[a]
Benzodiazepines					
Alprazolam	Xanax	0.25–8	8–16 mg × 42 days (est.)	8–24	2–3
Clorazepate	Tranxene	7.5–15	45–180 mg × 42–120 days (est.)	12–24	5–8
Diazepam	Valium	5–10	40–100 mg × 42–120 days	12–24	5–8
Flunitrazepam	Rohypnol	1–2	8–10 mg × 42 days (est.)	24–36	2–3
Barbiturates					
Amobarbital	Amytal	65–100	Same	8–12	2–5
Secobarbital	Seconal, Seco-8	100	800–2,200 mg × 35–37 days	6–12	2–3
Equal parts of secobarbital and amobarbital	Tuinal	100	Same	6–12	2–3
Pentobarbital	Nembutal	100	Same	6–12	2–3
Nonbarbiturate sedative-hypnotics					
Chloral hydrate	Noctec	250	Exact dose unknown; 12 g/day chronically has led to delirium upon sudden withdrawal	6–12	2–3
Meprobamate	Equanil, Miltown, Meprotabs	400	1.6–3.2 g × 270 days	8–12	3–8

[a]Withdrawal symptoms are tremor, tachycardia, diaphoresis, nausea, vomiting, elevated blood pressure, delirium, seizures, and hallucinations.

GHB as well as GHB analogs. Also available in gyms and health food stores, these substances include γ-butyrolactone (GBL) and 1,4-butanediol.[17] GBL is converted in the body to GHB. Labels of marketed products can use unfamiliar synonyms to disguise the actual content. GBL is also known by the names 2(3H)-furanone dihydro, butyrolactone, 4-butyrolactone, dihydro-2(3H)-furanone, 4-butanolide, 2(3H)-furanone, dihydro, tetrahydro-2-furanone, and butyrolactone-γ.

Withdrawal resulting in severe agitation, mental status changes, elevated blood pressure, and tachycardia has been reported hours after stopping chronic use of GHB. In one case the patient admitted to substantial GHB abuse on a daily basis for 2.5 years. Previous

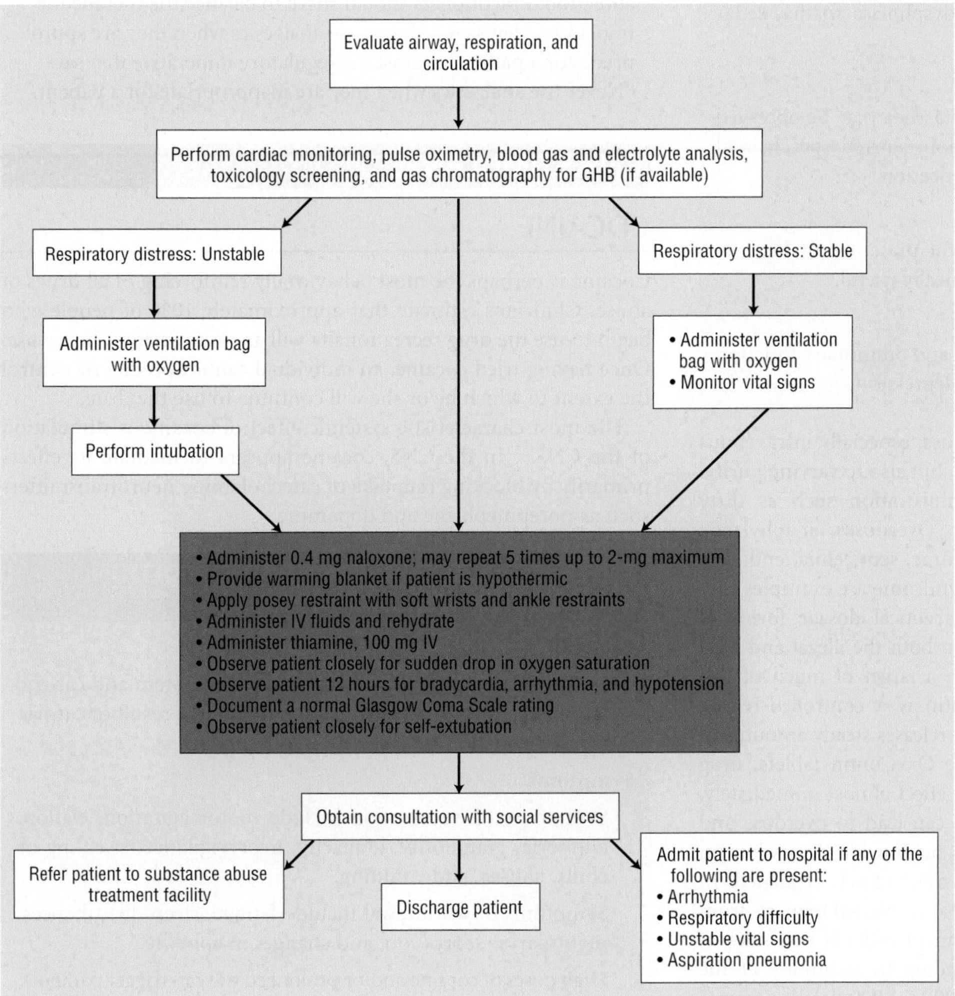

FIGURE 68-1. Protocol for treatment of suspected γ-hydroxybutyrate (GHB) overdose.

attempts at cessation reportedly resulted in diaphoresis, tremors, and agitation. The patient required 507 mg lorazepam and 120 mg diazepam over 90 hours to control agitation.[18]

OPIATES

Incidence and prevalence of opiate use are widely variable depending on the drug. In 2005, there were 136,000 current heroin users. Collectively, use of opiates other than heroin is far more common. An estimated 4.7 million people used narcotic pain relievers, and 3.1 million persons 12 years of age or older used what Substance Abuse and Mental Health Services Administration (SAMHSA) classified as "OxyContin" nonmedically at least once in their lifetime.[19]

PRESENTATION OF OPIOID INTOXICATION AND WITHDRAWAL

General

- Onset of the acute phase of withdrawal ranges from a few hours after stopping heroin to 3 to 5 days after stopping methadone. The duration of withdrawal ranges from 3 to 14 days.
- Opioid withdrawal is not fatal unless there is a concurrent medical problem of major concern.
- The presence of delirium should raise the question of concurrent withdrawal from another drug, such as alcohol, or another cause of delirium possibly secondary to drug use.

Symptoms

- During withdrawal, patients can experience piloerection, insomnia, muscle aches, and yawning. While intoxicated, patients can experience euphoria, dysphoria, apathy, sedation, or attention impairment.

Signs

- Fever, lacrimation, diaphoresis, or diarrhea may be observed during withdrawal. Motor retardation, slurred speech, and miosis may be observed during intoxication.

Laboratory Tests

- Treatment is based more on clinical presentation because plasma opioid levels may not be clinically useful.

Other Diagnostic Tests

- Arterial blood gases, pulse oximetry, and pulmonary function tests are useful to assess respiratory depression.

Many of the complications of opiate use, especially intravenous use, are related not only to the drug itself, but also to varying purity, contaminants, and techniques of administration such as dirty equipment and use of shared needles. Overdoses, anaphylactic reactions to impurities, nephrotic syndrome, septicemia, endocarditis, and acquired immune deficiency syndrome are examples.

Increased recreational use of pharmaceutical dosage forms of opiates has sparked nationwide debate on both the illegal and legal use of these drugs. OxyContin has been a target of much of this criticism. Introduced in 1995, OxyContin is a controlled-release dosage form of oxycodone that gradually releases steady amounts of narcotics for 12 hours. By crushing the OxyContin tablets, drug abusers can get the full 12-hour narcotic effect almost immediately. Snorting or injecting the crushed tablet can lead to overdose and death. Abuse of this drug has caused a nationwide discussion on whether drugs of this nature should be more closely regulated. In September 2003, a federal drug advisory panel rejected requests from members of Congress and drug enforcement officials that sales of OxyContin be severely restricted. According to testimony at the hearings, OxyContin is responsible for 500 to 1,000 deaths a year.[20] But, these data are refuted in a careful examination of data from an oxycodone postmortem database.[21] Created from 1,243 solicited cases from medical examiner and coroner offices in 23 states in the United States, the database included information collected from August 27, 1999, through January 17, 2002. Researchers examined records of the 919 deaths related to oxycodone and discovered that in only 12 of the cases was OxyContin the only agent found at autopsy. The remaining victims had taken either an overdose of other oxycodone-containing drugs (for example, Percocet [oxycodone + acetaminophen]) or a combination of drugs. In fact, 97% had at least three other drugs in their systems, mostly alcohol, benzodiazepines, cocaine, antidepressants, or other narcotics such as heroin. From these data, the authors concluded that oxycodone-related deaths overwhelmingly occur in drug-abusing individuals, and rarely is OxyContin an exclusive cause of death.

Various groups have weighed in on the pros and cons of prescribing opiates for chronic pain and the debate at times is emotional. Various position statements and points of view have been expressed, but the limited space here precludes an exhaustive review of the issues. An excellent review of the appropriate use of opioid therapy for chronic pain has recently been published, and the interested reader is directed there for more information.[22]

CLINICAL CONTROVERSY

There is considerable debate about the appropriate use of prescribed opiates and how this might contribute to the overuse or abuse of these same drugs for nonmedicinal purposes. Some clinicians believe that use of opiates in patients with chronic pain is inappropriate because it leads to physical dependence and addiction. Practitioners should strive to balance the therapeutic imperative that says "Always use analgesics when they are appropriate for a patient" against the regulatory imperative that says "Never use analgesics when they are inappropriate for a patient."

CNS STIMULANTS

COCAINE

Cocaine is perhaps the most behaviorally reinforcing of all drugs of abuse. Clinicians estimate that approximately 10% of people who begin to use the drug recreationally will go on to serious, heavy use. Once having tried cocaine, an individual cannot predict or control the extent to which he or she will continue to use the drug.

The most characteristic systemic effect of cocaine is stimulation of the CNS.[23] In the CNS, cocaine appears to mediate its effects primarily by blocking reuptake of catecholamine neurotransmitters such as norepinephrine and dopamine.

PRESENTATION OF COCAINE INTOXICATION AND WITHDRAWAL

General

- In overdoses, cocaine is a central nervous system and cardiac stimulant. Cocaine-related deaths are often a result of cardiac arrest or seizures followed by respiratory arrest.

Symptoms

- Symptoms of intoxication include motor agitation, elation, euphoria, grandiosity, loquacity, hypervigilance, sweating or chills, nausea, and vomiting.
- Symptoms of withdrawal include fatigue, sleep disturbances, nightmares, depression, and changes in appetite.
- High doses of cocaine and/or prolonged use can trigger paranoia.

Signs

- Tachycardia, mydriasis, and either elevated or lowered blood pressure may be observed with overdose. Cardiac abnormalities (e.g., arrhythmias) and respiratory depression may be observed with overdose. Bradyarrhythmias, myocardial infarction, and tremors may be observed in acute withdrawal. Prolonged cocaine snorting can result in ulceration of the mucous membranes of the nose and can damage the nasal septum enough to cause it to collapse.

Laboratory Tests

- Qualitative drugs of abuse urine screening tests are useful, followed by confirmatory testing if necessary. Levels of the primary metabolite, benzoylecgonine, may help diagnose acute cocaine toxicity.

Other Diagnostic Tests

- Abnormal electroencephalograms may be observed with patients in acute withdrawal.

Cocaine is absorbed rapidly from virtually all sites of application. For many years, cocaine has been administered as the hydrochloride salt form, usually by inhalation, but also by injection. In the last 15 to 18 years, as the purity of cocaine hydrochloride obtained on the street declined, many users converted the cocaine hydrochloride to cocaine base, also known as "crack" or "rock." Smoking the drug leads to almost instant absorption and intense euphoria. Peak plasma concentrations of more than 900 ng/mL have been achieved following inhalation of cocaine base vapors, compared with concentrations of only 150 to 200 ng/mL achieved after inhalation of similar amounts of pure cocaine hydrochloride powder.[23]

The high from snorting can last 15 to 30 minutes, whereas that from smoking can last 5 to 10 minutes. Increased use can reduce the period of stimulation. An appreciable tolerance to the high can be developed, and many addicts report that they seek but fail to achieve as much pleasure as they did from their first exposure. Scientific evidence suggests that the powerful neuropsychologic reinforcing property of cocaine is responsible for an individual's continued use despite harmful physical and social consequences.

Recent research has helped clarify certain patterns of cocaine use such as combining cocaine and alcohol. Such drug use would seem counterintuitive because cocaine is a CNS stimulant and alcohol a CNS depressant. In the presence of alcohol, cocaine is metabolized to cocaethylene, a longer-acting but potent psychoactive compound compared to the parent drug.[24] The risk of death from cocaethylene is greater than from cocaine.[25] The cocaine-alcohol combination is one of the most commonly identified among individuals who come to hospital emergency departments with acute substance abuse problems.

Cocaine is metabolized and eliminated rapidly. The elimination half-life of cocaine is approximately 1 hour, and the duration of effect is very short.[23] The short duration of effect provides a powerful incentive for repeated use of the drug. Many users experience intense drug use cycling, sometimes lasting days, characterized by rapidly repeating doses of cocaine until their supply is exhausted. Laboratory monkeys, given a choice between food and cocaine around the clock for 8 days, consistently choose cocaine.[26]

Complications of cocaine use frequently involve cardiovascular events.[27] Cocaine is a psychotomimetic drug, sometimes even at systemically nontoxic doses. A kindling phenomenon has been described with cocaine in which neuronal function becomes altered with each dose of the drug. The psychosis is qualitatively very similar to a paranoid schizophrenic psychosis.[28] Although there is some controversy as to whether cocaine is associated with physical withdrawal on abrupt discontinuation, most clinicians feel that there is a characteristic syndrome of withdrawal effects, although they are not life-threatening.[13,29]

AMPHETAMINE, METHAMPHETAMINE, AND OTHER STIMULANTS

During the 1940s the Japanese government distributed amphetamines to soldiers, sailors, and pilots, as well as to armament factory workers, to mobilize all their reserves for the war effort. Pilots routinely used the drug to remain awake and alert for long periods on long-distance bombing missions. After 1945 large quantities of the drug from looted military supplies flooded the market. In the United States in the 1950s and 1960s, legally manufactured tablets of methamphetamine were used nonmedically by college students, truck drivers, and athletes, who usually did not become severely addicted. This pattern changed drastically in the later 1960s with the increased availability of injectable methamphetamine.

There were an estimated 512,000 methamphetamine users in 2005, up from 149,000 in 1990.[3] Street methamphetamine is referred to by many names, such as "speed," "meth," and "crank." Methamphetamine hydrochloride, clear chunky crystals resembling ice, which can be inhaled by smoking, is referred to as "ice," "crystal," and "glass."

The physiologic and psychologic effects of amphetamines and other stimulants are qualitatively similar to those of cocaine—they diminish fatigue, increase alertness, and suppress appetite. Pharmacologically, amphetamines increase the activity of catecholamine neurotransmitters (e.g., norepinephrine and dopamine) by blocking reuptake, increasing release of neurotransmitters, and inhibiting the degradative enzyme monoamine oxidase.[30] The longer duration of effect of methamphetamine has led to a shift away from cocaine and toward the longer-acting drug.

Methamphetamine is used orally, intranasally, rectally, by intravenous injection, and by smoking. Immediately after inhalation or intravenous injection, the methamphetamine user experiences an intense sensation, called a "rush" or "flash," that lasts only a few minutes and is described as extremely pleasurable.

PRESENTATION OF AMPHETAMINE INTOXICATION AND WITHDRAWAL

General

- Amphetamine intoxication is an acute condition that may result in death. Pharmacotherapy may be indicated for symptomatic control of seizures.
- Patients may experience withdrawal symptoms for several days, but are usually not in acute distress. Treatment is supportive in nature. Pharmacotherapy is not effective to treat the symptoms of amphetamine withdrawal.

Symptoms

- Depression, altered mental status, drug craving, dyssomnia, and fatigue are all symptoms of withdrawal.
- Amphetamine intoxication may present as increased wakefulness, increased physical activity, decreased appetite, increased respiration, hyperthermia, and euphoria. Other CNS effects include irritability, insomnia, confusion, tremors, convulsions, anxiety, paranoia, chest pain, and aggressiveness. Hyperthermia and convulsions can result in death.

Signs

- Patients with amphetamine intoxication may present with tachycardia, hypertension, or stroke.

Laboratory Tests

- A qualitative drug of abuse urine screening is used for diagnostic purposes. Confirmatory blood tests with gas chromatography or mass spectrophotometry may be used for verification.

Because methamphetamine elevates mood, people who experiment with it tend to use it with increasing frequency and in increasing doses, although this was not their original intent. The timing and intensity of the "rush" that accompanies the use of methamphetamine, which is a result of the release of high levels of dopamine in the brain, depends in part on the method of administration. Specifically, the effect is almost instantaneous when smoked or injected, whereas it takes approximately 5 minutes after snorting or 20 minutes after oral ingestion. Prolonged use of methamphetamine can result in a tolerance for the drug and increased use at higher dosage levels, creating dependence. Such continual use of the drug with little or no sleep leads to an extremely irritable and paranoid state. Discontinuing use of methamphetamine often results in a state of depression, as well as fatigue, anergia, and some types of cognitive impairment that can last from 2 days to several months.[31]

Both short- and long-term health effects have also been documented. Negative consequences of methamphetamine abuse range from anxiety and insomnia to convulsions, paranoia, and brain damage. Methamphetamine-induced caries, or "Meth mouth" is a characteristic pattern of dental decay commonly observed in patients that smoke methamphetamine.[32]

In addition to the many direct effects on methamphetamine users are the indirect impacts on individuals and society. Flammable ingredients that include acetone, red phosphorous, ethyl alcohol, and lithium metal are used in methamphetamine cookers, often with disastrous results. Fires and explosions often ensue, resulting in severe burns, and uncovering laboratories to local law enforcement.[33] Children of methamphetamine abusers are at high risk of neglect and abuse, and pregnant women's use of methamphetamine can cause growth retardation, premature birth, and developmental disorders in neonates. Within this particular group, effective treatment for methamphetamine dependence can be one of the most important strategies in reducing the spread of HIV and other associated communicable diseases.[34] Treatment for methamphetamine dependence is very difficult, with a low success rate.[34]

The expanding global market is fed by an increase in clandestine manufacture of methamphetamine. Not only are there more laboratories in more countries, but their size and sophistication are also increasing. The number of clandestine methamphetamine laboratories seized nationwide by the U.S. Drug Enforcement Administration (DEA) increased from 263 in 1994 to 1,815 in 2000, a 590% increase.[35] In 2005, state and local police agencies seized almost 5,249 clandestine laboratories in the United States. So-called "kitchen" laboratories are still discovered, but today clandestine laboratories with 100-kilogram capacities per week are also found. Initially the clandestine manufacture of methamphetamine was based primarily in the West and Southwest. Today methamphetamine can be found in cities across the United States, although local law enforcement pressures have caused a decrease in "superlaboratories" capable of producing at least 10 pounds per production cycle.[35] Unfortunately, increased methamphetamine production by Mexican drug cartels has offset the decreased domestic production.

Methamphetamine is manufactured using the ephedrine or pseudoephedrine reduction method. In this process, ephedrine or pseudoephedrine is extracted from OTC cold and allergy tablets. Pharmacists should be wary of persons wishing to purchase large quantities of products containing nonprescription sympathomimetic products. As a precaution, most states have imposed restrictions on the quantities of OTC decongestants that can be purchased at one time. Many states require that pseudoephedrine-containing products be kept behind the counter as an additional precaution.

Prices for methamphetamine vary throughout different regions of the United States, ranging from $20 to $300 for 1 gram, $270 to $5,000 for 1 ounce, and $1,600 to $45,000 for 1 pound.[36]

ECSTASY AND OTHER METHAMPHETAMINE ANALOGS

Several dozen analogs of amphetamine and methamphetamine are hallucinogenic. Two methamphetamine analogs of most concern are 3,4-methylenedioxyamphetamine (MDA) and especially 3,4-methylenedioxymethamphetamine (MDMA or ecstasy). Popular among young people at all-night dance parties referred to as "raves," these are classified among the "club drugs." According to the MTFS data from 2005, among children aged 12 to 17, annual prevalence rates of ecstasy use are down by one-half to two-thirds since the peak observed in 2001.[5] The vast majority of ecstasy consumed domestically is produced in Europe. It costs as little as 25 to 50 cents to manufacture an ecstasy tablet in Europe, but the street value of that same ecstasy tablet can be as high as $40, with a tablet typically selling for between $20 and $30.

Patented in 1914 by Merck Pharmaceuticals, MDMA was never "legally" marketed.[37] MDMA is structurally similar to methamphetamine and mescaline. A mild, hallucinogenic effect is produced by stimulating the CNS. Known most commonly on the street as ecstasy, it is also called "Adam," "X," "X-TC," "Stacy," "beans," "e," or simply "pills." MDMA is usually taken by mouth in tablet, capsule, or powder form, but it also can be smoked, snorted, or injected.

The effects of MDMA usually last approximately 4 to 6 hours. Users of the drug say that it produces profoundly positive feelings, empathy for others, elimination of anxiety, and extreme relaxation. MDMA is also said to suppress the need to eat, drink, or sleep, enabling users to endure 2- to 3-day parties. Consequently, MDMA use sometimes results in severe dehydration or exhaustion. MDMA generally reduces inhibitions and creates a sense of euphoria, but it also can evoke anxiety and paranoia. Heavier doses generate depression, irrationality, and psychosis. Users claim they experience feelings of closeness with others and a desire to touch them.

MDMA use can result in a variety of acute psychiatric disturbances, including panic, anxiety, depression, and paranoid thinking.[37] Physical symptoms include muscle tension, nausea, blurred vision, faintness, chills, and sweating. MDMA also increases the heart rate and blood pressure. Other effects include hyperthermia, dehydration, vomiting, tremors, loss of control over body movements, insomnia, convulsions, rapid eye movements, and teeth and jaw clenching.

MDMA is perceived to be a harmless drug by many of its users, based in part on the fact that the risk of death is low compared with other drugs such as heroin and cocaine. However, mounting evidence points to neurotoxic effects of MDMA, involving a complex and incompletely understood mechanism. MDMA has been clearly shown to destroy serotonin-producing neurons in animals.[38] Doses of MDMA that produce neurotoxicity are only two or three times more than the minimum dose needed to produce a psychotropic response.

Researchers have found that heavy MDMA users have memory problems that persist for at least 2 weeks after they have stopped using the drug.[39] McCann and colleagues[40] conducted a study to determine the effects of MDMA use on cognitive performance. MDMA users and controls were found to perform similarly on several cognitive tasks. However, MDMA subjects had significant performance deficits on a sustained-attention task requiring arithmetic calculations, a task requiring complex attention and incidental learning, a task requiring short-term memory, and a task of semantic recognition and verbal reasoning. MDMA users also had significant selective decreases in cerebrospinal fluid (CSF) 5-hydroxyindoleacetic acid (5-HIAA). The authors believe that their data provide further evidence that MDMA is neurotoxic to brain serotonin neurons in humans, and the behavioral data suggest that brain serotonin injury is associated with subtle but significant cognitive deficits. Additional evidence has been accruing.[41]

Manufacturers of illicit drugs sometimes substitute other, potentially more dangerous substances for the one the buyer is expecting. Other suppliers produce products adulterated with chemical by-products of the incomplete synthesis of active ingredients. One such chemical, *para*-methoxyamphetamine, is a drastically more potent hyperthermic agent than MDMA.[42] Deaths from the drug likely will increase as a result of poor-quality tablets.

PHENCYCLIDINE AND KETAMINE

Phencyclidine (PCP), commonly referred to as "angel dust" and "crystal," was popular in the 1970s, but as its adverse effects became better known, use declined. PCP is most often a substitute for or contaminant of other drugs, and its most common pattern of use may now be unintentional. The actual extent of its use is unclear. It is often misrepresented as LSD or Δ^9-tetrahydrocannabinol (THC). With the exception of the pharmaceutical dosage form of dronabinol, THC is virtually unavailable on the street because it is highly unstable when isolated from the marijuana plant. When used intentionally, PCP is commonly smoked with marijuana and referred to as a "crystal joint," but it also can be taken orally or intravenously.

PCP has widely varied actions including CNS stimulation, depression, and hallucinogenic properties. Pharmacologically, it is known to block reuptake of serotonin, dopamine, and norepinephrine, but neurotransmitter antagonists do not effectively block its effects. In low doses, PCP causes sedation, ataxia, nystagmus, slurred speech, and paresthesias. At higher doses, users experience an increase in heart rate, blood pressure, temperature, diaphoresis, and muscle rigidity. At acutely toxic doses, coma and seizures can occur.[43]

Behavioral effects of PCP range from sleep to catatonic detachment to paranoid psychosis to violent hostility. Users are sometimes amnestic for events that occur under the influence of the drug. Psychoses sometimes last for weeks. Users with a previous history of schizophrenia are especially susceptible to the psychotomimetic effects of the drug. The only truly characteristic behavioral effect of PCP use is its high unpredictability. The signs and symptoms of PCP intoxication are summarized in Table 68–2.

Ketamine, a compound chemically related to PCP, is used primarily as a veterinary anesthetic but has gained popularity recently as a recreational drug.[44] Once used extensively in human medicine, it has fallen out of favor because of "emergence delirium," characterized by hallucinations, delirium, vivid dreams, and other psychiatric effects. This untoward effect as a medicinal agent is precisely the effect that recreational users are seeking.

Known as "special K," "jet," "green," and other names on the street, ketamine is sometimes injected but can be evaporated to solid crystals, powdered, and smoked, snorted, or swallowed. Marijuana cigarettes are sometimes soaked in the ketamine solution, allowed to dry, and then smoked. Ketamine has become popular as a "rave" club drug. Side effects include significant transient increases in blood pressure and heart rate, respiratory depression, airway obstruction, apnea, muscular hypertonia, psychomotor and psychotomimetic effects, and acute dystonic reactions. Following overdose, seizures, polyneuropathy, increased intracranial pressure, respiratory arrest, and cardiac arrest can occur.[45,46]

TABLE 68-2 Signs and Symptoms of Phencyclidine Intoxication

Nystagmus	Euphoria
Increased blood pressure	Motor agitation
Tachycardia	Anxiety and emotional lability
Paresthesias	Hostility
Ataxia	Delusions
Slurred speech	Hallucinations
Muscle rigidity	

The effects of a ketamine "high" usually last an hour, but they can last 4 to 6 hours, and 24 to 48 hours are generally required before the user will feel completely normal again. Effects of chronic use of ketamine can take from several months to 2 years to disappear completely. Low doses (25 to 100 mg) produce psychedelic effects quickly. Large doses can produce vomiting and convulsions and can lead to hypoxia of the brain and muscles; 1 g can cause death. Long-term effects include tolerance and possible physical and/or psychological dependence.

Since its emergence as a drug of abuse in the late 1960s, PCP has been described as one of the most dangerous of all synthetic hallucinogens. Its niche in the drug world is usually one characterized by abusers exhibiting hostile behavior that manifests itself in extremely violent episodes.[45,46]

Despite the negative effects associated with PCP, there remains an illicit market for the drug. Illicit organizations producing and distributing PCP are still active in the United States.[47] These organizations, operating mainly in Los Angeles and to a lesser extent in Houston, supply most of the PCP available in the nation. PCP production appears to be stable, in limited quantities since 2000. The DEA considers PCP a drug of abuse that is not readily available.[47]

HALLUCINOGENS

The drugs commonly classified as hallucinogens are LSD, psilocybin, dimethyltryptamine (DMT), mescaline, and other related compounds. LSD is one of the most potent mood-changing chemicals. It is manufactured from lysergic acid, which is found in ergot, a fungus that grows on rye and other grains.

Pharmacologically, LSD and related drugs stimulate both presynaptic (5-hydroxytryptamine $[HT]_{1A}$ and $5\text{-}HT_{1B}$) and postsynaptic ($5\text{-}HT_2$) serotonin recognition sites in the brain, which functionally can cause either agonist or antagonist effects on serotonin activity.[48] Precisely how the hallucinogens exert their effects remains unclear. LSD, often referred to as "acid," is an extraordinarily potent compound, producing observable CNS effects at doses as low as 25 mcg.[48]

LSD is sold on the street in tablets, capsules, and occasionally in liquid form. It is odorless, colorless, and tasteless and usually is taken by mouth. Often LSD is added to absorbent paper, such as blotter paper, and divided into small decorated squares, with each square representing one dose.

The DEA reports that the strength of LSD samples obtained recently from illicit sources ranges from 20 to 80 mcg of LSD per dose. This is considerably less than the levels reported during the 1960s and early 1970s, when the dosage ranged from 100 to 200 mcg or higher per unit.

The effects of LSD are unpredictable. They depend on the amount taken; the user's personality, mood, and expectations; and the surroundings in which the drug is used. Usually the user feels the first effects of the drug 30 to 90 minutes after taking it. The physical effects include dilated pupils, higher body temperature, increased heart rate and blood pressure, sweating, loss of appetite, sleeplessness, dry mouth, and tremors.

Sensations and feelings change much more dramatically than the physical signs. The user can feel several different emotions at once or swing rapidly from one emotion to another. If taken in a large enough dose, the drug produces delusions and visual hallucinations. The user's sense of time and self changes. Sensations can seem to "cross over," giving the user the feeling of hearing colors and seeing sounds. These changes can be frightening and can cause panic.

Many LSD users experience flashbacks, or recurrence of certain aspects of a person's experience, without the user having taken the drug again. A flashback occurs suddenly, often without warning, and can occur within a few days or more than a year after LSD use. Flashbacks usually occur in people who use hallucinogens chronically or have an underlying personality problem; however, otherwise healthy people who use LSD occasionally also can have flashbacks.

Most users of LSD voluntarily decrease or stop its use over time. LSD is not considered an addictive drug because it does not produce compulsive drug-seeking behavior. However, as with many of the addictive drugs, LSD use produces tolerance, so some users who take the drug repeatedly must take progressively higher doses to achieve the state of intoxication that they had achieved previously.

Psychologic symptoms of intoxication include a subjective intensification of perceptions, depersonalization, illusions, hallucinations, and synesthesias, the overflow of one sensory modality to another (colors are heard, sounds are seen). Among the hallucinogenic drugs, LSD is the most potent and long acting; it is hundreds of times more potent than both psilocybin and mescaline. DMT is inactive when ingested orally but can be smoked, inhaled, or injected. There is cross-tolerance among LSD, psilocybin, and mescaline. There is no observable physical withdrawal syndrome after abrupt discontinuation of hallucinogenic drugs.[49]

Complications from hallucinogen use are primarily psychologic. Users sometimes experience prolonged episodes of panic—the so-called "bad trip." The flashbacks noted above are common, occurring in approximately 15% of users and occurring episodically up to several years after the last exposure to the drug. Flashbacks can occur spontaneously but are also triggered by other drugs, including marijuana, and by anxiety-provoking stimuli. Contrary to a widely held notion in the 1960s and early 1970s, there is no reliable evidence that hallucinogen use causes chromosome damage or genetic defects.[48]

Few LSD laboratories have ever been seized in the United States because of infrequent and irregular production cycles. In 2000, the DEA seized one LSD laboratory that was located in a converted missile silo in Kansas. This was the largest LSD laboratory seizure ever made by the DEA, and agents seized approximately 41.3 kilograms (90.86 pounds) of LSD and approximately 23.6 kilograms (51.92 pounds) of iso-LSD, a by-product of the manufacture of LSD.[50]

MARIJUANA

Marijuana, referred to as "reefer," "pot," "grass," or "weed," remains the most commonly used illicit drug. In 2005, marijuana was used by nearly 75% of current illicit drug users. Of those, 54.5% used only marijuana, and 19.6% used marijuana and another illicit drug.[3] According to the 2005 data, 14.6 million past month users of marijuana were reported; a similar percentage was observed in the previous 4 years. In 2005, 59.1% of the 2.1 million first-time users of marijuana were younger than 18 years of age.[3] The rate of current marijuana users among youths 12 to 17 years of age decreased from 7.6% to 6.8% in 2005, a positive trend that hopefully will continue.

Most users smoke marijuana in hand-rolled cigarettes called joints, among other names; some use pipes or water pipes called bongs. Marijuana cigars called blunts have also become popular. To make blunts, users slice open cigars and replace the tobacco with marijuana, often combined with another drug, such as crack cocaine. Marijuana also is used to brew tea and is sometimes mixed into foods.[51]

Marijuana's effects begin immediately after the drug enters the brain and last from 1 to 3 hours. If marijuana is consumed in food or drink, the short-term effects begin more slowly, usually in 30 minutes to 1 hour, and last longer, for as long as 4 hours. Smoking marijuana deposits several times more THC into the blood than does eating or drinking the drug.[51]

PRESENTATION OF MARIJUANA INTOXICATION

General Symptoms

- Patients intoxicated with marijuana may experience euphoria, sensory intensification, increased appetite, apathy, hallucinations, and dry mouth. Occasionally, marijuana use produces anxiety, fear, distrust, or panic.[51]

Signs

- Tachycardia and conjunctival congestion may be observed in patients intoxicated with marijuana.

Laboratory Tests

- Although the duration of effect of marijuana may only be several hours, THC is detectable on toxicologic screening for up to 4 to 5 weeks, especially in chronic users.

Marijuana use impairs a person's ability to form memories, recall events, and shift attention from one thing to another.[52] THC also disrupts coordination and balance by binding to receptors in the cerebellum and basal ganglia. Through its effects on the brain and body, marijuana intoxication can cause accidents. Studies show that approximately 6% to 11% of fatal accident victims test positive for THC. In many of these cases alcohol is detected as well.

In a study conducted by the National Highway Traffic Safety Administration, a moderate dose of marijuana alone was shown to impair driving performance; however, the effects of even a low dose of marijuana combined with alcohol were markedly greater than for either drug alone. Driving indices measured included reaction time, visual search frequency (driver checking of side streets), and the ability to perceive and/or respond to changes in the relative velocity of other vehicles.[53]

The principal psychoactive component of marijuana is THC. Hashish, the dried resin of the top of the plant, is much more potent than the plant itself. Increasingly sophisticated growing techniques have resulted in plants of greater potency. In a recent study, the amount of Δ^9-THC found in the samples ranged from 1.41% to 12.62% by dry weight. The average Δ^9-THC content was 6.2%, which is almost identical to the 2002 value reported by the University of Mississippi's Potency Monitoring Project.[54]

Marijuana has been used widely and is believed by many to be a relatively harmless, nonaddictive intoxicant. Chronic low doses of marijuana usually are not associated with significant physical withdrawal on abrupt discontinuation, but many chronic users exhibit compulsive drug-seeking and drug-use behaviors characteristic of addiction or dependence. Acutely, marijuana has many of the effects of alcohol—sedation, a decrease in reactivity and ability to perform complex tasks, and disinhibition. Marijuana also causes hallucinations with high enough doses. Chronic use is associated with all the risks of tobacco smoking, although marijuana smokers are commonly also tobacco smokers, and thus differentiation of effects is often difficult. Endocrine effects including amenorrhea, decreased testosterone production, and inhibition of spermatogenesis have been demonstrated. Marijuana is associated with an amotivational syndrome characterized by a behavioral pattern of apathy, dullness, impaired judgment, decreased concentration and memory, loss of interest in personal hygiene, and a general reduction of goal-directed behavior.

Marijuana smoke is irritating to the lungs. Researchers have found that the daily use of one to three marijuana joints appears to produce approximately the same lung damage and potential cancer risk as smoking five times as many cigarettes.[55] The study results suggest that the way smokers inhale marijuana, in addition to its chemical composition, increases the adverse physical effects. The study findings refute the argument that marijuana is safer than tobacco because users smoke only a few joints a day.

Clearly, there is much more work to be done before the precise health and psychologic effects of marijuana use are well understood. In fact, many of these health issues remain the subject of much debate. Undoubtedly, opinions on its risks are polarized along the lines of proponents' views on what its legal status should be. This polarization of opinion has prevented the development of any consensus on what health information the medical profession should give to patients who are users or potential users of marijuana. There is conflicting evidence about many of the effects of marijuana use. Readers are referred to an excellent article that attempts to summarize in a dispassionate way the evidence on the most probable adverse health and psychologic consequences of acute and chronic use of marijuana.[56]

INHALANTS

Inhalants are a diverse group of substances that include volatile solvents, gases, and nitrites that are sniffed, snorted, huffed, or bagged to produce intoxicating effects similar to those of alcohol. These substances are found in common household products such as glues, lighter fluid, cleaning fluids, paint products, nail polish remover, gasoline, rubber glue, waxes, and varnishes. Chemicals found in these products include toluene, benzene, methanol, methylene chloride, acetone, methylethyl ketone, methylbutyl ketone, trichloroethylene, and trichloroethane. The gas used as a propellant in canned whipped cream and in small metallic containers called "whippets" (used to make whipped cream) is nitrous oxide or "laughing gas." Tiny cloth-covered ampules called "poppers" or "snappers" by abusers contain amyl nitrite, a medication used to dilate blood vessels. Butyl nitrite, sold as tape head cleaner and referred to as "rush," "locker room," or "climax," is often sniffed or huffed to get high.

The easy accessibility, low cost, legal status, and ease of transport and concealment make inhalants one of the first substances abused by children. Survey data from 2004 indicate increased inhalant use in all grades. In 2005, that increase in use continued in twelfth graders.[5] In 2005, there were 877,000 persons aged 12 or older who had used inhalants for the first time within the last 12 months—72.3 % were younger than age 18 when they first used.[3] Parents worry about alcohol, tobacco, and drug use, but can be unaware of the hazards associated with products found throughout their homes.

Inhalants can be sniffed directly from an open container or huffed from a rag soaked in the substance and held to the face. Alternatively, the open container or soaked rag can be placed in a bag where the vapors can concentrate before being inhaled. Although inhalant abusers might prefer one particular substance because of taste or odor, a variety of substances can be used because of similar effects, availability, and cost. Once inhaled, the extensive capillary surface area of the lungs allows rapid absorption of the substance, and blood levels peak rapidly. Entry into the brain is fast, and the intoxicating effects are intense but short-lived. Intoxication is often accompanied by headache and nausea, and users can experience hallucinations and delusions. The most serious physical risk of acute use is sudden death, usually from cardiac arrhythmias. Some users die from suffocation by plastic bags that contain the solvent. With chronic use, the drugs are toxic to virtually all organ systems. Psychologic impairment; impaired pulmonary, renal, and hepatic function; neuropathies; encephalopathy; and brain damage have all been observed.[57]

Inhalants depress the CNS, producing decreased respiration and blood pressure. Users report distortion in perceptions of time and space. Many users experience headaches, nausea, slurred speech, and loss of motor coordination. Mental effects can include fear, anxiety, or depression. A rash around the nose and mouth can be seen, and the abuser can start wheezing. An odor of paint or organic solvents on clothes, skin, and breath is sometimes a sign of inhalant abuse. Other indicators of inhalant abuse include slurred speech or staggering gait; red, glassy, watery eyes; and excitability or unpredictable behavior.

TREATMENT

Substance-Related Disorders

■ ACUTE DRUG INTOXICATIONS

Treatment of drug intoxication, summarized in Table 68–3, is primarily supportive. Vital functions are maintained while waiting for the drug to be eliminated. When absolutely necessary, physical restraints can be required temporarily while a diagnostic evaluation is initiated. Whenever possible, drug therapy should be avoided because psychotropic drug therapy has the potential for worsening a toxic reaction to another psychoactive agent; however, when patients are agitated, combative, assaultive, hallucinating, or delusional, drug therapy may be required. Drug therapy also may be indicated in the treatment of an acute, potentially fatal drug overdose. Toxicology screens are useful in the evaluation and treatment process, but knowledge of the metabolism of the suspected drug and its excretion patterns is important for proper interpretation of test results. When toxicology screens are desired, blood or urine should be collected immediately upon the patient's arrival.

TABLE 68-3 Pharmacologic Treatment of Substance Intoxication

Drug Class	Nonpharmacologic Therapy	Pharmacologic Therapy	Level of Evidence[a,b]
Benzodiazepines	Support vital functions	Flumazenil 0.2 mg/min IV initially, repeat up to 3 mg maximum	A1
Alcohol, barbiturates, and sedative-hypnotics (nonbenzodiazepines)	Support vital functions	None	B3
Opiates	Support vital functions	Naloxone 0.4–2 mg IV every 3 min	A1
Cocaine and other CNS stimulants	Monitor cardiac function	Lorazepam 2–4 mg IM every 30 min to 6 h as needed for agitation	B2
		Haloperidol 2–5 mg (or other antipsychotic agent) every 30 min to 6 h as needed for psychotic behavior	B3
Hallucinogens, marijuana, and inhalants	Reassurance; "talk-down therapy"; support vital functions	Lorazepam and/or haloperidol as above	B3
Phencyclidine	Minimize sensory input	Lorazepam and/or haloperidol as above	B3

[a]Strength of recommendations, evidence to support recommendation, A, good; B, moderate; C, poor.
[b]Quality of evidence: 1, evidence from more than 1 properly randomized, controlled trial; 2, evidence from more than 1 well-designed clinical trial with randomization, from cohort or case-controlled analytic studies or multiple time series; or dramatic results from uncontrolled experiments; 3, evidence from opinions of respected authorities, based on clinical experience, descriptive studies, or reports of expert communities.
Data from O'Brien,[57] Fudala et al.,[58] Smith and Seymour,[59] and Knapp et al.[60]

For alcohol and barbiturate intoxication, supportive treatment is the rule. For benzodiazepine intoxication, the benzodiazepine antagonist flumazenil can be used to reverse toxic effects. However, it is not indicated in all cases of suspected drug overdose, and is specifically contraindicated in cases in which cyclic antidepressant involvement is known or suspected because of the risk of seizures. In addition, it should be used with caution in patients when benzodiazepine physical dependence is suspected because of the risks of induction of benzodiazepine withdrawal. In the case of opiate intoxication, if the patient is unconscious and respiration is depressed, the opiate antagonist naloxone can be used to revive the patient. The usual dosage for naloxone in acute opiate toxicity is 0.4 to 2 mg intravenously, given approximately every 3 minutes as necessary.[58] Although naloxone is effective in reversing opiate overdose, it also can precipitate physical withdrawal in physically dependent patients. Patients who fail to respond to a total dosage of 10 mg naloxone probably have a cause of acute intoxication other than an opiate.

Intoxication with stimulants, including cocaine, is treated pharmacologically only if the patient is overtly psychotic and agitated. Injectable benzodiazepines, usually lorazepam 2 to 4 mg intramuscularly every 30 minutes to 6 hours as necessary, can be used for agitation. As a backup to lorazepam, antipsychotic drugs can be used on a short-term basis, primarily in patients with psychotic symptoms, and usually at relatively low doses, such as haloperidol 2 to 5 mg intramuscularly every 30 minutes to 6 hours as necessary, followed by 5 to 15 mg orally per day in single or divided doses if the patient is still psychotic after initial treatment.[28–30,59] Cardiovascular complications are treated symptomatically with antiarrhythmic agents or other interventions as necessary. Seizures generally are treated supportively. Intravenous lorazepam or diazepam can be used if seizures progress to status epilepticus.

Hallucinogen intoxication is treated in a manner similar to stimulant intoxication. Drug therapy often can be avoided because patients can respond to careful reassurance, or so-called talk-down therapy. When necessary, short-term antianxiety and/or antipsychotic drug therapy can be used, as described previously. The same approach applies to marijuana and inhalant intoxication.

PCP intoxication is more unpredictable and more difficult to treat than other psychosis-producing drugs. Most clinicians suggest that sensory input be minimized to the extent possible; thus talk-down therapy is not recommended and can, in fact, make the patient worse. If PCP intoxication is suspected, patients should be left alone in a quiet, dimly lit room. If behavior is uncontrollable, antianxiety and/or antipsychotic drug therapy can be necessary.

WITHDRAWAL

❷ Treatment of drug withdrawal is the primary indication for drug therapy in substance-related disorders. Goals of drug therapy include prevention of progression of withdrawal to life-threatening severity, enabling the patient to be sufficiently comfortable and functional to participate in a behavioral treatment program, and supportive drug therapy. The clinician should remember that withdrawal is usually part of a substance dependence disorder. Patients with drug dependence generally cope with almost any stress through the use of a drug. In drug therapy for withdrawal, it is important to avoid reinforcing the patient's drug-seeking and drug-use behavior to the extent possible. Drug withdrawal in the best of circumstances is uncomfortable. Patients must be educated to deal with the stress of withdrawal without seeking drugs. The use of drugs as needed for anxiety or insomnia should be avoided. A recent review on the management of drug and alcohol withdrawal has been published.[13] Treatment of drug withdrawal is summarized in Table 68–4.

TABLE 68-4 Treatment of Withdrawal from Some Common Drugs of Abuse

Drug or Drug Class	Pharmacologic Therapy	Level of Evidence[a,b]
Benzodiazepines		
Short- to intermediate-acting	Lorazepam 2 mg three to four times a day; taper over 5–7 days	A1
Long-acting	Lorazepam 2 mg three to four times a day; taper over additional 5–7 days	A1
Barbiturates	Pentobarbital tolerance test; initial detoxification at upper limit of tolerance test; decrease dosage by 100 mg every 2–3 days	B3
Opiates	Methadone 20–80 mg orally daily; taper by 5–10 mg daily or buprenorphine 4-32 mg orally daily, or clonidine 2 mcg/kg three times a day × 7 days; taper over additional 3 days	A1 (methadone and buprenorphine) B1 (clonidine)
Mixed-substance withdrawal		
Drugs are cross-tolerant	Detoxify according to treatment for longer-acting drug used	B3
Drugs are not cross-tolerant	Detoxify from one drug while maintaining second drug (cross-tolerant drugs), then detoxify from second drug	B3
CNS stimulants	Supportive treatment only; pharmacotherapy often not used; bromocriptine 2.5 mg three times a day or higher may be used for severe craving associated with cocaine withdrawal	B2

[a]Strength of recommendations, evidence to support recommendation, A, good; B, moderate; C, poor.
[b]Quality of evidence: 1, evidence from more than 1 properly randomized, controlled trial; 2, evidence from more than 1 well-designed clinical trial with randomization, from cohort or case-controlled analytic studies or multiple time series; or dramatic results from uncontrolled experiments; 3, evidence from opinions of respected authorities, based on clinical experience, descriptive studies, or reports of expert communities.
Data from Hajak et al.,[11] O'Brien,[12] and Kosten and O'Conner.[13]

CNS DEPRESSANT WITHDRAWAL

Benzodiazepines

❷ Treatment of benzodiazepine withdrawal is very similar to the treatment of alcohol withdrawal, and the same drugs and dosages can be used. The major difference in management is the length of treatment. The onset of withdrawal symptoms in patients physically dependent on the long-acting benzodiazepines can be delayed up to 7 days after discontinuation of the drug.[12] A common approach in detoxification of such patients is to initiate treatment at usual dosages (chlordiazepoxide orally 50 mg three times a day; lorazepam orally 2 mg three times a day) and to maintain the initial dosage for 5 days, with gradual tapering over an additional 5 days. Detoxification in patients physically dependent on shorter-acting benzodiazepines is similar to treatment of alcohol withdrawal. Among the benzodiazepines, alprazolam has been suggested to be more difficult to taper and discontinue than the other benzodiazepines. Whether the difficulty is related to a different patient population commonly treated with alprazolam (e.g., panic disorder) or to intrinsic differences between alprazolam and other benzodiazepines is not clear. A longer, more gradual taper of the benzodiazepine used for detoxification can be needed. With all benzodiazepines, protracted minor abstinence symptoms—such as anxiety, insomnia, irritability, sensitivity to light and sound, and muscle spasms—can remain for several weeks in patients with a history of long exposure, even after the acute phase of benzodiazepine withdrawal is complete.

Barbiturates and Other Sedative-Hypnotic Drugs

❷ Although once used extensively, barbiturates and other nonbenzodiazepine sedating medications have been largely replaced by safer and more effective medications. Abuse problems with barbiturates resemble those seen with benzodiazepines in many ways. Withdrawal from barbiturates should be handled similarly to interventions for the abuse of alcohol and benzodiazepines.[11,12]

Opiates

Opiate withdrawal syndrome is similar to a severe case of influenza.[13] Opiate withdrawal is not life-threatening unless there is a concurrent life-threatening medical condition. Although most patients complain of symptoms of withdrawal such as cramping or insomnia, these symptoms are tolerable, and initiation of drug therapy can be avoided in many cases. Because opiate withdrawal is not life-threatening, observable signs of withdrawal, such as mydriasis, pilomotor erection, diaphoresis, or diarrhea should be noted before initiation of drug therapy. Characteristic signs and symptoms of opiate withdrawal include pupillary dilatation, lacrimation, rhinorrhea, piloerection ("gooseflesh"), yawning, sneezing, anorexia, nausea, vomiting, and diarrhea. Seizures do not occur. Onset and duration of withdrawal symptoms and the time of peak occurrence depends on the half-life of the drug involved. Typically heroin withdrawal reaches a peak within 36 to 72 hours of discontinuation and can last for 7 to 10 days. For methadone, symptoms peak at 72 hours but can last for 2 weeks or more.[12]

The conventional drug therapy for opioid withdrawal has been methadone, a synthetic opiate. Recently, buprenorphine has been approved for opioid withdrawal and will be discussed in detail below. In detoxification treatment, methadone is administered in decreasing doses over a period not exceeding 30 days (short-term detoxification) or 180 days (long-term detoxification). There are many tapering schedules recommended in the literature. Most patients in withdrawal continue to complain of mild symptoms after detoxification is completed. Some patients who are unable to discontinue methadone completely or habitually return to drug use when methadone is discontinued are placed in methadone-maintenance treatment programs and receive methadone chronically.[60]

Levo-α-acetylmethadol (LAAM) was approved by the FDA in 1993 as a potential alternative to methadone maintenance. LAAM forms two long-acting metabolites that allow three-times-a-week dosing.[58]

Typically, opioid dependency is treated initially with detoxification, usually as an inpatient. Except in a few individuals who remain drug free, detoxification is followed by long-term maintenance therapy. In the past, opioid-dependent patients relied on methadone or LAAM, but federal restrictions limited distribution of these drugs to a small number of methadone clinics, which are not only inconvenient, but also expose patients to other drug users, and can stigmatize patients if friends, family, or coworkers are aware of their trips to the clinic. There were limited provisions for take-at-home dosing of methadone or levomethadyl because of concern about the diversion of these drugs to illicit use.

In October 2003, the FDA approved two new products for treatment of opiate dependence. These products represent two new formulations of buprenorphine. The first of these formulations, Subutex, contains only buprenorphine and is intended for use at the beginning of treatment for opiate abuse. The other, Suboxone, contains both buprenorphine and the opiate antagonist naloxone, and is intended to be the formulation used in maintenance treatment of opiate addiction. Naloxone has been added to Suboxone to guard against intravenous abuse of buprenorphine by individuals physically dependent on opiates.

These drugs represent the first therapy for in-office prescribing for opioid dependence under the federal Drug Addiction Treatment Act (DATA) of 2000.[61] Prior to the passage of the DATA, office-based management of opioid dependence was illegal because existing federal laws prohibited physicians from prescribing narcotics for the sole purpose of maintaining a patient in a narcotic-addicted state. However, not every physician is permitted to prescribe these new drugs.

To qualify, physicians must be board certified in addiction medicine/psychiatry or hold other special credentials, and physicians are required to obtain 8 hours of authorized training before they can prescribe medications for office-based treatment of opioid dependence. They also must agree to treat no more than 30 opioid-dependent patients at any one time, and they must obtain special DEA numbers indicating that they are authorized to prescribe under the provisions of the DATA.

The two formulations of the drug have been placed into schedule III by the DEA. Each product is available in two dosage strengths, 2 mg and 8 mg. Once-daily doses are titrated to a target of 16 mg/day of buprenorphine, but the dosing range extends from 4 mg/day to 24 mg/day.

Office-based maintenance therapy is well studied for patients who are already receiving treatment.[62–65] A recent systematic review and meta-analysis including 18 clinical trials (n = 1,356 patients) determined that buprenorphine was more effective than clonidine for the management of opioid withdrawal. This meta-analysis did not detect a significant difference between buprenorphine and methadone in terms of completion of treatment. Withdrawal symptoms resolved more quickly with buprenorphine, according to this systematic review.[64]

In a multicenter, randomized, placebo-controlled trial,[62] 326 opiate-addicted persons were assigned to office-based treatment with sublingual tablets consisting of buprenorphine (16 mg) in combination with naloxone (4 mg), buprenorphine alone (16 mg), or placebo given daily for 4 weeks. The primary outcome measures were the percentage of urine samples negative for opiates and the subjects' self-reported craving for opiates. Safety data were obtained on 461 opiate-addicted persons who participated in an open-label study of buprenorphine and naloxone (at daily doses of up to 24 mg and 6 mg, respectively), and another 11 persons who received this combination only during the trial. The double-blind trial was terminated early because buprenorphine and naloxone in combination and buprenorphine alone were found to have greater efficacy than placebo. The proportion of urine samples that were negative for opiates was greater in the combined-treatment and buprenorphine groups (17.8% and 20.7%, respectively) than in the placebo group (5.8%; P <0.001 for both comparisons); the active-treatment groups also reported less opiate craving (P <0.001 for both comparisons against placebo). Rates of adverse events were similar in the active-treatment and placebo groups. During the open-label phase, the percentage of urine samples negative for opiates ranged from 35.2% to 67.4%. Results from the open-label followup study indicated that the combined treatment was safe and well tolerated. The authors concluded that buprenorphine and naloxone in combination and buprenorphine alone are safe and reduce the use of opiates and the craving for opiates among opiate-addicted persons who receive these medications in an office-based setting.

To check to see if the prescriber is authorized to treat patients under the DATA, pharmacists can call 1-866-BUP-CSAT or send an e-mail message to *info@buprenorphine.samhsa.gov*. Physicians generally use Subutex during induction and give a small supply of the product directly to the patient (clinical studies used buprenorphine-only tablets for the first 2 days). If patients present prescriptions for either agent from more than one prescriber for the same time period, a pharmacist should assume that diversion or abuse is occurring, refuse to fill the prescriptions, and notify both prescribers. Likewise, prescriptions for Subutex should be verified with prescribers, as the Suboxone formulation is preferred for long-term therapy.[65]

A rapid detoxification technique has been developed that is designed to shorten detoxification by precipitating withdrawal through the administration of opioid antagonists such as naloxone hydrochloride or naltrexone.[66] This approach is thought to have the advantage of getting patients though detoxification rapidly, minimizing the risk of relapse, and initiating treatment more quickly with naltrexone maintenance combined with suitable psychosocial interventions. Ultrarapid detoxification represents a variant of this technique in which patients undergo opioid antagonist–precipitated withdrawal while under general anesthesia or heavy sedation. Although it is difficult to estimate the extent of their clinical use, these techniques are becoming increasingly available in response to increasing demand for opioid-dependence treatment services. In the United States there has been a rapid proliferation of programs offering ultrarapid detoxification, with some programs charging up to $15,000 per treatment.[67]

A meta-analysis was performed to assess the evidence for the efficacy of both rapid detoxification and ultrarapid detoxification to determine their role among the available treatment options for opioid dependence.[66] Analysis was performed on 12 studies of rapid detoxification and 9 studies of ultrarapid detoxification. The authors concluded that more research is needed using more rigorous research methods, longer-term outcomes, and comparisons with other methods of treatment for opioid dependence before these techniques can gain widespread acceptance.[66] Recently, a randomized, open label, head-to-head trial (n = 106) compared the efficacy of ultrarapid detoxification compared with buprenorphine-assisted rapid opioid detoxification with naltrexone induction, versus clonidine-assisted opioid detoxification with delayed naltrexone induction.[67] Outcome measures included severity of withdrawal symptoms, rates of completion of inpatient detoxification program (12 weeks), and percentage of opioid positive urine samples. Severity of withdrawal symptoms, percentage of opioid-positive urine samples, and rates of completion of treatment did not differ among the three groups. Three life-threatening adverse events occurred in the ultrarapid detoxification group.[67]

CLINICAL CONTROVERSY

Ultrarapid detoxification from opiates remains somewhat controversial in terms of its efficacy, safety, and cost. Before consenting to such treatment, patients should inquire about the practitioner's previous experience with this technique, including success rates of patients remaining drug-free and also rates of complications that have occurred.

WITHDRAWAL FROM OTHER SUBSTANCES

Withdrawal from other drugs, including cocaine and other stimulants, is primarily supportive. However, pharmacotherapy recently has assumed a greater role in treating cocaine withdrawal and dependence. Bromocriptine, a dopamine antagonist at low dosages and an agonist at high dosages, is usually used in the treatment of parkinsonism and hyperprolactinemia and has been used to treat cocaine withdrawal symptoms and to reduce the craving for cocaine. Use of bromocriptine is based on the hypothesis that chronic use of cocaine causes dopamine depletion; therefore higher dosages should be used (i.e., 2.5 mg three times daily or higher). Despite initially promising pilot studies, recent evidence does not support the efficacy of bromocriptine to reduce cocaine use or craving.[68]

A more likely efficacious approach is the use of the cocaine vaccine that is still in clinical trials.[69] This vaccine is an immunotherapeutic agent that treats cocaine dependence. In the presence of the vaccine, the immune system forms antibodies that prevent cocaine from crossing the blood-brain barrier, blocking access to receptor sites in the brain. Phase II clinical trials suggest the vaccine is well tolerated and effective to decrease the likelihood of cocaine use in patients that received five 400-mcg vaccinations over a 12-week period. Cocaine-specific antibodies were still present at the 6 month followup.[70]

SUBSTANCE DEPENDENCE

❸ The treatment of drug dependence is primarily behavioral. The patient generally is taught that complete abstinence is the only realistic alternative to a life of uncontrollable drug use and despair that ultimately will end in death, and that there is no intermediate, controllable level of drinking or use of another drug. However, complete and permanent abstinence as the sole route to recovery is controversial. There may be an extremely few individuals who can return to controllable levels of drinking alcohol, but it is impossible to predict who these individuals are; thus most treatment programs continue to advocate complete abstinence. The prospect of life without alcohol or other drugs is incomprehensible to many patients. Entry into treatment often is facilitated by some type of leverage that the drug-dependent person associates with negative consequences, such as potential loss of job, divorce, legal problems, or deteriorating physical health. Early treatment is directed at penetrating the denial of a problem that is always present. The patient must be educated as to the disease of addiction, the effects of drugs, and the permanence of the condition.

As evidenced by the approval of the two buprenorphine products, there has been a trend toward outpatient treatment for drug dependence, caused in part by cost-containment efforts. Inpatient treatment programs can cost as much as $20,000 for a 4-week stay. When withdrawal symptoms are mild to moderate and there are no other medical indications for hospitalization, outpatient treatment can be an attractive alternative to inpatient treatment. One critical criterion for outpatient treatment is the patient's compliance with complete abstinence from the dependence-producing drug during the treatment experience.

Families must be involved in treatment. The course of the patient's illness often has a devastating effect on other family members. Severely depleted self-esteem, denial of the family member's addiction, feelings of responsibility for the family member's drug use, and other behaviors that parallel the addiction process are often present.

❹ Treatment must be a lifelong process. Aftercare, or what is now being called *continued care,* should include regular and frequent treatment in some form. Most drug-dependence treatment programs embrace a treatment approach based on the twelve steps to recovery. AA is one of the most successful of all self-help groups. Associated groups include Al-Anon (a group for family members of alcoholics), NA (self-help groups based on the AA concept for users of other drugs), Overeaters Anonymous (a group for individuals with eating disorders), Gamblers Anonymous, and several other similar programs. Among chemically dependent healthcare professionals, treatment that incorporates both AA and peer-led self-help groups can be most effective.[71]

CONCLUSIONS

Substance use disorders remain one of the great public health issues of contemporary society. Dependence on drugs is a powerful emotional and political issue. Because we live in a chemically oriented society, everyone is affected in some way by drug abuse and drug dependence. Healthcare professionals must be particularly vigilant for problems associated with drug use, not only for our patients, but also for ourselves.

ABBREVIATIONS

AA: Alcoholics Anonymous

ATOD: alcohol, tobacco, and other drugs

CASA: Center on Addiction and Substance Abuse

CNS: central nervous system

CSF: cerebrospinal fluid

DATA: Drug Addiction Treatment Act

DAWN: Drug Abuse Warning Network

DEA: U.S. Drug Enforcement Administration

DMT: dimethyltryptamine

DSM-IV-TR: *Diagnostic and Statistical Manual of Mental Disorders, 4th Edition, Text Revision*

FDA: Food and Drug Administration

GBL: γ-butyrolactone

GHB: γ-hydroxybutyrate

5-HIAA: 5-hydroxyindoleacetic acid

LAAM: *levo*-α-acetylmethadol

LSD: lysergic acid diethylamide

MDA: 3,4-methylenedioxyamphetamine

MDMA: 3,4-methylenedioxymethamphetamine

MTFS: Monitoring the Future Study

NA: Narcotics Anonymous

NSDUH: National Survey on Drug Use and Health

PCP: phencyclidine

REM: rapid eye movement

SAMHSA: Substance Abuse and Mental Health Services Administration

THC: Δ^9-tetrahydrocannabinol

REFERENCES

1. Schneider Institute for Health Policy, Brandeis University. Substance Abuse: The Nation's Number One Health Problem. Key Indicators for Policy—Update. Princeton, NJ: Robert Wood Johnson Foundation, 2001:1–128.
2. Substance Abuse and Mental Health Services Administration. Overview of Findings from the 2003 National Survey on Drug Use and Health. Rockville, MD: Office of Applied Studies, 2004. NSDUH Series H–24 DHHS Publication No. SMA 04–3963.
3. Substance Abuse & Mental Health Services Administration. Results from the 2005 National Survey on Drug Use and Health: National Findings. Rockville, MD: Office of Applied Studies, 2006. NHSDA Series H-30 DHHS Publication No. SMA 06–4194, *http://www.oas.samhsa.gov/NSDUH/2k5NSDUH/2k5results.htm*.
4. Savage SR, Joranson DE, Covington EC, et al. Definitions related to the medical use of opioids: Evolution towards universal agreement. J Pain Symptom Manage 2003;26:655–667.
5. Johnston LD, O'Malley PM, Bachman JG, Schulenberg JE. Monitoring the Future: National Results on Adolescent Drug Use: Overview of Key Findings, 2005. Bethesda, MD: National Institute on Drug Abuse, 2006. NIH Publication Number 06–5882, *http://www.monitoringthefuture.org/pubs/monographs/overview2005.pdf*.
6. Drug Abuse Warning Network, 2004: National Estimates of Drug-Related Emergency Department Visits. Rockville, MD: Department of Health and Human Services, 2006. DAWN Series D-28 DHHS Publication No. (SMA) 06–4143, *https://dawninfo.samhsa.gov/pubs/edpubs/default.asp*.
7. National Center on Addiction and Substance Abuse at Columbia University. Shoveling Up: The Impact of Substance Abuse on State Budgets. January 2001:2–3.
8. Diagnostic and Statistical Manual of Mental Disorders, 4th ed., Text Revision. Washington, DC: American Psychiatric Press, 2000:191–198.
9. Cami J, Farre M. Drug addiction. N Engl J Med 2003;349:975–986.
10. Woods JH, Winger G. Abuse liability of flunitrazepam. J Clin Psychopharmacol 1997;17(Suppl 2):1S–57S.
11. Hajak G, Muller WE, Wittchen HU, et al. Abuse and dependence potential for the non-benzodiazepine hypnotics zolpidem and zopiclone: A review of case reports and epidemiological data. Addiction 2003;98:1371–1378.
12. O'Brien CP. Drug addiction and drug abuse. In: Brunton LL, Lazo JS, Parker KL, eds. Goodman and Gilman's The Pharmacological Basis of Therapeutics, 11th ed. New York: McGraw-Hill, 2006:614–615.
13. Kosten TR, O'Connor PG. Management of drug and alcohol withdrawal. N Engl J Med 2003;348:1786–1795.
14. Schwartz RH, Milteer R, LeBeau MA. Drug-facilitated sexual assault ("date rape"). South Med J 2000;93:558–561.
15. Centers for Disease Control and Prevention. γ-Hydroxy butyrate use—New York and Texas, 1995–1996. MMWR Morb Mortal Wkly Rep 1997;46:281–283.
16. Kam PC, Yoong FF. γ-Hydroxybutyric acid: An emerging recreational drug. Anaesthesia 1998;53:1195–1198.
17. Zvosec DL, Smith SW, McCutcheon JR, et al. Adverse events, including death, associated with the use of 1,4-butanediol. N Engl J Med 2001;344:87–94.
18. Craig K, Gomez HF, McManus JL, Bania TC. Severe γ-hydroxybutyrate withdrawal: A case report and literature review. J Emerg Med 2000;18:65–70.
19. Substance Abuse and Mental Health Services Administration. Nonmedical uses of pain relievers: Characteristics of recent initiatives. The NSDUH Report, 2006;22:1–4, *http://www.oas.samhsa.gov/2k6/pain/pain.pdf*.
20. Department of Health and Human Services, Food and Drug Administration, Center for Drug Evaluation and Research, Anesthetic and Life Support Drugs Advisory Committee. Risk Management Programs for Opioid Analgesics. September 9, 2003, *http://www.fda.gov/ohrms/dockets/ac/03/transcripts/3978T1.pdf*.
21. Cone EJ, Fant RV, Rohay JM, et al. Oxycodone involvement in drug abuse deaths: A DAWN-based classification scheme applied to an oxycodone postmortem database containing over 1000 cases. J Anal Toxicol 2003;27:57–67.
22. Ballantyne JC, Mao J. Opioid therapy for chronic pain. N Engl J Med 2003;349:1943–1953.
23. Repetto M, Gold MS. Cocaine and crack: Neurobiology. In: Lowinson JH, Ruiz P, Millman RB, Langrod JG, eds. Substance Abuse: A Comprehensive Textbook, 4th ed. Baltimore: Williams & Wilkins, 2005:196–218.
24. Hart CL, Jatlow P, Sevarino KA, McCance-Katz EF. Comparison of intravenous cocaethylene and cocaine in humans. Psychopharmacology (Berl) 2000;149:153–162.
25. McCance-Katz EF, Kosten TR, Jatlow P. Concurrent use of cocaine and alcohol is more potent and potentially more toxic than use of either alone: A multiple-dose study. Biol Psychiatry 1998;44:250–259.
26. Aigner TG, Balster RL. Choice behavior in rhesus monkeys: Cocaine versus food. Science 1978;201:534–535.
27. Pozner CN, Levine M, Zane R. The cardiovascular effects of cocaine. J Emerg Med 2005;29:173–178.
28. Harris D, Batki SL. Stimulant psychosis: Symptom profile and acute clinical course. Am J Addict 2000;9:28–37.
29. Carrera MR, Meijler MM, Janda KD. Cocaine pharmacology and current pharmacotherapies for its abuse. Bioorg Med Chem 2004;12:5019–5030.
30. King GR, Ellinwood EH. Amphetamines and other stimulants. In: Lowinson JH, Ruiz P, Millman RB, Langrod JG, eds. Substance Abuse: A Comprehensive Textbook, 4th ed. Baltimore: Williams & Wilkins, 2005:277–302.
31. Simon SL, Domier C, Carnell J, et al. Cognitive impairment in individuals currently using methamphetamine. Am J Addict 2000;9:222–231.
32. Klasser GD, Epstein J. Methamphetamine and its impact on dental care. J Can Dent Assoc 2005;71:759–762.
33. Lineberry TW, Bostwick M. Methamphetamine abuse: A perfect storm of complications. Mayo Clin Proc 2006;81:77–84.
34. Rawson RA, Gonzales R, Brethen P. Treatment of methamphetamine use disorders: An update. J Subst Abuse Treat 2002;23:145–150.

35. U.S. Drug Enforcement Administration. El Paso Intelligence Center National Clandestine Laboratory Seizure System, in "Methamphetamine: Strategic Findings, Overview, Availability, Production, Transportation, Distribution, and Demand." 2006, *http://www.usdoj.gov/dea/concern/18862/meth.htm*.
36. Dedel K, Scott MS. Clandestine Methamphetamine Labs, 2nd ed. Problem Oriented Guides for Police Series, Number 16. 2006, *http://www.cops.usdoj.gov*.
37. Morton J. Ecstasy: Pharmacology and neurotoxicity. Curr Opin Pharmacol 2005;5:79–86.
38. McCann UD, Eligulashvili V, Ricaurte GA. (±) 3,4-Methylenedioxymethamphetamine ("Ecstasy")-induced serotonin neurotoxicity: Clinical studies. Neuropsychobiology 2000;42:11–16.
39. Bolla KI, McCann UD, Ricaurte GA. Memory impairment in abstinent MDMA ("ecstasy") users. Neurology 1998;51:1532–1537.
40. McCann UD, Mertl M, Eligulashvili V, Ricaurte GA. Cognitive performance in (±)3,4-methylenedioxymethamphetamine (MDMA, "ecstasy") users: A controlled study. Psychopharmacology (Berl) 1999;143:417–425.
41. Ricaurte GA, McCann UD, Szabo Z, Scheffel U. Toxicodynamics and long-term toxicity of the recreational drug, 3,4-methylenedioxymethamphetamine (MDMA, "Ecstasy"). Toxicol Lett 2000;112–113, 143–146.
42. James RA, Dinan A. Hyperpyrexia associated with fatal paramethoxyamphetamine (PMA) abuse. Med Sci Law 1998;38:83–85.
43. Zukin SR, Sloboda Z, Javitt DC. Phencyclidine (PCP). In: Lowinson JH, Ruiz P, Millman RB, Langrod JG, eds. Substance Abuse: A Comprehensive Textbook, 4th ed. Baltimore: Williams & Wilkins, 2005:324–336.
44. Freese TE, Miotto K, Reback CJ. The effects and consequences of selected club drugs. J Subst Abuse Treat 2002;23:151–156.
45. Jansen KL. A review of the nonmedical use of ketamine: Use, users and consequences. J Psychoactive Drugs 2000;32:419–433.
46. Jansen KL, Darracot-Cankovic R. The nonmedical use of ketamine, part two: A review of problem use and dependence. J Psychoactive Drugs 2001;33:151–158.
47. U.S. Drug Enforcement Administration. Other Dangerous Drugs. 2006, *http://www.usdoj.gov/dea/concern/18862/odd.htm*.
48. Glennon RA. Classical hallucinogens: An introductory overview. NIDA Res Monogr 1994;146:4–32.
49. Pechnick RN, Ungerleider JT. Hallucinogens. In: Lowinson JH, Ruiz P, Millman RB, Langrod JG, eds. Substance Abuse: A Comprehensive Textbook, 4th ed. Baltimore: Williams & Wilkins, 2005:313–323.
50. U.S. Drug Enforcement Administration. LSD. Pickard and Apperson Convicted of LSD Charges, Largest LSD Lab Seizure in DEA History. March 31, 2003, *http://www.usdoj.gov/dea/concern/lsd.html*.
51. National Institute on Drug Abuse (NIDA) Research Report—Marijuana Abuse. NIH Publication No. 05–3859. 2005, *http://www.drugabuse.gov/PDF/RRMarijuana.pdf*.
52. Solowij N, Stephens RS, Roffman RA, et al. Cognitive functioning of long-term heavy cannabis users seeking treatment. JAMA 2002;287:1123–1131.
53. National Highway Traffic Safety Administration (NHSTA) Notes. Marijuana and alcohol combined severely impede driving performance. Ann Emerg Med 2000;35:398–399.
54. ElSohly MA, Ross SA, Mehmedic Z, et al. Potency trends of delta 9-THC and other cannabinoids in confiscated marijuana from 1980–1997. J Forensic Sci 2000;45:24–30.
55. Sarafian TA, Magallanes JA, Shau H, et al. Oxidative stress produced by marijuana smoke: An adverse effect enhanced by cannabinoids. Am J Respir Cell Mol Biol 1999;20:1286–1293.
56. Kalant H. Adverse effects of cannabis on health: An update of the literature since 1966. Prog Neuropsychopharmacol Biol Psychiatry 2004;28:849–863.
57. O'Brien CP. Drug addiction and drug abuse. In: Brunton LL, Lazo JS, Parker KL, eds. Goodman and Gilman's The Pharmacological Basis of Therapeutics, 11th ed. New York: McGraw-Hill, 2006:625–626.
58. Fudala PJ, Greenstein RA, O'Brien CP. Alternative pharmacotherapies for opiate addiction. In: Lowinson JH, Ruiz P, Millman RB, Langrod JG, eds. Substance Abuse: A Comprehensive Textbook, 4th ed. Baltimore: Williams & Wilkins, 2005:641–653.
59. Smith DE, Seymour RB. Benzodiazepines and other sedative-hypnotics. In: Galanter M, Kleber HD, eds. Textbook of Substance Abuse Treatment. Washington, DC: American Psychiatric Press, 1994:179–186.
60. Knapp CM, Ciraulo DA, Jaffe J. Opiates: Clinical aspects. In: Lowinson JH, Ruiz P, Millman RB, Langrod JG, eds. Substance Abuse: A Comprehensive Textbook, 4th ed. Baltimore: Williams & Wilkins, 2005:180–195.
61. Drug Addiction Treatment Act of 2000 (DATA), Title XXXV of the Children's Health Act of 2000 (Pub L No. 106–310, 116 Stat 1222).
62. Fudala PJ, Bridge TP, Herbert S, et al. Buprenorphine/Naloxone Collaborative Study Group. Office-based treatment of opiate addiction with a sublingual-tablet formulation of buprenorphine and naloxone. N Engl J Med 2003;349:949–958.
63. Fiellin DA, O'Connor PG. Office-based treatment of opioid-dependent patients. N Engl J Med 2002;347:817–823.
64. Gowing L, Ali R, White J. Buprenorphine for the management of opioid withdrawal. Cochrane Database Syst Rev 2006;(2):CD002025.
65. Food and Drug Administration. Information for pharmacists—Suboxone and Subutex. 2002, *http://www.fda.gov/cder/drug/infopage/subutex_suboxone/default.htm*.
66. O'Connor PG, Kosten TR. Rapid and ultrarapid opioid detoxification techniques. JAMA 1998;279:229–234.
67. Collins ED, Kleber HD, Whittington RA, Heitler NE. Anesthesia-assisted vs buprenorphine- or clonidine-assisted heroin detoxification and naltrexone induction: A randomized trial. JAMA 2005;294:903–913.
68. Gorelick DA, Wilkins JN. Bromocriptine treatment for cocaine addiction: Association with plasma prolactin levels. Drug Alcohol Depend 2006;81:189–195.
69. Hall W, Carter L. Ethical issues in using a cocaine vaccine to treat and prevent cocaine abuse and dependence. J Med Ethics 2004;30:337–340.
70. Martell BA, Mitchell E, Poling J, et al. Vaccine pharmacotherapy for the treatment of cocaine dependence. Biol Psychiatry 2005;58:158–164.
71. Talbott GD, Wilson PO. Physicians and other health professionals. In: Lowinson JH, Ruiz P, Millman RB, Langrod JG, eds. Substance Abuse: A Comprehensive Textbook, 4th ed. Baltimore: Williams & Wilkins, 2005:1187–1202.

CHAPTER 69 Substance-Related Disorders: Alcohol, Nicotine, and Caffeine

PAUL L. DOERING, W. KLUGH KENNEDY, AND LISA A. BOOTHBY

KEY CONCEPTS

1. Alcohol, nicotine, and caffeine use impose enormous social and economic costs on society.
2. Alcohol abuse causes numerous chronic diseases and injuries with an inordinate amount of mortality.
3. Pharmacogenomics studies have identified genotypic and functional phenotypic variants that either serve to protect patients or predispose them toward alcohol dependence.
4. Alcohol is a central nervous system depressant that affects the central nervous system in a dose-dependent fashion.
5. The metabolism of alcohol is considered to follow zero-order pharmacokinetics, and this has important implications for the time course in which alcohol can exert its effects.
6. Benzodiazepines are the treatment of choice for alcohol withdrawal.
7. Disulfiram, naltrexone, and acamprosate are FDA-approved drug therapies for the treatment of alcohol dependence. The clinical usefulness of these agents to improve sustained abstinence remains controversial, and relapse is common.
8. More than three-quarters of smokers are nicotine dependent. Tobacco dependence is a chronic condition that requires repeated interventions.
9. Use of nicotine replacement therapy along with behavioral counseling doubles cessation rates.
10. Bupropion is efficacious alone and in combination with nicotine replacement therapy for smoking cessation.
11. Varenicline is efficacious for smoking cessation, although it is not first-line therapy.
12. Caffeine's pharmacologic actions are similar to those of other stimulant drugs. As such, abstinence from caffeine induces a distinct withdrawal syndrome that includes headache, drowsiness, and fatigue.

Learning objectives, review questions, and other resources can be found at **www.pharmacotherapyonline.com.**

KEY MEDICAL TERMS

Caffeinism: *Caffeinism* is the term coined to describe the clinical syndrome produced by acute or chronic overuse of caffeine.

Euphoria: A mood state characterized by an exaggerated, superficial sense of well-being, characterized extreme happiness, sometimes more than is reasonable in a particular situation.

Intoxication: The development of a substance-specific syndrome after recent ingestion and presence in the body of a substance, and it is associated with maladaptive behavior during the waking state caused by the effect of the substance on the central nervous system.

Withdrawal: The development of a substance-specific syndrome after cessation of or reduction in intake of a substance that was used regularly by the individual to induce a state of intoxication.

❶ Alcohol, nicotine, and caffeine are considered by most to be socially acceptable drugs, yet they impose an enormous social and economic cost on our society. Approximately 438,000 deaths each year are attributable to tobacco use, making tobacco the number one preventable cause of death and disease in this country.[1] The three leading causes of death attributable to smoking include lung cancer, chronic obstructive pulmonary disease, and ischemic heart disease.[2]

❷ Approximately 12.9 million persons in the United States report current heavy use of alcohol or alcohol abuse.[3] Almost one-half of these persons meet *Diagnostic and Statistical Manual of Mental Disorders, 4th edition, Text Revision* (*DSM-IV-TR*) criteria for alcohol dependence,[4] and more than 700,000 persons are in treatment for alcoholism at any one time.[5] Population-based surveys of current drinkers have found rates of 7% to 16% for alcohol abuse or dependence.[6] The World Health Organization estimates that there are approximately 2 billion people worldwide who consume alcoholic beverages, and 76.3 million with diagnosable alcohol-use disorders.[7] Long-term alcohol abuse often leads to chronic disease. A causal relationship between alcohol abuse and at least 60 types of chronic disease or injury have been established (e.g., esophageal cancer, liver cancer, and cirrhosis of the liver, epileptic seizures, homicide, and motor vehicle accidents) worldwide.[7] Nationally, according to the Drug Abuse Warning Network 2002 survey, emergency department visits related to drug abuse most frequently involved alcohol, and included 31% of the observed cases.[8]

❷ Worldwide, alcohol abuse leads to 1.8 million deaths annually.[7] Nationally, an estimated 100,000 U.S. citizens die each year because of alcohol-related causes, including traffic collisions and cirrhosis of the liver.[9] Direct and indirect health and social costs of alcoholism to the nation are estimated to be $185 billion annually.[10]

Caffeine is currently the most widely used psychoactive substance in the world.[11] In the United States, 80% to 90% of adults regularly consume behaviorally active doses of caffeine.[11] Although research has shown that caffeine can cause a compulsive pattern of use, the prevalence of caffeine dependence and its clinical significance are difficult to determine.

The subjects of alcohol, tobacco, and caffeine abuse deserve much more attention than space permits in this chapter. Therefore the information here should serve as a brief overview of these topics, and the reader desiring more details is urged to consult one or more of the many textbooks and articles devoted to these subjects.

ALCOHOL

EPIDEMIOLOGY OF ALCOHOL USE

Roughly half (51.8%) of Americans ages 12 and older reported being current drinkers of alcohol according to the National Survey on Drug Use and Health (formerly called the National Household Survey on Drug Abuse).[3] This translates to 126 million people, which is higher than the 2004 estimate of 121 million people (50.3 %). Approximately one-fifth of persons 12 years of age and older (55 million people) participated in binge drinking, defined as having five or more drinks on the same occasion, at least once in the 30 days prior to the survey. In 2005 there were 16 million heavy drinkers, meaning that they drank five or more drinks on the same occasion on at least five different days in the past month.[3]

THE DISEASE MODEL OF ADDICTION AS APPLIED TO ALCOHOLISM

The disease concept of addiction, using alcoholism as a model, states that addiction is a disease and that individuals who suffer from the disease do not choose to contract the disease any more than someone who suffers from heart disease or diabetes mellitus chooses to contract that illness. A *disease* is defined as "any deviation from or interruption of the normal structure or function of any part, organ, or system (or combination thereof) of the body that is manifested by a characteristic set of symptoms and signs and whose etiology, pathology, and prognosis may be known or unknown."[4] Alcoholism, which is discussed as a prototype, meets all the definitional criteria. Diagnostic criteria for alcoholism do not specify frequency of drinking or amount of alcohol consumed. The key determinant is whether drinking is compulsive, out of control, and consequential when one drinks.

❸ It has long been recognized that alcoholism is heritable, as 50% to 60% of first-degree relatives of alcoholics become alcohol dependent themselves.[12] Past discussions have focused on whether this heritable risk is because of genetics, environment, or both. Recent research has identified several traits (or phenotypes), that attenuate one's risk of alcohol dependence. Initially based on data from preclinical studies, pharmacogenomics studies have identified genotypic and functional phenotypic variants that either serve to protect patients, or predispose them toward alcohol dependence.[13] Large-scale pharmacoepidemiologic studies have further elucidated the environmental risk factors that are associated with either protective effects or predisposition toward alcoholism.[14] This is referred to as the "genome x" environment interaction effect. The known susceptibility genes, phenotypic characteristics, and environmental risk factors are summarized in Table 69–1.[13–17] Further elucidation of the gene-environment interactions are needed before these data are used to (1) create alcohol abuse prevention programs that target high-risk populations, and (2) develop targeted treatments to prevent and treat alcohol dependence.[18]

PHARMACOLOGY AND PHARMACOKINETICS OF ALCOHOL

Alcohol as a Drug

❹ Alcohol is a central nervous system (CNS) depressant that affects the CNS in a dose-dependent fashion, producing sedation that progresses to sleep, unconsciousness, coma, surgical anesthesia, and finally fatal respiratory depression and cardiovascular collapse. Alcohol affects endogenous opiates and several neurotransmitter systems in the brain, including γ-aminobutyric acid (GABA), glutamine, and dopamine. Alcohol intake results in an increase in endogenous opioids,[19] and this can be responsible for the euphoria experienced with alcohol consumption.

TABLE 69-1 Genotypic, Phenotypic, and Environmental Factors That Increase Alcohol Dependence Risk

Susceptibility Genes	Phenotype	Environment
Regions on chromosomes 1 and 4 that code for the following receptors:	Personality traits that include:	Religious background
$GABA_A$	Novelty seeking	Urban residence (vs. rural)
Serotonin 1b	Impulsivity	History of sexual abuse
DRD4	Aggression	Being single
Tryptophan hydroxylase	Depression	Having deceased parents
Neuropeptide Y	Maximum number of alcoholic drinks consumed per day	
Gene that codes for:		
ALDH2		
5HTTLPR		

ALDH2, aldehyde dehydrogenase 2; DRD4, type 4 dopamine receptor gene; GABA, gamma aminobutyric acid; 5HTTLPR, 5 hydroxytryptamine transporter.
Data from Bierut et al.,[13] Heath et al.,[14] Luo et al.,[15] Boothby and Doering,[16] and Krystal et al.[17]

Alcohol is available in a variety of concentrations in various alcoholic beverages. There are approximately 14 g of alcohol in a 12-oz can of beer (approximately 5%), 4 oz of nonfortified wine (approximately 10% to 14%), or one shot (1.5 oz) of 80-proof whiskey (40%). Full consumption of this amount will cause an increase in blood alcohol level of approximately 20 to 25 mg/dL in a healthy 70-kg (154 lb) male, although this varies with the time frame over which the alcohol is consumed, the type of alcoholic beverage, whether food is consumed along with it, and many patient variables. The lethal dose of alcohol in humans is variable, but deaths generally occur when blood alcohol levels are greater than 400 to 500 mg/dL.[20]

CLINICAL CONTROVERSY

Moderate alcohol consumption has been suggested in some studies to improve health. The definition of moderate consumption is narrow—one drink or less per day for females and two drinks or less per day for males. Controversy stems from the limitations of the studies that support moderate alcohol consumption. The major limitations of this research thus far are the observational study designs that cannot demonstrate cause and effect relationships between alcohol consumption and positive health benefits.[21–24] Additional potential confounders in these studies include diet, exercise, disease states, other drug therapies known to promote or hinder cardiovascular health, and psychosocial factors such as stress management.

Pharmacokinetics

Absorption of alcohol begins in the stomach within 5 to 10 minutes of oral ingestion. The onset of clinical effects follows fairly rapidly. Peak serum concentrations of alcohol usually are achieved 30 to 90 minutes after finishing the last drink, although it is variable depending on the type of alcoholic beverage consumed, what and when the person last ate, and other factors.[25]

More than 90% of alcohol in the plasma is metabolized in the liver by three enzyme systems that operate within the hepatocyte. The remainder is excreted by the lungs and in urine and sweat. Alcohol is metabolized to acetaldehyde by alcohol dehydrogenase in the cell. In turn, acetaldehyde is metabolized to carbon dioxide and water by the enzyme aldehyde dehydrogenase. A second pathway for oxidation of alcohol uses catalase, an enzyme located in the peroxisomes and microsomes. The third enzyme system, the microsomal alcohol oxidase system, has a role in the oxidation of alcohol to acetaldehyde. These last two mechanisms are of lesser importance than the alcohol dehydrogenase-aldehyde dehydrogenase system.

5 The metabolism of alcohol generally is said to follow zero-order pharmacokinetics.[25] This can, in fact, be an oversimplification because at very high or very low concentrations of alcohol the metabolism can follow first-order pharmacokinetics.[26] On average, the blood alcohol concentration (BAC) is lowered from 15 to 22.2 mg/dL per hour in the nontolerant individual, assuming that the individual is in the postabsorptive state (Table 69–2). Alcohol has a volume of distribution of 0.6 to 0.8 L/kg, representing the total body water.[25]

CLINICAL INDICATORS OF CHRONIC ALCOHOL ABUSE

The CAGE questionnaire, when correctly administered, is a tool for detecting individuals more likely to be abusing alcohol and therefore at greater risk for alcohol withdrawal. It is simple as well as sensitive and specific. CAGE is a mnemonic for four questions: (1) Do you ever feel the need to *C*UT DOWN on your alcohol use? (2) Have you ever been *A*NNOYED by others telling you that you drink too much? (3) Have you ever felt *G*UILTY about your drinking or something you did while drinking? (4) Do you ever have an "*E*YE OPENER"? A positive response to two or more of these four questions suggests an increased likelihood of alcohol abuse with a sensitivity of 43% to 94% and a specificity of 73% to 90%.[27] This can translate into an increased risk of alcohol withdrawal syndrome for this group. In some settings this is a useful tool to identify that subset of patients who will benefit from increased monitoring.

Alcohol Poisoning

Acute alcohol poisoning usually occurs with rapid consumption of large quantities of alcoholic beverages, because this type of drinking delivers a bolus of alcohol to the gastrointestinal (GI) tract. Normally, the user passes out before a toxic dose of alcohol can be ingested, and/or the person vomits to rid the stomach of its toxic reservoir. With rapid drinking as described, the person may fall asleep or pass out without vomiting, allowing continued alcohol absorption from the GI tract, while the patient sleeps, until fatal BACs are achieved.

TABLE 69-2 Specific Effects of Alcohol Related to BAC

BAC (%)[a]	Effect
0.02–0.03	No loss of coordination, slight euphoria, and loss of shyness.
0.04–0.06	Feeling of well-being, relaxation, lower inhibitions, sensation of warmth. Euphoria. Some minor impairment of reasoning and memory, lowering of caution.
0.07–0.09	Slight impairment of balance, speech, vision, reaction time, and hearing. Euphoria. Judgment and self-control are reduced, and caution, reason, and memory are impaired. It is illegal to operate a motor vehicle in some states at this level.
0.10–0.125	Significant impairment of motor coordination and loss of good judgment. Speech can be slurred; balance, vision, reaction time, and hearing impaired. Euphoria. It is illegal to operate a motor vehicle at this level of intoxication.
0.13–0.15	Gross motor impairment and lack of physical control. Blurred vision and major loss of balance. Euphoria is reduced, and dysphoria is beginning to appear.
0.16–0.2	Dysphoria (anxiety, restlessness) predominates, nausea can appear. The drinker has the appearance of a "sloppy drunk."
0.25	Needs assistance in walking; total mental confusion. Dysphoria with nausea and some vomiting.
0.3	Loss of consciousness.
≥ 0.4	Onset of coma, possible death caused by respiratory arrest.

BAC, blood alcohol concentration.

[a]Grams of ethyl alcohol per 100 mL of whole blood.

Data from Federal Aviation Administration,[27] Brunton et al.,[28] Goldman,[29] Alcohol and Substance Awareness Program,[30] and Garriot.[31]

CLINICAL PRESENTATION OF ALCOHOL INTOXICATION AND WITHDRAWAL

General

- Acute alcohol detoxification and withdrawal after chronic alcohol abuse is a serious condition that can require hospitalization and adjunctive pharmacotherapy. If the BAC gets high enough, death is possible.

Symptoms

- The intoxicated patient can present with slurred speech and ataxia. The patient can be sedated or unconscious. As BACs decrease rapidly, nausea, vomiting, and hallucinations can ensue. Delirium and seizures are the most severe symptoms.

Signs

- The intoxicated patient can present with nystagmus.
- In withdrawal, the patient can present with tachycardia, diaphoresis, or hyperthermia.

Laboratory Tests

- In the emergency department, a BAC should be ordered when alcohol ingestion is suspected. Most laboratories report BAC in units of milligrams per deciliter. A whole blood alcohol level of 150 mg/dL reported in the hospital corresponds to 0.15% BAC obtained by law enforcement.
- A complete toxicologic screen to rule out the presence of other substances can be useful.

Other Diagnostic Tests

- Differentiate acute alcohol intoxication from other medical illnesses (e.g., head trauma).
- Use computed tomography (CT) on any patient with focal neurologic findings, failure to improve, new-onset seizures, or mental status out of proportion to degree of intoxication.

TREATMENT

Alcohol Withdrawal

Goals for alcohol-dependent persons trying to decrease or discontinue alcohol intake include: (1) the prevention and treatment of withdrawal symptoms (including seizures and delirium tremens) and medical or psychiatric complications, (2) long-term abstinence after detoxification, and (3) entry into ongoing medical and alcohol-dependence treatment.

■ PHARMACOLOGIC THERAPY

6 Symptom-triggered treatment with a benzodiazepine is the current standard of care in alcohol detoxification to manage and minimize symptoms and avoid progression to the more severe stages of withdrawal. A meta-analysis was performed to provide evidence-based recommendations on the pharmacologic management of alcohol withdrawal[27] and delirium tremens.[32] Trials comparing different benzodiazepines demonstrated that all appear similarly efficacious in reducing signs and symptoms of withdrawal.[27,32] Lorazepam is preferred by many clinicians because it can be administered intravenously, intramuscularly, or orally with predictable results. Another consideration in the choice of benzodiazepine is their potential for abuse during recovery. Agents with rapid onset of action, such as

diazepam or alprazolam, demonstrate higher abuse potential because of their reinforcing effects. Those with slower onset of action, such as chlordiazepoxide or oxazepam, are less likely to be abused. This consideration can be relevant in an outpatient setting or for patients with a history of benzodiazepine or other substance abuse.[33]

Although barbiturates are used by approximately 10% of detoxification programs in the United States, there is less evidence-based support for their use versus the benzodiazepines.[33] Clonidine, carbamazepine, vigabatrin, valproic acid, gabapentin, and topiramate can reduce symptoms of alcohol withdrawal.[34–37]

Treatment Regimens

Symptom-Triggered Therapy With symptom-triggered therapy, medication is given only when the patient has symptoms. This approach results in treatment that is shorter, potentially avoiding oversedation and allowing the clinician to focus on specific therapy for alcohol dependence.[27,32] A typical regimen would include lorazepam 2 mg administered every hour as needed when a structured assessment scale—such as the Clinical Institute Withdrawal Assessment–Alcohol, Revised—indicates that symptoms are moderate to severe (Table 69–3).[35]

Fixed-Schedule Therapy Over the years, benzodiazepines given regularly at a fixed dosing interval have been used for alcohol withdrawal. The major problem with this approach is underdosing of the benzodiazepine because of the phenomenon of cross-tolerance (see Table 69–3). Current guidelines take exception with this rigid approach, urging clinicians to allow for some degree of individualization within fixed-schedule therapy.[27] Patients should be monitored and given additional medication when indicated by symptoms.

Treatment of Alcohol Withdrawal Seizures

Alcohol withdrawal seizures do not require treatment with an anticonvulsant drug unless they progress to status epilepticus because seizures usually end before diazepam or another drug can be administered.[32–34] Phenytoin, which is not cross-tolerant to alcohol, does not prevent or treat withdrawal seizures, and without an intravenous loading dose, therapeutic blood levels of phenytoin are not reached until acute withdrawal is complete. Patients experiencing seizures should be treated supportively. An increase in the dosage and slowing of the tapering schedule of the benzodiazepine used in detoxification or a single injection of a benzodiazepine can be necessary to prevent further seizure activity. Patients with a history of withdrawal seizures can be predicted to experience an especially severe withdrawal syndrome. In such patients, a higher initial dosage of a benzodiazepine and a slower tapering period of 7 to 10 days are advisable.

Treatment of Nutritional Deficits and Electrolyte Abnormalities

Fluid status should be carefully assessed, and fluid, electrolyte, and vitamin abnormalities should be corrected. Often hydration is

TABLE 69-3 Pharmacologic Agents Used in the Treatment of Alcohol Withdrawal

Drug	Dose per Day (Unless Otherwise Stated)	Indication	Monitoring	Duration of Dosing	Level of Evidence[a]
Multivitamin	1 tablet	Malnutrition	Diet	At least until eating a balanced diet at caloric goal	B3
Thiamine	50–100 mg	Deficiency	CBC, WBC, nystagmus	Empiric × 5 days. More if evidence of deficiency	B2
Crystalloid fluids (typically D5-0.45 NS with 20 mEq of KCl per liter)	50–100 mL/hr	Dehydration	Weight, electrolytes, urine output, nystagmus if dextrose	Until intake and outputs stabilize and oral intake is adequate	A3
Clonidine oral	0.05–0.3 mg	Autonomic tone rebound and hyperactivity	Shaking, tremor, sweating, blood pressure	3 days or less	B2
Clonidine transdermal	TTS-1 to TTS-3	Autonomic tone rebound and hyperactivity	Shaking, tremor, sweating, blood pressure	1 week or less. One patch only	B3
Labetalol	20 mg IV every 2 hours as needed	Hypertensive urgencies and above	Blood pressure target	Individual doses as needed	B3
Antipsychotics, haloperidol	2.5 mg to 5 mg every four hours	Agitation unresponsive to benzodiazepines, hallucinations (tactile, visual, auditory or otherwise) or delusions	Subjective response plus rating scale (CIWA-Ar or equivalent)	Individual doses as needed	B1
Antipsychotics, atypical Quetiapine Aripiprazole	 25–200 mg 5–15 mg	Agitation unresponsive to benzodiazepines, hallucinations, or delusions in patients intolerant of conventional antipsychotics	Subjective response plus rating scale (CIWA-Ar or equivalent)	Individual doses as needed in addition to scheduled antipsychotic	C3
Benzodiazepines Lorazepam Chlordiazepoxide Clonazepam Diazepam	 0.5–2 mg 5 mg–25 mg 0.5–2 mg 2.5–10 mg	Tremor, anxiety, diaphoresis, tachypnea, dysphoria, seizures	Subjective response plus rating scale (CIWA-Ar or equivalent)	Individual doses as needed. Underdosing is more common than overdosing	A2
Alcohol oral		Prevent withdrawal	subjective signs of withdrawal	Wide variation	C3
Alcohol IV		Prevent withdrawal	subjective signs of withdrawal	Wide variation	C3

CBC, complete blood count; CIWA-Ar, Clinical Institute Withdrawal Assessment for Alcohol, revised; D5, dextrose 5%; KCl, potassium chloride; NS, normal saline; WBC, white blood cell count.

[a]Strength of recommendations, evidence to support recommendation: A, good; B, moderate; C, poor.

Quality of evidence: 1, evidence from more than 1 properly randomized, controlled trial; 2, evidence from more than 1 well-designed clinical trial with randomization, from cohort or case-controlled analytic studies or multiple time series; or dramatic results from uncontrolled experiments; 3, evidence from opinions of respected authorities, based on clinical experience, descriptive studies, or reports of expert communities.

Data from Mayo-Smith,[26] Mayo-Smith et al.,[32] and Reoux and Miller.[35]

TABLE 69-4 Pharmacologic Agents Used in the Treatment of Alcohol Dependence

Drug	Dosage Range per Day	Indication	Monitoring	Duration of Dosing	Level of Evidence[a]
Disulfiram	250 mg–500 mg	Deterrence	Facial flushing, liver enzymes	Indefinite	B2
Acamprosate	999 mg–1,998 mg and higher (333 mg tablets)	Craving	Patient-reported craving, renal function	Indefinite	A1
Naltrexone	50 mg–100 mg	Craving	Patient-reported craving	Indefinite	A1
Mood stabilizers (e.g., lamotrigine, topiramate, carbamazepine, valproic acid)	Seizure disorder doses	Craving	Patient-reported craving, plasma drug levels	Indefinite	B2
Antidepressants (e.g., clomipramine, bupropion, doxepin, maprotiline, fluoxetine)	Depression doses	Craving, depression, anxiety	Patient-reported craving	Indefinite	B2

[a]Strength of recommendations: A, B, C = good, moderate, and poor evidence to support recommendation, respectively.
Quality of evidence: 1, evidence from more than 1 properly randomized, controlled trial. 2, evidence from more than 1 well-designed clinical trial with randomization, from cohort or case-controlled analytic studies or multiple time series; or dramatic results from uncontrolled experiments. 3, evidence from opinions of respected authorities, based on clinical experience, descriptive studies, or reports of expert communities.
Data from Boothby and Doering,[38] Mason et al.,[39] Garbutt et al.,[40,43] Morris et al.,[41] Srisurapanont and Jarusuraisin,[42] and Johnson et al.[44]

unnecessary. Excessive hydration should be avoided in patients going through alcohol withdrawal because of increased vasopressin levels. Hydration can be necessary in patients with vomiting, diarrhea, increased body temperature, or severe agitation.

Alcoholics often have electrolyte imbalances because of inadequate nutrition and fluid volume related to antidiuretic hormone inhibition. Hypokalemia can be corrected with oral potassium supplementation as long as renal function is adequate. Hypophosphatemia is common but should be allowed to gradually correct with adequate nutrition if phosphorus levels are greater than 1 mg/dL. Hypomagnesemia is also common but routine magnesium replacement for alcohol withdrawal is not recommended. Only if symptoms of hypomagnesemia are present should magnesium replacement be considered.

Thiamine (vitamin B_1) is often depleted in alcoholics, particularly those with poor nutrition. Thiamine supplementation is standard therapy because it can prevent the development of the Wernicke-Korsikoff syndrome (e.g., mental confusion, eye movement disorders, and ataxia [poor motor coordination]), which may not be reversible once it develops. An initial dose of 100 mg IV or IM is commonly used. If the patient has evidence of thiamine deficiency replacement with 100 mg orally every day for 1 to 4 weeks is appropriate. Thiamine should not be continued unless there is evidence of a deficiency. Adverse effects associated with thiamine use are hypersensitivity reactions, cardiovascular effects, and CNS effects. If thiamine deficiency is suspected thiamine should always be given before dextrose administration because it is a cofactor necessary for glucose metabolism. In practice, thiamine is usually given 100 mg once daily orally, intravenously, or intramuscularly for 3 to 5 days. It is not necessary for thiamine to be continued empirically for longer than 5 days (see Table 69–3).

Other nutritional deficits can also occur with chronic alcohol abuse primarily caused by poor eating habits. A multivitamin is usually given once daily. If clotting factors are abnormal because of decreased liver function and a relative inability to produce vitamin K–dependent clotting factors, then 2.5 to 25 mg of vitamin K can also be prescribed.

Alcohol hypoglycemia usually occurs in the absence of overt liver disease, and it is more likely if the patient is fasting or exercising or is sensitive to alcohol; it is less likely if the patient is obese. The alcohol directly interferes with hepatic gluconeogenesis but not glycogenolysis. The energy required for metabolism of alcohol is diverted away from the energy needed to take up lactate and pyruvate—substrates for gluconeogenesis. So, patients who drink alcohol can become hypoglycemic once glycogen stores are depleted. Neurologic symptoms of hypoglycemia can be confused with alcohol intoxication, and in the inpatient setting, blood glucose should be monitored regularly.

Treatment Settings

Alcohol withdrawal treatment can take place in hospitals, inpatient detoxification units, or outpatient settings. Inpatient treatment can be necessary when there are coexisting acute or chronic medical (including pregnancy), surgical, or psychiatric conditions that would complicate alcohol withdrawal. Only patients with mild to moderate symptoms should be considered for outpatient treatment, and it is a good idea to have a responsible, sober person available to help the patient monitor symptoms and administer medications. Patients with a strong craving for alcohol, those concurrently using other drugs, and those with a history of seizures or delirium tremens are not good candidates for outpatient treatment. Pharmacologic agents used in the treatment of alcohol withdrawal are summarized in Table 69–3.

PHARMACOLOGIC MANAGEMENT OF ALCOHOL DEPENDENCE

❼ In the United States, disulfiram, naltrexone, and acamprosate are the only three drugs that are FDA-approved for the treatment of alcohol dependence. Disulfiram acts as a deterrent to the resumption of drinking, and naltrexone is a competitive opioid antagonist that has been shown to reduce cravings for alcohol. Acamprosate is a GABA-ergic agonist that modulates alcohol cravings (Table 69–4).[38–44] Other drugs, including nalmefene,[39] bupropion, various serotonergic agents (including selective serotonin reuptake inhibitors and vascular serotonin 5-HT3 receptor antagonists), and lithium also have been used either abroad or in the United States off-label for alcohol dependence.[40]

CLINICAL CONTROVERSY

The most difficult clinical problem in the treatment of alcohol related illness is helping patients remain abstinent after alcohol detoxification. Despite the availability of pharmacologic agents to decrease the craving post-acute detoxification, the usefulness of these pharmacologic agents (e.g., acamprosate, naltrexone, disulfiram) remains controversial. Acamprosate and naltrexone have been shown to be superior to nonpharmacologic therapy alone for maintenance of abstinence from alcohol; however, relapse during naltrexone and acamprosate therapy is still common. Disulfiram use has fallen out of favor. Studies have failed to prove it effective, and it is poorly tolerated. For this reason, most clinicians rarely recommend the use of disulfiram.

DISULFIRAM

Disulfiram deters a patient from drinking by producing an aversive reaction if the patient drinks. In the absence of alcohol, disulfiram has minimal effects. Note that although disulfiram appeared to be effective in a series of studies with a small sample size, these were largely uncontrolled.[40] Disulfiram inhibits the liver enzyme aldehyde dehydrogenase in the biochemical pathway for alcohol metabolism, allowing acetaldehyde to accumulate. The resulting increase in acetaldehyde causes severe facial flushing, throbbing headache, nausea and vomiting, chest pain, palpitations, tachycardia, weakness, dizziness, blurred vision, confusion, and hypotension. Severe reactions including myocardial infarction, congestive heart failure, cardiac arrhythmia, respiratory depression, convulsions, and death can occur, particularly in vulnerable individuals.

A rare but potentially fatal idiosyncratic hepatotoxicity can occur with disulfiram. As a result, baseline liver function tests should be obtained and the patient monitored for hepatotoxicity by monitoring for symptoms and by repeating the liver function tests at 2 weeks, 3 months, 6 months, and twice yearly thereafter. The prescriber should wait at least 24 hours after the last drink before starting disulfiram, usually at a dose of 250 mg/day. At this dose there are fewer side effects than at 500 mg, although some research suggests that higher doses are needed to reliably produce an aversive reaction if the patient drinks.[40]

NALTREXONE

Naltrexone, an opiate antagonist that has been available in the United States since 1984 for the treatment of opioid dependence blocks the effects of exogenous opioids. In 1994 the FDA approved its use in the treatment of alcohol dependence. Naltrexone is thought to attenuate the reinforcing effects of alcohol, and those who consume alcohol while taking naltrexone report feeling less intoxicated and having less craving for alcohol.[41]

Short-term treatment (up to 12 weeks) with naltrexone decreases the chance of alcohol relapse by 36% versus placebo (number needed to treat seven patients to prevent one relapse).[42] Naltrexone should not be given to patients currently dependent on opiates because it can precipitate a severe withdrawal syndrome. Naltrexone is associated with dose-related hepatotoxicity, but this generally occurs at doses higher than those recommended for treatment of alcohol dependence. Nevertheless, it is considered contraindicated in patients with hepatitis or liver failure, and liver function tests should be monitored monthly for the first 3 months and every 3 months thereafter.

Nausea is the most common side effect of naltrexone, occurring in approximately 10% of patients. Other side effects are headache, dizziness, nervousness, fatigue, insomnia, vomiting, anxiety, and somnolence. If dosed daily, naltrexone 50 mg per day is sufficient to effectively block μ-opioid receptors. A new long-acting depot formulation allows monthly administration to increase compliance and adherence. The usual effective dose is 380 mg IM each month.[43]

ACAMPROSATE

Acamprosate is a glutamate modulator at the N-methyl-D-aspartate (NMDA) receptor that reduces alcohol craving. Acamprosate was approved in the United States in the summer of 2004 but has been available in Europe for many years. Patients treated with acamprosate are more successful in maintaining abstinence from alcohol versus placebo.[38] In addition, the combination of acamprosate and naltrexone has been shown to be more efficacious than acamprosate alone for the maintenance of abstinence from alcohol, when combined with psychosocial interventions.[38] Acamprosate is well tolerated, with gastrointestinal adverse effects most common. See Table 69–4 for dosing information for this and the other options used in treating alcohol dependence.

Using the limited data on serotonergic agents in the evidence-based analysis,[40] these drugs were deemed not very promising, although most studies were confounded by high rates of comorbid mood disorders.

NICOTINE

Cigarette smoking is an enormous national health problem, and as healthcare professionals, we are not doing enough to help people quit smoking. Although research has determined that brief interventions by medical professionals help patients quit smoking,[45] these interventions do not occur frequently enough in primary care settings.[46] A telephone survey of adult cigarette smokers was conducted to determine the types of smoking cessation counseling interventions they received during their physician office visits in the past year. Approximately one-half of the current smokers surveyed reported that their doctors talked with them about their smoking, less than half were advised to stop smoking, 15% were offered smoking cessation assistance in the form of education and support groups, and only 9% were prescribed drug therapies to assist smoking cessation efforts.[46] A second observational study was conducted to determine the effects of community-based academic detailing interventions on the quit rates of a sample of smokers (n = 4295). Detailed interventions were delivered to physicians that encouraged smoking cessation efforts with patients to comply with the National Cancer Institute and the Agency for Healthcare Quality and Research smoking intervention standards.[47] A small, significant effect was observed in a subgroup of patients residing in the intervention area.[47] Other healthcare professionals did an even poorer job, with only 22% of dentists, 24% of nurses, and 4% of pharmacists helping their patients to quit smoking.[46]

EPIDEMIOLOGY OF TOBACCO USE

In 2005, an estimated 71.5 million Americans aged 12 or older were current (past month) users of a tobacco product, a prevalence rate of 30.4% for the population aged 12 or older.[3] In addition, 60.5 million persons (24.9% of the population) were current cigarette smokers; 13.6 million (5.6%) smoked cigars; 7.7 million (3.2%) used smokeless tobacco; and 2.2 million (0.9%) smoked tobacco in pipes.

The rate of lifetime cigarette use among youths aged 12 to 17 has remained between 29% and 39% for every year since 1965. Although the rate increased during the 1990s from 30.3% in 1990 to 37.8% in 1999, there was a significant decline from 2001 to 2002 (from 37.3% to 33.3%). One of the national health objectives for 2010 is to reduce the prevalence of cigarette smoking among adults to less than 12%.[48]

ECONOMIC IMPACT OF SMOKING

The direct medical costs associated with smoking total more than $75 billion per year, and the costs associated with lost productivity are estimated to be $80 billion. Approximately 14% of all Medicaid expenditures are for smoking-related illnesses. This estimate does not include the costs of smoking-related neonatal disorders.

HEALTH RISKS OF SMOKING

Each year more than 440,000 deaths, or 20% of the total deaths in the United States, are caused by smoking.[49] Cigarette smoking substantially increases the risk of (1) cardiovascular diseases such as stroke, sudden death, and heart attack; (2) nonmalignant respiratory diseases including emphysema, asthma, chronic bronchitis, and chronic obstructive pulmonary disease; (3) lung cancer; and (4) other cancers.

Exposure to environmental tobacco smoke (*passive exposure*) has been cited as the cause of 3,000 lung cancer deaths and 35,000 to 40,000 heart disease related deaths in the United States every year.[49] When children are exposed to environmental smoke, they have a higher risk of respiratory infection, asthma, and middle ear infections than those who are not exposed. Sudden infant death syndrome occurs more often in infants whose mothers smoked during pregnancy than in offspring of nonsmoking mothers.[49] The harmful effects of smoking on reproduction and pregnancy include reduced fertility and fetal growth, as well as increased risk of ectopic pregnancy and spontaneous abortion.[49]

PHARMACOLOGY OF NICOTINE

Nicotine is a ganglionic cholinergic receptor agonist with pharmacologic effects that are highly dependent on dose. These effects include central and peripheral nervous system stimulation and depression, respiratory stimulation, skeletal muscle relaxation, catecholamine release by the adrenal medulla, peripheral vasoconstriction, and increased blood pressure, heart rate, cardiac output, and oxygen consumption.[50] Cigarette smoking or low doses of nicotine produce an increased alertness and increased cognitive functioning by stimulating the cerebral cortex. At higher doses, nicotine stimulates the "reward" center in the limbic system of the brain.[50]

Chronic nicotine ingestion can lead to physical and psychologic dependence and tolerance to some of its pharmacologic effects. Abrupt smoking cessation in physically dependent smokers results in withdrawal symptoms. Onset of these symptoms usually occurs within 24 hours and can last for days, weeks, or longer. The craving for tobacco can last for years.

CLINICAL PRESENTATION OF NICOTINE WITHDRAWAL

General

- The patient may experience anxiety but may not be in acute distress. Symptoms can wax and wane over time.

Symptoms

- The patient may complain of cravings, difficulty concentrating, frustration, irritability, and impatience. Hostility, insomnia, and restlessness can also occur.

Signs

- Increased skin temperature can be present.

❽ Although some smokers do not develop physical or psychologic dependence, most people who smoke 10 to 15 cigarettes daily for several weeks or longer do. Between 77% and 92% of smokers are addicted to nicotine in cigarettes.[51]

According to a recent report by the Massachusetts Department of Public Health (MDPH),[52] the amount of nicotine in a cigarette has increased steadily over the past 6 years. The study found that, regardless of brand, the amount of nicotine that is actually delivered to the smoker's lungs has increased significantly over this time period. The data were collected from reports submitted to the MDPH from 1998 to 2004 by all tobacco companies that sell cigarettes in the state, as required by Massachusetts general law. The report found that overall, nicotine yields increased 10% from 1998–2004. As of 2004, 93% of all cigarette brands were rated high nicotine. Increased levels of nicotine can make it more difficult for the average smoker to quit. Increased levels of nicotine consumed by pregnant women can lead to developmental delays in childhood as well as low birth weight infants.

TREATMENT

Nicotine Dependence

■ AGENCY FOR HEALTHCARE RESEARCH AND QUALITY CLINICAL PRACTICE GUIDELINE: TREATING TOBACCO USE AND DEPENDENCE

The Agency for Healthcare Research and Quality (AHRQ) periodically convenes expert panels to develop clinical guidelines for healthcare practitioners when the need dictates. Because of the widespread prevalence of smoking-related illnesses, its related morbidity and mortality, and the economic burden imposed, the agency convened a panel of experts in 1994 to develop guidelines on the treatment of tobacco addiction. The resultant guideline for smoking cessation was released in 1996. In June 2000, an updated version of the 1996 Smoking Cessation Clinical Practice Guideline was issued by AHRQ.[53]

The revised guideline suggests strategies for providing appropriate treatments for every patient. The panel reminds us that effective treatments for tobacco dependence now exist and that every patient should receive at least minimal treatment every time he or she visits a clinician (Figs. 69–1 and 69–2).

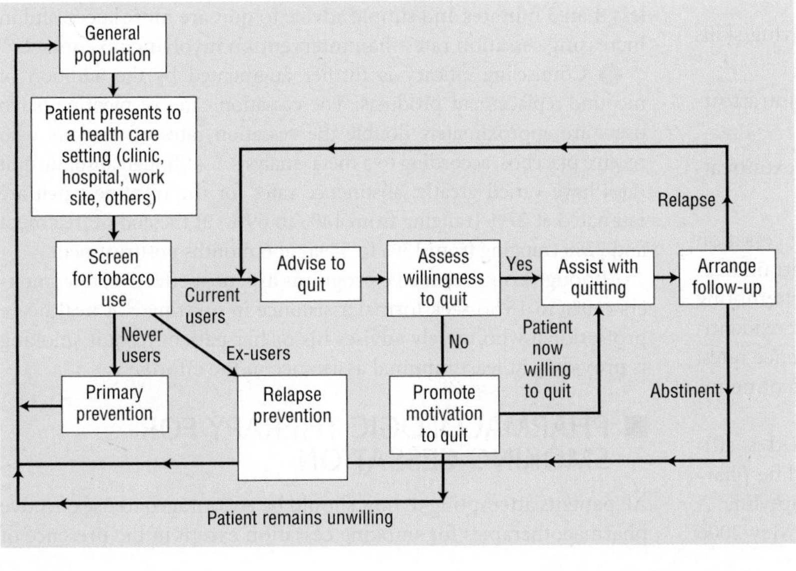

FIGURE 69-1. Model for treatment of tobacco use and dependence.

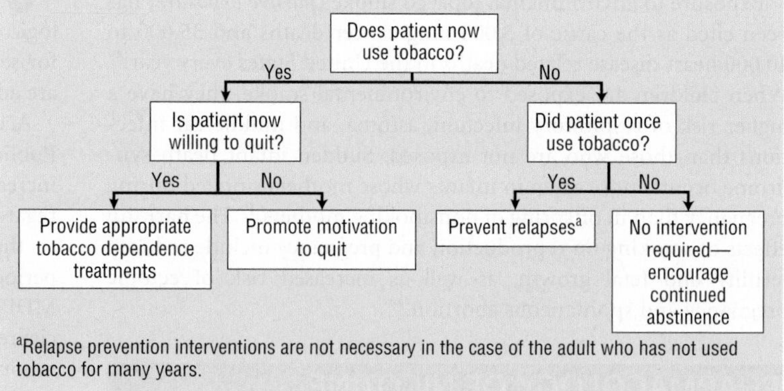

FIGURE 69-2. Algorithm for treating tobacco use.

The guideline identified a number of key findings that clinicians should use:

1. ❽ Tobacco dependence is a chronic condition that often requires repeated intervention. However, effective treatments exist that can produce long-term or even permanent abstinence.
2. Because effective tobacco dependence treatments are available, every patient who uses tobacco should be offered at least one of these treatments:
   - Patients willing to try to quit tobacco use should be provided with treatments that are identified as effective in the guideline.
   - Patients unwilling to try to quit tobacco use should be provided with a brief intervention that is designed to increase their motivation to quit.
3. It is essential that clinicians and healthcare delivery systems (including administrators, insurers, and purchasers) institutionalize the consistent identification, documentation, and treatment of every tobacco user who is seen in a healthcare setting.
4. Brief tobacco dependence treatment is effective, and every patient who uses tobacco should be offered at least brief treatment.
5. There is a strong dose-response relationship between the intensity of tobacco dependence counseling and its effectiveness. Treatments involving person-to-person contact (via individual, group, or proactive telephone counseling) are consistently effective, and their effectiveness increases with treatment intensity (e.g., minutes of contact).
6. Three types of counseling and behavioral therapies were found to be especially effective and should be used with all patients who are attempting tobacco cessation:
   - Provision of practical counseling (problem-solving/skills training).
   - Provision of social support as part of treatment (intratreatment social support).
   - Help in securing social support outside treatment (extratreatment social support).
7. Numerous effective pharmacotherapies for smoking cessation now exist (Table 69–5). Except in the presence of contraindications, these should be used with all patients who are attempting to quit smoking. Five first-line pharmacotherapies were identified that reliably increase long-term smoking abstinence rates: bupropion sustained-release (SR), nicotine gum, nicotine inhaler, nicotine nasal spray, and nicotine patch.

   Two second-line pharmacotherapies were identified as efficacious and can be considered by clinicians if first-line pharmacotherapies are not effective: clonidine and nortriptyline. A new drug, varenicline, was approved by the FDA in May 2006 as a smoking cessation aid. It has not yet been incorporated into Clinical Practice Guidelines.[54]
8. Tobacco dependence treatments are both clinically and cost-effective relative to other medical and disease-prevention interventions. As such, insurers and purchasers should ensure all insurance plans include as a reimbursed benefit the counseling and pharmacotherapeutic treatments that are identified as effective in this guideline, as well as clinician reimbursement for providing tobacco dependence treatment just as they are reimbursed for treating other chronic conditions.

■ OTHER FACTORS IMPORTANT TO THE SUCCESS OF A SMOKING-CESSATION STRATEGY

The AHRQ expert panel emphasized the importance of the type and intensity of the contact with the counselor to the success of the intervention. When interventions last for more than 10 minutes, the increase in cessation rates is much better than when interventions do not involve contact with a professional. Group and individual counseling is more effective than no intervention in increasing abstinence rates, but self-help materials (e.g., handouts, pamphlets, and brochures) are not. Interventions are more successful when they include social support and training in general problem-solving skills, stress management, and relapse prevention.[45] The number of treatment sessions offered is also important. Providing at least four to seven sessions significantly increased cessation rates, independent of the treatment's intensity.[53]

Comprehensive behavioral interventions are more effective in helping people quit smoking and remain abstinent, but less intensive treatments are beneficial as well. Even minimal contacts lasting less than 3 minutes and simple advice to quit are more successful in increasing cessation rates than intervention involving no contact.[53]

❾ Counseling efficacy is further augmented by the addition of nicotine-replacement products. The cessation rates of nicotine patch users are approximately double the cessation rates of smokers who receive placebos, according to a meta-analysis.[55] Although absolute quit rates have varied greatly, abstinence rates for the nicotine patch are estimated at 27% (ranging from 14% to 69%) at the end of treatment and 22% (ranging from 13% to 34%) at 6 months posttreatment.

Although comprehensive programs are most effective, few smokers (10% to 15%) seek formal assistance in quitting.[55] A healthcare professional who merely advises his or her patient to quit smoking is providing at least minimal assistance in the efforts.

■ PHARMACOLOGIC THERAPY FOR SMOKING CESSATION

All patients attempting to quit should be encouraged to use effective pharmacotherapies for smoking cessation except in the presence of special circumstances. Long-term smoking-cessation pharmacotherapy should be considered as a strategy to reduce the likelihood of relapse. As with other chronic diseases, the most effective treatment of tobacco dependence encompasses multiple modalities. Pharmacotherapy is a vital element of a multicomponent smoking cessation program that should also always include nonpharmacologic components. The clinician should encourage all patients initiating a quit attempt to use one or a combination of efficacious pharmacotherapies, although pharmacotherapy use requires special consideration with some patient groups (e.g., those with medical contraindications, those smoking fewer than 10 cigarettes a day, pregnant or breast-feeding women, and adolescent smokers). The role of pharmacotherapy is summarized in Table 69–5.

■ NICOTINE-REPLACEMENT THERAPY

A Systematic Review of Nicotine Replacement Therapy

In 2004 a systematic review[55] of published studies was performed to determine the effectiveness of the different forms of nicotine replacement therapy (NRT; e.g., chewing gum, transdermal patches, nasal spray, inhalers, and tablets) in achieving abstinence from cigarettes or a sustained reduction in the amount smoked. The review was also designed to determine whether the effect is influenced by the clinical setting in which the smoker is recruited and treated, the dosage and form of the NRT used, or the intensity of additional advice and support offered to the smoker; to determine whether combinations of NRT are more effective than one type alone; and to determine its effectiveness compared to other pharmacotherapies.

The review was limited to randomized trials in which NRT was compared to placebo or no treatment, or where different doses of NRT were compared. The main outcome measure was abstinence from smoking after at least 6 months of followup. For each trial, researchers used the most rigorous definition of abstinence, and confirmation with biochemical markers where available. The review includes 123 studies, 103 of which included a placebo or non–nicotine control arm. All of the commercially available forms of NRT were effective to aid smoking cessation. Use of nicotine replacement therapy doubled the odds of quitting. Higher doses of nicotine patch can produce additional small increases in quit rates compared to lower doses. Only one study directly compared NRT to another pharmacotherapy, in which bupropion was significantly more effective than nicotine patch or placebo.[55]

The AHRQ guidelines recommend use of NRT in the forms of transdermal nicotine patches, nicotine gum, nicotine sprays, and nicotine inhalers.[53] The use of NRT is relatively safe, but it is not recommended for all smokers. Although cardiovascular disease is not an independent risk factor for acute myocardial events in patients taking NRT, NRT should be used with caution among particular cardiovascular patient groups: those in the immediate (within 2 weeks) post–myocardial infarction period, those with serious arrhythmias, and those with serious or worsening angina pectoris.[53]

Nicotine Gum

Clinicians should offer 4-mg rather than 2-mg nicotine gum to highly dependent smokers.[55,56] The 2-mg gum is recommended for patients smoking less than 25 cigarettes per day, whereas the 4-mg gum is recommended for patients smoking 25 or more cigarettes per day. The 2-mg nicotine gum improves long-term abstinence rates by approximately 30% to 80% as compared with placebo. Generally, the gum should be used for up to 12 weeks, no more than 24 pieces chewed per day. The dosage and duration of therapy should be tailored to meet the needs of each patient.

Nicotine gum currently is available exclusively as an over-the-counter medication and is packaged with important instructions on correct use, including chewing instructions. There is currently little evidence to suggest that combined use of the patch and gum increases abstinence beyond 24 weeks.

Gum should be chewed slowly until a peppery or minty taste emerges and then "parked" between cheek and gums to facilitate nicotine absorption through the oral mucosa. It should be chewed slowly and intermittently and parked for about 30 minutes or until the

TABLE 69-5 Pharmacologic Agents Used for Smoking Cessation

Drug	Place in Therapy	Dosage Range	Duration	Comments/Monitoring Parameters	LOE[d]
Buproprion SR[a,b]	First-line	Titrate up to 150 mg orally twice daily.	3 to 6 months	Patients receiving both bupropion and a nicotine patch should be monitored for hypertension.	A1
Clonidine[b,c]	Second-line	Titrate to response. 0.2 to 0.75 mg per day	6 to 12 months	Monitor baseline electrolyte and lipid profiles, renal function, uric acid, complete blood count, and blood pressure.	B2
Nicotine polacrilex (gum)[a]	First-line	Initial dose depends on smoking history: 2 to 4 mg every 1 to 8 hours	12 weeks (taper down over time)	Heart rate and blood pressure should be monitored periodically during nicotine replacement therapy.	A1
Nicotine inhaler[a]	First-line	24 to 64 mg per day (total daily dose)	3 to 6 months (taper down over time)	Heart rate and blood pressure should be monitored periodically during nicotine replacement therapy.	A1
Nicotine nasal spray[a]	First-line	8 to 40 mg per day (total daily dose)	14 weeks (taper down over time)	Heart rate and blood pressure should be monitored periodically during nicotine replacement therapy.	A1
Nicotine patch[a]	First-line	Initial dose depends on smoking history: 7 to 21 mg topically once daily	6 weeks (taper down over time)	Heart rate and blood pressure should be monitored periodically during nicotine replacement therapy.	A1
Nortriptyline[b,c]	Second-line	Titrate up to 75 to 100 mg orally daily	6 to 12 months	Dry mouth, blurred vision, and constipation are dose-dependent adverse effects.	B2
Varenicline[b]	FDA-approved in 2006	Titrate up to 1 mg orally twice daily	3 to 6 months	Monitor renal function, especially in elderly patients. Nausea, headache, insomnia are dose-dependent adverse effects.	A1

LOE, level of evidence.

[a]Nicotine replacement therapies can be combined with each other and/or bupropion to increase long-term abstinence rates.

[b]Do not abruptly discontinue. Taper up initially, and taper off once therapy is complete.

[c]Clonidine and nortriptyline are not FDA-approved for smoking cessation.

[d]Strength of recommendations, evidence to support recommendation: A, good; B, moderate; C, poor.

Quality of evidence: 1, evidence from more than 1 properly randomized, controlled trial; 2, evidence from more than 1 well-designed clinical trial with randomization, from cohort or case-controlled analytic studies or multiple time series; or dramatic results from uncontrolled experiments; 3, evidence from opinions of respected authorities, based on clinical experience, descriptive studies, or reports of expert communities.

Data from Goldstein et al.[46,47] and U.S. Department of Health and Human Services.[48]

taste dissipates. Acidic beverages (e.g., coffee, juices, or soft drinks) interfere with the buccal absorption of nicotine, so eating and drinking anything except water should be avoided for 15 minutes before and during chewing. Patients often do not use enough gum to get the maximum benefit: they chew too few pieces per day, and they might not use the gum for a sufficient number of weeks. Instructions to chew the gum on a fixed schedule (at least one piece every 1 to 2 hours) for at least 1 to 3 months can be more beneficial than ad libitum use.

Nicotine Patch

9 The nicotine patch approximately doubles long-term abstinence rates over those produced by placebo interventions. The nicotine patch is available both as an over-the-counter medication and as a prescription medication. Treatment of 8 weeks or less has been shown to be as efficacious as longer treatment periods. The 16- and 24-hour patches are of comparable efficacy.[53] Clinicians should consider individualizing treatment based on specific patient characteristics, such as previous experience with the patch, amount smoked, and degree of addiction, among others. Finally, clinicians should consider starting treatment on a lower patch dose in patients smoking 10 or fewer cigarettes per day.[53]

At the start of each day, the patient should place a new patch on a relatively hairless location, typically between the neck and waist. There are no restrictions on activity while using the patch. Patches should be applied as soon as the patient wakes on the quit day. Patients who experience sleep disruption should remove the 24-hour patch prior to bedtime or use the 16-hour patch.

Nicotine Nasal Spray

Nicotine nasal spray more than doubles long-term abstinence rates when compared with a placebo spray. Nicotine nasal spray is available exclusively as a prescription medication. A dose of nicotine nasal spray consists of one 0.5-mg delivery to each nostril (1 mg total). Initial dosing should be one to two doses per hour, increasing as needed for symptom relief. The minimum recommended treatment is 8 doses per day, with a maximum limit of 40 doses per day (5 doses per hour). Each bottle contains approximately 100 doses. Recommended duration of therapy is 3 to 6 months. Patients should not sniff, swallow, or inhale through the nose while administering doses because this increases irritating effects. The spray is best delivered with the head tilted slightly back.[53]

Instructing Patients in the Use of NRT

Compliance with NRT improves when the patient is presented a clear rationale for its use and a realistic expectation about the response. It should be explained to the patient that nicotine is responsible for addiction and that discontinuation of the nicotine causes craving for cigarettes, tension, irritability, sadness, problems with sleep, and difficulty concentrating. These are partly because of nicotine withdrawal. The patient should be told that using the patch results in less desire to smoke and provides an opportunity for a new nonsmoker to practice all the new nonsmoking skills without being burdened by craving. The patient should understand that with smoking, there are naturally peaks and valleys in the amount of nicotine in the bloodstream. With the patch there is a steady gradual rise in the blood nicotine concentration that levels off and remains constant for much of the day and then gradually decreases while the person is asleep. Maintaining an adequate blood level of nicotine lessens withdrawal symptoms.

A similar rationale can be used if patients are using gum. It should be emphasized that NRT is not a "magic bullet" and that the use of coping skills is essential for abstinence. The patch or the gum only buys time by reducing withdrawal symptoms and giving individuals a chance to figure out alternatives that they can use in place of smoking.[56]

CLINICAL CONTROVERSY

Some clinicians are hesitant to prescribe NRT for smoking cessation during pregnancy because the safety and efficacy of NRT has not been established in controlled clinical trials in this population. This logic is somewhat counterintuitive in that continued smoking exposes the unborn child to much higher levels of nicotine and the harmful consequences of cigarette smoking during pregnancy are well documented.

Side Effects

Nicotine replacement products have relatively few side effects. Nausea and light-headedness are possible signs of nicotine overdose that warrant a reduction of the nicotine dose.

The most frequent side effect with the nicotine patch is skin irritation related to the adhesive or the medium containing nicotine and not to the nicotine itself. Approximately 50% of patients report skin irritation during the course of treatment with the patch. The patch site can be rotated to diminish this problem. The use of over-the-counter hydrocortisone cream (1%) or triamcinolone cream (0.5%) is recommended as a local treatment for patch-related skin irritations. Switching to a different brand of patch also can alleviate the problem because different products use different adhesives or media. The gum can be used instead of the patch when the skin irritation is severe. Less than 5% of patients were forced to discontinue therapy because of skin reactions.

Approximately 23% of patients using the patch report sleep disturbances, but the insomnia is hard to differentiate from the sleeplessness that often accompanies withdrawal itself, especially during the first few weeks of quitting.

More research regarding the safety and efficacy of pharmacotherapy during pregnancy is needed to define the risk-to-benefit profile of smoking cessation medications in this population.[57] Clearly, exposure of the fetus to nicotine delivered by smoking is known to be detrimental to the fetus. Because total nicotine levels are lower with NRT than smoking, if the alternative is active smoking, NRT is almost certainly safer if cessation can be achieved. Nicotine does cross the placenta, whether delivered by cigarette smoking or through nicotine replacement. Nicotine transdermal systems and inhalers are classified as FDA pregnancy risk category D, and nicotine gum is classified as FDA pregnancy category C, but there are conflicting data regarding pregnancy safety ratings of nicotine replacement products, and the pregnancy categories cannot be used in isolation from other information sources. Nicotine replacement is not contraindicated and could be appropriately used in well-selected pregnant patients.

A study[58] of women using various doses of transdermal nicotine while breast-feeding confirms that nicotine is transferred via milk to the infant. The absolute infant dose of nicotine and its metabolite cotinine decreased by about 70% while the mothers were using the 7-mg patch compared to when they were smoking or using the 21-mg patch. The use of the nicotine patch had no significant influence on milk intake by the breast-fed infant. The authors conclude that undertaking maternal smoking cessation with the nicotine patch is therefore a safer option than continued smoking. Ultimately, the choice of whether to use pharmacotherapy for smoking cessation should be made jointly by the pregnant or breast-feeding smoker and her healthcare provider.

Duration

Those who commit to quitting smoking using the nicotine patch should be told to expect a minimum of 6 to 8 weeks of treatment. Using the therapy beyond 8 weeks is not associated with better success rates.[53] However, some patients will experience severe withdrawal even beyond 8 weeks, and these people may need to use the patch longer.

The duration of therapy with the gum should be at least 1 to 3 months on a fixed schedule rather than when one has the urge to smoke.[55] Studies have found, however, that 15% to 20% of abstainers continue to use the gum for longer than 12 months. Patients should be encouraged to stick with the patch and/or gum for the minimally acceptable duration of treatment.

Economic and Pharmacoeconomic Considerations

Most health insurers provide coverage for the chronic illnesses caused by smoking (e.g., chronic obstructive pulmonary disease, cancer, and myocardial infarction), yet few provide coverage for treating the nicotine addiction that caused those ailments.[53] For each of the approximately 22 billion packs of cigarettes sold in the United States in 1999, $3.45 was spent on medical care attributable to smoking, and $3.73 in productivity losses were incurred, for a total cost of $7.18 per pack.[59] Even after adding the cost of the nicotine patch to physician counseling, costs from the standpoint of a third-party payer range from $1,441 to $3,445 per quality-adjusted life year saved for NRT (based on 15 minutes of physician counseling and 1 to 2 months of NRT).[59] Treating tobacco dependence is particularly important economically, in that it can prevent a variety of costly chronic diseases, including heart disease, cancer, and pulmonary disease. A recent meta-analysis conducted by the Cochrane Collaboration determined that a 36% reduction in risk of death from coronary heart disease was obtained by quitting smoking. This decrease in risk is comparable, if not greater, than that obtained from lowering low-density lipoprotein (LDL) cholesterol or blood pressure lowering.[60] The failure of a health plan to cover tobacco dependence treatment could reduce the number of people seeking and receiving these services.

BUPROPION

⑩ Bupropion inhibits neuronal reuptake and potentiates the effects of norepinephrine and dopamine. Although its precise mechanism in smoking cessation is not well understood, dopamine has been associated with the rewarding effects of addictive substances. Withdrawal symptoms can be decreased by virtue of bupropion inhibition of norepinephrine uptake. The AHRQ panel concluded that sustained-release (SR) bupropion is an efficacious smoking cessation treatment that patients should be encouraged to use.[53] Two large multicenter studies met selection criteria and were included in the meta-analysis comparing bupropion SR with placebo. The use of bupropion SR as a part of a comprehensive smoking cessation program approximately doubles long-term abstinence rates when compared with placebo.

One study compared the effects of 100, 150, or 300 mg/day of bupropion SR or placebo for 7 weeks in 615 patients who visited the clinic each week for evaluation and counseling.[61] When the study was concluded, smoking cessation rates were 19% with placebo and 28.8%, 38.6%, and 44.2% with the respective doses of the drug. The differences between the 150- and 300-mg doses and placebo were statistically significant. After 1 year, the respective rates were 12.4%, 19.6%, 22.9%, and 23.1%, indicating a fairly high rate of relapse in all groups.

Bupropion at a dose of 150 mg twice daily of sustained-release tablets was compared with the 21-mg nicotine patch separately and as combined therapy and with placebo in nearly 900 patients studied for 9 weeks. At the 10-week mark, smoking cessation had been accomplished in 20% of the placebo group, 32% of the group using the patch alone, 46% of the group using bupropion alone, and 51% of the group using combined therapy. All three active treatments were significantly better than placebo.[62] Unlike its use as an antidepressant, no seizures occurred with bupropion in smoking cessation trials. Insomnia and dry mouth were the most frequent adverse effects. Other side effects noted in the trials were tremor, rash, and a few anaphylactoid reactions characterized by pruritus, urticaria, angioedema, and dyspnea.[62]

⑩ For smoking cessation, the manufacturer recommends a dosage of 150 mg once daily for 3 days and then twice daily for 7 to 12 weeks or longer, with or without NRT. Patients are instructed to stop smoking during the second week of treatment and are encouraged to use counseling and support services along with the medication. For maintenance therapy, consider bupropion SR 150 mg twice daily for up to 6 months.[53] In addition, bupropion SR appears to be effective for smokeless tobacco cessation.[63] Cost per quality-adjusted life-year saved after smoking cessation ranged from $920 to $2,150 for bupropion alone, and $,1282 to $2,836 for NRT plus bupropion.[59]

SECOND-LINE MEDICATIONS

Second-line medications are pharmacotherapies for which there is evidence of efficacy for treating tobacco dependence but have a more limited role than first-line medications because (1) the FDA has not approved them for a tobacco-dependence treatment indication, and (2) there are more concerns about potential side effects than exist with first-line medications.[53] Second-line treatments should be considered for use on a case-by-case basis after first-line treatments have been used or considered.

Clonidine

Clonidine, a prescription drug, is an efficacious smoking cessation treatment. It can be used under a clinician's supervision as a second-line agent to treat tobacco dependence. A recent meta-analysis of six trials showed that clonidine increased smoking cessation rates by 11% (odds ratio [OR] 1.89; confidence interval [CI] 1.30 to 2.14). There was a high incidence of dose-dependent side effects, particularly dry mouth and sedation.[64] It should be noted that abrupt discontinuation of clonidine can result in symptoms such as nervousness, agitation, headache, and tremor, accompanied or followed by a rapid rise in blood pressure and elevated catecholamine levels.

Because clonidine is used primarily as an antihypertensive medication and has not been approved by the FDA as a smoking cessation medication, clinicians need to be aware of the specific warnings regarding this medication as well as its side-effect profile. Additionally, a specific dosing regimen for the use of clonidine in smoking cessation has not been established. Because of the warnings associated with clonidine discontinuation, the variability in dosages used to test this medication, and a lack of FDA approval, the guideline panel chose to recommend clonidine as a second-line agent. Doses used in various clinical cessation trials have varied significantly, from 0.15 to 0.75 mg/day orally to 0.1 to 0.2 mg/day transdermally, without a clear dose-response relation to cessation. Initial dosing typically is 0.1 mg orally twice daily or 0.1 mg/day transdermally, increasing by 0.1 mg/day each week if needed. The duration also varied across the clinical trials, ranging from 3 weeks to 12 months. Most commonly reported side effects include dry mouth, drowsiness, dizziness, sedation, and constipation. As an antihypertensive medication, clonidine can be expected to lower blood pressure in most patients. Therefore, clinicians should monitor blood pressure when using this medication.[53]

Nortriptyline

Nortriptyline is also considered to be efficacious as a second-line agent to treat tobacco dependence. Based on limited data, the use of nortriptyline appears to increase abstinence rates compared with placebo.

Nortriptyline should be considered for smoking cessation under a clinician's direction in patients unable to use first-line medications because of contraindications or in patients who failed using first-line medications. Therapy is initiated 10 to 28 days before the quit date to allow nortriptyline to reach steady state at the target dose. Smoking cessation trials have initiated treatment at a dose of 25 mg/day, increasing gradually to a target dose of 75 to 100 mg/day. Duration of treatment used in smoking cessation trials has been approximately 12 weeks. Most commonly reported side effects include sedation, dry mouth, blurred vision, urinary retention, light-headedness, and shaky hands.

Varenicline (Chantix)

⓫ A new and novel aid to smoking cessation was approved by the FDA on May 10, 2006. The drug, varenicline, acts at sites in the brain affected by nicotine and may help those who wish to give up smoking in two ways: by providing some nicotine effects to ease the withdrawal symptoms and by blocking the effects of nicotine from cigarettes if they resume smoking. Specifically, varenicline is a partial agonist that binds selectively to α_4-β_2-nicotinic acetylcholine receptors with a greater affinity than nicotine. When bound to the receptor, the drug blocks nicotine from binding and also evokes a response but to a lesser degree than nicotine. The stimulation of the receptor that occurs results in release of dopamine and thus provides a type of "reward" that can decrease craving and withdrawal symptoms.[65]

There have been five randomized double blind placebo-controlled studies of varenicline published to date. Three of these also included a bupropion SR arm.[66–68] In these three studies after 12 weeks of therapy, statistically higher rates of continuous smoking cessation were consistently observed for varenicline versus placebo as well as bupropion SR versus placebo. At the 12 month followup, the rates of continuous abstinence in the varenicline group remained statistically significantly different versus placebo. However, rates of continuous abstinence in the bupropion group were no longer statistically significantly different from placebo.[66–68] For each patient who achieved continuous abstinence at the 1-year followup, 14 patients needed to be treated with varenicline for 12 weeks.

Because this drug is so new to the market, its overall place in therapy is not known at this time. It has not been compared to the nicotine products but might be a reasonable choice for those who cannot tolerate NRT or for those who have failed therapy in the past.[68]

Future Treatments

Work has begun to develop a vaccine that would be used in treating nicotine addiction. One such product is called NicVAX (nicotine conjugate vaccine) and is designed to cause the immune system to produce antibodies that bind to nicotine and prevent it from entering the brain. As a result, the positive stimulus in the brain that is normally caused by nicotine is no longer present, thereby taking away the physical motivation for smoking, consequently helping people to quit.[69]

CAFFEINE

Caffeine is the most widely consumed behaviorally active substance in the world.[63] *Caffeinism* is the term coined to describe the clinical syndrome produced by acute or chronic overuse of caffeine.[70] The syndrome usually is characterized by CNS and peripheral manifestations, most notably anxiety, psychomotor alterations, sleep disturbances, mood changes, and psychophysiologic complaints.

CLINICAL PRESENTATION OF EXCESSIVE CAFFEINE INTAKE

General

- The patient may not be in acute distress.

Symptoms

- The patient may complain of nausea, vomiting, diarrhea, and psychomotor agitation, and can appear restless, nervous, and excited.

Signs

- The patient can present with facial flushing, diuresis, and muscle twitching.
- Tachycardia or cardiac arrhythmias can also occur

Laboratory Tests

- Caffeine serum concentrations are rarely used clinically.

As many as one in five adults consume doses of caffeine generally considered large enough to cause clinical symptoms.[71,72] Controlled double-blind studies demonstrate that caffeine has reinforcement properties in most people with a history of heavy prior use[73] and that this reinforcement is a function of dose and prior exposure.

Pharmacologically, the risk of developing some meaningful clinical manifestations becomes high when intake exceeds 500 mg/day. This places 20% to 30% of North Americans at risk.[71] Recognizing that there are individual variations and accepting a conservative approach, these data suggest that perhaps 10% to 20% of the North American adult population probably has meaningful clinical symptoms consistent with a diagnosis of caffeinism, a prevalence rate exceeding that of most other substances of abuse.

Caffeine has been proposed as a "model of drug abuse" despite the facts that its sale is largely unrestricted and that heavy consumption of caffeine-containing beverages is not considered to be drug abuse. An exhaustive review of caffeine dependence focused on the potential for abuse of caffeine and the nature of tolerance and withdrawal.[72] A second comprehensive review of human and animal data on coffee and caffeine consumption and caffeine dependence, withdrawal, and reinforcement also has been published.[71] The information below represents a broad overview of these topics, and the reader interested in more detail is urged to consult these two reviews.[71,72]

EPIDEMIOLOGY OF CAFFEINE USE AND ABUSE

Caffeine is used by 80% of the population of the United States,[74] and its use can be problematic for some people. In 1999 there were 108,000,000 coffee consumers in the United States spending approximately $9.2 billion in the retail sector and $8.7 billion in the food service sector every year.[75] The National Coffee Association found in 2001 that 52% of the adult population of the United States drinks coffee daily.[76]

Average caffeine consumption in humans can range in different cultures and nations from 80 to 400 mg per person per day. In the United States caffeine consumption exceeds several billion kilograms annually. Per capita intake for the entire world's population approximates 70 mg/day. In the United States this figure is considerably larger, at 210 to 238 mg. The majority of caffeine users progress to a pattern of frequent or daily consumption. Approximately one-fourth eventually begin consuming large quantities, exceeding 500 mg/day, and conservatively, 10% of all adults then progress to develop the syndrome of caffeinism. Mean daily consumption of caffeine in American children is surprisingly high. The Framingham Children's Study[77] investigated the amounts of caffeine consumed each day by children between the ages of 6 and 10 years (mean 8.4 years for boys and 8.1 years for girls). Mean intake of caffeine was 16 ± 9.6 mg/day. Caffeinated soft drinks and chocolate furnished almost all of the caffeine.

Caffeine is an added ingredient in approximately 70% of soft drinks consumed in the United States.[78] Soft drink manufacturers' justification to regulatory agencies and the public for adding caffeine to soft drinks is that caffeine is a flavoring agent. In a recent study, only 8% of a group of regular cola soft drink consumers could detect the taste effect of the caffeine concentration found in most cola soft drinks. Thus soft drinks serve as a major source of caffeine without any apparent purpose beyond its stimulant effects.[74]

DIFFERENTIAL DIAGNOSIS

Caffeine intoxication is the only official diagnosis associated with caffeinism in the *DSM-IV-TR*. Caffeine-induced anxiety can manifest as restlessness, nervousness, excitement, insomnia, diuresis, flushing, gastrointestinal disturbance, muscle twitching, irritability, and jitteriness. If caffeine-induced insomnia requires specific treatment, caffeine-induced sleep disorder (*DSM-IV-TR*) is an appropriate diagnosis.[4,70]

Because excessive caffeine consumption is so widespread, a thorough history of caffeine use should be included in the routine assessment of all new patients in primary care medical settings. In this manner, the practitioner can use the information gathered to uncover high levels of caffeine intake and then use the information to pinpoint the cause of clinical signs and symptoms typical of caffeinism. Clinical manifestations of caffeinism almost always will lessen in intensity or disappear completely within 1 to 2 weeks after removing the drug.[4]

PHARMACOLOGY OF CAFFEINE

Caffeine is rapidly and completely absorbed from the gastrointestinal tract, reaching a peak blood level within 30 to 45 minutes of oral ingestion. It easily crosses the blood–brain barrier, and levels achieved in the brain are proportional to the dose administered.

The half-life of caffeine in humans is approximately 3.5 to 5 hours. It is metabolized extensively by a complex metabolic pathway occurring primarily in the liver. Serious problems rarely result from overdoses of caffeine. In fact, the amount of caffeine needed to cause death in an average adult male is 5 to 10 g, the equivalent of 50 to 100 cups of regular brewed coffee. Thus the risk of overdose from dietary sources of caffeine is virtually nonexistent.

⓫ Caffeine increases the heart rate and force of contraction. It also has a strong diuretic effect. The key factor promoting caffeine use and dosage increases can be the drug's reinforcing effect on pleasure and reward centers of the brain. Caffeine's pharmacologic actions appear comparable (although less potent) in some aspects with those of other stimulants, such as amphetamines and cocaine. After years of uncertainty, it is apparent from both preclinical research and human studies that regular caffeine use does induce tolerance.

CAFFEINE DEPENDENCE

Research has shown that abstinence from caffeine induces a distinct withdrawal syndrome. Evidence for the existence of a caffeine dependence syndrome was presented by Strain and associates.[78] In a structured psychiatric interview, subjects self-identified as having problems with caffeine use were evaluated for features of a *DSM-IV-TR* diagnosis of drug dependence. Those judged as caffeine dependent manifested at least three of four criteria (i.e., tolerance, withdrawal, persistent desire, or an unsuccessful attempt to reduce consumption and persistent use despite adverse psychologic or physical consequences). Of 99 people screened, 27 were evaluated by means of a structured psychiatric interview modified for the diagnosis of caffeine dependence; 16 of those subjects (59%) met the criteria. In a second phase of the study, 11 of the 16 caffeine-dependent individuals participated in a 2-day double-blind crossover study of caffeine deprivation. Nine showed evidence of caffeine withdrawal during the placebo phase, a finding that validated one of the criteria for the diagnosis of dependence.

CAFFEINE WITHDRAWAL

⓬ The frequency of the caffeine withdrawal syndrome is not well known, but it may be common. Withdrawal can occur when individuals who previously have been consuming caffeine on a regular basis suddenly discontinue its intake.[4] When caffeine is reintroduced, relief of withdrawal symptoms tends to occur within 30 to 60 minutes. At present, this appears to be the most effective "treatment" for the caffeine-withdrawal syndrome.

CLINICAL PRESENTATION OF CAFFEINE WITHDRAWAL

General

- The patient may be uncomfortable but is not in acute distress.

Symptoms

- The patient can experience nausea, headache, drowsiness, and fatigue. The caffeine withdrawal headache is somewhat unique, starting with a sense of fullness in the head and progressing to throbbing and diffuse pain that is made worse by movement. The maximum intensity of the pain occurs 3 to 6 hours after beginning.
- The patient can also experience difficulty concentrating and impaired psychomotor performance.

EFFECT ON SLEEP

Caffeine interferes with sleep in most nontolerant individuals.[4,70] Once tolerance has developed, people are much less likely to self-report sleep abnormalities, or they may sense that the insomnia has disappeared altogether. To illustrate, 53% of those consuming less than 250 mg/day agreed that caffeine before bedtime would prevent sleep, compared with 43% of those consuming 250 to 749 mg/day, and only 22% of those taking 750 mg/day or more. Even though the higher-level consumers denied that caffeine interferes with their sleep, studies done in the sleep laboratory confirm that caffeine consumers do have greater sleep latency, more frequent awakenings, and altered sleep architecture, and that these effects are dose related.

TREATMENT

Caffeinism

Caffeinism is treated by reducing or discontinuing the drug. It can be necessary to wean the patient off the drug because going "cold turkey" can produce such serious symptoms that the drug must be restarted. Decaffeinated beverages can be substituted slowly for the caffeinated type. However, relapses are less likely to occur when the drug is discontinued all at once, probably because of the considerable self-discipline required to continue weaning the drug when one knows that an increase in dose will cause the symptoms to abate.

It can be possible for some individuals simply to reduce their dosage of caffeine rather than discontinue it altogether. Others can be particularly sensitive to the drug, and they may not be able to handle even reduced intake of caffeine. Patients with cardiovascular disease, especially arrhythmias, should refrain totally, as should people with prior stroke or transient ischemic attacks. Peptic ulcer patients and those with bipolar mood disorder and schizophrenia should be encouraged to avoid caffeine altogether.

An exhaustive review of recent research on coffee and its health effects has recently been published. The reader wishing more information is urged to consult this review.[79]

CONCLUSIONS

Use of alcohol, tobacco, and caffeine is so commonly accepted in our society that people take notice only when their use causes serious problems. When these problems do occur, the human and economic costs are enormous. Health professionals must be committed to helping people free themselves of the addictions that can occur with these common drugs.

ABBREVIATIONS

AHRQ: Agency for Healthcare Research and Quality

BAC: blood alcohol concentration

CT: computed tomography

DSM-IV-TR: *Diagnostic and Statistical Manual of Mental Disorders, 4th ed., Text Revision*

GABA: γ-aminobutyric acid

NRT: nicotine replacement therapy

REFERENCES

1. Annual smoking attributable mortality, years of potential life lost, and productivity losses—United States, 1997–2001. MMWR Morb Mortal Wkly Rep 2005;54:625–628.
2. Center for Disease Control and Prevention. The health consequences of smoking: A report from the surgeon general. Atlanta, GA: US Department of Health and Human Services, CDC, 2004.
3. Substance Abuse and Mental Health Services Administration. Results from the 2005 National Survey on Drug Use and Health: National Findings (Office of Applied Studies, NSDUH Series H-30 DHHS Publication No. SMA 06–4194). 2006, *http://www.oas.samhsa.gov/nsduh/2k5nsduh/2k5Results.htm#Ch3.*
4. Diagnostic and Statistical Manual of Mental Disorders, 4th ed., Text Revision. Washington DC: American Psychiatric Association, 2000:212–214.
5. National Institute on Alcohol Abuse and Alcoholism. Chapter 8: Treatment Research. Tenth Special Report to the U.S. Congress on Alcohol and Health, 2000. Washington, DC: U.S. Department of Health and Human Services. 2000, *http://pubs.niaaa.nih.gov/publications/10report/intro.pdf.*
6. Fiellin DA, Reid MC, O'Connor PG. Outpatient management of patients with alcohol problems. Ann Intern Med 2000;133:815–827.
7. World Health Organization Department of Mental Health and Substance Abuse, Geneva 2004. Global Status Report on Alcohol 2004. *http://www.who.int/substance_abuse/publications/global_status_report_2004_overview.pdf.*
8. Substance Abuse and Mental Health Services Administration, Office of Applied Studies. Emergency Department Trends from the Drug Abuse Warning Network, Final Estimates 1995–2002. DAWN Series: D-24 DHHS Publication No. (SMA) 03–3780. 2003, *http://dawninfo.samhsa.gov/pubs_94_02/.*
9. Center for Disease Control and Prevention. Alcohol, Injuries, and the Emergency Department. 2006, *http://www.cdc.gov/ncipc/fact_book/09_Alcohol_%20Injuries_%20ED.htm.*
10. Harwood, H. Updating Estimates of the Economic Costs of Alcohol Abuse in the United States: Estimates, Update Methods, and Data. Report prepared by The Lewin Group for the National Institute on Alcohol Abuse and Alcoholism. 2000, *http://pubs.niaaa.nih.gov/publications/economic-2000/index.htm.*
11. Griffiths RR, Juliano LM, Chausmer AL. Caffeine pharmacology and clinical effects. In: Graham AW, Schultz TK, Mayo-Smith MF, et al., eds. Principles of Addiction Medicine, 3rd ed. Chevy Chase, MD: American Society of Addiction, 2003:193–224. *http://www.caffeinedependence.org/caffeine_dependence.html.*
12. Enoch MA. Pharmacogenomics of alcohol response and addiction. Am J Pharmacogenomics 2003;3:217–232.
13. Bierut LJ, Saccone NL, Rice JP, et al. Defining alcohol-related phenotypes in humans. The Collaborative Study on the Genetics of Alcoholism. Alcohol Res Health 2002;26:208–213.
14. Heath AC, Nelson EC, National Institute of Alcohol Abuse and Alcoholism. Effects of the interaction between genotype and environment. Research into the genetic epidemiology of alcohol dependence. Alcohol Res Health 2002;26:193–201. *http://www.niaaa.nih.gov/publications/arh26-3/193–201.htm.*
15. Luo X, Kranzler HR, Zuo L, et al. Diplotype trend regression analysis of the ADH gene cluster and the ALDH2 gene: Multiple significant associations with alcohol dependence. Am J Hum Genet 2006;78:973–987.
16. Boothby LA, Doering PL. Health promotion and disease prevention. In: The Science and Practice of Pharmacotherapy. PSAP V, 2004, available at http://www.accp.com/strp5b05.php.
17. Krystal JH, Staley J, Mason G, et al. Gamma-aminobutyric acid type A receptors and alcoholism: Intoxication, dependence, vulnerability, and treatment. Arch Gen Psychiatry 2006;63:957–968.
18. Radel M, Goldman D. Pharmacogenetics of alcohol response and alcoholism: The interplay of genes and environmental factors in thresholds for alcoholism. Drug Metab Dispos 2001;29:489–494.
19. Hutchison KE, Wooden A, Swift RM, et al. Olanzapine reduces craving for alcohol: A DRD4 VNTR polymorphism by pharmacotherapy interaction. Neuropsychopharmacology 2003;28:1882–1888.
20. Jones AW, Holmgren P. Urine/blood ratios of ethanol in deaths attributed to acute alcohol poisoning and chronic alcoholism. Forensic Sci Int 2003;135:206–212.
21. Chiuve SE, McCullough ML, Sacks FM, Rimm EB. Healthy lifestyle factors in the primary prevention of coronary heart disease among men: Benefits among users and nonusers of lipid-lowering and antihypertensive medications. Circulation 2006;114:160–167.
22. Reid MC, Van Ness PH, Hawkins KA, et al. Light to moderate alcohol consumption is associated with better cognitive function among older male veterans receiving primary care. J Geriatr Psychiatry Neurol 2006;19:98–105.
23. Gronbaek M. Factors influencing the relation between alcohol and cardiovascular disease. Curr Opin Lipidol 2006;17:17–21.
24. Lucas DL, Brown RA, Wassef M, Giles TD. Alcohol and the cardiovascular system research challenges and opportunities. J Am Coll Cardiol 2005;45:1916–1924.
25. Ramchandani VA, Kwo PY, Li TK. Effect of food and food consumption on alcohol elimination rates in healthy men and women. J Clin Pharmacol 2001;41:1345–1350.
26. Norberg A, Jones AW, Hahn RG, Gabrielsson JL. Role of variability in explaining ethanol pharmacokinetics: Research and forensic applications. Clin Pharmacokinet 2003;42:1–31.
27. Mayo-Smith MF. Pharmacological management of alcohol withdrawal. A meta-analysis and evidence-based practice guideline. American Society of Addiction Medicine Working Group on Pharmacological Management of Alcohol Withdrawal. JAMA 1997;278:144–151.
28. Federal Aviation Administration. Alcohol and Flying: Deadly Combination. 2006, *http://www.faa.gov/pilots/safety/pilotsafetybrochures/media/alcohol.pdf.*
29. Brunton LL, Lazo JS, Parker KL, eds. Goodman and Gilman's The Pharmacological Basis of Therapeutics, 11th ed. [electronic version]. 2006, AccessMedicine. *http://www.accessmedicine.com/resourceTOC.aspx?resourceID=28.*
30. Goldman HH. Review of General Psychiatry, 5th ed. [electronic version]. 2000, StatRef. *http://onlinestatref.com.*
31. Alcohol and Substance Awareness Program. Blood alcohol level. 2006, *http://www.barnard.columbia.edu/asap/bal.html.*
32. Garriot JC, ed. Medical-Legal Aspects of Alcohol. Tucson, AZ: Lawyers and Judges Publishing, 2003:27.
33. Mayo-Smith MF, Beecher LH, Fischer TL, et al. Working Group on the Management of Alcohol Withdrawal Delirium, Practice Guidelines Committee, American Society of Addiction Medicine. Management of alcohol withdrawal delirium. An evidence-based practice guideline [erratum Arch Intern Med 2004;164:2068]. Arch Intern Med 2004;164:1405–1412.
34. Kosten TR, O'Connor PG. Management of drug and alcohol withdrawal. N Engl J Med 2003;348:1786–1795.

35. Hillbom M, Pieninkeroinen L, Leone M. Seizures in alcohol-dependent patients. CNS Drugs 2003;17:1013–1030.
36. Reoux JP, Miller K. Routine hospital alcohol detoxification practice compared to symptom triggered management with an objective withdrawal scale (CIWA-Ar). Am J Addict 2000;9:135–144.
37. Mariani JJ, Rosenthal RN, Tross S, et al. A randomized, open-label, controlled trial of gabapentin and phenobarbital in the treatment of alcohol withdrawal. Am J Addict 2006;15:76–84.
38. Book SW, Myrick H. Novel anticonvulsants in the treatment of alcoholism. Expert Opin Investig Drugs 2005;14:371–376.
39. Boothby LA, Doering PL. Acamprosate for the treatment of alcohol dependence. Clin Ther 2005;27:695–714.
40. Mason BJ, Salvato FR, Williams LD, et al. A double-blind, placebo-controlled study of oral nalmefene for alcohol dependence. Arch Gen Psychiatry 1999;56:719–724.
41. Garbutt JC, West SL, Carey TS, et al. Pharmacological treatment of alcohol dependence: A review of the evidence. JAMA 1999;281:1318–1325.
42. Morris PL, Hopwood M, Whelan G, et al. Naltrexone for alcohol dependence: A randomized controlled trial. Addiction 2001;96:1565–1573.
43. Srisurapanont M, Jarusuraisin N. Opioid antagonists for alcohol dependence. Cochrane Database Syst Rev 2005;2:CD001867.
44. Garbutt JC, Kranzler HR, O'Malley SS, et al. Vivitrex Study Group. Efficacy and tolerability of long-acting injectable naltrexone for alcohol dependence: A randomized controlled trial [erratum JAMA 2005;293:1978 and JAMA 2005 Jun 15:293(23):2864]. JAMA 2005;293:1617–1625.
45. Johnson BA, Ait-Daoud N, Bowden CL, et al. Oral topiramate for treatment of alcohol dependence: A randomized controlled trial. Lancet 2003;361:1677–1685.
46. Lancaster T, Stead L, Silagy C, Sowden A. Effectiveness of interventions to help people stop smoking: Findings from the Cochrane Library. BMJ 2000;321(7257):355–358.
47. Goldstein MG, Niaura R, Willey-Lessne C, et al. Physicians counseling smokers. A population-based survey of patients' perceptions of health care provider-delivered smoking cessation interventions. Arch Intern Med 1997;157:1313–1319.
48. Goldstein MG, Niaura R, Willey C, et al. An academic detailing intervention to disseminate physician-delivered smoking cessation counseling: Smoking cessation outcomes of the Physicians Counseling Smokers Project. Prev Med 2003;36:185–196.
49. U.S. Department of Health and Human Services. Healthy People 2010, 2nd ed. Understanding and Improving Health and Objectives for Improving Health (2 vols). Washington, DC: U.S. Department of Health and Human Services, 2000.
50. American Cancer Society. Cancer Facts and Figures 2004. 2004, *http://www.cancer.org/docroot/PED/ped_10.asp?sitearea=WHO&level=1*.
51. Balfour DJ. Neuroplasticity within the mesoaccumbens dopamine system and its role in tobacco dependence. Curr Drug Targets CNS Neurol Disord 2002;1:413–421.
52. Anonymous. Industry watch: Blowing smoke: How cigarette manufacturers argued that nicotine is not addictive. Tob Control 1999;8:210–213.
53. Change in nicotine yields 1998–2004 Massachusetts Department of Public Health, Data Submitted in Accordance with Massachusetts General laws, Chap. 94: Section 307B, 105 CMR 660.000. 2006, *http://www.mass.gov/dph/mtcp/reports/nicotine_yields_1998_2004_report.pdf*.
54. U.S. Department of Health and Human Services. Treating tobacco use and dependence: Clinical Practice Guideline. 2000, *http://www.surgeongeneral.gov/tobacco/treating_tobacco_use.pdf*.
55. Varenicline (Chantix) Official Labeling. May 2006, *http://www.fda.gov/cder/foi/label/2006/021928lbl.pdf*.
56. Silagy C, Lancaster T, Stead L, et al. Nicotine replacement therapy for smoking cessation. Cochrane Database Syst Rev 2004;3:CD000146.
57. Pierce JP, Gilpin EA. Impact of over-the-counter sales on effectiveness of pharmaceutical aids for smoking cessation. JAMA 2002;288:1260–1264.
58. Wisborg K, Henriksen TB, Jespersen LB, et al. Nicotine patches for pregnant smokers: A randomized controlled trial. Obstet Gynecol 2000;96:967–971.
59. Ilett KF, Hale TW, Page-Sharp M, et al. Use of nicotine patches in breast-feeding mothers: Transfer of nicotine and cotinine into human milk. Clin Pharmacol Ther 2003;74:516–524.
60. Song F, Raftery J, Aveyard P, et al. Cost-effectiveness of pharmacological interventions for smoking cessation: A literature review and a decision analytic analysis. Med Decis Making 2002;22:s26–s37.
61. Critchley J, Capewell S. Smoking cessation for the secondary prevention of coronary heart disease. Cochrane Database Syst Rev 2004(1):CD003041.
62. Hurt RD, Sachs DP, Glover ED, et al. A comparison of sustained release bupropion and placebo for smoking cessation. N Engl J Med 1997;337:1195–1202.
63. Jorenby DE, Leischow SJ, Nides MA, et al. A controlled trial of sustained-release bupropion, a nicotine patch, or both for smoking cessation. N Engl J Med 1999;340:685–691.
64. Glover ED, Glover PN, Sullivan CR, et al. A comparison of sustained-release bupropion and placebo for smokeless tobacco cessation. Am J Health Behav 2002;26:386–393.
65. Gourlay SG, Stead LF, Benowitz NL. Clonidine for smoking cessation. Cochrane Database Syst Rev 2004;(3):CD000058.
66. Coe JW, Brooks PR, Vetelino MG, et al. Varenicline: An alpha-4-beta-2 nicotinic receptor partial agonist for smoking cessation. Med Chem 2005;48:3474–3477.
67. Gonzales D, Rennard SI, Nides M, et al. Varenicline, an alpha-4-beta-2 nicotinic acetylcholine receptor partial agonist vs sustained-release bupropion and placebo for smoking cessation: A randomized controlled trial. JAMA 2006;296:47–55.
68. Jorenby DE, Hays JT, Rigotti NA, et al. Efficacy of varenicline, an alpha-4-beta-2 nicotinic acetylcholine receptor partial agonist vs placebo or sustained-release bupropion for smoking cessation: A randomized controlled trial. JAMA 2006;296:56–63.
69. Nides M, Oncken C, Gonzales D, et al. Smoking cessation with varenicline, a selective $alpha_4$ $beta_2$ nicotinic receptor partial agonist: Results from a 7-week, randomized, placebo- and bupropion-controlled trial with 1-year follow-up. Arch Intern Med 2006;166:1561–1568.
70. Boothby LA, Doering PL. What the pharmacist should know to help patients stop smoking. Drug Topics 2005;149:41–50.
71. Hughes JR, Oliveto AH, Liguori A, et al. Endorsement of DSM-IV dependence criteria among caffeine users. Drug Alcohol Depend 1998; 52:99–107.
72. Nehlig A. Are we dependent upon coffee and caffeine? A review of human and animal data. Neurosci Biobehav Rev 1999;23:563–576.
73. Daly JW, Fredholm BB. Caffeine: An atypical drug of dependence. Drug Alcohol Depend 1998;52:99–107.
74. Garrett BE, Griffiths RR. Physical dependence increases the relative reinforcing effects of caffeine versus placebo. Psychopharmacology (Berl) 1998;139:195–202.
75. Griffiths RR, Singer MR. Is caffeine a flavoring agent in cola soft drinks? Arch Fam Med 2000;9:727–734.
76. Gorman L. 2001 Specialty Coffee Market Research Report. The Gourmet Retailer 2001;98–106. *http://www.gourmetretailer.com/gourmetretailer/images/pdf/coffee.pdf*.
77. Associated Press. Java Joy in Coffee Study. 2006, *http://www.wired.com/news/medtech/0,1286,68677,00.html*.
78. Ellison RC, Singer MR, Moore LL, et al. Current caffeine intake of young children: Amount and sources. J Am Diet Assoc 1995;95:802–804.
79. Strain EC, Mumford GK, Silverman K, et al. Caffeine dependence syndrome: Evidence from case histories and experimental evaluations. JAMA 1994;272:1043–1048.
80. Higdon J, Frei B. Coffee and health: A review of recent human research. Crit Rev Food Sci Nutr 2006;46:101–123.

CHAPTER 70

Schizophrenia

M. LYNN CRISMON, TAMI R. ARGO, AND PETER F. BUCKLEY

KEY CONCEPTS

1. The pathophysiology of schizophrenia can occur in one or more different neurotransmitter systems.
2. The clinical presentation of schizophrenia is characterized by positive symptoms, negative symptoms, and impairment in cognitive functioning.
3. Comprehensive care for individuals with schizophrenia must occur in the context of a multidisciplinary mental health care environment that offers psychotropic medication management and comprehensive psychosocial services.
4. A thorough patient evaluation (e.g., history, mental status examination, physical examination, and laboratory analysis) should occur to establish a diagnosis of schizophrenia and to identify potential co-occurring disorders, including substance abuse and general medical disorders.
5. Given that it is challenging to differentiate among antipsychotics based on efficacy, side-effect profiles become important in choosing an antipsychotic for an individual patient.
6. Pharmacotherapy algorithms should emphasize monotherapies with antipsychotics of optimal efficacy: side-effect ratios and progress to medications with greater side-effect risks and then to combination regimens only in the most treatment-resistant patients.
7. Adequate time on a given medication at a therapeutic dose is the most important variable in predicting medication response.
8. Long-term maintenance antipsychotic treatment is necessary for the vast majority of patients with schizophrenia to prevent relapse.
9. Thorough patient and family psychoeducation should occur, including education about the illness, symptoms, prognosis, medication, psychosocial treatments, and methods to improve adaptive functioning.
10. Pharmacotherapy decisions should be guided by systematic monitoring of patient symptoms, preferably with the use of brief symptom rating scales.

Learning objectives, review questions, and other resources can be found at **www.pharmacotherapyonline.com.**

Schizophrenia is one of the most complex and challenging of psychiatric disorders. It represents a heterogeneous syndrome of disorganized and bizarre thoughts, delusions, hallucinations, inappropriate affect, and impaired psychosocial functioning. From the time that Kraepelin first described dementia praecox in 1896 until publication of the *Diagnostic and Statistical Manual of Mental Disorders, 4th edition, Text Revision (DSM-IV-TR)* in 2000, the description of this illness has continuously evolved.[1] Scientific advances that increase our knowledge of central nervous system (CNS) physiology, pathophysiology, and genetics will likely improve our understanding of schizophrenia in the future.

EPIDEMIOLOGY

According to the Epidemiologic Catchment Area Study, the U.S. lifetime prevalence of schizophrenia ranges from 0.6% to 1.9%, with an average of approximately 1%.[2] With only a few possible exceptions, the worldwide prevalence of schizophrenia is remarkably similar among all cultures. Schizophrenia most commonly has its onset in late adolescence or early adulthood and rarely occurs before adolescence or after the age of 40 years. Although the prevalence of schizophrenia is equal in males and females, the onset of illness tends to be earlier in males. Males most frequently have their first episode during their early twenties, whereas with females it is usually during their late twenties to early thirties.[1,2]

ETIOLOGY

Although the etiology of schizophrenia is unknown, research has demonstrated various abnormalities in brain structure and function.[3] However, these changes are not consistent among all individuals with a diagnosis of schizophrenia, and much has yet to be learned about its pathogenesis. The cause of schizophrenia is likely multifactorial; that is, multiple pathophysiologic abnormalities can play a role in producing the similar but varying clinical phenotypes we refer to as schizophrenia.

A neurodevelopmental model has been evoked as one possible explanation for the etiology of schizophrenia.[4] This model proposes that schizophrenia has its origins in some as yet unknown in-utero disturbance, possibly occurring during the second trimester of pregnancy. Evidence for this is provided by the abnormal neuronal migration demonstrated in most studies of schizophrenic brains. This "schizophrenic lesion" can result in abnormalities in cell shape, position, symmetry, connectivity, and functionally to the development of abnormal brain circuits.[3,4] Changes are consistent with a cell migration abnormality during the second trimester of pregnancy, and some studies associate upper respiratory infections during the second trimester of pregnancy with a higher incidence of schizophrenia.[5] Other studies show a relationship between obstetric complications or neonatal hypoxia and schizophrenia. Some studies also associate low birth-weight (less than 2.5 kg [5.5 lb]) with schizophrenia.[2] The resulting secondary "synaptic disorganization" associated with such insults is thought not to produce overt clinical manifestations of psychosis until adolescence or early adulthood because this is the corresponding time period of neuronal maturation.

Although studies have shown decreased cortical thickness and increased ventricular size in the brains of many patients with schizophrenia, this occurs in the absence of widespread gliosis.[3] Gliosis, or the proliferation of glial cells, is thought to occur as a compensatory change in degenerative diseases of the brain. One hypothesis is that obstetric complications and hypoxia, in combination with a genetic predisposition, could activate a glutamatergic cascade that results in increased neuronal pruning. It is hypothesized that this genetic predisposition may be related to genes controlling N-methyl-D-aspartate (NMDA) receptor activity. As a part of the normal neurodevelopmental process, pruning of dendrites occurs. In the normal individual, approximately 35% of the peak number of dendrites at 2 years of age are pruned by midadolescence. Some studies have shown a higher percentage of pruning in individuals with schizophrenia. Furthermore, synaptic pruning predominantly involves glutamatergic dendrites. Hypoxia or other prenatal insult can result in a decreased number of basal neurons from which to start, and glutamatergic activation can exaggerate the pruning process.[6]

Numerous studies have shown neuropsychologic abnormalities and impairment in reaching normal motor milestones and abnormal movements in young children who later develop schizophrenia.[2] Abnormalities in brain function occur long before the onset of psychotic symptomatology and provide empiric evidence for schizophrenia being a neurodevelopmental disorder.[4] However, the progressive clinical deterioration in many patients suggests that this illness can also have a neurodegenerative component. This is consistent with recent brain imaging studies that show deteriorative brain changes in patients with frequent relapses.[7,8] Schizophrenia may be neither neurodevelopmental or neurodegenerative in origin, but rather an illness exhibiting neurodegenerative propensity based on a vulnerable neurodevelopmental predisposition.[9,10]

GENETICS

Although a specific abnormality has not been discovered, evidence suggests a genetic basis for schizophrenia. Although the risk of developing schizophrenia is 0.6% to 1.9% in the general population, the risk is approximately 10% if a first-degree relative has the illness and 3% if a second-degree relative has the illness.[11] If both parents have schizophrenia, the risk of producing a schizophrenic offspring increases to approximately 40%. Twin studies in dizygotic twins report that the risk of the second twin developing schizophrenia if one twin has the illness is between 12% and 14%. However, in monozygotic twins the risk increases to 48%.[11] Numerous adoption studies indicate that the risk for schizophrenia lies with the biologic parents, and change in the environment during the child's developmental stages does not alter this. If schizophrenia occurs in siblings, the onset of illness tends to occur at the same age in each, thus lessening the possibility of an environmental precipitant. A search for a genetic linkage in schizophrenia has been difficult, and any genetic etiologies in schizophrenia are likely heterogeneous, but present with similar phenotypes. Potential loci have been identified on chromosomes 6, 8, 13, and 22.[11] Beyond traditional familial and twin association studies, the study of the genetics of schizophrenia has become increasingly molecular in focus.[3,11] Recent work has shown that polymorphism in the VAL/MET alleles of the catecholamine-O-methyl transferase gene can explain some of the frontal lobe functional deficits in a subset of individuals with schizophrenia.[11] Other recent studies have shown abnormalities in several genes that code for neurodevelopment and for trophic factors.[11–13] For example, dysbindin is a neurodevelopmental protein gene that is found on chromosome 6. Alleles associated with decreased dysbindin RNA in the dorsolateral prefrontal cortex have been reported in patients with schizophrenia and their families.[14] Another recent geno-wide linkage scan of a large pedigree showed increased signal at chromosome 8p, close to the gene that encodes for neuregulin—another neurodevelopmental gene.[15]

PATHOPHYSIOLOGY

Computed axial tomography (CAT) scans and magnetic resonance imaging (MRI) studies show increased ventricular size, particularly in the third and lateral ventricles, in subtypes of schizophrenics. Recent studies also show a small decrease in brain size compared to matched controls. These changes appear to be consistent with brain asymmetry, the ventricular enlargement being most pronounced in the left temporal horn, and the decreased cortical size being most obvious in the left temporal lobe.[3,7] Not only does premorbid lower hippocampal volume predict onset of symptoms in high-risk individuals, these structural changes can progress throughout the course of the illness. A reduction in medial temporal lobe volume has been reported in high-risk patients after they were scanned, indicating that some brain changes can be associated with the evolution of psychosis. In an extended analysis, high-risk subjects were compared with first-episode chronic schizophrenia and normal control groups according to hippocampal and amygdala volumes at baseline.[16] No difference in MRI volumes between the high-risk subjects and normal controls were observed, irrespective of whether the at-risk patients did or did not progress to overt psychosis. First-episode schizophrenia (but not other psychosis) groups had reduced (left) hippocampal volume. The implication that these changes occur during transition is intriguing and accords well with the notion of psychosis as a biologically toxic event. Changes in hippocampal volume may correspond with impairment in neuropsychologic testing, and these patients may have poorer response to first-generation antipsychotics (FGAs).[7] Rather than a decrease in the number of neurons in affected brain areas, a decrease in axonal and dendritic communications between cells can result in a loss of connectivity that can be important with respect to neuronal adaptivity and CNS homeostasis.[3] These changes are likely consistent with the evidence for abnormal neuronal pruning.[4]

Antipsychotic effects on the brain are complex, perhaps ranging from arrest of apoptotic (*cell-death*) responses, to boosting brain neurotrophins and promoting repair/regrowth of neurons (*neurogenesis*).[17–18] Human brain-imaging studies reveal that medications can influence brain structure in treated patients with repeated MRI brain scans.[19] The clinical relevance of these findings is not yet established.

NEUROTRANSMITTER CHANGES

Four dopaminergic tracts are of primary interest. Table 70–1 outlines the origin, innervation, and primary functional activity of each tract, as well as the effects of dopamine (DA) antagonists.[6]

Evidence supports the presence of a DA-receptor defect in schizophrenia. Numerous positron emission tomography (PET) studies have shown regional brain abnormalities, including increased glucose metabolism in the caudate nucleus, and decreased blood flow and glucose metabolism in the frontal lobe and left temporal lobe.[2,3] This can indicate dopaminergic hyperactivity in the head of the caudate nucleus and dopaminergic hypofunction in the frontotemporal regions. PET studies using Dopamine-2 (D_2)-specific ligands suggest increased densities of D_2 receptors in the head of the caudate nucleus with decreased densities in the prefrontal cortex.[2,3] PET studies

TABLE 70-1 Dopaminergic Tracts and Effects of Dopamine Antagonists

Dopamine Tract	Origin	Innervation	Function	Dopamine Antagonist Effect
Nigrostriatal	Substantia nigra (A9 area)	Caudate nucleus Putamen	Extrapyramidal system, movement	Movement disorders
Mesolimbic	Midbrain ventral tegmentum (A10 area)	Limbic areas (e.g., amygdala, olfactory tubercle, septal nuclei), cingulate gyrus	Arousal, memory, stimulus processing, motivational behavior	Relief of psychosis
Mesocortical	Midbrain ventral tegmentum (A10 area)	Frontal and prefrontal lobe cortex	Cognition, communication, social function, response to stress	Relief of psychosis Akathisia
Tuberoinfundibular	Hypothalamus	Pituitary gland	Regulates prolactin release	Increased prolactin concentrations

assessing Dopamine-1 (D_1) function suggest that subpopulations of schizophrenics may have decreased densities of D_1 receptors in the caudate nucleus and the prefrontal cortex. Hypofrontality can be associated with lack of volition and cognitive dysfunction, core features of schizophrenia. It is unknown whether these changes represent a primary event or secondary processes related to other pathophysiologic abnormalities in schizophrenia. Because of the heterogeneity in the clinical presentation of schizophrenia, it has been suggested that the DA hypothesis can be more applicable to "neuroleptic-responsive psychosis," with multiple different etiologies possibly being responsible for causing schizophrenia.[17] Attempts have been made to develop relationships between these abnormal findings and behavioral symptoms present in schizophrenic patients. The positive symptoms are possibly more closely associated with DA-receptor hyperactivity in the mesocaudate, whereas negative symptoms and cognitive impairment are most closely related to DA-receptor hypofunction in the prefrontal cortex. Presynaptic D_1 receptors in the prefrontal cortex are thought to be involved in modulating glutamatergic activity, and this can be important with regard to working memory in individuals with schizophrenia.[17]

The glutamatergic system is one of the most widespread excitatory neurotransmitter systems in the brain. Alterations in its function, either hypo- or hyperactivity, can result in toxic neuronal reactions.[2,3,17] Dopaminergic innervation from the ventral striatum decreases the limbic system's inhibitory activity (perhaps through γ-aminobutyric acid [GABA] interneurons); thus, dopaminergic stimulation increases arousal. The corticostriatal glutamate pathways have the opposite effect, inhibiting dopaminergic function from the ventral striatum, therefore allowing the limbic system to have increased inhibitory activity. Descending glutamatergic tracts interact with dopaminergic tracts directly as well as through GABA interneurons. Glutamatergic deficiency produces symptoms similar to those of dopaminergic hyperactivity and possibly those seen in schizophrenia. The overlap between schizophrenia and substance abuse can be of importance in understanding the neurobiology of schizophrenia.[20] This overlap may have a genetic basis, perhaps related to core dopaminergic deficits seen both in schizophrenia and addictive disorders.[20] Clinical support for this comes from the fact that phencyclidine, a potent psychotomimetic, is a noncompetitive antagonist at the NMDA receptor, a major glutamate receptor. Similarly, abuse of ketamine, a veterinary anesthetic, can resemble schizophrenia. Ketamine, a competitive antagonist at glutamatergic NMDA receptors, has been shown to lead to reduction in DA-D_1 neurotransmission through glutamatergic inhibition of DA release.[21] It is proposed that schizophrenia may involve some currently unknown in utero assault that leads to a developmental defect in NMDA receptor function—so-called NMDA hypofunction. This defect is proposed to have latent clinical expression with the psychotic manifestations from NMDA hypofunction not being seen until late adolescence or early adulthood. It has been shown that excess D_2 stimulation can impair NMDA transmission via GABAergic neurons. Thus the use of antipsychotic drugs could potentially enhance glutamatergic transmission.[17]

Serotoninergic receptors are present on dopaminergic axons, and stimulation of these receptors decreases DA release, at least in the striatum.[6] Although somewhat more diffuse, the distribution of serotonergic neurons is similar to that of dopaminergic neurons, thus allowing these two neurotransmitter systems to innervate the same areas. In fact, 5-hydroxytryptamine$_2$ (serotonin$_2$; 5-HT_2) receptors and D_4 receptors have been found to be colocalized in the cortex.[3,6] Patients with schizophrenia with abnormal brain scans have higher whole-blood 5-HT concentrations, and these concentrations are correlated with increased ventricular size.[22] Atypical antipsychotics with potent 5-HT_2 receptor antagonist effects reverse worsening of symptomatology induced by 5-HT agonists in patients with schizophrenia.[22]

❶ Schizophrenia is a complex disorder, and multiple etiologies likely exist. Based on current knowledge, it is naive to think that any currently proposed etiology can adequately explain the genesis of this complex disease. Molecular research involving genetically determined subtle changes in G proteins, protein metabolism, and other subcellular processes can eventually identify the biologic disturbances associated with schizophrenia.[3,7,17]

CLINICAL PRESENTATION

Schizophrenia is the most common functional psychosis, and great variability occurs in clinical presentation. Despite numerous attempts to portray a stereotype in movies and on television, the stereotypic schizophrenic essentially does not exist. Moreover, schizophrenia is not a "split personality." It is a chronic disorder of thought and affect with the individual having a significant disturbance in interpersonal relationships and ability to function in society.

The first psychotic episode can be sudden in onset with few premorbid symptoms, or commonly can be preceded by withdrawn, suspicious, peculiar behavior (schizoid). During acute psychotic episodes, the patient loses touch with reality, and in a sense, the brain creates a false reality to replace it. Acute psychotic symptoms can include hallucinations (especially hearing voices), delusions (fixed false beliefs), and ideas of influence (beliefs that one's actions are controlled by external influences). Thought processes are disconnected (loose associations), the patient may not be able to carry on logical conversation (alogia), and can have simultaneous contradictory thoughts (ambivalence). The patient's affect can be flat (no emotional expression), or it can be inappropriate and labile. The patient is often withdrawn and inwardly directed (autism). Uncooperativeness, hostility, and verbal or physical aggression can be seen because of the patient's misperception of reality. Self-care skills are impaired, and the patient is frequently dirty, unkempt, and in general has poor hygiene. Sleep and appetite are often disturbed. When the acute psychotic episode remits, the patient typically has residual features. This is an important point in differentiating schizophrenia from other psychotic disorders. Although residual symptoms and their severity vary, patients can have difficulty with anxiety management, suspiciousness, and lack of volition, motivation, insight, and judgment. Therefore, they often have difficulty living independently in the community. Because of poor anxiety management and suspiciousness, they are frequently withdrawn socially, and have difficulty forming close relationships with others. In addition, impaired volition and motivation contribute to poor self-care skills and make it difficult for the patient with schizophrenia to maintain employment.

Patients with schizophrenia frequently experience a lack of historicity, or difficulty in learning from their experiences. They can repeatedly make the same mistakes in social conduct and situations requiring judgment. They have difficulty understanding the importance of treatment, including medications, in maintaining their ability to function in society. Therefore they tend to discontinue medications and other treatments, and this increases the risk of relapse and rehospitalization. The co-occurrence of substance abuse (predominantly alcohol or polysubstance—alcohol, cannabis, cocaine) in patients with schizophrenia is very common and is another frequent reason for relapse and hospitalization.[20] This effect can be caused by direct toxic effects of these drugs on the brain[21] but is also caused by the medication nonadherence that is invariably associated with substance abuse.

Although the course of schizophrenia is variable, the long-term prognosis for many patients is poor. It is marked by intermittent acute psychotic episodes and impaired psychosocial functioning between acute episodes, with most of the deterioration in psychosocial functioning occurring within 5 years after the first psychotic episode.[17] By late life, the patient can appear "burned out," that is, the patient ceases to have acute psychotic episodes, but residual symptoms persist. However, functional skills can actually improve compared with earlier in the patient's life. In a subpopulation of patients, probably 5% to 15%, psychotic symptoms are nearly continuous, and response to antipsychotics is poor.[23]

Schizophrenia is a chronic disorder, and the patient's history must be carefully assessed for dysfunction that has persisted for longer than 6 months. After their first episode, patients with schizophrenia rarely have a level of adaptive functioning as high as before the onset of the disorder. Table 70–2 summarizes the *DSM-IV-TR* criteria.[1]

❷ The *DSM-IV-TR* classifies the symptoms of schizophrenia into two categories: positive and negative. Recently greater emphasis has been placed on a third symptom category, cognitive dysfunction (Table 70–3).[23] The areas of cognition found to be abnormal in schizophrenia include attention, working memory, and executive function. Positive symptoms have traditionally attracted the most attention and are the ones most improved by antipsychotics. However, negative symptoms and impairment in cognition are more closely associated with poor psychosocial function.

It has been suggested that symptom complexes can correlate with prognosis, cognitive functioning, structural abnormalities in the brain, and response to antipsychotic drugs. Negative symptoms and cognitive impairment can be more closely associated with prefrontal lobe dysfunction and positive symptoms with temporolimbic abnormalities. Many patients demonstrate both positive and negative symptoms. Patients with negative symptoms frequently have more antecedent cognitive dysfunction, poor premorbid adjustment, low level of educational achievement, and a poorer overall prognosis.[23]

TABLE 70-2 DSM-IV-TR Diagnostic Criteria for Schizophrenia

A. Characteristic symptoms: Two or more of the following, each persisting for a significant portion of at least a 1-month period:
  (1) Delusions
  (2) Hallucinations
  (3) Disorganized speech
  (4) Grossly disorganized or catatonic behavior
  (5) Negative symptoms
Note: Only one criterion A symptom is required if delusions are bizarre or if hallucinations consist of a voice keeping a running commentary on the person's behavior or two or more voices conversing with each other.
B. Social/occupational dysfunction: For a significant portion of the time since onset of the disorder, one or more major areas of functioning such as work, interpersonal relations, or self-care are significantly below the level prior to onset.
C. Duration: Continuous signs of the disorder for at least 6 months. This must include at least 1 month of symptoms fulfilling criterion A (unless successfully treated). This 6 months may include prodromal or residual symptoms.
D. Schizoaffective or mood disorder has been excluded.
E. Disorder is not due to a medical disorder or substance use.
F. If a history of a pervasive developmental disorder is present, there must be symptoms of hallucinations or delusions present for at least 1 month.

DSM-IV-TR, Diagnostic and Statistical Manual of Mental Disorders, 4th ed., text revision.
Adapted from American Psychiatric Association.[1]

TABLE 70-3 Schizophrenia Symptom Clusters

Positive	Negative	Cognitive
Suspiciousness	Affective flattening	Impaired attention
Unusual thought content (delusions)	Alogia	Impaired working memory
Hallucinations	Anhedonia	Impaired executive function
Conceptual disorganization	Avolition	

From American Psychiatric Association,[1] Lehman et al.,[23] and Velligan et al.[120]

TREATMENT

Schizophrenia

■ DESIRED OUTCOME

Pharmacotherapy is the mainstay of treatment in schizophrenia, and it is impossible in most patients to implement effective psychosocial rehabilitation programs in the absence of antipsychotic treatment.[23] ❸ A pharmacotherapeutic treatment plan should be developed that delineates drug-related aspects of therapy. Most deterioration in psychosocial functioning occurs during the first 5 years after the initial psychotic episode, and treatment should be particularly assertive during this period.[17] Explicit end points should be defined, including realistic goals for the target symptoms most likely to respond, and the relative time course for response.[2,23] Other goals include avoiding unwanted side effects, using the minimum effective dose, emphasizing adequate time as a primary variable in determining response, and limiting augmentation medications to nonresponsive patients.

■ NONPHARMACOLOGIC THERAPY

Psychosocial rehabilitation programs oriented toward improving patients' adaptive functioning are the mainstay of nondrug treatment for schizophrenia. These programs can include case management, psychoeducation, targeted cognitive therapy, basic living skills, social skills training, basic education, work programs, supported housing, and financial support. In particular, programs aimed at employment and housing have been the more effective interventions and are considered "best practices." Programs that involve families in the care and life of the patient have been shown to decrease rehospitalization and improve functioning in the community. For particularly low-functioning patients, assertive intervention programs, referred to as *active community treatment* (ACT), are effective in improving patients' functional outcomes. ACT teams are available on a 24-hour basis and work in the patient's home and place of employment to provide comprehensive treatment, including medication, crisis intervention, daily living skills, and supported employment and housing.[2,23] Medication treatment cannot be successful without proper attention to these other aspects of care. People with schizophrenia need comprehensive care, with coordination of services across psychiatric, addiction, medical, social, and rehabilitative services. The level of coordination in the

TABLE 70-4 Psychotherapeutic Approaches to the Treatment of Schizophrenia

Individual	Group	Cognitive Behavioral
Supportive/counseling	Interactive/social	Cognitive behavioral therapy
Personal therapy		Compliance therapy
Social skills therapies		
Vocational sheltered employment rehabilitation therapies		

United States is often insufficient, and patients become at risk to "fall through the cracks." Recent national policy documents have called for greater coordination of care.[24,25] Additionally, emphasis is growing on the role that the person him or herself plays in a recovery-based system of care, where the person's lifetime aspirations and goals become the center of care, rather than symptom reduction being the primary focus. A list of psychotherapeutic approaches to the treatment of schizophrenia is given in Table 70–4.

PHARMACOLOGIC THERAPY

Assessment Prior to Treatment

❹ The importance of initial accurate diagnostic assessment cannot be overemphasized. A thorough mental status examination, physical and neurologic examination, complete family and social history, and laboratory workup must be performed to confirm the diagnosis and exclude general medical or substance-induced causes of psychosis. Laboratory tests, biologic markers, and commonly available brain imaging techniques do not assist in diagnosis or selection of medication. A pretreatment patient workup is important in not only excluding other pathology, but in serving as a baseline for monitoring potential medication-related side effects, and should include: vital signs, complete blood count, electrolytes, hepatic function, renal function, electrocardiogram, fasting serum glucose, serum lipids, thyroid function, and urine drug screen.

ANTIPSYCHOTIC MEDICATION CHOICES

Second-Generation Antipsychotics

Second-generation antipsychotics (SGAs) (with the exception of clozapine) have become first-line agents in the treatment of schizophrenia.[23,26] No absolute criterion distinguishes atypical (second-generation) from typical (traditional, conventional, or first-generation) antipsychotics, and no universally accepted definition exists for an atypical antipsychotic.[22] In many respects, *second-generation antipsychotic* is a more appropriate term. Common to all definitions is the ability of the drug to produce antipsychotic response with few or no acutely occurring extrapyramidal side effects. Other attributes that have been ascribed to SGAs include enhanced efficacy, particularly for negative symptoms and cognition; absence or near absence of propensity to cause tardive dyskinesia; and lack of effect on serum prolactin.[22] To date, the only approved SGA that fulfills all of these criteria is clozapine.[22] Although conflicting, some evidence suggests that SGAs can have superior efficacy for the treatment of negative symptoms, cognition, and mood.[23,26] Whether these differences are a result of differences in core efficacy or differences in side-effect profile is unknown. The major advantage of atypical antipsychotics can be their lower risk of neurologic side-effects, particularly effects on movement. Results from the Clinical Antipsychotic Trials of Intervention Effectiveness (CATIE) study indicate that olanzapine, compared with quetiapine, risperidone, ziprasidone, and the FGA perphenazine, has modest superiority in maintenance therapy when treatment persistence is the primary clinical outcome.[27] No significant differences were apparent among the other compared antipsychotics. However, increased metabolic adverse effects occurred with olanzapine.

Risperidone has a low incidence of EPS at low to moderate doses. The mean optimal dose in parallel, fixed-dose studies was 4 to 6 mg daily. At doses greater than 6 mg daily, risperidone's profile is more similar to that of an FGA.[28] Because risperidone appears to lose its atypical profile at higher doses, the lowest possible dose should be used in treatment. This can include gradual dose titration downward if patients do not respond initially, rather than upward titration as has been the traditional approach to dosing antipsychotics.[23]

Paliperidone (9-hydroxyrisperidone), the major active metabolite of risperidone, is formulated in an extended-release osmotically controlled release system. EPS-related adverse effects with paliperidone appear at a dose threshold, increasing at doses greater than 9 mg daily.[29,30] Postmarketing pharmacovigilance studies are needed to further define the safety profile of paliperidone.

Olanzapine has a very low incidence of extrapyramidal side effects when used within the approved dose range of 10 to 20 mg daily.[2,23] However, many patients are being treated at doses above the currently recommended limit in the approved product labeling of 20 mg/day. Quetiapine is an efficacious antipsychotic with an excellent EPS profile.[23,31] Although contrary to efficacy studies, doses above 500 mg are often used to achieve optimal effects, with dose titration to 800 mg/day being a common occurrence. From a clinical perspective, the optimal daily quetiapine dose is unclear.

Ziprasidone 40 to 160 mg/day has efficacy similar to other SGAs, with response rates increasing at doses greater than 80 mg daily.[2,23,32] Aripiprazole has established efficacy at 15 to 30 mg/day.[23,33] Both aripiprazole and ziprasidone have significantly less potential to produce weight gain than other SGAs.

❺ Side-effect profiles differ among atypical antipsychotics, and this information in combination with individual patient characteristics should be used in deciding which drug to use in an individual patient. Information from the algorithm (Fig. 70–1) and the adverse effects sections should be used in arriving at this decision.

First-Generation (Typical) Antipsychotics

Maintenance effectiveness studies in individuals with chronic schizophrenia do not show any major overall clinical outcome differences between using the FGA perphenazine versus SGAs. However, in first-episode schizophrenia, SGAs are often considered first-line treatments because of the risk of tardive dyskinesia with FGAs.[23,26] This can be of particular significance in individuals with their first psychotic break, as they seem particular susceptible to extrapyramidal side effects.

No known differences exist in efficacy between low- and high-potency FGAs. Previous patient or family history of response to an antipsychotic is helpful in the selection of an agent. Traditional dosage equivalents (expressed in "chlorpromazine equivalent dosages"—the equipotent dosage of any traditional FGA compared with 100 mg of chlorpromazine) can assist in determining the effective dosage range if the need arises to treat a patient with a different FGA. However, because SGAs differ in mechanism of action, the dose equivalents have little relevance when comparing dosages of SGAs. Table 70–5 lists antipsychotics and their usual dosage ranges.

PHARMACOTHERAPEUTIC ALGORITHM

❻ Figure 70–1 outlines a suggested pharmacotherapeutic algorithm for schizophrenia.[26] Stage 1 of the treatment algorithm applies only to those patients experiencing their first episode of schizophrenia. In these patients, a majority of schizophrenia experts felt that SGAs should be used initially because of the risk of tardive dyskinesia with FGAs.[26] Treatment-naïve patients appear more sensitive to acutely occurring extrapyramidal side effects, and lower doses of antipsychotics should be used.[26] However, the tradeoff with SGAs is the increased risk of metabolic side effects, particularly weight gain with some SGAs,

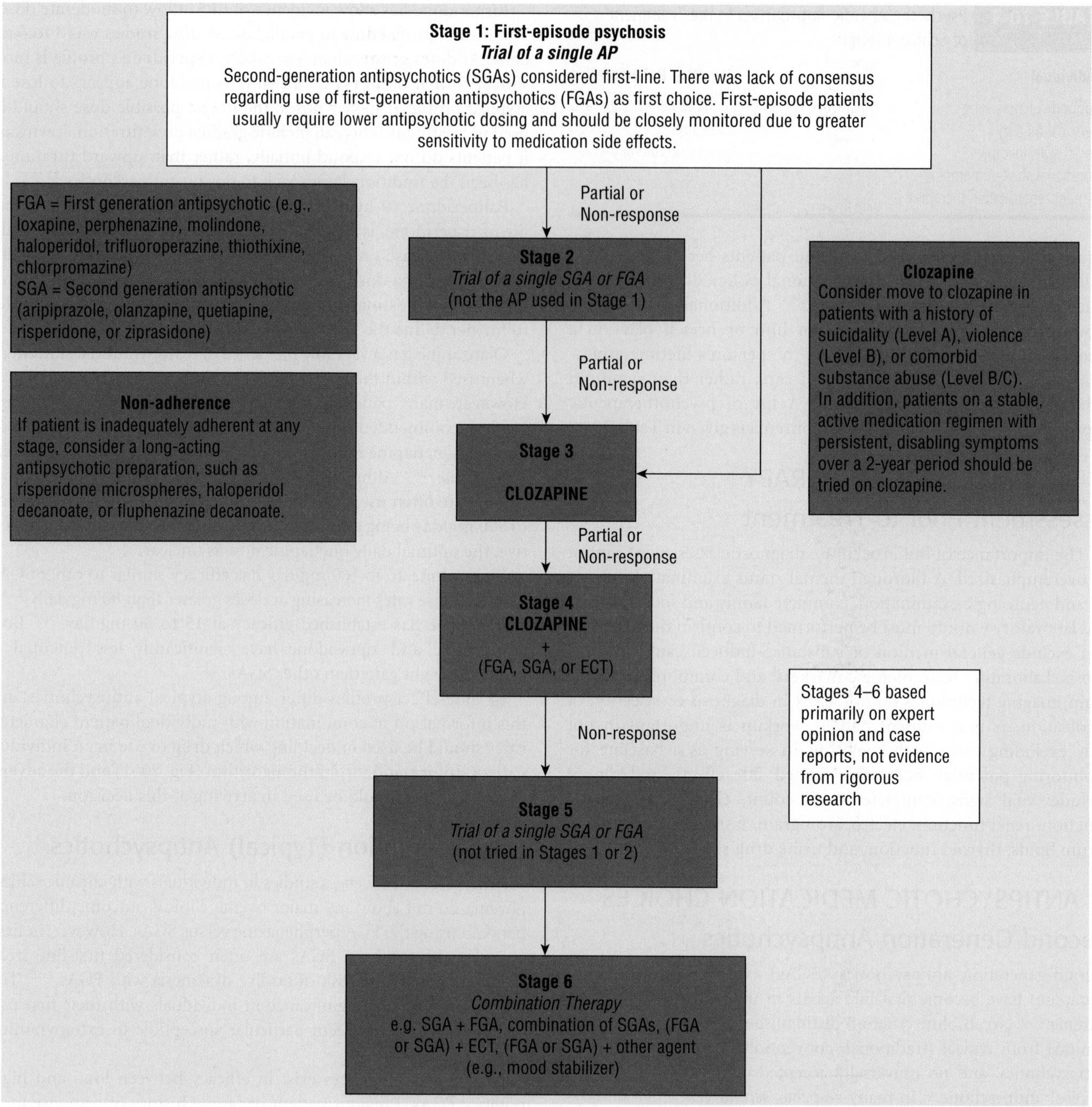
Stage 1: First-episode psychosis
Trial of a single AP
Second-generation antipsychotics (SGAs) considered first-line. There was lack of consensus regarding use of first-generation antipsychotics (FGAs) as first choice. First-episode patients usually require lower antipsychotic dosing and should be closely monitored due to greater sensitivity to medication side effects.
Partial or Non-response
FGA = First generation antipsychotic (e.g., loxapine, perphenazine, molindone, haloperidol, trifluoroperazine, thiothixine, chlorpromazine)
SGA = Second generation antipsychotic (aripiprazole, olanzapine, quetiapine, risperidone, or ziprasidone)
Stage 2
Trial of a single SGA or FGA
(not the AP used in Stage 1)
Clozapine
Consider move to clozapine in patients with a history of suicidality (Level A), violence (Level B), or comorbid substance abuse (Level B/C). In addition, patients on a stable, active medication regimen with persistent, disabling symptoms over a 2-year period should be tried on clozapine.
Partial or Non-response
Non-adherence
If patient is inadequately adherent at any stage, consider a long-acting antipsychotic preparation, such as risperidone microspheres, haloperidol decanoate, or fluphenazine decanoate.
Stage 3
CLOZAPINE
Partial or Non-response
Stage 4
CLOZAPINE
+
(FGA, SGA, or ECT)
Stages 4–6 based primarily on expert opinion and case reports, not evidence from rigorous research
Non-response
Stage 5
Trial of a single SGA or FGA
(not tried in Stages 1 or 2)
Stage 6
Combination Therapy
e.g. SGA + FGA, combination of SGAs, (FGA or SGA) + ECT, (FGA or SGA) + other agent
(e.g., mood stabilizer)

FIGURE 70-1. Patient entry into the algorithm is determined by individual patient history and clinical presentation. Only new onset patients with no history of antipsychotic treatment failure are treated at stage 1. Algorithm stages can be skipped if clinically appropriate, and one can go back stages if indicated. In general, inadequately responding patients should not remain in stages 1 or 2 longer than 12 weeks at therapeutic doses. Stage 3 can be up to 6 months. In stages 4, 5, and 6, a 12-week trial is recommended, and if there is greater than or equal to 20% improvement in positive symptoms at week 12, the medication trial warrants extension for an additional 12 weeks with dose titration as clinically warranted. The levels of evidence for algorithm recommendations are as follows: stage 1, level A for efficacy for both first-generation antipsychotics (FGAs) and second-generation antipsychotics (SGAs); level C for SGAs as first choice; stage 2, level A; stage 3, level A; stage 4, level C; stage 5, level C; stage 6, level C. Level A is supported by one or more randomized controlled trials. Level B is supported by large cohort studies, epidemiological studies, and so on. Level C is supported by case series, case reports, or expert opinion. (ECT, electroconvulsive therapy.) *(This figure is copyrighted by the Texas Department of State Health Services and may be reproduced with appropriate citation of the authors and source. Algorithm updates and user manuals can be obtained at http://www.mhmr.state.tx.us/centraloffice/medicaldirector/timasczman.pdf. Data from Moore et al.[26])*

especially olanzapine. Stage two applies to chronically ill patients who are newly started on antipsychotics, or it can involve a new onset patient who had inadequate clinical response at stage 1. Stage 2 recommends either FGAs or SGAs, with the exception of clozapine.[26]

Because of safety concerns and the need for white blood cell (WBC) monitoring, it is recommended that patients be tried on one newer SGA and one other SGA or FGA as monotherapy before proceeding to a trial of clozapine (stage 3).[26] Clozapine has superior efficacy in decreasing suicidal behavior, and it should also be considered as a higher treatment option in the suicidal patient.[26] Clozapine can also be considered earlier in treatment in patients with a history of violence or comorbid substance abuse.[26]

Stage 4 of the treatment algorithm includes clozapine and augmentation with either a FGA, SGA, or electroconvulsive therapy (ECT).[26] Combination treatment at this stage is supported by limited controlled and equivocal evidence.[26] Treatment algorithm recommendations after stage 3 (i.e., clozapine monotherapy) are based more on anecdotal experiences and expert opinion than on empirical

TABLE 70-5 Available Antipsychotics: Doses and Dosage Forms

Generic Name	Trade Name	Traditional Equivalent Dose (mg)	Usual Dosage Range (mg/day)	Manufacturer's Maximum Dose (mg/day)[a]	Dosage Forms[b]
Traditional antipsychotics (first-generation antipsychotics)					
chlorpromazine	Thorazine	100	100–800	2,000	T,L,LC,I,C-ER,S
fluphenazine	Prolixin	2	2–20	40	T,L,LC,I,LAI
haloperidol	Haldol	2	2–20	100	T,LC,I,LAI
loxapine	Loxitane	10	10–80	250	C,LC
molindone	Moban	10	10–100	225	T,LC
perphenazine	Trilafon	10	10–64	64	T,LC,I
thioridazine	Mellaril	100	100–800	800	T,LC
thiothixene	Navane	4	4–40	60	C,LC
trifluoperazine	Stelazine	5	5–40	80	T,LC,I
Atypical antipsychotics (second-generation antipsychotics)					
aripiprazole	Abilify	NA	15–30	30	T,O,L
clozapine	Clozaril	NA	50–500	900	T,O
olanzapine	Zyprexa	NA	10–20	20	T,I,O
paliperidone	Invega	NA	3–9	12	ER
quetiapine	Seroquel	NA	250–500	800	T
risperidone	Risperdal	NA	2–8	16	T,O,L
risperidone	Risperdal Consta	NA	25–50 mg every 2 weeks	50	LAI
ziprasidone	Geodon	NA	40–160	200	C,I

[a]NA. This parameter does not apply to atypical antipsychotics.

[b]C, capsule; ER or SR, extended or sustained release; I, injection; L, liquid solution, elixir, or suspension; LC, liquid concentrate; LAI, long-acting injectable; O, orally disintegrating tablets; R, rectal suppositories; T, tablet.

research.[26] In general, patients who experience poor improvement with clozapine do not respond well with other antipsychotic monotherapies (stage 5), thus one of the primary reasons that clozapine augmentation is recommended at stage 4. Stage 6 combination pharmacotherapy interventions should be implemented with time limited, careful evaluation of a patient's symptom response and discontinuation of the combination if improvement does not occur.[26]

If partial or poor adherence contributes to inadequate clinical improvement, then long-acting or depot injectable antipsychotics should be considered.[23,26] Risperidone microspheres is the only available long-acting injectable SGA, and long-acting FGAs include fluphenazine decanoate and haloperidol decanoate. In addition to individuals who are identified as partially adherent, some patients can elect for injections every 2 to 4 weeks instead of taking daily oral medications. A long-acting injectable antipsychotic can be substituted for an oral antipsychotic at any point in the algorithm where they are thought to be indicated.

CLINICAL CONTROVERSY

Efficacy and effectiveness studies demonstrate conflicting results with regard to the use of SGAs versus FGAs in schizophrenia. Although most studies have demonstrated a lower incidence of EPS with SGAs, weight gain is a significant trade-off adverse effect with some of the SGAs, particularly olanzapine. Tension exists between policy decision makers who are responsible for managing finite resources and clinicians who see clinical benefits of the SGAs in the patients they treat.

The use of antipsychotic combinations is controversial, as very limited evidence supports increased efficacy for combination antipsychotic treatment. Combination antipsychotics are frequently used by clinicians, and testimonies attest to clinical benefits when a second SGA is added.

PREDICTORS OF RESPONSE

Obtaining a thorough medication history is important, and previous antipsychotic treatment should help guide the selection of drug therapy, in that either a good prior response favors the use of the same agent or a negative prior response suggests the selection of a dissimilar drug. Nonprescription and illicit drug use can influence psychiatric presentation and thus diagnosis or antipsychotic response. Amphetamines and other CNS stimulants, cocaine, corticosteroids, digitalis glycosides, indomethacin, marijuana, pentazocine, phencyclidine, and other drugs can induce psychosis in susceptible individuals or exacerbate psychosis in patients with preexisting psychiatric illness.[34] Patients with schizophrenia who continue to abuse alcohol or drugs usually have a poor response to medications and a poor prognosis. Alcohol, caffeine, and nicotine use potentially results in drug interactions.

Individual differences in patient response have been either proposed or identified, which can be clinically useful predictors of response.[35] Acute onset and short duration of illness, presence of acute stressors or precipitating factors, later age of onset, family history of affective illness, and good premorbid adjustment as reflected in stable interpersonal relationships or employment are all predictors of good response.[35]

Although controversial, affective symptoms can correlate with an overall good response. Negative symptoms and neuropsychologic deficits related to cognition and neurologic soft signs can correlate with poor antipsychotic response.[35] A patient's subjective response within the first 48 hours after being administered an FGA can be associated with drug responsiveness.[36] An initial dysphoric response, demonstrated by stating a dislike of the medication, or feeling worse or zombie-like, combined with anxiety or akathisia-like symptoms, is associated with poor drug response, adverse effects, and nonadherence.

The importance of developing a therapeutic alliance between the patient and the clinician cannot be underestimated. Patients who form positive therapeutic alliances are more likely to be adherent with all aspects of therapy, experience a better outcome at 2 years, and require smaller antipsychotic doses.

A certain minority of patients fail to benefit from antipsychotic therapy, and their psychosocial functioning can actually worsen. Unfortunately, no accepted method is available to identify these people before treatment.[35] Recent evidence suggests that pharmacogenetics can play a role in predicting treatment response, both with respect to symptom improvement and with liability to develop side effects.[37–38] However, insufficient information is available to recommend routine clinical testing.

INITIAL TREATMENT IN AN ACUTE PSYCHOTIC EPISODE

The goals during the first 7 days of treatment should be decreased agitation, hostility, combativeness, anxiety, tension, and aggression, and normalization of sleep and eating patterns. The usual recommendation is to initiate therapy and to titrate dose over the first few days to an average effective dose, unless the patient's physiologic status or history indicates that this dose can result in unacceptable adverse effects. Table 70–5 lists the usual dosage range, and an average dose is typically midrange. Because of increased sensitivity to side effects, particularly extrapyramidal side effects, in first-episode psychotic patients, typical dosing ranges are approximately 50% of the doses used in chronically ill individuals.[26] If "cheeking" of medication is suspected, liquid formulations and orally disintegrating tablets of different antipsychotics are available (see Table 70–5). If a patient has shown absolutely no improvement after 3 to 4 weeks at therapeutic doses, then an alternative antipsychotic should be considered (i.e., moving to the next treatment stage in the algorithm; see Fig. 70–1).[20,22]

Although some clinicians believe that larger daily doses are necessary in more severely symptomatic patients, data are not available to support this practice. Some symptoms, such as agitation, tension, aggression, and increased motor activity, can respond more quickly, but side effects can be more common with higher doses. However, interindividual differences in dosage and patient response do occur. In partial but inadequate responders who are tolerating the chosen antipsychotic, it may be reasonable to titrate above usual dose ranges. However, this tactic should be time-limited (i.e., 2 to 4 weeks), and if the patient does not achieve further improvement, the dose should either be decreased, or an alternative treatment strategy tried.[39] In general, rapid titration of antipsychotic dosage is not indicated.[39] However, intramuscular antipsychotic administration (e.g., aripiprazole 5.25 to 9.75 mg IM, haloperidol 2 to 5 mg IM, olanzapine 2.5 to 10 mg IM, or ziprasidone 10 to 20 mg IM) can be used to assist in calming a severely agitated patient. Agitation can be manifested as loud, physically or verbally threatening behavior, motor hyperactivity, or physical aggression. Although this technique can assist in calming an acutely agitated psychotic patient, it does not improve the extent of or time to remission, or the length of hospitalization. If IM haloperidol is used, the occurrence of EPS can eliminate some of the advantages of using an oral SGA. If the patient is receiving an antipsychotic within the usual therapeutic range, the use of lorazepam 2 mg IM as needed in combination with the maintenance antipsychotic is a rational alternative to an injectable antipsychotic. Hypotension, respiratory depression, and CNS depression are possible when injectable lorazepam and olanzapine are used concomitantly; thus this parenteral combination is not recommended.

CLINICAL CONTROVERSY

Minimal research evidence supports the use of antipsychotic doses beyond the dose range in the Food and Drug Administration (FDA) approved product labeling. However, clinicians frequently titrate doses above the approved range, and frequently attest to symptom improvement when this is done.

STABILIZATION THERAPY

Improvement is usually a slow but steady process over 6 to 12 weeks or longer. During the first 2 to 3 weeks, goals should include increased socialization and improvement in self-care habits and mood. Improvement in formal thought disorder should follow and can take an additional 6 to 8 weeks to respond. Patients who are early in the course of their illness can experience a more rapid resolution of symptoms than individuals who are more chronically ill. In general, if a patient has no improvement with treatment after 3 to 4 weeks at therapeutic doses, or has achieved only a partial decrease in positive and negative symptoms within 12 weeks at adequate doses, then the next algorithm stage should be considered. In a more chronically ill patient, symptoms can continue to improve for 3 to 6 months. During acute stabilization, usual labeled doses of SGAs are recommended (see Table 70–5); with FGAs, a range of 300 to 1,000 mg of chlorpromazine equivalents daily is recommended.[23,26] An optimum dose of the chosen drug should be estimated in the initial treatment plan. If the patient begins to show adequate response before or at this dosage, then the patient should remain at this dosage as long as symptoms continue to improve. ❼ In general, adequate time on a therapeutic antipsychotic dose is the most important factor in predicting medication response. However, if necessary, dose titration can continue within the therapeutic range every week or two as long as the patient has no side effects.

Before changing medications in a poorly responding patient, the following should be considered: Were the initial target symptoms indicative of schizophrenia or did they represent manifestations of a different diagnosis, a long-standing behavioral problem, a substance abuse disorder, or a general medical condition? Is the patient adherent with pharmacotherapy? Are the persistent symptoms poorly responsive to antipsychotics (e.g., impaired insight or judgment, or fixed delusions)? How does the patient's current status compare with response during previous exacerbations? Would this patient potentially benefit from a change to a different treatment stage (see Fig. 70–1)? Does this patient have a treatment-refractory schizophrenic illness?

The conclusion that a partially responding patient has achieved as much symptomatic improvement as possible is one that must be made with great care and after considering all possible treatment alternatives. However, treatment goals must be realistic. Medications are effective at decreasing many of the symptoms of schizophrenia (and are thus referred to as palliative), but they are not curative, and all symptoms may not abate. This being said, the treatment approach should be assertive. Although one should aim to achieve none to minimal residual positive symptoms with effective treatment, it is still unclear what a realistic goal is with regard to maximum improvement in negative symptoms.

It is important to screen patients for co-occurring mental disorders, and their presence can become more apparent during the stabilization or maintenance phases of schizophrenia treatment. Examples include substance abuse disorders, depression, obsessive-compulsive disorder, and panic disorder. As co-occurring disorders will limit symptom and functional improvement and increase the risk of relapse, it is critical that pharmacologic and nonpharmacologic interventions for the co-occurring disorder be implemented in combination with evidence-based treatment for schizophrenia.

MAINTENANCE TREATMENT

Maintenance drug therapy prevents relapse, as shown in numerous double-blind studies. The average relapse rate after 1 year is 18% to 32% with active drug (including some nonadherent patients) versus 60% to 80% for placebo.[23,28,40]

After treatment of the first psychotic episode in a schizophrenic patient, medication should be continued for at least 12 months after remission.[23,39] ❽ Many schizophrenia experts recommend that patients with robust medication response be treated for at least 5 years. In chronically ill individuals, continuous or lifetime pharmacotherapy is necessary in the majority of patients to prevent relapse. This should be approached with the lowest effective dose of the antipsychotic that is likely to be tolerated by the patient.[23,39]

Antipsychotics should be tapered slowly before discontinuation. Abrupt discontinuation of antipsychotics, especially low-potency

FGAs and clozapine, can result in withdrawal symptoms, felt to be a manifestation of rebound cholinergic outflow. Insomnia, nightmares, headaches, gastrointestinal symptoms (e.g., abdominal cramps, stomach pain, nausea, vomiting, and diarrhea), restlessness, increased salivation, and sweating are reported. When switching from one antipsychotic to another, it is often recommended to taper and discontinue the first antipsychotic over at least 1 to 2 weeks after the second antipsychotic is initiated.[23,39] Tapering often needs to occur more slowly, especially with clozapine.[23,39]

Long-Acting or Depot Injectable Antipsychotics

Depot or long-acting antipsychotics are recommended for patients who are unreliable in taking oral medication on a daily basis, and thus are not usually used as first-line therapy. Before a long-acting antipsychotic is initiated, it should be determined whether the patient's medication nonadherence is because of side effects. If so, an alternative medication with a more favorable side-effect profile should be considered before a long-acting injectable antipsychotic.

The patient's motivation for treatment is a major factor influencing outcome. Conversion from oral therapy to a long-acting injectable is most successful in patients who have been stabilized on oral therapy. The ideal patient for a long-acting injectable is the individual who does not like the daily reminder of oral medication or is unreliable in taking medications. Risperidone is the only SGA available as a long-acting injectable.[26,41] Long-acting risperidone has demonstrated efficacy, with an optimum dose range likely between 25 and 50 mg given IM every 2 weeks. Doses above 50 mg every 2 weeks are not recommended, as results from one study showed no greater efficacy but more EPS.[41] The pattern of adverse effects, especially low propensity to induce EPS and tardive dyskinesia, is similar to that of oral risperidone, and it appears to be well tolerated by patients.[41]

Conversion from an oral antipsychotic to a long-acting medication should start with stabilization on an oral dosage form of the same agent, or at least a short trial (3 to 7 days), to determine whether the patient tolerates the medication without significant side effects. Long-acting risperidone is a suspension of drug in glycolic acid-lactate copolymer microspheres that must be reconstituted before administration. The microspheres are degraded via hydrolysis with significant risperidone serum concentrations being measurable approximately 3 weeks after single-dose administration. Thus it is important that the oral antipsychotic be administered for at least 3 weeks after beginning the injections. Dose adjustments are recommended to be made no more often than once every 4 weeks.[39,41] The recommended starting dose with the depot injection is 25 mg, and clinical experience suggests that titration to doses greater than or equal to 37.5 mg per injection may be necessary for maintenance treatment.

For fluphenazine decanoate, the simplest dosing conversion method recommends 1.2 times the oral fluphenazine daily dose for stabilized patients, rounding up to the nearest 12.5-mg interval, administered in weekly doses for the first 4 to 6 weeks; or 1.6 times the oral daily dose for more acutely ill patients.[42] Subsequently, fluphenazine decanoate can be administered once every 2 to 3 weeks. Oral fluphenazine can be overlapped for 1 week. For haloperidol decanoate, a factor of 10 to 15 times the oral haloperidol daily dose is commonly recommended, rounding up to the nearest 50-mg interval, administered in a once-monthly dose with an oral haloperidol overlap for the first month. A more assertive conversion method recommends 20 times the oral daily dose, but dividing the injection into consecutive doses of 100 to 200 mg every 3 to 7 days until the entire amount is given.[43] With this method, oral medication overlap is unnecessary. The haloperidol decanoate dose is decreased by 25% at the second and third months.

Injection site reactions have been reported with the haloperidol decanoate 100 mg/mL preparation, consisting of painful pruritic swelling at the injection site.[44] Acute EPS can be seen following injections of either fluphenazine or haloperidol decanoate. These effects are minimized with the use of risperidone microspheres. Both haloperidol and fluphenazine decanoate should be administered by a deep, "Z-tract" intramuscular method. Long-acting risperidone is injected by deep IM injection in the gluteus maximus, but Z-tracting is not necessary. An oral test dose of the medication is recommended before administering the first IM dose of the long-acting antipsychotic.

Methods to Enhance Patient Adherence

It is often a challenge for individuals with chronic illnesses to maintain high levels of medication adherence, and partial compliance is a reality in the treatment of all chronic illnesses.[45] Individuals with serious mental disorders have somewhat higher nonadherence rates than those with general medical disorders, with the following explanations provided: denial of illness, lack of insight, grandiosity or paranoia, no perceived need for medication, perceived lack of input into choice of medication or dosage, side effects, misperceived "allergies," or the number of medications prescribed or doses received daily. In fact, clinicians should expect partial compliance to be the norm with regard to medication-taking behavior. This should be approached in a nonjudgmental manner, with the clinician actively engaging the patient in care and using motivational interviewing techniques as mechanisms to enhance therapeutic alliance and patient adherence.

❾ Education geared toward patients becoming more informed about their illness and the effectiveness and risks of treatment can help to increase adherence.[46] These programs should be staged so that patients initially receive basic information about their disorder and its symptoms and basic information about their medication and self-monitoring techniques. As the patient is capable of dealing with more complex information, more detailed information regarding schizophrenia, psychosocial treatments, and prognosis should be discussed. Patients and families should be taught self-monitoring techniques and when to report symptom exacerbation or medication side effects to the clinician.[46] Psychoeducation strategies should include motivational interview techniques in individual counseling as well as group activities.

Recent evidence suggests that cognitive behavioral therapy focusing on medication adherence can improve patient outcome.[47] This approach is called compliance therapy. Groups facilitated by trained individuals who have the illness can be more effective in enhancing awareness and acceptance of schizophrenia and necessary treatment than groups led only by professionals. Active involvement of family members further increases the likelihood of patient adherence with treatment. In addition to programs provided by community mental health centers, support groups operated by consumer groups such as the National Alliance on Mental Illness (NAMI) are available in most urban areas. Contact information for local NAMI chapters can be accessed at http://www.nami.org/Template.cfm?Section=Your_Local_NAMI. In the hospital, self-medication administration can reinforce the patient's perception of their active role in their own treatment. When patients miss outpatient appointments, active outreach interventions must be implemented to enhance patient engagement in treatment.[23,46]

■ MANAGEMENT OF TREATMENT-RESISTANT SCHIZOPHRENIA

In general, "treatment resistant" describes a patient who has had inadequate symptom response from multiple antipsychotic trials.[23] Traditionally, treatment resistance has been defined as lack of improvement in positive symptoms, but it can be defined by poor improvement in negative symptoms, or even by medication intolerance. Between 10% and 30% of patients receive minimal symptomatic improvement after multiple FGA monotherapy trials.[23] An additional 30% to 60% of patients have partial but inadequate improvement in symptoms or unacceptable side effects associated with antipsychotic use.[23,26] In those patients failing two or more trials of pharmacotherapy, a treatment refractory evaluation should be performed to reexamine diagnosis, substance abuse, medication adherence, and psychosocial stressors. Targeted cognitive behavioral therapy or other psychosocial augmentation strategies should be considered.[26]

Clozapine

Only clozapine has shown superiority over other antipsychotics in randomized clinical trials for the management of treatment-resistant schizophrenia. Most other SGAs have either not been studied in treatment-refractory patients or evaluated in small open trials. In a seminal study, clozapine was effective in approximately 30% of patients with treatment-resistant schizophrenia, compared with only 4% treated with a combination of chlorpromazine and benztropine.[48] The criteria for treatment-resistance require two treatment failures, and includes both FGAs and SGAs. Other treatment candidates for clozapine include those patients who cannot tolerate even conservative doses of other antipsychotics.

Symptomatic improvement with clozapine in the treatment-resistant patient often occurs slowly, and as many as 60% of patients may improve if clozapine is used for up to 6 months.[39] This, in combination with clozapine's adverse effects profile, provides sufficient information to conclude that clozapine is not a panacea for schizophrenia. Polydipsia and hyponatremia (psychogenic water drinking) is a frequent problem among treatment-resistant patients, and clozapine reportedly decreases water drinking and increases serum sodium in such patients.[49]

Because of the risk of orthostatic hypotension, clozapine is usually titrated more slowly than other antipsychotics, particularly on an outpatient basis. If a 12.5 mg test dose does not produce hypotension, then clozapine 25 mg at bedtime is recommended, increased to 25 mg twice a day after 3 days, and then increased in 25- to 50-mg/day increments every 3 days until a dose of at least 300 mg/day is reached. Because high doses are associated with significantly increased side effects, including seizures, a clozapine serum concentration is recommended before exceeding 600 mg/day. Although some clinicians add valproate when exceeding this dose to prevent the occurrence of seizures, no evidence supports this intervention.

Augmentation and Combination Strategies

Little empirical evidence exists to guide treatment decisions for patients who do not respond to clozapine.[26,39] A small number of randomized trials have examined the efficacy of clozapine augmentation with SGAs, and the results have been inconsistent, but more negative than positive (see Fig. 70–1).[26] Augmentation therapy involves the addition of a nonantipsychotic drug to an antipsychotic drug in a poorly or partially responsive patient, whereas combination treatment involves using two antipsychotics simultaneously. Several guidelines should be followed regarding augmentation: (a) augmentation should be used only in inadequately responding patients; (b) augmentation agents are rarely effective for schizophrenic symptoms when used alone; (c) augmentation responders usually improve rapidly; and (d) if augmentation does not improve symptomatology, the augmenting agent should be discontinued.[39,50]

Mood stabilizers are frequently used as an augmentation strategy. Lithium does not enhance antipsychotic effect but can improve labile affect and agitated behavior in selected patients.[51] Valproic acid and carbamazepine have also been used. A large placebo-controlled trial supports faster symptom improvement, but no difference in maintenance treatment, when divalproex was used in combination with either olanzapine or risperidone.[52] Enzyme induction with carbamazepine can cause a decrease in antipsychotic serum concentrations and potentially worsen psychotic symptoms in some patients. Dosing of mood stabilizers in treatment-resistant schizophrenia is similar to dosing in bipolar disorder (Chap. 72).[23,39]

Selective serotonin reuptake inhibitors (SSRIs), particularly fluoxetine and fluvoxamine, have reasonable evidence for improving negative symptoms when used as augmentation of FGAs. Potential benefits of combining SSRIs with SGAs require more study.[53] Consistently positive results have been reported when using SSRIs to treat obsessive-compulsive symptoms that worsen or arise during clozapine treatment.

β-Blockers such as propranolol, pindolol, and nadolol have been reported to have an antiaggressive effect when used in a variety of psychiatric disorders, but particularly in the organic aggressive syndrome.[23] Doses are typically higher than those required for cardiovascular β-blockade, but patients should be monitored carefully for β-blocker–related side effects. Patients may need to be treated with adequate doses for 6 to 8 weeks to experience an antiaggression response.

Combining an FGA with an SGA and combining different SGAs have been suggested as intervention strategies for treatment-resistant patients. These treatments are based on the hypothesis that using antipsychotics with different mechanisms of action will result in greater efficacy than using any medication individually. Critics argue that combining an FGA with an SGA will negate the advantages of the SGA (e.g., fewer EPS). Pharmacodynamically, no clear rationale exists for explaining how combinations of antipsychotics would produce enhanced efficacy, and increased side effects, particularly increased EPS and hyperprolactinemia are possible results.[54] In general, a series of antipsychotic monotherapies, including clozapine, are preferred over antipsychotic combinations.[26,39] However, when this fails to produce desired outcomes, a time-limited combination trial can be attempted (see Fig. 70–1, stages 4 or 6).[23,26,29] Such antipsychotic combination treatment trials should be time limited (12 weeks) and the patient carefully evaluated with rating scales for changes in symptomatology. If no apparent improvement is observed, then one of the medications should be tapered and discontinued. However, if the patient has a partial response (greater than or equal to 20% improvement in positive symptoms) after 12 weeks with combination treatment in stages 4 or 6, medications should be titrated to doses at the upper end of the therapeutic range, and treatment should continue for an additional 12 weeks before a change in stage is considered.

■ ANTIPSYCHOTIC DRUG MECHANISMS OF ACTION

The exact mechanism of action of antipsychotics is unknown. It has been suggested that current antipsychotics be classified into three different categories: (a) typical or traditional (high D_2 antagonism and low 5-HT_{2A} antagonism); (b) atypical (moderate to high D_2 antagonism and high 5-HT_{2A} antagonism); and (c) atypical clozapine-like (low D_2 antagonism and high 5-HT_{2A} antagonism).[55,56] With the exception of aripiprazole, all current SGAs have a greater affinity for 5-HT_{2A} receptors than D_2 receptors.

Studies of antipsychotic receptor binding in humans have used PET scans to examine neurotransmitter receptor binding at steady-state, 12 hours postdose in small numbers of individuals. At least 60% to 65% occupation of D_2 receptors is necessary to decrease positive psychotic symptoms, whereas blockade of approximately 77% or more of D_2 receptors is associated with EPS.[55,57] FGAs are dopaminergic antagonists with high affinity for D_2 receptors. During chronic treatment with these agents, between 70% and 90% of D_2 receptors in the striatum are usually occupied. In contrast, during clozapine treatment only 38% to 47% of D_2 receptors are occupied, even with high doses. Newer SGAs have variable D_2 binding. With low-dose risperidone (2 to 5 mg/day), D_2 binding ranges from 60% to 79%, but with doses greater than 6 mg daily, binding commonly exceeds the 77% threshold associated with the development of EPS. Risperidone 2 mg/day produces $5\text{-}HT_{2A}$ binding greater than 70%, and with 4 mg/day it is nearly 100%.[55,58] The binding affinity of paliperidone to D_2 and $5\text{-}HT_{2A}$ receptors is yet to be characterized.

Olanzapine 10 to 20 mg/day produces D_2 binding ranging from 71% to 80%, whereas at 30 to 40 mg/day, it ranges from 83% to 88%. At 5 mg/day, $5\text{-}HT_{2A}$ receptors are near saturation of binding.[55] Ziprasidone has the highest $5\text{-}HT_{2A}$:D_2 affinity ratio of any of the currently available antipsychotics. It is also a potent $5\text{-}HT_{1A}$ agonist.[59]

Quetiapine has the lowest D_2 binding. At doses of 300 to 600 mg/day, D_2 binding ranges from 0% to 27%. Even at quetiapine 800 mg/day, only 30% of D_2 receptors are occupied. At these same daily doses, 45% to 90% of $5\text{-}HT_{2A}$ receptors are occupied. However, when quetiapine D_2 binding is examined 2 to 3 hours postdose, 58% and 64% of receptors were occupied with 400 mg and 450 mg, respectively. Transient blockade of dopamine receptors can be adequate to produce antipsychotic effect, but long-term D_2 blockade is required for production of EPS and sustained hyperprolactinemia. Low D_2 binding, and thus atypicality, can be directly associated with how rapidly the antipsychotic disassociates from the D_2 receptor.[55,58] The availability of aripiprazole, a partial agonist at D_2 receptors, represents a further elaboration of the dopamine hypothesis of antipsychotic action.[33,56] It is proposed that aripiprazole works as a functional partial agonist. Aripiprazole is a rather weak $5\text{-}HT_{2A}$ antagonist but a potent $5\text{-}HT_{1A}$ agonist.[33,56] It is clear that the SGAs differ in their mechanisms of action and most likely in the manner in which they produce an atypical clinical profile.

The primary therapeutic effects of FGAs are thought to occur in the limbic system, including the ventral striatum, whereas EPS are thought to be related to DA blockade in the dorsal striatum. Tolerance often develops to the acutely occurring EPS within a few weeks, but tolerance to the antipsychotic effects appears to be less common, if not rare. $5\text{-}HT_{2A}$ antagonism in combination with modest D_2 blockade leads to release of dopamine in the prefrontal cortex, and this is one explanation for the decrease in negative symptoms and improvement in cognition reported with atypical antipsychotics.

Antipsychotics vary in their effects on other neurotransmitter receptor systems.[55,56,58] Although the significance of these different mechanisms on efficacy is unclear, they do potentially explain differences in side-effect profiles. These differences in pharmacodynamic profiles also point out that the SGAs are not all alike, and that patients obtaining an inadequate clinical response (either efficacy or side effects) with one antipsychotic can have a superior response on an alternate drug. Thus serial SGA monotherapy trials should be tried in patients receiving a suboptimal clinical response (see Fig. 70–1).

■ PHARMACOKINETICS

As a class, antipsychotics are highly lipophilic and highly bound to membranes and plasma proteins. They distribute readily into most tissues with a high blood supply and can accumulate in tissues; therefore they have large volumes of distribution.[60] Most antipsychotics are largely metabolized, primarily through the cytochrome P450 (CYP) pathways in the liver, except for ziprasidone, which is largely metabolized by aldehyde oxidase. Risperidone is metabolized through CYP2D6, and thus is susceptible to polymorphic metabolism. In particular, 30% to 35% of Africans and Asians are slow to intermediate metabolizers, in addition to approximately 7% and 2%, respectively, who are poor metabolizers.[61] Thus approximately 40% of patients in these racial/ethnic groups can have increased sensitivity to side effects with drugs such as risperidone that are primarily metabolized through CYP2D6. Table 70–6 outlines the prominent metabolic pathways of selected antipsychotics.

Most antipsychotics have fairly long elimination half-lives, in the range of 20 to 40 hours, with the exception of quetiapine and ziprasidone, which have short half-lives.[33,60] After dosage stabilization most antipsychotics can be dosed once daily. Although not systematically studied, brain receptor kinetics are different than peripheral kinetics, and it may be possible to dose these SGAs less often than their plasma kinetics would suggest. Among the SGAs, only clozapine has an established therapeutic range, with efficacy being associated with a clozapine plasma concentration greater than 250 to 350 ng/mL. A 12-hour postdose clozapine serum concentration of at least 250 ng/mL is recommended if the patient is receiving divided clozapine doses, or 350 ng/mL if the patient is being dosed once daily. Whether a potential maximum therapeutic clozapine serum concentration exists is unknown. It is likely not cost effective to routinely monitor clozapine serum concentrations in all patients. However, they should be monitored before exceeding 600 mg daily; in patients who develop unusual or severe adverse side effects; in patients who are taking concomitant medications that can cause drug interactions; in patients who have age or pathophysiologic changes suggesting a change in pharmacokinetics; or for assessment of patient adherence.[39,40,60]

TABLE 70-6 Pharmacokinetic Parameters of Selected Antipsychotics

Drug	Bioavailability (%)	Half-Life (h)	Major Metabolic Pathways	Active Metabolites
Selected first-generation antipsychotics (FGAs)				
Chlorpromazine	10–30	8–35	FMO3, CYP3A4	7-hydroxy, others
Fluphenazine	20–50	14–24	CYP2D6	?
Fluphenazine decanoate		14.2 ± 2.2[a] days		
Haloperidol	40–70	12–36	CYP1A2, CYP2D6, CYP3A4	Reduced haloperidol
Haloperidol decanoate		21 days		
Perphenazine	20–25	8.1–12.3	CYP2D6	7-OH-perphenazine
Second-generation antipsychotics (SGAs)				
Aripiprazole	87	48–68	CYP3A4, CYP2D6	Dehydroaripiprazole
Clozapine	12–81	11–105	CYP1A2, CYP3A4, CYP2C19	Desmethylclozapine
Olanzapine	80	20–70	CYP1A2, CYP3A4, FMO3	N-glucuronide; 2-OH-methyl; 4-N-oxide
Paliperidone ER	28	23	Renal unchanged (59%) Multiple pathways	None known
Quetiapine	9 ± 4	6.88	CYP3A4	7-OH-quetiapine
Risperidone	68	3–24	CYP2D6	9-OH-risperidone
Risperidone Consta®		3–6 days	CYP2D6	9-OH-risperidone
Ziprasidone	59	4–10	Aldehyde oxidase, CYP3A4	None

[a]Based on multiple dose data. Single dose data indicate a β-half-life of 6–10 days.

Data from DeLeon et al.,[33] Harrison and Goa,[44] Ereshefsky et al.,[42,43] Mauri et al.,[60] and Spina and de Leon.[111]

TABLE 70-7 Relative Side-Effect Incidence of Commonly Used Antipsychotics[a,b]

	Sedation	EPS	Anticholinergic	Orthostasis	Weight Gain	Prolactin
Aripiprazole	+	+	+	+	+	+
Chlorpromazine	++++	+++	+++	++++	++	+++
Clozapine	++++	+	++++	++++	++++	+
Fluphenazine	+	++++	+	+	+	++++
Haloperidol	+	++++	+	+	+	++++
Olanzapine	++	++	++	++	++++	+
Perphenazine	++	++++	++	+	+	++++
Quetiapine	++	+	+	++	++	+
Risperidone	+	++	+	++	++	++++
Thioridazine	++++	+++	++++	++++	+	+++
Thiothixene	+	++++	+	+	+	++++
Ziprasidone	++	++	+	+	+	+

EPS, extrapyramidal side effects; Relative side-effect risk: ±, negligible; +, low; ++, moderate; +++, moderately high; ++++, high.
[a]Side effects shown are relative risk based on doses within the recommended therapeutic range.
[b]Individual patient risk varies depending on patient-specific factors.

Long-acting risperidone is a suspension of drug in glycolic acid-lactate copolymer microspheres.[41] After IM injection the polymer is slowly hydrolyzed, and significant risperidone begins being released after about 3 weeks. The apparent β-phase half-life is 3 to 6 days.[41] With dosing every 2 weeks, steady-state risperidone concentrations are achieved after approximately 2 months. The depot FGAs fluphenazine decanoate (also available in an enanthate salt) and haloperidol decanoate are esterified drugs formulated in sesame seed oil for deep intramuscular injection. Their absorption from the muscle and metabolism to the free base is sufficiently slow to cause absorption to be the rate-limiting step in determining their respective apparent half-lives.[42]

■ ADVERSE EFFECTS

Table 70–7 presents the relative incidence of common categories of antipsychotic side effects. Side effects are discussed below with respect to organ system affected. A general approach to monitoring and assessing side effects requires prospective monitoring by clinicians, preferably using a thorough review of systems approach. Patient-oriented self-rated side-effect scales can be helpful, as many patients with schizophrenia do not readily complain of side effects.

With the variety of antipsychotics currently available, using an alternative drug should be considered in patients who complain of poorly tolerated side effects. Because medication side effects are one of the primary predictors of patient nonadherence, the clinician should take advantage of the treatment options currently available in an attempt to improve patient outcomes. As new antipsychotics become available, side effects and risks associated with different drugs should be reevaluated. As we learn more about relative side-effect risks (e.g., weight gain, glucose intolerance, QTc prolongation, acute extrapyramidal side effects, and tardive dyskinesia), it will be necessary to regularly reconsider which antipsychotics should be considered first-line treatment alternatives.

Endocrine System

DA blockade in the tuberoinfundibular tract results in increased prolactin levels, because DA is the major prolactin-inhibiting factor. Galactorrhea can occur in up to 57% of women, and menstrual irregularities or amenorrhea in up to 97%. These effects can be dose related and are more common with the use of FGAs and risperidone. Gynecomastia and galactorrhea are reported in men as well. Tolerance does not appear to develop to these effects.[62] Switching to the SGAs olanzapine, quetiapine, ziprasidone, or aripiprazole, which have no appreciable sustained effect on prolactin, is the most reasonable treatment option.

Weight gain is frequently reported in both adults and children receiving antipsychotics.[63,64] Although the exact mechanism is uncertain, weight gain has been associated with antihistaminic effects, antimuscarinic effects, and blockade of 5-HT_{2C} receptors. However, dietary factors and activity levels can play a significant role in this population, as does renourishment after a period of poor self-care. In particular, significant weight gain, as defined by greater than or equal to 7% of the baseline body weight, is associated with clozapine and olanzapine therapy in 40% or more of patients.[63,65] Ziprasidone and aripiprazole both have been associated with minimal weight gain.

The clinical significance of weight gain during antipsychotic therapy is substantial. The risk of cardiovascular-related mortality is higher in individuals with schizophrenia,[66,67] and this is further aggravated by drug-related weight gain and the high prevalence of smoking.[68] Additionally, obesity is a risk factor for diabetes mellitus.[69] Weight gain during treatment is a major reason for poor patient medication adherence, and patients commonly report weight gain as being a concern.[70]

A number of pharmacologic interventions have been attempted for antipsychotic-related weight gain, but in general these should be discouraged. Switching patients to antipsychotics less likely to cause weight gain, dietary restriction, exercise, and behavior modification programs are reported to be successful in small short-term studies.[71] An American Diabetes Association consensus task force recommends consideration of a change in antipsychotic if a patient gains more than 5% of baseline body weight after starting the drug.[72]

Schizophrenic patients have a higher prevalence of type II diabetes than the nonschizophrenic population. Beyond this, antipsychotics may adversely affect glucose levels in diabetic patients. The extent to which these effects are related to drug-induced weight increase is unclear.[65,73] Data collected from the FDA MedWatch Drug Surveillance System for clozapine, olanzapine, quetiapine, and risperidone indicate that nearly 60% of the new-onset diabetes reported occurred within the first 6 months of treatment initiation.[74,75] New-onset diabetes has been reported during treatment with risperidone, olanzapine, quetiapine, and ziprasidone; aripiprazole has limited case reports linking its association with diabetes.[76,77] Although data are conflicting, evidence suggests a greater risk for the development of diabetes with clozapine and olanzapine.[75] In March 2004 the FDA issued a safety alert requiring revisions in the labeling of all SGAs, that describes the increased risk of diabetes mellitus in patients taking atypical antipsychotics.[78] Given the public health significance of diabetes, clarifying the diabetogenic effect of SGAs is a major focus of current research. Moreover, designing care models and standards for managing diabetes in patients with schizophrenia is another major consideration.

CLINICAL CONTROVERSY

The relative role of individual SGAs in precipitating diabetes mellitus is controversial. Clinicians are increasingly concerned about the escalating number of new cases of diabetes mellitus being reported in patients taking SGAs. It is clear, however, that obesity is associated with an increased risk of type II diabetes mellitus; olanzapine and clozapine cause more weight gain than other SGAs.

Cardiovascular System

Orthostatic Hypotension Postural or orthostatic hypotension, defined as a greater than 20-mm Hg drop in systolic pressure, is caused by α-adrenergic blockade.[79] Associated with lower potency FGAs and SGAs (especially on intramuscular or intravenous administration), orthostatic hypotension can occur in any patient, but diabetic patients with preexisting cardiovascular disease and the elderly seem particularly predisposed. Patient education should address slow changes in posture to allow for adaptation. For most patients, tolerance to this effect occurs within 2 to 3 months. If tolerance does not occur, lower doses or a change to an antipsychotic with less α-blockade can be attempted.

Electrocardiographic Changes Among the antipsychotics, thioridazine, clozapine, and ziprasidone are most likely to cause electrocardiogram (ECG) changes. ECG changes include increased heart rate (through sinus tachycardia from anticholinergic effects, or reflex tachycardia from α-adrenergic blockade), flattened T waves, ST segment depression, and prolongation of QT and PR intervals. The most clinically important of these potential changes is prolongation of the QTc, which has been associated with ventricular arrhythmias, including torsades de pointes syndrome. Thioridazine has been shown to prolong the QTc on average approximately 20 milliseconds (msec) longer than haloperidol, risperidone, olanzapine, or quetiapine.[65] Thioridazine's effects on QTc prolongation is dose related, and has led to a black box warning in the FDA-approved product labeling. In the same study, ziprasidone prolonged the QTc approximately 10 msec longer than about one-half of the effect of thioridazine.[65] Widespread clinical use suggests that ziprasidone's effects on the ECG are not associated with clinical sequelae, unless the patient has baseline risk factors.[65] Although the precise point at which QTc prolongation becomes clinically dangerous is unclear, it has been recommended to discontinue a medication associated with QTc prolongation if the interval consistently exceeds 500 msec.

Greater caution regarding antipsychotic choice and use is necessary in the elderly, in patients with preexisting cardiac or cerebrovascular disease, and in patients taking diuretics or medications that may prolong the QTc.[65] In patients older than 50 years of age, a pretreatment ECG is recommended, as are baseline serum potassium and magnesium levels. These factors should be considered in antipsychotic selection.

Lipid Changes

Treatment with at least some SGAs and phenothiazines appears associated with elevations in serum triglycerides and cholesterol. Among the SGAs, less risk for change in serum lipid or cholesterol levels can occur with risperidone, ziprasidone, or aripiprazole.[67] In the CATIE trial, olanzapine was associated with greater and significant adverse effects on metabolic parameters, including lipids, blood glucose, and body weight versus the other study treatments, but these differences in tolerability did not affect discontinuation rates.[80]

The occurrence of weight gain, diabetes, and lipid abnormalities during antipsychotic therapy is consistent with the development of metabolic syndrome (i.e., syndrome X). Metabolic syndrome consists of raised triglycerides (greater than or equal to 150 mg/dL), low HDL cholesterol (less than or equal to 40 mg/dL for males, less than or equal to 50 mg/dL for females), elevated fasting glucose (greater than or equal to 100 mg/dL), blood pressure elevation (greater than or equal to 130/85 mm Hg), and weight gain (abdominal circumference greater than 102 cm [40 in] for males, greater than 88 cm [34 in] in females).[67] These abnormalities dictate an important role for general health screening and monitoring in patients with schizophrenia, and prompt intervention when such abnormalities occur. The propensity of individual antipsychotics to produce metabolic disturbances should be considered in the context of individual patient risk factors at the time of drug selection.

Autonomic Nervous System

Patients receiving antipsychotics, or antipsychotics in combination with anticholinergics, can experience anticholinergic side effects (e.g., dry mouth, constipation, tachycardia, blurred vision, inhibition or impairment of ejaculation, urinary retention, or impaired memory). This is particularly so with low-potency FGAs, and the elderly are especially sensitive to these effects. Of the SGAs, clozapine and olanzapine have moderately high rates of causing anticholinergic effects. Constipation, caused by slowed peristaltic movement and decreased intestinal fluid content, should be closely monitored and treated, especially in the elderly. Paralytic ileus and necrotizing enterocolitis can also occur.

Central Nervous System

Extrapyramidal System

Dystonia. Dystonia is a state of abnormal tonicity, sometimes described simplistically as a severe "muscle spasm."[81] More accurately, they are prolonged tonic contractions, with a rapid onset, usually within 24 to 96 hours of dosage initiation or dosage increase. They can be life-threatening, as in the case of pharyngeal-laryngeal dystonias, and can contribute to patient nonadherence. Types of dystonic reactions include trismus, glossospasm, tongue protrusion, pharyngeal-laryngeal dystonia, blepharospasm, oculogyric crisis, torticollis, and retrocollis. Dystonic reactions occur primarily with FGAs. Risk factors include younger patients (especially males), the use of high-potency agents, and high dosage. The overall incidence from the 1960s through the mid-1970s ranged from 2.3% to 10%, but as higher-potency traditional antipsychotics became more widely used, the rate increased to as high as 64%.

Intramuscular or intravenous anticholinergics (Table 70–8) or benzodiazepines are the treatments of choice for dystonia. Benztropine mesylate 2 mg or diphenhydramine 50 mg can be given intramuscularly or intravenously. Diazepam 5 to 10 mg by slow IV push or lorazepam 1 to 2 mg intramuscularly are treatment alternatives. Relief is typically seen within 15 to 20 minutes of an intramuscular injection and within 5 minutes of intravenous administration. The antipsychotic can be continued, with concomitant short-term use of oral anticholinergic agents. In general, prophylactic anticholinergic medications are not recommended routinely with all FGAs. However, prophylaxis is reasonable when using high-potency FGAs (e.g., haloperidol or fluphenazine) in young men, and in patients with a history of dystonia.[81] Dystonias can also be minimized by the use of lower initial FGA doses. Anticholinergics are good choices for prophylaxis, whereas amantadine has not been proved effective for this purpose. The risk of dystonia is greatly reduced with SGAs.

Akathisia. Akathisia is defined as the inability to sit still and as being functionally motor restless. The most accurate diagnosis is made by combining subjective complaints with objective symptoms (pacing, shifting, shuffling, or tapping feet). Subjectively, patients may describe a feeling of inner restlessness or disquiet or a compulsion to move or remain in constant motion. Akathisia occurs in

TABLE 70-8 Agents Used to Treat Extrapyramidal Side Effects

Generic Name	Equivalent Dose (mg)	Daily Dosage Range (mg)
Antimuscarinics		
Benztropine[a]	1	1–8[b]
Biperiden[a]	2	2–8
Trihexyphenidyl	2	2–15
Antihistaminic		
Diphenhydramine[a]	50	50–400
Dopamine agonist		
Amantadine	NA	100–400
Benzodiazepines		
Lorazepam[a]	NA	1–8
Diazepam	NA	2–20
Clonazepam	NA	2–8
β-Blockers		
Propranolol	NA	20–160

NA, not applicable
[a]Injectable dosage form can be given intramuscularly for relief of acute dystonia.
[b]Dosage can be titrated to 12 mg/day with careful monitoring; nonlinear pharmacokinetics have been demonstrated.

20% to 40% of patients treated with high-potency FGAs.[81] Akathisia is frequently accompanied by dysphoria.

Treatment with anticholinergic agents, usually considered the standard treatment for acute extrapyramidal side effects, is disappointing for akathisia, but can be helpful in patients with concomitant pseudoparkinsonism.[81] Traditionally, reduction in antipsychotic dosage has been considered the best intervention; however, this might not be a realistic goal in an acutely psychotic patient. A logical alternative is to switch to an antipsychotic with a lower risk of akathisia, or an antipsychotic previously used in the patient without adverse effect. Akathisia can occasionally occur with SGAs. Quetiapine and clozapine appear to have the lowest risk of producing akathisia.[39]

Benzodiazepines have been used for treatment of akathisia, but the high prevalence of co-occurring substance abuse in schizophrenia discourages their prescribing.[81] The β-blockers (e.g., propranolol in doses up to 160 mg daily, nadolol in doses up to 80 mg daily, and metoprolol in β_2-selective doses of 100 mg daily or less) are reported as effective.[81]

Pseudoparkinsonism. Pseudoparkinsonism, produced by D_2 blockade in the nigrostriatum, resembles idiopathic Parkinson disease. A patient with pseudoparkinsonism can present with any of four cardinal symptoms: (1) akinesia, bradykinesia, or decreased motor activity including difficulty initiating movement, as well as extreme slowness, mask-like facial expression, micrographia, slowed speech, and decreased arm swing; (2) tremor, known as pill-rolling type, that is predominant at rest and decreases with movement, usually involving the fingers and hands, although tremors can also be seen in the arms, legs, neck, head, and chin; (3) cogwheel rigidity, seen as the patient's limbs yielding in jerky, ratchet-like fashion when passively moved by the examiner (a mild form can present as stiffness); and (4) postural abnormalities and instability manifested as stooped posture, difficulty in maintaining stability when changing body position, and a gait that ranges from slow and shuffling to festinating. Fatigue and weakness can be noted, as well as oral abnormalities including dysphagia, dysarthria, and abnormal palmomental and glabellar reflexes. The overall incidence of pseudoparkinsonism from FGAs ranges from 15.4% to 36%, depending on the drug and dose. Akinesia alone can be seen in 59% of patients on high-potency FGAs. Other risk factors include increasing age and possibly female gender. The onset of symptoms is typically 1 to 2 weeks after initiation of antipsychotic therapy or a dose increase.

The efficacy of anticholinergic medications in alleviating or attenuating symptoms of pseudoparkinsonism is well established.[81] Benztropine's long half-life allows once- to twice-daily dosing. Typical dosing is 1 to 2 mg twice a day up to a usual maximum dosage of 8 mg daily, although some patients will continue to respond to doses up to 12 mg. Trihexyphenidyl (2 to 5 mg three times a day), diphenhydramine (25 to 50 mg three times a day), and biperiden (2 mg three times a day) usually require thrice-daily administration. Diphenhydramine produces more sedation than the other agents. All of the anticholinergics have been abused for their euphoriant effects.[82] Symptoms typically begin to resolve within 3 to 4 days after initiation of treatment, but a minimum of at least 2 weeks of treatment is normally required for full response. Amantadine is generally as efficacious for pseudoparkinsonism as anticholinergics, with significantly less effect on memory function.[81] The need for prophylactic use of these agents against pseudoparkinsonism is less convincing than with dystonias, and is unnecessary when using SGAs.[81] The long-term treatment of pseudoparkinsonism with antiparkinsonism medication is somewhat controversial, and an attempt should be made to taper and discontinue these agents 6 weeks to 3 months after symptom resolution. If symptoms reappear, then switching to an SGA should be considered. The risk of pseudoparkinsonism with SGAs is extremely low. When risperidone is used in doses greater than 6 mg/day, the risk of pseudoparkinsonism symptoms approaches that with FGAs. Quetiapine, aripiprazole, or clozapine are reasonable alternatives in a patient experiencing extrapyramidal side effects with other SGAs.[33,39,81]

Tardive Dyskinesia. Tardive dyskinesia is a syndrome characterized by abnormal involuntary movements occurring late in onset in relation to initiation of antipsychotic therapy. Tardive dyskinesia is sometimes irreversible and continues to be a controversial issue.

The classic description of tardive dyskinesia is the buccal-lingual-masticatory (BLM) syndrome, or orofacial movements. The onset of BLM movements is usually insidious. Typically, they are the first detectable signs of tardive dyskinesia and begin with mild forward, backward, or lateral movements of the tongue. As the disorder progresses, more obvious or frank BLM movements appear, including tongue thrusting, rolling, or fly-catching movements, and chewing or lateral jaw movements. Tardive dyskinesia symptoms can interfere with the patient's ability to chew, speak, or swallow. Further complications include oral ulcerations, inability to wear dentures, and inflammation and loosening of mandibular joints. Eating difficulties and malnutrition can be primary physical complications of tardive dyskinesia. Weight loss can be seen in patients with esophageal or respiratory manifestations but not in those with truncal movements. Facial movements include frequent blinking, brow arching, grimacing, upward deviation of the eyes, and lip smacking. Involvement of the extremities sometimes occurs, with the appearance of restless choreiform (irregular spasmodic) and distal athetosis (slow, writhing movement) of limbs including twisting, spreading, flexion (bending) and extension of fingers, toe tapping, and toe dorsiflexion (upward turning). Unusual posture, hyperextension, pelvic thrusting, axial hyperkinesia (excessive muscular activity of head and trunk), ballismus (jerking or shaking), exaggerated lordosis (bending backward), rocking, and swaying are occasionally observed. Among the more common differential diagnoses are withdrawal dyskinesias occurring after short-term use of antipsychotics, spontaneous orofacial dyskinesias in the elderly, orofacial dyskinesias in the edentulous, stereotypic movements in schizophrenics, Huntington disease, and congenital torsion dystonia. Orofacial movements are reported more commonly in older patients, whereas the truncal axial movements are classically reported in young adults. Movements can worsen with stress, decrease with sedation, and disappear during sleep. Concentration on motor tasks or attempts to suppress the movements voluntarily can actually increase them.

Early signs of tardive dyskinesia can be reversible but if allowed to persist or if not detected in the early stages, they can become irreversible, even with drug discontinuation. When the antipsychotic dose is decreased or tapered and discontinued, worsening of abnormal movements can occur, followed by possible slow improvement after months or years if the patient remains on lower doses or discontinues treatment. No standardized diagnostic criteria for tardive dyskinesia are available. Abnormal involuntary movements can be detected early through physical assessment and the use of rating scales. Available rating scales include the Abnormal Involuntary Movements Scale (AIMS) and the Dyskinesia Identification System: Condensed User Scale (DISCUS).[81,83] Neither scale is diagnostic in itself.

Risk factors include increasing age, the occurrence of acute extrapyramidal side effects, poor antipsychotic drug response, diagnosis of organic mental disorder, diabetes mellitus, mood disorders, and possibly female gender.[84,85] Duration of antipsychotic therapy, daily dosage, and possibly total cumulative dosage are probably the most significant risk factors. Overall morbidity and mortality are greater in tardive dyskinesia patients.

With FGAs, the reported incidence of tardive dyskinesia ranges from 0.5% to 62%.[84] In a first episode of schizophrenia, the incidence is estimated at about 5% per year, with the overall prevalence ranging from 20% to 25% with long-term treatment. Among the elderly, the overall risk of tardive dyskinesia is higher.[85] Tardive dyskinesia is not always permanent, with remission of symptoms observed in 25% of patients after 5 years of continued treatment.[81,84,85]

The risk of tardive dyskinesia with SGAs is significantly lower. A systematic review of 11 studies with SGAs lasting 1 year or more found an overall risk of tardive dyskinesia to be approximately 0.8% per year in nonelderly (<65 years) adults and 5.3% per year in the elderly (≥65 years). For individual agents, the annual incidence rates ranged from zero to 0.5% for olanzapine to 0.6% to 0.7% for risperidone or quetiapine. To date, there are no reports of tardive dyskinesia with clozapine monotherapy.

Prevention of tardive dyskinesia is important, as treatment of the movements once they occur is difficult. One of the more compelling arguments for the first-line use of SGAs is their lower risk of tardive dyskinesia.[26,39,86] (see Fig. 70–1). Regular neurologic examinations (AIMS or other scales) should be performed at baseline and at least quarterly to assess for early signs of tardive dyskinesia. At the first signs of tardive dyskinesia, the need for continuing antipsychotic treatment should be reassessed. In such situations, if the patient is taking an FGA and continuing treatment is indicated, the medication should be switched to an SGA.

Numerous drugs have been used in an attempt to treat tardive dyskinesia, representing various strategies affecting CNS neurotransmission. In two controlled trials lasting 22 to 52 weeks, clozapine decreased abnormal involuntary movements.[85,87] Switching antipsychotic therapy to clozapine is a favored first-line pharmacotherapeutic strategy, particularly in patients with moderate to severe dyskinesias.[84,85,87]

Sedation and Cognition Sedation is as an antipsychotic side effect and not an indication of therapeutic effect. Chlorpromazine, thioridazine, mesoridazine, clozapine, olanzapine, and quetiapine are most frequently implicated. Administration of most or all of the daily dosage at bedtime (depending on the drug half-life) can decrease daytime sedation and in some patients eliminate the need for hypnotic agents. Sedation occurs early in treatment and can decrease over time.[79] Oversedation can play a large role in cognitive, perceptual, and motor dysfunction. However, positive effects of medication on cognition are seen with chronic administration, evidenced by improvements in tasks involving visual-motor skills, attention to task, and working memory. Compared with FGAs, several studies have shown cognitive benefits of SGAs. Comparative effects of different SGAs on cognition are as yet unclear, but available studies suggest that different SGAs can have effects on varying cognitive domains.[89] An algorithm-driven disease management program using SGAs as first-line treatment was shown to improve cognition over a 9-month period.[90]

Seizures An increased risk of drug-induced seizures occurs in all patients treated with antipsychotics. However, this risk is greater if the following predisposing factors are present: preexisting seizure disorder, history of drug-induced seizure, abnormal electroencephalogram (EEG), and preexisting CNS pathology or head trauma. Seizures are more closely associated with the use of higher doses, rapid dosage increases, and on initiation of treatment. When an isolated seizure occurs, a dosage decrease is first recommended; anticonvulsant therapy is not recommended. Although spontaneously occurring seizures have been reported with most antipsychotics, the highest potential risk for an antipsychotic-related seizure is with clozapine or chlorpromazine. If a change in antipsychotic therapy is required because of a drug-induced seizure, risperidone, molindone, thioridazine, haloperidol, pimozide, trifluoperazine, and fluphenazine are associated with the lowest potential.[91]

Thermoregulation Poikilothermia, the body temperature adjusting to the ambient temperature, can be a serious side effect of antipsychotic therapy in temperature extremes.[92] Hyperpyrexia can be a danger in hot weather or during exercise. Inhibition of sweating, a result of anticholinergic properties impairing the peripheral mechanisms of heat dissipation, can also contribute to this problem, which in its severest form can lead to heat stroke. Hypothermia is also a risk, particularly in the elderly (≥65 years) and in cold climates. All patients receiving antipsychotics should be educated about these potential problems. Thermoregulatory problems are reportedly more common with the use of low-potency FGAs and can occur with the more anticholinergic SGAs.

Neuroleptic Malignant Syndrome Neuroleptic malignant syndrome (NMS) occurs in 0.5% to 1% of patients receiving FGAs. The rate of NMS has diminished since the introduction of SGAs, and reliable current estimates of the incidence with SGAs are not available. NMS can occur more frequently in patients receiving high-potency FGAs, injectable or depot FGAs, and in patients who are dehydrated, with physical exhaustion, or organic mental disorders. Although less common than with FGAs, NMS has been reported with SGAs, including clozapine. The onset of symptoms varies from early in treatment to months later. It develops rapidly, over the course of 24 to 72 hours. NMS can occur after antipsychotic discontinuation, especially when depot agents are used. Possible mechanisms of NMS include disruption of the central thermoregulatory process or excess production of heat secondary to skeletal muscle contractions. The differential diagnosis includes heat stroke, lethal catatonia, anesthetic-associated malignant hyperthermia, anticholinergic toxicity, and monoamine oxidase inhibitor drug interactions. Cardinal signs and symptoms of NMS are body temperature exceeding 38°C (100.4°F), altered level of consciousness, autonomic dysfunction (tachycardia, labile blood pressure, diaphoresis, tach–ypnea, or urinary or fecal incontinence), and rigidity. Laboratory evaluation, although considered nonspecific, frequently shows leukocytosis with or without a left shift, increases in creatine kinase (CK), aspartate aminotransferase, alanine aminotransferase, lactate dehydrogenase, and myoglobinuria.[93]

Treatment should always begin with antipsychotic discontinuation and supportive care. In many cases that alone is effective. The role of adjunctive agents is unclear, yet they are often used in clinical settings. The DA agonist bromocriptine reduces rigidity, fever, or CK in up to 94% of patients, whereas the use of another DA agonist, amantadine, has been successfully used in up to 63% of patients. Dantrolene has been used as a skeletal muscle relaxant, with effects on temperature, heart rate, respiratory rate, and CK in up to 81% of patients.[93] Wide recognition and rapid antipsychotic discontinuation has drastically reduced mortality from 20% 15 years ago to 4% in the mid-1990s.

Many patients with schizophrenia, despite having had NMS, will require future antipsychotic pharmacotherapy. A review of antipsychotic rechallenges suggests that the risk of rechallenge is acceptable in most patients, provided that the patient is observed for an extended period of time (2 weeks or more is suggested) without antipsychotics, that there is careful monitoring and slow dose titration, and that the patient is maintained on the lowest possible dose.[93] Only SGAs should be used for rechallenge following an episode of NMS.

Psychiatric Side Effects Antipsychotic-induced akathisia, akinesia, and dysphoria can have unfortunate sequelae, resulting in what has been termed "behavioral toxicity."[36] Akinesia, characterized by "diminished spontaneity," results in symptoms of apathy and withdrawal, often mistaken for the negative symptoms of schizophrenia; these patients can actually appear depressed on formal evaluation.

Delirium and psychosis are reported with larger doses of FGAs or combinations of anticholinergics with FGAs. Chronic confusion and disorientation can occur in the elderly as a result of antipsychotic treatment.[94] Unfortunately, the link is not always made between initiation of antipsychotic therapy, and the patient can be misdiagnosed with an organic mental disorder. This clinical presentation, called a *pseudodementia*, is easily reversible on discontinuation of the antipsychotic.

Ophthalmologic Effects Anticholinergic effects of antipsychotics or concomitant antiparkinson medications can exacerbate narrow-angle (angle closure) glaucoma. Antipsychotics with low anticholinergic effects should be used in such individuals, and they should be appropriately monitored.[95]

Opaque deposits in the cornea and lens occur with chronic phenothiazine treatment, most frequently with chlorpromazine. Although visual acuity is not usually affected, periodic slit-lamp ophthalmologic examinations are frequently recommended in patients receiving long-term treatment with phenothiazines.

Because of cataract development and lenticular changes in animals, baseline and periodic eye examinations are recommended in the product labeling for patients receiving quetiapine.[96] However, clinical use of quetiapine since its marketing has not shown a significant risk of cataracts.[39,96] Retinitis pigmentosa can result from use of thioridazine doses greater than 800 mg daily. It is caused by melanin deposits and can result in permanent visual impairment or blindness. There is no evidence that it is a function of cumulative dose.[95]

Hepatic System

Cholestatic hepatocanalicular jaundice has been reported in up to 2% of patients receiving phenothiazines. Additionally, liver function test (LFT) abnormalities (elevated aminotransferases and alkaline phosphatase), often asymptomatic, were reported in up to 50% of patients.[97] If aminotransferases are greater than three times the upper limit of normal, antipsychotic therapy should be changed to a chemically unrelated antipsychotic.

Overall, LFT abnormalities are uncommon with SGAs. However, cholestatic hepatitis has been reported with risperidone,[98] and LFT abnormalities, mostly transient, have been reported with olanzapine and clozapine.[99]

Genitourinary System

Urinary hesitancy and retention is reported with low-potency FGAs and with clozapine. Anticholinergic effects cause smooth muscle slowing and paralyze the detrusor muscle of the bladder, requiring greater urine volume to evoke muscle contraction. Men with benign prostatic hypertrophy are especially prone to this effect.[94]

Urinary incontinence is thought to be caused by α-blockade, and among the SGAs, it appears to be particularly problematic with clozapine. The incidence has been reported to be as high as 44%, and it can be persistent in 25% of patients.[100]

Numerous different mechanisms have been suggested to cause sexual dysfunction, including dopaminergic blockade, hyperprolactinemia, histaminergic blockade (sedation), anticholinergic effects, and α-adrenergic blockade. This area is inadequately studied, and multiple mechanisms are likely responsible for producing sexual dysfunction. Unmedicated individuals with schizophrenia report decreased libido. Most but not all studies have shown a relationship between hyperprolactinemia and sexual dysfunction, including decreased libido, erectile dysfunction, difficulty achieving orgasm, and ejaculatory abnormalities. Although risperidone produces at least as much sexual dysfunction as FGAs, other SGAs, which have weak effects on prolactin or are "prolactin-sparing," produce less sexual dysfunction. It is unclear whether hyperprolactinemia directly impairs sexual functioning, reflects high dopaminergic blockade from risperidone and FGAs, or is associated with other mechanisms of producing sexual dysfunction. Patients experiencing sexual dysfunction with FGAs or risperidone should be switched to an SGA with less effect on prolactin.[101]

Hematologic System

Transient leukopenia can occur during initial treatment with antipsychotics; however, it typically does not progress to clinically significant parameters.[102] If the WBC count is less than 3,000 mm^3, or if the absolute neutrophil count (ANC) is less than 1,000 mm^3, the antipsychotic should be discontinued, and the WBC monitored closely until it returns to normal. Agranulocytosis reportedly occurs in 0.01% of patients receiving FGAs, and more frequently with chlorpromazine and thioridazine. The onset is usually within the first 8 weeks of therapy. Agranulocytosis can initially manifest clinically as a local infection, with sore throat, leukoplakia, erythema, and ulcerations of the pharynx. These symptoms in any patient receiving antipsychotics should signal the immediate need for a WBC count. If either the WBC count or ANC falls below these parameters, the drug should be discontinued immediately and the patient monitored closely for the development of secondary infections. Isolated rare cases of thrombocytopenia and eosinophilia have been reported.

Agranulocytosis with clozapine significantly limits the clinical usefulness of this agent. Data on the incidence since the release of clozapine in February 1990 following stringent monitoring guidelines reveal that the 1-year treatment risk of developing agranulocytosis with clozapine is approximately 0.8%, and the 18-month risk is 0.91%.[103] Increasing age and female gender are associated with greater risk. Based on available data, the time period for greatest risk appears to be between months 1 and 6 of treatment, and weekly WBC monitoring for the first 6 months of therapy is mandated in the FDA-approved product labeling. After the first 6 months, the labeling allows the frequency of WBC monitoring to be decreased to every 2 weeks for months 7 through 12 after which it can be decreased to monthly if all WBCs are normal. If the total WBC count drops to less than 2,000 mm^3, or the ANC is less than 1,000 mm^3, clozapine should be discontinued and the patient monitored closely. Some clinicians have used the granulocyte colony-stimulating factor filgrastim with hopes of improving the outcome by hastening resolution or decreasing morbidity. In cases of mild to moderate neutropenia (granulocytes between 2,000 mm^3 and 3,000 mm^3, or ANC between 1,000 mm^3 and 500 mm^3), which occurs in up to 2% of patients, clozapine should be discontinued with daily monitoring of complete blood counts until values return to normal.

Dermatologic System

Allergic reactions are rare and usually occur within 8 weeks of initiating therapy, manifesting as maculopapular, erythematous, pruritic rashes that are evident on the face, neck, trunk, or extremities. Drug discontinuation and topical steroids are recommended. Contact dermatitis, including the oral mucosa, can occur in patients or medical personnel. For patients, mixing the antipsychotic concentrate in a sufficient quantity of a nonacidic liquid and swallowing it quickly decreases problems in susceptible patients. Care should be taken in the handling and preparation of liquid FGAs.

Phenothiazine structures can absorb ultraviolet light and energy, resulting in the formation of free radicals, which can have damaging effects on the skin. Both SGAs and FGAs cause photosensitivity. Erythema and severe sunburns can occur. Exposure to sunlight should be limited, and patients should be educated about the use of a maximally blocking sunscreen, hats, protective clothing, and sunglasses.[104]

Blue-gray or purplish skin coloration in areas exposed to sunlight occurs in patients receiving higher doses of low-potency phenothiazines during long-term administration, especially with chlorpromazine. It commonly occurs with concurrent corneal or lens pigmentation.

Miscellaneous Adverse Effects

A particularly curious and sometimes troubling side effect with clozapine is sialorrhea, which can occur in up to 54% of patients taking clozapine. The mechanism of clozapine-induced drooling is unclear, although α-adrenergic blockade and muscarinic$_4$ receptor agonist have been suggested as potential etiologies. α-Agonists such as clonidine and antimuscarinics such as benztropine have been suggested as potential treatments.[105]

■ TOXICITY WITH OVERDOSE

Acute overdose with antipsychotics rarely results in serious symptomatology. Mild intoxication manifests as sedation, hypotension, and miosis, whereas with severe intoxication, agitation and delirium can typically progress to motor retardation, seizures, cardiac arrhythmias, respiratory arrest, and coma. Dystonias and pseudoparkinsonism symptoms also occur. Supportive measures, gastric lavage, and activated charcoal are recommended. Induction of emesis can be difficult because of effects on the chemoreceptor trigger zone, and dialysis is ineffective because of the degree of drug-protein binding. Phenytoin or sodium bicarbonate are useful in the treatment of quinidine-like cardiac conduction effects on the QRS or QTc. Physostigmine is not generally recommended to reverse anticholinergic toxicity because of deleterious effects on arrhythmias and seizure threshold.[106]

■ USE IN PREGNANCY AND LACTATION

Minimal data exist regarding the effects of pregnancy on schizophrenia. However, the disorganized thought processes, impaired cognition, and negative symptoms can have a detrimental effect on the functioning and self-care of the mother, and therefore adversely affect the fetus.[107] Currently available data assessing the risk of teratogenesis with antipsychotic agents are insufficient. Epidemiologic studies show a slightly increased risk of birth defects with low-potency FGAs. Haloperidol is the best studied of all antipsychotics, and no relationship between its use and teratogenicity has been found. SGAs have been inadequately studied. However, concern has been expressed regarding the use of clozapine in pregnancy.[108] The weight gain associated with olanzapine and clozapine and potential risk of gestational diabetes should be considered in drug selection.

The risk of antipsychotic use must be weighed against the benefits of pharmacotherapy in pregnant women who may be experiencing disorganized thoughts, delusions about change in body image or pregnancy, or who are unable to provide adequate prenatal care.[107]

Antipsychotics appear in breast milk with milk-to-plasma ratios of 0.5 to 1. However, 1 week after delivery, clozapine milk concentrations have been found to be as much as 279% of serum concentrations. Its use during breast-feeding is not recommended.[108] Overall, little is known about breast-feeding and the potential effects of antipsychotics on the neonate. Although not contraindicated, the lowest dosage should be used in the mother, and the infant should be carefully monitored.

■ DRUG INTERACTIONS

Most drug interactions occur because of pharmacodynamic or pharmacokinetic interactions. Common examples of pharmacodynamic interactions resulting in enhanced effect include the excess sedation that can occur when antipsychotics are used concomitantly with other medications that have sedative side effects. Additive antimuscarinic effects of antipsychotics used with other medications with antimuscarinic effects can result in urinary retention, constipation, blurred vision, or other anticholinergic side effects.[36,65] Both combined sedative and anticholinergic effects from multiple medications can result in impaired cognition, particularly in the elderly and other patients predisposed to such problems.[65] Patients can be more likely to experience symptomatic orthostatic hypotension when an antipsychotic is used with other medications that cause orthostasis. Although metoclopramide is prescribed for treating esophageal reflux, it is a DA antagonist, and patients are more likely to experience akathisia and other extrapyramidal side effects if it is used concomitantly with antipsychotics.[65] Although some SSRIs can interact with antipsychotics through enzyme inhibition, they can also interact through pharmacodynamic mechanisms. 5-HT$_2$ receptors are present on the presynaptic dopaminergic neuron, and their activation leads to decreased dopamine release from the presynaptic terminal. Increased availability of serotonin through SSRI effect can activate these receptors, decrease dopamine release, and add to the dopaminolytic effects of antipsychotic agents.[65] Thus in the absence of enzyme inhibition, SSRIs can still precipitate akathisia or extrapyramidal side effects when added to a patient stabilized on an antipsychotic medication. A potentially more dangerous interaction can occur when medications that slow myocardial conduction and thus prolong the QTc, are used in combination with antipsychotics that significantly prolong the QTc.[65,109] Medications that prolong the QTc should also be monitored carefully in patients taking concomitant diuretics.[65] These effects can all increase the risk of clinically significant side effects.

Although atypical antipsychotics can be affected to varying degrees by enzyme inhibitors and inducers, none of the available atypical antipsychotics have been shown to significantly affect the pharmacokinetics of other medications. Table 70–6 lists the major pathways thought to be involved in the metabolism of SGAs. Risperidone is metabolized primarily by CYP2D6 to its active metabolite, 9-OH-risperidone (paliperidone), which is thought to have a similar pharmacodynamic profile.[60,65] After single-dose administration, the mean bioavailability of quetiapine is 9% with significant interindividual variation.[110, 111]

Based on current information, inhibitors of CYP1A2 have the greatest potential for causing interactions with clozapine and olanzapine.[110] Examples include cimetidine, fluvoxamine, and fluoroquinolone antibiotics (e.g., ciprofloxacin) to varying degrees. To date, however, no serious inhibition interactions have been reported with olanzapine, which can be a result of olanzapine's wide therapeutic index. Carbamazepine has been reported to increase olanzapine elimination by as much as 50%.[112] Cigarette smoking is a potent inducer of CYP1A2, and one would expect lower mean olanzapine serum concentrations in smokers compared to nonsmokers.

Because of the risk of seizures with higher clozapine tissue concentrations, inhibition interactions with clozapine are potentially significant. In particular, fluvoxamine has been reported to increase clozapine serum concentrations by an average of two- to threefold and up to fivefold.[110,112] Fluoxetine and erythromycin can increase clozapine serum concentrations in some patients but to a lesser degree.[110,112] Mean clozapine serum concentrations are reported to be

32% lower in smokers compared with nonsmokers.[112] Carbamazepine can also induce clozapine metabolism and lead to lower serum concentrations.[112]

A study with the potent CYP3A4 inhibitor ketoconazole showed minimal effects on ziprasidone single-dose pharmacokinetics, with only a 33% mean increase in the ziprasidone area under the time-versus-concentration curve.[65] These results are consistent with data suggesting that aldehyde oxidase is the major metabolic pathway for ziprasidone, with only 30% to 35% being metabolized by CYP3A4.[113]

Modest elevations of aripiprazole serum concentration occur in the presence of ketoconazole or quinidine, which inhibit CYP2D6 and 3A4, respectively. Carbamazepine has been reported to decrease aripiprazole serum concentrations.[33,110] Recently, an FDA-approved gene chip analysis became available for evaluating metabolism through several P450 enzymes. The clinical usefulness of this technology in routine psychiatric pharmacotherapy is as yet unclear. Table 70–9 summarizes potential antipsychotic drug interactions.

■ PHARMACOECONOMIC CONSIDERATIONS

It is estimated that approximately 80% of individuals suffering their first schizophrenic break will have recurrent episodes and significant lifetime psychosocial dysfunction. In 1994, the direct cost of treating schizophrenia in the United States was estimated to be $45 billion.[113] The public mental healthcare sector provides the majority of services for individuals with schizophrenia. Mental healthcare costs for schizophrenia represent disproportionate expenditures for crisis intervention and hospitalization as compared to comprehensive outpatient services oriented toward maintaining remission and improving psychosocial functioning. The suboptimal or inadequate funding provided for efficient ambulatory mental health services further increases the demand for hospitalization, which diverts additional revenues that might be available for outpatient services. This has created a vicious revolving door cycle and is a major challenge facing public mental healthcare.

The advent of more expensive SGAs, accompanied by limited resources, has forced mental healthcare organizations to examine the outcomes and related economics of treating patients with the SGAs compared with the traditional, largely generic FGAs. Retrospective database studies have yielded conflicting results regarding the pharmacoeconomics of SGAs versus FGAs.[114] In the prospective effectiveness study, CATIE, differences in mental health costs between SGAs and the FGA perphenazine were driven by the higher acquisition costs of the SGAs.[115] Some studies have shown clozapine to result in lower overall mental healthcare costs, while others have shown no difference in costs compared to FGAs. Additionally, clozapine decreases suicidality more than comparator antipsychotics, and it is more effective in treatment-resistant schizophrenia.[116,117]

Significant differences in acquisition costs among the SGAs have produced controversy regarding formulary decisions in organized healthcare settings.[114] For example, although olanzapine has a higher acquisition cost, some studies have found no difference in total mental healthcare direct costs (i.e., medications plus services) when comparing olanzapine and risperidone.[114,118] However, these findings are inconsistent, and the comparative pharmacoeconomics of SGAs remain controversial.[114,115]

TABLE 70-9 Common Potential Drug Interactions with Antipsychotic Medications

Pharmacokinetic Drug Interactions with Antipsychotics

Mechanism of Interaction	***Interacting Drugs or Other Substances***	***Clinical Effect***
Muscarinic receptor blockade	*Anticholinergics*	↑ anticholinergic SE
	Benztropine	Blurred vision
	Diphenhydramine	Constipation
	Trihexyphenidyl	Impaired cognition
		Urinary retention
Additive or synergistic sedation	*Sedatives*	↑ sedation
	Benzodiazepines	Lethargy
	Concomitant AP	Impaired cognition
	Diphenhydramine	Impaired psychomotor activity
	Melatonin and melatonin agonists	↑ risk of accidents
	Mirtazapine	
	Trazodone	
	TCAs	
	Zaleplon	
	Zolpidem	
	Anticholinergics	
	Benztropine	
	Diphenhydramine	
	Trihexyphenidyl	
	Mirtazapine	
DA antagonist use for different indication	Metoclopramide	↑ EPS
Cardiovascular Interactions		
Additive effects on QTc	*TCA Antidepressants*	
	Amitriptyline	
	Clomipramine	
	Imipramine	
	Antiarrhythmics	
	Procainamide	
	Quinidine	
Electrolyte changes	Diuretics	↑ *risk of ECG changes and dysrhythmias*
Stimulation of presynaptic 5-HT receptors on DA neuron	SSRIs	↑ *EPS*
Sympatholytics: α blockade–↓ NE release	Clonidine	↑ hypotension
	Methyldopa	
	Prazosin	
↑ DA receptor binding	*Antipsychotics*	↑ SEs - particularly EPS

(continued)

TABLE 70-9 Common Potential Drug Interactions with Antipsychotic Medications (continued)

Pharmacokinetic Drug Interactions with Antipsychotics				
Mechanism of Interaction		***Interacting Drugs***		***Clinical Effect***
Aripiprazole				
Inhibition of AP metabolism (CYP2D6 & CYP3A4)	*Antidepressants* Bupropion Duloxetine Fluoxetine Fluvoxamine Paroxetine Sertraline *HIV Protease Inhibitors* Indinavir Nelfinavir Ritonavir	*Anti-infectives* Clarithromycin Erythromycin Fluconazole Ketoconazole Itraconazole	*Miscellaneous* Chlorpheniramine Diltiazem Quinidine Diphenhydramine Cimetidine Grapefruit juice Haloperidol Hydroxyzine Quinidine Verapamil	↑ AP effect ↑ SE
Induction of AP metabolism	*Antiepileptics* Carbamazepine Oxcarbazepine Phenobarbital Phenytoin	*Anti-infectives* Rifampin *Miscellaneous* Glucocorticoids Modafinil	*Herbals* St. John's wort	↓ AP effect
Clozapine				
Inhibition of AP metabolism (CYP3A4, CYP1A2, CYP2C19)	*Antidepressants* Fluoxetine Fluvoxamine *HIV Protease Inhibitors* Indinavir Nelfinavir Ritonavir	*Anti-infectives* Clarithromycin Erythromycin Fluconazole Ketoconazole Itraconazole	*Miscellaneous* Diltiazem Cimetidine Grapefruit juice Haloperidol Omeprazole Ticlopidine Topiramate Verapamil Cimetidine	↑ AP effect ↑ SE
Induction of AP metabolism	*Antiepileptics* Carbamazepine Phenobarbital Phenytoin	*Anti-infectives* Rifampin *Miscellaneous* Glucocorticoids Modafinil	*Herbals* St. John's wort	↓ AP effect
Haloperidol				
Inhibition of AP metabolism (CYP2D6, CYP3A4, CYP1A2)	*Antidepressants* Bupropion Duloxetine Fluoxetine Fluvoxamine Paroxetine Sertraline *HIV Protease Inhibitors* Indinavir Nelfinavir Ritonavir	*Anti-infectives* Clarithromycin Erythromycin Fluoconazole Fluoroquinolones Ketoconazole Itraconazole	*Miscellaneous* Chlorpheniramine Diltiazem Quinidine Diphenhydramine Cimetidine Grapefruit juice Hydroxyzine Quinidine Verapamil	↑ AP effect ↑ SE
Induction of AP metabolism	*Antiepileptics* Carbamazepine Oxcarbazepine Phenobarbital Phenytoin	*Anti-infectives* Rifampin *Miscellaneous* Broccoli Brussel sprouts Char-grilled meat Glucocorticoids Insulin Modafinil Omeprazole Modafinil	*Herbals* St. John's wort Tobacco smoking	↓ AP effect

(continued)

TABLE 70-9 Common Potential Drug Interactions with Antipsychotic Medications (continued)

Pharmacokinetic Drug Interactions with Antipsychotics				
Mechanism of Interaction		***Interacting Drugs***		***Clinical Effect***
Olanzapine				
Inhibition of AP metabolism (CYP3A4 & CYP1A2)	*Antidepressants*	*Anti-infectives*	*Miscellaneous*	↑ AP effect
	Fluvoxamine	Clarithromycin	Diltiazem	↑ SE
		Erythromycin	Cimetidine	
	HIV Protease Inhibitors	Fluconazole	Grapefruit juice	
	Indinavir	Fluoroquinolones	Verapamil	
	Nelfinavir	Ketoconazole		
	Ritonavir	Itraconazole		
Induction of AP metabolism	*Antiepileptics*	*Anti-infectives*	*Herbals*	↓ AP effect
	Carbamazepine	Rifampin	St. John's wort	
	Oxcarbazepine		Tobacco smoking	
	Phenobarbital	*Miscellaneous*		
	Phenytoin	Broccoli		
		Brussels sprouts		
		Char-grilled meat		
		Glucocorticoids		
		Modafinil		
		Omeprazole		
Paliperidone				
The bioavailability of paliperidone is significantly increased when it is taken with food. Although this could increase paliperidone effect, including adverse effects, the clinical significance is undetermined.				
Quetiapine				
Inhibition of AP metabolism (CYP3A4)	*Antidepressants*	*Anti-infectives*	*Miscellaneous*	↑ AP effect
	Fluvoxamine	Clarithromycin	Diltiazem	↑ SE
		Erythromycin	Cimetidine	
	HIV Protease Inhibitors	Fluconazole	Grapefruit juice	
	Indinavir	Ketoconazole	Verapamil	
	Nelfinavir	Itraconazole		
	Ritonavir			
Induction of AP metabolism	*Antiepileptics*	*Anti-infectives*	*Herbals*	↓ AP effect
	Carbamazepine	Rifampin	St. John's wort	
	Oxcarbazepine			
	Phenobarbital	*Miscellaneous*		
	Phenytoin	Glucocorticoids		
		Modafinil		
Perphenazine and Risperidone				
Note: Because risperidone's metabolite formed through CYP2D6 metabolism is active (paliperidone), the clinical significance of metabolic drug interactions with risperidone is undetermined.				
Inhibition of AP metabolis (CYP2D6)	*Antidepressants*	*Miscellaneous*		↑ AP effect
	Bupropion	Chlorpheniramine		↑ SE
	Duloxetine	Quinidine		
	Fluoxetine	Diphenhydramine		
	Paroxetine	Cimetidine		
		Haloperidol		
		Hydroxyzine		
		Quinidine		
Induction of AP metabolism	Dexamethasone			↓ AP effect
	Rifampin			
Ziprasidone				
The bioavailability of ziprasidone is increased twofold when it is taken with food. Consistent administration with food is recommended.				

AP, antipsychotic; DA, dopamine; EPS, extrapyramidal symptoms; 5-HT, serotonin; SE, side effect; SSRI, serotonin selective reuptake inhibitor; TCAs, tricyclic antidepressants.

The assistance of Jessica Wu, PharmD in preparing this table is acknowledged.

EVALUATION OF THERAPEUTIC OUTCOMES

Assessment of response has traditionally been done subjectively or empirically (a relative sense of how the clinician feels the patient is doing). A formal mental status examination (MSE) is used to structure the patient interview and focus on items related to appearance, mood, sensorium, intellectual functioning, and thought processes. However, the MSE is not specific for the measurement of drug response. ⑩ Clinicians should be trained to use simple, standardized psychiatric rating scales to assist in objectively rating patient drug responses.[39,119] The Brief Psychiatric Rating Scale (BPRS) and the Positive and Negative Symptom Scale (PANSS) were developed for use in clinical trials as research tools to quantify symptoms and improvement seen with antipsychotic treatment.[119] Objectively, the use of a numeric indicator (e.g., 20%, 30%, or 40% reduction in BPRS score) has been used to quantify overall symptom reduction and classify patients according to different degrees of response. However, these types of rating scales are too long and unwieldy to be routinely used within the time constraints of most clinical practices. Symptom scales used in clinical practice

TABLE 70-10 Brief Clinical Assessments for Monitoring Antipsychotic Response in Schizophrenia

4-Item Positive Symptom Rating Scale (PSRS)								
Use each item's anchor points to rate the patient.								
1. Suspiciousness	NA[a]	1	2	3	4	5	6	7
2. Unusual thought content	NA	1	2	3	4	5	6	7
3. Hallucinations	NA	1	2	3	4	5	6	7
4. Conceptual disorganization	NA	1	2	3	4	5	6	7
Each item is scored from 1 (not present) to 7 (extremely severe)							SCORE: ______	
Brief Negative Symptom Assessment (BNSA)								
Use each item's anchor points to rate the patient.								
1. Prolonged time to respond	1	2	3	4	5	6		
2. Emotion: Unchanging facial expression, blank, expressionless face	1	2	3	4	5	6		
3. Reduced social drive	1	2	3	4	5	6		
4. Poor grooming and hygiene	1	2	3	4	5	6		
Each item is scored from 1 (normal) to 6 (severe)					SCORE: ______			

[a]NA, not able to be assessed

To enhance consistency in ratings, the structured probes in the Administration Manual should be used each time the scales are used. The complete Administration Manual for the PSRS and the BNSA can be accessed from the appendices in the TIMA Procedure Manual: Schizophrenia Module at *http://www.mhmr.state.tx.us/centraloffice/medicaldirector/timasczman.pdf*.

This rating scale and the administration manual were created for the State of Texas, and they are in the public domain. They can be used with appropriate referencing and credit to the authors and the Texas Department of State Health Services.

Data from Miller et al.[39,119]

must be sufficiently brief to be used during an ordinary clinic visit (e.g., 15 to 30 minutes) while measuring both positive and negative symptoms, and being sufficiently representative of overall symptomatology. The four-item Positive Symptom Rating Scale and the Brief Negative Symptom Assessment are brief scales that meet such criteria (Table 70–10).[39,119] It is increasingly recognized that clinicians should be examining cognition as an outcome in treatment of schizophrenia. However, a brief cognition battery has recently been developed and validated, and it can be completed in 15 to 20 minutes.[120]

Similarly, the pharmacotherapeutic plan should include specific monitoring parameters for potential side effects. The plan should include how the potential side effect will be evaluated, and the frequency of assessment (e.g., daily or weekly). Given the risk of weight gain, diabetes, and lipid abnormalities associated with many of the SGAs, a consensus task force led by the American Diabetes Association recommends the following baseline parameters before beginning antipsychotics: family history, weight, height, body mass index, waist circumference, blood pressure, fasting plasma glucose, and fasting lipid profile.[72] They also recommend followup monitoring of these parameters after beginning or changing SGAs. Weight should be monitored monthly for the first 3 months, and quarterly thereafter. The other parameters should be assessed at the end of 3 months and then annually. If normal, serum lipids can be monitored less often. Self-assessments can be a useful adjunct in treating the patient. Although the patient with schizophrenia may not always be accurate in evaluating symptom severity, the use of patient self-assessments increases patient engagement in care, enhances therapeutic alliance, and gives the clinician an opportunity to identify misconceptions the patient can have regarding symptoms associated with the illness, medication side effects, and the like.[46,119] Traditionally, clinicians have often accepted partial symptom response in schizophrenia as success, and have not been aggressive in attempting to achieve greater symptomatic remission. The advent of multiple different SGAs with varying, but overall favorable, side-effect profiles should encourage clinicians to be more assertive in attempting to achieve symptom remission. This is also consistent with an increasing focus on remission as a goal of treatment and evolving recovery movements with an increasing emphasis on consumerism in the care of the severely mentally ill.[24,25]

CONCLUSIONS

Schizophrenia is a complex disease with multiple ramifications for patients and their families. Treatment issues remain clouded by the fact that the etiology of the illness is unknown. It is clear, however, that no single treatment modality is adequate to properly manage a patient with schizophrenia. Antipsychotics are the bedrock of treatment. SGAs have substantially advanced the care of people with schizophrenia. However, notwithstanding such advances, the SGAs are not a panacea and have multiple adverse effects in addition to the limitations of their efficacy. However, when used within the context of multidisciplinary treatment, SGAs improve positive and negative symptoms and cognition so that patients can appropriately participate in psychosocial rehabilitation programs. Scientific advances continue to expand our understanding of CNS physiology and the abnormalities present in schizophrenia. Advances in our understanding of the pathophysiology of schizophrenia should, in turn, result in the development of treatments that are more specific and more effective. In practice, it is mandatory that clinicians appropriately use their expanding armamentarium. It is important that clinicians appreciate the pharmacodynamic basis for treatment interventions so that they can effectively design and implement rational pharmacotherapeutic regimens. Finally, it is critical that clinicians more objectively evaluate individual patient response to medication so that treatment can be optimized. With these strategies, the gap between practice and science can be narrowed and patients' lives benefited.

ABBREVIATIONS

AIMS: abnormal Involuntary Movement Scale

ANC: absolute neutrophil count

BLM: buccal-lingual-masticatory

BPRS: Brief Psychiatric Rating Scale

CAT: computed axial tomography

CATIE: Clinical Antipsychotic Trials of Intervention Effectiveness study

CK: creatine kinase

CYP: cytochrome P450

CNS: central nervous system

DA: dopamine

DISCUS: Dyskinesia Identification System: Condensed User Scale

DSM-IV-TR: Diagnostic and Statistical Manual of Mental Disorders, 4th edition, Text Revision

ECG: electrocardiogram
ECT: electroconvulsive therapy
EEG: electroencephalogram
EPS: extrapyramidal side effect
FDA: Food and Drug Administration
FGA: first generation antipsychotic
GABA: γ-aminobutyric acid
5-HT: serotonin
LFT: liver function test
MRI: magnetic resonance imaging
MSE: mental status examination
msec: millisecond
NAMI: National Alliance for the Mentally Ill
NMDA: N-methyl-D-aspartate
NMS: neuroleptic malignant syndrome
PANSS: Positive and Negative Symptom Scale
PET: positron emission tomography
SGA: second-generation antipsychotic
SSRI: serotonin specific reuptake inhibitor
WBC: white blood cell

REFERENCES

1. American Psychiatric Association. Schizophrenia and other psychotic disorders. In: Diagnostic and Statistical Manual of Mental Disorders, 4th ed., Text Revision. Washington, DC: American Psychiatric Association, 2000:297–319.
2. Jones P, Buckley P. Schizophrenia. London: Mosby, 2006.
3. Harrison P. The neuropathology of schizophrenia. A critical review of the data and their interpretation. Brain 1999;122:593–624.
4. Weinberger D. Schizophrenia as a neurodevelopmental disorder. In: Weinberger DR, Hirsch SR, eds. Schizophrenia. Oxford: Blackwell Science, 2003:326–348.
5. Brown AS, Susser ES. In utero infection and adult schizophrenia. Ment Retard Dev Disabil Res Rev 2002;8:51–57.
6. Mahadik, SP, Evans DR. Is schizophrenia a metabolic brain disorder? Membrane phospholipid dysregulation and its therapeutic implications. Psychiatr Clin North Am 2003;26:41–63.
7. Mathalon DH, Sullivan EV, Lim KO, Pfefferbaum A. Progressive brain volume changes and the clinical course of schizophrenia in men: A longitudinal magnetic resonance imaging study. Arch Gen Psychiatry 2001;58:148–157.
8. Ho BC, Andreasen NC, Nopoulos P, et al. Progressive structural brain abnormalities and their relationships to clinical outcome: A longitudinal magnetic resonance imaging study early in schizophrenia. Arch Gen Psychiatry 2003;60:585–594.
9. McClure RK, Lieverman JA. Neurodevelopmental and neurodegenerative hypothesis of schizophrenia: A review and critique. Curr Opin Psychiatry 2003;16(Suppl 2):S15–S28.
10. Buckley PF, Mahadik S, Evans D, Stirewalt E. Causes, course, and neurodevelopment of schizophrenia. Current Psychosis and Therapeutic Reports 2003;1:41–49.
11. McDonald C, Murphy KC. The new genetics of schizophrenia. Psychiatr Clin North Am 2003;26:41–63.
12. Wei J, Jemmings GP. The NOTCH4 locus is associated with susceptibility to schizophrenia. Nat Genet 2002;25:376–377.
13. Novak G, Kim D, Seeman P, Tallerico T. Schizophrenia and Nogo: Elevated mRNA in cortex, and high prevalence of a homozygous CAA insert. Brain Res Mol Brain Res 2002;107:183–189.
14. Weickert, CS Straub RE, McClintock BW, et al. Human dysbindin (DTNBP1) gene expression in normal brain and in schizophrenia prefrontal cortex and midbrain. Arch Gen Psychiatry 2004:61;544–555.
15. Suarez BK, Duan J, Sanders AR, et al. Genomewide linkage scan of 409 European-ancestry and African American families with schizophrenia: Suggestive evidence of linkage at 8p23.3-p21.2 and 11p13.1-q14.1 in the combined sample. Am J Hum Genet 2006;78:315–333.
16. Velakoulis D, Wood SJ, Wong MT, et al. Hippocampal and amygdala volumes according to psychosis stage and diagnosis. A magnetic resonance imaging study of chronic schizophrenia, first-episode psychosis, and ultra-high risk individuals. Arch Gen Psychiatry 2006:63:139–149.
17. Lieberman JA, Bymaster F, Mahadik SP, Weinberger DR. Neurobiology of schizophrenia and antipsychotic effects. Biol Psychiatry, in press.
18. Mahadik SP, Pillai A. A Comparison of Typical versus Atypical Antipsychotic Drugs: Effects of Sub-chronic and Long-term Treatment of Neurotrophic Factors and Neurogenesis. Biol Psychiatry, in press.
19. Lieberman JA, Tollesfson GD, Zipursky R, et al. Antipsychotic drug effects on brain morphology in first-episode psychosis. Arch Gen Psychiatry 2005;62(4):361–70.
20. Buckley PF. Schizophrenia and substance abuse. J Clin Psychiatry, submitted for publication.
21. Narendran R, Frankle WG, Keefe R, et al. Altered prefrontal dopaminergic function in chronic recreational ketamine users. Am J Psychiatry 2005;162:2352–2359.
22. Meltzer HY. What's atypical about atypical antipsychotic drugs? Curr Opin Pharmacol 2004;4:53–57.
23. Lehman AF, Lieberman JA, Dixon LB, et al. American Psychiatric Association Practice Guidelines; Work Group on Schizophrenia. Practice guideline for the treatment of patients with schizophrenia, 2nd ed. Am J Psychiatry 2004;161(2 Suppl):1–56.
24. President's New Freedom Commission on Mental Health. Achieving the Promise: Transforming Mental Health Care in America. Final Report. DHHS Pub. No. SMA-03-3832. Rockville, MD: 2003.
25. Improving the Quality of Health Care for Mental and Substance-Use Conditions: Quality Chasm Series. Committe on Crossing the Quality Chasm: Adaptation to Mental Health and Addictive Disorders. Institute of Medicine, National Academies Press, Rockville, MD 2005.
26. Moore TA, Buchanan RW, Buckley PF, et al. The Texas Medication Algorithm Project antipsychotic algorithm for schizophrenia: 2006 update. J Clin Psychiatry 2007;68:1751–1762.
27. Lieberman JA, Stroup TS, McEvoy JP, et al. Effectiveness of antipsychotic drugs in patients with chronic schizophrenia. N Engl J Med 2005;353:1209–1223.
28. Csernansky JG, Mahmoud R, Brenner R. Risperidone-USA-7 group: A comparison of risperidone and haloperidol for the prevention of relapse in patients with schizophrenia. N Engl J Med 2002;346:16–22.
29. Kane J, Canas F, Kramer M, et al. Treatment of schizophrenia with paliperidone extended-release tablets: A 6-week placebo-controlled trial. Schizophr Res 2007;90:147–61.
30. Meltzer H, Kramer M, Gassmann-Mayer C, et al. Efficacy and tolerability of oral paliperidone extended-release tablets in the treatment of acute schizophrenia: Pooled data from three 6-week placebo-controlled studies [poster]. Presented at the Collegium Internationale Neuro-Psychopharmacologium Congress; July 9–13, 2006; Chicago, IL.
31. Small JG, Hirsch SR, Arvanitis LA, et al. Quetiapine in patients with schizophrenia. A high- and low-dose double-blind comparison with placebo. Arch Gen Psychiatry 1997;54:549–557.
32. Daniel DG, Zimbroff DL, Potkin SG, et al. Ziprasidone 80 mg/day and 160 mg/day in the acute exacerbation of schizophrenia and schizoaffective disorder: A 6-week placebo-controlled trial. Neuropsychopharmacology 1999;20:491–505.
33. De Leon A, Patel NC, Crismon ML. Aripiprazole: A comprehensive review of its pharmacology, clinical efficacy, and tolerability. Clin Ther 2004;26:649–666.
34. Green AL, Canuso CM, Brenner MJ, Wojcik JD. Detection and management of comorbidity in patients with schizophrenia. Psychiatr Clin North Am 2003;26:115–139.
35. Awad AG. Drug therapy in schizophrenia: Variability of outcome and prediction of response. Can J Psychiatry 1989;34:711–720.
36. Van Putten T, Marder SR. Behavioral toxicity of antipsychotic drugs. J Clin Psychiatry 1987;48(Suppl 9):13–19.
37. Lenz T, Robinson D, Su K, et al. DRD2 Promoter region variation as a predictor of sustained response to antipsychotic medication in first-episode schizophrenia. Am J Psychiatry 2006;163:529–536.

38. Miller D, Ellingrod V, Holman TL, et al. Clozapine-induced weight gain associated with 5HT2C receptor–759C/T polymorphism. Am J Med Genet B Neuropsychiatr Genet 2005;133:97–100.
39. Miller AL, Hall CS, Crismon ML, Chiles J. TIMA procedural manual: schizophrenia algorithm. Austin, TX, Texas Department of Mental Health and Mental Retardation. 2003, *http://www.dshs.state.tx.us/mhprograms/timasczman.pdf*.
40. Leucht S, Barnes TR, Kissling W, et al. Relapse prevention in schizophrenia with new-generation antipsychotics: A systematic review and exploratory meta-analysis of randomized, controlled trials. Am J Psychiatry 2003;160:1209–1222.
41. Harrison TS, Goa KL. Long-acting risperidone: A review of its use in schizophrenia. CNS Drugs 2004;18:113–132.
42. Ereshefsky L, Saklad SR, Jann MW, et al. Future of depot neuroleptic therapy: Pharmacokinetics and pharmacodynamic approaches. J Clin Psychiatry 1984;45(5 pt 2):50–59.
43. Ereshefsky L, Toney G, Saklad SR, Seidel DR. A loading dose strategy for converting from oral to depot haloperidol. Hosp Community Psychiatry 1993;44:1155–1161.
44. Hamann GL, Egan TM, Wells BG, et al. Injection site reactions after intramuscular administration of haloperidol decanoate 100 mg/mL. J Clin Psychiatry 1990;51:502–504.
45. Cramer JA, Rosenheck R. Compliance with medication regimens for mental and physical disorders. Psychiatr Serv 1998;49:196–201.
46. Toprac MG, Rush AJ, Conner TM, et al. The Texas Medication Algorithm Project patient and family education program: A consumer-guided initiative. J Clin Psychiatry 2000;61:477–486.
47. O'Donnell C, Donohoe G, Sharkey L, et al. Compliance therapy: A randomised controlled trial in schizophrenia. BMJ 2003;327:834.
48. Kane J, Honigfeld G, Singer J, et al. Clozapine for the treatment-resistant schizophrenic: A double-blind comparison with chlorpromazine. Arch Gen Psychiatry 1988;45:789–796.
49. Spears NM, Leadbetter RA, Shutty MS. Clozapine treatment in polydipsia and intermittent hyponatremia. J Clin Psychiatry 1996;57:123–128.
50. Canales PL, Olsen J, Miller AL, Crismon ML. The role of antipsychotic polypharmacotherapy in the treatment of schizophrenia. CNS Drugs 1999;12:179–188.
51. Leucht S, Kissling W, McGrath J. Lithium for schizophrenia revisited: A systematic review and meta-analysis of randomized controlled trials. J Clin Psychiatry 2004;65:177–186.
52. Casey DE, Daniel DG, Wassef AA, et al. Effect of divalproex combined with olanzapine or risperidone in patients with an acute exacerbation of schizophrenia. Neuropsychopharmacology 2003;28:182–192.
53. Silver H. Selective serotonin reuptake inhibitor augmentation in the treatment of negative symptoms of schizophrenia. Int Clin Psychopharmacol 2003;18:305–313.
54. Kapur S, Roy P, Daskalakis J, Remington G. Increased dopamine D_2 receptor occupancy and elevated prolactin level associated with addition of haloperidol to clozapine. Am J Psychiatry 2001;158:311–314.
55. Kapur S, Mamo D. Half a century of antipsychotics and still a central role for dopamine D_2 receptors. Prog Neuropsychopharmacol Biol Psychiatry 2003;27:1081–1090.
56. Meltzer L, Li Z, Kaneda Y, Ichikawa J. Serotonin receptors: Their key role in drugs to treat schizophrenia. Prog Neuropsychopharmacol Biol Psychiatry 2003;27:1159–1172.
57. Nyberg S, Eriksson B, Oxenstierna G, et al. Suggested minimal effective dose of risperidone based on PET measured D_2 and 5-HT_{2A} receptor occupancy in schizophrenic patients. Am J Psychiatry 1999;156:869–875.
58. Kapur S, Zipursky RB, Remington G. Clinical and theoretical implications of 5-HT_2 and D_2 receptor occupancy of clozapine, risperidone, and olanzapine in schizophrenia. Am J Psychiatry 1999;156:286–293.
59. Stahl SM, Shayegan DK. The psychopharmacology of ziprasidone: Receptor-binding properties and real-world psychiatric practice. J Clin Psychiatry 2003;64(Suppl 19):6–12.
60. Mauri MC, Volonteri LS, Colasanti A, et al. Clinical pharmacokinetics of atypical antipsychotics: a critical review of the relationship between plasma concentrations and clinical response. Clin Pharmacokinet 2007;46:359–388.
61. Bradford LD. CYP2D6 allele frequency in European Caucasians, Asians, Africans, and their descendants. Pharmacogenetics 2002;3:229–243.
62. Zito JM, Sofair JB, Jaeger J. Self-reported neuroendocrine effects of APs in women: A pilot study. DICP 1990;24:176–180.
63. Allison DB, Mentore JL, Heo M, et al. Antipsychotic induced weight gain: A comprehensive research synthesis. Am J Psychiatry 1999;156:1686–1696.
64. Patel NC, Kistler JL, James EB, Crismon ML. A retrospective analysis of olanzapine and quetiapine on weight and body mass index in children and adolescents. Pharmacotherapy 2004;24:824–830.
65. Miller AL, Dassori A, Ereshefsky L, Crismon ML. Recent issues and developments in antipsychotic use. In: Dunner DL, Rosenbaum JF, eds. Psychiatric Clinics of North America Annual Review of Drug Therapy 2001. Philadelphia, PA: WB Saunders, 2001;8:209–235.
66. Harris EC, Barraclough B. Excess mortality of mental disorder. Br J Psychiatry 1998;173:11–53.
67. Meyer JM. Cardiovascular illness and hyperlipidemia in patients with schizophrenia. In: Meyer JM, Nasarallah HA, eds. Medical Illness and Schizophrenia. Washington, DC: American Psychiatric Press, 2003:53–80.
68. Lasser K, Boyd JW, Woolhandler S, et al. Smoking and mental illness: A population-based prevalence study. JAMA 2000;284:2606–10.
69. Wirshing D, Boyd J, Meng LR, et al. The effects of novel antipsychotics on glucose and lipid levels. J Clin Psychiatry 2002;63:856–865.
70. Weiden PJ, Ross R. Why do patients stop their antipsychotic medications? A guide for family and friends. J Psychiatr Pract 2002;8:413–416.
71. Vreeland B, Minsky S, Menza M, et al. A program for managing weight gain associated with atypical antipsychotics. Psychiatr Serv 2003;54:1155–1157.
72. American Diabetes Association. Consensus development conference on antipsychotic drugs and obesity and diabetes. Diabetes Care 2004;27:596–601.
73. Newcomer JW. Second-generation (atypical) antipsychotics and metabolic effects: A comprehensive literature review. CNS Drugs 2005;19(S1):1–93.
74. Henderson DC, Cagliero E, Gray C, et al. Clozapine, diabetes mellitus, weight gain and lipid abnormalities: A five-year naturalistic study. Am J Psychiatry 2000;157:975–981.
75. Newcomer JW. Second-generation (atypical) antipsychotics and metabolic effects: A comprehensive literature review. CNS Drugs 2005;19(S1):1–93.
76. Church CO, Stevens DL, Fugate SE. Diabetic ketoacidosis associated with aripiprazole. Diabet Med 2005;22:1440–3.
77. Reddymasu S, Bahta E, Levine S, et al. Elevated lipase and diabetic ketoacidosis associated with aripiprazole. JOP 2006;7:303–5.
78. Zyprexa (olanzapine). MedWatch, U.S. Food and Drug Administration. 2004, *http://www.fda.gov/medwatch/SAFETY/2004/safety04.htm#zyprexa*.
79. Tandon R. Safety and tolerability: how do newer generation "atypical" antipsychotics compare? Psychiatr Q 2002;73:297–311.
80. Nasrallah HA. Metabolic findings from the CATIE trial and their relation to tolerability. CNS Spectr 2006;11(S7):32–9.
81. Holloman LC, Marder SR. Management of acute extrapyramidal effects induced by antipsychotic drugs. Am J Health Syst Pharm 1997;54:2461–2477.
82. Wells BG, Marken PA, Rickman LA, et al. Characterizing anticholinergic abuse in community mental health. J Clin Psychopharmacol 1989;9:431–435.
83. Sprague RL, Kalachnik JE. Reliability, validity, and a total score cutoff for the Dyskinesia Identification System Condensed User Scale (DISCUS) with mentally ill and mentally retarded populations. Psychopharmacol Bull 1991;27:51–58.
84. Egan MF, Apud J, Wyatt RJ. Treatment of tardive dyskinesia. Schizophr Bull 1997;23:583–609.
85. Tandon R, Kasper S, Kane J, Juncos J. The scourge of extrapyramidal side effects: Have atypical antipsychotics solved the problem? J Clin Psychiatry 2000;61:955–962.
86. Correll CU, Leucht S, Kane JM. Lower risk for tardive dyskinesia associated with second-generation antipsychotics: A systematic review of 1-year studies. Am J Psychiatry 2004;161:414–425.
87. Tamminga CA, Woerner MG. Clinical course and cellular pathology of tardive dyskinesia. In: Davis KL, Charney D, Coyle JT, Nemeroff C, eds. Neuropsychopharmacology: The Fifth Generation of Progress. Philadelphia, PA: Lippincott Williams & Wilkins, 2002:1831–1841.
88. Soares KV, McGrath JJ. Vitamin E for neuroleptic-induced tardive dyskinesia. Cochrane Database Syst Rev 2001;4:CD000209.

89. Bilder RM, Goldman RS, Volavka J, et al. Neurocognitive effects of clozapine, risperidone, and haloperidol in patients with chronic schizophrenia or schizoaffective disorder. Am J Psychiatry 2002;159:1018–1028.
90. Miller AL, Crismon ML, Rush AJ, et al. The Texas Medication Algorithm Project: clinical results for schizophrenia. Schizophr Bull 2004;30:627–47.
91. Pisani F, Oteri G, Costa C, et al. Effects of psychotropic drugs on seizure threshold. Drug Saf 2002;25:91–110.
92. Simpson GM, Pi EH, Sramek JJ. Adverse effects of antipsychotic agents. Drugs 1981;21:138–151.
93. Buckley PF, Adityanjee A, Sajatovic M. Neuroleptic malignant syndrome. In: Bashier Y, et al., eds. Textbook of Neuromuscular Disorders. Philadelphia, PA: Butterworth-Heinemann, 2001:1264–1278.
94. Crismon ML. Psychotropic drugs in the elderly: Principles of use. Am Pharm 1990;NS30:57–63.
95. Oshika T. Ocular adverse effects of neuropsychiatric agents: Incidence and management. Drug Saf 1995;12:256–263.
96. Shahzad S, Suleman MI, Shahab H, et al. Cataract occurrence with antipsychotic drugs. Psychosomatics 2002;43:354–359.
97. Regal RE, Billi JE, Glazer HM. Phenothiazine-induced cholestatic jaundice. Clin Pharm 1987;6:787–794.
98. Linares TF, Hernandez PC, Boscacoma RN. Acute cholestatic hepatitis associated with risperidone. Int J Psychiatry Med 2005;35:199–205.
99. Ozcanli T, Erdogan A, Ozdemir S, et al. Severe liver enzyme elevations after three years of olanzapine treatment: a case report and review of olanzapine associated hepatotoxicity Prog Neuropsychopharmacol Biol Psychiatry 2006;30:1163–1166.
100. Lin CC, Bai YM, Chen JY, et al. A retrospective study of clozapine and urinary incontinence in Chinese in-patients. Acta Psychiatr Scand 1999;100:158–161.
101. Knegtering H, van der Moolen AEGM, Castelein S, et al. What are the effects of antipsychotics on sexual dysfunctions and endocrine functioning? Psychoneuroendocrinology 2003;28(Suppl 2):109–123.
102. Hall RL, Smith AG, Ewards JG. Haematological safety of antipsychotic drugs. Expert Opin Drug Saf 2003;2:395–399.
103. Alvir JMJ, Lieberman JA, Safferman AZ, et al. Clozapine-induced agranulocytosis: Incidence and risk factors in the United States. N Engl J Med 1993;329:162–167.
104. Meltzer HY, Fatemi SH. Treatment of schizophrenia. In: Schatzberg AF, Nemeroff CB, eds. Textbook of Psychopharmacology, 2nd ed. Washington, DC: American Psychiatric Press, 1998:747–774.
105. Davydov L, Botts SR. Clozapine-induced hypersalivation. Ann Pharmacother 2000;34:662–665.
106. Perry PJ, Alexander B, Liskow B. Psychotropic Drug Handbook, 8th ed. Washington, DC: American Psychiatric Press, 2007:1–139.
107. American Academy of Pediatrics Committee on Drugs. Use of psychoactive medication during pregnancy and possible effects on the fetus and newborn. Pediatrics 2000;105:880–887.
108. Ernst CL, Goldberg JF. The reproductive safety profile of mood stabilizers, atypical antipsychotics, and broad-spectrum psychotropics. J Clin Psychiatry 2002;63(Suppl 4):42–55.
109. Hartigan-Go K, Bateman DN, Nyberg G, et al. Concentration-related pharmacodynamic effects of thioridazine and its metabolites in humans. Clin Pharmacol Ther 1996;60:543–553.
110. Spina E, de Leon J. Metabolic drug interactions with newer antipsychotics: a comparative review. Basic Clin Pharmacol Toxicol 2007; 100:4–22.
111. Ereshefsky L. Pharmacokinetics and drug interactions: Update for new antipsychotics. J Clin Psychiatry 1996;57(Suppl 11):12–25.
112. DeVane CL, Markowitz JS. Antipsychotics. In: Levy RH, Thummel KE, Trager WF, et al. Metabolic Drug Interactions. Philadelphia, PA: Lippincott Williams & Wilkins, 2000:245–258.
113. Prakash C, Kamel A, Cui D, et al. Identification of the major human liver cytochrome P450 isoform(s) responsible for the formation of the primary metabolites of ziprasidone and prediction of possible drug interactions. Br J Clin Pharmacol 2000;49(Suppl 1):35S–42S.
114. Liu GG, Sun SX, Christensen DB, Luo X. Cost comparisons of olanzapine and risperidone in treating schizophrenia. Ann Pharmacother 2004;38:134–141.
115. Rosenheck RA, Leslie DL, Sindelar J, et al. Cost-effectiveness of second-generation antipsychotics and perphenazine in a randomized trial of treatment for chronic schizophrenia. Am J Psychiatry 2006;163:2080–2089.
116. Hayhurst KP, Brown P, Lewis SW. The cost-effectiveness of clozapine: A controlled, population-based mirror-image study. J Psychopharmacol 2002;16:169–175.
117. Duggan A, Warner J, Knapp M, Kerwin R. Modeling the impact of clozapine on suicide in patients with treatment-resistant schizophrenia. Br J Psychiatry 2003;182:505–508.
118. Rascati KL, Johnsrud MT, Crismon ML, et al. Olanzapine versus risperidone in the treatment of schizophrenia: A comparison of costs among Texas Medicaid patients. Pharmacoeconomics 2003;21;683–697.
119. Miller AL, Chiles JA, Chiles JK, et al. The TMAP schizophrenia algorithms. J Clin Psychiatry 1999;60:649–657.
120. Velligan DI, DiCocco M, Bow-Thomas C, et al. A brief cognitive assessment (BCA) for use with schizophrenia patients in a community clinic. Schizophr Res 2004;71:273–283.

CHAPTER 71

Depressive Disorders

CHRISTIAN J. TETER, JUDITH C. KANDO, BARBARA G. WELLS, AND PEGGY E. HAYES

KEY CONCEPTS

1. Extensive treatment guidelines are available to assist in the treatment of major depressive disorder, including medication management. Clinicians treating individuals with major depressive disorder should be familiar with these guidelines.
2. When evaluating a patient for the presence of depression, it is essential to rule out medical causes of depression and drug-induced depression.
3. The goal of pharmacologic treatment of depression is the resolution of current symptoms (i.e., remission) and the prevention of further episodes of depression (i.e., relapse or recurrence).
4. When counseling patients with depression who are receiving antidepressant medications, the patient should be informed that adverse effects might occur immediately, whereas resolution of symptoms can take 2 to 4 weeks or longer. Adherence to the treatment plan is essential to a successful outcome, and tools to help increase medication adherence should be discussed with each patient.
5. Antidepressants are generally considered equally efficacious for the treatment of major depressive disorder. Therefore, other factors, such as age, side effects, and past history of response, are used to guide clinicians in their selection of medication management.
6. When determining if a patient has been nonresponsive to a particular pharmacotherapeutic intervention, it must be determined whether the patient has received an adequate dose for an adequate duration and whether the patient has been medication adherent.
7. When evaluating response to an antidepressant, in addition to target signs and symptoms, the clinician must consider quality-of-life issues such as role, social functioning, and occupational function. In addition, the tolerability of the agent should be assessed because the occurrence of side effects can lead to medication nonadherence, especially given the chronicity of the disease and need for long-term medication management.

A diagnosis of major depressive disorder is given when an individual experiences one or more major depressive episodes without a history of manic, mixed, or hypomanic episodes. A major depressive episode is defined by the criteria listed in the *Diagnostic and Statistical Manual of Mental Disorders, Fourth Edition, Text Revision* (*DSM-IV-TR*), published by the American Psychiatric Association.[1] Depression is associated with significant functional disability, morbidity, and mortality.

Newer generations of antidepressants have provided pharmacologic interventions that are effective and better tolerated than older agents such as the tricyclic antidepressants (TCAs) and the monoamine oxidase inhibitors (MAOIs). In addition, substantial efforts have been undertaken to improve the ability of clinicians to recognize and appropriately treat the signs and symptoms of depression. This chapter focuses exclusively on the diagnosis and treatment of major depressive disorder.

❶ In the absence of well-accepted evidence-based medicine for the medication management of major depressive disorder, the reader is referred to the *Practice Guideline for the Treatment of Patients with Major Depressive Disorder, Second Edition*, which is available at www.psych.org. This extensive document is a practical guide to the management of depression based on the best available data as well as clinical consensus.[2]

Learning objectives, review questions, and other resources can be found at **www.pharmacotherapyonline.com.**

EPIDEMIOLOGY

The true prevalence of depressive disorders in the United States is unknown. The National Comorbidity Survey Replication found that 16.2% of the population studied had a history of major depressive disorder in their lifetime, and more than 6.6% had an episode within the past 12 months.[3] Women are at increased risk of depression from early adolescence until their mid-50s, with a lifetime rate that is 1.7 to 2.7 times greater than for men.[4] Although depression can occur at any age, adults 18 to 29 years of age experience the highest rates of major depression during any given year.[3] The estimated lifetime prevalence of major depression in individuals aged 65 to 80 years recently was reported to be 20.4% in women and 9.6% in men.[5] Depressive disorders are common during adolescence, with comorbid substance abuse, suicide attempts, and deaths occurring frequently in these young patients.[6,7] Depressive disorders and suicide tend to occur within families. For example, approximately 8% to 18% of patients with major depression have at least one first-degree relative (father, mother, brother, or sister) with a history of depression, compared with 5.6% of the first-degree relatives of those without depression.[8] Furthermore, first-degree relatives of patients with depression are 1.5 to 3 times more likely to develop depression than normal controls.[1,8,9] A recent meta-analysis found that the heritability of liability for major depression was 37%, whereas the remaining 63% of the variance in liability was caused by individual-specific environment.[10] Therefore major depressive disorder is relatively common, occurs more frequently in women than men, and prevalence is influenced by both genetic and environmental factors.

ETIOLOGY

The etiology of depressive disorders is too complex to be totally explained by a single social, developmental, or biologic theory. Several factors appear to work together to cause or precipitate depressive disorders. The symptoms reported by patients with major depression consistently reflect changes in brain monoamine neurotransmitters, specifically norepinephrine (NE), serotonin (5-hydroxytryptamine [5-HT]), and dopamine (DA).[11–13]

PATHOPHYSIOLOGY

BIOGENIC AMINE HYPOTHESIS

Several years before the introduction of antidepressants, the cause of depression was linked to decreased brain levels of the neurotransmitters NE, 5-HT, and DA, although the actual cause remains unknown. This biogenic amine hypothesis evolved as a result of several observations made in the early 1950s. It was noted that the antihypertensive drug reserpine depleted neuronal storage granules of NE, 5-HT, and DA and produced clinically significant depression in 15% or more of patients.[14] Although the reuptake blockade of monoamines (e.g., NE and 5-HT) occurs immediately on administration of an antidepressant, the clinical antidepressant effects generally are not observed until after approximately 4 weeks of dosing.[15] This delay can be the result of a cascade of events from receptor occupancy to gene transcription.[16] This delay in onset of action has caused researchers to focus on the adaptive changes induced by antidepressants, as discussed below.[12]

THEORIES OF POSTSYNAPTIC CHANGES IN RECEPTOR SENSITIVITY

A more perplexing aspect of the observed effects of antidepressants is the discrepancy between monoamine reuptake blockade (immediate) and any measurable improvement in depressive symptoms (delayed therapeutic response).[11] Accordingly, theories that focus on adaptive (or chronic) changes in amine receptor systems compared with acute changes have emerged over the past decade.

In the mid-1970s it was recognized that chronic, but not acute, administration of antidepressants to animals caused desensitization of NE-stimulated cyclic adenosine monophosphate synthesis. In fact, for most antidepressants, downregulation of β-adrenergic receptors accompanies this desensitization.[17] Studies of many antidepressants have demonstrated that either desensitization or downregulation of NE receptors corresponds to a clinically relevant time course for antidepressant effects.[11] Other studies have revealed desensitization of presynaptic 5-HT_{1A} autoreceptors following chronic administration of antidepressants.[18] Thus a theory based on changes in receptor sensitivity provides a cogent explanation of the delayed onset of therapeutic response of antidepressant drugs.[11]

DYSREGULATION HYPOTHESIS

The dysregulation hypothesis incorporates the diversity of antidepressant activity with the adaptive changes occurring in receptor sensitization over several weeks.[19] In this theory, emphasis is placed on a failure of homeostatic regulation of neurotransmitter systems rather than on absolute increases or decreases in their activities. According to this hypothesis, effective antidepressant agents restore efficient regulation to the dysregulated neurotransmitter system.[19,20]

5-HT/NE LINK HYPOTHESIS

It is apparent that no single neurotransmitter theory of depression is adequate. The 5-HT/NE link hypothesis maintains that both the serotonergic and noradrenergic systems are involved in an antidepressant response.[17] This hypothesis is also consistent with the rationale of the postsynaptic alteration theory of depression, which emphasizes the importance of β-adrenergic receptor downregulation for achieving an antidepressant effect.[17] Furthermore, both serotonergic and noradrenergic medications downregulate β-adrenergic receptors, and there is a link between 5-HT and NE.[17] This implies that medications that are effective in the treatment of depression act at both of these neurotransmitter systems.

ROLE OF DA IN DEPRESSION

Traditional explanations of the biologic basis of depressive disorders have focused largely on NE and 5-HT; however, most of the evidence that coalesced into the biogenic amine hypothesis of depression does not clearly distinguish between NE and DA. There is an abundance of evidence suggesting that DA transmission is decreased in depression and that agents that increase dopaminergic transmission have been found to be effective antidepressants.[21] Specifically, studies suggest that increased DA transmission in the mesolimbic pathway account for at least part of the mechanism of action of antidepressant medications.[21] The mechanisms by which antidepressant drugs alter DA transmission remain unclear but can be mediated indirectly by primary actions at NE or 5-HT terminals. The complexity of the interaction between 5-HT, NE, and possibly DA is gaining greater appreciation, but a more in-depth understanding of the precise mechanism is needed.

BIOLOGIC MARKERS

Investigators continue to search for biologic or pharmacodynamic markers to assist in the diagnosis and treatment of depressed patients. Although no biologic marker has been discovered, several biologic abnormalities are present in many depressed patients. Approximately 45% to 60% of patients with major depression have a neuroendocrine abnormality, including hypersecretion of cortisol, lack of cortisol suppression after dexamethasone administration (i.e., a positive dexamethasone suppression test), or an abnormal or diminished thyroid-stimulating hormone response to the administration of thyrotropin-releasing hormone. The dexamethasone suppression test is the most specific measure of hypothalamic-pituitary-adrenal axis overactivity. Dexamethasone administration suppresses adrenal corticosteroid production in normal subjects for 24 hours. Failure of dexamethasone to suppress plasma cortisol concentrations indicates overactivity or dysregulation of the hypothalamic-pituitary-adrenal axis. Unfortunately, the high rate of false-positive and false-negative results limits the usefulness of testing for these markers, and has led to their relative lack of use in clinical practice.

Sleep studies conducted in a sleep laboratory in patients with major depression have identified several abnormalities that become more pronounced with advancing age. In depressed patients, the onset of rapid eye movement (REM) sleep occurs earlier during sleep (decreased REM latency), and there is a shift of REM sleep to the first half of the night. There also may be a decrease in the number of minutes spent in slow-wave sleep (stages 3 and 4), an increased number of awakenings during sleep, and early morning awakening.[22] However, sleep abnormalities occur in other psychiatric disorders as well and are not diagnostic for major depression.

TABLE 71-1 Common Medical Conditions, Substance Use Disorders, and Medications Associated with Depressive Symptoms

General medical conditions	Metabolic disorders	**Substance use disorders (including intoxication and withdrawal)**
Endocrine diseases	Electrolyte imbalance	Alcoholism
Hypothyroidism	Hypokalemia	Marijuana abuse and dependence
Addison or Cushing disease	Hyponatremia	Nicotine dependence
Deficiency states	Hepatic encephalopathy	Opiate abuse and dependence (e.g., heroin)
Pernicious anemia	Cardiovascular disease	Psychostimulant abuse and dependence (e.g., cocaine)
Wernicke encephalopathy	Coronary artery disease	**Drug therapy**
Severe anemia	Congestive heart failure	Antihypertensives
Infections	Myocardial infarction	Clonidine
AIDS	Neurologic disorders	Diuretics
Encephalitis	Alzheimer's disease	Guanethidine sulfate
Human immunodeficiency virus	Epilepsy	Hydralazine hydrochloride
Mononucleosis	Huntington's disease	Methyldopa
Sexually transmitted diseases	Multiple sclerosis	Propranolol
Tuberculosis	Pain	Reserpine
Collagen disorder	Parkinson's disease	**Hormonal therapy**
Systemic lupus erythematosus	Poststroke	Oral contraceptives
	Malignant disease	Steroids/adrenocorticotropic hormone
		Acne therapy
		Isotretinoin
		Other
		Interferon-β_{1a}

AIDS, acquired immune deficiency syndrome.
Data from American Psychiatric Association,[1] Sofuoglu et al.,[23] Patten and Barbui.[24]

CLINICAL PRESENTATION

❷ When a patient presents with depressive symptoms, it is necessary to investigate the possibility of a contributing medical or drug-induced etiology (Table 71–1). In fact, in the *DSM-IV-TR* there is a diagnostic category for both "Mood Disorder Due to a General Medical Condition" and "Substance-Induced Mood Disorder."[1] For example, up to 40% of patients with certain neurological disorders (e.g., stroke, Alzheimer's disease) develop depressive symptoms at some point during the course of their neurologic illness.[1] Furthermore, individuals experiencing withdrawal from substances of abuse (e.g., cocaine) can present with depressive symptoms.[23] All depressed patients should have a complete physical examination, mental status examination, and basic laboratory workup, including a complete blood count with differential, thyroid function tests, and electrolyte determinations to identify any potential medical problems. Lastly, a complete medication review should be performed because several medications can contribute to depressive symptoms (see Table 71–1).[24] Once a medical condition or concomitant medication has been ruled out as the cause of the depressive symptoms, the patient should be evaluated for a major depressive disorder.

According to the *DSM-IV-TR*, a single major depressive episode is characterized by five or more of the symptoms described in Table 71–2. At least one of the symptoms is depressed mood (often an irritable mood in children or adolescents) or loss of interest or pleasure in nearly all activities.[1] These symptoms must have been present nearly every day for at least 2 weeks and must represent a change from the patient's previous level of functioning. The clinician must consider presenting symptoms, their duration, and the patient's current level of social, occupational, or other important areas of functioning. Significant stressors or life events can trigger depression in some individuals but not others; and there can be an important precipitant at the beginning of the disorder.[1] A patient diagnosed with major depressive disorder may have one or more recurrent episodes of major depression during their lifetime.

EMOTIONAL SYMPTOMS

A major depressive episode is characterized by a persistent, diminished ability to experience pleasure. A loss of interest and pleasure in usual activities, hobbies, or work is common. Patients appear sad or depressed, and they are often pessimistic and believe that nothing will help them feel better. The presence of feelings of worthlessness or inappropriate guilt can identify patients at risk for suicide.[25] Anxiety symptoms are present in almost 90% of depressed outpatients. Patients often have guilt feelings that are unrealistic, and these can reach delusional proportions. Patients can feel that they deserve punishment and can view their present illness as a punishment. A patient suffering from major depression with psychotic

TABLE 71-2 *DSM-IV-TR* Criteria for Major Depressive Episode

A. Five (or more) of the following symptoms have been present during the same 2-week period and represent a change from previous functioning; at least one of the symptoms is either (1) depressed mood or (2) loss of interest or pleasure.
Note: Do not include symptoms that are clearly caused by a general medical condition or mood-incongruent delusions or hallucinations.
1. Depressed mood most of the day nearly every day
2. Markedly diminished interest or pleasure in all, or almost all, activities most of the day nearly every day
3. Significant weight loss when not dieting or weight gain (e.g., a change of more than 5% of body weight in a month), or decrease or increase in appetite nearly every day
4. Insomnia or hypersomnia nearly every day
5. Psychomotor agitation or retardation nearly every day (observable by others, not merely subjective feelings of restlessness or being slowed down)
6. Fatigue or loss of energy nearly every day
7. Feelings of worthlessness or excessive or inappropriate guilt nearly every day
8. Diminished ability to think or concentrate, or indecisiveness, nearly every day
9. Recurrent thoughts of death (not just fear of dying), recurrent suicidal ideation without a specific plan, or a suicide attempt or a specific plan for committing suicide

B. The symptoms cause clinically significant distress or impairment in social, occupational, or other important areas of functioning.
C. The symptoms are not due to the direct physiologic effects of a substance (e.g., a drug of abuse, a medication) or a general medical condition (e.g., hypothyroidism).
D. The symptoms are not better accounted for by bereavement (i.e., after the loss of a loved one), the symptoms persist for longer than 2 months or are characterized by marked functional impairment, morbid preoccupation with worthlessness, suicidal ideation, psychotic symptoms, or psychomotor retardation.

DSM-IV-TR, *Diagnostic and Statistical Manual of Mental Disorders*, 4th ed., text revision.
Modified and reprinted with permission from American Psychiatric Association.[1]

features can hear voices (auditory hallucinations) saying that he or she is a bad person and that he or she should commit suicide. Depression with psychotic features can require hospitalization, especially if the patient becomes a danger to self or others.

PHYSICAL SYMPTOMS

Physical symptoms often motivate patients, especially the elderly, to seek medical attention. Chronic fatigue is a common complaint, with a decreased ability to perform normal daily tasks. Fatigue often appears worse in the morning and does not improve with rest. Complaints of pain, especially headache, often accompany fatigue.

Sleep disturbances generally present as frequent early morning awakening with difficulty returning to sleep. This can coexist with difficulty falling asleep and frequent nighttime awakening. Less frequently, depressed patients complain of increased sleep (hypersomnia), although they experience daytime exhaustion or fatigue.

Appetite disturbances, including complaints of decreased appetite, often result in substantial weight loss, especially in the elderly.[26] Some patients lose 0.9 kg (2 lb) or more per week without dieting. Other patients, especially in the ambulatory setting, might overeat and gain weight, although they actually might not enjoy eating. They might crave specific foods. Some patients exhibit gastrointestinal complaints, others cardiovascular complaints, especially palpitations. Patients frequently present with a loss of sexual interest or libido.[27]

INTELLECTUAL OR COGNITIVE SYMPTOMS

Intellectual or cognitive symptoms include a decreased ability to concentrate, slowed thinking, and a poor memory for recent events. Patients can appear confused and indecisive. Depression should be considered when cognitive symptoms are present in the elderly.[26]

PSYCHOMOTOR DISTURBANCES

Patients can appear noticeably slowed or retarded in physical movements, thought processes, and speech (psychomotor retardation). Conversely, depression can be accompanied by psychomotor agitation, manifesting as purposeless, restless motion (e.g., pacing, wringing of hands, or outbursts of shouting).

SUICIDE RISK EVALUATION AND MANAGEMENT

The Center for Disease Control lists suicide as the third leading cause of death in those aged 15 to 24 years and the second leading cause of death in those aged 25 to 34 years.[28] All patients diagnosed with major depression should be assessed for suicidal thoughts. Widely held myths regarding suicide include the belief that people are more likely to commit suicide if they are asked about it, that people who attempt or talk about suicide are just looking for attention and are not serious, that suicidal people are crazy, and that most suicides are caused by a sudden traumatic event.

Factors that increase the risk for suicide include (in order of decreasing frequency), suicidal plans/attempts, being of male gender, being single or living alone, inpatient status, and having feelings of hopelessness.[29] Other identified risk factors include alcohol/substance abuse, having a general medical condition, more work hours missed in the past week, and relationship difficulties.[30] The presence of a very detailed plan with the intention and ability to carry it out indicates a high risk of suicide. Although women attempt suicide two to three times more often than men, men succeed about three times more frequently. Suicide is almost twice as common in the elderly as in the general population.[31] This appears to be a result of more determination, carefully planned acts, and fewer warning signs.[31] To assess the severity of suicidal thoughts, the clinician must be sensitive to hints of suicidal ideation, including a change in personality, a sudden decision to make a will or give away possessions, and any recent purchase of a gun or obtaining (or hoarding) a large supply of medications or other potentially toxic substances. It is important to remember that the risk of suicide in those recovering from major depression can increase as they develop the energy and capacity to act on a plan made earlier in a course of illness. It is not always possible to predict whether or when a depressed person will attempt suicide.

When suicidal intent is suspected, it is important to ask, "Are you thinking about harming or killing yourself?" If the risk is significant, the patient must be referred immediately to an appropriate healthcare professional.

TREATMENT

Depressive Disorders

■ DESIRED OUTCOME

The goals of treatment are to reduce the symptoms of acute depression, facilitate the patient's return to a level of functioning before the onset of illness, and prevent further episodes of depression. Whether or not to hospitalize the patient is often the first decision that is made in consideration of the patient's risk of suicide, physical state of health, social support system, and presence of a psychotic and/or catatonic depression.

■ GENERAL APPROACH TO TREATMENT

❸ There are three phases of treatment to consider when treating patients with major depressive disorder: (1) the *acute* phase lasting from 6 to 10 weeks in which the goal is remission (i.e., absence of symptoms); (2) the *continuation* phase lasting 4 to 9 months after remission is achieved, in which the goal is to eliminate residual symptoms or prevent relapse (i.e., return of symptoms within 6 months of remission); and (3) the *maintenance* phase lasting at least 12 to 36 months in which the goal is to prevent recurrence (i.e., a separate episode of depression).[2,32] The risk of recurrence increases as the number of past episodes increase. The duration of antidepressant therapy depends on the risk of recurrence. Some investigators recommend lifelong maintenance therapy for persons at greatest risk for recurrence (persons younger than 40 years of age with two or more prior episodes and persons of any age with three or more prior episodes).[2]

❹ Educating the patient and his or her support system (e.g., family and friends) regarding the delay in antidepressant effects and the importance of adherence should occur before and during the entire course of treatment. The treatment of major depressive disorder generally includes nonpharmacologic and pharmacologic strategies, which are discussed in further detail below.

■ NONPHARMACOLOGIC THERAPY

In addition to pharmacologic interventions, psychotherapy should be employed whenever the patient is able and willing to participate. Psychotherapy alone is not recommended for the acute treatment of patients with severe and/or psychotic major depressive disorder. However, if the depressive episode is mild to moderate in severity, psychotherapy can be the first-line therapy.[33] The effects of psychotherapy and antidepressant medications are considered to be additive. Combined treatment can be advantageous for patients with partial responses to either treatment alone and for those with a chronic course of illness. However, for uncomplicated, nonchronic major depressive disorder, combined treatment might provide no unique advantage.[33] Although not extensively evaluated, cognitive therapy, behavioral therapy, and interpersonal psychotherapy appear equally effective.[33] Maintenance psychotherapy as the sole treatment to prevent recurrence generally is not recommended. Often, medication alone might prevent a depressive recurrence during the maintenance phase.[33]

Electroconvulsive therapy (ECT) is a safe and effective treatment for certain severe mental illnesses, including major depressive disorder as well as other selected psychiatric illnesses. Patients with depression are candidates for ECT when a rapid response is needed, risks of other treatments outweigh potential benefits, there is a history of poor response to antidepressants and a history of good response to ECT, and the patient expresses a preference for ECT.[34] A course of ECT generally consists of either unilateral or bilateral ECT administered two to three times weekly for a total of 6 to 12 treatments. A rapid therapeutic response (10 to 14 days) has been reported. Although there are no absolute contraindications to the use of ECT, several conditions are associated with increased risk. These include increased intracranial pressure, cerebral lesions, recent myocardial infarction, recent intracerebral hemorrhage, bleeding, or otherwise unstable vascular condition. The use of an anesthetic as well as a nondepolarizing neuromuscular blocking agent decreases the morbidity associated with ECT.[34] Adverse effects of ECT include cognitive dysfunction, cardiovascular dysfunction, prolonged apnea, treatment-emergent mania, headache, nausea, and muscle aches. Cognitive changes associated with ECT include confusion immediately after the seizure and retrograde and anterograde memory disturbance. Most cognitive disturbances are transient, but some patients can report permanent loss of memory for events occurring over the months before, after, or during treatment.[34] Relapse rates during the year immediately following ECT are high unless maintenance antidepressant medication is prescribed. Guidelines developed by the American Psychiatric Association include indications and contraindications for the appropriate use of ECT, procedures for obtaining informed consent, and issues in administering ECT.[34]

Another nonpharmacologic treatment for depression is bright light therapy. Bright light therapy consists of the patient gazing into a 10,000-lux intensity light box, which is slanted downward toward the patient's face for approximately 30 minutes per day. It has shown effectiveness for treating both the winter "blues," also known as seasonal affective disorder (SAD), and for adjunctive use in major depressive disorder with seasonal exacerbations.[2] Light therapy is well tolerated, with minor visual complaints being the most frequently reported event.[35] Consequently, anyone undergoing light therapy should receive baseline and periodic eye examinations. The combination of bright light therapy and an antidepressant may provide additional benefit beyond either approach alone.[2]

PHARMACOLOGIC THERAPY

Antidepressants can be classified in several ways, including by chemical structure and the presumed mechanism of antidepressant activity. Although the link between the presumed mechanism of drug action and antidepressant response is tenuous, this classification has the advantage of being based on established pharmacology and clearly explains some of the common, but expected adverse effects. The knowledgeable clinician can use these facts to tailor treatment to individual patient needs and thereby optimize treatment outcome. Currently available antidepressants and initial dosages are shown in Table 71–3.

TABLE 71-3 Adult Dosages for Currently Available Antidepressant Medications[a]

Generic Name	Trade Name	Suggested Therapeutic Plasma Concentration (ng/mL)	Initial Dose (mg/day)	Usual Dosage Range (mg/day)
Selective serotonin reuptake inhibitors				
Citalopram	Celexa		20	20–60
Escitalopram	Lexapro		10	10–20
Fluoxetine	Prozac		20	20–60
Fluvoxamine	Luvox		50	50–300
Paroxetine	Paxil		20	20–60
Sertraline	Zoloft		50	50–200
Serotonin/norepinephrine reuptake inhibitors				
Venlafaxine	Effexor		37.5–75	75–225
Duloxetine	Cymbalta		30	30–90
Aminoketone				
Bupropion	Wellbutrin		150	150–300
Triazolopyridines				
Nefazodone	Serzone		100	200–600
Trazodone	Desyrel		50	150–300
Tetracyclics				
Mirtazapine	Remeron		15	15–45
Tricyclics				
Tertiary amines				
Amitriptyline	Elavil	120–250[b]	25	100–300
Clomipramine	Anafranil		25	100–250
Doxepin	Sinequan		25	100–300
Imipramine	Tofranil	200–350[c]	25	100–300
Secondary amines				
Desipramine	Norpramin	100–300[c]	25	100–300
Nortriptyline	Pamelor	50–150	25	50–200
Monoamine oxidase inhibitors				
Phenelzine	Nardil		15	30–90
Selegiline (transdermal)	Emsam		6[d]	6–12[d]
Tranylcypromine	Parnate		10	20–60

[a]Doses listed are total daily doses; elderly patients are usually treated with approximately one-half of the dose listed.
[b]Parent drug plus metabolite.
[c]It has been suggested that combined imipramine + desipramine concentrations should fall between 150–240 ng/mL.
[d]Transdermal delivery system designed to deliver stated dose continuously over a 24-hour period.
Data from American Psychiatric Association,[2] Baldessarini,[15] Mann,[32] Patkar et al.,[41] and Watanabe and Winter.[66]

5 Studies have found that antidepressants are of equivalent efficacy in groups of patients when administered in comparable doses. Because one cannot predict which antidepressant will be the most effective in an individual patient, the initial choice is made empirically. Factors that often influence the choice of an antidepressant include the patient's history of response, pharmacogenetics (history of familial antidepressant response), patient's concurrent medical history, presenting symptoms (e.g., fatigue as compared to psychomotor agitation), potential for drug-drug interactions, adverse events profile, patient preference, and drug cost.

Although the pathophysiology of major depression remains elusive, the clinician can now select from multiple approved drug therapies with different mechanisms of action.[2] Failure to respond to one antidepressant class or one antidepressant drug within a class does not predict a failed response to another drug class or another drug within the class. Approximately 65% to 70% of patients with varying types of depression improve with drug therapy, compared with 30% to 40% who are well-documented to improve with placebo.

MIXED SEROTONIN AND NOREPINEPHRINE REUPTAKE INHIBITORS

Although TCAs are effective in treating all depressive subtypes, their use has diminished greatly because of the availability of equally effective therapies that are much safer in overdose and better tolerated. All TCAs potentiate the activity of NE and 5-HT by blocking their reuptake. However, the potency and selectivity of TCAs for the inhibition of reuptake of NE and 5-HT vary greatly among these agents (Table 71–4). Because TCAs affect other receptor systems including the cholinergic, neurologic, and cardiovascular systems, adverse events are reported frequently during TCA therapy.[15]

Venlafaxine inhibits 5-HT reuptake at low doses, with additional NE reuptake at higher doses; thus, it is referred to as a *serotonin-norepinephrine reuptake inhibitor* (SNRI). Duloxetine is also an SNRI with both 5-HT and NE reuptake inhibition across all doses. Some studies suggest that the SNRIs can be associated with higher rates of response and remission than other antidepressants; however, most of these studies involved venlafaxine and not all studies support this conclusion.[36]

SELECTIVE SEROTONIN REUPTAKE INHIBITORS

The efficacy of selective serotonin reuptake inhibitors (SSRIs) is superior to placebo and comparable to other classes of antidepressants in treating patients with major depression.[2,32] SSRIs are generally chosen as *first-line antidepressants* because of their safety in overdose and improved tolerability.

TRIAZOLOPYRIDINES

Trazodone and nefazodone have dual actions on serotonergic neurons, acting as both 5-HT_2 receptor antagonists and 5-HT reuptake

TABLE 71-4 Relative Potencies of Norepinephrine and Serotonin Reuptake Blockade and Side-Effect Profile of Antidepressant Drugs

	Reuptake Antagonism		Anticholinergic Effects	Sedation	Orthostatic Hypotension	Seizures[a]	Conduction Abnormalities[a]
	Norepinephrine	***Serotonin***					
Selective serotonin reuptake inhibitors							
Citalopram	0	++++	0	+	0	++	0
Escitalopram	0	++++	0	0	0	0	0
Fluoxetine	0	+++	0	0	0	++	0
Fluvoxamine	0	++++	0	0	0	++	0
Paroxetine	0	++++	+	+	0	++	0
Sertraline	0	++++	0	0	0	++	0
Serotonin/norepinephrine reuptake inhibitors							
Venlafaxine[b]	++++	++++	+	+	0	++	+
Duloxetine[c]	++++	++++	+	0	+	0	0
Aminoketone							
Bupropion[d]	+	0	+	0	0	++++	+
Triazolopyridines							
Nefazodone	0	++	0	+++	+++	++	+
Trazodone	0	++	0	++++	+++	++	+
Tetracyclics							
Mirtazapine	0	0	+	++	++	0	+
Tricyclics							
Tertiary amines							
Amitriptyline	++	++++	++++	++++	+++	+++	+++
Clomipramine	++	+++	++++	++++	++	++++	+++
Doxepin	++	++	+++	++++	++	+++	++
Imipramine	+++	+++	+++	+++	++++	+++	+++
Secondary amines							
Desipramine	++++	+	++	++	++	++	++
Nortriptyline	+++	++	++	++	+	++	++
Monoamine oxidase inhibitors							
Phenelzine	++	++	+	++	++	+	
Selegiline	0	0	0	+	++	0	0
Tranylcypromine	++	+	+	+	++	+	+

++++, high; +++, moderate; ++, low; +, very low; 0, absent.

[a]These are uncommon side effects of antidepressant drugs, particularly when used at normal therapeutic doses.

[b]Primarily serotonin (5-HT) at lower doses, norepinephrine (NE) at higher doses, and dopamine (DA) at very high doses.

[c]Balanced 5-HT and NE reuptake inhibition.

[d]Also blocks dopamine reuptake.

Data from Baldessarini,[15] Mann,[32] Stahl et al.,[36] Horst and Preskorn,[38] and Patkar et al.[41]

inhibitors. They can also enhance 5-HT_{1A}-mediated neurotransmission.[15] Trazodone blocks α_1-adrenergic and histaminergic receptors leading to increased side effects (e.g., dizziness and sedation) that limit its use as an antidepressant. Nefazodone's use as an antidepressant has declined as well after reports of hepatic toxicity began to emerge. The FDA-approved nefazodone labeling includes a black box warning describing rare cases of liver failure.[37] The triazolopyridines are effective agents in treating major depression; however, they both carry risks that limit their usefulness as antidepressants.

■ AMINOKETONE

Bupropion has no appreciable effect on the reuptake of 5-HT, whereas having reuptake properties at both the NE and DA reuptake pumps.[18,38] These pharmacologic properties make bupropion unique among all currently available antidepressants.

■ MIXED SEROTONIN-NOREPINEPHRINE EFFECTS

Mirtazapine enhances central noradrenergic and serotonergic activity through the antagonism of central presynaptic α_2-adrenergic autoreceptors and heteroreceptors.[39] Furthermore, it antagonizes 5-HT_2 and 5-HT_3 receptors as well as histamine receptors. The antagonism of 5-HT_2 and 5-HT_3 receptors has been linked to lower anxiety and gastrointestinal side effects, respectively. Blockade of histamine receptors is associated with the sedative properties of mirtazapine.[18]

■ MONOAMINE OXIDASE INHIBITORS

MAOIs increase the concentrations of NE, 5-HT, and DA within the neuronal synapse through inhibition of the MAO enzyme. Studies have demonstrated that similarly to TCAs, chronic therapy causes changes in receptor sensitivity (i.e., downregulation of β-adrenergic, α-adrenergic, and serotonergic receptors).[40] The MAOIs phenelzine and tranylcypromine are nonselective inhibitors of MAO-A and MAO-B. Recently, a selegiline transdermal patch was approved by the FDA for treatment of major depressive disorder that allows inhibition of MAO-A and MAO-B in the brain, yet has reduced effects on MAO-A in the gut[41] (see tyramine interactions with MAOIs below).

■ ST. JOHN'S WORT

Increasingly, consumers are choosing alternative forms of therapy, such as herbal medications including St. John's wort. Evaluations have found mixed results regarding the efficacy of the active ingredient in St. John's wort, hypericum, when compared with placebo and other antidepressants.[42] St. John's wort is available as an over-the-counter medication. Although this can allow certain advantages such as reduced cost of therapy and self-treatment, it also has the potential to result in circumvention of the healthcare system. St. John's wort has been found to have significant drug interactions with commonly used medications.[42] Perhaps most disconcerting is the fact that herbal medications are not regulated by the FDA, and manufacturers are not required to adhere to good manufacturing practices or provide proof of safety and/or efficacy. If St. John's wort is to be used, it should be administered under the guidance of a clinician trained in the treatment of depression, and a single-source product should be used continuously from a reputable and trusted manufacturer.

■ ADVERSE EFFECTS

TCAs

The adverse effects of antidepressant medications are summarized in Table 71–4. The TCAs affect several neurotransmitters and produce a wide range of pharmacologic actions, including several unwanted, but expected, adverse effects. The most commonly occurring side effects are dose related and are associated with blockade of cholinergic receptors (anticholinergic effects) and include dry mouth, constipation, blurred vision, urinary retention, dizziness, tachycardia, memory impairment, and at higher doses, delirium.[40] Although some tolerance does develop to these adverse effects, they have the potential to impact patient adherence, particularly in the elderly and those receiving long-term maintenance therapy. Orthostatic hypotension is a common, dose-related, and potentially problematic adverse effect that has been attributed to the affinity of the TCAs for adrenergic receptors.[43] TCAs also cause cardiac conduction delays and can even induce heart block in patients with a preexisting conduction disorder. TCA overdose can produce severe arrhythmias.[43] Therefore, caution should be exercised when prescribing these agents, especially in higher doses, to patients with clinically significant cardiac disease. Other adverse effects that lead to patient nonadherence include weight gain and sexual dysfunction.[44] Abrupt withdrawal of TCAs is often associated with symptoms suggestive of cholinergic rebound (e.g., dizziness, nausea, diarrhea, insomnia, and restlessness), especially if the daily dose exceeds 300 mg.[45] Therefore, the dose should be tapered over several days.

Serotonin-Norepinephrine Reuptake Inhibitors

The most commonly reported adverse effects with venlafaxine are similar to those of the SSRIs and can be dose related; they include nausea, sexual dysfunction, and activation.[2] Venlafaxine can also cause a dose-related increase in diastolic blood pressure, and baseline blood pressure is not a useful predictor of the occurrence of this phenomenon. Blood pressure should be monitored regularly during venlafaxine therapy, and dosage reduction or discontinuation can be necessary if sustained hypertension occurs.[46] Duloxetine was relatively well tolerated in short-term clinical trials; however, experience with long-term studies and in a larger population of patients will more clearly define the risks and benefits of this newly approved antidepressant. The most commonly reported adverse events were nausea, dry mouth, constipation, decreased appetite, insomnia, and increased sweating.[36,47]

Selective Serotonin Reuptake Inhibitors

The SSRIs include fluoxetine, citalopram, sertraline, paroxetine, escitalopram, and fluvoxamine. These drugs have a low affinity for histaminergic, α_1-adrenergic, and muscarinic receptors, and therefore they produce fewer anticholinergic and cardiovascular adverse effects than the TCAs, and are not usually associated with significant weight gain.[48–50] The most common adverse effects, which generally are mild and short lived, are gastrointestinal symptoms (i.e., nausea, vomiting, and diarrhea), sexual dysfunction in both males and females, headache, and insomnia.[49] A discontinuation or withdrawal syndrome can occur if the SSRIs are abruptly discontinued. The longer the half-life of the drug and its active metabolite, the less likely a withdrawal syndrome will occur.[50,51] Although the SSRIs are known to improve the anxiety symptoms associated with depression, a few patients experience an increase in anxiety symptoms or agitation early in treatment.

Triazolopyridines

Trazodone and nefazodone have minimal anticholinergic effects and 5-HT agonist side effects, but they can cause orthostatic hypotension. Sedation, cognitive slowing, and dizziness are the most frequent dose-limiting side effects associated with trazodone.[40] Common adverse effects associated with nefazodone include light-headedness, dizziness, orthostatic hypotension, somnolence, dry mouth, nausea, and asthenia (weakness). Because of the potential for hepatic injury associated with nefazodone use (see black box warning above), treatment should not be initiated in individuals with active liver disease or with elevated baseline serum transaminases.[37] A rare but potentially serious adverse effect of trazodone is priapism, which is reported to occur in approximately 1 in 6,000 male patients. Some cases have required surgical intervention (1 in 23,000), and permanent impotence can result.[52] There have been no reports of priapism associated with nefazodone use in men, but there is a published case report of nefazodone-induced clitoral priapism.[53]

Aminoketone

Adverse effects associated with bupropion include nausea, vomiting, tremor, insomnia, dry mouth, and skin reactions. The occurrence of seizures in patients taking bupropion appears to be strongly dose-related, and can be increased by predisposing factors such as history of head trauma and CNS tumor. Additionally, bupropion use is contraindicated in patients with eating disorders such as bulimia and anorexia, as these patients are prone to electrolyte abnormalities and are therefore at higher risk for seizure activity. At daily doses of 450 mg (the FDA-approved maximum dose) or less, the incidence of seizures is 0.4%.[54] Because of its pharmacologic profile (i.e., pro-adrenergic) bupropion can cause activation or agitation in some patients.[18]

Mixed Serotonin-Norepinephrine Effects

The most common adverse effects of mirtazapine are somnolence, weight gain, dry mouth, and constipation. Interestingly, side effects such as weight gain can be less with larger mirtazapine doses because of different mechanisms of action at different doses,[50] such as increased noradrenergic transmission as the dose is increased.

TABLE 71-5 Dietary Restrictions for Patients Taking Monoamine Oxidase Inhibitors[a]

Aged cheeses[b]
Sour cream[c]
Yogurt[c]
Cottage cheese[c]
American cheese[c]
Mild Swiss cheese[c]
Wine[d] (especially Chianti and sherry)
Beer
Herring (pickled, salted, dry)
Sardines
Snails
Anchovies
Canned, aged, or processed meats
Monosodium glutamate
Liver (chicken or beef, more than 2 days old)
Fermented foods
Canned figs
Raisins
Pods of broad beans (fava beans)
Yeast extract and other yeast products
Meat extract (Marmite)
Soy sauce
Chocolate[e]
Coffee[e]
Ripe avocado
Sauerkraut
Licorice

[a]According to the FDA-approved prescribing information for the transdermal selegiline patch, patients receiving the 6 mg/24 h dose are not required to modify their diet. However, patients receiving the 9 or 12 mg/24 h are still required to follow the dietary restrictions similar to the other monoamine oxidase inhibitors (MAOIs).
[b]Clearly warrants absolute prohibition (e.g., English Stilton, blue, Camembert, cheddar).
[c]Up to 56 g (2 oz) daily is acceptable.
[d]An 88 mL (3 oz) white wine or a single cocktail is acceptable.
[e]Up to 56 g (2 oz) daily is acceptable: larger amounts of decaffeinated coffee are acceptable.
Recommended first-line drug and food interaction search engines: Lexi-Comp[101] and Thomson Micromedex.[102]

Monoamine Oxidase Inhibitors

The most common adverse effect of MAOIs is postural hypotension; this is more likely to occur with phenelzine than with tranylcypromine. Hypotensive reactions can be minimized through divided dosage scheduling. Other common adverse effects include weight gain and sexual side effects (e.g., decreased libido, anorgasmia).[2] Phenelzine, the most frequently prescribed MAOI, has mild to moderate sedating effects, whereas tranylcypromine can exert a stimulating effect, and therefore insomnia can occur. In addition, fever, myoclonic jerking, and brisk deep tendon reflexes can occur.[55]

Hypertensive crisis, a potentially serious and life-threatening but rare adverse reaction, can occur when MAOIs are taken concurrently with certain foods, especially those high in tyramine (Table 71–5), or medications (Table 71–6). Ten milligrams of tyramine can cause a marked pressor effect, and 25 mg can result in serious hypertensive crisis.[56] These incidents can culminate in cerebrovascular accident and death. Symptoms of hypertensive crisis include occipital headache, stiff neck, nausea, vomiting, sweating, and sharply elevated blood pressure. Hypertensive crises can be treated with antihypertensive agents such as captopril.[57] Education of patients taking MAOIs regarding dietary and medication restrictions is extremely important. Printed and verbal patient instructions should be provided. It is important that patients be instructed to consult a healthcare professional before taking any over-the-counter medications, including non-FDA approved items sold as herbal/dietary supplements. Patients should be taught to recognize the symptoms of hypertensive crisis and to seek immediate treatment should those symptoms occur.

CLINICAL CONTROVERSY

In recent years, there have been numerous reports from the Food and Drug Administration warning healthcare providers of adverse effects associated with the use of the antidepressants in various populations. Many of these warnings have been accompanied by product labeling changes, including *black box warnings*. However, some of the warnings have not been unequivocally supported in the scientific literature. Therefore, the reader is encouraged to examine and understand these reports, and consider them within the context of the scientific literature.

PHARMACOKINETICS

The pharmacokinetics of the antidepressants are summarized in Table 71–7. Bioavailability is low (30% to 70% for most TCAs) as a

TABLE 71-6 Medication Restrictions for Patients Taking Monoamine Oxidase Inhibitors (MAOIs)

Amphetamines	Local anesthetics containing sympathomimetic vasoconstrictors
Appetite suppressants	Meperidine
Asthma inhalants	Methyldopa
Buspirone	Methylphenidate
Carbamazepine	Other antidepressants[a]
Cocaine	Other MAOIs
Cyclobenzaprine	Reserpine
Decongestants (topical and systemic)	Rizatriptan
Dextromethorphan	Stimulants
Dopamine	Sumatriptan
Ephedrine	Sympathomimetics
Epinephrine	Tryptophan
Guanethidine	
Levodopa	

[a]Tricyclic antidepressants can be used with caution by experienced clinicians in treatment-resistant populations.
Recommended first-line drug interaction search engines: Lexi-Comp[101] and Thomson Micromedex.[102]

TABLE 71-7 Pharmacokinetic Properties of Antidepressants

Generic Name	Elimination Half-Life (h)[a]	Time of Peak Plasma Concentration (h)	Plasma Protein Binding (%)	Percentage Bioavailable	Clinically Important Metabolites
Selective serotonin reuptake inhibitors					
Citalopram	33	2–4	80	≥80	None
Escitalopram	27–32	5	56	80	None
Fluoxetine	4–6 days[b]	4–8	94	95	Norfluoxetine
Fluvoxamine	15–26	2–8	77	53	None
Paroxetine	24–31	5–7	95	[d]	None
Sertraline	27	6–8	99	36[c]	None
Serotonin/norepinephrine reuptake inhibitor					
Venlafaxine	5	2	27–30	45	O-Desmethylvenlafaxine
Duloxetine	12	6	90	50	None
Aminoketone					
Bupropion	10–21	3	82–88	[d]	Hydroxybupropion Threohydrobupropion Erythrohydrobupropion
Triazolopyridines					
Nefazodone	2–4	1	99	20	Meta-chlorophenylpiperazine
Trazodone	6–11	1–2	92	[d]	Meta-chlorophenylpiperazine
Tetracyclics					
Mirtazapine	20–40	2	85	50	None
Tricyclics					
Tertiary amines					
Amitriptyline	9–46	1–5	90–97	30–60	Nortriptyline
Clomipramine	20–24	2–6	97	36–62	Desmethylclomipramine
Doxepin	8–36	1–4	68–82	13–45	Desmethyldoxepin
Imipramine	6–34	1.5–3	63–96	22–77	Desipramine
Secondary amines					
Desipramine	11–46	3–6	73–92	33–51	2-Hydroxydesipramine
Nortriptyline	16–88	3–12	87–95	46–70	10-Hydroxynortriptyline

[a]Biologic half-life in slowest phase of elimination.
[b]4–6 days with chronic dosing; norfluoxetine, 4–16 days.
[c]Increases 30–40% when taken with food.
[d]No data available.
Data from Stahl et al.,[36] Hemeryck and Belpaire,[62] Kent,[69] DeVane.[70]

result of the first-pass hepatic effect, which shows great interindividual variation.[58] The TCAs have a large volume of distribution and concentrate in brain and cardiac tissue in laboratory animals. They are bound extensively and strongly to plasma albumin, erythrocytes, α_1-acid glycoprotein, and lipoprotein.[58] The major metabolic pathways are demethylation, aromatic and aliphatic hydroxylation, and glucuronide conjugation. Enterohepatic cycling has been described.[58,59] Metabolism of TCAs is linear within the usual dosage range. The elimination half-lives of the TCAs can vary greatly among individual patients.[58]

Venlafaxine is metabolized to an active metabolite, O-desmethylvenlafaxine, which contributes to the overall pharmacologic effect.[60] Venlafaxine has the lowest plasma protein binding of any antidepressant (27%–30%), which reduces the likelihood of drug interactions via this mechanism. As might be expected, different formulations of venlafaxine with different pharmacokinetic profiles have led to different adverse-effect profiles. For example, venlafaxine extended-release, with its sustained plasma concentrations, has been associated with higher rates of sexual dysfunction among men (37%) as compared to the immediate release formulation (6%).[60]

The diversity of the SSRIs is evident not only in their chemical structures but also in their pharmacokinetic profiles.[61,62] These unique pharmacokinetic attributes of each SSRI can be used to guide treatment. For example, the long half-life of fluoxetine and its active metabolite norfluoxetine can be beneficial in instances of partial nonadherence (e.g., missed doses). Conversely, caution must be taken to monitor for drug-drug interactions prior to combining another medication with fluoxetine. The SSRIs are extensively distributed to the tissues, and all, with the possible exception of citalopram and sertraline, can have a nonlinear pattern of drug accumulation with long-term administration.[48,61] Therefore, the relationship between the dose and observed effect (e.g., side effect) can change over time for the nonlinear SSRIs, and this needs to be considered during treatment.

Bupropion is metabolized to multiple active metabolites (see Table 71–7). There are currently three formulations of bupropion (immediate release, sustained release, and extended release), which are considered bioequivalent.[63] The bupropion peak plasma concentrations are lower for the sustained-release formulation of bupropion, and it is believed this can contribute to a lower seizure risk with that formulation.[64]

Mirtazapine undergoes extensive biotransformation to several metabolites[65] and is primarily eliminated in the urine (renal elimination). However, these metabolites are present at such low plasma concentrations as to minimally contribute to the overall pharmacologic profile of mirtazapine.

Altered Pharmacokinetics

Factors that influence TCA plasma concentrations include disease states, genetics, age, cigarette smoking, and concurrent drug administration. Hepatic disease can result in increased TCA plasma concentrations.[66] Renal failure does not alter nortriptyline metabolism, but the 10-hydroxy metabolite can accumulate, and protein binding can be diminished, with resulting enhanced sensitivity to the drug.[58] Clinicians should be alert to the possibility of higher-than-expected plasma concentrations of some TCAs in the elderly.

In cirrhotics, the half-lives of fluoxetine and norfluoxetine increased to 7.6 and 12 days, respectively.[61] Patients with hepatic impairment had a twofold increase in plasma concentrations of paroxetine.[67] Similarly, in patients with mild stable cirrhosis, the half-life of sertraline was 2.5 times greater than in patients without liver disease.[68] Patients with renal impairment had a two- to fourfold increase in paroxetine plasma concentrations compared with normal volunteers.[67] Plasma concentrations of SSRIs in the elderly are reported to be greater than in younger patients.[61]

The clearance of venlafaxine, mirtazapine, and their metabolites can be reduced among patients with hepatic or renal disease,[69] and doses should be adjusted accordingly. Elderly patients can require a dose reduction with mirtazapine.[69]

Plasma Concentration and Clinical Response

Studies in acutely depressed patients have demonstrated a correlation between antidepressant effect and plasma concentrations for some TCAs. The patient's clinical response, not plasma concentration, dictates dosage adjustments. Some patients with plasma concentrations outside the suggested therapeutic plasma concentration range respond, whereas others are nonresponsive regardless of their plasma concentration. See Table 71–3 for a listing of suggested therapeutic plasma concentration ranges. There are four TCAs (nortriptyline, desipramine, imipramine, and amitriptyline) with evidence to support an association between plasma concentrations and clinical response. However, the best established therapeutic range is for nortriptyline (50–150 ng/mL),[66] which appears to demonstrate a curvilinear plasma concentration-response relationship.

For the newer antidepressants, a correlation has not been established between plasma concentration and clinical response or adverse effects.

Plasma Concentration Monitoring

Because of interindividual variations in plasma concentrations achieved by a given dose, interpretation of plasma concentrations can be very difficult for the TCAs.[66] Although plasma level monitoring is not performed routinely, some indications include inadequate response, relapse, serious or persistent adverse effects, use of higher-than-standard doses, suspected toxicity, elderly patients, pregnant patients, cardiac disease, suspected nonadherence, suspected pharmacokinetic drug interactions, and when the manufacturer of the product changes. If plasma concentration monitoring is used to detect nonadherence, a cutoff as low as 30 ng/mL for the TCAs has been suggested to avoid confusion with low bioavailability or unusually rapid metabolism. Plasma concentrations should be obtained at steady state, usually after a minimum of 1 week at constant dosage. Sampling should be performed during the drug elimination phase, usually in the morning, 12 hours after the last dose. Samples collected in this manner are comparable for patients on once-, twice-, or thrice-daily regimens.[58]

■ DRUG INTERACTIONS

TCAs

Because the TCAs are metabolized in the liver through the cytochrome P450 system, they can interact with other drugs that modify hepatic enzyme activity or hepatic blood flow. TCAs are also extensively protein bound, which can cause drug interactions through displacement from protein-binding sites. Many commonly used medications can interact when given concurrently with TCAs. Pharmacokinetic and pharmacodynamic drug interactions involving TCAs are shown in Tables 71–8 and 71–9, respectively. Because of their frequent coadministration, a common drug interaction occurs between the TCAs and certain SSRIs, such as paroxetine and fluoxetine. These drugs are known to inhibit cytochrome P450 (e.g., CYP2D6) with the resultant increase in TCA plasma concentrations. Although MAOIs and TCAs can be coadministered safely in refractory patients with apparent increased efficacy compared with monotherapy, severe reactions (e.g., hypertensive crisis) and fatalities have occurred.[2,58] Therefore, this combination should be monitored extremely carefully.

TABLE 71-8 Pharmacokinetic Drug Interactions Involving Tricyclic Antidepressants

Elevates plasma concentrations of TCAs
Cimetidine
Diltiazem
Ethanol, acute ingestion
SSRIs
Haloperidol
Labetalol
Methylphenidate
Oral contraceptives
Phenothiazines
Propoxyphene
Quinidine
Verapamil
Lowers plasma concentrations of TCAs
Barbiturates
Carbamazepine
Ethanol, chronic ingestion
Phenytoin
Elevates plasma concentrations of interacting drug
Hydantoins
Oral anticoagulants
Lowers plasma concentrations of interacting drug
Levodopa

SSRI, selective serotonin reuptake inhibitor; TCA, tricyclic antidepressants.
Recommended first-line drug interaction search engines: Lexi-Comp[101] and Thomson Micromedex.[102]

SSRIs

Table 71–10 summarizes the drug interactions of newer-generation antidepressants. Drug-drug interactions can occur when an SSRI is

TABLE 71-9 Pharmacodynamic Drug Interactions Involving Tricyclic Antidepressants

Interacting Drug	Effect
Alcohol	Increased CNS depressant effects
Amphetamines	Increased effect of amphetamines
Androgens	Delusions, hostility
Anticholinergic agents	Excessive anticholinergic effects
Bepridil	Increased antiarrhythmic effect
Clonidine	Decreased antihypertensive efficacy
Disulfiram	Acute organic brain syndrome
Estrogens	Increased or decreased antidepressant response; increased toxicity
Guanadrel	Decreased antihypertensive efficacy
Guanethidine	Decreased antihypertensive efficacy
Insulin	Increased hypoglycemic effects
Lithium	Possible additive lowering of seizure threshold
Methyldopa	Decreased antihypertensive efficacy; tachycardia; CNS stimulation
Monoamine oxidase inhibitors	Increased therapeutic and possibly toxic effects of both drugs; hypertensive crisis; delirium; seizures; hyperpyrexia; serotonin syndrome
Oral hypoglycemics	Increased hypoglycemic effects
Phenytoin	Possible lowering of seizure threshold and reduced antidepressant response
Sedatives	Increased CNS depressant effects
Sympathomimetics	Increased pharmacologic effects of direct-acting sympathomimetics; decreased effects of indirect-acting sympathomimetics
Thyroid hormones	Increased therapeutic and possibly toxic effects of both drugs; CNS stimulation; tachycardia

Recommended first-line drug interaction search engines: Lexi-Comp[101] and Thomson Micromedex.[102]

TABLE 71-10 Selected Drug Interactions of Newer-Generation Antidepressants

Antidepressant	Interacting Drug/Drug Class	Effect
Serotonin/norepinephrine reuptake inhibitors		
Venlafaxine	MAOIs	Potential for hypertensive crisis, serotonin syndrome, delirium
	Sibutramine	Serotonin syndrome
	Triptans	Serotonin syndrome
Duloxetine	MAOIs	Potential for hypertensive crisis, serotonin syndrome, delirium
	Sibutramine	Serotonin syndrome
	Thioridazine	Thioridazine C_{max} increased; prolonged QTc interval
	Triptans	Serotonin syndrome
Selective serotonin reuptake inhibitors		
Citalopram & escitalopram	MAOIs	Potential for hypertensive crisis, serotonin syndrome, delirium
	Linezolid (*MAOI effects*)	Serotonin syndrome
	Sibutramine	Serotonin syndrome
	Triptans	Serotonin syndrome
Fluoxetine	Alprazolam	Increased plasma concentrations and half-life of alprazolam; increased psychomotor impairment
	Antipsychotics (e.g., haloperidol and risperidone)	Increased antipsychotic concentrations; increased extrapyramidal side effects
	β-Adrenergic blockers	Increased metoprolol serum concentrations; increased bradycardia; possible heart block
	Carbamazepine	Increased plasma concentrations of carbamazepine; symptoms of carbamazepine toxicity
	Linezolid (*MAOI effects*)	Serotonin syndrome
	MAOIs	Potential for hypertensive crisis, serotonin syndrome, delirium
	Phenytoin	Increased plasma concentrations of phenytoin; symptoms of phenytoin toxicity
	TCAs	Markedly increased TCA plasma concentrations; symptoms of TCA toxicity
	Sibutramine	Serotonin syndrome
	Triptans	Serotonin syndrome
	Thioridazine	Thioridazine C_{max} increased; prolonged QTc interval
Fluvoxamine	Alosetron	Increased alosetron AUC (sixfold) and half-life (threefold)
	Alprazolam	Increased AUC of alprazolam by 96%, increased alprazolam half-life by 71%; increased psychomotor impairment
	β-Adrenergic blockers	Fivefold increase in propranolol serum concentration; bradycardia and hypotension
	Carbamazepine	Increased plasma concentrations of carbamazepine; symptoms of carbamazepine toxicity
	Clozapine	Increased clozapine serum concentrations; increased risk for seizures and orthostatic hypotension
	Diltiazem	Bradycardia
	MAOIs	Potential for hypertensive crisis, serotonin syndrome, delirium
	Methadone	Increased methadone plasma concentrations; symptoms of methadone toxicity
	Ramelteon	Increased AUC (190-fold) and C_{max} (70-fold)
	Sibutramine	Serotonin syndrome
	TCAs	Increased TCA plasma concentration; symptoms of TCA toxicity
	Theophylline & caffeine	Increased serum concentrations of theophylline or caffeine; symptoms of theophylline or caffeine toxicity
	Thioridazine	Thioridazine C_{max} increased; prolonged QTc interval
	Warfarin	Increased hypoprothrombinemic response to warfarin
Paroxetine	Antipsychotics (e.g., haloperidol, perphenazine and risperidone)	Increased antipsychotic concentrations; increased central nervous system and extrapyramidal side effects
	β-Adrenergic blockers	Increased metoprolol serum concentrations; increased bradycardia; possible heart block
	Linezolid (MAOI effects)	Serotonin syndrome
	MAOIs	Potential for hypertensive crisis, serotonin syndrome, delirium
	TCAs	Markedly increased TCA plasma concentrations; symptoms of TCA toxicity
	Sibutramine	Serotonin syndrome
	Triptans	Serotonin syndrome
	Thioridazine	Thioridazine C_{max} increased; prolonged QTc interval
Sertraline	Linezolid (*MAOI effects*)	Serotonin syndrome
	MAOIs	Potential for hypertensive crisis, serotonin syndrome, delirium
	Sibutramine	Serotonin syndrome
	Triptans	Serotonin syndrome
Tetracyclics		
Mirtazapine	Carbamazepine	Mirtazapine concentration decrease (60%)
	MAOIs	Theoretically central serotonin syndrome could occur
Aminoketone		
Bupropion	MAOIs	Potential for hypertensive crisis
	Medications that lower seizure threshold	Increased incidence of seizures

AUC, area under the curve, C_{max}, maximum concentration; MAOI, monoamine oxidase inhibitor; TCA, tricyclic antidepressant.
Recommended first-line drug interaction search engines: Lexi-Comp[101] and Thomson Micromedex.[102]

coadministered with another drug metabolized through the cytochrome P450 system. Two of the isoenzymes of the cytochrome P450 system, CYP2D6 and CYP3A4, are responsible for the metabolism of over 80% of currently marketed drugs.[70] The ability of an SSRI, or any antidepressant, to inhibit or induce the activity of these enzymes will be a significant contributory factor in determining its capability to cause a pharmacokinetic drug interaction when administered concomitantly. Table 71–11 shows the cytochrome P450 enzyme inhibitory potential of the second- and third-generation antidepressant agents. In patients receiving a stable dose of any

TABLE 71-11 Second- and Third-Generation Antidepressants and Cytochrome (CYP) P450 Enzyme Inhibitory Potential

	CYP Enzyme			
Drug	***1A2***	***2C***	***2D6***	***3A4***
Bupropion	0	0	+	0
Citalopram	0	0	+	0
Escitalopram	0	0	+	0
Fluoxetine	0	++	++++	++
Fluvoxamine	++++	++	0	+++
Mirtazapine	0	0	0	0
Nefazodone	0	0	0	++++
Paroxetine	0	0	++++	0
Sertraline	0	++	+	+
Venlafaxine	0	0	0/+	0

++++, high; +++, moderate; ++, low; +, very low; 0, absent.
Data from Preskorn,[48] Hemeryck and Belpaire,[62] Kent,[69] DeVane.[70]

medication known to interact with the SSRIs, if an SSRI is to be initiated, the starting dose should be low and titrated carefully to evaluate the potential importance of the interaction.

Certain pharmacodynamic drug interactions that can occur with the SSRIs are concerning and require close monitoring. For example, the combination of an SSRI with another drug that augments serotonergic function (e.g., linezolid) can lead to the *serotonin syndrome*, which is characterized by symptoms such as clonus, hyperthermia, and mental status changes.[71] Therefore, a washout period of 2 to 5 weeks (depending on the half-life of the SSRI) can be necessary before the initiation of another serotonergic medication.

Other Agents

In contrast to the SSRIs, which have potential for both pharmacokinetic and pharmacodynamic interactions, other newer-generation antidepressants such as venlafaxine, duloxetine, mirtazapine, and bupropion have drug interactions that are primarily pharmacodynamic. This can be partly explained by the relative lack of cytochrome P450 inhibition among these newer agents as compared to the SSRIs (see Table 71–11). As nefazodone use has been severely limited because of its potential to induce liver toxicity, and trazodone is primarily used as a non-FDA approved hypnotic at low doses, neither of these agents are likely to be involved in clinically significant drug interactions. However, it should be noted that nefazodone is a potent inhibitor of cytochrome P450 3A4.[70]

■ SPECIAL POPULATIONS

Elderly Patients

Depression in the elderly is a major public health problem. Many elderly depressed patients are often inadequately treated, or depression is missed or mistaken for another disorder, such as dementia. In the elderly, depressed mood, the typical signature symptom of depression, can be less prominent than other depressive symptoms such as loss of appetite, cognitive impairment, sleeplessness, anergia, and loss of interest in and enjoyment of the normal pursuits of life.[72] Older adults might not recognize common symptoms associated with depression such as anhedonia (inability to experience pleasure), fatigue, and concentration difficulties. In fact, somatic (physical) complaints are quite frequently the presenting symptoms in elderly depressed patients. Appropriate recognition and treatment of depression in the elderly is extremely important. In fact, individuals 65 years of age and older have the highest rates of suicide as compared to any other age group.[73] The increased suicidal attempts present in the depressed elderly can be because of access to firearms, diminished cognitive functions, sleep disruptions, poor social interactions, and inattention among primary caregivers.[73]

Before initiating antidepressant treatment, a complete physical examination should be performed. In prescribing antidepressants, elderly patients can be either over- or undertreated. Overtreatment occurs when age-related pharmacokinetic and pharmacodynamic factors are overlooked. Undertreatment results from an overly conservative approach as a result of the patient's advanced age or concurrent medical problems. The SSRIs are usually selected as first-choice antidepressants in the elderly, and this can enable the clinician to avoid some of the problematic adverse effects commonly associated with the TCAs (e.g., sedative, anticholinergic, and cardiovascular-related side effects). Furthermore, there is evidence to suggest that the long-term use of antidepressants such as the SSRIs in the elderly, administered with either psychotherapy or clinical-management, can prevent a depressive relapse.[74] Bupropion and venlafaxine are often selected because of milder anticholinergic and less frequent cardiovascular side effects.[75]

Pediatric Patients

Accumulating evidence indicates that childhood depression occurs quite commonly. Symptoms of depression in the young can vary from accepted diagnostic criteria and include several nonspecific symptoms such as boredom, anxiety, failing adjustment, and sleep disturbance.[76]

Data collected under controlled conditions that support the efficacy of antidepressants in children and adolescents are sparse, and no antidepressant, except fluoxetine, is FDA-approved for the treatment of depression in patients younger than 18 years of age although other antidepressants (e.g., sertraline) have been studied in this population.[77]

The use of antidepressants in children and adolescents was complicated when, in March 2004, the FDA issued a black box warning in the product labeling for antidepressant medications warning clinicians and patients of the increased risk of suicidal ideation and behavior when antidepressants are used in this population. However, several retrospective longitudinal reviews of the use of antidepressants in children found no significant increase in the risk of suicide attempts or deaths.[78,79,80] Furthermore, adolescents suffering from depression who remain untreated may successfully commit suicide.[81,82] Further study is needed to resolve this controversy.

Several cases of sudden death have been reported in children and adolescents taking antidepressants, such as desipramine. A baseline electrocardiogram (ECG) is recommended before initiating treatment with a TCA in children and adolescents, and many clinicians recommend an additional ECG when steady-state plasma concentrations are achieved.[83]

The treatment of depression in children remains challenging, as depression can be difficult to diagnose and treat once identified. Antidepressants are used to treat depressed children and adolescents because no other definitive effective therapies are currently available. Also, demonstration of efficacy in this population, as well as in adults, is confounded by a high placebo response rate. However, the TCAs and several of the SSRIs remain viable treatment options when prescribed and monitored appropriately.

Pregnant and Lactating Patients

Approximately 14% of pregnant women develop a serious depression during pregnancy.[84] The data presented in several recent publications should be considered when making treatment decisions for pregnant women suffering from major depression.[84,85,86] The first evaluation looked at the risk of discontinuing antidepressant therapy in pregnant women suffering from depression and found a significant risk of relapse. In this study, women who discontinued antidepressant therapy were five times more likely to have a relapse during their pregnancy than were women who continued treatment.[86] Another study used population health data to determine whether exposure to SSRIs and depression in pregnant women differs from exposure to maternal depression alone. The authors found that prenatal exposure to SSRIs was associated with an increased risk of low birth weight and respiratory distress, and that this relationship remained after accounting for maternal illness severity.[84] A study by Chambers and colleagues reported a sixfold greater likelihood of the occurrence of persistent pulmonary hypertension of newborn infants exposed to an SSRI after the 20th week of gestation.[85] A recent editorial on the use of antidepressants in pregnancy lists four therapeutic principles to guide the clinician in treating women during pregnancy: (1) Pregnancy does not protect against the occurrence of depression, and the likelihood of relapse is very high in untreated women with recurrent illness; (2) Maternal depression adversely affects child development, and prenatal depression can adversely affect the offspring; (3) When attempting to balance benefit and risk, transient postnatal behavioral abnormalities in the offspring of treated mothers must not be assumed to portend long-term compromise; and (4) SSRIs, the most commonly used and best-tolerated treatment for depression, carry a small but significant risk for a serious medical consequence.[87]

In summary, the risks and benefits of drug therapy during pregnancy must always be weighed, and concerns about the risks of untreated depression during pregnancy should be considered. These include the possibility of low birth weight secondary to poor maternal weight gain, suicidality, potential for hospitalization, potential for marital discord, inability to engage in appropriate obstetric care, and difficulty caring for other children.[88] Several different approaches exist for dealing with pregnancy and antidepressant use. First, discontinuation of an antidepressant before conception is an option for women who are stable and appear likely to remain well while not taking antidepressant medication. Secondly, continuation of the antidepressant until conception can be reasonable. For those who have a history of depressive relapse after medication discontinuation, the antidepressant should be continued throughout pregnancy. Further evaluations of the newer antidepressant agents are needed to fully understand the risks associated with their use at various stages of the gestational period. Again, the risks of not treating depression in a pregnant woman should not be underestimated or minimized.

Refractory Patients

The majority of "treatment-resistant" depressed patients are likely the result of inadequate therapy (relative resistance). In fact, the ongoing National Institutes of Health (NIH)-sponsored study, Sequenced Treatment Alternatives to Relieve Depression (STAR* D), has shown that one in three depressed patients who previously did not achieve remission using an antidepressant became symptom-free with the help of an additional medication (e.g., bupropion sustained release [SR]) and one in four achieved remission after switching to a different antidepressant (e.g., venlafaxine extended release [XR]).[89]

❻ Issues to be addressed in assessing the patient who has not responded to treatment include the following:

1. Is the diagnosis correct?
2. Does the patient have a psychotic depression?
3. Has the patient received an adequate dose and adequate duration of treatment?
4. Do adverse effects preclude adequate dosing?
5. Has the patient adhered to the prescribed regimen?
6. Was a stepwise approach to treatment used?
7. Was treatment outcome adequately measured?
8. Is there a coexisting or preexisting medical or psychiatric disorder?
9. Are there other factors that interfere with treatment?

When a patient fails to respond, nondrug modalities including environmental manipulation, family counseling, cognitive therapy, or interpersonal psychotherapy are often beneficial.[2]

More than 40% of patients with major depressive disorder do not achieve remission even after two optimal antidepressant trials.[90] Although several different definitions for treatment-resistant depression (TRD) have been proposed, the most widely accepted is patients who do not achieve remission even after two optimal antidepressant trials.[90] Three primary pharmacologic approaches are used when dealing with treatment nonresponse. The current antidepressant can be stopped, and a trial with an unrelated agent initiated. For example, the patient can be switched from a TCA to an SSRI. Second, the current antidepressant can be augmented (potentiated) by the addition of another agent, such as lithium. For example, the STAR* D trial recently evaluated the addition of lithium or T_3 to current antidepressant treatment.[90] These patients had failed to respond to or been unable to tolerate at least two previous antidepressant trials. After approximately 10 weeks of treatment, T_3 augmentation resulted in higher remission rates (24.7%) compared to lithium (15.9%). However, these results were modest and not statistically significant, and the use of lithium was associated with a greater incidence of adverse events.[90] A second evaluation in the STAR* D trial, compared switching to mirtazapine (up to 60 mg per day) versus nortriptyline (up to 200 mg per day) after two, consecutive failed medication treatments.[91] This trial also found modest response rates that were not statistically significant. In the mirtazapine group, 12.3% of patients met the remission criteria of a score of seven or less on the Hamilton Depression (HAMD) scale, whereas 19.8% of nortriptyline patients met these criteria at the end of 14 weeks. There was no difference in tolerability between the two agents.

An additional strategy includes the use of atypical antipsychotic agents to augment the antidepressant response (antipsychotic medications are not FDA-approved for the treatment of depression). Risperidone has been shown to be effective in combination with fluvoxamine, paroxetine, or citalopram in TRD, with reported remission rates of 61% to 76%.[92,93] The combination of olanzapine and fluoxetine has also been found to be safe and effective in TRD.[92] Ziprasidone, aripiprazole, and quetiapine augmentation of SSRIs has been shown to be effective for TRD in open-label evaluations.[92]

The American Psychiatric Association practice guideline for the treatment of patients with major depressive disorder offers guidance for managing patients who fail to respond. These guidelines advise that if patients fail to respond to medication after 6 to 8 weeks, a reappraisal of the treatment regimen should be considered.[2] Partial responders should consider changing the dose, augmenting the antidepressant, or adding psychotherapy or ECT. For those with no response, options include changing to a second antidepressant or the addition of psychotherapy or ECT. Comorbid medical or psychiatric conditions should be identified and treated because they can complicate treatment. Before changing a patient's treatment, the clinician is advised to evaluate the adequacy of the medication dosage and adherence with the prescribed regimen. A combination of two drugs should not be used when one drug will suffice.

CLINICAL CONTROVERSY

There are no universally agreed on algorithms or guidelines for individuals experiencing treatment-resistant depression. Approaches include discontinuing the current antidepressant and initiating treatment with a different agent (i.e., "switching"), augmenting the current treatment, or beginning a trial of combination antidepressant therapy (Fig. 71–1).

■ CLINICAL APPLICATION

A suggested algorithm for the management of depression is shown in Figure 71–1.

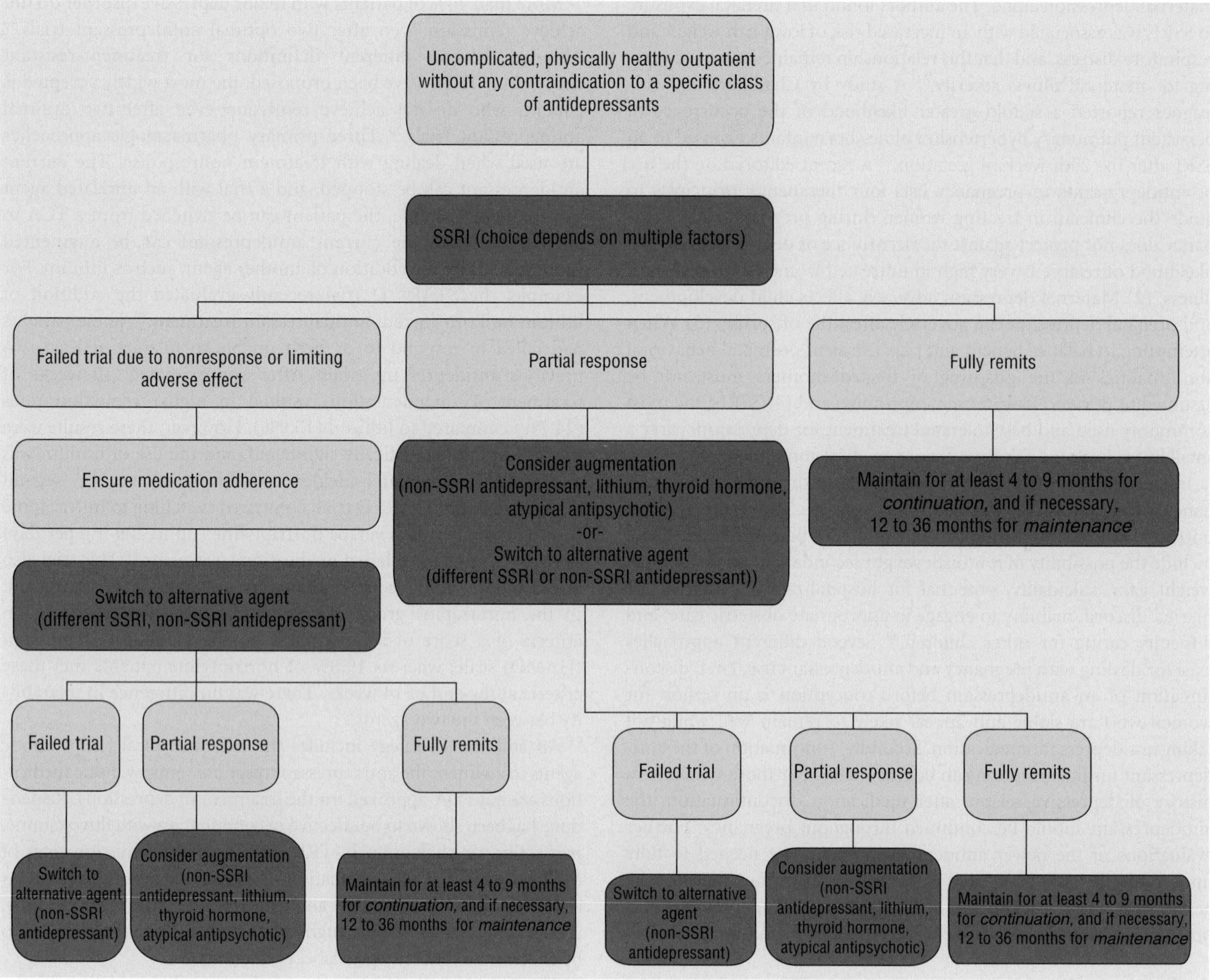

FIGURE 71-1. Algorithm for treatment of uncomplicated major depression. (SSRI, selective serotonin reuptake inhibitor.)

Dosing

Recommended initial doses and dosage ranges are shown in Table 71–3. In elderly patients, as a general rule, dosing is initiated at one-half the initial dose administered to younger adults, and the dose is increased at a slower rate.

The usual initial adult dose of most TCAs is 25 mg at bedtime, and the dose can be increased by 25 to 50 mg every third day. The recommended initial dose for the SSRIs, citalopram, fluoxetine, and paroxetine is 20 mg and 10 mg for escitalopram. The initial dose for fluvoxamine and sertraline is 50 mg/day. The doses are titrated upwards depending on symptom response and adverse effects.

The usual starting dose of venlafaxine is 75 mg/day and taken with food. Some patients can better tolerate a starting dose of 37.5 mg/day for a few days before beginning 75 mg/day. Depending on tolerability, the dose is then titrated to 150 mg/day. If needed, the dose can be further increased to 225 mg/day. Severely depressed patients can require doses as high as 375 mg/day. Both an immediate-release and extended release formulation of venlafaxine are now available. Duloxetine can be started at 30 mg and titrated upwards to 60 to 90 mg/day, given as a divided or single-daily dose. The recommended starting dose of mirtazapine is 15 mg/day administered in a single dose at bedtime, and the maximum recommended dose is 45 mg/day.

Bupropion is usually initiated at 75 mg twice daily, and this dose can be increased to 100 mg three times daily after a few days. Most patients will respond at 300 mg/day; however, an increase to 450 mg/day, given as 150 mg three times daily, can be considered in patients with no clinical response after several weeks of treatment at 300 mg/day. Additionally, both a 12-hour and 24-hour sustained release formulation are available, allowing for less frequent dosing.

Caution is urged when switching from one antidepressant to another. It is important to remember that 3 to 4 weeks is usually required before a mood-elevating response is seen. A 6-week trial at a maximum dosage is considered an adequate trial.[2] It is crucial to counsel the patient about the expected lag time before the onset of clinical response. Patients uneducated in this regard often fail to comply with their prescribed regimens.

■ PHARMACOECONOMIC CONSIDERATIONS

Cost of illness studies attempt to provide an estimation of the amount spent on a particular disease and to identify different components of the cost.[94] Ideally, direct, indirect, and intangible costs would be included. Direct costs include medical and nonmedical costs such as outpatient costs, inpatient costs, medication costs, transportation costs, and social services costs. Indirect costs include loss of productivity or reduced productivity. Intangible costs result from a decreased quality of life for the depressed individual and their family. Intangible costs are often not considered in pharmacoeconomic models because an accurate quantification in monetary terms is difficult.[94] Most published studies do not include all of the relevant aspects necessary for credible economic analyses.[95] In addition, there is wide variability among studies with regard to cost inclusion and evaluation of treatment withdrawals, relapses, toxicity, and adverse effects.[95]

When SSRIs were introduced, many managed care organizations restricted these medications to those who had failed treatment with the TCAs or who had been unable to tolerate these agents, with the belief that the SSRIs represented a more expensive approach to the treatment of depression. One of the major claims for SSRIs is the greater tolerability and safety profile in overdose when compared to the TCAs.[96] Studies including the costs associated with hospitalization following TCA overdoses as opposed to SSRI overdoses indicate that overdoses with TCAs are significantly more expensive.[96] All of the randomized clinical trials evaluating total expenditure of SSRIs versus TCAs indicate a cost advantage associated with SSRIs. Recently, several of the SSRIs have lost patent exclusivity, and generic versions of these medications are available at substantially lower prices than the brand name version. Several older studies and a more recent evaluation conducted in the United Kingdom found lower costs associated with the use of the SNRI, venlafaxine, when compared to SSRIs and TCAs.[97,98]

Additional longer-term studies in more diverse populations are necessary before judgments can be made regarding which of the newer antidepressant agents offers a cost advantage. It would be extremely useful if cost effective agents in various subpopulations and special populations (e.g., the elderly, those with comorbid substance abuse, those with comorbid anxiety disorders, and children) were identified. Also, the pharmacoeconomics of medication management of depressed patients in various healthcare environments such as public, private, psychiatry, or primary care, needs evaluation.

Pharmacoeconomic studies conducted to date are difficult to generalize, as there are no widely accepted uniform criteria and studies vary greatly in accounting for factors such as adherence, treatment withdrawals, relapses, toxicity, and adverse effects. There is also great variability in the type of costs included.[95]

EVALUATION OF THERAPEUTIC OUTCOMES

❼ Several monitoring parameters, in addition to plasma concentrations, are useful in managing patients. Patients must be monitored for adverse effects, such as sedation, anticholinergic effects, and sexual dysfunction, and for remission of previously documented target symptoms. The presence of side effects does not necessarily indicate adequate dosage. In addition, changes in social and occupational functioning should be assessed. Patients receiving venlafaxine should have their blood pressure monitored at regular intervals. Patients older than 40 years of age should receive a pretreatment ECG before starting TCA therapy, and followup ECGs should be performed periodically. Patients should be monitored for the emergence of suicidal ideation after initiation of any antidepressant. Weight gain and sexual dysfunction, common events associated with most antidepressants, are associated with nonadherence and should be monitored and discussed with the patient.

In addition to the clinical interview, psychometric rating instruments (e.g., patient-rated and clinician-rated scales) allow for rapid and reliable measurement of the nature and severity of depressive and associated symptoms (see Chap. 64). It is helpful to administer the rating scales prior to treatment, 6 to 8 weeks after initiation of therapy, and periodically thereafter. Interviewing a family member or friend (with the patient's permission) regarding symptoms and daily functioning also can assist in assessment of progress. Patients should be monitored at more frequent intervals early in treatment. Monitoring is then continued at regular intervals throughout the continuation and maintenance phases of treatment. Regular monitoring for reemergence of symptoms should be continued for several months after antidepressant therapy is discontinued.

Finally, one useful set of criteria that can be used with a variety of psychometric scales was suggested by Mann.[32] Following these criteria, the following definitions are used: (1) *nonresponse* is less than 25% decrease in baseline symptoms, (2) *partial response* is a 26% to 49% decrease in baseline symptoms, and (3) *partial remission or response* is greater than a 50% decrease in baseline symptoms. Consistent with other recommendations, *remission* is a return to baseline functioning with no symptoms present.[2]

COLLABORATIVE PRACTICE

Significant evidence exits to show that depression is common, chronic, and causes significant morbidity and mortality.[99] Pharmacists, in conjunction with other healthcare providers can play a crucial role in the screening, recognition, and treatment of this disorder. In fact, the United States Preventive Services Task Force has recommended that clinicians "maintain an especially high index of suspicion for depressive symptoms in adolescents and young adults, persons with a family history or personal history of depression, those with chronic illnesses, those who perceive or have experienced a recent loss, and those with sleep disorders, chronic pain, or multiple unexplained somatic complaints."[100] In addition, pharmacists and other healthcare clinicians play a crucial role in ensuring adherence to medication regimens through assessment of a patient's willingness and ability to take a medication, including an assessment of financial viability, and through patient education regarding dosing, side effects and drug interactions, and guidance regarding followup appointments with prescribing clinicians.[101]

CONCLUSIONS

Major depressive disorder remains one of the most commonly occurring mental illnesses in adults, and it is often undiagnosed and untreated. Pharmacologic intervention is the cornerstone of treatment for major depressive disorder. Antidepressant medications have a broad spectrum of neurochemical effects and influence a variety of receptors peripherally and centrally. Safe and effective use of antidepressants requires a thorough understanding of the pharmacology of these drugs and of the principles of monitoring efficacy and adverse effects. It also requires that the patient adhere to the prescribed antidepressant regimen. Clinicians must have a thorough understanding of antidepressant drug interactions and factors that can influence the pharmacokinetics of antidepressant drugs. Pharmacists are in an ideal position to accomplish these treatment goals. The search for more effective antidepressants with more favorable adverse-effect profiles must continue.

ABBREVIATIONS

DA: dopamine

DSM-IV-TR: Diagnostic and Statistical Manual of Mental Disorders, 4th ed., Text Revision

ECT: electroconvulsive therapy

5-HT: serotonin

HAMD: Hamilton Depression scale

MAOI: monoamine oxidase inhibitor

NE: norepinephrine

NIH: National Institutes of Health

REM: rapid eye movement

SNRI: serotonin-norepinephrine reuptake inhibitor

SSRI: serotonin-selective reuptake inhibitor

STAR* D: Sequenced Treatment Alternatives to Relieve Depression

TCA: tricyclic antidepressant

TRD: treatment-resistant depression

REFERENCES

1. American Psychiatric Association. Diagnostic and Statistical Manual of Mental Disorders, 4th ed., text revision. Washington, DC: American Psychiatric Association, 2000.
2. American Psychiatric Association. Practice guideline for the treatment of patients with major depressive disorder (revision). Am J Psychiatry 2000;157(4Suppl):1–45.
3. Kessler RC, Berglund P, Demler O. The epidemiology of major depressive disorders: Results from the National Comorbidity Survey Replication (NCS-R). JAMA 2003;289:3095–3105.
4. Burt VK, Stein K. Epidemiology of depression throughout the female life cycle. J Clin Psychol 2002;63(Suppl 7):9–15.
5. Steffens DC, Skoog I, Norton MC, et al. Prevalence of depression and its treatment in an elderly population. The Cache County study. Arch Gen Psychiatry 2000;57:601–607.
6. Kessler RC, Walters EE. Epidemiology of DSM-III-R major depression and minor depression among adolescents and young adults in the National Comorbidity Survey. Depress Anxiety 1998;7:3–14.
7. Larsson B, Ivarsson T. Clinical characteristics of adolescent psychiatric inpatients who have attempted suicide. Eur Child Adolesc Psychiatry 1998;7:201–208.
8. Weissman MM, Gershon ES, Kidd KK, et al. Psychiatric disorders in the relatives of probands with affective disorder. Arch Gen Psychiatry 1984;41:13–21.
9. Warner V, Weissman MM, Mufson L, Wickramaratne PJ. Grandparents, parents, and grandchildren at high risk for depression: A three-generation study. J Am Acad Child Adolesc Psychiatry 1999;38:289–296.
10. Sullivan PF, Neale MC, Kendler KS. Genetic epidemiology of major depression: Review and meta-analysis. Am J Psychiatry 2000;157:1552–1562.
11. Stahl SM. Blue genes and the mechanism of action of antidepressants. J Clin Psychiatry 2000;61:164–165.
12. Delgado PL. Depression: The case for a monoamine deficiency. J Clin Psychiatry 2000;61(Suppl 6):7–11.
13. Hirschfield RM. History and the evolution of the monoamine hypothesis of depression. J Clin Psychiatry 2000;61(Suppl 6):4–6.
14. Delgado PL, Moreno FA, Potter R, et al. Norepinephrine and serotonin in antidepressant action: Evidence from neurotransmitter depletion studies. In: Briley M, Montgomery SA, eds. Antidepressant Therapy at the Dawn of the Third Millennium. London: Marin Dunitz, 1997:141–163.
15. Baldessarini RJ. Drugs and the treatment of psychiatric disorders: Depression and anxiety disorders. In: Hardman JG, Limbrid LE, Goodman A, et al. eds. Goodman and Gilman's The Pharmacological Basis of Therapeutics, 10th ed. New York: McGraw-Hill, 2000:447–484.
16. Stahl SM. Blue genes and the monoamine hypothesis of depression. J Clin Psychiatry 2000;61:77–78.
17. Feighner JP. Mechanism of action of antidepressant medications. J Clin Psychiatry 1999;60(Suppl 4):4–11.
18. Stahl SM. Basic psychopharmacology of antidepressants, part 1: Antidepressants have seven distinct mechanisms of action. J Clin Psychiatry 1998;59(Suppl 4):5–14.
19. Bryant SG, Brown CS. Current concepts in clinical therapeutics: Major affective disorders, part 1. Clin Pharmacol 1986;5:304–318.
20. Siever LJ, Davis KL. Overview: Toward a dysregulation hypothesis of depression. Am J Psychiatry 1985;142:1017–1031.
21. Ordway GA, Klimek V, Mann JJ. Neurocircuitry of mood disorders. In: Davis KL, Charney D, Coyle JT, Nemeroff C, eds. Neuropsychopharmacology: The Fifth Generation of Progress. American College of Neuropsychopharmacology. Lippincott Williams and Wilkins: Philadelphia, 2002:1051–1064.
22. Thase ME, Fasiczka AL, Berman SR, et al. Electroencephalographic sleep profiles before and after cognitive behavior therapy of depression. Arch Gen Psychiatry 1998;55:138–144.
23. Sofuoglu M, Dudish-Poulsen S, Poling J, et al. The effect of individual cocaine withdrawal symptoms on outcomes in cocaine users. Addict Behav 2005;30:1125–1134.
24. Patten SB, Barbui C. Drug-induced depression: a systematic review to inform clinical practice. Psychoth Psychosom 2004;73:207–215.
25. McGirr A, Renaud J, Seguin M, et al. An examination of DSM-IV depressive symptoms and risk for suicide completion in major depressive disorder: A psychological autopsy study. J Affect Disord 2007;97:203–209.
26. Lebowitz BD, Pearson JL, Schneider LS, et al. Diagnosis and treatment of depression in late life: Consensus statement update. JAMA 1997;278:1186–1190.
27. Trivedi MH. The link between depression and physical symptoms. Prim Care Companion J Clin Psychiatry 2004;6(suppl 1):12–16.
28. Centers for Disease Control and Prevention, National Center for Injury Prevention and Control. Suicide: Fact Sheet. 2006, *http://www.cdc.gov/ncipc/factsheets/suifacts.htm*.
29. Coryell WH. Clinical assessment of suicide risk in depressive disorder. CNS Spectr 2006;11(6):137–142.
30. Claassen CA, Trivedi MH, Rush AJ, et al. Clinical differences among depressed patients with and without a history of suicide attempts: findings from the STAR*D trial. J Affect Disord 2007;97:77–84.
31. Alexopoulos GS, Bruce ML, Hull J, et al. Clinical determinant of suicidal ideation and behavior in geriatric depression. Arch Gen Psychiatry 1999;56:1048–1053.
32. Mann JJ. The Medical Management of Depression. N Engl J Med 2005;353:1819–1834.
33. Blackburn IM, Moore RG. Controlled acute and follow-up trial of cognitive therapy and pharmacotherapy in outpatients with recurrent depression. Br J Psychiatry 1997;171:328–334.
34. Klapheke MM. Electroconvulsive therapy consultation: An update. Convuls Ther 1997;13:227–241.
35. Lafer B, Sachs GS, Labbate LA, et al. Side effects induced by bright light therapy. Am J Psychiatry 1994;151:1081–1083.
36. Stahl SM, Grady MM, Moret C, Briley M. SNRIs: Their pharmacology, clinical efficacy, and tolerability in comparison with other classes of antidepressants. CNS Spectr 2005;10:732–747.
37. Ables AZ, Baughman III, OL. Antidepressants: Update on new agents and indications. Am Fam Physician 2003;67:547–554.
38. Horst WD, Preskorn SH. Mechanism of action and clinical characteristics of three atypical antidepressants: Venlafaxine, nefazodone, bupropion. J Affect Disord 1998;51:237–254.
39. Gorman JM. Mirtazapine: Clinical overview. J Clin Psychiatry 1999;60(Suppl 17):9–13.
40. Bryant SG, Brown CS. Current concepts in clinical therapeutics: Major affective disorders, part 2. Clin Pharm 1986;5:385–395.
41. Patkar AA, Pae C-U, Masand PS. Transdermal Selegiline: The New Generation of Monoamine Oxidase Inhibitors. CNS Spectr 2006;11:363–375.
42. Linde K, Mulrow CD, Berner M, Egger M. St. John's Wort for depression. Cochrane Database of Systematic Reviews 2005, Issue 2 Art. No.: CD000448.
43. Nemeroff CB. The burden of severe depression: a review of diagnostic challenges and treatment alternatives. J Psychiatr Res 2007;41:189–206.
44. Settle ED Jr. Antidepressant drugs: disturbing and potentially dangerous adverse effects. J Clin Psychiatry 1998;59(Suppl 16):25–30.
45. Haddad P. Antidepressant discontinuation reactions. In: Thompson C, chairperson. Discontinuation of antidepressant therapy: Emerging complications and their relevance [academic highlights]. J Clin Psychiatry 1998;59:541–548.
46. Feighner JP. Cardiovascular safety in depressed patients: Focus on venlafaxine. J Clin Psychiatry 1995;56:574–579.
47. Bauer M, Moller HJ, Schneider E. Duloxetine: a new selective and dual-acting antidepressant. Expert Opin Pharmacother 2006;7(4):421–427.
48. Preskorn SH. Clinically relevant pharmacology of selective serotonin reuptake inhibitors: An overview with emphasis on pharmacokinetics and effects on oxidative drug metabolism. Clin Pharmacokinet 1997;32(Suppl 1):1–21.
49. Goldstein BJ, Goodnick PJ. Selective serotonin reuptake inhibitors in the treatment of affective disorders: III. Tolerability, safety and pharmacoeconomics. J Psychopharmacol 1998;12(3 Suppl B):S55–S87.
50. Masand PS and Gupta S. Long-term side effects of newer-generation antidepressants: SSRIs, venlafaxine, nefazodone, bupropion, and mirtazapine. Ann Clin Psychiatry 2002;14:175–182.
51. Westenberg HG, Sander C. Tolerability and safety of fluvoxamine and other antidepressants. Int J Clin Pract 2006;60(4):482–491.

52. Aranoff GM. Trazodone associated with priapism. Lancet 1984;1:856.
53. Brodie-Meijer CC, Diemont WL, Buijs PJ. Nefazodone-induced clitoral priapism. Int Clin Psychopharmacol 1999;14:257–258.
54. Johnston JA, Lineberry CG, Ascher JA. A 102-center prospective study of seizures in association with bupropion. J Clin Psychiatry 1991;52:450–456.
55. Rabkin JG, Quitkin FM, McGrath P, et al. Adverse reactions to monoamine oxidase inhibitors: II. Treatment correlates and clinical management. J Clin Psychopharmacol 1985;5:2–9.
56. Neil JF, Licata SM, May SJ, Himmelhock JM. Dietary noncompliance during treatment with tranylcypromine. J Clin Psychiatry 1979;40:33–37.
57. Varon J, Marik PE. The diagnosis and management of hypertensive crises. Chest 2000;118:214–227.
58. Wells BG. Tricyclic antidepressants. In: Taylor WJ, Caviness MHD, eds. A Textbook for the Clinical Application of Therapeutic Drug Monitoring. Irving, TX: Abbott Laboratories, 1986:449–465.
59. Rudorfer MV, Potter WZ. Metabolism of tricyclic antidepressants. Cell Mol Neurobiol 1999;19:373–409.
60. Olver JS, Burrows GD, Norman TR. The treatment of depression with different formulations of venlafaxine: a comparative analysis. Hum Psychopharmacol 2004;19:9–16.
61. DeVane CL. Metabolism and pharmacokinetics of the selective serotonin reuptake inhibitors. Cell Mol Neurobiol 1999;19:443–466.
62. Hemeryck A, Belpaire FM. Selective serotonin reuptake inhibitors and cytochrome P450 mediated drug-drug interactions: An update. Curr Drug Metab 2002;3:13–37.
63. Jefferson JW, Pradko JF, Muir KT. Bupropion for major depressive disorder: Pharmacokinetic and formulation considerations. Clin Ther 2005;27:1685–1695.
64. Dunner DL, Zisook S, Billow AA, et al. A prospective safety surveillance study for bupropion sustained-release in the treatment of depression. J Clin Psychiatry 1998;59;366–373.
65. Timmer CJ, Sitsen JM, Delbressine LP. Clinical pharmacokinetics of mirtazapine. Clin Pharmacokinet 2000;38:461–474.
66. Watanabe MD, Winter ME. Tricyclic antidepressants: amitriptyline, desipramine, imipramine, and nortriptyline. In: Winter ME, ed. Basic Clinical Pharmacokinetics, 4th ed. Baltimore, MD: Lippincott Williams & Wilkins, 2004:423–437.
67. Krastev Z, Terzivoanov D, Vlahov V, et al. The pharmacokinetics of paroxetine in patients with liver cirrhosis. Acta Psychiatr Scand 1989;350(Suppl):91–92.
68. Demolis JL, Angebaud P, Grange JD, et al. Influence of liver cirrhosis on sertraline pharmacokinetics. Br J Clin Pharmacol 1996;42:394–397.
69. Kent JM. SNaRIs, NaSSAs, and NaRIs: New agents for the treatment of depression. Lancet 2000;355:911–918.
70. DeVane CL. Differential pharmacology of newer antidepressants. J Clin Psychiatry 1998;59(Suppl 20):85–93.
71. Boyer EW, Shannon M. Current Concepts: The Serotonin Syndrome. N Engl J Med 2005;352:1112–1120.
72. Otong D. The art of prescribing. Antidepressants in late-life depression: prescribing principles. Perspect Psychiatr Care May 2006;42(2):149–153.
73. Turvey CL, Conwell Y, Jones MP, et al. Risk factors for late-life suicide. A Prospective, Community-Based Study. Am J Geriatr Psychiatry 2002;10:398–406.
74. Reynolds CF 3rd, Dew MA, Pollock BG, Mulsant BH, et al. Maintenance treatment of major depression in old age. N Engl J Med 2006;354(11):1130–1138.
75. Kohn R, Epstein-Lubrow G. Course and outcomes of depression in the elderly Curr Psychiatry Rep 2006;8(1):34–40.
76. Cosgrave E, McGorry P, Allen N, Jackson H. Depression in young people: A growing challenge for primary care. Aust Fam Physician 2000;29:123–127.
77. Wagner KD, Ambrosini P, Rynn M, et al. Efficacy of sertraline in the treatment of children and adolescents with major depressive disorder. JAMA 2003;290:1033–1041.
78. Olfson M, Marcus SC, Shaffer D. Antidepressant drug therapy and suicide in severely depressed children and adults: A case-control study. Arch Gen Psychiatry 2006;63(8):865–872.
79. Valuck RJ, Libby AM, Sills MR, et al. Antidepressant treatment and risk of suicide attempt by adolescents with major depressive disorder: a propensity-adjusted retrospective cohort study. CNS Drugs 2004;18(15):1119–1132.
80. Simon GE, Savarino J, Operskalski B, Wang PS. Suicide risk during antidepressant treatment. Am J Psychiatry 2006;163(1):41–47.
81. Hallfors DD, Waller MW, Ford CA, et al. Adolescent depression and suicide risk: Association with sex and drug behavior. Am J Prev Med 2004;27(3):224–231.
82. Haavisto A, Sourander A, Ellila H, et al. Suicidal ideation and suicide attempts among child and adolescent psychiatric inpatients in Finland. J Affect Disord 2003;76(1–3):211–221.
83. Leonard HL, Meyer HC, Swedo SE, et al. Electrocardiographic changes during desipramine and clomipramine treatment in children and adolescents. J Am Acad Child Adolesc Psychiatry 1995;34:1460–1468.
84. Oberlander TF, Warburton W, Misri S, et al. Neonatal outcomes after prenatal exposure to selective serotonin reuptake inhibitor antidepressants and maternal depression using population-based linked health data. Arch Gen Psychiatry 2006;63:898–906.
85. Chambers CD, Hernandex-Diaz S, Van Marter LJ, et al. Selective Serotonin-reuptake inhibitors and risk of persistent pulmonary hypertension of the newborn. N Engl J Med 2006;354(6):579–587.
86. Cohen LS, Altshuler LL, Harlow BL, et al. Relapse of major depression during pregnancy in women who maintain or discontinue antidepressant treatment. JAMA 2006;295(5):499–507.
87. Rubinow, DR. Antidepressant treatment during pregnancy: Between Scylla and Charybdis. Am J Psychiatry 2006;163(6):954–955.
88. Hendrick V, Altshuler L. Management of major depression during pregnancy. Am J Psychiatry 2002;159:1667–1673.
89. Sequenced Treatment Alternatives to Relieve Depression (STAR*D) (Available at *http://www.edc.pitt.edu/std/*, accessed February 12, 2007).
90. Nierenberg AA, Fava M, Trivedi MH, et al. A comparison of lithium and T3 augmentation following two failed medication treatments for depression: A STAR*D Report. Am J Psychiatry 2006;163:1519–1530
91. Fava M, Rush AJ, Wisniewski SR, et al. A comparison of mirtazapine and nortriptyline following two consecutive failed medication treatments for depressed outpatients: a STAR*D report. Am J Psychiatry 2006;163(7):1161–1172.
92. Nemeroff CB. Use of atypical antipsychotics in refractory depression and anxiety. J Clin Psychiatry 2005:66(Suppl 8):13–21.
93. Rapaport MH, Gharabawi GM, Canuso CM, et al. Effects of risperidone augmentation in patients with treatment-resistant depression: results of open-label treatment followed by double-blind continuation. Neuropsychopharmacology 2006;31:2505–2513.
94. Luppa M, Heinrich S, Angermeyer MC, et al. Cost-of-illness studies of depression: A systematic review. J Affect Disord 2007;98:29–43.
95. Iqbal SU, Prashker M. Pharmacoeconomic evaluation of antidepressants. Pharmacoeconomics 2005;23(6):595–606.
96. Barbui C, Peercudani M, Hotopf M. Economic evaluation of antidepressive agents: A systematic critique of experimental and observational studies. J Clin Psychopharmacol 2003;23(2):145–154.
97. Lenox-Smith A, Conway P, Knight C. Cost effectiveness of representatives of three classes of antidepressants used in major depression in the UK. Pharmacoeconomics 2004;22(5):311–319.
98. Morrow TJ. The pharmacoeconomics of venlafaxine in depression. Am J Manag Care 2001;7:S386–S392.
99. American College of Physicians/American Society of Internal Medicine. Pharmacist scope of practice. Ann Intern Med 2002;136:79–85.
100. U.S. Preventive Services Task Force. Guide to Clinical Preventive Services, 2nd ed. Baltimore, MD: Williams & Wilkins, 1996:541–546.
101. Finely P, Rens HR, Pont JT, et al. Impact of a collaborative pharmacy practice model on the treatment of depression in primary care. Am J Health Syst Pharm 2002;59:1518–1526.
102. Lexi-Comp, Inc. Lexi-Comp Online. *http://online.lexi.com*.
103. Thomson MICROMEDEX Healthcare Series. *https://www.thomsonhc.com*.

CHAPTER 72 Bipolar Disorder

SHANNON J. DRAYTON AND BENJAMIN WEINSTEIN

KEY CONCEPTS

1. Bipolar disorder is a cyclic mental illness with recurrent mood episodes that occur over a person's lifetime. The symptoms, course, severity, and response to treatment differ among individuals.
2. Bipolar disorder is likely caused by genetic factors, environmental triggers, and the dysregulation of neurotransmitters, neurohormones, and second messenger systems in the brain.
3. The goal of therapy for bipolar disorder should be to improve functioning of the patient by reducing mood episodes. This is accomplished by maximizing adherence to therapy and limiting adverse effects.
4. Patients and family members should be educated about bipolar disorder and treatments. Long-term monitoring and adherence to treatment are major factors in obtaining stabilization of the disorder.
5. Lithium and valproate are the mainstays of treatment for both acute mania and prophylaxis for recurrent manic and depressive episodes. Anticonvulsants, such as lamotrigine, carbamazepine, and oxcarbazepine, and atypical antipsychotics, such as aripiprazole, olanzapine, risperidone, quetiapine, and ziprasidone are alternative or adjunctive treatments for bipolar disorder. Anticonvulsants can be more effective than lithium in several mood subtypes (e.g., mixed states and rapid cycling). Lamotrigine and lithium can be more effective for recurrent bipolar depression.
6. Some patients can be stabilized on one mood stabilizer, but others may require combination therapies or adjunctive agents during an acute mood episode. If possible, adjunctive agents should be tapered and discontinued when the acute mood episode remits and the patient is stabilized. Adjunctive agents can include antidepressants, additional mood stabilizers, antipsychotics, and benzodiazepines.
7. Baseline and followup laboratory tests are required for some medications to monitor for adverse effects.

(1) Bipolar disorder (manic-depressive illness) is one of the most common of the severe chronic psychiatric disorders. The cyclic mood disorder is characterized by recurrent fluctuations in mood, energy, and behavior encompassing the extremes of human experiences.[1–4] Bipolar disorder differs from recurrent major depression (or unipolar depression) in that a manic, hypomanic, or mixed episode occurs during the course of the illness.[2] Bipolar disorder is a lifelong illness with a variable course and requires both nonpharmacologic and pharmacologic treatments for mood stabilization.[2,3]

Learning objectives, review questions, and other resources can be found at **www.pharmacotherapyonline.com.**

EPIDEMIOLOGY

The lifetime prevalence of bipolar I disorder (one or more manic or mixed episodes) is 0.4% to 1.6%; that for bipolar II disorder (recurrent major depressive episodes with hypomanic episodes) is approximately 0.5%.[2,3] A national comorbidity survey reported that the lifetime prevalence rate of a manic episode is 1.6% ±0.3% for men and 1.7% ± 0.3% for women in the United States (approximately 4 million people).[5] Bipolar I disorder occurs equally in men and women, whereas bipolar II disorder is more common in women.[2,3] Of the 1.9 million Americans who have either bipolar I or II disorder, it is estimated that only 50% of these individuals are receiving any type of treatment for their illness.[1]

ETIOLOGY

(2) The exact etiology of bipolar disorder is unknown. Bipolar disorder is thought to be a complex genetic disease that is environmentally influenced and caused by a wide range of neurobiologic abnormalities. Stressful life events, alcohol or substance use, and changes in the sleep-wake cycle can elicit the expression of genetic or biologic vulnerabilities that cause dysregulation of neurotransmitters, neuroendocrine pathways, and second messenger systems.[4] Table 72–1 summarizes the etiologic theories of bipolar disorder.

PATHOPHYSIOLOGY

(2) Many theories have been proposed regarding the pathophysiology of mood disorders.[4] Family, twin, and adoption studies report an increased lifetime prevalence risk of having mood disorders among first-degree relatives of patients with bipolar disorder.[3,11] Genetic linkage studies suggest multiple gene loci can be involved in the heredity of mood disorders.[6–9,12] Neuroimaging studies have found neurochemical, anatomic, and functional abnormalities in bipolar patients.[12,13] Environmental or psychosocial stressors, nutritional deficiencies, infections, immunologic reactions, sleep deprivation, and disruption of circadian rhythms can cause dysregulation in neurotransmitters, hormones, endocrine function, neuropeptides, cations, intracellular second messengers, and signal transduction pathways.[3,4,7,12–18]

TABLE 72-1 Etiologic Theories of Bipolar Disorder

Genetic factors

80–90% of patients with bipolar disorder have a biologic relative with a mood disorder (e.g., bipolar disorder, major depression, cyclothymia, or dysthymia).

First-degree relatives of bipolar patients have a 15–35% lifetime risk of developing any mood disorder and a 5–10% lifetime risk for developing bipolar disorder.

The concordance rate of mood disorders is 60–80% for monozygotic twins and 14–20% for dizygotic twins.

Linkage studies suggest that certain loci on genes and the X chromosome may contribute to genetic susceptibility of bipolar disorder.

Nongenetic factors

Perinatal insult

Head trauma

Environmental factors

- Desynchronization of circadian or seasonal rhythms cause diurnal variations in mood and sleep patterns and can result in seasonal recurrences of mood episodes.
- Changes in the sleep-wake cycle or light-dark cycle can precipitate episodes of mania or depression.
- Bright light therapy can be used for the treatment of winter depression and can precipitate hypomania, mania, or mixed episodes.

Psychosocial or physical stressors

- Stressful life events often precede mood episodes and can increase recurrence rates and prolong time to recovery from mood episodes.

Nutritional factors

- Deficiency of essential amino acid precursors in the diet can cause a dysregulation of neurotransmitter activity (e.g., L-tryptophan deficiency causes a decrease in 5-HT and melatonin synthesis and activity).
- Deficiency in essential fatty acids (e.g., omega-3 fatty acids) can cause a dysregulation of neurotransmitter activity.

Neurotransmitter/neuroendocrine/hormonal theories

- Dysregulation between excitatory and inhibitory neurotransmitter systems; excitatory: NE, DA, glutamate, and aspartate; inhibitory: 5-HT and GABA.

Monoamine hypothesis

- An excess of catecholamines (primarily NE and DA) cause mania.
- Agents that decrease catecholamines are used for the treatment of mania (e.g., DA antagonists and α_2-adrenergic agonists).
- Deficit of neurotransmitters (primarily NE, DA, and/or 5-HT) cause depression.
- Agents that increase neurotransmitter activity are used for the treatment of depression (e.g., 5-HT and NE/DA reuptake inhibitors and MAOIs).

Dysregulation of amino acid neurotransmitters

- Deficiency of GABA or excessive glutamate activity causes dysregulation of neurotransmitters (e.g., increased DA and NE activity).
- Agents that increase GABA activity or decrease glutamate activity are used for the treatment of mania and for mood stabilization (e.g., benzodiazepines, lamotrigine, lithium, or valproic acid).

Cholinergic hypothesis

- Deficiency of acetylcholine causes an imbalance in cholinergic-adrenergic activity and can increase the risk of manic episodes.
- Agents that increase acetylcholine activity can decrease manic symptoms (e.g., use of cholinesterase inhibitors or augmentation of muscarinic cholinergic activity).
- Increased central acetylcholine levels can increase the risk of depressive episodes.
- Agents that decrease acetylcholine activity can alleviate depressive symptoms (i.e., anticholinergic agents).

Secondary messenger system dysregulation

- Abnormal G protein functioning dysregulates adenylate cyclase activity, phosphoinositide responses, sodium/potassium/calcium channel exchange, and activity of phospholipases. Abnormal cyclic adenosine monophosphate and phosphoinositide secondary messenger system activity.
- Abnormal protein kinase C activity and signaling pathways.

Hypothalamic-pituitary-thyroid axis dysregulation

- Hyperthyroidism can precipitate manic-like symptoms.
- Hypothyroidism can precipitate a depression and be a risk factor for rapid cycling; thyroid supplementation can be used for refractory rapid cycling and augmentation of antidepressants in unipolar depression.
- Positive antithyroid antibody titers reported in patients with bipolar disorder.
- Hormonal changes during the female life cycle can cause dysregulation of neurotransmitters (e.g., premenstrual, postpartum, and perimenopause).

Membrane and cation theories

- Abnormal neuronal calcium and sodium activity and homeostasis cause neurotransmitter dysregulation.
- Hypocalcemia has been associated with causing anxiety, mood irritability, mania, psychosis, and delirium.
- Hypercalcemia has been associated with causing depression, stupor, and coma.
- Extracellular and intracellular calcium concentrations may affect the synthesis and release of NE, DA, and 5-HT, as well as the excitability of neuronal firing.

Sensitization and kindling theories

- Recurrences of mood episodes causes behavioral sensitivity and electrophysiologic kindling (similar to the amygdala-kindling models for seizures in animals) and can result in rapid or continuous mood cycling.

DA, dopamine; GABA, γ-aminobutyric acid; 5-HT, serotonin; MAOI, monoamine oxidase inhibitor; NE, norepinephrine.

Data from Torrey and Knable,[1] Goldberg and Harrow,[4] Kelso,[6] Manji et al.,[7] Lenox et al.,[8] Baron,[9] Bezchlibnyk and Young,[10] Goodnick,[12] Soares,[13] Manji et al.,[14] Gould and Manji,[15] Sobczak et al.,[16] Freeman et al.,[17] Ketter and Wang,[18] White,[19] Rasgon et al.,[20] and Mahmood and Silverstone.[21]

NEUROCHEMICAL THEORIES

The kindling and behavioral sensitization model postulates that psychosocial stressors can result in manic or depressive episodes because various brain networks are sensitized for exaggerated and spontaneous reactions secondary to neurotransmitter imbalances or dysregulation and voltage-gated ion channel abnormalities.[4,19] Dysregulation between neurotransmitters, neuropeptides, hormones, and secondary messenger systems can produce a cyclic rhythm disturbance in the central nervous system.[1,4,7,12,19] Abnormal calcium, potassium, and sodium homeostasis can alter neurotransmitter release and the secondary messenger system.[7,19] Hormonal changes during the menstrual cycle, postpartum period, and perimenopausal phase can contribute to mood dysregulation.[17,20]

The "permissive serotonin hypothesis" proposes that serotonin (5-hydroxytryptamine or 5-HT) plays a critical role in modulating brain activity (e.g., stabilization of the catecholamine system and inhibition of dopamine [DA] release), and is low in both mania and depression.[12,21] The type of affective state that is expressed with the permissive hypothesis is determined secondarily by the level of norepinephrine (NE) (e.g., increased amounts of NE lead to mania, decreased amounts lead to depression). L-tryptophan or 5-HT deficiency and changes in the light–dark cycle may result in reduced melatonin secretion from the pineal gland that disrupts the sleep-wake cycle, alters circadian rhythms, and causes seasonal affective changes.[1,12,21]

The catecholamine hypothesis of mood disorders suggests that increased DA and norepinephrine activity contribute to hyperactivity and psychosis associated with the severe stages of mania, and reduced activity causes depression.[4,12] A γ-aminobutyric acid (GABA) deficiency theory has been proposed for mania as it inhibits NE and DA activity.[4,7,12] Glutamate and aspartate, excitatory amino acid neurotransmitters, may be overactive and involved in causing manic episodes.[7] Cholinergic underactivity has been proposed to cause mania and overactivity of acetylcholine to cause depression.[7,12] Acetylcholine is an antagonist of the catecholamine system and contributes to the interaction between phosphatidylinositol and phosphatidylcholine secondary messenger systems.[7]

DIAGNOSTIC DIFFICULTY

Several medical, medication-induced, or substance-related causes of mania and depression have been identified (see Table 72–2 for causes of mania and Table 71–1 in Chap. 71 for causes of depression).[1–3] A complete medical, psychiatric, and medication history; physical examination; and laboratory testing are necessary to rule out any organic causes of mania or depression.[3] An accurate diagnosis is important because some psychiatric and neurologic disorders present with manic-like or depressive-like symptoms.[3,4] For example, attention-deficit/hyperactivity disorder and a manic episode have similar characteristics; thus individuals with bipolar disorder can be misdiagnosed and prescribed central nervous system stimulants.[11,22] Use of any substance that affects the central nervous system (e.g., alcohol, antidepressants, caffeine, central nervous system stimulants, hallucinogens, or marijuana) can worsen symptoms of mania or depression and decrease response to treatment.[3,12,23–25]

Another disease state that has a similar presentation to bipolar disorder is schizoaffective disorder. This disease is a mix between schizophrenia and bipolar disorder. Patients with schizoaffective disorder have mood episodes, but the distinguishing factor from bipolar disorder is that these patients experience psychosis even between mood episodes during periods of euthymia. Clinicians must rely on family members or others that know the patient to determine if the patient is psychotic between mood episodes. It can be difficult for clinicians to obtain a full psychiatric history on patients, thus making schizoaffective disorder widely diagnosed. Schizoaffective disorder is treated with mood stabilizers and antipsychotics as maintenance therapy.

TABLE 72-2 Secondary Causes of Mania

Medical conditions that induce mania
• CNS disorders (brain tumor, strokes, head injuries, subdural hematoma, multiple sclerosis, systemic lupus erythematosus, temporal lobe seizures, Huntington's disease)
• Infections (encephalitis, neurosyphilis, sepsis, human immunodeficiency virus)
• Electrolyte or metabolic abnormalities (calcium or sodium fluctuations, hyper- or hypoglycemia)
• Endocrine or hormonal dysregulation (Addison's disease, Cushing's disease, hyper- or hypothyroidism, menstrual-related or pregnancy-related or perimenopausal mood disorders)
Medications or drugs that induce mania
• Alcohol intoxication
• Drug withdrawal states (alcohol, α_2-adrenergic agonists, antidepressants, barbiturates, benzodiazepines, opiates)
• Antidepressants (MAOIs, TCAs, 5-HT and/or NE and/or DA reuptake inhibitors, 5-HT antagonists)
• DA-augmenting agents (CNS stimulants: amphetamines, cocaine, sympathomimetics; DA agonists, releasers, and reuptake inhibitors)
• Hallucinogens (LSD, PCP)
• Marijuana intoxication precipitates psychosis, paranoid thoughts, anxiety, and restlessness
• NE-augmenting agents (α_2-adrenergic antagonists, β-agonists, NE reuptake inhibitors)
• Steroids (anabolic, adrenocorticotropic hormone, corticosteroids)
• Thyroid preparations
• Xanthines (caffeine, theophylline)
• Over-the-counter weight loss agents and decongestants (ephedra, pseudoephedrine)
• Herbal products (St. John's wort)
Somatic therapies that induce mania
• Bright light therapy
• Sleep deprivation

CNS, central nervous system; DA, dopamine; 5-HT, serotonin; LSD, lysergic acid diethylamide; MAOI, monoamine oxidase inhibitor; NE, norepinephrine; PCP, phencyclidine; TCA, tricyclic antidepressant.
Data from Torrey and Knable,[1] American Psychiatric Association,[2] American Psychiatric Association,[3] and Goodnick.[12]

CLINICAL PRESENTATION

❶ The essential feature of bipolar spectrum disorders are a history of mania or hypomania that is not caused by any other medical condition, substance, or psychiatric disorder (see Table 72–2 for secondary causes of mania).[2,3] The *Diagnostic and Statistical Manual of Mental Disorders, Fourth Edition, Text Revision (DSM-IV-TR)* of the American Psychiatric Association (APA) details the present understanding of mood disorders.[2] Bipolar disorder is divided into four subtypes based on the identification of specific mood episodes: bipolar I, bipolar II, cyclothymic disorder, and bipolar disorder not otherwise specified. See Table 72–3 for a definition of mood disorders by type of episode. The mood states are further separated into four subcategories to differentiate the current or most recent mood episode: major depressive, manic, hypomanic, or mixed. See Table 72–4 for the evaluation and diagnostic criteria of mood episodes. A new concept of "bipolar spectrum disorder" has been suggested that broadens the diagnosis to include dysthymia, cyclothymia, drug-induced hypomania, and recurrent unipolar depression.[4,26] Bipolar disorder is a cyclic mood disorder in which patients can move from one episode to another with or without a period of normal mood (euthymia) between. Persons with bipolar disorder can have mood fluctuations that continue for months, or after one episode they can sometimes go

TABLE 72-3 Mood Disorders Defined by Episodes

Disorder Subtype	Episode(s)[a]
Major depressive disorder, single episode	Major depressive episode
Major depressive disorder, recurrent	Two or more major depressive episodes
Bipolar disorder, type I[b]	Manic episode ± major depressive or mixed episode
Bipolar disorder, type II[c]	Major depressive episode + hypomanic episode
Dysthymic disorder	Chronic subsyndromal depressive episodes
Cyclothymic disorder[d]	Chronic fluctuations between subsyndromal depressive and hypomanic episodes (2 years for adults and 1 year for children and adolescents)
Bipolar disorder not otherwise specified	Mood states do not meet criteria for any specific bipolar disorder

[a]The length and severity of a mood episode and the interval between episodes varies from patient to patient. Manic episodes are usually briefer and end more abruptly than major depressive episodes. The average length of untreated manic episodes ranges from 4 to 13 months. Episodes can occur regularly (at the same time or season of the year) and often cluster at 12-month intervals. Women have more depressive episodes than manic episodes, whereas men have a more even distribution of episodes.
[b]For bipolar I disorder, 90% of individuals who experience a manic episode later have multiple recurrent major depressive, manic, hypomanic, or mixed episodes alternating with a normal mood state.
[c]Approximately 5–15% of patients with bipolar II disorder will develop a manic episode over a 5-year period. If a manic or mixed episode develops in a patient with bipolar II disorder, the diagnosis is changed to bipolar I disorder.
[d]Patients with cyclothymic disorder have a 15–50% risk of later developing a bipolar I or II disorder.
Data from American Psychiatric Association,[2] Goldberg and Harrow,[4] and Goodnick.[12]

years without recurrence of any type of mood episode. Comorbid psychiatric disorders associated with bipolar disorder include but are not limited to the following; alcohol and substance abuse, personality disorders, and anxiety disorders such as panic disorder, social anxiety disorder, and obsessive-compulsive disorder.[2–4,12,23,25,27,28]

MAJOR DEPRESSIVE EPISODE

Bipolar depression is often underdiagnosed and is frequently misdiagnosed as major depressive disorder.[3,29] Approximately 95% of patients with bipolar disorder experience episodes of depression during their lifetime.[2,4] Compared to manic episodes, depressive episodes are more frequent, longer lasting, and occur more often in bipolar II than in bipolar I disorder.[4,30] Over a person's lifetime, depressive episodes can account for up to 80% of all mood episodes. Recurrent depressive episodes are more common in women compared to men.[4] In bipolar depression, patients have an increased suicide risk and often have mood lability, hypersomnia, low energy, psychomotor retardation, cognitive impairment, anhedonia, decreased sexual activity, slowed speech, carbohydrate craving, and weight gain (also called atypical depressive features).[4,30,31] Delusions, hallucinations, and suicide attempts are more common in bipolar depression than in unipolar depression.[4]

MANIC EPISODE

For a diagnosis of mania, the symptoms must last at least 1 week, the mood must be elevated (expansive or irritable), and there must be an impairment in functioning.[2] Acute mania usually begins abruptly, and symptoms escalate over several days. Common symptoms of mania include grandiosity, decreased need for sleep or food, pressured speech, flight of ideas (racing thoughts), distractibility, increased activity, poor judgment, and involvement in pleasurable activities with potentially negative consequences.[2] Patients with acute mania often have psychotic symptoms, thus some patients are incorrectly diagnosed as having schizophrenia.[12] Mania symptoms that can resemble paranoid schizophrenia are bizarre behavior, hallucinations, and paranoid or grandiose delusions. Seasonal changes, stressors, sleep deprivation, antidepressants, central nervous system stimulants, or bright light can precipitate a manic episode.

HYPOMANIC EPISODE

Hypomania is a less severe form of mania, and by definition does not cause a marked impairment in social or occupational functioning, and no delusions or hallucinations are present.[2,4] Patients with hypomania often do not seek treatment until they have a depressive episode, thus hypomania may not be recognized or reported.[3] Symptoms found in hypomanic episodes are similar to those of cocaine- or antidepressant-induced mood disorders; thus the differential diagnosis should rule out any substance-induced or medical conditions that present with elevated mood.[25] Hypomanic states should be closely monitored, because 5% to 15% of patients can rapidly switch to a manic episode.[4]

MIXED EPISODE

Bipolar "mixed episode" (previously known as mixed state, dysphoric mania, or depressive mania) is defined as the simultaneous occurrence of manic and depressive symptoms.[2,4] Mixed mood states occur in up to 40% of all episodes and are more common in younger and older patients and in females.[4] Mixed episodes are often difficult to diagnose and treat because of the fluctuating clinical presentation. Patients with mixed states often have comorbid alcohol and substance abuse, severe anxiety symptoms, a higher suicide rate, and a poorer prognosis.[4,25]

COURSE OF ILLNESS

❶ Bipolar disorder is frequently not recognized and treated for many years because of its fluctuating course and episodic mood states.[3,4,12] The onset of bipolar disorder is rare before puberty, but its incidence increases during late adolescence and into early adulthood (usually between the ages of 15 and 30 years).[2] The average age of onset of a first manic episode is 21 years for both men and women.[3] The first episode in females is more likely to be a major depressive episode, whereas males are more likely to first experience a manic episode.[2,3] Women are more likely to have mixed states, depressive episodes, and rapid cycling compared to men.[2,3] Onset of manic episodes after the age of 60 years is rare and is likely caused by a medical or neurologic condition (e.g., stroke, tumor, or dementia), medications, or substance use.[3]

More than 80% of patients have more than 4 mood episodes during their lifetime; untreated patients can have 10 or more episodes during their lifetime.[3] Episodes can become longer in duration and more frequent with aging.[3] The kindling theory is used to explain why bipolar disorder progresses over one's life and why preventative treatment is imperative. Usually there is a period of normal functioning between episodes, but approximately 20% to 30% of patients with bipolar I disorder and 15% with bipolar II disorder have no period of euthymia because of mood lability, residual mood symptoms, or a direct switch to the opposite polarity.[2]

Rapid cycling (more than four mood episodes per year) is more common in females and occurs in approximately 10% to 20% of bipolar I and II disorder patients.[1–4,17,24] Frequent and severe episodes of depression appear to be the most common hallmark of rapid cycling. Use of alcohol, stimulants, antidepressants, sleep deprivation, hypothyroidism, and seasonal changes can play a role in rapid cycling.[4,24,32] Seasonal patterns of mania in the summer and depression during the winter have been observed.[1] Rapid-cycling patients have a poorer long-term prognosis and often require combination therapies.[4]

Bipolar disorder affects an estimated 1% of children and adolescents and is often harder to recognize, diagnose, and treat than in a

TABLE 72-4 Evaluation and Diagnostic Criteria of Mood Episodes

Diagnostic workup depends on clinical presentation and findings		• Mental status examination • Psychiatric, medical, and medication history • Physical and neurologic examination • Basic laboratory tests: complete blood count, blood chemistry screen, thyroid function, urinalysis, urine drug screen • Psychological testing • Brain imaging: magnetic resonance imaging and functional scan; alternative: computed tomography scan, positron emission tomography scan • Lumbar puncture • Electroencephalogram
Diagnosis Episode	**Impairment of Functioning or Need for Hospitalization**[a]	**DSM-IV-TR Criteria**[b]
Major depressive	Yes	>2-Week period of either depressed mood or loss of interest or pleasure in normal activities, associated with at least five of the following symptoms: • Depressed, sad mood (adults); can be irritable mood in children • Decreased interest and pleasure in normal activities • Decreased appetite, weight loss • Insomnia or hypersomnia • Psychomotor retardation or agitation • Decreased energy or fatigue • Feelings of guilt or worthlessness • Impaired concentration and decision making • Suicidal thoughts or attempts
Manic	Yes	>1-Week period of abnormal and persistent elevated mood (expansive or irritable), associated with at least three of the following symptoms (four if the mood is only irritable): • Inflated self-esteem (grandiosity) • Decreased need for sleep • Increased talking (pressure of speech) • Racing thoughts (flight of ideas) • Distractible (poor attention) • Increased activity (either socially, at work, or sexually) or increased motor activity or agitation • Excessive involvement in activities that are pleasurable but have a high risk for serious consequences (buying sprees, sexual indiscretions, poor judgment in business ventures)
Hypomanic	No	At least 4 days of abnormal and persistent elevated mood (expansive or irritable); associated with at least three of the following symptoms (four if the mood is only irritable): • Inflated self-esteem (grandiosity) • Decreased need for sleep • Increased talking (pressure of speech) • Racing thoughts (flight of ideas) • Increased activity (either socially, at work, or sexually) or increased motor activity or agitation • Excessive involvement in activities that are pleasurable but have a high risk for serious consequences (buying sprees, sexual indiscretions, poor judgment in business ventures)
Mixed	Yes	Criteria for both a major depressive episode and manic episode (except for duration) occur nearly every day for at least a 1-week period
Rapid cycling	Yes	>4 Major depressive or manic episodes (manic, mixed, or hypomanic) in 12 months

[a]Impairment in social or occupational functioning; need for hospitalization because of potential self-harm, harm to others, or psychotic symptoms.
[b]The disorder is not caused by a medical condition (e.g., hypothyroidism) or substance-induced disorder (e.g., antidepressant treatment, medications, electroconvulsive therapy).
Data from Torrey and Knable,[1] American Psychiatric Association,[2] American Psychiatric Association.[3]

typical adult patient.[2,3,24,33] Late adolescence (ages 15 to 19 years) is a period with increased vulnerability for the onset of bipolar disorder.[12] Approximately 10% to 15% of adolescents with recurrent major depressive episodes have a subsequent episode of mania or hypomania.[2] Early stressful experiences in childhood (e.g., physical or sexual abuse) can precipitate an earlier onset and result in faster cycling, increased suicide risk, and alcohol or substance abuse.[4,12] Before the onset of mania, adolescents can exhibit irritability, hyperactivity, impulsivity, emotional lability, poor judgment, marked anxiety, insomnia, depression, and psychosis.[2,12,22] Early-onset bipolar disorder (before age 7 years) often presents similarly to attention-deficit/hyperactivity disorder with extreme irritability or rages. A delay in diagnosing bipolar disorder can be a factor in causing treatment-refractory mixed states or rapid cycling.

Fluctuations in hormones and neurotransmitters during the luteal phase of the menstrual cycle, postpartum period, and during perimenopause (starting approximately 10 years before menopause) can precipitate mood changes and increase cycling.[2,17,20] Women with bipolar I disorder are at greater risk for relapse into mania or depression during the postpartum period.[3] If a severe mood episode occurs postpartum, there is an increased risk for recurrences during subsequent postpartum periods.[3]

Alcohol and substance abuse is common among patients with bipolar disorder and can have a significant impact on the age of onset, course of the illness, and response to treatment.[4,12,23,28] Alcohol and drug abuse or dependence has been reported in 46% and 41% of bipolar patients, respectively.[3,12] Patients with substance use disorders are more likely to have an earlier onset of their illness, mixed states, higher rates of relapse, a poorer response to treatment, comorbid personality disorders, increased suicide risk, and more psychiatric hospitalizations.[4] Bipolar patients can self-medicate with substances such as alcohol or cocaine during episodes, resulting in further impairment of judgment, poor impulse control, treatment nonadherence, and a worsening of the clinical course.[3,4,25]

More than one-half (55% to 65%) of bipolar I patients have some degree of functional disability after the onset of their illness, and approximately 10% to 20% of bipolar patients have severe impairment in their psychosocial and occupational functioning.[1–4,34] In a 1-year longitudinal study in 258 bipolar patients, two-thirds had four or more mood episodes a year despite comprehensive pharmacologic treatment, and approximately 33.2% of the year was spent being depressed compared to 10.8% of the time in a manic phase.[34]

Compared with the general population, individuals with bipolar disorder have a 2.3-times higher mortality rate.[1] Suicide attempts occur in up to 50% of patients with bipolar disorder, and approximately 10% to 19% of individuals with bipolar I disorder commit suicide.[2–4,35] Recent studies suggest patients with bipolar II disorder have more suicide attempts than bipolar I patients.[31] Suicidal ideation and attempts are most likely to occur in a depressive or mixed state and in patients with personality disorders, psychotic features, and/or a comorbid alcohol- and substance-use disorder.[3,4,36] Acutely manic or depressed patients can need hospitalization because they are suicidal, have violent or aggressive behavior, or lack appropriate judgment and insight.[3] Accidental deaths are more frequent during manic episodes when the person has grandiosity, hallucinations, or delusions that result in risk-taking behaviors.[1,3] In addition, bipolar patients have a higher mortality from endocrine, respiratory, and cardiovascular disease that can be related to higher rates of obesity, smoking, alcohol and substance abuse, infections, and lack of medical care.[1,3]

The best predictor for level of functioning during a person's lifetime is adherence with medication treatment. Medication discontinuation occurs in up to 50% of patients secondary to intolerance of drug-induced side effects.[37] Failure to recognize the disorder, reluctance to acknowledge it, or poor adherence with treatment are reasons an estimated two-thirds of patients with bipolar disorder do not receive appropriate treatment.[1] Nonadherence with pharmacologic treatment and substance abuse are major factors in relapse and hospitalizations.[3,4]

TABLE 72-5 General Principles for the Management of Bipolar Disorder

Goals of treatment
- Eliminate mood episode with complete remission of symptoms (i.e., acute treatment)
- Prevent recurrences or relapses of mood episodes (i.e., continuation phase treatment)
- Return to complete psychosocial functioning
- Maximize adherence with therapy
- Minimize adverse effects
- Use medications with the best tolerability and fewest drug interactions
- Treat comorbid substance use and abuse
- Eliminate alcohol, marijuana, cocaine, amphetamines, and hallucinogens
- Minimize nicotine use and stop caffeine intake at least 8 hours prior to bedtime
- Avoidance of stressors or substances that precipitate an acute episode

Monitor for
- Mood episodes: document symptoms on a daily mood chart (document life stressors, type of episode, length of episode, and treatment outcome); monthly and yearly life charts are valuable for documenting patterns of mood cycles
- Medication adherence (missing doses of medications is a primary reason for nonresponse and recurrence of episodes)
- Adverse effects, especially sedation and weight gain (manage rapidly and vigorously to avoid noncompliance)
- Suicidal ideation or attempts (suicide completion rates with bipolar I disorder are 10–15%; suicide attempts are primarily associated with depressive episodes, mixed episodes with severe depression or presence of psychosis)

Frequency of visits
- Severely ill patients should be seen more often (i.e., weekly) compared with less ill patients who are symptomatic (i.e., every 2 weeks)
- When starting new medications or switching therapies, frequent monitoring is recommended (e.g., every 2 weeks) to assess adherence, efficacy, dosing, and adverse effects
- When a patient is stabilized on medication, less frequent monitoring is possible during the continuation phase (e.g., every month for the first 3 months, then every 2–3 months)
- Patients should be encouraged to call their clinician if any problems or adverse events occur or if mood episodes occur between scheduled appointments; rapidly identifying and correcting potential problems or making dosage adjustments is essential in achieving mood stabilization

Data from Torrey and Knable,[1] American Psychiatric Association,[3] Goodnick,[12] and Suppes et al.[42]

TREATMENT

Bipolar Disorder

■ DESIRED OUTCOME

❸ The desired outcome for bipolar disorder is to prevent acute manic, hypomanic, or depressive episode, to maintain good functioning, and to prevent further episodes of mania or depression.[1,3,4] The general principles and goals for the management of bipolar disorder are found in Table 72–5.

■ GENERAL APPROACH TO TREATMENT

❹ Treatment of bipolar disorder must be individualized because the clinical presentation, severity, and frequency of episodes vary widely among patients. Treatment approaches should include both nonpharmacologic and pharmacologic strategies.[4] Patients and family members should be educated about bipolar disorder (e.g., symptoms, causes, and course) and treatment options. Long-term adherence to treatment is the most important factor in achieving stabilization of the disorder.

❺ The treatment of bipolar disorder can vary depending on what type of episode a patient is experiencing. Once diagnosed with bipolar disorder patients should remain on a mood stabilizer (e.g. lithium, valproate) for life. During acute episodes medications can be added and then tapered once a patient is stabilized and euthymic. For example, when treating a patient for mania with psychotic features, the patient should be on a mood stabilizer and antipsychotic. If the antipsychotic is the patient's maintenance therapy, the dose should be increased or perhaps changed altogether. If treating a patient for a severe depressive episode, add an antidepressant to the mood stabilizer and an antipsychotic if psychosis is also present.

Nonpharmacologic Therapy

❹ The basics of nonpharmacologic approaches should address issues of adequate nutrition, sleep, exercise, and stress reduction.[1,4] Sleep deprivation, high stress, and deficiencies in dietary essential amino acids, fatty acids, vitamins, and minerals can exacerbate mood episodes and result in poorer outcomes.[4] Mood charting is an effective strategy in detecting early signs and symptoms of mania and depression. Another effective treatment is to combine medications with adjunctive psychoeducational programs, supportive counseling, insight-oriented psychotherapy (individual or group), couples or family therapy, cognitive behavioral therapy, and communication enhancement training.[1,3,4,12,38]

Most communities have self-help, support groups, and mental health organizations that provide information, educational materials, and support. For public information, individuals can contact the Depression and Bipolar Support Alliance at 800–826–3632 and *www.dbsalliance.org*; the National Alliance on Mental Illness (NAMI) at 800–950–6264 (help line) and *www.nami.org*; Mental Health America (National Mental Health Association) 800–969–6642 (resource center) and *www.nmha.org*; and National Institute of Mental Health at 866–615–6464 or *www.nimh.nih.gov*.[1,3]

TABLE 72-6 Efficacy Ratings of Pharmacological Treatments Used in Bipolar I Disorder

Drug	Acute Mania or Mixed States	Acute Bipolar Depression	Continuation or Maintenance Therapy
Lithium			
Lithium carbonate	A+: monotherapy	A	A+
Anticonvulsants			
Carbamazepine	A: monotherapy	B	B
Divalproex	A+: monotherapy	C	A
Gabapentin	X: monotherapy and adjunctive	D	D
Lamotrigine	C: monotherapy B: rapid cycling	A	A+
Levetiracetam	D	D	D
Oxcarbazepine	B: monotherapy	D	B
Tiagabine	X: monotherapy D: adjunctive	D	D
Topiramate	C: monotherapy or adjunctive	C: adjunctive	C: adjunctive
Zonisamide	C: monotherapy	D	D
Antipsychotics			
Aripiprazole	A+: monotherapy	D	D
Clozapine	A: monotherapy for treatment-resistant patients	D	D
Haloperidol	A: monotherapy or adjunctive	D	D
Olanzapine	A+: monotherapy or adjunctive	B: adjunctive with fluoxetine	A+
Risperidone	A+: monotherapy or adjunctive	B: adjunctive	D
Quetiapine	A+: monotherapy or adjunctive	A+	D
Ziprasidone	A+: monotherapy	D	D

Definition of Ratings:

A = Efficacy established by two or more randomized, double-blind, placebo-controlled or comparator trials and/or recommended as a first-line agent by APA Practice Guidelines for the Treatment of Patients with Bipolar Disorder (Revision) or Texas Consensus Panel on Medication Treatment of Bipolar Disorder; + = approved by the FDA.

B = Efficacy suggested by one randomized, double-blind, placebo-controlled or comparator trial; recommended as a second-line (alternative) agent by APA Practice Guidelines for the Treatment of Patients with Bipolar Disorder (Revision) or Texas Consensus Panel on Medication Treatment of Bipolar Disorder; not approved by the FDA.

C = Efficacy suggested by two or more open-label and/or non–placebo-controlled trials; not approved by the FDA.

D = No controlled clinical trials and/or efficacy not established for monotherapy in bipolar disorder.

X = Not recommended due to negative results or no significant difference from placebo on a randomized, placebo-controlled or comparator trial.

APA, American Psychiatric Association, FDA, Food and Drug Administration.

Data from American Psychiatric Association,[3] Suppes et al.,[42] Sachs,[44] Keck and McElroy,[47] and Kusmakar.[48]

Several nonpharmacologic treatment strategies (e.g., electroconvulsive therapy [ECT], high-intensity bright light therapy, phase-advanced sleep schedule, and partial or complete sleep deprivation) have been used in the treatment of bipolar disorder.[1,3,4] The use of ECT for severe episodes of mania, depression, psychotic features (e.g., hallucinations or delusions), mixed episodes, or rapid cycling is still considered the best acute treatment approach for those patients who do not respond to first-line mood stabilizers such as lithium and valproate.[3,4] Repetitive transcranial magnetic stimulation has been reported to be effective in unipolar depression, but effectiveness in bipolar disorder is unknown.[3,4,39]

Pharmacologic Therapy

❺ Pharmacotherapy is crucial for the acute and maintenance treatment of bipolar disorder and includes lithium, valproate, carbamazepine, lamotrigine, atypical antipsychotics, and adjunctive agents such as antidepressants and benzodiazepines.

Medication Treatment of Choice

Published Guidelines and Treatment Protocols. Currently there are no published evidence-based studies that compare different agents and combination therapies for the treatment of acute mania, mixed states, and depression, and for the maintenance phase.[3,40–45] An example of efficacy ratings for various medications used in bipolar I disorder is found in Table 72–6.[3,42,44,47,48]

❺ The term *mood stabilizer* is often used to describe the class of medications used in the treatment of bipolar disorder, but this may not be accurate as some medications are more effective for acute mania, some for the depressive episode, and others for the maintenance phase.[3,47,49] Lithium, valproate (or divalproex sodium), aripiprazole, olanzapine, quetiapine, risperidone, and ziprasidone are currently approved by the Food and Drug Administration (FDA) for the treatment of acute mania in bipolar disorder; only lithium, olanzapine, and lamotrigine are approved for the maintenance treatment of bipolar disorder. Quetiapine is the only antipsychotic that is FDA approved for bipolar depression. Lithium is the drug of choice for bipolar disorder with euphoric mania, whereas valproate has better efficacy for mixed states, irritable/dysphoric mania, and rapid cycling compared to lithium.[3]

Combination therapies (e.g., lithium plus valproate or carbamazepine; lithium or valproate plus an atypical antipsychotic) can provide better acute response and long-term prevention of relapse and recurrence than monotherapy in some bipolar patients particularly those with mixed states or rapid cycling.[3,4,50] Controlled efficacy and safety studies addressing the combination of specific antidepressants with mood-stabilizing agents for acute versus long-term therapy are lacking.[3,4,46]

❻ Several guidelines and algorithms have been published regarding the treatment of bipolar disorder, and these are generally based on the best available data and the clinical consensus of experts. One excellent reference is the *Practice Guideline for the Treatment of Patients with Bipolar Disorder (Revision)* that was published in 2002 and revised in 2006 by the APA.[3] The APA guidelines address the diagnosis, clinical course, epidemiology, and treatment strategies for adults but are not intended to be used as a standard of psychiatric care. The Texas Department of Mental Health and Mental Retardation has developed and implemented algorithms in the public mental health system to improve treatment outcomes with bipolar I disorder.[42,51] Several other states have also adopted and implemented programs similar to the Texas algorithm project. In addition, an international task force of the World Federation of Societies of Biological Psychiatry has published guidelines for the treatment of bipolar depression and mania.[43,52]

Based on the APA guidelines,[3] the Texas algorithms for bipolar disorder,[42] available research, and current marketing of medications,

TABLE 72-7 Algorithm and Guidelines for the Acute Treatment of Mood Episodes in Patients with Bipolar I Disorder

Acute Manic or Mixed Episode		Acute Depressive Episode	
General guidelines Assess for secondary causes of mania or mixed states (e.g., alcohol or drug use) Taper off antidepressants, stimulants, and caffeine if possible Treat substance abuse Encourage good nutrition (with regular protein and essential fatty acid intake), exercise, adequate sleep, stress reduction, and psychosocial therapy Optimize the dose of mood stabilizing medication(s) before adding on benzodiazepines; if psychotic features are present, add on antipsychotic; ECT used for severe or treatment-resistant manic/mixed episodes or psychotic features		**General guidelines** Assess for secondary causes of depression (e.g., alcohol or drug use) Taper off antipsychotics, benzodiazepines or sedative-hypnotic agents if possible Treat substance abuse Encourage good nutrition (with regular protein and essential fatty acid intake), exercise, adequate sleep, stress reduction, and psychosocial therapy Optimize the dose of mood stabilizing medication(s) before adding on lithium, lamotrigine, or antidepressant (e.g., bupropion or an SSRI); if psychotic features are present, add on an antipsychotic; ECT used for severe or treatment-resistant depressive episodes or for psychosis or catatonia	
Hypomania	**Mania**	**Mild to Moderate Depressive Episode**	**Severe Depressive Episode**
First, optimize current mood stabilizer or initiate mood-stabilizing medication: lithium,[a] valproate,[a] or carbamazepine.[a] Consider adding a benzodiazepine (lorazepam or clonazepam) for short-term adjunctive treatment of agitation or insomnia if needed Alternative medication treatment options: carbamazepine[a]; If patient does not respond or tolerate, consider atypical antipsychotic (e.g., olanzapine, quetiapine, risperidone) or oxcarbazepine. Second, if response is inadequate, consider a two-drug combination: • Lithium[a] **plus** an anticonvulsant or an atypical antipsychotic • Anticonvulsant plus an anticonvulsant or atypical antipsychotic	First, two or three drug combinations: lithium[a] or valproate[a] **plus** a benzodiazepine (lorazepam or clonazepam) for short-term adjunctive treatment of agitation or insomnia; lorazepam is recommended for catatonia. If psychosis is present, initiate atypical antipsychotic in combination with above. Alternative medication treatment options: carbamazepine[a]; If patient does not respond or tolerate, consider oxcarbazepine. Second, if response is inadequate, consider a three-drug combination: • Lithium[a] **plus** an anticonvulsant **plus** an atypical antipsychotic • Anticonvulsant **plus** an anticonvulsant **plus** an atypical antipsychotic Third, if response is inadequate, consider ECT for mania with psychosis or catatonia[d]; or add clozapine for treatment-refractory illness	First, initiate and/or optimize mood-stabilizing medication: lithium[a] or lamotrigine[b] Alternative anticonvulsants: valproate,[a] carbamazepine,[a] or oxcarbazepine.	First, two or three drug combinations: lithium[a] or lamotrigine[b] **plus** an antidepressant[c]; lithium **plus** lamotrigine. If psychosis is present, initiate atypical antipsychotic in combination with above. Alternative anticonvulsants: valproate,[a] carbamazepine,[a] or oxcarbazepine. Second, if response is inadequate, consider adding an atypical antipsychotic (quetiapine). Third, if response is inadequate, consider a three drug combination: • Lamotrigine[b] **plus** an anticonvulsant **plus** an antidepressant • Lamotrigine[b] **plus** lithium[a] **plus** an antidepressant Fourth, if response is inadequate, consider ECT for treatment-refractory illness and depression with psychosis or catatonia[d]

ECT, electroconvulsive therapy; MAOI, monoamine oxidase inhibitor; SNRI, serotonin-norepinephrine reuptake inhibitor; SSRI, selective serotonin reuptake inhibitor; TCA, tricyclic antidepressant.

[a]Use standard therapeutic serum concentration ranges if clinically indicated; if partial response or breakthrough episode, adjust dose to achieve higher serum concentrations without causing intolerable adverse effects; valproate is preferred over lithium for mixed episodes and rapid cycling; lithium and/or lamotrigine is preferred over valproate for bipolar depression.

[b]Lamotrigine is not approved for the acute treatment of depression, and the dose must be started low and slowly titrated up to decrease adverse effects if used for maintenance therapy of bipolar I disorder. A drug interaction and a severe dermatologic rash can occur when lamotrigine is combined with valproate (i.e., lamotrigine doses must be halved from standard dosing titration).

[c]Antidepressant monotherapy is not recommended for bipolar depression. Bupropion, SSRIs, (e.g., citalopram, escitalopram, or sertraline), and SNRIs (e.g., venlafaxine) have shown good efficacy and fewer adverse effects in the treatment of unipolar depression; MAOIs and TCAs have more adverse effects (e.g., weight gain) and can have a higher risk of causing antidepressant-induced mania; fluoxetine, fluvoxamine, nefazodone, and paroxetine inhibit liver metabolism and should be used with caution in patients on concomitant medications that require cytochrome P450 clearance; paroxetine and venlafaxine have a higher risk for causing a discontinuation syndrome.

[d]ECT is used for severe mania or depression during pregnancy and for mixed episodes; prior to treatment, anticonvulsants, lithium, and benzodiazepines should be tapered off to maximize therapy and minimize adverse effects.

Data from American Psychiatric Association,[3] Suppes et al.,[42] Sachs,[44] Keck and McElroy,[47] and Kusmakar.[48]

an example treatment algorithm and guidelines for acute mood episodes in adult patients with bipolar I disorder are listed in Table 72–7.[42,44,47,48] Because newer anticonvulsants, atypical antipsychotics, and combination therapies are under investigation for bipolar disorder, published guidelines, algorithms, and decision trees can be out of date as new scientific knowledge evolves. Selection of treatments for acute mood episodes (e.g., manic or mixed, depressive, or rapid cycling) and for maintenance strategies to prevent relapses of mood episodes should be individualized. Treatment plans should be based on patient-specific characteristics, comorbid psychiatric and medical conditions, and avoidance of drug interactions and adverse effects.[3]

There are few controlled studies in children and adolescents with bipolar disorder, thus little is known about the long-term efficacy and safety of specific agents or for combination therapies in this population.[3,4,11,33,53] Published guidelines for treatment of bipolar disorder in children and adolescents include *Treatment Guidelines for Children and Adolescents with Bipolar Disorder: Child Psychiatric Workgroup on Bipolar Disorder*[54] and the *Practice Parameters for the Assessment and Treatment of Children and Adolescents with Bipolar Disorder* by the American Academy of Child and Adolescent Psychiatry.[11]

General Information Regarding Efficacy and Safety. Lithium was first used in 1949 as a treatment for mania and was approved in 1972 in the United States for the treatment of acute mania and for maintenance therapy. Lithium was the first established mood stabilizer, and is still considered a first-line agent for acute mania and continuation treatment of bipolar I and II disorder.[47,55,56] Lithium is the only bipolar medication approved for children and adults aged 12 years and older. Long-term lithium treatment has been shown to reduce suicide risk in several studies.[3,57] Patients with rapid cycling or mixed states may not respond as well to lithium monotherapy compared to some anticonvulsants.[32,54] Lithium requires regular assessment of renal and thyroid functioning and lithium blood level monitoring to minimize adverse effects.[3]

In the 1980s, anticonvulsants were investigated for manic-depressive illness as the disorder had similar characteristics to episodic neurologic disorders such as epilepsy and migraines. Divalproex sodium (known as sodium valproate) was marketed in 1995 for the acute treatment of mania in adults and is now the most prescribed mood stabilizer in the United States. Divalproex sodium is FDA approved only for the treatment of acute manic or mixed episodes; however it is commonly used in clinical practice as maintenance monotherapy for bipolar disorder. Although carbamazepine is commonly used for both acute and maintenance therapy, it is not approved in the United States for bipolar disorder. There are some data to support the use of oxcarbazepine, a 10-keto analogue of carbamazepine, in the treatment of bipolar disorder, however it is not approved for the treatment of bipolar disorder in the United States. Valproate, carbamazepine, and oxcarbazepine each have a wide range of neurologic, gastrointestinal, electrolyte, and hematologic adverse effects that requires regular assessment and routine blood work.

Lamotrigine, a newer anticonvulsant, was approved in 2003 in the United States for the maintenance treatment of bipolar I disorder.[58,59] Lamotrigine add-on or monotherapy has been used for treatment-refractory bipolar depression.[3,58] Lamotrigine is associated with causing hypersensitivity reactions and rare life-threatening skin rashes and requires slow dosage titration.[3]

Atypical antipsychotics such as aripiprazole, olanzapine, quetiapine, risperidone, and ziprasidone are effective as monotherapy or adjunctive therapy with lithium and valproate in the treatment of acute mania.[60] Some antipsychotics have the potential to cause adverse effects such as extrapyramidal reactions, sedation, emotional blunting, sexual dysfunction, metabolic syndrome, and orthostatic hypotension.[12,61] Prophylactic use of antipsychotics can be needed for some patients with recurrent mania or mixed states, but the risks versus benefits must be weighed because of long-term adverse effects (e.g., obesity, type 2 diabetes, hyperlipidemia, hyperprolactinemia, cardiac disease, and tardive dyskinesia).[48,62]

Alternative Drug Treatments ❻ Although monotherapy with an established mood stabilizer is preferred for long-term maintenance, combinations of different types of medications can be necessary for patients during an acute episode of depression, mania, or mixed episodes who have partial or nonresponse to monotherapy, and for those who experience rapid cycling.[3,48,63]

Benzodiazepines. High potency benzodiazepines such as clonazepam and lorazepam are commonly used as an alternative to or in combination with antipsychotics when patients are experiencing acute mania, agitation, anxiety, panic, and insomnia, or cannot take mood stabilizers (e.g., during the first trimester of pregnancy).[3,4,27,64,65] Lorazepam is available for intramuscular injection and is useful in the acute management of agitation. Benzodiazepines cause minimal adverse effects compared to antipsychotics, and at higher doses, rapidly sedate agitated patients.[4] Benzodiazepines can cause central nervous system depression, sedation, cognitive and motor impairment, dependence, and withdrawal reactions. Relative contraindications for long-term therapy with benzodiazepines are drug or alcohol abuse or dependency. When no longer required, benzodiazepines should be gradually tapered and discontinued to avoid withdrawal symptoms.

Antidepressants. Antidepressants are routinely added for the treatment of acute depression, but some studies have reported that specific classes such as the tricyclic antidepressants can carry an increased risk of inducing mania in bipolar I disorder and possibly cause rapid cycling.[3,4] Some guidelines recommend avoiding antidepressants in the treatment of bipolar depression or limiting their use to brief intervals, but recent evidence suggests that the coadministration of mood stabilizers can reduce the risk of antidepressant-induced switching.[49] It is very important that before initiating therapy with an antidepressant, the patient should be on a therapeutic dosage or blood level of a primary mood stabilizer.[3] Patients who have a history of mania after a depressive episode or who have frequent cycling should be treated cautiously with antidepressants.[3,4] In general, the antidepressant should be gradually withdrawn 2 to 6 months after remission, and the patient maintained on a mood-stabilizing agent.[30,41] For patients with recurrent depressive episodes, long-term adjunctive treatment with antidepressants can be required to avoid relapses, particularly in bipolar II disorder.[3,48,66] Treatment-resistant depression is often associated with using inadequate dosages and duration of treatment for mood-stabilizing agents and antidepressants, alcohol and substance abuse, poor compliance, and rapid cycling. For more information, see Chap. 71 for comparisons between antidepressants.

Calcium Channel Antagonists. Calcium channel antagonists inactivate voltage-sensitive calcium channels, thus inhibiting neurotransmitter synthesis and release and neuronal signal transmission.[7,12] Verapamil, a nondihydropyridine, has demonstrated mood stabilizing properties in some studies but negative results were found in other trials.[3,4,12,67] Nimodipine, a dihydropyridine, can be more effective than verapamil for rapid-cycling bipolar disorder because of its anticonvulsant properties, high lipid solubility, and good penetration into the brain.[3,4,7,12,32,67] Calcium channel blockers are generally well tolerated, and the most common adverse effects are bradycardia and hypotension. The low teratogenic effects of these agents can make them a preferable choice over lithium or anticonvulsants during pregnancy and breastfeeding.[12] These are seldom used in everyday clinical practice.

Newer Anticonvulsants. Third-generation anticonvulsants have been investigated for treating bipolar disorder with the hope that a different mechanism of action would be beneficial for mood stabilization.[1,68,69] Despite early reports of efficacy based on open-label trials, agents such as gabapentin and topiramate were not effective for acute mania in double-blind comparator trials.[70–72] There is negative data for topiramate monotherapy in the treatment of acute mania from two placebo-controlled trials and two placebo-controlled trials with active comparator (lithium).[73] Topiramate has been used as an add-on weight-reduction medication, but there are no randomized controlled trials supporting its use in bipolar disorder.[62,74] The effectiveness of gabapentin and topiramate as adjunctive agents for bipolar depression or for the maintenance phase still needs to be evaluated in controlled studies.[4,69–71]

Newer anticonvulsants such as levetiracetam and zonisamide have several published case reports or open trials showing efficacy in mania and treatment-refractory rapid cycling, but it is too early to predict whether they have a place in either acute or maintenance therapy.[46,69,71] Tiagabine has caused seizures in patients with bipolar disorder and has two negative open-label trials, thus there is little support for its safety and efficacy as a mood stabilizer.[69]

CLINICAL CONTROVERSY

The place in therapy of the newer anticonvulsants, such as gabapentin, levetiracetam, tiagabine, topiramate, and zonisamide, is controversial. Many clinicians consider these agents to be less effective than established mood stabilizers based on initial studies and avoid them for monotherapy in bipolar disorder.

No published algorithms and guidelines have addressed the long-term use of combination therapies; thus the concurrent use of psychotropic agents from different classes remains controversial. At present the best approach is to maximize the dose and/or blood levels of the established mood stabilizer, and if possible, to taper off any adjunctive agent once the mood episode has resolved.

Novel Agents and Dietary Intake. Disturbances in 5-HT neurotransmission secondary to inadequate dietary L-tryptophan or abnormalities in tryptophan hydroxylase, 5-HT transporters, and 5-HT receptors was implicated in the pathophysiology of manic-depressive illness as early as 1958.[12] Low 5-HT activity can be a trait marker for bipolar disorder.[21] If available 5-HT is low, the synthesis and secretion of melatonin can be disrupted, thus causing circadian rhythm changes.[12] Acute tryptophan depletion has been shown to reverse the antidepressant effects of 5-HT reuptake inhibitors in depressed patients in remission, but may not negatively affect mood in lithium-stabilized bipolar patients.[75] Randomized controlled studies of L-tryptophan or 5-hydroxytryptophan have shown positive results in the acute treatment and prophylaxis of bipolar disorder.[12] Because 5-HT synthesis in the brain is dependent on dietary L-tryptophan intake, the importance of adequate and regular ingestion of animal-derived protein should be discussed with patients.[12]

A dietary deficiency in essential fatty acids (found in certain fish oils and flaxseed oil that contains α-linolenic acid) has been proposed as a potential cause of mood disorders.[76,77] Omega-3 fatty acids have been shown to suppress neuronal pathways and inhibit kindling processes by several mechanisms (e.g., inhibition of phosphatidylinositol and G-protein secondary messengers and blocking L-type calcium channels). Seafood and fish are rich dietary sources of omega-3 essential fatty acids, specifically docosahexaenoic acid and eicosapentaenoic acid.[77] It seems that omega-3 fatty acids may have more antidepressant effects than antimanic.[77] Data reported by Keck and colleagues for bipolar depression and rapid cycling did not support the use of eicosapentaenoic acid.[78] The data supporting the use of omega-3 fatty acids is controversial and needs to be evaluated further.

Special Populations

The approach for treating bipolar disorder in special populations (e.g., comorbid medical or psychiatric disorders, pregnancy, or breast-feeding) can vary among clinicians. Patients with comorbid medical conditions or concomitant substance abuse, those older than 65 years of age, and pregnant patients can require different treatment approaches. Approximately 20% to 50% of women with bipolar disorder relapse postpartum; therefore prophylaxis with mood stabilizers is recommended immediately postpartum to decrease the risk of relapse.[79]

Prophylactic medications such as lithium or valproate can prevent postpartum episodes in women with bipolar disorder.[3] Pharmacotherapy during pregnancy is complicated, and the risk-to-benefit ratio must be weighed. Infants whose mothers took lithium during the first trimester of pregnancy may have a lower incidence of cardiovascular defects (particularly Epstein's anomaly) than was previously thought.[3,12] Initial estimates of Epstein's anomaly in infants exposed to lithium during the first trimester was 400 times higher than in the general population rate of approximately 1:20,000 live births.[80] Current estimates of this malformation during the first trimester are estimated between 1:1,000 and 1:2,000.[80] Lithium freely crosses the placenta and is found in equal concentrations in maternal and fetal blood.[81] When lithium is used during pregnancy, it should be tapered down to the lowest effective dose necessary to decrease the risk of relapse. Lithium can cause a "floppy" infant syndrome (e.g., low Apgar scores, lethargy, hypotonia, bradycardia, cyanosis, shallow respiration, and poor sucking), hypothyroidism, and nontoxic goiters. Milk concentrations of lithium range from 30% to 50% of the mother's serum concentration, and serum concentrations in the nursing infant are 10% to 50% of the mother's; thus breast-feeding is usually discouraged.[3,12,82]

The use of anticonvulsants also pose a teratogenic risk when used during pregnancy. Neural tube defects cause the most concern for clinicians treating pregnant patients during their first trimester of pregnancy. Carbamazepine's risk of neural tube defects is estimated to be 0.5% to 1% and valproate's risk is higher at 5% to 9%.[80] Carbamazepine is excreted in breast milk (the milk-to-maternal plasma ratio of carbamazepine is approximately 0.4).[4] Craniofacial, developmental delays, microcephaly, and other abnormalities are also of concern when using anticonvulsants. Lamotrigine's registry of 1,081 cases as of September 2003 shows 9 major defects in women treated with monotherapy.[80] Data thus far on lamotrigine shows major malformation rates similar to the general population, but data for lamotrigine is much more limited than for some older anticonvulsants.[80] Valproate is usually not recommended during the first trimester of pregnancy because of a 1% to 5% risk of neural tube birth defects, primarily spina bifida.[81,83] Administration of folate can reduce the risk of neural tube defects; therefore the risks versus benefits of using valproate during pregnancy must be discussed with the patient.[12] Valproic acid is excreted into human breast milk in low concentrations (less than 1% to 10% of the mother's serum level), so is considered to be compatible with breast-feeding.[4] One case report of thrombocytopenia and anemia from valproate exposure has been reported in a nursing infant. If the mother receives valproate during breast-feeding, mother and infant should have identical laboratory monitoring. Caution should be used when prescribing antipsychotics during pregnancy. There are far more data on the use of typical than atypical antipsychotics during pregnancy. The most data are available for chlorpromazine, and these data show no elevated rate of physical malformations during first trimester exposure.

Treatment of catatonia also varies from standard treatment in that mood stabilizers and antipsychotics have minimal effect. Catatonic features such as mutism, motor excitement, stereotypic movements, waxy flexibility, negativism, echopraxia, and echolalia are best treated with benzodiazepines, specifically lorazepam. The use of antipsychotics in catatonia should be minimized because of an increased risk of neuroleptic malignant syndrome. ECT is usually a treatment of choice in this patient population.

■ DRUG CLASS INFORMATION

Product information, dosing and administration, clinical use, and proposed mechanism of action for agents used in the treatment of bipolar disorder are found in Table 72–8.

❼ Recommendations for baseline and routine laboratory testing for patients receiving carbamazepine, lamotrigine, lithium, atypical antipsychotics, oxcarbazepine, and valproate are found in Table 72–9.

Antipsychotics

Pharmacology and Mechanism of Action Typical (conventional) antipsychotic agents that block DA_2 receptors and newer atypical antipsychotics that block both DA_2 and $5\text{-}HT_{2A}$ receptors are used to decrease DA activity in the treatment of mania and mixed states.

Pharmacokinetics A summary of the absorption, distribution, metabolism, and elimination data on antipsychotics can be found in Chap. 70.

Efficacy Typical antipsychotic agents (e.g., chlorpromazine and haloperidol) are effective in up to 70% of patients with acute mania, particularly those with psychosis and psychomotor agitation. Atypical antipsychotics have demonstrated similar efficacy and fewer side effects than typical antipsychotics for the treatment of acute mania associated with agitation, aggression, and psychosis.[3,60,61,84,85] Currently aripiprazole, olanzapine, quetiapine, risperidone, and ziprasidone are FDA approved for the treatment of acute manic episodes in bipolar I disorder. Depot antipsychotics (e.g., haloperidol decanoate, fluphenazine decanoate, and risperidone long-acting injection) can have a place in maintenance treatment of bipolar disorder patients with noncompliance or treatment-resistance.[3] Controlled studies in

TABLE 72-8 Product Formulations, Dosage and Administration, Clinical Use, and Proposed Mechanism of Action of Agents Used in the Treatment of Bipolar Disorder

Generic Name	Trade Name	Formulations	Dosage and Administration	Clinical Use	Proposed Mechanism of Action
Lithium salts: FDA-approved for bipolar disorder					
Lithium carbonate	Eskalith	Capsule: 300 mg	900–2,400 mg/day in 2–4 divided doses, preferably with meals. There is wide variation in the dosage needed to achieve therapeutic response and trough serum lithium concentration (i.e., 0.6–1.2 mEq/L for maintenance therapy and 1.0–1.2 mEq/L for acute mood episodes taken 8–12 hours after the last dose).	Use alone or in combination with other drugs (e.g., valproate, carbamazepine, antipsychotics) for the acute treatment of mania and for maintenance treatment.	Normalizes or inhibits secondary messenger systems (e.g., inhibits phosphoinositide and adenylate cyclase signaling; normalizes guanine nucleotide- binding protein [G protein] signal transduction system); Decreases 5-HT reuptake and increases postsynaptic 5-HT receptor sensitivity; Inhibits the synthesis of DA, decreases the number of β-adrenergic receptors and inhibits DA2 and β-adrenergic receptor supersensitivity; Enhances GABAergic activity and normalizes GABA levels; Reduces glutamatergic activity (e.g., increases glutamate uptake) with chronic therapy. Decreases Ca^+ transport into cells, interferes with Ca^+-Na^+ active transport system, increases renal tubular reabsorption of Ca^+ and increases serum Ca^+ and parathyroid concentrations; Increases choline in red blood cells and potentiates the cholinergic secondary messenger system.
	Eskalith CR	Extended-release tablet: 450 mg			
	Lithobid	Extended-release tablet: 300 mg			
	Generic	Tablet: 300 mg (scored) Capsule: 150, 300, 600 mg			
Lithium citrate	Cibalith-S	8 mEq/5 mL			
Anticonvulsants: FDA-approved for bipolar disorder					
Divalproex sodium	Depakote	Enteric-coated, delayed-release tablet: 125, 250, 500 mg Sprinkle capsule: 125 mg	750–3,000 mg/day (20–60 mg/kg per day) given once daily or in divided doses for delayed-release divalproex or valproic acid. Extended-release divalproex can be given once daily at bedtime after stabilization. A loading dose of divalproex (20–30 mg/kg per day) can be given, then 20 mg/kg per day and titrated to a serum concentration of 50–125 mcg/mL or clinical response.	Use alone or in combination with other drugs (e.g., lithium, carbamazepine, antipsychotics) for the acute treatment of mania and for maintenance treatment. Use caution when combining with lamotrigine because of potential drug interaction.	Increases GABA levels in plasma and CNS; inhibits GABA catabolism, increases synthesis, and release; can prevent GABA reuptake; enhances the action of GABA at the $GABA_A$ receptor; Normalizes Na^+ and Ca^+ channels; Reduces intracellular inositol and protein kinase C isozymes; Can modulate gene expression. Antikindling properties can decrease rapid cycling and mixed states.
	Depakote ER	Enteric-coated extended release tablet: 250, 500 mg			
Valproic acid	Depakene	Capsule: 250 mg	50–400 mg/day in divided doses. Dosage should be slowly increased (e.g., 25 mg/day for 2 weeks, then 50 mg/day for weeks 3 and 4, then 50-mg/day increments at weekly intervals up to 200 mg/day). When combined with valproate, initial and titration dosing should be decreased by 50% to minimize the risk of a serious rash.	Use alone or in combination with other drugs (e.g., lithium, carbamazepine) for long-term maintenance treatment for bipolar I disorder. Lamotrigine can have efficacy for prevention of bipolar depression	Blocks voltage-sensitive Na^+ and Ca^+ channels; Modulates or decreases presynaptic aspartate and glutamate release; Antikindling properties may decrease rapid cycling and mixed states.
Valproate sodium	Depakene	Syrup: 250 mg/5 mL			
Lamotrigine	Lamictal	Tablet: 25, 100, 150, 200 mg Chewable tablet: 2, 5, 25 mg			
Anticonvulsants: Not FDA-approved for bipolar disorder					
Carbamazepine	Tegretol, Epitol	Tablet: 200 mg	200–1,800 mg/day in 2–4 divided doses. Dosage should be slowly increased according to response and adverse effects (e.g., 100–200 mg twice daily and increase by 200 mg/day at weekly intervals). Dose can be increased rapidly for inpatients. Administer conventional tablets and suspension with meals. Extended-release tablets should be swallowed whole and not be broken or chewed. Carbatrol capsules can be opened and contents sprinkled over food.	Use alone or in combination with other medications (e.g., lithium, valproate, antipsychotics) for the acute and long-term maintenance treatment of mania or mixed episodes for bipolar I disorder. APA guidelines recommend reserving it for patients unable to tolerate or who have inadequate response to lithium or valproate.	Blocks voltage-sensitive Na^+ channels; Stimulates the release of antidiuretic hormone and decreases Na^+ serum concentrations; Blocks Ca^+ influx through the NMDA glutamate receptor and decreases Ca^+ serum concentrations; Modulates presynaptic aspartate and glutamate release; Antikindling properties may decrease rapid cycling and mixed states.
	Tegretol	Chewable tablet: 100 mg Suspension: 100 mg/5 mL			
	Tegretol-XR	Extended-release tablet: 100, 200, 400 mg			
	Carbatrol	Extended-release capsule: 200, 300 mg			
	Equetro	Extended-release capsule: 100, 200, 300 mg			

(continued)

TABLE 72-8 Product Formulations, Dosage and Administration, Clinical Use, and Proposed Mechanism of Action of Agents Used in the Treatment of Bipolar Disorder (continued)

Generic Name	Trade Name	Formulations	Dosage and Administration	Clinical Use	Proposed Mechanism of Action
Oxcarbazepine	Trileptal	Tablet: 150, 300, 600 mg Suspension: 300 mg/5 mL	300–1,200 mg/day in two divided doses. Dosage should be slowly adjusted up and down according to response and adverse effects (e.g., 150–300 mg twice daily and increase by 300–600 mg/day at weekly intervals). Dose can be increased rapidly for inpatients.	Can have fewer adverse effects and be better tolerated than carbamazepine	Oxcarbazepine and its monohydroxy metabolite increase K^+ conductance; modulates the activity of high-voltage activated Ca^+ channels; and blocks Na^+ channels.
Clonazepam	Klonopin	Tablet: 0.5, 1, 2 mg	0.5–20 mg/day in divided doses or one dose at bedtime. Dosage should be slowly adjusted up and down according to response and adverse effects.	Use in combination with other drugs (e.g., antipsychotics, lithium, valproate) for the acute treatment of mania or mixed episodes. Use as a short-term adjunctive sedative-hypnotic agent.	Binds to the benzodiazepine site and augments the action of $GABA_A$ by increasing the frequency of Cl^- channel opening, which causes hyperpolarization (a less excitable state) and inhibits neuronal firing.
Lorazepam	Ativan	Tablet: 0.5, 1, 2 mg Oral solution: 2 mg/mL Injection: 2, 4 mg/mL	2–40 mg/day in divided doses or one dose at bedtime. Dosage should be slowly adjusted up and down according to response and adverse effects.		
Atypical antipsychotics: FDA-approved for bipolar disorder					
Aripiprazole	Abilify	Tablet: 5, 10, 15, 20, 30 mg	10–30 mg/day once daily	Use in combination with lithium or valproate for the acute treatment of mania or mixed states (primarily with psychotic features) for bipolar I disorder. Only olanzapine is FDA-approved at this time for maintenance treatment and only quetiapine for bipolar depression.	Antagonist of postsynaptic DA_2 receptors; atypical agents also block $5\text{-}HT_{2A}$ receptors that increase the presynaptic release of DA, thus lowering the risk of extrapyramidal symptoms and prolactin release Receptor blockade varies by agent: DA_4, $5\text{-}HT_{2A\text{-}2C}$, α_{1-2}-adrenergic, muscarinic, and histamine$_1$.
Olanzapine	Zyprexa	Tablet: 2.5, 5, 7.5, 10, 15, 20 mg	5–20 mg/day once daily or in divided doses		
	Zyprexa Zydis	Tablet, orally disintegrating: 5, 10, 15, 20 mg			
Quetiapine	Seroquel	Tablet: 25, 50, 100, 200, 300, 400 mg	50–800 mg/day in divided doses or once daily when stabilized		
Risperidone	Risperdal	Tablet: 0.25, 0.5, 1, 2, 3, 4 mg Oral solution: 1 mg/mL	0.5–6 mg/day once daily or in divided doses		
	Risperdal M-Tab	0.5, 1, 2, 3, 4 mg			
Ziprasidone	Geodon	Capsule: 20, 40, 60, 80 mg	40–160 mg/day in divided doses		
Calcium channel blockers: Not FDA-approved for bipolar disorder					
Nimodipine	Nimotop	Capsule: 30 mg	30–120 mg/day	Use as third-line agent for combination with other drugs (e.g., carbamazepine, valproate, antipsychotics).	Blocks Ca^+ influx through L-type Ca^+ channels Alters Ca^+-Na^+ exchange Deacreases 5-HT, DA, and endorphin activity
Verapamil	Verelan	Capsule: 120, 180, 240, 360 mg	80–480 mg/day		
	Calan, Isoptin	Film-coated tablet: 40, 80, 120 mg Extended-release tablet: 120, 180, 240 mg			

APA, American Psychiatric Association; Ca^+, calcium; Cl^-, chloride; DA, dopamine; FDA, Food and Drug Administration; GABA, γ-aminobutyric acid; 5-HT, serotonin; K^+, potassium; Na^+, sodium; NMDA, N-methyl-D-aspartate; NE, norepinephrine.

Compiled data from Torrey and Knable,[1] American Psychiatric Association,[3] Goldberg and Harrow,[4] Manji et al.,[7,9] Goodnick,[12,17] and White.[19,24]

acute mania with lithium or valproate plus an antipsychotic suggest greater efficacy with combination therapies compared with any of these agents alone.[3,60] Adjunctive atypical antipsychotics can be beneficial in the treatment of breakthrough manic episodes or if there is incomplete response to monotherapy with lithium or valproate.

Olanzapine has shown efficacy in the treatment of acute manic, mixed, and depressive phases with or without psychotic features in double-blind trials (compared with placebo, lithium, valproate, and haloperidol).[60,84] Olanzapine is also efficacious for maintenance therapy in bipolar disorder. When compared to placebo, olanzapine increases time to symptomatic relapse of any mood episode (22 days, 174 days, respectively).[86] Olanzapine is the only antipsychotic that has FDA approval for bipolar maintenance therapy.

Risperidone, in combination with other mood-stabilizing agents (lithium or valproate), and as monotherapy (versus haloperidol, lithium, and placebo) has demonstrated efficacy in several double-blind acute mania trials.[3,12,60,87] Quetiapine at higher doses (e.g., 400 to 800 mg/day) has been reported to be effective for monotherapy and as an adjunctive agent with standard mood stabilizers in acute mania in double-blind, placebo-controlled trials.[88,89] Ziprasidone was more effective than placebo in a double-blind, placebo-controlled study for acute mania but has also been associated with inducing mania or hypomania.[90] Aripiprazole, has been evaluated in three randomized, placebo-controlled studies in bipolar I disorder patients with an acute manic or mixed episode.[91] Aripiprazole was statistically significantly better than placebo in one 3-week study at

TABLE 72-9 Guidelines for Baseline and Routine Laboratory Tests and Monitoring for Agents Used in the Treatment of Bipolar Disorder

	Baseline: Physical Examination & General Chemistry[a]	Hematologic Tests[b]		Metabolic Tests[c]		Liver Function Tests[d]		Renal Function Tests[e]		Thyroid Function Tests[f]		Serum Electrolytes[g]		Dermatologic[h]	
	Baseline	*Baseline*	*6–12 mo*	*Baseline*	*6–12 mo*	*Baseline*	*6–12 mo*	*Baseline*	*6–12 mo*	*Baseline*	*6–12 mo*	*Baseline*	*6–12 mo*	*Baseline*	*3–6 mo*
Atypical antipsychotics[i]	X			X	X										
Carbamazepine[j]	X	X	X			X	X	X				X	X	X	X
Lamotrigine[k]	X													X	X
Lithium[l]	X	X	X	X	X			X	X	X	X	X	X	X	X
Oxcarbazepine[m]	X											X	X		
Valproate[n]	X	X	X	X	X	X	X							X	X

[a]Screen for drug abuse and serum pregnancy.

[b]Complete blood cell count (CBC) with differential and platelets.

[c]Fasting glucose, serum lipids, weight.

[d]Lactate dehydrogenase, aspartate aminotransferase, alanine aminotransferase, total bilirubin, alkaline phosphatase.

[e]Serum creatinine, blood urea nitrogen, urinalysis, urine osmolality, specific gravity.

[f]Triiodothyronine, total thyroxine, thyroxine uptake, and thyroid-stimulating hormone.

[g]Serum sodium.

[h]Rashes, hair thinning, alopecia.

[i]Atypical antipsychotics: Monitor for increased appetite with weight gain (primarily in patients with initial low or normal body mass index); monitor closely if rapid or significant weight gain occurs during early therapy; cases of hyperlipidemia and diabetes reported.

[j]Carbamazepine: Manufacturer recommends CBC and platelets (and possibly reticulocyte counts and serum iron) at baseline, and that subsequent monitoring be individualized by the clinician (e.g., CBC, platelet counts, and liver function tests every 2 weeks during the first 2 months of treatment, then every 3 months if normal). Monitor more closely if patient exhibits hematologic or hepatic abnormalities or if the patient is receiving a myelotoxic drug; discontinue if platelets are <100,000/mm^3, if white blood cell (WBC) count is <3,000/mm^3 or if there is evidence of bone marrow suppression or liver dysfunction. Serum electrolyte levels should be monitored in the elderly or those at risk for hyponatremia. Carbamazepine interferes with some pregnancy tests.

[k]Lamotrigine: If renal or hepatic impairment, monitor closely and adjust dosage according to manufacturer's guidelines. Serious dermatologic reactions have occurred within 2–8 weeks of initiating treatment and are more likely to occur in patients receiving concomitant valproate, with rapid dosage escalation, or using doses exceeding the recommended titration schedule.

[l]Lithium: Obtain baseline electrocardiogram for patients older than 40 years or if preexisting cardiac disease (benign, reversible T-wave depression can occur). Renal function tests should be obtained every 2–3 months during the first 6 months, then every 6–12 months; if impaired renal function, monitor 24-hour urine volume and creatinine every 3 months; if urine volume >3 L/day, monitor urinalysis, osmolality, and specific gravity every 3 months. Thyroid function tests should be obtained once or twice during the first 6 months, then every 6–12 months; monitor for signs and symptoms of hypothyroidism; if supplemental thyroid therapy is required, monitor thyroid function tests and adjust thyroid dose every 1–2 months until thyroid function indices are within normal range, then monitor every 3–6 months.

[m]Oxcarbazepine: Hyponatremia (serum sodium concentrations <125 mEq/L) has been reported and occurs more frequently during the first 3 months of therapy; serum sodium concentrations should be monitored in patients receiving drugs that lower serum sodium concentrations (e.g., diuretics or drugs that cause inappropriate antidiuretic hormone secretion) or in patients with symptoms of hyponatremia (e.g., confusion, headache, lethargy, and malaise). Hypersensitivity reactions have occurred in approximately 25–30% of patients with a history of carbamazepine hypersensitivity and requires immediate discontinuation.

[n]Valproate: Weight gain reported in patients with low or normal body mass index. Monitor platelets and liver function during first 3–6 months if evidence of increased bruising or bleeding. Monitor closely if patients exhibit hematologic or hepatic abnormalities or in patients receiving drugs that affect coagulation, such as aspirin or warfarin; discontinue if platelets are <100,000/mm^3/L or if prolonged bleeding time. Pancreatitis, hyperammonemic encephalopathy, polycystic ovary syndrome, increased testosterone, and menstrual irregularities have been reported; not recommended during first trimester of pregnancy due to risk of neural tube defects.

Data from American Psychiatric Association,[3] Goodnick,[12] McEvoy et al.,[93] McEvoy et al.,[96] McEvoy et al.,[81] McEvoy et al.,[83] and McEvoy et al.[103]

doses of 30 mg/day, however clinical significance is low because there was only a five point difference between aripiprazole and placebo in rating scale scores.[92] Clozapine monotherapy has acute and long-term mood-stabilizing effects in refractory bipolar disorder, including conditions with mixed mania and rapid cycling, but requires regular white blood cell monitoring for agranulocytosis.[3,12,79] The long-term safety and efficacy of antipsychotics for monotherapy or as an adjunctive treatment for bipolar depression and as a prophylactic agent in bipolar disorder still needs to be evaluated.[3,49,84,85]

Adverse Effects A summary of adverse effects for antipsychotics can be found in Chap. 70.

Drug-Drug Interactions A summary of drug interactions with antipsychotics can be found in Chap. 70.

Dosing and Administration For acute mania, higher initial doses of antipsychotics can be required (e.g., olanzapine 20 mg/day in hospitalized patients). Once acute mania is controlled (usually within 7 to 28 days), the antipsychotic can be gradually tapered and discontinued, and the patient maintained on the mood stabilizer alone.

Carbamazepine

Pharmacology and Mechanism of Action Carbamazepine, a dibenzazepine derivative, is structurally related to the tricyclic antidepressants.[12,92] The precise mechanism of action of carbamazepine in affective disorders remains to be elucidated.[9] Proposed mechanisms of action for carbamazepine are listed in Table 72–8.

Pharmacokinetics A summary of the absorption, distribution, metabolism, and elimination data for carbamazepine can be found in Chap. 58.

Efficacy Carbamazepine is not a first-line agent for bipolar disorder, and is generally reserved for lithium-refractory patients, rapid cyclers, or for mixed states.[1,3,12] Carbamazepine has acute antimanic effects comparable to lithium and chlorpromazine, but its long-term effectiveness is unclear.[3,12] One comparison trial in hospitalized manic patients indicated that carbamazepine was less effective and needed more rescue adjunctive medications than valproate.[3] Other comparison studies with lithium have reported carbamazepine to be less effective than lithium for maintenance therapy.[3] In a double-blind, placebo-controlled crossover study and in an open study, carbamazepine showed efficacy in the treatment of bipolar depression.[3,12] Studies with treatment-refractory patients have reported that carbamazepine has both acute and long-term prophylactic effects.[4,12] A gradual loss of efficacy over time (similar to lithium and valproate) has been reported in some patients.[4,12]

The combination of carbamazepine with lithium, valproate, and antipsychotics is often used for treatment-resistant patients experiencing a manic episode.[12] Carbamazepine increases the hepatic metabolism of antidepressants, anticonvulsants, and antipsychotics; thus dosage increases can be necessary (see drug-drug interactions).[12,93] Calcium channel blockers (i.e., verapamil and diltiazem) increase carbamazepine blood levels; thus combination therapy should be closely monitored.[93] The combination of carbamazepine with nimodipine for treatment-refractory bipolar illness can have potential benefit.[94]

Adverse Effects A summary of adverse effects for carbamazepine can be found in Chap. 58. Acute overdoses of carbamazepine are potentially lethal, and serum levels above 15 mcg/mL are associated with ataxia, choreiform movements, diplopia, nystagmus, cardiac conduction changes, seizures, and coma.[3] Gastric lavage, hemoperfusion, and symptomatic treatment are recommended for the management of carbamazepine toxicity.

Drug-Drug Interactions Carbamazepine significantly induces the hepatic cytochrome P450 isoenzyme 3A4 and to a lesser degree 1A2, 2C9/10, and 2D6, which increases the metabolism of many medications.[3,4,93] Women who receive carbamazepine require higher dosages of oral contraceptives or alternative contraceptive methods.[4]

Carbamazepine is metabolized to an active 10,11-epoxide metabolite, thus medications that inhibit 3A4 isoenzymes can result in carbamazepine toxicity (e.g., cimetidine, diltiazem, erythromycin, fluoxetine, fluvoxamine, isoniazid, itraconazole, ketoconazole, nefazodone, propoxyphene, and verapamil).[3,4,12,93] When carbamazepine is combined with valproate, the carbamazepine dose should be reduced because valproate displaces carbamazepine from protein binding sites, thus increasing free levels.[4,12] Combining clozapine and carbamazepine is not recommended because of the possibility of bone marrow suppression with both agents.[12]

Dosing and Administration During an acute manic episode in most hospitalized patients, carbamazepine can be started at 400 to 600 mg/day in divided doses with meals and increased by 200 mg/day every 2 to 4 days up to 10 to 15 mg/kg per day. In outpatients the initial dose of carbamazepine should be lower and titrated gradually in order to avoid adverse effects. In clinical practice many patients are able to tolerate once daily dosing of carbamazepine once their mood episode has stabilized. The dose of carbamazepine should be gradually increased until response is achieved or there is evidence of toxicity. During the first month of therapy, serum concentrations of carbamazepine can decrease because of its autoinduction of cytochrome P450 3A4 enzymes, and the dose can need to be increased to maintain serum concentrations.[93]

Carbamazepine serum levels are usually obtained every 1 to 2 weeks during the first 2 months, and then every 3 to 6 months during maintenance therapy. Serum levels should be drawn 10 to 12 hours after the dose (trough levels) and at least 4 to 7 days after a dosage change. Although there is no correlation between carbamazepine serum concentration and degree of antimanic or antidepressant response, most clinicians attempt to maintain levels between 6 and 10 mcg/mL (although some treatment-resistant patients can require serum concentrations of 12 to 14 mcg/mL.[1] Recommended baseline and routine laboratory tests for carbamazepine are listed in Table 72–9.

Lamotrigine

Pharmacology and Mechanism of Action Lamotrigine blocks voltage-sensitive sodium channels, modulates or decreases glutamate and aspartate release, and has antikindling properties (see Table 72–8).[4,7,59,95,96]

Pharmacokinetics A summary of the absorption, distribution, metabolism, and elimination data for lamotrigine can be found in Chap. 58.

Efficacy The effectiveness of lamotrigine for the maintenance treatment of bipolar I disorder in adult patients was established in two multicenter double-blind, placebo-controlled studies.[3] Doses of 200 mg/day were more effective than lower doses, and there were no advantages to using 400 mg/day. Lamotrigine has both antidepressant and mood-stabilizing effects, it may have augmenting properties when combined with lithium or valproate, and has low rates of switching patients to mania.[95,97] Although lamotrigine is less effective for acute mania compared to standard mood stabilizers, it may be beneficial in the maintenance therapy of treatment-resistant bipolar I and II disorders, in rapid-cycling dysphoric mania, and in mixed states.[3,4,72,95] Lamotrigine seems to be most effective for the prevention of bipolar depression, therefore clinically it is often used in the treatment of patients with bipolar II. In a small 1-year outcome study of lamotrigine plus lithium, the combination did not show long-term prophylactic response.[98] There are case reports of possible lamotrigine induced mania when added to lithium, carbamazepine, and valproic acid.[99] In each of the cases reported the patients had depressive mood symptoms or rapid mood changes requiring additional therapy.[99]

Adverse Effects Common adverse effects include headache, nausea, dizziness, ataxia, diplopia, drowsiness, tremor, rash, and pruritus.[95,96] Approximately 10% of patients in premarketing clinical trials developed a maculopapular rash and required discontinuation of therapy.[95,96] Although most rashes are self-limiting and resolve with continued treatment, some cases progressed to life-threatening conditions such as Stevens-Johnson's syndrome. The incidence of rash appears to be greatest with coadministration of valproate, with higher than recommended initial doses, and with rapid dose escalation.[96] Patients should be warned about the rash, and the need for discontinuing lamotrigine if the rash is diffuse, involves mucosal membranes, and is accompanied by a fever or sore throat. For an in-depth discussion of the adverse effects of lamotrigine, see Chap. 58.

Drug-Drug Interactions Valproate decreases the clearance of lamotrigine (i.e., more than doubles the half-life), and lamotrigine must be administered at a reduced dosage (approximately half the standard dose).[96] For an in-depth discussion of drug-drug interactions with lamotrigine see Chap. 58.

Dosing and Administration For the maintenance treatment of bipolar disorder, the usual dosage range of lamotrigine is 50 to 300 mg/day. The target dose is generally 200 mg/day (100 mg/day in combination with valproate and 400 mg/day in combination with carbamazepine).[95,96] For patients not taking medications that affect lamotrigine's clearance, the dose is 25 mg/day for the first 2 weeks of therapy, 50 mg/day for weeks 3 and 4, 100 mg/day for week 5, and 200 mg/day for week 6 and beyond.[3,95,96] Patients who stop lamotrigine therapy for more than a few days should be restarted on the recommended dosage escalation titration schedule.

Lithium

Pharmacology and Mechanism of Action Despite numerous investigations into the biologic and clinical properties of lithium, there is no unified theory for its mechanism of action (see Table 72–8).[7,12,14,100] Chronic lithium administration may modulate gene expression and have neuroprotective effects.

Pharmacokinetics Lithium has unique pharmacokinetics because it is a monovalent cation. Lithium is rapidly absorbed, is widely distributed with no protein binding, is not metabolized, and is excreted unchanged in the urine and in other body fluids.[81]

Efficacy Early placebo-controlled studies with lithium reported up to a 78% response rate in aborting an acute manic or hypomanic episode, but more recent studies suggest a slower onset of action and a more moderate effectiveness when compared to other agents.[3,4,56] Lithium has displayed efficacy in acute mania trials similar to that of valproate, carbamazepine, risperidone, olanzapine, chlorpromazine, and other typical antipsychotics.[3] In placebo-controlled studies in bipolar depression, lithium has been found to have efficacy, but there can be a 6- to 8-week delay for its antidepressant effects.[3] Lithium is more effective for pure or elated (classic) mania, and can be less effective for mania with psychotic features, mixed episodes, rapid or continuous cycling, alcohol and drug abuse, and in organic-induced mood states.[3,4,55]

Long-term lithium therapy is more effective in patients with fewer prior episodes, with a history of euthymia or good functioning between episodes, and with a family history of bipolar illness with a positive response to lithium.[4,12] Lithium produces a prophylactic response in up to two-thirds of patients and reduces suicide risk by 8- to 10-fold.[3,55–57]

Patients maintained on standard serum concentrations of lithium (between 0.8 and 1 mEq/L) may have fewer relapses than patients maintained on lower serum concentrations (0.4 to 0.6 mEq/L).[3,4] Abrupt discontinuation or noncompliance with lithium therapy can increase the risk of relapse.[3,4] Discontinuation-induced refractoriness has been reported in approximately one-fifth of patients who previously were stabilized on lithium.[3,4]

Lithium augmentation of antidepressants, carbamazepine, lamotrigine, and valproate can improve treatment response in bipolar I disorder.[3,101] Concomitant use of lithium with valproate or carbamazepine appears to be well tolerated but can increase the risk of sedation, weight gain, gastrointestinal complaints, and tremor.

Lithium is frequently combined with both typical and atypical antipsychotics in euphoric acute mania with psychotic features. Case reports of neurotoxicity (e.g., delirium, cerebellar dysfunction, extrapyramidal symptoms, and severe tremors) have been reported in elderly patients receiving lithium and traditional antipsychotics.[81] Combining lithium with calcium channel blockers is not recommended because of reports of neurotoxicity and severe bradycardia with verapamil and diltiazem.[81] Acute neurotoxicity and delirium have been reported in patients receiving ECT with lithium (even at reduced dosages); therefore lithium should be withdrawn and discontinued at least 2 days before ECT and should not be resumed until 2 to 3 days after the last treatment.

Adverse Effects Approximately 35% to 93% of patients treated with lithium will experience adverse effects. These are divided into those that occur early in therapy but are generally innocuous and transient, those that occur with long-term therapy and are usually not dose-related, and toxic effects that occur with high serum concentrations.[1,3,81]

Initial side effects are often dose-related and are worse at peak serum concentrations (1 to 2 hours postdose).[3] Standard approaches for minimizing adverse effects include lowering the dose, taking smaller doses with food, using extended-release products, and trying once-daily dosing at bedtime.[3] Gastrointestinal distress (e.g., nausea, vomiting, dyspepsia, and diarrhea) can be minimized by the standard approaches or by adding antacids or antidiarrheal agents.[3] Diarrhea can sometimes be managed by switching from the tablet or capsule formulation to the liquid formulation. Diarrhea produced by lithium is commonly an osmotic diarrhea, and therefore switching to a formulation that clears the gut quickly can ameliorate symptoms. Muscle weakness and lethargy develop in about 30% of patients, but these symptoms are usually transient. Polydipsia with polyuria and nocturia occurs in up to 70% of patients and can be managed by changing to once-daily bedtime dosing.

As many as 40% of patients complain of headache, memory impairment, confusion, poor concentration, and impaired motor performance.[12] A fine hand tremor can be evident in up to 50% of patients. Stress, concomitant use of antidepressants or antipsychotics, caffeine, sympathomimetics, and impending toxicity can exacerbate the tremor. Strategies to reduce the tremor include standard approaches (e.g., switch to long acting preparation, lower dose if possible) or adding a β-adrenergic antagonist (e.g., propranolol 20 to 120 mg/day).

Lithium reduces the kidney's ability to concentrate urine and can cause a nephrogenic diabetes insipidus characterized by low urine specific gravity and a low osmolality polyuria (urine volumes greater than 3 L/day).[3,81] Lithium-induced nephrogenic diabetes insipidus is treated with loop diuretics, thiazide diuretics, or triamterene. If a thiazide diuretic is used (e.g., hydrochlorothiazide 50 mg/day), lithium doses should be decreased by 50%, and potassium levels need to be monitored.[3] Amiloride, a potassium-sparing diuretic, has weaker natriuretic effects than thiazides and appears to be relatively safe with minimal effect on lithium clearance. Potassium supplements have been suggested as another treatment for lithium-induced polyuria.[12] Fluid restriction is not recommended because dehydration increases the risk of lithium toxicity. If edema occurs, treatment approaches include lowering sodium intake or using a diuretic (e.g., spironolactone); close monitoring for lithium toxicity is necessary because these treatments often increase lithium concentrations.

Patients on long-term lithium therapy have a 10% to 20% risk of developing morphologic renal changes (e.g., glomerular sclerosis, tubular atrophy, and interstitial nephritis) that is associated with impairment of water resorption and increased serum creatinine concentrations.[3] Lithium rarely causes nephrotoxicity if patients are maintained on the lowest effective dose, if once-daily dosing is used, if adequate hydration is maintained, and if toxicity is avoided.[12] Lithium should be avoided in patients with preexisting renal disease unless there is frequent monitoring.

Lithium is concentrated in the thyroid gland, interferes with thyroid hormone synthesis and can induce the formation of thyroid antibodies.[81] Up to 30% of patients on maintenance lithium therapy develop transiently elevated thyroid-stimulating hormone concentrations, and 5% to 35% of patients develop a goiter and/or hypothyroidism.[3] Lithium-induced hypothyroidism is not dose-related, is observed 10 times more frequently in women (particularly in those with rapid cycling), and usually occurs after 6 to 18 months of therapy.[3] Hypothyroidism does not require discontinuation of lithium, because exogenous thyroid hormone (i.e., levothyroxine) can be added to the regimen. When lithium is discontinued, the need for exogenous thyroid hormone should be reassessed, because hypothyroidism can be reversible.

Lithium can cause a variety of benign and reversible cardiac effects, particularly T-wave flattening or inversion (in up to 30% of patients), atrioventricular block, and bradycardia.[3,12,81] Lithium rarely causes myocarditis, sinus node dysfunction, or sinoatrial block but can aggravate ventricular arrhythmias and atrial premature contractions. If a patient has significant preexisting cardiac disease, consultation with a cardiologist and an electrocardiogram is recommended at baseline and during lithium therapy.

Other late-appearing lithium side effects include benign reversible leukocytosis and a variety of dermatologic effects (e.g., acne and acneiform eruptions, alopecia, exacerbation of psoriasis, pruritic dermatitis, maculopapular rashes, and folliculitis).[3,12] Weight gain is common (approximately 20% of patients gain more than 10 kg) and can be related to fluid retention, the consumption of high-calorie beverages as a result of polydipsia, or to a decreased metabolic rate because of hypothyroidism.[12,74,102] Decreased libido, sexual dysfunction, dry mouth, alterations in taste, changes in glucose tolerance, hypercalcemia, and hyperparathyroidism have been reported.[3,12,81] Severe neurologic disturbances such as coarse hand tremors, ataxia, slurred speech, myasthenia gravis, extrapyramidal syndrome, pseudotumor cerebri, and papilledema are occasionally observed.

CLINICAL CONTROVERSY

The issue of medication-induced weight gain in psychiatric patients has received considerable attention in the literature because of the medical complications of obesity. The optimal management of weight gain and its consequences on physical and mental health remains controversial. Clinicians must strive to reduce weight gain because it decreases adherence to treatment and results in increased morbidity and mortality.

Lithium is an extremely toxic drug if accidentally or intentionally taken in overdose. Lithium toxicity can occur with blood levels greater than 1.5 mEq/L, but elderly patients can have symptoms at therapeutic levels.[3] Severe lithium intoxication occurs when concentrations are higher than 2 mEq/L, and there is a worsening in several key symptoms: *gastrointestinal* (e.g., vomiting, diarrhea, or incontinence); *coordination* (e.g., severe fine to coarse hand tremor, unstable gait, slurred speech, and muscle twitching); and *cognition* (e.g., poor concentration, drowsiness, disorientation, apathy, and coma).[3] Several reports of seizures, cardiac dysrhythmia, permanent neurologic impairments with ataxia and deficits in memory, and kidney damage with reduced glomerular filtration rate have been reported after lithium intoxication.[3]

Situations that predispose patients to lithium toxicity include: sodium restriction, dehydration, vomiting, diarrhea, and drug interactions that decrease lithium clearance. Heavy exercise, sauna baths, hot weather, and fever can promote sodium loss. Patients should be cautioned to maintain adequate sodium and fluid intake (2.5 to 3 quarts per day of fluids) and to avoid the excessive use of coffee, tea, cola, and other caffeine-containing beverages and alcohol.

If lithium toxicity is suspected, the person should go to an emergency room to be monitored, and lithium should be discontinued.[3] Gastric lavage and intravenous fluids can be needed, and the patient should be monitored for fluid balance, renal and electrolyte status, and neurologic changes. In cases of overdose with sustained-release lithium products, the development and duration of toxicity can be prolonged.[3] When lithium concentrations are above 3.5 to 4 mEq/L, intermittent hemodialysis (12 hours on and 12 hours off) can be started and continued until the lithium concentration is below 1 mEq/L when taken 12 hours after the last dialysis. Hemodialysis is generally required when serum lithium levels are above 4 mEq/L for patients on long-term treatment, and greater than 6 to 8 mEq/L after acute poisoning.[3] Rebound increases in serum lithium concentrations can occur 5 to 8 hours after dialysis, thus repeat dialysis can be needed.[3]

Drug-Drug Interactions Thiazide diuretics, nonsteroidal antiinflammatory drugs, cyclooxygenase-2 inhibitors, angiotensin-converting enzyme inhibitors, and salt-restricted diets can elevate lithium levels.[1,3] Neurotoxicity can occur when lithium is combined with carbamazepine, diltiazem, losartan, methyldopa, metronidazole, phenytoin, and verapamil.[3,81] Analgesics such as acetaminophen or aspirin and loop diuretics are less likely to interfere with lithium clearance. Caffeine and theophylline can enhance the renal elimination of lithium. Because lithium has no effect on hepatic metabolizing enzymes, it has fewer drug-drug interactions compared with carbamazepine, oxcarbazepine, and valproate.

Dosing and Administration Lithium dosing depends on the patient's age and weight, tolerance to adverse effects, and the acuity of the illness. Dosing is generally titrated up to achieve steady-state serum lithium concentrations of 0.6 to 1.2 mEq/L.[3] Lithium therapy is usually initiated with low to moderate doses (600 mg/day) for prophylaxis and higher doses (900 to 1,200 mg/day) for acute mania, using a two- to three-times daily dosing regimen.[3,81] Immediate-release lithium preparations should be given in two or three divided daily doses, whereas extended-release products can be given once or twice daily. In clinical practice many clinicians dose the immediate-release and extended-release preparations once daily. It can be best to initially begin a patient on divided dosing, but once stabilized many patients are able to switch to once daily dosing without decompensating.

Lithium levels are considered to be at steady state at approximately day 5, and serum samples should be drawn 12 hours postdose. Once a desired serum concentration has been achieved, levels should be drawn in 2 weeks and then if stable every 3 to 6 months or as clinically indicated. Maintenance lithium serum concentrations are usually measured every 3 months, but can be adjusted to every 6 months for stabilized patients, and every 1 to 2 months for patients with frequent mood episodes.[3] Lithium clearance rates increase by 50% to 100% during pregnancy and return to normal postpartum; thus lithium levels should be determined monthly during pregnancy and weekly the month before delivery. At delivery, rapid fluid changes can significantly increase lithium levels, thus a reduction to prepregnancy lithium doses and adequate hydration are recommended.[3]

The recommended guidelines for baseline and routine laboratory testing for lithium are listed in Table 72–9. The 12-hour postdose lithium serum concentration can be 12% to 33% higher with extended-release preparations and lower with regular-release tablets with divided dosage schedules. The dose should be adjusted based on the steady-state serum concentration drawn 12 hours (±30 minutes) after the last dose.[81] A therapeutic trial for outpatients should last a minimum of 4 to 6 weeks with lithium serum concentrations of 0.6 to 1.2 mEq/L. Acutely manic patients can require serum concentrations of 1 to 1.2 mEq/L, and some need up to 1.5 mEq/L to achieve a therapeutic response. Although serum concentrations less than 0.6 mEq/L are associated with higher rates of relapse, some patients can do well at 0.4 to 0.7 mEq/L.[3] For bipolar prophylaxis in elderly patients, serum concentrations of 0.4 to 0.6 mEq/L are recommended because of increased sensitivity to adverse effects.[3]

Oxcarbazepine

Pharmacology and Mechanism of Action Oxcarbazepine, a 10-keto analog of carbamazepine, blocks voltage-sensitive sodium channels, modulates voltage-activated calcium currents, and increases potassium conductance.[103]

Pharmacokinetics A summary of the absorption, distribution, metabolism, and elimination data for oxcarbazepine can be found in Chap. 58.[103]

Efficacy Initial trials suggested oxcarbazepine has mood-stabilizing effects similar to those of carbamazepine, with the advantages of milder adverse effects, no autoinduction of liver enzymes, and potentially fewer drug interactions.[3] There are currently less data supporting the use of oxcarbazepine than carbamazepine in the treatment of bipolar disorder. The APA treatment guidelines recommend the use of oxcarbazepine in any situation where one would use carbamazepine. However, many clinicians prefer to use oxcarbazepine only after a patient has failed treatment with carbamazepine because of an adverse reaction or side effects.[3] Genuine debate exists regarding drug interactions, side effects, and rates of hyponatremia with oxcarbazepine.

Adverse Effects Oxcarbazepine has dose-related adverse effects of dizziness, sedation, headache, ataxia, fatigue, vertigo, abnormal vision, diplopia, nausea, vomiting, and abdominal pain.[103] In one study hyponatremia was reported to occur in patients taking oxcarbazepine and carbamazepine at rates of 29.9% and 13.5% respectively.[104] Severe hyponatremia (sodium less than or equal to 128 mEq/L) was reported by Dong and coworkers as 12.4% and 2.8% of patients for oxcarbazepine and carbamazepine, respectively.[104] An in-depth discussion of adverse effects can be found in Chap. 58.

Drug-Drug Interactions Oxcarbazepine, a cytochrome P450 2C19 enzyme inhibitor and a 3A3/4 enzyme inducer, has the potential for causing drug interactions.[103] Oxcarbazepine induces the metabolism of oral contraceptives, thus alternative contraceptive measures are required.[3,105]

Dosing and Administration Initial dosing is usually 150 to 300 mg twice daily, and daily doses can be increased by 300 to 600 mg every 3 to 6 days up to 1,200 mg/day in divided doses (with or without food).[103]

Valproate Sodium and Valproic Acid

Pharmacology and Mechanism of Action The exact mechanism of action of valproic acid is not known (see Table 72–8).[7,12,14,83]

Pharmacokinetics A summary of the absorption, distribution, metabolism, and elimination data for valproate can be found in Chap. 58.

Efficacy Valproic acid is a branched chain fatty acid and was originally used as an organic solvent before it was discovered in the 1960s to have anticonvulsant properties. Valproate has antimigraine, mood-stabilizing, and antiaggressive effects.[83] In 1995 the enteric-coated formulation divalproex sodium (valproate) was approved for the acute treatment of mania. Several controlled studies have shown valproate to be as effective as lithium and olanzapine in patients with pure mania, and it can be more effective than lithium in certain subtypes of bipolar disorder (e.g., rapid cycling, mixed states, bipolar disorder, and comorbid substance abuse).[3,4,24,12,106]Placebo- and lithium-controlled and open studies report that valproate reduces or prevents recurrent manic, depressive, and mixed episodes.[3,4,12] Although valproate is not approved for bipolar disorder in children and adolescents, studies suggest that it is effective and well tolerated.[12,33]

Giving lithium, carbamazepine, antipsychotics, or benzodiazepines with valproate can augment its antimanic effects. The addition of valproate to lithium can have synergistic effects in treatment-refractory rapid cycling and mixed states, and the combination has demonstrated efficacy in maintenance therapy for bipolar I disorder.[24] Combinations of valproate and carbamazepine can have synergistic effects, but the potential drug interactions make blood level monitoring of both agents essential.[12] Adding adjunctive atypical antipsychotics to valproate can be effective for breakthrough mania or if there is incomplete or partial response to monotherapy. Clozapine, olanzapine, and quetiapine can increase the risk of sedation and weight gain when combined with valproate. The combination of valproate and lamotrigine can be effective, but there is an increased risk of rashes, ataxia, tremor, sedation, and fatigue.[83,95]

Adverse Effects The most frequent dose-related adverse effects with valproate are gastrointestinal complaints (anorexia, nausea, indigestion, vomiting, mild diarrhea, and flatulence), fine hand tremors, and sedation.[3,12,83] The gastrointestinal complaints are usually transient, but giving the drug with food, using lower initial doses with gradual increases in doses, switching to divalproex sodium extended-release tablets, or adding a histamine$_2$ antagonist such as famotidine or ranitidine can minimize them.[3,12] Reduction of the dose or the addition of a β-blocker can alleviate tremors, and giving the total daily dose at bedtime can minimize daytime sedation.[3,12]

Other adverse effects of valproate include ataxia, lethargy, alopecia, changes in the texture or color of hair, pruritus, prolonged bleeding because of inhibition of platelet aggregation, transient increases in liver enzymes, and hyperammonemia.[12,83] Increased appetite and weight gain occurs in approximately 50% of patients on long-term valproate therapy. Thrombocytopenia can occur at higher doses, and patients should be monitored for bleeding and bruising. Lowering the valproate dose can restore platelet counts to normal levels.[3] Fatal necrotizing hepatitis is a rare idiosyncratic, non–dose-related adverse effect that has occurred in children with epilepsy receiving multiple anticonvulsants.[12,83] A life-threatening hemorrhagic pancreatitis has been reported in both children and adults.[3,12,83] An in-depth discussion of adverse effects can be found in Chap. 58.

Drug-Drug Interactions A summary of drug-drug interactions for valproate can be found in Chap. 58.

Dosing and Administration For healthy inpatient adults with acute mania, the initial starting dosage of valproate is typically 20 mg/kg per day in divided doses over 12 hours. The daily dose is adjusted by 250 to 500 mg every 1 to 3 days based on clinical response and tolerability. Maximum recommended dosing is 60 mg/kg per day (see Table 72–8).[3,12,83] For outpatients who are hypomanic, euthymic, or for elderly patients, the initial starting dose is generally lower (5–10 mg/kg per day in divided doses) and gradually titrated to avoid adverse effects. Once an optimal dose has been achieved, the total daily dose can be given twice daily or at bedtime if tolerated.[3,12,83] Extended-release divalproex can be administered once daily, but bioavailability can be 15% lower than immediate-release products, thus requiring slightly higher doses.[3] In clinical practice patients with bipolar disorder who are stable can be switched between formulations without having to change the dose. This is not the case for patients with seizure disorder.

Recommended baseline and routine laboratory tests for valproate are listed in Table 72–9. Data from clinical trials in acutely manic patients indicated that there was an earlier response when trough serum levels were greater than 45 mcg/mL during the first week of treatment.[4] Although therapeutic serum concentrations of valproic acid have not been established in bipolar disorder, most clinicians use the anticonvulsant therapeutic serum range of 50 to 125 mcg/mL taken 12 hours after the last dose.[3,12] In one study patients with valproate levels greater than 94.1 mcg/mL had greater efficacy for bipolar mania.[107] Patients with cyclothymia or mild bipolar II disorder can have a therapeutic response to lower doses and blood levels, whereas some patients with a more severe form of bipolar disorder can require up to 150 mcg/mL. Serum valproic acid levels are most useful when assessing for compliance and toxicity.

CLINICAL CONTROVERSY[108]

In the treatment of seizure disorders monitoring serum concentrations are controversial for valproate, and the same is true in bipolar disorder. Some clinicians feel that therapeutic blood level monitoring is essential for the appropriate treatment of bipolar disorder, whereas others feel that blood level monitoring is overused and, in many cases, unwarranted. Antiepileptic blood level monitoring should be viewed as a tool to be used as part of overall treatment optimization. Achievement of a specific "therapeutic" level should not be an absolute goal in and of itself.

PHARMACOECONOMIC CONSIDERATIONS

Bipolar disorder is one of the leading causes of chronic disability worldwide and shares characteristics of both major depressive disorder and schizophrenia.[4,108] Bipolar disorder is primarily treated in the public mental health sector, and a majority of patients receive lifelong disability coverage because of compromised functioning.[4] The total cost to society for bipolar disorder is enormous and is exceeded only by the costs for treating individuals with schizophrenia.[12] It is estimated that the total annual economic impact of bipolar disorder in the United States is approximately $45 billion.[1]

Despite the prevalence, morbidity, mortality, and costs associated with the illness, there are few pharmacoeconomic or evidence-based outcome studies.[4,109,110] To address some of these issues, the Stanley

Foundation Bipolar Network was created to obtain longitudinal data (among five core sites and a number of affiliated sites) from double-blind, randomized controlled trials using consistent methodology and reliable and validated instruments.[111] A Systematic Treatment Enhancement Program for Bipolar Disorder (STEP-BD) is a 5-year outpatient study funded by the National Institute of Mental Health (*www.stepbd.org*) to determine which treatments or combination of treatments are most effective for bipolar disorder. The results from these controlled studies will help to provide the data for evidence-based outcomes and pharmacoeconomic considerations.

EVALUATION OF THERAPEUTIC OUTCOMES

❹ The establishment and maintenance of a therapeutic alliance with a clinician is essential in monitoring a patient's psychiatric status and safety; enhancing treatment adherence; promoting good nutrition, sleep, and exercise; identifying stressors; recognizing new mood episodes; and minimizing adverse reactions and drug interactions.[1,3] Patients who have a partial response or nonresponse to established bipolar therapies should be reassessed for an accurate diagnosis, concomitant medical or psychiatric conditions, and medications or substances that exacerbate mood symptoms. Nonadherence to medication treatment, delusional symptoms, alcohol or substance abuse, rapid cycling, or mixed states are often associated with poorer treatment outcomes.

The evaluation of therapeutic outcomes for bipolar disorder requires regular monitoring by a clinician. More frequent office visits, telephone calls, and intensive outpatient programs are first-line strategies to prevent hospitalization during the acute treatment phase of a manic or depressive episode.[3] Patients (and family members if needed) should be actively involved with their treatment and help to monitor target symptoms, efficacy of treatment, and adverse effects.[1,3]

Standardized rating scales for mania and depression are used to measure severity and changes in symptoms in clinical trials (e.g., Young Mania Rating Scale, brief bipolar disorder symptoms scale, Hamilton Rating Scale for Depression, and Montgomery-Asberg Depression Rating Scale). Patient-rated life mood charts, a timeline of stressful life events, and a graphic display of sleep patterns are helpful in recognizing early symptoms of mood episodes and in documenting patterns and lengths of episodes.[3] A mood disorder questionnaire, a 13-item self-reported screening tool, was developed to differentiate bipolar disorder from other mood disorders (*www.dbsalliance.org/questionnaire/screening_intro.asp*).[3,26] Health-related quality of life scales such as the Short Form (SF)-36 and the Psychological General Well Being Scale have been recommended to assess the quality of life in individuals with bipolar disorder.[112]

ACKNOWLEDGMENTS

The authors of the Bipolar Disorder chapter in the sixth edition of *Pharmacotherapy: A Pathophysiologic Approach* were Martha P. Fankhauser and Marlene P. Freeman.

ABBREVIATIONS

APA: American Psychiatric Association

DA: dopamine

DSM-IV-TR: Diagnostic and Statistical Manual, Fourth Edition, Text Revision

ECT: electroconvulsive therapy

FDA: Food and Drug Administration

GABA: γ-aminobutyric acid

5-HT: serotonin

NAMI: National Alliance on Mental Illness

NE: norepinephrine

STEP-BD: Systematic Treatment Enhancement Program for Bipolar Disorder

REFERENCES

1. Torrey EF, Knable MB. Surviving Manic Depression: A Manual on Bipolar Disorder for Patients, Families, and Providers. New York: Basic Books, 2002.
2. American Psychiatric Association. Diagnostic and Statistical Manual of Mental Disorders, 4th ed., Text Revision. Washington, DC: American Psychiatric Association, 2000:382–401.
3. American Psychiatric Association. Practice guideline for the treatment of patients with bipolar disorder (revision). Am J Psychiatry 2002;159:1–50.
4. Goldberg JF, Harrow M, eds. Bipolar Disorders: Clinical Course and Outcome. Washington, DC: American Psychiatric Press, 1999.
5. Kessler RC, McGonagle KA, Zhao S, et al. Lifetime and 12-month prevalence of DSM-III-R psychiatric disorders in the United States: Results from the national comorbidity survey. Arch Gen Psychiatry 1994;51:8–19.
6. Kelso JR. Arguments for the genetic basis of the bipolar spectrum. J Affect Disord 2003;73:183–197.
7. Manji HK, Bowden CL, Belmaker RH, eds. Bipolar Medications: Mechanisms of Action. Washington, DC: American Psychiatric Press, 2000.
8. Lenox RH, Gould TD, Manji HK. Endophenotypes in bipolar disorder. Am J Med Genet 2002;114:391–406.
9. Baron M. Manic-depressive genes and the new millennium: Poised for discovery. Mol Psychiatry 2002;7:342–358.
10. Bezchlibnyk Y, Young LT. The neurobiology of bipolar disorder: Focus on signal transduction pathways and the regulation of gene expression. Can J Psychiatry 2002;47:135–148.
11. Practice Parameters for the Assessment and Treatment of Children and Adolescents with Bipolar Disorder. J Am Acad Child Adolesc Psychiatry 1997;36:138–157.
12. Goodnick PJ, ed. Mania: Clinical and Research Perspectives. Washington, DC: American Psychiatric Press, 1998.
13. Soares JC. Can brain imaging studies provide a "mood stabilizer signature?" Mol Psychiatry 2002;7(Suppl 1):S64–S70.
14. Manji HK, Moore GJ, Chen G. Bipolar disorder: leads from the molecular and cellular mechanisms of action of mood stabilizers. Br J Psychiatry Suppl 2001;41:S107–S119.
15. Gould TD, Manji HK. Signaling networks in the pathophysiology and treatment of mood disorders. J Psychosom Res 2002;53:687–697.
16. Sobczak S, Honig A, van Duinen MA, Riedel WJ. Serotonergic dysfunction in bipolar disorders: A literature review of serotonergic challenge studies. Bipolar Disord 2002;4:347–356.
17. Freeman MP, Wosnitzer Smith K, Freeman SA, et al. The impact of reproductive events on the course of bipolar disorder in women. J Clin Psychiatry 2002;63:284–287.
18. Ketter TA, Wang PW. The emerging differential roles of GABAergic and antiglutamatergic agents in bipolar disorders. J Clin Psychiatry 2003;64(Suppl 3):15–20.
19. White HS. Mechanism of action of newer anticonvulsants. J Clin Psychiatry 2003;64(Suppl 8):5–8.
20. Rasgon N, Bauer M, Glenn T, et al. Menstrual cycle related mood changes in women with bipolar disorder. Bipolar Disord 2003;5:48–52.
21. Mahmood T, Silverstone T. Serotonin and bipolar disorder. J Affect Disord 2001;66:1–11.
22. Kim EY, Miklowitz DJ. Childhood mania, attention deficit hyperactivity disorder and conduct disorder: A critical review of diagnostic dilemmas. Bipolar Disord 2002;4:215–225.
23. Salloum IM, Thase ME. Impact of substance abuse on the course and treatment of bipolar disorder. Bipolar Disord 2000;2:269–280.
24. Calabrese JR, Shelton MD, Rapport DJ, et al. Current research on rapid cycling bipolar disorder and its treatment. J Affect Disord 2001;67:241–255.

25. Sherwood Brown E, Suppes T, Adinoff B, Rajan Thomas N. Drug abuse and bipolar disorder: Comorbidity or misdiagnosis? J Affect Disord 2001;65:105–115.
26. Hirschfeld RM. Bipolar spectrum disorder: improving its recognition and diagnosis. J Clin Psychiatry 2001;62(Suppl 14):5–9.
27. Freeman MP, Freeman SA, McElroy SL. The comorbidity of bipolar and anxiety disorders: Prevalence, psychobiology, and treatment issues. J Affect Disord 2002;68:1–23.
28. Cassidy F, Ahearn EP, Carroll BJ. Substance abuse in bipolar disorder. Bipolar Disord 2001;3:181–188.
29. Bowden CL. Strategies to reduce misdiagnosis of bipolar depression. Psychiatr Serv 2001;52:51–55.
30. Sachs GS, Koslow CL, Ghaemi SN. The treatment of bipolar depression. Bipolar Disord 2000;2:256–260.
31. Rihmer Z, Kiss K. Bipolar disorders and suicidal behavior. Bipolar Disord 2002;4(Suppl 1):21–25.
32. Barrios C, Chaudhry TA, Goodnick PJ. Rapid cycling bipolar disorder. Expert Opin Pharmacother 2001;2:1963–1973.
33. Chang KD, Ketter TA. Special issues in the treatment of pediatric bipolar disorder. Expert Opin Pharmacother 2001;2:613–622.
34. Post RM, Denicoff KD, Leverich GS, et al. Morbidity in 258 bipolar outpatients followed for 1 year with daily prospective ratings on the NIMH life chart method. J Clin Psychiatry 2003;64:680–690.
35. Jamison KR. Suicide and bipolar disorder. J Clin Psychiatry 2000;61(Suppl 9):47–51.
36. Dalton EJ, Cate-Carter TD, Mundo E, et al. Suicide risk in bipolar patients: The role of comorbid substance use disorders. Bipolar Disord 2003;5:58–61.
37. Lingam R, Scott J. Treatment non-adherence in affective disorders. Acta Psychiatr Scand 2002;105:164–172.
38. Otto MW, Reilly-Harrington N, Sachs GS. Psychoeducational and cognitive-behavioral strategies in the management of bipolar disorder. J Affect Disord 2003;73:171–181.
39. Hasey G. Transcranial magnetic stimulation in the treatment of mood disorder: A review and comparison with electroconvulsive therapy. Can J Psychiatry 2001;46:720–727.
40. Goldberg JF. Treatment guidelines: current and future management of bipolar disorder. J Clin Psychiatry 2000;61(Suppl 13):12–18.
41. Sachs GS, Printz DJ, Kahn DA, et al. The expert consensus guideline series: Medication treatment of bipolar disorder 2000. Postgrad Med 2000;Spec No:1–104.
42. Suppes T, Dennehy EB, Swann AC, et al. Report of the Texas Consensus Conference Panel on medication treatment of bipolar disorder 2000. J Clin Psychiatry 2002;63:288–299.
43. Grunze H, Kasper S, Goodwin G, et al. World Federation of Societies of Biological Psychiatry (WFSBP) guidelines for biological treatment of bipolar disorders. Part I. Treatment of bipolar depression. World J Biol Psychiatry 2002;3:115–124.
44. Sachs GS. Decision tree for the treatment of bipolar disorder. J Clin Psychiatry 2003;64(Suppl 80):35–40.
45. Möller JH, Nasrallah HA. Treatment of bipolar disorder. J Clin Psychiatry 2003;64(Suppl 6):9–17.
46. Mondimore FM, Fuller GA, DePaulo JR Jr. Drug combinations for mania. J Clin Psychiatry 2003;64(Suppl 5):25–31.
47. Keck PE Jr., McElroy SL. Redefining mood stabilization. J Affect Disord 2003;73:163–169.
48. Kusmakar V. Antidepressants and antipsychotics in the long-term treatment of bipolar disorder. J Clin Psychiatry 2002;63(Suppl 10):23–28.
49. Keck PE Jr., Nelson EB, McElroy SL. Advances in the pharmacologic treatment of bipolar depression. Biol Psychiatry 2003;53:671–679.
50. Keck PE Jr., McElroy SL. Carbamazepine and valproate in the maintenance treatment of bipolar disorder. J Clin Psychiatry 2002;63(Suppl 10):13–17.
51. Suppes T, Rush AJ, Dennehy EB, et al. Texas Medication Algorithm Project, phase 3 (TMAP-3): Clinical results for patients with a history of mania. J Clin Psychiatry 2003;64:370–382.
52. Grunze H, Kasper S, Goodwin G, et al. The World Federation of Societies of Biological Psychiatry (WFSBP) guidelines for the biological treatment of bipolar disorders, part ii. Treatment of mania. World J Biol Psychiatry 2003;4:5–13.
53. Weller EB, Danielyan AK, Weller RA. Somatic treatment of bipolar disorder in children and adolescents. Child Adolesc Psychiatr Clin N Am 2002;11:595–617.
54. Kowatch RA, Firstad M, Birmaher B, et al. Treatment guidelines for children and adolescents with bipolar disorder: Child psychiatric workgroup on bipolar disorder. J Am Acad Child Adolesc Psychiatry 2005;44:213–235.
55. Goodwin FK. Rationale for long-term treatment of bipolar disorder and evidence for long-term lithium treatment. J Clin Psychiatry 2002;63(Suppl 10):5–12.
56. Baldessarini RJ, Tondo L, Hennen J, Viguera AC. Is lithium still worth using? An update of selected recent research. Harv Rev Psychiatry 2002;10:59–75.
57. Baldessarini RJ, Tondo L, Hennen J. Lithium treatment and suicide risk in major affective disorders: Update and new findings. J Clin Psychiatry 2003;64(Suppl 5):44–52.
58. Calabrese JR, Shelton MD, Rapport DJ, et al. Long-term treatment of bipolar disorder with lamotrigine. J Clin Psychiatry 2002;63(Suppl 10):18–22.
59. Hurley SC. Lamotrigine update and its use in mood disorders. Ann Pharmacother 2002;36:860–873.
60. Perlis RH, Welge JA, Vornik LA, et al. Atypical antipsychotics in the treatment of mania: a meta-analysis of randomized, placebo-controlled trials. J Clin Psychiatry 2006;67:509–516.
61. Yatham LN. The role of novel antipsychotics in bipolar disorders. J Clin Psychiatry 2002;63(Suppl 3):10–14.
62. Nemeroff CB. Safety of available agents used to treat bipolar disorder: Focus on weight gain. J Clin Psychiatry 2003;64:532–539.
63. Goodwin FK. Rationale for using lithium in combination with other mood stabilizers in the management of bipolar disorder. J Clin Psychiatry 2003;64(Suppl 5):18–24.
64. McEvoy GK, Miller J, Snow EK, et al. Benzodiazepines. AHFS Drug Information 2004. Bethesda, MD: American Society of Health-System Pharmacists, 2004:2372–2380.
65. Alderfer BS, Allen MH. Treatment of agitation in bipolar disorder across the life cycle. J Clin Psychiatry 2003;64(Suppl 4):3–9.
66. Keck PE Jr., McElroy SL. New approaches in managing bipolar depression. J Clin Psychiatry 2003;64(Suppl 1):13–18.
67. Levy NA, Janicak PG. Calcium channel antagonists for the treatment of bipolar disorder. Bipolar Disord 2000;2:108–119.
68. White HS. Mechanism of action of newer anticonvulsants. J Clin Psychiatry 2003;64(Suppl 8):5–8.
69. Yatham LN. Newer anticonvulsants in the treatment of bipolar disorder. J Clin Psychiatry 2004;65(Suppl 10):28–35.
70. Macdonald KJ, Young LT. Newer antiepileptic drugs in bipolar disorder: Rationale for use and role in therapy. CNS Drugs 2002;16:549–562.
71. Yatham LN, Kusumakar V, Calabrese JR, et al. Third generation anticonvulsants in bipolar disorder: a review of efficacy and summary of clinical recommendations. J Clin Psychiatry 2002;63:275–283.
72. Calabrese JR, Shelton MD, Rapport DJ, Kimmel SE. Bipolar disorders and the effectiveness of novel anticonvulsants. J Clin Psychiatry 2002;63(Suppl 3):5–9.
73. Kushner SF, Kahn A, Lane R, et al. Topiramate monotherapy in the management of acute mania: Results of four double-blind placebo-controlled trial. Bipolar Disord 2006;8:15–27.
74. Aronne LJ, Segal KR. Weight gain in the treatment of mood disorders. J Clin Psychiatry 2003;64(Suppl 8):22–29.
75. Johnson L, El-Khoury A, Aberg-Wistedt A, et al. Tryptophan depletion in lithium-stabilized patients with affective disorder. Int J Neuropsychopharmacol 2001;4:329–336.
76. Noaghiul S, Hibbelm JR. Cross-national comparisons of seafood consumption and rates of bipolar disorders. Am J Psychiatry 2003;160:2222–2227.
77. Parker F, Gibson NA, Brotchie H, et al. Omega-3 fatty acids and mood disorders. Am J Psychiatry 2006;163:969–978.
78. Keck PE, Mintz J, McElroy SL, et al. Double-blind, randomized, placebo-controlled trials of ethyl-eicosapentaenoate in the treatment of bipolar depression and rapid cycling bipolar disorder. Biol Psychiatry 2006;60:1020–1022.
79. Viguera AC, Cohen LS, Baldessarini RJ, Nonacs R. Managing bipolar disorder during pregnancy: Weighing the risks and benefits. Can J Psychiatry 2002;47:426–436.

80. Yonkers KA, Wisner KL, Stowe Z, et al. Management of bipolar disorder during pregnancy and the postpartum period. Am J Psychiatry 2004;161:608–620.
81. McEvoy GK, Miller J, Snow EK, et al. Lithium salts. AHFS Drug Information 2004. Bethesda, MD: American Society of Health-System Pharmacists, 2004:2425–2434.
82. Ernst CL, Goldberg JF. The reproductive safety profile of mood stabilizers, atypical antipsychotics, and broad-spectrum psychotropics. J Clin Psychiatry 2002;63(Suppl 4):42–55.
83. McEvoy GK, Miller J, Snow EK, et al. Valproate sodium, valproic acid, divalproex sodium. AHFS Drug Information 2004. Bethesda, MD: American Society of Health-System Pharmacists, 2004:2152–2158.
84. Brambilla P, Barale F, Soares JC. Atypical antipsychotics and mood stabilization in bipolar disorder. Psychopharmacology Suppl 2003;166:315–332.
85. Strakowski SM, Del Bello MP, Adler CM, Keck PE Jr. Atypical antipsychotics in the treatment of bipolar disorder. Expert Opin Pharmacother 2003;4:751–760.
86. Tohen M, Calabrese JR, Sachs GS, et al. Randomized, placebo-controlled trial of olanzapine as maintenance therapy in patients with bipolar I disorder responding to acute treatment with olanzapine. Am J Psychiatry 2006;163:247–256.
87. Yatham LN, Grossman F, Augustyns I, et al. Mood stabilizers plus risperidone or placebo in the treatment of acute mania. Br J Psychiatry 2003;182:141–147.
88. Bowden CL, Grunze H, Mullen J, et al. A randomized, double-blind, placebo-controlled efficacy and safety study of quetiapine or lithium as monotherapy for mania in bipolar disorder. J Clin Psychiatry 2005;66:111–121.
89. Sachs G, Chengappa KNR, Suppes T, et al. Quetiapine with lithium or divalproex for the treatment of bipolar mania: A randomized, double-blind, placebo-controlled study. Bipolar Disord 2004;6:213–223.
90. Keck PE, Versiani M, Potkin S, et al. Ziprasidone in the treatment of acute bipolar mania: a three-week, placebo-controlled, double-blind, randomized trial. Am J Psychiatry 2003;160:741–748.
91. Perlis RH, Welge JA, Vornik LA, et al. Atypical antipsychotics in the treatment of mania: a meta-analysis of randomized, placebo-controlled trials. J Clin Psychiatry 2006;67:509–516.
92. Keck PE, Marcus R, Tourkodimitris S, et al. A placebo-controlled, double-blind study of the efficacy and safety of aripiprazole in patients with acute bipolar mania. Am J Psychiatry 2003;160:1651–1658.
93. McEvoy GK, Miller J, Snow EK, et al. Carbamazepine. AHFS Drug Information 2004. Bethesda, MD: American Society of Health-System Pharmacists, 2004:2122–2127.
94. Pazzaglia PJ, Post RM, Ketter TA, et al. Nimodipine monotherapy and carbamazepine augmentation in patients with refractory recurrent affective illness. J Clin Psychopharmacol 1998;18:404–413.
95. Bowden CL, Karren NU. Lamotrigine in the treatment of bipolar disorder. Expert Opin Pharmacother 2002;3:1513–1519.
96. McEvoy GK, Miller J, Snow EK, et al. Lamotrigine. AHFS Drug Information 2004. Bethesda, MD: American Society of Health-System Pharmacists, 2004:2134–2140.
97. Malhi GS, Mitchell PB, Salim S. Bipolar depression: Management options. CNS Drugs 2003;17:9–25.
98. Ghaemi SN, Schrauwen E, Klugman J, et al. Long-term lamotrigine plus lithium for bipolar disorder: one year outcome. J Psychiatr Pract 2006;12:300–305.
99. Raskin S, Teitelbaum A, Zislin J, Durst R. Adjunctive lamotrigine as a possible mania inducer in bipolar patients. Am J Psychiatry 2006;163:159–160.
100. Shaldubina A, Agam G, Belmaker RH. The mechanism of lithium action: state of the art, ten years later. Prog Neuropsychopharmacol Biol Psychiatry 2001;25:855–866.
101. Goodwin FK. Rationale for using lithium in combination with other mood stabilizers in the management of bipolar disorder. J Clin Psychiatry 2003;64(Suppl 5):18–24.
102. Altshuler LL, Frye MA, Gitlin MJ. Acceleration and augmentation strategies for treating bipolar depression. Biol Psychiatry 2003;53:691–700.
103. McEvoy GK, Miller J, Snow EK, et al. Oxcarbazepine. AHFS Drug Information 2004. Bethesda, MD: American Society of Health-System Pharmacists, 2004:2146–2147.
104. Dong Xiaoming, Leppik IE, White J, Rarick J. Hyponatremia from oxcarbazepine and carbamazepine. Neurology 2005;65:1976–1978.
105. Perucca E. Clinically relevant drug interactions with antiepileptic drugs. Br J Clin Pharmacol 2005;61:246–255.
106. Macritchie K, Geddes JR, Scott J, et al. Valproate for acute mood episodes in bipolar disorder. Cochrane Database Syst Rev 2003;1:CD004052.
107. Allen MH, Hirschfeld RM, Wozniak PJ, et al. Linear relationship of valproate serum concentration to response and optimal serum levels for acute mania. Am J Psychiatry 2006;163:272–275.
108. Gidal BE, WR Garnett. Epilepsy. In: Pharmacotherapy: A Pathophysiologic Approach, 6th ed. Dipiro JT, Talbert RL, Yee GC, et al., eds. New York: McGraw-Hill; 2005:1023–1048.
109. Baldessarini RJ. Treatment research in bipolar disorder: Issues and recommendations. CNS Drugs 2002;16:721–729.
110. Kusumakar V. Antidepressants and antipsychotics in the long-term treatment of bipolar disorder. J Clin Psychiatry 2002;63(Suppl 10):23–28.
111. Post RM, Nolen WA, Kupka RW, et al. The Stanley Foundation Bipolar Network. I. Rationale and methods. Br J Psychiatry Suppl 2001;41: S69–S76.
112. Namjoshi MA, Buesching DP. A review of the health-related quality of life literature in bipolar disorder. Qual Life Res 2001;10:105–115.

CHAPTER 73

Anxiety Disorders I: Generalized Anxiety, Panic, and Social Anxiety Disorders

CYNTHIA K. KIRKWOOD AND SARAH T. MELTON

KEY CONCEPTS

1. The long-term goal in generalized anxiety disorder is remission with minimal or no anxiety symptoms and no functional impairment.
2. Antidepressants are the agents of choice for the management of generalized anxiety disorder.
3. Antidepressants have a lag time of 2 to 4 weeks or longer before antianxiety effects occur in generalized anxiety disorder.
4. When monitoring the effectiveness of antidepressants in panic disorder, it is important to allow an adequate amount of time (8 to 12 weeks) to achieve full therapeutic response.
5. Clonazepam and alprazolam extended-release are alternatives to alprazolam immediate-release for patients with panic disorder having breakthrough panic symptoms at the end of a dosing interval.
6. The optimal duration of panic therapy is unknown; 12 to 24 months of pharmacotherapy is recommended before gradual drug discontinuation over 4 to 6 months is attempted.
7. Social anxiety disorder is a chronic long-term illness requiring extended therapy. After improvement, at least a 1-year medication maintenance period is recommended to maintain response and decrease the rate of relapse.
8. The selective serotonin reuptake inhibitors or venlafaxine are considered first-line pharmacotherapy for social anxiety disorder, especially in patients with comorbid depression, other anxiety disorders, or substance abuse.
9. An adequate trial of antidepressants in generalized social anxiety disorder lasts at least 8 weeks, and maximal benefit may not be seen until 12 weeks.
10. The three principal domains in which improvement should be observed in generalized social anxiety disorder are symptoms, functionality, and well being.

Anxiety is an emotional state commonly caused by the perception of real or perceived danger that threatens the security of an individual. It allows a person to prepare for or react to environmental changes. Everyone experiences a certain amount of nervousness and apprehension when faced with a stressful situation. This is an adaptive response and is transient in nature.

Learning objectives, review questions, and other resources can be found at **www.pharmacotherapyonline.com.**

Anxiety can produce uncomfortable and potentially debilitating psychologic (e.g., worry or feeling of threat) and physiologic arousal (e.g., tachycardia or shortness of breath) if it becomes excessive. Some individuals experience persistent, severe anxiety symptoms and possess irrational fears that significantly impair normal daily functioning. These persons often suffer from an anxiety disorder.[1]

Anxiety disorders are among the most frequent mental disorders encountered in clinical practice. Healthcare professionals often mistake anxiety disorders for physical illnesses, and only 23% of patients receive appropriate treatment.[2] Failure to diagnose and manage anxiety disorders results in negative outcomes including overuse of healthcare resources, increased morbidity, and mortality.[3] Individuals with anxiety disorders develop cardiovascular, cerebrovascular, gastrointestinal, and respiratory disorders at a significantly higher rate than the general population.[4]

To treat anxiety appropriately, the clinician must make a reliable diagnosis. It is essential that the distinction between short-term symptoms of anxiety and anxiety disorders be understood. Common or situational anxiety is a normal response to a stressful circumstance. Although symptoms can be severe, they are temporary and usually last no more than 2 or 3 weeks. Although short-term, "as needed" treatment with an anxiolytic agent such as a benzodiazepine is common and can provide some symptomatic relief, prolonged drug therapy is unnecessary.[5]

EPIDEMIOLOGY

Anxiety disorders, as a group, are the most commonly occurring psychiatric disorders. According to the National Comorbidity Survey Replication of the prevalence, severity, and comorbidity estimates of mental disorders in the United States, the 1-year prevalence rate for anxiety disorders was 18.1% in persons aged 18 years and older. Specific phobias were the most common anxiety disorder, with a 12-month prevalence of 8.7%. The 1-year prevalence of generalized anxiety disorder (GAD) was 3.1%, that of panic disorder was 2.7%, and that of social anxiety disorder (SAD) was 6.8%.[6]

In general, anxiety disorders are a group of heterogeneous illnesses that develop before age 30 years and are more common in women, individuals with social issues, and those with a family history of anxiety and depression. Patients often develop another anxiety disorder, major depression, or substance abuse.[1–3] The clinical picture of mixed anxiety and depression is much more common than an isolated anxiety disorder.[2]

ETIOLOGY

The differential diagnosis of anxiety disorders includes medical and psychiatric illnesses and certain drugs.[2] Family studies show that SAD can be inherited. The frequency of generalized SAD is mark-

TABLE 73-1 Common Medical Illnesses Associated with Anxiety Symptoms

Cardiovascular	Angina, arrhythmias, congestive heart failure, ischemic heart disease, myocardial infarction
Endocrine and metabolic	Cushing's disease, hyperparathyroidism, hyperthyroidism, hypothyroidism, hypoglycemia, hyponatremia, hyperkalemia, pheochromocytoma, vitamin B_{12} or folate deficiencies
Neurologic	Dementia, migraine, Parkinson's disease, seizures, stroke, neoplasms, poor pain control
Respiratory system	Asthma, chronic obstructive pulmonary disease, pulmonary embolism, pneumonia
Others	Anemias, systemic lupus erythematosus, vestibular dysfunction

Data from Roy-Byrne[2] and Chen et al.[10]

TABLE 73-2 Drugs Associated with Anxiety Symptoms

Anticonvulsants:	carbamazepine
Antidepressants:	selective serotonin reuptake inhibitors, tricyclic antidepressants
Antihypertensives:	felodipine
Antibiotics:	quinolones, isoniazid
Bronchodilators:	albuterol, theophylline
Corticosteroids:	prednisone
Dopa agonists:	levodopa
Herbals:	ma huang, ginseng, ephedra
Nonsteroidal anti-inflammatory drugs:	ibuprofen
Stimulants:	amphetamines, methylphenidate, caffeine, cocaine
Sympathomimetics:	pseudoephedrine
Thyroid hormones:	levothyroxine
Toxicity:	anticholinergics, antihistamines, digoxin
Withdrawal:	alcohol, sedatives

Data from American Psychiatric Association[1] and Chen et al.[10]

edly increased (approximately 10 times greater) among first–degree relatives of patients.[7] Behavioral inhibition (i.e., wariness, decreased social interaction, and withdrawal) is a genetic trait that can contribute to SAD.[7,8] Patients with SAD commonly report having overprotective parents. Parental dysfunction and abuse are potential risk factors for developing SAD.[8,9]

MEDICAL DISEASES ASSOCIATED WITH ANXIETY

Anxiety symptoms are an inherent part of the initial clinical presentation of several diseases, thus complicating the distinction between anxiety disorders and medical disorders.[2] If the anxiety symptoms are secondary to a medical illness, they usually will subside as the medical situation stabilizes. However, the knowledge that one has a physical illness (e.g., cancer or diabetes) can trigger anxious feelings and further complicate therapy. Persistent anxiety subsequent to a physical illness requires further assessment for an anxiety disorder. Symptoms of anxiety frequently present in medical disorders include palpitations, tachycardia, chest pain or tightness, shortness of breath, and hyperventilation. Medical disorders most closely associated with anxiety are listed in Table 73–1.[2,10] Approximately 50% of patients with GAD have irritable bowel syndrome.[2]

PSYCHIATRIC DISEASES ASSOCIATED WITH ANXIETY

Anxiety can be a presenting feature of several major psychiatric illnesses. Anxiety symptoms are extremely common in patients with mood disorders, schizophrenia, delirium, dementia, and substance-use disorders. Most psychiatric patients will have two or more concurrent psychiatric disorders (comorbidity) within their lifetime.[6] It is important to diagnose and treat all comorbid psychiatric conditions in patients with anxiety disorders.

DRUG-INDUCED ANXIETY

Drugs are a common cause of anxiety symptoms (Table 73–2). Anxiety occurs during the use of central nervous system (CNS) stimulating drugs in a dose-dependent manner, but ingestion of minimal amounts can result in marked anxiety, including panic attacks, in some individuals. The onset of drug-induced anxiety is usually rapid after the initiation of therapy; look for a recent drug or dosage change to rule out drug etiologies for anxiety.

Anxiety occurs occasionally during the use of CNS depressants, especially in children and the elderly; however, anxiety complaints are more common as complications of drug withdrawal after the abrupt discontinuation of these agents.[10,11]

PATHOPHYSIOLOGY

Data from biochemical and neuroimaging studies indicate that the modulation of normal and pathologic anxiety states is associated with multiple regions of the brain and abnormal function in several neurotransmitter systems, including norepinephrine (NE), γ-aminobutyric acid (GABA), serotonin (5-HT), corticotrophin-releasing factor (CRF), and cholesystokinin.[12] Current neuroanatomic models of fear (i.e., the response to danger) and anxiety (i.e., the feeling of fear that is disproportionate to the actual threat) include some key brain areas. The amygdala, a temporal lobe structure, plays a critical role in the assessment of fear stimuli and learned response to fear.[12] The locus ceruleus (LC), located in the brain stem, is the primary NE-containing site, with widespread projections to areas responsible for implementing fear responses (e.g., vagus, lateral and paraventricular hypothalamus). The hippocampus is integral in the consolidation of traumatic memory and contextual fear conditioning. The hypothalamus is the principal area for integrating neuroendocrine and autonomic responses to a threat.[12]

NEUROCHEMICAL THEORIES

Noradrenergic Model

The basic premise of the noradrenergic theory is that the autonomic nervous system of anxious patients is hypersensitive and overreacts to various stimuli. Many anxious patients clearly display symptoms of peripheral autonomic hyperactivity. In response to threat or fearful situations, the LC serves as an alarm center, activating NE release and stimulating the sympathetic and parasympathetic nervous systems. Chronic central noradrenergic overactivity downregulates α_2-adrenoreceptors in patients with GAD. This receptor is hypersensitive in some patients with panic disorder.[12] Patients with SAD appear to have a hyperresponsive adrenocortical response to psychologic stress.[13]

By administering drugs that have a relatively specific effect on the LC, researchers have further explored the NE theory of anxiety and panic disorder. Drugs with anxiogenic effects (e.g., yohimbine [an α_2-adrenergic receptor antagonist]) stimulate LC firing and increase noradrenergic activity. NE in turn increases glutamate release (an excitatory neurotransmitter).[12] This produces subjective feelings of anxiety and can precipitate a panic attack in those with panic disorder, but not in normal volunteers or those with other psychiatric illnesses.[14] Drugs with anxiolytic or antipanic effects (e.g., benzodiazepines, antidepressants, and clonidine) inhibit LC firing, decrease noradrenergic activity, and block the effects of anxiogenic drugs.[12]

GABA Receptor Model

There are two superfamilies of GABA protein receptors: $GABA_A$ and $GABA_B$. Drugs to reduce anxiety and produce sedation target the

$GABA_A$ receptor. The $GABA_B$ receptor is a G-protein coupled receptor postulated to be involved in the presynaptic inhibition of GABA release.[12] $GABA_A$ receptors are ligand-gated ion channels composed of five protein subunits. Several classes of subunits (i.e., α_{1-6}, β_{1-3}, γ_{1-3}, δ, ε, θ, π, ρ_{1-3}) surround a central pore and the receptor is connected to the cytoskeleton.[15] Benzodiazepine ligands enhance the inhibitory effects of GABA.[12] GABA, the major inhibitory neurotransmitter in the CNS, has a strong regulatory or inhibitory effect on the 5-HT, NE, and dopamine (DA) systems. When GABA binds to the $GABA_A$ receptor, neuronal excitability is reduced.

The specific role of the GABA receptors in anxiety disorders has not been established. The number of $GABA_A$ receptors can change with alterations in the environment (e.g., chronic stress), and the subunit expression can be altered by hormonal changes.[16] In patients with GAD, benzodiazepine binding in the left temporal lobe is reduced.[16] Abnormal sensitivity to antagonism of the benzodiazepine binding site and decreased binding was demonstrated in panic disorder.[12,16] This is consistent with the suggestion that panic disorder is secondary to a lack of central inhibition that results in uncontrolled elevations in anxiety during panic attacks.[16] Growth hormone response to baclofen in patients with generalized SAD suggests an abnormality of central $GABA_B$ receptor function.[17]

Serotonin Model

Although there are data suggesting that the 5-HT system is dysregulated in patients with anxiety disorders, definitive evidence that shows a clear abnormality in 5-HT function is lacking. 5-HT is primarily an inhibitory neurotransmitter that is used by neurons originating in the raphe nuclei of the brain stem and projecting diffusely throughout the brain (e.g., cortex, amygdala, hippocampus, and limbic system). The diverse actions of 5-HT are regulated by at least 14 different postsynaptic receptor subtypes.[12] Abnormalities in serotonergic functioning through release and uptake at the presynaptic autoreceptors ($5\text{-}HT_{1A/1D}$), the serotonin reuptake transporter (SERT) site, or effect of 5-HT at the postsynaptic receptors (e.g., $5\text{-}HT_{1A}$, $5\text{-}HT_{2A}$, and $5\text{-}HT_{2C}$) may play a role in anxiety disorders.[12] Preclinical models suggest that greater 5-HT function facilitates avoidance behavior; however, primate studies show that reducing 5-HT increases aggression.[12] It is postulated that greater 5-HT activity reduces NE activity in the LC, inhibits defense/escape response via the periaqueductal gray region, and reduces hypothalamic release of CRF. The selective serotonin reuptake inhibitors (SSRIs) acutely increase 5-HT levels by blocking the SERT to increase the amount of 5-HT available postsynaptically, and are efficacious in blocking the manifestations of panic and anxiety.[12] The precise role of 5-HT in panic disorder is unclear; however, 5-HT might play a role in anticipatory anxiety development.[14]

Low 5-HT activity may lead to a dysregulation of other neurotransmitters. NE and 5-HT systems are closely linked, and interactions between the two are reciprocal and vary. NE may act at presynaptic 5-HT terminals to decrease 5-HT release, and its activity at postsynaptic receptors can cause increased 5-HT release. Stimulation of the postsynaptic $5\text{-}HT_{2A}$ receptors in the limbic system results in anxiety and avoidance behavior.

Buspirone is a selective $5\text{-}HT_{1A}$ partial agonist that is effective for GAD but not for panic disorder. Because the selective $5\text{-}HT_{1A}$ partial agonists reduce serotonergic activity, GAD symptoms may reflect excessive 5-HT transmission or overactivity of the stimulatory 5-HT pathways. Patients with SAD have greater prolactin response to buspirone challenge compared with healthy controls, indicating an enhancement of central serotonergic response.[18] The comparable efficacy of the serotonin-norepinephrine reuptake inhibitor (SNRI), venlafaxine extended-release, at high and low dosages suggests that 5-HT (rather than NE) reuptake blockade contributes to the therapeutic effect in SAD.[19]

NEUROIMAGING STUDIES

Functional neuroimaging studies suggest that frontal and occipital brain areas are integral to the anxiety response. In GAD there is an abnormal increase in cortical activity and a decrease in basal ganglia activity. After benzodiazepine treatment, basal ganglia activity increases, and cortical activity is reduced.[14] Patients with panic disorder have abnormal activation of the parahippocampal region and prefrontal cortex at rest, and reduced GABA concentrations in the occipital region.[14] Panic anxiety is associated with activation of brain stem and basal ganglia areas.[14] Both pharmacotherapy and psychotherapy decreased cerebral blood flow in the amygdala, hippocampus, and surrounding cortical areas in patients with SAD.[7,19]

CLINICAL PRESENTATION

The *Diagnostic and Statistical Manual of Mental Disorders, Fourth Edition, Text Revision* classifies anxiety disorders into several categories: GAD, panic disorder (with or without agoraphobia), agoraphobia, SAD, specific phobia, obsessive-compulsive disorder, posttraumatic stress disorder, and acute stress disorder.[1] The characteristic features of these illnesses are anxiety and avoidance behavior. Anxiety symptoms must cause significant distress, and impairment in social, occupational, or other areas of functioning and should not be secondary to a drug or illicit substance or a general medical disorder, or occur solely as part of another psychiatric disorder.[1] Obsessive-compulsive disorder and posttraumatic stress disorder are discussed in Chap. 74.

GENERALIZED ANXIETY DISORDER

The diagnostic criteria for GAD require persistent symptoms for most days for at least 6 months.[1] The essential feature of GAD is unrealistic or excessive anxiety and worry about a number of events or activities.[1] The clinical presentation of GAD appears in Table 73–3. The anxiety or apprehensive expectation is accompanied by at least three psychologic or physiologic symptoms. Anxiety and worry are not confined to features of another psychiatric illness (e.g., having a panic attack, being embarrassed in public).[1]

The onset, course of illness, and comorbid conditions of GAD are important considerations. GAD has a gradual onset with an average age of 21 years; however, there is a bimodal distribution. If GAD is the primary disorder, the patient can present in their teens. GAD can be exacerbated or precipitated in later life by severe psychologic stressors. Most patients present between the ages of 35 and 45 years. GAD is the most common anxiety disorder in patients older than 55 years of age.[11] Tense life events also can play a role in the persistence of symptoms. The course of the illness is chronic (i.e., episodes can last

TABLE 73-3 Presentation of Generalized Anxiety Disorder

Psychologic and cognitive symptoms
• Excessive anxiety
• Worries that are difficult to control
• Feeling keyed up or on edge
• Poor concentration or mind going blank
Physical symptoms
• Restlessness
• Fatigue
• Muscle tension
• Sleep disturbance
• Irritability
Impairment
• Social, occupational, or other important functional areas
• Poor coping abilities

Data from American Psychiatric Association[1] and Baldwin et al.[20]

for a decade or longer); there is a high percentage of relapse and low rates of recovery. The likelihood of remission at 2 years is 25%.[1] Patients report substantial interference with their lives and have a high probability of seeking treatment.[3] The majority of patients with GAD eventually will develop another mental disorder. GAD is usually the primary disorder in patients with comorbid anxious depression.

PANIC DISORDER

Panic disorder begins as a series of unexpected (spontaneous) panic attacks involving an intense, terrifying fear similar to that caused by life-threatening danger. The unexpected panic attacks are followed by at least 1 month of persistent concern about having another panic attack, worry about the possible consequences of the panic attack, or a significant behavioral change related to the attacks.[1] During an attack, patients describe at least four physiologic and physical symptoms (Table 73–4).[1] Panic attacks usually last no more than 20 to 30 minutes, with the peak intensity of symptoms within the first 10 minutes. Often patients seek help at a physician's office or emergency department, only to have their symptoms resolve before or on arrival. Because panic symptoms mimic those present in several medical conditions, patients often are misdiagnosed, and multiple referrals are common.[1]

Secondary to the panic attacks, many patients develop agoraphobia. Agoraphobia is anxiety about being in places or situations in which escape might be difficult or where help might not be available in the event of a panic attack.[1] As a result, patients often avoid specific situations (e.g., being in a crowd or flying) in which they fear a panic attack might occur.[1]

Panic disorder has an adverse impact on the patient's quality of life (QOL), including a significant degree of social and work impairment. Complications include depression (10% to 65% have major depressive disorder), alcohol abuse, and high use of health services and emergency rooms.[1] Patients with panic disorder have a high lifetime risk for suicide attempts compared with the general population.[21] The usual course is chronic but waxing and waning.

SOCIAL ANXIETY DISORDER

SAD is characterized by an intense, irrational, and persistent fear of being negatively evaluated or scrutinized in at least one social or performance situation. Exposure to the feared circumstance usually provokes an immediate situation-related panic attack. Symptoms of SAD are found in Table 73–5. Blushing is the principal physical indicator and distinguishes SAD from other anxiety disorders. Adults with SAD usually recognize their fear is excessive and unreasonable; however, they are unable to overcome it without treatment. If necessary, the feared situation is avoided or endured with significant distress.[1] In individuals younger than 18 years of age, the duration of symptoms must be at least 6 months to meet the diagnostic criteria.[1]

The mean age of onset of SAD is during the mid-teens. Rates of SAD are slightly higher among women than men and more frequent in younger cohorts. It is a chronic disorder with a mean duration of 20 years.[1] People with social anxiety can be reluctant to seek professional help despite the existence of beneficial treatments because consultation with a clinician is perceived as a feared social interaction.[9,19]

Differentiating SAD from other anxiety disorders can be difficult. Panic attacks occur in both SAD and panic disorder, but the distinction between the two is the rationale behind fear; fear of anxiety symptoms is characteristic of panic disorder, whereas fear of embarrassment from social interaction typifies SAD.[1] GAD is likely the diagnosis if anxiety regarding social situations are part of a pattern of multiple worries. A majority of SAD patients eventually develop a concurrent mood, anxiety, or substance abuse disorder.[9,22]

TABLE 73-4 Symptoms of a Panic Attack

Psychological symptoms
- Depersonalization
- Derealization
- Fear of losing control
- Fear of going crazy
- Fear of dying

Physical symptoms
- Abdominal distress
- Chest pain or discomfort
- Chills
- Dizziness or light-headedness
- Feeling of choking
- Hot flushes
- Palpitations
- Nausea
- Paresthesias
- Shortness of breath
- Sweating
- Tachycardia
- Trembling or shaking

Data from American Psychiatric Association,[1] Baldwin et al.,[20] and Katon.[21]

TABLE 73-5 Presentation of Social Anxiety Disorder

Fears
- Being scrutinized by others
- Being embarrassed
- Being humiliated

Some feared situations
- Addressing a group of people
- Eating or writing in front of others
- Interacting with authority figures
- Speaking in public
- Talking with strangers
- Use of public toilets

Physical symptoms
- Blushing
- "Butterflies in the stomach"
- Diarrhea
- Sweating
- Tachycardia
- Trembling

Types
- Generalized type: fear and avoidance extend to a wide range of social situations
- Nongeneralized type: fear is limited to one or two situations

Data from American Psychiatric Association,[1] Schneier,[9] and Ballenger.[22]

SPECIFIC PHOBIA

Specific phobia is marked and persistent fear of a circumscribed object or situation (e.g., insects, heights, or injections). Apart from contact with the feared object or situation, the patient is usually free of symptoms. Most persons simply avoid the feared object and adjust to certain restrictions on their activities.[1]

TREATMENT

Generalized Anxiety Disorder

DESIRED OUTCOME

The goals of therapy in the acute management of GAD are to reduce the severity and duration of the anxiety symptoms and to improve overall functioning. ❶ The long-term goal in GAD is remission with minimal or no anxiety symptoms, no functional impairment,

TABLE 73-6 Drug Choices for Anxiety Disorders

Anxiety Disorder	First-Line Drugs	Second-Line Drugs	Alternatives
Generalized anxiety	Duloxetine Escitalopram Paroxetine Venlafaxine XR	Benzodiazepines Buspirone Imipramine Sertraline	Hydroxyzine Pregabalin
Panic disorder	SSRIs Venlafaxine XR	Alprazolam Clomipramine Clonazepam Imipramine	Phenelzine
Social anxiety disorder	Escitalopram Fluvoxamine Paroxetine Sertraline Venlafaxine XR	Citalopram Clonazepam	Buspirone Gabapentin Mirtazapine Phenelzine Pregabalin

SSRI, selective serotonin reuptake inhibitor; XR, extended-release.
Data from Schneier,[9] Baldwin et al.,[20] Ballenger,[22] Bandelow et al.,[24] and Work Group on Panic Disorder.[25]

TABLE 73-7 Benzodiazepine Antianxiety Agents

Generic Name	Brand Name	Approved Dosage Range (mg/day)[a]	Approximate Equivalent Dose (mg)
Alprazolam[b]	Niravam,[c] Xanax, Xanax XR	0.75–4 1–10[d]	0.5
Chlordiazepoxide[b]	Librium	25–100	10
Clonazepam[b]	Klonopin Klonopin Wafers[c]	1–4[d]	0.25
Clorazepate[b]	Tranxene	7.5–60	7.5
Diazepam[b]	Valium	2–40	5
Lorazepam[b]	Ativan	0.5–10	1
Oxazepam[b]	Serax	30–120	15

[a]Elderly patients are usually treated with approximately one-half of the dose listed.
[b]Available generically.
[c]Orally disintegrating formulation.
[d]Panic disorder dose.
Equivalent doses from Chouinard.[26]

and increased QOL.[23] Patients with comorbid depression should have minimal depressive symptoms.

GENERAL APPROACH TO TREATMENT

Once GAD is diagnosed, a patient-oriented treatment plan, which usually consists of both psychotherapy and drug therapy, is developed. The plan depends on the severity and chronicity of symptoms, age, drug history, and comorbid medical and psychiatric conditions.[20] Psychotherapy is the least invasive and safest treatment modality. Antianxiety medication is indicated for patients experiencing anxiety symptoms severe enough to produce functional disability. Table 73–6 lists drug choices for GAD, panic disorder, and SAD. Many questions remain unanswered regarding how to manage treatment-resistant GAD.

NONPHARMACOLOGIC THERAPY

Nonpharmacologic treatment modalities in GAD include psychoeducation, short-term counseling, stress management, psychotherapy, meditation, or exercise. Psychoeducation includes information on the etiology and management of GAD. Anxious patients should be instructed to avoid caffeine, nonprescription stimulants, diet pills, and excessive use of alcohol. Most patients with GAD require psychologic therapy, alone or in combination with antianxiety drugs, to overcome fears and to learn to manage their anxiety and worry.[5] Cognitive behavioral therapy (CBT) is the most effective psychologic therapy in GAD patients. Psychotherapy or medication alone have comparable efficacy in acute treatment.[20] The relapse rate with CBT is less than that of other types of psychologic modalities.[20] Controlled trials comparing the efficacy of combining drug and psychotherapy over long-term treatment are lacking.[20] The current literature is not clear regarding when to use CBT.

PHARMACOLOGIC THERAPY

The benzodiazepines are the most effective, safe, and commonly prescribed drugs for the rapid relief of acute anxiety symptoms (Table 73–7). All benzodiazepines are equally effective anxiolytics, and consideration of pharmacokinetic properties and the patient's clinical situation will assist in the selection of the most appropriate agent. Pharmacokinetic properties vary, and the clinician must monitor response to the initial treatment regimen after 2 to 4 weeks.[5]

Because of the lack of dependency and tolerable adverse effect profile, antidepressants have emerged as the treatment of choice for the management of chronic anxiety, especially in the presence of comorbid depressive symptoms. Buspirone is an additional anxiolytic option (Table 73–8) in patients without comorbid depression or other anxiety disorders (e.g., panic disorder and SAD). Because of the high risk of adverse effects and toxicity, barbiturates, antipsychotics, antipsychotic-antidepressant combinations, and antihistamines generally are not indicated in the treatment of GAD.[24] The benzodiazepines are more effective in treating the somatic and autonomic symptoms of GAD as opposed to the psychic symptoms (e.g., apprehension and worry), which are reduced by antidepressants.[5]

The most recent treatment guidelines from the British Society for Psychopharmacology and National Institute for Clinical Excellence are evidence-based.[20,33] An algorithm for the pharmacologic management of GAD is shown in Fig. 73–1, but the current literature is not conclusive on the optimal sequence of pharmacologic therapies.[20]

Alternative Drug Treatments

Hydroxyzine, kava kava, and pregabalin are alternatives. Patients with GAD demonstrated continued efficacy for 3 months with hydroxyzine or bromazepam (not marketed in the United States), but not with placebo.[34] Efficacy was maintained in 86% of the hydroxyzine group and 88% of the bromazepam group.[34] Analysis of data from a

TABLE 73-8 Nonbenzodiazepine Antianxiety Agents for Generalized Anxiety Disorder

Generic Name	Trade Name	Starting Dose	Dosage Range (mg/day)[a]
Antidepressants			
Duloxetine	Cymbalta	30 or 60 mg per day	60–120
Escitalopram[b]	Lexapro	10 mg per day	10–20
Imipramine[c]	Tofranil	50 mg per day	75–200
Paroxetine[b,c]	Paxil	20 mg per day	20–50
Venlafaxine[b]	Effexor XR	37.5 or 75 per day	75–225[d]
Azapirones			
Buspirone[b,c]	BuSpar	7.5 mg twice per day	15–60[d]
Diphenylmethane			
Hydroxyzine[b,c,e]	Vistaril, Atarax	25 or 50 mg four times daily	200–400
Anticonvulsant			
Pregabalin	Lyrica	50 mg three times daily	150–600

[a]Elderly patients are usually treated with approximately one-half of the dose listed.
[b]FDA approved for generalized anxiety disorder.
[c]Available generically.
[d]No dosage adjustment is required in elderly patients.
[e]FDA approved for anxiety and tension in children in divided daily doses of 50–100 mg.
Data from Bandelow et al,[24] Cymbalta package insert,[27] Lexapro package insert,[28] Paxil package insert,[29] Effexor XR package insert,[30] Vistaril package insert,[31] and Kavoussi.[32]

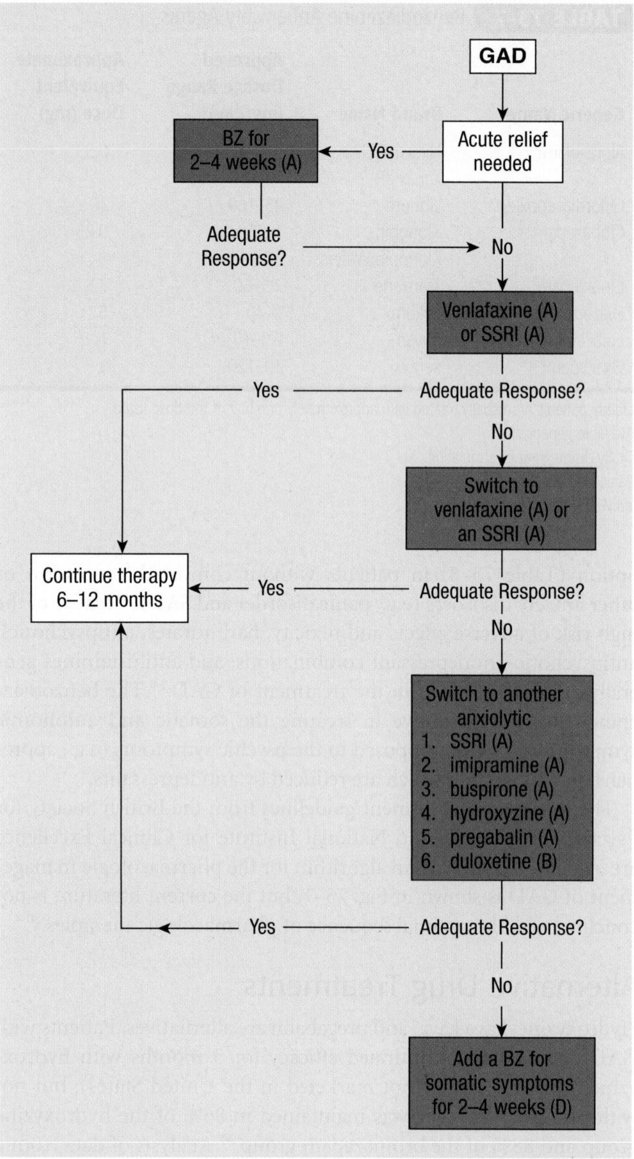

FIGURE 73-1. Algorithm for the pharmacotherapy of GAD. Strength of recommendations: A = directly based on category I evidence (i.e., meta-analysis of randomized clinical trials [RCT] or at least one RCT); B = directly based on category II evidence (i.e., at least one controlled study without randomization or one other type of quasi-experimental study); D = directly based on category IV evidence (i.e., expert committee reports or opinions and/or clinical experience of respected authorities). (BZ, benzodiazepine; SSRI, selective serotonin reuptake inhibitor.) *(Data from Baldwin et al.,[20] and NICE.[33])*

pooled sample of three placebo-controlled trials found kava kava to be no more effective than placebo.[34] Because of reports of hepatotoxicity, kava kava is not recommended as an anxiolytic.[35] Pregabalin, which binds to the $\alpha_2\delta$ subunit of voltage-gated calcium channels to reduce nerve terminal calcium influx, acts on "hyper-excited" neurons. Pregabalin produced anxiolytic effects similar to lorazepam, alprazolam, and venlafaxine in acute efficacy trials.[32] Sedation and dizziness were the most common adverse effects, and the dose should be tapered over a week on discontinuation.

Special Populations

The management of anxiety in pregnancy, children, elderly patients, and those with hepatic impairment requires special consideration in the choice of anxiolytic. The literature is unclear if the potential risks of anxiolytic therapy outweigh the benefits of treating anxiety during pregnancy. Clinical practice guidelines for anxiety disorders indicate that the use of SSRIs or tricyclic antidepressants (TCAs) in pregnancy does not pose increased teratogenic risk; however, perinatal syndromes (e.g., jitteriness, myoclonus, irritability) in the neonate and premature delivery were reported.[20,36]

Cleft lip, cleft palate, and other teratogenic effects are associated with benzodiazepine use, but a causal relationship is inconclusive. Clinicians should avoid benzodiazepine use during the first trimester, use the lowest dosage for the shortest period of time, divide the total daily dosage into two or three doses to prevent high peak plasma levels, and use the agent as monotherapy.[37] Benzodiazepine risks during the third trimester include sedation, withdrawal symptoms, and "floppy baby syndrome" (e.g., hypotonia, low Apgar scores, hypothermia). Alprazolam and lorazepam should be avoided during pregnancy because of neonatal withdrawal.[37] Diazepam is the benzodiazepine with the longest safety record. If drug therapy is required during pregnancy, the antidepressants are favored based on safety considerations.[36] Diazepam and clonazepam should not be used if the mother is nursing because infants can experience sedation, lethargy, and weight loss.[37]

In the elderly, secondary to a decreased capacity for oxidation and alterations in the volume of distribution, drug accumulation can result. Patients with hepatic disease also are at risk for drug accumulation and subsequent complications. Duloxetine use should be avoided in patients with hepatic insufficiency.[27] Therefore, intermediate- or short-acting benzodiazepines without active metabolites are preferred for chronic use. Elderly patients are also sensitive to the CNS adverse effects of benzodiazepines (regardless of half-life), and their use is associated with a high frequency of falls and hip fractures.[38] Venlafaxine and citalopram showed efficacy in elderly patients with GAD.[20,39]

There are few controlled clinical trials of drugs in children and adolescents with GAD. CBT alone or in conjunction with antidepressants can have long-term benefits.[40] Randomized controlled trials of sertraline and fluvoxamine, and open trials of alprazolam, clonazepam, and fluoxetine indicate short-term efficacy;[41] however, behavioral activation was reported with clonazepam.[40,41] To date, fluoxetine is FDA-indicated for treatment of both depression and obsessive-compulsive disorder (OCD), and fluvoxamine and sertraline are FDA-indicated for OCD in children and adolescents. Other SSRIs and SNRIs have not been proved safe and effective in children and adolescents. There are reports of hostility, suicidal ideation, and self-harm with paroxetine in children with major depression, young adults with psychiatric disorders, and venlafaxine in children with major depression or GAD.[29,30] Increased monitoring for behavioral activation with benzodiazepines and suicide-related adverse effects with antidepressants is necessary if these agents are prescribed for anxiety in children and adolescents. The FDA placed a black box warning on the use of all antidepressants in children and adolescents, and specific monitoring parameters were defined. The reader is referred to the official approved labeling for each antidepressant and to the FDA for additional information.

Antidepressant Therapy

❷ Antidepressants are considered first-line agents in the management of GAD. Venlafaxine extended-release, duloxetine, paroxetine, and escitalopram are FDA-approved antidepressants for GAD. Imipramine is considered when patients fail to respond to SSRIs or venlafaxine (see Table 73–8). ❸ The antianxiety response of antidepressants is delayed by 2 to 4 weeks or longer.[23] The pharmacokinetics and drug interactions of the antidepressants are reviewed in the chapter on depressive disorders (Chap. 71).

Efficacy Antidepressants are efficacious in the acute and long-term management of GAD. Data support the use of the SSRIs, escitalopram, paroxetine, sertraline, and the SNRIs, venlafaxine extended-release and duloxetine, for acute therapy (8–12 week trials). The acute response and remission rates were approximately 60% to 68% and 30%, respectively.[20,42] Preliminary data suggests that duloxetine 60 mg and 120 mg daily produces similar remission rates as other antidepressants.[43] In a comparative trial, there was no difference in efficacy between paroxetine and sertraline.[44] Escitalopram 10 mg was superior to paroxetine 20 mg in a fixed-dose study.[45]

Studies with continued treatment after acute response to SSRIs showed further improvement with escitalopram or paroxetine over 6 months (escitalopram group had fewer withdrawals).[46] Continued venlafaxine therapy was associated with a 61% rate of remission.[47] Relapse-prevention studies found that patients continued on paroxetine or escitalopram achieved remission rates of 73% and 65%, respectively.[47,48] In a four parallel-group comparison, diazepam and trazodone were found to be equivalent in anxiolytic activity (remission rates of 66% and 69%, respectively) compared with placebo (47% remission rate), but imipramine's rate of remission (73%) exceeded that of the other three treatments.[41]

Mechanism of Action The mechanism of action of antidepressants in anxiety disorders is not fully understood. Research indicates that antidepressants modulate receptor activation of neuronal signal transduction pathways connected to the neurotransmitters 5-HT, DA, and NE. As a result these cascades modify the expression of certain genes and the proteins that are produced (e.g., increase messenger RNA [mRNA] for glucocorticoid receptors and brain-derived neurotropic factor for tyrosine kinase type B [trkB] receptors, and reduce mRNA expression for corticotropin-releasing hormone).[49] It is theorized that by activating stress-adapting pathways, SSRIs and SNRIs reduce the somatic anxiety symptoms and the general distress experienced by patients.[49]

Adverse Effects Paroxetine was associated with a high rate of somnolence, nausea, abnormal ejaculation, dry mouth, decreased libido, and asthenia compared with placebo.[11,30] Escitalopram caused nausea, insomnia, fatigue, decreased libido, ejaculation disorders, and decreased libido at a higher rate than placebo in patients with GAD.[28] The most common adverse events of venlafaxine in patients with GAD were nausea, somnolence, and dry mouth.[30] The package insert warns of toxicity in venlafaxine overdose.[30] The use of TCAs can be limited by troublesome adverse events (e.g., sedation, orthostatic hypotension, anticholinergic effects, and weight gain) in some patients and the risk of toxicity in overdose.[5] However, in a meta-analysis of antidepressant trials there was no difference in dropout rates between antidepressants (e.g., paroxetine, venlafaxine, and imipramine) compared with placebo, suggesting equivalent tolerability between antidepressants.[41]

Dosing and Administration The antidepressants can be dosed once a day (see Table 73–8). Some patients require small initial daily doses for the first week of therapy. Paroxetine doses greater than 20 mg/day have not been found to be more effective, but it can be increased by 10 mg/day every week.[29]

Benzodiazepine Therapy

The benzodiazepines are the most frequently prescribed drugs for the acute treatment of anxiety. Although all benzodiazepines possess anxiolytic properties, only 7 of the 13 currently marketed agents have FDA approval for the treatment of GAD (see Table 73–7). Estazolam, flurazepam, temazepam, quazepam, and triazolam are marketed as sedative-hypnotic agents. Clonazepam is marketed as an antipanic agent and anticonvulsant,[50] and midazolam is labeled for preoperative sedation. Alprazolam is indicated for the treatment of panic disorder with or without agoraphobia, as well as GAD, and is also available in once-daily extended-release tablets.[51]

Pharmacology and Mechanism of Action The GABA receptor model of anxiety (described in the Pathophysiology section) theorizes that benzodiazepines ameliorate anxiety through potentiation of the inhibitory activity of GABA.[12] The GABA receptor is composed of protein subunits arranged in a pentamer with an ion channel in the center. Benzodiazepines bind on the $GABA_A$ receptor at the α_1, α_2, α_3, and α_5 subunits in combination with a β subunit and the γ_2 subunit.[15] The anxiolytic effects of benzodiazepines are mediated at the α_2 site while sedative effects result from binding at the α_1 subunit. The binding sites of benzodiazepines and GABA are at the receptor interfaces of α/β and α/γ_2, respectively. The GABA receptor controls tonic inhibition to reduce neuronal excitability.[15] Other neurotransmitters (e.g., 5-HT, NE, and DA) can be involved in benzodiazepine activity.

Pharmacokinetics A wide difference in milligram potency exists between the benzodiazepine compounds; however, when dosage adjustments are made, all agents share similar anxiolytic and sedative-hypnotic activity. The variations in lipid solubility between compounds influence the pharmacokinetic properties of benzodiazepines. Different pharmacokinetic and pharmacodynamic properties can assist the clinician in choosing an appropriate anxiolytic (Table 73–9). After a single dose, the onset, intensity, and duration of pharmacologic effects are important factors to consider when using benzodiazepines for the short-term, intermittent, or as-needed treatment of anxiety.

The primary determinant of a drug's onset of effect after a single oral dose is the rate of drug absorption. Because of high lipophilicity, diazepam and clorazepate are absorbed rapidly and distributed quickly into the CNS. Therefore the onset of anxiolytic effect occurs within 30 to 60 minutes, which results in a rapid and intense relief

TABLE 73-9 Pharmacokinetics of Benzodiazepine Antianxiety Agents

Generic Name	Time to Peak Plasma Level (h)	Elimination Half-Life, Parent (h)	Metabolic Pathway	Clinically Significant Metabolites	Protein Binding (%)
Alprazolam	1–2	12–15	Oxidation	–	80
Chlordiazepoxide	1–4	5–30	*N*-Dealkylation	Desmethylchlordiazepoxide	96
			Oxidation	Demoxepam	
				DMDZ[a]	
Clonazepam	1–4	30–40	Nitroreduction	–	85
Clorazepate	1–2	Prodrug	Oxidation	DMDZ	97
Diazepam	0.5–2	20–80	Oxidation	DMDZ	98
				Oxazepam	
Lorazepam	2–4	10–20	Conjugation	–	85
Oxazepam	2–4	5–20	Conjugation	–	97

[a]Desmethyldiazepam (DMDZ) half-life 50–100 h.

Data from Bailey et al.[52] and Facts and Comparisons.[53]

of anxiety. High lipophilicity also increases the extent of drug redistribution into the periphery, particularly adipose tissue, resulting in a shorter duration of effect after a single dose than indicated by single-dose elimination half-life studies.[52] Clinically, patients perceive a rapid onset of action, but some experience an unpleasant feeling of drowsiness or loss of control. This "rush" can be euphoric and contribute to abuse. Chlordiazepoxide's onset of action is much slower because of decreased lipophilicity, slower absorption, and delayed passage into the CNS.

Compared with diazepam, lorazepam, and oxazepam are relatively less lipophilic and have a slower onset of effect. These benzodiazepines have smaller volumes of distribution and a resulting longer duration of action.[52] Oxazepam absorption is slow, and peak levels are not obtained until 2 to 4 hours after a single dose; however, like lorazepam, oxazepam's anxiolytic effects are long lasting because extensive distribution does not occur.

Parenteral administration via the intramuscular route should be avoided with diazepam and chlordiazepoxide secondary to variability in the rate and extent of drug absorption. Intramuscular lorazepam provides rapid, reliable, and complete absorption.

After multiple dosing, the rate and extent of drug accumulation are functions of the drug's elimination half-life in relation to dosing intervals, clearance, and formation of active metabolites. Differences in clinical effects that occur during and after repeated dosages with the benzodiazepines are related in part to variability in metabolism and metabolite accumulation.[52]

The benzodiazepines undergo two primary metabolic processes, hepatic oxidation (catalyzed by cytochrome P450 3A4) and glucuronide conjugation. With the exception of lorazepam and oxazepam (which are conjugated only) and clonazepam (which undergoes nitroreduction), all benzodiazepines are oxidized first and then conjugated and excreted renally.[52] Diazepam's metabolism is also catalyzed by cytochrome P450 2C19. Oxidation can be impaired in patients with liver disease, in the elderly, and in those who simultaneously use drugs that inhibit oxidation resulting in higher levels of the parent drug and/or an active metabolite.

Many benzodiazepines are converted to desmethyldiazepam (DMDZ), an active metabolite with a long elimination half-life[52] (see Table 73–9). DMDZ is further oxidized to oxazepam and then conjugated and excreted. After multiple dosing, accumulation of DMDZ is slow and extensive, providing a long-lasting antianxiety effect. If oxidation of DMDZ is impaired, the half-life is prolonged, and drug accumulation can result with repeated dosing.

Clorazepate is a prodrug and possesses no anxiolytic effects until metabolized to DMDZ. Before absorption, clorazepate is metabolized rapidly in the stomach through a pH-dependent process under acidic conditions.

Benzodiazepines with shorter half-lives (e.g., alprazolam, lorazepam, and oxazepam) reach steady-state plasma concentrations rapidly, and drug accumulation after repeated dosing is minimal. Oxazepam and lorazepam are not converted into active metabolites.

Benzodiazepine protein binding is extensive, especially for the drugs with a long elimination half-life. After a single dose of a benzodiazepine with a long elimination half-life, the expected duration of clinical activity may not parallel the drug's pharmacokinetic half-life because of drug redistribution.[52] After multiple dosing, drugs with long elimination half-lives and active metabolites require 1 to 2 weeks to reach steady state.

Efficacy Clinical trials of benzodiazepines show that 65% to 75% of patients with GAD have a marked to moderate response, with most of the improvement occurring in the first 2 weeks of therapy. Benzodiazepines are more effective on the somatic symptoms of anxiety and fail to obviate the cognitive or psychic symptoms (e.g., worry).[11,23] Up to 50% of patients fail to reach remission with benzodiazepine therapy, and rates of relapse exceed that of the antidepressants.[23]

Adverse Effects The most common adverse events associated with benzodiazepine therapy involve CNS depression. This is manifested clinically as drowsiness, sedation, psychomotor impairment, and ataxia.[23] A transient mild drowsiness is experienced commonly by patients during the first few days of treatment; however, tolerance often develops. Disorientation, depression, confusion, irritability, aggression, and excitement are reported.[23]

Impairment of memory and recall also can occur during benzodiazepine treatment. The memory loss induced by the benzodiazepines typically is limited to events occurring after drug ingestion (anterograde amnesia).[23] Anterograde amnesia is secondary to disordered consolidation processes that store information and is not impairment in the perception or retrieval of information.[2] Benzodiazepines with high affinity for binding to the benzodiazepine receptor (e.g., lorazepam) appear to possess a higher potential for amnesia.[26]

Abuse, Dependence, Withdrawal, and Tolerance Two serious complications of benzodiazepine therapy are the potential for abuse and development of physical dependence. Benzodiazepine abuse is rare in the general population of users; however, individuals with a history of multiple drug abuse (e.g., alcohol or sedatives) are at the greatest risk for becoming benzodiazepine abusers.[5]

Because of the chronicity of illness, persons with GAD and panic disorder are at high risk of developing benzodiazepine dependence. Benzodiazepine dependence is a physiologic phenomenon demonstrated by the appearance of a predictable abstinence syndrome (withdrawal symptoms) on abrupt discontinuation of therapy.[26] Withdrawal symptoms can result because of the sudden dissociation of a benzodiazepine from its receptor site. After abrupt discontinuation, an acute decrease in GABA neurotransmission results, producing a less inhibited CNS.

Benzodiazepine Discontinuation After benzodiazepine therapy is discontinued suddenly, several events can occur. Rebound anxiety represents an immediate but transient return of original symptoms having an increased intensity compared with baseline. Recurrence or relapse is the return of original symptoms with similar intensity as before treatment.

Withdrawal symptoms are the emergence of new symptoms and a worsening of preexisting symptoms after benzodiazepine discontinuation. Symptoms can persist for days to weeks and resolve gradually over months.

Common symptoms of benzodiazepine withdrawal include anxiety, insomnia, restlessness, muscle tension, and irritability. Less frequently occurring symptoms are nausea, malaise, coryza, blurred vision, diaphoresis, nightmares, depression, hyperreflexia, and ataxia. Tinnitus, confusion, paranoid delusions, hallucinations, seizures, and psychosis occur rarely. Seizures can occur with both therapeutic and high doses of benzodiazepines with a short elimination half-life, usually within 3 days of drug discontinuation. They can occur approximately 1 week after discontinuation of agents with a long elimination half-life. High benzodiazepine doses, a long duration of therapy, and concurrent ingestion of drugs that lower the seizure threshold are risk factors for withdrawal seizures.

The onset of withdrawal symptoms in patients ingesting benzodiazepines with short elimination half-lives occurs much earlier (within 24 to 48 hours) than in those taking benzodiazepines with long elimination half-lives (within 3 to 8 days). Other factors associated with an increased incidence and severity of benzodiazepine withdrawal include high doses and long-term benzodiazepine therapy.

Several strategies to minimize the severity of benzodiazepine withdrawal include a 25% per week reduction in dosage until 50% of the dose is reached, and then dosage reduction by one-eighth every 4 to 7 days.[26] If therapy exceeds 8 weeks, a slow dosage taper over 2 to 3 weeks is recommended; however, if the duration of treatment is 6 months, a taper over 4 to 8 weeks should ensue.[5] Long-term use of benzodiazepines (i.e., 1 year or longer) requires a 2- to 4-month slow taper.[5] Tapering will not eliminate the emergence of withdrawal symptoms entirely but will prevent severe withdrawal. Slow drug taper is extremely important for the drugs with a short elimination half-life, because some individuals have greater difficulty with discontinuation. Adjunctive use of certain drugs (e.g., imipramine, valproic acid, or buspirone) or CBT can help to reduce withdrawal symptoms during the benzodiazepine taper.[5] If patients experience difficulties, especially with the agents with a short elimination half-life, then substitution of an agent with a long elimination half-life should be considered. Although tolerance develops to the sedative, muscle relaxant, and anticonvulsant activities, the benzodiazepines do not appear to lose anxiolytic or antipanic efficacy. The anxiolytic efficacy of benzodiazepines in long-term clinical trials (greater than 6 to 8 months of chronic use) has not been reported.[5]

Drug Interactions Drug interactions with the benzodiazepines generally fall into two categories: pharmacodynamic and pharmacokinetic (Table 73–10). Simultaneous use of alcohol and a benzodiazepine results in additive CNS depressant effects. In addition, concurrent use of a benzodiazepine and other drugs with CNS depressant properties (e.g., narcotic agonists, antipsychotics, and antihistamines) can potentiate the adverse sedative effects. When ingested alone in an overdose attempt, benzodiazepines are rarely life-threatening; however, the combination of benzodiazepines with alcohol or other CNS depressant agents is potentially fatal.

Dosing and Administration Benzodiazepine dosage requirements vary widely among patients and must be individualized. Therapy should be initiated using low doses (e.g., alprazolam 0.25 mg three times a day or equivalent doses of other benzodiazepines) and titrated upward to relieve anxiety symptoms and avoid adverse events. After an initial treatment response is achieved, agents with long elimination half-lives can be dosed at bedtime. Dosage adjustments should be made weekly. Three to four weeks of a daily dose at the maximum dose constitutes an adequate clinical trial (see Table 73–7).[5]

The duration of benzodiazepine therapy for the acute management of anxiety generally should not exceed 2 to 4 weeks. Benzodiazepines can be prescribed on an as-needed basis, and if several acute courses are necessary a benzodiazepine-free period of 2 to 4 weeks should be implemented between courses.[5] Individuals with persistent symptoms should be managed with antidepressants because of the risk of dependence with continued benzodiazepine therapy.[23]

Patient education should include the anticipated length of drug therapy, potential side effects, and consequences of the ingestion of alcohol and other CNS depressants. Patients should understand that benzodiazepines provide symptomatic relief but do not solve underlying psychologic problems. Patients should be instructed not to decrease or discontinue benzodiazepine usage without contacting their prescriber.

TABLE 73-10 Pharmacokinetic Drug Interactions with the Benzodiazepines

Drug	Effect
Carbamazepine	Decreased Cl of alprazolam
Ciprofloxacin	Decreased Cl of diazepam and increased $t_{1/2}$
Erythromycin	Decreased Cl of alprazolam
Fluoxetine	Decreased Cl of diazepam
Fluvoxamine	Decreased Cl of alprazolam and diazepam and prolonged $t_{1/2}$
Isoniazid	Decreased Cl of diazepam and increased $t_{1/2}$
Ketoconazole	Decreased Cl and Vd of chlordiazepoxide; increased AUC of alprazolam
Nefazodone	Decreased Cl of alprazolam, AUC doubled, and $t_{1/2}$ prolonged
Omeprazole	Decreased Cl of diazepam and prolonged $t_{1/2}$
Oral contraceptives	Decreased Cl and increased $t_{1/2}$ of diazepam and chlordiazepoxide; decreased $t_{1/2}$ of lorazepam and oxazepam
Paroxetine	Decreased Cl of alprazolam
Phenytoin	Increased Cl of clonazepam and reduced $t_{1/2}$
Propoxyphene	Decreased Cl of alprazolam and prolonged $t_{1/2}$
Propranolol	Decreased Cl of diazepam and prolonged $t_{1/2}$
Rifampin	Increased metabolism of diazepam
St. John's wort	Decreased AUC of alprazolam
Valproate	Decreased Cl of lorazepam

AUC, area under the plasma concentration curve; BZ, benzodiazepine; Cl, clearance; $t_{1/2}$, elimination half-life; Vd, volume of distribution.

Data from Drug Facts and Comparisons[53] and Madabushi.[54]

Buspirone Therapy

Buspirone is a nonbenzodiazepine anxiolytic that lacks anticonvulsant, muscle relaxant, hypnotic, motor impairment, and dependence properties. It is considered to be a second-line agent for GAD because of inconsistent reports of efficacy (particularly long term), delayed onset of effect (i.e., 2 weeks or longer), and lack of efficacy for other potential concurrent depressive and anxiety disorders.[20,23] Unlike benzodiazepines, buspirone is effective for the psychic symptoms of anxiety.[23]

Pharmacology and Mechanism of Action Buspirone's anxiolytic mechanism of action is unknown. It is thought to exert its anxiolytic effect through 5-HT_{1A} partial agonist activity at the presynaptic 5-HT receptors by reducing the firing of 5-HT neurons.[12]

Pharmacokinetics After an oral dose, buspirone is absorbed rapidly and completely and undergoes extensive first-pass metabolism. The mean elimination half-life is 2.5 hours, and it must be dosed two to three times daily, which adversely affects adherence to the drug regimen.[23]

Adverse Effects Adverse events include dizziness, nausea, and headaches.[23]

Drug Interactions Drugs that inhibit cytochrome P450 3A4 (e.g., verapamil, itraconazole, fluvoxamine) can increase buspirone levels. Rifampin caused a 10-fold reduction in buspirone levels. Buspirone reportedly increases haloperidol levels and elevates blood pressure in patients taking a monoamine oxidase inhibitor (MAOI).

Dosing and Administration The dose of buspirone can be titrated in increments of 5 mg/day every 2 to 3 days as needed.[23] The onset of improvement in psychic symptoms precedes the relief of somatic symptoms; maximum therapeutic benefit might not be evident for 4 to 6 weeks.

Buspirone is an agent of choice in the management of uncomplicated GAD, in patients who fail other anxiolytic therapies, or in patients with a history of substance abuse. It is not useful in clinical situations requiring immediate anxiolysis or for situations requiring as-needed anxiolytic therapy. The use of benzodiazepines within the month previous to initiation of buspirone therapy was associated with reduced efficacy of buspirone because of its delayed onset in the reduction of somatic symptoms.[23]

■ PHARMACOECONOMIC CONSIDERATIONS

The annual economic burden of anxiety disorders in the United States was estimated to be $42.3 billion in 1990 ($63.1 billion in 1998 dollars).[3] Nonpsychiatric medical treatment costs represented more than half of this figure, with expenses of $13.3 billion for psychiatric treatment, $4.1 billion for indirect workplace costs, and $1.2 billion in mortality costs.

GAD is associated with high rates of healthcare use and disability. The number of days missed from work increases when GAD is concurrent with one or more other psychiatric disorders. Patients with GAD tend to use family practitioners and gastroenterologists more frequently than healthy controls.[2] GAD ranks third among anxiety disorders in the rate of use of primary care physician time, and it is the leading cause of disability in the workplace in the United States.[2] Two decision analyses for GAD were published by researchers in the United Kingdom: venlafaxine was more cost-effective than diazepam,[55] and escitalopram was associated with higher treatment success, and lower discontinuation rates and costs than paroxetine.[56]

CLINICAL CONTROVERSIES

It is unclear if combining pharmacotherapy with CBT confers greater overall efficacy than treatment with either approach alone. CBT is an option if patients fail treatment with consecutive trials of antidepressants. Clinicians should be aware that many patients lack access to CBT and should take this into consideration during treatment planning.

■ EVALUATION OF THERAPEUTIC OUTCOMES

Initially, anxious patients should be monitored once every 2 weeks[33] for a reduction in the frequency, duration, and severity of anxiety symptoms and improvement in functioning. The clinician should assess the patient for response to treatment by asking about specific target symptoms of anxiety and emergence of adverse events. Ideally, the patient should have no or minimal anxiety or depressive symptoms and no functional impairment. Use of an objective measurement of remission of GAD (e.g., Hamilton Rating Scale for Anxiety score less than 7 to 10 and a Sheehan Disability Scale score less than or equal to 1 on each item) can assist in the evaluation of drug response.[23] If a patient has only a partial response, the dose should be increased after 4 to 6 weeks of antidepressant therapy (or 2 weeks of acute therapy with benzodiazepines). The length of therapy should be individualized, with some patients requiring up to 1 year of antidepressant therapy.[5,20,33]

TREATMENT

Panic Disorder

■ DESIRED OUTCOME

The goal of therapy in panic disorder is remission. Patients should be free of panic attacks, have no or minimal anticipatory anxiety and agoraphobic avoidance, and no functional impairment.[57] Naturalistic studies indicate that after pharmacotherapy, over 50% of patients have occasional panic attacks, 40% experience agoraphobic avoidance, and most continue to take medications.[58]

■ GENERAL APPROACH TO TREATMENT

Therapeutic options include single or combined pharmacologic agents, concurrent psychotherapy, or psychotherapy followed by pharmacotherapy. Most patients without agoraphobic avoidance will improve with pharmacotherapy alone; however, if avoidance is present, CBT typically is initiated concurrently. With all effective drug therapies, resolution of agoraphobic avoidance tends to occur slowly. A meta-analysis of 11 randomized clinical trials comparing the use of SSRIs, TCAs, and CBT showed the effect on global anxiety and response to be similar among all treatments.[59]

In the most comprehensive study to date, efficacy of imipramine alone and CBT alone were equivalent in acute therapy for 3 months and during 6 months of maintenance therapy. Combined imipramine and CBT therapy was not significantly better than CBT or imipramine alone for acute therapy but was significantly better during maintenance. At 6 months after discontinuation, only patients previously treated with CBT maintained improvement (4% relapse) compared with a 25% relapse rate in patients previously treated with imipramine.[60] Patients who failed to respond to CBT and had paroxetine added to therapy had a significant improvement in agoraphobic behavior and anxiety symptoms.[61]

■ NONPHARMACOLOGIC THERAPY

Patients should be educated to avoid substances that can precipitate panic attacks, including caffeine, drugs of abuse, and nonprescription stimulants.[1] CBT is associated with short-term improvement in 80% to 90% of patients and 6-month improvement in 75% of patients. A course of CBT for panic disorder is 16 to 20 hours in length conducted over a period of 4 months.[33] Bibliotherapy (the use of self-help books), exercise, and Internet-based CBT are other options.[20,33]

■ PHARMACOLOGIC THERAPY

Panic disorder is treated effectively with several drugs including the SSRIs, the TCA imipramine, and the benzodiazepines alprazolam and clonazepam[21,24,57] (Table 73–11). Alprazolam, clonazepam, sertraline, paroxetine, and venlafaxine are approved for this indication. SSRIs are the first-line agents because of their tolerability and efficacy in acute and long-term studies;[24,25,58] however, the benzodiazepines are the most commonly used drug for panic disorder.[57] In a meta-analysis of the pharmacotherapy of panic disorder, the effect size of SSRIs and TCAs did not differ; however, the number of dropouts in the TCA group (31%) was significantly higher than in the SSRI group (18%).[62] A second meta-analysis comparing efficacy of benzodiazepines, TCAs,

TABLE 73-11 Drugs Used in the Treatment of Panic Disorder

Class/Generic Name	Brand Name	Starting Dose	Antipanic Dosage[a] Range (mg)
Selective serotonin reuptake inhibitors			
Citalopram[b]	Celexa	10 mg per day	20–60
Escitalopram	Lexapro	5 mg per day	10–20
Fluoxetine[b]	Prozac	5 mg per day	10–30
Fluvoxamine[b]	Luvox	25 mg per day	100–300
Paroxetine[b]	Paxil	10 mg per day	20–60[c]
	Paxil CR	12.5 mg per day	25–75[c]
Sertraline[b]	Zoloft	25 mg per day	50–200[c]
Serotonin norepinephrine reuptake inhibitors			
Venlafaxine XR	Effexor XR	37.5 mg per day	75–225[c]
Benzodiazepines			
Alprazolam[b]	Xanax	0.25 mg three times a day	4–10[c]
	Xanax XR	0.5–1 mg per day	1–10[c]
Clonazepam[b]	Klonopin	0.25 mg once or twice per day	1–4[c]
Diazepam[b]	Valium	2–5 mg three times a day	5–20
Lorazepam[b]	Ativan	0.5–1 mg three times a day	2–8
Tricyclic antidepressant			
Imipramine[b]	Tofranil	10 mg per day	75–250
Monoamine oxidase inhibitor			
Phenelzine	Nardil	15 mg per day	45–90

[a]Dosage used in clinical trials but not FDA-approved.
[b]Available generically.
[c]Dosage is FDA approved.
Data from Katon,[21] Bandelow et al,[24] Work Group on Panic Disorder,[25] Effexor XR package insert.[28]

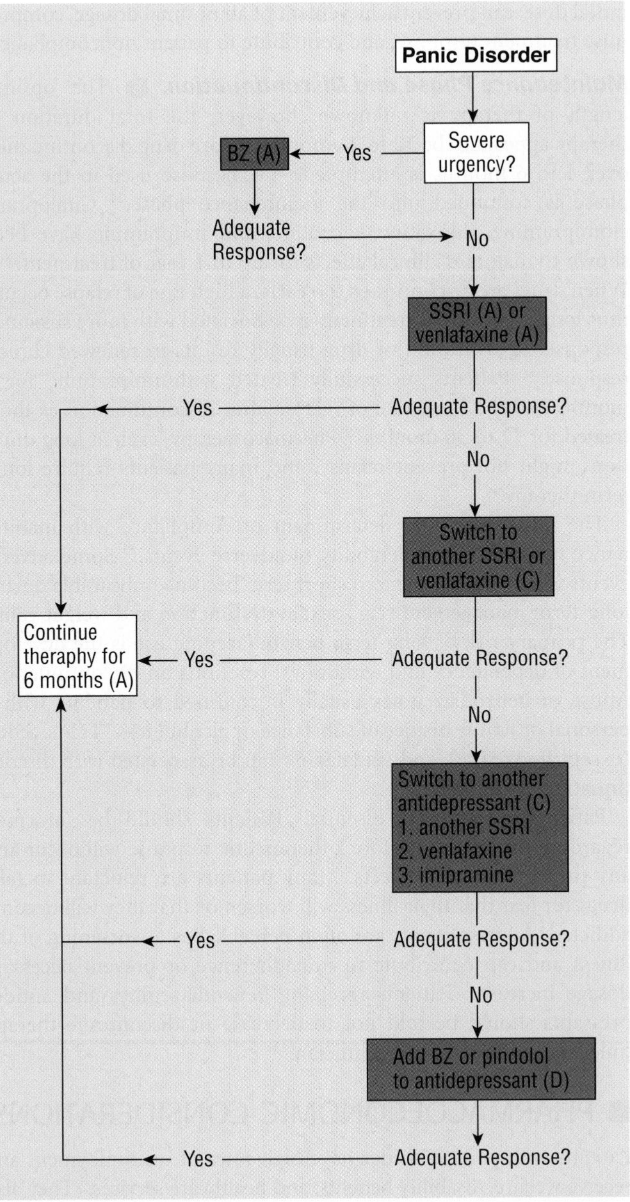

FIGURE 73-2. Algorithm for the pharmacotherapy of panic disorder. Strength of recommendations: A = directly based on category I evidence (i.e., meta-analysis of randomized clinical trials [RCT] or at least one RCT); B = directly based on category II evidence (i.e., at least one controlled study without randomization or one other type of quasi-experimental study); C = directly based on category III evidence (i.e., nonexperimental descriptive studies); D = directly based on category IV evidence (i.e., expert committee reports or opinions and/or clinical experience of respected authorities). (BZ, benzodiazepine; SSRI, selective serotonin reuptake inhibitor.) *(Data from Baldwin et al.[20] and NICE.[33])*

and SSRIs in panic disorder concluded that all treatments were equally efficacious with 50% to 80% of patients responding to treatment; however benzodiazepines were less effective for depression.[59] Four practice guidelines[24,25,33,58] are published. An algorithm for the pharmacologic therapy of panic disorder appears in Fig. 73–2.

The efficacy of antidepressants was demonstrated in acute and long-term trials. Three 12-week, acute trials compared antidepressants. Escitalopram, but not citalopram, reduced the frequency of panic attacks although both improved QOL and reduced disease severity.[63] There was no difference in outcomes between paroxetine 40 to 60 mg and sertraline 50 to 150 mg daily.[64] Venlafaxine extended-release (75 mg or 150 mg) and paroxetine 40 mg achieved a 44% remission rate compared with that of placebo (24%).[65] Double-blind trials indicated that continuing sertraline, citalopram, or imipramine from 3 months to 1 year improved response rates.[20] Relapse prevention trials with fluoxetine, imipramine, paroxetine, sertraline, and venlafaxine extended-release resulted in reduced relapse rates compared with placebo.[20,66]

Benzodiazepines are considered second-line agents. Because of the risk of dependency, benzodiazepines should be used only after several trials of antidepressants have failed.[24,25] Because of potential emergence of depressive symptoms during treatment, benzodiazepines should not be used as monotherapy in a patient who is clinically depressed or has a history of depression. In patients whose illness is complicated by a history of alcohol or drug abuse, benzodiazepine use should be avoided.[25] Limited data support the combined use of SSRIs and benzodiazepines in the first weeks of treatment to offset the delay in the SSRI effect.[20]

Alternative Drug Treatments

Buspirone, trazodone, bupropion, antipsychotics, antihistamines, and β-blockers are ineffective in panic disorder.[20,24,58] The majority of studies assessing the efficacy of MAOIs in treating panic disorder were open-labeled. These trials lacked sufficient dosage and duration of treatment, adequate sample size, and valid ratings of panic attacks. No maintenance trials of MAOIs are published. MAOIs are reserved for the most refractory or difficult patients.[24]

Special Populations

Elderly patients with panic disorder have fewer, less intense symptoms and avoidant behavior than younger patients.[67] Youth often present with fear that they are dying or being smothered, and agoraphobia can be manifested as a fear of leaving home.[68] Antidepressants, especially the SSRIs, are preferred for management of panic disorder,[67,68] and benzodiazepines are second-line agents because of potential problems with disinhibition in these two populations.

Antidepressant Therapy

Tricyclic Antidepressants

Efficacy. Imipramine is the most studied TCA, alleviating panic attacks in 75% of patients with panic disorder. Imipramine effectively blocks panic attacks within at least 4 weeks; however, maximal improvement (including antiphobic response) does not occur until 8 to 12 weeks.[25]

Adverse Effects. Up to 40% of patients experience stimulant-like side effects, including anxiety, insomnia, and jitteriness.[25] These side effects often affect patient compliance, prevent medication dosage increases, and interfere with the overall treatment outcome.

Problems with TCA use in panic disorder are well documented and include stimulatory side effects, anticholinergic effects, orthostatic hypotension, delayed onset of antipanic effects, and toxicity in overdose.[25] Approximately 25% of patients reportedly discontinue treatment because of side effects. Weight gain is problematic with long-term therapy.[25]

Dosing and Administration. When using imipramine, treatment should be slowly increased by 10 mg every 2 to 4 days as tolerated.

Selective Serotonin Reuptake Inhibitors

Efficacy. Clinical studies indicate that all SSRIs are effective in panic disorder.[20,21,58] The percentage of patients who become panic-free ranges between 60% and 80%.[25] ❹ The antipanic effect of SSRIs is delayed for at least 4 weeks, and some patients do not respond for 8 to 12 weeks.[25,33]

Adverse Effects. Typical antidepressant doses of SSRIs can cause side effects of insomnia, jitteriness, restlessness, and agitation, and lead to drug discontinuation in patients with panic disorder. Transient gastrointestinal disturbances occur more frequently with SSRIs than with TCAs. Thus low initial SSRI doses should be prescribed.[21,24,57] Sleep disturbances, headaches, and sexual dysfunction often are problematic.[24,57]

Dosing and Administration. Low initial doses of SSRIs are recommended (see Table 73–11) to avoid stimulatory side effects (e.g., insomnia or nervousness), and should be maintained for the first week of therapy. Doses at the upper end of the dosing range can be necessary to achieve response.[33]

Serotonin Norepinephrine Reuptake Inhibitors

Efficacy. Approximately 54% to 60% of patients were panic-free on venlafaxine-extended release 75 mg or 150 mg daily. The remission rates were 44% for both dosages in acute efficacy studies.[65]

Adverse Effects. The most common adverse effects of venlafaxine extended-release in panic trials were nausea, somnolence, tremors, sweating, and abnormal sexual functioning (ejaculation difficulties and anorgasmia).[30]

Dosing and Administration. The dosage of venlafaxine can be increased at weekly intervals. A dose-response relationship was not evident in clinical trials.[30]

Benzodiazepines

Efficacy. The high-potency benzodiazepines clonazepam and alprazolam are the preferred agents.[5,21] Diazepam and lorazepam are possibly effective in treating panic disorder when taken in sufficiently high doses.[25] Alprazolam is an ideal agent for patients who need rapid relief. Therapeutic response to benzodiazepines occurs in 1 to 2 weeks. Relapse rates of 50% or higher are common despite slow drug tapering.[25]

Adverse Effects. Patient acceptance of benzodiazepines usually is not a problem, and except for sedation, side effects are reported rarely.

Dosing and Administration. Doses of clonazepam can be increased by 0.25 or 0.5 mg every 3 days to 4 mg/day if needed.[50] Alprazolam can be slowly increased over several weeks to reach an ideal dose. ❺ The duration of action of immediate-release alprazolam can be as little as 4 to 6 hours with resulting breakthrough symptoms; use of the extended-release alprazolam or clonazepam will avoid this problem. Most patients require 3 to 6 mg/day of alprazolam, and some need higher doses to obtain a full therapeutic (antipanic and antiphobic) response.

Treatment Resistance. Common reasons for treatment failures are comorbid psychiatric disorders, rapid dosage increases with resulting intolerable side effects, and underdosage.[25] All standard treatments should be tried before using augmentation strategies. The most common strategy used in patients with a partial response to one agent is to augment it with low doses of another antipanic agent (e.g., a TCA, benzodiazepine, or an SSRI).[25]

Phases of Therapy

Acute Phase. The main goal of therapy in the acute phase is reduction of symptoms (e.g., resolution of panic attacks, reduction in anxiety and phobic fears, resumption of the patient's usual activities).[25] The duration of this phase is generally 1 to 3 months depending on the choice of drug. The duration of the acute phase with antidepressants is about 12 weeks.[25] Therapy should be altered if there is no response after 6 to 8 weeks of an adequate dose. The duration of the acute phase with benzodiazepines is approximately 1 month because response is rapid.

The guiding principle for using drugs in panic disorder is to start low, use an adequate dose, and treat for an appropriate period of time. Side effects with the antidepressants, often from too high an initial dose, can prevent achievement of an optimal dosage, compromise treatment response, and contribute to patient noncompliance.

Maintenance Phase and Discontinuation. ❻ The optimal length of therapy is unknown; however, the total duration of therapy appears to be 12 to 24 months before drug discontinuation over 4 to 6 months is attempted.[24,25] The dose used in the acute phase is continued into the maintenance phase.[24] Citalopram, clomipramine, fluoxetine, sertraline, and imipramine have been shown to maintain clinical effects for up to 1 year of treatment.[20,24] When drugs are discontinued too early, a high rate of relapse occurs; thus longer periods of treatment are associated with more sustained response. Reinstitution of drug usually results in renewed clinical response.[25] Patients successfully treated with imipramine for 6 months had the same rate of relapse after discontinuation as those treated for 12 to 30 months.[69] Pharmacotherapy, even at long duration, might not prevent relapse, and many patients require long-term therapy.

The most important determinant of compliance with maintenance therapy is the tolerability of adverse events.[25] Some adverse events which are experienced short term become unbearable during long-term management (e.g., sexual dysfunction and weight gain). The primary risk of long-term benzodiazepine use is the development of dependency and withdrawal reactions on discontinuation. Abuse of benzodiazepines usually is confined to patients with a personal or family history of substance or alcohol use.[5] TCAs, SSRIs (except fluoxetine), and venlafaxine can be associated with discontinuation symptoms.

Patient education is essential. Patients should be informed regarding the lag time before a therapeutic response will occur and any problematic side effects. Many patients are reluctant to take drugs for fear that their illness will worsen or that they will become addicted. Adverse events are often perceived as a worsening of the illness and can contribute to nonadherence or prevent necessary dosage increases. Patients receiving benzodiazepines and antidepressants should be told not to decrease or discontinue therapy unless authorized by their clinician.[33]

■ PHARMACOECONOMIC CONSIDERATIONS

Patients with panic disorder have high rates of unemployment and receive welfare, disability benefits, and healthcare services.[3] They also have impaired emotional and physical health status and experience poor marital and social functioning.[20,21] Measures of QOL improved with imipramine, clonazepam, sertraline, and venlafaxine. Treatment with clomipramine, paroxetine, or fluoxetine improved work, social, and family responsibilities. Improvements in anxiety and phobic avoidance were significantly associated with QOL improvements.[20,21] In a cost comparison, group CBT was more cost-beneficial than pharmacotherapy for the initial 4 months of therapy.[70]

CLINICAL CONTROVERSY

The optimal sequence of treatments for panic disorder is not well defined by the current literature. When initial SSRI therapy fails, there is no clear evidence on which alternative therapeutic treatment modality to initiate. Most clinicians will prescribe a second SSRI.

■ EVALUATION OF THERAPEUTIC OUTCOMES

During the first few weeks of the acute phase of therapy, patients with panic disorder should be seen every 2 weeks to adjust drug dosages based on improvement in panic symptoms and to monitor for adverse events.[33] Subsequently, visits every 2 months should suffice.[33] The patient should be counseled to maintain a diary to record the date, time, frequency, and duration of panic episodes and the severity of symptoms. Treatment outcomes can be assessed objectively by use of the Hamilton Rating Scale for Anxiety (with a desired score of less than or equal to 7 to 10).[71] At scheduled visits, the clinician can inquire about the level of disability experienced by the patient and have the patient complete the Sheehan Disability Scale (with a goal of less than or equal to 1 point on each item).[71] During drug discontinuation, the frequency of appointments should be increased to evaluate for emergence of withdrawal symptoms and monitor for relapse.

TREATMENT

Social Anxiety Disorder

DESIRED OUTCOME

The goals of therapy in the acute phase of treatment are to reduce physiologic symptoms of anxiety (e.g., tachycardia, flushing, and sweating), social anxiety, and phobic avoidance. The duration of this phase is 4 to 12 weeks, depending on the drug therapy.

The goals of therapy in the continuation phase (3 to 6 months) are to extend the therapeutic benefits, especially the patient's ability to participate in social activities, and improve QOL. Although the primary goal of treatment is to reduce anxiety symptoms to manageable levels, even modest reductions in avoidance and discomfort can be highly valued by patients.[9]

❼ SAD is a chronic, long-term illness. At least a 1-year maintenance period is recommended to maintain improvement and decrease the rate of relapse.[19,22] Situations suggesting a possible need for long-term treatment include the presence of unresolved symptoms or comorbidity, an early onset of disease, and a prior history of relapse.[19,22] The long-term goal in the treatment of SAD is remission with the disappearance of the core symptoms of social anxiety, little or no anxiety, and no functional impairment or concurrent depressive symptoms.[71]

GENERAL APPROACH TO TREATMENT

Generalized SAD is associated with significant morbidity, and patients should be treated aggressively. Obstacles to effective treatment include patient avoidance of therapy secondary to fear and shame, treatment directed toward somatic symptoms or concurrent conditions, and financial barriers.[72] Patients with SAD often respond to treatment more slowly and less completely than patients with other anxiety disorders. Therefore it is important to set reasonable expectations for response to therapy. The patient's symptoms, prior treatments, concurrent conditions, and history of substance abuse direct treatment selections.

CBT and pharmacotherapy are effective in the treatment of SAD.[9,19,73] Pharmacotherapy is often the most practical choice because CBT might not be available outside of large urban areas secondary to the lack of trained therapists and high treatment costs. Studies suggest the acute treatment outcomes for CBT and pharmacotherapy are equal.[9,19] Drug therapy tends to be superior in reducing subjective general anxiety in acute treatment, although CBT can lead to a greater likelihood of maintaining response after treatment termination.[9,19,74]

There are no data to predict which patients will respond best to pharmacotherapy, CBT, or a combination,[9] or maintain gains after discontinuing pharmacotherapy. The only significant predictor of treatment response in pharmacotherapy is duration of treatment.[75] Some patients elect lifelong therapy, and many are reluctant to attempt drug discontinuation because of fear of relapse. Discontinuation of drug therapy after only 2 to 3 months resulted in higher rates of relapse than when therapy was continued for 5 to 12 months.[9] Data show that relapse rates after discontinuation of CBT are significantly less than those after discontinuation of effective pharmacotherapy.[9,19,74] Sertraline is the only medication approved for the long-term treatment of SAD, although paroxetine, escitalopram, and venlafaxine prevented relapse.[76–78]

NONPHARMACOLOGIC THERAPY

Patients should be educated about SAD and effective therapeutic options. Support groups are helpful for some patients. Self-help group programs that focus on effective communication can benefit people with public-speaking phobia.

CBT for SAD consists of exposure therapy, cognitive restructuring, relaxation training techniques, and social skills training.[9] Through CBT, patients learn to overcome anxiety in social situations and change the beliefs and responses that maintain this behavior. Therapy usually lasts several months and often is conducted in a group setting. In clinical trials, one-half to two-thirds of patients responded at 12 weeks.[9]

PHARMACOLOGIC THERAPY

Special Populations

SAD can present in children of preschool to elementary school age. If the disorder is not treated, it can persist into adulthood and increase the risk of depression and substance abuse. CBT and social skills training are effective nonpharmacologic therapies in children.[8,9] Placebo-controlled and open-label trials have provided evidence of efficacy of pharmacotherapy with an SSRI or SNRI in children 6 to 17 years of age.[9,19] Children and adolescents prescribed an SSRI or SNRI for social anxiety (or for other purposes) should be closely monitored for increased risk of suicidal ideation. Headache, nausea, drowsiness, insomnia, jitteriness, and stomach aches were reported in children receiving antidepressants.[8]

Benzodiazepines should be reserved as the last-line agents in children with SAD.[8] If prescribed, they should be used for the shortest time period possible. The adverse effects of benzodiazepines in children include drowsiness, oppositional behavior, disinhibition, fatigue, and nausea.

Approximately one-fifth of patients with SAD also suffer from an alcohol use disorder. Many people with SAD report that they use alcohol to cope with their anxiety. Most clinical trials evaluating pharmacotherapy for SAD excluded patients with alcohol use disorder. Paroxetine significantly reduced social anxiety and decreased the frequency and severity of alcohol use in patients with SAD and an alcohol use disorder.[79] MAOIs and benzodiazepines are not appropriate therapy for patients with SAD and alcohol use disorder. The tyramine present in many alcoholic beverages can precipitate a hypertensive crisis in patients on an MAOI. People who abuse alcohol are at risk for abusing or becoming dependent on benzodiazepines. SSRI therapy is the treatment of choice in this patient population.

Antidepressant Therapy

❽ The SSRIs and venlafaxine have the benefits of antidepressant activity for concurrent depression and safety when used in patients with substance abuse. Paroxetine, sertraline, and venlafaxine extended-release are approved for the treatment of generalized SAD and are considered first-line agents because of their efficacy and tolerability (Table 73–12). Escitalopram has also been found to be effective in the treatment of generalized social anxiety.[20,80,81] Controlled trials comparing different SSRIs, or SSRIs and an SNRI, demonstrated equivalent efficacy between agents.[9] TCAs are not effective in SAD.[9] The International Consensus Group on Depression and Anxiety published a consensus statement on SAD,[22] and

TABLE 73-12 Drugs Used in the Treatment of Generalized Social Anxiety Disorder

Class/Generic Name	Brand Name	Starting Dose	Dosage Range[a] (mg/day)
Selective serotonin reuptake inhibitors			
Citalopram[b]	Celexa	20 mg per day	20–40
Escitalopram	Lexapro	5 mg per day	10–20
Fluvoxamine[b]	Luvox	50 mg per day	150–300
Paroxetine[b]	Paxil	10 mg per day	10–60[c]
Paroxetine CR	Paxil CR	12.5 mg per day	12.5–37.5[c]
Sertraline[b]	Zoloft	25–50 mg per day	50–200[c]
Serotonin-norepinephrine reuptake inhibitor			
Venlafaxine XR	Effexor XR	75 mg per day	75–225[c]
Benzodiazepine			
Clonazepam[b,d]	Klonopin	0.25 mg per day	1–4
Monoamine oxidase inhibitor			
Phenelzine	Nardil	15 mg at bedtime	60–90
Alternate agents			
Buspirone[b,d]	BuSpar	10 mg twice per day	45–60
Gabapentin[b]	Neurontin	100 mg three times a day	900–3600
Mirtazapine[a,b]	Remeron	15 mg at bedtime	30
Pregabalin	Lyrica	100 mg three times a day	600

[a]Dosage used in clinical trials but not FDA approved.
[b]Available generically.
[c]Dosage is FDA approved.
[d]Used as augmenting agent.
Data from Schneier,[9] Ballenger et al,[22] Paxil package insert,[27] Effexor XR package insert,[28] and Blanco et al.[73]

evidence-based guidelines for the treatment of SAD were published by the British Association for Psychopharmacology.[20] An algorithm for the pharmacotherapy of generalized SAD appears in Fig. 73–3.

Selective Serotonin Reuptake Inhibitors

Efficacy. The efficacy and safety of SSRIs in the treatment of SAD were established in large placebo-controlled trials.[80] Response rates to SSRIs ranged from 50% to 80% after 8 to 12 weeks of treatment.[80,81]

Patients treated with paroxetine, sertraline, escitalopram, and fluvoxamine showed improvement in anxiety and avoidance symptoms and a decrease in disability.[80] Daily doses up to 60 mg of paroxetine, 200 mg of sertraline, 20 mg of escitalopram, and 300 mg of fluvoxamine were well tolerated, and emergent adverse effects were similar to those of depression trials (e.g., nausea, sexual dysfunction, sweating, and somnolence). The onset of effect was delayed 4 to 8 weeks, and maximum benefit was often not observed until 12 weeks or longer. Sertraline was effective in disabled patients suffering from the marked to severe form of generalized SAD.[82] Limited data suggest that citalopram is also effective in treating SAD.[83] Fluoxetine was not effective in SAD.[84]

Dosing and Administration. SSRIs should be initiated at doses similar to those used for the treatment of depression and administered as a single daily dose (see Table 73–12). If the patient suffers from comorbid panic disorder, the SSRI dose should be started at one-fourth or one-half of the dose. Safety for paroxetine in SAD was demonstrated in doses up to 60 mg/day, but additional therapeutic benefits above 20 mg/day were not shown.[85]

The dose response curve for SSRIs tends to be relatively flat, but individual patients can require higher doses.[9,19] When discontinuing an SSRI, the dosage should be tapered monthly (i.e., decreasing sertraline by 50 mg or paroxetine by 10 mg) to reduce the risk of relapse and discontinuation symptoms. Escitalopram produced significantly fewer discontinuation symptoms compared with paroxetine in patients with SAD.[20]

Venlafaxine

Efficacy. Venlafaxine extended-release was significantly better than placebo in improving social interaction, performance, avoidance factors, and some fear factors (e.g., public speaking).[86] Beneficial effects were seen by week 3. Venlafaxine was effective in patients who failed to respond to therapy with SSRIs.[19]

Adverse Effects. Adverse effects included anorexia, dry mouth, nausea, insomnia, and sexual dysfunction.

Dosing and Administration. Additional therapeutic benefits of venlafaxine above 75 mg/day were not shown.[86] Venlafaxine should be tapered slowly (i.e., decreasing by 37.5 mg/mo) to decrease the risk of relapse during discontinuation.

Mirtazapine Mirtazapine reduced social anxiety and improved QOL in women with SAD over 10 weeks. The dose was 30 mg/day, and mirtazapine was well tolerated.[87]

Alternate Agents

Benzodiazepines Benzodiazepines are commonly used in the treatment of patients who cannot tolerate or fail to respond to antidepressants.[9] Benzodiazepines are not considered first-line therapy for SAD because of concerns over the adverse effects, potential for dependence, the possibility of rebound anxiety, and ineffectiveness in the treatment of depression.[19,20] Clonazepam is the most extensively studied benzodiazepine for the treatment of generalized SAD.[88] Clonazepam improved fear and phobic avoidance, interpersonal sensitivity, fears of negative evaluation, and disability measures.[88] Adverse effects included sexual dysfunction, unsteadiness, dizziness, and poor concentration.[88]

If clonazepam is prescribed, the acute phase of therapy is about 1 month. The initial dose of 0.25 mg/day can then be increased as tolerated over several weeks up to 3 mg/day. The average daily dose in clinical trials was 2.4 mg.[69,73] Patients should be instructed not to decrease or discontinue clonazepam without consulting their clinician because of the risks of rebound anxiety and withdrawal symptoms.

Benzodiazepines must be slowly tapered on discontinuation. Patients on clonazepam for 6 months who were slowly tapered over 5 months maintained their treatment response.[88] Clonazepam should be gradually tapered at a rate not to exceed 0.25 mg every 2 weeks.[9]

Anticonvulsants Anticonvulsants are another therapeutic option in SAD. Gabapentin, a nonbenzodiazepine GABA analog, was effective for SAD in a 14-week placebo-controlled trial.[9,19] The onset of effect occurred within 2 to 4 weeks. Patients reported dizziness and dry mouth. Pregabalin was superior to placebo in an 11-week, placebo-controlled trial. The effective dose was 600 mg/day and adverse effects included dizziness and somnolence.[89]

β-Blockers β-Blockers decrease the perception of anxiety by blunting the peripheral autonomic symptoms of arousal (e.g., rapid heart rate, sweating, blushing, and tremor), and they are often used to decrease anxiety in performance-related situations. For patients with specific SAD, 10 to 80 mg of propranolol or 25 to 100 mg of atenolol can be taken one hour before a performance as needed.[9,19] A test dose should be taken at home before the presentation to assure that β-blockade is sufficient and there are no adverse events. The effect of a single dose can last up to several hours. Controlled trials with β-blockers do not support daily use in generalized SAD.[19]

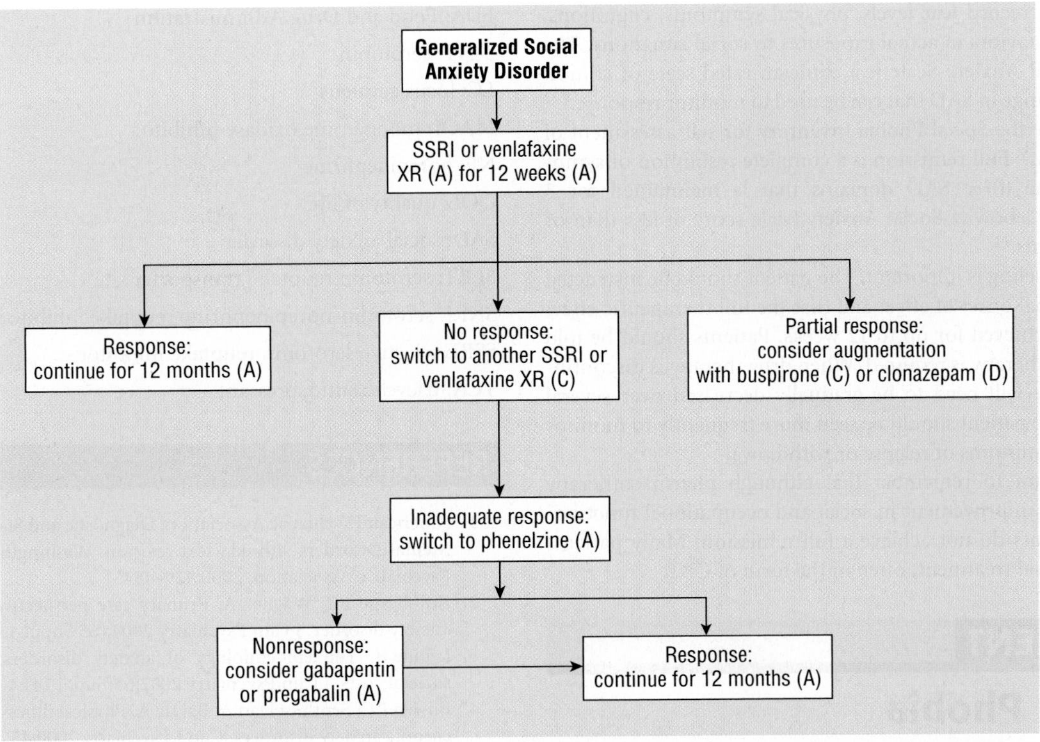

FIGURE 73-3. Algorithm for the pharmacotherapy of generalized social anxiety disorder. Strength of recommendations: A = directly based on category I evidence (i.e., meta-analysis of randomized clinical trials [RCT] or at least one RCT); B = directly based on category II evidence (i.e., at least one controlled study without randomization or one other type of quasi-experimental study); C = directly based on category III evidence (i.e., nonexperimental descriptive studies); D = directly based on category IV evidence (i.e., expert committee reports or opinions and/or clinical experience of respected authorities). (SSRI, selective serotonin reuptake inhibitor.) *(Data from reference Baldwin et al.[20])*

Treatment Resistance There are no data to guide clinicians in the choice of treatments if there is a lack of response to antidepressants. Patients who have an incomplete response to a first-line agent can benefit from augmentation with buspirone.[9,73] Clonazepam can be used as an augmenting agent in patients without a history of substance abuse.[20] When clonazepam was combined with paroxetine over 10 weeks in a placebo-controlled trial, clonazepam did not lead to more rapid resolution of SAD symptoms.[90] However, the group that received the combination therapy had a higher response rate.

❾ An adequate trial usually consists of 8 to 12 weeks (at maximum dosages) to determine if a drug will be effective. Subsequent options include a trial of a second SSRI or venlafaxine extended-release. Some patients experience clinical benefit during the first 4 weeks of therapy.[9,19] If nonresponsiveness continues, a trial of an alternative agent is warranted.

The MAOIs are reserved for treatment-resistant patients. Although phenelzine is effective in 77% of patients with SAD,[22,73] dietary restrictions, potential drug interactions and adverse effects (e.g., weight gain and hypertensive crisis) have limited its use. If a patient is switched from another antidepressant to phenelzine, an appropriate washout period should be followed.

■ PHARMACOECONOMIC CONSIDERATIONS

Generalized SAD is associated with lower health-related QOL, a higher rate of lifetime suicide attempts, diminished educational and occupational attainment, and increased use of healthcare resources.[22] Patients with SAD have a low employment status.

Early intervention is important in the treatment of SAD. Pharmacotherapy can dramatically improve QOL. Patients treated with fluvoxamine, sertraline, paroxetine, or escitalopram showed a significantly greater improvement in functioning, disability, and QOL compared with placebo-treated patients.[78,82,91,92] In a relapse prevention study, patients treated with escitalopram experienced a better health-related QOL and more cost-effective therapy than placebo.[92] The acquisition cost of escitalopram was more than offset by a decrease in total costs of care.[92] Healthcare professionals can assist patients who qualify for pharmaceutical manufacturer patient access-to-care programs to ease the burden of drug costs.

CLINICAL CONTROVERSY

The role of benzodiazepines in the treatment of SAD is controversial. Some clinicians prescribe benzodiazepines in combination with an antidepressant in the initial acute management of SAD, then taper the benzodiazepine after 3 to 4 weeks. Recent data indicate that the addition of a benzodiazepine to an SSRI during the acute treatment of SAD does not provide more rapid response, although these patients tended to have better outcomes at the end of the trial.

■ EVALUATION OF THERAPEUTIC OUTCOMES

❿ The pharmacotherapy of SAD can be monitored in three principal domains: SAD symptoms (e.g., fears and physical symptoms), functionality, and well-being or overall improvement.[22] Response to pharmacotherapy in SAD is defined as a stable, clinically meaningful improvement; patients no longer have the full range of symptoms but typically continue to experience more than minimal symptoms.[22]

During the acute phase of treatment, patients should be seen weekly while the drug dosage is titrated. Once the patient responds and the dosage is stabilized, the patient can be seen monthly. At each visit, the patient should be asked about adverse effects and improvement in symptoms. The patient should be instructed to keep a diary to record fear levels, physical symptoms, cognitions, and anxious behaviors in actual exposures to social situations. The Liebowitz Social Anxiety Scale is a clinician-rated scale of clinical severity and change in SAD that can be used to monitor response.[9,22] Patients can use the Social Phobia Inventory for self-assessment of SAD symptoms.[22] Full remission is a complete resolution of symptoms across the three SAD domains that is maintained for 3 months[22] or a Liebowitz Social Anxiety Scale score of less than or equal to 30 points.[71]

Patient counseling is important. The patient should be instructed about the gradual onset of effect and that the full therapeutic effect might not be achieved for up to 12 weeks. Patients should be told that long-term therapy is required. When drug therapy is discontinued, the dosage will need to be gradually decreased over several months, and the patient should be seen more frequently to monitor for signs and symptoms of relapse or withdrawal.

It is important to remember that although pharmacotherapy usually leads to improvement in social and occupational functioning, most patients do not achieve a full remission. Many patients require additional treatment, often in the form of CBT.

TREATMENT

Specific Phobia

Specific phobia is considered unresponsive to drug therapy, although highly responsive to CBT. The use of benzodiazepines or paroxetine in patients who failed CBT is supported by limited data. Benzodiazepines can be detrimental in patients with specific phobias treated with CBT.[20]

CONCLUSIONS

Anxiety disorders are common in the population and occur concurrently with other psychiatric disorders. The proper management of anxiety disorders begins with the correct diagnosis; not all patients should receive antianxiety agents. Nonpharmacologic interventions often are effective alone or when combined with drug therapy.

There are several subtypes of anxiety disorders, and the diagnosis determines the type of drug and nonpharmacologic intervention selected. Although benzodiazepines remain the drugs of choice for situational anxiety, antidepressants have emerged as first-line therapy for GAD, panic disorder, and SAD. Benzodiazepines are reserved for use in situations requiring immediate anxiety relief or for use on an as-needed basis. Antidepressants, including the SSRIs and SNRIs, and the benzodiazepines clonazepam and alprazolam, are used extensively in patients with GAD, panic disorder, and SAD.

The long-term goal of therapy for GAD, panic disorder, and SAD is remission of core anxiety symptoms with no impairment in functionality, minimal anxiety, and no depressive symptoms. Clinicians can use the pharmacologic armamentarium effectively to achieve this goal for patients.

ABBREVIATIONS

CBT: cognitive behavioral therapy

CNS: central nervous system

CRF: corticotrophic releasing factor

DA: dopamine

DMDZ: desmethyldiazepam

GABA: γ-aminobutyric acid

GAD: generalized anxiety disorder

FDA: Food and Drug Administration

5-HT: serotonin

LC: locus ceruleus

MAOI: monoamine oxidase inhibitor

NE: norepinephrine

QOL: quality of life

SAD: social anxiety disorder

SERT: serotonin reuptake transporter site

SNRI: serotonin-norepinephrine reuptake inhibitor

SSRI: selective serotonin reuptake inhibitor

TCA: tricyclic antidepressant

REFERENCES

1. American Psychiatric Association. Diagnostic and Statistical Manual of Mental Disorders, 4th ed., text revision. Washington, DC: American Psychiatric Association, 2000:429–484.
2. Roy-Byrne PR, Wagner A. Primary care perspectives on generalized anxiety disorder. J Clin Psychiatry 2004;(65 Suppl 13):20–26.
3. Lépine J. The epidemiology of anxiety disorders: Prevalence and societal costs. J Clin Psychiatry 2002;63(Suppl 14):4–8.
4. Bowen RC, Senthilselvan A, Barale A. Physical illness as an outcome of chronic anxiety disorders. Can J Psychiatry 2000;45:459–464.
5. Rickels K, Rynn M. Pharmacotherapy of generalized anxiety disorder. J Clin Psychiatry 2002;63(Suppl 14):9–16.
6. Kessler RC, Chiu WT, Demler O, et al. Prevalence, severity and comorbidity of 12-month DSM-IV disorders in the National Comorbidity Survey Replication. Arch Gen Psychiatry 2005;62:617–627.
7. Mathew SJ, Coplan JD, Gorman JM. Neurobiological mechanisms of social anxiety disorder. Am J Psychiatry 2001;158:1558–1567.
8. Mancini C, Van Amerigen M, Bennett M, et al. Emerging treatments for child and adolescent social phobia: A review. J Child Adolesc Psychopharmacol 2005;15(4):589–607.
9. Schneier FR. Social anxiety disorder. N Engl J Med 2006;355:1029–1036.
10. Chen J, Reich L, Chung H. Anxiety disorders. West J Med 2002;176:249–253.
11. Baldwin DS, Polkinghorn C. Evidence-based pharmacotherapy of generalized anxiety disorder. Int J Neuropsychopharmacol 2005;8:293–302.
12. Kent JM, Mathew SJ, Gorman JM. Molecular targets in the treatment of anxiety. Biol Psychiatry 2002;52:1008–1030.
13. Condren RM, O'Neill A, Ryan MC, et al. HPA axis response to a psychological stressor in generalised social phobia. Psychoneuroendocrinology 2002;27:693–703.
14. Gorman JM, Kent JM, Sullivan GM, Coplan JD. Neuroanatomical hypothesis of panic disorder, revised. Am J Psychiatry 2000;157:493–505.
15. Möhler H. GABAA receptor diversity and pharmacology. Cell Tissue Res 2006;326:505–516.
16. Malizia AL. Receptor binding and drug modulation in anxiety. Eur Neuropsychopharmacol 2002;12:567–574.
17. Condren RM, Lucey TV, Thakore JH. A preliminary study of baclofen-induced growth hormone release in generalised social phobia. Hum Psychopharmacol 2003;18:135–130.
18. Condren RM, Dinan TG, Thakore JH. A preliminary study of buspirone stimulated prolactin release in generalised social phobia: Evidence for enhanced serotonergic responsivity? Eur Neuropsychopharmacol 2002;12:349–354.
19. Muller JE, Koen L, Soraya S, et al. Social anxiety disorder: Current treatment recommendations. CNS Drugs 2005;19:377–391.
20. Baldwin DS, Anderson IM, Nutt DJ, et al. Evidence-based guidelines for the pharmacological treatment of anxiety disorders: Recommendations from the British Society for Psychopharmacology. J Psychopharmacology 2005;19:567–596.
21. Katon WJ. Panic disorder. N Engl J Med 2006;354:2360–2367.
22. Ballenger JC, Davidson JRT, Lecrubier Y, et al. Consensus statement on social anxiety disorder from the International Consensus Group on Depression and Anxiety. J Clin Psychiatry 1998;59(Suppl 17):54–60.

23. Goodman WK. Selecting pharmacotherapy for generalized anxiety disorder. J Clin Psychiatry 2004;65(Suppl 13):8–13.
24. Bandelow B, Zohar J, Hollander E, et al. Guidelines for the pharmacological treatment of anxiety, obsessive-compulsive and posttraumatic stress disorders. World J Biol Psychiatry 2002;3:171–199.
25. Work Group on Panic Disorder. Practice guideline for the treatment of patients with panic disorder. Am J Psychiatry 1998;155(Suppl 5):1–34.
26. Chouinard G. Issues in the clinical use of benzodiazepines: Potency, withdrawal and rebound. J Clin Psychiatry 2004;65(Suppl 5):7–12.
27. Duloxetine [package insert]. Indianapolis, IN: Eli Lily and Company, May 2007.
28. Lexapro [package insert]. St. Louis, MO: Forest Pharmaceuticals, Inc., September 2006.
29. Paxil [package insert]. Research Triangle Park, NC: GlaxoSmithKline, July 2006.
30. Effexor XR [package insert]. Philadelphia, PA: Wyeth Pharmaceuticals, Inc., August 2006.
31. Vistaril [package insert]. New York: Pfizer Labs, April 2004.
32. Kavoussi R. Pregabalin: From molecule to medicine. Eur Neuropsychopharmacol 2006;16:S128–S133.
33. National Institute for Clinical Excellence. The Management of Panic Disorder and Generalized Anxiety Disorder in Primary Care And Secondary Care: Clinical Guideline 22. London: National Collaborating Centre for Mental Health, December 2004.
34. Llorca P, Spadone C, Sol O, et al. Efficacy and safety of hydroxyzine in the treatment of generalized anxiety disorder: A 3-month double-blind study. J Clin Psychiatry 2002;63:1020–1027.
35. Connor KM, Payne V, Davidson JRT. Kava in generalized anxiety disorder: Three placebo-controlled trials. Int Clin Psychopharmacol 2006;21:249–253.
36. Rubinchik SM, Kablinger AS, Gardener JS. Medications for panic disorder and generalized anxiety disorder during pregnancy. Prim Care Companion J Clin Psychiatry 2005;7:100–105.
37. Ibqual MM, Sobhan T, Ryals T. Effects of commonly used benzodiazepines on the fetus, the neonate, and the nursing infant. Psychiatr Serv 2002;53:39–49.
38. Wang PS, Bohn RL, Glynn RJ, et al. Hazardous benzodiazepine regimens in the elderly: Effects of half-life, dosage, and duration on risk of hip fracture. Am J Psychiatry 2001;158:892–898.
39. Lenze EJ, Mulsant BH, Shear MK, et al. Efficacy and tolerability of citalopram in the treatment of late-life anxiety disorders: Results from an 8-week randomized, placebo-controlled trial. Am J Psychiatry 2005:162:146–150.
40. Wagner CD. Generalized anxiety disorder in children and adolescents. Psychiatr Clin North Am 2001;24:139–153.
41. Kapczinski F, Lima MS, Souza JS, et al. Antidepressants for generalized anxiety disorder Cochrane Database Syst Rev 2003;2:CD003592.
42. Brawman-Mintzer O, Knapp RG, Ryman M, et al. Sertraline treatment for generalized anxiety disorder: A randomized, double-blind, placebo-controlled study. J Clin Psychiatry 2006;67:874–881.
43. Koponen H, Allgulander C, Pritchett Y, et al. A fixed-dose study of the efficacy and safety of duloxetine for the treatment of generalized anxiety disorder [abstract]. 26th Annual Conference of the Anxiety Disorders Association of America, March 2006.
44. Ball SG, Kuhn, A, Wall D, et al. Selective serotonin reuptake inhibitor treatment for generalized anxiety disorder: A double-blind, prospective comparison between paroxetine and sertraline. J Clin Psychiatry 2005;66:94–99.
45. Baldwin DS, Huuson AKT, Mehuylum E. Escitalopram and paroxetine in the treatment of generalized anxiety disorder. Br J Psychiatry 2006;189:264–272.
46. Bielski RJ, Bose A, Chang CC. A double-blind comparison of escitalopram and paroxetine in the long-term treatment of generalized anxiety disorder. Ann Clin Psychiatry 2005;17:65–69.
47. Montgomery SA, Sheehan DV, Meoni P. Characterization of the longitudinal course of improvement in generalized anxiety disorder during long-term treatment with venlafaxine XR. J Psychiatr Res 2002;36:209–217.
48. Davidson JRT, Bose Wang Q. Safety and efficacy of escitalopram in the long-term treatment of generalized anxiety disorder. J Clin Psychiatry 2005;66:1441–1446.
49. Shelton RC, Brown LL. Mechanisms of action in the treatment of anxiety. J Clin Psychiatry 2001;62(Suppl 12):10–15.
50. Klonopin [package insert]. Nutley, NJ: Roche Laboratories, July 2001.
51. Xanax XR [package insert]. Kalamazoo, MI: Pharmacia & Upjohn Company, April 2004.
52. Bailey L, Ward M, Musa M. Clinical pharmacokinetics of benzodiazepines. J Clin Pharmacol 1994;34:804–811.
53. Benzodiazepines. Facts and Comparisons 4.0 Online. Wolters Kluwer Health, Inc. 2005, *http://online.factsandcomparisons.com*.
54. Madabushi R, Frank B, Drewelow B, et al. Hyperforin in St. John's wort drug interactions. Eur J Clin Pharmacol 2006;62:225–233.
55. Guest J, Russ J, Lenox-Smith A. Cost-effectiveness of venlafaxine XL compared with diazepam in treatment of generalized anxiety disorder in the United Kingdom. Eur J Health Econ 2005;6:136–145.
56. Jørgensen TR, Stein DJ, Despiegel N, et al. Cost-effectiveness analysis of escitalopram compared with paroxetine in the treatment of generalized anxiety disorder in the United Kingdom. Ann Pharmacotherapy 2006;40:1752–1758.
57. Pollack MH. The pharmacotherapy of panic disorder. J Clin Psychiatry 2005;66(Suppl 4):23–27.
58. Royal Australian and New Zealand College of Psychiatrists Clinical Practice Guidelines Team for Panic Disorder and Agoraphobia. Australian and New Zealand clinical practice guidelines for the treatment of panic disorder and agoraphobia. Aust N Z J Psychiatry 2003;37:641–656.
59. Mitte K. A meta-analysis of the efficacy of psycho- and pharmacotherapy in panic disorder with and without agoraphobia. J Affect Disord 2005;88:27–45.
60. Barlow DH, Gorman JM, Shear MK, Woods SW. Cognitive-behavioral therapy, imipramine, or their combination for panic disorder. JAMA 2000;283:2529–2536.
61. Kampman M, Keijsers GPJ, Hoogduin CAL, Hendriks G. A randomized, double-blind, placebo-controlled study of the effects of adjunctive paroxetine in panic disorder patients unsuccessfully treated with cognitive-behavioral therapy alone. J Clin Psychiatry 2002;63:772–777.
62. Bakker A, van Balkom AJ, Spinhoven P. SSRIs vs. TCAs in the treatment of panic disorder: A meta-analysis. Acta Psychiatr Scand 2002;106:163–167.
63. Stahl SM, Gergel I, Li D. Escitalopram in the treatment of panic disorder: A randomized, double-blind, placebo-controlled trial. J Clin Psychiatry 2003:64:1322–1327.
64. Bandelow B, Behnke K, Lenior S, et al. Sertraline versus paroxetine in the treatment of panic disorder: An acute double-blind noninferiority trial. J Clin Psychiatry 2004;65:405–413.
65. Pollack MH, Lepola U, Koponen H, et al. A double-blind study of the efficacy of venlafaxine extended-release, paroxetine and placebo in the treatment of panic disorder. Depress Anxiety 2007;24:1–14.
66. Ferguson JM, Khan A, Mangano R, et al. Relapse prevention of panic disorder in adult outpatient responders to treatment with venlafaxine extended-release. J Clin Psychiatry 2007;68:58–68.
67. Flint AJ, Gagnon N. Diagnosis and management of panic disorder in older adults. Drugs Aging 2003;20:881–891.
68. Varley C, Smith CJ. Anxiety disorders in the child and teen. Pediatr Clin North Am 2003:50:1107–1138.
69. Mavissakalian MR, Perel JM. Duration of imipramine therapy and relapse in panic disorder with agoraphobia. J Clin Psychopharmacol 2002;22:294–299.
70. Otto MW, Deveney C. Cognitive-behavioral therapy and the treatment of panic disorder: Efficacy and strategies. J Clin Psychiatry 2005;66(Suppl 4):28–32.
71. Doyle AC, Pollack MH. Establishment of remission criteria for anxiety disorders. J Clin Psychiatry 2003;64(Suppl 15):40–45.
72. Olfson M, Guardino M, Struening E, et al. Barriers to the treatment of social anxiety. Am J Psychiatry 2000;157:521–527.
73. Blanco C, Muhammad SR, Schneier FR, et al. The evidence-based pharmacological treatment of social anxiety disorder. Int J Neuropsychopharmacol 2003;6:427–442.
74. Prasko J, Dockery C, Horacke J, et al. Moclobemide and cognitive behavioral therapy in the treatment of social phobia. A 6-month controlled study and 24-months follow up. Neuro Endocrinol Lett 2006;27(4):473–481.
75. Stein DJ, Versiani M, Hair T, Kumar R. Efficacy of paroxetine for relapse prevention in social anxiety disorder: A 24-week study. Arch Gen Psychiatry 2002;59:1111–1118.
76. Montgomery SA. Escitalopram: Treatment shows better cost-effectiveness and improved quality of life versus placebo in social anxiety

disorder [poster]. The 23rd Annual Congress of the Anxiety Disorder Association of America, Toronto, May 2003.
77. Stein DJ, Stein MB, Pitts CD, et al. Predictors of response to pharmacotherapy in social anxiety disorder: An analysis of three placebo-controlled paroxetine trials. J Clin Psychiatry 2002;63:152–155.
78. Stein DJ, Versiani M, Hair T, et al. Efficacy of paroxetine for relapse prevention in social anxiety disorder: A 24-week study. Arch Gen Psychiatry 2002;59(12):1111–1118.
79. Randall CL, Johnson MR, Thevos AK, et al. Paroxetine for social anxiety and alcohol use in dual-diagnosed patients. Depress Anxiety 2001;14(4):255–262.
80. Hedges DW, Brown BL, Shwalb DA, et al. The efficacy of selective serotonin reuptake inhibitors in adult social anxiety disorder: A meta-analysis of double-blind, placebo-controlled trials. J Psychopharmacol 2007;21:102–111.
81. Stein DJ, Ipser JC, Van Balkom AJ. Pharmacotherapy for social anxiety disorder. Cochrane Database Syst Rev 2000;4:CD001206.
82. Liebowitz MR, DeMartinis NA, Weihs K, et al. Efficacy of sertraline in severe generalized social anxiety disorder: Results of a double-blind, placebo-controlled study. J Clin Psychiatry 2003;64:785–792.
83. Schneier FR, Blanco C, Campeas R, et al. Citalopram treatment of social anxiety disorder with comorbid major depression. Depress Anxiety 2003;17:191–196.
84. Kobak KA, Greist JH, Jefferson JW, Katzelnick DJ. Fluoxetine in social phobia: A double-blind, placebo-controlled pilot study. J Clin Psychopharmacol 2002;22:257–262.
85. Liebowtiz MR, Stein MB, Tancer M, et al. A randomized, double-blind, fixed-dose comparison of paroxetine and placebo in the treatment of generalized social anxiety disorder. J Clin Psychiatry 2002;63:66–74.
86. Stein MB, Pollack MH, Bystritsky A, et al. Efficacy of low and higher dose extended-release venlafaxine in generalized social anxiety disorder: A 6-month randomized controlled trial. Psychopharmacology (Berl) 2005;177(3):280–288.
87. Muehlbacher M, Nickel MK, Nickel C, et al. Mirtazapine treatment of social phobia in women—a randomized, double-blind, placebo-controlled study. J Clin Psychopharmacol 2005;25:580–583.
88. Jefferson JW. Benzodiazepines and anticonvulsants for social phobia (social anxiety disorder). J Clin Psychiatry 2001;62:50–53.
89. Pande AC, Feltner DE, Jefferson JN, et al. Efficacy of the novel anxiolytic pregabalin in social anxiety disorder: A placebo-controlled, multicenter study. J Clin Psychopharmacol 2004;24:141–149.
90. Seedat S, Stein MB. Double-blind, placebo-controlled assessment of combined clonazepam with paroxetine compared with paroxetine monotherapy for generalized social anxiety disorder. J Clin Psychiatry 2004;65(2):244–248.
91. Davidson J, Yaryura-Tobias J, Dupont R, et al. Fluvoxamine controlled-release formulation for the treatment of generalized social anxiety disorder. J Clin Psychopharmacol 2004;24:118–125.
92. Montgomery SA, Nil R, Durr-Pal N, et al. A 24-week randomized, double-blind, placebo controlled study of escitalopram for the prevention of generalized social anxiety disorder. J Clin Psychiatry 2005;66:1270–1278.

CHAPTER 74

Anxiety Disorders II: Posttraumatic Stress Disorder and Obsessive-Compulsive Disorder

CYNTHIA K. KIRKWOOD, EUGENE H. MAKELA, AND BARBARA G. WELLS

KEY CONCEPTS

1. The short-term goal in posttraumatic stress disorder is reduction in core symptoms, whereas the long-term goal is remission.
2. Cognitive behavioral therapy and eye movement desensitization and reprocessing are the most effective nonpharmacologic methods to reduce symptoms of posttraumatic stress disorder.
3. The selective serotonin reuptake inhibitors are considered first-line treatment for posttraumatic stress disorder.
4. An adequate trial of selective serotonin reuptake inhibitors in posttraumatic stress disorder requires appropriate dosing, titration, and duration of treatment.
5. Posttraumatic stress disorder compares with depression in the level of disability it imposes on patients.
6. The selective serotonin reuptake inhibitors are the drugs of choice for the treatment of obsessive-compulsive disorder.
7. Clomipramine should be considered after two or three failed selective serotonin reuptake inhibitor trials for obsessive-compulsive disorder.
8. Typically, a taper of antidepressants and discontinuation can be considered after 1 to 2 years of treatment for obsessive-compulsive disorder.
9. Long-term or lifetime prophylactic maintenance medication is recommended for obsessive-compulsive disorder after two to four severe relapses or three to four mild to moderate relapses.

Recent world events (e.g., wars, terrorist attacks, hurricanes, and tsunamis) have placed a renewed focus on posttraumatic stress disorder (PTSD). Initially diagnosed in veterans of war, PTSD is now acknowledged as a significant psychiatric illness in the civilian population.[1] PTSD continues to be poorly recognized and diagnosed in clinical practice.[2] Because of its co-occurrence with other anxiety disorders, depression, and substance abuse, the overlapping symptoms can lead to diagnostic uncertainty. Advances in the science and treatment of PTSD can assist clinicians in all fields of healthcare to screen patients for a history of trauma and effectively manage PTSD if it is present.

Patients with obsessive-compulsive disorder (OCD) experience significant impairment in their quality of life (QOL) with reductions in social, family, and occupational functioning.[3,4] OCD affects far more individuals than was thought in the past. Because of the nature and potential severity of signs and symptoms and the resultant negative effects on QOL, OCD is considered a major medical condition. Clinicians should be able to identify OCD and understand the current treatment options.

Learning objectives, review questions, and other resources can be found at **www.pharmacotherapyonline.com.**

EPIDEMIOLOGY

The prevalence data on anxiety disorders were recently revised to encompass clinically significant cases in the community.[5] According to the modified prevalence estimates of mental disorders in the United States, the prevalence of PTSD is 3.6%.[5] The prevalence of OCD is 2.4% in persons aged 18 to 54 years and 1.5% in those older than age 55 years.[5]

The epidemiology of PTSD is associated with the incidence of trauma. It is estimated that approximately 50% of men and 60% of women are exposed to a life-threatening traumatic event. Of these individuals 8.2% of men and 20% of women will develop PTSD.[6] Previous exposure to a trauma and the intensity of response to the event increase the risk of PTSD.[6] Individuals with a history of childhood sexual abuse are at higher risk of developing PTSD as adults.[7] Men tend to be assaulted more frequently, but women have a higher rate of PTSD after assault. The incidence of PTSD is equal between men and women after rape (i.e., 50%) and natural disasters (i.e., less than 5%).[6] Genetic factors can increase vulnerability to PTSD if an individual is exposed to a traumatic event. Offspring of Holocaust survivors had a higher lifetime prevalence rate of PTSD compared with a control group.[6]

OCD usually begins early in life, with 20% of cases occurring in childhood, 29% in adolescence, and 49% of cases occurring by age 20. The onset of illness is earlier in men than women.[1] The average patient first reports minor symptoms at age 12 years, meets diagnostic criteria at age 18 years, and receives initial treatment at 29 years of age. Individuals with early-onset OCD report more first-degree relatives with a probable diagnosis of OCD and higher rates of panic disorder, eating disorders, and obsessive-compulsive personality disorder.[8] Twin studies revealed significantly higher concordance rates in monozygotic versus dizygotic twins, but there is probably nongenetic as well as genetic influences over expression of OCD, because the concordance rate for monozygotic twins is less than 100%. Individuals have an 11% to 12% risk of developing the illness if a first-degree relative has OCD; however, this familial relationship may be age-sensitive. In one epidemiologic study, no cases of OCD were found in relatives of patients developing the illness after 18 years of age.[9]

Irritable bowel syndrome is more common in individuals with anxiety and depressive disorders. Approximately 35% of patients with OCD meet criteria for irritable bowel syndrome compared with 2.5% of a control group.[10]

ETIOLOGY

The exact etiologies of PTSD and OCD are not known. It is likely that abnormalities in several areas of brain functioning interact to cause these chronic anxiety disorders. Genetics may play a role in expression of PTSD and OCD, but environmental factors likely are also involved.

OCD has been characterized as a pediatric autoimmune neuropsychiatric disorder associated with streptococcal infections. In response to streptococcal infection, antibodies are produced in some individuals that temporally precipitate sudden onset or exacerbation of symptoms of OCD. Neuroimaging studies suggest that in these patients the antibodies produce inflammation of the basal ganglia. This leads to increased volumes of the caudate, putamen, and the globus pallidus, and subsequently to smaller caudate volumes potentially reflective of scarring or atrophy related to streptococcal infection.[11] Although most patients with OCD do not have a streptococcal etiology, an accurate medical history regarding onset of illness is imperative because specific treatment strategies are indicated.

PATHOPHYSIOLOGY

Research findings in the areas of neuroendocrinology, neurobiology, and neuroimaging have advanced a number of theories on the pathophysiology of anxiety disorders. Neuroendocrine changes in the hypothalamic-pituitary-adrenal (HPA) axis are implicated in the pathophysiology of PTSD.[6] As reviewed in the previous chapter (Chap. 73), data from neurochemical and neuroimaging studies indicate that the modulation of normal and pathologic anxiety states is associated with multiple regions of the brain (e.g., amygdala, hippocampus, thalamus, and prefrontal cortex). Abnormal function in several neurotransmitter systems, including norepinephrine (NE), γ-aminobutyric acid (GABA), glutamate, dopamine (DA), and serotonin (5-HT) may affect the manifestations of anxiety disorders.[6,13]

NEUROENDOCRINE THEORIES

Neuroendocrine studies provide data that abnormalities occurring pretrauma, during trauma, and posttrauma contribute to PTSD.[6] Normally the immediate reaction to stress occurs as an automatic response from the amygdala to the sympathetic and parasympathetic systems and the HPA axis. The release of corticotropin-releasing factor stimulates cortisol secretion from the adrenal gland. Both catecholamines and cortisol levels rise in tandem. Cortisol reduces the stress response by tempering the sympathetic reaction through negative feedback on the pituitary and hypothalamus.[6] These systems return to normal after a few hours.

Patients with PTSD have a hypersecretion of corticotropin-releasing factor but demonstrate subnormal levels of cortisol at the time of trauma and chronically.[6] Dysregulation of the HPA axis is postulated to be a risk factor for eventual development of PTSD.[6]

NEUROCHEMICAL THEORIES

Several neurotransmitters may be involved in the pathophysiology of PTSD. 5-HT and NE are associated with the processing of emotional and somatic contents of memories in the amygdala. The cortex and hippocampus are involved in storing the facts and related cues of memory.[14] The noradrenergic theory posits that the autonomic nervous system of anxious patients is hypersensitive and overreacts to stimuli. The alarm center, the locus ceruleus, releases NE to stimulate the sympathetic and parasympathetic nervous systems. Patients with PTSD tend to experience sustained elevated heart rates during trauma and enhanced startle effects starting a month after trauma exposure. Patients with chronic central noradrenergic overactivity have downregulated α_2-adrenoreceptors.[15] Dysregulation of the processing of sensory input and memories may contribute to the dissociative and hypervigilant symptoms in PTSD. Preliminary data indicate that the 5-HT and 5-HT_2 antagonist *meta*-chlorophenylpiperazine (*m*-CPP) causes increased anxiety symptoms in patients with PTSD.[14] Abnormalities of GABA inhibition may lead to increased awareness or response to stress, as seen in PTSD.[14]

Both 5-HT and DA are implicated in the pathogenesis of OCD. Selective and potent serotonergic reuptake inhibitors have consistently been shown be effective for symptoms of the illness. Results of challenge studies using 5-HT agonists support a role for this neurotransmitter as well. However, to date there is no specific identified abnormality in the 5-HT system with OCD.[13] DA dysregulation may contribute to some forms of OCD. Neurologic symptoms (e.g., tics) are part of the clinical presentation in some patients with OCD. Tourette's disorder, a disorder of DA dysfunction, is often a concurrent disease.[1] Patients with OCD and tics benefit from the addition of an antipsychotic drug to their treatment regimen.[13]

NEUROIMAGING STUDIES

Neuroimaging studies suggest that certain areas of the brain are altered by psychologic trauma. In PTSD most functional neuroimaging studies have involved amygdala, ventromedial prefrontal cortex (vmPFC), and the hippocampus. Findings of increased activation of the amygdala after symptom provocation (e.g., via personal trauma script, visual imagery, or audio tape of combat sounds) indicate that this structure plays a role in the formation of emotional memory.[16] Hypofunctioning of the vmPFC is theorized to prevent extinction in patients with PTSD.[16,17] The most consistent findings are decreased hippocampal volumes and *N*-acetylaspartate levels in patients with PTSD.[17] In twin studies, the unaffected twin of patients with PTSD also demonstrated smaller hippocampi compared with twins without PTSD.[17] These findings suggest that lower hippocampal volumes in patients with PTSD are likely a precursor associated with vulnerability for subsequent development of PTSD.[12]

Recent neuroimaging studies support the roles of 5-HT and DA in the pathophysiologic expression of OCD.[18] The reader is referred to Friedlander and Desrocher for a review of neuroimaging abnormalities in patients with OCD.[19]

CLINICAL PRESENTATION

The *Diagnostic and Statistical Manual of Mental Disorders, Fourth Edition, Text Revision* classifies anxiety disorders into several categories: generalized anxiety disorder, panic disorder (with or without agoraphobia), social anxiety disorder, specific phobia, OCD, PTSD, and acute stress disorder (ASD).[1] The characteristic features of these illnesses are anxiety and avoidance behavior. Generalized anxiety disorder, panic disorder, and social anxiety disorder are discussed in Chap. 73.

POSTTRAUMATIC STRESS DISORDER

Exposure to a traumatic event is required for a diagnosis of PTSD.[1] The person must have witnessed, experienced, or have been confronted with a situation that involved definite or threatened death or serious injury, or possible harm to themselves or others. The patient's response to the trauma must include intense fear, helplessness, or horror.[1] Some examples of traumatic events include physical attacks by an intimate partner, motor vehicle accidents, natural disasters, rape, being held hostage, child sexual abuse, and witnessing a murder or injury of another.

The resulting PTSD symptoms include persistent reexperiencing of the traumatic event, avoidance of stimuli associated with the

TABLE 74-1 Presentation of Posttraumatic Stress Disorder

Reexperiencing symptoms
- Recurrent, intrusive distressing memories of the trauma
- Recurrent, disturbing dreams of the event
- Feeling that the traumatic event is recurring (e.g., dissociative flashbacks)
- Physiologic reaction to reminders of the trauma

Avoidance symptoms
- Avoidance of conversations about the trauma
- Avoidance of thoughts or feelings about the trauma
- Avoidance of activities that are reminders of the event
- Avoidance of people or places that arouse recollections of the trauma
- Inability to recall an important aspect of the trauma
- Anhedonia
- Estrangement from others
- Restricted affect
- Sense of a foreshortened future (e.g., does not expect to have a career, marriage)

Hyperarousal symptoms
- Decreased concentration
- Easily startled
- Hypervigilance
- Insomnia
- Irritability or angry outbursts

Subtypes
- Acute: duration of symptoms is less than 3 months
- Chronic: symptoms last for longer than 3 months
- With delayed onset: onset of symptoms is at least 6 months posttrauma

Screening questions
- Have you ever experienced a significant trauma in your life?
- Did this experience have a lasting negative impact or change your life?

Data from American Psychiatric Association[1] and Ballenger et al.[12]

TABLE 74-2 Presentation of Obsessive-Compulsive Disorder

Obsessions
- Repetitive thoughts (e.g., feeling contaminated after touching an object, doubting whether the stove was turned off)
- Repetitive images (e.g., recurrent sexually explicit pictures)
- Repetitive impulses (e.g., need for symmetry or putting things in specific order, impulse to shout out obscenities in a church)

Compulsions
- Repetitive activities (e.g., hand washing, checking, ordering, need to ask, need to confess)
- Repetitive mental acts (e.g., counting, repeating words silently, praying)

Screening questions
- Do you have repetitive thoughts that make you anxious and that you cannot get rid of?
- Do you check things excessively?
- Do you feel the need to wash your hands frequently?
- Do you keep things exceptionally clean?

Data from American Psychiatric Association[1] and Jenike.[20]

trauma, numbing of general responsiveness, and persistent symptoms of hyperarousal (Table 74–1). Patients must have at least one reexperiencing symptom, at least three signs or symptoms of persistent avoidance of stimuli associated with the trauma, and at least two symptoms of increased arousal.[1] Symptoms from each category need to be present for longer than 1 month and cause significant distress or impairment in functioning. Most persons diagnosed with PTSD also meet criteria for another mental disorder.[1]

Anxiety and dissociative symptoms (e.g., sense of numbing or absence of emotional responsiveness, derealization, depersonalization, inability to recall important features of the event) emerging within 1 month after exposure to a traumatic stressor are classified as ASD. Symptoms of ASD are experienced during or immediately after the trauma, last for at least 2 days and resolve within 4 weeks.[1]

The age of onset and course of PTSD are variable. PTSD can occur at any age. The presentation is not predictable because symptoms are related to the duration and intensity of the trauma, the presence of other psychiatric disorders, and how the patient deals with the trauma. The average duration of symptoms in patients in treatment is approximately 36 months. In those not receiving treatment, symptoms can last for a mean of 5 years. Approximately one-third of patients with PTSD have a poor prognosis for recovery.[7] Approximately 80% of patients with PTSD have a concurrent depression or anxiety disorder.[7] More than one-half of men with PTSD suffer from comorbid alcohol abuse or dependence.[7] Approximately 20% of patients with PTSD attempt suicide.[7]

OBSESSIVE-COMPULSIVE DISORDER

Patients with OCD exhibit a great variety of symptoms on presentation to clinicians (Table 74–2). The diversity and oddity of symptoms that manifest can obscure accurate diagnosis and delay appropriate treatment of the disorder. Patients can be secretive about symptoms and purposefully refuse to report or deny symptoms.[20] Patients can present in a seemingly incongruous manner to nonpsychiatrists for other complaints—dermatologists for eczema or chapped skin, pediatricians for parental concerns over a child's compulsive hand washing, neurologists for tics, or dentists for gum lesions from compulsive teeth brushing.

The diagnostic criteria for OCD requires the presence of either obsessions and/or compulsions (although most patients have both) that are severe enough to cause marked distress, to be time-consuming (occupy more than 1 hour per day), or to cause significant impairment in social or occupational functioning.[1] An obsession is a recurrent, persistent idea, thought, impulse, or image that is experienced as intrusive and inappropriate and produces marked anxiety. Common obsessions involve thoughts about contamination (e.g., concern with germs or dirt), repeated doubts, and needing to have things in a particular order.[1]

Individuals must recognize that their obsessions or compulsions are excessive or unreasonable. Obsessions must be acknowledged as products of the individual's own mind and attempts must be made to ignore or suppress them. The obsessions produce marked feelings of anxiety and are not simply excessive worry about a real life situation.[1]

A compulsion is defined as a repetitive behavior or mental act generally performed in response to an obsession. The most common compulsions involve washing and cleaning, counting, checking, and requesting or demanding assurances. Diagnostically, compulsive behavior is not pleasurable and is designed to prevent discomfort or the occurrence of a dreaded event that is often unknown. For example, many patients are obsessed with feelings of doubt (e.g., whether a door was left unlocked), causing them marked distress, and leading to repetitive checking (or compulsive behaviors). These behaviors are usually performed according to certain rules or in a stereotyped fashion. Because patients recognize their compulsive behavior as silly or senseless, they become extremely adept at denying symptoms, disguising their rituals, and concealing their illness from friends and family.[1]

Patients with OCD often have concurrent depression, anxiety disorders, and alcohol abuse or dependence.[20] It is a chronic illness in most patients, with severity of symptoms varying in intensity over time. Many patients with OCD have significantly impaired QOL and ability to function.[20]

TREATMENT

Posttraumatic Stress Disorder

■ DESIRED OUTCOME

❶ The short-term goal of therapy in the management of PTSD is reduction in core symptoms (i.e., intrusive reexperiencing, avoidance, and hyperarousal). Patients should also have improvements in disability, concurrent psychiatric conditions, and QOL. The long-term goal in PTSD is remission.[21]

■ GENERAL APPROACH TO TREATMENT

In general, patients who seek treatment acutely after a trauma and are in intense distress should receive therapy based on their presenting symptoms (e.g., a nonbenzodiazepine hypnotic for difficulty sleeping). Short courses of trauma-focused cognitive behavioral therapy (TFCBT) can be helpful to prevent chronic PTSD in patients who present during the first 3 months of the event.[22] If symptoms (e.g., hyperarousal, avoidance, dissociation, sleep difficulties, or depressed mood) persist for 3 to 4 weeks and the patient experiences marked social, occupational, and/or interpersonal impairment, they can be treated with pharmacotherapy, psychotherapy, or both. Many patients with PTSD will improve substantially with pharmacotherapy but retain some symptoms. Treatment regimens usually combine psychoeducation, psychosocial support and/or treatment, and pharmacotherapy.[12]

■ NONPHARMACOLOGIC THERAPY

Psychotherapy can be used when a patient suffers from mild symptoms, in patients who prefer not to use medications, or in conjunction with drugs in patients with severe symptoms to improve response.[12] Patients who have experienced trauma should be educated that they can experience anxiety, depression, nightmares, and even flashbacks as a normal reaction to the event.[12] Brief courses of cognitive behavioral therapy (CBT) in close proximity to the traumatic event resulted in lower rates of PTSD 3 and 6 months later.[12] Single-session critical incident stress debriefing was not shown to be effective in preventing development of PTSD and actually can cause harm.[12,22]

❷ Psychotherapies for treating PTSD include stress management, TFCBT and eye movement desensitization and reprocessing (EMDR), and psychoeducation.[22,23] Short-term reductions in symptoms can be achieved with stress management, group therapy, hypnosis, or psychodynamic therapy.[23] Cognitive and behavioral approaches are more effective than stress management or group therapy to reduce symptoms of PTSD.[24] Either TFCBT or EMDR can be used if symptoms are evident for longer than 3 months postevent.[22] Followup studies after a 3-month course of CBT demonstrated continued benefit for 3 to 12 months.[24] An 8-week comparison found EMDR more successful in maintaining improvements in PTSD scores than fluoxetine or placebo.[25] Psychoeducation includes information about the disease state, treatment options, and avoidance of excessive use of alcohol, nicotine, and other substances of abuse.

■ PHARMACOLOGIC THERAPY

❸ Antidepressants are the major pharmacotherapeutic treatment for PTSD. In addition to their efficacy in PTSD, these agents are also effective for concurrent depression and anxiety disorders. The selective serotonin reuptake inhibitors (SSRIs) are the first-line pharmacotherapy of PTSD.[26] Other antidepressants (e.g., venlafaxine, tricyclic antidepressants [TCAs] and monoamine oxidase inhibitors [MAOIs]) can also be effective, but they have less favorable side-effect profiles (Table 74–3). Sertraline and paroxetine are both approved for the acute treatment of PTSD,[29,30] and sertraline is approved for the long-term (i.e., 52 weeks) management of PTSD.[30] A number of drugs can be used as augmentation agents (e.g., antiadrenergic drugs and atypical antipsychotics).[27] Benzodiazepines are not effective for PTSD.[12,28] Four practice guidelines[22,23,27,28] and one consensus statement for the treatment of PTSD are published.[12] An algorithm for the treatment of PTSD appears in Fig. 74–1.

TABLE 74-3 Antidepressants Used in the Treatment of Posttraumatic Stress Disorder

Class/Generic Name	Starting Dose	Dosage Range[a] (mg/day)
Selective serotonin reuptake inhibitors		
Citalopram[c]	20 mg per day	20–60
Escitalopram	10 mg per day	10–20
Fluoxetine[c]	10–20 mg per day	10–80
Fluvoxamine[c]	50 mg per day	100–250
Paroxetine[c]	10–20 mg per day	20–50[b]
Sertraline[c]	25–50 mg per day	50–200[b]
Other agents		
Amitriptyline[c]	25–50 mg per day	50–300
Imipramine[c]	25–50 mg per day	50–300
Mirtazapine[c]	15 mg at bedtime	15–45
Phenelzine	15 mg every night	15–90
Venlafaxine extended-release	37.5 mg per day	37.5–225

[a]Dosage used in clinical trials but not FDA approved.
[b]Doasge is FDA approved.
[c]Available generically.
Data from Ballenger et al.,[12] Baldwin et al.,[27] Bandelow et al.,[28] Paxil package insert,[29] Zoloft package insert,[30] and Schoenfeld et al.[31]

Special Populations

Children who experience stress and trauma (e.g., sexual or physical abuse or loss of a parent) are predisposed to develop mood and anxiety disorders. The SSRIs are the initial pharmacologic agents of choice in this patient population. Psychotherapy is also a treatment option (e.g., play therapy).[32]

Antidepressant Therapy

Selective Serotonin Reuptake Inhibitors The SSRIs act pharmacologically to enhance serotonergic functioning. Large prospective studies documented the efficacy of sertraline and paroxetine in the acute management of PTSD. In a 12-week trial sertraline (mean dose 146 mg/day) was effective across the spectrum of PTSD-specific, global, and functional outcome measures. Approximately 60% of the patients improved on symptom clusters of arousal and avoidance/numbing but not on reexperiencing.[33] Sixty percent of patients with PTSD receiving a paroxetine dose of 20 mg/day and 54% of patients receiving 40 mg/day responded; response was not related to dose.[34] In a flexible-dose trial, paroxetine significantly improved all three PTSD symptom clusters and disability compared with placebo at 12 weeks.[35] Fluoxetine showed efficacy in a placebo-controlled trial,[36] and fluvoxamine was efficacious in an open trial in acute PTSD.[37] In a comparison between sertraline and citalopram, PTSD symptoms improved significantly in both groups, but sertraline was significantly better in reducing avoidance/numbing than citalopram.[38] In general, the SSRIs reduced the numbing symptoms of PTSD, whereas other drugs have not. Adverse reactions reported in patients with PTSD treated with SSRIs include gastrointestinal symptoms, sexual dysfunction, insomnia, and agitation. The results of two long-term trials indicate that sertraline (12 months) and fluoxetine (9 months) were effective in preventing relapse.[36,39]

Other Antidepressants Other antidepressants have been studied in controlled trials. Mirtazapine was effective on global ratings of symptoms in 64% of patients with PTSD in doses up to 45 mg/day.[40] In a 12-week, placebo-controlled trial comparing venlafaxine extended-release and sertraline, venlafaxine was effective in reducing the avoidance/numbing and hyperarousal clusters of PTSD, whereas sertraline improved all PTSD symptom clusters.[41] The remission rates for venlafaxine extended release were 30.2% after 12

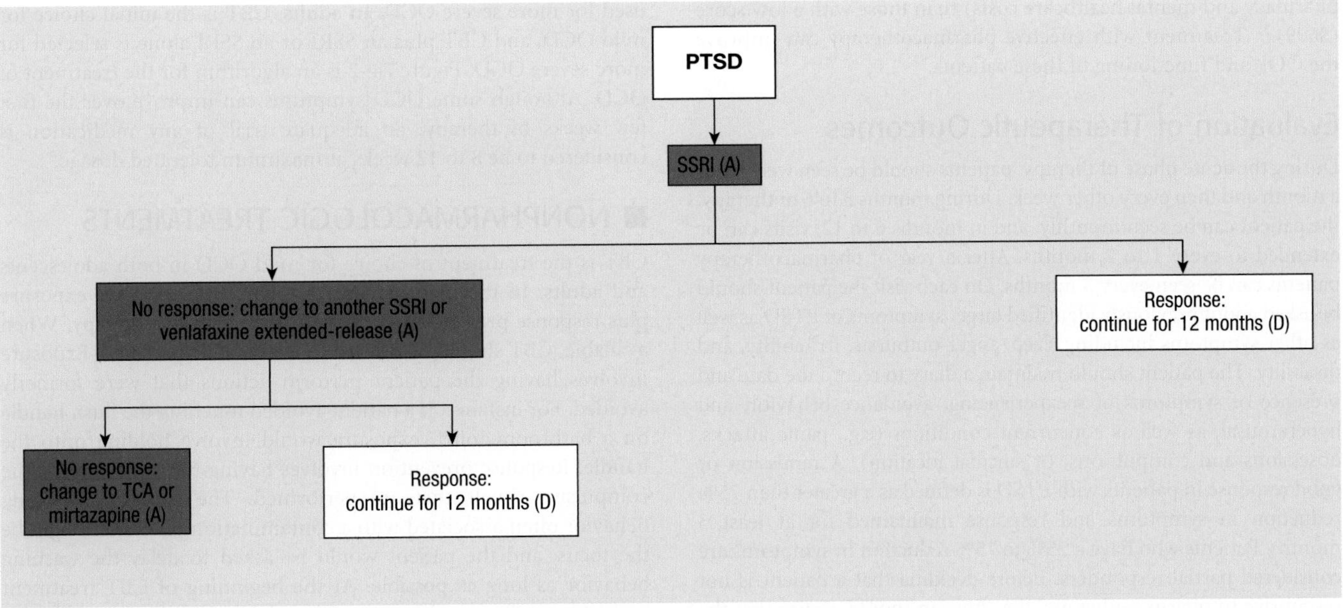

FIGURE 74-1. Algorithm for the pharmacotherapy of posttraumatic stress disorder. Strength of recommendations: A = directly based on category I evidence (i.e., meta-analysis of randomized clinical trials [RCT] or at least one RCT); D = directly based on category IV evidence (i.e., expert committee reports or opinions and/or clinical experience of respect authorities). (PTSD, posttraumatic stress disorder; SSRI, selective serotonin reuptake inhibitor; TCA, tricyclic antidepressant.) *(Data from Ballenger et al.,[12] Baldwin et al.,[27] and Bandelow et al.[28])*

weeks[41] and 50.1% after 6 months.[42] Bupropion sustained release was not effective in patients with chronic PTSD.[43]

The TCAs amitriptyline and imipramine and the MAOI phenelzine can be considered second- or third-line antidepressants if therapeutic trials of SSRIs have failed. Phenelzine decreased insomnia, nightmares, and flashbacks. TCAs are associated with a higher burden of adverse effects compared with SSRIs (e.g., daytime drowsiness, toxicity in overdose, and poor compliance).[28,31]

Alternative Drug Treatments

Atypical antipsychotics can be used as augmentation therapy in cases of partial response to SSRI therapy.[27] Risperidone reduced PTSD symptoms in combat veterans on antidepressants with and without psychosis.[44,45] Quetiapine (mean dose 216 mg/day) reduced core PTSD symptoms over a 8-week period when added to concurrent therapy.[46] Olanzapine (mean dose 15 mg/day) added adjunctively to SSRIs decreased PTSD symptoms and significantly improved sleep compared with placebo. Patients gained an average of 13.2 pounds (6 kg) over the course of the 8-week trial.[47]

Prazosin, an α_1-adrenergic antagonist, can be useful in some patients with PTSD. Prazosin decreased nightmares and sleep disturbances, and improved the core PTSD symptoms in daily doses of 1 to 4 mg. Its presumed mechanism of action is reduction of noradrenergic transmission.[48]

Dosage and Administration

Acute Phase PTSD symptoms respond slowly to pharmacotherapy, and some patients might never experience full resolution. SSRIs should be started 3 to 4 weeks after exposure to a trauma in patients with no improvement in their acute stress response.[12] The initiation of an SSRI should be at a low dose with gradual titration upward toward antidepressant doses. ❹ Eight to twelve weeks is an appropriate duration of antidepressant therapy to determine response.[49]

The dose of sertraline can be increased in weekly intervals by 50 mg/day up to a maximum dosage of 200 mg/day. Paroxetine can be increased by 10 mg/day in weekly intervals to a target dose of 40 mg/day. The dosing of other antidepressants is shown in Table 74–3.

Continuation Phase Many patients are undergoing psychotherapy during the continuation phase of therapy, and dosages can vary as patients deal with past traumatic experiences. During this phase symptoms continue to improve, and the maximal drug benefit (i.e., improvement of disability) accrues.[49] Six-month relapse prevention trials in patients responsive to fluoxetine or sertraline indicate low rates of relapse with SSRI therapy compared with placebo.[27,49]

Maintenance and Discontinuation Patients with PTSD who respond to pharmacotherapy should continue treatment for at least 12 months.[28,49] If residual symptoms persist, drug therapy should be continued. The decision about when to discontinue therapy is based on response to therapy, presence of ongoing stresses, and adverse effects. The patient must be confident in the discontinuation plan and can require extra support throughout the process. Drug therapy should be withdrawn and tapered slowly over a period of at least 1 month to reduce the potential for relapse.

CLINICAL CONTROVERSY

The use of propranolol immediately after a traumatic event is postulated to prevent PTSD symptoms (e.g., hyperarousal secondary to traumatic memories).[27,49] Study results are conflicting as to whether propranolol actually prevents the emergence of PTSD symptoms.

■ PHARMACOECONOMIC CONSIDERATIONS

❺ PTSD compares with depression in the level of disability it imposes on patients with the disorder.[50] Individuals fail to realize their potentials for career development, marriage, and education. Decreased productivity leads to a financial loss of more than $3 billion per year, and this figure does not include economic loss associated with the failure of PTSD patients to achieve their educational or career goals.[50] Women in a healthcare maintenance organization with high scores on the Posttraumatic Stress Disorder Checklist had more than twice the adjusted total annual median cost ($1,283) of care (i.e., outpatient, specialty care, primary care, pharmacy and mental healthcare costs) than those with a low score ($609).[51] Treatment with effective pharmacotherapy can improve the QOL and functioning of these patients.[52]

Evaluation of Therapeutic Outcomes

During the acute phase of therapy, patients should be seen weekly for a month and then every other week. During months 3 to 6 of therapy, the patient can be seen monthly, and in months 6 to 12, visits can be extended to every 1 to 2 months. After a year of pharmacotherapy patients can be seen every 3 months. On each visit the patient should be asked about previously identified target symptoms of PTSD as well as other symptoms including sleep, anger outbursts, irritability, and disability. The patient should maintain a diary to record the date and presence of symptoms of reexperiencing, avoidance behavior, and hyperarousal, as well as concurrent conditions (e.g., panic attacks, obsessions and compulsions, or suicidal ideation). A remission or good response in patients with PTSD is defined as a greater than 75% reduction in symptoms and response maintained for at least 3 months. Patients who have a 25% to 75% reduction in symptoms are considered partial responders. Before deciding that a patient is not responsive to pharmacotherapy, the clinician should ensure that the medication trial has been adequate in both dose and duration. Use of an objective measurement of remission of PTSD (e.g., a Treatment Outcome PTSD Scale [TOPS-8] score less than or equal to 5 points and a Sheehan Disability Scale less than or equal to 1 point on each item) can assist in the evaluation of drug response.[21]

Many patients with PTSD are sensitive to the adverse effects of drugs. They should be monitored carefully for adverse reactions that can delay the escalation of drug dosages or cause the patient distress. When pharmacotherapy is discontinued, patients should be seen more frequently and monitored carefully for signs of relapse or withdrawal.

TREATMENT

Obsessive-Compulsive Disorder

■ DESIRED OUTCOMES

Goals of therapy for OCD include reduction in the frequency of obsessive thoughts and in the time spent performing compulsive acts and reduction in the degree of anxiety. Treatment for OCD might not completely eliminate obsessions or compulsions, but patients can feel remarkably improved with partial resolution of their symptoms. Treatment should provide the patient with an optimal level of psychosocial and occupational functioning and an overall improved QOL. Efforts should be made to minimize adverse drug events and prevent drug interactions.

■ GENERAL APPROACH TO TREATMENT

It is important at the outset of therapy to identify and document the specific target symptoms for pharmacotherapy. Rating scales can be used to measure symptom severity at baseline and during treatment to ascertain the degree of improvement. The Yale-Brown Obsessive-Compulsive Scale (YBOCS) is the most widely used clinician-administered scale. The Padua Inventory is a useful self-report questionnaire.[53] A QOL scale can assist the clinician in identifying other areas to target for treatment (e.g., depression and reduced physical well-being).[54]

The Food and Drug Administration (FDA) has approved five antidepressants for the management of OCD: clomipramine, fluoxetine, fluvoxamine, paroxetine, and sertraline. In adolescents with OCD, CBT is generally selected first for mild OCD, but CBT plus an SSRI (e.g., fluoxetine, fluvoxamine, sertraline, or paroxetine) are used for more severe OCD. In adults, CBT is the initial choice for mild OCD, and CBT plus an SSRI or an SSRI alone is selected for more severe OCD. Figure 74–2 is an algorithm for the treatment of OCD. Although some OCD symptoms can improve over the first few weeks of therapy, an adequate trial of any medication is considered to be 8 to 12 weeks at maximum tolerated dosage.

■ NONPHARMACOLOGIC TREATMENTS

CBT is the treatment of choice for mild OCD in both adolescents and adults. In the management of OCD, CBT involves exposure plus response prevention combined with cognitive therapy. When available, CBT should be offered to every OCD patient.[55] Exposure involves having the patient perform actions that were formerly avoided. For instance, if a patient avoided touching the flush handle on a bathroom toilet, exposure would involve holding onto the handle. Response prevention involves having the patient resist the compulsive rituals that are performed. The ritualistic washing behavior often associated with a contamination obsession might be the focus, and the patient would be asked to delay the washing behavior as long as possible. At the beginning of CBT treatment patients are often unable to perform these activities, and imaginal exposure is used as the first step in the treatment process. Over time in a gradual manner the patient is exposed to feared objects/activities and is trained to resist rituals for longer periods of time.

Most patients who continue in CBT therapy generally respond. CBT should be added to the regimen when a patient is a nonresponder or a partial responder to SSRI or clomipramine monotherapy. CBT should be used alone if the patient is intolerant to adverse drug effects, is pregnant, or has a medical condition that contraindicates medication.[55] Behavioral therapy appears to have stronger effects on compulsive rituals than for the associated obsessions.

Exposure and response prevention therapies, applied individually or in groups, have longer-lasting effects after discontinuation, and produce greater improvement compared with drug therapy.[57–59] Techniques such as teaching patients to prevent relapse through self-exposure and self-imposed ritual prevention are suggested to foster optimal nonpharmacologic therapy.[57] Exposure with response prevention is particularly helpful for contamination or other fears, symmetry rituals, counting/repeating, hoarding, and aggressive urges. Cognitive therapy is beneficial for scrupulosity, moral guilt, and pathologic doubt. Thirteen to twenty sessions are typically required to treat uncomplicated OCD.[55]

A major barrier to the application of nonpharmacologic therapy is availability and cost of treatment. CBT requires specific training. Many psychiatrists are not adequately trained and/or do not have the time or desire necessary to apply this therapy. Some psychologists and social workers are skilled in this discipline; however, availability can be restricted in some areas.

■ PHARMACOLOGIC THERAPY

❻ The Expert Consensus Panel report reflects comprehensive opinions of a large number of leading authorities in the field of OCD treatment.[55] New consensus guidelines from the American Psychiatric Association are expected in late 2007. The SSRIs are considered to be the drugs of choice in the treatment of OCD. Drug therapy is reserved for patients with moderate to severe symptoms. Antidepressants can be combined with CBT or used alone in adults with moderate to severe symptoms. An SSRI should be added when there has been no response or partial response to CBT alone. Generally, an SSRI is selected before clomipramine, and whenever anticholinergic, cardiovascular, sexual, sedative, or weight-gain adverse effects are a major concern. If one SSRI is ineffective, then another SSRI should be tried. Treatment resistance can be defined as failure to achieve at least a 25% reduction in baseline scores on

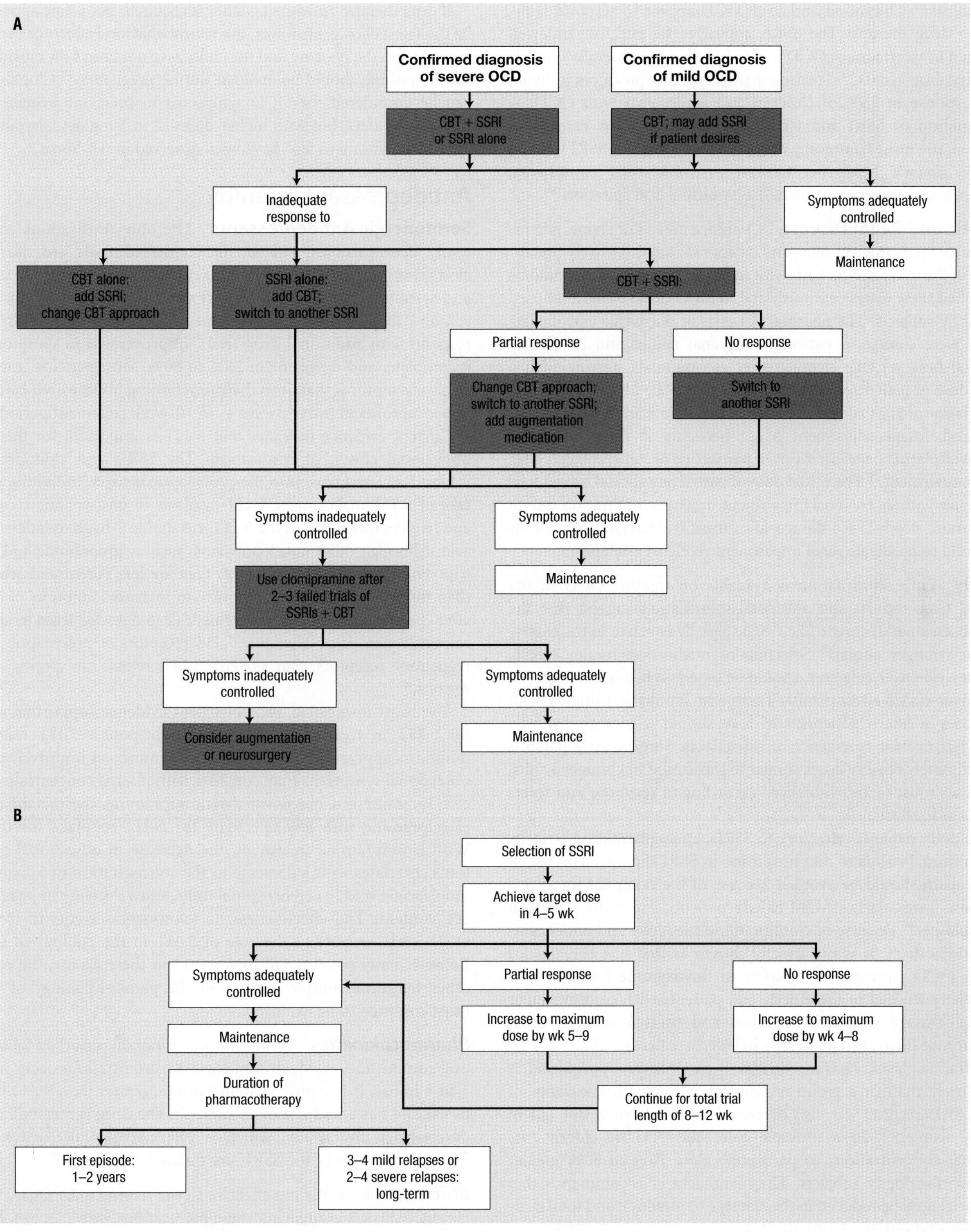

FIGURE 74-2. Algorithm for management of obsessive-compulsive disorder in adults. *A.* Overall approach to treatment. *B.* Pharmacotherapeutic approach to treatment. (CBT, cognitive behavioral therapy; OCD, obsessive-compulsive disorder; SSRI, selective serotonin reuptake inhibitor. *(Derived from Expert Consensus Panel for Obsessive-Compulsive Disorder*[55] *and American Pharmaceutical Association.*[56]*)*

the YBOCS.[20,55] ❼ Clomipramine can be selected after two to three failed SSRI trials. Clomipramine can be used to augment an SSRI in partially responsive or nonresponsive patients.[55]

Special Populations

Children and Adolescents OCD affecting children and adolescents is prevalent. There are symptom and treatment similarities and differences between OCD developing earlier in life and that which develops later. Younger patients exhibit poorer insight regarding obsessions, have more obsessions involving fear of harm and separation, and possess more rituals involving family members.[60] CBT provided in the group setting has been shown to be effective and is an alternative to individual CBT or medication treatment.[61] Clomipramine, fluvoxamine, sertraline, and fluoxetine are approved by the FDA for treatment of OCD in children and adolescents.[62] Childhood and adult OCD appear to respond similarly to drug therapy. The SSRIs appear to be effective and well tolerated in treatment of OCD in children and are generally considered first-line agents.[63] Treatment with an SSRI produces a favorable response in 75% of children and adolescents with OCD. A combination of SSRI and CBT is preferred in most cases.[64] In children, the most commonly described side effects of SSRI therapy include nausea, headache, tremor, gastrointestinal complaints, drowsiness, akathisia, insomnia, disinhibition, and agitation.[64]

Hepatic and Renal Disease Clomipramine, fluoxetine, sertraline, paroxetine, fluvoxamine, and citalopram are extensively metabolized in the liver, and patients with significant liver disease should be prescribed these drugs cautiously and in lower doses than those used in healthy subjects. The pharmacokinetics of fluoxetine and fluvoxamine were similar in patients with renal failure and in healthy subjects; however, the manufacturer recommends starting with a lower dose in patients with renal impairment. The pharmacokinetics of sertraline are not altered in patients with significant renal dysfunction, and dosage adjustment is not necessary in these patients.[30] Increased plasma concentrations of paroxetine occur in subjects with renal impairment.[29] The initial dose of paroxetine should be reduced in patients with severe renal impairment, and upward titration should occur more slowly.[29] No dosage adjustment is necessary for patients with mild to moderate renal impairment receiving citalopram.

Elderly Little information is available on treating OCD in the elderly. Case reports and anecdotal information suggest that the anti-obsessional drugs are likely to be equally effective in the elderly and in younger adults.[65] Selection of medication for an elderly person with OCD, however, should be based on history of response and adverse side-effect profile. Treatment should be initiated with low doses in elderly patients, and doses should be increased slowly, with vigilance for emergence of side effects. Some elderly patients can ultimately require doses similar to those used in younger adults, but doses must be individualized according to response and tolerance of side effects.

In elderly patients refractory to SSRIs, an augmentation strategy with minimal risk is to add buspirone to SSRI therapy. The use of clonazepam should be avoided because of the potential for excess sedation, particularly in frail elderly patients and those with gait disturbances.[66] Because of clomipramine's sedative and anticholinergic side effects, it is not usually chosen as first-line therapy for elderly OCD patients.[66] The safety of fluvoxamine has not been adequately studied in the elderly and patients with cardiovascular disease. Dosage should be reduced and titrated slowly during initiation of fluvoxamine therapy in elderly patients.

Sertraline plasma clearance in elderly patients was approximately 40% lower than in a group of younger individuals. Clearance of desmethylsertraline was also decreased in elderly men but not in elderly women.[30] In a multiple-dose study in the elderly, the minimal concentrations of paroxetine were 70% to 80% greater than in nonelderly subjects. The manufacturer recommends that the initial dose be reduced in the elderly (10 mg/day), and total daily doses should not exceed 40 mg.[29]

Pregnancy In general, CBT alone should be used for pregnant patients except in cases in which the risks of untreated OCD outweigh the risks of drug use (e.g., a pregnant woman who will not eat because of contamination fears).[55] Women with a history of OCD should be informed that OCD can worsen during pregnancy and during the postpartum period. OCD symptoms can exacerbate during the first trimester, especially if pharmacotherapy is discontinued just before conception or early in pregnancy. Symptoms often improve during the second trimester and worsen during the third trimester. The use of SSRIs in pregnancy and lactation is discussed in the chapter on depression (Chap. 71).

If drug therapy during pregnancy is required, fluoxetine appears to be the safest choice. However, the neurobehavioral effects of prenatal exposure on the neonate and the child have not been fully elucidated. Clomipramine should be avoided during pregnancy.[67] Clonazepam can be considered for OCD symptoms in pregnant women with disabling anxiety, but with higher doses (2 to 5 mg/day), hypotonia, apnea, and failure to feed have been observed in newborns.[67]

Antidepressant Therapy

Serotonergic Antidepressants The only medications consistently demonstrating efficacy in controlled trials are the TCA clomipramine and the SSRIs fluoxetine, fluvoxamine, paroxetine, and sertraline. Sixty-five to seventy percent of patients with OCD respond to their first SSRI treatment, and up to 90% ultimately respond with additional drug trials. Improvement in symptoms is incomplete, and ranges from 25% to 60%. Most patients continue to have symptoms that limit their functioning.[62] Obsessive-compulsive symptoms improve over a 4- to 10-week treatment period.[68]

Current evidence indicates that 5-HT is important for the anti-obsessional effects of medication. The SSRIs and clomipramine inhibit 5-HT reuptake into the presynaptic neuron. Inhibiting reuptake of 5-HT makes more 5-HT available to postsynaptic receptors and reduces formation of the 5-HT metabolite 5-hydroxyindoleacetic acid. Although other antidepressants, such as imipramine and amitriptyline, inhibit 5-HT reuptake, they are less potent and selective than the SSRIs. Prolonged exposure to increased amounts of 5-HT after chronic antidepressant treatment (2 to 3 weeks) leads to altered responsiveness of postsynaptic 5-HT receptors or presynaptic autoregulatory receptors that govern 5-HT release in specific brain regions.[68]

The most impressive and consistent evidence supporting a role for 5-HT in treating OCD is that only potent 5-HT reuptake inhibitors appear to be effective. Furthermore, an improvement in obsessional symptoms may correlate with plasma concentrations of clomipramine but not desmethylclomipramine, the metabolite of clomipramine with less selectivity for 5-HT reuptake inhibition. With clomipramine treatment, the decrease in obsessional symptoms correlates with a decrease in the concentration of 5-hydroxyindoleacetic acid in cerebrospinal fluid, and a decrease in platelet 5-HT content. The effectiveness of serotonergic agents in treating OCD lends support to the role of 5-HT in the etiology of OCD. Because many patients fail to respond to these agents, the role of other neurotransmitter systems in the pathophysiology of OCD must continue to be explored.

Pharmacokinetics. Clomipramine is rapidly absorbed following oral administration. Maximum plasma concentrations occur within 3 to 8 hours. It is highly protein-bound (greater than 90%) in the blood and has a half-life of 15 hours.[69] The drug is metabolized to desmethylclomipramine, which is pharmacologically active. The pharmacokinetics of the SSRIs are discussed in Chap. 71.

Efficacy. The SSRIs are effective in the treatment of OCD. Well-conducted trials comparing these medications with placebo, head-to-head comparative trials, and meta-analyses have established that fluoxetine, fluvoxamine, paroxetine, sertraline, and citalopram are equally effective and that clomipramine may be somewhat more effective.[70]

Most experts agree that the SSRIs are better tolerated than clomipramine. The SSRIs are less likely to cause cardiovascular, sedative, anticholinergic, and weight-gain side effects. Clomipramine is less likely than the SSRIs to cause insomnia, akathisia, nausea, and diarrhea. Side effects can be more severe when larger doses are used and with faster dose escalation. Tolerance to adverse effects often develops over 6 to 8 weeks of treatment, and tolerance is more likely to develop to nausea, diarrhea, sedation, diminished libido and/or orgasm, anxiety, restlessness, insomnia, and anticholinergic side effects than to akathisia.[55,70]

Other Antidepressants Venlafaxine, which acts as a serotonin and norepinephrine reuptake inhibitor, can be effective for OCD.[70]

Alternative Drug Treatments

If there is no response or partial response to combined CBT and three adequate antidepressant trials (one of which is clomipramine), augmentation with another drug and more intensive CBT can be tried. Augmentation of SSRI treatment with low doses of risperidone, quetiapine, and olanzapine may be helpful, but more research is needed. Typical antipsychotics are generally not recommended because of an increased likelihood of extrapyramidal symptoms.[70,71] It is suggested that attempts at augmentation be conducted with the use of rating scales or careful symptom severity assessment so that the benefit of the added drug therapy is clearly assessed and documented.

Dosage and Administration

Table 74–4 summarizes dosing guidelines for the SSRIs and clomipramine. If there is inadequate response to an average dose, then it should be incrementally increased to the maximum dose within 4 to 9 weeks from the start of treatment. If there is an inadequate response after 4 to 6 weeks at the maximum dose, then another SSRI should be tried. Eight to thirteen weeks is considered an adequate trial before changing to another drug or augmenting with another agent.

After patients have responded to the acute phase of treatment, treatment gains are maintained with maintenance-phase strategies. ❽ Monthly followup visits are recommended for at least 3 to 6 months, and a medication taper can be considered after 1 to 2 years of treatment. Medication should not be rapidly discontinued, and booster CBT sessions can reduce the risk of relapse when medication is withdrawn. The drug dosage can be decreased by 25%, and then 2 months should lapse before again decreasing the dose, depending on response.

❾ Long-term or lifelong prophylaxis with pharmacotherapy is recommended after two to four severe relapses or three to four mild relapses.[55] Although the appropriate maintenance dose of antidepressants is unknown, it is notable that one investigator was successful in reducing the dose of clomipramine from a mean of 270 mg/day to 165 mg/day in the maintenance phase. Mundo and colleagues studied patients successfully treated with clomipramine or fluvoxamine and reduced their doses by 33% to 66% for maintenance therapy, with clear advantages for tolerability and compliance. However, the study duration was only 102 days.[72]

CLINICAL CONTROVERSY

The use of atypical antipsychotics for patients having both schizophrenia and OCD can be problematic. Some studies have shown that atypical antipsychotics worsen symptoms of OCD in this patient population, but other studies report benefits from atypical antipsychotic use. Patients with schizophrenia have a higher incidence of OCD than patients without schizophrenia. Therefore, OCD symptoms should be monitored closely when changing antipsychotic medication or adjusting the dosage.

Pharmacoeconomic Considerations

The annual outpatient direct costs for patients seeking treatment for OCD in the United States in 1995 were $5.1 billion. In 1990, the total cost to the economy was $8 billion, which includes expenditures for direct ($2.1 billion) and indirect costs. Direct costs include costs of hospitalization, outpatient professional services, and drugs. Indirect costs include costs associated with lost productivity, work

TABLE 74-4 Dosing of Serotonin Reuptake Inhibitors in Treatment of OCD

Generic Name	Usual Initial Daily Dose (mg)	Daily Dosage Range (mg)	Usual Target Daily Dose (mg)
Citalopram[a]	20	20–60	40
Clomipramine	10	100–250	150–200
Fluoxetine	20	20–80	40–60
Fluvoxamine	50	100–300	200
Paroxetine	20	20–60	40
Sertraline	50	75–200	150

OCD, obsessive-compulsive disorder.
[a]Not FDA approved for treatment of OCD. Optimal dosing guidelines are not well established.
Data from Expert Consensus Panel for Obsessive-Compulsive Disorder[55] and Ellingrod.[68]

loss, early retirement, and absenteeism. As OCD frequently has its onset in childhood or adolescence, loss of income over a lifetime is substantial.[73]

Another pharmacoeconomic consideration that impacts the provision of optimal treatment for patients with OCD relates to inability to pay for nonpharmacologic therapy. Although CBT has been shown to be a very effective modality, very often the patient cannot afford this therapy or does not have medical insurance that helps pay the associated costs.

Evaluation of Therapeutic Outcomes

Target symptoms of OCD should be monitored closely. The degree of response can indicate a need to modify dosage, change drug, or augment therapy. Rating scales can be used to monitor symptom response to therapy for OCD and changes in QOL. The clinician should inquire about and address problematic adverse effects (including the emergence of suicidal ideation) reported by the patient. Drug interactions should be monitored. Changes in social and occupational functioning should be assessed.

Patients older than 40 years of age should receive a pretreatment electrocardiogram before starting clomipramine. In patients with liver disease, baseline and periodic liver function tests are recommended when clomipramine is used. If clomipramine is given concurrently with sympatholytic antihypertensive agents, blood pressure should be regularly monitored. Patients receiving clomipramine who develop fever and sore throat should have leukocyte and differential white blood cell counts assessed to evaluate for agranulocytosis.

CONCLUSIONS

The past decade has brought a renewed interest in the recognition and management of PTSD. Healthcare workers are sensitized to the devastating effects that PTSD can have on patient functioning, QOL, and use of healthcare resources. Adequately detecting and appropriately managing PTSD is important to improving the lives of patients who suffer from this illness. Data on the efficacy of the SSRIs supports their use for both acute and long-term management of the symptoms of PTSD. The SSRIs are the first-line pharmacotherapy of PTSD and OCD. Research in OCD has resulted in new pharmacologic treatment strategies, especially with augmentation therapies.

ABBREVIATIONS

ASD: acute stress disorder

CBT: cognitive behavioral therapy

DA: dopamine

EMDR: eye movement desensitization and reprocessing

FDA: Food and Drug Administration
5-HT: serotonin
GABA: γ-aminobutyric acid
HPA: hypothalamic-pituitary-adrenal axis
MAOI: monoamine oxidase inhibitor
m-CPP: *meta*-chlorophenylpiperazine
NE: norepinephrine
OCD: obsessive-compulsive disorder
PTSD: posttraumatic stress disorder
QOL: quality of life
SSRI: selective serotonin reuptake inhibitor
TCA: tricyclic antidepressant
TFCBT: trauma-focused cognitive behavioral therapy
TOPS-8: Treatment Outcome PTSD Scale (8 items)
vmPFC: ventromedial prefrontal cortex
YBOCS: Yale-Brown Obsessive Compulsive Scale

REFERENCES

1. American Psychiatric Association. Diagnostic and Statistical Manual of Mental Disorders, Fourth Edition, Text Revision. Washington, DC: American Psychiatric Association, 2000:429–484.
2. Lecrubier Y. Posttraumatic stress disorder in primary care: A hidden diagnosis. J Clin Psychiatry 2004;65(Suppl 1):49–54.
3. Eisen JL, Mancebo MA, Pinto A, et al. Impact of obsessive compulsive disorder on quality of life. Compr Psychiatry 2006;47:270–275.
4. Stein DJ, Allen A, Bobes J, et al. Quality of life in obsessive-compulsive disorder. CNS Spectr 2000;5(Suppl 4):37–39.
5. Narrow WE, Rae DS, Robins LN, Regier DA. Revised prevalence estimates of mental disorders in the United States: Using a clinical significance criterion to reconcile 2 surveys' estimates. Arch Gen Psychiatry 2002;59:115–123.
6. Yehuda R. Risk and resilience in posttraumatic stress disorder. J Clin Psychiatry 2004;65(Suppl 1):29–36.
7. Grinage BD. Diagnosis and management of post-traumatic stress disorder. Am Fam Physician 2003;68:2401–2408.
8. Pinto A, Mancebo MC, Eisen JL, et al. The Brown Longitudinal Obsessive Compulsive Study: Clinical features and symptoms of the sample at intake. J Clin Psychiatry 2006;67:703–711.
9. Pato MT, Schindler KM, Pato CN. The genetics of obsessive-compulsive disorder. Curr Psychiatry Rep 2001;3:163–168.
10. Masand PS, Keuthen NJ, Gupta S, et al. Prevalence of irritable bowel syndrome in obsessive-compulsive disorder. CNS Spectr 2006;11:21–25.
11. Snider LA, Swedo SE. PANDAS: Current status and directions for research. Mol Psychiatry 2004;9:900–907.
12. Ballenger JC, Davidson JRT, Lecrubier Y, et al. Consensus statement update on posttraumatic stress disorder from the International Consensus Group on Depression and Anxiety. J Clin Psychiatry 2004;65(Suppl 1):55–62.
13. Stein DJ. Neurobiology of the obsessive-compulsive spectrum disorders. Biol Psychiatry 2000;47:296–304.
14. Nutt DJ. The psychobiology of posttraumatic stress disorder. J Clin Psychiatry 2000;61(Suppl 5):24–29.
15. Kent JM, Mathew SJ, Gorman JM. Molecular targets in the treatment of anxiety. Biol Psychiatry 2002;52:1008–1030.
16. Hull AM. Neuroimaging findings in posttraumatic stress disorder: Systematic review. Br J Psychiatry 2002;181:102–110.
17. Rauch SL, Shin LM, Phelps EA. Neurocircuitry models of posttraumatic stress disorder and extinction: Human neuroimaging research—Past, present and future. Biol Psychiatry 2006;60:376–382.
18. Hesse S, Muller U, Lincke T, Barthel H, et al. Serotonin and dopamine transporter imaging in patients with obsessive-compulsive disorder. Psychiatry Res 2005;140:63–72.
19. Friedlander L, Desrocher M. Neuroimaging studies of obsessive-compulsive disorder in adults and children. Clin Psychol Rev 2006;26:32–49.
20. Jenike MA. Obsessive-compulsive disorder. N Engl J Med 2004;350:259–265.
21. Doyle AC, Pollack MH. Establishment of remission criteria for anxiety disorders. J Clin Psychiatry 2003;64(Suppl 15):40–45.
22. National Institute for Clinical Excellence. Post-traumatic stress disorder (PTSD): The management of PTSD in adults and children in primary and secondary care. Clinical Guideline 26 March 2005, *http://www.nice.org.uk/CG26/guidance/pdf/English*.
23. Work Group on ASD and PTSD. Practice guideline for the treatment of patients with acute stress disorder and posttraumatic stress disorder. Am J Psychiatry 2004;161(11 Suppl):1–61.
24. Bisson J, Andrew M. Psychological treatment of post-traumatic stress disorder (PTSD). Cochrane Database Syst Rev 2005;2:CD003388. DOI:10.1002/1465/14651858.CD003388.pub2.
25. van der Kolk BA, Spinazzola J, Blaustein ME, et al. A randomized clinical trial of eye movement desensitization and reprocessing (EMDR), fluoxetine, and pill placebo in the treatment of posttraumatic stress disorder: Treatment effects and long-term maintenance. J Clin Psychiatry 2007;68:37–46.
26. Stein DJ, Ipser JC, Seedat S. Pharmacotherapy for post traumatic stress disorder (PTSD). Cochrane Database Syst Rev 2006;1:CD002795. DOI:10.1002/1264/1858.CD002795.pub2.
27. Baldwin DS, Anderson IM, Nutt DJ, et al. Evidence-based guidelines for the pharmacological treatment of anxiety disorders: Recommendations from the British Association for Pharmacology. J Psychopharmacol 2005;19:567–596.
28. Bandelow B, Zohar J, Hollander E, et al. Guidelines for the pharmacological treatment of anxiety, obsessive-compulsive and posttraumatic stress disorders. World J Biol Psychiatry 2002;3:171–199.
29. Paxil [package insert]. Research Triangle Park, NC: GlaxoSmithKline, July 2006.
30. Zoloft [package insert]. New York: Pfizer, September 2006.
31. Schoenfeld FB, Marmar CR, Neylan TC. Current concepts in pharmacotherapy for posttraumatic stress disorder. Psychiatr Serv 2004;55:519–531.
32. Donnelly CL. Pharmacologic treatment approaches for children and adolescents with posttraumatic stress disorder. Child Adolesc Psychiatr Clin N Am 2003;12:251–269.
33. Brady K, Pearlstein T, Asnis GM, et al. Efficacy and safety of sertraline treatment of posttraumatic stress disorder: A randomized controlled trial. JAMA 2000;283:1837–1844.
34. Marshall RD, Beebe KL, Oldham M, Zaninelli R. Efficacy and safety of paroxetine treatment for chronic PTSD. A fixed-dose, placebo-controlled study. Am J Psychiatry 2001;158:1982–1988.
35. Tucker P, Zaninelli R, Yehuda R, et al. Paroxetine in the treatment of chronic posttraumatic stress disorder: Results of a placebo-controlled, flexible-dosage trial. J Clin Psychiatry 2001;62:860–868.
36. Martenyi F, Brown EB, Zhang H, et al. Fluoxetine versus placebo in posttraumatic stress disorder. J Clin Psychiatry 2002;63:199–206.
37. Tucker P, Smith KL, Marx B, et al. Fluvoxamine reduces physiologic reactivity to trauma scripts in posttraumatic stress disorder. J Clin Psychiatry 2000;20:367–372.
38. Tucker P, Potter-Kimball R, Wyatt DB, et al. Can physiologic assessment and side effects tease out differences in PTSD trials? A double-blind comparison of citalopram, sertraline, and placebo. Psychopharmacol Bull 2003;37:135–149.
39. Davidson JRT, Pearlstein T, Londborg P, et al. Efficacy of sertraline in preventing relapse of posttraumatic stress disorder: Results of a 28-week double-blind, placebo-controlled study. Am J Psychiatry 2001;158:1974–1981.
40. Davidson JRT, Weisler RH, Butterfield MI, et al. Mirtazapine versus placebo in posttraumatic stress disorder: A pilot study. Biol Psychiatry 2003;53:188–191.
41. Davidson J, Rothbaum BO, Tucker P, et al. Venlafaxine extended release in posttraumatic stress disorder: A sertraline- and placebo-controlled study. J Clin Psychopharmacol 2006;26:259–267.
42. Davidson J, Baldwin D, Stein DJ, et al. Treatment of posttraumatic stress disorder with venlafaxine extended release: A 6-month randomized controlled trial. Arch Gen Psychiatry 2006;63:1158–1165.
43. Becker ME, Hertzberg MA, Moore SD, et al. A placebo-controlled trial of bupropion SR in the treatment of chronic posttraumatic stress disorder. J Clin Psychopharmacol 2007;27:193–7.

44. Hamner MB, Deitsch SE, Brodrick PS, et al. Quetiapine treatment in patients with posttraumatic stress disorder: An open trial of adjunctive therapy. J Clin Psychopharmacol 2003;23:15–20.
45. Bartzokis G, Lu PH, Turner J, et al. Adjunctive risperidone in the treatment of chronic combat-related posttraumatic stress disorder. Biol Psychiatry 2005;57:474–479.
46. Ahern EP, Mussey M, Johnson C, et al. Quetiapine as an adjunctive treatment for post-traumatic stress disorder: An 8-week open-label study. Int Clin Psychopharmacol 2006;21:29–33.
47. Stein MB, Kline NA, Matloff JL. Adjunctive olanzapine for SSRI-resistant combat-related PTSD. A double-blind, placebo-controlled study. Am J Psychiatry 2002;159:1777–1779.
48. Raskind MA, Peskind ER, Kanter ED, et al. Reduction of nightmares and other PTSD symptoms in combat veterans by prazosin: A placebo-controlled study. Am J Psychiatry 2003;160:371–373.
49. Davidson JRT. Pharmacologic treatment of acute and chronic stress following trauma. J Clin Psychiatry 2006;67(Suppl 2):34–39.
50. Friedman MJ, Davidson JRT, Mellman TA, Southwick SM. Pharmacotherapy. In: Foa EB, Keane TM, Friedman MJ, eds. Effective Treatments of Posttraumatic Stress Disorder. New York: Guilford Press, 2000:84–105.
51. Walker EA, Katon W, Russo J, et al. Health care costs associated with posttraumatic stress disorder symptoms in women. Arch Gen Psychiatry 2003;60:369–374.
52. Seedat S, Lochner C, Vythilingum B, Stein DJ. Quality of life in posttraumatic stress disorder: Impact of drug treatment. Pharmacoeconomics 2006;24:989–998.
53. American Psychiatric Association. Handbook of Psychiatric Measures. Washington, DC: American Psychiatric Association, 2000:572–576.
54. Moritz S, Rufer M, Fricke S, Karow A, et al. Quality of life in obsessive-compulsive disorder before and after treatment. Compr Psychiatry 2005;46:453–459.
55. Expert Consensus Panel for Obsessive-Compulsive Disorder. Obsessive-compulsive disorder executive summary: Recommendations for first-line treatments by clinical situation. J Clin Psychiatry 1997;58(Suppl 4):2–72.
56. American Pharmaceutical Association. Management of obsessive-compulsive disorder. In: APhA Guide to Drug Treatment Protocols: A Resource for Creating and Using Disease-Specific Pathways. Washington, DC: American Pharmaceutical Association, 1997:OCDi–OCDii.
57. Marks I. Behavior therapy for obsessive-compulsive disorder: A decade of progress. Can J Psychiatry 1997;42:1021–1027.
58. Braga DT, Cordioli AV, Niederauer K, Manfro GG. Cognitive-behavioral group therapy for obsessive-compulsive disorder: A 1-year follow-up. Acta Psychiatr Scand 2005;112:180–186.
59. Tenneij NH, van Megen HJ, Denys DA, Westenberg HG. Behavior therapy augments response of patients with obsessive-compulsive disorder responding to drug treatment. J Clin Psychiatry 2005;66:1169–1175.
60. Geller DA. Obsessive-compulsive and spectrum disorders in children and adolescents. Psychiatr Clin North Am 2006;29:353–370.
61. Asbahr FR, Castillo AR, Ito LM, et al. Group cognitive-behavioral therapy versus sertraline for the treatment of children and adolescents with obsessive-compulsive disorder. J Am Acad Child Adolesc Psychiatry 2005 ;44:1128–1136.
62. Hollander E, Pallanti S. Current and experimental therapeutics of OCD. In: Davis KL, Charney D, Coyle JT, Nemeroff C, eds. Neuropsychopharmacology: The Fifth Generation of Progress. Philadelphia, PA: Lippincott Williams & Wilkins, 2002:1647–1664.
63. King RA, Leonard H, March J, et al. Practice parameters for the assessment of children and adolescents with obsessive-compulsive disorder. J Am Acad Child Adolesc Psychiatry 1998;37(Suppl 10):27S–45S.
64. Thomsen PH. Obsessive-compulsive disorder: Pharmacologic treatment. Eur Child Adolesc Psychiatry 2000;9(Suppl 1):176–184.
65. Sheikh JL, Salzman C. Anxiety in the elderly. Psychiatr Clin North Am 1995;18:871–883.
66. Pollard CA, Carmin CN, Ownby R. Obsessive-compulsive disorder in later life. In: Dickstein LJ, Riba MB, et al., eds. OCD Across the Life Cycle. Section III of Review of Psychiatry, vol. 16. Washington, DC: American Psychiatric Press, 1997:57–72.
67. Diaz SF, Grush LR, Sichel DA, Cohen LS. Obsessive-compulsive disorder in pregnancy and the puerperium. In: Dickstein LJ, Riba MB, et al., eds. OCD Across the Life Cycle. Section III of Review of Psychiatry, vol. 16. Washington, DC: American Psychiatric Press, 1997:97–112.
68. Ellingrod VL. Pharmacotherapy of primary obsessive-compulsive disorder: Review of the literature. Pharmacotherapy 1998;18:936–960.
69. Clomipramine. LexiComp online. 2007, *http://www.crlonline.com/crlsql/servlewt/crlonline*.
70. Denys D. Pharmacotherapy of obsessive-compulsive disorder and obsessive-compulsive spectrum disorders. Psychiatr Clin North Am 2006;29:553–584.
71. Blier P, Habib R, Flament MF. Pharmacotherapies in the management of obsessive-compulsive disorder. Can J Psychiatry 2006;51:417–430.
72. Mundo E, Bareggi SR, Pirola R, et al. Long-term therapy of obsessive-compulsive disorder: A double-blind controlled study. J Clin Psychiatry 1997;17:4–10.
73. Hollander E, Stein DJ, Kwon JH, et al. Psychosocial function and economic costs of obsessive-compulsive disorder. CNS Spectr 1997;2:16–25.

CHAPTER 75

Sleep Disorders

JOHN M. DOPP AND BRADLEY G. PHILLIPS

KEY CONCEPTS

1. Common causes of insomnia include concomitant psychiatric disorders, significant psychosocial stressors, excessive alcohol use, caffeine intake, and nicotine use.
2. Good sleep hygiene, including relaxing before bedtime, exercising regularly, establishing a regular bedtime and wake-up time, and discontinuing alcohol, caffeine, and nicotine, alone and in combination with drug therapy should be part of patient education and treatments for insomnia.
3. Long-acting benzodiazepines should be avoided in the elderly.
4. Benzodiazepine tolerance and dependence are avoided by using low-dose therapy for the shortest possible duration.
5. Obstructive sleep apnea can be an independent risk factor for the development of hypertension. When hypertension is present, it is often refractory to drug therapy until sleep disordered breathing is alleviated.
6. Nasal continuous positive airway pressure is the first-line therapy for obstructive sleep apnea, and weight loss should be encouraged in all obese patients.
7. Pharmacologic management of narcolepsy is focused on two primary areas: treatment of excessive daytime sleepiness and cataplexy.
8. Short-acting benzodiazepine receptor agonists or melatonin taken at appropriate target bedtimes for east or west travel reduce jet lag and shorten sleep latency.
9. Dopamine agonists are effective for restless legs syndrome and have replaced levodopa as first-line therapy.

Approximately 70 million Americans suffer with a sleep-related problem, and as many as 60% of those experience a chronic disorder.[1] In a study by the National Institute of Aging, of 9,000 patients age 65 years and older, more than 80% report a sleep-related disturbance.[1]

INTRODUCTION TO SLEEP

SLEEP CYCLES

Sleep is divided into two phases: nonrapid eye movement (NREM) sleep and rapid eye movement (REM) sleep. Humans typically experience four to six cycles of NREM and REM sleep, with each cycle lasting between 70 and 120 minutes.[2]

There are four stages of NREM sleep. Healthy sleep will typically progress through the four stages of NREM sleep prior to the first REM period. From wakefulness, sleep typically progresses quickly through stages 1 and 2. Stage 1 of NREM sleep is the stage between wakefulness and sleep, and individuals describe this experience as being awake, being drowsy, or as being asleep. During stages 3 and 4 NREM, both metabolic activity and brain waves slow. This slow-wave sleep occurs most frequently early in the sleep period. Stage 3 and stage 4 sleep is called *delta sleep* as the sleep is characterized by high-amplitude slow activity known as delta waves (0.5 to 3 Hz). In this stage eye movements are absent and muscle tone is atonic.[3]

REM sleep involves a dramatic physiologic change from NREM sleep, to a state in which the brain becomes electrically and metabolically activated.[2] REM occurs in bursts, and is accompanied by a 62% to 173% increase in cerebral blood flow, generalized muscle atonia, bursts of bilateral rapid eye movements, poikilothermia, dreaming, and fluctuations in respiratory and cardiac rate.[2] REM cycles tend to lengthen in the later stages of the sleep cycle.[2]

CIRCADIAN RHYTHM

At birth human infants spend up to 20 hours a day sleeping. At 3 to 6 months of age there is a differentiation between REM and NREM sleep: By age 3 the ultradian sleep-wake rhythm changes to a circadian pattern. The suprachiasmatic nucleus of the brain serves as the biologic clock and paces the circadian rhythm. Although the length of a day is 24 hours, in environments devoid of light cues, the sleep-wake cycle lasts 24.2 hours.[3] In midlife, there is a gradual decline in sleep efficiency and sleep time.[2] The elderly have lighter and more fragmented sleep, with intermittent arousals, shifts in the sleep stages, and a gradual reduction of slow wave sleep.

NEUROCHEMISTRY

The neurochemistry of sleep is complex as sleep cannot be localized to either a specific area of the brain or neurotransmitter. NREM sleep appears to be controlled by the basal forebrain, the area surrounding the solitary tract in the medulla and the dorsal raphe nucleus, which is primarily serotonergic.[3] Sleep is reduced when there are decreases in serotonin or destruction of the dorsal raphe nucleus in the brainstem, which contains most of the brain's serotonergic bodies. REM sleep appears to be turned on by cholinergic cells in the mesencephalic, medullary, and pontine gigantocellular regions. REM sleep appears to be turned off by the dorsal raphe nucleus, the locus coeruleus, and the nucleus parabrachialis lateris, the latter two of which are primarily noradrenergic. The ascending reticular activating system and the posterior hypothalamus facilitate arousal and wakefulness.[4] Dopamine has an alerting effect: Decreases in dopamine promote sleepiness.[5] Neurochemicals

Learning objectives, review questions, and other resources can be found at **www.pharmacotherapyonline.com.**

involved in wakefulness include norepinephrine and acetylcholine in the cortex and histamine and neuropeptides such as substance P and corticotropin-releasing factor in the hypothalamus.[5,6]

POLYSOMNOGRAPHY

Sleep is typically measured and observed in sleep laboratories using an electroencephalogram (EEG), electro-oculograms of each eye, electrocardiogram, electromyogram, air thermistors, abdominal and thoracic strain belts, and oxygen saturation monitor. This study is named polysomnography (PSG) and is used to assess and record variables that characterize sleep and aid in diagnosis of sleep disorders. Variables obtained during PSG include sleep onset, arousals, sleep stages, eye movements, leg and jaw movements, arrhythmias, airflow during sleep, respiratory effort, and oxygen desaturations.

CLASSIFICATION OF SLEEP DISORDERS

The *Diagnostic and Statistical Manual of Mental Disorders, Fourth Edition, Text Revision (DSM-IV-TR)* classifies sleep disorders into four categories based on etiology (Table 75–1) and requires a minimum of 1 month before a sleep disorder can be diagnosed.[7,8] Primary sleep disorders are those disorders in which there is no other etiology (mental disorder, substance-related disorder, or medical condition) responsible for the disorder. Primary sleep disorders appear to be based on an endogenous abnormality of the sleep-wake cycle, or circadian rhythm, and they are divided into dyssomnias or parasomnias.

TABLE 75-1 *DSM-IV-TR* Classification of Sleep Disorders

Primary sleep disorders
Dyssomnias – abnormality in the amount, quality, or timing of sleep
Primary insomnia
Primary hypersomnia
Narcolepsy
Breathing-related sleep disorder
Circadian rhythm sleep disorder
Delayed sleep phase type
Jet lag type
Shift work type
Unspecified type
Dyssomnia not otherwise specified
Parasomnias – abnormal behavioral or physiologic events associated with sleep
Nightmare disorder
Sleep terror disorder
Sleepwalking disorder
Parasomnia not otherwise specified
Sleep disorders related to another mental disorder
Insomnia or hypersomnia related to another mental disorder

Data from American Psychiatric Association[8] with permission.
DSM-IV-TR, Diagnostic and Statistical Manual of Mental Disorders, 4th ed., text revision.

INSOMNIA

Insomnia is the most common complaint in general medical practice.[9] It causes distress, frequently because of a fear or a feeling of not being able to fall asleep at bedtime and can impair work-related productivity because of daytime fatigue or drowsiness. Insomnia is subjectively characterized as a complaint of difficulty falling asleep, difficulty maintaining sleep, or experiencing nonrestorative sleep.[8] Insomnia lasting two or three nights because of jet lag, for example, is considered to be transient insomnia, whereas short-term insomnia usually resolves in less than 3 weeks. Insomnia, according to the *DSM-IV-TR*, is considered to be chronic when it lasts longer than 1 month.[8]

Epidemiology

Primary insomnia usually begins in early or middle adulthood and is rare in childhood or adolescence. More than 50% of the population complains of insomnia in their lifetime.[1] A 1-year prevalence study of insomnia in the United States reports that one-third of the individuals surveyed complained of insomnia, and 17% reported that the symptoms were serious.[1] Conservative estimates of chronic insomnia range from 9% to 12% in adulthood and up to 20% in the elderly.[1,10] Although young adults are more likely to complain that they have difficulty falling asleep, middle-aged and elderly adults are more likely to complain that they have middle-of-the-night awakening or early morning awakening. Women complain of insomnia twice as frequently as men. Individuals who are elderly, unemployed, separated or widowed, and those with a lower socioeconomic status reported a significantly higher incidence of insomnia than the general population. Forty percent of individuals with insomnia also had a concurrent psychiatric disorder (anxiety, depression, or substance abuse).[9]

Despite the prevalence of insomnia, only 5% of individuals seek medical attention for management of their insomnia. Approximately 10% to 20% use nonprescription drugs or alcohol to self-treat. Of the 3% of the population who are prescribed sedative–hypnotics for insomnia, 11% report use exceeding 1 year.[11]

Differential Diagnosis

Primary insomnia is considered to be an endogenous disorder caused by either a neurochemical or structural disorder affecting the sleep-wake cycle. Individuals with primary insomnia can be light sleepers who are easily aroused by noise, temperature, or anxiety. Some studies suggest that primary insomnia is a "hyperarousal state," in that insomnia patients have increased metabolic rates compared with controls, and thus, take longer to fall asleep.[2] Evaluation of patients with a complaint of transient or short-term insomnia should focus on recent stressors, such as a separation, a death in the family, a job change, or college exams.

❶ Chronic insomnia is frequently associated with psychiatric or medical conditions. A complete diagnostic examination should be completed in these individuals and include routine laboratory tests, physical and mental status examinations, as well as ruling out any medication- or substance-related causes.[12] Special consideration should also be given to other sleep disorders that can have a similar presentation, including restless legs syndrome, periodic limb movements of sleep, and sleep apnea. Common causes of insomnia are listed in Table 75–2.

TABLE 75-2 Common Etiologies of Insomnia

Situational
Work or financial stress, major life events, interpersonal conflicts
Jet lag or shift work
Medical
Cardiovascular (angina, arrhythmias, heart failure)
Respiratory (asthma, sleep apnea)
Chronic pain
Endocrine disorders (diabetes, hyperthyroidism)
Gastrointestinal (gastroesophageal reflux disease, ulcers)
Neurologic (delirium, epilepsy, Parkinson's disease)
Pregnancy
Psychiatric
Mood disorders (depression, mania)
Anxiety disorders (e.g., generalized anxiety disorder, obsessive-compulsive disorder)
Substance abuse (alcohol or sedative-hypnotic withdrawal)
Pharmacologically induced
Anticonvulsants
Central adrenergic blockers
Diuretics
Selective serotonin reuptake inhibitors
Steroids
Stimulants

TREATMENT

Insomnia

Therapeutic management of insomnia is initially based on whether the individual has experienced a transient, short-term, or chronic sleep disturbance. Clinical history should assess the onset, duration, and frequency of the symptoms, effect on daytime functioning, sleep hygiene habits, and history of previous symptoms or treatment.[13] Management of all patients with insomnia should include identifying the cause of the insomnia, patient education on sleep hygiene, and stress management. Any unnecessary pharmacotherapy should be eliminated.[10] Transient insomnia, which occurs as a result of an acute stressor, is expected to resolve quickly, and should be treated with good sleep hygiene and careful use of sedative-hypnotics.[14] Short-term insomnia, lasting up to 3 weeks, associated with situational, personal, or medical stress can be treated similarly.[13] Chronic insomnia requires careful assessment for possible underlying medical causes, nonpharmacologic techniques, and careful use of sedative-hypnotics.[12]

■ NONPHARMACOLOGIC THERAPY

❷ In many cases insomnia can be treated without sedative-hypnotics. Education about normal sleep and habits for good sleep hygiene are often sufficient interventions.[2] Nonpharmacologic interventions for insomnia frequently consist of short-term cognitive behavioral therapies, most commonly stimulus control therapy, sleep restriction, relaxation therapy, cognitive therapy, paradoxical intention, and education on good sleep hygiene (Table 75–3).[10,15,16] In patients age 55 and older, a recent study indicates that cognitive behavioral therapy may be more effective than pharmacologic therapy at improving certain measures of insomnia.[17]

CLINICAL CONTROVERSY

Pharmacologic treatment is indicated for transient and short-term insomnia. Historically, the use of sedative hypnotic agents for greater than 1 month was frowned on and discouraged in fear of the patient developing drug dependence. Experts now agree that clinicians should encourage hypnotic therapy using the lowest effective dose for short-term periods whenever possible. However, long-term use of hypnotics is not contraindicated unless the patient has another contraindication (e.g., history of substance abuse, pregnancy, etc.).

TABLE 75-3 Nonpharmacologic Recommendations for Insomnia

Stimulus control procedures

1. Establish regular times to wake up and to go to sleep (including weekends).
2. Sleep only as much as necessary to feel rested.
3. Go to bed only when sleepy. Avoid long periods of wakefulness in bed. Use the bed only for sleep or intimacy; do not read or watch television in bed.
4. Avoid trying to force sleep; if you do not fall asleep within 20–30 minutes, leave the bed and perform a relaxing activity (e.g., read, listen to music, or watch television) until drowsy. Repeat this as often as necessary.
5. Avoid daytime naps.
6. Schedule worry time during the day. Do not take your troubles to bed.

Sleep hygiene recommendations

1. Exercise routinely (three to four times weekly) but not close to bedtime because this can increase wakefulness.
2. Create a comfortable sleep environment by avoiding temperature extremes, loud noises, and illuminated clocks in the bedroom.
3. Discontinue or reduce the use of alcohol, caffeine, and nicotine.
4. Avoid drinking large quantities of liquids in the evening to prevent nighttime trips to the restroom.
5. Do something relaxing and enjoyable before bedtime.

■ PHARMACOLOGIC THERAPY

Miscellaneous Agents

Antihistamines exhibit sedating properties and are included in many over-the-counter sleep agents. They are effective in the treatment of mild insomnia and are generally safe.[13] Diphenhydramine and doxylamine are more sedating than pyrilamine. Increasing the dose of antihistamines will not produce a linear increase in response. The safety and efficacy of antihistamines over placebo have been documented in several studies. Antihistamines are considered to be less effective than benzodiazepines, and have the disadvantages of anticholinergic side effects, which are especially troublesome in the elderly.[13,18]

Antidepressants are alternatives for patients with nonrestorative sleep who should not receive benzodiazepines, especially those who have depression, pain, or a risk of substance abuse. Using antidepressants for insomnia without depression is common but not well studied.[18] Sedating antidepressants such as amitriptyline, doxepin, and nortriptyline are effective for inducing sleep continuity, although daytime sedation and side effects can be significant.[18] Anticholinergic activity, adrenergic blockage, and cardiac conduction prolongation can be problematic, especially in the elderly and in overdose situations.[18] Some of the new generation of antidepressants such as mirtazapine and nefazodone are also sedating. Mirtazapine can cause daytime sedation and weight gain.

Trazodone in doses of 25 to 100 mg at bedtime is sedating and can improve sleep continuity.[11] Trazodone is popular for the treatment of insomnia in patients prone to substance abuse, as dependence is not a problem. Trazodone is frequently used in patients with selective serotonin reuptake inhibitor (SSRI) and bupropion-induced insomnia.[11] Caution should be used to avoid serotonin syndrome when used in these combinations. Other side effects include carryover sedation and α-adrenergic blockade. Orthostasis can occur at any age, but it is more dangerous in the elderly. Priapism is a rare but serious side effect.[19]

Ramelteon is a melatonin receptor agonist that has recently been approved for the treatment of sleep onset insomnia. Ramelteon is selective for the MT1 and MT2 melatonin receptors that are thought to regulate the circadian rhythm and sleep onset. The recommended dose is 8 mg taken at bedtime to induce sleep and although generally well-tolerated, the most common adverse events reported are headache, dizziness, and somnolence. Ramelteon is not a controlled substance and can be a viable option for patients with a history of substance abuse.

Valerian is an herbal sleep remedy that has been studied for its sedative-hypnotic properties in patients with insomnia. The mechanism of action is not fully understood but may involve increasing concentrations of γ-aminobutyric acid (GABA). The recommended dose for insomnia ranges from 300 to 600 mg. An equivalent dose of dried herbal valerian root is 2 to 3 g soaked in 1 cup of hot water for 20 to 25 minutes.[20]

CLINICAL CONTROVERSY

The over-the-counter supplement melatonin is a popular treatment for insomnia. Although melatonin has demonstrated efficacy for inducing sleep, its use for the treatment of insomnia is not well-supported by clinical studies. Further research is needed before melatonin can be recommended for the treatment of insomnia.

Benzodiazepine Receptor Agonists

The most commonly used treatments for insomnia have been the benzodiazepine receptor agonists. All benzodiazepine receptor agonists are effective as sedative-hypnotics, and are Food and Drug

TABLE 75-4 Pharmacokinetics of Benzodiazepine Receptor Agonists

Generic Name (Brand Name)	t_{max} (hours)[a]	Half-Life[b] (hours)	Daily Dose Range (mg)	Metabolic Pathway	Clinically Significant Metabolites
Estazolam (ProSom)	2	12–15	1–2	Oxidation	–
Eszopiclone (Lunesta)	1–1.5	6	2–3	Oxidation	–
Flurazepam (Dalmane)	1	8	15–30	Demethylation Oxidation *N*-dealkylation	Hydroxyethylflurazepam, Flurazepam aldehyde N-desalkylflurazepam[c]
Quazepam (Doral)	2	39	7.5–15	Oxidation, *N*-dealkylation	2-Oxo-quazepam, N-desalkylflurazepam[c]
Temazepam (Restoril)	1.5	10–15	15–30	Conjugation	–
Triazolam (Halcion)	1	2	0.125–0.25	Oxidation	–
Zaleplon (Sonata)	1	1	5–10	Oxidation	–
Zolpidem (Ambien)	1.6	2–2.6	5–10	Oxidation	–

[a]Time to peak plasma concentration.
[b]Half-life of parent drug.
[c]*N*-desalkylflurazepam, mean half-life 47 to 100 hours.

Administration (FDA) labeled for the treatment of insomnia (Table 75–4). The benzodiazepine receptor agonists consist of the newer nonbenzodiazepine $GABA_A$ agonists and the traditional benzodiazepines. All benzodiazepine receptor agonists bind to $GABA_A$ receptors in the brain resulting in stimulatory effects on GABAergic transmission and hyperpolarization of neuronal membranes. Traditional benzodiazepines have sedative, anxiolytic, muscle relaxant, and anticonvulsant properties; newer nonbenzodiazepine GABA agonists possess only sedative properties.

Benzodiazepine Hypnotics

Benzodiazepines relieve insomnia by reducing sleep latency and increasing total sleep time. Benzodiazepines increase stage 2 sleep while decreasing REM, stage 3, and stage 4 sleep.[11] Benzodiazepines are very safe, and fatal overdoses are rare unless they are taken in combination with central nervous system (CNS) depressants or alcohol.[11] Benzodiazepine hypnotics should not be prescribed for individuals with sleep apnea, a history of substance abuse, or during pregnancy. Patients should be instructed to avoid alcohol and other CNS depressants.

Pharmacokinetics The choice of a particular benzodiazepine can be based on its pharmacokinetic profile. When used as a single dose, the extent of distribution and elimination half-life is important in predicting the duration of action. However, after multiple doses, the elimination half-life and formation of active metabolites determine the extent of drug accumulation and resultant clinical effects.[11] Elderly patients, liver dysfunction, and drug interactions can prolong drug effects. The pharmacokinetic profiles of benzodiazepine receptor agonists are summarized in Table 75–4.

Adverse Effects Side effects are dose dependent and vary according to the pharmacokinetics of the individual benzodiazepine. High doses with long or intermediate elimination half-lives have a greater potential for producing daytime sedation and performance impairment. These effects include excessive drowsiness, psychomotor incoordination, decreased concentration, and cognitive deficits. Tolerance to benzodiazepine hypnotic effects develops sooner with triazolam (after 2 weeks of continuous use) than with other benzodiazepine hypnotics.[11] Most traditional benzodiazepines maintain hypnotic efficacy for 1 month. However, tolerance can develop with time. Rapidly eliminated benzodiazepines have less potential for daytime sedation.[11]

Anterograde amnesia, an impairment of memory and recall of events occurring after the dose is taken, has been reported with most benzodiazepine receptor agonists.[11] Rebound insomnia is characterized by increased wakefulness beyond baseline amounts that last for one to two nights after abrupt discontinuation of benzodiazepine receptor agonists. Rebound insomnia occurs more frequently after high doses of triazolam, even when ingested intermittently.[11] The lowest effective dosage should be used to minimize rebound insomnia and avoid adverse effects on memory.

❸ Benzodiazepine half-lives are prolonged in older patients, increasing the potential for drug accumulation and the incidence of CNS side effects. Prolonged sedation and cognitive and psychomotor impairment are concerns in the elderly. Benzodiazepine receptor agonists with long elimination half-lives are generally not first-line agents. There is an association between falls and hip fractures and the use of benzodiazepines with long elimination half-lives; thus flurazepam and quazepam should be avoided in elderly patients.[21]

Non-Benzodiazepine $GABA_A$ Agonists

Zolpidem, zaleplon and eszopiclone are nonbenzodiazepine hypnotics that selectively bind to $GABA_A$ receptors and effectively induce sleepiness. Zolpidem, an imidazopyridine chemically unrelated to benzodiazepines or barbiturates, has a duration of action of 6 to 8 hours.[22] It is comparable in efficacy to benzodiazepine hypnotics, and is effective for reducing sleep latency and nocturnal awakenings and increasing total sleep time. It does not appear to have significant effects on next-day psychomotor performance. A sustained release formulation of zolpidem is now available that is effective at increasing total sleep time and reducing wakefulness after sleep onset without significant carryover sedation.

The safety and efficacy of zolpidem for insomnia is similar to that of the benzodiazepines. As with other sedative medications, treatment optimally should not exceed 4 weeks to minimize tolerance and dependence. Zolpidem is less disruptive of sleep stages than benzodiazepines. Adverse effects are dose related and can include drowsiness, amnesia, dizziness, headache, and gastrointestinal complaints.[22] Several cases of brief psychotic reactions have been reported in women, and recent reports of sleep-eating during zolpidem therapy have caused significant weight gain.[22] The recommended daily dose of zolpidem is 10 mg or 5 mg in elderly patients and those with hepatic impairment. The dosage can be increased to 20 mg per night.[22] Because food decreases its absorption, zolpidem should be taken on an empty stomach.[23]

Zaleplon is a pyrazolopyrimidine and has a rapid onset of action, a half-life of 1 hour, and is metabolized to inactive metabolites.[24] It is effective for decreasing time to sleep onset but not for reducing nighttime awakening or for increasing total sleep time.[25] Because of its short half-life, zaleplon has no effect on next-day psychomotor performance and can be best used as a sleep aid for middle-of-the-night awakenings.[26] The recommended dose is 10 mg in adults and 5 mg in the elderly.[24] The most common adverse effects with zaleplon are dizziness, headache, and somnolence. There are two drug interactions of note: zaleplon plasma levels are increased when combined with cimetidine and decreased with rifampin.[22]

Eszopiclone is a pyrrolopyrazine hypnotic with a rapid onset of action and a half-life of 5 to 6 hours.[27] It is effective at reducing time to sleep onset, wake time after sleep onset, number of awakenings and increasing total sleep time and sleep quality. Eszopiclone's duration of action is up to 6 hours,[27] so it can be a better option for treatment of sleep maintenance insomnia or early morning awakenings than zaleplon. The most common adverse effects with eszopiclone are somnolence, unpleasant taste, headache, and dry mouth.[28] Eszopiclone is labeled for long-term use and may be taken nightly for up to 6 months.[28]

Other Considerations

Rebound effects, withdrawal, and tolerance with prolonged use are minimal with zolpidem; however, theoretical concerns about abuse exist.[22] Zaleplon does not appear to cause rebound insomnia, and development of tolerance does not appear to be significant.[22] The incidence of rebound insomnia, tolerance, and withdrawal to eszopiclone has been reported to be minimal when taken nightly for 6 months.[28] In general, the nonbenzodiazepine hypnotics seem to be associated with less withdrawal, tolerance, and rebound insomnia than the benzodiazepine hypnotics. None of the $GABA_A$ agonists has significant active metabolites.

■ EVALUATION OF THERAPEUTIC OUTCOMES

An algorithm for the evaluation and treatment of sleep disorders is shown in Figure 75–1. Patients with short-term or chronic insomnia should be evaluated after 1 week of therapy to assess for drug efficacy, adverse effects, and adherence to nonpharmacologic recommendations. Patients should be instructed to keep a sleep diary. The diary requires daily recording of bedtime, wake time, latency of sleep onset, number and duration of awakenings, medication ingestion, naps, and an index of sleep quality. For patients with chronic insomnia, possible medical, psychiatric, and pharmacologic causes should be identified and managed.[11] Patients with insomnia should receive education about possible medication side effects and their management. Prescriptions for benzodiazepine receptor agonists should be accompanied by printed information and verbal counseling on precautions.

❹ Clinicians should educate patients about the concepts of tolerance, withdrawal, and rebound insomnia. Tolerance and dependence can be avoided by using hypnotics at the lowest possible dose, intermittently, and for the shortest duration possible. Patients should receive instruction on the initiation of therapy about frequency of drug use and the expected duration of therapy, to help prevent development of dependence. Withdrawal symptoms can be diminished by tapering the dosage gradually.

SLEEP APNEA

Approximately 15 million Americans have sleep-disordered breathing.[29] The prevalence of sleep apnea in the U.S. adult population is 4% in males and 2% in females.[30] It appears to be more common in African Americans and less common in Asian populations. Sleep apnea also occurs in children and adolescents. It is characterized by repetitive episodes of cessation of breathing during sleep followed by brief arousal from sleep to restart breathing. Blood oxygen desaturation can occur with these apneic episodes. As a result, individuals with sleep apnea experience fragmented sleep, poor sleep architecture, and

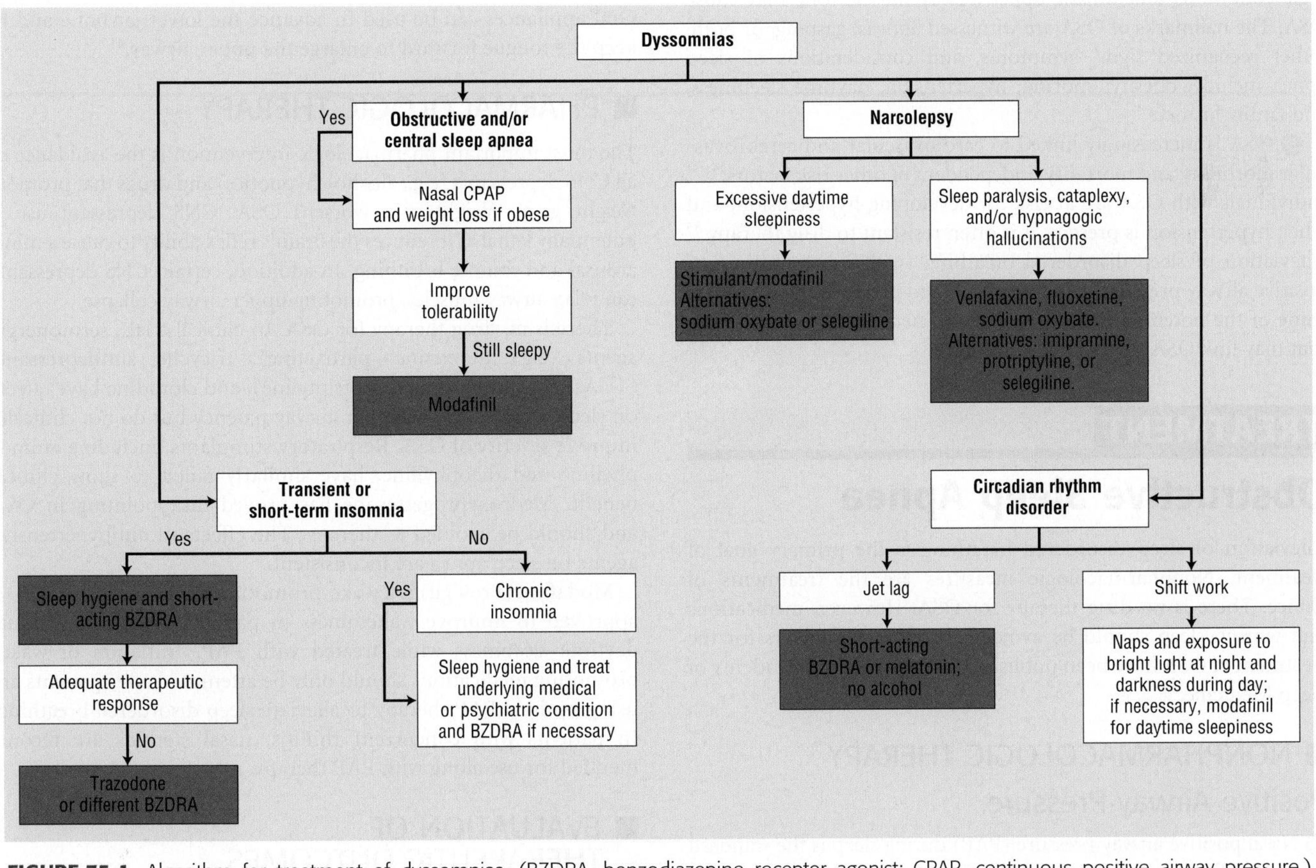

FIGURE 75-1. Algorithm for treatment of dyssomnias. (BZDRA, benzodiazepine receptor agonist; CPAP, continuous positive airway pressure.) *(Adapted with permission from the American College of Clinical Pharmacy. Jermaine DM. Sleep Disorders. In: Carter BL, Angaren DM, Lake KD, Raebel MA, eds. Pharmacotherapy Self-Assessment Program, 2nd ed. Psychiatry module. Kansas City: American College of Clinical Pharmacy, 1995:139–154.)*

periods of apnea and hypopnea. Polysomnography (PSG) is used to diagnose and quantify sleep apnea as central, obstructive, or mixed. Central sleep apnea (CSA) involves impairment of the respiratory drive, whereas obstructive sleep apnea (OSA) is caused by upper airway collapse and obstruction. Patients with mixed sleep apnea experience both central and obstructive sleep apnea. Severity of sleep apnea is determined by the number of apnea (total cessation of airflow) and hypopnea (partial airway closure with blood oxygen desaturation) episodes documented by PSG and is expressed by calculating the respiratory disturbance index (RDI). Mild sleep apneics have an RDI between 5 and 15 episodes per hour, moderate 15 to 30, whereas individuals with severe OSA can exhibit more than 30 episodes per hour.

Sleep apnea can affect behavior, cognitive abilities, and systemic disease.[31] Neurocognitive sequelae are important factors in motor vehicle accidents, loss of work-related productivity, and personality changes.[31,32] Alleviation of sleep disordered breathing can have a beneficial impact on both cardiovascular and neurobehavioral conditions.[33]

OBSTRUCTIVE SLEEP APNEA

OSA is characterized by partial or complete closure of the upper airway, posterior from the nasal septum to the epiglottis, during inspiration. The reason for the loss of upper airway patency is not fully understood and is likely caused by several competing factors. Anatomical factors including neck obesity, narrow airway, and fixed upper airway lesions (e.g., polyps, enlarged tonsils) can narrow the upper airway. Intraluminal negative pressure generated during each inspiration also promotes collapse of the upper airway. Airway anatomy and intraluminal negative pressure that tend to collapse the airway compete with dilating forces, primarily the pharyngeal dilator muscle. Acromegaly, amyloidosis, hypothyroidism as well as neurologic conditions that impair upper airway muscle tone may cause OSA. The hallmarks of OSA are witnessed apneas, gasping, or both. Other recognized signs, symptoms, and considerations of sleep apnea include, obesity, snoring, hypertension, daytime sleepiness, and family history.

❺ OSA is increasingly linked to cardiovascular and cerebrovascular morbidity and mortality, independent of other risk factors.[33,34] Individuals with OSA are at risk for developing hypertension, and when hypertension is present, it is often resistant to drug therapy.[35] Alleviation of sleep disordered breathing (with nasal continuous positive airway pressure) can improve blood pressure and attenuate some of the potential hemodynamic and neurohumoral responses that may link OSA to systemic disease.[36,37]

TREATMENT

Obstructive Sleep Apnea

Alleviation of sleep disordered breathing is the primary goal of treatment. Nonpharmacologic measures are the treatments of choice. There is no drug therapy for OSA. However, medications that worsen sleep should be avoided. Practice parameters for the treatment of OSA have been published by the American Academy of Sleep Medicine.[38]

■ NONPHARMACOLOGIC THERAPY

Positive Airway Pressure

❻ Nasal positive airway pressure (PAP) during sleep is the standard treatment for most patients with OSA. PAP produces a positive pressure column in the upper airway using room air to maintain patency. PAP can be continuous (CPAP) or bi-level PAP providing a reduced applied pressure during expiration. During PSG, the pressure setting is increased until sleep-disordered breathing is eliminated. Each pressure setting (range 1 to 20 cm H20) is individualized. Barriers to PAP adherence, such as ill-fitted mask and nasal dryness, can be managed. Nonadherence for one night results in a complete reversal of the gains made in daytime alertness.[39] CPAP machines are small enough to be transportable and sit at the bedside. A flexible tube connects the CPAP machine to a mask that covers the nose.

Weight Reduction

Obesity can worsen sleep apnea, and weight management should be implemented for all overweight patients with OSA. OSA can itself predispose to weight gain and in obese patients with mild OSA weight loss alone can be effective.[40] Individuals who are morbidly obese and have severe OSA can undergo gastric stapling for weight loss.

Surgery

Surgical therapy (uvulopalatopharyngoplasty) opens the upper airway by removing the tonsils, trimming and reorienting the posterior and anterior tonsillar pillars, and removing the uvula and posterior portion of the palate. This is not a first-line option because it is invasive. In very severe cases tracheostomy can be necessary. This procedure can be indicated for select individuals that are morbidly obese, have severe facial skeletal deformity, experience severe drops in oxygen saturation (e.g., less than 70%), or have significant cardiac arrhythmias associated with their OSA.

Other Therapies

For individuals that experience OSA only during certain position (e.g. on their back) during sleep, positional therapies can be effective alone but usually are used in conjunction with PAP therapy. Oral appliances can be used to advance the lower jawbone and to keep the tongue forward to enlarge the upper airway.[41]

■ PHARMACOLOGIC THERAPY

The most important pharmacologic intervention is the avoidance of all CNS depressants (e.g., alcohol, hypnotics) and drugs that promote weight gain. Weight gain worsens OSA. CNS depressant use is potentially lethal as it reduces the brain's reflex ability to cause a mini-arousal and resume breathing. In addition, certain CNS depressants can relax airway muscles, promoting upper airway collapse.

There is no drug therapy for OSA. In clinical trials, serotonergic agents (e.g., fluoxetine, paroxetine), tricyclic antidepressants (TCAs) (i.e., imipramine, protriptyline), and clonidine have effects on sleep architecture or upper airway patency but do not clinically improve severity of OSA. Respiratory stimulants, including aminophylline and theophylline, have similarly failed to show clinical benefit. Medroxyprogesterone has proved disappointing in OSA and should be avoided as therapy. The effects of antihypertensive agents on sleep apnea are inconsistent.[42]

Modafinil (Provigil) is a wake-promoting medication and is FDA approved to improve wakefulness in patients who have residual daytime sleepiness while treated with PAP. Initiation of wake-promoting medications should only be attempted after patients are using optimal PAP therapy to alleviate sleep disordered breathing. In patients with concurrent rhinitis, nasal steroids are recommended for use along with PAP therapy.

■ EVALUATION OF THERAPEUTIC OUTCOMES

Individuals with sleep apnea should be evaluated after 1 to 3 months of treatment for improvement in alertness and daytime symptoms (improvement in memory and decreased irritability) and weight reduction. Individuals experiencing symptoms (e.g., daytime sleepiness, snoring) despite PAP therapy should have PSG repeated. Symptoms can recur if patients gain weight, requiring a higher pressure setting. Conversely, PAP pressure settings can be decreased if weight loss is achieved. Patient adherence to PAP therapy can be monitored by assessing the built-in compliance meter that measures the hours used at effective pressure.

CENTRAL SLEEP APNEA

CSA causes fragmented sleep and consequent daytime somnolence. However, unlike OSA, arousals from sleep are not required to initiate airflow. During PSG, there is an absence of airflow out of the mouth and nose with no activation of the inspiratory muscles. The prevalence of CSA is not well established and is less than OSA. CSA can be idiopathic but more commonly is caused by underlying autonomic nervous system lesions (e.g., cervical cordotomy), neurologic diseases (e.g., poliomyelitis, encephalitis, and myasthenia gravis), high altitudes, and congestive heart failure.[42]

Potential underlying causes for CSA should be evaluated and treated. For example, worsening CSA in heart failure patients can signal the need to optimize heart failure therapies. Several medications for CSA have been studied. For example, acetazolamide induces a metabolic acidosis that stimulates respiratory drive. It has been shown to be beneficial in a small number of studies for high altitude, heart failure, and idiopathic CSA.[43,44] Currently, the primary treatment approach for CSA is PAP therapy with or without supplemental oxygen.[45]

NARCOLEPSY

Narcolepsy is a severely debilitating neurologic disease that affects approximately 140,000 Americans.[46] Despite the debilitating nature of the disease, it can be undiagnosed or misdiagnosed for years. Prevalence estimates differ between studies and range from 0.03% to 0.06% in the adult population.[46] It is equal or somewhat higher in men compared to women, and it has been noted in children and adolescents. However, it is commonly recognized in the second decade of life and increases in severity through the third and fourth decade.[46] Individuals with narcolepsy complain of excessive daytime sleepiness, with sleep attacks that last up to 30 minutes. In the sleep laboratory, individuals with narcolepsy exhibit impairment of both the onset and offset of REM and NREM sleep and have multiple arousals and disturbed sleep during the night.

Four characteristic symptoms differentiate narcolepsy from other sleep disorders and are known as the *narcolepsy tetrad*: sleep attacks, cataplexy, hypnagogic hallucinations, and sleep paralysis. Cataplexy, a sudden bilateral loss of muscle tone of varying severity and duration without the loss of consciousness, occurs in 70% to 80% of people with narcolepsy.[46] Patients can suffer subtle changes, such as jaw or head slumping, or severe weakness, such as knee buckling or collapsing to the ground. Cataplexy is often precipitated by situations characterized by high emotion (e.g., laughter, anger, excitement). Cataleptic episodes can be brief, lasting seconds or can last for several minutes. Sleep paralysis is an episodic loss of voluntary muscle tone that occurs when the individual is falling asleep or waking. Individuals are conscious but not able to move or speak. Hallucinations while falling asleep (i.e., hypnagogic) and on awakening (i.e., hypnopompic) are brief, dream-like experiences that intrude into wakefulness. Nearly 70% of narcoleptics experience these hallucinations. Unfortunately, these symptoms sometimes lead to an incorrect diagnosis of mental illness.[46] Cataplexy, sleep paralysis, and hypnagogic hallucinations can be caused by REM sleep disturbances.[47]

TABLE 75-5 Drugs Used to Treat Narcolepsy

Generic Name	Trade Name	Daily Dosage Range (mg)
Excessive daytime somnolence		
Dextroamphetamine	Dexedrine	5–60
Dextroamphetamine/Amphetamine salts[a]	Adderall	5–60
Methamphetamine[b]	Desoxyn	5–15
Methylphenidate	Ritalin	30–80
Modafinil	Provigil	200–400
Sodium oxybate[c]	Xyrem	4.5–9 grams per night
Adjunct agents for cataplexy		
Fluoxetine	Prozac	20–80
Imipramine	Tofranil	50–250
Nortriptyline	Aventyl, Pamelor	50–200
Protriptyline	Vivactil	5–30
Selegiline	Eldepryl	20–40

[a]Dextroamphetamine sulfate, dextroamphetamine saccharate, amphetamine aspartate, and amphetamine sulfate.
[b]Not available in some states.
[c]Also is effective at treating cataplexy.
Compiled from U.S. Modafinil in Narcolepsy Multicenter Study Group and Standard of Practice Committee of the American Sleep Disorders Association. Practice parameters for the use of stimulants in the treatment of narcolepsy. Sleep 1994;17:348–351.

The primary cause of narcolepsy is not known and can be caused by multiple external and internal factors. There can be a genetic component, as 3% of patients have a first-degree relative with the disorder.[47] The onset of disease in adolescence or adulthood, but not at birth, suggests that environmental influences might play a role. Molecular studies of human leukocyte antigen (HLA) have found a high prevalence of the HLA-DR2 and HLA-DQ6/DQB1 haplotypes in narcoleptics.[48] However, the HLA-DR2 haplotype is also common in the non-narcoleptic population and is not diagnostic.[47] The hypocretin-orexin neurotransmitter system has been implicated and can play a central role in narcolepsy. Neurons containing hypocretin-orexin are found in the lateral hypothalamus and project to various parts of the brain that are thought to regulate sleep. In 75% of narcoleptic patients, hypocretin-orexin is undetectable in cerebrospinal fluid.[48] Because narcoleptic patients have deficiencies in hypocretin-orexin–producing neurons,[49] an autoimmune process may be responsible for the destruction of hypocretin-producing cells.[50,51]

TREATMENT

Narcolepsy

Nonpharmacologic management of narcolepsy includes counseling the patient and family concerning the illness to alleviate misconceptions around the individual's behavior. Good sleep hygiene should be encouraged as well as two or more scheduled daytime naps. Daytime naps lasting 15 minutes each can help the individual with narcolepsy stay refreshed for several hours.

7 Pharmacologic management of narcolepsy is focused on two primary areas: treatment of excessive daytime sleepiness (EDS) and cataplexy. Drug therapy for narcolepsy is summarized in Table 75–5.

CLINICAL PRESENTATION OF NARCOLEPSY

Symptoms

- Patients may complain of excessive daytime sleepiness and disrupted nighttime sleep; often they have some accompanying REM sleep abnormality, sleep paralysis, cataplexy, and/or hallucinations.

Laboratory Tests

- Although not routinely tested, there is a high incidence of HLA haplotypes DR2 and HLA-DQ6/DQB1 in narcolepsy.

Other Diagnostic Tests

- Narcolepsy is definitively diagnosed using the multiple sleep latency test (nap test). The patient takes four to five naps in a day, and narcolepsy is diagnosed if the patient falls asleep quickly (within less than 5 minutes) and goes into REM sleep in two of those nap periods.

Modafinil, a racemic compound unrelated to psychostimulants, is a recognized standard treatment for EDS.[52] The precise mechanism of action of modafinil is not fully understood. It is readily absorbed, reaches peak plasma concentrations in 2 to 4 hours, and has a half-life of 15 hours. Common adverse effects are usually mild and include headache, nausea, nervousness, anxiety, and insomnia. The dose is between 200 and 400 mg/day.[53] Although modafinil is effective in treating EDS, it lacks efficacy for the treatment of cataplectic symptoms.[54]

EDS can also be treated with stimulants to improve alertness and to increase daytime performance. Dextroamphetamine and methylphenidate also have FDA approval for the treatment of narcolepsy. Methamphetamine has also been used on an off-label basis. Methylphenidate and amphetamines have a fast onset of action and durations of 6 to 10 and 3 to 4 hours, respectively. The dose can range from 5 to 60 mg daily. Many clinicians prescribe both immediate-release and sustained-release stimulants to increase alertness throughout the day. Sustained-release stimulants are prescribed with scheduled administration times, and immediate release stimulants can be taken as needed when the patient requires alertness (e.g., driving, etc.).

Stimulants improve alertness, increase daytime performance, can elevate mood and prevent sleep. Side effects can include insomnia, hypertension, palpitations, and irritability. Tolerance to long-term stimulant therapy can occur, necessitating dosage increases. Amphetamine use is associated with more likelihood of abuse and tolerance, especially when prescribed in high doses.

The most effective treatments for cataplexy are TCAs, venlafaxine, and fluoxetine. The mechanism of antidepressants in relieving cataplexy, hypnagogic hallucinations, and sleep paralysis can be mediated through blockade of serotonin and norepinephrine reuptake in the locus coeruleus and raphe and subsequent suppression of REM sleep.[55] Imipramine, protriptyline, clomipramine, fluoxetine, and nortriptyline are effective in approximately 80% of patients. Selegiline improves hypersomnolence and cataplexy through REM suppression and an increase in REM latency. The cost of the medication is high, and experience with the high doses needed for narcolepsy is limited. Methylphenidate and amphetamines alone are usually ineffective for cataplexy.

Sodium oxybate (γ-hydroxybutyrate, Xyrem) improves symptoms of EDS and decreases episodes of sleep paralysis, cataplexy, and hypnagogic hallucinations. Nightly administration of sodium oxybate changes sleep architecture to resemble normal sleep. It increases slow-wave sleep, decrease nighttime awakenings, and increases REM efficiency.[56] Sodium oxybate is available only as a liquid and is taken as two doses; one is taken at bedtime and the second dose is taken 2.5 to 4 hours later. Sodium oxybate is a potent sedative hypnotic and should not be used concomitantly with any other sedating medications. The most common side effects include nausea, somnolence, confusion, dizziness, and incontinence.

EVALUATION OF THERAPEUTIC OUTCOMES

The primary objective of pharmacologic treatment of narcolepsy is to reduce symptoms that adversely impact quality of life. The goal is to produce the fullest possible return of normal function for patients at work, school, home, and socially. Patients with narcolepsy should keep a diary of the frequency and severity of cataplexy, sleep paralysis, and sleep hallucinations. Patients should be evaluated regularly during medication titrations and then every 6 to 12 months to assess for adverse drug effects (e.g., sleep disturbances, and cardiovascular abnormalities). The health care provider should consider the benefit-to-risk ratio for the individual patient, the cost of medication, the convenience of administration, and cost of laboratory tests when selecting narcolepsy therapies.[52] One wake-promoting agent can work better than another in an individual patient. If the first agent is not successful at adequate doses, a trial with another agent should be attempted.

CIRCADIAN RHYTHM DISORDERS

The sleep-wake cycle is under the circadian control of oscillators and can be disrupted by misalignment between an individual's biologic clock and external demands on the sleep cycle. Circadian rhythm sleep disorders usually present with either insomnia or hypersomnia, depending on the individual's performance requirements. Two commonly occurring circadian rhythm sleep disorders are jet lag and shift work sleep problems.

JET LAG

Jet lag occurs when a person travels across time zones, and the external environmental time is mismatched with the internal circadian clock. Sleep disturbances typically last for 2 to 3 days, but can last as long as 7 to 10 days if the time zone changes are greater than 8 hours. Compared to westward travel, eastward travel is associated with a longer duration of jet lag. Jet lag leads to increased incidence of gastrointestinal disturbances and a decrease in alertness and performance.

❽ Treatment of jet lag includes nonpharmacologic approaches alone or in combination with drug therapy. Jet lag can be minimized in coast-to-coast travel in the United States if the duration is less than 7 days and the normal sleep-wake cycle is observed. For travel lasting longer than 7 days, jet lag severity can be lessened by 1- to 2-hour adjustments in sleep and wake times prior to departure to the destination time zone. Short-acting benzodiazepine receptor agonists or 0.5 to 5 mg melatonin taken at appropriate target bedtimes for east or west travel reduce jet lag and shorten sleep latency.[57]

SHIFT WORK SLEEP DISORDER

Shift workers comprise approximately 20% of the work force.[58] Night shift work causes a misalignment in the sleep-wake cycle and circadian rhythm that is associated with a decrease in alertness, performance, and quality of daytime sleep. More than 65% of workers on rotating shifts complain of insomnia, compared with only 20% who work one shift.[58] Shift workers ultimately are at risk of developing shift work sleep disorder (SWSD). SWSD is a complaint of insomnia or excessive sleepiness that occurs because of working shifts during normal sleep time.[7,59] Shift workers have a higher injury rate, rate of divorce, occurrence of on-the-job sleepiness, and incidence of substance use. Shift workers can also be at increased risk of developing peptic ulcers, heart disease, depression, breast cancer, and sleepiness-related accidents.[59–61] Night shift workers are usually in a state of permanent circadian misalignment because of the tendency to revert to conventional sleep schedules on their days off.[58]

Treatment for shift work sleep problems includes optimizing sleep hygiene, extending daytime sleep by sleeping in the afternoon, scheduling a 2- to 3-hour nap on days off from work, or switching to a day shift job. Short-acting benzodiazepine receptor agonists can consolidate sleep during day sleep periods and reduce lost sleep time.

Modafinil is FDA approved to improve wakefulness in patients with excessive daytime sleepiness associated with SWSD. Scheduled exposure to bright lights at night and darkness in the daytime improves adaptation to night work and daytime sleep.[58] Melatonin has also been used successfully.

RESTLESS LEGS SYNDROME

Restless legs syndrome (RLS), or Ekbom syndrome, is characterized by paresthesias that are usually felt deep in the calf muscles but also can appear in the thighs and arms with the urge to keep limbs in motion. RLS occurs in both males and females, and occurs more frequently in the elderly. It has been associated with chronic kidney disease, iron deficiency anemia, and pregnancy. Caffeine, stress, alcohol, and fatigue can worsen symptoms. Recent data suggest that RLS can be caused by iron deficiency in the substantia nigra in the CNS.[62] The diagnosis of RLS is based on patient or bed partner reported symptoms and specific diagnostic criteria. Criteria required to diagnose RLS are: (1) desire to move the limbs that is associated with paresthesias, (2) symptoms are worse in the evening or night, (3) symptoms are worsened by inactivity and are relieved by moving the affected limb, and (4) accompanying motor restlessness. The discomfort returns when the person tries to sleep, resulting in insomnia.[63]

❾ Dopamine agonists are effective for RLS and have replaced levodopa as first-line therapy.[64] Ropinirole and pramipexole are FDA approved for RLS, but rotigotine may also be effective.[64] Lower doses of dopamine agonists are used when treating RLS compared to Parkinson's disease. Levodopa therapy is associated with a high incidence of symptom augmentation and because of a short half-life, might not provide relief over the entire night. Augmentation is a worsening in symptom severity, increase in symptom distribution, or emergence of symptoms earlier in the evening. Sedative hypnotic agents can be effective in patients who have frequent awakenings from their RLS symptoms. Clonazepam at doses ranging from 0.5 mg to 2 mg has been most frequently studied, however, patients frequently experience carryover sedation because of its long duration of action. Shorter half-life sedative hypnotics (e.g., zolpidem, zaleplon, triazolam) can improve sleep and reduce daytime sleepiness without carryover sedation. Opiates such as methadone 5 to 20 mg, codeine 30 to 120 mg, and oxycodone 2.5 mg are very effective for patients with painful RLS. The potential for tolerance and dependence on opiate therapy should be considered. Gabapentin 300 to 900 mg near bedtime can also be considered for those with paresthetic or painful RLS symptoms.[65] Iron studies should be completed in patients with RLS and iron supplementation initiated in those that are iron deficient. In patients with ferritin concentrations less than 50 mcg/L, iron supplementation improves RLS symptoms. Patients with RLS or periodic limb movements of sleep should be evaluated regularly to monitor for excessive daytime somnolence, tolerance, efficacy, and adverse effects of the medication.

PERIODIC LEG MOVEMENTS OF SLEEP

RLS patients commonly have periodic limb movements during sleep (PLMS): approximately one-third of patients with PLMS have RLS.[64] PLMS are stereotypic, repetitive, periodic movements of the legs that occur during sleep every 20 to 40 seconds and last 10 minutes to several hours.[64] The movements usually involve the big toe, but the ankle, knee, and hip can also flex. They can be terminated by a violent kick or other body movement. Often patients will be unaware of these movements and only recognize consequent insufficient sleep and morning leg cramps. A bed partner can describe PLMS. PLMS is diagnosed in the sleep laboratory using electromyogram recordings. Bursts of muscle activity lasting 0.5 to 5 seconds that reoccur at least 40 times within 8 hours of sleep is diagnostic.[64]

PLMS can occur with RLS or alone because of systemic disease (e.g., renal failure) or drug therapy.[66] TCAs, SSRIs, dopaminergic antagonists, xanthines, nicotine, alcohol, and caffeine can all worsen PLMS. The treatment approach for PLMS is similar to that of RLS. If PLMS do not cause disruptions for the patient or bedpartner or daytime symptoms, they might not require treatment. Symptomatic or problematic PLMS should be treated with dopaminergic medications to suppress limb movements or sedative hypnotics to reduce awakenings and consolidate sleep.

PARASOMNIAS

Parasomnias are abnormal behavior or physiologic events that either occur during sleep or are exaggerated by sleep. Many of these disorders are considered to be disorders of partial arousal from various sleep stages. Parasomnias can be categorized as disorders of arousal (sleepwalking, sleep terrors), sleep-wake transition disorders (sleeptalking), rhythmic movement disorder, REM parasomnias (REM-behavior disorder), and miscellaneous parasomnias (enuresis, bruxism). Sleepwalking, sleep terrors and sleeptalking predominantly occur during NREM sleep whereas others (REM-behavior disorder) occur during REM sleep.

Sleepwalking and sleep terrors are found normally in children between the ages of 4 and 12 years and usually resolve in adolescence. These disorders are associated with psychopathology only if they persist into adulthood.[67] Sleep terrors can begin in adults between the ages of 20 and 30 years. Onset of sleepwalking in adults without a history of sleepwalking as children should prompt a search for a neurologic or substance-use condition.[67] Sleepwalking and sleep terror disorder involve intrusions of wakefulness into NREM sleep during the first third of the night. In sleepwalking, individuals become ambulatory, are difficult to awaken, and are amnestic for the event. Sleep terrors involve intense fear and autonomic arousal. Individuals are difficult to awaken, inconsolable, and amnestic for the event.[67]

Treatment of sleepwalking involves protecting the individual from harm by putting safety latches on doors and windows, removing hazardous objects from bedrooms, and covering glass doors with heavy curtains. In adult patients, benzodiazepines, SSRIs, or TCAs can be beneficial therapies for sleepwalking or other NREM disorders of arousal.[68] Benzodiazepines can also be helpful in curtailing sleep terrors in adults.[67] Nightmares are anxiety-provoking dreams characterized by vivid recall. Treatment is directed at reducing stress, anxiety, and sleep deprivation. In extreme cases, low-dose benzodiazepines can be indicated. Clonazepam is the treatment of choice for REM behavior disorder. Melatonin (3–12 mg at bedtime) can also be an effective therapy for REM behavior disorder.[69]

PHARMACOECONOMIC CONSIDERATIONS

Despite the prevalence of sleep disorders, most cases go undiagnosed and untreated. The direct cost of insomnia alone adds an estimated $13.9 billion to the national health care bill each year.[1,70] The direct and indirect costs of sleep disorders is estimated to be between $92.5 and $107.5 billion annually. Improvements in recognition and treatment can decrease the economic burden and prevent progression to both medical and psychiatric disorders.[70]

Quality of life can be improved by appropriate treatment. For example, treatment of OSA with PAP improves the number of years of good health by 5.5 quality-adjusted life years. Hypnotic therapy has also been found to markedly improve both the disorder and quality of life in shift workers.[70]

CONCLUSIONS

Disturbances of sleep affect approximately one-third of the population. Patients with sleep disorders should be accurately identified and diagnosed. Patients can have one or more concomitant sleep disorders. Unrecognized and poorly treated sleep disorders can worsen severity of and ability to effectively treat underlying systemic diseases. Effective management of sleep disorder(s) involves combined nonpharmacologic and pharmacologic treatment.

ACKNOWLEDGMENT

This chapter was authored by Cherry W. Jackson and Judy L. Curtis in the sixth edition of *Pharmacotherapy: A Pathophysiologic Approach*.

ABBREVIATIONS

CPAP: continuous positive airway pressure
CNS: central nervous system
CSA: central sleep apnea
EDS: excessive daytime sleepiness
EEG: electroencephalogram
FDA: Food and Drug Administration
GABA: γ-aminobutyric acid
HLA: human leukocyte antigen
NREM: nonrapid eye movement (sleep)
OSA: obstructive sleep apnea
PAP: positive airway pressure
PLMS: periodic limb movement during sleep
PSG: polysomnography
RDI: respiratory disturbance index
REM: rapid eye movement (sleep)
RLS: restless legs syndrome
SSRI: selective serotonin reuptake inhibitor
SWSD: shift work sleep disorder
TCA: tricyclic antidepressant

REFERENCES

1. Walsh JK, Engelhardt CL. The direct economic costs of insomnia in the United States for 1995. Sleep 1999;22:S386–S393.
2. Neylan TC, Reynolds CF, Kupfer DJ. Sleep disorders. In: Yudofsky SC, Hales RE, eds. American Psychiatric Press Textbook of Neuropsychiatry, 3rd ed. Washington, DC: American Psychiatric Press, 2000:583–606.
3. Gillin CJ, Seifritz E, Zoltoski RK, et al. Basic science of sleep. In: Sadock BJ, Sadock VA, eds. Kaplan and Sadock's Comprehensive Textbook of Psychiatry, 7th ed. Philadelphia, PA: Lippincott Williams & Wilkins, 2000:199–209.
4. Dagan Y, Abadi J. Sleep-wake disorder disability: A lifelong untreatable pathology of the circadian time structure. Chronobiol Int 2001;18:1019–1027.
5. Franken P. Long-term versus short-term processes regulating REM sleep. J Sleep Res 2002;11:17–28.
6. Stickgold R, Hobson JA, Fosse R, Fosse M. Sleep, learning and dreams: Off-line memory reprocessing. Science 2001;294:1052–1058.
7. American Sleep Disorders Association. International Classification of Sleep Disorders: Diagnostic and Coding Manual: Revised Addition. Rochester, MN: American Sleep Disorders Association, 1997.
8. American Psychiatric Association. Sleep disorders. In: Diagnostic and Statistical Manual of Mental Disorders, 4th ed., text revision. Washington, DC: American Psychiatric Press, 2000:597–644.
9. Shocat T, Umphress J, Isreal AG, Ancoli-Israel S. Insomnia in primary care patients. Sleep 1999;22(Suppl 2):S359–S365.
10. Chesson AL, Anderson WM, Littner M, et al. Practice parameters for the nonpharmacologic treatment of chronic insomnia. Sleep 1999;8:1–6.
11. Kirkwood CK. Management of insomnia. J Am Pharm Assoc 1999;39:688–696.
12. Sateia MJ, Doghramji K, Hauri PJ, et al. Evaluation of chronic insomnia. Sleep 2000;23:1–39.
13. Lippmann S, Mazour I, Shabab H. Insomnia: Therapeutic approach. South Med J 2001;94:866–874.
14. Vaughn-McCall W. A psychiatric perspective on insomnia. J Clin Psychiatr 2001;62(Suppl 10):27–32.
15. Espie C. Insomnia: Conceptual issues in the development, persistence and treatment of sleep disorders in adults. Annu Rev Psychol 2002;53:215–243.
16. Chesson A, Hartse K, McDowell-Anderson W. Practice parameters for the evaluation of chronic insomnia. Sleep 2000;23:1–5.
17. Sivertsen B, Omvik S, Pallesen S, et al. Cognitive behavioral therapy vs zopiclone for treatment of chronic primary insomnia in older adults: A randomized controlled trial. JAMA 2006;295:2851–2858.
18. Hauri PJ. Insomnia. Clin Chest Med 1998;19:157–168.
19. Jackson CW. Mood disorders. In: Mueller BA, ed. Pharmacotherapy Self Assessment Program (PSAP). Kansas City, MO: American College of Clinical Pharmacy, 2002:203–250.
20. Schulz V, Hansel R, Tyler VE. Rational Phytotherapy. A Physician's Guide to Herbal Medicine. Berlin: Springer, 1998:81.
21. Ancoli-Isreal S. Insomnia in the elderly: A review for the primary care practitioner. Sleep 2000;23:S23–S30.
22. Terzano MG, Rossi M, Palomba V, et al. New drugs for insomnia: Comparative tolerability of zopiclone, zolpidem and zaleplon. Drug Saf 2003;26:261–282.
23. Ambien, zolpidem [product information]. Bridgewater, NJ: Sanofi-Aventis, 2006.
24. Elie R, Ruteher E, Farr IK, et al. Sleep latency is shortened during 4 weeks of treatment with zaleplon, a novel nonbenzodiazepine hypnotic. J Clin Psychiatry 1999;60:536–544.
25. Walsh JK, Fry J, Erwin CS, et al. Efficacy and tolerability of 14-day administration of zaleplon 5 mg and 10 mg for the treatment of primary insomnia. Clin Drug Investig 1998;16:347–354.
26. Walsh JK, Pollack CP, Shark MMB, et al. Lack of residual sedation following middle-of-the-night zaleplon administration in sleep maintenance insomnia. Clin Neuropharmacol 2000;23:17–21.
27. Lunesta, eszopiclone [product information]. Marlborough, MA: Sepracor, 2005.
28. Krystal AD, Walsh JK, Laska E, et al. Sustained efficacy of eszopiclone over 6 months of nightly treatment: results of a randomized, double-blind, placebo-controlled study in adults with chronic insomnia. Sleep 2003;26:793–797.
29. Young T, Peppard PE, Gottlieb DJ. Epidemiology of obstructive sleep apnea: a population health perspective. Am J Respir Crit Care Med 2002;165:1217–1239.
30. Young T, Palta M, Dempsey J, et al. The occurrence of sleep-disordered breathing among middle-aged adults. N Engl J Med 1993;328:1230–1235.
31. Peppard PE, Szklo-Coxe M, Hla KM, Young T. Longitudinal Association of Sleep-Related Breathing Disorder and Depression. Arch Intern Med 2006;166:1709–1715.
32. Terán-Santos J, Jimenez-Gomez A, Cordero-Guevara J for The Cooperative Group Burgos–Santander. The association between sleep apnea and the risk of traffic accidents. N Engl J Med 1999;340:847–851.
33. Marin JM, Carrizo SJ, Vicente E, et al. Long-term cardiovascular outcomes in men with obstructive sleep apnoea-hypopnoea with or without treatment with continuous positive airway pressure: an observational study. Lancet 2005;365:1046–1053.
34. Yaggi HK, Concato J, Kernan WN, et al. Obstructive sleep apnea as a risk factor for stroke and death. N Engl J Med 2005;353:2034–2041.
35. Phillips BG, Somers VK. Sleep disordered breathing and risk for cardiovascular disease. Curr Opin Pulm Med 2002;8:516–520.

36. Becker HF, Jerrentrup A, Ploch T, et al. Effect of nasal continuous positive airway pressure treatment on blood pressure in patients with obstructive sleep apnea. Circulation 2003;107:68–73.
37. Kato M, Roberts-Thomson P, Phillips BG, et al. Impairment of endothelium dependent vasodilation of resistance vessels in patients with obstructive sleep apnea. Circulation 2000;102:2607–2610.
38. Morganthaler TI, Kapen S, Lee-Chiong T, et al. Practice parameters for the medical therapy of obstructive sleep apnea. Sleep 2006;29:1031–1035.
39. Kribbs NB, Pack AJ, Kline LR, et al. Effects of one night without nasal CPAP treatment on sleep and sleepiness in patients with obstructive sleep apnea. Am Rev Respir Dis 2003;147:1162–1168.
40. Peppard PE, Young T, Palta M, et al. Longitudinal study of moderate weight change and sleep-disordered breathing. JAMA 2000;284:3015–3021.
41. Gotsopoulos H, Chen C, Qian J, et al. Oral appliance therapy improves symptoms in obstructive sleep apnea: A randomized, controlled trial. Am J Respir Crit Care Med 2002;166:743–748.
42. Grunstein RR, Hedner J, Grote L. Treatment options for sleep apnea. Drugs 2001;61:237–251.
43. Javaheri S. Acetazolamide improves central sleep apnea in heart failure: A double-blind, prospective study. Am J Respir Crit Care Med 2006;172:234–237.
44. White DP, Zwillich CS, Pickett CK, et al. Central sleep apnea improvement with acetazolamide therapy. Arch Intern Med 1982;182:1816–1819.
45. Naughton MT, Bradley TD. Sleep apnoea in congestive heart failure. Clin Chest Med 1998;19:99–113.
46. Mitler M, Hayduk R. Benefits and risks of pharmacotherapy for narcolepsy. Drug Saf 2002;25:791–809.
47. Nakayama J, Miura M, Honda M, et al. Linkage of human narcolepsy with HLA association to chromosome 4p-13-q21. Genomics 2000;65:84–86.
48. Nishin S, Ripley B, Overeem S, et al. Low cerebrospinal fluid hypocretin (orexin) and altered energy homeostasis in human narcolepsy. Ann Neurol 2001;50:381–388.
49. Thannicakal TC, Moore RY, Nienhuis R, et al. Reduced number of hypocretin neurons in human narcolepsy. Neuron 2000;27:469–474.
50. Lin L, Hungs M, Mignot E. Narcolepsy and the HLA region. J Neuroimmunol 2001;117:9–20.
51. Mignot E, Thorsby E. Narcolepsy and the HLA system (letter). N Engl J Med 2001;344:692.
52. Littner M, Johnson SF, McCall WV, et al. Practice parameters for the treatment of narcolepsy: An update for 2000. Sleep 2001;24:451–466.
53. Robertson P, Hellriegel ET. Clinical pharmacokinetic profile of modafinil. Clin Pharmacokinet 2003;42:123–127.
54. Feldman N. Narcolepsy. South Med J 2003;96:277–287.
55. Rosenthal MS. Physiology and neurochemistry of sleep. Am J Pharm Educ 1998;62:204–208.
56. Mamelak M, Black J, Montplaisir J, et al. A pilot study of the effects of sodium oxybate on sleep architecture and daytime alertness in narcolepsy. Sleep 2004;27:1327–1334.
57. Herxheimer A, Petrie KJ, Cochrane Depression, Anxiety and Neurosis Group. Melatonin for the prevention and treatment of jet lag. [systematic review]. Cochrane Database Syst Rev 2005;4.
58. Garbarino S, Nobili L, Beelke, M, et al. Sleep disorders and daytime sleepiness in state police shiftworkers. Arch Environ Health 2002;57:167–175.
59. Drake CL, Roehrs T, Richardson G, et al. Shift work sleep disorder: Prevalence and consequences beyond that of symptomatic day workers. Sleep 2004;27:1453–1462.
60. Knutsson A. Health disorders of shift workers. Occup Med (Lond) 2003;53:103–108.
61. Kawachi I, Colditz GA, Stampfer MJ, et al. Prospective study of shift work and risk of coronary heart disease in women. Circulation 1995;92:3178–3182.
62. Connor JR, Boyer PJ, Menzies SL, et al. Neuropathological examination suggests impaired brain iron acquisition in restless legs syndrome. Neurology 2003;61:304–309.
63. Saletu M, Anderer P, Saletu G, et al. Acute placebo-controlled sleep laboratory studies and clinical follow-up with pramipexole in restless legs syndrome. Eur Arch Psychiatry Clin Neurosci 2002;252:185–194.
64. Hening WA, Allen RP, Earley CJ, et al., Restless Legs Syndrome Task Force of the Standards of Practice Committee of the American Academy of Sleep Medicine. An update on the dopaminergic treatment of restless legs syndrome and periodic limb movement disorder. Sleep 2004;27:560–583.
65. Garcia-Borreguero D, Larrosa O, de la Llave Y, et al. Treatment of restless legs syndrome with gabapentin: A double-blind, cross-over study. Neurology 2002;59:1573–1575.
66. Montplaisir J, Nicolas A, Denesle R, Gomez-Mancilla B. Restless legs syndrome improved by pramipexole: A double-blind randomized trial. Neurology 1999;52:938–943.
67. Schenck CH, Mahowald MW. Parasomnias managing bizarre sleep-related behavior disorders. Postgrad Med 2000;107:145–156.
68. Mahowald MW. NREM sleep-arousal parasomnias. In: Kryger MH, Roth T, Dement WC, eds. Principles and Practice of Sleep Medicine, 4th ed. Philadelphia, PA: Elsevier Saunders, 2005:889–896.
69. Mahowald MW, Schenck CH. REM sleep parasomnias. In: Kryger MH, Roth T, Dement WC, eds. Principles and Practice of Sleep Medicine, 4th ed. Philadelphia, PA: Elsevier Saunders, 2005:897–916.
70. Leger D. Public health and insomnia: Economic impact. Sleep 2000;23(Suppl 3):S69–S76.

CHAPTER 76 Developmental Disabilities

NANCY BRAHM, JERRY MCKEE, AND ROBERT C. BROWN

KEY CONCEPTS

1. Behavioral therapies, education, and pharmacologic treatment are complementary and should be integrated as part of a multimodal treatment approach in persons with developmental disabilities and concomitant behavioral issues.
2. Persons diagnosed with Down syndrome can be at increased risk for medical and psychiatric comorbidities.
3. When treating autism, objective and measurable outcome monitoring of psychoactive medication-responsive target behaviors is critical because of the variable response of individuals to medication therapy.
4. Many purported treatments for autism have limited or no evidence supporting their use. The use of such strategies should be discouraged, as many effective treatments exist.
5. Goals of treatment in persons with autism are to increase social interactions, improve verbal and nonverbal communication, and minimize the occurrence or impact of ritualistic repetitive behaviors and other related mood and behavior problems (e.g., overactivity, irritability, self-injury).
6. A structured approach to teaching, which focuses on increasing social communication and understanding and fosters integration with peers, is the treatment most highly correlated with improvement in persons with autism.
7. Although no medication has been shown to be universally effective, psychopharmacologic treatment in autism is effective and should be targeted at specific well-defined behavioral symptoms.
8. Rett's syndrome is characterized by the onset of developmental regression that occurs in four stages.

INTRODUCTION

Developmental disabilities and mental retardation can be identified in childhood or adolescence. Current criteria for a diagnosis of mental retardation are based on deficiencies in intellectual and adaptive functioning with an onset prior to 18 years of age.[1,2] This diagnosis is made regardless of the presence or absence of concomitant medical or psychiatric disorders. In the case of mild mental retardation, deficiencies may not be initially apparent. Problems can be noted when the chronologic age of the child and the developmental milestones achieved by peers with similar backgrounds, cultures, and socioeconomic and psychosocial settings differ significantly.[1] These gaps widen as the individual ages.

The complete chapter, learning objectives, and other resources can be found at **www.pharmacotherapyonline.com.**

❶ Adaptive functioning deficits pose a number of challenges in treating those with a developmental disability (DD). This population can be four to five times more likely to experience mental health problems compared to the general population.[3] Until recently, little attention was given to this population and the need to evaluate them for psychiatric illnesses, leading to underrecognition of psychopathology. This oversight is a function of several factors, including limited, population-specific training for clinicians and a general lack of clinical contact with developmentally disabled individuals during training.[3] Additional barriers are patient-related deficits in expressive and receptive language, combined with a lack of mental health screening and diagnostic testing instruments specific to developmentally disabled adults.[3]

Those with developmental disabilities often have fewer social interactions and less integration into the community. In the absence of stimulation and interaction with peers that typically shapes behaviors in persons with normal intellect, a different set of coping skills can functionally evolve. An example is self-talk, which can represent such a coping mechanism in some persons with DD. This behavior can be misinterpreted by some as psychosis. Another potential problem for the clinician assessing persons with DD is a significant deficit between receptive language skills and expressive language skills. If not readily recognized, intellectual capabilities can be overestimated, and coping skills can be inadequate to deal with demands placed on the individual. This can result in anxiety-induced decompensation.[3]

In the general population, features of psychiatric illnesses are more readily identifiable, and the clinician is able to interview and evaluate the patient, as indicated. The term "diagnostic overshadowing" has been used to refer to clinician perception of behavioral problems thought to be secondary to mental retardation, which can actually be caused by a mental illness. Diagnostic overshadowing can therefore result in underestimating the clinical significance of the emotional and behavioral presentation as the deficits are inaccurately associated with a diagnosis of mental retardation.[3] This chapter will focus on three syndromes that are commonly seen in persons with developmental disabilities: Down syndrome, autistic disorder, and Rett's syndrome. In discussing these three syndromes, a broader perspective of issues encountered in persons with DD will be reviewed.

SECTION 8
ENDOCRINOLOGIC DISORDERS

CHAPTER 77

Diabetes Mellitus

CURTIS L. TRIPLITT, CHARLES A. REASNER, AND WILLIAM L. ISLEY

KEY CONCEPTS

1. Diabetes mellitus is a group of metabolic disorders of fat, carbohydrate, and protein metabolism that results from defects in insulin secretion, insulin action (sensitivity), or both.

2. The incidence of type 2 diabetes mellitus (DM) is increasing. This has been attributed in part to a Western style diet, increasing obesity, sedentary lifestyle, and an increasing minority population.

3. The two major classifications of DM are type 1 (insulin deficient) and type 2 (combined insulin resistance and relative deficiency in insulin secretion). They differ in clinical presentation, onset, etiology, and progression of disease. Both are associated with microvascular and macrovascular disease complications.

4. Diagnosis of diabetes is made by three criteria: fasting plasma glucose ≥126 mg/dL, a 2-hour value from a 75-g oral glucose tolerance test ≥200 mg/dL, or a casual plasma glucose level of ≥200 mg/dL with symptoms of diabetes; with results confirmed by any of the three criteria on a separate day.

5. Goals of therapy in diabetes mellitus are directed toward attaining normoglycemia, reducing the onset and progression of retinopathy, nephropathy, and neuropathy complications, intensive therapy for associated cardiovascular risk factors, and improving quality and quantity of life.

6. Metformin should be included in the therapy for all type 2 DM patients, if tolerated and not contraindicated, as it is the only oral antihyperglycemic medication proven to reduce the risk of total mortality, according to the United Kingdom Prospective Diabetes Study (UKPDS).

7. Intensive glycemic control is paramount for reduction of microvascular complications (neuropathy, retinopathy, and nephropathy) as evidenced by the Diabetes Control and Complications Trial (DCCT) in type 1 DM and the UKPDS in type 2 DM. The UKPDS also reported that control of hypertension in patients with diabetes will not only reduce the risk of retinopathy and nephropathy but also reduce cardiovascular risk.

8. Knowledge of the patient's quantitative and qualitative meal patterns, activity levels, pharmacokinetics of insulin preparations, and pharmacology of oral and injected antihyperglycemic agents are essential to individualize the treatment plan and optimize blood glucose control while minimizing risks for hypoglycemia and other adverse effects of pharmacologic therapies.

9. Type 1 treatment necessitates insulin therapy. Currently, the basal-bolus insulin therapy or pump therapy in motivated individuals often leads to successful glycemic outcomes. Basal-bolus therapy includes a basal insulin for fasting and postabsorptive control, and rapid-acting bolus insulin for mealtime coverage. Addition of pramlintide in patients with uncontrolled or erratic postprandial glycemia can be warranted, if the patient is willing to inject additional times before each meal.

10. Treatment of type 2 DM often necessitates use of multiple therapeutic agents (combination therapy), including oral and/or injected antihyperglycemics and insulin to obtain glycemic goals.

11. Aggressive management of cardiovascular disease risk factors in type 2 DM is necessary to reduce the risk for adverse cardiovascular events or death. Smoking cessation, use of antiplatelet therapy as a primary prevention strategy, aggressive management of dyslipidemia minimally toward a goal of low-density lipoprotein-cholesterol (LDLC) at <100 mg/dL and secondarily to increase high-density lipoprotein-cholesterol (HDLC) to ≥40 mg/dL, and treatment of hypertension (again often requiring multiple drugs) minimally to attain a blood pressure of <130/80 mm Hg are vital.

12. Prevention strategies for type 1 DM have been unsuccessful. Prevention strategies for type 2 DM are established. Lifestyle changes, dietary restriction of fat, aerobic exercise for 30 minutes five times a week, and weight loss, form the backbone of successful prevention. No medication is currently FDA approved for prevention of diabetes, although several, including metformin and rosiglitazone, have evidence of potential delay of the onset of diabetes.

Learning objectives, review questions, and other resources can be found at **www.pharmacotherapyonline.com.**

13 Patient education and ability to demonstrate self-care and adherence to therapeutic lifestyle and pharmacologic interventions are crucial to successful outcomes. Multidisciplinary teams of healthcare professionals including physicians (primary care, endocrinologists, ophthalmologists, and vascular surgeons), podiatrists, dietitians, nurses, pharmacists, social workers, behavioral health specialists, and certified diabetes educators are needed to optimize these outcomes in persons with diabetes mellitus.

1 DM is a group of metabolic disorders characterized by hyperglycemia. It is associated with abnormalities in carbohydrate, fat, and protein metabolism and results in chronic complications including microvascular, macrovascular, and neuropathic disorders. Nearly 20.8 million Americans have DM, yet only approximately two-thirds of them have been diagnosed.[1] The economic burden of DM approximated $132 billion in 2002, including direct medical and treatment costs as well as indirect costs attributed to disability and mortality.[1] DM is the leading cause of blindness in adults aged 20 to 74 years, and the leading contributor to development of end-stage renal disease. It also accounts for approximately 82,000 lower extremity amputations annually.[1] Finally, a cardiovascular event is responsible for two-thirds of deaths in individuals with type 2 DM.[1]

Although efforts to control hyperglycemia and associated symptoms are important, the major challenges in optimally managing the patient with DM are targeted at reducing or preventing complications, and improving life expectancy and quality of life. Research and drug development efforts over the past several decades have provided valuable information that applies directly to improving outcomes in patients with DM and have expanded the therapeutic armamentarium. Additionally, interventions in an attempt to prevent disease in high-risk populations have been reported for type 1 and 2 DM.

EPIDEMIOLOGY

Typical type 1 DM is an autoimmune disorder developing in childhood or early adulthood, although some latent forms do occur. Type 1 DM accounts for 5% to 10% of all cases of DM and is likely initiated by the exposure of a genetically susceptible individual to an environmental agent.[2] Candidate genes and environmental factors are reportedly prevalent in the general population, but development of β-cell autoimmunity occurs in less than 10% of the genetically susceptible population and progresses to type 1 DM in less than 1% of the population.[3]

The prevalence of β-cell autoimmunity appears proportional to the incidence of type 1 DM in various populations. For instance, the countries of Sweden, Sardinia, and Finland have the highest prevalence of islet cell antibody (3% to 4.5%) and are associated with the highest incidence of type 1 DM, 22 to 35 per 100,000.[4]

Markers of autoimmunity have been detected in 14% to 33% of persons with type 2 DM in some populations and manifest with early failure of oral agents and insulin dependence. This type of DM has also been referred to as latent autoimmune diabetes of adults (LADA).[4]

Type 1 DM idiopathic is a nonimmune form of diabetes frequently seen in minorities with intermittent insulin requirements.[5] The prevalence of type 1 DM has been increasing over the last 100 years.[6] Maturity-onset diabetes of youth (MODY), which can be caused by one of at least six genetic defects, and endocrine disorders such as acromegaly and Cushing syndrome, can be secondary causes of DM.[7] These unusual etiologies, however, only account for 1% to 2% of the total cases of type 2 DM. See the section on Other Specific Types of Diabetes later in this chapter for further discussion.

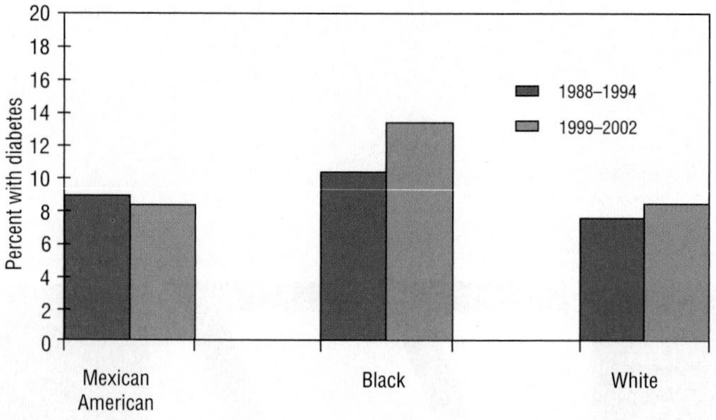

FIGURE 77-1. National Health and Nutrition Evaluation Survey (NHANES) prevalence of diabetes by race among adults ≥20 years of age: United States, 1988–1994 and 1999–2002. *(Adapted from Cowie et al.[9])*

2 The prevalence of type 2 DM is increasing. Type 2 DM accounts for as much as 90% of all cases of DM, and the overall the prevalence of type 2 DM in the United States is approximately 9.6% in persons age 20 years or older. However, there is likely one person undiagnosed for every three persons currently diagnosed with the disease.[1] Multiple risk factors for the development of type 2 DM have been identified, including family history (i.e., parents or siblings with diabetes); obesity (i.e., ≥20% over ideal body weight, or body mass index [BMI] ≥25 kg/m^2); habitual physical inactivity; race or ethnicity; previously identified impaired glucose tolerance or impaired fasting glucose (see Diagnosis of Diabetes section); hypertension (≥140/90 mm Hg in adults); high-density lipoprotein (HDL) cholesterol ≤35 mg/dL and/or a triglyceride level ≥250 mg/dL; history of gestational DM (see Classification of Diabetes section) or delivery of a baby weighing >4 kg (9 lb); history of vascular disease; presence of acanthosis nigricans; and polycystic ovary disease.[8] The prevalence of type 2 DM increases with age, it is more common in women than in men in the United States, and varies widely among various racial and ethnic populations, being especially increased in some groups of Native Americans, Hispanic American, Asian American, African American, and Pacific Island people[9] (Fig. 77–1). Although the prevalence of type 2 DM increases with age (Fig. 77–2),[9] the disorder is increasingly being recognized in adolescence. Much of the increase in adolescent type 2 DM is related to an increase in adiposity and sedentary lifestyle, in addition to an inheritable predisposition.[10] Most cases of type 2 DM do not have a well-known cause; therefore it is uncertain whether it represents a few or many independent disorders manifesting as hyperglycemia.[11]

Gestational diabetes mellitus (GDM) complicates roughly 7% of all pregnancies in the United States.[12] Most women will return to

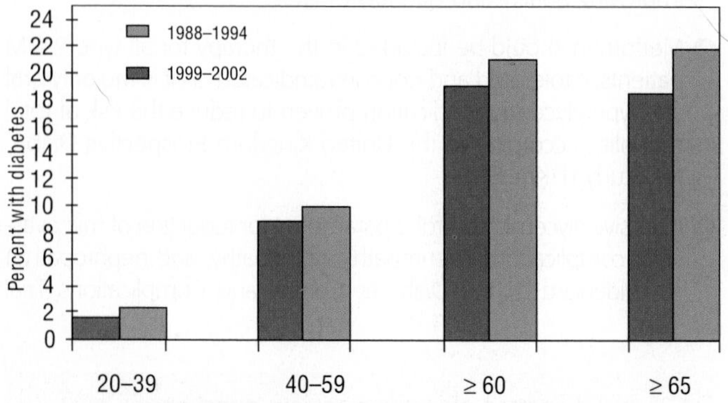

FIGURE 77-2. National Health and Nutrition Evaluation Survey (NHANES) prevalence of diabetes mellitus in United States by age (≥20 years of age) 1988–1994 and 1999–2002. *(Adapted from Cowie et al.[9])*

normoglycemia postpartum, but 30% to 50% will develop type 2 DM or glucose intolerance later in life.

PATHOGENESIS, DIAGNOSIS, AND CLASSIFICATION

CLASSIFICATION OF DIABETES

Diabetes is a metabolic disorder characterized by resistance to the action of insulin, insufficient insulin secretion, or both.[13] The clinical manifestation of these disorders is hyperglycemia. The vast majority of diabetic patients are classified into one of two broad categories: type 1 diabetes caused by an absolute deficiency of insulin, or type 2 diabetes defined by the presence of insulin resistance with an inadequate compensatory increase in insulin secretion. Women who develop diabetes because of the stress of pregnancy are classified as having gestational diabetes. Finally, uncommon types of diabetes caused by infections, drugs, endocrinopathies, pancreatic destruction, and known genetic defects are classified separately (Table 77–1).

Type 1 Diabetes

❸ This form of diabetes results from autoimmune destruction of the β cells of the pancreas. Markers of immune destruction of the β cell are present at the time of diagnosis in 90% of individuals and include islet cell antibodies, antibodies to glutamic acid decarboxylase, and antibodies to insulin. Although this form of diabetes usually occurs in children and adolescents, it can occur at any age. Younger individuals typically have a rapid rate of β-cell destruction and present with ketoacidosis, whereas adults often maintain sufficient insulin secretion to prevent ketoacidosis for many years, which is often referred to as LADA.[4]

Type 2 Diabetes

❸ This form of diabetes is characterized by insulin resistance and a relative lack of insulin secretion, with progressively lower insulin secretion over time. Most individuals with type 2 diabetes exhibit abdominal obesity, which itself causes insulin resistance. In addition, hypertension, dyslipidemia (high triglyceride levels and low HDL-cholesterol levels), and elevated plasminogen activator inhibitor type 1 (PAI-1) levels are often present in these individuals. This clustering of abnormalities is referred to as the *insulin resistance syndrome* or the *metabolic syndrome*. Because of these abnormalities, patients with type 2 diabetes are at increased risk of developing macrovascular complications. Type 2 diabetes has a strong genetic predisposition and is more common in all ethnic groups other than those of European ancestry. At this point the genetic cause of most cases of type 2 diabetes is not well defined.[14]

TABLE 77-1 Etiologic Classification of Diabetes Mellitus

1. Type 1 diabetes[a] (β-cell destruction, usually leading to absolute insulin deficiency)
- Immune mediated
- Idiopathic

2. Type 2 diabetes[a] (can range from predominantly insulin resistance with relative insulin deficiency to a predominantly insulin secretory defect with insulin resistance)

3. Other specific types
- Genetic defects of β-cell function
  - Chromosome 20q, HNF-4α (MODY1)
  - Chromosome 7p, glucokinase (MODY2)
  - Chromosome 12q, HNF-1β (MODY3)
  - Chromosome 13q, insulin promoter factor (MODY4)
  - Chromosome 17q, HNF-1β (MODY5)
  - Chromosome 2q, neurogenic differentiation 1/b-cell e-box transactivator 2 (MODY6)
  - Mitochondrial DNA
  - Others
- Genetic defects in insulin action
  - Type 1 insulin resistance
  - Leprechaunism
  - Rabson-Mendenhall syndrome
  - Lipoatrophic diabetes
  - Others
- Diseases of the exocrine pancreas
  - Pancreatitis
  - Trauma/pancreatectomy
  - Neoplasia
  - Cystic fibrosis
  - Hemochromatosis
  - Fibrocalculous pancreatopathy
  - Others
- Endocrinopathies
  - Acromegaly
  - Cushing's syndrome
  - Glucagonoma
  - Pheochromocytoma
  - Hyperthyroidism
  - Somatostatinoma
  - Aldosteronoma
  - Others
- Drug- or chemical-induced
  - Vacor (pyriminil)
  - Pentamidine
  - Nicotinic acid
  - Glucocorticoids
  - Thyroid hormone
  - Diazoxide
  - β-Adrenergic agonists
  - Thiazides
  - Phenytoin
  - Interferon alpha
  - Others
- Infections
  - Congenital rubella
  - Cytomegalovirus
  - Others
- Uncommon forms of immune-mediated diabetes
  - "Stiff-man" syndrome
  - Anti-insulin receptor antibodies
  - Others
- Other genetic syndromes sometimes associated with diabetes
  - Down's syndrome
  - Klinefelter's syndrome
  - Turner's syndrome
  - Wolfram's syndrome
  - Friedreich's ataxia
  - Huntington's chorea
  - Laurence-Moon-Biedel syndrome
  - Myotonic dystrophy
  - Porphyria
  - Prader-Willi syndrome
  - Others

4. Gestational diabetes mellitus (GDM)

[a]Patients with any form of diabetes can require insulin treatment at some stage of their disease. Such use of insulin does not in itself classify the patient.

Adapted with permission from Report of the Expert Committee.[13]

Gestational Diabetes Mellitus

GDM is defined as glucose intolerance that is first recognized during pregnancy. Gestational diabetes complicates approximately 7% of all pregnancies. Clinical detection is important, as therapy will reduce perinatal morbidity and mortality.

Other Specific Types of Diabetes

Genetic Defects MODY is characterized by impaired insulin secretion with minimal or no insulin resistance. Patients typically exhibit mild hyperglycemia at an early age. The disease is inherited in an autosomal dominant pattern with at least six different loci identified to date. Genetic inability to convert proinsulin to insulin results in mild hyperglycemia and is inherited in an autosomal dominant pattern. Similarly, the production of mutant insulin molecules has been identified in a few families and results in mild glucose intolerance.

Several genetic mutations have been described in the insulin receptor and are associated with insulin resistance. Type A insulin resistance refers to the clinical syndrome of acanthosis nigricans, virilization in women, polycystic ovaries, and hyperinsulinemia. In contrast, type B insulin resistance is caused by autoantibodies to the insulin receptor. Leprechaunism is a pediatric syndrome with specific facial features and severe insulin resistance because of a defect in the insulin receptor gene. Lipoatrophic diabetes probably results from postreceptor defects in insulin signaling.

SCREENING

Type 1 Diabetes Mellitus

There is still a low prevalence of type 1 DM in the general population and because of the acuteness of symptoms, screening for type 1 DM is not recommended.[8]

Type 2 Diabetes Mellitus

Based on expert opinion, and not uniformly accepted by all guidance organizations, the American Diabetes Association (ADA) recommends screening for type 2 DM every 3 years in all adults beginning at age 45 years.[8] Testing should be considered at an earlier age and more frequently in individuals with risk factors. The recommended screening test is the fasting plasma glucose (FPG). An oral glucose tolerance test (OGTT) (more costly, less convenient, less reproducible) can be performed alternatively or in addition to FPG when a high index of suspicion for the disease is present.[5]

Children and Adolescents

Despite a lack of clinical evidence to support widespread testing of children for type 2 DM, it is clear that more children and adolescents are developing type 2 DM. The ADA, by expert opinion, recommends that overweight (defined as BMI >85th percentile for age and sex, weight for height >85th percentile, or weight >120% of ideal [50th percentile] for height) youths with at least two of the following risk factors: a family history of type 2 diabetes in first- and second-degree relatives; Native Americans, African Americans, Hispanic Americans, and Asians/South Pacific Islanders; and those with signs of insulin resistance or conditions associated with insulin resistance (acanthosis nigricans, hypertension, dyslipidemia, or polycystic ovary syndrome) be screened. Testing should be done every 2 years starting at 10 years of age or at the onset of puberty if it occurs at a younger age.[8]

Gestational Diabetes

Risk assessment for GDM should occur at the first prenatal visit. Women at high risk (positive family history, history of GDM, marked obesity, or member of a high-risk ethnic group) should be screened as soon as feasible. If the initial screening is negative, they should undergo retesting at 24 to 28 weeks of gestation, as should all other pregnant women with the possible exception of low-risk primigravidas. Evaluation for GDM can be done in one of two ways. The one-step approach involves a 3-hour, 100 gram-OGTT and can be cost-effective in high-risk patient populations. The two-step approach uses a screening test to measure plasma or serum glucose concentration 1 hour after a 50 gram oral glucose load (glucose challenge test), followed by a diagnostic 3-hour OGTT on the subset of women exceeding a glucose threshold of either ≥140 mg/dL (80% sensitive) or ≥130 mg/dL (90% sensitive). The diagnosis of GDM is based on a 75-gram (not as well validated) or 100-gram OGTT. Criteria for diagnosis of GDM based on the OGTT are summarized in Table 77–2.

TABLE 77-2 Diagnosis of Gestational Diabetes Mellitus with a 100-g or 75-g Glucose Load

Time	Plasma Glucose
100-g Glucose load	
Fasting	≥95 mg/dL (5.3 mmol/L)
1 hour	≥180 mg/dL (10.0 mmol/L)
2 hours	≥155 mg/dL (8.6 mmol/L)
3 hours	≥140 mg/dL (7.8 mmol/L)
75-g Glucose load	
Fasting	≥95 mg/dL (5.3 mmol/L)
1 hour	≥180 mg/dL (10.0 mmol/L)
2 hours	≥155 mg/dL (8.6 mmol/L)

Two or more values must be met or exceeded for a diagnosis of diabetes to be made. The test should be done in the morning after an 8- to 14-hour fast.

DIAGNOSIS OF DIABETES

❹ The diagnosis of diabetes requires the identification of a glycemic cut point, which discriminates normal persons from diabetic patients (Table 77–3). The present cut points reflect the level of glucose above which microvascular complications have been shown to increase. Cross-sectional studies from Egypt, in Pima Indians, and in a representative sample from the United States have shown a consistent increase in the risk of developing retinopathy at a fasting glucose level above 99 to 116 mg/dL (5.5 to 6.4 mmol/L), at a 2-hour postprandial level above 125 to 185 mg/dL (6.9 to 10.3 mmol/L), and a hemoglobin A_{1c} (HbA_{1c}) above 5.9 to 6.0% (Fig. 77–3).[13,15,16]

The ADA recommends using the fasting glucose test as the principal tool for the diagnosis of DM in nonpregnant adults. In addition, as shown in Table 77–4, they defined a new category of glycemia, impaired fasting glucose (IFG). IFG is a plasma glucose of at least 100 mg/dL (5.6 mmol/L) but less than 126 mg/dL (7.0

TABLE 77-3 Criteria for the Diagnosis of Diabetes Mellitus[a]

Symptoms of diabetes plus casual[b] plasma glucose concentration ≥200 mg/dL (11.1 mmol/L)
or
Fasting[c] plasma glucose ≥126 mg/dL (7.0 mmol/L)
or
2-hour postload glucose ≥200 mg/dL (11.1 mmol/L) during an OGTT[d]

OGTT, oral glucose tolerance test.

[a]In the absence of unequivocal hyperglycemia, these criteria should be confirmed by repeat testing on a different day. The third measure is not recommended for routine clinical use.

[b]Casual is defined as any time of day without regard to time since last meal. The classic symptoms of diabetes include polyuria, polydipsia, and unexplained weight loss.

[c]Fasting is defined as no caloric intake for at least 8 hours.

[d]The test should be performed as described by the World Health Organization, using a glucose load containing the equivalent of 75 g anhydrous glucose dissolved in water.

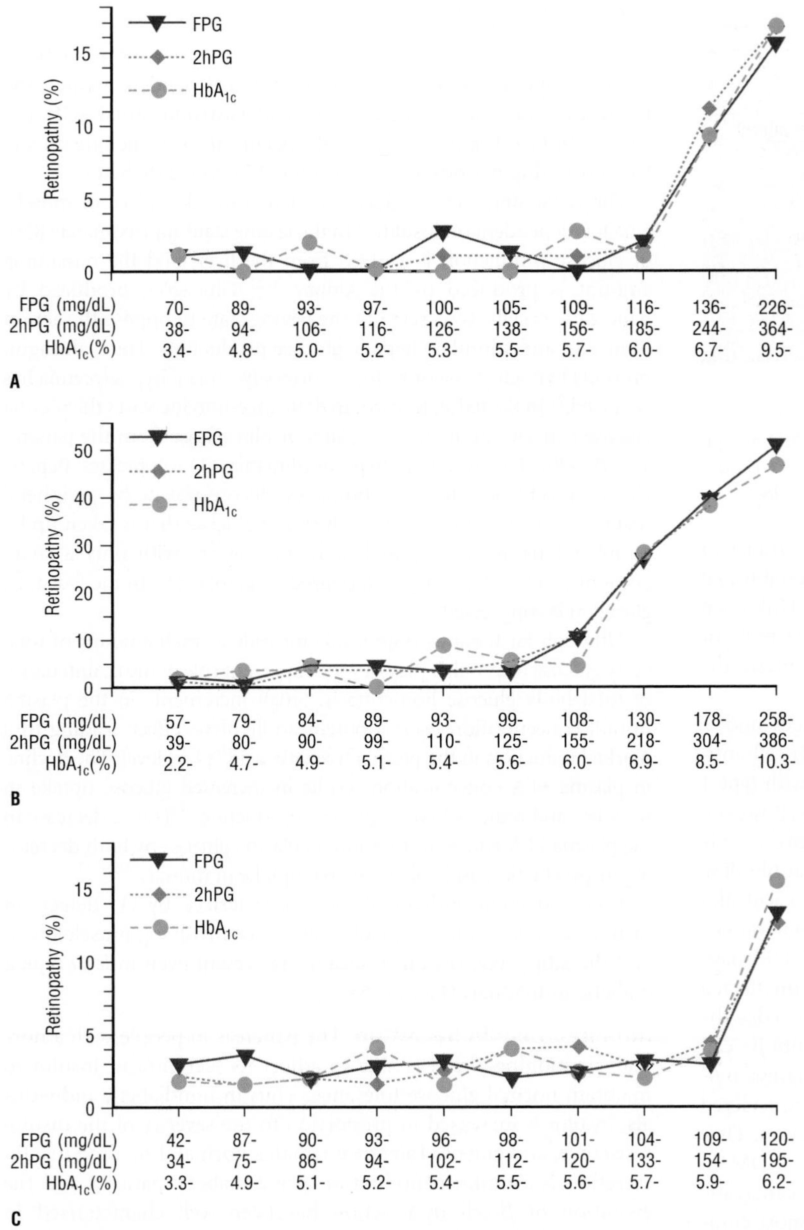

FIGURE 77-3. Prevalence of retinopathy by deciles of the distribution of fasting plasma glucose (FPG), 2-hour postprandial glucose (2-h PG), and hemoglobin A_{lc} (HbA_{lc}) in *(A)* Pima Indians,[12] *(B)* Egyptians,[11] and *(C)* in 40- to 74-year old participants in National Health and Nutrition Examination Survey (NHANES) III.[13] The *X*-axis labels indicate the lower limit of each decile group. Note that these deciles and the prevalence rates of retinopathy differ considerably among the studies, especially the Egyptian study, in which diabetic subjects were oversampled. Retinopathy was ascertained by different methods in each study; therefore the absolute prevalence rates are not comparable between studies, but their relationships with FPG, 2-h PG, and HbA_{lc} are very similar within each population.

mmol/L). Impaired glucose tolerance (IGT), is defined as a 2-hour glucose value ≥140 mg/dL (7.8 mmol/L), but less than 200 mg/dL (11.0 mmol/L) during an OGTT. Patients with either IFG or IGT are now commonly referred to as having "prediabetes" because of a higher risk of developing diabetes in the future.

TABLE 77-4 Categorization of Glucose Status

Fasting plasma glucose (FPG)
Normal
- FPG <100 mg/dL (5.6 mmol/L)

Impaired fasting glucose (IFG)
- 100–125 mg/dL (5.6–6.9 mmol/L)

Diabetes mellitus[a]
- FPG ≥126 mg/dL (7.0 mmol/L)

2-Hour postload plasma glucose (oral glucose tolerance test)
Normal
- Postload glucose <140 mg/dL (7.8 mmol/L)

Impaired glucose tolerance (IGT)
- 2-hour postload glucose 140–199 mg/dL (7.8–11.1 mmol/L)

Diabetes mellitus[a]
- 2-hour postload glucose ≥200 mg/dL (11.1 mmol/L)

[a]Provisional diagnosis of diabetes (diagnosis to be confirmed; see Table 77–3).

The fasting and postprandial glucose levels do not measure the same physiologic processes and do not identify the same individuals as having diabetes. The fasting glucose reflects hepatic glucose production, which depends on insulin secretory capacity of the pancreas. The postprandial glucose reflects uptake of glucose in peripheral tissues (muscle and fat) and depends on insulin sensitivity of these tissues.

The ADA recommends use of HbA_{1c} determinations to monitor glycemic control in known diabetic patients. Because there is no gold standard assay and several countries do not have ready access to the test, a HbA_{1c} determination is not recommended to diagnose diabetes at the present time.

PATHOGENESIS

Type 1 Diabetes Mellitus

Type 1 DM is characterized by an absolute deficiency of pancreatic β-cell function. Most often this is the result of an immune-mediated destruction of pancreatic β cells, but rare unknown or idiopathic processes can contribute. What is evident are four main features: (1) a long preclinical period marked by the presence of immune markers when β-cell destruction is thought to occur; (2) hypergly-

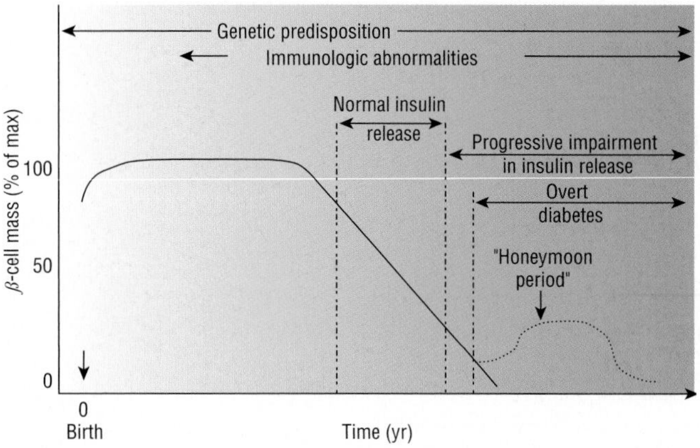

FIGURE 77-4. Scheme of the natural history of the β-cell defect in type 1 diabetes mellitus. *(From ADA Medical Management of Type 1 Diabetes, 3rd ed. American Diabetes Association, Alexandria, VA, 1998.)*

cemia when 80% to 90% of β cells are destroyed; (3) transient remission (the so-called *honeymoon* phase); and (4) established disease with associated risks for complications and death. Unknown is whether there is one or more inciting factors (e.g., cow's milk, or viral, dietary, or other environmental exposure) that initiate the autoimmune process (Fig. 77–4).[2]

The autoimmune process is mediated by macrophages and T lymphocytes with circulating autoantibodies to various β-cell antigens. The most commonly detected antibody associated with type 1 DM is the islet cell antibody. The test for islet cell antibody, however, is difficult to standardize across laboratories. Other more readily measured circulating antibodies include insulin autoantibodies, antibodies directed against glutamic acid decarboxylase, insulin antibodies against islet tyrosine phosphatase, and several others. More than 90% of newly diagnosed persons with type 1 DM have one or another of these antibodies, as will 3.5% to 4% of unaffected first-degree relatives. Preclinical β-cell autoimmunity precedes the diagnosis of type 1 DM by up to 9 to 13 years. Autoimmunity can remit in some perhaps less-susceptible persons, or can progress to β-cell failure in others. These antibodies are generally considered markers of disease rather than mediators of β-cell destruction. They have been used to identify individuals at risk for type 1 DM in evaluating disease-prevention strategies. Other nonpancreatic autoimmune disorders are associated with type 1 DM, most commonly Hashimoto thyroiditis, but the extent of organ involvement can range from no other organs to polyglandular failure.[17]

There are strong genetic linkages to the DQA and B genes, and certain human leukocyte antigens (HLAs) can be predisposing (DR3 and DR4) or protective (DRB1*04008-DQB1*0302 and DRB1*0411-DQB1*0302) on chromosome 6.[17] Other candidate gene regions have been identified on several other chromosomes as well. Because twin studies do not show 100% concordance, environmental factors such as infectious agents, chemical agents, and dietary agents are likely contributing factors in the expression of the disease.

Destruction of pancreatic β-cell function causes hyperglycemia because of an absolute deficiency of both insulin and amylin.[18] Insulin lowers blood glucose by a variety of mechanisms including: stimulation of tissue glucose uptake, suppression of glucose production by the liver, and suppression of free fatty acid release from fat cells.[19] The suppression of free fatty acids plays an important role in glucose homeostasis. Increased levels of free fatty acids inhibit the uptake of glucose by muscle and stimulate hepatic gluconeogenesis.[20] Amylin, a glucoregulatory peptide hormone cosecreted with insulin, plays a role in lowering blood glucose by slowing gastric emptying, suppressing glucagon output from pancreatic α cells, and increasing satiety.[21] In type 1 DM amylin production, caused by β-cell destruction, is very low.

Type 2 Diabetes Mellitus

Normal Insulin Action In the fasting state 75% of total body glucose disposal takes place in non–insulin-dependent tissues: the brain and splanchnic tissues (liver and gastrointestinal [GI] tissues).[22] In fact, brain glucose uptake occurs at the same rate during fed and fasting periods and is not altered in type 2 diabetes.

The remaining 25% of glucose metabolism takes place in muscle, which is dependent on insulin.[23] In the fasting state approximately 85% of glucose production is derived from the liver, and the remaining amount is produced by the kidney.[22–24] Glucagon, produced by pancreatic α cells, is secreted in the fasting state to oppose the action of insulin and stimulate hepatic glucose production. Thus, glucagon prevents hypoglycemia or restores normoglycemia if hypoglycemia has occurred.[25] In the fed state, carbohydrate ingestion increases the plasma glucose concentration and stimulates insulin release from the pancreatic β cells. The resultant hyperinsulinemia (1) suppresses hepatic glucose production and (2) stimulates glucose uptake by peripheral tissues.[22,26] The majority (~80%–85%) of glucose that is taken up by peripheral tissues is disposed of in muscle,[22,26] with only a small amount (~4%–5%) being metabolized by adipocytes. In the fed state, glucagon is suppressed.[25]

Although fat tissue is responsible for only a small amount of total body glucose disposal, it plays a very important role in the maintenance of total body glucose homeostasis. Small increments in the plasma insulin concentration exert a potent antilipolytic effect, leading to a marked reduction in the plasma free fatty acid (FFA) level. The decline in plasma FFA concentration results in increased glucose uptake in muscle[27] and reduces hepatic glucose production.[28] Thus a decrease in the plasma FFA concentration lowers plasma glucose by both decreasing its production and enhancing the uptake in muscle.[20,29]

Type 2 diabetic individuals are characterized by (1) defects in insulin secretion; and (2) insulin resistance involving muscle, liver, and the adipocyte. Insulin resistance is present even in *lean* type 2 diabetic individuals (Fig. 77–5).

Impaired Insulin Secretion The pancreas in people with a normal-functioning β cell is able to adjust its secretion of insulin to maintain normal glucose tolerance. Thus in nondiabetic individuals, insulin is increased in proportion to the severity of the insulin resistance, and glucose tolerance remains normal. Impaired insulin secretion is a uniform finding in type 2 diabetic patients and the evolution of β-cell dysfunction has been well characterized in diverse ethnic populations.

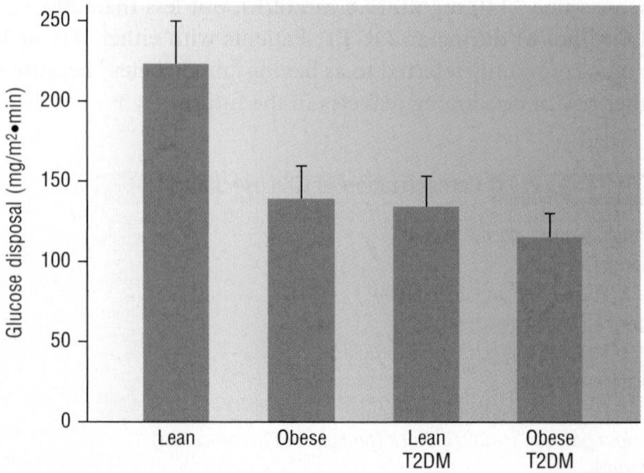

FIGURE 77-5. Whole body glucose disposal, a measure of insulin resistance, is reduced 40% to 50% in obese nondiabetic and lean type 2 diabetic individuals. Obese diabetic individuals are slightly more resistant than lean diabetic patients. (T2DM, type 2 diabetes mellitus.) *(Copyright © 1988 American Diabetes Association. From Diabetes, Vol. 37, 1988;667–687. Reprinted with permission from The American Diabetes Association.)*

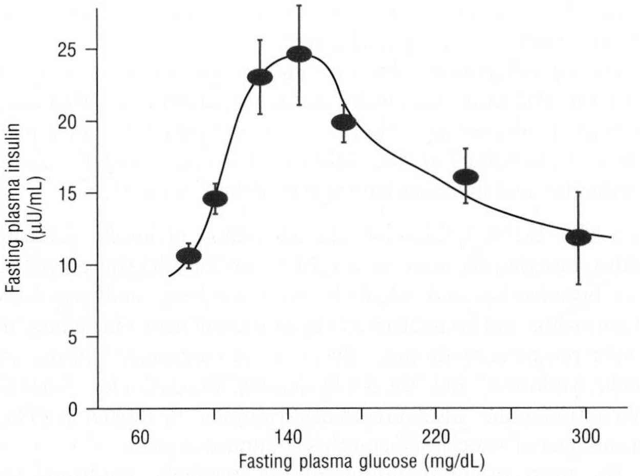

FIGURE 77-6. The relationship between fasting plasma insulin and fasting plasma glucose in 177 normal weight individuals. Plasma insulin and glucose increase together up to a fasting glucose of 140 mg/dL. When the fasting glucose exceeds 140 mg/dL, the β cell makes progressively less insulin, which leads to an overproduction of glucose by the liver and results in a progressive increase in fasting glucose. *(Adapted from DeFronzo,[30] with permission.)*

DeFronzo and colleagues[30] measured the fasting plasma insulin concentration and performed OGTTs in 77 normal-weight type 2 diabetic patients and more than 100 lean subjects with normal or impaired glucose tolerance (Fig. 77–6). The relationship between the FPG concentration and the fasting plasma insulin concentration resembles an inverted U or horseshoe. As the FPG concentration increases from 80 to 140 mg/dL, the fasting plasma insulin concentration increases progressively, peaking at a value that is 2- to 2.5-fold greater than in normal weight nondiabetic controls. When the FPG concentration exceeds 140 mg/dL, the β cell is unable to maintain its elevated rate of insulin secretion, and the fasting insulin concentration declines precipitously. This decrease in fasting insulin leads to an increase in hepatic glucose production overnight, which results in an elevated FPG concentration.[30]

In the type 2 diabetic patient, decreased postprandial insulin secretion is caused by both impaired pancreatic β-cell function and a reduced stimulus for insulin secretion from gut hormones. The role gut hormones play in insulin secretion is best shown by comparing the insulin response to an oral glucose load versus an isoglycemic intravenous glucose infusion.[31] In nondiabetic control individuals 73% more insulin is released in response to an oral glucose load compared to the same amount of glucose given intravenously (Fig. 77–7, left panel). This increased insulin secretion in response to an oral glucose stimulus is referred to as *the incretin effect* and suggests that gut derived hormones when stimulated by glucose lead to an increase in pancreatic insulin secretion. In type 2 diabetic patients this incretin effect is blunted, with the increase in insulin secretion to only 50% of that seen in nondiabetic control individuals (Fig. 77–7).[31] It is now known that two hormones, glucagon-like peptide-1 (GLP-1) and glucose-dependent insulin-releasing peptide (GIP), are responsible for more than 90% of the increased insulin secretion seen in response to an oral glucose load. In patients with type 2 diabetes GLP-1 levels are reduced whereas GIP levels are increased.[32]

GLP-1 is secreted from the L-cells in the distal intestinal mucosa in response to mixed meals. Because GLP-1 levels increase within minutes of food ingestion, neural signals initiated by food entry in the proximal gastrointestinal tract must simulate GLP-1 secretion.[33] The insulinotropic action of GLP-1 is glucose-dependent, and for GLP-1 to enhance insulin secretion, glucose concentrations must be higher than 90 mg/dL.[32] In addition to stimulating insulin secretion, GLP-1 suppresses glucagon secretion, slows gastric emptying and reduces food intake by increasing satiety. These effects of GLP-1 combine to limit postprandial glucose excursions. GIP is secreted by K-cells in the intestine and like GLP, increase insulin secretion.[34] However, GIP has no effect on glucagon secretion, gastric motility, or satiety.[35] The half-life of GLP-1 and GIP are short (<10 minutes). Both hormones are rapidly inactivated by removal of two N-terminal amino acids by the enzyme, dipeptidyl peptidase IV (DPP-IV).[36]

Site of Insulin Resistance in Type 2 Diabetes

Liver In type 2 diabetic subjects with mild to moderate fasting hyperglycemia (140 to 200 mg/dL, 7.8 to 11.1 mmol/L), basal hepatic glucose production is increased by ~0.5 mg/kg per minute. Consequently, during the overnight sleeping hours the liver of an 80-kg diabetic individual with modest fasting hyperglycemia adds an additional 35 g of glucose to the systemic circulation. This increase in fasting hepatic glucose production is the cause of fasting hyperglycemia.[22]

Following glucose ingestion, insulin is secreted into the portal vein and carried to the liver, where it suppresses glucagon secretion and reduces hepatic glucose output. Type 2 diabetic patients fail to suppress glucagon in response to a meal and can even have a paradoxical rise in glucagon levels.[36,37] Thus, hepatic insulin resistance and hyperglucagonemia result in continued production of glucose by the liver. Therefore, type 2 diabetic patients have two sources of glucose in the postprandial state, one from the diet and one from continued glucose production from the liver. These sources of glucose in combination with a shortened gastric emptying time can result in marked hyperglycemia.

Peripheral (Muscle) Muscle is the major site of glucose disposal in man, and approximately 80% of total body glucose uptake occurs

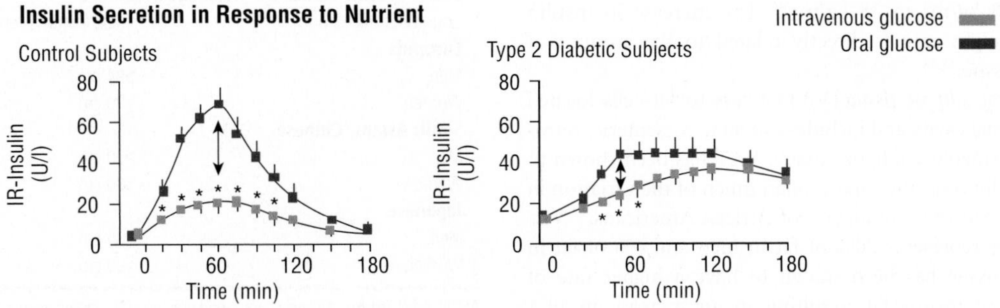

FIGURE 77-7. The loss of the incretin effect in type 2 diabetes mellitus. The plasma insulin responses to oral and intravenous glucose in nondiabetic subjects *(left figure)*, compared to patients with diabetes *(right figure)*. *(Adapted from Nauck M, Stockmann F, Ebert R, Creutzfeldt W. Reduced incretin effect in type 2 [non-insulin dependent] diabetes. Diabetologia 1986;29:46–52.)*

in skeletal muscle.[22] In response to a physiologic increase in plasma insulin concentration, muscle glucose uptake increases linearly, reaching a plateau value of 10 mg/kg per minute. In contrast, in lean type 2 diabetic subjects, the onset of insulin action is delayed for ~40 minutes, and the ability of insulin to stimulate leg glucose uptake is reduced by 50%. Therefore the primary site of insulin resistance in type 2 diabetic subjects resides in muscle tissue.

Peripheral (Adipocyte) In obese nondiabetic and diabetic humans, basal plasma FFA levels are increased and fail to suppress normally after glucose ingestion. FFAs are stored as triglycerides in adipocytes and serve as an important energy source during conditions of fasting. Insulin is a potent inhibitor of lipolysis, and restrains the release of FFAs from the adipocyte by inhibiting the hormone-sensitive lipase enzyme. It is now recognized that chronically elevated plasma FFA concentrations can lead to insulin resistance in muscle and liver,[20,22,27,38] and impair insulin secretion.[29,39,40] In addition to FFAs that circulate in plasma in increased amounts, type 2 diabetic and obese nondiabetic individuals have increased stores of triglycerides in muscle[41,42] and liver,[43,44] and the increased fat content correlates closely with the presence of insulin resistance in these tissues.

In summary, insulin resistance involving both muscle and liver are characteristic features of the glucose intolerance in type 2 diabetic individuals. In the basal state, the liver represents a major site of insulin resistance, and this is reflected by overproduction of glucose. This accelerated rate of hepatic glucose output is the primary determinant of the elevated FPG concentration in type 2 diabetic individuals. In the fed state, both decreased muscle glucose uptake and impaired suppression of hepatic glucose production contribute to the insulin resistance. In obese individuals and in the majority (>80%) of type 2 diabetic subjects, there is an expanded fat cell mass, and the adipocytes are resistant to the antilipolytic effects of insulin. Most obese and diabetic individuals are characterized by expanded visceral adiposity, discussed in detail later in the chapter, which is especially refractory to insulin effects and results in a high lipolytic rate. Not surprisingly, both type 2 diabetes and obesity are characterized by an elevation in the mean 24-hour plasma FFA concentration. Elevated plasma FFA levels, as well as increased triglyceride/fatty acyl coenzyme A (CoA) content in muscle, liver, and β cells, lead to the development of muscle/hepatic insulin resistance and impaired insulin secretion.

Cellular Mechanisms of Insulin Resistance

Insulin resistance and the components of the insulin resistance syndrome are described below.

Obesity and Insulin Resistance Weight gain leads to insulin resistance, and obese nondiabetic individuals have the same degree of insulin resistance as lean type 2 diabetic patients.[45] In 1,146 nondiabetic, normotensive individuals, Ferrannini and associates showed a progressive loss of insulin sensitivity when the BMI increased from 18 kg/m^2 to 38 kg/m^2.[46] The increase in insulin resistance with weight gain is directly related to the amount of visceral adipose tissue.[47,48]

The term *visceral adipose tissue* (VAT) refers to fat cells located within the abdominal cavity and includes omental, mesenteric, retroperitoneal, and perinephric adipose tissue. VAT has been shown to correlate with insulin resistance and explain much of the variation in insulin resistance seen in a population of African Americans.[49] Visceral adipose tissue represents 20% of fat in men and 6% of fat in women. This fat tissue has been shown to have a higher rate of lipolysis than subcutaneous fat, resulting in an increase in FFA production. These fatty acids are released into the portal circulation and drain into the liver, where they stimulate the production of very-low-density lipoproteins and decrease insulin sensitivity in peripheral tissues.[47] VAT also produces a number of cytokines that cause insulin resistance. These factors drain into the portal circulation and reduce insulin sensitivity in peripheral tissues.[50]

The fat cell also has the capability of producing at least one hormone that improves insulin sensitivity: adiponectin. This factor is made in decreasing amounts as an individual becomes more obese.[51,52] In animal models, adiponectin decreases hepatic glucose production and increases fatty acid oxidation in muscle.[53,54]

The Metabolic Syndrome The association of insulin resistance with a clustering of cardiovascular risk factors including hyperinsulinemia, hypertension, abdominal obesity, dyslipidemia, and coagulation abnormalities has been referred to by a variety of names including "the insulin resistance syndrome," "the metabolic syndrome," "the dysmetabolic syndrome," and "the deadly quartet," to name a few. Since the description of the "insulin resistance syndrome" by Reaven in 1988,[55] the number of associated factors has continued to grow.

The most recent definition of the metabolic syndrome was adopted by the International Diabetes Federation (IDF) in 2005 (Table 77–5).[56]

In the IDF definition of the metabolic syndrome, central obesity is recognized as an important causative factor and is a prerequisite component for the diagnosis. Central obesity can be easily assessed

TABLE 77-5 NCEP ATP III: Five Components of the Metabolic Syndrome (Individuals Having at Least Three Components Meet the Criteria for Diagnosis)

Risk Factor	Defining Level
Abdominal obesity	Waist circumference
Men	>102 cm (>40 in)
Women	>88 cm (>35 in)
Triglycerides	≥150 mg/dL
High-density–lipoprotein C	
Men	<40 mg/dL
Women	<50 mg/dL
Blood pressure	≥130/≥85 mm Hg
Fasting glucose	≥110 mg/dL
The 2005 IDF definition of metabolic syndrome	
For a person to be defined as having the metabolic syndrome they must have: *Central obesity* (defined as waist circumference >94 cm for Europid men and >80 cm for Europid women, with *ethnicity specific values for other groups*)	
Plus any two of the following four factors:	
1. Raised TG level: >150 mg/dL (1.7 mmol/L), or specific treatment for this lipid abnormality	
2. Reduced HDL cholesterol: <40 mg/dL (1.03 mmol/L) in males and <50 mg/dL (1.29 mmol/L) in females, or specific treatment for this lipid abnormality	
3. Raised blood pressure: systolic BP >130 or diastolic BP >85 mm Hg, or treatment of previously diagnosed hypertension	
4. Raised FPG >100 mg/dL (5.6 mmol/L), or previously diagnosed type 2 diabetes	
If above 5.6 mmol/L or 100 mg/dL, OGTT is strongly recommended but is not necessary to define the presence of the syndrome.	
Ethnic specific values for waist circumference	
Country/Ethnic Group	Waist Circumference
Europids	
Men	>94 cm
Women	>80 cm
South Asians, Chinese	
Men	>90 cm
Women	>80 cm
Japanese	
Men	>85 cm
Women	>90 cm

ASP III, Adult Treatment Panel III; BP, blood pressure; FPG, fasting plasma glucose; HDL, high-density lipoprotein; OGTT, oral glucose tolerance test; TG, triglyceride.
In the United States, the ATP III values (102 cm male, 88 cm female) are still being used. European cut points are recommended for sub-Saharan Africans and Eastern Mediterranean and Middle East (Arab) populations. South Asian values are recommended for South and Central Americans.
Reproduced from Expert Panel on Detection.[159]

using waist circumference. The IDF has made a "first attempt" to provide ethnic group specific cut points for waist circumference. At the present time these are pragmatic estimates taken from various data sources. As more complete data becomes available these values can be modified. Table 77–5 lists the ethnic specific values for waist circumference.

The evolution of definitions of the metabolic syndrome is a result of accumulating data correlating degree of risk and specific metabolic abnormalities in various populations. As more robust data sets become available, future changes in the component cut points will be warranted.

Prevalence. Regardless of the definition used, large numbers of U.S. adults have the metabolic syndrome. The National Health and Nutrition Examination Survey (NHANES) 1999 to 2002 is the most scientifically rigorous sample of the U.S. population.[57] A total of 3,601 men and women aged >20 years were included in the survey. Using the National Cholesterol Education Program (NCEP) definition, the prevalence of metabolic syndrome was 33.7% of men and 35.4% of women. In comparison the prevalence using the IDF definition was 39.9% of men and 38.1% of women. The largest difference in prevalence was found in Mexican American men among whom the age-adjusted prevalence was 40.3% using the NCEP definition and 50.6% using the IDF definition. The percent agreement between the two definitions was 89.8% among men and 96% among women.

In a sample of 4,060 predominantly European adults from South Australia, the metabolic syndrome was present in 19.4% of men and 14.4% of women using the Adult Treatment Panel III (ATP III) definition.[58] Using the IDF definition, the metabolic syndrome was identified in 26.4% of men and 15.7% of women. In this population the IDF, using a smaller waist circumference, categorized 15 to 20% more individuals as having the metabolic syndrome. Although the prevalence of the metabolic syndrome in these surveys is staggering, these data are now more than 8 years old, and the prevalence has almost certainly increased as these populations age and become more obese.

The impact of treating the clinical components of the metabolic syndrome was demonstrated in the Steno-2 Study.[59] In this prospective study, 63 patients with diabetes and microalbuminuria were randomized to the usual therapy group, and 67 patients were treated intensively. Intensive therapy consisted of diet and exercise and pharmacologic intervention aimed at hyperglycemia, hypertension, dyslipidemia, microalbuminuria, and increased coagulopathy (aspirin therapy). Treatment goals for intensive therapy included a blood pressure <130/80 mm Hg, HbA_{1c} <6.5%, total cholesterol <175 mg/dL, and triglycerides <150 mg/dL. All patients in the intensive treatment group were given an aspirin and treated with an angiotensin-converting enzyme (ACE) inhibitor. Patients in the intensively treated group showed a 53% relative risk reduction in cardiovascular disease and a 61% relative risk reduction in nephropathy. In this small study, the magnitude of this reduction is greater than has been demonstrated with individual interventions, stressing the importance of targeting all the components of the metabolic syndrome. The study design did not allow conclusions regarding which interventions had the most impact.

CLINICAL PRESENTATION

The clinical presentations of type 1 DM and type 2 DM are very different (Table 77–6). Autoimmune type 1 DM can occur at any age. Approximately 75% will develop the disorder before age 20 years, but the remaining 25%, including relatives of index patients, develop the disease as adults. Individuals with type 1 DM are often thin and are prone to develop diabetic ketoacidosis if insulin is withheld, or under conditions of severe stress with an excess of counterregulatory hormones.[2] Twenty to forty percent of patients with type 1 DM present with diabetic ketoacidosis after several days of polyuria, polydipsia, polyphagia, and weight loss. Occasionally, patients are diagnosed as short of "metabolic bankruptcy" when they have blood tests drawn for other reasons or for early symptoms. Because newly diagnosed patients with type 1 DM often have a small amount of residual pancreatic β-cell function, they can enter a "honeymoon" phase, when their blood glucose concentrations are relatively easy to control and small amounts of insulin are needed. Once this residual insulin secretion wanes, the patients are completely insulin deficient and tend to have more labile glycemia.

TABLE 77-6 Clinical Presentation of Diabetes Mellitus[a]

Characteristic	Type 1 DM	Type 2 DM
Age	<30 years[b]	>30 years[b]
Onset	Abrupt	Gradual
Body habitus	Lean	Obese or history of obesity
Insulin resistance	Absent	Present
Autoantibodies	Often present	Rarely present
Symptoms	Symptomatic[c]	Often asymptomatic
Ketones at diagnosis	Present	Absent[d]
Need for insulin therapy	Immediate	Years after diagnosis
Acute complications	Diabetic ketoacidosis	Hyperosmolar hyperglycemic state
Microvascular complications at diagnosis	No	Common
Macrovascular complications at or before diagnosis	Rare	Common

DM, diabetes mellitus.

[a]Clinical presentation can vary widely.

[b]Age of onset for type 1 DM is generally <20 years of age but can present at any age. The prevalence of type 2 DM in children, adolescents, and young adults is increasing. This is especially true in ethnic and minority children.

[c]Type 1 can present acutely with symptoms of polyuria, nocturia, polydipsia, polyphagia, and weight loss.

[d]Type 2 children and adolescents are more likely to present with ketones but after the acute phase can be treated with oral agents. Prolonged fasting can also produce ketones in individuals.

Patients with type 2 DM often present without symptoms, even though complications tell us that they may have had type 2 DM for several years.[10] Often these patients are diagnosed secondary to unrelated blood testing. Lethargy, polyuria, nocturia, and polydipsia can be seen at diagnosis in type 2 diabetes, but significant weight loss at diagnosis is less common.

TREATMENT

DM

■ DESIRED OUTCOME

❺ The primary goals of DM management are to reduce the risk for microvascular and macrovascular disease complications, to ameliorate symptoms, to reduce mortality, and to improve quality of life.[8] Near-normal glycemia will reduce the risk for development of microvascular disease complications, but aggressive management of traditional cardiovascular risk factors (i.e., smoking cessation, treatment of dyslipidemia, intensive blood pressure control, and antiplatelet therapy) are needed to reduce the likelihood of development of macrovascular disease. Evidence-based guidelines, as published by the ADA, can help in the attainment of these goals (Table 77–7).

Hyperglycemia not only increases the risk for microvascular disease, but contributes to poor wound healing, compromises white blood cell function, and leads to classic symptoms of DM. Diabetic ketoacidosis and hyperosmolar hyperglycemic state are severe manifestations of poor diabetes control, invariably requiring hospitaliza-

TABLE 77-7 Selected American Diabetes Association Evidence-Based Recommendations[a]

Recommendation Area	Specific Recommendation	Evidence Level[a]
Screening for diabetes	Screen overweight at 45 years old, repeat at 3-year intervals	E
	Screen with fasting plasma glucose or 2-hour 75-g OGTT	B
Monitoring	Home blood-glucose monitoring is needed if on insulin	A
	Subjects on other therapeutic interventions, including oral agents may need home blood glucose monitoring	E
	Quarterly HbA1c in individuals not meeting glycemic goals, twice yearly in individuals meeting glycemic goals should be performed	E
Glycemic goals	HbA1c goal for patients in general is <7%	B
	HbA1c goal for individuals is as close to normal (<6%) as possible without significant hypoglycemia	E
Treatment		
Medical nutrition therapy	Weight loss is recommended for all insulin-resistant/overweight or obese individuals	A
	Saturated fat should be <7% of total calories	A
	Monitoring carbohydrate intake by carbohydrate counting or exchanges is recommended.	A
	Glycemic index can give modest benefits over total carbohydrate intake.	B
	Low-carbohydrate diets (<130 g of carbohydrate) are not currently recommended as long-term effects are unknown	B
Physical activity	150 min/wk of moderate intensity exercise is recommended or 90 minutes of vigorous exercise per week	A
	Resistance-train large muscle groups 3 times per week	A
Blood pressure	Systolic blood pressure should be treated to <130 mm Hg	C
	Diastolic blood pressure should be treated to <80 mm Hg	B
	Initial drug therapy should be with an ACE inhibitor, angiotensin receptor blocker, diuretic, β-blocker, or calcium channel blocker	A
Nephropathy	Type 1 DM with any degree of albuminuria–ACE inhibitor	A
	Type 2 DM with microalbuminuria–ACE inhibitor or angiotensin receptor blocker	A
	Type 2 DM with macroalbuminuria–angiotensin receptor blocker	A
Dyslipidemia	The primary goal is an LDL<100 mg/dL	A
	If 40 years of age or older, statin therapy to reduce LDL 30–40%, regardless of baseline LDL, is recommended	A
	LDL<70 mg/dL is an optional goal in individuals with overt cardiovascular (CV) disease	C
	Triglycerides should be lowered to <150 mg/dL	C
	Increase HDL to >40 mg/dL in men and >50 mg/dL in women	C
Antiplatelet	Use aspirin (75–162 mg daily) for secondary cardioprotection	A
	Use aspirin (75–162 mg) for primary prevention in *type 2 DM* if the subject is >40 years old or has additional CV risks	A
	Use aspirin (75–162 mg) for primary prevention in *type 1 DM* if the subject is >40 years old or has additional CV risks	C

ACE, angiotensin-converting enzyme; DM, diabetes mellitus; HbA_{1c}, glycosylated hemogloblin; HDL, hight-density lipoprotein; LDL, low-density lipoprotein; OGTT, oral glucose tolerance test.
[a]Evidence levels: A, Clear evidence from well-conducted, generalizable, randomized controlled trials that are adequately powered; B, supportive evidence from well-conducted cohort studies or well-conducted case-control study; C, supportive evidence from poorly controlled or uncontrolled studies or conflicting evidence with weight of evidence supporting intervention; and E, expert consensus or clinical experience.
Based on American Diabetes Association Practice Recommendations.[8]

tion. Reducing the potential for microvascular complications is targeted at adherence to therapeutic lifestyle intervention (i.e., diet and exercise programs) and drug-therapy regimens, as well as at maintaining blood pressure as near normal as possible.

GENERAL APPROACH TO TREATMENT

Appropriate care requires goal setting for glycemia, blood pressure, and lipid levels, regular monitoring for complications, dietary and exercise modifications, medications, appropriate self-monitored blood glucose (SMBG), and laboratory assessment of the aforementioned parameters.[8] Glucose control alone does not sufficiently reduce the risk of macrovascular complications in persons with DM.

GLYCEMIC GOAL SETTING AND THE HEMOGLOBIN A_{1C}

Controlled clinical trials provide ample evidence that glycemic control is paramount in reducing microvascular complications in both type 1 DM[60] and type 2 DM.[61] HbA_{1c} measurements are the gold standard for following long-term glycemic control for the previous 2 to 3 months.[62] Hemoglobinopathies, anemia, and red cell membrane defects can affect HbA_{1c} measurements. Other strategies such as measurement of fructosamine, which measures glycated plasma proteins and correlates to glucose control over the last 2 to 3 weeks, can be necessary to assess diabetes control in these patients. Unless the risk outweighs the benefit (as in elderly patients, patients with advanced complications, and patients with other advanced disease), a HbA_{1c} target of <7% is appropriate (Table 77–8), and lower values should be targeted if significant hypoglycemia and/or weight gain can be avoided.[8]

MONITORING COMPLICATIONS

The ADA recommends initiation of complications monitoring at the time of diagnosis of DM.[8] Current recommendations continue to advocate yearly dilated eye examinations in type 2 DM, and an initial eye examination in the first 3 to 5 years in type 1 DM, then yearly thereafter. Less frequent testing (every 2 to 3 years) can be implemented on the advice of an eye care specialist. The feet should be examined and the blood pressure assessed at each visit. A urine test for microalbumin once yearly is appropriate. Yearly testing for lipid abnormalities, and more frequently if needed to achieve lipid goals, is recommended.

TABLE 77-8 Glycemic Goals of Therapy

Biochemical Index	ADA	ACE and AACE
Hemoglobin A_{1c}	<7%[a]	≤6.5%
Preprandial plasma glucose	90–130 mg/dL (5.0–7.2 mmol/L)	<110 mg/dL
Postprandial plasma glucose	<180 mg/dL[b] (<10 mmol/L)	<140 mg/dL

ADA, American Diabetes Association; ACE, American College of Endocrinology; AACE, American Association of Clinical Endocrinologists; DCCT, Diabetes Control and Complications Trial.
[a]Referenced to a nondiabetic range of 4.0–6.0% using a DCCT-based assay. More stringent glycemic goals (i.e., a normal HbA1c, <6%) can further reduce complications at the cost of increased risk of hypoglycemia (particularly in those with type 1 diabetes).
[b]Postprandial glucose measurements should be made 1–2 hours after the beginning of the meal, generally the time of peak levels in patients with diabetes.

SELF-MONITORING OF BLOOD GLUCOSE

The advent of SMBG in the early 1980s revolutionized the treatment of DM, enabling patients to know their blood glucose concentration at any moment easily and relatively inexpensively. Frequent SMBG is necessary to achieve near-normal blood glucose concentrations and to assess for hypoglycemia, particularly in patients with type 1 DM.[62] The more intense the pharmacologic regimen is, the more intense the SMBG needs to be (four or more times daily in patients on multiple insulin injections or pump therapy). The optimal frequency of SMBG for patients with type 2 DM is unresolved. Frequency of monitoring in type 2 DM should be sufficient to facilitate reaching glucose goals. The role of SMBG in improving glycemic control in type 2 DM patients is controversial but has shown to reduce the HbA_{1c} ~0.4%.[63] What is clear is that patients must be empowered to change their therapeutic regimen (lifestyle and medications) in response to test results, or no meaningful glycemic improvement is likely to be effected.

CLINICAL CONTROVERSY

SMBG improves glycemic control when insulin is used, but few well-conducted studies have shown significant glycemic reductions with increasing use of home blood-glucose testing for type 2 DM patients not on insulin. In a recent review, the average HbA_{1c} reduction with use of SMBG in type 2 DM patients not on insulin was 0.4%, although others have reported no glycemic improvement.[63] Patients must be empowered to change their therapeutic regimen (lifestyle and medications) in response to test results, or no meaningful glycemic improvement is likely to be effected, and thus the money spent on the strip is wasted.

NONPHARMACOLOGIC THERAPY

Diet

Medical nutrition therapy is recommended for all persons with DM.[64] Paramount for all medical nutrition therapy is the attainment of optimal metabolic outcomes and the prevention and treatment of complications. For individuals with type 1 DM, the focus is on regulating insulin administration with a balanced diet to achieve and maintain a healthy body weight. A meal plan that is moderate in carbohydrates and low in saturated fat (<7% of total calories), with a focus on balanced meals is recommended. The amount (grams) and type (via the glycemic index, although controversial) of carbohydrates, whether accounted for by exchanges or carbohydrate counting, should be considered.[64] It is imperative that patients understand the connection between carbohydrate intake and glucose control. In addition, patients with type 2 DM often require caloric restriction to promote weight loss. Rather than a set diabetic diet, advocate a diet using foods that are within the financial reach and cultural milieu of the patient. As most patients with type 2 DM are overweight or obese, bedtime and between-meal snacks are not needed if pharmacologic management is appropriate.

CLINICAL CONTROVERSY

The recommended daily carbohydrate intake for type 2 DM, and even type 1 DM, has become controversial since low-carbohydrate diets such as the Atkins, South Beach, and Carbohydrate Addict's Diets have become exceptionally popular. Currently, the ADA recommends that approximately 45% to 65% of daily caloric intake should come from carbohydrates and does not recommend restricting diets to <130 grams of carbohydrate a day. Many clinicians are trying to increase the monounsaturated fat percentage and decrease the carbohydrate percentage in a patient's diet to accomplish improved glycemic control. Recent studies have documented short-term success for weight loss on low-carbohydrate diets (~6 months), without deleterious effects on the lipid panel. Weight loss can reduce cardiovascular risk factors in type 2 DM.

Activity

In general, most patients with DM can benefit from increased activity.[65] Aerobic exercise improves insulin resistance and glycemic control in the majority of individuals, and reduces cardiovascular risk factors, contributes to weight loss or maintenance, and improves well-being. The patient should choose an activity that she or he is likely to continue. Start exercise slowly in previously sedentary patients. Older patients, patients with long-standing disease (age >35 years, or >25 years with DM ≥10 years), patients with multiple cardiovascular risk factors, presence of microvascular disease, and patients with previous evidence of atherosclerotic disease should have a cardiovascular evaluation, probably including an electrocardiogram and graded exercise test with imaging, prior to beginning a moderate to intense exercise regimen. In addition, several complications (autonomic neuropathy, insensate feet, and retinopathy) can require restrictions on the activities recommended. Physical activity goals include at least 150 minutes/week of moderate (50%–70% maximal hear rate) intensity exercise. In addition, resistance training, in patients without retinal contraindications, is recommended for 30 minutes three times per week.

PHARMACOLOGIC THERAPY

Until 1995, only two options for pharmacologic treatment were available for patients with diabetes; sulfonylureas (for type 2 DM only) and insulin (for type 1 or 2). Since 1995, a number of new oral agents, injectables, and insulins have been introduced in the United States.

Currently, six classes of oral agents are approved for the treatment of type 2 diabetes: α-glucosidase inhibitors, biguanides, meglitinides, peroxisome proliferator-activated receptor γ-agonists (which are also commonly identified as thiazolidinediones [TZDs] or glitazones), DPP-IV inhibitors, and sulfonylureas. Oral antidiabetic agents are often grouped according to their glucose-lowering mechanism of action. Biguanides and TZDs are often categorized as insulin sensitizers because of their ability to reduce insulin resistance. Sulfonylureas and meglitinides are often categorized as insulin secretagogues because they enhance endogenous insulin release.

New options for implementation of insulin therapy are now available. Detemir has given an additional option for choice of basal insulin for type 1 and 2 DM patients. Exubera, the first inhaled prandial insulin, was FDA approved, but has been withdrawn from the market due to poor sales. The subsequent sections describe the current antidiabetic medications that are available to treat type 1 and type 2 DM.

Drug Class Information

Insulin *Pharmacology.* Insulin is an anabolic and anticatabolic hormone. It plays major roles in protein, carbohydrate, and fat metabolism. For a complete review of insulin action, the reader is referred to a diabetes physiology text.[66] Endogenously produced insulin is cleaved from the larger proinsulin peptide in the β cell to the active peptide of insulin and C-peptide, which can be used as a marker for endogenous insulin production. All commercially available insulin preparations contain only the active insulin peptide.

TABLE 77-9 Available Injectable and Insulin Preparations

Trade/Generic Name	Manufacturer	Analog[a]	Administration Options	Room Temperature[b] Expiration
Rapid-acting insulins				
Humalog (insulin lispro)	Lilly	Yes	Insulin pen 3-mL, vial, and 3-mL pen cartridge	28 days
NovoLog (insulin aspart)	Novo-Nordisk	Yes	Insulin pen 3-mL, vial, or 3-mL pen cartridge	28 days
Apidra (insulin glulisine)	Sanofi-Aventis	Yes	3-mL, pen cartridge or Opticlick pen system	28 days
Exubera (inhaled human insulin)	Pfizer	No	1 and 3-mg blister packs	3 months once foil overwrap opened
Short-acting insulins				
Humulin R (regular; human insulin rDNA)	Lilly	No	100 units, 10-mL vial 500 units, 20-mL vial	28 days
Novolin R (regular; human insulin rDNA)	Novo-Nordisk	No	Insulin pen, vial, or 3-mL pen cartridge, and InnoLet[d]	Vial: 30 days; others: 28 days
Intermediate-acting insulins				
NPH				
Humulin N	Lilly	No	Vial, prefilled pen	Vial: 28 days; pen: 14 days
Novolin N	Novo-Nordisk	No	Vial, prefilled pen, and InnoLet[d]	Vial: 30 days; others: 14 days
Long-acting insulins				
Lantus (insulin glargine)	Sanofi-Aventis	Yes	Vial, 3-mL Opticlick pen cartridge	28 days
Levemir (insulin detemir)	Novo-Nordisk	Yes	Vial, 3-mL pen cartridge and pen, InnoLet[d]	42 days
Pre-mixed insulins				
Premixed insulin analogs				
Humalog Mix 75/25 (75% neutral protamine lispro, 25% lispro)	Lilly	Yes	Vial, prefilled pen	Vial: 28 days; pen: 10 days
NovoLog Mix 70/30 (70% aspart protamine suspension, 30% aspart)	Novo-Nordisk	Yes	Vial, prefilled pen, 3-mL pen cartridge	Vial: 28 days; others: 14 days
Humalog Mix 50/50 (50% neutral protamine lispro/ 50% lispro)	Lilly	Yes	3-mL pen	10 days
NPH-regular combinations				
Humulin 70/30	Lilly	No	Vial, prefilled pen	Vial: 28 days; pen: 10 days
Novolin 70/30	Novo-Nordisk	No	Vial, pen cartridge, InnoLet[c]	Vial: 30 days; others: 10 days
Humulin 50/50	Lilly	No	Vial	28 days
Other injectables				
Byetta (exenatide)	Amylin/Lilly	No	5 mcg and 10 mcg pen, ~60 injections (doses)/ pen	Pen in use can be used at room temperature (< 25°C [< 77° F])
Symlin (pramlintide)	Amylin	Yes	5-mL vial	28 days

NPH, neutral protamine Hagedern.
[a]All insulins available in the United States are now made by human recombinant DNA technology. An insulin analog is a modified human insulin molecule that imparts particular pharmacokinetic advantages.
[b]Room temperature defined as 15–30°C (59–86°F).
[c]InnoLet: A prefilled insulin pen with a "kitchen timer" type of dial for determining the number of insulin units. Can be useful in patients with impaired eyesight or dexterity.
Adapted from the Texas Diabetes Council.

Characteristics. Characteristics that are commonly used to categorize insulins include source, strength, onset, and duration of action. Additionally, insulins can be characterized as analogs, defined as insulins that have had amino acids within the insulin molecule modified to impart particular physiochemical and pharmacokinetic advantages. Table 77–9 summarizes available insulin preparations.

The strengths of injectable insulin currently available in the United States are 100 units/mL (U-100) and 500 units/mL (U-500). For individuals who require large doses of insulin to control their diabetes, 500 units/mL regular insulin is available. In the United States, all other insulins are available only in 100 units/mL strength. For some type 1 diabetes patients who require extremely low doses of insulin, dilution of 100 units/mL insulin to obtain accurate insulin doses can be necessary. Diluents and empty bottles can be obtained from the manufacturers for dilution.

Historically, insulin came from either beef or pork sources. Beef insulin differs by three amino acids and pork by one amino acid when compared to human insulin. Manufacturers in the United States have discontinued production of beef and pork source insulins as of December 2003, and now exclusively use recombinant DNA (rDNA) technology to manufacture insulin. Eli Lilly, Pfizer, and Sanofi-Aventis currently use a non–disease-producing strain of *Escherichia coli* for synthesis of insulin, whereas Novo Nordisk uses *Saccharomyces cerevisiae*, or bakers' yeast, for synthesis.

Purity of insulin refers to the amount of proinsulin and other impurities present in a given insulin product. Prior to 1980, most insulin contained enough impurities (300 to 10,000 ppm) to cause local reactions on injection, as well as systemic adverse effects from antibody production. Modern technology has provided less expensive techniques to purify insulin. As a result, all insulin products contain ≤10 ppm of proinsulin, with purified preparations (all rDNA human insulin and insulin analogs) containing <1 ppm of proinsulin.

Regular crystalline insulin naturally self-associates into a hexameric (six insulin molecules) structure when injected subcutaneously. Before absorption through a blood capillary can occur, the hexamer must dissociate first to dimers, and then to monomers. This principle is the premise for additives such as protamine and zinc described below, and modification of amino acids for insulin analogs. Lispro, aspart, and glulisine insulins dissociate rapidly to monomers, thus absorption is rapid. Lispro (B-28 lysine and B-29 proline human insulin; monomeric) insulin with two amino acids transposed, aspart (B-28 aspartic acid human insulin; mono- and dimeric) insulin with replacement of one amino acid, and glulisine (B-3 lysine and B-29 glutamic acid) are rapidly absorbed, peak faster, and have shorter durations of action when compared to regular insulin. In comparison to human insulin, with an isoelectric point of 5.4, the analog glargine insulin (A-21 glycine, B-30a-arginine, B-30a L-arginine, and B-30b L-arginine human insulin) has an isoelectric point of 6.8. In the bottle, glargine is buffered to a pH of 4, a level at which it is completely soluble, resulting in a clear colorless solution. When injected into the neutral pH of the body, it rapidly forms microprecipitates that slowly dissolve into monomers and dimers which are then subsequently absorbed. The result is a long-acting, peakless, 24-hour duration insulin analog. Detemir, in contrast, attaches a C14 fatty acid (a 14 carbon fatty acid) at the B-29 position and removes the B-30 amino acid. This allows the fatty acid side chain to bind to interstitial albumin at the subcutaneous injection site. Also, the formulation allows stronger hexamer (six molecules of insulin associated together) associations, which prolong absorption. Once detemir dissociates from the interstitial albumin, it is free to enter a capillary, where it is again bound to albumin. It then travels to a site of action and interacts, after dissociation from albumin, with insulin receptors.

Insulin analogs are modified human insulin molecules, and safety is paramount for FDA approval. Key factors that should be considered in the approval process include local injection reactions, antigenicity, efficacy compared to human insulin, insulin receptor binding affinity, and insulin-like growth factor 1–receptor affinity (which is compared to that of human insulin to determine mitogenic potential).

Pharmacokinetics. Subcutaneous injection kinetics are dependent on onset, peak, and duration of action, and are summarized in Table 77–10. The pharmacokinetic considerations for Exubera will be discussed later in the section. Absorption of insulin from a subcutaneous depot is dependent on several factors, including: source of insulin, concentration of insulin, additives to the insulin preparations (e.g., zinc, protamine, etc.), blood flow to the area (rubbing of injection area, increased skin temperature, and exercise in muscles near the injection site can enhance absorption), and injection site. Regular or neutral protamine Hagedorn (NPH) insulin is commonly injected in (from most rapid to slowest absorption): abdominal fat, posterior upper arms, lateral thigh area, and superior buttocks area. Insulin analogs, unlike regular or NPH insulin, appear to retain their kinetic profile at all sites of injection. When compared to 100 units/mL insulin, 500 units/mL regular insulin has a delayed onset, peak, and a longer duration of action. Addition of protamine (NPH, insulin lispro protamine [NPL], and aspart protamine suspension) or excess zinc (historically lente or ultralente insulin) will delay onset, peak, and duration of the insulin's effect. Variability in absorption, inconsistent suspension of the insulin by the patient or healthcare provider when drawing up a dose, and inherent insulin action based on the pharmacokinetics of the products can all contribute to a labile glucose response. NPH should be inverted or rolled gently at least 10 times to fully resuspend the insulin prior to each use.

As detemir has a unique mechanism to prolong absorption, it should not be surprising that its pharmacokinetics are unique. The onset of detemir is consistent across doses, but the peak is delayed slightly with higher dosing. Also, at low dose (0.2 units/kg) the duration of action is approximately 14 hours, whereas at higher doses it is close to 24 hours.

The half-life of an intravenous (IV) injection of regular insulin is approximately 9 minutes. Thus the effective duration of action of a single IV injection is short, and changes in IV insulin rates will reach steady state in approximately 45 minutes. Intravenous pharmacokinetics of other soluble insulins (lispro, aspart, glulisine, and even glargine) appear similar to IV regular insulin, but they have no advantages over IV regular insulin and are more expensive.

Insulin is degraded in the liver, muscle, and kidney. Liver deactivation is 20% to 50% in a single passage. Approximately 15% to 20% of insulin metabolism occurs in the kidney. This can partially explain the lower insulin dosage requirements in patients with end-stage renal disease.

Human Insulin (rDNA Origin) Inhalation Powder (Exubera)

Due to poor sales, Exubera was recently discontinued, and subjects were asked to be switched to alternative treatments. Exubera was the first inhaled insulin, and was formulated to easily reach the alveolar space. Bronchial tubes are impermeable to insulin, but it is easily absorbed across the alveoli. The onset and peak of Exubera insulin after inhalation is similar to rapid-acting insulin analogs, but the duration of action is similar to regular insulin (see Table 77–10). Exubera consists of blister packets labeled as 1 mg or 3 mg of human insulin inhalation powder, which are administered using the Exubera inhaler. After an Exubera blister is inserted into the inhaler, the patient pumps the handle of the inhaler. When the patient presses a "fire" button, the insulin blister is pierced and the insulin inhalation powder is dispersed into the chamber, allowing inhalation. Normally, up to 45% of the 1 mg blister contents and up to 25% of the 3 mg blister contents can be retained in the blister. The 1 mg blister packet is equal to ~3 units of subcutaneously injected insulin and the 3 mg blister packet is equal to ~8 units. One puff of a 3 mg blister is not equivalent to three 1 mg blisters, which will deliver a higher dose of insulin than the one 3 mg blister. Human insulin inhalation powder should be given as prandial insulin, and the efficacy is equivalent to rapid-acting injected insulin analogs. Human insulin inhalation powder can be used in type 1 or type 2 DM, though the smallest increment between inhaled doses is equivalent to 2 to 3 units injected subcutaneously. This can restrict the usefulness in many patients with type 1 DM, who may have large reductions in glucose with a single unit of insulin. The following patient populations have relative contraindications to Exubera: chronic smoking in last 6 months, which increases

TABLE 77-10 Pharmacokinetics of Various Insulins Administered Subcutaneously or Inhaled

Type of Insulin	Onset (Hours)	Peak (Hours)	Duration (Hours)	Maximum Duration (Hours)	Appearance
Rapid-acting					
Aspart	15–30 min	1–2	3–5	5–6	Clear
Lispro	15–30 min	1–2	3–4	4–6	Clear
Glulisine	15–30 min	1–2	3–4	5–6	Clear
Inhaled human insulin	15–30 min	1–2	6	8	Powder
Short-acting					
Regular	0.5–1.0	2–3	3–6	6–8	Clear
Intermediate-acting[a]					
NPH	2–4	4–6	8–12	14–18	Cloudy
Long-acting					
Detemir	2 hours	6–9	14–24[b]	24	Clear
Glargine	4–5	–	22–24	24	Clear

NPH, neutral protamine Hagedorn.
[a]Lente and ultralente insulin has been discontinued.
[b]See text for further discussion.
Adapted from the Texas Diabetes Council.

absorption two- to fivefold when compared to nonsmokers; chronic passive smoke, which reduces absorption of insulin inhalation; asthma, which decreases Exubera absorption, but bronchodilator use prior to insulin inhalation can increase absorption; chronic obstructive pulmonary disease (COPD), which increases the absorption of insulin inhalation; and other chronic lung diseases. A dry cough near inhalation, increased sputum, and dyspnea are the three most common drug-related side effects. Hypoglycemia rates are similar to regular insulin. There was a small, but statistically significant decrease in forced expiratory volume in the first second of expiration (FEV_1) and diffusing capacity of the lung for carbon monoxide (DLCO) in type 1 DM (T1DM) patients treated with Exubera. Two-year safety data indicate that in both T1DM and type 2 DM (T2DM) changes in FEV_1 and DLCO are small (<1%–2% from baseline), occur within the first 3 months of initiation, and the defect is reversible with discontinuation of therapy. A decline in FEV_1 or DLCO of ≥20% occurred in 1.5% versus 1.3%, and 5.1% versus 3.6% for Exubera and the comparator group, respectively. Pulmonary function testing is recommended at baseline, after 6 months of therapy, and annually thereafter, even if no symptoms are present. If the FEV1 or DLCO declines by ≥20% on followup testing, the test should be repeated, and if confirmed, Exubera should be discontinued other inhaled insulin systems are in development.[67] Other inhaled insulin systems are in development.

Efficacy. The efficacy of traditional insulins (e.g., regular and NPH insulins) is unequivocal. Insulin analog efficacy is measured via the same ways as traditional insulins. Insulin analogs in most studies have not shown superior HbA_{1c} levels when compared to traditional insulins but are often preferred by patients and practitioners because of their ability to more closely mimic normal insulin secretion profiles. Lispro, aspart, glulisine, and Exubera are advantageous because of the ability to administer within 10 minutes of a meal, as compared to the recommendation to inject regular insulin approximately 30 minutes prior. Rapid-acting analogs have shown superior postprandial lowering of glucose when compared to regular insulin. Both detemir and glargine insulin injected at bedtime have shown significantly less nocturnal hypoglycemia when compared to NPH injected at bedtime.

An educated patient in conjunction with a skilled practitioner can achieve excellent glycemic control with insulin therapy. Efficacy with insulin therapy is related to achieving glycemic control while minimizing the risk of potential side effects, specifically hypoglycemia and weight gain. Insulin is recommended in patients with: extremely high FPG levels (>280 to 300 mg/dL) or HbA1c, patients with ketonuria or ketonemia, symptomatic patients (weight loss with polyuria, polydipsia, and/or nocturia), GDM, and if deemed appropriate by the clinician and patient.[68–71]

Microvascular Complications. Insulin has been shown to be as efficacious as any oral agent for treating DM. The UKPDS, which used sulfonylureas or insulin, showed equal efficacy in lowering the risk of microvascular events in newly diagnosed type 2 DM.[61] Similarly, in type 1 DM the DCCT showed efficacy in reducing microvascular complications.[60]

Macrovascular Complications. The connection between high insulin levels (hyperinsulinemia), insulin resistance, and cardiovascular events incorrectly leads some clinicians to believe that insulin therapy can cause macrovascular complications. The UKPDS and DCCT found no differences in macrovascular outcomes with intensive insulin therapy. One study, the Diabetes Mellitus, Insulin Glucose Infusion in Acute Myocardial Infarction study,[72] reported reductions in mortality with insulin therapy. This group assessed the effect of an insulin-glucose infusion in type 2 DM patients who had experienced an acute myocardial infarction. Those randomized to insulin infusion followed by intensive insulin therapy lowered their absolute mortality risk by 11% over a mean followup period of approximately 3 years. This was most evident in subjects who were insulin-naïve or had a low cardiovascular risk prior to the acute myocardial infarction.[72] The importance of glycemic control in hospitalized patients is covered later in the chapter.

Adverse Effects. The most common adverse effects reported with insulin are hypoglycemia and weight gain. Hypoglycemia is more common in patients on intensive insulin therapy regimens versus those on less-intensive regimens. Also, patients with type 1 DM tend to have more hypoglycemic events compared to type 2 DM patients. In the UKPDS, performed over 10 years, the percentage of diabetic patients who needed assistance (third-party or hospitalization) because of a hypoglycemic reaction was 2.3%. The UKPDS reported a rate of 36.5% for risk of any hypoglycemic event, including mild, self-treated events. In the DCCT, tighter control produced a risk three times higher for severe hypoglycemia compared to conventional therapy. Glycemic goals should incorporate hypoglycemic risk versus the benefit of lowering the glucose when HbA_{1c} levels are near normal, especially in type 1 DM.

Minimization of risk for patients on insulin should include education about the signs and symptoms of hypoglycemia, proper treatment of hypoglycemia, and blood glucose monitoring. Blood glucose monitoring is essential for those on insulin, and is particularly of value in patients with hypoglycemia unawareness. Patients with hypoglycemia unawareness do not experience the normal sympathetic symptoms of hypoglycemia (tachycardia, tremulousness, and often, sweating). Initial hypoglycemia symptoms are neuroglycopenic in nature (confusion, agitation, loss of consciousness, and/or progression to coma). Patients with hypoglycemia unawareness often should at least temporarily raise their glycemic goals (requiring a reduction in insulin dose) and check their blood glucose level prior to any activities that can be dangerous with a low blood sugar (e.g., driving and certain sports, among others). Proper treatment of hypoglycemia dictates ingestion of carbohydrates, with glucose being preferred. Unconsciousness is an indication for either IV glucose, or glucagon injection, which increases glycogenolysis in the liver. Glucagon use would be appropriate in any situation in which the patient does not have or cannot have ready IV access for glucose administration. Education for reconstitution and injection of glucagon is recommended for close friends and family of a patient who has recurrent neuroglycopenic events. The patient and close contacts should be informed that it can take 10 to 15 minutes for the injection to start increasing glucose levels, and patients often vomit during this time. Proper positioning to avoid aspiration should be emphasized.

Weight gain is predominantly from increased truncal fat, and tends to be related to daily dose and plasma insulin levels present. Weight gain is undesirable in most type 2 DM patients, but can be seen as beneficial in underweight patients with type 1 DM. Weight gain appears to be related to intensive insulin therapy, and can be somewhat minimized by physiologic replacement of insulin.

Two forms of lipodystrophy, although much less common today in people with diabetes, still occur. Lipohypertrophy is caused by many injections into the same injection site. Because of insulin's anabolic actions, a raised fat mass is present at the injection site with resultant variable insulin absorption. Lipoatrophy, in contrast, is thought to be caused by insulin antibodies, with destruction of fat at the site of injection. Injection away from the site with more purified insulin is recommended, although several reports of lipoatrophy with lispro have been reported.

Drug-Drug Interactions. There are no significant drug-drug interactions with injected insulin, although other medications that can affect glucose control can be considered. Detemir does not appear to have albumin binding interactions, as it occupies only a small percent of albumin binding sites. Table 77–11 lists common medications known to affect blood glucose levels.

TABLE 77-11 Medications That Can Affect Glycemic Control[a]

Drug	Effect on Glucose	Mechanism/Comment
Angiotensin-converting enzyme inhibitors	Slight reduction	Improves insulin sensitivity
Alcohol	Reduction	Reduces hepatic glucose production
Interferon alfa	Increase	Unclear
Diazoxide	Increase	Decreases insulin secretion, decreases peripheral glucose use
Diuretics	Increase	Can increase insulin resistance
Glucocorticoids	Increase	Impairs insulin action
Nicotinic acid	Increase	Impairs insulin action, increases insulin resistance
Oral contraceptives	Increase	Unclear
Pentamidine	Decrease, then increase	Toxic to β cells; initial release of stored insulin, then depletion
Phenytoin	Increase	Decreases insulin secretion
β-Blockers	Can increase	Decreases insulin secretion
Salicylates	Decrease	Inhibition of I-kappa-B kinase-beta (IKK-beta) (only high doses, e.g., 4–6 g/day)
Sympathomimetics	Slight increase	Increased glycogenolysis and gluconeogenesis
Clozapine and olanzapine	Increase	Decrease insulin sensitivity; weight gain

[a]This list is not inclusive of all medications reported to cause glucose changes.

Dosing and Administration. The dose of insulin for any person with altered glucose metabolism must be individualized. In type 1 DM, the average daily requirement for insulin is 0.5 to 0.6 units/kg, with approximately 50% being delivered as basal insulin, and the remaining 50% dedicated to meal coverage. During the honeymoon phase it can fall to 0.1 to 0.4 units/kg. During acute illness or with ketosis or states of relative insulin resistance, higher dosages are warranted. In type 2 DM a higher dosage is required for those patients with significant insulin resistance. Dosages vary widely depending on underlying insulin resistance and concomitant oral insulin sensitizer use. Strategies on how to initiate and monitor insulin therapy will be described later in the therapeutics section.

Storage. It is recommended that unopened injectable insulin be refrigerated (2.2° to 7.7°C [36° to 46°F]) prior to use. The manufacturer's expiration date printed on the insulin is used for unopened, refrigerated insulin. Once the insulin is in use, the manufacturer-recommended expiration dates will vary based on the insulin and delivery device. Table 77–9 outlines manufacturer-recommended expiration dates for room temperature (15° to 30°C [59° to 86°F]) insulin, including Exubera. For financial reasons, patients can attempt to use insulins longer than their expiration dates, but careful attention must be paid to monitoring for glycemic control deterioration and signs of insulin decay (clumping, precipitates, discoloration, etc.) if this is attempted.

Exenatide *Pharmacology.* Exendin-4 is a 39-amino acid peptide isolated from the saliva of the Gila monster (*heloderma suspectum*) and shares approximately 50% amino acid sequence with human GLP-1. Exenatide is the synthetic analog to exendin-4. Exenatide (Byetta) has been shown to bind to GLP-1 receptors in many parts of the body including the brain and pancreas. Exenatide and GLP-1 have common glucoregulatory actions. Exenatide enhances glucose dependent insulin secretion while suppressing inappropriately high postprandial glucagon secretion in the presence of elevated glucose concentrations, resulting in a reduction in hepatic glucose production. Exenatide reduces food intake, which can result in weight loss, and slows gastric emptying so that the rate of glucose appearance into the plasma better matches the glucose disposition. Unlike GLP-1, exenatide does not increase gastric secretions.

Pharmacokinetics. Exenatide concentrations are detectable in plasma within 10 to 15 minutes after subcutaneous injection, and the drug has a time of maximal concentration (t_{max}) of ~2 hours and a plasma half life of ~3.3 to 4.0 hours. Exenatide plasma concentrations increase in a dose-dependent manner and plasma exenatide concentrations are detectable for up to 10 hours postinjection, although pharmacodynamically, effects last for approximately 6 hours. Bioavailability of exenatide after injection in the abdomen, upper arm, or the thigh is similar. Elimination of exenatide is primarily by glomerular filtration with subsequent proteolytic degradation. When exenatide is administered to subjects with worsening degrees of renal insufficiency, there is a progressive prolongation of the half-life, and in dialysis patients, plasma clearance of exenatide is markedly reduced. The incidence of GI side effects appears to be increased in individuals with impaired renal function, possibly because of higher plasma levels, thus caution is advised.

No significant differences in exenatide pharmacokinetics have been observed with obesity, race, gender, or advancing age (up to 73 years old).

Efficacy. The average HbA_{1c} reduction is approximately 0.9% with exenatide, although, similar to oral agents, it is dependent on the baseline HbA_{1c} values. Three phase III trials reported similar HbA_{1c} reduction in patients on metformin, sulfonylureas, or both. Exenatide significantly decreases postprandial glucose excursions but has only a modest effect on FPG values. If a patient has significant elevations in FPG levels, these should be corrected with other agents, and the exenatide added on. Exenatide can allow some patients to lose weight. The average weight loss in controlled trials was 1 to 2 kg over 30 weeks, without dietary advice being given to the patients, although long-term, open-label followup on 10 mcg twice daily shows continued weight loss for at least 2.5 years. Exenatide, through decreasing appetite and slowing gastric emptying, can reduce the number of calories a patient eats at a meal.

Microvascular Complications. Exenatide reduces the HbA_{1c} level, which have been shown to be related to the risk of microvascular complications.

Macrovascular Complications. No published clinical trials have examined the effect of exenatide on cardiovascular outcomes. However, improvements in several cardiovascular risk factors have been reported. Plasma triglycerides (–37 ± 10 mg/dL) decreased and, plasma HDL cholesterol (+4.5 ± 0.4 mg/dL) increased on exenatide 10 mcg twice daily. Nonsignificant reductions in systolic and diastolic blood pressure were observed. The greatest improvement in cardiovascular risk factors was seen in subjects who had the greatest weight loss.[73]

Adverse Effects. The most common adverse effects associated with exenatide are GI in nature. Nausea occurs in ~40% of subjects on 5 mcg, and ~45% to 50% of subjects on 10 mcg twice daily. Vomiting or diarrhea occurs in approximately 10% of patients placed on exenatide. GI adverse effects appear to decrease over time, but approximately 1 in 20 patients can have prolonged problems with one of the above side effects, possibly requiring discontinuation. As these adverse effects appear to be dose-related, the patient should be started on 5 mcg twice daily and titrated to 10 mcg twice daily only if the adverse effects are mostly gone. Also, when the patient is increased to the 10 mcg twice daily dose, these adverse effects can recur for a short period of time. Many episodes of nausea would be better characterized as stomach fullness, and patients should be instructed to eat slow and stop eating when full, or risk nausea and vomiting. Also, weight loss appears not to be related to adverse effects but rather to a reduction in calories consumed. Exenatide provides glucose-dependent insulin secretion, thus hypoglycemic rates when combined with metformin or a TZD are not increased, but when combined with a sulfonylurea or insulin, significant hypoglycemia can occur. Although exenatide reduces glucagon when the glucose is high, no suppression of counter-regulatory hormones has been noted during hypoglycemia. Exenatide antibodies can occur, but generally decrease over time and do not affect glycemic control. In approximately 5% of patients, titers can increase over time, resulting in a blunting of glycemic control in approximately one-half of these patients.

Drug Interactions. Exenatide delays gastric emptying, thus it can delay the absorption of other medications. Examples of medications that can be affected include oral pain medications and antibiotics dependent on threshold levels for efficacy. If rapid absorption of the medication is necessary, it is best to take the medication 1 hour before, or at least 3 hours after the injection of exenatide. In addition, if the patient has gastroparesis, exenatide is not recommended.

Dosing and Administration. Exenatide dosing should be started with 5 mcg twice daily, and titrated to 10 mcg twice daily in 1 month or when tolerability allows and if warranted. Exenatide should be injected 0 to 60 minutes before the morning and evening meals. If the patient does not eat breakfast, they can take the first injection of the day at lunch. The peak effect of exenatide is at approximately 2 hours, so anecdotally the patient can get better appetite suppression if injected 30 minutes to 1 hour prior to the meal. Storage and dosage availability information can be found in Table 77–9.

Pramlintide *Pharmacology.* Pramlintide (Symlin) is an antihyperglycemic agent used in patients currently treated with insulin. Pramlintide is a synthetic analog of amylin (amylinomimetic), a neurohormone co-secreted from the β cells with insulin. Pramlintide suppresses inappropriately high postprandial glucagon secretion, reduces food intake, which can result in weight loss, and slows gastric emptying so that the rate of glucose appearance into the plasma better matches the glucose disposition.

Pharmacokinetics. The absolute bioavailability of pramlintide after subcutaneous injection is 30% to 40%. The t_{max} is approximately 20 minutes, but the maximal drug concentration (C_{max}) is dose dependent and appears to be linear. The half-life ($t_{1/2}$) is approximately 45 minutes, thus the pharmacodynamic duration of action is approximately 3 to 4 hours. Pramlintide does not extensively bind to albumin, and should not have significant binding interactions. Metabolism is primarily by the kidneys, and one active metabolite (2–37 pramlintide) has a similar half-life as the parent compound. No accumulation has been seen in renal insufficiency, but caution is advised. Injection into the arm can increase exposure and variability of absorption, so injection into the abdomen or thigh is recommended.

Efficacy. The average HbA_{1c} reduction is approximately 0.6% with pramlintide, although optimization of the insulin and pramlintide doses can result in further drops in HbA_{1c}. If the 120 mcg dose is used in type 2 DM patients on insulin, it can also result in 1.5 kg weight loss. In type 1 DM patients, the average reduction in HbA_{1c} was 0.4% to 0.5%. Pramlintide decreases prandial glucose excursions but has little effect on the FPG concentration. The main advantage of pramlintide is in type 1 DM, where it helps to stabilize wide postprandial glycemic swings. The average weight loss in controlled trials was 1 to 2 kg, without dietary advice being given to the patients. Pramlintide, through decreasing appetite and slowing gastric emptying, can reduce the number of calories a patient eats at a meal.

Microvascular Complications. Pramlintide reduces the HbA_{1c} level, which has been shown to be related to the risk of microvascular complications.

Macrovascular Complications. No published clinical trials have examined the effect of pramlintide on cardiovascular outcomes.

Adverse Effects. The most common adverse effects associated with pramlintide are GI in nature. Nausea occurs in ~20% of type 2 DM patients, and vomiting or anorexia occurs in approximately 10% of type 1 or type 2 DM patients. Nausea is more common in type 1 DM, occurring in ~40% to 50% of patients. GI adverse effects appear to decrease over time and are dose related, thus starting at a low dose and slowly titrating as tolerated is recommended. Pramlintide alone does not cause hypoglycemia, but it is indicated for use in patients on insulin, thus hypoglycemia can occur. The risk of severe hypoglycemia early in therapy is higher in type 1 DM than in type 2 DM patients. A twofold increase in severe hypoglycemic reactions in type 1 DM patients has been reported.

Drug Interactions. Pramlintide delays gastric emptying, thus it can delay the absorption of other medications. Examples of medications that can be affected include oral pain medications and antibiotics dependent on threshold levels for efficacy. If rapid absorption of the medication is necessary, it is best to take the mediation 1 hour before, or at least 3 hours after the injection of pramlintide.

Dosing and Administration. Pramlintide dosing varies in type 1 and type 2 DM. It is imperative that the prandial insulin dose, if used, be reduced 30% to 50% when pramlintide is started to minimize severe hypoglycemic reactions. Basal insulin may need to be adjusted only if the FPG is close to normal. In type 2 DM, the starting dose is 60 mcg prior to major meals, and can be titrated to the maximally recommended 120 mcg dose as tolerated and warranted based on postprandial plasma glucose concentrations. In type 1 DM dosing starts at 15 mcg prior to each meal and can be titrated up to a maximum of 60 mcg prior to each meal if tolerated and warranted. Pramlintide comes in a vial, allowing individualization of titration at even smaller increments (by units) than the package insert recommends. Each 2.5 units on a 100 units/mL insulin syringe equals 15 mcg of pramlintide. In addition, pramlintide has a pH of 4, and it is not recommended that pramlintide be mixed with any other insulin, thus this potentially adds two to four additional injections a day. Storage information can be found in Table 77–9.

Sulfonylureas *Pharmacology.* The primary mechanism of action of sulfonylureas is enhancement of insulin secretion. Sulfonylureas bind to a specific sulfonylurea receptor (SUR) on pancreatic β cells. Binding closes an adenosine triphosphate–dependent potassium ion (K^+) channel, leading to decreased potassium efflux and subsequent depolarization of the membrane. Voltage-dependent calcium ion (Ca^{+2}) channels open and allow an inward flux of Ca^{+2}. Increases in intracellular Ca^{+2} cause translocation of secretory granules of insulin to the cell surface and resultant exocytosis of the granule of insulin. Elevated secretion of insulin from the pancreas travels via the portal vein and subsequently suppresses hepatic glucose production.

Classification. Sulfonylureas are classified as first-generation and second-generation agents. The classification scheme is largely derived from differences in relative potency, relative potential for selective side effects, and differences in binding to serum proteins (i.e., risk for protein-binding displacement drug interactions). First-generation agents consist of acetohexamide, chlorpropamide, tolazamide, and tolbutamide. Each of these agents is lower in potency relative to the second-generation drugs: glimepiride, glipizide, and glyburide (Table 77–12). It is important to recognize that all sulfonylureas are equally effective at lowering blood glucose when administered in equipotent doses.

Pharmacokinetics. All sulfonylureas are metabolized in the liver; some to active, others to inactive metabolites (see Table 77–12).

TABLE 77-12 Oral Agents for the Treatment of Type 2 Diabetes Mellitus

Generic Name (generic version available? Y = yes, N = no)	Brand	Dose (mg)	Recommended Starting Dosage (mg/day) *Nonelderly*	Recommended Starting Dosage (mg/day) *Elderly*	Equivalent Therapeutic Dose (mg)	Maximum Dose (mg/day)	Duration of Action	Metabolism or Therapeutic Notes
Sulfonylureas								
Acetohexamide (Y)	Dymelor	250, 500	250	125–250	500	1,500	Up to 16 hours	Metabolized in liver; metabolite potency equal to parent compound; renally eliminated
Chlorpropamide (Y)	Diabinese	100, 250	250	100	250	500	Up to 72 hours	Metabolized in liver; also excreted unchanged renally
Tolazamide (Y)	Tolinase	100, 250, 500	100–250	100	250	1,000	Up to 24 hours	Metabolized in liver; metabolite less active than parent compound; renally eliminated
Tolbutamide (Y)	Orinase	250, 500	1,000–2,000	500–1,000	1,000	3,000	Up to 12 hours	Metabolized in liver to inactive metabolites that are renally excreted
Glipizide (Y)	Glucotrol	5, 10	5	2.5–5	5	40	Up to 20 hours	Metabolized in liver to inactive metabolites
Glipizide (Y)	Glucotrol XL	2.5, 5, 10, 20	5	2.5–5	5	20	24 hours	Slow-release form; do not cut tablet
Glyburide (Y)	DiaBeta Micronase	1.25, 2.5, 5	5	1.25–2.5	5	20	Up to 24 hours	Metabolized in liver; elimination 1/2 renal, 1/2 feces
Glyburide, micronized (Y)	Glynase	1.5, 3, 6	3	1.5–3	3	12	Up to 24 hours	Equal control, but better absorption from micronized preparation
Glimepiride (Y)	Amaryl	1, 2, 4	1–2	0.5–1	2	8	24 hours	Metabolized in liver to inactive metabolites
Short-acting insulin secretagogues								
Nateglinide (N)	Starlix	60, 120	120 with meals	120 with meals	NA	120 mg three times a day	Up to 4 hours	Metabolized by cytochrome P450 (CYP450), CYP2C9, and CYP3A4 to weakly active metabolites; renally eliminated
Repaglinide (N)	Prandin	0.5, 1, 2	0.5–1 with meals	0.5–1 with meals	NA	16	Up to 4 hours	Metabolized by CYP3A4 to inactive metabolites; excreted in bile
Biguanides								
Metformin (Y)	Glucophage	500, 850, 1,000	500 mg twice a day	Assess renal function	NA	2,550	Up to 24 hours	No metabolism; renally secreted and excreted
Metformin extended-release (Y)	Glucophage XR	500, 750, 1,000 mg	500–1,000 mg with evening meal	Assess renal function	NA	2,550	Up to 24 hours	Take with evening meal or may split dose; can consider trial if intolerant to immediate-release
Thiazolidinediones								
Pioglitazone (N)	Actos	15, 30, 45	15	15	NA	45	24 hours	Metabolized by CYP2C8 and CYP3A4; two metabolites have longer half-lives than parent compound
Rosiglitazone (N)	Avandia	2, 4, 8	2–4	2	NA	8 mg/day or 4 mg twice a day	24 hours	Metabolized by CYP2C8 and CYP2C9 to inactive metabolites that are renally excreted
α-Glucosidase inhibitors								
Acarbose (N)	Precose	25, 50, 100	25 mg one to three times a day	25 mg one to three times a day	NA	25–100 mg three times a day	1–3 hours	Eliminated in bile
Miglitol (N)	Glyset	25, 50, 100	25 mg one to three times a day	25 mg one to three times a day	NA	25–100 mg three times a day	1–3 hours	Eliminated renally
Dipeptidyl peptidase-IV inhibitors (DPP-IV inhibitors)								
Sitagliptin (N)	Januvia	25, 50, 100	100 mg daily	25 to 100 mg daily based on renal function	NA	100 mg daily	24 hours	50 mg daily if: creatinine clearance >30 to <50 mL/minute 25 mg if: creatinine clearance < 30 mL/min

(continued)

TABLE 77-12 Oral Agents for the Treatment of Type 2 Diabetes Mellitus (continued)

Generic Name (generic version available? Y = yes, N = no)	Brand	Dose (mg)	Recommended Starting Dosage (mg/day) *Nonelderly*	Recommended Starting Dosage (mg/day) *Elderly*	Equivalent Therapeutic Dose (mg)	Maximum Dose (mg/day)	Duration of Action	Metabolism or Therapeutic Notes
Combination products								
Glyburide/metformin (Y)	Glucovance	1.25/250 2.5/500 5/500	2.5–5/500 twice a day	1.25/250 twice a day; assess renal function	NA	20 of glyburide, 2,000 of metformin	Combination medication	Use as initial therapy: 1.25/250 mg twice a day
Glipizide/metformin (N)	Metaglip	2.5/250 2.5/500 5/500	2.5–5/500 twice a day	2.5/250; assess renal function	NA	20 of glipizide, 2,000 of metformin	Combination medication	Use as initial therapy: 2.5/250 mg twice a day
Rosiglitazone/metformin (N)	Avandamet	1/500 2/500 4/500 2/1,000 4/1,000	1–2/500 twice a day	1/500 twice a day; assess renal function	NA	8 of rosiglitazone; 2,000 of metformin	Combination medication	Past manufacturing problems but recently reintroduced to market. Can use as initial therapy
Rosiglitazone/glimepiride (N)	Avandaryl	4/1 4/2 4/4	4/1 or 4/2 once a day	4/1 daily	NA	8 mg of rosiglitazone, 8 mg of glimepiride	Combination medication	Recent labeling that it can increase cardiovascular events in patients with concomitant heart failure—caution
Pioglitazone/metformin (N)	ACTOplus Met	15/500 15/850	15/500 to 15/850 once or twice daily	15/500 daily to twice daily; assess renal function	NA	45 mg of pioglitazone, 2,550 mg of metformin	Combination medication	
Pioglitazone/glimepiride (N)	Duetact	30/2 30/4	30/2 or 30/4 daily	30/2 daily to avoid hypoglycemia	NA	45 mg pioglitazone, 8 mg glimepiride	Combination medication	Maximum dose cannot be given of either medication because of formulations available
Sitagliptin/metformin (N)	Janumet	50/500 50/1,000	50/500 twice daily with meals up to 50/1,000 twice daily with meals	Either given twice daily; assess renal function prior to use	NA	100 mg sitagliptin daily	Combination medication	Follow renal precautions for metformin.

Data from Gerich JE. Oral hypoglycemic agents. N Engl J Med 1989;321:1231–1245.

Cytochrome P450 (CYP) 2C9 is involved with the hepatic metabolism of the majority of sulfonylureas. Agents with active metabolites or parent drug that are renally excreted require dosage adjustment or use with caution in patients with compromised renal function. The half-life of the sulfonylurea also relates directly to the risk for hypoglycemia. The hypoglycemic potential is therefore higher with chlorpropamide and glyburide. The long duration of effect of chlorpropamide can be particularly problematic in elderly individuals, whose renal function declines with age, and therefore it has great potential for accumulation, resulting in severe and protracted hypoglycemia. Individuals at high risk for hypoglycemia (e.g., elderly individuals and those with renal insufficiency or advanced liver disease) should be started at a very low dose of a sulfonylurea with a short half-life. Hypoglycemia on low-dose sulfonylureas can dictate a short-acting insulin secretagogue (nateglinide or repaglinide) in lieu of a sulfonylurea.

Efficacy. As mentioned earlier, when given in equipotent doses, all sulfonylureas are equally effective at lowering blood glucose. On average, HbA_{1c} will decrease 1.5% to 2%, with FPG reductions of 60 to 70 mg/dL. A majority of patients will not reach glycemic goals with sulfonylurea monotherapy. Patients who fail sulfonylurea usually fall into two groups: Those with low C-peptide levels and high (>250 mg/dL) FPG levels. These patients are often primary failures on sulfonylureas (<30 mg/dL drop of FPG) and have significant glucose toxicity or slow-developing type 1 DM. The other group is those with a good initial response (>30 mg/dL drop of FPG), but which is insufficient to reach their glycemic goals. More than 75% of patients fall into the second group. Factors that portend a positive response include newly diagnosed patients with no indicators of type 1 DM, high fasting C-peptide levels, and moderate fasting hyperglycemia (<250 mg/dL). If glycemic goals are met, a secondary failure rate of approximately 5% to 7% per year can be expected.

Microvascular Complications. Sulfonylureas showed a reduction of microvascular complications in type 2 DM patients in the UKPDS.[61] A more in-depth discussion follows later in the chapter.

Macrovascular Complications. In the largest study to date, the UKPDS, no significant benefit or harm was seen in newly diagnosed type 2 DM patients given sulfonylureas over 10 years. The University Group Diabetes Program study documented higher rates of coronary artery disease in type 2 patients given tolbutamide, when compared to patients given insulin or placebo, although this study has been widely criticized.[74,75] Some sulfonylureas bind to the SUR-2A receptor that is found in cardiac tissue. Binding to the SUR-2A receptor has been implicated in blocking ischemic preconditioning via K^+ channel closure in the heart. Ischemic preconditioning is the premise that prior ischemia in cardiac tissue can provide greater tolerance of subsequent ischemia. Thus patients with heart disease potentially have one compensatory mechanism to protect the heart from ischemia blocked. Conclusions are controversial, and readers are referred to the pertinent articles for further discussion.[76–78]

Adverse Effects. The most common side effect of sulfonylureas is hypoglycemia. The pretreatment FPG is a strong predictor of hypoglycemic potential. The lower the FPG is on initiation, the higher the potential for hypoglycemia. Also, in addition to the high-risk individuals outlined in the pharmacokinetics section, those who skip meals, exercise vigorously, or lose substantial amounts of weight are also more likely to experience hypoglycemia.

Hyponatremia (serum sodium <129 mEq/L) is reportedly associated with tolbutamide, but it is most common with chlorpropamide and occurs in as many as 5% of individuals treated. An increase in antidiuretic hormone secretion is the mechanism for hyponatremia. Risk factors include age >60 years, female gender, and concomitant use of thiazide diuretics.

Weight gain is common with sulfonylureas. In essence, patients who are no longer glycosuric and who do not reduce caloric intake with improvement of blood glucose will store excess calories. Other notable, although much less common, adverse effects of sulfonylureas are skin rash, hemolytic anemia, GI upset, and cholestasis. Disulfiram-type reactions and flushing have been reported with tolbutamide and chlorpropamide when alcohol is consumed.

Drug Interactions. Several drugs are thought to interact with sulfonylureas, and Table 77–13 summarizes them by proposed mechanisms of action.[79] Drug interactions from protein-binding changes should occur shortly after the interacting medication is given, as the concentration of free (thus active) sulfonylurea will acutely increase. First-generation sulfonylureas, which bind to proteins ionically, are more likely to cause drug-drug interactions than second-generation sulfonylureas, which bind nonionically.[80] The clinical importance of protein-binding interactions has been questioned, as the majority of these drug interactions have been found to truly be caused by hepatic metabolism. Drugs that are inducers or inhibitors of CYP2C9 should be monitored carefully when used with a sulfonylurea. Additionally, other drugs known to alter blood glucose should be considered (see Table 77–11).

Dosing and Administration. The usual starting dose and maximum dose of sulfonylureas are summarized in Table 77–12. Lower dosages are recommended for most agents in elderly patients and those with compromised renal or hepatic function. The dosage should be titrated every 1 to 2 weeks (use a longer interval with chlorpropamide) to achieve glycemic goals. This is possible because of the rapid increase of insulin secretion in response to the sulfonylurea. Of note, immediate-release glipizide's maximal dose is 40 mg/day, but its maximal effective dose is about 10 to 15 mg/day. The maximal effective dose of sulfonylureas tends to be approximately 60% to 75% of their stated maximum dose.

Short-Acting Insulin Secretagogues *Pharmacology.* Although the binding site is adjacent to the binding site of sulfonylureas, nateglinide and repaglinide stimulate insulin secretion from the β cells of the pancreas, similarly to sulfonylureas. Repaglinide, a benzoic acid derivative, and nateglinide, a phenylalanine amino acid derivative, both require the presence of glucose to stimulate insulin secretion. As glucose levels diminish to normal, stimulated insulin secretion diminishes.

TABLE 77-13 Drug Interactions with Sulfonylureas

Interaction	Drugs
Displacement from protein binding sites[a]	Warfarin, salicylates, phenylbutazone, sulfonamides
Alters hepatic metabolism (cytochrome P450)	Chloramphenicol, monoamine oxidase inhibitors, cimetidine, rifampin[b]
Altered renal excretion	Allopurinol, probenecid

[a]Many of these drug interactions may be metabolism-based.
[b]Inducer.
Reproduced from Gerich.[79]

Pharmacokinetics. Both nateglinide and repaglinide are rapid-acting insulin secretagogues that are rapidly absorbed (~0.5 to 1 hour) and have a short half-life (1 to 1.5 hours). Nateglinide is highly protein-bound, primarily to albumin, but also to α_1-acid glycoprotein. Nateglinide is predominantly metabolized by CYP2C9 (70%) and CYP3A4 (30%) to less active metabolites. Glucuronide conjugation then allows rapid renal elimination. Repaglinide is mainly metabolized by the CYP3A4 system to inactive metabolites that are excreted in the bile.

Efficacy. In monotherapy, both significantly reduce postprandial glucose excursions and reduce HbA_{1c} levels. Repaglinide, dosed 4 mg three times a day, when compared to glyburide in diet-treated drug-naïve patients reduced HbA_{1c} levels less (1% vs. 2.4%, from baseline, respectively).[81] Nateglinide, dosed 120 mg three times a day in a similar population reduced HbA_{1c} values by 0.8%.[82] The lower efficacy of these agents versus sulfonylureas should be considered when patients are >1% above their HbA_{1c} goal. These agents can be used to provide increased insulin secretion during meals, when it is needed, in patients close to glycemic goals. Also, it should be noted that addition of either agent to a sulfonylurea will not result in any improvement in glycemic parameters.

Adverse Effects. Hypoglycemia is the main side effect noted with both agents. Hypoglycemic risk appears to be less than with sulfonylureas. In part, this is because of the glucose-sensitive release of insulin. If the glucose concentration is normal, less glucose-stimulated release of insulin will occur. In two separate studies, nateglinide rates of hypoglycemia were 3% and repaglinide 15% versus glyburide and glipizide rates of 15% and 19%, respectively. Weight gain of 2 to 3 kg has been noted with repaglinide, whereas weight gain with nateglinide appears to be <1 kg.

Drug Interactions. Glycemic control and hypoglycemia should be closely monitored when inducers or inhibitors of CYP3A4 are given with repaglinide. Gemfibrozil, a common medication used to treat hypertriglyceridemia in DM, more than doubles the half-life of repaglinide and has resulted in prolonged hypoglycemic reactions. Nateglinide appears to be a weak inhibitor of CYP2C9 based on tolbutamide metabolism, although no significant drug-drug interactions have been reported.

Dosing and Administration. Nateglinide and repaglinide should be dosed prior to each meal (up to 30 minutes prior). The recommended starting dose for repaglinide is 0.5 mg in subjects with HbA_{1c} <8% or treatment-naïve patients, increased weekly to a total maximum daily dose of 16 mg (see Table 77–12). The maximal effective dose of repaglinide is likely 2 mg with each meal, as a dose of 1 mg prior to each meal provides approximately 90% of the maximal glucose-lowering effect. Nateglinide should be dosed at 120 mg prior to meals, and does not require titration. A 60-mg dose is available, but the HbA_{1c} decrement is small (0.3% to 0.5%). If a meal is skipped, the medication can be skipped, and meals extremely low in carbohydrate content may not need a dose. Both agents can be used in patients with renal insufficiency and offer an excellent alternative in patients experiencing hypoglycemia with low-dose sulfonylurea. Caution is advised for patients with moderate to severe hepatic impairment, as nateglinide has not been studied and the half-life is prolonged with use of repaglinide.

Biguanides *Pharmacology.* Metformin is the only biguanide available in the United States. Metformin has been used clinically for 45 years and has been approved in the United States since 1995. Metformin enhances insulin sensitivity of both hepatic and peripheral (muscle) tissues. This allows for an increased uptake of glucose into these insulin-sensitive tissues. The exact mechanisms of how metformin accomplishes insulin sensitization are still being investigated, although adenosine 5-monophosphate–activated protein kinase activity, tyrosine kinase activity enhancement, and glucose transporter-4 all play a part. Metformin has no direct effect on the β cells, although insulin levels are reduced, reflecting increases in insulin sensitivity.

Pharmacokinetics. Metformin has approximately 50% to 60% oral bioavailability, low lipid solubility, and a volume of distribution that approximates body water. Metformin is not metabolized and does not bind to plasma proteins. Metformin is eliminated by renal tubular secretion and glomerular filtration. The average half-life of metformin is 6 hours, although pharmacodynamically, metformin's antihyperglycemic effects last >24 hours.

Efficacy. Metformin consistently reduces HbA_{1c} levels by 1.5% to 2.0%, FPG levels by 60 to 80 mg/dL, and retains the ability to reduce FPG levels when they are extremely high (>300 mg/dL). The sulfonylureas' ability to stimulate insulin release from β cells at extremely high glucose levels is often impaired, a concept commonly referred to as *glucose toxicity*. Metformin also has positive effects on several components of the insulin resistance syndrome. Metformin decreases plasma triglycerides and LDL-C by approximately 8% to 15%, as well increasing HDL-C very modestly (2%). Metformin reduces levels of plasminogen activator inhibitor-1 and causes a modest reduction in weight (2 to 3 kg).

Microvascular Complications. Metformin ($n = 342$) was compared to intensive glucose control with insulin or sulfonylureas in the UKPDS. No significant differences were seen between therapies with regard to reducing microvascular complications.

❻ ***Macrovascular Complications.*** Although normal weight type 2 DM subjects may not receive benefit, metformin reduced macrovascular complications in obese subjects in the UKPDS.[83] Metformin significantly reduced all-cause mortality and risk of stroke versus intensive treatment with sulfonylureas or insulin. Metformin also reduced diabetes-related death and myocardial infarctions as opposed to the conventional treatment arm of the UKPDS. Metformin should be included in the therapy for all type 2 DM patients, if tolerated and not contraindicated, as it is the only oral antihyperglycemic medication proven to reduce the risk of total mortality and is generic.

Adverse Effects. Metformin causes GI side effects, including abdominal discomfort, stomach upset, and/or diarrhea in approximately 30% of patients. Anorexia and stomach fullness is likely part of the reason loss of weight is noted with metformin. These side effects are usually mild and can be minimized by slow titration. GI side effects also tend to be transient, lessening in severity over several weeks. If encountered, make sure patients are taking metformin with or right after meals and reduce the dose to a point at which no GI side effects are encountered. Increases in the dose can be tried again in several weeks. Anecdotally, extended-release metformin (Glucophage-XR) can lessen some of the GI side effects. Metallic taste, interference with vitamin B_{12} absorption, and hypoglycemia during intense exercise have been documented but are clinically uncommon.

Metformin therapy rarely (3 cases per 100,000 patient-years) causes lactic acidosis. Any disease state that can increase lactic acid production or decrease lactic acid removal can predispose to lactic acidosis. Tissue hypoperfusion, such as that caused by congestive heart failure, hypoxic states, shock, or septicemia, via increased production of lactic acid; and severe liver disease or alcohol, through reduced removal of lactic acid in the liver, all increase the risk of lactic acidosis. The clinical presentation of lactic acidosis is often nonspecific flu-like symptoms, thus the diagnosis is usually made by laboratory confirmation. Metformin use in renal insufficiency, defined as a serum creatinine of 1.4 mg/dL in women and 1.5 mg/dL in men or greater, is contraindicated, as it is renally eliminated. Elderly patients, who often have reduced muscle mass, should have their glomerular filtration rate estimated by a 24-hour urine creatinine collection. If the estimated glomerular filtration rate is less than 70 mL/min, metformin should not be given. Because of the risk of acute renal failure during intravenous dye procedures, metformin therapy should be withheld starting the day of the procedure and resumed in 2 to 3 days, after normal renal function has been documented.

Drug Interactions. Cimetidine competes for renal tubular secretion of metformin and concomitant administration leads to higher metformin serum concentrations. At least one case report of lactic acidosis with metformin therapy implicates cimetidine. Other cationic drugs may interact similarly such as procainamide, digoxin, quinidine, trimethoprim, and vancomycin.[84]

Dosing and Administration. Metformin immediate-release is usually dosed 500 mg twice a day with the largest meals to minimize GI side effects. Metformin can be increased by 500 mg weekly until glycemic goals or 2,000 mg/day is achieved (see Table 77–12). Metformin 850 mg can be dosed daily and then increased every 1 to 2 weeks to the maximum dose of 850 mg three times a day (2,550 mg/day). Approximately 80% of the glycemic-lowering effect can be seen at 1,500 mg, and 2,000 mg/day is the maximal effective dose.

Extended-release metformin can be initiated at 500 mg a day with the evening meal and titrated weekly by 500 mg as tolerated to a single evening dose of 2,000 mg/day. Twice daily to three times a day dosing of extended-release metformin can help minimize GI side effects and improve glycemic control. Metformin extended-release 750 mg tablets can be titrated weekly to the maximum dose of 2,250 mg/day, although as stated above, 1,500 mg/day provides the majority of the glycemic-lowering effect.

Thiazolidinediones *Pharmacology.* Thiazolidinediones are also referred to as TZDs or glitazones. Pioglitazone and rosiglitazone are the two currently approved TZDs for the treatment of type 2 DM (see Table 77–12). TZDs work by binding to the peroxisome proliferator-activated receptor-γ (PPAR-γ), which are primarily located on fat cells and vascular cells. The concentration of these receptors in the muscle is very low; thus this is unlikely to be the main site of action. TZDs enhance insulin sensitivity at muscle, liver, and fat tissues indirectly. TZDs cause preadipocytes to differentiate into mature fat cells in subcutaneous fat stores. Small fat cells are more sensitive to insulin and more able to store FFAs. The result is a flux of FFAs out of the plasma, visceral fat, and liver into subcutaneous fat, a less insulin-resistant storage tissue. Muscle intracellular fat products, which contribute to insulin resistance, also decline. TZDs also affect adipokines, (e.g., angiotensinogen, tissue necrosis factor-α, interleukin-6, plasminogen activator inhibitor-1), which can positively affect insulin sensitivity, endothelial function, and inflammation. Of particular note, adiponectin is reduced with obesity and/or diabetes but is increased with TZD therapy, which improves endothelial function, insulin sensitivity, and has a potent antiinflammatory effect.

Pharmacokinetics. Pioglitazone and rosiglitazone are well absorbed with or without food. Both are highly (>99%) protein bound to albumin. Pioglitazone is primarily metabolized by CYP2C8, and to a lesser extent by CYP3A4 (17%), with the majority being eliminated in the feces. Rosiglitazone is metabolized by CYP2C8, and to a lesser extent by CYP2C9, then conjugated with two-thirds found in urine and one-third in feces. The half-life of pioglitazone and rosiglitazone is 3 to 7 hours and 3 to 4 hours, respectively. Two active metabolites of pioglitazone with longer half-lives deliver the majority of activity at steady state. Both medications have a duration of antihyperglycemic action of more than 24 hours.

Efficacy. Pioglitazone and rosiglitazone, given for approximately 6 months, reduce HbA_{1c} values ~1.5% and reduce FPG levels by approximately 60 to 70 mg/dL at maximal doses. Glycemic-lowering onset is slow, and maximal glycemic-lowering effects may not be seen until 3 to 4 months of therapy. It is important to inform patients of this fact and that they should not stop therapy even if minimal glucose lowering is initially encountered. The efficacy of both drugs is dependent on sufficient insulinemia. If there is insufficient endogenous insulin production (β-cell function) or exogenous insulin delivery via injections, neither will lower glucose concentrations efficiently. Interestingly, patients who are more obese, or who gain weight on either medication tend to have a larger reduction in HbA_{1c} values. Pioglitazone consistently decreases plasma triglyceride levels by 10% to 20%, whereas rosiglitazone tends to have a neutral effect. LDL-C concentrations tend to increase with rosiglitazone 5% to 15% but do not significantly increase with pioglitazone. Both appear to convert small, dense low-density lipoprotein (LDL) particles, which have been shown to be highly atherogenic, to large, fluffy LDL particles that are less dense. Large, fluffy LDL particles may be less atherogenic, but any increase in LDL must be of concern. Both drugs increase HDL similarly, up to 3 to 9 mg/dL. TZDs also affect several components of the insulin resistance syndrome. PAI-1 levels are decreased, and many other adipocytokines are affected, endothelial function improves, and blood pressure can decrease slightly.

Microvascular Complications. TZDs reduce HbA_{1c} levels, which have been shown to be related to the risk of microvascular complications.

Macrovascular Complications. Macrovascular complications with TZDs are controversial. In the Prospective Pioglitazone Clinical Trial in Macrovascular Events (PROactive) study, pioglitazone 45 mg was added to standard therapy in patients who had experienced a macrovascular event or had peripheral vascular disease.[85] The two groups were well matched at baseline, and the reported average observation time period was approximately 3 years. The primary end point (reduction in death, myocardial infarction, stroke, acute coronary syndrome, coronary revascularization, leg amputation, and leg revascularization) was reduced 10% ($P = 0.095$). The main secondary end point (all-cause mortality, nonfatal myocardial infarction, or stroke) was reduced 16% ($P = 0.027$). The seemingly dichotomous results relate to the inclusion of leg revascularization, which were increased in the pioglitazone group. Reasons for the increase are speculative, but can relate to more testing and inspection because of peripheral edema. Also of note, the pioglitazone group had 209 nonadjudicated admissions for heart failure occur versus 153 in the placebo group ($P = 0.007$), although fatal heart failure was not increased. Several nonpublished meta-analyses of rosiglitazone reported higher myocardial infarction rates with rosiglitazone. Recently, a hazard ratio of 1.43 (95% confidence intervals 1.03–1.98; $P = 0.03$) for the risk of a myocardial infarction with rosiglitazone versus other oral agents was reported, but has been widely criticized.[86] A prospective cardiovascular outcome trial with rosiglitazone is underway, but the FDA will likely require a black box warning about cardiovascular events with rosiglitazone.

Adverse Effects. Troglitazone, the first TZD approved, caused idiosyncratic hepatotoxicity and had 28 deaths from liver failure, which prompted removal from the U.S. market in March, 2000. Approximately 1.9% of patients placed on troglitazone had alanine aminotransferase (ALT) levels more than three times the upper limit of normal. The incidence, using these criteria for elevated liver enzymes, with pioglitazone (0.25%) and rosiglitazone (0.2%) has been low. No evidence of hepatotoxicity was reported in an analysis of more than 5,000 patients given rosiglitazone or pioglitazone.[87] Several case reports of hepatotoxicity with rosiglitazone or pioglitazone have been reported, but improvement in ALT was consistently noted when the drug was discontinued. Prior to therapy, it is recommended that an ALT be checked. ALT monitoring vigilance has been lowered, and it is now recommended that the ALT be checked periodically at the practitioner's discretion. Patients with ALT levels >2.5 times the upper limit of normal should not start either medication, and if the ALT is >3 times the upper limit of normal the medication should be discontinued.

Retention of fluid leads to many different possible side effects with rosiglitazone and pioglitazone. The etiology of the fluid retention has not been fully elucidated but appears to include peripheral vasodilation and/or improved insulin sensitization with a resultant increase in renal sodium and water retention. A reduction in plasma hemoglobin (2% to 4%), attributed to a 10% increase in plasma volume, can result in a dilutional anemia, which does not require treatment. Edema is also commonly (4% to 5% in mono- or combination therapy) reported. When a TZD is used in combination with insulin, the incidence of edema (~15%) is increased. TZDs are contraindicated in patients with New York Heart Association class III and IV heart failure, and great caution should be exercised when given to patients with class I and II heart failure or other underlying cardiac disease, as pulmonary edema and heart failure have been reported. Edema tends to be dose related and if not severe, a reduction in the dose as well as use of diuretics (anecdotally spironolactone appears to help selected patients) will allow the continuation of therapy in the majority of patients.[88] In addition, rarely, TZDs have been reported to worsen macular edema in the eye.

Weight gain, which is also dose related, can be seen with both rosiglitazone and pioglitazone. Mechanistically, both fluid retention and fat accumulation play a part in explaining the weight gain. TZDs, besides stimulating fat cell differentiation, also reduce leptin levels, which stimulate appetite and food intake. Average weight gain varies, but a 1.5- to 4-kg weight gain is not uncommon. Rarely, a patient will gain large amounts of weight in a short period of time, and this may necessitate discontinuation of therapy. Weight gain positively predicts a larger HbA_{1c} reduction but must be balanced with the well documented effects of long-term weight gain.

TZDs have also been associated with an increased fracture rate in the upper and lower limbs in postmenopausal women, but not men. As opposed to comparative diabetes therapy, TZDs can double the risk of fracture in this population. The underlying pathophysiology is speculative but can relate to the effect of TZD in bone marrow, with a reduction in osteoblast activity and an increase in bone marrow fat. It would be prudent to consider a patient's risk factors for fractures if prescribed a TZD and possibly have a lower threshold for additional assessment in postmenopausal women.

As a caution, anovulatory patients can resume ovulation on TZDs. Adequate pregnancy and contraception precautions should be explained to all women capable of becoming pregnant, as both agents are pregnancy category C.

Drug Interactions. No significant drug interactions have been noted with either medication. Neither pioglitazone nor rosiglitazone appear to be inhibitors or inducers of CYP3A4 and CYP2C8 or CYP2C8 and CYP2C9, respectively, although drugs that are strong inhibitors or inducers of these pathways (e.g., gemfibrozil or rifampin) necessitate close monitoring.

Dosing and Administration. The recommended starting dosages of pioglitazone and of rosiglitazone are 15 to 30 mg once daily and 2 to 4 mg once daily, respectively. Dosages can be increased slowly based on therapeutic goals and side effects. The maximum dose and maximum effective dose of pioglitazone is 45 mg, and rosiglitazone is 8 mg once daily, although 4 mg twice a day can reduce HbA_{1c} by 0.2% to 0.3% more as opposed to 8 mg once daily.

α-Glucosidase Inhibitors *Pharmacology.* Currently, there are two α-glucosidase inhibitors available in the United States (acarbose and miglitol). α-Glucosidase inhibitors competitively inhibit enzymes (maltase, isomaltase, sucrase, and glucoamylase) in the small intestine, delaying the breakdown of sucrose and complex carbohydrates.[89,90] They do not cause any malabsorption of these nutrients. The net effect from this action is to reduce the postprandial blood glucose rise.

Pharmacokinetics. The mechanism of action of α-glucosidase inhibitors is limited to the luminal side of the intestine. Some metabolites of acarbose are systemically absorbed and renally excreted, whereas the majority of miglitol is absorbed and renally excreted unchanged.

Efficacy. Postprandial glucose concentrations are reduced (40 to 50 mg/dL), whereas fasting glucose levels are relatively unchanged (~10% reduction). Efficacy on glycemic control is modest (average reductions in HbA_{1c} of 0.3% to 1%), affecting primarily postprandial glycemic excursions. Thus patients near target HbA_{1c} levels with near-normal FPG levels, but high postprandial levels, might be candidates for therapy.

Microvascular Complications. α-Glucosidase inhibitors modestly reduce HbA_{1c} levels, which have been shown to be related to the risk of microvascular complications.

Macrovascular Complications. The Study to Prevent Non–Insulin-Dependent Diabetes Mellitus (STOP-NIDDM), in subjects with impaired glucose tolerance, reported a significant reduction in the risk of cardiovascular events, although the total number of events were small.[91,92] No large cardiovascular study confirming these preliminary results has been done in prediabetes or diabetes patients.

Adverse Effects. The GI side effects, such as flatulence, bloating, abdominal discomfort, and diarrhea, are very common and greatly limit the use of α-glucosidase inhibitors. Mechanistically, these side effects are caused by distal intestinal degradation of undigested carbohydrate by the microflora, which results in gas (carbon dioxide [CO_2] and methane) production. α-Glucosidase inhibitors should be initiated at a low dose and titrated slowly to reduce GI intolerance. Beano, an α-glucosidase enzyme, can help to decrease GI side effects but can decrease efficacy slightly.[93]

If a patient develops hypoglycemia within several hours of ingesting an α-glucosidase inhibitor, oral glucose is advised because the drug will inhibit the breakdown of more complex sugar molecules. Milk, with lactose sugar, can be used as an alternative when no glucose is available, as acarbose only slightly (10%) inhibits lactase.

Rarely, elevated serum aminotransferase levels have been reported with the highest doses of acarbose. It appeared to be dose and weight related and is the premise for the weight-based maximum doses.

Dosing and Administration. Dosing for both miglitol and acarbose are similar. Initiate with a very low dose (25 mg with one meal a day); increase very gradually (over several months) to a maximum of 50 mg three times a day for patients ≤60 kg or 100 mg three times a day for patients >60 kg (see Table 77–12). Both α-glucosidase inhibitors should be taken with the first bite of the meal so that drug may be present to inhibit enzyme activity. Only patients consuming a diet high in complex carbohydrates will have significant reductions in glucose levels. α-Glucosidase inhibitors are contraindicated in patients with short-bowel syndrome or inflammatory bowel disease, and neither should be administered in patients with serum creatinine >2 mg/dL, as this population has not been studied.

DPP-IV inhibitors Sitagliptin is currently approved for use in the United States, whereas vildagliptin has received an approvable letter from the FDA.

Pharmacology. DPP-IV inhibitors prolong the half-life of an endogenously produced glucagon-like peptide-1 (GLP-1). It has clearly been shown that in type 2 DM, GLP-1 levels are deficient. DPP-IV inhibitors partially reduce the inappropriately elevated glucagon postprandially and stimulate glucose-dependent insulin secretion. As these agents block nearly 100% of the DPP-IV enzyme activity for at least 12 hours, near normal, nondiabetic GLP-1 levels are achieved. These drugs do not alter gastric emptying.

Pharmacokinetics. Sitagliptin appears to have rapid absorption, with t_{max} and C_{max} of approximately 1.5 hours. Absolute bioavailability after oral intake is approximately 87%. The $t_{1/2}$ of sitagliptin is approximately 12 hours, and 79% of the dose of sitagliptin is excreted unchanged in the urine by active tubular secretion. Sitagliptin exposure is increased by approximately 2.3-, 3.8-, and 4.5-fold relative to healthy subjects for patients with moderate renal insufficiency (creatinine clearance 30 to <50 mL/min), severe renal insufficiency (creatinine clearance <30 mL/min), and end-stage renal disease (on dialysis), respectively. Pharmacodynamically, DPP-IV inhibition appeared to mirror directly the plasma concentration of sitagliptin. Doses of 50 mg produced at least 80% inhibition of DPP-IV enzyme activity at 12 hours, and 100 mg produced 80% inhibition of DPP-IV enzyme activity at 24 hours. Food had no effect on absorption kinetics of sitagliptin or vildagliptin.

Vildagliptin is rapidly and almost completely (85%) absorbed after oral intake. Within 1 to 2 hours, t_{max} is achieved. The plasma $t_{1/2}$ varies with dose and is approximately 1.5 to 4.5 hours over a range or 25 mg to 200 mg. Approximately 55% of the drug is metabolized by hydrolysis, with the majority of the remaining drug eliminated unchanged by the kidneys. Vildagliptin dose-dependently inhibits the DPP-IV enzyme activity, approximately a 70% inhibition at 50 mg and 90% inhibition at 100 mg at 12 hours, with a continued 40% inhibition at 24 hours.

Efficacy. The average reduction in HbA_{1c} with vildagliptin or sitagliptin is approximately 0.7% to 1% at a dose of 100 mg a day. The HbA_{1c} decrement is dependent on the baseline value, with a larger reduction being seen with a higher baseline HbA_{1c}. As they are well tolerated, adjustment in the dose for adverse effects is unlikely.

Microvascular and Macrovascular Complications. HbA_{1c} levels are reduced, which have been related to a reduction in microvascular complications, but no outcome data are available to date.

Drug-Drug Interactions. Both are unlikely to have significant drug-drug interactions. Sitagliptin is metabolized approximately 20% by CYP3A4 with some CYP2C8 involvement but is neither an inhibitor nor inducer of any CYP450 enzyme system. Sitagliptin is a p-glycoprotein substrate, but had negligible effects on digoxin kinetics, and cyclosporine A increased the area under the curve (AUC) by only 30%. Neither drug is extensively plasma protein bound. Vildagliptin is neither an inhibitor nor inducer of CYP450 enzymes.

Adverse Effects. Both drugs are very well tolerated, weight neutral, and do not cause GI side effects. Mild hypoglycemia appears to be the only significant adverse effect, and the rate is similar to metformin. No significant increases in peripheral edema, hypertension, or cardiac outcomes have been noted to date. In regards to long-term safety, DPP-IV enzymes metabolize a wide variety of peptides (peptide YY [PYY], neuropeptide Y, growth hormone releasing hormone, and vasoactive intestinal polypeptide, and others) potentially affecting other regulatory systems. DPP-IV (also known as CD26) plays an important role for T-cell activation and theoretically the inhibition of DPP-IV could be associated with adverse immunologic reactions. Additionally DPP-8/9 inhibition in animals produced multiple toxicities. Both compounds have explored their binding to DPP-8/9, and have found minimal binding to these subtypes. Long-term safety data is still limited, but to date no adverse effects have been clearly linked to this issue.

Dosing and Administration. Vildagliptin will be dosed orally, likely at 50 mg to 100 mg daily. Sitagliptin is dosed orally at 100 mg daily unless renal insufficiency is present. The 50 mg dose is recommended if the creatinine clearance is 30 to less than 50 mL/min, or 25 mg if less than 30 mL/min. Equivalent serum creatinine levels are: sitagliptin 50 mg daily in men, greater than 1.7 to 3.0 mg/dL, women, greater than 1.5 to 2.5 mg/dL; 25 mg daily in men, greater than 3.0 mg/dL, women, greater than 2.5 mg/dL. No short-term adverse effects have been noted with increased exposure. Because of their excellent tolerability profile and a fairly flat dose-response curve, it seems logical that these drugs should be maximally dosed, unless cautions exist.

PIVOTAL TRIALS

Diabetes Control and Complications Trial

7 Much of the last century in diabetes care was dominated by the debate over whether glycemic control actually was causative in complications of DM. Animal studies and some human studies suggested that the worse the glycemia the greater the risk of complications. But "the glucose hypothesis" was not ultimately accepted as proven until the publication of the DCCT in 1993.[60] One thousand four hundred forty-one patients with type 1 DM were divided into two groups: those without complications (726 subjects, primary prevention), and those with early microvascular complications (715 subjects, secondary prevention). These two groups were then again divided into two groups, one randomized to receive conventional therapy (one or two shots of insulin daily and infrequent SMBG with no attempt to change therapy based on home blood glucose readings), and the other to receive intensive therapy (three or more injections of insulin daily or insulin pump, with frequent SMBG and alteration of insulin therapy based on SMBG results, plus frequent contact with a health professional). After 6.5 years mean followup with a difference in HbA_{1c} between the two groups being ~2% (~9% vs. ~7%), retinopathy was decreased by 76% in the primary prevention cohort, with retinopathy progression reduced 54% in the secondary prevention group. Neuropathy was decreased by 60% in both groups combined. Microalbuminuria was decreased 39%, whereas macroproteinuria was reduced 54% with intensive therapy. Hypoglycemia was more common and weight gain greater with intensive therapy. A nonstatistically significant reduction in coronary events was seen in the intensively treated group as compared to the conventional group. Followup studies 8 years after the DCCT ended continued to show an advantage of good glycemic control over what was previously considered conventional therapy.[94] The DCCT revolutionized therapy of DM, demanding that stricter glycemic control be the goal. Long-term followup of former DCCT subjects in the Epidemiology of Diabetes Interventions and Complications (EDIC) trial reported that, despite similar HbA_{1c} values 11 years later, renal and cardiovascular outcomes continued to be lower in intensively treated subjects from the DCCT as opposed to those who received conventional treatment.[95]

Implications of the United Kingdom Prospective Diabetes Study

The UKPDS was a landmark study for the care of patients with type 2 DM, confirming the importance of glycemic control for reducing the risk of microvascular complications.[61] More than 5,000 patients with newly diagnosed type 2 DM were entered into the study. Patients were followed for an average of 10 years. The major portion of the study assessed "conventional therapy" (no drug therapy unless the patient was symptomatic or had FPG >270 mg/dL), versus intensive therapy starting with either sulfonylureas or insulin, aimed at keeping the FPG <108 mg/dL. A subset of obese patients was studied using metformin as the primary therapeutic agent.

CLINICAL CONTROVERSY

Preservation of β-cell function, and thus arresting the progression of type 2 diabetes, appears to be the future goal of treatment. The UKPDS clearly showed that sulfonylureas, metformin, and insulin are ineffective in stopping the progressive β-cell failure. In animal models TZDs, exenatide, and DPP-IV inhibitors have been able to arrest β-cell failure, and in humans, short-term indirect β-cell function measures have improved. Confirmatory human data showing arrest or delay of the progressive β-cell decline in type 2 DM is needed. Rosiglitazone data in prediabetes and newly diagnosed diabetes, although measured by the homeostatic model assessment (HOMA)-β, has not shown significant preservation of β-cell function. Long-term data is underway with incretin based therapies.

Significant findings from the study include:

- Microvascular complications (predominantly the need for laser photocoagulation on retinal lesions) are reduced by 25% when median HbA_{1c} is 7% as compared to 7.9%.[53]
- A continuous relationship exists between glycemia and microvascular complications, with a 35% reduction in risk for each 1% decrement in HbA_{1c}. No glycemic threshold for microvascular disease exists.[96]
- Glycemic control has minimal effect on macrovascular disease risk.[61] Excess macrovascular risk appears to be related to conventional risk factors such as dyslipidemia and hypertension.[97]
- Sulfonylureas and insulin therapy do not increase macrovascular disease risk.[61]
- Metformin reduces macrovascular risk in obese patients.[84]
- Vigorous blood pressure control reduces microvascular and macrovascular events.[97] There was no evidence for a threshold systolic blood pressure above 130 mm Hg for protection against complications. β-Blockers and ACE inhibitors appear to be equally efficacious.[98]

THERAPEUTICS

8 Knowledge of the patient's quantitative and qualitative meal patterns, activity levels, pharmacokinetics of insulin preparations and other injectables, and pharmacology of oral and antidiabetic agents for type 2 DM are essential to individualize the treatment plan and optimize blood glucose control while minimizing risks for hypoglycemia and other adverse effects of pharmacologic therapies.

Type 1 DM

The choice of therapy for type 1 DM is simple: All patients need insulin. However, how that insulin is delivered to the patient is a matter of considerable practice difference among patients and clinicians. Historically, after the discovery of insulin by Banting and Best in 1921, frequent injections of regular insulin (initially the only insulin available) were given. Modifications of insulin led to longer-acting insulin suspensions and the use by many patients of one or two shots of longer-acting insulin each day. Because SMBG and HbA_{1c} testing were not available at that time, patients and practitioners had no idea how well their patients' blood glucose concentrations were controlled, other than a vague sense from an indirect method, measurement of glucose in the urine. Although the renal threshold for glucose is relatively predictable in young healthy subjects, it is highly variable in older patients and patients with renal disease. The advent of SMBG and HbA_{1c} testing in the 1980s revolutionized the care of diabetes, enabling patients and practitioners to directly access blood glucose for assessment, and enabling the patient to make instantaneous changes in the insulin regimen if need be. Modern diabetes management would be impossible without these two tools.

Contemporary management of type 1 DM attempts to match carbohydrate intake with glucose-lowering processes, most commonly insulin, as well as with exercise. Diet is still the cornerstone of diabetes therapy, but unlike in previous years, attempts are made to allow the patient to live as normal a life as possible. Understanding the principles of glucose input and glucose egress from the blood will allow the practitioner and the patient great latitude in the management of patients with type 1 DM.

Simplistically speaking, one can break down normal insulin secretion into a relatively constant background level of insulin (*basal*) for the fasting and postabsorptive period, and prandial spikes of insulin after eating (*bolus*) (Fig. 77–8).[99] Insulin sensitivity and insulin secretion are not constant throughout the day, rendering the basal concept inaccurate. However, in most clinical situations, this approach provides a useful paradigm for understanding and applying insulin treatment for type 1 DM. The other basic principle to consider is that the timing of insulin onset, peak, and duration of effect must match meal patterns and exercise schedules to achieve near-normal blood glucose values throughout the day.

Historically, complexity of insulin regimens has usually been related to the number of injections of insulin administered per day.

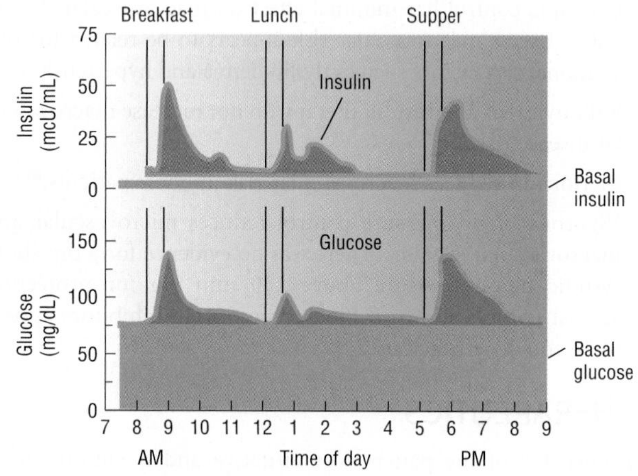

Intensive insulin therapy regimens

	7AM	11AM	5PM	Bedtime
1. 2 doses,[a] R or rapid acting + N	R, L, A, E, GLU + N		R, L, A, E, GLU + N	
2. 3 doses, R or rapid acting + N	R, L, A, E, GLU + N	R, L, A, E, GLU	R, L, A, E, GLU + N	
3. 4 doses, R or rapid acting + N	R, L, A, E, GLU	R, L, A, E, GLU	R, L, A, E, GLU	N
4. 4 doses R or rapid acting + N	R, L, A, E, GLU + N	R, L, A, E, GLU	R, L, A, E, GLU	N
5. 4 doses,[b] R or rapid acting + long acting	R, L, A, E, GLU	R, L, A, E, GLU	R, L, A, E, GLU	G or D[b] (G may be given anytime every 24 hours)
	←	Adjusted Basal	→	
6. CS-II pump	Bolus	Bolus	Bolus	

[a]Many clinicians may not consider this intensive insulin therapy
[b] May be given BID in type 1 DM= 5 doses

FIGURE 77-8. Relationship between insulin and glucose over the course of a day and how various insulin regimens could be given. (A, aspart; CS-II, continuous subcutaneous insulin infusion; D, detemir; E, Exubera; G, glargine; GLU, glulisine; L, lispro; N, NPH; R, regular.)

This is a reasonable classification. Clearly one injection of any insulin preparation daily will in no way mimic normal physiology, and therefore is unacceptable. Similarly, two injections of any insulin daily will fail to replicate normal insulin release patterns. Injection regimens that begin to approximate physiologic insulin release start with "split-mixed" injections of a morning dose of NPH and regular insulin before breakfast, and again before the evening meal. The presumption is made that the morning NPH insulin gives basal insulin for the day and covers the midday meal, the morning regular insulin covers breakfast, the evening NPH insulin gives basal insulin for the rest of the day, and the evening regular covers the evening meal. If patients are very compulsive about consistency of timing of their injections and meals and intake of carbohydrate, such a strategy can be successful. However, most patients are not sufficiently predictable in their schedule and food intake to allow "tight" glucose control with such an approach.

The first modification that is frequently made to such a regimen is the movement of the evening NPH to bedtime (now three total injections per day) because the fasting glucose in the morning is too high. This approach improves glycemic control and reduces hypoglycemia, sufficiently intensifying the insulin therapy for some patients.[100] However, many patients need a more intense approach that also allows greater flexibility in their lifestyle.

❾ The basal-bolus concept is an attempt to replicate normal insulin physiology with a combination of intermediate- or long-acting insulin to give the basal component, and short-acting insulin to give the bolus component. Various strategies have been used for the former, including once- or twice-daily NPH or detemir, or once-daily insulin glargine. Most type 1 DM patients require two shots of all of the above insulins except insulin glargine. Also, all of the above insulins, with the exception of insulin glargine, have some degree of peak effect that must be considered in planning meals and activity. Insulin glargine or insulin detemir is a feasible basal insulin supplement for most patients with type 1 DM. The bolus insulin component is given before meals with regular insulin, insulin lispro, insulin aspart, or insulin glulisine. The rapid onset of action and short time course of rapid-acting insulin analogs more closely replicate normal physiology. This approach allows the patient to vary the amount of insulin injected, depending on the preprandial SMBG level, the anticipated activity (upcoming exercise can reduce insulin requirement), and anticipated carbohydrate intake. Most patients will have a prescribed dose of insulin preprandially that they vary by use of a *sliding scale*. This type of adjusted scale insulin is intended to optimize the insulin regimen. In light of the negative connotation of the term *sliding scale* (usually referring to giving insulin only after the blood glucose increases, rather than treating the underlying disorder), a better descriptor for the adjusted-dose insulin is *variable-dose prandial insulin, correction factor*, or *insulin algorithm*. A rough correction factor can be calculated by taking 1,500 divided by the total daily dose of insulin. This gives the approximate glucose lowering (mg/dL) effect of one unit of insulin. Carbohydrate counting is a very effective tool for determining the amount of insulin to be injected preprandially. Although general algorithms give rough guidelines, each patient will have to adjust the prescribed preprandial insulin dosage to achieve optimal glucose control. A rough estimate of how much carbohydrate (grams) one unit of rapid-acting insulin will cover is to divide 500 by the total daily dose of insulin.

Empirically, patients can begin on ~0.6 unit/kg per day with basal insulin 50% of total dose and prandial insulin 20% of total dose prebreakfast, 15% prelunch, and 15% presupper. Type 1 DM patients generally require between 0.5 and 1 unit/kg per day. The need for significantly higher amounts of insulin suggests the presence of insulin antibodies or insulin resistance (coexistent endocrinopathy or type 2 DM).

Obviously, insulin pump therapy (continuous subcutaneous insulin infusion [CSII], generally using lispro or aspart insulin to diminish aggregation) is the most sophisticated form of basal bolus insulin delivery system. CSII can be slightly more efficacious in achieving good glycemic control than multiple-dose insulin injections.[101,102] Extensive discussion of this mode of therapy is beyond the scope of this text.[103] Nevertheless, the basic principles for implementation are the same. The one advantage of pump therapy is that the basal insulin dose can be varied, consistent with changes in insulin requirements throughout the day. In selected patients, this feature will allow greater glycemic control with CSII. However, insulin pumps require even greater attention to detail and frequency of SMBG than four injections daily.[104] In appropriately selected patients willing to pay sufficient attention to detail of SMBG and insulin administration, CSII can be a very useful form of therapy.

Intensive therapy (basal-bolus) to all adult patients with type 1 DM at the time of diagnosis is recommended to reinforce the importance of glycemic control from the outset rather than change strategies over time after lack of control. Occasional patients with an extended honeymoon period may need less intense therapy initially but should be converted to basal-bolus therapy at the onset of glycemic lability. For patients insisting on two injections daily, NPH and regular insulin (starting at 0.6 units/kg with two-thirds in the morning, two-thirds of morning dose as NPH, and one-half of evening dose as NPH) may be sufficient. Regardless of the regimen chosen, gross adjustments in the total insulin dose can be made based on HbA_{1c} measurements and symptoms such as polyuria, polydipsia, and weight gain or loss. Finer insulin adjustments can be determined on the basis of the results of frequent SMBG.

All patients receiving insulin should have extensive education in the recognition and treatment of hypoglycemia. Yearly (or more often) questioning about the recognition of hypoglycemia is warranted. Documentation of frequency of hypoglycemia, particularly that requiring assistance of another person, visit to an emergent or urgent care facility, or hospitalization, should be recorded. In type 1 DM, the development of hypoglycemia unawareness is common. It can result from progression of disease with autonomic neuropathy. Loss of adrenergic warning signs in such a situation is a relative contraindication to intensive insulin therapy. More commonly, type 1 DM patients have loss of warning signs because of a presumed lower set point for release of counterregulatory hormones as a result of frequent episodes of hypoglycemia ("hypoglycemia begets hypoglycemia").[105] In such situations, more normal hypoglycemia awareness can be restored by reduction or redistribution of the insulin dose to eliminate significant hypoglycemic episodes. A recent publication has found that short-term treatment with theophylline will improve hypoglycemia awareness.[106] This therapy should not routinely be employed but can be considered in refractory cases.

Children and pubescent adolescents are relatively protected from microvascular complications and must be managed with consideration of what is practical. Therefore it is not unreasonable to use less intense management (two shots per day, premixed insulins) until the patient is postpubertal.[107]

Occasional patients have antibodies to injected insulin, but the significance of the antibodies is usually minimal.[108] Human insulin therapy has not totally eliminated insulin allergies, although most patients have a local reaction that will dissipate over time. If the allergic reaction does not improve or is systemic, insulin desensitization can be carried out.[109] Protocols for desensitization are available from major insulin manufacturers. Although more common in the animal insulin era, lipohypertrophy is still seen in some patients with long-standing type 1 DM. Such patients give their insulin injections in the same site to minimize discomfort. Because insulin absorption from an area of lipohypertrophy is unpredictable, avoidance of injections into these areas is mandatory.

Several common errors can occur in the therapy of patients with type 1 DM, causing erratic glucose fluctuations:

- Failure to take into account peaks of insulin action when using a peaking insulin and planning meals and/or activity. Eating should be planned around the peaks of the insulin.
- Random rotation of insulin injection sites. There is sufficient variability of insulin absorption from site to site that this practice alone can cause wide glucose swings. The most consistent absorption of insulin is from the abdominal wall. We try to get our patients to take all their injections in the abdomen. If the patient is unable or unwilling to follow this advice, then systematic site rotation is the next preferable option. The patient always gives the insulin injection in the same region of the body the same time of the day each day. For instance, the arms are always used every morning. Needless to say, the patient would not inject in a limb and then go out and exercise that limb, increasing blood flow and insulin absorption.
- Overinsulinization is a very common problem. The answer to all high blood glucose is not necessarily more insulin, as the patient may be insulinopenic, or may be "rebounding" from a previous low glucose and treating it with excessive amounts of carbohydrate. Fastidious SMBG, particularly during the night (or selected use of continuous glucose monitoring) will help sort this out. Also, practitioners sometimes do not adequately differentiate type 1 DM from type 2 DM when using insulin. Patients with type 1 DM are insulinopenic but have normal insulin sensitivity. Patients with type 2 DM have varying degrees of insulin resistance. Therefore one unit change in the dose of insulin for a patient with type 1 DM can have a dramatic effect on glucose concentrations, whereas in some patients with type 2 DM 10 to 20 times that amount of insulin can have little effect on glucose. Large changes in insulin dose in patients with type 1 DM are not usually indicated unless the patient's blood glucose control is very poor. Widely erratic SMBG results and/or weight gain often suggest overinsulinization.
- When in doubt, always double check the patient's technique for insulin dosing, insulin injection, and SMBG. Sometimes the simplest of errors results in miserable glycemic control.

Pramlintide in type 1 DM patients who continue to have erratic postprandial control despite consideration or implementation of the above strategies can be appropriate. It is imperative at initiation of therapy with pramlintide that each dose of prandial insulin (rapid acting analog or regular insulin) be reduced by 30% to 50%, or severe hypoglycemic reactions have occurred. Pramlintide should be judiciously titrated based on GI adverse effects and postprandial glycemic goals. As pramlintide is not recommended for mixing, you are adding an additional prandial injection at each meal. A patient who is cognizant of the hypoglycemic risk, GI side effects, and effective strategies to reduce both is needed.

Islet cell and whole pancreas transplantation are occasionally used in patients, usually renal transplants, who require immunosuppressive therapy for other reasons.[110] There has been considerable interest in islet cell transplantation since investigators in Edmonton reported success without using glucocorticoids as immunosuppressive agents.[111] Some of these patients are able to come off insulin altogether.

Type 2 DM

Pharmacotherapy for type 2 DM has changed dramatically in the last few years with the addition of several new drug classes and recommendations to achieve more stringent glycemic control. Symptomatic patients may initially require treatment with insulin or combination oral therapy to reduce glucose toxicity (which can reduce β-cell insulin secretion and worsen insulin resistance). Patients with HbA_{1c} ~7% or less are usually treated with therapeutic lifestyle measures and an agent that will not cause hypoglycemia. Those with HbA_{1c} >7% but <8% could be initially treated with single oral agents, or low dose combinations. Patients with higher initial HbA_{1c} can benefit from initial therapy with two oral agents, or even insulin.

⑩ Depending on patient motivation and adherence to therapeutic lifestyle changes, most patients with HbA_{1c} greater than 9% to 10% will likely require therapy with two or more agents to reach glycemic goals. Treatment of type 2 DM often necessitates use of multiple therapeutic agents (combination therapy), to obtain glycemic goals.

The best initial oral therapy for patients with type 2 DM is widely debated. Based on the results of the UKPDS and safety record, obese patients (>120% ideal body weight) without contraindications should be started on metformin titrated to ~2,000 mg/day.[112] Near-normal weight patients can be treated with insulin secretagogues. Failure of initial therapy should result in addition rather than substitution (reserve substitution for intolerance to a drug because of side effects) of another class of drug. For cost and glycemic efficacy reasons, metformin and an insulin secretagogue are often first- and second-line therapy, although combination with other agents for potential cardioprotection or potential β-cell preservation may be preferred. Initial oral combination therapy for patients with HbA_{1c} >9% to 10% should be considered, and several oral combination products are available. Oral combination agents that have metformin in combination with a sulfonylurea are often very effective in lowering initially high HbA_{1c} levels. Figure 77–9 is an algorithm developed by the Texas Diabetes Council for glycemic control. TZDs can be substituted in situations in which a patient is intolerant of, or has a contraindication to, metformin as an insulin sensitizer, understanding that TZDs should be used with caution in heart failure.

The paradigm of treatment is slowly changing, as potentially preserving β-cell function, thus arresting the progressive nature of type 2 DM, is becoming a priority. In the UKPDS, insulin, metformin, or sulfonylureas did not halt β-cell failure. TZDs, exenatide, vildagliptin, and sitagliptin can potentially preserve β-cell function.[113,114] Despite long-term success at preventing diabetes or treating newly diagnosed diabetes, HOMA-β measures have not shown β-cell benefit with rosiglitazone. Long-term β-cell studies with pioglitazone are underway. If positive human results are found long-term, any of these medications could become potential first-line therapy. For dual therapy, HbA_{1c} reductions vary according to the medication added to the current therapy (Table 77–14). After a patient has inadequate control on two drugs, adding a third drug can be considered. Triple therapy with a TZD is often instituted, but a significant number of patients either have inadequate glycemic improvement or significant side effects. An alternative is to add exenatide, DPP-IV inhibitor, basal insulin, or even the prandial inhaled insulin, Exubera. Therapy should be guided by the HbA_{1c}, FPG, cost, additional benefits (such as weight loss), and avoidance of contraindications and side effects. If the HbA_{1c} is >8.5% to 9% on multiple therapies, insulin therapy should be considered first. If the patient is obese and the HbA_{1c} is ≤8.5%, addition of exenatide or potentially a DPP-IV inhibitor can be considered. Sulfonylureas are often stopped when insulin is added, but continuing the sulfonylurea is permissible until multiple daily injections are started, at which time it should definitely be discontinued.

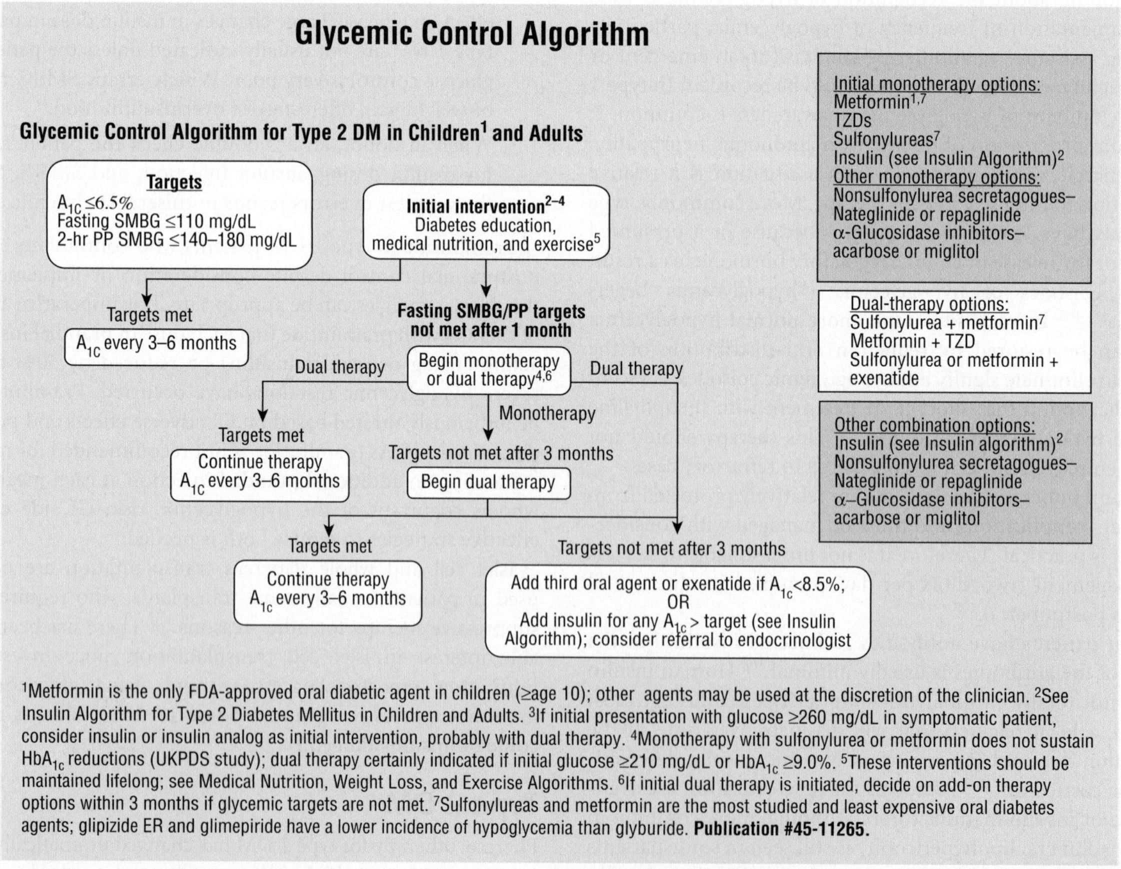

FIGURE 77-9. Glycemic control algorithm for type 2 diabetes mellitus (DM) in children and adults. See *www.texasdiabetescouncil.org* for current algorithms. (A_{1c}, glycosylated hemoglobin; ER, extended release; PP, postprandial; SMBG, self-monitoring of blood glucose; TZD, thiazolidinedione; UKPDS, United Kingdom Prospective Diabetes Study.) *(Reprinted with permission from the Texas Diabetes Council.)*

TABLE 77-14 Add-On Dual Therapy: Average HbA_{1c} Reductions[a]

Drug Combination	Change in HbA_{1c} (%)	Number of Studies	Number of Subjects
Sulfonylurea + metformin	−2.2	8	458
Sulfonylurea + insulin	−1.9	17	88
Meglitinide + thiazolidinedione	−1.7	1	434
Metformin + insulin	−1.7	8	138
Sulfonylurea + α-glucosidase inhibitor	−1.6	3	177
Metformin + meglitinide	−1.4	3	226
Insulin + α-glucosidase inhibitor	−1.2	1	20
Insulin + thiazolidinedione	−1.2	7	850
Sulfonylurea + thiazolidinedione	−1.1	12	1,315
Metformin + exenatide	−0.8	2	1,070
Metformin + vildagliptin	−0.7	1	416
Metformin + thiazolidinedione	−0.9	3	284
Metformin + α-glucosidase inhibitor	−0.4	3	173

HbA_{1c}, glycosolated hemoglobin.

[a]Reductions are averages and do not imply superiority or inferiority of a combination.

Adapted from American Diabetes Association. Dyslipidemia management in adults with diabetes. Diabetes Care 2004;27:568-571.

Exenatide and DPP-IV inhibitors add a new mechanistic way to lower blood glucose. Exenatide is advantageous because it can allow weight loss in type 2 DM patients, but is a twice-a-day injection and has some GI adverse effects. DPP-IV inhibitors are advantageous because they are orally active, weight neutral, and are very well tolerated but lack long-term safety data. It should be remembered that both classes work mainly to lower postprandial glucose excursions and have only a modest effect on the FPG. Thus, if the patient's fasting glucose is significantly elevated, additional therapy to lower the FPG will often be needed. Metformin, sulfonylureas, repaglinide, TZDs, and basal insulin all effectively lower the FPG.

Virtually all patients with type 2 DM ultimately become relatively insulinopenic and will require insulin therapy. Insulin therapy for type 2 DM has changed dramatically in the last few years. Specifically, patients are often "transitioned" to insulin by using a bedtime injection of an intermediate- or long-acting insulin, and using oral agents primarily for control during the day.[115,116] This strategy leads to less hyperinsulinemia during the day and is associated with less weight gain than the more traditional insulin strategies. Because most patients are insulin resistant, insulin sensitizers are commonly used with insulin therapy. Patients with type 2 DM are usually well buffered against hypoglycemia. Patients should be monitored for hypoglycemia by asking about nocturnal sweating, nightmares (both indicative of nocturnal hypoglycemia), palpitations, tremulousness, and neuroglycopenic symptoms, as well as SMBG. When bedtime insulin plus daytime oral medications fail to achieve glycemic goals, a conventional multiple daily dose insulin regimen while continuing the insulin sensitizers is often tried. Alternatively, off-label use of exenatide for prandial control can be considered, if covered by insurance. Concerns and problems with insulin administration as addressed in the section on type 1 DM generally relate to the therapy of type 2 DM. However, patients with type 2 DM rarely have hypoglycemia unawareness. Also, the variability of insulin resistance means that insulin doses can range from 0.7 to 2.5 units/kg or more. Figure 77–10 is an algorithm for insulin therapy options in type 2 diabetes developed by the Texas Diabetes Council.

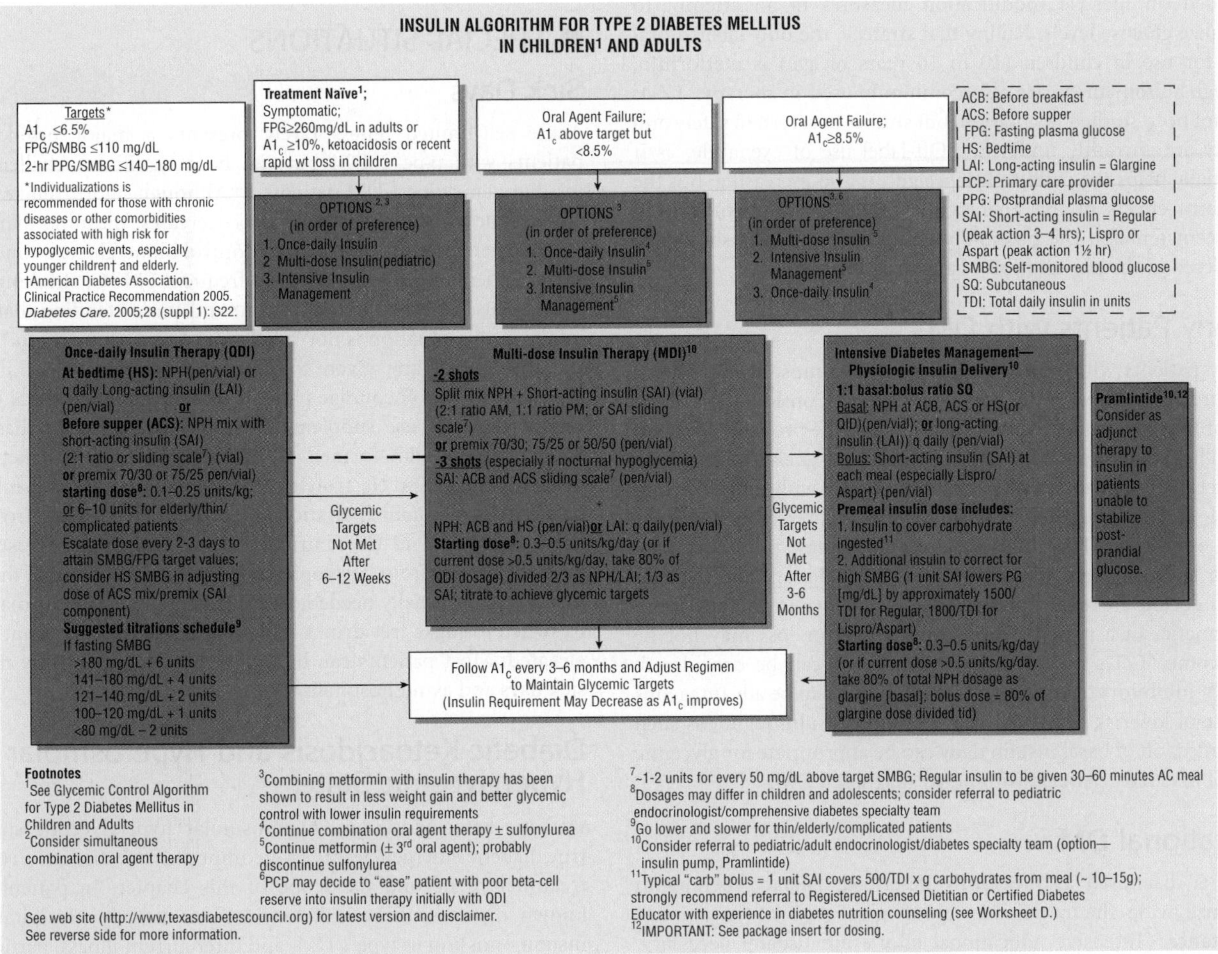

FIGURE 77-10. Insulin algorithm for type 2 diabetes mellitus (DM) in children and adults. See *www.texasdiabetescouncil.org* for current algorithms. *(Reprinted with permission from the Texas Diabetes Council.)*

The availability of short-acting insulin secretagogues, rapid-acting insulin analogs, human insulin inhalation powder, exenatide, DPP-IV inhibitors, and α-glucosidase inhibitors, all of which target postprandial glycemia, has reminded practitioners that glycemic control is a function of fasting and preprandial glycemia and postprandial glycemic excursions.[117] Therefore postprandial glucose measurements may need more emphasis if the HbA_{1c} is near the glycemic goal. Currently, it remains controversial whether targeting after-meal glucose excursions will have more of an effect on complications risk than more conventional strategies. Importantly, postprandial excursions proportionally contribute more than the FPG to the HbA_{1c} percentage when the HbA_{1c} nears goals, and thus will need to be targeted for optimal glycemic control in many patients. Also controversial are the American College of Endocrinology/American Association of Clinical Endocrinologists postprandial glycemic goals (see Table 77–8). These guidelines use epidemiologic studies with post–glucose challenge glucose measurements in diabetic and nondiabetic subjects to state that postprandial glycemia is a better predictor of macrovascular disease risk in DM.[118] In contrast, the ADA continues to recommend peak postprandial blood glucose levels less than 180 mg/dL.

■ SPECIAL POPULATIONS

Children and Adolescents with Type 2 DM

Type 2 DM is increasing in adolescence.[10] Obesity and physical inactivity seem to be particular culprits in the pathogenesis of this disease. Given the many years that the patient will have to live with diabetes, and recent evidence that the timeline for complications may mimic that of older adults, extraordinary efforts should be expended on lifestyle modification measures in an attempt to normalize glucose levels. Failing that strategy, the only labeled oral agent for use in children (10 to 16 years of age) is metformin, although sulfonylureas are also commonly used in therapy. TZDs have not been studied in children, but studies to ascertain safety and efficacy are currently underway. Off-label use of exenatide, as it potentially helps the child to lose weight, is also increasing, but the long-term effects of this therapeutic modality are unknown. In adolescent females, the possibility of future pregnancy should be considered in the prescription of any drug regimen.

Elderly Patients with DM

Elderly patients with newly diagnosed DM (almost always type 2 DM) present a different therapeutic challenge. Consideration of the risks of hypoglycemia in this population and the probable life span should help determine if less-stringent glycemic goals should be set. Thinner, older patients can primarily be treated with shorter-acting insulin secretagogues, low-dose sulfonylureas (preferably not long-acting ones), DPP-IV inhibitors, or α-glucosidase inhibitors. The risk for lactic acidosis, which increases with older age and the age-related decline in renal function, makes metformin therapy more problematic. In a patient whom weight gain or loss may not be unwelcome, TZDs or exenatide, respectively, can be considered. DPP-IV inhibitors or α-glucosidase inhibitors can be advantageous because of low risk of hypoglycemia. Simple insulin regimens such as an injection of basal insulin daily can be appropriate for glycemic control in elderly patients with newly diagnosed DM.

Gestational DM

GDM is diagnosed as previously described. Dietary therapy to minimize wide fluctuations in blood glucose is of paramount importance.[5] Intensive educational efforts are usually necessary. Pregnant women without DM maintain plasma glucose concentrations between 50 and 130 mg/dL. Frequent SMBG is needed to tell whether dietary interventions are successful. If FPG is >105 mg/dL, or 1-hour postprandial plasma glucose levels are >155 mg/dL, or if 2-hour postprandial plasma glucose levels are >130 mg/dL, insulin therapy is usually begun. One shot of NPH or a mixture of NPH and regular insulin in a 2:1 ratio given before breakfast may be adequate to reach glucose targets. Titration of insulin and switching to more complicated regimens is guided by SMBG results. Use of basal insulins other than NPH is still debated, but with the ease of use of detemir or glargine insulin, their use in GDM will likely increase. In addition, pump therapy for the duration of the pregnancy is often instituted, as it can obtain excellent glycemic control and is quickly adjustable. In spite of the long-standing labeling of sulfonylureas as contraindicated in pregnancy, one randomized, open-label, controlled trial evaluated the efficacy of glyburide as compared to insulin initiated after 11 weeks' gestation.[119] Adequate control of blood glucose was achieved as compared to traditional insulin therapy, with less hypoglycemia in the glyburide group. No evidence of any difference in complications, specifically cord-serum insulin concentrations, incidence of macrosomia (birth weight of 4 kg or more), cesarean delivery, or neonatal hypoglycemia between regimens were noted. Glyburide was not detected in the cord serum of any infant. As the study limited enrollment beyond 11 weeks' gestation, no conclusions regarding teratogenicity can be made from this study. The ADA cites this study in a position paper and mentions its usefulness, but also warns that it is not a labeled use of the drug and suggests further studies are needed to establish its safety.[12] Patients with GDM should be evaluated 6 weeks after delivery to ensure that normal glucose tolerance has returned. Because these patients' long-term risk for the development of type 2 DM is considerable, periodic assessment after that is warranted.

■ SPECIAL SITUATIONS

Sick Days

Acute self-limited illness rarely presents a major problem for patients with type 2 DM but can be a significant challenge for insulinopenic type 1 DM patients.[120] Although caloric intake generally declines, insulin sensitivity also decreases, meaning that it can take greater amounts of insulin to control blood glucose concentrations. Patients need to be adept at frequent SMBG, checking urine ketones, use of short-acting insulin, and understanding that sugar intake in this situation is not "bad" but can be necessary to "cover" the insulin therapy given to keep the patient out of diabetic ketoacidosis. We encourage patients to continue their usual insulin regimen and to use supplemental rapid-acting insulin based on SMBG results, with further additional insulin given if ketonuria develops. Sugar and electrolyte solutions, such as sports drinks, can be used to maintain hydration, to provide needed electrolytes if there are significant GI or urinary losses, and to provide sugar to keep the patient from developing hypoglycemia because of the extra insulin that is usually needed. In contrast, type 2 patients may need to switch to sugar-free drinks if blood glucose levels are continually elevated. Most patients can be taught how to sufficiently manage sick days and avoid hospitalization.

Diabetic Ketoacidosis and Hyperosmolar Hyperglycemic State

Diabetic ketoacidosis and hyperosmolar hyperglycemic state are true diabetic emergencies.[121,122] A comprehensive discussion of their treatment is beyond the scope of this chapter. In patients with known diabetes, diabetic ketoacidosis is usually precipitated by insulin omission in type 1 DM, and intercurrent illness, particularly infection, in both type 1 and type 2 DM. However, patients with type 1 or type 2 DM (the latter being usually nonwhites or Hispanics) can present at initial presentation.[123] It is possible that some of the patients deemed to have type 2 DM actually have type 1 idiopathic DM. Patients with diabetic ketoacidosis can be alert, stuporous, or comatose at presentation. The hallmark diagnostic laboratory values include hyperglycemia, anion gap acidosis, and large ketonemia or ketonuria. Afflicted patients have fluid deficits of several liters and sodium and potassium deficits of several hundred milliequivalents. Restoration of intravascular volume acutely with normal saline, followed by hypotonic saline to replace free water, potassium supplements, and constant infusion insulin restore the patient's metabolic status relatively quickly. A flow sheet is often helpful in tracking the fluid and insulin therapies and laboratory parameters in these patients. Bicarbonate administration is generally not needed and may be harmful, especially in children.[124] Treatment of the inciting medical condition is also vital. Hourly bedside monitoring of glucose and frequent monitoring (every 2 to 4 hours) of potassium is essential. Metabolic improvement is manifested by an increase in the serum bicarbonate or pH. Serum phosphorus usually starts high and plummets to lower-than-normal levels, although replacing phosphorus, although not unreasonable, is of questionable benefit in most patients. Fluid administration alone will reduce the glucose concentration, so a decrement in glucose values does not necessarily mean that the patient's metabolic status is improving. Rare patients will require larger amounts of insulin than those usually given (5 to 10 units/h). We double the patient's insulin dose if the serum bicarbonate has not improved after the first 4 hours of insulin therapy. Constant infusion of a fixed dose of insulin and the administration of intravenous glucose when the blood glucose level decreases to <250 mg/dL is preferable to titration of the insulin infusion based on the glucose level. The latter strategy may delay clearance of the ketosis and prolong treatment. The insulin infusion should be continued until the urine ketones clear and the anion gap closes. Long-acting insulin should be given 1 to 3 hours prior to discontinuing the insulin infusion. Intramuscular regular insulin or subcutaneous insulin lispro or aspart given every 1 to 2 hours can be used rather than an insulin infusion in patients without hypoperfusion. Patients can develop hyperchloremic metabolic acidosis with treatment if they have been given large volumes of normal saline in the course of their treatment. Such a situation does not require any specific treatment.

Hyperosmolar hyperglycemic state usually occurs in older patients with type 2 DM, at times undiagnosed, or in younger patients with prolonged hyperglycemia and dehydration or significant renal insufficiency. Large ketonemia is usually not seen, as residual insulin secretion suppresses the production of ketones. Infection or another medical illness is the usual precipitant. Fluid deficits are usually greater and blood glucose concentrations higher (at times >1,000 mg/dL) in these patients than in patients with diabetic ketoacidosis. Blood glucose levels should be lowered very gradually with hypotonic fluids and low-dose insulin infusions (1 to 2 units/h). Rapid correction of the glucose levels, a drop greater than 75 to 100 mg/dL per hour, is not recommended, as it can result in cerebral edema. This is especially true for children with diabetic ketoacidosis. Mortality is high with the hyperosmolar hyperglycemic state.

Hospitalization for Intercurrent Medical Illness

Patients on oral agents can need transient therapy with insulin to achieve adequate glycemic control. In patients requiring insulin, patients should receive scheduled doses of insulin with additional short-acting insulin. "Sliding-scale" insulin is to be discouraged, as it is notorious for not controlling glucose and for sometimes resulting in therapeutic misadventures, with wide swings in the blood glucose as the patient "bounces" from hypoglycemia to hyperglycemia.[125] In-hospital mortality is increased in many hyperglycemic conditions. At least one study documented a reduction in mortality in type 2 diabetes patients with acute myocardial infarctions[126] who receive constant intravenous insulin during the acute phase of the event to maintain near-normal glucose concentrations. Similar mortality results have been documented in some intensive care unit settings using intravenous insulin and tight glucose control.[127,128] Currently the American College of Endocrinology recommends preprandial levels <110 mg/dL, and postprandial level <180 mg/dL, but the ADA lists these data as evidence based level B.[129] Many protocols for IV insulin infusion are currently available, and implementation for an inpatient setting should use a well established protocol. It is prudent to stop metformin in all patients who arrive in acute care settings until full elucidation of the reason for presentation can be ascertained, as contraindications to metformin are prevalent in hospitalized patients.[130]

Perioperative Management

Surgical patients can experience worsening of glycemia for reasons similar to those listed above for intercurrent medical illness.[131] Patients on oral agents can need transient therapy with insulin to control blood glucose. In patients requiring insulin, scheduled doses of insulin or continuous insulin infusions are preferred. For patients who can eat soon after surgery, the time-honored approach of giving one-half of the usual morning NPH insulin dose with dextrose 5% in water intravenously is acceptable, with resumption of scheduled insulin, perhaps at reduced doses, within the first day. For patients requiring more prolonged periods without oral nutrition and for major surgery, such as coronary artery bypass grafting and major abdominal surgery, constant infusion intravenous insulin is preferred. Use of intravenous insulin infusion has been shown to reduce deep sternal wound infections in patients undergoing coronary artery bypass grafting. Metformin should be discontinued temporarily after any major surgery until it is clear that the patient is hemodynamically stable and normal renal function is documented.

Reproductive-Age Women and Preconception Care for Women

An increasing prevalence of DM has been noted in reproductive-age women.[132,133] Prepregnancy planning is absolutely mandatory, as organogenesis is largely completed within 8 weeks, so good glycemic control should be obtained prior to conception. Unfortunately, major congenital malformations because of poor glucose control remain the leading cause of mortality and serious morbidity in infants of mothers with type 1 or type 2 diabetes. For women with DM controlled by lifestyle measures alone, conversion to insulin as soon as the pregnancy is confirmed is appropriate. For women with polycystic ovary disease who ovulate and become pregnant with insulin sensitizer therapy, conversion to insulin is mandatory as soon as pregnancy is confirmed. Insulin is the only acceptable pharmacologic therapy during pregnancy for women with DM in the United States. In Europe, metformin and glyburide are sometimes used in pregnancy for type 2 DM, but their use is controversial in the United States. Patients previously treated with insulin can need intensification of their regimen to achieve therapeutic goals. Normal pregnancy is associated with a decrease in the blood glucose concentration as fuel is diverted to the fetus. Pregnant patients will be ingesting both meals and snacks daily. SMBG is generally intensified to try to reach glycemic targets and reduce fetal and maternal morbidity. Whether preprandial or postprandial glucose concentrations should be the target of therapy is hotly debated. Ketosis should be avoided, requiring urine monitoring for ketones in the morning and if the blood sugar is >200 mg/dL.

There has been some concern about the safety of insulin analogs in pregnancy, both for fetal development and advancement of microvascular complications. One study has shown no increase in retinopathy or progression of same with the use of insulin lispro in pregnancy.[134]

SPECIAL TOPICS

Prevention of DM

⓬ Efforts to prevent type 1 DM with immunosuppressives[135] or injected[136] or oral insulin therapy[137] have been unsuccessful. The Diabetes Prevention Program[138] confirmed that modest weight loss in association with exercise can have a dramatic impact on insulin sensitivity and the conversion from impaired glucose tolerance to type 2 diabetes. In this study approximately 2,000 individuals with impaired glucose tolerance were randomized to lifestyle changes (diet, exercise, and weight loss) as opposed to usual care. The study, which was originally planned to be ongoing for 5 years, was stopped after 2.8 years because the results were so conclusive. The usual care group developed diabetes at the rate of 11% each year. The lifestyle arm developed diabetes at a rate of 5% per year, a 58% reduction in the risk of developing diabetes.[138] Surprisingly, a modest amount of diet and exercise yielded impressive results. The exercise program in the lifestyle group was walking 30 minutes, 5 days each week. The mean weight loss over the 2.8 year study period was only 3.6 kg (8 lb). Similar results were seen in the Finnish Diabetes Study.[139] In the Diabetes Prevention Program[138] discussed above, approximately 1,000 of the study patients were randomized to metformin therapy. The metformin-treated patients showed a 1.8-kg (4-lb) weight loss [138] Interestingly, young and overweight individuals on metformin had a greater reduction in the risk of developing diabetes than normal weight and older study patients.[138]

Metformin and acarbose[92] appear to mostly be treating early diabetes, because when the drugs were stopped, diabetes rates were close to the conversion rates for placebo. In contrast, the Troglitazone in the Prevention of Diabetes (TRIPOD) study[140] evaluated the ability of troglitazone to prevent the development of diabetes in women with a history of gestational diabetes. The rate of development of diabetes in the placebo arm of the study was approximately 12% per year, compared to about 5% in the treatment group. Total preservation of β-cell function was demonstrated over a 5-year period in women who had near normal β-cell function at baseline and who initially responded to the drug.[140] The preservation of β-cell function was observed for at least 8 months after the drug had been discontinued. The Diabetes Reduction Assessment with Ramipril and Rosiglitazone Medication (DREAM) trial evaluating rosiglitazone and/or ramipril treatment for the delay or prevention of type 2 DM in impaired glucose tolerant subjects was recently published.[141,142] Rosiglitazone 8 mg daily, over approximately 3 years, reduced the incidence of type 2 diabetes by 60%. In addition, a 37% nonsignificant increase in cardiovascular events was reported. Ramipril 15 mg daily did not significantly prevent the conversion to diabetes. It is possible that longer exposure could have made a difference, but the study was stopped prematurely. It should be noted that no pharmacologic agents are currently FDA approved or recommended for prevention of type 2 diabetes, though the ADA recommends metformin in conjunction with lifestyle changes if the patient is younger, obese, has a family history of diabetes, dyslipidemia, hypertension, or a HbA_{1c} above 6%.[143] Prevention studies are still underway using pioglitazone, nateglinide, and valsartan.

CLINICAL CONTROVERSY

DM is associated with a substantially higher risk of morbidity and mortality. Pharmacologic prevention or delay of type 2 DM has been widely discussed since the release of the Diabetes Prevention Program results. Although lifestyle changes were effective, with a 58% lower relative risk of progression to diabetes, metformin 850 mg twice a day reduced the risk by 31%, and was essentially as effective as diet and exercise in young/obese subjects. Rosiglitazone, acarbose, and even orlistat all have, to one extent or another, been able to delay the onset of type 2 DM. Despite these data, there are no FDA-approved drugs for the delay or prevention of diabetes. The ADA-recommended medications, in conjunction with lifestyle, for the delay or prevention of type 2 DM include metformin. It should be remembered that medications require monitoring and can have serious side effects. Many feel they are simply treating diabetes early, as β-cell dysfunction can be documented in early impaired glucose tolerant subjects. Other than troglitazone, which is not on the market, no medication has clearly shown β-cell preservation. It is logical to try to use medications if they alter the decline of β-cell function, but this is currently off-label use and any attempt to use medication in these situations should be clearly and frankly discussed with the patient.

Patient Education

⓭ It is not satisfactory to give patients with DM brief instructions with a few pamphlets and expect them to manage their disease adequately. Thinking that diabetes education is limited to one or two encounters is misguided; education is a lifetime exercise. Successful treatment of DM involves lifestyle changes for the patient (e.g., medical nutrition therapy, physical activity, self-monitoring of blood glucose and possibly of urine for ketones, and taking prescribed medications). The patient must be involved in the decision-making process and must learn as much about the disease and associated complications as possible. Emphasis should be placed on the evidence that indicates that complications can be prevented or minimized with glycemic control and management of risk factors for cardiovascular disease. Recognition of the need for proper patient education to empower them into self-care has generated programs for certification in diabetes education. Certified diabetes educators must document their patient education hours and sit for a certification examination that assesses the knowledge, tasks, and skills of an educator in order to become certified. An increasing number of nurses, pharmacists, dietitians, and physicians are becoming certified diabetes educators to document to the public that they meet a minimum standard for diabetes education and to fulfill quality initiatives in meeting guidelines for education recognition.[144]

TREATMENT OF CONCOMITANT CONDITIONS AND COMPLICATIONS

Retinopathy

Patients with established retinopathy should see an ophthalmologist or optometrist trained in diabetic eye disease.[145] A dilated eye examination is required to fully evaluate diabetic eye disease. Early background retinopathy can reverse with improved glycemic control. More advanced retinopathy will not regress with improved glycemia and can actually worsen with short-term improvements in glycemia. Studies are underway to determine whether medical therapy independent of glucose control will prevent the development of advanced retinopathy. Laser photocoagulation has markedly improved sight preservation in diabetic patients.

Neuropathy

Peripheral neuropathy is the most common complication seen in type 2 DM patients in outpatient clinics.[146] Paresthesias, numbness, or pain can be the predominant symptom. The feet are involved far more often than the hands. Improved glycemic control can alleviate some of the symptoms. If neuropathy is painful, symptomatic therapy is empiric, including low-dose tricyclic antidepressants, anticonvulsants (gabapentin, pregabalin, carbamazepine, and maybe phenytoin), duloxetine, venlafaxine, topical capsaicin, and various pain medications, including tramadol and nonsteroidal antiinflammatory drugs. Recently, another anticonvulsant, topiramate, has shown promise in the reduction of symptoms, with the positive side effect of weight loss in type 2 diabetes patients, although tolerability is problematic. The numb variant of peripheral neuropathy is not treated with medication. Clinical manifestations of diabetic autonomic neuropathy include resting tachycardia, exercise intolerance, orthostatic hypotension, constipation, gastroparesis, erectile dysfunction, sudomotor dysfunction (anhidrosis, heat intolerance, gustatory sweating, and/or dry skin), impaired neurovascular function, and hypoglycemic autonomic failure. Gastroparesis can be a severe and debilitating complication of DM. Improved glycemic control, discontinuation of medications that slow gastric motility, and the use of metoclopramide (preferably for only a few weeks at a time) or erythromycin can be helpful. Gastric pacemakers as therapeutic hardware are rarely used, although available. Orthostatic hypotension can require pharmacologic management with mineralocorticoids or adrenergic agonist agents. In severe cases, supine hypertension is extreme, mandating that the patient sleep in a sitting or semirecumbent position. Patients with cardiac autonomic neuropathy are at a higher risk for silent myocardial infarction and mortality. The hallmark of diabetic diarrhea is its nocturnal occurrence. Diabetic diarrhea frequently responds to a 10- to 14-day course of an antibiotic such as doxycycline or metronidazole. In more unresponsive cases, octreotide can be useful. Erectile dysfunction is common in diabetes, and initial treatment should include a trial of one of the oral medications currently available to treat erectile dysfunction. People with diabetes often require the highest doses of these medications to have an adequate response. Sudomotor dysfunction, as earlier defined, results in loss of sweating and resultant dry, cracked skin. Use of hydrating creams and ointments is needed.

Microalbuminuria and Nephropathy

DM, and particularly type 2 DM, is the biggest contributor statistically to the development of end-stage renal disease in the United States.[147] The ADA recommends a screening urinary analysis for albumin at diagnosis in persons with type 2 DM. Precise onset of type 2 DM can rarely be ascertained, and patients will often present at diagnosis with microvascular complications. In type 1 DM, microalbuminuria rarely occurs with short duration of disease or before puberty. Screening individuals with type 1 DM should begin with puberty and after 5 years' disease duration. There are three methods for assessing microalbuminuria: (1) measurement of the urine albumin-to-creatinine ratio in a random spot collection (preferably the first morning void); (2) 24-hour timed collection; and (3) timed (e.g., 4-hour or 10-hour overnight) collection. Microalbuminuria on a spot urine specimen is defined as a ratio of 30 to 300 mg/g albumin-to-creatinine. On timed collections, microalbuminuria is defined as 30 to 300 mg/24 hours or an albumin excretion rate of 20 to 200 mcg/min. Because of day-to-day variability, microalbuminuria should be confirmed on at least two of three samples over 3 to 6 months. Additionally, when assessing urine protein or albumin, conditions that can cause transient elevations in urinary albumin excretion should be excluded. These conditions include: intense exercise, recent urinary tract infections, hypertension, short-term hyperglycemia, heart failure, and acute febrile illness.[147]

In type 2 DM, the presence of microalbuminuria is a strong risk factor for macrovascular disease and is frequently present at the time of diagnosis. Microalbuminuria is a weaker predictor for future kidney disease in type 2 versus type 1 DM.

Glucose and blood pressure control are most important for the prevention of nephropathy, and blood pressure control is the most important for retarding the progression of established nephropathy. ACE inhibitors and angiotensin receptor blockers, considered first-line recommended treatment modalities, have shown efficacy in preventing the clinical progression of renal disease in patients with type 2 DM.[148–150] Diuretics frequently are necessary because of the volume-expanded state of the patient and are recommended second-line therapy. The ADA and the National Kidney Foundation blood pressure goal of $<130/80$ mm Hg can be difficult to achieve. Three or more antihypertensives are often needed to treat to goal blood pressures.

Peripheral Vascular Disease and Foot Ulcers

Claudication and nonhealing foot ulcers are common in type 2 DM patients.[151] Smoking cessation, correction of lipid abnormalities, and antiplatelet therapy are important strategies in treating claudicants. Pentoxifylline or cilostazol can be useful in selected patients. Revascularization is successful in selected patients. Local débridement and appropriate footwear and foot care are vitally important in the early treatment of foot lesions. In more advanced lesions, topical treatments can be of benefit. Diabetic foot care is an excellent example of the adage, "an ounce of prevention is worth a pound of cure."

Coronary Heart Disease

⓫ The risk for coronary heart disease (CHD) is two to four times greater in diabetic patients than in nondiabetic individuals. CHD is the major source of mortality in patients with DM. Recent studies suggest that multiple risk-factor intervention (lipids, hypertension, smoking cessation,[152] and antiplatelet therapy)[153] will reduce the burden of excess macrovascular events. Epidemiologic data suggest that CHD prevention guidelines for type 2 DM apply equally to patients with type 1 DM.[154] β-Blocker therapy supplies an even greater protection from recurrent CHD events in diabetic patients than in nondiabetic subjects. Masking of hypoglycemic symptoms is a greater problem in type 1 DM patients than in patients with type 2 DM.

Lipids The Collaborative Atorvastatin Diabetes Study (CARDS) randomized diabetes subjects with no documented cardiovascular disease to atorvastatin 10 mg daily ($n = 1,428$) or placebo ($n = 1,410$). The trial was stopped 2 years early (mean duration of followup was 3.9 years) after meeting the primary efficacy end point of major cardiovascular events, which were reduced by 37% ($P = 0.001$). All-cause death was reduced 27% ($P = 0.059$) and potentially could have had its significance influenced by the early stoppage of the trial.[155] The Heart Protection Study randomized 5,963 patients age >40 years with diabetes and total cholesterol >135 mg/dL. A significant 22% reduction (95% confidence interval [CI], 13–30) in the event rate for major cardiovascular events was seen with simvastatin 40 mg per day. This was evident even at lower LDL levels (<116 mg/dL), and suggests that ~30% reduction in LDL levels regardless of starting LDL levels can be appropriate.[156] The proper use of fibrates in diabetes continues to be controversial. The diabetic subgroup in the Veterans Administration HDL Intervention Trial (VA-HIT) of CHD patients with low HDL-C and low LDL-C showed approximately 22% reduction in CHD events in diabetic patients with known CHD when HDL-C was increased by approximately 6% by gemfibrozil.[157] The Fenofibrate Intervention and Event Lowering in Diabetes (FIELD) was conducted in 9,795 subjects (22% with previously documented cardiovascular disease) with type 2 DM given fenofibrate 200 mg daily or placebo. A relative reduction of 11% ($P = 0.16$) was seen in any coronary event in conjunction with a slight increase in the risk of all-cause mortality. (0.7%, $P = 0.18$). Reasons for this have been speculated on, including the increased use of statins in the placebo group, but it continues to be controversial.[158]

The National Cholesterol Education Program Adult Treatment Panel III (NCEP-ATP III)[159] guidelines classify the presence of DM

TABLE 77-15 Classification of Lipid and Lipoprotein Levels in Adults

Parameter	Goal		Treatment (in order of preference)
LDL cholesterol	<100 mg/dL <70 mg/dL[a]		Lifestyle; HMG-CoA reductase inhibitors; cholesterol absorption inhibitor; niacin or fenofibrate
HDL cholesterol	Men >40 mg/dL	Women >50 mg/dL	Lifestyle; nicotinic acid; fibric acid derivatives
Triglycerides	<150 mg/dL		Lifestyle; glycemic control; fibric acid derivatives; high-dose statins (in those with high LDL)

HDL, high-density lipoprotein; HMG-CoA, 3-hydroxy-3-methylglutaryl coenzyme A; LDL, low-density lipoprotein.

[a]Can be optimal goal in patients with preexisting cardiovascular disease.

Data from American Diabetes Association. Dyslipidemia managment in adults with diabetes. Diabetes Care 2004;27:568–571.

as a CHD risk equivalent, and therefore recommend that LDL-C be lowered to <100 mg/dL. An optional LDL goal in high-risk DM patients, such as those who already have CHD, has been updated to be <70 mg/dL.[160] Unlike previous guidelines, more consideration is now given to HDL-C and triglycerides. The primary target is the treatment of LDL-C. After the LDL-C goal is reached (usually with a statin), triglycerides are possibly considered for pharmacologic management, assuming unresponsiveness to glycemic control efforts, weight management, and exercise. In such situations, a non-HDL-C goal is established (a surrogate for all apolipoprotein B–containing particles). The non-HDL-C goal for patients with DM is <130 mg/dL. Niacin or a fibrate can be added to reach that goal if triglycerides are 201 to 499 mg/dL. Niacin or a fibrate can also be added if the LDL-C goal is reached, but the patient has low HDL-C (<40 mg/dL). Patients with marked hypertriglyceridemia (≥500 mg/dL) are at risk for pancreatitis. Efforts to reduce triglycerides with glycemic control, elimination of other secondary causes (including medications), and drug therapy (fibrate and/or niacin) are effective treatment strategies. The ADA also recommends similar LDL goals but places raising HDL as the second priority (Table 77–15). The definitive role of pharmacologic therapy of HDL-C and/or hypertriglyceridemia in type 2 DM patients (beyond that seen with statin therapy) has yet to be proven in clinical trials.

Hypertension

The role of hypertension in increasing microvascular and macrovascular risk in patients with DM has been confirmed in the UKPDS[97] and Hypertension Optimization Treatment[161] trials. The ADA recommends aggressive goals for blood pressure (<130/80 mm Hg) in patients with DM.[8] ACE inhibitors and angiotensin receptor blockers are generally recommended for initial therapy. The National Kidney Foundation also suggests that the blood pressure goal be less than 130/80 mm Hg, as well as recommending diuretics as second-line therapy in patients with diabetic kidney disease.[162] Many patients require multiple agents, on average three agents, to obtain goals, so diuretics, calcium channel blockers, and β-blockers frequently are useful as second and third agents. Blood pressure goals are generally more difficult to achieve than glycemic goals or lipid goals in most diabetic patients.[163]

CLINICAL CONTROVERSY

Initial therapy choices for hypertension in DM usually include ACE inhibitors or an angiotensin receptor blocker because of their well documented renoprotective effects. Currently, angiotensin receptor blockers have less robust data to support cardiovascular reduction compared to other therapeutic choices, yet the data that exists appears to be positive in patients with type 2 DM. Also, in the diabetic subset of the Antihypertensive and Lipid-Lowering Treatment to Prevent Heart Attack Trial (ALLHAT), diuretics have shown equivalent results to an ACE inhibitor. The ADA currently recommends the use of any class (ACE inhibitors, angiotensin receptor blockers, β-blockers, diuretics, or calcium channel blockers) of antihypertensive medication that has shown benefit in prevention of poor cardiovascular outcomes. Choice of monotherapy may not be important, as an average of two to three antihypertensive medications are needed to reach blood pressure goals.

Transplantation

Whole pancreas and islet cell transplantation are still relatively experimental procedures in patients with type 1 DM; those with end-stage renal disease also receive kidney transplantation.[164]

PHARMACOECONOMIC CONSIDERATIONS

As described in the introduction, the direct and indirect costs of DM are substantial. Much of the indirect costs are related to loss of productivity because of the significant morbidity (hospitalizations, loss of vision, lower extremity amputations, kidney failure, and cardiovascular events) associated with the disease. For a disease that affects about 9% of the population, it is responsible for 11% to 12% of health expenditures. With evidence from the DCCT and UKPDS to support intensive blood glucose control to reduce the risk of complications, the question of cost effectiveness comes into play.

An economic model based on the DCCT approximates that 120,000 persons in the United States would meet criteria for intensive intervention. The cost of implementing intensive therapy over the lifetime of the population is estimated at $4 billion dollars. The benefits of this strategy are net gains of 920,000 years of sight, 691,000 years free from end-stage renal disease, and 678,000 years free from lower extremity amputations. The incremental cost per year of life gained is $28,661.[165] This is well within the limits of a cost-effective strategy and compares favorably to treatment of high blood pressure or hypercholesterolemia.

Economic analysis of intensive therapy for type 2 DM is more complex. Outcomes must also factor in the burden of cardiovascular disease as the major cause of mortality. One model analyzed the health benefits and economics of treating type 2 DM with the goal of achieving normoglycemia but using outcomes based on the DCCT trial results. Accounting for the prevalence of cardiovascular disease in type 2 DM, an estimate of $16,002 incremental cost per quality-adjusted life year gained was obtained. The limitation of this analysis is that although the UKDPS did demonstrate an improvement in diabetes-related outcomes, the overall efficacy on microvascular disease complications was not mirrored by the DCCT.

Two economic analyses were performed on data generated from the UKPDS, one assessing cost effectiveness of an intensive blood glucose control policy in type 2 DM, and the other assessing improved blood pressure control in hypertensive patients with type 2 DM. In the first analysis, outcome was measured as the incremental cost per event-free year gained within the trial. Based on trial outcomes and assumptions, the incremental cost in the intensive treatment group per event-free year gained is $1,366. Although intensive treatment costs were higher, the cost per event-free year gained appears cost-effective. The second analysis showed the incremental cost per extra year free from microvascular and macrovascular end points from intensive blood pressure control in a standard clinical practice model to be $1,498. The incremental cost per life year gained was estimated at $619, again demonstrating the cost-effectiveness of intensive intervention.[166,167]

EVALUATION OF THERAPEUTIC OUTCOMES

MONITORING OF THE PHARMACEUTICAL CARE PLAN

A comprehensive pharmaceutical care plan for the patient with DM will integrate considerations of goals to optimize blood glucose control and protocols to screen for, prevent, or manage microvascular and macrovascular complications. In terms of standards of care for persons with DM, one can review the document published by the ADA that outlines initial and ongoing assessments for patients with DM.[8] For quality-of-care measures, one can refer to the National Diabetes Quality Improvement Alliance website at *www.nationaldiabetesalliance.org*, whose members include many of the governmental and physician organizations concerned with diabetes quality-of-care measures.

The major performance measures, such as Health Plan Employer Data and Information Set (HEDIS), should assess the ability to meet current standards of care and recognize the minimal treatment goals for glycemia, lipids, and hypertension, and provide targets for monitoring and adjusting pharmacotherapy as discussed in various sections above. Publicly reported quality measures continue to move closer to current guidelines. Glycemic control (percentage of patients with HbA_{1c} <7%), lipid (percentage of patients with LDL <100 mg/dL), and hypertension (percentage of patients with blood pressure <130/80 mm Hg) are now quality measures congruent with the current goals recommended by the ADA. Glycemic control is paramount in managing type 1 or type 2 DM but as readily identified from the above discussion, it requires frequent assessment and adjustment in diet, exercise, and pharmacologic therapies. Minimally, HbA_{1c} should be measured twice a year in patients meeting treatment goals on a stable therapeutic regimen. Quarterly assessments are recommended for those whose therapy has changed or who are not meeting glycemic goals. Fasting lipid profiles should be obtained as part of an initial assessment and thereafter at each followup visit if not at goal, annually if stable and at goal, or every 2 years if the lipid profile suggests low risk. Documenting regular frequency of foot exams (each visit), urine albumin assessment (annually), dilated ophthalmologic exams (yearly or more frequently with identified abnormalities), and office visits for followup are also important. Assessment for pneumococcal vaccine administration, annual administration of influenza vaccine, and routine assessment for and management of other cardiovascular risks (i.e., smoking and antiplatelet therapy) are components of preventive medicine strategies. The multiplicity of assessments for each patient visit are likely to be better facilitated using an integrative computer program and electronic medical record, standardized progress note forms, or flow sheets, which assist the clinician in identifying whether the patient has met standards of care in the frequency of monitoring and achievement of defined targets of therapy.

ABBREVIATIONS

ACE: angiotensin-converting enzyme

ADA: American Diabetes Association

ALLHAT: Antihypertensive and Lipid-Lowering Treatment to Prevent Heart Attack Trial

ALT: alanine aminotransferase

BMI: body mass index

CHD: coronary heart disease

CSII: continuous subcutaneous insulin infusion

CYP450: cytochrome P450

DCCT: Diabetes Control and Complications Trial

DM: diabetes mellitus

DPP-IV: dipeptidyl peptidase IV

DREAM: Diabetes Reduction Assessment with Ramipril and Rosiglitazone Medication (study)

FFA: free fatty acid

GDM: gestational diabetes mellitus

GIP: glucose-dependent insulin-releasing peptide

GLP-1: glucagon-like peptide-1

HbA_{1c}: hemoglobin A_{1c}

HDLC: high-density lipoprotein cholesterol

IFG: impaired fasting glucose

IGT: impaired glucose tolerance

LADA: latent autoimmune diabetes in adults

LDLC: low-density lipoprotein cholesterol

MODY: maturity onset diabetes of youth

NCEP-ATP: National Cholesterol Education Program Adult Treatment Panel

NHANES III: The Third National Health and Nutrition Evaluation Survey

NPH: neutral protamine Hagedorn

OGTT: oral glucose tolerance test

PAI-1: activator-1 plasminogen-inhibitor

PPAR-γ: peroxisome proliferator activator receptor-γ

PROactive: Prospective Pioglitazone Clinical Trial in Macrovascular Events

SMBG: self-monitored blood glucose

STOP-NIDDM: Study to Prevent Non–Insulin-Dependent Diabetes Mellitus

SUR: sulfonylurea receptor

TRIPOD: Troglitazone in the Prevention of Diabetes

TZD: thiazolidinedione

UKPDS: United Kingdom Prospective Diabetes Study

VAT: visceral adipose tissue

REFERENCES

1. American Diabetes Association. Diabetes facts and figures. 2007, *http://www.diabetes.org/diabetes-statistics.jsp.*
2. Daneman D. Type 1 diabetes. Lancet 2006;367:847–858.
3. Raffel LJ, Scheuner MT, Rotter JI. Genetics of diabetes. In: Porte D Jr, Sherwin RS, eds. Ellenberg & Rifkin's Diabetes Mellitus, 5th ed. Stamford, CT: Appleton & Lange, 1997:401–454.
4. Bennett P, Rewers M, Knowler W. Epidemiology of diabetes mellitus. In: Porte D Jr, Sherwin RS, eds. Ellenberg & Rifkin's Diabetes Mellitus, 5th ed. Stamford, CT: Appleton & Lange, 1997:373–400.
5. American Diabetes Association. Diagnosis and classification of diabetes mellitus. Diabetes Care 2007;30(Suppl 1):S42–S47.
6. Gale EA. The rise of childhood type 1 diabetes in the 20th century. Diabetes 2002;51:3353–3361.
7. Froguel P, Zouali H, Vionnet N, et al. Familial hyperglycemia due to mutations in glucokinase. Definition of a subtype of diabetes mellitus. N Engl J Med 1993;328:697–702.

8. American Diabetes Association. Standards for medical care in diabetes—2007. Diabetes Care 2007;30(Suppl 1):S4–S41.
9. Cowie CC, Rust KF, Byrd-Holt DD, et al. Prevalence of diabetes and impaired fasting glucose in adults in the U.S. population. Diabetes Care 2006;29:1263–1268.
10. American Diabetes Association. Type 2 diabetes in children and adolescents. Diabetes Care 2000;23:381–389.
11. Kahn SE, Porte D Jr. The pathophysiology of type II (non-insulin dependent) diabetes mellitus: Implications for treatment. In: Porte D Jr, Sherwin RS, eds. Ellenberg & Rifkin's Diabetes Mellitus, 5th ed. Stamford, CT: Appleton & Lange, 1997:487–512.
12. American Diabetes Association. Gestational diabetes mellitus. Diabetes Care 2004;27(Suppl 1):S88–S90.
13. Report of the expert committee on the diagnosis and classification of diabetes mellitus. Diabetes Care 1997;20:1183–1197.
14. van Tilburg J, van Haeften TW, Pearson P, Wijimenga C. Defining the genetic contribution of type 2 diabetes mellitus. J Med Genet 2001;38:569–578.
15. Engelgau MM, Thompson TJ, Herman WH, et al. Comparison of fasting and 2-hour glucose and HbA_{1c} levels for diagnosing diabetes: Diagnostic criteria and performance revisited. Diabetes Care 1997;20:785–791.
16. McCance DR, Hanson RL, Charles MA, et al. Comparison of tests for glycated haemoglobin and fasting and two hour plasma glucose concentrations as diagnostic methods for diabetes. BMJ 1994;308:1323–1328.
17. Janeway CA. Immunology relevant to diabetes. In: Porte D Jr, Sherwin RS, eds. Ellenberg & Rifkin's Diabetes Mellitus, 5th ed. Stamford, CT: Appleton & Lange, 1997:287–300.
18. Edelman SV, Weyer C. Unresolved challenges with insulin therapy in type 1 and type 2 diabetes: Potential benefit of replacing amylin, a second β-cell hormone. Diabetes Technol Ther 2002;4:175–189.
19. Cherrington AD. Banting Lecture 1997: Control of glucose uptake and release by the liver in vivo. Diabetes 1999;48:1198–1214.
20. McGarry JD. Banting Lecture 2001: Dysregulation of fatty acid metabolism in the etiology of type 2 diabetes. Diabetes 2002;51:7–18.
21. Nogid A, Pham DQ. Adjunctive therapy with pramlintide in patients with type 1 or type 2 diabetes mellitus. Pharmacotherapy 2006;26:1626–1640.
22. DeFronzo RA. Pathogenesis of type 2 diabetes mellitus: Metabolic and molecular implications for identifying diabetes genes. Diabetes 1997;5:117–269.
23. Gerich JE, Meyer C, Woerle HJ, Stumvoll M. Renal gluconeogenesis. Its importance in human glucose homeostasis. Diabetes Care 2001;24:382–391.
24. Ekberg K, Landau BR, Wajngot A, et al. Contributions by kidney and liver to glucose production in the postabsorptive state and after 60 h of fasting. Diabetes 1999;48:292–298.
25. Unger RH, Orci L. Glucagon and the α cell: Physiology and pathophysiology (first two parts). N Engl J Med 1981;304:1518–1524.
26. Mandarino L, Bonadonna R, McGuinness O, Wasserman D. Regulation of muscle glucose uptake in vivo. In: Jefferson LS, Cherrington AD, eds. Handbook of Physiology, Section 7, the Endocrine System, vol. II, the Endocrine Pancreas and Regulation of Metabolism. Oxford: Oxford University Press, 2001:803–848.
27. Santomauro A, Boden G, Silva M, et al. Overnight lowering of free fatty acids with acipimox improves insulin resistance and glucose tolerance in obese diabetic and non-diabetic subjects. Diabetes 1999;48:1836–1841.
28. Bergman RN. Non-esterified fatty acids and the liver: Why is insulin secreted into the portal vein? Diabetologia 2000;43:946–952.
29. Boden G. Role of fatty acids in the pathogenesis of insulin resistance and NIDDM. Diabetes 1997;46:3–10.
30. DeFronzo RA, Ferrannini E, Simonson DC. Fasting hyperglycemia in non-insulin-dependent diabetes mellitus: Contributions of excessive hepatic glucose production and impaired tissue glucose uptake. Metabolism 1989;38:387–395.
31. Nauck M, Stockmann F, Ebert R, Creutzfeldt W. Reduced incretin effect in type 2 (non-insulin-dependent) diabetes. Diabetologia 1986;291:46–52.
32. Jolst JJ, Gromada J. Role of incretin hormones in the regulation of insulin secretion in diabetic and nondiabetic humans. Am J Physiol Endocrinol Metab 2004;287:E199-E206.
33. Vilsboll T, Holst JJ. Incretins, insulin secretion and type 2 diabetes mellitus. Diabetologia 2004;47:357–366.
34. Meier JJ, Nauck MA, Schmidt WE, Gallwitz B. Gastric inhibitory polypeptide: The neglected incretin revisited. Regul Pept 2002;107:1–13.
35. Nauck MA, Heimesaat MM, Orskov C, et al. Preserved incretin activity of glucagon-like peptide-1 [7–36amide] but not of synthetic human gastric inhibitory polypeptide in patients with type 2 diabetes mellitus. J Clin Invest 1993;91:301–307.
36. Deacon CF, Nauck MA, Tolf-Nielsen M, et al. Both subcutaneously and intravenously administered glucagon-like peptide I are rapidly degraded from the NH2-terminus in type II diabetic patients and in healthy subjects. Diabetes 1995;44:1126–1131.
37. Unger RH, Aguilar-Parada E, Muller WA, Eisentraut AM. Studies of pancreatic α cell function in normal and diabetic subjects. J Clin Invest 1970;49:837–848.
38. Kelley DE, Mandarino LJ. Fuel selection in human skeletal muscle in insulin resistance. A reexamination. Diabetes 2000;49:677–683.
39. Kashyap S, Belfort R, Gastaldelli A, et al. A sustained increase in plasma free fatty acids impairs insulin secretion in nondiabetic subjects genetically predisposed to develop type 2 diabetes. Diabetes 2003;52:2461–2474.
40. Carpentier A, Mittelman SD, Bergman RN, et al. Prolonged elevation of plasma free fatty acids impairs pancreatic beta-cell function in obese nondiabetic humans but not in individuals with type 2 diabetes. Diabetes 2000;49:399–408.
41. Goodpaster BH, Thaete FL, Kelley BE. Thigh adipose tissue distribution is associated with insulin resistance in obesity and in type 2 diabetes mellitus. Am J Clin Nutr 2000;71:885–892.
42. Greco AV, Mingrone G, Giancaterini A, et al. Insulin resistance in morbid obesity. Reversal with intramyocellular fat depletion. Diabetes 2002;51:144–151.
43. Ryysy L, Hakkinen AM, Goto T, et al. Hepatic fat content and insulin action on free fatty acids and glucose metabolism rather than insulin absorption are associated with insulin requirements during insulin therapy in type 2 diabetic patients. Diabetes 2000;49:749–758.
44. Miyazaki Y, Mahankali A, Matsuda M, et al. Effect of pioglitazone on abdominal fat distribution and insulin sensitivity in type 2 diabetic patients. J Clin Endocrinol Metab 2002;87:2784–2791.
45. DeFronzo RA. Pathogenesis of type 2 diabetes: Metabolic and molecular implications for identifying diabetes genes. ADA 1997;4:177–269.
46. Ferrannini E, Natali A, Bell P, et al. On behalf of the European Group for the Study of Insulin Resistance (EGIR). Insulin resistance and hypersecretion in obesity. J Clin Invest 1997;100:1166–1173.
47. Montague CT, O'Rahilly S. The perils of portliness: Causes and consequences of visceral adiposity. Diabetes 2000;49:883–888.
48. Kelley DE, Williams KV, Price JC, et al. Plasma fatty acids, adiposity and variance of skeletal muscle insulin resistance in type 2 diabetes mellitus. J Clin Endocrinol Metab 2001;86:5412–5419.
49. Banerji MA, Lebowitz J, Chaiken RL. Relationship of visceral adipose tissue and glucose disposal is independent of sex in black NIDDM subjects. Am J Physiol 1997;273:E425–E432.
50. Kelley DE. The impact of obesity, regional adiposity and ectopic fat on the pathophysiology of type 2 diabetes. Council on Obesity Diabetes Education 2003;12–20.
51. Weyer C, Funahashi T, Tanaka S, et al. Hypoadiponectinemia in obesity and type 2 diabetes: Close association with insulin resistance and hyperinsulinemia. J Clin Endocrinol Metab 2000;86:1930–1935.
52. Arita Y, Kihara S, Ouchi N, et al. Paradoxical decrease of an adipose-specific protein, adiponectin, in obesity. Biochem Biophys Res Commun 1999;257:79–83.
53. Berg AH, Combs TP, Du X, et al. The adipocyte-secreted protein Acrp30 enhances hepatic insulin action. Nat Med 2001;7:947–953.
54. Yamauchi T, Kamon J, Waki H, et al. The fat-derived hormone adiponectin reverses insulin resistance associated with both lipoatrophy and obesity. Nat Med 2001;7:941–946.
55. Reaven GM. Role of insulin resistance in human disease. Diabetes 1988;37:1595–1607.
56. International Diabetes Federation: The IDF consensus worldwide definition of the metabolic syndrome. 2007, *http://www.idf.org/webdata/docs/MetS_def_update2006.pdf.*
57. Ford ES. Prevalence of the metabolic syndrome defined by the International Diabetes Federation among adults in the U.S. Diabetes Care 2005;28:2745–2749.
58. Adams RJ, Appleton S, Wilson DH, et al. Population comparison of two clinical approaches to the metabolic syndrome: Implications of the new International Diabetes Federation consensus definition. Diabetes Care 2005;28:2777–2779.

59. Gaede P, Vedel P, Larsen N, et al. Multifactorial intervention and cardiovascular disease in patients with type 2 diabetes. N Engl J Med 2003;348:383–393.
60. Diabetes Control and Complications Trial Research Group. The effect of intensive treatment of diabetes on the development and progression of long-term complications in insulin-dependent diabetes mellitus. N Engl J Med 1993;329:977–986.
61. UK Prospective Diabetes Study Group. Intensive blood-glucose control with sulphonylureas or insulin compared with conventional treatment and risk of complications in patients with type 2 diabetes (UKPDS 33). Lancet 1998;352:837–853.
62. American Diabetes Association. Self-monitoring of blood glucose. Diabetes Care 1994;17:81–86.
63. Welschen LMC, Bloemendal E, Nijpels G, et al. Self-monitoring of glucose in patients with type 2 diabetes who are not using insulin. Diabetes Care 2005;28:1510–1517.
64. American Diabetes Association. Nutrition recommendations and interventions for diabetes. Diabetes Care 2007;30(Suppl 1):S48–S65.
65. American Diabetes Association. Diabetes mellitus and exercise. Diabetes Care 2004;27(Suppl 1):S58–S62.
66. Alberti KGMM, Zimmet P, DeFronzo RA, Keen H, eds. International Textbook of Diabetes Mellitus, 2nd ed., vol. 1. New York: Wiley, 1997:469–610.
67. Insulin human (rDNA origin) inhalation Powder (Exubera) [package insert]. New York: Pfizer Labs, Pfizer Inc., 2006.
68. Dewitt DE, Dugdale DC. Using new insulin strategies in the outpatient treatment of diabetes: Clinical applications. JAMA 2003;289:2265–2269.
69. DeWitt DE, Hirsch IB. Outpatient insulin therapy in type 1 and type 2 diabetes mellitus: scientific review. JAMA 2003;289:2254–2264.
70. Gerich JE. Novel insulins: Expanding options in diabetes management. Am J Med 2002;113:308–316.
71. Lepore M, Pampanelli S, Fanelli C, et al. Pharmacokinetics and pharmacodynamics of subcutaneous injection of long-acting human insulin analog glargine, NPH insulin, and ultralente human insulin and continuous subcutaneous infusion of insulin lispro. Diabetes 2000;49:2142–2148.
72. Malmberg K, for the DIGAMI Study Group. Prospective randomised study of intensive insulin treatment on long term survival after acute myocardial infarction in patients with diabetes mellitus. BMJ 1997;314:1512–1515.
73. Kendall DM, Kim D, Poon T, et al. Improvements in cardiovascular risk factors accompanied sustained effects on glycemia and weight reduction in patient with type 2 diabetes treated with exenatide for 82 weeks. Diabetes 2005;54(Suppl 1):A4–5.
74. Schor S. The University Group Diabetes Program. A statistician looks at the mortality results. JAMA 1971;217:1673–1675.
75. Kilo C, Miller L, Williamson J. The crux of the UGDP. Spurious results and biologically inappropriate data analysis. Diabetologia 1980;18:179–185.
76. Brady PA, Jovanovic A. The sulfonylurea controversy: Much ado about nothing or cause for concern? J Am Coll Cardiol 2003;42:1022–1025.
77. Klamann A, Sarfert P, Lanhardt V, et al. Myocardial infarction in diabetic vs. non-diabetic subjects: Survival and infarct size following therapy with sulfonylureas (glibenclamide). Eur Heart J 2000;21:220–229.
78. Riddle MC. Sulfonylureas differ in effects on ischemic preconditioning—Is it time to retire glyburide? J Clin Endocrinol Metab 2003;88:528–530.
79. Gerich JE. Oral hypoglycemic agents. N Engl J Med 1989;321:1231–1245.
80. Triplitt C. Drug interactions of medications commonly used in diabetes. Diabetes Spectr 2006;19:202–211.
81. Wolffenbuttel BH, Landgraf R, for the Dutch and German repaglinide study group. A 1-year multicenter randomized double-blind comparison of repaglinide and glyburide for the treatment of type 2 diabetes. Diabetes Care 1999;22:463–467.
82. Horton ES, Clinkingbeard C, Gatlin M, et al. Nateglinide alone and in combination with metformin improves glycemic control by reducing mealtime glucose levels in type 2 diabetes. Diabetes Care 2000;23:1660–1665.
83. UK Prospective Diabetes Study (UKPDS) Group. Effect of intensive blood-glucose control with metformin on complications in overweight patients with type 2 diabetes (UKPDS 34). Lancet 1998;352:854–865.
84. Dawson D, Conlon C. Case study: Metformin associated lactic acidosis: Could orlistat be relevant? Diabetes Care 2003;26:2471–2472.
85. Dormandy JA, Charbonnel B, Eckland DJA, et al. Secondary prevention of vascular events in patients with type 2 diabetes in the PROactive study prospective pioglitazone clinical trial in macrovascular events: a randomized controlled trial. Lancet 2005;366:1279–1289.
86. Nissen SE, Wolski K. The effect of rosiglitazone on the risk of myocardial infarction and death from cardiovascular causes. N Engl J Med 2007;356:1–15.
87. Lebovitz HE, Kreider M, Freed MI. Evaluation of liver function in type 2 diabetic patients during clinical trials: Evidence that rosiglitazone does not cause hepatic dysfunction. Diabetes Care 2002;25:815–821.
88. Nesto RW, Bell D, Bonow RO, et al. Thiazolidinedione use, fluid retention, and congestive heart failure. A consensus statement from the American Heart Association and the American Diabetes Association. Diabetes Care 2004;27:256–263.
89. Mooradian AD, Thurman JE. Drug therapy of postprandial hyperglycemia. Drugs 1999;57:19–29.
90. Campbell LK, Baker DE, Campbell RK. Miglitol: Assessment of its role in the treatment of patients with diabetes mellitus. Ann Pharmacother 2000;34:1291–1301.
91. Chiasson JL, Josse RG, Gomis R, et al. Acarbose for prevention of type 2 diabetes mellitus: The STOP-NIDDM randomized trial. Lancet 2002;359:2072–2077.
92. Chiasson JL, Josse RG, Gomis R, et al. Acarbose treatment and the risk of cardiovascular disease and hypertension in patients with impaired glucose tolerance: The STOP-NIDDM trial. JAMA 2003;290:486–494.
93. Lettieri JT, Dain B. Effects of beano on the tolerability and pharmacodynamics of acarbose. Clin Ther 1998;20:497–504.
94. EDIC writing group. Sustained effect of intensive treatment of type 1 diabetes mellitus on development and progression of diabetic nephropathy: The Epidemiology of Diabetes Interventions and Complications of Study. JAMA 2003;290:2159–2167.
95. DCCT/EDIC Study Research Group. Intensive diabetes treatment and cardiovascular disease in patients with type 1 diabetes. N Engl J Med 2005;353:2643–2653.
96. Stratton IM, Adler AI, Neil HA. Association of glycaemia with macrovascular and microvascular complications of type 2 diabetes (UKPDS 35): Prospective observational study. BMJ 2000;321:405–412.
97. Adler AI, Stratton IM, Neil HA. Association of systolic blood pressure with macrovascular and microvascular complications of type 2 diabetes (UKPDS 36): Prospective observational study. BMJ 2000;321:412–419.
98. UK Prospective Diabetes Study Group. Efficacy of atenolol and captopril in reducing risk of macrovascular and microvascular complications in type 2 diabetes: UKPDS 39. BMJ 1998;317:713–720.
99. Strowig S, Raskin P. Intensive management of insulin-dependent diabetes mellitus. In: Porte D Jr., Sherwin RS, eds. Ellenberg & Rifkin's Diabetes Mellitus, 5th ed. Stamford, CT: Appleton & Lange, 1997:709–733.
100. Fanelli CG, Pampanelli S, Porcellati F, et al. Administration of neutral protamine Hagedorn insulin at bedtime versus with dinner in type 1 diabetes mellitus to avoid nocturnal hypoglycemia and improve control. A randomized, controlled trial. Ann Intern Med 2002;136:504–514.
101. DeVries JH, Snoek FJ, Kostense PJ, et al. on behalf of the Dutch Insulin Pump Study Group. A randomized trial of continuous subcutaneous insulin infusion and intensive injection therapy in type 1 diabetes for patients with long-standing poor glycemic control. Diabetes Care 2002;25:2074–2080.
102. Pickup J, Mattock M, Kerry S. Glycaemic control with continuous subcutaneous insulin infusion compared with intensive insulin injections in patients with type 1 diabetes: Meta-analysis of randomised controlled trials. BMJ 2002;324:705.
103. Lenhard MJ, Reeves GD. Continuous subcutaneous insulin infusion: A comprehensive review of insulin pump therapy. Arch Intern Med 2001;161:2293–2300.
104. Schade DS, Valentine V. To pump or not to pump. Diabetes Care 2002;25:2100–2102.
105. Cryer PE. Hypoglycemia is the limiting factor in the management of diabetes. Diabetes Metab Res Rev 1999;15:42–46.
106. de Galan BE, Tack CJ, Lenders JW, et al. Theophylline improves hypoglycemia unawareness in type 1 diabetes. Diabetes 2002;51:790–796.
107. Rosenbloom AL, Schatz DA, Krischer JP, et al. Therapeutic controversy: Prevention and treatment of diabetes in children. J Clin Endocrinol Metab 2000;85:494–522.

108. Binder C, Brange J. Insulin chemistry and pharmacokinetics. In: Porte D Jr, Sherwin RS, eds. Ellenberg & Rifkin's Diabetes Mellitus, 5th ed. Stamford, CT: Appleton & Lange, 1997:689–708.
109. Kelly DB, ed. Management of Type 1 Diabetes Mellitus, 3rd ed. Alexandria, VA: American Diabetes Association, 1998:211–222.
110. Halvorsen T, Levine F. Diabetes mellitus-cell transplantation and gene therapy approaches. Curr Mol Med 2001;1:273–286.
111. Shapiro AM, Lakey JR, Ryan EA, et al. Islet transplantation in seven patients with type 1 diabetes mellitus using a glucocorticoid-free immunosuppressive regimen. N Engl J Med 2000;343:230–238.
112. DeFronzo RA. Pharmacologic therapy for type 2 diabetes mellitus. Ann Intern Med 1999;131:281–303.
113. Higa M, Zhou YT, Ravazzola M, et al. Troglitazone prevents mitochondrial alterations, beta cell destruction, and diabetes in obese prediabetic rats. Proc Natl Acad Sci USA 1999;96:11513–11518.
114. Wang Q, Brubaker PL. Glucagon-like peptide-1 treatment delays the onset of diabetes in 8 week-old db/db mice. Diabetologia 2002:45;1263–1273.
115. Shank ML, Del Prato S, DeFronzo RA. Bedtime insulin/daytime glipizide. Effective therapy for sulfonylurea failures in NIDDM. Diabetes 1995;44:165–172.
116. Yki-Jarvinen H, Ryysy L, Nikkila K. Comparison of bedtime insulin regimens in patients with type 2 diabetes mellitus. A randomized, controlled trial. Ann Intern Med 1999;130:389–396.
117. Bastyr EJ, Stuart CA, Brodows RG. Therapy focused on lowering postprandial glucose, not fasting glucose, may be superior for lowering HbA1C. IOEZ Study Group. Diabetes Care 2000;23:1236–1241.
118. European Diabetes Epidemiology Group. Glucose tolerance and mortality. Comparison of WHO and American Diabetes Association diagnostic criteria. The DECODE study group. Diabetes Epidemiology: Collaborative analysis of diagnostic criteria in Europe. Lancet 1999;354:617–621.
119. Langer O, Conway DL, Berkus MD, et al. A comparison of glyburide and insulin in women with gestational diabetes mellitus. N Engl J Med 2000;343:1134–1138.
120. Laffel L. Sick-day management in type 1 diabetes. Endocrinol Metab Clin North Am 2000;29:707–723.
121. Kitabchi AE, Umpierrez GE, Murphy MB, et al. Management of hyperglycemic crises in patients with diabetes. Diabetes Care 2001;24:131–153.
122. Kitabchi AE, Umpierrez GE, Murphy MB, Kreisburg RA. Hyperglycemic crises in adult patients with diabetes. A consensus statement from the American diabetes association. Diabetes Care 2006;29:2739–2748.
123. Balasubramanyam A, Zern JW, Hyman DJ, Pavlik V. New profiles of diabetic ketoacidosis: Type 1 vs. type 2 diabetes and the effect of ethnicity. Arch Intern Med 1999;159:2317–2322.
124. Glaser N, Barnett P, McCaslin I, et al. Pediatric Emergency Medicine Collaborative Research Committee of the American Academy of Pediatrics. N Engl J Med 2001;344:264–269.
125. Sawin CT. Action without benefit. The sliding scale of insulin use. Arch Intern Med 1997;157:489.
126. Malmberg K, Norhammar A, Wedel H. Glycometabolic state at admission: Important risk marker of mortality in conventionally treated patients with diabetes mellitus and acute myocardial infarction: Long-term results from the Diabetes and Insulin-Glucose Infusion in Acute Myocardial Infarction (DIGAMI) Study. Circulation 1999;99:2626–2632.
127. van den Berghe G, Wouters P, Weekers F, et al. Intensive insulin therapy in the critically ill patients. N Engl J Med 2001;345:1359–1367.
128. Montori VM, Bistrian BR, McMahon MM. Hyperglycemia in acutely ill patients. JAMA 2002;288:2167–2169.
129. Clement S, Braithwaite SS, Magee MF, et al. Management of diabetes and hyperglycemia in hospitals. Diabetes Care 2004;27:553–591.
130. Dumo P, Knapp E, Wesley G. Inappropriate metformin use in hospitalized patients [abstract 503-P], ADA 63rd Annual Scientific Sessions, New Orleans, LA, 2002.
131. Jacober SJ, Sowers JR. An update on perioperative management of diabetes. Arch Intern Med 1999;159:2405–2411.
132. American Diabetes Association. Preconception care of women with diabetes. Diabetes Care 2004;27(Suppl 1):S76–S78.
133. Ryan EA. Pregnancy in diabetes. Med Clin North Am 1998;82:823–845.
134. Buchbinder A, Miodovnik M, McElvy S, et al. Is insulin lispro associated with the development or progression of diabetic retinopathy during pregnancy? Am J Obstet Gynecol 2000;183:1162–1165.
135. Schernthaner G. Progress in the immunointervention of type 1 diabetes mellitus. Horm Metab Res 1995;27:547–554.
136. Diabetes Prevention Trial-Type 1 Diabetes Study Group. Effects of insulin in relatives of patients with type 1 diabetes mellitus. N Engl J Med 2002;346:1685–1691.
137. Kakka R, Koda-Kimble MA. Can insulin therapy delay or prevent insulin-dependent diabetes mellitus? Pharmacotherapy 1997;17:38–44.
138. Diabetes Prevention Program Research Group. Reduction in the incidence of type 2 diabetes with lifestyle intervention or metformin. N Engl J Med 2002;346:393–403.
139. Tuomilehto J, Lindstrom J, Eriksson JG, et al. for the Finnish Diabetes Prevention Study Group. Prevention of type 2 diabetes mellitus by changes in lifestyle among subjects with impaired glucose tolerance. N Engl J Med 2001;344:1343–1350.
140. Buchanan TA, Xiang AH, Peters RK, et al. Preservation of pancreatic β-cell function and prevention of type 2 diabetes by pharmacological treatment of insulin resistance in high-risk Hispanic women. Diabetes 2002;51:2796–2803.
141. The DREAM Trial Investigators. The effect of ramipril on the incidence of diabetes. N Engl J Med 2006;355:1551–1562.
142. The DREAM Trial Investigators. The effect of rosiglitazone on the frequency of diabetes in patients with impaired glucose tolerance or impaired fasting glucose. A randomised controlled trial. Lancet 2006;368:1096–1105.
143. Nathan DM, Davidson MB, Defronzo RA, et al. Impaired fasting glucose and impaired glucose tolerance. Implication for care. Diabetes Care 2007;30:753–759.
144. Mensing C, Boucher J, Cypress M, et al. National standards for diabetes self-management education. Diabetes Care 2000;23:682–689.
145. Fong DS, Aiello LP, Ferris FL III, Klein R. Diabetic retinopathy. Diabetes Care 2004;27:2540–2553.
146. Boulton AJ, Malik RA, Arezzo JC, Sosenko JM. Diabetic somatic neuropathies. Diabetes Care 2004;27:1458–1486.
147. American Diabetes Association. Diabetic nephropathy. Diabetes Care 2004;27(Suppl 1):S79–S83.
148. Lewis EJ, Hunsicker LG, Clarke WR, et al. Renoprotective effect of the angiotensin-receptor antagonist irbesartan in patients with nephropathy due to type 2 diabetes. N Engl J Med 2001;345:851–860.
149. Brenner BM, Cooper ME, deZeeuw D, et al. Effects of losartan on renal and cardiovascular outcomes in patients with type 2 diabetes and nephropathy. N Engl J Med 2001;345:861–869.
150. Parving HH, Lehnert H, Brochner-Mortensen J, et al. The effect of irbesartan on the development of diabetic nephropathy in patients with type 2 diabetes. N Engl J Med 2001;345:870–878.
151. American Diabetes Association. Consensus development conference on diabetic foot wound care, April 7–8, 1999 Boston, MA. Diabetes Care 1999;22:1354–1360.
152. Haire-Joshu D, Glasgow RE, Tibbs TL. Smoking and diabetes (technical review). Diabetes Care 1999;22:1887–1898.
153. American Diabetes Association. Aspirin therapy. Diabetes Care 2004;27(Suppl 1):S72–S73.
154. Orchard TJ, Forrest KY, Kuller LH, Becker DJ. Lipid and blood pressure treatment goals for type 1 diabetes: 10-Year incidence data from the Pittsburgh Epidemiology of Diabetes Complications Study. Diabetes Care 2001;24:1053–1059.
155. Colhoun HM, Betteridge DJ, Durrington PN, et al. Primary prevention of cardiovascular disease with atorvastatin in type 2 diabetes in the collaborative atorvastatin diabetes study (CARDS): A multicentre, randomised placebo-controlled trial. Lancet 2004;364:685–696.
156. Heart Protection Study Collaborative Group. MRC/BHF Heart Protection Study of cholesterol-lowering with simvastatin in 5963 people with diabetes: A randomised placebo-controlled trial. Lancet 2003;361:2005–2016.
157. Rubins HB, Robins SJ, Collins D, et al. Gemfibrozil for the secondary prevention of coronary heart disease in men with low levels of high-density lipoprotein cholesterol. Veterans Affairs High-Density Lipoprotein Cholesterol Intervention Trial Study Group. N Engl J Med 1999;341:410–418.
158. The FIELD Study Investigators. Effects of long-term fenofibrate therapy on cardiovascular events in 9795 people with type 2 diabetes mellitus (the FIELD study): Randomised controlled trial. Lancet 2005;366:1849–1861.

159. Expert Panel on Detection, Evaluation, and Treatment of High Blood Cholesterol in Adults. Executive summary of the third report of the National Cholesterol Education Program (NCEP) expert panel on detection, evaluation, and treatment of high blood cholesterol in adults (Adult Treatment Panel III). JAMA 2001;285:2486–2496.
160. Grundy SM, Cleeman JI, Merz CN. Implications of recent clinical trials for the national cholesterol education program adult treatment panel III guidelines. Circulation 2004;110:227–239.
161. Hansson L, Zanchetti A, Carruthers SG. Effects of intensive blood-pressure lowering and low-dose aspirin in patients with hypertension: Principal results of the Hypertension Optimal Treatment (HOT) randomised trial. HOT Study Group. Lancet 1998;351:1755–1762.
162. Bakris GL, Williams M, Dworkin L, et al. Preserving renal function in adults with hypertension and diabetes: A consensus approach. National Kidney Foundation Hypertension and Diabetes Executive Committees Working Group. Am J Kidney Dis 2000;36:646–661.
163. Deedwania PC. Hypertension and diabetes: New therapeutic options. Arch Intern Med 2000;160:1585–1594.
164. Robertson RP, Davis C, Larsen J, et al. Pancreas and islet transplantation for patients with diabetes mellitus (technical review). Diabetes Care 2000;23:112–116.
165. Herman WH, Eastman RC. The effects on treatment on the direct costs of diabetes. Diabetes Care 1998;21(Suppl 3):C19-C24.
166. Gray A. Raikou M, McGuire A, et al. Cost effectiveness of an intensive blood glucose control policy in patient with type 2 diabetes: Economic analysis alongside randomized controlled trial (UKPDS 41). BMJ 2000;320:1373–1378.
167. Anonymous. Cost effectiveness analysis of improved blood pressure control in hypertensive patients with type 2 diabetes: UKPDS 40. BMJ 1998;317:720–726.
168. American Diabetes Association. Dyslipidemia management in adults with diabetes. Diabetes Care 2004;27:S68–S71.

CHAPTER 78

Thyroid Disorders

STEVEN I. SHERMAN AND ROBERT L. TALBERT

KEY CONCEPTS

1. The molecular biology of the thyroid hormones and their receptors has provided an in-depth understanding of the various mutations that give rise to hyper- and hypothyroidism.

2. Thyrotoxicosis is most commonly caused by Graves' disease, which is an autoimmune disorder in which thyroid-stimulating antibody (TSAb) directed against the thyrotropin receptor elicits the same biologic response as thyroid-stimulating hormone (TSH).

3. Hyperthyroidism can be treated with antithyroid drugs such as propylthiouracil (PTU) or methimazole (MMI), radioactive iodine (RAI; e.g., iodine-131 [^{131}I]), or surgical removal of the thyroid gland; selection of the initial treatment approach is based on patient characteristics such as age, concurrent physiology (e.g., pregnancy), comorbidities (e.g., chronic obstructive lung disease), and convenience.

4. PTU and MMI reduce the synthesis of thyroid hormones and are similar in efficacy and adverse effects, but their dosing ranges differ by 10-fold.

5. Response to PTU and MMI is seen in 4 to 6 weeks with a maximal response in 4 to 6 months; treatment usually continues for 1 to 2 years, and therapy is monitored by clinical signs and symptoms and by measuring the serum concentrations of TSH and free thyroxine (T_4).

6. Many patients choose to have ablative therapy with ^{131}I rather than undergo repeated courses of PTU or MMI; most receiving RAI eventually become hypothyroid and require thyroid hormone supplementation.

7. Adjunctive therapy with β-blockers controls the adrenergic symptoms of thyrotoxicosis but does not correct the underlying disorder; iodine can also be used adjunctively in preparation for surgery and acutely for thyroid storm.

8. Hypothyroidism is most often caused by an autoimmune disorder known as Hashimoto's thyroiditis, and the drug of choice for replacement therapy is levothyroxine.

9. Monitoring of levothyroxine replacement therapy is done by clinical signs and symptoms and by measuring the TSH (elevated for under-replacement, suppressed for overreplacement).

Thyroid hormones affect the function of virtually every organ system. In the child, thyroid hormone is critical for normal growth and development. In the adult, the major role of thyroid hormone is to maintain metabolic stability. Substantial reservoirs of thyroid hormone in the thyroid gland and blood provide constant thyroid hormone availability. In addition, the hypothalamic-pituitary-thyroid axis is exquisitely sensitive to small changes in circulating thyroid hormone concentrations, and alterations in thyroid hormone secretion maintain peripheral free thyroid hormone levels within a narrow range. Patients seek medical attention for evaluation of symptoms because of abnormal thyroid hormone levels or because of diffuse or nodular thyroid enlargement.

THYROID HORMONE PHYSIOLOGY

THYROID HORMONE SYNTHESIS

The thyroid hormones thyroxine (T_4) and triiodothyronine (T_3) are formed on thyroglobulin, a large glycoprotein synthesized within the thyroid cell (Fig. 78–1). Because of the unique tertiary structure of this glycoprotein, iodinated tyrosine residues present in thyroglobulin are able to bind together to form active thyroid hormones.[1]

Iodide is actively transported through the basolateral membrane via a sodium/iodine (Na^+/I^-) symporter from the extracellular space into the thyroid follicular cell against an electrochemical gradient, driven by the coupled transport of sodium.[2] Structurally related anions such as thiocyanate (SCN^-), perchlorate (ClO_4^-), and pertechnetate (TcO_4^-) are competitive inhibitors of iodine transport.[3] In addition, bromine, fluorine, and lithium block iodide transport into the thyroid (Table 78–1). Inorganic iodide that enters the thyroid follicular cell is ushered through the cell to the apical membrane, where it is transported into the follicular lumen by at least two efflux channels.[4,5] Located on the luminal side of the apical membrane, thyroid peroxidase oxidizes iodide and covalently binds the organified iodide to tyrosine residues of thyroglobulin (Fig. 78–2). It is interesting that although salivary glands and the gastric mucosa are able to actively transport iodide, they are unable to effectively incorporate iodide into proteins given the lack of similar oxidizing machinery. Similarly, when tyrosine molecules are iodinated on proteins other than thyroglobulin, they lack the proper tertiary structure needed to allow the formation of active thyroid hormones.

The iodinated tyrosine residues monoiodotyrosine (MIT) and diiodotyrosine (DIT) combine to form iodothyronines (Fig. 78–3). Thus, two molecules of DIT combine to form T_4, whereas MIT and DIT constitute T_3. In addition to its role in iodine organification, the hemoprotein thyroid peroxidase also catalyzes the formation of iodothyronines (coupling).

Iodine deficiency causes an increase in the ratio of MIT to DIT in thyroglobulin and leads to a relative increase in the production of T_3.[6] Because T_3 is more potent than T_4, the increase in T_3 production in

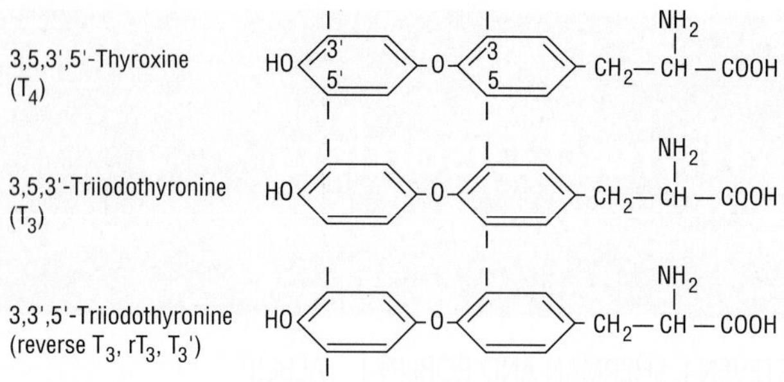

FIGURE 78-1. Structure of thyroid hormones.

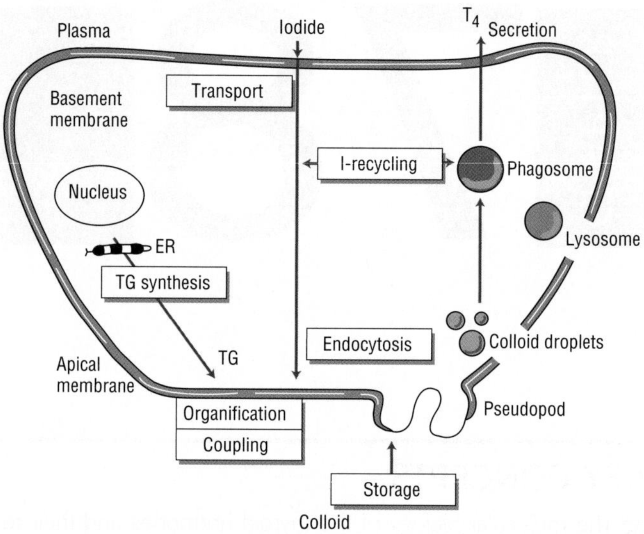

FIGURE 78-2. Thyroid hormone synthesis. Iodide is transported from the plasma, through the cell, to the apical membrane where it is organified and coupled to the thyroglobulin (TG) synthesized within the thyroid cell. Hormone stored as colloid reenters the cell through endocytosis and moves back toward the basal membrane, where T_4 is secreted. (T_4, thyroxine.)

iodine-depleted areas can be beneficial. The thionamide drugs used to treat hyperthyroidism inhibit thyroid peroxidase and thus block thyroid hormone synthesis.

Thyroglobulin is stored in the follicular lumen and must reenter the cell, where the process of proteolysis liberates thyroid hormone into the bloodstream. Thyroid follicles active in hormone synthesis are identified histologically by columnar epithelial cells lining follicular lumens, which are depleted of colloid. Inactive follicles are lined by cuboidal epithelial cells and are replete with colloid. Both iodide and lithium block the release of preformed thyroid hormone through poorly understood mechanisms.

T_4 and T_3 are transported in the bloodstream primarily by three proteins: thyroxine-binding globulin (TBG), transthyretin (TTR), and albumin.[7] It is estimated that 99.96% of circulating T_4 and 99.5% of T_3 are bound to these proteins. However, only the unbound (free) thyroid hormone is able to diffuse into the cell, elicit a biologic effect, and regulate thyroid-stimulating hormone (TSH; also known as thyrotropin) secretion from the pituitary. Multiple functions have been ascribed to these transport proteins, including (1) assuring minimal urinary loss of iodide, (2) providing a mechanism for uniform tissue distribution of free hormone, and (3) transport of hormone into the central nervous system.

Whereas T_4 is secreted solely from the thyroid gland, less than 20% of T_3 is produced in the thyroid. The majority of T_3 is formed from the breakdown of T_4 catalyzed by the enzyme 5-monodeiodinase found in extrathyroidal peripheral tissues. Because the binding affinity of nuclear thyroid hormone receptors is 10 to 15 times higher for T_3 than T_4, the deiodinase enzymes play a pivotal role in determining overall metabolic activity. Three different monodeiodinase enzymes are present in the body.[8] Of the enzymes that catalyze 5'-monodeiodination, type I enzymes are present in peripheral tissues, whereas type II enzymes are found in the central nervous system, pituitary, and thyroid. Type III enzymes, found in the placenta, skin, and developing brain, inactivate T_4 and T_3 by deiodinating the inner ring at the 5'-position. The principal characteristics of these enzymes are listed in Table 78–2. T_4 may also be acted on by the enzyme 5'-monodeiodinase to form reverse T_3, but this accounts for a small component of hormone metabolism. Reverse T_3 has no known significant biologic activity. T_3 is removed from the body by deiodinative degradation and through the action of sulfotransferase enzyme systems to T_3 sulfate and 3,3-diiodothyronine sulfates, thus facilitating enterohepatic clearance.

TABLE 78-1 Thyroid Hormone Synthesis and Secretion Inhibitors

Mechanism of Action	Substance
Blocks iodide transport into the thyroid	Bromine
	Fluorine
	Lithium
Impairs organification and coupling of thyroid hormones	Thionamides
	Sulfonylureas
	Sulfonamide (?)
	Salicylamide (?)
	Antipyrine (?)
Inhibits thyroid hormone secretion	Lithium iodide (large doses)

The growth and function of the thyroid are stimulated by activation of the thyrotropin receptor by TSH.[9] The receptor belongs to the family of G-protein–coupled receptors. The thyrotropin receptor is coupled to the α subunit of the stimulatory guanine-nucleotide–binding protein ($G_s\alpha$), activating adenylate cyclase and increasing the accumulation of cyclic adenosine monophosphate. Through this mechanism, TSH stimulates the expression of thyroglobulin and thyroid peroxidase genes as well as increases apical iodide efflux. Somatic activating mutations in the receptor are commonly seen in autonomously functioning thyroid nodules.[10] Rarely, germline activating mutations of the TSH receptor have been reported in kindreds with Leclère's syndrome, and thyrotoxicosis can also result from germline-activating mutations in G protein signaling in McCune-

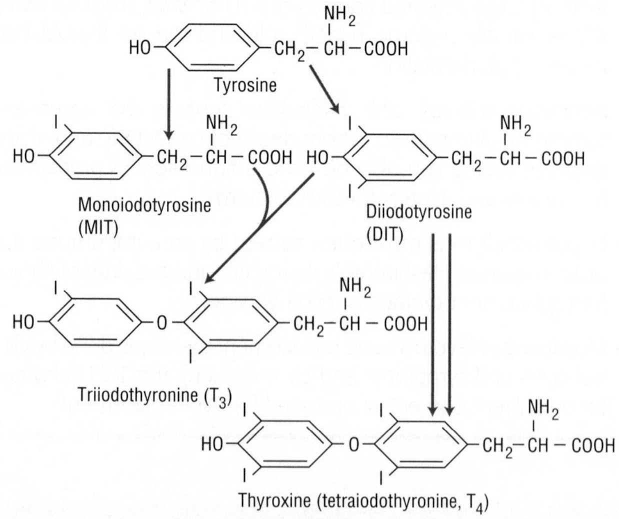

FIGURE 78-3. Scheme of coupling reactions. After tyrosine is iodinated to form monoiodotyrosine (MIT) or diiodotyrosine (DIT) (organification of the iodine), MIT and DIT combine to form triiodothyronine (T_3), or two molecules of DIT form thyroxine (T_4).

TABLE 78-2 Properties of Iodothyronine 5′-Deiodinase Isoforms

Property	Type I	Type II	Type III
Effect of propylthiouracil	Increase	Decrease	Increase
Tissue localization	Thyroid, liver, kidney	Pituitary, thyroid, CNS, brown adipose tissue	Placenta, developing brain, skin
Preferred substrate	$rT_3 > T_4 > T_3$	$T_4 > T_3$	T_3 (sulfate) $> T_4$
Physiologic role	Extracellular T_3 production for peripheral tissue	Intracellular T_3 production, especially for brain in hypothyroidism or iodine deficiency	Inactivation of T_4 and T_3
Developmental expression	Expressed latest in development; predominant deiodinase in adult	Expressed second; especially high in brain and brown adipose tissue	Expressed first; high in developing brain; may be important for fetal thyroid hormone metabolism

rT_3, reverse T_3; T_3, triiodothyronine; T_4, thyroxine.

Albright's syndrome.[9,11–13] Conversely, thyrotropin resistance would result from point mutations that prevent TSH binding, leading to abnormalities in the thyrotropin receptor–adenylate cyclase system and congenital hypothyroidism.[14,15] Individuals with this abnormality have high levels of TSH, but decreased thyroglobulin levels and a normal or small gland.

Thyroid hormone receptors regulate the transcription of target genes in the presence of physiologic concentrations of T_3.[16] Unlike most other nuclear receptors, thyroid hormone receptors also actively regulate gene expression in the absence of hormone, typically resulting in an opposite effect. Thyroid receptors translocate from the cytoplasm to the nucleus, interact in the nucleus with T_3, and target genes and other proteins required for basal and T_3-dependent gene transcription. Thyroid receptors exist in three isoforms, $TR\beta_2$, $TR\beta_1$, and $TR\alpha_1$, with variation in the expression of each in differing tissues.

The production of thyroid hormone is regulated in two main ways. First, thyroid hormone is regulated by TSH secreted by the anterior pituitary. The secretion of TSH is itself under negative feedback control by the circulating level of free thyroid hormone and the positive influence of hypothalamic thyrotropin-releasing hormone (TRH). Second, extrathyroidal deiodination of T_4 to T_3 is regulated by a variety of factors including nutrition, nonthyroidal hormones, drugs, and illness.

THYROTOXICOSIS

Thyrotoxicosis results when tissues are exposed to excessive levels of T_4, T_3, or both.[17] In the National Health and Nutrition Examination Survey III (NHANES III), 0.7% of those surveyed who were not taking thyroid medications and had no history of thyroid disease had subclinical hyperthyroidism (TSH <0.1 mIU/L; and T_4 normal), and 0.5% had "clinically significant" hyperthyroidism (TSH <0.1 mIU/L; and T_4 >13.2 mcg/dL).[18] The prevalence of suppressed TSH peaked in people aged 20 to 39 years, declined in those 40 to 79 years of age, and increased again in those 80 years of age or older. Abnormal TSH levels were more common among women than among men.

CLINICAL PRESENTATION OF THYROTOXICOSIS

General

- Patients can have symptoms for an extended time period before the diagnosis of hyperthyroidism is made.

Symptoms

- The typical clinical manifestations of thyrotoxicosis include nervousness, anxiety, palpitations, emotional lability, easy fatigability, menstrual disturbances, and heat intolerance. A cardinal symptom is loss of weight concurrent with an increased appetite.

Signs

- A variety of physical signs can be elicited including warm, smooth, moist skin, exophthalmos (in Graves' disease only), pretibial myxedema (in Graves' disease only), and unusually fine hair. Separation of the end of the fingernails from the nail beds (onycholysis) may be noted. Ocular signs that result from thyrotoxicosis include retraction of the eyelids and lagging of the upper lid behind the globe when the patient looks downward (lid lag). Physical signs of a hyperdynamic circulatory state are common and include tachycardia at rest, a widened pulse pressure, and a systolic ejection murmur. Gynecomastia is sometimes noted in men. Neuromuscular examination often reveals a fine tremor of the protruded tongue and outstretched hands. Deep tendon reflexes are generally hyperactive. Thyromegaly is usually present.

Diagnosis

- Low TSH serum concentration. Elevated free and total T_3 and T_4 serum concentrations, particularly in more severe disease.
- Elevated radioactive iodine uptake (RAIU) by the thyroid gland when hormone is being overproduced; suppressed RAIU in thyrotoxicosis caused by thyroid inflammation (thyroiditis)

Other Tests

- Thyroid stimulating antibodies (TSAb)
- Thyroglobulin
- Thyrotropin receptor antibodies
- Thyroid biopsy
- Thyroperoxidase antibodies (TPO antibodies)

In the elderly (>65 years old) patient and in the patient with very severe disease, anorexia can be present as well. Elderly patients are also more likely to develop atrial fibrillation with thyrotoxicosis than younger patients. The frequency of bowel movements can increase, but frank diarrhea is unusual. Palpitations are a prominent and distressing symptom, particularly in the patient with preexisting heart disease. Proximal muscle weakness is common and is noted on climbing stairs or in getting up from a sitting position. Women might note their menses are becoming scanty and irregular. Extremely thyrotoxic (thyrotoxic storm) patients can have tachycardia, heart failure, psychosis, hyperpyrexia, and coma.[19]

DIFFERENTIAL DIAGNOSIS

If the clinical history and examination do not provide pathognomonic clues to the etiology of the patient's thyrotoxicosis, measurement of the RAIU is critical in the evaluation (Table 78–3). The normal 24-hour RAIU ranges from 10% to 30% with some regional variation because of differences in iodine intake. An elevated RAIU indicates true hyperthyroidism, that is, the patient's thyroid gland is actively overproducing T_4, T_3, or both. Conversely, a low RAIU, in the absence of iodine excess, indicates that high levels of thyroid hormone are not a consequence of thyroid gland hyperfunction but likely caused by thyroiditis or hormone ingestion. The importance

TABLE 78-3 Differential Diagnosis of Thyrotoxicosis

Increased RAIU	Decreased RAIU
TSH-induced hyperthyroidism	Inflammatory thyroid disease
TSH-secreting tumors	Subacute thyroiditis
Selective pituitary resistance to T_4	Painless thyroid
Thyroid stimulators other than TSH[a]	Ectopic thyroid tissue
TSAb (Graves' disease)	Struma ovarii
hCG (trophoblastic diseases)	Metastatic follicular carcinoma
Thyroid autonomy	Exogenous sources of thyroid hormone
Toxic adenoma	Medication
Multinodular goiter	Food

hCG, human chorionic gonadotropin; RAIU, radioactive iodine uptake; TSAb, thyroid-stimulating antibodies; TSH, thyroid-stimulating hormone; T_3, triiodothyrine; T_4, thyroxine.
[a]The RAIU can be decreased if the patient has been recently exposed to excess iodine.

of differentiating true hyperthyroidism from other causes of thyrotoxicosis lies in the widely different prognosis and treatment of the diseases in these two categories. Therapy of thyrotoxicosis associated with thyroid hyperfunction is mainly directed at decreasing the rate of thyroid hormone synthesis, secretion, or both. Such measures are ineffective in treating thyrotoxicosis that is not the result of true hyperthyroidism, because hormone synthesis and regulated hormone secretion are already at a minimum.

CAUSES OF THYROTOXICOSIS ASSOCIATED WITH ELEVATED RAIU

TSH-Induced Hyperthyroidism

To better understand these syndromes we must first review TSH biosynthesis and secretion. TSH is synthesized in the anterior pituitary as separate α- and β-subunit precursors. The α subunits from luteinizing hormone (LH), follicle-stimulating hormone (FSH), human chorionic gonadotropin (hCG), and TSH are similar, whereas the β subunits are unique and confer immunologic and biologic specificity. Free β-subunits are devoid of receptor binding and biologic activity and require combination with an α-subunit to express their activity. Criteria for the diagnosis of TSH-induced hyperthyroidism include (1) evidence of peripheral hypermetabolism, (2) diffuse thyroid gland enlargement, (3) elevated free thyroid hormone levels, and (4) elevated or inappropriately "normal" serum immunoreactive TSH concentrations. Because the pituitary gland is extremely sensitive to even minimal elevations of free T_4, a "normal" or elevated TSH level in any thyrotoxic patient indicates the inappropriate production of TSH.

TSH-Secreting Pituitary Adenomas

TSH-secreting pituitary tumors occur sporadically and release biologically active hormone that is unresponsive to normal feedback control.[20] The mean age at diagnosis is approximately 40 years of age, with women being diagnosed more commonly than men (8:7). These tumors can cosecrete prolactin or growth hormone; therefore the patients can present with amenorrhea/galactorrhea or signs of acromegaly. Most patients present with classic symptoms and signs of thyrotoxicosis. Visual-field defects can be present because of impingement of the optic chiasm by the tumor. Tumor growth and worsening visual-field defects have been reported following treatment of thyrotoxicosis, because of loss of feedback inhibition from high thyroid hormone levels.

Diagnosis of a TSH-secreting adenoma should be made by demonstrating lack of TSH response to TRH stimulation, inappropriate TSH levels, elevated α-subunit levels, and radiologic imaging; given the lack of routine availability of TRH, the other three criteria are essential. Note that some small tumors are not identified by magnetic resonance imaging (MRI). Moreover, 10% of "normal" individuals can have pituitary tumors or other benign focal lesions noted on pituitary imaging.

Transsphenoidal pituitary surgery is the treatment of choice for TSH-secreting adenomas. Pituitary gland irradiation is often given following surgery to prevent tumor recurrence. Bromocriptine and octreotide have been used to treat tumors, especially those that cosecrete prolactin.

Pituitary Resistance to Thyroid Hormone

Pituitary resistance to thyroid hormone (PRTH) refers to selective resistance of the pituitary thyrotrophs to thyroid hormone.[21] Approximately twice as many women as men have been reported with this rare, probably familial syndrome. Multiple abnormalities have been reported in the initial 50 reported cases including schizophrenia (three patients), mental retardation (two patients), short fourth metacarpals (one patient), and Marfanoid habitus (one patient). Approximately 90% of patients studied have an appropriate increase in TSH in response to TRH; conversely, the TSH will be suppressed by T_3 administration.

Patients with PRTH require treatment to reduce their elevated thyroid hormone levels. Determining the appropriate serum T_4 level is difficult because TSH cannot be used to evaluate adequacy of therapy. Any reduction in thyroid hormone carries the risk of inducing thyrotroph hyperplasia. Ideally, agents that suppress TSH secretion could be used to treat these individuals. Glucocorticoid, dopaminergic drugs, somatostatin and its analog, and thyroid hormone analogs with reduced metabolic activity have all been tried; given the ability of retinoid X receptor ligands to inhibit TSH production, drugs such as bexarotene can have therapeutic benefit in PRTH.[22]

THYROID STIMULATORS OTHER THAN TSH

Graves' Disease

Graves' disease is an autoimmune syndrome that usually includes hyperthyroidism, diffuse thyroid enlargement, and exophthalmos, and less commonly pretibial myxedema and thyroid acropachy (Fig. 78–4).[17,23,24] Graves' disease is the most common cause of hyperthyroidism, with a prevalence estimated to be 3 per 1,000 in the U.S. population. Hyperthyroidism results from the action of TSAbs, which are directed against the thyrotropin receptor on the surface of the thyroid cell.[14,15] When these immunoglobulins bind to the receptor, they activate downstream G-protein signaling and adenylate cyclase in the same manner as TSH. Autoantibodies that react with orbital muscle and fibroblast tissue in the skin are responsible for the extrathyroidal manifestations of Graves' disease, and these autoantibodies are encoded by the same germline genes that encode for other autoantibodies for striated muscle and thyroid peroxidase.[25] Clinically, the extrathyroidal disorders might not appear at the same time that hyperthyroidism develops.

There is now compelling evidence that heredity predisposes the susceptible individual to development of clinically overt autoimmune thyroid disease in the setting of appropriate environmental and hormonal triggers. A role for gender in the emergence of Graves' disease is suggested by the fact that hyperthyroidism is approximately eight times more common in women than men. Other lines of evidence support a role for heredity. First, there is a well-recognized clustering of Graves' disease within some families. Twin studies in Graves' disease have revealed that a monozygotic twin has a 35% likelihood of ultimately developing the disease compared with a 3% likelihood for a dizygotic twin, resulting in estimation that the 79% of the predisposition to Graves' disease is genetic.[26] Second, the occurrence of other autoimmune diseases, including Hashimoto's thyroiditis, is also increased in families of patients with Graves' disease. Third, several

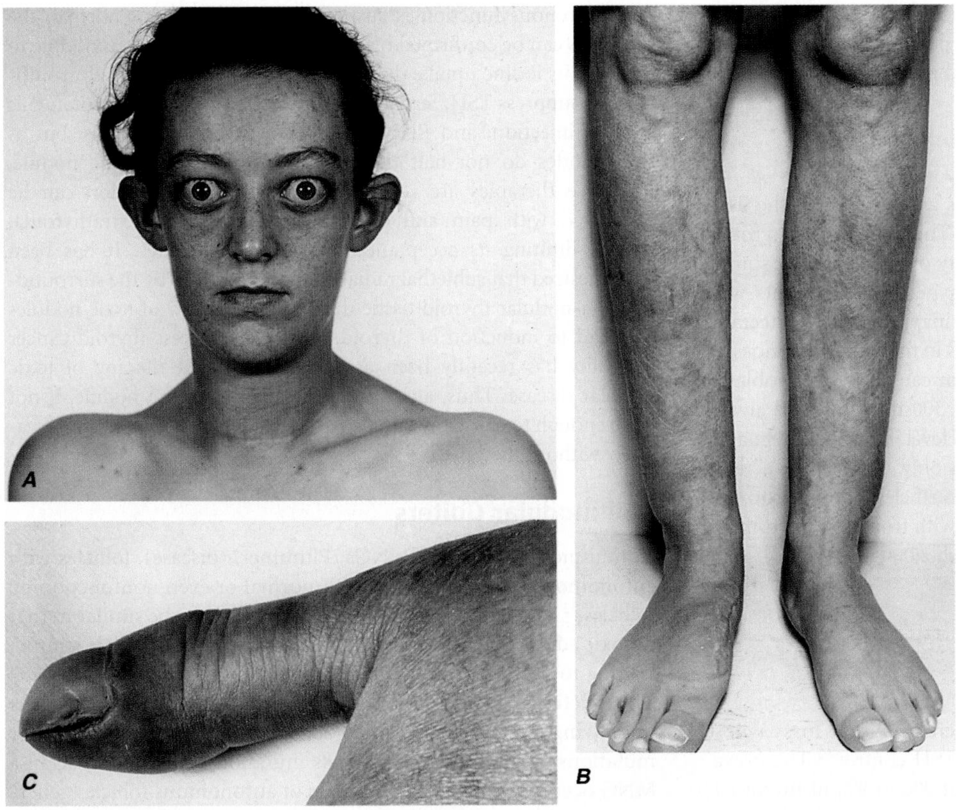

FIGURE 78-4. Features of Graves' disease. *(A)* Facial appearance in Graves' disease; lid retraction, periorbital edema, and proptosis are marked. *(B)* Thyroid dermopathy over the lateral aspects of the shins. *(C)* Thyroid acropachy. *(Reproduced with permission from Kasper DL, et al., eds. Harrison's Principles of Internal Medicine, 16th ed. New York: McGraw-Hill, 2005:2114.)*

studies have demonstrated an increased frequency of certain human leukocyte antigens (HLAs) in patients with Graves' disease. Differing HLA associations have been identified in the various ethnic groups studied. In whites, for example, the relative risk of Graves' disease in carriers of the HLA-DR3 haplotype is between 2.5 and 5, whereas lesser associations have been reported for HLA-B8 and the HLA-DQA*0501 allele.[27,28] As with other autoimmune conditions, certain polymorphisms of the T-cell immunoregulatory protein CTLA-4 have also been associated with Graves' disease. Despite these statistical associations, however, even detailed molecular genetic linkage studies have failed to identify specific genes responsible for the disease.[29]

The thyroid gland is diffusely enlarged in the majority of patients and is commonly 40 to 60 g (two to three times the normal size). The surface of the gland is either smooth or bosselated, and the consistency varies from soft to firm. In patients with severe disease, a thrill may be felt and a systolic bruit may be heard over the gland, reflecting the increased intraglandular vascularity typical of hyperplasia. Whereas the presence of any of the extrathyroidal manifestations of this syndrome, including exophthalmos, thyroid acropachy, or pretibial myxedema, in a thyrotoxic patient is pathognomonic of Graves' disease, most patients can be diagnosed on the basis of their history and examination of their diffuse goiter (see Fig. 78–4). An important clinical feature of Graves' disease is the occurrence of spontaneous remissions, albeit uncommon. The abnormalities in TSAb production can decrease or disappear over time in many patients.

The results of laboratory tests in thyrotoxic Graves' disease include an increase in the overall hormone production rate with a disproportionate increase in T_3 relative to T_4 (Table 78–4). In an occasional patient, the disproportionate overproduction of T_3 is exaggerated, with the result that only the serum T_3 concentration is increased (T_3 toxicosis). The saturation of TBG is increased because of the elevated levels of serum T_4 and T_3, which is reflected in elevated values for the T_3 resin uptake. As a result, the concentration of free T_4, free T_3, and the free T_4 and T_3 indices are increased to an even greater extent than are the measured serum total T_4 and T_3 concentrations. The TSH level will be undetectable because of negative feedback by elevated levels of thyroid hormone at the pituitary.

In the patient with manifest disease, measurement of the serum free T_4 concentration (or total T_4 and T_3 resin uptake), total T_3, and the TSH value will confirm the diagnosis of thyrotoxicosis. If the patient is not pregnant, a 24-hour RAIU should be obtained if there is any diagnostic uncertainty, for example, recent onset of symptoms or other factors suggestive of thyroiditis. An increased RAIU documents that the thyroid gland is inappropriately using the iodine to produce more thyroid hormone at a time when the patient is thyrotoxic.

Hypokalemic periodic paralysis is a rare complication of hyperthyroidism more commonly observed in Asian and Hispanic populations.[30] It presents as recurrent proximal muscle flaccidity ranging from mild weakness to total paralysis. The paralysis can be asymmetric and usually involves muscle groups that are strenuously exercised before the attack. Cognition and sensory perception are spared, whereas deep tendon reflexes are commonly markedly diminished. Hypokalemia results from a sudden shift of potassium from extracellular to intracellular sites, rather than reduced total body potassium.

TABLE 78-4 Thyroid Function Test Results in Different Thyroid Conditions

	Total T_4	Free T_4	Total T_3	T_3 Resin Uptake	Free Thyroxine Index	TSH
Normal	4.5–10.9 mcg/dL	0.8–2.7 ng/dL	60–181 ng/dL	22% to 34%	1.0–4.3 units	0.5–4.7 mIU/L
Hyperthyroid	↑↑	↑↑	↑↑↑	↑	↑↑↑	↓↓
Hypothyroid	↓↓	↓↓	↓	↓↓	↓↓↓	↑↑
Increased TBG	↑	Normal	↑	↓	Normal	Normal

TBG, thyroid-binding globulin; TSH, thyroid-stimulating hormone; T_3, triiodothyrine; T_4, thyroxine.

High carbohydrate loads and exercise provoke the attacks. Treatment includes correcting the hyperthyroid state, potassium administration, spironolactone to conserve potassium, and propranolol to minimize intracellular shifts.

Trophoblastic Diseases

Human chorionic gonadotropin (hCG) is a stimulator of the TSH receptor and can cause hyperthyroidism.[31] The basis for the thyrotropic effect of hCG is the structural similarity of hCG to TSH (similar α-subunits and unique β subunits). In hyperthyroid patients with very high hCG levels, serum TSH can be inappropriately detectable because of the weak cross-reactivity of hCG in the radioimmunoassay for TSH. In patients with hyperthyroidism caused by trophoblastic tumors, serum hCG levels usually exceed 300 units/mL and always exceed 100 units/mL. The mean peak hCG level in normal pregnancy is 50 units/mL. On a molar basis, hCG has only 1/10,000 the activity of pituitary TSH in mouse bioassays. Nevertheless, this thyrotropic activity can be very substantial in patients with trophoblastic tumors, whose serum hCG concentrations can reach 2,000 units/mL.

THYROID AUTONOMY

Toxic Adenoma

An autonomous thyroid nodule is a discrete thyroid mass whose function is independent of pituitary and TSH control.[32] The prevalence of toxic adenoma ranges from about 2% to 9% of thyrotoxic patients, and depends on iodine availability and geographic location. Toxic adenomas arise from gain-of-function somatic mutations of the TSH receptor, or less commonly the $G_s\alpha$ protein; more than a dozen TSH receptor mutations have been described.[10] These nodules can be referred to as a toxic adenoma or a "hot" nodule because of their persistent uptake on a radioiodine thyroid scan, despite suppressed uptake in the surrounding non-nodular gland (Fig. 78–5). The amount of thyroid hormone produced by an autonomous nodule is mass related. Therefore hyperthyroidism usually occurs with larger nodules (i.e., those >3 cm in diameter). Older patients (>60 years of age) are more likely (up to 60%) to be thyrotoxic from autonomous nodules than are younger (<60 years of age) patients (12%). There are many reports of isolated elevation of serum T_3 in patients with autonomously functioning nodules. Therefore if the T_4 level is normal, a T_3 level must be measured to rule out T_3 toxicosis.

If autonomous function is suspected, but the TSH is normal, the diagnosis can be confirmed by a failure of the autonomous nodule to decrease its iodine uptake during exogenous T_3 administration sufficient to suppress TSH. Surgical resection, thionamides, percutaneous ethanol injection, and RAI ablation are treatment options, but as thionamides do not halt the proliferative process in the nodule, definitive therapies are recommended.[33] Ethanol ablation can be associated with pain and damage to surrounding extrathyroidal tissues, limiting its acceptance in the United States. It has been hypothesized that sublethal radiation doses received by the surrounding non-nodular thyroid tissue during RAI therapy of toxic nodules can lead to induction of thyroid cancer, and excess thyroid cancer mortality has recently been associated with RAI therapy of toxic nodular disease. Thus, an autonomously functioning nodule, if not large enough to cause thyrotoxicosis, can often be observed conservatively without therapy.

Multinodular Goiters

In multinodular goiters (MNGs; Plummer's disease), follicles with autonomous function coexist with normal or even nonfunctioning follicles.[32] The pathogenesis of MNG is thought to be similar to that of toxic adenoma: diffuse hyperplasia caused by goitrogenic stimuli, leading to mutations and clonal expansion of benign neoplasms.[34] The functional status of the nodule(s) depends on the nature of the underlying mutations, whether activating such as TSH-receptor mutations or inhibitory such as ras mutations. Thyrotoxicosis in a MNG occurs when a sufficient mass of autonomous follicles generates enough thyroid hormone to exceed the needs of the patient. It is not surprising that this type of hyperthyroidism develops insidiously over a period of several years and predominantly affects older individuals with long-standing goiters. The patient's complaints of weight loss, depression, anxiety, and insomnia might be attributed to old age. Any unexplained chronic illness in an elderly patient presenting with a MNG calls for the exclusion of hidden thyrotoxicosis.[35] Third-generation TSH assays and T_3 suppression testing can be useful in detecting subclinical hyperthyroidism.[36]

A thyroid scan will show patchy areas of autonomously functioning thyroid tissue intermixed with hypofunctioning areas. When the patient is euthyroid, therapy is based on the need to reduce goiter size because of mass-related symptoms such as dysphagia. Doses of thyroid hormone sufficient to suppress TSH levels can slow goiter growth or cause some degree of shrinkage, but in general suppression

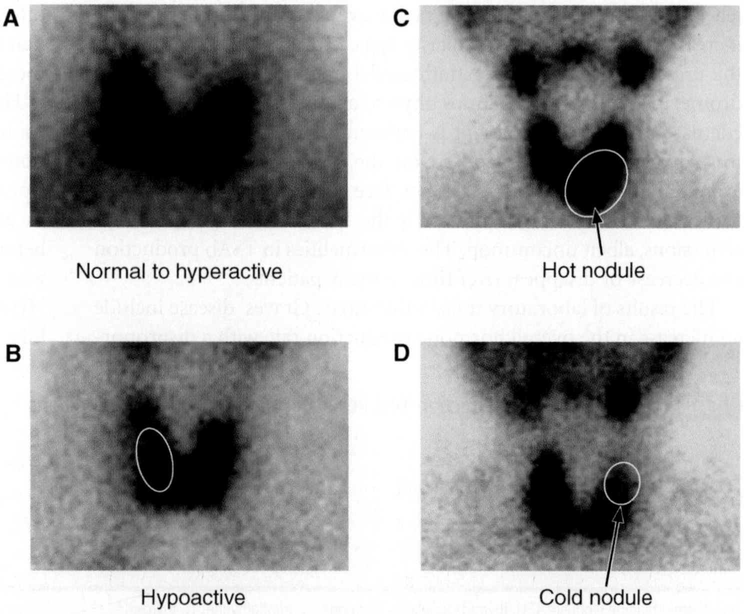

FIGURE 78-5. Radioiodine thyroid scans. *(A)* Normal to increased thyroid uptake of iodine-125 (^{125}I). *(B)* Thyroid with marked decrease in ^{125}I uptake in a large palpable mass. *(C)* Increased ^{125}I uptake isolated to a single nodule, the "hot nodule." *(D)* Decreased thyroid ^{125}I uptake in an isolated region, the "cold nodule." *(Reproduced with permission from Molina PE. Endocrine Physiology, 2nd ed. New York: McGraw-Hill, 2006:90. Images courtesy of Dr. Luis Linares, Memorial Medical Center, New Orleans, LA.)*

therapy for nodular disease is inadequate to address mass effect.[37] The preferred treatment for toxic MNG is RAI or surgery. Surgery is usually selected for younger (<60 years old) patients and patients in whom large goiters impinge on vital organs. Alternatively, percutaneous injection of 95% ethanol has also been used to destroy single or multinodular adenomas with a 5-year success rate approaching 80%.

CAUSES OF THYROTOXICOSIS ASSOCIATED WITH SUPPRESSED RAIU

Inflammatory Thyroid Disease

Subacute Thyroiditis Painful subacute (granulomatous or de Quervain's) thyroiditis often develops after a viral syndrome but rarely has a specific virus been identified in thyroid parenchyma.[38] A genetic predisposition exists with markedly higher risk for developing subacute thyroiditis in patients with HLA-Bw35. Systemic symptoms often accompany the syndrome, including fever, malaise, and myalgia, in addition to those symptoms caused by thyrotoxicosis. Typically, patients complain of severe pain in the thyroid region, which often extends to the ear on the affected side.[39] With time, the pain can migrate from one side of the gland to the other. On physical examination, the thyroid gland is firm and exquisitely tender. Signs of thyrotoxicosis are present.

Thyroid function tests typically run a triphasic course. Initially, serum T_4 levels are elevated because of release of preformed thyroid hormone from disrupted follicles. The 24-hour RAIU during this time is less than 2% because of thyroid inflammation and TSH suppression by the elevated T_4 level. As the disease progresses, intrathyroidal hormone stores are depleted, and the patient can become mildly hypothyroid with an appropriately elevated TSH level. During the recovery phase thyroid hormone stores are replenished, and serum TSH elevation gradually returns to normal. Recovery is generally complete within 2 to 6 months. Most patients remain euthyroid, and recurrences of painful thyroiditis are extremely rare. The patient with painful thyroiditis should be reassured that the disease is self-limited and is unlikely to recur. Thyrotoxic symptoms can be relieved with β-blockers. Aspirin (650 mg orally every 6 hours) will usually relieve the pain. Occasionally, prednisone (20 mg orally three times a day) must be used to suppress the inflammatory process. Antithyroid drugs are not indicated because they do not decrease the release of preformed thyroid hormone.

Painless Thyroiditis Since its description in 1975, painless (silent, lymphocytic) thyroiditis has been recognized as a common cause of thyrotoxicosis and can represent up to 15% of cases of thyrotoxicosis in North America.[40] In the setting of development of lymphocytic thyroiditis during the first 12 months after the end of pregnancy, the condition is also called "postpartum thyroiditis."[41] The etiology is not fully understood and may be heterogeneous, but evidence indicates that autoimmunity underlies most cases. There is an increased frequency of HLA-DR3 and DR5 in patients with subacute thyroiditis; nonendocrine autoimmune diseases are also more common. Histologically, diffuse lymphocytic infiltration is generally identified. The triphasic course of this illness mimics that of subacute thyroiditis. Most patients present with mild thyrotoxic symptoms. Lid retraction and lid lag are present, but exophthalmos is absent. The thyroid gland can be diffusely enlarged, but thyroid tenderness is absent.

The 24-hour RAIU will typically be suppressed to less than 2% during the thyrotoxic phase of painless thyroiditis. Antithyroglobulin and antimicrosomal antibody levels are elevated in more than 50% of patients. Patients with mild hyperthyroidism and painless thyroiditis should be reassured that they have a self-limited disease, although patients with postpartum thyroiditis can experience recurrence of the disease with subsequent pregnancies. As with other thyrotoxic syndromes, adrenergic symptoms can be ameliorated with propranolol or metoprolol. Antithyroid drugs, which inhibit new hormone synthesis, are not indicated because they do not decrease the release of preformed thyroid hormone.

Ectopic Thyroid Tissue

Struma Ovarii Struma ovarii is a teratoma of the ovary that contains differentiated thyroid follicular cells and is capable of making thyroid hormone.[42] This extremely rare cause of thyrotoxicosis is suggested by the absence of thyroid enlargement in a thyrotoxic patient with a suppressed RAIU in the neck and no findings to suggest thyroiditis. The diagnosis is established by localizing functioning thyroid tissue in the ovary with whole-body radioactive iodine (^{131}I) scanning. Interestingly, struma ovarii without associated hyperthyroidism is much more common than struma ovarii associated with hyperthyroidism. Because the tissue is neoplastic and potentially malignant, combined surgical and radioiodine treatment of malignant struma ovarii for both monitoring and therapy of relapse is the recommended treatment.

Follicular Cancer In widely metastatic differentiated papillary or follicular carcinomas with relatively well-preserved function, sufficient thyroid hormone can be synthesized and secreted to produce thyrotoxicosis.[43,44] In most instances, a previous diagnosis of thyroid malignancy has been made. The diagnosis can be confirmed by whole-body ^{131}I scanning. Treatment with ^{131}I is generally effective at ablating functioning thyroid metastases.

Exogenous Sources of Thyroid Hormone

Thyrotoxicosis factitia is produced by the ingestion of exogenous thyroid hormone.[45] Obesity is the most common nonthyroidal disorder for which thyroid hormone is inappropriately used, but thyroid hormone has been used for almost every conceivable problem from menstrual irregularities and infertility to hypercholesterolemia and baldness. Despite there being little evidence to suggest that these patients benefit from treatment with thyroid hormone, the physician or patient can gradually increase the dose of hormone employed in an attempt to gain the desired effect. Obviously, thyrotoxicosis factitia can also occur when too large a dose of thyroid hormone is employed for conditions in which it is likely to be beneficial, such as differentiated thyroid carcinoma. Rarely, thyrotoxicosis factitia is caused by the purposeful and secretive ingestion of thyroid hormone by disturbed patients (usually with a medical background) who wish to obtain attention or lose weight.

Thyrotoxicosis factitia should be suspected in a thyrotoxic patient without evidence of increased hormone production, thyroidal inflammation, or ectopic thyroid tissue. The RAIU uptake is at low levels because the patient's thyroid gland function is suppressed by the exogenous thyroid hormone.[46] Measurement of plasma thyroglobulin (TG) is a valuable laboratory aid in the diagnosis of thyrotoxicosis factitia. TG is normally secreted in small amounts by the thyroid gland; however, when thyroid hormone is taken orally, very low amounts of thyroglobulin are detectable in the plasma. In other entities characterized by a low RAIU, such as thyroiditis, leakage of preformed thyroid hormone results in elevated thyroglobulin levels. If a history of thyroid hormone ingestion is elicited or deduced, exogenous thyroid hormone should be withheld for between 4 and 6 weeks and thyroid function tests repeated to document that the euthyroid state has been restored. Rarely, thyroid hormone analogues or metabolites can be the drug of abuse, specific detection of which can be difficult with standard thyroid hormone assays. For example, tiratricol (3,5,3-triiodothyroacetic acid [TRIAC]), an endogenous metabolite of T_3 that has been used for weight loss and paradoxically by body builders, will suppress TSH at high enough doses and may cross-react in many T_3 immunoassays; thus, thyrotoxicosis factitia because of tiratricol abuse can be misinterpreted as T_3-toxicosis.[47]

Amiodarone can induce thyrotoxicosis (2% to 3% of patients), hypothyroidism, or euthyroid hyperthyroxinemia, depending on the underlying thyroid pathology or lack thereof.[48] Because amiodarone contains 37% iodine by weight, approximately 6 mg/day of iodine is released for each 200 mg of amiodarone, 1,000 times greater than the recommended daily amount of iodine of 200 mcg/day. As a result of this iodine overload, iodine-exacerbated thyroid dysfunction commonly occurs among those patients with preexisting thyroid disease: thyrotoxicosis in patients with hyperthyroidism or euthyroid nodular autonomy, and hypothyroidism in patients with autoimmune thyroid disease. In contrast to hyperthyroidism induced by amiodarone (type I), destructive thyroiditis with loss of thyroglobulin and thyroid hormones also occurs (type II), typically among individuals with otherwise normal glands. The two types of amiodarone-induced thyrotoxicosis can be differentiated using color flow Doppler ultrasonography. Such distinction is critically important, given the therapeutic implications of the two syndromes: type I amiodarone-induced hyperthyroidism responds somewhat to thionamides, whereas type II can require glucocorticoids or iopanoic acid.[49–51] Obviously, RAI therapy is inappropriate, in type I because of the drug-induced iodine excess and in type II because of lack of increased hormone synthesis. The manifestations of amiodarone-induced thyrotoxicosis can be atypical symptoms such as ventricular tachycardia and exacerbation of underlying chronic obstructive pulmonary disease, both of which are even more significant given the severe underlying cardiac pathology which led to the use of the drug in the first place. Amiodarone also directly interferes with type I 5'-deiodinase, leading to reduced conversion of T_4 to T_3 and hyperthyroxinemia without thyrotoxicosis.

TREATMENT

Hyperthyroidism

DESIRED OUTCOMES

❸ Three common treatment modalities are used in the management of hyperthyroidism: surgery, antithyroid medications, and RAI (Table 78–5). The overall therapeutic objectives are to eliminate the excess thyroid hormone and minimize the symptoms and long-term consequences of hyperthyroidism. Therapy must be individualized based on the type and severity of hyperthyroidism, patient age and gender, existence of nonthyroidal conditions, and response to previous therapy.[52,53] Clinical guidelines for the treatment of hyperthyroidism have been published by various groups.[54–56]

NONPHARMACOLOGIC THERAPY

Surgical removal of the hypersecreting thyroid gland became feasible in 1923 when Plummer discovered that iodine reduced the gland's vascularity, making this definitive procedure possible. Surgery should be considered in patients with a large thyroid gland (>80 g), severe ophthalmopathy, and a lack of remission on antithyroid drug treatment. In case of cosmetic or pressure symptoms, the choice in MNG stands between surgery, which is still the first choice, and radioiodine if uptake is adequate (hot). In addition to surgery, the solitary nodule, whether hot or cold, can be treated with percutaneous ethanol injection therapy. If hot, radioiodine is the therapy of choice.[57] Traditional preparation of the patient for thyroidectomy includes PTU or MMI until the patient is biochemically euthyroid (usually 6 to 8 weeks), followed by the addition of iodides (500 mg/day) for 10 to 14 days before surgery to decrease the vascularity of the gland. Levothyroxine can be added to maintain the euthyroid state while the thionamides are continued. Iodine supplementation in iodine-deficient areas of the country can lead to a greater reduction in remnant volume in nontoxic goiter.[58] Propranolol for several weeks preoperatively and 7 to 10 days after surgery has also been used to maintain a pulse rate of less than 90 beats/min. Combined pretreatment with propranolol and 10 to 14 days of potassium iodide also has been advocated.

The overall morbidity rate with surgery is 2.7%. Hyperthyroidism persists or recurs in 0.6% to 17.9% of patients after thyroidectomy for Graves' disease and is more common in children. The most common complications of surgery include hypothyroidism (up to about 49%), hypoparathyroidism (up to 3.9%), and vocal cord abnormalities (up to 5.4%). The frequent occurrence of hypothyroidism following surgery requires periodic followup for identification and treatment of these patients.[59,60]

PHARMACOLOGIC THERAPY

Antithyroid Medications

Thiourea Drugs Two drugs within this category, PTU and MMI, are approved for the treatment of hyperthyroidism in the United States.[61] They are classified as thioureylenes (thionamides), which incorporate a N—C—S = N group into their ring structures.

Mechanism of Action. PTU and MMI share several mechanisms to inhibit the biosynthesis of thyroid hormone.[17] These drugs serve as preferential substrates for the iodinating intermediate of thyroid peroxidase and divert iodine away from potential iodination sites in thyroglobulin. This prevents subsequent incorporation of iodine into

TABLE 78-5 Treatments for Hyperthyroidism Caused by Graves' Disease

Treatment	Advantages	Disadvantages	Comment
Antithyroid drugs	Noninvasive Lower initial cost Low risk of permanent hypothyroidism Possible remissions because of immune effects	Low cure rate (30–80%; average 40–50%) Adverse drug reactions Drug compliance	First-line treatment in children, adolescents, and in pregnancy Initial treatment in severe cases or preoperative preparation
Radioactive iodine (^{131}I)	Cure of hyperthyroidism Most cost effective	Permanent hypothyroidism almost inevitable Might worsen ophthalmopathy Pregnancy must be deferred for 6–12 months; no breast-feeding Small potential risk of exacerbation of hyperthyroidism	Best treatment for toxic nodules and toxic multinodular goiter
Surgery	Rapid, effective treatment, especially in patients with large goiters	Most invasive Potential complications (recurrent laryngeal nerve damage, hypoparathyroidism) Most costly Permanent hypothyroidism Pain, scar	Potential in pregnancy if major side-effect from antithyroid Useful when coexisting suspicious nodule present Option for patients who refuse radioiodine

iodotyrosines and ultimately iodothyronine (*organification*). Second, they inhibit coupling of monoiodotyrosine and diiodotyrosine to form T_4 and T_3. The coupling reaction can be more sensitive to these drugs than the iodination reaction. Experimentally, these drugs exhibit immunosuppressive effects, although the clinical relevance of this finding is unclear. In patients with Graves' disease, antithyroid drug treatment has been associated with lower TSAb titers and restoration of normal suppressor T-cell function. However, perchlorate, which has a different mechanism of action, also decreases TSAbs, suggesting that normalization of the thyroid hormone level can itself improve the abnormal immune function. PTU inhibits the peripheral conversion of T_4 to T_3. This effect is acutely dose related and occurs within hours of PTU administration. MMI does not have this effect. Over time, depletion of stored hormone and lack of continuing synthesis of thyroid hormone results in the clinical effects of these drugs.

Pharmacokinetics. Both antithyroid drugs are well absorbed (80% to 95%) from the gastrointestinal tract, with peak serum concentrations approximately 1 hour after ingestion. The plasma half-life ranges of PTU and MMI are 1 to 2.5 hours and 6 to 9 hours, respectively, and are not appreciably affected by thyroid status. Urinary excretion is approximately 35% for PTU and less than 10% for MMI. These drugs are actively concentrated in the thyroid gland, which can account for the disparity between their relatively short plasma half-lives and the effectiveness of once-daily dosing regimens even with PTU. Approximately 60% to 80% of PTU is bound to plasma albumin, whereas MMI is not protein-bound. MMI readily crosses the placenta and appears in breast milk. Older studies suggested that PTU crosses the placental membranes only one-tenth as well as MMI; however, these studies were done in the course of therapeutic abortion early in pregnancy. Newer studies show little difference between fetal concentrations of PTU and MMI, and both are associated with elevated TSH in approximately 20% and low T_4 in approximately 7% of the fetuses.[62]

Dosing and Monitoring. PTU is available as 50-mg tablets and MMI as 5- and 10-mg tablets. MMI is approximately 10 times more potent than PTU. Initial therapy with PTU ranges from 300 to 600 mg daily, usually in three or four divided doses. MMI is given in three divided doses totaling 30 to 60 mg/day. Although the traditional recommendation is for divided doses, evidence exists that both drugs can be given as single daily doses. Patients with severe hyperthyroidism can require larger initial doses, and some might respond better at these larger doses if the dose is divided. The maximal blocking doses of PTU and MMI are 1,200 and 120 mg daily, respectively. Once the intrathyroidal pool of thyroid hormone is reduced, and new hormone synthesis is sufficiently blocked, clinical improvement should ensue. Usually within 4 to 8 weeks of initiating therapy, symptoms are diminished, and circulating thyroid hormone levels are returning to normal. At this time the tapering regimen can be started. Changes in dose for each drug should be made on a monthly basis, because the endogenously produced T_4 will reach a new steady-state concentration in this interval. Typical ranges of daily maintenance doses for PTU and MMI are 50 to 300 mg and 5 to 30 mg, respectively.

If the objective of therapy is to induce a long-term remission, the patient should remain on continuous antithyroid drug therapy for 12 to 24 months. Antithyroid drug therapy induces permanent remission rates of 10% to 98%, with an overall average of about 40% to 50%.[63] This is much higher than the remission rate seen with propranolol alone, which is reported to range from 22% to 36%. Patient characteristics for a favorable outcome include older patients (>40 years of age), low ratio of T_4 to T_3 (<20), a small goiter (<50 g), short duration of disease (<6 months), no previous history of relapse with antithyroid drugs, duration of therapy 1 to 2 years or longer, and low TSAb titers at baseline or a reduction with treatment.[17] It is important that patients be followed every 6 to 12 months after remission occurs.

❻ If a relapse occurs, alternate therapy with RAI is preferred to a second course of antithyroid drugs. Relapses seem to plateau after approximately 5 years, and eventually 5% to 20% of patients will develop spontaneous hypothyroidism.

Concurrent administration of T_4 with thionamide therapy for thyrotoxicosis and subclinical hyperthyroidism can reduce autoantibodies directed toward the thyroid gland and improve the remission rate; however, these effects have not been consistently observed in all studies.[63,64] In a Japanese study, adjunctive treatment with T_4 was associated with a 20-fold reduction in the recurrence rate of Graves' disease compared with the recurrence rate seen in patients treated with antithyroid drugs alone. Attempts to reproduce these results in American and European patients with Graves' disease have failed to show any delay or reduction in the recurrence of Graves' disease with T_4 administration.[65]

Adverse Effects. Minor adverse reactions to PTU and MMI have an overall incidence of 5% to 25% depending on the dose and the drug, whereas major adverse effects occur in 1.5% to 4.6% of patients receiving these drugs.[61,66] Pruritic maculopapular rashes (sometimes associated with vasculitis based on skin biopsy), arthralgias, and fevers occur in up to 5% of patients and can occur at greater frequency with higher doses and in children. Rashes often disappear spontaneously, but if persistent, can be managed with antihistamines.

Perhaps one of the most common side effects is a benign transient leukopenia characterized by a white blood cell (WBC) count of less than 4,000/mm^3. This condition occurs in up to 12% of adults and 25% of children, and sometimes can be confused with mild leukopenia seen in Graves' disease. This mild leukopenia is not a harbinger of the more serious adverse effect of agranulocytosis, so therapy can usually be continued. If a minor adverse reaction occurs with one antithyroid drug, the alternate thiourea can be tried, but cross-sensitivity occurs in approximately 50% of patients.[61]

Agranulocytosis is the most serious adverse effect of thiourea drug therapy and is characterized by fever, malaise, gingivitis, oropharyngeal infection, and a granulocyte count less than 250/mm^3.[61] These drugs are concentrated in granulocytes, and this reaction can represent a direct toxic effect rather than hypersensitivity. This toxic reaction has occurred with both thioureas, and the incidence varies from 0.5% to 6%. It is higher in patients older than age 40 years receiving a MMI dose greater than 40 mg/day or the equivalent dose of PTU, and is linked to HLA class II genes containing the DRB1*08032 allele.[67] Agranulocytosis almost always develops in the first 3 months of therapy. Because the onset is sudden, routine monitoring is not recommended. Colony-stimulating factors have been used with some success to restore cell counts to normal, but it is unclear how effective this form of therapy is to routine supportive care.[68,69] Peripheral lymphocytes obtained from patients with PTU-induced agranulocytosis undergo transformation in the presence of other thioamides, suggesting that these severe reactions are immunologically mediated, and patients should not receive other thionamides. Aplastic anemia has been reported with MMI and can be associated with an inhibitor to colony-forming units. Once antithyroid drugs are discontinued, clinical improvement is seen over several days to weeks. Patients should be counseled to discontinue therapy and contact their physician when flu-like symptoms such as fever, malaise, or sore throat develop.

Arthralgias and a lupus-like syndrome (sometimes in the absence of antinuclear antibodies) have been reported in 4% to 5% of patients. This generally occurs after 6 months of therapy. Uncommonly, polymyositis, presenting as proximal muscle weakness and elevated creatine phosphokinase, has been reported with PTU administration. Gastrointestinal intolerance is also reported to occur in 4% to 5% of patients. Hepatotoxicity, which usually occurs within the first 3 months of therapy, can be seen with both MMI and PTU with a prevalence of approximately 1.3%.[70] In mice, MMI undergoes epoxidation of the C-4,5 double bond by cytochrome P450 enzymes, and after being hydrolyzed, the resulting epoxide is decomposed to form *N*-methylthiourea, a proximate toxicant.[71] At moderate doses, some authors have found that initial enzyme elevations eventually normalize in most patients with continued therapy.[72] High doses of PTU are more likely to produce severe hepatitis and even death. Discontinuation of therapy usually results in complete resolution of hepatitis. Patients receiving interferon products for hepatitis C or other disorders can develop hyper- or hypothyroidism along with liver enzyme abnormalities.[73] Although older reports suggested that congenital skin defects (aplasia cutis) can be caused by MMI and carbimazole, a registry review from the Netherlands could not find an association between maternal use of these drugs and skin defects.[74] Hypoprothrombinemia is a rare complication of thionamide therapy. Patients who have experienced a major adverse reaction to one thiourea drug should not be converted to the alternate drug because of cross-sensitivity.

Iodides Iodide was the first form of drug therapy for Graves' disease. Its mechanism of action is to acutely block thyroid hormone release, inhibit thyroid hormone biosynthesis by interfering with intrathyroidal iodide use (the Wolff-Chaikoff effect), and decrease the size and vascularity of the gland. This early inhibitory effect provides symptom improvement within 2 to 7 days of initiating therapy, and serum T_4 and T_3 concentrations can be reduced for a few weeks. Despite the reduced release of T_4 and T_3, thyroid hormone synthesis continues at an accelerated rate, resulting in a gland rich in stored hormones. The normal and hyperfunctioning thyroid soon escapes from this inhibitory effect within 1 to 2 weeks by decreasing the active transfer of iodide into the gland. Iodides are often used as adjunctive therapy to prepare a patient with Graves' disease for surgery, to acutely inhibit thyroid hormone release and quickly attain the euthyroid state in severely thyrotoxic patients with cardiac decompensation, or to inhibit thyroid hormone release following radioactive iodine therapy. However, large doses of iodine can exacerbate hyperthyroidism or indeed precipitate hyperthyroidism in some previously euthyroid individuals (Jod-Basedow's disease).[75] This Jod-Basedow's phenomenon is most common in iodine-deficient areas, particularly in patients with preexisting nontoxic goiter. Iodide is contraindicated in toxic MNG.

Potassium iodide is available either as a saturated solution (saturated solution of potassium iodide [SSKI]), which contains 38 mg of iodide per drop, or as Lugol solution, which contains 6.3 mg of iodide per drop. The typical starting dose of SSKI is 3 to 10 drops daily (120 to 400 mg) in water or juice. There is no documented advantage to using doses in excess of 6 to 8 mg/day. When used to prepare a patient for surgery, it should be administered 7 to 14 days preoperatively. As an adjunct to RAI, SSKI should not be used before, but rather 3 to 7 days after RAI treatment, so that the radioactive iodide can concentrate in the thyroid. The most frequent toxic effect with iodide therapy is hypersensitivity reactions (skin rashes, drug fever, rhinitis, and conjunctivitis); salivary gland swelling; "iodism" (metallic taste, burning mouth and throat, sore teeth and gums, symptoms of a head cold, and sometimes stomach upset and diarrhea); and gynecomastia.

Other compounds containing organic iodide have also been used therapeutically for hyperthyroidism. These include various radiologic contrast media that share a triiodo- and monoaminobenzene ring with a propionic acid chain (e.g., iopanoic acid and sodium ipodate). The effect of these compounds is a result of the iodine content inhibiting thyroid hormone release as well as competitive inhibition of 5'-monodeiodinase conversion related to their structures, which resemble thyroid analogs.[76]

Adrenergic Blockers 7 Because many of the manifestations of hyperthyroidism are mediated by β-adrenergic receptors, β-blockers (especially propranolol) have been used widely to ameliorate thyrotoxic symptoms such as palpitations, anxiety, tremor, and heat intolerance. Although β-blockers are quite effective for symptom control, they have no effect on the urinary excretion of calcium, phosphorus, hydroxyproline, creatinine, or various amino acids, suggesting a lack of effect on peripheral thyrotoxicosis and protein metabolism. Furthermore, β-blockers do not reduce TSAb nor prevent thyroid storm. Propranolol and nadolol partially block the conversion of T_4 to T_3, but this contribution to the overall therapeutic effect is small in magnitude. Inhibition of conversion of T_4 to T_3 is mediated by *d*-propranolol, which is devoid of β-blocking activity, and *l*-propranolol, which is responsible for the antiadrenergic effects and has little effect on the conversion.

β-Blockers are usually used as adjunctive therapy with antithyroid drugs, RAI, or iodides when treating Graves' disease or toxic nodules; in preparation for surgery; or in thyroid storm. The only conditions for which β-blockers are primary therapy for thyrotoxicosis are thyroiditis and iodine-induced hyperthyroidism. The dose of propranolol required to relieve adrenergic symptoms is variable, but an initial dose of 20 to 40 mg four times daily is effective (heart rate <90 beats/min) for most patients. Younger or more severely toxic patients can require as much as 240 to 480 mg/day because there seems to be an increased clearance rate in these patients. β-Blockers are contraindicated in patients with decompensated heart failure unless it is caused solely by tachycardia (high output). Nonselective agents and those lacking intrinsic sympathomimetic activity should be used with caution in patients with asthma and bronchospastic chronic obstructive lung disease. β-Blockers that are cardioselective and have intrinsic sympathomimetic activity may have a slight margin of safety in these situations. Other patients in whom contraindications exist are those with sinus bradycardia, those receiving monoamine oxidase inhibitors or tricyclic antidepressants, and those with spontaneous hypoglycemia. β-Blockers can also prolong gestation and labor during pregnancy. Other side effects include nausea, vomiting, anxiety, insomnia, light-headedness, bradycardia, and hematologic disturbances.

Antiadrenergic agents such as centrally acting sympatholytics and calcium channel antagonists may have some role in the symptomatic treatment of hyperthyroidism. These drugs might be useful when contraindications to β-blockade exist. When compared to nadolol 40 mg twice daily, clonidine 150 mcg twice daily reduced plasma catecholamines, whereas nadolol increased both epinephrine and norepinephrine after 1 week of treatment. Diltiazem 120 mg given every 8 hours reduced heart rate by 17%; fewer ventricular extrasystoles were noted after 10 days of therapy, and diltiazem has been shown to be comparable to propranolol in lowering heart rate and blood pressure.

Radioactive Iodine Although other radioisotopes have been used to ablate thyroid tissue, sodium iodide 131 (^{131}I) is considered to be the agent of choice for Graves' disease, toxic autonomous nodules, and toxic MNGs.[77,78] RAI is administered as a colorless and tasteless liquid that is well absorbed and concentrates in the thyroid. Sodium iodide 131 is a β- and γ-emitter with a tissue penetration of 2 mm and a half-life of 8 days. Other organs take up ^{131}I, but the thyroid gland is the only organ in which organification of the absorbed iodine takes place. Initially, RAI disrupts hormone synthesis by incorporating into thyroid hormones and thyroglobulin. Over a period of weeks, follicles that have taken up RAI and surrounding follicles develop evidence of cellular necrosis, breakdown of follicles, development of bizarre cell forms, nuclear pyknosis, and destruction of small vessels within the gland, leading to edema and fibrosis of the interstitial tissue. Pregnancy is an absolute contraindication to the use of RAI.

β-Blockers can be given any time without compromising RAI therapy, accounting for their role as a mainstay of adjunctive therapy to RAI treatment. If iodides are administered, they should be given 3 to 7 days after RAI to prevent interference with the uptake of RAI in the thyroid gland. Because thyroid hormone levels will transiently increase following RAI treatment because of release of preformed thyroid hormone, patients with cardiac disease and elderly patients are often treated with thionamides prior to RAI ablation. Occasionally, in patients with underlying cardiac disease, it can be necessary to reinstitute antithyroid drug therapy following radioactive iodine ablation. The standard practice is to withdraw the thionamide 4 to 6 days prior to RAI treatment and to reinstitute it 4 days after therapy is concluded. Administering antithyroid drug therapy following RAI treatment can result in a higher rate of posttreatment recurrence or persistent hyperthyroidism.[78]

Corticosteroid administration will blunt and delay the increase in antibodies to the TSH receptor, thyroglobulin, and thyroid peroxidase while reducing T_3 and T_4 concentrations following RAI. Bartalena and associates found no progression in ophthalmopathy in patients receiving prednisone after RAI compared with MMI (2% to 3% worsened), or no other treatment (5% with persistent worsening).[46] Theoretically, if shared thyroidal and orbital antigen is involved in the pathogenesis of Graves' ophthalmopathy, antigen released with RAI treatment could aggravate preexisting eye disease. Note also that thyroid ablation can decrease eye disease in the long term by removing the source of antigen, but it is unclear if RAI differs from surgery or thionamide for the risk of worsening eye disease.[79]

Destruction of the gland attenuates the hyperthyroid state, and hypothyroidism commonly occurs months to years following RAI.[80] The goal of therapy is to destroy overactive thyroid cells, and a single dose of 4,000 to 8,000 rads results in a euthyroid state in 60% of patients at 6 months or less. The remaining 40% become euthyroid within 1 year, requiring two or more doses. It is advisable that a second dose of RAI be given 6 months after the first RAI treatment if the patient remains hyperthyroid. Variables that influence the outcome of RAI include gender (men are less likely to develop hypothyroidism), race (blacks are more resistant to ^{131}I), the size of the thyroid, severity of disease, and perhaps the level of TSAb. The acute, short-term side effects of ^{131}I therapy are minimal and include mild thyroidal tenderness and dysphagia. Concern over the development of thyroid carcinoma and leukemia and increased risk of mutations and congenital defects now appears to be unfounded because long-term followup studies have not revealed increased risk for these complications.[81] Although RAI is very effective in the treatment of hyperthyroidism, long-term followup from Great Britain suggests that among patients with hyperthyroidism treated with RAI, mortality from all causes and mortality resulting from cardiovascular and cerebrovascular disease and fracture are increased.[82]

A common approach to Graves' hyperthyroidism is to administer a single dose of 5 to 15 mCi (80 to 200 microCi/g of tissue).[78] The optimal method for determining ^{131}I treatment doses for Graves' hyperthyroidism is unknown, and techniques have varied from a fixed dose to more elaborate calculations based on gland size, iodine uptake, and iodine turnover. In a trial of 88 patients with Graves' disease, no difference in outcome was seen among high or low, fixed or adjusted doses.[83] Thyroid glands estimated to weigh >80 g can require larger doses of RAI. Larger doses are likely to induce hypothyroidism and are seldom given outside the United States because of the imposition of stringent safety restrictions. For example, in the United Kingdom, a nursery school teacher is advised to stay out of school for 3 weeks following a 15-mCi dose of ^{131}I.[84]

EVALUATION OF THERAPEUTIC OUTCOMES: HYPERTHYROIDISM

After therapy (surgery, thionamides, or RAI) for hyperthyroidism has been initiated, patients should be evaluated on a monthly basis until they reach a euthyroid condition. Clinical signs of continuing thyrotoxicosis (tachycardia, weight loss, and heat intolerance, among others) or the development of hypothyroidism (bradycardia, weight gain, and lethargy, among others) should be noted. β-Blockers can be used to control symptoms of thyrotoxicosis until the definitive treatment has returned the patient to a euthyroid state. Once T_4 replacement is initiated, the goal is to maintain both the free T_4 level and the TSH concentration in the normal range. Once a stable dose of T_4 is identified, the patient can be followed up every 6 to 12 months.

Finally, a common, potentially confusing clinical situation should be mentioned. Why are the TSH concentrations suppressed in some patients who are clinically hypothyroid and who have a low free T_4 level? In patients with long-standing hyperthyroidism, the pituitary thyrotrophs responsible for making TSH become atrophic. The average amount of time required for these cells to resume normal functioning is 6 to 8 weeks.[85] Therefore if a thyrotoxic patient has his or her free T_4 concentration lowered rapidly, before the thyrotrophs resume normal function, a period of "transient central hypothyroidism" will be observed.

SPECIAL CONDITIONS

Graves' Disease and Pregnancy[86]

Inappropriate production of hCG is a cause of abnormal thyroid function tests during the first half of pregnancy, and hCG can cause either subclinical (normal T_4, suppressed TSH) or overt hyperthyroidism.[87,88] This is because of the homology of hCG and TSH, leading to hCG-mediated stimulation through the TSH receptor. Hyperthyroidism during pregnancy is almost solely caused by Graves' disease, with approximately 0.1% to 0.4% of pregnancies affected. Although the increased metabolic rate is usually well tolerated in pregnant women, two symptoms suggestive of hyperthyroidism during pregnancy are failure to gain weight despite good appetite, and persistent tachycardia. There is no increase in maternal mortality or morbidity in well-controlled patients; however, postpartum thyroid storm has been reported in about 20% of untreated individuals. Fetal loss is also more common, because spontaneous abortion and premature delivery are more common in untreated pregnant women, as are low-birth-weight infants and eclampsia. Transplacental passage of thyroid-stimulating antibodies can occur, causing fetal as well as neonatal hyperthyroidism.[89] An uncommon cause of hyperthyroidism is molar pregnancy; women present with a large-for-date uterus, and evacuation of the uterus is the preferred management approach.[90]

Because RAI is contraindicated in pregnancy and surgery is usually not recommended (especially during the first trimester), antithyroid drug therapy is usually the treatment of choice. MMI readily crosses the placenta and appears in breast milk.

PTU is considered to be the drug of choice in pregnancy, with the lowest possible doses used to maintain the maternal T_4 level in the high-normal range, but as described previously, there appears to be little difference between PTU and MMI.[89,91] To prevent fetal goiter and suppression of fetal thyroid function, PTU is usually prescribed in daily doses of 300 mg or less and tapered to 50 to 150 mg daily after 4 to 6 weeks. PTU doses of less than 200 mg daily are unlikely to produce fetal goiter.[91] Thioamide doses should be adjusted to maintain free T_4 within 10% of the upper normal limit of the nonpregnant reference range.[86] During the last trimester, TSAbs fall spontaneously, and some patients will go into remission so that antithyroid drug doses can be reduced. A rebound in maternal hyperthyroidism occurs in approximately 10% of women and can require more intensive treatment postpartum than in the last trimester of pregnancy.[89]

Neonatal and Pediatric Hyperthyroidism

Following delivery, some babies will be hyperthyroid because of placental transfer of TSAbs, which stimulates thyroid hormone production in utero and postpartum.[92,93] This is likely if the maternal TSAb titers were quite high. The disease is usually expressed 7 to 10 days postpartum, and treatment with antithyroid drugs (PTU 5 to 10 mg/kg per day or MMI 0.5 to 1 mg/kg per day) can be needed for as long as 8 to 12 weeks until the antibody is cleared (immunoglobulin G half-life is approximately 2 weeks). Iodide (potassium iodide 1 drop/day or Lugol solution 1 to 3 drops/day) and sodium ipodate can be used for the first few days to acutely inhibit hormone release.

Childhood hyperthyroidism is usually managed with either PTU or MMI. Long-term followup studies suggest that this form of therapy is quite acceptable, with 25% of a cohort experiencing remission every 2 years.[94]

Thyroid Storm

Thyroid storm is a life-threatening medical emergency characterized by decompensated thyrotoxicosis, high fever (often >39.4°C [103°F]), tachycardia, tachypnea, dehydration, delirium, coma, nausea, vomiting, and diarrhea.[19] Although Graves' disease and less commonly toxic nodular goiter are usually the underlying thyrotoxic pathology, at least two cases of subacute thyroiditis leading to thyroid storm have been reported.[95–97] Precipitating factors for thyroid storm include infection, trauma, surgery, RAI treatment, and withdrawal from antithyroid drugs. Although the duration of clinical decompensation lasts for an average duration of 72 hours, symptoms can persist up to 8 days. With aggressive treatment, the mortality rate has been lowered to 20%. The following therapeutic measures should be instituted promptly: (1) suppression of thyroid hormone formation and secretion, (2) antiadrenergic therapy, (3) administration of corticosteroids, and (4) treatment of associated complications or coexisting factors that precipitated the storm. Specific agents used in thyroid storm are outlined in Table 78–6. PTU in large doses is the preferred thionamide because it interferes with the production of thyroid hormones and blocks the peripheral conversion of T_4 to T_3. If patients are unable to take medications orally, the tablets can be crushed into suspension and instilled by gastric or rectal tube.[98] Iodides, which rapidly block the release of preformed thyroid hormone, should be administered after PTU is initiated to inhibit iodide use by the overactive gland. If iodide is administered first, it could theoretically provide substrate for even higher levels of hormone.

Antiadrenergic therapy with the short-acting agent esmolol is preferred, both because it can be used in the patient with pulmonary disease or at risk for cardiac failure and because its effects can be rapidly reversed.[99] Corticosteroids are generally recommended, although there is no convincing evidence of adrenocortical insufficiency in thyroid storm, and the benefits derived from steroids can be caused by their antipyretic action and their effect of stabilizing blood pressure.[19] General supportive measures, including acetaminophen as an antipyretic (do not use aspirin or other nonsteroidal antiinflammatory agents because they can displace bound-thyroid hormone), fluid and electrolyte replacement, sedatives, digitalis, antiarrhythmics, insulin, and antibiotics should be given as indicated. Plasmapheresis and peritoneal dialysis have been used to remove excess hormone (and to remove thyroid-stimulating immunoglobulins in Graves' disease) when the patient has not responded to more conservative measures, although these measures do not always work.[100]

TABLE 78-6 Drug Dosages Used in the Management of Thyroid Storm

Drug	Regimen
Propylthiouracil	900–1200 mg/day orally in four or six divided doses
Methimazole	90–120 mg/day orally in four or six divided doses
Sodium iodide	Up to 2 g/day IV in single or divided doses
Lugol solution	5–10 drops three times a day in water or juice
Saturated solution of potassium iodide	1–2 drops three times a day in water or juice
Propranolol	40–80 mg every 6 h
Dexamethasone	5–20 mg/day orally or IV in divided doses
Prednisone	25–100 mg/day orally in divided doses
Methylprednisolone	20–80 mg/day IV in divided doses
Hydrocortisone	100–400 mg/day IV in divided doses

HYPOTHYROIDISM

Hypothyroidism is defined as the clinical and biochemical syndrome resulting from decreased thyroid hormone production.[101] Overt hypothyroidism occurs in 1.5% to 2% of women and 0.2% of men, and its incidence increases with age. In the Third National Health and Nutrition Examination Survey, levels of serum TSH and total T_4 were measured in a representative sample of adolescents and adults (age 12 years or older). Among 16,533 people who neither were taking thyroid medication nor reported histories of thyroid disease, 3.9% had subclinical hypothyroidism (serum TSH >4.5 mIU/L; and T_4 normal), and 0.2% had "clinically significant" hypothyroidism (TSH >4.5 mIU/L; and T_4 <4.5 mcg/dL).[18] The vast majority of patients have primary hypothyroidism because of thyroid gland failure caused by chronic autoimmune thyroiditis. Special populations with higher risk of developing hypothyroidism include postpartum women, individuals with a family history of autoimmune thyroid disorders and patients with previous head and neck or thyroid irradiation or surgery, other autoimmune endocrine conditions (e.g., type 1 diabetes mellitus, adrenal insufficiency, and ovarian failure), some other nonendocrine autoimmune disorders (e.g., celiac disease, vitiligo, pernicious anemia, Sjögren's syndrome, and multiple sclerosis), primary pulmonary hypertension, and Down's and Turner's syndromes. Secondary hypothyroidism caused by pituitary failure is uncommon, but should be suspected in a patient with decreased levels of T_4 and inappropriately normal or low TSH levels. Most patients with secondary hypothyroidism because of inadequate TSH production will have clinical signs of more generalized pituitary insufficiency, such as abnormal menses and decreased libido, or evidence of a pituitary adenoma, such as visual field defects, galactorrhea, or acromegaloid features, but isolated TSH deficiency can be congenital or acquired as a result of autoimmune hypophysitis.[102] Generalized (peripheral and central) resistance to thyroid hormone is extremely rare.

Thyroid hormone is essential for normal growth and development during embryonic life. Uncorrected thyroid hormone deficiency during fetal and neonatal development results in mental retardation and/or cretinism. There is loss of physical and mental activity, as well as of cardiovascular, gastrointestinal, and neuromuscular function.

CLINICAL PRESENTATION OF HYPOTHYROIDISM

General

- Hypothyroidism can lead to a variety of end-organ effects with a wide range of disease severity, from entirely asymptomatic individuals to patients in coma with multisystem failure. In the adult, manifestations of hypothyroidism are varied and nonspecific. In the child, thyroid hormone deficiency can manifest as growth or intellectual retardation.

Symptoms

- Common symptoms of hypothyroidism include dry skin, cold intolerance, weight gain, constipation, and weakness. Complaints of lethargy, depression, fatigue or loss of ambition and energy are also common but are less specific. Muscle cramps, myalgia, and stiffness are frequent complaints of hypothyroid patients. Menorrhagia and infertility can present commonly in women.

Signs

- Objective weakness is common, with proximal muscles being affected more than distal muscles. Slow relaxation of deep tendon reflexes is common. The most common signs of decreased levels of thyroid hormone include coarse skin and hair, cold or dry skin, periorbital puffiness, and bradycardia. Speech is often slow as well as hoarse. Reversible neurologic syndromes such as carpal tunnel syndrome, polyneuropathy, and cerebellar dysfunction can also occur. Galactorrhea can be found in women.

Diagnosis

- In primary hypothyroidism, TSH serum concentration should be elevated. In secondary hypothyroidism, TSH levels can be within or below the reference range; when TSH bioactivity is altered, the levels reported by immunoassay can even be elevated.
- Free and/or total T_4 and T_3 serum concentrations should be low.

Other Tests

- Antithyroid peroxidase antibodies and antithyroglobulin antibodies are likely to be elevated in autoimmune thyroiditis.
- An increase in the TSH level is the first evidence of primary hypothyroidism. Many patients will have a free T_4 level within the normal range (compensated hypothyroidism) and few, if any, symptoms of hypothyroidism. As the disease progresses the free T_4 concentration will drop below the normal level. Interestingly, as a result of TSH stimulation, thyroidal production will shift toward greater amounts of T_3, and thus T_3 concentrations will often be maintained in the normal range in spite of a low T_4. The RAIU is not a useful test in the evaluation of a hypothyroid patient, as it can be low, normal, or even elevated.

CAUSES OF HYPOTHYROIDISM

Table 78–7 outlines the causes of hypothyroidism.

Chronic Autoimmune Thyroiditis

8 Autoimmune thyroiditis (Hashimoto's disease) is the most common cause of spontaneous hypothyroidism in the adult.[103] Patients can present with either goitrous thyroid gland enlargement and mild hypothyroidism, or thyroid gland atrophy and more severe thyroid hormone deficiency. Both forms of autoimmune thyroiditis probably result from cell- and antibody-mediated thyroid injury. The bulk of evidence suggests that the presence of specific defects in suppressor T-lymphocyte function leads to the survival of a randomly mutating clone of helper T lymphocytes, which are directed against normally occurring antigens on the thyroid membrane. Once these T lymphocytes interact with thyroid membrane antigen, B lymphocytes are stimulated to produce thyroid antibodies.[104]

TABLE 78-7 Causes of Hypothyroidism

Primary hypothyroidism
Hashimoto's disease
Iatrogenic hypothyroidism
Others
Iodine deficiency
Enzyme defects
Thyroid hypoplasia
Goitrogens
Secondary hypothyroidism
Pituitary disease
Hypothalamic disease

Antimicrosomal antibodies are present in virtually all patients with Hashimoto's thyroiditis and appear to be directed against the enzyme thyroid peroxidase.[105] These antibodies are capable of fixing complement and inducing cytotoxic changes in thyroid cells. Antibodies that are capable of stimulating thyroid growth through interaction with the TSH receptor can occasionally be found particularly in goitrous hypothyroidism; conversely, antibodies that inhibit the trophic effects of TSH are present in the atrophic type.

Iatrogenic Hypothyroidism

Iatrogenic hypothyroidism follows exposure to excessive amounts of radiation (radioiodine or external radiation) or surgery. Hypothyroidism occurs within 3 months to a year after ^{131}I therapy in most patients treated for Graves' disease. Thereafter it occurs at a rate of approximately 2.5% each year. External radiation therapy to the region of the thyroid using doses of greater than 2,500 cGy for therapy of neck carcinoma also causes hypothyroidism. This effect is dose-dependent, and more than 50% of patients who receive more than 4,000 cGy to the thyroid bed develop hypothyroidism. Total thyroidectomy causes hypothyroidism within 1 month.

Other Causes of Primary Hypothyroidism

Iodine deficiency, enzymatic defects within the thyroid gland, thyroid hypoplasia, and maternal ingestion of goitrogens during fetal development can cause cretinism. Early recognition and treatment of the resultant thyroid hormone deficiency is essential for optimal mental development.[106,107] Large-scale neonatal screening programs in North America, Europe, Japan, and Australia are now in place.[108] The frequency of congenital hypothyroidism in North America and Europe is 1 per 3,500 to 4,000 live births. In the United States, there are racial differences in the incidence of congenital hypothyroidism, with whites being affected seven times as frequently as blacks.

In the adult, hypothyroidism can rarely be caused by iodine deficiency and goitrogens. Rarely, iodine ingestion in the form of expectorants can lead to hypothyroidism. In sensitive persons (particularly those with autoimmune thyroiditis), the iodide blocks the synthesis of thyroid hormone, leading to an increased secretion of TSH and thyroid enlargement. Thus both iodine excess and iodine deficiency can cause decreased secretion of thyroid hormone.

Causes of Secondary Hypothyroidism

Pituitary Disease TSH is required for normal thyroid secretion. Thyroid atrophy and decreased thyroid secretion follow pituitary failure. Pituitary insufficiency can be caused by destruction of thyrotrophs by either functioning or nonfunctioning pituitary tumors, surgical therapy, external pituitary radiation, postpartum pituitary necrosis (Sheehan's syndrome), trauma, and infiltrative processes of the pituitary such as metastatic tumors, tuberculosis, histiocytosis, and autoimmune mechanisms.[109,110] In all these situations, TSH deficiency most often occurs in association with other pituitary hormone deficiencies. The identification of secondary hypothyroidism because of bexarotene use has led to recognition of the role of rexinoids and retinoids to cause dysregulation of TSH production.[22,111]

In most hypothyroid patients with pituitary disease, serum TSH concentrations are generally low or normal. A serum TSH concentration in the normal range is clearly inappropriate if the patient's T_4 is low.

Note that pituitary enlargement in hypothyroidism does not invariably indicate the presence of a primary pituitary tumor. Pituitary enlargement is seen in patients with severe primary hypothyroidism because of compensatory hyperplasia and hypertrophy of the thyrotrophs.[112] With thyroid hormone replacement therapy, serum TSH concentrations decline, indicating that the TSH secretion is not autonomous, and the pituitary resumes a more normal configuration. These patients are easily separated from patients with primary pituitary failure by measuring a TSH level.

Hypothalamic Hypothyroidism TRH deficiency also causes a rare form of central hypothyroidism. In both adults and children it can occur as a result of cranial irradiation, trauma, infiltrative diseases, or neoplastic diseases.

TREATMENT

Hypothyroidism

■ PHARMACOLOGIC THERAPY

Desired Outcomes

The goals of therapy are to restore normal thyroid hormone concentrations in tissue, provide symptomatic relief, prevent neurologic deficits in newborns and children, and reverse the biochemical abnormalities of hypothyroidism.

General Approach

Any of the commercially available thyroid preparations accomplish this goal (Table 78–8); however, levothyroxine (L-thyroxine; T_4) is considered to be the drug of choice. The thyroid preparations are either natural (i.e., desiccated thyroid and thyroglobulin) or synthetic (levothyroxine, liothyronine, and liotrix) in origin. The availability of sensitive and specific assays for total and free hormone levels as well as TSH now allow more definitive dose titration to allow adequate replacement without inadvertent overdose. The response of TSH to TRH had been advocated for use by some for "fine-tuning" thyroid replacement, but this is not necessary if the sensitive immunoradiometric assays for TSH are used. Minimum clinical guidelines for the treatment of hypothyroidism have been published by the American Thyroid Association[56] and the American Association of Clinical Endocrinologists.[113]

Natural Thyroid Hormones

Desiccated thyroid is derived from hog, beef, or sheep thyroid gland. The *United States Pharmacopeia, 23rd Edition*, requires thyroid USP to contain 38 mcg (±15%) of levothyroxine and 9 mcg (±10%) of liothyronine for each 65 mg (1 grain) of the labeled content of thyroglobulin. Thyroglobulin USP should contain 36 mcg (±15%) of levothyroxine and 12 mcg (±10%) of liothyronine for each 65 mg (1 grain) of the labeled content of thyroglobulin. Not all generic brands can be bioequivalent, and switching among brands in patients stabilized on one product should be discouraged. Thyroid USP, as an animal protein–derived product, can be antigenic in allergic or sensitive patients. Even though desiccated thyroid is inexpensive, its limitations preclude it from being considered as a drug of choice for hypothyroid patients. Thyroglobulin is a purified hog-gland extract, but it has no clinical advantages and is not widely used.

Synthetic Thyroid Hormones

Levothyroxine (T_4; L-thyroxine) is the drug of choice for thyroid replacement and suppressive therapy because it is chemically stable, relatively inexpensive, and free of antigenicity, and has uniform potency. Whereas T_3 and not T_4 is the biologically more active form of thyroid hormone, levothyroxine administration results in a pool of thyroid hormone that is readily and consistently converted to T_3; in this regard levothyroxine can be thought of as a prohormone. The half-life of levothyroxine is approximately 7 days. This long half-life is responsible for a stable pool of prohormone and the need for only once-daily dosing with levothyroxine. Older studies with levothyroxine suggested that bioavailability was low and erratic; however, this product has been reformulated, and the average bioavailability is now approximately 80%.[114–116] The bioavailability of Synthroid, Levoxine, and generic levothyroxine preparations were compared in a blinded, randomized, four-way crossover trial.[117] The study was sponsored by the manufacturers of Synthroid, who have challenged the authors' conclusions that the levothyroxine preparations are bioequivalent and should be interchangeable for the majority of patients. However, because the relationship between T_4 concentration and TSH is not linear, very small changes in T_4 concentration can lead to substantial changes in TSH, which is a more accurate reflection of hormone replacement status. Currently, the Food and Drug Administration mandates that levothyroxine bioequivalency testing be done in normal volunteers (600 mcg in the fasted state) and three baseline free-T_4 concentrations be used to correct for endogenous T_4 production. Bioequivalency is based on the area under the curve (AUC) and

TABLE 78-8 Thyroid Preparations Used in the Treatment of Hypothyroidism

Drug/Dosage Form	Content	Relative Dose	Comments/Equivalency
Thyroid USP			
Armour Thyroid (T_4:T_3 ratio) 9.5 mcg:2.25 mcg, 19 mcg:4.5 mcg, 38 mcg:9 mcg, 57 mcg:13.5 mcg, 76 mcg:18 mcg, 114 mcg:27 mcg, 152 mcg:36 mcg, 190 mcg:45 mcg tablets	Desiccated beef or pork thyroid gland	1 grain (equivalent to 60 mcg of T_4)	Unpredictable hormonal stability, inexpensive generic brands may not be bioequivalent
Thyroglobulin			
Proloid 32-mg, 65-mg, 100-mg, 130-mg, 200-mg tablets	Partially purified pork thyroglobulin	1 grain	Standardized biologically to give T_4:T_3 ratio of 2.5:1; more expensive then thyroid extract; no clinical advantage
Levothyroxine			
Synthroid, Levothroid, and other generics 25-, 50-, 75-, 88-, 100-, 112-, 125-, 137-, 150-, 175-, 200-, 300-mcg tablets; 200- and 500-mcg/vial injection	Synthetic T_4	50–60 mcg	Stable; predictable potency; generics are bioequivalent; when switching from natural thyroid to L-thyroxine, lower dose by 1/2 grain; variable absorption between products; half-life = 7 days, so daily dosing; considered to be drug of choice
Levoxyl, Thyro-Tabs, Unithroid			
Liothyronine			
Cytomel 5-, 25-, and 50-mcg tablets	Synthetic T_3	15–37.5 mcg	Uniform absorption, rapid onset; half-life = 1.5 days, monitor TSH assays
Liotrix			
Thyrolar 1/4-, 1/2-, 1-, 2-, and 3-strength tablets	Synthetic T_4:T_3 in 4:1 ratio	50–60 mcg T_4 and 12.5–15 mcg T_3	Stable; predictable; expensive; lacks therapeutic rationale because T_4 is converted to T_3 peripherally

TSH, thyroid-stimulating hormone; T_3, triiodothyrine; T_4, thyroxine.

maximum concentration (C_{max}) of T_4 out to 48 hours. Approximately 70% of the AUC is derived from endogenous production. TSH is not considered, and it is now very clear that T_4 is too insensitive as a measure of bioequivalency.[118,119] To avoid over- and undertreatment, once a product is selected, therapeutic interchange should be discouraged. Currently, there are nine levothyroxine products available, and a number of permutations for interchange are available considering that there are AB1, AB2, AB3 and BX products available as no reference listed drug is mandated in bioequivalency testing. The time to maximal absorption is 2 hours, and this should be considered when T_4 and TSH concentrations are determined. Mucosal diseases such as sprue, diabetic diarrhea, and ileal bypass surgery can also reduce absorption. Cholestyramine, calcium carbonate, sucralfate, aluminum hydroxide,[120] ferrous sulfate,[121] soybean formula,[122] and dietary fiber supplements[123] can also impair the absorption of levothyroxine from the gastrointestinal tract. Acid suppression with histamine blockers and proton pump inhibitors can also reduced levothyroxine absorption. Drugs that increase T_4 clearance include rifampin, carbamazepine, and possibly phenytoin. Selenium deficiency and amiodarone can block the conversion of T_4 to T_3.

Liothyronine (T_3) is chemically pure with known potency and has a shorter half-life of 1.5 days. Although it is widely used diagnostically in the T_3-suppression test, T_3 has some clinical disadvantages, including a higher incidence of cardiac adverse effects, higher cost, and difficulty in monitoring with conventional laboratory tests. Liotrix is a combination of synthetic T_4 and T_3 in a 4:1 ratio that attempts to mimic natural hormonal secretion. It is chemically stable and pure and has a predictable potency. The major limitations to this product are high cost and lack of therapeutic rationale because approximately 35% of T_4 is peripherally converted T_3.

Trials comparing levothyroxine alone to a combination of levothyroxine plus partial replacement with liothyronine (T_3) have generally shown that combinations of T_4 plus T_3 are no better than T_4 alone.[124,125] Clyde and colleagues in a trial of combination therapy, when compared with levothyroxine alone, treatment of primary hypothyroidism with combination levothyroxine plus liothyronine demonstrated no beneficial changes in body weight, serum lipid levels, hypothyroid symptoms as measured by a health-related quality of life questionnaire, and standard measures of cognitive performance.[125]

Dosing and Monitoring During the mid-1980s the average dose of levothyroxine was approximately 160 mcg/day. With the advent of more sensitive assay methods for TSH and the reformulation of levothyroxine, it is now apparent that many patients have been treated with excessive amounts of levothyroxine. More recent studies suggest that the average maintenance dose for most adults should be closer to about 125 mcg per day.[101] Indeed, as many as one-third of patients receiving levothyroxine 150 mcg daily will be over-replaced. There is, however, a wide range of replacement doses, necessitating individualized therapy and appropriate TSH monitoring to determine an adequate but not excessive dose.

The initial dose of levothyroxine is dependent on the patient's age, and the presence of associated disorders, as well as the severity and duration of hypothyroidism.[126] Most patients will require approximately 1.7 mcg/kg/day once they reach steady state for full replacement. In young patients with long-standing disease and patients older than 45 years of age without known cardiac disease, therapy should be initiated with 50 mcg daily of levothyroxine and increased to 100 mcg daily after 1 month. The recommended initial daily dose for older patients or those with known cardiac disease is 25 mcg per day titrated upward in increments of 25 mcg at monthly intervals to prevent stress on the cardiovascular system. Some patients can experience an exacerbation of angina with higher doses of thyroid hormone. Although the TSH is very sensitive for under- or overreplacement, clinicians often fail to alter the dose of T_4 based on TSH clearly outside of the normal range.[127,128]

Patients with subclinical or mild hypothyroidism (seen more commonly in the elderly and women) have no or few signs or symptoms, normal serum T_3 and T_4 concentrations, and an elevated basal TSH concentration.[129,130] The prevalence of this disorder in the NHANES III study was found to be 4.3%.[18] Although the treatment of subclinical hypothyroidism is controversial, patients presenting with marked elevations in TSH (>10 mIU/L) and high titers of thyroperoxidase antibody (TPO Ab) or prior treatment with ^{131}I can be most likely to benefit from treatment. Other patients who can improve with replacement include those with mild symptoms of hypothyroidism and depression. It should be noted that some studies find that only one of four treated patients experienced improvement.[131] Conservative treatment goals in this situation would be to maintain serum T_4 and T_3 levels in the normal range and reduce TSH to a value of 1 mIU/L.

Once euthyroidism is attained, the daily maintenance dose of levothyroxine does not fluctuate greatly. As patients age, the dosing requirement can need to be reduced.[113] The ability to measure serum TSH concentrations has improved the accuracy with which thyroid hormone replacement can be monitored. Many clinicians now consider serum TSH concentration to be the most sensitive and specific monitoring parameter for adjustment of levothyroxine dose. Plasma TSH concentrations begin to fall within hours and are usually normalized within 2 weeks but can take up to 6 weeks in some patients, depending on the baseline value. TSH and T_4 concentrations are both used to monitor therapy, and they should be checked every 6 weeks until a euthyroid state is achieved. Serum T_4 concentrations can be useful in detecting noncompliance, malabsorption, or changes in levothyroxine product bioequivalence. An elevated TSH concentration indicates insufficient replacement. The appropriate dose maintains the TSH concentration in the normal range. T_4 disposal is accelerated by nephritic syndrome, other severe systemic illnesses, and several antiseizure medications (phenobarbital, phenytoin, and carbamazepine) and rifampin. Pregnancy increases the T_4 dose requirement in 75% of women, probably because of increased degradation by the placental deiodinase. Initiating postmenopausal hormone replacement therapy increases the dose needed in 35% of women, perhaps because of an increased circulating T_4-binding globulin level. Patient noncompliance with prescribed T_4, the most common cause of inadequate treatment, might be suspected in patients with a dose that is higher than expected, variable thyroid function test results that do not correlate well with prescribed doses, and an elevated serum thyrotropin concentration with serum-free T_4 at the upper end of the normal range, which can suggest improved compliance immediately before testing because of a lag in the thyrotropin response. The metabolism of other pharmacologic agents can be altered in patients with hypothyroidism. The mechanism might be decreased expression of hepatic enzymes involved in drug metabolism, as seen in hypothyroid rats. As a result, increased sensitivity to anesthetic and sedative agents and higher serum levels of phenytoin have been reported. Hypothyroidism can also cause higher serum digoxin values, an effect attributed to a decreased volume of drug distribution. Conversely, hypothyroidism might decrease sensitivity to warfarin because of slowed metabolism of the vitamin K–dependent clotting factors, and restoration of euthyroidism can then increase the warfarin dose requirement.

In patients with hypothyroidism caused by hypothalamic or pituitary failure, alleviation of the clinical syndrome and restoration of serum T_4 to the normal range are the only criteria available for estimating the appropriate replacement dose of levothyroxine. Concurrent use of dopamine, dopaminergic agents (bromocriptine), somatostatin or somatostatin analogs (octreotide), and corticosteroids suppresses TSH concentrations and can confound the interpretation of this monitoring parameter.[113]

TSH-suppressive levothyroxine therapy can also be given to patients with nodular thyroid disease and diffuse goiter, to patients with a history of thyroid irradiation, and to patients with thyroid cancer. The rationale for suppression therapy is to reduce TSH secretion, which promotes growth and function in abnormal thyroid tissue. In patients with solitary nodules who have not received radiation, TSH should be suppressed to 0.05 to 0.1 mIU/L in premenopausal women and in men <60 years old. A dose of levothyroxine of 100 to 150 mcg per day is usually sufficient. In men older than 60 years of age and postmenopausal women, TSH levels should be reduced to 0.1 to 0.3 mIU/L because of the risk of more serious adverse effects in this population and reduced clearance of levothyroxine with advanced age. Levothyroxine can be given in nontoxic MNG to suppress the TSH to low-normal levels of 0.5 to 1 mIU/L if the baseline TSH is >1 mIU/L. Goiter size and thyroid volume can be reduced with suppression therapy. Diffuse goiter associated with autoimmune thyroiditis can also be treated with levothyroxine to reduce goiter size and thyroid volume. In patients with follicular or papillary thyroid cancer, current recommendations are to suppress the TSH to <0.02 mIU/L. Doses of levothyroxine of up to 2.2 to 2.5 mcg/kg can be needed to provide TSH levels of <0.02 mIU/L in this population, and free T_3 and T_4 levels are useful in detecting hyperthyroidism.[132]

Adverse Effects Serious untoward effects are unusual if dosing is appropriate and the patient is carefully monitored during initial treatment. Levothyroxine replacement in athyrotic hypothyroid patients restores systolic and diastolic left ventricular performance within 2 weeks, and the use of levothyroxine can increase the frequency of atrial premature beats but not necessarily ventricular premature beats. Excessive doses of thyroid hormone can lead to heart failure, angina pectoris, and myocardial infarction; rarely, the latter can be caused by coronary artery spasm. Allergic or idiosyncratic reactions can occur with the natural animal-derived products such as desiccated thyroid and thyroglobulin, but these are extremely rare with the synthetic products used today. The 0.05-mg Synthroid tablet is the least allergenic (caused by a lack of dye and few excipients) and should be tried in the patient suspected to be allergic to thyroid hormone.

Hyper-remodeling of cortical and trabecular bone caused by hyperthyroidism leads to reduced bone density and can increase the risk of fracture. Compared with normal controls, excess exogenous thyroid hormone results in histomorphometric and biochemical changes similar to those observed in osteoporosis and untreated hyperthyroidism; however, at routinely used replacement doses, bone mineral density loss is less than that seen with untreated hyperthyroidism and only slightly greater than in controls.[133,134] The risk for this complication of therapy seems to be related to the dose of levothyroxine, patient age, and gender. Markers for bone turnover include urinary cross-linked *N*-telopeptides, pyridinoline of type I collagen, osteocalcin, and bone-specific alkaline phosphatase. When doses of levothyroxine are used to suppress TSH concentrations to below-normal values (less than 0.3 mIU/L) in postmenopausal women, this adverse effect is more likely to be seen. Cortical bone is affected to a greater degree than trabecular bone at suppressive doses of 1-thyroxine. In contrast, it appears to be much less likely in men and in premenopausal women. Maintaining the TSH between 0.7 and 1.5 mIU/L with approximately 150 mcg/day of levothyroxine does not alter bone mineral density in premenopausal women.

SPECIAL CONDITIONS

Myxedema Coma

Myxedema coma is a rare consequence of decompensated hypothyroidism.[135,136] Clinical features include hypothermia, advanced stages of hypothyroid symptoms, and altered sensorium ranging from delirium to coma. Mortality rates of 60% to 70% necessitate immediate and aggressive therapy. Traditionally, the initial treatment has been intravenous bolus levothyroxine 300 to 500 mcg. However, as deiodinase activity is markedly reduced, impairing T_4 to T_3 conversion, initial treatment with intravenous T_3 or a combination of both hormones has also been advocated.[136] Glucocorticoid therapy with intravenous hydrocortisone 100 mg every 8 hours should be given until coexisting adrenal suppression is ruled out. Consciousness, lowered TSH concentrations, and normal vital signs are expected within 24 hours. Maintenance doses of levothyroxine are typically 75 to 100 mcg given intravenously until the patient stabilizes and oral therapy is begun. Supportive therapy must be instituted to maintain adequate ventilation, euglycemia, blood pressure, and body temperature. Any underlying disorder, such as sepsis or myocardial infarction, obviously must be diagnosed and treated.

Congenital Hypothyroidism[137]

In congenital hypothyroidism, full maintenance therapy should be instituted early to improve the prognosis for mental and physical development.[138] The average maintenance dose in infants and children depends on the age and weight of the child. Several studies demonstrate that aggressive therapy with levothyroxine is important for normal development and current recommendations are for initiation of therapy within 45 days of birth at a dose of 10 to 15 mcg/kg per day.[108] This dose is used to keep T_4 concentrations at about 10 mcg/dL within 30 days of starting therapy and is associated with improved intelligence quotients (IQs) in treated infants. The dose is progressively decreased to a typical adult dose as the child ages, the adult dose being given in the age range of 11 to 20 years.

Hypothyroidism in Pregnancy[86]

Hypothyroidism during pregnancy leads to an increased rate of stillbirths and possibly lower psychologic scores in infants born of women who received inadequate replacement during pregnancy.[139] Thyroid hormone is necessary for fetal growth and must come from the maternal side during the first 2 months of gestation. Although liothyronine can cross the placental membrane slightly better than levothyroxine, the latter is considered to be the drug of choice. The objective of treatment is to decrease TSH to 1 unit/mL and maintain free T_4 concentrations in the normal range. Based on elevated TSH levels during pregnancy, it was found that the mean dose of levothyroxine had to be increased by 36 mcg/day to suppress TSH into the normal range. Increased production of binding proteins, a marginal decrease in free hormone concentration, modification of peripheral thyroid hormone metabolism, and increased T_4 metabolism by the fetal-placental unit also contributes to increased thyroid hormone demand and the need for increased doses decreases after delivery.[87] Up to 60% of women need to have levothyroxine dose adjustment during pregnancy. Upward adjustment will be needed by week 8 of pregnancy. After delivery the levothyroxine can need to be reduced based on T_3 concentrations and measurement of TSH, typically approximately 6 to 8 weeks after delivery.[86]

Effects of Hypothyroidism on Selected Medications

Hypothyroidism can affect the metabolism and clinical efficacy of several medications. Digitalis preparations have a decreased volume of distribution in the hypothyroid state, resulting in increased sensitivity to the digitalis effect. Therefore, many hypothyroid patients achieve a therapeutic effect at lower digitalis doses. Insulin degradation can be delayed in hypothyroidism, thereby requiring a lower insulin dose. Hypothyroidism delays the catabolism of clotting factors, and if a patient stabilized on warfarin is made euthyroid with levothyroxine, the patient can become excessively anticoagulated. Respiratory depressants such as barbiturates, phenothiazines, and opioid analgesics should be avoided, because increased sensitivity can increase carbon dioxide retention and precipitate myxedema coma.

RECOMBINANT TSH IN THYROID CANCER

Patients with previously treated differentiated (papillary, follicular, or their respective variants) thyroid carcinoma require lifelong monitoring for recurrent disease.[140,141] Two diagnostic tests that play a central role in followup of these patients—serum thyroglobulin measurement and radioiodine whole body scanning—are most accurate during TSH stimulation. Temporary discontinuation of thyroid hormone therapy was previously the sole effective approach for TSH-stimulated testing. However, hormone withdrawal is associated with the morbidity of hypothyroidism and occasional tumor progression. The introduction of recombinant TSH (rTSH)-stimulated testing offers an alternative therapy. Recent clinical trials have shown that the sensitivity of combined rTSH-stimulated radioiodine scanning and serum thyroglobulin measurement has nearly equivalent sensitivity to testing after thyroid hormone withdrawal.[111,142] Furthermore, measurement of the rTSH-stimulated thyroglobulin concentration is a more sensitive way to detect residual thyroid cancer or normal tissue than thyroglobulin measurement or thyroid hormone therapy alone. Post-thyroidectomy adjuvant radioiodine therapy can also be administered following rTSH, instead of thyroid hormone withdrawal, with equivalent rates of remnant ablation.[143] Patients in whom thyroid hormone withdrawal would be contraindicated can also be successfully treated with radioiodine following rTSH.[144]

NONTHYROIDAL ILLNESS

A wide variety of abnormalities of hypothalamic-pituitary-thyroid function, serum thyroid hormone binding, and extrathyroidal thyroid hormone metabolism occur in patients with nonthyroidal illness.[11,12] These abnormalities frequently result in decreased serum T_3 concentrations and, with more severe nonthyroidal disease, lead to a decreased serum free T_4 concentration as well. Serum TSH concentrations are usually within the normal range, although low levels can occur with severe or critical illness. The presence of coexisting primary hypothyroidism can be recognized in patients who have other illnesses by an elevation in the TSH concentration.

The degree and extent of the abnormality in thyroid function generally correlates with the severity of the nonthyroidal illness. These conditions are frequently referred to as the "euthyroid sick syndrome." However, it is likely that these changes represent adaptive forms of hypothyroidism that serve to reduce the availability of thyroid hormones to lessen the catabolic impact of the nonthyroidal illness.

Decreased serum T_3 concentrations occur in patients with both acute and chronic illnesses. The fundamental cause of decreased serum T_3 concentrations in these situations is decreased extrathyroidal conversion of T_4 to T_3, normally mediated by T_4–5'-deiodinase. A circulating inhibitor of this enzyme, perhaps interleukin-6, is present in patients with nonthyroidal illness.[145] Serum total and free T_4 concentrations are usually normal in mild illness. The serum reverse T_3 concentration is characteristically high because the same enzyme, 5'-deiodinase, that is necessary to convert T_4 to T_3, is necessary to convert reverse T_3 to its breakdown products.

Low serum T_4 is seen in most critically ill patients.[146–148] This change is caused by diminished serum T_4 synthesis as well as impaired binding to serum transport proteins, resulting either from decreased serum concentrations of thyroid-binding globulin, thyroid-binding prealbumin, or albumin, or from inhibitors of T_4 binding. The free T_4 concentration is generally normal early in critical illness but also declines with more severe disease. This more severe degree of hypothyroidism, which occurs in severely ill patients, produces a greater reduction in thyroid hormone availability. The low serum T_4 concentrations in patients with nonthyroidal illness indicates a grave prognosis. In two studies, more than 60% of hospitalized patients with a low serum free T_4 index died. Although controversial, T_4 or T_3 supplementation has been of no benefit in this situation and in fact has increased morbidity.

To confuse matters, some patients with nonthyroidal illness have elevation of their serum T_4 concentration. Most commonly, this is seen in patients with psychiatric disorders during acute psychotic breaks. Thyroid hormone levels return to normal within 2 weeks after successful treatment of the underlying psychiatric disease. The occurrence of these abnormalities requires that care be taken in diagnosing hypothyroidism or hyperthyroidism in patients who have nonthyroidal illnesses.

GOITROUS THYROID DISEASE

Endemic goiter is the major thyroid disease throughout the world, affecting more than 200 million people. Many goitrous glands contain one or more nodules. The introduction of iodide supplementation has eliminated goiter as a major medical problem in developed countries, although it continues to be a problem in developing countries with geographic positions that make them more susceptible to iodide deficiency. In 1924, Marine postulated that periods of iodide deficiency resulted in cyclic hyperplasia and involution of thyroid follicular cells with eventual development of nodular hyperplasia.[44,149] This hypothesis is still used to explain goiter formation today. Whatever the specific cause, the final common pathway appears to result from an inadequate thyroid hormone secretion with compensatory TSH secretion and eventual thyroid gland enlargement. The essential factor for the conversion of a hyperplastic iodine-deficiency goiter into a colloid goiter appears to be an acute reduction of TSH stimulation; therefore, any situation that would result in a cyclical increase and decrease in TSH secretion might eventually result in the production of a nodular goiter.

There has been an interest in the possibility that growth factors other than TSH play a role in the development of a goiter. Immunoglobulin fractions capable of stimulating thyroid growth have been found in patients with nontoxic goiter and Graves' disease. In these patients, thyroid growth–promoting immunoglobulin titers correlate with goiter size rather than with the thyroid hormone concentration.

Sporadic goiter is defined as a goiter occurring in a nonendemic goiter region. Although a number of known goitrogens and errors in thyroid hormone biosynthesis can cause goiter, the majority of cases of sporadic goiter have no known etiology.

Treatment of all goiters is a trial of thyroid hormone suppression in an effort to eliminate TSH as a possible stimulus for continued thyroid growth. Large, long-standing goiters seldom undergo significant reduction in size. If the patient is symptomatic (with dysphagia or dyspnea) or there is a question of malignant thyroid involvement, surgery is recommended.

PHARMACOECONOMIC CONSIDERATIONS

Although the initial expense of surgery would seem to make it the most expensive treatment option, the relapse rates for thionamides and RAI are higher and in longer-term followup, there is not much difference between treatment options nor patients' opinions concerning treatment preferences.[150] The cost proportion between the medical and surgical treatment in younger patients is 1:2.5 (1 = US $1126) before and 1:1.3 (1 = US $2284) after inclusion of the relapse costs. The proportion between the medical, surgical, and ^{131}I treatment in older patients is 1:2.5:1.6 (1 = US $1164) before and 1:1.6:1.4 (1 = US $1972) after inclusion of the relapse costs.

CLINICAL CONTROVERSIES

Although the current FDA standards of bioavailability for T_4 products suggest that several products are bioequivalent, the relationship between T_4 serum concentration and TSH response suggests that the products are not truly bioequivalent. New standards of bioequivalency might need to be developed for drug products such as T_4.

Combination therapy of T_4 plus T_3 for hypothyroidism seems to improve cognitive function over monotherapy with T_4; however, there are not corresponding improvements in biochemical markers of thyroid hormone nor differences in TSH response.

Multiple studies have addressed the role of thyroid supplementation in critically ill patients with cardiac disease, sepsis, pulmonary disease (e.g., acute respiratory distress syndrome), or severe infection, or with burn and trauma patients. In spite of a very large number of published studies, it is very difficult to form clear recommendations for treatment with thyroid hormone in the intensive care unit.

EVALUATION OF THERAPEUTIC OUTCOMES

Patients on optimal thyroid hormone replacement therapy should have TSH and free T_4 serum concentrations in the normal range with idiopathic hypothyroidism and Hashimoto's thyroiditis. Those who are being treated for thyroid cancer should have TSH suppressed to very low levels and thyroglobulin should be undetectable. Given the half-life of 7 days of T_4, the appropriate monitoring interval is no more often than 4 weeks. The signs and symptoms of hypothyroidism should be improved or absent (see clinical presentation of hypothyroidism, above), although this can take several months for most to improve.

ABBREVIATIONS

ClO_4^-: perchlorate

DIT: diiodotyrosine

FSH: follicle-stimulating hormone

$G_s\alpha$: α subunit of the stimulatory guanine-nucleotide-binding protein

hCG: human chorionic gonadotropin

HLA: human leukocyte antigen

^{131}I: sodium iodide 131

L-Thyroxine: levothyroxine

LH: luteinizing hormone

MIT: monoiodotyrosine

MMI: methimazole

MNG: multinodular goiter

PRTH: pituitary resistance to thyroid hormone

PTU: propylthiouracil

RAI: radioactive iodine

RAIU: radioactive iodine uptake

rTSH: recombinant thyroid-stimulating hormone

SCN^-: thiocyanate

SSKI: saturated solution of potassium iodide

T_3: triiodothyronine

T_4: thyroxine

TBG: thyroid-binding globulin

TG: thyroglobulin

TPO Ab: thyroperoxidase antibody

$TR\beta_2$, $TR\beta_1$, $TR\alpha_1$: thyroid hormone receptors

TRH: thyrotropin-releasing hormone

TSAb: thyroid-stimulating antibody

TSH: thyroid-stimulating hormone

REFERENCES

1. Nilsson M. Iodide handling by the thyroid epithelial cell. Exp Clin Endocrinol Diabetes 2001;109:13–17.
2. Dohan O, De la Vieja A, Paroder V, et al. The sodium/iodide symporter (NIS): Characterization, regulation, and medical significance. Endocr Rev 2003;24:48–77.
3. Clewell RA, Merrill EA, Narayanan L, Gearhart JM, Robinson PJ. Evidence for competitive inhibition of iodide uptake by perchlorate and translocation of perchlorate into the thyroid. Int J Toxicol 2004;23:17–23.
4. Delange F, de Benoist B, Pretell E, Dunn JT. Iodine deficiency in the world: Where do we stand at the turn of the century? Thyroid 2001;11:437–447.
5. Dunn JT, Dunn AD. Update on intrathyroidal iodine metabolism. Thyroid 2001;11:407–414.
6. Obregon MJ, Escobar del Rey F, Morreale de Escobar G. The effects of iodine deficiency on thyroid hormone deiodination. Thyroid 2005;15:917–929.
7. Schussler GC. The thyroxine-binding proteins. Thyroid 2000;10:141–149.
8. Bianco AC, Kim BW. Deiodinases: Implications of the local control of thyroid hormone action. J Clin Invest 2006;116:2571–2579.
9. Kopp P. The TSH receptor and its role in thyroid disease. Cell Mol Life Sci 2001;58:1301–1322.
10. Krohn K, Paschke R. Somatic mutations in thyroid nodular disease. Mol Genet Metab 2002;75:202–208.
11. Peeters RP, Debaveye Y, Fliers E, Visser TJ. Changes within the thyroid axis during critical illness. Crit Care Clin 2006;22:41–55, vi.
12. Peeters RP, van der Deure WM, Visser TJ. Genetic variation in thyroid hormone pathway genes; polymorphisms in the TSH receptor and the iodothyronine deiodinases. Eur J Endocrinol 2006;155:655–662.
13. Gillam MP, Kopp P. Genetic defects in thyroid hormone synthesis. Curr Opin Pediatr 2001;13:364–372.
14. Ando T, Latif R, Davies TF. Thyrotropin receptor antibodies: New insights into their actions and clinical relevance. Best Pract Res Clin Endocrinol Metab 2005;19:33–52.
15. Davies TF, Ando T, Lin RY, Tomer Y, Latif R. Thyrotropin receptor-associated diseases: From adenomata to Graves' disease. J Clin Invest 2005;115:1972–1983.
16. Harvey CB, Williams GR. Mechanism of thyroid hormone action. Thyroid 2002;12:441–446.
17. Cooper DS. Hyperthyroidism. Lancet 2003;362:459–468.
18. Hollowell JG, Staehling NW, Flanders WD, et al. Serum TSH, T(4), and thyroid antibodies in the United States population (1988 to 1994): National Health and Nutrition Examination Survey (NHANES III). J Clin Endocrinol Metab 2002;87:489–499.
19. Nayak B, Burman K. Thyrotoxicosis and thyroid storm. Endocrinol Metab Clin North Am 2006;35:663–686 vii.
20. Socin HV, Chanson P, Delemer B, et al. The changing spectrum of TSH–secreting pituitary adenomas: Diagnosis and management in 43 patients. Eur J Endocrinol 2003;148:433–442.
21. Beck-Peccoz P, Persani L, Calebiro D, Bonomi M, Mannavola D, Campi I. Syndromes of hormone resistance in the hypothalamic-pituitary-thyroid axis. Best Pract Res Clin Endocrinol Metab 2006;20:529–546.
22. Golden WM, Weber KB, Hernandez TL, Sherman SI, Woodmansee WW, Haugen BR. Single-dose rexinoid rapidly and specifically suppresses serum thyrotropin in normal subjects. J Clin Endocrinol Metab 2007;92:124–130.
23. Weetman AP. Controversy in thyroid disease. J R Coll Physicians Lon 2000;34:374–380.
24. Fung S, Malhotra R, Selva D. Thyroid orbitopathy. Aust Fam Physician 2003;32:615–620.

25. Garrity JA, Bahn RS. Pathogenesis of Graves' ophthalmopathy: Implications for prediction, prevention, and treatment. Am J Ophthalmol 2006;142:147–153.
26. Brix TH, Kyvik KO, Christensen K, Hegedus L. Evidence for a major role of heredity in Graves'' disease: A population-based study of two Danish twin cohorts. J Clin Endocrinol Metab 2001;86:930–934.
27. Ban Y, Concepcion ES, Villanueva R, Greenberg DA, Davies TF, Tomer Y. Analysis of immune regulatory genes in familial and sporadic Graves' disease. J Clin Endocrinol Metab 2004;89:4562–4568.
28. Ban Y, Davies TF, Greenberg DA, et al. Arginine at position 74 of the HLA-DR beta1 chain is associated with Graves'' disease. Genes Immun 2004;5:203–208.
29. Taylor JC, Gough SC, Hunt PJ, et al. A genome-wide screen in 1119 relative pairs with autoimmune thyroid disease. J Clin Endocrinol Metab 2006;91:646–653.
30. Kung AW. Clinical review: Thyrotoxic periodic paralysis: A diagnostic challenge. J Clin Endocrinol Metab 2006;91:2490–2495.
31. Rodien P, Jordan N, Lefevre A, et al. Abnormal stimulation of the thyrotrophin receptor during gestation. Hum Reprod Update 2004;10:95–105.
32. Siegel RD, Lee SL. Toxic nodular goiter. Toxic adenoma and toxic multinodular goiter. Endocrinol Metab Clin North Am 1998;27:151–168.
33. Freitas JE. Therapeutic options in the management of toxic and nontoxic nodular goiter. Semin Nucl Med 2000;30:88–97.
34. Krohn K, Fuhrer D, Bayer Y, et al. Molecular pathogenesis of euthyroid and toxic multinodular goiter. Endocr Rev 2005;26:504–524.
35. Campbell AJ. Thyroid disorders in the elderly. Difficulties in diagnosis and treatment. Drugs 1986;31:455–461.
36. Papi G, Pearce EN, Braverman LE, Betterle C, Roti E. A clinical and therapeutic approach to thyrotoxicosis with thyroid-stimulating hormone suppression only. Am J Med 2005;118:349–361.
37. Sdano MT, Falciglia M, Welge JA, Steward DL. Efficacy of thyroid hormone suppression for benign thyroid nodules: Meta-analysis of randomized trials. Otolaryngol Head Neck Surg 2005;133:391–396.
38. Luotola K, Hyoty H, Salmi J, Miettinen A, Helin H, Pasternack A. Evaluation of infectious etiology in subacute thyroiditis—Lack of association with coxsackievirus infection. APMIS 1998;106:500–504.
39. Fatourechi V, Aniszewski JP, Fatourechi GZ, Atkinson EJ, Jacobsen SJ. Clinical features and outcome of subacute thyroiditis in an incidence cohort: Olmsted County, Minnesota, study. J Clin Endocrinol Metab 2003;88:2100–2105.
40. Pearce EN, Farwell AP, Braverman LE. Thyroiditis [erratum appears in N Engl J Med 2003;349(6):620]. N Engl J Med 2003;348:2646–2655.
41. Stagnaro-Green A. Postpartum thyroiditis. Best Pract Res Clin Endocrinol Metab 2004;18:303–316.
42. DeSimone CP, Lele SM, Modesitt SC. Malignant struma ovarii: A case report and analysis of cases reported in the literature with focus on survival and I131 therapy. Gynecol Oncol 2003;89:543–548.
43. Als C, Gedeon P, Rosler H, Minder C, Netzer P, Laissue JA. Survival analysis of 19 patients with toxic thyroid carcinoma. J Clin Endocrinol Metab 2002;87:4122–4127.
44. Delange F. Iodine deficiency in Europe and its consequences: An update. Eur J Nucl Med Mol Imaging 2002;29:S404–416.
45. Meurisse M, Gollogly L, Degauque C, Fumal I, Defechereux T, Hamoir E. Iatrogenic thyrotoxicosis: Causal circumstances, pathophysiology, and principles of treatment—Review of the literature. World J Surg 2000;24:1377–1385.
46. Bartalena L, Marcocci C, Bogazzi F, et al. Relation between therapy for hyperthyroidism and the course of Graves' ophthalmopathy. N Engl J Med 1998;338:73–78.
47. Ferner RE, Burnett A, Rawlins MD. Triiodothyroacetic acid abuse in a female body builder [letter]. Lancet 1986;1:383.
48. Basaria S, Cooper DS. Amiodarone and the thyroid. Am J Med 2005;118:706–14.
49. Bartalena L, Bogazzi F, Braverman LE, Martino E. Effects of amiodarone administration during pregnancy on neonatal thyroid function and subsequent neurodevelopment. J Endocrinol Invest 2001;24:116–130.
50. Bogazzi F, Bartalena L, Gasperi M, Braverman LE, Martino E. The various effects of amiodarone on thyroid function. Thyroid 2001;11:511–519.
51. Martino E, Bartalena L, Bogazzi F, Braverman LE. The effects of amiodarone on the thyroid. Endocr Rev 2001;22:240–254.
52. Biondi B, Palmieri EA, Klain M, Schlumberger M, Filetti S, Lombardi G. Subclinical hyperthyroidism: Clinical features and treatment options. Eur J Endocrinol 2005;152:1–9.
53. Bartalena L, Tanda ML, Bogazzi F, Piantanida E, Lai A, Martino E. An update on the pharmacological management of hyperthyroidism due to Graves' disease. Expert Opin Pharmacother 2005;6:851–861.
54. Franklyn JA. Management guidelines for hyperthyroidism. Baillieres Clin Endocrinol Metab 1997;11:561–571.
55. Surks MI Oe, Daniels GH, Sawin CT, et al. Subclinical thyroid disease: Scientific review and guidelines for diagnosis and management. JAMA 2004;291:228–238.
56. Singer PA, Cooper DS, Levy EG, et al. Treatment guidelines for patients with hyperthyroidism and hypothyroidism. Standards of Care Committee, American Thyroid Association. JAMA 1995;273:808–812.
57. Hegedus L, Bonnema SJ, Bennedbaek FN. Management of simple nodular goiter: Current status and future perspectives. Endocr Rev 2003;24:102–132.
58. Carella C, Mazziotti G, Rotondi M, et al. Iodized salt improves the effectiveness of L-thyroxine therapy after surgery for nontoxic goitre: A prospective and randomized study. Clin Endocrinol (Oxf) 2002;57:507–513.
59. Boger MS, Perrier ND. Advantages and disadvantages of surgical therapy and optimal extent of thyroidectomy for the treatment of hyperthyroidism. Surg Clin North Am 2004;84:849–874.
60. Zambudio AR, Rodriguez J, Riquelme J, Soria T, Canteras M, Parrilla P. Prospective study of postoperative complications after total thyroidectomy for multinodular goiters by surgeons with experience in endocrine surgery [see comment]. Ann Surg 2004;240:18–25.
61. Cooper D. Drug therapy: Antithyroid drugs. N Engl J Med 2005;352:905–917.
62. Momotani N, Noh JY, Ishikawa N, Ito K. Effects of propylthiouracil and methimazole on fetal thyroid status in mothers with Graves' hyperthyroidism. J Endocrinol Metab 1997;82:3633–3636.
63. Raber W, Kmen E, Waldhausl W, Vierhapper H. Medical therapy of Graves'' disease: Effect on remission rates of methimazole alone and in combination with triiodothyronine. Eur J Endocrinol 2000;142:117–124.
64. Rittmaster RS, Abbott EC, Douglas R, et al. Effect of methimazole, with or without L-thyroxine, on remission rates in Graves'' disease. J Clin Endocrinol Metab1998;83:814–818.
65. McIver B, Rae P, Beckett G, Wilkinson E, Gold A, Toft A. Lack of effect of thyroxine in patients with Graves'' hyperthyroidism who are treated with an antithyroid drug. N Engl J Med 1996;334:220–224.
66. Bartalena L, Bogazzi F, Martino E. Adverse effects of thyroid hormone preparations and antithyroid drugs. Drug Saf 1996;15:53–63.
67. Tamai H, Sudo T, Kimura A, et al. Association between the DRB1*08032 histocompatibility antigen and methimazole-induced agranulocytosis in Japanese patients with Graves' disease. Ann Intern Med 1996;124:490–494.
68. Tamai H, Mukuta T, Matsubayashi S, et al. Treatment of methimazole-induced agranulocytosis using recombinant human granulocyte colony-stimulating factor (rhG-CSF). J Clin Endocrinol Metab1993;77:1356–1360.
69. Fukata S, Kuma K, Sugawara M. Granulocyte colony-stimulating factor (G-CSF) does not improve recovery from antithyroid drug-induced agranulocytosis: A prospective study. Thyroid 1999;9:29–31.
70. Woeber KA. Methimazole-induced hepatotoxicity. Endocr Pract 2002;8:222–224.
71. Mizutani T, Yoshida K, Murakami M, Shirai M, Kawazoe S. Evidence for the involvement of *N*-methylthiourea, a ring cleavage metabolite, in the hepatotoxicity of methimazole in glutathione-depleted mice: Structure-toxicity and metabolic studies. Chem Res Toxicol 2000;13:170–176.
72. Gurlek A, Cobankara V, Bayraktar M. Liver tests in hyperthyroidism: Effect of antithyroid therapy. J Clin Gastroenterol 1997;24:180–183.
73. Monzani F, Caraccio N, Dardano A, Ferrannini E. Thyroid autoimmunity and dysfunction associated with type I interferon therapy. Clin Exp Med 2004;3:199–210.
74. Van Dijke CP, Heydendael RJ, De Kleine MJ. Methimazole, carbimazole, and congenital skin defects. Ann Intern Med 1987;106:60–61.
75. Stanbury JB, Ermans AE, Bourdoux P, et al. Iodine-induced hyperthyroidism: Occurrence and epidemiology. Thyroid 1998;8:83–100.
76. Wolf J. Perchlorate and the thyroid gland. Pharmacological Reviews 1998;50:89–105.

77. Wartofsky L. Radioiodine therapy for Graves' disease: Case selection and restrictions recommended to patients in North America. Thyroid 1997;7:213–216.
78. Kaplan MM, Meier DA, Dworkin HJ. Treatment of hyperthyroidism with radioactive iodine. Endocrinol Metab Clin North Am1998;27:205–223.
79. Tallstedt L, Lundell G. Radioiodine treatment, ablation, and ophthalmopathy: A balanced perspective. Thyroid 1997;7:241–245.
80. Lazarus JH, Clarke S. Use of radioiodine in the management of hyperthyroidism in the UK. development of guidelines. Thyroid 1997;7:229–231.
81. Franklyn JA, Maisonneuve P, Sheppard M, Betteridge J, Boyle P. Cancer incidence and mortality after radioiodine treatment for hyperthyroidism: A population-based cohort study. Lancet 1999;353:2111–2115.
82. Franklyn JA, Maisonneuve P, Sheppard MC, Betteridge J, Boyle P. Mortality after the treatment of hyperthyroidism with radioactive iodine. N Engl J Med 1998;338:712–718.
83. Leslie WD, Ward L, Salamon EA, Ludwig S, Rowe RC, Cowden EA. A randomized comparison of radioiodine doses in Graves' hyperthyroidism. J Clin Endocrinol Metab 2003;88:978–983.
84. Franklyn JA. The management of hyperthyroidism. N Engl J Med 1994;330:1731–1738.
85. Uy HL, Reasner CA, Samuels MH. Pattern of recovery of the hypothalamic-pituitary-thyroid axis following radioactive iodine therapy in patients with Graves' disease. Am J Med 1995;99:173–179.
86. Chan GW, Mandel SJ. Therapy insight: Management of Graves'' disease during pregnancy. Nat Clin Pract Endocrinol Metab 2007;3:470–478.
87. Glinoer D. Management of hypo- and hyperthyroidism during pregnancy. Growth Horm IGF Res 2003;13:S45–54.
88. Lazarus JH, Kokandi A. Thyroid disease in relation to pregnancy: A decade of change. Clin Endocrinol (Oxf) 2000;53:265–278.
89. Momotani N, Noh J, Ishikawa N, Ito K. Relationship between silent thyroiditis and recurrent Graves'' disease in the postpartum period. J Clin Endocrinol Metab1994;79:285–289.
90. Coukos G, Makrigiannakis A, Chung J, Randall TC, Rubin SC, Benjamin I. Complete hydatidiform mole. A disease with a changing profile. J Reprod Med 1999;44:698–704.
91. Momotani N, Yamashita R, Makino F, Noh JY, Ishikawa N, Ito K. Thyroid function in wholly breast–feeding infants whose mothers take high doses of propylthiouracil. Clin Endocrinol (Oxf) 2000;53:177–181.
92. Polak M, Le Gac I, Vuillard E, et al. Fetal and neonatal thyroid function in relation to maternal Graves'' disease. Best Pract Res Clin Endocrinol Metab 2004;18:289–302.
93. Zimmerman D, Lteif AN. Thyrotoxicosis in children. Endocrinol Metab Clin North Am1998;27:109–126.
94. Segni M, Leonardi E, Mazzoncini B, Pucarelli I, Pasquino AM. Special features of Graves'' disease in early childhood. Thyroid 1999;9:871–877.
95. Swinburne JL, Kreisman SH. A rare case of subacute thyroiditis causing thyroid storm. Thyroid 2007;17:73–76.
96. Sherman RG, Lasseter DH. Pharmacologic management of patients with diseases of the endocrine system. Dent Clin North Am 1996;40:727–752.
97. Sherman SI, Simonson L, Ladenson PW. Clinical and socioeconomic predispositions to complicated thyrotoxicosis: A predictable and preventable syndrome? Am J Med 1996;101:192–198.
98. Zweig SB, Schlosser JR, Thomas SA, Levy CJ, Fleckman AM. Rectal administration of propylthiouracil in suppository form in patients with thyrotoxicosis and critical illness: Case report and review of literature. Endocr Pract 2006;12:43–47.
99. Duggal J, Singh S, Kuchinic P, Butler P, Arora R. Utility of esmolol in thyroid crisis. Can J Clin Pharmacol 2006;13:e292–295.
100. Ozbey N, Kalayoglu-Besisik S, Gul N, Bozbora A, Sencer E, Molvalilar S. Therapeutic plasmapheresis in patients with severe hyperthyroidism in whom antithyroid drugs are contraindicated. Int J Clin Pract 2004;58:554–558.
101. Roberts CG, Ladenson PW. Hypothyroidism. Lancet 2004;363:793–803.
102. LaFranchi S. Thyroid hormone in hypopituitarism, Graves' disease, congenital hypothyroidism, and maternal thyroid disease during pregnancy. Growth Horm IGF Res 2006;16(Suppl A):S20–24.
103. Roberts HJ. Aspartame disease: A possible cause for concomitant Graves' disease and pulmonary hypertension [comment]. Tex Heart Inst J 2004;31:105–6.
104. Sinclair D. Clinical and laboratory aspects of thyroid autoantibodies. Ann Clin Biochem 2006;43:173–183.
105. Stassi G, De Maria R. Autoimmune thyroid disease: New models of cell death in autoimmunity. Nat Rev Immunol 2002;2:195–204.
106. Mitchell ML, Klein RZ. The sequelae of untreated maternal hypothyroidism. Eur J Endocrinol 2004;151.
107. Morreale de Escobar G, Obregon MJ, Escobar del Rey F. Role of thyroid hormone during early brain development. Eur J Endocrinol 2004;151.
108. Buyukgebiz A. Newborn screening for congenital hypothyroidism. J Pediatr Endocrinol Metab 2006;19:1291–1298.
109. Prabhakar VK, Shalet SM. Aetiology, diagnosis, and management of hypopituitarism in adult life. Postgrad Med J 2006;82:259–266.
110. Urban RJ. Hypopituitarism after acute brain injury. Growth Horm IGF Res 2006;16 Suppl A.S25–29.
111. Sherman SI, Gopal J, Haugen BR, et al. Central hypothyroidism associated with retinoid X receptor-selective ligands. N Engl J Med 1999;340:1075–1079.
112. Joshi AS, Woolf PD. Pituitary hyperplasia secondary to primary hypothyroidism: A case report and review of the literature. Pituitary 2005;8:99–103.
113. Baskin HJ, Cobin RH, Duick DS, Gharib H, et al. American Association of Clinical Endocrinologists Medical guidelines for clinical practice for evaluation and treatment of hyperthyroidism and hypothyroidism. Endocr Pract 2002;8:457–469.
114. Blouin RA, Clifton GD, Adams MA, Foster TS, Flueck J. Biopharmaceutical comparison of two levothyroxine sodium products. Clin Pharm 1989;8:588–592.
115. Berg JA, Mayor GH. A study in normal human volunteers to compare the rate and extent of levothyroxine absorption from Synthroid and Levoxine. J Clin Pharmacol 1992;32:1135–1140.
116. Gottwald R, Lorkowski G, Petersen G, Schnitzler M, Lucker PW. Bioequivalence of two commercially available levothyroxine-Na preparations in athyreotic patients. Methods Find Exp Clin Pharmacol 1994;16:645–650.
117. Dong BJ, Hauck WW, Gambertoglio JG, et al. Bioequivalence of generic and brand-name levothyroxine products in the treatment of hypothyroidism. JAMA 1997;277:1205–1213.
118. Blakesley V, Awni W, Locke C, Ludden T, Granneman GR, Braverman LE. Are bioequivalence studies of levothyroxine sodium formulations in euthyroid volunteers reliable? Thyroid 2004;14:191–200.
119. Hennessey JV. Levothyroxine dosage and the limitations of current bioequivalence standards. Nat Clin Pract Endocrinol Metab2006;2:474–475.
120. Liel Y, Sperber AD, Shany S. Nonspecific intestinal adsorption of levothyroxine by aluminum hydroxide. Am J Med 1994;97:363–365.
121. Shakir KM, Chute JP, Aprill BS, Lazarus AA. Ferrous sulfate-induced increase in requirement for thyroxine in a patient with primary hypothyroidism. South Med J 1997;90:637–639.
122. Jabbar MA, Larrea J, Shaw RA. Abnormal thyroid function tests in infants with congenital hypothyroidism: The influence of soy-based formula. J Am Coll Nutr 1997;16:280–282.
123. Liel Y, Harman-Boehm I, Shany S. Evidence for a clinically important adverse effect of fiber-enriched diet on the bioavailability of levothyroxine in adult hypothyroid patients. J Clin Endocrinol Metab1996;81:857–859.
124. Appelhof BC, Fliers E, Wekking EM, et al. Combined therapy with levothyroxine and liothyronine in two ratios, compared with levothyroxine monotherapy in primary hypothyroidism: A double-blind, randomized, controlled clinical trial. J Clin Endocrinol Metab2005;90:2666–2674.
125. Clyde PW, Harari AE, Getka EJ, Shakir KM. Combined levothyroxine plus liothyronine compared with levothyroxine alone in primary hypothyroidism: A randomized controlled trial [see comment]. JAMA 2003;290:2952–2958.
126. Kabadi UM. Influence of age on optimal daily levothyroxine dosage in patients with primary hypothyroidism grouped according to etiology. South Med J 1997;90:920–924.
127. De Whalley P. Do abnormal thyroid stimulating hormone level values result in treatment changes? A study of patients on thyroxine in one general practice. Br J Gen Pract 1995;45:93–95.
128. Parle JV, Franklyn JA, Cross KW, Jones SR, Sheppard MC. Thyroxine prescription in the community: Serum thyroid stimulating hormone level assays as an indicator of undertreatment or overtreatment [see comment]. Br J Gen Pract 1993;43:107–109.

129. Garber JR, Hennessey JV, Liebermann JA, 3rd, Morris CM, Talbert RL. Clinical update. Managing the challenges of hypothyroidism. J Fam Pract 2006;55.
130. Vanderpump MP, Tunbridge WM. Epidemiology and prevention of clinical and subclinical hypothyroidism. Thyroid 2002;12:839–847.
131. Vanderpump M. Subclinical hypothyroidism: The case against treatment. Trends Endocrinol Metab 2003;14:262–266.
132. Cooper DS, Doherty GM, Haugen BR, et al. Management guidelines for patients with thyroid nodules and differentiated thyroid cancer. Thyroid 2006;16:109–142.
133. Vestergaard P, Mosekilde L. Hyperthyroidism, bone mineral, and fracture risk—A meta-analysis. Thyroid 2003;13:585–593.
134. Uzzan B, Campos J, Cucherat M, Nony P, Boissel JP, Perret GY. Effects on bone mass of long term treatment with thyroid hormones: A meta-analysis. J Clin Endocrinol Metab1996;81:4278–4289.
135. Sarlis NJ, Gourgiotis L. Thyroid emergencies. Rev Endocr Metab Disord 2003;4:129–136.
136. Wartofsky L. Myxedema coma. Endocrinol Metab Clin North Am 2006;35:687–698, vii–viii.
137. American Academy of P, Rose SR, Section on E, et al. Update of newborn screening and therapy for congenital hypothyroidism. Pediatrics 2006;117:2290–303.
138. Rovet J, Daneman D. Congenital hypothyroidism: A review of current diagnostic and treatment practices in relation to neuropsychologic outcome. Paediatr Drugs 2003;5:141–149.
139. Haddow JE, Palomaki GE, Allan WC, et al. Maternal thyroid deficiency during pregnancy and subsequent neuropsychological development of the child [see comment]. N Engl J Med 1999;341:549–555.
140. Sherman SI. Etiology, diagnosis, and treatment recommendations for central hypothyroidism associated with bexarotene therapy for cutaneous T-cell lymphoma. Clin Lymphoma 2003;3:249–252.
141. Sherman SI. Thyroid carcinoma. Lancet 2003;361:501–511.
142. Haugen BR, Pacini F, Reiners C, et al. A comparison of recombinant human thyrotropin and thyroid hormone withdrawal for the detection of thyroid remnant or cancer. J Clin Endocrinol Metab1999;84:3877–3885.
143. Pacini F, Ladenson PW, Schlumberger M, et al. Radioiodine ablation of thyroid remnants after preparation with recombinant human thyrotropin in differentiated thyroid carcinoma: Results of an international, randomized, controlled study. J Clin Endocrinol Metab 2006;91:926–932.
144. Robbins RJ, Driedger A, Magner J. Recombinant human thyrotropin-assisted radioiodine therapy for patients with metastatic thyroid cancer who could not elevate endogenous thyrotropin or be withdrawn from thyroxine. Thyroid 2006;16:1121–1130.
145. Torpy DJ, Tsigos C, Lotsikas AJ, Defensor R, Chrousos GP, Papanicolaou DA. Acute and delayed effects of a single-dose injection of interleukin-6 on thyroid function in healthy humans. Metabolism 1998;47:1289–1293.
146. Burman KD, Wartofsky L. Thyroid function in the intensive care unit setting. Crit Care Clin 2001;17:43–57.
147. Stathatos N, Levetan C, Burman KD, Wartofsky L. The controversy of the treatment of critically ill patients with thyroid hormone. Best Pract Res Clin Endocrinol Metab 2001;15:465–478.
148. Langton JE, Brent GA. Nonthyroidal illness syndrome: Evaluation of thyroid function in sick patients. Endocrinol Metab Clin North Am 2002;31:159–172.
149. Simescu M, Varciu M, Nicolaescu E, et al. Iodized oil as a complement to iodized salt in schoolchildren in endemic goiter in Romania. Horm Res 2002;58:78–82.
150. Ljunggren JG, Torring O, Wallin G, et al. Quality of life aspects and costs in treatment of Graves' hyperthyroidism with antithyroid drugs, surgery, or radioiodine: Results from a prospective, randomized study. Thyroid 1998;8:653–659.

CHAPTER 79 Adrenal Gland Disorders

JOHN G. GUMS AND SHAWN ANDERSON

KEY CONCEPTS

1. Glucocorticoid secretion from the adrenal cortex is stimulated by corticotropin or adrenocorticotropic hormone (ACTH) that is released from the anterior pituitary in response to hypothalamic-mediated release of corticotropin-releasing hormone (CRH).
2. To ensure the proper treatment of Cushing's syndrome, diagnostic procedures should (1) establish the presence of hypercortisolism and (2) discover the underlying etiology of the disease.
3. The rationale for treating Cushing's syndrome is to reduce the morbidity and mortality resulting from disorders such as diabetes mellitus, cardiovascular disease, and electrolyte abnormalities.
4. The treatment of choice for both ACTH-dependent and ACTH-independent Cushing's syndrome is surgery, whereas pharmacologic agents are reserved for adjunctive therapy, refractory cases, or inoperable disease.
5. Pharmacologic agents that can be used to manage the patient with Cushing's syndrome include: steroidogenic inhibitors, adrenolytic agents, neuromodulators of ACTH release, and glucocorticoid-receptor blocking agents.
6. Spironolactone, a competitive inhibitor of aldosterone, is the drug of choice in bilateral adrenal hyperplasia (BAH)-dependent hyperaldosteronism.
7. Addison's disease (primary adrenal insufficiency) is a deficiency in cortisol, aldosterone, and various androgens resulting from the loss of function of all regions of the adrenal cortex.
8. Secondary adrenal insufficiency usually results from exogenous steroid use, leading to hypothalamic-pituitary-adrenal (HPA)-axis suppression followed by a decrease in ACTH release, and low levels of androgens and cortisol.
9. Virilism results from the excessive secretion of androgens from the adrenal gland and is usually seen as hirsutism in females.

The adrenal glands were first characterized by Eustachius in 1563. After Addison identified a case of adrenal insufficiency in humans, adrenal anatomy and physiology flourished. Most of the work done in the early and mid-1900s centered on the glucocorticoid cortisol. With the discovery of aldosterone by Simpson and Tait in 1952, adrenal pharmacology turned toward the mineralocorticoid. Conn[1] followed with his classical description of primary aldosteronism in 1955, and numerous clinicians and investigators have continued the discovery of the variety of disease processes promoted through the adrenal gland.

Learning objectives, review questions, and other resources can be found at **www.pharmacotherapyonline.com.**

PHYSIOLOGY, ANATOMY, AND BIOCHEMISTRY

There are two adrenal glands located extraperitoneally to the upper poles of each kidney (Fig. 79–1). On average, each adrenal gland weighs 4 g and is 2 to 3 cm in width and 4 to 6 cm in length. The gland is fed by small arteries from the abdominal aorta and renal and phrenic arteries. Drainage of the adrenal gland occurs via the renal vein on the left and the inferior vena cava on the right.

The adrenal medulla occupies 10% of the total gland and is responsible for the secretion of catecholamines. The adrenal cortex accounts for the remaining 90% and is responsible for the secretion of three types of hormones (Fig. 79–2) from three separate zones.[2]

The zona glomerulosa, 15% of the total adrenal cortex, is responsible for mineralocorticoid production, of which aldosterone is the principal end product. Aldosterone maintains electrolyte and volume homeostasis by altering potassium and magnesium secretion and renal tubular sodium reabsorption. The zona fasciculata, the middle zone, makes up 60% of the cortex, is high in cholesterol, and is responsible for basal and stimulated glucocorticoid production. Glucocorticoids, mainly cortisol, are responsible for the regulation of fat, carbohydrate, and protein metabolism. The zona reticularis occupies 25% of the adrenal cortex, and is responsible for all adrenal androgen production. The androgens, testosterone and estradiol, are the major end products and have influence within the reproductive system as well as affecting primary and secondary sex characteristics.

HORMONE PRODUCTION AND METABOLISM

Cortisol production is accomplished via two successive hydroxylations: the first at the 21-position by 21-hydroxylase (yielding 11-deoxycortisol) and the second at the 11-position by 11-hydroxylase, yielding cortisol or hydrocortisone.

Aldosterone is a by-product of the 21-hydroxylation of pregnenolone to form deoxycorticosterone. The oxidation of 18-hydroxycorticosterone to aldosterone is a unique feature of the zona glomerulosa, explaining why aldosterone is not affected during disease processes limited to the fasciculata and/or reticularis.

Androgens have a 19-carbon nucleus and serve as precursors to more potent analogs produced in the periphery. The adrenal gland can synthesize estradiol and estrone from testosterone and androstenedione, respectively; however, the quantities are extremely small. The rates of production for the various steroids produced by the adrenal gland are listed in Table 79–1.

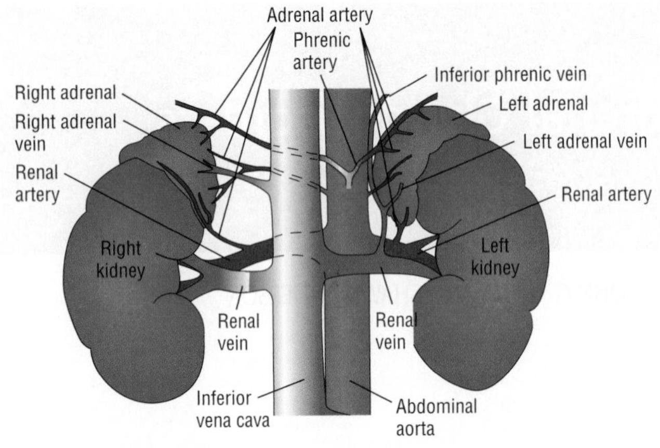

FIGURE 79-1. Anatomy of the adrenal gland.

Metabolism of glucocorticoids occurs in the liver and is responsible for converting inactive steroids to active metabolites, as well as deactivating the active steroids to less active or inactive metabolites. Most pharmaceutical steroid products are active; however, in the case of prednisone and cortisone, metabolism is necessary for the conversion to the active prednisolone and cortisol, respectively. Following metabolic conversion, glucocorticoids are excreted renally as less active or inactive metabolites.

After metabolism, glomerular filtration is primarily responsible for the elimination of endogenously produced glucocorticoids. The half-life of cortisol is 70 to 120 minutes; with aldosterone, the half-life is only 15 minutes because of an extremely high intrinsic clearance.

Metabolism and conversion of the various steroids can be altered by a variety of disease states and medicinal compounds. Drugs and diseases known to result in enhanced clearance of steroids include phenytoin, phenobarbital, rifampin, mitotane, aminoglutethimide, hyperthyroidism, and renal disease (dexamethasone only). Drugs and diseases known to result in reduced clearance of steroids include estrogens and estrogen-containing oral contraceptives, liver disease, age, pregnancy, hypothyroidism, anorexia nervosa, protein-calorie malnutrition, and renal disease (prednisolone only). Plasma glucocorticoids are bound to one of three plasma proteins in varying degrees. Corticosteroid-binding globulin (CBG), albumin, and α_1-glycoprotein are capable of binding glucocorticoids, with CBG being the principal binding protein.

The function of steroid binding is to serve as a reservoir of steroids in their inactive state. This binding can change the availability of glucocorticoids to receptor-activating sites. Therefore, a final but important variable in altered plasma concentration of free (active) steroids is concentration of plasma proteins.

REGULATION OF HORMONE SECRETION

❶ The regulation of glucocorticoid secretion is accomplished by the pituitary hormone, ACTH. Under normal conditions, ACTH is released from the anterior pituitary in response to CRH, which is secreted by the median eminence of the hypothalamus (Fig. 79–3). Vasopressin and oxytocin have weak ACTH-releasing activity through binding to the inferior V_3 receptor. CRH, in combination with vasopressin and oxytocin, stimulates greater ACTH secretion than each hormone individually.

Additionally, histochemical studies have demonstrated that certain neurotransmitters have the unique ability to stimulate production of CRH or ACTH directly. 5-Hydroxytryptamine and norepinephrine have both been shown to increase levels of ACTH. 5-Hydroxytryptamine causes a release of CRH through excitation of a cholinergic intervention. Norepinephrine can cause direct stimulation of ACTH release, although this effect is still controversial. After release, ACTH stimulates the adrenal gland to release cortisol and to a lesser extent aldosterone and androgens. The rising cortisol concentration inhibits the secretion of CRH and ACTH through a negative-feedback mechanism. In addition, leptin, an adipocyte hormone, can have inhibitory effects on HPA activity.

Regulation of adrenal androgens is accomplished in a manner similar to cortisol regulation. When plasma androgen reaches sufficient concentrations, production is terminated via a negative-feedback loop. Androgen release is increased during puberty and in women with hirsutism. Adrenal androgen release is decreased in fasting, anorexia nervosa, and aging.

Regulation of aldosterone secretion is considerably more complex. The renin-angiotensin system has the ability to respond to electrolyte and volume changes to increase or decrease aldosterone secretion. Renin production and subsequent aldosterone secretion is stimulated by blood pressure lowering, erect posture, salt depletion, β-adrenergic stimulation, and central nervous system excitation. Renin production is inhibited by salt loading, angiotensin II, vasopressin, potassium, calcium, blood pressure increases, and a variety of drugs. The conversion of renin substrate angiotensinogen

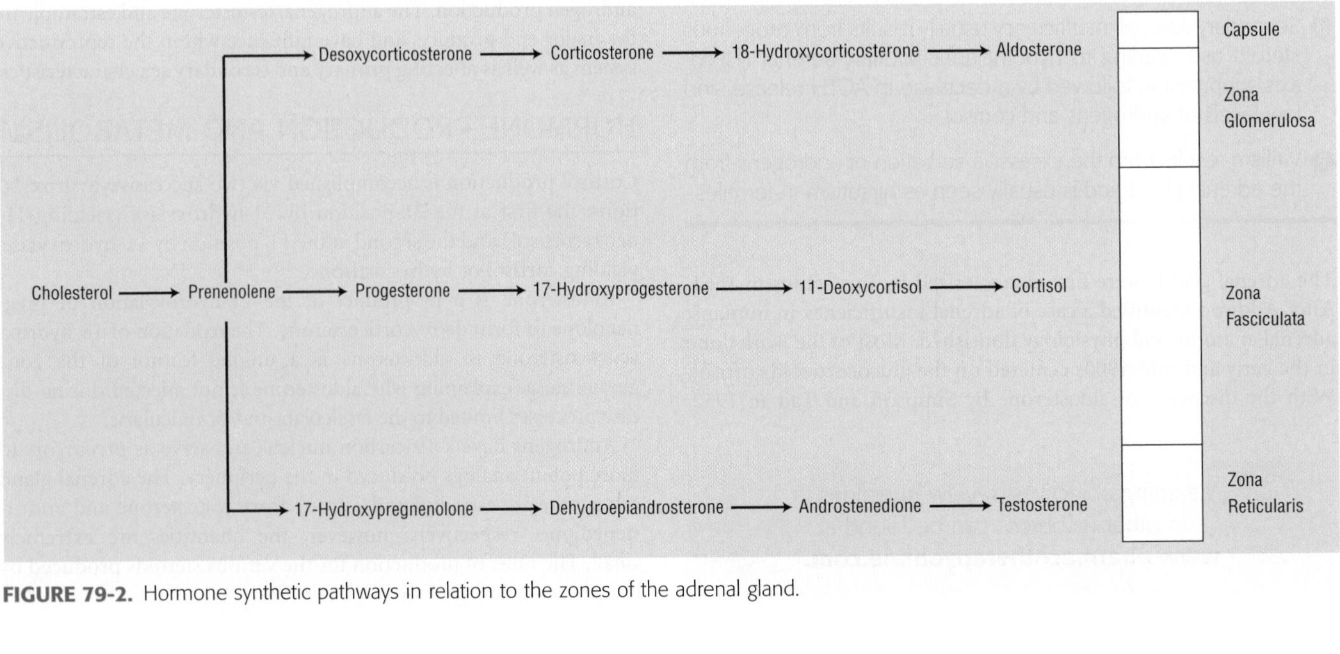

FIGURE 79-2. Hormone synthetic pathways in relation to the zones of the adrenal gland.

TABLE 79-1 Rates of Adrenal Production and Plasma Concentrations of Various Steroids

Steroid	24-Hour Secretion (mg)	Plasma Concentration (ng/dL)
Aldosterone	0.15	2–9 (supine, normal-sodium diet)
Androstenedione	2.2–2.5	50–250
Corticosterone	1–4	2.4 ± 1.5 (female) 4.2 ± 2.2 (male)
Cortisol	8–25	0–25 mcg/DL
11-Deoxycorticosterone	0.60	2–19
11-Deoxycortisol	0.40	12–158
Progesterone	0.0	<20 (female)[a] 300–2,000 (female)[b] <20–140 (male)
Testosterone (total)	0.23 (female)	6–86 (female) 270–1070 (male)

[a]Follicular phase of menstrual cycle
[b]Luteal phase of menstrual cycle
From Kratz A, Ferraro M, Sluss PM, Lewandrowski KB. Laboratory reference values. N Engl J Med 2004;351(15):1548–1563.

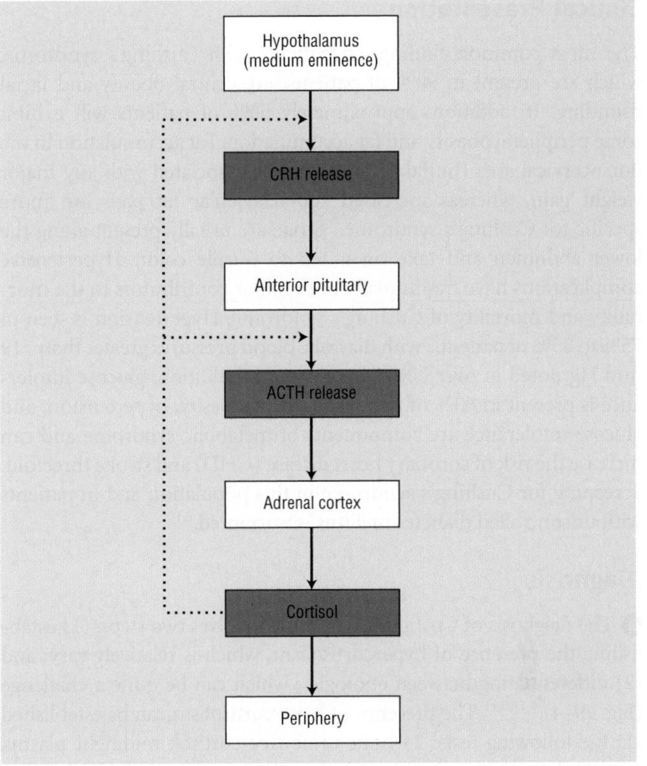

FIGURE 79-3. Negative feedback system involved in the regulation of cortisol secretion under normal conditions. (ACTH, adrenocorticotropic hormone; CRH, corticotropin-releasing hormone.)

to angiotensin I and subsequently to angiotensin II is the initial stimulus for aldosterone synthesis. Angiotensin II is acted on by aminopeptidase and converted to angiotensin III. Angiotensin II and III are both capable of stimulating the zona glomerulosa to secrete aldosterone. Following aldosterone secretion, increases in renal sodium and water retention as well as blood pressure are seen, thereby turning off the stimulus for renin release.

HYPERFUNCTION OF THE ADRENAL GLAND

CUSHING'S SYNDROME

In 1932, Cushing first described a syndrome of pituitary basophilism that attracted national attention. It was not until this time that patients with unexplained central obesity, cutaneous striae, osteoporosis, weakness, hypertension, diabetes mellitus, and congestion had a definite diagnosis. Cushing emphasized that the disease was of pituitary origin. Ten years later, Albright focused his attention on the sugar hormone, which he believed originated from the adrenal cortex.[3]

After the development of the method for measuring urinary steroids, Daughaday discovered elevated steroids in the urine of patients with Cushing's disease. Finally, the end product was identified, and Cushing's syndrome was correctly explained as an excess of cortisol in the plasma (hypercortisolism).

Etiology

Cushing's syndrome results from the effects of supraphysiologic levels of glucocorticoids originating either from exogenous administration or from endogenous overproduction by the adrenal glands (ACTH-dependent) or by abnormal adrenocortical tissues (ACTH-independent). ACTH-dependent Cushing's syndrome is usually (≈70% of Cushing's cases) caused by overproduction of ACTH by the pituitary gland, causing adrenal hyperplasia (Cushing's disease). Pituitary adenomas account for approximately 85% of these cases. Ectopic ACTH-secreting tumors and non-neoplastic corticotropin hypersecretion, possibly secondary to excess CRH production, are thought to be responsible for the remaining 20% of ACTH-dependent causes.[4] Ectopic ACTH syndrome refers to excessive ACTH production resulting from an endocrine or nonendocrine tumor, usually of the pancreas, thyroid, or lung. Small-cell carcinoma of the lung will lead to ectopic ACTH secretion in 0.5% to 2% of cases, whereas bronchial carcinoid tumors are usually the most common.[5] To distinguish between the various etiologies, a careful history and some pertinent laboratory work are required (Table 79–2).

The remaining 20% of Cushing's syndrome cases are ACTH-independent and are almost equally divided between adrenal adenomas and adrenal carcinomas, with rare cases caused by macronodular hyperplasia, primary pigmented nodular adrenal disease, and McCune-Albright syndrome.[4,6,7] The majority of adrenal cortex tumors are benign adenomas. Adrenal carcinoma is found more often in children than in adults with Cushing's syndrome.

TABLE 79-2 Various Etiologies of Cushing's Syndrome and Their Respective Differences

	Pituitary-Dependent	Ectopic ACTH Syndrome	Adrenal Adenoma	Adrenal Carcinoma
Course	Slow	Rapid	Slow	Rapid
Symptoms	Mild to moderate	Atypical	Mild to moderate	Severe
Dominant sex/age	Female/male	Male	None noted	Children
Virilization	+	+	+	+++
Abdominal mass	0	0	0	++
Plasma ACTH concentration	Slightly elevated	High	0	0
Dexamethasone suppression test	≥50% Suppression	No suppression	No suppression	No suppression
Iodocholesterol scan	Bilateral uptake	Bilateral uptake	Unilateral	None

ACTH, adrenocorticotropic hormone.

Clinical Presentation

The most common findings in patients with Cushing's syndrome, which are present in 90% of patients, are central obesity and facial rounding. In addition, approximately 50% of patients will exhibit some peripheral obesity and fat accumulation. Fat accumulation in the dorsocervical area (buffalo hump) can be associated with any major weight gain, whereas increased supraclavicular fat pads are more specific for Cushing's syndrome.[7] Striae are usually present along the lower abdomen and take on a red to purple color. Hypertensive complications have traditionally been major contributors to the morbidity and mortality of Cushing's syndrome. Hypertension is seen in 75% to 85% of patients, with diastolic blood pressures greater than 119 mm Hg noted in over 20% of patients.[8] In addition, glucose intolerance is present in 60% of patients. Central obesity, hypertension, and glucose intolerance are components of metabolic syndrome and can increase the risk of coronary heart disease (CHD) and stroke threefold. Screening for Cushing's syndrome in this population and in patients with uncontrolled diabetes mellitus is warranted.[9,10]

Diagnosis

❷ The diagnosis of Cushing's syndrome involves two steps: (1) establishing the presence of hypercortisolism, which is relatively easy; and (2) differentiating between etiologies, which can be quite a challenge (Fig. 79–4).[6,7,10,11] The presence of hypercortisolism can be established via the following tests: 24-hour urine free cortisol, midnight plasma cortisol, late-night salivary cortisol, and/or the low-dose dexamethasone suppression test (DST) (using 1 mg for the overnight test or 0.5 mg/6 h for the classic 2-day study). However, because these tests cannot determine the etiology of Cushing's syndrome, other tests and procedures subsequently will be employed. They can include any of the following: high-dose DST; plasma ACTH via immunoradiometric assay (IRMA) or radioimmunoassay (RIA); adrenal vein catheterization; metyrapone stimulation test; adrenal, chest, or abdominal computed tomography (CT); CRH stimulation test; inferior petrosal sinus sampling (IPSS); jugular venous sampling (JVS); cavernous sinus sampling; and pituitary magnetic resonance imaging (MRI). Other possible tests and procedures include insulin-induced hypoglycemia; somatostatin receptor scintigraphy; the desmopressin stimulation test; naloxone CRH stimulation test; loperamide test; the hexarelin stimulation test; and radionuclide imaging.[6–8,10–16] Table 79–3 summarizes some of the tests used to diagnose Cushing's syndrome.

Elevated urinary free cortisol concentrations are highly suggestive of Cushing's syndrome, especially values fourfold greater than the upper limit of normal.[4,13] Normal reference values for urinary free cortisol are 20 to 90 mcg per 24-hour period. It is not unusual to detect a twofold or threefold increase in urine cortisol in the patient with hyperfunction of the adrenal gland. Starvation, topical steroid application, hydration from water loading, alcoholism, and acute stress all are capable of elevating urine cortisol concentrations. Conversely, renal impairment (glomerular filtration rate [GFR] of less than 30 mL/min) can falsely lower urinary free cortisol concentrations. Because other pathologic conditions can increase the amount of free cortisol, additional tests should be performed to confirm the diagnosis, or the diagnostic evaluation should be repeated when the acute stress has resolved. Of all urinary measures, urinary free cortisol is the most useful for assessment of any patient with suspected Cushing's syndrome.[10,11,13]

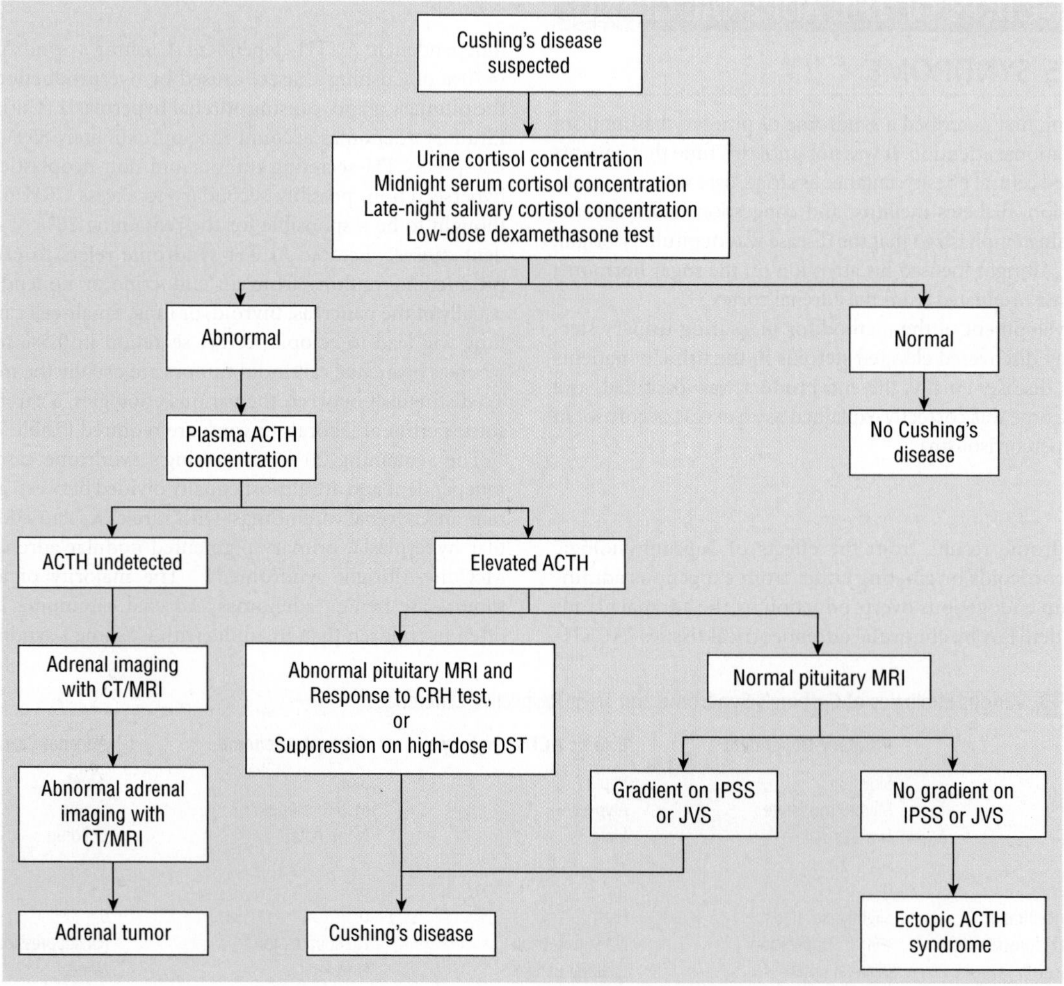

FIGURE 79-4. Algorithm for diagnosing Cushing's syndrome. (ACTH, adrenocorticotropic hormone.)

TABLE 79-3 Summary of Tests Used to Diagnose Cushing's Syndrome

Test	Normal	Hyperplasia	Adenoma	Carcinoma
Plasma				
Cortisol (mcg/dL, AM/PM)	5–25/5–15	↑/↑↑	↑↑/↑↑	↑↑↑/↑↑↑
After low-dose DST	↓	↔	↔	↔
After high-dose DST	↓	↓/↔	↔	↔
ACTH (pg/mL)	6–76	↑↑	↓	↓
Urine				
Cortisol (mcg/24 h)	20–90	↑↑	↑↑	↑↑↑
Saliva				
Cortisol (mcg/dL, PM)	Assay dependent	↑↑	↑↑	↑↑↑

ACTH, adrenocorticotropic hormone; DST, dexamethasone suppression test.

From Kratz A, Ferraro M, Sluss PM, Lewandrowski KB. Laboratory reference values. N Engl J Med 2004;351(15):1548-1563.

CLINICAL PRESENTATION: CUSHING'S SYNDROME

General

- The most common findings, which are present in 90% of patients, are central obesity and facial rounding.

Symptoms

- Approximately 65% and 58% of patients complain of myopathies and muscular weakness, respectively.

Signs

- Peripheral obesity and fat accumulation is found in 50% of patients.
- Facial plethora is caused by an underlying atrophy of the skin and connective tissue and is seen in approximately 84% of patients.
- Patients often are described as having moon facies with a buffalo hump.
- Hypertension is seen in 75% to 85% of patients.
- Psychiatric changes can occur in as many as 55% of patients.
- Approximately 50% to 60% of patients will develop Cushing-induced osteoporosis. Of these, 40% will present with back pain and 20% will progress to compression fractures of the spine.
- Gonadal dysfunction is common with amenorrhea seen in up to 75% of females.
- Excess androgen secretion is responsible for 80% of females presenting with hirsutism.

Laboratory Tests

- A midnight plasma cortisol, late-night salivary cortisol, 24-hour urine free cortisol, and/or low-dose DST will establish the presence of hypercortisolism.

Other Diagnostic Tests

- The high-dose DST, plasma ACTH test, metyrapone stimulation test, CRH stimulation test, or inferior petrosal sinus sampling will help determine the etiology.

The normal circadian rhythm of cortisol will demonstrate a 60% to 80% decline between 8:00 AM and 11:00 PM. This rhythm is lost in the Cushing's syndrome patient. Although many patients with Cushing's syndrome will have serum cortisol values in the high normal range if the serum is assayed in the morning, only 3.4% will have normal values if measured late at night.[17] Thus, a midnight serum cortisol greater than 7.5 mcg/dL is a highly sensitive assay for Cushing's syndrome. However, this test requires that patients be admitted for more than 48 hours to avoid false-positive responses secondary to the stress of hospitalization. Also if a patient is sleeping, a lower serum cortisol value (>1.8 mcg/dL) should be used. An alternative assay is the measurement of late-night salivary cortisol. Salivary cortisol is highly correlated with free serum cortisol independent of salivary flow rates. This test is used in a similar manner to midnight plasma cortisol, with the exception of an 11 PM sample collection. Salivary cortisol can be considered as an acceptable alternative to urinary free cortisol because of its convenience, stability (1 week), accuracy, and reproducibility. Unfortunately, normal reference ranges are assay-dependent, and cutoff points vary among institutions.[18,19]

In the overnight DST, 1 mg of dexamethasone is administered at 11:00 PM. The following morning at 8:00 AM fasting plasma cortisol is obtained for analysis. The Cushing's syndrome patient will not exhibit a suppressed cortisol concentration via the negative-feedback loop, and the morning cortisol concentration will be elevated above 5 mcg/dL. However, some Cushing's patients administered the overnight DST can slightly suppress cortisol and using 1.8 mcg/dL as a cutoff can increase sensitivity .[7,20] The overnight DST is useful only as a screening tool for Cushing's syndrome, not because of high sensitivity, but rather low specificity. Phenytoin, rifampin, phenobarbital, and other drugs that induce liver enzymes can cause an increase in the clearance rate of the dexamethasone, causing decreased levels leading to a false-positive suppression test. In addition, increased concentration of CBG noted in pregnancy and with estrogen use can also illicit a false-positive suppression test.[13] Plasma dexamethasone measured at the conclusion of this test can clarify results clouded by differences in metabolism from these drug interactions, individual variability, or patient noncompliance.

The first test used to determine the etiology of Cushing's syndrome is the plasma ACTH test. Plasma ACTH concentrations can be measured via RIA or IRMA.[12] In ACTH-dependent Cushing's syndromes, ACTH can be normal or elevated. Very high levels of ACTH favor ectopic production. ACTH values are low (<5 pg/mL) in ACTH-independent (adrenal) Cushing's syndrome. ACTH levels can appear artificially low in some ectopic ACTH-producing tumors because ACTH can be secreted as an active prohormone that is not detected by the assay.

The high-dose DST operates under the same principle as the low-dose test.[4,12,13] The high-dose test has its main application in differentiating the Cushing's disease patient from the patient with another form of hypercortisolism. The Cushing's disease patient will generally demonstrate a 50% reduction in urinary steroids over baseline, whereas the others will generally not suppress. The high-dose test is based on the principle that patients with Cushing's syndrome not caused by adrenal tumors or ectopic ACTH production will suppress their hypothalamic-pituitary axis in the presence of glucocorticoids, but it takes much higher-than-normal doses. An overnight high-dose DST has been developed, whereby the patient has a baseline serum cortisol drawn at 8:00 AM and dexamethasone 8 mg is taken at 11:00 PM. The next morning, at 8:00 AM, another serum cortisol is drawn.[17] The high-dose test is most useful when the low-dose test and other diagnostic studies have confirmed the diagnosis of Cushing's syndrome. The high-dose DST has been studied in combination with ACTH and metapyrone testing, and results in better specificity than either test alone. In addition, specificity of high-dose DST can be increased by using an 80% reduction in urinary steroids over baseline.[13]

IPSS offers the highest sensitivity and specificity of any test to confirm Cushing's syndrome. This technique requires catheterization of both petrosal sinuses with serial measurements of ACTH in each sinus and a peripheral vein after administration of CRH. A central-to-peripheral ACTH gradient is diagnostic for Cushing's syndrome whereas no gradient indicates ectopic ACTH production.

Complications, such as venous thromboembolism and brain stem vascular damage, cost, and testing expertise can limit use.[12] JVS uses the same concept as IPSS, is less invasive, and produces fewer complications; however, sensitivity is compromised.

Abnormal adrenal anatomy is effectively identified using high-resolution CT scanning and perhaps MRI.[21] Nodules as small as 1 to 1.5 cm on the adrenal cortex are easily identified by CT. With the use of thin-section scanning, nodules as small as 3 to 5 mm can be visualized.[22,23] In ACTH-dependent Cushing's syndrome, a pituitary MRI should be performed prior to inferior petrosal sinus sampling detecting 40% to 52% of tumors.[11,12]

Differential Diagnosis

Although the diagnosis of Cushing's disease is not a difficult one, at times the clinician will need to differentiate it from syndromes that mimic Cushing's. Pseudo-Cushing's syndrome refers to a group of diseases that can mimic Cushing's disease. Patients with obesity, chronic alcoholism, depression, and acute illness of any type can cloud the diagnosis of Cushing's disease. Depressed patients, although mimicking the urinary steroid abnormalities of Cushing's disease, will not resemble a cushingoid patient in appearance. The chronic alcoholic will have his or her laboratory panel returned to baseline after he or she stops drinking. The obese patient often will have normal cortisol concentrations on both serum and urinary screening. Iatrogenic Cushing's syndrome, induced by pharmacologic agents, often is indistinguishable from Cushing's disease. This syndrome can occur from administration of oral, inhaled, intranasal, intra-articular, and topical glucocorticoids, as well as progestins such as medroxyprogesterone acetate and megestrol acetate.[24] Patients taking an inhibitor of cytochrome P450 3A4 concomitantly with a glucocorticoid can be at higher risk of developing iatrogenic Cushing's syndrome.[25,26] A careful history and serum determination in a basal state can aid the clinician in making the diagnosis. If exogenous glucocorticoids are being taken, plasma cortisol levels can increase, while corticosterone levels remain low.[17,27]

TREATMENT

Cushing's Syndrome

❸ If left untreated, Cushing's syndrome is associated with a high percentage of morbidity and mortality owing to associated disorders such as diabetes mellitus, cardiovascular disease, and electrolyte abnormalities. These disorders limit the survival of the Cushing's disease patient to 4 to 5 years following initial diagnosis. The desired outcomes of treatment are to limit the morbidity and mortality and return the patient to a normal functional state by removing the source of hypercortisolism without causing any pituitary or adrenal deficiencies.

❹ Once the etiology of the disease is identified, the treatment of choice for both ACTH-dependent and ACTH-independent Cushing's syndrome is surgical resection of any offending tumors.[4,11] However, several secondary pharmacologic treatment plans are available, depending on the etiology of the disease (Table 79–4).[28–30]

■ PHARMACOLOGIC THERAPY

❺ Pharmacotherapy of Cushing's syndrome (dosing can be found in Table 79–4)[31] can be divided into four categories based on the anatomic site of action of the agent: (1) steroidogenic inhibitors; (2) adrenolytic agents; (3) neuromodulators of ACTH release; and (4) glucocorticoid-receptor blocking agents.[28–30]

Steroidogenic inhibition can be accomplished with the following agents: metyrapone, aminoglutethimide, ketoconazole, and etomidate. Aminoglutethimide used alone has limited efficacy, with relapse occurring after discontinuation of therapy. In addition, steroidogenic inhibitors should not be used after successful surgery. Their use is mainly in preparation for surgery, as adjunctive treatment after unsuccessful surgery or radiotherapy, or for the refractory patient who is not a surgical candidate. Combination therapy with metyrapone and aminoglutethimide appears more effective than either alone and can cause fewer side effects.

Metyrapone inhibits 11-hydroxylase activity, resulting in inhibition of cortisol synthesis. Initially, patients can demonstrate an increase in plasma ACTH concentrations because of a sudden drop in cortisol. As such, increased ACTH concentrations can cause an increase in androgenic and mineralocorticoid hormones resulting in hypertension, acne, and hirsutism. Metyrapone is biologically active following oral administration. Nausea, vomiting, vertigo, headache, dizziness, abdominal discomfort, and allergic rash have been reported following administration.[28–30,32]

Initially, aminoglutethimide was used to treat refractory forms of epilepsy, but it was later discovered to be a potent inhibitor of cortisol synthesis. Aminoglutethimide inhibits the conversion of cholesterol to pregnenolone early in the cortisol pathway.[33] Plasma cortisol concentrations are reduced by up to 50% following aminoglutethimide therapy. Side effects include severe sedation, nausea, ataxia, and skin rashes.[28–30] Most of these reactions are dose-depen-

TABLE 79-4 Possible Treatment Plans in Cushing's Syndrome Based on Etiology

		Treatment			
			Dosing		
Etiology	*Nondrug*	*Generic (Brand) Drug Name*	*Initial*	*Usual*	*Max*
Ectopic ACTH syndrome	Surgery, chemotherapy, irradiation	Metyrapone (Metopirone) 250-mg capsules	0.5–1 g/day, divided every 4–6 h	1–2 g/day, divided every 4–6 h	6 g/day
		Aminoglutethimide (Cytadren) 250-mg tabs	0.5–1 g/day, divided two to four times a day for 2 weeks	1 g/day, divided every 6 h	2 g/day
Pituitary-dependent	Surgery, irradiation	Cyproheptadine (Periactin) 2 mg/5 mL syrup or 4-mg tabs	4 mg twice a day	24–32 mg/day, divided four times a day	32 mg/day
		Mitotane (Lysodren) 500-mg tabs	0.5–1 g/day, increased by 0.5–1 g/day every 1–4 weeks	1–4 g daily, with food to decrease GI effects	12 g/day
		Metyrapone	See above	See above	See above
Adrenal adenoma	Surgery, postoperative replacement	Ketoconazole (Nizoral) 200-mg tabs	200 mg once or twice a day	200–1200 mg/day, divided twice a day	1600 mg/day divided four times a day
Adrenal carcinoma	Surgery	Mitotane	See above	See above	See above

ACTH, adrenocorticotropic hormone.

dent and limit the use of aminoglutethimide in most patients. Aminoglutethimide can decrease the anticoagulant effect of warfarin. As aminoglutethimide can induce the metabolism of exogenous glucocorticoids, careful titration is required with steroid replacement. Aminoglutethimide also blocks the synthesis of thyroxine, which can result in elevated thyroid-stimulating hormone (TSH) levels and hypothyroidism.[29]

Alone, aminoglutethimide is indicated for short-term use in inoperable Cushing's disease with ectopic ACTH syndrome as the suspected underlying etiology. Aminoglutethimide can be used in combination with metyrapone. Smaller doses of both drugs can be used, thereby minimizing the toxicity associated with either agent. The combination therapy appears effective for various etiologies of Cushing's disease and is useful in the inoperable patient.

The imidazole derivative antifungal ketoconazole is highly effective in lowering cortisol in Cushing's disease, resulting in normal corticosteroid values in 84% of patients, with an additional 11% of patients reporting improvement.[28–30] Patients can be maintained successfully for months to years on ketoconazole therapy. In addition to lowering serum cortisol levels, ketoconazole can cause gynecomastia and lower plasma testosterone values. All of these effects are attributed to its inhibition of a variety of cytochrome P450 enzymes, including 11-hydroxylase and 17-hydroxylase.[29] In some patients, ACTH levels actually decrease suggesting ketoconazole has a secondary inhibitory effect on ACTH. The most common adverse effects are reversible elevation of hepatic transaminases, gynecomastia, and gastrointestinal upset.[28–30]

The anesthetic etomidate is an imidazole derivative similar to ketoconazole that inhibits 11-hydroxylase.[29] Etomidate is only available in a parenteral formulation; therefore, use is limited to patients with acute hypercortisolemia awaiting surgery.

The adrenolytic agent mitotane is a cytotoxic drug that structurally resembles the insecticide dichlorodiphenyltrichloroethane (DDT). Mitotane inhibits the 11-hydroxylation of 11-desoxycortisol and 11-desoxycorticosterone in the cortex. The net result is a reduced synthesis of cortisol and corticosterone. It decreases the cortisol secretion rate, plasma cortisol concentrations, urinary free cortisol, and plasma concentrations of the 17 substituted steroids.[31] This drug appears to selectively inhibit adrenocortical function without causing cellular destruction. Degeneration of cells within the zona fasciculata and reticularis occurs with resultant atrophy of the adrenal cortex. The zona glomerulosa is minimally affected during acute therapy but can become damaged following long-term treatment.[28,31,34]

Because mitotane can severely reduce cortisol production, the patient should be hospitalized before initiating therapy. Mitotane should be continued as long as clinical benefits occur. Mitotane increases production of corticosteroid binding globulin resulting in elevated plasma cortisol; thus, urinary free cortisol, and urinary steroid production should be monitored to assess response to therapy.[29] If necessary, steroid replacement therapy can be given. Nausea and diarrhea are common adverse effects that occur at doses greater than 2 g/day and can be avoided by gradually increasing the dose and/or administering the agent with food. Approximately 80% of mitotane-treated patients develop lethargy and somnolence, and other central nervous system adverse drug reactions occur in approximately 40% of patients. Furthermore, significant but reversible hypercholesterolemia can result from mitotane use.[29,30]

Neuromodulatory agents include cyproheptadine, ritanserin, bromocriptine, cabergoline, valproic acid, octreotide, lanreotide, rosiglitazone, and tretinoin. None of the neuromodulatory agents has demonstrated consistent clinical efficacy in the treatment of Cushing's disease. The existence of a bromocriptine-responsive subset of patients remains controversial.[28,29] Combination therapy with these agents can prove more efficacious than any one agent alone. For example, cabergoline plus lanreotide successfully normalized urinary free cortisol in one patient when treatment failed on either agent alone.[35]

Cyproheptadine can decrease ACTH secretion in the Cushing's disease patient. Morning plasma cortisol concentrations, as well as 24-hour urinary cortisol (free) concentrations should be monitored. Side effects are minor and include sedation and hyperphagia. Cyproheptadine should be reserved for nonsurgical candidates who fail more conventional therapy. Because the response rate is no more than 30%, patients should be followed closely for relapses.

Tretinoin, also known as all-*trans*-retinoic acid, is a derivative of vitamin A that has been used for the treatment of acute promyelocytic leukemia. Tretinoin can reduce the secretion of ACTH through inhibition of transcriptional activities.[36] In addition to ACTH suppression, tretinoin inhibits tumor growth, which is consistent with its use as an antineoplastic agent. The use of this agent has been limited to animal models; thus, efficacy in humans is yet undetermined.

Glucocorticoid receptor antagonism can be accomplished via RU-486 (mifepristone). RU-486 is a progesterone-, androgen-, and glucocorticoid-receptor antagonist that inhibits dexamethasone suppression and increases endogenous cortisol and ACTH values in normal subjects.[29,32] Limited clinical experience in Cushing's suggests that RU-486 is highly effective in reversing the manifestation of hypercortisolism. Because of its novel site of action as a receptor antagonist leading to higher cortisol and ACTH levels, the diagnosis of treatment-induced glucocorticoid insufficiency must rest on clinical signs only. The efficacy and long-term effects of RU-486 remain to be determined.

Spironolactone has been used for its competitive antagonism of aldosterone in the treatment of Cushing's syndrome. Spironolactone can provide symptomatic relief of the hypertension and hypokalemia often seen in Cushing's syndrome.

Close monitoring of 24-hour urinary free cortisol levels and serum cortisol levels are essential to monitor for adrenal insufficiency. Steroid secretion should be monitored with all of these drugs and steroid replacement given as needed. Whatever the choice, pharmacologic therapy in pituitary-dependent disease is mainly centered around patient stabilization prior to surgery or in patients waiting for potential response to other therapies.

■ NONPHARMACOLOGIC THERAPY

Surgery

During the last decade, the treatment of choice for Cushing's disease has been transsphenoidal resection of the pituitary microadenoma.[4,11,32,37] The advantages to this procedure include preservation of pituitary function, low complication rate, and high clinical improvement rate. The overall cure rate of histologically proven tumors approaches 98%.

Bilateral adrenalectomy surgery had been the mainstay of therapy for years. Laparoscopic surgery is now the treatment of choice in patients for whom transsphenoidal surgery and pituitary radiotherapy have failed or cannot be used, with primary pigmented nodular adrenal disease, and with macronodular adrenal hyperplasia.[4,11,32,38] Bilateral adrenalectomy rapidly reverses hypercortisolism. However, patients can develop Nelson syndrome, which involves sella turcica enlargement and hyperpigmentation, caused by postoperative hypothalamic stimulation. Therefore if bilateral adrenalectomy is used it should be accompanied by some form of hypothalamic inhibition, such as cyproheptadine or pituitary radiation.

Irradiation of the pituitary has provided clinical improvement in approximately 50% of patients. Improvement is usually not seen until 6 to 12 months after therapy and can create pituitary-dependent hormone deficiencies (hypopituitarism). Most clinicians will reserve pituitary radiotherapy for the patient with persistent hypercortisolemia after transsphenoidal surgery.[4,39]

TABLE 79-5 Alternative Steroid Replacement Regimens in the Adrenal Adenoma Patient

	Hydrocortisone Dose (mg)		
Time	***IV***	***IM***	***PO***
Operation day	300	50 before surgery and 50 after surgery	
Postoperative day 1	200	50 every 12 h	
Postoperative day 2	150	50 every 12 h	
Postoperative day 3	100	50 every 12 h	
Postoperative day 4		50 every 12 h	25 every 6 h
Postoperative day 5		25 every 12 h	25 every 6 h[a]
Postoperative day 7			25 every 6 h
Postoperative days 8–10			25 every 8 h
Postoperative days 11–20			25 every 12 h
Postoperative days 21+			20 at 8 AM 10 at 4 PM

PO, orally.

[a]Add fludrocortisone 0.05–2 mg orally once daily starting on postoperative day 5. Adjust dose based on blood pressure, body weight, and serum electrolytes.

Adrenal Adenoma

Surgical resection of benign adrenal adenoma is associated with relatively few side effects and a high cure rate (95%). The contralateral gland in the patient with adrenal adenoma is usually atrophic, therefore steroid replacement is needed both perioperatively and postoperatively. Table 79–5 outlines an approach to steroid replacement for three separate routes of hydrocortisone. Therapy should be continued for 6 to 12 months following surgery. Before replacement therapy is discontinued, recovery of the adrenal axis can be assessed by measuring the morning (8 AM) cortisol level. Cortisol levels should exceed 20 mcg/dL before discontinuance of the exogenous steroids.[24]

Adrenal Carcinoma

Unlike the benign adenoma patient, patients with adrenal carcinoma have an unpredictable and unfavorable outcome with surgical resection.[11] Often the complete tumor cannot be excised, leaving the patient with some degree of symptomatology and extra-adrenal involvement. Radiotherapy can be used if metastases are discovered. In the patient with adrenal carcinoma who is not a surgical candidate, the focus of treatment is on palliative pharmacologic intervention (e.g., mitotane).

Mitotane appears to be the drug of choice in inoperable functional and nonfunctional adrenal carcinoma. Tumor regression is seen in approximately 35% to 50% of patients, with most regression occurring between the second and fourth month of therapy. Seventy-five percent of patients will exhibit a 30% decrease in urinary steroids, with 50% of patients showing an improved clinical response after 5 months of treatment. Patient survival appears prolonged, although no adequate clinical trials are available to support this assumption.

Metyrapone, aminoglutethimide, and ketoconazole can be given to attempt control of steroid hypersecretion. 5-Fluorouracil has also been used in combination therapy.

Ectopic ACTH Syndrome

In the ectopic ACTH syndrome, multiple sites of tumors exist, and locating the ectopic sites are essential but often difficult. Therefore only approximately 10% to 30% of patients are cured following surgery, and the remaining 70% to 90% receive postoperative medication.

Surgical excision remains optimal in these patients. Pharmacologic management with metyrapone and ketoconazole is effective in ectopic ACTH syndrome. Aminoglutethimide is an alternative agent but is more effective when combined with other inhibitors, usually metyrapone.[5,29,40] Mitotane has been tried in patients with ectopic ACTH syndrome; however, its side-effect profile generally limits its use. RU-486 and the somatostatin analog octreotide have been reported to reduce the clinical signs of the ectopic ACTH syndrome.[28] Bilateral adrenalectomy is performed when surgical excision of the tumor and pharmacologic treatments fail.

HYPERALDOSTERONISM

Excess aldosterone is categorized as either primary or secondary hyperaldosteronism.[41–46]

Primary Aldosteronism

Etiology Primary aldosteronism (PAL) implies that the physiologic abnormality is within the adrenal cortex. The most common causes include BAH (70%) and aldosterone-producing adenoma (APA) (30%). Historically, APA was the most common cause, but screening normokalemic, hypertensive patients has detected less severe forms of PAL more commonly diagnosed as BAH.[47] Other rare causes include unilateral adrenal hyperplasia, adrenal cortex carcinoma, primary adrenocortical hyperplasia, renin-responsive adrenocortical adenoma, and two forms of familial hyperaldosteronism (FH): FH type 1, or glucocorticoid-remediable aldosteronism (GRA), and FH type II.[41,42,44]

Clinical Presentation The incidence of primary aldosteronism is disputed, with estimates ranging from approximately 3% to 32%, depending on the selection of hypertensive populations.[41,43] The disease is more common in women aged 30 to 50 years. Signs and symptoms can include arterial hypertension, muscle weakness, fatigue, and headache, although many patients are asymptomatic.

Diagnosis The absolute diagnosis is obtainable through screening, confirmatory tests, and subtype differentiation by skilled clinicians. As in Cushing's disease, the discovery of the underlying etiology is mandatory to ensure proper treatment. Table 79–6 lists the various abnormalities that must be ruled out when suspicion of hyperaldosteronism is high.

CLINICAL PRESENTATION: PRIMARY ALDOSTERONISM

Symptoms

- Patients may complain of muscle weakness, fatigue, paresthesias, and headache.
- Signs
- Hypertension
- Tetany/paralysis
- Polydipsia/nocturnal polyuria

Laboratory Tests

- A plasma-aldosterone–to–plasma-renin-activity ratio (PA:PRA), or aldosterone-to-renin ratio (ARR) greater than 20 is suggestive of primary aldosteronism
- Common laboratory findings include suppressed renin activity, elevated plasma aldosterone concentrations, hypernatremia (>142 mEq/L), hypokalemia, hypomagnesemia, elevated bicarbonate concentration (>31 mEq/L), and glucose intolerance

Confirmatory Tests

- Oral or intravenous saline loading, fludrocortisone suppression test (FST), and genetic testing

TABLE 79-6 Differential Diagnosis of Primary Aldosteronism

Disease	Plasma Renin Concentration	Plasma Aldosterone Concentration	Blood Pressure
Primary aldosteronism	Low	High	High
Edematous disorders	High	High	Normal
Malignant hypertension	High	High	High
Congenital adrenal hyperplasia	Low	Low	High
Cushing's syndrome	Low to normal	Low to normal	High
Liddle's syndrome	Low	Low	High
Bartter's syndrome	High	High	Low to normal
Licorice ingestion	Low	Low	High
Low-renin essential hypertension	Low	Low to normal	High

Although serum potassium concentration of less than 3.5 mEq/L with a concurrent urinary potassium content greater than 30 mEq per 24 hours is suggestive of primary aldosteronism, normokalemia can be present in up to 80% of diagnosed patients.[48] Initial diagnosis is made through proper screening of patients with suspected primary aldosteronism, such as resistant hypertensives with or without hypokalemia. Some institutions choose to screen patients with stage 2 hypertension realizing that the prevalence of PAL increases with hypertensive severity.[47,49] Screening for primary aldosteronism is most often done by using the plasma-aldosterone-concentration–to–plasma-renin-activity ratio (PAC:PRA), or aldosterone-to-renin ratio (ARR). An elevated ARR is highly suggestive of PAL; however, an optimal cutoff level is nonexistent because of testing conditions (posture, time, drug therapy), patient characteristics, and variable levels of specificity and sensitivity. For example, Hirohara and colleagues[50] found an ARR greater than 32 to be 100% sensitive and 61% specific in patients with aldosterone-producing adenomas, whereas Giacchetti and colleagues[51] determined that a supine ARR cutoff of 25 was 98% sensitive and 67% specific and an upright ARR cutoff of 40 was 100% sensitive and 84% specific in patients with confirmed PAL and hypertension. ARR cutoffs of 20 to 40 or 20 with an aldosterone level greater than 15 ng/dL are most commonly used.[43,52,53]

Confirmatory testing must be done after a positive ARR screening test. Oral or intravenous saline loading and the FST are the most widely used, with FST being the most reliable.[43,47] Positive tests demonstrate autonomous aldosterone secretion under inhibitory pressures and are diagnostic for PAL. After diagnosis, all patients should undergo genetic testing to properly identify GRA or FH type I.[42]

Differentiating between an APA and BAH is imperative to formulate a proper treatment plan. A majority of the adenomas are singular and small, less than 1 cm. The left adrenal gland is affected at a higher rate than the right. Patients with APA generally have more severe hypertension, more profound hypokalemia, and higher plasma and urinary aldosterone levels compared to patients with BAH. CT scanning can usually detect most adenomas, although an incidentaloma can occasionally cause confusion. If CT scanning is inconclusive, adrenal venous sampling (AVS) is performed to indicate lateralization, or aldosterone secretion from one adrenal gland.[43,47,49,54,55]

The underlying abnormality in BAH remains a mystery, but some investigators believe that a hormone factor stimulates the zona glomerulosa, resulting in increased sensitivity to angiotensin II. In contrast to APA patients, patients with BAH are able to maintain control of the renin-angiotensin system, with little effect following doses of ACTH.

Therapeutic Management

6 ***BAH-Dependent Aldosteronism.*** Spironolactone, the drug of choice in BAH-dependent aldosteronism, competitively inhibits aldosterone biosynthesis within the adrenal gland, making it extremely useful in overstimulated BAH patients.[43,56,57] It is available in oral form, with most patients responding to doses of 25 to 400 mg/day. The clinician should wait 4 to 8 weeks before reassessing the patient for urinary electrolytes and blood pressure control. Adverse effects of spironolactone include gastrointestinal discomfort, impotence, gynecomastia, and menstrual irregularities, and are dose-dependent. Additionally, because salicylates increase the renal secretion of canrenone, the active metabolite, patients should be advised to avoid concomitant therapy with salicylates. Because spironolactone blocks testosterone biosynthesis, it often is not used in men. In patients intolerant of spironolactone, eplerenone and amiloride are options.[43,49,56–58] Eplerenone, an aldosterone antagonist with high affinity for the aldosterone receptor and low affinity for androgen and progesterone receptors, has been approved for the treatment of hypertension. It appears to be more beneficial than spironolactone because of its limited progestational and antiandrogenic side effects. Dosing starts at 50 mg daily, with titration to 50 mg twice a day.[49] Again, titration should occur at 4 to 8 week intervals. In addition, eplerenone is a substrate of CYP3A4 and should not be taken with potent CYP3A4 inhibitors. Eplerenone has been proven effective in low-renin hypertension; however, its role in the management of hyperaldosteronism has not been established.[59]

The usual dose of amiloride is 5 mg twice a day up to 30 mg/day if necessary. Unfortunately, amiloride is not as effective as aldosterone antagonists in BAH; thus second-line therapy is often required to control the blood pressure. Agents useful as second-line choices include the calcium channel blockers, angiotensin-converting enzyme inhibitors, and low-dose diuretics such as hydrochlorothiazide.[55,56]

APA-Dependent Aldosteronism. The treatment of choice for APA-dependent aldosteronism remains laparoscopic resection of the adenoma.[60] Nearly 100% of patients show blood pressure improvement with 30% to 60% resulting in long-term cure.[57,61] If no primary lesion is found, resection of one and a half of the adrenal glands can be attempted, followed by supplemental spironolactone therapy. However, a recent retrospective analysis of patients with aldosterone-producing adenomas who chose medical management instead of surgical resection, revealed medical management to be efficacious in this population and should be considered as an alternative in patients in whom surgery is contraindicated.[62]

Glucocorticoid-Remediable Aldosteronism. Glucocorticoids are very effective in treating GRA.[42] Low doses are typically used (0.125 to 0.5 mg/day of dexamethasone or 2.5 to 5 mg/day of prednisone) because complete suppression of ACTH-stimulated aldosterone release is unnecessary. Spironolactone, eplerenone, and amiloride are alternative treatment options.[43]

Summary The diagnosis of primary aldosteronism is made through proper screening of suspected patients and confirmatory testing. Differentiating between the various etiologies is mandatory (Fig. 79–5). Patients with adrenal adenomas can be distinguished from patients with hyperplasia by CT scan, but adrenal venous sampling provides increased sensitivity and specificity. Treatment depends on the etiology with surgical resection, well accepted as the treatment of choice in adenomas, and spironolactone, eplerenone, or amiloride plus second-line agents in patients with hyperplasia.

Secondary Aldosteronism

Secondary aldosteronism results from stimulation of the zona glomerulosa by an extra-adrenal factor, usually the renin-angiotensin system. Excessive potassium intake can create a physiologic increase in aldosterone, as can oral contraceptive use, pregnancy (10 times normal by the third trimester), and menses. Congestive heart failure, cirrhosis, renal artery stenosis, and Bartter syndrome also can lead to elevated aldosterone concentrations.

Treatment of secondary aldosteronism is dictated by etiology. Control or correction of the extra-adrenal stimulation of aldosterone secretion should resolve the disorder. Medical therapy with spironolactone is the mainstay of treatment until an exact etiology can be located.

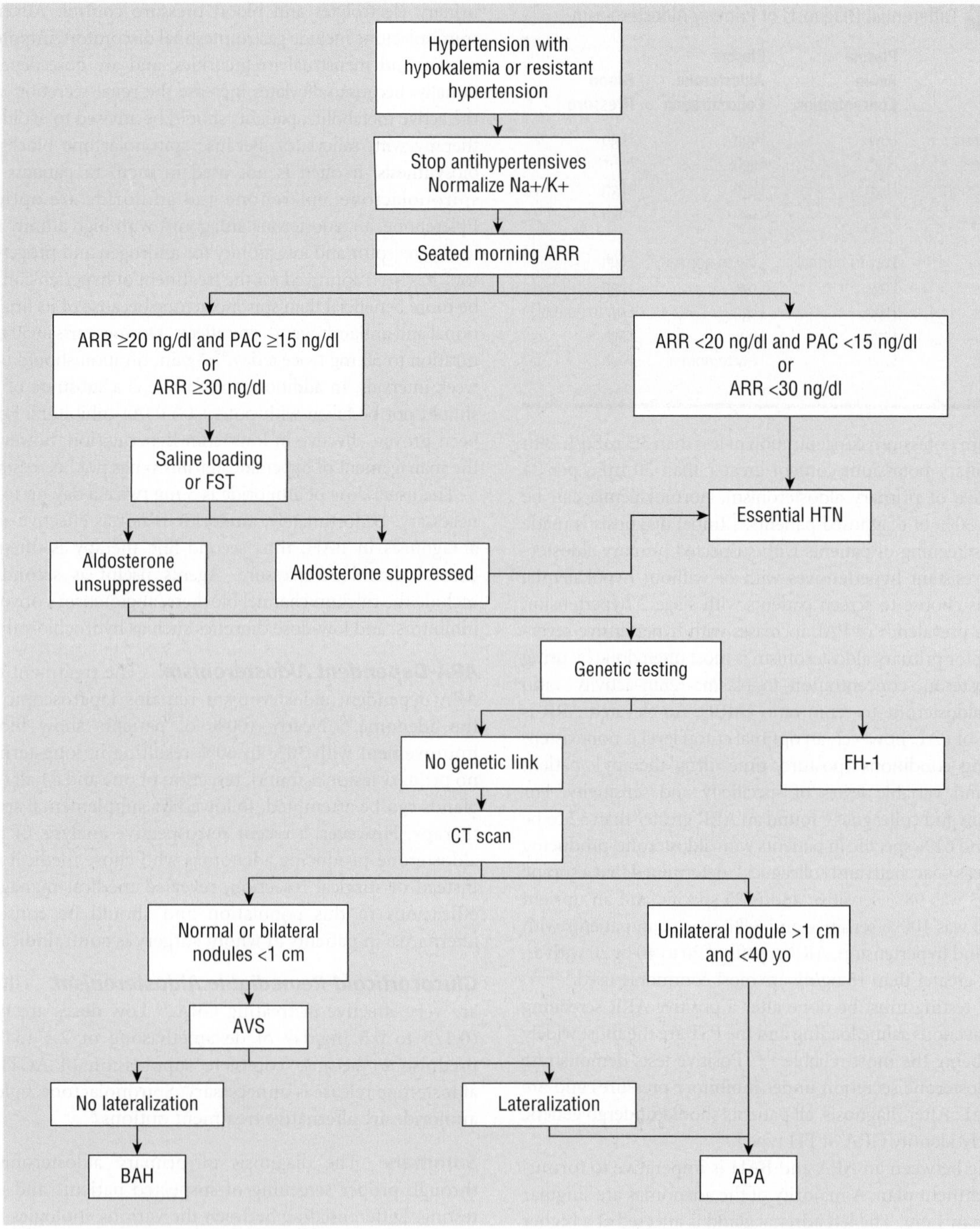

FIGURE 79-5. Algorithm for the diagnosis of primary aldosteronism.

HYPOFUNCTION OF THE ADRENAL GLAND

❼ Primary adrenal insufficiency, or Addison's disease, most often involves the destruction of all regions of the adrenal cortex. Deficiencies arise in cortisol, aldosterone, and the various androgens. Approximately 40% to 53% of patients with idiopathic primary adrenal insufficiency present with one or more clinical disorders involving multiple endocrine organs. The organs involved can include ovary, thyroid, pancreas, and parathyroid gland. This polyglandular failure syndrome is associated with the idiopathic etiology only and has not been seen with adrenal insufficiency associated with tuberculosis or other invasive diseases. Medications that inhibit cortisol synthesis (ketoconazole), or accelerate cortisol metabolism (phenytoin, rifampin, phenobarbital) can also cause primary adrenal insufficiency.[63,64]

❽ Secondary insufficiency most commonly results from exogenous steroid use, leading to suppression of the HPA axis and decreased release of ACTH, resulting in impaired androgen and cortisol production. This has been reported from oral, inhaled, intranasal, and topical glucocorticoid administration.[65–67] Moreover, mirtazapine and progestins, such as medroxyprogesterone acetate and megestrol acetate have been reported to induce secondary adrenal insufficiency.[68,69] Chronic suppression also can result in atrophy

TABLE 79-7 Etiologies of Primary and Secondary Adrenal Insufficiency

Primary Insufficiency	Secondary Insufficiency
Slow onset	Craniopharyngioma
Acquired immunodeficiency syndrome	Cure of Cushing's syndrome
Adrenomyeloneuropathy	Empty sella syndrome
Adrenoleukodystrophy	Tumors of the third ventricle
Amyloidosis	Histiocytosis
Autoimmune adrenalitis[a]	Hypothalamic tumors
Bilateral adrenalectomy	Hypopituitarism
Congenital adrenal hypoplasia	Long-term corticosteroid administration
Hemochromatosis	Lymphocytic hypophysitis
Isolated glucocorticoid deficiency	Pituitary surgery, radiation, or tumor
Metastatic neoplasia	Sarcoidosis
Systemic fungal, bacterial, or viral infections	Medications–progestins and glucocorticoid discontinuation
Tuberculosis[b]	Postpartum pituitary necrosis
Medications–ketoconazole, etomidate, rifampin, phenytoin, phenobarbital	Necrotic or bleeding pituitary macroadenoma
Fast onset	Head trauma, lesions of the pituitary stalk
Adrenal thrombosis, hemorrhage, sepsis, trauma, or necrosis	Pituitary or adrenal surgery for Cushing's syndrome

[a]Accounts for approximately 70% of cases.
[b]Accounts for approximately 20% of cases.

of the anterior pituitary and hypothalamus, impairing recovery of function if the exogenous steroid is reduced. Secondary disease classically presents with normal concentrations of mineralocorticoids.

Approximately 90% of the adrenal cortex must be destroyed before adrenal insufficiency symptoms will occur.[70] Specific etiologies for both primary and secondary insufficiency are listed in Table 79–7. Adrenal hemorrhage can result from multiple etiologies including traumatic shock, coagulopathies, ischemic disorders, and other situations of severe stress, but septicemia is the most common. Symptoms include truncal pain, fever, shaking, chills, hypotension preceding shock, anorexia, headache, vertigo, vomiting, rash, psychiatric symptoms, abdominal rigidity or rebound, and death in 6 to 48 hours if not treated. The most common organisms found on autopsy are *Neisseria meningitidis, Pseudomonas aeruginosa, Streptococcus pneumoniae,* Group A *Streptococcus,* and *Haemophilus influenzae.*[70,71]

ADDISON'S DISEASE

Distinguishing Addison's disease from secondary insufficiency is difficult; however, the following guidelines may be helpful:

1. Hyperpigmentation usually is not seen in secondary adrenal insufficiency because of low amounts of melanocyte-stimulating hormone. Low amounts of melanocyte-stimulating hormone are present owing to a deficient pituitary secretion of ACTH and β-lipotropin, all of which are synthesized together in a common precursor peptide, proopiomelanocortin (POMC).
2. Aldosterone secretion usually is preserved in secondary insufficiency.
3. Weight loss, dehydration, hyponatremia, hyperkalemia, and elevated blood urea nitrogen are common in Addison's disease.
4. Addison's disease will have an abnormal response to the rapid ACTH-stimulation test. Plasma ACTH levels are usually 400 to 2000 pg/mL in primary insufficiency, versus normal to low (0 to 50 pg/mL; see Table 79–3) in secondary insufficiency. A normal cosyntropin-stimulation test does not rule out secondary adrenal insufficiency.

The short cosyntropin-stimulation test can be used to assess patients suspected of hypocortisolism. Patients are given 250 mcg of synthetic ACTH intravenously or intramuscularly, with serum cortisol levels drawn at baseline and 30 to 60 minutes after the injection. An increase to a cortisol level ≥18 mcg/dL (500 mmol/L) rules out adrenal insufficiency.[72] Although this test remains the most commonly used method, in some patients with secondary adrenal insufficiency or mild primary adrenal insufficiency, this test will be normal. This result can be owing to the high dose of corticotropin given. Thus some suggest that higher cutoff values (≥22 to 25 mcg/dL) should be used.[73] Alternatively, studies have demonstrated that equivalent results can be seen using 1 mcg of cosyntropin. The normal response is an increase to a cortisol level ≥18 mcg/dL 30 minutes after the injection. Other tests include the insulin hypoglycemia test, the metyrapone test, and the corticotropin-releasing hormone stimulation test.[63,72,74]

Cortisol levels greater than 18 to 20 mcg/dL 30 minutes after a cosyntropin-stimulation test are not useful in patients who are acutely ill.[75] Severe infection, trauma, burns, illnesses, or surgery can increase cortisol production by as much as a factor of six, making the recognition of adrenal insufficiency in this population extremely difficult. In the critically ill, a random cortisol level below 15 mcg/dL is indicative of adrenal insufficiency, whereas a level greater than 34 mcg/dL suggests that adrenal insufficiency is unlikely.[75] For patients who fall between these two values, a poor response to corticotropin (less than 9 mcg/dL increase in plasma cortisol from baseline at 30 or 60 minutes) indicates the possibility of adrenal insufficiency and a need for corticosteroid supplementation.[75] A severe hypoproteinemic patient (albumin <2.5 g/L) will have markedly lower CBG, which can falsely underestimate the free fraction of cortisol. These patients can benefit from retesting as an outpatient to prevent indefinite glucocorticoid therapy.[63]

Treatment of Addison's disease must include adequate patient education, so that the patient is aware of treatment complications, expected outcome, missed doses, and drug side effects. The agents of choice are hydrocortisone, cortisone, and prednisone, administered twice daily with the treatment objective being the establishment of the lowest effective dose while mimicking the normal diurnal adrenal rhythm.[63] Usually a twice-daily dosing schedule is adequate with the dose depending on the agent used.

Endogenous cortisol production varies between 5 and 10 mg/m^2 per day.[76] Hence, the classic 12- to 15-mg/m^2 per day rule for cortisol supplementation can be excessive in most patients. Recommended starting doses to properly mimic endogenous cortisol production is 15 mg of hydrocortisone daily, which is roughly equal to 20 mg of cortisone acetate or 2.5 mg of prednisone.[63,76] The majority of the dose (67%) is given in the morning, whereas the remainder (33%) is given in the evening to duplicate the normal circadian rhythm of cortisol production. The patient's symptoms should be monitored every 6 to 8 weeks to assess proper glucocorticoid replacement. To replace mineralocorticoid loss, fludrocortisone acetate can be used. A dose of 0.05 to 0.2 mg by mouth once a day is adequate. If parenteral therapy is needed, 2 to 5 mg of deoxycorticosterone trimethylacetate in oil intramuscularly every 3 to 4 weeks can be used. The main reason for adding the mineralocorticoid is to minimize the development of hyperkalemia. Adverse effects must be monitored closely. Symptoms include gastric upset, edema, hypertension, hypokalemia, insomnia, excitability, and diabetes mellitus. In addition, patient weight, blood pressure, and electrocardiogram should be monitored regularly.[74]

In women, the primary source of dehydroepiandrosterone (DHEA) and androgens is the adrenal cortex, specifically the zona reticularis. As such, women with adrenal insufficiency can have decreased libido. Although clinical trials are conflicting, 25 to 50 mg DHEA can increase energy levels and libido. Currently, the use of DHEA, a dietary supplement, is an option for female patients with adrenal insufficiency complaining of decreased libido and low energy.[77]

Most adrenal crises occur secondary to glucocorticoid dose reduction or lack of stress-related dose adjustments. It is recommended that patients receiving corticosteroid-replacement therapy add 5 to 10 mg hydrocortisone to their normal daily regimen shortly before strenuous activities such as hiking.[74] Likewise, during times of severe physical stress such as febrile illnesses or after accidents, patients should be instructed to double their daily dose until recovery.[78,79]

The end point of therapy is difficult to assess in most patients, but a reduction in excess pigmentation is a good clinical marker. The development of features of Cushing's syndrome indicates excessive replacement. Treatment of secondary adrenal insufficiency is identical to primary disease treatment with the exception that mineralocorticoid replacement usually is not necessary. Patient education still should be stressed with emphasis placed on establishing an alternate-day regimen.

Acute Adrenal Insufficiency

Adrenal crisis, or Addisonian crisis, is characterized by an acute adrenocortical insufficiency. Adrenal crisis represents a true endocrine emergency. Anything that increases adrenal requirements dramatically can precipitate an adrenal crisis. Stressful situations, surgery, infection, and trauma all are potential triggering events, especially in the patient with some underlying adrenal or pituitary insufficiency. The most common cause of adrenal crisis is HPA-axis suppression brought on by chronic use of exogenous glucocorticoids and abrupt withdrawal.

Treatment of adrenal crisis involves the administration of parenteral glucocorticoids. Hydrocortisone is the agent of choice owing to its combined mineralocorticoid and glucocorticoid activity. Hydrocortisone is started at 100 mg intravenously through rapid infusion, and followed by a continuous infusion or intermittent bolus of 100 to 200 mg every 24 hours.[80] Intravenous administration is continued for 24 to 48 hours, at which time if the patient is stable, oral hydrocortisone can be started at a dose of 50 mg every 8 hours for another 48 hours. Following oral maintenance therapy, a hydrocortisone taper is initiated until the dosage is 30 to 50 mg/day in divided doses. Fluid replacement often is required and can be accomplished with dextrose 5% in normal saline solution (D_5NS) at a rate to support blood pressure. If hyperkalemia is present after the hydrocortisone maintenance phase, additional mineralocorticoid usually is required. Fludrocortisone acetate in a dose of 0.1 mg by mouth daily is the agent of choice.

Patients with adrenal insufficiency should be instructed to carry a card or wear a bracelet or necklace, such as MedicAlert, that contains information about their condition. Patients should also have easy access to injectable hydrocortisone or glucocorticoid suppositories in case of an emergency or during times of physical stress, such as febrile illness or injury.[74]

CLINICAL PRESENTATION: ADRENAL INSUFFICIENCY

Symptoms

- Patients commonly complain of weakness, weight loss, gastrointestinal symptoms, craving for salt, headaches, memory impairment, depression, and postural dizziness.
- Early symptoms of acute adrenal insufficiency also include myalgias, malaise, and anorexia. As the situation progresses, vomiting, fever, hypotension, and shock will develop.

Signs

- Increased pigmentation
- Hypotension (postural)
- Fever
- Decreased body hair
- Vitiligo
- Features of hypopituitarism (amenorrhea and cold intolerance)

Laboratory Tests

- The short cosyntropin stimulation test can be used to assess patients suspected of hypercortisolism.

Other Diagnostic Tests

- Other tests include the insulin hypoglycemia test, the metyrapone test, and the corticotropin-releasing hormone stimulation test.

HYPOALDOSTERONISM

Hypoaldosteronism is rare and usually is associated with low renin status, diabetes, complete heart block, or severe postural hypotension, or it can occur postoperatively following tumor removal.[2] Hypoaldosteronism can be part of a larger adrenal insufficiency or be the only defect the patient has. In nonselective hypoaldosteronism, the etiology of the low aldosterone is most likely generalized adrenocortical insufficiency (see Addison's Disease). In selective hypoaldosteronism, the etiology is usually a specific defect in the stimulation of adrenal aldosterone secretion (21-hydroxylase deficiency being most common) or a defect in peripheral aldosterone action (decreased aldosterone receptors).

Laboratory analysis reveals low serum sodium and high serum potassium concentrations. Patients often will present with hyperchloremic metabolic acidosis. Because the deficiency is in the mineralocorticoid, replacement with fludrocortisone in a dose of 0.1 to 0.3 mg is usually effective. Patients should be followed for blood pressure response as well as electrolyte status.

CONGENITAL ADRENAL HYPERPLASIA

Because many enzyme systems are needed to complete the complex cholesterol-to-cortisol pathway, enzyme deficiencies can lead to disruptions of the normal cascade of events (see Fig. 79–2). This group of enzyme disorders is known as congenital adrenal hyperplasia, mainly because of the resultant chronic adrenal gland stimulation that occurs following enzyme deficiency.[81,82] The most frequent is steroid 21-hydroxylase deficiency, accounting for more than 90% of cases. Any enzyme deficiency is capable of affecting any one or all three of the steroid pathways. Therefore, treatment should be focused on replacement of the deficient hormone, psychologic support, and surgical repair of the external genitalia in most female patients.[83] In Table 79–8, six of the most common enzyme deficiencies are briefly outlined.

ADRENAL VIRILISM

9 Virilism, excessive secretion of androgens from the adrenal gland, is more commonly seen in females, with hirsutism being the dominant feature. Women who present with hirsutism also can have voice deepening, acne, increased muscle mass, menstrual abnormalities, clitoral enlargement, redistribution of body fat and loss of female body contour, breast atrophy, and hair recession and crown balding.[84] Although virilism can be easy to diagnose based on clinical symptoms, making the diagnosis on a biochemical basis is difficult.[85] The most common etiology of adrenal virilism involves one of many possible congenital enzyme defects. Depending on the enzyme deficiency, accumulation of a variety of androgens, notably testosterone, can develop.

Treatment of virilism centers around suppression of the pituitary-adrenal axis with exogenous glucocorticoids. Choice of steroids is variable. In adults, the usual steroids used are dexamethasone (0.25 to 0.5 mg), prednisone (2.5 to 5 mg), or hydrocortisone (10 to 20 mg).[86] Antiandrogen use can allow lower steroid doses to be used.

TABLE 79-8 Congenital Adrenal Hyperplasia (CAH)

Enzyme Deficiency (Disorder)	Symptoms	Laboratory Tests	Comments
21-Hydroxylase (nonvirilizing CAH)	Enlarged female genitalia and adrenal gland (caused by cholesterol)	All steroids are low in blood and urine	Poor prognosis for infants
17-Hydroxylase (nonvirilizing CAH)	Hypertension usually present	Low concentrations of cortisol and estrogens	Mineralocorticoid replacement not necessary
21-Hydroxylase (virilizing CAH)	Pubertal irregularities (acne, early pubic hair, voice lowering, and increased muscularity); mature normally with replacement	High progesterone, renin, 17-hydroxyprogesterone and ACTH; low cortisol, sodium, and aldosterone	Most common form of CAH (90% of total), incidence of 1:10,000; monitor growth velocity, bone age, renin, and 17-hydroxyprogesterone
11-Hydroxylase (virilizing CAH)	Hypertension secondary to high deoxycortisol and virilism from androgen excess; mistaken for Cushing's, but no glucose intolerance	Low plasma cortisone and aldosterone; high ACTH and MSH concentrations	Second most common form of CAH (9% of total), incidence of 1:100,000; final step in biosynthesis of corticosterone and cortisol; found only in adrenal cortex
3-Hydroxysteroid dehydrogenase (mixed CAH)	Both cortisol and aldosterone deficiencies	Decreased aldosterone, cortisol, estrogens, and androgens; increased pregnenolone and cholesterol	Defect affects both adrenals and gonads
18-Hydroxysteroid dehydrogenase (corticosterone methyloxidase deficiency)	Hypotension	Restricted to zona glomerulosa; sole aldosterone defect; hyponatremia, hyperkalemia, increased renin	Mineralocorticoid replacement without glucocorticoid replacement

ACTH, adrenocorticotropic hormone; MSH, melanocyte-stimulating hormone.

HIRSUTISM

Hirsutism is defined as excessive male pattern terminal hair growth in women, which is distinguishable for hypertrichosis, or nonspecific excessive hair growth.[86] Common causes of hypertrichosis are genetic predisposition or the use drugs such as minoxidil, phenytoin, cyclosporine, methyldopa, danazol, metoclopramide, phenothiazines, reserpine, and diazoxide. The majority of cases of hirsutism occur in women with some degree of excess androgen production. Androgen excess can be derived from either the ovaries or the adrenal glands, with a small fraction coming from pituitary disorders. Ovarian excess is described as polycystic ovarian syndrome (PCOS) and can manifest as obesity, insulin resistance, and menstrual abnormalities. In the patient with hirsutism, congenital adrenal hyperplasia, adrenal tumors, and ovarian tumors should be ruled out.[86,87]

Cosmetic approaches are generally tried first, with laser photothermodestruction offering the greatest long-term success. Only when cosmetic surgery is ineffective should suppressive therapy be used. Eflornithine hydrochloride, an ornithine decarboxylase inhibitor, is a topical cream that is applied as a thin layer to the affected area twice daily, at least 8 hours apart. Reduction in unwanted hair can be noted as soon as 4 weeks with a maximal effect at 8 to 24 weeks.[86,88] Skin irritation can occur that resolves on discontinuation. Glucocorticoids, such as dexamethasone, can be used if the androgen source is adrenal, but can induce cushingoid symptoms even in doses of 0.5 mg/day. Oral contraceptives can be used in patients who require contraception concurrently. If oral contraceptives are used, a progestin with low androgen activity (norethindrone, ethynodiol diacetate, or drospirenone) should be employed. Gonadotropin-releasing hormone can be an effective adjunct or alternative to oral contraceptives if the source of androgen is ovarian. In addition, insulin sensitizers, such as metformin or thiazolidinediones, can show moderate improvement in women with PCOS. Antiandrogens are often added to the more specific therapies. The most common include spironolactone, flutamide, and finasteride, although none of these is approved by the Food and Drug Administration for the treatment of hirsutism. It can take 6 to 12 months for the antiandrogens to alleviate hirsutism, and treatment should be continued for 2 years. Subsequently, a slow reduction in the dose should be achieved.[87]

CLINICAL CONTROVERSY

Some clinicians believe that the usual starting doses for glucocorticoid supplementation are high and unnecessarily increase a patient's risk for adverse outcomes such as osteoporosis.

PRINCIPLES OF GLUCOCORTICOID ADMINISTRATION

Originally, the term *glucocorticoid* was given to these agents to describe their glucose-regulating properties. However, carbohydrate metabolism is only one of a multitude of effects that steroids can exhibit. The activity produced is a function of the receptor activated (glucocorticoid versus mineralocorticoid) as well as the agent and dose prescribed.

The mechanism of glucocorticoids is complex and not fully known. The glucocorticoid enters the cell through passive diffusion and binds to its specific receptor. There are between 5,000 and 100,000 receptors per cell. Steroids exhibit various binding affinities to the vast number of receptors in almost every tissue and therefore elicit a wide variety of biologic effects.

After binding to the receptor, there is a structural change that occurs in the receptor, known as *activation*. After activation, the receptor-steroid complex binds to deoxyribonucleic acid sites in the cell called *glucocorticoid response elements* (GREs). This binding to the GREs stimulates or inhibits transcription of nearby genes.

The pharmacokinetics of the glucocorticoids varies with the agent given and the route of administration. In general, most steroids given by the oral route are well absorbed. Water-soluble agents are more rapidly absorbed following intramuscular injection than are lipid-soluble agents. Intravenous administration is recommended when a quick onset of action is needed. A summary of the steroids is provided in Table 79–9.

In addition to systemic steroids causing iatrogenic Cushing's syndrome, they also can lead to increased susceptibility to infection, osteoporosis, sodium retention with resultant edema, hypokalemia, hypomagnesemia, cataracts, peptic ulcer disease, seizures, and generalized suppression of the HPA-axis. Long-term complications tend to be insidious and less likely to respond to steroid withdrawal.

TABLE 79-9 Relative Potencies of Glucocorticoids

Glucocorticoid	Anti-Inflammatory Potency	Equivalent Potency (mg)	Approximate Half-Life (min)	Sodium-Retaining Potency
Cortisone	0.8	25	30	2
Hydrocortisone	1	20	90	2
Prednisone	3.5	5	60	1
Prednisolone	4	5	200	1
Triamcinolone	5	4	300	0
Methylprednisolone	5	4	180	0
Betamethasone	25	0.6	100–300	0
Dexamethasone	30	0.75	100–300	0

Suppression of the HPA-axis is a major concern whenever systemic steroids are tapered or withdrawn. Single doses of glucocorticoids can prevent the axis from responding to major stressors for several hours. In general, the longer the steroid is administered and the higher the dose used, the more suppression of the axis occurs. However, the possibility of suppression occurs any time the patient is exposed to supraphysiologic doses of a steroid.[24,89] Symptoms of steroid withdrawal resemble those seen in a patient with adrenocortical deficiency.

A variety of recommendations for steroid tapering are available.[24,90–92] In general, patients who have been on long-term steroid therapy will need to be gradually withdrawn toward physiologic doses over months. On average, the normal adult produces approximately 10 to 30 mg of cortisol per day with the peak concentration occurring around 8:00 AM. As the steroid or steroid-equivalent dose approaches the 20- to 30-mg level, the taper should be slowed and the patient checked for axis function. The primary modes to test HPA integrity are the ACTH test, either high- or low-dose, or a morning (8:00 AM) serum cortisol. A normal morning serum cortisol (>20 mcg/dL) or a normal ACTH test would indicate that daily steroid maintenance therapy is not needed. If morning serum cortisol is between 3 and 20 mcg/dL, an ACTH test or an CRH stimulation test can be useful in the assessment of pituitary-adrenal function.[24] A morning cortisol less than 3 mcg/dL indicates axis suppression and the need for continued replacement therapy. Suppression can be noted for up to a year in some patients. Caution should be used to prevent disease exacerbation during the steroid taper to prevent the need for rebolusing the patient with another course of high-dose steroids. The dilemma of prolonged steroid administration is sometimes lessened by the use of an alternate day therapy (ADT) regimen.[24,92] ADT theoretically minimizes the hypothalamic-pituitary suppression as well as some of the adverse effects seen with once-daily therapy. This can be especially important in the treatment of the child and young adult, in whom growth suppression is a major concern. ADT is not recommended for initial management, but rather in the management of the stabilized patient who needs long-term therapy. The patient will be exposed to "on" and "off" days, with the "on" day dose gradually increased with concurrent reduction in the "off" day dose over a period of 14 days. By the day 14, the patient will be consuming medication only on the "on" day. It should be noted that not all patients will have equivalent disease control on ADT, and it should be avoided in certain indications.[24,92]

EVALUATION OF THERAPEUTIC OUTCOMES

Successful glucocorticoid therapy involves counseling the patient, monitoring the patient, and recognizing complications of therapy (Table 79–10). The risk-to-benefit ratio of glucocorticoid administration should always be considered, especially with concurrent disease states such as hypertension, diabetes mellitus, peptic ulcer disease, and uncontrolled systemic infections.

TABLE 79-10 Factors in Successful Glucocorticoid Therapy

Monitoring	Glucose concentrations (serum and urine) Electrolytes (serum and urine) Ophthalmologic examinations Stool tests for occult blood loss Growth and development (children and adolescents)
Counseling	Take with food to minimize gastrointestinal discomfort Never discontinue medication on your own; check with your physician; gradual dose reduction is usually necessary Carry or wear medical identification indicating that you are on long-term glucocorticoid therapy Dosage increases can be necessary at times of increased stress (surgery or emergency treatments) Be aware of potential side effects (i.e., visual disturbances, bruising, and delayed wound healing) What to do if you miss a dose: If your dosing schedule is *Every other day:* Take as soon as possible if remembered that morning. If not remembered until later, skip that day. Take the next morning, then skip the following day. *Every day:* Take as soon as possible, but skip if almost time for the next dose. Never double doses.
Recognizing complications	Early in therapy and essentially unavoidable: insomnia, enhanced appetite, weight gain Common in patients with underlying risk factors: hypertension, diabetes mellitus, peptic ulcer disease Long-term intense treatment: cushingoid habitus, hypothalamic-pituitary-adrenal suppression, impaired wound healing Delayed and insidious: cataracts, atherosclerosis Rare and unpredictable: psychosis, glaucoma, pancreatitis

From United States Pharmacopeial Convention[94] and Barlow.[95]

CLINICAL CONTROVERSY

Some clinicians believe that twice-daily administration of glucocorticoids in patients with adrenal insufficiency is not as effective as three-times daily. If a twice-daily regimen is used, the second dose should be administered 6 to 8 hours after the first.

ABBREVIATIONS

ACTH: adrenocorticotropic hormone
ADT: alternate day therapy
APA: aldosterone-producing adenoma
ARR: aldosterone-to-renin ratio
AVS: adrenal venous sampling
BAH: bilateral adrenal hyperplasia
CBG: corticosteroid-binding globulin
CRH: corticotropin-releasing hormone
CT: computed tomography
D_5NS: dextrose 5% in normal saline solution
DDT: dichlorodiphenyltrichloroethane
DST: dexamethasone suppression test
FH: familial hyperaldosteronism
FST: fludrocortisone suppression test
GRA: glucocorticoid-remediable aldosteronism
GRE: glucocorticoid response element
HPA: hypothalamic-pituitary-adrenal
IPSS: inferior petrosal sinus sampling
IRMA: immunoradiometric assay
JVS: jugular venous sampling

MRI: magnetic resonance imaging

PAC:PRA: plasma-aldosterone-concentration–to–plasma-renin-activity (ratio)

PAL: primary aldosteronism

RIA: radioimmunoassay

RU-486: mifepristone

REFERENCES

1. Conn JW. Primary aldosteronism, a new clinical syndrome. J Lab Clin Med 1955;45:6–17.
2. Orth DN, Kovacs WJ. The adrenal cortex. In: Wilson JD, Foster DW, Kronenberg HM, Larsen PR, eds. Williams' Textbook of Endocrinology. Philadelphia, PA: Saunders, 1998:517–664.
3. Albright F. Cushing syndrome. Harvey Lect 1942–1943;38:123–186.
4. Newell-Price J, Bertagna X, Grossman AB, Nieman LK. Cushing's syndrome. Lancet 2006;367:1605–1617.
5. Isidori AM, Kaltsas GA, Pozza C, et al. The ectopic adrenocorticotropin syndrome: Clinical features, diagnosis, management, and long-term follow-up. J Clin Endocrinol Metab 2006;91:371–377.
6. Boscaro M, Barzon L, Sonino N. The diagnosis of Cushing's syndrome: Atypical presentations and laboratory shortcomings. Arch Intern Med 2000;160:3045–3053.
7. Orth DN. Cushing's syndrome. N Engl J Med 1995;332:791–803.
8. Williams GH, Duly RG. Diseases of the adrenal cortex. In: Isselbacher KJ, Braunwald E, Wilson JD, et al., eds. Harrison's Principles of Internal Medicine, 13th ed. New York: McGraw-Hill, 1994:1953–1976.
9. Catargi B, Rigalleau V, Poussin A, et al. Occult Cushing's syndrome in type-2 diabetes. J Clin Endocrinol Metab 2003;88:5808–5813.
10. Findling JW, Raff H. Screening and diagnosis of Cushing's syndrome. Endocrinol Metab Clin North Am 2005;34:385–402.
11. Nieman LK, Ilias I. Evaluation and treatment of Cushing's syndrome. Am J Med 2005;118:1340–1346.
12. Lindsay JR, Nieman LK. Differential diagnosis and imaging in Cushing's syndrome. Endocrinol Metab Clin North Am 2005;34:403–421.
13. Arnaldi G, Angeli A, Atkinson AB, et al. Diagnosis and complications of Cushing's syndrome: A consensus statement. J Clin Endocrinol Metab 2003;88:5593–5602.
14. Jackson RV, Hockings GI, Torpy DJ, et al. New diagnostic tests for Cushing's syndrome: Uses of naloxone, vasopressin and alprazolam. Clin Exp Pharmacol Physiol 1996;23:579–581.
15. Ambrosi B, Bochicchio D, Colombo P, et al. Loperamide to diagnose Cushing's syndrome. JAMA 1993;270:2301–2302.
16. Arvat E, Giordano R, Ramunni J, et al. Adrenocorticotropin and cortisol hyperresponsiveness to hexarelin in patients with Cushing's disease bearing a pituitary microadenoma, but not in those with macroadenoma. J Clin Endocrinol Metab 1998;83:4207–4211.
17. Newell-Price J, Trainer P, Besser M, Grossman A. The diagnosis and differential diagnosis of Cushing's syndrome and pseudo-Cushing's states. Endocr Rev 1998;19:647–672.
18. Papanicolaou DA, Mullen N, Kyrou I, Nieman LK. Nighttime salivary cortisol: A useful test for the diagnosis of Cushing's syndrome. J Clin Endocrinol Metab 2002;87:4515–4521.
19. Viardot A, Huber P, Puder JJ, et al. Reproducibility of nighttime salivary cortisol and its use in the diagnosis of hypercortisolism compared with urinary free cortisol and overnight dexamethasone suppression test. J Clin Endocrinol Metab 2005;90:5730–5736.
20. Findling JW, Raff H, Aron DC. The low-dose dexamethasone suppression test: A reevaluation in patients with Cushing's syndrome. J Clin Endocrinol Metab 2004;89:1222–1226.
21. Rockall AG, Babar SA, Sohaib SA, et al. CT and MR imaging of the adrenal glands in ACTH-independent Cushing syndrome. Radiographics 2004;24:435–452.
22. Peppercorn PD, Reznek RH. State-of-the-art CT and MRI of the adrenal gland. Eur Radiol 1997;7:822–836.
23. Sosa JA, Udelsman R. Imaging of the adrenal gland. Surg Oncol Clin N Am 1999;8:109–127.
24. Hopkins RL, Leinung MC. Exogenous Cushing's syndrome and glucocorticoid withdrawal. Endocrinol Metab Clin North Am 2005;34:371–384.
25. Bolland MJ, Bagg W, Thomas MG, et al. Cushing's syndrome due to interaction between inhaled corticosteroids and itraconazole. Ann Pharmacother 2004;38:46–49.
26. Samaras K, Pett S, Gowers A, et al. Iatrogenic Cushing's syndrome with osteoporosis and secondary adrenal failure in human immunodeficiency virus-infected patients receiving inhaled corticosteroids and ritonavir-boosted protease inhibitors: Six cases. J Clin Endocrinol Metab 2005;90:43944398.
27. Cizza G, Chrousos GP. Adrenocorticotrophic hormone-dependent Cushing's syndrome. Cancer Treat Res 1997;89:25–40.
28. Morris D, Grossman A. The medical management of Cushing's syndrome. Ann N Y Acad Sci 2002;970:119–133.
29. Nieman LK. Medical therapy of Cushing's disease. Pituitary 2002;5:77–82.
30. Labeur M, Arzt E, Stalla GK, Paez-Pereda M. New perspectives in the treatment of Cushing's syndrome. Curr Drug Targets—Immune Endocri Metabol Disord 2004;4:335–342.
31. McEvoy GK, ed. American Hospital Formulary Service (AHFS) Drug Information. American Society of Health-System Pharmacists 2005;15–16, 510–516, 1116–1118.
32. Utz AL, Swearingen B, Biller BM. Pituitary surgery and postoperative management in Cushing's disease. Endocrinol Metab Clin North Am 2005;34:459–478.
33. Cocconi G. First generation aromatase inhibitors-aminoglutethimide and testololactone. Breast Cancer Res Treat 1994;30:57–80.
34. Sonino N, Boscaro M. Medical therapy for Cushing's disease. Endocrinol Metab Clin North Am 1999;28:211–222.
35. Pivonello R, Ferone D, Lamberts SW, Colao A. Cabergoline plus lanreotide for ectopic Cushing's syndrome. N Engl J Med 2005;352:2457–2458.
36. Paez-Pereda M, Kovalovsky D, Hopfner U, et al. Retinoic acid prevents experimental Cushing syndrome. J Clin Invest 2001;108:1123–1131.
37. Semple PL, Vance ML, Findling J, Laws ER. Transsphenoidal surgery for Cushing's disease: Outcome in patients with a normal magnetic resonance imaging scan. Neurosurgery 2000;46:553–558.
38. Young WF, Thompson GB. Laparoscopic adrenalectomy for patients who have Cushing's syndrome Endocrinol Metab Clin North Am 2005;34:489–499.
39. Vance ML. Pituitary radiotherapy. Endocrinol Metab Clin North Am 2005;34:479–487.
40. Ilias I, Torpy DJ, Pacak K, et al. Cushing's syndrome due to ectopic corticotrophin secretion: Twenty years' experience at the National Institutes of Health. J Clin Endocrinol Metab 2005;90:4955–4962.
41. Young WF. Minireview: Primary aldosteronism—Changing concepts in diagnosis and treatment. Endocrinology 2003;144:2208–2213.
42. Stowasser M, Gordon RD. Primary aldosteronism: From genesis to genetics. Trends Endocrinol Metab 2003;14:310–317.
43. Stowasser M, Gordon RD. Primary aldosteronism. Best Pract Res Clin Endocrinol Metab 2003;17:591–605.
44. Fardella CE, Mosso L. Primary aldosteronism. Clin Lab 2002;48:181–190.
45. Corry DB, Tuck ML. Secondary aldosteronism. Endocrinol Metab Clin North Am 1995;24:511–529.
46. Bope ET, Rakel RE, ed. Conn's Current Therapy 2005. Philadelphia, PA: Elsevier Saunders, 2005:745–747.
47. Mulatero P, Dluhy RG, Giacchetti G, et al. Diagnosis of primary aldosteronism: From screening to subtype differentiation. Trends Endocrinol Metab 2005;16:114–119.
48. Stowasser M, Gordon RD. Primary aldosteronism—Careful investigation is essential and rewarding. Mol Cell Endocrinol 2004;217:33–39.
49. Nishizaka MK, Calhoun DA. Primary aldosteronism: Diagnostic and therapeutic considerations. Curr Cardiol Rep 2005;7:412–417.
50. Hirohara D, Nomura K, Okamoto T, et al. Performance of the basal aldosterone to renin ratio and of the renin stimulation test by furosemide and upright posture in screening for aldosterone-producing adenoma in low renin hypertensives. J Clin Endocrinol Metab 2001;86:4292–4298.
51. Giacchetti G, Ronconi V, Lucarelli G, et al. Analysis of screening and confirmatory tests in the diagnosis of primary aldosteronism: Need for a standardized protocol. J Hypertens 2006;24:737–745.
52. Schwartz GL, Turner ST. Screening for primary aldosteronism in essential hypertension: Diagnostic accuracy of the ratio of plasma aldosterone concentration to plasma renin activity. Clin Chem 2005;51:386–394.
53. Stowasser M, Gordon RD, Gunasekera TG, et al. High rate of detection of primary aldosteronism, including surgically treatable forms, after "non-

selective" screening of hypertensive patients. J Hypertens 2003;21:2149–2157.
54. Young WF, Stanson AW, Thompson GB, et al. Role for adrenal venous sampling in primary aldosteronism. Surgery 2004;136:1227–1235.
55. Nwariaku FE, Miller BS, Auchus R, et al. Primary hyperaldosteronism: Effect of adrenal vein sampling on surgical outcome. Arch Surg 2006;141:497–502.
56. Young WF Jr. Primary aldosteronism: Management issues. Ann N Y Acad Sci 2002;970:61–76.
57. Young WF. Primary aldosteronism—Treatment options. Growth Horm IGF Res 2003;13:S102–108.
58. Stewart PM. Mineralocorticoid hypertension. Lancet 1999;353:1341–1347.
59. Weinberger MH, White WB, Ruilope LM, et al. Effects of eplerenone versus losartan in patients with low-renin hypertension. Am Heart J 2005;150:426–433.
60. Meria P, Kempf BF, Hermieu JF, et al. Laparoscopic management of primary aldosteronism: Clinical experience with 212 cases. J Urol 2003;169:32–35.
61. Meyer A, Brabant G, Behrend M. Long-term follow-up after adrenalectomy for primary aldosteronism. World J Surg 2005;29:155–159.
62. Ghose RP, Hall PM, Bravo EL. Medical management of aldosterone-producing adenomas. Ann Intern Med 1999;131:105–108.
63. Salvatori R. Adrenal insufficiency. JAMA 2005;294:2481–2488.
64. Ten S, New M, Maclaren N. Addison's disease 2001. J Clin Endocrinol Metab 2001;86:2909–2922.
65. Levin C, Maibach HI. Topical corticosteroid-induced adrenocortical insufficiency: Clinical implications. Am J Clin Dermatol 2002;3:141–147.
66. Bello CE, Garrett SD. Therapeutic issues in oral glucocorticoid use. Lippincotts Prim Care Pract 1999;3:333–341.
67. Sizonenko PC. Effects of inhaled or nasal glucocorticosteroids on adrenal function and growth. J Pediatr Endocrinol Metab 2002;15:5–26.
68. Goodman A, Cagliero E. Megestrol-induced clinical adrenal insufficiency. Eur J Gynaecol Oncol 2000;21:117–118.
69. Schule C, Baghai T, Bidlingmaier M, et al. Endocrinological effects of mirtazapine in healthy volunteers. Prog Neuropsychopharmacol Biol Psychiatry 2002;26:1253–1261.
70. Alevritis EM, Sarubbi FA, Jordan RM, Peiris AN. Infectious cause of adrenal insufficiency. South Med J 2003;96:888–890.
71. Torrey SP. Recognition and management of adrenal emergencies. Emerg Med Clin North Am 2005;23:687–702.
72. Dorin RI, Qualls CR, Crapo LM. Diagnosis of adrenal insufficiency. Ann Intern Med 2003;139:194–204.
73. Oelkers W. The role of high- and low-dose corticotropin tests in the diagnosis of secondary adrenal insufficiency. Eur J Endocrinol 1998;139:567–570.
74. Arlt W, Allolio B. Adrenal insufficiency. Lancet 2003;361:1881–1893.
75. Cooper MS, Stewart PM. Corticosteroid insufficiency in acutely ill patients. N Engl J Med 2003;348:727–734.
76. Crown A, Lightman S. Why is the management of glucocorticoid deficiency still controversial: A review of the literature. Clin Endocrinol (Oxf) 2005;63:483–492.
77. Arlt W. Dehydroepiandrosterone replacement therapy. Semin Reprod Med 2004;22:379–388.
78. Coursin DB, Wood KE. Corticosteroid supplementation for adrenal insufficiency. JAMA 2002;287:236–240.
79. Nieman LK, Turner MC. Addison's disease. Clin Dermatol 2006;24:276–280.
80. Jacobi J. Corticosteroid replacement in critically ill patients. Crit Care Clin 2006;22:245–253.
81. Speiser PW, White PC. Congenital adrenal hyperplasia. N Engl J Med 2003;349:776–788.
82. Forest MG. Recent advances in the diagnosis and management of congenital adrenal hyperplasia due to 21-hydroxylase deficiency. Hum Reprod Update 2004;10:469–485.
83. Merke DP, Bornstein SR. Congenital adrenal hyperplasia. Lancet 2005;365:2125–2136.
84. Yildiz BO. Diagnosis of hyperandrogenism: Clinical criteria. Best Psract Res Clin Endocrinol Metab 2006;20:167–176.
85. Stanczyk FZ. Diagnosis of hyperandrogenism: biochemical criteria. Best Pract Res Clin Endocrinol Metab 2006;20:177–191.
86. Rosenfield RL. Hirsutism. N Engl J Med 2005;353:2578–2588.
87. Azziz R. The evaluation and management of hirsutism. Obstet Gynecol, 2003;101:995–1007.
88. Moghetti P. Treatment of hirsutism and acne in hyperandrogenism. Best Pract Res Clin Endocrinol Metab 2006;20:221–234.
89. Henzen C, Suter A, Lerch E, et al. Suppression and recovery of adrenal response after short-term, high-dose glucocorticoid treatment. Lancet 2000;355:542–545.
90. Krasner AS. Glucocorticoid-induced adrenal insufficiency. JAMA 1999;282:671–676.
91. Kountz DS, Clark CL. Safely withdrawing patients from chronic glucocorticoid therapy. Am Fam Physician 1997;55:521–552.
92. Baxter JD. Advances in glucocorticoid therapy. Adv Intern Med 2000;45:317–349.
93. Kratz A, Ferraro M, Sluss PM, Lewandrowski KB. Laboratory reference values. N Engl J Med 2004;351:1548–1563.
94. United States Pharmacopeial Convention Inc. USPDI. Advice for the patient: Drug Information in Lay Language, vol. II, 19th ed. Taunton, MA: Rand-McNally, 1999:612–616.
95. Barlow JE. Complications of therapy. In: Boumpas DT, moderator. Glucocorticoid therapy for immune mediated diseases: Basic and clinical correlates. Ann Intern Med 1993;119:1198–1208.

CHAPTER 80 Pituitary Gland Disorders

AMY HECK SHEEHAN, JACK A. YANOVSKI, AND KARIM ANTON CALIS

KEY CONCEPTS

1. Pharmacologic therapy for acromegaly should be considered when surgery and irradiation are contraindicated, when rapid control of symptoms is needed, or when other treatments have failed to normalize growth hormone (GH) and insulin-like growth factor-1 (IGF-1) concentrations.

2. Pharmacotherapy for acromegaly using dopamine agonists provide advantages of oral dosing and reduced cost compared to somatostatin analogs and pegvisomant. However, dopamine agonists effectively normalize IGF-1 concentrations in only 10% of patients.

3. Octreotide therapy for acromegaly should be initiated using the short-acting subcutaneous formulation. Patients who have been maintained on subcutaneous octreotide for at least 2 weeks and have shown response to therapy can be converted to the long-acting depot form of octreotide.

4. Blood glucose concentrations should be monitored frequently in the early stages of octreotide therapy in all acromegalic patients.

5. Pegvisomant appears to be the most effective agent for normalizing IGF-1 concentrations. However, further study is needed to determine the long-term safety and efficacy of this agent for the treatment of acromegaly.

6. Recombinant GH is currently considered the mainstay of therapy for treatment of children with growth hormone-deficient (GHD) short stature. Prompt diagnosis of GHD and initiation of replacement therapy with recombinant GH is crucial for optimizing final adult heights.

7. All GH products are generally considered to be equally efficacious. The recommended dose for treatment of GHD short stature in children is 0.3 mg/kg/wk.

8. Pharmacologic agents that antagonize dopamine or increase the release of prolactin can induce hyperprolactinemia. Discontinuation of the offending medication and initiation of an appropriate therapeutic alternative usually normalize serum prolactin concentrations.

9. Cabergoline appears to be more effective than bromocriptine for the medical management of prolactinomas and offers the advantage of less-frequent dosing and decreased adverse events.

10. Although preliminary data do not suggest cabergoline has significant teratogenic potential, cabergoline is not recommended for use during pregnancy, and patients receiving cabergoline who plan to become pregnant should discontinue the medication or substitute bromocriptine for cabergoline at least 1 month before planned conception.

11. Pharmacologic treatment of panhypopituitarism consists of glucocorticoids, thyroid hormone preparations, sex steroids, and recombinant GH, where appropriate, as lifelong replacement therapy.

Learning objectives, review questions, and other resources can be found at **www.pharmacotherapyonline.com.**

In the 1950s, Geoffrey Harris and his colleagues uncovered the physiologic importance of pituitary hormones and proposed the theory of neurohormonal regulation of the pituitary by the hypothalamus.[1] Today the pituitary gland is recognized for its essential role in body homeostasis, and for this reason it often is referred to as the "master gland." The hypothalamus and the pituitary gland are closely connected, and together they provide a means of communication between the brain and many of the body's endocrine organs. The hypothalamus uses nervous input and metabolic signals from the body to control the secretion of pituitary hormones that regulate growth, thyroid function, adrenal activity, reproduction, lactation, and fluid balance.

ANATOMY AND PHYSIOLOGY

The hypothalamus (Fig. 80–1) is a small region at the base of the brain that receives autonomic nervous input from different areas of the body to regulate limbic functions, food and water intake, body temperature, cardiovascular function, respiratory function, and diurnal rhythms. In addition, the hypothalamus controls the release of hormones from the anterior and posterior regions of the pituitary gland. Neurons in the hypothalamus produce vasopressin and oxytocin and make many hormone-releasing factors that stimulate or inhibit the release of trophic hormones. At the base of the hypothalamus, a projection known as the *median eminence* is rich with nerve axons and blood vessels and provides both chemical and physical connections between the hypothalamus and the pituitary gland.

The pituitary gland, also referred to as the *hypophysis,* is located at the base of the brain in a cavity of the sphenoid bone known as the *sella turcica.* The pituitary is separated from the brain by an extension of the dura mater known as the *diaphragma sella.* The pituitary is a very small gland, weighing between 0.4 and 1 g in adults. It is divided into two distinct regions, the anterior lobe, or adenohypophysis, and the posterior lobe, or the neurohypophysis (see Fig. 80–1).

The posterior pituitary gland secretes two major hormones: oxytocin and vasopressin (antidiuretic hormone) (Table 80–1). Oxyto-

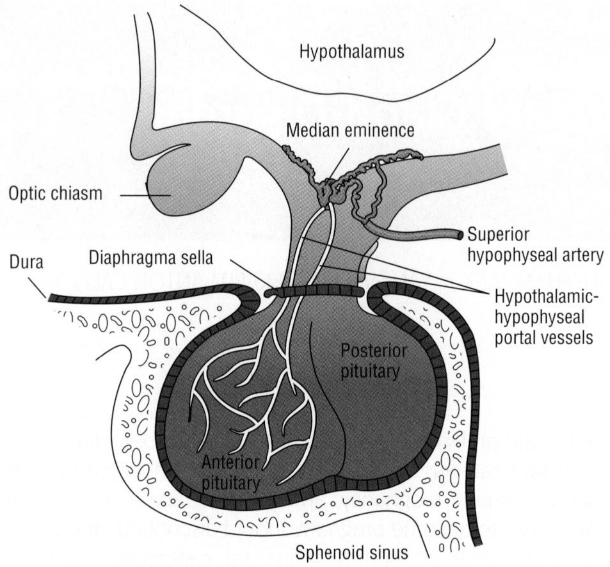

FIGURE 80-1. Pituitary gland.

cin release from the posterior pituitary causes contraction of the smooth muscles in the breast during lactation. It also plays a role in uterine contraction during parturition. Vasopressin is essential for proper fluid balance and acts on the renal collecting ducts to conserve water. Oxytocin and vasopressin are synthesized in the paraventricular and supraoptic nuclei of the hypothalamus. The posterior pituitary gland contains the terminal nerve endings of these two nuclei as well as specialized secretory granules that release hormones in response to appropriate signals. Loss of anterior pituitary function does not necessarily affect the release of vasopressin or oxytocin because these hormones actually are synthesized in the hypothalamus.

Unlike the posterior pituitary, the release of anterior pituitary hormones is not regulated by direct nervous stimulation but rather is controlled by specific hypothalamic-releasing and inhibitory hormones. The median eminence of the hypothalamus contains a large number of capillaries that converge to form a network of veins known as the *hypothalamic–hypophysial portal circulation.* Inhibiting and releasing hormones synthesized in the neurons of the hypothalamus reach the anterior pituitary via the hypothalamic–hypophysial portal vessels to control release of anterior pituitary hormones. Although there is a direct arterial blood supply to the anterior pituitary lobe, the hypothalamic–hypophysial portal vessels provide the primary blood supply (see Fig. 80–1). In contrast to the posterior pituitary, the anterior pituitary lobe is extremely vascular and has the highest rate of blood flow of all body organs.

The specialized secretory cells of the anterior pituitary lobe secrete six major polypeptide hormones (see Table 80–1). These include growth hormone (GH) or somatotropin, adrenocorticotropic hormone (ACTH) or corticotropin, thyroid-stimulating hormone (TSH) or thyrotropin, prolactin, follicle-stimulating hormone (FSH), and luteinizing hormone (LH). The release of these hormones is regulated primarily by hypothalamic-releasing and inhibiting hormones. Thyrotropin-releasing hormone (TRH) stimulates anterior pituitary release of TSH and prolactin, corticotropin-releasing hormone (CRH) stimulates anterior pituitary release of ACTH, growth hormone-releasing hormone (GHRH) stimulates anterior pituitary release of GH, and gonadotropin-releasing hormone (GnRH) stimulates anterior pituitary release of LH and FSH. Hypothalamic release of somatostatin inhibits release of GH, and hypothalamic release of dopamine (prolactin inhibitory hormone) inhibits the secretion of prolactin. Prolactin differs from the other anterior lobe hormones in that an inhibiting factor, rather than a stimulating factor, is primarily responsible for controlling its secretion. In the absence of hypothalamic input, an excess of prolactin is produced, whereas a deficiency state of other anterior pituitary hormones results. Physiologic regulation and action of anterior and posterior pituitary hormones are summarized in Table 80–1.[2–4]

Destruction of the pituitary gland may result in secondary hypothyroidism, hypogonadism, adrenal insufficiency, GH deficiency, and hypoprolactinemia. The formation of certain types of pituitary tumors may result in pituitary hormone excess. Pituitary tumors may physically compress the pituitary and prevent the release of trophic hypothalamic factors that regulate pituitary hormones. In this chapter, the pathophysiology and role of pharmacotherapy in the treatment of acromegaly, short stature, hyperprolactinemia, and panhypopituitarism are discussed.

GROWTH HORMONE

GH has direct antiinsulin effects on lipid and carbohydrate metabolism. GH decreases utilization of glucose by peripheral tissues, increases lipolysis, and increases muscle mass. GH also stimulates gluconeogenesis in hepatocytes, impairs tissue glucose uptake, decreases insulin-receptor sensitivity, and impairs postreceptor insulin action. The growth-promoting effects of GH are largely mediated by insulin-like growth factors (IGFs) also known as *somatomedins.* GH stimulates the formation of insulin-like growth factor-1 (IGF-1) in the liver as well as in other peripheral tissues. This anabolic peptide acts as a direct stimulator of cell proliferation and growth. There are two types of insulin-like growth factors: IGF-1 and IGF-2. IGF-1 regulates growth to some extent before, and largely after, birth. In contrast, IGF-2 is thought to primarily regulate growth in utero.[5] GH is secreted by the anterior pituitary in a pulsatile fashion, with several short bursts that occur mostly at night. Because of the short half-life of GH in the plasma (approximately 30 minutes), measurements of circulating GH concentrations throughout the waking hours usually are very low or undetectable. Daytime GH pulses are most likely to occur after meals, following exercise, or during periods of stress. The greatest amount of GH secretion occurs during the night within the first 1 to 2 hours of slow-wave sleep (stage III or IV). Secretion of GH is lowest during infancy, increases slightly during childhood, reaches its peak during adolescence, and then begins to gradually decline during the middle-age years.[3]

GROWTH HORMONE EXCESS

Acromegaly is a pathologic condition characterized by excessive production of GH. This is a rare disorder that affects approximately 50 to 70 adults per million.[6] Gigantism, which is even more rare than acromegaly, is the excess secretion of GH prior to epiphyseal closure in children.[7] Patients diagnosed with acromegaly are reported to have a twofold to threefold increase in mortality, usually related to cardiovascular, respiratory, or neoplastic disease.[8–10] Most patients are middle-aged at the time of diagnosis, and this disorder does not appear to affect one gender to a greater extent than the other. The most common cause of excess GH secretion in acromegaly is a GH-secreting pituitary adenoma, accounting for approximately 98% of all cases.[8] Rarely, acromegaly is caused by ectopic GH-secreting adenomas, GH cell hyperplasia, or excess GHRH secretion, or is one of the manifestations of multiple endocrine neoplasia syndrome type 1, McCune-Albright's syndrome, or the Carney complex, all very rare hypersecretory endocrinopathies.[8]

The clinical signs and symptoms of acromegaly develop gradually over an extended period of time. In fact, because of the subtle and slowly developing changes in physical appearance caused by GH excess, most patients are not definitively diagnosed with acromegaly

TABLE 80-1 Pituitary Hormones

Hormone	Stimulation	Inhibition	Physiologic Effects
Anterior pituitary hormones			
Growth hormone (GH)	*Physiologic* GH-releasing hormone Ghrelin ADH GABA Norepinephrine Dopamine Serotonin Estrogen Sleep Stress Exercise *Pharmacologic* α-Adrenergic agonists (e.g., clonidine) β-Adrenergic antagonists (e.g., propranolol) Dopamine agonists (e.g., bromocriptine) GABA agonists (e.g., muscimol)	*Physiologic* Somatostatin Elevated IGF-1 Growth hormone Progesterone Glucocorticoids Postprandial hyperglycemia Elevated free fatty acids *Pharmacologic* Dopamine antagonists (e.g., phenothiazines) α-Adrenergic antagonists (e.g., phentolamine) β-Adrenergic agonists (e.g., isoproterenol) Serotonin antagonists (e.g., methysergide)	Stimulates IGF-I production IGF-I and GH promote growth in all body tissues
Prolactin	*Physiologic* TRH VIP Estrogen Serotonin Histamine Endogenous opioids Pregnancy and nursing *Pharmacologic* Dopamine antagonists (e.g., phenothiazines, haloperidol, methyldopa) Opiates Estrogens H_2-antagonists (e.g., cimetidine) MAO inhibitors	*Physiologic* Dopamine GABA *Pharmacologic* Dopamine agonists (e.g., L-dopa, bromocriptine, pergolide, cabergoline)	Lactation
Adrenocorticotropic hormone (ACTH)	CRH	Elevated cortisol	Glucocorticoid effects Pigmentation
Thyroid-stimulating hormone (TSH)	TRH Estrogens Norepinephrine Serotonin	Thyroxine Triiodothyronine Somatostatin Glucocorticoids Dopamine	Iodine uptake and thyroid hormone synthesis
Luteinizing hormone (LH)	*Physiologic* GnRH *Pharmacologic* Clomiphene	Estradiol Testosterone Fasting	Ovulation Maintains corpus luteum
Follicle-stimulating hormone (FSH)	*Physiologic* GnRH Menopause Ovarian disorders *Pharmacologic* Clomiphene	Estradiol Inhibin Fasting	Ovarian follicle development Stimulates estradiol and progesterone
Posterior pituitary hormones			
Vasopressin (antidiuretic hormone [ADH])	Hyperosmolality Volume depletion	Hypervolemia Hypoosmolality	Acts on renal collecting ducts to prevent diuresis
Oxytocin	Parturition Suckling		Uterine contraction Milk ejection

CRH, corticotropin-releasing hormone; GABA, γ-aminobutyric acid; GnRH, gonadotropin-releasing hormone; IGF-1, insulin-like growth factor-1; MAO, monoamine oxidase; TRH, thyrotropin-releasing hormone; VIP, vasoactive intestinal peptide.

From Amar and Weiss,[2] Cuttler,[3] and Molitch.[4]

until 7 to 10 years after the presumed onset of excessive GH secretion.[9] Excessive secretion of GH and IGF-1 adversely affects several organ systems. Almost all acromegalic patients will present with physical signs and symptoms of soft-tissue overgrowth. Table 80–2 summarizes the classic clinical presentation of patients with acromegaly.[8–13] Some patients with acromegaly present with only a few of these classic signs and symptoms, making recognition of this disease extremely difficult.

TABLE 80-2 Clinical Presentation of Acromegaly

General
The patient will experience slow development of soft-tissue overgrowth affecting many body systems. Signs and symptoms may gradually progress over 7 to 10 years.
Symptoms
The patient may complain of symptoms related to local effects of the growth hormone (GH)-secreting tumor, such as headache and visual disturbances. Other symptoms related to elevated GH and insulin-like growth factor-1 (IGF-1) concentrations include excessive sweating, neuropathies, joint pain, and paresthesias.
Signs
The patient may exhibit coarsening of facial features, increased hand volume, increased ring size, increased shoe size, an enlarged tongue, and various dermatologic conditions.
Laboratory tests
The patient's GH concentration will be >1 mcg/L following an oral glucose tolerance test (OGTT) and IGF-1 serum concentrations will be elevated. Glucose intolerance may be present in up to 50% of patients.
Additional clinical sequelae
• Cardiovascular diseases such as hypertension, coronary heart disease, cardiomyopathy, and left ventricular hypertrophy are common in patients with acromegaly.
• Osteoarthritis and joint damage develops in up to 90% of acromegalic patients.
• Respiratory disorders and sleep apnea occur in up to 60% of acromegalic patients.
• Type 2 diabetes develops in approximately 25% of acromegalic patients.
• Patients with acromegaly may have an increased risk for development of esophageal, colon, and stomach cancer.

From Ben-Shlomo and Melmed,[8] Melmed,[9] Kauppinen-Makelin et al.,[10] Fatti et al.,[11] Vitale et al.,[12] and Webb et al.[13]

The diagnosis of acromegaly is based on a combination of diagnostic tests and clinical signs and symptoms. Random measures of plasma GH levels are not usually dependable because of the pulsatile pattern of release. The oral glucose tolerance test (OGTT) is commonly used as an important diagnostic tool. Postprandial hyperglycemia inhibits the secretion of GH for at least 1 to 2 hours. Therefore, an oral glucose load would be expected to suppress GH concentrations. However, patients with acromegaly continue to secrete GH during the OGTT. Because GH stimulates the production of IGF-1, serum IGF-1 concentrations can also be measured to aid in the diagnosis of acromegaly. Circulating IGF-1 is cleared from the body at a much slower rate than is GH, and measurements can be collected at any time of the day to identify patients with GH excess.[9] Current criteria for the diagnosis of acromegaly include failure of GH suppression <1 mcg/L following an OGTT in the presence of elevated IGF-1 serum concentrations.[14,15] With the development of more sensitive GH and IGF-1 assays, the cutoff value for diagnosis of acromegaly will likely decrease in the future. Insulin-like growth factor-1 binding protein-3 (IGFBP-3) also can be measured because it is positively regulated by GH and binds to circulating IGF-1 with high affinity. This test may be useful in monitoring response to therapy.[8] Computed tomography and magnetic resonance imaging of the pituitary are important diagnostic tests to confirm the presence of a pituitary adenoma.[9,14,15]

TREATMENT

Acromegaly

The primary treatment goals for patients diagnosed with acromegaly are to reduce GH and IGF-1 concentrations, improve the clinical signs and symptoms of the disease, and decrease mortality.[15–17] Many clinicians define cure of acromegaly as suppression of GH concentrations to <1 mcg/L after a standard OGTT in the presence of normal IGF-1 serum concentrations.[16] The treatment of choice for most patients with acromegaly is transsphenoidal surgical resection of the GH-secreting adenoma.[9,15,17,18] Postsurgical cure rates have been reported to range from 50% to 90%, depending on the type of adenoma and the expertise of the neurosurgeon.[8,17,18] Complications of transsphenoidal surgery are relatively infrequent and include cerebrospinal fluid leak, meningitis, arachnoiditis, diabetes insipidus, and pituitary failure.[8] For patients who are poor surgical candidates, those who have not responded to surgical interventions, or others who refuse surgical treatment, radiation therapy may be considered. Radiation, however, may take several years to relieve the symptoms of acromegaly.

Because neither radiation therapy nor surgery will cure all patients with acromegaly, adjuvant drug therapy is often needed to control symptoms.[9,17,18]

PHARMACOLOGIC THERAPY

❶ Drug therapy should be considered for acromegalic patients in whom surgery and irradiation are contraindicated, when rapid control of symptoms is indicated, or when other treatments have failed to normalize GH and IGF-1 concentrations. Pharmacologic treatment options include dopamine agonists, somatostatin analogs, and the GH receptor antagonist pegvisomant. Dopamine agonists such as bromocriptine and cabergoline are effective in a small subset of patients and provide the advantages of oral dosing and reduced cost. Somatostatin analogs are more effective than dopamine agonists, reducing GH concentrations and normalizing IGF-1 in approximately 50% to 60% of patients. Pegvisomant, a GH receptor antagonist, is highly effective in normalizing IGF-1 concentrations in up to 97% of patients. However, additional long-term data are needed to establish the safety and efficacy of pegvisomant in the management of acromegaly.

DOPAMINE AGONISTS

❷ In normal healthy adults, dopamine agonists cause an increase in GH production. However, when these agents are given to patients with acromegaly, there is a paradoxical decrease in GH production. Most clinical experience with the use of dopamine agonists in acromegaly is with bromocriptine. Other agents such as pergolide, cabergoline, and lisuride also have been used. Bromocriptine is a semisynthetic ergot alkaloid that acts as a dopamine-receptor agonist. Most trials assessing the efficacy of bromocriptine in the treatment of acromegaly were conducted in the 1970s and early 1980s. These studies determined that certain subsets of acromegalic patients have a favorable response to drug therapy with bromocriptine. These patients include individuals with high circulating concentrations of prolactin and patients who experience GH suppression following a single 2.5-mg dose of bromocriptine, known as a *bromocriptine challenge*.[19] A review evaluating 34 studies concluded that therapy with bromocriptine was effective in suppressing mean serum GH levels to <5 mcg/L in approximately 20% of patients.[20] Only 10% of patients experience normalization of IGF-1 concentrations with bromocriptine therapy, but >50% of patients treated with bromocriptine experience improvement in acromegalic symptoms.[9,21]

In the United States, bromocriptine is commercially available as 2.5-mg oral tablets and 5-mg oral capsules. In acromegalic patients, significant reductions in GH concentrations are observed within 1 to 2 hours of oral dosing. This effect persists for at least 4 to 5 hours. An overall clinical response in acromegalic patients typically occurs after 4 to 8 weeks of continuous bromocriptine therapy. For treatment of acromegaly, bromocriptine is initiated at a dose of 1.25 mg at bedtime and is increased by 1.25-mg increments every 3 to 4 days as needed.[19,20] Doses as high as 80 mg/day have been used for treatment of acromegaly, but clinical studies have shown that dosages >20 or 30 mg daily do not offer additional benefits in the suppression of GH.[18,20,21] When used for treatment of acromegaly, the duration of action of bromocriptine is shorter than that for treatment of hyperprolactinemia. Therefore, the total daily dose of bromocriptine should be divided into three or four doses.[18,19,21]

The most common adverse effects of bromocriptine therapy include central nervous system (CNS) symptoms such as headache, lightheadedness, dizziness, nervousness, and fatigue. Gastrointestinal effects such as nausea, abdominal pain, or diarrhea also are very common. Some patients may need to take bromocriptine with food to decrease the incidence of adverse gastrointestinal effects. Most adverse effects are seen early in the course of therapy and tend to decrease with continued treatment.[18,21] Bromocriptine may cause thickening of bronchial secretions and nasal congestion. Rare cases of psychiatric disturbances, pleural diseases, and an erythromelalgic syndrome (painful paroxysmal dilation of the blood vessels in the skin of the feet and lower extremities) have been reported with bromocriptine use. These conditions appear to be associated with higher doses and prolonged duration of therapy.[20,21]

Bromocriptine generally should be discontinued if a woman becomes pregnant while taking the drug. Surveillance of women who took bromocriptine throughout pregnancy does not suggest that bromocriptine is associated with an increased risk for birth defects.[21] If a woman becomes pregnant while taking bromocriptine, the risks and benefits of therapy should be fully considered. In most cases, the benefits of successful therapy outweigh the risks, and bromocriptine therapy should be continued if it is effective in improving symptoms and reducing elevated GH concentrations.

Other dopamine agonists that have been used to treat acromegaly include pergolide, cabergoline, lisuride, and quinagolide. Cabergoline may be especially useful in patients with pituitary tumors that secrete both prolactin and GH.[21,22] Quinagolide, a dopamine agonist available in Europe, has been shown to be more effective than both bromocriptine and cabergoline in normalizing GH and IGF-1 values in acromegalic patients.[19] Because of the potential cost advantages and convenience of oral administration, dopamine agonists are often considered for treatment of acromegaly prior to initiation of somatostatin analogs. However, the availability of long-acting somatostatin analogs has made these agents more attractive for first-line treatment of acromegaly.

SOMATOSTATIN ANALOGS

Octreotide is a long-acting somatostatin analog that is approximately 40 times more potent in inhibiting GH secretion than is endogenous somatostatin.[23,24] It also suppresses the LH response to GnRH; decreases splanchnic blood flow; and inhibits the secretion of insulin, vasoactive intestinal peptide (VIP), gastrin, secretin, motilin, serotonin, and pancreatic polypeptide. Lanreotide is another somatostatin analog, currently not available in the United States, which is a slow-release depot formulation administered twice monthly.[23] See Addendum at end of chapter.

Octreotide (Sandostatin) injection is commercially available in the United States for subcutaneous or intravenous administration. A long-acting intramuscular formulation of octreotide (Sandostatin LAR) is available for monthly administration. In addition to the treatment of acromegaly, octreotide has many other therapeutic uses, including the treatment of carcinoid tumors, vasoactive intestinal peptide-secreting tumors (VIPomas), gastrointestinal fistulas, variceal bleeding, diarrheal states, and irritable bowel syndrome.

The efficacy of octreotide for treatment of acromegaly has been determined by two major multicenter trials.[25,26] These studies determined that drug therapy with octreotide suppresses mean serum GH concentrations to <5 mcg/L and normalizes serum IGF-1 concentrations in 50% to 60% of acromegalic patients. Octreotide also is beneficial in reducing the clinical signs and symptoms of acromegaly. In a 6-month multicenter trial, 70% of patients experienced significant relief of headaches.[26] In some patients, relief of headache symptoms occurred within minutes of octreotide administration. In addition, middle-finger circumference was reduced significantly, and 50% to 75% of patients experienced improvement in symptoms of excessive perspiration, fatigue, joint pain, and cystic acne. A 2-year followup of 103 patients treated with octreotide showed that octreotide therapy is safe and effective for long-term use in acromegalic patients.[27] Octreotide also has been shown to improve the cardiovascular manifestations of acromegaly, including left ventricular hypertrophy and cardiac performance.[28–31] Data from two major multicenter trials indicate that pituitary tumor growth is halted during octreotide treatment, and a small number of patients experience tumor regression.[25,26] Data from more recent studies indicate that shrinkage of pituitary tumor mass during octreotide therapy occurs in approximately 50% of patients.[32]

The pharmacodynamic effects of long-acting octreotide are similar to those of subcutaneously administered octreotide. Single monthly doses of long-acting octreotide have been shown to be at least as effective as daily doses of 300 or 600 mcg of subcutaneous octreotide administered in divided doses three times daily in normalizing IGF-1 levels and maintaining suppression of mean serum GH concentrations.[33] A large multicenter trial evaluating the efficacy of long-acting octreotide in acromegalic patients who previously had responded to subcutaneously administered octreotide reported suppression of GH concentrations to <5 mcg/L in 94% of patients and normalization of IGF-1 in 66% of patients following 1 year of therapy.[34]

Response to long-term therapy with octreotide is related to the presence and increased quantity of functioning somatostatin receptors located in the pituitary adenoma.[26,27] Identification of patients who most likely will respond to octreotide, prior to initiation of therapy, is important when considering the high cost of this medication and the inconvenience of subcutaneous or intramuscular drug administration. Suppression of serum GH concentrations after a single 50-mcg dose of octreotide has been used to predict a favorable long-term response to octreotide therapy.[35,36]

❸ The initial dose of octreotide for treatment of acromegaly is 100 mcg administered every 8 hours.[17,20,24] Some clinicians recommend a starting dose of 50 mcg every 8 hours, then increasing the dose to 100 mcg every 8 hours after 1 week, to improve the patient's tolerance of adverse gastrointestinal effects.[14,18] The dose can be increased by increments of 50 mcg every 1 to 2 weeks based on mean serum GH and IGF-1 concentrations. Patients who experience a significant rise in GH prior to the end of the 8-hour dosing interval may benefit from decreasing the dosing interval to every 4 to 6 hours. Although doses as high as 1,500 mcg/day have been used, doses >600 mcg daily generally do not offer additional benefits, and most patients are adequately managed with 100 to 200 mcg three times daily.[18,25–27] Patients who have been maintained on subcutaneous octreotide for at least 2 weeks and have shown response to therapy can be converted to the long-acting depot form of octreotide. The initial dose of long-acting octreotide is 20 mg administered intramuscularly in the gluteal region every 28 days. Steady-state serum concentrations are not obtained until after 3 months of therapy. Therefore, dosage adjustments for long-acting octreotide should not be considered until after this time. Some patients may require additional subcutaneous injections during the initial dose-titration phase in order to control symptoms. Long-acting octreotide doses >30 mg every 4 weeks have not been studied.

The most common adverse effects of octreotide therapy are gastrointestinal disturbances such as diarrhea, nausea, abdominal cramps, malabsorption of fat, and flatulence.[17,18,23] These effects are dose dependent and can be seen within a few hours of the first octreotide injection. Gastrointestinal adverse effects occur in approximately 75% of patients but usually subside within 10 to 14 days of continued treatment.[17,18,23] Octreotide has been reported to cause injection-site pain (4% to 31%), conduction abnormalities and arrhythmias (9%), biochemical hypothyroidism (2% to 12%), biliary tract disorders (4% to 50%), and abnormalities in glucose metabolism (2% to 18%).[20,23]

Octreotide also inhibits cholecystokinin release and gallbladder motility, predisposing patients to the development of cholelithiasis.[17,18,23] The development of gallstones is a long-term adverse effect of octreotide use and is largely dependent on geographic factors, dietary habits, and length of therapy.[20,24] The incidence of gallstones in acromegalic patients receiving octreotide increases with length of therapy and has been reported to range from 20% to 50%.[24–27] However, most patients are asymptomatic, and the diagnosis of cholelithiasis usually is made following an ultrasonographic study that is not prompted by patient symptoms. It has been estimated that only 1% of patients will develop symptomatic gallstones during 1 year of octreotide treatment.[24] Because octreotide-induced gallstones usually are present without clinical symptoms, the latest International Acromegaly Consensus recommends that treatment of octreotide-induced gallstones be the same as that for gallstones in the general population.[9,15] Prophylactic cholecystectomy or medical therapy with ursodeoxycholic acid for acromegalic patients with asymptomatic gallstones usually is not recommended. A small number of studies have suggested that the incidence of gallstone development may be lower with long-acting octreotide compared to subcutaneous octreotide.[33,34] However, further studies are needed to confirm this observation.

❹ The effect of octreotide on glucose metabolism in patients with acromegaly is multifactorial. Decreases in serum GH concentrations induced by octreotide should result in decreased hepatic gluconeogenesis and increased insulin-receptor sensitivity. However, octreotide also decreases insulin secretion and increases IGFBP-1, which is known to inhibit the insulin-like effects of IGF-1. In addition, octreotide delays the gastrointestinal absorption of glucose, which may further alter glucose metabolism in acromegalic patients.[37] Small studies conducted in acromegalic patients receiving octreotide have reported improvement in insulin sensitivity as well as impaired insulin secretion.[37,38] Risk factors associated with worsening glucose tolerance included female gender and elevated baseline insulin values. Although octreotide appears to have a beneficial effect on glucose tolerance in most patients, glucose determinations should be obtained frequently in the early stages of octreotide therapy in all acromegalic patients.

GROWTH HORMONE RECEPTOR ANTAGONIST

❺ Pegvisomant (Somavert) is a genetically engineered GH derivative that binds to GH receptors in the liver and inhibits IGF-1. This agent is different from other medications used in the management of acromegaly because it does not inhibit GH production; rather, it blocks the physiologic effects of GH on target tissues. Therefore, GH concentrations remain elevated during therapy, and response to treatment is evidenced by a reduction in IGF-1 concentrations. Unlike somatostatin analogs, the pharmacologic activity of pegvisomant does not depend on the presence and quantity of somatostatin receptors in the pituitary tumor.[39] Studies evaluating the clinical efficacy of pegvisomant in acromegalic patients have reported a dose-dependent normalization of IGF-1 concentrations in 54% to 89% of patients after 12 weeks of therapy and in 97% of patients after 1 year of therapy.[40,41] Significant improvements in the clinical signs and symptoms of acromegaly were reported and persisted throughout the 1-year treatment period.[41] Adverse effects appeared to be minimal and included injection-site pain, gastrointestinal complaints such as nausea and diarrhea, and flu-like symptoms. Significant elevations in hepatic aminotransferase concentrations, which were reversible upon discontinuation of the drug, were reported in two patients.[40] As a result, hepatic function tests should be monitored very closely during therapy as outlined in the product labeling, and the drug should be used with caution in patients with baseline elevations in hepatic aminotransferase concentrations. GH concentrations increased significantly during the first 6 months of therapy. Although tumor size did not change significantly during clinical trials, there are theoretical concerns that persistently elevated GH concentrations may stimulate tumor growth or result in other unfavorable long-term effects.

Pegvisomant is commercially available in the United States for daily subcutaneous use. The first dose should be administered under the supervision of a physician as a 40-mg loading dose. Subsequent doses are self-administered by the patient starting at a dose of 10 mg daily. The dose can be adjusted in 5-mg increments based on serum IGF-1 concentrations every 4 to 6 weeks, up to a maximum daily dose of 30 mg.[42]

Based on the available data, pegvisomant appears to be among the most effective agents for normalizing IGF-1 serum concentrations. However, given the limited clinical data, further study is needed to determine the long-term safety and efficacy of pegvisomant in the treatment of acromegaly. Pegvisomant is licensed in the European Union for treatment of acromegaly as a third-line agent, for patients with an inadequate response to surgery and/or radiation therapy, and in patients in whom appropriate medical treatment with somatostatin analogs did not normalize IGF-1 concentrations. Use of pegvisomant after failure of other modalities appears to be a reasonable approach to therapy for acromegaly.

COMBINATION THERAPY

Several small studies have suggested that combination therapy with octreotide and dopamine agonists (bromocriptine or cabergoline) or octreotide and pegvisomant may be more beneficial than monotherapy with either drug alone.[20,23,43,44] Because of the potential for additive adverse effects, combination therapy should be considered as a therapeutic option only for refractory patients who have not fully responded to monotherapy.

PHARMACOECONOMIC CONSIDERATIONS

Cost-effectiveness comparisons of the various treatment options for patients with acromegaly have not been performed. Considering that approximately 40% of patients are not completely cured after transsphenoidal surgery, pharmacologic treatment often becomes necessary. Bromocriptine and cabergoline are considerably less expensive than octreotide and pegvisomant. However, these agents are not effective in the majority of patients. Long-acting octreotide offers a convenient method of octreotide administration for acromegalic patients. Although this formulation is approximately twice the cost of subcutaneous octreotide, it may result in improved patient compliance, quality of life, and overall disease management. Pegvisomant appears to the most effective agent for normalizing IGF-1 concentrations and may be useful in patients who are intolerant to or have not responded to therapy with dopamine agonists or somatostatin analogs. However, pegvisomant is significantly more expensive than long-acting octreotide and requires daily subcutaneous injections. Long-term studies evaluating the safety of pegvisomant are needed to clearly define its role in the management of acromegaly. The drug therapy of choice for an acromegalic patient should be determined by careful consideration of several patient-specific factors, including clinical response, compliance, tolerability, and cost of therapy.

CLINICAL CONTROVERSY

Some clinicians advocate the use of somatostatin analogs as primary therapy for acromegaly in place of surgery. However, others believe that sufficient long-term safety and efficacy data are lacking.

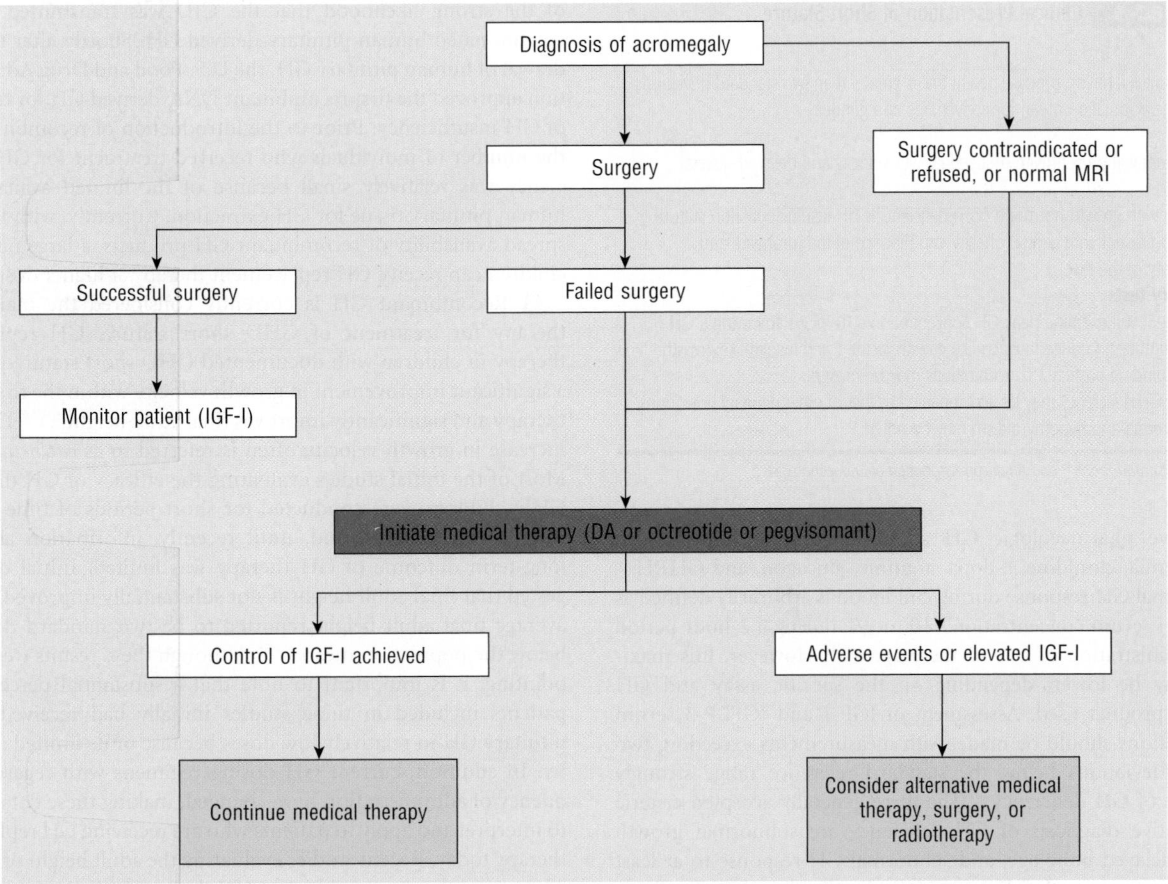

FIGURE 80-2. Treatment algorithm for acromegaly. (DA, dopamine agonist; IGF-I, insulin-like growth factor type I; MRI, magnetic resonance imaging.) *(Modified from Clemmons DR, Chihara K, Freda PU, et al. Optimizing control of acromegaly: integrating a growth hormone receptor antagonist into the treatment algorithm. J Clin Endocrinol Metab 2003;88:4759–4767. Copyright 2003, The Endocrine Society.)*

■ CONCLUSIONS

Acromegaly is a chronic debilitating disease characterized by excess GH secretion most commonly caused by a GH-secreting pituitary adenoma. Transsphenoidal surgical resection of the adenoma is the current treatment of choice for most patients with acromegaly. Patients who are poor surgical candidates may receive radiation therapy or long-term pharmacologic therapy. Drug therapy options within the United States for acromegaly include dopamine agonists, the somatostatin analog octreotide, and pegvisomant. Figure 80–2 shows a treatment algorithm for the management of acromegaly.[9,39]

GROWTH HORMONE DEFICIENCY

Short stature is a condition that is commonly defined by a physical height that is more than two standard deviations below the population mean and lower than the third percentile for height in a specific age group.[45–47] It has been estimated that more than 1.8 million children in the United States can be characterized as having short stature.[47] Short stature is a very broad term describing a condition that may be the result of many different causes. A true lack of GH is among the least common causes and is known as growth hormone-deficient (GHD) short stature. Absolute GH deficiency is a congenital disorder that can result from various genetic abnormalities, such as GHRH deficiency, GH gene deletion, and developmental disorders including pituitary aplasia or hypoplasia.[45,46] GH insufficiency is an acquired condition that can result secondary to hypothalamic or pituitary tumors, cranial irradiation, head trauma, pituitary infarction, and various types of CNS infections. In addition, psychosocial deprivation, hypothyroidism, poorly controlled diabetes mellitus, treatment of precocious puberty with LH-releasing hormone agonists, and pharmacologic agents such as glucocorticoids, methylphenidate, and dextroamphetamine may induce transient GH insufficiency.[45]

Short stature also occurs with several conditions that are not associated with a true GH deficiency or insufficiency. These conditions include intrauterine growth restriction; constitutional growth delay; malnutrition; malabsorption of nutrients associated with inflammatory bowel disease, celiac disease, and cystic fibrosis; chronic renal failure; skeletal and cartilage dysplasia; and genetic syndromes such as Turner's syndrome.[45,46,48] In addition, many children are diagnosed with idiopathic or normal variant short stature. These patients have heights that are significantly lower than the third percentile but present with normal GH serum concentrations and no specific underlying explanation for short stature.[47]

Children with GHD short stature usually are born with an average birth weight. Decreases in growth velocity generally become evident between the ages of 6 months and 3 years.[45] In contrast, GH insufficiency may arise at any age during growth and development. The clinical characteristics of GHD or GH-insufficient children are listed in Table 80–3.[45,46]

Several factors must be considered in the diagnosis of GH deficiency or insufficiency. Standard epidemiologic growth charts developed by the National Center for Health Statistics typically are used to determine the percentile of anthropometric measurements, such as height, weight, and head circumference. Pubertal stage typically is determined using the Tanner method. Bone age is determined according to published standards, and growth velocity is calculated to determine the patient's height velocity percentile using standard growth-velocity charts.[45,46,48] GH deficiency is rarely seen in the absence of delayed skeletal maturation and decreased growth velocity. In addition, several different provocative stimuli that induce GH secretion are used diagnostically to determine GH status. Common

TABLE 80-3 Clinical Presentation of Short Stature

General
- The patient will have a physical height that is greater than two standard deviations below the population mean for a given age and gender.

Signs
- The patient will present with reduced growth velocity and delayed skeletal maturation.
- Children with growth hormone (GH)-deficient or GH-insufficient short stature may also present with central obesity, prominence of the forehead, and immaturity of the face.

Laboratory tests
- The patient will exhibit a peak GH concentration <10 mcg/L following a GH provocation test. Reduced insulin-like growth factor-1 and insulin-like growth factor-1 binding protein-3 concentrations may be present.
- Because GH deficiency may be accompanied by loss of other pituitary hormones, hypoglycemia and hypothyroidism may be noted.

From Hindmarsh and Brook[45] and American Association of Endocrinologists.[46]

provocative pharmacologic GH stimuli include insulin-induced hypoglycemia, clonidine, L-dopa, arginine, glucagon, and GHRH.[46] A subnormal GH response during childhood is arbitrarily defined as a peak GH serum concentration <10 mcg/L during a 2-hour period after administration of one of these agents.[46] However, this maximum may be lower, depending on the specific assay and GH reference product used. Assessment of IGF-1 and IGFBP-3 serum concentrations should be made, with measurements exceeding two standard deviations below the standard reference range strongly suggestive of GH deficiency.[46] The three generally accepted criteria for definitive diagnosis of GH deficiency are subnormal growth velocity, delayed bone age, and subnormal GH response to at least two provocative stimuli.[49] For prepubertal and early pubertal patients (Tanner stage less than III), priming with sex hormones to improve the specificity of GH provocation tests is often considered. Some patients exhibit clinical signs of GH deficiency, subnormal growth velocity, and delayed bone age despite GH levels that are within normal limits after provocative testing. This makes diagnosis in this group of patients very difficult. Diagnosis based on GH stimulation tests becomes further complicated because of the paucity of data reporting the normal range of GH concentrations after provocative testing in healthy children and the fact that commercial GH assays currently available may not be equivalent. One study comparing several different GH assays found a significant variation between measured GH serum concentrations.[49] Because of these limitations, careful consideration of multiple factors by a pediatric endocrinology specialist is required to correctly diagnose GH deficiency.

TREATMENT

Growth Hormone Deficiency

■ PHARMACOLOGIC THERAPY

The treatment of GH deficiency with pituitary-derived human GH was first reported in the late 1950s. The National Hormone and Pituitary Program was founded by the National Institutes of Health in 1963 to coordinate the collection of human pituitary glands and purification of GH for administration to children with GH deficiency. In 1985, three deaths linked to Creutzfeldt-Jakob's disease (CJD) were identified in young individuals who were previously treated with human pituitary GH. An evaluation of National Hormone and Pituitary Program data identified 26 cases of fatal CJD in a cohort of 6,107 patients who received treatment with human pituitary-derived GH in the United States between 1963 and 1985.[50] Human pituitary GH was withdrawn from the U.S. market because of the strong likelihood that the CJD was transmitted through contaminated human pituitary-derived GH. Shortly after the withdrawal of human pituitary GH, the U.S. Food and Drug Administration approved the first recombinant DNA-derived GH for treatment of GH insufficiency. Prior to the introduction of recombinant GH, the number of individuals who received treatment for GH insufficiency was relatively small because of the limited availability of human pituitary tissue for GH extraction. Currently, with the widespread availability of recombinant GH products, a large number of children can receive GH replacement therapy at higher doses.

❻ Recombinant GH is currently considered the mainstay of therapy for treatment of GHD short stature. GH replacement therapy in children with documented GHD short stature produces a significant improvement in growth velocity within the first year of therapy and significantly improves final adult height.[51–54] The initial increase in growth velocity often is referred to as *catch-up growth*. Most of the initial studies evaluating the efficacy of GH therapy in GHD children were conducted for short periods of time in small numbers of patients, and, until recently, information about the long-term outcome of GH therapy was limited. Initial data suggested that final adult height is not substantially improved, with an average final adult height reported to be two standard deviations below the population mean.[55–58] Although these results were disappointing, it is important to note that a substantial percentage of patients included in these studies initially had received human pituitary GH in relatively low doses because of its limited availability. In addition, current GH dosing regimens with regard to frequency of administration have changed, making these data difficult to interpret and apply to patients who are receiving GH replacement therapy today. Recent studies evaluating the adult height of children who received only recombinant GH therapy with currently recommended dosing regimens suggest that current recombinant GH therapy has a greater impact on final adult height than previously reported.[51–54] These studies have reported average final adult heights ranging from 0.5 to 1.7 standard deviations below the population mean. Initiation of therapy at an early chronologic age, prior to the onset of puberty, is associated with a more favorable increase in final height.[46,52,53] Therefore, prompt diagnosis of GH deficiency and early initiation of replacement therapy with recombinant GH are crucial factors in optimizing the final adult height of children with GH deficiency.

Recombinant GH has been shown to increase the short-term growth rate in pediatric patients with chronic renal insufficiency, intrauterine growth restriction, Turner's syndrome, idiopathic short stature, and Prader-Willi's syndrome and is approved by the FDA for treatment of growth failure associated with these conditions.[46] GH is also FDA approved for treatment of adult GH deficiency, short bowel syndrome in patients receiving specialized nutritional support, and acquired immunodeficiency syndrome wasting syndrome. When used in adult patients, the recommended dosage of recombinant GH is significantly lower than the dosage used in pediatric patients. Adult patients with GH deficiency during childhood must have the diagnosis of GH deficiency confirmed when they are adults. Long-term GH therapy in GHD adults significantly decreases body fat, increases muscle mass, and improves exercise capacity.[46] GH therapy in adults has been shown to improve the cardiac risk profile, bone mineral density, and psychological well-being.[59–61] In addition, GH currently is being investigated for a variety of disorders, including infertility, chronic fatigue, obesity, and natural aging.[46] Use of GH as an anabolic agent for management of acute catabolism is not recommended.[46]

The majority of short children in the United States do not have an identifiable medical cause for their condition, but with widespread availability of several recombinant GH formulations, many children have received GH therapy regardless of the underlying etiology of their short stature. The use of recombinant GH therapy in children with non-GHD short stature, also referred to as *idiopathic short stature,* has been studied by many investigators and was approved by the FDA in 2003. However, the use of GH therapy in this patient population remains controversial. A metaanalysis of 38 clinical studies evaluating the efficacy of GH treatment in children with idiopathic short stature reported average increases in final adult height of 4 to 5 cm (1.6 to 2 inches) following a mean duration of therapy of 4.7 years.[62] This corresponded to an increase above the predicted final adult height of 0.56 to 0.63 standard deviations of the population mean. A more recently published randomized, double-blind, placebo-controlled trial with a mean GH treatment duration of 4.4 years reported an increase in final adult height of 3.7 cm (1.5 inches).[63] The slightly smaller height increase reported in the later study may be explained by the more stringent study design, lower mean GH doses, and GH treatment initiation at an older age (peripubertal) compared to the studies included in the metaanalysis.

CLINICAL CONTROVERSY

Most pediatric endocrinologists in the United States believe that GH therapy is appropriate treatment in certain patients with non-GHD short stature. However, given the high cost of therapy and small increases in height, use of GH in this patient population remains controversial.

7 Eleven different recombinant GH products currently are available for use in the United States (Genotropin, Humatrope, Norditropin, Nutropin, Nutropin AQ, Nutropin Depot, Omnitrope, Saizen, Serostim, Tev-Tropin, and Zorbtive) Each of these products contains somatropin. Somatropin is composed of the same amino acid sequence as human pituitary GH. Recombinant GH formulations must be administered by intramuscular or subcutaneous injection. Nutropin AQ, Norditropin, and Serostim LQ are the only GH products available as liquid formulations. The remaining products are formulated as lyophilized powders for injection, and patients must be instructed regarding proper administration. A long-acting depot form of GH, Nutropin Depot, is available for once- or twice-monthly subcutaneous injection. This product may be particularly useful for patients who are noncompliant or experience significant adverse effects from frequent injections. The potency of GH products is expressed as international units per milligram (international units/mg), with 1 mg containing approximately 2.6 international units of GH. Direct comparisons between the different recombinant GH products have not been published. However, all GH products are generally considered to be equally efficacious. The recommended dose for treatment of GHD short stature in children is 0.3 mg/kg/wk.[46] Recombinant GH can be administered daily or in equal doses six times per week, depending on the specific GH product used.[46] Dosing regimens with greater frequency of administration have been shown to provide more favorable short-term growth responses.[46] GH replacement therapy should be initiated as early as possible after diagnosis of GH insufficiency and continued until a desirable height is reached or growth velocity has decreased to <2.5 cm per year after the pubertal growth spurt. However, the suitable time point for discontinuation of therapy with growth-promoting doses remains controversial. Glucocorticoids may inhibit the growth-promoting effects of recombinant GH, and concomitant administration of androgens, estrogens, thyroid hormones, or anabolic steroids may accelerate epiphyseal closure and compromise final height.

Three large databases, the National Cooperative Growth Study, the Kabi International Growth Study, and the Australian and New Zealand growth database (OZGROW), have been developed to collect postmarketing adverse effect data or reports associated with recombinant GH. Development of these databases was prompted by the unexpected and tragic cases of CJD reported in patients treated with human pituitary GH. These databases are maintained by pharmaceutical companies that manufacture GH products.[64] Recombinant GH is generally well tolerated in children, and adverse effects are relatively uncommon.[64,65] A small number of patients may complain of injection-site pain or arthralgias. Idiopathic intracranial hypertension, also known as *pseudotumor cerebri,* has been reported in a very small number of children receiving GH therapy. This condition usually develops within the first 8 to 12 of weeks of treatment and presents with symptoms such as headache, blurred vision, diplopia, nausea, and vomiting.[64] The symptoms of idiopathic intracranial hypertension usually resolve after discontinuation of GH therapy, and long-term complications are rare. Cases of slipped capital femoral epiphysis have been reported in children with GH deficiency who are receiving GH therapy.[64] This condition is thought to occur as a result of the increased width of the femoral plate during GH treatment, but it also has been reported in GHD children who are not receiving GH replacement. Patients with this condition typically complain of hip or knee pain. Slipped capital femoral epiphysis can be managed by an orthopedic surgeon, and GH therapy does not need to be withdrawn. Because GH is known to cause decreased insulin sensitivity, hyperglycemia and diabetes mellitus may develop.[66] Patients who have specific predisposing risk factors for diabetes mellitus are at greatest risk for this adverse effect.[64–66] Glycosylated hemoglobin concentrations should be monitored in all patients receiving GH products.[46] GH may promote the growth of various types of neoplasms and increase tumor recurrence rates in patients with a history of malignancy.[46,64,65] For this reason, GH should not be administered to patients with an active malignant tumor or a history of recurrent tumor growth. In 1988, a Japanese report indicated that children receiving GH therapy were twice as likely to develop leukemia as children who were not receiving the hormone.[67] A more recent analysis of all collected reports of leukemia associated with GH therapy determined that these children had other leukemia risk factors (Fanconi's anemia, Bloom's syndrome, or history of cancer).[68] GH therapy in children without these risk factors does not appear to predispose children to develop leukemia.[64,65,68] Some patients may develop antibodies to recombinant GH. The development of antibodies during replacement therapy with recombinant GH products has been reported to be relatively low, affecting approximately 15% to 20% of patients.[69,70] More importantly, the presence of GH antibodies has not been shown to adversely affect growth response and appears to be clinically insignificant except in patients with GH gene deletions. Finally, recent postmarketing reports suggest an increased risk of death associated with long-term GH treatment in children with Prader-Willi's syndrome who are severely obese or have severe respiratory impairment. GH treatment is contraindicated in patients with Prader-Willi's syndrome who have any of these risk factors.

RECOMBINANT INSULIN-LIKE GROWTH FACTOR-1

Recombinant IGF-1 products, consisting of either IGF-1 alone (mecasermin [Increlex]) or IGF-1 in combination with IGFBP-3 (mecasermin rinfabate [Iplex]), have been recently approved by the FDA for the treatment of children with short stature due to severe primary IGF-1 deficiency (defined as children with height standard deviation score ≤–3.0 plus basal IGF-1 standard deviation score ≤–3.0, plus normal or elevated GH concentration) or GH gene deletion with neutralizing antibodies to GH. Recombinant IGF-1 products are not intended for use in subjects with secondary forms of IGF-1 deficiency, such as GH deficiency, malnutrition, hypothyroidism, or chronic treatment with pharmacologic doses of antiinflammatory steroids. Recombinant IGF-1 products have been shown to increase growth velocity in children with short stature who have low IGF-1 serum concentrations and resistance to GH.[70–72] However, the efficacy of these agents is less than that reported with GH products in patients with GH deficiency.

The recommended dose of mecasermin is 0.04 to 0.12 mg/kg administered by subcutaneous injection twice daily. Mecasermin rinfabate is administered by once-daily injections at a dose of 1 to 2 mg/kg. Because of the insulin-like effects of these products, patients should be monitored very closely for hypoglycemia, and the drug should be initiated at a dose at the lower end of the dosage range and administered with a meal or snack. The incidence of hypoglycemia may be less frequent with mecasermin rinfabate because of the longer half-life of the combination product.[70] Additional adverse effects experienced by patients receiving recombinant IGF-1 products include injection-site reactions, tonsillar/adenoidal hypertrophy, lymphoid hypertrophy, coarsening facial features, headache, dizziness, and arthralgia.[71,72] Intracranial hypertension has been reported in a small number of patients.[72] Additional studies are needed to elucidate the exact role of recombinant IGF-1 products in the management of short stature not caused by GH gene deletion or GH receptor defects.

■ GROWTH HORMONE-RELEASING HORMONE

A synthetic GHRH product known as sermorelin (Geref) currently is FDA approved for the treatment of idiopathic GH deficiency in children. Sermorelin [GH-RH(1–29)-NH_2] is composed of 29 amino acid residues that are identical to the amino-terminal segment of human GHRH. Although not as effective as recombinant GH therapy, sermorelin has been shown to increase short-term growth velocity in children with idiopathic GH deficiency.[73] This product also has been shown to increase growth velocity in children who have GH deficiency secondary to hypothalamic damage rather than pituitary abnormalities, as is observed with radiation-induced GH deficiency.[74] In most cases of radiation-induced GH deficiency, pituitary somatotropes are capable of secreting endogenous GH, and stimulation of these cells by exogenously administered GHRH may restore the natural pulsatile secretion of GH and result in increased growth rate.

The recommended dose of sermorelin is 0.03 mg/kg administered daily by subcutaneous injection. No serious adverse events have been identified. The most common adverse effect reported by patients receiving sermorelin therapy is injection-site pain. Because normal pituitary function is needed for sermorelin to stimulate GH secretion, children should not receive GHRH therapy with sermorelin unless adequate capacity to secrete GH is documented by provocative GH stimulation testing. Sermorelin may prove to be a beneficial therapeutic option in the treatment of various types of non-GHD short stature. However, because of its mechanism of action, sermorelin does not have a role in the treatment of most cases of true GHD short stature.

■ EVALUATION OF THERAPEUTIC OUTCOMES

Appropriate monitoring of therapy for GHD and non-GHD short stature includes regular assessments of height, weight, growth velocity, serum alkaline phosphatase, and bone age every 6 to 12 months. Additional laboratory tests to monitor for potential adverse effects include serum glucose concentration and thyroid function. The dose of GH will periodically need to be increased as weight increases in growing children.

■ PHARMACOECONOMIC CONSIDERATIONS

The treatment of short stature with recombinant GH is expensive. Despite the prohibitive cost, recombinant GH remains the mainstay of therapy for children with GHD short stature. However, treatment of non-GHD short stature with recombinant GH is not widely accepted. The benefits in final adult height and increases in growth velocity, particularly in children with true GH deficiency, are associated with significant psychosocial benefits. Many clinicians believe that GH therapy can improve quality of life and should be made available to all children with short stature, regardless of whether or not they are GH deficient.[75] Until studies using recombinant GH more definitively demonstrate improvements in both final adult height and quality of life, the cost-effectiveness of GH, particularly for non-GHD short stature, remains uncertain.

■ CONCLUSIONS

GH deficiency during childhood results in short stature. Replacement with recombinant GH is considered the mainstay of therapy for patients with GHD short stature, but its use for treatment of non-GHD short stature remains controversial, albeit such treatment is FDA approved. Recombinant GH has proven to be safe for use in children and is associated with few adverse effects. The synthetic GHRH sermorelin and other GH-releasing peptides and preparations of IGF-1 may provide benefit for patients with non-GHD short stature. GH regimens can be particularly demanding and inconvenient for pediatric patients because they must be administered by subcutaneous injection. Knowledge of the long-term benefits and risks is critical to the development of rational, cost-effective treatments for patients with short stature.

PROLACTIN

PHYSIOLOGIC EFFECTS

Prolactin is secreted in a pulsatile fashion by the lactotroph cells of the anterior pituitary, with the highest peak concentrations observed during sleep.[4] The secretion of prolactin is regulated primarily by tonic hypothalamic inhibitory effects of dopamine. As described earlier in this chapter and as listed in Table 80–1, many factors can affect prolactin secretion. During pregnancy, prolactin serum concentrations rise substantially above normal. All other conditions characterized by excess prolactin serum concentrations, known as *hyperprolactinemia,* are considered pathologic.

HYPERPROLACTINEMIA

Hyperprolactinemia is a state of persistent serum prolactin elevation. Prolactin concentrations >20 mcg/L observed on multiple occasions are generally considered indicative of hyperprolactinemia.[76,77] Hyperprolactinemia usually affects women of reproductive age.[76,78] The incidence of hyperprolactinemia in the general population is reported to be <1%.[77]

Hyperprolactinemia has several etiologies. The most common causes are benign prolactin-secreting pituitary tumors, known as *prolactinomas,* and various medications. Prolactinomas are classified according to size. Prolactin-secreting microadenomas are <10 mm in diameter and often do not increase in size.[4,77] In contrast, macroadenomas are tumors with a diameter >10 mm that continue to grow and can cause invasion of surrounding tissues.[4,77] In the presence of a prolactinoma, prolactin serum concentrations may remain normal or may be markedly elevated to thousands of micrograms per liter.

❽ Any pharmacologic agent that antagonizes dopamine or increases the release of prolactin can induce hyperprolactinemia (Table 80–4). Serotonin is a strong stimulator of prolactin secretion, and selective serotonin reuptake inhibitors (SSRIs) such as fluoxetine, paroxetine, sertraline, and fluvoxamine are the medications

TABLE 80-4 Drug-Induced Hyperprolactinemia

Dopamine antagonists
Antipsychotics
Phenothiazines
Metoclopramide
Domperidone
Prolactin stimulators
Methyldopa
Reserpine
Selective serotonin reuptake inhibitors (SSRIs)
Dexfenfluramine
Estrogens
Progestins
Protease inhibitors
Gonadotropin-releasing hormone analogs
Benzodiazepines
Tricyclic antidepressants
Monoamine oxidase inhibitors
H_2-Receptor antagonists
Opioids
Other
Verapamil

From Molitch,[4] Mah and Webster,[77] Gillam et al.,[78] and Davies.[79]

most frequently associated with hyperprolactinemia.[79] Prior to the increased use of SSRIs, antipsychotic medications with potent dopamine-receptor blockade, such as the phenothiazine derivatives and haloperidol, were most often identified as the cause of drug-induced hyperprolactinemia.[80] Metoclopramide and domperidone, an antiemetic available in Europe, are potent dopamine-receptor antagonists reported to induce hyperprolactinemia.[79] Hormones such as estrogen and progesterone, commonly prescribed as oral contraceptives, can stimulate lactotroph growth to promote prolactin secretion and have been implicated in drug-induced hyperprolactinemia. Although the exact mechanism of action remains to be determined, the calcium channel-blocking agent verapamil has been associated with cases of hyperprolactinemia.[4,79] Methyldopa and reserpine, although not used frequently in clinical practice today, are antihypertensive agents that can stimulate prolactin secretion.[79] Prolactin concentrations may increase with administration of GnRH analogs such as leuprolide or goserelin.[79] Other medications rarely reported to cause hyperprolactinemia include H_2-receptor blocking agents, benzodiazepines, tricyclic antidepressants, dexfenfluramine, opioids, protease inhibitors, and monoamine oxidase inhibitors.[4,77,79] Prolactin levels do not typically rise to >150 mcg/L in cases of drug-induced hyperprolactinemia. Measurement of serum prolactin concentrations prior to the initiation of therapy with medications known to cause prolactin elevation may obviate the need for extensive examination of pituitary function and aid with the appropriate diagnosis of drug-induced hyperprolactinemia.

Less common etiologies include CNS lesions that physically compress the pituitary stalk and interrupt tonic hypothalamic dopamine secretion, resulting in hyperprolactinemia.[77] Increased TRH concentrations in hypothyroidism can stimulate prolactin secretion and cause hyperprolactinemia. During conditions of renal or hepatic compromise, the clearance of prolactin is decreased, resulting in elevated prolactin concentrations.[4] Despite vigorous diagnostic effort, the cause of hyperprolactinemia cannot always be determined. This is known as *idiopathic hyperprolactinemia* and most likely is a result of the presence of very small tumors that are not detected by standard imaging techniques.[76] It should be noted that many physiologic factors, such as stress (including the stress of phlebotomy), sleep, exercise, coitus, and eating, also can induce transiently elevated prolactin levels.[4,76] This emphasizes the importance of obtaining multiple prolactin measurements to confirm the diagnosis. Ideally, after an intravenous line is placed in the patient's arm, the patient should rest in a supine position or in a chair for 2 hours before prolactin samples are collected.

TABLE 80-5 Clinical Presentation of Hyperprolactinemia

General

Hyperprolactinemia most commonly affects women and is very rare in men.

Signs and symptoms

- The patient may complain of symptoms related to local effects of the prolactin-secreting tumor, such as headache and visual disturbances, that result from tumor compression of the optic chiasm.
- Female patients experience oligomenorrhea, amenorrhea, galactorrhea, infertility, decreased libido, hirsutism, and acne.
- Male patients experience decreased libido, erectile dysfunction, infertility, reduced muscle mass, galactorrhea, and gynecomastia.

Laboratory tests

Prolactin serum concentrations at rest will be >20 mcg/L on multiple occasions.

Additional clinical sequelae

- Prolonged suppression of estrogen in premenopausal women with hyperprolactinemia leads to decreases in bone mineral density and significant risk for development of osteoporosis.
- Risk for ischemic heart disease may be increased with untreated hyperprolactinemia.

From Molitch,[4] Schlechte,[76] and Mah and Webster.[77]

Elevated prolactin serum concentrations inhibit gonadotropin secretion and sex-steroid synthesis.[76] Because prolactin concentrations >60 mcg/L are associated with anovulation, women with hyperprolactinemia typically present with menstrual irregularities such as oligomenorrhea or amenorrhea and infertility.[7,76,77] In addition, approximately 40% to 80% of women with hyperprolactinemia will have galactorrhea.[76,77] The clinical presentation of patients with hyperprolactinemia is summarized in Table 80–5.[4,76,77]

The diagnosis of hyperprolactinemia, as defined by multiple prolactin serum concentrations >20 mcg/L, is relatively simple. However, identifying the underlying cause of this abnormality may be more challenging. Patients with modest prolactin elevations should have multiple prolactin serum determinations to minimize the potential for detecting only transient increases in prolactin. A careful medication history is essential, and the presence of hypothyroidism, renal failure, or hepatic dysfunction should be evaluated. If the cause of hyperprolactinemia remains ambiguous, a computed tomography scan or magnetic resonance imaging study should be performed to determine the presence of a pituitary tumor.[76,77] If an underlying cause of elevated prolactin serum concentration is not determined, the hyperprolactinemia is considered to be idiopathic.

TREATMENT

Hyperprolactinemia

The treatment of hyperprolactinemia depends on the underlying cause of the abnormality. In cases of drug-induced hyperprolactinemia, discontinuation of the offending medication and initiation of an appropriate therapeutic alternative usually normalizes serum prolactin concentrations.[79] In cases for which an appropriate therapeutic alternative does not exist, medical therapy with dopamine agonists is warranted. Sex-steroid replacement also should be considered.[77] Treatment options for the management of prolactinomas include clinical observation, medical therapy with dopamine agonists, radiation therapy, and transsphenoidal surgical removal of the tumor.[4,76–78] Because prolactin-secreting microadenomas are very small and typically do not increase in size, treatment of these tumors is primarily directed toward alleviating symptoms.[76–78] The goal of therapy is to normalize prolactin serum concentrations and reestablish gonadotropin secretion to restore fertility and reduce the risk of osteoporosis. In patients with asymptomatic elevations in serum prolactin, observation and close followup are appropriate.[76–78]

Treatment goals are more aggressive in patients with prolactin-secreting macroadenomas because these tumors are larger and can cause invasion of local tissues with significant visual defects.[78] Therefore, in addition to normalizing prolactin concentrations, tumor shrinkage and correction of visual defects are primary goals of treatment.

Medical therapy with dopamine agonists usually is more effective than transsphenoidal surgery for both types of pituitary prolactinomas.[4,76–78] Postsurgical cure rates differ depending on tumor type and expertise of the neurosurgeon. Long-term cure rates are reported to be approximately 60% for microprolactinomas and only 25% for macroprolactinomas.[4] Transsphenoidal surgery for removal of prolactinomas usually is reserved for patients who are refractory to or cannot tolerate therapy with dopamine agonists and for patients with very large tumors that cause severe compression of adjacent tissues.[4,76–78] Radiation therapy may require several years for effective tumor shrinkage and reduction in serum prolactin concentrations and usually is used only in conjunction with surgery.[4]

■ PHARMACOLOGIC THERAPY

Medical therapy with dopamine agonists has proven to be very effective in normalizing prolactin serum concentrations, restoring menstruation, and reducing tumor size in approximately 80% to 90% of patients within 3 to 6 months of therapy.[4,77] Bromocriptine has been the mainstay of therapy since the 1970s. Cabergoline is a long-acting dopamine agonist that offers the advantage of less-frequent dosing. In recent years cabergoline has replaced bromocriptine as the agent of choice for the medical management of prolactinomas.

■ BROMOCRIPTINE

Bromocriptine was the first D_2-receptor agonist to be used in the treatment of hyperprolactinemia and has been the mainstay of therapy for over 20 years. It inhibits the release of prolactin by directly stimulating postsynaptic dopamine receptors in the hypothalamus. Hypothalamic release of dopamine (prolactin-inhibitory hormone) inhibits the release of prolactin. Decreases in serum prolactin concentrations occur within 2 hours of oral administration, with maximal suppression occurring after 8 hours and suppressive effects persisting for up to 24 hours. Medical therapy with bromocriptine normalizes prolactin serum concentrations, restores gonadotropin production, and shrinks tumor size in approximately 90% of patients with microprolactinomas and 70% of patients with macroprolactinomas.[78]

For the management of hyperprolactinemia, bromocriptine therapy typically is initiated at a dose of 1.25 to 2.5 mg once daily at bedtime to minimize adverse effects.[76,77] The dose can be gradually increased by 1.25-mg increments every week to obtain desirable serum prolactin concentrations. Usual therapeutic doses of bromocriptine range from 2.5 to 15 mg/day, although some patients may require doses as high as 40 mg/day.[77] Bromocriptine usually is administered in two or three divided doses, but once-daily dosing has also been shown to be effective.[78]

The most common adverse effects associated with bromocriptine therapy include CNS symptoms such as headache, lightheadedness, dizziness, nervousness, and fatigue. Gastrointestinal effects such as nausea, abdominal pain, and diarrhea also are common. Bromocriptine should be administered with food to decrease the incidence of adverse gastrointestinal effects. Although most of these adverse effects diminish with continued treatment, approximately 12% of patients will not tolerate the adverse effects associated with bromocriptine therapy.[78] Vaginal preparations of bromocriptine have been studied in an effort to decrease the incidence of adverse effects associated with oral dosage forms.[4,77,81]

Because most patients with hyperprolactinemia are women with a principal complaint of infertility, the safety of bromocriptine in pregnancy must be considered. One report of 100 pregnancies in women who received bromocriptine throughout gestation did not detect an increase in the risk for spontaneous abortion or incidence of congenital anomalies.[78] Although bromocriptine does not appear to be teratogenic, most clinicians discontinue therapy as soon as pregnancy is detected because the effects of in utero exposure to bromocriptine on gonadal function and fertility of the offspring remain unknown.[4,76–78] In patients with macroprolactinomas undergoing rapid tumor expansion, bromocriptine therapy may need to be continued throughout pregnancy.

■ PERGOLIDE

Pergolide is a dopamine-receptor agonist with affinity for both D_1- and D_2-receptors. This agent is 10 to 1,000 times more potent than bromocriptine on a per milligram basis. In the United States, pergolide was never FDA approved for treatment of hyperprolactinemia. However, it was used for many years as an effective alternative to bromocriptine in the management of patients with hyperprolactinemia and offered the advantage of once-daily dosing.[4,78] In 2007, pergolide was withdrawn from the U.S. market because of cases of cardiac valvulopathy.[82] Pathologic assessment suggested that the valvulopathy associated with pergolide appeared to be similar to that reported with other ergot alkaloids.

■ CABERGOLINE

❾ Cabergoline is a long-acting dopamine agonist with high selectivity and affinity for dopamine D_2-receptors. This agent is approved for treatment of hyperprolactinemia and has been shown to effectively reduce serum prolactin concentrations in 80% to 90% of hyperprolactinemic patients.[83–85] Cabergoline also effectively reduces tumor size in patients with both microprolactinomas and macroprolactinomas.[83–86] In a multicenter randomized trial comparing the efficacy of cabergoline and bromocriptine, serum prolactin levels were normalized in 83% of patients receiving cabergoline and 58% of patients receiving bromocriptine after 6 months of therapy.[87] Cabergoline also has proved effective in patients who are intolerant of or resistant to bromocriptine, and recent data suggest that cabergoline is as effective in men as in women with microprolactinomas and macroprolactinomas.[85,88,89]

Cabergoline is commercially available as 0.5-mg oral tablets. The initial dose of cabergoline for treatment of hyperprolactinemia is 0.5 mg once weekly or in divided doses twice weekly. This dose may be increased by 0.5-mg increments at 4-week intervals based on serum prolactin concentrations. The usual dose is 1 to 2 mg weekly; however, doses as high as 4.5 mg weekly have been used.[90] The efficacy of a vaginal dosage form of cabergoline to reduce the adverse effects associated with oral therapy has been evaluated.[91]

Following oral administration, peak serum concentrations are obtained within 2 hours, and food does not affect absorption. Data from animal studies indicate that cabergoline is widely distributed to well-perfused organs, including the pituitary gland.[90] The elimination of cabergoline from the pituitary appears to be very slow; this rate may explain the long duration of action. Cabergoline is extensively metabolized in the liver by hydrolysis, and the dose should be reduced in patients with severe hepatic failure. This drug is eliminated primarily in the feces, and the elimination half-life ranges from 79 to 155 hours in hyperprolactinemic patients.[90]

The most common adverse effects reported with use of cabergoline are nausea, vomiting, headache, and dizziness.[78,90] These effects are similar to the adverse effects reported with bromocriptine and pergolide. However, in a large comparative study evaluating bromocriptine and cabergoline, fewer patients receiving cabergoline reported adverse effects than did patients receiving bromocriptine, and only 3% of the patients in the cabergoline group withdrew from the study because of adverse effects versus 12% of patients taking bromocriptine.[87] Other adverse events associated with use of cabergoline include gastrointestinal complaints, drowsiness, fatigue, paresthesias, dyspnea, suffocation sensation, and epistaxis.[78,90] As with other dopamine agonists, adverse events usually occur early in therapy and subside with continued treatment. However, in one study 15% to 20% of patients receiving cabergoline experienced a recurrence of early symptoms or an onset of new symptoms after several weeks of treatment.[87] Mild-to-moderate decreases in blood pressure have been observed in up to 50% of patients taking cabergoline; however, the incidence of symptomatic orthostatic hypotension has not been significant.[83,84,87] Transient increases in serum alkaline phosphatase, bilirubin, and aminotransferases have been reported in small numbers of patients receiving cabergoline.[87] Pleuropulmonary disease[78] and newly diagnosed cardiac valve regurgitation[82] have been reported with cabergoline use at the larger doses used in the treatment of Parkinson's disease.

⑩ Use of cabergoline in pregnancy has not been extensively studied. However, several case reports of women who received cabergoline therapy during the first and second trimesters of pregnancy have not documented an increased risk of spontaneous abortion, congenital abnormalities, or tubal pregnancy.[90] However, prospective data in large numbers of pregnancies are lacking. Because of the long half-life and limited data on cabergoline use in pregnancy, most clinicians recommend that women receiving cabergoline therapy who plan to become pregnant should discontinue the medication 1 month before planned conception.[92]

Other dopamine agonists that have been used in the treatment of hyperprolactinemia but are not commercially available in the United States include lisuride, terguride, metergoline, dihydroergocristine, and quinagolide.[78] Quinagolide, a D_2-receptor agonist used frequently in Europe, is dosed once daily. Quinagolide has been shown to be as effective as bromocriptine for the management of hyperprolactinemia and may be effective in the treatment of patients who are resistant to or intolerant of bromocriptine.[78]

EVALUATION OF THERAPEUTIC OUTCOMES

Prolactin serum concentrations should be monitored every 3 to 4 weeks after the initiation of any dopamine-agonist therapy to assess efficacy and appropriately titrate medication dosage.[76] In addition, symptoms such as headache, visual disturbances, menstrual cycles in women, and sexual function in men should be evaluated to assess clinical response to therapy. Once prolactin concentrations have normalized and clinical symptoms of hyperprolactinemia have resolved with dopamine-agonist therapy, prolactin serum concentrations should be monitored every 6 to 12 months. In patients receiving long-term treatment, the dose of the dopamine agonist can be gradually reduced or discontinued in some patients. For patients with microprolactinomas who have normal serum prolactin concentrations and at least a 50% reduction in tumor size, medical therapy may be withdrawn every 2 to 5 years to assess if remission has been achieved. In the case of macroprolactinomas, the dose of the dopamine agonist can be gradually reduced in some cases, but complete drug discontinuation should be attempted only if careful monitoring for renewed tumor growth can be ensured.[76,77,93]

PHARMACOECONOMIC CONSIDERATIONS

Medical therapy with dopamine agonists is more effective than transsphenoidal surgery or radiation for the management of hyperprolactinemia. Because most patients receive therapy for long periods, the medical management of hyperprolactinemia may result in considerable cost. Cabergoline has been shown to be more effective than bromocriptine and offers additional advantages such as a decreased incidence of adverse effects and improved patient compliance. Most clinicians agree that cabergoline is the most efficacious dopamine agonist currently available. However, the cost of cabergoline therapy is approximately two times greater than that of bromocriptine. Pharmacoeconomic studies are needed to assess whether the higher cost of cabergoline therapy is balanced by the potential added benefits.

CONCLUSIONS

Hyperprolactinemia is a common disorder that can have a significant impact on fertility. Hyperprolactinemia is most commonly caused by the presence of prolactin-secreting pituitary tumors and various medications that antagonize dopamine or increase the secretion of prolactin. Available treatment options for this disorder include medical therapy with dopamine agonists, radiation therapy, and transsphenoidal surgery. In most cases, medical therapy with dopamine agonists is considered the most effective treatment. Cabergoline has replaced bromocriptine as the mainstay of medical therapy because it appears to be better tolerated and more effective. However, because of limited data regarding the safety of cabergoline during pregnancy, bromocriptine remains the preferred agent when fertility is the primary purpose for treatment.

PANHYPOPITUITARISM

⑪ Panhypopituitarism is a condition of complete or partial loss of anterior and posterior pituitary function resulting in a complex disorder characterized by multiple pituitary hormone deficiencies. Patients with panhypopituitarism may have ACTH deficiency, gonadotropin deficiency, GH deficiency, hypothyroidism, and hyperprolactinemia. Panhypopituitarism can be classified as either primary or secondary depending on the etiology. Primary panhypopituitarism involves an abnormality within the secretory cells of the pituitary, whereas secondary panhypopituitarism is caused by a lack of proper external stimulation needed for normal release of pituitary hormones. Some of the most common causes of panhypopituitarism include primary pituitary tumors, ischemic necrosis of the pituitary, surgical trauma, irradiation, and various types of CNS infections. Pharmacologic treatment of panhypopituitarism is essential and consists of replacement of specific pituitary hormones after careful assessment of individual deficiencies. Replacement most often consists of glucocorticoids, thyroid hormone preparations, and sex steroids. Administration of recombinant GH also may be necessary. Patients with panhypopituitarism will need lifelong replacement therapy and constant monitoring of multiple homeostatic functions.

ABBREVIATIONS

ACTH: adrenocorticotropic hormone

CJD: Creutzfeldt-Jakob's disease

CRH: corticotropin-releasing hormone

FSH: follicle-stimulating hormone

GH: growth hormone

GHD: growth hormone deficient

GHRH: growth hormone-releasing hormone

GnRH: gonadotropin-releasing hormone

IGF: insulin-like growth factor

IGFBP-3: insulin-like growth factor-1 binding protein-3

LH: luteinizing hormone
OGTT: oral glucose tolerance test
SSRI: selective serotonin reuptake inhibitor
TRH: thyrotropin-releasing hormone
TSH: thyroid-stimulating hormone
VIP: vasoactive intestinal peptide

ADDENDUM

In August 2007, the US FDA approved a depot formulation of the somatostatin analog, lanreotide (Somatuline Depot), for treatment of acromegaly in patients who have failed or are not candidates for surgery or radiation. This agent is currently designated as an orphan drug.

REFERENCES

1. Raisman G. An urge to explain the incomprehensible: Geoffrey Harris and the discovery of the neural control of the pituitary gland. Ann Rev Neurosci 1997;20:533–566.
2. Amar AP, Weiss MH. Pituitary anatomy and physiology. Neurosurg Clin North Am 2003;14:11–23.
3. Cuttler L. The regulation of growth hormone secretion. Endocrinol Metab Clin North Am 1996;25:541–571.
4. Molitch ME. Disorders of prolactin secretion. Endocrinol Metab Clin North Am 2001;30:585–610.
5. Le Roith D. Insulin-like growth factors. N Engl J Med 1997;336:633–640.
6. Holdaway M, Rajasoorya C. Epidemiology of acromegaly. Pituitary 1999;2:29–41.
7. Eugster EA, Pescovitz OH. Gigantism. J Clin Endocrinol Metab 1999;84:4379–4384.
8. Ben-Shlomo A, Melmed S. Acromegaly. Endocrinol Metab Clin North Am 2001;30:565–583.
9. Melmed S. Acromegaly. N Engl J Med 2006;355:2558–2573.
10. Kauppinen-Makelin R, Sane T, Reunanen A, et al. A nationwide survey of mortality in acromegaly. J Clin Endocrinol Metab 2005;90:4081–4086.
11. Fatti LM, Scacchi M, Pincelli AI, et al. Prevalence and pathogenesis of sleep apnea and lung disease in acromegaly. Pituitary 2001;4:259–262.
12. Vitale G, Pivonello R, Galderisi M, et al. Cardiovascular complications in acromegaly: Methods of assessment. Pituitary 2001;4:251–257.
13. Webb SM, Casanueva F, Wass JA. Oncological complications of excess GH in acromegaly. Pituitary 2002;5:21–25.
14. Bonadonna S, Doga M, Gola M, et al. Diagnosis and treatment of acromegaly and its complications: Consensus guidelines. J Endocrinol Invest 2005;28(11 Suppl):43–47.
15. Doga M, Bonadonna S, Gola M, et al. Diagnostic and therapeutic consensus on acromegaly. J Endocrinol Invest 2005;28(5 Suppl):56–60.
16. Melmed S, Casanueva F, Cavagnini F, et al. Consensus statement: Medical management of acromegaly. Eur J Endocrinol 2005;153:737–740.
17. Sheppard MC. Primary medical therapy for acromegaly. Clin Endocrinol 2003;58:387–399.
18. Melmed S, Vance ML, Barkan AL, et al. Current status and future opportunities for controlling acromegaly. Pituitary 2002;5:185–196.
19. Colao A, Ferone D, Marzullo P, et al. Effect of different dopaminergic agents in the treatment of acromegaly. J Clin Endocrinol Metab 1997;82:518–523.
20. Jaffe CA, Barkan AL. Acromegaly recognition and treatment. Drugs 1994;47:425–445.
21. Orrego JJ, Barkan AL. Pituitary disorders. Drugs 2000;59:93–106.
22. Abs R, Verhelst J, Maiter D, et al. Cabergoline in the treatment of acromegaly: A study of 64 patients. J Clin Endocrinol Metab 1998;83:374–378.
23. Freda PU. Somatostatin analogs in acromegaly. J Clin Endocrinol Metab 2002;87:3013–3018.
24. Lamberts SE, Van der Lely A, de Herder WW, Hofland LJ. Drug therapy: Octreotide. N Engl J Med 1996;334:246–254.
25. Vance ML, Harris AG. Long-term treatment of 189 acromegalic patients with the somatostatin analog octreotide. Results of the international multicenter acromegaly study group. Arch Intern Med 1991;151:1573–1578.
26. Ezzat S, Snyder PJ, Young WF, et al. Octreotide treatment of acromegaly: A randomized, multicenter study. Ann Intern Med 1992;117:211–218.
27. Newman CB, Melmed S, Snyder PJ, et al. Safety and efficacy of long term octreotide therapy of acromegaly: Results of a multicenter trial in 103 patients—A clinical research center study. J Clin Endocrinol Metab 1995;80:2768–2775.
28. Colao A, Marzullo P, Ferone D, et al. Cardiovascular effects of depot long-acting somatostatin analog Sandostatin LAR in acromegaly. J Clin Endocrinol Metab 2000;85:3132–3140.
29. Colao A, Cuocolo A, Marzullo P, et al. Is the acromegalic cardiomyopathy reversible? Effect of a 5-year normalization of growth hormone and insulin-like growth factor I levels on cardiac performance. J Clin Endocrinol Metab 2001;86:1551–1557.
30. Gilbert J, Ketchen M, Kane P, et al. The treatment of de novo acromegalic patients with octreotide-LAR: Efficacy, tolerability and cardiovascular effects. Pituitary 2003;6:11–18.
31. Tolis, G, Angelopoulos NG, Katounda E, et al. Medical treatment of acromegaly: Comorbidities and their reversibility by somatostatin analogs. Neuroendocrinology 2006;83:249–257.
32. Melmed S, Sternberg R, Cook D, et al. A critical analysis of pituitary tumor shrinkage during primary medical therapy in acromegaly. J Clin Endocrinol Metab 2005;90:4405–4410.
33. McKeage K, Cheer S, Wagstaff AJ. Octreotide long-acting release (LAR): A review of its use in the management of acromegaly. Drugs 2003;63:2473–2499.
34. Lancranjan L, Brew Atkinson A, and the Sandostatin LAR Group. Results of European multicentre study with Sandostatin LAR in acromegaly patients. Pituitary 1999;1:105–114.
35. Gilbert JA, Miell JP, Chambers SM, et al. The nadir growth hormone after an octreotide test dose predicts the long-term efficacy of somatostatin analogue therapy in acromegaly. Clin Endocrinol 2005;62:742–747.
36. Coloa A, Ferone D, Lastoria S, et al. Prediction of efficacy of octreotide therapy in patients with acromegaly. J Clin Endocrinol Metab 1996;81:2356–2362.
37. Pereira AM, Biermasz NR, Roelfsema F, et al. Pharmacologic therapies for acromegaly: A review of their effects on glucose metabolism and insulin resistance. Treat Endocrinol 2005;4:43–53.
38. Baldelli R, Battista C, Leonetti F, et al. Glucose homeostasis in acromegaly: Effects of long-acting somatostatin analogues treatment. Clin Endocrinol 2003;59:492–499.
39. Clemmons DR, Chihara K, Freda PU, et al. Optimizing control of acromegaly: Integrating a growth hormone receptor antagonist into the treatment algorithm. J Clin Endocrinol Metab 2003;88:4759–4767.
40. Trainer PJ, Drake WM, Katznelson L, et al. Treatment of acromegaly with the growth hormone-receptor antagonist Pegvisomant. N Engl J Med 2000;342:1171–1177.
41. Van Der Lely AJ, Hutson R, Trainer PJ, et al. Long-term treatment of acromegaly with pegvisomant, a growth hormone receptor antagonist. Lancet 2001;358:1754–1759.
42. Anonymous. Pegvisomant (Somavert) for acromegaly. Med Lett Drugs Ther 2003;45:55–56.
43. Cozzi R, Attanasio R, Lodrini S, et al. Cabergoline addition to depot somatostatin analogues in resistant acromegalic patients: efficacy and lack of predictive value of prolactin status. Clin Endocrinol 2004;61:209–215.
44. Feenstra J, Herder WW, ten Have SM, et al. Combined therapy with somatostatin analogues and weekly pegvisomant in active acromegaly. Lancet 2005;365:1644–1646.
45. Hindmarsh PC, Brook CGD. Short stature and growth hormone deficiency. Clin Endocrinol 1995;43:133–142.
46. American Association of Clinical Endocrinologists. Medical guidelines for clinical practice for growth hormone use in adults and children—2003 Update. Endocr Pract 2003;9:64–76.
47. Pasquino AM, Albanese A, Bozzola M, et al. Idiopathic short stature. J Pediatr Endocrinol Metab 2001;(Suppl 2):967–974.

48. Hindmarsh PC, Dattani MT. Use of growth hormone in children. Nat Clin Pract Endocrinol Metab 2006;2:260–268.
49. Lawson Wilkins Pediatric Endocrine Society Executive Committee. Guidelines for the use of growth hormone in children with short stature. A report by the drug and therapeutics committee of the Lawson Wilkins Pediatric Endocrine Society. J Pediatr 1995;127:857–867.
50. Mills JL, Schonberger LB, Wysowski DK, et al. Long-term mortality in the United States cohort of pituitary-derived growth hormone recipients. J Pediatr 2004;144:430–436.
51. Blethen SL, Bapitista J, Kuntze J, et al. Adult height in growth hormone (GH)-deficient children treated with biosynthetic GH. J Clin Endocrinol Metab 1997;82:418–420.
52. August GP, Julius JR, Blethen SL. Adult height in children with growth hormone deficiency who are treated with biosynthetic growth hormone: The national cooperative growth study experience. Pediatrics 1998;102:512–516.
53. Frinkik JP, Baptista J. Adult height in growth hormone deficiency: Historical perspective and examples from the nation cooperative growth study. Pediatrics 1999;104:1000–1004.
54. Thomas M, Massa G, Bourguignon JP, et al. Final height in children with idiopathic growth hormone deficiency treated with recombinant human growth hormone: The Belgian experience. Horm Res 2001;55:88–94.
55. Rikken B, Massa GG, Wit JM, and the Dutch Growth Hormone Working Group. Final height in a large cohort of Dutch patients with growth hormone deficiency treated with growth hormone. Horm Res 1995;43:136–137.
56. Chipman JJ, Hicks JR, Holcombe JH, Draper MW. Approaching final height in children treated for growth hormone deficiency. Horm Res 1995;43:129–131.
57. Serveri F. Final height in children with growth hormone deficiency. Horm Res 1995;43:138–140.
58. Coste J, Letrait M, Carel JC, et al. Long term results of growth hormone treatment in France in children of short stature: Population, register based study. BMJ 1997;315:708–713.
59. Cuneo RC, Judd S, Wallace JD, et al. The Australian multicenter trial of growth hormone (GH) treatment in GH-deficient adults. J Clin Endocrinol Metab 1998;83:107–116.
60. Bravenboer N, Holzmann PJ, ter Maaten JC, et al. Effect of long-term growth hormone treatment on bone mass and bone metabolism in growth hormone-deficient men. J Bon Miner Res 2005;20:1778–1784.
61. Rosilio M, Blum WF, Edwards DJ, et al. Long-term improvement of quality of life during growth hormone (GH) replacement therapy in adults with GH deficiency, as measured by questions on life satisfaction-hypopituitarism (QLS-H). J Clin Endocrinol Metab 2004;89:1684–1693.
62. Finkelstein BS, Imperiale TF, Speroff T, et al. Effect of growth hormone therapy on height in children with idiopathic short stature. Arch Pediatr Adolesc Med 2002;156:230–240.
63. Werber E, LeschekS, Yanovski JA, et al. Effect of growth hormone treatment on adult height in peripubertal children with idiopathic short stature: A randomized, double-blind, placebo-controlled trial. J Clin Endocrinol Metab 2004;89:3140–3148.
64. Blethen SL, MacGillivray MH. A risk-benefit assessment of growth hormone use in children. Drug Saf 1997;17:303–316.
65. Thorner MO and the Growth Hormone Research Society. Critical evaluation of the safety of recombinant human growth hormone administration. J Clin Endocrinol Metab 2001;86:1868–1870.
66. Jeffcoate W. Growth hormone therapy and its relationship to insulin resistance, glucose intolerance and diabetes mellitus. Drug Saf 2002;25:199–212.
67. Wantanabe S, Tsunematsu Y, Fujimoto J, et al. Leukaemia in patients treated with growth hormone. Lancet 1988;1:1159–1160.
68. Ogilvy-Stuart A, Gleeson H. Cancer risk following growth hormone use in childhood: Implications for current practice. Drug Saf 2004;24:369–382.
69. Pirazzoli P, Cacciari E, Mandini M, et al. Follow-up of antibodies to growth hormone in 210 growth hormone-deficient children treated with different commercial preparations. Acta Paediatr 1995;84:1233–1236.
70. Backeljauw PF, Underwood LE, and the GHIS Collaborative Group. Therapy for 6.5–7.5 years with recombinant insulin-like growth factor I in children with growth hormone insensitivity syndrome: A clinical research center study. J Clin Endocrinol Metab 2001;86:1504–1510.
71. Kemp SF, Thrailkill KM. Investigational agents for the treatment of growth hormone-insensitivity. Expert Opin Investig Drugs 2006;4:409–415.
72. Chernausek SD, Backeljauw PF, Frane J, et al. Long-term treatment with recombinant insulin-like growth factor (IGF)-1 in children with severe IGF-I deficiency due to growth hormone insensitivity. J Clin Endocrinol Metab 2007;992:902–910.
73. Thorner M, Rochiccioli P, Colle M, et al. Once daily subcutaneous growth hormone-releasing hormone accelerates growth in growth-hormone deficient children during the first year of therapy. J Clin Endocrinol Metab 1996;81:1189–1196.
74. Ogilvy-Stuart AL, Stirling HF, Kelnart CJH, et al. Treatment of radiation-induced growth hormone deficiency with growth hormone-releasing hormone. Clin Endocrinol 1997;46:571–578.
75. American Academy of Pediatrics Committee on Drugs and Committee on Bioethics. Considerations related to the use of recombinant human growth hormone in children. Pediatrics 1997;99:122–129.
76. Schlechte JA. Prolactinoma. N Engl J Med 2003;349:2035–2041.
77. Mah PM, Webster J. Hyperprolactinemia: Etiology, diagnosis and management. Semin Reprod Med 2002;20:365–373.
78. Gillam MP, Molitch ME, Lombardi, et al. Advances in the treatment of prolactinomas. Endocr Rev 2006;27:485–534.
79. Davies PH. Drug-related hyperprolactinaemia. Adverse Drug React Toxicol Rev 1997;16:83–94.
80. Haddad PM, Wieck A. Antipsychotic-induced hyperprolactinemia: Mechanisms, clinical features and management. Drugs 2004;64:2291–2314.
81. Darwish AM, Hafez E, El-Gelbali I, et al. Evaluation of a novel vaginal bromocriptine mesylate formulation: A pilot study. Fertil Steril 2005;83:1053–1055.
82. Schade R, Andersohn F, Suissa S, et al. Dopamine agonists and the risk of cardiac-valve regurgitation. N Engl J Med 2007;356:29–38.
83. Verhelst J, Abs R, Maiter D, et al. Cabergoline in the treatment of hyperprolactinemia: A study in 455 patients. J Clin Endocrinol Metab 1999;84:2518–2522.
84. Cannavo S, Curto L, Squadrito S, et al. Cabergoline: A first-choice treatment in patients with previously untreated prolactin-secreting pituitary adenoma. J Endocrinol Invest 1999;22:354–359.
85. Colao A, DiSarno A, Landi ML, et al. Macroprolactinoma shrinkage during cabergoline treatment is greater in naïve patients than in patients pretreated with other dopamine agonists: A prospective study in 110 patients. J Clin Endocrinol Metab 2000;85:2247–2252.
86. Ferrari CI, Abs R, Bevan JS, et al. Treatment of macroprolactinoma with cabergoline: A study of 85 patients. Clin Endocrinol 1997;46:409–413.
87. Webster J, Piscitelli G, Polli A, et al. A comparison of cabergoline and bromocriptine in the treatment of hyperprolactinemic amenorrhea. N Engl J Med 1994;331:904–909.
88. DiSarno A, Landi ML, Cappabianca P, et al. Resistance to cabergoline as compared with bromocriptine in hyperprolactinemia: Prevalence, clinical definition, and therapeutic strategy. J Clin Endocrinol Metab 2001;86:5256–5261.
89. Colao A, Vitale G, Cappabianca P, et al. Outcome of cabergoline treatment in men with prolactinoma: Effects of a 24-month treatment on prolactin levels, tumor mass, recovery of pituitary function, and semen analysis. J Clin Endocrinol Metab 2004;89:1704–1711.
90. Rains CP, Bryson HM, Fitton A. Cabergoline: A review of its pharmacological properties and therapeutic potential in the treatment of hyperprolactinaemia and inhibition of lactation. Drugs 1995;49:255–279.
91. Motta T, Colombo N, DeVincentiis S, et al. Vaginal cabergoline in the treatment of hyperprolactinemic patients intolerant to oral dopaminergics. Fertil Steril 1996;65:440–442.
92. Colao A, di Sarno A, Pivonello R, et al. Dopamine receptor agonists for treating prolactinomas. Expert Opin Investig Drugs 2002;11:787–800.
93. Colao A, DiSarno A, Cappabianca P, et al. Withdrawal of long-term cabergoline therapy for tumoral and nontumoral hyperprolactinemia. N Engl J Med 2003;349:2023–2033.

SECTION 9
GYNECOLOGIC DISORDERS

CHAPTER 81

Pregnancy and Lactation: Therapeutic Considerations

DENISE L. WALBRANDT PIGARELLI, CONNIE K. KRAUS, AND BETH E. POTTER

KEY CONCEPTS

1. Altered drug pharmacokinetics during pregnancy can influence drug selection and dosing. Physiologic changes during pregnancy result in changes in absorption, protein binding, distribution, and elimination.

2. Although drug-induced teratogenicity is a serious concern during pregnancy, most drugs required by pregnant women can be used safely. Informed selection of drug therapy is essential.

3. Healthcare practitioners must know where to find and how to evaluate evidence related to the safety of drugs used during pregnancy.

4. Pregnancy-influenced health issues, such as constipation, gastroesophageal reflux disease, and nausea/vomiting, have been treated safely and effectively with carefully selected drug therapy. Some acute and chronic illnesses pose special risks during pregnancy and should be treated with appropriately selected and monitored drug therapies to avoid harm to both the woman and the fetus.

5. Understanding the physiology of lactation and pharmacokinetic factors affecting drug distribution, metabolism, and elimination can assist the clinician in selecting safe and effective medications used during lactation.

Drug use in pregnancy and lactation is a critically important topic that is underemphasized in the education of health professionals. This subject encompasses a dichotomous discussion of the benefits of drug therapy for the mother and the potential risks for the embryo/fetus. Drug use in pregnancy and lactation is a controversial and emotionally charged area because of medicolegal and ethical implications.

Learning objectives, review questions, and other resources can be found at **www.pharmacotherapyonline.com.**

It is the clinician's responsibility to ensure safe and effective therapy before conception, during pregnancy, and after delivery. The patient's active participation is essential. Both acute and chronic illnesses must be managed during pregnancy, and optimal treatments sometimes are different from those used in the nonpregnant patient. Pharmacotherapeutic issues also apply to selection of drugs used during parturition and the postpartum period. Principles of drug use during lactation, although similar, are not the same as those applicable during pregnancy.

In many instances, medication dosing recommendations for acute or chronic illnesses in pregnant women are the same as for the general population. However, in some instances the dosing and selection of medications are quite different.

PHYSIOLOGY OF PREGNANCY

Because of the complexity of fertilization and subsequent pregnancy events, approximately 50% of embryos do not survive.[1] Most losses occur in the first 2 weeks after fertilization before many women realize they were pregnant. About 15% of pregnancies that survive the first 2 weeks of gestation are lost spontaneously later in the course of the pregnancy.

Fertilization occurs when a sperm attaches to a receptor on the outer protein layer of the egg, the zona pellucida.[1] Immediately, the egg becomes unresponsive to other sperm. The attached sperm releases enzymes that cause the egg's chromosomes to mature, allowing the sperm to fully penetrate the zona pellucida and contact the egg's cell membrane. The membranes of the sperm and egg then are fused to create a new, single cell. Male and female chromosomes join in the new cell, fuse to create a single nucleus, and organize to set the stage for cell division.

Fertilization usually occurs in the fallopian tube.[1] Cell division continues for the first 2 days while the fertilized egg travels down the fallopian tube, reaching the uterine cavity on the third day. Cell division continues for another 2 to 3 days in the uterine cavity before implantation begins. Approximately 6 days after fertilization, the cell mass is termed a *blastocyst.* Human chorionic gonadotropin now is produced in amounts that may be detected by commercial laboratories. The blastocyst sloughs the zona pellucida and rests directly on the endometrium, which now responds to the denuded blastocyst by allowing it to begin to grow into the endometrial wall.

After 6 days of this growth, the blastocyst lies implanted under the surface of the endometrium and begins to receive nutrition from maternal blood.[1] Now it is called an *embryo.*[2]

The embryonic period lasts from approximately 2 weeks after fertilization until 8 weeks after fertilization, when the conceptus is renamed a *fetus.*[2] Most body structures are formed during the embryonic period, and they continue to grow and mature during the fetal period. The fetal period continues until the pregnancy reaches term, approximately 40 weeks after the last menstrual period.

Gravidity refers to the number of times that a woman experiences pregnancy.[2] A multiple birth is counted as a single pregnancy. *Parity* refers to the number of a woman's pregnancies that exceeded 20 weeks of gestation and relates information regarding the outcome of each pregnancy. In sequence, the numbers reflect (1) term deliveries, (2) premature deliveries, (3) aborted and/or ectopic pregnancies, and (4) number of living children. A woman who has been pregnant four times; has experienced two term deliveries, one premature delivery, and one ectopic pregnancy; and has three living children would be designated by G_4P_{2113}.

Pregnancy Dating

Approximately 280 days (about 40 weeks or 9 months) constitute the duration of a pregnancy; this time period extends from the first day of the last menstrual period to birth.[2] *Gestational age* or *menstrual age* refers to the age of the embryo or fetus beginning with the first day of the last menstrual period, which is about 2 weeks prior to fertilization. To calculate an approximate pregnancy due date, the clinician adds 7 days to the first day of the last menstrual period and subtracts 3 months. For simple description purposes, pregnancy is divided into three periods of 3 calendar months, and each period of 3 months is called a *trimester.*

Pregnancy Signs and Symptoms

Early symptoms of pregnancy include fatigue and increased frequency of urination.[3] At approximately 6 weeks' gestation, the pregnant woman may experience nausea and vomiting. This is commonly known as *morning sickness* but can occur at any time of the day. Nausea and vomiting usually resolve at 12 to 18 weeks' gestation. Fetal movement is detected in the woman's lower abdomen at 16 to 20 weeks of gestation. Signs of pregnancy may include sudden cessation of menses, changes in consistency of the cervical mucus, bluish discoloration of the vaginal mucosa, increased skin pigmentation, and anatomic breast changes.

MATERNAL PHARMACOKINETIC CHANGES IN PREGNANCY

❶ Normal physiologic changes that occur during pregnancy may alter medication effects, resulting in the need to monitor and, sometimes, adjust therapy.[4] Physiologic changes begin in the first trimester and peak during the second trimester. For medications that can be monitored by blood or serum concentration measurements, monitoring should occur throughout pregnancy.

During pregnancy, maternal plasma volume, cardiac output, and glomerular filtration increase by 30% to 50%, potentially lowering the concentration of renally cleared drugs.[5] As body fat increases during pregnancy, the volume of distribution of fat-soluble drugs may increase. Plasma albumin concentration decreases, which increases the volume of distribution of drugs that are highly protein bound. However, these unbound drugs are more rapidly cleared by the liver and kidney during pregnancy, resulting in little change in concentration. Nausea and vomiting, as well as delayed gastric emptying, may alter the absorption of drugs. Likewise, a pregnancy-induced increase in gastric pH may affect the absorption of weak acids and bases. Higher levels of estrogen and progesterone alter liver enzyme activity and increase the elimination of some drugs but result in accumulation of others.

TRANSPLACENTAL DRUG TRANSFER

Although once thought to be a barrier to drug transfer, the placenta is fundamentally the organ of exchange for a number of substances, including drugs, between the mother and fetus.[6] Most drugs move from the maternal circulation to the fetal circulation by diffusion.[5] Certain chemical properties, such as lipid solubility, electrical charge, molecular weight, and degree of protein binding of medications, may influence the rate of transfer across the placenta.[5,6]

Drugs with molecular weights less than 500 Da readily cross the placenta, whereas larger molecules (600–1,000 Da) cross more slowly.[5,6] Drugs with molecular weights greater than 1,000 Da, such as insulin and heparin, do not cross the placenta in significant amounts.[5] Lipophilic drugs, such as opiates and antibiotics, cross the placenta more easily than do water-soluble drugs.[5,6] Maternal plasma albumin progressively decreases while fetal albumin increases during the course of pregnancy, which may result in higher concentrations of certain protein-bound drugs in the fetus.[5] Fetal pH is slightly more acidic than maternal pH, permitting weak bases to more easily cross the placenta. Once in the fetal circulation, however, the molecule becomes more ionized and less likely to diffuse back into the maternal circulation.

DRUG SELECTION DURING PREGNANCY

❷ Although some drugs have the potential to cause teratogenic effects, most medications required by pregnant women can be used safely. There are many misconceptions about the association of medications and birth defects.

The overall incidence of congenital malformations is approximately 3% to 5%.[7,8] It is estimated that medication exposure accounts for less than 1% of all birth defects.[8] Genetic causes are responsible for 15% to 25%, other environmental issues (e.g., maternal conditions and infections) account for 10%, and the remaining 65% to 75% of congenital malformations result from unknown causes.

Despite the greater potential of harm with certain drugs, not every exposure results in a birth defect. Factors such as the stage of pregnancy when the exposure occurred, the route of administration, and the dose all can influence outcomes.[7] In the first 2 weeks after conception, exposure to a teratogen may result in an "all-or-nothing" effect, which could either destroy the embryo or cause no problems. In the period from 18 to 60 days postconception (organogenesis), organ systems are developing, and teratogenic exposures may result in structural anomalies. In the remainder of the pregnancy, exposure to teratogenic agents may result in retardation of growth, central nervous system abnormalities, or death. Examples of medications associated with teratogenic effects in the period of organogenesis include chemotherapy drugs (e.g., methotrexate, cyclophosphamide), sex hormones (e.g., diethylstilbestrol), lithium, retinoids, thalidomide, certain antiepileptic drugs, and coumarin derivatives. Other medications such as nonsteroidal antiinflammatory drugs and tetracycline derivatives are more likely to exhibit effects in the second or third trimester.

In summary, a small number of medications have the potential to cause congenital malformations. Many of these agents can be avoided during pregnancy. In situations where a drug may be harmful to the developing child but is necessary for maternal care, considerations related to route of administration and dosing may lessen the risk of congenital malformations.

METHODS OF DETERMINING SAFETY OF DRUGS IN PREGNANCY

❸ Information about medication safety in pregnancy comes from a variety of sources. One of the most important questions for the clinician is how to evaluate the quality of the evidence related to the safety of medications used during pregnancy.

Randomized, controlled trials form the basis for some of the most reliable assessments of drug safety, but pregnant women usually are not eligible for participation in clinical trials. Other types of data often used to estimate the risk associated with medication use during pregnancy are animal studies, case reports, case-control studies, prospective cohort studies, historical cohort studies, and voluntary reporting systems.

Although animal studies are a required component of drug testing, extrapolation of the results of animal testing to humans is not always accurate.[9] One example is thalidomide, which was found to be safe in some animal models but proved to have teratogenic effects in human offspring.

Case reports may be of limited value because an isolated occurrence of a birth defect in the infant of a woman who used a medication during her pregnancy may have occurred by chance.[9] Case-control studies identify an outcome (congenital anomaly), match subjects with and without that outcome, and report how often exposure to a suspected agent occurred. The concern with this type of study is recall bias, as a woman with an affected pregnancy may be more likely to recall drugs used during the pregnancy than would a woman who had a normal outcome.

Cohort studies look at the intervention (use of a particular drug) in a group of persons and compare outcomes in a similar group of subjects without the intervention.[9] Prospective studies eliminate some of the problems with recall bias. This approach has several potential disadvantages, however, such as the need for large numbers of participants, time involved, and potential loss to followup. Despite these disadvantages, cohort studies are used often for evaluating the effects of a drug exposure on pregnancy outcomes. An example of a cohort study is the Michigan Medicaid Study, which consisted of data collected from 229,101 pregnancies over 7 years.

Teratology information services provide pregnant women with information about potential exposures during pregnancy and, in turn, follow these women throughout the pregnancy to assess the outcomes of the pregnancy.[9] These services may report pooled data to facilitate information sharing about medications used during pregnancy. Some pharmaceutical companies have organized voluntary reporting systems for drugs used during pregnancy.

RESOURCES

❸ Computerized databases (e.g., the Canadian database, *www.motherisk.org*) and textbooks with information from large cohorts of treated women offer valuable assistance. New information regarding drug use in pregnancy can be obtained from searches of the primary literature for cohort and case studies.

One commonly used source of information about drug safety is the category system of the Food and Drug Administration (FDA).[10] The FDA created drug categories to provide guidance on the risk versus benefit for drug use during pregnancy. However, when the FDA categories were compared with two other risk classification systems from other countries, only 61 (26%) of 236 drugs common to all three systems were ranked in the same risk category. Certain agents (e.g., oral contraceptives) classified as teratogenic in the FDA ratings are not considered harmful by other sources. The FDA ranks very few drugs as safe during pregnancy (category A) because the FDA has a requirement for a controlled trial to establish safety, leaving an impression that few drugs are safe.

In summary, drug safety categorizations may provide a rough estimate of risks for medication related adverse fetal outcomes,[11] but they must be used in conjunction with other information sources to make decisions about an individual pregnant woman's need for medication therapy.

GENERAL RECOMMENDATIONS FOR OPTIMIZING USE OF MEDICATIONS IN PREGNANCY

❷ Many women require medications during pregnancy for treatment of acute and chronic conditions.[4] Strategies to optimize use of medications during pregnancy include identifying patterns of medication use before conception, eliminating nonessential medications and discouraging self-medication, minimizing exposure to medications known to be harmful, and adjusting doses of necessary medications to optimize the health of the mother while minimizing the risk to the fetus.

PRECONCEPTION PLANNING

Pregnancy outcomes are influenced by maternal health status, lifestyle, and history prior to conception.[12] In the United States, more than 60% of pregnancies are unintended, and many women do not receive prenatal care. Of those who receive prenatal care, 18% do not access care before the end of the first trimester. Preconception care, including evidence-based screening, health promotion, and interventions, should be received by all women of child-bearing age.[13] Prenatal interventions related to ongoing treatment of chronic conditions and acute treatment of other illnesses are covered in other parts of this chapter.

Neural tube defects, cleft palate and lip, and cardiac anomalies are the most common major congenital anomalies.[14] Approximately 2,500 infants are born with neural tube defects each year in the United States. Neural tube defects occur within 1 month of conception, and folic acid supplementation has been shown to reduce the incidence and recurrence. In women with no history of neural tube defect, four of five studies reported a 40% to 100% decrease in the incidence of neural tube defects with administration of folic acid. The outcome data for women with a history of neural tube defect who received supplementation are similar. Because neural tube closure occurs in the first month of pregnancy and many pregnancies are unplanned and may not be recognized until after the first month, folic acid intake should be encouraged throughout a woman's reproductive years. For women at low risk, folic acid 400 mcg/day is recommended.[15] It should be taken as a supplement because nutritional sources are not sufficient. For women at high risk or who have had a previously affected pregnancy, folic acid 4 mg/day is recommended. Higher doses of folic acid should not be achieved by taking multivitamins because of risk for vitamin A toxicity.

Use of alcohol and recreational drugs during pregnancy is associated with birth defects.[13] Smoking is associated with preterm birth, low birth weight, and other adverse outcomes. These negative outcomes can be prevented if smoking is discontinued early in pregnancy. A systematic review of 64 trials revealed data on smoking cessation and perinatal outcomes.[16] Incidences of low birth weight and preterm birth were reduced, and birth weight increased by 33 g with smoking cessation. An intervention strategy of rewards plus social support resulted in higher rates of smoking cessation than did other strategies. For women who cannot stop smoking with behavioral interventions alone, nicotine replacement therapies can be used in combination with behavioral therapy.[17] Although the efficacy of nicotine replacement in pregnancy has not been substantiated by clinical trials, this intervention appears to be safe. Intermittent delivery formulations are recommended in order to deliver a smaller daily dose than received from the topically applied patch. If patches are necessary because of poor tolerability of other agents, they should be applied for 16 rather than 24 hours per day. The initial dose of the patch should be similar or higher than that used for nonpregnant women. Therapeutic drug monitoring of cotinine levels may be considered for dosing nicotine. Bupropion is an alternative to nicotine replacement for women who have not quit smoking with behavioral therapy. The efficacy of this agent for smoking cessation in pregnancy has not been determined. Bupropion use during pregnancy should be reported to the GlaxoSmithKline pregnancy registry.

Prevention of infectious diseases during pregnancy is important for ensuring positive outcomes. Influenza vaccination is generally offered to women who will be in their second or third trimester during influenza season.[18] Women with comorbid conditions that increase risks of complications from influenza should receive vaccine regardless of time of gestation.

PREGNANCY-INFLUENCED ISSUES

❹ Pregnant women commonly experience health issues that are either caused by or exacerbated by the pregnant state. Constipation, gastroesophageal reflux, hemorrhoids, and nausea and vomiting may affect many women during pregnancy. Gestational diabetes, gestational hypertension, and venous thromboembolism have the potential to cause adverse pregnancy consequences. Gestational thyrotoxicosis usually is a self-limiting condition.

GASTROINTESTINAL TRACT

Constipation occurs commonly in pregnancy. Therapy should be instituted first with nondrug modalities, such as education, physical exercise, biofeedback, and increased intake of dietary fiber and fluid.[19] If additional therapy is warranted, use of supplemental fiber and/or a stool softener is appropriate. Lactulose, sorbitol, and bisacodyl are acceptable treatments but should be reserved for occasional rather than routine use. Senna can be used occasionally. Castor oil and mineral oil should be avoided.

Gastroesophageal reflux disease occurs in up to 80% of pregnant women.[20] Therapy includes lifestyle and dietary modifications (e.g., small, frequent meals; alcohol and tobacco avoidance; food avoidance prior to bedtime; elevation of the head of the bed). Pharmacologic therapy is reserved for patients who do not receive adequate relief from nondrug therapies. Drug therapy can be initiated with aluminum, calcium, or magnesium antacid preparations; sodium bicarbonate should be avoided. Sucralfate is another option, and evidence supports the use of ranitidine and cimetidine. Literature on the use of famotidine and nizatidine is limited. If a patient does not respond to lifestyle changes and histamine-2 receptor blockers, metoclopramide, omeprazole, and lansoprazole are viable options.[20,21]

The exact prevalence of hemorrhoids during pregnancy is unknown.[19] Therapy is generally conservative; high intake of dietary fiber, adequate oral fluid intake, and use of sitz baths are helpful. Topical anesthetics, skin protectants, and astringents can be used. Other options for refractory hemorrhoids include rubber band ligation, sclerotherapy, and surgery.

Nausea and vomiting affect up to 80% of pregnant women; however, hyperemesis gravidarum (i.e., unrelenting vomiting causing weight loss of more than 5% prepregnancy weight and ketonuria) occurs in only about 1% to 3% of women.[22] Dietary modifications, such as eating frequent, small, bland meals and avoiding fatty foods, may be helpful. Lifestyle changes including shorter work days and taking frequent naps. Acupressure and acustimulation may be beneficial.

A number of pharmacotherapeutic approaches have been tried for treatment of nausea and vomiting.[22] Multivitamins, pyridoxine (vitamin B_6), and cyanocobalamin (vitamin B_{12}) have shown efficacy. Antihistamines (including doxylamine) have not proved to be toxic and have shown efficacy. Phenothiazines and metoclopramide have been used widely and are generally considered safe. Efficacy and safety information on ondansetron use are limited, but ondansetron can be considered when other options fail. Corticosteroids (dexamethasone and prednisolone) have shown efficacy for hyperemesis gravidarum, but a small increase in the risk of oral clefts may be associated with use during the first trimester. Ginger has shown efficacy for hyperemesis in five randomized, controlled trials and probably is safe.

GESTATIONAL DIABETES

About 4% of pregnant women develop gestational diabetes (defined as glucose intolerance first identified during pregnancy), although the prevalence may range from 1% to 14%.[23] Whether or not to screen for gestational diabetes is an issue of significant controversy. The U.S. Preventative Services Task Force Independent Expert Panel has concluded that there is a lack of evidence proving that screening for gestational diabetes decreases adverse maternal and fetal outcomes.[24] However, the American Diabetes Association recommends screening at her first prenatal visit any woman who has risk factors for developing gestational diabetes mellitus (e.g., obesity, history of the condition, glycosuria, or strong family history of diabetes).[23] If this screening is normal, testing should be repeated between weeks 24 and 28 of gestation. Pregnant women without these risk factors should undergo screening for gestational diabetes mellitus between weeks 24 and 28 of gestation unless they are considered low risk. To be considered low risk, a woman must fulfill *all* the following criteria: (1) age younger than 25 years, (2) normal body weight, (3) no known diabetes in first-degree relatives, (4) no history of abnormal glucose tolerance, (5) no history of adverse obstetric results, and (6) not a member of an ethnic group with a high prevalence of gestational diabetes mellitus (e.g., African Americans, Native Americans, Asian Americans, Latino Americans, Pacific Islanders). Initial screening for hyperglycemia in pregnancy is similar to that in the general population and is described in the American Diabetes Association practice guidelines.[23]

First-line therapy for gestational diabetes mellitus includes nutritional interventions for all women and caloric restriction for obese women.[25] Daily self-monitoring of blood glucose is necessary for all women with the condition. If nutritional interventions do not result in a fasting plasma glucose concentration ≤105 mg/dL, 1-hour postprandial plasma glucose concentration ≤155 mg/dL, or 2-hour postprandial plasma glucose concentration ≤130 mg/dL, insulin therapy with recombinant human insulin should be instituted. Glyburide may be a reasonable alternative for some women.[26] Metformin also may be a practical alternative, but it is less well studied than insulin or glyburide.[26,27] For women who require insulin therapy, some evidence supports use of postprandial blood glucose monitoring.[25] Goals for self-monitored blood glucose are preprandial plasma glucose concentration 80 to 110 mg/dL and 2-hour postprandial plasma glucose concentration <155 mg/dL.[28]

Conversely, Cochrane Reviews have revealed that evidence is insufficient to recommend dietary, exercise, or pharmacologic interventions for women with abnormal glucose tolerance in pregnancy.[29,30] However, a randomized clinical trial revealed that nutritional education, self-monitoring of blood glucose, and insulin therapy as required resulted in reductions in serious perinatal morbidity (death, nerve palsy, bone fracture, and shoulder dystocia).[31]

CLINICAL CONTROVERSY

Despite a lack of evidence for the benefit of screening for gestational diabetes or for implementation of dietary interventions as therapy for gestational diabetes, many clinicians offer screening and dietary guidelines for women with impaired glucose tolerance results.

HYPERTENSION

Broadly stated, hypertension in pregnancy includes gestational hypertension (pregnancy-induced hypertension defined as hypertension without proteinuria), preeclampsia (hypertension with proteinuria), and chronic hypertension (hypertension diagnosed prior to pregnancy with or without overlying preeclampsia).[32] Ten percent of pregnancies are complicated by elevated blood pressure at some time during the pregnancy, and 2% to 8% are complicated by preeclampsia. Outcomes of pregnancies complicated by mild-to-moderate hypertension (defined as systolic blood pressure 140–169 mm Hg or diastolic blood pressure 90–109 mm Hg) are similar to normotensive pregnancies; however, blood pressure elevation can become severe (systolic blood pressure 160–170 mm Hg or higher, or diastolic blood pressure 110 mm Hg or higher) and result in maternal complications, hospital admission, and potential premature delivery. Preeclampsia can cause poorer outcomes, including eclampsia (seizures in addition to preeclampsia), renal failure, blood coagulation complications for the mother, preterm delivery, and intrauterine growth limitation for the fetus.

Calcium supplementation may help prevent hypertension in pregnancy. Supplemental calcium 1 g/day has been found to decrease the relative risk of preeclampsia by 50% (range 31%–67%).[33] Although the greatest effect was seen in patients at highest risk and lowest initial calcium intake, even women with baseline adequate dietary calcium intake had a 38% decreased risk of preeclampsia. Therefore, 1 g/day of supplemental calcium is recommended for all pregnant women.

Prevention of preeclampsia in at-risk women includes daily low-dose aspirin therapy after 12 weeks' gestation.[34] Factors considered to place a pregnancy at high risk include previous severe preeclampsia, renal disease, autoimmune disease, diabetes, and chronic hypertension. Features associated with moderate risk for preeclampsia include first pregnancy, maternal age 13 to 19 years, mild increase in blood pressure without proteinuria, abnormal uterine artery Doppler scan, family history of severe preeclampsia, and multiple fetuses. Administration of low-dose aspirin therapy has been found to decrease the risk of preeclampsia by 19% in at-risk women. Stated differently, treatment of 69 women will result in prevention of one case of preeclampsia. Pre-term birth may be reduced by 7%, and fetal or neonatal death may be reduced by 16%.

Nondrug therapeutic approaches traditionally have focused on activity restriction, psychosocial therapy, and biofeedback. Currently no evidence indicates that any of these approaches improves pregnancy outcome, and prolonged bed rest may increase the risk of venous thromboembolic disease.

Antihypertensive drug therapy for mild-to-moderate hypertension in pregnancy has not been conclusively shown to positively affect potential negative pregnancy outcomes attributed to hypertension, except for prevention of hypertensive crisis.[32] Pregnant women are advised to carefully discuss with their healthcare providers the risks and benefits of treating mild-to-moderate hypertension. No evidence recommends one pharmacologic agent over another. Commonly used drugs include methyldopa, labetalol, and calcium channel blockers.[35] Angiotensin-converting enzyme inhibitors should probably be avoided throughout pregnancy.[36]

Drug therapy is appropriate for women with very high blood pressure, although no conclusive evidence recommends one agent over another.[37] Agents to avoid include magnesium sulfate (unless indicated for eclampsia prevention), high-dose diazoxide, nimodipine, and chlorpromazine.

Preeclampsia may progress rapidly to eclampsia, which is a medical emergency, so signs and symptoms of preeclampsia must be monitored carefully.[35] Signs and symptoms include blood pressure elevation, proteinuria, ongoing severe headache, ongoing new epigastric pain, visual changes, vomiting, hyperreflexia, sudden and severe swelling of hands, face, or feet, low platelet count, hemolytic anemia, and elevated liver enzyme tests. The only cure for preeclampsia is timely delivery of the fetus. Drug therapy for hypertension in preeclampsia includes therapy as mentioned previously (i.e., methyldopa, labetalol, calcium channel blockers). Magnesium sulfate is recommended to prevent eclampsia as well as treat eclamptic seizures. Diazepam and phenytoin should be avoided.

THYROID ABNORMALITIES

Human chorionic gonadotropin may stimulate the thyroid gland because the structure of human chorionic gonadotropin is similar to that of thyrotropin.[38] Pregnant patients with excessive thyroid gland stimulation have gestational transient thyrotoxicosis. Such thyrotoxic patients usually present with vomiting, which can be severe, an increased serum level of free thyroxine, and a depressed thyrotropin level. No other findings support the diagnosis of true thyrotoxicosis. Gestational transient thyrotoxicosis resolves with declining human chorionic gonadotropin concentrations at the completion of the first trimester. Nausea and vomiting can be treated as for patients without this pseudohyperthyroid state.

Within 1 to 4 months postpartum, about 4% of women may experience transient thyrotoxicosis due to extreme secretion of thyroid hormone.[38] Although most cases resolve spontaneously, β-blockers (propranolol or labetalol) can be provided for symptomatic relief; patients should be monitored carefully because transient hypothyroidism may follow. About 2% to 5% of women develop hypothyroidism between 4 and 8 months after delivery, and levothyroxine replacement is suggested for a total of 6 to 12 months.

THROMBOEMBOLISM

The actual incidence of venous thromboembolism during pregnancy is not known but is greater than in nonpregnant women.[39]

❹ Therapy to prevent or treat venous thromboembolism during pregnancy must not include warfarin after the first 6 weeks of gestation because this drug may cause fetal bleeding, malformations of the nose, stippled epiphyses, and central nervous system anomalies.[39] For treatment of acute thromboembolism, adjusted-dose low-molecular-weight heparin or unfractionated heparin should be used for the duration of pregnancy and for 6 weeks after delivery. Patients who should receive antepartum and postpartum anticoagulation therapy include women who have a history of a single episode of thromboembolism and who have thrombophilia or a strong family history of thrombosis and are not currently receiving chronic anticoagulation therapy; women with two or more episodes of thromboembolism; and women receiving long-term anticoagulation. Pregnant women with antiphospholipid antibodies and a history of pregnancy complications should receive antepartum aspirin in addition to unfractionated heparin or low-molecular-weight heparin. Women with antiphospholipid antibodies but no history of thromboembolism or pregnancy complications can be treated with careful observation, heparin, low-molecular-weight heparin, and/or low-dose aspirin (up to 325 mg/day).

Women with prosthetic heart valves should receive low-molecular-weight heparin or unfractionated heparin during pregnancy.[39] Alternatively, a heparin product can be used until week 13 of gestation, at which time it can be replaced with warfarin until the middle of the third trimester when a heparin product should again be used. High-risk women with prosthetic heart valves may also receive aspirin therapy in doses of 75 to 162 mg/day.

CONCLUSION

Many women with pregnancy-influenced gastrointestinal issues can be treated safely with lifestyle modification or medications, many of them nonprescription. Gestational diabetes, hypertension, and thyrotoxicosis may or may not require drug therapy. Venous thromboembolism treatment or prevention usually will require therapy with a low-molecular-weight heparin or unfractionated heparin.

ACUTE CARE ISSUES IN PREGNANCY

❹ Acute illnesses that occur in pregnant women may present challenges for providers. In some cases, such as asymptomatic bacteriuria, the risks associated with the illness are magnified during pregnancy, and early screening and treatment become critical. In other cases, such as during treatment of certain sexually transmitted diseases, the urgency regarding treatment comes from an increased likelihood of infection leading to preterm labor. Occasionally, common acute care issues, such as migraine headache, actually improve during pregnancy.

URINARY TRACT INFECTION

❹ Urinary tract infections are the most common type of bacterial infections in pregnancy.[40] The incidence of asymptomatic bacteriuria is 2% to 10% and acute cystitis is 1% to 4%. Twenty to forty percent of pregnant women with asymptomatic bacteriuria develop pyelonephritis later in pregnancy, illustrating the importance of early detection. Pyelonephritis may lead to complications such as premature delivery, low infant birth weight, fetal death, preeclampsia, pregnancy-induced hypertension, anemia, thrombocytopenia, and transient renal failure.

With regard to screening for urinary tract infections in pregnant women, the American College of Obstetrics and Gynecology recommends a urine culture both at the initial prenatal visit and during the third trimester.[40] In contrast, the U.S. Preventive Task Force recommends a urine culture between 12 and 16 weeks' gestation. A urine culture is the preferred method for screening because other methods, such as dipsticks that measure nitrites or leukocyte esterase, require high concentrations of bacteria and may lead to underdiagnosis.

In 95% of cases, *Escherichia coli* is the principal infecting organism.[40] Other gram-negative rods, such as *Proteus mirabilis* and *Klebsiella pneumoniae,* account for some infections. Group B *Streptococcus* bacteriuria is present in 5% of pregnant women. The presence of group B *Streptococcus* in the urine also may correspond to heavy colonization of the genitourinary tract, increasing the risk for group B *Streptococcus* infection in the newborn.

Treatment of asymptomatic bacteriuria is necessary to reduce the risk of development of pyelonephritis and premature delivery.[40] The incidence of *E. coli* resistance to ampicillin, amoxicillin, and trimethoprim-sulfa has limited the use of these agents. Cephalexin is considered safe and effective. Nitrofurantoin should not be used after week 37 due to concern for hemolytic anemia in the newborn. Sulfa-containing drugs may increase the risk for kernicterus in the newborn and should be avoided during the last weeks of gestation. Folate antagonists, such as trimethoprim, are relatively contraindicated during the first trimester of pregnancy because of associations with cardiovascular malformations. Fluoroquinolones and tetracyclines are contraindicated. The optimal duration of therapy for asymptomatic bacteriuria in pregnancy has not been determined. Courses of 7 to 10 days are common, but some studies have demonstrated that shorter courses of 3 days may be sufficient. A repeat culture 10 days after completion of treatment is recommended.

Signs and symptoms of acute cystitis include urgency, frequency, hematuria, pyuria, and dysuria.[40] Treatment of acute cystitis is similar to that of asymptomatic bacteriuria. A duration of 7 to 10 days may reduce the risk of recurrence more than 3-day courses of therapy.

A Cochrane Review using outcomes of cure rates, recurrent infection, incidence of preterm delivery or rupture of membranes, admission to neonatal intensive care, need for change of antibiotic, or incidence of prolonged fever demonstrated that antibiotic treatment was effective for symptomatic urinary tract infections (including pyelonephritis) in pregnancy.[41] No specific treatment appeared superior to other commonly used treatments.

Acute pyelonephritis complicates 1% to 2% of pregnancies.[40] Patients usually present with bacteriuria and systemic symptoms of fever, flank pain, nausea, and vomiting. Hospitalization has been the standard of practice for pregnant women. Inpatient therapy has included parenteral administration of cephalosporins (e.g., cefazolin), ampicillin or cefazolin with gentamicin, or ceftriaxone. Outpatient antibiotic therapy can be considered if the woman has been afebrile for 48 hours and symptoms have resolved; cephalexin has been used. The total duration of antibiotic therapy for acute pyelonephritis is 10 to 14 days. Because up to 23% of women may experience recurrence, suppression therapy with nitrofurantoin 100 mg nightly is recommended for the duration of the pregnancy.

SEXUALLY TRANSMITTED DISEASES

❹ Sexually transmitted diseases in pregnant women range from infections that may be transmitted across the placenta and infect the infant prenatally (e.g., syphilis) to organisms that may be transmitted during birth and cause neonatal infection (e.g., *Chlamydia trachomatis, Neisseria gonorrhoeae,* or herpes simplex virus) to infections that pose a threat for preterm labor (e.g., bacterial vaginosis). Screening is essential for early detection of most sexually transmitted diseases but may not be beneficial in other instances (e.g., bacterial vaginosis in low-risk patients). Sexual partners of women with certain infections (e.g., syphilis, *N. gonorrhoeae, C. trachomatis*) also will require treatment to prevent recurrence of infection.

Syphilis

It is recommended that all women take a serologic test for syphilis at the first prenatal visit.[42] Additional testing may be warranted for women who live in areas with a high prevalence of syphilis, are at high risk, have not been tested previously, or had positive serology in the first trimester. Penicillin is the drug of choice and is effective in preventing transmission to the fetus and in treating the fetus, if already infected. The dose and route of administration are determined by the stage of syphilis and are the same for pregnant women as for other patients. No alternatives for penicillin are acceptable for pregnant women allergic to penicillin; therefore, penicillin skin testing and desensitization are required.

Women who receive treatment during the second half of pregnancy may be at risk for premature labor and/or fetal distress if treatment results in the Jarisch-Herxheimer reaction.[42] All women should have serologic titers repeated at 28 to 32 weeks' gestation, at delivery, and as dictated by recommendations for the stage of disease.

Neisseria gonorrhoeae

Perinatal gonococcal infection results from exposure to the infected cervix during birth.[42] Symptoms generally start within 2 to 5 days of birth. Milder manifestations include rhinitis, vaginitis, urethritis, and infection at the site of fetal monitoring. More severe presentations include ophthalmia neonatorum and sepsis.

N. gonorrhoeae cervicitis coinfection with *C. trachomatis* is common, and treatment of most *N. gonorrhoeae* infections includes treatment for *C. trachomatis.*[42] Cotreatment regimens for presumptive or diagnosed *C. trachomatis* infection are described in the

TABLE 81-1 Recommended Regimens for Treatment of Cervical Infections Due to *Chlamydia* in Pregnancy

First-line treatment
Azithromycin 1 g orally in a single dose *or*
Amoxicillin 500 mg orally three times daily for 7 days
Alternative regimens
Erythromycin base 500 mg orally four times per day for 7 days *or*
Erythromycin base 250 mg mg orally four times per day for 14 days
Erythromycin ethylsuccinate 800 mg orally four times per day for 7 days *or*
Erythromycin ethylsuccinate 400 mg orally four times per day for 14 days

Data from Centers for Disease Control and Prevention, Workowski KA, Berman SM.[42]

following section. The treatment of choice for *N. gonorrhoeae* cervical infection is ceftriaxone 125 mg intramuscularly as a single dose or cefixime 400 mg orally in a single dose. For women unable to use a cephalosporin, spectinomycin 2 g intramuscularly as a single dose is appropriate. Quinolones or tetracyclines should not be used.

Chlamydia trachomatis

C. trachomatis infection of the newborn occurs during movement through the birth canal and exposure to the infected cervix.[42] Perinatal infection most commonly causes conjunctivitis. A subacute, afebrile pneumonia with an onset at ages 1 to 3 months may occur.

The recommended treatment of *C. trachomatis* cervicitis is azithromycin 1 g orally as a single dose or amoxicillin 500 mg three times daily for 7 days.[42] Erythromycin base or ethylsuccinate regimens can be considered as alternatives. Erythromycin estolate should be avoided because of an increased risk for hepatitis (Table 81–1).

Genital Herpes

❹ Neonatal herpes often occurs in infants born of women lacking clinical evidence of genital herpes.[42] For women who initially acquire genital herpes near the time of delivery, the risk of transmission is 30% to 50%. For women with a history of recurrent herpes at term or who have an initial episode during the first half of the pregnancy, the risk of transmission is less than 1%. However, because recurrent herpes is more common than initial episodes during pregnancy, it remains the cause for most cases of neonatal transmission.

Prevention strategies include counseling uninfected women to avoid intercourse during the third trimester with partners having known or suspected genital herpes infection.[42] Women with no history of orolabial herpes should avoid receptive oral sex during the third trimester with partners having orolabial herpes. The usefulness of antiviral agents for preventing transmission of genital herpes to pregnant women has not been studied.

All women should be asked about symptoms of genital herpes at the time of delivery and examined for lesions.[42] Women who have no symptoms or lesions can deliver vaginally. Those who have evidence of outbreak at the time of delivery generally deliver by cesarean section to reduce the risk of transmission to the infant.

Of the agents available for treatment, acyclovir has been used the longest and has not demonstrated an increased risk for birth defects with first-trimester use.[42] Safety data for valacyclovir and famciclovir are limited. Most women receive oral acyclovir therapy for first or recurrent episodes. Intravenous acyclovir can be used for severe infections. Acyclovir use during late pregnancy has been associated with a reduced frequency of cesarean section because of fewer recurrences. No data suggest benefit of treatment for women who are seropositive for herpes simplex virus but have not experienced a clinical episode. For women with an initial outbreak late in pregnancy, treatment may consist of acyclovir, cesarean section, or a combination of the two.

CLINICAL CONTROVERSY

Although there is evidence that use of antiviral therapy during the last month of pregnancy in women with recurrent genital herpes reduces outbreaks and therefore the need for cesarean section, there is no evidence that use of these agents reduces perinatal transmission.[43] Because transmission rates for recurrent herpes are low, the sample size for a study would need to be very large. Several guidelines suggest that prophylactic use of acyclovir during the last month of pregnancy may be warranted.

Bacterial Vaginosis

Although not a sexually transmitted disease, bacterial vaginosis is a risk factor for premature rupture of membranes, preterm labor, preterm birth, spontaneous abortion, and postpartum endometritis.[44] It is found in 9% to 23% of pregnant women.

Women with a history of preterm delivery should undergo screening for asymptomatic bacterial vaginosis at the first prenatal visit.[42] If the infection is present, the recommended regimen is metronidazole 500 mg orally twice per day for 7 days, metronidazole 250 mg three times per day for 7 days, or clindamycin 300 mg twice per day for 7 days.

Conflicting data exist with regard to treating women at low risk for preterm labor.[42] Symptomatic women should be treated using the metronidazole or clindamycin regimen. Vaginal creams have not been found to be effective in reducing the risk of adverse pregnancy outcomes associated with bacterial vaginosis. Use of intravaginal clindamycin cream during the second half of pregnancy has been associated with adverse neonatal effects.

HEADACHE

❹ Headaches in pregnant women can be classified as primary (tension, migraine) or secondary (trauma, infection).[45] Migraine and tension headaches are the most common types.

For more than 60% to 70% of women with a history of migraine headaches, symptoms improve during pregnancy.[46] The largest improvements in symptoms usually occur in the second and third trimesters.[45] Women with a history of menstrual migraine are less likely to have remission of symptoms during pregnancy and are more likely to experience postpartum recurrence. Women who have migraine headache without aura are more likely to experience improvement.[46]

Rest, reassurance, and ice packs should be used to initially treat migraine attacks.[46] Acetaminophen (with or without codeine), codeine, or other narcotic analgesics can be used to treat headaches that do not respond to nonpharmacologic treatment. Nonsteroidal antiinflammatory drugs are considered safe during the first trimester but are generally contraindicated in late pregnancy. Salicylates and indomethacin are potent inhibitors of prostaglandin synthesis and should be avoided throughout the pregnancy if possible, but especially during the third trimester. Use of sumatriptan is controversial, but some clinicians continue the drug in women who have not responded to other agents for treatment of migraine headaches.[45] Patients who have nausea associated with migraine headaches can be treated with metoclopramide.[46] Both ergotamine and dihydroergotamine should be avoided. Chronic, preventive treatment can be considered for women who have three to four severe episodes per month that are not responsive to other treatments. β-Blockers, such as propranolol, are commonly used for this purpose but may be associated with side effects, including intrauterine growth retardation.

Tension headaches have been less studied.[45] Most women report no change in the frequency or intensity of tension headaches.

Tension headaches may be difficult to distinguish from secondary headaches. Primary treatments for tension headache are nonpharmacologic interventions, including exercise, biofeedback, and massage. Simple analgesics such as acetaminophen, ibuprofen, or caffeine can be used if nonpharmacologic treatments fail. Narcotics and benzodiazepines should be avoided.[46]

CHRONIC ILLNESSES IN PREGNANCY

❹ For the majority of women and their healthcare providers, pregnancy is a new consideration for a previously diagnosed health condition. Medications used to treat the chronic illness often can be used throughout the pregnancy and during breast-feeding.

ALLERGIC RHINITIS AND ASTHMA

❹ Asthma and rhinitis are two of the most common chronic illnesses in pregnancy. Although rhinitis itself is unlikely to cause harm to the mother or fetus, untreated rhinitis may be associated with diminished quality of life. Asthma control may change, and worsening asthma may have significant health consequences to both the mother and the fetus.

Asthma affects approximately 4% of pregnancies.[47] Asthma severity can change during pregnancy; almost equal proportions of patients have symptoms that worsen, improve, or remain unchanged. Asthma symptoms may worsen during the third trimester but may improve in the last month of pregnancy.

Appropriate treatment is critical to the health of the mother and the infant.[47] In the mother, undertreated asthma is associated with placenta previa, oligohydramnios, preterm labor, maternal hypertension, preeclampsia, uterine hemorrhage, and need for cesarean section. In the infant, poor maternal asthma control may result in premature birth, low birth weight, and stillbirth.

The treatment goal is to control symptoms in order to maintain maternal health and well-being and promote normal fetal development.[48] Optimal control is described as (1) minimal use of short-acting β_2-agonists, (2) achievement of normal or near-normal pulmonary function, (3) lack of adverse effects of treatment, (4) control of symptoms during both day and night, (5) ability to continue normal activities, and (6) avoidance of acute exacerbations.

Treatment of asthma should include (1) assessment and monitoring of asthma (including pulmonary function testing); (2) identifying, controlling, or avoiding allergens and irritants (e.g., tobacco smoke); (3) patient education; and (4) stepwise approach to use of medications.[48] Treatment of asthma with medications is considered safer than the risks to the fetus from untreated asthma.

All patients with asthma should have access to a short-acting β_2-agonist for quick relief of symptoms.[48] Women with mild intermittent asthma require only a short-acting, inhaled β_2-agonist; albuterol is the preferred agent.

Low-dose inhaled corticosteroids are the treatment of choice for women with mild persistent asthma.[48] Although budesonide is the preferred agent, other inhaled corticosteroids that were effective prior to pregnancy can be continued. Cromolyn, leukotriene receptor antagonists, and theophylline are considered alternative treatments but are not preferred because of less efficacy (cromolyn), less experience (leukotriene receptor antagonists), and more potential toxicity (theophylline) than inhaled corticosteroids.

For moderate persistent asthma, either a combination of low-dose inhaled corticosteroids with a long-acting β_2-agonist or an increase in the dose of the inhaled corticosteroids is the recommended treatment option.[48] Because long-acting bronchodilators have similar pharmacologic and safety profiles compared to short-acting agents, they appear to be safe for use during pregnancy.

For severe persistent asthma, the inhaled corticosteroid dose should be increased to the high-dose range.[48] Addition of systemic corticosteroids may be warranted if symptoms continue.

As with asthma, allergic rhinitis may improve, worsen, or remain the same during pregnancy.[49] Treatment strategies include avoidance of allergens, immunotherapy, and pharmacotherapy. World Health Organization standards state that immunotherapy is not contraindicated in pregnancy but advises against dose increases during pregnancy to lessen risk for anaphylaxis.

Intranasal corticosteroids are the most effective treatment for allergic rhinitis during pregnancy and have a low risk of systemic effect.[48] Beclomethasone and budesonide have been most widely studied.[49] Nasal cromolyn and first-generation antihistamines (chlorpheniramine, tripelennamine, and hydroxyzine) are also considered first-line choices. The second-generation antihistamines loratadine and cetirizine do not appear to increase risk to the fetus but have not been studied as extensively as the first-generation products. Oral decongestants, such as pseudoephedrine, may be associated with an increased risk for the rare birth defect gastroschisis.[48] Use of an external nasal dilator, short-term topical oxymetazoline, or inhaled corticosteroids may be preferable to use of oral decongestants, especially during early pregnancy.

DERMATOLOGIC CONDITIONS

❹ Treatment of dermatologic conditions often can be delayed until after the delivery.[50] If implementation of treatment during pregnancy is necessary, topical agents with minimal pregnancy risk include bacitracin, benzoyl peroxide, ciclopirox, clindamycin, erythromycin, metronidazole, mupirocin, permethrin, and terbinafine. Topical corticosteroids are thought to be safe for use but should be applied at the lowest possible dose for the shortest time. Systemic agents considered safe include acyclovir, amoxicillin, azithromycin, cephalosporins, cyproheptadine, dicloxacillin, diphenhydramine, erythromycin (except estolates), nystatin, and penicillins. Lidocaine and lidocaine with epinephrine can be used topically during pregnancy. Dermatologic drugs with teratogenic potential that should be avoided include acitretin, fluorouracil, isotretinoin, methotrexate, and thalidomide.

DIABETES

❹ Women with diabetes should defer pregnancy until the condition is under control with medication and lifestyle interventions because of increased fetal loss and malformations resulting from suboptimally controlled diabetes.[28] In addition, diabetic retinopathy may worsen, hypertension may develop, and renal function may deteriorate during pregnancy. Enhanced monitoring for these target-organ problems is essential.

Insulin is the drug treatment of choice for patients with both type 1 and type 2 diabetes.[26,28] However, use of glyburide after week 11 of gestation in patients with type 2 diabetes may be acceptable.[26] Metformin is another option. Medical nutrition therapy and supervised physical activity programs should continue.[26,28] Goals for self-monitored blood glucose are the same as for gestational diabetes.[28]

EPILEPSY

❹ Maternal epilepsy complicates 1% of pregnancies.[51] About 35% of women experience an increase in seizure frequency during pregnancy, 55% have no change, and 10% experience a decrease in frequency. Seizures may become more frequent because of changes in maternal hormones, sleep schedule, antiepileptic drug pharmacokinetics, and medication adherence problems (because of perceived teratogenic risk of antiepileptic drug therapy). In addition, free serum concentrations of the antiepileptic drug may change as a result of maternal increased volume of distribution, decreased protein binding because of hypoalbuminemia, increased hepatic drug metabolism, and increased renal drug clearance. A woman's clinical condition and the free serum concentrations of antiepileptic drug should be the bases for any adjustments in antiepileptic drug dosage. If a woman chooses to breast-feed, her antiepileptic drug requirements will not change until breast-feeding stops.

Major malformations occur in 4% to 6% of offspring of epileptic women taking benzodiazepines, carbamazepine, phenobarbital, phenytoin, or valproic acid.[51] Lamotrigine has been associated with an incidence of oral cleft palate and/or lip of one case per 113 exposed infants.[52] Minor malformations occur in 6% to 20% of pregnancies affected by epilepsy, which is twice the rate in the general population. The malformations are considered to result from fetal exposure to antiepileptic drug therapy rather than from maternal epilepsy.[51,53] Combination regimens of antiepileptic drugs are associated with higher malformation rates.[51]

Recommendations are use of antiepileptic drug monotherapy, if possible, and optimization of any drug therapy prior to conception.[54] Medication change exclusively to minimize teratogenic risk, such as the prior recommendation to switch to phenobarbital from other antiepileptic drugs, is *no longer* recommended. Drug withdrawal, if planned, should be attempted at least 6 months before conception is attempted. To correct vitamin K deficiency in newborns, the mother should receive supplementation with 10 mg oral vitamin K_1 daily during the last month of gestation.[54] In addition, all women with epilepsy should take folic acid supplementation of 0.4 to 5 mg daily.[51,54]

HUMAN IMMUNODEFICIENCY VIRUS INFECTION

❹ Zidovudine is the mainstay of antiretroviral therapy and is recommended for use during pregnancy (after the first trimester), labor, and delivery, as well as during the postpartum period.[55] If a woman has received prior antiretroviral therapy, continuation should be strongly considered. Without prior therapy, the regimen should be selected from those suggested for nonpregnant adults. If therapy is discontinued during the first trimester because of nausea, vomiting, or other reasons, the woman should wait to resume therapy until her ability to tolerate all medications is determined with certainty. Additionally, all medications should be restarted at the same time to decrease risk of resistance. The current zidovudine dosing recommendation during pregnancy is 100 mg five times daily, 200 mg three times daily, or 300 mg twice daily. Zidovudine should be initiated at the beginning of the second trimester and continued for the duration of the pregnancy. Intravenous zidovudine is recommended during labor, and the infant should receive the drug beginning 8 to 12 hours after birth and continuing for the first 6 weeks of life.

HYPERTENSION

❹ For women with stage 1 or 2 chronic hypertension (blood pressure 140–179 mm Hg systolic or 90 to 109 mm Hg diastolic), the decision of whether to continue or stop antihypertensive therapy is controversial because most of the increases in adverse fetal and maternal outcomes are due to preeclampsia superimposed on chronic hypertension.[56] Therapy should be restarted if medication is discontinued and women are monitored closely but blood pressure exceeds 150 to 160 mm Hg systolic or 100 to 110 mm Hg diastolic or if target-organ damage is present. Alternatively, antihypertensive drugs may be continued (except for angiotensin-converting enzyme inhibitors and angiotensin II receptor blockers) at the lowest effective dose. Use of diuretics is controversial but may be considered for chronic hypertension. For women with severe hypertension (diastolic blood pressure ≥100 mm Hg), the benefit of drug therapy may outweigh the risks. No evidence exists for superior efficacy of one agent versus another for blood pressure reduction.[32,37,56]

MENTAL HEALTH CONDITIONS

❹ An estimated 500,000 pregnancies each year involve women with psychiatric illnesses (either newly or previously diagnosed).[57] Although depression is the most studied mental health condition during pregnancy, it is not the most common.

Anxiety disorders, including panic disorder, obsessive–compulsive disorder, generalized anxiety disorder, posttraumatic stress disorder, social anxiety disorder, and phobias, are the most commonly occurring psychiatric illnesses in the general population.[57] Little information is available regarding the incidence and clinical course of these illnesses during pregnancy.

Depression occurs in 10% to 16% of pregnant women.[57] Maternal depression is associated with greater risk for premature birth and low birth weight. Bipolar disorder affects 1.5% of Americans, but the incidence in pregnancy is unknown. Relapse in bipolar patients may be more likely during pregnancy, especially if pharmacologic treatment is stopped. In addition to the potential impact of maternal depression on obstetric complications, untreated depression may have long-term implications for normal infant development.

Schizophrenia occurs in 1% to 2% of women, but the incidence in pregnancy is unknown.[57] Because of the risk for decompensation of symptoms during pregnancy and during the postpartum period, drug therapy is often necessary. Maternal schizophrenia is associated with increased risk of perinatal death, low birth weight, preterm delivery, stillbirth, and infant death.

Five percent of Americans, mostly women, suffer from eating disorders.[57] Some evidence indicates that women with eating disorders may have a more benign course during pregnancy, but common comorbid conditions such as depression and anxiety deserve attention. Eating disorders may pose problems during the postpartum period.

A number of nonpharmacologic options can be used for treatment of psychiatric illness in pregnant women. Both cognitive behavioral therapy and interpersonal psychotherapy have been shown to be beneficial in the treatment of anxiety disorders and depression.[57] Light therapy also has been effective in treatment of depression. Electroconvulsive therapy is considered safe and effective treatment of major depression and bipolar disorder.

Because many of the psychotropic medications are used to treat more than one condition, the reader should refer to other sources for information about treatment of specific mental health diagnoses. The following section describes medications commonly used for treatment of mental illness, along with implications for use in pregnant women.

Antidepressants have been used with relative safety for more than 40 years.[57] The selective serotonin reuptake inhibitors are the drugs of first choice in the general population and are widely used by pregnant women. Research findings have revealed adverse events in newborns exposed to selective serotonin reuptake inhibitors in utero.[58] About one to two babies per 1,000 develop persistent pulmonary hypertension. A study found this risk was six times greater in infants born to women who took selective serotonin reuptake inhibitors after week 20 of pregnancy. Another risk associated with use of selective serotonin reuptake inhibitors late in pregnancy is a withdrawal reaction in the infant consisting of irritability and difficulty with feeding and breathing. Finally, an epidemiologic study suggests that first-trimester use of paroxetine may be associated with an increased risk for cardiac defects in the infant. Despite the concerns about adverse effects in infants born to women who used selective serotonin reuptake inhibitors during pregnancy, a study indicated that pregnant women who stopped taking antidepressant medications were five times more likely to have a relapse than women who completed treatment, which has implications for the well-being of the infant.

Benzodiazepines are used to treat a number of mental health conditions.[57] Early studies of benzodiazepine use during pregnancy warned of an increased risk for oral clefts in infants who were exposed to these agents during pregnancy. Later studies did not have the same findings. A meta-analysis estimated an increase in the absolute risk of oral cleft of 0.01% from 6:10,000 to 7:10,000. Benzodiazepine use in the third trimester can be associated with infant sedation and withdrawal symptoms, which are considered more significant than those seen with selective serotonin reuptake inhibitors.[59] A "floppy baby syndrome," consisting of low Apgar scores, hypothermia, poor muscle tone, and poor temperature adaptation, has been described.[59]

Mood stabilizers, such as lithium, lamotrigine, carbamazepine, and valproic acid, are often used to treat bipolar disorder.[57] The reader can find information related to the use of the seizure medications used for mood stabilization in the section on Epilepsy.

Lithium is considered the first-line treatment of bipolar disorder during pregnancy.[57] Lithium's place in therapy has been controversial because of concerns about cardiovascular anomalies, especially Ebstein anomaly, in exposed infants. A systematic review calculated that the risk ratio for cardiac malformations was 1.2:7.7 and for all congenital malformations was 1.5:3. Stated differently, the risk for Ebstein anomaly would rise from 1:20,000 to 1:1,000. Other reported side effects in the newborn include "floppy baby syndrome," nephrogenic diabetes insipidus, hypoglycemia, cardiac arrhythmias, thyroid dysfunction, polyhydramnios, and premature delivery. Several case reports describe adverse effects in infants thought to be due to lithium use by lactating mothers.[6] During lactation, the infant's lithium levels and thyroid function should be monitored.

Chlorpromazine, haloperidol, and perphenazine have long histories of use during pregnancy, with no reported significant increase in congenital malformations.[57] Atypical antipsychotics are now more widely used for treatment of schizophrenia because of their more favorable side-effect profiles compared to the older agents.[60] However, use of atypical antipsychotics in pregnant women is controversial. Although olanzapine and clozapine have not been associated with increased risk for congenital malformation, they have been associated with weight gain and an increased incidence of glucose intolerance, which have implications for poorer obstetric outcomes. Other agents, such as quetiapine, risperidone, aripiprazole, and ziprasidone, have been used less in pregnancy, so only limited information is available. At present, atypical antipsychotics do not appear to be safer than the typical agents.

THYROID DISORDERS

❹ Hypothyroidism affects between 1 and 3 per 1,000 pregnancies.[38] Untreated hypothyroidism increases the risk of preeclampsia, premature birth, and low birth weight. Causes of hypothyroidism include autoimmune diseases such as Hashimoto thyroiditis, iodine deficiency (uncommon in the United States), and thyroid dysfunction following surgery or ablative therapy for previous hyperthyroidism. Thyroid replacement therapy should be instituted with levothyroxine if hypothyroidism is diagnosed; the goal is to attain normal thyrotropin concentrations. Women who receive thyroid replacement therapy prior to pregnancy may have an increased dosage requirement during pregnancy; any dose change should follow thyroid function testing. After delivery, maternal thyroid supplementation should be returned to prepregnancy doses, with laboratory followup in 6 to 8 weeks.

Hyperthyroidism affects approximately 2 of every 1,000 pregnancies and may precipitate outcomes of fetal death, low birth weight, malformations, and maternal heart failure. Graves disease is the most common cause of hyperthyroidism in pregnancy.[38] Therapy includes thioamides (e.g., propylthiouracil, methimazole) and surgery. Methimazole crosses the placenta less than propylthiouracil, but both drugs are commonly used to treat the disorder. Iodine-131 is contraindicated because of the risk of thyroid damage in the fetus. The goal of therapy is to attain free thyroxine concentrations in the upper end of the normal range; this allows for minimization of the thioamide dose.

LABOR AND DELIVERY

PRETERM LABOR

Preterm labor is defined as cervical changes and uterine contractions that occur before 37 weeks' gestation.[61] In the United States, the incidence of preterm births is 11% and is a leading cause of infant morbidity and mortality.[61,62] Risk factors for preterm delivery include previous preterm delivery, infections, multiple gestation, poverty, nonwhite race, maternal complication factors (e.g., smoking and use of illicit drugs or alcohol), uterine functional causes (e.g., incompetent cervix and uterine septum), and fetal causes (e.g., congenital anomalies and growth retardation).[61]

Despite knowledge of the risk factors for preterm labor, no good tests are available for monitoring and preventing preterm labor. No evidence supports the use of routine cervical assessments or home monitoring of uterine activity to improve outcomes.[61] The presence of fetal fibronectin, an extracellular protein in cervical and vaginal secretions, in the cervix or vagina after 20 weeks is associated with a threefold risk of preterm delivery.[63] A cervical length less than 30 mm is associated with increased risk of preterm delivery. Fetal fibronectin determinations and cervical ultrasonography have not helped to prevent preterm labor but have been useful for their negative predictive value.[64]

Tocolytic Therapy

The purpose of tocolytic therapy is to postpone delivery long enough to allow for administration of antenatal corticosteroids to improve pulmonary maturity and for transportation of the mother to a facility equipped to deal with high-risk deliveries.[61] Tocolytics have not been shown to reduce the number of premature deliveries. The criteria for starting tocolysis are regular uterine contractions with cervical change; however, tocolytic therapy is less effective when cervical dilatation is greater than 3 cm. Tocolytic therapy should not be used in cases of intrauterine infection, fetal distress, severe preeclampsia, vaginal bleeding, or maternal hemodynamic instability.[63]

Five classes of tocolytic therapy are available in the United States: β-adrenergic agents, magnesium, calcium channel blockers, nonsteroidal antiinflammatory drugs, and ethanol.[62] The first four therapies have similar effectiveness in prolonging pregnancy from 48 hours to 1 week. Ethanol has not been shown to be effective.

The β-adrenergic agents terbutaline and ritodrine have been used for tocolytic therapy.[62] (Of the two, only ritodrine had FDA approval for this use but has been withdrawn from the market.) Relative to other agents, β-agonists have a higher incidence of maternal side effects, including hyperkalemia, arrhythmias, hyperglycemia, hypotension, and pulmonary edema. Recommended terbutaline doses range from 250 to 500 mcg subcutaneously every 3 to 4 hours.[63]

Magnesium sulfate has been used as a tocolytic agent in intravenous infusion form. A Cochrane meta-analysis demonstrates that magnesium sulfate is ineffective as a tocolytic agent and that an association exists between magnesium sulfate use and increased mortality in infants.[65] Maternal side effects are rare but can include pulmonary edema. At toxic levels, hypotension, muscle paralysis, tetany, cardiac arrest, and respiratory depression may occur.[63]

Nifedipine is associated with fewer side effects than magnesium or β-agonist therapy.[62] A few studies have suggested that calcium channel blockers are better than β-agonists at prolonging labor. One concern with the use of nifedipine is the potential negative effect on blood flow between the placenta and the uterus. However, a meta-analysis has not shown increased harm to infants. With the initial diagnosis of preterm labor, 5 to 10 mg nifedipine can be administered sublingually every 15 to 20 minutes for three doses. Once the patient is stabilized and no evidence of continuing cervical dilation is seen, 10 to 20 mg nifedipine can be administered by mouth every 4 to 6 hours for preterm contractions.[63]

Nonsteroidal antiinflammatory drugs such as indomethacin have been used for tocolysis.[63] The drug is first given orally or rectally in a dose of 50 to 100 mg, followed by an oral dose of 25 to 50 mg every 6 hours. An increased rate of premature constriction of the ductus arteriosus has been noted in infants when indomethacin has been used as tocolytic therapy.[62]

Other Methods for Preterm Labor Prevention

Because infection has been thought to play a role in the etiology of preterm labor, antibiotics have been used, in addition to tocolytics and corticosteroids, to improve the outcome of preterm labor.[66] Most studies of antibiotic use do not demonstrate a reduction in the incidence of preterm delivery, and a meta-analysis showed a trend toward neonatal mortality in patients who received antibiotics. Therefore, routine use of antibiotics is not recommended.

A low level of maternal serum progesterone has been associated with miscarriage and preterm labor. Several small trials using progesterone and progesterone-like drugs have shown inconclusive results in the prevention of preterm labor. However, studies using 17α-hydroxyprogesterone caproate have shown some success. In women at high risk for preterm delivery of a singleton pregnancy, administration of 17α-hydroxyprogesteron caproate as early as 20 weeks' gestation has shown some reduction in preterm delivery.[67] Additional randomized trials are needed.

CLINICAL CONTROVERSY

Continuation of tocolytic therapy after acute tocolysis has been achieved is controversial. Maintenance therapy with tocolytics has not been shown conclusively to be of value.[62] However, some clinicians use maintenance tocolytics such as β-agonists or nifedipine to treat patients who experience frequent contractions without cervical change.

Antenatal Corticosteroids

❹ A Cochrane meta-analysis demonstrates the benefit of administering antenatal corticosteroids for fetal lung maturation in order to prevent respiratory distress syndrome, intraventricular hemorrhage, and death in infants delivered prematurely.[68] The current clinical recommendation is to administer betamethasone 12 mg intramuscularly every 24 hours for two doses or dexamethasone 6 mg intramuscularly every 12 hours for four doses to pregnant women between 26 and 34 weeks' gestation who are at risk for preterm delivery within the next 7 days. Benefits from antenatal corticosteroids are believed to begin within 24 hours. A meta-analysis in 2000 did not show a clear benefit to repeat doses of steroids.

GROUP B *STREPTOCOCCUS* INFECTION

❹ Maternal infection with group B *Streptococcus* is associated with invasive disease in the newborn.[69] Women colonized with group B *Streptococcus* have an increased risk for premature delivery and transmission of the bacteria to the infant during delivery. Between 10% and 30% of pregnant women are colonized with group B *Streptococcus*.

With active prevention efforts in the 1990s, the incidence of early-onset disease now is 0.5 cases per 1,000 births, down from 1.8 cases per 1,000 births.[69] No change has occurred in the incidence of late-onset group B *Streptococcus* disease, which remains consistent at 0.35 cases per 1,000 births. The consequences of neonatal infections include bacteremia, pneumonia, and meningitis in the newborn. The case-fatality rate is approximately 4%.

The recommendations for prevention of group B *Streptococcus* infection were revised in 2002.[69] Universal prenatal screening for group B *Streptococcus* colonization now is recommended instead of risk-based screening. Antibiotics are given if the woman previously gave birth to an infant with invasive group B *Streptococcus* disease or if the woman had group B *Streptococcus* bacteriuria. In all other pregnant women at 35 to 37 weeks' gestation, a vaginal/rectal culture should be obtained. If negative, no antibiotics are given. If a woman presents in labor and no screening information is available, antibiotics are given for fever ≥100.4°F (38°C), membrane rupture ≥18 hours, or gestation <37 weeks.

The currently recommended regimen for group B *Streptococcus* disease is 5 million units of penicillin G given intravenously, followed by 2.5 million units given every 4 hours until delivery.[69] Alternatively, ampicillin 2 g can be given intravenously, followed by 1 g every 4 hours. If the patient is allergic to penicillin and is not at risk for anaphylaxis, cefazolin 2 g intravenously, followed by 1 g every 8 hours, should be used. In patients at high risk for anaphylaxis, clindamycin 900 mg intravenously every 8 hours or erythromycin 500 mg intravenously every 6 hours should be used. For penicillin-allergic women, the group B *Streptococcus* cultures should be sent for sensitivities. If the group B *Streptococcus* is resistant to clindamycin or erythromycin, the woman should receive vancomycin 1 g intravenously every 12 hours until delivery.

CERVICAL RIPENING AND LABOR INDUCTION

Throughout most of pregnancy, the cervix is closed and firm.[70] During the last few weeks of pregnancy, the cervix becomes softer and thinner in order to facilitate labor. This process is mediated by hormonal changes, including final mediation by prostaglandins E_2 and $F_2\alpha$, which cause increased collagenase activity in the cervix leading to thinning and dilation.

The rate of pregnancy induction ranges from 9.5% to 33.5%.[70] The most common reason for induction is postdatism (>42 weeks), which occurs in 10% of all pregnancies.[71] Other reasons for induction include suspected fetal growth retardation, maternal hypertension, premature rupture of membranes with no active onset of labor, and social factors. Contraindications for induction include placenta previa, oblique or transverse lie, pelvic structure abnormality, prolapsed umbilical cord, and active herpes. Concerns associated with induction of labor are ineffective labor and side effects, such as uterine hyperstimulation, that may adversely affect the infant, increasing the likelihood of cesarean section.

A scoring system has been used to determine the likelihood of successful labor induction.[70] The most commonly used system is the Bishop scoring system, which is based on five parameters: cervical dilation, cervical effacement (thinning), station of the baby's head, consistency of the cervix, and position of the cervix. A Bishop score <6 means that a patient requires cervical ripening, and a score >8 means that the patient most likely will have a successful vaginal delivery.

A number of nonpharmacologic methods are used for cervical ripening. Castor oil, hot baths, sexual intercourse, and nipple stimulation all have been recommended for labor induction.[70] However, minimal evidence supports the efficacy of these methods. Use of a Foley catheter placed in an unfavorable cervix for ripening has been found as effective as prostaglandin E_2. Membrane stripping is safe and inexpensive.

Herbal supplements have been used to induce labor. The most commonly used agents are evening primrose oil, black haw, black and blue cohosh, and red raspberry leaves.[70] Currently, no evidence supports the safety and efficacy of herbal agents.

Prostaglandin E_2 analogs (e.g., dinoprostone [Prepidil, Cervidil]) are pharmacologic agents commonly used for cervical ripening. Prepidil gel is administered intracervically at a dose of 500 mcg.[70] This can be repeated after 6 hours with up to three doses in 24 hours. After administration, the patient remains supine for 30 minutes. Cervidil, a vaginal insert, contains 10 mg dinoprostone with a slower, more constant release of medication than the gel. The insert can be removed when labor begins or after a maximum of 24 hours. Patients must be attached to a fetal heart rate monitor for the duration of Cervidil use and for 15 minutes after its removal.

Misoprostol, a prostaglandin E_1 analog, is an effective and inexpensive drug for cervical ripening and labor induction.[72] Intravaginal administration of 25 mcg misoprostol every 4 hours for up to six doses is more effective than other prostaglandin agents and results in a shorter time to delivery. The most commonly encountered side effects are uterine hyperstimulation and meconium-stained amniotic fluid. Use of misoprostol is contraindicated in women with a previous uterine scar because of its association with uterine rupture, a catastrophic medical event. Despite its efficacy and lack of expense, some hospitals have decided not to use misoprostol as an induction agent due to concerns for uterine rupture and lack of FDA indication for cervical ripening.

Mifepristone is an antiprogesterone agent that is being studied as an induction agent.[70] Preliminary studies show that mifepristone compared with placebo results in a shorter time to delivery and fewer cesarean sections.[73] Little information on fetal and maternal outcomes is available because of the small sample sizes.

Oxytocin is the most commonly used agent for labor induction after cervical ripening. By the end of pregnancy, the number of oxytocin receptors has increased by 300-fold.[70] A solution of 10 milliunits/mL is used for infusion. Oxytocin has been shown to be effective in both low-dose (physiologic) and high-dose (pharmacologic) regimens.

LABOR ANALGESIA

During the first phase of labor, women perceive visceral pain associated with uterine contractions. During the second phase of labor, the pain is associated with perineal stretching.[74,75] Pain perception is variable among women as a result of physiologic, psychosocial, cultural, and environmental influences.[74]

Nonpharmacologic Approaches to Analgesia

A number of nonpharmacologic strategies have been used to reduce the pain of childbirth. Women who receive continuous support from a doula, a laywoman trained in labor support, have fewer operative vaginal deliveries, cesarean deliveries, and requests for pain medication.[74] Intermittent support from a caregiver and continuous support from nursing staff have not been shown to affect birth outcomes. Warm water baths provide temporary pain relief but have not been shown to decrease the use of pharmacologic pain treatments. Intradermal injections of sterile water in the sacral area have been shown to decrease back pain during labor for 45 to 90 minutes. However, requests for pain medication did not decrease. Acupuncture is another modality for pain relief. One study of acupuncture versus no acupuncture showed that women required less analgesia but were no more satisfied with this mode of pain control. Methodologically sound studies on acupuncture are sparse.[76]

Pharmacologic Approaches to Labor Pain Management

A joint position statement on pain in labor published in 2000 stated that labor is a medical indication for women to receive pain relief upon request.[77] The two main types of pharmacologic methods in the United States are parenteral opioids and epidural analgesia.

Between 39% and 56% of women receive parenteral narcotics to alleviate labor pain.[77] Meperidine, morphine, and fentanyl are the most commonly used agents. In comparison with epidural analgesia, parenteral opioids have lower rates of oxytocin augmentation, result in shorter stages of labor, and require fewer instrumental deliveries.

Approximately 60% of women choose an epidural for pain relief during labor and report better pain relief than with other analgesic modalities.[75] Epidural analgesia involves introducing a catheter into the epidural space and administering an opioid and/or an anesthetic (e.g., fentanyl and/or bupivacaine) to provide pain relief during labor. Another method is a combined spinal–epidural, which consists of injection of a single bolus of an opioid into the subarachnoid space, providing instant pain relief, and placement of an epidural catheter with a local anesthetic. Side effects of the regional anesthesia include hypotension, pruritus, and inability to void. One study showed difficulty breast-feeding in women who had received labor epidurals.[78] Epidural analgesia is associated with prolongation of the first and second stages of labor, higher numbers of instrumental deliveries, and maternal fever. A rare complication of epidural anesthesia is puncture of the subarachnoid space leading to a severe headache, which occurs in approximately 2% of women.[75] Other complications include hypotension, nausea, vomiting, itching, and urinary retention. Low back pain has not been shown to be associated with the use of epidural analgesia.

Paracervical blocks using local anesthesia may decrease pain associated with the first phase of labor.[77] However, these types of blocks have been associated with fetal bradycardia and are used rarely in clinical practice.

CLINICAL CONTROVERSY

Many clinicians believe that epidural analgesia is associated with a higher number of cesarean deliveries. To the contrary, two systematic reviews have not substantiated an increased rate of cesarean delivery with epidural analgesia compared with parenteral opioids. However, one of the reviews did caution that data are not sufficient to rule out such an association.[77]

POSTPARTUM HEMORRHAGE

The third stage of labor occurs after delivery of the baby. During this stage, the placenta is delivered. Postpartum hemorrhage is defined as loss of more than 500 mL of blood within 24 hours of delivery.[79] There are few identifiable risk factors for postpartum hemorrhage. In the United States, the postpartum hemorrhage rate is approximately 3.9% in vaginal deliveries.

Active management of the third stage of labor involves administration of a uterotonic medication (intramuscular oxytocin, ergotamine, or combination) before delivery of the placenta; early clamping and cutting of the umbilical cord; and controlled traction of the cord.[79] Instituting active management of labor after all uncomplicated vaginal deliveries results in reduced maternal blood loss, fewer cases of postpartum hemorrhage, and a lower incidence of prolonged third stage of labor. However, use of ergotamines is associated with an increased risk of maternal elevated blood pressure, nausea, and vomiting.

POSTPARTUM ISSUES

DRUG USE DURING LACTATION

5 Although most drugs diffuse into breast milk, breast-feeding may be continued in most circumstances. Healthcare providers should encourage breast-feeding women who require medications to continue breast-feeding whenever possible. Medications that require the mother to pump and discard milk are few.

Extensive research has demonstrated the wide variety of benefits (health, nutritional, immunologic, psychological, economic, developmental, and social) imparted by breast-feeding to infants, mothers, families, and society.[80] It is recommended that women breast-feed exclusively for 6 months and continue until at least infant age 12 months while other foods are introduced. Healthy People 2010 set a target of 75% of neonates being breast-fed at the time of birth and 50% of infants continued being breast-fed at 6 months of age.[6,80]

A number of drug-related factors influence transfer of drug from maternal circulation into breast milk, including (1) degree of protein binding in maternal circulatory system, (2) molecular weight of the drug, (3) lipid solubility of drug and fat content of milk, (4) maternal plasma concentration, (5) half-life of the drug, and (6) pH of the drug.[80] The degree to which a drug is bound to maternal plasma is one of the most significant factors in transfer to breast milk; highly bound medications transfer in low amounts. Low-molecular-weight (<200 kDa) drugs passively diffuse into breast milk, but larger molecules are not likely to transfer in large amounts. Higher lipid solubility of drugs also increases the likelihood of transfer. Colostrum is lower in fat content than mature milk, so a drug with high lipid solubility will achieve a higher concentration in mature milk. The higher the concentration of drug in the mother's serum, the higher the concentration will be in the breast milk. As mother's serum concentration drops from metabolism and excretion of drug, the concentration of drug in the breast milk may redistribute back into the mother's bloodstream. Maternal plasma pH is 7.4, but the pH of breast milk varies between 6.8 and 7.[6] Weak bases are un-ionized in the maternal circulation and easily transfer to breast milk. However, upon encountering the lower pH of breast milk, molecules become ionized and less likely to diffuse back into maternal circulation. Likewise, drugs with longer half-lives are more likely to maintain higher levels in breast milk, resulting in greater exposure to the infant.

Infant-related factors also may influence the amount of drug ingested through breast-feeding.[80] Both the frequency of feedings and the amount of milk ingested are important considerations. Exclusively breast-fed younger infants are more likely to ingest larger amounts of drugs than older infants who receive other foods. Drugs that denature in gastric acid (aminoglycosides, omeprazole, heparin, insulin) are less likely to be absorbed by infants. Finally, infants may vary in their ability to metabolize and excrete ingested medication. Premature and full-term infants may not have full renal and liver function.

Strategies for reducing the amount of drug transferred to the infant may include selection of medicines that would be considered safe for use in the infant.[6] Medications that have shorter half-lives tend to accumulate less, and those that are more protein bound do not cross into breast milk as well as those that are less protein bound. Drugs with lower oral bioavailability and lower lipid solubility are good choices. If the mother is using a once-daily medication, administration before the infant's longest sleep period may be advised to increase the interval to the next feeding. For medications taken multiple times per day, administration immediately after a breast-feeding session will give the longest interval to allow back diffusion of drug from the breast milk as the mother's serum concentration decreases.

Because of the scarcity of industry-based research on transfer of drugs into breast milk, information from drug manufacturers is generally a poor source of information for the provider.[80] Information from expert committees (e.g., American Academy of Pediatrics Committee on Drugs) and evidence-based textbooks may be of assistance in providing reassurance regarding the safe use of medications in the lactating mother.

MASTITIS

Mastitis is an infection in one breast.[81] Women who experience mastitis note breast tenderness, redness, and warmth and have flu-like symptoms. About 1% to 2% of women who breast-feed will experience mastitis, and the highest incidence of mastitis occurs within 1 to 2 weeks of beginning breast-feeding. Mastitis usually is caused by a break in the skin, often a cracked nipple. Risk factors for developing mastitis include breast engorgement, plugged milk ducts, and cracked nipples.

Staphylococcus aureus, E. coli, and *Streptococcus* are the most common organisms associated with mastitis.[81] Antibiotics used for treatment of mastitis include penicillinase-resistant penicillins (e.g., cloxacillin, dicloxacillin, and oxacillin) and cephalosporins (e.g., cephalexin).[81]Antibiotics are often given for 10 to 14 days.[81,82] Antiinflammatory drugs, such as ibuprofen, also can be given for pain. Nondrug therapies that may be helpful are application of warm or cold pack and wearing a bra.[82] Affected women should be counseled to continue breast-feeding from both breasts throughout treatment and to pump if breasts are not emptied completely with feedings.

POSTPARTUM DEPRESSION

Mood disorders in the postpartum period may include postpartum blues, postpartum depression, and postpartum psychosis.[83] Postpartum blues is common, usually affecting 50% to 80% of new mothers within the first 10 days of delivery. Symptoms such as anxiety, anger, and sadness generally resolve within 2 weeks postpartum. Postpartum psychosis is more severe but is rare, affecting one in 1,000 new mothers.

Postpartum depression usually begins within the first 3 months after delivery and affects 8% to 15% of women.[83] As many as 50% of women diagnosed with postpartum depression may have symptoms that began during pregnancy, emphasizing the need for screening.[83,84] Treatment is important for women with postpartum depression, because without treatment 30% to 70% of women may experience depression for 1 year or longer.[83] Psychotherapy, including individual interpersonal psychotherapy, cognitive behavioral therapy, and group/family therapy, has been shown to be effective treatment of moderate depression.

In cases where pharmacotherapy is warranted, selection of medication with low transfer to breast milk is desired.[83] Antidepressants such as nortriptyline, paroxetine, amitriptyline, clomipramine, desipramine, fluvoxamine, and bupropion appear to be undetectable in breast milk. Treatment should continue for a minimum of 29 weeks, consistent with treatment guidelines for a single episode of depression.[84]

RELACTATION

Declining serum prolactin concentrations cause a decrease in or cessation of lactation. This can be problematic, as well as distressing, for mothers who desire to breast-feed their infants. Relactation is the process of increasing the breast milk supply for such women.[85] Lactation also can be induced in women who have not recently delivered a baby, such as adoptive mothers. The mainstay of therapy for this condition involves nipple stimulation either by the infant's nursing or by pumping of the breast with a mechanical pump or the hand.

Recommended pharmacologic therapy in the United States for relactation is metoclopramide, which should be used only if non-drug therapy is ineffective.[85] The most commonly used dose is 10 mg taken orally three times daily for 7 to 14 days. Breast milk production can be increased up to 100% or more in women who are 1 month postpartum or less. In mothers who are 8 to 12 weeks postpartum, milk production may be increased up to 40%. Breast milk production may decrease after metoclopramide therapy is stopped, but production will continue if lactation has been established successfully.

CONCLUSION

Providing pharmacologic care to women during pregnancy can be rewarding and, at times, difficult. Many women perceive a high inherent risk of birth defects with drug exposure during pregnancy. This perception, linked with a high rate of unplanned pregnancies, may create anxiety because of drug exposure prior to the discovery of pregnancy.

Some medications are considered safe for use in pregnancy because of frequent use with no apparent increase in the rate of congenital problems. Women using these medications should be reassured that these choices are unlikely to increase the risk of birth defects. In some cases, ensuring the health of the mother and, in some instances, of the fetus will require selection or continuation of medications that have been associated with a higher risk of adverse effects to the fetus. In these instances, realistic information about the types and likelihood of adverse effects will aid the patient and her family in making decisions.

Healthcare providers who care for pregnant women must work in collaboration to seek, evaluate, and present the most contemporary and accurate information to their patients. Use of technology to access evidence-based resources, databases related to drug use in pregnancy, and primary and secondary literature may assist healthcare practitioners in accessing relevant medication information to manage drug therapy needs during pregnancy and lactation.

ABBREVIATION

FDA: Food and Drug Administration

REFERENCES

1. Namnoun AB, Hatcher RA. The menstrual cycle. In: Hatcher RA, Trussell J, Stewart F, et al., eds. Contraceptive Technology, 17th ed. New York: Ardent Media, 1998:69–76.
2. Fetal growth and development. In: Cunningham FG, Gant NF, Leveno KJ, et al., eds. Williams' Obstetrics, 21st ed. New York: McGraw-Hill, 2001:129–166.
3. Bovone S, Pernoll ML. Normal pregnancy and prenatal care. In: DeCherney AH, Nathan L, eds. Current Obstetric Gynecologic Diagnosis and Treatment, 9th ed. New York: McGraw-Hill, 2003:193–212.
4. Cragan JD, Friedman JM, Holmes LB, et al. Ensuring the safe and effective use of medications during pregnancy: Planning and prevention through preconception care. Matern Child Health J 2006;10:S129–S135.
5. McCarter-Spaulding DE. Medications in pregnancy and lactation. MCN Am J Matern Child Nurs 2005:30:10–17.
6. Della-Giustina K, Chow G. Medications in pregnancy and lactation. Emerg Med Clin North Am 2003;21:585–613.
7. Polifka JE, Friedman JM. Medical genetics: 1. Clinical teratology in the age of genomics. Can Med Assoc J 2002;167:265–273.
8. Brent RL. Immunization of pregnant women: Reproductive, medical and societal risks. Vaccine 2003;21:3414–3421.
9. Irl C, Hasford J. Assessing the safety of drugs in pregnancy. Drug Saf 2000;22:169–177.
10. Addis A, Sharabi S, Bonati M. Risk classifications systems for drug use during pregnancy: Are they a reliable source of information? Drug Saf 2000;23:245–253.
11. Malm H, Martikainen J, Klaukka T, Neuvonen PJ. Prescription of hazardous drugs during pregnancy. Drug Saf 2004;27:899–908.
12. Korenbrot CC, Steinberg A, Bender C, Newberry S. Preconception care: A systematic review. Matern Child Health J 2002;6:75–88.
13. Center for Disease Control and Prevention. Preconception care questions and answers. *http://www.cdc.gov/ncbddd/preconception/QandA_providers.htm#1.*
14. Toriello HV. ACMG Practice guideline. Folic acid and neural tube defects. Genet Med 2005;7:283–284.
15. American College of Obstetrics and Gynecology (ACOG). ACOG Practice Bulletin 44: Neural Tube Defects. Washington, DC: American College of Obstetrics and Gynecology, 2003.
16. Lumley J, Oliver SS, Chamberlain C, Oakley L. Interventions for promoting smoking cessation during pregnancy. Cochrane Database Syst Rev 2004;4:CD001055.
17. Benowitz NL, Dempsey DA. Pharmacotherapy for smoking cessation during pregnancy. Nicotine Tob Res 2004;6:S189–S202.
18. Kirkham C, Harris S, Grzybowski S. Evidence-based prenatal care: Part II. Third-trimester care and prevention of infectious diseases. Am Fam Physician 2005;71:1555–1560,1561–1562.
19. Wald A. Constipation, diarrhea, and symptomatic hemorrhoids during pregnancy. Gastroenterol Clin 2003;32:309–322.
20. Richter JE. Review article: The management of heartburn in pregnancy. Aliment Pharmacol Ther 2005;22:749–757.
21. Nava-Ocampo AA, Velazquez-Armenta EY, Han J-Y, Koren G. Use of proton pump inhibitors during pregnancy and breastfeeding. Can Fam Physician 2006;52:853–854.
22. Badell ML, Ramin SM, Smith JA. Treatment options for nausea and vomiting during pregnancy. Pharmacotherapy 2006;26:1273–1287.
23. American Diabetes Association. Diagnosis and classification of diabetes mellitus. Diabetes Care 2006;29(Suppl 1):S43–S48.
24. U.S. Preventive Services Task Force (USPSTF). Screening for gestational diabetes mellitus: Recommendations and rationale. Obstet Gynecol 2003;101:393–395.
25. American Diabetes Association. Gestational diabetes mellitus. Diabetes Care 2004;27(Suppl 1):S88–S90.
26. Langer O. Management of gestational diabetes: Pharmacologic treatment options and glycemic control. Endocrinol Metab Clin North Am 2006;35:53–78.
27. Gilbert C, Valois M, Koren G. Pregnancy outcome after first-trimester exposure to metformin: A meta-analysis. Fertil Steril 2006; 86:658–663.
28. American Diabetes Association. Preconception care of women with diabetes. Diabetes Care 2004;27(Suppl 1):S76–S78.
29. Tuffnell DJ, West J, Walkinshaw SA. Treatments for gestational diabetes and impaired glucose tolerance in pregnancy. Cochrane Database Syst Rev 2003;3:CD003395.
30. Ceysens G, Rouiller D, Boulvain M. Exercise for diabetic pregnant women. Cochrane Database Syst Rev 2006;3:CD004225.
31. Crowther CA, Hiller JE, Joss JR, et al. Effect of treatment of gestational diabetes mellitus on pregnancy outcomes. N Engl J Med 2005;352:2477–2486.
32. Abalos E, Duley L, Steyn DW, Henderson-Smart DJ. Antihypertensive drug therapy for mild to moderate hypertension during pregnancy. Review. Cochrane Database Syst Rev 2001;2:CD002252.
33. Hofmeyr GJ, Atallah AN, Duley L. Calcium supplementation during pregnancy for preventing hypertensive disorders and related problems. Cochrane Database Syst Rev 2006;3:CD001059.
34. Duley L, Henderson-Smart DJ, Knight M, King JF. Antiplatelet agents for preventing pre-eclampsia and its complications. Cochrane Database Sys Rev 2004;1:CD004659.
35. Duley L, Meher S, Abalos E. Management of pre-eclampsia. BMJ 2006;332:463–468.
36. Cooper WO, Hernandez-Diaz S, Arbogast PG, et al. Major congenital malformations after first-trimester exposure to ACE inhibitors. N Engl J Med 2006;354:2443–2451.
37. Duley L, Henderson-Smart DJ, Meher S. Drugs for treatment of very high blood pressure during pregnancy: Review. Cochrane Database Syst Rev 2006;3:CD001449.

38. Casey BM, Leveno KJ. Thyroid disease in pregnancy. Obstet Gynecol 2006;108:1283–1292.
39. Bates SM, Greer IA, Hirsh J, Ginsberg JS. Use of antithrombotic agents during pregnancy. Chest 2004;126:627S-644S.
40. Le J, Briggs GG, McKeown A, Bustillo G. Urinary tract infections during pregnancy. Ann Pharmacother 2004;38:1692–1701.
41. Vazquez JC, Villar J. Treatments for symptomatic urinary tract infections during pregnancy. Cochrane Database Syst Rev 2003;4:CD002256.
42. Centers for Disease Control and Prevention. Sexually transmitted diseases treatment guideline, 2006. MMWR Recomm Rep 2006;55(RR-11):1–94.
43. Wenner C, Nashelsky J. Antiviral agents for pregnancy women with genital herpes. Am Fam Physician 2005;72:9.
44. Guise JM, Mahon SM, Aickin M, et al. Screening for bacterial vaginosis in pregnancy. Am J Prevent Med 2001;20:67–72.
45. Martin SR, Foley MR. Approach to the pregnant patient with headache. Clin Obstet Gynecol 2005;48:2–11.
46. Silberstein SD. Headaches in pregnancy. Neurol Clin 2004:22:727–756.
47. Blaiss MS. Management of asthma during pregnancy. Allergy Asthma Proc 2004;25:375–376.
48. National Asthma Education and Prevention Program. Quick reference from the Working Group Report on Managing Asthma During Pregnancy: Recommendations for pharmacologic treatment. NIH Publication no. 05–5246. Washington, DC: U.S. Department of Health and Human Services, National Institutes of Health National Heart, Lung, and Blood Institute, 2005.
49. Gilbert C, Mazzotta P, Loebstein R, Koren G. Fetal safety of drugs used in the treatment of allergic rhinitis. Drug Saf 2005;28:707–719.
50. Leachman SA, Reed BR. The use of dermatologic drugs in pregnancy and lactation. Dermatol Clin 2006;24:167–197.
51. Morrell MJ. Reproductive and metabolic disorders in women with epilepsy. Epilepsia 2003;44(Suppl 4):11–20.
52. Holmes LB, Wyszynski DF, Baldwin EJ, et al. Increased risk for non-syndromic cleft palate among infants exposed to lamotrigine during pregnancy [abstract]. Birth Defects Res A Clin Mol Teratol 2006;76:318.
53. Fried S, Kozer E, Nulman I, et al. Malformation rates in children of women with untreated epilepsy. A meta-analysis. Drug Saf 2004;27: 197–202.
54. Practice parameter: Management issues for women with epilepsy (summary statement). Report of the Quality Standards Subcommittee of the American Academy of Neurology. Neurology 1998;51:944–948.
55. Public Health Service Task Force. Recommendations for the use of antiretroviral drugs in pregnant HIV-1-infected women for maternal health and interventions to reduce perinatal HIV-1 transmission in the United States. *http://www.aidsinfo.nih.gov*.
56. National High Blood Pressure Education Program Working Group on High Blood Pressure in Pregnancy. Report of the National High Blood Pressure Education Program Working Group on high blood pressure in pregnancy. Am J Obstet Gynecol 2000;183:S1–S22.
57. Levey L, Ragan K, Hower-Hartley A, et al. Psychiatric disorders in pregnancy. Neurol Clin 2004:22:863–893.
58. U.S. Food and Drug Administration. Treatment challenges of depression in pregnancy. *http://www.fda.gov/cder/drug/advisory/SSRI_PPHN200607.htm.*
59. Rubinchik SM, Kablinger AS, Gardner JS. Medications for panic disorder and generalized anxiety disorder during pregnancy. Prim Care Companion J Clin Psychiatry 2005:7:100–105.
60. Gentile S. Clinical utilization of atypical antipsychotics in pregnancy and lactation. Ann Pharmacother 2004;38:1265–1271.
61. Slattery MM, Morrison JJ. Preterm delivery. Lancet 2002;360:1489–1497.
62. Berkman ND, Thorp JM, Lohr KN, et al. Tocolytic treatment for the management of preterm labor: A review of the evidence. Am J Obstet Gynecol 2003;188:1648–1659.
63. Weismiller DG. Preterm labor. Am Fam Physician 1999;59:593–602.
64. Iams JD. Prediction and early detection of preterm labor. Obstet Gynecol 2003;101:402–412.
65. Crowther CA, Hiller JE, Doyle LW. Magnesium sulphate for preventing preterm birth in threatened preterm labour: Review. Cochrane Database Syst Rev 2002;4:CD001060.
66. King J, Flenady V. Prophylactic antibiotics for inhibiting preterm labor with intact membranes. Cochrane Database Syst Rev 2002;3:CD001807.
67. Meis PJ, Connors N. Progesterone treatment to prevent preterm birth. Clin Obstet Gynecol 2004;47:784–795.
68. Roberts D, Dalziel S. Antenatal corticosteroids for accelerating fetal lung maturation for women at risk of preterm birth. Cochrane Database Syst Rev 2006;3:CD004454.
69. Centers for Disease Control and Prevention. Prevention of perinatal Group B streptococcal disease. *http://www.cdc.gov/mmwr/preview/mmwrhtml/rr5111al.htm.*
70. Tenore JL. Methods for cervical ripening and induction of labor. Am Fam Physician 2003;67:2213–2218.
71. Rand L, Robinson JN, Economy KE, Norwitz ER. Post-term induction of labor revisited. Obstet Gynecol 2000;96:779–783.
72. Hofmeyr GJ, Gulmezoglu AM. Vaginal misoprostol for cervical ripening and induction of labor. Cochrane Database Syst Rev 2003;1:CD000941.
73. Neilson JP. Mifepristone for induction of labour. Cochrane Database Syst Rev 2000;4:CD002865.
74. Leeman L, Fontaine P, King V, et al. The nature and management of labor pain: I. Nonpharmacologic pain relief. Am Fam Physician 2003;68:1109–1112.
75. Eltzschig HK, Lieberman ES, Camann W. Regional anesthesia and analgesia for labor and delivery. N Engl J Med 2003;348:319–322.
76. Althaus J, Wax J. Analgesia and anesthesia in labor. Obstet Gynecol Clin North Am 2005;32:231–244.
77. Leeman L, Fontaine P, King V, et al. The nature and management of labor pain: II. Pharmacologic pain relief. Am Fam Physician 2003;68:1115–1120.
78. Buamgarder DJ, Muehl P, Fischer M, et al. Effect of labor epidural anesthesia on breast-feeding healthy full-term newborns delivered vaginally. J Am Board Fam Pract 2003;16:7–13.
79. Prendiville WJ, Elbourne D, McDonald S. Active versus expectant management in the third stage of labour. Cochrane Database Syst Rev 2000;3:CD000007.
80. Marks JM, Spatz DL. Medications and lactation: What PNPs need to know. J Pediatr Health Care 2003;17:311–317.
81. Mass S. Breast pain: Engorgement, nipple pain, and mastitis. Clin Obstet Gynecol 2004:47:676–682.
82. Marchant DJ. Inflammation of the breast. Obstet Gynecol Clin North Am 2002;29:89–102.
83. Perfetti J, Clark R, Fillmore CM. Postpartum depression: Identification, screening, and treatment. Wis Med J 2006;103:56–63.
84. Tcheremissine OV, Lieving LM. Pharmacotherapy of postpartum depression: Current practice and future directions. Expert Opin Pharmacother 2005;6:1999–2005.
85. Anderson PO, Valdes V. Therapy consultation: Increasing breast milk supply. Clin Pharmacol Ther 1993;12:479–480.

CHAPTER 82 Contraception

LORI M. DICKERSON, SARAH P. SHRADER, AND VANESSA A. DIAZ

KEY CONCEPTS

1. The attitude of both the patient and the sexual partner toward various contraceptive methods, the reliability of the patient in using the method correctly (which may affect the effectiveness of the method), and the patient's ability to pay must be considered carefully when selecting a contraceptive method.
2. Patient-specific factors (e.g., frequency of intercourse, age, smoking status, and concomitant diseases, conditions, or medications) that may prove to be a consideration or precaution for use of a specific method must be evaluated when selecting a contraceptive method.
3. Adverse effects or difficulties using the chosen method should be monitored carefully and managed in consideration of patient-specific factors.
4. Accurate and timely counseling on the optimal use of the contraceptive method and strategies for minimizing sexually transmitted diseases must be provided to all patients when contraceptive pharmacotherapy is initiated and on an ongoing basis.
5. Certain oral contraceptives in high doses can be used as emergency contraception to prevent pregnancy after unprotected intercourse.

Unintended pregnancy is a significant public health problem with economic, health, personal, and social consequences. In the United States, approximately 62 million women are of childbearing age (15–44 years), and approximately six million become pregnant each year.[1] The most recent data reveal that 31% of pregnancies are unintended, with the highest rates occurring in women aged 25 to 44 years (38%).[1] About half of all unintended pregnancies end in abortion, and half also occurred in sexually active couples who claimed they used some method of contraception.[2] If the goal of contraception—for pregnancies to be planned and desired—is to be realized, education on the use and efficacy of contraceptive methods must be improved.

ETIOLOGY AND PATHOPHYSIOLOGY

Comprehension of the hormonal regulation of the normal menstrual cycle is essential to understanding contraception in women (Fig. 82–1).

Learning objectives, review questions, and other resources can be found at **www.pharmacotherapyonline.com.**

The cycle of menstruation begins with menarche, usually around age 12 years, and continues to occur in nonpregnant women until menopause, usually around age 50 years.[3,4] The cycle includes the vaginal discharge of sloughed endometrium called *menses* or *menstrual flow*. The menstrual cycle comprises three phases: follicular (or preovulatory), ovulatory, and luteal (or postovulatory).

THE MENSTRUAL CYCLE

The first day of menses is referred to as *day 1 of the menstrual cycle* and marks the beginning of the follicular phase.[3,4] The follicular phase continues until ovulation, which typically occurs on day 14. The time after ovulation is referred to as the *luteal phase*, which lasts until the beginning of the next menstrual cycle. The median menstrual cycle length is 28 days, but it can range from 21 to 40 days. Generally, variation in length is greatest in the follicular phase, particularly in the years immediately after menarche and before menopause.[4]

The menstrual cycle is influenced by the hormonal relationships among the hypothalamus, anterior pituitary, and ovaries.[3] In response to epinephrine and norepinephrine stimulation, the hypothalamus secretes gonadotropin-releasing hormone (GnRH) in a pulsatile fashion every 60 to 90 minutes.[3,4] These GnRH bursts stimulate the anterior pituitary to secrete bursts of gonadotropins, follicle-stimulating hormone (FSH), and luteinizing hormone (LH). The gonadotropins FSH and LH direct events in the ovarian follicles that result in the production of a fertile ovum.

Follicular Phase

In the first 4 days of the menstrual cycle, FSH levels rise and allow the recruitment of a small group of follicles for continued growth and development (see Fig. 82–1).[3,4] Between days 5 and 7, one follicle becomes dominant and later ruptures, releasing the oocyte. The dominant follicle develops increasing amounts of estradiol and inhibin, which cause a negative feedback on the hypothalamic secretion of GnRH and pituitary secretion of FSH, causing atresia of the remaining follicles recruited during the cycle.

Once the follicle has received FSH stimulation, it must receive continued FSH stimulation or it will die.[3,4] Gonadotropin-dependent growth allows the follicle to enlarge, produce other layers of receptors for FSH and LH, and synthesize estradiol, progesterone, and androgen. Estradiol serves to stop the menstrual flow from the previous cycle, thickening the endometrial lining of the uterus to prepare it for embryonic implantation. Estrogen is responsible for increased production of thin, watery cervical mucus, which will enhance sperm transport during fertilization. FSH regulates the aromatase enzymes that convert androgens to estrogens in the follicle. If a follicle has insufficient aromatase, androgen will accumulate, and the follicle will not survive. Therefore, follicles with the most FSH stimulation have the lowest ratios of androgen to estrogen.

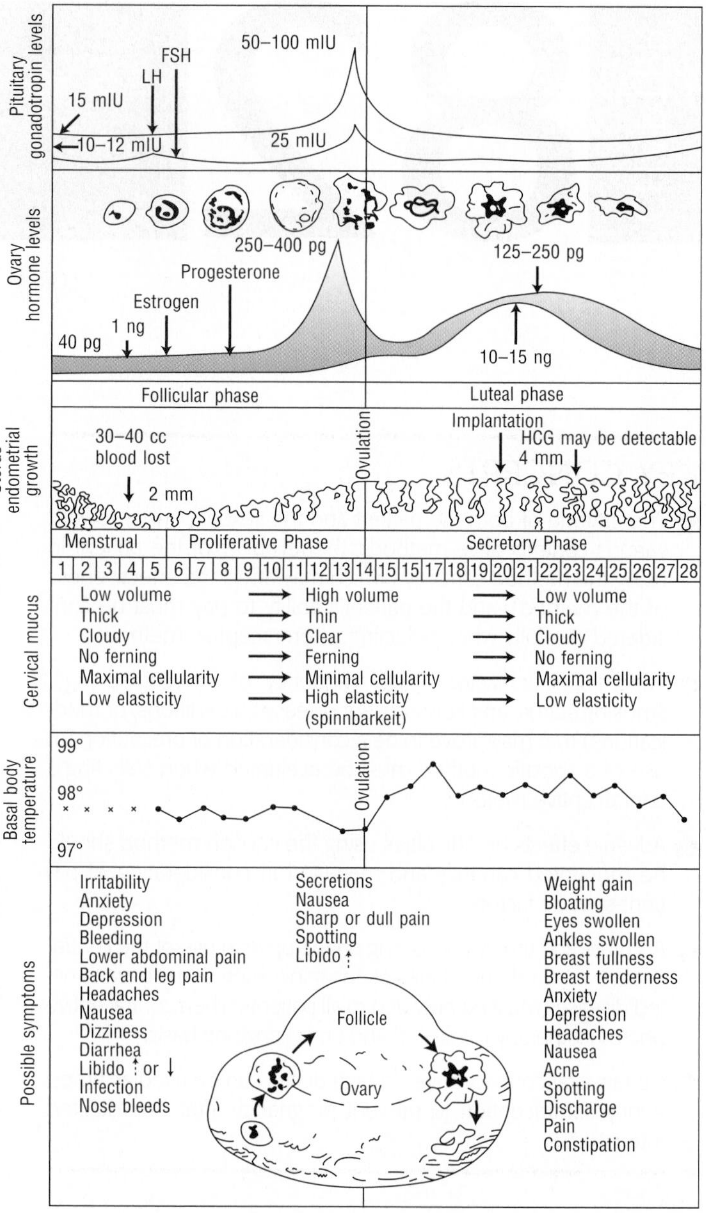

FIGURE 82-1. Menstrual cycle events, idealized 28-day cycle. (FSH, follicle-stimulating hormone; HCG, human chorionic gonadotropin, LH, luteinizing hormone.) *(From Hatcher et al.[3] This figure may be reproduced at no cost to the reader.)*

Ovulation

When estradiol levels remain elevated for a sustained period of time (200 pg for at least 50 hours), the pituitary releases a midcycle LH surge (see Fig. 82–1).[3,4] This LH surge stimulates the final stages of follicular maturation and ovulation (follicular rupture and release of the oocyte). On average, ovulation occurs 24 to 36 hours after the estradiol peak and 10 to 16 hours after the LH peak. The LH surge, which occurs 28 to 32 hours before a follicle ruptures, is the most clinically useful predictor of approaching ovulation. After ovulation, the oocyte is released and travels to the fallopian tube, where it can be fertilized and transported to the uterus for embryonic implantation. Conception is most successful when intercourse takes place from 2 days before ovulation to the day of ovulation.

Luteal Phase

After rupture of the follicle and release of the ovum, the remaining luteinized follicles become the corpus luteum, which synthesizes androgen, estrogen, and progesterone (see Fig. 82–1).[3,4] Progesterone helps to maintain the endometrial lining, which sustains the implanted embryo and maintains the pregnancy. It also inhibits GnRH and gonadotropin release, preventing the development of new follicles. If pregnancy occurs, human chorionic gonadotropin (hCG) prevents regression of the corpus luteum and stimulates continued production of estrogen and progesterone secretion to maintain the pregnancy until the placenta is able to fulfill this role (usually 6–8 weeks' gestation).

If fertilization or implantation does not occur, the corpus luteum degenerates, and progesterone production declines.[3,4] The life span of the corpus luteum depends on the continuous presence of small amounts of LH, and its average duration of function is 9 to 11 days. As progesterone levels decline, endometrial shedding (menstruation) occurs, and a new menstrual cycle begins. At the end of the luteal phase, when estrogen and progesterone levels are low, FSH levels start to rise, and follicular recruitment for the next cycle begins.

EPIDEMIOLOGY

Contraception generally implies the prevention of pregnancy following sexual intercourse by inhibiting viable sperm from coming into contact with a mature ovum (i.e., methods that act as barriers or prevent ovulation) or by preventing a fertilized ovum from implanting successfully in the endometrium (i.e., mechanisms that create an unfavorable uterine environment).

Commonly used methods of reversible contraception include oral, transdermal, and vaginal ring contraceptives, injectable and implantable progestins, intrauterine devices (IUDs), condoms, spermicides, diaphragms, cervical caps, sponges, withdrawal, and periodic abstinence.[3–5] These methods differ in their relative effectiveness, safety, and patient acceptability.

The actual effectiveness of any contraceptive method is difficult to determine because many factors affect contraceptive failure. A failure in patients who use the contraceptive agent properly is considered a method failure or perfect-use failure. User failure or typical use failure takes into account the user's ability to follow directions correctly and consistently.[3,4] In a survey of women who had abortions in 2000 to 2001, 46% had not used a contraceptive method in the month they conceived owing to a perceived low risk of pregnancy (33%) and concerns about the use of contraceptives (32%).[6] The male condom was the most commonly used method (28%), with inconsistent use the cited cause of pregnancy in 49% of cases. Oral contraceptives (OCs) were used by 14% of women, 76% of whom reported inconsistent use resulting in pregnancy.[6]

CLINICAL PRESENTATION

For many young women, a major reason for visiting a clinician is to obtain contraception. Clinicians may use this opportunity to provide health maintenance/disease prevention by counseling about reproductive health and sexually transmitted diseases (STDs). Most health maintenance annual visits should include assessment of and counseling about reproductive health. Traditionally, hormonal contraception is provided subsequent to clinical breast and pelvic examinations. However, the need for the physical examination may delay access to contraception, resulting in unintended pregnancies and other health risks. In addition, requiring the breast and pelvic examinations prior to prescription of hormonal contraception reinforces the incorrect perception that these methods of pregnancy prevention are harmful or dangerous. Therefore, the American College of Obstetrics and Gynecology (ACOG) and other national organizations allow provision of hormonal contraception after a simple medical history and blood pressure measurement.[7] Other preventive measures, such as pelvic and breast examinations, provision of the human papillomavirus vaccine, screening for cervical neoplasia, and counseling for prevention of STDs, can be accomplished during routine annual office visits.[8–10]

TREATMENT

DESIRED OUTCOME

The obvious goal of treatment with all methods of contraception is to prevent pregnancy. However, many health benefits are associated with contraceptive methods, including prevention of STDs (with condoms), improvements in menstrual cycle regularity (with hormonal contraceptives), prevention of malignancies and other health conditions (with OCs), and management of perimenopause.[3]

NONPHARMACOLOGIC THERAPY

Periodic Abstinence

❶ ❷ Highly motivated couples may use the abstinence (rhythm) method of contraception, avoiding sexual intercourse during the days of the menstrual cycle when conception is likely to occur. These women rely on physiologic changes, such as basal body temperature and cervical mucus, during each cycle to determine the fertile period. The major reasons for the lack of acceptance are the relatively high pregnancy rates among users and the need to avoid intercourse for several days during each menstrual cycle. To overcome these drawbacks, many women use barrier methods or spermicides during the fertile period.[3,4]

Barrier Techniques

❶ ❷ The effectiveness of barrier methods and spermicides depends almost exclusively on a couple's motivation to use them consistently and correctly.[3,4] These methods include condoms, diaphragms, cervical caps, and sponges (Table 82–1). A major disadvantage is higher failure rates than with most hormonal contraceptives; thus, provision of counseling and an advanced prescription for emergency contraception (EC) are recommended for all patients using barrier methods as their primary means of contraception.

Condoms are devices that create a mechanical barrier, preventing direct contact of the vagina with semen, genital lesions and discharges, and infectious secretions.[3,4] Most condoms in the United States are made of latex rubber, which is impermeable to viruses. A small proportion (5%) are made from young lamb intestine, which is not impermeable to viruses. Condoms are used worldwide as protection from STDs. When condoms are used in conjunction with any other barrier method, their effectiveness theoretically approaches 98%. Spillage of semen or perforation and tearing of the condom can occur, but proper use minimizes these problems.[4] Mineral oil–based vaginal drug formulations (e.g., Cleocin vaginal cream, Premarin vaginal cream, Vagistat 1, Femstat, and Monistat Vaginal suppositories), lotions, or lubricants can decrease the barrier strength of latex by 90% in just 60 seconds, thus making water-soluble lubricants (e.g., Astroglide, K-Y Jelly) preferable.[4] Condoms with spermicides are no longer recommended at all because they provide no additional protection against pregnancy or STDs and may increase vulnerability to human immunodeficiency virus (HIV) infection.[4]

The female condom (Reality) is a prelubricated, soft, loose-fitting polyurethane sheath, closed at one end, with flexible rings at both ends.[3,4] Properly positioned, the ring at the closed end covers the cervix, and the sheath lines the walls of the vagina. The outer ring remains outside the vagina, covering the labia; this may make the female condom more effective than the male condom in preventing transmission of STDs because it protects the labia from contact with the base of the penis. However, the pregnancy rate is reported to be 21% in the first year of use.

The diaphragm, a reusable dome-shaped rubber cap with a flexible rim that is inserted vaginally, fits over the cervix in order to decrease access of sperm to the ovum. The diaphragm requires a prescription from a physician who has fitted the patient for the correct size.[3,4] Its effectiveness depends on its function as a barrier and on the spermicidal cream or jelly placed in the diaphragm before insertion. The diaphragm may be inserted up to 6 hours before intercourse and must be left in place for at least 6 hours afterward. With subsequent acts of intercourse, the diaphragm should be left in place, and a condom should be used for additional protection.[3] Users of diaphragms appear to have a lower incidence of cervical neoplasia, which may be attributed to the adjunctive spermicide and the diaphragm's barrier effect against the human papillomavirus.

The cervical cap is a soft, deep cup with a firm round rim that is smaller than a diaphragm and fits over the cervix like a thimble.[3,4] Currently, two latex-free cervical caps are available by prescription in the United States: the FemCap and the Lea's Shield.[3] The FemCap is available in three sizes and should be filled with spermicide prior to insertion.[3,4] It is held in place against the cervix until the cap is removed. The Lea's Shield is available in only one size and is held in place by the vaginal wall; therefore, cervical size is not a factor.[3] Both caps can be inserted 6 hours prior to intercourse and remain in place for multiple episodes of intercourse without adding more spermicide.

TABLE 82-1 Comparison of Methods of Nonhormonal Contraception

Method	Absolute Contraindications	Advantages	Disadvantages	Percent of Women with Pregnancy[a] Perfect Use	Percent of Women with Pregnancy[a] Typical Use
Condoms, male	Allergy to latex or rubber	Inexpensive STD protection, including HIV (latex only)	High user failure rate Poor acceptance Possibility of breakage Efficacy decreased by oil-based lubricants Possible allergic reactions to latex in either partner	2	15
Condoms, female (Reality)	Allergy to polyurethane History of TSS	Can be inserted just before intercourse or ahead of time STD protection, including HIV	High user failure rate Dislike ring hanging outside vagina Cumbersome	5	21
Diaphragm with spermicide	Allergy to latex, rubber, or spermicide Recurrent UTIs History of TSS Abnormal gynecologic anatomy	Low cost Decreased incidence of cervical neoplasia Some protection against STDs	High user failure rate Decreased efficacy with increased frequency of intercourse Increased incidence of vaginal yeast UTIs, TSS Efficacy affected by oil-based lubricants Cervical irritation	6	16
Cervical cap (FemCap, Leah's Shield)	Allergy to spermicide History of TSS Abnormal gynecologic anatomy Abnormal Papanicolaou smear	Low cost Latex-free Some protection against STDs FemCap reusable for up to 2 years	High user failure rate Decreased efficacy with parity Cannot be used during menses	9	16[b]
Spermicides alone	Allergy to spermicide	Inexpensive	High user failure rate Must be reapplied before each act of intercourse May enhance HIV transmission No protection against STDs	18	29
Sponge (Today)	Allergy to spermicide Recurrent UTIs History of TSS Abnormal gynecologic anatomy	Inexpensive	High user failure rate Decreased efficacy with parity Cannot be used during menses No protection against STDs	9	16

HIV, human immunodeficiency virus; STD, sexually transmitted disease; TSS, toxic shock syndrome; UTI, urinary tract infection.
[a]Failure rates in the United States during first year of use.
[b]Failure rate with FemCap reported to be 29% per package insert.
Data from Hatcher et al.[3,4] and Dickey.[5]

They should not be worn for more than 48 hours at a time to reduce the risk of toxic shock syndrome. Failure rates are higher than with other methods, perhaps due to difficulty in fitting the cap. Some studies have shown an increased risk of cervical dysplasia, so users must have a repeat Papanicolaou (Pap) smear 3 months after starting to use a cervical cap. Followup data showed no increase in dysplasia at 1 year.[3]

PHARMACOLOGIC THERAPY

Spermicides

❶ ❷ Spermicides, most of which contain nonoxynol-9, are chemical surfactants that destroy sperm cell walls and act as barriers that prevent sperm from entering the cervical os.[4] They are available as creams, films, foams, gels, suppositories, sponges, and tablets.[3,4] Unfortunately, spermicides offer no protection against STDs. In fact, when used frequently (more than two times per day), spermicides containing nonoxynol-9 may increase the risk of transmission of HIV by causing small disruptions in the vaginal epithelium.[11,12] The World Health Organization (WHO) and the Centers for Disease Control and Prevention (CDC) do not promote products containing nonoxynol-9 for protection against STDs. Women at high risk for HIV infection or who are HIV infected should not use spermicides.[3,13]

Spermicide-Implanted Barrier Techniques

❶ ❷ The vaginal contraceptive sponge (Today) is pillow shaped and contains 1 g of the spermicide nonoxynol-9.[4] It has a concave dimple on one side (to fit over the cervix and decrease the risk of dislodgement during intercourse) and a loop on the other side (to facilitate removal). After being moistened with tap water, the sponge is inserted into the vagina up to 6 hours before intercourse. The sponge provides protection for 24 hours, regardless of the frequency of intercourse during this time. After intercourse, the sponge must be left in place for at least 6 hours before removal. Sponges should not be left in place for more than 24 to 30 hours in order to reduce the risk of toxic shock syndrome. After use, sponges should be discarded (they are not effective for reuse). The sponge comes in one size and is available over the counter (OTC).[4]

Hormonal Contraception

Hormonal contraceptives contain either a combination of estrogen and progestin or a progestin alone. OC preparations first became available in the 1960s, but options have expanded to include a transdermal patch, a vaginal contraceptive ring, and long-acting injectable, implantable, and intrauterine contraceptives.

Components Combined hormonal contraceptives (CHCs) work primarily before fertilization to prevent conception. Progestins provide most of the contraceptive effect, by thickening cervical mucus to prevent sperm penetration, slowing tubal motility and delaying sperm transport, and inducing endometrial atrophy. Progestins block the LH surge, therefore inhibiting ovulation. Estrogens suppress FSH release from the pituitary, which may contribute to blocking the LH surge and preventing ovulation. However, the primary role of estrogen in hormonal contraceptives is to stabilize the endometrial lining and provide cycle control.[3–5]

Estrogens. Two synthetic estrogens found in hormonal contraceptives available in the United States, ethinyl estradiol (EE) and mestranol, differ only by the presence of a methyl group attached to mestranol at the C-3 site. Mestranol, which must be converted by the liver to ethinyl estradiol before it is pharmacologically active, is estimated to be 50% less potent than EE.[3–5] Most combined OCs contain estrogen at doses of 20 to 50 mcg of EE, and the transdermal patch releases approximately 20 mcg of EE daily. The contraceptive ring produces half the serum concentration of EE derived from a 30-mcg OC.[4]

Progestins. Progestins currently used in OCs include desogestrel, drospirenone, ethynodiol diacetate, norgestimate, norethindrone, norethindrone acetate, norethynodrel, norgestrel, and levonorgestrel, the active isomer of norgestrel. The transdermal patch contains norelgestromin, the active metabolite of norgestimate. The vaginal ring contains etonogestrel, the metabolite of desogestrel.[4,5]

Progestins vary in their progestational activity and differ with respect to inherent estrogenic, antiestrogenic, and androgenic effects.[3–5] Estrogenic and antiestrogenic properties are secondary to the extent of progestins' metabolism to estrogenic substances, whereas androgenic activity results from the structural similarity of the progestin to testosterone (receptor binding and activity) and the ability to affect free testosterone concentrations through impact on sex hormone-binding globulin, a major carrier protein for testosterone.[5]

Considerations with Combined Hormonal Contraceptive Use ❶ When selecting a CHC, clinicians are challenged by the many formulations, weighing benefits and evaluating potential risks associated with their use. The clinician also must determine if the form of contraception fits the patient's lifestyle and if the patient will be compliant. As previously stated, a complete medical examination and Pap smear are not necessary before a CHC is prescribed. A medical history and blood pressure measurement should be obtained before a patient begins using CHC, and the benefits, adverse effects, and risks should be discussed.[3–5,14,15,16] For example, OCs are associated with numerous noncontraceptive benefits, including relief from menstruation-related problems (e.g., decreased menstrual cramps, decreased ovulatory pain [mittelschmerz], and decreased menstrual blood loss), improvement in menstrual regularity, increased hemoglobin concentrations, and an improvement in acne. Women who take combination OCs have a reduced risk of ovarian and endometrial cancer, which is detectable within 1 year and persists for years after discontinuation. Combination OCs reduce the risk of ovarian cysts, ectopic pregnancy, pelvic inflammatory disease, and benign breast disease. The CHC transdermal patch is convenient because it is applied only once weekly, and it may be associated with less breast discomfort and dysmenorrhea than OCs. The CHC vaginal ring also has the advantage of convenience, being inserted for 3 weeks at a time.

❷ ❸ Adverse effects may hinder compliance and therefore efficacy, so they should be discussed prior to initiating a hormonal contraceptive agent (Table 82–2). Estrogen excess can cause nausea and bloating, and low-dose estrogen CHCs can cause early or midcycle breakthrough bleeding and spotting. Progestins may be associated with fatigue and changes in mood. Low-dose progestin CHCs may cause late-cycle breakthrough bleeding and spotting. Androgenic activity derived from progestins may cause increased appetite and acne.[3–5] The CHC vaginal ring may be uncomfortable and cause some vaginal discharge.

The main safety concern about the use of CHC is their lack of protection against STDs. Because of their high efficacy in preventing pregnancy, patients may choose not to use condoms, which do protect against STDs. In addition to public health awareness, at every office visit clinicians must encourage their sexually active patients to use condoms for prevention of STDs. OCs have an extensive history of safety concerns, which traditionally were related to high-dose estrogen in early pills. To replace the traditional absolute and relative contraindications to the use of OCs, the WHO developed a graded list of precautions for clinicians to consider when they are initiating OCs and other methods of CHC (Table 82–3).[4,13] For specific clarifications and explanations, please refer to the complete WHO document.[13]

TABLE 82-2 Adverse Effects of Combined Hormonal Contraception and Management[a]

Adverse Effects	Management
Estrogen excess	
Nausea, breast tenderness, headaches, cyclic weight gain due to fluid retention	Decrease estrogen content in CHC Consider progestin-only methods or IUD
Dysmenorrhea, menorrhagia, uterine fibroid growth	Decrease estrogen content in CHC Consider extended-cycle or continuous regimen OC Consider progestin-only methods or IUD NSAIDs for dysmenorrhea
Estrogen deficiency	
Vasomotor symptoms, nervousness, decreased libido	Increase estrogen content in CHC
Early-cycle (days 1–9) breakthrough bleeding and spotting	Increase estrogen content in CHC
Absence of withdrawal bleeding (amenorrhea)	Exclude pregnancy Increase estrogen content in CHC if menses is desired Continue current CHC if amenorrhea acceptable
Progestin excess	
Increased appetite, weight gain, bloating, constipation	Decrease progestin content in CHC
Acne, oily skin, hirsutism	Decrease progestin content in CHC Choose less androgenic progestin in CHC
Depression, fatigue, irritability	Decrease progestin content in CHC
Progestin deficiency	
Dysmenorrhea, menorrhagia	Increase progestin content in CHC Consider extended-cycle or continuous regimen OC Consider progestin-only methods or IUD NSAIDs for dysmenorrhea
Late-cycle (days 10–21) breakthrough bleeding and spotting	Increase progestin content in CHC

CHC, combined hormonal contraceptive; IUD, intrauterine device; NSAID, nonsteroidal antiinflammatory drug; OC, oral contraceptive.

[a]CHC regimens should be continued for at least 3 months before adjustments are made based on adverse effects.

Data from Hatcher et al.[3,4] and Dickey.[5]

In addition to the WHO precautions, the ACOG provides information for clinicians to use when selecting CHCs for women with coexisting medical conditions.[16] Overall, the health risks associated with pregnancy, the specific health risks associated with CHCs, and the noncontraceptive benefits of CHCs should be factored into risk-to-benefit considerations.

Women Older Than 35 Years. Generally, CHCs containing less than 50 mcg EE are an acceptable form of contraception for nonsmoking women up to the time of menopause. Population-based case-control studies have not demonstrated an increased risk of myocardial infarction (MI) and stroke in healthy nonsmoking women older than 35 years using low-dose OCs. As women approach the perimenopausal stage, CHCs may confer a benefit with respect to bone mineral density (BMD), reduction in vasomotor symptoms, and reduced risk of endometrial and ovarian cancer. However, these benefits must be weighed against the risk of cardiovascular disease in women with risk factors. If women choose to use hormone therapy, they should switch from CHCs to hormone therapy in the perimenopausal period.[4,16,17]

Smoking. In early studies, OCs with 50 mcg EE or more were associated with MI in women who smoked cigarettes.[4,14,16,17] United States case-control studies have found that both nonsmoking and

TABLE 82-3 World Health Organization Precautions in the Provision of Combined Hormonal Contraceptives (CHCs)

Category 4: Refrain from providing CHCs for women with the following diagnoses

- Thrombophlebitis or thromboembolic disorder, or a history of these conditions
- Cerebrovascular disease, coronary artery disease, peripheral vascular disease
- Valvular heart disease with thrombogenic complications (e.g., pulmonary hypertension, atrial fibrillation, history of endocarditis)
- Diabetes with vascular involvement (e.g., nephropathy, retinopathy, neuropathy, other vascular disease or diabetes >20 years' duration)
- Migraine headaches with focal aura
- Migraine headaches without aura in women ≥35 years old should discontinue CHC
- Uncontrolled hypertension (≥160 mm Hg systolic or ≥90 mm Hg diastolic)
- Major surgery with prolonged immobilization
- Thrombogenic mutations (e.g., factor V Leiden, protein C or S deficiency, antithrombin III deficiency, prothrombin deficiency)
- Breast cancer
- Acute or chronic hepatocellular disease with abnormal liver function, cirrhosis, hepatic adenomas, or hepatic carcinomas
- Age >35 years and currently smoking ≥15 cigarettes per day
- Known or suspected pregnancy
- Breast-feeding women <6 weeks postpartum

Category 3: Conditions may be adversely impacted by CHCs, and the risks generally outweigh the benefits; providers should exercise caution if combined CHCs are used in these situations and carefully monitor for adverse effects

- Multiple risk factors for arterial cardiovascular disease
- Known hyperlipidemia
- Migraine headache without aura in women ≥35 years old
- History of hypertension (systolic 140–159 mm Hg or diastolic 90–99 mm Hg)
- History of cancer, but no evidence of current disease for 5 years
- Cirrhosis, mild and compensated
- Symptomatic gallbladder disease
- Cholestatic jaundice with prior pill use
- Age >35 years and currently smoking <15 cigarettes per day
- Postpartum <21 days, not breast-feeding
- Breast-feeding women 6 weeks to 6 months postpartum
- Commonly used drugs that induce liver enzymes (rifampin, phenytoin, carbamazepine, barbiturates, primidone, topiramate) and reduce efficacy of CHC

Category 2: Some conditions may trigger potential concerns with CHCs, but benefits usually outweigh risks

- Family history of thromboembolism
- Superficial thrombophlebitis
- Uncomplicated valvular heart disease
- Diabetes without vascular disease
- Sickle cell disease
- Migraine headaches without aura in women <35 years old
- Nonmigrainous headaches at any age should discontinue CHC
- Hypertension during pregnancy, resolved postpartum
- Major surgery without prolonged immobilization
- Gallbladder disease (symptomatic and treated by cholecystectomy or asymptomatic)
- Cholestatic jaundice of pregnancy
- Undiagnosed breast mass
- Undiagnosed abnormal genital bleeding
- Cervical intraepithelial neoplasia or cervical cancer
- Obesity (body mass index ≥30 kg/m^2)
- Age <35 years and currently smoking
- Breastfeeding women ≥6 months postpartum
- Age ≥40 years
- Drugs that may induce metabolism of CHC and reduce efficacy (griseofulvin, antiretroviral therapy)

Category 1: Do not restrict use of combined oral contraceptives for the following conditions

- Varicose veins
- History of gestational diabetes
- Nonmigrainous headaches
- Thyroid disease
- Thalassemia
- Iron deficiency anemia
- Depression
- Epilepsy
- Infectious diseases (HIV, schistosomiasis, tuberculosis, malaria)
- Minor surgery without immobilization
- Benign ovarian tumors
- Endometriosis
- Irregular or heavy vaginal bleeding, severe dysmenorrhea
- Sexually transmitted diseases
- Uterine fibroids
- Pelvic inflammatory disease
- Endometrial cancer
- Ovarian cancer
- History of pelvic surgery
- Trophoblast disease
- History of ectopic pregnancy
- Postabortion
- Postpartum women ≥21 weeks, not breast-feeding
- Menarche to 40 years of age
- Drug interactions with antibiotics other than rifampin and griseofulvin

CHC, combined hormonal contraception; HIV, human immunodeficiency virus.

Data from Hatcher et al.,[3,4] Dickey,[5] World Health Organization,[13] Roddey et al.,[14] and Petitti.[16]

smoking women, regardless of age, taking OCs with less than 50 mcg EE did not have an increased risk of MI or stroke. However, these studies included few women older than 35 years who were smokers. European studies, with a higher population of older smoking women, demonstrated an increased risk of MI in this population. Therefore, practitioners should prescribe CHC with caution, if at all, to women older than 35 years who smoke. The WHO precautions further state that smoking 15 or more cigarettes per day by women in this age group is a contraindication to CHC, and that the risks generally outweigh the benefits of CHC in those who smoke fewer than 15 cigarettes per day.[13] Progestin-only contraceptive methods should be considered for women in this group.

Hypertension. CHCs, even those containing less than 35 mcg of estrogen, can cause small increases (i.e., 6–8 mm Hg) in blood pressure.[4,14,16,17] This has been documented in both normotensive and mildly hypertensive women given a 30-mcg EE OC. In case-control studies of women with hypertension, OCs have been associated with an increased risk of MI and stroke. Use of low-dose CHC is acceptable in women younger than 35 years with well-controlled and frequently monitored hypertension. If a CHC-related increase in blood pressure occurs, discontinuing the CHC usually restores blood pressure to pretreatment values within 3 to 6 months.[4] Hypertensive women who have end-organ vascular disease or who smoke should not use CHCs. Women with hypertension who are taking potassium-sparing diuretics, angiotensin-converting enzyme inhibitors, angiotensin-receptor blockers, or aldosterone antagonists may have increased serum potassium concentrations if they are also using an OC-containing drospirenone (e.g., Yasmin), which has antialdosterone properties.[4] Progestin-only pills and depot medroxyprogesterone acetate (DMPA) have not been shown to increase blood pressure or increase the risk of vascular events in normotensive or hypertensive women and therefore are choices for women with hypertension.

Dyslipidemia. Generally, synthetic progestins adversely affect lipid metabolism by decreasing high-density lipoprotein (HDL) and increasing low-density lipoprotein (LDL).[4,16,17] Estrogens tend to have more beneficial effects by enhancing removal of LDL and increasing HDL levels. Estrogens also may moderately increase triglycerides. As a net result, most low-dose CHCs have no significant impact on HDL, LDL, triglycerides, or total cholesterol. CHCs containing more androgenic progestins (e.g., levonorgestrel) may result in lower HDL levels in some patients. Although the lipid effects of CHCs theoretically can influence cardiovascular risk, the mechanism of increased cardiovascular disease in CHC users is believed to be due to thromboembolic and thrombotic changes, not atherosclerosis. Women with controlled dyslipidemia can use low-dose CHCs, although periodic fasting lipid profiles are recommended. Women with uncontrolled dyslipidemia (LDL >160 mg/dL, HDL <35 mg/dL, triglycerides >250 mg/dL) and additional risk factors (e.g., coronary artery disease, diabetes, hypertension, smoking, or positive family history) should use an alternative method of contraception.

Diabetes. Any effect of CHCs on carbohydrate and lipid metabolism is thought to be due to the progestin component.[4,17] However, with the exception of some levonorgestrel-containing products, formulations containing low doses of progestins do not significantly alter insulin, glucose, or glucagon release after a glucose load in healthy women or in those with a history of gestational diabetes. The new progestins are believed to have little, if any, effect on carbohydrate metabolism. CHCs do not appear to alter the hemoglobin A_{1c} values or accelerate the development of microvascular complications in women with type 1 diabetes. In the Nurses' Health Study, women who used OCs did not demonstrate any increased risk of developing type 2 diabetes.[17] Therefore, nonsmoking women younger than 35 years with diabetes but no associated vascular disease can safely use CHCs. Diabetic women with vascular disease (e.g., nephropathy, retinopathy, neuropathy, or other vascular disease or diabetes of more than 20 years' duration) should not use CHCs. Copper and progestin-releasing IUDs have not been associated with impaired metabolic control in women with uncomplicated diabetes.

Migraine Headaches. Women in their reproductive years frequently experience headaches, primarily tension headaches. Women with migraine headaches (with and without aura) may experience a decreased or an increased frequency of migraine headaches when using CHCs.[4,14,16,17] Headaches may even occur during the hormone-free interval (during menses). Most studies have demonstrated a higher risk of stroke in women experiencing migraine with aura compared to women with simple migraines (without aura). In population-based studies, the risk of stroke in women with migraines has been elevated twofold to threefold. However, given the low absolute risk of stroke in young women (age <35 years), the ACOG recommends considering CHCs in healthy, nonsmoking women with migraine headaches if they do not have focal neurologic signs.[16] Women of any age who have migraine with aura should not use CHC. Women who develop migraines (with or without aura) while receiving CHC should discontinue use immediately. Progestin-only, intrauterine, or barrier contraceptives should be considered in these patients.

Breast Cancer. Worldwide epidemiologic data from 54 studies in 25 countries (many of which studied high-dose OCs) were collected to assess the relationship between OCs and breast cancer.[17] Overall, investigators noted a small increased risk of breast cancer associated with current or recent use, but OCs did not further increase risk in women with a history of benign breast disease or a family history of breast cancer. A more recent U.S.–based case-control study found no association between overall breast cancer and current or past OC use.[17] This study also found no association between DMPA and breast cancer. Although some studies have found differences in risk of breast cancer based on the presence of *BRCA1* and *BRCA2* mutations, the most recent cohort study found no association with low-dose OCs and the presence of either mutation. Therefore, the choice to use CHCs should not be affected by the presence of benign breast disease or a family history of breast cancer with either mutation. The WHO precautions state that women with a recent personal history of breast cancer should not use CHCs, but that CHCs can be considered in women without evidence of disease for 5 years.[13]

Thromboembolism. Estrogens increase hepatic production of factor VII, factor X, and fibrinogen in the coagulation cascade, therefore increasing the risk of thromboembolic events (e.g., deep-vein thrombosis, pulmonary embolism). These risks are increased in women who have underlying hypercoagulable states (e.g., deficiencies in antithrombin III, protein C, and protein S; factor V Leiden mutations, prothrombin G2010 A mutations) or who have acquired conditions (e.g., obesity, pregnancy, immobility, trauma, surgery, and certain malignancies) that predispose them to coagulation abnormalities.[4,14,16,17] In U.S. case-control studies, the risk of venous thromboembolism (VTE) in women currently using low-dose OCs (<50 mcg EE with norethindrone or levonorgestrel) was four times the risk in nonusers.[4,16,17] However, this risk is less than the risk of thromboembolic events incurred during pregnancy. OCs containing desogestrel have been associated with a 1.7 to 19 times higher risk of VTE than OCs containing levonorgestrel. Some clinicians argue that this difference reflects preferential prescribing of the newer, and perceived safer, progestin products for women at greater risk for VTE. Estrogen exposure in women using transdermal CHC may be greater than that in women taking OCs or using the vaginal contraceptive ring, but the absolute risk of VTE in this population is unknown. Therefore, CHCs are contraindicated in women with a history of thromboembolic events and in those at risk due to prolonged immobilization with major surgery unless they are currently taking anticoagulants. Women with familial coagulopathies are at particular risk during pregnancy, given the risk of VTE and of fetal exposure to warfarin. CHCs reduce menstrual blood loss and are safe for use by women with appropriate anticoagulation. DMPA and levonorgestrel IUDs are also recommended for this population. EC has not been associated with an increased risk of thromboembolic events.

Obesity. As the proportion of women who are obese (body mass index [BMI] >30 mg/kg^2) has increased, the issue of contraception in this population has become more important. Obese women (weight >90 kg) taking OCs or using transdermal contraceptives are at increased risk for contraceptive failure compared to women with a normal BMI.[4,17] These women who use CHCs also are at increased risk of VTE. Because increased pregnancy rates have not been documented in obese women using DMPA as the method of contraception, this or intrauterine methods of contraception should be considered. Given that the intrauterine levonorgestrel system improves dysfunctional uterine bleeding, a particular problem in obese women, and that DMPA may increase irregular bleeding patterns, the levonorgestrel IUD may be preferred for this population.

Systemic Lupus Erythematosus. Contraception is important in women with systemic lupus erythematosus (SLE) because the risks associated with pregnancy are high in this population. Historically, clinicians have thought that CHCs exacerbated the symptoms of SLE.[4,17,18] However, randomized controlled trials have shown that OCs do not increase the risk of flare among women with stable SLE and without antiphospholipid/anticardiolipin antibodies. Because 25% of women with SLE who become pregnant choose to terminate the pregnancy, effective contraception is essential for these patients. CHCs should be avoided in women with SLE and antiphospholipid antibodies or vascular complications; progestin-only contraceptives can be used in this situation.

Sickle Cell Disease. Two controlled trials have demonstrated a reduction in risk of vasoocclusive crises in women with sickle cell disease using DMPA as the method of contraception.[17] Theoretical concerns about the effects of CHCs on platelet activation and red cell deformity, for example, led clinicians to avoid their use in women with sickle cell disease. Because pregnancy carries such a high risk in this population, contraception with DMPA should be considered.

Oral Contraceptives ❶ ❷ When OCs are used correctly, their effectiveness approaches that of surgical sterilization.[3–5] With perfect use, their efficacy is greater than 99%, but with typical use, up to 8% of women may experience unintended pregnancy.[4] The low-dose combination OCs currently available are modifications of the original products introduced in 1960, containing significantly less estrogen and progestin than the earlier pills.[3–5,14] High-dose formulations were associated with vascular and embolic events, cancers, and significant side effects, but reductions in estrogen and progestin doses have been associated with fewer complications.

Monophasic OCs contain the same amounts of estrogen and progestin for 21 days, followed by 7 days of placebo pills (Table 82–4). Biphasic and triphasic pills contain variable amounts of estrogen and progestin for 21 days, also followed by a 7-day placebo phase. Over the past decade, combination multiphasic formulations have further lowered the total monthly hormonal dose without clearly demonstrating any significant clinical differences.[3,4,14] Monophasic, biphasic, and triphasic OCs attempted to reduce breakthrough bleeding and other side effects, but reviews from the Cochrane Library found no important differences in bleeding patterns based on phasic composition.[19,20]

Extended-cycle pills and continuous combination regimens are new developments that may offer some benefits for patients in terms of side effects. Extended-cycle OCs increase the number of hormone-containing pills from 21 to 84 days, followed by a 7-day placebo phase, resulting in four menstrual cycles per year. One unique product provides hormone-containing pills daily throughout the year.[15] Continuous combination regimens provide OCs for 21 days, then very-low-dose estrogen and progestin for an additional 4 to 7 days (during the traditional placebo phase).

OCs containing newer progestins (e.g., desogestrel, drospirenone, gestodene, and norgestimate) are sometimes referred to as *third-generation* OCs. These progestins are potent progestational agents that appear to have no estrogenic effects and are less androgenic compared with levonorgestrel on a weight basis. Therefore, these agents are thought to have improved side-effect profiles, such as improving mild to moderate acne.[3–5] Drospirenone also has antimineralocorticoid and antialdosterone activities, which may result in less weight gain compared to use of OCs containing levonorgestrel.[3–5] Unfortunately, few clinical trials have compared OCs and sample sizes are small, so the actual relevance of these differences in progestational selectivity and lower androgenic activity remains unknown. For example, a review by the Cochrane Library concluded that there was no evidence supporting a causal association between combination OCs or combination skin patches and weight gain.[21] Table 82–4 lists available OCs products by brand name and specifies hormonal composition.

Also introduced in 1960, the progestin-only "minipills" (28 days of active hormone per cycle) still are available.[3–5,14] Progestin-only pills tend to be less effective than combination OCs and are associated with irregular and unpredictable menstrual bleeding.[3–5] Minipills must be taken every day of the menstrual cycle at approximately the same time to maintain contraceptive efficacy. If a progestin-only pill is taken more than 3 hours late, patients should use a backup method of contraception for 48 hours.[4] Because minipills may not block ovulation (nearly 40% of women continue to ovulate normally), the risk of ectopic pregnancy is higher with their use than with use of other hormonal contraceptives.

Initiating an Oral Contraceptive. ❹ Historically, women were instructed to initiate OCs at some point after the next menstrual period occurred, several weeks after childbirth, or after a breast-feeding infant was weaned.[21] However, these recommendations to delay initiation of contraception resulted in many unintended pregnancies. This practice began in an effort to avoid exposing an unknown pregnancy to hormones. Because a large body of evidence shows that combined estrogens and progestins do not cause birth defects, delaying initiation of OCs is unnecessary.

In the "quick start" method for initiating OCs, the patient takes the first pill on the day of her office visit (after a negative urine pregnancy test).[3,4,22] Women should be instructed to use a second method of contraception for at least 7 days and informed that the menstrual period will be delayed until completion of the active pills in the current OC pill pack. The quick start method has been shown to be more successful in getting women to start OCs and to continue using OCs through the third cycle of use. No evidence shows increased bleeding irregularities with this method of OC initiation.

In the first-day start method, women take the first pill on the first day of the next menstrual cycle.[3,4,22] The Sunday start method was the most common method of initiating OCs for years. Women started OCs on the first Sunday after starting the menstrual cycle. Sunday start methods result in "period-free" weekends but may affect compliance if obtaining refills on weekends is difficult.

In the postpartum phase, there is concern about use of OCs because of the mother's hypercoagulability and the effects on lactation. The WHO precautions state that, in the first 21 days postpartum (when the risk of thrombosis is higher), estrogen-containing hormonal contraceptives should be avoided if possible (Table 82–3).[13] If contraception is required during this period, progestin-only pills and IUDs (progesterone or copper) are acceptable choices. Although a review by the Cochrane Library indicated that existing randomized, controlled trials were insufficient to establish an effect of CHC, if any, on milk quality and quantity, the WHO recommends that women who are breast-feeding avoid CHC in the first 6 weeks postpartum.[13,23] WHO precautions cite concerns about hormonal exposure in the newborn and diminished quality and quantity of breast milk due to early exposure to CHCs. Progestin-only pills do not adversely affect milk production, so they can be used after 6 weeks postpartum. Once effective lactation has been established, particularly in women who are not exclusively breast-feeding, estrogen-containing hormonal contraceptives can be safely used.

Choice of Oral Contraceptive. ❶ ❷ Because all combined OCs are similarly effective in preventing pregnancy, the initial choice is based on the hormonal content and dose, preferred pattern of pill use, and coexisting medical conditions (Table 82–3). In women without coexisting medical conditions, an OC containing 35 mcg or less of EE and less than 0.5 mg of norethindrone is recommended (Table 82–4).[5] This strategy is based on evidence that complications and side effects from CHC (i.e., thromboembolic events, stroke, or MI) result from excessive hormonal content.[3–5,14] Adolescents, underweight women (<110 lb [50 kg]), women older than 35 years, and those who are perimenopausal may have fewer side effects with OCs containing 20 to 25 mcg of EE. Risk of noncompliance with OCs is greater in women taking OCs containing less than 35 mcg of EE and thus should be considered, particularly in adolescents. Women weighing more than 160 lb (72.7 kg) may have higher contraceptive failure rates with low-dose OCs and may benefit from pills containing 35–50 mcg of EE. Women with regular heavy menses initially may benefit from a 50-mcg EE OC as well because of their higher endometrial activity. On the other hand, women with regular light menses can be started on 20-mcg EE OCs. Women with oily skin, acne, and hirsutism should be given low androgenic OCs.[5]

Conventional regimens (21 days of active pills, 7 days of placebo) provide predictable menses. Because monophasic OCs may be easier to take, easier to identify and manage side effects, and easier to manipulate to alter the timing of the menstrual cycle, they are preferred over conventional biphasic or triphasic OCs.[3–5] Extended-cycle OCs either eliminate the menstrual cycle or result in only four

TABLE 82-4 Composition of Commonly Prescribed Oral Contraceptives[a]

Product	Estrogen	Micrograms[b]	Progestin	Milligrams[b]	Spotting and Breakthrough Bleeding
50 mcg estrogen					
Necon, Nelova, Norethin, Norinyl, Ortho-Novum 1/50	Mestranol	50	Norethindrone	1	10.6
Norlestrin 1/50	Ethinyl estradiol	50	Norethindrone acetate	1	13.6
Ovcon 50	Ethinyl estradiol	50	Norethindrone	1	11.9
Ovral, Ogestrel	Ethinyl estradiol	50	Norgestrel	0.5	4.5
Demulen 50, Zovia 1/50	Ethinyl estradiol	50	Ethynodiol diacetate	1	13.9
Sub-50 mcg estrogen monophasic					
Alesse, Aviana, Lessina, Levlite	Ethinyl estradiol	20	Levonorgestrel	0.1	26.5
Brevicon, Modicon, Necon, Nortrel 0.5/30	Ethinyl estradiol	35	Norethindrone	0.5	24.6
Demulen, Zovia 1/35	Ethinyl estradiol	37.4	Ethynodiol diacetate	1	37.4
Apri, Desogen, Ortho-Cept	Ethinyl estradiol	30	Desogestrel	0.15	13.1
Levlen, Levora, Nordette, Portia	Ethinyl estradiol	30	Levonorgestrel	0.15	14
Loestrin 1/20 (check)	Ethinyl estradiol	20	Norethindrone acetate	1	29.7
Microgestin 1/20 (check)	Ethinyl estradiol	20	Norethindrone acetate	1	29.7
Loestrin, Microgestin 1.5/30	Ethinyl estradiol	30	Norethindrone acetate	1.5	25.2
Cryselle, Lo-Ovral, Low-Ogestrel	Ethinyl estradiol	30	Norgestrel	0.3	9.6
Necon, Nelova, Norinyl, Norethin, Nortrel, Ortho-Novum 1/35	Ethinyl estradiol	35	Norethindrone	1	14.7
Ortho-Cyclen, Sprintec	Ethinyl estradiol	35	Norgestimate	0.25	14.3
Ovcon-35	Ethinyl estradiol	35	Norethindrone	0.4	11
Yasmin	Ethinyl estradiol	30	Drospirenone	3	14.5
Sub-50 mcg estrogen monophasic extended cycle					
Loestrin-24 FE[c]	Ethinyl estradiol	20	Norethindrone	1	
Lybrel	Ethinyl estradiol	20	Levonorgestrel	0.09	52[e]
Seasonale[d]	Ethinyl estradiol	30	Levonorgestrel	0.15	58.5%[e]
YAZ[c]	Ethinyl estradiol	20	Drospirenone	3	
Sub-50 mcg estrogen multiphasic					
Cyclessa	Ethinyl estradiol	25 (7)	Desogestrel	0.1 (7)	11.1
		25 (7)		0.125 (7)	
		25 (7)		0.15 (7)	
Estrostep	Ethinyl estradiol	20 (5)	Norethindrone acetate	1 (5)	21.7
	Ethinyl estradiol	30 (7)	Norethindrone acetate	1 (7)	
	Ethinyl estradiol	35 (9)	Norethindrone acetate	1 (9)	
Kariva, Mircette	Ethinyl estradiol	20 (21)	Desogestrel	0.15 (21)	19.7
	Ethinyl estradiol	10 (5)	Desogestrel		
Necon, Nelova, Ortho-Novum 10/11	Ethinyl estradiol	35 (10)	Norethindrone	0.5 (10)	17.6
	Ethinyl estradiol	35 (11)	Norethindrone	1 (11)	
Nortrel, Ortho-Novum 7/7/7	Ethinyl estradiol	35 (7)	Norethindrone	0.5 (7)	14.5
	Ethinyl estradiol	35 (7)	Norethindrone	0.75 (7)	
	Ethinyl estradiol	35 (7)	Norethindrone	1 (7)	
Ortho Tri-Cyclen	Ethinyl estradiol	35 (7)	Norgestimate	0.18 (7)	17.7
	Ethinyl estradiol	35 (7)	Norgestimate	0.215 (7)	
	Ethinyl estradiol	35 (7)	Norgestimate	0.25 (7)	
Ortho Tri-Cyclen LO	Ethinyl estradiol	25 (7)	Norgestimate	0.18 (7)	11.5
	Ethinyl estradiol	25 (7)	Norgestimate	0.215 (7)	
	Ethinyl estradiol	25 (7)	Norgestimate	0.25 (7)	
Tri-Norinyl	Ethinyl estradiol	35 (7)	Norethindrone	0.5 (7)	25.5
	Ethinyl estradiol	35 (9)	Norethindrone	1 (9)	
	Ethinyl estradiol	35 (5)	Norethindrone	0.5 (5)	
Sub-50 mcg estrogen multiphasic extended cycle					
Seasonique	Ethinyl estradiol	30 (84)	Levonorgestrel	0.15 (84)	42.5[e]
	Ethinyl estradiol	10 (7)	Levonorgestrel	0.15 (7)	
Progestin only					
Camila, Errin, Micronor, Nor-QD	Ethinyl estradiol	–	Norethindrone	0.35	42.3
Ovrette	Ethinyl estradiol	–	Norgestrel	0.075	34.9

[a]28-day regimens (21-day active pills, then 7-day pill-free interval) unless otherwise noted.
[b]Number in parentheses refers to the number of days the dose is received in multiphasic oral contraceptives.
[c]28-day regimen (24-day active pills, then 4-day pill-free interval).
[d]91-day regimen (84-day active pills, then 7-day pill-free interval).
[e]Percent reporting after 6–12 months of use.
Data from Hatcher et al.,[3,4] Dickey,[5] and Anonymous.[14]

menstrual cycles per year, so they may be associated with less dysmenorrhea and menstrual migraines. Commercially available extended-cycle OCs are available, or monophasic 28 day OCs can be cycled by skipping the 7-day placebo phase for two to three cycles (sometimes referred to as *bicycling* and *tricycling*). With continued use of extended-cycle OCs for 1 year, no significant changes in blood pressure, weight, or hemoglobin compared with cyclic users have been noted. However, long-term studies have not been performed to assess the risk of cancer, VTE, or changes in fertility. Continuous regimens provide a shortened pill-free interval, from the traditional 7 days to 2 to 4 days. These regimens may be beneficial for women with dysmenorrhea and menstrual migraines.

Coexisting medical conditions and their impact on CHC use have been previously addressed. Women with migraine headaches, history of thromboembolic disease, heart disease, cerebrovascular disease, SLE with vascular disease, and hypertriglyceridemia are good candidates for progestin-only methods (pills, DMPA, and the levonorgestrel intrauterine system). Women older than 35 years who are smokers or are obese, or who have hypertension or vascular disease should use progesterone-only methods.[13,17]

Managing Oral Contraceptive Side Effects. ❸ Many symptoms occurring with early OC use (e.g., nausea, bloating, breakthrough bleeding) improve spontaneously by the third cycle of use after adjusting to the altered hormone levels.[3–5] However, 59% to 81% of women who stopped OCs in one study did so because of the side effects. Therefore, patient education and early reevaluation (i.e., within 3–6 months) are necessary to identify and manage adverse effects, in an effort to improve compliance and prevent unintentional pregnancies. A list of OC-related side effects and their management is given in Table 82–2.

If the patient has symptoms related to OC use, it is necessary to determine if the symptom indicates the presence or potential development of a serious illness (Table 82–5).[4,5] Patients should be instructed to immediately discontinue CHCs if they experience warning signs, sometimes described as ACHES (abdominal pain, chest pain, headaches, eye problems, and severe leg pain).[4]

CLINICAL CONTROVERSY

There is a widely held belief that antibiotics reduce the efficacy of OCs, increasing the risk of pregnancy. However, few data support this drug interaction with most antibiotics, with the exception of rifampin. Because of this potential risk and considering the fact that OCs are not 100% effective, many practitioners still counsel patients about this issue. The Council on Scientific Affairs at the American Medical Association recommends that women be informed about the small risk of interactions with antibiotics and, if desired, provided with additional nonhormonal contraceptive agents.

Managing Oral Contraceptive Drug Interactions. ❸ The effectiveness of an OC is sometimes limited by drug interactions that interfere with gastrointestinal absorption, increase intestinal motility by altering gut bacteriologic flora, and alter the metabolism, excretion, or binding of the OC (Table 82–6).[4,17,24] The lower the dose of hormone in the OC, the greater the risk that a drug interaction will compromise its efficacy. Women should be instructed to use an alternative method of contraception (e.g., condoms) if there is a possibility of a drug interacting altering the efficacy of the OC.[4] Although less well documented, these recommendations generally also apply to patients receiving transdermal and vaginal CHC products.

TABLE 82-5 Serious Symptoms That May Be Associated with Combined Hormonal Contraception

Serious Symptoms	Possible Underlying Problem
Blurred vision, diplopia, flashing lights, blindness, papilledema	Stroke, hypertension, temporary vascular problem of many possible sites, retinal artery thrombosis
Numbness, weakness, tingling in extremities, slurred speech	Hemorrhagic or thrombotic stroke
Migraine headaches	Vascular spasm, stroke
Breast mass, pain, or swelling	Breast cancer
Chest pain (radiating to left arm or neck), shortness of breath, coughing up blood	Pulmonary embolism, myocardial infarction
Abdominal pain, hepatic mass or tenderness, jaundice, pruritus	Gallbladder disease, hepatic adenoma, pancreatitis, thrombosis of abdominal artery or vein
Excessive spotting, breakthrough bleeding	Endometrial, cervical, or vaginal cancer
Severe leg pain (calf, thigh), tenderness, swelling, warmth	Deep-vein thrombosis

Data from Hatcher et al.[4] and Dickey.[5]

TABLE 82-6 Interactions of Oral Contraceptives with Other Drugs

Interacting Drugs	Outcome and Recommendation
Anticonvulsants (barbiturates, including phenobarbital and primidone; carbamazepine; felbamate; phenytoin; topiramate; vigabatrin)	Decreased contraceptive effect Use OCs containing 50 mcg ethinyl estradiol and a second method of contraception or IUD
Griseofulvin (Fulvicin, Grifulvin V, and others)	Possible decreased contraceptive effect Use second method of contraception
Nonnucleoside reverse transcriptase inhibitors (delavirdine, efavirenz, nevirapine)	Possible decreased contraceptive effect Use IUD
Protease inhibitors (amprenavir, atazanavir, indinavir, lopinavir, nelfinavir, ritonavir, saquinavir)	Increased or decreased contraceptive effect Use IUD
Rifampin	Decreased contraceptive effect Use second method of contraception or alternate method (IUD) if concomitant use is long term

IUD, intrauterine device; OC, oral contraceptives.
Data from Hatcher et al.,[4] World Health Organization,[13] ACOG Practice Bulletin,[17] Dickenson et al.,[24] and Archer and Archer.[25]

Several reviews of the interaction between antibiotics and OCs have documented a true pharmacokinetic interaction with rifampin in which the efficacy of OCs is impaired. Pharmacokinetic studies of other antibiotics have not shown any consistent interaction, but case reports of individual patients have shown a reduction in EE levels when OCs are taken with tetracyclines and penicillin derivatives.[24,25] The ACOG states that ampicillin, doxycycline, fluconazole, metronidazole, miconazole, fluoroquinolones, and tetracyclines do not decrease steroid levels in women taking OCs.[17] The Council on Scientific Affairs at the American Medical Association recommends that women taking rifampin should be counseled about the risk of OC failure and advised to use an additional nonhormonal contraceptive agent during the course of rifampin therapy. The council also recommends that women be informed about the small risk of interactions with other antibiotics, and, if desired, appropriate additional nonhormonal contraceptive agents should be considered. In addition, women who develop breakthrough bleeding during concomitant use of antibiotics and OCs (and other CHCs) should be advised to use an alternate method of contraception during the period of concomitant use.[24]

Women receiving anticonvulsants for a seizure disorder require special attention with regard to hormonal contraception. Some anticonvulsants (mainly phenobarbital, carbamazepine, phenytoin) induce the metabolism of estrogen and progestin, inducing breakthrough bleeding and potentially reducing contraceptive efficacy. In addition, some anticonvulsants (i.e., phenytoin) are known teratogens. Use of condoms in conjunction with high-estrogen OCs or IUDs can be considered for these women.[17]

Patient Instructions with Oral Contraceptives. ❹ Many women who take OCs are poorly informed about the proper use of these medications. The patient first should be given the package insert that accompanies all estrogen products and instructed to read it carefully. The written information in the package insert should be supplemented with verbal information describing the way the medication works (primarily by thickening cervical mucus to prevent sperm penetration), both common and serious side effects, and management of side effects (Table 82–4). Although several transient self-limiting side effects often occur, the patient should be aware of the danger signals that require immediate medical attention (Table 82–5). The benefits and risks should be discussed in terms that the patient can understand, including the fact that OCs provide no physical barrier to the transmission of STDs, including HIV. Detailed instructions on when to start taking the OC, such as the "Quick Start" method, should be provided. Patients should be told the importance of routine daily administration to ensure consistent plasma concentrations and improve compliance, and specific instructions should be given regarding what to do if a pill is missed (Table 82–7). Use of an additional contraceptive method is advisable if the patient misses taking a pill or experiences severe diarrhea or vomiting for several days. Important drug interactions should be discussed. The patient taking combination OCs should expect her menses to start within 1 to 3 days after taking the last active pill. She should start another pack of pills immediately after finishing a 28-day pack (no days between) or 1 week after finishing the previous 21-day pack, even if her menses is not completed.[3–5]

Discontinuing Oral Contraceptives and Return of Fertility. The average delay in ovulation after discontinuing OCs is 1 to 2 weeks, but delayed ovulation is more common in women with a history of irregular menses. Post-OC amenorrhea rarely lasts 6 months.[3–5] Traditionally, women are counseled to allow two to three normal menstrual periods before becoming pregnant to permit the reestablishment of menses and ovulation. However, in several large cohort and case-control studies, infants conceived in the first month after discontinuation of an OC had no greater chance of miscarriage or being born with a birth defect than those born in the general population.

TABLE 82-7 Recommendations for Missed Oral Contraceptive Doses

Number of Pills Missed	Week in Which Pills Were Missed	Recommendation	Use of 7-Day Back Up Method
1	1	Take two pills as soon as possible Finish the pill pack Use emergency contraception if necessary	Yes
1	2–3	Take two pills as soon as possible Finish the pill pack	No
1	4	Skip placebo pills Finish the pill pack	No
2–4	1	Take two pills as soon as possible[a] Finish the pill pack Use emergency contraception if necessary	Yes
2–4	2	Take two pills as soon as possible[a] Finish the pill pack Use emergency contraception if necessary	Yes
2–4	3	Start a new pill pack[a]	No
2–4	4	Skip placebo pills Finish the pill pack	No
5	Any	Take two pills as soon as possible Start a new pill pack Use emergency contraception if necessary	Yes

[a]Alternative recommendation is to take one of the missed pills every 12 hours until caught up, then continue the rest of the pill pack.

Data from Hatcher et al.[3,4] and Dickey.[5]

Transdermal Contraceptives ❶ ❷ A CHC is available as a transdermal patch (Ortho Evra), which includes 0.75 mg of EE and 6 mg of norelgestromin, the active metabolite of norgestimate.[3–5] Comparative trials have shown the transdermal patch to be as effective as combined OCs in patients weighing less than 90 kg (198 pounds). Of the 15 pregnancies reported in the clinical trials, five were among women weighing more than 198 lb (90 kg); therefore, this product is not recommended as a first-line option for these women.[3,4,26] Some patients experience application-site reactions, but other side effects are similar to those experienced with OCs (e.g., breast discomfort, headache, and nausea).

❸ A warning from the manufacturer states that women using the patch are exposed to approximately 60% more estrogen than from a typical OC containing 35 mcg of EE, due to the transdermal system eliminating first-pass metabolism. Whether this increased estrogen exposure leads to increased cardiovascular or thromboembolic events is unclear. The Ortho Evra package insert provides preliminary data indicating a higher incidence of thromboembolic events with the patch.[26] Another case-control study compared the patch to a 35-mcg norgestimate-containing OC and found no significant difference in thromboembolism occurrence.[27] Currently, the Food and Drug Administration (FDA) is monitoring this risk because more consistent data are needed.

The patch should be applied to the abdomen, buttocks, upper torso, or upper arm at the beginning of the menstrual cycle and replaced every week for 3 weeks (the fourth week is patch-free).[3,4] The patch releases estrogen and progestin for 9 days. If the woman forgets to change her patch or restarts the active patches after the ninth day, a backup method should be used for 7 days. Approximately 5% of patches will need to be replaced because they become partly detached or fall off altogether, so single replacements are available. If the patch is detached for more than 24 hours, a new 4-week cycle should be restarted and backup method used for 7 days.[3,4] Users have demonstrated greater compliance with the patch than with an OC, but whether this results in reduced pregnancy rates remains to be seen.[28] The benefits of compliance must be weighed against of the risk of increased estrogen exposure and possibility of thromboembolic events.

Vaginal Rings ❶ ❷ The vaginal ring containing EE and etonogestrel (NuvaRing) currently is the only product available using vaginal delivery for hormonal contraception.[29] It is a 54-mm flexible ring, 4 mm in thickness.[3] Over a 3-week period, the ring releases approximately 15 mcg/day of EE and 120 mcg/day of etonogestrel. Comparative trials have shown the vaginal ring to be as effective as combined OCs. On the first cycle of use, the ring should be inserted on or before the fifth day of the menstrual cycle, remain in place for 3 weeks, then removed for 1 week to allow for withdrawal bleeding. The new ring should be inserted on the same day of the week as it was during the last cycle, similar to starting a new OC pack on the same day of the week. A second method of contraception should be used if the ring has been expelled accidentally for more than 3 hours.[3,29]

❸ Side effects, precautions, and contraindications for use of the hormonal ring are similar to those for all CHCs. The most commonly reported reasons for discontinuation of use were device-related issues, such as foreign-body sensation, device expulsion, and vaginal symptoms. Cycle control with the vaginal ring appears to be as good as or better than with combined OCs, with a low incidence of breakthrough bleeding and spotting after the second cycle of use, presumably due to increased compliance and release of steady levels of estrogen and progestin.[29,30] Patient acceptability of the delivery system has been studied, and the majority of women do not complain of discomfort in general or during intercourse.[31]

The ring should be inserted vaginally. In contrast to diaphragms and cervical caps, precise placement is not an issue because the estrogen and progestin are absorbed anywhere in the vagina.

Women should be in a comfortable position, and compress the ring between the thumb and index finger and push it into the vagina. There is no danger of inserting the ring too far because the cervix will prevent it from traveling up the genital tract. Removal of the ring is performed in a similar manner; pulling it out with the thumb and index finger, and discarding into the foil patch (the ring should not be flushed down the toilet).[29] Patients should be discouraged from douching, but other vaginal products, including antifungal creams and spermicides, can be used.[3,4,29]

Long-Acting Injectable and Implantable Contraceptives Steroid hormones provide long-term contraception when injected or implanted into the skin. Progestins are used in existing injectable and implantable contraceptives.[3–5] Sustained progestin exposure blocks the LH surge, thus preventing ovulation. Should ovulation occur, progestins reduce ovum motility in the fallopian tubes. Even if fertilization occurs, progestins thin the endometrium, reducing the chance of implantation. Progestins also thicken the cervical mucus, producing a barrier to sperm penetration. These long-acting methods of contraception do not provide any protection from STDs.

❶ ❷ Women who particularly benefit from progestin-only methods are those who are breast-feeding, those who are intolerant to estrogens (i.e., have a history of estrogen-related headache, breast tenderness, or nausea), and those with concomitant medical conditions in which estrogen is not recommended (Table 82–3). Additionally, injectable and implantable contraceptives are beneficial for women with compliance issues. Pregnancy failure rates with long-acting progestin contraceptives are comparable to the rates with female sterilization.[3–5] Reports have stated an increased risk of ectopic pregnancies while using progestin-only methods, but no evidence supports this finding with use of recent injectable and implantable products.

Injectable Progestins. ❶ ❷ Medroxyprogesterone acetate is similar in structure to naturally occurring progesterone. DMPA 150 mg (Depo-Provera) is administered by deep intramuscular injection in the gluteal or deltoid muscle within 5 days of onset of menstrual bleeding and inhibits ovulation for more than 3 months.[32] Additionally, a new formulation approved by the FDA contains 104 mg of DMPA (Depo-SubQ Provera 104), which is injected subcutaneously into the abdomen or thigh.[33] With perfect use, the efficacy of DMPA is more than 99%; however, with typical use, 3% of women experience unintended pregnancy.[4] Although these injections may inhibit ovulation for up to 14 weeks, the dose should be repeated every 3 months (12 weeks) to ensure continuous contraception. The manufacturer recommends excluding pregnancy in women with a lapse of 13 or more weeks between injections for the intramuscular formulation or 14 or more weeks between injections for the subcutaneous formulation. Depo-Provera is available as a 150 mg/mL injection vial or prefilled syringe and Depo-SubQ Provera 104 is available as a prefilled syringe.[32,33]

Although no adverse effects have been documented in infants exposed to DMPA through breast milk, the manufacturer recommends not initiating DMPA until 6 weeks postpartum in breast-feeding women. Women who are not breast-feeding but require contraception can receive DMPA immediately postpartum.[13,32] Women with sickle cell disease are good candidates for DMPA, as studies have demonstrated a reduction in sickle cell pain crises in women using DMPA.[13] In addition, women with seizure disorders may experience fewer seizures when taking DMPA for contraception.[4] The subcutaneous DMPA formulation has been FDA approved for treatment of endometriosis-associated pain.[33] The incidence of *Candida* vulvovaginitis, ectopic pregnancy, and pelvic inflammatory disease, as well as endometrial and ovarian cancer, is decreased in women using DMPA for contraception compared with women using no contraception.[3,32]

Because return of fertility may be delayed after discontinuation of DMPA, it should not be recommended to women desiring pregnancy in the near future. The median time to conception from the first omitted dose is 10 months. Sixty-eight percent of women will be able to conceive within 12 months, 83% within 15 months, and 93% within 18 months of the last injection.[32,33]

❸ Menstrual irregularities, including irregular, unpredictable spotting or, more rarely, continuous heavy bleeding, are the most frequent adverse effects of both formulations of DMPA. In some cases, bleeding is severe enough to cause a significant drop in hemoglobin. Women who cannot tolerate prolonged bleeding may benefit from a short course of estrogen (e.g., 7 days of 2-mg estradiol or 1.25-mg conjugated estrogen given orally).[3,4] The incidence of irregular bleeding decreases from 30% in the first year to 10% thereafter. After 12 months of therapy with either formulation, 55% of women report amenorrhea, with the incidence increasing to 68% after 2 years.[32,33] Bleeding patterns after 1 year of the subcutaneous formulation have not been established.[33,34]

Other adverse effects, including breast tenderness, weight gain, and depression, occur less commonly (<5%). However, data suggest that DMPA may actually improve depression, and use of DMPA in women with depression may be appropriate with close monitoring.[13] Weight gain averages 1 kg annually and may not resolve until 6 to 8 months after the last injection.[32,33]

CLINICAL CONTROVERSY

Both formulations of DMPA have a black box warning that addresses the association between DMPA use and decreased BMD, specifically in adolescent and young women. The clinical significance of this finding is unknown, and current evidence suggests osteoporosis or fractures do not occur more frequently in women who use DMPA. Many clinicians have adopted the policy, recommended by the manufacturer, of dual-energy x-ray absorptiometry (DXA) studies to monitor BMD. In contrast, WHO and ACOG guidelines recommend against the use of DXA in short- and long-term DMPA users due to the limited clinical utility of monitoring BMD in this population.

Concern has been raised over DMPA use and the development of osteoporosis because DMPA suppresses ovarian production of estradiol and has been associated with a reduction in BMD.[4,17] However, DMPA has not been associated with the development of osteoporosis or fractures, and discontinuation of DMPA results in return to baseline BMD values within 12 to 30 months. In 2004, the FDA added a black box warning to DMPA, recommending continued use of more than 2 years only if other contraceptive methods were inappropriate.[17,32,33] However, current data do not provide a clear rationale for this time limit, as evidence suggests the rate of BMD loss may slow after 1 to 2 years of DMPA use.[35]

Many clinicians have adopted the policy, recommended by the manufacturer, of DXA studies to monitor BMD in DMPA users. Bone loss with DMPA can be prevented by providing supplemental estrogen (0.625-mg conjugated equine estrogen daily or 5-mg intramuscular estradiol cypionate), but because reductions in BMD have not been linked to the development of osteoporosis, the utility of this finding is questionable. In addition, most women use DMPA because they are unable to use estrogen-containing contraceptives, or adolescents use DMPA because of compliance issues. The WHO does not recommend a restriction on the use of DMPA in women aged 18 to 45 years and states that the benefits of use outweigh the potential risks.[36] Appropriate counseling regarding prevention of osteoporosis should be provided for women using DMPA, including the use of 1,200 to 1,500 mg of elemental calcium plus 400 international units of vitamin D and a regular regimen of weight-bearing exercise.[3]

Subdermal Progestin Implants. ❶ ❷ Norplant, developed by the Population Council, was the first subdermal progestin implant approved for use in the United States in 1990.[4] The Norplant contraceptive system was a set of six implantable, nonbiodegradable, soft silicone rubber capsules, each filled with 36-mg crystalline levonorgestrel, that provided continuous contraception for up to 5 years. Although extremely effective, Norplant was removed from the U.S. market in 2003 due to difficulty with insertion and removal.

Implanon is the progestin implant currently available in the United States.[37] Implanon is a single 4-cm-long implant, containing 68 mg of etonogestrel, that is placed under the skin of the upper arm using a preloaded inserter.[37,38] Implanon releases etonogestrel at a rate of 60 mcg daily for the first month, then decreases to an average of 30 mcg daily at the end of the 3 years of recommended use. Etonogestrel suppresses ovulation in 97% of cycles. When ovulation is not suppressed, etonogestrel still is effective as the progestin thickens the cervical mucus and produces an atrophic endometrium. With perfect use, efficacy approaches 100% but may be reduced in women weighing more than 130% of their ideal body weight. Because only one rod is used, the difficulties experienced with insertion and removal of Norplant hopefully will be avoided.

❹ The etonogestrel implant should be inserted between days 1 and 5 of the menstrual cycle in women who have not previously used hormonal contraception.[37,38] Women currently taking OCs can have the implant inserted within 7 days after taking the last active OC tablet. Women currently taking progestin-only pills should have the implant inserted without skipping any days, on the same day that the progestin-only IUD is removed, or on the day that the DMPA injection is due. After removal, fertility returns within 30 days.

❸ The major adverse effect associated with Implanon is irregular menstrual bleeding, which led to discontinuation of the implant in 11% of patients in clinical trials.[37,38] Like the bleeding pattern seen with other progestins, some women (22%) became amenorrheic with continued use, but many continued to have prolonged bleeding and spotting (18%) and frequent bleeding (7%). Other adverse effects include headache, vaginitis, weight gain, acne, and breast and abdominal pain. Implanon does not appear to affect BMD. Concomitant administration of drugs that induce hepatic enzymes (Table 82–6) may decrease the efficacy of etonogestrel, necessitating use of a different method of contraception while these potentially interacting drugs are used. Implanon is contraindicated in women who are pregnant or have active liver disease, a history of thromboembolic events, or a history of breast cancer.

Implanon is a unique implantable contraceptive agent that provides enhanced compliance and prolonged efficacy. Therefore, it may be a good choice for women with a history of noncompliance, who do not plan to have children for at least 3 years, and who have estrogen-related adverse effects or contraindications. Because fertility returns soon after removal and Implanon does not affect bone health, it may be preferred over DMPA. Women should be counseled about the risk of irregular bleeding patterns so that patients will not request early removal of Implanon.

Intrauterine Devices

❶ ❷ The low-grade intrauterine inflammation and increased prostaglandin formation caused by IUDs and endometrial suppression caused specifically by the progestin-releasing IUD appear to be primarily spermicidal, although interference with implantation is a backup mechanism.[3,4,39] Efficacy rates with IUDs are greater than 99% with both perfect and typical use.[4] Although increasing in popularity, the IUD still has several contraindications. The risk of pelvic inflammatory disease among IUD users ranges from 1% to 2.5%. Because the increased risk of infection appears to be related to introduction of bacteria into the genital tract during IUD insertion, the risk is highest during the first 20 days after the procedure.[40] Ideal patients for IUD use include nulligravid women who are monogamous and are not at risk for STDs or pelvic inflammatory disease. Two IUDs currently are marketed in the United States; all are T-shaped and are medicated, one with copper (ParaGard) and one with levonorgestrel (Mirena).[3,4]

❸ ParaGard provides better contraceptive effectiveness than previous copper devices and can be left in place for 10 years.[3,4] A disadvantage of ParaGard is increased menstrual blood flow and dysmenorrhea; average monthly blood loss among users increased by 35% in clinical trials. Initially, Mirena releases 20 mcg of levonorgestrel daily, but release decreases to 10 mcg daily over the 5 years of use.[3,4,39] Systemically absorbed levonorgestrel is minimal and considerably less than with OCs. However, the levonorgestrel IUD produces its effects locally via suppression of the endometrium, causing a reduction in menstrual blood loss. In contrast to the copper IUD, menstrual flow in users of the levonorgestrel IUD is decreased, and development of amenorrhea has been observed in 20% of users in the first year and 60% in the fifth year. A disadvantage of the levonorgestrel IUD is increased spotting in the first 6 months of use, and women should be counseled that the spotting will decline gradually over time.[3,4,39]

IUDs should be considered because they require no compliance once inserted and result in immediate return of fertility once removed. The levonorgestrel IUD is a good choice for women with menorrhagia or dysmenorrhea because of its benefits with regard to menstrual blood loss. IUDs, in general, are an alternative for women who cannot tolerate estrogen-containing contraceptive agents.

CLINICAL CONTROVERSY

Pharmacists who refuse to fill valid prescriptions for emergency contraception have been highly publicized in the media. Position statements published by the American Pharmaceutical Association and American College of Clinical Pharmacy support pharmacists' rights to decline filling a valid prescription if doing so conflicts with moral, ethical, or religious beliefs. However, it is the pharmacists' professional responsibility to refer the patient to another pharmacist who will fill the prescription in a timely, confidential, and nonjudgmental manner so that no harm is caused to the patient.

Emergency Contraception

❺ EC is used to prevent unwanted pregnancy after unprotected sexual intercourse (e.g., condom breakage, diaphragm dislodging, or sexual assault). Higher doses of combined estrogen and progestin or progestin-only containing products can be used.[3–5] Insertion of copper IUD is an option, although it is not an FDA approved or a widely used method of EC. Exact mechanisms of action of oral EC are being studied and vary according to the product used. EC may prevent the fertilized egg from implanting into the endometrium; however, studies contradict this potential mechanism. Additional mechanisms include impaired sperm transport and corpus luteum function. Pregnancy occurs when the fertilized egg is implanted into the endometrial lining. After intercourse, implantation of the fertilized egg typically takes approximately 5 days. Oral EC will not disrupt the fertilized egg after implantation has occurred.[40,41] Currently, one progestin-containing pill is approved and marketed specifically for EC in the United States. Commercially available OCs in specific dosages can be used as an alternative.[3–5,41]

Plan B is the only product specifically approved for EC and is the regimen of choice. It contains two white tablets, each containing

0.75 mg of levonorgestrel. The first dose is taken within 72 hours of unprotected intercourse (although the sooner, the more effective); the second dose is taken 12 hours later.[3–5,41–43] One study found that 1.5 mg of levonorgestrel (two tablets of Plan B) taken as a single dose was as effective as taking the doses 12 hours apart and did not cause an increased incidence of adverse effects. Although this single-dose regimen is not FDA approved, it is a reasonable option, especially in women who may not be compliant with the two-dose regimen.[41,44] Plan B was approved by the FDA in 2006 for OTC sales to women 18 years of age or older. A prescription is required for patients aged 17 years and younger. It is sold only in pharmacies and must be stocked behind the counter. Patients must provide proof of age prior to purchasing the product. The manufacturer is continuing its efforts in gaining OTC status for provision to minors.[45]

Despite the availability of Plan B, use of regular combined contraceptives for EC (i.e., Yuzpe method) still is permissible, although some studies suggest that they may not be as effective and may be associated with more adverse effects.[41,42] Specifically, the FDA has declared the following regimens containing the progestins norgestrel and levonorgestrel safe and effective methods of EC: Ovral (two tablets per dose); Nordette, Levlen, Levora, Lo/Ovral, Triphasil, Tri-Levlen, or Trivora (four tablets per dose); and Alesse or Levlite (five tablets per dose).[3–5,41] Additionally, regular progestin-only pills can be used as EC, but many tablets must be taken (i.e., Ovrette, 20 tablets per dose).[3,4,41] Patients should be counseled to take the appropriate number of tablets as soon as possible after unprotected sexual intercourse and to repeat the dose in 12 hours.

The efficacy of all EC regimens declines if they begin more than 72 hours after intercourse.[3,4,41] However, one study suggests that EC may still be effective when used up to 120 hours after intercourse and should be considered in some women when use is delayed.[41,46] It is recommended that women have an advanced prescription on hand to maximize the effectiveness of EC.

Common adverse effects include nausea, vomiting, and irregular bleeding. Nausea and vomiting occur significantly less when Plan B is administered. If the Yuzpe method is prescribed, antiemetics given 1 hour before the dose is taken may be warranted. Many women will experience irregular bleeding regardless of which EC method is used, with the menstrual period usually occurring 1 week before or after the expected time. No current data regarding the safety of repeated use EC are available, but current consensus suggests the risks are low, and women can receive multiple regimens if warranted. Pharmacists have a key role in providing patient counseling regarding EC. Appropriate counseling should be provided regarding timing of the dose, common adverse effects, and use of a regular contraceptive method (backup barrier methods should be used after EC for at least 7 days).[41]

PHARMACOECONOMIC CONSIDERATIONS

More than half of all pregnancies in the United States are unintended.[4] Not all unintended pregnancies are unwanted; many are just "mistimed." Nevertheless, the United States has a higher rate of induced abortions than most other industrialized western nations. Whatever method is used, preventing unintended pregnancy is highly cost effective. With regard to the acquisition cost of reversible contraception, spermicides alone are the least expensive method, followed by use of spermicides with condoms. The diaphragm and cervical cap (with spermicide) are midrange in cost; the female condom is slightly more expensive than the other female barrier methods. Injectable and implantable methods (Depo-Provera, Implanon, ParaGard, Mirena) carry a higher initial cost that can be prohibitive for some women, and the annual cost is greater if the products are removed prior to their expiration. OCs, the contraceptive patch, and the vaginal ring are the most expensive forms of reversible contraception. These cost estimates are based on the assumption of 100 acts of intercourse annually. However, with regard to direct medical costs (e.g., method use, side effects, and unintended pregnancies) over 5 years, IUDs, vasectomy, Depo-Provera, and now Implanon are the most cost effective. OCs are more cost effective than methods with high failure rates (e.g., barrier methods, spermicides, withdrawal, and periodic abstinence), but even these methods are more cost effective than no method.[47]

EVALUATION OF THERAPEUTIC OUTCOMES

❹ Patients should receive both verbal and written instructions on the chosen method of contraception. Followup appointments can increase compliance, allow time for the patient to ask questions, and provide opportunities to address other health maintenance issues (e.g., self-breast examination, Pap smears, human papillomavirus vaccines, STD risk).[4]

At least annual blood pressure monitoring is recommended for all users of CHC. When a patient with a history of glucose intolerance or overt diabetes mellitus begins or discontinues the use of CHC, glucose levels must be monitored closely for deterioration of the condition. Contraceptive users should receive at least annual (more frequent if they are at risk for STDs) cytologic screening. Women should undergo annual examination for clinical problems possibly relating to the CHC (e.g., breakthrough bleeding, amenorrhea, weight gain, and acne).

Women using Implanon should be monitored annually for menstrual cycle disturbances, weight gain, local inflammation or infection at the implant site, acne, breast tenderness, headaches, and hair loss. Women using DMPA should be asked at 3-month followup visits about weight gain, menstrual cycle disturbances, and STD risks. Patients taking DMPA should be weighed, undergo blood pressure checks, and receive annual examinations as indicated based on the patient's age.

Choosing a contraceptive method most suited to the patient's needs will reduce significantly the chance of unintended pregnancy. A medical and sexual history and a thorough physical examination are essential when evaluating the various methods available. Understanding the risks and precautions associated with the methods available is essential for both patients and clinicians.

ABBREVIATIONS

ACOG: American College of Obstetrics and Gynecology

BMD: bone mineral density

BMI: body mass index

CDC: Centers for Disease Control and Prevention

CHC: combined hormonal contraception

DMPA: depot medroxyprogesterone acetate

DXA: dual-energy x-ray absorptiometry

EC: emergency contraception

EE: ethinyl estradiol

FDA: Food and Drug Administration

FSH: follicle-stimulating hormone

GnRH: gonadotropin-releasing hormone

hCG: human chorionic gonadotropin

HDL: high-density lipoprotein

HIV: human immunodeficiency virus

IUD: intrauterine device

LDL: low-density lipoprotein

LH: luteinizing hormone
MI: myocardial infarction
OC: oral contraceptive
OTC: over the counter
Pap: papanicolaou (smear)
SLE: systemic lupus erythematosus
STD: sexually transmitted disease
VTE: venous thromboembolism
WHO: World Health Organization

REFERENCES

1. Chandra A, Martinez GM, Mosher WD, et al. Fertility, Family Planning, and Reproductive Health of U.S. Women: Data from the 2002 National Survey of Family Growth. National Center for Health Statistics. Vital Health Stat 23. 2005, *http://www.cdc.gov/nchs/data/series/sr_23/sr23_025.pdf, September 12, 2006*.
2. Get "In the Know": 20 Questions About Pregnancy, Contraception and Abortion. 2006, *http://www.guttmacher.org/in-the-know/index.html*.
3. Hatcher RA, Zieman M, Cwiak C et al. A Pocket Guide to Managing Contraception. Tiger, GA: Bridging the Gap Foundation, 2005.
4. Hatcher RA, Trussel J, Stewart F, et al. Contraceptive Technology, 18th ed. New York: Ardent Media, 2004.
5. Dickey RP. Managing Contraceptive Pill Patients, 12th ed. Dallas, TX: Essential Medical Information Systems, 2004.
6. Jones RK, Darroch JE, Henshaw SK. Contraceptive use among US women having abortions in 2000–2001. Perspect Sex Reprod Health 2002;34:294–303.
7. Stewart FH, Harper CC, Ellertson CE, et al. Clinical breast and pelvic examination requirements for hormonal contraception: Current practice versus evidence. JAMA 2001;285:2232–2239.
8. Steinbrook R. The potential of human papillomavirus vaccines. N Engl J Med 2006;354:1109–1112.
9. Centers for Disease Control and Prevention. CDC's Advisory Committee Recommends Human Papillomavirus Virus Vaccination. *http://www.cdc.gov/od/oc/media/pressrel/r060629.htm*.
10. Meckstroth KR. Physical examination before initiating hormonal contraception: What is necessary? Am Fam Physician 2006;74:32–33.
11. Roddy RE, Zekeng L, Ryan KA, et al. A controlled trial of nonoxynol 9 film to reduce male-to-female transmission of sexually transmitted diseases. N Engl J Med 1998;339:504–510.
12. Van Damme L, Ramjee G, Alary M, et al. Effectiveness of COL-1492, a nonoxynol-9 vaginal gel, on HIV-1 transmission in female sex workers: A randomised controlled trial. Lancet 2002;360:971–977.
13. World Health Organization. Medical Eligibility Criteria for Contraceptive Use, 3rd ed. 2004, *http://www.who.int/reproductive-health/publications/mec/index.htm*.
14. Anonymous. Choice of contraceptives. Treat Guidel Med Lett 2004;2:55–62.
15. Lybrel package insert. *http://www.wyeth.com/content/ShowLabeling.asp?id=489*.
16. Petitti DB. Combination estrogen-progestin oral contraceptives. N Engl J Med 2003;349:1443–1450.
17. Use of hormonal contraception in women with coexisting medical conditions. ACOG Practice Bulletin No 73. American College of Obstetricians and Gynecologists. Obstet Gynecol 2006;107:1453–1472.
18. Petri M, Kim MY, Kalunian KC, et al. Combined oral contraceptives in women with systemic lupus erythematosus. N Engl J Med 2005;353:2550–2558.
19. Van Vliet HAAM, Grimes DA, Helmerhorst FM, Schulz KF. Biphasic versus monophasic oral contraceptives for contraception. Cochrane Database Syst Rev 2006;3:CD002032.
20. Van Vliet HAAM, Grimes DA, Helmerhorst FM, Schulz KF. Biphasic versus triphasic oral contraceptives for contraception. Cochrane Database Syst Rev 2006;3:CD003283.
21. Gallo MF, Lopez LM, Grimes DA, Schulz KF, Helmerhorst FM. Combination contraceptives: Effects on weight. Cochrane Database Syst Rev 2006;1:CD003987.
22. Lesnewski R, Prine L. Initiating hormonal contraception. Am Fam Physician 2006;71:105–12.
23. Truitt ST, Fraser AB, Grimes DA, et al. Combined hormonal versus nonhormonal versus progestin-only contraception in lactation. Cochrane Review Syst Rev 2003;3:CD003988.
24. Dickinson BD, Altman RD, Neilsen NH, Sterling ML. Drug interactions between oral contraceptives and antibiotics. Obstet Gynecol 2001;98:853–860.
25. Archer JS, Archer DF. Oral contraceptive efficacy and antibiotic interaction: A myth debunked. J Am Acad Dermatol 2002;46:917–923.
26. Ortho Evra Package Insert. *http://www.orthoevra.com/active/janus/en_US/assets/common/company/pi/orthoevra.pdf#zoom=100*.
27. Jick SS, Kaye JA, Russman S, Jick H. Risk of nonfatal venous thromboembolism in women using a contraceptive transdermal patch and oral contraceptives containing norgestimate and 35 mcg ethinyl estradiol. Contraception 2006;73:223–228.
28. Audet MC, Moreau M, Koltun WD, et al. Evaluation of contraceptive efficacy and cycle control of a transdermal contraceptive patch vs an oral contraceptive. A randomized controlled trial. JAMA 2001;285:2347–2354.
29. NuvaRing package insert. *http://www.nuvaring.com/Authfiles/Images/309_76063.pdf*.
30. Bjarnadottir RI, Tuppurainen M, Killick SR. Comparison of cycle control with a combined contraceptive vaginal ring and oral levonorgestrel/ethinyl estradiol. Am J Obstet Gynecol 2002;186:389–395.
31. Dieben T, Roumen F, Apter D. Efficacy, cycle control, and user acceptability of a novel combined contraceptive vaginal ring. Obstet Gynecol 2002;100:585–593.
32. Depo-Provera Contraceptive Injection package insert. *http://www.contracept.info/docs/depo-doctors.pdf*.
33. Depo-SubQ Provera 104 Package Insert. *http://www.pfizer.com/pfizer/download/uspi_depo_subq_provera.pdf*.
34. Jain J, Jakimiuk AJ, Bode PR, et al. Contraceptive efficacy and safety of DMPA-SC. Contraception 2004;70:269–275.
35. Society for Adolescent Medicine. Depot medroxyprogesterone acetate and bone mineral density in adolescents: The Black Box Warning: A position paper of the Society for Adolescent Medicine. J Adolesc Health 2006;39:296–301.
36. WHO statement on hormonal contraception and bone health. 2005, *http://www.who.int/reproductive-health/family_planning/docs/hormonal_contraception_bone_health.pdf*.
37. Anonymous. A new progestin implant for long-term contraception. Med Lett Drugs Ther 2006;48:83–84.
38. Implanon package insert. *http://www.implanon-usa.com/authfiles/images/543_174733.pdf*.
39. Jensen JT. Contraceptive and therapeutic effects of the levonorgestrel intrauterine system: An overview. Obstet Gynecol Surv 2005;60:604–612.
40. Grimes DA. Intrauterine device and upper-genital-tract infection. Lancet 2000;356:1013–1019.
41. American College of Obstetricians and Gynecologists (ACOG). Emergency contraception. Washington (DC): American College of Obstetricians and Gynecologists (ACOG). 2005, *http://www.guideline.gov/summary/pdf.aspx?doc_id=9006&stat=1&string=*.
42. Westhoff C. Emergency contraception. N Engl J Med 2003:349:1830–1835.
43. Plan B package insert. *http://www.go2planb.com/PDF/PlanBPI.pdf*.
44. Von Hertzen H, Piaggo G, Ding J, et al. Low dose mifepristone and two regimens of levonorgestrel for emergency contraception: A WHO multicentre randomized trial. Lancet 2002;360:1803–1810.
45. FDA Approves Over-the-Counter Access for Plan B for Women 18 and Older. Prescription Remains Required for Those 17 and Under. *http://www.fda.gov/bbs/topics/NEWS/2006/NEW01436.html*.
46. Rodrigues I, Grou F, Joly J. Effectiveness of emergency contraceptive pills between 72 and 120 hours after unprotected sexual intercourse. Am J Obstet Gynecol 2001;184:531–537.
47. Chiou CF, Trussell J, Reyes E, et al. Economic analysis of contraceptives for women. Contraception 2003;68:3–10.

CHAPTER 83

Menstruation-Related Disorders

ELENA M. UMLAND, LARA C. WEINSTEIN, AND EDWARD M. BUCHANAN

KEY CONCEPTS

1. Unrecognized pregnancy is the most common cause of amenorrhea. A urine pregnancy test should be one of the first steps in evaluating this disorder.
2. For hypoestrogenic conditions associated with primary and secondary amenorrhea, estrogen (along with a progestin) is provided.
3. Causes of menorrhagia can be divided into systemic disorders and specific uterine abnormalities.
4. Pregnancy, including intrauterine pregnancy, ectopic pregnancy, and miscarriage, must be at the top of the differential diagnosis for any woman presenting with heavy menses.
5. The reduction in menorrhagia-related blood loss with use of nonsteroidal antiinflammatory drugs and oral contraceptives is directly proportional to the amount of pretreatment blood loss.
6. Intrauterine devices (IUDs) are considered therapeutic options in a variety of menstruation-related disorders. Guidelines from the American College of Obstetricians and Gynecologists indicate that both nulliparous and multiparous women at low risk of sexually transmitted diseases are good candidates for IUD use.
7. Anovulatory bleeding is the standard terminology used to describe bleeding from the uterine endometrium as a result of a dysfunctioning menstrual system, specifically excluding an anatomic lesion of the uterus.
8. Polycystic ovarian syndrome can present as a variety of menstruation disorders, including amenorrhea, menorrhagia, and anovulatory bleeding. Although its definition continues to evolve, it is generally considered to be a disorder of androgen excess that often includes polycystic ovarian morphology and ovulatory dysfunction.
9. Use of metformin and the thiazolidinediones for anovulatory bleeding associated with polycystic ovarian syndrome is beneficial not only for anovulatory bleeding and fertility but also for improving glucose tolerance and decreasing overall, long-term cardiovascular risk.
10. The selective serotonin reuptake inhibitors are first-line pharmacologic treatment options for premenstrual dysphoric disorder.

Learning objectives, review questions, and other resources can be found at **www.pharmacotherapyonline.com.**

Problems related to the menstrual cycle are exceedingly common in women of reproductive age. This chapter discusses the most frequently encountered menstruation-related difficulties: amenorrhea, menorrhagia, anovulatory bleeding, dysmenorrhea, premenstrual syndrome (PMS), and premenstrual dysphoric disorder (PMDD). The need for effective treatments of these disorders stems from their impact on any or all of the following: a reduced quality of life, negative effects on reproductive health, and potential for long-term detrimental health effects, such as osteoporosis in the case of amenorrhea and cardiovascular disease in the case of polycystic ovarian syndrome (PCOS).

AMENORRHEA

Amenorrhea is traditionally described as either primary or secondary in nature. Primary amenorrhea is the absence of menses by age 16 years in the presence of normal secondary sexual development or the absence of menses by age 14 in the absence of normal secondary sexual development. Secondary amenorrhea is the absence of menses for three cycles or for 6 months in a previously menstruating woman. In clinical practice there is a significant amount of overlap between the two. The initial evaluation of amenorrhea often is the same, regardless of age of onset, except in unusual clinical situations.[1]

EPIDEMIOLOGY

The incidence of primary amenorrhea is less than 0.1% in the general population. Secondary amenorrhea, on the other hand, has an incidence of 0.7% to 4% in the general population and occurs more frequently in women younger than 25 years with a history of menstrual irregularities.[2]

ETIOLOGY

1 Unrecognized pregnancy is the most common cause of amenorrhea. A urine pregnancy test should be one of the first steps in evaluating this disorder. In organizing an approach to diagnosis and treatment, it is helpful to consider the organs involved in the menstrual cycle, which include the uterus, ovaries, anterior pituitary, and hypothalamus.

After excluding pregnancy, the five most common causes of secondary amenorrhea, in descending order of prevalence, are hypothalamic suppression (33%), chronic anovulation (28%), hyperprolactinemia (14%), ovarian failure (12%), and uterine disorders (7%).[3]

PATHOPHYSIOLOGY

Each organ in the hypothalamic–pituitary–ovarian–uterine axis must be considered in determining the etiology and pathophysiology of amenorrhea. Beginning with the uterus/outflow tract and pro-

TABLE 83-1 Pathophysiology of Selected Menstrual Bleeding Disorders

Organ System	Condition	Pathophysiology/Laboratory Findings
Amenorrhea		
Uterus	Asherman's syndrome	Postcurettage/postsurgical uterine adhesions
	Congenital uterine abnormalities	Abnormal uterine development
Ovaries	Turner's syndrome	Lack of ovarian follicles
	Gonadal dysgenesis	Other genetic abnormalities
	Premature ovarian failure	Early loss of follicles
	Chemotherapy/radiation	Gonadal toxins
Anterior pituitary	Pituitary prolactin-secreting adenoma	↑ Prolactin suppresses HPO axis
	Hypothyroidism	TRH causes ↑ prolactin, other abnormalities
	Medication (antipsychotics, verapamil)	↑ Prolactin suppresses HPO axis
Hypothalamus	"Functional" hypothalamic amenorrhea	↓ Pulsatile GnRH secretion in the absence of other abnormalities
	Eating disorder	↓ Pulsatile GnRH secretion, ↓ FSH and LH secondary to weight loss
	Exercise	↓ Pulsatile GnRH secretion, ↓ FSH and LH secondary to low body fat
	Anovulation/PCOS	Asynchronous gonadotropin and estrogen production, abnormal endometrial growth
Anovulatory bleeding		
Physiologic causes	Adolescence	Immaturity of the HPO axis: no LH surge
	Perimenopause	Declining ovarian function
Pathologic causes	Hyperandrogenic anovulation (PCOS)	Hyperandrogenism: high testosterone, high LH, hyperinsulinemia, and insulin resistance
	Hypothalamic dysfunction (physical or emotional stress, exercise, weight loss)	Suppression of pulsatile GnRH secretion and estrogen deficiency: low LH, low FSH
	Hyperprolactinemia (pituitary gland tumor, psychiatric medications)	High prolactin
	Hypothyroidism	High TSH
	Premature ovarian failure	High FSH
Menorrhagia		
Hematologic	von Willebrand's disease	Factor VII defect causing impaired platelet adhesion and increased bleeding time
	Idiopathic thrombocytopenic purpura	Decrease in circulating platelets, can be acute or chronic
Hepatic	Cirrhosis	Decreased estrogen metabolism, underlying coagulopathy
Endocrine	Hypothyroidism	Alterations in HPO axis
Uterine	Fibroids	Alteration of endometrium, changes in uterine contractility
	Adenomyosis	Alteration of endometrium, changes in uterine contractility
	Endometrial polyps	Alteration of endometrium
	Gynecologic cancers	Various dysplastic alterations of endometrium, uterus, cervix

FSH, follicle-stimulating hormone; GnRH, gonadotropin-releasing hormone; HPO, hypothalamic–pituitary–ovarian axis; LH, luteinizing hormone; PCOS, polycystic ovary disease; TSH, thyroid stimulating hormone; TRH, thyrotropin-releasing hormone.
Data from references 1, 2, 4, and 5.

gressing caudally will result in a comprehensive differential diagnosis. Table 83–1 lists the pathophysiology of amenorrhea relative to the organ system(s) involved as well as the specific condition(s) that results in amenorrhea.

Uterus/Outflow Tract

For menstruation to occur, a uterus, functional endometrium, and patent vagina must be present. Several anatomic abnormalities of the female genital tract may cause amenorrhea. If primary amenorrhea is the presenting symptom, a congenital anomaly such as imperforate hymen or uterine agenesis may be present and often can be determined by physical examination. In the case of secondary amenorrhea, an acquired condition of the genital tract, such as Asherman's syndrome or cervical stenosis, is more likely.

Ovaries

Normal ovarian function is critical for menstruation to occur. The ovaries must respond appropriately to follicle-stimulating hormone (FSH) and luteinizing hormone (LH) by secreting estrogen and progesterone in proper sequence to influence growth and shedding of the endometrium (Fig. 83–1).

Premature ovarian failure occurs when no viable follicles remain in the ovaries. As in menopause, estrogen will not be produced in sufficient quantity to stimulate endometrial growth in the absence of follicles. In a woman younger than 30 years, amenorrhea due to premature ovarian failure may be the result of genetic anomalies.[1]

The ovaries may play a role in amenorrhea through anovulation. Ovulation is required for the follicle (an estrogen-secreting body) to become a corpus luteum (a progesterone-secreting body). Without ovulation, the proper sequence of estrogen production, progesterone production, and estrogen/progesterone withdrawal will not occur. This can result in amenorrhea. Anovulation can occur secondary to thyroid disease, androgen excess (PCOS), or chronic illness.

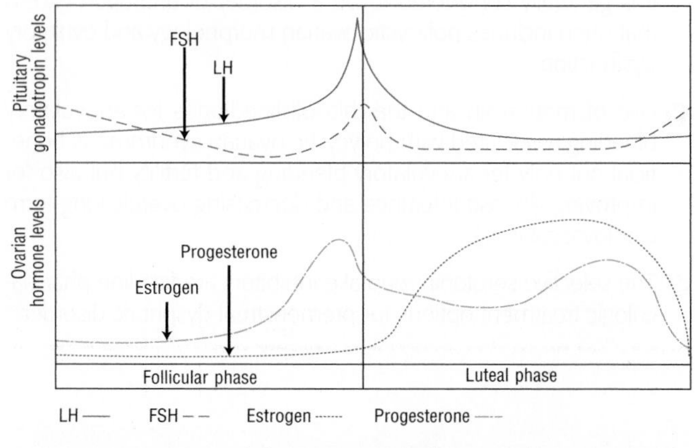

FIGURE 83-1. Hormonal fluctuations with the normal menstrual cycle. *(Courtesy of Hatcher RA, Nelson AL, Zieman M, et al. A Pocket Guide to Managing Contraception. Tiger GA: Bridging the Gap Foundation, 2003:1-146. This figure may be reproduced at no cost to the reader.)*

Pituitary Gland

The anterior pituitary gland secretes FSH and LH in sequential fashion in response to stimulation by the hypothalamus and a complex feedback mechanism from the ovaries. Normal secretion of FSH and LH can be altered by several endocrinologic and iatrogenic conditions, including thyroid disease, hyperprolactinemia, and dopaminergic drug administration.

Hypothalamus

The hypothalamus secretes cyclic gonadotropin-releasing hormone (GnRH), which causes the pituitary to produce FSH and LH. A disruption of this cyclic excretion will interrupt the hormonal cascade that results in normal menstruation. Anorexia nervosa, bulimia, intense exercise, and stress may cause hypothalamic amenorrhea.

CLINICAL PRESENTATION OF AMENORRHEA

General

- Although patients may be concerned about cessation of menses and implications for fertility, patients are generally not in acute distress.

Symptoms

- Patient will note cessation of menses.
- Patients may complain of infertility, vaginal dryness, or decreased libido.

Signs

- Cessation of menses for more than 6 months in women with established menstruation, absence of menses by age 16 in the presence of normal secondary sexual development, or absence of menses by age 14 in the absence of normal secondary sexual development
- Recent significant weight loss or weight gain
- Presence of acne, hirsutism, hair loss, or acanthosis nigrans may suggest androgen excess

Laboratory Tests

- Pregnancy test
- Thyroid-stimulating hormone
- Prolactin
- If PCOS is suspected, consider free or total testosterone, 17-hydroxyprogesterone, fasting glucose, fasting lipid panel.
- If suspect premature ovarian failure, consider FSH, LH.

Other Diagnostic Tests

- Progesterone challenge
- Pelvic ultrasound to evaluate for polycystic ovaries

TREATMENT

Just as the causes of amenorrhea are varied, so are the nonpharmacologic and pharmacologic treatment options.

Desired Outcome

Therapeutic modalities for amenorrhea are used to restore the normal menstrual cycle. Treatment goals include preservation of bone density, prevention of bone loss, and restoration of ovulation, thus improving fertility as desired. Amenorrhea resulting from hypoestrogenism may affect quality of life via induction of hot flashes (premature ovarian failure), dyspareunia, and, in prepubertal females, lack of secondary sexual characteristics and absence of menarche. Treatment of these patients would be targeted at reversing these effects.

General Approach to Treatment

The overall success of any intervention to treat amenorrhea is dependent on proper identification of the underlying cause(s) of the disorder. Once the cause is identified, the appropriate intervention(s) can be made. For patients experiencing amenorrhea secondary to hypoestrogenic states, a diet rich in calcium and vitamin D is essential to avoid negative impact on bone health.

Nonpharmacologic Therapy

Nonpharmacologic therapy for amenorrhea varies depending upon the underlying cause. Amenorrhea secondary to anorexia may respond to weight gain. In young women for whom excessive exercise is an underlying cause, a reduction in exercise is recommended.

Pharmacologic Therapy

❷ For hypoestrogenic conditions associated with primary or secondary amenorrhea, estrogen (along with a progestin) is provided. It can be administered in the form of an oral contraceptive (OC), conjugated equine estrogen, or estradiol patch. The purpose of estrogen therapy in this patient population is twofold: to reduce the risk of osteoporosis and to improve quality of life.[7,8] Table 83–2 lists a variety of therapeutic agents for treatment of amenorrhea, including recommended doses. Figure 83–2 illustrates a treatment algorithm for management of amenorrhea.

If hyperprolactinemia is identified as the cause of amenorrhea, use of bromocriptine or cabergoline, dopamine agonists, results in a reduction in prolactin concentrations and the resumption of menses. Bromocriptine requires multiple doses per day, but cabergoline is dosed twice weekly. Bromocriptine has been observed in head-to-head clinical trials to be less effective in normalizing prolactin levels and has a higher incidence of adverse events leading to treatment discontinuation compared to cabergoline.[15,16]

Amenorrhea related to anovulation resulting from PCOS may respond to agents that reduce insulin resistance. Metformin and the thiazolidinediones for this purpose are discussed in the section on anovulatory bleeding.

Progestins have long been used to induce withdrawal bleeding in women with secondary amenorrhea. Several factors predict the efficacy of progesterone for this purpose.[10] These factors include estrogen concentrations ≥35 pg/mL and endometrial thickness (the greater the thickness, the greater the amount of withdrawal bleeding).

The efficacy of progestins for secondary amenorrhea varies depending upon the formulation used. Progesterone in oil administered intramuscularly results in withdrawal bleeding in 70% of treated patients, whereas oral medroxyprogesterone acetate (MPA) induces withdrawal bleeding in 95% of treated patients.[10] Table 83–2 identifies the types and doses of progesterones used for treatment of secondary amenorrhea. Figure 83–2 illustrates when to consider progesterone use for amenorrhea treatment.

Special Populations Amenorrhea in the adolescent population is of particular concern because this is the time in the female life cycle when peak bone mass is achieved. The cause of amenorrhea, whether primary or secondary, must be promptly identified in this population, as amenorrhea and its related hypoestrogenism contribute negatively to bone development. In addition to treating or eliminating the underlying cause of the amenorrhea, ensuring that the patient is receiving adequate amounts of calcium and vitamin D is imperative. Estrogen replacement, typically via an OC, is important.

Drug class information Table 83–3 identifies the significant pharmacologic properties, common adverse events, and clinically significant drug–drug and drug–food interactions of the agents used for management of amenorrhea.

TABLE 83-2 Therapeutic Agents for Selected Menstrual Disorders

Specific Menstrual Disorder(s)	Agent(s)	Dose Recommended
Amenorrhea (primary or secondary)	CEE	0.625–1.25 mg by mouth daily on days 1–25 of the cycle[8]
	Ethinyl estradiol patch	50 mcg/24 hours[10]
	Combination OC	30–40 mcg formulations[7]
Amenorrhea (secondary)	Oral MPA	5–10 mg by mouth on days 14–25 of the cycle[8]
Amenorrhea related to hyperprolactinemia	Bromocriptine[15,16]	2.5 mg by mouth 2–3 times daily
	Cabergoline[15,16]	0.25 mg by mouth 2 times weekly (maximum 1 mg by mouth 2 times weekly)
Anovulatory bleeding	Combination OC	Optimal dose unknown[5]
Dysmenorrhea	Combination OC	Less than 35 mcg formulations + norgestrel or levonorgestrel[11]; use of extended-cycle formulations is beneficial for this indication
	Depo MPA	150 mg intramuscularly every 12 weeks
	Levonorgestrel IUD[12]	20 mcg released daily
	NSAIDs (any are acceptable); the most commonly studied/cited are included in this table	Diclofenac 50 mg by mouth 3 times daily; ibuprofen 800 mg by mouth 3 times daily; mefenamic acid 500 mg by mouth as a loading dose, then 250 mg by mouth up to 4 times daily as needed[9]
		Naproxen 550-mg loading dose by mouth started 1–2 days prior to menses followed by 275 mg by mouth every 6–12 hours as needed[11]
		Treatment should begin 1–2 days prior to the suspected onset of menses[9]
Menorrhagia	Combination OC	Optimal dose unknown
	Levonorgestrel IUD	20 mcg released daily
	Oral MPA	5–10 mg by mouth on days 5–26 of the cycle or during the luteal phase[12]
	NSAIDs	Doses as recommended for dysmenorrhea may be used; therapy should be initiated with the onset of menses[12]
PCOS-related amenorrhea and/or anovulatory bleeding	Clomiphene[5]	50 mg by mouth daily for 5 days starting 3–5 days after the start of menses; dose can be increased in 50 mg increments to a maximum dose of 250 mg daily
	Depo MPA	150 mg intramuscularly every 12 weeks
	Oral MPA	10 mg by mouth for 10 days[5]
	Metformin	1,500–2,000 mg by mouth daily[15]
	Thiazolidinediones (pioglitazone, rosiglitazone)[5]	Pioglitazone 15–45 mg by mouth daily; rosiglitazone 4–8 mg by mouth daily
PMDD	Clomipramine[14]	25–75 mg by mouth daily taken either continuously or only during the luteal phase
	Drospirenone	3 mg (+ 30 mcg ethinyl estradiol) by mouth on days 1–21 of the menstrual cycle[13]
	Leuprolide	3.75 mg intramuscularly[14]
	SSRIs (citalopram, escitalopram, fluoxetine, fluvoxamine, paroxetine, sertraline)	Citalopram 10–30 mg; escitalopram 10–20 mg[59]; fluoxetine 10–20 mg; fluvoxamine 50 mg; paroxetine 10–30 mg; sertraline 25–150 mg; all agents are given by mouth daily and can be dosed either continuously or during the luteal phase only[14]

CEE, conjugated equine estrogen; IUD, intrauterine device; MPA, medroxyprogesterone acetate; NSAID, nonsteroidal antiinflammatory drug; OC, oral contraceptive; PCOS, polycystic ovarian syndrome; PMDD, premenstrual dysphoric disorder; SSRI, selective serotonin reuptake inhibitors.
Data from references 5 and 7–16.

PHARMACOECONOMIC CONSIDERATIONS

The largest price gap among agents used for management of amenorrhea occurs when comparing the dopamine agonists bromocriptine and cabergoline in the treatment of hyperprolactinemia. Cabergoline is slightly more effective, with fewer side effects and less frequent dosing, but its monthly cost is significantly greater than that of bromocriptine. Given this, it is reasonable to reserve its use for patients who do not achieve treatment success with bromocriptine or for whom the side effects of bromocriptine are responsible for drug discontinuation.

EVALUATION OF THERAPEUTIC OUTCOMES

Table 83–4 lists the expected outcomes and specific monitoring parameters for treatment modalities used in the management of amenorrhea.

MENORRHAGIA

The traditional definition of menorrhagia is menstrual blood loss greater than 80 mL per cycle. This definition has been questioned because of several factors, including difficulty quantifying menstrual loss in clinical practice. Additionally, many women with "heavy menses" but blood loss less than 80 mL merit treatment consideration because of problems with flow containment, unpredictably heavy flow days, or other associated symptoms.[21,28]

EPIDEMIOLOGY

Rates of menorrhagia in healthy women range from 9% to 14%.[4]

ETIOLOGY

❸ Causes of menorrhagia can be divided into systemic disorders and specific uterine abnormalities. ❹ Pregnancy, including intrauterine pregnancy, ectopic pregnancy, and miscarriage, must be at the top of the differential diagnosis for any woman presenting with heavy menses. In several studies of adolescents with acute menorrhagia, underlying bleeding disorders accounted for 3% to 13% of emergency room presentations. Although von Willebrand's disease has an incidence of 1% in the general population,[29] its prevalence in women with menorrhagia may be as high as 20%.[30] It initially may present as heavy menses in the adolescent.[29] Hypothyroidism also may be associated with heavy menses. Specific uterine causes of menorrhagia are more common in older childbearing women and include fibroids, adenomyosis, endometrial polyps, and gynecologic malignancies.

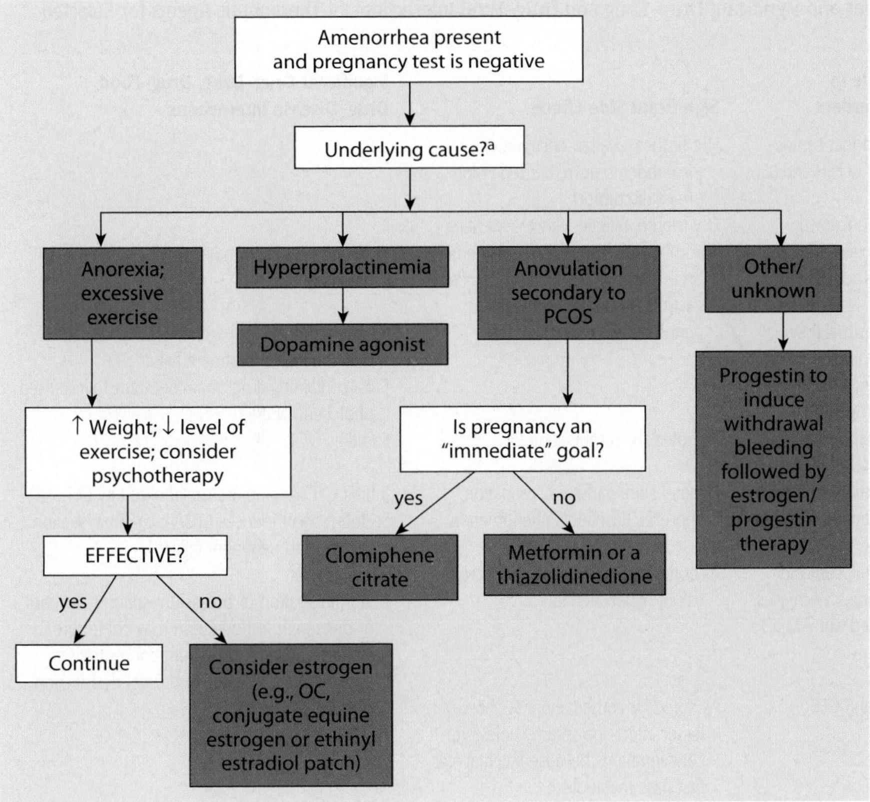

FIGURE 83-2. Treatment algorithm for amenorrhea. [a]Regardless of cause, adequate calcium and vitamin D intake must be ensured. (OC, oral contraceptive; PCOS, polycystic ovarian syndrome.)

PATHOPHYSIOLOGY

Table 83–1 lists the pathophysiology of menorrhagia relative to the organ system(s) involved and the specific conditions that result in menorrhagia.

CLINICAL PRESENTATION OF MENORRHAGIA

General

- Patient may or may not be in acute distress.

Symptoms

- Patients may complain of heavy/prolonged menstrual flow. They also may have signs of fatigue and lightheadedness in cases of severe blood loss. These symptoms may or may not occur with dysmenorrhea.

Signs

- Orthostasis, tachycardia, and pallor may be noted, especially in cases of significant acute blood loss.

Laboratory Tests

- Complete blood count and ferritin levels; hemoglobin and hematocrit results may be low.
- If the history dictates, testing may be performed to identify coagulation disorder(s) as a cause.

Other Diagnostic Tests

- Pelvic ultrasound
- Pelvic magnetic resonance imaging
- Papanicolaou (Pap) smear
- Endometrial biopsy
- Hysteroscopy
- Sonohysterogram

TREATMENT

Initial treatment choice for menorrhagia is influenced by whether or not the woman desires to become pregnant.

Desired Outcome

Menorrhagia therapy should reduce menstrual blood flow, improve the patient's quality of life, and defer the need for surgical intervention. Table 83–2 lists the various agents and their recommended dosing for management of menorrhagia. Figure 83–3 illustrates how to decide which treatment(s) to use and when.

General Approach to Treatment

Several treatment options exist for menorrhagia. The initial and, if needed, subsequent treatment options should be thoughtfully chosen in an effort to avoid the need for surgery.

Nonpharmacologic Therapy

Nonpharmacologic interventions for menorrhagia include surgical interventions that are generally reserved for patients who do not respond to pharmacologic treatment. These interventions may vary from conservative endometrial ablation to hysterectomy.[31]

Pharmacologic Therapy

Among the agents used to treat menorrhagia, the nonsteroidal antiinflammatory drugs (NSAIDs) have the advantage of being taken only during menses. NSAID use is associated with a 20% to 50% reduction in blood loss in 75% of treated women.[12] In some patients, as much as an 80% reduction in blood loss has been observed.[12]

For women who wish to avoid pregnancy, use of OCs is beneficial for menorrhagia and can be considered. A 43% to 53% reduction in menstrual blood loss has been observed in 68% of menorrhagia patients treated with OCs containing ≥35 mcg of estradiol.[12] ❺ The reduction in

TABLE 83-3 Significant Pharmacologic Properties and Significant Drug–Drug and Drug–Food Interactions of Therapeutic Agents for Selected Menstrual Disorders

Therapeutic Agent/ Drug Class	Mechanism of Action/Role in Particular Menstrual Disorders	Significant Side Effects	Significant Drug–Drug, Drug–Food, Drug–Disease Interactions
Clomiphene	Estrogen receptor antagonist that contributes to a compensatory ↑ in FSH and LH to induce ovulation	Hot flashes, ovarian enlargement, thromboembolism, blurred vision, breast discomfort	
Clomipramine	Exact mechanism in PMDD unknown	Dry mouth, fatigue, vertigo, sweating	
Combination OCs	Exogenous estrogen and progesterone that suppresses FSH and LH production and thus inhibits ovulation Can be used to reduce menstrual flow (menorrhagia, dysmenorrhea), and control menstrual cycle (anovulatory bleeding secondary to hypoestrogenism)	Thromboembolism, breast enlargement, breast tenderness, bloating, nausea, gastrointestinal upset, headache, peripheral edema	St. John's wort contributes to altered menstrual bleeding Rifampin induces estrogen metabolism, possibly contributing to treatment failure Sulfa-containing drugs may contribute to increased photosensitivity
CEE	Estrogen replacement for hypoestrogenic states leading to anovulatory bleeding	As noted for combination OC	Same as OCs
Dopamine agonists (bromocriptine, cabergoline)	Suppresses prolactin production from pituitary tumors such that resumption of normal FSH and LH production occurs	Hypotension, nausea, constipation, anorexia, Raynaud's phenomenon	Inhibit CYP3A4 and are metabolized by CYP3A4[17] St. John's wort induces CP3A4; coadministration may lead to treatment failure
Drospirenone-containing OCs	Progesterone with antimineralocorticoid and antiandrogenic properties; decreases emotional lability associated with PMDD	As noted for combination OC; increased risk of hyperkalemia	Same as OCs Coadministration of potassium-sparing diuretics or diets high in potassium may contribute to increased serum potassium concentrations, particularly in women with renal dysfunction
Ethinyl estradiol transdermal patch	Same as combination OCs and CEE	As noted for combination OC; however, lesser effects on serum cholesterol concentrations because patch avoids first-pass metabolism	Same as OCs
Leuprolide	GnRH agent that contributes to suppression of FSH and LH and ultimately a reduction in estrogen and progesterone, inhibiting the normal menstrual cycle/hormonal fluctuations	Hot flashes, night sweats, headache, nausea	
Levonorgestrel-containing IUD	Suppresses FSH and LH and ultimately estrogen and progesterone, inhibiting the usual growth of the endometrium	Irregular menses, amenorrhea	
MPA (oral and depot)	Suppresses FSH and LH and ultimately estrogen and progesterone, inhibiting the usual growth of the endometrium	Edema, anorexia, depression, insomnia, weight gain or loss, increase in serum total and LDL cholesterol, may reduce HDL cholesterol	
Metformin	Inhibits hepatic glucose production and increases sensitivity of tissues to insulin, thus reducing insulin resistance	Anorexia, nausea, vomiting, diarrhea, flatulence, lactic acidosis (rare)	IV contrast dye may increase the risk of lactic acidosis; stop metformin 1 day prior and restart when renal function is normal and stabilized following the IV dye
NSAIDs	Inhibits prostaglandin release that occurs with menses, thus reducing inflammatory response contributing to dysmenorrhea	Gastrointestinal upset, stomach ulcer, nausea, vomiting, heartburn, indigestion, rash, dizziness	
SSRIs	Exact mechanism in PMDD unknown	Sexual dysfunction (reduced libido, anorgasmia), insomnia, sedation, hypersomnia, nausea, diarrhea	
Thiazolidinediones	Increases peripheral tissue sensitivity to insulin, thus reducing insulin resistance	Weight gain, increase in total, LDL, and HDL cholesterol, edema, headache, fatigue, hepatic injury (rare)	
Venlafaxine	Exact mechanism in PMDD unknown		

CEE, conjugated equine estrogen; FSH, follicle-stimulating hormone; GnRH, gonadotropin-releasing hormone; HDL, high-density lipoprotein; IUD, intrauterine device; LDL, low-density lipoprotein; LH, luteinizing hormone; MPA, medroxyprogesterone acetate; NSAID, nonsteroidal antiinflammatory drug; OC, oral contraceptive; PMDD, premenstrual dysphoric disorder; SSRI, selective serotonin reuptake inhibitor.
Data from references 7, 9, 12, 14, 15, and 17–20.

menorrhagia-related blood loss with use of NSAIDs and OCs is directly proportional to the amount of pretreatment blood loss.[12]

Menorrhagia also can be treated with the levonorgestrel-releasing intrauterine device (IUD). This is a very effective treatment that has consistently reduced menstrual flow by at least 90%.[12,32] In particular, a reduction in blood loss by as much as 86% has been observed after 3 months of use and as much as 97% after 12 months.[33] Its use has also resulted in the postponement or cancellation of scheduled endometrial resection surgery or hysterectomy. Specifically, 60% of treated patients have been able to avoid hysterectomy.[32,34,35]

Progesterone therapy either during the luteal phase of the menstrual cycle or for 21 days, starting on day 5 after onset of menses, results in a 32% to 50% reduction in menstrual blood loss.[12] However, progesterone use has not been shown to be superior to other medical treatments, including the NSAIDs.[12] Progesterone use is not associated with any contraceptive benefit.[26]

TABLE 83-4 Expected Outcome Measures for Select Menstrual Bleeding Disorders

Menstrual Disorder	Expected Outcome Measures: Specific Monitoring Parameters and Frequency of Monitoring
Amenorrhea	Patient should return after one month of treatment to evaluate whether menses has resumed. Menses should resume within 1–2 months of therapy. If amenorrhea has been long-standing and secondary to a hypoestrogenic condition, preservation/improvement of BMD is warranted. A baseline BMD test may be desirable; repeat test no sooner than 1–2 years. If amenorrhea is secondary to high prolactin levels, serum prolactin levels should be measured at baseline and weekly with dosage increases until response (resumption of menses) is observed; consider discontinuation of therapy after 6–12 months of menses and serum prolactin concentrations have normalized. In young women who have primary amenorrhea, normal breast development should occur over a time frame of several months of therapy.
Menorrhagia	Amount of blood lost with menses should be reduced (monitor decline in number of times feminine hygiene products such as pads and tampons require changing during menses) as observed within 1–2 menstrual cycles of therapy. Patient should return for evaluation after one full menstrual cycle of therapy. Hemoglobin/hematocrit should be measured at baseline and within 3 months of beginning therapy. Annual gynecologic examination should be performed in women receiving hormonal agents for treatment of menorrhagia. Serum lipid concentrations should be measured within 3–6 months of starting the hormonal regimen and repeated per national lipid guidelines as appropriate. Blood pressure should be measured at baseline and within 4–6 weeks of beginning any hormonal agents; repeat blood pressure measurements per national hypertension guidelines as appropriate.
Anovulatory bleeding	Patients should return for follow up within 1 week to evaluate alleviation of acute bleeding when present. Acute severe bleeding should decline within 10 days of therapy onset. Ovulation, if desired, can be measured via daily basal body temperature evaluation, use of home ovulation predictor kits, and serum FSH/LH measurements at the time of suspected ovulation. If ovulation has not occurred after 2–3 months of initial clomiphene dosing, the dose can be increased in 50 mg increments. If resumption of ovulation is desired by women receiving metformin, the same monitoring parameters as noted for clomiphene can be used. Metformin may contribute to resumption of ovulation after 3–6 months of therapy. In women with PCOS, baseline and repeat measurements of blood pressure, serum lipids, and blood glucose should be taken per national guidelines to monitor for the development, presence, or progression of hypertension, hyperlipidemia, and diabetes. When OCs are used for control of abnormal uterine bleeding, improvement in the pattern of abnormal bleeding should occur within 1–2 menstrual cycles of therapy. Annual gynecologic examinations should be performed; serum lipid concentrations should be measured within 3–6 months of starting the OC and repeated per national lipid guidelines. Blood pressure should be measured at baseline and within 4–6 weeks of beginning any hormonal agents; repeat blood pressure measurements per national hypertension guidelines as appropriate.
Dysmenorrhea	Patient should return for evaluation of reduction in or absence of pelvic pain related to menses after 1–2 menstrual cycles of therapy. In addition, reduction in time lost from work/school and improved quality of life should be observed after a full 1–3 menstrual cycles of OC therapy. If NSAIDs are used, improvement in pain should be observed within hours of the dose.
PMDD	Reduction in or absence of initial symptoms and improved quality of life may be observed within 1–3 menstrual cycles of therapy. SSRIs have resulted in significant improvement after one cycle of treatment. If an OC containing drospirenone is used, serum potassium should be monitored within the first month of use if the woman is also receiving agents that predispose her to increased serum potassium concentrations. An annual gynecologic examination should be performed; serum lipid concentrations should be measured within 3–6 months of starting the OC and repeated per national lipid guidelines as appropriate. Blood pressure should be measured at baseline and within 4–6 weeks of beginning any hormonal agents; repeat blood pressure measurements per national hypertension guidelines as appropriate.

BMD, bone mineral density; FSH, follicle-stimulating hormone; LH, luteinizing hormone; NSAID, nonsteroidal antiinflammatory drug; OC, oral contraceptive; PCOS, polycystic ovary syndrome; PMDD, premenstrual dysphoric disorder; SSRI, selective serotonin reuptake inhibitor.
Data from references 4, 5, 18, and 21–27.

Drug Treatments of First Choice For women who have menorrhagia associated with ovulatory cycles and do not desire hormonal therapy and/or contraception, NSAIDs during menses is a reasonable choice, in the absence of any contraindications or gastrointestinal illnesses such as peptic ulcer disease or gastroesophageal reflux disease. This choice is convenient (only taken during menses) and comparatively inexpensive. For women who do desire contraception, it would be reasonable to start with either an OC or the levonorgestrel-releasing IUD. Either choice is acceptable for both nulligravid and multiparous women who desire a long-term reversible form of contraception.[32] Given cost-effectiveness data, the levonorgestrel-releasing IUD would be the best first-line choice for women desiring contraception.[36] Clinical trial data illustrate a higher failure rate with the OCs as the primary treatment method (62.5%) compared to the levonorgestrel-releasing IUD as the primary treatment method (34%).[36]

Alternative Drug Treatments Given their side effects, reduced efficacy compared to the first-line agents, and/or cost, use of oral progesterone and depot medroxyprogesterone acetate should be reserved. Tranexamic acid may be considered, in particular, as a treatment option for women with identified coagulopathies. In comparison to luteal phase oral progesterone, tranexamic acid results in a significantly greater reduction in menstrual blood loss and greater relief of patient-reported symptoms.[12]

Special Populations Although in the past it was believed that IUD use should be avoided in nulliparous women, the American College of Obstetricians and Gynecologists (ACOG) currently supports its use in such women who are at low risk for developing sexually transmitted diseases (see Clinical Controversy).[32] As such, any of the treatment options discussed could be used in any female presenting with menorrhagia.

Drug Class Information Table 83–3 identifies the significant pharmacologic properties, common adverse events, and clinically significant drug–drug and drug–food interactions of the agents used for management of menorrhagia.

PHARMACOECONOMIC CONSIDERATIONS

Use of the levonorgestrel-releasing IUD was observed to be the most cost effective compared to both surgical management and OCs in women who were naïve to OCs and women who had received OCs with or without a response.[36]

CLINICAL CONTROVERSY

Fear of pelvic inflammatory disease and subsequent infertility has been the primary reason why use of IUDs in nulliparous women has been considered controversial. ACOG guidelines state that any woman at low risk for contracting sexually transmitted diseases is a good candidate for IUD use.[32] ACOG specifically recommends the levonorgestrel IUD as a treatment option for idiopathic amenorrhea.[33] ❻ IUDs are considered therapeutic options for a variety of menstruation-related disorders.

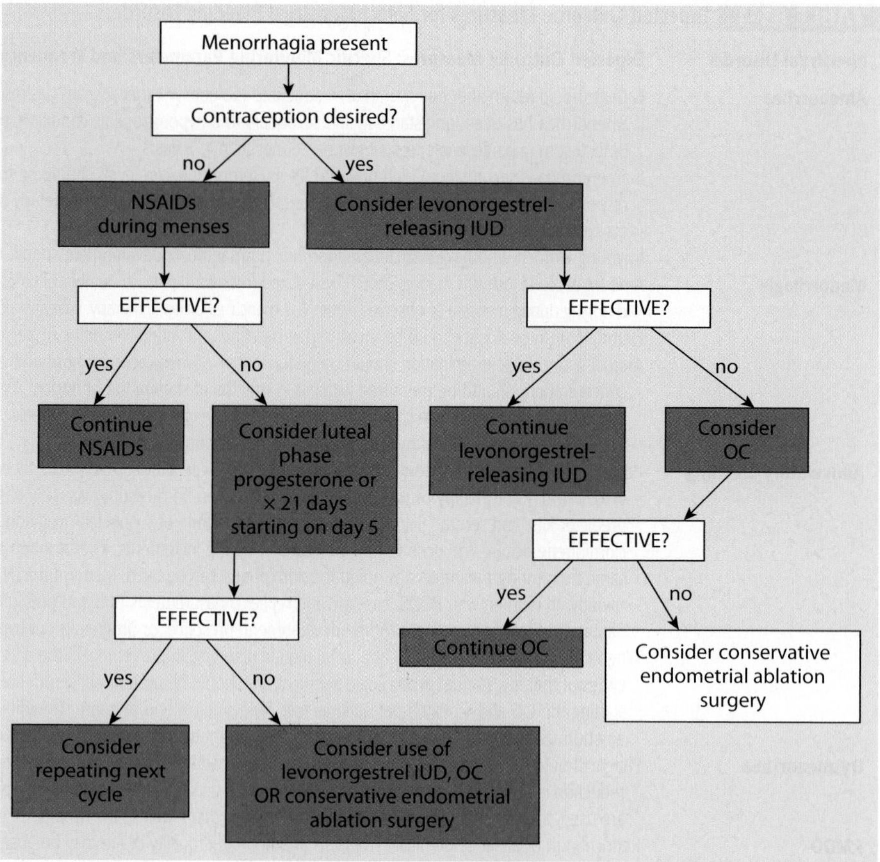

FIGURE 83-3. Treatment algorithm for menorrhagia. (IUD, intrauterine device; NSAIDs, nonsteroidal antiinflammatory drugs; OC, oral contraceptive.)

EVALUATION OF THERAPEUTIC OUTCOMES

Table 83–4 illustrates the expected outcomes and specific monitoring parameters for the treatment modalities used in the management of menorrhagia.

ANOVULATORY BLEEDING

❼ Anovulatory bleeding is the standard terminology used to describe bleeding from the uterine endometrium as a result of a dysfunctioning menstrual system, specifically excluding an anatomic lesion of the uterus.[1,22] Anovulatory bleeding also is referred to as *dysfunctional* or *irregular uterine bleeding.*

EPIDEMIOLOGY

Anovulatory bleeding is the most common form of noncyclic uterine bleeding.[22] PCOS is by far the most common cause, with prevalence rates ranging from 4% to 8% in various reports, depending on the diagnostic criteria used (e.g., PCOS-NIH[37] or PCOS-Rotterdam[38]).[1,5,39,40] In fact, PCOS is the most common endocrine abnormality among U.S. women of reproductive age.[41] ❽ PCOS can present as a variety of menstruation disorders, including amenorrhea, menorrhagia, and anovulatory bleeding. Although its definition continues to evolve, it is generally considered to be a disorder of androgen excess that often includes polycystic ovarian morphology and ovulatory dysfunction. It is a significant risk factor for the metabolic syndrome, type 2 diabetes, dyslipidemia, hypertension, and possibly cardiovascular disease.[42] Approximately 70% of ovulatory dysfunction cases in adult women are secondary to PCOS.[40] Other common causes in adult women include hyperprolactinemia (approximately 10% of cases), hypothalamic amenorrhea, also known as hypogonadotropic hypogonadism (approximately 10% of cases), and premature ovarian failure (approximately 10% of cases).[40] Thyroid disease can contribute to anovulation, and approximately 23% of hypothyroidism cases and 21% of hyperthyroidism cases are associated with menstrual irregularities.[43]

ETIOLOGY

When considering the etiology of anovulatory bleeding, it is helpful to consider the patient's age. All patients who present with abnormal bleeding should be evaluated for pregnancy. Most adolescents will experience physiologic anovulatory cycles in the first few years following menarche because their hypothalamic–pituitary–gonadal axis is still maturing. However, if an adolescent has not developed regular menstrual cycles within 5 years of menarche, further evaluation for the cause, such as PCOS, should be considered.[44] Anovulatory cycles may "unmask" an underlying bleeding disorder. When irregular menses is associated with significant bleeding, it is important to consider an inherited bleeding disorder as the cause, especially in adolescence.[22,45] Women who experience anovulation in their reproductive years should be evaluated for pathologic causes, including PCOS, thyroid dysfunction, hyperprolactinemia, primary pituitary disease, premature ovarian failure, hypothalamic dysfunction, disordered eating, adrenal disease, and androgen-producing tumors. Women in their perimenopausal years may experience "physiologic" anovulatory cycles because of intermittently declining estrogen levels. Regardless of age, evaluation for endometrial hyperplasia and/or endometrial cancer should be considered any time a woman experiences excessive bleeding with anovulatory cycles. When considering the etiology of anovulation, it is not unusual for several conditions to coexist (e.g., PCOS and hypothyroidism), each contributing to the woman's constellation of symptoms. All common etiologies should be considered when beginning an evaluation for anovulation.[1]

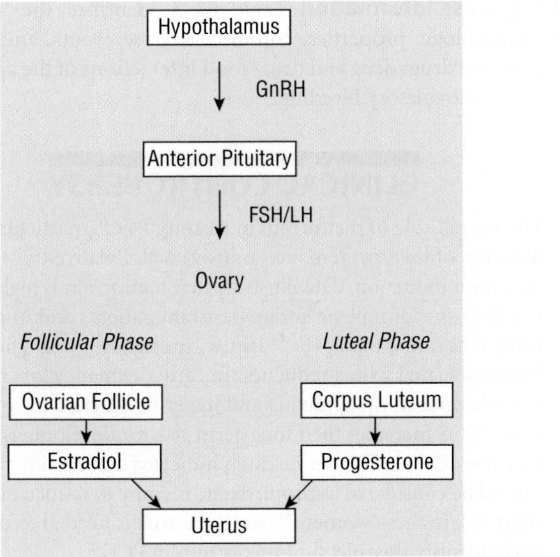

FIGURE 83-4. Summary of the normal menstrual cycle. (FSH, follicle-stimulating hormone; GnRH, gonadotropin-releasing hormone; LH, luteinizing hormone.)

PATHOPHYSIOLOGY

Normal menstrual cycles occur through a complex interaction of the hypothalamus, pituitary gland, ovaries, and endometrium (Fig. 83–4). In an ovulatory cycle, the ovary produces a mature, estrogen-secreting follicle in response to FSH release from the pituitary. The endometrium proliferates under the influence of this estrogen production. At a critical level of estrogen concentration, the pituitary is induced to produce an "LH surge," which creates a cascade of events in the ovaries, culminating in ovulation. Upon release of the oocyte, the follicle becomes a progesterone-producing corpus luteum. The endometrium "organizes" into secretory endometrium in the presence of adequate progesterone. If conception and implantation do not occur, involution of the corpus luteum causes a decline in estrogen and progesterone leading to predictable, organized menstrual flow as the endometrium sloughs.

If ovulation does not occur, progesterone will not be produced, and the endometrium will continue to proliferate in an "unorganized" fashion under the influence of continued estrogen production. Eventually the endometrium will become so thick that it cannot be supported by continued estrogen production. This results in unorganized, sporadic sloughing of the endometrium, characteristic of the unpredictable and heavy bleeding of anovulation. Anovulation can be caused by several etiologies. In adolescence, hypothalamic–pituitary axis immaturity contributes to the absence of the LH surge required for ovulation. In the anorexic patient, the hypothalamus loses much of its pulsatile GnRH release, leading to production of low levels of FSH and LH, enough for estrogen production but not enough to induce ovulation.

CLINICAL PRESENTATION OF ANOVULATORY BLEEDING

General

- Patients may or may not be in acute distress.

Symptoms

- Irregular, heavy, or prolonged vaginal bleeding, perimenopausal symptoms (hot flashes, nights sweats, vaginal dryness.)

Signs

- Acne, hirsutism, obesity

Laboratory Tests

- If PCOS is suspected, consider free or total testosterone, fasting glucose, fasting lipid panel.
- If perimenopause is suspected, measure FSH.
- Thyroid-stimulating hormone

Other Diagnostic Tests

- If the patient is older than 35 years, endometrial biopsy
- Pelvic ultrasound to evaluate for polycystic ovaries
- If perimenopause is suspected, measure FSH.

TREATMENT

The optimal treatment choice for anovulatory bleeding depends on accurate identification of the cause(s). As such, the treatment options for anovulatory bleeding are wide and varied.

Desired Outcome

The need to control excessive bleeding in the short term is paramount. The long-term goals of therapy include preventing future episodes of noncyclic bleeding, decreasing the complications of anovulation (e.g., osteopenia, infertility), and improving overall quality of life.[22] Table 83–2 identifies the agents used to manage anovulatory bleeding and their recommended doses.

General Approach to Treatment

Although the appropriate primary treatment choice for anovulatory bleeding depends on the accurate diagnosis of its cause and identification of desired outcomes, additional treatment may be necessary to manage other signs and symptoms. In addition to initiating treatment to resolve the anovulatory bleeding, underlying menorrhagia may need to be addressed.

Nonpharmacologic Therapy

Nonpharmacologic treatment options for anovulatory bleeding depend on the underlying cause. In a woman of reproductive age with PCOS, weight loss may be beneficial. In women who have completed childbearing or who have not responded to medical management, endometrial ablation or resection and hysterectomy are surgical options. The choice of procedure should be based on shared decision making with the patient. In the short term, ablation appears to result in less morbidity and shorter recovery periods. However, a significant number of women eventually undergo hysterectomy in the subsequent 5 years.[22]

Pharmacologic Therapy

Estrogen is the recommended treatment for managing acute severe bleeding episodes because it promotes endometrial stabilization.[22] Following initial use of estrogen for controlling acute bleeding episodes, continuation of therapy may be necessary to prevent future occurrences. OC use fulfills this role and contributes to predictable menstrual cycles.

The OCs help to prevent recurrent anovulatory bleeding by providing a progestin and by suppressing ovarian hormones and adrenal androgen production. They also, indirectly, increase sex hormone–binding globulin (SHBG). SHBG binds to androgens and reduces their circulating concentrations. For women with high androgen levels and its related signs (e.g., hirsutism), OCs containing ≤35 mcg of ethinyl estradiol are the treatment of choice.[22] Theoretically, use of an OC with a progesterone that has a larger impact on increasing SHBG can be considered, but to date there is no best contraceptive choice for these women (e.g., those with PCOS).[5]

In women with contraindication(s) to estrogen or in whom the side effects are unacceptable, progesterone-only products may be considered. They should be strongly considered for women experiencing menorrhagia associated with anovulatory bleeding.[46] In women with PCOS, use of depot and intermittent oral MPA suppresses pituitary gonadotropins and circulating androgens.[5] Use of cyclic progesterone may benefit women older than 40 years in whom anovulatory bleeding occurs.[22] In particular, if pregnancy is not a desired outcome of treatment, another progesterone option is placement of a levonorgestrel-containing IUD.[46]

Use of metformin and the thiazolidinediones, including pioglitazone, results in improved insulin sensitivity. In patients with PCOS, this is associated with reduced circulating androgen concentrations, increased ovulation rates,[5,47,48] and improved glucose tolerance.[5] These improvements can be attributed to the SHBG increase that occurs via increased insulin sensitivity. ❾ Metformin and thiazolidinedione use for anovulatory bleeding associated with PCOS is beneficial not only for anovulatory bleeding and fertility but also for improving glucose tolerance and decreasing overall long-term cardiovascular risk.[5] For women who have pregnancy as a desired outcome, metformin is pregnancy category B, and pioglitazone and rosiglitazone are category C.

If the goal of treatment is to improve fertility via ovulation induction, then clomiphene citrate is an option. Treatment with 50 mg/day for 5 days can be initiated between days 3 and 5 of the menstrual cycle. This often occurs after induction of withdrawal bleeding with a progesterone such as MPA 10 mg daily orally for 10 days. If ovulation does not occur with this dose of clomiphene, the dose may need to be increased to 100 mg/day. In rare instances, it may be increased in 50 mg increments up to 250 mg/day.

Drug Treatments of First Choice As with many menstruation-related disorders, there is not one universal treatment option of first choice for anovulatory bleeding. Rather, the treatment(s) chosen depends on accurate diagnosis of the etiology as well as identification of the desired treatment outcome(s).

ACOG recommends OCs as the first-choice treatment in women with anovulatory bleeding.[22] Based on consensus and expert opinion, the ACOG recommends the temporary use of conjugated equine estrogen not for anovulatory bleeding per se but for its efficacy in controlling severe abnormal uterine bleeding.[22]

Relative to anovulation in women with PCOS, the ACOG recommends using insulin-sensitizing agents including metformin and the thiazolidinediones to improve ovulatory frequency. The ACOG also recommends clomiphene because it frequently results in pregnancy in these patients.[5]

More recent data appear to support even further the use of metformin compared to the use of clomiphene for ovulation induction.[47,48] Its use for ovulation induction[47] as well as its use throughout pregnancy[49] in women with PCOS has been associated with reduced miscarriage rates in this population of patients (see Clinical Controversy).

Special Populations Anovulatory cycles are not unusual in the perimenarchal reproductive years. Ovulation typically is established 1 year or more following menarche. Anovulatory bleeding that occurs in this population may be excessive. If excessive bleeding occurs, the patient should be evaluated for bleeding disorders. The prevalence of bleeding disorders, including von Willebrand's disease, prothrombin deficiency, and idiopathic thrombocytopenia purpura, in this population ranges from 5% to 20%.[22]

In the adolescent population, specific bleeding disorders should be treated. Acute severe bleeding can be managed with high-dose estrogen. OCs containing ≤35 mcg of ethinyl estradiol are the treatment of choice in adolescents with chronic anovulation.[22]

Drug Class Information Table 83–3 identifies the significant pharmacologic properties, common adverse events, and clinically significant drug–drug and drug–food interactions of the agents used to treat anovulatory bleeding.

CLINICAL CONTROVERSY

The overall role of metformin in treating PCOS, particularly its duration of therapy, remains controversial. Relative to its use for ovulation induction, data illustrate that metformin is highly effective in both clomiphene citrate–resistant patients and in patients using it as initial therapy.[47,48] Its use throughout pregnancy has been associated with a reduction in early pregnancy loss rates.[49] The presence of dyslipidemia and hyperinsulinemia in women with PCOS increases their long-term risk for developing cardiovascular disease. Current research indicates that metformin use should be considered as prophylactic therapy to reduce cardiovascular risk in these women.[50] More research is needed to definitively identify the role(s) of metformin in PCOS.

EVALUATION OF THERAPEUTIC OUTCOMES

Table 83–4 lists the expected outcomes and specific monitoring parameters for the treatment modalities used to manage anovulatory bleeding.

DYSMENORRHEA

Dysmenorrhea is one of the most commonly encountered gynecologic complaints. It is defined as crampy pelvic pain occurring with or just prior to menses. Primary dysmenorrhea implies pain in the setting of normal pelvic anatomy and physiology. Secondary dysmenorrhea is associated with underlying pelvic pathology.[9]

EPIDEMIOLOGY

Rates of dysmenorrhea range from 20% to 90%.[9,23,51] Its presence may be associated with significant interference in work and school attendance. Risk factors include young age, heavy menses, nulliparity, early menarche, and cigarette smoking.[9,11]

ETIOLOGY

For most patients, dysmenorrhea is associated with normal ovulatory cycles and normal pelvic anatomy. This is referred to as *primary*, or *functional, dysmenorrhea.* However, in approximately 10% of the adolescents and young adults who present with painful menses, an underlying anatomic or physiologic cause is found.[11]

PATHOPHYSIOLOGY

The most significant mechanism for primary dysmenorrhea is the release of prostaglandins and leukotrienes into the menstrual fluid, initiating an inflammatory response and possibly vasopressin-mediated vasoconstriction.[9,11,29] Causes of secondary dysmenorrhea include cervical stenosis, endometriosis, pelvic infections, pelvic congestion syndrome, uterine or cervical polyps, uterine fibroids, genital outflow tract obstructions, and pelvic adhesions.[11,24] Pregnancy and miscarriage must be considered in the presentation of dysmenorrhea.

CLINICAL PRESENTATION OF DYSMENORRHEA

General

- Patient may or may not be in acute distress, depending on the level of menstrual pain experienced.

Symptoms

- Patients complain of crampy pelvic pain beginning shortly before or at the onset of menses. Symptoms typically last from 1 to 3 days.

Laboratory Tests

- Pelvic examination should be performed to screen for sexually transmitted diseases as a cause of the pain in sexually active females.
- Gonorrhea, *Chlamydia* cultures or polymerase chain reaction, wet mount

Other Diagnostic Tests

- Pelvic ultrasound can be used to identify potential anatomic abnormalities such as masses/lesions or to detect ovarian cysts and endometriomas.

TREATMENT

Initial choice of treatment is influenced by whether or not the woman desires to become pregnant. Nonpharmacologic options have been studied and observed to be as effective as some existing pharmacologic options.

Desired Outcome

Medical management of dysmenorrhea should relieve the related pelvic pain and, as applicable, should result in reducing lost school and work days. Table 83–2 identifies the agents used to manage dysmenorrhea and their recommended doses. Figure 83–5 shows a treatment algorithm for the management of dysmenorrhea.

General Approach to Treatment

There are several effective treatment options for dysmenorrhea. They include nonhormonal and hormonal pharmacologic options and other noninvasive nonpharmacologic options. Treatment choice may be influenced by the desire for contraception, the patient's level of sexual activity, potential for adverse effects, and cost.

Nonpharmacologic Therapy

Several nonpharmacologic interventions are used for managing dysmenorrhea. Among these, topical heat therapy, exercise, and a low-fat vegetarian diet all have been shown to reduce the intensity of dysmenorrhea.[9,11] Dietary changes may shorten the duration of dysmenorrhea. Application of topical heat via an abdominal patch for 12 consecutive hours/day has been proven to be as effective as 400 mg of ibuprofen dosed three times daily.[52] Because topical heat, exercise, and dietary changes do not impart any systemic effects, they are associated with little to no risk compared to the available pharmacologic options. Other nonpharmacologic options that are reserved for use following a failed trial of pharmacologic interventions include transcutaneous electric nerve stimulation, acupressure, and acupuncture.[9]

Pharmacologic Therapy

Given the role of prostaglandins in the pathophysiology of dysmenorrhea, NSAIDs are the initial treatment of choice. These agents do appear to be different in terms of efficacy. The most commonly used agents are naproxen and ibuprofen.

All NSAIDs have a propensity for causing gastrointestinal distress and ulceration, so they should be taken with food or milk to minimize these effects. Choice of one agent over another may be based on cost, convenience, and patient preference.[9] It has been suggested that a loading dose (twice the usual single dose) of the NSAID be used, followed by the usually recommended dose until symptoms resolve.[11] An alternate recommendation is to begin the NSAID at the onset of menses or perhaps even the day before and continue treatment around the clock instead of waiting until symptom onset. For patients in whom NSAID use is contraindicated, hormonal agents should be considered. Acetaminophen is inferior to NSAID in treatment of this disorder.[9]

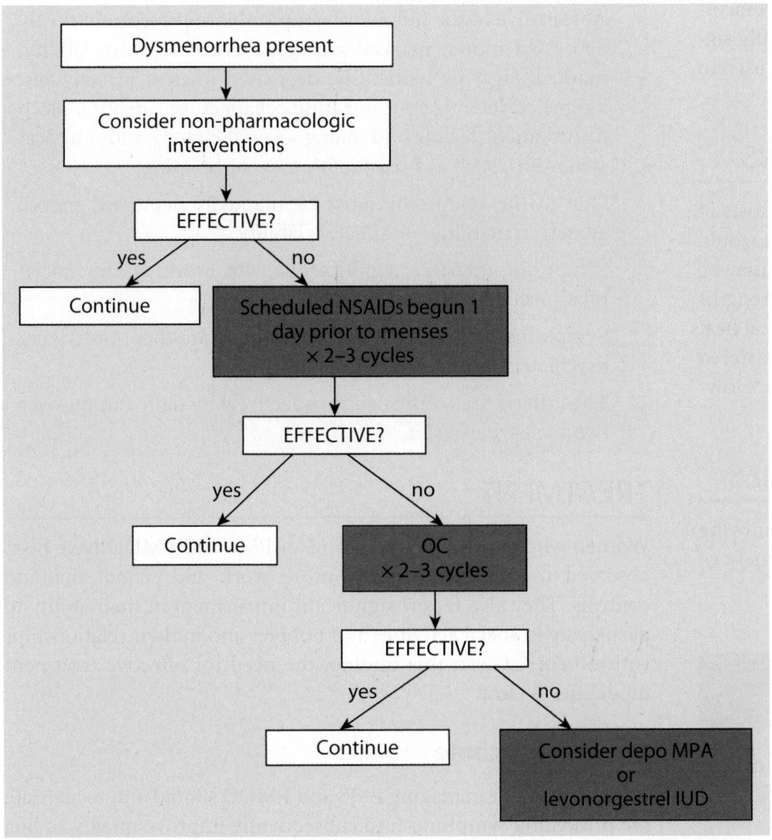

FIGURE 83-5. Treatment algorithm for dysmenorrhea. (IUD, intrauterine device; MPA, medroxyprogesterone acetate; NSAIDs, nonsteroidal antiinflammatory drugs; OC, oral contraceptive.)

OCs are effective in improving dysmenorrhea by inhibiting endometrial tissue proliferation. This reduction in tissue contributes to a reduction in endometrial-derived prostaglandins that cause the pelvic pain.[11] A trial of 2 to 3 months of OC dosing is required to establish whether the patient will respond to therapy.[27] Significant improvements in mild, moderate, and severe dysmenorrhea have been noted with the use of OCs. These agents have other benefits, such as prevention of pregnancy, improving acne, and reducing ovarian cancer risk. Although monophasic formulations may be more efficacious for this indication, the supporting evidence is limited.[9]

Depot MPA can be considered for dysmenorrhea treatment. Its efficacy is secondary to its ability to render most patients amenorrheic within 1 year of use.[9] Because the pelvic pain of dysmenorrhea is related to the prostaglandins released during menses, in the setting of amenorrhea the underlying cause of dysmenorrhea is removed.

Another progesterone product to be considered in managing dysmenorrhea is the levonorgestrel-releasing IUD. Observational data indicate its ability to reduce dysmenorrhea from 60% to 29% after 3 years of use.[9] As observed with depot MPA, this reduction likely is secondary to its effect in reducing menstrual flow.

Drug Treatments of First Choice Several factors influence the first-line treatment option chosen to treat dysmenorrhea. If contraception is desired, then a hormonal option may be considered using the same rationale for choosing it as would be used for choosing contraception (cost, adherence issues, side effects). If contraception is not desired, then a scheduled-dose NSAID started 1 day before menses would be desirable from both cost and convenience standpoints. If NSAIDs are contraindicated or the patient has a history of gastrointestinal disorders that would preclude their use, topical heat should be recommended.

Special Populations Dysmenorrhea is common in adolescent females. Any of the treatment measures used for adult patients would be appropriate in the adolescent population. Although NSAIDs, topical heat, and OCs are among the top choices, use of the levonorgestrel IUD is also an option.[32]

Drug Class Information Table 83–3 identifies the pharmacology, pharmacokinetics, common adverse events, and clinically significant drug–drug and drug–food interactions of the agents used to treat dysmenorrhea.

PHARMACOECONOMIC CONSIDERATIONS

For women with third-party coverage for prescriptions, the costs of OCs and the higher doses of NSAIDs used for dysmenorrhea would be covered. For women without such coverage, the OC cost may be prohibitive. Generic forms of NSAIDs in over-the-counter strengths can be considered and are less expensive than marketed topical heat products, such as Therma Care. Topical heat can be administered inexpensively via a reusable heating pad or hot water bottle. However, these products are generally not convenient to use.

EVALUATION OF THERAPEUTIC OUTCOMES

Table 83–4 lists the expected outcomes and specific monitoring parameters for the treatment modalities used in the management of dysmenorrhea.

PREMENSTRUAL SYNDROME AND PREMENSTRUAL DYSPHORIC DISORDER

PMS is a constellation of symptoms including mild mood disturbance and physical symptoms that occur prior to menses and resolve with initiation of menses. It is distinct from PMDD.

EPIDEMIOLOGY

It is estimated that up to 75% of menstruating women experience symptoms of PMS.[53] However, a spectrum of premenstrual mood disturbances exists, and the most severe is PMDD. Approximately 3% to 8% of women have PMDD.[53]

ETIOLOGY AND PATHOPHYSIOLOGY

PMDD is a complex psychiatric disorder with multiple biological, psychological, and sociocultural determinants.[54] Although cyclic hormonal changes are in some way related to PMS and PMDD, the association is neither linear nor simple. When ovulation is suppressed medically or surgically, symptoms improve. Some evidence suggests that PMS and PMDD symptoms are related to low levels of the centrally active progesterone metabolite allopregnanolone in the luteal phase and/or lower cortical γ-aminobutyric acid levels in the follicular phase.[54] Women with PMS and PMDD may have enhanced sensitivity to progesterone.[25] Studies of the relationship between PMS and PMDD and testosterone levels are conflicting.[54] A number of studies suggest a link between PMS and PMDD and low serotonin levels.[25,54] A study suggests that, despite similar affective symptoms, hypothalamic–pituitary–adrenal (HPA) axis function in PMS and PMDD is distinct from that seen in major depressive disorder. Specifically, women with PMS show a decrease in stimulated HPA axis response, whereas this response is increased in women with major depressive disorder.[55] Although several cross-cultural studies suggest that the physical symptoms of PMS are consistent across cultures, the negative affective symptoms are part of the negative "menstrual socialization" in western culture.[1,54]

CLINICAL PRESENTATION OF PMDD

A summary of the American Psychiatric Association's criteria for PMDD is as follows[1,54]:

- Symptoms are temporally associated with the last week of the luteal phase and remit with onset of menses.
- At least five of the following symptoms are present: markedly depressed mood, marked anxiety, marked affective lability, marked anger or irritability, decreased interest in activities, fatigue, difficulty concentrating, changes in appetite, sleep disturbance, feelings of being overwhelmed, and physical symptoms, such as breast tenderness or bloating.
- One of the symptoms must be markedly depressed mood, anxiety, irritability, or affective lability.
- Symptoms interfere significantly with work and/or social relationships.
- Symptoms are not an exacerbation of another underlying psychiatric disorder.
- The criteria are confirmed prospectively by daily ratings over two menstrual cycles.

TREATMENT

Women who experience symptoms of PMS and PMDD have been observed to miss significantly more work and school than do controls. They also report significant impairment of their ability to participate in social activities and hobbies and in their relationships with others.[56] Given this finding, the need for effective treatment modalities is clear.

Desired Outcome

Interventions for managing PMS and PMDD should aim to alleviate the presenting symptoms and subsequently improve quality of life.

Table 83–2 lists the various agents used in the management of this disorder and their recommended dosing.

General Approach to Treatment

As with any disorder or disease state, a treatment modality that is minimally invasive or without systemic effects is desired for initial therapy. Key to the successful choice of pharmacologic therapy for PMS and PMDD is having the patient chart her specific symptoms for at least 2 months.

Nonpharmacologic Therapy

Lifestyle interventions should be started and followed for 2 months while the patient charts her symptoms. Although these interventions lack significant supporting clinical trial data, anecdotal efficacy reports exist. Some lifestyle changes for women with mild-to-moderate premenstrual symptoms include minimizing intake of caffeine, refined sugar, and sodium and increasing exercise.[14,53] Vitamin and mineral supplements, such as vitamin B_6 (50–100 mg daily) and calcium carbonate (1,200 mg daily), have been observed to help reduce the physical symptoms associated with PMS.[14,53] A review of clinical trials concludes that the following options lack efficacy and safety data and therefore should not be recommended: herbal medicines, homeopathic remedies, dietary supplements, relaxation, massage therapy, reflexology, chiropractic treatments, and biofeedback.[57]

Pharmacologic Therapy

If symptoms persist after 2 months of symptom charting and lifestyle modifications, pharmacologic therapy can be considered for PMDD management. Over the past decade, use of the selective serotonin reuptake inhibitors (SSRIs) for this disorder has been studied significantly.[58–63] Studies have revealed very positive results relative to most of the symptoms associated with PMDD. Other agents that have been studied and are alternatives include the selective serotonin–norepinephrine reuptake inhibitor venlafaxine, as well as OCs, tricyclic antidepressants, and GnRH agonists.

Drug Treatments of First Choice ⑩ The first-line pharmacologic treatment options for PMDD are the SSRIs.[53] Among this class of agents, data support the use of citalopram, escitalopram, fluoxetine, fluvoxamine, paroxetine, and sertraline. They can be given either continuously or only during the luteal phase of the menstrual cycle. The ideal time for initiating therapy is unknown (see Clinical Controversy), and new evidence suggests efficacy when they are started at the onset of symptoms.

The SSRIs are efficacious in more than half of the treated patients compared to less than 30% of those receiving placebo.[14,58,61–63] Several studies report 50% or greater symptom reduction with SSRI treatment compared to baseline.[14,59,60] Improvement is noted to occur during the first cycle of use.[14]

Alternative Drug Treatments The tricyclic antidepressant clomipramine has been studied for treatment of PMDD. In placebo-controlled trials, both continuous daily dosing and luteal phase administration proved effective.[14] Compared to the SSRIs, however, clomipramine has a less desirable side-effect profile with low tolerability. Venlafaxine has been studied on a continuous daily basis[64] and during the luteal phase.[65] Both venlafaxine regimens resulted in significant symptom improvement (compared to placebo) in more than 60% of the women treated.

If treatment with an SSRI or another antidepressant such as clomipramine is not successful, hormonal treatment with a GnRH agonist, such as leuprolide, can be considered.[14] Leuprolide improves premenstrual emotional symptoms as well as some physical symptoms, such as bloating and breast tenderness. However, its cost, the need for intramuscular administration, and its hypoestrogenism side effects (e.g., vaginal dryness and hot flashes) limit its use.

A randomized, double-blind, placebo-controlled trial evaluating the use of a monophasic OC containing 30 mcg of ethinyl estradiol and 3 mg of drospirenone, a progesterone with antiandrogenic effects, showed improvement in the treatment arm compared to placebo.[13] In particular, appetite, food cravings, and acne improved. However, active treatment was not associated with a statistically significant improvement in the overall outcome measure, the Calendar of Premenstrual Experiences (COPE) scale, perhaps because of the small sample size (n = 82).

Drug Class Information Table 83–3 lists the pharmacology, pharmacokinetics, common adverse events, and clinically significant drug–drug and drug–food interactions of the agents used to treat PMDD.

PHARMACOECONOMIC CONSIDERATIONS

The SSRIs as first-line treatment options for PMDD management are comparably priced overall; however, a generic formulation of fluoxetine is available. Emerging data on the most appropriate dosing regimens (see Clinical Controversy) may contribute even further to a reduction in the cost of managing this disorder.

CLINICAL CONTROVERSY

Current evidence supports SSRI use, either dosed continuously or during the luteal phase, as first-line treatment of PMDD. Some evidence suggests that dosing at symptom onset also may be effective.[63] The bulk of studies evaluating the SSRIs include women over the age of 18 years and had durations not longer than 3 to 6 months.[53] The most effective dosing strategy (continuous, luteal phase, or symptom onset), the most efficacious treatments in the adolescent and perimenopausal populations, and the optimal duration of treatment all warrant further investigation.

EVALUATION OF THERAPEUTIC OUTCOMES

Table 83–4 lists the expected outcomes and specific monitoring parameters for the treatment modalities used in the management of PMDD.

CONCLUSIONS

Treatment success for the various menstruation-related disorders can be measured by the degree to which the care plan (1) relieves or reverses symptoms of the disorder, (2) prevents or reverses the complications of the disorder (e.g., osteoporosis, anemia, and infertility as noted with amenorrhea, menorrhagia, and anovulatory bleeding, respectively), and (3) minimizes side effects. The return of a regular menstrual cycle with minimal premenstrual symptoms or symptoms of dysmenorrhea is desirable. Depending on the desire for conception and subsequent therapy, this cycle may be ovulatory or anovulatory.

Once optimal therapy has been identified, the regimen can be continued as long as is deemed necessary. In amenorrhea, discontinuation of therapy may be warranted once menses resumes. In anovulatory bleeding, therapy may be discontinued once ovulatory menstrual cycles return. In menorrhagia, dysmenorrhea, and PMDD, optimal therapy may be continued for years or until other health factors affect its continuation. For example, a woman taking OCs for menorrhagia or dysmenorrhea may discontinue them when she is trying to become pregnant.

Symptom relief in dysmenorrhea should occur within hours of starting an NSAID or within the next menstrual cycle/menses if using OCs. Evaluate the patient for improvement of symptoms associated with amenorrhea, menorrhagia, anovulatory bleeding, or PMDD within one to two menstrual cycles. Ask patients at this visit about the type, frequency, and severity of current symptoms compared to their initial presenting symptoms. Refer patients with persistent symptoms for further medical evaluation to identify other underlying issues or complications.

Assess the effectiveness of therapy in resuming normal menstrual cycles with minimal related pain after an appropriate treatment interval (1–2 months). Assess improvement in quality of life measures such as physical, psychological, and social functioning and well-being. Evaluate the patient for adverse drug reactions, drug allergies, and drug interactions. Table 83–3 lists the common side effects that may occur and the monitoring required. Table 83–4 lists the specific expected outcome measures for each of the menstruation-related disorders discussed in this chapter.

ABBREVIATIONS

COPE: Calendar of Premenstrual Experiences
FSH: follicle-stimulating hormone
GnRH: gonadotropin-releasing hormone
HPA: hypothalamic–pituitary axis
IUD: intrauterine device
LH: luteinizing hormone
MPA: medroxyprogesterone acetate
NSAID: nonsteroidal antiinflammatory drug
OC: oral contraceptive
PCOS: polycystic ovarian syndrome
PID: pelvic inflammatory disease
PMDD: premenstrual dysphoric disorder
PMS: premenstrual syndrome
SHBG: sex hormone–binding globulin
SSRI: selective serotonin reuptake inhibitor

REFERENCES

1. Speroff L, Fritz MA. Clinical Gynecologic Endocrinology and Infertility, 7th ed. Philadelphia: Lippincott Williams & Wilkins, 2005:187–232, 401–463.
2. Stenchever MA, Droegemueller W, Herbst AL, Mishell DR. Primary and secondary amenorrhea. In Comprehensive Gynecology, 4th. St. Louis: Mosby, 2001:1099–1119.
3. Reindollar RH, Novak M, Thomas SP, McDonough PG. Adult-onset amenorrhea: A study of 262 patients. Am J Obstet Gynecol 1986;292;155:531–543.
4. Stenchever MA, Droegemueller W, Herbst AL, Mishell DR. Abnormal uterine bleeding: Ovulatory and anovulatory dysfunctional uterine bleeding, management of acute and chronic excessive bleeding. In: Comprehensive Gynecology, 4th ed. St. Louis: Mosby, 2001:1079–1097.
5. Polycystic ovary syndrome. ACOG Practice Bulletin Number 41. American College of Obstetricians and Gynecologists. Obstet Gynecol 2002;100:1389–1402.
6. Harmon KG. Evaluating and treating exercise related menstrual irregularities. The Physician and Sports Medicine. 2002, *http://www.physsportsmed.com/issues/202/03_02/harmon.htm.*
7. Gordon CM, Nelson LM. Amenorrhea and bone health in adolescents and young women. Curr Opin Obstet Gynecol 2003;15:377–384.
8. Pletcher JR, Slap GB. Menstrual disorders—amenorrhea. Pediatr Clin North Am 1999;46:505–518.
9. French L. Dysmenorrhea. Am Fam Physician 2005;71:285–291.
10. Simon JA. Progestogens in the treatment of secondary amenorrhea. J Reprod Med 1999;44(2 Suppl):185–189.
11. Harel Z. A contemporary approach to dysmenorrhea in adolescents. Pediatr Drugs 2002;4:797–805.
12. Roy SN, Bhattacharya S. Benefits and risks of pharmacological agents used for the treatment of menorrhagia. Drug Saf 2004;27:75–90.
13. Freeman EW, Kroll R, Rapkin A, et al. Evaluation of a unique oral contraceptive in the treatment of premenstrual dysphoric disorder. J Womens Health Gend Based Med 2001;10:561–569.
14. Grady-Weliky TA. Premenstrual dysphoric disorder. N Engl J Med 2003;348:433–438.
15. European Multicentre Study Group for Cabergoline in Lactation Inhibition. Single dose cabergoline versus bromocriptine for inhibition of puerperal lactation: Randomized, double-blind, multicenter study. Br Med J 1991;302:1367–1371.
16. Webster J, Piscitelli G, Polli A, et al. A comparison of cabergoline and bromocriptine in the treatment of hyperprolactinemic amenorrhea. N Engl J Med 1994;331:904–909.
17. Kvernmo T, Hartter S, Burger E. A review of the receptor-binding and pharmacokinetic properties of dopamine agonists. Clin Ther 2006;28:1065–1078.
18. Eng PM, Seeger JD, Loughlin J, et al. Serum potassium monitoring for users of ethinyl estradiol/drospirenone taking medications predisposing to hyperkalemia: physician compliance and survey of knowledge and attitudes. Contraception 2007;75:101–107.
19. Schurmann R, Blode H, Benda N, et al. Effect of drospirenone on serum potassium and drospirenone pharmacokinetics in women with normal or impaired renal function. J Clin Pharmacol 2006;46:867–875.
20. Bent S, Ko R. Commonly used herbal medicines in the United States: A review. Am J Med 2004;116:478–485.
21. Warner PE, Critchley HO, Lumsden MA, et al. Menorrhagia I. Measured blood loss, clinical features, and outcome in women with heavy periods: A survey with follow-up data. Am J Obstet Gynecol 2004;190:1216–1223.
22. ACOG Practice Bulletin Management of Anovulatory Bleeding Number 14, March 2000. International Journal of Gynecology and Obstetrics; 72(2001):263–271.
23. Davis AR, Westhoff CL. Primary dysmenorrhea in adolescent girls and treatment with oral contraceptives. J Pediatr Adolesc Gynecol 2001;14:3–8.
24. Stenchever MA, Droegemueller W, Herbst AL, Mishell DR. Primary and secondary dysmenorrhea and premenstrual syndrome etiology, diagnosis, and management. In: Comprehensive Gynecology, 4th ed. St. Louis: Missouri: Mosby, 2001:1065–1078.
25. Dickerson LM, Mazyck PJ, Hunter MH. Premenstrual syndrome. Am Fam Physician 2003;67:1743–1752.
26. Prentice A. Fortnightly review: Medical management of menorrhagia. BMJ 1999;319:1343–1345.
27. Schroeder B, Sanfilippo JS. Dysmenorrhea and pelvic pain in adolescents. Pediatr Clin North Am 1999;46:555–571.
28. Warner PE, Critchley HO, Lumsden MA, et al. Menorrhagia II. Is the 80-mL blood loss criterion useful in management of complaint of menorrhagia? Am J Obstet Gynecol 2004;190:1224–1229.
29. Adams Hillard PJ, Deitch HR. Menstrual disorders in the college age female. Pediatr Clin North Am 2005;52:179–197.
30. James AH, Ragni MV, Picozzi VJ. Bleeding disorders in premenopausal women: (another) public health crisis for hematology? Hematol Am Soc Hematol Educ Program 2006;2006:474–485.
31. Neuwirth RS. Cost effective management of heavy uterine bleeding: ablative methods versus hysterectomy. Curr Opin Obstet Gynecol 2001;13:407–410.
32. Intrauterine device. ACOG Practice Bulletin No. 59. American College of Obstetricians and Gynecologists. Obstet Gynecol 2005;105:223–232.
33. ACOG Committee Opinion No. 337. Noncontraceptive uses of the levonorgestrel intrauterine system. Obstet Gynecol 2006;107:1479–1482.
34. Hurskainen R, Paavonen J. Levonorgestrel-releasing intrauterine system in the treatment of heavy menstrual bleeding. Curr Opin Obstet Gynecol 2004;16:487–490.
35. Hurskainen R, Teperi J, Rissanen P, et al. Clinical outcomes and costs with the levonorgestrel-releasing intrauterine system or hysterectomy for treatment of menorrhagia: Randomized trial 5-year follow-up. JAMA 2004;291:1456–1463.

36. Blumenthal PD, Trussell J, Singh RH, et al. Cost-effectiveness of treatments for dysfunctional uterine bleeding in women who need contraception. Contraception 2006;74:249–258.
37. Zawadski JK, Dunaif A. Diagnostic criteria for polycystic ovary syndrome: Towards a rational approach. In: Dunaif A, Givens JR, Haseltine FP, eds. Polycystic Ovary Syndrome. Boston: Blackwell Scientific Publications, 1992;377–384.
38. Rotterdam ESHRE/ASRM-Sponsored PCOS Consensus Workshop Group. Revised 2003, consensus on diagnostic criteria and long-term health risks related to polycystic ovary syndrome. Fertil Steril 2004;81:19–25.
39. Carmina E, Azziz R. Diagnosis, phenotype and prevalence of polycystic ovary syndrome. Fertil Steril 2006;86(Suppl 1):S7–S8.
40. Management of infertility caused by ovulatory dysfunction. ACOG Practice Bulletin No. 34, American College of Obstetricians and Gynecologists. Obstet Gynecol 2002;99:347–358.
41. Azziz R, Woods KS, Reyna R, et al. The prevalence and features of the polycystic ovary syndrome in an unselected population. J Clin Endocrinol Metab 2004;89:2745–2749.
42. Azziz R, Carmina E, Didier D, et al. Position statement: Criteria for defining polycystic ovarian syndrome: An Androgen Excess Society Guideline. J Clin Endocrinol Metab 2006;91:4237–4245.
43. Krassas GE. Thyroid disease and female reproduction. Fertil Steril 2000;74:1063–1070.
44. Matytsina LA, Zoloto EV, Sinenko LV, et al. Dysfunctional uterine bleeding in adolescents: Concept of pathophysiology and management. Prim Care 2006;33:503–515.
45. Dilley A, Drews C, Miller C, et al. von Willebrand's disease and other inherited bleeding disorders in women with diagnosed menorrhagia. Obstet Gynecol 2001;97:630–636.
46. Ely JW, Kennedy CM, Clark EC, et al. Abnormal uterine bleeding: A management algorithm. J Am Board Fam Med 2006;19:590–602.
47. Palomba S, Orio F, Falbo A, et al. Prospective parallel randomized, double-blind, double-dummy controlled clinical trial comparing clomiphene citrate and metformin as the first-line treatment for ovulation induction in nonobese anovulatory women with polycystic ovary syndrome. J Clin Endocrinol Metab 2005;90:4068–4074.
48. Siebert TI, Kruger TF, Steyn DW, et al. Is the addition of metformin efficacious in the treatment of clomiphene citrate-resistant patients with polycystic ovary syndrome? A structured literature review. Fertil Steril 2006;86:1432–1437.
49. Khattab S, Mohsen IA, Foutouh IA, et al. Metformin reduces abortion in pregnant women with polycystic ovary syndrome. Gynecol Endocrinol 2006;22:680–684.
50. Banaszewska B, Duleba AJ, Spaczynski RZ, et al. Lipids in polycystic ovary syndrome: Role of hyperinsulinemia and effects of metformin. Am J Obstet Gynecol 2006;194:1266–1272.
51. Banikarim C, Chacko MR, Kelder SH. Prevalence and impact of dysmenorrhea on Hispanic female adolescents. Arch Pediatr Adolesc Med 2000;154:1226–1229.
52. Akin MD, Weingand KW, Hengehold DA, et al. Continuous low-level topical heat in the treatment of dysmenorrhea. Obstet Gynecol 2001;97:343–349.
53. Steiner M, Pearlstein T, Cohen LS, et al. Expert guidelines for the treatment of severe PMS, PMDD, and comorbidities: The role of SSRIs. J Womens Health 2006;15:57–69.
54. Ross LE, Steiner M. A biopsychosocial approach to premenstrual dysphoric disorder. Psychiatr Clin North Am 2003;26:529–546.
55. Roca CA, Schmidt PJ, Altemus M, et al. Differential menstrual cycle regulation of hypothalamic-pituitary-adrenal axis in women with premenstrual syndrome and controls. J Clin Endocrinol Metab 2003;88:3057–3063.
56. Mishell DR. Premenstrual disorders: Epidemiology and disease burden. Am J Manag Care 2005;11:S473–S479.
57. Stevinson C, Ernst E. Complementary/alternative therapies for premenstrual syndrome: A systematic review of randomized clinical trials. Am J Obstet Gynecol 2001;185:227–235.
58. Freeman EW, Rickels K, Sondheimer SJ, et al. Differential response to antidepressants in women with premenstrual syndrome/premenstrual dysphoric disorder: A randomized controlled trial. Arch Gen Psychiatry 1999;56:932–939.
59. Freeman EW, Sondheimer SJ, Sammel MD, et al. A preliminary study of luteal phase versus symptom-onset dosing with escitalopram for premenstrual dysphoric disorder. J Clin Psychiatry 2005;66:769–773.
60. Steiner M, Hirschberg AL, Begeron R, et al. Luteal phase dosing with paroxetine controlled release (CR) in the treatment of premenstrual dysphoric disorder Am J Obstet Gynecol 2005;193:352–360.
61. Yonkers KA, Holthausen GA, Poschman K, et al. Symptom-onset treatment for women with premenstrual dysphoric disorder. J Clin Psychopharmacol 2006;26:198–202.
62. Halbreich U, Bergeron R, Yonkers KA, et al. Efficacy of intermittent, luteal phase sertraline treatment of premenstrual dysphoric disorder. Obstet Gynecol 2002;100:1219–1229.
63. Kornstein SG, Pearlstein TB, Fayyad R, et al. Low-dose sertraline in the treatment of moderate-to-severe premenstrual syndrome: efficacy of 3, dosing strategies. J Clin Psychiatry 2006;67:124–132.
64. Freeman EW, Rickels K, Yonkers KA, et al. Venlafaxine in the treatment of premenstrual dysphoric disorder. Obstet Gynecol 2001;98(5 Pt 1):737–744.
65. Cohen LS, Soares CN, Lyster A, et al. Efficacy and tolerability of premenstrual use of venlafaxine (flexible dose) in the treatment of premenstrual dysphoric disorder. J Clin Psychpharmacol 2004;24:540–543.

CHAPTER 84

Endometriosis

DEBORAH A. STURPE

KEY CONCEPTS

1. The etiology of endometriosis likely is due to multiple factors, with no single theory satisfactory to explain all cases.
2. Endometriosis should be suspected in any woman of reproductive age, including adolescents, with recurring cyclic or acyclic pelvic pain and/or subfertility.
3. No physical examination findings or laboratory tests are considered diagnostic for endometriosis. A definitive diagnosis can be made only via surgical visualization of lesions. Confirmation of diagnosis is not necessary in all cases.
4. Treatment goals of endometriosis include improvement of painful symptoms and maintenance or improvement of fertility. Therapy is considered successful based on resolution of the patient's symptoms or achievement of pregnancy.
5. All medical therapies are equally efficacious in treating endometriosis-related pain based on available evidence. Choice among agents is determined primarily by side-effect profile, cost, and individual patient response.
6. Endometriosis-related pain can be treated by medical or surgical therapy. Empirical medical therapy likely is more cost effective and is recommended based on consensus guidelines.
7. Recurrence rates of endometriosis-related pain are high after both medical and surgical therapies. Extended use of medical therapy or postoperative use of medical therapy may be needed to maintain efficacy.
8. Endometriosis-related infertility is unresponsive to medical therapy. Conservative surgical therapy is the preferred treatment.

Endometriosis is a common cause of chronic pelvic pain in women and is associated with infertility. Characterized by the presence of endometrial tissue outside the uterus, endometriosis is a chronic, recurring disease. Therapy is targeted at relieving symptoms and improving fertility.

EPIDEMIOLOGY

Prevalence of endometriosis in the general population is estimated at approximately 6% to 10% of women.[1,2] An estimated 35% to 50% of women presenting with chronic pelvic pain have endometriosis, and approximately 38% of women with infertility have the disorder.[1,2] The disease typically presents during the reproductive years but has been documented over a wide age range from 8 to 76 years, with some cases occurring prior to menarche.[3,4] A genetic predisposition for endometriosis has been noted, as evidenced by disease rates that are six times higher in primary relatives of affected women compared to the general population.[2]

Learning objectives, review questions, and other resources can be found at **www.pharmacotherapyonline.com.**

ETIOLOGY

1 The etiology of endometriosis is unknown. Multiple mechanisms for development of lesions are likely, including theories of retrograde menstrual flow, coelomic metaplasia, lymphatic and vascular spread, and immunologic abnormalities.[1,2,5,6] Although retrograde menstruation is the most popular theory of endometriosis development, the low percentage of women with this disorder who develop endometriosis along with rare occurrence of disease in prepubertal girls supports other mechanisms of pathogenesis.[3] Involvement of immune system factors in the development and progression of endometriosis is recognized. Findings of abnormal B- and T-cell function, decreased apoptosis, and altered levels of prostanoids, cytokines, growth factors, and interleukins in endometrial lesions and peritoneal fluid of affected women support this theory.[6,7] Based on these findings, it has been hypothesized that an underlying immunologic disorder is responsible for development of endometriosis in most women.[6]

PATHOPHYSIOLOGY

Endometriosis-associated pain is secondary to structural and/or inflammatory causes. Endometrial lesions may cause pain or dyspareunia by direct compression of nerve fibers or increased pressure within endometriomas (cysts within the ovary).[6,8] Endometrial lesions also generate local inflammation, resulting in prostaglandin release and development of adhesions.[6,8] Endometrial lesions contain estrogen and progesterone receptors; thus, symptoms may correlate with the cyclic release of hormones during the menstrual cycle. In severe endometriosis, infertility may result from distortion of the pelvic structure secondary to endometrial lesions, inflammation, and adhesions.[6,8,9] In milder disease, the cause-and-effect relationship is more controversial. Decreased oocyte viability and/or production resulting from the altered uterine environment may be a contributing factor.[8]

CLINICAL PRESENTATION

Symptoms

- The patient may be asymptomatic or complain of symptoms such as dyspareunia, chronic pelvic pain (cyclic or acyclic), premenstrual spotting, gastrointestinal disturbances, urinary disturbances (dysuria, hematuria), low back pain, painful defecation, or infertility.

Signs

- Findings on physical examination may include cul-de-sac or uterosacral ligament tenderness, adnexal enlargement or tenderness, or a pelvic mass.
- Findings on laparoscopic examination may include red "flame" lesions (early disease), blue/brown/gray "powder burn" lesions, "white lesions" (healed or inactive disease), or "chocolate cysts" (endometriomas containing blood).

Data from Valle[6] and Child and Tan.[8]

❷ ❸ Endometriosis should be suspected in women, including adolescents, with subfertility, dysmenorrhea, dyspareunia, or chronic pelvic pain. A definitive diagnosis can be made only by direct surgical visualization of endometrial lesions; however, most treatment guidelines allow for nondefinitive diagnosis in patients presenting with chronic pelvic pain provided that other causes of pain are ruled out and pain responds to first-line empiric therapies.[3,10–12] Severity of disease can be classified according to the American Association of Reproductive Medicine staging system (stage I = mild to stage IV = severe), but this staging system is not useful in clinical practice because the size, location, and number of lesions do not correlate with painful symptoms, nor does the staging system predict pregnancy rates.[1,6] In addition, disease severity may be underestimated.[10]

TREATMENT

The treatment of endometriosis varies depending on presenting symptoms, patient age, and desired outcome.

DESIRED OUTCOME

❹ Treatment goals for endometriosis depend on the patient's presentation. Only women with active symptoms (pelvic pain, infertility, or both) require therapy. Depending on the primary complaint, goals of endometriosis treatment include (1) minimization or removal of endometrial deposits, (2) prevention of disease progression, (3) minimization of associated pain, and (4) prevention or correction of associated infertility.

GENERAL APPROACH TO TREATMENT

❺ The treatment of an asymptomatic patient with endometriosis consists of expectant management (watchful waiting) only because therapy is not indicated unless symptoms develop. For symptomatic patients, the foundation of therapy includes medical treatment, surgical treatment, or both. To date, no studies have directly compared medical and surgical treatment as first-line therapy. Furthermore, determining the optimal medical or surgical approach is difficult secondary to a paucity of well-designed, randomized, controlled trials. All commonly prescribed medical therapies relieve endometriosis-related pain by regressing lesions via induction of a pseudopregnancy or pseudomenopausal state but do not eradicate lesions or improve fertility. Therefore, choice of initial therapy depends on multiple factors such as the patient's primary complaint, location and extent of disease, desire for future fertility, cost of therapy, contraindications to therapy, and potential side effects or complications of therapy.

❻ Guidelines recommend empirical treatment of chronic pelvic pain suspected to be secondary to endometriosis with nonsteroidal antiinflammatory drugs (NSAIDs) and/or combined hormonal contraceptives (CHCs) for 3 months.[3,10–12] If symptoms fail to improve with such therapy, empiric therapy with a gonadotropin-releasing hormone (GnRH) agonist can be considered. Other pharmacologic agents (e.g., danazol, progestins) also can be considered for use in selected patients. Conservative surgical therapy is recommended for treatment of painful symptoms in women who do not respond to, or have contraindications to, medical therapy or patients with other compelling reasons for surgery. Of note, ❼ 30% to 75% of women will experience recurrence of pain within 6 to 24 months after initial treatment with either medical or surgical means, and extended use of medical therapy or postoperative adjunctive medical therapy may be necessary.[2,6,13] Definitive treatment for endometriosis involves nonconservative surgical therapy via bilateral salpingo-oophorectomy, with or without hysterectomy. This therapy should be reserved for women not desiring future fertility who accept the potential complications of surgically induced menopause. A general treatment algorithm for endometriosis-related pain is shown in Fig. 84–1.

❽ For women presenting with infertility as a primary complaint, first-line therapy involves surgical resection of endometrial lesions to restore normal anatomy, followed by watchful waiting.[10,11,14] Medical therapy is ineffective for endometriosis-related infertility and should be avoided.[8,10,11,14–17] For women in whom surgical intervention does not result in pregnancy within 6 months, controlled ovarian stimulation with intrauterine insemination or in vitro fertilization is commonly used.[18] Pretreatment with a GnRH agonist prior to in vitro fertilization cycles may increase success rates.[18,19] No clear guidelines or recommendations exist to guide the choice of one therapy or technique over another.

NONPHARMACOLOGIC THERAPY: SURGERY

❽ Surgical intervention in endometriosis can be used as both a diagnostic and a therapeutic tool. Laparoscopic procedures are highly effective in treating endometriosis pain and are preferred over laparotomy because of lower complication rates, lower incidence of postoperative adhesions, and more rapid patient recovery.[1,6,20] Unfortunately, up to 44% of women will experience recurrence of painful symptoms at 1 year, so use of adjunctive medical therapy postoperatively is sometimes recommended in order to extend the pain-free interval.[1,6,13,19] Current data best support use of danazol or a GnRH agonist for this purpose.[10] Conservative surgical therapy is also primary treatment of endometriosis-associated infertility, and patients with advanced disease causing distortion of the pelvic structure may benefit most from surgical intervention.

PHARMACOLOGIC THERAPY

Typically, pharmacologic therapy is the first choice for treatment of endometriosis-related pain in order to minimize risks from surgery. However, drug therapy will not treat endometriosis-related infertility.

Drug Treatments of First Choice

❺ First-line therapy for endometriosis-associated pain includes NSAIDs or CHCs.[3,10–12] These two drug classes are considered as effective as, and less costly than, other endometriosis treatments. Choice of agent depends on patient characteristics, such as desire for contraception, pain patterns, and contraindications. Long-term maintenance therapy with these agents may be considered for women achieving a good therapeutic response.

Efficacy of NSAIDs in patients with endometriosis has not been evaluated in a large number of controlled trials. However, NSAIDs have proven efficacy in treating primary dysmenorrhea and likely have benefit in endometriosis as well.[10–12]

Use of CHCs for treatment of endometriosis pain is desirable because of the potential for long-term use without significant side effects. A low-dose combined oral contraceptive administered cyclically was compared with a GnRH agonist in a randomized trial.[21] Both groups showed overall improvement in dyspareunia, nonmen-

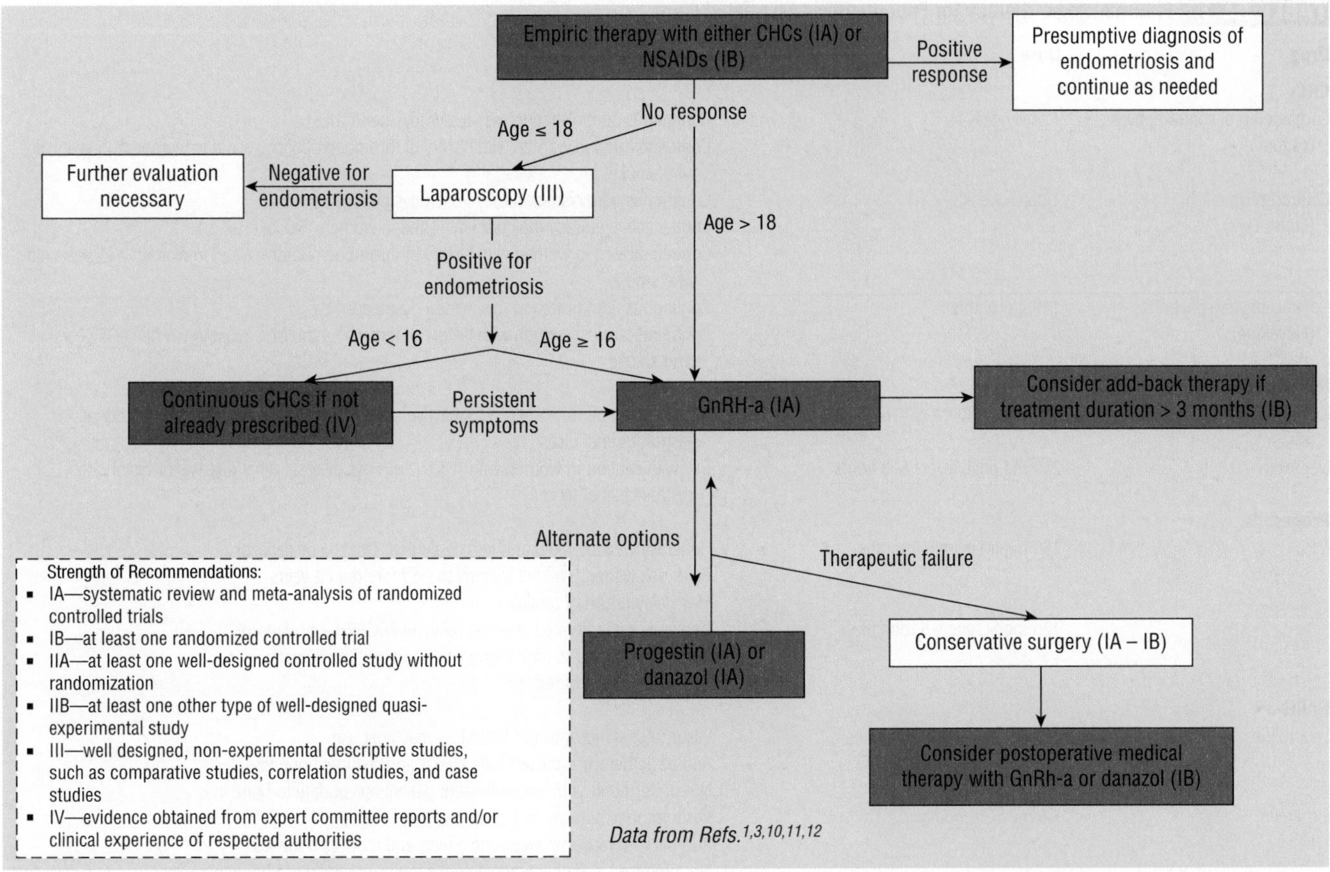

FIGURE 84-1. Treatment algorithm for cyclic/acyclic chronic pelvic pain and suspected endometriosis. (CHC, combined hormonal contraceptive; GnRH-a, gonadotropin-releasing hormone agonist.)

strual pain, and dysmenorrhea at 6 months. The rate of recurrent symptoms 6 months after cessation of therapy was equal between groups. Combined oral contraceptives can be administered on a continuous basis if desired. Studies on the efficacy of other formulations of CHCs (vaginal ring and transdermal patch) for treatment of endometriosis pain have not been conducted; however, use of these agents in endometriosis is reasonable.

Alternative Drug Treatments

Adolescents (age less than 18 years) experiencing chronic pelvic pain despite therapy with NSAIDs or CHCs should undergo evaluative laparoscopy prior to initiation of additional pharmacotherapy.[3]

In adolescents with endometriosis diagnosed by laparoscopy or in adults with chronic pelvic pain unresponsive to NSAIDs or CHCs, advanced medical therapy for endometriosis pain may be considered.[3,10–12] Agents that can be used as advanced medical therapy include progestins, danazol, or GnRH agonists. Systematic reviews have concluded that all three classes are effective choices, and no class has been proven superior to another.[19,22–24] The primary difference between treatments is the side-effect profile and available dosage forms; therefore, choice of agent depends on patient age, preference, and tolerance of side effects. A 2-month trial of the agent should be used, and treatment should be continued for a minimum of 6 months if relief is obtained.[12] For women treated with a GnRH agonist, add-back therapy with estrogens or progestins should be considered to minimize vasomotor side effects and bone mineral density loss.[3,10–12]

Surgical therapy for endometriosis pain should be considered for women who do not respond to advanced medical therapy, women with contraindications to medical therapy, and women unable to tolerate side effects caused by medical therapy.[12]

Special Populations: Adolescents

❹ Treatment goals for endometriosis in adolescent patients include pain control, minimization of disease progression, and preservation of fertility.[3] Medical therapy is preferred over surgical therapy in this population in order to minimize adhesion development from repeated surgeries.[25] A treatment algorithm that includes therapy for adolescent patients is shown in Fig. 84–1.

The effect of drugs on bone mineral density is of particular concern in young women who have not achieved peak bone mass; thus, add-back therapy should be considered for all adolescents receiving GnRH agonist therapy.[3,4,25] Although progestins are likely to be well tolerated by the adolescent population, efficacy has not been clearly established, and concerns regarding long-term effects on bone mineral density and lipid profile are not clearly defined.[3,25] Danazol is not likely to be well tolerated by the adolescent population and generally is not recommended for use.[3,4,25]

Drug Class Information

When selecting therapy for endometriosis related pain, choice of drug within a class often depends on strength of evidence for efficacy in endometriosis or specific patient factors.

Nonsteroidal Antiinflammatory Drugs NSAIDs treat the painful symptoms of endometriosis by interfering with prostaglandin production but do not directly affect the structure of endometrial lesions.[6] Long-term use of these agents may be limited by gastrointestinal or renal toxicity. They also may aggravate reactive airway disease and should be used with caution in such patients. The NSAIDs most commonly used for treatment of gynecologic pain are ibuprofen and naproxen.[13] Dosing may be intermittent or

TABLE 84-1 Pharmacologic Therapy for Endometriosis-Associated Pain

Drug	Dose	Comments
CHCs		
Combined oral contraceptives (various)	1 orally daily	Continuous administration may lessen dysmenorrhea Contraindicated in women with history of thromboembolism; avoid in women >35 years old who smoke
Contraceptive patch (Ortho-Evra)	1 patch weekly	Continuous administration may lessen dysmenorrhea Contraceptive efficacy may be diminished in women >90 kg (198 lb) Contraindicated in women with history of thromboembolism; avoid in women >35 years old who smoke
Contraceptive vaginal ring (NuvaRing)	1 ring monthly	Continuous administration may lessen dysmenorrhea Contraindicated in women with history of thromboembolism; avoid in women >35 years old who smoke
NSAIDs		
Ibuprofen	400 mg orally every 4–6 hours	Use with caution in women with reactive airways disease, renal disease, or history of gastrointestinal ulcer
Naproxen	250 mg orally every 6–8 hours	Use with caution in women with reactive airways disease, renal disease, or history of gastrointestinal ulcer
Progestins		
MPA	150 mg IM every 3 months	Generally well tolerated and less costly than GnRH-a or danazol Black box warning to limit therapy to no more than 2 years May delay return of fertility
	120 mg SC every 3 months	Generally well tolerated and less costly than GnRH-a or danazol Black box warning to limit therapy to no more than 2 years May delay return of fertility
GnRH-a		
Leuprolide	11.25 mg IM every 3 months	Vasomotor symptoms and bone loss may limit use Add-back therapy improves side effects and reduces bone loss Not preferred in younger adolescent patients secondary to bone loss
Goserelin	3.6 mg SC monthly	Vasomotor symptoms and bone loss may limit use Add-back therapy improves side effects and reduces bone loss Not preferred in younger adolescent patients secondary to bone loss
Nafarelin	200 mcg (one spray) intranasally twice daily	Vasomotor symptoms and bone loss may limit use Add-back therapy improves side effects and reduces bone loss Not preferred in younger adolescent patients secondary to bone loss
Other		
Danazol	600–800 mg orally daily in divided doses	Androgenic side effects limit use; not preferred in adolescent patients secondary to side-effect profile

CHC, combined hormonal contraceptive; MPA, medroxyprogesterone acetate; IM, intramuscular; GnRH-a, gonadotropin-releasing hormone agonists; SC, subcutaneous; NSAID, nonsteroidal antiinflammatory drug.
Data from references 1, 3, 10, 11, 12, 43, and 44.

continuous, depending on whether the pain is cyclic or acyclic.[12] Specific dosing information is listed in Table 84–1.

Combined Hormonal Contraceptives CHCs treat the pain of endometriosis by decreasing menstrual flow and regressing endometrial implants through induction of an anovulatory and/or hypoestrogenic state.[3,26] Continuous therapy also can be used to suppress menstruation and induce a "pseudopregnancy"-like state.[3] Studies suggest that combined oral contraceptives likely are equal in efficacy to GnRH agonists and medroxyprogesterone for relieving endometrial pain.[27] Combined oral contraceptives also are effective in preventing recurrence of pain after surgical intervention for endometriosis.[28] No evidence suggests that one combined oral contraceptive is superior to another. Additionally, although no specific studies have examined the efficacy of the contraceptive patch or vaginal ring in endometriosis, effects of these agents likely are similar to those of the oral formulations.[3] Thus, choice between CHCs should be guided by patient preference, likelihood of adherence, and cost.

Side effects of CHCs typically are mild and may include nausea, bloating, headache, and breakthrough bleeding. However, all CHCs can increase risk of thromboembolism, so they should not be used in women with a history of thromboembolism or in smokers over age 35 years.

Administration of CHCs may be cyclic (includes a placebo or nondrug week) or continuous. Although no studies have directly compared the two methods, continuous administration is more likely to induce amenorrhea and, therefore, may be more beneficial in treating dysmenorrhea.[3,13,19]

Progestins Multiple progestins have been studied for the treatment of endometriosis. Agents available in the United States include oral medroxyprogesterone, depot medroxyprogesterone (both subcutaneous and intramuscular), megestrol, norethindrone, and the levonorgestrel-releasing intrauterine device (IUD). The progestins treat endometriosis via atrophy and decidualization of endometrial tissue. They tend to be less expensive and better tolerated than other advanced medical endometriosis treatments.

Despite a paucity of well-designed, controlled trials examining use of progestins in endometriosis, a systematic review concluded that continuous therapy with progestins is no more or less effective than other therapies for treatment of endometriosis-associated pain.[24] More recent studies have examined the use of the subcutaneous form of depot medroxyprogesterone for treatment of endometriosis-associated pain.[29,30] Both studies compared subcutaneous medroxyprogesterone to the GnRH agonist leuprolide, and in each study the progestin showed statistically equivalent improvement in symptoms. Studies examining the use of the levonorgestrel-releasing IUD also suggest some efficacy in the treatment of endometriosis-associated pain.[31–33]

Common side effects of systemic progestins include breakthrough bleeding, weight gain, fluid retention, and mood swings. For women desiring immediate future fertility after cessation of therapy, progestins may not be optimal secondary to prolonged amenorrhea and anovulation. Also of concern are unknown long-term effects on bone mineral density associated with these agents. Both depot medroxyprogesterone products carry black box warnings against use for more than 2 years.[34,35] However, in the studies that directly compared the subcutaneous form of depot medroxyprogesterone to leuprolide over a treatment period of 6 months, the extent and degree of bone loss were less severe with the progestin.[29,30] Specific progestin dosing information is given in Table 84–1.

Gonadotropin-Releasing Hormone Agonists GnRH agonists create a functional oophorectomy via inhibition of follicle-stimulating hormone (FSH) and luteinizing hormone (LH) secretion. This, in turn, diminishes endometrial implants. When first initiated, GnRH agonists create an initial gonadotropin flare prior to receptor downregulation that may cause a temporary increase in pain. Initiating therapy during the midluteal phase may minimize such effects.

Therapy with a GnRH agonist is superior to placebo and comparable with danazol for relief of endometriosis-associated pain.[23] Response rates are approximately 85% to 100% after 6 months of therapy, but recurrence rates at 5 years are 53%.[1,19,23,27] Although a GnRH agonist typically is taken for 6 months, one comparative study has shown equivalent efficacy and recurrence rates between 3 and 6 months of GnRH agonist therapy.[36] Therapy may be extended beyond 6 months to maintain efficacy, although data regarding such extended usage are limited.

The three GnRH agonists currently available in the United States are goserelin, leuprolide, and nafarelin. These agents differ primarily by route of administration; therefore, choice of therapy depends on patient preference. Specific dosing information for the GnRH agonists is given in Table 84–1.

Side effects are the primary limitation of GnRH agonist use. The pharmacologically induced hypoestrogenic environment results in bone loss and vasomotor symptoms such as hot flashes, vaginal dryness, and insomnia. Loss of bone mineral density is estimated at 4% to 6% over 6 months of GnRH agonist therapy and occurs at both the hip and spine, but this loss is partially to fully recoverable upon cessation of the drug.[37] Bone loss is progressive as use of the drugs is extended beyond 6 months, and whether reversibility is maintained after such longer treatment periods is unknown.[38] Add-back therapy with estrogens, progestins, or bisphosphonates has been studied for treatment of vasomotor symptoms and prevention of bone loss while maintaining drug efficacy.[3,10,11]

Women receiving GnRH agonist therapy should be encouraged to take supplemental calcium and to exercise. One small study suggests that women who exercise (walking and aerobic sessions) during 6 months of GnRH agonist therapy sustain similar bone mineral loss during therapy but have better recovery of bone mineral density after cessation of therapy compared to women who do not exercise.[39]

CLINICAL CONTROVERSY

Add-back therapy alleviates the vasomotor symptoms and bone density loss associated with GnRH agonist therapy. Controversy exists as to when to initiate such therapy. Some practitioners believe that add-back therapy should be prescribed only after 6 months of GnRH agonist treatment because bone loss until this point is believed to be reversible. However, recent data suggest that this may not be entirely true. Consequently, some clinicians recommend immediate use of add-back therapy to minimize side effects and improve adherence, especially because some evidence suggests that use of immediate add-back therapy can completely eliminate bone mineral density loss. Consideration for use of immediate add-back therapy may be of particular importance in women younger than 30 years because bone mineral density is still building.

Danazol Danazol is a synthetic steroid analog of 17-ethinyl testosterone. It induces anovulation, amenorrhea, and endometrial atrophy through pituitary suppression of the midcycle LH and FSH surge and induction of a high-androgen, low-estrogen environment. The drug also has immunosuppressive activity that may contribute to its efficacy. Formerly the "gold standard" of endometriosis treatment, the popularity of danazol has decreased with the development of agents with more favorable side-effect profiles.

Danazol has proven effective as empirical therapy as well as postoperative therapy. Symptomatic improvement has been reported in up to 80% to 90% of women using the drug, with the best results seen in women achieving amenorrhea.[13] A systematic review concluded that 6 months of danazol therapy is superior to placebo in relieving painful symptoms.[22] Therapy for only 3 months has not been as successful, especially when used postoperatively.[1,12,13]

The primary limitation of danazol therapy is the high occurrence of androgenic side effects, including weight gain, acne, hot flashes, decreased breast size, hirsutism, and increased low-density lipoprotein cholesterol. Lowering the dose of danazol may alleviate some of these side effects, but drug efficacy is compromised.[13] Danazol should not be initiated in women with hyperlipidemia or liver disease. Danazol is teratogenic, and barrier forms of contraception must be used. The dose of danazol ranges from 200 to 800 mg/day; most studies have used doses of 600 to 800 mg. Specific dosing information is given in Table 84–1.

PHARMACOECONOMIC CONSIDERATIONS

Several cost considerations must be made when choosing endometriosis therapy. Cost of medical therapy must be weighed against the cost of surgical therapy, and the costs of each type of medical therapy must be weighed against another.

❻ Two studies have determined that empirical pain therapy with a GnRH agonist is less expensive than empirical surgical therapy by laparotomy. Cost savings estimates from these studies range from $1,000 to $2,500 per treated patient, although the results of these studies are limited by the lack of consideration of the cost of add-back therapy and/or postoperative medical therapy.[40–42] Because the rate of recurrence of symptoms is high for both conservative surgical therapy and medical therapy, empirical medical therapy appears to be the most reasonable option. Generally, GnRH agonists are the most expensive agents and CHCs and progestins are the least expensive.

CLINICAL CONTROVERSY

Several of the drug therapies used for treatment of endometriosis may lead to decreases in bone mineral density. Unfortunately, the role of routine bone mineral density testing as a monitoring parameter for these drug therapies is not yet determined. Some clinicians choose to routinely measure bone mineral density in order to follow changes over time. However, the accuracy of bone mineral density results in predicting fracture risk in younger patients has not been well established, nor has a threshold of loss been established for discontinuation of therapy. Thus, some clinicians may decide that the cost of routine testing is not justified.

EVALUATION OF THERAPEUTIC OUTCOMES

❹ Monitoring of endometriosis therapy is focused on subjective relief of symptoms.[12,13] Although objective confirmation of lesion regression by laparotomy is feasible, the results typically are misleading because the number and size of lesions do not correlate well with patient symptoms.[13]

Endometriosis-related pain should be relieved within 2 months of initiating medical therapy. If symptoms persist, consideration should be given to different medical and/or surgical therapy. For endometriosis-related infertility, most experts recommend 6 months of watchful waiting after surgical intervention. If pregnancy is not achieved within that time, assisted reproductive techniques can be considered.

Careful monitoring of the patient for side effects to recommended drug therapy is important. Most of the monitoring can be accomplished by eliciting any subjective complaints from the patient at routine followup visits. However, certain drug therapies may require additional objective monitoring, such as fasting lipid profile and blood pressure measurements.

ABBREVIATIONS

CHCs: combined hormonal contraceptives
FSH: follicle-stimulating hormone
GnRH: gonadotropin-releasing hormone
IUD: intrauterine device
LH: leuteinizing hormone
NSAID: nonsteroidal antiinflammatory drug

REFERENCES

1. Bulletins-Gynecology ACoP. ACOG practice bulletin: Medical management of endometriosis. Int J Gynaecol Obstet 2000;71:183–196.
2. Giudice LC, Kao LC. Endometriosis. Lancet 2004;364:1789–1799.
3. American College of Obstetricians and Gynecologists. ACOG committee opinion: Endometriosis in adolescents. Obstet Gynecol 2005;105:921–927.
4. Laufer MR, Sanfilippo J, Rose G. Adolescent endometriosis: Diagnosis and treatment approaches. J Pediatr Adolesc Gynecol 2003;16:S3–S11.
5. Lessey BA. Medical management of endometriosis and infertility. Fertil Steril 2000;73:1089–1096.
6. Valle RF. Endometriosis: Current concepts and therapy. Int J Gynaecol Obstet 2002;78:107–119.
7. Kim JG, Suh CS, Kim SH, et al. Insulin-like growth factors (IGFs), IGF-binding proteins (IGFBPs), and IGFBP-3 protease activity in the peritoneal fluid of patients with and without endometriosis. Fertil Steril 2000;73:996–1000.
8. Child TJ, Tan SL. Endometriosis: Aetiology, pathogenesis and treatment. Drugs 2001;61:1735–1750.
9. Jacobson TZ, Barlow DH, Koninckx PR, et al. Laparoscopic surgery for subfertility associated with endometriosis. Cochrane Database of Systematic Reviews 2002;4:CD001398.
10. Kennedy S, Bergqvist A, Chapron C, et al. Eshre guideline for the diagnosis and treatment of endometriosis. Hum Reprod 2005;20:2698–2704.
11. Royal College of Obtetricians and Gynecologists. The investigation and management of endometriosis. 2006, *http://www.rcog.org.uk/resources/Public/pdf/endometriosis_gt_24_2006.pdf.*
12. Gambone JC, Mittman BS, Munro MG, et al. Consensus statement for the management of chronic pelvic pain and endometriosis: Proceedings of an expert-panel consensus process. Fertil Steril 2002;78:961–972.
13. Mahutte NG, Arici A. Medical management of endometriosis-associated pain. Obstet Gynecol Clin North Am 2003;30:133–150.
14. Olive DL, Pritts EA. Treatment of endometriosis. N Engl J Med 2001;345:266–275.
15. Farquhar CM. Extracts from the "clinical evidence": Endometriosis. BMJ 2000;320:1449–1452.
16. Hughes E, Fedorkow D, Collins J, Vandekerckhove P. Ovulation suppression for endometriosis. Cochrane Database of Systematic Reviews 2000l2:CD000155.
17. Adamson GD, Pasta DJ. Surgical treatment of endometriosis-associated infertility: Meta-analysis compared with survival analysis. Am J Obstet Gynecol 1994;171:1488–1504.
18. Surrey ES, Schoolcraft WB. Management of endometriosis-associated infertility. Obstet Gynecol Clin North Am 2003;30:193–208.
19. Olive DL, Pritts EA. The treatment of endometriosis: A review of the evidence. Ann N Y Acad Sci 2002;955:360–372.
20. Jacobson TZ, Barlow DH, Garry R, Koninckx P. Laparoscopic surgery for pelvic pain associated with endometriosis. Cochrane Database of Systematic Reviews 2001;4:CD001300.
21. Vercellini P, Trespidi L, Colombo A, et al. A gonadotropin-releasing hormone agonist versus a low-dose oral contraceptive for pelvic pain associated with endometriosis. Fertil Steril 1993;60:75–79.
22. Selak V, Farquhar C, Prentice A, Singla A. Danazol for pelvic pain associated with endometriosis. Cochrane Database of Systematic Reviews 2000;2:CD000068.
23. Prentice A, Deary AJ, Goldbeck-Wood S, et al. Gonadotrophin-releasing hormone analogues for pain associated with endometriosis. Cochrane Database of Systematic Reviews 2000;2:CD000346.
24. Prentice A, Deary AJ, Bland E. Progestagens and anti-progestagens for pain associated with endometriosis. Cochrane Database of Systematic Reviews 2000;2:CD002122.
25. Attaran M, Gidwani GP. Adolescent endometriosis. Obstet Gynecol Clin North Am 2003;30:379–390.
26. Rice VM. Conventional medical therapies for endometriosis. Ann N Y Acad Sci 2002;955:343–352.
27. Winkel CA, Scialli AR. Medical and surgical therapies for pain associated with endometriosis. J Womens Health Gend -Based Med 2001;10:137–162.
28. Muzii L, Marana R, Caruana P, et al. Postoperative administration of monophasic combined oral contraceptives after laparoscopic treatment of ovarian endometriomas: A prospective, randomized trial. Am J Obstet Gynecol 2000;183:588–592.
29. Schlaff WD, Carson SA, Luciano A, et al. Subcutaneous injection of depot medroxyprogesterone acetate compared with leuprolide acetate in the treatment of endometriosis-associated pain. Fertil Steril 2006;85:314–325.
30. Crosignani PG, Luciano A, Ray A, Bergqvist A. Subcutaneous depot medroxyprogesterone acetate versus leuprolide acetate in the treatment of endometriosis-associated pain. Hum Reprod 2006;21:248–256.
31. Lockhat FB, Emembolu JO, Konje JC. The evaluation of the effectiveness of an intrauterine-administered progestogen (levonorgestrel) in the symptomatic treatment of endometriosis and in the staging of the disease. Hum Reprod 2004;19:179–184.
32. Lockhat FB, Emembolu JO, Konje JC. The efficacy, side-effects and continuation rates in women with symptomatic endometriosis undergoing treatment with an intra-uterine administered progestogen (levonorgestrel): A 3 year follow-up. Hum Reprod 2005;20:789–793.
33. Petta CA, Ferriani RA, Abrao MS, et al. Randomized clinical trial of a levonorgestrel-releasing intrauterine system and a depot GnRH analogue for the treatment of chronic pelvic pain in women with endometriosis. Hum Reprod 2005;20:1993–1998.
34. Depo-provera package insert. Pharmacia and Upjohn Co. November 2004.
35. Depo-subQ provera 104 package insert. Pharmacia and Upjohn Co. March 2005.
36. Hornstein MD, Yuzpe AA, Burry KA, et al. Prospective randomized double-blind trial of 3 versus 6 months of nafarelin therapy for endometriosis associated pelvic pain. Fertil Steril 1995;63:955–962.
37. Surrey ES. Add-back therapy and gonadotropin-releasing hormone agonists in the treatment of patients with endometriosis: Can a consensus be reached? Fertil Steril 1999;71:420–424.
38. Hornstein MD, Surrey ES, Weisberg GW, Casino LA. Leuprolide acetate depot and hormonal add-back in endometriosis: A 12-month study. Lupron add-back study group. Obstet Gynecol 1998;91:16–24.
39. Bergstrom I, Freyschuss B, Jacobsson H, Landgren B-M. The effect of physical training on bone mineral density in women with endometriosis treated with GnRH analogs: A pilot study. Acta Obstet Gynecol Scand 2005;84:380–383.
40. Winkel CA. A cost-effective approach to the management of endometriosis. Curr Opin Obstet Gynecol 2000;12:317–320.
41. Winkel CA. Modeling of medical and surgical treatment costs of chronic pelvic pain: New paradigms for making clinical decisions. Am J Manag Care 1999;5:S276–S290.
42. Kephart W. Evaluation of lovelace health systems chronic pelvic pain protocol. Am J Manag Care 1999;5:S309–S315.
43. DRUGDEX System [Internet database]. Greenwood Village, CO: Thomson Micromedex.
44. Drug Facts and Comparisons 4.0, 2005. Available from Wolters Kluwer Health.

CHAPTER 85

Hormone Therapy in Women

SOPHIA N. KALANTARIDOU, SUSAN R. DAVIS, AND KARIM ANTON CALIS

KEY CONCEPTS

1. Estrogen-based postmenopausal hormone therapy should be used for treatment of menopausal symptoms (e.g., vasomotor and urogenital symptoms) and, when specifically indicated, for osteopenia and osteoporosis prevention.
2. A progestogen should be added for endometrial protection when estrogen therapy is prescribed. Thus, women with an intact uterus should not receive unopposed estrogen, whereas women who have undergone hysterectomy always should receive estrogen alone.
3. Lower doses of hormone therapy than previously used should be considered as standard initial therapy. Clinicians should prescribe hormone therapy at the lowest effective dose for the shortest duration, carefully and individually weighing treatment goals and risks for each woman.
4. The major indication for estrogen-containing hormone therapy is the relief of menopausal symptoms. The benefits of short-term perimenopausal and postmenopausal hormone therapy for the relief of severe menopausal symptoms outweigh the risks in many women.
5. Osteoporosis prevention remains an approved indication for estrogen-based hormone therapy, but alternative strategies are available and should be considered as first-line agents for asymptomatic women. Vitamin D deficiency should be excluded before any other treatment is prescribed for the prevention or treatment of bone loss, and adequate calcium intake should be ensured.
6. Postmenopausal hormone treatment with oral combined estrogen plus progestogen has no benefit for cardiovascular disease prevention and increases the risk of breast cancer, coronary heart disease events, stroke, and venous thromboembolic events. However, it reduces the rates of hip fracture.
7. Hormone therapy improves mood and well-being primarily in women with hot flushes, night sweats, and sleep disturbance, but it does not improve gross quality-of-life measures in postmenopausal women who do not experience vasomotor symptoms.
8. Evaluation of each individual woman is essential in determining the appropriateness of perimenopausal and postmenopausal hormone therapy, and collaboration between a woman and her primary care provider in the decision-making process is essential. The benefits and risks of hormone therapy should be reassessed annually.
9. Results from randomized trials of hormone therapy in postmenopausal women cannot be extrapolated to premenopausal women with ovarian dysfunction. Women with premature ovarian failure (i.e., those younger than 40 years) need exogenous sex steroids to compensate for the decreased production by their ovaries.

Learning objectives, review questions,
and other resources can be found at
www.pharmacotherapyonline.com.

Menopause is the permanent cessation of menses following the loss of ovarian follicular activity.[1] By definition, it is a physiologic event that occurs after 12 consecutive months of amenorrhea, so the time of the final menses is determined retrospectively. Women who have undergone hysterectomy must rely on their symptoms to estimate the actual time of menopause.

Many women seek therapy for alleviation of symptoms that arise from loss of ovarian function at the time of menopause. However, since 2002, use of hormone therapy (estrogen with or without progestogen) for the prevention of diseases of aging has attracted considerable public attention as a result of the premature termination of the estrogen–progestogen arm of the Women's Health Initiative (WHI) trial due to increased risk of coronary heart disease and breast cancer.[2] The estrogen-alone arm of the trial also was discontinued after 7 years of followup because the study found that estrogen alone did not affect (either increase or decrease) heart disease.[3] Breast cancer risk was not increased during the study period.[3]

The median age at the onset of menopause in the United States is 51 years, whereas the average life expectancy for women is 81 years. Thus, American women can expect to be postmenopausal for more than one third of their lives.

Although the age at menarche has declined steadily throughout the centuries, probably as a result of improved nutrition, the age at menopause onset appears to be relatively stable. However, on average, cigarette smokers experience menopause 2 years earlier than do nonsmokers. Women who have undergone hysterectomy also are more likely to have an earlier menopause despite preservation of their ovaries.

Since the publication of the WHI trial results, many women have either stopped or become reluctant to use hormone therapy.[4] The WHI trial was a chronic disease prevention trial designed to evaluate the role of hormone therapy in reducing the risks of cardiovascular disease in older women and at the same time to investigate the effects on the risk of breast cancer.[2,3] The trial was conducted in a total of 16,607 mainly asymptomatic women who were an average 12 to 13 years postmenopausal (mean age 63 ± 7.11 years).[2,3] No randomized controlled clinical trials of the population of women normally targeted for hormone therapy (i.e., symptomatic perimenopausal or early postmenopausal women) have been reported. Although hormone therapy is not indicated for prevention of chronic diseases of aging, it remains the most effective treatment for vasomotor symptoms, impaired sleep quality, and urogenital symptoms of menopause. Regulatory authorities expressed major concerns about hormone therapy use following the results of the WHI trial.[5,6]

Approved indications of postmenopausal hormone therapy include treatment of menopausal symptoms (e.g., hot flushes, night sweats, and urogenital atrophy) and osteoporosis prevention.[5] Although it has been proposed that hormone therapy should be prescribed at the lowest possible dose for the shortest possible time,[5] evidence that new low-dose regimens are safer than traditionally prescribed doses is lacking. Weighing the risks and benefits, the Food and Drug Administration (FDA) mandated the addition of new safety warnings to the labels of all systemic estrogens (regardless of route or dosage form), including estrogen-only and combined estrogen–progestogen products.[6] The labels now caution that use of estrogen-containing hormone therapy regimens by postmenopausal women may be associated with an increased risk of myocardial infarction, stroke, breast cancer, and thromboembolism.[6]

MENOPAUSE AND PERIMENOPAUSAL AND POSTMENOPAUSAL HORMONE THERAPY

PHYSIOLOGY

Characteristics of the human menstrual cycle throughout reproductive life are well described.[7] A woman is born with approximately two million primordial follicles in her ovaries. During a normal reproductive life span, she ovulates fewer than 500 times. The vast majority of follicles undergo atresia.

The hypothalamic–pituitary–ovarian axis dynamically controls reproductive physiology throughout the reproductive years. The pituitary is regulated by pulsatile secretion of gonadotropin-releasing hormone (GnRH) from the hypothalamus. Follicle-stimulating hormone (FSH) and luteinizing hormone (LH), produced by the pituitary in response to GnRH, regulate ovarian function. These gonadotropins also are influenced by negative feedback from estradiol and progesterone. Ovarian follicular activity is reflected by the circulating concentrations of sex steroids and by peptide hormones (e.g., inhibin and activin). The sex steroids include estradiol, produced by the dominant follicle; progesterone, produced by the corpus luteum after maturation of the dominant ovarian follicle; and androgens, primarily testosterone and androstenedione, secreted by the ovarian stroma. Sex steroids are important for the healthy functioning of many organs, including the bones, brain, skin, and reproductive and urogenital tracts. They act primarily by regulating gene expression.

Pathophysiologic changes associated with menopause are caused by loss of ovarian follicular activity.[1] Ovarian primordial follicle numbers decrease with advancing age, and at the time of the menopause, few follicles remain in the ovary. Hence the postmenopausal ovary is no longer the primary site of estradiol or progesterone synthesis. The postmenopausal ovary secretes primarily androstenedione and testosterone. In contrast to the acute fall in circulating estrogen at the time of menopause, the decline in circulating androgens commences in the decade leading up to the average age of natural menopause and closely parallels increasing age.[8] Androgens are secreted by both the ovaries and the adrenal glands. Following menopause, direct ovarian androgen secretion appears to account for as much as 50% of testosterone production, with the adrenal gland being a less important source. Hypertrophy of the ovarian stroma may develop after menopause, probably secondary to high LH concentrations, thereby resulting in increased ovarian testosterone production. Alternatively, the ovaries may become fibrotic and a poor source of sex steroids.

No endocrine event clearly signals the time just prior to final menses.[9] Nonetheless, as women age, a progressive rise in circulating FSH[10] and a concomitant decline in ovarian inhibin[9] are observed. In women who continue to experience menstrual bleeding, FSH determinations on day 2 or 3 of the menstrual cycle are considered elevated when concentrations exceed 10 to 12 international units/L, an indication of diminished ovarian reserve. Clear elevations in serum FSH are seen in women at age approximately 40 years.[9] When ovarian function has ceased, serum FSH concentrations are greater than 40 international units/L.

The perimenopause is the period immediately prior to the menopause and the first year after menopause. The menopausal transition is the period of time when the endocrinologic, biologic, and clinical features of the approaching menopause commence.[9] The menopausal transition usually begins approximately 4 years prior to menopause and is characterized by menstrual cycle irregularity caused by increased frequency of anovulatory cycles. Vasomotor symptoms (hot flushes and night sweats), psychological symptoms (anxiety, mood swings, and depression), and disturbances of sexuality are increased markedly in the perimenopause. Menopause is characterized by a 10- to 15-fold increase in circulating FSH concentrations compared with concentrations of FSH in the follicular phase of the cycle, a fourfold to fivefold increase in LH, and a greater than 90% decrease in circulating estradiol concentrations.[9] During the perimenopause, FSH concentrations may rise to the postmenopausal range during some cycles but return to premenopausal levels during subsequent cycles. Thus, high concentrations of FSH should not be used to diagnose menopause in perimenopausal women. However, vasomotor symptoms in perimenopausal women may require treatment despite the presence of menstrual bleeding. Abnormal thyroid function and other conditions that may cause similar symptomatology should be excluded first. Dysfunctional uterine bleeding may occur during the perimenopausal years because of anovulatory cycles, but other gynecologic causes also should be considered. Treatment options for dysfunctional uterine bleeding include progestogens or low-dose oral contraceptives.

An observational study of more than 9,000 postmenopausal women examined the relationship between endogenous estrogens and bone mineral density, bone loss, fractures, and breast cancer.[11–14] Women with detectable serum estradiol concentrations (5–25 pg/mL) had a 6% to 7% higher bone mineral density at the total hip and spine compared with women with undetectable levels (less than 5 pg/mL).[11] They also had significantly less bone loss at the hip than women with undetectable levels.[12] Women with undetectable serum estradiol concentrations had a relative risk of 2.5 for subsequent hip and vertebral fractures.[13] However, women with the highest estradiol serum concentrations had the greatest risk of developing breast cancer.[14]

CLINICAL PRESENTATION OF PERIMENOPAUSE AND MENOPAUSE

Symptoms

- Vasomotor symptoms (hot flushes and night sweats)
- Sleep disturbances
- Mood changes
- Sexual dysfunction
- Problems with concentration and memory
- Vaginal dryness and dyspareunia

Signs

- *Perimenopause:* Dysfunctional uterine bleeding as a result of anovulatory cycles (other gynecologic disorders should be excluded)
- *Menopause:* Signs of urogenital atrophy

Laboratory Tests

- *Perimenopause:* FSH on day 2 or 3 of the menstrual cycle greater than 10–12 international units/L
- *Menopause:* FSH greater than 40 international units/L

Other Relevant Diagnostic Tests

- Thyroid function tests
- Iron stores

CLINICAL PRESENTATION OF MENOPAUSE

Vasomotor symptoms, hot flushes, and night sweats are common symptoms of estrogen withdrawal. Hot flushes are the classic sign of menopause and the major clinical complaint of American women during the perimenopausal and early menopausal years. Hot flushes are a sensation of warmth, frequently accompanied by skin flushing and perspiration. A chill may follow as the core body temperature drops. Hot flushes may occur in women of any age who experience acute estrogen withdrawal. They can be occasional or frequent, can last from seconds to 1 hour, and are characterized by symptoms ranging from mild warmth to profuse sweating. For some women, hot flushes are a minor nuisance, but for other women, they are a disturbing symptom that disrupts their sense of well-being and causes problems in their social and professional lives. They usually occur spontaneously but often are increased in frequency or severity in hot or humid weather or after ingestion of caffeine, alcohol, or spicy foods. The prevalence of hot flushes is higher in the first 2 postmenopausal years. Women who have undergone surgical menopause tend to have more intense menopausal symptoms than those who experience a natural menopause.

Vaginal dryness is directly related to estrogen insufficiency, but some women can find adequate relief from nonestrogenic vaginal creams. Most women with significant vaginal dryness require local or systemic estrogen therapy to replenish moisture. Vaginal dryness should be differentiated from lack of lubrication during sexual stimulation. The latter is an impaired arousal response and may not improve with simple vaginal estrogen therapy.

Although some accept a range of other symptoms to be typical of estrogen deficiency (e.g., mood swings, tiredness, poor concentration, depression, insomnia, migraines, formication, arthralgia, myalgia, and urinary frequency), the relationship between these symptoms and the absolute decline in estrogen is more controversial. Many women, nonetheless, experience relief of such symptoms with estrogen therapy.

TREATMENT

Menopause

Postmenopausal hormone therapy is a subject of major interest in the field of women's health. In some women, menopausal symptoms can be managed effectively with lifestyle modifications, including exercise, weight control, smoking cessation, and a healthful diet. More recently, however, dietary supplements and nonpharmacologic therapies have been promoted as "complementary medicine" alternatives to hormone therapy. To date, little evidence supports the use of such nonprescription products, which include various herbal remedies and soy-based supplements.

PHYTOESTROGENS

Phytoestrogens have physiologic effects in humans.[15] They are plant compounds with estrogen-like biologic activity and relatively weak estrogen receptor–binding properties. Epidemiologic studies suggest that consumption of a phytoestrogen-rich diet, which is common in traditional Asian societies, is associated with a lower risk of breast cancer.[16]

The biologic potencies of phytoestrogens vary. Most of these compounds are nonsteroidal and are less potent than synthetic estrogens. The three main classes of phytoestrogens are isoflavones, lignans, and coumestans, all of which are found in plants or their seeds.[15] The most commonly studied phytoestrogen is the isoflavone class. Genistein and daidzein are the most abundant active components of isoflavones. The concentration of isoflavones per gram of soy protein varies considerably among preparations. Also, a single plant often contains more than one class of phytoestrogen. Common food sources of phytoestrogens include soybeans (isoflavones), cereals, oilseeds such as flaxseed (lignans), and alfalfa sprouts (coumestans).

Mild estrogenic effects have been seen in postmenopausal women,[15] but current data suggest that phytoestrogen supplementation is no more effective than placebo in relieving hot flushes or other symptoms of menopause in postmenopausal women.[17]

Phytoestrogens decrease low-density lipoprotein (LDL) cholesterol and triglyceride concentrations with no significant change in high-density lipoprotein (HDL) cholesterol concentrations.[18] Furthermore, phytoestrogens have the ability to inhibit LDL oxidation and normalize vascular reactivity in estrogen-deprived primates.[18] In addition, bone density may be improved by phytoestrogens.[15] Common adverse effects include constipation, bloating, and nausea.[19]

Larger, long-term studies are needed to document the effects of phytoestrogens on the breast, bone, and endometrium. Furthermore, differences among classes of phytoestrogens must be identified clearly, including dosing and biologic activity, before phytoestrogens can be considered an alternative to conventional hormone therapy in postmenopausal women.

Black cohosh (*Cimicifuga racemosa*), a widely used herbal supplement, may not offer substantial benefits for relief of vasomotor symptoms as suggested by earlier trials.[20] This substance does not appear to have strong intrinsic estrogenic properties but may act through the serotonergic system. Long-term effects of black cohosh are unknown.

HORMONAL REGIMENS

Approved indications of hormone therapy include treatment of menopausal symptoms and osteoporosis prevention. Therapy directed at menopausal symptoms, such as hot flushes, often is short term. However, therapy directed at prevention of osteoporosis should be long term. For osteoporosis prevention, the advantages of hormone therapy must be weighed against the risks, including thrombosis and the increased incidence of cardiovascular disease and breast cancer,[2] and consideration should be given to approved nonestrogen alternatives.

In women with an intact uterus, hormone therapy consists of an estrogen plus a progestogen. In women who have undergone hysterectomy, estrogen therapy is given unopposed by a progestogen.

The WHI randomized controlled trial was a chronic disease prevention trial designed to evaluate the role of hormone therapy in diseases of aging.[2,3] The continuous combined oral estrogen–progestogen arm of the WHI trial was terminated prematurely. This arm included 16,608 relatively healthy postmenopausal women aged 50 to 79 years at enrollment (mean age 63.2 years). The primary outcome was coronary heart disease events, defined as nonfatal myocardial infarction and coronary artery disease death, with invasive breast cancer as the primary adverse outcome.[2] The study also examined secondary outcomes, including stroke, thromboembolic disease, fractures, colon cancer, and endometrial cancer.[2] After a mean followup of 5.2 years (planned duration 8.5 years), the Data and Safety Monitoring Board recommended stopping this arm of the trial because of the occurrence of a prespecified level of invasive breast cancer. That is, women who received the active drug had an increased risk of invasive breast cancer (hazard ratio [HR] 1.26, 95% confidence interval [CI] 1–1.59), and the overall risks exceeded benefits.[2] The study also found increased coronary disease events (HR 1.29, 95% CI 1.02–1.63), stroke (HR 1.41, 95% CI 1.07–1.85), and pulmonary embolism (HR 2.13, 95% CI 1.39–3.25). Beneficial effects included decreases in hip fracture (HR 0.66, 95% CI 0.45–0.98) and colorectal cancer (HR 0.63, 95% CI 0.43–0.92).[2] Results from this study indicated that short-term use (<1 year) has risks for coronary heart disease and thromboembolic disease events. The number of deaths was similar among the groups.

After a mean followup of 7 years, the Data and Safety Monitoring Board also recommended stopping the oral estrogen-alone arm of the study. This arm consisted of 10,739 women who had undergone hysterectomy. Estrogen-only therapy had no effect on coronary heart disease risk and was not associated with increased breast cancer risk.[3]

Among women in the estrogen–progestogen arm, one serious adverse event occurred in every 100 women treated for 5 years. Specifically, the study suggested that for every 10,000 women taking combined hormone therapy, there would be eight more cases of breast cancer, seven more cases of myocardial infarctions, eight more cases of stroke, and eight more cases of pulmonary embolism. However, six fewer colorectal cancers and five fewer hip fractures would be expected.[2] For the majority of women who had never used hormone therapy before enrolling in the study (6,280 treated with estrogen–progestogen and 6,024 treated with placebo), the HR for breast cancer was 1.06 (95% CI 0.81–1.38), indicating that the burden of risk for breast cancer resulted from use of hormone therapy for more than 5 years. Subsequently, a large epidemiologic study reported a greater risk estimate for combined estrogen–progestogen use as well as increased risk for estrogen-only therapy and tibolone.[21] However, interpretation of these findings is limited by selection bias because the risk profiles of women who used hormone therapy were significantly different from the those of nonusers.[21] Whether the type of estrogen compound or the dose, route, or administration method could be at least partly responsible for the risks observed in the WHI trial is unclear.

■ ESTROGEN AND PROGESTOGEN TREATMENT

Estrogens

❶ The primary accepted indication for estrogen-based hormone therapy is the relief of vasomotor symptoms, and the initial dose should be the lowest effective dose for symptom control. Estrogens are naturally occurring hormones or synthetic steroidal or nonsteroidal compounds with estrogenic activity. Various systemically administered estrogens (typically oral and transdermal) are suitable for replacement therapy (Table 85–1). Estrogens can be administered orally, transdermally (patches and other topical products), intravaginally (creams, tablets, or rings), intranasally, intramuscularly, and even subcutaneously in the form of implanted pellets. The choice of estrogen delivery (product, route, and method) should be determined in consultation with the patient to ensure acceptability and enhance compliance. In general, the oral and transdermal routes are used most frequently, with oral conjugated equine estrogens (CEEs) particularly popular in the United States. No evidence indicates that one estrogen compound is more effective than another in relieving menopausal symptoms or preventing osteoporosis.

Oral Estrogen Oral CEE has been available for more than 50 years. CEE is prepared from the urine of pregnant mares and is composed of estrone sulfate (50%–60%) and multiple other equine estrogens such as equilin and 17α-dihydroequilin.[22]

Estradiol is the predominant and most active form of endogenous estrogens. A micronized form of estradiol (produced by a technique that yields extremely small particles of the pure hormone) is readily absorbed from the small intestines.[22] When given orally, estradiol is metabolized by the intestinal mucosa and the liver during the first hepatic passage, and only 10% reaches the circulation as free estradiol. Metabolism of estrogen is partly mediated by the cytochrome P450 3A4 isoenzyme. Gut and liver metabolism converts a large proportion of estradiol to the less potent estrone. Thus, measurement of serum estradiol is not useful for monitoring oral estrogen replacement. The principal metabolites of micronized estradiol are estrone and estrone sulfate. Administration of estradiol via the oral route results in estrone concentrations that are three to six times those of estradiol. Ethinyl estradiol is a highly potent semisynthetic estrogen that has similar activity following administration by the oral or parenteral route.

Orally administered estrogens stimulate the synthesis of hepatic proteins and increase the circulating concentrations of sex hormone–binding globulin, which, in turn, may compromise the bioavailability of androgens and estrogens.

Other Routes Parenteral estrogens (including transdermal, intranasal, and vaginal) bypass the gastrointestinal tract and thereby avoid first-pass liver metabolism. Parenteral routes of estrogen delivery result in a more physiologic estradiol-to-estrone ratio (estradiol con-

TABLE 85-1 Selected Systemic Estrogen Products[a,b]

Estrogen	Dosage Strength	Comments
Oral estrogens		
Conjugated equine estrogens	0.3, 0.45, 0.625, 0.9, 1.25 mg	Orally administered estrogens stimulate synthesis of hepatic proteins and increase circulating concentrations of sex hormone–binding globulin, which, in turn, may compromise the bioavailability of androgens and estrogens
Synthetic conjugated estrogens	0.3, 0.45, 0.625, 0.9, 1.25 mg	
Esterified estrogens	0.3, 0.625, 1.25, 2.5 mg	
Estropipate (piperazine estrone sulfate)	0.625, 1.25, 2.5, 5 mg	
Micronized estradiol	0.5, 1, 1.5, 2 mg	
Estradiol acetate	0.45, 0.9, 1.8 mg	
Parenteral estrogens		
Transdermal 17β-estradiol (patch)	14, 25, 37.5, 50, 60, 75, 100 mcg per 24 h	Women with elevated triglyceride concentrations or significant liver function abnormalities may benefit from parenteral therapy
Estradiol vaginal ring	0.05, 0.1 mg per 24 h (replaced every 3 months)	
Estradiol topical emulsion	4.35 mg of estradiol hemihydrate per foil-laminated pouch	Single approved dose is 8.7 mg of estradiol hemihydrate per day (two pouches)
Estradiol topical gel	0.25 to 1 mg of estradiol per dose	Apply to skin once daily
Estradiol topical solution	1.53 mg of estradiol per spray	Spray on inner surface of forearm once daily
Intranasal estradiol[c]	One spray per nostril delivers 150 mcg	

[a]Systemic oral and transdermal estrogen and progestogen combination products are available in the United States.
[b]Systemic oral estrogen and androgen combination products are available in the United States.
[c]Not available in the United States.

TABLE 85-2 Estrogen for Treatment of Menopausal Symptoms and Osteoporosis Prevention

Regimen	Standard Dose	Low Dose	Route	Frequency
Conjugated equine estrogens	0.625 mg	0.3 or 0.45 mg	Oral	Once daily
Synthetic conjugated estrogens	0.625 mg	0.3 mg	Oral	Once daily
Esterified estrogens	0.625 mg	0.3 mg	Oral	Once daily
Estropipate (piperazine estrone sulfate)	1.5 mg	0.625 mg	Oral	Once daily
Ethinyl estradiol	5 mcg	2.5 mcg	Oral	Once daily
Micronized 17β-estradiol	1–2 mg	0.25–0.5 mg	Oral	Once daily
Transdermal 17β-estradiol	50 mcg	25 mcg	Transdermal (patch)	Once or twice weekly
Intranasal 17β-estradiol[a]	150 mcg per nostril	–	Intranasally	Once daily
Implanted 17β-estradiol	50–100 mg pellets	25-mg pellets	Pellets implanted subcutaneously	Every 6 months
Percutaneous 17β-estradiol	0.04 mg (gel) 0.05 mg (emulsion)		Transdermal (emulsion, gel)	Once daily

[a]Not available in the United States.

centrations greater than estrone concentrations), as seen in the normal premenopausal state. Parenteral estrogen therapy also is less likely to affect sex hormone–binding globulin compared with oral therapy. Parenteral regimens produce little or no change in circulating lipids, coagulation parameters, or C-reactive protein levels.[23]

Transdermal estrogens share the advantages of other parenteral estrogen routes. Transdermal systems have the added advantage of delivering estradiol to the general venous circulation at a continuous rate. Reactions at the application site occur in approximately 10% of women who use reservoir (alcohol-based) patches. The newer matrix systems (estrogen in adhesive) generally are better tolerated, and fewer than 5% of women experience skin reactions.[24] The incidence of skin irritation diminishes when the application site is rotated. Topical antiinflammatory products can be applied for managing the rashes, and switching to another transdermal patch is often a viable option.

Percutaneous preparations (gels, creams, and emulsions) are convenient, but variability in drug absorption is common. This form of estrogen is used for systemic therapy. Topical emulsion and gel formulations are approved for use in the United States.

Estradiol pellets (implants) containing pure crystalline 17β-estradiol have been available for more than 50 years. They are inserted subcutaneously into the anterior abdominal wall or buttock. Pellets are difficult to remove and may continue to release estradiol for a long time after insertion. Implantation should not be repeated until serum estradiol concentrations have fallen to values similar to those at the midfollicular phase of the menstrual cycle. Estradiol pellets have not gained popularity in the United States.

Intranasal 17β-estradiol spray, which enables single-daily or twice-daily dosing, has been shown to have clinical therapeutic equivalence to oral and transdermal estradiol and is associated with significantly lower reports of mastalgia.[25]

Vaginal creams, tablets, and rings are used for treatment of urogenital (vulval and vaginal) atrophy. However, this route of administration can have more than just a local effect. Systemic estrogen absorption is lower with the vaginal tablets and rings (specifically Estring) compared with the vaginal creams. Nonetheless, local application of the cream at low doses can reverse atrophic vaginal changes and avoid significant systemic exposure. Nonestrogen vaginal moisturizers and lubricants also may provide local symptom relief. These products can be used alone or in combination with locally acting vaginal estrogens. Vaginal rings are a sustained-release delivery system composed of a biologically inert liquid polymer matrix with pure crystalline estradiol that can maintain adequate estradiol concentrations. One such vaginal ring product (Femring) is designed to achieve systemic concentrations of estrogen and is indicated for treatment of moderate-to-severe vasomotor symptoms.

The standard dose of estrogen previously believed to be effective in alleviating vasomotor symptoms is equivalent to 0.625 mg CEE,[26] but new evidence indicates that lower doses of estrogen also are effective in controlling postmenopausal symptoms and reducing bone loss (Table 85–2).[27–30] Even ultralow doses of 17β-estradiol delivered by a vaginal ring (Estring) improved serum lipid profiles and prevented bone loss in elderly women.[31] In general, if adverse effects such as breast tenderness occur with initial doses, lowering the dose may resolve the problem and improve patient compliance. Alternatively, if vasomotor symptoms are not controlled adequately with a lower-dose regimen, increasing the estrogen dose may be a reasonable option.

Adverse Effects Common adverse effects of estrogen include nausea, headache, breast tenderness, and heavy bleeding. More serious adverse effects include increased risk for coronary heart disease, stroke, venous thromboembolism, breast cancer, and gallbladder disease.

Initiating therapy with low doses of estrogen often will minimize breast tenderness, unscheduled bleeding, and potentially other adverse effects. Transdermal estrogen is less likely than oral estrogen to cause nausea and headache. Also, transdermal estrogen is associated with a lower incidence of breast tenderness and deep-vein thrombosis than is oral estrogen.[32,33] In many cases changing from one estrogen regimen to another can alleviate certain adverse effects.

Progestogens

❷ Because of the increased risk of endometrial hyperplasia and endometrial cancer with estrogen monotherapy (unopposed estrogen), women who have not undergone hysterectomy should be treated concurrently with a progestogen in addition to the estrogen.[34] Progestogens reduce nuclear estradiol receptor concentrations, suppress DNA synthesis, and decrease estrogen bioavailability by increasing the activity of endometrial 17-hydroxysteroid dehydrogenase, an enzyme responsible for converting estradiol to estrone.[35]

Several progestogen regimens designed to prevent endometrial hyperplasia are available (Table 85–3). Progestogens must be taken for a sufficient period of time during each cycle. A minimum of 12 to 14 days of progestogen therapy each month is required for complete protection against estrogen-induced endometrial hyper-

TABLE 85-3 Progestogen Doses for Endometrial Protection (Oral Cyclic Administration)

Progestogen	Dose
Dydrogesterone[a]	10–20 mg for 12–14 days per calendar month
Medroxyprogesterone acetate	5–10 mg for 12–14 days per calendar month
Micronized progesterone	200 mg for 12–14 days per calendar month
Norethisterone[a]	0.7–1 mg for 12–14 days per calendar month
Norethindrone acetate	5 mg for 12–14 days per calendar month
Norgestrel[a]	0.15 mg for 12–14 days per calendar month
Levonorgestrel[a]	150 mcg for 12–14 days per calendar month

[a]Not available in a progestogen-only oral dosage form in the United States.

plasia.[36] Of note, use of even low-dose estrogen, including some vaginal preparations, requires progestogen coadministration for endometrial protection in women with an intact uterus.[37] However, rarely is progestogen administration needed in women who have undergone hysterectomy.

Four combination estrogen and progestogen regimens currently in use are continuous-cyclic (sequential), continuous-combined, continuous long-cycle (or cyclic withdrawal), and intermittent-combined (or continuous-pulsed) hormone therapy.[38] The latter two were introduced during the past decade. Sequential hormone therapy results in scheduled vaginal withdrawal bleeding but often is scant or completely absent in older women. For many women, the scheduled withdrawal bleeding is one of the main reasons for avoiding or discontinuing hormone therapy. Because there is no physiologic need for bleeding, new hormone therapy regimens that reduce monthly bleeding (e.g., continuous long-cycle regimens) or prevent monthly bleeding (e.g., continuous-combined and intermittent-combined regimens) have been developed. Various hormone therapy regimens that combine an estrogen and a progestogen are available (Table 85–4).

The first generation of progestogens included the C-19 androgenic progestogens norethisterone, norgestrel, and levonorgestrel. More recent preparations have included the C-21 progestogens dydrogesterone and medroxyprogesterone acetate, which are less androgenic. Drospirenone, a synthetic progestogen analog of the potassium-sparing diuretic spironolactone, has both antiandrogenic and antialdosterone properties. Micronized progesterone also has become available for use in postmenopausal women. The most commonly used oral progestogens are medroxyprogesterone acetate, micronized progesterone, and norethisterone acetate. The latter now can be administered transdermally in the form of a combined estrogen–progestogen patch.

Adverse Effects Common adverse effects of progestogens include irritability, depression, and headache. Changing from a cyclic to a continuous-combined regimen or changing from one progestogen to another may decrease the incidence or severity of untoward effects. Adverse effects of progestogens are difficult to evaluate and can vary with the agent administered. Some women experience "premenstrual-like" symptoms, such as mood swings, bloating, fluid retention, and sleep disturbance. New methods and routes of progestogen delivery (e.g., parenterally by an intranasal spray or locally by an intrauterine device that releases levonorgestrel or a progesterone-containing bioadhesive vaginal gel) may be associated with fewer adverse effects. Women who are unable to tolerate a progestogen may be given unopposed estrogen if they are informed of the significant increased risk for endometrial cancer and have endometrial biopsy annually or whenever breakthrough vaginal bleeding occurs.

TABLE 85-4 Common Combination Postmenopausal Hormone Therapy Regimens

Regimen	Doses
Oral continuous-cyclic regimens	
CEE + MPA[a]	0.625 mg + 5 mg; 0.625 mg + 10 mg
Oral continuous-combined regimens	
CEE + MPA	0.625 mg + 2.5 mg; 0.625 mg + 5 mg; 0.45 mg + 2.5 mg; 0.3 mg + 1.5 mg/day
17β-Estradiol + NETA	1 mg + 0.1 mg;1 mg + 0.25 mg; 1 mg + 0.5 mg/day
Ethinyl estradiol + NETA	1 mcg + 0.2 mg; 2.5 mcg + 0.5 mg; 5 mcg + 1 mg; 10 mcg + 1 mg/day
Transdermal continuous-cyclic regimens	
17β-Estradiol + NETA[a]	50 mcg + 0.14 mg; 50 mcg + 0.25 mg
Transdermal continuous-combined regimens	
17β-Estradiol + NETA	50 mcg + 0.14 mg; 50 mcg + 0.25 mg; 25 mcg + 0.125 mg

CEE, conjugated equine estrogens; MPA, medroxyprogesterone acetate; NETA, norethindrone acetate.
Other oral (drospirenone and norgestimate) and transdermal (levonorgestrel) progestogens also are available in combination with an estrogen.
[a]Estrogen alone for days 1–14, followed by estrogen–progestogen on days 15–28.

Methods of Estrogen and Progestogen Administration

Continuous Cyclic Estrogen/Progestogen (Sequential) Treatment Estrogen typically is administered continuously (daily). A progestogen is coadministered with the estrogen for at least 12 to 14 days of a 28-day cycle.[36] The progestogen causes scheduled withdrawal bleeding in approximately 90% of women. With this regimen, bleeding usually begins 1 to 2 days after the last progestogen dose. Occasionally, bleeding begins during the latter phase of progestogen administration.

Continuous Combined Estrogen–Progestogen Treatment Continuous-combined estrogen–progestogen administration results in endometrial atrophy and the absence of vaginal bleeding. However, initially it causes unpredictable spotting or bleeding, which usually resolves within 6 to 12 months. Decreasing the estrogen dose or increasing the progestogen dose usually decreases or stops the spotting. Occasionally, a drug-free period of 1 or 2 weeks is useful to stop the bleeding.

Women who recently have undergone menopause have a higher risk for excessive, unpredictable bleeding while receiving continuous therapy; thus, this regimen is best reserved for women who are at least 2 years postmenopause. Continuous-combined hormone therapy is more acceptable than traditional cyclic therapy.

Continuous Long-Cycle Estrogen–Progestogen Treatment To decrease the incidence of uterine bleeding, a modified sequential regimen has been developed.[38] In the continuous long-cycle (or cyclic-withdrawal) estrogen–progestogen regimen, estrogen is given daily, and progestogen is given six times per year, every other month for 12 to 14 days, resulting in six periods per year. Bleeding episodes may be heavier and last for more days than withdrawal bleeding with continuous-cyclic regimens. The effect of continuous long-cycle estrogen–progestogen treatment on endometrial protection is unclear.

Intermittent Combined Estrogen–Progestogen Treatment The intermittent combined estrogen–progestogen regimen, also called *continuous-pulsed estrogen–progestogen* or *pulsed-progestogen*, consists of 3 days of estrogen therapy alone, followed by 3 days of combined estrogen and progestogen, which is then repeated without interruption.[38] This regimen is designed to lower the incidence of uterine bleeding. It is based on the assumption that pulsed-progestogen administration will prevent downregulation of progesterone receptors that can be produced by continuous-combined regimens. The lower progestogen dose induces fewer side effects and can be better tolerated. The long-term effect of intermittent-combined regimens in endometrial protection is undetermined.

CLINICAL CONTROVERSY

Although some clinicians believe that estrogen can be used safely at lower doses to treat postmenopausal women with severe and protracted vasomotor symptoms, others caution that such long-term therapy, even with lower doses of estrogen, may be associated with unacceptable risks.

Low-Dose Hormone Therapy

❸ Increasingly, it has become recognized that use of hormone therapy at doses lower than prescribed historically is effective in the management of menopausal symptoms (see Table 85–2). The Women's Health, Osteoporosis, Progestin, Estrogen (HOPE) trial demonstrated equivalent symptom relief and bone density preservation without an increase in endometrial hyperplasia using lower doses of hormone therapy (CEE 0.45 mg/day and medroxyprogesterone acetate 1.5 mg/day).[27–31] Whether lower doses of estrogen will be safer (lower incidence of venous thromboembolism and breast cancer) remains to be proven. Nonetheless, evidence of harm associated with a standard dose of hormone therapy[2,3] has prompted many patients to either discontinue such therapy or taper to lower doses.

ANDROGENS

Pathophysiologic states affecting ovarian and adrenal function, along with aging, have been associated with androgen deficiency in women.[39] Therapeutic use of testosterone in women, although controversial, is becoming more widespread despite the lack of accurate clinical or biochemical findings of androgen deficiency.[39] Androgens have important biologic effects in women, acting both directly via androgen receptors in tissues, such as bone, skin fibroblasts, hair follicles, and sebaceous glands, and indirectly via the aromatization of testosterone to estrogen in the ovaries, bone, brain, adipose tissue, and other tissues.

A cluster of symptoms that characterizes androgen insufficiency in women, manifested as diminished sense of well-being, persistent or unexplained fatigue, and sexual function changes such as decreased libido, decreased sexual receptivity, and decreased pleasure, has been reported.[39] However, studies designed to evaluate this have shown no relationships between serum total and free testosterone levels and either sexual function[40] or well-being[41] in women. Thus, as data supporting an androgen deficiency syndrome are lacking, in 2006 the American Endocrine Society recommended against making a diagnosis of androgen deficiency in women at the present time.[40] Evidence of short-term efficacy of testosterone is seen in selected populations, such as surgically menopausal women.[42] Studies with adequate followup are necessary to assess long-term safety and efficacy of androgen therapy in women.

Absolute contraindications to androgen therapy include pregnancy or lactation and known or suspected androgen-dependent neoplasia. Relative contraindications include concurrent use of CEEs (for parenteral testosterone therapy), low sex hormone–binding globulin level, moderate–to-severe acne, clinical hirsutism, and androgenic alopecia.

Adverse effects from excessive dosage include virilization, fluid retention, and potentially adverse lipoprotein lipid effects, which are more likely with oral administration.

Testosterone is available as oral methyltestosterone in the United States and as testosterone implants in the United Kingdom. Of the available oral preparations, methyltestosterone in combination with esterified estrogen (either 0.625 mg esterified estrogen plus 1.25 mg methyltestosterone or 1.25 mg esterified estrogen plus 2.5 mg methyltestosterone) is the most widely studied.

Testosterone replacement for women is available in a variety of formulations (Table 85–5). Most of the earlier studies showing clinical improvement with testosterone therapy reported supraphysiologic levels. More recent studies using transdermal patch therapy have shown efficacy with free testosterone levels in the upper normal range for young women. The availability of testosterone regimens specifically designed for women has the potential to maintain testosterone levels within the normal range and help to clarify whether the apparent beneficial effects of testosterone therapy are physiologic or pharmacologic.[42,43] In general, testosterone treatment should not be administered to postmenopausal women who are not receiving concurrent estrogen therapy until completion of studies on the use of testosterone without estrogen. At present, generalized use of testosterone is not recommended because the indications are inadequate, and evidence from long-term studies evaluating safety is lacking.[44]

SELECTIVE ESTROGEN RECEPTOR MODULATORS

Selective estrogen receptor modulators (SERMs) are a group of nonsteroidal compounds that are chemically distinct from estradiol. They act as estrogen agonists in some tissues, such as bone, and as estrogen antagonists in other tissues, such as breast, through specific, high-affinity binding to the estrogen receptor.

The ideal SERM would protect against osteoporosis and decrease the incidence of breast, endometrial, and colorectal cancer and coronary heart disease without exacerbating menopausal symptoms or increasing the risk of venous thromboembolism or gallbladder disease. To date, no SERM meets these ideals. Tamoxifen, the first-generation SERM (a nonsteroidal triphenylethylene derivative), has estrogen antagonist activity on the breast and estrogen-like agonist activity on bone and endometrium. The second generation of SERMs, most notably raloxifene (a nonsteroidal benzothiophene derivative), has become available for prevention of osteoporosis. Raloxifene does not alleviate, and may even exacerbate, vasomotor symptoms.

Raloxifene decreases bone loss in recently menopausal women without affecting the endometrium and has estrogen-like actions on lipid metabolism.[45] Raloxifene generally is well tolerated. Its adverse effects include leg cramps and hot flushes.

The Multiple Outcomes of Raloxifene Evaluation (MORE), a multicenter randomized, blinded, placebo-controlled trial, showed that raloxifene increases bone mineral density in the spine and femoral neck and reduces the risk of vertebral fractures.[45] More important, the same study[46] and the Continuing Outcomes Relevant to Evista (CORE) trial[47] suggest that raloxifene use is associated with a significantly lower incidence of breast cancer compared with placebo. This benefit is primarily due to a reduced risk of estrogen receptor–positive invasive breast cancers.[47,48] A prospective randomized study (Raloxifene Use for the Heart [RUTH]) of 10,101 postmenopausal women (mean age 67.5 years) with coronary heart disease or multiple risk factors for coronary heart disease showed that raloxifene did not significantly affect the risk of coronary heart disease.[48] Nonetheless, raloxifene use increases the risk of venous thromboembolism[45–48] and stroke[48] to a degree similar to that of oral estrogen.

TABLE 85-5 Androgen Regimens Used for Women

Regimen	Dose	Frequency	Route
Methyltestosterone in combination with esterified estrogen	1.25–2.5 mg	Daily	Oral
Mixed testosterone esters	50–100 mg	Every 4–6 weeks	Intramuscular
Testosterone pellets	50 mg	Every 6 months	Subcutaneous (implanted)
Transdermal testosterone system[a]	150–300 mcg/day	Every 3–4 days	Transdermal patch
Nandrolone decanoate	50 mg	Every 8–12 weeks	Intramuscular

[a]Undergoing clinical trials in the United States.

TIBOLONE

Tibolone is a gonadomimetic synthetic steroid in the norpregnane family with combined estrogenic, progestogenic, and androgenic activity.[49] Tibolone has been used for almost 2 decades in Europe for treatment of menopausal symptoms and prevention of osteoporosis. The hormonal effects of this synthetic steroid depend on its metabolism and activation in peripheral tissues. The parent compound has been described as a prodrug that is metabolized quickly in the gastrointestinal tract. It has several active metabolites, including a $\Delta 4$-isomer and 3α-OH and 3β-OH compounds.[49] The $\Delta 4$-isomer metabolite confers significant progestogenic and androgenic properties. Tibolone has beneficial effects on mood and libido and improves menopausal symptoms and vaginal atrophy. Tibolone protects against bone loss and reduces the risk of vertebral fractures in postmenopausal women with osteoporosis.[50] Tibolone use in elderly women has been reported to be associated with an increased risk of stroke.[50]

Tibolone reduces concentrations of total cholesterol, triglycerides, and lipoprotein (a) but significantly decreases HDL cholesterol and thus may increase overall cardiovascular risk.[22] Long-term safety data are lacking. The Million Women Study, a cohort study, suggested that current users of tibolone may be at increased risk for breast cancer (adjusted relative risk 1.45, 95% CI 1.25–1.68).[21] This study had multiple limitations, including biased prescribing of tibolone in the community to women at greater risk for breast cancer. The Million Women Study also indicated a greater risk of endometrial cancer (adjusted relative risk 1.79, 95% CI 1.43–2.25).[51] However, other controlled studies contradict this finding and suggest that tibolone has an endometrial safety profile similar to continuous-combined CEE and medroxyprogesterone acetate.[52]

The major adverse effects of tibolone include weight gain and bloating. Additional studies are necessary to identify the true risk-to-benefit ratio of tibolone with respect to its overall effect on coronary artery disease and breast cancer.

TREATMENT CONSIDERATIONS

In the absence of contraindications, hormone therapy is appropriate mainly for women with hot flashes and vulvar or vaginal atrophy.[53] It is contraindicated in women with endometrial cancer, breast cancer, undiagnosed vaginal bleeding, coronary heart disease, thromboembolism (including recent spontaneous thrombosis or in the presence of a thrombophilia), stroke or transient ischemic attack, and active liver disease.[53] Relative contraindications include uterine leiomyoma, migraine headaches, and seizure disorder. In addition, oral estrogen should be avoided in women with hypertriglyceridemia, liver disease, and gallbladder disease. For these women, transdermal administration is a safer approach. The main reasons for discontinuing hormone therapy are side effects such as bleeding, breast tenderness, bloating, and "premenstrual-like symptoms." Reducing the dose or changing the regimen or the route of administration can minimize these effects.

Pretreatment Assessment

The initial visit of a perimenopausal or postmenopausal woman is the most appropriate time to obtain a complete medical history, perform a physical examination, and educate the patient. Medical history should include a personal or family history of coronary heart disease and thrombotic problems. The physical examination should include a complete cardiovascular examination, clinical assessment of thyroid status, and breast and pelvic examinations. Papanicolaou cervical cytologic examination and screening mammography negative for malignancy are required before initiating hormone therapy. Thyroid function tests and lipoprotein lipid profile also are performed at the discretion of the clinician.

Each patient should be evaluated for the presence of indications (i.e., menopausal symptoms such as hot flushes or vaginal dryness) and possible contraindications. The risks and benefits of hormone therapy should be discussed with the patient so that she can weigh the risks and benefits versus alternatives and make a rational decision about whether to use hormone therapy.

BENEFITS OF HORMONE THERAPY

Relief of Menopausal Symptoms

Vasomotor Symptoms ❹ The major indication for postmenopausal hormone therapy is management of vasomotor symptoms. Most women with vasomotor symptoms require hormone treatment for fewer than 5 years, so the risk appears to be small.

Fewer than 25% of women experience a menopausal transition without symptoms, whereas more than 25% suffer severe menopausal symptoms, most commonly hot flushes and night sweats.[54]

Without treatment, hot flushes in most women typically disappear within 1 to 2 years, but in some untreated women hot flashes continue for more than 20 years.[32] Women with mild vasomotor symptoms often experience relief by lifestyle modification (e.g., wearing layered clothing that can be removed or added as necessary); reduction in intake of hot spicy foods, caffeine, and hot beverages; exercise; and other good general health practices. At least 25% of women in clinical trials reported significant improvement of vasomotor symptoms when taking placebo. However, no therapy has been shown to be as effective as estrogen therapy in alleviating significant vasomotor symptoms. Estrogens diminish hot flushes in most women, and all types and routes of administration of estrogen are equally effective.[55] A dose-dependent relationship between estrogen administration and suppression of hot flushes is well established. Some women, especially younger women, may require a higher than average dose of estrogen to suppress symptoms. On the other hand, many women with hot flushes at the time of menopause require lower dose of estrogen.[55] Hormone therapy for menopausal symptoms can be stopped about 2 or 3 years after starting. If treatment can be tapered and stopped within 5 years, no evidence of increased risk of breast cancer is seen.[2]

Alternatives to estrogen for treatment of hot flushes include tibolone, selective serotonin reuptake inhibitors (e.g., paroxetine, fluoxetine), dual serotonin and noradrenaline reuptake inhibitors (e.g., venlafaxine), medroxyprogesterone acetate, megestrol acetate, clonidine, and gabapentin (Table 85–6).[56] Progestogens alone may be an option for some women (e.g., those with a history of breast cancer or venous thrombosis), but weight gain, vaginal bleeding, and other adverse effects often limit their use. Tibolone and progestogens cannot be considered nonhormonal agents for treatment of hot flushes in women for whom hormone therapy is contraindicated. For this group of patients, selective serotonin reuptake inhibitors and venlafaxine are considered by some to be a first-line therapy.[56,57] However, the efficacy of venlafaxine for treatment of hot flushes has not been shown to extend beyond 12 weeks.[58] Furthermore, in breast cancer patients, evidence suggests that selective serotonin reuptake inhibitors could interfere with metabolism of endocrine therapies, such as tamoxifen.[59] Clonidine often is effective for symptom control but is not always well tolerated by women.

Randomized, placebo-controlled trials of nonhormonal therapies have been equivocal and have not established the safety and efficacy of herbal remedies, homeopathic treatments, or acupuncture for prevention or treatment of hot flushes.

Vaginal Atrophy Estrogen receptors have been demonstrated in the lower genitourinary tract, and at least 50% of postmenopausal women suffer symptoms of urogenital atrophy caused by estrogen deficiency.[60] Atrophy of the vaginal mucosa results in vaginal dryness

TABLE 85-6 Alternatives to Estrogen for Treatment of Hot Flushes

Drug	Dose (Oral)	Interval	Comments
Tibolone	2.5–5 mg	Once daily	Tibolone is not recommended during the perimenopause because it may cause irregular bleeding
Venlafaxine	37.5–150 mg	Once daily	Side effects include dry mouth, decreased appetite, nausea, and constipation
Paroxetine	12.5–25 mg	Once daily	12.5 mg is an adequate, well-tolerated starting dose for most women; adverse effects include headache, nausea, and insomnia
Fluoxetine	20 mg	Once daily	Modest improvement seen in hot flushes
Megestrol acetate	20–40 mg	Once daily	Progesterone may be linked to breast cancer etiology; also, there is concern regarding the safety of progestational agents in women with preexisting breast cancer
Clonidine	0.1 mg	Once daily	Can be administered orally or transdermally; drowsiness and dry mouth can occur, especially with higher doses
Gabapentin	900 mg	Divided in three daily doses	Adverse effects include somnolence and dizziness; these symptoms often can be obviated with a gradual increase in dosing

and dyspareunia. Lower urinary tract symptoms include urethritis, recurrent urinary tract infection, urinary urgency, and frequency. Most women with significant vaginal dryness because of vaginal atrophy require local or systemic estrogen therapy for symptom relief. Such treatment also reduces the risk of recurrent urinary tract infections, possibly by modifying the vaginal flora.[61] Vaginal dryness and dyspareunia can be treated with a topical estrogen cream, tablet, or vaginal ring. In clinical trials, topical estrogen appears to be better than systemic estrogen for relieving these symptoms and avoids high levels of circulating estrogen. Concomitant progestogen therapy generally is unnecessary if women are using low-dose micronized 17β-estradiol. However, regular use of CEE vaginal creams and other products that potentially promote endometrial proliferation in women with an intact uterus requires intermittent progestogen challenges (i.e., for 10 days every 12 weeks). This is an important caveat because vaginal atrophy requires long-term estrogen treatment.[61]

Urinary incontinence, which becomes more prevalent with increasing age, usually is not improved by estrogen therapy. In one large clinical trial, estrogen–progestogen therapy actually increased incontinence.[62]

Osteoporosis Prevention

❺ Postmenopausal osteoporosis is a serious age-related disease that affects millions of women throughout the world. The WHI randomized trial was the first study to demonstrate that hormone therapy reduces the risk of fractures at the hip, spine, and wrist.[2,63] Hip and clinical vertebral fractures are reduced by 34%, and total osteoporotic fractures are reduced by 24%.[63] These findings are in agreement with observational data and several meta-analyses of the efficacy of hormone therapy for reducing fractures in postmenopausal women.[64]

Menopause is accompanied by accelerated bone loss, and the central role of estrogen deficiency in postmenopausal osteoporosis is well established. Osteoporosis is characterized by reduced bone mass associated with architectural deterioration of the skeleton and increased risk for fracture.[65] Estrogen deficiency results in bone loss through its actions in accelerating bone turnover and uncoupling bone formation from resorption. Annual decrements in bone mass of 3% to 5% are common in the years soon after the menopause, and decrements of 0.5% to 1% are seen after age 65 years.[66] Estrogen therapy reduces bone turnover and increases bone density in postmenopausal women of all ages. Nonetheless, the protective effect persists as long as the treatment is maintained. With cessation of therapy, postmenopausal bone loss resumes at the same rate as in untreated women. The standard bone-sparing daily estrogen dose is equivalent to 0.625 mg CEE[26] (see Table 85–2). Even low doses of estrogen may increase bone mass when they are supplemented with adequate calcium intake.[26]

Osteoporosis prevention remains an indicated use of estrogen products; however, nonestrogen products, such as raloxifene and bisphosphonates, are as effective as hormone therapy for preventing osteoporosis (Table 85–7). The FDA has withdrawn the "osteoporosis treatment" indication from estrogen products.

Raloxifene decreases the risk of vertebral fracture by 30% to 50%, although it has not been shown to decrease the risk of hip fracture.[46] The bisphosphonates reduce the risk of both hip and vertebral fractures by 30% to 50%.[65] Bisphosphonates are analogs of pyrophosphate that inhibit bone resorption. Drugs in this class include alendronate, etidronate, pamidronate, risedronate, tiludronate, and zoledronate. Bisphosphonates have no known impact on the incidence of cardiovascular disease or breast or endometrial cancer. Adverse effects include upper gastrointestinal side effects, especially if not taken properly. A few trials have shown improved bone density over single therapy when a bisphosphonate is combined with estrogen or raloxifene, but no fracture data are available.[67]

Tibolone can prevent bone loss and vertebral fractures in postmenopausal women with osteoporosis.[50]

TABLE 85-7 Alternatives to Hormone Therapy for Osteoporosis Prevention

Drug	Dose	Comments
Raloxifene	60 mg/day	Raloxifene reduces the risk of vertebral fractures. Adverse effects include hot flushes and leg cramps. Slowly increasing the dose of raloxifene may help reduce the incidence and severity of hot flushes.
Tibolone	1.25 mg or 2.5 mg/day	Tibolone prevents bone loss. No data regarding fracture rates are available.
Alendronate	5 mg/day or 35 mg/wk	A 50% reduction in the risk of fractures is observed in women with osteoporosis. In younger postmenopausal women without osteoporosis, therapy with alendronate protected all women from bone loss for up to 4 years. Side effects include upper gastrointestinal symptoms, especially if the drug is not taken as directed.
Risedronate	5 mg/day or 35 mg/wk	A 40% reduction in vertebral and nonvertebral fractures is observed in women with osteoporosis. In postmenopausal women without osteoporosis, risedronate increases bone mineral density over 2 years. Significant side effects were not observed.
Etidronate	Intermittent administration of 400 mg/day (in 2-wk cycles); dose repeated every 3 months	Calcium is taken between the cycles of etidronate. Continuous daily use may cause abnormalities in bone mineralization. A 37% reduction is observed in the risk of vertebral fractures (but not nonvertebral fractures) in women with osteoporosis. Therapy in women without osteoporosis prevents bone loss over 2 years. Side effects include diarrhea and nausea.
Zoledronic acid	4 mg as a single intravenous infusion once yearly	Effects on bone turnover and bone density were similar to those with daily oral bisphosphonates. Adverse effects include myalgia and pyrexia.

General protective measures, such as adequate calcium intake (1,200 mg/day),[68] regular weight-bearing exercise, and avoidance of detrimental lifestyle habits such as smoking and alcohol abuse, are appropriate for all women. Most women require calcium supplementation to their dietary intake. Adequate exposure to sunlight is believed to protect against vitamin D deficiency, but many western women are deficient in this vitamin. The current recommended dietary intake for vitamin D is 400 international units/day for women aged 51 to 70 years and 600 international units/day for women older than 70 years.[68]

Low bone density is the most important risk factor for osteoporosis. According to the World Health Organization, a woman with a bone mineral density >2.5 SD below the mean peak density has osteoporosis.[65] The rates of osteoporosis vary with ethnicity; it is more common in whites and those of Asian descent and less common in blacks.[65] In the United States, approximately 20% of white women 50 years and older have osteoporosis.[65]

Bone mass measurement accurately determines the bone density in the spine and hip. The current "gold standard" method of bone density testing is dual-energy x-ray absorptiometry (DEXA).[65] In the United States, bone density testing is recommended for all women with medical causes of bone loss and for all women 65 years or older. Bone density testing should be assessed in conjunction with clinical risk profile evaluation. For women at high risk for fracture (i.e., T-score <2, previous nonspine fracture, family history of hip or spine fracture, and low body weight), bisphosphonates are the treatment of choice because of demonstrated fracture protection.[65] There are no clear indications for treating women at low risk for fracture (T-score >2), but raloxifene, tibolone, and bisphosphonates can be used. Long-term hormone therapy is no longer an appropriate first-choice option for osteoporosis prevention because of the risks associated with its long-term use. Therefore, hormone therapy should be considered for osteoporosis prevention only in women at significant risk for osteoporosis who cannot take nonestrogen regimens.

Colon Cancer Risk Reduction

Colorectal cancer is the fourth most common cancer and the second leading cause of cancer death in the United States (see Chapter 133). The estrogen-progestogen arm of the WHI study was the first randomized, controlled trial to confirm that combined estrogen–progestogen therapy reduces colon cancer risk. Compared with placebo, six fewer colorectal cancers are reported per year in every 10,000 women taking hormone therapy.[2]

Other

Diabetes In healthy postmenopausal women, hormone therapy appears to have a beneficial effect on fasting glucose levels in women with elevated fasting insulin concentrations.[69] Also, in women with coronary artery disease, hormone therapy reduces the incidence of diabetes by 35%.[70] These findings provide important insights into the metabolic effects of hormone therapy but are insufficient to recommend the long-term use of hormone therapy in women with diabetes.

Body Weight A meta-analysis of randomized controlled trials showed that unopposed estrogen or estrogen combined with a progestogen has no effect on body weight, suggesting that hormone therapy does not cause weight gain in excess of that normally observed at the time of menopause.[71]

■ RISKS OF HORMONE THERAPY

Cardiovascular Disease

❻ Cardiovascular disease, including coronary artery disease, stroke, and peripheral vascular disease, is the leading cause of death among women. The American Heart Association recommends that postmenopausal hormone therapy should not be used for reducing the risk of coronary heart disease.[72]

In the last decade, an expectation of coronary benefit had been a major reason for use of postmenopausal hormone because observational studies indicated that women who use hormone therapy have a 35% to 50% lower risk of coronary heart disease than do nonusers.[73] In addition, previous studies have shown that estrogen exerts protective effects on the cardiovascular system, including lipid-lowering,[74] antioxidant,[75] and vasodilating effects.[76] Nevertheless, recent randomized clinical trials have provided no evidence of cardiovascular disease protection and even some evidence of harm with hormone therapy.[2,77–80]

The primary findings of the estrogen-progestogen arm of the WHI trial showed an overall increase in the risk of coronary heart disease (HR 1.24, 95% CI 1–1.54) among healthy postmenopausal women 50 to 79 years old receiving combined estrogen–progestogen hormone therapy compared with those receiving placebo.[2,80] The primary findings of the estrogen-only arm of the WHI trial show no effect (either increase or decrease) on the risk of coronary heart disease in women taking estrogen alone.[3] However, recent analysis revealed that women in this cohort who initiated hormone therapy closer to the time of menopause tended to have decreased coronary heart disease risk compared to the increased risk noted among women who were more distant from menopause when estrogen therapy was initiated.[81,82]

In the estrogen–progestogen arm of the WHI trial, the elevation in coronary heart disease risk was most apparent at 1 year (HR 1.81, 95% CI 1.09–3.01). The increased risk for stroke and venous thromboembolism continued throughout the 5 years of therapy.[2] Increased risk was observed only for ischemic stroke and not for hemorrhagic stroke.[83] In the estrogen-alone arm of the study, a similar increased risk for stroke was observed.[3] Recent evidence suggests that hormone therapy has different effects on coronary heart disease risk in women when initiated in the early menopausal years (50–59 years of age) versus long after the menopause (i.e., menopausal for more than a decade), emphasizing the importance of timing of hormone therapy initiation.[81,82,84]

Raloxifene therapy does not significantly affect the risk for coronary heart disease.[48]

In the WHI trial, it is unclear whether the cardiovascular effects of hormone therapy during the perimenopause/early menopause and late menopause differ. There is a need for a long-term randomized controlled study of low-dose hormone therapy started around the time of menopause.[85] Hormone therapy should not be initiated or continued for the prevention of cardiovascular disease. Adherence to a healthful lifestyle (cessation of smoking, regular exercise, healthy diet, and body mass index <25) may prevent the onset of cardiovascular disease in postmenopausal women.[86,87]

Breast Cancer

The WHI trial found that combined estrogen–progestogen therapy has an increased risk of invasive breast cancer (HR 1.26, 95% CI 1.0–1.59) and a trend toward increasing risk with increasing duration of therapy.[2] The estrogen-only arm of the WHI trial found no increased risk for breast cancer during the 7-year followup period. [3] In the estrogen–progestogen arm, the increased breast cancer risk did not appear until after 3 years of study participation.[2] The breast cancers diagnosed in women in the hormone therapy group had similar histology and grade but were more likely to be in an advanced stage compared with women in the placebo group.[88] In an unselected postmenopausal population, the Million Women Study found that current use of hormone therapy increased breast cancer risk and breast cancer mortality (relative risk 1.66 and 1.22, respectively). Increased incidence was observed for estrogen-only use (relative risk 1.30), for estrogen–progestogen (relative risk 2), and for tibolone (relative risk 1.45).[21]

The lifetime risk of developing breast cancer in the United States is approximately one in eight women,[89] and the greatest incidence occurs in women older than 60 years (see Chapter 131). In a collaborative reanalysis of data from 51 studies evaluating more than 52,000 women with breast cancer and 108,000 controls, less than 5 years of therapy with estrogen combined with progestogen was associated with a 15% increase in the risk of breast cancer, and the increase was greater with longer duration (relative risk 1.53 after ≥5 of use).[90] However, 5 years after discontinuation of hormone replacement therapy, the risk of breast cancer was no longer increased.[90]

Addition of progestogens to estrogen may increase breast cancer risk beyond that observed with estrogen alone.[91] The Iowa Women's Health Study showed that exposure to hormone therapy is associated with an increased risk of breast cancer that has a favorable prognosis.[92] These findings have been attributed to an increased breast cancer screening in women taking hormone therapy. A study of the effects of hormone therapy in women with a family history of breast cancer found that those who currently were receiving hormone therapy had approximately the same increased relative risk compared with those who did not have a family history.[93] The overall mortality for women with a family history of breast cancer from all causes was reduced significantly among hormone therapy users.[93] These data suggest that hormone therapy use in women with a family history of breast cancer is not associated with a significantly increased incidence of the disease.

Sex steroid deficiency during menopause results in lipomatous involution of the breast, which is seen as decreased mammographic breast density and markedly improved radiotransparency of breast tissue. Thus, mammographic changes indicating breast cancer can be recognized more easily and earlier after the menopause. Conversely, combination hormone therapy results in increased mammographic breast density, and increased density on mammography has been associated with higher breast cancer risk.[94] Of note, increased mammographic density is not observed with estrogen-only therapy.[95]

Although raloxifene is not approved for prevention or treatment of breast cancer, a 4-year trial of raloxifene in women with osteoporosis (who were not at increased risk for breast cancer) showed a 76% risk reduction for estrogen receptor–positive breast cancer[46] (relative risk 0.24, 95% CI 0.13–0.44). Furthermore, the CORE trial, a study evaluating the efficacy of an additional 4 years of raloxifene therapy in women with osteoporosis, showed that the reduction in incidence of estrogen receptor–positive breast cancer continues for up to 8 years (HR 0.24, 95% CI 0.15–0.40).[47] Importantly, a prospective randomized double-blinded trial of 19,747 women at high risk for breast cancer (Study of Tamoxifen and Raloxifene [STAR]) showed that raloxifene is as effective as tamoxifen in reducing the risk of invasive breast cancer and has a lower risk of thromboembolic events.[96]

Endometrial Cancer

The WHI trial suggests that combined hormone therapy does not increase endometrial cancer risk compared with placebo (HR 0.81, 95% CI 0.48–1.36).[97] Estrogen alone given to women with an intact uterus significantly increases uterine cancer risk.[35] With unopposed estrogen therapy, the risk of endometrial cancer increases within 2 years.[35] The excess risk increases with dose and duration of estrogen (10 years of unopposed estrogen increases the risk 10-fold), is apparent within 2 years of the start of treatment, and persists for many years after estrogen replacement is discontinued. Estrogen-induced endometrial cancer usually is of a low stage and grade at the time of diagnosis,[32] and it can be prevented almost entirely by progestogen coadministration. The sequential addition of progestogen to estrogen for at least 10 days of the treatment cycle or continuous combined estrogen–progestogen does not increase the risk of endometrial cancer.[98]

Lower doses of estrogen may be associated with a lower risk of endometrial hyperplasia.[99] Raloxifene does not result in endometrial hyperplasia, has no effect on endometrial thickness, is not associated with polyp formation, and has virtually no proliferative effect on the endometrium.[100] A 4-year trial of raloxifene in women with osteoporosis showed no increased risk of endometrial cancer.[48]

Ovarian Cancer

Lifetime risk of ovarian cancer is low (1.7%). The WHI trial suggests that combined hormone therapy may increase the risk of ovarian cancer (HR 1.58, 95% CI 0.77–3.24).[97] However, a study reported an increased risk of ovarian cancer in women taking postmenopausal estrogen therapy for more than 10 years (relative risk 1.8, 95% CI 1.1–3.0) but no increased risk of ovarian cancer among women receiving combination estrogen–progestogen therapy.[101] Additional large, controlled studies are needed to confirm these findings.

Venous Thromboembolism

Venous thromboembolism, including thrombosis of the deep veins of the legs and embolism to the pulmonary arteries, is uncommon in the general population. The absolute risk of venous thromboembolism in nonhormone therapy users is approximately 1 in 10,000 women.[102] Women taking combined estrogen–progestogen hormone therapy have a twofold increased risk for thromboembolic events, with the highest risk occurring in the first year of use.[103] The absolute increase in risk is small, with 1.5 venous thromboembolic events per 10,000 women in 1 year.[103] Lower doses of estrogen are associated with a decreased risk for thromboembolism as compared with higher doses.[102] Oral administration of estrogen increases the risk of venous thromboembolism compared to the transdermal route.[104] Also, the norpregnane progestogens, unlike micronized progesterone and pregnane derivatives (e.g., medroxyprogesterone acetate), appear to be thrombogenic.

Currently, there is no indication for thrombophilia screening before initiating hormone therapy. However, hormone therapy should be avoided in women at high risk for thromboembolic events.

Gallbladder Disease

Gallbladder disease is a commonly cited complication of oral estrogen use. A randomized trial showed an increased risk for cholecystitis, cholelithiasis, and cholecystectomy among women taking oral estrogen or estrogen–progestogen therapy.[105] Transdermal estrogen is an alternative to oral therapy for women at high risk for cholelithiasis.

CLINICAL CONTROVERSY

Some clinicians believe that hormone therapy improves well-being and quality of life of postmenopausal women, whereas others believe that hormone therapy, at best, has no effect. Hormone therapy improves mood and well-being mainly in women with vasomotor symptoms and sleep disturbance.

■ OTHER EFFECTS OF HORMONE THERAPY

Quality of Life, Mood, Cognition, and Dementia

❼ Hormone therapy improves depressive symptoms in symptomatic menopausal women, most probably by relieving flushing and improving sleep.[106] Women with vasomotor symptoms receiving hormone therapy have improved mental health and fewer depressive symptoms compared with women receiving placebo; however, hormone therapy may worsen quality of life in women without flushes.[107]

There is no evidence that hormone therapy improves quality of life or cognition in older, asymptomatic women.[106–110]

More than 33% of women 65 years and older will develop dementia during their lifetime.[111] Several observational studies have suggested that estrogen therapy may be protective against Alzheimer's disease (see Chapter 67). The WHI Memory Study (an ancillary study of WHI trial) evaluated the effect of combined hormone therapy on dementia and cognition in 4,532 women 65 years and older.[110] The study found that postmenopausal women 65 years and older taking estrogen plus progestogen therapy had twice the rate of dementia, including Alzheimer's disease, than women taking placebo (HR 2.05, 95% CI 1.21–3.48).[110] In addition, estrogen plus progestogen therapy in these women did not prevent mild cognitive impairment, a cognitive and functional state between normal aging and dementia that frequently progresses to dementia.[110] The estrogen-alone arm of the WHI trial showed similar findings.[112,113]

Raloxifene does not have a significant effect on cognitive function; however, there is a trend toward a smaller decline in verbal memory and attention scores among women receiving raloxifene.[114]

Hormone therapy does not improve quality of life in postmenopausal women who do not have vasomotor symptoms. Hormone therapy does not improve cognitive function compared with placebo and, more importantly, produces an increased risk (albeit small) of clinically meaningful cognitive decline among women 65 years and older taking hormone therapy.[107–110,112,113]

■ INDIVIDUALIZING HORMONE THERAPY

❽ Menopause is a natural life event, not a disease. The decision to take hormone therapy must be individualized and based on several parameters, including menopausal symptoms, osteoporosis risk, coronary artery disease risk, breast cancer risk, and thromboembolism risk. Recommendations should be specific to each woman and her background (Table 85–8). Thus, menopausal treatment should be based on each woman's clinical profile and concerns. Approved indications of hormone therapy include treatment of vasomotor symptoms and urogenital atrophy and prevention of osteoporosis. Weighing risks and benefits, the FDA determined that the indication for vasomotor symptoms (hot flushes and night sweats) should remain unchanged, but the other two indications for hormone therapy should be revised. For treatment of vasomotor symptoms, systemic hormone therapy remains the most effective pharmacologic intervention (Fig. 85–1). For symptoms of urogenital atrophy, such as vaginal dryness, topical products should be considered. In addition, although prevention of postmenopausal osteoporosis remains an indicated use of hormone therapy, consideration should be given to approved nonestrogen products, such as raloxifene and bisphosphonates (Fig. 85–1). Clinicians should prescribe the lowest effective dose of hormone therapy for the shortest duration, weighing the potential benefits and risks for the individual woman. Measures to reduce the risks of cardiovascular disease (e.g., treating hypertension and avoiding smoking) and osteoporosis (e.g., taking calcium supplements and vitamin D, changing diet, and performing weight-bearing exercise) should be addressed.

TABLE 85-8 Evidence-Based Hormone Therapy Guidelines for Menopausal Symptom Management

Recommendation	Recommendation Grade[a]
In the absence of contraindications, estrogen-based postmenopausal hormone therapy should be used for treatment of moderate-to-severe vasomotor symptoms	A1
Systemic or vaginal estrogen therapy should be used for treatment of urogenital symptoms and vaginal atrophy	A1
Hormone therapy should be prescribed at the lowest effective dose and for the shortest duration	B2
Postmenopausal women taking estrogen-based therapy should be followed-up every year, taking into account findings from new clinical trials	A1
Postmenopausal women taking estrogen-based therapy for longer than 5 years should be informed about potential risks	A1
Safety and tolerability may vary substantially with the type and regimen of hormone therapy	B2
Breast cancer risk increases after use of continuous combined hormone therapy for longer than 5 years	A1
Breast cancer risk does not increase after long-term estrogen-only therapy (6.8 years) in postmenopausal women with hysterectomy	A1
Hormone therapy should not be used for primary or secondary prevention of coronary heart disease	A1
Oral hormone therapy increases risk of venous thromboembolism	A1
Parenteral hormone therapy may be safer for postmenopausal women at risk for venous thromboembolism who choose to take hormone therapy	B2
Oral hormone therapy increases risk of ischemic stroke	A1
Although hormone therapy decreases risk of osteoporotic fractures, it cannot be recommended as a first-line therapy for the treatment of osteoporosis	A1
Potential harm (cardiovascular disease, breast cancer, and thromboembolism) from long-term hormone therapy (use greater than 5 years) outweighs potential benefits	A1
Young women with premature ovarian failure have severe menopausal symptoms and increased risk for osteoporosis and cardiovascular disease. Decisions on whether and how these young women must be treated should not be based on studies of hormone therapy in women older than 50 years	B3

Quality of evidence: 1 = evidence from more than one properly randomized, controlled trial; 2 = evidence from more than one well-designed clinical trial with randomization, from cohort or case-controlled analytic studies or multiple time series; or dramatic results from uncontrolled experiments; 3 = evidence from opinions of respected authorities, based on clinical experience, descriptive studies, or reports of expert communities.

[a]Strength of recommendations: A, B, C = good, moderate, and poor evidence to support recommendation, respectively.

EVALUATION OF THERAPEUTIC OUTCOMES

After the menopausal woman begins hormone therapy, a brief followup visit 6 weeks later may be useful to discuss patient concerns about hormone therapy and to evaluate the patient for symptom relief, adverse effects, and patterns of withdrawal bleeding. The FDA recommends that women who choose estrogen-based therapy should have yearly breast examinations, perform monthly breast self-examinations, and receive periodic mammograms (scheduled based on their age and risk factors). Also, women receiving hormone therapy should undergo annual monitoring, including a medical history, physical examination, pelvic examination, blood pressure measurement, and routine endometrial cancer surveillance, as indicated. Additional followup is determined based on the patient's initial response to therapy and the need for any modification of the regimen. Endometrial biopsy should be considered in women taking cyclic hormone therapy if vaginal bleeding occurs at any time other than the expected time of withdrawal bleeding or when heavier or more prolonged withdrawal bleeding occurs. In women taking continuous combined hormone therapy, endometrial evaluation should be considered when irregular bleeding persists for more than 6 months after initiating therapy. Endovaginal ultrasonography also has been used for evaluation of abnormal uterine bleeding in women receiving hormone therapy. However, there is no universal agreement that endovaginal ultrasonography is adequate for excluding endometrial pathology.

The main indication for hormone therapy is relief of menopausal symptoms, and hormone therapy should be used only as long as symptom control is necessary (typically 2–3 years). When hormone

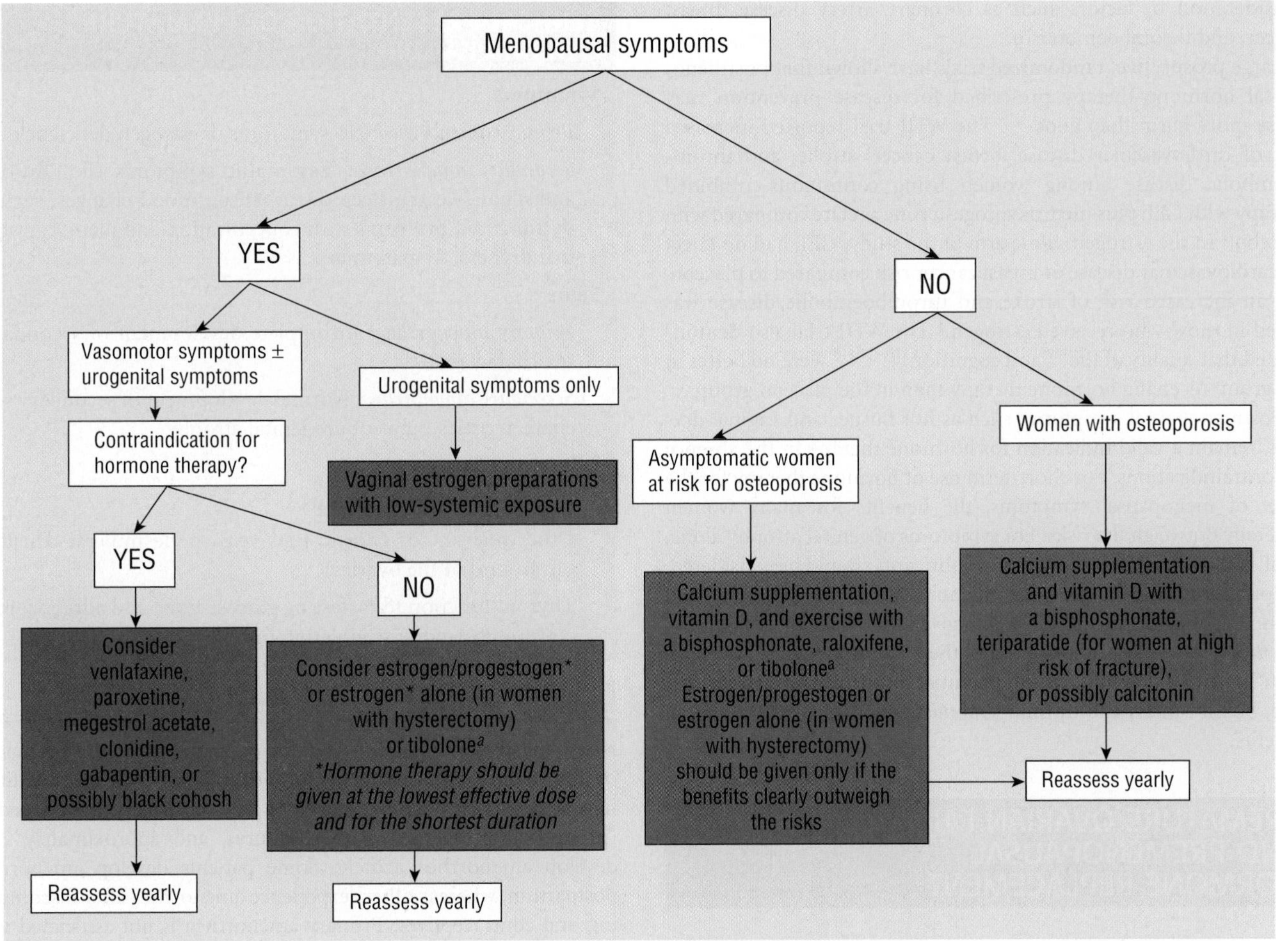

FIGURE 85-1. Algorithm for management of postmenopausal women. [a]Tibolone is currently not approved for use in the United States.

therapy is used under such conditions, the absolute risk of harm to an individual woman is very small.[2]

Many women have no difficulty abruptly stopping hormone therapy; others develop vasomotor symptoms after discontinuation. Although these symptoms usually are mild and resolve over a few months, in some women the symptoms are severe and intolerable. Few studies have addressed the appropriate method for discontinuing use of hormone therapy. There is no evidence that gradual discontinuation of hormone therapy reduces the recurrence of hot flushes compared with sudden discontinuation. Studies determining effective ways to reduce symptoms of estrogen withdrawal are needed.

Bone mineral density should be measured in women older than 65 years and in women younger than 65 years with risk factors for osteoporosis. Although bone densitometry has been shown to predict fractures, at present there are no guidelines for followup bone mineral density testing. However, in women with significant bone loss, repeat testing should be performed as clinically indicated.

PHARMACOECONOMIC CONSIDERATIONS

Estrogens and progestogens used for postmenopausal hormone therapy still are prescribed commonly in the United States, especially for the management of menopausal vasomotor symptoms. Even before publication of the WHI trial findings, only a fraction of women filled their hormone therapy prescriptions, and only 25% to 40% continued to take postmenopausal hormone therapy for more than 1 year.[115] This may be due to women's attitudes toward hormone therapy or a result of fear about adverse effects and associated risks. Hormone therapy use in the United States declined substantially after dissemination of the WHI trial results.[116]

Use of hormone therapy for the management of vasomotor symptoms is cost effective, and data supporting the use of nonhormonal alternatives are limited. The cost of hormone therapy varies depending on the route and method of delivery. Transdermal preparations are about twice as expensive as their equivalent oral preparations.[117] Women who have undergone hysterectomy use hormone therapy more frequently than do women with an intact uterus (58.7% vs 19.6%).[5]

Raloxifene adversely affects hot flushes, but it is likely to be used for osteoporosis prevention. For women with a history of breast cancer or thromboembolic disease, alternative means of reducing the risk of osteoporosis, such as bisphosphonates, should be considered.

The results of randomized trials suggest that hormone therapy should not be used for cardiovascular disease prevention. Women with coronary disease risk factors (e.g., hypertension, lipid abnormalities) can benefit from reduction of these risk factors through interventions such as weight loss, lipid-lowering therapy, use of aspirin, use of antioxidants, and physical activity.

CONCLUSIONS

During the past decade, postmenopausal hormone therapy became one of the most frequently prescribed therapies in the United States. Menopause is a natural life event, not a disease. Therefore, the decision to use hormone therapy must be individualized based on the severity of menopausal symptoms, risk of osteoporosis, and consideration of factors such as coronary artery disease, breast cancer, and thromboembolism.

Large prospective, randomized trials have shown that postmenopausal hormone therapy prescribed for disease prevention may cause more harm than good.[2,77] The WHI trial reported increased risk of cardiovascular disease, breast cancer, stroke, and thromboembolic disease among women using continuous-combined therapy with CEE plus medroxyprogesterone acetate compared with placebo.[2] In the estrogen-alone arm of the study, CEE had no effect on cardiovascular disease or breast cancer risk compared to placebo, but an increased risk of stroke and thromboembolic disease was noted in those who received estrogen.[3] The WHI trial also demonstrated that quality of life[109] and cognition[110,112,113] were no better in the group receiving hormone therapy than in the placebo group.

Postmenopausal symptoms, such as hot flushes and vaginal dryness, remain a valid indication for hormone therapy in the absence of contraindications. For short-term use of hormone therapy for the relief of menopausal symptoms, the benefits for many women generally outweigh the risks. For symptoms of genital atrophy alone, local estrogen and/or nonhormonal lubricants should be considered.

Long-term use of hormone therapy cannot be recommended routinely for osteoporosis prevention given the availability of alternative therapies, such as raloxifene and the bisphosphonates. For long-term hormone therapy use, the potential harm (cardiovascular disease, breast cancer, and thromboembolism) outweighs the potential benefits.

PREMATURE OVARIAN FAILURE AND PREMENOPAUSAL HORMONE REPLACEMENT

PATHOPHYSIOLOGY

Premature ovarian failure is a condition characterized by sex-steroid deficiency, amenorrhea, and infertility in women younger than 40 years.[118] It affects 1% of women by age 40 years.[119] Premature ovarian failure once was considered irreversible and was described as "premature menopause." Premature ovarian failure is not an early natural menopause. Normal menopause results from ovarian follicle depletion, whereas premature ovarian failure is characterized by intermittent ovarian function in half of affected women.[118] For this reason, the term "primary ovarian insufficiency" may be a more accurate term to describe this condition. These women produce estrogen intermittently and may ovulate despite the presence of high gonadotropin concentrations. Pregnancies have occurred in 5% to 10% of women after the diagnosis of premature ovarian failure, even in women with no follicles observed on ovarian biopsy.

Premature ovarian failure may occur as a result of ovarian follicle dysfunction or ovarian follicle depletion and may present as either primary amenorrhea (absence of menses in a girl who has reached age 16 years) or secondary amenorrhea (cessation of menses in a woman previously menstruating for at least 6 months).

In most cases, the etiology cannot be identified (Table 85–9). In the majority of patients, ovarian failure develops after the establishment of regular menses. Young women with premature ovarian failure who develop ovarian dysfunction before they achieve peak adult bone mass sustain sex steroid deficiency for more years than do naturally menopausal women. This deficiency can result in a significantly higher risk for osteoporosis[120] and cardiovascular disease.[121,122] Importantly, a survey of more than 19,000 women between the ages of 25 and 100 years suggests that ovarian failure occurring before age 40 years is associated with significantly increased mortality, with an age-adjusted odds ratio for all-cause mortality of 2.14 (95% CI 1.15–3.99).[123]

CLINICAL PRESENTATION OF PREMATURE OVARIAN FAILURE

Symptoms

- *Primary amenorrhea*: No symptoms of estrogen deficiency
- *Secondary amenorrhea*: Vasomotor symptoms (hot flushes and night sweats), sleep disturbances, mood changes, sexual dysfunction, problems with concentration and memory, vaginal dryness, dyspareunia

Signs

- *Primary amenorrhea*: Incomplete development of secondary sex characteristics
- *Secondary amenorrhea*: Normal development of secondary sex characteristics, signs of urogenital atrophy

Laboratory Tests

- FSH >40 international units/L
- Other relevant diagnostic tests (e.g., bone mineral density, ultrasound of the ovaries)
- Thyroid function tests, fasting glucose level, and adrenocorticotropic hormone stimulation test

CLINICAL PRESENTATION

No characteristic menstrual pattern or history precedes premature ovarian failure. Approximately 50% of patients with this condition have a history of oligomenorrhea or dysfunctional uterine bleeding (prodromal premature ovarian failure), and approximately 25% develop amenorrhea acutely. Some patients develop amenorrhea postpartum, whereas others experience amenorrhea after discontinuing oral contraceptives. Primary amenorrhea is not associated with symptoms of estrogen deficiency. In cases of secondary amenorrhea, symptoms may include hot flushes, night sweats, fatigue, and mood changes. Prodromal premature ovarian failure may present with hot flushes even in women who menstruate regularly. Incomplete development of secondary sex characteristics may occur in women with primary amenorrhea, whereas these characteristics typically are normal in women with secondary amenorrhea. In general, women with premature ovarian failure have normal fertility before the disorder develops.

Approximately 50% of women with premature ovarian failure have documented ovarian follicle function.[118]

Premature ovarian failure is defined by the presence of at least 4 months of amenorrhea and at least two serum FSH concentrations measuring >40 international units/L (obtained at least 1 month apart) in women younger than 40 years. A complete history should be taken, considering other factors that can affect ovarian function such as prior ovarian surgery, chemotherapy, radiation, and autoimmune disorders. In patients with primary amenorrhea, particular

TABLE 85-9 Etiology of Premature Ovarian Failure

Idiopathic: *Karyotypically normal spontaneous premature ovarian failure*
Autoimmunity: (A) isolated autoimmune premature ovarian failure or (B) as a component of an autoimmune polyglandular syndrome in association with Addison's disease, hypothyroidism, hypoparathyroidism, or mucocutaneous candidiasis
Iatrogenic: *Chemotherapy, radiation, extensive ovarian surgery*
X-chromosome abnormalities
Gonadotropin and gonadotropin-receptor abnormalities: Signal defects
Enzyme deficiencies: Cholesterol desmolase, 17α-hydroxylase, 17, 20-desmolase
Galactosemia
Blepharophimosis, ptosis, and epicanthus inversus syndrome type 1: Rare autosomal dominant syndrome in which premature ovarian failure is the predominant syndrome
Perrault's syndrome: Familial autosomal recessive premature ovarian failure in association with deafness

attention should be paid to breast and pubic hair development according to Tanner stages. Short stature, stigmata of Turner's syndrome, and other dysmorphic features of gonadal dysgenesis should be considered. Ideally, a pelvic examination is performed but is not always clinically appropriate. Alternatively, transabdominal ultrasonography can be performed in patients with primary amenorrhea to confirm the presence of normal anatomic structures. In the majority of cases, physical examination is completely normal. A karyotype should be performed in all patients experiencing premature ovarian failure. Women with ovarian failure and a karyotype containing a Y chromosome should undergo bilateral gonadectomy because of substantial risk for gonadal germ cell neoplasia.[124] Ovarian biopsy and antiovarian antibody testing are investigational procedures with no proven clinical benefit in premature ovarian failure. As clinically indicated, the workup should include tests for the diagnosis of other possible associated autoimmune disorders, such as hypothyroidism, diabetes mellitus, and Addison disease.

Young women find the diagnosis of premature ovarian failure particularly traumatic and frequently need extensive emotional and psychological support. Although most of these women will, in fact, be infertile, it is important to emphasize that premature ovarian failure can be transient and that spontaneous pregnancies have occurred even years after diagnosis.

TREATMENT

Premature Ovarian Failure

9 Postmenopausal women who take hormone therapy prolong their exposure to estrogen beyond the average age of completion of their reproductive phase. In contrast, women with premature ovarian failure need exogenous sex steroids to compensate for the decreased production by their ovaries. Importantly, 47% of young women with premature ovarian failure have significantly reduced bone mineral density within 1.5 years of their diagnosis despite taking standard hormone therapy.[120]

The goal of therapy in young women with premature ovarian failure is to provide a hormone replacement regimen that maintains sex steroid status as effectively as the normal, functioning ovary.

PHARMACOLOGIC THERAPY: HORMONAL REGIMENS

Optimal hormone therapy depends on whether the patient has primary or secondary amenorrhea. Young women with primary amenorrhea in whom secondary sex characteristics have failed to develop initially should be given very low doses of estrogen in an attempt to mimic the gradual pubertal maturation process. A typical regimen is 0.3 mg CEE unopposed (i.e., no progestogen) daily for 6 months, with incremental dose increases at 6-month intervals until the required maintenance dose is achieved. Gradual dose escalation often results in optimal breast development and allows time for the young woman to adjust psychologically to her physical maturation. Cyclic progestogen therapy, given 12 to 14 days per month, should be instituted toward the end of the second year of treatment.

Women with secondary amenorrhea who have been estrogen deficient for 12 months or longer also should be given low-dose estrogen replacement initially to avoid adverse effects such as mastalgia and nausea. However, the dose can be titrated up to maintenance levels over a 6-month period, and progestogen therapy can be instituted with the initiation of estrogen therapy. Women with a brief history of secondary amenorrhea are less likely to experience undesired effects from hormone therapy if they are given a reduced dose for the first month of therapy, followed by a full dose from the second month onward.

TABLE 85-10 Premenopausal Hormone Replacement Therapy for Young Women with Premature Ovarian Failure

Regimen	Dose	Frequency	Route
Estrogen therapy			
Conjugated equine estrogen	1.25 mg	Daily	Oral
Piperazine estrone sulfate	2.5 mg	Daily	Oral
Micronized 17β-estradiol	4 mg	Daily	Oral
Transdermal estrogen system	100 mcg/24 h	Once or twice weekly	Transdermal patch
Progestogen therapy			
Medroxyprogesterone acetate	10 mg	12–14 days[a]	Oral
Dydrogesterone[b]	20 mg	12–14 days[a]	Oral
Norethindrone acetate	10 mg	12–14 days[a]	Oral
Norethisterone[b]	1 mg	12–14 days[a]	Oral
Micronized progesterone	200 mg	12–14 days[a]	Oral
Transdermal norethindrone[c]	250 mcg/24 h	Twice weekly for 14 days per calendar month	Transdermal patch

[a]Per calendar month.
[b]Not available in a progestogen-only oral dosage form in the United States.
[c]Available only in combination with estradiol.

An estrogen dose equivalent to at least 1.25 mg CEE (or 100 mcg transdermal estradiol) is needed to achieve adequate estrogen replacement in young women. A progestogen should be given for 12 to 14 days per calendar month to prevent endometrial hyperplasia (Table 85–10). Estrogens given in usual replacement doses do not suppress spontaneous follicular activity or ovulation. Because women with premature ovarian failure can have spontaneous pregnancies, hormone therapy should produce regular, predictable menstrual flow patterns (i.e., only cyclic regimens should be used). Patients who miss an expected menses should be tested for pregnancy and should discontinue hormone therapy. Because most young women negatively associate hormone therapy with menopause in older women, some clinicians prefer to prescribe oral contraceptives for hormone replacement in premenopausal women with hypogonadism. However, oral contraceptives may not inhibit ovulation or effectively prevent pregnancy in young women with elevated gonadotropin levels.

Women with premature ovarian failure have testosterone deficiency.[125] In these young women, testosterone replacement, in addition to estrogen, may be important.[43] However, preliminary analysis of a prospective study at the National Institutes of Health suggests that long-term "physiologic" testosterone supplementation (150 mcg/day), in addition to standard hormone replacement, did not significantly improve bone density and sexual function in these young women.[126,127]

Importantly, all women with premature ovarian failure should understand that hormone therapy generally should be continued until the average age of natural menopause and that long-term follow up is necessary.

EVALUATION OF THERAPEUTIC OUTCOMES

Young women with premature ovarian failure should be monitored annually for their response to treatment, and their compliance with hormone therapy should be assessed regularly. Patients should be evaluated continuously for the presence of signs and symptoms of associated autoimmune endocrine disorders, such as hypothyroidism, adrenal insufficiency, and diabetes mellitus. Baseline bone mineral density testing should be performed in all women with premature ovarian failure. Mammography should be performed annually after age 40 years in accordance with accepted guidelines. Additional mammography screening in premenopausal women younger than 40 years who are receiving physiologic hormone therapy is not warranted. Other tests should be performed as clinically indicated.

CONCLUSIONS

Approximately 1% of women spontaneously develop ovarian failure before age 40 years.[5] Premature ovarian failure is not an early natural menopause. Most affected women produce estrogen intermittently and may ovulate despite the presence of high gonadotropin concentrations. However, these women sustain sex steroid deficiency for more years than do naturally menopausal women, resulting in a significantly higher risk for osteoporosis[120] and cardiovascular disease.[121,122]

Women with premature ovarian failure need exogenous sex steroids to compensate for the decreased production by their ovaries. Thus, premenopausal hormone therapy is required at least until these women reach the age of "natural menopause."

The goal of therapy is to provide a hormone replacement regimen that maintains sex steroid status as effectively as the normal, functioning ovary. This usually requires the administration of estrogen at a dose greater than the standard dose given to older women experiencing natural menopause.

Because women with premature ovarian failure can have spontaneous pregnancies, hormone therapy should produce regular, predictable menstrual flow patterns. Patients who miss an expected menses should be tested for pregnancy and promptly discontinue the hormone treatment.

Annual followup should include assessment of adherence with the prescribed hormone therapy regimen and evaluation for signs and symptoms of associated endocrine disorders.[118]

ABBREVIATIONS

CEE: conjugated equine estrogens

CORE: Continuing Outcomes Relevant to Evista

FDA: Food and Drug Administration

FSH: follicle-stimulating hormone

GnRH: gonadotropin-releasing hormone

HDL: high-density lipoprotein

LDL: low-density lipoprotein

LH: luteinizing hormone

MORE: Multiple Outcomes of Raloxifene Evaluation

NETA: norethindrone acetate

SERM: selective estrogen receptor modulator

WHI: Women's Health Initiative

REFERENCES

1. Richardson SJ, Senikas JF, Nelson JF. Follicular depletion during the menopausal transition: Evidence for accelerated loss and ultimate exhaustion. J Clin Endocrinol Metab 1987;65:1231–1237.
2. Writing Group for the Women's Health Initiative Investigators. Risks and benefits of estrogen plus progestin in healthy postmenopausal women: Principal results from the Women's Health Initiative randomized controlled trial. JAMA 2002;288:321–333.
3. Anderson GL, Limacher M, Assaf AR, et al. Effects of conjugated equine estrogen in postmenopausal women with hysterectomy: The Women's Health Initiative randomized controlled trial. JAMA, 2004;291:1701–1712.
4. Hersh AL, Stefanick ML, Stafford RS. National use of postmenopausal hormone therapy: annual trends and response to recent evidence. JAMA 2004;291:47–53.
5. American College of Obstetricians and Gynecologists Women's Health Care Physicians. Executive Summary. Hormone Therapy. Obstet Gynecol 2004;104(4 Suppl):1–4.
6. Stephenson J. FDA orders estrogen safety warnings: Agency offers guidance for HRT use. JAMA 2003;289:537–538.
7. Treloar AE, Boynton RE, Behn BG, Brown BW. Variation of the human menstrual cycle through reproductive life. Int J Fertil 1967;12:77–126.
8. Zumoff B, Strain GW, Miller LK, Rosner W. Twenty-four-hour mean plasma testosterone concentration declines with age in normal premenopausal women. J Clin Endocrinol Metab 1995;80:1429–1430.
9. Burger HG. The endocrinology of the menopause. J Steroid Biochem Mol Biol 1999;69:31–35.
10. Lee SJ, Lenton EA, Sexton L, Cooke ID. The effect of age on the cyclical patterns of plasma LH, FSH, oestradiol and progesterone in women with regular menstrual cycles. Hum Reprod 1988;3:851–855.
11. Ettinger B, Pressman A, Sklarin P, et al. Associations between low concentrations of serum estradiol, bone density, and fractures among elderly women: The study of osteoporotic fractures. J Clin Endocrinol Metab 1998;83:2239–2243.
12. Stone K, Bauer DC, Black DM, et al. Hormonal predictors of bone loss in elderly women: A prospective study. J Bone Miner Res 1998;13:1167–1174.
13. Cummings SR, Browner WS, Bauer D. Endogenous hormones and the risk of hip and vertebral fractures among older women. N Engl J Med 1998;339:733–738.
14. Cauley JA, Lucas FL, Kuller LH, et al. Elevated serum estradiol and testosterone concentrations are associated with a high risk for breast cancer. Ann Intern Med 1999;130:270–277.
15. Murkies AL, Wilcox G, Davis SR. Phytoestrogens: Clinical review. J Clin Endocrinol Metab 1998;83:297–303.
16. Yamamoto S, Sobue T, Kobayashi M, et al., for the Japan Public Health Center–Based Prospective Study on Cancer and Cardiovascular Diseases (JPHC) Study Group. Soy, isoflavones, and breast cancer risk in Japan. J Natl Cancer Inst 2003;95:906–913.
17. Tice JA, Ettinger B, Ensrud K, et al. Phytoestrogen supplements for the treatment of hot flashes: The isoflavone clover extract (ICE) study. A randomized, controlled trial. JAMA 2003;290:207–214.
18. Wroblewski-Lissin L, Cooke JP. Phytoestrogens and cardiovascular health. J Am Coll Cardiol 2000;35:1403–1410.
19. Albertazzi P, Pansini F, Bonaccorsi G, et al. The effect of dietary soy supplementation on hot flushes. Obstet Gynecol 1998;91:6–11.
20. Newton KM, Reed SD, LaCroix AZ, et al. Treatment of vasomotor symptoms of menopause with black cohosh, multibotanicals, soy, hormone therapy, or placebo: A randomized trial. Ann Intern Med 2006;145:869–879.
21. Beral V, Million Women Study Collaborators. Breast cancer and hormone-replacement therapy in the Million Women Study. Lancet 2003;362:419–427.
22. Sturdee DW. Newer HRT regimens. Br J Obstet Gynaecol 1997;104:1109–1115.
23. Lowe G, Upton M, Rumley A, et al. Different effects of oral and transdermal hormone replacement regimens on factor IX, APC-resistance, t-PA, PAI and C-reactive protein: A cross-sectional population survey. Thromb Haemost 2001;86:550–556.
24. Greendale GA, Lee NP, Arriola ER. The menopause. Lancet 1999;353:571–580.
25. Mattsson LA, Christiansen C, Colau J, et al. Clinical equivalence of intranasal and oral 17β-estradiol for postmenopausal symptoms. Am J Obstet Gynecol 2000;182:545–552.
26. Lindsay R, Hart DM, Clark DM. The minimum effective dose of estrogen for postmenopausal bone loss. Obstet Gynecol 1984;63:759–763.
27. Bachmann GA, Schaefers M, Uddin A, Utian WH. Lowest effective transdermal 17-beta-estradiol dose for relief of hot flushes in postmenopausal women: A randomized controlled trial. Obstet Gynecol 2007;110:771–779.
28. Lindsay R, Gallagher JC, Kleerekoper M, Pickar JH. Effect of lower doses of conjugated equine estrogens with and without medroxyprogesterone acetate on bone in early postmenopausal women. JAMA 2002;287:2668–2676.
29. Pickar JH, Wheeler JE, Cunnane MF, Speroff L. Endometrial effects of lower doses of conjugated equine estrogens and medroxyprogesterone acetate. Fertil Steril 2001;76:25–31.
30. Utian WH, Shoupe D, Bachmann G, et al. Relief of vasomotor symptoms and vaginal atrophy with lower doses of conjugated equine estrogens and medroxyprogesterone acetate. Fertil Steril 2001;75:1065–1079.
31. Naessen T, Rodriguez-Macias K, Lithell H. Serum lipid profile improved by ultra-low doses of 17β-estradiol in elderly women. J Clin Endocrinol Metab 2001;86:2757–2762.

32. Barrett-Connor E. Hormone-replacement therapy. Br Med J 1998; 317:457–461.
33. Scarabin PY, Oger E, Genevieve PB, on behalf of the Estrogen and Thromboembolism Risk (ESTHER) Study Group. Differential association of oral and transdermal oestrogen-replacement therapy and venous thromboembolism risk. Lancet 2003;362:428–432.
34. Lethaby A, Farquhar C, Sarkis A, et al. Hormone-replacement therapy in postmenopausal women: Endometrial hyperplasia and irregular bleeding. Cochrane Database Syst Rev 2000;2:CD000402.
35. Casper RF. Estrogen with interrupted progestin HRT. A review of experimental and clinical studies. Maturitas 2000;34:97–108.
36. The Writing Group for the Postmenopausal Estrogen/Progestin Interventions (PEPI) Trial. Effects of hormone-replacement therapy on endometrial histology in postmenopausal women. JAMA 1996;275:370–375.
37. Cushing KL, Weiss NS, Voight LF, et al. Risk of endometrial cancer in relation to use of low-dose, unopposed estrogens. Obstet Gynecol 1998;91:35–39.
38. North American Menopause Society. Role of progestogen in hormone therapy for postmenopausal women: Position statement of the North American Menopause Society. Menopause 2003;10:113–132.
39. The North American Menopause Society. The role of testosterone therapy in postmenopausal women: Position statement of the North American Menopause Society. Menopause, 2005;12:497–511.
40. Davis SR, Davison SL, Donath S, Bell RJ. Circulating androgen levels and self-reported sexual function in women. JAMA 2005;294:91–96.
41. Bell RJ, Donath S, Davison SL, Davis SR. Endogenous androgen levels and well-being: Differences between premenopausal and postmenopausal women. Menopause 2006;13:65–71.
42. Shifren JL, Braunstein GD, Simon JA, et al. Transdermal testosterone treatment in women with impaired sexual function after oophorectomy. N Engl J Med 2000;343:682–688.
43. Kalantaridou SN, Calis KA, Mazer NA, et al. A pilot study of an investigational transdermal testosterone patch system in young women with spontaneous premature ovarian failure. J Clin Endocrinol Metab 2005;90:6549–6552.
44. Wierman ME, Basson R, Davis SR, et al. Androgen therapy in women: An Endocrine Society Clinical Practice guideline. J Clin Endocrinol Metab 2006;91:3697–3710.
45. Ettinger B, Black DM, Mitlak BH, et al. Reduction of vertebral fracture risk in postmenopausal women with osteoporosis treated with raloxifene: Results from a 3-year randomized clinical trial. Multiple Outcomes of Raloxifene Evaluation (MORE) investigators. JAMA 1999;282:637–645.
46. Cummings SR, Eckert S, Krueger KA, et al. The effect of raloxifene on risk of breast cancer in postmenopausal women: Results from the MORE randomized trial. JAMA 1999;281:2189–2197.
47. Martino S, Cauley JA, Barrett-Connor E, et al., for the CORE Investigators. Continuing outcomes relevant to Evista: Breast cancer incidence in postmenopausal osteoporotic women in a randomized trial of raloxifene. J Natl Cancer Inst 2004;96:1751–1761.
48. Barrett-Connor E, Mosca L, Collins P, et al. Effects of raloxifene on cardiovascular events and breast cancer in postmenopausal women. N Engl J Med 2006;355:125–137.
49. Kenemans P, Speroff L for the International Tibolone Consensus Group. Tibolone: Clinical recommendations and practice guidelines. A report of the International Tibolone Consensus Group. Maturitas 2005;51:21–28.
50. Cummings SR. LIFT study is discontinued. BMJ 2006;332:667.
51. Million Women Study Collaborators. Endometrial cancer and hormone-replacement therapy in the Million Women Study. Lancet 2005;365:1543–1551.
52. Langer RD, Landgren BM, Rymer J, et al. Effects of tibolone and continuous combined conjugated equine estrogen/medroxyprogesterone acetate on the endometrium and vaginal bleeding: Results of the OPAL study. Am J Obstet Gynecol 2006;195:1320–1327.
53. Ettinger B, Barrett-Connor E, Hoq LA, et al. When is it appropriate to prescribe postmenopausal hormone therapy? Menopause 2006;13:404–410.
54. Porter M, Penney GC, Russell D, et al. A population based survey of women's experience of the menopause. Br J Obstet Gynaecol 2002;103:1025–1028.
55. Ettinger B. Vasomotor symptom relief versus unwanted effects: Role of estrogen dosage. Am J Med 2005;118:74S-78S.
56. Hickey M, Davis SR, Sturdee DW. Treatment of menopausal symptoms: What shall we do now? Lancet 2005;366:409–421.
57. Loprinzi CL, Kugler JW, Sloan JA, et al. Venlafaxine in management of hot flashes in survivors of breast cancer: A randomized, controlled trial. Lancet 2000;356:2059–2063.
58. Evans ML, Pritts E, Vittinghoff E, et al. Management of postmenopausal hot flushes with venlafaxine hydrochloride: A randomized, controlled trial. Obstet Gynecol 2005;105:161–166.
59. Stearns V, Johnson MD, Rae JM, et al. Active tamoxifen metabolite plasma concentrations after coadministration of tamoxifen and the selective serotonin reuptake inhibitor paroxetine. J Natl Cancer Inst 2003;95:1758–1764.
60. Bachmann GA. A new option for managing urogenital atrophy in postmenopausal women. Cont Obstet Gynecol 1997;42:13–28.
61. Davis SR. Hormone-replacement therapy: Indications, benefits and risks. Aust Fam Physician 1999;28:437–445.
62. Grady D, Brown JS, Vittinghoff E, et al. Postmenopausal hormones and incontinence: The Heart and Estrogen/Progestin Replacement Study. Obstet Gynecol 2001;97:116–120.
63. Cauley JA, Robbins J, Chen Z, et al. Effects of estrogen plus progestin on risk of fracture and bone mineral density: The Women's Health Initiative Randomized Trial. JAMA 2003;290:1729–1738.
64. Wells G, Tugwell P, Shea B, et al. Meta-analysis of the efficacy of hormone replacement therapy in treating and preventing osteoporosis in postmenopausal women. Endocr Rev 2002;23:529–539.
65. North American Menopause Society. Management of postmenopausal osteoporosis: Position statement of the North American Menopause Society. Menopause 2002;9:84–101.
66. Greenspan SL, Maitland LA, Myers ER, et al. Femoral bone loss progresses with age: A longitudinal study in women over age 65. J Bone Miner Res 1994;9:1959–1965.
67. Lindsay R, Cosman F, Lobo RA, et al. Addition of alendronate to ongoing hormone replacement therapy in the treatment of osteoporosis: A randomized controlled clinical trial. J Clin Endocrinol Metab 1999;84:3076–3081.
68. North American Menopause Society. The role of calcium in peri- and postmenopausal women: Consensus opinion of the North American Menopause Society. Menopause 2001;8:84–95.
69. Espeland MA, Hogan PE, Fineberg SE, et al., for the PEPI investigators. Effect of postmenopausal hormone therapy on glucose and insulin concentrations. Diabetes Care 1998;21:1589–1595.
70. Kanaya AM, Herrington D, Vittinghoff E, et al. Glycemic effects of postmenopausal hormone therapy: The Heart and Estrogen/Progestin Replacement Study. A randomized, double-blind, placebo-controlled trial. Ann Intern Med 2003;138:1–9.
71. Norman RJ, Flight IH, Rees MC. Oestrogen and progestogen hormone replacement therapy for perimenopausal and post-menopausal women: Weight and body fat distribution. Cochrane Database Syst Rev 2000;2:CD001018.
72. Mosca L, Collins P, Herrington DM, et al. Hormone replacement therapy and cardiovascular disease: A statement for healthcare professionals from the American Heart Association. Circulation 2001;104:499–503.
73. Grodstein F, Manson JE, Colditz GA, et al. A prospective observational study of postmenopausal hormone therapy and primary prevention of cardiovascular disease. Ann Intern Med 2000;133:933–941.
74. The Writing Group for the Postmenopausal Estrogen/Progestin Interventions (PEPI) Trial. Effects of estrogen or estrogen/progestin regimens on heart disease risk factors in postmenopausal women. JAMA 1995;273:199–208.
75. Sack MN, Rader JR, Cannon RO. Oestrogen and inhibition of oxidation of low-density lipoproteins in postmenopausal women. Lancet 1994;343:269–270.
76. Koh KK, Jin DK, Yang SH, et al. Vascular effects of synthetic or natural progestogen combined with conjugated equine estrogen in healthy postmenopausal women. Circulation 2001;103:1961–1966.
77. Hulley S, Grady D, Bush T, et al. Randomized trial of estrogen plus progestin for secondary prevention of coronary heart disease in postmenopausal women. JAMA 1998;280:605–613.
78. Herrington DM, Reboussin DM, Brosnihan KB, et al. Effects of estrogen replacement on the progression of coronary artery atherosclerosis. N Engl J Med 2000;343:522–529.
79. Viscoli CM, Brass LM, Kernan WN, et al. A clinical trial of estrogen-replacement therapy after ischemic stroke. N Engl J Med 2001;345:1243–1249.

80. Vickers MR, MacLennan AH, Lawton B, et al. Main morbidities recorded in the women's international study of long duration oestrogen after menopause (WISDOM): A randomized controlled trial of hormone replacement therapy in postmenopausal women. BMJ 2007;335(7613):239. Epub 2007 Jul 11.
81. Rossouw JE, Prentice RL, Manson JE, et al. Postmenopausal hormone therapy and risk of cardiovascular disease by age and years since menopause. JAMA 2007;297:1465–1477.
82. Manson JE, Allison MA, Rossouw JE, et al. Estrogen therapy and coronary-artery calcification. N Engl J Med 2007;356:2591–2602.
83. Wassertheil-Smoller S, Hendrix S, Limacher M, et al. Effect of estrogen plus progestin on stroke in postmenopausal women: The Women's Health Initiative. JAMA 2003;289:2673–2684.
84. Mendelsohn ME, Karas RH. HRT and the young at heart. N Engl J Med 2007;356:2639–2641.
85. Harman SM, Brinton EA, Cedars M, et al. KEEPS. The Kronos Ealry Estrogen Prevention Trial. Climacteric 2005;8:3–12.
86. Hu FB, Stampfer MJ, Manson JE, et al. Trends in the incidence of coronary heart disease and changes in diet and lifestyle in women. N Engl J Med 2000;343:530–537.
87. Stampfer MJ, Hu FB, Manson JE, et al. Primary prevention of coronary heart disease in women through diet and lifestyle. N Engl J Med 2000;343:16–22.
88. Chlebowski RT, Hendrix SL, Langer RD, et al. Influence of estrogen plus progestin on breast cancer and mammography in healthy postmenopausal women. The Women's Health Initiative Randomized Trial. JAMA 2003;289:3243–3253.
89. Swanson GM. Breast cancer risk estimation: A translational statistic for communication to the public. J Natl Cancer Inst 1993;85:848–849.
90. Collaborative Group on Hormonal Factors in Breast Cancer. Breast cancer and hormone replacement therapy: Collaborative reanalysis of data from epidemiological studies of 52,705 women with breast cancer and 108,411 women without breast cancer. Lancet 1997;350:1047–1059.
91. Schairer C, Lubin J, Troisi R, et al. Menopausal estrogen and estrogen-progestin replacement therapy and breast cancer risk. JAMA 2000;283:485–491.
92. Gapstur SM, Morrow M, Sellers TA. Hormone replacement therapy and risk of breast cancer with a favorable histology. JAMA 1999;281:2091–2097.
93. Sellers TA, Mink PJ, Cerhan JR, et al. The role of hormone replacement therapy in the risk of breast cancer and total mortality in women with a family history of breast cancer. Ann Intern Med 1997;127:973–980.
94. McTiernan A, Martin CF, Peck JD, et al. Estrogen-plus-progestin use and mammographic density in postmenopausal women: Women's Health Initiative Randomized Trial. J Natl Cancer Inst 2005;97:1366–1376.
95. Stefanick ML, Anderson GL, Margolis KL, et al. Effects of conjugated equine estrogens on breast cancer and mammography screening in postmenopausal women with hysterectomy. JAMA 2006;295:1647–1657.
96. Vogel VG, Constantino JP, Wickerham DL, et al. Effects of tamoxifen vs raloxifene on the risk of developing invasive breast cancer and other disease outcomes: The NSABP Study of Tamoxifen and Raloxifene (STAR) P-2 trial. JAMA 2006;295:2727–2741.
97. Anderson GL, Judd HL, Kaunitz AM, et al. Effects of estrogen plus progestin on gynecologic cancers and associated diagnostic procedures. The Women's Health Initiative randomized trial. JAMA 2003;290:1739–1748.
98. Pike MC, Peters RK, Cozen W, et al. Estrogen-progestin replacement therapy and endometrial cancer. J Natl Cancer Inst 1997;89:1110–1116.
99. Genant HK, Lucas J, Weiss S, et al. Low-dose esterified estrogen therapy: Effects on bone, plasma estradiol concentrations, endometrium, and lipid concentrations. Estratab/Osteoporosis Study Group. Arch Intern Med 1997;157:2609–2615.
100. Goldstein SR, Scheele WH, Rajagopalan SK, et al. A 12-month comparative study of raloxifene, estrogen, and placebo on the postmenopausal endometrium. Obstet Gynecol 2000;95:95–103.
101. Lacey JV, Mink PJ, Lubin JH, et al. Menopausal hormone replacement therapy and risk of ovarian cancer. JAMA 2002;288:3343–3341.
102. Jick H, Derby LE, Myers MW, et al. Risk of hospital admission for idiopathic venous thromboembolism among users of postmenopausal oestrogens. Lancet 1996;348:981–983.
103. Nelson HD, Humphrey LL, Nygren P, et al. Postmenopausal hormone replacement therapy: Scientific review. JAMA 2002;288:872–881.
104. Canonico M, Oger E, Plu-Bureau G, et al. Hormone therapy and venous thromboembolism among postmenopausal women—Impact of the route of estrogen administration and progestogens: The ESTHER study. Circulation 2007;115:840–845.
105. Cirillo DJ, Wallace RB, Rodabough RJ, et al. Effect of estrogen therapy on gallbladder disease. JAMA 2005;293:330–339.
106. Schmidt PJ, Nieman L, Danaceau MA, et al. Estrogen replacement in perimenopause-related depression: A preliminary report. Am J Obstet Gynecol 2000;183:414–420.
107. Hlatky MA, Boothroyd D, Vittnghoff E, et al., for the HERS research group. Quality of life and depressive symptoms in postmenopausal women after receiving hormone therapy: Results from the Heart and Estrogen/Progestin Replacement Study (HERS) Trial. JAMA 2002;287:591–597.
108. Hays J, Ockene JK, Brunner RL, et al. Effects of estrogen plus progestin on health-related quality of life. N Engl J Med 2003;348:1839–1854.
100. Shumaker SA, Legault C, Rapp SR, et al. Estrogen plus progestin and the incidence of dementia and mild cognitive impairment in postmenopausal women. The Women's Health Initiative Memory Study: A randomized, controlled trial. JAMA 2003;289:2651–2662.
110. Rapp SR, Espeland MA, Shumaker SA, et al. Effect of estrogen plus progestin on global cognitive function in postmenopausal women. The Women's Health Initiative Memory Study: A randomized, controlled trial. JAMA 2003;289:2663–2672.
111. Ott A, Breteler MM, Van Harskamp F, et al. Incidence and risk of dementia: The Rotterdam Study. Am J Epidemiol 1998;147:574–580.
112. Espeland MA, Rapp SR, Shumaker SA, et al. Conjugated equine estrogens and global cognitive function in postmenopausal women: Women's Health Initiative Memory Study. JAMA 2004;291:2959–2968.
113. Shumaker SA, Legault C, Kuller L, et al. Conjugated equine estrogens and incidence of probable dementia and mild cognitive impairment in postmenopausal women: Women's Health Initiative Memory Study. JAMA 2004;291:2947–2958.
114. Yaffe K, Krueger K, Sarkar S, et al. Cognitive function in postmenopausal women treated with raloxifene. N Engl J Med 2001;344:1207–1213.
115. Ettinger B, Pressman A. Continuation of postmenopausal hormone replacement therapy in a large health maintenance organization: Transdermal matrix versus oral estrogen therapy. Am J Manag Care 1999;7:779–785.
116. Majumdar SR, Almasi EA, Stafford RS. Promotion and prescribing of hormone therapy after report of harm by the Women's Health Initiative. JAMA 2004;292:1983–1988.
117. Torgerson DJ, Reid DM. The Pharmacoeconomics of hormone replacement therapy. Pharmacoeconomics 1999;16:9–16.
118. Kalantaridou SN, Davis SR, Nelson LM. Premature ovarian failure. Endocrinol Metab Clin North Am 1998;27:989–1006.
119. Coulam CB, Adamson SC, Annegers JF. Incidence of premature ovarian failure. Obstet Gynecol 1986;67:604–606.
120. Anasti JN, Kalantaridou SN, Kimzey LM, et al. Bone loss in young women with karyotypically normal spontaneous premature ovarian failure. Obstet Gynecol 1998;91:12–15.
121. Van Der Schouw YT, Van Der Graaf Y, Steyerberg EW, et al. Age at menopause as a risk for cardiovascular mortality. Lancet 1996;347:714–717.
122. Kalantaridou SN, Naka KK, Papanikolaou E, et al. Impaired endothelial function in young women with premature ovarian failure: Normalization with hormone therapy. J Clin Endocrinol Metab 2004;89:3907–3913.
123. Snowdon DA, Kane RL, Beeson WL, et al. Is early natural menopause a biologic marker of health and aging? Am J Public Health 1989;79:709–714.
124. Davis SR. Premature ovarian failure. Maturitas 1996;28:1–8.
125. Kalantaridou SN, Calis KA, Vanderhoof VH, et al. Testosterone deficiency in young women with 46,XX spontaneous premature ovarian failure. Fertil Steril 2006;86:1475–1482.
126. Popat VB, Kalantaridou SN, Vanderhoof VH, Calis KA, Nelson LM. Effect of long-term physiologic transdermal testosterone (150 mcg/day) replacement therapy on femoral neck bone density in women with spontaneous premature ovarian failure: Results of a 3-year double-blind placebo controlled clinical trial. P1–349. Abstract presented at the Annual Meeting of the Endocrine Society, June 2–5, 2007. Toronto, Canada.
127. Kalantaridou SN, Vanderhoof VH, Calis KA, Popat V, Bakalov VK, Troendle JF, Nelson LM. Physiologic transdermal testosterone replacement (150 mcg/day) does not significantly improve sexual function in women with 46,XX spontaneous premature ovarian failure: A placebo-controlled randomized study. OR27-4. Abstract presented at the Annual Meeting of the Endocrine Society, June 2–5, 2007. Toronto, Canada.

SECTION 10
UROLOGIC DISORDERS

CHAPTER 86
Erectile Dysfunction

MARY LEE

KEY CONCEPTS

1. The incidence of erectile dysfunction is low in men younger than 40 years. The incidence increases as men age, likely as a result of concurrent medical conditions that impair the vascular, neurologic, psychogenic, and hormonal systems necessary for a normal penile erection.
2. Many commonly used drugs have sympatholytic, anticholinergic, sedative, or antiandrogenic effects that may exacerbate or contribute to the development of erectile dysfunction. Clinicians should be familiar with these agents and be prepared to make adjustments in drug regimens to minimize adverse effects of these drugs on a patient's erectile function.
3. The first step in clinical management of erectile dysfunction is to identify and, if possible, reverse the underlying causes. Risk factors for erectile dysfunction, including hypertension, diabetes mellitus, smoking, and chronic ethanol abuse, should be addressed and minimized.
4. Specific treatments for erectile dysfunction include vacuum erection devices, pharmacologic treatments, psychotherapy, and surgery.
5. The ideal treatment of erectile dysfunction should have a fast onset, be effective, be convenient to administer, be cost effective, have a low incidence of serious adverse effects, and be free of serious drug interactions.
6. Specific treatment is first initiated with the least invasive forms of treatment, including vacuum erection devices or oral phosphodiesterase inhibitors, followed by intracavernosal injections or intraurethral inserts, and finally by surgical insertion of a penile prosthesis.
7. Vacuum erection devices can have a slow onset of action (30 minutes) and are not discreet; therefore, they are most effective for a couple in a stable relationship.
8. Although phosphodiesterase inhibitors are convenient and effective regardless of the etiology of erectile dysfunction, they fail in 30% to 40% of patients. Also, phosphodiesterase inhibitors are contraindicated in patients taking any dosage formulation of nitrate.
9. Testosterone supplementation should be reserved for patients with primary or secondary hypogonadism who have erectile dysfunction as a consequence of a decreased libido. Testosterone supplementation should not be used by patients with erectile dysfunction who have normal serum testosterone levels.
10. Although intracavernosal injections and intraurethral pellets of alprostadil are effective independent of the etiology of erectile dysfunction, they fail in one third of patients. To self-administer medication by these routes, patients require training to minimize administration-related adverse effects.

Learning objectives, review questions, and other resources can be found at **www.pharmacotherapyonline.com.**

The National Institutes of Health Consensus Development Panel on Impotence defines erectile dysfunction as the failure to achieve a penile erection to allow for satisfactory sexual intercourse.[1] Patients may refer to it as impotence.

Erectile dysfunction must be distinguished from disorders of libido, ejaculatory disorders, and infertility, which are caused by different pathophysiologic mechanisms and are treated with alternative agents (Table 86–1). A patient may suffer from one or more disorders of sexual dysfunction. For example, an elderly man with primary hypogonadism may suffer from decreased libido and erectile dysfunction. Diagnosis of the type of sexual disorder that a patient has is a key to initiating the most appropriate treatment.

EPIDEMIOLOGY

1 The incidence of erectile dysfunction is low in men younger than 40 years but increases as men age.[2–4] The Massachusetts Male Aging Study, a cross-sectional survey of a random sample of 1,290 men in the Boston area, was conducted during the period from 1987 to 1989. The study reported an overall prevalence of 52% for any degree of erectile dysfunction in men aged 40 to 70 years, with an age-related increase in incidence ranging from 12.4% in men aged 40 to 49 years, up to 46.4% in men aged 60 to 69 years.[1,2] In the most

TABLE 86-1 Types of Sexual Dysfunction in Men

Type of Dysfunction	Definition
Decreased libido	Decreased sexual drive or desire
Increased libido	Precocious puberty; inappropriate and excessive sexual drive or desire
Erectile dysfunction (impotence)	Failure to achieve a penile erection suitable for satisfactory sexual intercourse
Delayed ejaculation	Commonly referred to as "dry sex"; ejaculation is delayed or absent
Retrograde ejaculation	Ejaculate passes retrograde into the bladder, instead of toward the anterior urethra (antegrade) and out of the penis
Infertility	Sperm are insufficient in number or have inadequate motility and fail to fertilize the ovum

recent Health Professional Follow-Up Study of more than 31,000 male health professionals aged 53 to 90 years, the prevalence of erectile dysfunction was 33%.[3]

Although erectile dysfunction is sometimes assumed to be a symptom of the aging process in men, it likely results from concurrent medical conditions of the patient (e.g., hypertension, arteriosclerosis, hyperlipidemia, diabetes mellitus, or psychiatric disorders) or from medications that patients may be taking for these diseases.[2–5] For example, up to 50% of patients with diabetes mellitus develop erectile dysfunction, and medications such as β-blockers are associated with a high incidence of erectile dysfunction.

PHYSIOLOGY OF A NORMAL PENILE ERECTION

A normal penile erection requires full functioning of several physiologic systems: vascular, nervous, and hormonal. The patient also must be psychologically receptive to sexual stimuli.

VASCULAR SYSTEM

The penis comprises two corpora cavernosa on the dorsal side and one corpus spongiosum on the ventral side. The corpus spongiosum surrounds the urethra and forms the glans penis. The corpora are composed of multiple interconnected sinuses, which can fill with blood to produce an erection. The corpora are encased by the tunica albuginea, a fibrous tissue membrane, which has limited distensibility. In the flaccid state, arterial flow into and venous outflow from the corpora are balanced. During the erectile phase, arterial blood flow increases and blood fills the sinusoids within the corpora, which causes penile swelling and elongation. The erection is prolonged by a decrease in venous outflow from the corpora, which is caused by compression of subtunical venules against the tunica albuginea by the swollen corpora (Fig. 86–1).

Arterial flow into the corpora is enhanced by acetylcholine-mediated vasodilation. Acetylcholine does not directly enhance arterial flow to the corpora or increase sinusoidal filling of the corporal tissue. Rather, acetylcholine is a coneurotransmitter, which works along with other nonpeptidinergic intracellular neurotransmitters—

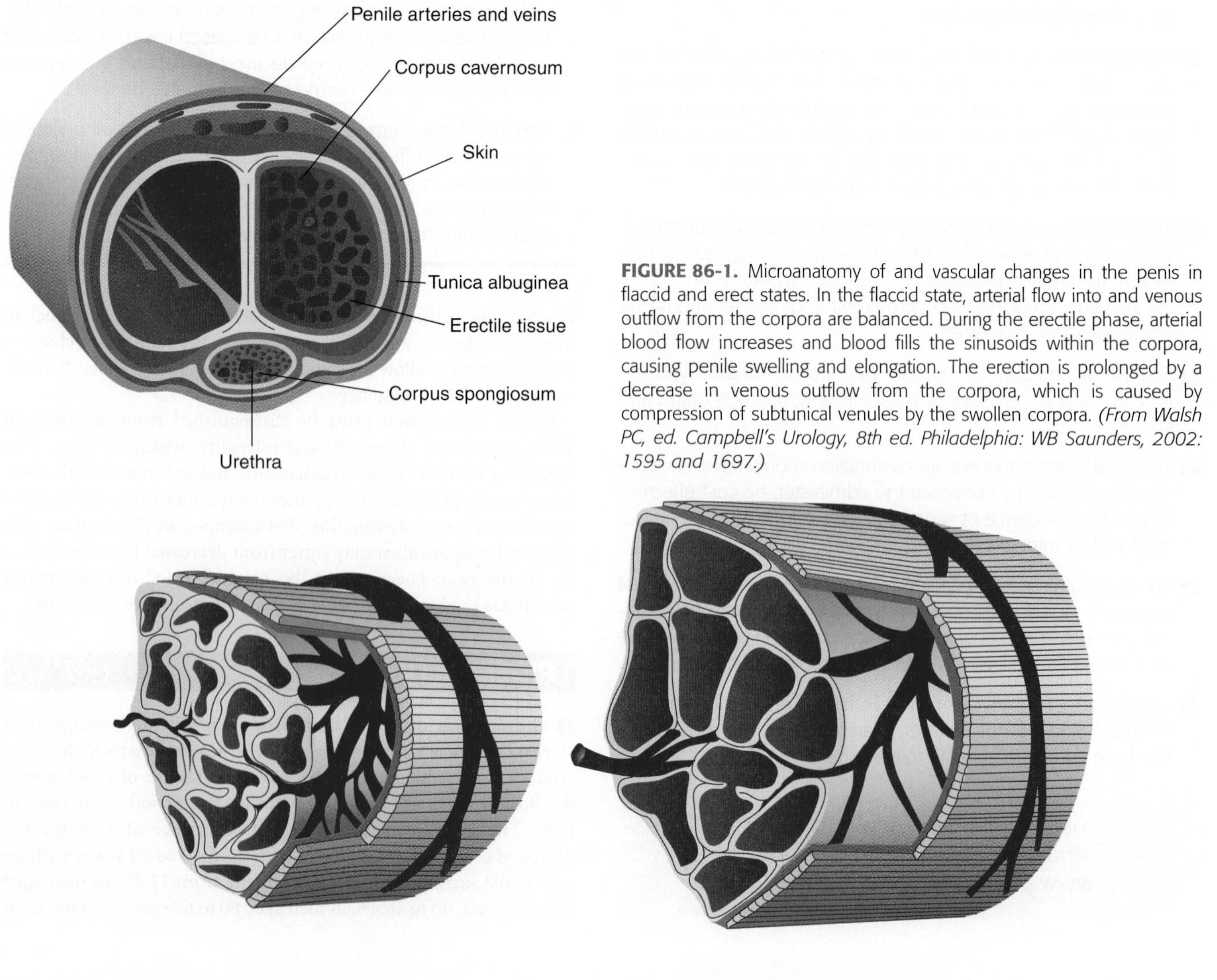

FIGURE 86-1. Microanatomy of and vascular changes in the penis in flaccid and erect states. In the flaccid state, arterial flow into and venous outflow from the corpora are balanced. During the erectile phase, arterial blood flow increases and blood fills the sinusoids within the corpora, causing penile swelling and elongation. The erection is prolonged by a decrease in venous outflow from the corpora, which is caused by compression of subtunical venules by the swollen corpora. *(From Walsh PC, ed. Campbell's Urology, 8th ed. Philadelphia: WB Saunders, 2002: 1595 and 1697.)*

including cyclic guanosine monophosphate (cGMP), cyclic adenosine monophosphate (cAMP), or vasoactive intestinal polypeptide—to produce vasodilation. In effect, cGMP and cAMP are secondary messengers that direct desired effects in target tissues.[6]

Acetylcholine produces an erection probably through two different pathways. Through one pathway, in the presence of sexual stimulation to genital tissue, acetylcholine enhances the production of nitric oxide by endothelial cells and nonadrenergic–noncholinergic neurons. Nitric oxide enhances the activity of guanylate cyclase, which increases the conversion of cyclic guanosine triphosphate to cGMP. cGMP decreases intracellular calcium concentrations in smooth muscle cells of penile arteries and cavernosal sinuses. As a result, smooth muscle relaxation occurs, which enhances arterial blood flow to and blood filling of the corpora.[5] An erection results.

In an alternative pathway, acetylcholine stimulates a smooth muscle cell membrane receptor to enhance the activity of adenyl cyclase. Adenyl cyclase increases the conversion of cyclic adenosine triphosphate to cAMP, a potent muscle relaxant. Similarly to cGMP, cAMP decreases intracellular calcium concentrations to produce smooth muscle relaxation in cells of the arteries and cavernosal sinuses. Arterial blood flow to and blood filling of the corpora are enhanced, and a penile erection results.[5]

NERVOUS SYSTEM AND PSYCHOGENIC STIMULI

Some erections are mediated by a sacral nerve reflex arc (e.g., erections can occur while the patient is sleeping). However, in the conscious patient, sensory sexual stimulation mediates erections via the central nervous system. That is, when a patient sees an attractive partner, hears sweet words, smells a particular scent, or tastes or touches a pleasant object, these situations can result in an erection. In this case, the patient's brain processes this information and the nervous impulse is carried down the spinal cord to peripheral cholinergic nerves that innervate the vascular supply to the corpora, resulting in an erection.

The medial preoptic area of the hypothalamus is thought to be that portion of the brain responsible for integrating external stimuli. Here dopamine exerts a proerectogenic effect, whereas, α_2-adrenergic stimulation causes the penis to become and/or remain flaccid. After moving down the spinal cord, nerve impulses travel to the penis by efferent peripheral nerves, including inhibitory sympathetic neurons (T11 through L2), proerectogenic parasympathetic neurons (S2 through S4), and proerectogenic somatic neurons (S2 through S4).

In summary, acetylcholine produces an erection by working along with other coneurotransmitters, including cGMP and cAMP. Thus, an erection is initiated by the action of nerves, maintained by arterial blood filling of the corpora, and sustained by occlusion of venous outflow from the corpora.

Detumescence, or the progression of an erect penis to a flaccid state, results from the actions of norepinephrine, which contracts vascular smooth muscle to decrease arterial inflow to the corpora and contracts sinusoidal tissue in the corpora. As a result, venous outflow from the corpora increases.

HORMONAL SYSTEM

Testosterone stimulates libido or sexual drive in males. Within the normal physiologic serum concentration range (normal 300–1,100 ng/dL), sexual drive is normal. Approximately one third of men older than 50 years have hypogonadism, which is characterized by subphysiologic serum testosterone levels. Patients complain of loss of energy, loss of muscle strength, depressive mood, and decreased libido.

When libido is decreased, a patient may not develop erections. Thus, erectile dysfunction is considered secondary to a decreased libido. The relationship between erectile dysfunction and serum testosterone levels is complicated. Patients with normal serum testosterone levels may have erectile dysfunction, and patients with subnormal serum testosterone levels may have normal sexual function.[5]

PATHOPHYSIOLOGY

Erectile dysfunction can result from any single abnormality or combination of abnormalities of the four systems necessary for a normal penile erection. Vascular, neurologic, or hormonal etiologies of erectile dysfunction are collectively referred to as *organic erectile dysfunction*. Approximately 80% of patients with erectile dysfunction have the organic type. Patients who do not respond to psychogenic stimuli have *psychogenic erectile dysfunction*.

Diseases that compromise vascular flow to the corpora cavernosum (e.g., peripheral vascular disease, arteriosclerosis, and essential hypertension) are associated with an increased incidence of erectile dysfunction. Diseases that impair nerve conduction to the brain (e.g., spinal cord injury or stroke) or conditions that impair peripheral nerve conduction to the penile vasculature (e.g., diabetes mellitus) can result in erectile dysfunction.

Diseases associated with hypogonadism, primary or secondary, result in subphysiologic levels of testosterone, which cause diminished sexual drive (decreased libido) and secondary erectile dysfunction. Primary hypogonadism can be associated with the normal aging process in men or surgical removal of the testes for treatment of prostate or testicular cancer. Secondary hypogonadism may result from hypothalamic or pituitary disorders of luteinizing hormone–releasing hormone or luteinizing hormone, respectively; or elevated prolactin levels, which can result from pituitary tumors or can occur in patients with chronic renal failure.

Patients must be in the proper mental frame of mind to be receptive to sexual stimuli. Patients who suffer from malaise, have reactive depression or performance anxiety, are sedated, have Alzheimer's disease, have hypothyroidism, or have mental disorders, commonly complain of erectile dysfunction. In most studies, patients with psychogenic erectile dysfunction generally exhibit a higher response rate to various interventions than do patients with organic erectile dysfunction because the former have less severe disease.

Social habits of patients have been linked to erectile dysfunction. The vasoconstrictor effect of cigarette smoking may compromise blood flow to the corpora and decrease cavernosal filling. Excessive ethanol intake may lead to androgen deficiency, peripheral neuropathy, or chronic liver disease, all of which can contribute to erectile dysfunction.

❷ Medications may cause erectile dysfunction through similar pathophysiologic mechanisms (Table 86–2).[7,8] Medications are estimated to be responsible for approximately 10% to 25% of cases of erectile dysfunction.

CLINICAL PRESENTATION: ERECTILE DYSFUNCTION

General

- Men are affected emotionally in many different ways
- Depression
- Performance anxiety
- Marital difficulties and avoidance of sexual intimacy (patients are often brought to a physician by their partners)
- Nonadherence to medications patient believes are causing erectile dysfunction

Symptoms

- Impotence or inability to have sexual intercourse

TABLE 86-2 Medication Classes That Can Cause Erectile Dysfunction

Drug Class	Proposed Mechanism by Which Drug Causes Erectile Dysfunction	Special Notes
Anticholinergic agents (antihistamines, antiparkinsonian agents, tricyclic antidepressants, phenothiazines)	Anticholinergic activity	• Second-generation nonsedating antihistamines (e.g., loratadine) are not associated with erectile dysfunction • Selective serotonin reuptake inhibitor antidepressants can be substituted for tricyclic antidepressants if erectile dysfunction is a problem • Phenothiazines with less anticholinergic effect (e.g., chlorpromazine) can be substituted in some patients if erectile dysfunction is a problem
Dopamine agonists (e.g., metoclopramide, phenothiazines)	Inhibit prolactin inhibitory factor, thereby increasing prolactin levels	• Increased prolactin levels are associated with blocking testosterone production from the testes; depressed libido results
Estrogens, antiandrogens (e.g., luteinizing hormone–releasing hormone superagonists, digoxin, spironolactone, ketoconazole, cimetidine)	Suppress testosterone-mediated stimulation of libido	• In the face of a decreased libido, a secondary erectile dysfunction develops
Central nervous system depressants (e.g., barbiturates, narcotics, benzodiazepines, short-term use of large doses of alcohol)	Suppress perception of psychogenic stimuli	
Agents that decrease penile blood flow (e.g., diuretics, peripheral β-adrenergic antagonists, or central sympatholytics [methyldopa, clonidine, guanethidine])	Reduce arteriolar flow to corpora	• Any diuretic that produces a significant decrease in intravascular volume can decrease penile arteriolar flow • Safer antihypertensives include angiotensin-converting enzyme inhibitors, postsynaptic α_1-adrenergic antagonists (terazosin, doxazosin), calcium channel blockers, and angiotensin II receptor antagonists

From Thomas et al.[7] *and Lee and Sharifi.*[8]

Signs

- If completing an International Index of Erectile Dysfunction survey, results are consistent with low satisfaction with the quality of erectile function.
- Medical history may identify concurrent medical illnesses, past surgical procedures that interfere with good vascular flow to the penis or damage nerve function to the corpora, or mental disorders associated with decreased reception of sexual stimuli.
- Medication history may reveal prescription or nonprescription medications that could cause erectile dysfunction.
- Physical examination may reveal signs of hypogonadism (e.g., gynecomastia, small testicles, decreased body hair, decreased muscle mass), which may contribute to erectile dysfunction. The patient may have signs of an abnormally curved penis when erect, decreased pulses in the pelvic region (suggesting impaired vascular flow to the penis), or decreased anal sphincter tone (suggesting impaired nerve function to the corpora). Men older than 50 years should undergo a digital rectal examination to determine whether an enlarged prostate is be contributing to the patient's erectile dysfunction.

Laboratory Tests

- If patient has signs of hypogonadism and complains of decreased libido, a serum testosterone concentration may be below the normal, which would be consistent with the disorder.
- If the patient has an enlarged prostate noted on digital rectal examination, a blood sample for prostate specific antigen should be obtained. If elevated, the patient should be evaluated for a prostate disorder, which could contribute to erectile dysfunction.

DIAGNOSIS

With the availability in the late 1990s of effective medications for erectile dysfunction independent of the etiology, diagnostic evaluation of erectile dysfunction became streamlined.[9,10] Key assessments include a description of the severity of erectile dysfunction, complete medical and surgical histories, review of concurrent medications, physical examination, and selected clinical laboratory tests.[10]

To assess the severity of erectile dysfunction, the patient should be asked about the quality of sexual intercourse for the last 4 weeks to 6 months. A self-administered standardized questionnaire, such as the International Index of Erectile Dysfunction (IIEF), is often used. It is administered before initiation of any treatment and repeated at regular intervals during treatment. It includes 15 questions about the quality of erectile function and satisfactoriness of sexual intercourse.[11] Questions include the following: How often were you able to maintain an erection? How difficult was it to sustain an erection? How satisfied are you with your sexual life? The physician should carefully assess the expectations for erectile function of the patient and the partner to ensure that the expectations are reasonable. Shorter versions of the IIEF and other self-reporting questionnaires are also used in clinical practice.

A medical history should be obtained to identify concurrent medical illnesses or surgical procedures that are risk factors for or are associated with organic or psychogenic erectile dysfunction. Underlying diseases that do not optimally respond to treatment should be addressed before specific treatment for erectile dysfunction is initiated. If the patient smokes cigarettes, drinks excessive amounts of ethanol, or uses recreational drugs, these social habits should be discontinued before specific treatment for erectile dysfunction is started.

A complete listing of the patient's prescription and nonprescription medications and dietary supplements should be reviewed by the clinician, who should identify drugs that may be contributing to erectile dysfunction. If possible, causative agents should be discontinued or the dose should be reduced.

A physical examination of the patient should include a check for hypogonadism (i.e., signs of gynecomastia, small testicles, and decreased body hair). The penis should be evaluated for diseases associated with abnormal penile curvature (e.g., Peyronie's disease), which are associated with erectile dysfunction. Femoral and lower extremity pulses should be assessed to provide an indication of vascular supply to the genitals. Anal sphincter tone and other genital reflexes should be checked for the integrity of the nerve supply to the penis. A digital rectal examination in patients 50 years or more is needed to rule out benign prostatic hyperplasia, which may contribute to erectile dysfunction.

Selected laboratory tests should be obtained to identify the presence of underlying diseases that could cause erectile dysfunction. They include a fasting serum blood glucose and lipid profile. Serum testosterone levels should be checked in patients older than 50 years and in younger patients who complain of decreased libido. Serum testosterone levels follow a circadian pattern of secretion, with the highest levels occurring during the morning hours. To interpret serum testosterone levels properly, serum samples should be obtained in the mornings. At least two serial serum testosterone levels are needed to confirm the presence of hypogonadism.[12]

Finally, erectile dysfunction is a potential marker for arteriosclerosis. Therefore, patients who present with erectile dysfunction should undergo a cardiovascular risk assessment to identify treatable medical conditions.[13]

TREATMENT

Erectile Dysfunction

DESIRED OUTCOMES

The goal of treatment is improvement in the quantity and quality of penile erections suitable for satisfactory intercourse. Simple as this may sound, healthcare providers must ensure that patients and their partners have reasonable expectations for any therapies that are initiated. Furthermore, only patients with erectile dysfunction should be treated. Patients who have normal sexual function should not seek—or be encouraged to seek—treatment in an effort to enhance sexual function or enable increased activity.[14]

GENERAL APPROACH TO TREATMENT

❸ The Second Princeton Consensus Conference is a widely accepted multidisciplinary approach to managing erectile dysfunction that maps out a stepwise treatment plan.[15–17] The first step in clinical management of erectile dysfunction is to identify and, if possible, reverse underlying causes. Risk factors for erectile dysfunction, including hypertension, diabetes mellitus, smoking, or chronic ethanol abuse, should be addressed and minimized. Patients should follow a heart-healthy lifestyle, which includes physical fitness, weight loss to achieve a normal body mass index, low-cholesterol diets, no excessive ethanol intake, and no smoking.[18,19] In some cases, these types of interventions are sufficient to restore erectile function. However, if erectile dysfunction does not respond to these measures, specific treatment is indicated.

For patients with psychogenic erectile dysfunction, psychotherapy can be used as monotherapy or as an adjunct to specific treatments for the disorder. To enhance the relevance of psychotherapy, both the patient and the partner should be included in the counseling sessions. Treatment should be individualized and should address immediate factors that may be causing performance anxiety or depression, rather than the remote, deep-seated reasons for psychological disorders.[20] The effectiveness of psychotherapy is generally low, and long-term psychotherapy is often necessary.

❹ ❺ ❻ Specific treatments of erectile dysfunction include vacuum erection devices (VEDs), pharmacologic treatments, and surgery. The ideal treatment of this disorder should have a fast onset, be effective, be convenient to administer, be cost effective, have a low incidence of serious adverse effects, and be free of serious drug interactions (Table 86–3). Generally, when choosing from among treatment approaches, those that are least invasive are selected first; more invasive therapies are reserved for patients who do not respond to first-line agents. A sample algorithm that guides selection of treatment is shown in Fig. 86–2.

TABLE 86-3 Dosing Regimens for Selected Drug Treatments for Erectile Dysfunction

Route of Administration	Generic Name (Brand Name)	Dosage Form	Common Dosing Regimen
Oral	Yohimbine (Aphrodyne, Yocon, Yohimex)	5.4-mg tablet or capsule	5.4 mg three times per day
	Sildenafil (Viagra)	25-mg, 50-mg, 100-mg tablet	25–100 mg 1 hour before intercourse
	Apomorphine (Uprima)[a]	10-mg sublingual tablet, 25-mg tablet and capsule	10–40 mg daily
	Fluoxymesterone (Halotestin)	2-mg, 5-mg, 10-mg, 50-mg tablet	5–20 mg daily
	Trazodone (Desyrel)	100-mg, 150-mg, 300-mg tablet	50–150 mg daily
	Vardenafil (Levitra)	2.5-mg, 5-mg, 10-mg, 20-mg tablet	5–10 mg 1 hour before intercourse
	Tadalafil (Cialis)	5-mg, 10-mg, 20-mg tablet	5–20 mg before intercourse
Topical	Testosterone patch (Testoderm)	4 mg/patch, 6 mg/patch	4–6 mg/day; apply to scrotum
	Testosterone patch (Testoderm TTS)	4 mg/patch, 6 mg/patch	4–6 mg/day; apply to arm, buttock, back
	Testosterone patch (Androderm)	2.5 mg/patch	2.5–5 mg/day; apply to arm, back, abdomen, thigh
	Testosterone gel (AndroGel 1%)	5 g/pkt, 10 g/pkt	5–10 g/day; apply to shoulders, upper arms, abdomen
Intramuscular	Testosterone cypionate (Depo-Testosterone)	100 mg/mL, 200 mg/mL	200–400 mg every 2–4 weeks
	Testosterone enanthate (Delatestryl)	100 mg/mL, 200 mg/mL	200–400 mg every 2–4 weeks
Subcutaneous implant	Testosterone (Testopel)	75-mg pellet	150–450 mg every 3–4 months
Intraurethral	Alprostadil (MUSE)	125-mcg, 250-mcg, 500-mcg, 1,000-mcg pellet	125–1,000 mcg 5–10 minutes before intercourse
Intracavernosal	Alprostadil (Caverject)	5-mcg, 10-mcg, 20-mcg injection	2.5–60 mcg 5–10 minutes before intercourse
	Alprostadil (Edex)	5-mcg, 20-mcg, 40-mcg injection	2.5–60 mcg 5–10 minutes before intercourse
	Papaverine[b]	30 mg/mL injection	Variable, usually used in combination with alprostadil and phentolamine
	Phentolamine[b]	2.5 mg/mL injection	Variable, usually used in combination with alprostadil and papaverine

[a]Not commercially available in the United States as a sublingual formulation; only available in United States as subcutaneous injection that is FDA approved for Parkinson's disease.
[b]Not FDA approved for this use.

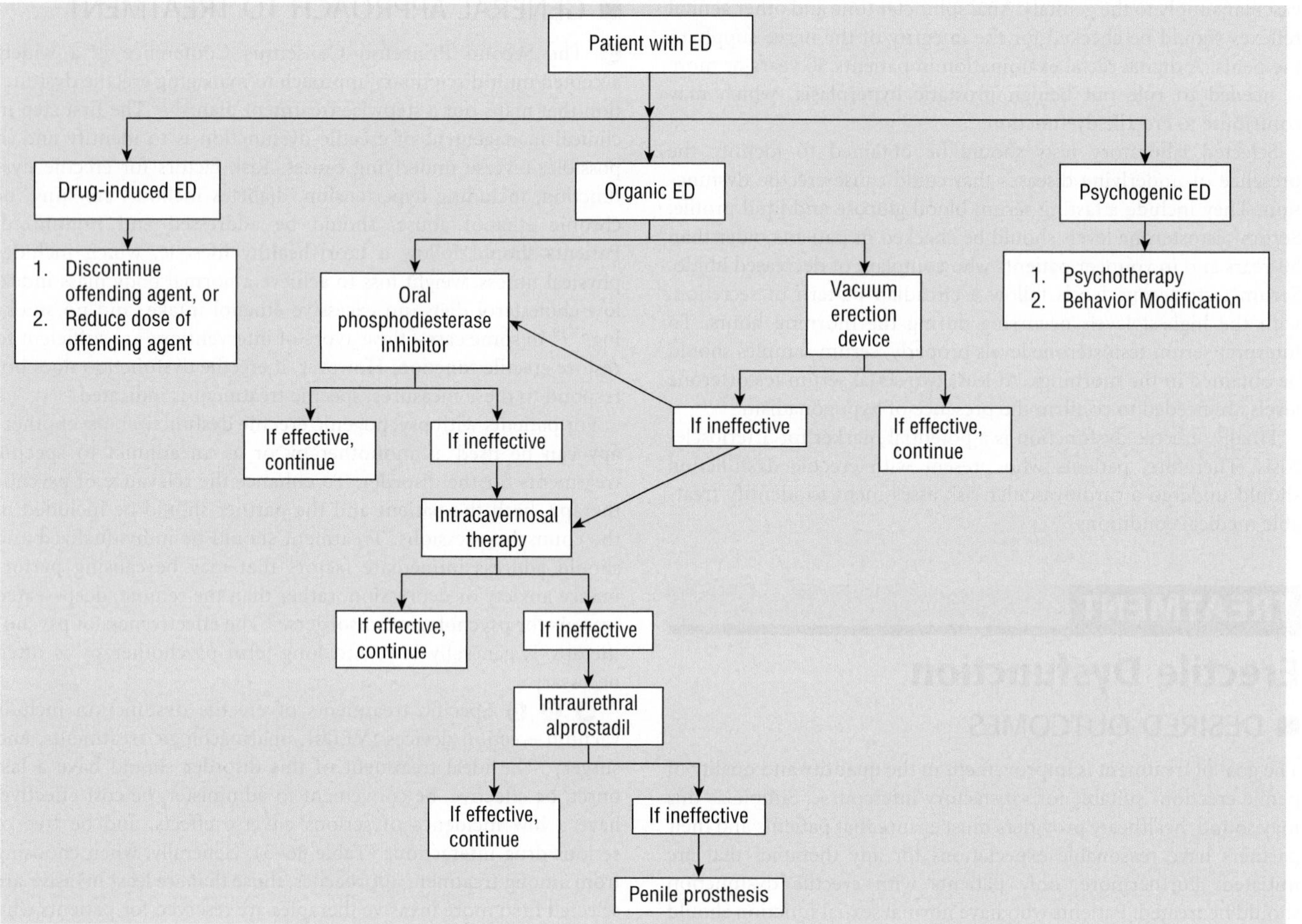

FIGURE 86-2. Algorithm for selecting treatment for erectile dysfunction. For organic erectile dysfunction (ED), oral agents are first-line therapy for younger patients, and vacuum erection devices are generally used first in older patients who are married or otherwise have a stable sexual relationship. These two approaches are sometimes used together in an effort to avoid surgical implantation of penile prostheses.

■ VACUUM ERECTION DEVICE

A VED has three parts: a pump, which generates a negative vacuum pressure; a cylinder, which is closed at one end and into which the penis is inserted; and tubing, which connects the pump to the cylinder. The patient inserts his penis into the open end of the cylinder, which is then pushed up flush against his lower abdomen to create a vacuum chamber. Then the patient activates the pump to produce a vacuum pressure, which draws arteriolar blood into the corpora cavernosa. To prolong the erection, the patient can use constriction bands or tension rings, which are placed at the base of the penis, to keep the arteriolar blood in and to reduce venous outflow from the penis. With the assistance of loading cones to protect the glans, these bands or rings can be rolled over the glans penis and up the erect penile shaft. Alternatively, they can be first threaded onto the plastic cylinder before the penis is inserted. Once the penis is erect, the band or ring can be rolled off the cylinder onto the base of the penis (Fig. 86–3).

❼ The onset of action of the VED is comparatively slow (30 minutes), which requires patience from both the patient and the sexual partner. VEDs are not discreet. That is, a patient's use of a VED is evident to the partner. For this reason, VEDs appear to work best in older patients who are married or have stable sexual relationships. In this group, VEDs are considered first-line therapy, and the overall satisfaction rate is 60% to 80%.[5,14] However, 6% to 11% of partners complain that the penis is cool to the touch or is discolored (bluish) in appearance, particularly when constriction bands are used.

VEDs may be used as second-line therapy in patients who do not respond to oral or injectable drug treatments for erectile dysfunction. The combination of a VED with intracavernosal or intraurethral alprostadil is associated with a higher efficacy rate than use of the VED alone. As a result, combination therapy sometimes is attempted before penile prosthesis surgery is considered in the patient who fails VED monotherapy.

VEDs are available with manual or battery-operated pumps. The latter offer greater convenience, particularly in patients with arthritis of the hands, who find the manual pumps too difficult and tiring to operate. The American Urological Association recommends the use of commercially available VEDs by prescription only.[21]

Pain or injury from VEDs most often is caused by the constriction bands used to sustain an erection. Because these rings trap blood in the corpora and reduce arteriolar flow into the penis, the penile shaft may feel cold and numb. If the constriction bands are applied for longer than 30 to 60 minutes, the penile shaft may turn blue and hurt. Patients may complain that a hinge-like erection is produced in that the penis pivots on the rubber ring or tension band. Patients sometimes fail to ejaculate.

VEDs are contraindicated in patients with sickle cell disease. These patients are prone to priapism, which can be exacerbated by the use of constriction bands with VEDs. The devices also should be used cautiously by patients taking oral anticoagulants because warfarin, through a poorly understood and idiosyncratic mechanism, can cause priapism.

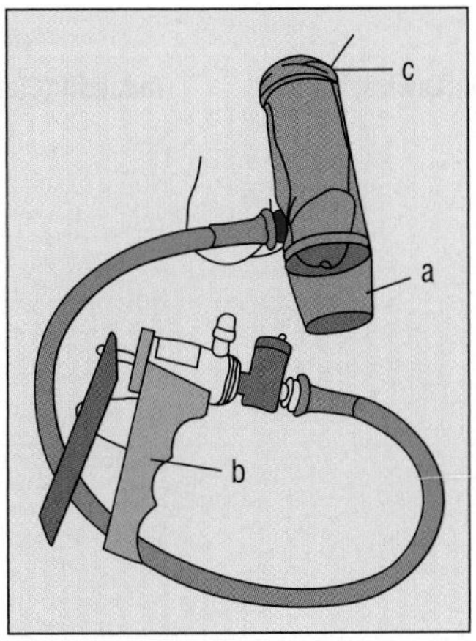

FIGURE 86-3. Technique for using a vacuum erection device with tension band or rubber constriction ring. The patient inserts his penis into the cylinder, which is then pushed up flush against his lower abdomen to create a vacuum chamber. The patient activates the pump to produce a vacuum pressure, which draws arteriolar blood into the corpora cavernosa. To prolong the erection, the patient can use constriction bands or tension rings, which are placed at the base of the penis, to keep the arteriolar blood in and reduce venous outflow from the penis. *(From http://kidney.niddk.nih.gov/kudiseases/pubs/impotence.)*

■ PHOSPHODIESTERASE INHIBITORS

Mechanism

In the presence of sexual stimulation, nitric oxide is released by neurons or endothelial cells in penile tissue, thereby enhancing the activity of guanylate cyclase, the enzyme responsible for conversion of guanylate triphosphate to cGMP (Fig. 86–4).[22] cGMP is a vasodilatory secondary messenger that enhances arterial flow to the corpora cavernosa and enhances blood filling of cavernosal sinuses. Catabolism of cGMP is mediated by phosphodiesterase.

Three selective inhibitors of the phosphodiesterase isoenzyme type 5 found in genital tissue are marketed for erectile dysfunction in the United States (Table 86–4). They act by decreasing catabolism of cGMP. However, phosphodiesterase isoenzyme type 5 is also found in peripheral vascular tissue, tracheal smooth muscle, and platelets. Inhibition of phosphodiesterase in these nongenital tissues can produce unwanted effects.

The three marketed phosphodiesterase inhibitors differ in their degree of selectivity in inhibiting other phosphodiesterase isoenzymes, pharmacokinetic profiles, drug–food interactions, and adverse effects (see Table 86–4).

Efficacy

Because of their apparent effectiveness, convenient route of administration, and comparatively low incidence of serious adverse effects, phosphodiesterase inhibitors are considered first-line therapy for erectile dysfunction, particularly in younger patients. They allow for discreet use. All three commercially available phosphodiesterase inhibitors are equally effective.[23,24]

In the presence of sexual stimulation and in doses of 25 to 100 mg, sildenafil produces satisfactory erections in 56% to 82% of patients, independent of the etiology of erectile dysfunction. Similar results are documented in the product labeling for the other two agents in this class (65%–80% for vardenafil and 62%–77% for tadalafil). Response rates in the lower range for phosphodiesterase inhibitors have been documented in patients with diabetes mellitus or in patients after radical prostatectomy, probably due to postoperative nerve damage.[22,25] The effectiveness of the drugs appears to be dose related.

8 Approximately 30% to 40% of patients do not respond to phosphodiesterase inhibitors.[13] At least half of nonresponders can benefit from education on proper use of the drugs, and this likely will prove true for the other agents used for erectile dysfunction. Education of patients should include the following points: (1) patients must engage in sexual stimulation (foreplay) for the best response; (2) sildenafil should be taken on an empty stomach, at least 2 hours before meals, for the fastest response, but the other two agents can be taken without regard to meals; (3) taking sildenafil or vardenafil with a fatty meal can decrease the absorption rate, but the absorption rate of tadalafil is not affected[26]; (4) patients who do not respond to the first dose should continue with the phosphodiesterase inhibitor for at least five to eight doses before failure is declared, as increasing success rates are reported with sequential dose administration[27]; and (5) some patients require dosage titration up to 100 mg sildenafil, 20 mg vardenafil, or 20 mg tadalafil for a response.[27–29]

The effectiveness of switching from one phosphodiesterase inhibitor to another when the patient does not respond to an initial agent is controversial. In two small studies, vardenafil was beneficial in patients who did not respond to sildenafil.[26,30] However, controlled clinical trials in larger patient groups are needed before this strategy is used as routine treatment.

The phosphodiesterase inhibitors should not be used by patients with normal erectile function. Also, according to Food and Drug

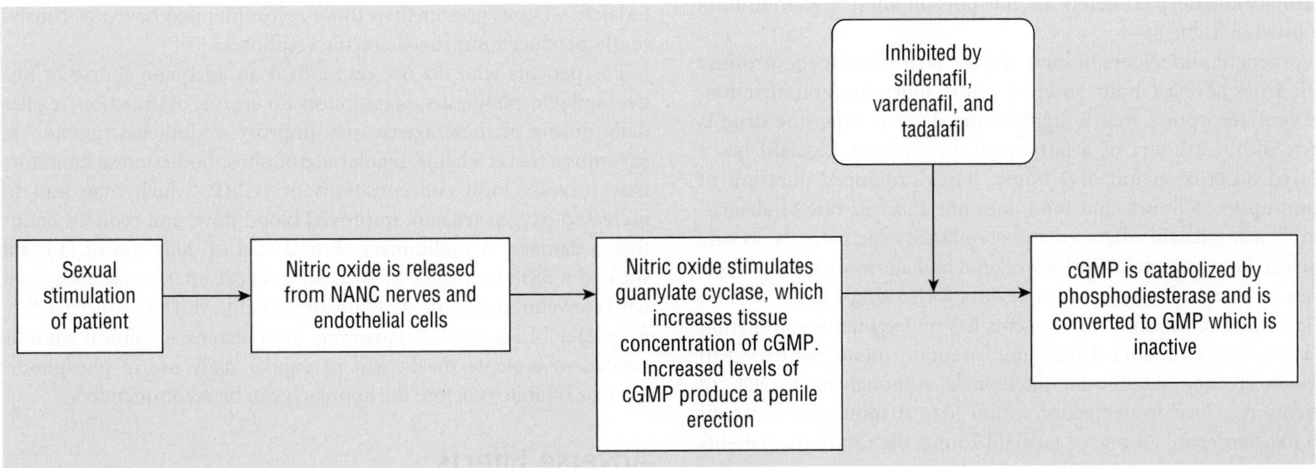

FIGURE 86-4. Mechanism of action of phosphodiesterase inhibitors. All inhibit catabolism of cGMP, a vasodilatory secondary messenger. (cGMP, cyclic guanosine monophosphate; NANC, nonadrenergic noncholinergic.)

TABLE 86-4 Pharmacodynamics and Pharmacokinetics of Phosphodiesterase Inhibitors

	Sildenafil (Viagra)[a]	Vardenafil (Levitra)[a]	Tadalafil (Cialis)[a]
Inhibits PDE-5	Yes	Yes	Yes
Inhibits PDE-6	Yes	Minimally	No
Inhibits PDE-11	No	No	Yes
Time to peak plasma level (h)	0.5–1	0.7–0.9	2
Fatty meal decreases rate of oral absorption?	Yes	Yes	No
Mean plasma half-life (h)	3.7	4.4–4.8	18
Percentage of dose excreted in feces	80	91–95	61
Percentage of dose excreted in urine	13	2–6	36
Duration (h)	4	4	24–36
Usual daily dose (mg)	25–100	5–20	5–20
Daily dose in patients ≥65 years (mg)	25	5	5–20
Daily dose in moderate renal impairment (mg)	25–100	5–20	5
Daily dose in severe renal impairment (mg)	25	5–20	5
Daily dose in mild hepatic impairment (mg)	25–100	5–20	10
Daily dose in moderate hepatic impairment (mg)	25–100	5–10	10
Daily dose in severe hepatic impairment (mg)	25	Not evaluated	Not recommended
Dose in patients taking cytochrome P450 3A4 inhibitors[a]	25 mg daily	2.5–5 mg every 24–72 hours	10 mg every 72 hours

[a]Sildenafil doses should be decreased when any potent cytochrome P450 3A4 inhibitor (e.g., cimetidine, erythromycin, clarithromycin, ketoconazole, itraconazole, ritonavir, and saquinavir) is used. Vardenafil doses vary according to the agent used (2.5 mg every 72 hours for ritonavir; 2.5 mg every 24 hours for indinavir, ketoconazole 400 mg daily, and itraconazole 400 mg daily; and 5 mg every 24 hours for ketoconazole 200 mg daily, itraconazole 200 mg daily, and erythromycin). Tadalafil doses are reduced only when the drug is used with the most potent cytochrome P450 3A4 inhibitors (e.g., ketoconazole, ritonavir).
PDE, phosphodiesterase.

Administration (FDA)-approved labeling, the drugs should not be used in combination with other forms of therapy for erectile dysfunction because prolonged erections may result.[31]

■ SELECTIVITY OF OTHER PHOSPHODIESTERASE ISOENZYMES

More than 25 different phosphodiesterase isoenzymes have been identified; however, the physiologic effects of stimulation and inhibition of some of these isoenzymes remain to be elucidated. Of note, phosphodiesterase isoenzyme type 6 is localized to the rods and cones of the eye. Inhibition of this isoenzyme has been associated with blurred vision and cyanopsia. Sildenafil is the most potent inhibitor of phosphodiesterase isoenzyme type 6, vardenafil is an intermediate inhibitor, and tadalafil is the least potent inhibitor.[26] Likewise, phosphodiesterase isoenzyme type 11 is localized to striated muscle. Inhibition of this isoenzyme has been associated with myalgia and muscle pain. Tadalafil exerts the greatest inhibitory activity against phosphodiesterase type 11.[6]

Pharmacokinetics and Drug–Food Interactions

Pharmacokinetic parameters of the phosphodiesterase inhibitors are listed in Table 86–4.

Vardenafil and sildenafil have similar pharmacokinetic profiles. Both drugs have a 1-hour onset of action, short duration of action, and oral absorption that is significantly delayed when the drug is taken within 2 hours of a fatty meal. In contrast, tadalafil has a delayed onset of action of 2 hours, has a prolonged duration of action up to 36 hours, and food does not affect its rate of absorption. Thus, tadalafil offers greater spontaneity for patients, as one dose can last through an entire weekend and allow for multiple acts of sexual intercourse over multiple days with a single dose.[32–35]

The onset of action of these agents has undergone reexamination to assess how soon after drug administration patients can expect to have an erection suitable for intercourse. Although up to 50% of patients may develop an erection within 20 to 30 minutes of sildenafil 100 mg, vardenafil 20 mg, or tadalafil 20 mg, the rest of the patients may require a full hour to achieve an adequate erectile response.[26,36] Therefore, patients should be instructed to allow adequate time for the drug to work.

Concomitant ingestion of ethanol with phosphodiesterase inhibitors can result in orthostatic hypotension. Therefore, the manufacturer recommends that patients avoid ethanol when taking these medications.

All three phosphodiesterase inhibitors are hepatically catabolized by the cytochrome P450 3A4 microsomal isoenzyme as well as by other P450 isoenzymes (minor routes) and/or other hepatic enzymes. The drugs and their metabolites (some of which are active) are excreted primarily in the feces, but also in the urine to varying degrees (see Table 86–4).

Dosing

The usual oral doses of the phosphodiesterase inhibitors are listed in Table 86–4. Sildenafil and vardenafil should be taken on demand or at least 30 to 60 minutes before sexual intercourse. Tadalafil should be taken at least 2 hours before sexual intercourse. The durations of action for sildenafil and vardenafil are 4 to 5 hours, whereas the effects of tadalafil last for 36 hours. The agents vary as to whether doses must be adjusted for patients 65 years and older and those with compromised hepatic or renal function. Patients should be advised to take no more than the amount prescribed and to use only one dose per day (or less often in the case of some patients taking tadalafil). Doses greater than those recommended have not consistently produced improved erectile responses.

For patients who do not respond to an adequate course of on-demand phosphodiesterase inhibitors for erectile dysfunction, regular daily dosing of these agents may improve endothelial function in cavernosal tissue. That is, regular use of phosphodiesterase inhibitors may increase local concentrations of cGMP, which may lead to increased oxygen tension, improved blood flow, and reduced endothelial damage. A preliminary clinical trial of daily use of tadalafil showed a 58% frequency of successful sexual intercourse compared with conventional on-demand use of tadalafil, which produced a 21% frequency of success.[13,36] However, more extensive clinical study is needed to evaluate the benefit of regular daily use of phosphodiesterase inhibitors before the approach can be recommended.

Adverse Effects

Most adverse effects of the phosphodiesterase inhibitors are mild or moderate and are self-limited, and patients often become tolerant to them with continued use.[37] The rates of drug discontinuation caused by adverse effects are low, ranging from 2.1% to 2.5%, and are similar for all three agents. In usual doses the most common adverse effects are headache (11%), facial flushing (12%), dyspepsia (5%), nasal congestion (3.4%), and dizziness (3%),[22] all of which result from vasodilation or smooth muscle relaxation secondary to inhibition of phosphodiesterase isoenzyme type 5 in extragenital tissues.[14]

Sildenafil and vardenafil produce an 8- to 10-mm Hg decrease in systolic and a 5- to 6-mm Hg decrease in diastolic blood pressure starting approximately 1 hour after a dose is taken and lasting for 4 hours. Most patients are asymptomatic as a result of these blood pressure changes, but some patients, particularly those taking multiple antihypertensives or nitrates or those with baseline hypotension, may develop clinical symptoms as a consequence of these peripheral vascular effects. Tadalafil does not produce decreases in blood pressure, but it must be used with caution in patients with cardiovascular disease because of the cardiac risk inherent to sexual activity. A management approach for such patients, developed based on an analysis of deaths in men who were using sildenafil and commonly referred to as the recommendations of the Princeton Consensus Guideline Conference II,[15] should be applied to all the phosphodiesterase inhibitors (Table 86–5).

Sildenafil and vardenafil cause increased sensitivity to light, blurred vision, or loss of blue–green color discrimination in 2% to 3% of patients. These effects result from inhibition of phosphodiesterase type 6 in the photoreceptor cells of in retinal rods and cones, particularly at doses larger than 100 mg.[39] Visual adverse effects commonly occur at the time of peak serum concentrations. Although visual adverse effects are mild and reversible, caution regarding use is recommended for airplane pilots, who rely on green and blue lights for landing planes. Tadalafil has minimal to no inhibitory activity against type 6 phosphodiesterase, and no visual adverse effects have been reported. Nevertheless, according to current product labeling, all phosphodiesterase inhibitors should be used cautiously in patients at risk for retinitis pigmentosa, a genetic disease associated with retinal phosphodiesterase deficiency.[40]

Isolated cases of nonarteritic anterior ischemic optic neuropathy (NAION) have been associated with phosphodiesterase inhibitor use.[41] Although a cause-and-effect relationship has not been definitively established, the blood pressure–lowering effects of these medications may decrease blood flow to the optic nerve and lead to sudden unilateral decrease in vision. Because NAION may lead to permanent vision loss, the FDA has required inclusion of warnings on the product labeling of phosphodiesterase inhibitors. Specifically, before receiving these agents, patients at risk for NAION should be evaluated by an ophthalmologist. Patients at risk include those with glaucoma, macular degeneration, and diabetic retinopathy, and those who have undergone eye surgery or have experienced eye trauma. A patient who experiences sudden vision loss while taking a phosphodiesterase inhibitor should be evaluated for NAION before continuing treatment.

Tadalafil inhibits type 11 phosphodiesterase, which is found in skeletal muscle. This may explain the symptoms of lower back and limb muscle pain, which occur in a dose-related fashion in 7% to 30% of patients treated with doses of 10 to 100 mg.[32]

Sildenafil inhibits phosphodiesterase isoenzyme type 5 in platelets, which theoretically could inhibit platelet aggregation. However, in vitro and in vivo studies show no significant effect of sildenafil on platelets.[36]

Priapism is a rare adverse effect of phosphodiesterase inhibitors, particularly sildenafil and vardenafil, which have shorter plasma half-lives than tadalafil. Priapism has been associated with excessive doses of the phosphodiesterase inhibitor or concomitant therapy involving other erectogenic drugs.

Drug Interactions

Patients taking organic nitrates may develop severe hypotension if they are taken with phosphodiesterase inhibitors as a result of two major factors: (1) organic nitrates on their own produce hypotension, and (2) organic nitrates are nitric oxide donors, which can stimulate the activity of guanylate cyclase and increase tissue levels of cGMP. For this reason, use of the three phosphodiesterase inhibitors is contraindicated in patients taking nitrates given by any route at scheduled times or intermittently.[15,42] Furthermore, nitrates should be withheld for 24 hours after sildenafil or vardenafil administration and for 48 hours after tadalafil administration.[42] Finally, if a patient who has taken a phosphodiesterase inhibitor requires medical treatment of angina, non–nitrate-containing agents (e.g., calcium channel blocker, β-adrenergic antagonist, morphine) should be used.

If severe hypotension occurs after exposure to nitrates and a phosphodiesterase inhibitor, the patient should be placed in a

TABLE 86-5 Recommendations of the Second Princeton Consensus Conference for Cardiovascular Risk Stratification of Patients Being Considered for Phosphodiesterase Inhibitor Therapy

Risk Category	Description of Patient's Condition	Management Approach
Low risk	Has asymptomatic cardiovascular disease with <3 risk factors for cardiovascular disease Has well-controlled hypertension Has mild, stable angina Has mild congestive heart failure (NYHA class I) Has mild valvular heart disease Had a myocardial infarction >6 weeks ago	Patient can be started on phosphodiesterase inhibitor
Intermediate risk	Has ≥3 risk factors for cardiovascular disease Has moderate, stable angina Had a recent myocardial infarction or stroke within the past 6 weeks Has moderate congestive heart failure (NYHA class II)	Patient should undergo complete cardiovascular workup and treadmill stress test to determine tolerance to increased myocardial energy consumption associated with increased sexual activity
High risk	Has unstable or symptomatic angina, despite treatment Has uncontrolled hypertension Has severe congestive heart failure (NYHA class III or IV) Had a recent myocardial infarction or stroke within past 2 weeks Has moderate or severe valvular heart disease Has high-risk cardiac arrhythmias Has obstructive hypertrophic cardiomyopathy	Phosphodiesterase inhibitor is contraindicated; sexual intercourse should be deferred

NYHA, New York Heart Association.
From Rosen et al.[15] and Kostis et al.[17]

Trendelenburg position and aggressive fluid administration initiated. If severe hypotension continues, parenteral α-adrenergic agonists (e.g., dopamine) should be administered cautiously.

Interestingly, dietary sources of nitrates, nitrites, or L-arginine (a precursor for nitrates) do not interact with the phosphodiesterase inhibitors. This is because dietary sources do not increase circulating levels of nitric oxide in humans.

Sildenafil does not appear to interact with antihypertensive medications. In retrospective analyses of patients taking sildenafil in combination with α-adrenergic antagonists, β-adrenergic antagonists, diuretics, angiotensin-converting enzyme inhibitors, angiotensin receptor blockers, or calcium channel blockers, the incidence of hypotension was similar to that reported in patients taking sildenafil alone.[43,44] This finding was confirmed by a retrospective analysis of pooled data on more than 4,800 patients in 35 clinical trials.[31]

Small decreases in blood pressure with clinically symptomatic hypotension have been described in some patients taking sildenafil and tadalafil and immediate-release formulations of terazosin and doxazosin.[45] In contrast, concurrent administration of extended-release alfuzosin or tamsulosin, which produce lower peak serum concentrations than immediate-release formulations after administration, show no decrease in blood pressure.[46,47] Until more data become available, manufacturers of phosphodiesterase inhibitors recommend a 4-hour interval between doses of phosphodiesterase inhibitors and α-adrenergic antagonists when these drugs are prescribed concomitantly in the same patient.

Hepatic metabolism of all three phosphodiesterase inhibitors can be inhibited by cytochrome P450 hepatic microsomal enzyme inhibitors of CYP 3A4, including cimetidine, erythromycin, clarithromycin, ketoconazole, itraconazole, ritonavir, and saquinavir.[48] Lower starting doses should be used in these patients (see Table 86–4).

CLINICAL CONTROVERSY

Some clinicians believe that tachyphylaxis may develop with continuous use of sildenafil, but others believe that a lack of responsiveness may be due to worsening of underlying diseases that may contribute to the development of erectile dysfunction.[14] Positive treatment response despite continuous use of these agents for up to 6 years suggests that tachyphylaxis does not occur.[26,38,49]

■ TESTOSTERONE REPLACEMENT REGIMENS

Mechanism

9 Testosterone replacement regimens supply exogenous testosterone and restore serum testosterone levels to the normal range (300–1,100 ng/dL). In so doing, testosterone replacement regimens correct symptoms of hypogonadism, which include malaise, loss of muscle strength, depressed mood, and decreased libido. Testosterone can directly stimulate androgen receptors in the central nervous system and is thought to be responsible for maintaining normal sexual drive. In addition, testosterone may stimulate nitric oxide synthase, thereby increasing cavernosal concentrations of nitric oxide,[13,50,51] or enhance the effects of phosphodiesterase type 5 in cavernosal tissue.[52]

Indications

Testosterone replacement regimens are indicated in symptomatic patients with primary or secondary hypogonadism, as confirmed by the presence of a decreased libido and low serum concentrations of testosterone.[14] Serum testosterone concentrations typically are measured in the early morning because the secretion pattern of this hormone follows a circadian pattern, with highest serum concentrations in the morning hours. Simultaneous serum luteinizing hormone levels help to distinguish patients with primary hypogonadism, who have elevated luteinizing hormone levels, from those with secondary hypogonadism, who have decreased luteinizing hormone levels. Primary hypogonadism can be a characteristic of aging men who undergo andropause, in which the Leydig cells of the testes slowly and progressively decrease testosterone production.[50]

Testosterone replacement regimens should never be administered to men with normal serum testosterone levels.

Efficacy

Testosterone replacement regimens restore muscle strength and sexual drive and improve mood in patients with hypogonadism. Improvements are generally observed within days or weeks of the start of testosterone replacement. Administration of testosterone will correct the serum testosterone level to the normal range. No additional benefit has been demonstrated for large doses of testosterone, which increase the serum testosterone level from the low end to the upper end of the normal range or to the above-normal range.[7] Testosterone replacement regimens do not directly correct erectile dysfunction; instead, they improve libido, thereby correcting secondary erectile dysfunction.

Testosterone replacement regimens can be administered orally, parenterally, or transdermally (Table 86–6). Injectable testosterone replacement regimens are the preferred treatment for symptomatic patients with primary or secondary hypogonadism because they are effective, inexpensive, and not associated with the bioavailability problems or hepatotoxic adverse effects of oral androgens.[5,50] Although convenient for the patient, testosterone patches and gels are much more expensive than other forms of androgen replacement; therefore, they should be reserved for patients who refuse injectable testosterone.

In the ideal testosterone replacement regimen, the medication would mimic the normal circadian pattern of serum testosterone concentrations such that peak and trough concentrations occur in the early morning and late afternoon, respectively; produces serum concentrations in the normal range; produces serum concentrations of dihydrotestosterone and estradiol, which are metabolites of testosterone that mimic the normal physiologic pattern; and produces minimal adverse effects.[50] Table 86–6 compares commercially available testosterone replacement regimens for these characteristics and shows that an ideal regimen has yet to be identified.

Pharmacokinetics

Natural testosterone has poor oral bioavailability because of extensive first-pass hepatic metabolism; therefore, large doses must be taken. To improve oral bioavailability, alkylated derivatives were formulated. Of these derivative, methyltestosterone and fluoxymesterone are more resistant to hepatic catabolism and can be taken in smaller daily doses, which are potentially safer. However, oral alkylated derivatives of testosterone are associated with a higher incidence of serious hepatotoxicity and therefore are not preferred for management of hypogonadism.

An alternative to oral administration is the testosterone buccal system (Striant), which is applied to the gum above the upper incisor teeth twice per day. Over time it forms a gel from which testosterone is absorbed. One advantage of this route of administration is that the drug bypasses first-pass hepatic catabolism, which allows for increased bioavailability of testosterone.

Several testosterone esters have been formulated for intramuscular injection, with different durations of action (see Table 86–3). The shorter-acting testosterone propionate, which requires dosing three times per week, has largely completely replaced with testosterone cypionate or enanthate, which can be dosed every 2, 4, or 6 weeks in most patients. An even longer-acting parenteral testoste-

TABLE 86-6 Comparison of Testosterone Replacement Regimens and Ideal Testosterone Replacement Regimen

	Achieves Serum Testosterone Concentrations in Normal Range?	Produces Normal Circadian Pattern of Serum Testosterone Concentrations?	Produces Normal Pattern of Serum Concentrations of Androgen Metabolites?	Adverse Effects
Oral testosterone	No	No	No	Hyperlipidemia Sodium retention
Oral alkylated androgens	Yes	No	No	Hyperlipidemia Sodium retention Hepatotoxicity
Intramuscular testosterone cypionate or enanthate	Yes	No; produces supraphysiologic serum concentrations for several days after injection	No, excess testosterone is converted to estradiol	Mood swings Gynecomastia Polycythemia Hyperlipidemia
Transdermal nonscrotal skin patch	Yes	Yes, provided the patch is placed at night	Yes	Dermatitis due to permeation enhancers in formulation
Transdermal scrotal skin patch	Yes	Yes provided the patch is applied in the morning	No; 5α-reductase in scrotal skin metabolizes testosterone and increases serum concentrations of dihydrotestosterone	Dermatitis due to permeation enhancers in formulation
Transdermal gel	Yes	Yes	Yes	May be inadvertently transferred to others who rub up against the patient's skin treated area
Testosterone subcutaneous implant	Yes	No	No; produces elevated concentrations of dihydrotestosterone	Pellet may be extruded accidentally, resulting in loss of drug effect
Buccal system	Yes	No	Yes	Gum irritation, bitter taste

Data from Gore JL, Swerdloff RS, Rajfer J. Androgen deficiency in the etiology and treatment of erectile dysfunction. Urol Clin N Am 2005;32:457–468.

rone is available as a subcutaneous implant for dosing every 4 to 6 months. Although this schedule minimizes repeat visits to the clinician's office for repeated dosing, the implant must be administered by a physician, and the implanted pellet may be extruded after administration. This extrusion has been reported in up to 8.5% of treated patients and results in loss of drug effect. However, these testosterone formulations produce suprapharmacologic patterns of serum testosterone during the dosing interval, which have been linked to mood swings in some patients.

Topical testosterone replacement regimens can be delivered as once-daily patches or gel. Testosterone patches increase serum testosterone levels into the normal range in 2 to 6 hours. Serum testosterone levels return to baseline 24 hours after patch administration. However, unlike oral or injectable supplements, transdermal testosterone patches applied at bedtime or testosterone gel applied each morning produce physiologic patterns of serum testosterone levels throughout the day. The clinical importance of this biochemical effect is unknown.[50]

The original Testoderm brand patch was formulated for scrotal application. Scrotal skin is thinner and has a richer vascular supply than does the skin on the arms or thighs. Therefore, application of Testoderm patches produces excellent absorption of the hormone. However, the patch can fall off when the scrotum becomes damp or moist, when the patient exercises, or if the scrotum is excessively hairy.

For improved convenience, Androderm and Testoderm TTS patches were formulated for application to the arms, buttocks, or back; Androderm can also be applied to the thighs. The addition of absorption enhancers and different adhesives has been linked to a higher incidence of contact dermatitis with Androderm patches compared with the original Testoderm scrotal patch.

Testosterone gel 1% formulation (AndroGel) is applied in much larger doses—5 or 10 g each day—to the skin of the shoulders, upper arms, or abdomen. The hormone is absorbed quickly, within 30 minutes, but several hours may be required for complete absorption of the dose. For this reason, the patient should be reminded to wait at least 5 to 6 hours after application before showering. To prevent inadvertent transfer of testosterone gel to others, the patient should thoroughly wash his hands with soap and water after administration of a dose.

Dosing

Table 86–3 lists the usual doses for testosterone replacement regimens. Two to three months is considered an adequate treatment trial with a particular dose. Thus, a dose should not be increased until the patient has used one particular dose for at least this time period.[52]

Before initiating any testosterone replacement regimen in patients 40 years and older, patients should be screened for benign prostatic hyperplasia and prostate cancer. Both of these diseases are testosterone-dependent conditions and theoretically could be worsened by exogenous administration of testosterone. Prostate cancer is a contraindication to androgen supplementation. To screen for these conditions, a prostate-specific antigen serum concentration should be obtained and a digital rectal examination of the prostate performed. These tests are generally repeated at 1-year intervals after treatment is started.[50]

Adverse Effects

Testosterone replacement regimens can cause sodium retention, which can cause weight gain, or exacerbate hypertension, congestive heart failure, and edema. Gynecomastia can occur as a result of conversion of testosterone to estrogen in peripheral tissues. This has been reported most often in patients with liver cirrhosis.

Deleterious serum lipoprotein changes have been reported, including decreasing high-density lipoprotein cholesterol levels. However, no cases of cardiovascular disease have been reported with testosterone replacement regimens.

Large doses of parenteral testosterone can produce adverse metabolic effects. Thus, patients on long-term testosterone replacement regimens must undergo clinical laboratory testing for a serum testosterone level, lipid profile, and hematocrit before starting treatment and every 6 to 12 months during treatment.[50] Repeated serum testosterone levels that exceed the normal range require a dosage reduction or increased interval between drug doses. An abnormal lipid profile may require lifestyle and dietary modification and, if necessary, antihyperlipidemic drug therapy. If the hematocrit exceeds 55%, the testosterone replacement regimen should be withheld to avoid polycythemia and its consequences.

Oral alkylated testosterone replacement regimens have caused hepatotoxicity, ranging from mild elevations of hepatic transaminases to serious liver diseases, including peliosis hepatis (hemorrhagic liver cysts), hepatocellular and intrahepatic cholestasis, and benign or malignant tumors. For this reason, parenteral testosterone replacement regimens are preferred.

Topical testosterone patches may cause contact dermatitis, which responds well to topical corticosteroids. This adverse effect has been associated with the presence of permeation enhancers, which are added to patch formulations. If the dermatitis becomes problematic, an alternative is testosterone gel formulations, which are associated with a lower incidence of contact dermatitis compared with patches.

■ ALPROSTADIL

Mechanism

Alprostadil, also known as prostaglandin E_1, stimulates adenyl cyclase, resulting in increased production of cAMP, a secondary messenger that causes smooth muscle relaxation of the arterial blood vessels and sinusoidal tissues in the corpora. This results in enhanced blood flow to, and blood filling of the corpora.

Alprostadil is commercially available as an intracavernosal injection (Caverject and Edex) and as an intraurethral insert (medicated urethral system for erection [MUSE]).

Indications

Both commercially available formulations of alprostadil are FDA approved as monotherapy for management of erectile dysfunction. Alprostadil is more effective by the intracavernosal route than the intraurethral route.

The enhanced efficacy of the intracavernosal injection may be related to the excellent bioavailability of the drug when injected directly into the corpora cavernosum. In contrast, intraurethral alprostadil doses generally are several hundred times larger than intracavernosal doses. This is because intraurethral alprostadil must be absorbed from the urethra, through the corpus spongiosum, and into the corpus cavernosum, where it exerts its full proerectogenic effect.

Although several other agents, including papaverine, phentolamine, and atropine, have been used off-label for intracavernosal therapy, alprostadil is preferentially prescribed. This is because intracavernosal alprostadil has been FDA approved for erectile dysfunction, it does not require extemporaneous compounding, and it has a low potential for causing prolonged erections and priapism.

Both formulations of alprostadil are considered more invasive than VEDs or phosphodiesterase inhibitors. For this reason, intracavernosal alprostadil is generally prescribed after patients do not respond to or cannot use the less invasive interventions. Intracavernosal alprostadil is preferred over intraurethral alprostadil because of its greater effectiveness. Intracavernosal alprostadil may be preferred in patients with diabetes mellitus, who are accustomed to injectable drug therapy and may suffer from peripheral neuropathies, which decrease the patient's perception of pain upon injection. Intraurethral alprostadil is generally reserved as a treatment of last resort for patients who do not respond to other less invasive and more effective forms of therapy and who refuse surgery.

Intracavernosal Alprostadil

Efficacy The overall efficacy of intracavernosal alprostadil is 70% to 90%.[5] Three characteristics of intracavernosal alprostadil are the following:

1. The effectiveness of alprostadil is dose related over the range from 2.5 to 20 mcg. The mean duration of erection is directly related to the dose of alprostadil administered and ranges from 12 to 44 minutes.
2. A higher percentage of patients with psychogenic and neurogenic erectile dysfunction respond to alprostadil at a lower dose compared to patients with vasculogenic erectile dysfunction.
3. Tolerance does not appear to develop with continued use of intracavernosal alprostadil at home.

⑩ Although 70% to 75% of patients respond to intracavernosal alprostadil, a high proportion of patients elect to discontinue its use over time. Depending on the study and the length of observation, 30% to 50% of patients voluntarily discontinue therapy, usually during the first 6 to 12 months. Common reasons for discontinuation include lack of perceived effectiveness; inconvenience of administration; an unnatural, nonspontaneous erection; needle phobia; loss of interest; and cost of therapy.[5,53]

Approximately one third of patients do not respond to usual doses of intracavernosal alprostadil. In these patients, intracavernosal alprostadil has been used successfully along with VEDs. Such combination therapy can be attempted by patients before transitioning to more invasive surgical procedures.[54,55] Alternatively, intracavernosal injections of synergistic combinations of vasoactive agents that act by different mechanisms have been used.[54] Intracavernosal drug combinations typically produce an erection that lasts longer than an erection produced by any one of the agents in the mixture. In addition, because of the low dosage of each agent in the combination, fewer systemic and local fibrotic adverse effects develop compared with high-dose monotherapy. For example, when used in low-dose combination regimens, papaverine is less likely to induce hypotension and liver dysfunction, and phentolamine is less likely to induce tachycardia and hypotension.[55] However, as previously mentioned, such intracavernosal drug combinations are not commercially available and must be extemporaneously compounded.

Pharmacokinetics Intracavernosal injection should be administered into only one corpus cavernosum. From this injection site, the drug will reach the other corpus cavernosum through vascular communications between the two corpora. Alprostadil acts rapidly, with an onset in 5 to 15 minutes. The duration is directly related to the dose. Within the usual dosage range of 2.5 to 20 mcg, the duration of erection is no more than 1 hour. Higher doses are expected to exhibit a longer duration of action. Local enzymes in the corpora cavernosum quickly metabolize alprostadil. Any alprostadil that escapes into the systemic circulation is deactivated on first pass through the lungs.[5] Hence, the plasma half-life of alprostadil is approximately 1 minute, and the potential for systemic adverse effects is negligible. Dose modification is not necessary in patients with renal or hepatic disease.

Dosing The usual dose of intracavernosal alprostadil is 10 to 20 mcg, with a maximum recommended dose of 60 mcg. Doses greater than 60 mcg have not produced any greater improvement in penile erection but may cause prolonged erections lasting more than 1 hour or systemic hypotension.[5] The dose should be administered 5 to 10 minutes before intercourse. The manufacturer recommends that patients be slowly titrated up to the minimally effective dosage. Under a physician's supervision, patients should be started with a 1.25-mcg dose, which can be increased in increments of 1.25 to 2.50 mcg at 30-minute intervals up to the lowest dose that produces a firm erection for 1 hour and does not produce adverse effects. In clinical practice, this process is rarely done because it is time consuming. Thus, many physicians start the patient on 10 mcg and move quickly up the dosage range to identify the best dose for the patient. To avoid adverse effects, patients should receive no more than one injection per day and not more than three injections per week.

Intracavernosal injections should be performed using a 0.5-inch, 27- or 30-gauge needle. A tuberculin syringe or a syringe prefilled with diluent as supplied by the manufacturer should be used to

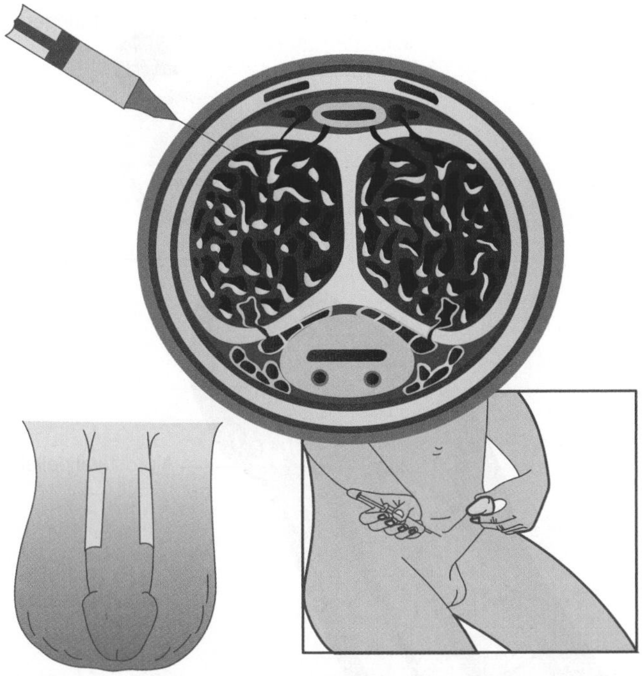

FIGURE 86-5. Technique for administration of intracavernosal injections. *(From package insert for Caverject, Pharmacia & Upjohn company, Kalamazoo, MI. Revised October 2003. Data from http://pfizer.com/pfizer/do/medicines/mn_uspi.jsp. Web site accessed 3/27/2007.)*

ensure precise measurement of doses. Patients with needle phobia, poor vision, or poor manual dexterity can use commercially available autoinjectors (e.g., PenInject) to facilitate administration of intracavernosal alprostadil.

Intracavernosal injections require that the patient or the sexual partner practice good aseptic technique (to avoid infection), have good manual skills and visual ability, and be comfortable with injection techniques. When practicing self-injection, the patient should use one hand to firmly hold the glans penis against his thigh to expose the lateral surface of the shaft. The injection should be made at right angles into one of the lateral surfaces of the proximal third of the penis. The injection should never be made into the dorsal or ventral surface of the penis. This will prevent inadvertent injection of the drug into arteries on the dorsal surface or the urethra on the ventral surface. After the injection, the penis should be massaged to help distribute the drug into the opposite corpus cavernosum. Injection sites should be rotated with each dose. Finally, manual pressure should be applied to the injection site for 5 minutes to reduce the likelihood of hematoma formation (Fig. 86–5).

Once the optimal dosage of intracavernosal alprostadil is established, the patient should return for routine medical followup every 3 to 6 months. Some patients subsequently require dosage adjustment, largely attributed to worsening of the underlying disease that is contributing to the erectile dysfunction.

Adverse Effects Intracavernosal alprostadil is most commonly associated with local adverse effects, which occur most often during the first year of therapy. However, improved administration technique with continued use is believed to account for the lower frequency of adverse effects during subsequent treatment periods.

Intracavernosal injections are associated with several local adverse effects. Cavernosal plaques or areas of fibrosis at injection sites form in approximately 2% to 12% of patients. When they occur, the patient should suspend further injections until the plaques resolve. These plaques may cause penile curvature, similar to Peyronie disease, which makes sexual intercourse difficult or impossible. The cause of corporal fibrosis and plaque formation is unknown. This adverse effect may be caused by poor injection technique[56] or by alprostadil itself. Although patients have developed corporal fibrosis, alprostadil may be less likely to cause this adverse effect compared to other intracavernosal drug combinations, such as phentolamine or papaverine. Unlike cavernosal fibrosis associated with large doses and repeated administration of papaverine, penile scarring secondary to alprostadil appears to be unpredictable.

Alprostadil causes penile pain in approximately 10% to 44% of patients. The pain has been described as a burning discomfort or dull pain near the injection site or during the erection, which generally does not persist after the penis becomes flaccid. The pain usually is mild, generally does not require discontinuation of therapy, and often abates even with continued treatment. However, 2% to 5% of patients discontinue taking alprostadil because of severe pain. The pain can be managed by oral analgesics (e.g., acetaminophen), if necessary. One investigator has recommended adding procaine to intracavernosal alprostadil, but this may mask the signs of more serious adverse effects of the drug or of penile injury during intercourse and is not recommended.[58] The mechanism of this adverse reaction is poorly understood. Alprostadil may intrinsically produce pain. Also, the pain may be a result of the pH of the parenteral solution. Alprostadil is acidic, and the commercially available Caverject formulation is buffered with sodium citrate, a weak base, to reduce pain on injection.[5]

Priapism, a prolonged, painful erection lasting more than 1 hour, occurs in 1% to 15% of treated patients.[5] It occurs most often during the dose titration period and is rare thereafter. Blood sludging in the corpora can lead to tissue hypoxia and cavernosal fibrosis and scarring. The risk for this complication is greatest for erections that persist beyond 4 hours. Patients are advised to seek medical attention immediately when drug-induced erections last more than 1 hour, as this is considered a urologic emergency. Its management includes supportive care, including analgesics for pain and sedatives for anxiety. In addition, needle aspiration of sludged blood in the corpora or intracavernosal injection of α-adrenergic agonists (e.g., phenylephrine) has been used.[5] These procedures facilitate venous drainage of the corpora, allowing venous outflow to "catch up" with arterial inflow.

The likelihood of prolonged erections with intracavernosal alprostadil is dose related. Therefore, to prevent this adverse effect, the lowest effective dose should be used, and the dose should be titrated to ensure that the duration of the erection is no more than 1 hour.

Other local adverse effects include injection site hematomas and bruising. These effects are largely the result of unskillful injection technique. To minimize the risk of injection site hematomas, patients should be advised to apply pressure to the injection site for 5 minutes after each dose. Similarly, infection at the injection site has been reported. Meticulous aseptic technique is recommended to prevent this complication.

Intracavernosal alprostadil rarely causes systemic adverse effects, owing to the agent's localized injection and rapid catabolism. However, large doses greater than 20 mcg are associated with dizziness and hypotension in some patients and is one reason why such large doses are not commonly used.

Intracavernosal injection therapy should be used cautiously by patients at risk for priapism, including patients with sickle cell disease or lymphoproliferative disorders. It should be used cautiously by patients who may develop bleeding complications secondary to injections, including patients with thrombocytopenia or those taking anticoagulants. It also should be used cautiously by patients who use poor-quality injection technique, including patients with psychiatric disorders, obese patients (who may not be able to reach or see the penile injection site), patients who are blind, and patients with severe arthritis.

Intraurethral Alprostadil

Efficacy ⑩ Intraurethral alprostadil inserts are marketed as MUSE, which contains a medication pellet inside a prefilled urethral applicator. Multiple studies show this product has an overall effectiveness rate of 43% to 60%[5] compared with 70% to 90% for intracavernosal alprostadil. Its decreased effectiveness and inconvenient administration method have resulted in this product being considered a third-line treatment option for patients with erectile dysfunction. However, some patients respond to intraurethral alprostadil even though they did not respond to intracavernosal alprostadil.[58]

Intraurethral alprostadil has been combined with an adjustable penile constriction band to improve treatment response.[59]

Pharmacokinetics Following intraurethral instillation, alprostadil is absorbed quickly through the urethra, into the corpus spongiosum, and then into the corpora cavernosum. As much as 90% of each dose is absorbed by the urethra and corpus spongiosum in less than 10 minutes, with peak absorption occurring in 20 to 25 minutes. An estimated 20% of each dose is delivered to the corpora cavernosum. As with intracavernosal injections of alprostadil, any drug absorbed into the systemic circulation is rapidly metabolized on first pass through the lungs.

The onset after intraurethral insertion is similar to that of intracavernosal injection, 5 to 10 minutes.

Dosing The usual dose of intraurethral alprostadil is 125 to 1000 mcg. The dose should be administered 5 to 10 minutes before sexual intercourse. No more than two doses per day are recommended. Before administration, the patient should be advised to empty his bladder, voiding completely.

Similar to intracavernosal injection treatments, intraurethral insertion of alprostadil requires good manual and visual skills to minimize the risk of urethral injuries. Intraurethral alprostadil is supplied in a prefilled intraurethral applicator. The patient should void first. With one hand the patient holds the glans penis, and with the other hand the patient inserts the intraurethral applicator 0.5 inch into the urethra. The drug pellet is then pushed into the urethra. The penis should be massaged to enhance drug dissolution in the urethral fluids and drug absorption (Fig. 86–6).

Adverse Effects The urethra can be injured because of improper administration technique. Injuries can lead to urethral stricture and difficulty voiding. Patients should receive complete education about optimal administration procedures before starting treatment.

Urethral pain has been reported in 24% to 32% of patients. Usually it is mild and does not require discontinuation of treatment. Female sexual partners may experience vaginal burning, itching, or pain, which probably is related to transfer of alprostadil from the man's urethra to the woman's vagina during intercourse. However, the resumption of sexual intercourse also could produce such symptoms.

Prolonged painful erections (priapism) have been rarely reported.[5]

Syncope and dizziness have been reported rarely (only 2% to 3% of patients) and likely are related to use of excessively large doses.

CLINICAL CONTROVERSY

Although combinations of proerectogenic drugs (e.g., sildenafil plus alprostadil intracavernosal injection) may be used by some patients,[13] such combinations are not recommended by the FDA and may lead to prolonged erections and priapism.

■ UNAPPROVED AGENTS

A variety of other commercially available and investigational agents have been used for management of erectile dysfunction. Although it is beyond the scope of this chapter to discuss all of them, some of the more commonly used agents are discussed here.

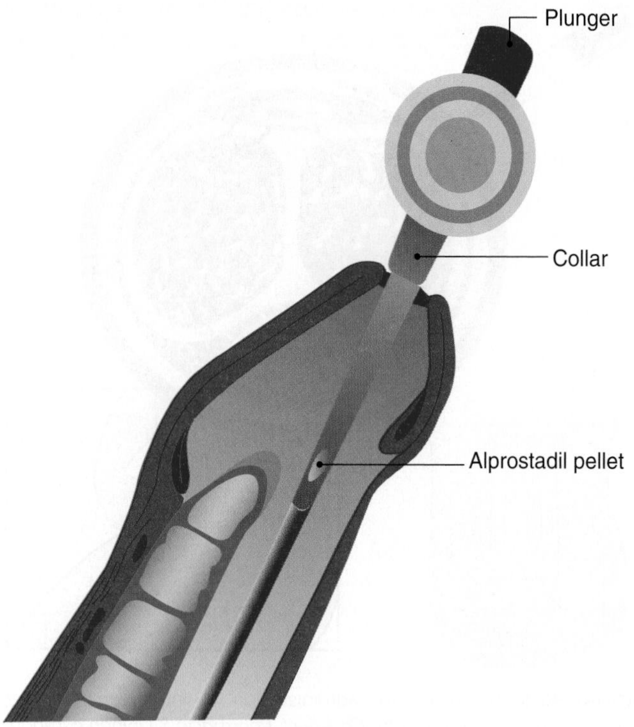

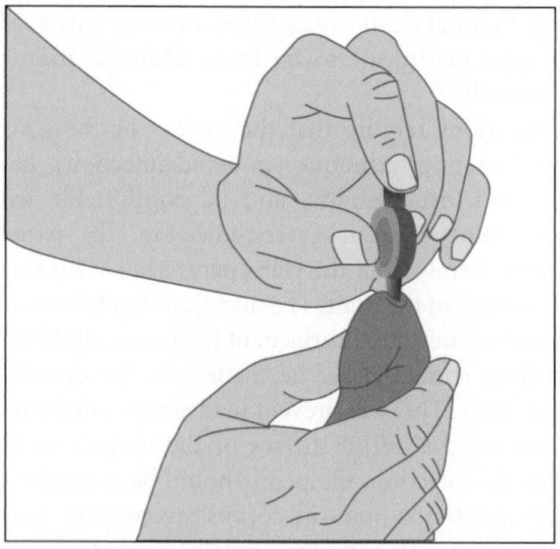

FIGURE 86-6. Technique for administration of intraurethral alprostadil with a medicated urethral system for erection applicator. *(From package insert for Muse, Vivus, Inc., Mountain View, CA. Data from http://www.vivus.com. Web site accessed 3/27/2007.)*

Trazodone

The mechanism by which trazodone produces an erection is not clear. It likely acts peripherally to antagonize α-adrenergic receptors. As a result, a predominant cholinergic effect results, which causes peripheral arteriolar vasodilation and relaxation of cavernosal tissues, enhancing blood filling of the corpora. Intracavernosal injection of trazodone in experimental studies supports this likely mechanism.[60]

Although some clinical trials suggested that trazodone 50 to 200 mg daily by mouth might be effective in the management of erectile dysfunction, these trials were generally poorly controlled, were nonrandomized, included small samples treated for short time periods, and did not include validated objective parameters of response.[60,61]

The adverse effects of trazodone, when used for erectile dysfunction, are similar to those reported with trazodone when used to treat depression and include dry mouth, sedation, and dizziness.

Yohimbine

Yohimbine, a tree-bark derivative also known as *yohimbe*, is widely used as an aphrodisiac. Yohimbine is a central α_2-adrenergic antagonistic that increases catecholamines and improves mood. Some investigators believe that yohimbine has peripheral proerectogenic effects. Yohimbine may reduce peripheral α-adrenergic tone, thereby permitting a predominant cholinergic tone, which could result in a vasodilatory response.[5,62] The usual oral dose is 5.4 mg three times per day.

A controlled clinical trial has shown that high-dose yohimbine (100 mg daily) is no more effective than placebo.[63] Based on a meta-analysis of published studies that came to the same conclusion, the American Urological Association has cautioned against the use of yohimbine.[21] In addition, yohimbine can cause many systemic adverse effects, including anxiety, insomnia, tachycardia, and hypertension. In a 2004 article on "12 supplements you should avoid," *Consumer Reports* called yohimbine "likely hazardous" and reported that deaths and cardiovascular adverse effects had been associated with its use.

Papaverine

Papaverine is a nonspecific phosphodiesterase inhibitor that decreases metabolic catabolism of cAMP in cavernosal tissue. As a result of enhanced tissue levels of cAMP, smooth muscle relaxation occurs. Cavernosal sinusoids fill with blood, and a penile erection results.[5]

Papaverine is not FDA approved for erectile dysfunction. Intracavernosal papaverine alone is not commonly used for management of erectile dysfunction because the large doses required produce dose-related adverse effects, such as priapism, corporal fibrosis, hypotension, and hepatotoxicity.[55,64] Papaverine is more often administered in lower doses combined with phentolamine and/or alprostadil. A variety of formulas have been used, but no one mixture has been proven better than other mixtures (see Table 86–6). Combination formulations are considered safer and are associated with the potential for fewer serious adverse effects than high doses of any one of these agents.

A portion of each papaverine dose is systemically absorbed, and its prolonged plasma half-life of 1 hour contributes to adverse effects. The usual dose of papaverine is 7.5 to 60 mg when used as a single agent for intracavernosal injection. When used in combination, the dose decreases to 0.5 to 20 mg.

If treated with papaverine, patients with a history of underlying liver disease or alcohol abuse should undergo liver function tests at baseline and every 6 to 12 months during continued treatment.

Phentolamine

Phentolamine is a competitive nonselective α-adrenergic blocking agent. It reduces peripheral adrenergic tone and enhances cholinergic tone. As a result, it improves cavernosal filling and is proerectogenic.

Phentolamine has most often been administered as an intracavernosal injection. Monotherapy is avoided because large doses are required for an erection, and at these large doses systemic hypotensive adverse effects would be prevalent. Most often, phentolamine has been used in combination with other vasoactive agents for intracavernosal administration. A ratio of 30 mg papaverine to 0.5 to 1 mg phentolamine is typical, and the usual dose ranges from 0.1 to 1 mL of the mixture. Such a mixture promotes local effects of phentolamine and minimizes systemic hypotensive adverse effects.[5]

Hypotension is the most common adverse effect of intracavernosal phentolamine. It is more common and more severe with large

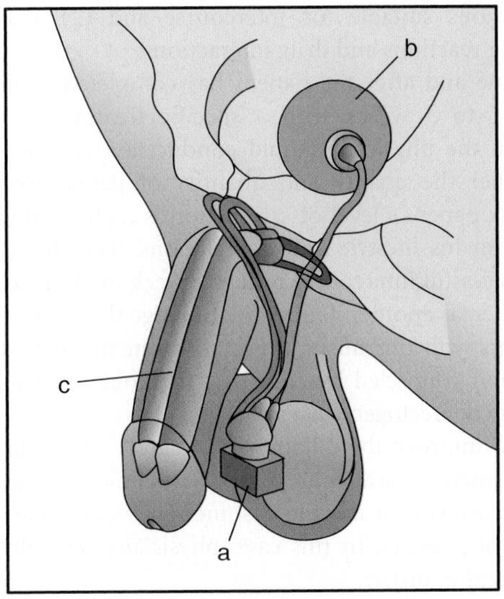

FIGURE 86-7. Example of surgically implanted penile prosthesis. (a, activation mechanism; b, reservoir with fluid for inflating prosthesis; c, inflatable rods in corpora.) *(From http://kidney.niddk.nih.gov/kudiseases/pubs/impotence.)*

doses or in patients with poor injection technique who have injected into a vein (rather than the cavernosa). Prolonged erections have been reported in patients who used excessive doses of combination intracavernosal therapy.

■ PENILE PROSTHESES

Surgical insertion of a penile prosthesis is the most invasive treatment of erectile dysfunction. It is reserved for patients who do not respond to or who are not candidates for less invasive oral or injectable treatments.

Prosthesis insertion requires anesthesia and skilled urologists. Two prostheses are widely used: malleable and inflatable. Malleable prostheses consist of two bendable rods that are inserted into the corpora cavernosa. The patient appears to have a permanent erection after the procedure; the patient is able to bend the penis into position at the time of intercourse.

The inflatable prosthesis has several mechanical parts. The inflatable prosthesis produces a more natural erection. The patient develops an erection only when the device is activated. Some newer advances in inflatable prosthesis technology have resulted in devices with fewer mechanical parts. These devices can be placed during shorter surgical procedures and are less likely to malfunction than are the original inflatable prostheses (Fig. 86–7).

Penile prostheses provide penile rigidity suitable for vaginal intercourse and are associated with a greater than 90% patient satisfaction rate, which is generally higher than that observed with any other drug treatment or VED.[65] The surgical success rate after insertion is 82% to 98%.[5]

Adverse effects of prosthesis insertion can occur early or late after the surgical procedure. The most common early complication is infection. Late complications include mechanical failure of the prosthesis, particularly when an inflatable prosthesis has been inserted. With improved technology, the mechanical failure rate has decreased to 5%.[5] Other late complications include erosion of the rods through the penis or late-onset infection. Although some salvage procedures have been devised, in many cases the prosthesis requires removal.

EVALUATION OF THERAPEUTIC OUTCOMES

The primary therapeutic outcomes of specific treatments for erectile dysfunction include (1) improvement in the quantity and quality of penile erections suitable for intercourse and (2) avoidance of adverse drug reactions and drug interactions.

At baseline and after the patient has completed a clinical trial period of 1 to 3 weeks with a specific treatment for erectile dysfunction, the physician should conduct assessments to determine whether the quality and quantity of penile erections has improved. A patient's level of satisfaction is highly individualized, depending on his lifestyle and expectations. Therefore, a patient who has successful intercourse once per week might be completely satisfied, whereas another patient might judge this to be unsatisfactory. Patients with unrealistic expectations in this regard must be identified and counseled by clinicians to avoid adverse effects of excessive use of erectogenic agents.

Failure to improve the quality and quantity of penile erections suitable for intercourse after an appropriate clinical trial period with a specific treatment for erectile dysfunction occurs in a significant percentage of patients. In this case, physicians generally take the following steps in order:

1. Ensure that the patient has been prescribed a maximum tolerated dose and has an adequate clinical trial of a specific treatment before discarding it as ineffective.
2. Switch to another drug, usually one with a greater potential for adverse effects and complications than the first drug initiated (see Fig. 86–4).
3. Reserve surgical treatment for patients who do not respond to drug treatment.

CONCLUSIONS

Erectile dysfunction is a common disorder of aging men. Its incidence is higher in patients with underlying medical disorders that compromise the vascular, neurologic, hormonal, or psychogenic systems necessary for a normal penile erection. Medications are common causes of erectile dysfunction. By correcting the underlying etiology, erectile dysfunction can often be reversed without the use of specific treatments.

When treatments of erectile dysfunction are needed, the least invasive forms of treatment should be used first because they produce the lowest incidence of serious adverse effects. VEDs or phosphodiesterase inhibitors are considered first-line treatments. If these treatments fail, intracavernosal alprostadil injection therapy can be initiated. If this treatment fails, the patient can attempt a combination of intracavernosal alprostadil plus VED, combination intracavernosal therapy, or intraurethral alprostadil. If this treatment fails, the patient may require insertion of a penile prosthesis.

Some insurance companies do not reimburse for drug treatments for erectile dysfunction, so cost is an important issue for some patients.

Clinicians should provide clear and simple advice. Patient confidentiality and privacy, which are extremely important to men with erectile dysfunction, should be maintained at all times.

ABBREVIATIONS

cAMP: cyclic adenosine monophosphate

cGMP: cyclic guanosine monophosphate

VED: vacuum erection device

REFERENCES

1. NIH Consensus Conference. NIH Consensus Development Panel on Impotence. Impotence. JAMA 1993;270:83–90.
2. Johannes CB, Aranjo AB, Feldman HA, et al. Incidence of erectile dysfunction in men 40–69 years old: Longitudinal results from the Massachusetts Male Aging Study. J Urol 2000;163:460–463.
3. Bacon CG, Mittleman MA, Kawach I, et al. Sexual function in men older than 50 years of age: Results from the Health Professionals Follow-up Study. Ann Intern Med 2003;139:161–168.
4. Bertel ME, Weidner W, Brahler E. Epidemiology of sexual dysfunction in the male population. Andrologia 2006;38:115–121.
5. Lue TF. Erectile dysfunction. N Engl J Med 2000;342:1802–1813.
6. Carrier S. Pharmacology of phosphodiesterase inhibitors. Can J Urol 2003;10(Suppl 1):12–16.
7. Thomas A, Woodard C, Rovner ES, Wein AJ. Urologic complications of nonurologic medications. Urol Clin North Am 2003;30: 123–131.
8. Lee M, Sharifi R. Sexual dysfunction in males. In Tisdale JE, Miller DA, eds. Drug-Induced Diseases: Prevention, Detection, and Management. Bethesda, MD: ASHP, 2005:455–467.
9. Carson CC, Burnett AL, Levine LA, et al. The efficacy of sildenafil citrate (Viagra) in clinical populations: An update. J Urol 2002;60(Suppl 2B): 12–27.
10. Lobo JR, Nehra A. Clinical evaluation of erectile dysfunction in the era of PDE-5 inhibitors. Urol Clin North Am 2005;32:447–455.
11. Rosen RC, Riley A, Wagner G, et al. The International Index of Erectile Function (IIEF): A multidimensional scale for assessment of erectile dysfunction. Urology 1997;49:822–830.
12. Buvat J, Lemaire A. Endocrine screening in 1,022 men with erectile dysfunction: Clinical significance and cost-effective strategy. J Urol 1997;158:1764–1767.
13. McMahon CN, Smith CJ, Shabsigh R. Treating erectile dysfunction when PDE5 inhibitors fail. BMJ 2006;332:589–792.
14. Burnett AL. Erectile dysfunction. J Urol 2006;175:S25–S31.
15. Rosen RC, Jackson G, Kostis JB. Erectile dysfunction and cardiac disease: Recommendations of the Second Princeton Conference. Curr Urol Rep 2006;7:490–496.
16. Rosen RC, Friedman M, Kostis JB. Lifestyle management of erectile dysfunction: The role of cardiovascular and concomitant risk factors. Am J Cardiol 2005;96(Suppl):76M–79M.
17. Kostis JB, Jackson G, Rosen R, et al. Sexual dysfunction and cardiac risk (the Second Princeton Consensus Conference). Am J Cardiol 2005;96:313–321.
18. Bacon CG, Mittleman MA, Kawachi I, et al. A prospective study of risk factors for erectile dysfunction. J Urol 2006;176:217–221.
19. Bacon CG, Mittleman MA, Kawachi I, et al. Sexual function in men older than 50 years of age: Results from the health professionals follow-up study. Ann Intern Med 2003;139:161–168.
20. Masters WH, Johnson VE. Human Sexual Inadequacy. Boston: Little Brown, 1970.
21. Montague DK, Barada JH, Belker AM, et al. Clinical guidelines panel on erectile dysfunction: Summary report on the treatment of organic erectile dysfunction. J Urol 1996;156:2007–2011.
22. Fink HA, Mac Donald R, Rutks IR, et al. Sildenafil for male erectile dysfunction: A systematic review and meta-analysis. Arch Intern Med 2002;162;1349–1360.
23. Curran MP, Keathing GM. Tadalafil. Drugs 2004;63:2203–2212.
24. Keating GM, Scott LJ. Vardenafil. Drugs 2003;63:2673–2703.
25. Gonzalgo ML, Brotzman M, Trock BJ, et al. Clinical efficacy of sildenafil citrate and predictors of long-term response. J Urol 2003; 170:503–506.
26. Carson CC. PDE5 inhibitors: Are there differences? Can J Urol 2006;13(Suppl 1):34–39.
27. McCullough AR, Barada JH, Fawzy A, et al. Achieving treatment optimization with sildenafil citrate (Viagra) in patients with erectile dysfunction. Urology 2002;60(Suppl 2B):28–38.
28. Guay AT. Optimizing response to phosphodiesterase therapy: Impact of risk-factor management. J Androl 2003;24(Suppl):S59–S62.
29. Jackson G. Erectile dysfunction: The right to be treated. Int J Clin Pract 1999;53:323.
30. Brisson TE, Broderick GA, Thiel DD, et al. Vardenafil rescue rates of sildenafil nonresponders: Objective assessment of 327 patients with erectile dysfunction. Urology 2006;68:397–401.
31. Padma-Nathan H, Eardley I, Kloner RA, et al. A 4-year update on the safety of sildenafil citrate (Viagra). Urology 2002;60(Suppl 2B):67–90.

32. Gresser U, Gleiter CH. Erectile dysfunction: Comparison of efficacy and side effects of the PDE-5 inhibitors sildenafil, vardenafil, and tadalafil—Review of the literature. Eur J Med Res 2002;7:435–446.
33. Porst H, Padma-Nathan H, Giuliano F, et al. Efficacy of tadalafil for the treatment of erectile dysfunction at 24 and 36 hours after dosing: A randomized controlled trial. Urology 2003;62:121–126.
34. Ormrod D, Easthope SE, Figgett DP. Vardenafil. Drugs Aging 2002;19:217–227.
35. Young JM. Vardenafil. Expert Opin Invest Drugs 2002;11:1487–1496.
36. Shabsigh R, Seftel AD, Rosen RC, et al. Review of time of onset and duration of clinical efficacy of phosphodiesterase type 5 inhibitors in treatment of erectile dysfunction. *Urology* 2006;68:689–696.
37. Hellstrom WJG, Kendirci M. Type 5 phosphodiesterase inhibitors: Curing erectile dysfunction. Eur Urol 2006;49:942–945.
38. Carson CC. Long-term use of sildenafil. Expert Opin Pharmacother 2003;4:397–405.
39. Marmor MF, Kessler R. Sildenafil (Viagra) and ophthalmology. Surv Ophthalmol 1999;44:153–162.
40. Padma-Nathan H. Sildenafil citrate (Viagra) treatment for erectile dysfunction: An updated profile of response and effectiveness. Int J Impot Res 2006;18:423–431.
41. Laties A, Sharlip I. Ocular safety in patients using sildenafil citrate therapy for erectile dysfunction. J Sex Med 2006;3:12–27.
42. Kloner RA, Hutter AM, Emmick JT. Time course of the interaction between tadalafil and nitrates. J Am Coll Cardiol 2003;42:1855–1860.
43. Tran D, Howles LG. Cardiovascular safety of sildenafil. Drug Saf 2003;26:453–460.
44. Kloner RA. Pharmacology and drug interaction effects of the phosphodiesterase 5 inhibitors: Focus on α blocker interactions. Am J Cardiol 2005;96(Suppl):42M–46M.
45. Kloner RA, Jackson G, Emmick JT, et al. Interaction between the phosphodiesterase 5 inhibitor, tadalafil, and 2 alpha-blockers, doxazosin and tamsulosin in healthy normotensive men. J Urol 2004;172:1935–1940.
46. Giuliano F, Kaplan SA, Cabanis MJ, Astruc B. Hemodynamic interaction study between the $alpha_1$ blocker alfuzosin and the phosphodiesterase-5 inhibitor tadalafil in middle-aged healthy male subjects. Urology 2006;67:1199–1204.
47. Carson CC. Combination of phosphodiesterase-5 inhibitors and α blockers in patients with benign prostatic hyperplasia: Treatments of lower urinary tract symptoms, erectile dysfunction, or both? BJU Int 2006;97(Suppl 2):39–43.
48. Muirhead GJ, Wulff MB, Fielding H, et al. Pharmacokinetic interactions between sildenafil and saquinavir/ritonavir. Br J Clin Pharmacol 2000;59:99–197.
49. Hall MCS, Ahmad S. Interaction with sildenafil and HIV-1 combination therapy. Lancet 1999;353:2071–2072.
50. Gore JL, Swerdloff RS, Rajfer J. Androgen deficiency in the etiology and treatment of erectile dysfunction. Urol Clin North Am 2005;32:457–468.
51. Jordan WP. Allergy and topical irritation associated with transdermal testosterone administration: A comparison of scrotal and nonscrotal transdermal systems. Am J Contact Dermatol 1997;8:108–113.
52. Morales A, Tenover JL. Androgen deficiency in the aging male: When, who, and how to investigate and treat. Urol Clin North Am 2002;29:975–982.
53. Mulhall JP, Jahoda AE, Cairney M, et al. The causes of patient dropout from penile self-injection therapy for impotence. J Urol 1999;162:1291–1294.
54. Israilov S, Niv E, Livine PM, et al. Intracavernosal injections for erectile dysfunction in patients with cardiovascular diseases and failure or contraindications for sildenafil citrate. Int J Impot Res 2002;14:38–43.
55. Leungwattanakij S, Flynn V, Hellstrom WJG. Intracavernosal injection and intraurethral therapy for erectile dysfunction. Urol Clin North Am 2001;28:343–353.
56. The European Alprostadil Study Group. The long-term safety of alprostadil (prostaglandin-E1) in patients with erectile dysfunction. Br J Urol 1998;82:538–543.
57. Engel JD, McVary KT. Transurethral alprostadil as therapy for patients who withdrew from or failed prior intracavernous injection therapy. Urology 1998;51:687–692.
58. Moriel EZ, Rajfer J. Sodium bicarbonate alleviates penile pain induced by intracavernous injections for erectile dysfunction. J Urol 1993;149 (5 part 2):1299–1300.
59. Bodner PR, Haas CA, Krueger B, Seftel AD. Intraurethral alprostadil for treatment of erectile dysfunction in patients with spinal cord injury. Urology 1999;53:199–202.
60. Fink HA, MacDonald R, Rutks IR, Wilt TJ. Trazodone for erectile dysfunction: A systematic review and meta analysis. BJU Int 2003;92:441–446.
61. Vitezic D, Pelcic JM. Erectile dysfunction: Oral pharmacotherapy options. Int J Clin Pharmacol Ther 2002;40:393–403.
62. Morales A. Yohimbine in erectile dysfunction: Would an orphan drug ever be properly assessed. World J Urol 2001;19:251–255.
63. Teloken C, Rhoden EL, Sogari P, et al. Therapeutic effects of high-dose yohimbine hydrochloride on organic erectile dysfunction. J Urol 1998;159:122–124.
64. Brown SL, Haas CA, Koehler M, et al. Hepatotoxicity related to intracavernous pharmacotherapy with papaverine. Urology 1998;52: 844–847.
65. Rajpurkar A, Dhabuwala CB. Comparison of satisfaction rates and erectile function in patients treated with sildenafil, intracavernous prostaglandin E1 and penile implant surgery for erectile dysfunction in urology practice. J Urol 2003;2003;170:159–163.

CHAPTER 87

Management of Benign Prostatic Hyperplasia

MARY LEE

KEY CONCEPTS

1. Although symptomatic benign prostatic hyperplasia (BPH) is rare in men younger than 50 years, it is very common in men 60 years and older as a result of androgen-driven growth in the size of the prostate. Symptoms commonly result from both static and dynamic factors.

2. BPH symptoms may be exacerbated by medications, including antihistamines, phenothiazines, tricyclic antidepressants, and anticholinergic agents. In these cases, discontinuing the causative agent can relieve symptoms.

3. Specific treatments for BPH include watchful waiting, drug therapy, and surgery.

4. For patients with mild disease who are asymptomatic or have mildly bothersome symptoms and no complications of BPH disease, no specific treatment is indicated. These patients can be managed with watchful waiting. Watchful waiting includes behavior modification and return visits to the physician at 12-month intervals for assessment of worsening symptoms or signs of BPH.

5. If symptoms progress to a moderate or severe level, drug therapy or surgery is indicated. Drug therapy with an α_1-adrenergic antagonist is an interim measure that relieves voiding symptoms. In selected patients with prostates of at least 40 g, 5α-reductase inhibitors delay symptom progression and reduce the incidence of BPH-related complications.

6. All α_1-adrenergic antagonists are equally effective in relieving BPH symptoms. Older second-generation α_1-adrenergic antagonists (e.g., terazosin, doxazosin) can cause adverse cardiovascular effects, mainly first-dose syncope, orthostatic hypotension, and dizziness. In patients who cannot tolerate hypotensive effects of the second-generation agents, the third-generation, pharmacologically uroselective agent tamsulosin is a good alternative. An extended-release formulation of alfuzosin, a second-generation functionally uroselective agent, has fewer cardiovascular adverse effects than terazosin or doxazosin; however, whether alfuzosin has the same cardiovascular safety profile as tamsulosin is unclear.

7. 5α-Reductase inhibitors are useful primarily in patients with large prostates greater than 40 g who wish to avoid surgery and cannot tolerate the side effects of α_1-adrenergic antagonists. 5α-Reductase inhibitors have a slow onset of action, taking up to 6 months to exert maximal clinical effects, which is a disadvantage of their use. In addition, decreased libido, erectile dysfunction, and ejaculation disorders are common adverse effects, which may be troublesome problems in sexually active patients.

8. Surgery is indicated for moderate to severe symptoms of BPH in patients who do not respond to or do not tolerate drug therapy, or in patients with complications of BPH. It is the most effective mode of treatment in that it relieves symptoms in the greatest number of men with BPH. However, the two most widely used techniques, transurethral resection of the prostate and open prostatectomy, are associated with the highest rates of complications, including retrograde ejaculation and erectile dysfunction. Therefore, minimally invasive surgical procedures are often desired by patients. These relieve symptoms and are associated with a lower rate of adverse effects and a higher reoperation rate than the gold standard procedures.

9. Although widely used in Europe for treatment of BPH, phytotherapy should be avoided. Studies of these herbal medicines are inconclusive, and the purity of available products is questionable.

Learning objectives, review questions, and other resources can be found at **www.pharmacotherapyonline.com.**

Benign prostatic hyperplasia (BPH) is the most common benign neoplasm of American men. A nearly ubiquitous condition among elderly men, BPH is of major societal concern, given the large number of men affected, the progressive nature of the condition, and the healthcare costs associated with it.

This chapter discusses BPH and its available treatments: watchful waiting, α_1-adrenergic antagonists, 5α-reductase inhibitors, and surgery. The limitations of phytotherapy are described.

EPIDEMIOLOGY

1 According to the results of autopsy studies, approximately 80% of elderly men develop microscopic evidence of BPH. About half of the patients with microscopic changes develop an enlarged prostate gland and as a result have difficulty emptying the contents of the urinary bladder. Approximately half of symptomatic patients eventually require treatment.

The peak incidence of clinical BPH occurs at 63 to 65 years of age. Symptomatic disease is uncommon in men younger than 50 years, but some urinary voiding symptoms are present by the time men turn 60 years of age. The Boston Area Normative Aging Study estimated that the cumulative incidence of clinical BPH was 78% in patients at age 80 years.[1] Similarly, the Baltimore Longitudinal Study of Aging projected that approximately 60% of men at least 60 years old develop clinical BPH.[2]

NORMAL PROSTATE PHYSIOLOGY

Located anterior to the rectum, the prostate is a small heart-shaped, chestnut-sized gland located below the urinary bladder. It surrounds the proximal urethra like a doughnut.

Round, soft, symmetric, and mobile on palpation, a normal prostate gland in an adult man weighs 4 to 20 g. Physical examination of the prostate must be done by digital rectal examination (i.e., the prostate is manually palpated by inserting a finger into the rectum). Thus, the prostate is examined through the rectal mucosa.

The prostate has two major functions: (a) to secrete fluids that make up a portion (20%–40%) of the ejaculate volume; and (b) to provide secretions with possible antibacterial effect related to its high concentration of zinc.[2]

At birth, the prostate is the size of a pea and weighs approximately 1 g. The prostate remains that size until the boy reaches puberty. At that time, the prostate undergoes its first growth spurt, growing to its normal adult size of 15 to 20 g by the time the young man is 25 to 30 years of age. The prostate remains this size until the patient reaches age 40 years, when a second growth spurt begins and continues until the man is 70 to 80 years. During this period, the prostate can quadruple in size or grow even larger.

The prostate gland comprises three types of tissue: epithelial tissue, stromal tissue, and the capsule. Epithelial tissue, also known as *glandular tissue*, produces prostatic secretions. These secretions are delivered into the urethra during ejaculation and contribute to the ultimate ejaculate volume. Androgens stimulate epithelial tissue growth. Stromal tissue, also known as *smooth muscle tissue*, is embedded with α_1-adrenergic receptors. Stimulation of these receptors by norepinephrine causes smooth muscle contraction, which results in an extrinsic compression of the urethra, reduction of the urethral lumen, and decreased urinary bladder emptying. The normal prostate is composed of a higher amount of stromal tissue than epithelial tissue, as reflected by a stromal-to-epithelial tissue ratio of 2:1. This ratio is exaggerated to 5:1 in patients with BPH, which explains why α_1-adrenergic antagonists are quickly effective in symptomatic management and why 5α-reductase inhibitors reduce an enlarged prostate gland by only 25%.[2,3] The capsule, or outer shell of the prostate, is composed of fibrous connective tissue and smooth muscle, which also is embedded with α_1-adrenergic receptors. When stimulated with norepinephrine, the capsule contracts around the urethra (Fig. 87–1).

Testosterone is the principal testicular androgen in males, whereas androstenedione is the principal adrenal androgen. These two hormones are responsible for penile and scrotal enlargement, increased muscle mass, and maintenance of the normal male libido. These androgens are converted by 5α-reductase in target cells to dihydrotestosterone (DHT), an active metabolite. Two types of 5α-reductase exist. Type I enzyme is localized to hair follicles, sebaceous glands in the frontal scalp, liver, and skin. DHT produced at these target tissues causes acne, increased body and facial hair, and male pattern baldness. Type II enzyme is localized to the prostate, genital tissue, and scalp. In the prostate, DHT induces growth and enlargement of the gland.[3]

In prostate cells, DHT has greater affinity for intraprostatic androgen receptors than for testosterone, and DHT forms a more stable complex with the androgen receptor. Thus, DHT is considered a more potent androgen in the prostate than is testosterone. Of note, despite the decrease in testicular androgen production in the aging male, intracellular DHT levels in the prostate remain normal, probably due to increased activity of intraprostatic 5α-reductase.

Estrogen, a product of peripheral metabolism of androgens, is believed to stimulate the growth of the stromal portion of the prostate gland. Estrogens are produced when testosterone and androstenedione are converted by aromatase enzymes in adipose tissues. In addition, estrogens may induce the androgen receptor.[2] As men age, the ratio of serum levels of testosterone to estrogen decreases as a result of a decline in testosterone production by the testes and increased adipose tissue conversion of androgen to estrogen.

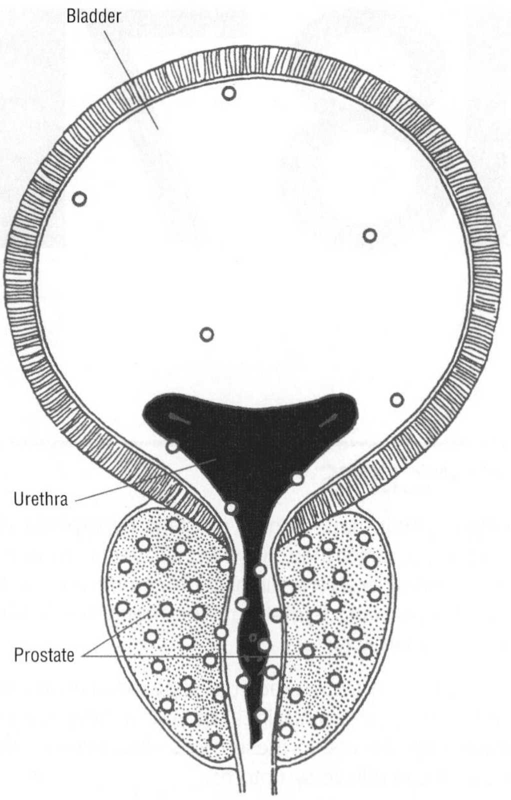

FIGURE 87-1. Representation of the anatomy of and α-adrenergic receptor distribution in the prostate, urethra, and bladder. *(From the Western Journal of Medicine 1994;161:501. Reproduced with permission from the BMJ Publishing Group.)*

PATHOPHYSIOLOGY

Although the precise pathophysiologic mechanisms causing BPH remain unclear, the role of intraprostatic DHT and type II 5α-reductase in the development of BPH is evidenced by several observations:

- BPH does not develop in men who are castrated before puberty.
- Castration causes an enlarged prostate to shrink.
- Patients with type II 5α-reductase enzyme deficiency do not develop BPH.
- Administration of testosterone to orchiectomized dogs of advanced age produces BPH.

The pathogenesis of BPH is often described as resulting from both static and dynamic factors. Static factors relate to anatomic enlargement of the prostate gland, which produces a physical block at the bladder neck and thereby obstructs urinary outflow. Enlargement of the gland depends on androgen stimulation of epithelial tissue and estrogen stimulation of stromal tissue in the prostate. Dynamic factors relate to excessive α-adrenergic tone of the stromal component of the prostate gland, bladder neck, and posterior urethra, which results in contraction of the prostate gland around the urethra and narrowing of the urethral lumen.

Symptoms of BPH disease may result from static and/or dynamic factors, and this must be recognized when drug therapy is considered. For instance, some patients may present with obstructive voiding symptoms but have prostates of normal size. In these patients, dynamic factors likely are responsible for the symptoms. However, in patients with enlarged prostate glands, static and dynamic factors likely are working in concert to produce the observed symptoms.

Static factors may be accentuated by environmental factors. Patients who are stressed or in pain may experience an exacerbation of voiding difficulty. In these situations, increased α-adrenergic tone may precipitate excessive contraction of prostatic stromal tissue. When the stressful event resolves, voiding symptoms often disappear.[2]

MEDICATION-RELATED SYMPTOMS

❷ Medications in several pharmacologic categories should be avoided in patients with BPH because they may exacerbate symptoms. Testosterone replacement regimens, used to treat primary or secondary hypogonadism, deliver additional substrate that can be metabolized to DHT by the prostate. Although no cases of BPH have been reported as a result of exogenous testosterone administration, cautious use is advised in patients with prostatic enlargement. α-Adrenergic agonists, used as oral or intranasal decongestants (e.g., pseudoephedrine, ephedrine, or phenylephrine), can stimulate α-adrenergic receptors in the prostate, resulting in muscle contraction. By decreasing the caliber of the urethral lumen, bladder emptying may be compromised. Drugs with significant anticholinergic adverse effects (e.g., antihistamines, phenothiazines, tricyclic antidepressants, or anticholinergic drugs used as antispasmodics or to treat Parkinson's disease) may decrease contractility of the urinary bladder detrusor muscle. For patients with BPH who have a narrowed urethral lumen, loss of effective detrusor contraction could result in acute urinary retention, particularly in patients with significantly enlarged prostate glands. Diuretics, particularly in large doses, can produce polyuria, which may present as urinary frequency, similar to that experienced by patients with BPH.

CLINICAL PRESENTATION

Patients with BPH can present with a variety of symptoms and signs of disease. All symptoms of BPH can be divided into two categories: obstructive and irritative.

CLINICAL PRESENTATION OF BENIGN PROSTATIC HYPERPLASIA

General

- Patient is in no acute distress unless he has moderate to severe symptoms or complications of BPH

Symptoms

- Urinary frequency, urgency, intermittency, nocturia, decreased force of stream, hesitancy, and straining

Signs

- Digital rectal examination reveals an enlarged prostate (>20 g) with no nodules or area of induration; prostate is soft, symmetric, and mobile

Laboratory Tests

- Increased blood urea nitrogen (BUN) and serum creatinine, elevated prostate-specific antigen (PSA) level

Other Diagnostic Tests

- Increased American Urological Association (AUA) Symptom Score, decreased urinary flow rate (<10 mL/s), and increased postvoid residual (PVR) urine volume

Obstructive symptoms, also known as *prostatism* or *bladder outlet obstruction*, result when dynamic and/or static factors reduce bladder emptying. The force of the urinary stream becomes diminished, urinary flow rate decreases, and bladder emptying is incomplete and takes a long time. Patients report urinary hesitancy and straining and a weak urine stream. Urine dribbles out of the penis, and the urinary bladder always feels full, even after patients have voided. Some patients state that they need to press on their bladder to force out the urine. In severe cases, patients may go into urinary retention when bladder emptying is not possible. In these cases, suprapubic pain can result from bladder overdistension.

Approximately 50% to 80% of patients have irritative voiding symptoms, which typically occur late in the disease course. Irritative voiding symptoms result from long-standing obstruction at the bladder neck. To compensate, the bladder muscle undergoes hypertrophy so that it can generate a greater contractile force to empty urine past the anatomic obstruction at the bladder neck. Although initially helpful, decompensation eventually occurs, and the hypertrophied bladder muscle is no longer able to generate adequate contractile force as it becomes hypersensitive and ineffective in storing urine. As a result, small amounts of urine irritate the bladder and initiate a bladder emptying response. Patients complain of urinary frequency and urgency. Bedwetting or clothes wetting occurs. Patients report waking up every 1 to 2 hours at night to void (nocturia), which significantly reduces quality of life.

Symptoms of BPH vary over time. Symptoms may improve, remain stable, or worsen spontaneously. Thus, BPH is not necessarily a progressive disease; in fact, some patients experience symptom regression. Between one and two thirds of men with mild disease stabilize or improve without treatment over 2.5 to 5 years.[2] However, other patients experience a slow progression of disease.

Collectively, obstructive and irritative voiding symptoms and their impact on a patient's quality of life are referred to as *lower urinary tract symptoms* (LUTS). However, LUTS is not pathognomonic for BPH and may be caused by other diseases, such as neurogenic bladder and urinary tract infection.[4]

Another characteristic of BPH is silent prostatism. Patients have obstructive or irritative voiding symptoms but adapt to them and do not voluntarily complain about them. Such patients do not present for medical treatment until complications of BPH disease arise or a spouse brings in a symptomatic patient for medical care.

BPH can be a progressive disease, although the rate of progression is variable among patients.[2,4] When BPH progresses, it can produce complications that include the following:

- Acute, painful urinary retention, which can lead to acute renal failure
- Persistent gross hematuria when tissue growth exceeds its blood supply
- Overflow urinary incontinence or unstable bladder
- Recurrent urinary tract infection that results from urinary stasis
- Bladder diverticula
- Bladder stones
- Chronic renal failure from long-standing bladder outlet obstruction

Approximately 17% to 20% of patients with symptomatic BPH require treatment because of disease complications.[5] Older men with large prostates greater than 40 g were three times more likely to have severe symptoms or suffer from acute urinary retention and to require prostatectomy than patients with smaller prostates.[6–8] Thus, a serum PSA level of 1.4 ng/mL has been used as a surrogate marker for an enlarged prostate gland to identify patients at risk for developing complications of BPH disease[6] and has been used to guide selection of the most appropriate treatment modality in some patients.[9,10]

DIAGNOSTIC EVALUATION

Because the common obstructive and irritative voiding symptoms associated with BPH are not unique to the disease and can be presenting symptoms of other genitourinary tract disorders, including prostate or bladder cancer, neurogenic bladder, prostatic calculi, or urinary tract infection, the patient presenting with signs and symptoms of BPH must be thoroughly evaluated.

A careful medical history should be taken to ensure that a complete listing of symptoms is collected as well as to identify concomitant disorders that may be contributing to voiding symptoms. The medical history should be followed by a thorough medication history, including all prescription and nonprescription medications and dietary supplements that the patient is taking. Any drugs that could be causing or exacerbating the patient's symptoms should be identified. If possible, the suspected drugs should be discontinued or the dosing regimen modified to ameliorate the voiding symptoms.

The patient should undergo a physical examination, including a digital rectal examination, although the size of the prostate gland does not correspond to symptoms. BPH usually presents as an enlarged, soft, smooth, symmetric gland, greater than 20 g in size. Some patients have only a slightly enlarged gland and yet have bothersome or even serious voiding difficulties, usually the result of dynamic factors. Other patients have an intravesical enlargement of the prostate gland (i.e., the gland grows into the urinary bladder and produces a ball-valve blockage of the bladder neck). This type of prostate enlargement is not palpable on manual examination.

The patient's perception of the severity of BPH symptoms guides selection of a particular treatment modality in a patient. To evaluate perceptions objectively, validated instruments, such as the AUA Symptom Score, are commonly used. Using the AUA index, the patient rates the "bothersomeness" of seven obstructive and irritative voiding symptoms.[2,11] Each item is rated for severity on a scale from 0 to 5, such that 35 is the maximum score and is consistent with the most severe symptoms.

The only clinical laboratory test that must be performed is a urinalysis. Because many of the voiding symptoms of BPH could be caused by other urologic disorders, a urinalysis can help screen for hematuria due to bladder cancer, stones, and infection. Other clinical laboratory tests include BUN and serum creatinine to check for renal impairment as a result of bladder outlet obstruction and PSA to screen for prostate cancer, another common cause of glandular enlargement. The latter test should be performed only in patients with at least a 10-year life expectancy in whom the cost of the test will be outweighed by the potential benefit of diagnosing the disorder.[12]

Additional objective measures of bladder emptying should be performed if surgical treatment is being considered. Measures include peak and average urinary flow rate (normal is at least 10 mL/s). These measures are determined using a uroflowmeter, which checks the rate of urine flow out of the bladder. This is a quick noninvasive outpatient procedure in which the patient is instructed to drink water until his bladder feels full and then the patient's urinary flow is clocked during voiding. A low urinary flow rate (<12 mL/s) implies failure of bladder emptying, but the degree of bladder outlet obstruction correlates poorly with peak urinary flow rate.[12]

Another objective measure is PVR urine volume (normal is 0 mL). This is a simple outpatient procedure and is determined after the patient has attempted to empty his bladder. A straight catheter is inserted to drain any urine remaining in the bladder. A high PVR urine volume (>25–30 mL) implies failure of bladder emptying and a predisposition for urinary tract infections. Because of a weak correlation among voiding symptoms, prostate size, and urinary flow rate, most physicians use a combination of measures, including the patient's assessment of symptoms along with objective evaluation of urinary outflow and presence of complications of BPH to determine the need for treatment.

Many other tests can be performed if additional information is needed to assess the severity of BPH disease and its complications, to assist in the preoperative assessment of the patient, or to distinguish prostate enlargement due to BPH from prostate cancer. Tests include a voiding cystometrogram, transrectal ultrasound of the prostate, intravenous pyelogram, renal ultrasound, and prostate biopsy.

TREATMENT

Benign Prostatic Hyperplasia

As a disease of symptoms, BPH is treated by relieving bothersome symptoms. Patients usually are stratified into three severity groups for the purposes of deciding a treatment modality (Table 87–1). However, literature about the natural history of BPH and the significant risk of disease complications suggests that physicians also should consider prevention of serious complications of BPH and decreasing the need for surgery as goals of treatment in selected patients. This is a controversial topic complicated by many issues, including the variable costs of treatment options, the inability to clearly distinguish patients who experience spontaneous regression or disease stabilization from those in whom symptoms progress, and the potential benefit that may occur in a comparatively small number of treated patients.

The AUA Guidelines on Management of Benign Prostatic Hyperplasia is the principal tool used in the United States,[11] and the AUA recommendations are similar to the European[13] and Canadian Practice Guidelines (Fig. 87–2).[14]

❸ Management options include watchful waiting, drug treatment, and surgical intervention. Although phytotherapy is used by some patients alone or along with conventional medications for BPH, head-to-head comparisons with FDA-approved treatments are lacking, so such herbals cannot be recommended at this time.

❹ Patients with mild disease are asymptomatic or have mildly bothersome symptoms and have no complications of BPH disease. In these patients, no specific treatment is indicated. These patients can be managed with watchful waiting, which entails having the patient return for reassessment at yearly intervals. At each return visit, the patient should complete a standardized, validated survey tool to assess severity of symptoms. Watchful waiting should be accompanied by patient education about the disease and behavior modification to avoid practices that exacerbate voiding symptoms. Behavior modification includes fluid restriction close to bedtime, avoiding caffeine and alcohol intake, frequent emptying of the bladder during waking hours (to avoid overflow incontinence and urgency), and avoiding drugs that could exacerbate voiding symptoms.[15] At each visit, physicians should assess the patient's risk of developing acute

TABLE 87-1 Categories of BPH Disease Severity Based on Symptoms and Signs

Disease Severity	AUA Symptom Score	Typical Symptoms and Signs
Mild	≤7	Asymptomatic Peak urinary flow rate <10 mL/s Postvoid residual urine volume >25–50 mL Increased BUN and serum creatinine
Moderate	8–19	All of the above signs plus obstructive voiding symptoms and irritative voiding symptoms (signs of detrusor instability)
Severe	≥20	All of the above plus one or more complications of BPH

AUA, American Urological Association; BPH, benign prostatic hyperplasia; BUN, blood urea nitrogen.

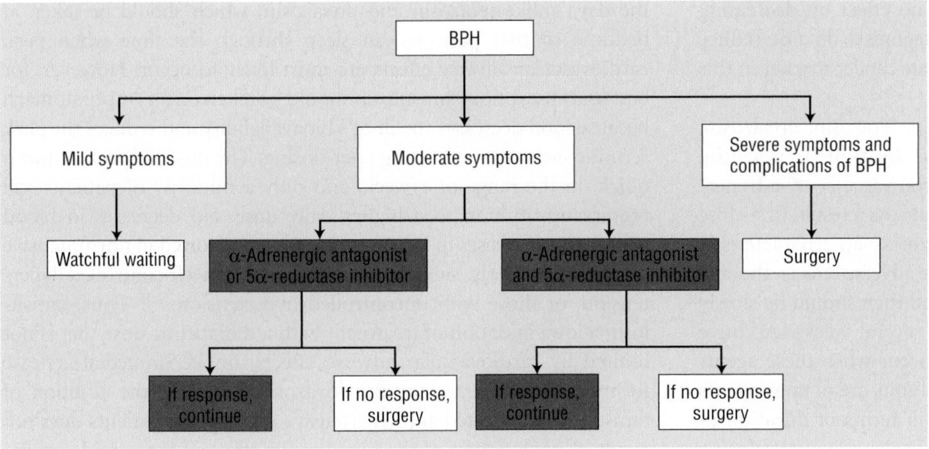

FIGURE 87-2. Management algorithm for benign prostatic hyperplasia (BPH).

urinary retention by evaluating the patient's prostate size or using PSA as a surrogate marker of prostate enlargement.[12]

❺ If symptoms progress to the moderate or severe level or the patient perceives his symptoms to be bothersome, the patient should be offered specific treatment. In these patients, watchful waiting delays—but does not decrease—the need for prostatectomy. In symptomatic patients, watchful waiting can lead to intractable urinary retention, increased PVR urine volumes, and significant voiding symptoms.[16] Recommended treatment options include drug therapy with an α_1-adrenergic antagonist or 5α-reductase inhibitor, a combination of an α_1-adrenergic antagonist and a 5α-reductase inhibitor, or surgery.

❺ Patients with serious complications of BPH should be offered surgical correction (transurethral or open prostatectomy, or a minimally invasive surgical procedure). Drug therapy is considered an interim measure in such patients because it likely only delays worsening of complications and the need for surgical intervention.[11,16]

PHARMACOLOGIC THERAPY

Drug therapy for BPH can be categorized into three types: agents that relax prostatic smooth muscle (reducing the dynamic factor), agents that interfere with testosterone's stimulatory effect on prostate gland enlargement (reducing the static factor), and combination therapy of an α_1-adrenergic antagonist and a 5α-reductase inhibitor (Table 87–2).[17,18] Of the agents that relax prostatic smooth muscle, second- and third-generation α_1-adrenergic antagonists have been most widely used. These agents relax the intrinsic urethral sphincter and prostatic smooth muscle, thereby enhancing urinary outflow from the bladder. α_1-Adrenergic antagonists do not reduce prostate size. Of the agents that interfere with testosterone's stimulatory effect on prostate gland size, the only agents approved by the U.S. Food and Drug Administration (FDA) are 5α-reductase inhibitors (e.g., finasteride, dutasteride). Other agents that interfere with androgen stimulation of the prostate have not been popular in the United States because of the many adverse effects associated with their use. The luteinizing hormone-releasing hormone superagonists leuprolide and goserelin decrease libido and can cause erectile dysfunction, gynecomastia, and hot flashes. Antiandrogens (e.g., bicalutamide, flutamide) produce nausea, diarrhea, and hepatotoxicity.[19]

TABLE 87-2 Summary of Medical Treatment Options for Benign Prostatic Hyperplasia

Category	Mechanism	Drug (Brand Name)
Reduces dynamic factor	Blocks α_1-adrenergic receptors in prostatic stromal tissue	Prazosin (Minipress) Alfuzosin (Uroxatral) Terazosin (Hytrin) Doxazosin (Cardura)
	Blocks α_{1A}-receptors in the prostate	Tamsulosin (Flomax)
Reduces static factor	Blocks 5α-reductase enzyme	Finasteride (Proscar) Dutasteride (Avodart)
	Blocks dihydrotestosterone at its intracellular receptor	Bicalutamide (Casodex) Flutamide (Eulexin)
	Blocks pituitary release of luteinizing hormone	Leuprolide (Lupron) Nafarelin
	Blocks pituitary release of luteinizing hormone and blocks androgen receptor	Megestrol acetate

Selection of a medical treatment for a patient should be determined on a case-by-case basis after patient and provider discussion of risks, benefits, and costs of various treatments. With drug therapy for BPH, patients must understand that the benefits continue only as long as the medication is taken.[11,19]

If possible, drug therapy should be initiated with a single agent, usually an α_1-adrenergic antagonist, which is faster acting and more effective than a 5α-reductase inhibitor. In addition, α_1-adrenergic antagonists are effective in reducing LUTS independent of prostate size, have no effect on PSA, and are associated with less sexual dysfunction than are 5α-reductase inhibitors. A 5α-reductase inhibitor is a good first-choice agent in patients with a significantly enlarged prostate (>40 g) who cannot tolerate the cardiovascular adverse effects of α_1-adrenergic antagonists. In patients at risk for developing complications of BPH, specifically patients with an enlarged prostate gland greater than 40 g[5,11,20] and an elevated PSA ≥1.4 ng/mL, combination drug therapy with an α_1-adrenergic antagonist and a 5α-reductase inhibitor is more beneficial than single drug therapy. The pharmacologic rationale for such a combination is that using two drugs with different mechanisms of action can be more effective than either drug alone. The clinical benefit of combination therapy is that it delays disease progression and reduces the need for surgical intervention.

α-Adrenergic Antagonists

Three generations of α-adrenergic antagonists have been used to treat BPH. They all relax smooth muscle in the prostate and bladder neck. Because of their antagonism of presynaptic α_2-adrenergic receptors that results in tachycardia and arrhythmias, first-generation agents such as phenoxybenzamine have been replaced by the second-generation postsynaptic α_1-adrenergic antagonists and third-generation uroselective postsynaptic α_1-adrenergic antagonists.

❻ The second- and third-generation α_1-adrenergic antagonists are considered equally effective for treatment of BPH.[11,21,22] These agents generally improve AUA Symptom Score by 30% to 40%, increase urinary flow rate by 2 to 3 mL/s in 60% to 70% of treated patients, and reduce PVR urine volume. They have no effect on decreasing prostate volume. Finally, α_1-adrenergic antagonists do not reduce PSA levels, preserving the utility of this prostate cancer marker in this high-risk population.[11]

Second-generation agents include prazosin, terazosin, doxazosin, and alfuzosin. At the usual doses used to treat BPH, prazosin, terazosin, and doxazosin antagonize peripheral vascular α_1-adrenergic receptors in addition to those in the prostate. As a result, first-dose syncope, orthostatic hypotension, and dizziness are characteristic adverse effects. To improve tolerance to these adverse effects, therapy should start with a low dose of 1 mg daily and then should be slowly titrated up to a full therapeutic dose over several weeks. Additive blood pressure lowering effects commonly occur when these agents are used with antihypertensive agents, which limits use of these agents in some patients. These three agents differ in terms of duration of action and dosage formulation. Whereas prazosin requires dosing two to three times per day, terazosin, doxazosin, and alfuzosin offer more convenient once-daily dosing. Because prazosin requires twice- to thrice-daily dosing and has significant cardiovascular adverse effects, it is not recommended in the current AUA guidelines for treatment of BPH.[11] Extended-release dosage formulations are available for doxazosin and alfuzosin. These offer the convenience of once-daily dosing, treatment initiation with a full therapeutic dose, and decreased dose-related hypotension as the formulation produces lower peak serum concentrations than immediate-release products.[6,23,24] An α_1-adrenergic antagonist is not preferred as single-drug therapy for treatment of both BPH and hypertension in a patient. In the Antihypertensive and Lipid-Lowering Treatment to Prevent Heart Attack Trial (ALLHAT) of 24,000 patients with hypertension, doxazosin produced more congestive heart failure than amlodipine, lisinopril, or chlorthalidone.[25] Thus, both the AUA and the Joint National Committee on Prevention, Detection, Evaluation and Treatment of High Blood Pressure[26] recommend that patients with BPH and hypertension be treated with separate and appropriate drug treatment initiated for each medical condition.[27]

Alfuzosin is considered functionally and clinically uroselective in that usual doses used to treat BPH are less likely than other second-generation agents to cause cardiovascular adverse effects in animal or human models.[28] This clinical observation has been seen more often with the once-daily, extended-release formulation of alfuzosin, which is the only commercially available formulation in the United States, compared to the immediate-release formulation that is dosed three times per day, which is available in Europe.[29] It has been postulated to be due to higher concentrations of alfuzosin achieved in the prostate versus serum after usual doses,[30] decreased blood–brain barrier penetration of alfuzosin,[19] absence of high peak serum levels with the extended-release formulation,[31] and fixed dosing schedule of the extended-release formulation. Extended-release alfuzosin dosing is FDA approved for 10 mg daily, with no dose titration increase.[29,32] This is convenient for physician prescribers and patients who are starting to take the medication.

Tamsulosin is the only third-generation α_1-adrenergic antagonist available in the United States. It is an advance over second-generation agents in that it is selective for prostatic α_{1A}-adrenergic receptors, which compose approximately 70% of the adrenergic receptors in the prostate gland.[33] Blockade of these receptors results in smooth muscle relaxation of the prostate and bladder neck without causing peripheral vascular smooth muscle relaxation. Tamsulosin has low affinity for vascular α_{1B}-adrenergic receptors, which explains why hypotension is not a common adverse effect and why the agent has not been studied as a therapy for hypertension.

Tamsulosin's selectivity for α_{1A}-adrenergic receptors has multiple implications. Dose titration is minimal; therefore, patients can begin therapy with the lowest effective maintenance dose of 0.4 mg/day taken orally. Patients can be instructed to take the dose anytime during the day, unlike terazosin and doxazosin, which should be taken at bedtime so that patients can sleep through the time when peak cardiovascular adverse effects are most likely to occur. However, for best oral absorption, tamsulosin should be taken on an empty stomach because food decreases the drug's bioavailability and reduces the peak serum concentration of drug after dosing. The onset of peak action is quick, in the range of 1 week, and only a minority of patients will require up-titration to a higher daily dose. No decreases in blood pressure or increases in heart rate have been reported in normotensive patients, the elderly, subgroups of patients with well-controlled hypertension, or those with uncontrolled hypertension.[34,35] Thus, tamsulosin allows initiation of treatment with a therapeutic dose that is not limited by cardiovascular adverse effects, unlike immediate-release formulations of terazosin and doxazosin.[36] Finally, the addition of tamsulosin to selected antihypertensive regimens of patients does not result in potentiation of the hypotensive effect of furosemide, enalapril, nifedipine, and atenolol.[35,37] Therefore, tamsulosin is a good choice, particularly for patients who cannot tolerate hypotension; have severe coronary artery disease, volume depletion, cardiac arrhythmias, severe orthostasis, or liver failure; are taking multiple antihypertensives; or when the titration would be too complicated for the patient or produce an unacceptable delay in onset for a particular patient.

The usual doses of α_1-adrenergic antagonists are summarized in Table 87–3.

When using the second-generation α_1-adrenergic antagonists terazosin and doxazosin, slow titration up to a therapeutic maintenance dose is necessary to minimize orthostatic hypotension and first-dose syncope. Conservatively, dosages should be increased in an orderly stepwise process, at 2- to 7-day intervals, depending on the patient's response to the medication. A faster titration schedule can be used as long as the patient does not develop orthostatic hypotension or dizziness. Two sample titration schedules for terazosin are as follows:

- **Schedule 1: Slow titration**
  Days 4 to 14: 2 mg at bedtime
  Weeks 2 to 6: 5 mg at bedtime
  Weeks 7 and on: 10 mg at bedtime
- **Schedule 2: Quicker titration**
  Days 1 to 3: 1 mg at bedtime
  Days 4 to 14: 2 mg at bedtime
  Weeks 2 to 3: 5 mg at bedtime
  Weeks 4 and on: 10 mg at bedtime

TABLE 87-3 Dosing Schedule of α_1-Adrenergic Antagonists in Patients with Benign Prostatic Hyperplasia

Drug	Half-Life (h)	Usual Daily Dosage	Time to Peak Effect on BPH Symptoms[a]
Prazosin (Minipress)	2–3	2–10 mg in two to three divided doses	2–6 weeks
Terazosin (Hytrin)	11–14	1–10 mg as a single dose; maximum 20 mg	2–6 weeks
Doxazosin (Cardura)	15–19	1–4 mg as a single dose; maximum 8 mg	2–6 weeks
Doxazosin GTS (Cardura XL)	15–19	4 or 8 mg as a single dose, maximum 8 mg	Several days
Alfuzosin (Uroxatral)		10 mg as a single dose	Several days
Tamsulosin (Flomax)	14–15	0.4 or 0.8 mg as a single dose	Several days

[a]Time to peak effect on benign prostatic hyperplasia (BPH) symptoms is dependent on the titration period to achieve full therapeutic doses.

Patients should continue taking the drug as long as they continue to respond to it. Durable responses for 6 and 10 years have been reported for tamsulosin[38] and doxazosin,[39] respectively. If BPH symptoms worsen despite maximum tolerable drug doses, surgery should be considered.

No dosage adjustments are recommended for α_1-adrenergic antagonists in patients with renal failure. Because these drugs are hepatically catabolized, the lowest effective dose should be used in patients with hepatic dysfunction, and patients should be monitored carefully for adverse effects. No specific dosing guidelines for this patient population are available.

Approximately 10% to 12% of patients discontinue taking second-generation α_1-adrenergic antagonists because of adverse effects, especially those that affect the cardiovascular system (e.g., syncope, dizziness, hypotension).[40] Patients who tolerate hypotension poorly should avoid second-generation α_1-adrenergic antagonists. This includes patients with poorly controlled angina, serious cardiac arrhythmias, patients with reduced circulating volume, and patients taking multiple antihypertensives.[40] These patients are candidates for tamsulosin or finasteride, if drug therapy is deemed necessary. Whether extended-release alfuzosin is a good choice remains to be elucidated in controlled comparison trials with tamsulosin.[27,41]

Tiredness and asthenia, ejaculatory dysfunction, flu-like symptoms, and nasal congestion are the most common dose-related adverse effects of tamsulosin.[42] These adverse effects are extensions of its α-adrenergic antagonist activity and are unavoidable, but with proper education patients likely will not discontinue treatment. Floppy iris syndrome has been associated with tamsulosin use. Tamsulosin blocks α_{1A}-receptors in the iris dilator muscles. As a result, during cataract surgery, papillary constriction occurs and the iris billows out (floppy iris), both of which complicate the procedure. Tamsulosin should be discontinued 1 week before elective cataract surgery.[43–45] Patients with severe sulfa allergy should avoid tamsulosin.

Caution is needed when cimetidine or diltiazem is used with tamsulosin or other α_1-adrenergic antagonists because a drug–drug interaction leads to decreased metabolism of the latter agents. In contrast, carbamazepine and phenytoin may increase hepatic catabolism of α_1-adrenergic antagonists.

Phosphodiesterase inhibitors (e.g., sildenafil, vardenafil, tadalafil) may produce systemic hypotension if used in large doses along with α_1-adrenergic antagonists. The mechanisms for this interaction are related to the intrinsic vasodilatory effects of phosphodiesterase inhibitors and the higher susceptibility of elderly patients to venous pooling because of autonomic incompetence.[27,46] Therefore, package labeling for these drugs includes a warning to avoid α_1-adrenergic antagonists for 4 hours after taking a dose of one of these phosphodiesterase inhibitors. The exception is tadalafil, which can be taken together with tamsulosin 0.4 mg.

CLINICAL CONTROVERSY

Among the α_1-adrenergic antagonists, tamsulosin and extended-release alfuzosin have been associated with the highest and lowest incidences of ejaculatory dysfunction, respectively. Although some clinicians claim that this difference should be considered when selecting one agent over another, this adverse effect is of variable clinical significance. Some patients complain of decreased sexual satisfaction because of ejaculatory dysfunction, whereas other patients do not.

5α-Reductase Inhibitors

❼ Finasteride competitively inhibits type II 5α-reductase, suppresses intraprostatic DHT by 80% to 90%, and decreases serum DHT levels by 70%.[47] Dutasteride is a nonselective inhibitor of type I and II 5α-reductase. It more quickly and completely suppresses intraprostatic DHT production and decreases serum DHT levels by 90%.[48] However, direct comparison clinical trials showed no advantages of these pharmacodynamic actions of dutasteride compared to finasteride.[49] These agents are indicated for management of moderate to severe BPH disease in patients with enlarged prostate glands of at least 40 g.[49] In such patients, 5α-reductase inhibitors may slow disease progression and decrease the risk of disease complications, thereby decreasing the ultimate need for surgical intervention.[50] When taken continuously for 4 years, finasteride has been shown to decrease the risk of acute urinary retention and prostatectomy.[51] In patients with severe disease, these agents generally can be used with a 6-month short course of an α_1-adrenergic antagonist, which will provide fast symptom relief until the 5α-reductase inhibitor starts to work. 5α-Reductase inhibitors may be preferred in patients with BPH and an enlarged prostate gland who have uncontrolled arrhythmias, have poorly controlled angina, are taking multiple antihypertensive agents, or are unable to tolerate hypotensive adverse effects of second-generation α_1-adrenergic antagonists.

5α-Reductase inhibitors reduce prostate size by 25%, increase peak urinary flow rate by 1.6 to 2.0 mL/s, improve voiding symptoms in approximately 30% of treated patients, and produce few serious adverse effects. Compared to α_1-antagonists, 5α-reductase inhibitors have several disadvantages. 5α-Reductase inhibitors have a delayed peak onset of clinical effect, which is undesirable in patients with bothersome symptoms, and an adequate clinical trial is 6 to 12 months. In addition, the percentage of patients who experience objective improvement is less with 5α-reductase inhibitors than with α_1-adrenergic antagonists. 5α-Reductase inhibitors cause more sexual dysfunction than α_1-adrenergic receptor antagonists; therefore, physicians consider 5α-reductase inhibitors to be second-line agents for treatment of BPH (Table 87–4).[11]

Patients with BPH who are concerned about developing prostate cancer can be prescribed finasteride, which has been shown to reduce the 7-year prevalence of prostate cancer by 25% in the Prostate Cancer Prevention Trial.[42,50] However, in this study, finasteride use was associated with a small increased risk of developing a higher-grade prostate cancer, which has a greater potential for invasiveness. The ongoing Reduction by Dutasteride in Prostate Cancer Events (REDUCE) trial[51] should provide additional information on the value of 5α-reductase inhibitors in preventing prostate cancer.[52–54]

TABLE 87-4 Comparison of α_1-Adrenergic Antagonists and 5α-Reductase Inhibitors

	α_1-Adrenergic Antagonists	5α-Reductase Inhibitors
Decreases prostate size	No	Yes
Halts disease progression	No	Yes
Peak onset	1–6 weeks	3–6 months
Efficacy	++	++ (in patients with enlarged prostates)
Frequency of dosing	1–2 times per day, depending on the agent	Once per day
Decreases prostate-specific antigen	No	Yes
Sexual dysfunction adverse effects	+	++
Cardiovascular adverse effects	Yes	No

CLINICAL CONTROVERSY

Dutasteride is a nonselective 5α-reductase inhibitor that more quickly and effectively lowers intraprostatic DHT production and lowers plasma DHT levels than finasteride. Whether these hormonal changes result in clinical advantages over finasteride remains to be elucidated.[49,55]

Finasteride is well absorbed from the gastrointestinal tract (95%), and its absorption is unaffected by food. Peak serum concentrations are reached 1 to 2 hours after the dose. Finasteride is highly protein bound. The liver extensively metabolizes finasteride to inactive metabolites, which are largely excreted in stool. The plasma half-life is 4.7 to 7.1 hours, but its biologic half-life probably is longer, as decreased serum DHT levels persist for up to 2 weeks after finasteride dosing is stopped.[47]

For BPH, finasteride is given in doses of 5 mg by mouth daily. The dose can be taken with meals or on an empty stomach. No dosage adjustment is needed in patients with renal dysfunction. Although no dosage reduction is recommended in patients with hepatic insufficiency, patients should be monitored carefully. Maximal reductions in prostate volume or symptom improvement may not be evident for 12 months, but noticeable changes from baseline should occur after 6 months of continuous treatment. No clinically relevant drug interactions have been reported with 5α-reductase inhibitors.

Patients must continue to take 5α-reductase inhibitors as long as they respond. Durable responses to finasteride and dutasteride have been reported with continued treatment for 6 years[52] and 4 years,[49] respectively. Upon discontinuation of the drug, prostate size and voiding symptoms generally return to baseline.

5α-Reductase inhibitors can produce sexual dysfunction, and this has led to discontinuation of therapy in up to 12% of treated patients in one pooled analysis.[22] Ejaculation disorders (dry sex or delayed ejaculation) have been reported in 3% to 8% of treated patients.[56] These disorders, which are possible results of decreased prostatic secretion, are reversible with drug discontinuation.

Erectile dysfunction has been reported in 3% to 16% of patients.[19,22] It may be secondary to ejaculation disorders or may be due to drug-induced inhibition of nitric oxide synthase (which is needed to produce nitric oxide, a vasodilatory substance) in cavernosal tissue.[57] The role of 5α-reductase inhibitors in causing erectile dysfunction is not clear, as elderly men with BPH commonly develop erectile dysfunction as they age or have concurrent medical illnesses or concomitant drug therapies that may predispose to the development of sexual dysfunction.[56] Decreased libido has been reported in 2% to 10% of treated patients.[19,22]

Other minor adverse effects include nausea, abdominal pain, asthenia, dizziness, flatulence, headache, rash, muscle weakness, and gynecomastia.

5α-Reductase inhibitors are in FDA pregnancy category X, which means that they are contraindicated in pregnant females. Exposure of the male fetus to finasteride may produce pseudohermaphroditic offspring with ambiguous genitalia, similar to those of patients with a rare genetic deficiency of type II 5α-reductase. Because of this teratogenic effect, women who are pregnant or seeking to become pregnant should not handle 5α-reductase inhibitor tablets and should not have contact with semen from men being treated with 5α-reductase inhibitors. Women pharmacists of childbearing age should handle this product with rubber gloves if there is any chance that they are pregnant.

Usual doses of 5α-reductase inhibitors reduce serum PSA levels by 50%. For this reason, PSA levels must be measured before treatment begins, and the patient should have a digital rectal examination. After 6 months of therapy, the patient should have a repeat PSA. If the level does not decline by 50% and the patient has been adherent to the 5α-reductase inhibitor regimen, he should be evaluated for prostate cancer. Annually thereafter, the patient should have a PSA assay and digital rectal examination, and patients with any increase in PSA levels should be evaluated for prostate cancer or noncompliance to the prescribed regimen. To interpret a PSA level in a patient being treated with a 5α-reductase inhibitor, it is generally recommended that the actual measured level be doubled to get an estimate of the true level.[11,58,59]

CLINICAL CONTROVERSY

5α-Reductase inhibitors have been shown to delay disease progression, which is linked to shrinkage of an enlarged prostate gland. This benefit of treatment remains to be demonstrated for α_1-adrenergic antagonists.

Combination Therapy

Combination therapy with an α_1-adrenergic antagonist and a 5α-reductase inhibitor is ideal in patients with severe symptoms, who also have an enlarged prostate gland of at least 40 g and PSA of at least 1.4 ng/mL.[5,11,59] Such patients appear to be at high risk for disease progression, as evidenced by symptom worsening and development of disease complications.[6] A regimen of finasteride and doxazosin for 5 years was shown to prevent symptom progression by 66%, decrease the risk of developing acute urinary retention by 81%, and decrease the need for prostate surgery by 67%.[6] Although not proven by direct comparison trials, any combination of 5α-reductase inhibitor and α_1-adrenergic antagonist probably is similarly effective in patients with the aforementioned characteristics.[11] The disadvantages of a combination regimen include increased medication cost to the patient and an increased incidence of adverse drug effects.

Use of Anticholinergic Agents in Patients with BPH

Treatment with an α_1-adrenergic antagonist, 5α-reductase inhibitor, or surgery may improve urinary flow rate and bladder emptying; however, the patient may still complain of irritative voiding symptoms (e.g., urinary frequency, urgency). Oxybutynin and tolterodine have been used to relieve these symptoms. By blocking muscarinic receptors in the detrusor muscle, these agents can reduce uninhibited detrusor contractions, a sequela of prolonged bladder outlet obstruction from BPH. Thus, they can reduce urinary frequency and urgency. Because elderly patients are sensitive to the central nervous system adverse effects and dry mouth associated with anticholinergic agents, patients should be started on the lowest effective dose and then slowly titrated up.[59–61] Similarly in the presence of BPH, anticholinergic agents can cause acute urinary retention. Therefore, prescribing anticholinergic agents should be done cautiously and patients monitored closely.

■ SURGICAL INTERVENTION

❽ The gold standard for treatment of patients with complications of BPH is prostatectomy performed either transurethrally or suprapubically.[16] Surgical intervention is also used in patients with moderate to severe symptoms, who are not responsive to drug therapy, who are noncompliant with drug therapy, or who prefer surgical intervention. Surgical removal of the prostate offers the highest rate of symptom improvement, but it also has the highest complication rate.

With transurethral resection of the prostate (TURP), an endoscopic resectoscope inserted through the urethra is used to remove the inside core of the prostate. This enlarges the urethral opening at the bladder neck. TURP is performed only in men with enlarged prostates that are less than 50 g so that the resection can be completed in less than 1 hour. Often performed as outpatient surgery, this procedure produces on average a peak urinary flow rate increase of 125% and improvement of voiding symptoms by almost 90% in approximately 90% of patients.[6] A common complication of TURP is retrograde ejaculation, occurring in up to 75% of patients. Significant bleeding, urinary incontinence, and erectile dysfunction occur in smaller but significant numbers of patients (2%–15%).[62,63] Approximately 2% to 10% and 12% to 15% of patients require second surgeries within 5 and 8 years, respectively.[62]

Men with larger prostates (>50 g) require an open surgical procedure (open prostatectomy), which can be performed retropubically or suprapubically. This necessitates hospitalization for at least a few days, anesthesia, and a longer recuperation time. Adverse effects of open prostatectomy include bleeding, urinary and soft-tissue infection, retrograde ejaculation in 77% of patients, erectile dysfunction in 16% to 33% of patients, and urinary incontinence in 2% of patients. The reoperation rate is 3% to 5% at 10 years.[4,11]

Transurethral incision of the prostate (TUIP) is an alternative surgical procedure for patients with moderate to severe voiding symptoms who have an enlarged prostate gland less than 30 g in size. TUIP is as effective as TURP but requires less operation time, causes less blood loss, and produces fewer adverse effects.[11] TUIP involves using an endoscopic resectoscope to make two or three incisions at the bladder neck to widen the opening. Finally, transurethral vaporization of the prostate uses laser energy under direct visualization to ablate prostate tissue.[11]

Minimally invasive surgical procedures are highly desirable by patients. The procedures are short (lasting minutes), have a lower potential to produce adverse effects, are less expensive than continuous drug therapy lasting years, and may be particularly useful in debilitated patients who are poor surgical candidates. The ideal candidates have moderate to severe voiding symptoms with smaller-sized prostate glands.[12] These procedures typically use heat energy from microwaves, water, or laser to destroy prostate tissue.[64] Commonly used procedures include transurethral needle ablation of the prostate and transurethral microwave thermotherapy of the prostate.[4,65] A disadvantage of all minimally invasive surgical procedures is that a higher percentage of patients may develop acute urinary retention in the immediate postoperative period and may require reoperation after an initial improvement in symptoms than patients who undergo TURP or open prostatectomy.[64,65]

■ PHYTOTHERAPY

❾ Although phytotherapy is widely used in Europe for the management of BPH, the published data on herbal agents are largely inconclusive and conflicting. Studies often lack placebo controls, which are essential for assessing treatments of BPH because spontaneous regression of symptoms can occur. Furthermore, because these agents are marketed under the Dietary Supplements Health and Education Act, their efficacy, safety, and quality are not regulated by the FDA. For these reasons, herbal products—including saw palmetto berry (*Serenoa repens*), stinging nettle (*Urtica dioica*), South African stargrass (Hypoxis rooperi), pumpkin seed (*Cucurbita pepo*), and African plum (*Pygeum africanum*)—are not recommended for treatment of BPH.[11,66–70] An excellent review on phytotherapy for BPH has been published.[69]

EVALUATION OF THERAPEUTIC OUTCOMES

The primary therapeutic outcome of BPH therapy is improvement of voiding symptoms with minimal treatment-related adverse effects. As a disease for which therapy is directed at the voiding symptoms that the patient finds most bothersome, assessment of outcomes depends on the patient's perceptions of the effectiveness of therapy. Use of a validated, standardized instrument, such as the AUA Symptom Score, for assessing patient's voiding symptoms is important in this process.[2,11]

In patients being considered for surgical treatment, objective measures of bladder emptying are useful and include the urinary flow rate and PVR urine volume (see Diagnostic Evaluation above).

Because this patient population is at high risk for prostate cancer, PSA should be measured and a digital rectal examination performed annually if the patient has a life expectancy of at least 10 years. For patients taking 5α-reductase inhibitors, a second PSA taken after 6 months of treatment should be compared with baseline measurements. If the patient is suspected to have developed renal impairment as a consequence of long-standing bladder outlet obstruction, then BUN and serum creatinine should be evaluated at regular intervals.

SUMMARY

A ubiquitous disease of aging men, symptomatic BPH requires medical attention to preserve the patient's quality of life and to prevent disease complications, many of which can be life threatening in this patient population. In men who have no or mildly bothersome symptoms, watchful waiting and behavior modification are the best treatment approach, as BPH remains stable or even regresses in approximately half of these men.

For patients with voiding symptoms that are moderate to severely bothersome, pharmacotherapy is indicated. An α_1-adrenergic antagonist is the agent of first choice. Second-generation agents include terazosin, doxazosin, and alfuzosin, and a third-generation agent is tamsulosin. Terazosin and doxazosin cause more cardiovascular adverse effects than do extended-release alfuzosin and tamsulosin. Whether extended-release alfuzosin is as well tolerated as tamsulosin in patients at risk for hypotension or hypotension-related morbidity remains to be elucidated. 5α-Reductase inhibitors are preferred drug treatment in patients with enlarged prostates who poorly tolerate the hypotensive adverse effects of α_1-adrenergic antagonists. However, 5α-reductase inhibitors have a slow onset of action. For patients who do not respond to monotherapy, combination drug therapy could be attempted. Such regimens have been found to be most effective in patients with enlarged prostates greater than 40 g. Alternatively, surgery is an option.

In patients who have complications of BPH, surgery is required. Although it has more adverse complications than does pharmacotherapy or watchful waiting, TURP is considered the gold standard.

ABBREVIATIONS

AUA: American Urological Association

BPH: benign prostatic hyperplasia

BUN: blood urea nitrogen

DHT: dihydrotestosterone

LUTS: lower urinary tract symptoms

PSA: prostate-specific antigen

PVR: postvoid residual

TUIP: transurethral incision of the prostate

TURP: transurethral resection of the prostate

REFERENCES

1. Glynn RJ, Campion EW, Bouchard GR, Silbert JE. The development of benign prostatic hyperplasia among volunteers in the normative aging study. Am J Epidemiol 1985;131:79–90.

2. Roehrborn CG, McConnell JD. Etiology, pathophysiology, epidemiology and natural history of benign prostatic hyperplasia. In: Walsh PC, Retik AB, Vaughan ED Jr, Wein AJ, eds. Campbell's Urology, 8th ed. Philadelphia: WB Saunders, 2002:1297–2002.
3. Steers WD. 5α reductase activity in the prostate. Urology 2001;58(Suppl 1):17–24.
4. Thorpe A, Neal D. Benign prostatic hyperplasia. Lancet 2003;361:1359–1367.
5. McConnell JD, Roehrborn CG, Bautista OM, et al. The long term effect of doxazosin, finasteride, and combination therapy on the clinical progression of benign prostatic hyperplasia. N Engl J Med 2003;349:2387–2398.
6. Trachtenberg J. Treatment of lower urinary tract symptoms suggestive of benign prostatic hyperplasia in relation to the patient's risk profile for progression. BJU Int 2005;95(Suppl 4):6–11.
7. Marberger MJ, Andersen JT, Nickel JC, et al. Prostate volume and serum prostate specific antigen as predictors of acute urinary retention. Combined experience from three large multicenter national placebo-controlled trials. Eur Urol 2000;38:563–568.
8. Marks LS, Roehrborn CG, Andriole GL. Prevention of benign prostatic hyperplasia disease. J Urol 2006;176:1299–1306.
9. Marks LS. Use of 5-α reductase inhibitors to prevent benign prostatic hyperplasia disease. Curr Urol Rep 2006;4:293–303.
10. Crawford ED. Management of lower urinary tract symptoms suggestive of benign prostatic hyperplasia: The central role of the patient risk profile. BJU Int 2005;95(Suppl 4):1–5.
11. American Urological Association Practice Guidelines Committee. AUA guidelines on management of benign prostatic hyperplasia (2003). Chapter 1: Diagnosis and treatment recommendations. J Urol 2003;170:530–547.
12. Burnett AL, Wein AJ. Benign prostatic hyperplasia in primary care: What you need to know. J Urol 2006;175(Suppl):S19–S24.
13. Chatelain C, Denis L, Foo JK, et al. Evaluation and treatment of lower urinary tract symptoms (LUTS) in older men. Benign prostatic hyperplasia. 5th International Consultation on Benign Prostatic Hyperplasia, June 25–28, 2000 Paris. Plymouth: Plymbridge Distributors, 2001;519–534.
14. Nickel JC, Herschorn S, Corcos J, et al. Canadian guidelines for the management of benign prostatic hyperplasia. Can J Urol 2005;12:2677–2683.
15. Ranjan P, Dalela D, Sankhwar S. Diet and benign prostatic hyperplasia: Implications for prevention. Urology 2006;68:470–476.
16. Wasson JH, Reda DJ, Bruskewitz RC, et al.; for the Veterans Affairs Cooperative Study Group on Transurethral Resection of the Prostate. A comparison of transurethral surgery with watchful waiting for moderate symptoms of benign prostatic hyperplasia. N Engl J Med 1995;332:75–79.
17. Beckman TJ, Mynderse LA. Evaluation and medical management of benign prostatic hyperplasia. Mayo Clin Proc 2005;80:1356–1362.
18. Chapple CR. Pharmacological therapy of benign prostatic hyperplasia/lower urinary tract symptoms: An overview for the practicing clinician. BJU Int 2004;94:738–744.
19. Dutkiewics S. Efficacy and tolerability of drugs for treatment of benign prostatic hyperplasia. Int Urol Nephrol 2001;32:423–432.
20. Kirby RS, Roehrborn C, Boyle P, et al. Efficacy and tolerability of doxazosin and finasteride alone or in combination in treatment of symptomatic benign prostatic hyperplasia—The Prospective European Doxazosin Combination Therapy (PREDICT) Trial. Urology 2003;61:119–126.
21. Milani S, Djavan B. Lower urinary tract symptoms suggestive of benign prostatic hyperplasia: Latest update on α_1 adrenoceptor antagonists. BJU Int 2005;95(Suppl 4):29–36.
22. Lowe F. Treatment of lower urinary tract symptoms suggestive of benign prostatic hyperplasia: Sexual function. BJU Int 2005;95(Suppl 4):12–18.
23. Hernandez C, Duran R, Jara J, et al. Controlled release doxazosin in the treatment of benign prostatic hyperplasia. Prostate Cancer Prostatic Dis 2005;8:375–380.
24. Goldsmith DR, Plosker GL. Doxazosin gastrointestinal therapeutic system. Drugs 2006;65:2037–2047.
25. Major cardiovascular events in hypertensive patients randomized to doxazosin vs chlorthalidone: The Antihypertensive and Lipid-Lowering Treatment to Prevent Heart Attack Trial (ALLHAT). ALLHAT Collaborative Research Group [erratum appear in JAMA 2002;288:2976]. JAMA 2000;283:1967–1975.
26. White WB, Moon T. Treatment of benign prostatic hyperplasia in hypertensive men. J Clin Hypertens 2005;7:212–217.
27. Kaplan SA, Neutel J. Vasodilatory factors in treatment of older men with symptomatic benign prostatic hyperplasia. Urology 2006;67:225–231.
28. MacDonald R, Wilt TJ. Alfuzosin for treatment of lower urinary tract symptoms compatible with benign prostatic hyperplasia: A systematic review of efficacy and adverse effects. Urology 2005;66:780–788.
29. Elhilali MM. Alfuzosin: An α_1 receptor blocker for the treatment of lower urinary tract symptoms associated with benign prostatic hyperplasia. Expert Opin Pharmacother 2006;7:583–596.
30. Mottet N, Bressolle F, Delmas V, et al. Prostatic tissue distribution of alfuzosin in patients with benign prostatic hyperplasia following repeated oral administration. Eur Urol 2003;44:101–105.
31. Roehrborn CG for the ALFUS Study Group. Efficacy and safety of once daily alfuzosin in the treatment of lower urinary tract symptoms and clinical benign prostatic hyperplasia: A randomized, placebo-controlled trial. Urology 2001;58:953–959.
32. Roehrborn CG. Are all α-blockers created equal? An update. Urology 2002;59(Suppl 2A):3–6.
33. Chapple CR. Pharmacotherapy for benign prostatic hyperplasia—The potential for α1-adrenoceptor subtype-specific blockade. Br J Urol 1998;81(Suppl):34–47.
34. Chapple CR, Baert L, Thind P, et al. Tamsulosin 0.4 mg once daily: Tolerability in older and young patients with lower urinary tract symptoms suggestive of benign prostatic obstruction. The Europ Tamsulosin Study Group. Eur Urol 1997;32:462–470.
35. Lowe FC. Coadministration of tamsulosin and three antihypertensive agents in patients with benign prostatic hyperplasia: Pharmacodynamic effect. Clin Ther 1997;19:730–742.
36. Djavan B, Chapple C, Milani S. State of the art on the efficacy and tolerability of alpha$_1$ adrenoceptor antagonists in patients with lower urinary tract symptoms suggestive of benign prostatic obstruction. Urology 2004;64:1081–1088.
37. DeMey C. Cardiovascular effects of alpha blockers used for the treatment of symptomatic BPH. Impact on safety and well being. Eur Urol 2998;34(Suppl 2):18–28.
38. Narayan P, Evans CP, Moon T. Long-term safety and efficacy of tamsulosin for the treatment of lower urinary tract symptoms associated with benign prostatic hyperplasia. J Urol 2003;170:498–502.
39. Dutkiewicz S. Long term treatment with doxazosin in men with benign prostatic hyperplasia: 10 year follow up. Int Urol Nephrol 2004;36:169–173.
40. Kaplan SA, D'Alisera PM. Tolerability of α-blockade with doxazosin as a therapeutic option for symptomatic benign prostatic hyperplasia in the elderly: A pooled analysis of seven double-blind, placebo-controlled studies. Gerontology 1998;53A:M201–M206.
41. Barendrecht MM, Koopman RP, De La Rosette JJ, Michel MC. Treatment of lower urinary tract symptoms suggestive of benign prostatic hyperplasia: The cardiovascular system. BJU Int 2005;95(Suppl 4):19–28.
42. Hellstrom WJG, Sikka SC. Effects of acute treatment with tamsulosin versus alfuzosin on ejaculatory function in normal volunteers. J Urol 2006;176:1529–1533.
43. Chang DF, Campbell JR. Intraoperative floppy iris syndrome associated with tamsulosin. J Cataract Refract Surg 2005;31:664–673.
44. Lawrentschuk N, Bylsma GW. Intraoperative floppy iris syndrome and its relationship to tamsulosin: A urologist's guide. BJU Int 2006;97:2–4.
45. Schwinn DA, Afshari NA. α_1 Adrenergic receptor antagonists and the iris: New mechanistic insights into floppy iris syndrome. Surv Ophthalmol 2006;51:501–512.
46. Nieminen T, Tammela TLJ, Koobi T, Kahonen M. The effects of tamsulosin and sildenafil in separate and combined regimens on detailed hemodynamics in patients with benign prostatic hyperplasia. J Urol 2006;175:2551–2556.
47. Roehrborn CG, Boyle P, Nickel JC, Hoefner K, Andriole G, ARIA3001 ARIA3002 and ARIA3003 Study Investigators. Efficacy and safety of a dual inhibitor of types 1 and 2 (dutasteride) in men with benign prostatic hyperplasia. Urology 2002;60:434–441.

48. Anonymous. Dutasteride (Avodart) for benign prostatic hyperplasia. Med Lett Drugs Ther 2002;44:109–110.
49. Andriole GL, Kirby R. Safety and tolerability of the dual 5α-reductase inhibitor dutasteride in the treatment of benign prostatic hyperplasia. Eur Urol 2003;44:82–88.
50. Thompson IM, Goodman PJ, Tangen CN, et al. The influence of finasteride on the development of prostate cancer. N Engl J Med 2003;349:215–224.
51. Andriole GL, Roehrborn CG, Schulman C, et al. Effect of dutasteride on the detection of prostate cancer in men with benign prostatic hyperplasia. Urology 2004;64:537–541.
52. Roehrborn CG, Bruskewitz R, Nickel JC, et al. Sustained decrease in incidence of acute urinary retention and surgery with finasteride for 6 years in men with benign prostatic hyperplasia. J Urol 2004;171:1194–1198.
53. Thompson IM. New sights and developments from the Prostate Cancer Prevention Trial: The promise of SELECT. *http://webcasts.prous.com/aua2005*.
54. Andriole GL, Roehrborn CG, Schulman C, et al. Effect of dutasteride on the detection of prostate cancer in men with benign prostatic hyperplasia. Urology 2004;64:537–543.
55. Edwards JE, Moore RA. Finasteride in the treatment of clinical benign prostatic hyperplasia: A systematic review of randomized trials. BMC Urol 2002;2:14.
56. Rosen R, O'Leary M, Altwein J, et al. Ejaculatory disorders are frequent and bothersome in aging males with LUTS. A worldwide survey (MSAM-7) [abstract]. J Urol 2003;169(Suppl 1):365.
57. Park KH, Kim SW, Kim KD, et al. Effects of androgens on the expression of nitric oxide synthase mRNA in rat corpus cavernosum. BJU Int 1999;83:327–333.
58. Andriole GL, Marberger M, Roehrborn CG. Clinical usefulness of serum prostate specific antigen for the detection of prostate cancer is preserved in men receiving the dual 5α reductase inhibitor dutasteride. J Urol 2006;175:1657–1662.
59. Patel A, Chapple CR. Benign prostatic hyperplasia: Treatment in primary care. BMJ 2006;333:535–539.
60. Dmochowski R. Antimuscarinic therapy in men with lower urinary tract symptoms: What is the evidence. Curr Urol Rep 2006;7:462–467.
61. Ruggieri MR Sr, Braverman AS, Pontari MA. Combined use of alpha-adrenergic and muscarinic antagonists for the treatment of voiding dysfunction. J Urol 2005;174:1743–1748.
62. Rassweiler J, Teber D, Kuntz R, Hofmann R. Complications of transurethral resection of the prostate (TURP): Incidence, management, and prevention. Eur Urol 2006;50:969–980.
63. Kassabian VS. Sexual function in patients treated for benign prostatic hyperplasia. Lancet 2003;361:60–62.
64. Larson TR. Rationale and assessment of minimally invasive approaches to benign prostatic hyperplasia therapy. Urology 2002;59(Suppl 2A):2–16.
65. Tanuguntla HS, Evans CP. Minimally invasive therapies for benign prostatic hyperplasia. World J Urol 2002;20:197–206.
66. Debruyne F, Koch G, Boyle P, et al. Comparison of phytotherapeutic agent (Permixon) with an α-blocker (tamsulosin) in the treatment of benign prostatic hyperplasia: A 1-year randomized international study. Eur Urol 2002;41:497–507.
67. Gerber GS, Kuznetsov D, Johnson BC, et al. Randomized double blind controlled trial of saw palmetto in men with lower urinary tract symptoms. Urology 2001;58:960–964.
68. Avins AL, Bent S. Saw palmetto and lower urinary tract symptoms: What is the latest evidence. Curr Urol Rep 2006;7:260–265.
69. Bent S, Kane C, Shinohara K, et al. Saw palmetto for benign prostatic hyperplasia. N Engl J Med 2006;354:557–566.
70. Chapple C, Artibani W, Berges R, et al. New medical developments in the treatment of LUTS in adult men (World Health Organization report, committee 6). In: McConnell J, Abrams P, Dens L, Khoury S, Roehrborn C, eds. Male lower urinary tract dysfunction. Jersey, United Kingdom: Health Publications, 2006:143–194.

CHAPTER 88 Urinary Incontinence

ERIC S. ROVNER, JEAN WYMAN, THOMAS LACKNER, AND DAVID GUAY

KEY CONCEPTS

1. In evaluating urinary incontinence, drug-induced or drug-aggravated etiologies must be ruled out.
2. Accurate diagnosis and classification of urinary incontinence type are critical to the selection of appropriate pharmacotherapy.
3. Nonpharmacologic, nonsurgical therapy is the cornerstone of management of several types of urinary incontinence, often should be the first therapy initiated, and should be continued even when drug therapy is initiated.
4. Anticholinergic/antispasmodic agents are the pharmacologic therapies of choice for bladder overactivity (urge incontinence).
5. Duloxetine (not yet approved for treatment of urinary incontinence in the United States), α-adrenergic receptor agonists, and topical (vaginal) estrogens (alone or together) are the pharmacologic therapies of choice in urethral underactivity (stress incontinence).
6. Patient-specific treatment goals should be identified. They are not static and may change over time. Choice of therapy may be influenced by characteristics such as patient age, comorbidities, concurrent medications, and ability to adhere to the prescribed regimen. If therapeutic goals are not achieved with a given agent at optimal dosage, addition of a second agent or switching to an alternative single agent should be considered.

Urinary incontinence (UI) is defined as involuntary leakage of urine.[1] It is frequently accompanied by other bothersome lower urinary tract symptoms, such as urgency, increased daytime frequency, and nocturia. It is a common yet underdetected and underreported health problem that can significantly affect quality of life. Patients with UI may have depression as a result of the perceived lack of self-control, loss of independence, and lack of self-esteem, and they often curtail their activities for fear of an "accident." UI also may have serious medical and economic ramifications for untreated or undertreated patients, including perineal dermatitis, worsening of pressure ulcers, urinary tract infections, and falls.

This chapter highlights the epidemiology, etiology, pathophysiology, and treatment of stress, urge, mixed, and overflow UI in men and women.

Learning objectives, review questions, and other resources can be found at **www.pharmacotherapyonline.com.**

EPIDEMIOLOGY

Determining the true prevalence of UI is difficult because of problems with definition, reporting bias, and other methodologic issues.[2] Epidemiologic studies have not historically used a standard definition of the condition or a standard methodology for data recording, with some studies including "postvoid dribbling," while other studies specify "urinary leakage causing a social or hygienic problem." Many people suffer from UI, and the impact of this condition is substantial, crossing all racial, ethnic, and geographic boundaries. Compared with continent controls, patients with UI have an overall poorer quality of life.[3] Several studies have objectively shown that UI is associated with reduced levels of social and personal activities, increased psychological distress, and overall decreased quality of life as measured by numerous indices.[4,5] The condition can affect people of all age groups, but the peak incidence of UI, at least in women, appears to occur around the age of menopause, with a slight decrease in the age group 55 to 60 years, and then a steadily increasing prevalence after age 65 years.

One of the earliest comprehensive epidemiologic studies on UI was conducted by Diokno et al.[6] using a standardized survey questionnaire. The Medical, Epidemiologic, and Social Aspects of Aging survey found that the prevalence of UI in noninstitutionalized women 60 years of age and older was approximately 38%. Almost one third of those surveyed noted urine loss at least once weekly and 16% noted UI daily. A publication from a National Institutes of Health working group conference estimated the median level of UI prevalence to be approximately 20% to 30% during young adult life, with a broad peak around middle age (30%–40% prevalence) and an increase in the elderly (30%–50% prevalence).[7]

In the United States, chronic UI is one of the most common reasons cited for institutionalization of the elderly, and the condition is frequently encountered in the nursing home setting.[8] Little is known about the basic differences in clinical and epidemiologic characteristics of incontinence across racial or ethnic groups. Some studies report a higher incidence of UI overall in white populations[9,10] as compared with African Americans, but differences in access to healthcare as well as cultural attitudes and mores may contribute to these differences.

Consistent across all studies of unselected, noninstitutionalized populations is that UI is at least half as common in men as in women.[11,12] Overall, the prevalence of UI in men has been estimated to be approximately 9%.[13] Unlike in women, the prevalence of UI in men increases with age across most studies, with the highest prevalence recorded in the oldest patient cohorts.[13]

ETIOLOGY AND PATHOPHYSIOLOGY

ANATOMY

The lower urinary tract consists of the bladder, urethra, urinary or urethral sphincter, and surrounding musculofascial structures, including connective tissue, nerves, and blood vessels. The urinary bladder is a hollow organ composed of smooth muscle and connective tissue located deep in the bony pelvis in men and women. The urethra is a hollow tube that acts as a conduit for urine flow out of the bladder. The interior surface of both the bladder and urethra is lined by an epithelial cell layer termed the *transitional epithelium,* which is in constant contact with urine. Previously considered inert and inactive, transitional epithelium may play an active role in the pathophysiology of many lower urinary tract disorders, including interstitial cystitis and UI. The urinary or urethral sphincter is a combination of smooth and striated muscle within and surrounding the most proximal portion of the urethra adjacent to the bladder in both men and women. This is a functional but not anatomic sphincter that includes a portion of the bladder neck or outlet as well as the proximal urethra.

URINARY CONTINENCE

To prevent incontinence during the bladder filling and storage phase of the micturition cycle, the urethra, or more accurately the urethral sphincter, must maintain adequate closure in order to resist the flow of urine from the bladder at all times until voluntary voiding is initiated. Urethral closure or resistance to flow is maintained to a large degree by the proximal (under involuntary control) and distal (under both voluntary and involuntary control) urinary sphincters, a combination of smooth and striated muscles within and external to the urethra. Variable contributions to urethral closure may also come from the urethral mucosa, submucosal spongy tissue, and the overall length of the urethra. During bladder filling and storage, the bladder accommodates increasing volumes of urine flowing in from the upper urinary tract without a significant increase in bladder (intravesical) pressure. The maintenance of a low intravesical pressure despite increasing volumes of urine is a unique property of the bladder and is termed *compliance.* In addition, bladder or detrusor smooth muscle activity normally is suppressed during the filling phase by centrally mediated neural reflexes. Normal bladder emptying occurs with opening of the urethra concomitant with a volitional bladder contraction. Bladder contraction occurs in a coordinated fashion, resulting in a rise in intravesical pressure. The rise in intravesical pressure is ideally of adequate magnitude and duration to empty the bladder to completion. Opening and funneling of the bladder outlet results in urine flow into the urethra until the bladder is emptied to near completion.

The primary motor input to the detrusor muscle of the bladder is along the pelvic nerves emanating from spinal cord segments S2 to S4. Parasympathetic impulses travel to the bladder along the efferent fibers of the pelvic nerves. The impulses pass through ganglia situated in the bladder wall before reaching their target. Acetylcholine appears to be the primary neurotransmitter at the neuromuscular junction in the human lower urinary tract. Both volitional and involuntary contractions of the detrusor muscle are mediated by activation of postsynaptic muscarinic receptors by acetylcholine. Of the five known subtypes of muscarinic receptors, the majority of bladder smooth muscle cholinergic receptors are of the M_2 variety. In humans, the ratio of M_2/M_3 receptor numbers is approximately 3:1. However, M_3 receptors are the subtype responsible for both emptying contraction of normal micturition as well as involuntary bladder contractions that may result in UI.[14] Thus, most pharmacologic antimuscarinic therapy is primarily anti-M_3 based.

This description of the mechanisms of urinary continence is a bit simplistic. Many other neurohumoral pathways and mechanisms, both within and outside the urinary tract, may play substantial roles in urinary continence (and voiding dysfunction) and may be future therapeutic options for treatment of voiding dysfunction and UI. Examples include adrenergic, purinergic, serotoninergic, and dopaminergic pathways, tachykinin receptor antagonists, and calcium and potassium channel modulators.[14]

The bladder and urethra normally operate in unison during the bladder filling and storage phase, as well as the bladder emptying phase of the micturition cycle. The smooth and striated muscles of the bladder and urethra are organized during the micturition cycle by a number of reflexes coordinated at the pontine micturition center in the midbrain. Disturbances in the neural regulation of micturition at any level (brain, spinal cord, or pelvic nerves) often lead to characteristic changes in lower urinary tract function that may result in UI.

Mechanisms of Urinary Incontinence

Simply stated, UI may occur only as a result of abnormalities of the urethra (including the bladder outlet and urinary sphincter), the bladder, or a combination of both.[15] Abnormalities may result in either overfunction or underfunction of the bladder and/or urethra, with resulting development of UI. Although this simple classification scheme excludes extremely rare causes of UI such as congenital ectopic ureters and urinary fistulas, it is useful for gaining a working understanding of the condition.

Urethral Underactivity (Stress Urinary Incontinence) Some patients characteristically note UI during exertional activities such as exercise, running, lifting, coughing, and sneezing. This implies that the compromised urethral sphincter is no longer able to resist the flow of urine from the bladder during periods of physical activity. In essence, increases in intraabdominal pressure during physical activity are transmitted to the bladder (an intraabdominal organ), compressing it and forcing urine through the weakened sphincter.

This type of UI is known as *stress urinary incontinence* (SUI). Although the exact etiology of urethral underactivity and SUI in women is incompletely understood, clearly identifiable risk factors include pregnancy, childbirth, menopause, cognitive impairment, obesity, and age.[16,17] The prevalence of SUI in women appears to peak during or after the onset of menopause. This implies that hormonal factors are important in maintaining continence.

In men, SUI is most commonly the result of prior lower urinary tract surgery or injury, with resulting compromise of the sphincter mechanism within and external to the urethra. Radical prostatectomy for treatment of adenocarcinoma of the prostate probably is the most common setting in which surgical manipulation leads to UI. Overall, SUI in the male is uncommon and, in the absence of prior prostate surgery, severe trauma, or neurologic illness, is extraordinarily rare. Transurethral resection of the prostate for benign prostatic hyperplasia (BPH; see Chap. 87) may lead to SUI in men.

Bladder Overactivity (Urge Urinary Incontinence) Bladder overactivity, including bladder filling and urinary storage characterized by involuntary bladder contractions, is termed *urge urinary incontinence* (UUI). Symptoms of bladder overactivity occur because the detrusor muscle is overactive and contracts inappropriately during the filling phase. The terms *overactive bladder* and *detrusor overactivity* are distinct and should not be used interchangeably, as they frequently are in the medical lexicon. The International Continence Society defines *overactive bladder* as a symptom syndrome characterized by urinary urgency, with frequency and nocturia, with or without associated UI in the absence of a known pathologic condition that may result in similar symptoms (e.g., urinary tract infection or bladder cancer).[1]

Therefore, a diagnosis of overactive bladder does not require urodynamic testing for confirmation but is a diagnosis based on patient symptoms. Conversely, detrusor overactivity is a specific urodynamic diagnosis referring to the finding of involuntary detrusor contractions during the filling phase of a urodynamic study. Therefore, invasive urodynamic testing is required to make the diagnosis. Up to 40% of patients with overactive bladder do not demonstrate detrusor overactivity on urodynamic testing. The clinical significance of this finding is unknown. However, the effectiveness of pharmacologic therapy appears to be independent of the presence or absence of detrusor overactivity. This distinction between overactive bladder (a symptom syndrome) and detrusor overactivity (a urodynamic diagnosis) is essential in fully understanding the patient population under study and the effects of pharmacologic therapy reported in the literature.

Symptoms characteristic of overactive bladder are urinary frequency and urgency, with or without urge incontinence. *Frequency* is defined as micturition more than eight times per day. *Urgency* is described as a sudden compelling desire to urinate that is difficult to delay. People suffering from overactive bladder typically have to empty their bladders frequently, and, when they experience a sensation of urgency, they may leak urine if they are unable to reach the toilet quickly or if the sensation of urgency is very strong. Many patients have associated nocturia (>1 micturition per night) and/or nocturnal incontinence (enuresis). Nocturia and enuresis are particularly disruptive to sleep. For patients with incontinence, the amount of urine lost may be large, as the bladder may empty completely.

Most patients with overactive bladder and UUI have no identifiable underlying etiology. The most common cause of overactive bladder and UUI is "idiopathic." Clearly identifiable risk factors for UUI include normal aging, neurologic disease (including stroke, Parkinson's disease, multiple sclerosis, and spinal cord injury), and bladder outlet obstruction (e.g., due to BPH or prostate cancer).

The mechanism for overactive bladder and UUI must be either neurogenic or myogenic. The neurogenic hypothesis ascribes the condition to disease-related changes within the central or peripheral nervous system.[18] The myogenic hypothesis states that overactive bladder and UUI result from changes within the smooth muscle of the bladder wall itself.[19] Precipitating factors, such as bladder outlet obstruction, can cause partial denervation of smooth muscle, leading to a state of decreased responsiveness to activation of intrinsic nerves but supersensitivity to contractile agonists and direct electrical activation.[20] In practice, UUI is difficult to categorize as either neurogenic or myogenic in origin, as these etiologies often seem to be interconnected and complementary.

Urethral Overactivity and/or Bladder Underactivity (Overflow Incontinence) Overflow incontinence, the result of urethral overactivity and/or bladder underactivity, is an important but uncommon type of UI in both men and women. Overflow incontinence results when the bladder is filled to capacity at all times but is unable to empty, causing urine to leak from a distended bladder past a normal or even overactive outlet and sphincter.

In the setting of urethral overactivity, resistance to the flow of urine during volitional voiding is increased, resulting in functional or anatomic obstruction and incomplete bladder emptying. Clinically and practically, the most common causes of urethral overactivity in men are anatomic urethral obstruction, including that due to BPH and prostate cancer. In women, urethral overactivity is rare but may result from cystocele formation (with resultant kinking or obstruction of the urethra) or surgical overcorrection (iatrogenic obstruction) following anti-SUI surgery. In both men and women, overflow UI may be associated with systemic neurologic dysfunction or diseases, such as spinal cord injury or multiple sclerosis.

Bladder underactivity may result in overflow incontinence. Under certain circumstances, the detrusor muscle of the bladder may become progressively weakened and eventually lose the ability to voluntarily contract. In the absence of adequate contractility, the bladder is unable to empty completely, and large volumes of residual urine are left after micturition. Both myogenic and neurogenic factors have been implicated in producing the impaired contractility seen in this condition. Clinically, overflow incontinence is most commonly seen in the setting of long-term chronic bladder outlet obstruction in men, such as that due to BPH or prostate cancer, diabetes mellitus, or denervation due to radical pelvic surgery, such as abdominopelvic resection or radical hysterectomy.

Mixed Incontinence and Other Types of Urinary Incontinence Various types of UI may coexist in the same patient. The combination of bladder overactivity and urethral underactivity is termed *mixed incontinence*. The diagnosis often is difficult because of the confusing array of presenting symptoms. Bladder overactivity may also coexist with impaired bladder contractility. This occurs most commonly in the elderly and is termed *detrusor hyperactivity with impaired contractility*.[21]

Functional incontinence is not caused by bladder- or urethra-specific factors. Rather, in patients with conditions such as dementia or cognitive or mobility deficits, the UI is linked to the primary disease process more than any extrinsic or intrinsic deficit of the lower urinary tract. An example of functional incontinence occurs in the postoperative orthopedic surgery patient. Following extensive orthopedic reconstructions such as total hip arthroplasty, patients often are immobile secondary to pain or traction. Therefore, patients may be unable to access toileting facilities in a reasonable amount of time and may become incontinent as a result. Treatment of this type of UI may involve simple interventions such as placing a urinal or commode at the bedside that allows for uncomplicated access to toileting.

Many localized or systemic illnesses may result in UI because of their effects on the lower urinary tract or the surrounding structures:

- Dementia/delirium
- Depression
- Urinary tract infection (cystitis)
- Postmenopausal atrophic urethritis or vaginitis
- Diabetes mellitus
- Neurologic disease (e.g., stroke, Parkinson disease, multiple sclerosis, spinal cord injury)
- Pelvic malignancy
- Constipation
- Congenital malformations

❶ Many commonly used medications may precipitate or aggravate existing voiding dysfunction and UI (Table 88–1).

TABLE 88-1 Medications That Influence Lower Urinary Tract Function

Medication	Effect
Diuretics, acetylcholinesterase inhibitors	Polyuria, frequency, urgency
α-Receptor antagonists	Urethral relaxation and stress urinary incontinence in women
α-Receptor agonists	Urethral constriction and urinary retention in men
Calcium channel blockers	Urinary retention
Narcotic analgesics	Urinary retention from impaired contractility
Sedative hypnotics	Functional incontinence caused by delirium, immobility
Antipsychotics	Anticholinergic effects and urinary retention
Anticholinergics	Urinary retention
Antidepressants, tricyclic	Anticholinergic effects, α-antagonist effects
Alcohol	Polyuria, frequency, urgency, sedation, delirium
Angiotensin-converting enzyme inhibitors (ACEIs)	Cough as a result of ACEIs may aggravate stress urinary incontinence by increasing intra-abdominal pressure

CLINICAL PRESENTATION

CLINICAL PRESENTATION OF URINARY INCONTINENCE RELATED TO URETHRAL UNDERACTIVITY

General

- The patient usually notes UI during activities such as exercise, running, lifting, coughing, and sneezing. Occurs much more commonly in women (seen only in men with lower urinary tract surgery or injury compromising the sphincter).

Symptoms

- Urine leakage with physical activity (volume is proportional to activity level). No UI with physical inactivity, especially when supine (no nocturia). May develop urgency and frequency as a compensatory mechanism (or as a separate component of bladder overactivity).

Diagnostic Tests

- Observation of urethral meatus while patient coughs or strains.

CLINICAL PRESENTATION OF URINARY INCONTINENCE RELATED TO BLADDER OVERACTIVITY

General

- Can have bladder overactivity and UI without urgency if sensory input from the lower urinary tract is absent.

Symptoms

- Urinary frequency (>8 micturitions per day), urgency with or without urge incontinence; nocturia (≥1 micturition per night) and enuresis may be present.

Diagnostic Tests

- Urodynamic studies are the gold standard for diagnosis. Urinalysis and urine culture should be negative (rule out urinary tract infection as cause of frequency).

CLINICAL PRESENTATION OF URINARY INCONTINENCE RELATED TO URETHRAL OVERACTIVITY AND/OR BLADDER UNDERACTIVITY

General

- Important but rare type of UI in both men and women. Urethral overactivity usually is due to prostatic enlargement (males) or cystocele formation or surgical overcorrection following stress incontinence surgery in women.

Symptoms

- Lower abdominal fullness, hesitancy, straining to void, decreased force of stream, interrupted stream, sense of incomplete bladder emptying. May have urinary frequency and urgency. Abdominal pain if acute urinary retention is present.

Signs

- Increased postvoid residual urine volume.

Diagnostic Tests

- Digital rectal examination or transrectal ultrasound to rule out prostatic enlargement. Renal function tests to rule out renal failure due to acute urinary retention.

❷ UI may present in a number of ways, depending on the underlying pathophysiology. Generally, SUI is considered the most common type of UI and probably accounts for at least a portion of UI in more than half of all incontinent women. Some studies have found that mixed UI (SUI + UUI) is the most common type of UI.[6] However, the proportions of SUI versus UUI versus mixed UI vary considerably with age group and sex of patients studied, study methodology, and a variety of other factors. A complete medical history, including an assessment of symptoms and a physical examination, is essential for correctly classifying the type of incontinence and thereby assuring appropriate therapy.

URINE LEAKAGE

UI represents a spectrum of severity in terms of both volume of leakage and degree of bother to the patient. To carefully consider the level of patient discomfort when discussing urine leakage, the clinician must probe during the patient interview to accurately determine the precise nature of the problem.

Use of absorbent products, such as panty liners, pads, or briefs, is an obvious point of discussion, but the clinician must keep in mind that use of these products varies among patients. The number and type of pads may not relate to the amount or type of incontinence, as their use is a function of personal preference and hygiene. A high number of absorbent pads may be used every day by a patient with severe, high-volume UI or, alternatively, by a fastidiously hygienic patient with low-volume leakage who simply changes pads often to prevent wetness or odor. Nevertheless, a large number of pads that are described by the patient as "soaked" is indicative of high-volume urine loss.

Regardless of the volume of urine loss, the desire to seek evaluation and therapy for UI in all patients almost always is elective and contingent on the degree of bother to the individual patient. As with use of absorbent products, patients differ with regard to the amount of urine loss they will tolerate before considering the condition bothersome enough to seek assistance.

SYMPTOMS

Under the best of circumstances, UI is difficult to categorize based on symptoms alone (Table 88–2).[22] In a study of patients who appeared to have SUI based on symptoms and patient history, urodynamics showed that only 72% of patients had SUI as the sole cause of incontinence.[23]

Patients with urethral underactivity or SUI characteristically complain of urinary leakage with physical activity. Volume of leakage is proportional to the level of activity. They will often leak urine during periods of exercise, coughing, sneezing, lifting, or even

TABLE 88-2 Differentiating Bladder Overactivity from Urethral Underactivity

Symptoms	Bladder Overactivity	Urethral Underactivity
Urgency (strong, sudden desire to void)	Yes	Sometimes
Frequency with urgency	Yes	Rarely
Leaking during physical activity (e.g., coughing, sneezing, lifting)	No	Yes
Amount of urinary leakage with each episode of incontinence	Large if present	Usually small
Ability to reach the toilet in time following an urge to void	No or just barely	Yes
Nocturnal incontinence (presence of wet pads or undergarments in bed)	Yes	Rare
Nocturia (waking to pass urine at night)	Usually	Seldom

when rising from a seated to a standing position. Patients with pure SUI will not have leakage when physically inactive, especially when they are supine. Often they will have little or no UI at night, will not awaken to void during the night (nocturia), will not wet the bed, and often do not even wear absorbent products at bedtime. Urinary urgency and frequency may be associated with SUI, either as a separate component caused by bladder overactivity (mixed incontinence) or as a compensatory mechanism wherein the patient with SUI learns to toilet frequently to prevent large-volume urine loss during physical activity.

Typical symptoms of bladder overactivity include frequency, urgency, and urge incontinence. Nocturia and nocturnal incontinence are often present. Urine leakage is unpredictable, and the volume loss may be large. Patients often wear protection both day and night. Urinary frequency can be affected by a number of factors unrelated to bladder overactivity, including excessive fluid intake (polydipsia) and bladder hypersensitivity states such as interstitial cystitis and urinary tract infection, and should be ruled out. In some patients, bladder overactivity manifests as UI without awareness in the absence of a sense of urinary urgency or frequency. *Urinary urgency*, a sensation of impending micturition, requires intact sensory input from the lower urinary tract. In patients with spinal cord injury, sensory neuropathies, and other neurologic diseases, a diminished ability to perceive or process sensory input from the lower urinary tract may result in bladder overactivity and UI without urgency or urinary frequency. When bladder contraction occurs without warning and sensation is absent, the condition is referred to as *reflex incontinence*.

Patients with overflow incontinence may present with lower abdominal fullness as well as considerable obstructive urinary symptoms, including hesitancy, straining to void, decreased force of urinary stream, interrupted stream, and a vague sense of incomplete bladder emptying. These patients may also have a significant component of urinary frequency and urgency. In patients with acute urinary retention and overflow incontinence, lower abdominal pain may be present. Although these symptoms are not specific for overflow incontinence, they may warrant further investigation, including an assessment of postvoid residual urine volume.

SIGNS

A presenting complaint of UI mandates a directed physical examination and a brief neurologic assessment. The workup ideally includes an abdominal examination to exclude a distended bladder, neurologic assessment of the perineum and lower extremities, pelvic examination in women (looking especially for evidence of prolapse or hormonal deficiency), and genital and prostate examination in men.

SUI usually can be objectively demonstrated by having the patient cough or strain during the examination and observing the urethral meatus for a sudden spurt of urine. In women, SUI may be associated with varying degrees of vaginal prolapse, including cystourethrocele (bladder and urethral prolapse), enterocele (small bowel prolapse), rectocele (rectal prolapse), and uterine prolapse. These conditions may have important implications for therapy.

Perineal skin maceration, erythema, breakdown, and ulceration may be indicative of chronic, severe UI. Patients with chronic incontinence may manifest fungal infections of the skin of the perineum and upper thighs.

In both men and women, digital rectal examination provides an opportunity to check ambient rectal tone and the integrity of the sacral reflex arc (e.g., anal wink) as well as assess the patient's ability to perform a voluntary pelvic floor muscle contraction (i.e., Kegel exercise), which may be an important factor in deciding on appropriate therapy. In men, a digital examination of the prostate assesses for the presence of prostate cancer, inflammation, and BPH.

A targeted neurologic examination includes assessment of reflexes, rectal tone, and sensory or motor deficits in the lower extremities, which might be indicative of systemic or localized neurologic disease. Neurologic diseases have the potential to affect bladder and sphincter function and thus may have significant implications in the incontinent patient.

PRIOR MEDICAL OR SURGICAL ILLNESS

UI may present in the setting of concurrent, seemingly unrelated illnesses. New-onset UI may be the initial manifestation of systemic illnesses such as diabetes mellitus, metastatic malignancies, multiple sclerosis, and other neurologic illnesses. Central nervous system disease, or injury above the level of the pons, generally results in symptoms of bladder overactivity and UUI. Spinal cord injury or disease may manifest as bladder overactivity and UUI or as overflow incontinence, depending on the spinal level and completeness of the injury or disease.

Medications may have wide-ranging effects on lower urinary tract function (see Table 88–1). A thorough inquiry into the use of new medications in the setting of recent-onset UI may show a relationship.

Acute UI manifesting in the immediate postoperative setting may be secondary to a number of factors, including surgical manipulation and immobility, and to a number of medications, especially opioid analgesics. In the postoperative setting, acute urinary retention and overflow incontinence are commonly related to the administration of anesthetic agents and/or opioid analgesics in the perioperative period. These agents may have profound effects on bladder contractility that are completely reversible once the agents are metabolized and excreted.

Prior surgery may have effects on lower urinary tract function. UI following prostate surgery in men is highly suggestive of injury to the sphincter and resultant SUI. Pelvic surgery for benign and malignant conditions may result in denervation or injury to the lower urinary tract. This includes bowel surgery and gynecologic procedures. For example, new-onset total UI following gynecologic surgery suggests intraoperative bladder injury and subsequent development of a postoperative vesicovaginal fistula. Radiation therapy to the pelvis for malignant disease (e.g., prostate cancer or cervical cancer) may result in injury to the bladder or urethra and subsequent UI.

In women, UI may be related to several gynecologic factors, including childbirth, hormonal status, and prior gynecologic surgery. Pregnancy and childbirth, particularly vaginal delivery, are associated with SUI and pelvic prolapse. Significant SUI in the nulliparous woman is uncommon. UI that becomes progressive at or around menopause suggests a hormonal component that may be responsive to estrogen or hormone replacement therapy.

UI may present in the setting of other significant pelvic floor disorders, signs, and symptoms. Constipation, diarrhea, fecal incontinence, dyspareunia, sexual dysfunction, and pelvic pain may be related to UI. A history of gross hematuria in the setting of UI mandates further urologic investigation, including radiologic imaging of the upper urinary tract and cystoscopy. Acute dysuria with or without hematuria in the setting of UI suggests cystitis. Urinalysis and urine culture should be performed in these patients.

TREATMENT

Urinary Incontinence

■ NONPHARMACOLOGIC TREATMENT

❸ Nonpharmacologic treatment of UI commonly constitutes the initial form of incontinence management at a primary care level. For patients in whom pharmacologic or surgical management is inappropriate or undesired, nondrug treatment is the only option. Examples of patients who fulfill these criteria include patients who are not medically fit for surgery, those who plan future pregnancies (which may adversely affect long-term surgical outcomes), those with overflow incontinence whose condition is not amenable to surgery or drug therapy, those with comorbid conditions that place them at high risk for adverse effects from drug therapy, those who are delaying surgery or do not want to undergo surgery, and those with mild to moderate symptoms who do not want to take medication.

For additional information on nonpharmacologic interventions for UI, readers are referred to comprehensive literature reviews and consensus opinions of treatment guidelines on nonpharmacologic interventions by multidisciplinary experts.[24] Table 88–3 summarizes the basic nondrug approaches.

Behavioral interventions are the first line of treatment for SUI, UUI, and mixed UI. Interventions include lifestyle modifications, toilet scheduling regimens, and pelvic floor muscle rehabilitation. Because the key to success with any type of behavioral intervention is motivation of patients or caregivers, these individuals must be active participants in developing a treatment plan. Regular followup is needed to help motivate patients and caregivers, provide reassurance and support, and monitor treatment outcomes.

■ PHARMACOLOGIC TREATMENT

Urge Urinary Incontinence

Pharmacotherapy is useful when UUI symptoms are not adequately controlled with nonpharmacologic therapies, particularly in patients with low functional bladder capacity, especially individuals who frequently attempt to toilet and are independent or require only limited assistance in toileting. In many cases, the combined use of pharmacotherapy with nonpharmacologic therapy produces a better response than either intervention alone.

❹ Anticholinergic/antispasmodic drugs have proved to be the most effective agents for suppressing premature detrusor contractions, enhancing bladder storage, and relieving UUI symptoms and complications and constitute the pharmacotherapy of first choice for treatment of UUI (Tables 88–4 and 88–5).[25–44] Drugs with anticholinergic activity act by antagonizing muscarinic cholinergic receptors, through which efferent parasympathetic nerve impulses evoke detrusor contraction. Anticholinergics have been demonstrated to improve quality of life, with no significant differences between agents.[45] Women with mixed UI or UUI plus urethritis or vaginitis may benefit from a topical estrogen (alone or in combination with an anticholinergic drug). Patients with irritative symptoms of BPH that persist despite specific BPH treatment may benefit from anticholinergic therapy as well (caution is warranted because these agents may precipitate acute urinary retention).

Immediate-Release Oxybutynin Even though a substantial proportion of patients may discontinue oxybutynin immediate-release (IR) therapy because of its nonurinary antimuscarinic effects, oxybutynin IR remains the drug of first choice for treatment of UUI and the gold standard against which other drugs are compared. In addition to antimuscarinic effects (e.g., dry mouth, constipation, vision impairment, confusion, cognitive dysfunction, and tachycardia), oxybutynin IR is associated with orthostatic hypotension secondary to α-adrenergic receptor blockade as well as sedation and weight gain from histamine H_1-receptor blockade.[26,31,46–50] Furthermore, adverse effects jeopardize medication adherence and can prevent dose escalation to that needed for optimal benefit.

Emerging evidence suggests that the high incidence of adverse effects, especially dry mouth, with use of oxybutynin IR is largely due to the active metabolite *N*-desethyloxybutynin (DEO), which is generated during extensive first-pass metabolism in the liver and upper gastrointestinal tract.[51] The lower DEO plasma concentrations seen with long-acting forms of oxybutynin (which are due to reduced first-pass metabolism) compared with those of oxybutynin IR may explain the lesser propensity of the long-acting formulations to cause dry mouth and other anticholinergic adverse effects.

Another factor associated with the adverse effects of oxybutynin IR, especially in older patients, is the transient high peak serum oxybutynin plasma concentrations.[52] Oxybutynin IR is best tolerated when the dose is gradually escalated from no more than 2.5 mg twice daily to start, to 2.5 mg three times daily after 1 month, then further increased in increments of 2.5 mg/day every 1 to 2 months until the desired response or the maximum recommended or tolerated dose is attained. The optimal response usually requires no more than 5 mg three times daily (see Table 88–4).[26,53]

Adverse effects of oxybutynin IR can sometimes be managed by a dose reduction if this does not significantly compromise drug efficacy. Dry mouth can be relieved by use of sugarless hard candy, gum, or a saliva substitute. Constipation can be minimized by increasing the intake of water, dietary fiber, physical activity such as walking, or laxative therapy. The need for multiple daily dosing of oxybutynin IR can further jeopardize adherence, especially in people who take multiple medications or those who are cognitively impaired.

Extended-Release Oral Oxybutynin Because of the problems noted with oxybutynin IR, an extended-release (XL) formulation of oxybutynin was developed. It can be considered an alternative first-line therapy of UUI (see Table 88–5).[54]

Unlike oxybutynin IR, oxybutynin XL delivers a controlled amount of oxybutynin continuously throughout the gastrointestinal tract over a 24-hour period, reducing first-pass metabolism by cytochrome P450 (CYP) isoenzyme 3A4, which is present in higher concentrations in the upper portion of the small intestine than in the lower gastrointestinal tract.[54,55] This results in relative bioavailabilities of oxybutynin and DEO of 153% and 69%, respectively, for oxybutynin XL compared with oxybutynin IR.[56] The greater ratio of parent drug concentration to active metabolite concentration after oxybutynin XL administration and, probably less importantly, the lower peak plasma drug concentration are believed to be the reasons for fewer dose- and concentration-dependent adverse effects and better patient tolerance with the XL preparation compared with oxybutynin IR.[57] Elimination of oxybutynin XL is not known to be altered in patients with renal or hepatic impairment or in geriatric patients (up to age 78 years).[54] The absence of an effect of advanced age on oxybutynin XL pharmacokinetics is unexpected because clearance of oxybutynin IR is significantly lower (by approximately 50%) in older patients compared with younger individuals.

Controlled studies have demonstrated that oxybutynin XL is significantly more effective than placebo and is as effective as oxybutynin IR in terms of reducing the mean number of UI episodes, restoring continence, decreasing the number of micturitions per day, and increasing urine volume voided per micturition (see Table 88–5).[30,31,46–48,58–60]

In short-term studies of up to 12 weeks' duration, oxybutynin XL was better tolerated than oxybutynin IR, with approximately 7% of patients discontinuing treatment because of adverse effects (compared with approximately 27% of those taking oxybutynin IR).[26,31,46,47,53,54] The rate and severity of adverse effects did not differ significantly between elderly persons (≥65 years old) and younger adults using the XL preparation. A 12-week study demonstrated the superiority of oxybutynin XL over tolterodine IR in reducing the mean number of weekly incontinent episodes and micturitions.[39]

In the Overactive Bladder: Performance of Extended-Release Agents (OPERA) trial, oxybutynin XL and tolterodine long-acting (LA) were equally effective in decreasing the mean number of incontinence episodes, but oxybutynin XL was superior in reducing weekly micturition frequency and achieving total dryness.[61] In another study

TABLE 88-3 Nonpharmacologic Management of Urinary Incontinence

Intervention	Description	Patient Characteristics
Lifestyle modifications	Self-management strategies targeted toward reducing or eliminating risk factors that cause or exacerbate urinary incontinence	Smoking cessation for patients with cough-induced stress incontinence; weight reduction for obese patients with stress and urge incontinence; prevention of constipation; caffeine reduction, selected dietary and fluid modifications for patients with urge incontinence (e.g., eliminate aspartame, spicy foods, citrus fruits, carbonated beverages)
Scheduling regimens		
Timed voiding	Toileting on a fixed schedule at interval does not change, typically every 2 hours during waking hours	Used for stress, urge, and mixed incontinence in patients with cognitive or physical impairments; used in patients without impairments who have infrequent voiding patterns
Habit retraining	Scheduled toiletings with adjustments of voiding intervals (longer or shorter) based on patient's voiding pattern	Used for institutionalized or homebound patients with cognitive or physical impairments; may be used in patients who have diuretic-induced incontinence
Prompted voiding	Scheduled toiletings that require prompts to void from a caregiver, typically every 2 hours; patient assisted in toileting only if response is positive; used in conjunction with operant conditioning techniques for rewarding patients for maintaining continence and appropriate toileting	Used for patients who are functionally able to use toilet or toilet substitute, able to feel urge sensation, and able to request toileting assistance appropriately; primarily used in institutional settings or in homebound patients with an available caregiver
Bladder training	Scheduled toiletings with progressive voiding intervals; includes teaching urge control strategies using relaxation and distraction techniques, self-monitoring, and use of reinforcement techniques; sometimes combined with drug therapy	Used for stress, urge, and mixed incontinence in patients who are cognitively intact, able to toilet, and motivated to comply with training program
Pelvic floor muscle rehabilitation		
Pelvic floor muscle exercises (e.g., Kegel exercises)	Regular practice of pelvic floor muscle contractions; may involve use of pelvic floor muscle contraction for prevention of stress leakage and urge inhibition	Used for stress, urge, and mixed incontinence in patients who can correctly contract pelvic floor muscles without using accessory muscles; requires cognitively intact and highly motivated patient
Biofeedback	Use of electronic or mechanical instruments to display visual or auditory information about neuromuscular or bladder activity; used to teach correct pelvic floor muscle contraction and/or urge inhibition	Used for stress, urge, and mixed incontinence in patients who have the capability to learn voluntary control through observation and are motivated; used in conjunction with pelvic floor muscle exercises
Vaginal weight training	Active retention of increasing vaginal weights (e.g., Kegel Kones, Milex, Chicago, IL); typically used in combination with pelvic floor muscle exercises at least twice per day	Women with stress incontinence who are cognitively intact, can correctly contract pelvic floor muscles, able to stand, and have sufficient vaginal vault and introitus to retain cone and are highly motivated; contraindicated in patients with moderate to severe pelvic organ prolapse
Acupuncture	Involves insertion of disposable sterile stainless steel needles into points on the skin that are thought to suppress or stimulate spinal and/or supraspinal reflexes to the bladder and/or urethra	Used for urge and mixed incontinence and urinary incontinence due to spinal cord injury
Nonimplantable electrical stimulation	Application of electrical current to sacral or pudendal afferent fibers through vaginal, anal, surface, or needle electrodes; used to inhibit bladder overactivity and improve awareness, contractility, and efficacy of pelvic floor muscle contraction	Used for stress, urge, and mixed incontinence in patients who are highly motivated; contraindicated in patients with diminished sensory perception, moderate or severe pelvic organ prolapse; urinary retention, history of cardiac arrhythmia, or demand cardiac pacemaker
Extracorporeal magnetic innervation	Pulsed magnetic stimulation to pelvic floor musculature causing depolarization of motor neurons, thus inducing pelvic floor muscle contraction; stimulation is provided through a specially designed chair that contains a device for producing a pulsing magnetic field (e.g., Neotonus, Inc., Marietta, GA)	Used for treatment of stress, urge, and mixed incontinence; contraindicated in patients with demand cardiac pacemakers or metallic joint replacements; may be useful treatment option when other approaches fail or are not feasible
Antiincontinence devices		
Pessaries	Intravaginal devices designed to support the bladder neck, relieve minor to moderate pelvic organ prolapse, and change pressure transmission to the urethra (e.g., Milex; Mentor Corporation, Santa Barbara, CA; Adamed, Inc., Rutherford, NJ)	Used for female stress incontinence and mild to moderate pelvic organ prolapse; in postmenopausal women, topical estrogen therapy typically is prescribed to prevent ulceration and breakdown of vaginal tissue; requires good manual dexterity to manipulate device
Bed or pant alarms	Sensor devices that respond to wetness; used to awaken or alert individuals via noise or vibrating mechanism (e.g., Nite Train-r, Koregon Enterprises, Inc., Beaverton, OR; Healthshield Incontinence Detectors, Jonas Inc., Wilmington, DE)	Primarily used for nocturnal enuresis in children; system available for monitoring incontinence in home care and institutional environments
Urethral compression device (men only)	Penile clamp (e.g., Cunningham Incontinence Clamp, Bard Medical, Covington, GA; ActiCuf, GT Urological, Minneapolis, MN; Cook Continence, Cook Wound/Ostomy/Continence, Spencer, IN)	Used in male stress incontinence patients who are intact and have good manual dexterity
Intraurethral occlusive device (urethral plug) (women only)	Small, single-use device worn in the urethra to provide mechanical obstruction to prevent urine leakage; removed for voiding (e.g., FemSoft Insert, Rochester Medical Corp., Stewartville, MN)	Used for female stress incontinence patients who are cognitively intact with good manual dexterity; contraindicated with primary urge incontinence, urinary tract infection, urethral stricture, and any anatomic or pathologic condition that makes catheter passage difficult
External collection devices (men only)	Condom catheter with leg bag	Used in men with urge, stress, and overflow incontinence and in those with functional impairments
Catheters	Disposable, intermittent urethral catheters and indwelling urethral and suprapubic catheters	Used for overflow incontinence; used in patients who are bed-bound or with significant mobility impairments and severe incontinence; those with terminal illness; those with sacral pressure ulcers until healing occurs

(continued)

TABLE 88-3 Nonpharmacologic Management of Urinary Incontinence (continued)

Intervention	Description	Patient Characteristics
Supportive interventions		
Toileting substitutes and other environmental modifications	Female and male urinals, bedside commodes, elevated toilet seats	Used for patients with mobility impairments that make reaching a toilet in timely fashion difficult
Absorbent products	Variety of reusable and disposable pads and pant systems; some products contain a polymer that absorbs and wicks urine away from the body	Used for all types of incontinence
Physical therapy	Gait and/or strength training	Used for frail elderly patients with mobility impairments that make reaching a toilet in timely fashion difficult

that pooled results of two open-label studies, tolterodine LA was associated with significantly greater patient-perceived improvement in bladder control and fewer withdrawals due to adverse effects than oxybutynin XL. However, the treatments were similar in terms of patients' or physicians' perception of benefit over baseline and proportions of withdrawals due to lack of efficacy. However, the lack of blinding may have introduced patient and observer bias.[62]

Oxybutynin XL, available only in a tablet formulation, is administered once daily, with or without food, and should not be crushed or chewed (see Table 88–4). Like oxybutynin IR, the dosage does not require adjustment in patients of advanced age or in patients with renal or hepatic impairment. However, treatment should be initiated at the smallest recommended dosage in the elderly (5 mg once daily).[32,54] The maximum benefit of oxybutynin XL may not be realized for up to 4 weeks after starting therapy or after dose escalation. No known clinically relevant drug–drug interactions with either oxybutynin XL or oxybutynin IR have been identified. However, other drugs with anticholinergic activity may increase overall anticholinergic effects (i.e., produce an additive or synergistic pharmacodynamic interaction), as might be expected.[54] Another potential pharmacodynamic interaction involves the mutual antagonism of anticholinergic agents and cholinergic stimulants, such as the acetylcholinesterase inhibitors used to treat dementia.

Extended-Release Transdermal Oxybutynin The oxybutynin transdermal system (TDS), which delivers 3.9 mg/day, is applied twice weekly (every 3 or 4 days). Transdermal absorption of oxybutynin from this formulation bypasses first-pass hepatic and gut metabolism, resulting in similar plasma oxybutynin but lower plasma DEO concentrations compared with levels achieved after administration of an equivalent dose via the oral route.[51,63,64] No dosage adjustment of the TDS product for advancing age is necessary.[44]

Oxybutynin TDS is superior to placebo in reducing the number of incontinence episodes and micturitions and increasing the volume voided per micturition.[43,44] It is similar to oxybutynin IR in reducing the frequency of UUI episodes and improving patient-perceived urinary leakage.[65] Oxybutynin TDS and tolterodine LA are significantly superior to placebo and similar to each other in reducing the frequency of UUI episodes, increasing the volume voided per micturition, attaining complete continence, and improving quality of life.[43]

TABLE 88-4 Pharmacotherapeutic Options in Patients with Urinary Incontinence

Type	Drug Class	Drug Therapy (Usual Dose)	Comments
Overactive bladder	Anticholinergic agents/ antispasmodics	Oxybutynin IR (2.5–5 mg two, three or four times daily), oxybutynin XL (5–30 mg daily), oxybutynin TDS (3.9 mg/day); (apply one patch twice weekly), tolterodine IR (1–2 mg twice daily), tolterodine LA (2–4 mg daily), trospium chloride (20 mg once or twice daily), solifenacin (5–10 mg daily), darifenacin (7.5–15 mg daily)	Anticholinergics are first-line drug therapy (oxybutynin or tolterodine is preferred)
	Tricyclic antidepressants (TCAs)	Imipramine, doxepin, nortriptyline, or desipramine (25–100 mg at bedtime)	TCAs are generally reserved for patients with an additional indication (e.g., depression, neuropathic pain)
	Topical estrogen (only in women with urethritis or vaginitis)	Conjugated estrogen vaginal cream (0.5 g) three times per week for up to 8 months. Repeat course if symptom recurrence, or use estradiol vaginal insert/ring [2 mg (one ring)] and replace after 90 days if needed.	Marginally effective; few adverse effects with vaginal cream and insert
Stress	Duloxetine[a]	40–80 mg/day (one or two doses)	Even though not FDA approved, duloxetine is first-line therapy; most adverse events diminish with time, so support patient during initial period of use
	α-Adrenergic agonists	Pseudoephedrine (15–60 mg three times daily) with food, water, or milk Phenylephrine (10 mg four times daily)	Pseudoephedrine and phenylephrine are alternative first-line therapies for women with no contraindication (notably hypertension); phenylpropanolamine was the preferred agent in the class until its removal from the U.S. market in 2000.
	Estrogen	See estrogens (above). Works best if urethritis or vaginitis are present.	Considered a less-effective alternative to α-adrenergic agonists and duloxetine. Combined α-adrenergic agonist and estrogen may be somewhat more effective than α-adrenergic agonist alone in postmenopausal women.
	Imipramine	25–100 mg at bedtime	Imipramine is an optional therapy when first-line therapy is inadequate.
Overflow (atonic bladder)	Cholinomimetics	Bethanechol (25–50 mg three or four times daily) on an empty stomach	Avoid use if patient has asthma or heart disease. Short-term use only. Never give IV or IM because of life-threatening cardiovascular and severe gastrointestinal reactions.

IR, immediate-release; LA, long-acting; TDS, transdermal system; XL, extended-release.
[a]Investigational. Doses provided are those best supported by clinical trials to date.

TABLE 88-5 Adverse Event Incidence Rates with First-Line Drugs for Bladder Overactivity[a]

Drug	Dry Mouth	Constipation	Dizziness	Vision Disturbance
Oxybutynin IR	85	40	32	20
Oxybutynin XL	35	7	5	2
Oxybutynin TDS	7	3	1	1
Tolterodine	61	13	6	8
Tolterodine LA	23	6	2	1
Trospium chloride	20	10	1	1
Solifenacin	11	5	2	4
Darifenacin	20	15	2	2

IR, immediate-release; LA, long-acting; TDS, transdermal system; XL, extended-release.

[a]All values constitute mean data, predominantly using product information from the manufacturers. Due to the absence of information regarding dizziness for oxybutynin IR in the product information, pooled data from references 48 and 65 have been used.

A combined analysis of two phase III studies demonstrated a significant decrease in the number of UUI episodes and urinary frequency and increase in the volume voided per micturition from baseline with oxybutynin TDS in a study population, half of whom were elderly. These results were similar to those achieved in other studies with younger adults.[66] A subgroup analysis of combined placebo-controlled and open-label studies found similar reductions in numbers of UUI episodes and daily micturitions in patients 65 years and older compared with younger adults.[67]

The most common adverse effects with the TDS formulation are pruritus (15%) and erythema (9%) at the application site. Dry mouth (7%), constipation (3%), dizziness (1%), and abnormal vision (1%) occur less frequently with the TDS formulation than with the IR formulation and with similar frequency compared to oxybutynin XL and tolterodine IR/LA.[39,44]

In a study population in which approximately half were elders, the incidences of total adverse events, dry mouth, constipation, abnormal vision, dizziness, and somnolence with oxybutynin TDS were similar to those observed in younger adults.[66] A subgroup analysis of combined placebo-controlled and open-label studies showed that the incidence of adverse events with oxybutynin TDS in patients 65 years and older was similar to that in younger adults. The rates of pruritus and overall treatment discontinuation were lower in elders compared with younger adults.[67]

Immediate-Release Tolterodine Tolterodine is a competitive muscarinic receptor antagonist that can be considered first-line therapy for UI in patients with symptoms of urinary frequency, urgency, or urge incontinence (see Table 88–4).[33]

Controlled studies demonstrated that tolterodine was significantly more effective than placebo and as effective as oxybutynin IR in decreasing the mean daily number of micturitions and increasing the mean volume voided per micturition.[27,34–38,68,69] Although three controlled trials showed a significant decrease in the mean number of incontinence episodes per 24 hours compared with placebo, most other studies have not confirmed the finding, and the manufacturer's package insert does not claim a significant improvement in this parameter.[28,34–38,69] The only controlled study of the ability of tolterodine to restore urinary continence reported an insignificant effect size of 9% over placebo.[34]

Extended-Release Tolterodine In a controlled study of 1,529 adult outpatients with urinary frequency and UUI, tolterodine LA, an extended-release formulation of tolterodine, significantly decreased the mean number of weekly incontinence episodes (23% effect size over placebo and 7% effect size over tolterodine IR). Premature study withdrawal rates did not differ significantly between the two active treatments, but dry mouth was observed significantly less often in patients taking the LA formulation than among those receiving the IR formulation.[40]

Tolterodine LA was significantly superior to placebo and similar in elderly and young patient populations in reducing the frequencies of incontinence episodes and micturitions, increasing the volume voided per micturition and ability to complete tasks before voiding, and enhancing patient perception of benefit. Adverse effect types and frequencies were similar in the two age groups.[70]

A major consideration in using tolterodine is its pharmacokinetics, specifically its metabolism. The agent is predominantly eliminated by hepatic metabolism, which is partially under the control of genetic polymorphism.[33] The principal metabolic pathway in extensive metabolizers involves oxidation of the parent drug by CYP isoenzyme 2D6 to the active 5-hydroxymethyl metabolite (DD01), followed by further oxidation and dealkylation. In poor metabolizers who lack the CYP 2D6 (approximately 7% of the U.S. population), the principal metabolic pathway involves CYP 3A4, with dealkylation of the amino group, oxidation to a dealkylated hydroxy metabolite, and further oxidation to a dealkylated acid metabolite that undergoes glucuronidation. Because tolterodine is principally metabolized by CYP 3A4 in this case, its elimination may be impaired by inhibitors of this isoenzyme (e.g., fluoxetine, sertraline, fluvoxamine, macrolide antibiotics, azole antifungals, and grapefruit juice). For example, fluoxetine, an inhibitor of CYP 2D6 and 3A4, decreases the metabolism of tolterodine to DD01. The result is a mean 4.8-fold increase in the tolterodine area under the plasma concentration–time curve (AUC), mean 52% decrease in peak plasma concentration, and mean 20% decrease in the AUC of DD01.[33] Whether tolterodine significantly alters the pharmacokinetics of drugs metabolized by CYP 2D6 is unknown, so caution is advised with concurrent use with agents metabolized by CYP 2D6.

Single-dose interaction studies have demonstrated that concurrent administration of tolterodine LA with antacid leads to rapid release of drug (70% within 4 hours) and a mean 1.5-fold elevation in tolterodine peak plasma concentration compared with placebo. The same studies showed that the pharmacokinetics of oxybutynin XL were unaltered by concurrent antacid administration.[71] Another single-dose study showed that concurrent administration of tolterodine LA with omeprazole 20 mg once daily resulted in significantly increased peak plasma tolterodine concentrations compared with tolterodine LA given without prior omeprazole use. Conversely, no significant differences in peak plasma concentration of oxybutynin were evident when the XL formulation was administered with or without omeprazole. However, the AUCs of both agents were not significantly affected by omeprazole administration.[72] The clinical implication of this interaction is unclear. Whether a similar interaction exists with histamine H_2-receptor antagonists is unknown.

One of two phase I pharmacokinetic studies comparing tolterodine pharmacokinetics in healthy elderly volunteers (age 64–80 years) with those in healthy volunteers younger than 40 years found no significant differences in pharmacokinetic parameters between the groups. However, in the second phase I study, the mean serum concentrations of tolterodine and DD01 were 20% and 50% greater in elderly volunteers than in young healthy volunteers, respectively. Despite possibly altered pharmacokinetics in elderly individuals, no differences in the incidences and severity of adverse events between these age groups have been noted in clinical trials, so no dosage adjustment is recommended on the basis of age alone.[33]

Tolterodine elimination is diminished in patients with impaired hepatic function. Patients with hepatic cirrhosis who are extensive metabolizers exhibit a significantly higher mean AUC of DD01, higher serum tolterodine and DD01 concentrations, and longer terminal disposition half-life of tolterodine and DD01 than do healthy subjects who are extensive metabolizers. The tolterodine AUC is higher in cirrhotic patients who are poor metabolizers than in healthy people who are poor metabolizers.[33] If use of tolterodine cannot be avoided in patients with hepatic impairment or in those receiving inhibitors of CYP 3A4 (and possibly inhibitors of CYP 2D6), the initial dose should be reduced by 50% to tolterodine IR 1 mg twice daily or tolterodine LA 2 mg once daily.[33] No formal tolterodine dosage recommendation is possible based on available information for individuals who concurrently have hepatic impairment and are taking a CYP 3A4 and/or 2D6 inhibitor. Intuitively, the initial dose should not exceed 1 mg twice daily (IR) or 2 mg once daily (LA).

Elimination of tolterodine has not been evaluated in patients with impaired renal function; therefore, the drug should be used more cautiously in such individuals (i.e., starting dose of IR product is 1 mg twice daily with gradual dose escalation, if needed, to the usual maximum of 2 mg twice daily or a starting dose of the LA formulation is 2 mg once daily with gradual dose escalation, if needed, to the usual maximum of 4 mg once daily).[33]

Tolterodine is better tolerated than oxybutynin IR, with approximately 8% of patients discontinuing treatment prematurely (compared with approximately 27% of individuals taking oxybutynin IR).[26,28,34,35,37,46,72] The most common adverse effects of tolterodine are dry mouth, dyspepsia, headache, constipation, and dry eyes.[33]

Tolterodine, available only as a tablet formulation, can be taken with or without food. The LA product should not be crushed or chewed or taken less than 2 hours before or 4 hours after antacid administration. The maximum benefit from tolterodine may not be realized for up to 8 weeks after starting therapy or dose escalation.

Trospium Chloride Trospium chloride is a quaternary ammonium anticholinergic. It was approved in 2004 by the U.S. Food and Drug Administration (FDA) for the management of overactive bladder but has been available for many years in other countries. Trospium chloride has been comprehensively reviewed. [73] The data discussed here derive from that review, supplemented with detailed clinical trial data.

Preclinical studies have demonstrated that trospium chloride is an antimuscarinic agent in bladder and gastrointestinal tract tissues. It is poorly absorbed after oral administration (<10%), and food reduces bioavailability by 70% to 80%. It is principally cleared by the renal route (70%), with 80% of urinary excretion accounted for by the parent compound. The mean terminal disposition half-life in the presence of normal renal function is 10 to 12 hours. Advancing age and mild to moderate hepatic impairment do not affect trospium chloride pharmacokinetics to a clinically significant degree. In contrast, renal impairment does significantly reduce drug clearance. When creatinine clearance is less than 30 mL/min, AUC is increased by a mean of 4.5-fold, peak plasma concentration by a mean of two-fold, and terminal disposition half-life by a mean of two- to three-fold.

Eleven English-language publications on the efficacy/tolerability of trospium chloride for treatment of UUI are available. Except for the two trials (one published) described in the product information, clinical trials have emphasized cystometric, not clinical, endpoints.[74–83]

The paucity of clinical outcome data makes difficult the evaluation of trospium chloride compared with other approved anticholinergics. Although trospium chloride is statistically superior to placebo, the absolute differences in results between trospium chloride and placebo call into question the clinical relevance of such differences. In the four trials with active controls, results with trospium chloride were statistically equivalent to those with oxybutynin IR and tolterodine IR.[79–82] No comparative data with LA formulations of these two agents are available.

In a study involving a large proportion of elders (mean age 63 years), the decreases in the number of UUI episodes and daily micturitions and increase in volume voided per micturition were significantly lower in trospium chloride recipients compared with placebo recipients.[83]

The expected anticholinergic adverse effects occur with trospium chloride as well. Of interest, the frequency of these events is increased in patients 75 years and older compared with younger subjects. This occurrence is believed to be pharmacodynamic (i.e., increased sensitivity) and not pharmacokinetic in nature. No data at present support the hypothesis that trospium chloride is less neurotoxic than nonquaternary ammonium anticholinergics (based on the hypothesis of reduced transit across the blood–brain barrier of trospium chloride due to its positive electrical charge on the quaternary nitrogen). Available drug–drug interaction data are clearly inadequate.

The usual dosage regimen is 20 mg twice daily. The drug should be taken on an empty stomach. Dosage reduction (by 50% of the daily dose) is recommended when creatinine clearance is less than 30 mL/min. In patients 75 years and older, dose reduction to 20 mg once daily should be considered based upon tolerability. At this time, trospium chloride does not appear to be a significant advance over oxybutynin and tolterodine in managing UUI.

Solifenacin Succinate Solifenacin succinate was approved by the FDA in late 2004 for treatment of overactive bladder with urge incontinence, urgency, and urinary frequency. Solifenacin succinate has been comprehensively reviewed.[84] The data discussed here derive from that review, supplemented with detailed clinical trial data.

Preclinical studies demonstrated that solifenacin is an antagonist at M_1, M_2, and M_3 muscarinic cholinergic receptors. Based on comparative ex vivo and animal studies with solifenacin and oxybutynin, solifenacin is believed to be a "uroselective" agent. The drug is well absorbed (mean absolute bioavailability 88%), and food has no clinically relevant effect on absorption.[85,86] It is principally eliminated via metabolism and renal excretion of metabolites, with renal excretion of parent compound less than 10% of the dose. With a mean terminal disposition half-life of 50 to 60 hours, the drug can be dosed once daily.[87] Results of two placebo-controlled and two placebo- and active (tolterodine)-controlled clinical trials in UUI are available. Like oxybutynin and tolterodine, solifenacin significantly reduced the number of incontinence episodes, urge episodes, and micturitions per day and increased the volume voided per micturition in a dose-dependent fashion compared with placebo. In the active-controlled trials, solifenacin was statistically superior to tolterodine. However, neither of these two studies directly compared solifenacin and tolterodine.[88,89] Surprisingly, the effect of tolterodine in these trials was no better than that of placebo. A direct comparative trial of tolterodine ER demonstrated that the effect of solifenacin was significantly greater than that of tolterodine in terms of reducing the number of UUI episodes and pad usage and in patients' perception of their bladder condition.[90] An analysis of pooled data from two phase III studies showed that solifenacin recipients had significant improvement in five of 10 quality of life domains from baseline compared with placebo recipients.[91]

No comparative efficacy/tolerability data with oxybutynin are available. The effect sizes (solifenacin effect minus placebo effect) in these studies were similar to those noted with oxybutynin.

A retrospective analysis of pooled data from elders (mean age 72 years) in four phase III studies showed that compared with baseline, solifenacin recipients achieved a significantly greater decrease in number of UUI episodes, number of urgency episodes, and number of micturitions per day and a greater increase in the proportion of patients who became totally dry compared with placebo recipients.[92]

The recommended dose of solifenacin is 5 mg once daily. If the drug is well tolerated but the effectiveness is not optimal, the dose can be increased to 10 mg once daily. Little additional benefit is generally achieved with doses exceeding 5 mg daily. Solifenacin can be administered with or without food. For patients with creatinine clearance rates less than 30 mL/min or with moderate hepatic impairment (Child-Pugh class B), the daily dosage should not exceed 5 mg. If the patient has severe hepatic impairment (Child-Pugh class C), the drug should not be used. If the patient is receiving concurrent therapy with one or more potent CYP 3A4 inhibitors, the daily dose should not exceed 5 mg. In contrast to findings of preclinical studies, solifenacin behaves like a nonselective anticholinergic in humans, causing dry mouth, constipation, blurred vision, and other anticholinergic effects to a similar extent as tolterodine in clinical trials and oxybutynin in pharmacokinetic trials. At this time, solifenacin does not appear to be a significant advance over existing anticholinergics in managing UUI.

Darifenacin The data on darifenacin discussed here derive from a review,[93] supplemented with detailed clinical trial data.

Preclinical studies have demonstrated that darifenacin is an antagonist at M_1, M_3, and M_5 muscarinic cholinergic receptors. As with solifenacin, darifenacin is believed to be "uroselective" on the basis of preclinical data. The mean absolute bioavailabilities of the 7.5-, 15-, and 30-mg extended-release (ER) formulations are 15%, 19%, and 25%, respectively. Bioavailability is affected by formulation, CYP 2D6 genotype, dose, and race. Bioavailability is enhanced using an ER formulation (70%–110% higher than IR), in heterozygous CYP 2D6 extensive metabolizers and poor metabolizers (40%–90% higher than homozygous extensive metabolizers), and white race (56% higher than Japanese). Darifenacin is extensively metabolized, with cumulative urinary excretion of the parent compound less than 10%. The 2D6 and 3A4 isoenzymes of CYP are responsible for darifenacin metabolism. With a mean terminal disposition half-life of 3 to 5 hours (depending on CYP 2D6 metabolizer status), an ER formulation is needed to allow once-daily dosing. Results of four placebo-controlled clinical trials (one published) on UUI are available. Although a comparative study of darifenacin with oxybutynin IR showed that both agents significantly decreased the number of UUI episodes, the number of micturitions, urinary urgency and their severity compared with placebo, the active treatments were not directly compared.[94] A comparison with tolterodine IR and placebo showed that darifenacin 15 mg and 30 mg significantly decreased the number of UUI episodes from baseline after 2 weeks compared with placebo, but only the 30-mg daily dose continued to be superior to placebo after 12 weeks. Compared to placebo, tolterodine IR did not significantly decrease the number of UUI episodes from baseline at either time point. Darifenacin 30 mg once daily achieved a significantly greater decrease in the number of UUI episodes compared with tolterodine IR at both time points. At 12 weeks, both darifenacin and tolterodine IR produced significant improvements from baseline in the number of micturitions per day and volume voided per micturition compared with placebo.[95]

A large pooled subanalysis of patients 65 years and older from three phase III studies demonstrated that darifenacin produced a significant decrease in the number of UUI episodes, urgency episodes, and micturition frequency and an increase in volume voided per micturition compared with placebo.[96] No comparative efficacy/tolerability data with anticholinergics other than tolterodine IR and oxybutynin IR are available.

The recommended daily dose of darifenacin is 7.5 to 15 mg once daily of the ER oral formulation. As with solifenacin, darifenacin behaves like a nonselective anticholinergic in humans, causing dry mouth, constipation, and other well-known anticholinergic adverse effects. Dry mouth was significantly more common with oxybutynin IR than either darifenacin or placebo.[97] In one study, the rates of treatment discontinuation and adverse events in elderly recipients of darifenacin were similar to those seen in other studies of darifenacin conducted in younger adults.[96] At this time, darifenacin does not appear to be a significant advance over existing anticholinergics in managing UUI.

CLINICAL CONTROVERSY

Should anticholinergic pharmacotherapy be used to treat UUI in patients with mild cognitive impairment or mild or moderate dementia?

Other Anticholinergics and Antispasmodics Other drugs for treatment of UUI are less effective, are no safer, or have not been adequately studied.[24,98] Thus, their use is not recommended. Tricyclic antidepressants are generally no more effective than oxybutynin IR and exhibit a high incidence of bothersome and potentially serious adverse effects (e.g., orthostatic hypotension, cardiac conduction abnormalities, dizziness, confusion, and potentially life threatening in overdose). Therefore, their use should be limited to individuals who have one or more additional medical indications for these agents (e.g., depression or neuropathic pain); patients with mixed UI (because of their effect of decreasing bladder contractility and increasing outlet resistance); and possibly those with nocturnal incontinence associated with altered sleep patterns.[24,98–101] Because of the lower incidence of adverse effects, desipramine and nortriptyline may be preferred over imipramine and doxepin. However, due to their lower anticholinergic activity, they may not be as effective.

Propantheline, a quaternary ammonium anticholinergic and potential treatment, produces a high incidence of adverse effects and is only modestly effective for UUI.[102–106] When used, propantheline appears to be best tolerated at a dose no more than 15 mg three times daily plus 60 mg at bedtime.[102]

Flavoxate is a tertiary amine that relaxes smooth muscle in vitro. Four controlled trials revealed that flavoxate is no more effective than placebo for treatment of UUI; therefore, flavoxate is not recommended.[24]

Dicyclomine hydrochloride, an anticholinergic agent that relaxes smooth muscle, produced minimal benefit as well as bothersome adverse effects in two small studies.[107,108]

Hyoscyamine, an anticholinergic and antispasmodic drug related to atropine, has been suggested for treatment of UUI, but data recommending its use are insufficient.[24]

In a systematic review and pooled analysis of 32 controlled trials of anticholinergic therapy for overactive bladder (January 2002 database), the agents discussed were found to be modestly effective clinically and urodynamically. Although the clinical relevance of the small improvements in clinical and urodynamic parameters were questioned, the effects of these agents were still considered positive.[109]

It is hoped that an improved understanding of the pathophysiology of UUI will lead to the development of safer and more effective pharmacotherapy.

CLINICAL CONTROVERSY

Which anticholinergic agent should be used as first-line pharmacotherapy of UUI (oxybutynin, tolterodine, trospium chloride, solifenacin, or darifenacin) and which formulation of oxybutynin (oral IR, oral XL, or topical) or tolterodine (oral IR, oral LA) is unclear. Financial considerations currently favor generic oxybutynin IR, and this is the initial choice of many clinicians.

Botulinum Toxin A Enthusiasm is considerable for the application of botulinum toxin A for treatment of both neurogenic and nonneurogenic detrusor overactivity. Direct injection of botulinum toxin A into the muscle of interest results in paralysis. Both smooth and striated muscle are affected. In the United States, botulinum toxin A currently is approved for use for the treatment of a variety of conditions associated with muscle spasticity. It also is widely used to reduce skin wrinkles (cosmetic use).

In the lower urinary tract, botulinum toxin A is useful for treating neurogenic spasm of the external sphincter (due to striated sphincter dyssynergia in the patient with spinal injury) and detrusor overactivity. The usual dose for detrusor overactivity is 100 to 300 units. It is delivered directly into bladder muscle via a long needle through a cystoscope, usually in 10-unit increments with or without anesthesia. The toxin is distributed symmetrically using a series of submucosal injections throughout the bladder, usually avoiding the trigone and openings for the ureters. Preliminary studies suggest good efficacy and tolerability.[110] Although the effects appear to be dose dependent; the optimal dosing regimen has not yet been defined. Delivery of too much toxin may lead to detrusor underactivity and urinary retention. Durability of effect ranges from 3 to 9 months, at which time repeat administration is necessary to maintain effect.[111] Extensive studies of botulinum toxin A are ongoing in the United States and Europe.

Catheterization Combined with Medications Patients with UUI and an elevated postvoid residual urine volume due to retention may require intermittent self-catheterization along with frequent voiding between catheterizations.

If intermittent catheterization is not possible, surgical placement of a suprapubic catheter may be necessary. Use of a chronic indwelling catheter should be avoided because of the increased occurrence of urinary tract infections and nephrolithiasis.

Regardless of catheterization status, patients may experience symptom relief with oxybutynin (IR, XL, or TDS formulations), tolterodine (IR or LA formulations), trospium chloride, solifenacin, or darifenacin, as these agents relax the detrusor muscle and enhance bladder storage. Patients with UUI and symptoms of retention also may benefit from an α-adrenergic receptor antagonist that relaxes the internal bladder sphincter (e.g., prazosin, terazosin, doxazosin, tamsulosin, and alfuzosin). Although theoretically of benefit, bethanecol, a cholinergic agonist, has not been demonstrated effective in improving bladder emptying in well-done trials. In addition, it causes numerous bothersome (e.g., muscle and abdominal cramping and diarrhea) and potentially life-threatening adverse effects and should not be used in patients with asthma or heart disease.[24]

Urethral Underactivity

❺ Urethral underactivity, or SUI, may be aggravated by agents with α-adrenergic receptor blocking activity, including prazosin, terazosin, doxazosin, tamsulosin, alfuzosin, methyldopa, clonidine, guanfacine, guanadrel, and labetalol. The goal of therapy is to improve the urethral closure mechanism by stimulating α-adrenergic receptors in the smooth muscle of the bladder neck and proximal urethra, enhancing the supportive structures underlying the urethral epithelium, or enhancing the positive effects of serotonin and norepinephrine in the afferent and efferent pathways of the micturition reflex. There is no role for medications in the management of SUI after radical prostatectomy.[112]

Estrogens Local and systemic estrogens have been considered the mainstays of pharmacologic management of SUI since the 1940s. Estrogens are believed to work via several mechanisms, including enhancement of the proliferation of urethral epithelium, local circulation, and numbers and/or sensitivity of urogenital α-adrenergic receptors.[113] However, a trial has questioned whether estrogens exert a stimulatory effect on vaginal collagen production, at least over the short term.[114]

Open trials support the use of a variety of estrogens in the management of SUI: transdermal estradiol, conjugated estrogen vaginal cream, Estring, oral-conjugated estrogen, oral quinestradol, oral estriol, intramuscular estrogens, estriol vaginal suppositories, and oral estradiol.[115] Variable effects of estrogen treatment on urodynamic parameters, such as maximum urethral closure pressure, functional urethral length, and pressure transmission ratio, have been noted in these studies.

Results of four placebo-controlled comparative trials have not been as favorable, finding no significant clinical or urodynamic effects for oral estrogen compared with placebo.[116–119] In fact, observational studies have documented that estrogen use is associated with an increased risk of UI compared with that in nonusers.[120–123] Systemic estrogen therapy is associated with numerous adverse effects, including mastodynia, uterine bleeding, nausea, thromboembolism, cardiac and cerebrovascular ischemic events, and enhancement of the risk of certain cancers.[98] If estrogens are to be used for treatment of SUI, only topical products should be administered. Estrogen use is best justified when SUI exists with urethritis or vaginitis due to estrogen deficiency.

α-Adrenergic Receptor Agonists Numerous open trials have supported the use of a variety of α-adrenergic receptor agonists in SUI, including ephedrine, norfenefrine, phenylpropanolamine, and midodrine.[115] Phenylpropanolamine was withdrawn from the U.S. market in late 2000 because of a risk for stroke in women using the agent.[124] Some patients may have leftover supplies of this agent or may obtain it from international sources. If so, individuals with the contraindications listed below (especially coronary artery disease and/or cardiac arrhythmias) should be warned against self-treatment with this or other α-adrenergic receptor agonists.

Placebo-controlled comparative trials with phenylpropanolamine, norfenefrine, and norephedrine support the modest efficacy of these agents for treatment of mild or moderate SUI.[115,125] These agents have been found to variably affect maximum urethral closure pressure and functional urethral length.

Adverse effects include hypertension, headache, dry mouth, nausea, insomnia, and restlessness.[98] Contraindications to the use of these agents include the presence of hypertension, tachyarrhythmias, coronary artery disease, myocardial infarction, cor pulmonale, hyperthyroidism, renal failure, and narrow-angle glaucoma.

Usual doses are ephedrine 25 to 50 mg four times daily (25 mg twice daily in elders), pseudoephedrine 60 mg three times daily (15–30 mg three times daily in elders), and phenylephrine 10 mg four times daily (see Table 88–4).

Several studies have evaluated whether the clinical and urodynamic effects of a combination of estrogen and an α-adrenergic receptor agonist exceed those of the individual therapies in SUI.[126–130] In general, combination therapy has resulted in somewhat superior clinical and urodynamic responses compared with monotherapy, including severity of complaints, amount of urine lost per episode, number of daily voluntary micturitions, number of leakage episodes per day, patient preference, pad use, maximum urethral closure pressure, functional urethral length, and pressure transmission ratio.

Duloxetine Duloxetine, a dual inhibitor of serotonin and norepinephrine reuptake, was approved in 2004 for treatment of depression and painful diabetic neuropathy.[131] Its use for treatment of SUI (for which the drug is approved by European authorities but not by the U.S. FDA) is based on studies in rats and cats demonstrating that central serotoninergic and noradrenergic regions are involved in ascending and descending control of urethral smooth muscle and the external urethral sphincter. These mechanisms facilitate the bladder-to-sympathetic reflex pathway, increasing urethral and external urethral sphincter muscle tone during the storage phase. Data documenting this control mechanism in humans are limited. The mean terminal disposition half-life, clearance, and volume of distribution of duloxetine in healthy volunteers are 10 to 12 hours, 114 to 119 L/h, and 1787 to 1,943 L, respectively. The drug is extensively metabolized to inactive metabolites (via oxidation at the 4, 5, and/or 6 positions in the naphthyl ring, followed by further oxidation or via methylation) with elimination in the urine as conjugated metabolites. CYP 2D6 and 1A2 are involved in the ring oxidations. This involvement was demonstrated in studies of the interaction of duloxetine with the CYP 2D6 substrate desipramine (wherein desipramine's peak plasma concentration, AUC, and terminal disposition half-life were increased 1.7-, 2.9-, and 1.9-fold, respectively, and clearance fell by 66% during concurrent therapy) and the CYP

2D6 inhibitor paroxetine (wherein duloxetine's peak plasma concentration, AUC, and terminal disposition half-life increased 1.6-, 1.6-, and 1.3-fold, respectively, and clearance fell 37% during concurrent therapy). Fluvoxamine, a CYP 1A2 inhibitor, increased duloxetine's peak plasma concentration, AUC, and terminal disposition half-life by over 5-fold, 2.5-fold, and 3-fold, respectively. Thus, clinicians must be careful when prescribing duloxetine concurrently with CYP 2D6 and 1A2 substrates or inhibitors. The effect of advancing age on duloxetine pharmacokinetics is not clinically significant. Moderate hepatic dysfunction (Child-Pugh class B) significantly affects duloxetine disposition, increasing mean AUC and terminal disposition half-life by 5-fold and 3-fold, respectively, and reducing clearance 85% compared with controls. Mild or moderate renal impairment (creatinine clearance 30–80 mL/min) does not affect drug disposition. In severe renal impairment (hemodialysis patients), mean peak plasma concentration and AUC both are increased 100%, whereas metabolite concentrations are increased up to 900%.

Results of six large clinical trials with duloxetine in SUI have been published. All were double-blinded, randomized, placebo-controlled, and parallel group in design. Compared with placebo, duloxetine therapy produced significant reductions in incontinence episode frequency and number of micturitions per day, improvement in Incontinence Quality of Life questionnaire scores and patient self-assessment, and increase in mean micturition interval. Results were independent of baseline UI severity (severity based on incontinent episode frequency). Significant intergroup differences were seen by week 4. However, cure rates were generally not improved by duloxetine. When evaluating the absolute differences between treatments, the actual benefit of duloxetine was generally quite modest.

A randomized, placebo-controlled clinical trial evaluated the effects of duloxetine (80 mg daily), pelvic floor muscle training (PFMT), and the combination of both modalities on incontinent episode frequency, incontinence-related quality of life, pad use, and patient global impression of change. Sham PFMT was used in the placebo group. Results indicated that duloxetine plus PFMT probably were additive in effect and that combination therapy afforded greater improvement than either monotherapy.[132]

Although duloxetine is an encouraging development in the pharmacologic management of SUI, its adverse event profile may make adherence problematic. In the SUI trials, treatment/emergent adverse events occurred in 68% to 93% of duloxetine and 50% to 72% of placebo recipients. Premature study withdrawal rates (due to adverse events) were 12% to 33% for duloxetine and 2% to 8% for placebo. The frequencies of individual events in duloxetine recipients were nausea 9% to 46%, headache 7% to 27%, insomnia 13% to 14%, constipation 4% to 27%, dry mouth 4% to 22%, dizziness 8% to 16%, fatigue 10% to 18%, somnolence 8% to 13%, vomiting 6% to 13%, and diarrhea 4% to 6%. Of interest, the drug may be associated with small increases in blood pressure (like venlafaxine, another dual reuptake inhibitor) and withdrawal symptoms (sleep disturbances).

Despite these negatives, duloxetine is the first drug approved by a regulatory agency for treating SUI. Based on studies conducted to date, a dosage regimen of 40 to 80 mg/day (in one or two doses) appears reasonable. Initiating therapy with 40 mg daily for 2 weeks and then increasing to 80 mg daily (rather than initiating therapy with 80 mg daily) reduces the risks of nausea, dizziness, and premature drug discontinuation.[133] If the drug is to be stopped, it should be withdrawn slowly, reducing the dose by 50% for 2 weeks before discontinuation.[133]

Overflow Incontinence

Overflow incontinence secondary to benign or malignant prostatic hyperplasia may be amenable to pharmacotherapy. For management of malignant prostatic disease, see Chap. 134. The pharmacotherapy of BPH is discussed in Chap. 87.

CURRENT CONTROVERSY

The optimal approach to pharmacotherapy of SUI is unclear. Although not supported by evidence-based medicine, many clinicians initiate a trial of topical estrogen, followed by addition of an α-adrenergic receptor agonist in estrogen nonresponders unless contraindicated. Based on available data, duloxetine is the drug of choice for treatment of SUI, provided it is tolerated.

SURGICAL TREATMENT

Only rarely does surgery play a role in the initial management of UI.[134] In the absence of secondary complications from UI (e.g., skin breakdown or infection), the decision to surgically treat symptomatic UI should be based on the premise that the degree of bother or lifestyle compromise to the patient is great enough to warrant an elective operation, and that nonoperative therapy either is undesired or has been ineffective.

Successful application of surgery depends most on defining the underlying abnormalities responsible for UI (bladder vs urethra, underactivity vs overactivity). Once the underlying factors are determined, other considerations come into play: renal function, sexual function, severity of leakage, history of abdominal or pelvic surgery, presence of concurrent abdominal or pelvic pathology requiring surgical correction, and finally the patient's suitability for, and willingness to accept the risks of, surgery.

When patients with uncomplicated SUI become dissatisfied with the initial management approaches of pelvic floor exercises, medications, and/or behavioral modification,[134] surgical treatment assumes the primary role.

Surgical correction of female SUI (urethral underactivity) is directed toward either (1) repositioning the urethra and/or creating a backboard of support, or otherwise stabilizing the urethra and bladder neck in a well-supported retropubic (intraabdominal) position that is receptive to changes in intraabdominal pressure; or (2) creating coaptation and/or compression or otherwise augmenting the urethral resistance provided by the intrinsic sphincteric unit, with (i.e., sling) or without (i.e., periurethral collagen and other injectables) urethral and bladder neck support.

In men, SUI can be treated surgically with collagen or the artificial urinary sphincter. The vast majority of collagen injections in men are performed in a retrograde fashion under direct vision through a cystoscope. However, a transabdominal, transvesical, suprapubic antegrade approach also has been used.[135] The artificial urinary sphincter is generally considered to be the gold standard for treatment of male SUI. Placement of this manually operated silicone device has been associated with very high long-term success and satisfaction rates.[136]

Most patients with UUI are managed nonsurgically with a combination of behavioral modification, pelvic floor exercises, and pharmacologic therapy. Only rarely is surgery applied to the problem of UUI. Surgery of UUI may involve bladder denervation, implantation of a sacral nerve stimulator (neuromodulation), or augmentation (enlargement) cystoplasty.

Few surgical treatments for bladder underactivity are effective. After an appropriate evaluation for reversible causes is performed, the most effective management of this condition is intermittent self-catheterization performed by the patient or a caregiver three or four times per day. Sacral nerve stimulation (neuromodulation) has shown some efficacy in this patient population, but success rates for detrusor underactivity (nonobstructive urinary retention) are inferior to those seen with urinary frequency and urgency. Proper patient selection for this therapy remains poorly defined. Alternative methods of management that are less satisfactory or more invasive include indwelling urethral or suprapubic catheters and urinary diversion.

Urethral overactivity is most commonly caused by anatomic obstruction. Anatomic obstruction in men is most often caused by benign prostatic enlargement (see Chap. 87).

Rarely, bladder outlet obstruction is caused by a functional obstruction at the level of the bladder neck. Hypertrophy of the smooth muscle fibers at the level of the bladder neck in men and women may result in obstruction to the flow of urine. In patients who do not respond to pharmacologic therapy with α-adrenergic receptor antagonists, endoscopic incision using the cystoscope is highly effective in treating this very uncommon condition.

EVALUATION OF THERAPEUTIC OUTCOMES

❻ During long-term management of UI, patient-specific clinical signs and symptoms of most distress ("bother") to the individual must be monitored. A daily diary may be useful in this regard. Some of the short-form instruments used in incontinence research for measuring symptom impact and condition-specific quality of life can be used in clinical monitoring. In addition, quantitating the use of ancillary supplies, such as pads, may be useful. The goal of therapy is to minimize the signs and symptoms of most bother to the patient, as well as the use of pads and other ancillary supplies or devices. Total elimination of UI signs and symptoms may not be possible, and patients and practitioners need to mutually establish realistic goals of therapy. Because the therapies for UI frequently have nuisance adverse effects (e.g., anticholinergic effects such as xerostomia, xerophthalmia, and constipation) that may compromise regimen adherence, the presence and severity of adverse effects must be carefully elicited at each visit to the healthcare practitioner. Emergence of adverse effects may necessitate drug dosage adjustment or use of alternative strategies (e.g., chewing sugarless gum, sucking on hard sugarless candy, or use of saliva substitutes in xerostomia) or even drug discontinuation.

ABBREVIATIONS

AUC: area under the plasma or serum concentration-versus-time curve

BPH: benign prostatic hyperplasia

CYP: cytochrome P450

DD01: 5-hydroxymethyl metabolite of tolterodine

DEO: *N*-desethyloxybutynin

IR: immediate-release

LA: long-acting

SUI: stress urinary incontinence

TDS: transdermal system

UI: urinary incontinence

UUI: urge urinary incontinence

XL: extended-release

REFERENCES

1. Abrams P, Cardozo L, Fall M, et al. The standardization of terminology of lower urinary tract function: Report from the standardization sub-committee of the International Continence Society. Neurourol Urodyn 2002;21:167–178.
2. Arnold EP, Burgio K, Diokno AC, et al. Epidemiology and natural history of urinary incontinence (UI). In: Abrams P, Khoury S, Wein AJ, eds. Incontinence. Plymouth, United Kingdom: Plymbridge Distributors, 1999:199–226.
3. Simeonova Z, Milsom I, Kullendorff AM, et al. The prevalence of urinary incontinence and its influence on the quality of life in women from an urban Swedish population. Acta Obstet Gynecol Scand 1999;78:546–551.
4. Kobelt F, Kirchberger I, Malone-Lee J. Quality-of-life aspects of the overactive bladder and the effect of treatment with tolterodine. BJU Int 1999;83:583–590.
5. DuBeau CF, Kiely DK, Resnick NM. Quality of life impact of urge incontinence in older persons: A new measure and conceptual structure. J Am Geriatr Soc 1999;47:989–994.
6. Diokno AC, Brock BM, Brown MB, et al. Prevalence of urinary incontinence and other urological symptoms in the noninstitutionalized elderly. J Urol 1986;136:1022–1025.
7. Brown JS, Nyberg LM, Kusek JW, et al. Proceedings of the National Institute of Diabetes, Digestive and Kidney Diseases International Symposium on Epidemiologic Issues in Urinary Incontinence in Women. Am J Obstet Gynecol 2003;188:S77–S88.
8. Ouslander JG, Kane RL, Abrass IB. Urinary incontinence in elderly nursing home patients. JAMA 1982;248:1194–1198.
9. Bump RC. Racial comparisons and contrasts in urinary incontinence and pelvic organ prolapse. Obstet Gynecol 1993;81:421–425.
10. Burgio KL, Matthews KA, Engel BT. Prevalence, incidence and correlates of urinary incontinence in healthy, middle-aged women. J Urol 1991;146:1255–1259.
11. Fliegner JR, Glenning PP. Seven years experience in the evaluation and management of patients with urge incontinence of urine. Aust N Z J Obstet Gynecol 1979;19:42–44.
12. Breakwell SL, Walker SN. Differences in physical health, social interaction and personal adjustment between continent and incontinent homebound aged women. J Community Health Nurs 1988;5:19–31.
13. Malmsten UG, Milsom I, Molander U, Norlen LJ. Urinary incontinence and lower urinary tract symptoms: An epidemiological study of men aged 45–99 years. J Urol 1997;158:1733–1737.
14. Andersson K-E, Wein AJ. Pharmacology of the lower urinary tract: basis for current and future treatments of urinary incontinence. Pharmacol Rev 2004;56:581–631.
15. Blaivas JG, Heritz DM. Classification, diagnostic evaluation and treatment overview. In: Blaivas JG, ed. Topics in Clinical Urology—Evaluation and Treatment of Urinary Incontinence. New York: Igaku-Shoin, 1996:22–45.
16. Kuh D, Cardozo L, Hardy R. Urinary incontinence in middle-aged women: Childhood enuresis and other lifetime risk factors in a British prospective cohort. J Epidemiol Community Health 1999;53:453–458.
17. Groutz A, Gordon D, Keidar R, et al. Stress urinary incontinence: Prevalence among nulliparous compared with primiparous and grand multiparous premenopausal women. Neurourol Urodyn 1999;18:419–425.
18. deGroat WC. A neurologic basis for the overactive bladder. Urology 1997;50(6A Suppl):36–52.
19. Brading AF. A myogenic basis for the overactive bladder. Urology 1997;50(6A Suppl):57–67.
20. Turner WH, Brading AF. Smooth muscle of the bladder in the normal and the diseased state: Pathology, diagnosis and treatment. Pharmacol Ther 1997;75:77–110.
21. Resnick NM, Yalla S. Detrusor hyperactivity with impaired contractile function. An unrecognized but common cause of incontinence in the elderly patient. JAMA 1987;257:3076–3081.
22. Rovner ES, Wein AJ. Today's treatment of overactive bladder and urge incontinence. Womens Health Prim Care 2000;3:179–192.
23. James M, Jackson S, Shepard A, Abrams P. Pure stress leakage symptomatology: Is it safe to discount detrusor instability? Br J Obstet Gynaecol 1999;106:1255–1258.
24. Abrams P, Cardozo L, Khoury S, Wein A, eds. Incontinence. Second International Consultation on Incontinence, 2nd ed. Plymouth, United Kingdom: Health Publications Ltd., 2002.
25. Ouslander JG, Schnelle JF, Uman G, et al. Does oxybutynin add to the effectiveness of prompted voiding for urinary incontinence among nursing home residents? A placebo-controlled trial. J Am Geriatr Soc 1995;43:610–617.
26. Burgio KL, Locher JL, Goode PS, et al. Behavioral vs drug treatment for urge urinary incontinence in older women: A randomized controlled trial. JAMA 1998;280:1995–2000.

27. Drutz HP, Appell RA, Gleason D, et al. Clinical efficacy and safety of tolterodine compared to oxybutynin and placebo in patients with overactive bladder. Int Urogynecol 1999;10:283–289.
28. Abrams P, Freeman R, Anderstrom C, Mattiasson A. Tolterodine, a new antimuscarinic agent: As effective but better tolerated than oxybutynin in patients with an overactive bladder. Br J Urol 1998;81:801–810.
29. Tapp AJ, Cardozo LD, Versi E, Cooper D. The treatment of detrusor instability in post-menopausal women with oxybutynin chloride: A double blind placebo controlled study. Br J Obstet Gynaecol 1990;97:1063–1064.
30. Riva D, Casolati E. Oxybutynin chloride in the treatment of female idiopathic bladder instability. Clin Exp Obstet Gynecol 1984;11:37–42.
31. Schmidt RA, The Oxybutynin XL Study Group. Efficacy of controlled-release, once-a-day oxybutynin chloride for urge urinary incontinence. Jerusalem, International Continence Society, Sept. 14–17, 1998:188.
32. ALZA Corporation. Ditropan XL (oxybutynin chloride) extended-release tablets. Data on file. Palo Alto, CA, 1999.
33. Pharmacia & Upjohn. Detrol (tolterodine) package insert. Kalamazoo, MI, October 2005.
34. Pharmacia & Upjohn. Detrol (tolterodine). Data on file. Kalamazoo, MI, 1998.
35. Appell RA. Clinical efficacy and safety of tolterodine in the treatment of overactive bladder: A pooled analysis. Urology 1997;50(Suppl 6A):90–96.
36. Chancellor M, Freedman S, Mitcheson HD, et al. Tolterodine, an effective and well tolerated treatment for urge incontinence and other overactive bladder symptoms. Clin Drug Invest 2000;19:83–91.
37. Rentzhog L, Stanton SL, Cardozo L, et al. Efficacy and safety of tolterodine in patients with detrusor instability: A dose-ranging study. Br J Urol 1998;81:42–48.
38. Millard R, Tuttle J, Moore K, et al. Clinical efficacy and safety of tolterodine compared to placebo in detrusor overactivity. J Urol 1999;161:1551–1555.
39. Appell RA, Sand P, Dmochowski R, et al. Prospective randomized controlled trial of extended-release oxybutynin chloride and tolterodine tartrate in the treatment of overactive bladder: Results of the OBJECT study. Mayo Clin Proc 2001;76:358–363.
40. Van Kerrebroeck P, Kreder K, Jonas U, et al. Tolterodine once daily: Superior efficacy and tolerability in the treatment of the overactive bladder. Urology 2001;57:414–421.
41. Malone-Lee JG, Walsh JB, Maugourd M-F. Tolterodine: A safe and effective treatment for older patients with overactive bladder. J Am Geriatr Soc 2001;49:700–705.
42. Dmochowski RR, Sand PK, Zinner NR, et al. Comparative efficacy and safety of transdermal oxybutynin and oral tolterodine versus placebo in previously treated patients with urge and mixed urinary incontinence. Urology 2003;62:237–242.
43. Dmochowski RR, Davila GW, Zinner NR, et al. Efficacy and safety of transdermal oxybutynin in patients with urge and mixed urinary incontinence. J Urol 2002;168:580–586.
44. Watson Pharma, Oxytrol (oxybutynin transdermal system) package insert. Morristown, NJ, June 2005.
45. Khullar V, Chapple C, Gabriel Z, Dooley JA. The effects of antimuscarinics on health-related quality of life in overactive bladder: A systematic review and meta-analysis. Urology 2006;68(Suppl 2A):38–48.
46. Nilsson CG, Lukkari E, Haarala M, et al. Comparison of a 10-mg controlled release oxybutynin tablet with a 5-mg oxybutynin tablet in urge incontinent patients. Neurourol Urodyn 1997;16:533–542.
47. Birns J, Malone Lee JG, and the Oxybutynin CR Study Group. Controlled-release oxybutynin maintains efficacy with a 43% reduction in side effects compared with conventional oxybutynin treatment. Neurourol Urodyn 1997;16:429–430.
48. Anderson RU, Mobley D, Blank B, et al. Once daily controlled versus immediate-release oxybutynin chloride for urge urinary incontinence. OROS Oxybutynin Study Group. J Urol 1999;161:1809–1812.
49. Katz IR, Sands LP, Bilker E, et al. Identification of medications that cause cognitive impairment in older people: The case of oxybutynin chloride. J Am Geriatr Soc 1998;46:8–13.
50. Kelleher CJ, Cardozo LD, Khullar S. A medium term analysis of the subjective efficacy of treatment for women with detrusor instability and low bladder compliance. Obstet Gynecol 1997;104:988–993.
51. Appell RA, Chancellor MB, Zobrist RH, et al. Pharmacokinetics, metabolism, and saliva output during transdermal and extended-release oxybutynin administration in healthy subjects. Mayo Clin Proc 2003;78:696–702.
52. Hughes KM, Lang JCT, Lazare R, et al. Measurement of oxybutynin and its N-desethyl metabolite in plasma and its application to pharmacokinetic studies in young, elderly and frail elderly volunteers. Xenobiotica 1992;22:859–869.
53. Amarenco G, Marquis P, McCarthy C, Richard F. Efficacy of oxybutynin on health related quality of life (HRQL) in 1701 women suffering from urinary urge incontinence (UUI). Eur Urol 1998;33(Suppl 1):32–38.
54. Ortho-McNeil Pharmaceuticals. Ditropan XL (oxybutynin chloride) extended-release tablets package insert. Raritan, NJ, June 2004.
55. Paine MF, Khalighi M, Fisher JM, et al. Characterisation of interintestinal and intraintestinal variations in human CYP3A-dependent metabolism. J Pharmacol Exp Ther 1997;283:1552–1562.
56. Gupta SK, Sathyan G. Pharmacokinetics of an oral once-a-day controlled-release oxybutynin formulation compared with immediate-release oxybutynin. J Clin Pharmacol 1999;39:289–296.
57. Buyse G, Waldeck K, Ver C, et al. Intravesical oxybutynin for neurogenic bladder: Less systemic side effects due to reduced first-pass metabolism. J Urol 1998;160:892–896.
58. Gleason DM, Susset J, White C. Evaluation of a new once-daily formulation of oxybutynin for the treatment of urinary urge incontinence. Urology 1999;54:420–423.
59. Susset JG, Gleason DM, White CF, et al. Open-label safety and dose conversion/determination of once-daily OROS oxybutynin chloride for urge urinary incontinence. J Urol 1998;159(Suppl):36.
60. Moore KH, Hay DM, Imrie AE, et al. Oxybutynin hydrochloride (3 mg) in the treatment of women with idiopathic detrusor instability. Br J Urol 1990;66:479–485.
61. Diokno AC, Appell RA, Sand PK, et al. Prospective, randomized, double-blind study of the efficacy and tolerability of the extended-release formulations of oxybutynin and tolterodine for overactive bladder: Results of the OPERA trial. Mayo Clin Proc 2003;78:687–695.
62. Sussman D, Garely A. Treatment of overactive bladder with once-daily extended-release tolterodine or oxybutynin: The Antimuscarinic Clinical Effectiveness Trial (ACET). Curr Med Res Opin 2002;18:177–184.
63. Guay DRP. Clinical pharmacokinetics of drugs used to treat urge incontinence. Clin Pharmacokinet 2003;42:1243–1285.
64. Zobrist RH, Schmid B, Feick A, et al. Pharmacokinetics of the R- and S-enantiomers of oxybutynin and N-desethyloxybutynin following oral and transdermal administration of the racemate in healthy volunteers. Pharm Res 2001;18:1029–1034.
65. Davila GW, Daugherty CA, Sanders SW. A short-term, multicenter, randomized double-blind dose titration study of the efficacy and anticholinergic side effects of transdermal compared to immediate release oral oxybutynin treatment of patients with urge urinary incontinence. J Urol 2001;166:140–145.
66. Dmochowski RR, Nitti V, Staskin D, Luber K, Appell R, Davila GW. Transdermal oxybutynin in the treatment of adults with overactive bladder: Combined results of two randomized clinical trials. World J Urol 2005;23:263–270.
67. Davila GW, Dmochowski RR, Sanders SW. Influence of age on improvements in overactive bladder symptoms and adverse events during oxybutynin transdermal system treatment [abstract]. Obstet Gynecol 2002;99(Suppl 1):103S-104S.
68. Leung HY, Yip SK, Cheon C, et al. A randomized trial of tolterodine and oxybutynin on tolerability and clinical efficacy for treating Chinese women with an overactive bladder. BJU Int 2002;90:375–380.
69. Malone-Lee J, Shaffu B, Anand C, Powell C. Tolterodine: Superior tolerability than and comparable efficacy to oxybutynin in individuals 50 years old or older with overactive bladder. A randomized controlled trial. J Urol 2001;165:1452–1456.
70. Zinner NR, Mattiason A, Stanton SL. Efficacy, safety, and tolerability of extended-release once-daily tolterodine treatment for overactive bladder in older versus younger patients. J Am Geriatr Soc 2002; 50:799–807.
71. Dmochowski R, Sathyan G, Ye C, et al. The pH effect of drug release from extended-release formulations of oxybutynin and tolterodine. Proceedings of the Second International Consultation on Incontinence. Paris, France, July 2001.
72. Dmochowski R, Chen A, Sathyan G, MacDiarmid S, Gidwani S, Gupta S. Effect of the proton pump inhibitor omeprazole on the pharmaco-

kinetics of extended-release formulations of oxybutynin and tolterodine. J Clin Pharmacol 2005;45:961–968.
73. Guay DRP. Trospium chloride: An update on a quaternary anticholinergic for treatment of urge urinary incontinence. Ther Clin Risk Manage 2005;1:157–166.
74. Rudy D, Cline K, Harris R, Goldberg K, Dmochowski R. Multicenter phase III trial studying trospium chloride in patients with overactive bladder. Urology 2006;67:275–280.
75. Esprit Pharma. Sanctura (trospium chloride) tablets package insert. East Brunswick, NJ, May 2004.
76. Cardozo L, Chapple CR, Toozs-Hobson P, et al. Efficacy of trospium chloride in patients with detrusor instability: a placebo-controlled, randomized, double-blind, multicentre clinical trial. BJU Int 2000;85:659–664.
77. Frohlich G, Bulitta M, Strosser W. Trospium chloride in patients with detrusor overactivity: meta-analysis of placebo-controlled, randomized, double-blind, multi-center clinical trials on the efficacy and safety of 20 mg trospium chloride twice daily. Int J Clin Pharmacol Ther 2002;40:295–303.
78. Junemann K-P, Fusgen I. Placebo-controlled, randomized, double-blind, multicentre clinical trial on the efficacy and tolerability of 1 × 40 mg and 2 × 40 mg trospium chloride (Spasmo-Lyt®) daily for 3 weeks in patients with urge-syndrome [abstract]. Neurourol Urodyn 1999;18:375–376.
79. Hofner K, Halaska M, Primus G, Al-Shukri S, Jonas U. Tolerability and efficacy of trospium chloride in a long-term treatment (52 weeks) in patients with urge-syndrome: A double-blind, controlled, multicentre clinical trial [abstract]. Neurourol Urodyn 2000;19:487–488.
80. Madersbacher H, Stohrer M, Richter R, Burgdorfer H, Hachen HJ, Murtz G. Trospium chloride versus oxybutynin: a randomized, double-blind, multicentre trial in the treatment of detrusor hyper-reflexia. Br J Urol 1995;75:452–456.
81. Junemann KP, Al-Shukri S. Efficacy and tolerability of trospium chloride and tolterodine in 234 patients with urge-syndrome: A double-blind, placebo-controlled, multicentre clinical trial [abstract]. Neurourol Urodyn 2000;19:488–490.
82. Halaska M, Ralph G, Wiedemann A, et al. Controlled, double-blind, multicentre clinical trial to investigate long-term tolerability and efficacy of trospium chloride in patients with detrusor instability. World J Urol 2003;20:392–399.
83. Zinner N, Gittelman M, Harris R, et al. Trospium chloride improves overactive bladder symptoms: a multicenter phase III trial. J Urol 2004;171:2311–2315.
84. Guay DRP. Drug forecast: Solifenacin: An investigational anticholinergic for overactive bladder. Consult Pharm 2004;19:437–444.
85. Kuipers ME, Krauwinkel WJ, Mulder H, Visser N. Solifenacin demonstrates high absolute bioavailability in healthy men. Drugs R D 2004;5:73–81.
86. Uchida T, Krauwinkel WJ, Mulder H, Smulders RA. Food does not affect the pharmacokinetics of solifenacin, a new muscarinic receptor antagonist: Results of a randomized crossover trial. Br J Clin Pharmacol 2004;58:4–7.
87. Smulders RA, Krauwinkel WJ, Swart PJ, Huang M. Pharmacokinetics and safety of solifenacin succinate in healthy young men. J Clin Pharmacol 2004;44:1023–1033.
88. Chapple CR, Arano P, Bosch JLHR, DeRidder D, Kraemer AEJL, Ridder AM. Solifenacin appears effective and well tolerated in patients with symptomatic idiopathic detrusor overactivity in a placebo- and tolterodine-controlled phase 2 dose-finding study. BJU Int 2004;93:71–77.
89. Chapple CR, Rechberger T, Al-Shukri S, et al. Randomized, double-blind placebo- and tolterodine-controlled trial of the once-daily antimuscarinic agent solifenacin in patients with symptomatic overactive bladder. BJU Int 2004;93:303–310.
90. Chapple CR, Martinez-Garcia R, Selvaggi L, et al. A comparison of the efficacy and tolerability of solifenacin succinate and extended release tolterodine at treating overactive bladder syndrome: results of the STAR trial. Eur Urol 2005;48:464–470.
91. Kelleher CJ, Cardozo L, Chapple CR, Haab F, Ridder AM. Improved quality of life in patients with overactive bladder symptoms treated with solifenacin. BJU Int 2005;95:81–85.
92. Wagg A, Wyndaele JJ, Sieber P. Efficacy and tolerability of solifenacin in elderly subjects with overactive bladder syndrome: a pooled analysis. Am J Geriatr Pharmacother 2006;4:14–24.
93. Guay DRP. Drug forecast: Darifenacin: Another investigational antimuscarinic for overactive bladder. Consult Pharm 2005;20:424–431.
94. Steers W, Corcos J, Foote F, Kralidis G. An investigation of dose titration with darifenacin, an M3-selective receptor antagonist. BJU Int 2005;95:580–586.
95. Foote J, Elhilali M. A multicenter, randomized, double-blind study of darifenacin versus tolterodine in the treatment of overactive bladder (OAB) [abstract]. Presented at the British Geriatrics Society meeting, Harrogate, UK, October 6–8, 2004:32.
96. Foote J, Glavind K, Kralidis G, Wyndaele JJ. Treatment of overactive bladder in the older patient: Pooled analysis of three phase III studies of darifenacin, an M_3 selective receptor antagonist. Eur Urol 2005;48:471–477.
97. Zinner N, Tuttle J, Marks L. Efficacy and tolerability of darifenacin, a muscarinic M3 selective receptor antagonist (M3SRA), compared with oxybutynin in the treatment of overactive bladder (OAB) [abstract]. World J Urol 2005;23:248–252.
98. Owens RG, Karram MM. Comparative tolerability of drug therapies used to treat incontinence and enuresis. Drug Saf 1998;2:123–139.
99. Milner G, Hills NF. A double-blind assessment of antidepressants in the treatment of 212 enuretic patients. Med J Aust 1968;1:943–947.
100. Castleden CM, George CF, Renwick AG, Asher MJ. Imipramine—A possible alternative to current therapy for urinary incontinence in the elderly. J Urol 1981;125:318–320.
101. Lose G, Jorgenson L, Thuriedborg P. Doxepin in the treatment of female detrusor overactivity: A randomized double-blind crossover study. J Urol 1989;142:1024–1026.
102. Deguecker J. Drug treatment of urinary incontinence in the elderly: Controlled trial with vasopressin and propantheline bromide. Gerontol Clin 1965;7:311–317.
103. Zorzitto ML, Jewett MAS, Fernie GR, et al. Effectiveness of propantheline bromide in the treatment of geriatric patients with detrusor instability. Neurourol Urodyn 1986;5:133–140.
104. Blaivas JG, Labib AB, Michalik SJ, Zayed AAH. Cystometric response to propantheline in detrusor hyperreflexia: Therapeutic implications. J Urol 1980;124:259–262.
105. Holmes DM, Montz FJ, Stanton SL. Oxybutynin versus propantheline in the management of detrusor instability: A patient-regulated variable dose trial. Br J Obstet Gynaecol 1989;96:607–612.
106. Thuroff JW, Bunke B, Ebner A, et al. Randomized, double-blind, multicentre trial on treatment of frequency, urgency and incontinence related to detrusor hyperactivity: Oxybutynin versus propantheline versus placebo. J Urol 1991;145:813–817.
107. Beck RP, Arnusch D, King C. Results in treating 210 patients with detrusor overactivity incontinence of urine. Am J Obstet Gynecol 1976;125:593–596.
108. Castleden CM, Duffin HM, Millar AW. Dicyclomine hydrochloride in detrusor instability: A controlled clinical pilot study. J Clin Exp Gerontol 1987;9:265–270.
109. Herbison P, Hay-Smith J, Ellis G, Moore K. Effectiveness of anticholinergic drugs compared with placebo in the treatment of overactive bladder: systematic review. BMJ 2003;326:841–844.
110. Schurch B, DeSeze M, Denys P, et al. Botulinum toxin type A is a safe and effective treatment for neurogenic urinary incontinence: results of a single treatment, randomized, placebo controlled 6-month study. J Urol 2005;174:196–200.
111. Grosse J, Kramer G, Stohrer M. Success of repeat detrusor injections of botulinum A toxin in patients with severe neurogenic detrusor overactivity and incontinence. Eur Urol 2005;47:653–659.
112. Peyromaure M, Ravery V, Boccon-Gibod L. The management of stress urinary incontinence after radical prostatectomy. BJU Int 2002;90:155–161.
113. Schreiter F, Fuchs P, Stockamp K. Estrogenic sensitivity of α-receptors in the urethral musculature. Urol Int 1976;31:13–19.
114. Jackson S, James M, Abrams P. The effect of oestradiol on vaginal collagen metabolism in postmenopausal women with genuine stress incontinence. BJOG 2002;109:339–344.
115. Guay DRP. Incontinence. Clin Trends Pharm Pract 2002;June:entire issue.
116. Samsioe G, Jansson I, Mellstrom D, Svanborg A. Occurrence, nature, and treatment of urinary incontinence in a 70-year-old female population. Maturitas 1985;7:335–342.

117. Wilson PD, Faragher B, Butler B, et al. Treatment with oral piperazine oestrone sulphate for genuine stress incontinence in postmenopausal women. Br J Obstet Gynaecol 1987;94:568–574.
118. Jackson S, Shepherd A, Brookes S, Abrams P. The effect of oestrogen supplementation on post-menopausal urinary stress incontinence: A double-blind placebo-controlled trial. Br J Obstet Gynaecol 1999;106:711–718.
119. Jackson S, Shepherd A, Abrams P. Does oestrogen supplementation improve the symptoms of postmenopausal urinary stress incontinence? [abstract] Neurourol Urodyn 1997;16:350–351.
120. Brown JS, Seeley DG, Fong J, et al. Urinary incontinence in older women: Who is at risk? Study of Osteoporotic Fractures Research Group. Obstet Gynecol 1996;87:715–721.
121. Thom DH, van den Eeden SK, Brown JS. Evaluation of parturition and other reproductive variables as risk factors for urinary incontinence in later life. Obstet Gynecol 1997;90:983–989.
122. Diokno AC, Brock BM, Herzog AR, Bromberg J. Medical correlates of urinary incontinence. Urology 1990;36:129–138.
123. Grady D, Brown JS, Vittinghoff E, et al., and HERS Research Group. Postmenopausal hormones and incontinence: The Heart & Estrogen/Progestin Replacement Study. Obstet Gynecol 2001;97:116–120.
124. Kernan WN, Viscoli CM, Brass LM, et al. Phenylpropanolamine and the risk of hemorrhagic stroke. N Engl J Med 2000:343:1826–1832.
125. Alhasso A, Glazener CM, Pickard R, N'dow J. Adrenergic drugs for urinary incontinence in adults. Cochrane Databse Syst Rev 2005;3:CD001842.
126. Ahlstrom K, Sandahl B, Sjoberg B, et al. Effect of combined treatment with phenylpropanolamine and estriol, compared with estriol treatment alone, in postmenopausal women with stress urinary incontinence. Gynecol Obstet Invest 1990;30:37–43.
127. Kinn A-C, Lindskog M. Estrogens and phenylpropanolamine in combination for stress urinary incontinence in postmenopausal women. Urology 1988;32:273–280.
128. Ek A, Andersson K-E, Gullberg B, Ulmsten U. Effects of oestradiol and combined norephedrine and oestradiol treatment on female stress incontinence. Zentralbl Gynakol 1980;102:839–844.
129. Kiesswetter H, Hennrich F, Englisch M. Clinical and urodynamic assessment of pharmacologic therapy of stress incontinence. Urol Int 1983;38:58–63.
130. Beisland HO, Fossberg E, Moer A, Sander S. Urethral sphincteric insufficiency in postmenopausal females: Treatment with phenylpropanolamine and estriol separately and in combination. Urol Int 1984; 39:211–216.
131. Guay DRP. Duloxetine in the management of stress urinary incontinence. Am J Geriatr Pharmacother 2005;3:25–38.
132. Ghoneim GM, VanLeeuwen JS, Elser DM, et al. A randomized controlled trial of duloxetine alone, pelvic floor muscle training alone, combined treatment and no active treatment in women with stress urinary incontinence. J Urol 2005;173:1647–1653.
133. Bump R, Yalcin I, Voss S. The effect of duloxetine dose escalation and tapering on the incidence of adverse events (AE) in women with stress urinary incontinence (SUI) [abstract]. Neurourol Urodyn 2005;24: 582.
134. Urinary Incontinence Guideline Panel. Urinary Incontinence in Adults: Clinical Practice Guideline. AHCPR Pub. No. 92–0038. Agency for Health Care Policy and Research, Public Health Service, U.S. Department of Health and Human Services: Rockville, MD, 1992.
135. Klutke CG, Tiemann DD, Nadler RB, Andriole GL. Early results with antegrade collagen injection for post-radical prostatectomy stress urinary incontinence. J Urol 1996;156:1703–1706.
136. Litwillwer SE, Kim KB, Fone PD, et al. Post-prostatectomy incontinence and the artificial urinary sphincter: A long-term study of patient satisfaction and criteria for success. J Urol 1996;156:1975–1980.

SECTION 11
IMMUNOLOGIC DISORDERS

CHAPTER 89

Function and Evaluation of the Immune System

PHILIP D. HALL AND NICOLE A. WEIMERT

KEY CONCEPTS

1. After activation, dendritic cells express higher concentrations of major histocompatibility complex (MHC) class II molecules B7–1, B7–2, CD40, ICAM-1, and LFA-3 and produce more interleukin-12 than other antigen-presenting cells. This may explain why in vitro dendritic cells are the most efficient antigen-presenting cell.

2. A T lymphocyte expresses hundreds of T-cell receptors. All T-cell receptors expressed on the surface of an individual T lymphocyte have the same antigen specificity.

3. A B lymphocyte can simultaneously express membrane immunoglobulin as immunoglobulin (Ig)M (monomeric) or IgD with the same variable region (i.e., antigen binding site). The B lymphocyte then can secrete different isotypes (e.g., IgM [pentamer], IgA, IgG, IgE) with the same variable region as the membrane immunoglobulin.

4. A serum protein electrophoresis determines the total concentration of circulating immunoglobulins (i.e., IgG, IgA, IgM, IgD, and IgE). To determine the concentration of the individual isotypes, isotype quantification is necessary. Most clinical laboratories quantitate only IgG, IgM, and IgA because they are the most prevalent isotypes in the bloodstream. In patients with allergic disorders, quantification of IgE may be useful. Depending on the clinical laboratory, results may come back in international units per milliliter or milligrams per deciliter for IgE.

5. An understanding of the mechanism by which immunomodulators act and of the immune system allows the clinician to anticipate potential adverse effects. The benefit of manipulating immune responses must be balanced with the potential consequences and long-term sequelae of such manipulation.

The primary function of the immune system is to protect the body against invading pathogens. The immune system evolves and adapts based on its exposure environment. To undergo these processes, the immune system exhibits specificity, memory, mobility, replicability, and redundancy. *Specificity* indicates the immune system can distinguish between non–cross-reacting antigens. *Memory* ensures a quicker and more vigorous response to a subsequent but similar pathogen. *Mobility* of the elements of the immune system enables local reactions to provide systemic protection. *Replication* of the cellular components of the immune system amplifies the immune response. *Redundancy* refers to the immune system's ability to produce components with the same biologic effect but produced from multiple cell lines, such as inflammatory cytokines. These characteristics make the immune system a formidable defense against offending pathogens. They also make the immune system difficult to control with pharmacotherapy.

Learning objectives, review questions, and other resources can be found at **www.pharmacotherapyonline.com.**

The immune system includes two functional divisions: (a) the *innate* or nonspecific, which encodes evolutionary genes aimed at providing rapid responses against nonmammalian targets; and (b) the *adaptive* or specific, which utilizes cells that can genetically rearrange their DNA to create specific structures that bind individual antigens or proteins (Table 89–1).[1] Despite this simple separation, these divisions heavily interact.[2] Awareness of each component of the immune system and the consequences of disrupting homeostasis must be understood in order to appropriately dose, administer, and monitor the effect of medications given to manipulate immune responses.

METHODS TO DISTINGUISH SELF FROM NONSELF

The immune system is designed to attack and destroy a broad spectrum of foreign antigens/pathogens. However, the immune system must be able to distinguish self from nonself, termed self-*tolerance*, in order to avoid unleashing its components onto self tissues.[3] The body uses many tactics to avoid attacking itself; failure of self-tolerance may lead to the development of an autoimmune disease.

INNATE IMMUNE SYSTEM

Physical Defense

Physical and chemical defenses are the most rudimentary form of innate immunity and the first line of defense against invading pathogens. The skin, the largest organ of the body, has the primary

TABLE 89-1 Functional Divisions of the Immune System

	Innate	Adaptive
Exterior defenses	Skin, mucus, cilia, normal flora, saliva, low pH of the stomach, skin, genitourinary tract	None
Specificity	Limited and fixed	Extensive
Memory	None	Yes
Time to response	Hours	Days
Soluble factors	Lysozymes, complement, C-reactive protein, interferons, mannose-binding lectin, antimicrobial peptides[a]	Antibodies, cytokines
Cells	Neutrophils, monocytes, macrophages, natural killer cells, eosinophils	B lymphocytes, T lymphocytes

[a]Cathelicidins, α-defensins, β-defensins.

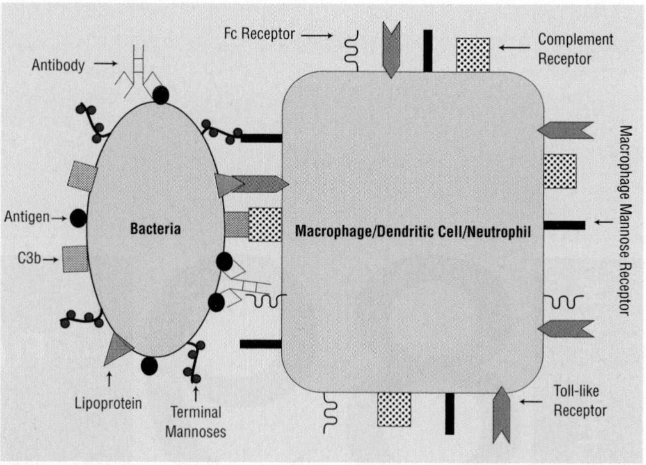

FIGURE 89-1. Phagocytosis of bacteria by macrophages, dendritic cells, and neutrophils. Macrophages, dendritic cells, and neutrophils recognize bacteria opsonized (coated) with antibody or complement (C3b). On the surface of macrophages, dendritic cells, and neutrophils reside receptors for antibody (Fc receptors) and complement (CR1, CR3, CR4). In addition, these cells may recognize the bacteria by pattern recognition receptors on the surface of macrophages, dendritic cells, and neutrophils. Pattern recognition receptors include toll-like receptors, scavenger receptors, and mannose receptors.

role of providing a physical defense. Alterations in the skin, such as burns and abrasions, allow an easy portal of entry for pathogens. The gastrointestinal tract also provides physical defense. The low pH of the stomach (pH 1–2) is inhospitable to most organisms. The rapid turnover of intestinal cells limits systemic infection as cells, including infected cells, are sloughed frequently. Drugs, such as cell-cycle specific antineoplastics that disrupt the sloughing process, leave the patient at increased risk for infections. Likewise, the respiratory tract has its forms of physical defense. The mucus coating the epithelial cells serves in part to prevent microorganisms from adhering to cell surfaces, and the cilia lining the epithelium of the lungs help to repel inhaled organisms. The combination of cilia, mucus, and reactive coughing provides a natural barrier to invasion via the respiratory tract. Other examples of mechanical or nonspecific defenses include normal urine flow, lysozymes in tears and saliva, and the normal flora in the throat, lower gastrointestinal tract, and genitourinary tract. Disruption of the normal physical defense system through mechanical ventilation can, for example, place the host at substantial risk for penetration by a pathogenic organism.[4]

Innate Immune Response

If an infectious pathogen invades and is able to infiltrate through a host's physical defense system, innate immunity is used to halt progression of the infection. Innate immunity is present from birth and utilizes a preexisting but limited repertoire of receptors to recognize and destroy pathogens. Innate immune cells include subgroups of leukocytes, specifically, monocytes/macrophages, neutrophils, basophils, mast cells, and eosinophils. When stimulated by a foreign pathogen, mast cells and basophils secrete inflammatory mediators. Monocytes/macrophages, neutrophils, mast cells, and eosinophils act as phagocytes, which allow them to recognize, internalize, and destroy invading pathogens. This process may occur in two ways: opsonin-dependent or opsonin-independent phagocytosis. For opsonin-dependent phagocytosis, antibody (e.g., immunoglobulin [Ig]G), complement (e.g., C3b), or lectin (e.g., C-reactive protein) coat, or opsonize, the infectious pathogens. Once the pathogen is opsonized, the antibody, complement, or lectin binds to the receptors on the phagocyte (Fig. 89–1) and activates the phagocytic process. For opsonin-independent phagocytosis, innate leukocytes utilize pattern recognition receptors. Pattern recognition receptors recognize highly conserved structures present on a large number of microorganisms. These highly conserved structures are essential for the microorganism's survival or pathogenicity. The pattern recognition receptors include the macrophage mannose receptor, macrophage scavenger receptor, and members of the toll-like receptor family. Pattern recognition receptors on the phagocytes directly recognize ligands (Table 89–2) on the surfaces of infectious pathogens, leading to immediate phagocytosis of the pathogen (Fig. 89–1). Toll-like receptors are a family of pattern recognition receptors on the cell surface of innate leukocytes. To date, 11 toll-like receptors have been identified in humans. They recognize a broad spectrum of antigens ranging from lipopolysaccharide and flagellin on bacteria to zymosan on yeast to double-stranded RNA from RNA viruses (Table 89–2). Binding of the ligand to the toll-like receptors allows the phagocyte to recognize and engulf the pathogen. This binding of toll-like receptors to its ligand also results in secretion of chemokines, inflammatory cytokines, and antimicrobial peptides as well as increased expression of costimulatory proteins (e.g., B7) and the major histocompatibility complex (MHC) proteins by the phagocyte. This leads to the recruitment and activation of antigen-specific lymphocytes.[2,5,6] Other pattern recognition receptors that mediate phagocytosis include MARCO and DEC205.

Cells of the Innate Immune System

Neutrophils, eosinophils, and basophils are considered granulocytes because of the presence of numerous cytoplasm granules in these cells that contain inflammatory mediators or digestive enzymes. Neutrophils compose the majority of leukocytes in the bloodstream. They are polymorphonuclear cells, which serve as the primary human defense against invasive bacteria. Neutrophils migrate from the bloodstream into infected or inflamed tissue in response to chemotactic factors such as interleukin (IL)-8 and C3a and C5a, breakdown products of complement. In this migration, a process termed *chemotaxis*, neutrophils reach the site of inflammation and then recognize, adhere to, and phagocytose pathogens. Via the complement and antibody receptors located on its surface, neutro-

TABLE 89-2 Ligands for Pattern Recognition Receptors

Pathogen Ligand	Type of Organism
Lipoteichoic acid	Gram-positive organisms
Lipopolysaccharide	Gram-negative organisms
Mannose	Fungi, gram-positive, gram-negative
Double-stranded RNA	RNA viruses
Triacyl lipopeptides	Gram-positive, gram-negative
Peptidoglycans	Gram-positive
Bacterial flagella	Various

phils can recognize and engulf pathogens opsonized with complement or IgG (antibody). During phagocytosis, the engulfed pathogen is internalized within the phagocyte into a cytoplasmic lysosome. The neutrophil then releases its granular contents into lysosomes and generates the release of oxidative metabolites that destroy the engulfed pathogens.[7] Neutrophils also can recognize pathogens via toll-like receptors.

Eosinophils are also granulocytic cells involved in innate immunity. They exhibit motility and migrate from the blood into the tissues. Eosinophils play a less significant role in combating bacterial infections, but they play a major role against nonphagocytable multicellular pathogens, such as parasites. After activation via high-affinity receptor for IgE (i.e., Fc), eosinophils exocytose their granules, which release basic proteins or reactive oxygen species into the microenvironment, causing lysis of the parasite. In addition to Fc receptors, eosinophils express lower levels of complement receptor 3 and Fcγ for IgG than neutrophils. The high affinity of eosinophils for IgE contribute to their role in the pathogenesis of allergic disorders (i.e., allergic asthma).[8]

Macrophages and monocytes are mononuclear cells capable of phagocytosis. Tissue macrophages arise from the migration of monocytes from the bloodstream into the tissues. Macrophages differ from monocytes by possessing an increased number of Fc and complement receptors. Macrophages are found within specific tissues, such as the liver, spleen, gastrointestinal tract, lymph nodes, brain, bone, and connective tissue. These specific types of macrophages often are called *histiocytes* or are referred to by a specialized name depending on where they are found (e.g., Kupffer cells in the liver, osteoclasts in the bone, microglial cells in the central nervous system). The term *reticuloendothelial system* was commonly used to refer to macrophages found in reticular connective tissue, but the preferred nomenclature now is the *mononuclear phagocyte system*.[9]

Despite the first description in 1868 of Langerhans cells, a type of dendritic cell found in the skin, our current understanding of the biologic function of dendritic cells did not develop until the 1990s. Before pathogen recognition, most dendritic cells are in an immature/resting state with limited ability to activate T lymphocytes, but they express numerous receptors (e.g., Fc receptors of IgG and IgE, macrophage mannose receptor, toll-like receptors) enabling rapid antigen recognition. Following antigen recognition and particle engulfment, dendritic cells become activated and dramatically increase their expression of the MHC class II, B7, CD40, and adhesion molecules. Dendritic cells then begin to migrate through the tissues toward lymphoid organs (e.g., spleen, lymph nodes) to present antigen to T lymphocytes, which activates the adaptive immune system.[10]

❶ In addition to phagocytosing pathogens, macrophages and dendritic cells act as antigen-presenting cells (APCs) to stimulate the adaptive (specific) system. Macrophages and dendritic cells internalize the organism, digest it into small peptide fragments, and then combine these antigenic fragments together with MHC proteins. Once the APC has formed the antigen/MHC complex, the APC places the complex on its surface. This surface complex then can be recognized by the T-cell receptor (TCR) on the surface of a T lymphocyte. Recognition of the antigen/MHC complex by the TCR is the first step in activation of the T lymphocyte (Fig. 89–2). Other cells (B lymphocytes and mast cells) also can act as APCs (Fig. 89–3).[9–11]

Mast cells and basophils act primarily by releasing inflammatory mediators. Mast cells are tissue cells predominately associated with

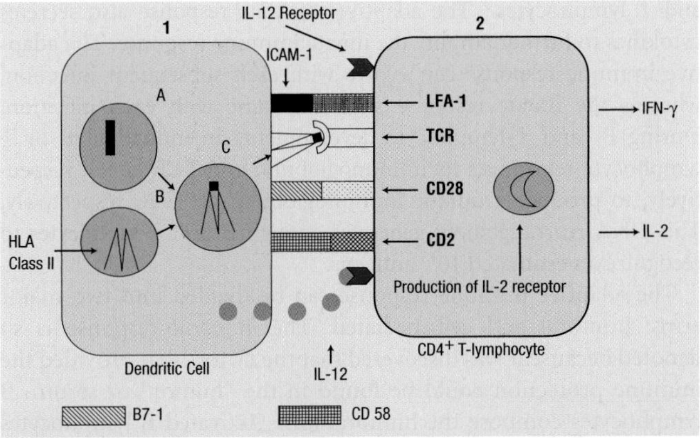

FIGURE 89-2. Induction of T-helper type 1 (TH_1) response. *1.* The antigen-presenting cell, in this case a dendritic cell, engulfs the pathogen by any of numerous cell surface receptors (see Fig. 89–1). After phagocytosis of the bacteria by the dendritic cell (A), the pathogen is digested into small peptides and become associated with major histocompatibility (MHC) class II within the endosome (B). Finally, the MHC class II plus peptide is expressed on the surface of the dendritic cell (C). The activated dendritic cell also secretes interleukin (IL)-12. *2.* Naive $CD4^+$ T-lymphocyte activation requires the T-cell receptor (TCR) to recognize the antigenic peptide in association with MHC class II as well as the B7-1 (CD80) binding to CD28. The binding of CD2-CD58 and LFA-1 (CD11a/CD18) allows adherence between the T lymphocyte and dendritic cell. Upon activation, the TH_1 $CD4^+$ T lymphocyte secretes IL-2 and interferon (IFN)-γ and increases the production and expression of the IL-2 receptor. (ICAM, intercellular adhesion molecule.)

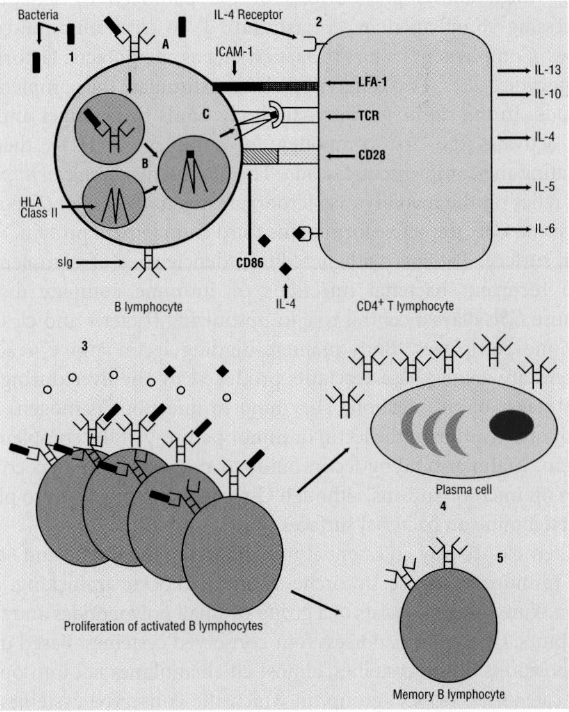

FIGURE 89-3. Induction of T-helper type 2 (TH_2) response. *1A,* A B lymphocyte recognizes invading bacteria via its surface immunoglobulin (sIg). *1B,* The bound bacteria are phagocytosed into an endosome, where the bacteria are broken down into small peptide fragments. *1C,* The small peptide fragments are placed within major histocompatibility complex (MHC) class II molecules and transported to the surface of the B lymphocyte for antigen presentation to a $CD4^+$ T lymphocyte. *2,* $CD4^+$ T-lymphocyte recognition requires antigen recognition within the MHC class II peptide groove by the T-cell receptor (TCR) and a secondary signal from B7-2 from the antigen-presenting cell, in this case a B lymphocyte binding to CD28 on the T lymphocyte. When both signals are delivered to the $CD4^+$ T lymphocyte becomes activated. In the TH_2 environment (see text), the naive $CD4^+$ T lymphocyte develops into a TH_2 subtype and secretes interleukin (IL)-4, IL-5, IL-6, IL-10, and IL-13, which promote a TH_2 response. *3,* In the presence of these cytokines plus antigen binding to the sIg, the B lymphocyte becomes activated. The activated B lymphocyte becomes a plasma cell *(4),* which produces and secretes immunoglobulin or becomes a memory B lymphocyte *(5).* A minority of B lymphocytes become memory B lymphocytes.

IgE-mediated inflammation. They are especially abundant in the skin, lungs, nasal mucosa, and connective tissue. Granules within the mast cells contain large amounts of preformed mediators that include histamine, heparin, and serotonin. Mast cells can also phagocytize, destroy, and present bacterial antigens to T lymphocytes.[10] Basophils are similar to mast cells because they contain granules filled with histamine, but they usually circulate in the blood and are not found in connective tissue. Like mast cells, basophils express high-affinity IgE Fc receptors (Fc). IgE-mediated anaphylaxis (type I hypersensitivity; see Chap. 91) is caused by stimulation of mast cell and/or basophil degranulation and release of preformed mediators after allergen binds to IgE bound to the Fc receptor on the surface of mast cells or basophils.[11]

Soluble Mediators of the Innate Immune System

Soluble mediators of innate immunity include the complement system, mannose-binding lectin, antimicrobial peptides, and C-reactive protein.[1] The complement system consists of more than 30 proteins in the plasma and on cell surfaces that play a key role in immune defense. The four major functions of the complement system include: (a) to lyse certain microorganisms and cells; (b) to stimulate the chemotaxis of phagocytic cells; (c) to coat or opsonize foreign pathogens, which allows phagocytosis of the pathogen by leukocytes expressing complement receptors; and (d) to clear immune complexes. Complement factors (C3a, C5a) act as chemotactic factors for phagocytic cells.[12] Two different pathways stimulate the complement cascade. In the *classic pathway*, antibody binds to its target antigen and activates the first component of complement (C1), thereby initiating the complement cascade. The *alternative complement pathway* relies on the inability of microorganisms to clear spontaneously produced C3b, the active form of the third complement protein, from their surface. Patients with hereditary deficiencies of complement have recurrent bacterial infections or immune complex disease because C3b plays a central role in opsonizing bacteria and clearing immune complexes. Both mannan-binding lectin and C-reactive protein are acute phase reactants produced by the liver during the early stages of an infection. They bind to infectious pathogens that result in activation of the lectin or minor pathway of the complement system. Mannan-binding lectin binds to mannose-rich glycoconjugates on microorganisms, although C-reactive protein binds to phosphorylcholine on bacterial surfaces.[1,12]

Chemokines play an essential role in linking the innate and adaptive immune response by orchestrating leukocyte trafficking. The chemokine system consists of a group of small polypeptides and their receptors. Chemokines possess four conserved cysteines. Based upon the positions of the cysteines, almost all chemokines fall into one of two categories: (a) CC group, in which the conserved cysteines are contiguous, or (b) CXC subgroup, in which the cysteines are separated by some other amino acid ("X"). As with all ligand–receptor interactions, a cell can respond to a chemokine only if the cell possesses a receptor that recognizes the chemokine. Chemokine receptors are unique in that they traverse the membrane seven times. CC receptors (CCRs) and CXC receptors (CXCRs) bind CC ligands (CCLs) and CXC ligands (CXCLs), respectively (Table 89–3).

Binding of infectious pathogens to pattern recognition receptors stimulates the release of chemokines such as macrophage inflammatory protein (MIP)-1α, MIP-1β, MIP-3α, and IP-10 from macrophages and dendritic cells embedded in the tissues. These chemokines attract more immature dendritic cells to the site of inflammation/infection. Immature dendritic cells constitutively express CCR1, CCR5, and CCR6. The interaction between pattern recognition receptors on the dendritic cell to the infectious pathogen causes the activation and maturation of the dendritic cell. After activation, dendritic cells downregulate the expression of CCR1, CCR5, and CCR6 and upregulate the expression of CCR7. This switch in chemokine receptor expression results in the antigen-loaded dendritic cell leaving the tissue and migrating toward the lymph nodes.[13]

TABLE 89-3 Common Chemokines

Receptor	Cell Expression	Ligand
CCR1	Immature DC	MIP-1α, MIP-1β, MCP-2, RANTES
CCR3	Eosinophils, basophils	Eotaxin-1, eotaxin-2, eotaxin-3, MCP-4
CCR6	Immature DC	Exodus-1
CCR7	Activated DC	CCL21 (SLC), CCL19 (ELC)
CXCR1/2	Neutrophils	IL-8
CXCR3	Natural killer cells, activated T lymphocytes	IP-10

DC, dendritic cell; MCP, monocyte chemoattractant protein; RANTES, regulated upon activation normal T lymphocyte expressed and secreted.

Naturally occurring antimicrobial peptides include α-defensins, β-defensins, and cathelicidins. These peptides exhibit antibacterial, antifungal, and antiviral activity. Human antimicrobial peptides range in length from 29 to 37 amino acid residues. Neutrophils are a rich source of both α- and β-defensins as well as cathelicidins. Other sources of the human antimicrobial peptides include keratinocytes, Paneth cells of the intestinal and genital tracts, and epithelial cells of the pancreas and the kidney. These peptides can be induced at sites of inflammation or can be constitutively produced. The clinical interest in human antimicrobial peptides centers on their broad spectrum activity and their rapid onset of killing. They are believed to work by disrupting microbial membranes. An active area of research is how these peptides discriminate between microbial and host membranes.[14]

ADAPTIVE IMMUNE SYSTEM

Adaptive Immune Response: Antigen Recognition

Generally, the body uses both innate and adaptive immune responses to rapidly kill foreign pathogens.[1] The greatest difference between the innate and adaptive immune responses is in specificity and memory, characterized by antigen-specific receptors located on the surface of B and T lymphocytes.[3] The adaptive immune response also secretes cytokines to further amplify the innate immune response. The adaptive immune response can evolve with each subsequent infection, whereas the innate response stays the same with each infection. During B- and T-lymphocyte development, an individual B or T lymphocyte rearranges its immunoglobulin and TCR genes, respectively, to produce a unique immunoglobulin or TCR, respectively. This DNA rearrangement generates enough B or T lymphocytes to recognize an estimated 10^{15} antigens.

The adaptive immune response can be divided into two major arms: humoral and cell-mediated. The *humoral* response is so denoted because it was discovered that the factors that provided the immune protection could be found in the "humor" or serum. B lymphocytes compose the humoral arm. Activated B lymphocytes can differentiate into plasma cells that secrete immunoglobulin or memory B cells specific for each pathogen. T lymphocytes constitute the cell-mediated arm of the adaptive system. The immune protection provided by T lymphocytes cannot be transferred by serum alone. Rather, it is essential to actually have T lymphocytes present, thus the term *cell-mediated* immunity. T lymphocytes are specially tailored to defend against infections that are intracellular, such as viral infections, whereas B lymphocytes secrete antibodies that can neutralize pathogens prior to their entry into host cells.

Adaptive Immune Response: Cells That Mediate Antigen Recognition

The role of the T lymphocyte is to search and destroy pathogens that infect and replicate intracellularly. When these pathogens enter a cell, they are no longer vulnerable to innate host defenses. Therefore, it is critical that T lymphocytes be able to distinguish which cells are infected and which cells are not. ❷ T lymphocytes do not recognize intact antigens, such as bacterial cell walls. T lymphocytes only recognize processed antigens in association with MHC.

Major Histocompatibility Complex

The MHC, a cluster of genes found on chromosome 6 in humans, is also known as the *human leukocyte antigen (HLA) complex.* The MHC is used by the immune system to distinguish self from nonself and provides a so-called immunologic "fingerprint." The genes from this complex encode for molecules that play a pivotal role in immune recognition and response. The MHC complex is divided into three different classes: I, II and III. The molecules encoded by class I HLA genes include HLA-A, HLA-B, and HLA-C antigens. These molecules can be found on all nucleated cells within the body as well as on platelets. Class I antigens are not found on mature red blood cells. Molecules encoded by class II HLA genes include HLA-DP, HLA-DQ, and HLA-DR. The expression of these molecules is more restricted and can be found primarily on cells of the immune system, namely, APCs such as macrophages, dendritic cells, and B lymphocytes. Class III HLA antigens encode for soluble factors, complement, and tumor necrosis factors.[15] In order for a $CD4^+$ T lymphocyte to become activated, the $CD4^+$ T lymphocyte must recognize the antigenic peptide in association with MHC class II (Figs. 89–2 and 89–3). $CD8^+$ T lymphocytes recognize antigenic peptide in association with class I molecules. Class I molecules generally contain endogenous peptides from within the cell, such as those derived from viruses, although class II molecules contain exogenous peptides from antigen that has been phagocytized and digested, such as bacterial peptides (Fig. 89–2). For it to destroy a virally infected cell, a $CD8^+$ cytotoxic T lymphocyte requires two steps. First, its TCR must recognize the antigenic fragment, such as a viral protein, in association with MHC class I. The second step involves the costimulatory step of B7–CD28 binding. Because any cell can become infected, it is advantageous that $CD8^+$ cytotoxic T lymphocytes recognize the MHC class I molecule that is expressed on all cells except red blood cells. The ability of MHC class I to present endogenous peptides allows $CD8^+$ cytotoxic T lymphocytes to constantly screen cells for infections.[15,16] Dendritic cells and macrophages demonstrate the unique capacity to direct exogenous antigens toward MHC class I molecules, a process termed *cross-presentation.*[17]

APCs (e.g., macrophages, dendritic cells) engulf the pathogen, digest it, and express its peptide fragments on their cell surface in association with their MHC. T lymphocytes use a specific antigen receptor (TCR) to propagate the immune response. The TCR is composed of two chains, and each chain has a variable and a constant region. The variation of the amino acid sequence within the variable domain of TCR gives the cell its unique antigen specificity. Linked to the TCR is a complex of single chains known as the *CD3 complex.*[1,11]

Naive T lymphocytes are cells that have not been previously exposed to an antigen specific for their TCR. These cells require two signals for activation. The first signal for activation involves the T lymphocyte recognizing both the processed antigen and the MHC molecule complex. The second signal involves the interaction of the B7-1 (CD80) or B7-2 (CD86) molecule on the APC with the CD28 molecule on the surface of the T lymphocyte (Figs. 89–2 and 89–3). Without the second signal, the naive T lymphocyte becomes anergic or inactive. Memory T lymphocytes are less dependent on the second signal than are naive T lymphocytes. CD28 is expressed on both resting and activated T lymphocytes, although CTLA-4, a second ligand for B7 on T lymphocytes, is expressed only on activated T lymphocytes. CTLA-4 binding B7 transduces a negative signal so it plays a role in downregulating a T-lymphocyte response.[18] After the two activation signals, a message is sent through the TCR to the CD3 complex into the cell. Then a calcium influx occurs with subsequent activation of the T lymphocyte. Activated $CD4^+$ T lymphocytes begin to express the high-affinity IL-2 receptor and to release multiple soluble factors (e.g., IL-2) to stimulate T lymphocytes and other cells of the immune system (Fig. 89–2). Autocrine stimulation by IL-2 leads to proliferation of activated T lymphocytes.

Cell surface markers delineate the functional activity of T-lymphocyte populations. All T lymphocytes express the CD3 protein. Typically, T lymphocytes are further divided into helper cells ($CD4^+$), suppressor cells ($CD8^+$), and cytotoxic cells ($CD8^+$). Each of the subclasses appears to play a distinct role in the cell-mediated immune response. Naive T lymphocytes express CD45RA, a high-molecular-weight isoform of CD45, whereas memory T lymphocytes express CD45RO, a lower-molecular-weight isoform of CD45.[19] The primary role of $CD4^+$ cells is to stimulate other cells in the immune response. Functionally, $CD4^+$ cells can be divided into TH_1 and TH_2. This functional system was first described in mice. TH_1 cells secrete IL-2 and interferon-γ and stimulate $CD8^+$ cytotoxic cells, whereas TH_2 cells secrete IL-4, IL-5, and IL-10 and stimulate B-lymphocyte production of antibody.[20] Multiple factors determine whether a naive $CD4^+$ T lymphocyte develops into a TH_1 or a TH_2 cell. The cytokine microenvironment plays an important role in this development. IL-12 secreted by the APCs promotes TH_1 development, whereas IL-4 promotes TH_2 development. Other factors that promote TH_1 development include B7-1 (CD80), high-affinity of the TCR for the antigen, interferon-γ, and interferon-α. Factors that promote TH_2 development include B7-2 (CD86), low-affinity of the TCR for the antigen, IL-10, and IL-1.[21]

$CD8^+$ T lymphocytes recognize antigen in association with MHC class I. $CD8^+$ cytotoxic cells are instrumental in killing cells recognized as foreign, such as those that have become infected by a virus. $CD8^+$ cytotoxic T lymphocytes play an important beneficial role in the eradication of tumor cells, but they also are responsible for rejection of transplanted organs.[11] Classically, a second type of $CD8^+$ T lymphocytes was a suppressor cell. It is clear that some T lymphocytes help suppress the immune responses, but whether this subset is $CD8^+$ is debatable. Emerging evidence is leading away from $CD8^+$ T lymphocytes and toward $CD4^+CD25^+$ T lymphocytes in maintaining self-tolerance. The preferred term for these suppressive T lymphocytes is *regulatory T lymphocytes.*[22]

To fully activate the $CD8^+$ cytotoxic T lymphocyte requires $CD4^+$ T-lymphocyte activation, namely, the TH_1 subset, and its subsequent secretion of IL-2 (Fig. 89–4A). This model of $CD8^+$ cytotoxic T-lymphocyte activation requires the close proximity of two rare antigen-specific T lymphocytes. In addition, some $CD8^+$ cytotoxic T-lymphocyte responses can occur in the absence of $CD4^+$ T lymphocytes. New data suggest that $CD4^+$ T lymphocytes can activate/prime APCs through CD40, which primes the APC (e.g., dendritic cell) to fully activate $CD8^+$ cytotoxic T lymphocytes (Fig. 89–4B).[23] Remember that the classification of $CD4^+$ lymphocytes as T-helper lymphocytes and $CD8^+$ lymphocytes as T-cytotoxic lymphocytes is not an absolute. Some $CD8^+$ T lymphocytes secrete cytokines similar to a T-helper lymphocyte, whereas some $CD4^+$ T lymphocytes can act as cytotoxic cells.

Unlike neutrophils and macrophages, cytotoxic T lymphocytes are unable to ingest their targets. They destroy target cells by two different mechanisms: the *perforin system* and the *Fas ligand pathway*. After recognition by the cytotoxic T lymphocyte, cytoplasmic granules containing perforins and granzymes are rapidly oriented toward the target cell, and the contents of the granules are released into the intracellular space. Like the membrane attack complex formed after complement activation, perforins form a pore in the target cell membrane. Besides a direct cytotoxic effect on the target

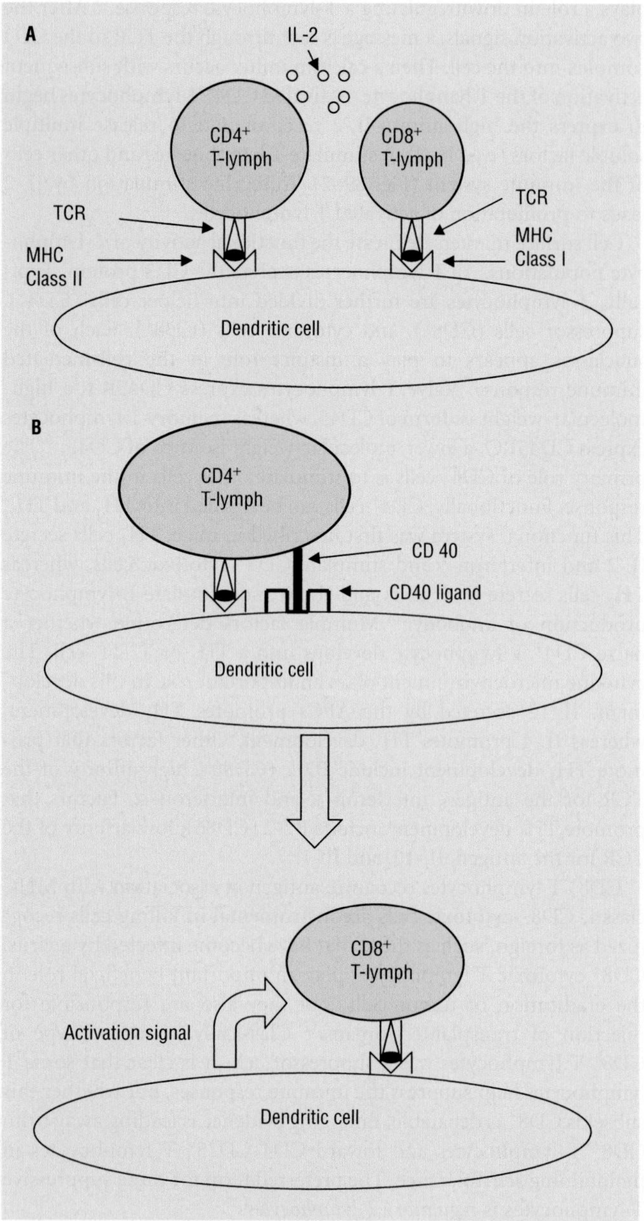

FIGURE 89-4. In the classic model of CD8+ T-lymphocyte activation *(A)*, CD4+ and CD8+ T lymphocytes recognize antigen on the same dendritic cell. In the presence of interleukin (IL)-2 from the activated CD4+ T lymphocyte and the recognition of antigen in association with major histocompatibility complex (MHC) class I, the CD8+ T lymphocyte becomes activated. In the new model *(B)*, activated CD4+ T lymphocytes activate dendritic cells via CD40 ligand binding to CD40. The activated dendritic cell then migrates through the tissues to present antigen to CD8+ T lymphocytes. If recognition via the T-cell receptor (TCR) on the CD8+ T lymphocyte occurs, the dendritic cell can fully activate the CD8+ T lymphocyte without the presence of CD4+ T lymphocytes.

cell, the pores produced by perforins allow the granzymes to penetrate into the target cell to induce apoptosis. The second mechanism of cytotoxicity involves the binding of Fas ligand on the cytotoxic T lymphocyte to the Fas receptor on the target cell. The Fas ligand is predominately expressed on CD8+ cytotoxic T lymphocytes and natural killer (NK) cells, and its expression increases after activation. After destroying that target cell by either mechanism, the cytotoxic T lymphocyte detaches from the target cell and attacks other targets.[24]

A B lymphocyte recognizes antigen via its antibody or immunoglobulin located on its cell surface (Fig. 89–3). The antibody on the surface can recognize an intact pathogen, such as bacteria, and present antigen to T lymphocytes (i.e., acts as an APC). However, the major function of B lymphocytes is to produce antibody to bind to the invading pathogen, a process that first entails activation of the B lymphocyte. Activation of B lymphocytes requires two steps: (a) recognition of antigen by the surface immunoglobulin and (b) presence of B-lymphocyte growth factors (IL-4, IL-5, IL-6) secreted by activated CD4+ T lymphocytes. Once activated, the B lymphocyte becomes a plasma cell, a differentiated cell capable of producing and secreting antibody. A fraction of activated B lymphocytes do not differentiate into plasma cells but rather form a pool of memory cells. The memory cells will respond to subsequent encounters with the pathogen, generating a quicker and more vigorous response to the pathogen. Some B lymphocytes can become activated without help from T lymphocytes, but these responses are generally weak and do not invoke memory.[1,11]

NK cells, often referred to as *large granular lymphocytes*, are defined functionally by their ability to lyse target cells without prior sensitization and without restriction by MHC. Resting NK cells express the intermediate-affinity IL-2 receptor CD122. Upon exposure to IL-2, NK cells exhibit greater cytotoxic activity against a wide variety of tumors. NK cells recognize target cells by two mechanisms. First, NK cells express the IgG Fc receptor CD16, which allows recognition of IgG-coated cells. Second, NK cells express killer-activating and killer-inhibiting receptors. The killer-activating receptors recognize multiple targets on normal cells, but the binding of MHC class I to the killer-inhibitor receptor blocks release of perforins and granzymes. Therefore, cells (e.g., tumor cells, virally infected cells) that downregulate MHC class I expression are susceptible to NK cell cytolysis. NK cells play important roles in the surveillance and destruction of tumors and virally infected host cells and in the regulation of hematopoiesis.[1,25]

Soluble Mediators of the Adaptive Immune Response: Immunoglobulins

❸ When a specific antigen binds to the surface immunoglobulin receptor of the B lymphocyte, the B lymphocyte matures into a plasma cell and produces large quantities of antibody that can bind to the inciting antigen. The secreted antibodies may be of five different isotypes. On primary exposure to the pathogen, the plasma cell will secrete IgM, but eventually it switches to predominately IgG. On second exposure, the memory B lymphocytes will predominately produce IgG. Isotype switching from IgM to IgG, IgA, or IgE is controlled by T lymphocytes.

An antibody or immunoglobulin is a glycoprotein composed of two different chains, heavy and light (Fig. 89–5). The basic structure of every immunoglobulin consists of four peptide chains: two identical heavy chains and two identical light chains held together by disulfide bonds. The basic structure of the antibody is a Y-shaped figure. Each arm of the Y is formed by the linkage of the end of the light chain to its heavy chain partner. These arms contain the portions described as the *fragments of antigen binding (Fab)*. The stem of the Y contains the heavy chains, which compose the *fragment crystallizable (Fc fragment)* portion of the antibody. It is within the Fc portion that complement is activated once the antibody has bound its target. Likewise, it is the Fc portion of the antibody that is recognized by Fc receptors on the surface of phagocytes (Fig. 89–1). The amino acid composition of the same isotype is homogenous except in the variable regions of the light (V_L) and heavy chains (V_H). The variation in amino acid composition of the variable region gives the antibody its unique specificity (Fig. 89–5)

IgG, the most prevalent of the antibody classes, composes approximately 80% of serum antibody. IgG usually is the second isotype of antibody produced in an initial humoral immune response. IgG is the only isotype of antibody that can cross the

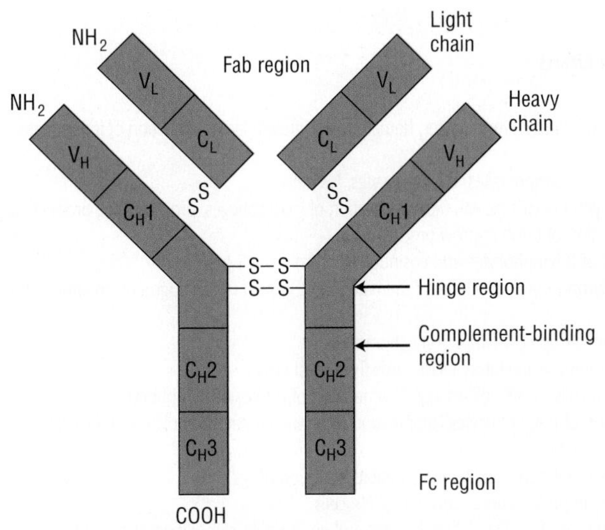

FIGURE 89-5. Schematic diagram of the structure of the immunoglobulin G (IgG) molecule. IgG molecule consists of two heavy (H) and two light (L) chains covalently linked by disulfide bonds. Each chain is composed of variable (V) and constant (C) regions. A light chain consists of one variable (V_L) and one constant (C_L) region. Heavy chains consist of one variable (V_H) and three or four constant (C_H) regions, depending on the isotype. The variable regions (V_L and V_H) compose the antigen-binding region of the IgG molecule, or fragment antigen binding (Fab). The constant regions provide the structure to the IgG molecule as well as binding the first component of complement (C_H2) and binding to Fc receptors via the Fc portion of the molecule (C_H3).

placenta. Therefore, early maternal humoral protection of neonates is primarily due to maternal IgG that crossed the placenta in utero.

Four different subclasses of IgG have been described: IgG1, IgG2, IgG3, and IgG4. These subclasses differ slightly in their constant amino acid sequences. IgG1 constitutes the majority (60%) of the subclasses. It appears that different subclasses recognize different types of antigen. IgG1 and IgG3 are principally responsible for recognition of protein antigens, although IgG2 and IgG4 commonly bind to carbohydrate antigens. Another difference in the subclasses is the ability to activate complement. IgG3 and IgG1 are the most efficient, and IgG4 is unable to activate the complement system.

IgM can be found on the surface of B lymphocytes as a monomeric Y-shaped structure. In contrast, secreted IgM is a pentamer in which five of the monomers are joined together by a joining chain (J chain). IgM is the first class of antibody produced on initial exposure to an antigen. Because the pentameric form of IgM has no Fc portions exposed, phagocytic cells cannot bind pathogens opsonized by IgM. However, IgM is an excellent activator of the complement cascade by the classic pathway.

IgA is found primarily in the fluid secretions of the body (tears, saliva, nasal fluids) and in the gastrointestinal, genitourinary, and respiratory tracts. IgA functions by preventing pathogens from adhering to and infecting the epithelial cells at these sites. IgA is also secreted in a nursing mother's breast milk, as are IgG and IgM but in lower concentrations. In bodily secretions, IgA is in a dimeric form in which a J chain and a secretory chain hold two monomers together. The dimeric form is resistant to proteolysis in mucosal secretions.

IgD is the least understood isotype. IgD is found on the surface of B lymphocytes at different stages of maturation and may be involved in the differentiation of these cells. The main function of circulating IgD has not yet been determined. However, mice treated with exogenous anti–IgD antibody display a marked increase in immunoreactivity and secretion of all types of immunoglobulins and several T-cell–specific cytokines. High levels of anti–IgD autoantibodies of various subtypes have been observed in most autoimmune diseases (frequencies >50%), suggesting that IgD plays an important role in the etiology of these diseases.[26]

IgE is the least common of the serum antibody isotypes. Most of the IgE in the body is bound to the IgE Fc receptors on mast cells. When the IgE on the surface of mast cells binds antigen, it causes the release of various inflammatory substances (e.g., histamine) from the mast cell. The overall effect is stimulation of inflammation. Asthma and hay fever are two examples of allergic reactions primarily due to antigen binding to IgE.[21]

Soluble Mediators of the Adaptive Immune Response: Cytokines

Cytokines are soluble factors released or secreted by cells that affect the activity of other cells (paracrine) or the secreting cell itself (autocrine). For example, activated $CD4^+$ T lymphocytes secrete IL-2, which activates itself as well as $CD8^+$ T lymphocytes and NK cells. Research has shown that many cytokines (Table 89–4) have a broad spectrum of effects depending on their concentration, the presence of other factors, and the target cell. New cytokine families and their roles in disease processes are being discovered daily. Cytokines provide communication between the divisions of the immune system. Cytokines produced from APCs generally promote chemotaxis of other cells and induce a state of inflammation.[27] Monocytes, as previously mentioned, use pattern recognition receptors, enabling the immune system to distinguish pathogenic proteins from nonpathogenic proteins through toll-like receptors stimulating T-lymphocyte activation.[27] Cytokines can also prevent activation or response of immunologic cells. For example, IL-10 is an antiinflammatory cytokine that is produced in the respiratory tract to prevent IgE synthesis and activation of eosinophils when exposed to benign inhaled particles.[27] In vivo cytokines do not act alone but in combination with other cytokines. For example, activated $CD4^+$ T lymphocytes secrete both IL-2 and interferon-γ, which are synergistic in activating NK cells. Cytokines are broadly classified as regulatory or hematopoietic growth factors (Table 89–4).[11,28–32] This classification does not describe all their activities. Granulocyte-macrophage colony-stimulating factor (GM-CSF) released by activated T lymphocytes acts as a hematopoietic growth factor but also activates granulocytes and macrophages to phagocytize foreign pathogens.

The division of the immune system into the two functional groups does not imply that the divisions do not interact. In order to generate a vigorous immune response, both soluble mediators (e.g., complement, antibody, and cytokines) and cells (e.g., neutrophils, macrophages, dendritic cells, T lymphocytes, and B lymphocytes) are needed. The innate system usually responds first. Dendritic cells, macrophages, and neutrophils in the tissues recognize pathogen via surface receptors (Fig. 89–1). In order to amplify the immune response, APCs present antigen to $CD4^+$ T lymphocytes (Figs. 89–2 and 89–3). The activated $CD4^+$ T lymphocytes then secrete cytokines to activate B lymphocytes, $CD8^+$ T lymphocytes, NK cells, macrophages, and neutrophils.

DISEASES OF THE IMMUNE SYSTEM

This chapter is not intended to detail the diseases of the immune system, but a review of the terminology and specific examples of diseases of the immune system are necessary to understand the role of monitoring and possible intervention with pharmacotherapy. Diseases of the physical defense immune system are not often thought of as diseases of the immune system, but the loss of normal physical defenses is the most common cause of impaired immunity resulting in infectious sequelae. For example, thick respiratory secretions secondary to altered chloride transport in cystic fibrosis lead to pathogen airway colonization. Primary immunodeficiency

TABLE 89-4 Cytokines

Cytokines	Sources	Principal Effects
Regulatory		
IL-1	Macrophages, fibroblasts, endothelial cells	Activation of T and B lymphocytes, hematopoietic growth factor, induction of inflammatory events
IL-2	$CD4^+$ T lymphocytes (TH_1 subset)	Activation of T lymphocytes, B lymphocytes, NK cells
IL-4	$CD4^+$ T lymphocytes (TH_2 subset), mast cells, basophils, eosinophils	B- and T-lymphocytes growth factor, activation of macrophages, promotes IgE production, proliferation of bone marrow precursors
IL-5	$CD4^+$ T lymphocytes (TH_2 subset), mast cells	Activation of B lymphocytes and eosinophils, promotes IgE production
IL-6	$CD4^+$ T lymphocytes (TH_2 subset), macrophages, mast cells, fibroblasts	T- and B-lymphocyte growth factor, hematopoietic growth factor, augments inflammation
IL-8	T lymphocytes, monocytes, endothelial cells, fibroblasts	Neutrophil, basophil, T-lymphocyte chemotaxis
IL-10	T and B lymphocytes, macrophages	Cytokine synthesis inhibitory factor, growth of mast cells
IL-12	Macrophages, neutrophils, dendritic cells	Induce TH_1 cells, ↑ NK cell activity, ↑ generation of cytotoxic T lymphocytes
IL-13	Activated T lymphocytes	Proliferation of B lymphocytes, suppression of proinflammatory cytokines, directs IgE isotype switching
IL-14	T lymphocytes	Induces B-lymphocyte proliferation, inhibits secretion of Igs
IL-15	Macrophages, fibroblasts, dendritic cells, epithelial cells	T-lymphocyte proliferation, activation of NK cells
IL-16	$CD8^+$ T lymphocytes, epithelial cells	Chemoattractant for $CD4^+$ T lymphocytes and eosinophils; stimulation of secondary cytokine secretion from and proliferation of $CD4^+$ T lymphocytes
IL-18	Macrophages	Induces IFN-γ production
IL-28, IL-29[a]	Antigen-presenting cells, but proposed that all nucleated cells may produce	Alternative to IFN-α/IFN-β to provide immunity against viral infections by inhibiting viral replication
IL-31	Activated T lymphocytes	Involved in recruitment of polymorphonuclear cells, monocytes, and T cells to site of inflammation
IL-32	NK cells, T lymphocytes, epithelial cells	Induces proinflammatory cytokines including TNF-α and IL-8
TNF-α	Macrophages, NK cells, T and B lymphocytes, mast cells	Activation of neutrophils, endothelial cells, lymphocytes, liver cells to produce acute phase proteins
TNF-β	T lymphocytes	Tumoricidal
IFN α	Monocytes, other cells	Antiviral, activation of NK cells and macrophages, upregulation of MHC class I
IFN γ	T lymphocytes, NK cells	Activation of macrophages, NK cells, upregulation of MHC class I and II
Hematopoietic growth factors		
IL-3	T lymphocytes, macrophages	Maturation and differentiation of hematopoietic and mast cells
IL-7	Bone marrow stromal cells	Lymphopoietin
IL-9	T lymphocytes	Maturation and proliferation of T lymphocytes and mast cells
IL-11	Bone marrow stromal cells	Maturation of B lymphocytes and megakaryocytes
G-CSF	Macrophages, endothelial cells, fibroblasts	Maturation and activation of neutrophils
GM-CSF	T lymphocytes, macrophages, endothelial cells, fibroblasts	Maturation and activation of granulocytes, monocytes/macrophages, and eosinophils
M-CSF	Macrophages, endothelial cells, fibroblasts	Maturation and activation of monocytes/macrophages
Erythropoietin	Kidney, liver	Maturation of red blood cells
Stem cell factor	Bone marrow stromal cells, hepatocytes	Activation of mast cells, early-acting growth factor for myeloid and lymphoid precursors
c-MPL ligand (thrombopoietin)	Bone marrow stromal cells, liver, kidney	Lineage-specific growth factor for megakaryocytes (platelets)
FLT3 ligand	Bone marrow stromal cells	Early-acting growth factor

G-CSF, granulocyte colony-stimulating factor; GM-CSF, granulocyte-macrophage colony-stimulating factor; IFN, interferon; Ig, immunoglobulin; IL, interleukin; M-CSF, macrophage cology-stimulating factor; MHC, major histocompatibility complex; NK, natural killer; TNF, tumor necrosis factor.

[a]Also known as the new type III IFN λ family.

diseases are characterized as either a genetic inability to produce components of the immune system (e.g., severe combined immunodeficiency or hypogammaglobulinemia) or acquired (e.g., human immunodeficiency virus infection). Autoimmune diseases result from a dysregulation of a component or a combination of components of the immune system (e.g., rheumatoid arthritis, systemic lupus erythematosus).[33] Autoimmune diseases are often characterized by production of autoantibodies against a particular host structure that is critical for normal function or by loss of tolerance or anergy to a ubiquitous antigen (e.g., gluten in celiac sprue).[33] Often medications that suppress the immune system are necessary to control symptoms and halt autoimmune disease progression. Exposure to immunosuppressive agents in the setting of autoimmune disease or organ transplantation may reduce disease symptoms but at the cost of the host's ability to fight off infection or cancer. Exogenous regulation of the immune system must be done judiciously, and we must continue to discover new methods for the appropriate evaluation of immune responses.

EVALUATION OF IMMUNE FUNCTION

Assessment of a patient's immune function requires knowledge and understanding of multiple components, including mechanical defenses, cell phenotypes and cell numbers, and soluble components. Recent developments in biotechnology have allowed for progress in further characterization of immune system components and their functions. This is important because upregulation and downregulation of immune responses is necessary to treat various disease states. Therefore, pharmacotherapeutic considerations must balance the risk of disrupting normal immunologic homeostasis. Improvements in immune monitoring are necessary for the goal of patient-specific immunologic pharmacotherapy. Despite the technologic advances, careful patient evaluations are required to accurately assess the structure and function of the immune system. Specific methods for assessment of patient immune status are discussed here.

INNATE IMMUNITY: EVALUATION OF MECHANICAL IMMUNODEFENSES

The mechanical aspects of host defense are extremely important in protection from infection; therefore, assessment of mechanical defenses is critical. Much of the assessment of mechanical immunodefense is accomplished by recognizing situations where such defense is compromised. Careful patient examination usually reveals the extent of compromise, and laboratory tests are generally not necessary for evaluation of this component. To assess the extent of compromise in mechanical immunodefenses, the clinician should carefully examine the patient and identify the specific types of risks present. Specific examples of altered mechanical defenses are listed in Table 89–5.

INNATE AND ADAPTIVE IMMUNITY: GROSS EVALUATION OF CELLULAR COMPONENTS

A major aspect of the assessment of immune function relates to the cells of the immune system. Assessment of cells in the clinical setting includes determination of cell type, cell number, and/or function. Generally, determination of cell types and quantification of cell numbers are performed first because of the ease of obtaining these results and the common correlation with the clinical situation.

To quickly screen cell numbers, a *white blood (cell) count* (WBC) with differential is performed. Normal cell counts are given in Table 89–6.[34] This simple test often steers the differential diagnosis. In interpreting a WBC with differential, the clinician must consider several factors. A normal cell count does not mean that a leukocyte disorder does not exist. For example, in chronic granulomatous disease, a child has a normal neutrophil count, but the neutrophils are unable to destroy the bacteria. Second, a differential is reported as percentage of the WBC; therefore, the absolute number as well as the percentage of white cell subtypes must be assessed. For example, a patient admitted to the hospital with pneumonia has an elevated WBC (15,000 cells/mm^3) with a manual differential of 70% mature neutrophils (segs), 10% immature neutrophils (bands), 15% lymphocytes, and 5% monocytes. The WBC is predominately neutrophils: segs or mature neutrophils (70%) and bands or immature neutrophils (10%). The percentage of lymphocytes appears low at 15% (Table 89–6), but the absolute number of lymphocytes is normal at 2,250 cells/mm^3 (15,000 cells × 0.15). A third factor to consider is that most lymphocytes are in secondary lymphoid organs (e.g., lymph nodes, spleen), and changes in peripheral blood lymphocytes do not always reflect changes in secondary lymphoid organs. Similarly, most granulocytes, macrophages, and mast cells are in the tissues, not the bloodstream.

TABLE 89-5 Examples of Alteration in Mechanical Immunodefenses That Result in Impaired Immune Status

- Reduced gastric pH
  - Achlorhydria
  - Use of histamine-2 blockers and proton pump inhibitors
  - Patients with acquired immune deficiency syndrome (AIDS)
- Break in skin barrier
- Burns
  - Surgical incision
  - Penetrating trauma
  - Vascular access devices
- Impaired mucociliary function of the lungs
  - Smoking
- Impaired esophageal or epiglottal function
  - Endotracheal intubation
  - Stroke
  - Recumbent position
- Altered urine flow
  - Urinary stones
  - Anatomic deformities obstructing flow
  - Bladder catheter
- Anatomic alterations of the heart resulting in turbulent blood flow and endocarditis

TABLE 89-6 Leukocyte Counts in Adults

Cell	Absolute Count (Range)[a]	Percent (Range)
White blood cells	7.5 (4.5–11.0)	100
Neutrophils	4.5 (2.3–7.7)	60 (50–70)
Eosinophils	0.2 (0.0–0.45)	3 (0–5)
Basophils	0.04 (0.0–0.2)	1 (0–2)
Monocytes	0.3 (0.0–0.8)	4 (0–10)
Lymphocytes	2.1 (1.6–2.4)	32 (28–39)
T lymphocytes	1.4 (1.1–1.7)	72 (67–76)[b]
CD4$^+$	0.8 (0.7–1.1)	42 (38–46)[b]
CD8$^+$	0.7 (0.5–0.9)	35 (31–40)[b]
B lymphocytes	0.3 (0.2–0.4)	13 (11–16)[b]
Natural killer cells	0.3 (0.2–0.4)	14 (10–19)[b]
CD4/CD8 ratio	1.2 (1.0–1.5)	

[a] × 10^3 cells/mm^3.
[b] Percent of lymphocyte subpopulations expressed as percentage of total lymphocyte population.

The numbers of granulocytes (neutrophils, basophils, eosinophils) and monocytes usually can be assessed by a WBC with differential. It has long been recognized that the lower the absolute neutrophil count, the greater the risk of infection. Drugs (e.g., chemotherapy) and diseases (e.g., collagen vascular disorders) may lower the neutrophil count and make the patient more susceptible to infections. Patients with a neutrophil count <1,500 cells/mm^3 are considered to have neutropenia. Functional analysis of these cell types is rarely done in routine clinical practice. Patients with suspected functional deficits in these cell types generally are referred to tertiary medical centers for evaluation and treatment.

A routine WBC with differential can determine the total lymphocyte count. Total lymphocyte count has been used as a measure of nutritional status, which rapidly changes with nutrient loss or repletion. This is a relatively gross measure of a patient's immune status, although it has been correlated to patient outcome and risk of infection.

Lymphocyte populations with different functions or in various stages of activation can be enumerated based on their cell surface markers. These cell surface markers are known as *clusters of differentiation* (CD). The CD is usually a protein or glycoprotein on the surface of the cell. CD followed by a number designates the marker. Hundreds of monoclonal antibodies have been designed to recognize these cell surface markers. Monoclonal antibodies can be labeled with a fluorescent marker. The labeled monoclonal antibodies are then incubated with the patient's cells. The antibodies will recognize and bind to the cells expressing the CD of interest, and the cells are counted with flow cytometry. For flow cytometry, the cell suspension is put under pressure such that the cells flow past a laser in a stream of single cells. The laser excites the fluorescently labeled antibodies bound to the lymphocytes. A light detector counts the labeled cell as the fluorescent tag emits light and determines the size of the cell based on its light scatter. These evaluations are valuable for assessment of patients with immune deficiency states such as acquired immunodeficiency syndrome (AIDS) or leukemia, and for patients who have received organ transplants. For example, clinically quantification of CD3$^+$ and CD4$^+$ cells is used to monitor muromonab, a monoclonal antibody directed against the CD3 receptor. The number of CD4$^+$ cells in human immunodeficiency virus (HIV)-positive patients correlates with the risk of opportunistic infection and delineates the time to initiate antiviral therapy. Some of the more common CD antigens and their respective cellular distributions are listed

TABLE 89-7 Cluster of Differentiation (CD) Guide: Characterization of Human Leukocyte Antigens

CD	Predominant Cellular Distribution
CD3	All T lymphocytes
CD4	Helper T lymphocytes, either TH_1 or TH_2
CD5	T lymphocytes, B-lymphocyte subset
CD8	Cytotoxic/suppressor T lymphocytes
CD14	Monocytes, neutrophils
CD20	B lymphocytes
CD25	Activated T lymphocytes, B lymphocytes, interleukin-2 receptor α-chain (Tac)
CD33	Committed myeloid progenitor cells
CD34	Hematopoietic progenitor cells that include the stem cell
CD56	Natural killer cells
CD83	Dendritic cells

in Table 89–7.[35] Flow cytometry can be used for leukocyte phenotyping, tumor cell phenotyping, and for some types of DNA analysis.

INNATE AND ADAPTIVE IMMUNITY: FUNCTIONAL EVALUATION

Several disease states are characterized by an adequate number of cells, but either the cells are nonfunctional or they do not produce cytokines to communicate effectively. No single test can predict the function of the immune system with 100% accuracy. However, tests are available to measure the viability of certain cell lines and communication between cells. Historically, the most common in vivo assay of lymphocyte function is the delayed hypersensitivity skin test. This test specifically evaluates the presence of delayed-type hypersensitivity or the presence of memory T lymphocytes. Specifically, a small amount of antigen, of which the patient is known to have been previously exposed, is administered. Under normal immunologic host conditions, exposure to this amount of antigen in the skin should produce lymphocytic infiltrate into the area within a few hours, followed by additional lymphocyte recruitment and phagocyte (e.g., macrophages, neutrophils) translocation. The maximal intensity of the inflammatory reaction occurs within 24 to 72 hours. This reaction often is referred to as type IV hypersensitivity (i.e., cell-mediated; see Chap. 91). A delayed-type hypersensitivity reaction is a test of cell-mediated immunity used to assess immunocompetency. The most common method for assessing delayed-type hypersensitivity is intradermal administration of a panel of recall antigens. Commonly used antigens include *Candida albicans*, mumps, trichophyton, tetanus toxoid, and purified protein derivative of tuberculin.[36] Measurements in millimeters of induration at the site of injection should be taken 48 to 72 hours after placement of the antigens. A reaction is considered positive if the diameter of induration is 2 mm or greater. The degree of sensitivity correlates to the area of induration.[35] Reaction to even a single antigen indicates a functioning cell-mediated immunity. The majority of immunocompetent individuals show a positive reaction to at least one of these antigens. Possible reasons for not mounting a response to these antigens include congenital T-lymphocyte deficiency, cancer, HIV, or immunosuppressive drug therapy.[36] Sometimes, no response is mounted because the individual being tested has not been previously exposed to a particular test antigen, although this is rare.

Global assessment of the in vivo immunologic response is used commonly in patients with solid organ transplantation during the diagnosis and assessment of acute rejection. For example, cellular rejection is detected on gross tissue biopsy by counting the number of lymphocytes present in the tissue and correlating their presence with other clinical findings, such as increasing serum creatinine level in patients with kidney transplant.

In vivo assessment of B-lymphocyte function involves immunizing the patient with a protein (e.g., tetanus toxoid) and a polysaccharide (e.g., pneumococcal polysaccharide vaccine) antigen to elicit and measure antibody responses after immunization. Two to three weeks after immunization, the patient's serum is tested for antibodies specific for the immunized antigen. This test measures B-lymphocyte responsiveness to the inoculated antigens but is reserved for patients who are suspected of having impaired B-lymphocyte function.[34]

A number of specific lymphocyte functional in vitro assays are used in the research setting. A few assays are performed at specialized clinical laboratories. One of these tests is the lymphocyte proliferation assay. In this assay, lymphocytes are obtained from a patient's peripheral blood and cultured in vitro. The cells are exposed to nonspecific mitogens such as pokeweed mitogen, phytohemagglutinin, or concanavalin A. Then the cells are incubated in growth media containing tritium-labeled (^3H) thymidine, a nucleotide used in the synthesis of DNA. Normally in the presence of the mitogens, lymphocytes are stimulated to proliferate. Proliferating lymphocytes incorporate ^3H thymidine as they replicate DNA. The level of radioactivity of the cells can be measured on a β-scintillation counter and is proportional to the degree of proliferation. The patient sample must be compared to lymphocytes from normal, healthy controls. Patients with immune deficiencies (AIDS, cancer, etc.) have fewer active or less active lymphocytes, as detected by this test.

A modification of the lymphocyte proliferation assay can be used in allogeneic hematopoietic stem cell transplantation to evaluate how closely a donor and host are "matched" in order to predict a patient's risk for developing graft-versus-host disease. A mixed lymphocyte culture (MLC) can be used to assess the potential of the donor cells to attack the host cells, a condition known as graft-versus-host disease (see Chap. 142). In this test, donor cells and host cells are incubated in vitro. The host lymphocytes are irradiated prior to the incubation so that they cannot proliferate. In vitro, ^3H thymidine is provided to the cells and uptake is measured. The degree of uptake correlates to level of proliferation of donor lymphocytes. If the cells are well matched, proliferation is minimal. If the cells are mismatched, proliferation is noted, with the level of proliferation predictive of the potential extent of graft-versus-host disease. With the introduction of DNA-based molecular typing of HLA antigens, the MLC is rarely used today. However, the MLC may play a role in selecting not completely histocompatible donors.[36]

The Cylex immune cell function assay is FDA approved as a novel test for determining the magnitude of suppression of $CD4^+$ cells.[37] Briefly, activity of $CD4^+$ cells is measured by quantification of the amount of ATP produced and characterized as high, medium, or low. Initial retrospective experience in the solid organ transplant population has been reported.[38] Although this assay is in its clinical infancy, it is one of the first functional assays aimed at assessing individual patient response to immunosuppressive therapy. This type of testing may allow for tailoring of immunosuppression. In addition to the Cylex immune cell function assay, a number of other tests have been devised to evaluate the function of $CD8^+$ T lymphocytes, NK cells, and monocytes/macrophages. Although these evaluations are not commonly performed, they may be helpful in some specific diseases. A thorough discussion of these tests is available.[39]

EVALUATION OF CYTOKINES AND CHEMOKINES

Disease states involving the loss or upregulation of cytokines and chemokines are often overlooked as diseases of the immune system. However, as just reviewed, cytokines and chemokines are essential components of both the innate and adaptive immune systems and provide the communication linking them together. Assays of humoral components may be either quantitative, to determine the absolute concentration of the factor, or qualitative, to determine the function of the component.

TABLE 89-8 Potential Indications for Measurement of Antigen-Specific Antibody

Environmental or drug allergy
Exposure to or infection with bacteria
Streptococci (ASO titer)
Staphylococcus aureus (teichoic acid antibody)
Neisseria gonorrhoeae
Legionella pneumophila
Exposure to or infection with viruses
Human immunodeficiency virus
Cytomegalovirus
Epstein-Barr virus
Hepatitis A, B, or C
Rubella
Exposure to or infection with other pathogens
Syphilis
Lyme disease
Typhoid
Chlamydia
Immune disorders
Rheumatoid factor antibody, rheumatoid arthritis
Antinuclear antibodies, systemic lupus erythematosus
Platelet-associated immunoglobulin G, idiopathic thrombocytopenic purpura
Blood typing and crossmatching
Transplantation
Human leukocyte antigen (HLA) antibodies

IMMUNOGLOBULINS

Measurement of immunoglobulins is a direct measure of B-cell function. The most common evaluation of immunoglobulins is the estimation of total immunoglobulin. This is estimated by subtracting the albumin concentration from the total protein concentration in serum. This difference provides a gross estimate of the total immunoglobulin concentration. Total immunoglobulin concentration can be more accurately determined by serum protein electrophoresis. Five separate zones are detected by this method: albumin, α_1-globulin, α_2-globulin, β-globulin, and γ-globulin.

❹ The γ-globulin fraction contains the five isotypes of immunoglobulin (IgG, IgA, IgM, IgE, and IgD). A normal total immunoglobulin or γ-globulin concentration ranges from 0.8 to 1.6 g/dL. This test is used to determine if patients have hypogammaglobulinemia (i.e., primary and secondary immunodeficiencies), a monoclonal peak (e.g., multiple myeloma, Waldenstrom's macroglobulinemia), or a polyclonal hypergammaglobulinemia (e.g., chronic inflammatory condition, such as systemic lupus erythematosus or chronic active hepatitis). Total immunoglobulin or γ-globulin concentrations cannot be used to measure antigen-specific antibodies or specific isotypes, although other tests are available for this purpose.

In a patient suspected of having humoral immune deficiency or B-lymphocyte failure (i.e., primary and secondary hypogammaglobulinemia), specific immunoglobulin isotypes in the plasma should be measured.

There are many indications for the measurement of antigen-specific antibody. Some common indications are listed in Table 89–8. Methods for performing these measurements include enzyme-linked immunosorbent assay (ELISA), radioimmunoassay (RIA), and radioallergosorbent test (RAST; Fig. 89–6). The most common reason for measuring antigen-specific antibody is to determine whether a patient has been exposed to an infectious agent. Generally, IgM antibodies directed against the pathogen indicate an active or recent infection, whereas IgG antibodies directed against the pathogen indicate prior exposure. This interpretation is based on our understanding of B-lymphocyte responses in which plasma cells produce IgM initially in response to an infection but later switches to IgG. Therefore, IgM antibodies will be present during an active infection and shortly after recovery from the infection. IgG concentrations will increase at the end of the primary exposure but predominate after a second exposure. IgG predominates after a second exposure because memory B lymphocytes predominately secrete IgG in the serum. Other uses of antigen-specific antibody include determining if a patient has been exposed and is likely to be protected from infection (e.g., hepatitis A virus) or to determine adequate response to vaccination (e.g., hepatitis B vaccine).

Antigen-specific IgE is commonly measured in patients with allergies. Because the presence of antigen-specific IgE is related to clinical allergy, measurement of this antibody can be helpful in diagnosing allergies and determining offending substances. A standard method for determining allergen-specific IgE is the RAST. The basic technique involves adding the antigen of interest, which is bound to beads or disks, to the patient's serum. After precipitation and several washings, the antibody bound to the bead or disk is isolated. Finally, a radiolabeled antibody that binds to IgE is added. After further washings, the radiolabeled antibody bound to IgE, which is bound to the antigen on the bead or disk, is counted on a γ-counter.

Antigen skin testing is the preferred method for determining the presence of allergen-specific IgE. When produced, IgE binds to high-affinity IgE Fc receptors on basophils or mast cells. Contact of an allergen with the specific IgE on the basophil or mast cell surface causes activation of these cells and release of inflammatory mediators (e.g., histamine). When this process occurs systemically, it can cause anaphylaxis. When it occurs in a confined area such as the skin, erythema and induration are observed within a few minutes of allergen injection. This is the principle used for detection of penicillin allergy as well as for environmental or food allergies. A positive skin reaction (≥5 mm of induration) within 15 to 20 minutes is indicative of the presence of allergen-specific IgE.

IgG1, IgG2, IgG3, and IgG4 (the four subclasses of IgG) make up 65%, 20%, 10%, and 5% of total plasma IgG, respectively. Concentrations of the subclasses are often measured in patients with suspected primary and secondary hypogammaglobulinemia. IgG2

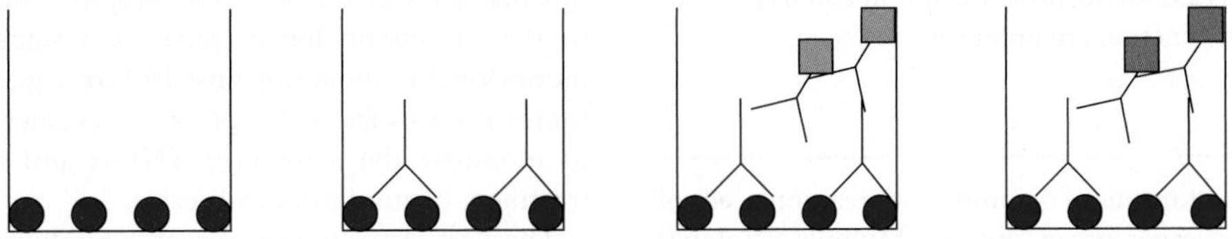

FIGURE 89-6. Enzyme-linked immunosorbent assay (ELISA). ELISA is a commonly used method for measuring concentrations of a wide variety of substances. To measure the concentration of antibodies to a particular antigen, the antigen is coated onto a solid phase, such as a microtiter plate or beads. If the purpose of the assay is to measure the concentration of antigen in solution, an antibody to the antigen is coated on the solid phase. The biologic fluid, often sera, is added to the wells. An enzyme-labeled anti-human antibody is added next. Finally, the chromogenic substrate for the enzyme is added. The intensity of the color as measured spectrophotometrically is proportional to the concentration of the antibody in the biologic fluid.

and IgG4 deficiencies are associated with chronic infections. IgG4 deficiencies are also associated with autoimmune disorders.

COMPLEMENT SYSTEM

The complement system consists of a group of more than 30 different proteins involved in lysing and opsonizing invading pathogens as well as serving as chemotactic factors. Numbers following the letter C (e.g., C1, C2) name the various proteins of the complement system. A test for the global assessment of the complement system is the CH_{50}, the total hemolytic complement test. This test is based on the premise that complement is needed for a rabbit anti-sheep antibody to lyse sheep red blood cells. The source of the complement is the patient's serum. Each laboratory standardizes the test so normal ranges vary, but a standard curve is developed by adding titrated amounts of sera and measuring the amount of hemolysis. The hemolysis is determined with a spectrophotometer to measure the amount of hemoglobin released. The patient's serum is then tested, and the amount of serum that is needed to lyse 50% of the red blood cells is reported as the CH_{50}. This test does not provide an indication of the function of any specific complement component but is used as a screening test for any complement system defects. If a defect is found, individual complement proteins can be evaluated by functional or immunochemical methods. Assessment of the complement system is important in patients suspected of having humoral immune deficiencies (i.e., recurrent infections).[35]

Several disease states can alter complement concentrations. Low complement concentrations are frequently found during states of acute inflammation (e.g., systemic lupus erythematosus, rheumatoid arthritis, collagen vascular disorders, poststreptococcal glomerulonephritis, and subacute bacterial endocarditis). These states of apparently low complement concentrations are generally due to high rates of complement utilization or consumption that cannot be compensated for by increased complement synthesis.[12]

The liver is the primary source of several components of the complement system (i.e., C2, C3, C4, factors B and D); therefore, a global decrease in complement factors occurs in severe liver failure. Inherited complement deficiencies have been described in patients with systemic lupus erythematosus, autoimmune diseases, recurrent gonococcal and meningococcal infections, membranoproliferative glomerulonephritis, and hereditary angioedema.[12]

Clinically, the complement system has been used to diagnose and treat solid organ rejection. Antibody-mediated or humoral rejection is evaluated by quantifying the amount of donor MHC-specific antibody present in the recipient's serum. The presence of donor-specific antibodies is correlated with evidence of antibody-mediated rejection on tissue samples. This is characterized by the presence of complement split products, namely, C4d, which is present after complement dependent antibody-mediated rejection. C4d covalently binds to the allograft tissue and can be stained for on biopsy samples. Unfortunately, unless biopsy findings can be correlated with a clinical finding consistent with rejection, the presence of C4d and its prognosis on long-term allograft function are unknown.

CYTOKINES

Cytokines are an important means of communication among cells of the immune system and other organ systems. Multiple cytokines with overlapping and redundant functions have been identified. Methods for detecting and measuring cytokines in biologic samples have been developed. Commercial kits are available to measure nearly all currently identified endogenous and exogenously administered cytokines. The most common and preferable methods for measuring cytokines are the ELISA and RIA. ELISA and RIA are easy to run, and they measure immunoactivity but not biologic activity (Fig. 89–6). Bioassays measure biologic activity, but are cumbersome and extremely variable. ELISA can measure only how much cytokine was produced by the cells in the culture. The enzyme-linked immunosorbent spot (ELISPOT) is an enzyme-linked assay that detects and enumerates cytokine-producing leukocytes.[40] In contrast to conventional ELISA, ELISPOT allows the user to detect absolute numbers and frequencies of cytokine-secreting leukocytes.

Interpretation of the clinical relevance of endogenous cytokine concentrations is still in the early stages. Not only is the immune system affected by cytokines such as IL-1, IL-6, and tumor necrosis factor-α (TNF-α), but other systems (e.g., skeletal, endocrine, central nervous system) also are affected. Therefore, measurement of cytokine concentrations may be important in the evaluation of other systems as well as the immune system.

Administration of pharmacologic doses of recombinant cytokines in clinical practice may change not only the concentration of that particular cytokine but also the resultant concentration of other cytokines. For example, systemic administration of GM-CSF to patients increases concentrations not only of GM-CSF but also of TNF-α, IL-6, IL-8, macrophage colony-stimulating factor, and erythropoietin.[41,42] Secondary endogenous cytokine release should be taken into account when evaluating the therapeutic effects of these agents and monitoring cytokine concentrations.

In the future, tissue concentrations as well as blood concentrations may be measured. For example, many centers currently measure cyclosporine concentrations to estimate the potential for immunosuppressive effects, but monitoring IL-2 concentrations may be advantageous. One of the primary actions of cyclosporine is inhibition of IL-2 production. Furthermore, measuring tissue concentrations of IL-2 in the transplanted organ may be beneficial in obtaining a better estimate of the extent of immunologic suppression.

SOLUBLE RECEPTORS AND RECEPTOR ANTAGONISTS

The inflammatory response is highly regulated. The activity of cytokines, their receptors, and their antagonists are in a delicate balance. Although cytokine receptors usually are found on the surface of the target cell, soluble cytokine receptors can modulate the activity of cytokines in at least two ways: (a) acting as antiinflammatory agents by binding cytokines with high affinity but without biologic activity,[43] and (b) augmenting cytokine activity by prolonging the cytokine plasma half-life and even maintaining agonist activity on cells that do not inherently respond to the cytokine.[44] Finally, antagonists to cytokine receptors have been identified.

TNF-α plays a central role in the inflammatory response by both increasing the expression of adhesion molecules in the tissues and stimulating production of proinflammatory cytokines (e.g., IL-2, IL-8), prostaglandins, and nitric oxide. Soluble tumor necrosis factor receptors act primarily as inhibitors of TNF-α by preventing TNF-α from binding to the membrane-bound TNF-α receptor or by causing the cells to shed the receptor from the surface of the cell so that it can no longer serve as a signaling molecule.[45] Both monoclonal antibodies against TNF-α (e.g., infliximab) and soluble tumor necrosis factor receptors (e.g., etanercept) have been shown to modulate the activity of TNF-α and are used clinically for treatment of autoimmune diseases.

The best characterized receptor-binding antagonist is the IL-1 receptor antagonist (IL-1RA). IL-1RA blocks the binding of IL-1 to its receptor by competing for the same binding site, but IL-1RA does not possess agonist activity.[46] Anakinra, a recombinant IL-1RA, is used clinically for treatment of severe rheumatoid arthritis.[47]

Our developing understanding of soluble receptors and receptor antagonists allows us to better mimic natural mechanisms for minimizing the toxicity of exogenously administered cytokines (e.g., IL-1, IL-2, TNF-α) as well as for immunomodulating of various diseases (e.g., solid organ transplant rejection, collagen vascular disorders, sepsis).

MODULATION OF THE IMMUNE RESPONSE

5 Modulation of the immune response through administration of pharmacologic agents or with blood product components does not come without risks. Providing supplementation to the immune system, for example, during periods of sepsis with recombinant activated protein C (drotrecogin alfa), provides increased levels of protein C that decrease levels of proinflammatory IL-6, potentially limiting the effects of the immune reaction and preventing end-organ damage at the cost of bleeding for overexposure to protein C. Although interfering with the immune system to halt the damage of an autoimmune disorder may suppress symptoms, this strategy may place the patient at risk for opportunistic viral infections, as observed for agents such as etanercept for rheumatoid arthritis. Many of the newer biologic agents directed at a pathway in the immune system are genetically engineered from animals and humanized to increase their biologic effectiveness. As a result, these agents can serve as antigens to the immune system and display variable effectiveness between and among patients over time. For example, an agent commonly used in solid-organ transplantation is rabbit antithymocyte globulin, which is a polyclonal antibody directed against lymphocytes that is given at the time of transplant or to treat rejection. Patients with previous exposure to this agent may have developed antibodies against the rabbit epitope of the drug. This results in either a decrease in the effectiveness of the drug because it is bound by antibody or production of an immunologic reaction, commonly manifested by antibody–antigen complex deposition in the kidneys and joints producing high fevers and renal failure. Based on the few examples presented here, one can understand why manipulation of the immune system must be carefully assessed and appropriate patient instruction given.

IMMUNOSUPPRESSION

Immunosuppression was first developed and used to allow transplantation of foreign tissues or to treat malignancies of the immune system. Today, the number of compounds and disease states in which the immune system is implicated is virtually unquantifiable. Therefore, a thorough review of these drugs is beyond the scope of this chapter. Immunosuppressants often are very expensive and must be administered through an injection. Immunosuppressants block critical steps of the immune response, and patients must be counseled on their risk of infection and the plan to monitor effectiveness of the immunosuppressant. Some key concepts and questions can be used to help clinicians discern the potential benefits and ramifications of administering any immunosuppressant: (a) what is its mechanism of action, (b) what arm of the immune system does it effect, (c) when is its onset of action, (d) how was this compound derived and does it have the potential to stimulate antibody production if the patient is reexposed, (e) is this compound's effect dose or duration related, (f) what type of infection is the patient at risk for and does the clinician need to administer prophylactic medications, and (g) how does the clinician monitor the biologic effect of this compound?

IMMUNOPOTENTIATION

Immunopotentiators are often used in an attempt to restore normal immune system function or to activate the immune system. The best example of immunopotentiation of the immune system is the practice of immunizations. Active immunization with a vaccine or toxoid induces the host's immune system to confer protection against a pathogen (e.g., hepatitis A, hepatitis B, diphtheria toxoid). This process requires the uptake of the immunogenic epitope by APCs, followed by presentation to $CD4^+$ T lymphocytes and subsequent development of either a cellular or humoral immune response.

In contrast to active immunization, passive immunity entails the administration of human immunoglobulin to provide short-term protection to individuals who will be or have been exposed to a pathogen. Intravenous immunoglobulin (IVIG) consists of >90% polyclonal IgG that is prepared from donated plasma. In patients with primary or secondary hypogammaglobulinemia, IVIG restores circulating IgG concentrations, thus decreasing the incidence of infections in these patients. In addition to restoring IgG concentrations, IVIG can potentially immunomodulate the immune response. For example, in idiopathic thrombocytopenic purpura, an autoantibody directed against platelets leads to destruction of the platelets by antibody-dependent cellular cytotoxicity. IVIG saturates the Fc receptors on phagocytic cells, preventing the engulfment of autoantibody-opsonized platelets. IVIG also can contain antiidiotype antibodies to immunomodulate an immune response. Antiidiotype antibodies are directed against the idiotype or hypervariable region of a native antibody. After administration of IVIG, the antiidiotypes bind to the hypervariable region of the autoantibody and prevent the autoantibody from opsonizing circulating platelets. In addition, the antiidiotypes directed against the autoantibody can bind to the surface immunoglobulin on the B lymphocyte producing the autoantibody that leads to destruction of the B lymphocyte.[48]

SUMMARY

Our understanding of the immune system has increased dramatically over the last decade. An immune response encompasses dynamic events involving both immunologic cells (e.g., phagocytes, lymphocytes) and soluble mediators (e.g., complement, cytokines, antibodies). A better understanding of the normal immune response allows us to investigate the pathophysiology of diseases in which the immune response is inappropriate. All clinicians need a basic understanding of the immune system and a familiarity with parameters to monitor immune system function in order to refine the development of immunologic treatments for diseases ranging from diabetes mellitus to collagen vascular disorders to cancer.

REFERENCES

1. Delves PJ, Roitt IM. The immune system, first of two parts. N Engl J Med 2000;343:37–49.
2. Medzhitov R, Janeway C. Innate immunity. N Engl J Med 2000;343:338–344.
3. Chaplin DD. Overview of the human immune response. J Allergy Clin Immunol 2006;117:S430-S435.
4. Rennard SI, Romberger DJ. Host defenses and pathogenesis. Semin Respir Infect 2000;15:7–13.
5. Modlin RL. Mammalian toll-like receptors. Ann Allergy Asthma Immunol 2002;88:543–548.
6. Janeway CA, Medzhitov R. Innate immune recognition. Annu Rev Immunol 2002;20:197–216.
7. Witko-Sarsat V, Rieu P, Descamps-Latscha B, Lesavre P, Halbwachs-Mecarelli L. Neutrophils: Molecules, functions, and pathophysiological aspects. Lab Invest 2000;80:617–653.
8. Rothenberg ME, Hogan SP. The eosinophil. Annu Rev Immunol 2006;24:147–174.
9. Aderem A, Underhill DM. Mechanisms of phagocytosis in macrophages. Annu Rev Immunol 1999;17:593–623.
10. Banchereau J, Steinman RM. Dendritic cells and the control of immunity. Nature 1998;392:245–252.
11. Delves PJ, Roitt IM. The immune system, second of two parts. N Engl J Med 2000;343:108–117.

12. Walport MJ. Complement, first of two parts. N Engl J Med 2001;344:1058–1066.
13. Luster AD. The role of chemokines in linking innate and adaptive immunity. Curr Opin Immunol 2002;14:129–135.
14. Izadpanah A, Gallo RL. Antimicrobial peptides. J Am Acad Dermatol 2005;52:381–390.
15. Klein J, Sato A. The HLA system, first of two parts. N Engl J Med 2000;343:702–709.
16. Klein J, Sato A. The HLA system, second of two parts. N Engl J Med 2000;343:782–786.
17. Hartgers FC, Figdor CG, Adema GJ. Towards a molecular understanding of dendritic cell immunobiology. Immunol Today 2000;21:542–545.
18. Reiser H, Stadecker MJ. Costimulatory B7 molecules in the pathogenesis of infectious and autoimmune diseases. N Engl J Med 1996;335:1396–1377.
19. Dutton RW, Bradley LM, Swain SL. T cell memory. Annu Rev Immunol 1998;16:201–223.
20. Farrar JD, Asnagli H, Murphy KM. T helper subset development: Role of instruction, selection and transcription. J Clin Invest 2002;109:431–435.
21. Constant SL, Bottomly K. Induction of TH1 and TH2 CD4+ T cell responses: The alternative approaches. Annu Rev Immunol 1997;15:297–322.
22. Bach JF. Regulatory T cells under scrutiny. Nat Rev Immunol 2003;3:189–198.
23. Lanzavecchia A. License to kill. Nature 19989:413–414.
24. Liu CC, Young LHY, Young JDE. Lymphocyte-mediated cytolysis and disease. N Engl J Med 1996;335:1651–1659.
25. Lanier LL. NK cell receptors. Annu Rev Immunol 1998;16:359–393.
26. Preud'homme JL, Petit I, Barra A, Morel F, Lecron JC, Lelievre E. Structural and functional properties of membrane and secreted IgD. Mol Immunol 2000;15:871–887.
27. Steinke JW, Borigh L. Cytokines and chemokines. J Allergy Clin Immunol 2006;117:S441-S445.
28. Anonymous. Cytokines. In: Goldsby RA KT, Obsborne BA, Kuby J, eds: Immunology. New York: WH Freeman and Company, 2003:277–298.
29. Trinchieri G. Interleukin-12: A cytokine at the interface of inflammation and immunity. Adv Immunol 1998;70:83–243.
30. Wynn TA. IL-13 effector functions. Annu Rev Immunol 2003;21:425–456.
31. Kennedy MK, Park LS. Characterization of interleukin-15 (IL-15) and the IL-15 receptor complex. J Clin Immunol 1996;16:134–143.
32. Okamura H, Tsutsui J, Kashiwamura SI, Yoshimota T, Nakanishi K. Interleukin-18: A novel cytokine that augments both innate and acquired immunity. Adv Immunol 1998;70:281–312.
33. Lee SJ, Kavanaugh A. Autoimmunity, vasculitis, and autoantibodies. J Allergy Clin Immunol 2006;117:S445–S450.
34. Elliott MB. Interpretation of clinical laboratory test results. In: Boh LE, ed. Pharmacy Practice Manuel A guide to clinical experience. Baltimore: Lippincott, Williams & Wilkins, 2001:136–212.
35. Fleisher TA, Tomar RH. Introduction to diagnostic laboratory immunology. JAMA 1997;278:1823–1834.
36. Folds JD, Schmitz JL. Clinical and laboratory assessment of immunity. J Allergy Clin Immunol 2003;111:S702–S711.
37. United States Department of Health and Human Services. K013169; Cylex Immune Cell Function Assay, April 2002.
38. Zeevi A, Britz JA, Bentlejewski CA, et al. Monitoring immune function during tacrolimus tapering in small bowel transplant recipients. Transplant Immunol 2005;15:17–24.
39. Lowell C. Section II. Immunological laboratory tests. In: Parslow TG, Stites DP, Terr AI, Imboden JB, eds. Medical Immunology. New York: Lange Medical Books/McGraw-Hill Medical, 2001.
40. Helms T, Boehm BO, Asaad RJ, Trezza RP, Lehmann PV, Tary-Lehmann M. Direct visualization of cytokine-producing recall antigen-specific CD4 memory T cells in healthy individuals and HIV patients. J Immunol 2000;164:3723–3732.
41. Rabinowitz J, Petros W, Stuart A, Peters W. Characterization of endogenous cytokine concentrations after high-dose chemotherapy with autologous bone marrow support. Blood 1993;81:2452–2459.
42. van Pelt L, Huisman M, Weening R, von dem Borne A, Roos D, van Oers R. A single dose of granulocyte-macrophage colony-stimulating factor induces systemic interleukin-8 release and neutrophil activation in healthy volunteers. Blood 1996;87:5305–5313.
43. Opal SM, DePalo VA. Anti-Inflammatory cytokines. Chest 2000;117:1162–1172.
44. Jones SA, Horiuchi S, Topley N, Yamamoto N, Fuller GM. The soluble interleukin 6 receptor: Mechanisms of production and implications in disease. FASEB J 2001;15:43–58.
45. Dinarello CA. Proinflammatory cytokines. Chest 2000;118:503–508.
46. Choy EH, Panayi GS. Cytokine pathways and joint inflammation in rheumatoid arthritis. N Engl J Med 2001;344:907–916.
47. Cohen S, Hurd E, Cush J, et al. Treatment of rheumatoid arthritis with anakinra, a recombinant human interleukin-1 receptor antagonist, in combination with methotrexate: Results of a twenty-four-week, multicenter, randomized, double-blind, placebo-controlled trial. Arthritis Rheum 2002;46:614–624.
48. Kazatchkine MD, Kaveri SV. Immunomodulation of autoimmune and inflammatory diseases with intravenous immune globulin. N Engl J Med 2001;345:747–755.

CHAPTER 90

Systemic Lupus Erythematosus and Other Collagen-Vascular Diseases

JEFFREY C. DELAFUENTE AND KIMBERLY A. CAPPUZZO

KEY CONCEPTS

1. Systemic lupus erythematosus (SLE) is a disease that predominantly occurs in women.
2. The hallmark of SLE is the development of autoantibodies to cellular nuclear components, resulting in chronic inflammatory autoimmune disease. Symptoms and organ involvement depend on the nature of the autoantibodies.
3. SLE has a large spectrum of symptoms and organ system involvement, making therapy highly patient specific. In addition, the signs and symptoms will fluctuate over time.
4. The large spectrum of symptoms and organ system involvement makes pharmacotherapy difficult because therapy must be individualized based on each patient's disease activity.
5. There is a paucity of quality evidence for the treatment of SLE except for lupus nephritis.
6. Almost all classes of medications, including antiinflammatory and immunosuppressive agents, are reported to cause vasculitis in most major organ systems.

The collagen–vascular diseases are a heterogeneous group of diseases that can involve the musculoskeletal system, integument, and blood vessels. Each collagen–vascular disease has its own set of diagnostic criteria, although diagnosis can be difficult because of overlapping and nonspecific clinical presentations. The etiology of the various collagen–vascular diseases is often unknown, but the immune system usually is involved in the pathogenesis and manifestations of the disease. Therefore, pharmacotherapy usually includes antiinflammatory agents with or without immunosuppressive drugs.

Although the prevalence of other collagen–vascular diseases may be greater than that of systemic lupus erythematosus (SLE) (e.g., polymyalgia rheumatica), SLE is discussed most extensively in this chapter because it is a major collagen–vascular disease with numerous clinical manifestations, its pharmacotherapy can be complex, and a plethora of data is available on the therapy of SLE. As all the diseases discussed in this chapter have an immune-mediated pathogenesis, the therapeutic principles of SLE can be applied to other autoimmune collagen–vascular diseases. The collagen–vascular diseases discussed include systemic sclerosis, polymyositis/dermatomyositis, polymyalgia rheumatica, and drug-induced vasculitis; these were chosen because they are seen in general practice.

Learning objectives, review questions, and other resources can be found at **www.pharmacotherapyonline.com.**

SYSTEMIC LUPUS ERYTHEMATOSUS

SLE is a fluctuating multisystem disease with a diversity of clinical presentations. Abnormal immunologic function and formation of antibodies against "self" antigens underlie the pathogenesis of SLE.

The term *lupus erythemateux* was first used in 1851 by Cazenave, a Frenchman who described an illness in a patient with manifestations occurring in the skin. It is not surprising that SLE was first recognized as a skin disorder because cutaneous manifestations constitute one of the most common clinical features of the disease. Further descriptions by Kaposi in 1872 and Osler in 1895 led to the concept of a multisystem disease as it became recognized that patients developed complications in other organ systems.[1,2]

The hallmark of SLE is the development of autoantibodies to cellular nuclear components that leads to a chronic inflammatory autoimmune disease. Recognition of SLE as an autoimmune disease of multisystemic nature led the American College of Rheumatology to develop criteria for identifying lupus patients (Table 90–1). These criteria were developed in 1971, revised in 1982, and modified slightly in 1997. The criteria do not include all the clinical manifestations of the disease and are used primarily for distinguishing SLE from other collagen–vascular diseases.[3] If 4 or more of the 11 criteria are documented at any time in a patient's medical history, the diagnosis of SLE can be made with approximately 95% specificity and 85% sensitivity.[4] Although these criteria may be helpful, diagnosis requires additional serologic, immunopathologic, and clinical evaluations.

EPIDEMIOLOGY

(1) The incidence of SLE varies among ethnic groups with the annual incidence in adults ranging from 1.9 to 5.6 per 100,000 persons per year, with a prevalence of 124 cases per 100,000 persons.[5,6] The disease occurs predominantly in women, with a reported female-to-male ratio approaching 10:1. Those afflicted with SLE are usually diagnosed between the ages of 15 and 45.[7,8] SLE is reported to be less prevalent in whites than in other ethnic groups, including blacks, Hispanics, Native Americans, and Asians.[7,8] Although the most typical SLE patient is a young adult woman, the disease can occur in people of any age or race and either gender.

ETIOLOGY

The etiology of abnormal autoantibody production and development of SLE is still unknown. Genetic, environmental, and hormonal factors all may play a role in loss of "self" tolerance and expression of disease. A popular theory is that autoimmune disease such as SLE

TABLE 90-1 Revised Criteria for Classification of Systemic Lupus Erythematosus[a]

Criterion	Definition
Malar rash	Fixed erythema, flat or raised, over the malar eminences, tending to spare the nasolabial folds
Discoid rash	Erythematous raised patches with adherent keratotic scaling and follicular plugging; atrophic scarring may occur in older lesions
Photosensitivity	Skin rash as a result of unusual reaction to sunlight, by patient history or physician observations
Oral ulcers	Oral or nasopharyngeal ulceration, usually painless, observed by a physician
Arthritis	Nonerosive arthritis involving two or more peripheral joints, characterized by tenderness, swelling, or effusion
Serositis	Pleuritis—convincing history of pleuritic pain or rub heard by a physician or evidence of pleural effusion *or* Pericarditis—documented by electrocardiogram or rub or evidence of pericardial effusion
Renal disorder	Persistent proteinuria greater than 0.5 g/day or greater than 3+ if quantitation not performed *or* Cellular casts—may be red cell, hemoglobin, granular, tubular, or mixed
Neurologic disorder	Seizures—in the absence of offending drugs or known metabolic derangements, e.g., uremia, ketoacidosis, or electrolyte imbalance *or* Psychosis—in the absence of offending drugs or known metabolic derangements, e.g., uremia, ketoacidosis, or electrolyte imbalance
Hematologic disorder	Hemolytic anemia—with reticulocytosis *or* Leukopenia—fewer than 4,000/mm^3 total on two or more occasions *or* Lymphopenia—fewer than 1,500/mm^3 on two or more occasions *or* Thrombocytopenia—fewer than 100,000/mm^3 in the absence of offending drugs
Immunologic disorder	Anti-DNA; antibody to native DNA in abnormal titer *or* Anti-Smith (Sm) antigen; presence of antibody to Sm nuclear antigen *or* Positive finding of antiphospholipid antibodies based on (a) an abnormal serum level of immunoglobulin (Ig)G or IgM anticardiolipin antibodies, (b) a positive test result for lupus anticoagulant using a standard method, or (c) a false-positive serologic test for syphilis known to be positive for at least 6 months and confirmed by *Treponema pallidum* immobilization or fluorescent treponemal antibody absorption test
Antinuclear	An abnormal titer of antinuclear antibody by immunofluorescence or an antibody equivalent assay at any point in time in the absence of drugs known to be associated with "drug-induced lupus" syndrome

[a]The proposed classification is based on 11 criteria. For the purpose of identifying patients in clinical studies, a person shall be said to have systemic lupus erythematosus if any 4 or more of the 11 criteria are present, serially or simultaneously, during any interval of observation.

From Tan EM, Cohen AS, Fries JF, et al. The 1982 revised criteria for the classification of systemic lupus erythematosus. Arthritis Rheum 1982;25:1274; and Hochberg MC. Updating the American College of Rheumatology Revised Criteria for the Classification of Systemic Lupus Erythematosus. Arthritis Rheum 1997;40;1725, with permission.

develops in genetically susceptible individuals after exposure to a triggering agent, possibly something in the environment.[8–10]

Genetic analysis shows that at least four susceptibility genes are required for the expression of lupus in humans.[10] Familial and twin studies indicate a genetic predisposition for the development of SLE. First-degree relatives of SLE patients are about 20 times more likely to develop SLE than the general population; more than 5% of cases are familial. The concordance rate among identical twins ranges from 24% to 58%, compared with 3% to 10% for nonidentical twins.[11] Multiple genes contribute to SLE susceptibility, and at least 100 genes have been linked to SLE in humans. Evidence indicates that major histocompatibility complex genes, particularly several human leukocyte antigen genes, may be important in lupus. However, nonmajor histocompatibility complex genes, such as immunoglobulin receptor genes and mannose-binding protein genes, also may contribute to disease susceptibility.[10,11] Environmental agents that may induce or activate SLE include sunlight (i.e., ultraviolet light), drugs, chemicals such as hydrazine (found in tobacco) and aromatic amines (found in hair dyes), diet, environmental estrogens, and infection with viruses or bacteria.[10] A number of viruses have been implicated as causative agents in genetically susceptible people, but much of the evidence is circumstantial.[12] Additionally, androgen may inhibit and estrogen may enhance the expression of autoimmunity, and elevated circulating prolactin levels have been associated with lupus in males and females.[10,13]

PATHOPHYSIOLOGY

❷ SLE represents a clinical syndrome rather than a discrete disease with a unique pathogenesis.[14] SLE has a large spectrum of symptoms and organ system involvement. A major event in the development of SLE is excessive and abnormal autoantibody production and the formation of immune complexes. Patients may develop autoantibodies against multiple nuclear, cytoplasmic, and surface components of multiple types of cells in various organ systems in addition to soluble markers such as immunoglobulin G and coagulation factors; these autoantibodies account for the multiple-organ system involvement of the disease.[10]

Excessive autoantibody production results from hyperactive B lymphocytes. Multiple mechanisms likely lead to B-cell hyperactivity, including loss of immune "self" tolerance and high antigenic load consisting of environmental and self antigens presented to B cells by other B cells or specific antigen-presenting cells, a shift of T-helper type 1 cells to T-helper type 2 cells that further enhance B-cell antibody production, and defective B-cell suppression. Impairment in other immune regulatory processes involving T lymphocytes (suppressor T cells), cytokines (e.g., interleukins, interferon-γ tumor necrosis factor-α, transforming growth factor-β), and natural killer cells also may be involved.[10,15]

Many autoantibodies are directed against nuclear constituents of the cell; collectively, they are called *antinuclear antibodies*. Several antinuclear antibodies are important because their presence or absence may aid in the diagnostic and clinical evaluation of patients with SLE. The SLE patient may have more than one antigen-specific antinuclear antibody in the patient's serum and tissues.[16] These are antibodies against such nuclear constituents as double-stranded, or native, DNA (dsDNA); single-stranded, or denatured, DNA (ssDNA); and RNA. Four RNA-associated antigens frequently occurring in SLE are the Smith (Sm) antigen, the small nuclear ribonucleoprotein (snRNP), the Ro (SS-A) antigen, and the La (SS-B) antigen.[17,18] Histone, a basic component of chromatin and nucleosomes, is another important nuclear component against which antinuclear antibodies are formed in lupus patients. Antibodies to Ro, La, Sm, or RNP antigens plus antibodies to dsDNA will detect most patients with SLE.[17] Antibodies also may be directed against the phospholipid moiety of the prothrombin activator complex (lupus anticoagulant) and against cardiolipin. The lupus anticoagulant and anticardiolipin antibodies constitute the two main types in a group of autoantibodies called *antiphospholipid antibodies*.

These autoantibodies often are present many years before the diagnosis of SLE.[19] The appearance of these autoantibodies follows a predictable pattern, with accumulation of specific autoantibodies before the onset of clinical illness. For example, antinuclear, anti-La,

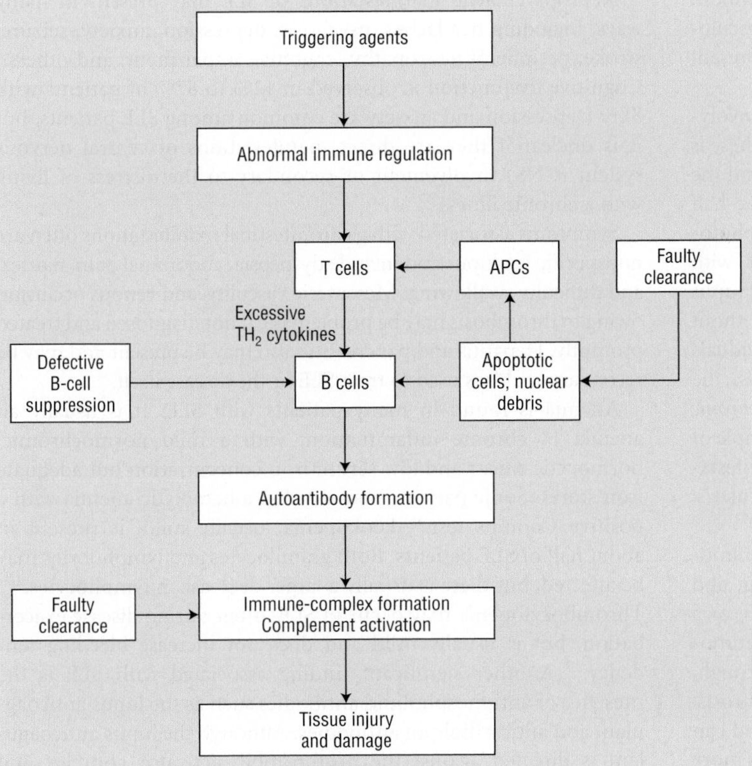

FIGURE 90-1. Pathogenesis of systemic lupus erythematosus. Environmental factors, such as infectious organisms, drugs, and chemicals, serve as triggering agents in genetically and hormonally susceptible individuals to induce a state of immune dysregulation. These abnormal immune responses lead to hyperactive T-helper type 2 lymphocyte and B-lymphocyte function. Suppressor T-lymphocyte function, cytokine production, faulty clearance mechanisms, and other immune regulatory mechanisms also are abnormal and fail to downregulate autoantibody formation from hyperactive B lymphocytes. The autoantibodies formed from this immune dysregulation become pathogenic, form immune complexes, and activate complement that leads to damage of host tissue. (APCs, antigen-presenting cells; TH_2, T-helper type 2.)

anti-Ro, and antiphospholipid antibodies often precede the onset of SLE by many years, whereas anti-Sm and anti-snRNP antibodies appear only months before diagnosis, usually when clinical symptoms begin to manifest.

Immune dysregulation leading to B-cell hyperactivity and subsequent production of pathogenic autoantibodies, coupled with defective clearance of apoptotic cells, followed by immune-complex formation, complement activation, and defective clearance of immune complexes all lead to inflammatory reactions that ultimately result in tissue injury and damage. Figure 90–1 is an overview of the pathogenesis of SLE.[10]

CLINICAL PRESENTATION

❸ As mentioned previously, SLE is a multisystem disease. Below are many of the signs and symptoms and incidences in patients with SLE.[20–22] Although certain of these may be more common than others, each patient presents differently, and the course of the disease is highly unpredictable. Furthermore, SLE is not static, and most patients have fluctuations or flare-ups during the course of the disease.

CLINICAL PRESENTATION OF SYSTEMIC LUPUS ERYTHEMATOSUS

Sign/Symptom	Incidence (%)
■ Musculoskeletal	
Arthritis and arthralgia	53–95
■ Constitutional	
Fatigue	81
Fever	41–86
Weight loss	31–71
■ Mucocutaneous	55–85
Butterfly rash	10–61
Photosensitivity	11–45
Raynaud's phenomenon	10–44
Discoid lesions	9–29
■ Central nervous system	13–59
Psychosis	5–37
Seizures	6–26
■ Pulmonary	
Pleuritis	31–57
Pleural effusion	12–40
■ Cardiovascular	
Pericarditis	2–45
Myocarditis	3–40
Heart murmur	1–44
Hypertension	23–46
■ Renal	13–65
■ Gastrointestinal	
Nausea	7–53
Abdominal pain	8–34
Bowel hemorrhage (vasculitis)	1–6
■ Hematologic	
Anemia	30–78
Leukopenia	35–66
Thrombocytopenia	7–30
■ Lymphadenopathy	10–59

Nonspecific signs and symptoms such as fatigue, fever, anorexia, and weight loss are seen frequently in patients with active disease. Musculoskeletal involvement (e.g., arthralgia, myalgia, and arthritis) is very common in SLE,[20,22,23] with arthritis and arthralgia frequently the chief complaint on initial presentation of the disease.[22] All major and minor joints may be affected, and the pattern of arthritis is often recurrent and of short duration, presenting mainly as joint stiffness, pain, and sometimes inflammation.[24] Objective evidence of musculoskeletal disease often is missing, although a few patients may present with deforming arthritis or subcutaneous nodules.

Manifestations in the skin are nearly as common as those involving the musculoskeletal system.[2,20,22] The most well known of these is the butterfly rash, which occurs over the bridge of the nose and the malar eminences. The classic butterfly rash is seen in about one-half of patients and often is observed after sun exposure. In fact, photosensitivity is common to many SLE patients who present with cutaneous manifestations. Skin lesions characteristic of discoid lupus occur in 10% to 20% of patients with SLE and may occur without other clinical or serologic evidence of lupus.[20,21,25] Some individuals are said to develop *subacute cutaneous lupus erythematosus,* the nature of whose lesions falls between discoid (one type of *chronic cutaneous lupus erythematosus*) and the butterfly rash (an example of *acute cutaneous lupus erythematosus*).[25] Other cutaneous manifestations include vasculitis (which may be ulcerative), livedo reticularis, periungual erythema, Raynaud's phenomenon, and alopecia.[2,22]

Another common source of symptomatology in SLE is the pulmonary system, with manifestations such as pleurisy, coughing, and dyspnea. Pleurisy may present as pleuritic pain, a pleural rub, or a pleural effusion that usually is exudative in nature. Lupus pneumonitis may present acutely with fever, dyspnea, tachypnea, cough, rales, and patchy infiltrates or chronically with interstitial fibrosis. Lupus pneumonitis is an uncommon manifestation of SLE and can be difficult to distinguish from infectious pneumonia, which is more common in SLE patients and should be the primary consideration when evaluating new pulmonary infiltrates.[26] Pulmonary hypertension associated with SLE is more common than previously thought, which is likely a result of asymptomatic increases in pulmonary artery pressures being more common than symptomatic increases. Patients with SLE-associated pulmonary hypertension have a poor prognosis. Pulmonary embolism also should be ruled out in any SLE patient presenting with pleuritic chest pain and dyspnea.

Cardiac manifestations of SLE often present as pericarditis, myocarditis, electrocardiographic changes, or valvular heart disease, including the classic cardiac lesion of Libman-Sacks endocarditis (nonbacterial verrucous endocarditis).[26] Coronary artery disease (CAD) is being seen in SLE with increasing frequency as the life expectancy of SLE patients increases.[27] The development of heart disease in these patients is probably multifactorial, and traditional CAD risk factors are common in patients with SLE.

Corticosteroid therapy and underlying renal disease are also believed to be contributing factors in the development of these cardiac risk factors.[26] Although hypertension, obesity, and hyperlipidemia are common in SLE patients, these traditional risk factors do not account for the strikingly high cardiovascular event rate found in some recent studies.[28,29] Other SLE-related risk factors highlight the importance of autoimmunity and inflammation in the pathogenesis of accelerated atherosclerotic cardiovascular disease.[29,30] Additionally, two studies reported that long-term corticosteroid therapy was not associated with a significantly increased risk of accelerated atherosclerosis.[31,32] In fact, one of the studies[31] found that patients with higher mean daily doses of prednisone and more frequent use of other common therapies for SLE exhibited less plaque formation, which suggests that more aggressive control of disease activity actually may help to prevent CAD.[30,31]

CLINICAL CONTROVERSY

Some research suggests that long-term corticosteroid therapy is responsible for the increased incidence of coronary heart disease, whereas other data suggest that it has no effect on atherosclerosis.

Neuropsychiatric manifestations of SLE may present in many ways, including headaches, psychosis, depression, anxiety, seizure, stroke, peripheral neuropathy, cognitive impairment, and others.[5] Cognitive dysfunction is observed in 12% to 87% of patients with SLE. Depression and anxiety are common among SLE patients, but it is unclear if they are direct manifestations of central nervous system (CNS) involvement or secondary to the distress of living with a chronic illness.[33]

Symptoms associated with gastrointestinal manifestations often are nonspecific for lupus and include dyspepsia, abdominal pain, nausea, and difficulty swallowing. Mesenteric vasculitis and venous occlusion owing to thrombosis may be problematic if not diagnosed and treated promptly. Hepatitis and pancreatitis also may be present and may be secondary to drugs used to treat SLE or the disease itself.[34]

Anemia is found in many patients with SLE. It is usually an anemia of chronic inflammation, with a mild normochromic, normocytic smear and low serum iron concentration but adequate iron stores. Some patients may develop a hemolytic anemia with a positive Coombs test.[35] Leukopenia, usually mild, is present in about half of SLE patients. Both granulocytes and lymphocytes may be affected, but there is usually a larger decrease in lymphocytes.[2,22] Thrombocytopenia may occur in SLE, often during disease exacerbation, but is usually mild and does not increase bleeding tendency.[35] Another significant finding associated with SLE is the presence of antiphospholipid antibodies such as the lupus anticoagulant and anticardiolipin antibodies. Although the lupus anticoagulant is directed against the prothrombin activator complex and implies potential bleeding complications, this is not the case. In fact, the presence of lupus anticoagulant, anticardiolipin, or other antiphospholipid antibodies may be associated with thrombosis, neurologic disease, thrombocytopenia, and fetal loss.[23,36] Thrombotic events occur in more than 10% of patients with SLE.[36] Not all patients with antiphospholipid syndrome have lupus. If a patient has no concomitant autoimmune disease, the syndrome is *primary.* If a patient has accompanying SLE, the syndrome is *secondary.*[37,38]

Clinical evidence of renal involvement, such as a rising serum creatinine or proteinuria level, generally is associated with a poorer outcome compared with patients without renal involvement. Progression to end-stage renal disease is a major cause of morbidity and mortality in SLE. However, the extent and course of renal disease are quite variable, and many lupus nephritis patients do very well. The World Health Organization has classified lupus nephritis on the basis of histologic characteristics observed following renal biopsy. A revision of this system by the International Society of Nephrology and Renal Pathology Society recommends modifying the lupus nephritis classifications as minimal mesangial (class I), mesangial proliferative (class II), focal (class III), diffuse (class IV), membranous (class V), and advanced sclerosing (class VI).[39] Many patients progress from one form of nephritis to another during the course of the disease. Predictors of poorer outcome in lupus nephritis include African American race, increased serum creatinine level, poor initial response to immunosuppressive drugs, hypertension, and persistent nephrotic syndrome.[40]

DIAGNOSIS

As mentioned earlier, the diagnostic criteria listed in Table 90–1 should not be the primary means for diagnosing SLE, although many of the criteria may be valuable in the diagnostic process. Epidemiologic characteristics, clinical signs and symptoms, and common laboratory abnormalities all are used in the diagnosis of SLE.

Once the disease is suspected, serologic tests may be helpful in making the diagnosis. A serologic test used extensively to aid in the diagnosis of SLE is the fluorescent antinuclear antibody (ANA) test. Nearly all SLE patients are ANA-positive, but other diseases also can be associated with

TABLE 90-2 Antinuclear Antibody Test: Patterns, Antigens, and Specificities

Pattern	Antigen	Disease
Peripheral	dsDNA	SLE
Speckled	Acidic nuclear protein	Rheumatoid arthritis
	Ribonucleoprotein	SLE
	Extractable nuclear antigen	Scleroderma; mixed connective tissue disease
Homogeneous	dsDNA, ssDNA	Rheumatoid arthritis
	Histones	SLE; drug-induced lupus
Nucleolar	Nucleolar RNA	Progressive systemic sclerosis

ds, double-stranded; SLE, systemic lupus erythematosus; ss, single-stranded.

a positive test (Table 90–2). However, in other diseases, many of the positive ANA tests are of a lower titer. The pattern of immunofluorescence of the ANA test also may be of diagnostic value (Table 90–2), with a peripheral (also called *rim*) pattern being specific for SLE. Detecting antibodies to specific nuclear constituents also may be useful diagnostically. Antibodies to native DNA (dsDNA) and to Sm antigen are quite specific for and are considered diagnostic of SLE.[10,17,41,42]

PROGNOSIS

In earlier years, SLE was associated with a poor prognosis. For example, three decades ago 5-year survival was approximately 83% and 76% at 10 years.[5] Today, as a result of improved treatment and improved diagnostic techniques that allow earlier diagnosis, the 5-year survival rate exceeds 96%, and 20-year survival rates approach 70%.[43,44] The natural course of SLE has changed dramatically not only because of improved therapies but also because of improvement in ability to manage patients with kidney disease (e.g., dialysis), infection, and CAD.[40,44,45] However, CAD and infection are still among the leading causes of death among SLE patients.

TREATMENT

Systemic Lupus Erythematosus

Desired treatment outcomes for the patient with SLE are twofold: (a) management of symptoms and induction of remission during times of disease flare and (b) maintenance of remission for as long as possible between disease flares. Figure 90–2 outlines an approach to the management of the patient with SLE. Because of the variability in clinical presentation of disease, treatment will vary accordingly and should be highly individualized. Optimal care of the patient with SLE will include education and support services in addition to the nonpharmacologic and pharmacologic treatments discussed below. Numerous lupus organizations exist throughout the world and can be located by contacting the Lupus Foundation of America[46] (*www.lupus.org*), the Arthritis Foundation[47] (*www.arthritis.org*), and Lupus Canada[48] (*www.lupuscanada.org*).

■ NONPHARMACOLOGIC THERAPY

Several nonpharmacologic measures can be employed to manage symptoms and help maintain remission. Fatigue is a common symptom in patients with lupus.[43] A balanced routine of rest and exercise, while avoiding overexertion, is essential in managing fatigue.[49] Avoidance of smoking may be particularly important because hydrazines in tobacco smoke may be an environmental trigger of lupus and likely contribute to accelerated CAD.[10] Smoking also has been associated with increased disease activity in SLE patients.[50] No specific dietary measures are known to clearly affect the clinical course of lupus. However, fish-oil derivatives might prevent miscarriages in pregnant women with antiphospholipid antibodies,[51] but alfalfa sprouts should be avoided because they contain the amino acid L-canavanine, which has been linked to the development of lupus-like symptoms in

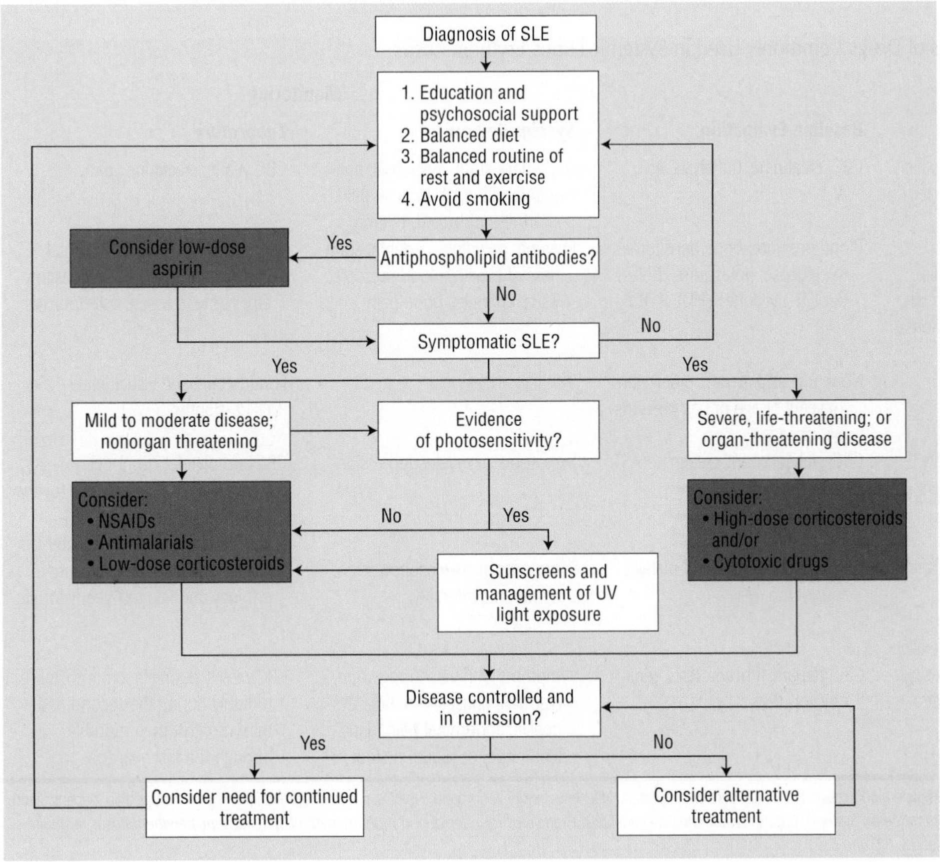

FIGURE 90-2. General approach to the management of systemic lupus erythematosus (SLE). (NSAIDs, nonsteroidal antiinflammatory drugs; UV, ultraviolet.)

TABLE 90-3 Drug Treatment of Systemic Lupus Erythematosus

Drug Class	Drug and Dose	Indication
NSAID	Various agents Antiinflammatory dose	Mild disease: fever, arthritis, skin rash, serositis
Antimalarial	Hydroxychloroquine 200–400 mg po daily Chloroquine 250–500 mg po daily	Mild disease: arthritis, skin rash, serositis
Corticosteroid	Prednisone 1–2 mg/kg/day po (or equivalent)	Initial control of severe disease
	<1 mg/kg/day (or equivalent)	Control of mild disease or maintenance after disease suppression with higher doses
	Methylprednisolone 500–1,000 mg IV daily × 3–6 day	Life-threatening disease
Cytotoxic	Cyclophosphamide 0.5–1 g/m² IV monthly for 6 months; then every 3 months for 2 years or for 1 year after remission Azathioprine 1–3 mg/kg po daily Cyclophosphamide 1–3 mg/kg po daily Mycophenolate mofetil 1–3 g po daily	Most commonly used in severe lupus nephritis; may be necessary for other severe disease manifestations

IV, intravenously; NSAID, nonsteroidal antiinflammatory drugs; po, orally.

numerous case reports.[10] Many patients with SLE will need to limit exposure to sunlight and use sunscreens to block the possible exacerbating effects of ultraviolet light.[51] The amount of sunlight exposure limitation should be individualized.

■ PHARMACOLOGIC THERAPY

❺ Drug therapy for SLE is often designed to suppress the immune response and inflammation. Except for lupus nephritis, large controlled clinical trials comparing treatment options for SLE are needed. Table 90–3 lists common agents and doses used to control SLE. In general, the choice of drug therapy depends on the extent and severity of disease. Table 90–4 describes selected monitoring parameters and adverse events for many of the drugs used to treat collagen-vascular diseases.

Nonsteroidal Antiinflammatory Drugs

As discussed earlier, signs and symptoms such as fever, arthritis, and serositis are among the most common in patients with active disease. Therefore, in many patients with mild disease, initial treatment with a nonsteroidal antiinflammatory drug (NSAID) is a logical choice. The choice of NSAIDs in SLE is empirical. The dose used should be adequate to provide antiinflammatory effects, although low-dose aspirin may be useful in the management of patients with antiphospholipid syndrome.[36]

Nonselective cyclooxygenase NSAIDs significantly increase the risk of gastric irritation and peptic ulceration. Coprescribing with a gastroprotective agent such as a proton pump inhibitor may be beneficial.[38] Patients with SLE taking NSAIDs may experience a decline in renal function because of drug effects and not the underlying disease. NSAIDs can decrease renal blood flow and glomerular filtration rates, and should be used cautiously in patients with nephritis. Awareness of this adverse effect is important because declining renal function may be attributed mistakenly to progression of lupus nephritis. Patients with SLE have a higher incidence of hepatotoxicity than do other patients taking traditional NSAIDs. The use of NSAIDs is also associated with aseptic meningitis in SLE patients.[4,23,51]

Antimalarial Drugs

Antimalarial agents such as chloroquine and hydroxychloroquine have been used successfully in the management of discoid lupus and SLE. A few controlled trials provide evidence for the role of antimalarial therapy in controlling disease exacerbations and as steroid-sparing agents.[54] In general, the manifestations of SLE that can be managed with antimalarials are cutaneous manifestations, arthralgia,

TABLE 90-4 Monitoring Adverse Effects of Drugs Commonly Used in Systemic Lupus Erythematosus

			Monitoring	
Drug	**Toxicities to Monitor**	**Baseline Evaluation**	***System Review***	***Laboratory***
Salicylates, NSAIDs	Gastrointestinal bleeding, hepatic toxicity, renal toxicity, hypertension	CBC, creatinine, urinalysis, AST, ALT	Dark/black stool, dyspepsia, nausea/vomiting, abdominal pain, shortness of breath, edema	CBC yearly, creatinine yearly
Corticosteroids	Hypertension, hyperglycemia, hyperlipidemia, hypokalemia, osteoporosis, avascular necrosis, cataract, weight gain, infections, fluid retention	Blood pressure, bone densitometry, glucose, potassium, cholesterol, triglycerides (HDL, LDL)	Polyuria, polydipsia, edema, shortness of breath, blood pressure, visual changes, bone pain	Glucose every 3–6 months, total cholesterol yearly, bone densitometry yearly to assess osteoporosis
Hydroxychloroquine	Macular damage	None unless patient is older than 40 years of age or has previous eye disease	Visual changes	Funduscopic and visual fields every 6–12 months
Azathioprine	Myelosuppression, hepatoxicity, lymphoproliferative disorders	CBC, platelet count, creatinine, AST or ALT	Symptoms of myelosuppression	CBC and platelet count every 1–2 weeks with changes in dose (every 1–3 months thereafter), AST yearly, Pap test at regular intervals
Cyclophosphamide	Myelosuppression, myeloproliferative disorders, malignancy, immunosuppression, hemorrhagic cystitis, secondary infertility	CBC and differential and platelet count, urinalysis	Symptoms of myelosuppression, hematuria, infertility	CBC and urinalysis monthly, urine cytology and Pap test yearly for life
Mycophenolate mofetil	Myelosuppression, hepatotoxicity, lymphoproliferative disorders, malignancy	CBC, hepatic function tests, renal function tests	Symptoms of myelosuppression, diarrhea, nausea/vomiting, dyspepsia, abdominal pain, dark/black stool or blood in stool	CBC weekly during first month, twice monthly during the second and third months, then monthly through the first year

ALT, alanine transaminase; AST, aspartate transaminase; CBC, complete blood count; HDL, high-density lipoprotein; LDL, low-density lipoprotein; NSAIDs, nonsteroidal anti-inflammatory drugs; Pap, papanicolaou.
Modified from American College of Rheumatology Ad Hoc Committee on Systemic Lupus Erythematosus Guidelines. Guidelines for referral and management of systemic lupus erythematosus in adults. Arthritis Rheum 1999;42:1790, with permission. Other references 23, 52, and 53.

pleuritis, mild pericardial inflammation, fatigue, and leukopenia.[23,38] Because these drugs are not effective immediately, they are best used in long-term management. Response to chloroquine occurs within 1 to 3 months, whereas the maximal effect of hydroxychloroquine may not occur for 3 to 6 months.[25] Hydroxychloroquine is probably safer than chloroquine and is considered the antimalarial of first choice.

The mechanism of action of the antimalarial drugs is uncertain. It has been proposed that antimalarials interfere with T-lymphocyte activation.[23] Other effects of antimalarials that may benefit patients with SLE include inhibition of cytokines, decreased sensitivity to ultraviolet light, antiinflammatory activity, antiplatelet effects, and antihyperlipidemic activity.[23,30]

Dosage and duration of therapy depend on patient response, tolerance of side effects, and development of retinal toxicity, which is a potentially irreversible adverse reaction associated with long-term therapy, especially with chloroquine. Current recommended doses of antimalarials in SLE are hydroxychloroquine 200 to 400 mg/day and chloroquine 250 to 500 mg/day. After 1 or 2 years of treatment, gradual tapering of dosage can be attempted. Some patients may require only 1 or 2 tablets per week to suppress cutaneous manifestations.[23,55]

Side effects of these drugs include CNS effects (e.g., headache, nervousness, insomnia, and others), rashes, dermatitis, pigmentary changes of the skin and hair, gastrointestinal disturbance (e.g., nausea), and reversible ocular toxicities such as cycloplegia and corneal deposits. Potentially serious retinal toxicity is uncommon when the currently recommended doses are used and is least common with hydroxychloroquine.[56] However, because of the possibility of permanent damage associated with the retinopathy, an ophthalmologic evaluation should be done at baseline and every 3 months when chloroquine is used and every 6 to 12 months when hydroxychloroquine is used. If retinal abnormalities are noted, antimalarial therapy should be discontinued or the dose reduced.[23]

Corticosteroids

Corticosteroid therapy is commonplace in therapeutic regimens for SLE. Although evidence for improved survival with corticosteroid therapy is inadequate, these agents are known to suppress the clinical expression of disease and are considered by many to be a major factor in the improved prognosis in recent years. Most controlled trials of corticosteroid therapy have been conducted in patients with severe lupus nephritis, but evidence suggests that corticosteroids are also effective in the management of severe cases of CNS disease, pneumonitis, polyserositis, vasculitis, thrombocytopenia, and other clinical manifestations.[23]

A patient with the diagnosis of SLE does not automatically require corticosteroid therapy. Mild disease with such manifestations as fever, arthralgia, pleuritis, or skin manifestations may respond adequately to NSAIDs or antimalarials, but patients with clinical manifestations that are more serious or unresponsive to other drugs usually require corticosteroids. Some patients with lupus dermatitis may benefit from topical or intralesional administration of corticosteroids.[23]

The goal of treatment with corticosteroids in SLE is to suppress and maintain suppression of active disease with the lowest dose possible. In patients with mild disease, low-dose therapy (prednisone 10 to 20 mg/day) is adequate,[38,42] but in patients with more severe disease (severe hemolytic anemia or cardiac involvement), higher doses, such as prednisone 1 to 2 mg/kg daily, may be required. Once adequate suppression of disease is achieved, the dose should be tapered to the minimum amount required for continued disease suppression. When analyzing the need to treat with corticosteroids, the clinician should consider other conditions that may increase the risk of corticosteroid therapy, such as infection, hypertension, atherosclerotic disease, diabetes, obesity, osteoporosis, and psychiatric disease.[4,23,38]

Steroid pulse therapy is the administration of short-term, high-dose intravenous corticosteroids with the goal of inducing remission in SLE patients with serious, life-threatening disease, such as severe active nephritis, CNS involvement, or hemolytic disease. A standard pulse regimen consists of intravenous methylprednisolone 500 to 1000 mg for 3 to 6 consecutive days. Pulse therapy usually is followed by high-dose prednisone (1 to 1.5 mg/kg per day) therapy that is tapered rapidly to low-dose maintenance therapy.[23] Potential advantages of pulse therapy over high-dose oral steroids include a quicker response and avoidance of side effects associated with the longer duration of therapy required with oral steroids. Although generally well tolerated, methylprednisolone pulse therapy may result in significant adverse effects, including infection, gastrointestinal disturbances, rapid increases in blood pressure, arrhythmias, seizures, and sudden death. Furthermore, there are insufficient data from controlled clinical trials to clearly define the role of pulse steroids in the management of SLE. Thus pulse therapy represents an alternative mode of treatment for patients with life-threatening disease or disease unresponsive to other pharmacotherapy.

Cytotoxic Drugs

A considerable amount of literature exists describing the use of cytotoxic and immunosuppressive drugs in SLE, although few of these are reports of controlled clinical trials. Included in this category are the alkylating agent cyclophosphamide and the antimetabolite azathioprine. These agents, usually used in combination with corticosteroids, have been the mainstays of immunosuppressive therapy. Although both are known to suppress and stabilize extrarenal disease activity, much of the evaluation of these agents has focused on lupus nephritis, a major factor associated with morbidity and mortality in SLE.

Evidence supporting the use of cyclophosphamide in lupus nephritis has been collected over the last several decades. Controlled clinical trials have shown that cyclophosphamide improves long-term outcomes in lupus nephritis.[38,57,58] Based on controlled trials, combination prednisone and cyclophosphamide has become standard treatment for focal and diffuse proliferative lupus nephritis (World Health Organization classes III/IV) and is superior to prednisone alone.[14] No studies have evaluated cyclophosphamide in earlier stages of nephritis (World Health Organization classes II/III), and therefore, corticosteroids remain the treatment of choice for these less severe forms of nephritis.[57] Pulse intravenous cyclophosphamide plus prednisone is more effective at slowing progression to end-stage renal disease than either prednisone alone or prednisone plus azathioprine.[59] Cyclophosphamide plus corticosteroids, the current standard of care, decreases the risk of developing end-stage renal failure requiring dialysis and renal transplantation.[14,60] Intermittent pulse administration of intravenous cyclophosphamide is preferred over daily oral therapies because of reduced adverse effects. However, pulse cyclophosphamide plus prednisone is not always effective.

When used in combination with corticosteroids, cyclophosphamide is dosed at 1 to 3 mg/kg for oral therapy and 0.5 to 1 g/m^2 of body surface area for intravenous therapy. The most common route of cyclophosphamide administration is intravenous, although there is little evidence that this is better than oral administration.[57,58] Likewise, there is no evidence to suggest the optimal duration of treatment. Based on empirical experience, cyclophosphamide generally is dosed monthly for 6 months and then every 3 months for a period of either 2 years or for 1 year after the nephritis is in remission.[40,57,58] Of course, cyclophosphamide therapy is not without risk. Serious toxic effects include suppression of hematopoiesis, opportunistic infections, bladder complications (e.g., hemorrhagic cystitis and cancer), sterility, and teratogenesis. White blood cell counts must be monitored during cyclophosphamide therapy, and if the nadir is less than 1,500/mm^3, the dose must be adjusted to keep the white cell count above 1,500/mm^3. Nausea and vomiting associated with cyclophosphamide can be controlled with oral ondansetron plus dexamethasone.[57]

Azathioprine can be used as a "steroid-sparing" agent, allowing for the reduction of corticosteroid doses.[38,42] Azathioprine has not been studied as extensively as cyclophosphamide for lupus nephritis. Additionally, azathioprine is only slightly more effective than prednisone alone.[40] Azathioprine may be useful in treating early onset and less-severe nephritis.[38,40] Long-term maintenance azathioprine therapy also may prevent renal flares after successful induction with cyclophosphamide.[58] Azathioprine is given orally in doses of 1 to 3 mg/kg per day, often in combination with corticosteroids for severe disease.[23] Azathioprine generally is less toxic than cyclophosphamide, but adverse reactions may be serious and include myelosuppression, opportunistic infections including herpes zoster, cancer, hepatotoxicity, and ovarian failure.

Cyclophosphamide often is administered intravenously in intermittent pulse doses to minimize toxicity. To decrease the risk of bladder toxicity, patients should be well hydrated with oral or intravenous fluids, and urinary output should be monitored. Mesna may be used to prevent hemorrhagic cystitis. Mesna is dosed at 20% of the total cyclophosphamide dose and is administered immediately before cyclophosphamide therapy and 3, 6, and 9 hours after therapy.[61]

Cyclophosphamide may be of benefit to some patients with other serious, refractory manifestations of lupus, including neurologic manifestations.[62] Reports of the use of other cytotoxic drugs for lupus in recent years include methotrexate,[23] mycophenolate mofetil,[6,23,38,58] mechlorethamine (nitrogen mustard), chlorambucil, and cyclosporine.[6,23,38,58]

Because of the adverse effects of cyclophosphamide, other approaches to treating lupus nephritis have been attempted. Mycophenolate mofetil is an immunosuppressive agent that has become an established treatment of severe renal and nonrenal lupus refractory to conventional cytotoxic agents.[38,58] Mycophenolate mofetil has been investigated as an alternative to cyclophosphamide for induction of remission. In an open-label trial, mycophenolate mofetil was more effective than standard cyclophosphamide therapy, achieving a higher rate of complete and partial remissions.[60] Prednisone was used in both treatment arms. Mycophenolate mofetil was also better tolerated. In this study, mycophenolate mofetil was initially dosed at 500 mg twice daily and was increased to 750 mg twice daily after 2 weeks; the dose continued to be increased weekly to a maximum of 1,000 mg three times daily. A larger study with longer followup is needed before any definitive conclusion can be drawn about the superiority of mycophenolate mofetil as induction therapy. Patients with the most severe forms of lupus nephritis should receive the standard boluses of intravenous cyclophosphamide plus corticosteroid therapy, but mycophenolate mofetil plus corticosteroid therapy may be a reasonable option for patients with mild-to-moderate nephritis and good renal function.[63]

Alternatives to cyclophosphamide for maintenance therapy have also been studied. Following induction therapy with the standard cyclophosphamide protocol, patients were assigned to either intravenous cyclophosphamide, 0.5 to 1 g/m^2; 1 to 3 mg/kg per day of oral azathioprine; or 500 to 3,000 mg of oral mycophenolate mofetil per day, with dose titrations. All groups received prednisone.[64] This open-label study showed that standard cyclophosphamide induction therapy followed by mycophenolate mofetil or azathioprine was more effective and better tolerated than standard cyclophosphamide bolus therapy. Although these data need to be interpreted cautiously because of study design limitations, azathioprine and mycophenolate mofetil are good options for maintenance therapy in lupus nephritis.[65]

Cytotoxic therapy is useful in combination with corticosteroids, allowing for lower steroid doses and improved efficacy compared with steroids alone. However, cytotoxic therapy must be monitored closely for adverse effects, and maximum response may take 6 months or longer in some patients. No data from controlled trials are available to support the combination of two or more cytotoxic agents; however, this approach has been used in patients refractory to standard therapies.[14,57]

ALTERNATIVE AND EXPERIMENTAL TREATMENTS

As the pathogenesis of SLE continues to be elucidated, new and promising treatments are being developed. Table 90–5 lists several alternative treatments reportedly successful in managing various manifestations of SLE[49,59,66–69]; however, many of these reports are uncontrolled trials. Furthermore, in addition to reports of success, the literature contains reports of unsuccessful or controversial treatments for many of these therapies (e.g., plasmapheresis or immunoglobulin for lupus nephritis). A number of newer agents are being evaluated and include various biologic therapies that interfere with immune response, ablative chemotherapy with hematopoietic stem cell transplantation, and combination chemotherapy.[14,51,70,71]

SPECIAL POPULATIONS

Pregnancy

Pregnancy in SLE patients is associated with exacerbation of disease during pregnancy, exacerbation during the early postpartum period, a greater incidence of spontaneous abortion, and a greater chance of developing preeclampsia or pregnancy-induced hypertension (particularly in patients with nephritis).

Lupus flares during pregnancy are associated with prematurity. Whether there is an increased risk for lupus flares during pregnancy versus those who are not pregnant is controversial, but exacerbation of lupus during pregnancy seems to be less likely if the disease is in remission at conception.[6,72,73] Disease exacerbations can be managed aggressively with corticosteroids, if needed, with little concern about harm to the fetus.[72] The decision to use other classes of drug therapy to control disease exacerbation should be highly individualized, although hydroxychloroquine is safe during pregnancy.[74–76] In fact, it may be safer to continue hydroxychloroquine during pregnancy than to discontinue it.[38,72] The decision to use cytotoxic drugs during pregnancy should be made with extreme caution because of potential harmful effects (e.g., teratogenesis, fetal loss) to the fetus.[77] Azathioprine may be the safest of the cytotoxic drugs if needed during pregnancy.[72,74]

Antiphospholipid antibodies may be associated with a greater likelihood of spontaneous abortion.[6,38] Corticosteroids, intravenous immunoglobulin, aspirin, and heparin, alone and in various combinations, have been used to try to improve fetal outcome.[42] Fetal survival increases with all these therapies, and none has been shown to be superior.[23] The optimal treatment regimen for pregnant patients with antiphospholipid antibodies is yet to be determined, although it has been recommended that women with antiphospholipid antibodies and no prior fetal losses should receive low-dose daily aspirin. High-risk women with a history of recurrent fetal loss

TABLE 90-5 Alternative and Experimental Treatments for Systemic Lupus Erythematosus

Treatment	Symptom	Reference
Mycophenolate mofetil	Nephritis	69
Dehydroepiandrosterone (DHEA)	Multiple symptoms	59
Abetimus sodium	Reduction in anti-dsDNA titers	67
	Nephritis	68
Anti-CD20 monoclonal antibody (Rituximab)	Multiple symptoms	69
Thalidomide	Cutaneous lesions	71
Cladribine	Nephritis	71

dsDNA, double-stranded DNA.

should be treated with low-dose subcutaneous heparin with or without aspirin.[23,72] Low-molecular-weight heparin may be an effective alternative to low-dose heparin in the treatment of antiphospholipid syndrome-related pregnancy loss.[6,23,72]

Although there is an increased chance of a high-risk pregnancy in women with SLE, appropriate planning and disease management will result in a high likelihood of a successful pregnancy and a healthy child.

Contraception

Estrogen-containing oral contraceptives have been avoided in women with SLE because of the link between estrogens and disease activity. Uncontrolled trials suggest that oral contraceptives exacerbate SLE, but this issue was only recently rigorously examined. There are good reasons to prescribe oral contraceptives in SLE: (a) outcomes of pregnancy are better when pregnancies are planned and conception occurs during disease remission; (b) women with very active disease or receiving teratogenic medications should use a very reliable method of birth control and; (c) estrogen-containing oral contraceptives may have a beneficial effect counteracting glucocorticoid-induced osteoporosis.[78]

The use of a combined oral contraceptive (ethinyl estradiol plus levonorgestrel), a progestin-only contraceptive (levonorgestrel), and an intrauterine device were compared in women with SLE.[79] This 12-month study showed comparable rates of disease flares and no clinically significant differences among all three groups during the trial. A placebo-controlled trial of ethinyl estradiol plus norethindrone also showed no difference in disease activity between the two groups over 12 months.[80] Neither of these two trials studied combined oral contraceptives in severe active SLE, leaving the issue of oral contraceptives in these patients unanswered. Because of the risk of thrombotic events in estrogen-treated women and the risk of thrombosis in SLE, antiphospholipid antibodies should be measured before oral contraceptives are started, and oral contraceptives should probably be avoided if these antibodies are present.[78]

Antiphospholipid Syndrome and Thrombosis

As mentioned earlier, the presence of antiphospholipid antibodies may result in several clinical manifestations, including thrombosis. There is no agreement on prophylaxis of patients with antiphospholipid antibodies without a history of thromboembolism.[36] In such patients, low-dose aspirin (100 to 325 mg/day) may be used prophylactically, although efficacy has not been established.[36] Patients with an acute thrombotic event should receive standard treatment with anticoagulants (e.g., heparin). Followup treatment with warfarin to prevent recurrence may require an international normalized ratio of 3 or greater in patients with antiphospholipid syndrome.[6,42] However, there is no consensus on the intensity of anticoagulation or duration of secondary prophylaxis, but as recurrence is common, patients usually are treated with oral anticoagulants indefinitely.[42]

CLINICAL CONTROVERSY

The optimal dose of aspirin and the intensity of anticoagulation therapy have not been well established, and clinicians will use various strategies for prevention of thrombosis in the presence of antiphospholipid antibodies.

Drug-Induced Lupus

Up to 10% of SLE cases may be drug-induced.[81] More than 80 drugs have been implicated as causing drug-induced lupus (DIL), although the incidence for most of these drugs is low.[81,82] Procainamide and hydralazine are associated most commonly with DIL (Table 90–6). A consensus on diagnostic criteria for DIL does not exist. To meet criteria for DIL, a patient should have exposure to a suspected drug, no prior history of idiopathic SLE prior to the use of the drug, development of ANAs (usually antihistone antibodies) and at least one clinical feature of SLE, and rapid improvement of symptoms with a gradual decline in ANAs following drug discontinuation.[81,82,84,85] The epidemiologic characteristics of DIL are different from those of idiopathic SLE. In general, patients with procainamide- or hydralazine-induced lupus develop the disease much later in life compared with idiopathic SLE probably because most people who use these drugs are older. There is also an absence of female predominance when compared with idiopathic SLE.

TABLE 90-6 Medications Implicated in Drug-Induced Lupus[a]

Acebutolol	Interleukin 2	Pindolol
Amiodarone	**Isoniazid**	Primidone
Anti-tumor necrosis factor therapies	Labetalol	**Procainamide**
Atenolol	Lisinopril	Propranolol
Captopril	Lithium	Propylthiouracil
Carbamazepine	Lovastatin	**Quinidine**
Chlorpromazine	Mephenytoin	Reserpine
Ciprofloxacin	Methimazole	Simvastatin
Clobazam	**Methyldopa**	Streptomycin
Clonidine	Metoprolol	Sulfasalazine
Clozapine	**Minocycline**	Tetracycline
Diltiazem	Nifedipine	Thiazide diuretics
Ethosuximide	Oral contraceptives	Ticlopidine
Fluvastatin	Para-aminosalicylate	Timolol
Gold salts	Penicillamine	Tocainide
Griseofulvin	Penicillin	Valproate
Hydralazine	Phenytoin	Verapamil
Hydroxyurea	Phenylbutazone	Zafirlukast
Interferon (α, γ)	Phenelzine	

[a]Drugs in **boldface** represent those with best evidence of association.
Data from references 81 to 85.

Patients of the slow acetylator phenotype may have a greater risk for developing DIL, particularly with procainamide and hydralazine.[10,81] Procainamide-induced lupus can present as early as 1 month or even after years of therapy. Hydralazine-induced lupus is dose-related, leading to the recommended maximum dose of 100 mg/day for men and 50 mg/day for women to minimize the risk of DIL.[86]

Musculoskeletal symptoms are the most common clinical manifestations, while renal manifestations and CNS involvement are rare. Other common features of DIL include fever, fatigue, pericarditis, pleurisy, and weight loss.[85] The classic malar rash is rare in DIL and skin manifestations are generally less frequent than idiopathic SLE.[81] A positive ANA test is found in nearly all (~90%) hydralazine-induced cases and in 50% to 90% of procainamide-induced disease. The immunofluorescence pattern usually is homogeneous, and antibodies are primarily against ssDNA and not dsDNA as in idiopathic SLE. Antihistone antibodies are specific for DIL but might be found in only 20% of patients with idiopathic SLE.[81]

If signs and symptoms of SLE appear in a patient and are suspected to be drug-related, the drug should be discontinued. If the lupus is drug-induced, the clinical manifestations should disappear in days to weeks, although it may take up to 1 year or longer for symptoms and serologic abnormalities to resolve completely.[38] A NSAID might be useful in treating musculoskeletal manifestations. Other, more aggressive drug therapy should not be necessary unless manifestations are deemed more serious.

PHARMACOECONOMIC CONSIDERATIONS

Treating patients with SLE is costly, requiring frequent visits to physician offices for monitoring therapy and treating adverse reactions from therapy and hospitalization for disease exacerbation and adverse drug effects. Therefore, it is particularly important in the management of a potentially debilitating chronic disease such as SLE to achieve desired treatment outcomes in an optimal manner to minimize the impact on use of healthcare resources. Costs of treating patients with SLE are slightly higher in the United States compared to Canada and the United Kingdom, but outcomes are similar.[87] The estimated annual direct cost in the United States is about $4,200, with mediations contributing approximately 29% of direct costs.[88]

Lupus patients with poor physical or poor psychological functioning have been shown to incur higher direct medical costs, whereas patients with the poorest psychological functioning and those with the most severe pain incur higher indirect costs (costs associated with loss of productivity such as days of work missed).[89] Higher direct, indirect, and total costs also are associated with higher education level, greater disease activity, and lower physical functioning in another study.[89] Specific treatment strategies that incorporate therapies to improve physical and psychological functioning, as well as reduce disease activity and end-organ damage, might reduce use of healthcare resources.

SYSTEMIC SCLEROSIS

CLINICAL MANIFESTATIONS

Systemic sclerosis is characterized by alteration of the microvasculature and by massive deposition of collagen. This disease can present as a spectrum of differing manifestations depending on affected areas and the extent of disease. Sclerosis of the skin is a hallmark for this disease, but other manifestations include a proximal diffuse (truncal) sclerosis, with skin tightness and marked skin thickening involving most of the body. Internal organs can also be involved, such as the gastrointestinal tract, lung, kidney, or heart, and can result in death. *Scleroderma* refers to patients with only skin involvement. Disease that affects only the fingers and toes is referred to as *sclerodactyly*.

CLINICAL PRESENTATION OF SYSTEMIC SCLEROSIS

General

- Sclerosis of the skin

Symptoms

- Raynaud's phenomenon
- Dyspepsia
- Constipation
- Diarrhea
- Steatorrhea
- Esophageal dysmotility

Most patients with systemic sclerosis have Raynaud's phenomenon, where the digits turn white, followed by a bluish color, which is then followed by reddening in response to an appropriate stimulus. The precipitating event is usually cold temperature or emotion. The pallor is caused by vasospasm, the bluish color is from ischemia, and the reddish color is caused by a reactive hyperemia. Raynaud's phenomenon is a common manifestation of other syndromes, and most patients with Raynaud's phenomenon do not have systemic sclerosis. Approximately 50% to 80% of patients with systemic sclerosis have gastrointestinal symptoms, and 75% to 90% of patients have esophageal dysmotility.[90,91]

Survival rates are highly variable depending on the extent of disease presentation, organ involvement, and other factors. In general, the 5-year survival rate is greater than 60%, which diminishes to approximately 50% at 10 years.[92,93]

ETIOLOGY AND PREVALENCE

The cause of systemic sclerosis is unknown. Ninety-five percent of patients have identifiable autoantibodies. There are two major subsets of the disease: limited cutaneous and diffuse systemic sclerosis. Patients with limited cutaneous involvement often have the CREST syndrome (*c*alcinosis, *R*aynaud's phenomenon, *e*sophageal dysmotility, *s*clerodactyly, and *t*elangiectasias), whereas patients with diffuse systemic sclerosis have a more aggressive disease with renal, cardiac, or pulmonary involvement. The prevalence of the disease is estimated to be between 138 and 286 cases per 1 million population.[93] The wide range may be a result of differences in diagnostic criteria, regional variation, or sample sizes used to estimate the prevalence.

TREATMENT

Systemic Sclerosis

Treatment is empirical because there are no well-controlled trials evaluating and comparing various forms of therapy. Available data are difficult to interpret because of the heterogeneity of the disease, spontaneous remissions that can occur, and lack of objective measures to assess changes in clinical status. D-Penicillamine has been used for skin involvement. When started within the first 2 years of the disease, this drug does seem to improve the skin manifestations and prolong survival.[94] The initial dose of D-penicillamine is 250 mg/day, with gradual increases in dose every 2 to 3 months to an optimal dose of 750 to 1,000 mg/day. Response occurs over many months, and the drug is not always effective. The high incidence of severe adverse events and the increased dropout rates for D-penicillamine limit its usefulness. Methotrexate appears promising as an effective therapy for skin involvement.[95] Other agents currently used are cyclophosphamide and mycophenolate mofetil, although there are no controlled trials to support their use.[96] Antiinflammatory agents and corticosteroids have not been effective in systemic sclerosis.

Angiotensin-converting enzyme (ACE) inhibitors have improved survival dramatically in patients with renal involvement and improve outcomes in patients with disease-associated pulmonary hypertension or myocardial involvement.[97,98] Patients with sclerosis of the kidneys develop hypertension, leading to a renal crisis. In these patients, plasma renin activity and angiotensin concentrations can be more than twice normal. Renal involvement should be anticipated in all systemic sclerosis patients who develop hypertension. Patients with systemic sclerosis and hypertension should be treated and maintained with an ACE inhibitor regardless of renal involvement. ACE inhibitors should be used in patients on dialysis, and have allowed some dialysis-dependent systemic sclerosis patients to discontinue dialysis.[96,97] Angiotensin receptor blockers are less effective than ACE inhibitors, but may have an additive effect to ACE inhibitors in refractory cases.[96] Treatment of Raynaud's phenomenon requires patient education and sometimes drug therapy. Patients must maintain their peripheral extremity and core body temperatures. Wearing appropriate clothing in cold environments is essential. Reaching into a freezer with unprotected hands should be avoided. Drugs that can cause peripheral vasoconstriction, such as pseudoephedrine and β-blockers, should be avoided in patients with Raynaud's phenomenon or systemic sclerosis. Smoking causes cutaneous vasoconstriction and should be eliminated, including passive smoke. When preventive measures are insufficient, calcium channel blocking agents have become the agents of choice for Raynaud's phenomenon. Nifedipine (10 to 20 mg three or four times per day) decreases the frequency and duration of attacks; diltiazem (60 mg three or four times per day) also can be used. The sustained-release formulations of these agents may enhance patient adherence. Although there are limited data, other agents that may be beneficial for Raynaud's are selective serotonin reuptake inhibitors and angiotensin II receptor antagonists.[91]

POLYMYOSITIS AND DERMATOMYOSITIS

CLINICAL MANIFESTATIONS

Polymyositis (PM) and dermatomyositis (DM) are chronic inflammatory diseases of skeletal muscle and skin of unknown etiology. DM is distinguished from PM by a typical rash, which is red, scaly, and plaque-like over the knuckles, wrists, elbows, and knees. A blue-purple discoloration on the upper eyelids with edema also can occur in dermatomyositis.

There is an increase in serum creatine kinase concentration and electromyography abnormalities. Other serum enzymes, such as the alanine transaminase, aspartate transaminase, and lactate dehydrogenase, also may be increased.[99] Muscle biopsies show a necrotizing inflammatory process. The skin lesions of DM show an immune-complex-mediated necrosis of the microvasculature. PM appears to be related to cytotoxic T-cell activity, and up to 20% of patients with inflammatory myopathies have ANAs and cytoplasmic antibodies.

CLINICAL PRESENTATION OF POLYMYOSITIS AND DERMATOMYOSITIS

General

- Inflammation of skeletal muscle and skin

Symptoms

- Muscle weakness in shoulder and hip girdles and trunk
- Insidious onset
- Arthritis, Raynaud's phenomenon, and other symptoms of connective tissue diseases

TREATMENT

Polymyositis and Dermatomyositis

Large, controlled trials of drug therapy have not been conducted. The goal of therapy is to increase muscle strength so as to improve function in activities of daily living (e.g., bathing, dressing, feeding, and toileting). Treatment consists of physical therapy during periods of remission and rest during periods of disease activity. Prednisone is the first line of drug therapy for PM and DM. Although the optimal dose of prednisone is not clear, most clinicians use prednisone at a starting dose of 60 to 100 mg/day or about 1 mg/kg per day as a single morning dose.[99–101] Higher prednisone doses of 1.5 mg/kg per day can be used if needed.[102] The initial dose of prednisone is continued for 1 to 2 months or until maximum benefit is achieved or a remission is induced. The full effect of prednisone may not be evident for several months. After 4 months of treatment, approximately 85% of patients treated with prednisone will have normal muscle strength. The prednisone dose is tapered when muscle strength improves and serum creatine kinase concentrations decrease. If the patient is responding to prednisone and there are no serious side effects, the drug is tapered slowly. One expert advocates using prednisone for 3 to 4 weeks and then tapering the dose over 10 weeks to an every-other-day regimen.[99] The dose that maintains a good clinical response can be used as maintenance. Tapering too quickly can cause an exacerbation of disease activity. Monitoring serum creatine kinase concentrations is useful because they tend to increase several weeks before clinical symptoms become apparent. Some clinicians will treat patients with daily prednisone for 1 or more years, whereas others may use every-other-day therapy for many years.

One complication from corticosteroid use is the development of a myopathy. Based on symptoms, it is difficult to know if increased muscle weakness is caused by the corticosteroid or to worsening disease status. Lowering the prednisone dose may be useful. If patients get better on a lower dose of prednisone, then most likely the muscle weakness was caused by the drug. It may take 2 to 8 weeks for this to become evident clinically. Use of serum creatine kinase concentration also may be helpful because this does not increase with steroid myopathy. It is possible that a steroid myopathy and worsening disease can coexist.

Although most patients with PM or DM improve with prednisone, some will not, and some will develop corticosteroid resistance. In these patients, azathioprine has been used at a dose of 2 to 3 mg/kg per day in divided doses, with a maintenance dose of 0.5 mg/kg per day.[101] Clinical response may take 3 to 6 months. Another alternative is methotrexate at a dose of 5 to 20 mg once weekly.[101] In patients resistant to these therapies, cyclophosphamide, cyclosporine, or chlorambucil can be tried. Intravenous immunoglobulin at a dose of 2 g/kg per month for 3 months may be effective in patients with refractory disease.[102] Alternative therapies are often used in PM or DM, but there is no convincing evidence to support their use. These alternative therapies also may be beneficial in patients who cannot take corticosteroids because of serious adverse effects.

POLYMYALGIA RHEUMATICA AND GIANT CELL ARTERITIS

CLINICAL MANIFESTATIONS

Polymyalgia rheumatica (PMR) and giant cell arteritis are closely related diseases, and some experts consider them to be different phases of the same disease.[103,104]

Giant cell arteritis is a vasculitis of large and medium-size vessels. The most frequent symptom is headache, with pain usually in the temporal or occipital areas; signs of systemic inflammation are also usually present.[103,105] Giant cell arteritis was referred to previously as "temporal arteritis" or "granulomatous arteritis." Both PMR and giant cell arteritis occur in people older than 50 years of age, and the incidence increases with age, peaking between ages 70 and 80 years.[101] Some patients go from exhibiting no symptoms to overt clinical manifestations overnight, whereas others have a gradual onset of symptoms over a number of weeks. The etiology is unknown.

CLINICAL PRESENTATION OF POLYMYALGIA RHEUMATICA AND GIANT CELL ARTERITIS

General

- Aching and morning stiffness of neck, shoulder, and pelvic girdle musculature and torso.

Symptoms

- Pain and morning stiffness lasting 1 to 6 hours
- Fatigue, malaise, and weight loss are usually present
- Anorexia
- Headache in giant cell arteritis

Signs

- Low-grade fever

Laboratory Tests

- Erythrocyte sedimentation rate is generally >40 mm/h and often >100 mm/h

TREATMENT

Polymyalgia Rheumatica and Giant Cell Arteritis

The treatment of choice for PMR is prednisone at a dose of 10 to 20 mg/day, and giant cell arteritis requires doses of 40 to 60 mg/day. Pulse therapy with intravenous methylprednisolone, 1,000 mg/day for 3 days, may be used in patients experiencing visual loss.[103,104] Corticosteroid therapy is so effective that if improvement does not occur within a week, another diagnosis should be considered. The erythrocyte sedimentation rate (ESR) should decrease by 2 weeks and become normal after 4 weeks of therapy. The prednisone should be tapered beginning several weeks following control of symptoms. The rate of tapering is based on clinical response. A taper of 2.5 mg/day at 2- to 4-week intervals to 5 to 10 mg/day followed by a slower tapering of 1 mg/day at monthly intervals has been suggested.[106,107] The lowest dose of prednisone that controls symptoms should be used for maintenance, which is usually between 7 and 15 mg/day. Maintaining the ESR and C-reactive protein concentration in the normal range is a good monitoring approach. For elderly patients, the normal ESR may be slightly higher than that usually given as a reference value by the clinical laboratory. PMR is a self-limited disease, and patients usually continue maintenance therapy for 2 to 5 years. Patients may experience a relapse when the prednisone is discontinued. Every-other-day prednisone has not been as successful as daily therapy. Because these are diseases of the elderly, it is particularly important to use calcium and vitamin D supplements to prevent corticosteroid-induced osteoporosis. Prophylactic bisphosphonate therapy also should be considered. Unlike most other autoimmune diseases, other forms of immunosuppressive therapy are not as effective as corticosteroids in PMR and giant cell arteritis.[105]

DRUG-INDUCED VASCULITIS

CLINICAL MANIFESTATIONS

❻ Drugs are common causes of vasculitis, often occurring in the skin, but other organ involvement can occur. The pathogenesis of inflammation of small and medium-size blood vessel walls caused by drugs is poorly understood.[108] Even drugs used to treat inflammatory and immune-mediated disease, such as NSAIDs, sulfasalazine, and etanercept, can cause vasculitis.

CLINICAL PRESENTATION OF DRUG-INDUCED VASCULITIS

General

- Signs and symptoms depend on organ involvement

Symptoms

- Rash
- Glomerulonephritis
- Hepatitis
- Fatigue
- Myalgia
- Arthralgia

Signs

- Fever

Symptoms can occur within hours of drug administration or after more than 15 years of using a drug.[109] Most classes of medications have been reported to cause vasculitis. Although there are no specific diagnostic tests for drug-induced vasculitis, antineutrophil cytoplasmic autoantibodies have been identified in many cases of drug-induced vasculitis.[108,109] Eosinophilia, leukocytosis, and elevated ESR also may occur.

TREATMENT

Drug-Induced Vasculitis

The first step in therapy of drug-induced vasculitis is to discontinue the suspected inducing agent. This may be all that is necessary to abate symptoms in mild cases. For more serious cases, corticosteroids may be used, and where life-threatening organ involvement occurs, immunosuppressive therapy with agents such as cyclophosphamide may be used.[109] Following therapy, symptoms resolve within a few weeks to a few months.

EVALUATION OF THERAPEUTIC OUTCOMES

The diversity of clinical features and disease severity associated with the collagen–vascular diseases leads to a number of possible clinical outcomes with a broad range of desired therapeutic outcomes. Achieving desired therapeutic outcomes for most of the collagen–vascular diseases is highly variable. Currently, it is not possible to predict which patients will have a satisfactory therapeutic response and which will have unrelenting progressive disease. These diseases often have fluctuating courses, necessitating frequent changes in drug therapy and drug doses.

Evaluation of drug therapy of several of the collagen–vascular diseases often only requires monitoring for resolution of symptoms such as rash or muscle pain. However, patients with life-threatening disease receiving aggressive pharmacotherapy may require intensive monitoring and evaluation of therapy. For example, the patient receiving cytotoxic drug therapy for severe lupus nephritis requires close monitoring of laboratory indices of renal function, as well as monitoring of symptomatology and laboratory indices for possible bone marrow suppression, infection, cystitis, or other potential adverse effects.

Evaluation of therapeutic outcomes also should include an awareness of the possibility of drug therapy mimicking signs and symptoms of disease, such as the lupus patient receiving NSAID therapy and presenting with renal insufficiency or the patient with PM receiving prednisone and presenting with an exacerbation of muscle weakness.

As patients live longer, as is the case with SLE, outcome measures other than mortality will be needed to assess the effect of treatment. Clinicians and researchers working with lupus patients have developed and continue to refine some of these alternative outcome measures. Three important domains for assessing lupus patients are disease activity, accumulated damage, and quality of life.[110] Table 90–7 lists several instruments useful for assessing patients with SLE. Increased use of these and similar instruments for assessment of treatment outcomes in patients with SLE can be expected.

CONCLUSION

SLE is a disease that affects multiple organ systems and consists of abnormal immunologic function and the development of autoantibodies. The disease is quite variable in clinical presentation and progression. The cause of lupus is unknown, although several factors (e.g., genetics, environment, and hormones) may predispose an individual to the development of the disease. Although SLE was

TABLE 90-7 Instruments Used for Assessing Outcome Measures in Patients with Systemic Lupus Erythematosus

Outcome Domain	Instrument
Disease activity	Systemic Lupus Activity Measure (SLAM)/SLAM Revised (SLAM-R)
	Systemic Lupus Erythematosus Disease Activity Index (SLEDAI)
	European Community Lupus Activity Index (ECLAM)
	British Isles Lupus Activity Group (BILAG)
Accumulated damage	Systemic Lupus International Collaborating Clinics/American College of Rheumatology (SLICC/ACR) damage index
Quality of life	Health Assessment Questionnaire (HAQ) functional ability index
	Medical Outcome Survey short form (MOS SF-20) and (MOS SF-36)

Data from reference 110.

once thought to be rapidly fatal, today nearly 90% of patients survive 10 years.

Drug therapy is nonspecific and is aimed at suppressing the inflammation and abnormal immune response associated with active disease. Clinical trials with various agents often have been inadequate and contradictory, and the therapeutic management of lupus is not optimal. Nevertheless, drug therapy of recent years probably has contributed significantly to the improved survival of these patients. As the understanding of SLE progresses and advances in molecular biology occur, we can expect to see the development of more specific and optimal treatment and further improvement in survival.

Each of the collagen–vascular diseases has its own recommended form of therapy. For most of these diseases, there are few well-controlled clinical trials evaluating pharmacotherapy. Treatment of most of these diseases requires antiinflammatory or immunosuppressive drugs. Monitoring therapeutic outcomes is essential because drugs and drug doses may need to be modified frequently.

ABBREVIATIONS

ACE: angiotensin-converting enzyme

ANA: antinuclear antibodies

CAD: coronary artery disease

DIL: drug-induced lupus

DM: dermatomyositis

DNA: deoxyribonucleic acid

dsDNA: double-stranded DNA

ESR: erythrocyte sedimentation rate

NSAID: nonsteroidal anti-inflammatory drug

PM: polymyositis

PMR: polymyalgia rheumatica

RNP: ribonucleoprotein

SLE: systemic lupus erythematosus

ssDNA: single-stranded DNA

RNA: ribonucleic acid

REFERENCES

1. Benedek TG. Historical background of discoid and systemic lupus erythematosus. In: Wallace DJ, Hahn BH, eds. Dubois' Lupus Erythematosus, 6th ed. Philadelphia: Lippincott Williams & Wilkins, 2002:3–16.
2. Edworthy SM. Clinical manifestations of systemic lupus erythematosus. In: Ruddy S, Harris ED, Sledge CB, eds. Kelley's Textbook of Rheumatology, 6th ed. Philadelphia: WB Saunders, 2001:1105–1123.
3. Tan EM, Cohen AS, Fries JF, et al. The 1982 revised criteria for the classification of systemic lupus erythematosus. Arthritis Rheum 1982;25:1271–1277.
4. Hochberg MC, for the Diagnostic and Therapeutic Criteria Committee of the American College of Rheumatology. Updating the American College of Rheumatology revised criteria for the classification of systemic lupus erythematosus [letter]. Arthritis Rheum 1997;40:1725.
5. Benseler SM, Silverman ED. Systemic lupus erythematosus. Pediatr Clin North Am 2005;52:443–467.
6. Ruiz-Irastorza G, Khamashta MA, Castellino G, Hughes GRV. Systemic lupus erythematosus. Lancet 2001;357:1027–1032.
7. D'Cruz DP. Systemic lupus erythematosus. BMJ 2006;332:890–894.
8. Lupus Foundation of America. Statistics about lupus. Available at *www.lupus.org/index.html*.
9. Riemekasten G, Hahn BH. Key autoantigens in SLE. Rheumatology 2005;44:975–982.
10. Mok CC, Lau CS. Pathogenesis of systemic lupus erythematosus. J Clin Pathol 2003;56:481–490.
11. Perdriger A, Werner-Leyval S, Rollot-Elamrani K. The genetic basis for systemic lupus erythematosus. Joint Bone Spine 2003;70:103–108.
12. Denman AM. Systemic lupus erythematosus: Is a viral aetiology a credible hypothesis? J Infect 2000;40:229–233.
13. McMurray RW, May W. Sex hormones and systemic lupus erythematosus. Arthritis Rheum 2003;48:2100–2110.
14. Balow JE, Boumpas DT, Austin HA III. New prospects for treatment of lupus nephritis. Semin Nephrol 2000;20:32–39.
15. Lauwerys BR, Houssiau FA. Involvement of cytokines in the pathogenesis of systemic lupus erythematosus. Adv Exp Med Biol 2003;520:237–251.
16. Rahman A. Autoantibodies, lupus and the science of sabotage. Rheumatology (Oxford) 2004;43:1326–1336.
17. Enger W. The use of laboratory tests in the diagnosis of SLE. J Clin Pathol 2000;53:424–432.
18. Shmerling RH. Autoantibodies in systemic lupus erythematosus: There before you know it. N Engl J Med 2003;349:1499–1500.
19. Arbuckle MR, McClain MT, Rubertone MV, et al. Development of auto-antibodies before the clinical onset of systemic lupus erythematosus. N Engl J Med 2003;349:1526–1533.
20. Lupus Foundation of America. Lupus fact sheet. Available at *www.lupus.org/index.html*.
21. National Institute of Arthritis and Musculoskeletal and Skin Diseases. Lupus: A Patient Care Guide for Nurses and Other Health Professionals, Chapter 1: Lupus Erythematosus, May 2001. 2001, *http://www.niams.nih.gov/hi/topics/lupus/lupusguide/chp1.htm#chp1_symp*.
22. Wallace DJ. The clinical presentation of systemic lupus erythematosus. In: Wallace DJ, Hahn BH, eds. Dubois' Lupus Erythematosus, 6th ed. Philadelphia: Lippincott Williams & Wilkins, 2002:621–628.
23. Hahn BH. Management of systemic lupus erythematosus. In: Ruddy S, Harris ED, Sledge CB, eds. Kelley's Textbook of Rheumatology, 6th ed. Philadelphia: WB Saunders, 2001:1125–1143.
24. Wallace DJ. The musculoskeletal system. In: Wallace DJ, Hahn BH, eds. Dubois' Lupus Erythematosus, 6th ed. Philadelphia: Lippincott Williams & Wilkins, 2002:629–644.
25. Patel P, Werth V. Cutaneous lupus erythematosus: A review. Dermatol Clin 2002;20:373–385.
26. Kao AH, Manzi S. How to manage patients with cardiopulmonary disease? Best Pract Res Clin Rheumatol 2002;16:211–227.
27. Hall FC, Dalbeth N. Disease modification and cardiovascular risk reduction: Two sides of the same coin? Rheumatology (Oxford) 2005;44:1473–1482.
28. Esdaile JM, Abrahamowicz M, Grodzicky T, et al. Traditional Framingham risk factors fail to fully account for accelerated atherosclerosis in systemic lupus erythematosus. Arthritis Rheum 2001;44:2331–2337.
29. Shattner A, Liang MH. The cardiovascular burden of lupus: A complex challenge. Arch Intern Med 2003;163:1507–1510.
30. Hahn BH. Systemic lupus erythematosus and accelerated atherosclerosis. N Engl J Med 2003;349:2379–2380.
31. Roman MJ, Shanker B, Davis A, et al. Prevalence and correlates of accelerated atherosclerosis in systemic lupus erythematosus. N Engl J Med 2003;349:2399–2406.
32. Asanuma Y, Oeser A, Shintani AK, et al. Premature coronary-artery atherosclerosis in systemic lupus erythematosus. N Engl J Med 2003;349:2407–2415.
33. Harrison MJ, Ravdin LD. Cognitive dysfunction in neuropsychiatric systemic lupus erythematosus. Curr Opin Rheumatol 2002;14:510–514.

34. Hallegua DS, Wallace DJ. Gastrointestinal manifestations of systemic lupus erythematosus. Curr Opin Rheumatol, 2000;12:379–385.
35. Quismorio FP. Hematologic and lymphoid abnormalities in systemic lupus erythematosus. In: Wallace DJ, Hahn BH, eds. Dubois' Lupus Erythematosus, 6th ed. Philadelphia: Lippincott Williams & Wilkins, 2002:793–819.
36. Wahl DG, Bounameaux H, de Moerlosse P, Sarasin FP. Prophylactic antithrombotic therapy for patients with systemic lupus erythematosus with or without antiphospholipid antibodies: Do the benefits outweigh the risks? Arch Intern Med 2000;160:2042–2048.
37. Lockshin MD, Sammaritano LR, Schwartzman S. Validation of the Sapporo criteria for antiphospholipid syndrome. Arthritis Rheum 2000;43:440–443.
38. Ioannou Y, Isenberg DA. Current concepts for the management of systemic lupus erythematosus in adults: A therapeutic challenge. Postgrad Med J 2002;78:599–606.
39. Weening JJ, D'Agati VD, Schwartz MM, et al. The classification of glomerulonephritis in systemic lupus erythematosus revisited. J Am Soc Nephrol 2004;15:241–250.
40. Austin HA, Balow JE. Treatment of lupus nephritis. Semin Nephrol 2000;20:265–276.
41. Shmerling RH. Diagnostic tests for rheumatic disease: Clinical utility revisited. South Med J 2005;98:704–711.
42. Brasington RD Jr, Kahl LE, Ranganathan P, et al. Immunologic rheumatic disorders. J Allergy Clin Immunol 2003;111:S593–601.
43. Urowitz MD, Gladman DD. How to improve morbidity and mortality in systemic lupus erythematosus. Rheumatology 2000;39:238–244.
44. Manger K, Manger B, Repp R, et al. Definition of risk factors for death, end stage renal disease, and thromboembolic events in a monocentric cohort of 338 patients with systemic lupus erythematosus. Ann Rheum Dis 2002;61:1065–1070.
45. Petri M. Hopkins lupus cohort: 1999 update. Rheum Dis Clin North Am 2000;26:199–213.
46. Lupus Foundation of America, Inc., 2000 L Street, N.W., Suite 710, Washington, DC 20036; 800–558–0121.
47. Arthritis Foundation, 1330 West Peachtree Street, Atlanta, GA; 404–872–7100.
48. Lupus Canada, 590 Alden Road, Suite 211 Markham, Ontario L3R 8N2 Canada; 800–661–1468.
49. Wallace DJ. Principles of therapy and local measures. In: Wallace DJ, Hahn BH, eds. Dubois' Lupus Erythematosus, 6th ed. Philadelphia: Lippincott Williams & Wilkins, 2002:1131–1140.
50. Ghaussy NO, Sibbitt WL, Bankhurst AD, Qualls CR. Cigarette smoking and disease activity in systemic lupus erythematosus. J Rheumatol 2003;30:1215–1221.
51. Solsky MA, Wallace DJ. New therapies in systemic lupus erythematosus. Best Pract Res Clin Rheumatol 2002;16:293–312.
52. Stein CM. Immunoregulatory drugs. In: Ruddy S, Harris ED, Sledge CB, eds. Kelley's Textbook of Rheumatology, 6th ed. Philadelphia: WB Saunders, 2001:879–898.
53. CellCept (mycophenolate mofetil). Package insert. Nutley, NJ: Roche Laboratories, October 2005.
54. Gordon DA, Klinkhoff AV. Second line agents. In: Harris ED Jr, Budd RC, Genovese MC, et al. eds. Kelley's Textbook of Rheumatology, 7th ed. Philadelphia: Elsevier/Saunders, 2005:877–899.
55. Wallace DJ. Antimalarial therapies. In: Wallace DJ, Hahn BH, eds. Dubois' Lupus Erythematosus, 6th ed. Philadelphia: Lippincott Williams & Wilkins, 2002:1149–1172.
56. Rynes RI. Antimalarial drugs. In: Ruddy S, Harris ED, Sledge CB, eds. Kelley's Textbook of Rheumatology, 6th ed. Philadelphia: WB Saunders, 2001:859–867.
57. Ortmann RA, Klippel JH. Update on cyclophosphamide for systemic lupus erythematosus. Rheum Dis Clin North Am 2000;26:363–375.
58. Mok CC, Wong RWS, Lai KN. Treatment of severe proliferative lupus nephritis: The current state. Ann Rheum Dis 2003;62:799–804.
59. Ginzler EM, Dvorkina O. Newer therapeutic approaches for systemic lupus erythematosus. Rheum Dis Clin North Am 2005;315–328.
60. Ginzler EM, Dooley MA, Aranow C, et al. Mycophenolate mofetil or intravenous cyclophosphamide for lupus nephritis. N Engl J Med 2005;353:2219–2228.
61. Davis JC, Klippel JH. Antimalarials and immunosuppressive therapies. In: Lahita RG, ed. Systemic Lupus Erythematosus, 4th ed. New York: Elsevier, 2004:1273–1293.
62. Gold R, Fontana A, Zierz S. Therapy of neurological disorders in systemic vasculitis. Semin Neurol 2003;23:207–214.
63. McCune WJ. Mycophenolate mofetil for lupus nephritis. N Engl J Med 2005;353:2282–2284.
64. Contreras G, Pardo V, Leclercq B, et al. Sequential therapies for proliferative lupus nephritis. N Engl J Med 2004;350:971–980.
65. Balow JE, Austin HA. Maintenance therapy for lupus nephritis—Something old, something new. N Engl J Med 2004;350:1044–1046.
66. Goldblatt F, Isenberg DA. New therapies for systemic lupus erythematosus. Clin Exp Immunol 2005;140:205–212.
67. Furie RA, Cash JM, Cronin ME, et al. Treatment of systemic lupus erythematosus with LJP 394. J Rheumatol 2001;28:257–265.
68. Alarcon-Segovia D, Tumlin JA, Furie RA, et al. LJP 394 for the prevention of renal flare in patients with systemic lupus erythematosus: Results form a randomized, double-blind, placebo-controlled study. Arthritis Rheum 2003;48:442–454.
69. Leandro MJ, Edwards JC, Cambridge G, et al. An open study of B lymphocyte depletion in systemic lupus erythematosus. Arthritis Rheum 2002;46:2673–2677.
70. Gescuk BD, Davis JC Jr. Novel therapeutic agents for systemic lupus erythematosus. Curr Opin Rheumatol 2002;14:515–521.
71. Strand V. New therapies for systemic lupus erythematosus. Rheum Dis Clin North Am 2000;26:389–406.
72. Mok CC, Wong RWS. Pregnancy in systemic lupus erythematosus. Postgrad Med J 2001;77:157–165.
73. Cervera R, Font J, Carmona F, Balasch J. Pregnancy outcome in systemic lupus erythematosus: Good news for the new millennium. Autoimmun Rev 2002;1:354–359.
74. Mosca M, Ruiz-Irastorza G, Khamashta MA, Hughes GRV. Treatment of systemic lupus erythematosus. Int Immunopharmacol 2001;1:1065–1075.
75. Costedoat-Chalumeau N, Amoura Z, Duhaut P, et al. Safety of hydroxychloroquine in pregnant patients with connective tissue diseases: A study of one hundred thirty-three cases compared with a control group. Arthritis Rheum 2003;48:3207–3211.
76. Levy RA, Vilela VS, Cataldo MJ, et al. Hydroxychloroquine (HCQ) in lupus pregnancy: Double-blind and placebo-controlled study. Lupus 2001;10:401–404.
77. Petri M. Immunosuppressive drug use in pregnancy. Autoimmunity 2003;36:51–56.
78. Bermas BL. Oral contraceptives in systemic lupus erythematosus—A tough pill to swallow? N Engl J Med 2005;353:2602–2604.
79. Sanchez-Guerrero J, Uribe AG, Jimenez-Santana L, et al. A trial of contraceptive methods in women with systemic lupus erythematosus. N Engl J Med 2005;353:2539–2549.
80. Petri M, Kim MY, Kalunian KC, et al. Combined oral contraceptives in women with systemic lupus erythematosus. N Engl J Med 2005;353:2550–2558.
81. Antonov D, Kazandjieva J, Etugov D, Gospodinov D, Tsankov N. Drug-induced lupus erythematosus. Clin Dermatol 2004;22:157–166.
82. Rubin RL. Drug-induced lupus. Toxicology 2005;209:135–147.
83. Spiera RF, Berman RS, Werner AJ, Spiera H. Ticlopidine-induced lupus: A report of 4 cases. Arch Intern Med 2002;162:2240–2243.
84. Brogan BL, Olsen NJ. Drug-induced rheumatic syndromes. Curr Opin Rheumatol 2003;15:76–80.
85. di Fazano CS, Berrin P, Vergne P, et al. The pharmacological management of drug-induced rheumatic disorders. Expert Opin Pharmacother 2001;2:1623–1631.
86. Finks SW, Finks AL, Self TH. Hydralazine-induced lupus: Maintaining vigilance with increased use in patients with heart failure. South Med J 2006;99:18–22.
87. Clarke AE, Petri MA, Manzi S, et al. The systemic lupus erythematosus Tri-nation Study: Absence of a link between health resource use and health outcome. Rheumatology (Oxford) 2004;43:1016–1024.
88. Brunner HI, Sherrard TM, Klein-Gitelman MS. Cost of treatment of childhood-onset systemic lupus erythematosus. Arthritis Rheum 2006;55:184–188.

89. Sutcliffe N, Clarke AE, Taylor R, et al. Total costs and predictors of costs in patients with systemic lupus erythematosus. Rheumatology 2001;40:37–47.
90. Cossio M, Menon Y, Wilson W, deBoisblanc BP. Life-threatening complications of systemic sclerosis. Crit Care Clin 2002;18:819–839.
91. Leighton C. Drug treatment of scleroderma. Drugs 2001;61:419–427.
92. Steen VD, Medsger TA Jr. Severe organ involvement in systemic sclerosis with diffuse scleroderma. Arthritis Rheum 2000;43:2437–2444.
93. Mayers MD, Lacey JV Jr, Beebe-Dimmer J, et al. Prevalence, incidence, survival, and disease characteristics of systemic sclerosis in a large US population. Arthritis Rheum 2003;48:2246–2255.
94. Steen VD, Medsger TA Jr. Improvement in skin thickening in systemic sclerosis associated with improved survival. Arthritis Rheum 2001;44:2828–2835.
95. Charles C, Clements P, Furst DE. Systemic sclerosis: Hypothesis-driven treatment strategies. Lancet 2006;367:1683–1691.
96. Ong VH, Brough G, Denton CP. Management of systemic sclerosis. Clin Med 2005;5:214–219.
97. Lin ATH, Clements PJ, Furst DE. Update on disease-modifying anti-rheumatic drugs in the treatment of systemic sclerosis. Rheum Dis Clin North Am 2003;29:409–426.
98. Maddison P. Prevention of vascular damage in scleroderma with angiotensin-converting enzyme (ACE) inhibition. Rheumatology 2002;41:965–971.
99. Dalakas MC, Hohlfeld R. Polymyositis and dermatomyositis. Lancet 2003;362:971–982.
100. Choy EHS, Isenberg DA. Treatment of dermatomyositis and polymyositis. Rheumatology 2002;41:7–13.
101. Ghate J, Katsambas A, Augerinou G, Jorizzo JL. A therapeutic update on dermatomyositis/polymyositis. Int J Dermatol 2000;39:81–87.
102. Koler RA. Dermatomyositis. Am Fam Physician 2001;64:1565–1572.
103. Salvarani C, Cantini F, Boiardi L, Hunder GG. Polymyalgia rheumatica and giant-cell arteritis. N Engl J Med 2002;347:261–271.
104. Weyand CM, Goronzy JJ. Giant-cell arteritis and polymyalgia rheumatica. Ann Intern Med 2003;139:505–515.
105. Weyand CM, Goronzy JJ. Medium- and large-vessel vasculitis. N Engl J Med 2003;349:160–169.
106. Epperly TD, Moore KE, Harrover JD. Polymyalgia rheumatica and temporal arteritis. Am Fam Physician 2000;62:789–796, 801.
107. Evans JM, Hunder GG. Polymyalgia rheumatica and giant cell arteritis. Rheum Dis Clin North Am 2000;26:493–515.
108. Merkel PA. Drug-induced vascuitis. Rheum Dis Clin North Am 2001;27:849–862.
109. tan Holder SM, Joy MS, Falk RJ. Cutaneous and systemic manifestations of drug-induced vasculitis. Ann Pharmacother 2002;36:130–147.
110. Haq I, Isenberg DA. How does one assess and monitor patients with systemic lupus erythematosus in daily clinical practice? Best Pract Res Clin Rheumatol, 2002;16:181–194.

CHAPTER 91

Allergic and Pseudoallergic Drug Reactions

JOSEPH T. DIPIRO

KEY CONCEPTS

1. Allergic reactions are responsible for 6% to 10% of adverse reactions to medications. Although some reactions are relatively well defined, the majority are due to mechanisms that are either unknown or poorly understood.

2. The following criteria suggest that a drug reaction may be immunologically mediated: (a) the reaction occurs in a small percentage of patients receiving the drug, (b) the observed reaction does not resemble the drug's pharmacologic effect, (c) the type of manifestation is similar to that seen with other allergic reactions (anaphylaxis, urticaria, serum sickness), (d) there is a lag time between first exposure of the drug and reaction, (e) the reaction is reproduced even by minute doses of the drug, (f) the reaction is reproduced by agents with similar chemical structures, (g) eosinophilia is present, or (h) the reaction resolves after the drug has been discontinued. Exceptions to each of these criteria are observed commonly.

3. Anaphylaxis is an acute, life-threatening allergic reaction involving multiple organ systems that generally begins within 30 minutes but almost always within 2 hours after exposure to the inciting allergen. Anaphylaxis requires prompt treatment to restore respiratory and cardiovascular function. Epinephrine is administered as primary treatment to counteract bronchoconstriction and vasodilation. Intravenous fluids should be administered to restore intravascular volume.

4. Factors that influence the likelihood of allergic drug reactions are the dose of the allergen, the route of exposure, and the sensitivity of the individual as determined by age, genetics, or environmental factors. For many drugs, the severity of a reaction is determined by the dose and duration of exposure.

5. Patients with a history of a reaction to penicillin are advised not to receive cephalosporins if they can be avoided. Patients who have negative penicillin skin tests or experienced only mild cutaneous reactions, such as maculopapular rashes, have a low risk of serious reactions to cephalosporins.

6. Less than 1% of patients receiving nonionic radiocontrast agents experience some type of adverse reaction. Of the variety of reactions reported, approximately 90% are allergic-like, mostly urticarial, with severe reactions occurring as infrequently as 0.02%.

7. Aspirin and other nonsteroidal antiinflammatory drugs (NSAIDs) can produce two general types of reactions, urticaria/angioedema and rhinosinusitis/asthma, in susceptible patients. About 20% of asthmatics are sensitive to aspirin and other NSAIDs.

8. Adverse reactions to trimethoprim–sulfamethoxazole occur much more frequently in patients with acquired immune deficiency syndrome (AIDS) compared with those without AIDS (50% to 80% of AIDS patients compared with 10% in other immunocompromised patients).

9. The basic principles of management of allergic reactions to drugs or biologic agents include (a) discontinuation of the medication or agent when possible, (b) treatment of the adverse clinical signs and symptoms, and (c) substitution, if necessary, of another agent.

10. One of the most helpful tests to evaluate risk of penicillin allergy is the skin test. Skin testing can demonstrate the presence of penicillin-specific immunoglobulin E and predict a relatively high risk of immediate hypersensitivity reactions. Skin testing does not predict the risk of delayed reactions or most dermatologic reactions.

Learning objectives, review questions, and other resources can be found at **www.pharmacotherapyonline.com.**

❶ *Allergic drug reactions* are adverse medication effects that involve immunologic mechanisms. Adverse drug effects not proven to be immune mediated but resembling allergic reactions in their clinical presentation are referred to as *allergic-like* or *pseudoallergic reactions.* Immunologically mediated adverse drug reactions account for 6% to 10% of all adverse drug reactions and even up to 15% by some estimates.[1,2] Examples of allergic drug reactions are anaphylaxis from β-lactam antibiotics, halothane hepatitis, dermatitis from sulfonamides, hypotension after protamine, and serum sickness from phenytoin.[3] Examples of pseudoallergic reactions are shock after radiocontrast media, aspirin-induced asthma, opiate-related urticaria, and flushing after vancomycin infusion.[3]

The true frequency of allergic drug reactions is difficult to determine because many reactions may not be reported, and others may be difficult to distinguish from nonallergic adverse events. Dermatologic reactions represent the most frequently recognized and reported form of allergic drug reaction.[4]

MECHANISMS OF ALLERGIC DRUG REACTIONS

Drugs can cause allergic reactions by a variety of immunologic mechanisms. Although some reactions are relatively well defined, most are due to mechanisms that are either unknown or poorly understood.[2,3]

TABLE 91-1 Classification of Allergic Drug Reactions

Type	Descriptor	Characteristics	Typical Onset	Drug Causes
I	Anaphylactic (IgE mediated)	Allergen binds to IgE on basophils or mast cells, resulting in release of inflammatory medicators.	Within 30 min	Penicillin immediate reaction Blood products Polypeptide hormones Vaccines Dextran
II	Cytotoxic	Cell destruction occurs because of cell-associated antigen that initiates cytolysis by antigen-specific antibody (IgG or IgM). Most often involves blood elements.	Typically 5–12 h	Penicillin, quinidine, phenylbutazone, thiouracils, sulfonamides, methyldopa
III	Immune complex	Antigen–antibody complexes form and deposit on blood vessel walls and activate complement. Result is a serum sickness-like syndrome.	3–8 h	May be caused by penicillins, sulfonamides, radiocontrast agents, hydantoins
IV	Cell-mediated (delayed)	Antigens cause activation of lymphocytes, which release inflammatory mediators.	24–48 h	Tuberculin reaction

❷ The following criteria suggest that a drug reaction may be immunologically mediated[2]: (a) the observed reaction does not resemble the drug's pharmacologic effect, (b) there is a lag time between first exposure of the drug and reaction unless the recipient has been sensitized by prior exposure to the drug, which can lead to immediate reactions, (c) the reaction may occur even by minute doses of the drug, (d) the symptoms are characteristic of an allergic reaction (e.g., anaphylaxis, urticaria, serum sickness), (e) the reaction resolves after the drug has been discontinued, and (f) the reaction may be reproduced by agents with similar chemical structures. Exceptions to each of these criteria are observed commonly. Many allergic reactions can be classified into one of four immunopathologic categories: type I, II, III, or IV (Table 91–1 and Fig. 91–1).[2,3,5]

EFFECTORS OF ALLERGIC DRUG REACTIONS

Allergic drug reactions can involve most of the major components of the immune system, including the cellular elements, immunoglobulins, complement, and cytokines. Most immunoglobulin isotypes have been implicated in immunologically mediated drug reactions. Immunoglobulin E (IgE) bound to basophils or mast cells mediates immediate (anaphylactic-type) reactions. IgG or IgM antibodies also may be involved in allergic reactions, resulting in destruction of cells and tissues. T lymphocytes are important in some types of allergic reactions.[2,5]

CELLULAR ELEMENTS

A variety of cells are involved in immunologic drug reactions. Basophils, mast cells, eosinophils, and lymphocytes are involved most frequently. Platelets and vascular endothelial cells are important because they also can release a number of inflammatory mediators.[6] Most cells of the body, including nerve cells, can become involved directly or indirectly in allergic drug reactions.

MEDIATORS OF ALLERGIC REACTIONS

The release of a number of preformed, pharmacologically active chemical mediators (e.g., histamine, heparin, proteases such as tryptase and chymase, and a variety of other enzymes) is triggered when antigens cross-link IgE molecules on the surface of circulating basophils and tissue mast cells. Newly formed mediators include platelet-activating factor and arachidonic acid metabolites (e.g., prostaglandins, thromboxanes, and leukotrienes).

Histamine is a low-molecular-weight amine compound formed by decarboxylation of histidine and is stored in basophil and mast cell granules.[7] Release of histamine from these cells is triggered by antigen cross-linking IgE bound to specific receptors on the surface membranes of mast cells and basophils. The tissue effects of histamine are evident within 1 to 2 minutes, but it is rapidly metabolized within 10 to 15 minutes. The major effects of histamine on target tissues include increased capillary permeability, contraction of bronchial and vascular smooth muscle, and hypersecretion of mucus glands. Four classes of histamine receptors (H_1–H_4) are present to varying degrees in organs and tissues. H_1 receptors are most prominent in blood vessels and bronchial and intestinal smooth muscle.

Platelet-activating factor (PAF) is a glyceride-derived substance that is released by mast cells, alveolar macrophages, neutrophils, platelets, and other cells but not by basophils. It has potent bronchoconstrictor effects and causes platelet aggregation and lysis. It attracts neutrophils and causes their activation. PAF enhances vascular permeability and can cause pain, pruritus, and erythema.

The leukotrienes (LTs) are metabolites of arachidonic acid produced through the 5-lipoxygenase pathway that have potent effects on bronchial and vascular smooth muscle. Three important leukotrienes,

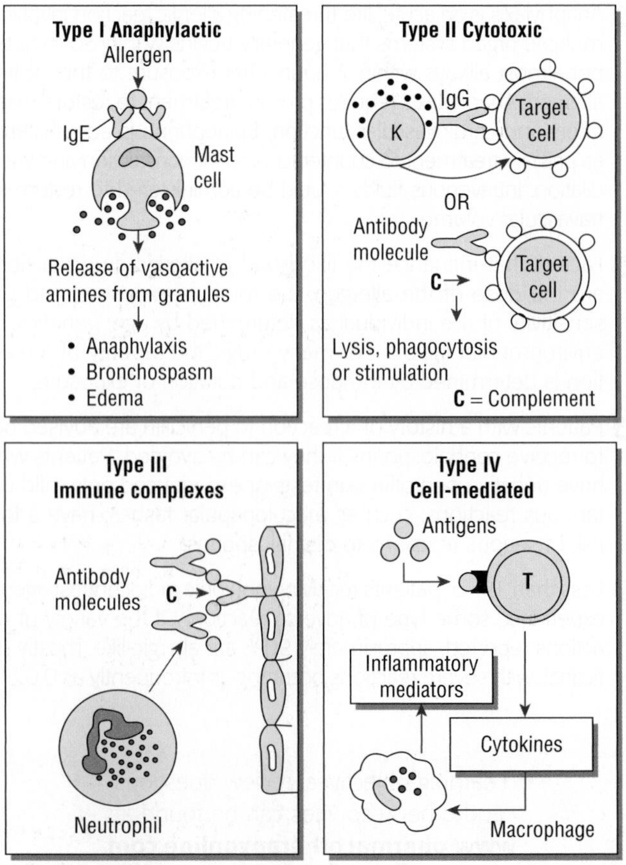

FIGURE 91-1. Types of hypersensitivity reactions.

LTC_4, LTD_4, and LTE_4, are produced by basophils or mast cells. These three substances are also referred to as *cysteinyl leukotrienes* and in older literature as *slow-reacting substances of anaphylaxis.* The LTs have more potent and longer-lasting bronchoconstrictor effects than histamine and can increase vascular permeability and cause arteriolar vasoconstriction followed by vasodilation. Their effects are slower in onset but longer lasting than those of histamine. Another product, LTB_4, is a potent chemoattractant, particularly for neutrophils. It is also produced by neutrophils, macrophages, and monocytes.

Prostaglandins (PGs) and thromboxanes are metabolites of arachidonic acid produced through the cyclooxygenase pathway. Some PGs have vasoconstrictive and/or bronchodilatory properties, whereas others are vasodilatory and/or bronchoconstrictive. PGD_2 is the major PG product of mast cells. It is a potent inhibitor of platelet aggregation and is a bronchoconstrictor. Thromboxanes cause platelet aggregation and are important regulators of coagulation.

The complement system consists of approximately 30 plasma proteins and is involved in hypersensitivity through a variety of immunologic responses, including enhancement of phagocytosis (opsonization of target cells), cell lysis, and generation of anaphylatoxins (C3a, C4a, and C5a), which can cause non–IgE-mediated activation of mast cells and release of inflammatory mediators.

CLASSIFICATION OF IMMUNOPATHOLOGIC DRUG REACTIONS

Immunologic mechanisms have been identified for some drug reactions, and many can be classified into one of four immunopathologic reactions, first described by Coombs and Gell. Small-molecular-weight molecules (<10,000 MW) are not usually immunogenic. Most drugs are <1,000 MW. To become immunogenic, these small compounds must first combine with carrier proteins in plasma or tissue. The combination of the drug bound to a carrier protein can be recognized as foreign, leading to an immune response. The more likely that large amounts of the drug become chemically bound to a protein, the greater the risk of producing an allergic reaction. Penicillin G (356 MW) is an example of a drug that binds covalently to serum proteins through amide or disulfide linkages. For drugs such as the sulfonamides, the parent compound first must be converted to a metabolite before it can combine with the macromolecule. The species that combines with the carrier macromolecule is referred to as a *hapten* or an *incomplete antigen.*[8] Some macromolecular drugs such as insulin are referred to as *complete antigens* because they are large enough to initiate an immune response without binding to another protein. Drugs may also interact directly with T cells with or without the involvement of antigen-presenting cells.[5]

TYPE I

Type I reactions require the presence of IgE specific for the drug or the portion of the drug that becomes a hapten. IgE specific for the drug allergen is produced on initial exposure to the drug. It then binds to basophils and mast cells through high-affinity receptors. On repeat exposure to the drug, two or more IgE molecules on the basophil or mast cell surface may bind to one multivalent antigen molecule (referred to as *cross-linking;* see Fig. 91–1), initiating an activation of the cell. Activation causes the extracellular release of granules with preformed inflammatory mediators, including histamine, heparin, proteases (tryptase in the mast cell), as well as generation of newly formed mediators, as previously discussed, such as LTs, PGs, thromboxanes, and PAF, among others.

Generation of a type I reaction can be evident as an immediate hypersensitivity reaction, or anaphylaxis. Immediate reactions may be limited to single organs, typically in the nasal mucosa (rhinitis), respiratory tract (acute asthma), skin, or gastrointestinal tract, or they can involve multiple organs simultaneously, termed *anaphylaxis.*

TYPE II

Type II immunopathologic reactions involve destruction of host cells (usually blood cells) through cytotoxic antibodies by one of two mechanisms (see Fig. 91–1). First, the drug binds to the cell as a hapten (e.g., the platelet or red blood cell). Antibodies (IgG or IgM) specific for the bound drug or to a component of the cell surface that has been altered by the drug then bind, initiating a cytolytic reaction. Cell destruction may be mediated by complement or by phagocytic cells that have antibody Fc receptors on their surfaces. Activation of complement near the cell surface can result in loss of cell membrane integrity and cell death. Alternatively, neutrophils, monocytes, or macrophages may bind to an antibody-coated cell through IgG Fc receptors on their cell surfaces, resulting in phagocytosis of the target cell. The process of enhancement of phagocytosis by antibody binding to cell surfaces or other particles is referred to as *opsonization.* In addition, cell-bound IgG may direct the nonphagocytic action of T cells or natural killer cells, which results in cell destruction by a process called *antibody-dependent cellular cytotoxicity.* This process can proceed in a nonspecific fashion as T cells bind to the target cell through IgG Fc receptors on the T-cell surface. Contact between the target and effector cells is necessary.

Cells commonly affected by these types of reactions include erythrocytes, leukocytes, and platelets, resulting in hemolytic anemia, agranulocytosis, or thrombocytopenia, respectively. This process may be initiated by drugs such as penicillin, quinidine, quinine, phenacetin, cephalosporins, and sulfonamides.

Another type of reaction that may affect the formed elements in blood is the "innocent bystander" reaction. With this type of reaction, antigen–antibody complexes formed in blood adhere nonspecifically to cells. Complement is then activated, resulting in cell lysis.

TYPE III

Type III immunologic reactions are caused by antigen–antibody complexes that are formed in blood. The complexes form with drug allergen and antibody in varying ratios and may deposit in tissues, resulting in local or disseminated inflammatory reactions. Antigen–antibody complex formation can result in platelet aggregation, complement activation, or macrophage activation. Chemotactic substances such as C4a also are produced. These substances cause the influx of neutrophils and result in the release of a number of toxic substances from the neutrophil (e.g., proteinases, collagenases, kinin-generating enzymes, and reactive oxygen and nitrogen substances), which can cause local tissue destruction.

Platelet aggregation may occur as a result of immune-complex formation, resulting in the formation of microthrombi and the release of vasoactive mediators. Also, insoluble complexes may be phagocytized by macrophages and activate these cells.

The formation of antigen–antibody complexes can lead to clinical syndromes such as the Arthus reaction. In this model, a high level of preformed specific IgG antibody combines with antigen to produce a localized edematous, erythematous reaction within 5 to 8 hours. The reaction involves local formation of insoluble antigen–antibody complexes, complement activation with release of C3a and C5a collectively referred to as *anaphylatoxins,* mast cell degranulation, and influx of polymorphonuclear cells.

TYPE IV

Type IV reactions are delayed hypersensitivity reactions that typically are demonstrated as dermatologic reactions and are mediated by T cells ($CD4^+$ or $CD8^+$).[9] Four subclasses of type IV reactions have been described.[5] Type IV reactions require memory T cells specific for the antigen in question. On exposure to the antigen, T cells become activated and produce an inflammatory response. Although these reactions may be associated with adverse effects (e.g., contact dermatitis, maculopapular exanthemas, bullous exanthemas, eczema, or pustular exanthemas), they also may be useful for diagnostic purposes. Examples of the latter include the purified protein derivative (PPD) antigen from *Mycobacterium tuberculosis* used in the tuberculin skin test and other recall skin test antigens, such as mumps. After intradermal injection, these antigens produce a local reaction (erythema and induration) within 48 to 72 hours. Delayed contact hypersensitivity also can be caused by a wide variety of chemicals and drugs.

OTHER ALLERGIC REACTIONS

The precise mechanism of many drug reactions is not known, although the reactions are believed to be immune mediated. Perhaps most common are the delayed dermatologic reactions that occur with a variety of drugs (especially penicillins and sulfonamides).[5,9] These reactions may be evident as macropapular, morbilliform, or erythematous rashes; exfoliative dermatitis; photosensitivity reactions; or eczema. These reactions also may be manifest as pruritus, urticaria, and angioedema.

Other serious dermatologic syndromes may be the result of immunologic reactions. Erythema multiforme is an acute syndrome characterized by a variety of skin lesions. The skin lesions typically start as a maculopapular eruption that may progress to irregular lesions with central clearing (target lesions), mostly on the extremities. The rash may be accompanied by bullous lesions that break down into erosions involving more of the body, especially mucous membranes. This more extensive disease usually associated with fever and extensive purpura is called *erythema multiforme major* or *Stevens-Johnson syndrome* (SJS). Some have termed these types of reactions *febrile mucocutaneous syndromes.* If the skin lesions progress to sloughing of large portions of the skin, resembling third-degree burns, the term *toxic epidermal necrolysis* (TEN) is applied. Mortality from TEN can be as high as 40%.[10] Drugs commonly associated with these syndromes include the penicillins, sulfonamides, nonsteroidal antiinflammatory drugs (NSAIDs), and anticonvulsants such as phenytoin and phenobarbital, as well as a number of other agents. Drug-induced fever also may involve immunologic mechanisms. Other general types of reactions believed to be immune mediated in some cases include hepatic drug reactions (cholestatic or hepatocellular) and pulmonary reactions, for example, interstitial pneumonitis, which has been associated with nitrofurantoin.

ANAPHYLACTOID REACTIONS

Various drugs and other substances can produce anaphylactoid (anaphylaxis-like) reactions that are similar to anaphylaxis in clinical signs and symptoms. The substances causing these reactions can produce the direct release of inflammatory mediators from cells by a pharmacologic or physical effect rather than through cell-bound IgE. These reactions are sometimes referred to as *pseudoallergic,* but not all pseudoallergic reactions are anaphylactoid. Drugs that can produce anaphylactoid reactions include vancomycin, opiates, iodinated radiocontrast agents, amphotericin B, and D-tubocurarine. The "red man syndrome" is a common example of an anaphylactoid reaction from vancomycin. If vancomycin is infused too rapidly, it can cause the direct release of histamine and other mediators from cutaneous mast cells, producing a typical clinical picture of itching, flushing, and hives, first around the neck and face and then progressing to the chest and other parts of the body usually beginning shortly after the infusion has begun. Most patients who have had "red man syndrome" will tolerate vancomycin if the rate of infusion is slowed. A number of other agents (including aspirin) may produce anaphylactoid reactions by altering the metabolism of inflammatory mediators such as PGs or kinins.

CLINICAL MANIFESTATIONS OF ALLERGIC AND ALLERGIC-LIKE REACTIONS

ANAPHYLAXIS

❹ Anaphylaxis is an acute, life-threatening allergic reaction involving multiple organ systems that occurs in 10 to 20 per 100,000 population per year.[11,12] Approximately 1,500 deaths from anaphylaxis occur annually in the United States.[13] From 1.2% to 15% of the U.S. population may be at risk for anaphylactic reactions.[14] Although many drugs may cause anaphylaxis (or anaphylactoid) reactions, the most commonly reported are aspirin and other NSAIDs, penicillins, and insulins.[11] The manifestations of anaphylaxis may include signs and symptoms referable to the skin (flushing, pruritus, urticaria, angioedema), respiratory tract (tightness of the throat and chest, dysphagia, dysphonia and hoarseness, cough, stridor, shortness of breath, dyspnea, congestion, rhinorrhea, sneezing), gastrointestinal tract (nausea, crampy abdominal pain, vomiting, diarrhea), cardiovascular system (hypotension, syncope, altered mental status, chest pain, dysrhythmia), or any combination of these systems.[12]

A consensus panel has constructed a definition of anaphylaxis as follows.[12,15] Anaphylaxis is highly likely when any one of the following three criteria are fulfilled:

1. Acute onset of an illness (minutes to several hours) with involvement of the skin, mucosal tissue, or both (e.g., generalized hives, pruritus or flushing, swollen lips/tongue/uvula) AND at least one of the following:
   - Respiratory compromise (e.g., dyspnea, wheeze/bronchospasm, stridor, reduced peak expiratory flow, hypoxemia)
   - Reduced blood pressure or associated symptoms of end-organ dysfunction (e.g., hypotonia, syncope, incontinence)
2. Two or more of the following that occur rapidly after exposure to a likely allergen (minutes to several hours):
   - Involvement of skin/mucosal tissue (as above)
   - Respiratory compromise (as above)
   - Reduced blood pressure or associated symptoms
   - Persistent gastrointestinal symptoms (e.g., crampy abdominal pain, vomiting)
3. Reduced blood pressure after exposure to known allergen (minutes to several hours)

The panel indicated that other presentations may indicate anaphylaxis and that the potential exists for false-positive results.

Anaphylactic reactions generally begin within 30 minutes but almost always within 2 hours of exposure to the inciting allergen. The risk of fatal anaphylaxis is greatest within the first few hours. After apparent recovery, anaphylaxis may recur 6 to 8 hours after antigen exposure. Because of the possibility of these "late-phase" reactions, patients should be observed for at least 12 hours after an anaphylactic reaction. Fatal anaphylaxis most often results from asphyxia due to airway obstruction either at the larynx or within the lungs. Cardiovascular collapse may occur as a result of asphyxia in some cases, whereas in others cases cardiovascular collapse may be the dominant manifestation from the release of mediators within the heart muscles and coronary blood vessels.

SERUM SICKNESS

Serum sickness is a clinical syndrome resulting from the effects of soluble circulating immune complexes that form under conditions of antigen excess. The reaction commonly results from the use of antisera containing foreign (donor) antigens such as equine serum in the form of antitoxins or antivenins. The onset of serum sickness usually occurs 7 to 14 days after antigen administration. The onset may be more rapid with reexposure to the same agent in an individual with prior serum sickness. Fever, malaise, and lymphadenopathy are the most common clinical manifestations. Arthralgias, urticaria, and morbilliform skin eruption also may be present. Although often associated with administration of heterologous antisera, serum sickness also may be caused by drugs, including sulfonamides, hydantoins, penicillins, minocycline, and cephalosporins (especially cefaclor). In addition, immune complex–mediated systemic lupus erythematosus (SLE)-like syndrome has been attributed to reactions from drugs such as hydralazine, procainamide, isoniazid, and phenytoin.

DRUG FEVER

Fever may occur in response to an inflammatory process or develop as a manifestation of a drug reaction. Drug fever occurs in as many as 10% of hospital inpatients.[16] Many drugs have been reported to cause fever, including methyldopa, procainamide, phenytoin, barbiturates, quinidine, and a variety of antibiotics. These drugs may affect the central nervous system directly to alter temperature regulation or stimulate the release of endogenous pyrogens (e.g., interleukin-1 and tumor necrosis factor) from white blood cells. Drugs also may cause fever as a result of their pharmacologic effects on tissues, for example, fever resulting from massive tumor cell destruction caused by chemotherapy. However, the mechanism of drug fever remains unknown for agents such as amphotericin B and radiographic contrast agents.

The temperature pattern of drug-induced fever is quite variable and therefore of little help in the diagnosis. It may be low grade and continuous or spiking and intermittent. A temporal relationship between drug administration and occurrence of fever has been noted for some medications. Generally, withdrawal of the causative agent results in prompt defervescence as soon as the drug is eliminated completely. Fever usually recurs on readministration of the causative agent.

DRUG-INDUCED AUTOIMMUNITY

Autoimmune diseases have been associated with drugs and may involve a variety of tissues and organs. A commonly recognized drug-related autoimmune disorder is SLE induced by procainamide, hydralazine, quinidine, or isoniazid.[17] Exposure of susceptible persons to these agents appears to alter normal body proteins, RNA, or DNA in such a way as to make these components antigenic, leading to the formation of autoreactive antibodies and cells. The most common clinical manifestations include arthralgias, myalgias, and polyarthritis. Facial rash, ulcers, and alopecia occur less frequently. Renal or pulmonary involvement also may occur. These reactions typically develop several months after beginning the drug and generally resolve soon after the drug is discontinued.[18]

Other syndromes believed to involve autoimmune mechanisms include drug-induced hemolytic anemia attributed to methyldopa, renal interstitial nephritis produced by methicillin, and hepatitis caused by phenytoin and halothane. Interstitial nephritis is characterized by fever, rash, and eosinophilia associated with proteinuria and hematuria. Hepatic damage due to drugs generally is manifested as either hepatocellular necrosis or cholestatic hepatitis. Drug-induced hepatitis has been associated with phenothiazines, sulfonamides, halothane, phenytoin, and isoniazid (see Chap. 40). Hepatocellular destruction is evidenced by elevations in serum transaminases. Hepatomegaly and jaundice sometimes may be evident. Cholestasis may be manifested by jaundice and elevations in serum alkaline phosphatase and sometimes by rash, fever, and eosinophilia.

VASCULITIS

Vasculitis is a clinicopathologic process characterized by inflammation and necrosis of blood vessels walls. The vasculitic process may be limited to the skin, or it may involve multiple organs, including the liver or kidney, joints, or central nervous system. Characteristically, cutaneous vasculitis is manifested by purpuric lesions that vary in size and number. Vasculitis also may be manifested as papules, nodules, ulcerations, or vesiculobullous lesions, generally occurring on the lower extremities but sometimes involving the upper extremities, including the hands. Drugs associated with vasculitis include allopurinol, β-lactam antibiotics, sulfonamides, thiazide diuretics, and phenytoin.

DERMATOLOGIC REACTIONS

A wide variety of dermatologic drug reactions have been reported to have an immunologic basis.[2,19] Cutaneous reactions are the most common manifestations of allergic drug reactions. Although most dermatologic reactions are mild and resolve promptly after discontinuing the drug, some may progress to serious or even life-threatening reactions (e.g., TEN or SJS). SJS is a serious dermatologic reaction characterized by blistering of the mucous membranes (mouth, eyes, vagina) and patchy rashes that can cover most of the body. Patients may experience fever, headache, and cough. TEN is a syndrome similar to SJS, characterized by blistering of skin and mucous membranes in response to administration of a drug. Large areas of skin may peel off.

Cutaneous adverse reactions were reported to occur in 2.7% of hospitalized patients.[20] Serious dermatologic drug reactions are estimated to occur in 1.9 cases per one million people per year and can have a mortality rate as high as 40%.[21,22] Table 91–2 lists drugs and agents associated most commonly with cutaneous reactions.[23] Antimicrobials are implicated most frequently with reaction rates ranging from 1% to 8%. In a report of almost 6,000 children, approximately 12% developed rashes with cefaclor compared with 7.4% with penicillins and 8.5% with sulfonamides.[24]

RESPIRATORY REACTIONS

Drugs may produce upper or lower respiratory tract reactions, including rhinitis and asthma. Respiratory tract manifestations may result from direct injury to the airways or may occur as a component of a systemic reaction (e.g., anaphylaxis). Asthma may be

TABLE 91-2 Top 10 Drugs or Agents Reported to Cause Skin Reactions

	Reactions per 1,000 Recipients
Amoxicillin	51.4
Trimethoprim–sulfamethoxazole	33.8
Ampicillin	33.2
Iopodate	27.8
Blood	21.6
Cephalosporins	21.1
Erythromycin	20.4
Dihydralazine hydrochloride	19.1
Penicillin G	18.5
Cyanocobalamin	17.9

Data from Roujeau JC, Stern RS. New Engl J Med 1994;331:1272–1285.

induced by aspirin and other NSAIDs or by sulfites used as preservatives in foods and medications. Other pulmonary drug reactions believed to be immunologic include acute infiltrative and chronic fibrotic pulmonary reactions. The latter is often caused by antineoplastic agents such as bleomycin. For a more detailed discussion of drug-induced pulmonary disease, see Chap. 31.

HEMATOLOGIC REACTIONS

Most formed elements and soluble components of the hematopoietic system may be affected by immunologic drug reactions. Eosinophilia is a common manifestation of drug hypersensitivity and may be the only presenting sign. Hemolytic anemia may result from hypersensitivity to drugs. Other hematologic reactions include thrombocytopenia, granulocytopenia, and agranulocytosis. For a detailed discussion of hematologic drug reactions, see Chap. 107.

FACTORS RELATED TO THE OCCURRENCE OR SEVERITY OF ALLERGIC DRUG REACTIONS

❸ Among the factors that influence the likelihood of allergic drug reactions are the dose of the drug, how the drug is metabolized, the degree to which the drug and metabolites bind to human proteins, the route of exposure, and the sensitivity of the individual as determined by age, genetics, and environmental factors. For many drugs, the severity of a reaction is determined by the dose and the duration of exposure. A relatively larger dose or longer duration of treatment encourages development of drug sensitivity. The route of administration also influences drug sensitivity. The topical route of drug administration appears to be the most likely to sensitize and predispose to drug reactions. The oral route is the safest, and the parenteral route is the most hazardous for administration of drugs in sensitive individuals. Relatively few cases of immediate hypersensitivity-associated deaths with oral β-lactam antimicrobials have been reported. Although intravenous administration is more likely to result in severe immediate reactions in a sensitized individual, it may be the least likely route for initially inducing sensitivity. One possible explanation is that intravenous administration results in systemic drug exposure for the shortest period of time.

Individual host factors are important in determining drug sensitivity. There may be a genetic predisposition for some types of allergic reactions. For example, slow acetylators of procainamide and hydralazine are at increased risk for SLE.

Drug allergies appear to develop with equal frequency in atopic and nonatopic individuals. In addition, patients with a history of drug allergy appear to be at increased risk for adverse reactions to other pharmacologic agents.[3] Age seems to be related to the risk of allergic reactions, as they occur less frequently in children. This may be related to immaturity of the immune system or decreased exposure. The presence of some concurrent diseases, particularly viral infections, predisposes to drug reactions. Examples include the morbilliform rash that occurs after ampicillin administration to patients with infectious mononucleosis and the reactions that occur with trimethoprim-sulfamethoxazole in patients with acquired immune deficiency syndrome (AIDS).

DRUGS COMMONLY CAUSING ALLERGIC OR ALLERGIC-LIKE DRUG REACTIONS

β-LACTAM ANTIMICROBIALS

Allergy to β-lactam antibiotics is commonly reported by patients in healthcare settings.[25] Allergic reactions to penicillin occur in 0.7% to 8% of treatment courses but was as high as 15% in one retrospective report of hospitalized patients treated with penicillin.[26,27] Although most patients reporting penicillin allergy do not have allergy, a reported history is associated with a higher likelihood of positive skin test reactivity.[28] Only 10% to 20% of patients reporting penicillin allergy are found to be allergic by skin testing.[28] Patients with a history of penicillin allergy who have a negative penicillin skin test are unlikely to react on subsequent courses of penicillins.[29]

The most common reactions to penicillin include urticaria, pruritus, and angioedema. All four of the major types of hypersensitivity reactions have been reported with penicillin, as well as some reactions that do not fit into these categories. A wide variety of idiopathic reactions occur, such as maculopapular eruptions, eosinophilia, SJS, and exfoliative dermatitis. Cutaneous reactions can occur in up to 4.4% of treatment courses of penicillin[30] and in up to 8% with aminopenicillins.[31] The incidence of ampicillin rash is close to 100% in patients with viral infections such as infectious mononucleosis.[22]

Some aspects of the mechanism of penicillin immunogenicity have been determined. Because benzylpenicillin is a relatively small molecule (356 MW), it must combine with macromolecules (presumably proteins) to elicit an immune response. Penicillin may bind covalently to the lysine residues of proteins such as albumin through an amide linkage involving the β-lactam ring (Fig. 91–2). This is the penicilloyl–protein conjugate and is referred to as the *major antigenic determinant.* In addition, a number of other penicillin metabolites may bind covalently to proteins. These are referred to as *minor antigenic determinants.* The terms *major* and *minor* refer to the relative proportions of these conjugates that are formed and not to the clinical severity of the reactions generated. Immediate hypersensitivity reactions may be mediated by IgE for both minor and major determinants. In fact, the minor antigenic determinants are more likely to cause life-threatening anaphylactic reactions.

Patients who are allergic to penicillins also may be sensitive to other β-lactams.[32] The exact incidence of cross-reactivity between cephalosporins and penicillins is not known but is believed to be low.[33] Patients who report penicillin allergy and a positive penicillin skin test have an eightfold greater risk of allergic reaction to cephalosporins compared with patients not reporting penicillin allergy. One to eight percent of patients with penicillin-specific IgE may develop an immediate-type hypersensitivity reaction to cephalosporins.[33] In contrast, patients with reported penicillin allergy and negative skin test are at no greater risk.[34]

❺ Most allergists would not administer cephalosporins to patients with a history of hives or other immediate hypersensitivity reactions from penicillin, although some studies have suggested there is little risk of an allergic response to a cephalosporin even in a person with a positive skin test to penicillin.[35–37] One postmarketing surveillance report states there was no increase in allergic reactions to second- and third-generation cephalosporins in patients with histories of penicillin allergy.[35] Results of skin testing with cephalosporins are not reliable because the mechanism of cephalosporin sensitivity has not been clearly defined. At present, patients with positive penicillin skin tests are advised not to receive cephalosporins if they can be avoided. Patients who have negative penicillin skin tests or experienced only mild cutaneous reactions from penicillin, such as maculopapular rashes, may receive cephalosporins with caution.

Aztreonam only weakly cross-reacts with penicillin and can be administered safely to most patients who are penicillin allergic.[38] In contrast, there is considerable cross-reactivity between imipenem (a carbapenem) and penicillin. Therefore, imipenem (and other carbapenems) should not be administered to patients who have positive penicillin skin tests.

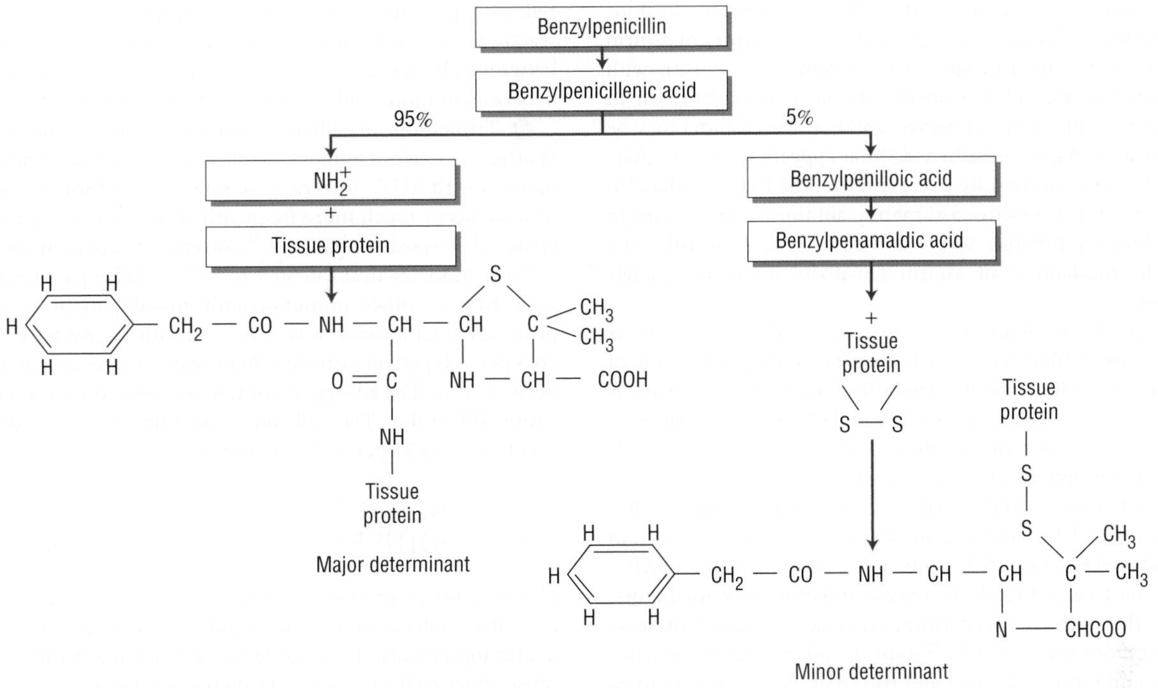

FIGURE 91-2. Formation of a benzylpenicilloyl hapten–protein complex.

RADIOCONTRAST MEDIA

❻ Radiocontrast agents frequently cause allergic-like reactions because these agents are used commonly in medical practice and are administered as large, rapidly infused intravenous boluses. From <1% to >3% of patients receiving nonionic contrast media experienced an adverse reaction, with reports as high as 12.7% for mild reactions.[39,40] Delayed skin reactions occur in 1% to 3% of patients over 5 to 7 days. Severe, immediate anaphylactic reactions occur in 0.01% to 0.04% of patients.[39] In addition, radiocontrast agents may cause dose-dependent toxic reactions that can produce renal impairment, cardiovascular effects, and arrhythmias.[39,41] The older, high-osmolar agents that are now used less commonly have a greater frequency of reactions compared with the newer, low-osmolar agents.[39]

The mechanism of reactions to radiocontrast agents is not clearly understood. Histamine release and mast cell triggering have been documented in severe immediate reactions, suggesting an IgE-mediated mechanism.[42] The older, high-osmolar radiocontrast agents can activate mast cells and basophils directly (IgE-independent mechanism), resulting in the release of inflammatory mediators. The low-osmolar contrast agents appear to result in fewer anaphylactoid reactions.

Patients at risk for reactions to radiocontrast agents are difficult to identify. History is helpful because a patient who previously experienced reactions is more likely to experience subsequent reactions. The risk of allergic reactions to radiocontrast media is greater in women and in patients with a history of atopy or asthma.[43,44] Other recognized risk factors include a history of previous reaction, severe allergy, cardiac disease, and treatment with β-blockers.[40] Despite a common misconception, a seafood allergy does not predispose to radiocontrast media reactions. Neither skin tests nor oral tests are useful for predicting reactions to these agents. Some regimens have been recommended to prevent reactions in patients who have experienced them previously; however, the value of these preventive regimens has not been proven.[45] One consensus guideline recommends oral prednisone (30 mg) or methylprednisolone (32 mg) 12 and 2 hours before exposure in high-risk patients to prevent immediate reactions. Ephedrine has also been recommended for premedication.[46] Other studies have examined the use of H_1- and H_2-antihistamines, clemastine, or cimetidine, respectively.[45]

INSULIN

Insulin is capable of producing allergic reactions through a variety of immunologic mechanisms. A protein molecule, insulin is a complete antigen. Allergic reactions have been reported with beef, pork, and recombinant human insulin, although the frequency of reactions with human insulin appears low. Reactions to insulin may involve the insulin molecule itself or other substances that have been added to insulin (e.g., protamine). Most patients have anti-insulin IgG antibodies after a few months of therapy.

Insulin reactions may be limited to the site of injection, or they may produce systemic reactions. Local reactions present most often as a wheal and flare at the injection site and may occur immediately after injection or up to 8 to 12 hours later. Generally, these reactions are mild, do not require treatment, and resolve with continued insulin administration. If a patient does not tolerate the local reaction well, antihistamines may be given or a different insulin source (or product of higher purity) may be substituted. Rarely, systemic reactions to insulin (e.g., urticaria or anaphylaxis) occur. IgE-mediated reactions to insulin allergy appear to be declining with greater use of human insulins.[47] Skin testing with various products can aid in selecting the type of insulin least likely to cause a systemic reaction. Human insulin appears to be least allergenic but occasionally may cause reactions. In some patients, insulin desensitization may be indicated.

ASPIRIN AND NONSTEROIDAL ANTIINFLAMMATORY DRUGS

❼ Aspirin and other NSAIDs can produce eight general types of reactions, four of which are related to cyclooxygenase inhibition.[48,49] These reactions can involve asthma and rhinitis, urticaria/angioedema, anaphylaxis and anaphylactoid reactions, aseptic meningitis, or pneumonitis. Approximately 9% to 20% of asthmatics are sensitive to aspirin and other NSAIDs.[48,50]

The rhinosinusitis/asthma syndrome typically develops in middle-aged patients who are nonatopic and have no history of aspirin intolerance. Generally, it progresses from rhinitis to sinusitis with nasal polyps and steroid-dependent asthma. It is uncommon in children and young adults. However, children with asthma may be aspirin sensitive. Aspirin-sensitive asthma appears to be an inherited disorder characterized by overexpression of LTC_4 synthase in airways.[51] In aspirin-sensitive asthmatics, administration of aspirin and NSAIDs may provoke severe and sometimes fatal asthmatic attacks. The mechanism of aspirin sensitivity is not completely understood.

One suspected mechanism of aspirin and NSAID sensitivity is cyclooxygenase-1 blockade, which may facilitate production of alternative arachidonic acid metabolites (e.g., LTs).[48] This is supported by the observed correlation between the degree of cyclooxygenase-1 blockade and the risk of a reaction; thus, agents such as acetaminophen, which minimally block cyclooxygenase-1, rarely cause reactions. Additional support is found in the clinical observation that LT-modifying drugs can reduce the severity of aspirin-induced reactions.[48] It is possible that aspirin and NSAIDs stimulate mast cells directly to release inflammatory mediators. Subjects with aspirin-induced asthma also have a marked increase in airway responsiveness to LTs.[52] Aspirin and the cyclooxygenase-2–selective inhibitors celecoxib and rofecoxib do not appear to be cross-reactive.[53–55]

In patients with asthma or those suspected of being sensitive to aspirin, an oral challenge can be performed. Protocols to detect aspirin or NSAID sensitivity have been recommended, but the risk for anaphylaxis cannot be reliably predicted.[48] The challenge should be performed with great caution in a hospital setting with resuscitation equipment at hand. For patients known to be aspirin-sensitive, the major preventive measure is avoidance. Other agents reported to be cross-reactive with aspirin include tartrazine dye, indomethacin, and phenylbutazone.

NSAIDs have been associated with pulmonary infiltrates and eosinophilia syndrome. Pulmonary infiltrates and eosinophilia syndrome is associated with fever, cough, dyspnea, infiltrates on chest roentgenogram, and a peripheral eosinophilia that develop 2 to 6 weeks after initiating treatment. Pulmonary infiltrates and eosinophilia syndrome occurs more frequently for naproxen compared with other NSAIDs and is noted to resolve rapidly after discontinuation of the offending agent.[56]

SULFONAMIDES

Sulfonamide drugs, including antimicrobials, diuretics, oral hypoglycemics, and carbonic anhydrase inhibitors, are a common cause of allergic reactions. Allergic reactions were recognized in 4.8% of 20,226 patients who received a sulfonamide antibiotic and in 2% of patients who received a nonantibiotic sulfonamide.[57] Although immediate IgE-mediated reactions such as anaphylaxis can occur, sulfonamides typically cause delayed cutaneous reactions, often beginning with fever and then followed by a rash (e.g., morbilliform eruptions, erythema multiforme, or, less frequently, SJS/toxic epidermal necrolysis).[1] Other reactions to sulfonamides may include mucocutaneous, gastrointestinal, hepatic, renal, or hematologic complications, which may be fatal. Immune-mediated sulfonamide reactions involve the production of reactive metabolites (hydroxylamines).[58] Patients with the slow acetylator phenotype may be at increased risk for these reactions.[4]

Although allergic reactions to sulfonamides can occur with a wide variety of chemical entities, cross-reactivity between sulfonamide antibiotics and nonantibiotics appears to be minimal, with cross-reactivity characterized as "highly unlikely."[59] The occurrence of allergic reactions after receipt of nonantibiotic sulfonamides may reflect a predisposition to allergic reactions rather than cross-reactivity with sulfonamide antibiotics.[57] In fact, the cross-reactivity between sulfonamide antibiotics and penicillin appears higher than between antibiotic and nonantibiotic sulfonamides.[58]

❽ Trimethoprim–sulfamethoxazole is used frequently for preventive or active treatment of *Pneumocystis carinii* pneumonia in patients with AIDS. Adverse reactions to trimethoprim–sulfamethoxazole occur much more frequently in human immunodeficiency virus (HIV)-positive patients.[60] Adverse effects to trimethoprim–sulfamethoxazole occur in 50% to 80% of AIDS patients compared with 10% of other immunocompromised patients.[61] Trimethoprim–sulfamethoxazole was associated with an adverse event rate of 26.3 per 100 person-years and hypersensitivity events at 22 per 100 person-years. The adverse event rate was related to lower $CD4^+$ cell count. When the $CD4^+$ cell count was $<100/mm^3$, the adverse drug event rate was 31 per 100 person-years.[62]

PHARMACEUTICAL EXCIPIENTS AND ADDITIVES

Pharmaceutical products contain a number of "inert" additives (e.g., dyes, fillers, buffers, and stabilizers) in addition to the therapeutic ingredients. These additives are not always inert and may cause adverse effects, including allergic reactions.

The azo dye tartrazine (FD&C Yellow No. 5) is associated with anaphylactoid reactions, acute bronchospasm, urticaria, rhinitis, and contact dermatitis.[63,64] Although the immunologic mechanisms are unclear, approximately 10% of aspirin-sensitive asthmatics are also intolerant to tartrazine,[65] suggesting a role for tartrazine as a cyclooxygenase inhibitor. As little as 0.85 mcg or as much as 25 mg tartrazine has provoked positive responses.[65]

Sulfites (including sulfur dioxide, sodium sulfite, sodium and potassium bisulfite, and sodium and potassium metabisulfite) are used commonly as antioxidants in pharmaceutical products and some foods. Many cases of adverse reactions associated with ingestion of sulfites (usually in foods) have been reported to the Food and Drug Administration (FDA),[66] including wheezing, dyspnea, chest tightness, urticaria, angioedema, flushing, weakness, nausea, anaphylaxis, and death.

IgE-mediated and nonimmunologic sulfite hypersensitivity has been demonstrated in children with a history of chronic asthma. Adverse reactions to sulfite-preserved injectables, such as gentamicin, metoclopramide, lidocaine, and doxycycline, have been reported. In contrast to reactions caused by foods, these reactions do not occur more frequently in steroid-dependent asthmatics and do not always coincide with a positive oral sulfite challenge.[67] Blunted bronchodilation may be observed in asthmatics following inhalation of sulfite-containing nebulizer solutions. Although many nebulizer solutions contain sulfites, metered-dose inhalers do not. Many aqueous epinephrine products also contain sulfites. The FDA labeling states that in emergency situations when sulfite-free preparations are not available, sulfite-containing epinephrine should not be withheld from a sulfite-intolerant individual because small subcutaneous doses of sulfites usually are well tolerated. However, an increased risk of anaphylaxis exists after subcutaneous injection in rare patients with a positive oral challenge to 5 to 10 mg sulfite.

Parabens (including methyl-, ethyl-, propyl-, and butylparaben) are used widely in pharmaceutical products as a biocidal agent. Most allergic reactions to parabens are observed after topical exposure.[68] Delayed hypersensitivity contact dermatitis occurs more often in individuals with preexisting dermatitis.[65] Immediate hypersensitivity after parenteral administration is rare. Although these agents are chemically related to benzoic acid and *p*-aminobenzoic acid, the evidence for cross-sensitivity is lacking.[65]

CANCER CHEMOTHERAPY AGENTS

Chemotherapy agents are implicated in hypersensitivity reactions in 5% to 15% of patients who receive them.[69] Up to 65% of patients receiving L-asparaginase experience immediate hypersensitivity reactions such as urticaria and anaphylaxis.[70]

The combination regimen of paclitaxel (or docetaxel) and carboplatin frequently is responsible for producing hypersensitivity reactions. Each agent precipitates a distinct reaction, allowing for differentiation between causative factors. Hypersensitivity reactions have been observed with paclitaxel and docetaxel as frequently as 34% of patients.[1,71,72] The reaction, typically occurring shortly after initiation of the first dose, is due to Cremophor EL, the polyoxyethylated castor oil vehicle for paclitaxel. Severe reactions are characterized by dyspnea, bronchospasm, urticaria, and hypotension. Minor reactions include flushing and rashes. In patients receiving a 3-hour infusion, the incidence of severe reactions is reduced to 1.3%, and the incidence of minor reactions is 42%.[73] To reduce the risk of hypersensitivity reaction, patients are routinely premedicated with corticosteroids and H_1- and H_2-receptor antagonists. A protein-bound formulation of paclitaxel (Abraxane) is available that avoids most of the hypersensitivity reactions.

Carboplatin hypersensitivity develops after six or more courses of carboplatin or its parent compound cisplatin.[74] Reactions typically develop shortly after completing the infusion or up to 3 days after therapy.[75] Symptoms of severe reaction include tachycardia, dyspnea, facial swelling, rigors, and hypotension. Mild reactions include itching, erythema, and facial flushing. Desensitization with carboplatin usually is not successful owing to previous prolonged exposure. Skin testing is useful because a negative test has a high predictive value for nonreactivity.[76]

Oxaliplatin hypersensitivity has been reported in as many as 12% of patients. Symptoms range from facial flushing to dyspnea. Management strategies include decreasing the rate of infusion and administration of corticosteroids and H_1- and H_2-receptor antagonists.[77] Desensitization has been successful in patients desiring to continue treatment after experiencing a hypersensitivity reaction.[78,79]

ANTICONVULSANTS

Many anticonvulsant drugs produce a variety of hypersensitivity reactions and pseudoallergic reactions. Drugs such as phenytoin, phenobarbital, carbamazepine, and lamotrigine can cause an "anticonvulsant hypersensitivity syndrome" characterized by fever, rash, lymphadenopathy, and internal organ involvement. Eosinophilia is frequently present. Onset usually occurs several weeks into therapy.[80] In some cases, morbilliform rash develops into exfoliative dermatitis. Concomitant use of valproate with lamotrigine significantly increases the risk of hypersensitivity as a result of reduced lamotrigine metabolism, leading to a prolonged elimination half-life.[81]

TREATMENT

Allergic Reactions

❾ The basic principles for management of allergic reactions to drugs or biologic agents include (a) discontinuation of the medication or agent when possible, (b) treatment of the adverse clinical signs and symptoms, and (c) substitution, if necessary, of another agent.[82]

Identification of patients at high risk for allergic drug reactions requires a careful history and, where appropriate, performance of drug provocation tests to evaluate sensitivity.[83,84] One of the most helpful tests for evaluating risk is the allergen skin test. For some drugs, skin testing can demonstrate the presence of drug-specific IgE and predict a relatively high risk of immediate hypersensitivity reactions. Note that skin testing does not predict the risk of delayed or most dermatologic reactions.

A higher proportion of patients report an "allergic reaction" to penicillin than actually experience a reaction. However, patients with a history of penicillin allergy are recognized to have a fourfold to sixfold greater risk of subsequent reactions.[26] In addition, a negative history of penicillin allergy does not eliminate the risk of immediate reactions because many serious and even fatal allergic reactions to β-lactam antibiotics occur in patients who have no history of penicillin allergy.[26]

❿ Skin testing can reduce the uncertainty of penicillin sensitivity and should be performed in all patients who have a history of penicillin allergy and require treatment with these agents. Penicillin skin testing in advance of need for penicillin treatment in patients with a history of penicillin allergy does not appear to induce sensitization.[85] Testing for the major penicillin determinant is accomplished with penicilloyl-polylysine (PPL; Pre-Pen), but this product is not currently available in the United States. If this agent is used alone, patients reacting only to minor determinants will be missed. At present, there is also no commercially available product that can be used to test for most of the minor determinants. Benzylpenicillin (at a concentration of 10,000 units/mL) has been used, but some reactive patients still will be missed. When commercially available β-lactams are used for skin testing, as many as 15% of patients with β-lactam allergies will be missed.[86] Penicillin skin testing can facilitate the safe use of penicillin in 90% of patients with a history of penicillin allergy.[87] The incidence of penicillin skin test positive reactivity is low (<1%) in patients with a negative history and up to 72% in patients with a convincing positive history of penicillin allergy.[88] Even in patients who report a history of penicillin allergy but are skin test negative, penicillin treatment does not appear to cause resensitization.[89] The procedure for performing penicillin skin testing is given in Table 91–3.

A negative penicillin skin test indicates that the risk of life-threatening reactions is extremely low with administration of penicillin or other β-lactams. Patients occasionally may experience systemic reactions after skin testing. Also, certain types of patients (e.g., those with dermatographism or taking antihistamines) may be unsuitable for skin testing because a false-positive or false-negative test may result. Penicillin is the only drug for which the predictive value of skin testing has been well established. The value of skin testing for evaluating the risk of adverse reactions to other drugs is largely unknown, but these tests are recommended in selected patients with histories of immediate reactions to nonpenicillin antibiotics.[84]

■ ANAPHYLAXIS

Anaphylaxis requires prompt treatment to minimize the risk of serious morbidity or death. On presentation, attention should be given first to stopping the likely offending agent, if possible, and restoring respiratory and cardiovascular function. A protocol for treatment of anaphylaxis is presented in Table 91–4. Epinephrine is administered as primary treatment to counteract bronchoconstriction and vasodilation. Epinephrine should be administered intramuscularly in the lateral aspect of the thigh.[90] If blood pressure is not restored by epinephrine, crystalloid intravenous fluids should be administered to restore intravascular volume. Typically, 1 L of 0.9% sodium chloride or lactated Ringer solution is administered over 10 to 15 minutes. This can be repeated if the patient is still believed to be volume depleted. A maintenance intravenous fluid then is initiated. Intravenous fluids should be given early in the course of treatment in an attempt to prevent shock. An immediate priority is to establish and maintain an airway by the use of

TABLE 91-3 Procedure for Performing Penicillin Skin Testing

A. Percutaneous (prick) Skin Testing	
Materials	**Volume**
Pre-Pen 6 × 10^6M (currently not commercially available in the United States)	1 drop
Penicillin G 10,000 units/mL	1 drop
β-Lactam drug 3 mg/mL	1 drop
0.03% albumin-saline control	1 drop
Histamine control (1 mg/mL)	1 drop

1. Place a drop of each test material on the volar surface of the forearm.
2. Prick the skin with a sharp needle inserted through the drop at a 45° angle, gently tenting the skin in an upward motion.
3. Interpret skin responses after 15 minutes.
4. A wheal at least 2 × 2 mm with erythema is considered positive.
5. If the prick test is nonreactive, proceed to the intradermal test.
6. If the histamine control is nonreactive, the test is considered uninterpretable.

B. Intradermal Skin Testing	
Materials	**Volume**
Pre-Pen 6 × 10^6M (currently not commercially available in the United States)	0.02 mL
Penicillin G 10,000 units/mL	0.02 mL
β-Lactam drug 3 mg/mL	0.02 mL
0.03% albumin-saline control	0.02 mL
Histamine control (0.1 mg/mL)	0.02 mL

1. Inject 0.02–0.03 mL of each test material intradermally (amount sufficient to produce a small bleb).
2. Interpret skin responses after 15 minutes.
3. A wheal at least 6 × 6 mm with erythema and at least 3 mm greater than the negative control is considered positive.
4. If the histamine control is nonreactive, the test is considered uninterpretable.

Antihistamines may blunt the response and cause false-negative reactions.

From Sullivan TJ. Current Therapy in Allergy. St. Louis: Mosby, 1985:57–61, with permission.

TABLE 91-4 Treatment of Anaphylaxis

1. Place patient in recumbent position and elevate lower extremities.
2. Monitor vital signs frequently (every 2–5 minutes) and stay with the patient.
3. Administer epinephrine 1:1,000 into nonoccluded site: (adults: 0.01 mL/kg up to a maximum of 0.2–0.5 mL every 10 to 15 minutes as needed, children: 0.01 mL/kg up to a maximum dose of 0.2–0.5 mL) subcutaneously or intramuscularly. If necessary, repeat every 15 minutes, up to 2 doses.
4. Administer oxygen, usually 8–10 L/min; however, lower concentrations may be appropriate for patients with chronic obstructive pulmonary disease. Maintain airway with oropharyngeal airway device.
5. Administer the antihistamine diphenhydramine (Benadryl, adults 25–50 mg; children 1–2 mg/kg) usually given parenterally. Apply tourniquet proximal to site of antigen injection; remove every 10–15 minutes.
6. If anaphylaxis is caused by an injection, administer aqueous epinephrine 1:1,000 into site of antigen injection; 0.15–0.3 mL into the injection site.
7. Treat hypotension with IV fluids or colloid replacement, and consider use of a vasopressor such as dopamine.
8. Treat bronchospasm with a β_2-agonist given intermittently or continuously, consider the use of aminophylline 5.6 mg/kg as an IV loading dose, given over 20 minutes, or to maintain a blood level of 8–15 mcg/mL.
9. Give hydrocortisone, 5 mg/kg, or approximately 250 mg IV (prednisone 20 mg orally can be given in mild cases) to reduce the risk of recurring or protracted anaphylaxis. These doses can be repeated every six hours as required.
10. In refractory cases not responding to epinephrine because a β-adrenergic blocker is complicating management, glucagon 1 mg IV as a bolus may be useful. A continuous infusion of glucagon, 1–5 mg/h, may be given if required.

Reprinted and adapted from J Allerg Cli Immunol 1998;101:S465–528.

endotracheal intubation if necessary. When a patient with anaphylaxis is hypotensive, vasopressors will be needed in addition to crystalloids. Norepinephrine is the vasoconstrictor agent of choice for treatment of anaphylactic shock, although dopamine also may be useful. Patients in shock should remain supine with raised legs.[29]

Other agents may be required for treatment of anaphylactic reactions. Corticosteroids (hydrocortisone sodium succinate intravenously) can reduce the risk of late-phase reactions. Aminophylline can be used as adjunctive therapy for bronchospasm. Histamine (H_1) receptor blockers (e.g., diphenhydramine) can be administered to reduce some of the symptoms associated with anaphylaxis, but these agents are not effective as primary therapy.

DESENSITIZATION

For some patients allergic to penicillin, no reasonable alternatives exist, and penicillin therapy may be necessary for treatment of severe, life-threatening infection. In this situation, penicillin desensitization should be considered. Desensitization can reduce the risk of anaphylaxis but does not influence the likelihood of other types of reactions such as exfoliative dermatitis or SJS.

Penicillin desensitization should be performed by a physician experienced in the risks and management of severe allergic reactions. Desensitization should be performed in a hospital setting with resuscitation equipment available. The potential risks and benefits should be discussed with the patient. Prior to initiating the protocol, the patient should be stabilized and fluid, pulmonary, and cardiovascular function optimized. The use of premedications (antihistamines or corticosteroids) is controversial because these agents may mask the early signs of acute reactions and do not reliably reduce the severity of acute reactions. Approximately one third of patients who have undergone desensitization experience mild, transient allergic reaction either during the desensitization procedure or during penicillin therapy.[26] Patients who can take oral medication should undergo desensitization with oral penicillin. Protocols for oral and intravenous penicillin desensitization are given in Tables 91–5 and 91–6. Once the desensitization protocol is begun, it should not be interrupted except for severe reactions. Antihistamines or epinephrine can be administered to treat reactions. In addition, if the patient completes the desensitization regimen and then undergoes penicillin treatment, a lapse between doses of as few as 24 hours can allow for reemergence of sensitivity. Protocols are available for desensitization of other β-lactam antibiotics.[91]

Desensitization of trimethoprim–sulfamethoxazole can be achieved within 2 days in most AIDS patients.[1,92] This can be accomplished by

TABLE 91-5 Protocol for Oral Desensitization

	Phenoxymethyl Penicillin			
Step[a]	***Concentration (units/mL)***	***Volume (mL)***	***Dose (units)***	***Cumulative Dose (units)***
1	1,000	0.1	100	100
2	1,000	0.2	200	300
3	1,000	0.4	400	700
4	1,000	0.8	800	1,500
5	1,000	1.6	1,600	3,100
6	1,000	3.2	3,200	6,300
7	1,000	6.4	6,400	12,700
8	10,000	1.2	12,000	24,700
9	10,000	2.4	24,000	48,700
10	10,000	4.8	48,000	96,700
11	80,000	1.0	80,000	176,700
12	80,000	2.0	160,000	336,700
13	80,000	4.0	320,000	656,700
14	80,000	8.0	640,000	1,296,700
		Observe for 30 min		
15	500,000	0.25	125,000	
16	500,000	0.5	250,000	
17	500,000	1.0	500,000	
18	500,000	2.25	1,125,000	

[a]The interval between steps is 15 min.

Reprinted from Weiss ME, Adkinson NF. Immunol Allerg Clin North 1998;18:731–734.

TABLE 91-6 Parenteral Desensitization Protocol

Injection No.	Benzylpenicillin Concentration (units)	Volume (mL)	Route
1[a,b]	100	0.1	ID
2	100	0.2	SC
3	100	0.4	SC
4	100	0.8	SC
5[b]	1,000	0.1	ID
6	1,000	0.3	SC
7	1,000	0.6	SC
8[b]	10,000	0.1	ID
9	10,000	0.2	SC
10	10,000	0.4	SC
11	10,000	0.8	SC
12[b]	100,000	0.1	ID
13	100,000	0.3	SC
14	100,000	0.6	SC
15[b]	1,000,000	0.1	ID
16	1,000,000	0.2	SC
17	1,000,000	0.2	IM
18	1,000,000	0.4	IM
19	Continuous IV infusion at 1,000,000 units/h		

[a]Administer doses at intervals of not less than 20 min.
[b]Observe and record skin wheal-and-flare response.
ID, intradermally; IM, intramuscularly; SC, subcutaneously.
Reprinted from Weiss ME, Adkinson NF. Immunol Allerg Clin North 1998;18:731–734.

using the following schedule of doses (milligrams of sulfamethoxazole–trimethoprim): day 1: 9 AM, 4 and 0.8 mg; 11 AM, 8 and 1.6 mg; 1 PM, 20 and 4 mg; 5 PM, 40 and 8 mg; day 2: 9 AM, 80 and 16 mg; 3 PM, 160 and 32 mg; 9 PM, 200 and 40 mg; day 3: 9 AM, 400 and 80 mg, and 400 and 80 mg daily thereafter. Other investigators have described a 6-hour graded challenge in HIV-infected patients.[93]

Skin tests often become negative during and shortly after desensitization. The mechanism by which desensitization is protective is unclear. It does not appear that penicillin-specific IgE is neutralized or that IgG as "blocking antibody" is produced. One possible explanation is that basophils and mast cells attain some degree of tolerance on exposure to the antigen.

ABBREVIATIONS

IgE: immunoglobulin E
LT: leukotriene
NSAID: nonsteroidal antiinflammatory drug
PAF: platelet-activating factor
PG: prostaglandin
PPD: purified protein derivative
SLE: systemic lupus erythematosus
TEN: toxic epidermal necrolysis

REFERENCES

1. Gruchalla RS. Drug allergy. J Allerg Clin Immunol 2003;111:S548–S559.
2. Demoly P, Hillaire-Buys D. Classification and epidemiology of hypersensitivity drug reactions. Immunol Allergy Clin North Am 2004;24:345–356.
3. Adkinson NF. Drug allergy. In: Adkinson NF, Yunginger JW, Busse WW, Bochner BS, Holgate ST, Simous FER, eds. Middleton's Allergy: Principles and Practice, 6th ed. St. Louis: Mosby, 2003.
4. Svensson CK, Cowen EW, Gaspari AA. Cutaneous drug reactions. Pharmacol Rev 2000;53:357–379.
5. Pichler WJ. Immune mechanism of drug hypersensitivity. Immunol Allergy Clin North Am 2004;24:373–397.
6. Barnes PJ. Pathophysiology of allergic inflammation. In: Adkinson NF, Yunginger JW, Busse WW, Bochner BS, Holgate ST, Simous FER, eds. Middleton's Allergy: Principles and Practice, 6th ed. St. Louis: Mosby, 2003.
7. MacGlashan D. Histamine: A mediator of inflammation. J Allerg Clin Immunol 2003;112:S53–S59.
8. Solensky R, Mendelson LM. Systemic reactions to antibiotics. Immunol Allergy Clin North Am 2001;21:679–697.
9. Pichler WJ. Delayed drug hypersensitivity reactions. Ann Intern Med 2003;139:683–693.
10. Auquier-Dunant A, Mockenhaupt M, Naldi L, Correia O, Schroder W, Roujeau JC. Correlations between clinical patterns and causes of erythema multiforme major, Stevens-Johnson syndrome, and toxic epidermal necrolysis: Results of an international prospective study. Arch Dermatol 2002;138:1019–1024.
11. Tang AW. A practical guide to anaphylaxis. Am Family Physician 2003;68:1325–1332.
12. Sampson HA, Munoz-Furlong A, Bock A, et al. Symposium on the definition and management of anaphylaxis: Summary report. J Allerg Clin Immunol 2005;115:584–591.
13. Matasar MJ, Neugut AI. Epidemiology of asthma. Curr Allerg Asthma Reports 2003;3:30–35.
14. Neuqut AI, Ghatak AT, Miller RL. Anaphylaxis in the United States: An investigation into its epidemiology. Ann Intern Med 2001;161:15–21.
15. Sampson HA, Munoz-Furlong A, Campbell RL, et al. Second symposium on the definition and management of anaphylaxis: Summary report—Second National Institute of Allergy and Infectious Diseases/Food Allergy and Anaphylaxis Network Symposium. J Allerg Clin Immunol 2006;117:391–397.
16. Johnson DH, Cuhna BA. Drug fever. Infect Dis Clin North Am 1996;10:85–91.
17. Rubin RL. Drug-induced lupus. Toxicology 2005;209:135–147.
18. Sarzi-Puttini P, Atzeni F, Capsoni F, Lubrano E, Doria A. Drug-induced lupus erythematosus. Autoimmunity 2005;38:507–518.
19. Roujeau JC, Stern RS. Severe adverse cutaneous reactions to drugs. N Engl J Med 1994;331:1272–1285.
20. Hunziker T, Kunzi U, Braunschweig S, et al. Comprehensive hospital drug monitoring: Adverse drug reactions—A 20-year survey. Allergy 1997;52:388–393.
21. Mockenhaupt M, Schopf E. Epidemiology of drug-induced severe skin reactions. Semin Cutan Med Surg 1996;15:236–243.
22. McKenna JK, Leiferman KM. Dermatologic drug reactions. Immunol Allergy Clin North Am 2004;24:399–423.
23. Bigby M. Rates of cutaneous reactions to drugs. Arch Dermatol 2001;137:765–770.
24. Ibia EO, Schwartz RH, Wiederman BL. Antibiotic rashes in children: A survey in a private practice setting. Arch Dermatol 2000;136:849–854.
25. Thethi AK, Van Dellen RG. Dilemmas and controversies in penicillin allergy. Immunol Allergy Clin North Am 2004;24:445–461.
26. Weiss ME, Adkinson NF. Immediate hypersensitivity reactions to penicillin and related antibiotics. Clin Allergy 1988;18:515–540.
27. Lee CE, Zembower TR, Fotis MA, et al. The incidence of antimicrobial allergies in hospitalized patients. Arch Intern Med 2000;160:2819–2822.
28. Salkind AR, Cuddy PG, Foxworth JW. Is this patient allergic to penicillin? An evidence-based analysis of the likelihood of penicillin allergy. JAMA 2001;285:2498–2505.
29. Sicherer SH, Leung DYM. Advances in allergic skin disease, anaphylaxis, and hypersensitivity reactions to foods, drugs, and insect stings. J Allerg Clin Immunol 2004;114:118–124.
30. Hunziker T, Kunzi UP, Braunschweig S, et al. Comprehensive hospital drug monitoring (CHDM): Adverse skin reactions, a 20-year survey. Allergy 1997;52:388–393.
31. Bigby M. Rates of cutaneous reactions to drugs. Arch Dermatol 2001;137:765–770.
32. Baldo BA. Penicillins and cephalosporins as allergens: Structural aspects of recognition and cross-reactions. Clin Exp Allergy 1999;29:744–749.
33. Madaan A, Li JTC. Cephalosporin allergy. Immunol Clin North Am 2004;24:463–476.
34. Kelkar PS, Lu JT. Cephalosporin allergy. N Engl J Med 2001;345:804–809.
35. Anne S, Reisman RE. Risk of administering cephalosporin antibiotics to patients with histories of penicillin allergy. Ann Allergy Asthma Immunol 1995;74:167–170.
36. Wickern GM, Nish WA, Bitner AS, Freeman TM. Allergy to β-lactams: A survey of current practices. J Allerg Clin Immunol 1994;94:725–731.
37. Ponvert C, Le Clainche L, de Blic J, et al. Allergy to β-lactam antibiotics in children. Pediatrics 1999;104:45.

38. Kishiyama JL, Adelman DC. The cross-reactivity of β-lactam antibiotics. Drug Saf 1994;10:318–327.
39. Christiansen C. X-ray contrast media—An overview. Toxicology 2005;209:185–187.
40. Brochow K, Christiansen C, Kanny G, et al. Management of hypersensitivity reactions to iodinated contrast media. Allergy 2005;60:150–158.
41. Idee JM, Pines E, Pringent P, Coror C. Allergy-like reactions to iodinated contrast agents. A critical analysis. Fundam Clin Pharmacol 2005;19:263–281.
42. Gueant-Rodriguez RM, Romano A, Barbaud A, Brucknow K, Gueant JL. Hypersensitivity reactions to iodinated contrast media. Curr Pharmaceut Design 2006;12:3359–3372.
43. Murphy KJ, Brunberg JA, Cohan RH. Adverse reactions to gadolinium contrast media: A review of 36 cases. AJR Am J Roentgenol 1996;167:847–849.
44. Marshall GD, Lieberman PL. Anaphylactoid reactions to radiocontrast agents. Immunol Allergy Clin North Am 1998;18:799–807.
45. Tramer MP, von Elm E, Loubeyre P, Hauser C. Pharmacologic prevention of serious anaphylactic reactions due to iodinated contrast media: Systematic review. BMJ 2006;333:663–664.
46. Hagan JB. Anaphylactoid and adverse reactions to radiocontrast agents. Immunol Allergy Clin North Am 2004;24:507–519.
47. Castera V, Dutor-Meyer A, Koeppel MC, Petitjean C, Darmon P. Systemic allergy to human insulin and its rapid and long acting analogs: Successful treatment by continuous subcutaneous insulin lispro infusion. Diabetes Metab 2005;31:391–400.
48. Stevenson DD, Simon RA, Zuraw BL. Sensitivity to aspirin and nonsteroidal anti-inflammatory drugs. In: Adkinson NF, Yunginger JW, Busse WW, Bochner BS, Holgate ST, Simous FER, eds.: Middleton's Allergy: Principles and Practice, 6th ed. St. Louis: Mosby, 2003.
49. Stevenson DD. Aspirin and NSAID sensitivity. Immunol Allergy Clin North Am 2004;24:491–505.
50. Babu KS, Salvi SS. Aspirin and asthma. Chest 2000;118:1470–1466.
51. Sanak M, Szczeklik A. Genetics of aspirin induced asthma. Thorax 2000;55(Suppl 2):S45–S47.
52. Lee TH. Mechanisms of aspirin sensitivity. Am Rev Respir Dis 1992;145:S34–S36.
53. Stevenson DD, Simon RA. Lack of cross-reactivity between rofecoxib and aspirin in aspirin-sensitive patients with asthma. J Allergy Clin Immunol 2001;108:47–51.
54. Woessner KM, Simon RA, Stevenson DD. The safety of celecoxib in patients with aspirin-sensitive asthma. Arthritis Rheum 2002;46:2201–2206.
55. Gyllfors P, Bochenek G, Overholt J, et al. Biochemical and clinical evidence that aspirin-intolerant asthmatic subjects tolerate the cyclo-oxygenase 2-selective analgesic celecoxib. J Allerg Clin Immunol 2003;111:1116–1121.
56. Goodwin SD, Glenny RW. Nonsteroidal anti-inflammatory drug–associated pulmonary infiltrates with eosinophilia. Arch Intern Med 1992;152:1521–1524.
57. Strom BL, Schinnar R, Apter AJ, et al. Absence of cross-reactivity between sulfonamide antibiotics and sulfonamide nonantibiotics. N Engl J Med 2003;349:1628–1635.
58. Slatore CG, Tilles SA. Sulfonamide hypersensitivity. Immunol Allergy Clin North Am 2004;24:477–490.
59. Brackett CC, Singh H, Block JR. Likelihood and mechanisms of cross-allergenicity between sulfonamide antibiotics and other drugs containing a sulfonamide functional group. Pharmacotherapy 2004;24:856–870.
60. Temesgen Z, Beri G. HIV and drug allergy. Immunol Allergy Clin North Am 2004;24:521–531.
61. Santomauro JT, Stover DE. *Pneumocystis carinii* pneumonia. Med Clin North Am 1997;81:299–318.
62. Moore RD, Fortgang I, Keruly J, Chaisson RE. Adverse events from drug therapy for human immunodeficiency virus disease. Am J Med 1996;101:34–40.
63. Bhatia MS. Allergy to tartrazine in psychotropic drugs. J Clin Psychiatry 2000;61:473–476.
64. Ardern KD, Ram FS. Tartrazine exclusion for allergic asthma. Cochrane Database Syst Rev 2001;4:CD000460.
65. American Academy of Pediatrics Committee on Drugs. "Inactive" ingredients in pharmaceutical products. Pediatrics 1985;76:635–642.
66. Timbo B, Koehler KM, Wolyniak C, Klontz KC. Sulfites—A food and drug administration review of recalls and reported adverse events. J Food Protect 2004;67:1806–1811.
67. Campbell JR, Maestrello CL, Campbell RL. Allergic responses to metabisulfite in lidocaine anesthetic solution. Anesth Prog 2001;48:21–26.
68. Mowad CM. Allergic contact dermatitis caused by parabens: Two case reports and a review. Am J Contact Dermat 2000;11:53–56.
69. Weiss RB. Hypersensitivity reactions. Semin Oncol 1992;19:458–477.
70. Shepherd GM. Hypersensitivity reactions to chemotherapeutic drugs. Clin Rev Allergy Immunol 2003;24:253–262.
71. Markman M, Kennedy A, Webster K, et al. Combination chemotherapy with carboplatin and docetaxel in the treatment of cancers of the ovary and fallopian tube and primary carcinoma of the peritoneum. J Clin Oncol 2001;19:1901–1905.
72. Bookman MA, Kloth DD, Kover PE, et al. Intravenous prophylaxis for paclitaxel-related hypersensitivity reactions. Semin Oncol 1997;24:S19-13–S19-15.
73. Eisenhauer EA, ten Bokkel Huinink WW, Swenerton KD, et al. European-Canadian randomized trial of paclitaxel in relapsed ovarian cancer: High-dose versus low-dose and long versus short infusion. J Clin Oncol 1994;12:2654–2666.
74. Hendrick AM, Simmons D, Cantwell BMJ. Allergic reactions to carboplatin. Ann Oncol 1992;3:239–240.
75. Markman M, Kennedy A, Webster K, et al. Clinical features of hypersensitivity reactions to carboplatin. J Clin Oncol 1999;17:1141–1145.
76. Markman M, Zanotti K, Peterson G, et al. Expanded experience with an intradermal skin test to predict for the presence or absence of carboplatin hypersensitivity. J Clin Oncol 2003;21:4611–4614.
77. Saif MW. Hypersensitivity reactions associated with oxaliplatin. Expert Opin Drug Saf 2006;5:687–694.
78. Mis L, Fernando NH, Hurwitz HI, Morse MA. Successful desensitization to oxaliplatin. Anna Pharmacother 2005;39:966–969.
79. Gammon D, Bhargava P, McCormick MJ. Hypersensitivity reactions to oxaliplatin and the application of a desensitization protocol. Oncologist 2004;9:546–549.
80. Sullivan JR, Shear NH. The drug hypersensitivity syndrome: What is the pathogenesis? Arch Dermatol 2001;137:357–364.
81. Schlienger RG, Knowles SR, Shear NH. Lamotrigine-associated anticonvulsant hypersensitivity syndrome. Neurology 1998;51:1172–1175.
82. Anderson JA. Allergic reactions to drugs and biologic agents. JAMA 1992;268:2845–2857.
83. Weiss ME, Adkinson NF. Diagnostic testing for drug hypersensitivity. Immunol Allergy Clin North Am 1998;18:731–734.
84. Aberer W, Bircher A, Romaro A, et al. Drug provocation testing in the diagnosis of drug hypersensitivity reactions: General considerations. Allergy 2003;58:854–863.
85. Macy E, Mangat R, Burchetts RJ. Penicillin skin testing in advance of need: Multiyear follow-up in 568 test result-negative subjects exposed to oral penicillins. J Allerg Clin Immunol 2003;111:1111–1115.
86. Bousquet PJ, Co-Minh HB, Amoux B, Daures JP, Demoly P. Importance of mixture of minor determinants and benzylpenicilloyl poly-L-lysine skin testing in the diagnosis of beta-lactam allergy. J Allerg Clin Immunol 2005;115:1314–1316.
87. Gadde J, Spence M, Wheeler B, Adkinson NF. Clinical experience with penicillin skin testing in a large inner-city STD clinic. JAMA 1993;270:2456–2463.
88. Kalogeromitros D, Rigopoulos D, Gregoriou S, et al. Penicillin hypersensitivity: Value of clinical history and skin testing in daily practice. Allerg Asthma Proc 2004;25:157–160.
89. Solensky R, Earl HS, Gruchalla RS. Lack of penicillin resensitization in patients with a history of penicillin allergy after receiving repeated penicillin courses. Arch Intern Med 2002;162:822–826.
90. Lieberman P. Use of epinephrine in the treatment of anaphylaxis. Curr Opin Allerg Clin Immunol 2003;3:313–318.
91. Solensky R. Drug desensitization. Immunol Allergy Clin North Am 2004;24:425–443.
92. Caumes E, Guermonprez G, Lecomte C, et al. Efficacy and safety of desensitization with sulfamethoxazole and trimethoprim in 48 previously hypersensitive patients infected with human immunodeficiency virus. Arch Dermatol 1997;133:465–469.
93. Demoly P, Messaad D, Sahla H, et al. Six-hour trimethoprim-sulfamethoxazole-graded challenge in HIV-infected patients. J Allerg Clin Immunol 1998;102:1033–1036.

CHAPTER 92

Solid-Organ Transplantation

KRISTINE S. SCHONDER AND HEATHER J. JOHNSON

KEY CONCEPTS

1. Acute allograft rejection is primarily due to the activation of T cells, which is mediated, to a large degree, by interleukin (IL)-2.

2. A combination of two to four immunosuppressive drugs is used to target different levels of the immune cascade to prevent allograft rejection and to allow lower doses of individual agents to be used to minimize toxicity.

3. The goals of immunosuppression are to decrease the incidence of acute and chronic rejection while minimizing adverse events associated with immunosuppressive medications.

4. Calcineurin inhibitors (CIs), such as cyclosporine and tacrolimus, are the backbone of immunosuppressive regimens because they inhibit IL-2 and thereby block T-cell activation. However, they are associated with significant adverse effects, namely, nephrotoxicity and neurotoxicity.

5. Calcineurin inhibitor-induced nephrotoxicity is one of the most common side effects observed in transplant recipients and is the leading cause of renal dysfunction in nonrenal transplant patients.

6. Corticosteroids are a key component of immunosuppressive regimens because they block the initial steps in allograft rejection. However, the adverse effects associated with long-term use of corticosteroids have prompted the investigation of corticosteroid-free immunosuppressive protocols.

7. Antiproliferative agents such as azathioprine and mycophenolate inhibit T-cell proliferation by altering purine synthesis to prevent acute rejection. Bone marrow suppression is the most significant adverse effect associated with these agents.

8. Sirolimus exerts its activity by inhibiting the mTOR (mammalian target of rapamycin) receptor, which alters T-cell response to IL-2. The adverse effects associated with sirolimus include thrombocytopenia, anemia, and hyperlipidemia.

9. The effect of antibody preparations on T cells depends on the specific target receptors on the surface of T cells. Most antibody preparations are associated with significant infusion-related reactions.

10. Long-term allograft and patient survival is limited by chronic rejection, cardiovascular disease, and long-term immunosuppressive complications, such as malignancy.

Learning objectives, review questions, and other resources can be found at **www.pharmacotherapyonline.com.**

Solid-organ transplantation provides a lifesaving treatment for patients with end-stage cardiac, kidney, liver, lung, and intestinal disease. In 2004, the most recent year for which data is available, 26,539 solid organ transplants were performed. Kidney transplants remain the most common; 9,025 were from cadaveric donors and 6,646 from living donors. The next most frequently transplanted organ was the liver, with 5,457 from cadaveric donors and 323 from living donors. Heart and pancreas (or combined kidney-pancreas) transplants account for almost 2,000 and 1,500 transplants, respectively.[1] Despite the demand for transplantation, the number of cadaveric donors has remained relatively stable during the past decade. In 2006, more than 90,000 persons in the United States were waiting for a transplant (almost 70,000 people were awaiting a kidney, 17,000 a liver, and almost 3,000 were on the list for a heart transplant). Median waiting time for a cadaveric kidney is more than 3 years. For liver transplantation the median time to transplant is more than 2 years, whereas for heart transplantation it is approximately 6 months. For heart, liver, and lung transplantation clinical status is an important factor affecting waiting times, with the sickest patients receiving priority for available organs.

To increase the number of organs available for transplantation, several strategies have been employed in the past several years. The use of living donors for renal transplantation represents almost half of all kidney transplants, more than any other organ. Living-donor transplantation is also becoming increasingly important for those with end stage liver and lung disease. Efforts to expand the cadaveric donor pool have included relaxation of age restrictions, development of better preservation solutions, use of "extended-criteria" and non–heart-beating donors, and the transplantation of one liver to more than one recipient, as well as the implantation of only a segment of a liver.

Despite all these efforts, patients continue to die awaiting transplantation. In 2004, more than 7,000 people died who were on transplantation waiting lists. In all areas, efforts have been made to improve organ allocation, moving toward allocation based primarily on "medical necessity" versus time-on-waiting-list. Although dialysis can be used for an extended period of time to partially replace the function of the kidneys, such options are not readily available for most liver and heart transplantation candidates. Left ventricular assist devices are now used commonly as a bridge to transplantation for many heart transplantation candidates, however, hepatocyte transplantation and artificial liver support remain investigational alternatives or bridges to liver transplantation.[2]

Patient and graft survival rates following transplantation have improved significantly over the past 30 years as a result of advances

TABLE 92-1 Organ-Specific Patient and Graft Survival Rates

	Patient Survival (%)		Graft Survival (%)	
Organ	*1 Year*	*5 Years*	*1 Year*	*5 Years*
Kidney				
Living donor	97.9	90.2	95.1	66.7
Cadaveric donor	94.6	81.1	89	66.7
Liver				
Living donor	87.7	77.4	81.7	69.7
Cadaveric donor	86.8	73.1	82.2	66.9
Heart	87.5	72.8	86.8	71.8

Data from reference 1.

in pharmacotherapy, surgical techniques, organ preservation, and the postoperative management of patients (Table 92–1). In fact, the number of people living with transplants exceeded 110,000 in 2004. In this chapter the epidemiology of endstage kidney, liver and heart disease is briefly reviewed, the pathophysiology of organ rejection is reviewed, the pharmacotherapeutic options for individualized immunosuppressive regimens are critiqued and the unique complications of these regimens along with the therapeutic challenges they present are discussed.

EPIDEMIOLOGY AND ETIOLOGY

KIDNEY

Renal transplantation is the preferred long-term therapeutic option for most patients with end-stage renal disease because it provides patients with the greatest potential improvement in quality of life. Dialysis catheter-related infections, peritoneal dialysis-associated peritonitis, and scheduled dialysis treatments are avoided, and dietary restrictions are fewer. Patients who receive a renal transplant before the initiation of dialysis have markedly improved quality of life and prolonged life expectancy. The use of living-donor transplantation has made this increasingly possible. Although the analysis of quality of life is complex, patients generally report improved quality of life following transplantation as compared with patients on maintenance dialysis.[3]

Diabetes mellitus, hypertension, and glomerulonephritis are the most common causes of end-stage renal disease leading to kidney transplantation, accounting for more than 70% of patients (see Chapters 47 and 48).[4] Patients with medical conditions such as unstable cardiac disease or recently diagnosed malignancy, for whom the risk of surgery or chronic immunosuppression would be greater than the risks associated with chronic dialysis, are generally excluded from consideration for transplantation.

LIVER

Noncholestatic cirrhosis (hepatitis C, alcoholic cirrhosis, hepatitis B, cryptogenic cirrhosis, and autoimmune hepatitis) is the primary cause of end-stage liver disease and more than 70% of liver transplant recipients have been diagnosed with one of these conditions.[1] Hepatitis C remains the most common indication leading to liver transplantation, accounting for 40% of all cases. Livers are allocated based on a United Network for Organ Sharing-adapted, Model for End-stage Liver Disease (MELD) score. This score, which is based on serum creatinine concentration, total serum bilirubin concentration, international normalization ratio, and etiology of cirrhosis, has been demonstrated to be a useful tool to predict impending mortality.

There are few absolute contraindications to liver transplantation. Patients should be free from active alcohol or substance abuse. Although hepatitis B and C can recur in the transplanted liver, these are not absolute contraindications to liver transplantation.[2,5]

CLINICAL CONTROVERSY

Retransplantation for hepatitis C recurrence after liver transplantation often depends on the time frame in which recurrence occurs. If recurrence occurs within 6 months of transplantation, retransplantation is contraindicated. If recurrence occurs after 1 year, some clinicians may consider retransplantation. However, other clinicians consider recurrence at any point to be a contraindication for another transplant.

HEART

Cardiac transplant candidates typically are patients with end-stage heart failure who have New York Heart Association class III or IV symptoms despite maximal medical management and have an expected 1-year mortality risk of 25% or greater without a transplant.[6] Idiopathic cardiomyopathy and ischemic heart disease account for heart failure in more than 90% of heart transplantation recipients.[1] Other etiologies include valvular disease, retransplantation for graft atherosclerosis or dysfunction, and congenital heart disease. Chapters 16 and 20 discuss the role of heart transplantation as a therapeutic option for patients with heart failure.

Absolute contraindications to orthotopic cardiac transplantation include the presence of an active infection (except in the case of an infected ventricular assist device, which is an indication for urgent transplantation) or the presence of other diseases (i.e., malignancy) that may limit survival and/or rehabilitation and severe, irreversible pulmonary hypertension.

CLINICAL CONTROVERSY

Many clinicians do not consider patients infected with human immunodeficiency virus (HIV) to be appropriate candidates for transplantation, although some transplant centers will transplant organs to HIV-infected patients. A similar debate exists with regards to elderly patients, who are in otherwise good health.

SURGICAL PROCEDURES

Kidney transplantation is generally performed by placing the allograft retroperitoneally in the right iliac fossa. The renal artery and vein are anastomosed to the external iliac artery and vein, respectively, and the donor ureter is connected directly to the bladder. If the donor kidney has not undergone prolonged ischemia, the production of urine immediately follows revascularization. For the most part, native kidneys are not removed.[7]

The transplanted liver, in contrast to the kidney, is placed orthotopically; the recipient's own liver must be removed. Liver transplantation occurs in several phases: removal of recipient liver, donor graft revascularization, and biliary reconstruction. During the anhepatic phase, the patient is placed on venovenous bypass to preserve venous return from the kidney and lower extremities. Size may be a limiting factor in liver transplantation. Donor and recipient are usually matched for size to prevent splinting of the diaphragm and pulmonary complications that would result from transplantation of an excessively large liver.[8]

Heart transplantation is usually an orthotopic procedure. Leaving most of the atria and septum of the recipient, the patient is placed on cardiopulmonary bypass. The donor heart is implanted by anastomosis of the left atrium to the residual left atrial wall and joining the right atrial wall and septum. The main pulmonary artery is connected to the ascending aorta.[9]

PHYSIOLOGIC CONSEQUENCES OF TRANSPLANTATION

Transplantation is truly lifesaving for heart, liver, and lung transplantation recipients, whereas renal transplantation is associated with improved quality of life and survival when compared with dialysis.[10] Most heart transplantation patients return to New York Heart Association functional class I following transplantation. Although not all return to work, 89.9% of patients consider themselves to have no limitations on activity at 1-year followup.[11] The specific physiologic consequences of kidney, liver, and heart transplantation are discussed below.

KIDNEY TRANSPLANTATION

The glomerular filtration rate of a successfully transplanted kidney may be near normal almost immediately after transplantation. In some patients, however, the concentration of standard biochemical indicators of renal function, such as serum creatinine and blood urea nitrogen, may remain elevated for several days. Standard formulas used to predict drug dosing rely on a stable serum creatinine and may be inaccurate immediately following transplantation (see Chap. 44).

Although the allograft is able to remove uremic toxins from the body, it may take several weeks for other physiologic complications of chronic renal failure, such as anemia, calcium and phosphate imbalance, and altered lipid profiles, to resolve. The renal production of erythropoietin and 1-hydroxylation of vitamin D may return toward normal early in the postoperative period. Because the onset of physiologic effects may be delayed, continuation of pretransplantation calcitriol, calcium supplementation, and/or phosphate binders may be warranted in some patients.

Primary nonfunction of a renal allograft or delayed graft function (DGF) is characterized by the need for dialysis in the first 7 postoperative days or the failure of the serum creatinine to fall below 4 mg/dL or by 30% of the pretransplantation value. The incidence of DGF in primary cadaveric renal transplantation ranges from 8% to 50% and results in a slower return of the kidney's excretory, metabolic, and synthetic functions. DGF is associated with prolonged hospital stays, higher costs, difficult management of immunosuppressive therapy, slower patient rehabilitation, and poor graft survival. Urinary complications, such as ureteral obstruction, thrombosis, or leak or vascular complications, including arterial or venous stenosis or thrombosis, also may result in early graft dysfunction.

The primary cause of DGF is acute tubular necrosis (ATN). The incidence of ATN increases when kidneys are harvested from donors who recently experienced a cardiac arrest, from donors who were hypotensive or on vasopressors, or from older donors (age >55 years). Prolonged periods of ischemia can increase the risk of ATN. The management of patients with ATN may be difficult (see Chap. 45). Cyclosporine and tacrolimus may be implicated in the prolongation of ATN, but a clear cause-and-effect relationship has not been established. DGF predisposes patients to acute rejection, possibly as a consequence of decreased calcineurin inhibitor levels.

LIVER TRANSPLANTATION

The physiologic consequences of liver transplantation are complex, involving changes in both metabolic and synthetic function. Postoperatively, the liver transplant recipient likely will have many fluid, electrolyte, and nutritional abnormalities. Biliary tract dysfunction may alter the absorption of fats and fat-soluble drugs.[12] Poor absorption of the lipid-soluble drug cyclosporine improves after successful liver transplantation and reestablishment of bile flow. Vitamin E deficiency and its neurologic complications in liver failure patients are reversed after successful liver transplantation. In stable adult liver transplant patients, the concentrations of retinol and tocopherol are similar to those seen in normal healthy subjects, indicating recovery of transplanted liver production and excretion of bile salts needed for fat-soluble vitamin absorption. Table 92–2 summarizes the effects of liver transplantation on metabolism and renal elimination which are seen in the immediate postoperative period. Most of these changes resolve as liver function normalizes.

TABLE 92-2 Perioperative Changes in Drug Disposition and Elimination following Liver Transplantation

	Result	Comment
Serum proteins		
↓ Albumin	↑ Free fraction of drugs usually bound to albumin	Diazepam, salicylic acid binding greater in liver transplant than chronic liver disease because of endogenous binding inhibitors (up to 45 days post-transplant)
↑ alpha-1-Acid glycoprotein	Lower free fraction of drugs	Lidocaine
Metabolism/elimination		
Microsomal enzymes	↑ CYP2E1 activity	Increased drug metabolism (induction)
	↔CYP2D6	Unaffected
	↓ CYP activity	Decreased drug elimination (inhibition)
Oxidation	Stable	
Conjugation	Normalizes after transplant	
Biliary function	↓ Absorption of lipophilic compounds	
	↑ Cyclosporine metabolites in blood	
Renal elimination	Elimination of gentamicin, vancomycin, cephalosporins less than predicted by serum creatinine	Renal elimination of metabolites limited

Adapted from reference 12.

The newly transplanted liver fails to function in 10% to 15% of recipients as the result of several different mechanisms. Early graft failure can result from preexisting disease in the donor, and even coagulation defects have been acquired through donor organs. The technical complexity of the operation can produce flaws in revascularization that also lead to graft nonfunction. Surgical complications encountered include portal vein thrombosis, hepatic artery thrombosis, and bile duct leaks. Ischemic injury to the donor liver through preservation is difficult to predict and can result in early graft dysfunction. Perioperative immune events rarely lead to the classic picture of hyperacute rejection in liver transplantation, but graft failure in the first 2 postoperative weeks may indicate antibody-mediated graft destruction.

HEART TRANSPLANTATION

The orthotopically transplanted heart is denervated and no longer responds to physiologic stimuli and pharmacologic agents in a normal manner (Table 92–3).[13] Patients, for example, do not experience angina. In situations requiring an increased heart rate (e.g., exercise or hypotension), the denervated heart is unable to acutely increase heart rate but instead relies on increasing the stroke volume. Later in the course of exercise or hypotension, heart rate increases in response to circulating catecholamines. While the maximum exercise capacity of heart transplant recipients is below normal, most patients are able to resume normal lifestyles and reasonably vigorous activity levels. Partial reinnervation may occur

TABLE 92-3 Altered Responses to Cardiac Drugs in the Denervated Transplanted Heart

Drug	Effect	Mechanism	Comment
Digitalis	Normal inotropic effect; minimal effect on AV node	Direct myocardial effect; denervation	
Atropine	No effect on AV node	Denervation	
Adrenaline/ noradrenaline	Increased contractility; increased chronotropy	Denervation; hypersensitivity	Increased cardiac output mediated by increased heart rate
Isoproterenol	Normal increase in contractility; normal increase in chronotropy	No neuronal uptake	
Quinidine	No vagolytic effect	Denervation	
Verapamil	AV block	Direct effect	
Nifedipine	No reflex tachycardia	Denervation	
Hydralazine	No reflex tachycardia	Denervation	
β-Blocker	Increased antagonist effect	Denervation	Impaired heart rate response, use sparingly
Adenosine	Negative chronotropic effect	Hypersensitivity; effect on sinus node of denervated heart	Life-threatening asystole (>0.5 min) may occur if used to treat supraventricular arrhythmia or stress testing
Acetylcholine	Negative chronotropic effect	Hypersensitivity; effect on sinus node of denervated heart	

AV, atriovenous node.

Deng MC. Heart failure: Cardiac transplantation. Heart 2002;87:177–184. Reproduced with permission from the BMJ Publishing Group.

over time, thereby facilitating more normal physiologic and pharmacologic responses and better exercise capacity.[14]

In the first 6 weeks after transplantation, a number of autoregulatory, anatomic, and physiologic responses present in the normal heart are interrupted or blunted. The donor sinus node function may be impaired by preservation injury, direct surgical trauma at excision, the presence of long-acting antiarrhythmics (e.g., amiodarone) taken prior to transplant by the recipient, and a lack of "conditioning" responsiveness to catecholamines.[14] Consequently, the transplanted heart generally requires chronotropic support with either milrinone or pacing in the perioperative period to maintain a heart rate of 90 to 110 beats per minute and satisfactory hemodynamics (i.e., blood pressure, urine output, and tissue perfusion). Approximately 10% to 20% of transplant patients will have persistent chronotropic incompetence requiring either short courses of medications, such as terbutaline or theophylline, or permanent cardiac pacing.

Right ventricular function frequently is impaired, presumably as a result of preservation injury and elevated pulmonary vascular resistance. A "restrictive" hemodynamic pattern may be present initially, but it usually improves over the 6 weeks following transplantation. Donor–recipient size mismatch may contribute to early post-transplantation hemodynamic abnormalities characterized by higher right and left ventricular end-diastolic pressures. Supraventricular arrhythmias are usually transient and may result from overvigorous use of catecholamines or milrinone. If this type of arrhythmia occurs after the perioperative period, the astute clinician should consider the possibility of acute rejection.

Myocardial depression frequently occurs and generally requires inotropic support with agents such as dobutamine, milrinone, and epinephrine. On occasion, intra- or postoperative administration of vasodilators, including nitric oxide, and inotropic agents may be necessary to treat right-sided failure in the transplant patient; milrinone and isoproterenol are preferred in this setting.

Persistent abnormalities of diastolic function are often noted in the transplanted heart such that intracardiac pressures increase in an exaggerated fashion in response to exercise and/or volume infusion.[14] These abnormalities are due in part to denervation, but also to acute rejection or to the scarring secondary to previously treated rejection episodes, hypertension, or cardiac allograft vasculopathy.

Hypertension may occur following surgery secondary to the effect of elevated catecholamine levels and systemic vascular resistance as the residual effects of end-stage heart failure on the healthy heart. Systolic blood pressure should be maintained at 110 to 120 mm Hg to enhance cardiac function. In the acute post-transplantation period, intravenous nitroprusside or nitroglycerin may be needed, whereas oral angiotensin-converting enzyme inhibitors (ACEIs) and/or amlodipine are commonly used once the patient can ingest oral medications.

PATHOPHYSIOLOGY OF REJECTION

GENERAL CONCEPTS

❶ Rejection of any transplanted organ is primarily mediated by activation of alloreactive T cells and antigen-presenting cells such as B lymphocytes, macrophages, and dendritic cells. Acute allograft rejection is caused primarily by the infiltration of T cells into the allograft, which triggers inflammatory and cytotoxic effects on the graft. Complex interactions between the allograft and cellular cytokines, cell-to-cell interactions, CD4+ and CD8+ T cells, and B cells ultimately lead to chronic rejection and graft loss if adequate immunosuppression is not maintained.[15]

The sequence of events that underlies graft rejection is recognition of the donor's histocompatibility differences by the recipient's immune system, recruitment of activated lymphocytes, initiation of immune effector mechanisms, and finally graft destruction.

Class I and II antigens of the major histocompatibility complex (MHC) are important for histocompatibility in transplantation.[16] Class I antigens are present on virtually all nucleated cells in the body, whereas the class II antigens are located primarily on B lymphocytes, antigen-presenting cells, and vascular endothelium.[16] T-helper cells, specialized to direct the immune system, can only recognize foreign antigen in the presence of MHC type II. Cytotoxic T cells, specialized to destroy, can only recognize antigen in the presence of MHC type I antigens. Lymphocytes are the only cells in the body that can recognize specific antigens and are central to allograft rejection.

T-cell activation is caused by interactions between T-cell receptors, the MHC, cellular adhesion molecules, and costimulatory molecules. Among the series of events is calcineurin activation, which ultimately promotes interleukin (IL)-2 proliferation. After initial T-cell activation, the process of clonal expansion and immunologic progression is mediated by cytokines. IL-2 is released from T cells and activates T lymphocytes locally and in other regions of the body. Undifferentiated T-helper cells can be induced to develop along two lines: T-helper type 1 cells secrete IL-2, interferon-γ, and IL-12 and favor cytotoxicity, whereas T-helper type 2 cells secrete IL-4, IL-5, IL-10, and IL-13, which stimulate B-cell and immunoglobulin development. A predominance of T-helper type 2 cells is associated with tolerance (the ability of the body to

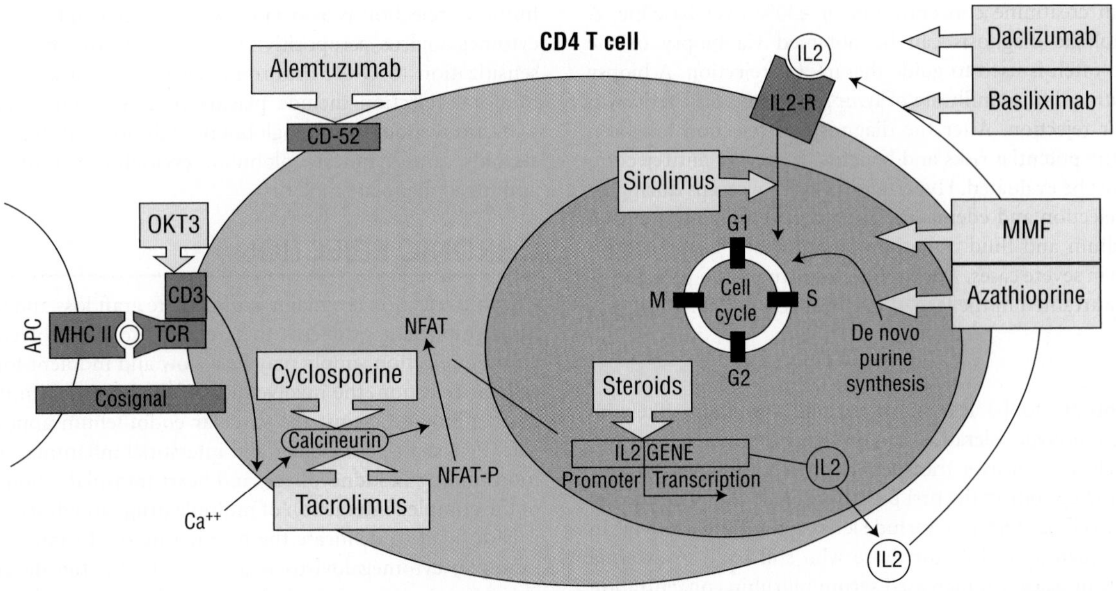

FIGURE 92-1. Stages of CD4 T-cell activation and cytokine production with identification of the sites of action of different immunosuppressive agents. Antigen major histocompatibility complex (MHC) II molecule complexes are responsible for initiating the activation of CD4 T cells. These MHC-peptide complexes are recognized by the T-cell recognition complex (TCR). A costimulatory signal initiates signal transduction with activation of second messengers, one of which is calcineurin. Calcineurin removes phosphates from the nuclear factors (NFAT-P) allowing them to enter the nucleus. These nuclear factors specifically bind to an interleukin (IL)-2 promoter gene facilitating IL-2 gene transcription. Interaction of IL-2 with the IL-2 receptor (IL-2R) on the cell membrane surface induces cell proliferation and production of cytokines specific to the T cell. (APC, antigen-presenting cells; MMF, mycophenolate mofetil.) *(With permission from reference 17.)*

recognize the transplanted allograft as "self") in some experimental models. The complex nature of these cytokine interactions makes it very difficult to design drugs with exclusive actions (Fig. 92–1). Allograft inflammation is thus the result of specific T-cell interactions with antigen-presenting cells and nonspecific immunologic mechanisms (natural killer cell chemotaxis, release of vasoactive substances). Rejection of the transplanted tissue can take place at any time following surgery and is classified clinically as hyperacute rejection, acute cellular rejection, and/or humoral or chronic rejection.

Efforts are made to allocate well-matched, according to human leukocyte antigens (HLA)-A, -B, and -DR, kidneys to minimize rejection and enhance survival rates. However, the benefit of having no recipient donor mismatches may be negated by excessive cold ischemia time (>36 hours) and donor age older than 60 years. HLA tissue matching is not performed routinely before transplantation for livers and hearts because organ availability is more limited and the optimal cold ischemia time is shorter. However, if the potential recipient is reactive against a panel of random donor antigens (i.e., patient has a positive panel reactive antibody [PRA] >10% to 20%), a negative T-cell crossmatch is required prior to transplantation. Transplanted organs must be matched for ABO blood group compatibility with the recipient as ABO mismatching will result in hyperacute rejection. Liver transplantation may be carried out in emergency situations across ABO blood groups, but survival is lower, because of the risks of acute and chronic complications.

HYPERACUTE REJECTION

Hyperacute rejection may be evident within minutes of the transplantation procedure when preformed donor-specific antibodies are present in the recipient at the time of the transplant. Hyperacute rejection can also be induced by immunoglobulin G antibodies that bind to antigens on the vascular endothelium, such as class I MHC, ABO, and vascular endothelial cell antigens. Tissue damage can be mediated through antibody-dependent, cell-mediated cytotoxicity or through activation of the complement cascade. The ischemic damage to the microvasculature rapidly results in tissue necrosis.

Hyperacute rejection has become uncommon in kidney and heart transplants because transplant donors are matched for ABO blood groups and crossmatch testing is done to determine the presence of donor-specific lymphocytotoxic antibodies. A positive crossmatch presents a serious risk for graft failure even if hyperacute rejection does not occur. A negative lymphocytotoxicity crossmatch does not entirely rule out the possibility of hyperacute rejection because non-MHC antigens on the vascular endothelium can serve as targets of donor-specific antibodies. Early graft dysfunction is treated with supportive care and retransplantation if possible. Hyperacute rejection however rarely occurs in patients receiving a liver transplant. The reason for this is not fully understood, but the local release of cytokines may alter the immunologic reaction in the liver.

ACUTE CELLULAR REJECTION

Acute rejection is most common in the first few months following transplantation but can occur at any time during the life of the allograft. Acute rejection generally is reversible within 1 to 3 days, if treated. Acute cellular rejection is mediated by alloreactive T-lymphocytes that appear in the circulation and infiltrate the allograft through the vascular endothelium. After the graft is infiltrated by lymphocytes, the cytotoxic cells specifically target and kill the functioning cells in the allograft. At the same time local release of lymphokines attracts and stimulates macrophages to produce tissue damage through a delayed hypersensitivity-like mechanism. These immunologic and inflammatory events lead to the nonspecific signs and symptoms of acute rejection: pain and tenderness over the graft site, fever, and lethargy.

Kidney

Acute rejection, which may affect up to 20% of patients during the first 6 months following transplantation, is evidenced by an abrupt rise in serum creatinine concentration of ≥30% over baseline. A specific histologic diagnosis can be obtained via biopsy of the allograft and often is used to guide therapy for rejection. A biopsy specimen with a diffuse infiltrate of lymphocytes is consistent with acute cellular rejection. After the diagnosis of rejection has been confirmed, the potential risks and benefits of specific antirejection therapies must be evaluated. Hypertension often worsens during an episode of rejection and edema and weight gain are common as a result of sodium and fluid retention. Symptomatic azotemia also may develop in severe cases. Appropriate adjustments in pharmacotherapy are warranted in the face of diminished renal function.

Liver

The liver appears to be less immunogenic and more likely to promote immunologic tolerance than the other vascularized organs. Approximately 18% of liver transplantation recipients will experience a rejection episode in the first post-transplant year. The clinical signs of acute cellular rejection include leukocytosis and a change in the color or quantity of bile for those who still have an external drainage tube in place. An increased serum bilirubin concentration and increases in hepatic enzymes are sensitive markers of rejection. Although a liver biopsy provides definitive evidence of the diagnosis of rejection, a prompt response to antirejection medication also has proven useful as a means to differentiate rejection from other causes of hepatic dysfunction.

Heart

Acute rejection is a major determinant of survival following cardiac transplantation and accounts for approximately 17% of all deaths.[17] More than 60% of heart transplantation recipients will experience at least one episode of rejection during the first year. The incidence of rejection is substantially higher during the early months following transplantation, with 90% of all rejections occurring within the first 6 months. Because the incidence of acute rejection is highest during this time period, endomyocardial biopsies are often performed at regularly scheduled intervals following transplantation because rejection of the cardiac allograft is not necessarily accompanied by overt clinical signs or symptoms. A typical biopsy schedule would be weekly for the first postoperative month, biweekly for the next 2 months, and monthly to bimonthly through the remainder of the first post-transplant year. Biopsy frequency subsequently decreases based on patient clinical status. Nonspecific findings may include low-grade fever, malaise, and mild reduction in exercise capacity, whereas heart failure or atrial arrhythmias may reflect more severe rejection. The "gold standard" for detection of rejection is histologic confirmation after examination of the endomyocardial biopsy specimens. The majority of rejection episodes are characterized histologically by lymphocytic infiltrates with or without myocyte degeneration.[18] Cardiac function is assessed by either echocardiography or measurement of right-sided heart and pulmonary wedge pressures and cardiac output by pulmonary artery catheterization at the time of each biopsy.

HUMORAL REJECTION

Humoral rejection, sometimes referred to as vascular rejection, is an antibody-mediated process directed against HLA antigens present on the donor vascular endothelium. It can be characterized by capillary deposition of immunoglobulins, complement, and fibrinogen on immunofluorescence staining. Circulating immune complexes often precede humoral rejection. This form of rejection is less common than cellular rejection and generally occurs in the first 3 months after transplantation. It is associated with an increased fatality rate and appears to be more common when antilymphocyte antibodies are used for rejection prophylaxis. An increased risk of humoral rejection is associated with female gender, elevated PRA, cytomegalovirus seropositivity, a positive crossmatch, and prior sensitization to OKT3 (muromonab CD3).[19] Strategies to reverse humoral rejection include plasmapheresis, often in combination with intravenous immunoglobulin, high-dose intravenous corticosteroids, antithymocyte globulin, cyclophosphamide, rituximab, and mycophenolate mofetil.

CHRONIC REJECTION

Chronic rejection is a major cause of late graft loss and is one of the most important problems that remains to be resolved. Although chronic rejection simply may be a slow and indolent form of acute cellular rejection, the involvement of the humoral immune system and antibodies against the vascular endothelium appear to play a role. Persistent perivascular and interstitial inflammation is a common finding in kidney, liver, and heart transplantation. As a result of the complex interaction of multiple drugs and diseases over time, it is difficult to delineate the true nature of chronic rejection. For example, cytomegalovirus is associated with the development of chronic rejection in both liver and heart transplant recipients. Unlike acute rejection, chronic rejection is not reversible with any of the immunosuppressive agents currently available.

Kidney

Advances in the management of acute rejection during the last decade have increased the duration of functioning grafts from living and cadaveric donors by more than 70%.[20] Chronic allograft nephropathy remains the most common cause of graft loss in the late post-transplantation period (>1 year). The histopathologic characteristics of chronic allograft nephropathy include vascular intimal hyperplasia, tubular atrophy, interstitial fibrosis, and chronic transplant glomerulopathy. Structural changes associated with chronic allograft nephropathy are seen in as many as 40% of kidney transplantation patients 1 year after transplantation, and may present as early as 3 months.[21] Hypertension, proteinuria, and a progressive decline in renal function represent the classic clinical triad of chronic allograft nephropathy. Factors that contribute to the development of chronic allograft nephropathy include calcineurin inhibitor nephrotoxicity, polyomavirus infection, hypertension, chronic rejection, which results from slowly progressing immunologic activity, donor-related factors including ischemia time and undetected kidney disease in the donor kidney, and recurrence of the primary kidney disease in the recipient.

Liver

Chronic rejection, which affects approximately 3% to 5% of transplanted livers, is characterized by an obliterative arteriopathy and the gradual loss of bile ducts, often referred to as the vanishing bile duct syndrome. Initially patients experience an asymptomatic rise in the alkaline phosphatase and γ-glutamyl transpeptidase. As levels of bilirubin increase, patients become jaundiced and may experience itching. These changes are considered the result of immunologic and ischemic injury and can be seen in patients who have not responded adequately to therapy for acute rejection.

Heart

Cardiac allograft vasculopathy, characterized by accelerated intimal thickening or development of atherosclerotic plaques, is the leading cause of graft failure and death in heart transplant recipients.[22] Endothelial injury, caused by both cell-mediated and humoral responses, is the first step in the process. Vasculopathy is restricted to the transplanted allograft and rarely affects the recipient's native vessels. Lipid abnormalities and cytomegalovirus have been linked to the development of vasculopathy. Routine surveillance with coronary angiography, intravascular ultrasound, or other procedures can aid in the diagnosis of vasculopathy. Evidence of cardiac allograft vasculopathy can be seen in as many as 14% of patients within 1 year of transplantation and in as many as 50% of patients within 5 years.[22] β-Hydroxy-β-methylglutaryl-coenzyme A (HMG-CoA) reductase inhibitors and ACEIs have been used to decrease the incidence of vasculopathy.[22] More recently, sirolimus and everolimus have been shown to reduce the incidence and slow progression of cardiac allograft vasculopathy.[23] Percutaneous transluminal coronary angioplasty and coronary artery bypass grafting have been used in severe cases of vasculopathy; these procedures, however, are limited by significantly increased mortality compared with the general population.[22]

TREATMENT

Immunosuppression

DESIRED OUTCOME

The goals of immunosuppression vary depending on the time interval since transplantation. Immediately following surgery, the primary goal of therapy is to prevent hyperacute and acute rejection. The high doses of immunosuppressants required to achieve this goal, if maintained long-term, may result in serious complications (e.g., nephrotoxicity, infection, thrombocytopenia, and drug-induced diabetes). Therefore rapid dosage reductions are frequently used to minimize these effects. Transplant immunosuppression must be balanced in terms of graft and patient survival (the prevention of rejection versus the risk of adverse effects associated with therapy, including life-threatening infection or malignancy).

GENERAL APPROACH TO TREATMENT

❷ A multidrug approach is rational from an immunomechanistic viewpoint because the many agents have overlapping and potentially synergistic mechanisms of action. Furthermore, the use of a multidrug immunosuppression regimen may allow the use of lower doses of individual agents, thus reducing the severity of dose-related adverse effects (Fig. 92–2). The protocols and individual drug regimens tend to be center specific; although induction therapy may not be uniformly used, in almost every setting, patients receive IV methylprednisolone during the perioperative period. The patient will then begin the maintenance immunosuppressive regimen. The center-specific protocols generally combine a drug from two or three of the following classes: calcineurin inhibitors; antimetabolites or sirolimus; and corticosteroids.

If rejection is suspected, a biopsy can be done for definitive diagnosis or the patient may be empirically treated for rejection. Empiric treatment generally involves administration of high-dose corticosteroids, usually 500 to 1,000 mg of methylprednisolone intravenously for one to three doses. If signs and symptoms of rejection are resolved with empiric therapy, the maintenance immunosuppressive regimen is generally modified to provide a greater level of overall immunosuppression. If rejection is confirmed by biopsy, treatment may be based on the severity of rejection with polyclonal and monoclonal antibodies being reserved for moderate to severe rejections or those which have not responded to a course of corticosteroids.

Induction Therapy

Induction therapy involves the use of a high level of immunosuppression at the time of transplantation with or without the immediate introduction of cyclosporine or tacrolimus (see Fig. 92–2). Induction historically included the use of polyclonal or monoclonal antibodies in addition to triple therapy of azathioprine, high-dose corticosteroids, and a calcineurin inhibitor at the time of transplantation. Today, induction therapy consists of one of two perioperative immunosuppressive strategies: (a) the provision of a highly intense level of immunosuppression, either universally or on the basis of patient-specific risk factors such as age and race, or (b) the use of antibody therapy to provide enough immunosuppression to delay the initiation of therapy with the nephrotoxic calcineurin inhibitors. The rationale for delayed calcineurin inhibitor administration varies slightly depending on the type of transplant. In renal transplantation, the newly transplanted kidney is very susceptible to nephrotoxic injury, whereas in liver and heart transplantation, the idea is to protect patients with pre-existing renal insufficiency from further insults during the perioperative period. Additionally, calcineurin inhibitor dosage adjustment to maintain target concentrations is quite difficult in the perioperative period.

CLINICAL CONTROVERSY

Some clinicians use induction therapy with IL-2 receptor antagonists, such as daclizumab or basiliximab or antithymocyte globulin for all transplant recipients. Others reserve induction therapy for patients who are at a higher risk for rejection, such as those who have a high PRA, had a previous transplant or multiple pregnancies, or are of nonwhite race.

Acute Rejection

The primary goal of acute rejection therapy is to minimize the intensity of the immune response and prevent irreversible injury to the allograft. The available options include (a) increasing the doses of current immunosuppressive drugs, (b) "pulse" corticosteroids with subsequent dose taper, (c) addition of an another immunosuppressant indefinitely, or (d) short-term treatment with a polyclonal or monoclonal antibody. The treatment of acute rejection varies among transplant centers and by type of allograft, but almost always begins with "pulse" corticosteroid therapy for several days (oral or intravenously). Recent data in renal transplantation indicate, however, that African Americans do not respond as well to corticosteroids as non–African Americans. Other therapies, such as antithymocyte globulin, thus may be preferable for this patient population.[24]

Cytolytic agents are often reserved for those with corticosteroid-resistant rejection, signs of hemodynamic compromise (heart), or more severe rejections. Other innovative forms of therapy for persistent or intractable rejection have been investigated, including mycophenolate mofetil, tacrolimus, low-dose methotrexate, sirolimus, total lymphoid irradiation, and plasmapheresis and intravenous immunoglobulin. Prophylactic agents such as valganciclovir, nystatin, trimethoprim-sulfamethoxazole, H_2-receptor antagonists or proton-pump inhibitors, and/or antacids may be used to minimize adverse effects associated with these intensive immunosuppression regimens.

Maintenance Therapy

❸ The goal of maintenance immunosuppression is to prevent acute and chronic rejection while minimizing drug-related toxicity. As patients progress through the post-transplant course, the risk of acute rejection decreases; thus allowing the clinician to gradually reduce, the doses of immunosuppressants or in some cases totally withdraw them over a period of 6 to 12 months in an effort to minimize adverse effects. It is important to recognize that while the goal of transplant immunosuppression is universal, protocols for immunosuppressive therapy vary widely among institutions.

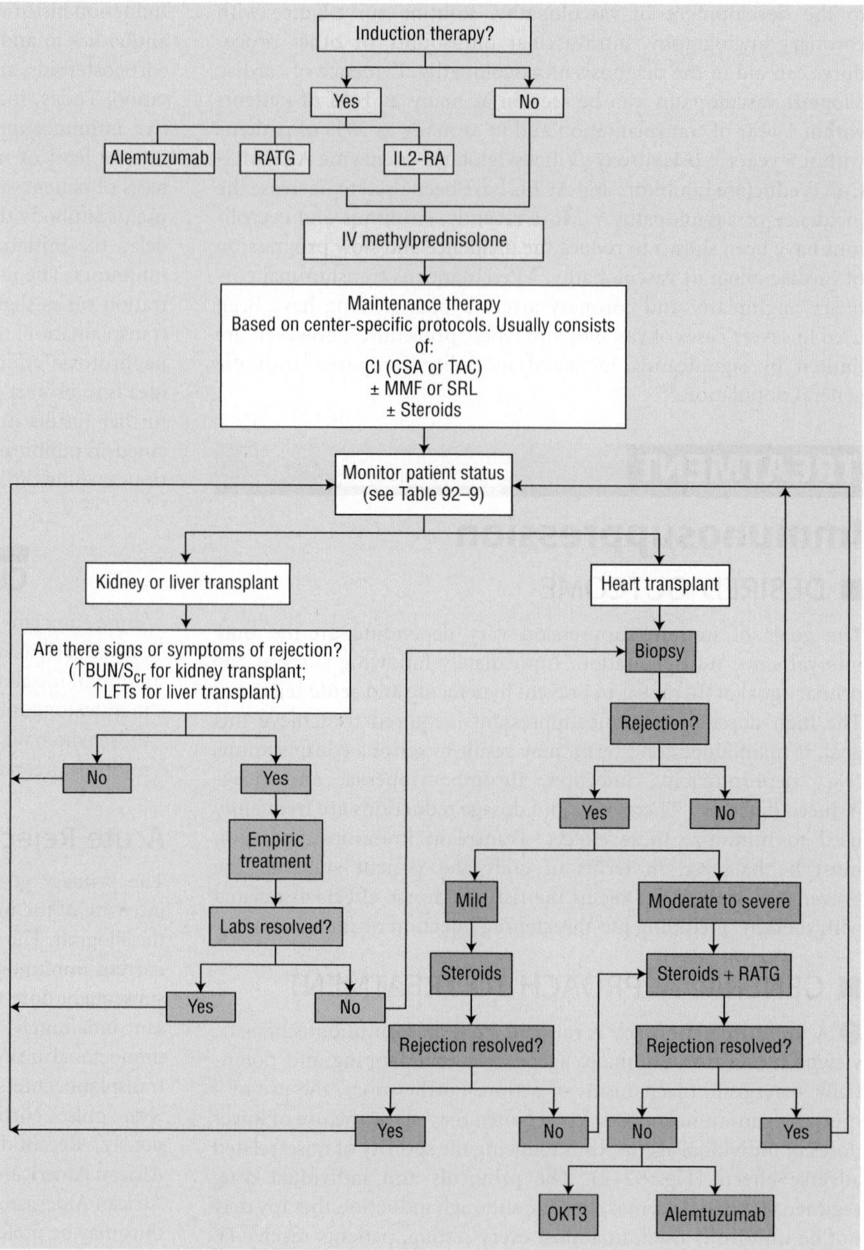

FIGURE 92-2. General approach to solid-organ transplant immunosuppression. (BUN, blood urea nitrogen; CI, calcineurin inhibitor; CSA, cyclosporine; IL2RA, interleukin-2 receptor antagonist; LFTs, liver function tests; MMF, mycophenolate mofetil; OKT3, muromonab CD3; RATG, rabbit antithymocyte immunoglobulin; S_{cr}, serum creatinine; SRL, sirolimus; TAC, tacrolimus.)

Transplant organ and type (cadaveric versus living-donor), the degree of HLA mismatch, time after transplantation, post-transplantation complications (including the number of acute rejections), previous immunosuppressive adverse reactions, compliance, and financial considerations are among the patient-specific factors considered in individualizing maintenance immunosuppression. Calcineurin inhibitors generally are a central component in most maintenance regimens, although calcineurin inhibitor-free immunosuppression remains the "Holy Grail" of transplantation immunology as this is the most direct way to decrease the complications associated with calcineurin inhibitor-induced nephropathy. Ideally, immunosuppression should be optimized to prevent acute rejection episodes and minimize the occurrence of chronic rejection. However, the changes seen with chronic rejection are not reversible with current immunosuppressive therapies.

■ CALCINEURIN INHIBITORS

❹ Cyclosporine and tacrolimus are the two calcineurin inhibitors currently used for most solid-organ transplant recipients. The introduction of cyclosporine dramatically improved the outcomes of transplantation significantly with a lower incidence of acute rejection episodes and severe infectious complications. A decade later, tacrolimus produced similar results, solidifying calcineurin inhibitors as the backbone of the transplant immunosuppression. Today, tacrolimus is used more commonly than cyclosporine by most transplant centers. However, despite the reduction in the incidence and severity of acute rejection, the incidence of chronic rejection and long-term complications, including hypertension and compromised kidney function, have not changed with the use of calcineurin inhibitors.

Pharmacology/Mechanism of Action

Calcineurin inhibitors block T-cell proliferation by inhibiting the production of IL-2 and other cytokines by T cells (see Fig. 92–1). The drugs bind to unique cytoplasmic immunophilins: cyclosporine binds to cyclophilin and tacrolimus binds to FK-binding protein-12 (FKBP12). In both cases, the drug–immunophilin complex inhibits the action of calcineurin, an enzyme that activates the nuclear factor of activated T cells, which is, in turn, responsible for the transcription of several key cytokines necessary for T-cell activity, including IL-2. IL-2 is a potent growth factor for T cells and ultimately is responsible for activation and clonal expansion.

Pharmacokinetics

The calcineurin inhibitors are highly lipophilic compounds, with variable but generally low bioavailability of approximately 30% for both drugs (range: 5% to 60%). Unlike tacrolimus, cyclosporine depends on bile for intestinal absorption, which lends to more interpatient and intrapatient variability. Liver recipients with a T-tube for diversion of bile may thus experience incomplete and erratic absorption of cyclosporine.

Because of the significant variability in absorption of cyclosporine, peak concentrations are reached within 2 to 6 hours of oral administration. To overcome the pharmacokinetic problems of cyclosporine, a microemulsion formulation was developed. Both forms are available commercially in the United States and are referred to as "cyclosporine, USP" and "cyclosporine, USP [MODIFIED]." The two formulations are not bioequivalent and should not be used interchangeably. The microemulsion formulation is self-emulsifying and forms a microemulsion spontaneously with aqueous fluids in the gastrointestinal tract, making it less dependent on bile for absorption. The result is a significantly greater rate and extent of absorption and decreased intraindividual variability in pharmacokinetic parameters. Bioavailability is enhanced owing to better dispersion and absorption and does not require bile excretion. The relative bioavailability of the microemulsion formulation is 60%. Peak concentrations generally are reached within 1.5 to 2 hours after oral administration and decline in a log linear fashion with a terminal half-life of about 8 hours. Tacrolimus, on the other hand, has a more predictable absorption pattern, reaching peak concentrations within 1 to 3 hours.

Following oral absorption, both cyclosporine and tacrolimus are highly protein bound. Ninety percent of cyclosporine is bound to lipoproteins in the blood. In contrast, 99% of tacrolimus is bound primarily to albumin and α_1-acid glycoprotein. Cyclosporine is distributed widely into tissue and body fluids, resulting in a large and variable volume of distribution, ranging from 3 to 5 L/kg. Because of the high concentration of FKBP12 that is found in red blood cells, tacrolimus is distributed primarily in the vasculature, with a volume of distribution of 0.8 to 1.9 L/kg. Both drugs are extensively metabolized by the cytochrome P450 3A4 (CYP3A4) system in both the gut and the liver, which accounts for both the poor bioavailability and numerous drug interactions (see Chap. 6). Children have an increased rate of metabolism, which results in a shorter half-life for both drugs. The terminal half-life is approximately 8.5 hours for the cyclosporine microemulsion and tacrolimus, but can be as long as 19 hours for the conventional formulation of cyclosporine.

Efficacy

The introduction of the calcineurin inhibitors significantly improved the outcomes of solid-organ transplantation in terms of patient and graft survival. Both cyclosporine and tacrolimus are currently approved for prophylaxis of organ rejection in kidney, liver, and heart transplantations. When compared with the standard formulation, the microemulsion formulation of cyclosporine has demonstrated equivalent or superior efficacy in kidney, liver, and heart transplantation recipients. Studies comparing tacrolimus with either formulation of cyclosporine as primary immunosuppression demonstrate equivalent efficacy between the two agents in kidney, liver, and heart transplantations.

Monotherapy with calcineurin inhibitors has been described.[25,26] The avoidance of long-term corticosteroids is the primary advantage of calcineurin inhibitor monotherapy, whereas the primary disadvantage is the higher incidence of rejection. As a result, calcineurin inhibitors are rarely used as monotherapy.

Adverse Effects

Table 92–4 summarizes the adverse effects of calcineurin inhibitors, cyclosporine and tacrolimus, and other immunosuppressants. Nephrotoxicity is often evidenced by an increase in serum creatinine concentration, decrease in glomerular filtration rate, proteinuria, and hyperkalemia. The nephrotoxic potential of both drugs is equal and is often related to the dose and duration of exposure. Neurotoxicity typically manifests as tremors, headache, and peripheral neuropathy; occasionally, however, seizures have been observed. Tacrolimus may be associated with an increased occurrence of neurologic complications compared to cyclosporine.

Cyclosporine appears to have a greater propensity to cause or worsen hypertension and hyperlipidemia compared to tacrolimus.[27–30] On the other hand, hyperglycemia is more common with tacrolimus than cyclosporine, but is often reversible when doses of tacrolimus and/or corticosteroids are reduced.[28] Cyclosporine is associated with cosmetic changes, such as hirsutism and gingival hyperplasia, which may be managed by converting from cyclosporine to tacrolimus or by proper hygiene in patients who cannot be switched to tacrolimus. Tacrolimus, in contrast, has been reported to cause alopecia, which is usually self-limiting and reversible.

Drug–Drug and Drug–Food Interactions

Drug interactions occur frequently with the calcineurin inhibitors because they are substrates for CYP3A4 and P-glycoprotein.[31–33] The most commonly administered drugs that are known to significantly alter cyclosporine and tacrolimus levels are highlighted in Table 92–5. Inhibitors of CYP3A4, such as diltiazem or erythromycin, can increase drug concentrations significantly, whereas drugs that induce CYP3A4 activity, such as phenytoin or rifampin, can decrease drug concentrations significantly. Some centers take advantage of these interactions by routinely prescribing CYP3A4 inhibitors to reduce the dosage and cost of calcineurin inhibitor therapy while maintaining the same therapeutic concentrations.[34] One distinct drug interaction with tacrolimus that differs from cyclosporine is an interaction with antacids. In vitro data suggest that drugs that increase the pH of the GI tract, such as magnesium-, aluminum-, or calcium-containing antacids, sodium bicarbonate, and magnesium oxide, can cause a pH-mediated degradation of tacrolimus by physically adsorbing to tacrolimus in the GI tract.[35,36] Such compounds should be separated from tacrolimus administration by at least 2 hours to prevent the physical interaction.

TABLE 92-4 Comparison of Common Adverse Effects of Maintenance Immunosuppressants

AZA	MMF	SIR	Steroids	CSA	TAC
Nausea, vomiting	Diarrhea, nausea	Hyperlipidemia	GI bleeding	Hyperlipidemia	Diarrhea, nausea
Thrombocytopenia	Leukopenia	Thrombocytopenia	Hyperlipidemia	Nephrotoxicity	Hepatotoxicity
Leukopenia		Leukopenia	Leukocytosis	Tremor	Nephrotoxicity
			Hypertension	Hypertension	Tremor, headache
			Hyperglycemia	Hyperglycemia	Hypertension
			Weight gain	Gingival hyperplasia	Hyperglycemia
			Mood changes	Hirsutism	Hyperkalemia, hypomagnesemia

AZA, azathioprine; CSA, cyclosporine; MMF, mycophenolate mofetil; SIR, sirolimus; TAC, tacrolimus.

TABLE 92-5 Effect of Concomitant Drug Administration on Cyclosporine, Tacrolimus, and Sirolimus

Cyclosporine Levels		Tacrolimus Levels		Sirolimus Levels	
Increase	***Decrease***	***Increase***	***Decrease***	***Increase***	***Decrease***
Ketoconazole	Rifampicin	Ketoconazole	Rifampin	Ketoconazole	Rifampin
Fluconazole	Phenytoin	Fluconazole	Dexamethasone	Fluconazole	Phenytoin
Itraconazole	Phenobarbital	Itraconazole	Phenytoin	Itraconazole	
Voriconazole	Carbamazepine	Voriconazole		Voriconazole	
Erythromycin	Sulfadimidine	Erythromycin		Erythromycin	
Levofloxacin	Trimethoprim	Levofloxacin		Clarithromycin	
Diltiazem		Diltiazem		Diltiazem	
Verapamil		Verapamil		Verapamil	
Danazol		Danazol		Atorvastatin	
Nicardipine		Cimetidine		Cyclosporine	
Metoclopramide		Omeprazole		Protease inhibitors	
Methylprednisolone		Clotrimazole			
Norethisterone		Nefazodone			
Sirolimus		Corticosteroids			
Tacrolimus		Cyclosporine			
Protease inhibitors		Basiliximab			
		Protease inhibitors			

Adapted from references 31, 32, 43, and 47.

Cyclosporine and to a lesser extent, tacrolimus are inhibitors of CYP3A4.[38] The inhibitory effects of cyclosporine and tacrolimus on CYP3A4 can be seen with weaker substrates, such as the HMG-CoA reductase inhibitors. Concomitant administration of a calcineurin inhibitor with an HMG-CoA reductase inhibitor results in an increase in the HMG-CoA reductase inhibitor levels, which increases the risk of HMG-CoA reductase inhibitor adverse effects, most notably myopathy.[39] Patients should be monitored for clinical signs of myopathy when receiving HMG-CoA reductase inhibitors in combination with cyclosporine and tacrolimus.

Consistency in administration of the calcineurin inhibitors with regard to meals and food intake is important to sustain an effective concentration time profile. High-fat meals can enhance both plasma clearance and the volume of distribution of cyclosporine by more than 60%.[40] Food reduces the rate and extent of tacrolimus absorption and a high-fat meal may further delay gastric emptying and further reduce tacrolimus concentrations and pharmacokinetics, including maximum serum concentration (C_{max}), time of maximal concentration (t_{max}), and the area under the concentration–time curve (AUC).[33] Grapefruit juice increases both cyclosporine and tacrolimus concentrations significantly. Furocoumarins, such as quercetin, naringin, and bergamottin, found in grapefruit juice, are potent inhibitors of CYP3A4. The AUC and C_{max} of cyclosporine have been reported to be increased by more than 55% and 35%, respectively.[41]

Dosing and Administration

Starting doses of calcineurin inhibitors are often weight-based; subsequent doses are then adjusted based on serum concentrations. Initial oral cyclosporine doses range from 8 to 18 mg/kg per day divided into two doses administered every 12 hours. Higher doses of cyclosporine are used more commonly in two-drug regimens, whereas lower doses are part of triple-drug regimens. Oral tacrolimus doses range from 0.1 to 0.3 mg/kg per day given in two divided doses every 12 hours. If oral administration is not possible, both drugs can be administered intravenously at one-third the oral dosage, to account for first-pass metabolism. The usual intravenous dose of cyclosporine is 2 to 5 mg/kg per day, given as a continuous infusion or, more commonly, as a single or twice-daily injection. Intravenous tacrolimus doses range from 0.05 to 0.1 mg/kg per day, and must be administered by continuous infusion. Children require higher doses to maintain therapeutic drug concentrations, up to 14 to 18 mg/kg per day for cyclosporine and 0.3 mg/kg per day for tacrolimus, which is often two- to four-fold higher than adults on a milligram per kilogram basis for both drugs.

Calcineurin inhibitor serum concentrations are measured routinely in an attempt to optimize therapy. The most common and practical method for monitoring calcineurin inhibitors is by measuring trough blood concentrations. Radioimmunoassay (RIA) and fluorescence polarization immunoassay are the most commonly used methods to measure cyclosporine concentrations. Tacrolimus concentrations are most commonly measured by microparticle enzyme immunoassays or enzyme-linked immunoassays. Both drugs can be measured by high-performance liquid chromatography (HPLC), which is recognized as the reference procedure.[42] It is important to determine which assay methodology the laboratory is using because target ranges vary between nonspecific assays, such as RIA and microparticle enzyme immunoassay, which quantitate parent plus metabolite concentration, and specific assays, such as HPLC using mass spectrometry, which quantitate only the parent compound. Thus, the target concentrations will be lower for the specific assays (HPLC) compared to nonspecific assays (RIA and microparticle enzyme immunoassays) by approximately 20% to 25%. The therapeutic range for whole-blood cyclosporine concentration is 375 to 400 ng/mL for RIA and 100 to 300 ng/mL for HPLC. In serum or plasma, the therapeutic range for RIA or HPLC is 150 to 250 ng/mL and 75 to 150 ng/mL, respectively. The therapeutic range for tacrolimus for RIA is 5 to 20 ng/mL and 8 to 13 ng/mL for HPLC. The specific goal level for both drugs is dependent on transplant type, time after transplantation, concomitant immunosuppression, and transplantation center. One review of the role of tacrolimus in renal transplantation suggests that target 12-hour whole blood concentrations for tacrolimus are 15 to 20 ng/mL (0 to 1 month after transplantation), 10 to 15 ng/mL (1 to 3 months after transplantation), and 5 to 12 ng/mL (>3 months after transplantation).[27] Serum drug concentrations should be measured frequently (daily or three times per week) following initiation of the drug and during the stabilization period after transplantation. As the time increases after transplantation, serum concentrations are measured less frequently, usually monthly.

Studies have revealed lack of predictive value of trough cyclosporine concentrations and rejection.[43] Alternative strategies, including AUC and peak concentration, have been suggested to better correlate with rejection.[44] Limited sampling techniques using two to five blood samples within the first 4 hours after an oral dose have been used. AUC levels >4,400 mcg/L per hour correlate with a reduction in rejection.[44] Peak concentrations measured 2 hours after an oral dose (C_2) have a better predictive value in terms of rejection compared with trough concentrations.[45] Some transplantation centers have adopted this strategy to manage cyclosporine levels because of the convenience of a single blood sample. The suggested therapeutic range for C_2 cyclosporine levels is 1,500 to 2,000 ng/mL for the first few months after transplant and 700 to 900 ng/mL after 6 to 12 months.[43] The predictive value of trough concentrations and rejection is also being questioned with tacrolimus. As a result, pharmacokinetic profiling with AUC and peak concentrations to determine alternative monitoring strategies are also being explored with tacrolimus.[43]

Calcineurin Inhibitor Nephrotoxicity

❺ A common side effect observed in all transplantation recipients who are receiving maintenance cyclosporine or tacrolimus therapy is nephrotoxicity. Two types of toxicity can occur. Acute nephrotoxicity frequently is seen early and is dose dependent and reversible, but chronic nephropathy is more common. Clinical manifestations of calcineurin inhibitor nephrotoxicity include elevated serum creatinine and blood urea nitrogen levels, hyperkalemia, hyperuricemia, mild proteinuria, and a decreased fractional excretion of sodium. Calcineurin inhibitor nephrotoxicity is recognized as the leading cause of renal dysfunction following nonrenal solid-organ transplant.

The predominant mechanism for calcineurin inhibitor nephrotoxicity is renal vasoconstriction, primarily of the afferent arteriole, resulting in increased renal vascular resistance, decreased renal blood flow by up to 40%, reduced glomerular filtration rate by up to 30%, and increased proximal tubular sodium reabsorption with a reduction in urinary sodium and potassium excretion. A number of other mechanisms have been implicated, including changes in the renin–angiotensin–aldosterone system, prostaglandin synthesis, nitrous oxide production, sympathetic nervous system activation, and calcium handling.[45]

Measures to reduce calcineurin inhibitor nephrotoxicity include delaying administration immediately postoperatively in patients at high risk for nephrotoxicity (using alternative induction protocols including an IL-2 receptor antagonist or antilymphocyte globulin), monitoring calcineurin inhibitor trough blood levels and reducing the calcineurin inhibitor dosage if the vasoconstrictive effects are problematic, and avoiding other nephrotoxins (e.g., aminoglycosides, amphotericin B, and nonsteroidal antiinflammatory agents) when possible. Currently, no proven therapies consistently prevent or reverse the nephrotoxic effects ofcyclosporine.[46]

In patients who have received a kidney transplant, it is often difficult to differentiate calcineurin inhibitor nephrotoxicity from renal allograft rejection. Because the clinical features of acute renal allograft rejection and calcineurin inhibitor nephrotoxicity may overlap considerably, a renal biopsy continues to be the diagnostic "gold standard" (Table 92–6). However, differentiating between chronic renal allograft rejection and calcineurin inhibitor nephrotoxicity may be more difficult because, in addition to clinical signs and symptoms, biopsy findings also may be similar.

CLINICAL CONTROVERSY

Although calcineurin inhibitors are the mainstay of immunosuppressive protocols, some clinicians attempt to use calcineurin inhibitor-sparing protocols to avoid the significant adverse effects associated with calcineurin inhibitors. Others will delay the initiation of calcineurin inhibitors to avoid the dose-related adverse effects associated with their use during the early posttransplantation period.

TABLE 92-6 Differential Diagnosis of Acute Rejection and Cyclosporine or Tacrolimus Nephrotoxicity

	Acute Rejection	CSA or TAC Nephrotoxicity
History	Often <4 weeks postoperatively	Often >6 weeks postoperatively
Clinical presentation	Fever Hypertension Weight gain Graft swelling/tenderness Decreased daily urine volume	Afebrile Hypertension Graft nontender Good urine output
Laboratory biopsy	Rapid rise in serum Cr (0.3 mg/dL/day) Normal CSA or TAC concentration Interstitial lymphocytic infiltrates	Gradual rise in serum Cr (>0.15 mg/dL/day) Elevated CSA or TAC concentration Interstitial fibrosis, tubular atrophy, glomerular thrombosis, arterial inflammation

Cr, creatinine; CSA, cyclosporine; TAC, tacrolimus.

CORTICOSTEROIDS

Corticosteroids have been used since the beginning of the modern transplantation era. Despite their many adverse events, they continue to be a cornerstone of immunosuppression regimens in many transplant centers. The most commonly used corticosteroids in transplantation are methylprednisolone and prednisone.

Pharmacology/Mechanism of Action

Corticosteroids block cytokine activation by binding to corticosteroid response elements, thereby inhibiting IL-1, IL-2, IL-3, IL-6, γ-interferon, and tumor necrosis factor-α synthesis (see Fig. 92–1). Additionally, corticosteroids interfere with cell migration, recognition, and cytotoxic effector mechanisms.[47]

Pharmacokinetics

Prednisone is converted to active prednisolone in the body and has multiple effects on the immune system. Prednisone is very well absorbed from the gastrointestinal (GI) tract and has a long biologic half-life, so it can be dosed once daily.

Efficacy

❻ Animal models of transplantation in the 1950s and 1960s used corticosteroids empirically in combination with azathioprine. Corticosteroids subsequently became a part of the immunosuppressive regimens used in the first human transplantations[48] and continue to be used in immunosuppressive protocols today. The efficacy of corticosteroids is irrefutable based on the decades of clinical experience. Systematic studies comparing corticosteroid-free immunosuppressive agent combinations with conventional therapy are difficult to perform because of the hundreds of potential combinations that now exist. However, recent studies of corticosteroid-free immunosuppressive agent combinations with newer, more specific immunosuppressants suggests that corticosteroids may in the future have less of a role in maintenance immunosuppression.[26,27]

Adverse Effects

Adverse effects of prednisone that occur in more than 10% of patients include increased appetite, insomnia, indigestion (bitter taste), and mood changes. Side effects that occur less often but which are seen with high doses or prolonged therapy include cataracts, hyperglycemia, hirsutism, bruising, acne, sodium and water retention, hypertension, bone growth suppression, and ulcerative esophagitis (see Table 92–4).

Drug–Drug and Drug–Food Interactions

Barbiturates, phenytoin, and rifampin induce hepatic metabolism of prednisone and thus decrease the effectiveness of prednisone. Prednisone decreases the effectiveness of vaccines and toxoids.[47]

Dosing and Administration

An intravenous corticosteroid, commonly high-dose methylprednisolone, is given during the perioperative period. The dose of methylprednisolone is tapered rapidly and discontinued within days, and oral prednisone is initiated. Prednisone doses are tapered progressively over time, depending on the type of additional immunosuppression and organ function. As doses are tapered, it is preferable to administer corticosteroids every other day and between 7 AM and 8 AM to mimic the body's diurnal release of cortisol. Although conversion to alternate-day regimens or complete withdrawal of prednisone in patients with stable post-transplantation courses has been used with success in some transplantation centers, corticosteroids often are continued for the entire life of the functional graft. Long-term corticosteroid use and its associated deleterious effects are well recognized and particularly troublesome in transplantation patients (see Table 92–4).

The first-line therapy for the treatment of acute graft rejection is high-dose intravenous methylprednisolone (250 to 1,000 mg) daily for 3 days or oral prednisone (200 mg). Doses of oral prednisone are then tapered over 5 days to 20 mg/day. Prednisone should be taken with food to minimize GI upset. The dose of prednisone varies with the transplant center's protocol but usually is highest immediately following transplantation and during treatment for acute rejection. It is becoming a frequent practice to taper prednisone, with the goal of discontinuation over a period of months. Corticosteroids never should be discontinued abruptly; tapering should be gradual because of suppression of the hypothalamic–pituitary–adrenal axis. Corticosteroids slow the growth rates in children, prompting clinicians to use alternate-day dosing or to withhold corticosteroids until rejection occurs.

■ ANTIMETABOLITES

❼ Antimetabolites have been used since the early days of transplantation because they prevent proliferation of lymphocytes. Azathioprine has been considered a part of the "gold standard" regimen with cyclosporine and corticosteroids, to which all newer regimens have traditionally been compared. However, mycophenolate is more specific in its effects on lymphocytes and has fewer side effects. Because each agent is unique in its profile and actions, they are discussed separately.

Mycophenolate

Mycophenolic acid (MPA) was first isolated from the *Penicillium glaucum* mold. Two formulations of MPA are currently available in the United States: mycophenolate mofetil is the morpholinoethyl ester of MPA, whereas mycophenolate sodium is available as an enteric-coated formulation of the sodium salt of MPA.

Pharmacology/Mechanism of Action The immunosuppressive effect of MPA is exerted through noncompetitive binding to inosine monophosphate dehydrogenase, the key enzyme responsible for guanosine nucleotide synthesis via the de novo pathway. Inhibition of inosine monophosphate dehydrogenase results in decreased nucleotide synthesis and diminished DNA polymerase activity, ultimately reducing lymphocyte proliferation.[49] The actions of MPA are more specific for T and B cells, which use only the de novo pathway for nucleotide synthesis (see Fig. 92–1). Other cells within the body have a salvage pathway by which they can synthesize nucleotides, making them less susceptible to the actions of MPA and thereby reducing, but not eliminating, the potential for the hematologic adverse effects seen with azathioprine, which affects both the de novo and salvage pathways. In addition to the decreasing lymphocyte proliferation, MPA also may downregulate activation of lymphocytes.[50]

Pharmacokinetics Because MPA is unstable in an acidic environment, mycophenolate mofetil acts as a prodrug that is readily absorbed from the GI tract, after which it is rapidly and completely converted to MPA by first-pass metabolism. The enteric coating of mycophenolate sodium protects MPA from the acidic gastric pH and allows for MPA to be released directly into the small intestine for absorption. The absolute bioavailability of MPA when delivered from mycophenolate mofetil and mycophenolate sodium is 94% and 72%, respectively. Peak concentrations of MPA are reached within 1 hour following administration of either preparation.

A total of 97% of MPA is bound to albumin in the blood. MPA is eliminated by the kidney and also undergoes glucuronidation in the liver to an inactive glucuronide metabolite (MPAG) that is excreted in the bile and urine. Enterohepatic cycling of MPAG can lead to deconjugation, thereby recirculating MPA into the bloodstream. The half-life of MPA is 18 hours.

Efficacy Currently, mycophenolate mofetil is approved for use in kidney, liver, and heart transplantations. Mycophenolate sodium was approved in 2004 for use in kidney transplantations only. Early studies comparing mycophenolate to azathioprine in patients receiving cyclosporine and corticosteroids demonstrated a statistically significant difference in patient and graft survival at 1 and 3 years.[51] Subsequent studies have confirmed the efficacy of mycophenolate combined with tacrolimus.

Mycophenolate has also demonstrated efficacy in the treatment of acute rejection. Kidney transplantation recipients converted to mycophenolate mofetil after the first acute rejection episode had fewer subsequent rejections compared with those who continued with azathioprine after rejection treatment. The change in therapy was associated with no increase in adverse effects or malignancies and a trend toward better graft function and survival.[52]

Mycophenolate is a key component of calcineurin inhibitor-sparing protocols. Although mycophenolate monotherapy has been investigated, patients experienced an unacceptable increase in rejection. Combination of mycophenolate with sirolimus, on the other hand, resulted in improved renal function with no change in acute rejection and patient and graft survival.[51]

Adverse Effects Unlike cyclosporine and tacrolimus, mycophenolate is not associated with nephrotoxicity, neurotoxicity, or hypertension. The most common side effects are related to the GI tract, including nausea, vomiting, diarrhea, and abdominal pain (see Table 92–4), which occur with similar frequency during intravenous and oral therapy. Clinically, GI symptoms may be alleviated in some patients by reducing the dose, dividing the total daily dose into three or four doses, administration with food, or titrating upward from lower doses during initial therapy. Mycophenolate also has hematologic effects, such as leukopenia and anemia, particularly with higher doses. Because peripheral intravenous mycophenolate administration is associated with local edema and inflammation, central venous administration may be the preferred route.

Drug–Drug and Drug–Food Interactions Food has no effect on MPA AUC, but delays the absorption and decreases MPA C_{max} by 40% and 33% when mycophenolate mofetil and mycophenolate sodium, respectively, are administered. Administration with aluminum- and magnesium-containing antacids or cholestyramine, significantly decreases the AUC of MPA and should be avoided.[49] It has been suggested that administration of iron may produce similar results, but this has not been tested.

Acyclovir, commonly used in renal transplant recipients for the treatment and prevention of viral infections, competes with MPAG for renal tubular secretion. AUCs of both entities are increased with concomitant acyclovir and mycophenolate administration.[49] Single-dose intravenous ganciclovir in combination with mycophenolate produced no change in the disposition of ganciclovir, MPA, or MPAG.[53] Although no pharmacokinetic interaction in a single-dose study was demonstrated, there is potential for additive pharmacodynamic effects such as bone marrow suppression.

Decreased MPA trough concentrations have been reported when mycophenolate is administered with cyclosporine compared with those achieved when mycophenolate is given with tacrolimus or sirolimus. This interaction is most likely a result of cyclosporine interference with the enterohepatic recycling of MPAG, which results in decreased MPA concentrations.[54] To achieve equivalent MPA and MPAG serum concentrations, it may be necessary to administer higher doses of mycophenolate with cyclosporine compared to tacrolimus.

Dosing and Administration Mycophenolate mofetil is currently available in both oral and intravenous formulations. Although intravenous administration of equal doses closely mimics oral administration, the two cannot be considered bioequivalent.[55] Mycophenolate sodium is only available as an oral formulation. Unlike other immunosuppressive agents, there is no compelling indication that mycophenolate should be dosed in adult patients on a milligram per kilogram basis given the weak correlation between MPA *AUC* and body weight.[49] To optimize immunosuppression and minimize adverse effects, mycophenolate is administered in two divided doses given every 12 hours. The total daily dose for kidney and liver transplants is 2 g/day for mycophenolate mofetil and 1.44 g/day for mycophenolate sodium. A higher level of immunosuppression is required for heart transplants, thus for these patients a total daily dose of 3 g/day for mycophenolate mofetil and 2.16 g/day for mycophenolate sodium is recommended. The recommended pediatric dose is 600 mg/m^2 for mycophenolate mofetil and 400 mg/m^2 for mycophenolate sodium, in two divided doses.

Plasma appears to be the most appropriate medium in which to measure MPA for therapeutic drug monitoring. Trough concentrations are not accurate in predicting total drug exposure during a 12-hour interval and AUC monitoring has been proposed as the most appropriate measure of MPA drug exposure to predict therapeutic outcomes.[43] Better outcomes are associated with MPA AUC levels of greater than 42.8 mcg/mL per hour (by HPLC),[56] although a reference range of 30 to 60 mcg/mL per hour has been proposed.[57] However, the correlation between MPA AUC levels and adverse effects is low. Further studies are required to determine the best means to evaluate MPA levels, the acceptable targets for each, and the appropriate strategy to monitor MPA levels.[56,57]

Azathioprine

Azathioprine, a prodrug for 6-mercaptopurine, has been used as an immunosuppressant in combination with corticosteroids since the earliest days of the modern transplantation era. It is associated with substantial toxicities, however, and its use has dramatically declined with the availability of newer, less-toxic immunosuppressants.

Pharmacology/Mechanism of Action Azathioprine is an inactive compound that is converted rapidly to 6-mercaptopurine (6-MP) in the blood and is subsequently metabolized by three different enzymes. Xanthine oxidase, found in the liver and GI tract, converts 6-MP to the inactive final end product, 6-thiouric acid. Thiopurine *S*-methyltransferase, found in hematopoietic tissues and red blood cells, methylates 6-MP to an inactive product, 6-methylmercaptopurine. Finally, hypoxanthine-guanine phosphoribosyltransferase is the first step responsible for converting 6-MP to 6-thioguanine nucleotides (6-TGNs), the active metabolites, which are incorporated into nucleic acids, ultimately disrupting both the salvage and de novo pathways of DNA, RNA, and protein synthesis. This process is toxic to the cell and renders the cell unable to proliferate (see Fig. 92–1). 6-TGNs eventually are catabolized by xanthine oxidase and thiopurine *S*-methyltransferase to inactive products.

Pharmacokinetics Oral bioavailability of azathioprine is approximately 40%. Metabolism of 6-MP is primarily by xanthine oxidase to inactive metabolites, which are excreted by the kidneys. The half-life of azathioprine, the parent compound, is very short, approximately 12 minutes. The half-life of 6-MP is longer, ranging from 0.7 to 3 hours. However, it is the activity of the 6-TGNs that determines the pharmacodynamic half-life of the drug. The half-life of 6-TGNs has been estimated to be 9 days.[58]

Adverse Effects Dose-limiting adverse effects of azathioprine are often hematologic (see Table 92–4). Leukopenia, anemia, and thrombocytopenia can occur within the first few weeks of therapy and can be managed by dose reduction or discontinuation of azathioprine. Other common adverse effects include nausea and vomiting, which can be minimized by taking azathioprine with food. Alopecia, hepatotoxicity and pancreatitis are less-common adverse effects of azathioprine; they generally are reversible on dose reduction or discontinuation.

Drug–Drug and Drug–Food Interactions Allopurinol inhibits xanthine oxidase and can increase the bioavailability of azathioprine and 6-MP concentrations by as much as fourfold. The metabolic pathways shift to favor production of 6-TGNs, which ultimately results in increased bone marrow suppression and pancytopenia. Doses of azathioprine should be reduced by 50% to 75% when allopurinol is added. Additional clinically significant drug interactions include other bone marrow-suppressing agents such as ganciclovir, trimethoprim-sulfamethoxazole, and sirolimus, and other drugs that irritate the GI tract.

Dosing and Administration Initial doses of azathioprine are 3 to 5 mg/kg per day intravenously or orally. Individualization to maintain the white blood cell count between 3,500 and 6,000 cells/mm may be accomplished in some with doses as low as 0.25 mg/kg per day.[2] Patients often are instructed to take azathioprine in the evening when initiating or titrating therapy to allow for dose adjustments based on morning determinations of their white blood cell count.

■ MAMMALIAN TARGET OF RAPAMYCIN INHIBITORS

❽ The newest class of immunosuppressive agents consists of drugs that target the mammalian target of rapamycin and are collectively known as mTOR inhibitors. Currently, sirolimus is the only drug approved in this class, but a second agent, everolimus, is currently being studied in kidney transplantation. Sirolimus, also known as rapamycin, is an immunosuppressive macrolide antibiotic that is structurally similar to tacrolimus, and is effective in reducing the risk of acute rejection. Sirolimus is thought to have potential to reduce chronic rejection, but this remains to be proven.

Pharmacology/Mechanism of Action Sirolimus binds to FKBP12, but the resulting complex does not inhibit the activity of calcineurin. Whereas the tacrolimus-FKBP12 complex inhibits cytokine production, the sirolimus-FKBP12 complex binds to mTOR, which inhibits the response to these cytokines (see Fig. 92–1). IL-2 stimulates mTOR to activate kinases that ultimately advance the cell cycle from G_1 to the S phase. Thus sirolimus inhibits T-cell proliferation by inhibiting the cellular response to IL-2 and progression of the cell cycle.[59]

Pharmacokinetics Bioavailability after oral administration is low, only 15%, with peak concentrations being reached within 1 to 2 hours.[61] Sirolimus has a high volume of distribution, readily distributing into most tissues of the body, even though it binds extensively to erythrocytes because of the high FKBP12 concentration found in red blood cells. Metabolism occurs primarily by CYP3A4 both in the gut and in the liver. The half-life is reported to be 60 hours but can be as long as 110 hours in patients with liver dysfunction.[60]

Efficacy Currently, sirolimus is only approved for the prevention of rejection in kidney transplant recipients when given in combination with corticosteroids and cyclosporine or after withdrawal of cyclosporine in patients with low to moderate immunologic risk. Sirolimus has also been demonstrated to be effective in combination with tacrolimus or mycophenolate in kidney transplants, with patient survival rates >99% and graft survival rates >96%.[61–64] Combination therapy with sirolimus and mycophenolate can be used to avoid the use of calcineurin inhibitors and decrease the risk of nephrotoxicity.

Two clinical trials evaluated the use of sirolimus in kidney transplants. All patients in both studies received cyclosporine and corticosteroids and were randomly assigned to one of three groups: (a) Sirolimus in a fixed dose—a 6-mg loading dose followed by 2 mg daily; (b) a 15-mg loading dose followed by 5 mg daily; or (c) azathioprine in the U.S. trial or placebo in the global trial. The results of both studies showed similar patient and graft survival in all groups at 12 months but lower rates of acute rejection in the sirolimus arms compared with azathioprine and placebo.[65,66]

Early cyclosporine withdrawal has been studied in patients receiving sirolimus-based immunosuppressive protocols. Patients receiving sirolimus who did not have a recent or severe rejection episode and adequate renal function 3 months after transplant were enrolled. Patients were randomly assigned to continue triple-drug therapy with sirolimus (adjusted to trough concentrations of greater than 5 ng/mL), cyclosporine, and corticosteroids or to double-drug therapy with sirolimus (adjusted to trough concentrations of 20 to 30 ng/mL) and corticosteroids. The results showed a low risk of acute rejection following cyclosporine discontinuation (5.6%) and no difference in graft survival. Long-term followup (2 years) showed improved renal function and blood pressure without an increase in acute rejection or graft loss in patients who discontinued cyclosporine.[67]

Currently, because the safety and efficacy of sirolimus has not been established in liver or lung transplants, it is recommended that its use be avoided in these populations immediately following transplant. In contrast, limited data on the use of sirolimus in heart transplantation indicate benefit in reversing acute rejection in patients who do not respond to antilymphocyte therapy.[68] Furthermore, sirolimus may slow the progression of vasculopathy, which may have an impact on chronic rejection and long-term patient survival after heart transplantation.[23]

Adverse Effects Myelosuppression associated with sirolimus appears to be dose-related. Thrombocytopenia is usually seen within the first 2 weeks of sirolimus therapy but generally improves with continued treatment; leukopenia and anemia are also typically transient.[69] Sirolimus trough serum concentrations greater than 15 ng/mL have been correlated with thrombocytopenia and leukopenia.[70] Hypercholesterolemia and hypertriglyceridemia are quite common in patients receiving sirolimus. It is postulated that the mechanism of this adverse effect is related to an overproduction of lipoproteins or inhibition of lipoprotein lipase. Peak cholesterol and triglyceride levels are often seen within 3 months of starting sirolimus but usually decrease after 1 year of therapy and can be managed by reducing the dose, discontinuing sirolimus, or by initiating therapy with an HMG-CoA reductase inhibitor or fibric acid derivative. One study suggests that the dyslipidemia associated with sirolimus is not a major risk factor for early cardiovascular complications following kidney transplantation.[71] Delayed wound healing and dehiscence could be a result of inhibition of smooth muscle proliferation and intimal thickening.[72] Mouth ulcers also have been reported with sirolimus, more commonly with the oral solution. The cause may be a direct effect of the drug or secondary to activation of herpes simplex virus.[73] Reversible interstitial pneumonitis has been described in kidney, liver, and heart-lung transplantation recipients.[60] Other adverse effects reported with sirolimus include increased liver enzymes, hypertension, rash, acne, diarrhea, and arthralgia (see Table 92–4).

Drug–Drug and Drug–Food Interactions The major metabolic pathway for sirolimus is CYP3A4; thus the drug interactions mediated by induction or inhibition of the CYP3A4 enzyme system are similar to those seen with cyclosporine and tacrolimus (see Table 92–5). Administration of the microemulsion formulation of cyclosporine with sirolimus significantly increases the AUC and trough sirolimus levels. The same is not seen with the standard formulation of cyclosporine. Conversely, cyclosporine concentrations and AUC are also increased when it is given concomitantly with sirolimus. The mechanism is proposed to be competitive binding to CYP3A4 and P-glycoprotein.[60] It is recommended that patients separate the dose of sirolimus and cyclosporine by 4 hours to minimize the interaction.[74] Concomitant administration of tacrolimus does not affect sirolimus levels.[75]

As with cyclosporine and tacrolimus, grapefruit juice increases sirolimus levels. Administration of sirolimus with a high-fat meal is associated with a delayed rate of absorption, decreased C_{max}, and increased AUC, indicating an increased drug exposure, whereas the half-life remained unchanged.[76] The clinical significance of this is unknown.

Dosing and Administration A fixed sirolimus dosing regimen is approved for concomitant use with cyclosporine that includes a loading dose of 6- or 15-mg followed by 2 or 5 mg daily, respectively. Therapeutic monitoring of sirolimus is advocated using whole-blood concentrations measured by HPLC, which is specific for the parent compound. The target concentration range is 10 to 15 ng/mL when used in combination with a calcineurin inhibitor, or 15 to 25 ng/mL, when used in regimens that do not. When RIA is used, which measures the parent compound and metabolites, reference ranges of 15 to 20 ng/mL and 20 to 30 ng/mL should be used, respectively.

CLINICAL CONTROVERSY

Routine therapeutic drug monitoring of sirolimus therapy is not recommended in patients who are receiving triple-drug therapy with cyclosporine and corticosteroids. However, many clinicians now believe that sirolimus drug levels should be monitored in all patients, although there is no universally accepted therapeutic range.

■ POLYCLONAL ANTIBODIES (ANTITHYMOCYTE GLOBULINS)

❾ There are currently two antithymocyte globulins available in the United States: ATG (Atgam, Pfizer, NY, NY), an equine polyclonal antibody, and RATG (Thymoglobulin, Genzyme, Cambridge, MA), a rabbit polyclonal antibody. The rabbit preparation is less immunogenic and may have other advantages over the equine preparation. Both ATG and RATG are currently approved only for the treatment of rejection; however, the drugs are used often as induction therapy to prevent acute rejection.

Pharmacology/Mechanism of Action Because of their polyclonal antibody nature, both ATG and RATG exert their immunosuppressive effect by binding to a wide array of lymphocyte receptors, including CD2, CD3, CD4, CD8, CD25, and CD45. Binding of ATG or RATG to the various receptors results in complement-mediated lysis and subsequent lymphocyte depletion. T cells are the major lymphocytic target for the compounds; however, other blood cell components are also affected, including B cells and other leukocytes (see Fig. 92–1). Damaged T cells are removed subsequently by the spleen, liver, and lungs.

Pharmacokinetics ATG is poorly distributed into lymphoid tissue and binds primarily to circulating lymphocytes, granulocytes, and platelets. The terminal half-life of ATG is 5.7 days. RATG has a volume of distribution of 0.12 L/kg and its terminal half-life in renal transplant recipients is significantly longer than ATG at 30 days.[77] Peak plasma concentrations are reached after 5 to 7 days of ATG or RATG infusions. Antiequine antibodies can form in up to 78% of patients who are receiving ATG therapy. Similarly, antirabbit antibodies have been reported in up to 68% of patients who are receiving RATG therapy. The effects of preformed antibodies on the efficacy and safety of these preparations has not been studied adequately.

Efficacy ATG and RATG are used most commonly for the treatment of acute allograft rejection or as induction therapy to prevent acute rejection. ATG is currently approved for both indications in kidney transplants. RATG is approved only for the treatment of acute allograft rejection in kidney transplantations. However, both drugs have been studied extensively for both indications. A meta-analysis revealed that polyclonal antibodies demonstrated a significantly higher reversal rate for first acute rejection episodes compared to corticosteroids. However, there was no difference between the two groups in preventing subsequent rejections.[78] Accordingly, polyclonal antibodies are most often reserved for the treatment of corticosteroid-resistant or moderate to severe acute rejection episodes.

The efficacy of ATG and RATG induction therapy has been described in liver and heart transplantation recipients. Use of RATG as part of quadruple therapy in liver transplantation is associated with similar rates of patient and graft survival and acute rejection compared with dual therapy; however, a significant increase in the number of cytomegalovirus infections was noted.[79] Quadruple-drug therapy results in similar rates of patient and graft survival and malignancy in heart transplantations, but a significantly lower rate of acute rejection and infection episodes is seen at 1 year compared with triple-drug therapy.[80]

Adverse Effects Most adverse effects reported with ATG and RATG are related to the lack of specificity for T cells owing to their polyclonal nature. Dose-limiting myelosuppression, including leukopenia, anemia, and thrombocytopenia, occurs frequently. Other adverse effects include anaphylaxis, hypotension, hypertension, tachycardia, dyspnea, urticaria, and rash. Serum sickness is seen more frequently with ATG than RATG. Nephrotoxicity has been reported but is rare in the absence of serum sickness. Infusion-related febrile reactions are most common with the first few doses and can be managed by premedicating the patient with acetaminophen, diphenhydramine, and corticosteroids. Finally, as with any immunosuppressive agent, ATG and RATG are associated with an increased risk of infections, particularly viral infections, and malignancy.

Drug–Drug and Drug–Food Interactions Administration of ATG or RATG can interfere with the immune response to live vaccines, such as varicella vaccine. If a live vaccine is administered within 2 months of receiving one of these immunoglobulins, protection may not be conferred.

Dosing and Administration ATG doses range from 10 to 30 mg/kg per day as a single dose for 7 to 14 days. RATG is a more potent compound and is administered at doses of 1 to 1.5 mg/kg per day as a single dose for 7 to 14 days for acute rejection or for 5 to 10 days for induction of immunosuppression. Although literature reports now support peripheral administration of both agents it is recommended that both ATG and RATG be administered through a central line or through a high-flow vein with an in-line 0.22-micron filter over at least 4 hours to minimize phlebitis and thrombosis whenever possible.[81,82]

MONOCLONAL ANTIBODIES

Monoclonal antibodies are more specific than the polyclonal antibodies for targeting a single receptor on the T cells. The result of their actions varies, depending on the nature of and target of the antibody.

Interleukin-2 Receptor Antagonists

There are currently two available IL-2 receptor antagonists: basiliximab, a chimeric monoclonal antibody (25% murine), and daclizumab, a humanized monoclonal antibody (90% human, 10% murine). Daclizumab contains a greater proportion of human sequences, making it theoretically less immunogenic. The percentage of murine component determines the antibody's affinity for the epitope. Consequently, the chimeric antibody basiliximab has a higher affinity than daclizumab.[83]

Pharmacology/Mechanism of Action Both basiliximab and daclizumab exert their immunosuppressive effect by specifically binding to the α-chain (CD25) on the surface of activated T lymphocytes (see Fig. 92–1). Binding of either basiliximab or daclizumab to the IL-2 receptor prevents IL-2-mediated activation and proliferation of T cells, a critical step in clonal expansion of T cells and the development of allograft rejection. Saturation of the IL-2 receptor occurs rapidly and confers an immunosuppressive effect immediately.[83]

Pharmacokinetics Most of the pharmacokinetic data available for both basiliximab and daclizumab are in renal transplantation patients. Caution must be used when extrapolating these data to nonrenal transplantation recipients. The volume of distribution is approximately 5.3 L for daclizumab and 8 L for basiliximab. Basiliximab and daclizumab saturate CD25 in vivo at serum concentrations of 0.2 and 1 mg/L or greater, respectively.[84] The terminal half-life of daclizumab is about 20 days in renal transplantation patients compared with 3 to 4 days in bone marrow transplant recipients. Basiliximab has a shorter half-life of approximately 7 days in renal transplant recipients. Clearance of both drugs is increased in patients who have received a liver transplant, primarily as a consequence of drainage of ascites. It is recommended that patients with greater than 10 L of ascites receive an additional dose of basiliximab on postoperative day 8.[85] Therapeutic concentrations of daclizumab range from 5 to 10 mg/L.

Efficacy Both basiliximab and daclizumab are approved for use in kidney transplantation in combination with cyclosporine and corticosteroids, although induction therapy has also been studied extensively in liver and heart transplantation recipients. A meta-analysis of daclizumab and basiliximab in renal transplantation concluded that IL-2 receptor antagonists reduced the risk of rejection significantly with no increases in graft loss, infectious complications, malignancy, or death.[86] Similar results were seen in liver and heart transplantation.[87,88]

IL-2 receptor antagonists offer a reasonable addition to calcineurin inhibitor- or corticosteroid-sparing protocols. Although calcineurin inhibitor therapy can not be completely avoided in most cases,[84] IL-2 receptor antagonists allow for delayed use or reduced doses of calcineurin inhibitors, thus minimizing the risk of nephrotoxicity in the early post-transplantation period. Similar rates of rejection and corticosteroid-resistant rejection were seen in patients with DGF who received an IL-2 receptor antagonist in conjunction with lower tacrolimus doses compared with patients without DGF who received standard tacrolimus doses and no IL-2 receptor inhibitor induction.[83]

Adverse Effects Few adverse effects have been reported with basiliximab and daclizumab. In contrast to polyclonal antibody preparations and OKT3, basiliximab and daclizumab have not been associated with infusion-related reactions. However, since the marketing of basiliximab, an increased number of hypersensitivity reactions have been reported. Of note, only one patient developed anti-idiotypic antibodies to the murine portion during clinical trials.[85] The manufacturer of basiliximab reported an increase in mortality in a placebo-controlled trial, which was associated with an increase in severe infections. No increased risk of malignancy as has been noted with standard immunosuppression has been reported.

Drug–Drug and Drug–Food Interactions Reports of increased cyclosporine and tacrolimus levels in patients receiving concomitant basiliximab were recently published.[89,90] Both authors hypothesized a potential interaction with the cytochrome P450. No drug interactions have been reported with daclizumab.

Dosing and Administration Basiliximab is administered as two 20-mg intravenous doses: intraoperatively and again on postoperative day 4. Basiliximab is compatible with both 0.9% sodium chloride and 5% dextrose and can be administered either centrally or peripherally over 20 to 30 minutes in a volume of 50 mL. This regimen results in saturation of the IL-2 receptor for 30 to 45 days. The approved daclizumab dosing regimen for renal transplantation is 1 mg/kg every 2 weeks from the time of transplant for a total of 5 doses. Daclizumab should be diluted in 50 mL of sterile 0.9% sodium chloride and administered peripherally or centrally over 15 minutes. This regimen saturates the IL-2 receptors for approximately 90 to 120 days after renal transplantation.[47,83] Alternative dosing regimens have been proposed for daclizumab in combination with tacrolimus, mycophenolate, and corticosteroids: 1 mg/kg every 2 weeks for 5 doses, 2 mg/kg every 2 weeks for 2 doses, or 2 mg/kg on day 0 followed by 1 mg/kg on day 5.[91,92]

Muromonab-CD3

Pharmacology/Mechanism of Action OKT3 is a murine monoclonal antibody to the CD3 receptor on mature human T cells (see Fig. 92–1). Minutes following the administration of OKT3, T-cell concentrations decrease dramatically, as measured by CD3 levels. Cells reappear after a few days but bear no CD3 receptors. After cessation of OKT3 therapy, T-cell function normalizes in a week.[93]

Pharmacokinetics OKT3 has a volume of distribution of 6.5 L and half-life of about 18 hours. Concentrations above 0.9 mcg/mL are considered therapeutic. An OKT3 concentration of 0.8 mcg/mL or greater in combination with a CD3+ T-cell count of <25 cells/mL is also a reasonable therapeutic target. If CD3 levels begin to rise, this may signify the presence of antimurine antibodies antagonizing the actions of OKT3. Administration of mycophenolate mofetil has been suggested to reduce the formation of antimurine antibodies during OKT3 administration. Although T-cell depletion is achieved within minutes of administration, resolution of rejection takes 3 to 4 days.

Efficacy OKT3 has been used as induction therapy at doses of 5 mg/day for 7 to 14 days. OKT3 can be used safely and successfully as an acute rejection therapy in patients who have undergone previous OKT3 induction.[93] Specifically, these studies confirm that the presence of low anti-OKT3 antibody titers (≤1:100) does not preclude successful retreatment with OKT3 for rejection. However, today, OKT3 is generally reserved for treatment of corticosteroid-resistant rejection.

Adverse Effects OKT3 administration is associated with significant first-dose adverse reactions. The cytokine-release syndrome related to OKT3, including fever, chills, rigors, pruritus, and alterations in blood pressure, may occur with the first several doses. Methylprednisolone, acetaminophen, diphenhydramine, indomethacin, and pentoxifylline have been used as premedications to prevent or minimize the severity of this syndrome. Other adverse effects include capillary leak syndrome and pulmonary edema, especially in fluid overloaded patients. It is recommended that patients be within 3% of their dry weight and have chest radiographs evaluated prior to administration. Aseptic meningitis is another potential complication of OKT3 therapy. If encephalitic symptoms develop, OKT3 should be discontinued and appropriate care initiated. Other adverse effects include encephalopathy, nephrotoxicity, infection, and post-transplantation lymphoproliferative disorder.[47]

Drug–Drug and Drug–Food Interactions No drug or food interactions have been reported with OKT3.

Dosing and Administration OKT3 should be filtered with a 0.2- to 0.22-micron filter and then administered as an intravenous push over 1 minute. The dose of OKT3 usually is 5 mg/day for 5 to 14 days. Induction with 2.5 mg/day also has been used effectively.[93] Vital signs should be assessed frequently during the first few doses, and it is advisable to have a physician present for the first dose. A high proportion of patients treated with OKT3 form antibodies to one of the components of OKT3 and may not be able to receive or adequately respond to retreatment.[93] The dosages of other immunosuppressant drugs often need to be decreased while administering corticosteroids, OKT3, or antithymocyte globulin therapy.

Alemtuzumab

Alemtuzumab is approved for use in B-cell chronic lymphocytic leukemia. However, its effects on depleting both T and B lymphocytes make it useful in solid-organ transplants. Although alemtuzumab use in solid-organ transplantation is considered to be investigational, it is increasingly recognized as a viable therapeutic option and, consequently, its use is increasing despite the lack of sound clinical evidence.

Pharmacology/Mechanism of Action Alemtuzumab is a humanized monoclonal antibody directed at cells that express the CD52 surface antigen, which is found on both T and B lymphocytes, as well as macrophages, monocytes, eosinophils, and natural killer cells. When alemtuzumab binds to the CD52 surface antigen, antibody-dependent lysis occurs, which removes both T and B lymphocytes from the blood, bone marrow, and organs, resulting in complete lymphocyte depletion.

Pharmacokinetics The pharmacokinetics of alemtuzumab in solid-organ transplantation patients has not been investigated. Data from patients with B-cell chronic lymphocytic leukemia indicate that the volume of distribution of alemtuzumab after repeated dosing was 0.18 L/kg. The mean half-life after the first 30 mg dose was 11 hours, but increased to 6 days after 12 weeks of therapy. The extrapolation of this data to solid-organ transplantation is difficult because of the differences in dosing strategies (single or double doses in solid-organ transplantation versus weekly to three times weekly dosing in B-cell chronic lymphocytic leukemia). One or two doses of alemtuzumab result in complete and prolonged lymphocyte depletion. Following administration, B lymphocyte counts return to normal within 3 to 12 months. T lymphocytes, however, remain depressed for as long as 3 years following administration.[94]

Efficacy Recent data suggests that alemtuzumab is effective as induction therapy for the prevention of acute rejection in kidney, liver, pancreas, intestinal, and lung transplants.[95] Additionally, alemtuzumab has been used to successfully treat acute rejection following transplantation and is effective for corticosteroid- and antibody-resistant rejection.[95] The most promising role of alemtuzumab in solid-organ transplantation is its use in corticosteroid-sparing protocols, which allow for calcineurin inhibitor monotherapy following transplantation. Tacrolimus appears to be the optimal calcineurin inhibitor to use for monotherapy immunosuppression in patients who receive alemtuzumab induction.

Adverse Effects The adverse effects of alemtuzumab include infusion-related reactions, hematologic effects, and infections. Infusion-related reactions include rigors, hypotension, fever, shortness of breath, bronchospasms, and chills. The potential for developing these reactions can be reduced by administering premedications, including corticosteroids, diphenhydramine, and acetaminophen, or by administering smaller doses and escalating the dose gradually. Hematologic effects include pancytopenia, neutropenia, thrombocytopenia, and lymphopenia. Dose modifications are recommended based on the degree of thrombocytopenia.

Drug–Drug and Drug–Food Interactions No drug or food interactions have been reported with alemtuzumab.

Dosing and Administration Several dosing regimens have been proposed for alemtuzumab in solid-organ transplantation. The most commonly recommended dosing strategy for alemtuzumab is 30 mg as a single dose; some centers administer a second dose 1 to 5 days after transplantation.[95] Other studied dosing strategies include 0.3 mg/kg per dose, as a single- or multiple-dose regimen, and, finally, two 20-mg doses given on the day of transplantation and the first postoperative day.[96]

EVALUATION OF THERAPEUTIC OUTCOMES

⑩ The success of transplantation can be measured in terms of length of graft and patient survival or quality of life. Several donor and recipient factors that have an impact on graft and patient survival have been identified (Table 92–7). The greatest risk to short-term graft survival is acute rejection. Routine surveillance of appropriate biochemical markers and serum drug concentrations are essential to minimize the potential for acute rejection. These parameters should be assessed daily to weekly for the first 1 to 3 months after transplantation. Monitoring should include complete blood counts, serum electrolyte concentrations, serum creatinine and blood urea nitrogen concentrations, and the appropriate serum drug concentrations. Liver function tests should also be evaluated using the same schedule in liver transplantation recipients. Routine biopsies are necessary to monitor for acute rejection in heart transplantation recipients. As the time after transplantation increases, the frequency of monitoring decreases. Once 3 months have elapsed after transplantation, monitoring of these parameters can be reduced to biweekly or monthly for most patients.

TABLE 92-7 Factors Negatively Affecting Allograft and Patient Survival

	Kidney	Liver	Heart
Donor factors	Decreased HLA matching Increased age Increased serum creatinine Cardiac instability Prolonged ischemia time History of hypertension	Size mismatch Age (youngest, oldest)	Size mismatch Increased age Prolonged ischemia time
Recipient factors	Age <15, >50 years Retransplantation African race Elevated PRA Multiparous women Poor drug compliance	Increased age Retransplantation African race ICU pretransplant ABO blood type Poor drug compliance	Age <5, >60 years ICU pretransplant Mechanical ventilation LVAD IABP Poor drug compliance

HLA, human leukocyte antigens; IABP, intraaortic balloon pump; LVAD, left ventricular assist device; PRA, panel of reactive antibodies.

Long-term graft survival is limited by chronic rejection. Overall survival rates for solid-organ transplantations are described in terms of half-life, or the time after transplantation at which only 50% of transplanted organs are still functioning. Estimated half-lives for kidneys are 26.9 years for HLA-identical grafts and 12.2 and 10.8 years, respectively, for grafts from a sibling or parent who are 1-haplotype matches. The estimated half-life for HLA-matched grafts was 17.3 years while a markedly lower value of 7.8 years has been noted with mismatched kidneys.[20] The overall median patient survival time for heart transplantation recipients is 9.8 years, but in these patients surviving the first year after transplantation, the median survival increases to 12 years.[1] The highest rate of mortality occurs within the first year after liver transplantation due to the risks of surgery and early postoperative complications. Table 92–8 depicts a typical post-transplantation laboratory monitoring plan.

IMMUNOSUPPRESSION-RELATED COMPLICATIONS

Comorbidities such as cardiovascular disease and malignancy, recurrent disease, drug toxicities (namely nephrotoxicity), and chronic

TABLE 92-8 Laboratory Monitoring after Transplantation as a Function of Time Post-Transplant

	1–2 Weeks	1 Month	2–4 Months	4–12 Months	>12 Months
SCr/BUN	Daily	1–2 times per week	Every 1–2 weeks	Monthly	Every 1–2 months
Chemistries[a]	Daily	1–2 times per week	Every 1–2 weeks	Monthly	Every 1–2 months
Liver function tests[b]					
Kidney or heart recipient	Once	Once	Monthly	Every 1–3 months	Every 1–3 months
Liver recipient	Daily	1–3 times per week	Every 1–2 weeks	Monthly	Every 1–2 months
Immunosuppressant level	Daily	1–2 times per week	Every 1–2 weeks	Monthly	Every 1–2 months
Complete blood count[c]	Daily	1–2 times per week	Every 1–2 weeks	Monthly	Every 1–2 months
Lipid panel[d]	Once	Every 3 months	Every 3 months	Every 3 months	Every 3 months
HbA_{1c}	Once	Every 3 months	Every 3 months	Every 3 months	Every 3 months

BUN, blood urea nitrogen; HbA_{1c}, hemoglobin A1c; SCr infusion, serum creatinine.

[a]Chemistries include sodium, potassium, chloride, CO2 content, magnesium, calcium, phosphorus and blood glucose.

[b]Liver function tests include total bilirubin, aspartate transaminase (AST), alanine transaminase (ALT), gamma glutamyl transpeptidase (GGTP), alkaline phosphatase.

[c]Complete blood count includes white blood cells (WBC), red blood cells (RBC), platelets and/or differential.

[d]Lipid panel includes total cholesterol, low-density lipoprotein (LDL), high-density lipoprotein (HDL), triglyceride and/or very low-density lipoprotein (VLDL).

TABLE 92-9 Special Pharmacotherapy Considerations in Transplant Recipients

Problem	Pharmacotherapy	Special Considerations
Infection		
Perioperative prophylaxis		Donor culture results Penicillin allergy: vancomycin
	Bowel decontamination	
Pneumocystis carinii pneumonia prophylaxis	TMP-SMX 400/80 daily or thrice weekly Pentamidine 300 mg inhaled monthly or dapsone 50–100 mg po daily or atovaquone 750–1,500 mg po daily	Sulfa allergy
Fungal		
Prophylaxis	Nystatin, clotrimazole	
Treatment	Fluconazole, itraconazole, voriconazole	Inhibit P450 3A4; monitor CSA and TAC levels; decrease doses
	Amphotericin B	Consider liposomal products; decrease or stop CSA or TAC to minimize nephrotoxicity Remember to adjust doses of renally eliminated drugs, e.g., acyclovir, ganciclovir, TMP-SMX, valganciclovir
Hyperkalemia	Restrict dietary intake; dialysis	May be exacerbated by CSA or TAC or ACEIs, acidosis or RI; fludrocortisone acetate 0.1 mg PO once daily or twice daily for refractory hyperkalemia
Hyperglycemia		
Diabetes pretransplant	Insulin, oral hypoglycemics	Corticosteroids, TAC, and CSA also increase hypoglycemic requirements Insulin requirements will increase with improving renal function
	Metformin	Avoid in those with RI
Post transplant diabetes	Insulin	Risk factors: obesity, family history, African American race, cadaveric kidney, TAC > CSA
	Oral hypoglycemics	May resolve/improve as immunosuppressive doses decrease
Ulcer prophylaxis	H_2-receptor antagonists	Adjust dose in those with RI
	Sucralfate	Decreased TAC absorption If RI: caution aluminum content No RI: caution hypophosphatemia
	Proton pump inhibitors	
Hyperlipidemia	Diet	CSA > TAC; consider switch to TAC; discontinue or hold SRL
	HMG-CoA reductase inhibitors ("statins")	CSA/TAC may increase "statin" levels; start at lowest dose Monitor for muscle cramps, CPK levels and LFTs
	Gemfibrozil	Adjust dose in those with RI Caution with concomitant "statin"
Hypertension	Calcium channel blockers	Diltiazem, verapamil inhibit CSA/TAC metabolism Dihydropyridines may potentiate CSA-gingival hyperplasia
	ACEIs; angiotensin II receptor antagonists	May exacerbate hyperkalemia Monitor K+, S_{cr} to assess for renal allograft vascular disease; may be useful in post-transplant erythrocytosis (HCT >55%)
Osteoporosis	Oral calcium supplementation (1,000–1,500 mg/day)	If daily intake <1,000 mg elemental calcium
	Oral vitamin D	Documented deficiency
	Calcifediol (1,000 international units/day)	If kidney functioning
	Calcitriol (0.5 mcg/day)	If kidney not functioning
	Hormone-replacement therapy	Postmenopausal women without contraindications
	Calcitonin or oral bisphosphonates	Documented loss in bone mineral density >3% Data lacking for bisphosphonates in patients with RI
Malignancy		
Prevention	Minimize immunosuppressant doses; avoid sun exposure (sun block, hats, clothing); routine self-examinations (skin, lymph nodes); yearly gynecologic/prostate exams	AZA particularly associated with skin cancers CSA/TAC may be associated with lymphoproliferative disorders (lymphomas)
Treatment	Discontinue or minimize immunosuppressants Surgical, radiologic, or antineoplastic therapy	Do not abruptly withdraw corticosteroids

ACEI, ACE inhibitor; CMV, cytomegalovirus; CPK, creatinine phosphokinase enzymes; CSA, cyclosporine; HCT, hematocrit; K+, potassium; LFTs, liver function tests; RI, renal insufficiency; S_{cr}, serum creatinine; SRL, sirolimus; TAC, tacrolimus; TMP-SMX, trimethoprim-sulfamethoxazole.

rejection are the primary causes of mortality in patients who have a functioning graft 5 or more years after transplantation.[1] Special considerations for the management of these conditions in transplant patients are discussed below and summarized in Table 92–9.

CARDIOVASCULAR DISEASE

Cardiovascular disease is a leading cause of morbidity and mortality in transplant patients.[97] Preexisting cardiovascular disease, which is common in end-stage organ failure, is not reversed with transplantation. Additionally, hypertension, hyperlipidemia, and diabetes are common complications in transplantation recipients and are independent risk factors that contribute significantly to cardiovascular disease. Chronic rejection has been linked to hypertension and hyperlipidemia.[98,99]

HYPERTENSION

Corticosteroids, cyclosporine, tacrolimus, and impaired kidney graft function may cause post-transplantation hypertension. The primary mechanism of calcineurin inhibitor-associated hypertension in heart transplantation recipients may be related to the calcineurin inhibitor-induced stimulation of intact renal sympathetic nerves and the absence of reflex cardiac inhibition of the sympathetic nervous system, but a number of other mechanisms, including decreased prostacyclin and nitric oxide production, also have been proposed.[45,100,101] In addition to the propensity to cause peripheral vasoconstriction, calcineurin inhibitors promote sodium retention, resulting in extracellular fluid volume expansion. Tacrolimus appears to have less potential to induce hypertension following transplantation than cyclosporine.[29] Most classes of antihypertensive medications effectively reduce blood pressure in transplantation patients.[102]

Calcium channel blockers traditionally have been the first-line agents to treat hypertension after transplantation.[103] In addition to their ability to control blood pressure, calcium channel blockers may ameliorate the nephrotoxic effects of cyclosporine, improve renal hemodynamics, decrease the incidence of delayed graft function and the development of allograft atherosclerosis, and provide some immunosuppression. Calcium channel blockers, however, also may contribute to gingival hyperplasia that is often associated with cyclosporine-based immunosuppression.[98] CYP3A4 interactions with cyclosporine and tacrolimus are of concern with this class of medications, particularly with diltiazem, verapamil, and nicardipine, and cyclosporine or tacrolimus concentrations must be monitored to ensure proper dosage adjustments.

ACEIs and angiotensin II receptor blockers traditionally have been avoided in kidney transplantation recipients, especially in the perioperative phase, because of the potential for hyperkalemia and their potentially negative influence on glomerular filtration rate. ACEIs and angiotensin II receptor blockers are now considered to be an equivalent alternative to calcium channel blockers for the treatment of hypertension in all transplant recipients. When ACEIs or angiotensin II receptor blockers are used in patients after transplantation, serum creatinine and potassium levels should be monitored closely. If the increase in serum creatinine is greater than 30% within 1 to 2 weeks after initiating ACEIs or angiotensin II receptor blockers, the drug should be discontinued and other measures used to control blood pressure (see Chap. 49).

CLINICAL CONTROVERSY

Many clinicians avoid using ACEIs in kidney transplantation recipients because of the potential to decrease the glomerular filtration rate by promoting efferent arteriole vasodilation in the presence of calcineurin inhibitor-induced afferent arteriole vasoconstriction. Emerging evidence suggests that this situation does not occur.

Multiple antihypertensive agents usually are necessary to achieve the goal blood pressure in transplant recipients; consequently, the addition of a β-blocker, diuretic, or centrally acting antihypertensive is usually necessary. β-Blockers generally are considered to be second-line therapy in solid-organ transplantation recipients, because of the potential to worsen metabolic disturbances caused by immunosuppressants, such as hyperkalemia and dyslipidemia. Calcineurin inhibitor-induced hypertension is often salt-sensitive, making it very responsive to diuretics. Central-acting agents (e.g., clonidine) are used often as adjunctive therapy in transplantation recipients who are unable to achieve blood pressure control with calcium channel blockers or ACEIs.

HYPERLIPIDEMIA

Hyperlipidemia may be exacerbated by corticosteroids, calcineurin inhibitors, sirolimus, diuretics, and β-blockers.[104] Corticosteroids promote insulin resistance and a decrease in lipoprotein lipase activity, as well as excessive triglyceride production. The mechanism of calcineurin inhibitor-induced hyperlipidemia is not well understood. Calcineurin inhibitors may decrease the activity of the low-density lipoprotein (LDL) receptor or lipoprotein lipase, altering LDL catabolism.[99] Tacrolimus appears to have less potential to induce hyperlipidemia than cyclosporine.[27,28,30] post-transplantation hyperlipidemia is characterized by elevated LDL, very-low-density lipoprotein, triglyceride apolipoprotein B, and lipoprotein(a) levels.[99] It is controversial whether the management of hyperlipidemia in transplantation recipients should be more aggressive than current guidelines for the general population established by the National Cholesterol Education Program.[105] Aggressive lipid lowering may not only arrest the progress or prevent the complications of atherosclerosis but also may promote graft survival in the kidney and heart transplantation population. With the use of lipid-lowering agents, potential interactions with immunosuppressive regimens must be considered.

Dietary intervention, although safe, may be relatively ineffective for the treatment of hyperlipidemia in the transplant population. Along with dietary modification, dose reduction or withdrawal of cyclosporine and/or corticosteroids may assist in minimizing hyperlipidemia. For most patients, the combination of dietary intervention and an HMG-CoA reductase inhibitor should be considered the treatment of choice. HMG-CoA reductase inhibitors are highly effective in the treatment of hyperlipidemia, especially increased LDL, in transplantation patients. HMG-CoA reductase inhibitors as a class have immunomodulatory effects on MHC expression and T-cell activation and reduce cardiac allograft rejection.[99,106]

HMG-CoA reductase inhibitors should be used with caution in transplantation recipients because of several reports of rhabdomyolysis when these agents are combined with calcineurin inhibitors.[39,106,107] Safety measures, including the use of low HMG-CoA reductase inhibitor doses and avoiding inappropriately high cyclosporine or tacrolimus concentrations. The concurrent use of medications known to increase the risk of myopathy (such as gemfibrozil) should be avoided.[99] Patients should be informed of the signs and symptoms of rhabdomyolysis. Baseline and followup creatine phosphokinase measurements (every 6 months) have been used to identify patients who develop subclinical rhabdomyolysis when cholesterol-lowering therapy is used. Pravastatin may be preferred as a result of its lower interactive potential with calcineurin inhibitors because it is not metabolized by CYP3A4. The potential for hepatotoxicity from HMG-CoA reductase inhibitors warrants close monitoring of liver function in all transplantation recipients.[104]

Bile acid-binding resins may be used to lower cholesterol in transplant patients, but adequate doses are difficult to achieve without the development of GI adverse effects. Because the absorption of cyclosporine is dependent on the presence of bile in the GI tract, patients should be instructed to separate dosing of bile acid-binding resins and cyclosporine by at least 2 hours. Bile acid-binding resins also should be separated from other immunosuppressants by at least 2 hours to avoid physical adsorption in the GI tract. For transplantation patients who have hypertriglyceridemia refractory to dietary intervention, fish oil and fibric acid derivatives are well-tolerated, effective alternatives (see Chap. 23). Fibric acid derivatives are most effective in lowering serum triglyceride concentrations.

POST-TRANSPLANTATION DIABETES MELLITUS

Corticosteroids and calcineurin inhibitors can impair glucose control in previously diabetic patients, as well as cause new-onset post-transplantation diabetes mellitus (PTDM) in 4% to 20% of patients. Corticosteroids induce insulin resistance and impair peripheral glucose uptake, whereas calcineurin inhibitors appear to inhibit insulin production.[108] Tacrolimus seems to be more diabetogenic than cyclosporine, although recent studies have failed to show a statistical difference.[27] Other possible risk factors that have been identified for PTDM include ethnicity (African American or Hispanic), age (>40 years), pretransplant diabetes status, family history, and weight.[109]

Patients with PTDM should be referred for nutritional counseling and advised on the merits of weight loss (if appropriate). There are, however, some special considerations in transplantation patients. Up to 40% of patients with PTDM will require insulin therapy.[108] In diabetic patients who can be managed with an oral hypoglycemic agent, glipizide, which is metabolized extensively by the liver, may be preferred over renally eliminated agents such as glyburide. Metformin should be used with extreme caution because of the risk of accumulation and lactic acidosis in those with moderate renal impairment. Regardless of therapy, frequent blood glucose monitoring is imperative in the early postoperative phase both to improve glucose control and to identify those with PTDM. Changes in renal function secondary to calcineurin inhibitor nephrotoxicity or delayed graft function or acute rejection in kidney transplantation recipients affects the elimination of many hypoglycemic agents, including insulin, and may result in hyper- or hypoglycemia. Patients and clinicians also should be aware that dose changes of immunosuppressant drugs also affect glycemic control. Tapering of immunosuppressive medications may result in reduced insulin requirements, whereas corticosteroid pulses for the treatment of rejection may result in increased insulin requirements.

INFECTION

Both the severity and incidence of infections and deaths caused by infections have decreased dramatically since the introduction of cyclosporine and the use of lower corticosteroid dosages. Nonetheless, infection and rejection remain the most frequently encountered complications associated with immunosuppression in the first year after transplantation.[110] The risk of infection is related directly to the overall level of immunosuppression and is greatest during the first 3 postoperative months, as well as following treatment of acute rejection episodes.[111] Infectious complications following transplantation generally are classified according to the causative organism, site of infection, and time of appearance following surgery. Bacterial infections occur most frequently within the first month after transplantation and generally affect the urinary tract, wound, or vascular access sites. Viral infections are caused most commonly by herpes simplex (early transplantation), herpes zoster (late post-transplantation), or cytomegalovirus (CMV). Chapter 126 discusses the treatment of infection in the immunocompromised host. Special considerations for CMV, herpes, and *Pneumocystis carinii* infections in transplant patients are described in the following paragraphs.

CMV is the most important viral pathogen affecting transplant patients; 50% to 60% of patients are infected with the virus. Following transplantation, patients may develop symptomatic primary or secondary CMV infections. A previously CMV-seronegative patient who receives an organ or blood product from a CMV-seropositive donor is considered to have primary CMV infection. A secondary infection is characterized by reactivation of the latent virus or reinfection in a previously seropositive patient. Patients with primary infections generally are more symptomatic than patients with secondary infections.

The incidence and severity of CMV infections in transplant recipients are related to the intensity of immunosuppression required to prevent graft rejection. Patients treated on multiple occasions with high-dose corticosteroids or patients receiving antilymphocyte preparations or OKT3 and patients with poor HLA matching, cadaveric allografts, and CMV-positive donor serology tend to have more severe CMV disease. Transplantation centers use different strategies for managing CMV, which often are based on the risk of CMV infection. Prophylactic strategies may include oral or intravenous antiviral or immunoglobulin preparations to prevent the reactivation or emergence of CMV. Prophylaxis is used most often in high-risk patients (i.e., donor–recipient CMV–serology mismatch or for those receiving antilymphocyte preparations). Some centers routinely screen transplantation recipients for CMV via blood tests (i.e., pp65 antigenemia, polymerase chain reaction) and use preemptive therapy in patients who have a positive test. Treatment is given to all patients who have evidence of active CMV infection. Ganciclovir and valganciclovir have been used prophylactically and pre-emptively in transplant patients. Other treatment strategies include intravenous immunoglobulin and CMV hyperimmune immunoglobulin. Ganciclovir and CMV hyperimmune immunoglobulin are the mainstays for treatment of CMV infection. CMV has been linked to chronic rejection and cardiac allograft vasculopathy.

CLINICAL CONTROVERSY

Some clinicians use CMV prophylaxis for all patients receiving a transplant. Others will reserve prophylaxis for only those patients who are at a high risk for CMV infection, such as those with donor–recipient CMV–serology mismatch or recipients who have received induction therapy or rejection treatment with antithymocyte globulin. A third strategy is to pre-emptively treat patients who have laboratory evidence of CMV infection.

Herpes simplex virus infections in transplant patients are most commonly the result of reactivation of a previous infection. Symptomatic herpes simplex virus infection usually presents as labial or oral lesions in the first 1 to 3 months after transplantation, but patients also may present with reactivation of varicella-zoster as "shingles." Prophylactic therapy with low-dose oral acyclovir delays the development of herpes simplex virus infections in patients following transplantation.

The incidence of *P. carinii* pneumonia within the first year after transplantation is reported to be 3% to 5%.[113] Low-dose trimethoprim-sulfamethoxazole (400 mg/80 mg three times weekly) is effective in the prevention of *P. carinii* pneumonia infections. Alternative agents include aerosolized pentamidine (300 mg every month), dapsone, and atovaquone. The duration of *P. carinii* pneumonia prophylaxis is unclear. Because the risk of infection caused by *P. carinii* is likely to decrease as immunosuppression is reduced, prophylaxis in patients requiring treatment for acute rejection may be appropriate.

Polyomavirus infection is a common cause of kidney allograft dysfunction. The specific polyomavirus that infects kidney allografts is the BK virus. Primary infection with BK virus occurs in childhood as an asymptomatic infection in 50% to 90% of the general population. The precise mechanism of transmission is not clear, but is suspected to be via the oral or respiratory routes. The virus then remains latent primarily in the genitourinary tract. Reactivation of BK virus is limited to people with compromised immune function and is most common in kidney transplant recipients. Reactivation can be detected as the presence of BK virus in the urine of approximately 30% to 40% of kidney transplant recipients, although it does not progress to nephropathy in the majority of patients. However, BK viremia if it develops has been noted to progresses to allograft nephropathy in 50% of patients.[115] The development of BK virus nephropathy results in graft loss in as many as 45% to 67% of affected patients.[115]

Nephropathy associated with BK virus is definitively diagnosed by kidney allograft biopsy, although it is easily mistaken for acute rejection to the pathologist who does not recognize the presence of BK virus inclusions in renal tubular cells. It is important to differentiate the two because treatment of acute rejection with increased immunosuppression can worsen BK virus nephropathy. The mainstay of treatment is a reduction in immunosuppression, which should be instituted when BK viremia is detected. The risks of acute rejection resulting from decreased immunosuppression must be weighed against the potential benefits of resolving BK viremia. Cidofovir, a potent nephrotoxic antiviral used for the treatment of CMV retinitis, has also been used for the treatment of BK virus in very low doses (0.25 mg/kg administered every 1 to 3 weeks).[114]

Hepatitis C recurs almost universally following liver transplantation, resulting in chronic hepatitis or cirrhosis in 90% of patients by 5 years. These patients tend to experience a much more aggressive course than that observed in immunocompetent patients. While short-term survival is not affected, hepatitis C virus infection recurrence results in the need for retransplantation in more than 10% of patients originally transplanted for hepatitis C virus. Pegylated interferons as monotherapy or in combination with ribavirin have been used after liver transplantation, in both the acute and chronic phases of hepatitis C virus infection and as prophylactic or preemptive therapy. Although some patients do achieve sustained viral responses, the rates are generally lower than for immunocompetent patients, 10% to 30% versus 30% to 70%, respectively, for combination therapy. Preexisting anemia and renal dysfunction make it difficult to maintain ribavirin at effective doses. Combination of immunosuppressive drugs and interferon may result in dose-limiting neutropenia. Administration of hematopoietic growth factors may be needed to allow administration of adequate doses of interferons and ribavirin. Even with these adjunctive therapies high rates of therapy discontinuation are still reported.[116,117]

In the absence of preventative therapy, hepatitis B recurs in approximately 80% of patients. Initial studies with short-term intravenous administration of hepatitis B immunoglobulin (HBIg) showed equally high rates of recurrence upon discontinuation of therapy. However, strategies that employ the long-term administration of HBIg with or without antiviral therapy report much lower recurrence rates, 15% to 30% and 20% to 40%, for nonreplicative and replicative hepatitis B virus, respectively. Common strategies include intravenous HBIg 10,000 units during the anhepatic phase followed by 10,000 units daily for 6 days. Antihepatitis B surface titer should be monitored weekly to ensure adequate levels for protection, as well as optimize HBIg use. HBIg has been typically dosed to maintain titers >100 to 500 international units/L. Monotherapy with lamivudine is insufficient. Treatment for active hepatitis B virus graft infection should include HBIg, antiviral therapy such as lamivudine or adefovir, and concomitant reduction in immunosuppression.[117]

MALIGNANCY

Advances in immunosuppression have decreased the incidence of acute rejection and increased patient survival, thus increasing the patient's lifetime exposure to immunosuppression. Although the precise mechanism is unclear, post-transplantation malignancy seems to be related to the overall level of immunosuppression, as evidenced by a difference in the rates of malignancy associated with quadruple versus triple versus dual immunosuppressant regimens. The risk of malignancy in transplantation recipients is increased three- to fourfold over the general population. Although the risk of lung, breast, colon, and prostate cancers does not appear to increase, a number of cancers that are uncommon in the general population often occur with a higher prevalence in transplantation recipients: post-transplantation lymphomas and lymphoproliferative disorders (PTLD), Kaposi sarcoma, renal carcinoma, in situ carcinomas of the uterine cervix, hepatobiliary tumors, and anogenital carcinomas. Skin cancers are the most common tumors, accounting for 38% of all malignancies. Factors that may predispose transplant recipients to skin cancers include copious sun exposure and therapy with azathioprine, possibly as a result of azathioprine's metabolite, nitroimidazole, which causes significant photosensitivity.[118] Azathioprine therapy is associated with a 2:1 predominance of squamous over basal cell carcinomas, whereas basal cell carcinoma occurs more frequently in the general population. Azathioprine-induced cutaneous squamous cell carcinoma is also associated with more metastatic disease and accounts for 6% of all deaths in comparison with less than 1% with cyclosporine. Patients must be encouraged to use effective techniques to reduce sun exposure.[118]

PTLD encompasses a broad spectrum of disorders, ranging from benign polyclonal hyperplasias to malignant monoclonal lymphomas. Factors that predispose patients to PTLD include Epstein-Barr virus seronegativity at transplantation and intense immunosuppression, particularly with OKT3 and antithymocyte globulin. Nonrenal transplantation recipients are more likely to develop PTLD secondary to the heavy immunosuppression used to reverse rejection. Administration of ganciclovir or acyclovir pre-emptively during antilymphocyte therapy may decrease the risk of eventual PTLD. Treatment of life-threatening PTLD generally includes severe reduction or cessation of immunosuppression. Other options include systemic chemotherapy or rituximab.[119]

Post-transplantation malignancies appear an average of 5 years after transplantation and increase with the length of followup. As many as 72% of patients surviving greater than 20 years may be affected. Malignancy accounts for 11.8% of deaths after cardiac transplantation and is the single most common cause of death in the sixth to the tenth post-transplant years.[113]

CONCLUSIONS

Transplantation is a lifesaving therapy for several types of end-organ failure. Advances in the understanding of transplant immunology have produced an unprecedented number of choices in terms of immunosuppression. The increasing number of effective immunosuppressive medications and therapies offer clinicians diverse ways to prevent allograft rejection in a patient-specific manner. However, the vast array and efficacy of currently available immunosuppressive agents make it increasingly difficult to evaluate their long-term efficacy. Clinicians must be keenly aware of the adverse effects of immunosuppressive medications and their treatment in order to optimize the care of the transplanted patient.

ABBREVIATIONS

6-MP: 6-mercaptopurine

ACEI: angiotensin-converting enzyme inhibitor

ATG: antithymocyte globulin

ATN: acute tubular necrosis

AUC: area under the concentration curve

C_2: concentration 2 hours after dose

C_{max}: peak concentration

CMV: cytomegalovirus

CYP: cytochrome P450 liver enzyme system

DGF: delayed graft function

FKBP: FK-binding protein

GI: gastrointestinal

HBIg: hepatitis B immunoglobulin

HIV: human immunodeficiency virus

HLA: human leukocyte antigen

HPLC: high-performance liquid chromatography

IL: interleukin
LDL: low-density lipoprotein
MELD: model for end-stage liver disease
MHC: major histocompatibility complex
MPA: mycophenolic acid
MPAG: mycophenolic acid glucuronide
mTOR: mammalian target of rapamycin
OKT3: muromonab-CD3
PRA: panel of reactive antibodies
PTDM: post-transplantation diabetes mellitus
PTLD: post-transplantation lymphoproliferative disorder
RIA: radioimmunoassay
t_{max}: time to peak concentration

REFERENCES

1. 2004 Annual Report of the U.S. Organ Procurement and Transplantation Network and the Scientific Registry of Transplant Recipients: Transplant Data 1994–2003. Rockville, MD: Department of Health and Human Services, Health Resources and Services Administration, Healthcare Systems Bureau, Division of Transplantation; Richmond, VA: United Network for Organ Sharing; Ann Arbor, MI: University Renal Research and Education Association.
2. Wiesner RH, Rakela J, Ishitani MB, et al. Recent advances in liver transplantation. Mayo Clin Proc 2003;78:197–210.
3. Pablo R, Ortega F, Baltar JM, et al. Health-related quality of life (HRQOL) of kidney transplanted patients: Variables that influence it. Clin Transplant 2000;14:199–207.
4. U.S. Renal Data System. USRDS 2004 Annual Data Report. Bethesda, MD: National Institutes of Health, National Institute of Diabetes and Digestive and Kidney Diseases, 2004.
5. Saab S, Wang V. Recurrent hepatitis C following liver transplant: Diagnosis, natural history and therapeutic options. J Clin Gastroenterol 2003;37:155–163.
6. Keck BM, Bennett LE, Rosendale J, et al. Worldwide Thoracic Organ Transplantation: A report from the UNOS/ISHLT International Registry for Thoracic Organ Transplantation. In: JM Cecka, PI Terasaki, eds. Clinical Transplants 1999. Los Angeles: UCLA Immunogenetics Center, 1999:35–49.
7. Merion RM, Magee JC. Renal transplantation. In: Greenfield LJ, ed. Surgery: Scientific Principles and Practice. Philadelphia: Lippincott Williams & Wilkins, 2001:568–576.
8. Campbell DA, Magee JC, Rudich SM, Punch JD. Hepatic transplantation. In: Greenfield LJ, ed. Surgery: Scientific Principles and Practice. Philadelphia: Lippincott Williams & Wilkins, 2001:577–597.
9. Pierson RN. Cardiac transplantation. In: Greenfield LJ, ed. Surgery: Scientific Principles and Practice. Philadelphia: Lippincott Williams & Wilkins, 2001:597–608.
10. Wolfe RA, Ashby VB, Milford EL, et al. Comparison of mortality in all patients on dialysis, patients on dialysis awaiting transplantation and recipients of a first cadaveric transplant. N Engl J Med 1999;341:1725–1730.
11. Hosenpud JD, Bennett LE, Keck BM, et al. The Registry of the International Society for Heart and Lung Transplantation: Fifteenth official report—1998. J Heart Lung Transplant 1998;17:656–668.
12. Venkataramanan R, Habucky K, Burckart GJ, et al. Clinical pharmacokinetics in organ transplant patients. Clin Pharmacokinet 1989;16:134–161.
13. Deng MC. Heart failure: Cardiac transplantation. Heart 2002;87:177–184.
14. Braith RW, Edwards DG. Exercise following heart transplantation. Sports Med 2000;30:171–192.
15. LeMoine A, Goldman M, Abramawicz D. Multiple pathways to allograft rejection. Transplantation 2002;73:1373–1381.
16. Mueller XM. Drug immunosuppressive therapy for adult heart transplantation. Part I. Immune response to allograft and mechanism of action of immunosuppressants. Ann Thorac Surg 2004;77:354–362.
17. Kobashigawa JA, Kirklin JK, Naftel DC, et al. Pretransplantation risk factors for acute rejection after heart transplantation: A multiinstitutional study. The Transplant Cardiologists Research Database Group. J Heart Lung Transplant 1993;12:355–366.
18. Stewart S, Winters GL, Fishbein MC, et al. Revision of the 1990 working formulation for the standardization of nomenclature in the diagnosis of heart rejection. J Heart Lung Transplant 2005;24:1710–1720.
19. Michaels PJ, Espejo ML, Kobashigawa J, et al. Humoral rejection in cardiac transplantation: Risk factors, hemodynamic consequences and relationship to transplant coronary artery disease. J Heart Lung Transplant 2003;22:58–69.
20. Hariharan S, Johnson CP, Bresnahan BA, et al. Improved graft survival after renal transplantation in the U.S., 1988 to 1996. N Engl J Med 2000;342:605–612.
21. Merville P. Combating chronic renal allograft dysfunction: Optimizing immunosuppressive regimens. Drugs 2005;65:615–631.
22. Behrendt D, Ganz P, Fang JC. Cardiac allograft vasculopathy. Curr Opin Cardiol 2000;15:422–429.
23. Eisen H, Ross H. Optimizing the immunosuppressive regiment in heart transplantation. J Heart Lung Transplant 2004;23(Suppl):S207–S231.
24. Vasquez EM, Benedetti E, Pollak R. Ethnic differences in clinical response to corticosteroid treatment of acute allograft rejection. Transplantation 2001;71:229–233.
25. Andreu J, Campistol JM, Oppenheimer F, et al. Cyclosporine monotherapy as primary immunosuppression in renal transplantation: Five-year experience. Transplant Proc 1994;26:337–340.
26. Squifflet JP, Vanrenterghem Y, van Hooff JP, et al. Safe withdrawal of corticosteroids or mycophenolate mofetil: Results of a large, prospective, multicenter, randomized study. Transplant Proc 2002;34:1584–1586.
27. Scott LJ, McKeage K, Keam SJ, Plosker GL. Tacrolimus: A further update of its use in the management of organ transplantation. Drugs 2003;63:1247–1297.
28. Laskow DA, Neylan JF III, Shapiro RS, et al. The role of tacrolimus in adult kidney transplantation: A review. Clin Transplant 1998;12:489–503.
29. Keogh A. Calcineurin inhibitors in heart transplantation. J Heart Lung Transplant 2004;23:S203–S206.
30. Vincenti F, et al. Tacrolimus (FK506) in kidney transplantation: Five-year survival results of the U.S. multicenter, randomized, comparative trial. Transplant Proc 2001;33:1019–1020.
31. Kahan BD. Cyclosporine. N Engl J Med 1989;321:1725–1738.
32. Lake KD, Canafax DM. Important interactions of drugs with immunosuppressive agents used in transplant recipients. J Antimicrob Chemother 1995;36:11–22.
33. Staatz CE, Tett SE. Clinical pharmacokinetics and pharmacodynamics of tacrolimus in solid organ transplantation. Clin Pharmacokinet 2004;43:623–653.
34. Jones TE. The use of other drugs to allow a lower dosage of cyclosporine to be used: Therapeutic and pharmacoeconomic considerations. Clin Pharmacokinet 1999;32:357–367.
35. Steeves M, Abdallah HY, Venkataramanan R, et al. In-vitro interaction of a novel immunosuppressant, FK506 and antacids. J Pharm Pharmacol 1991;43:574–577.
36. Mignat C. Drug interactions with new immunosuppressive agents. Drug Saf 1997;16:267–278.
37. van Gelder T. Drug interactions with tacrolimus. Drug Saf 2002;25:707–712.
38. Christians U, Jacobsen W, Benet LZ, Lampen A. Mechanisms of clinically relevant drug interactions associated with tacrolimus. Clin Pharmacokinet 2002;41:813–851.
39. Asberg A. Interactions between cyclosporine and lipid-lowering drugs: Implications for organ transplant recipients. Drugs 2003;63:367–378.
40. Gupta SK, Benet LZ. High-fat meals increase the clearance of cyclosporine. Pharm Res 1990;7:46–68.
41. Edwards DJ, Fitzsimmons ME, Schuetz EG, et al. 6,7-Dihydroxybergamottin in grapefruit juice and Seville orange juice: Effects on cyclosporine disposition, enterocyte CYP3A4 and *p*-glycoprotein. Clin Pharmacol Ther 1999;65:237–244.
42. Dumont RJ, Ensom MH. Methods for clinical monitoring on cyclosporine in transplant patients. Clin Pharmacokinet 2000;38:427–447.
43. Kuypers DRJ. Immunosuppressive drug monitoring—what to use in clinical practice today to improve renal graft outcome. Transpl Intl 2005;18:140–150.

44. Keown PA. New concepts in cyclosporine monitoring. Curr Opin Nephrol Hypertens 2002;11:61.
45. Olyaei AJ, de Mattos AM, Bennett WM. Immunosuppressant-induced nephropathy: Pathophysiology, incidence and management. Drug Saf 1999;21:471–488.
46. Rodicio JL. Calcium antagonists and renal protection from cyclosporine nephrotoxicity: Long-term trial in renal transplantation patients. J Cardiovasc Pharmacol 2000;35:S7–11.
47. Bush WW. Overview of transplantation immunology and the pharmacotherapy of adult solid organ transplant recipients: Focus on immunosuppression. AACN Clin Issues 1999;10:253–269.
48. Halloran PF. Immunosuppressive drugs for kidney transplantation. N Engl J Med 2004;351:2715–2729.
49. Bullingham RES, Nicholls AJ, Kamm BR. Clinical pharmacokinetics of mycophenolate mofetil. Clin Pharmacokinet 1998;34:429–455.
50. Weigel G, Griesmacher A, Karimi A, et al. Effect of mycophenolate mofetil therapy on lymphocyte activation in heart transplant recipients. J Heart Lung Transplant 2002;21:1074–1079.
51. Ciancio G, Miller J, Gonwa TJ. Review of major clinical trials with mycophenolate mofetil in renal transplantation. Transplantation 2005;80(2S):S191–S200.
52. The Mycophenolate Mofetil Acute Renal Rejection Study Group. Mycophenolate mofetil for the treatment of a first acute renal allograft rejection: Three-year follow-up. Transplantation 2001;71:1091–1097.
53. Wolfe EJ, Mathur V, Tomlanovich S, et al. Pharmacokinetics of mycophenolate mofetil and intravenous ganciclovir alone and in combination in renal transplant recipients. Pharmacotherapy 1997;17:591–598.
54. van Gelder T, Klupp J, Barten MJ, et al. Comparison of the effects of tacrolimus and cyclosporine on the pharmacokinetics of mycophenolic acid. Ther Drug Monit 2001;23:119–128.
55. Pescovitz MD, Conti D, Dunn J, et al. Intravenous mycophenolate mofetil: Safety, tolerability, and pharmacokinetics. Clin Transplant 2000;14:179–188.
56. Cox VC, Ensom MHH. Mycophenolate mofetil for solid organ transplantation: Does the evidence support the need for clinical pharmacokinetic monitoring? Ther Drug Monit 2003;25:137–157.
57. Shaw LM, Korecka M, Venkataramanan R, et al. Mycophenolic acid pharmacodynamics and pharmacokinetics provide a basis for rational monitoring strategies. Am J Transplant 2003;3:534–542.
58. Lancaster DL, Patel N, Lennard L, Lilleyman JS. 6-Thioguanine in children with acute lymphoblastic leukemia: Influence of food on parent drug pharmacokinetics and 6-thioquanine nucleotide concentrations. Br J Clin Pharmacol 2001;51:531–539.
59. Ingle GR, Sievers TM, Hold CD. Sirolimus: Continuing the evolution of transplant immunosuppression. Ann Pharmacother 2000;34:1044.
60. Kahan BD, Camardo JS. Rapamycin: Clinical results and future opportunities. Transplantation 2001;72:1181.
61. van Hooff JP, Squifflett JP, Wlodarczyk Z, et al. A prospective, randomized multicenter study of tacrolimus in combination with sirolimus in renal transplant recipients. Transplantation 2003;75:1934–1939.
62. Pham SM, Qi XS, Mallon SM, et al. Sirolimus and tacrolimus in clinical cardiac transplantation. Transplant Proc 2002;34:1839–1842.
63. Flechner SM, Goldfard D, Moldin C, et al. Kidney transplantation without calcineurin inhibitor drugs: A prospective, randomized trial of sirolimus versus cyclosporine. Transplantation 2002;74:1070–1076.
64. Kreis H, Cisterne JM, Land W, et al. Sirolimus in association with mycophenolate mofetil induction for the prevention of acute graft rejection in renal allograft recipients. Transplantation 2000;69:1252–1260.
65. Kahan BD. Efficacy of sirolimus compared with azathioprine for reduction of acute renal allograft rejection: A randomized multicentre study. Lancet 2000;356:194–202.
66. MacDonald AS. A worldwide, phase III, randomized, controlled, safety and efficacy study of a sirolimus/cyclosporine regiment for prevention of acute rejection in recipients of primary mismatched renal allografts. Transplantation 2001;71:271–280.
67. Oberbauer R, Kreis H, Johnson RWG, et al. Long-term improvement in renal function with sirolimus after early cyclosporine withdrawal in renal transplant recipients: 2-year results of the Rapamune maintenance regimen study. Transplantation 2003;76:364–370.
68. Ankersmit HJ, Roth G, Zuckermann A, et al. Rapamycin as rescue therapy in a patient supported by biventricular assist device to heart transplantation with consecutive ongoing rejection. Am J Transplant 2003;3:231–234.
69. Saunders RN, Metcalfe MS, Nicholson ML. Rapamycin in transplantation: A review of the evidence. Kidney Int 2001;59:3.
70. Kahan BD, Napoli KL, Kelly PA, et al. Therapeutic drug monitoring of sirolimus: Correlations with efficacy and toxicity. Clin Transplant 2000;14:97–109.
71. Chueh SCJ, Kahan BD. Dyslipidemia in renal transplant recipients treated with a sirolimus and cyclosporine-based immunosuppressive regimen: Incidence, risk factors, progression, and prognosis. Transplantation 2003;76:375–382.
72. Guilbeau JM. Delayed wound healing with sirolimus after liver transplant. Ann Pharmacother 2002;36:1391–1395.
73. van Gelder T, ter Meulen CG, Hené R, et al. Oral ulcers in kidney transplant recipients treated with sirolimus and mycophenolate mofetil. Transplantation 2003;75:788–791.
74. Kaplan B, Meier-Kriesche HU, Napoli KL, Kahan BD. The effects of relative timing of sirolimus and cyclosporine microemulsion formulation coadministration on the pharmacokinetics of each agent. Clin Pharmacol Ther 1998;63:48.
75. McAlister VC, Mahalati K, Peltekian KM, et al. A clinical pharmacokinetic study of tacrolimus and sirolimus combination immunosuppression comparing simultaneous to separated administration. Ther Drug Monit 2002;23:346–350.
76. Zimmerman JJ, Ferron GM, Lim HK, Parker V. The effect of a high-fat meal on the oral bioavailability of the immunosuppressant sirolimus (rapamycin). J Clin Pharmacol 1999;39:1155–1161.
77. Bunn D, Lea CK, Bevan DJ, et al. The pharmacokinetics of anti-thymocyte globulin (ATG) following intravenous infusion in man. Clin Nephrol 1996;45:29–32.
78. Webster AC, Pankhurst T, Rinaldi F, Chapman JR, Craig JC. Monoclonal and polyclonal antibody therapy for treating acute rejection in kidney transplant recipients: A systematic review of randomized trial data. Transplantation 2006;81:953–965.
79. Neuhaus P, Klupp J, Langrehr JM, et al. Quadruple tacrolimus-based induction therapy including azathioprine and ALG does not significantly improve outcome after liver transplantation when compared with standard induction with tacrolimus and steroids: Results of a prospective, randomized trial. Transplantation 2000;69:2343–2353.
80. Carrier M, White M, Perrault LP, et al. A 10-year experience with intravenous Thymoglobulin in induction of immunosuppression following heart transplantation. J Heart Lung Transplant 1999;18:1218–1223.
81. Marvin MR, Drogan C, Sawinski D, et al. Administration of rabbit antithymocyte globulin (Thymoglobulin) in ambulatory renal-transplant patients. Transplantation 2003;75:488–489.
82. Rahman GF, Hardy MA, Cohen DJ. Administration of equine anti-thymocyte globulin via peripheral vein in renal transplant recipients. Transplantation 2000;69:1958–1960.
83. Cibrik DM, Kaplan B, Meier-Kriesche H. Role of anti-interleukin-2 receptor antibodies in kidney transplantation. BioDrugs 2001;15:655–666.
84. Carswell CI, Plosker GL, Wagstaff AJ. Daclizumab: A review of its use in the management of organ transplantation. BioDrugs 2001;15:745–773.
85. Kovarik J, Breidenbach T, Gerveau C, et al. Disposition and immunodynamics of basiliximab in liver allograft recipients. Clin Pharmacol Ther 1998;64:66–72.
86. Adu D, Cockwell P, Ives NJ, et al. Interleukin-2 receptor monoclonal antibodies in renal transplantation: Meta-analysis of randomized trials. BMJ 2003;326:789–794.
87. Moser, MAJ. Options for induction immunosuppression in liver transplant recipients. Drugs 2002;62:995–1011.
88. Beniaminovitz A, Itescu S, Letiz K, et al. Prevention of rejection in cardiac transplantation by blockade of the interleukin-2 receptor with a monoclonal antibody (see comments). N Engl J Med 2000;342:613–619.
89. Strehlau J, Pape L, Offner G, et al. Interleukin-2 receptor antibody-induced alterations of ciclosporin dose requirements in paediatric transplant recipients. Lancet 2000;356:1327–1328.
90. Sifontis NM, Benedetti E, Vasquez EM. Clinically significant drug interaction between basiliximab and tacrolimus in renal transplant recipients. Transplant Proc 2002;34:1730–1732.
91. Stratta RJ, Alloway RR, Lo A, Hodge E. Two-dose daclizumab regimen in simultaneous kidney-pancreas transplant recipients: Primary end

point analysis of a multicenter, randomized study. Transplantation 2003;75:1260–1266.

92. Eckhoff DE, McGuire G, Sellers M, et al. The safety and efficacy of a two-dose daclizumab (Zenapax) induction therapy in liver transplant recipients. Transplantation 2000;69:1867–1872.
93. Wilde MI, Goa KL. Muromonab-CD3: A reappraisal of it pharmacology and use as prophylaxis of solid organ transplant rejection. Drugs 1996;51:865–894.
94. Bloom DD, Hu H, Fechner JH, Knechtle SJ. T-lymphocyte alloresponses of Campath-1H-treated kidney transplant patients. Transplantation 2006;81:81–87.
95. Morris PJ and Russell NK. Alemtuzumab (Campath-1H): A systematic review in organ transplantation. Transplantation 2006;81:1361–1367.
96. Calne R, Moffatt SD, Friend PJ, et al. Campath-IH allows low-dose cyclosporine monotherapy in 31 cadaveric renal allograft recipients. Transplantation 1999;68:1613.
97. Bostom AD, Brown RS, Chavers BM, et al. Prevention of post-transplant cardiovascular disease: Report and recommendations of an ad hoc group. Am J Transplant 2002;2:491–500.
98. Zhang R, Leslie B, Boudreaux P, et al. Hypertension after kidney transplantation: Impact, pathogenesis and therapy. Am J Med Sci 2003;325:202–208.
99. Moore R, Hernandez D, Valantine H. Calcineurin inhibitors and post-transplant hyperlipidemias. Drug Saf 2001;24:755–766.
100. Textor SC, Taler SJ, Canzanello VJ, Schwartz L. Cyclosporine, blood pressure and atherosclerosis. Cardiol Rev 1997;5:141–151.
101. Ventura HO, Malik FS, Mehra MR, et al. Mechanisms of hypertension in cardiac transplantation and the role of cyclosporine. Curr Opin Cardiol 1997;12:375–381.
102. Chobanian AV, Bakris GL, Black HR, et al. The seventh report of the Joint National Committee on Prevention, Detection, Evaluation, and Treatment of High Blood Pressure: The JNC 7 report. JAMA 2003:289;2560–2572.
103. Tylicki L, Habicht A, Watchinger B, Hörl WH. Treatment of hypertension in renal transplant recipients. Curr Opin Urol 2003;13:91–98.
104. Kasiske B, Cosio FG, Beto J, et al. Clinical practice guidelines for managing dyslipidemias in kidney transplant patients: A report from the managing dyslipidemias in chronic kidney disease work group of the national kidney foundation kidney disease outcomes quality initiative. Am J Transplant 2004;4 Suppl 7:13–53.
105. Executive Summary of the Third Report of the National Cholesterol Education Program (NCEP). Expert Panel on Detection, Evaluation, and Treatment of High Blood Cholesterol in Adults (Adult Treatment Panel III). JAMA 2001;285:2486–2497.
106. Mach F. Statins as immunomodulators. Transpl Immunol 2002;9:197–200.
107. Kotanko P, Kirisits W, Skrabal F. Rhabdomyolysis and acute renal graft impairment in a patient treated with simvastatin, tacrolimus, and fusidic acid [letter]. Nephron 2002;90:234–235.
108. Jindal RM, Sidner RA, Milgrom ML. Post-transplant diabetes mellitus: The role of immunosuppression. Drug Saf 1997;16:242–257.
109. Reisæter AV, Hartmann A. Risk factors and incidence of post-transplant diabetes mellitus. Transplant Proc 2001;33:8–18S.
110. Fishman JA, Rubin RH. Infection in organ-transplant recipients. N Engl J Med 1998;338:1741–1751.
111. Thaler SJ, Rubin RH. Opportunistic infections in the cardiac transplant patients. Curr Opin Cardiol 1996;11:191–203.
112. Sagedal S, Hartmann A, Rollag H. The impact of early cytomegalovirus infection and disease in renal transplant recipients. Clin Microbiol Infect 2005;11:518–530.
113. Higgins RM, Bloom SL, Hopkin JM, Morris PJ. The risks and benefits of low-dose cotrimoxazole prophylaxis for *Pneumocystis* pneumonia in renal transplantation. Transplantation 1989;47:558–560.
114. de Bruyn G and Limaye AP. BK-virus associated nephropathy in kidney transplant recipients. Rev Med Virol 2004;14:193–205.
115. Kazory A and Ducloux D. Renal transplantation and polyomavirus infection: Recent clinical facts and controversies. Transpl Infect Dis 2003;5:65–71.
116. Fredrick RT, Hassanein TI. Role of growth facotors in the treatment of patients with HIV/HCV coinfection and patients with recurrent hepatitis C following liver transplantation. J Clin Gastroenterol 2005;39:S14-S22.
117. Roche B, Samuel D. Treatment of hepatitis B and C after liver transplantation. Part 2 hepatitis C. Transpl Int 2005;17:759–766.
118. Penn I. Post-transplant malignancy: The role of immunosuppression. Drug Saf 2000;23:101–113.
119. Berney T, Delis S, Kato T, et al. Successful treatment of post-transplant lymphoproliferative disease with prolonged rituximab treatment in intestinal transplant recipients. Transplantation 2002;74:1000–1006.

SECTION 12
RHEUMATOLOGIC DISORDERS

CHAPTER 93

Osteoporosis and Other Metabolic Bone Diseases

MARY BETH O'CONNELL AND SHERYL F. VONDRACEK

KEY CONCEPTS

1. Postmenopausal women, men older than age 65 years, and those with potential disease- or drug-induced bone loss should be assessed for osteoporosis. Patients with premature or severe osteoporosis should be evaluated for secondary causes of bone loss.
2. Central bone densitometry can determine bone mass, predict fracture risk, and influence patient and provider treatment decisions. Portable equipment can be used for screening in the community to determine the need for further testing.
3. Vitamin D insufficiency and deficiency, which sometimes causes osteomalacia, can be insidious and coexist with osteoporosis. A serum 25(OH) vitamin D concentration should be obtained in patients with decreased oral vitamin D intake, limited or no sun exposure, or unexplained muscle weakness or pain.
4. All people, regardless of age, should incorporate a bone-healthy lifestyle beginning at birth, which emphasizes regular exercise, nutritious diet, tobacco avoidance, minimal alcohol use, and fall prevention to prevent and treat osteoporosis.
5. The adequate intake for calcium in American adults is 1,000 to 1,500 mg of elemental calcium daily in divided doses from diet or supplements. The adequate intake for American adults, especially seniors, is 600 to 1,000 units of vitamin D daily from mainly supplements, with some experts recommending even higher doses.
6. Bisphosphonates decrease vertebral, hip, and nonvertebral fractures and are considered the drug of choice for osteoporosis treatment.
7. Raloxifene is an alternative treatment option to prevent vertebral fractures, particularly in women who cannot tolerate, should not, or will not take bisphosphonates. Postmenopausal women at high risk for breast cancer might choose this medication to obtain dual actions.
8. Male osteoporosis is often secondary to specific diseases and drugs and responds well to a bone-healthy lifestyle, bisphosphonate therapy, and in some cases, testosterone replacement.
9. Patients taking chronic oral glucocorticoids (e.g., rheumatoid arthritis, cystic fibrosis, transplantation, bowel disorders, cancer) need to be identified and started on a bone-healthy lifestyle, higher doses of calcium and vitamin D, and bisphosphonate therapy to prevent or treat osteoporosis.
10. Patients with certain diseases such as gastrectomy, celiac disease, inflammatory bowel disease, and organ transplantation, or taking medications known to influence vitamin D and/or bone metabolism should be evaluated for disease and drug induced osteopenia and osteoporosis.

Learning objectives, review questions, and other resources can be found at **www.pharmacotherapyonline.com.**

Osteoporosis is a major public health threat for an estimated 44 million Americans, or 55% of the people 50 years of age and older.[1] In the United States, 8 million women and 2 million men are estimated to have the disease. Osteoporosis is defined as a "skeletal disorder characterized by compromised bone strength predisposing a person to an increased risk of fracture."[2] The development of osteoporosis and osteoporotic fractures is multifactorial, beginning with genetics and unhealthy bone lifestyles, along with other skeletal factors, which lead to compromised bone strength, and nonskeletal factors that lead to falls (Fig. 93–1). President Clinton declared 2002 to 2011 to be the Decade of the Bone and Joint. To coincide with this initiative, the Surgeon General released a report in 2004 on Bone Health and Osteoporosis, providing information, challenges, and opportunities for change.[3] Healthcare practitioners must take an active role in educating people of all ages and healthcare providers on healthy bone habits and osteoporosis treatment options.

EPIDEMIOLOGY

Osteopenia (low bone mass), osteoporosis, and osteoporotic fractures are very common and affect all ethnic groups. Almost 34 million Americans are estimated to have low bone mass (osteopenia),[1]

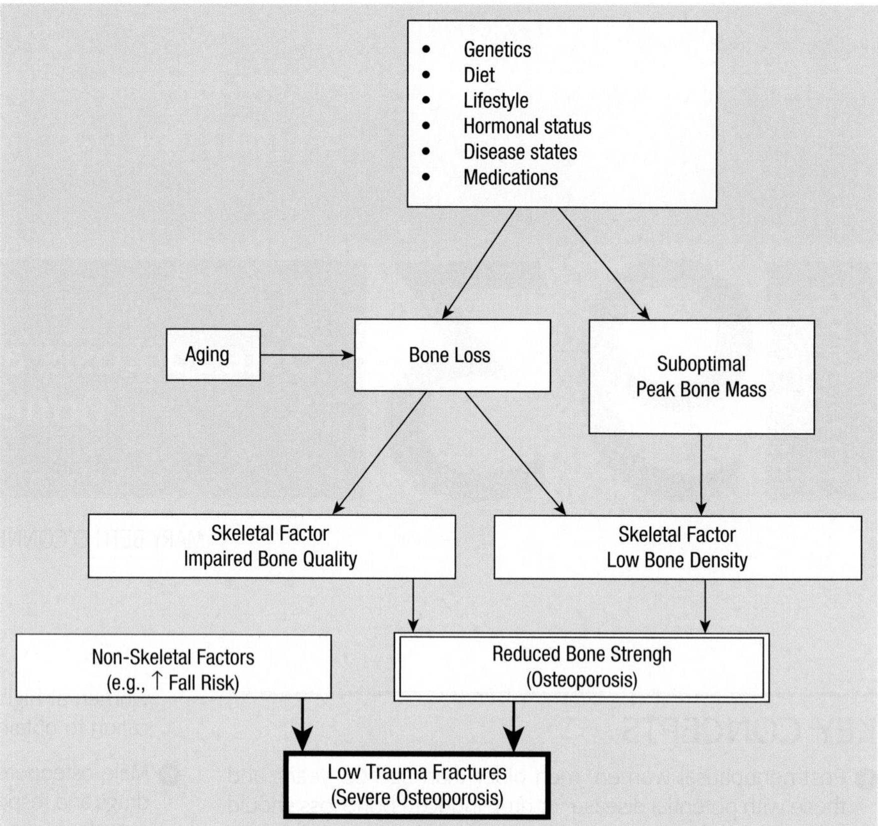

FIGURE 93-1. Etiology of osteoporosis.

including 50% of Asian, 47% of Hispanic, 45% of Native American, 40% of white, and 28% of black women.[4] Osteoporosis affects 12% of Native American, 10% of Asian, 10% of Hispanic, 7% of white, and 4% of black women. Disease prevalence greatly increases with age; from 4% in women 50 to 59 years of age to 44% to 52% in women 80 years of age and older.[5,6] Fragility or low trauma wrist and vertebral fractures are common throughout adulthood, whereas hip fractures are more common in seniors. Fracture incidence was estimated to be 2 million (71% in women, 29% in men) in 2005, with an estimated total medical cost of $17 billion.[7] Fractures in women accounted for 75% of the costs and in seniors 87% of the costs. Hip fractures represented 72% of these costs. Forecasting predicts 3 million fractures at a cost of $25 billion in 2025. In a women's lifetime, hip fracture risk is 17% for whites, 14% for Hispanics, and 6% for African Americans.[5] In a man's lifetime, hip fracture risk is 6% to 11%.[8]

BONE PHYSIOLOGY

Bone is made of collagen and mineral components. The collagen component gives bone its flexibility and energy-absorbing capability.[9] The mineral component gives bone its stiffness and strength. The correct balance of these substances is needed for bone to adequately accommodate to stress and strain and resist fractures. Imbalances can impair bone quality and lead to reduced bone strength.

Bone strength reflects the integration of bone quality and bone mineral density (bone mass). Bone mass increases rapidly throughout childhood and adolescence. Ninety percent of peak bone mass is attained by age 18 to 20 years, with small gains until approximately age 30 years. Peak bone mass is highly dependent on genetic factors that account for approximately 60% to 80% of the variability.[5,10,11] The remaining 20% to 40% is influenced by modifiable factors such as nutritional intake (e.g., calcium, vitamin D, and protein), exercise, adverse lifestyle practices (e.g., smoking), hormonal status, and certain diseases and medications. Optimizing peak bone mass is important for preventing osteoporosis. The higher the peak bone mass, the more bone one can lose before being at an increased fracture risk.

The skeleton is composed of mostly cortical bone (80%) with some trabecular bone (20%), which varies by bone site. The forearm is predominantly cortical bone (95%), the spine is predominantly trabecular bone (66% to 75%), and the femoral neck of the hip and wrist are mostly cortical bone (50% to 75%, respectively).[12] Of note, trabecular bone has a 5 to 10 times higher metabolic turnover rate than cortical bone.

Bone remodeling is a dynamic process that occurs continuously throughout life. One to two million tiny sections of bone are in the process of remodeling at any given time. The complete physiology of bone remodeling is not fully known but appears to begin with signals from lining cells or osteocytes (bone communication cells) that are triggered by stress, microfractures, biofeedback systems, and potentially certain diseases and medications (Fig. 93–2, step 1).[12,13] Many cytokines, growth factors, and hormones influence each remodeling step. A major stimulus for hematopoietic stem cell (monocyte–macrophage lineage) differentiation to become mature osteoclasts (bone resorbing cells) is the receptor activator of nuclear factor kappa B ligand (RANKL), which is emitted from the osteoblast (bone-forming cells) in step 2. RANKL also stimulates mature osteoclast activation and bone adherence via integrins to resorb bone. Proteinases are secreted to resorb the protein matrix, and hydrogen ions are secreted to dissolve the mineralized component (step 3). After bone is resorbed and a cavity is created, additional cytokines and growth factors are released that first mature osteoblasts from mesenchymal stem cells and then stimulate osteoblast bone formation (step 4). Mature osteoblasts produce osteoprotegerin (OPG) that binds (step 4) to RANKL, thereby stopping bone resorption.

Bone formation occurs over two phases. First, osteoblasts fill the resorption cavity with osteoid and then mineralization occurs (step 5). Once bone formation is complete, mature osteoblasts undergo

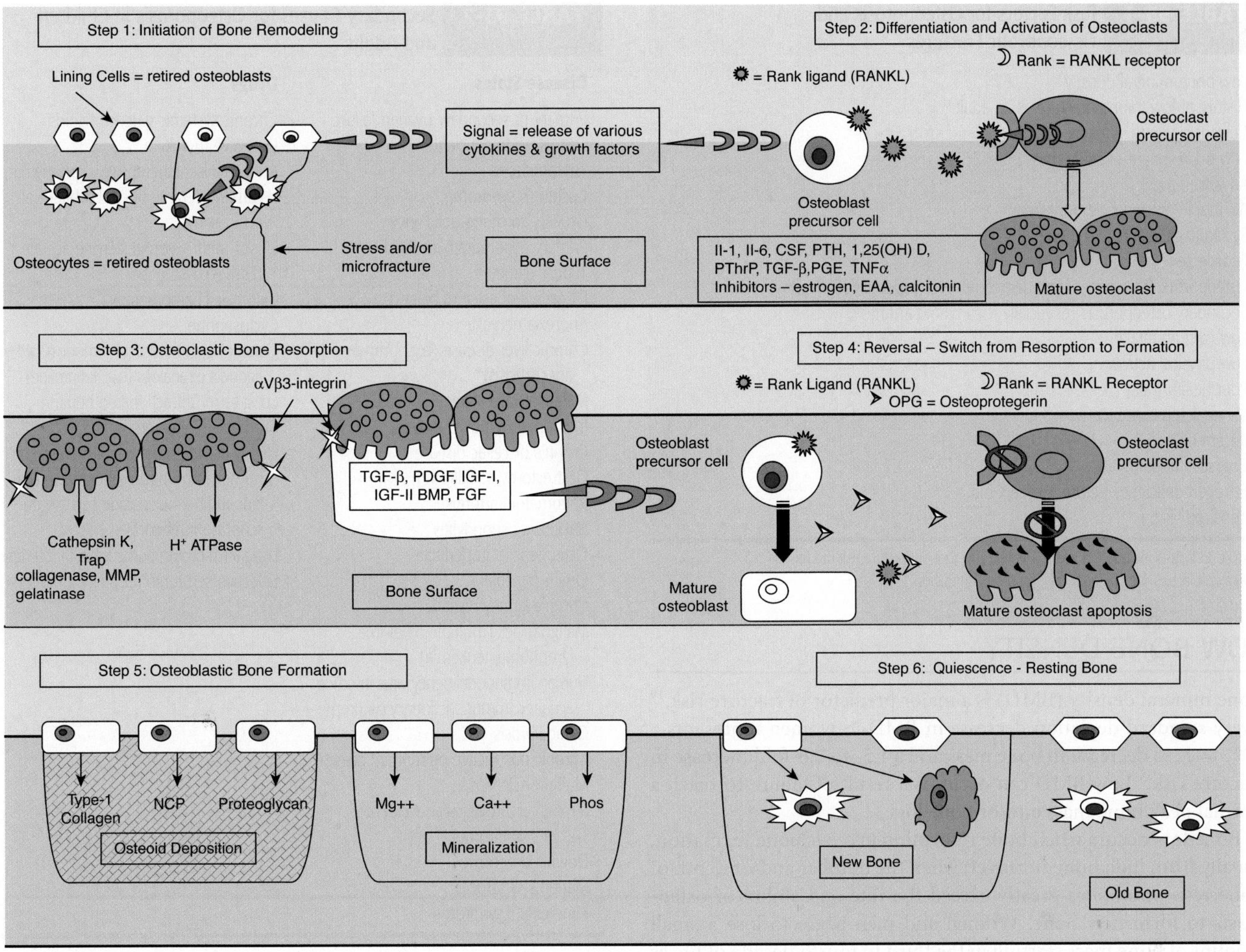

FIGURE 93-2. Bone remodeling cycle.[12,13] (1α,25(OH)D_2, calcitriol/1,25(OH)$_2$ vitamin D; BMP, bone morphogenetic protein; Ca, calcium; CSF, colony-stimulating factors; EAA, estrogen agonist/antagonist; FGF, fibroblast growth factor; IGF, insulin-like growth factor; Il, interleukin; Mg, magnesium; MMP, matrix metalloproteases; NCP, noncollagenous proteins; OPG, osteoprotegerin; PDGF, platelet-derived growth factor; PG, prostaglandin; Phos, phosphorous; PTH, parathyroid hormone; PTHrP, parathyroid hormone-related protein; SERM, selective estrogen receptor modulator; TGF, transforming growth factor; TNF, tumor necrosis factor; Trap, tartrate-resistant acid phosphate.)

apoptosis or become lining cells or osteocytes (step 6). Quiescence is the phase when bone is at rest until another remodeling cycle is initiated at that site.

Estrogen has many positive effects on the bone remodeling process, with most of its actions helping to maintain a normal bone resorption rate. Estrogen suppresses the proliferation and differentiation of osteoclasts and increases osteoclast apoptosis. Estrogen decreases the production of several cytokines that are potent stimulators of osteoclasts including interleukins 1 and 6, and tumor necrosis factor-α. Estrogen also decreases the production of RANKL and increases the production of OPG; both of which reduce osteoclastogenesis.[14]

VITAMIN D, PARATHYROID HORMONE, AND CALCIUM

Vitamin D and parathyroid hormone (PTH) maintain calcium homeostasis.[15] The most abundant source of vitamin D is the endogenous production from exposure to ultraviolet B light. The sun's ultraviolet B light converts 7-dehydrocholesterol in the skin to cholecalciferol (vitamin D_3). Maximal skin production occurs within 20 minutes for whites and 60 to 120 minutes for blacks or darker-skin individuals.[16] Dietary vitamin D sources include cholecalciferol and ergocalciferol (vitamin D_2). Subsequent conversion of cholecalciferol and ergocalciferol to 25-hydroxyvitamin D [25(OH) D] (calcidiol) occurs in the liver and then PTH stimulates conversion of 25(OH) D via 25(OH) D-1α-hydroxylase to its final active form, 1α,25-dihydroxyvitamin D (calcitriol), in the kidney.[15] Calcitriol binds to the intestinal vitamin D receptor and then increases calcium binding protein. As a result, calcium and phosphorous intestinal absorption is increased. Vitamin D receptors are also found in many tissues, such as bone, intestine, brain, heart, stomach, pancreas, lymphocytes, skin, and gonads.

Calcium absorption under normal conditions is approximately 30% to 40%, decreasing to 10% to 15% with low vitamin D concentrations.[15] Calcium absorption is predominantly rate limited through vitamin D controlled intestinal transport with less than 23% absorbed through passive paracellular diffusion, which is not rate limited.[17] Elevated PTH concentrations secondary to hypocalcemia increase kidney calcitriol production and calcium reabsorption by the kidney. PTH concentrations also increase when vitamin D concentration falls below around 30 ng/mL, the minimum normal therapeutic vitamin D concentration.[18] Sometimes the increased fractional calcium absorption is insufficient and thus bone resorption is needed. Together, PTH and calcitriol increase osteoclast activity, thereby releasing calcium from bone to restore calcium homeostasis.

ETIOLOGY

❶ Figure 93–1 depicts a model describing the etiology of osteoporosis and fractures. Table 93–1 lists risk factors for osteoporosis and Table 93–2 lists secondary causes.

TABLE 93-1 Risk Factors for Osteoporosis and Osteoporotic Fractures

Low bone mineral density[a]
History of low trauma fracture as an adult[a,b]
Current cigarette smoking[a,b]
Low body weight or body mass index[a,b]
Advanced age[a]
Alcohol in amounts >2 drinks/day[a]
Systemic glucocorticoid therapy[a]
Female sex
Osteoporotic fracture in a first-degree relative (especially hip fracture)[a,b]
Secondary osteoporosis (especially rheumatoid arthritis[a])
Low calcium intake
Low physical activity
Poor health/frailty
Minimal sun exposure
Recent falls
Cognitive impairment
Estrogen deficiency before 45 years old
Impaired vision

[a]Proposed factors included in World Health Organization fracture risk model.
[b]Major risk factors per National Osteoporosis Foundation.

LOW BONE DENSITY

Bone mineral density (BMD) is a major predictor of fracture risk.[19] Every standard deviation decrease in BMD in women represents a 10% to 12% decrease in bone mass and a 1.5- to 2.6-fold increase in fracture risk.[5] Low BMD can occur as a result of failure to reach a normal peak bone mass and/or bone loss.

Bone loss occurs when bone resorption exceeds bone formation, usually from high bone turnover; when the number and/or depth of bone resorption sites greatly exceed the rate and ability of osteoblasts to form new bone. Women and men begin to lose a small amount of bone mass starting in the third to fourth decade of life as a consequence of a slight reduction in bone formation.[9] During perimenopause and for up to 5 to 7 years after menopause, women can experience an accelerated rate of bone loss because of the drop in circulating estrogen and an increase in bone resorption. The rate and duration of loss can vary greatly, with up to 3% to 5% of bone density lost per year, and can differ depending on the skeletal site measured. Seniors steadily lose bone mass at approximately 0.5% to 1% per year as a consequence of an accelerated rate of bone remodeling combined with reduced bone formation.

The major factors (see Tables 93–1 and 93–2) influencing bone losses are hormonal status, exercise, aging, nutrition, lifestyle, disease states, medications, and some genetic influences. Nonhormonal risk factors are similar between women and men.

IMPAIRED BONE QUALITY

In addition to BMD, the strength of bone is highly impacted by the quality of the bone's material properties and its structure.[9] For example, accelerated bone turnover can result in bone loss, but also can impair bone quality and the structural integrity of bone by increasing the quantity of immature bone that is not yet adequately mineralized. Bone quality assessment is important because changes in bone quality effect bone strength much more than bone mass changes. Future osteoporosis diagnostic testing will assess both bone quality and density.

FALLS

Although up to 50% of vertebral fractures can occur spontaneously with minimal to no trauma, most wrist fractures and greater than 90% of hip fractures result from a fall from standing height or less.[20]

TABLE 93-2 Secondary Causes for Osteoporosis in Children and Adults

Disease States	Drugs
Primary or secondary ovarian failure	Chronic systemic glucocorticoids
Testosterone deficiency	Excessive thyroxine
Thyrotoxicosis	Anticonvulsant therapy (e.g., phenytoin, carbamazepine, phenobarbital, valproic acid)
Cushing's syndrome	Depot medroxyprogesterone acetate (DMPA)
Growth hormone deficiency	Cytotoxic chemotherapy
Primary hyperparathyroidism	Cyclosporine
Type 1 diabetes	Gonadotropin-releasing hormone (GnRH) agonists or analogs (e.g., leuprolide)
Disorders of calcium balance	Long-term unfractionated heparin
Anorexia nervosa	Aromatase inhibitors
Chronic liver disease (e.g., primary biliary cirrhosis)	Highly-active antiretroviral therapy for human immunodeficiency virus (e.g., zidovudine, nucleoside reverse transcriptase inhibitors)
Malabsorptive states	Long-term proton pump inhibitor therapy
Inflammatory bowel disease	Selective serotonin reuptake inhibitors
Crohn's or celiac disease	
Gastrectomy or Billroth I	
Rheumatoid arthritis	
Ankylosing spondylitis	
Osteogenesis imperfecta	
Organ transplant	
Chronic kidney disease	
Malignancies (multiple myeloma, lymphoma, leukemia)	
Human immunodeficiency virus infection/acquired immunodeficiency syndrome	
Cystic fibrosis	
Chronic obstructive pulmonary disease	
Multiple sclerosis	
Stroke/cerebrovascular accident	
Turner's syndrome	
Down's syndrome	
Marfan's syndrome	
Klinefelter's syndrome	

One-third to one-half of all seniors fall each year with 50% falling more than once. Up to 5% of all falls will result in a fracture. In 2003, more than 1.8 million seniors were treated in the emergency department, and more than 400,000 were hospitalized for a fall-related injury.

Risk of falling increases with advanced age predominantly as a result of balance, gait, and mobility problems, poor vision, reduced muscle strength, impaired cognition, multiple medical conditions (e.g., stroke, Alzheimer's dementia, Parkinson's disease), and polypharmacy. Psychoactive medications such as benzodiazepines, antidepressants, antipsychotics, sedative hypnotics, and narcotics have been strongly associated with falls. The ability to adapt to falls also decreases with aging. Seniors are more likely to sustain a hip or pelvic fracture because they tend to fall backwards or sideways instead of forward.

PATHOPHYSIOLOGY

Osteoporosis pathophysiology depends on gender, age, and presence of secondary causes.

POSTMENOPAUSAL OSTEOPOROSIS

The accelerated bone loss during perimenopause and postmenopause results from enhanced resorption mainly as a result of the loss in ovarian hormone production, specifically estrogen. Estrogen deficiency increases proliferation, differentiation, and activation of new osteoclasts and prolongs survival of mature osteoclasts.[14] The number of remodeling sites increases and resorption pits are deeper and inadequately filled by normal osteoblastic function. Significant bone density is lost and bone architecture is compromised. Trabecular bone is most susceptible leading to vertebral and wrist fractures.

MALE OSTEOPOROSIS

Men are at a lower risk for developing osteoporosis and osteoporotic fractures because of larger bone size, greater peak bone mass, and fewer falls.[21] Men also do not undergo a period of accelerated bone resorption similar to menopause. However, men have a higher mortality rate after fractures.

The etiology of male osteoporosis tends to be multifactorial with secondary causes (see Table 93–2) and aging being the most common contributing factors. In young and middle-age men, a secondary cause for bone loss is usually identified, with hypogonadism being the most common. Idiopathic osteoporosis (no known cause) can occur and is probably a result of genetic factors that have yet to be determined.

AGE-RELATED OSTEOPOROSIS

Age-related osteoporosis occurs in seniors mainly as a result of hormone, calcium, and vitamin D deficiencies leading to an accelerated bone turnover rate in combination with reduced osteoblast bone formation. Hip fracture risk rises dramatically in seniors as a consequence of the cumulative loss of cortical and trabecular bone and an increased risk for falls.

SECONDARY CAUSES OF OSTEOPOROSIS

1 A secondary cause (see Table 93–2) is identified in more than half of premenopausal and perimenopausal women, about one-third of postmenopausal women, and more than two-thirds of men.[22] The two most common secondary causes for osteoporosis are vitamin D deficiency and glucocorticoid therapy, which are discussed in Osteomalacia and Glucocorticoid-Induced Osteoporosis sections later. A potential drug-induced cause of bone loss in premenopausal women is depot medroxyprogesterone acetate (DMPA or Depo-Provera), a long-acting progestin-only contraceptive injection. This drug contains a "black box" warning based on data from several studies that demonstrated significant bone loss or impaired bone mass accrual.[23] Some women will recover some or all bone loss after discontinuation, especially if the agent has been used for a short time. Although more information is needed to fully understand the risks associated with depot medroxyprogesterone acetate, more than 2 years' use warrants consideration of BMD testing using central dual-energy x-ray absorptiometry (DXA).

CLINICAL PRESENTATION

Table 93–3 outlines the clinical presentation of osteoporosis.

Osteoporosis is diagnosed by BMD measurement or presence of a low trauma fracture. Two-thirds of patients with a vertebral fracture are asymptomatic or attribute mild lower back pain to "old age." The other third present with moderate to severe back pain that radiates down their leg after a new vertebral fracture. The pain usually subsides significantly after 2 to 4 weeks; however, residual chronic lower back pain may persist. Multiple vertebral fractures decrease height and sometimes curve the spine (kyphosis or lordosis) with or without significant back pain. Patients who have experienced a nonvertebral fracture frequently present with severe pain, swelling, and reduced function and mobility at the fracture site.

TABLE 93-3 Clinical Presentation of Osteoporosis

General
- Many patients are unaware they have osteoporosis and only present after fracture
- Fractures can occur after bending, lifting, or falling, or independent of any activity

Symptoms
- Pain
- Immobility
- Depression, fear, and low self-esteem from physical limitations and deformities
- Two-thirds of vertebral fractures are asymptomatic

Signs
- Shortened stature (>1.5" loss), kyphosis, or lordosis
- Vertebral, hip, wrist, or forearm fracture
- Low bone density on radiography

Laboratory tests
- Routine tests to detect a possible secondary cause: complete blood count, liver function tests, creatinine, urea nitrogen, calcium, phosphorous, alkaline phosphatase, albumin, thyroid-stimulating hormone, free testosterone, 25(OH) vitamin D, and 24-hour urine concentrations of calcium and phosphorous.
- Urine or serum biomarkers (e.g., NTX, osteocalcin) are sometimes used, especially to determine if high bone turnover exists. Additional testing might be necessary if the patient's history, physical examination, or the initial investigation suggests a specific secondary cause.

Other diagnostic tests
- Spine and hip bone-density measurement using DXA
- Radiograph to confirm vertebral fracture

DXA, dual-energy x-ray absorptiometry; NTX, N-terminal crosslinking telopeptide of type 1 collagen.

CONSEQUENCES OF OSTEOPOROSIS

A fragility or low-trauma fracture is defined as one that occurs as a result of a fall from standing height or less or with minimal to no trauma. The most common osteoporosis-related fractures are those of the vertebrae, proximal femur, and distal radius (wrist or Colles fracture).[24] Fractures of the face, skull, fingers, and toes are typically not considered osteoporosis-related. Osteoporotic fractures can lead to increased morbidity and mortality and decreased quality of life. Depression is common because of fear, pain, loss of self-esteem from physical deformity, and loss of independence and mobility.

Symptomatic vertebral fractures can cause significant pain, physical deformity, and adverse health consequences. Patients with severe kyphosis can experience respiratory problems as a result of compression of the thoracic region and gastrointestinal complications, such as poor nutrition, from intraabdominal compression. Women and men who suffer a symptomatic vertebral fracture have a lower 5-year survival rate compared to those without a fracture history.

Wrist fractures occur more commonly in younger postmenopausal women and are frequently a result of a fall on an outstretched hand. Negative outcomes include prolonged pain and weakness, and decreased advanced activities of daily living (such as cooking and shopping).

Hip fractures are associated with the greatest increase in morbidity and mortality. In 1999, hip fractures resulted in approximately 340,000 hospital admissions.[25] After a hip fracture, only 33% to 40% of patients regain their ability to perform basic activities of daily living, while 20% become nonambulatory. Three to 4% of patients die during the initial hospitalization for hip fracture, and 14% to 36% will die within 1 year either from complications of the hip fracture or other comorbid disease processes. Men have a twofold higher 1-year mortality rate after hip fracture than women.

Once a low-trauma fracture has occurred, the risk for subsequent fractures goes up exponentially. In subjects with one clinical vertebral fracture, the chance of experiencing any new fracture was 2.8-fold higher, and with two or more vertebral fractures it was 12-fold higher, than for subjects who did not have baseline fractures.[26]

PATIENT ASSESSMENT

Bone pain, postural changes (i.e., kyphosis), and loss of height are simple useful physical examination findings. Height loss greater than

1.5 inches from the tallest mature height is considered significant and warrants further investigation. Height should be routinely measured using a wall-mounted stadiometer. A spine radiograph can confirm vertebral fractures. Low bone density or osteopenia reported on routine radiographs requires an evaluation for osteoporosis. In addition to physical examination and laboratory studies (see Table 93–3), patients can be assessed with risk factor assessment, osteoporosis questionnaires, peripheral and central DXA, and biomarkers.

RISK FACTOR ASSESSMENT

The aim of an initial fracture risk assessment (see Table 93–1) is to identify those patients who are at highest risk for low bone density and who would benefit from further evaluation. Many risk factors for osteoporosis have been identified and are similar for both sexes. The majority of risk factors are predictors of either low BMD (e.g., female gender, ethnicity) or an increased fall risk (e.g., cognitive impairment, previous falls). The most important risk factors are those associated with fracture risk independent of BMD and fall risk. These major risk factors, in combination with BMD, are used to determine which patient will benefit most from pharmacologic intervention. Current smoker, low body weight (<127 lb in postmenopausal women), history of osteoporotic fracture in a first-degree relative, and personal history of low-trauma fracture as an adult are all considered major risk factors by the National Osteoporosis Foundation.[27] Other identified independent risk factors include age, high bone turnover, low body mass index (<19 kg/m^2), rheumatoid arthritis, and glucocorticoid use.

RISK ASSESSMENT TOOLS

Several clinical predication tools help clinicians determine who should undergo BMD testing. The Osteoporosis Risk Assessment Instrument (ORAI) decision tool for postmenopausal women is based on age range, weight range, and current estrogen therapy, with high sensitivity (93%) but low specificity (61%). The Simple Calculated Osteoporosis Risk Estimation (SCORE) decision tool, also for postmenopausal women, assesses race, rheumatoid arthritis, use of estrogen therapy (ever), number of osteoporotic fractures, age, and weight, with a sensitivity and specificity similar to that of the Osteoporosis Risk Assessment Instrument. Both the Osteoporosis Risk Assessment Instrument and Simple Calculated Osteoporosis Risk Estimation performed well when compared to other prediction rules.[28,29] Other tools are the Osteoporosis Self-Assessment Tool, Osteoporosis Self-Assessment Tool for Asians, and the FRACTURE index.

A fracture prediction model is being developed by the World Health Organization (WHO) to determine which patients would benefit most from therapy, not to determine which patient should undergo BMD testing.[29] The WHO model uses the following risk factors: age, previous fracture, family history of hip fracture, body mass index, glucocorticoid use (ever), current smoking, alcohol use >2 units/day, and rheumatoid arthritis with or without BMD to predict an individual's percent absolute probability of fracturing in the next 10 years.

SCREENING USING PERIPHERAL BONE MINERAL DENSITY DEVICES

❷ Peripheral bone density devices that utilize x-ray absorptiometry or quantitative ultrasonometry are helpful as screening tools to determine which patients require further evaluation with central DXA. They should not be used for diagnosis or monitoring response to therapy. Peripheral DXA of the forearm, heel, and finger uses a low amount of radiation. Heel quantitative ultrasonometry uses sound waves without radiation or need for specialty training. Because peripheral devices are considerably less expensive than central DXA, easy to use, portable, fast (<5 minutes), and can predict general fracture risk, they are very popular for screening patients at health fairs, community pharmacies, and clinics.[30] No guidelines specifically address who should undergo peripheral bone density screening.[31] However, the best population to screen is younger postmenopausal women without major risk factors for osteoporosis. A low peripheral BMD value for postmenopausal women would warrant further testing. The specific T-score threshold for referral is not universally defined and varies by device.[31] Healthy premenopausal women and patients already identified as being at high risk for osteoporosis based on risk factors, fragility fracture, or secondary causes for osteoporosis, should not be screened but rather referred to a physician for central DXA testing.

CLINICAL CONTROVERSY

The use of peripheral BMD screenings for older men and perimenopausal women with risk factors for osteoporosis is controversial. Data supporting fracture risk predication with these devices are either lacking or not as robust in older men and perimenopausal women. The T-score thresholds for referral in these populations are unknown. In addition, many peripheral devices do not have a male reference database. More data are needed on the predictive value of peripheral screening devices in these populations before routine use.

CENTRAL DUAL-ENERGY X-RAY ABSORPTIOMETRY

❷ BMD measurements at the hip or spine can be used to assess fracture risk, establish the diagnosis and severity of osteoporosis, and sometimes confirm osteoporosis as causative for low-trauma fractures. Central DXA is considered the gold standard for measuring BMD because of its high precision, short scan times, low radiation dose (comparable to the average daily dose from natural background), and stable calibration. Measurement of both lumbar spine and proximal femur or total hip BMD are recommended with the lowest BMD value used for diagnosis. Newer methods, such as micromagnetic resonance imaging, are undergoing investigation to provide measurements of bone quality in addition to bone density.

❶ ❷ Several consensus guidelines or position statements are available that discuss which women should undergo central DXA.[5,27,32,33] Most are consistent in recommending central BMD testing for all senior women aged 65 years or older, postmenopausal women younger than 65 years of age with risk factors for fracture, women with a low-trauma fracture, and women with an identified secondary cause for bone loss. The United States Preventive Services Task Force recommends screening all senior women and women 60 to 64 years of age who are at increased risk for osteoporotic fractures.[34] The International Society for Clinical Densitometry recommends central BMD testing using a male database in all men older than age 70 years, men with a history of a low-trauma fracture as an adult, and men with an identified secondary cause for bone loss.[35] Ethnic-specific reference databases are not recommended at this time. In the absence of a suspected or known secondary cause for osteoporosis or a history of a low trauma fracture, central BMD testing is not recommended for premenopausal or perimenopausal women.

A central DXA BMD report provides the actual bone density value, T-score, and Z-score. The actual bone density value (g/cm^2) is most useful for serial monitoring of drug therapy response. The T-score is a comparison of the patient's measured BMD to the mean BMD of a healthy, young (20- to 29-year-old), sex-matched white reference population. The T-score is the number of standard deviations from the mean of the reference population. The Z-score compares the patient's BMD to the mean BMD for a healthy, sex, and age-matched white population and is usually low when secondary causes of osteoporosis are present.

LABORATORY TESTS

Laboratory testing (see Table 93–3) is used to identify secondary causes of bone loss. If a preliminary investigation indicates a possible secondary cause, additional testing might be needed.

❸ Serum 25(OH) D is the best indicator of total body vitamin D status.[15] Data suggest that serum 25(OH) D concentrations of at least 30 ng/mL are necessary to maximize intestinal calcium absorption, minimize secondary hyperparathyroidism, and reduce fracture risk.[15,36] Osteomalacia can occur at concentrations less than 8 to 10 ng/mL.[18] Although no consensus exists, a reasonable definition for vitamin D deficiency can be considered a 25(OH) D concentration of ≤10 ng/mL, insufficiency as a concentration between 11 and 29 ng/mL, and sufficiency as ≥30 ng/mL (1 ng/mL = 2.5 nmol/L).

Vitamin D insufficiency and deficiency are common in all age groups, especially in seniors and individuals who are malnourished, living in an institution (e.g., nursing home), or living in extreme northern latitudes.[15,18,36] Low vitamin D concentrations result from insufficient intake, decreased sun exposure, decreased skin production, or decreased liver and renal metabolism. Endogenous synthesis of vitamin D can be decreased by factors that impact exposure to or decrease skin penetration of ultraviolet B light. Sunscreen use, full body coverage with clothing (e.g., women wearing veiled dress), and darkly pigmented skin can all cause a decrease in vitamin D production. Seasonal variations in vitamin D concentrations are also seen with nadirs in late winter and peaks in late summer.

Because vitamin D assays are expensive and large interlab assay variability exists, routine vitamin D screening cannot be recommended.[15] A 25(OH) D concentration should be considered in anyone at high risk for vitamin D deficiency (e.g., seniors with minimal sun exposure, insufficient intake, dark pigmented skin), low bone density, history of a low-trauma fracture or frequent falls, on medications known to affect vitamin metabolism, or with a history of unexplained muscle and/or bone pain.[15]

BONE TURNOVER MARKERS

Urine and serum bone turnover markers are either enzymes or proteins produced during bone formation or breakdown. Bone-specific alkaline phosphatase, osteocalcin and procollagen type 1 propeptides are examples of bone formation markers. Hydroxypyridinium crosslinks of collagen pyridinoline and deoxypyridinoline, C-terminal crosslinking telopeptide of type 1 collagen and N-terminal crosslinking telopeptide of type 1 collagen are examples of bone resorption markers. Increased concentrations of bone resorption markers (≥2 standard deviations above the premenopausal range) have been shown in some studies to predict fracture risk; however, results have been inconsistent.[19] Although not diagnostic, these tests my be helpful in identifying accelerated bone turnover and increased fracture risk or in monitoring response to therapy.

DIAGNOSIS OF OSTEOPOROSIS

The diagnosis of osteoporosis is based on a low-trauma fracture or central hip and/or spine DXA using WHO T-score thresholds. Osteopenia or low bone mass is a T-score of −1 to −2.4 and osteoporosis is a T-score at or below −2.5. Although these definitions are based on data from postmenopausal white women, they are applied to other racial/ethnic groups and senior men. The International Society for Clinical Densitometry recommends the presence of risk factors in addition to a low T-score before the diagnosis of osteoporosis can be made in men ages 50 to 65 years.

PREVENTION AND TREATMENT

Osteoporosis

Osteoporosis prevention and treatment begins with a bone-healthy lifestyle and uses nonprescription and prescription medications as needed.

■ DESIRED OUTCOMES

The primary goal of osteoporosis management should be prevention. Optimizing skeletal development and peak bone mass accrual in childhood, adolescence, and early adulthood will ultimately reduce the future incidence of osteoporosis. Once osteopenia or osteoporosis develops, the objective is to stabilize or improve bone mass and strength and prevent fractures. In patients who have already suffered osteoporotic fractures, reducing future falls and fractures, improving functional capacity, reducing pain and deformity, and improving quality of life are the main goals.

■ GENERAL APPROACH TO PREVENTION AND TREATMENT

A bone-healthy lifestyle should begin at birth and continue throughout life. Insuring adequate intakes of calcium and vitamin D along with other bone healthy lifestyle practices are the first steps in prevention and treatment. Prescription medication use for osteopenia (T-score −1 to −2.4) remains controversial. The National Osteoporosis Foundation recommends considering prescription therapy in any postmenopausal woman with a T-score less than −2.0 or less than −1.5 if they have one or more major osteoporosis risk factors.[27] Prescription medications, with bisphosphonates being the drug of choice, are recommended for men and women with osteoporosis (T-score of −2.5 or lower or presence of low-trauma fracture). Figure 93–3 provides an osteoporosis management algorithm that incorporates both nonpharmacologic and pharmacologic approaches.

■ NONPHARMACOLOGIC THERAPY

Nonpharmacologic therapy, referred to as bone-healthy lifestyle changes, includes diet, smoking cessation, exercise, fall prevention, and hip protectors.

Diet

❹ Overall, a diet well balanced in nutrients and minerals is important for bone health. In addition, limiting intakes of caffeine, alcohol, sodium, cola, and other carbonated beverages.

Although results are conflicting, excessive caffeine consumption is associated with increased calcium excretion, increased rates of bone loss, and a modest increased risk for fracture.[37] Ideally, caffeine consumption should be limited to two servings or less per day. Moderate caffeine intake (two to four servings per day) should not be a concern if adequate calcium intake is achieved daily. For excessive caffeine use, intake should be decreased. Alcohol consumption in moderation is not associated with an increased risk for osteoporosis or fractures. Excessive alcohol intake can increase risk because of poor nutrition, impaired calcium and vitamin D metabolism, and an increased risk for falls. According to 2005 dietary guidelines, alcohol consumption should not exceed one drink per day for women and two drinks per day for men.[38]

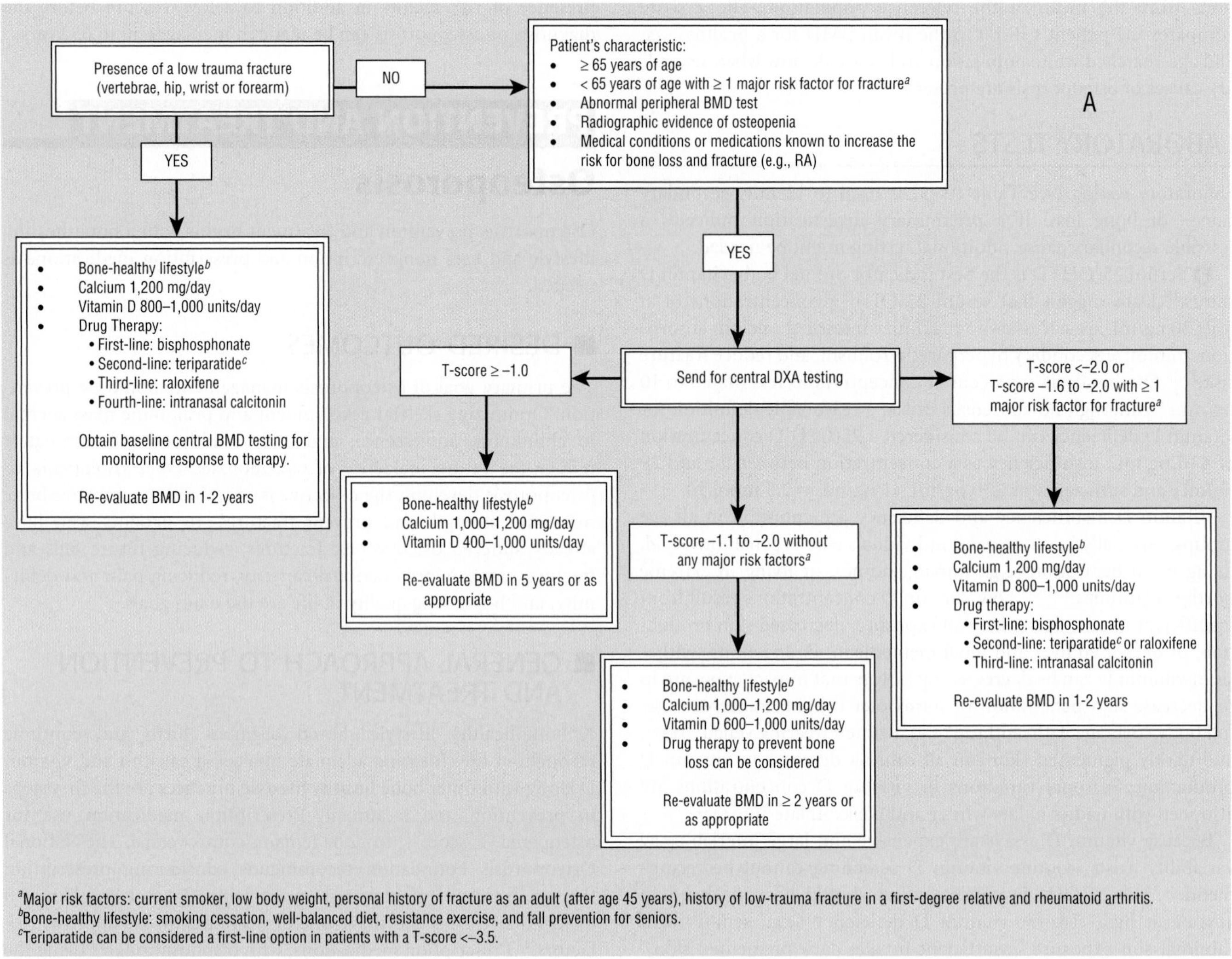

FIGURE 93-3. Algorithm for the management of osteoporosis in postmenopausal women (*A*) and men (*B*). (BMD, bone mineral density; DXA, dual-energy x-ray absorptiometry, RA, rheumatoid arthritis.)

Sodium intake increases calcium excretion.[39] In patients with low intakes of calcium, excessive sodium intake can lead to increased bone resorption and lower BMD. To minimize calcium loss secondary to increased sodium intake, an individual can consume higher amounts of daily calcium and potassium and decrease sodium intake to <2.4 g/day.

Consumption of cola beverages with or without caffeine is associated with decreased BMD and increased fracture risk; however, data are conflicting.[40] Caffeine and phosphoric acid content of cola beverages might cause bone loss by altering calcium balance. This effect is compounded by decreased milk consumption with a consequent reduction in calcium intake and simultaneous increased carbonated beverage intake in the United States.[41]

Calcium ❹ ❺ Data clearly indicate that adequate calcium intake is necessary for the development of bone mass during growth and for its maintenance throughout life. Adequate calcium intake is an essential component of all osteoporosis prevention and treatment strategies.

Table 93–4 summarizes the recommended adequate intakes for calcium based on age. Achieving daily calcium requirements from calcium-containing foods, which also contain other essential nutrients, is preferred (Table 93–5). Some food sources are absorbed well but have low elemental calcium content (e.g., broccoli), or contain oxalic acid (e.g., spinach) or phytic acid (e.g., wheat bran) that bind calcium within the food and decrease its absorption.[42] Approximately 25% of the U.S. population has some level of lactose intolerance, with the incidence in Asian (80%) and African American (50%) populations being much higher than in whites (10%).[42] For lactose-intolerant patients, lactose-reduced milk, lactose-free milk, yogurt with active cultures or Lactaid, along with other nondairy calcium-fortified products (e.g., orange juice, breakfast cereals, and energy bars) can be recommended.

Vitamin D ❹ ❺ Table 93–4 lists the Institute of Medicine's adequate intakes for Vitamin D.[43] The National Osteoporosis Foundation guidelines recommend 800 to 1,000 units vitamin D daily for adults age 50 years and older.[27] Several experts believe at least 800 to 2,000 units of vitamin D daily are needed, especially in seniors.[18] The three main sources of vitamin D are sunlight, diet, and supplements. Because few foods are naturally high or fortified with vitamin D (Table 93–6), most people, especially seniors, require supplementation.

Other Nutrients and Minerals Vitamin K is a cofactor for carboxylation (activation) of proteins, such as osteocalcin, which are involved in bone formation.[18,39,44] Several studies have demonstrated that vitamin K deficiency can contribute to bone loss and an increased risk for fractures.[44] Data suggest that the current recommended adequate intakes for vitamin K might be too low for optimal bone health.[44] More data are needed before recommending routine supplementation.

Minimal to no data exist for other nutrients and minerals such as boron and magnesium.[45] Until more data are available, taking a

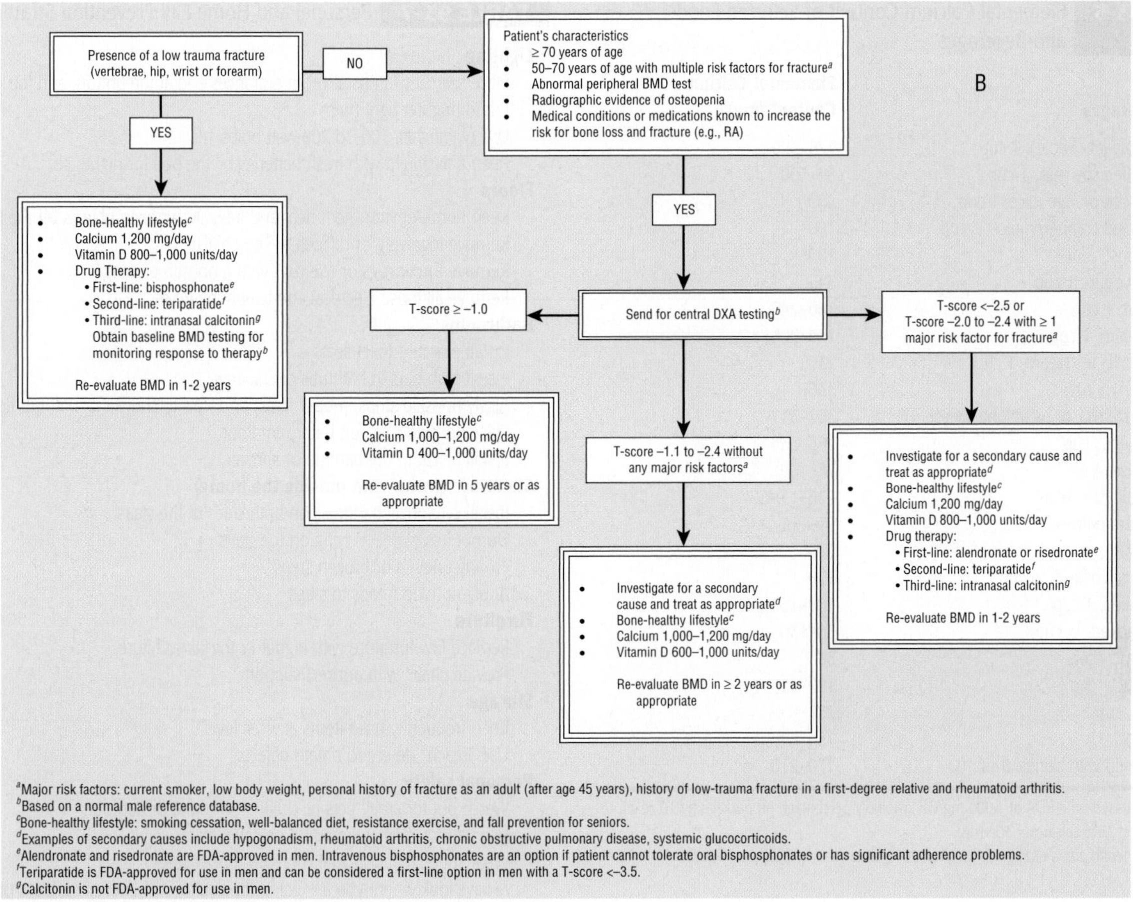

FIGURE 93-3. *(Continued)*

multivitamin once daily and consuming a healthy diet, following the United States Department of Agriculture food pyramid recommendations for daily fruit and vegetable intake, should provide an adequate intake of these vitamin and minerals for general bone health.

Protein Dietary protein represents a key nutrient for bone health.[46] High protein intakes (especially animal protein) were thought to be detrimental to bone health by increasing urinary calcium excretion. However, evidence suggests that low protein intakes increase osteoporosis risk and that higher protein intakes are protective against bone loss and fractures. The increased calciuria seen with higher intakes of protein is more likely an indicator of an increased absorption of dietary calcium rather than increased bone resorption as proposed.

TABLE 93-4 Calcium and Vitamin D Recommendations

	Institute of Medicine Adequate Intake	
Group and Ages	***Elemental Calcium (mg)[a]***	***Vitamin D (units)[a,b]***
Infants		
Birth to 6 months	210	200
6–12 months	270	200
Children		
1–3 years	500	200
4–8 years	800	200
9–13 years	1,300	200
Adolescents/young adults		
14–18 years	1,300	200
Adults		
19–30 years	1,000	200
31–50 years	1,000	200
51–70 years	1,200	400
>70 years	1,200	600

[a]U.S. Institute of Medicine of the National Academy of Sciences recommends no more than 2500 mg/day elemental calcium and 2000 units/day vitamin D.
[b]Most experts believe the recommended Adequate Intakes for Vitamin D are too low.

Dietary Soy Isoflavone phytoestrogens are plant-derived compounds that possess weak estrogenic agonist and antagonist effects. The most common source for isoflavone is dietary soy products. Genistein is the most abundant and biologically active isoflavone in soybeans. The evidence supporting a positive bone benefit from soy protein (isoflavone) intake is conflicting, with some positive data with larger isoflavone intakes (76 mg daily).[47] In the Chinese diet, higher soy protein intake was significantly associated with a lower risk of fractures, especially within 10 years of menopause and in women taking at least 21 mg isoflavone per day.[48] Since isoflavones are safe, patients can be encouraged to increase their intake, but true benefits on fracture are not clear.

Smoking Cessation

❹ Counseling patients of all ages on smoking cessation can help to optimize peak bone mass, minimize bone loss, and ultimately reduce fracture risk. Cigarette smoking is an independent risk factor for osteoporosis and is associated with up to an 80% increased relative risk for hip fracture.[49] The effect is dose and duration dependent. A decrease in sex hormone concentrations, reduced intestinal calcium absorption, a direct toxic effect on osteoblasts, and detrimental effects of smoking on neurovascular function have been implicated for the negative bone effects.

Exercise

❹ Physical activity or exercise is an important nonpharmacologic approach to preventing osteoporotic fractures. Exercise can decrease

TABLE 93-5 Elemental Calcium Content of Selected Foods and Beverages

Foods/Beverages	Elemental Calcium Content (mg)[a]
Milk (skim, low-fat, whole), 1 cup	276–309
Calcium-fortified soy milk, 1 cup	80–300
Calcium-fortified orange juice, 1 cup	300
Calcium-fortified cranberry juice, 1 cup	100
7UP Plus, 1 cup	100
Low-fat fruit yogurt, 1 cup	345
Frozen yogurt, 1 cup	180–240
Vanilla ice cream, 1 cup	176–200
Soft-serve vanilla ice cream, 1 cup	236
Swiss cheese, 1.5 oz.	336
Cheddar, mozzarella, or provolone cheese, 1.5 oz.	307–311
Ricotta cheese, 1/2 cup	255–335
Cottage cheese, 4 oz.	78–100
Fortified breakfast cereals	236–1,043
Fortified instant oatmeal	99–110
Figs, dried, 10	270
Collard greens, cooked, 1/2 cup	178
Broccoli, cooked, 1 cup	100–180
Soybeans, cooked, 1/2 cup	88–130
Okra, cooked, 1/2 cup	88
Bok choy, raw, 1 cup	160–250
Tofu, firm, 1/2 cup	253
Almonds, 1 oz.	75
Salmon, canned with bones, 3 oz.	170–210

[a]Food labels are based on a RDA of 1,000 mg/day; multiply percentage on package by 10 (e.g., product containing 30% calcium = 300 mg).
Data from www.health.gov/dietaryguidelines/dga2005/document/html/appendixB.htm.

the risk of falls and fractures by improving muscle strength, coordination, balance, and mobility. Physical activity is especially important early in life as lack of exercise during growth can lead to suboptimal loading/straining, decreased stimulation of bone deposition, and a subsequently reduced peak bone mass. All patients who are medically fit should be encouraged to perform a moderate-intensity weight-bearing activity (e.g., walking, jogging, golf, stair climbing) for at least 30 minutes most days of the week and a resistance activity (e.g., weight machines, free weights, or elastic bands) at least twice per week for 20 to 30 minutes.[3,27,38]

Fall Prevention

❹ Because of the link between falls and fractures, homes should be made safe and potentially harmful medications eliminated.[3,5] Table 93–7 provides solutions for commonly observed personal and home safety problems.[50] Medication profiles should be reviewed for any medications that can affect cognition and balance and potentially

TABLE 93-6 Vitamin D Content of Selected Foods and Beverages

Foods/Beverages	Vitamin D (international units)[a]
Salmon, 3.5 oz	360
Mackerel, 3.5 oz	345
Tuna fish, canned in oil, 3 oz	200
Sardines, canned in oil, 1.75 oz	250
Cow's milk (all forms), 1 cup	100
Vitamin D fortified orange juice	100
Ready-to-eat-cereal (fortified), 1 cup	40
Margarine, 1 tablespoon	60
Egg, 1 whole (or egg yolk)	20
Liver, beef, cooked, 3.5 oz	15

[a]Food labels are based on a RDA of 400 units/day; multiply percentage on package by 4 (e.g., product containing 20% vitamin D = 80 units).
Data from http://dietary-supplements.info.nih.gov/factsheets/vitamind.asp.

TABLE 93-7 Personal and Home Fall Prevention Strategies

Lighting
Place switches/lamps at room entrances and at the bottom and top of stairs
Put in brighter light bulbs
Use nightlights, 100- to 200-watt bulbs
Keep a flashlight with fresh batteries by the bed for night use
Floors
Keep home environment neat and tidy; always keep objects off the floor
Remove low-lying or difficult-to-see objects
Remove throw rugs or use rugs with a nonslip backing
Remove all loose electrical and telephone wires
Bathrooms
Install elevated toilet seats
Install grab bars in bathtubs or showers
Apply nonskid strips, rubber mats, or decals to shower or bathtub floor
Place nonskid mats on bathroom floor
Install a seat in the bathtub or shower
Stairways (inside and outside the home)
Install cylindrical handrails on both sides of the stairs
Do not leave objects lying on the stairs
Fix any uneven or broken steps
Apply nonskid treads to steps
Furniture
Replace low furniture with higher or thicker furniture
Provide chairs with armrest support
Storage
Keep frequently used items at waist level
Use "reach" device to obtain objects
Personal safety
Watch out for small pets or children in home or outdoors
Use handrails when going up or down stairs
Wear shoes that grip well (nonskid rubber soles)
Always look where you are going (be cautious of uneven surfaces or icy spots)
Clean up spills immediately so you do not slip
Rise slowly from a seated position
Visit ophthalmologist annually (ensure adequate vision correction)
Exercise regularly to improve strength, balance, and coordination

Modified from reference 50. Also available in Spanish and Chinese.

increase fall risk and that are unneeded or can be replaced with a safer alternative. Maintenance of a regular exercise program, such as Tai Chi, should be recommended to improve body strength, balance, and agility.

Hip Protectors

External hip protectors are specialized undergarments designed to pad the area surrounding the hip decreasing the force of impact from a sideways fall. Conflicting results and poor adherence limit their use.[5,51]

■ PHARMACOLOGIC THERAPY

Because nonpharmacologic interventions alone frequently are insufficient to prevent or treat osteoporosis, drug therapy is often necessary. Table 93–8 describes fracture and BMD effects and Table 93–9 describes important aspects of common osteoporosis medications. These medications should always be combined with a bone-healthy lifestyle.

Drug Treatments of First Choice

Currently, bisphosphonates are the prescription drug of choice with teriparatide, raloxifene, and calcitonin considered alternative agents. Duration of bisphosphonate therapy has not been defined, but safety data exist for periods of 7–10 years.[52] Short-term (18 to 24 months) teriparatide is used for severe osteoporosis and then followed by bisphosphonate therapy. The algorithm (see Fig. 93–3) helps determine for whom drug therapy should be used. Osteoporosis prescrip-

TABLE 93-8 Fracture and Bone Mineral Density Effects of FDA-Indicated Osteoporosis Medications in Postmenopausal Women[a]

Product	Vertebral Fracture Reduction *Absolute Risk/Relative Risk*	Nonvertebral Fracture Reduction *Absolute Risk/Relative Risk*	Hip Fracture Reduction *Absolute Risk/Relative Risk*	Lumbar Spine BMD	Femoral Neck BMD	Ref
Bisphosphonates						5,58,59
Alendronate	1.7%–3.7%/44%–48%	1.5%–2.8%/12%–21%	0.2%–1.1%/21%–51%	8.8%	5.9%	
Ibandronate (oral)	4.9%/38%	NS	NS	5.2%	4.1%	
Risedronate	4%–11%/41%–65%	3.2%–5.1%/33%–39%	1.3%/40%[b]	4.3%	2.8%	
Zoledronic acid (IV)	7.6%/70%	2.7%/25%	1.1%/41%	6.7%	5.1%	
Raloxifene	2.2%–6.5%/30%–50%	NS	NS	2.6%	2.1%	5,58,68
Calcitonin	8%/33%	NS	NS	3%	NS	5,58
Teriparatide	9.3%/65%	2.9%/53%	NS	6%–14%	1.5%–3.5%	5,58,78
Estrogen[c]	NA/36%[d]	0.53%/29%	0.07%/35%	7.1%	1.8%	72
Estrogen with progestin[e]	NA/35%[d]	0.47%/25%	0.05%/33%	7.6%	3.7%	71

BMD, bone mineral density; NA, not available; NS, not significant; Ref, reference.

[a]Only the pivotal trials with daily oral or yearly intravenous therapy were powered for fracture evaluation. Fracture data not available for weekly, monthly, and quarterly oral bisphosphonate therapy. For estrogen and estrogen/progestin, only the Women's Health Initiative Trials were used.

[b]Only seen in women 70 to 79 years old, not those ≥80 years old.

[c]Conjugated equine estrogen 0.625 mg daily.

[d]Only clinical vertebral fracture data given.

[e]Conjugated equine estrogen 0.625 mg and medroxyprogesterone 2.5 mg daily.

tion medications in children and pre- and perimenopausal women are controversial and undergoing further investigation.

Published Guidelines and Treatment Protocols

Osteoporosis diagnosis and treatment guidelines exist but none are universally accepted. Two North American guidelines are evidence based: the 2003 update of the American Association of Clinical Endocrinologists evidence-based guidelines for prevention and treatment of postmenopausal osteoporosis and the 2002 Canadian osteoporosis guidelines for women, men, and special populations.[33,53] The 2006 North American Menopause Society's position statement used both evidence and consensus to develop recommendations on the management of postmenopausal osteoporosis.[5] In 2003, the National Osteoporosis Foundation updated its consensus guidelines for postmenopausal women.[27] The National Institutes of Health held an osteoporosis consensus conference in 2001 and published the findings, recommendations, and research needs.[2] Guidelines are being updated to reflect newer diagnostics (e.g., WHO fracture risk assessment), agents (e.g., teriparatide), and monitoring (e.g., biomarkers, osteonecrosis of the jaw). Subspecialty guidelines continue to be developed (e.g., osteoporosis and gastrointestinal [GI] diseases, rheumatology and glucocorticoid-induced osteoporosis). Based on these guidelines and newer information, an algorithm reflecting current suggested practice is presented (see Fig. 93–3). Even with guidelines and algorithms, many patients are neither being evaluated nor receiving appropriate osteoporosis therapy.[54]

Antiresorptive

Antiresorptive therapies include calcium, vitamin D, bisphosphonates, estrogen agonists/antagonists (known previously as selective estrogen receptor modulators or SERMs), and calcitonin.

Calcium Supplementation ❺ Calcium imbalance can result from inadequate dietary intake, decreased fractional calcium absorption, or enhanced calcium excretion. Adequate calcium intake (see Table 93–4) is considered the minimal standard for osteoporosis prevention and treatment and should be combined with vitamin D and osteoporosis medications when needed. Supplemental calcium intake (Table 93–10) will be needed in the majority of people with or at risk for osteoporosis as survey data indicate that the average U.S. diet contains only 600 mg calcium per day.[42]

Efficacy. Although calcium increases BMD, fracture prevention is minimal. More than 150 studies have evaluated calcium's effect on BMD with almost all trials and observational studies showing that higher calcium intake in children and adults produced greater increases or maintenance of BMD compared to BMD losses with placebo.[17] Calcium's BMD effects are less than other antiresorptive and formation osteoporosis medications. If fracture prevention was documented, concomitant vitamin D therapy was usually given. Nonbone benefits of calcium intake include decreased

TABLE 93-9 Medications Used to Prevent and Treat Osteoporosis

Drug	Adult Dosage	Pharmacokinetics	Adverse Effects	Drug Interactions
Calcium	Adequate intake (Table 93–4) in divided doses	Absorption—predominantly active transport with some passive diffusion, fractional absorption 10%–60%, fecal elimination for the unabsorbed and renal elimination for the absorbed calcium	Constipation, gas, upset stomach, rare kidney stones	Carbonate salts—decreased absorption with proton pump inhibitors Decrease absorption of iron, tetracycline, quinolones, bisphosphonates, phenytoin, and fluoride when given concomitantly Might antagonize verapamil Might induce hypercalcemia with thiazide diuretics Fiber laxatives (variable), oxalates, phytates, and sulfates can decrease calcium absorption if given concomitantly

(continued)

TABLE 93-9 Medications Used to Prevent and Treat Osteoporosis (continued)

Drug	Adult Dosage	Pharmacokinetics	Adverse Effects	Drug Interactions
D_3 (cholecalciferol)	Adequate intake (Table 93-4); if malabsorption or multiple anticonvulsants might require higher doses (~ ≥4,000 or more units daily)	Hepatic metabolism to 25(OH) vitamin D and then renal metabolism to active compound $1,25(OH)_2$ vitamin D, other active and inactive metabolites	Hypercalcemia, (weakness, headache, somnolence, nausea, cardiac rhythm disturbance), hypercalciuria	Phenytoin, barbiturates, carbamazepine, rifampin increase vitamin D metabolism
D_2 (ergocalciferol)	For vitamin D deficiency, 50,000 units once weekly or once monthly; dosed dependent on serum calcium			Cholestyramine, colestipol, orlistat, or mineral oil decrease vitamin D absorption
$1,25(OH)_2$ vitamin D (calcitriol, Rocaltrol PO, Calcijex IV)	0.25–0.5 mcg orally or 1–2 mcg/mL intravenously daily for renal osteodystrophy, hypoparathyroidism, and refractory rickets			Might induce hypercalcemia with thiazide diuretics in hypoparathyroid patients
Oral bisphosphonates		Poorly absorbed–<1% decreasing to zero with food or beverage intake–long $T_{1/2}$ (<10 years); renal elimination (of absorbed) and fecal elimination (unabsorbed)	Nausea; heartburn; GI pain, irritation, perforation, ulceration, and/or bleeding; transient flu-like illness; muscle pains; black box warning for rare osteonecrosis of the jaw	Do not coadminister with any other medication or supplements (including calcium and vitamin D)
Alendronate (Fosamax, Fosamax plus D)	5 mg daily, 35 mg weekly (prevention) 10 mg daily, 70 mg tablet, 70 mg tablet with vitamin D 2,800 or 5,600 units, or 75 mL liquid weekly (treatment)			
Risedronate (Actonel)	5 mg daily, 35 mg weekly, 75 mg on two consecutive days once monthly 150 mg monthly, 3 mg intravenous quarterly			
Intravenous bisphosphonates			Muscle pains, transient flu-like illness, redness or swelling at injection site, black-box warning for rare osteonecrosis of the jaw	
Ibandronate (Boniva)	5 mg intravenous infusion yearly			
Zoledronic acid[a] (Reclast)				
Mixed estrogen agonist/antagonist		Hepatic metabolism	Hot flushes, leg cramps, venous thromboembolism, peripheral edema, rare cataracts and gallbladder disease; black box warning for fatal stroke	None
Raloxifene (Evista)	60 mg daily			
Calcitonin (Miacalcin)	200 units intranasal daily, alternating nares every other day	Renal elimination 3% nasal availability	Rhinitis, epistaxis	None
Teriparatide (1–34 units, Forteo)	20 mcg subcutaneously daily for up to 2 years	95% bioavailability T_{max} ~30 minutes $T_{1/2}$ ~60 minutes Hepatic metabolism	Pain at injection site, nausea, dizziness, leg cramps, rare increase in uric acid, slightly increased calcium	None
Testosterone products		10% gel absorption (5 mg absorbed from 50 mg testosterone in 5 g of gel)	Weight gain, acne, hirsutism, dyslipidemia, hepatic consequences, gynecomastia, priapism, prostate disorders, testicular atrophy, sleep apnea, and skin reactions with patches	
Transdermal patch (Testoderm TTS, Androderm, Testim)	5 mg patch applied to arm, back, or thigh every evening (patches 2.5, 4, 5, & 6 mg)[a]			
Testoderm (R) with or without adhesive)	6 mg applied to scrotal skin every evening			
Gel (AndroGel 1%, Testim 1%)	5 gm gel applied to shoulder, upper arm, or abdomen every morning			
Buccal system (Striant 30 mg)	Place one system in gum area twice a day. Alternate sides of mouth. Do not crush or swallow			
Injection				
Cypionate (100 or 200 mg/mL) or enanthate (200 mg/mL) salt	200–300 mg IM every 2–3 weeks			
Methyltestosterone (for women)	1.25–2.5 mg with esterified estrogen			

GI, gastrointestinal; IM, intramuscular; T_{max}, time to maximum concentration; $T_{1/2}$, half life.
[a]No abdomen patch placement for Testim; none of these patches can be applied to the genitals.

blood pressure, cholesterol, and colorectal cancer risk, the last being controversial.[17]

Adverse Events/Precautions. Calcium's most common adverse reaction, constipation, can first be treated with increased water intake, dietary fiber, and exercise. If still unresolved, smaller and more frequent administration or lower total daily dose can be tried. Calcium carbonate can create gas and cause stomach upset, which might resolve with calcium citrate, a product with fewer GI side effects.

Calcium rarely causes kidney stones. Some patients with a history of kidney stones can still ingest adequate amounts of calcium depending on the type of stones and/or will require increased fluid intake and decreased salt intake with their calcium supplementation.

Administration. Most children and adults of all ethnic backgrounds do not ingest sufficient (see Table 93–4) dietary calcium (see Table 93–5) and require supplements (see Table 93–10).[17,55] To insure adequate calcium absorption, 25(OH) D concentrations should be maintained in the normal range. Because fractional calcium absorption is dose-limited, maximum single doses of 600 mg or less of elemental calcium are recommended. Calcium carbonate is the salt of choice as it contains the highest amount of elemental calcium and is the least expensive (see Table 93–10). Calcium carbonate tablets should be taken with meals to enhance absorption. Calcium citrate absorption is acid-independent and need not be administered with meals. Although tricalcium phosphate contains 39% calcium, calcium-phosphate complexes could limit overall calcium absorption compared to other products. This product might be helpful in the 10% of seniors with hypophosphatemia that cannot be resolved with increased dietary intake. Disintegration and dissolution rates vary significantly between products and lots. Products labeled "USP Verified" for United States Pharmacopeia, which guarantees the identity, strength, purity, and quality of the product, should be recommended. Oyster shell (other than the OsCal brand) or coral calcium should not be recommended because of concerns for high concentrations of lead and other heavy metals. "Bone designer" nonprescription products continue to be developed by combining calcium and vitamin D with other nutrients, some of which are associated with bone physiology (e.g., magnesium, manganese, boron, vitamin K).[45] Minimal BMD and no fracture data exist for these combination products. Because product labeling is confusing, patients might not realize they need 4 to 6 tablets per day to obtain adequate calcium intakes. These products are also more expensive. Combining too many vitamins and supplements might lead to upper-tolerable nutrient limits being exceeded and a concern for toxicities.

TABLE 93-10 Calcium and Vitamin D Product Selection

Product (% calcium)[a]	Elemental Calcium (mg)	Vitamin D (units)
Calcium carbonate[b] (40%)		
Trade and generic products	200–600	100–200
Mylanta Supreme liquid (5 mL)	160	
Tums Chewable	200	
E-X	300	
Ultra	400	
Rolaids chewable	471	
Os-Cal sugar-free chewable	500	400
Viactiv chews[c]	500	200
CalMax powder (10 mL)	400	
Bayer's Women[d]	300	
Ensure high calcium[c] (8 oz)	400	140
Calcium citrate (24%)		
Generic	315	200
Citracal + Vit D	200–315	200
Citracal chew	500	200
Tricalcium phosphate (39%)		
Posture-D	600	125
Vitamin D_3 (cholecalciferol)	0	400, 700, 800, or 1,000
Multivitamin (D_3)[c]	40–250	400
Ergocalciferol (D_2)[e]		
Liquid (1 mL)		8,000
Tablets/capsules		25,000 or 50,000
Intramuscular (1 mL)		500,000

[a]Many products are adding magnesium, boron, zinc, copper, vitamin K, and/or manganese; sometimes adding "Plus" or "Ultra" to their name. These "bone designer" products are not listed here, see reference 45.
[b]There are many trade-name products for calcium carbonate (e.g., Calel-D, Caltrate, and Os-Cal). Only calcium carbonate alternative dosage forms (i.e., chewable, liquid, powder) are specifically listed.
[c]Contains vitamin K.
[d]Contains aspirin 81 mg.
[e]Prescription products.

Vitamin D Supplementation ❺ Vitamin D intake is critical for the prevention and treatment of osteoporosis because it maximizes intestinal calcium absorption. Given the safety, low cost, and other benefits of vitamin D, no patient should have an inadequate intake.

Efficacy. Two meta-analyses evaluated the efficacy of cholecalciferol with or without calcium supplementation on fracture risk and falls in seniors. Higher doses of vitamin D (700 to 800 units/day) demonstrated a significant 26% relative risk reduction in hip fractures, a 23% relative risk reduction in any nonvertebral fracture, and a 22% relative risk reduction in falls.[36,56] While several studies have demonstrated a beneficial effect of vitamin D on fractures and falls, not all studies have demonstrated a beneficial effect.[56] Conflicting results between studies are thought to be a result of differences in vitamin D dosing, concomitant calcium administration, adherence, and baseline vitamin D status of subjects.

Vitamin D has other potential nonskeletal benefits. Improvement in muscle strength and cardiovascular function, decreased cancer risk (e.g., breast, colon, and prostate cancers), and positive immunomodulatory effects (e.g., multiple sclerosis, type 1 diabetes, rheumatoid arthritis) have been proposed.[15,36]

Administration. Seniors and patients being treated for osteoporosis should take at minimum 800 units of vitamin D through food and supplementation with a goal to maintain their 25(OH) D concentration within the sufficient range.[18,36] Cholecalciferol (vitamin D_3) is more efficient than ergocalciferol (vitamin D_2) at raising 25(OH) D concentrations and is the preferred form of vitamin D supplementation. Usual supplementation is with daily nonprescription vitamin D products (see Table 93–10). However, higher-dose prescription oral or intramuscular regimens administered weekly, monthly, or quarterly have been studied in seniors residing in the community or nursing home environments.[56] In patients with measured insufficient 25(OH) D concentrations, higher daily intakes of vitamin D may be needed. More than one multivitamin or large doses of cod liver oil daily are no longer advocated because of the risk of hypervitaminosis A, which increases bone loss. Because the half-life of vitamin D is about 1 month, approximately 3 months of therapy are required before a new steady state is achieved and a repeat 25(OH) D concentration can be obtained.[16]

Individuals with deficient concentrations of vitamin D are at risk for osteomalacia. Their management is discussed in Other Metabolic Bone Diseases below. In patients with disorders affecting vitamin D absorption (e.g., celiac disease, cystic fibrosis, or Crohn's disease), higher doses and more frequent monitoring. In patients with severe hepatic or renal disease, the activated form of vitamin D (calcitriol) might be more appropriate.

CLINICAL CONTROVERSY

Some experts believe that the upper tolerable limit for vitamin D should be raised and that the recommended daily allowance for vitamin D should be 2,000 units per day. This is the amount of vitamin D that would be needed for approximately 90% of the population to maintain 25(OH) D concentrations at ≥30 ng/mL with a low risk for toxicity.[18,36]

Bisphosphonates ❼ Bisphosphonates mimic pyrophosphate, an endogenous bone resorption inhibitor. Bisphosphonate antiresorptive activity results from blocking prenylation and inhibiting guanosine triphosphatase-signaling proteins, which lead to decreased osteoclast maturation, number, recruitment, bone adhesion, and life span. Their various R2 side chains produce different bone binding, persistence, and affinities; however, the resulting clinical significances are not clearly known.[57] All bisphosphonates become incorporated into bone, giving them long biologic half-lives of up to 10 years. Alendronate, risedronate, and oral ibandronate are currently FDA indicated for the prevention and treatment of postmenopausal osteoporosis (see Table 93–9). Intravenous ibandronate and zoledronic acid are indicated only for treatment of postmenopausal women. Risedronate and alendronate are also FDA indicated in male and glucocorticoid-induced osteoporosis. Clinical trials with ibandronate and zoledronic acid are ongoing for these indications.

Efficacy. Of the antiresorptive agents, bisphosphonates consistently provide the greatest fracture risk reductions and BMD increases (see Table 93–8). Fracture data trials used daily oral bisphosphonate or annual intravenous therapy, not weekly, monthly, or quarterly regimens.[5,58,59] Although hip fracture reduction was not seen with daily oral ibandronate, the hip fracture incidence in the placebo group was low. Furthermore, not all studies for alendronate and risedronate have documented hip fracture prevention. Fracture reductions are demonstrated as early as 6 months,[60] with the greatest fracture reduction seen in patients with lower initial BMD and in those with the greatest BMD changes with therapy. (Note added in poof: Secondary fracture prevention has been documented after a hip fracture with annual intravenous zoledronic acid [Lyles KW, Colōn-Emeric CS, Magaziner JS, et al. Zoledronic acid and clinical fractures and mortality after hip fracture. N Engl J Med 2007;357(18):1799-1809.])

BMD increases with bisphosphonates are dose dependent and greatest in the first 6 to 12 months of therapy. Small increases continue over time at the lumbar spine, but plateau after 2 to 5 years at the hip. After discontinuation, the increased BMD is sustained for a prolonged period of time that varies depending on the bisphosphonate used. Weekly alendronate and risedronate therapy produce equivalent BMD changes to their respective daily regimens. Weekly alendronate therapy increases BMD more than weekly risedronate therapy; however, there is no evidence that this difference would equate to greater fracture efficacy.[60] Monthly oral and quarterly intravenous ibandronate therapies produce greater BMD changes than daily therapy.[61]

The BMD increases with alendronate and risedronate in men are similar to postmenopausal women.[62] Because of a lack of fracture data in men, bisphosphonates are only FDA indicated to increase BMD, not to reduce fracture risk in men.

CLINICAL CONTROVERSY

Women without evidence of a low-trauma fracture and who have responded well to alendronate therapy, with BMD increasing into the osteopenic range, are being considered for a "drug holiday." Patients are taken off their alendronate therapy and followed serially with bone turnover markers and central DXA BMD. Studies demonstrate prolonged suppression of bone turnover and maintenance of BMD in some women after discontinuation.[63] The impact of this practice on fracture risk and application to other bisphosphonates is unknown.

Adverse Events/Precautions. Bisphosphonate GI adverse effects are minimal if the medication is taken correctly. Weekly and monthly therapies have similar common but less-serious GI effects (perforation, ulceration, GI bleeding) than daily therapy. The GI event rates were not increased with concomitant nonsteroidal anti-inflammatory drug use. Patients should be encouraged to discuss GI complaints with a healthcare provider. Intravenous ibandronate and zoledronic acid can be used for patients with contraindications or intolerances to oral bisphosphonates.

The most common adverse effects of intravenous bisphosphonates include fever, flu-like symptoms, and local injection-site reactions.[59,60]

Osteonecrosis of the jaw has been increasingly reported as a rare side effect of bisphosphonate therapy.[64] Most cases occur in patients who are receiving high-dose intravenous bisphosphonate therapy for multiple myeloma and metastatic carcinoma of the skeleton and after tooth extraction, mouth trauma, or oral surgery. Additional risk factors include advanced age and concomitant estrogen or glucocorticoid therapy. The incidence of osteonecrosis of the jaw in women taking alendronate has been estimated at 0.7 cases per 100,000 person-years of exposure.[65] Although the mechanism is incompletely understood, oversuppression of bone turnover is thought to play a primary role. Controversy exists about preventing and treating this condition. Routine dental care and good oral hygiene should be encouraged in anyone beginning bisphosphonate therapy. In addition, major dental work probably should be completed prior to beginning bisphosphonates if possible. There is no evidence that discontinuing bisphosphonate therapy prior to major dental work is beneficial. If osteonecrosis of the jaw develops, oral chlorhexidine washes, systemic antibiotics, and systemic analgesics are used based on severity.

Administration. Because bioavailability is very poor for bisphosphonates (<1% to 5%) and to minimize GI side effects, each oral dose should be taken with at least 6 ounces of plain tap water (not coffee, juice, mineral water, or milk) at least 30 (60 for ibandronate) minutes before consuming any food, supplement (including calcium and vitamin D), or medication. The weekly, raspberry flavored, oral solution only needs to be taken with 2 ounces of water and can be used for patients with swallowing difficulties (e.g., after stroke, tube feeding). The patient should also remain upright (i.e., either sitting or standing) for at least 30 minutes after alendronate and risedronate and 1 hour after ibandronate administration.

Before intravenous bisphosphonates are used, the patient's serum calcium level must be normal. The quarterly ibandronate injection comes as a prefilled syringe (3 mg/mL) kit with a butterfly needle. The injection is given intravenously over 15 to 30 seconds. The injection can also be diluted with dextrose 5% in water or normal saline and used with a syringe pump. Once-yearly administration of zoledronic acid should be infused over at least 15 minutes. Acetaminophen or ibuprofen can be given to decrease adverse effects.

Although these medications are effective, adherence is poor. In one study, oral bisphosphonate adherence for 1 year was only 58% to 61% with only approximately 20% continuing therapy for at least 1 year.[66] Most patients prefer once-weekly or once-monthly bisphosphonate administration to daily therapy. If a patient misses a weekly dose, they can take it the next day. If more than 1 day has lapsed, that dose is skipped until the next scheduled ingestion. If a patient misses a monthly dose, they can take it up to 7 days before the next administration. For patients with adherence issues, the monthly e-mails or postcards sent by the ibandronate manufacturer might be helpful. Intravenous ibandronate could be used as replacements. Alendronate plus vitamin D can potentially help to ensure better adherence with vitamin D intake.

Mixed Estrogen Agonists/Antagonists ❼ Raloxifene, a second-generation mixed estrogen agonist/antagonist (EAA) approved for prevention and treatment of postmenopausal osteoporosis, is an estrogen agonist on bone but an antagonist on the breast and uterus (see Table 93–9). Newer second-generation EAAs will be approved soon. Bazedoxifene (Viviant) received an approvable letter for the prevention of osteoporosis and lasofoxifene (Oporia) is under review.

Efficacy. Raloxifene decreases vertebral fractures and increases spine and hip BMD, but to a lesser extent than bisphosphonates (see Table 93–8).[58,60] Eight-year data support long-term effects and safety. After raloxifene discontinuation, the medication effect is lost, with bone loss returning to age- or disease-related rates. For women with severe osteoporosis, particularly when hip fracture risk reduction is desired, a bisphosphonate is likely a better choice.

Raloxifene decreased invasive estrogen receptor positive breast cancer similarly to tamoxifen in the STAR (Study of Tamoxifen and Raloxifene) trial; however, tamoxifen had fewer (not significantly different) noninvasive breast cancer cases in women at high risk for breast cancer.[67] Raloxifene has an FDA-approved indication for invasive breast cancer risk reduction. Thus in a subset of women, this additional benefit might warrant raloxifene use for dual osteoporosis and breast cancer prevention.

Raloxifene causes some positive lipid effects (decreased total and low-density lipoprotein cholesterol, neutral effect on high-density lipoprotein cholesterol, slightly increased triglycerides); however, no reduction in cardiovascular effects was demonstrated in the RUTH (Raloxifene Use for the Heart)[68] or MORE-CORE (Multiple Outcomes with Raloxifene study and its continuation) trials.[69]

Adverse Events/Precautions. Hot flushes occur with a greater likelihood in women recently finishing menopause or discontinuing estrogen therapy. Raloxifene rarely causes endometrial bleeding. Raloxifene is contraindicated for women with an active or past history of venous thromboembolic event. Therapy should be stopped if a patient anticipates extended immobility.

In large trials, no change in overall death, cardiovascular death, or overall stroke incidence was seen; however, a slight increase in fatal stroke was documented.[68] Women at high risk for a stroke or coronary events and those with known coronary artery disease, peripheral vascular disease, atrial fibrillation, or a prior history of cerebrovascular events might not be good candidates for this medication.

Administration. Similar to bisphosphonates, adherence and persistence problems exist. At 1 year, adherence was 54% and persistence was only 6%.[66]

Calcitonin Calcitonin is released from the thyroid gland when serum calcium is elevated. Salmon calcitonin is more potent and longer lasting than the mammalian form. Calcitonin is FDA indicated for osteoporosis treatment for women who are at least 5 years past menopause (see Table 93–9). Although limited data document some benefits in men and concomitantly with glucocorticoids, these indications are not approved. Because efficacy is less robust than the other antiresorptive therapies, calcitonin is reserved as third-line treatment. Intermittent nasal regimens and an oral product are being explored.

Efficacy. Only vertebral fractures have been documented to decrease with intranasal calcitonin therapy (see Table 93–8).[5,60] Calcitonin does not consistently affect hip BMD and does not decrease hip fracture risk.

Calcitonin might provide pain relief to some patients with acute vertebral fractures, about a 2.5-point change on a visual analog scale. [70] If used, calcitonin should be prescribed for short-term (4 weeks) treatment and should not be used in place of other more effective and less expensive analgesics nor should it preclude the use of more appropriate osteoporosis therapy.

Administration. Subcutaneous administration with 100 units daily is available but rarely used because of adverse effects and costs.

Estrogen Therapy Although estrogens are FDA indicated for prevention of osteoporosis, they should only be used short-term in women who need estrogen therapy for the management of menopausal symptoms such as hot flushes. The risks of estrogen therapy outweigh the bone benefits.[60] Even though the Women's Health Initiative trials only assessed one dose of conjugated equine estrogens, most clinicians extrapolate the results to all postmenopausal estrogen therapies until data indicate otherwise.

Efficacy. Estrogen with (HT)[71] or without (ET)[72] progestin therapy significantly decreases fracture risk (see Table 93–8).[5] Increases in BMD are less than bisphosphonates or teriparatide, but greater than raloxifene and calcitonin. Oral and transdermal estrogens at equivalent doses and continuous or cyclic HT regimens have similar BMD effects. Effect on BMD is dose dependent with some benefit seen with lower estrogen doses. Fracture risk reduction has not been demonstrated with lower dose therapy. When ET or HT is discontinued, bone loss accelerates and fracture protection is lost.

Adverse Events/Precautions/Administration. The lowest effective dose of ET and HT should still be used for preventing and controlling menopausal symptoms with use discontinued with symptom abatement. A complete discussion of adverse events, precautions, and administration for all estrogen and estrogen and progestin combination products can be found in Chap. 85.

Testosterone ❽ Decreased testosterone concentrations are seen with certain gonadal diseases, eating disorders, glucocorticoid therapy, oophorectomy, menopause, and andropause. Testosterone replacement is not approved for the prevention or treatment of osteoporosis.

Efficacy. A few studies of testosterone replacement in women have demonstrated increases in BMD.[73] Testosterone, in various salt forms, was associated with increased BMD in some studies when given to hypogonadal men and senior men with normal or mild hormonal deficiency.[74,75] The impact of testosterone replacement on fracture risk in women and men have not been prospectively evaluated. Testosterone replacement should not be used solely for the prevention or treatment of osteoporosis, but might be beneficial to reduce bone loss in patients needing therapy for hypogonadal symptoms.

Adverse Events/Precautions. Patients using these products should be evaluated within 1 to 2 months of initiation and then every 3 to 6 months thereafter.[76] Testosterone and methyltestosterone are in pregnancy category X, indicating that the agents are contraindicated.

Administration. Testosterone products are schedule III drugs. The gel products can rub off and be absorbed by the patient's partner.

Thiazide Diuretics Thiazide diuretics increase urinary calcium reabsorption. Observational studies suggest that patients who receive thiazide diuretics have a greater bone mass, lower rates of bone loss, and fewer fractures.[77] Two prospective, controlled trials demonstrated small increases in bone mass over placebo. Prescribing thiazide diuretics solely for osteoporosis is not recommended but is a reasonable choice for the patient with osteoporosis who requires a diuretic and for patients on glucocorticoids with greater than 300 mg of calcium excreted in the urine over 24 hours.

Anabolic Therapies

Currently teriparatide is the only available medication that increases bone formation.

Teriparatide Teriparatide is a recombinant product representing the first 34 amino acids in human PTH (see Table 93–9). Teriparatide increases bone formation, the bone remodeling rate, and osteoblast number and activity. Both bone mass and architecture are improved. Teriparatide is FDA indicated for postmenopausal women and men who are at high risk for fracture. Patients who have a history of osteoporotic fracture, multiple risk factors for fracture, very low bone density (e.g., T-score < –3.5), or have failed or are intolerant of previous bisphosphonate therapy are candidates for PTH therapy. Human PTH (1–84), PTH analog (1–31), oral PTH, and intranasal, transdermal, and once-weekly subcutaneous teriparatide administration are being investigated.

Efficacy. Teriparatide reduces fracture risk in postmenopausal women (see Table 93–8); however, no fracture data are available in men. Lumbar spine BMD increases are higher than any other osteoporosis therapy.[60,78] Although wrist BMD is decreased, wrist fractures are not increased. Discontinuation of teriparatide therapy results in a decrease in BMD, although some antifracture efficacy appears to be maintained.[78] Sequential therapy with PTH followed by an antiresorptive agent (e.g., bisphosphonates) should be considered to maintain BMD gains.[60]

Adverse Events/Precautions. Transient hypercalcemia rarely occurs. A trough serum calcium concentration is recommended 1 month after initiation of therapy. If high (>10.6 mg/mL), calcium intake should be decreased to 1,000 mg daily. If the serum calcium is still high, lowering the dose by 25% or switching to every-other-day calcium therapy can be tried.[78]

Because of an increased incidence of osteosarcoma in rats, teriparatide contains a black box warning against use in patients at increased baseline risk for osteosarcoma (e.g., Paget's bone disease, unexplained elevations of alkaline phosphatase, pediatric patients, young adults with open epiphyses, or patients with prior radiation therapy involving the skeleton). In addition, teriparatide should not be used in patients with hypercalcemia, metabolic bone diseases other than osteoporosis, metastatic or skeletal cancers, or premenopausal women of child-bearing potential. Therapy is not recommended beyond 2 years because of a lack of efficacy and safety data.

Administration. Teriparatide is commercially available as a prefilled 3-mL "pen" delivery device that administers subcutaneous injections in the thigh or abdominal area. The administration of the initial dose should take place with the patient either sitting or lying down in case orthostatic hypotension occurs. The patient should be reeducated with each refill. The pen must be kept refrigerated and can be used immediately after removing from the refrigerator. The pen must be discarded 28 days after the initial injection. Teriparatide is the most expensive antiosteoporosis therapy.

Combination Therapy

Greater increases in BMD have been demonstrated in some small studies of combination antiresorptive therapy in postmenopausal women.[60] Greater fracture risk reduction has not been demonstrated. Combination antiresorptive and anabolic therapies have been evaluated with conflicting results.[78] Greater increases in BMD were demonstrated when a less-potent antiresorptive agent, raloxifene or HT, was used with PTH, whereas a blunting of the BMD effect was seen when combination therapy included alendronate. The effects of other bisphosphonates in combination with PTH are unknown. Because of lack of a clear benefit and potential for increased cost, side effects, and nonadherence, combination therapy is not recommended at this time.

Investigational Therapies

Besides the above mentioned investigational products, new drug classes are also being developed.

Denosumab Denosumab is a promising new antiresorptive agent with a unique mechanism of action. It is a fully human monoclonal antibody (immunoglobulin G_2) that binds to RANKL, blocking its ability to bind to its receptor activator of nuclear factor kappa B on the surface of osteoclast precursor cells and mature osteoclasts. Thus denosumab inhibits osteoclastogenesis and increases osteoclast apoptosis.[79–81] In a phase II study, greater increases in total hip and distal radius BMD were demonstrated in the intermittent (every 3 to 6 months) denosumab subcutaneous groups compared to once-weekly alendronate.[79]Adverse effects were similar between all groups. The 60-mg subcutaneous injection every 6 months is being evaluated in a phase III trial of postmenopausal women with osteoporosis.

Other Investigational Drug Classes Additional new classes of medications are beginning to show promise.[13] Although injectable OPG, a competitive inhibitor of RANKL, blocked osteoclastic differentiation and decreased bone resorption biomarkers in phases I and II, further development has ceased. Agents to enhance endogenous OPG, decrease RANKL production, or block RANKL binding to receptor activator of nuclear factor kappa B are being developed. Agents to block osteoclast attachment ($\alpha V\beta_3$ integrin receptor antagonists—preclinical), inhibit bone matrix degradation (cathepsin K inhibitors—phase I; nitrosylated nonsteroidal antiinflammatory drugs—phase II), or change osteoclast cell structure (Src inhibitors—preclinical) have been effective in animal studies, and for some, in early human studies. Strontium ranelate and tibolone (Canada as well) are approved in Europe but most likely will not be marketed in the United States.

■ VERTEBROPLASTY AND KYPHOPLASTY

Sometimes patients with debilitating pain between 6 and 52 weeks after a vertebral fracture might undergo vertebroplasty or kyphoplasty during which bone cement is injected into the fractured vertebral space.[82] The procedure stabilizes the damaged vertebrae and reduces pain in 70% to 95% of patients. Cement leakage into the spinal column can result in complicating nerve damage. Long-term benefits are unknown, but some vertebral fracturing around the cement has been documented.

SPECIAL POPULATIONS

Osteoporosis is a threat to all age groups and in some subgroups because of genetic abnormalities, diseases, and medications.

CHILDREN

Although rare, osteoporosis in children and adolescents can lead to significant pain, deformity, and chronic disability. The main causes of osteoporosis in children are secondary, such as chronic medications, genetic defects (e.g., osteogenesis imperfecta, cystic fibrosis), chromosomal defects (e.g., Turner's or Klinefelter's syndromes), endocrine disorders (e.g., growth hormone deficiency), malabsorptive or nutritional disorders (e.g., celiac sprue), malignancies, other chronic diseases (e.g., juvenile rheumatoid arthritis), and conditions associated with disuse (e.g., paralysis, muscular dystrophy).[83] Idiopathic juvenile osteoporosis is a condition that can develop in previously healthy children and is only diagnosed after the exclusion of all other possible causes of osteoporosis. It can spontaneously resolve after 3–5 years, but sequelae can persist into adulthood. Although the pathogenesis is unknown, reduced osteoblastic bone formation mainly in trabecular regions appears to play a primary role.

The diagnosis and treatment of osteoporosis in children and adolescents is challenging. No guidelines or consensus recommendations exist. The International Society for Clinical Densitometry suggests that the diagnosis of osteoporosis in children (<20 years of age) should not be made on bone density results alone.[35] Central spine and total body DXA using an ethnic-matched reference database is recommended with a Z-score below –2.0 indicating low bone density.[83]

After correcting any underlying causes (e.g., hypogonadism therapy, gluten free diet) and instituting a bone-healthy lifestyle, most experts recommend pharmacologic treatment when the Z-score is less than –2.0, with or without the presence of a low-trauma fracture.[83,84]

Small studies, mostly evaluating the intravenous bisphosphonate pamidronate (cancer hypercalcemia therapy), have been promising.[85] Research with oral bisphosphonates is ongoing. A major concern with bisphosphonates is their effect on longitudinal bone growth and modeling; however, fracture healing, skeletal growth/maturation, or the appearance of growth plates does not appear to be impaired.[84] Teriparatide should not be used because of an increased risk for osteosarcoma.

PREMENOPAUSAL WOMEN

Because of increased accessibility to peripheral and central BMD testing, more premenopausal women are being screened for osteoporosis. The relationship between low bone density and future fracture risk in healthy premenopausal women is not well established nor is the efficacy and safety of pharmacologic therapy.[86,87] Most premenopausal women with documented low bone density have an identifiable secondary cause (see Table 93–2). Approximately 15% of healthy premenopausal women will have low BMD as a normal variation of peak bone mass.[11,87] Low peak bone mass is a major risk factor for postmenopausal osteoporosis and fractures, but it has thus far not predicted an increased risk for fractures in the premenopausal years.[87] This might be a result of better bone architecture contributing to better bone strength in younger women.[35]

Routine bone density testing is not cost effective and should not be performed in healthy premenopausal women.[34] No evidence supports that identifying low bone density in healthy premenopausal women results in a better bone-healthy lifestyle compared to education alone. Nor does any evidence exist to support that pharmacologic treatment will reduce fracture risk in this population. Oral bisphosphonates and teriparatide are in pregnancy category C (zoledronic acid is category D) and are not recommended in women with childbearing capability. Long-term effects of bisphosphonates (>10 years) are unknown.

THE "OLDER" SENIOR

Age is an independent risk factor for osteoporosis and osteoporotic fractures, with the prevalence increasing dramatically with age. Seniors are living longer. The average additional life span for an 85-year-old was 6.8 years in 2003 and it is estimated that the number of people in the United States age 85 years and older will increase from 5.1 million in 2004 to 7.3 million by 2020. The number of "older" seniors with osteoporosis is on the rise and many do not realize they have the disease. According to National Health and Nutritional Examination Surveys data, only 12.1% and 9.7% of women and 1.3% and 1.6% of men ages 75 to 84 years and 85 years and older, respectively, reported they had osteoporosis.[3] However, when tested, 32.5% and 50.5% of women and 6.4% and 13.7% of men, respectively, had the disease. Central DXA should be performed and is cost-effective in this population.[88] The United States Preventive Services Task Force estimated that only 75 women between 75 and 79 years of age would need to be screened to prevent one vertebral fracture and 143 would need to be screened to prevent one hip fracture.[34]

Older seniors should practice a bone-healthy lifestyle, ingest adequate calcium and vitamin D, and implement measures to prevent falls (see Table 93–7). When deciding whether or not to use prescription medications in "older" seniors, the following factors need to be taken into consideration: remaining life span, ability to take and afford medications, cognitive function, GI disorders, polypharmacy, desire for more medications, and regimen complexity. Although efficacy and safety data are limited in the older senior, evidence consistently shows that those at highest risk for fracture benefit most from pharmacologic therapy.[89–91]

GLUCOCORTICOID-INDUCED OSTEOPOROSIS

9 Glucocorticoids are the most common secondary cause of osteoporosis and the third most common cause of osteoporosis overall.[92] Approximately 30% to 50% of patients taking chronic oral glucocorticoids will experience a fracture. Bone losses are rapid, with the greatest decrease occurring in the first 6 to 12 months of therapy. Low to medium doses of inhaled glucocorticoids have no appreciable effect on bone density and fracture risk.[93,94] The impact of long-term, high-dose inhaled glucocorticoids needs further evaluation.

The pathophysiology of glucocorticoid-induced osteoporosis (GIO) is multifactorial. Glucocorticoids decrease bone formation through decreased proliferation and differentiation, and enhanced apoptosis of osteoblasts.[92] They can interfere with the bone's natural repair mechanism through increased apoptosis of osteocytes, the bone's communication cells. Glucocorticoids increase bone resorption by increasing RANKL and decreasing OPG. They can reduce estrogen and testosterone concentrations and create a negative calcium balance by decreasing calcium absorption and increasing urinary calcium excretion.[92,95] The underlying disease processes might also contribute negatively to bone metabolism.

Guidelines on the management of GIO are available from the American College of Rheumatology.[95,96] A baseline BMD using central DXA is recommended for all patients starting on 5 mg or more daily of prednisone equivalent for at least 6 months. BMD testing should also be considered at baseline in patients being started on shorter durations of systemic glucocorticoids if they are at high risk for low bone mass and fractures based on risk factors (e.g., age >65 years, postmenopausal, current smoker, and personal history of a low trauma fracture as an adult). Because of the rapid loss of bone that can occur with oral glucocorticoid therapy, central DXA can be repeated every 6 to 12 months if needed. Patients using high-dose inhaled corticosteroids should be evaluated for osteopenia or osteoporosis.

All patients starting or receiving long-term systemic glucocorticoid therapy should receive at least 1,500 mg elemental calcium and 800 to 1,200 units of vitamin D daily, and practice a bone-healthy lifestyle. Both alendronate and risedronate have documented efficacy and are FDA indicated for GIO.[96] The American College of Rheumatology guidelines recommend all patients newly starting on systemic glucocorticoids (≥5 mg/day of prednisone equivalent) for an anticipated duration of at least 3 months should receive preventative bisphosphonate therapy. A more conservative approach might be considered in premenopausal women of child-bearding potential. Patients starting or receiving long-term glucocorticoid therapy with documented low bone density (T-score below –1.0) or evidence of a low trauma fracture should also receive bisphosphonate treatment. Teriparatide is the only anabolic therapy commercially available that increases bone formation. Teriparatide can be used if bisphosphonates are not tolerated or contraindicated. Testosterone replacement therapy should be considered in men, and high-dose hormonal oral contraceptives can be considered for premenopausal women with documented hypogonadism.

TRANSPLANTATION OSTEOPOROSIS

⑩ Patients undergoing solid-organ transplantation (e.g., kidney, lung, cardiac, and liver) have a high risk for osteoporosis and osteoporotic fractures.[97] Prior to transplantation, many patients have osteoporosis or low BMD because of osteoporosis risk factors (see Table 93–1) and negative bone effects from their underlying diseases (e.g., alcoholism, cachexia, impaired liver or kidney function, hypogonadism, and deconditioning). After transplantation, bone loss and fracture risk increase dramatically within the first 6 to 12 months, mainly as a consequence of high-dose systemic glucocorticoid exposure and the use of calcineurin inhibitors (e.g., cyclosporine).[97] Sometimes bone loss slows or improves within 1 year of transplant.

Before transplantation, patients should be evaluated for metabolic bone disease with lab tests and physical examination for secondary causes (see Table 93–2), radiographs for vertebral fractures, and central DXA.[97] Regardless of BMD results, patients should be counseled on a bone-healthy lifestyle and instructed to take 1,500 mg of elemental calcium and 800 to 1,200 units of vitamin D daily. Calcitriol (1,25-dihydroxyvitamin D) at a dose of 0.25 to 0.5 mcg daily might be needed for renal and/or liver dysfunction. Pretransplant patients with osteoporosis or a low trauma fracture, except patients with end-stage renal disease awaiting kidney transplantation, should be started on bisphosphonate therapy indefinitely. In patients with normal BMD prior to transplant, short-term bisphosphonate therapy (6 to 12 months) can be used to prevent bone loss after transplant. Parathyroid hormone has not been studied in the transplant population and is contraindicated in transplant patients with secondary hyperparathyroidism. Testosterone replacement might be considered for men, and high-dose hormonal oral contraceptives are options for premenopausal women with hypogonadism. Central DXA can be repeated as early as 6 to 12 months to evaluate bone loss and the effects of treatment.

CHRONIC KIDNEY DISEASE

Chronic kidney disease is defined as kidney damage for at least 3 months with or without a decrease in glomerular filtration rate (GFR) or a GFR less than 60 mL/min/1.73 m^2 for at least 3 months with or without kidney damage.[98] Most seniors have a GFR of less than 30 to 60 mL/min/1.73 m^2 without any kidney damage.[99] Consequently, to make osteoporosis treatment decisions, the origin of chronic kidney disease, either intrinsic kidney damage or aging needs to be determined. Patients with a GFR or creatinine clearance greater than 30 mL/min can be managed routinely (see Fig. 93–3). Bisphosphonates are not recommended for patients with creatinine clearances less than 30 or 35 mL/min because of potential drug accumulation. Based on large retrospective or pooled studies, oral bisphosphonates in patients with severe kidney impairment (creatinine clearance as low as 15 mL/min)[100] and teriparatide in patients with moderate kidney impairment (creatinine clearance 30 to 49 mL/min)[101] appear safe and efficacious in patients with age-related declines in renal function.

Renal osteodystrophy describes a constellation of metabolic bone disorders that develop in patients with stages 4 and 5 chronic kidney disease (GFR <30 mL/min/1.73 m^2) and end-stage renal disease as a consequence of intrinsic kidney damage. Bone biopsy is essential to differentiate the different types of renal osteodystrophy from osteoporosis in this population. Antiresorptive therapies would be appropriate for the management of osteoporosis; however, they are contraindicated in patients with osteomalacia or adynamic bone and ineffective for osteitis fibrosa cystica. In patients with stage 5 chronic kidney disease (creatinine clearance below 15 mL/min) and documented osteoporosis, 50% of the oral bisphosphonate dose is frequently recommended.

GASTROINTESTINAL DISEASES

⑩ The three most common gastrointestinal disorders associated with increased osteoporosis risk are inflammatory bowel disease, celiac disease, and postgastrectomy states.[102] Impaired absorption of key nutrients and minerals, chronic systemic glucocorticoid use and increased levels of inflammatory cytokines also are implicated. The prevalence of osteoporosis in patients with inflammatory bowel disease, Crohn's disease or ulcerative colitis is approximately 15%.[103] When glucocorticoids are used, the GIO prevention and treatment guidelines should be followed.[95,96] The role of proinflammatory cytokines needs further investigation.

Celiac disease is an inherited autoimmune disorder in which the ingestion of the protein gluten triggers an immune reaction that damages the mucosal lining of the small intestine and leads to impaired nutrient absorption.[104] The incidence of celiac disease in the United States is estimated at 1 in 133, and at 1 in 22 for primary degree relatives. Patients newly diagnosed with celiac disease have an estimated prevalence of osteoporosis of approximately 28% at the spine and 15% at the hip. Long-term fracture risk is estimated to be double that of the general population. Impaired nutrient absorption, especially calcium and vitamin D, plays a central role in the bone loss requiring 25(OH) D monitoring. Celiac disease management requires a gluten-free diet, which can significantly increase BMD by approximately 5% within 1 year.[102]

Patients undergoing total or partial gastrectomy are at high risk for the development of osteoporosis. The incidence of osteoporosis may be as high as 32% to 42% with a 30-year cumulative risk for fracture of 72% in women and 48% in men.[102] Although the pathophysiology of bone disease postgastrectomy is unknown, reduced nutritional intake of protein might play a role. Bone density evaluation using central DXA should be considered in all patients who are more than 10 years postgastrectomy.

PHARMACOECONOMIC CONSIDERATIONS

The estimated burden for fractures in 2005 was $17 billion and is expected to increase to $25 billion by 2025.[7] Consequently, determining who should be screened and treated for osteoporosis and fracture prevention is important. Various studies use different assumptions in their models. One study used the following mean annual costs for fractures; $19,200 to $25,300 for hip fracture; $5,300 to $6,800 for nonvertebral, nonhip fracture; and $2,700 to $3,000 for vertebral fractures.[105] Preventing osteoporosis in postmenopausal women with normal or osteopenic BMD is not cost-effective.[106] However, screening older women and only using a bisphosphonate for those with osteoporosis is cost-effective.[88] The cost per quality-adjusted life-year decreased from $40,100 for women 65 to 74 years old to a cost savings for women 85 years and older. In seniors, bisphosphonates were found to produce the greatest quality-adjusted life-years gain at the lowest cost (i.e., 0.637; $4,200), followed by PTH (0.0574; $6,833), calcitonin (0.0348; $5,761), and raloxifene (0.0339; $5,676).[105] In this model, bisphosphonates had the greatest hip and nonvertebral, nonhip fracture reduction. Calcitonin was assumed to have better vertebral fracture prevention than raloxifene, and both were assumed to have no hip or nonvertebral, nonhip prevention.

EVALUATION OF THERAPEUTIC OUTCOMES

Besides monitoring for efficacy and safety, adherence evaluation should also be conducted.

MONITORING OF THE PHARMACEUTICAL CARE PLAN

Central DXA BMD measurements can be obtained every 1 to 2 years for monitoring bone loss and treatment response. In patients with conditions associated with higher rates of bone loss (e.g., glucocorticoid use, after transplantation), more frequent monitoring might be warranted.

To minimize test variability, BMD testing must be performed on the same DXA machine and ideally with the same operator (technician). Any change in absolute BMD that exceeds the precision error of the machine at that site (approximately 3% spine and 4% hip) is considered clinically significant, and if below precision error, is considered a no response. Because changes in BMD do not entirely explain changes in fracture risk, many experts believe that decisions on whether or not to continue a particular therapy should not be based solely on BMD response.

Biochemical markers of bone turnover have been evaluated for use in monitoring early responses to drug therapy, especially for identifying therapy nonresponders or possibly promoting adherence. Bone resorption markers, with the first or second morning void for urinary N-terminal crosslinking telopeptide of type 1 collagen or morning for serum C-terminal crosslinking telopeptide of type 1 collagen, are typically performed after an overnight fast at baseline and repeated after 3 to 6 months of therapy. These parameters will decrease with effective therapy. Circadian variability, seasonal variations, food intake, and recent exercise can all impact results. As no consensus on result interpretation and high test variability exists, these tests are not yet considered routine.

PHARMACY SERVICES

Pharmacists play an important role in screening and monitoring for osteoporosis. Community pharmacy ultrasonography screenings identify patients who are at risk and, with pharmacist or other professional consultation, increase use of calcium and vitamin D, and physician referrals for osteoporosis.[107] (Note added in proof: This practice is financially sustainable in the community pharmacy setting [Liu Y, Nevins JC, Carruthers KM, et al. Osteoporosis risk screening for women in a community pharmacy. J Am Pharm Assoc 2007;47:521-526]). Patients should be frequently assessed for correct bisphosphonate ingestion. Specialty clinic practices have increased prevention and treatment of steroid-induced osteoporosis.[108] Hospital-based programs help increase the number of patients who, after a hip fracture, receive testing and treatment.

OTHER METABOLIC BONE DISEASES

Because of increased interest in bone diseases and newer medications, better therapies are being explored and developed for other bone diseases.

OSTEOMALACIA

Osteomalacia, meaning "soft bones," is a condition seen in adults in which the bone is significantly undermineralized. Rickets is the childhood equivalent of osteomalacia. The most common cause of osteomalacia is severe, prolonged vitamin D deficiency. Disorders that cause hypocalcemia or hypophosphatemia and, rarely, long-term anticonvulsant therapy can also cause osteomalacia. Phenytoin, phenobarbital, and carbamazepine are most commonly associated with severe vitamin D deficiency through cytochrome P450 system induction that increases vitamin D conversion to inactive metabolites. Oral doses of vitamin D_3 from 1,000 to 4,000 units per day might be needed to prevent vitamin D deficiency in patients on these medications.[109]

Patients with osteomalacia present with pathologic fractures and/or deep bone pain or no obvious symptoms but low BMD.[22] Patients with osteomalacia will have an extremely low 25(OH) D concentration (<10 ng/mL) and might have an elevated bone-specific alkaline phosphate and hypocalcemia. The treatment of osteomalacia caused by vitamin D deficiency is high-dose vitamin D replacement therapy. Prescription oral ergocalciferol 50,000 units once to twice weekly for at least 8 weeks is a regimen that is frequently used to raise vitamin D concentrations into the sufficient range. High-dose oral and intramuscular regimens have also been used. Once 25(OH) D concentrations are greater than 30 ng/mL, chronic maintenance vitamin D therapy can be instituted. Oral ergocalciferol 50,000 units once or twice a month or nonprescription cholecalciferol at least 1,000 units up 2,000 units once daily are reasonable maintenance options.

PAGET'S DISEASE

Unlike osteoporosis, which is a systemic disorder affecting the entire skeleton, Paget's disease is a disorder of bone remodeling in discrete sections of bone. The main areas affected are the skull, spine, pelvis, femur, and tibia.[110] The osteoclasts are abnormally large and have heightened activity, increasing bone turnover rate and affecting both bone resorption and formation. The accelerated bone formation does not allow for proper layering of collagen leading to disorganized or woven collagen. The disease is usually asymptomatic; however, patients can experience bone pain, fractures, skeletal deformities, and, rarely, malignant transformation into osteosarcoma.

Paget's disease tends to occur in adults older than age 55 years with a slight predominance in men and patients of north European ancestry. The disease affects approximately 1% of adults age 40 years and older.[110] Various environmental and genetic factors cause Paget's disease with viral causes a controversial pathogenesis. Paget's disease is typically discovered because of an unexplained elevation in serum alkaline phosphatase. A bone scan can be performed to determine the extent of skeletal involvement.

Bisphosphonates are the drug of choice for managing Paget's disease because they work directly on osteoclasts to slow down bone turnover, allowing more time for proper bone formation.[111] Four regimens are FDA-indicated: risedronate 30-mg tablet orally once daily for 2 months; pamidronate 30-mg intravenous infusion for 3 days; alendronate 40-mg tablet orally once daily for 6 months; or a one-time intravenous infusion of 5 mg zoledronic acid. Zoledronic acid and risedronate regimens were compared in a head-to-head study, with zoledronic acid demonstrating a superior and more rapid therapeutic response.[112] Therapy can be repeated if symptoms return or serum alkaline phosphatase increases by 25% or more. Subcutaneous or intramuscular salmon calcitonin can be used if bisphosphonates therapy is contraindicated.

OSTEOGENESIS IMPERFECTA

Osteogenesis imperfecta is a genetic disorder characterized by low trabecular and cortical bone density.[83] Bone formation and mineralization are disturbed leading to impaired bone strength and an increased risk for fractures. Up to seven different clinical types of this disease have been described, ranging in severity from mild disease with no major bone deformities (type I) to lethal in the perinatal period (type II).[113] Nonpharmacologic management, mostly physical therapy, is the mainstay of therapy for osteogenesis imperfecta. Orthopedic surgery is sometimes needed to help stabilize the brittle bones. Observational studies and case reports suggested intravenous pamidronate for moderate to severe osteogenesis imperfecta can increase BMD, reduce bone pain, and decrease fracture incidence.[84] Oral bisphosphonates and teriparatide are being evaluated in clinical trials.

CONCLUSIONS

Osteoporosis is currently a public health priority with the prevalence of both the disease and fracture incidence expected to increase in the next 10 to 20 years. Osteoporosis prevention begins at birth and continues throughout life by practicing a bone-healthy lifestyle (adequate calcium and vitamin intake, exercise, no smoking, and minimal alcohol use). Generally osteoporosis occurs in postmenopausal women and senior men; however, the disease can occur in all ages as a result of secondary causes such as genetics, diseases, and medications. Portable ultrasonography machines can screen for osteoporosis but central bone densitometry is used for diagnosis and monitoring. Bisphosphonates are the drug of choice because they decrease hip, nonvertebral, and vertebral fractures, are relatively safe, and are affordable. Teriparatide is the only medication that can build bone; however, cost and subcutaneous administration limit its use. New agents and drug classes to prevent and treat osteoporosis show promise. As osteoporosis management becomes more streamlined for postmenopausal women, practitioners are now focusing on identifying other special populations at risk for osteoporosis (e.g., men, transplantation patients, glucocorticoid therapy, cancer therapies).

Because vitamin D insufficiency and deficiency are very common, adequate intake of vitamin D is essential for everyone, generally requiring nonprescription vitamin D supplementation. Osteomalacia is a disease of decreased bone mineralization. Eliminating or treating any underlying causes of osteomalacia is the first step. In most cases, pharmacologic doses of vitamin D are required.

ABBREVIATIONS

25(OH) D: calcidiol/25-hydroxyvitamin D

BMD: bone mineral density

DXA: dual-energy x-ray absorptiometry

EAA: estrogen agonist/antagonist

ET: estrogen therapy

GFR: glomerular filtration rate

GI: gastrointestinal

GIO: glucocorticoid-induced osteoporosis

HT: hormone therapy (estrogen plus progestin)

OPG: osteoprotegerin

PTH: parathyroid hormone

RANKL: receptor activator of nuclear factor-kappa B ligand

SERM: selective estrogen receptor modulator

WHO: World Health Organization

REFERENCES

1. National Osteoporosis Foundation. About Osteoporosis: Fast facts. 2003, *http://www.nof.org/osteoporosis/diseasefacts.htm.*
2. NIH Consensus Development Panel on Osteoporosis Prevention Diagnosis and Treatment. Osteoporosis prevention, diagnosis, and therapy. JAMA 2001;285(6):785–795.
3. U.S. Department of Health and Human Services. Bone Health and Osteoporosis: A Report of the Surgeon General Rockville, MD: U.S. Department of Health and Human Services, Office of the Surgeon General, 2004:1–436.
4. Barrett-Connor E, Siris ES, Wehren LE, et al. Osteoporosis and fracture risk in women of different ethnic groups. J Bone Miner Res 2005;20(2):185–194.
5. North American Menopause Society. Management of osteoporosis in postmenopausal women: 2006 position statement of The North American Menopause Society. Menopause 2006;13(3):340–367; quiz 368–349.
6. Department of Health and Human Services Centers for Disease Control and Prevention and National Center for Health Statistics. National Health and Nutrition Examination Survey: Osteoporosis. 2007, *http://www.cdc.gov/nchs/data/nhanes/databriefs/osteoporosis.pdf.*
7. Burge R, Dawson-Hughes B, Solomon DH, et al. Incidence and economic burden of osteoporosis-related fractures in the United States, 2005–2025. J Bone Miner Res 2007;22(3):465–475.
8. Orwig DL, Chan J, Magaziner J. Hip fracture and its consequences: Differences between men and women. Orthop Clin North Am 2006;37(4):611–622.
9. Seeman E, Delmas PD. Bone quality—The material and structural basis of bone strength and fragility. N Engl J Med 2006;354(21):2250–2261.
10. Gourlay ML, Brown SA. Clinical considerations in premenopausal osteoporosis. Arch Intern Med 2004;164(6):603–614.
11. Lewiecki EM. Premenopausal bone health assessment. Curr Rheumatol Rep 2005;7(1):46–52.
12. Dempster DW. Anatomy and functions of the adult skeleton. In: Favus MJ, Bikle DD, Christakos S, et al., eds. Primer on the Metabolic Bone Diseases and Disorders of Mineral Metabolism, 6th ed. Washington, DC: Cadmus, 2006:7–11.
13. Vondracek SF, Chen JT, Csako G. Osteoporosis pathophysiology and new drug development. Clin Rev Bone Miner Metab 2004;2(4):293–313.
14. Reid IR. Menopause. In: Favus MJ, ed. Primer on the Metabolic Bone Diseases and Disorders of Mineral Metabolism, 6th ed. Washington, DC: Cadmus, 2006:68–70.
15. Holick MF. High prevalence of vitamin D inadequacy and implications for health. Mayo Clin Proc 2006;81(3):353–373.
16. Vieth R. Vitamin D supplementation, 25-hydroxyvitamin D concentrations, and safety. Am J Clin Nutr 1999;69(5):842–856.
17. O'Connell MB, Stamm PL. Calcium prevention and treatment of osteoporosis. Clin Rev Bone Miner Metab 2004;2(4):357–371.
18. Hanley DA, Davison KS. Vitamin D insufficiency in North America. J Nutr 2005;135(2):332–337.
19. Miller PD, Hochberg MC, Wehren LE, et al. How useful are measures of BMD and bone turnover? Curr Med Res Opin 2005;21(4):545–554.
20. Close JC, Lord SL, Menz HB, Sherrington C. What is the role of falls? Best Pract Res Clin Rheumatol 2005;19(6):913–935.
21. Seeman E, Bianchi G, Khosla S, et al. Bone fragility in men—Where are we? Osteoporos Int 2006;17(11):1577–1583.
22. Kelman A, Lane NE. The management of secondary osteoporosis. Best Pract Res Clin Rheumatol 2005;19(6):1021–1037.
23. Cromer BA, Scholes D, Berenson A, et al. Depot medroxyprogesterone acetate and bone mineral density in adolescents—The black box warning: A position paper of the Society for Adolescent Medicine. J Adolesc Health 2006;39(2):296–301.
24. Stone KL, Seeley DG, Lui LY, et al. BMD at multiple sites and risk of fracture of multiple types: Long-term results from the Study of Osteoporotic Fractures. J Bone Miner Res 2003;18(11):1947–1954.
25. Popovic JR. 1999 National hospital discharge survey: Annual summary with detailed diagnosis and procedure data. National Center for Health Statistics. Vital Health Stat 13 2001;13(152):23,154.
26. Klotzbuecher CM, Ross PD, Landsman PB, et al. Patients with prior fractures have an increased risk of future fractures: A summary of the literature and statistical synthesis. J Bone Miner Res 2000;15(4):721–739.
27. National Osteoporosis Foundation. Physician's guide to prevention and treatment of osteoporosis. 2003, *http://www.nof.org/physguide/index.asp*
28. Cadarette SM, Jaglal SB, Murray TM, et al. Evaluation of decision rules for referring women for bone densitometry by dual-energy x-ray absorptiometry. JAMA 2001;286(1):57–63.

29. Kanis JA, Oden A, Johnell O, et al. The use of clinical risk factors enhances the performance of BMD in the prediction of hip and osteoporotic fractures in men and women. Osteoporos Int 2007;18(8):1033–1046.
30. Miller PD, Siris ES, Barrett-Connor E, et al. Prediction of fracture risk in postmenopausal white women with peripheral bone densitometry: Evidence from the National Osteoporosis Risk Assessment. J Bone Miner Res 2002;17(12):2222–2230.
31. Raisz LG. Clinical practice. Screening for osteoporosis. N Engl J Med 2005;353(2):164–171.
32. Indications and reporting for dual-energy x-ray absorptiometry. J Clin Densitom 2004;7(1):37–44.
33. Hodgson SF, Watts NB, Bilezikian JP, et al. American Association of Clinical Endocrinologists medical guidelines for clinical practice for the prevention and treatment of postmenopausal osteoporosis: 2001 edition, with selected updates for 2003. Endocr Pract 2003;9(6):544–564.
34. Nelson HD, Helfand M, Woolf SH, Allan JD. Screening for postmenopausal osteoporosis: A review of the evidence for the U.S. Preventive Services Task Force. Ann Intern Med 2002;137(6):529–541.
35. Writing Group for the ISCD Position Development Conference. Diagnosis of osteoporosis in men, premenopausal women, and children. J Clin Densitom 2004;7(1):17–26.
36. Bischoff-Ferrari HA, Giovannucci E, Willett WC, et al. Estimation of optimal serum concentrations of 25-hydroxyvitamin D for multiple health outcomes. Am J Clin Nutr 2006;84(1):18–28.
37. Hallstrom H, Wolk A, Glynn A, Michaelsson K. Coffee, tea and caffeine consumption in relation to osteoporotic fracture risk in a cohort of Swedish women. Osteoporos Int 2006;17(7):1055–1064.
38. U.S. Department of Agriculture. Dietary guidelines for Americans 2005. 2005, *http://www.health.gov/dietaryguidelines/dga2005/recommendations.htm*.
39. Nieves JW. Osteoporosis: The role of micronutrients. Am J Clin Nutr 2005;81(5):1232S–1239S.
40. Tucker KL, Morita K, Qiao N, et al. Colas, but not other carbonated beverages, are associated with low bone mineral density in older women: The Framingham Osteoporosis Study. Am J Clin Nutr 2006;84(4):936–942.
41. Beverage Marketing Corporation. What Americans drink: Our favorite beverages. 2005, *http://www.ameribev.org/all-about-beverage-products-manufacturing-marketing--consumption/what-america-drinks/index.aspx*.
42. National Institute of Health Office of Dietary Supplements. Dietary supplement fact sheet: Calcium. 2005, *http://dietary-supplements.info.nih.gov/factsheets/calcium.asp*.
43. Standing Committee on the Scientific Evaluation of Dietary Reference Intakes, Food and Nutrition Board, Institute of Medicine. Dietary Reference Intakes for Calcium, Phosphorous, Magnesium, Vitamin D, and Fluoride. Washington, DC: National Academy Press, 1997.
44. Adams J, Pepping J. Vitamin K in the treatment and prevention of osteoporosis and arterial calcification. Am J Health Syst Pharm 2005;62(15):1574–1581.
45. O'Neill CK, Evans E. Beyond calcium and vitamin D. Is there a role for other vitamins, minerals, and nutrients in osteoporosis? Clin Rev Bone Miner Metab 2004;2(4):325–340 .
46. Bonjour JP. Dietary protein: An essential nutrient for bone health. J Am Coll Nutr 2005;24(6 Suppl):526S–536S.
47. Whelan AM, Jurgens TM, Bowles SK. Natural health products in the prevention and treatment of osteoporosis: Systematic review of randomized controlled trials. Ann Pharmacother 2006;40(5):836–849.
48. Zhang X, Shu XO, Li H, et al. Prospective cohort study of soy food consumption and risk of bone fracture among postmenopausal women. Arch Intern Med 2005;165(16):1890–1895.
49. Kanis JA, Johnell O, Oden A, et al. Smoking and fracture risk: A meta-analysis. Osteoporos Int 2005;16(2):155–162.
50. Department of Health and Human Services Center for Disease Control and Prevention. Check for Safety: A Home Fall Prevention Checklist for Older Adults. 2005, *http://www.cdc.gov/ncipc/duip/fallsmaterial.htm#Brochures*.
51. Sawka AM, Boulos P, Beattie K, et al. Do hip protectors decrease the risk of hip fracture in institutional and community-dwelling elderly? A systematic review and meta-analysis of randomized controlled trials. Osteoporos Int 2005;16(12):1461–1474.
52. Bone HG, Hosking D, Devogelaer JP, et al. Ten years' experience with alendronate for osteoporosis in postmenopausal women. N Engl J Med 2004;350(12):1189–1199.
53. Brown JP, Josse RG, Scientific Advisory Council of the Osteoporosis Society of C. 2002 clinical practice guidelines for the diagnosis and management of osteoporosis in Canada. CMAJ 2002;167(10 Suppl):S1–S34.
54. Solomon DH, Brookhart MA, Gandhi TK, et al. Adherence with osteoporosis practice guidelines: A multilevel analysis of patient, physician, and practice setting characteristics. Am J Med 2004;117(12):919–924.
55. Stafford RS, Drieling RL, Johns R, Ma J. National patterns of calcium use in osteoporosis in the United States. J Reprod Med 2005;50(11 Suppl):885–890.
56. Boonen S, Vanderschueren D, Haentjens P, Lips P. Calcium and vitamin D in the prevention and treatment of osteoporosis—A clinical update. J Intern Med 2006;259(6):539–552.
57. Russell RG. Bisphosphonates: From bench to bedside. Ann N Y Acad Sci 2006;1068:367–401.
58. Hamdy RC, Chesnut CH, 3rd, Gass ML, et al. Review of treatment modalities for postmenopausal osteoporosis. South Med J 2005;98(10):1000–1014.
59. Black DM, Delmas PD, Eastell R, et al. Once-yearly zoledronic acid for treatment of postmenopausal osteoporosis. N Engl J Med 2007;356(18): 1809–1822.
60. Epstein S. Update of current therapeutic options for the treatment of postmenopausal osteoporosis. Clin Ther 2006;28(2):151–173.
61. Delmas PD, Adami S, Strugala C, et al. Intravenous ibandronate injections in postmenopausal women with osteoporosis: One-year results from the dosing intravenous administration study. Arthritis Rheum 2006;54(6):1838–1846.
62. Orwoll E, Ettinger M, Weiss S, et al. Alendronate for the treatment of osteoporosis in men. N Engl J Med 2000;343(9):604–610.
63. Colon-Emeric CS. Ten vs five years of bisphosphonate treatment for postmenopausal osteoporosis: Enough of a good thing. JAMA 2006;296(24):2968–2969.
64. Woo SB, Hellstein JW, Kalmar JR. Narrative [corrected] review: Bisphosphonates and osteonecrosis of the jaws. Ann Intern Med 2006;144(10):753–761.
65. American Dental Association Council on Scientific Affairs. Dental management of patients on oral bisphosphonate therapy: Expert panel recommendations. J Am Dent Assoc 2006;137(8):1144–1150.
66. Downey TW, Foltz SH, Boccuzzi SJ, et al. Adherence and persistence associated with the pharmacologic treatment of osteoporosis in a managed care setting. South Med J 2006;99(6):570–575.
67. Vogel VG, Costantino JP, Wickerham DL, et al. Effects of tamoxifen vs raloxifene on the risk of developing invasive breast cancer and other disease outcomes: The NSABP Study of Tamoxifen and Raloxifene (STAR) P-2 trial. JAMA 2006;295(23):2727–2741.
68. Barrett-Connor E, Mosca L, Collins P, et al. Effects of raloxifene on cardiovascular events and breast cancer in postmenopausal women. N Engl J Med 2006;355(2):125–137.
69. Ensrud K, Genazzani AR, Geiger MJ, et al. Effect of raloxifene on cardiovascular adverse events in postmenopausal women with osteoporosis. Am J Cardiol 2006;97(4):520–527.
70. Knopp JA, Diner BM, Blitz M, et al. Calcitonin for treating acute pain of osteoporotic vertebral compression fractures: A systematic review of randomized, controlled trials. Osteoporos Int 2005;16(10):1281–1290.
71. Cauley JA, Robbins J, Chen Z, et al. Effects of estrogen plus progestin on risk of fracture and bone mineral density: The Women's Health Initiative randomized trial. JAMA 2003;290(13):1729–1738.
72. Jackson RD, Wactawski-Wende J, LaCroix AZ, et al. Effects of conjugated equine estrogen on risk of fractures and BMD in postmenopausal women with hysterectomy: Results from the women's health initiative randomized trial. J Bone Miner Res 2006;21(6):817–828.
73. The role of testosterone therapy in postmenopausal women: Position statement of The North American Menopause Society. Menopause 2005;12(5):497–511.
74. Tracz MJ, Sideras K, Bolona ER, et al. Testosterone use in men and its effects on bone health. A systematic review and meta-analysis of randomized placebo-controlled trials. J Clin Endocrinol Metab 2006;91(6):2011–2016.
75. Allan CA, McLachlan RI. Age-related changes in testosterone and the role of replacement therapy in older men. Clin Endocrinol (Oxf) 2004;60(6):653–670.

76. Rhoden EL, Morgentaler A. Risks of testosterone-replacement therapy and recommendations for monitoring. N Engl J Med 2004;350(5):482–492.
77. Follin SL, Hansen LB. Current approaches to the prevention and treatment of postmenopausal osteoporosis. Am J Health Syst Pharm 2003;60(9):883–901.
78. Hodsman AB, Bauer DC, Dempster DW, et al. Parathyroid hormone and teriparatide for the treatment of osteoporosis: A review of the evidence and suggested guidelines for its use. Endocr Rev 2005;26(5):688–703.
79. McClung MR, Lewiecki EM, Cohen SB, et al. Denosumab in postmenopausal women with low bone mineral density. N Engl J Med 2006;354(8):821–831.
80. Lewiecki EM. RANK ligand inhibition with denosumab for the management of osteoporosis. Expert Opin Biol Ther 2006;6(10):1041–1050.
81. Close P, Neuprez A, Reginster JY. Developments in the pharmacotherapeutic management of osteoporosis. Expert Opin Pharmacother 2006;7(12):1603–1615.
82. Eichholz KM, O'Toole JE, Christie SD, Fessler RG. Vertebroplasty and kyphoplasty. Neurosurg Clin N Am 2006;17(4):507–518.
83. Baroncelli GI, Bertelloni S, Sodini F, Saggese G. Osteoporosis in children and adolescents: Etiology and management. Paediatr Drugs 2005;7(5):295–323.
84. Bianchi ML. How to manage osteoporosis in children. Best Pract Res Clin Rheumatol 2005;19(6):991–1005.
85. Thornton J, Ashcroft DM, Mughal MZ, et al. Systematic review of effectiveness of bisphosphonates in treatment of low bone mineral density and fragility fractures in juvenile idiopathic arthritis. Arch Dis Child 2006;91(9):753–761.
86. Khan AA, Syed Z. Bone densitometry in premenopausal women: Synthesis and review. J Clin Densitom 2004;7(1):85–92.
87. Lewiecki EM. Low bone mineral density in premenopausal women. South Med J 2004;97(6):544–550.
88. Schousboe JT, Ensrud KE, Nyman JA, et al. Universal bone densitometry screening combined with alendronate therapy for those diagnosed with osteoporosis is highly cost-effective for elderly women. J Am Geriatr Soc 2005;53(10):1697–1704.
89. Hochberg MC, Thompson DE, Black DM, et al. Effect of alendronate on the age-specific incidence of symptomatic osteoporotic fractures. J Bone Miner Res 2005;20(6):971–976.
90. Boonen S, Marin F, Mellstrom D, et al. Safety and efficacy of teriparatide in elderly women with established osteoporosis: Bone anabolic therapy from a geriatric perspective. J Am Geriatr Soc 2006;54(5):782–789.
91. Boonen S, McClung MR, Eastell R, et al. Safety and efficacy of risedronate in reducing fracture risk in osteoporotic women aged 80 and older: Implications for the use of antiresorptive agents in the old and oldest old. J Am Geriatr Soc 2004;52(11):1832–1839.
92. Mazziotti G, Angeli A, Bilezikian JP, et al. Glucocorticoid-induced osteoporosis: An update. Trends Endocrinol Metab 2006;17(4):144–149.
93. van Staa TP, Leufkens HG, Cooper C. Use of inhaled corticosteroids and risk of fractures. J Bone Miner Res 2001;16(3):581–588.
94. Lau E, Mamdani M, Tu K. Inhaled or systemic corticosteroids and the risk of hospitalization for hip fracture among elderly women. Am J Med 2003;114(2):142–145.
95. American College of Rheumatology Task Force on Osteoporosis Guidelines. Recommendations for the prevention and treatment of glucocorticoid-induced osteoporosis. Arthritis Rheum 1996;39(11):1791–1801.
96. Recommendations for the prevention and treatment of glucocorticoid-induced osteoporosis: 2001 update. American College of Rheumatology Ad Hoc Committee on Glucocorticoid-Induced Osteoporosis. Arthritis Rheum 2001;44(7):1496–1503.
97. Maalouf NM, Shane E. Osteoporosis after solid organ transplantation. J Clin Endocrinol Metab 2005;90(4):2456–2465.
98. K/DOQI clinical practice guidelines for chronic kidney disease: Evaluation, classification, and stratification. Am J Kidney Dis 2002;39(2 Suppl 1):S1–S266.
99. Clase CM, Garg AX, Kiberd BA. Prevalence of low glomerular filtration rate in nondiabetic Americans: Third National Health and Nutrition Examination Survey (NHANES III). J Am Soc Nephrol 2002;13(5):1338–1349.
100. Miller PD, Roux C, Boonen S, et al. Safety and efficacy of risedronate in patients with age-related reduced renal function as estimated by the Cockroft and Gault method: A pooled analysis of nine clinical trials. J Bone Miner Res 2005;20(12):2105–2115.
101. Miller PD, Schwartz EN, Chen P, et al. Teriparatide in postmenopausal women with osteoporosis and mild or moderate renal impairment. Osteoporos Int 2007;18(1):59–68.
102. Bernstein CN, Leslie WD, Leboff MS. AGA technical review on osteoporosis in gastrointestinal diseases. Gastroenterology 2003;124(3):795–841.
103. Lichtenstein GR, Sands BE, Pazianas M. Prevention and treatment of osteoporosis in inflammatory bowel disease. Inflamm Bowel Dis 2006;12(8):797–813.
104. Celiac Disease Foundation. Celiac disease. 2007, *http://www.celiac.org/cd-main.php*.
105. Pfister AK, Welch CA, Lester MD, et al. Cost-effectiveness strategies to treat osteoporosis in elderly women. South Med J 2006;99(2):123–131.
106. Schousboe JT, Nyman JA, Kane RL, Ensrud KE. Cost-effectiveness of alendronate therapy for osteopenic postmenopausal women. Ann Intern Med 2005;142(9):734–741.
107. Goode JV, Swiger K, Bluml BM. Regional osteoporosis screening, referral, and monitoring program in community pharmacies: Findings from Project IMPACT: Osteoporosis. J Am Pharm Assoc 2004;44(2):152–160.
108. Joy MS, Neyhart CD, Dooley MA. A multidisciplinary renal clinic for corticosteroid-induced bone disease. Pharmacotherapy 2000;20(2):206–216.
109. Petty SJ, O'Brien T J, Wark JD. Anti-epileptic medication and bone health. Osteoporos Int 2007;18(2):129–142.
110. Whyte MP. Clinical practice. Paget's disease of bone. N Engl J Med 2006;355(6):593–600.
111. Siris ES, Lyles KW, Singer FR, Meunier PJ. Medical management of Paget's disease of bone: Indications for treatment and review of current therapies. J Bone Miner Res 2006;21 Suppl 2:P94–P98.
112. Reid IR, Miller P, Lyles K, et al. Comparison of a single infusion of zoledronic acid with risedronate for Paget's disease. N Engl J Med 2005;353(9):898–908.
113. Rauch F, Glorieux FH. Osteogenesis imperfecta. Lancet 2004;363(9418):1377–1385.

CHAPTER 94 Rheumatoid Arthritis

ARTHUR A. SCHUNA

KEY CONCEPTS

1. Rheumatoid arthritis is a systemic disease characterized by symmetrical inflammation of joints yet may involve other organ systems.
2. Control of inflammation is the key to slowing or preventing disease progression as well as managing symptoms.
3. Drug therapy should be only part of a comprehensive program for patient management which would also include physical therapy, exercise, and rest. Assistive devices and orthopedic surgery may be necessary in some patients.
4. Disease-modifying antirheumatic drugs (DMARDs) or biologic agents should be started within 3 months of the diagnosis of rheumatoid arthritis.
5. Nonsteroidal antiinflammatory drugs and/or corticosteroids should be considered adjunctive therapy early in the course of treatment and as needed if symptoms are not adequately controlled with DMARDs.
6. When DMARDs used singly are ineffective or not adequately effective, combination therapy with two or more DMARDs or a DMARD plus biologic agents may be used to induce a response.
7. Patients require careful monitoring for toxicity and therapeutic benefit for the duration of treatment.

Rheumatoid arthritis is the most common systemic inflammatory disease characterized by symmetrical joint involvement. Extraarticular involvement, including rheumatoid nodules, vasculitis, eye inflammation, neurologic dysfunction, cardiopulmonary disease, lymphadenopathy, and splenomegaly, can be manifestations of the disease. Although the usual disease course is chronic, some patients will enter a remission spontaneously.

EPIDEMIOLOGY

Rheumatoid arthritis is estimated to have a prevalence of 1% to 2% and does not have any racial predilections. It can occur at any age, with increasing prevalence up to the seventh decade of life. The disease is three times more common in women. In people ages 15 to 45 years, women predominate by a ratio of 6:1; the sex ratio is approximately equal among patients in the first decade of life and in those older than age 60 years.

Epidemiologic data suggest that a genetic predisposition and exposure to unknown environmental factors may be necessary for expression of the disease. The major histocompatibility complex molecules, located on T lymphocytes, appear to have an important role in most patients with rheumatoid arthritis. These molecules can be characterized using human lymphocyte antigen (HLA) typing. A majority of patients with rheumatoid arthritis have HLA-DR4, HLA-DR1, or both antigens in the major histocompatibility complex region. Patients with HLA-DR4 antigen are 3.5 times more likely to develop rheumatoid arthritis than those patients who have other HLA-DR antigens.[1] Although the major histocompatibility complex region is important, it is not the sole determinant, because patients can have the disease without these HLA types. Rheumatoid arthritis is six times more common among dizygotic twins and nontwin children of parents with rheumatoid factor-positive, erosive rheumatoid arthritis when compared with children whose parents do not have the disease. If one of a pair of monozygotic twins is affected, the other twin has a 30 times greater risk of developing the disease.[2,3]

Learning objectives, review questions, and other resources can be found at **www.pharmacotherapyonline.com.**

PATHOPHYSIOLOGY

1 Chronic inflammation of the synovial tissue lining the joint capsule results in the proliferation of this tissue. The inflamed, proliferating synovium characteristic of rheumatoid arthritis is called *pannus*. This pannus invades the cartilage and eventually the bone surface, producing erosions of bone and cartilage and leading to destruction of the joint. The factors that initiate the inflammatory process are unknown.

The immune system is a complex network of checks and balances designed to discriminate self from non-self (foreign) tissues. It helps rid the body of infectious agents, tumor cells, and products associated with the breakdown of cells. In rheumatoid arthritis, this system no longer can differentiate self from non-self tissues and attacks the synovial tissue and other connective tissues.

The immune system has both humoral and cell-mediated functions (Fig. 94–1). The humoral component is necessary for the formation of antibodies. These antibodies are produced by plasma cells, which are derived from B lymphocytes. Most patients with rheumatoid arthritis form antibodies called *rheumatoid factors*. Rheumatoid factors have not been identified as pathogenic, nor does the quantity of these circulating antibodies always correlate with disease activity. Seropositive patients tend to have a more aggressive course of their illness than do seronegative patients. Immunoglobulins can activate the complement system. The complement system amplifies the immune response by encouraging chemotaxis, phagocytosis, and the release of lymphokines by mononuclear cells, which are then presented to T lymphocytes. The processed antigen is recognized by major histocompatibility complex proteins on the

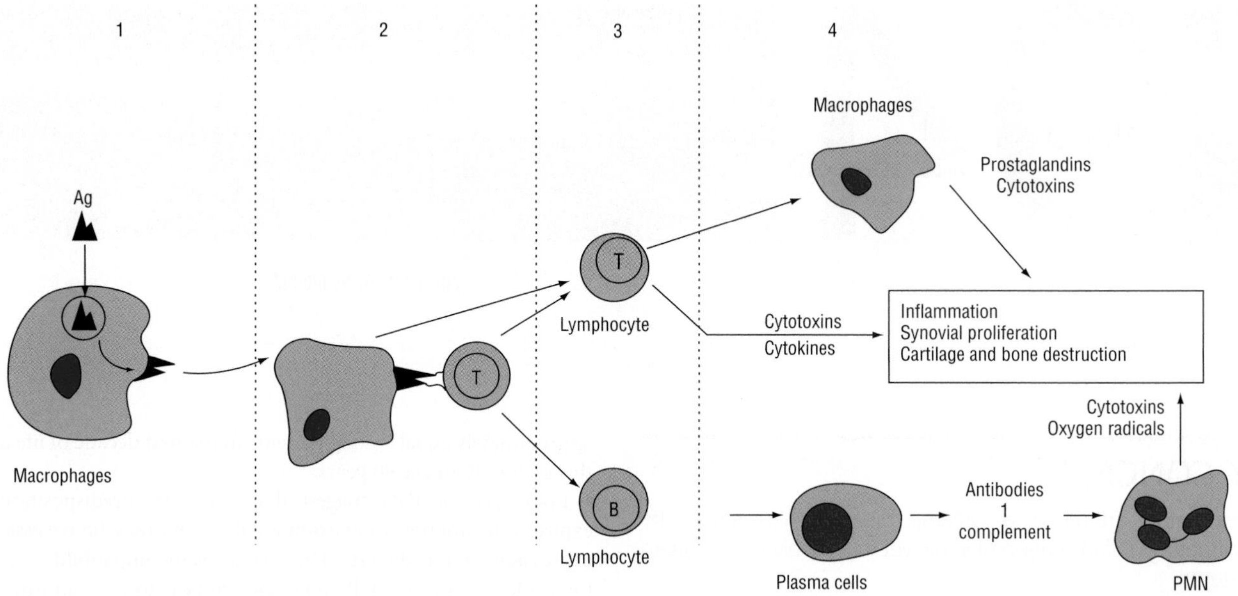

FIGURE 94-1. Pathogenesis of the inflammatory response. Phase 1: Antigen-presenting cell phagocytizes antigen. Phase 2: Antigen is presented to a T lymphocyte. The T lymphocyte attaches to antigen at the major histocompatibility complex portion of cell wall causing activation. Phase 3: An activated T cell stimulates T and B lymphocyte production, promoting inflammation. Phase 4: Activated T cells and macrophages release factors that promote tissue destruction, increase blood flow, and result in cellular invasion of synovial tissue and joint fluid. (Ag, antigen; PMN, polymorphonuclear leukocyte.)

lymphocyte, which activates it to stimulate the production of T and B cells. The proinflammatory cytokines tumor necrosis factor (TNF), interleukin (IL)-1 and IL-6 are key substances in the initiation and continuance of rheumatoid inflammation. Lymphocytes may be either B cells (derived from bone marrow) or T cells (derived from thymus tissue). T cells may be either CD4+ (T-helper) or CD8+ (cytotoxic or killer) T cells. There are two subtypes of T-helper cells, TH_1, which promote inflammation by producing interferon-γ, tumor necrosis factor, and interleukin-2, and TH_2, which produce the antiinflammatory cytokines IL-4, IL-5 and IL-10. CD8+ killer T cells have a regulatory effect on the immune process by suppressing activity of CD4+ cells through release of antiinflammatory cytokines and promoting apoptosis (cell death). Activated T cells produce cytotoxins, which are directly toxic to tissues, and cytokines, which stimulate further activation of inflammatory processes and attract cells to areas of inflammation. Macrophages are stimulated to release prostaglandins and cytotoxins.[4]

Although it has been suggested that T cells play a key role in the pathogenesis of rheumatoid arthritis, B cells clearly have an equally important role. Evidence for this importance may be found in the effectiveness of B-cell depletion using rituximab in controlling rheumatoid inflammation. Activated B cells produce plasma cells, which form antibodies. These antibodies in combination with complement result in the accumulation of polymorphonuclear leukocytes, which release cytotoxins, oxygen free radicals, and hydroxyl radicals that promote cellular damage to synovium and bone. B cells also produce cytokines that may alter the function of other immune cells, and they also have the ability to process antigens and act as antigen-presenting cells, which interact with T cells to activate the immune process.[5,6]

In the synovial membrane, CD4+ T cells are abundant and communicate with macrophages, osteoclasts, fibroblasts and chondrocytes either through direct cell–cell interactions using cell surface receptors or through proinflammatory cytokines such as TNF-α, IL-1, and IL-6. These cells produce metalloproteinases and other cytotoxic substances, which lead to the erosion of bone and cartilage.[1,7,8]

Vasoactive substances also play a role in the inflammatory process. Histamine, kinins, and prostaglandins are released at the site of inflammation. These substances increase both blood flow to the site of inflammation and the permeability of blood vessels. These substances cause the edema, warmth, erythema, and pain associated with joint inflammation and make it easier for granulocytes to pass from blood vessels to the site of inflammation.

The end results of the chronic inflammatory changes are variable. Loss of cartilage may result in a loss of the joint space. The formation of chronic granulation or scar tissue can lead to loss of joint motion or bony fusion (called *ankylosis*). Laxity of tendon structures can result in a loss of support to the affected joint, leading to instability or subluxation. Tendon contractures also may occur, leading to chronic deformity.[1,3,9,10]

CLINICAL PRESENTATION OF RHEUMATOID ARTHRITIS

Symptoms

- Joint pain and stiffness of more than 6 weeks' duration. May also experience fatigue, weakness, low-grade fever, loss of appetite. Muscle pain and afternoon fatigue may also be present. Joint deformity is generally seen late in the disease.

Signs

- Tenderness with warmth and swelling over affected joints usually involving hands and feet. Distribution of joint involvement is frequently symmetrical. Rheumatoid nodules may also be present.

Laboratory Tests

- Rheumatoid factor (RF) detectable in 60% to 70%.
- Anticyclic citrullinated peptide (anti-CCP) antibodies have similar sensitivity to RF (50% to 85%) but are more specific (90% to 95%) and are present earlier in the disease.
- Elevated erythrocyte sedimentation rate and C-reactive protein are markers for inflammation.
- Normocytic normochromic anemia is common as is thrombocytosis.

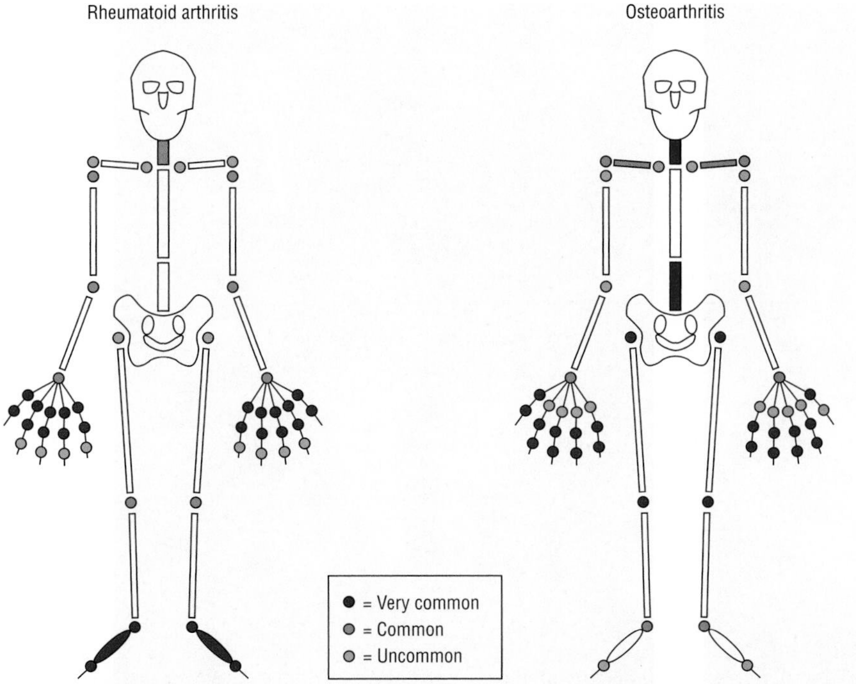

FIGURE 94-2. Patterns of joint involvement in rheumatoid arthritis and osteoarthritis.

Other Diagnostic Tests

- Joint fluid aspiration may show increased white blood cell counts without infection, crystals.
- Joint radiographs may show periarticular osteoporosis, joint space narrowing, or erosions.

The symptoms of rheumatoid arthritis usually develop insidiously over the course of several weeks to months. Prodromal symptoms include fatigue, weakness, low-grade fever, loss of appetite, and joint pain. Stiffness and muscle aches (myalgias) may precede the development of joint swelling (synovitis). Fatigue may be more of a problem in the afternoon. During disease flares, the onset of fatigue begins earlier in the day and subsides as disease activity lessens. Most commonly, joint involvement tends to be symmetrical; however, early in the disease some patients present with an asymmetrical pattern involving one or a few joints that eventually develops into the more classic presentation. Approximately 20% of patients develop an abrupt onset of their illness with fevers, polyarthritis, and constitutional symptoms (e.g., depression, anxiety, fatigue, anorexia, and weight loss).[2,3]

No single test or physical finding can be used to make the diagnosis of rheumatoid arthritis. In early disease the diagnosis can be particularly challenging as radiographic findings are usually not found and rheumatoid factor test can be undetectable. Duration of joint pain and swelling and morning stiffness lasting more than 1 hour and involvement of three or more joints are important predictors of the development of persistent erosive rheumatoid arthritis.[11]

JOINT INVOLVEMENT

The joints affected most frequently by rheumatoid arthritis are the small joints of the hands, wrists, and feet (Fig. 94–2). In addition, elbows, shoulders, hips, knees, and ankles may be involved. Patients usually experience joint stiffness that typically is worse in the morning. The duration of stiffness tends to be correlated directly with disease activity, usually exceeds 30 minutes, and may persist all day. Chronic inflammation with lack of an adequate exercise program results in loss of range of motion, atrophy of muscles, weakness, and deformity (Figs. 94–3 and 94–4).

On examination, the swelling of the joints may be visible or may be apparent only by palpation. The swelling feels soft and spongy because it is caused by proliferation of soft tissues or fluid accumulation within the joint capsule. The swollen joint may appear erythematous and feel warmer than nearby skin surfaces, especially early in the course of the disease. In contrast, the swelling associated with osteoarthritis usually is bony (caused by osteophytes) and infrequently is associated with signs of inflammation.

Involvement of the hands and wrists is common in rheumatoid arthritis. Hand involvement is manifested by pain, swelling, tenderness, and grip weakness during the acute phase and by subluxation, instability, deformity, and muscle atrophy in the chronic phase of the disease. Functional difficulties with clasp, grasp, and pinch alter both strength and fine motor movement.

Deformity of the hand may be seen with chronic inflammation. These changes may alter the mechanics of hand function reducing grip strength and making it difficult to perform usual daily activity.

Pain in the elbow and shoulder may be the result of true joint involving or inflammation of soft-tissue structures such as tendons

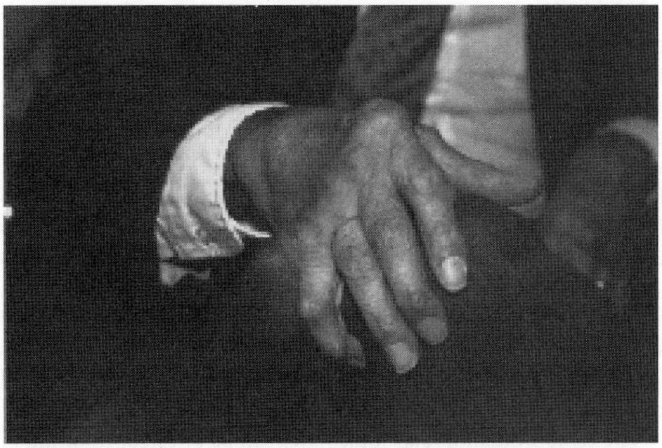

FIGURE 94-3. Deformities of rheumatoid arthritis, with marked ulnar deviation, swan-neck deformity, active synovitis, and nodules. *(Reproduced with permission from Brunicardi FC, Anderson DK, Billiar TR, Dunn DL, Hunter JG, Matthews JB, Pollock RE, Schwartz SI. Schwartz's Principles of Surgery. 8th ed, The McGraw-Hill Companies, 2005.)*

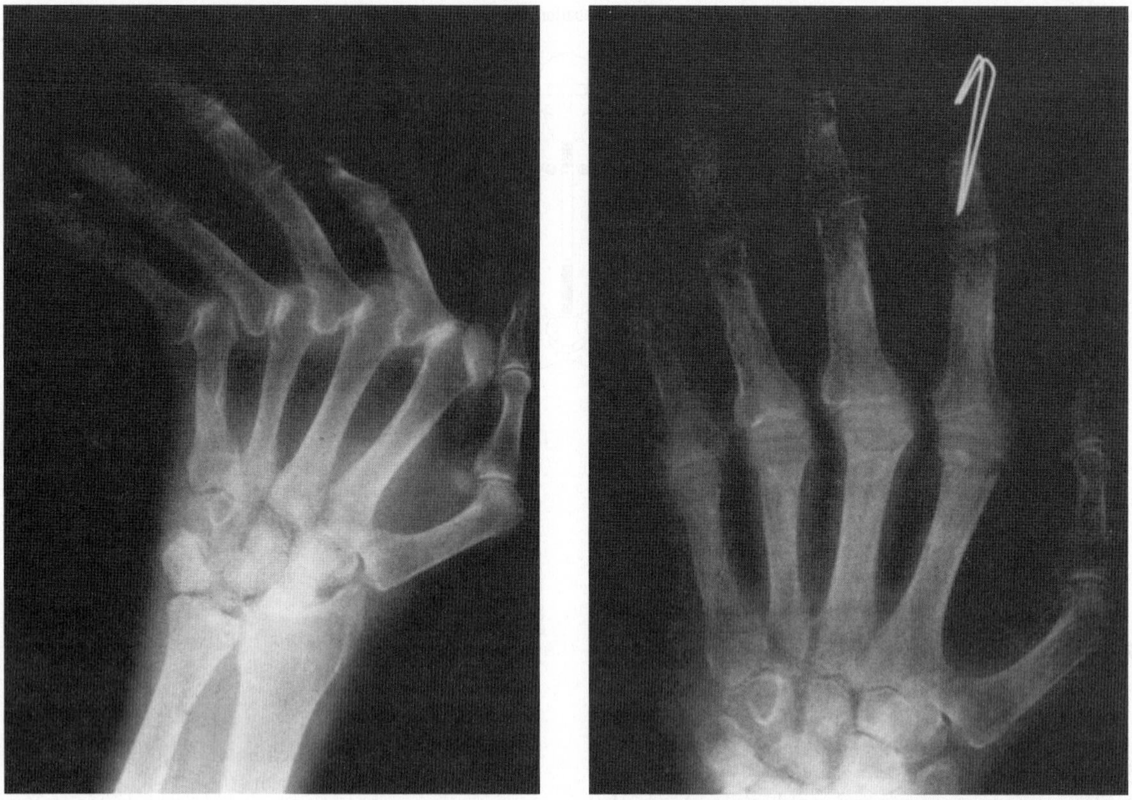

A B

FIGURE 94-4. *A.* Preoperative view of metacarpophalangeal joint in rheumatoid arthritis. *B.* Following resection arthroplasty. *(Reproduced with permission from Skinner H, ed. Current Diagnosis & Treatment in Orthopedics, 4th ed. New York: McGraw-Hill, 2006:592.)*

(tendonitis) or the bursa (bursitis). The knee also can be involved, with loss of cartilage, instability, and joint pain. Synovitis of the knee may cause the formation of a cyst behind the knee called a *popliteal* or *Baker cyst.* These cysts may become painful as they get tense, or they may rupture, producing a clinical picture similar to thrombophlebitis secondary to the release of inflammatory components into the area of the calf muscle. Chronic joint pain leads to muscle atrophy, which can result in a laxity of the ligamentous structures that support the knee, causing instability. Maintenance of an adequate range of motion of the knee is essential to normal gait.

Foot and ankle involvement in rheumatoid arthritis is common. The metatarsophalangeal joints are involved frequently in rheumatoid arthritis, making walking difficult. Subluxation of the metatarsal heads leads to "cock-up" or hammer toe deformities. Subluxation also may cause a flexion deformity at the proximal interphalangeal proximal interphalangeal joint of the toe, leading to pressure necrosis of the skin over the joint secondary to irritation caused by shoes. Hallux valgus (lateral deviation of the digit) and bunion or callus formation may occur at the great toe. A widening of the foot occurs commonly with long-standing disease.

Involvement of the spine usually occurs in the cervical vertebrae; lumbar vertebral involvement is rare. Involvement of the first and second cervical vertebrae (C1–C2) can lead to instability of this joint. Patients with this problem are at a greater risk for spinal cord compression, although this complication is rare.

The temporomandibular joint (jaw) can be affected, resulting in malocclusion and difficulty in chewing food. Inflammation of cartilage in the chest can lead to chest wall pain. Hip pain may occur as a result of destructive changes in the hip joint, soft-tissue inflammation (e.g., bursitis), or referred pain from nerve entrapment at the lumbar vertebrae.

EXTRAARTICULAR INVOLVEMENT

Rheumatoid Nodules

Rheumatoid nodules occur in 20% of patients with rheumatoid arthritis. These nodules are seen most commonly on the extensor surfaces of the elbows, forearms, and hands but also may be seen on the feet and at other pressure points. They also may develop in the lung or pleural lining of the lung and, rarely, in the meninges. Rheumatoid nodules usually are asymptomatic and do not require any special intervention. Nodules are observed more commonly in patients with erosive disease.[12]

Vasculitis

Vasculitis usually is seen in patients with long-standing rheumatoid arthritis. Vasculitis may result in a wide variety of clinical presentations. Invasion of blood vessel walls by inflammatory cells results in an obliteration of the vessel, producing infarction of tissue distal to the area of involvement. Most commonly, small-vessel vasculitis produces infarcts near the ends of the fingers or toes, especially around the nail beds. These infarcts are usually of little consequence.

Vasculitis also may cause the breakdown of skin, especially in the lower extremities, producing ulcers that may be indistinguishable in appearance from stasis ulcers. However, these ulcers do not heal with the usual modes of treatment used for stasis ulcers. Involvement of larger vessels with vasculitis can result in life-threatening complications. Infarction of vessels supplying blood to nerves can cause irreversible motor deficits. Involvement of vessels supplying other organ systems can lead to visceral involvement and a polyarteritis nodosa-like illness. Aggressive treatment of the inflammatory process is necessary in these patients. Fortunately, the more serious vasculitic picture is seen rarely.

Pulmonary Complications

Rheumatoid arthritis may involve the pleura of the lung, which is often asymptomatic, although pleural effusions may result. Pulmonary fibrosis also may develop as a result of rheumatoid involvement; smoking appears to increase the risk of this complication. Rheumatoid nodules may develop in lung tissue and appear similar to neoplasms on chest radiographs. Interstitial pneumonitis and arteritis are rare, potentially life-threatening complications of rheumatoid arthritis.

Ocular Manifestations

Ocular manifestations include keratoconjunctivitis sicca and inflammation of the sclera, episclera, and cornea. Atrophy of the lacrimal duct may result in a decrease in tear formation, causing dry and itchy eyes, termed *keratoconjunctivitis sicca.* When this is observed in association with rheumatoid arthritis, it is referred to as *Sjögren's syndrome.* Artificial tears may be used to relieve symptoms. The salivary glands may also be involved in Sjögren's syndrome. Inflammation of the superficial layers of the sclera (episcleritis) is generally self-limiting. Involvement of deeper tissues (scleritis) usually results in a more serious, painful, and chronic inflammation. Rheumatoid nodules may develop on the sclera.

Cardiac Involvement

The heart is sometimes affected by rheumatoid arthritis. Rheumatoid arthritis is associated with an increased risk of cardiovascular mortality. This risk appears to be higher in those with more active inflammation and is reduced with treatment, particularly with methotrexate.[13,14] Pericarditis may occur, resulting in the accumulation of fluid. Although many patients show evidence of previous pericarditis at autopsy, the development of clinically evident pericarditis with tamponade is a rare complication. Cardiac conduction abnormalities and aortic valve incompetence, caused by aortic root dilation, may occur. Myocarditis is a rare complication of rheumatoid arthritis.

Felty's Syndrome

Rheumatoid arthritis in association with splenomegaly and neutropenia is known as *Felty's syndrome.* Thrombocytopenia also may be a manifestation of the syndrome. Patients with Felty's syndrome and severe leukopenia are more susceptible to infection. The decrease in granulocytes appears to be mediated by the immune system because splenectomy does not result in improvement of the patient.[12]

Other Complications

Lymphadenopathy may occur in patients with rheumatoid arthritis, particularly in nodes proximal to more actively involved joints. Renal involvement is rare but can be associated with treatment, including nonsteroidal antiinflammatory drugs (NSAIDs), gold salts, and penicillamine. Amyloidosis is a rare complication of long-standing rheumatoid arthritis. It appears to be more common in Europe than in the United States.

LABORATORY FINDINGS

Hematologic tests often reveal a mild to moderate anemia with normocytic, normochromic indices. The hematocrit may fall as low as 30%. The anemia is usually inversely related to inflammatory disease activity and is referred to as an *anemia of chronic disease.* This type of anemia does not respond to iron therapy and can present a diagnostic dilemma because NSAIDs may induce gastritis and chronic blood loss, leading to iron-deficiency anemia. Laboratory tests useful in differentiating these anemias include stool guaiac (or other stool tests for occult blood), serum iron-to-iron-binding capacity ratio (decreased in iron deficiency), ferritin (decreased in iron deficiency), and mean corpuscular volume (more likely to be decreased in iron deficiency). Other causes of anemia also must be considered in the differential diagnosis (see Chap. 105).

Thrombocytosis is another common hematologic finding with active rheumatoid arthritis. Platelet counts rise and fall in direct correlation with disease activity in many patients. Thrombocytopenia may result from toxicity of gold salts, penicillamine, or immunosuppressive therapy. Thrombocytopenia also may be observed in Felty's syndrome or vasculitis.

Although leukopenia is associated with Felty's syndrome, it also may result from toxicity of methotrexate, gold, sulfasalazine, penicillamine, and immunosuppressive drugs. Leukocytosis is seen commonly as a result of corticosteroid treatment.

The erythrocyte sedimentation rate is usually elevated in patients with rheumatoid arthritis and other inflammatory diseases. This test is very nonspecific, and although the erythrocyte sedimentation rate usually falls as patients respond to therapy, there is a large variability among patients in response to treatment. C-reactive protein is another nonspecific marker for inflammatory arthritis when it is elevated. This protein is produced by the liver in response to certain cytokines.

Rheumatoid factor is present in 60% to 70% of patients with rheumatoid arthritis. The usual laboratory test for rheumatoid factor is an antibody specific for immunoglobulin (Ig) M rheumatoid factor. Patients with rheumatoid arthritis and a negative test for rheumatoid factor may have IgG or IgA rheumatoid factors, but tests for these are not routinely available. Rheumatoid factor tests may be reported positive at a specific serum dilution. Serum is diluted to a standard series of dilutions; the greatest dilution that yields a positive test result will be reported (e.g., rheumatoid factor positive at 1:640). Some laboratories quantify rheumatoid factor rather than using titers. Higher dilutional titers or serum concentrations of rheumatoid factors usually indicate a more severe disease, but like the erythrocyte sedimentation rate, the large interpatient variability makes this test unreliable as a means of assessing patient progress. Rheumatoid factor may be positive in patients without rheumatoid arthritis (Table 94–1).

Anticyclic citrullinated peptide antibody has similar sensitivity for rheumatoid arthritis, being found in 50% to 85% of patients with the disease, but is more specific (90% to 95%) and is detectable

TABLE 94-1 Diseases Associated with a Positive Rheumatoid Factor

Rheumatic diseases
Rheumatoid arthritis
Sjögren's syndrome (with or without arthritis)
Systemic lupus erythematosus
Progressive systemic sclerosis
Polymyositis/dermatomyositis
Infectious diseases
Bacterial endocarditis
Tuberculosis
Syphilis
Infectious mononucleosis
Infectious hepatitis
Leprosy
Other causes
Aging
Interstitial pulmonary fibrosis
Cirrhosis of the liver
Chronic active hepatitis
Sarcoidosis

very early in the disease. Many rheumatologists will do both tests in evaluating new patients.

Antinuclear antibodies are detected in 25% of patients with rheumatoid arthritis. These antibodies usually have a diffuse pattern of immunofluorescence. Tests for antibodies to double-stranded DNA (usually positive in systemic lupus erythematosus) are negative. Serum complement is usually normal, although complement concentrations of joint fluid often are depressed from consumption secondary to the inflammatory process. In patients with vasculitis, serum complement concentrations may be low.[15,16]

Synovial fluid usually is turbid because of the large number of leukocytes in inflammatory fluid. White cell counts of 5,000 to 50,000/mm^3 are not uncommon in inflamed joints. The fluid is usually less viscous than that in normal joints or in fluid associated with osteoarthritis. Glucose concentrations of joint fluid are normal or low compared with those in serum drawn at the same time as synovial aspirates. The decrease is not as profound as the decrease associated with joint infection or systemic lupus erythematosus.

Early radiographic manifestations of rheumatoid arthritis include soft-tissue swelling and osteoporosis near the joint (periarticular osteoporosis). Joint space narrowing occurs as a result of cartilage degradation. Erosions tend to occur later in the course of the disease and usually are seen first in the metacarpophalangeal and proximal interphalangeal joints of the hands and the metatarsophalangeal joints of the feet. Periodic joint radiographs are a useful way of evaluating disease progression.

Seronegative Inflammatory Arthritis

Although rheumatoid arthritis may have a negative rheumatoid factor titer, a number of other systemic inflammatory arthritic conditions exist including psoriatic arthritis, ankylosing spondylitis, and arthritis associated with inflammatory bowel disease. These conditions often tend to be less aggressive than what is typically seen with rheumatoid arthritis. Detailed discussion about these conditions is beyond the scope of this chapter, but further information may be found elsewhere.[2] Management principles are similar to those for rheumatoid arthritis.

TREATMENT

Rheumatoid Arthritis

■ DESIRED OUTCOME

❷ The primary objective is to improve or maintain functional status, thereby improving quality of life. Treatment of rheumatoid arthritis is a multifaceted approach that includes pharmacologic and nonpharmacologic therapies. Recent emphasis has been placed on aggressive treatment early in the disease course. The ultimate goal is to achieve complete disease remission, although this goal may be difficult to achieve in some patients. Additional goals of treatment include controlling disease activity and joint pain, maintaining the ability to function in daily activities or work, improving the quality of life, and slowing destructive joint changes.

■ NONPHARMACOLOGIC THERAPY

❸ Rest, occupational therapy, physical therapy, use of assistive devices, weight reduction, and surgery are the most useful types of nonpharmacologic therapy used in patients with rheumatoid arthritis. Rest is an essential component of a nonpharmacologic treatment plan. It relieves stress on inflamed joints and prevents further joint destruction. Rest also aids in alleviation of pain. Too much rest and immobility, however, may lead to decreased range of motion and, ultimately, muscle atrophy and contractures.

Occupational and physical therapy can provide the patient with skills and exercises necessary to increase or maintain mobility. These disciplines also may provide patients with supportive and adaptive devices such as canes, walkers, and splints.

Other nonpharmacologic therapeutic options include weight loss and surgery. Weight reduction helps to alleviate inflamed joint stress. This should be instituted and monitored with close supervision of a healthcare professional. Tenosynovectomy, tendon repair, and joint replacements are surgical options for patients with rheumatoid arthritis. Such management is reserved for patients with severe disease.[17,18]

■ PHARMACOLOGIC THERAPY

❹ ❺ A disease-modifying antirheumatic drug (DMARD) should be started within the first 3 months of symptom onset (Fig. 94–5).[17] Early introduction of DMARDs results in a more favorable outcome.[19–25] NSAIDs and/or corticosteroids may be used for symptomatic relief if needed. They provide relatively rapid improvement in symptoms compared with DMARDs, which may take weeks to months before benefit is seen; however, NSAIDs have no impact on disease progression and the long-term complication risk of corticosteroids make them less desirable.[24]

Early treatment with DMARDs can reduce mortality. Patients with rheumatoid arthritis have increased mortality compared to people without the disease. In one trial, methotrexate reduced risk of mortality.[13] Early treatment with DMARDs in patients followed for up to 10 years had mortality rates similar to patients without the disease.[26]

DMARDs including biologic agents should be used in all patients except those with limited disease. DMARDs commonly used include methotrexate, hydroxychloroquine, sulfasalazine, and leflunomide. The biologic agents that have disease-modifying activity include the anti-TNF drugs (etanercept, infliximab, adalimumab), the IL-1 receptor antagonist anakinra, the costimulation modulator abatacept, and rituximab, which depletes peripheral B cells. Less frequently used are azathioprine, D-penicillamine, gold (including auranofin), minocycline, cyclosporine and cyclophosphamide. This is due to either less efficacy, high toxicity, or both. The order in which the first-line agents are used is not clearly defined, although methotrexate is often chosen because long-term data suggests superior outcomes with methotrexate than with other DMARDs and a lower cost than biologic agents. Leflunomide appears to have similar long-term efficacy as that of methotrexate.[27]

The biologics have proven effective for patients who fail treatment with other DMARDs. Infliximab should be given in combina-

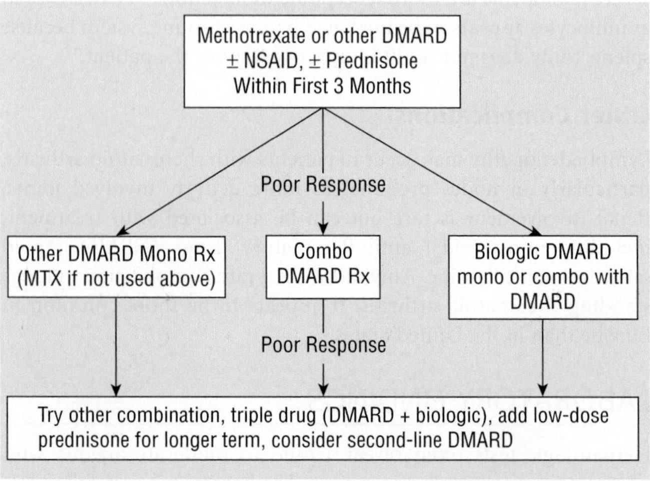

FIGURE 94-5. Algorithm for treatment of rheumatoid arthritis. (DMARD, disease-modifying antirheumatic drug; MTX, methotrexate; NSAID, nonsteroidal antiinflammatory drug.)

TABLE 94-2 Usual Doses and Monitoring Parameters for Antirheumatic Drugs

Drug	Usual Dose	Initial	Maintenance
Nonsteroidal antiinflammatory drugs	See Table 95-2 in Chap. 95	Scr or BUN, CBC q 2–4 weeks p starting therapy × 1–2 months salicylates: serum salicylate levels if therapeutic dose & no response	Same as initial plus stool guaiac q 6–12 months
Methotrexate	Oral or IM: 7.5–15 mg q week	Baseline: AST, ALT, alk phos, alb, t. bili, hep B & C studies, CBC w/plt, Scr	CBC w/plt, AST, alb q 1–2 months
Leflunomide	Oral: 100 mg daily for 3 days then 10–20 mg daily or 10–20 mg daily without loading dose	Baseline: ALT, CBC with platelets	CBC with platelets and ALT monthly initially and then every 6–8 weeks
Hydroxychloroquine	Oral: 200–300 mg bid, after 1–2 months may ↓ to 200 mg bid or daily	Baseline: color fundus photography & automated central perimetric analysis	Ophthalmoscopy q 9–12 months and Amsler grid at home q 2 weeks
Sulfasalazine	Oral: 500 mg bid, then ↑ to 1 g bid max	Baseline: CBC w/plt, then q week × 1 month	Same as initial–q 1–2 months
Etanercept	50 mg SC weekly	Tuberculin skin test	None
Infliximab	3 mg/kg IV at 0, 2, 6 weeks then q 8 weeks	Tuberculin skin test	None
Adalimumab	40 mg SC q 2 weeks	Tuberculin skin test	None
Anakinra	100 mg SC daily	None	None
Rituximab	1,000 mg twice 2 weeks apart	None	None
Abatacept	<60 kg–500 mg 60–100 kg–750 mg >100 kg–1,000 mg	None	None
Auranofin	Oral: 3 mg daily to bid	Baseline: UA, CBC w/plt	Same as initial–q 1–2 months
Gold thiomalate	IM: 10 mg test dose, then weekly dosing 25–50 mg, after response may ↑ dosing interval	Baseline & until stable: UA, CBC w/plt preinjection	Same as initial–every other dose
Azathioprine	Oral: 50–150 mg daily	CBC w/plt, AST q 2 weeks × 1–2 months	Same as initial–q 1–2 months
D-Penicillamine	Oral: 125–250 mg daily, may ↑ by 125–250 mg q 1–2 months, max 750 mg daily	Baseline: UA, CBC w/plt, then q week × 1 month	Same as initial–q 1–2 months, but q 2 weeks if dose change
Cyclophosphamide	Oral: 1–2 mg/kg/day	UA, CBC w/plt q week × 1 month	Same as initial–q 2–4 weeks
Cyclosporine	Oral: 2.5 mg/kg/day	S_{cr}, blood pressure q month	Same as initial
Corticosteroids	Oral, IV, IM, IA, and soft-tissue injections: variable	glucose, blood pressure q 3–6 months	Same as initial

alb, albumin; alk phos, alkaline phosphatase; ALT, alanine aminotransferase; AST, aspartate aminotransferase; BUN, blood urea nitrogen; CBC, complete blood count; hep, hepatitis; IA, intraarticular; IM, intramuscular; IV, intravenous; p, after; plt, platelet; q, every; S_{cr}, serum creatinine; t. bili, total bilirubin; UA, urinalysis.

tion with methotrexate to prevent development of antibodies that may reduce drug efficacy or induce allergic reactions.

❻ Combination therapy with two or more DMARDs may be effective when single-DMARD treatment is unsuccessful.[24,28–34] The combinations of cyclosporine plus methotrexate and methotrexate plus sulfasalazine and hydroxychloroquine are particularly effective.[33] One study suggests that the initial combination therapy with either methotrexate, sulfasalazine plus prednisone, or infliximab plus methotrexate were superior to more conventional sequential monotherapy or step-up combinations of DMARDs in early rheumatoid arthritis.[30]

Corticosteroids can be used in various ways. They are valuable in controlling symptoms before the onset of action of DMARDs. A burst of corticosteroids can be used in acute flares. Continuous low doses may be adjuncts when DMARDs do not provide adequate disease control. Corticosteroids may be injected into joints and soft tissues to control local inflammation. Corticosteroids seldom should be used as monotherapy. There are data to suggest they have disease-modifying activity;[35,36] however, it is preferable to avoid chronic use when possible to avoid long-term complications. NSAIDs and DMARDs have steroid-sparing properties that permit reductions of corticosteroid doses.

❼ Tables 94–2, 94–3, and 94–4 provide monitoring parameters and dosing guidelines for DMARDs and NSAIDs used in rheumatoid arthritis.

TABLE 94-3 Clinical Monitoring of Drug Therapy in Rheumatoid Arthritis

Drug	Toxicities Requiring Monitoring	Symptoms to Inquire About[a]
NSAIDs and salicylates	GI ulceration and bleeding, renal damage	Blood in stool, black stool, dyspepsia, nausea/vomiting, weakness, dizziness, abdominal pain, edema, weight gain, SOB
Corticosteroids	Hypertension, hyperglycemia, osteoporosis[b]	Blood pressure if available, polyuria, polydipsia, edema, SOB, visual changes, weight gain, headaches, broken bones or bone pain
Azathioprine	Myelosuppression, hepatotoxicity, lymphoproliferative disorders	Symptoms of myelosuppression (extreme fatigue, easy bleeding or bruising, infection), jaundice
Gold (intramuscular or oral)	Myelosuppression, proteinuria, rash, stomatitis	Symptoms of myelosuppression, edema, rash, oral ulcers, diarrhea
Hydroxychloroquine	Macular damage, rash, diarrhea	Visual changes including a decrease in night or peripheral vision, rash, diarrhea
Methotrexate	Myelosuppression, hepatic fibrosis, cirrhosis, pulmonary infiltrates or fibrosis, stomatitis, rash	Symptoms of myelosuppression, SOB, nausea/vomiting, lymph node swelling, coughing, mouth sores, diarrhea, jaundice
Leflunomide	Hepatitis, GI distress, alopecia	Nausea/vomiting, gastritis, diarrhea, hair loss, jaundice
Penicillamine	Myelosuppression, proteinuria, stomatitis, rash, dysgeusia	Symptoms of myelosuppression, edema, rash, diarrhea, altered taste perception, oral ulcers
Sulfasalazine	Melosuppression, rash	Symptoms of myelosuppression, photosensitivity, rash, nausea/vomiting
Etanercept, adalimumab, anakinra	Local injection-site reactions, infection	Symptoms of infection
Infliximab, rituximab, abatacept	Immune reactions, infection	Postinfusion reactions, symptoms of infection

GI, gastrointestinal; NSAIDs, nonsteroidal antiinflammatory drugs; SOB, shortness of breath.

[a]Altered immune function increases infection which should be considered particularly in those patients taking azathioprine, methotrexate, and corticosteroids or other drugs as a symptom of myelosuppression.

[b]Osteoporosis is unlikely to manifest itself early in treatment, but all patients should be taking appropriate steps to prevent bone loss.

From American College of Rheumatology Ad Hoc Committee on Clinical Guidelines. Guidelines for monitoring drug therapy in rheumatoid arthritis. Arthritis Rheum 1996;39:723-731.

TABLE 94-4 Dosage Regimens for Nonsteroidal Antiinflammatory Drugs

	Recommended Antiinflammatory Total Daily Dosage		
Drug	***Adult***	***Children***	**Dosing Schedule**
Aspirin	2.6–5.2 g	60–100 mg/kg	Four times daily
Celecoxib	200–400 mg	–	Daily to twice daily
Diclofenac	150–200 mg	–	Three times per day to four times daily Extended release–twice daily
Diflunisal	0.5–1.5 g	–	Twice daily
Etodolac	0.2–1.2 g (max. 20 mg/kg)	–	Twice daily to four times daily
Fenoprofen	0.9–3.0 g	–	Four times daily
Flurbiprofen	200–300 mg	–	Twice daily to four times daily
Ibuprofen	1.2–3.2 g	20–40 mg/kg	Three times per day to four times daily
Indomethacin	50–200 mg	2–4 mg/kg (max. 200 mg)	Twice daily to four times daily Extended release–daily
Meclofenamate	200–400 mg	–	Three times per day to four times per day
Meloxicam	7.5–15 mg	–	Daily
Nabumetone	1–2 g	–	Daily to twice daily
Naproxen	0.5–1.0 g	10 mg/kg	Twice daily Extended release–daily
Naproxen sodium	0.55–1.1 g	–	Twice daily
Nonacetylated salicylates	1.2–4.8 g	–	Twice daily to six times per day
Oxaprozin	0.6–1.8 g (max. 26 mg/kg)	–	Daily to three times a day
Piroxicam	10–20 mg	–	Daily
Sulindac	300–400 mg	–	Twice daily
Tolmetin	0.6–1.8 g	15–30 mg/kg	Twice daily to four times daily

Nonsteroidal Antiinflammatory Drugs

NSAIDs should seldom be used as monotherapy for rheumatoid arthritis because they do not alter the course of the disease; instead, they should be viewed as adjuncts to DMARD treatment. NSAIDs possess both analgesic and antiinflammatory properties and reduce stiffness associated with rheumatoid arthritis. NSAIDs mainly inhibit prostaglandin synthesis, which is only a small portion of the inflammatory cascade (see Fig. 94–1). For details on these agents see Chap. 95.

Methotrexate

Methotrexate is now considered the DMARD of choice by many rheumatologists for treating rheumatoid arthritis. In psoriatic arthritis it not only treats the joint symptoms but also improves the skin disease for most patients. Methotrexate is contraindicated in pregnant and nursing women. It is also contraindicated in patients with chronic liver disease, immunodeficiency, pleural or peritoneal effusions, leukopenia, thrombocytopenia, preexisting blood disorders, and a creatinine clearance of less than 40 mL/min.

Absorption of methotrexate is variable and averages approximately 70% of an oral dose. Methotrexate is 35% to 50% bound to albumin; it may be displaced by highly protein-bound drugs such as NSAIDs, but the clinical importance of this interaction is unknown. Methotrexate is extensively metabolized intracellularly to polyglutamated derivatives. It is excreted by the kidney, 80% unchanged, by glomerular filtration and active transport. Some methotrexate may be reabsorbed, but this transport process may be saturated even with low doses, resulting in increased renal clearance.

Methotrexate inhibits cytokine production, inhibits purine biosynthesis, and may stimulate release of adenosine, all of which may lead to its antiinflammatory properties. The drug has a fairly rapid onset of action; results may be seen as early as 2 to 3 weeks after starting therapy. Some 45% to 67% of patients remain on methotrexate therapy in studies ranging from 5 to 7 years.[37,38] Methotrexate may be given intramuscularly, subcutaneously, or orally. Doses greater than 15 mg per week generally are given parenterally because of decreased oral bioavailability of larger doses.

The toxicities of methotrexate therapy are mainly gastrointestinal, hematologic, pulmonary, and hepatic. Stomatitis occurs in 3% to 10% of patients and may be painful or painless. Diarrhea, nausea, and vomiting may occur in up to 10% of patients. The most common hematologic toxicity is thrombocytopenia in 1% to 3% of patients. Leukopenia also may occur, but in a smaller number of patients. Although pulmonary fibrosis and pneumonitis can be severe adverse effects, they are rare.

Elevated liver enzymes may occur in up to 15% of patients; cirrhosis is rare. Liver function tests, aspartate aminotransferase or alanine aminotransferase, should be performed periodically. Methotrexate should be discontinued if these test values show sustained results greater than twice the upper limits of normal. An albumin blood level also should be checked periodically as a sign of liver toxicity because some patients may not have liver inflammation manifested by aspartate aminotransferase or alanine aminotransferase elevation. Liver biopsy is now recommended before beginning methotrexate therapy only for patients with a history of excessive alcohol use, ongoing hepatitis B or C infection, or recurring elevation of aspartate aminotransferase. Biopsies during methotrexate therapy are recommended only for patients who develop consistently abnormal liver function tests.[17]

Because the drug is teratogenic, patients should use contraception to avoid pregnancy and discontinue the drug if conception is planned.

Because it is a folic acid antagonist, methotrexate can induce a folic acid deficiency. This deficiency is thought to be partly responsible for methotrexate toxicity, and supplementation with folic acid does alleviate some adverse effects. Addition of folic acid to a methotrexate regimen for rheumatoid arthritis does not compromise drug efficacy.[17,39–42]

Leflunomide

Leflunomide is a DMARD that inhibits pyrimidine synthesis, leading to a decrease in lymphocyte proliferation and modulation of inflammation. It is given as a loading dose of 100 mg daily for 3 days, followed by a maintenance dose of 20 mg daily. Lower doses may be used if patients have gastrointestinal intolerance, complain of hair loss, or have other signs of dose-related toxicity. The loading dose allows the patient to achieve a therapeutic response, usually within the first month. The long elimination half-life of the drug (14 to 16 days) would require the patient to take the drug for several months to achieve steady state without a loading dose. Some rheumatologists prefer to begin with maintenance dosing as the loading dose may put the patient at risk for toxicity.

Leflunomide has efficacy similar to methotrexate for treating rheumatoid arthritis. The drug may cause liver toxicity and is contraindicated in patients with preexisting liver disease. Patients taking the drug should have alanine aminotransferase monitored monthly initially and periodically thereafter as long as they continue treatment. Leflunomide may cause bone marrow toxicity and complete blood count with platelets is recommended monthly for 6 months and then every 6 to 8 weeks thereafter.

The drug is teratogenic, and appropriate contraceptive measures are recommended to avoid pregnancy for all sexually active male and female patients who are taking leflunomide. If conception is desired, leflunomide must be discontinued. Because leflunomide undergoes enterohepatic circulation, the drug takes many months to drop to a plasma concentration considered safe during pregnancy (<0.02 mcg/mL). Cholestyramine may be used to rapidly clear the drug from plasma. In addition to pregnancy, cholestyramine use may be warranted to rapidly clear the drug in the event of severe toxicity.[27,43–46]

Hydroxychloroquine

The pharmacokinetics of hydroxychloroquine are poorly understood. It is well absorbed orally and widely distributed to body tissues. Hydroxychloroquine is partially metabolized in the liver and is excreted by the kidney. The onset of action of hydroxychloroquine may be delayed up to 6 weeks, but the drug is considered a therapeutic failure only when 6 months of therapy without a response has elapsed.

The main advantage of hydroxychloroquine is the lack of myelosuppressive, hepatic, and renal toxicities that may be seen with other DMARDs, which simplifies monitoring. Short-term toxicities of hydroxychloroquine include gastrointestinal effects such as nausea, vomiting, and diarrhea, which can be managed by taking doses with food. Ocular toxicity includes accommodation defects, benign corneal deposits, blurred vision, scotomas (small areas of decreased or absent vision in the visual field), and night blindness. Although the risk of true retinopathy with hydroxychloroquine approaches zero, preretinopathy may occur in 2.7% of patients. All patients must understand the importance of adhering to hydroxychloroquine monitoring guidelines, as delineated in Table 94–2. Any visual change must be reported immediately. Dermatologic toxicities include rash, alopecia, and increased skin pigmentation; neurologic adverse effects such as headache, vertigo, and insomnia usually are mild.[34,47,48]

Sulfasalazine

Sulfasalazine, a prodrug, is cleaved by bacteria in the colon into sulfapyridine and 5-aminosalicylic acid. It is believed that the sulfapyridine moiety is responsible for the agent's antirheumatic properties, although the exact mechanism of action is unknown. Once the colonic bacteria have cleaved sulfasalazine, sulfapyridine and 5-aminosalicylic acid are absorbed rapidly from the gastrointestinal tract. Sulfapyridine distributes rapidly throughout the body, but higher concentrations are found in certain tissues such as serous fluid, liver, and intestines. Both sulfasalazine and its metabolites are excreted in the urine. Antirheumatic effects should be seen in 2 months.

Use of sulfasalazine is often limited by its adverse effects. Gastrointestinal adverse effects such as nausea, vomiting, diarrhea, and anorexia are the most common. These can be minimized by initiating therapy with low doses and titrating gradually to higher doses, dividing the dose more evenly throughout the day, or using enteric-coated preparations. Rash, urticaria, and serum sickness-like reactions can be managed with antihistamines and, if indicated, corticosteroids. If a hypersensitivity reaction occurs, therapy should be stopped immediately and another DMARD substituted. Sulfasalazine is associated with leukopenia, alopecia, stomatitis, and elevated hepatic enzymes. It also may cause the patient's urine and skin to turn a yellow-orange color, which is of no clinical consequence however; patients should be educated about this to avoid premature discontinuance.

Sulfasalazine's absorption can be decreased when antibiotics are used that destroy the colonic bacteria. Sulfasalazine also binds iron supplements in the gastrointestinal tract that can lead to a decreased absorption of sulfasalazine. The administration of these two agents should be separated temporally to avoid this interaction. Sulfasalazine can potentiate warfarin's effects by displacing it from protein-binding sites. Close monitoring of the patient's international normalized ratio is indicated.[49,50]

Other Disease-Modifying Antirheumatic Drugs

Gold salts, azathioprine, D-penicillamine, cyclosporine, cyclophosphamide, and minocycline have all been used to treat rheumatoid arthritis. Although these drugs can be effective and they may be of value in certain clinical settings, they are used less frequently today because of toxicity, lack of long-term benefit, or both. Tables 94–2 and 94–3 provide dosing information and toxicity information.

Biologic Agents

Biologic agents are genetically engineered protein molecules that block the proinflammatory cytokines TNF-α (infliximab, etanercept, adalimumab) and IL-1 (anakinra), deplete peripheral B cells (rituximab), or bind to CD80/86 on T-cells to prevent the costimulation needed to fully activate T cells (abatacept). These drugs may be effective when other DMARDs fail to achieve adequate responses but are considerably more expensive to use. They have no toxicity that requires laboratory monitoring, but have a small increased risk for infection. There is an increased incidence of tuberculosis in patients treated with these agents. Tuberculin skin testing is recommended prior to treatment with these drugs.[51–54] Patients with a history of significant tuberculosis exposure or recurrent infection may not be good candidates for these drugs. Those who develop infections while on biologic agents should at least temporarily discontinue them until the infection is cured. Additionally, congestive heart failure is a relative contraindication for infliximab and etanercept. Increased cardiac mortality has been seen in patients treated with infliximab and etanercept-associated heart failure exacerbations have been documented.[46,55,56] It is postulated that TNF inhibitors may predispose patients to increased cancer risk as TNF plays a role in ridding the body of cancer cells. The reported incidence of malignancy is similar to that of patients with rheumatoid arthritis who are not on these drugs; however, long-term surveillance studies are lacking.[57,58]

Etanercept Etanercept is a fusion protein consisting of two p75-soluble TNF receptors linked to an Fc fragment of human IgG_1. The drug binds to TNF, making it biologically inactive and preventing it from interacting with the cell-surface TNF receptors that would lead to cell activation.

The drug is given by subcutaneous injection, 50 mg once weekly or 25 mg twice weekly, usually through self-injections or administration by a caregiver. Aside from local injection-site reactions, adverse effects are rare. There are case reports of pancytopenia and neurologic demyelinating syndromes like multiple sclerosis associated with use of etanercept, but these are rare. Patients with multiple sclerosis should avoid use of this drug. The infection and congestive heart failure precautions are discussed above. No laboratory monitoring is required.

Most clinical trials have used etanercept in patients who failed DMARDs. Response was seen in 60% to 75% of patients. The drug has also been FDA approved for the treatment of juvenile rheumatoid arthritis, ankylosing spondylitis, psoriatic arthritis and moderate to severe psoriasis. Clinical trials have shown that it slows erosive disease progression to a greater degree than oral methotrexate therapy.[59–67]

Infliximab Infliximab is a chimeric antibody combining portions of mouse and human IgG_1. An anti-TNF antibody was created by exposing mice to human TNF. The binding portion of that antibody was fused to a human constant-region IgG_1 to reduce the antigenicity of the foreign protein. This antibody, when injected in humans, binds to TNF and prevents its interaction with TNF receptors on inflammatory cells.

Infliximab is given by intravenous infusion at a dose of 3 mg/kg at 0, 2, and 6 weeks and then every 8 weeks. To prevent the formation of antibodies to this foreign protein, methotrexate should be given orally in doses typically used to treat rheumatoid arthritis for as long as the patient continues on infliximab. Antibodies develop in 7% to 15% of patients, which leads to a greater risk of infusion reactions and also may reduce the efficacy of the drug. Loss of response may be seen in patients with rheumatoid arthritis who have good initial response requiring increased doses or shorter intervals between doses to maintain response. Infusion reactions may occur in any patient treated with the drug. Both acute (within 24 hours of infusion) and delayed (24 hours to 14 days) reactions following infusion have been identified. An acute infusion reaction with symptoms including fever, chills, pruritus, and rash may occur during infusion or within 1 to 2 hours after giving the drug. Treatment includes slowing infusion rates and administering acetaminophen, diphenhydramine, or corticosteroids, depending on the severity of symptoms. Fortunately these reactions are rarely severe or anaphylactic in nature.[68] The drug may increase risk of infection as noted above. Autoantibodies and lupus-like syndrome also have been reported. In clinical trials, the combination of methotrexate plus infliximab halted progression of joint damage in patients and was superior to methotrexate monotherapy.[63,69–71] In addition to rheumatoid arthritis, infliximab is indicated for the treatment of psoriatic arthritis and ankylosing spondylitis.[69,72]

Adalimumab Adalimumab is a human IgG_1 antibody to TNF. Because it has no foreign protein components, it is less antigenic than infliximab. The drug is provided as either premixed syringes or injection pens containing 40 mg, which is administered by subcutaneous injection every 14 days. It has similar response rates to those seen with the other TNF inhibitors. Local injection-site reactions were the most common adverse reactions noted in clinical trials. It has the same precautions regarding tuberculosis and other infections as the other biologics. To date, congestive heart failure exacerbations have not been reported.[73–78]

Interleukin-1 Receptor Antagonist Anakinra is an IL-1 receptor antagonist (IL-1ra) which is a naturally occurring antiinflammatory. By binding to IL-1 receptors on target cells, it prevents the interaction between IL-1 and the cell.

IL-1 is very important in the pathogenesis of rheumatoid arthritis. It stimulates release of chemotactic factors and adhesion molecules, and these promote migration of inflammatory leukocytes to tissues. It also causes release of factors known to dilate blood vessels and direct cytotoxins that produce connective tissue damage.

In a double-blind, placebo-controlled trial, IL-1ra 150 mg given by daily subcutaneous injection had a response rate of 43%, compared with 27% for placebo-treated patients. Less radiographic progression of joint damage was noted in those patients receiving IL-1ra. Injection-site reactions were the most common adverse effect noted. Infection risk and precautions are similar to those for the TNF inhibitors. Limited trials combining anakinra with anti-TNF therapy failed to demonstrate better outcomes and increased infection risk and combination therapy is not recommended. When anakinra was added in patients who were not getting adequate response from methotrexate alone, nearly half of the patients had at least a 20% reduction in disease activity with the combination. The short half-life of the drug requires daily subcutaneous injections of 100 mg. Most rheumatologists feel anakinra has a less-robust response than the TNF inhibitors and reserve it for use in patients who fail these agents.[79–83]

Abatacept Abatacept is a costimulation modulator approved for the treatment of rheumatoid arthritis in patients with moderate to severe disease who fail to achieve an adequate response from one or more DMARDs. By binding to CD80/CD86 receptors on antigen-presenting cells, abatacept inhibits interactions between the antigen-presenting cells and T cells, preventing the T cell from activating to promote the inflammatory process, which results in reductions in cytokines, T-cell proliferation, and other consequences of T-cell activation. Abatacept is a fusion protein made using the extracellular domain of human cytotoxic T-lymphocyte antigen 4 (the binding portion of the drug) and a fragment of the Fc domain of human IgG modified to prevent complement fixation. The drug is given by intravenous infusion based on patient weight (<60 kg: 500 mg; 60 to 100 kg: 750 mg; >100 kg: 1,000 mg) every 2 weeks for two doses after the initial dose and then every 4 weeks. The drug is well tolerated, with headache, nasopharyngitis, dizziness, cough, back pain, hypertension, dyspepsia, urinary tract infection, rash, and extremity pain reported more frequently in clinical trials. Infusion reactions were 50% more likely with abatacept than with placebo and there was a slightly higher rate of serious infections with active treatment.[84,85] In patients who failed to achieve adequate responses with TNF-α inhibitors, half had a clinical response to abatacept.[86]

Rituximab Rituximab is a monoclonal chimeric antibody consisting of mostly human protein with the antigen-binding region derived from a mouse antibody to CD20 protein found on the cell surface of mature B lymphocytes. The binding of rituximab to B cells results in nearly complete depletion of peripheral B cells, with a gradual recovery over several months. The prolonged effect on B cells results in a duration of action that allows for intermittent therapy which varies based on reactivation of arthritis symptoms. Rituximab is useful in patients who failed methotrexate or TNF inhibitors.[87–90] Two infusions of 1,000 mg are given 2 weeks apart. Methylprednisolone 100 mg should be given 30 minutes prior to rituximab to reduce the incidence and severity of infusion reactions. Acetaminophen and antihistamines may also be of benefit in patients who have a history of reactions. Methotrexate should be given concurrently in the usual doses used for rheumatoid arthritis, as the combination has proved to provide the best therapeutic outcomes. Duration of benefit is variable after a course of rituximab and patients will need retreatment with reactivation of their disease. The drug is currently FDA approved for TNF inhibitor treatment failures.

Corticosteroids

Corticosteroids are used in rheumatoid arthritis for their antiinflammatory and immunosuppressive properties. They interfere with antigen presentation to T lymphocytes, inhibit prostaglandin and leukotriene synthesis, and inhibit neutrophil and monocyte superoxide radical generation. Corticosteroids also impair cell migration and cause redistribution of monocytes, lymphocytes, and neutrophils, thus blunting the inflammatory and autoimmune responses.

Oral corticosteroids are absorbed rapidly and completely from the gastrointestinal tract. They are metabolized and inactivated primarily by the liver and excreted in the urine. The elimination half-life of most corticosteroids is sufficiently long that once-daily dosing is possible.

Oral corticosteroids can be used in several ways. They can be used in bridging therapy, continuous low-dose therapy, and short-term high-dose bursts to control flares. Oral steroids (e.g., prednisone, methylprednisolone) can be used to control pain and synovitis while DMARDs are taking effect. This is termed *bridging therapy* and is often used in patients with debilitating symptoms when DMARD therapy is initiated. Patients with difficult-to-control disease may be placed on low-dose, long-term corticosteroid therapy to control their symptoms. Prednisone doses below 7.5 mg daily are well tolerated but are not devoid of the long-term adverse effects associated with corticosteroids. The lowest dose of corticosteroid that controls symptoms should be used to reduce adverse effects. Alternate-day dosing of low-dose oral corticosteroids usually is ineffective in rheumatoid arthritis; symptoms usually flare on days without medication. High-dose corticosteroid bursts often are used to suppress disease flares. High doses are sustained for several days until symptoms are controlled, followed by a taper to the lowest effective dose.

Corticosteroids also may be delivered by injection. The intramuscular route is preferable in patients with compliance problems. Long-acting depot forms of corticosteroids include triamcinolone acetonide, triamcinolone hexacetonide, and methylprednisolone acetate. This provides the patient with 2 to 6 weeks of symptomatic control. The depot effect provides a physiologic taper, avoiding withdrawal reaction associated with hypothalamic–pituitary axis suppression. Intravenous corticosteroids may be used to provide the patient with large amounts of drug during a steroid burst to control severe symptoms. Intraarticular injections of depot forms of corticosteroids can be useful in treating synovitis and pain when a small number of joints are affected. The onset and duration of symptomatic relief are similar to those of intramuscular injection. The intraarticular route often is preferred because it is associated with the fewest number of systemic adverse effects. If efficacious, intraarticular injections may be repeated every 3 months. No one joint should be injected more than two to three times per year because of the risk of accelerated joint destruction and atrophy of tendons. Soft tissues such as tendons and bursae also may be injected. This may help control the pain and inflammation associated with these structures. The onset and duration of symptomatic relief are similar to those of intramuscular and intraarticular injections.

The major limitation to the long-term use of corticosteroids is adverse effects. They include hypothalamic-pituitary–adrenal suppression, Cushing's syndrome, osteoporosis, myopathies, glaucoma, cataracts, gastritis, hypertension, hirsutism, electrolyte imbalances, glucose intolerance, skin atrophy, and increased susceptibility to infections. To minimize these effects, use the lowest effective corticosteroid dose and limit the duration of use. Patients on long-term therapy should be given calcium and vitamin D to minimize bone loss. Alendronate is effective in preventing bone loss and might be considered prophylactically for patients when long-term corticosteroid is anticipated, particularly for patients who are at high risk (e.g., post-menopausal females, elderly) for bone loss.[91,92] There is no evidence that corticosteroids alone increase the risk of gastrointestinal ulcerations, although they often have been implicated. Consequently, gastrointestinal protective measures usually are not indicated.[93,94]

PHARMACOECONOMIC CONSIDERATIONS

The total cost of treating a patient with rheumatoid arthritis is estimated to be between $7,500 and $11,000 annually (1991 dollars). Of this, drugs account for roughly 10% of the total, excluding monitoring costs. These costs are approximately three times the cost of medical care for patients of similar age and gender without rheumatoid arthritis. However, if biologic agents are used, the cost of this drug therapy alone may be $12,000 or more annually. The costs must be balanced against the high cost of disability on earning potential in these patients. Men with rheumatoid arthritis have average annual wages 50% lower than those of men of similar age without rheumatoid arthritis. In women with the disease, average annual wages are only 25% of the wages of those women without the disease. The costs of disability make treatment worth the price if disability can be prevented or delayed and patients can continue to function as productive members of society.[95]

CLINICAL CONTROVERSIES

1. The order of DMARD or biologic agent choice is not clearly defined.
2. Should combination DMARD be tried before biologic agents?
3. Even the best therapy available today does not completely eliminate all signs and symptoms of disease for most patients. How much treatment is enough?
4. Some patients show evidence of disease progression in spite of apparent control of clinical symptoms. How can these patients be identified and treatment course changed before progression occurs?

EVALUATION OF THERAPEUTIC OUTCOMES

The evaluation of therapeutic outcomes is based primarily on improvements of clinical signs and symptoms of rheumatoid arthritis. Clinical signs of improvement include a reduction in joint swelling, decreased warmth over actively involved joints, and decreased tenderness to joint palpation. Improvement in rheumatoid arthritis symptoms includes reduction in perceived joint pain and morning stiffness, longer time to onset of afternoon fatigue, and improvement in ability to perform activities of daily living. Improvement of activities of daily living may be assessed objectively using a Health Assessment Questionnaire score. Joint radiographs may be of some benefit in assessing the progression of the disease and should show little or no evidence of disease progression if treatment is effective.

Laboratory monitoring is of little value in monitoring individual patient response to therapy. Tables 94–2 and 94–3 provide monitoring of drug toxicity information. Routine monitoring of patients is essential to the safe use of these drugs. In addition, patients should be questioned about symptoms of the adverse effects outlined in the drug section of this chapter.

CONCLUSIONS

Rheumatoid arthritis is the most common inflammatory arthritis, affecting approximately 1% of the population. The disease is characterized by symmetrical swelling and stiffness of the involved joints. The stiffness is usually more prominent in the morning. Extraarticular features of rheumatoid arthritis include rheumatoid nodules, vasculitis, and ocular, cardiac, and pulmonary complications. The course of the disease is highly variable. Treatment is aimed at relieving pain and inflammation and maintaining and preserving joint function. Nondrug therapy, including exercise and adequate rest periods, should also be used early in the course of treatment. Early use of a DMARD or biologic agent results in better patient outcomes. Methotrexate, sulfasalazine, and hydroxychloroquine are often considered for initial therapy. Biologics have also been shown to be effective in these patients but may be considered second choice because of cost considerations; however, they are effective in patients who fail to achieve adequate response from older DMARDs. Combination DMARDs or biologics may be considered in those who fail adequate trials of single-agent therapy. Corticosteroids and NSAIDs may be useful adjuncts for treatment, but because of adverse effects and limited impact on long-term outcomes, they should not be considered as sole treatment for most patients.

ABBREVIATIONS

DMARD: disease-modifying antirheumatic drug
HLA: human lymphocyte antigen
Ig: immunoglobulin
IL: interleukin
NSAID: nonsteroidal antiinflammatory drug
TNF-α: tumor necrosis factor α

REFERENCES

1. Smith JB, Haynes MK. Rheumatoid arthritis—A molecular understanding. Ann Intern Med. 2002;136(12):908–922.
2. Klippel JH CL, Stone JH, Weyand CM, eds. Primer on the Rheumatic Diseases, 12th ed. Atlanta, GA: Arthritis Foundation, 2001.
3. Harris ED. The clinical features of rheumatoid arthritis. In: Harris ED, Budd RC, Firestein GS, et al, eds. Textbook of Rheumatology, 7th ed. Philadelphia: Elsevier/Saunders, 2005:1043–1078.
4. Jiang H, Chess L. Regulation of immune response by T cells. N Engl J Med 2006;354:1166–1176.
5. Tsokos GC. B cells, be gone—B-cell depletion in the treatment of rheumatoid arthritis. N Engl J Med 2004;350(25):2546–2548.
6. Weinstein E, Peeva E, Putterman C, Diamond B. B-cell biology. Rheum Dis Clin North Am 2004;30(1):159–174.
7. Choy EH, Panayi GS. Cytokine pathways and joint inflammation in rheumatoid arthritis. N Engl J Med 2001;344(12):907–916.
8. Arend WP. Physiology of cytokine pathways in rheumatoid arthritis. Arthritis Care Res 2001;45:101–106.
9. Choy E, Panayi GS. Cytokine pathways and joint inflammation in rheumatoid arthritis. N Engl J Med 2001;344:907–916.
10. Firestein GS. Etiology and pathogenesis of rheumatoid arthritis. In: Harris ED, Budd RC, Firestein GS, eds. Textbook of Rheumatology, 7th ed. Philadelphia: Elsevier/Saunders, 2005:996–1042.
11. Visser H. Early diagnosis of rheumatoid arthritis. Best Pract Res Clin Rheumatol 2005;19(1):55–72.
12. Hard ER. Extraarticular manifestations of rheumatoid arthritis. Semin Arthritis Rheum 1979;8:151–176.
13. Choi HK, Hernan MA, Seeger JD, et al. Methotrexate and mortality in patients with rheumatoid arthritis: A prospective study. Lancet 2002;359:1173–1177.
14. Wallberg-Jonsson S, Johansson H, Ohman ML, Rantapaa-Dahlqvist S. Extent of inflammation predicts cardiovascular disease and overall mortality in seropositive rheumatoid arthritis. A retrospective cohort study from disease onset. J Rheumatol 1999;26(12):2562–2571.
15. Colglazier CL, Sutej PG. Laboratory testing in rheumatic diseases: A practical review. South Med J 2005;98(2):185–191.
16. Shmerling RH. Diagnostic tests for rheumatic disease: Clinical utility revisited. South Med J 2005;98(7):704–711.
17. American College of Rheumatology Subcommittee on Rheumatoid Arthritis G. Guidelines for the management of rheumatoid arthritis: 2002 Update. Arthritis Rheum 2002;46(2):328–346.
18. Genovese MC, Harris ED. The treatment of rheumatoid arthritis. In: Ruddy S, Harris ED, Sledge CB, eds. Textbook of Rheumatology, 7th ed. Philadelphia: WB Saunders, 2005. Accessed online, *www.mdconsult.com* December 12, 2007.
19. Anderson JJ, Wells G, Verhoeven AC, Felson DT. Factors predicting response to treatment in rheumatoid arthritis: The importance of disease duration. Arthritis Rheum 2000;43(1):22–29.
20. Fries JF. Current treatment paradigms in rheumatoid arthritis. Rheumatology 2000;39(Suppl 1):30–35.
21. Mottonen T, Hannonen P, Korpela M, et al. Delay to institution of therapy and induction of remission using single-drug or combination-disease-modifying antirheumatic drug therapy in early rheumatoid arthritis. Arthritis Rheum 2002;46(4):894–898.
22. Tsakonas E, Fitzgerald AA, Fitzcharles MA, et al. Consequences of delayed therapy with second-line agents in rheumatoid arthritis: A 3-year followup on the Hydroxychloroquine in Early Rheumatoid Arthritis (HERA) study. J Rheumatol 2000;27(3):623–629.
23. Verstappen SM, Jacobs JW, Bijlsma JW, et al. Five-year followup of rheumatoid arthritis patients after early treatment with disease-modifying antirheumatic drugs versus treatment according to the pyramid approach in the first year. Arthritis Rheum 2003;48(7):1797–1807.
24. Goldbach-Mansky R, Lipsky PE. New concepts in the treatment of rheumatoid arthritis. Annu Rev Med 2003;54:197–216.
25. O'Dell JR. Therapeutic strategies for rheumatoid arthritis. N Engl J Med 2004;350(25):2591–2602.
26. Kroot EJ, VanLeeuwen MA, VanRijswijk MH, et al. No increased mortality in patients with rheumatoid arthritis: Up to 10 years of follow up from disease onset. Ann Rheum Dis 2000;59:954–958.
27. Kalden JR, Schattenkirchner M, Sorensen H, et al. The efficacy and safety of leflunomide in patients with active rheumatoid arthritis: A five-year followup study. Arthritis Rheum 2003;48(6):1513–1520.
28. Bingham S, Emery P. Combination therapy in rheumatoid arthritis. Springer Semin Immunopathol 2001;23(1–2):165–183.
29. Dougados M, Combe B, Cantagrel A, et al. Combination therapy in early rheumatoid arthritis: A randomised, controlled, double blind 52 week clinical trial of sulphasalazine and methotrexate compared with the single components. Ann Rheum Dis 1999;58(4):220–225.
30. Goekoop-Reuterman YP, deVries-Bouwstra JK, Allaart CF, et al. Comparison of treatment strategies in early rheumatoid arthritis: A randomized trial. Ann Intern Med 2007;146:406–415.
31. O'Dell JR. Combinations of conventional disease-modifying antirheumatic drugs. Rheum Dis Clin North Am 2001;27(2):415–426, x.
32. Pincus T, O'Dell JR, Kremer JM. Combination therapy with multiple disease-modifying antirheumatic drugs in rheumatoid arthritis: A preventive strategy. Ann Intern Med 1999;131(10):768–774.
33. Verhoeven AC, Boers M, Tugwell P. Combination therapy in rheumatoid arthritis: Updated systematic review [comment]. Br J Rheumatol 1998;37(6):612–619.
34. Kremer JM. Rational use of new and existing disease-modifying agents in rheumatoid arthritis. Ann Intern Med 2001;134(8):695–706.
35. Bijlsma JW, Van Everdingen AA, Huisman M, De Nijs RN, Jacobs JW. Glucocorticoids in rheumatoid arthritis: Effects on erosions and bone. Ann N Y Acad Sci 2002;966:82–90.
36. Rau R, Wassenberg S, Zeidler H. Low dose prednisolone therapy (LDPT) retards radiographically detectable destruction in early rheumatoid arthritis—Preliminary results of a multicenter, randomized, parallel, double blind study. Z Rheumatol 2000;59 Suppl 2:II/90–II/96.
37. Pincus T, Ferraccioli G, Sokka T, et al. Evidence from clinical trials and long-term observational studies that disease-modifying anti-rheumatic drugs slow radiographic progression in rheumatoid arthritis: Updating a 1983 review. Rheumatology 2002;41(12):1346–1356.
38. Wolfe F, Hawley DJ, Cathey MA. Termination of slow acting antirheumatic therapy in rheumatoid arthritis: A 14-year prospective evaluation of 1017 consecutive starts. J Rheumatol 1990;17:994–1002.
39. Kremer JM. Methotrexate and emerging therapies. Rheum Dis Clin North Am 1998;24(3):651–658.
40. O'Dell JR. Methotrexate use in rheumatoid arthritis. Rheum Dis Clin North Am1997;23(4):779–796.
41. Borchers AT, Keen CL, Cheema GS, Gershwin ME. The use of methotrexate in rheumatoid arthritis. Semin Arthritis Rheum 2004;34(1):465–483.
42. Suarez-Almazor ME, Belseck E, Shea BJ, Tugwell P, Wells G. Methotrexate for treating rheumatoid arthritis. Cochrane Database Syst Rev 1998(2):CD000959.
43. Prakash A, Jarvis B. Leflunomide: A review of its use in active rheumatoid arthritis. Drugs 1999;58(6):1137–1164.
44. Strand V, Cohen S, Schiff M, et al. Treatment of active rheumatoid arthritis with leflunomide compared with placebo and methotrexate. Leflunomide Rheumatoid Arthritis Investigators Group. Arch Intern Med 1999;159(21):2542–2550.
45. Osiri M, Shea BJ, Robinson V, et al. Leflunomide for treating rheumatoid arthritis. Cochrane Database Syst Rev 2002:CD002047.
46. Cush JJ. Safety overview of new disease-modifying antirheumatic drugs. Rheum Dis Clin North Am 2004;30(2):237–255, v.
47. Maturi RK, Folk JC, Nichols B, Oetting TT, Kardon RH. Hydroxychloroquine retinopathy. Arch Ophthalmol 1999;117(9):1262–1263.
48. Suarez-Almazor ME, Belseck E, Shea B, Homik J, Wells G, Tugwell P. Antimalarials for treating rheumatoid arthritis. update of Cochrane Database Syst Rev 2000;(2):CD000959]. Cochrane Database Syst Rev 2000(4):CD000959.

49. Weinblatt ME, Reda D, Henderson W, et al. Sulfasalazine treatment for rheumatoid arthritis: A metaanalysis of 15 randomized trials. J Rheumatol 1999;26(10):2123–2130.
50. Rains CP, Noble S, Faulds D. Sulfasalazine: A review of its pharmacological properties and therapeutic efficacy in the treatment of rheumatoid arthritis. Drugs 1995;50:137–156.
51. Gomez-Reino JJ, Carmona L, Valverde VR, Mola EM, Montero MD. Treatment of rheumatoid arthritis with tumor necrosis factor inhibitors may predispose to significant increase in tuberculosis risk: A multicenter active-surveillance report. Arthritis Rheum 2003;48(8):2122–2127.
52. Keane J, Gershon S, Wise RP, et al. Tuberculosis associated with infliximab, a tumor necrosis factor alpha-neutralizing agent [comment]. N Engl J Med 2001;345(15):1098–1104.
53. Myers A, Clark J, Foster H. Tuberculosis and treatment with infliximab. N Engl J Med 2002;346(8):623–626.
54. Weisman MH. What are the risks of biologic therapy in rheumatoid arthritis? An update on safety. J Rheumatol Suppl 2002;65:33–38.
55. Chung ES, Packer M, Lo KH, Fasanmade AA, Willerson JT. Randomized, double-blind, placebo-controlled, pilot trial of infliximab, a chimeric monoclonal antibody to tumor necrosis factor-alpha in patients with moderate-to-severe heart failure: Results of the anti-TNF Therapy Against Congestive Heart Failure (ATTACH) trial. Circulation 2003;107(25):3133–3140.
56. Kwon HJ, Cote TR, Cuffe MS, Kramer JM, Braun MM. Case reports of heart failure after therapy with a tumor necrosis factor antagonist. Ann Intern Med 2003;138(10):807–811.
57. Beauparlant P, Papp K, Haraoui B. The incidence of cancer associated with the treatment of rheumatoid arthritis. Semin Arthritis Rheum 1999;29(3):148–158.
58. Cohen RB, Dittrich KA. Anti-TNF therapy and malignancy—A critical review. Can J Gastroenterol 2001;15(6):376–384.
59. Bathon JM, Martin RW, Fleischmann RM, et al. A comparison of etanercept and methotrexate in patients with early rheumatoid arthritis [comment] [erratum appears in N Engl J Med 2001;344(3):240]. N Engl J Med2000;343(22):1586–1593.
60. Genovese MC, Bathon JM, Martin RW, et al. Etanercept versus methotrexate in patients with early rheumatoid arthritis: Two-year radiographic and clinical outcomes. Arthritis Rheum 2002;46(6):1443–1450.
61. Moreland LW. Inhibitors of tumor necrosis factor for rheumatoid arthritis. J Rheumatol 1999;26(Suppl 57):7–15.
62. Moreland LW, Schiff MH, Baumgartner SW, et al. Etanercept therapy in rheumatoid arthritis. A randomized, controlled trial. Ann Intern Med 1999;130(6):478–486.
63. Maini RN, Taylor PC. Anti-cytokine therapy for rheumatoid arthritis. Annu Rev Med 2000;51:207–229.
64. Jarvis B, Faulds D. Etanercept: A review of its use in rheumatoid arthritis. Drugs 1999;57(6):945–966.
65. Genovese MC, Kremer JM. Treatment of rheumatoid arthritis with etanercept. Rheum Dis Clin North Am 2004;30(2):311–328, vi–vii.
66. Nanda S, Bathon JM. Etanercept: A clinical review of current and emerging indications. Expert Opin Pharmacother 2004;5(5):1175–1186.
67. Blumenauer B, Judd MG, Cranney A, et al. Etanercept for the treatment of rheumatoid arthritis. Cochrane Database Syst Rev 2003(3):CD004525.
68. Cheifitz A, Mayer L. Monoclonal antibodies, immunogenicity, and associated infusion reactions. Mt Sinai J Med 2005;72:250–256.
69. Blumenauer B, Judd M, Wells G, et al. Infliximab for the treatment of rheumatoid arthritis. Cochrane Database Syst Rev 2002(3):CD003785.
70. Maini R, St Clair EW, Breedveld F, et al. Infliximab (chimeric antitumour necrosis factor alpha monoclonal antibody) versus placebo in rheumatoid arthritis patients receiving concomitant methotrexate: A randomised phase III trial. ATTRACT Study Group. Lancet 1999; 354(9194):1932–1939.
71. Lipsky PE, van der Heijde DM, St Clair EW, et al. Infliximab and methotrexate in the treatment of rheumatoid arthritis. Anti-Tumor Necrosis Factor Trial in Rheumatoid Arthritis with Concomitant Therapy Study Group [comment]. N Engl J Med 2000;343(22):1594–1602.
72. Maini SR. Infliximab treatment of rheumatoid arthritis. Rheum Dis Clin North Am 2004;30(2):329–347, vii.
73. Navarro-Sarabia F, Ariza-Ariza R, Hernandez-Cruz B, Villanueva I. Adalimumab for treating rheumatoid arthritis. Cochrane Database Syst Rev 2005(3):CD005113.
74. den Broeder A, van de Putte L, Rau R, et al. A single dose, placebo controlled study of the fully human anti-tumor necrosis factor-alpha antibody adalimumab (D2E7) in patients with rheumatoid arthritis. J Rheumatol 2002;29(11):2288–2298.
75. Weinblatt ME, Keystone EC, Furst DE, et al. Adalimumab, a fully human anti-tumor necrosis factor alpha monoclonal antibody, for the treatment of rheumatoid arthritis in patients taking concomitant methotrexate: The ARMADA trial [erratum appears in Arthritis Rheum 2003;48(3):855]. Arthritis Rheum 2003;48(1):35–45.
76. Bang LM, Keating GM. Adalimumab: A review of its use in rheumatoid arthritis. BioDrugs 2004;18(2):121–139.
77. Ebell M, Kripke C. Adalimumab for rheumatoid arthritis? Am Fam Physician 2006;73(3):435–436.
78. Keystone E, Haraoui B. Adalimumab therapy in rheumatoid arthritis. Rheum Dis Clin North Am 2004;30(2):349–364, vii.
79. Calabrese LH. Anakinra treatment of patients with rheumatoid arthritis. Ann Pharmacother 2002;36(7–8):1204–1209.
80. Cohen S, Hurd E, Cush J, et al. Treatment of rheumatoid arthritis with anakinra, a recombinant human IL-1 receptor antagonist, in combination with methotrexate: Results of a twenty-four-week, multicenter, randomized, double-blind, placebo-controlled trial [comment]. Arthritis Rheum 2002;46(3):614–624.
81. Fleischmann RM, Schechtman J, Bennett R, et al. Anakinra, a recombinant human IL-1 receptor antagonist (r-metHuIL-1ra), in patients with rheumatoid arthritis: A large, international, multicenter, placebo-controlled trial. Arthritis Rheum 2003;48(4):927–934.
82. Jiang Y, Genant HK, Watt I, et al. A multicenter, double-blind, dose-ranging, randomized, placebo-controlled study of recombinant human IL-1 receptor antagonist in patients with rheumatoid arthritis. Arthritis Rheum 2000;43:1001–1009.
83. Cohen SB. The use of anakinra, an IL-1 receptor antagonist, in the treatment of rheumatoid arthritis. Rheum Dis Clin North Am 2004;30(2):365–380, vii.
84. Kremer JM. Selective costimulation modulators: A novel approach for the treatment of rheumatoid arthritis. J Clin Rheumatol 2005;11(3 Suppl):S55–S62.
85. Hervey PS, Keam SJ. Abatacept. BioDrugs 2006;20(1):53–61; discussion 62.
86. Genovese MC, Becker JC, Schiff M, et al. Abatacept for rheumatoid arthritis refractory to tumor necrosis factor alpha inhibition. N Engl J Med 2005;353(11):1114–1123.
87. Cohen SB, Emery P, Greenwald MW, et al. Rituximab for rheumatoid arthritis refractory to anti-tumor necrosis factor therapy: Results of a multicenter, randomized, double-blind, placebo-controlled, phase III trial evaluating primary efficacy and safety at twenty-four weeks. Arthritis Rheum 2006;54(9):2793–2806.
88. De Vita S, Quartuccio L. Treatment of rheumatoid arthritis with rituximab: An update and possible indications. Autoimmun Rev 2006;5(7):443–448.
89. Emery P, Fleischmann R, Filipowicz-Sosnowska A, et al. The efficacy and safety of rituximab in patients with active rheumatoid arthritis despite methotrexate treatment: Results of a phase IIB randomized, double-blind, placebo-controlled, dose-ranging trial. Arthritis Rheum 2006;54(5):1390–1400.
90. Smolen JS, Emery P, Keystone EC, et al. Consensus statement on the use of rituximab in patients with rheumatoid arthritis. Ann Rheum Dis 2007;66:143–150.
91. Adachi JD, Saag KG, Delmas PD, et al. Two-year effects of alendronate on bone mineral density and vertebral fracture in patients receiving glucocorticoids: A randomized, double-blind, placebo-controlled extension trial. Arthritis Rheum 2001;44(1):202–211.
92. McIlwain HH. Glucocorticoid-induced osteoporosis: Pathogenesis, diagnosis, and management. Prev Med 2003;36(2):243–249.
93. Morand EF. Corticosteroids in the treatment of rheumatologic diseases. Curr Opin Rheumatol 1998;10(3):179–183.
94. Criswell LA, Saag KG, Sems KM, et al. Moderate-term, low-dose corticosteroids for rheumatoid arthritis. Cochrane Database Syst Rev 1998(3):CD001158.
95. Gabriel SE, Coyle D, Moreland LW. A clinical and economic review of disease-modifying antirheumatic drugs. Pharmacoeconomics 2001;19(7): 715–728.

CHAPTER 95

Osteoarthritis

LUCINDA M. BUYS AND MARY ELIZABETH ELLIOTT

KEY CONCEPTS

1. Approximately 46 million Americans have osteoarthritis (OA). OA prevalence increases with age, with women more commonly affected than men.
2. Contributors to OA are systemic (age, genetics, hormonal status, obesity, occupational or recreational activity) and/or local (injury, overloading of joints, muscle weakness, or joint deformity).
3. OA is primarily a disease of cartilage that reflects a failure of the chondrocyte to maintain proper balance between cartilage formation and destruction. This leads to loss of cartilage in the joint, local inflammation, pathologic changes in underlying bone, and further damage to cartilage triggered by the affected bone.
4. The most common symptom associated with OA is pain, which leads to decreased function and motion. Pain relief is the primary objective of medication therapy.
5. Manifestations of OA are local, affecting one or a few joints, usually the knees, hips, and hands. Osteophytes (bony proliferation of affected joints) are often found, in contrast to the soft-tissue swelling of rheumatoid arthritis.
6. Nonpharmacologic therapy is the foundation of the pharmaceutical care plan and should be initiated before or concurrently with pharmacologic therapy.
7. Based upon efficacy, safety, and cost considerations, scheduled acetaminophen, up to 4 g/day, should be tried initially for pain relief in OA. If this fails, a nonsteroidal antiinflammatory drug (NSAID) may be tried, if there are no contraindications
8. Strategies to reduce NSAID-induced GI toxicity include the use of nonacetylated salicylates, COX-2 selective inhibitors, or the addition of misoprostol or a proton pump inhibitor. COX-2 selective inhibitors vary in their ability to prevent GI toxicity, and concomitant use of aspirin largely negates their gastroprotective effects.
9. COX-2 selective inhibitors can increase the risk of cardiovascular events. This may be a class effect, but the extent of this risk varies among COX-2 selective inhibitors, and traditional NSAIDs may also pose risks. This hazard, in addition to the GI toxicity possible with all NSAIDs, underscores the importance of using NSAIDs only as needed and after assessing the individual patient's risk.
10. NSAIDs are associated with GI, renal, cardiovascular, liver, and central nervous system toxicity. Monitoring with complete blood count, serum creatinine, and hepatic transaminase levels can be valuable in detecting potential toxicity.
11. Other agents useful in treating OA include topical NSAIDs or capsaicin, opioids, glucosamine and chondroitin in combination, and intraarticular injections of corticosteroids or hyaluronic acid.

Learning objectives, review questions, and other resources can be found at **www.pharmacotherapyonline.com.**

Osteoarthritis (OA) is extremely common and poses tremendous personal, societal, and economic costs. Although OA has been defined in different ways, one definition created by a consensus panel reads

> OA diseases are a result of both mechanical and biologic events that destabilize the normal coupling of degradation and synthesis of articular cartilage, chondrocytes, and extracellular matrix, and subchondral bone. Although they may be initiated by multiple factors, including genetic, developmental, metabolic, and traumatic, OA diseases involve all of the tissues of the diarthrodial joint. Ultimately, OA diseases are manifested by morphologic, biochemical, molecular, and biomechanical changes of both cells and matrix which lead to a softening, fibrillation, ulceration, loss of articular cartilage, sclerosis and eburnation of subchondral bone, osteophytes, and subchondral cysts, when clinically evident, OA diseases are characterized by joint pain, tenderness, limitation of movement, crepitus, occasional effusion, and variable degrees of inflammation without systemic effects.[1]

This chapter first amplifies and clarifies the issues included in the above definition and summarizes the basics of OA diagnosis. It then focuses on pharmacologic and nonpharmacologic treatments currently in use for OA, as well as investigational agents. Because millions of persons take medications for OA, the overall risks posed by medications deserve thorough consideration, particularly by clinicians who treat and/or advise their patients on drug therapy for OA. This chapter examines the risks and benefits of OA treatments, with emphasis on those individuals who have the highest risk for adverse events, so as to help clinicians maximize benefit and reduce risks to their patients with OA.

EPIDEMIOLOGY

OA is the most prevalent of the rheumatic diseases and is responsible for enormous disability and loss of productivity.[2–4] As the U.S. population continues to age, the economic impact of the lost productivity and the quality of life limitations from disability will become even more pronounced.

PREVALENCE BY AGE, SEX, AND RACE

❶ The prevalence of clinician-diagnosed arthritis is estimated at 46 million in the United States and is projected to increase to nearly 67 million by 2030, of which 25 million are expected to report arthritis-related activity limitations.[5] The prevalence of OA is higher in older age groups than in younger groups. In those younger than age 45 years, about one-fifth have OA of the hands, whereas of those ages 75 to 79 years, 85% have OA of the hands. OA of the knee occurs in less than 0.1% of those ages 25 to 34 years, but in 10% to 20% of those ages 65 to 74 years.

OA severity also increases with age.[2–4] In persons between 65 and 74 years of age, 33% have moderate to severe knee OA, and 50% have moderate to severe hip OA. Women are more often affected by OA, with older women being twice as likely as men to have OA of the knee and hands.[3] Women are also more likely to have inflammatory OA of the proximal and distal interphalangeal joints of the hands, giving rise to the formation of Bouchard and Heberden nodes, respectively (Fig. 95–1). Knee OA appears to be twice as prevalent in black as opposed to white women. Chinese, East Indian, and Native American people have lower incidences of hip OA than do whites.

INCIDENCE

The overall incidence of hip or knee OA is approximately 200 per 100,000 person-years. Approximately one-half million symptomatic new cases of OA are estimated to occur annually in the United States.

ETIOLOGY

❷ The etiology of OA is multifactorial. Many patients have more than one risk factor for the development of OA. The most common risk factors for the development of OA include obesity, previous occupation, participation in certain sports, history of joint trauma, and a genetic predisposition to OA. Patients with osteoarthritis are less likely to have osteoporosis because heavy individuals have higher bone density as a result of weight-bearing, but an increased risk of OA as a consequence of excessive joint loading.[3]

OBESITY

Increased body weight is strongly associated with hip, knee, and hand OA, and obesity is regarded as the number one preventable risk factor for OA.[6–8] Obesity often precedes OA and contributes to its development, rather than occurring as a result of inactivity from joint pain. In a three-decade Framingham Study, the highest quintile of body mass was associated with a higher relative risk of knee OA (relative risk of 1.5 to 1.9 for men and 2.1 to 3.2 for women). Another study of 1,108 men in their twenties showed that a high body mass index was associated with later development of knee OA.[8] The risk of developing OA increases by approximately 10% with each additional kilogram of weight, and in obese persons without OA, weight loss of even 5 kg decreases the risk of future knee OA by half. In addition to being a risk factor for OA, obesity is also a predictor for eventual prosthetic joint replacement.

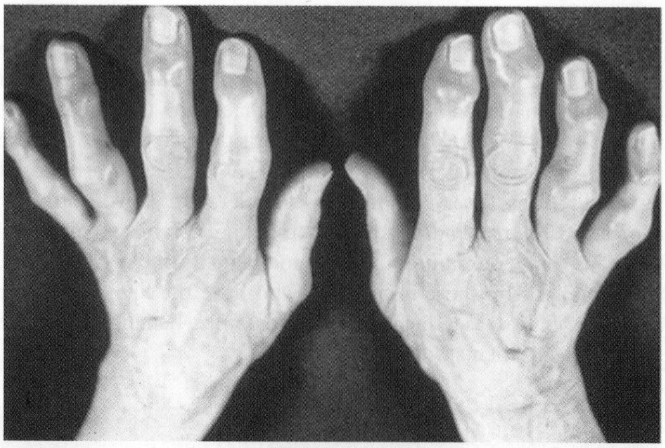

FIGURE 95-1. Heberden nodes (distal interphalangeal joint) noted on all fingers and Bouchard nodes (proximal interphalangeal joint) noted on most fingers. *(From Johnson BE. Arthritis: Osteoarthritis, Gout and Rheumatoid Arthritis. In: South-Paul JE, Matheny SC, Lewis EL, eds. Current Diagnosis and Treatment in Family Medicine. New York: McGraw-Hill; 2004, p. 266, p. 267.)*

OCCUPATION, SPORTS, AND TRAUMA

Those participating in activities involving repetitive motion or injury are at increased risk for developing OA.[6,10] Workers exposed to repetitive stress of the hands or lower limbs (e.g., shipyard workers, carpenters, and agricultural workers) are at higher risk for OA of the stressed joints.

OA is associated with participation in activities such as wrestling, boxing, baseball pitching, cycling, and football, although recreational participants may not have the increased risk seen in the professional athlete. Risk for OA also depends on the type and intensity of physical activity. The Framingham Study showed that heavy physical activity increases knee OA risk, especially in the obese, whereas moderate or light activity does not.[11] Interestingly, long-distance runners are not at higher risk of developing OA.[12]

Age at injury does matter, because older individuals who damage ligaments tend to develop OA more rapidly than young people with a similar injury. However, trauma that occurs early in life is significant: The incidence of knee OA by age 65 years was more than doubled for men who sustained a knee injury in adolescence compared to those who had not.[13]

Quadriceps strength is also related to knee OA and disability. Quadriceps weakness, once thought to result from disuse atrophy in OA patients, may precede and contribute to the development of OA, possibly through decreased knee stability.[14]

GENETIC FACTORS

OA is a multifactorial disease in which many genes are considered to play a role. Genetics may play different roles in different types of arthritis.[4] Heberden nodes are 10 times more prevalent in women than in men, for example, with a twofold higher risk if the woman's mother had them. Genetic links also have been shown with OA of the first metatarsophalangeal joint and with generalized OA. Twin studies indicate that OA can be attributed substantially to genetic factors (39% to 65%, 60%, and 70% for hand, hip, and spine OA, respectively).[15]

Genome-wide linkage studies (associating OA with a specific region out of the total human genome) also have been used to search for the genetic bases for OA.[16] These studies have been carried out for persons with OA who were all from unrelated families. These studies, carried out in the United Kingdom (481 pedigrees), Finland (27 pedigrees), Iceland (329 pedigrees), and the United States (296 pedigrees) show that there are dozens of loci that may include OA-linked genes. Searches for candidate genes (known proteins that are plausibly connected to OA, such as structural proteins in cartilage, or proteins that regulate chondrocyte function, such as interleukins and other signaling molecules) within the identified loci has provided some promising clues. Variants in the interleukin-1 family (in interleukin-1, in an interleukin-1 receptor antagonist, and in the interleukin-1 receptor), in the interleukin-4 receptor, and in the secreted frizzled-related protein (involved in regulation of chondrogenesis) all showed very significant associations with OA. Since then, one major collaborative research group used the more powerful technique of genome-wide association studies.[16] This group identified the gene which codes for asporin, an extracellular matrix protein, as being significant in OA. This was true as well for the gene coding for calmodulin, an intracellular regulator that has a large number of physiologic roles, including expression of the gene for type II collagen. In vitro functional studies accompanying these genetic studies provided additional evidence of the importance of these genetic findings in OA.

Rapid progress in identifying and understanding the contributions of genetic variation to the development of OA is being made. Especially for relatively common alleles coding for proteins that regulate cartilage function, there is exciting potential for new drugs that affect these regulatory proteins so as to prevent, mitigate, or treat OA.

PATHOPHYSIOLOGY

OA falls into two major etiologic classes. *Primary (idiopathic) OA,* the most common type, has no identifiable cause. Subclasses of primary OA are *localized OA,* involving one or two sites, and *generalized OA,* affecting three or more sites. *Erosive osteoarthritis* is used to describe the presence of erosion and marked proliferation in the proximal and distal interphalangeal joints of the hands. *Secondary OA* is that associated with a known cause such as rheumatoid or another inflammatory arthritis, trauma, metabolic or endocrine disorders, and congenital factors.[3,4,17,18]

Although OA was previously considered a wear-and-tear disease, increased knowledge about articular cartilage physiology has led to a more dynamic understanding of OA. Some changes in the OA joint may reflect compensatory processes to maintain function in the face of ongoing joint destruction. Not only biomechanical forces, but also inflammatory, biochemical, and immunologic factors are involved.[17–19] To aid in understanding the pathophysiology of OA, a brief review of the biochemistry and function of normal cartilage and of the diarthrodial joint is provided.

NORMAL CARTILAGE

Function, Structure, and Composition of Cartilage

Articular cartilage is a unique substance, with viscoelastic properties that provide lubrication with motion, shock absorbency during rapid movements, and load support. In synovial joints, articular cartilage is found between the synovial cavity on one side, and a narrow layer of calcified tissue overlying subchondral bone, on the other side (Fig. 95–2).[20] The layer of cartilage is narrow, with medial femoral articular cartilage being approximately 2 to 3 mm thick in humans. Despite this, healthy articular cartilage in weight-bearing joints withstands millions of cycles of loading and unloading each year. Another key feature of cartilage is that it is almost frictionless; for example, in comparison to articular cartilage, Teflon produces 20 times as much friction (has a 20-fold higher coefficient of sliding friction).[21] Articular cartilage is also far superior to artificial joints in regard to friction.[9] Articular cartilage enables movement in the joint, distributes load across joint tissues to prevent damage, and stabilizes the joint. Cartilage is easily compressed, losing up to 40% of its original height when a load is applied. Compression increases the area of contact and disperses force more evenly to underlying bone, tendons, ligaments, and muscles.

The robustness of articular cartilage, its extremely low coefficient of friction, its compressibility, and other exceptional features are a function of its unique structure. Cartilage is comprised of a complex, hydrophilic, extracellular matrix. It is approximately 75% to 85% water, 2% to 5% chondrocytes (the only cells in cartilage), and contains collagen proteins, smaller amounts of several other proteins, proteoglycans, and long hyaluronic acid molecules.[20] The proteoglycans combine with long hyaluronic acid molecules to form large complexes, which are located within a meshwork of collagen fibers. Five types of collagen are located in cartilage, approximately 95% being type II collagen.

The collagen network supports and holds together the extracellular matrix in which proteoglycan–hyaluronic complexes are held and in which chondrocytes are embedded. Cross-linking of type II collagen fibrils with other matrix proteins also provides tensile strength to cartilage and maintains its volume and shape. It is due to the hydrophilic and anionic nature of the proteoglycan–hyaluronate complexes in the collagen network that cartilage possesses the viscoelastic properties required for resiliency and load bearing.

Collagens also contribute to the function of joint cartilage in other ways, with orientation of collagen fibers being critical: superficial fibers are parallel to the surface, reducing friction and allowing forces to be dissipated; basal layer collagen fibers are perpendicular to the surface to anchor cartilage to the calcified zone or subchondral bony end plate.[17]

It is not clear exactly how biomechanical signals, such as stress, strain, or cyclic loading and unloading during walking, translate into biochemical signals which affect chondrocyte metabolism and cartilage turnover. Regulation of chondrocyte function and cartilage metabolism is complex.[17–19] Insulin-like growth factor, epidermal growth factor, fibroblast growth factor, and other agents enhance chondrocyte proliferation and proteoglycan synthesis. By contrast, interleukin-1 and tumor necrosis factor-α promote enzymes that degrade matrix proteins and suppress proteoglycan and collagen synthesis in the extracellular matrix. In healthy adult cartilage, as opposed to OA or during development, anabolic and catabolic influences are in homeostatic balance, resulting in a low metabolic rate and very slow turnover of cartilage.[9,20,22,23]

Finally, it is important to note that adult articular cartilage is avascular, with chondrocytes nourished by synovial fluid. With movement and cyclic loading and unloading of joints, nutrients

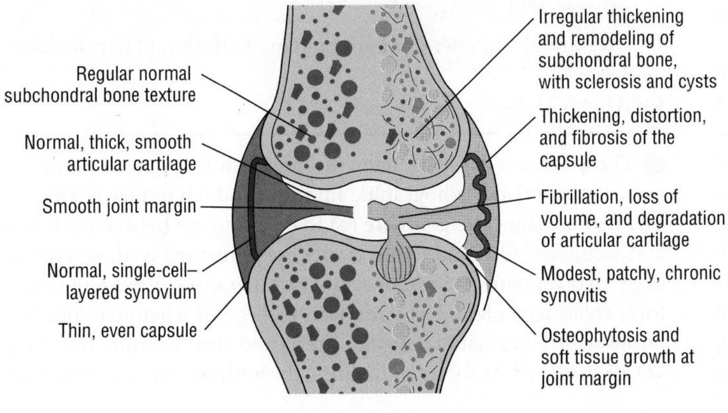

FIGURE 95-2. Characteristics of osteoarthritis in the diarthrodial joint. *(Courtesy of Dr. D. Gotlieb.)*

flow into the cartilage, whereas immobilization reduces nutrient supply. This is one of the reasons that normal physical activity is beneficial for joint health.

OSTEOARTHRITIC CARTILAGE

❸ Important contributors to the development of OA are local mechanical influences, genetic factors, inflammation, and aberrant chondrocyte function leading to loss of articular cartilage. At a molecular level, OA pathophysiology involves the interplay of dozens, if not hundreds, of extracellular and intracellular molecules with roles including chondrocyte regulation, proteolytic degradation of cartilage components, and interactions between articular cartilage, underlying subchondral bone, and the joint synovium.

OA most commonly begins with damage to articular cartilage, through trauma or other injury, excess joint loading from obesity or other reasons, or instability or injury of the joint that causes abnormal loading.[15] Although normal cartilage is in a state of slow turnover (see Normal Cartilage section), damage to cartilage dramatically increases the metabolic activity of chondrocytes. This leads to increased synthesis of matrix constituents, with swelling of cartilage. This hypertrophic phase is thought to represent a reparative response to damage, stimulated by the peptide annexin, parathyroid hormone-related protein, and other effectors.[9] This hypertrophic response, however, does not restore the cartilage to normal, but instead is the first step in a process ultimately leading to further loss of cartilage.

Following the hypertrophic phase, there is increased turnover (increased collagen synthesis and destruction), but with destruction outpacing formation, with net loss of cartilage. Key players in this destruction are the matrix metalloproteinases (MMPs), specifically MMPs 1, 3, 13, and 28.[9] In normal cartilage, activities of these enzymes are blocked by tissue inhibitors of metalloproteinases. In OA cartilage, however, there is increased expression and synthesis of MMPs, resulting in the MMP–tissue inhibitors of metalloproteinase balance tilting toward proteolysis. In addition, chondrocytes contribute to loss, secreting MMPs in response to inflammatory mediators present in OA (interleukin-1 and tumor necrosis factor-α). Also, chondrocytes in OA cartilage undergo apoptosis, likely as a result of induction of nitric oxide synthase and production of toxic metabolites.[15,20] This leaves fewer chondrocytes to synthesize matrix components. In addition, OA chondrocytes are hyporesponsive to the anabolic stimulus transforming growth factor-β.[20] The net result of all of these processes is that there is a progressive cycle of cartilage destruction and loss of chondrocytes.

In addition to changes taking place in OA cartilage, there is also a role in OA for the subchondral bone adjacent to articular cartilage. Subchondral bone undergoes pathologic changes that may precede, coincide with, or follow damage to the articular cartilage. This damage to subchondral bone may play an essential role in allowing damage to articular cartilage to progress.[9,18,24,25] In OA, subchondral bone releases vasoactive peptides and MMPs. Neovascularization and subsequent increased permeability of the adjacent cartilage also occurs and contributes further to cartilage loss.[18,25]

Substantial loss of cartilage causes joint space narrowing and leads to a painful, deformed joint. Furthermore, the remaining cartilage softens and develops fibrillations (vertical clefts into the cartilage), and there is splitting, further loss of cartilage, and exposure of underlying bone.[26] As cartilage is destroyed and the adjacent subchondral bone undergoes pathologic changes, cartilage is eroded completely, leaving denuded subchondral bone, which becomes dense, smooth, and glistening (eburnation). A more brittle, stiffer bone results, with decreased weight-bearing ability and development of sclerosis and microfractures. New bone formations, or osteophytes also appear at joint margins distant from cartilage destruction, and are thought to arise from local and humoral factors. There is direct evidence that osteophytes can help stabilize osteoarthritic joints.[27]

Accompanying the changes in cartilage and subchondral bone, local inflammatory changes and pathologic changes can occur in the joint capsule and synovium. Infiltration of the synovium with T cells with T-helper type 1 phenotype occurs, as well as the appearance of immune complexes.[15] Contributors to this inflammation may include crystals or cartilage shards in synovial fluid. With increased levels of interleukin-1, prostaglandin E_2, tumor necrosis factor-α, and nitric oxide observed in synovial fluid, these agents could also play a role.[27] With inflammatory changes in the synovium, effusions and synovial thickening occur.

❹ The pain of OA is not related to the destruction of cartilage, but arises from the activation of nociceptive nerve endings within the joint by mechanical and chemical irritants.[3] OA pain may result from distension of the synovial capsule by increased joint fluid, microfracture, periosteal irritation, or damage to ligaments, synovium, or the meniscus.

CLINICAL PRESENTATION

CLINICAL PRESENTATION OF OSTEOARTHRITIS

General

- The patient may have mild symptoms for months to years prior to seeking medical care; self-treatment is common for mild symptoms.
- Typical age at presentation is usually >50 years.

Symptoms

- Nearly all patients have pain in the affected joints, with the hands, knees, and hips being the most common locations.
- Pain is most commonly associated with motion, but pain in late disease can occur with rest.
- Joint stiffness resolves with motion; recurs with rest.

Signs

- Joint stiffness with or without joint enlargement.
- Crepitus, a crackling or grating sound heard with joint movement that is caused by irregularity of joint surfaces may be present.
- Limited range of motion that may be accompanied by joint instability.
- Late-stage disease is associated with joint deformity (Fig. 95–3).

Laboratory Tests

- There are no specific laboratory tests useful in the diagnosis.

Other Radiologic Tests—Plain Radiographic Films

- Joint space narrowing, appearance of osteophytes in moderate disease (Fig. 95–4).
- Abnormal alignment of joints and joint effusion in late disease.

DIAGNOSIS

❺ The diagnosis of OA is made through history, physical examination, characteristic radiographic findings, and laboratory testing.[3,24] The major diagnostic goals are (a) to discriminate between primary and secondary OA, and (b) to clarify the joints involved, severity of joint involvement, and response to prior therapies, providing a basis for a treatment plan. The American College of Rheumatology has published traditional diagnostic criteria and also "decision trees" for OA diagnosis.[24] As for all guidelines, the authors stress these are for

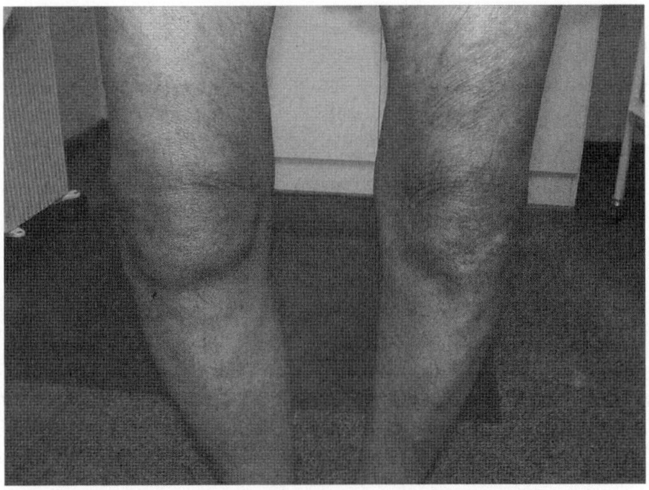

FIGURE 95-3. Physical findings of joint enlargement and genu varum of the knees. *(Courtesy of Dr. D. Gotlieb.)*

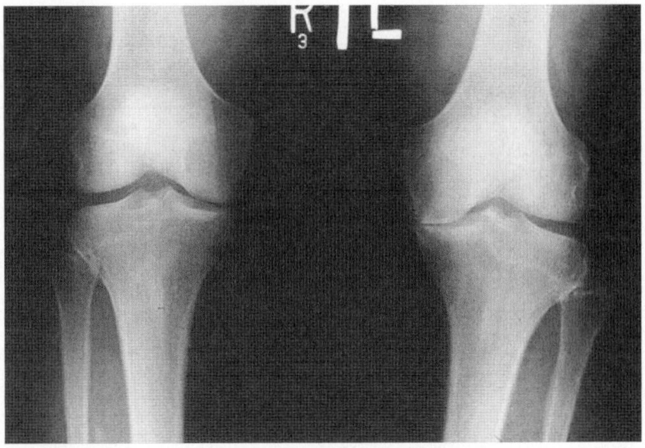

FIGURE 95-4. Plain x-ray films of the knee demonstrating joint space narrowing. *(From Johnson BE. Arthritis: Osteoarthritis, Gout and Rheumatoid Arthritis. In: South-Paul JE, Matheny SC, Lewis EL, eds. Current Diagnosis and Treatment in Family Medicine. New York: McGraw-Hill, 2004, p. 267.)*

assisting the clinician rather than replacing clinical judgment. For example, traditional criteria are as follows: (a) For hip OA, a patient must have pain in the hip and at least two of the following three: an erythrocyte sedimentation rate <20 mm/h, femoral or acetabular osteophytes on radiography, or joint space narrowing on radiography. This provides a sensitivity of 89% and a specificity of 91%. (b) For knee OA, a patient must have pain at the knee and osteophytes on radiography plus one of the following: age older than 50 years, morning stiffness no more than 30 minutes, crepitus on motion, bony enlargement, bony tenderness, or palpable warmth. This provides a sensitivity of 95% and a specificity of 69%. The addition of laboratory or radiographic data further improves accuracy of diagnosis. Criteria for hand OA have also been published.

PROGNOSIS

The prognosis for patients with primary OA is variable and depends on the joint involved. If a weight-bearing joint or the spine is involved, considerable morbidity and disability are possible. In the case of secondary OA, the prognosis depends on the underlying cause. Treatment of OA may relieve pain or improve function, but does not reverse preexisting damage to the articular cartilage.

TREATMENT

Osteoarthritis

■ DESIRED OUTCOME

Management of the patient with OA begins with a diagnosis based on a careful history, physical examination, radiographic findings, and an assessment of the extent of joint involvement. Treatment should be tailored to each individual. Goals are (a) to educate the patient, caregivers, and relatives; (b) to relieve pain and stiffness; (c) to maintain or improve joint mobility; (d) to limit functional impairment; and (e) to maintain or improve quality of life.[7,28–31]

■ GENERAL APPROACH TO TREATMENT

Treatment for each OA patient depends on the distribution and severity of joint involvement, comorbid disease states, concomitant medications, and allergies (Fig. 95–5). Management for all individuals with OA should begin with patient education, and physical and/or occupational therapy, and weight loss or assistive devices if appropriate.[7,28–33]

The primary objective of medication is to alleviate pain.[28–32] Scheduled acetaminophen, up to 4 g/day, should be tried initially. If this is ineffective, nonsteroidal antiinflammatory drugs (NSAIDs) are prescribed, or possibly a cyclooxygenase (COX)-2 selective inhibitor (celecoxib) if warranted. Application of capsaicin or methylsalicylate topical creams over specific joints can sometimes be helpful adjuncts for pain control. Glucosamine and chondroitin in combination can be helpful for those with moderate to severe arthritis. Joint aspiration followed by glucocorticoid or hyaluronate injection can relieve pain, and is offered concomitantly with oral analgesics or after their lack of efficacy, depending on the practitioner's style. Opioid analgesics are a final medication to prescribe if other therapies are unsuccessful. When symptoms are intractable or there is significant loss of function, joint replacement may be appropriate if the patient is a surgical candidate.

Finally, for patients interested in clinical trials, investigational strategies with oral doxycycline, matrix metalloproteinase inhibitors, disease-modifying osteoarthritis drugs, or cartilage transplantations may be considered.

For management of patients with OA, the Third Canadian Consensus Conference Group recently summarized evidence-based recommendations (Table 95–1).[34] As for all guidelines, these are for assisting the clinician rather than replacing the clinician's judgment based on the patient, other evidence, and other recommendations. The American College of Rheumatology recommends acetaminophen as the drug of first choice. In patients with risk factors for GI complications, selection of a nonselective NSAID plus a proton pump inhibitor, or a COX-2 selective inhibitor plus a proton pump inhibitor is supported by much recent evidence, as described in this chapter.

■ NONPHARMACOLOGIC THERAPY

❻ The first step in OA treatment is patient education about the disease process, the extent of OA, the prognosis, and treatment options. Education is paramount, in that OA is often seen as a "wear-and-tear" disease, an inevitable consequence of aging for which nothing helps. Even worse, patients may resort to the use of alternative but unproven medications or quackery. Patients should be warned about these and encouraged to access information from local or national units of the Arthritis Foundation.[35] The Arthritis Foundation provides literature about OA and OA medications and information about local clinics and agencies offering physical and economic assistance. The Arthritis Foundation also sponsors support groups and public education programs.

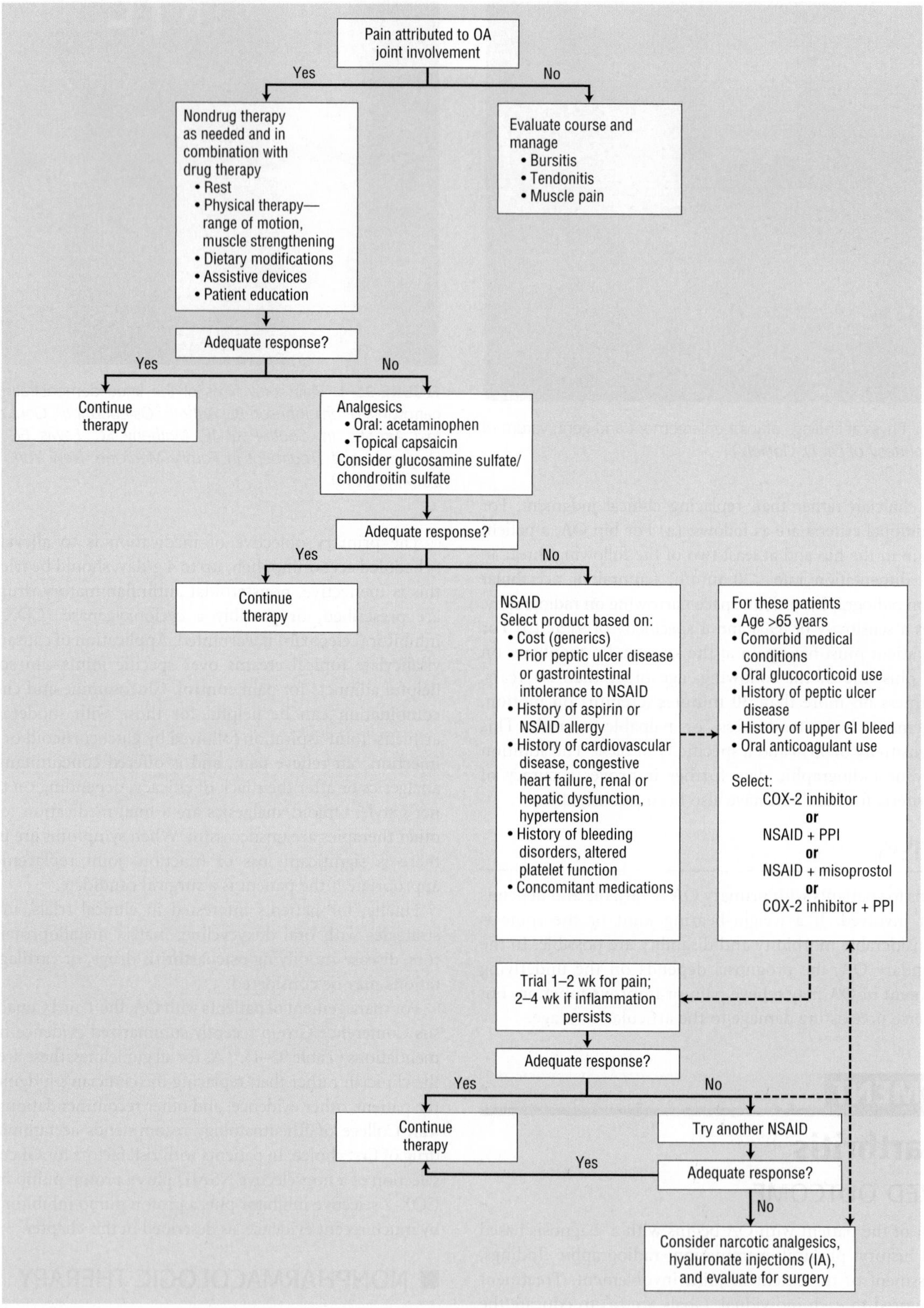

FIGURE 95-5. Treatment algorithm for osteoarthritis. (COX, cyclooxygenase; GI, gastrointestinal; IA, intraarticular; NSAID, nonsteroidal antiinflammatory drug; OA, osteoarthritis; PPI, proton pump inhibitor.)

The benefits of patient education have been documented in a variety of programs, including those using monthly telephone contact between trained volunteers and individuals with OA.[2] Volunteers speak with patients about symptoms, function, drugs, and clinic visits, resulting in improved pain and functional status at low cost. Likewise, OA patients participating in the program report decreases in joint pain and OA-related clinic visits, and improved physical activity and quality of life.

Diet

Excess weight increases the biomechanical load on weight-bearing joints and is the single best predictor of need for eventual joint replacement.[4,8,33,36] Even a 5-kg weight loss can decrease the load on a weight-bearing joint. Weight loss is associated with decreased symptoms and disability, although results are variable.[36,37] At least one randomized, controlled trial has demonstrated improvement in

TABLE 95-1 Summary of Recommendations for Osteoarthritis

Recommendation		Level of Evidence[a]	Grade of Recommendation[b]
1. Patient–physician communication	Patients should be fully informed about evolving information regarding the benefits and risks of their treatment options.	3	C
2. Indications	NSAIDs and coxibs are generally more effective and preferred by patients over acetaminophen, although a trial of the latter is warranted for some patients. Topical NSAID formulations may confer benefit in knee OA.	1	A
3. GI toxicity	In patients with risk factors for PUB, a coxib is still the antiinflammatory drug of choice, depending on the patient's cardiovascular risks. High-risk patients who must use nonselective NSAIDs should have a PPI.	1	A
4. Renal	Before starting an NSAID or coxib, determine renal status and creatinine clearance in patients older than 65 years and in those with comorbid conditions that may affect renal function.	3	C
	Advise patients that if they cannot eat or drink that day, they should withhold that day's dose of NSAID/coxib.	4	D
5. Hypertension	In patients receiving antihypertensive drugs, measure blood pressure within a few weeks after initiating NSAID/coxib therapy and monitor appropriately; drug doses may need adjustment.	1	A
6. Cardiovascular	Patients taking rofecoxib have been shown to have an increased risk of CV events. Current data suggest that this increased CV risk may be an effect of the NSAID/coxib class. Physicians and patients should weigh the benefits and risks of NSAID/coxib therapy.	1	A
7. Geriatric consideration	NSAIDs/coxibs should be used with caution in elderly patients, who are at the greatest risk for serious GI, renal, and CV side effects.	3	C
8. Pharmacoeconomics	Although the data are ambiguous, coxibs may be more cost-effective than traditional NSAID + proprietary PPI in high-risk patients.	3	C

CV, cardiovascular; GI, gastrointestinal; NSAID, nonsteroidal anti-inflammatory drug; OA, osteoarthritis; PPI, proton pump inhibitor; PUB, perforations, ulcers, and bleeds.

[a]Levels of evidence: 1A, meta-analysis of randomized, controlled trial; 1B, at least one randomized, controlled trial; 2A, at least one controlled study without randomization; 3, descriptive studies, such as comparative, correlation, or case-control studies; 4, expert committee reports or opinions and/or clinical experience of respected authorities.

[b]Grades of recommendation: A, Category 1 evidence; B, Category 2 evidence or extrapolated recommendation from Category 1 evidence; C, Category 3 evidence or extrapolated recommendation from Category 1 or 2 evidence; D, Category 4 evidence or extrapolated recommendation from Category 2 or 3 evidence.

From Tannenbaum H, Bombardier C, Davis P, Russell AS, Third Canadian Consensus Conference Group. An evidence-based approach to prescribing nonsteroidal antiinflammatory drugs. Third Canadian Consensus Conference. J Rheumatol 2006;33:140–157. Reprinted with permission from the Journal of Rheumatology and the author.

pain and self-reported physical function using a combination of modest weight loss (5%) and exercise.[38] Although dietary intervention for overweight OA patients is reasonable, weight loss usually requires a motivated patient and a structured weight-loss program.

Physical and Occupational Therapy

Physical therapy—with heat or cold treatments and an exercise program—helps to maintain and restore joint range of motion and to reduce pain and muscle spasms. Warm baths or warm water soaks may decrease pain and stiffness. Heating pads should be used with caution, especially in the elderly. Patients should be warned not to fall asleep on the heat source or to lie on it for more than brief periods to avoid burns.

Exercise programs and quadriceps strengthening can improve physical functioning and can decrease disability, pain, and analgesic use by OA patients.[2,38,39] Isometric exercise is preferred over isotonic exercise because the latter can aggravate affected joints. Exercises should be taught and then observed before the patient exercises at home, ideally three to four times daily. The patient should be instructed to decrease the number of repetitions if severe pain develops with exercise.

The decision about whether to encourage walking should be made on an individual basis. With weak or deconditioned muscles, the load is transmitted excessively to the joints, so weight-bearing activities can exacerbate symptoms. However, avoidance of activity by those with hip or knee OA leads to further deconditioning or weight gain. A program of patient education, muscle stretching and strengthening, and supervised walking can improve physical function and decrease pain in patients with knee OA.[2,38,39] Referral to the physical and/or occupational therapist is especially helpful for patients with functional disabilities. The therapist can assess muscle strength and joint stability, and recommend exercises and methods of protecting the affected joint from excessive forces. The therapist can also provide assistive and orthotic devices, such as canes, walkers, braces, heel cups, splints, or insoles for use during exercise or daily activities.

Surgery

Surgery can be recommended for OA patients with functional disability and/or severe pain unresponsive to conservative therapy. Criteria for total joint replacement (arthroplasty) of the knee were developed at an National Institutes of Health consensus conference.[40] Likewise, criteria for total hip replacement, as well as a summary of clinical outcomes resulting from this procedure have been published.[41] These hip and knee replacement recommendations have been based on critical review of the literature as well as on expert opinion. For patients with advanced disease, a partial or total arthroplasty can relieve pain and improve motion, with the best outcomes after hip or knee arthroplasty.

Other surgical options are also available. Arthrodesis (joint fusion) can reduce pain but will restrict motion, and may be appropriate for smaller joints that are causing intractable pain. For patients with mild knee OA, an osteotomy (removal of bony tissue) may correct the misalignment of genu varum ("bowlegged" knees) or genu valgum ("knock-knees"). In addition, osteotomies of the pelvis or femur can ameliorate joint misalignment in hip OA, subsequently slowing progression of disease. Although knee arthroscopy or lavage have been recommended for short-term relief of pain, these procedures appear to be equivalent to sham surgery.[39] Experimental but potentially restorative approaches involve soft-tissue grafts, chondrocyte transplantation, gene therapy, and use of growth factors or artificial matrices.[42] Cartilage-restoration approaches are investigational, and results regarding pain control and joint function have been mixed.

■ PHARMACOLOGIC THERAPY

Drug therapy in OA is targeted at relief of pain. OA is commonly seen in older individuals who have other medical conditions, and

OA treatment is often long-term. As such, a conservative approach to drug treatment, focusing on the needs of the individual patient, is warranted (see Fig. 95–5). For mild or moderate pain, topical analgesics or acetaminophen can be used. If these measures fail, or if there is inflammation, NSAIDs may be useful. Even when drug therapy is initiated, appropriate nondrug therapies should be continued and reinforced. Nondrug modalities are the cornerstone of OA management and may provide as much relief as drug therapy.

Acetaminophen

7 Place in Therapy The American College of Rheumatology recommends acetaminophen as first-line drug therapy for pain management in OA because of its relative safety, efficacy, and lower cost compared to NSAIDs.[2,34,43] Pain relief with acetaminophen has been reported as similar to that obtained with aspirin, naproxen, ibuprofen, and other NSAIDs, although many patients respond better to NSAIDs.[2,43,44] In addition to guidelines from the American College of Rheumatology, recommendations for OA management have been published by The European League Against Rheumatism, and a review of the evidence and suggestions for OA management have been formulated by rheumatology faculty in the Medical Research Council (UK) Environmental Epidemiology Unit.[2,45,46] These guidelines stress the importance of acetaminophen as first-line drug therapy for OA.

Pharmacology and Mechanism of Action Acetaminophen is understood to act within the central nervous system by inhibiting synthesis of prostaglandins, agents that enhance pain sensations. Acetaminophen prevents prostaglandin synthesis by blocking the action of central cyclooxygenase. Acetaminophen is well absorbed after oral administration, with a bioavailability of 60% to 98%. It achieves peak concentrations within 1 to 2 hours, is inactivated in the liver by conjugation with sulfate or glucuronide, and its metabolites are renally excreted.

Efficacy Comparable relief of mild to moderate OA pain has been demonstrated for acetaminophen at 2.6 to 4 g/day, aspirin 650 mg four times daily, and NSAIDS, including ibuprofen at 1,200 or 2,400 mg daily, and naproxen 750 mg daily.[2,43,47] Although studies have shown comparable efficacy for acetaminophen and NSAIDs, several others have reported that patients experience better pain control with NSAIDs than with acetaminophen.[2,44,47] Patients with OA have been shown to prefer NSAIDs compared to acetaminophen in clinical trials, but when queried using a questionnaire that included considerations of side effects, NSAIDs were less preferred by patients.[48]

Adverse Effects Although acetaminophen is one of the safest analgesics, its use carries some risks, primarily hepatotoxicity, and possibly renal toxicity with long-term use.[2,7,43,49] With acetaminophen overdose, serious hepatotoxicity, including fatalities, have been well documented. (See Chap. 10 for treatment of acetaminophen overdose.) In a study of normal, healthy volunteers administered acetaminophen 4 g/day (1 g every 6 hours), alone or with concomitant opioid therapy, for 14 days, elevations of alanine aminotransferase at levels above three times the upper limits of normal were found in 31% to 44% of patients, depending on treatment group.[50] None of these participants had clinical symptoms of acute liver disease. Although the results of this study are not robust enough to alter the current standard dosing recommendations, it serves as an important reminder that the maximum dose of acetaminophen should be not be exceeded in any patient population, and that chronic use of even the maximum 4 g/day can affect the liver. Acetaminophen should be used cautiously in patients with liver disease or in those who abuse alcohol. Acute liver failure has been reported in patients taking less than 4 g/daily.[51] The most common risk factor for liver failure in these patients was chronic alcohol intake. The FDA has recommended that chronic alcohol users (three or more drinks daily) should be warned regarding an increased risk of liver damage or GI bleeding with acetaminophen. Other individuals do not appear to be at increased risk of GI bleeding.

The National Kidney Foundation strongly discourages the use of nonprescription combination analgesic products (e.g., acetaminophen and NSAIDs) because this is associated with an increased prevalence of renal failure.[49] Finally, patients should be warned about potential toxicity if they inadvertently ingest more than the recommended dose when using both nonprescription and prescription products containing acetaminophen.

Recent prospective cohort studies in women and in men have suggested that regular long-term use of acetaminophen is associated with development of hypertension, although the risk appears less for men.[52,53] However, these studies were not designed to evaluate the effects of analgesics on the risk of developing hypertension, but were part of the Nurses' Health Study and Physicians' Health Study. Furthermore, patients taking analgesics for OA or other pain may have other risk factors for the development of hypertension, including advanced age, uncontrolled pain, use of other medications, obesity, and comorbid medical illness. Prospectively designed trials are needed to determine if the risk of developing hypertension is definitively linked to analgesic use, including acetaminophen.

Drug–Drug Interactions and Drug–Food Interactions Drug interactions with acetaminophen can occur; for example, isoniazid can increase the risk of hepatotoxicity. Chronic ingestion of maximal doses of acetaminophen may intensify the anticoagulant effect in patients taking warfarin; such individuals may need closer monitoring. Although food decreases the maximum serum concentration of acetaminophen by approximately half, the overall efficacy is unchanged.

Dosing and Administration When used for chronic OA, acetaminophen should be administered in a scheduled manner. It may be taken with or without food. Acetaminophen can be taken at 325 to 650 mg every 4 to 6 hours, but total dose must not exceed 4 g daily (see Adverse Effects above). If acetaminophen is used in the setting of chronic alcohol intake or in those with underlying disease, the duration should be limited and the dose should not exceed 2 g daily.

Nonsteroidal Antiinflammatory Drugs

Place in Therapy The American College of Rheumatology recommends consideration of NSAIDs for OA patients in whom acetaminophen is ineffective. NSAIDs have analgesic properties at lower doses and antiinflammatory effects at higher doses. NSAIDs all display comparable analgesic and antiinflammatory efficacy and are similarly beneficial in OA (Table 95–2).[54,55]

Pharmacology and Mechanism of Action Blockade of prostaglandin synthesis by inhibiting cyclooxygenase enzymes (COX-1 and COX-2) is thought to account for the ability of NSAIDs to relieve pain and inflammation (Fig. 95–6).[47,55–57] Because nonspecific NSAIDs and COX-2 selective inhibitors have similar efficacy, drug selection often depends on toxicity and cost. Increasing concern regarding safety of all NSAIDs, and particularly COX-2 selective inhibitors, has made patient safety paramount in drug selection. The next section will review the differences between nonspecific NSAIDs and COX-2 selective inhibitors.[47,55–57]

Nonspecific NSAIDs and COX-2 Selective Inhibitors The COX-1 enzyme participates in "housekeeping" or routine physiologic functions such as generation of gastroprotective prostaglandins to promote gastric blood flow and bicarbonate generation (see Fig. 95–6).[47,55–57] COX-1 is expressed constitutively not only in gastric mucosa, but also in vascular endothelial cells, platelets, and renal collecting tubules, so that COX-1–generated prostaglandins and

TABLE 95-2 Medications Commonly Used in the Treatment of Osteoarthritis

Medication	Dosage and Frequency	Maximum Dosage (mg/day)
Oral analgesics		
Acetaminophen	325–650 mg every 4–6 hours or 1 g three to four times/day	4,000
Tramadol	50–100 mg every 4–6 hours	400
Acetaminophen/codeine	300–1,000 mg/15–60 mg every 4 hours as needed	4,000 mg/360 mg[a]
Acetaminophen/oxycodone	325–650 mg/2.5–10 mg every 6 hours as needed	4,000 mg/40 mg[a]
Topical analgesics		
Capsaicin 0.025% or 0.075%	Apply to affected joint 3–4 times per day	–
Nutritional supplements		
Glucosamine HCl/chondroitin sulfate	500 mg/400 mg three times/day	1,500/1,200
Nonsteroidal antiinflammatory drugs (NSAIDs)		
Carboxylic acids		
Acetylated salicylates		
Aspirin, plain, buffered, or enteric-coated	325–650 mg every 4–6 hours for pain; antiinflammatory doses start at 3,600 mg/day in divided doses	3,600[b]
Nonacetylated salicylates		
Salsalate	500–1,000 mg two to three times a day	3,000[b]
Diflunisal	500–1,000 mg two times a day	1,500
Choline salicylate[c]	500–1,000 mg two to three times a day	3,000[c]
Choline magnesium salicylate	500–1,000 mg two to three times a day	3,000[c]
Acetic acids		
Etodolac	800–1,200 mg/day in divided doses	1,200
Diclofenac	100–150 mg/day in divided doses	200
Indomethacin	25 mg two to three times a day; 75 mg SR once daily	200; 150
Ketorolac[d]	10 mg every 4–6 hours	40
Nabumetone[e]	500–1,000 mg one to two times a day	2,000
Propionic acids		
Fenoprofen	300–600 mg three to four times a day	3,200
Flurbiprofen	200–300 mg/day in two to four divided doses	300
Ibuprofen	1,200–3,200 mg/day in three to four divided doses	3,200
Ketoprofen	150–300 mg/day in three to four divided doses	300
Naproxen	250–500 mg twice a day	1,500
Naproxen sodium	275–550 mg twice a day	1,375
Oxaprozin	600–1,200 mg daily	1,800
Fenamates		
Meclofenamate	200–400 mg/day in three to four divided doses	400
Mefenamic acid[f]	250 mg every 6 hours	1,000
Oxicams		
Piroxicam	10–20 mg daily	20
Meloxicam	7.5 mg daily	15
Coxibs		
Celecoxib	100 mg twice daily or 200 mg daily	200 (400 for RA)

RA, rheumatoid arthritis; SR, sustained release.
[a]Maximum dosage in combination product limited by acetaminophen maximum of 4,000 mg/day.
[b]Monitor serum salicylate levels over 3–3.6 g/day.
[c]Only available as a liquid; 870 mg salicylate/5 mL.
[d]Not approved for treatment of osteoarthritis for more than 5 days.
[e]Nonorganic acid but metabolite is an acetic acid.
[f]Not approved for treatment of osteoarthritis.

thromboxane also participate in hemostasis and renal blood flow. In contrast, the COX-2 enzyme is not as widely expressed in most body tissues, but is rapidly induced by inflammatory mediators, local injury, and cytokines, including interleukins, interferon, and tumor necrosis factor (see Fig. 95–6).[47,55–57] Prostaglandins made by COX-2 contribute to pain sensations in OA and other conditions. Prostaglandins made by the COX-2 enzyme, including prostacyclin (prostaglandin I_2) are also implicated in some physiologic processes, including renal function, tissue repair, reproduction, and development.

Nonspecific NSAIDs block both COX-1 and COX-2 enzymes. In view of the above roles of the COX enzymes, COX-1 blockade that occurs with nonspecific NSAIDs is potentially undesirable and can lead to GI ulcers and increased bleeding risk by inhibiting platelet aggregation.[47,55–58] Specific blockade of COX-2 activity could thus reduce prostaglandins, inflammation, and pain, without blocking effects of COX-1. This desirable quality led to development of specific COX-2 selective agents ("coxibs"). These agents are efficacious in relieving OA and other pain and some do have improved GI safety. Celecoxib and rofecoxib were the first two COX-2 selective agents marketed and have been widely used for pain relief in OA and other conditions.

It is now appreciated that the COX-2 enzyme may play an important physiologic role in normal hemostasis. The COX-2 enzyme, found in blood vessel endothelial cells, leads to production of prostaglandin I_2 (prostacyclin), which has antithrombotic effects. The COX-1 found in platelets forms thromboxane A_2 a prothrombotic molecule. As far back as 1999, and continuing today, some researchers postulate that blocking COX-2 alone could upset the hemostatic balance, in favor of thromboxane A_2, with prothrombotic events possible.[57,59] Although this explanation is plausible and is appealing in its simplicity, it has not been proven. Thus, whether the "prothrombotic imbalance" explanation accounts for the increased cardiovascular risk seen with COX-2 selective inhibitors is unknown.[57,59,60]

Rofecoxib was withdrawn from the market in 2004 because of increased cardiovascular events, and celecoxib is less often used now and carries a black box warning for cardiovascular and GI risks, as

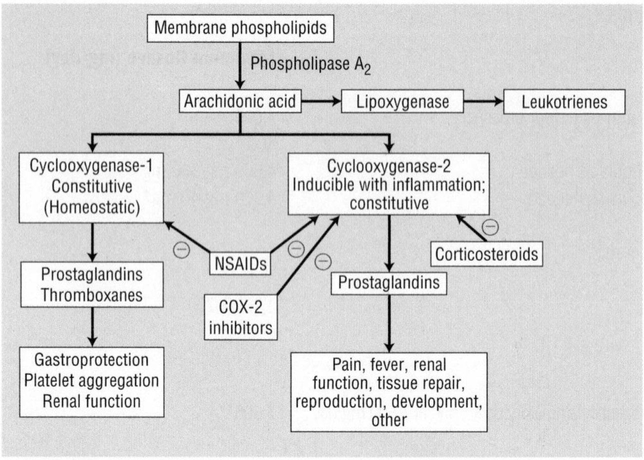

FIGURE 95-6. Pathway of synthesis for prostaglandins and leukotrienes. COX-1 and COX-2 are cyclooxygenase 1 and 2 enzymes. The minus (–) sign indicates inhibitory influence. Prostaglandins include PGE_2 and PGI_2, the latter also known as prostacyclin.

do other NSAIDs at this time. Although new coxibs are in development and some are in use in Canada and Europe, celecoxib is the only remaining coxib available in the United States.

Pharmacokinetics The various NSAIDs exhibit several pharmacokinetic similarities, including high oral availability, high protein binding, and absorption as active drugs (except for sulindac and nabumetone, which require hepatic conversion for activity). The most important difference in NSAIDs is a serum half-life ranging from 1 hour for tolmetin to 50 hours for piroxicam, impacting the frequency of dosing and, potentially, compliance with therapy.[47] Elimination of NSAIDs largely depends on hepatic inactivation, with a small fraction of active drug being renally excreted. NSAIDs penetrate joint fluid, reaching approximately 60% of blood levels.[47]

Efficacy Prescription-strength NSAIDs are often prescribed for OA patients after treatment with acetaminophen proves ineffective or for patients with inflammatory OA.[61] All NSAIDs and aspirin have similar analgesic and antiinflammatory effects, but these agents are only modestly more effective than acetaminophen.[34,47,54,61,62] In evaluating efficacy in OA studies, commonly used end points include pain on the visual analog scale (0 to 100), and the patient's global assessment of disease activity and functional status, assessed using the Western Ontario and McMaster Universities Osteoarthritis Index questionnaire.[63] Because of differences among study designs and patient populations, comparisons between efficacies of treatments are best made within the same study.

A systematic review of studies of NSAIDs for OA found no evidence to support a definitive ranking of NSAID efficacy.[62] However, individual patient response does differ among NSAIDs. The prescriber often relies on personal experience in choosing an NSAID. To assess efficacy in the individual patient, a trial that is adequate in time (2 to 3 weeks) and dose is needed. If the first trial fails, another NSAID in the same or another chemical class can be tried until an effective agent is found (see Table 95–2).[34,47,54,61,62] Patients must understand this approach, appreciate the necessity of adherence to medication therapy throughout this trial period, and actively participate in assessment of drug efficacy. Combining two NSAIDs increases adverse effects without providing additional benefit.

COX-2 selective inhibitors demonstrate similar analgesic benefits to traditional NSAIDs and to each other.[64] Newer COX-2 selective inhibitors in development have also shown similar efficacy to traditional NSAIDs. Lumiracoxib 100 to 400 mg/day[65–67] and etoricoxib 30 to 90 mg/day[68–70] provided significant relief in OA compared to placebo and showed efficacy similar to other comparator NSAIDs (ibuprofen 2,400 mg/day, naproxen 1,000 mg/day, or diclofenac 150 mg/day). The newer COX-2 selective inhibitors have also been compared to older COX-2 selective inhibitors: Etoricoxib 30 mg/day and celecoxib 200 mg/day were similarly efficacious in OA and superior to placebo.[71] Lumiracoxib 100 to 200 mg/day was similarly efficacious as celecoxib 200 mg/day in treating OA.[65,66,72]

Given that no proven efficacy differences exist among all traditional and COX-2 selective NSAIDs in OA, it is especially important that potential toxicities of these agents be rigorously examined. These safety issues are reviewed below.

⑧ Adverse Effects

Gastrointestinal Effects of Nonselective NSAIDs. The most common adverse effects of NSAIDs involve the GI tract, contributing to many treatment failures.[55] Minor complaints—nausea, dyspepsia, anorexia, abdominal pain, flatulence, and diarrhea—affect 10% to 60% of patients. To minimize these symptoms, NSAIDs should be taken with food or milk, except for enteric-coated products, which should *not* be taken with milk or antacids.

All NSAIDs have the potential to cause GI bleeding.[55] Un-ionized NSAIDs enter gastric mucosal cells, release hydrogen ions, and are concentrated ("ion trapped") within cells, with cell death or damage. Gastric mucosal injury can also result from NSAID inhibition of gastroprotective prostaglandins.

The most common sites of GI injury are the gastric and duodenal mucosae.[55] The incidence of gastric ulcers with NSAID use is approximately 11% to 13%, and that for duodenal ulcers is 7% to 10%. Serious GI complications are associated with NSAIDs, including perforations, gastric outlet obstruction, and bleeding. These important GI complications occur in 1.5% to 4% of patients per year. NSAIDs are so widely used that these small percentages translate into substantial morbidity and mortality.[2,55] Moreover, the risk increases to 9% per year for patients with the risk factors of advanced age, history of peptic ulcer or GI bleeding, or cardiovascular disease. Consequently, about 16,500 deaths are associated annually with NSAID use in rheumatoid arthritis or OA patients. A recent review that included a total of 1.3 million patients taking traditional NSAIDS for at least 2 months showed that 1 in 5 developed endoscopically evident ulcers, 1 in 70 had ulcer symptoms, 1 in 150 developed a GI tract perforation, and 1 in 1,200 died.[34]

A key part of the clinician's decision regarding starting NSAID therapy for an OA patient is the patient's risk for GI toxicity. Increased GI risk is seen for those with a history of complicated ulcer (relative risk [RR] 13.5), use of multiple NSAIDs, including aspirin (RR = 9), use of high-dose NSAID (RR = 7), use of anticoagulant (RR = 6.4), age older than 70 years (RR = 5.6), and concomitant use of corticosteroids (RR = 2.2).[34]

For patients taking NSAIDs, there is a poor correlation between GI ulceration and GI symptoms. The American College of Rheumatology recommends a complete blood count yearly to detect a silent bleeding ulcer characterized by an asymptomatic decline in hematocrit.[73] Fecal occult blood is an unreliable predictor of complications.

Medications are available for the treatment or prevention of ulcers in high-risk patients.[2,74] Misoprostol protects against both gastric and duodenal NSAID-induced ulcers, and more importantly, their associated serious GI complications (perforations, gastric outlet obstruction, and bleeding).[74] Unfortunately, misoprostol frequently causes diarrhea and abdominal cramps. Because of its abortifacient properties, misoprostol is contraindicated in pregnancy and in women of childbearing age who are not maintaining adequate contraception. It must be dispensed in its original container, which carries a warning for these individuals. Misoprostol is also available in a combination product with diclofenac, which bears the same restrictions as misoprostol alone.

Other agents have been evaluated in attempts to prevent NSAID-induced gastropathy. Proton pump inhibitors (PPIs) appear to be effective, although neither sucralfate or H_2 antagonists have been shown to be protective. In a recent meta-analysis that included 156 studies, misoprostol, COX-2 selective NSAIDs, and probably PPIs, were judged to significantly reduce the risk of symptomatic ulcers. Further work is required to strengthen the case for PPI's ability to reduce the risk of serious NSAID-induced GI complications. A new randomized, controlled trial has lent weight to this idea by showing that for persons who have experienced a prior GI bleed, the combination of a PPI with celecoxib substantially decreased the risk of future bleeding ulcers compared to celecoxib alone.[75]

At present, use of either a COX-2 selective inhibitor, or an NSAID in combination with either a proton pump inhibitor or misoprostol is recommended for treatment of OA patients who are at high risk for GI complications by OA authorities in the United States, Canada, and Europe.[24,34,45]

Gastrointestinal Effects of COX-2 Selective Inhibitors. Celecoxib, rofecoxib, and all COX-2 selective inhibitors studied to date have demonstrated fewer endoscopically observed ulcers compared to traditional NSAIDs. Such ulcers are relatively common with NSAIDs and are often asymptomatic. Data regarding the rare but serious GI complications of perforation, obstruction, or bleeding are more difficult to obtain as very large numbers of patients are required for such studies.

To evaluate the risk of serious GI complications with celecoxib, Celecoxib Long-term Arthritis Safety Study (CLASS) investigators used celecoxib (400 mg twice daily, or twice the highest FDA-approved dose) compared to diclofenac and ibuprofen at standard dose. Celecoxib use was reported to be associated with a reduced incidence for the combined end point of symptomatic ulcers and ulcer complications (perforations, gastric outlet obstruction, or bleeding) after 6 months.[76] However, this difference was not seen at 1 year and was not seen in patients taking aspirin. Furthermore, there was no reduction in the category of "perforations, gastric outlet obstruction, or bleeding" itself, but only if "symptomatic ulcers" were also included. Concerns have been raised by the FDA, which concluded that although there were trends favoring celecoxib, this drug did not show clear statistical superiority over nonspecific NSAIDs for clinically significant upper GI events.

In celecoxib's favor, its use was associated with decreased outpatient physician claims for upper GI symptoms compared with other prescription nonspecific NSAIDs. Celecoxib was also comparable to a combination of diclofenac and misoprostol in reducing the risk of recurrent GI bleeding in patients who had a prior GI bleed.[77] Celecoxib remains on the market and is an alternative to traditional NSAIDs for those at high risk for GI toxicity.

GI safety for rofecoxib was evaluated in the Vioxx Gastrointestinal Outcomes Research (VIGOR) study, where patients were randomized to receive rofecoxib 50 mg daily or naproxen 500 mg twice daily; use of concomitant aspirin was prohibited. Those randomized to rofecoxib experienced a 50% lower risk of serious GI events.[78] These findings led to its approval by the FDA, but rofecoxib was withdrawn from the worldwide market in 2004 because of increased risk of cardiovascular events, as discussed in Cardiovascular Inhibitors: Traditional NSAIDs section.

Lumiracoxib was evaluated in the Therapeutic Arthritis Research and Gastrointestinal Event Trial (TARGET), in which more than 18,000 patients were randomized to lumiracoxib 400 mg/day compared to naproxen 1,000 mg/day or ibuprofen 2,400 mg/day.[79] With lumiracoxib, there was a significant reduction in the risk of serious GI events (perforation, gastric outlet obstruction, bleeding) compared to naproxen (hazard ratio 0.34 [0.22 to 0.52], $P < 0.0001$ overall; hazard ratio 0.21 [95% confidence interval (CI) 0.12 to 0.37], $P < 0.0001$ in those not taking aspirin). However, in those taking aspirin, there was no difference in risk. Lumiracoxib is currently approved for use in Canada and the United Kingdom and is awaiting FDA approval.

Etoricoxib was evaluated in the Multinational Etoricoxib and Diclofenac Arthritis Long-term Program (MEDAL) study, in which more than 34,000 patients were randomized to etoricoxib 60 to 90 mg/day compared to diclofenac 150 mg/day.[80] With etoricoxib, there was a significant reduction in the risk of *clinical* GI events (perforation, gastric outlet obstruction, ulcers, bleeding) compared to diclofenac (hazard ratio 0.69, 95% CI 0.57 to 0.83; $P = 0.0001$). However, there was no advantage for etoricoxib when complicated GI events alone (perforation, gastric outlet obstruction, bleeding) were evaluated (hazard ratio 0.91, CI 0.67 to 1.24; $P = 0.561$). The interpretation was that there were significantly fewer upper gastrointestinal clinical events with etoricoxib than with diclofenac because of a decrease in uncomplicated events, but not in the more serious complicated events. Although etoricoxib is currently sold in 63 countries in Europe, Latin America, the Asia-Pacific region, and Middle East/North Africa, this drug received an FDA nonapproval letter on May 1, 2007. The FDA indicated further data was necessary to demonstrate a favorable risk-to-benefit ratio.

In summary, there is variable evidence that COX-2 inhibitors pose a decreased risk of GI toxicity compared to nonspecific NSAIDs, an especially important consideration when treating those at risk for clinically significant GI adverse effects. Proof that all COX-2 inhibitors are equally GI safe is lacking; this may reflect intrinsic differences among agents, or be a result of differences in study design, patient population, or concomitant medication use. Trends favor the GI safety of celecoxib, although GI complications were not convincingly decreased compared to traditional NSAIDs. Rofecoxib (since withdrawn) did decrease clinically significant GI complications. Lumiracoxib significantly decreases the risk of serious GI complications, although aspirin negates this advantage. Etoricoxib demonstrated some gastroprotection, but was not proven to decrease the number of serious GI complications (perforation, gastric outlet obstruction, and bleeding).

9 ***Cardiovascular Risk of COX-2 Inhibitors and Traditional NSAIDs.*** In 2004, rofecoxib was withdrawn from the market after analysis of the Adenomatous Polyp Prevention on Vioxx (APPROVe) trial, where rofecoxib appeared to double the risk of cardiovascular events compared to placebo.[81] Further concern about COX-2 selective inhibitors was raised when celecoxib use in the Adenoma Prevention with Celecoxib (APC) trial also increased cardiovascular risk.[82] These observations raised questions about the cardiovascular safety of all COX-2 selective NSAIDs, and even about traditional NSAIDs. These concerns have triggered new FDA regulations and new labeling on all NSAIDs and have prompted meta-analyses of randomized controlled trials of COX-2 selective inhibitors and of NSAIDs.[83] Case control and cohort studies of patients using these agents have also examined cardiovascular risks involved with their use. As of this writing, much remains to be defined about these risks, regarding class effects, effect of dose and duration, and the population studied, but certain trends have taken shape.

The increased cardiovascular risk posed by rofecoxib was clearly demonstrated in the APPROVe trial, and the VIGOR trial also showed this risk.[34] For celecoxib, other data on cardiovascular risk, especially when used at the approved OA dose, is much less certain. The CLASS trial showed a small but not significantly increased risk. As noted above, the APC study did show increased risk, but this was for doses greater than 400 mg daily. The Prevention of Spontaneous Polyps (PreSAP) study, with celecoxib used at 400 mg/day, and the Alzheimer's Disease Antiinflammatory Prevention Trial (ADAPT) study, using 200 mg twice daily, did not show increased cardiovascular risk. More recently, in a meta-analysis of randomized trials including more than 100,000 patients, rofecoxib was shown to increase risk of arrhythmias, relative to placebo and to other NSAIDs, and also in comparison to celecoxib, which did not significantly increase arrhythmias.[84] Taken as a whole, these data suggested that although there might be a "class effect" of coxibs (celecoxib and rofecoxib both posing risk), that this risk existed for rofecoxib at any dose, but to celecoxib when used at higher doses.[34]

The cardiovascular safety of lumiracoxib was evaluated in the Therapeutic Arthritis Research and Gastrointestinal Event Trial (TARGET) study.[85] In this study of more than 18,000 patients, cardiovascular risk showed a nonsignificant increase relative to ibuprofen (but no increase relative to naproxen), and this increase was only seen in those not taking aspirin. One potential drawback to this study is that cardiovascular events were low (59 for lumiracoxib, 50 for ibuprofen). The cardiovascular safety of etoricoxib was evaluated in the MEDAL study.[86] In this study, more than 34,000 subjects were randomly assigned to etoricoxib (60 mg or 90 mg daily) or diclofenac (150 mg daily). Very similar rates for thrombotic cardiovascular events occurred for the etoricoxib group and for the diclofenac group (event rates of 1.24 and 1.30 per 100 patient-years, respectively, with a hazard ratio of 0.95 [95% CI 0.81 to 1.11]) for etoricoxib compared with diclofenac. The number of events in each arm was more than 300, which lends reassurance to the results. Despite these clear results, some investigators have indicated that diclofenac, having some COX-2 selectivity (almost as selective as celecoxib) should not be used as the comparator drug. Ibuprofen or naproxen are nonselective and may be better comparator drugs for determining if a COX-2 selective inhibitor possesses risk relative to nonspecific NSAIDs. Although the TARGET study for lumiracoxib and the MEDAL study for etoricoxib are somewhat reassuring, given the study limitations, further confirmation of their cardiovascular safety would be welcome.

In addition to controlled trials, analysis of cohort or case control studies can also contribute to information about risk, but such studies have confounders and do not necessarily produce consistent findings. Some studies have shown increased risk for coxibs and for nonspecific NSAIDs. Recently, in a systematic review of observational studies of COX-2 inhibitors and traditional NSAIDs, including an approximate 1 million patients, risk for cardiovascular events were calculated in comparison to nonusers or those with remote use of NSAIDs.[87] The summary relative risk was 1.33 (95% CI 1.00 to 1.79) for rofecoxib 25 mg/day, and 2.19 (95% CI 1.64 to 2.91) with more than 25 mg/day, with risk apparent within the first month of treatment. Celecoxib summary relative risk was 1.06 (95% CI 0.91 to 1.23) (but without enough information to dose stratify). Other summary relative risks were also reassuring, with naproxen at 0.97 (95% CI 0.87 to 1.07), piroxicam at 1.06 (95% CI 0.70 to 1.59), and ibuprofen at 1.07 (95% CI 0.97 to 1.18). Diclofenac, however, showed an increased summary relative risk of 1.40 (CI 1.16 to 1.70), which is concerning.[87]

Taken together, the above data, both from controlled trials and from observational studies, confirm the increased cardiovascular risk seen with rofecoxib. Celecoxib 200 mg/day or even 400 mg/day does not appear to increase risk, but cardiovascular risk is likely increased with doses above 400 mg/day. Although studies with lumiracoxib and etoricoxib are somewhat reassuring and do not point to substantially increased cardiovascular risk, further work is needed on this issue. The balance of the evidence also suggests that, for the traditional NSAIDs which have been examined, with the exception of diclofenac, there is no significant or substantial increase in risk.[6]

CLINICAL CONTROVERSY

Controversy has arisen regarding both the gastroprotective effects of COX-2 selective inhibitors and the cardiovascular risk they may pose. Are all COX-2 selective inhibitors GI protective? Do they all pose cardiovascular risk? Is there a relationship between these two features for different coxibs? Although both rofecoxib and celecoxib are COX-2 selective inhibitors, rofecoxib demonstrated more robust reduction in GI complications. However, rofecoxib posed *greater* cardiovascular risk than celecoxib.

These differences may depend on the degree of selectivity of specific COX-2 inhibitors for COX-2 versus COX-1 enzymes. COX-2 selectivity is relative: Some traditional NSAIDs, such as diclofenac, possess some COX-2 selectivity, and even among the formally labeled COX-2 inhibitors, COX-2 selectivity varies. Interestingly, rofecoxib is more COX-2 selective than celecoxib. It is possible that rofecoxib's greater selectivity is responsible both for better GI protection *and* for increased cardiovascular risk. Such a connection is plausible, given the effects of COX-1 and COX-2 enzymes on the formation of thromboxane A_2 and prostacyclin. A highly selective COX-2 inhibitor may tilt the balance in favor of thromboxane A_2, thus promoting platelet aggregation (beneficial for preventing GI bleeds, but posing a prothrombotic risk to the cardiovascular system).

Several other COX-2 selective inhibitors are in development, and two key issues will be their degree of gastroprotection and what, if any, cardiovascular risk they pose. Further study will be needed to determine if one or more of these agents will be safe for the cardiovascular system and also gastroprotective, or whether the degree of gastroprotection is inextricably linked to the extent of cardiovascular risk for all COX-2 selective inhibitors.

Considerations for Patients at Risk for Both GI and Cardiovascular Events. For those without increased GI or cardiovascular risk, a nonspecific NSAID is reasonable. For patients with elevated GI risk or cardiovascular risk who need treatment with an NSAID, careful consideration of risk and benefit is warranted.[34] Recommendations for those with increased GI risk but not on aspirin include consideration of a COX-2 selective inhibitor or a traditional NSAID taken with a PPI. For those taking regular low-dose aspirin for cardiovascular risk (with or without increased GI risk), a traditional NSAID taken with a PPI, or a COX-2 selective inhibitor taken with a PPI can be considered. Given the current concerns regarding cardiovascular risk with COX-2 selective inhibitors or possibly any NSAIDs, and continuing concern about GI events, treatment with the lowest dose possible for the shortest duration possible is warranted.

⑩ ***Other Toxicities Associated with NSAIDs.*** NSAIDs may cause kidney diseases, including acute renal insufficiency, tubulointerstitial nephropathy, hyperkalemia, and renal papillary necrosis.[88] Clinical features of these NSAID-induced renal syndromes include increased serum creatinine and blood urea nitrogen, hyperkalemia, elevated blood pressure, peripheral edema, and weight gain. Mechanisms of NSAID injury include direct toxicity, and inhibition of local prostaglandins that promote vasodilation of renal blood vessels and preserve renal blood flow. Patients at high risk are those with conditions associated with decreased renal blood flow or taking certain medications. Examples are those with chronic renal insufficiency, congestive heart failure, severe hepatic disease, nephrotic syndrome, advanced age, or taking diuretics, angiotensin-converting enzyme inhibitors, cyclosporine, or aminoglycosides (Fig. 95–7).

Close monitoring is advisable for high-risk patients taking an NSAID, with monitoring of serum creatinine at baseline and within 3 to 7 days of drug initiation. For those with impaired renal function, the National Kidney Foundation recommends acetaminophen as the drug of choice.[49]

Coxibs can also pose renal risks, and there is neither evidence nor rationale why this class of drugs would be safer than nonspecific NSAIDs. In a meta-analysis of randomized trials of NSAIDs including more than 100,000 patients, rofecoxib was shown to significantly increase risk of renal toxicity in comparison to placebo, celecoxib, and nonspecific NSAIDs.[84] Although rofecoxib is now off the market, this study provides an important caution as new coxibs are approved: renal safety of coxibs may differ substantially. Keeping in mind that many OA patients may not be as healthy as trial participants, it is prudent to prescribe all coxibs and other NSAIDs with caution in patients who are at increased risk for renal dysfunction.[89]

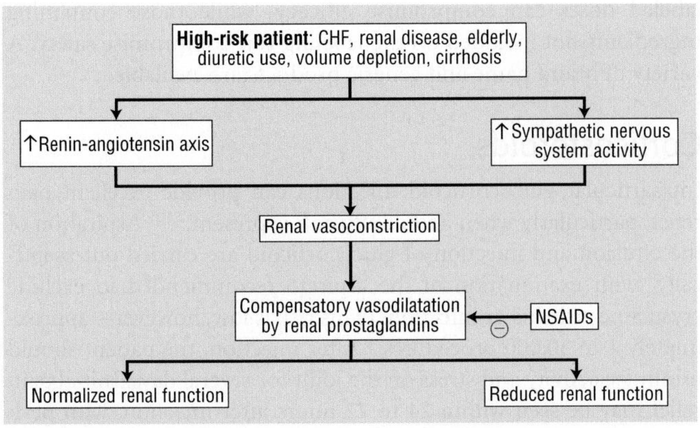

FIGURE 95-7. Mechanisms implicated in NSAID-induced renal injury. The minus (–) sign indicates inhibitory influence. (CHF, congestive heart failure; NSAIDs, nonsteroidal antiinflammatory drugs.)

Coxibs and NSAIDs uncommonly cause drug-induced hepatitis; the two NSAIDs most frequently implicated are diclofenac and sulindac. Patient monitoring should include periodic liver enzymes (aspartate aminotransferase and alanine aminotransferase), with cessation of therapy if these values exceed two to three times the normal range.

Other toxic effects of NSAIDs include hypersensitivity reactions, rash, and central nervous system complaints of drowsiness, dizziness, headaches, depression, confusion, and tinnitus.[47] Although NSAIDs are generally avoided in patients with asthma who are aspirin-intolerant, studies indicate that celecoxib is well tolerated in aspirin-sensitive asthma, providing a viable option for these patients.[90] Celecoxib is a sulfonamide and is thus contraindicated for those with sulfa allergies. However, some patients with sulfa allergies have shown no reaction to celecoxib, and in a meta-analysis including more than 11,000 patients, allergic reactions for those who did have sulfonamide allergies were similar in those taking celecoxib compared to those taking other NSAIDs.[91]

All nonspecific NSAIDs inhibit COX-1–dependent thromboxane production in platelets and thus increase bleeding risk. Importantly, aspirin inhibition is irreversible, and bleeding time requires 5 to 7 days to normalize after cessation of therapy, as new platelets enter the circulation. Other nonspecific NSAIDs inhibit thromboxane formation reversibly, with normalization of platelet function 1 to 3 days after the drug is stopped. The nonacetylated salicylate products and nabumetone, which have partial COX-2 selectivity, may be preferable to nonspecific NSAIDs.[47] COX-2 selective inhibitors do not block thromboxane synthesis and should pose even less bleeding risk. However, because warfarin and celecoxib are metabolized by the cytochrome P450 isoenzyme CYP2C9, patients receiving warfarin and COX-2 inhibitors should be followed closely.

Finally, NSAIDs should be used only with great caution and only if definitely necessary during pregnancy because of the risk to the fetus posed by the bleeding problems. In late pregnancy, all NSAIDs should be avoided because they may enhance premature closure of the ductus arteriosus. NSAIDs have a pregnancy risk factor of C/D (third trimester). Aspirin is also listed as C/D (D in third trimester if used at full dose). Acetaminophen has a pregnancy risk factor of B.

Drug–Drug and Drug–Food Interactions Important drug interactions with NSAIDs can be pharmacokinetic or pharmacodynamic in origin and have been reviewed.[47,92] The most potentially serious interactions include the use of NSAIDs with lithium, warfarin, oral hypoglycemics, high-dose methotrexate, antihypertensives, angiotensin-converting enzyme inhibitors, β-blockers, and diuretics. Anticipation and careful monitoring often can prevent serious events when these drugs are used together.

Another recent drug interaction has been noted for those taking some NSAIDs and cardioprotective doses of aspirin. Ibuprofen, used at doses of 400 mg or more, may block aspirin's antiplatelet effect if it is taken prior to aspirin. Patients are advised to take a single dose of ibuprofen at least 30 minutes after taking aspirin, or they should take their aspirin at least 8 hours after taking ibuprofen.[93] It is possible that other nonselective NSAIDs, such as naproxen, also may cause such interactions. Acetaminophen does not appear to interfere with the antiplatelet effect of aspirin.

Specific drug interactions are also seen with coxibs. Celecoxib metabolism is primarily via CYP2C9.[92] In clinical studies, increased celecoxib levels were seen with fluconazole administration. Cytochrome P450 inducers such as rifampin, carbamazepine, and phenytoin have the potential to reduce celecoxib levels. However, no clinically significant interactions have been documented with celecoxib and methotrexate, glyburide, ketoconazole, phenytoin, or tolbutamide. Because celecoxib inhibits CYP2D6, it has the potential to increase concentrations of a variety of agents, including antidepressants. Celecoxib increases lithium levels, as do other NSAIDs, thus caution is needed when using coxibs or NSAIDs with lithium.

Dosing and Administration Administration of NSAIDs must be tailored to the individual patient with OA. For the OA patient who has failed an adequate trial of acetaminophen, trial with an NSAID is warranted, if no contraindications exist. Selection of an NSAID depends on the prescriber's experience, medication cost, patient preference, allergies, toxicities, and adherence issues. Individual patient response differs among NSAIDs (see Table 95–2), so if an inadequate response is obtained with one NSAID, another NSAID may yet provide benefit.[2,47,54]

Topical Therapies

⓫ Topical products can be used alone or in combination with oral analgesics or NSAIDs. Capsaicin, isolated from hot peppers, releases and ultimately depletes substance P from afferent nociceptive nerve fibers. Substance P has been implicated in the transmission of pain in arthritis, and capsaicin cream has been shown in four placebo-controlled studies to provide pain relief in OA when applied over affected joints.[2,94] Data comparing topical capsaicin to other effective pharmacologic treatments for OA is lacking.

Adverse events associated with capsaicin are primarily local, with 1 in 3 patients experiencing burning, stinging, and/or erythema that usually subsides with repeated application. Some patients may experience coughing associated with application. Capsaicin is a nonprescription product available as a cream, gel, or lotion in concentrations ranging from 0.025% to 0.075%.

To be effective, capsaicin must be used regularly, and it may take up to 2 weeks to take effect. Although use is recommended four times a day, a twice-daily application may enhance long-term adherence and still provide adequate pain relief.[94] Patients should be warned not to get the cream in their eyes or mouth and to wash their hands after application. When patients were queried using an electronic questionnaire that considered possible toxicities of treatments, as well as route of administration and cost, capsaicin was the most preferred by patients, even when it was portrayed as being less effective than NSAIDs.[48]

Topical diclofenac in a dimethyl sulfoxide (DMSO) carrier (Pennsaid) is a safe and effective treatment for pain associated with OA.[95] Pennsaid is available in Canada and other European countries and is currently under review at the FDA. The mechanism of action of topical NSAIDs is thought to be primarily by local inhibition of COX-2 enzymes. This mode of delivery minimizes systemic exposure and may decrease the risk of the serious adverse events associated with oral NSAIDs.

Although not well studied in a controlled setting, the use of topical rubefacients, containing methylsalicylate, trolamine salicylate, and other salicylates, may have modest, short-term efficacy in the treatment of acute pain associated with musculoskeletal conditions, including OA.[96] These agents act by providing topical counterirritation to the affected joint area, rather than by local inhibition of COX-2 enzymes. Chronic OA pain may respond less favorably than acute pain. Clinically significant adverse events are local skin reactions that occur rarely. There are no reports of systemic toxicity associated with topical rubefacients.

Glucosamine and Chondroitin

Interest in chondroitin and glucosamine was spurred initially by anecdotal reports of benefit in animals and humans, and by the ability of these substances to stimulate proteoglycan synthesis from articular cartilage in vitro. The excellent safety profile of these agents makes them especially appealing for use in those at high risk for adverse events, such as elderly patients, and in those with multiple morbidities. Recently, enthusiasm for these agents has waned somewhat as additional efficacy data has become available.[97–99]

A meta-analysis of glucosamine and chondroitin had indicated that both agents had efficacy in reducing pain and improving mobility, and that glucosamine reduced joint space narrowing.[98] Use of glucosamine or chondroitin sulfate was associated with slower loss of cartilage than placebo in knees of OA patients.[100] Further support for the objective benefits of these compounds was seen in a followup survey carried out 5 years after completion of a 3-year study comparing glucosamine and placebo. This survey showed that rates of lower limb joint replacement were twofold higher in subjects given placebo, compared with subjects given glucosamine. In addition, subjects treated with glucosamine had lower rates of pain, joint space narrowing, and limitations of physical function.[99]

In contrast to earlier reports, a recent large, well-controlled National Institutes of Health-sponsored study demonstrated no significant clinical response to glucosamine therapy alone, chondroitin therapy alone, or combination glucosamine–chondroitin therapy when compared to placebo across all patients.[97] In subgroup analyses, however, patients with moderate to severe knee pain showed a response to combination glucosamine–chondroitin therapy superior to placebo. This finding did not reach the predetermined threshold for pain reduction. The safety of the glucosamine and chondroitin therapy was similar to that of placebo.

The exact role of glucosamine, chondroitin, or a combination of the two products is still unclear. Because of the relative safety of these agents, a trial of glucosamine–chondroitin may be reasonable in patients considering alternatives to traditional OA treatments. Dosing should be at least 1,500 mg/day of glucosamine and 1,200 mg/day of chondroitin. The glucosamine component should be the sulfate salt rather than the hydrochloride salt, as nearly all positive efficacy studies used the better-absorbed sulfate salt. Glucosamine-related adverse events are generally mild and include gastrointestinal symptoms (gas, bloating, cramps). If made from shellfish, however, glucosamine should not be used in patients with shellfish allergies. The initial concerns regarding glucosamine-induced hyperglycemia had likely been overstated as later safety data in both healthy subjects and those with type 2 diabetes mellitus did not show significant elevations in blood glucose. Chondroitin is extremely well tolerated with the most common adverse effect being nausea. Depending on the source of chondroitin (cattle, pig, or shark), this compound could also pose risk to persons who are allergic to shark.

Because glucosamine and chondroitin are marketed in the United States as dietary supplements, neither the products nor their purity is adequately regulated by the FDA. The potential consequences related to the lack of regulatory oversight for these products can affect both efficacy and safety. Products containing less-than-labeled doses can compromise efficacy, while those containing ingredients not included on the labeling can compromise safety. A variety of brand name and generic products are available.

Corticosteroids

Intraarticular glucocorticoid injections can provide excellent pain relief, particularly when a joint effusion is present.[2,101] Aspiration of the effusion and injection of glucocorticoid are carried out aseptically, with examination of the aspirate recommended to exclude crystalline arthritis or infection. (This risk is low, however—approximately 1 in 50,000 procedures.) After injection, the patient should minimize activity and stress on the joint for several days. Initial pain relief may be seen within 24 to 72 hours after injection, with peak pain relief about 1 week after injection and lasting up to 4 to 8 weeks.

Several randomized, placebo-controlled, double-blind studies have shown that intraarticular corticosteroids are superior to placebo in alleviating knee pain and stiffness caused by OA.[101] The branched esters of triamcinolone and methylprednisolone are preferred by practitioners because of the reduced solubility that allows the agents to remain in the joint space longer. There is no evidence of a clinically superior corticosteroid for intraarticular use, with equipotent doses of methylprednisolone acetate and triamcinolone hexacetonide having similar efficacy.[102] Average doses for injection of large joints in adults are 10 to 20 mg of triamcinolone hexacetonide or 20 to 40 mg of methylprednisolone acetate. The therapy is generally limited to three or four injections per year because of the potential systemic effects of steroids, and because the need for more frequent injections indicates little response to the therapy.

Adverse events associated with intraarticular injection of corticosteroids can be local or systemic in nature. Systemic adverse events are the same as with any other systemic corticosteroid and can include hyperglycemia, edema, elevated blood pressure, dyspepsia, and, rarely, adrenal suppression with continuous, repeated injections. Local adverse effects can include infection in the affected joint, osteonecrosis, tendon rupture, and skin atrophy at the injection site. It has long been thought that intraarticular corticosteroids can hasten cartilage loss, but the potential risk of cartilage destruction with steroid injections has not been substantiated. The rate of cartilage loss tends to be similar between treated and control groups.

Systemic corticosteroid therapy is not recommended in OA, given the lack of proven benefit and the well-known adverse effects with long-term use.

Hyaluronate Injections

Agents containing hyaluronic acid (HA; sodium hyaluronate) are available for intraarticular injection for treatment of knee OA.[103,104] High-molecular-weight HA is an important constituent of synovial fluid. Endogenous HA may also have antiinflammatory effects. Because the concentration and molecular size of synovial HA decrease in OA, administration of exogenous HA products has been studied, with the theory that this could reconstitute synovial fluid and reduce symptoms. In fact, HA injections temporarily and modestly increase viscosity. Although HA injections were reported to decrease pain, most studies were short-term and poorly controlled, and placebo injections also reduced OA pain dramatically. A study of patients who received two series of injections of HA demonstrated efficacy for 27 weeks after the first series of injections.[103]

HA products are injected once weekly for either 3 or 5 weeks, depending on the specific agent administered. There are four commercially available preparations, Hyalgan (20 mg sodium hylaronate/2 mL), Supartz (25 mg sodium hylaronate/2.5 mL), (16 mg hylan polymers/2 mL), and Orthovisc (30 mg hyaluronan/2 mL). Hyalgan and Supartz are administered weekly for five injections, whereas Synvisc and Orthovisc are administered weekly for three injections.

One study has demonstrated that a series of three injections of Hyalgan was as effective as a longer series of six injections.[103] Injections are well tolerated, although acute joint swelling and local skin reactions, including rash, ecchymoses, and pruritus have been reported.

HA injections may be beneficial for patients with knee OA unresponsive to other therapies. These agents are expensive because the treatment includes both drug costs and administration costs. As a result, HA injections are often used after less-expensive therapies have demonstrated a lack of efficacy.

Opioid Analgesics

Low-dose opioid analgesics can be useful in patients who experience no relief with acetaminophen, NSAIDs, intraarticular injections, or topical therapy. These agents are particularly useful in patients who cannot take NSAIDs because of renal failure, and for patients in whom all other treatment options have failed and who are at high surgical risk, precluding joint arthroplasty. Low-dose opioids are the initial intervention, usually given in combination with acetaminophen.

Sustained-release compounds usually offer better pain control throughout the day, and are used when simple opioids are ineffective. A recent randomized, double-blind, placebo-controlled study showed that extended-release oxycodone (20 to 120 mg twice daily) was superior to placebo in reducing pain and improving both function and quality of life, although a high number of patients (36%) did not complete the study as a consequence of adverse events.[105] Nearly all (93%) patients in the oxycodone group experienced a typical opioid-related (nausea, somnolence, constipation, and dizziness) adverse event in this 90-day study. Although this is not an unexpected finding, it serves as a reminder to use opioids cautiously in elderly patients who may be more susceptible to adverse effects.

If pain is intolerable and limits activities of daily living, and the patient has sufficiently good cardiopulmonary health to undergo major surgery, joint replacement may be preferable to continued reliance on opioids.

Tramadol

Tramadol, with or without acetaminophen has modest analgesic effects in patients with OA when compared to placebo.[106] Tramadol is also modestly effective as add-on therapy in patients taking concomitant NSAIDs or COX-2 selective inhibitors.[107] As with opioid analgesics, tramadol may be helpful for patients who cannot take NSAIDs or COX-2 selective inhibitors. Tramadol should be initiated at a lower dose (100 mg per day) and may be titrated as needed for pain control to a dose of 200 mg per day. Tramadol is available in a combination tablet with acetaminophen and as a sustained-release tablet.

Opioid-like adverse effects such as nausea, vomiting, dizziness, constipation, headache, and somnolence are common with tramadol. These occur in 60% to 70% of treated patients, and 40% discontinue tramadol because of an adverse effect.[106] Although the frequency of adverse effects is high, the severity of adverse effects is less than with NSAIDs, as tramadol use is not associated with life-threatening gastrointestinal bleeding or with renal failure.

Novel Therapies and Disease-Modifying Drugs

Disease-modifying drugs are targeted not at pain relief but at preventing, retarding, or reversing damage to articular cartilage. Thus far, OA is a progressive disease that can only be treated symptomatically. Because of this, clinicians were very interested in the possible ability of chondroitin and/or glucosamine to slow joint damage, although those findings require further study (see Glucosamine and Chondroitin above).

New approaches to slow progression of OA are being investigated, but most products have been tested in animal models, and limited human data are available. One approach involves pharmacologic agents that could mimic tissue inhibitors of metalloproteinases and thus potentially decrease cartilage destruction. Some studies have explored the use of tetracycline or doxycycline, which appear to inhibit metalloproteinases.[108] In knee OA, doxycycline has been seen to delay loss of articular cartilage (joint space narrowing) in humans when compared with placebo.[109] Other agents that act as inhibitors of metalloproteinase gene expression, are also under consideration in developing drugs to inhibit joint damage in OA.[21]

Another agent being studied is diacerein, an interleukin-1β inhibitor. In a meta-analysis including a total of 2,069 OA patients, this agent decreased pain to a modest but statistically significant extent compared to placebo. In long-term studies, diacerein appeared to show a significant slowing of progression of joint space narrowing at the hip, but not at the knee.[110]

Aside from agents that may prevent disease progression, attempts to find new agents or methods to treat symptoms of OA are being made. There is recent interest in the potential of cyclooxygenase-inhibiting nitric oxide-donor compounds to relieve OA pain while sparing GI adverse effects. There are two lipid-based nontraditional therapies that have received some attention for treatment of symptoms related to OA; avocado/soy unsaponifiables and fish oil (particularly n-3 PUFA). Several short-term studies have demonstrated that the use of avocado/soy unsaponifiables at a dose of 300 mg to 600 mg daily led to decreases in the use of NSAIDS for pain control, but one long-term (2 years) study failed to replicate these results.[111] It is theorized that the oily fractions of avocado unsaponifiables decrease production of nitric oxide and stimulate production of plasminogen activator inhibitor-1 that can decrease MMPs. The n-3 PUFA fractions of fish oils have been shown to decrease proinflammatory cytokines, MMPs, and tumor necrosis factor-α in vitro. The administration of 1.6 to 3.2 g per day of eicosapentaenoic acid is an effective adjunct to the treatment of rheumatoid arthritis.[112] The role of n-3 PUFAs in the symptomatic treatment of OA is less-well defined, possibly owing to the differences in the pathophysiology between the two types of arthritis.

In addition to pharmacologic agents, acupuncture has been examined in OA. In a systematic analysis of 18 randomized, controlled trials of manual or electroacupuncture, 10 showed positive effects for acupuncture.[113] However, in a recent, large, randomized, and well-controlled study, acupuncture was not seen to be any more effective than sham controls.[114]

CLINICAL CONTROVERSY

The role of herbal and supplement therapies in the treatment of OA is a source of continuing controversy. A variety of herbal therapies, including ginger, devil's claw, methylsulfonylmethane, flavonoids, willow bark, green tea polyphenols, bromelain, hyperimmune milk, and *Boswellia serrata* are purported to have efficacy in the treatment of pain associated with OA. Many patients encounter advertising and other publications in the lay press extolling the benefits of these products. Unfortunately, the lack of scientific trials evaluating these agents makes it difficult to determine their role in therapy. Key questions to be answered before recommendations about the safe use of these agents include the following: (a) Do these agents provide pain relief to a greater degree than placebo? (b) Are there safety issues? (c) Is the manufacturing process reliable? (d) Is it important to know the pharmacology, pharmacodynamics, and pharmacokinetics of these agents? Until additional efficacy and safety information becomes available, recommendations regarding the routine use of these products should be tempered by known drug safety data (if available) and other related safety issues, including costs of therapy, delays in seeking known, effective treatments, and potential exposure to products produced without standard manufacturing processes.

PHARMACOECONOMIC CONSIDERATIONS

There are substantial economic ramifications with OA, as the disease is extremely common, and OA ranks second in causes of disability in the United States.[2–4]

One of the highest costs associated with OA is hospitalization for joint replacement or for treatment of NSAID-related complications, particularly serious GI adverse events. To provide perspective on patient care costs for GI complications of NSAIDs, one study on more than 10,000 OA patients followed in a managed care setting showed that the mean annual cost of care per patient was $543, with hospital costs accounting for 46%, medications 32%, and ambulatory care 22%.[115] Consequently, intense focus has emerged on the cost-to-benefit ratio of medications to prevent ulcer complications, and the use of coxibs, which cause fewer ulcer complications.

For example, analysis of the cost-effectiveness of using NSAIDS or COX-2 selective inhibitors with or without concomitant PPI therapy in both high-risk and low-risk patients was reported, based on estimates of the risk of GI complications in these settings.[116] The cost of avoiding one serious GI complication would be $61,933 if all NSAID patients were given a PPI, but only $4,355 if PPIs were limited to high-risk patients. In the same analysis, the cost of avoiding one serious GI complication would be $62,467 if all NSAID patients were given a COX-2 selective inhibitor. The cost-effectiveness of an NSAID plus a PPI in high-risk patients has been demonstrated by others as well.[117] Gastroprotective therapy or the use of COX-2 selective inhibitors in low-risk patients is not cost-effective because of the large number needed to treat to prevent serious events. Additionally, the use of COX-2 selective inhibitors to protect gastric mucosa in aspirin users is not cost-effective, because aspirin negates most, if not all, of the gastroprotective effects of these agents.[116,117]

Pharmacoeconomic considerations for OA involve the selection of therapy for the initial treatment of patients with OA. Use of the nonprescription analgesic acetaminophen as initial therapy has greatly reduced medication costs in comparison with the use of NSAIDs, many of which are by prescription only. NSAID costs range from $20 to $120 per month, depending on the medication, daily dose, and regimen selected. As NSAIDs as a class are therapeutically similar, use of less-expensive NSAIDs, such as nonprescription ibuprofen or naproxen, may minimize the cost of medicine to the patient. More expensive NSAIDs can be prescribed if neither of these offers benefit after a 2-week trial at sufficient doses.

Nearly all elderly patients are eligible for prescription drug coverage through Medicare Part D insurance programs to assist with the costs of prescription medications for the treatment of OA. The use of nonformulary or noncovered medications can significantly reduce potential cost-savings to the patient. Careful attention to selection of appropriately covered medications will increase the affordability of medication for patients receiving drug therapy for OA.

EVALUATION OF THERAPEUTIC OUTCOMES

Pharmacotherapy monitoring in OA is patient-specific. It should be guided by aspects of disease that are most troubling to the patient, such as pain or decreased function, as well as the patient's risk of adverse effects. To monitor efficacy, the patient's baseline pain can be assessed with a visual analog scale, and range of motion for affected joints can be assessed, providing baseline measures to monitor the success of therapy. Baseline radiographs are helpful to document the extent of joint involvement and follow progression of disease with therapy. Additional tests of OA severity may include measurement of grip strength, 50-foot walking time, patient and physician global assessment of OA severity, and the Western Ontario and McMaster Universities Arthrosis Index or Stanford Health Assessment Questionnaire to monitor ability to perform activities of daily living. A decrease in the use of analgesics or NSAIDs would suggest a beneficial effect of nonpharmacologic interventions. Lastly, disease-specific quality of life is valuable in assessing clinical response to interventions.

Adverse events with acetaminophen are uncommon but are more problematic with NSAIDs, and avoiding toxicity requires individual attention. Each patient's GI, cardiovascular, renal, and other risks, as well as age and comorbidities, should be assessed. When assessing toxicity of therapy, patients should be asked first if they are having any "problems" with their medications. This open-ended question can be followed with more direct questions relating to the most common adverse effects associated with the respective medication. Symptoms of abdominal pain, heartburn, nausea, or change in stool color provide valuable clues to the presence of GI complications, although serious GI complications can occur without warning. Patients also should be monitored for the development of hypertension, weight gain, edema, skin rash, and central nervous system adverse effects such as headaches and drowsiness. Baseline serum creatinine, complete blood count, and serum transaminases are repeated at 6- to 12-month intervals to identify GI, renal, hepatic, and hematologic toxicities.

For patients receiving intraarticular corticosteroids, improvement should begin with 2 to 3 days and last 4 to 8 weeks. Patients should be advised about possible injection site reactions, as well as possible systemic effects, especially for those with hypertension or diabetes, as there is a potential for increased blood pressure or blood glucose (more likely for higher doses given more frequently). For patients receiving intraarticular hyaluronic acid, improvement can begin within 3 to 4 weeks and can last several months, and patients should be advised about possible injection-site reactions and allergic reactions. For patients receiving opioids or tramadol, relief from pain is expected to occur rapidly. Patients, especially if frail or elderly, should be monitored carefully and cautioned about sedation, dysphoria, nausea, risk of falls, constipation, and development of tolerance.

CONCLUSIONS

OA is a very common, slowly progressive disorder that affects diarthrodial joints and is characterized by progressive deterioration of articular cartilage, subchondral sclerosis, and osteophyte production. Clinical manifestations include gradual onset of joint pain, stiffness, and limitation of motion. The primary treatment goals are to reduce pain, maintain function, and prevent further destruction. An individualized approach based on education, rest, exercise, weight loss as needed, and analgesic medication can succeed in meeting these goals. Recommended drug treatment starts with acetaminophen ≤4 g/day and topical analgesics as needed. If acetaminophen is ineffective, NSAIDs may be used, often providing satisfactory relief of pain and stiffness. Individuals at increased risk for toxicity from NSAIDs, especially for GI, cardiovascular, or renal events, deserve special attention. Coxibs may have advantages in some OA patients, but their safety relative to other NSAIDS and their role in OA remain in a state of flux. Glucosamine–chondroitin may be useful in moderate to severe arthritis and is safe. Experimental therapy aimed at preventing the progression of OA requires further clinical investigation before entering widespread clinical use.

ABBREVIATIONS

APC: Adenoma Prevention with Celecoxib

APPROVe: Adenomatous Polyp Prevention on VIOXX

CLASS: Celecoxib Long-term Arthritis Safety Study

COX: cyclooxygenase

HA: hyaluronic acid

MEDAL: Multinational Etoricoxib and Diclofenac Arthritis Long-term Program

MMP: matrix metalloproteinase

NSAID: nonsteroidal antiinflammatory drug

OA: osteoarthritis

TARGET: Therapeutic Arthritis Research and Gastrointestinal Event Trial

VIGOR: Vioxx Gastrointestinal Outcomes Research Study

REFERENCES

1. Sharma L, Kapoor D. Epidemiology of osteoarthritis. In: Moscowitz RW, Altman, RD, Hochberg MC, Buckwalter JA, Goldberg VM, eds. Osteoarthritis: Diagnosis and Medical/Surgical Management, 4th ed. Philadelphia: Lippincott, Williams, & Wilkins, 2007:3–26.
2. ACR Subcommittee on Osteoarthritis Guidelines. Recommendations for the medical management of osteoarthritis of the hip and knee: 2000 update. Arthritis Rheum 2000;43:1905–1915.
3. Solomon L. Clinical features of osteoarthritis. In: Kelly WN, Harris ED, Ruddy S, Sledge CB, eds. Textbook of Rheumatology, 6th ed. Philadelphia: WB Saunders, 2001:1409–1418.
4. Felson DT, Lawrence RC, Dieppe PA, Hirsch R, et al. Osteoarthritis: New insights. Part 1: The disease and its risk factors. Ann Intern Med 2000;133:635–646.
5. Hootman JM, Helmick CG. Projections of U.S. prevalence of arthritis and associated activity limitations. Arthritis Rheum 2006;54:226–229.
6. Garstang SV, Stitik TP. Osteoarthritis: Epidemiology, risk factors, and pathophysiology. Am J Phys Med Rehabil 2006;85(Suppl):S2–S11.
7. Felson DT. Osteoarthritis of the knee. N Engl J Med 2006;354:841–848.
8. Gelber AC, Hochberg MC, Mead LA, et al. Body mass index in young men and the risk of subsequent knee and hip osteoarthritis. Am J Med 1999;107:542–548.
9. Poole AR, Guilak F, Abramson SB. Etiopathogenesis of osteoarthritis. In: Moscowitz RW, Altman, RD, Hochberg MC, Buckwalter JA, Goldberg VM, eds. Osteoarthritis: Diagnosis and Medical/Surgical Management, 4th ed. Philadelphia: Lippincott, Williams, & Wilkins, 2007:27–50.
10. Schouten JS, de Bie RA, Swaen G. An update on the relationship between occupational factors and osteoarthritis of the hip and knee. Curr Opin Rheumatol 2002;14:89–92.
11. McAlindon TE, Wilson PWF, Aliabadi P, et al. Level of physical activity and the risk of radiographic and symptomatic knee osteoarthritis in the elderly: The Framingham study. Am J Med 1999;106:151–157.
12. Lane NE, Oehlert JW, Bloch DA, Fries JF. The relationship of running to osteoarthritis of the knee and hip and bone mineral density of the lumbar spine: A 9-year longitudinal study. J Rheumatol 1998;25:334–341.
13. Gelber AC, Hochberg MC, Mead LA, et al. Joint injury in young adults and risk for subsequent knee and hip osteoarthritis. Ann Intern Med 2000;133:321–328.
14. Hurley MV. The role of muscle weakness in the pathogenesis of osteoarthritis. Rheum Dis Clin North Am 1999;25:283–298.
15. Sun BH, Christopher WW, Kalunian KC. New Developments in Osteoarthritis. Rheum Dis Clin North Am 2007;33:135–148.
16. Loughlin J, Chapman K. Molecular genetics of osteoarthritis. In: Moscowitz RW, Altman, RD, Hochberg MC, Buckwalter JA, Goldberg VM, eds. Osteoarthritis: Diagnosis and Medical/Surgical Management, 4th ed. Philadelphia: Lippincott, Williams, & Wilkins, 2007:127–136.
17. Mankin HJ, Brandt KD. Pathogenesis of osteoarthritis. In: Kelly WN, Harris ED, Ruddy S, Sledge CB, eds. Textbook of Rheumatology, 6th ed. Philadelphia: WB Saunders, 2001:1391–1408.
18. Lajeunesse D, Reboul P. Subchondral bone in osteoarthritis: A biologic link with articular cartilage leading to abnormal remodeling. Curr Opin Rheumatol 2003;15:628–633.
19. Freemont AJ, Byers RJ, Taiwo YO, et al. In situ zymographic localisation of type II collagen degrading activity in osteoarthritic human articular cartilage. Ann Rheum Dis 1999;58:357–365.
20. Sandell LJ, Heinegard D, Hering TH. Cell biology, biochemistry, and molecular biology of articular cartilage in osteoarthritis. In: Moscowitz RW, Altman, RD, Hochberg MC, Buckwalter JA, Goldberg VM, eds. Osteoarthritis: Diagnosis and Medical/Surgical Management, 4th ed. Philadelphia: Lippincott, Williams, & Wilkins, 2007:73–106.
21. *http://www.engineershandbook.com/Tables/frictioncoefficients.htm.*
22. Mix KS, Sporn MB, Brinckerhoff CE, et al. Novel inhibitors of matrix metalloproteinase gene expression as potential therapies for arthritis. Clin Orthop Relat Res 2004;427(Suppl):S129–S137.
23. Hayami T, Pickarski M, Zhuo Y, et al. Characterization of articular cartilage and subchondral bone changes in the rat anterior cruciate ligament transection and meniscectomized models of osteoarthritis. Bone 2006;38:234–243.
24. *http://www.rheumatology.org/publications/.*
25. Goldring SR, Goldring MB. The role of cytokines in cartilage matrix degeneration in osteoarthritis. Clin Orthop Relat Res 2004;427(Suppl):S27–S36.
26. Hough AB. Pathology of osteoarthritis. In: Moscowitz RW, Altman, RD, Hochberg MC, Buckwalter JA, Goldberg VM, eds. Osteoarthritis: Diagnosis and Medical/Surgical Management, 4th ed. Philadelphia: Lippincott, Williams, & Wilkins, 2007:51–72.
27. Altman RD. Laboratory findings in osteoarthritis. In: Moscowitz RW, Altman, RD, Hochberg MC, Buckwalter JA, Goldberg VM, eds. Osteoarthritis: Diagnosis and Medical/Surgical Management, 4th ed. Philadelphia: Lippincott, Williams, & Wilkins, 2007:201–214.
28. Dieppe PA, Lohmander LS. Pathogenesis and management of pain in osteoarthritis. Lancet 2005;365:965–973.
29. Chard J, Lohmander S, Smith C, Scott D. Osteoarthritis. Clin Evid 2003;10:1402–1430.
30. Roddy E, Zhang W, Doherty M, et al. Evidence-based recommendations for the role of exercise in the management of osteoarthritis of the hip or knee—The MOVE consensus. Rheumatology (Oxford) 2005;44:67–73.
31. Hunter DJ, Felson DT. Osteoarthritis. BMJ 2006;332:639–642.
32. Juni P, Reichenbach S, Dieppe P. Osteoarthritis: Rational approach to treating the individual. Best Pract Res Clin Rheumatol 2006;20:721–740.
33. Lievense AM, Bierma-Zeinstra SM, Verhagen AP, et al. Influence of obesity on the development of osteoarthritis of the hip: A systematic review. Rheumatology 2002;41:1155–1162.
34. Tannenbaum H, Bombardier C, Davis P, Russell AS. Third Canadian Consensus Conference Group. An evidence-based approach to prescribing nonsteroidal antiinflammatory drugs. Third Canadian Consensus Conference. J Rheumatol 2006;33:140–157.
35. *http://www.arthritis.org/disease-center.php?disease_id=32&df=treatments*
36. Reijman M, Pols HA, Bergink AP, et al. Body mass index associated with onset and progression of osteoarthritis of the knee but not of the hip: The Rotterdam Study. Ann Rheum Dis 2007;66:158–162.
37. Christensen R, Bartels EM, Astrup A, Bliddal H. Effect of weight reduction in obese patients diagnosed with knee osteoarthritis: A systematic review and meta-analysis. Ann Rheum Dis 2007;66:433–439.
38. Messier SP, Loeser RF, Miller GD, et al. Exercise and dietary weight loss in overweight and obese older adults with knee osteoarthritis: The Arthritis, Diet, and Activity Promotion Trial. Arthritis Rheum 2004;50:1501–1510.
39. Fransen M, McConnell S, Bell M. Exercise for osteoarthritis of the hip or knee. Cochrane Database Syst Rev 2003;3:CD004286.
40. National Institutes of Health (NIH) Consensus Development Panel on Total Knee Replacement. National Institutes of Health Consensus Statement on Total Knee Replacement December 8–10. Final Statement. Rockville (MD): U.S. Department of Health and Human Services, 2004.
41. Fitzpatrick R, Shortall E, Sculpher M, et al. Primary total hip replacement surgery: A systematic review of outcomes and modeling of cost-effectiveness associated with different prosthesis. Health Technol Assess 1998; 2:1–64.
42. Kuo CK, Li WJ, Mauck RL, Tuan RS. Cartilage tissue engineering: Its potential and uses. Curr Opin Rheumatol 2006;8:64–73.
43. Towheed TE. Acetaminophen for osteoarthritis. Cochrane Database Syst Rev, 2006;(1):CD004257.
44. Towheed TE, Judd MJ, Hochberg MC, Wells G. Acetaminophen for osteoarthritis. Cochrane Database Syst Rev 2003;2:CD004257.
45. Zhang W, Doherty M, Arden N, et al. EULAR evidence based recommendations for the management of hip osteoarthritis: Report of a task force of the EULAR Standing Committee for International Clinical Studies Including Therapeutics (ESCISIT). Ann Rheum Dis 2005;64:669–681.

46. Jordan K, Arden N, Doherty M, et al. EULAR Recommendations 2003: An evidence based approach to the management of knee osteoarthritis: Report of a Task Force of the Standing Committee for International Clinical Studies Including Therapeutic Trials (ESCISIT). Ann Rheum Dis 2003;62:1145–1155.
47. Pepper GA. Nonsteroidal anti-inflammatory drugs: New perspectives on a familiar drug class. Rheumatology 2000;35:223–244.
48. Fraenkel L, Bogardus ST, Concato J, Wittink DR. Treatment options in knee osteoarthritis: The Patient's Perspective. Arch Intern Med 2004;164:1299–1304.
49. Henrich WL, Agodoa LE, Barrett B, et al. Analgesics and the kidney: Summary recommendations to the Scientific Advisory Board of the National Kidney Foundation from an ad hoc committee of the National Kidney Foundation. Am J Kidney Dis 1996;27:162–165.
50. Watkins PB, Kaplowitz N, Slattery JT, et al. Aminotransferase elevations in healthy adults receiving 4 grams of acetaminophen daily: A randomized controlled trial. JAMA 2006;296:87–93.
51. Larson AM, Polson J, Fontana RJ, et al. Acetaminophen-induced acute liver failure: Results of a United States Multicenter, Prospective Study. Hepatology 2005;42:1364–1372.
52. Forman JP, Stampfer MJ, Curhan GC. Non-narcotic analgesic dose and risk of incident hypertension in U.S. women. Hypertension 2005;46:500–507.
53. Forman JP, Rimm EB, Curhan GC. Frequency of analgesic use and risk of hypertension among men. Arch Intern Med 2007;167:394–399.
54. Eccles M, Freemantle N, Mason J, for the North of England Non-Steroidal Anti-Inflammatory Drug Guideline Development Group. North of England Evidence Based Guideline Development Project: Summary guideline for nonsteroidal anti-inflammatory drugs versus basic analgesia in treating the pain of degenerative arthritis. BMJ 1998;317:526–530.
55. Wolfe MM, Lichenstein DR, Singh G. Medical progress: Gastrointestinal toxicity of nonsteroidal anti-inflammatory drugs. N Engl J Med 1999;340:1888–1899.
56. Crofford LJ, Lipsky PE, Brooks P, et al. Basic biology and clinical application of specific cyclooxygenase-2 inhibitors. Arthritis Rheum 2000;43:4–13.
57. Grosser T, Fries S, FitzGerald GA. Biological basis for the cardiovascular consequences of COX-2 inhibition: Therapeutic challenges and opportunities. J Clin Invest 2006;116:4–15.
58. Lipsky PE, Abramson SB, Breedveld FC, et al. Analysis of the effect of COX-2 specific inhibitors and recommendations for their use in clinical practice. J Rheumatol 2000;27:1338–1340.
59. Grosser T. The pharmacology of selective inhibition of COX-2. Thromb Haemost 2006;96:393–400.
60. Simon LS, Strand V. Perception of risk: The state of COX-2 selective inhibitors. Curr Rheumatol Rep 2005;7:163–166.
61. Wegman A, van der Windt D, van Tulder M, et al. Nonsteroidal antiinflammatory drugs or acetaminophen for osteoarthritis of the hip or knee? A systematic review of evidence and guidelines. J Rheumatol 2004;31:344–354.
62. Towheed T, Shea B, Wells G, et al. Analgesia and nonaspirin, nonsteroidal anti-inflammatory drugs of osteoarthritis of the hip. Cochrane Database Syst Rev. 2000;(2):CD000517.
63. Angst F, Ewert T, Lehmann S, et al. The factor subdimensions of the Western Ontario and McMaster Universities Osteoarthritis Index (WOMAC) help to specify hip and knee osteoarthritis. a prospective evaluation and validation study. J Rheumatol 2005;32:1324–1330.
64. Gibofsky A, Williams GW, McKenna F, Fort JG. Comparing the efficacy of cyclooxygenase 2-specific inhibitors in treating osteoarthritis: Appropriate trial design considerations and results of a randomized, placebo-controlled trial. Arthritis Rheum 2003;48:3102–3111.
65. Lyseng-Williamson KA, Curran MP. Lumiracoxib. Drugs 2004;64:2237–2246; discussion 2247–2248.
66. Fleischmann R, Sheldon E, Maldonado-Cocco J, Lumiracoxib is effective in the treatment of osteoarthritis of the knee: A prospective randomized 13-week study versus placebo and celecoxib. Clin Rheumatol 2006;25:42–53.
67. Berenbaum F, Grifka J, Brown JP, et al. Efficacy of lumiracoxib in osteoarthritis: A review of nine studies. J Int Med Res 2005;33:21–41.
68. Curtis SP, Bockow B, Fisher C, et al. Etoricoxib in the treatment of osteoarthritis over 52-weeks: A double-blind, active-comparator controlled trial [NCT00242489]. BMC Musculoskelet Disord 2005;6:58.
69. Wiesenhutter CW, Boice JA, Ko A, et al. Evaluation of the comparative efficacy of etoricoxib and ibuprofen for treatment of patients with osteoarthritis: A randomized, double-blind, placebo-controlled trial. Mayo Clin Proc 2005;80(4):470–479.
70. Cochrane DJ, Jarvis B, Keating GM. Etoricoxib. Drugs 2002;62:2637–2651.
71. Bingham CO 3rd, Sebba AI, Rubin BR, et al. Efficacy and safety of etoricoxib 30 mg and celecoxib 200 mg in the treatment of osteoarthritis in two identically designed, randomized, placebo-controlled, non-inferiority studies. Rheumatology (Oxford) 2007;46:496–507.
72. Sheldon E, Beaulieu A, Paster Z, et al. Efficacy and tolerability of lumiracoxib in the treatment of osteoarthritis of the knee: A 13-week, randomized, double-blind comparison with celecoxib and placebo. Clin Ther 2005;27:64–77.
73. American College of Rheumatology Ad Hoc Committee on Clinical Guidelines. Guidelines for monitoring drug therapy in rheumatoid arthritis. Arthritis Rheum 1996;39:723–731.
74. Maetzel A, Ferraz MB, Bombardier C. The cost-effectiveness of misoprostol in preventing serious gastrointestinal events associated with the use of nonsteroidal anti-inflammatory drugs. Arthritis Rheum 1998;41:16–25.
75. Chan FKL, Wong VWS, Suen BY, et al. Combination of a cyclooxygenase-2 inhibitor and a proton-pump inhibitor for prevention of recurrent ulcer bleeding in patients at very high risk: A double-blind, randomised trial. Lancet 2007;369:1621–1626.
76. Silverstein FE, Faich G, Goldstein JL, et al. Gastrointestinal toxicity with celecoxib vs nonsteroidal anti-inflammatory drugs for osteoarthritis and rheumatoid arthritis: The CLASS study. A randomized, controlled trial. JAMA 2000;284:1247–1255.
77. Chan FK, Hung LC, Suen BY, et al. Celecoxib versus diclofenac and omeprazole in reducing the risk of recurrent ulcer bleeding in patients with arthritis. N Engl J Med 2002;347:2104–2110.
78. Bombardier C, Laine L, Reicin A, et al. Comparison of upper gastrointestinal toxicity of rofecoxib and naproxen in patients with rheumatoid arthritis. N Engl J Med 2000;343:1520–1528.
79. Schnitzer TJ, Burmester GR, Mysler E, et al. for the TARGET Study Group. Comparison of lumiracoxib with naproxen and ibuprofen in the Therapeutic Arthritis Research and Gastrointestinal Event Trial (TARGET), reduction in ulcer complications: Randomised controlled trial. Lancet 2004;364:665–674.
80. Laine L, Curtis SP, Cryer B, et al. MEDAL Steering Committee. Assessment of upper gastrointestinal safety of etoricoxib and diclofenac in patients with osteoarthritis and rheumatoid arthritis in the Multinational Etoricoxib and Diclofenac Arthritis Long-term (MEDAL) programme: A randomised comparison. Lancet 2007;369:465–473.
81. Bresalier RS, Sandler RS, Quan H, et al. Cardiovascular events associated with rofecoxib in a colorectal adenoma chemoprevention trial. N Engl J Med 2005;352:1092–1102.
82. Solomon SD, McMurray JJ, Pfeffer MA, et al. Cardiovascular risk associated with celecoxib in a clinical trial for colorectal adenoma prevention. N Engl J Med 2005;352:107.
83. *http://www.fda.gov/cder/drug/infopage/COX2/NSAIDdecisionMemo.pdf.*
84. Zhang J, Ding EL, Song T. Adverse effects of cyclooxygenase 2 inhibitors on renal and arrhythmia events. Meta-analysis of randomized trials. JAMA 2006;296:1619–1632.
85. Farkouh ME, Kirshner H, Harrington RA, et al. Comparison of lumiracoxib with naproxen and ibuprofen in the Therapeutic Arthritis Research and Gastrointestinal Event Trial (TARGET), cardiovascular outcomes: Randomised controlled trial. Lancet 2004;364:675–684.
86. Cannon CP, Curtis SP, FitzGerald GA, et al. MEDAL Steering Committee. Cardiovascular outcomes with etoricoxib and diclofenac in patients with osteoarthritis and rheumatoid arthritis in the Multinational Etoricoxib and Diclofenac Arthritis Long-term (MEDAL) programme: A randomised comparison. Lancet 2006;368:1771–1781.
87. McGettigan P, Henry D. Cardiovascular risk and inhibition of cyclooxygenase: A systematic review of the observational studies of selective and nonselective inhibitors of cyclooxygenase 2. JAMA 2006;296:1633–1644.
88. Epstein M. Non-steroidal anti-inflammatory drugs and the continuum of renal dysfunction J Hypertens 2002;20(Suppl):S17–S23.
89. Brader DC. Anti-inflammatory agents and renal function. Semin Arthritis Rheum 2002;32(Suppl):33–42.
90. Martin-Garcia C, Hinjosa M, Berges P, et al. Safety of cyclooxygenase-2 inhibitor in patients with aspirin-sensitive asthma. Chest 2002;121:1812–1817.

91. Patterson R, Bello AE, Lefkowith J. Immunologic tolerability profile of celecoxib. Clin Ther 1999;21:2065–2079.
92. Garnett WR. Clinical implications of drug interactions with coxibs. Pharmacotherapy 2001;21:1223–1232.
93. *http://www.fda.gov/medwatch/safety/2006/safety06.htm#aspirin.*
94. Mason L, Moore RA, Derry S, et al. Systematic review of topical capsaicin for the treatment of chronic pain. BMJ 2004;328:991.
95. Towheed TE. Pennsaid therapy for osteoarthritis of the knee: A systematic review and meta-analysis of randomized controlled trials. J Rheumatol 2006;33:567–573.
96. Mason L, Moore Ra, Edwards JE, et al. Systemic review of efficacy of topical rubefacients containing salicylates for the treatment of acute and chronic pain. BMJ 2004;328:995.
97. Clegg DO, Glucosamine, chondroitin sulfate, and the two in combination for painful knee osteoarthritis. N Engl J Med 2006;354:795–808.
98. Richy F, Bruyere O, Ethgen O, et al. Structural and symptomatic efficacy of glucosamine and chondroitin in knee osteoarthritis: A comprehensive meta-analysis. Arch Intern Med 2003;163:1514–1522.
99. Bruyere O, Compere S, Rovati LC, et al. Five-year follow up of patients from a previous 3-year randomized, controlled trial of glucosamine sulfate in knee osteoarthritis. Arthritis Rheum 2003;48:S80.
100. Reginster JY, Bruyere O, Lecart MP, Henrotin Y. Naturocetic (glucosamine and chondroitin sulfate) compounds as structure-modifying drugs in the treatment of osteoarthritis. Curr Opin Rheumatol 2003;15:651–655.
101. Bellamy N, Intraarticular corticosteroid for treatment of osteoarthritis of the knee. Cochrane Database Syst Rev 2006;(2):CD005328.
102. Pyne D, Ioannou Y, Mootoo R, Bhanji A. Intra-articular steroids in knee osteoarthritis: A comparative study of triamcinolone hexacetonide and methylprednisolone acetate. Clin Rheumatol 2004;23:116–120.
103. Petrella RJ, Petrella M. A prospective, randomized, double-blind, placebo-controlled trial to evaluate the efficacy of intraarticular hyaluronic acid in osteoarthritis of the knee. J Rheumatol 2006:33:951–956.
104. Bellamy N, Viscosupplementation for the treatment of osteoarthritis of the knee. Cochrane Database Syst Rev 2006;(2):CD005321.
105. Markenson JA, Croft J, Zhang PG, Richard P. Treatment of persistent pain associated with osteoarthritis with controlled-release oxycodone tablets in a randomized controlled clinical trial. Clin J Pain 2005;21:524–535.
106. Cepeda MS, Camargo F, Zea C, Valencia L. Tramdol for Osteoarthritis: A systematic review and metaanalysis. J Rheumatol 2007;34:543–555.
107. Silverfield JC, Kamin M, Wu SC, Rosenthal N. Tramadol/acetaminophen combination tablets for the treatment of osteoarthritis flare pain: A multicenter, outpatient, randomized, double-blind, parallel-group, add-on study. Clin Ther 2002;24:282–297.
108. Cawston TE, Wilson AJ. Understanding the role of tissue degrading enzymes and their inhibitors in development and disease. Best Pract Res Clin Rheumatol 2006;20:983–1002.
109. Brandt KD, Mazzuca SA, Katz BP, et al. Effects of doxycycline on progression of osteoarthritis: Results of a randomised, placebo-controlled, double-blind trial. Arthritis Rheum 2005;52:2015–2025.
110. Fidelix TS, Soares BG, Trevisani VF. Diacerein for osteoarthritis. Cochrane Database Syst Rev 2006;(1):CD005117.
111. Ameye LG, Chee WSS. Osteoarthritis and nutrition. From nutraceuticals to functional foods: A systematic review of the scientific evidence. Arthritis Res Ther 2006;8:R127.
112. Goldberg RJ, Katz J. A meta analysis of the analgesic effects of omega-3 polyunsaturated fatty acid supplementation for inflammatory joint pain. Pain 2007;129:210–223.
113. Kwon YD, Pittler MH, Ernst E. Acupuncture for peripheral joint osteoarthritis: A systematic review and meta-analysis. Rheumatology (Oxford) 2006;45:1331–1337.
114. Scharf HP, Mansmann U, Streitberger K, et al. Acupuncture and knee osteoarthritis: A three-armed randomized trial. Ann Intern Med 2006;134:12–20.
115. Lanes SF, Lanza LL, Radensky PW, et al. Resource utilization and cost of care for rheumatoid arthritis and osteoarthritis in a managed care setting: The importance of drug and surgery costs. Arthritis Rheum 1997;40:1475–1481.
116. Spiegel B, Chiou CF, Ofman J. Minimizing complications from nonsteroidal antiinflammatory drugs: Cost-effectiveness of competing strategies in varying risk groups. Arthritis Rheum 2005;53:185–197.
117. Hur C, Chan AT, Tramontano AC, Gazelle GS. Coxibs versus combination NSAID and PPI therapy for chronic pain: An exploration of the risks, benefits, and costs. Ann Pharmacother 2006;40:1052–1063.

CHAPTER 96

Gout and Hyperuricemia

MICHAEL E. ERNST, ELIZABETH C. CLARK, AND DAVID W. HAWKINS

KEY CONCEPTS

1. Asymptomatic hyperuricemia does not require treatment.
2. Acute gouty arthritis may be treated effectively with short courses of high-dose nonacetylated nonsteroidal antiinflammatory drugs (NSAIDs).
3. Colchicine is highly effective at relieving acute attacks of gout but has the lowest benefit-to-toxicity ratio of the available pharmacotherapy for gout. When employed, it should only be used orally.
4. Individuals with contraindications to NSAIDs (e.g., active peptic ulcer disease, severe renal impairment, uncompensated congestive heart failure, or history of hypersensitivity) or colchicine, or who do not respond to these therapies may be treated with corticosteroids.
5. Uric acid nephrolithiasis should be treated with adequate hydration (2 to 3 L/day), a daytime urine-alkalinizing agent, and 60 to 80 mEq/day of potassium bicarbonate or potassium citrate.
6. Treatment with urate-lowering drugs to reduce risk of recurrent attacks of gouty arthritis is considered cost-effective in patients having two or more attacks of gout per year.
7. Allopurinol is efficacious for prophylaxis of recurrent gout attacks in both underexcretors and overproducers of uric acid. Start with a low dose (100 mg/day) after the acute attack has resolved, and titrate by 100 mg/day at 1-week intervals until the goal serum urate of <6 mg/dL is achieved. Many clinicians give colchicine (0.5 mg twice daily) during the first 3 months of therapy, to minimize the risk of acute attacks that may occur during initiation of uric acid-lowering therapy. Allopurinol should be discontinued if rash develops or liver function tests become abnormal.
8. Uricosuric agents should be avoided in patients with renal impairment (a creatinine clearance below 50 mL/min), a history of renal calculi, or overproduction of uric acid.
9. Patients with hyperuricemia or gout should be evaluated for signs of cardiovascular disease and appropriate risk reduction measures (weight loss, reduction of alcohol intake, control of blood pressure) undertaken.

Learning objectives, review questions, and other resources can be found at **www.pharmacotherapyonline.com.**

The term *gout* describes a heterogeneous clinical spectrum of diseases including elevated serum urate (hyperuricemia), recurrent attacks of acute arthritis associated with monosodium urate crystals in synovial fluid leukocytes, deposits of monosodium urate crystals (tophi) in tissues in and around joints, interstitial renal disease, and uric acid nephrolithiasis.[1]

The core metabolic disorder of gout is hyperuricemia, defined physiochemically as serum supersaturated with monosodium urate. At 37°C (98.6°F), serum urate concentrations above (or around) 7 mg/dL begin to exceed the limit of solubility for monosodium urate.[1] For determination of the risk of gout, hyperuricemia is defined statistically as serum urate concentrations greater than two standard deviations above the population means for age-and-sex-matched healthy populations, usually 7.0 mg/dL for men and 6.0 mg/dL for women.[1,2] Although hyperuricemia is fundamental to the development of gout, the mere presence of hyperuricemia itself is often an asymptomatic condition.

EPIDEMIOLOGY

Gout has been referred to as both the "king of diseases" and the "disease of kings."[1] Since ancient times, it has often been associated with affluent societies and lifestyles of overindulgence, gluttony, and intemperance.[3] The incidence and prevalence of gout continue to increase in Western industrialized countries, but the disease is not limited strictly to populations with a high standard of living.[3–5] Recent epidemiologic data indicate that the prevalence of gout is also increasing in less-industrialized Eastern countries.[6,7] Numerous factors may explain the rising prevalence of gout, including increased longevity, dietary habits, and increasing prevalence of obesity and the metabolic syndrome.[4]

There is a direct correlation between serum uric acid concentration and both the incidence and prevalence of gout. Population studies have shown that serum urate concentration correlates with increasing age, serum creatinine, blood urea nitrogen, male gender, blood pressure, body weight, and alcohol intake.[8] In several epidemiologic studies, the incidence of gout is consistently higher in individuals who are obese, or who consume large amounts of alcohol, or who consume higher amounts of meat or fish.[9–12]

The 5-year cumulative risk of gout in patients with serum urate <7 mg/dL is 0.6%, compared with a risk of 30.5% for those with urate levels >10 mg/dL.[13] Although serum urate levels are the single most important risk factor for the development of gout, hyperuricemia and gout are not always concurrently present.[14] Sustained elevation of serum urate is virtually essential for the development of gout; however, hyperuricemia does not always lead to gout, and most patients with hyperuricemia remain asymptomatic.[2] Conversely, acute gouty arthritis can occur in the presence of normal serum uric acid concentrations.[15]

Gout affects men about seven to nine times more often than women.[16] The incidence of gout increases with age, peaking at 30 to 50 years of age, with an annual incidence ranging from 1 in 1,000 for men ages 40 to 44 years and 1.8 in 1,000 for those ages 55 to 64 years.[12] The lowest rates of gout are observed in young women, approximately 0.8 cases per 10,000 patient-years.[17] Serum uric acid levels in women approach those of men once menopause has occurred; thus, in older age groups the gender gap narrows, and approximately half of newly diagnosed cases of gout are found in women.[2,5] Gout in men younger than 30 years of age, or in premenopausal women may indicate an inherited enzyme defect or the presence of renal disease.[18] Although no genetic marker has been isolated for gout, the familial nature of gout strongly suggests an interaction between genetic and environmental factors.

ETIOLOGY AND PATHOPHYSIOLOGY

In humans, uric acid is the end product of the degradation of purines. Because uric acid serves no known physiologic purpose, it is regarded as a waste product.[19] Normal uric acid levels are near the limits of urate solubility, because of the delicate balance that exists between the amount of urate produced and excreted.[20] Humans have higher uric acid levels than other mammals because they do not express the enzyme uricase, which converts uric acid to the more soluble allantoin.[3,21]

Gout occurs exclusively in humans in whom a miscible pool of uric acid exists. Under normal conditions, the amount of accumulated uric acid is about 1,200 mg in men and about 600 mg in women. The size of the urate pool is increased severalfold in individuals with gout. This excess accumulation may result from either overproduction or underexcretion of uric acid. Several conditions are associated with either decreased renal clearance or an overproduction of uric acid, leading to hyperuricemia. Table 96–1 lists some of these conditions.

OVERPRODUCTION OF URIC ACID

The purines from which uric acid is produced originate from three sources: dietary purine, conversion of tissue nucleic acid to purine nucleotides, and de novo synthesis of purine bases. The purines derived from these three sources enter a common metabolic pathway leading to the production of either nucleic acid or uric acid. Under normal circumstances, uric acid may accumulate excessively if production exceeds excretion. The average human produces about 600 to 800 mg of uric acid each day. Dietary purines play an unimportant role in the generation of hyperuricemia in the absence of some derangement in purine metabolism or elimination. However, diet modifications are important in patients with such problems who develop symptomatic hyperuricemia.

TABLE 96-1 Conditions Associated with Hyperuricemia

Primary gout	Obesity
Diabetic ketoacidosis	Sarcoidosis
Myeloproliferative disorders	Congestive heart failure
Lactic acidosis	Renal dysfunction
Lymphoproliferative disorders	Down syndrome
Starvation	Lead toxicity
Chronic hemolytic anemia	Hyperparathyroidism
Toxemia of pregnancy	Acute alcoholism
Pernicious anemia	Hypoparathyroidism
Glycogen storage disease type 1	Acromegaly
Psoriasis	Hypothyroidism
Hypoxanthine-guanine phosphoribosyltransferase deficiency	Phosphoribosylpyrophosphate synthetase overactivity
Polycythemia vera	Berylliosis
Renal transplantation	

Several enzyme systems regulate purine metabolism. Abnormalities in these regulatory systems can result in overproduction of uric acid.[22] Uric acid also may be overproduced as a consequence of increased breakdown of tissue nucleic acids and excessive rates of cell turnover, as with myeloproliferative and lymphoproliferative disorders, polycythemia vera, psoriasis, and some types of anemias. Cytotoxic medications used to treat these disorders can also result in overproduction of uric acid secondary to lysis and breakdown of cellular matter.[23]

Two enzyme abnormalities resulting in an overproduction of uric acid have been well described (Fig. 96–1). The first is an increase in the activity of phosphoribosyl pyrophosphate (PRPP) synthetase, which leads to an increased concentration of PRPP. PRPP is a key determinant of purine synthesis and thus uric acid production. The second is a deficiency of hypoxanthine-guanine phosphoribosyltransferase (HGPRT). HGPRT is responsible for the conversion of guanine to guanylic acid and hypoxanthine to inosinic acid. These two conversions require PRPP as the cosubstrate and are important reuse reactions involved in the synthesis of nucleic acids. A deficiency in the HGPRT enzyme leads to increased metabolism of guanine and hypoxanthine to uric acid, and more PRPP to interact with glutamine in the first step of the purine pathway.[24] Complete absence of HGPRT results in the childhood Lesch-Nyhan syndrome, characterized by choreoathetosis, spasticity, mental retardation, and markedly excessive production of uric acid. A partial deficiency of the enzyme may be responsible for marked hyperuricemia in otherwise normal, healthy individuals.

UNDEREXCRETION OF URIC ACID

The vast majority of patients (80% to 90%) with gout have a relative decrease in the renal excretion of uric acid for an unknown reason (primary idiopathic hyperuricemia).[2] Normally, uric acid does not accumulate as long as uric acid production is balanced with elimination. Uric acid is eliminated in two ways. About two-thirds of the uric acid produced each day is excreted in the urine. The rest is eliminated through the gastrointestinal tract after enzymatic degradation by colonic bacteria.

A decline in the urinary excretion of uric acid to a level below the rate of production leads to hyperuricemia and an increased miscible

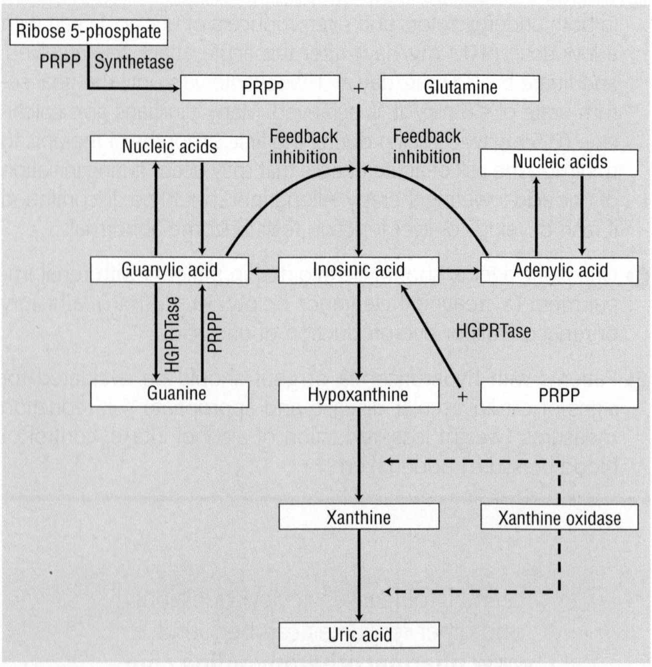

FIGURE 96-1. Purine metabolism. (HGPRT, hypoxanthine-guanine phosphoribosyltransferase; PRPP, phosphoribosyl pyrophosphate.)

TABLE 96-2 Drugs Capable of Inducing Hyperuricemia and Gout

Diuretics	Ethanol	Ethambutol
Nicotinic acid	Pyrazinamide	Cytotoxic drugs
Salicylates (<2 g/day)	Levodopa	Cyclosporine

pool of sodium urate. Almost all the urate in plasma is freely filtered across the glomerulus. The concentration of uric acid appearing in the urine is determined by multiple renal tubular transport processes in addition to the filtered load. Evidence favors a four-component model including glomerular filtration, tubular reabsorption, tubular secretion, and postsecretory reabsorption.

Approximately 90% of filtered uric acid is reabsorbed in the proximal tubule, probably by both active and passive transport mechanisms. There is a close linkage between proximal tubular sodium reabsorption and uric acid reabsorption, so conditions that enhance sodium reabsorption (e.g., dehydration) also lead to increased uric acid reabsorption. The exact site of tubular secretion of uric acid has not been determined; this too appears to involve an active transport process. Postsecretory reabsorption occurs somewhere distal to the secretory site. Table 96–2 lists the drugs that decrease renal clearance of uric acid through modification of filtered load or one of the tubular transport processes. By enhancing renal urate reabsorption, insulin resistance is also associated with gout.[25]

The pathophysiologic approach to the evaluation of hyperuricemia requires determining whether the patient is overproducing or underexcreting uric acid. This can be accomplished by placing the patient on a purine-free diet for 3 to 5 days and then measuring the amount of uric acid excreted in the urine in 24 hours. As it is very difficult in clinical practice to maintain someone on a purine-free diet for several days, this test is done infrequently in clinical practice. Nevertheless, when it is performed, individuals who excrete more than 600 mg on a purine-free diet may be considered overproducers. Hyperuricemic individuals who excrete less than 600 mg of uric acid per 24 hours on a purine-free diet may be classified as underexcretors of uric acid. However, on a regular diet, excretion of greater than 1,000 mg per 24 hours reflects overproduction; less than this is probably normal.

CLINICAL PRESENTATION

❶ Gout is a disease diagnosed by symptoms rather than laboratory tests of uric acid. In fact, asymptomatic hyperuricemia discovered incidentally generally requires no therapy because many individuals with hyperuricemia will never have an attack of gout. Nevertheless, these patients should still be encouraged to implement lifestyle measures to reduce serum urate.

CLINICAL PRESENTATION OF ACUTE GOUTY ARTHRITIS

General

- Gout classically presents as an acute inflammatory monoarthritis. The first metatarsophalangeal joint is often involved ("podagra"), but any joint of the lower extremity can be affected and occasionally gout will present as a monoarthritis of the wrist or finger. The spectrum of gout also includes nephrolithiasis, gouty nephropathy, and aggregated deposits of sodium urate (tophi) in cartilage, tendons, synovial membranes, and elsewhere (Fig. 96–2).

Signs and Symptoms

- Fever; intense pain, erythema, warmth, swelling, and inflammation of involved joints

Laboratory Tests

- Elevated serum uric acid levels; leukocytosis

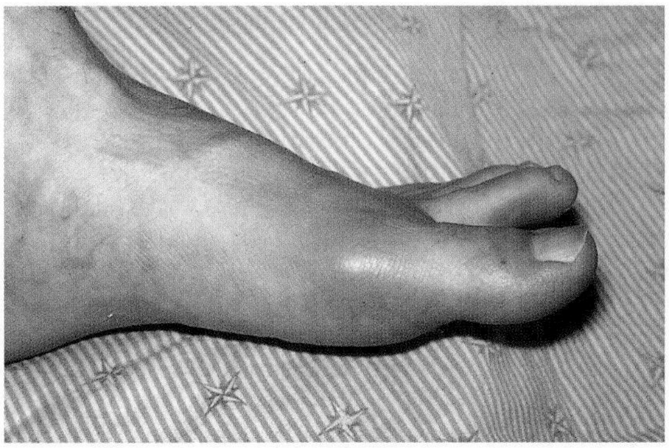

FIGURE 96-2. Acute gout attack of the first metatarsophalangeal joint. *(From Imboden J, Hellmann DB, Stone JH. Current Rheumatology Diagnosis & Treatment, 2d ed. New York: McGraw-Hill, 2004:316.)*

Other Diagnostic Tests

- Observation of monosodium urate crystals in synovial fluid or a tophus (Fig. 96–3)
- In patients with long-standing gout, radiographs may show asymmetric swelling within a joint or subcortical cysts without erosions

ACUTE GOUTY ARTHRITIS

Acute attacks of gouty arthritis are characterized by rapid onset of excruciating pain, swelling, and inflammation. The attack typically is monarticular at first, most often affecting the first metatarsophalangeal joint (great toe) and then, in order of frequency, the insteps, ankles, heels, knees, wrists, fingers, and elbows. In one-half of initial attacks, the first metatarsophalangeal joint is affected, a condition known as *podagra*. Up to 90% of patients with gout will experience attacks in the great toe at some point in the course of their disease.[19]

Atypical presentations of gout also occur. In elderly patients, gout can present as a chronic polyarticular arthritis that can be confused with rheumatoid arthritis or osteoarthritis.[4] Additionally, the onset of gout may be less dramatic than the typical acute attack and have fewer clinical findings. Multiple small joints in the hands may be involved, especially in elderly women.[2,19] Table 96–3 summarizes the different clinical manifestations of gout.

The predilection of acute gout for peripheral joints of the lower extremity is probably related to the low temperature of these joints combined with high intraarticular urate concentration. Synovial effusions are likely to occur transiently in weight-bearing joints in

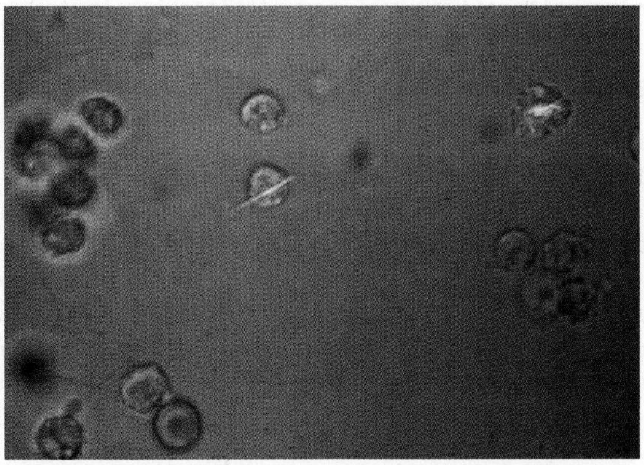

FIGURE 96-3. Urate crystal ingested by a polymorphonuclear leukocyte in synovial fluid. *(From Imboden J, Hellmann DB, Stone JH. Current Rheumatology Diagnosis & Treatment, 2d ed. New York: McGraw-Hill, 2004:317.)*

TABLE 96-3 Clinical Manifestations of Gout

Classic acute gout ("podagra")	Monoarticular arthritis Frequently attacks the first metatarsophalangeal joint although other joints of the lower extremities are also frequently involved Affected joint is swollen, erythematous, and tender
Interval or intercritical gout	Asymptomatic period between attacks
Tophaceous gout	Deposits of monosodium urate crystals in soft tissues Complications include soft-tissue damage, deformity, joint destruction, and nerve compression syndromes such as carpal tunnel syndrome
Atypical gout	Polyarthritis affecting any joint, upper or lower extremity May be confused with rheumatoid arthritis or osteoarthritis
Renal effects	Nephrolithiasis Acute and chronic gouty nephropathy

the course of a day with routine activity. At night, water is reabsorbed from the joint space, leaving behind a supersaturated solution of monosodium urate, which can precipitate attacks of acute arthritis. Attacks generally begin at night with the patient awakened from sleep by excruciating pain.

The development of crystal-induced inflammation involves a number of chemical mediators causing vasodilation, increased vascular permeability, complement activation, and chemotactic activity for polymorphonuclear leukocytes.[26] Phagocytosis of urate crystals by the leukocytes results in rapid lysis of cells and a discharge of lysosomal and proteolytic enzymes into the cytoplasm. The ensuing inflammatory reaction is associated with intense joint pain, erythema, warmth, and swelling. Fever is common, as is leukocytosis. Untreated attacks may last from 3 to 14 days before spontaneous recovery.

Although acute attacks of gouty arthritis may occur without apparent provocation, a number of conditions may precipitate an attack. These include stress, trauma, alcohol ingestion, infection, surgery, rapid lowering of serum uric acid by ingestion of uric acid-lowering agents, and ingestion of certain drugs known to elevate serum uric acid concentrations (see Table 96–2). Other crystal-induced arthropathies that may resemble gout on clinical presentation are caused by calcium pyrophosphate dihydrate crystals (pseudogout) and calcium hydroxyapatite crystals, which are associated with calcific periarthritis, tendinitis, and arthritis.[27,28]

Acute flares of gouty arthritis may occur infrequently, although with time the period between attacks may shorten if appropriate measures to correct hyperuricemia are not undertaken.[19] Later in the disease, tophaceous deposits of monosodium urate crystals in the skin or subcutaneous tissues may be found. These tophi can be anywhere but are often found on the hands, wrists, elbows, or knees. It is estimated to take 10 or more years for tophi to develop.[19]

Diagnostic Evaluation

Table 96–4 lists the differential diagnosis of an acute monoarthritis.[29] A definitive diagnosis of gout requires aspiration of synovial fluid from the affected joint and identification of intracellular crystals of monosodium urate monohydrate in synovial fluid leukocytes.[2,30] Identification of monosodium urate crystals is highly dependent on the experience of the observer. Crystals are needle shaped and when examined under polarizing light microscopy they are strongly negatively birefringent. Crystals can be observed in synovial fluid during asymptomatic periods.[31] If an affected joint is tapped, the resulting synovial fluid may have white cells and appear purulent. Such findings should always raise the question of infection. If any clinical features of infection are present, such as high fever, elevated white blood cell count, multiple joints affected, or an identified source of infection, proper diagnosis and treatment are critical. Patients with

TABLE 96-4 Differential Diagnosis of Acute Monoarthritis

1. Pseudogout (pyrophosphate crystal-related arthritis)
2. Palindromic rheumatism
3. Seronegative inflammatory arthritis
4. Trauma or hemarthrosis
5. Septic arthritis
6. Cellulitis
7. Type II dyslipidemia
8. Unrelated hyperuricemia (as in psoriasis, hypertension) when joint pain is not caused by gout

gout can have septic arthritis. Diabetes, alcohol abuse, and advanced age increase the likelihood of septic arthritis.

In lieu of obtaining a synovial fluid sample from an affected joint to inspect for urate crystals, the clinical triad of inflammatory monoarthritis, elevated serum uric acid level, and response to colchicine can be used to diagnose gout. However, this approach has limitations, including a failure to recognize atypical gout presentations and the fact that serum uric acid levels can be normal or even low during an acute gout attack.[13,32] In addition, use of colchicine as a diagnostic tool for gout is limited by lack of sensitivity and specificity for the disease. Other conditions such as psoriatic arthritis, sarcoidosis, and Mediterranean fever can respond to colchicine therapy. Table 96–5 shows the American College of Rheumatology classification criteria for an acute gouty arthritis attack.[33]

In patients with long-standing gout, radiographs may show punched-out marginal erosions and secondary osteoarthritic changes; however, in an acute first attack radiographs will be unremarkable.[14,29,34] Alternatively, the presence of chondrocalcinosis on radiographs may indicate pseudogout. Some studies have recently looked at the use of magnetic resonance imaging and computed tomography for imaging gout; however, this is not currently considered part of normal practice.

URIC ACID NEPHROLITHIASIS

Clinicians should be suspicious of hyperuricemic states in patients who present with kidney stones, as nephrolithiasis occurs in 10% to 25% of patients with gout.[35] The frequency of urolithiasis depends on serum uric acid concentrations, acidity of the urine, and urinary uric acid concentration. Typically, patients with uric acid nephrolithiasis have a urinary pH of less than 6.0. Uric acid has a negative logarithm of the acid ionization constant of 5.5. Therefore when the urine is acidic, uric acid exists primarily in the unionized, less-soluble form. At a urine pH of 5.0, urine is saturated at a uric acid level of 15 mg/dL. When the urine pH is 7.0, the solubility of uric acid in urine is increased to 200 mg/dL.[1] In patients with uric

TABLE 96-5 American College of Rheumatology Criteria for the Clinical Diagnosis of Gout[a]

1. More than one attack of acute arthritis
2. Maximum inflammation developed within 1 day
3. Monoarthritis attack
4. Redness observed over joints
5. First metatarsophalangeal joint painful or swollen
6. Unilateral first metatarsophalangeal joint attack
7. Unilateral tarsal joint attack
8. Tophus (proven or suspected)
9. Hyperuricemia
10. Asymmetric swelling within a joint on x-ray
11. Subcortical cysts without erosions on x-ray
12. Monosodium urate monohydrate microcrystals in joint fluid during attack
13. Joint fluid culture negative for organisms during attack

[a]The combination of crystals, tophi, and/or six or more criteria is highly suggestive of gout.
Data from Wallace SL, Robinson H, Masi AT, et al. Preliminary criteria for the classification of the acute arthritis of primary gout. Arthritis Rheum 1977; 20:895–900.

acid nephrolithiasis, urinary pH typically is less than 6.0 and frequently less than 5.5. When an acidic urine is saturated with uric acid, spontaneous precipitation of stones may occur.

Other factors that predispose individuals to uric acid nephrolithiasis include excessive urinary excretion of uric acid and a highly concentrated urine. The risk of renal calculi approaches 50% in individuals whose renal excretion of uric acid exceeds 1100 mg/day. In addition to pure uric acid stones, hyperuricosuric individuals are at increased risk for mixed uric acid–calcium oxalate stones and pure calcium oxalate stones. Uric acid stones are usually small, round, and radiolucent. Uric acid stones containing calcium are radiopaque.[35]

GOUTY NEPHROPATHY

There are two types of gouty nephropathy: acute uric acid nephropathy and chronic urate nephropathy.[36] In acute uric acid nephropathy, acute renal failure occurs as a result of blockage of urine flow secondary to massive precipitation of uric acid crystals in the collecting ducts and ureters. This syndrome is a well-recognized complication in patients with myeloproliferative or lymphoproliferative disorders and is a result of massive malignant cell turnover, particularly after initiation of chemotherapy.

Chronic urate nephropathy is caused by the long-term deposition of urate crystals in the renal parenchyma. Microtophi may form, with a surrounding giant cell inflammatory reaction. A decrease in the kidneys' ability to concentrate urine and the presence of proteinuria may be the earliest pathophysiologic disturbances. Hypertension and nephrosclerosis are common associated findings. Although renal failure occurs in a higher percentage of gouty patients than expected, it is not clear that hyperuricemia per se has a harmful effect on the kidneys. The chronic renal impairment seen in individuals with gout may result largely from the concurrence of hypertension, diabetes mellitus, and atherosclerosis.

TOPHACEOUS GOUT

Tophi (urate deposits) are uncommon in the general population of gouty subjects and are a late complication of hyperuricemia. The most common sites of tophaceous deposits in patients with recurrent acute gouty arthritis are the base of the great toe, helix of the ear, olecranon bursae, Achilles tendon, knees, wrists, and hands (Fig. 96–4).[2] Eventually, even the hips, shoulders, and spine may be affected. In addition to causing obvious deformities, tophi may damage surrounding soft tissue, cause joint destruction and pain, and even lead to nerve compression syndromes including carpal tunnel syndrome.

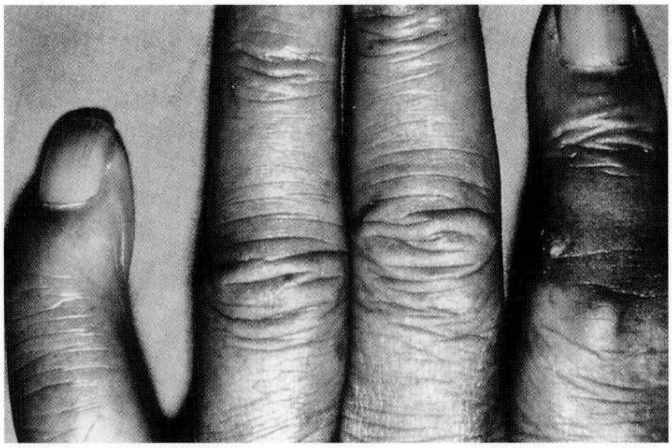

FIGURE 96-4. Tophaceous gout with subcutaneous nodule almost breaking through the skin. *(From South-Paul JE, Matheny SC, Lewis EL. Current Diagnosis & Treatment in Family Medicine. New York: McGraw-Hill, 2004:275.)*

TREATMENT

Gout and Hyperuricemia

The goals in the treatment of gout are to terminate the acute attack, prevent recurrent attacks of gouty arthritis, prevent complications associated with chronic deposition of urate crystals in tissues, and prevent or reverse features commonly associated with the illness including obesity, elevated triglycerides, and hypertension.[1] This can be accomplished through a combination of nonpharmacologic and pharmacologic methods. Table 96–6 summarizes the available pharmacotherapy for gout.

■ ACUTE GOUTY ARTHRITIS

❷ In most patients without contraindications, acute attacks of gouty arthritis may be treated successfully with short courses of high-dose nonsteroidal antiinflammatory drugs (NSAIDs) (Fig. 96–5).[37]

Nonsteroidal Antiinflammatory Drugs

Nonsteroidal antiinflammatory drugs are the mainstay of therapy for acute attacks of gouty arthritis because of their excellent efficacy and minimal toxicity with short-term use. Indomethacin has been historically favored as the NSAID of choice for acute gout flares, but there is little evidence to support one NSAID as more efficacious than another, and three (indomethacin, naproxen, and sulindac) have actual United States Food and Drug Administration (FDA)-approved labeling for this indication, among several that have been studied (see Table 96–6).[2] The most important determinant of therapeutic success with NSAIDs appears not to be which one is chosen, but rather how soon it is initiated.[18] Therapy should be initiated with maximum dosages at the onset of symptoms and continued for 24 hours after complete resolution of an acute attack, then tapered quickly over 2 to 3 days.[30] Resolution of an acute attack for most patients generally occurs within 5 to 8 days after initiating therapy.

All NSAIDs have the potential to cause similar adverse effects. The most common areas affected include the gastrointestinal system (gastritis, bleeding, and perforation), kidneys (renal papillary necrosis, reduced creatinine clearance), cardiovascular system (sodium and fluid retention, increased blood pressure), and central nervous system (impaired cognitive function, headache, dizziness). Caution should be exercised when using NSAIDs in individuals with a history of peptic ulcer disease, congestive heart failure, uncontrolled hypertension, renal insufficiency, coronary artery disease, or if they are receiving anticoagulants concurrently. Patients with active peptic ulcer disease, uncompensated congestive heart failure, severe renal impairment, or a history of hypersensitivity to aspirin or other NSAIDs should not be prescribed an NSAID.

Although the risk for gastric ulceration and bleeding is relatively small with short-term therapy normally employed when treating acute gout flares, consideration should be given to administering a proton pump inhibitor to protect from NSAID-induced gastric problems in elderly patients and in others who are at risk for these complications (e.g., presence of multiple comorbidities, alcoholism, previous history of ulcer, or concurrent anticoagulant use).[38,39] The efficacy and safety of selective cyclooxygenase-2 inhibitors have not been assessed in patients with gouty arthritis, but they are more costly than older NSAIDs and unlikely to result in fewer gastrointestinal complications because of the short courses of therapy routinely used to treat acute attacks.

Colchicine

❸ Colchicine is an antimitotic drug that is highly effective at relieving acute attacks of gout but has the lowest benefit/toxicity

TABLE 96-6 Pharmacotherapy of Acute and Chronic Gout

Therapeutic Agent	Typical Regimen	Considerations
Acute gout		
NSAIDs		
Etodolac	300 mg twice daily	Avoid in patients with peptic ulcer disease, active bleeding. May cause renal dysfunction, gastritis (worse with concurrent aspirin), fluid retention, hypertension. Use caution in congestive heart failure. Consider coadministration with a proton pump inhibitor in patients at risk for gastrointestinal bleeding.
Fenoprofen	300–600 mg three times per day to four times per day	
Ibuprofen	800 mg four times per day	
Indomethacin[a]	25–50 mg four times per day initially for 3 days, then taper to twice daily for 4–7 days	
Ketoprofen	75 mg four times per day	
Naproxen[a]	500 mg twice daily initially for 3 days, then 250–500 mg daily for 4–7 days	
Piroxicam	20 mg daily or divided twice daily	
Sulindac[a]	200 mg twice daily for 7–10 days	
Oral colchicine	0.5–0.6 mg q hour until side effects occur or maximum dosage of 8 mg is reached	Dose reduction necessary in patients with renal insufficiency. Dose-dependent gastrointestinal side effects (diarrhea, nausea, vomiting). Intravenous dosing not recommended because of toxicities.
Corticosteroids		
Oral	30–60 mg prednisone-equivalent daily × 3–5 days, then taper in 5-mg decrements spread over 10–14 days until discontinuation	Use with caution in diabetics. Avoid long-term use. May cause fluid retention, impaired wound healing. Intraarticular administration is preferred for monoarticular involvement; avoid use if joint sepsis is not excluded.
Intramuscular	Triamcinolone acetonide 60 mg IM once, or methylprednisolone 100–150 mg/day × 1–2 days	
Intraarticular	Triamcinolone acetonide 10–40 mg (large joints), 5–20 mg (small joints)	
Corticotropin	25 USP units subcutaneously for acute small-joint monoarticular gout; 40 USP units IM or IV for larger joints or polyarticular involvement	Repeat injections (every 6–8 hours for 2–3 days) may be needed. Requires intact pituitary–adrenal axis. Less effective in patients receiving long-term oral corticosteroid therapy.
Intercritical gout		
NSAIDs	Lowest effective dosage	NSAID gastropathy; see above.
Oral colchicine	0.6–1.2 mg daily to every other day	Reversible axonal neuromyopathy and rhabdomyolysis.
Xanthine oxidase inhibitor		
Allopurinol	50–300 mg daily	Can be used in both urate overproduction and urate underexcretion. Side effects include rash, gastrointestinal symptoms, potential for fatal hypersensitivity syndrome. Dose reduction necessary in patients with renal insufficiency.
Uricosurics		
Probenecid	250 mg twice daily, titrated up to 500–2,000 mg/day (target serum urate <6 mg/dL)	Useful in urate underexcretion. Avoid in patients with history of urolithiasis.
Sulfinpyrazone	50 mg twice daily, titrated to 100–400 mg/day (target serum urate <6 mg/dL)	

IM, intramuscular; IV, intravenous; NSAID, nonsteroidal antiinflammatory drug.
[a]FDA approved for treatment of acute gouty arthritis.

ratio of the available pharmacotherapy for gout.[40] When begun within the first 24 hours of an acute attack, colchicine produces a response in two-thirds of patients within hours of administration.[41] If the initiation of colchicine is delayed longer than 48 hours after the onset of acute symptoms, the probability of success with the drug diminishes substantially. Although it is a highly effective therapy, oral colchicine can cause dose-dependent gastrointestinal adverse effects, including nausea, vomiting, and diarrhea, in 50% to 80% of patients before the relief of the attack.[2] Other important nongastrointestinal adverse effects include neutropenia and axonal neuromyopathy, which may be worsened in patients taking other myopathic drugs such as β-hydroxy-β-methylglutaryl-coenzyme A reductase inhibitors, or in those with renal insufficiency.[19,22]

As a consequence of the high incidence of adverse effects and the low benefit-to-toxicity ratio, colchicine is used less often than NSAIDs in the United States.[19] Colchicine should be reserved for patients with intolerance or contraindications to NSAID use, or in whom ineffective relief with NSAIDs is obtained. Colchicine should not be used concurrently with macrolide antibiotics, particularly clarithromycin, because biliary excretion of colchicine may be reduced leading to increased plasma levels of colchicine.[42] Deaths caused by agranulocytosis are attributed to this interaction.[43–45]

Colchicine is available in both oral and parenteral formulations. It is usually dosed orally with 1 mg initially, followed by 0.5 mg every 1 hour until the joint symptoms subside, until the patient develops abdominal discomfort or diarrhea, or until a total dose of 8 mg has been administered. In patients with renal dysfunction (creatinine clearances of 10 to 50 mL/min) or hepatic dysfunction, there is no specific recommendation for adjustment of the dose of colchicine in an acute attack; however, the dose of oral colchicine should be reduced to no more than 0.6 mg daily to every other day when used as prophylaxis following an acute attack. Colchicine is contraindicated in patients with blood dyscrasias, severe cardiac or gastrointestinal disease, hepatic failure, and severe renal disease (creatinine clearance <10 mL/min).

Intravenous colchicine is associated with serious adverse effects, including bone marrow suppression, tissue necrosis from local extravasation, disseminated intravascular coagulation, hepatocellular toxicity, and renal failure. As safer alternatives exist, intravenous colchicine should generally be avoided. Intravenous colchicine is not dialyzable, and exceeding the recommended maximum cumulative dose of 2 to 4 mg during a course of therapy has resulted in fatalities.[46] If rare or unusual circumstances necessitate using colchicine parenterally, it should be overseen by experienced clinicians. Recommended guidelines suggest a dose of 2 mg diluted in 10 to 20 mL of normal saline administered slowly over 10 to 20 minutes in a secure free-flowing intravenous line to avoid extravasation, followed by two additional doses of 1 mg each at 6-hour intervals, with the total dose not exceeding 4 mg.[47] After a full intravenous course, patients should not receive colchicine from any route for at least 7 days.

Corticosteroids

❹ Corticosteroids may be used to treat acute attacks of gouty arthritis, but they are reserved primarily for patients with a contra-

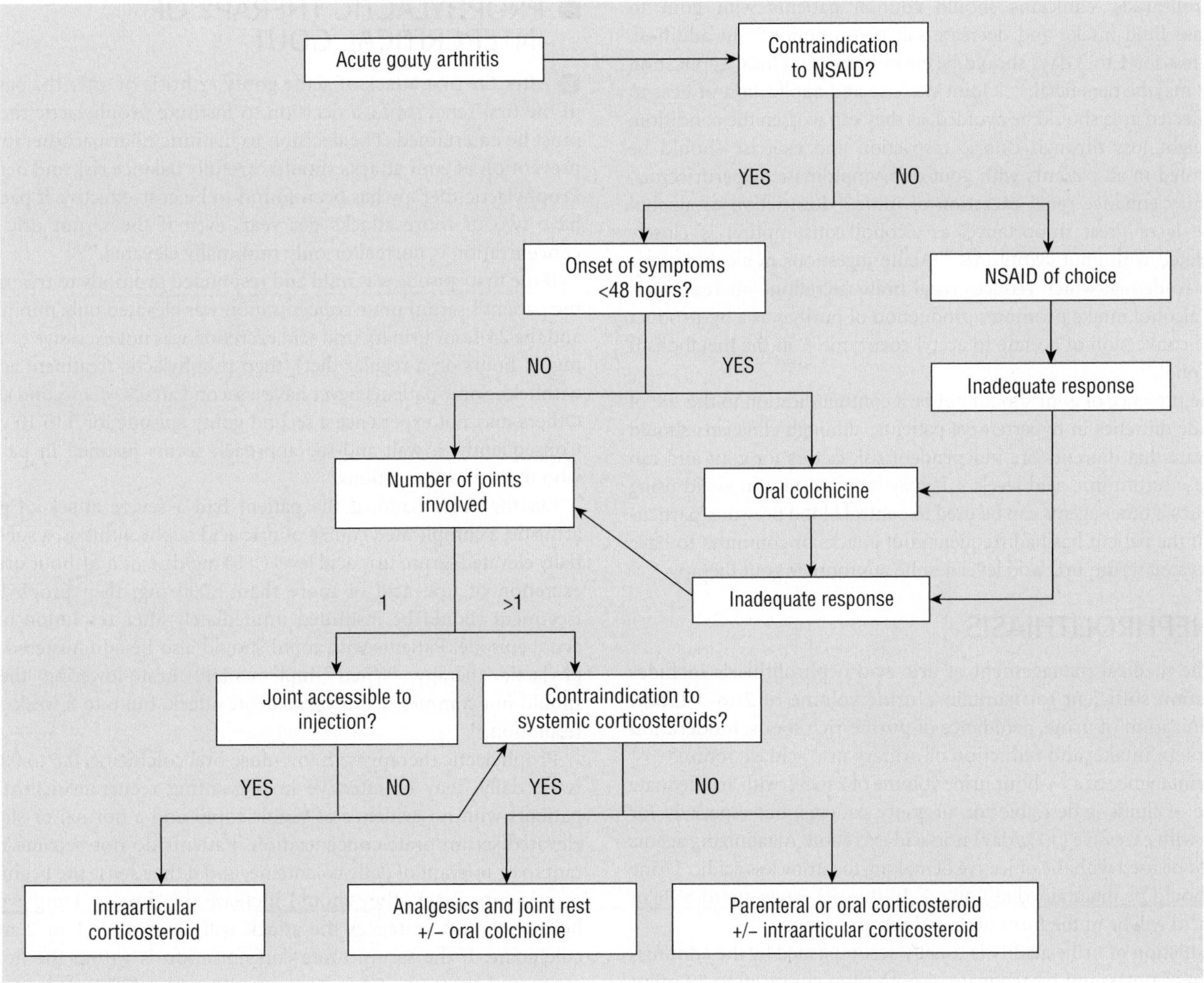

FIGURE 96-5. Treatment algorithm for acute gouty arthritis. (NSAID, nonsteroidal antiinflammatory drug.)

indication or who are unresponsive to NSAID or colchicine therapy.[2] Patients with polyarticular involvement may also benefit from corticosteroids. They can be used either systemically or by intraarticular injection. Oral corticosteroids may be administered in doses of 30 to 60 mg of prednisone-equivalent for 3 to 5 days in patients with multiple-joint involvement.[2] Because rebound attacks may occur upon steroid withdrawal, the dose should be tapered gradually in 5-mg decrements spread over 10 to 14 days and then discontinued. Intraarticular administration of triamcinolone acetonide in a dose of 20 to 40 mg may be useful in treating acute gout limited to one or two joints.[48] Injection should be done under aseptic technique in a joint determined not to be infected. A single intramuscular injection of a long-acting corticosteroid, such as methylprednisolone, can be used as an alternative to the oral route if patients are unable to take oral therapy.[2] If not contraindicated, low-dose colchicine can be used as adjunctive therapy to injectable corticosteroids to prevent rebound flare-ups.

Corticosteroids can have a number of adverse effects, and should be used with caution in patients with diabetes as they can increase blood sugar. In addition, patients with a history of gastrointestinal problems, bleeding disorders, cardiovascular disease, and psychiatric disorders should be monitored closely. Long-term corticosteroid use should be avoided because of the risk for osteoporosis, hypothalamic–pituitary axis suppression, cataracts, and muscle deconditioning that can occur with their use.

Corticotropin, or adrenocorticotropic hormone (ACTH), which stimulates the adrenal cortex to produce cortisol and corticosterone, can be administered in acute gout. Doses of 40 to 80 USP units are given intramuscularly every 6 to 8 hours for 2 to 3 days, and then discontinued. Studies with ACTH are limited, but it appears to provide similar efficacy to systemic antiinflammatory doses of corticosteroids.[49] When administered alone or in combination with colchicine, ACTH may provide earlier efficacy compared with indomethacin but with fewer adverse effects.[50] Unfortunately, ACTH is often difficult to obtain in the United States as a result of manufacturing problems. Because the studies have several limitations, the regimen should be considered only as an alternative, especially in patients with comorbidities where other regimens are contraindicated.[51] Examples of patients where ACTH has been used safely when other first-line gout therapies were contraindicated include those with congestive heart failure, chronic renal failure, and history of gastrointestinal bleeding.[52]

Nonpharmacologic Therapies

Gout is influenced by several dietary factors, including obesity, alcohol intake, hyperlipidemia, and insulin resistance syndrome.[53] Because of the elevated risk for development of gout that exists with hyperuricemia, even the asymptomatic patient should receive interventions directed toward modifying or correcting some of these underlying contributors.

Patients suffering from acute gouty arthritis should be advised to reduce their dietary intake of saturated fats and meats high in purines (e.g., organ meats).[54] Some consideration may be given to a rigid purine-free diet, although they may only be moderately effective in lowering serum uric acid levels and they can rarely be sustained for long periods of time.[53] Because of the increased risk of developing nephrolithiasis, clinicians should counsel patients with gout to increase fluid intake and decrease salt consumption.[55] In addition, joint rest for 1 to 2 days should be encouraged, and local application of ice may be beneficial.[53,56] Joint exercise and application of heat to the affected area should be avoided, as they can worsen the condition.

Weight loss through caloric restriction and exercise should be promoted in all patients with gout or asymptomatic hyperuricemia, and may enhance renal excretion of urate.[57] Restriction of alcohol intake is of great importance, as alcohol consumption is closely correlated with gout symptoms.[10] Acute ingestions of alcohol cause lactic academia, which reduces renal urate excretion, whereas long-term alcohol intake promotes production of purines as a by-product of the conversion of acetate to acetyl coenzyme A in the metabolism of alcohol.[53]

The presence of gout should not be a contraindication to the use of thiazide diuretics in hypertensive patients, although clinicians should be aware that diuretics are independent risk factors for gout and can increase serum uric acid levels.[11] It may be important to avoid using diuretics if other agents can be used to control blood pressure, particularly if the patient has had frequent gout attacks or continues to have an elevated serum uric acid level despite appropriate gout therapy.

NEPHROLITHIASIS

5 The medical management of uric acid nephrolithiasis includes hydration sufficient to maintain a urine volume of 2 to 3 L/day, alkalinization of urine, avoidance of purine-rich foods, moderation of protein intake, and reduction of urinary uric acid excretion.

Maintenance of a 24-hour urine volume of 2 to 3 L with an adequate intake of fluids is desirable for all gouty patients, but especially for those with excessive (>1 g/day) uric acid excretion. Alkalinizing agents should be used with the objective of making the urine less acidic. Urine pH should be maintained at 6 to 6.5. In this pH range, up to 85% of uric acid will be in the form of the soluble urate ion.

Reduction of urine acidity is usually accomplished by the administration of potassium bicarbonate or potassium citrate 60 to 80 mEq/day.[58,59] Administration of alkali via sodium salts is a less desirable option for two reasons. First, the sodium-induced volume expansion will increase sodium excretion and can secondarily cause hypercalcemia because calcium passively follows the reabsorption of sodium in the proximal tubule and loop of Henle. In the presence of uric acid, the resultant hypercalcemia can lead to calcium oxalate stone formation. Secondly, one must keep in mind that older patients with uric acid kidney stones also may have hypertension, congestive heart failure, or renal insufficiency, and obviously should not be overloaded with alkalinizing sodium salts or unlimited fluid intake. Acetazolamide, a carbonic anhydrase inhibitor, produces rapid and effective urinary alkalinization and sometimes is used in conjunction with alkali therapy. When a 250-mg dose of acetazolamide is given at bedtime, the excretion of an acidic urine in the early morning hours is avoided. The usual tachyphylaxis (rapid tolerance) to this drug is obviated by a daily repletion dose of bicarbonate.

Since the advent of allopurinol, a low-purine, low-protein diet in the patient with uric acid nephrolithiasis is no longer as critical as it once was; however, it is still advisable to instruct the patient to avoid foods rich in purine and to limit protein to no more than 90 g/day. Such a diet is still palatable and reduces appreciably the amount of uric acid in the urine.

The mainstay of drug therapy for recurrent uric acid nephrolithiasis is allopurinol. It is effective in reducing both serum and urinary uric acid levels, thus preventing the formation of calculi. Allopurinol is also recommended as prophylactic treatment in patients who will receive cytotoxic agents for the treatment of lymphoma or leukemia. The marked increase in uric acid production associated with cytolysis of a neoplasm predisposes a patient to the development of uric acid nephrolithiasis.

PROPHYLACTIC THERAPY OF INTERCRITICAL GOUT

6 After the first attack of acute gouty arthritis or after the passage of the first renal stone, a decision to institute prophylactic therapy must be entertained. The decision to institute pharmacotherapy for prevention of gout attacks should carefully balance risk and benefit. Prophylactic therapy has been found to be cost-effective if patients have two or more attacks per year, even if the serum uric acid concentration is normal or only minimally elevated.[60,61]

If the first episode was mild and responded promptly to treatment, the patient's serum urate concentration was elevated only minimally, and the 24-hour urinary uric acid excretion was not excessive (<1,000 mg/24 hours on a regular diet), then prophylactic treatment can be withheld. Some patients never have a second attack or a second stone. Others may not experience a second gouty episode for 5 to 10 years. Consequently, a wait-and-see approach seems justified in patients who meet these conditions.[62]

On the other hand, if the patient had a severe attack of gouty arthritis, a complicated course of uric acid nephrolithiasis, a substantially elevated serum uric acid level (>10 mg/dL), or a 24-hour urinary excretion of uric acid of more than 1,000 mg, then prophylactic treatment should be instituted immediately after resolution of the acute episode. Patients with tophi should also be administered prophylactic therapy. When implemented, urate-lowering therapy should not commence during an acute attack, but 6 to 8 weeks after resolution.[14]

Prophylactic therapy with low-dose oral colchicine, 0.5 to 0.6 mg twice daily, may be effective in preventing recurrent arthritis in patients with no evidence of visible tophi and a normal or slightly elevated serum urate concentration. Patients do not become resistant to or tolerant of daily colchicine, and if they sense the beginning of an acute attack, they should increase the dose to 1 mg every 2 hours; in most instances the attack will abort after 1 or 2 mg of colchicine. If the serum urate concentration is within the normal range and the patient has been symptom-free for 1 year, maintenance colchicine may be discontinued. The patient should be advised, however, that discontinuation of the treatment program may be followed by an exacerbation of acute gouty arthritis.

Patients with a history of recurrent acute gouty arthritis and a significantly elevated serum uric acid concentration probably are best managed with uric acid-lowering therapy. The goal of initiating urate-lowering therapies is to achieve and maintain a serum uric acid concentration of less than 6 mg/dL, and preferably below 5 mg/dL.[22,62] Reduction of the serum urate concentration can be accomplished pharmacologically by decreasing the synthesis of uric acid (xanthine oxidase inhibitors), or by increasing the renal excretion of uric acid (uricosurics). Colchicine at a dose of 0.5 mg twice daily is sometimes administered during the first 6 to 12 months of antihyperuricemic therapy to minimize the risk of acute attacks that may occur during initiation of uric acid–lowering therapy.

Xanthine Oxidase Inhibitor

7 Currently, allopurinol is the only drug approved in the United States for use in inhibiting uric acid synthesis. Because allopurinol is efficacious for prophylaxis of recurrent gout attacks in both underexcretors and overproducers of uric acid, it is the most widely prescribed agent for the long-term management of gout.[48] Both allopurinol and its major metabolite, oxypurinol, are xanthine oxidase inhibitors and thus impair the conversion of hypoxanthine to xanthine and xanthine to uric acid. Allopurinol also lowers the intracellular concentration of PRPP.

Allopurinol lowers uric acid levels in a dose-dependent manner. Because of the long half-life of its metabolite, allopurinol can be given once daily. It is typically initiated at a dose of 100 mg/day, and titrated by 100 mg/day at 1-week intervals to achieve a serum uric acid level of 6 mg/dL or less, which will promote shrinkage of tophi.[63] Serum uric acid levels can be checked approximately 1 week after initiating or modifying the dose of allopurinol. Typical doses of 100 to 300 mg/day are used, although tophaceous gout may require doses of 400 to 600 mg/day and the maximum recommended dose of allopurinol is 800 mg/day. Allopurinol should be considered for long-term use when prescribed, as intermittent administration has been found to be less effective in controlling gouty attacks.[64]

Although allopurinol is the most effective urate-lowering agent available, up to 5% of patients are unable to tolerate it because of adverse effects, and long-term persistence with allopurinol therapy may be less than optimal.[65] Mild adverse effects such as skin rash, leukopenia, gastrointestinal problems, headache, and urticaria can occur with allopurinol administration. More severe adverse reactions including severe rash (toxic epidermal necrolysis, erythema multiforme, or exfoliative dermatitis), hepatitis, interstitial nephritis, and eosinophilia reportedly occur in approximately 2% of patients, and are associated with a 20% mortality.[22,66] This "allopurinol hypersensitivity syndrome" is dose related (200 to 400 mg/daily) and occurs more commonly in the presence of renal insufficiency.[66] The dose of allopurinol should be reduced in patients with renal insufficiency (200 mg/day for creatinine clearance of 60 mL/min, and 100 mg/day for creatinine clearance of 30 mL/min). However, some evidence exists that allopurinol can be safely used at higher doses than traditionally recommended in patients with renal impairment.[67]

CLINICAL CONTROVERSY

To reduce the risk of developing the allopurinol hypersensitivity syndrome, some experts believe that the dose of allopurinol should be adjusted based on the patient's creatinine clearance.

A desensitization protocol (Table 96–7) is recommended for gout patients who have experienced maculopapular eruptions or mild rashes on allopurinol.[68] In addition, it is recommended for patients with gout and renal insufficiency (where uricosurics are contraindicated), gout caused by urate overproduction, intolerance or allergic reactions to uricosuric agents, and malignancy-associated hyperuricemia.[22,68] Unfortunately, not all patients are successfully able to be desensitized, and desensitization should not be attempted in patients who have previously experienced the allopurinol hypersensitivity syndrome.[69]

Uricosuric Drugs

Uricosuric drugs increase the renal clearance of uric acid by inhibiting postsecretory renal proximal tubular reabsorption of uric acid. The drugs used most widely to increase uric acid excretion are probenecid and sulfinpyrazone. Several other uricosuric drugs are available in Europe, but they have not been approved for use in the United States.

TABLE 96-7 Protocol for Desensitizing Patients Unable to Tolerate Allopurinol

Daily Allopurinol Dose	Preparation	Days
50 mcg	0.25 mL (1 mg/5 mL)	1–3
100 mcg	0.5 mL (1 mg/5 mL)	4–6
200 mcg	1 mL (1 mg/5 mL)	7–9
500 mcg	2.5 mL (1 mg/5 mL)	10–12
1 mg	5 mL (1 mg/5 mL)	13–15
5 mg	2.5 mL (10 mg/5 mL)	16–18
10 mg	5 mL (10 mg/5 mL)	19–21
25 mg	12.5 mL (10 mg/5 mL)	22–24
50 mg	$^1/_2$ of 100-mg tablet	25–27
100 mg	100-mg tablet	28 and beyond

Therapy with uricosuric drugs should be started at a low dose to avoid marked uricosuria and possible stone formation. They should be used only in patients with documented underexcretion of urate (less than 800 mg in 24 hours on a regular diet, or 600 mg on a purine-restricted diet). The maintenance of adequate urine flow and alkalinization of the urine during the first several days of uricosuric therapy further diminish the possibility of uric acid stone formation. Probenecid is given initially at a dose of 250 mg twice a day for 1 to 2 weeks and then 500 mg twice a day for 2 weeks. Thereafter the daily dose is increased by 500-mg increments every 1 to 2 weeks until satisfactory control is achieved or a maximum dose of 2 g is reached. The initial dose of sulfinpyrazone is 50 mg twice a day for 3 to 4 days and then 100 mg twice a day, increasing the daily dose by 100-mg increments each week up to 800 mg/day.

The major adverse effects associated with uricosuric therapy are gastrointestinal irritation, rash and hypersensitivity, precipitation of acute gouty arthritis, and stone formation. Of the two agents, probenecid is the most frequently used uricosuric as sulfinpyrazone is associated with more severe adverse effects. A disadvantage of uricosurics is that salicylates may interfere with this mechanism and result in treatment failure;[22] however, low-doses (325 mg/day or less) of enteric-coated aspirin may be used cautiously.[70] In addition, probenecid can inhibit the tubular secretion of other organic acids; thus, increased plasma concentrations of penicillins, cephalosporins, sulfonamides, and indomethacin can occur. Because it is chemically related to phenylbutazone, sulfinpyrazone can act as an antiplatelet agent and should be used with great caution in anticoagulated patients, or those with peptic ulcer disease.

❽ Uricosuric drugs are contraindicated in patients who are allergic to them and in patients with impaired renal function (a creatinine clearance <50 mL/min), a history of renal calculi, and in patients who are overproducers of uric acid; for such patients, allopurinol should be used.

Miscellaneous Agents

Several other medications have been effective in gout. Benzbromarone is a uricosuric that is efficacious in patients with renal insufficiency, but it is not available in the United States.[2] Oxypurinol, a metabolite of allopurinol, is not commercially available in the United States, but can be obtained through the manufacturer on a compassionate basis.[53] Several newer medications, such as uric acid oxidase (uricase), and febuxostat, are currently under investigation and may offer additional options in the future.[4,53] Of these agents, febuxostat has demonstrated superior efficacy to allopurinol in reducing serum urate, but had an increase in rebound gout flares.[71] It has received an approvable letter from the United States FDA, pending completion of a currently ongoing phase III clinical trial. A recombinant form of uricase (rasburicase) is currently available and indicated for use in the management of hyperuricemia in children with leukemia, lymphoma, or solid-tumor malignancies who are likely to experience tumor lysis syndrome. The efficacy of rasburicase has not been assessed outside of the oncology setting in adults with acute gouty arthritis.

Lipid-lowering agents, in particular fenofibrate, can also be prescribed for patients with gout. Although dyslipidemia is common in gout patients, the fibrates are believed to exert their effects as an ancillary benefit by increasing the clearance of hypoxanthine, and xanthine, leading to a sustained reduction in serum urate. Reductions of 20% to 30% in urate levels are observed with fenofibrate use.[72,73] Importantly, fenofibrate does not appear to not cause an acute gout flare when initiated, and is well tolerated overall.[74,75]

Losartan, an angiotensin II receptor antagonist, has also demonstrated benefit in reducing serum urate independent of angiotensin receptor antagonism.[76] Losartan inhibits renal tubular reabsorption of uric acid and increases urinary excretion, and this effect seems to be a unique property of losartan that is not shared with other angiotensin II receptor antagonists.[77] In addition, it alkalinizes the urine, which helps reduce the risk for stone formation.

■ ASYMPTOMATIC HYPERURICEMIA

Questions are often raised regarding the indications for drug therapy for asymptomatic hyperuricemia. The purported benefits from treatment include prevention of acute gouty arthritis, tophi formation, nephrolithiasis, and chronic urate nephropathy. The first three complications are easily controlled should they develop; therefore antihyperuricemic therapy is not warranted to prevent these conditions. The prevention of urate nephropathy might be a stronger indication because it is irreversible even with proper treatment. Available data indicate, however, that gouty nephropathy is extremely rare in the absence of clinical gout, and evidence that elevation of uric acid by itself may cause renal disease is weak and inconclusive.[18] As discussed previously, renal impairment is very rare in the absence of concurrent hypertension and atherosclerosis. In addition, it is unclear whether uric acid–lowering therapy protects renal function in such individuals. Thus, the routine treatment of asymptomatic hyperuricemia on the grounds of reducing renal complications is presently not recommended.

The relationship between elevated serum urate and cardiovascular disease is controversial. In observational studies, hyperuricemia has been shown to be a risk factor for ischemic heart disease.[78–81] However, as hyperuricemia is also associated with other known risk factors for cardiovascular disease, such as diabetes mellitus, dyslipidemia, and hypertension, the individual contribution of hyperuricemia on the risk for cardiovascular disease is difficult to separate from these associated factors. No studies have examined whether drug treatment of asymptomatic hyperuricemia is protective against coronary artery disease, and the available data at this time do not justify routine therapy for patients with asymptomatic hyperuricemia for this indication.

CLINICAL CONTROVERSY

Although asymptomatic hyperuricemia is not generally treated, some clinicians have begun recommending treatment to reduce the risk of coronary artery disease. Hyperuricemia is associated with both hypertension and coronary artery disease, and patients with elevated uric acid levels and hypertension may have an increased risk of cardiovascular morbidity and mortality.

■ PHARMACOECONOMIC CONSIDERATIONS

Assuming patients with asymptomatic hyperuricemia are not treated with pharmacologic therapy, pharmacoeconomic considerations apply only to the management of the acute and chronic clinical manifestations of gout.

In a cost-effectiveness analysis in patients with nontophaceous recurrent gouty arthritis, urate-lowering therapy was found to reduce costs if patients experienced two or more recurrent attacks per year.[60] Generic allopurinol was associated with a lower incremental cost-effectiveness ratio than were either probenecid or sulfinpyrazone.

In the case of chronic tophaceous gout, a need to continue long-term therapy with a urate-lowering drug clearly exists. Allopurinol generally is less expensive than uricosuric therapy and may be more effective. Comparative trials are lacking. For severe cases, combination therapy may be indicated. Many clinicians will add colchicine to the regimen to reduce the likelihood of precipitating acute gouty arthritis, but this does not appear to be a cost-effective measure.

■ EVALUATION OF THERAPEUTIC OUTCOMES

Followup of the gout sufferer depends on the frequency of attacks and on the medications used to treat symptoms. For a patient who is experiencing a first attack of gout, long-term therapy is generally not indicated. As mentioned previously, most experts agree that treatment should be started only after two or three attacks of gout, because the treatment is long-term and relatively expensive, the drugs used are potentially toxic, and adherence in patients without symptoms is generally poor.[61,65] Patients having a first attack should be educated about the likelihood of recurrence and what to do if another attack occurs. Approximately 60% of patients have a second attack within the first year, and 78% have a second attack within 2 years. Only 7% of patients do not have a recurrence within a 10-year period.[82]

Baseline blood work for patients receiving hypouricemic medications chronically should include renal function (serum creatinine, blood urea nitrogen), liver enzymes (aspartate aminotransferase, alanine aminotransferase), complete blood count, and electrolytes. There is generally no need to recheck these laboratory parameters for patients undergoing acute therapy with an NSAID or colchicine of limited duration. However, in patients requiring long-term therapy or prophylaxis, they should be rechecked every 6 to 12 months, or as clinically indicated. In patients without evident tophi, consideration can be given to discontinuing long-term therapy 6 to 12 months after normal serum urate levels are obtained.

For patients suspected of having an acute attack of gouty arthritis, it is reasonable to check a serum uric acid level, particularly if it is not the first attack and a decision is to be made regarding initiation of prophylactic therapy. However, clinicians should be mindful that acute gouty arthritis can occur in the presence of normal serum uric acid concentrations.[15] Repeat serum uric acid levels do not need to be routinely monitored in patients, with the exception of during the titration phase of allopurinol to achieve a goal serum urate of <6 mg/dL.[83]

❾ Because of comorbidity with diabetes mellitus, lipid abnormalities, hypertension, and stroke, elevated uric acid levels or gout should prompt evaluations for signs of cardiovascular disease and the need for appropriate risk reduction measures.[37] Additionally, clinicians should look for a possible correctable cause of hyperuricemia, such as medications (e.g., thiazide diuretics, niacin, cyclosporine), obesity, malignancy, and alcohol abuse. Patients should be encouraged to exercise, lose weight, reduce alcohol intake, and control blood pressure and have periodic followup to address these conditions.

CONCLUSIONS

Hyperuricemia may lead to acute arthritis, chronic gout, or kidney stones, or to no sequelae at all. Asymptomatic hyperuricemia need not be treated, although lifestyle modifications (e.g., weight loss, reduction of alcohol intake, control of blood pressure) should be encouraged to help reduce serum urate and overall cardiovascular health.

Acute gouty arthritis responds well to short courses of NSAIDs to treat the underlying inflammatory condition. Colchicine is also highly effective, but has the lowest benefit-to-toxicity ratio of the available pharmacotherapy for acute gouty arthritis. If contraindications to NSAIDs or colchicine exist, or there is lack of response to these agents, or polyarticular involvement is noted, intraarticular or oral corticosteroids may be used. The management of uric acid nephrolithiasis includes hydration and alkalinization of the urine. Prevention of recurrent gouty arthritis or recurrent nephrolithiasis and treatment of chronic gout require hypouricemic therapy with either a uricosuric drug or allopurinol. Allopurinol is effective in both underexcretors and overproducers of uric acid, making it the hypouricemic drug of choice in most patients with gout.

ABBREVIATIONS

ACTH: adrenocorticotropic hormone

HGPRT: hypoxanthine guanine phosphoribosyl transferase
NSAID: nonsteroidal antiinflammatory drug
PRPP: phosphoribosyl pyrophosphate (synthetase)

REFERENCES

1. Wortmann RL, Kelley WN. Gout and hyperuricemia. In: Harris ED, Budd RC, Genovese MC, et al., eds. Kelley's Textbook of Rheumatology. Philadelphia: WB Saunders, 2005:1402–1429.
2. Rott KT, Agudelo CA. Gout. JAMA 2003;289:2857–2860.
3. Johnson RJ, Rideout BA. Uric acid and diet—Insights into the epidemic of cardiovascular disease. N Engl J Med 2004;350:1071–1073.
4. Bieber JD, Terkeltaub RA. Gout: On the brink of novel therapeutic options for an ancient disease. Arthritis Rheum 2004;50:2400–2414.
5. Wallace KL, Riedel AA, Joseph-Ridge N, Wortmann R. Increasing prevalence of gout and hyperuricemia over 10 years among older adults in a managed care population. J Rheumatol 2004;31:1582–1587.
6. Zeng Q, Wang Q, Chen R, et al. Primary gout in Shantou: A clinical and epidemiological study. Chin Med J 2003;116:66–69.
7. Chen SY, Chen CL, Shen ML, Kamatani N. Trends in the manifestations of gout in Taiwan. Rheumatology 2003;42:1529–1533.
8. Chang HY, Pan WH, Yeh WT, Tsai KS. Hyperuricemia and gout in Taiwan: Results of the nutritional and health survey in Taiwan (1993–96). J Rheumatol 2001;28:1640–1646.
9. Choi HK, Curhan G. Gout: Epidemiology and lifestyle choices. Curr Opin Rheumatol 2005;17:341–345.
10. Choi HK, Atkinson K, Karlson EW, et al. Alcohol intake and risk of incident gout in men: A prospective study. Lancet 2004;363:1277–1281.
11. Choi HK, Atkinson K, Karlson EW, Curhan G. Obesity, weight change, hypertension, diuretic use, and risk of gout in men: The health professionals follow-up study. Arch Intern Med 2005;165:742–748.
12. Choi HK, Atkinson K, Karlson EW, et al. Purine-rich foods, dairy and protein intake, and the risk of gout in men. N Engl J Med 2004;350:1093–1103.
13. Campion EW, Glynn RJ, DeLabry LO. Asymptomatic hyperuricemia. Risks and consequences in the Normative Aging Study. Am J Med 1987;82:421–426.
14. Pittman JR, Bross MH. Diagnosis and management of gout. Am Fam Physician 1999;59:1799–1806.
15. McCarty DJ. Gout without hyperuricemia. JAMA 1994;271:302–303.
16. Kramer HM, Curhan G. The association between gout and nephrolithiasis: The National Health and Nutrition Examination Survey III, 1988–1994. Am J Kidney Dis 2002;40:37–42.
17. Mikuls TR, Farrar JT, Bilker WB, et al. Gout epidemiology: Results from the UK General Practice Research Database, 1990–1999. Ann Rheum Dis 2005;64:267–272.
18. Harris MD, Siegel LB, Alloway JA. Gout and hyperuricemia. Am Fam Physician 1999;59:925–934.
19. Kim KY, Schumacher HR, Hunsche E, et al. A literature review of the epidemiology and treatment of acute gout. Clin Ther 2003;25:1593–1617.
20. Terkeltaub RA. Gout. N Engl J Med 2003;349:1647–1655.
21. Choi HK, Mount DB, Reginato AM. Pathogenesis of gout. Ann Intern Med 2005;143:499–516.
22. Wortmann RL. Gout and hyperuricemia. Curr Opin Rheumatol 2002;14:281–286.
23. Monu JU, Pope TL, Jr. Gout: A clinical and radiologic review. Radiol Clin North Am 2004;42:169–184.
24. Wilson JM, Young AB, Kelley WN. Hypoxanthine-guanine phosphoribosyltransferase deficiency. N Engl J Med 1983;309:900–910.
25. Agedelo CA, Wise CM. Gout: Diagnosis, pathogenesis, and clinical manifestations. Curr Opin Rheumatol 2001;13:234–239.
26. Beutler A, Schumacher HR. Gout and "pseudogout": When are arthritis symptoms caused by crystal deposition? Postgrad Med 1994;95:103–116.
27. McGill NW. Gout and other crystal arthropathies. Med J Aust 1997;166:33–38.
28. Schumacher HR. Crystal-reduced arthritis: An overview. Am J Med 1996;100(Suppl 2A):46S–52S.
29. Pal B, Foxall M, Dysart T, et al. How is gout managed in primary care? A review of current practice and proposed guidelines. Clin Rheumatol 2000;19:21–25.
30. Schlesinger N, Baker DG, Schumacher HR, Jr. How well have diagnostic tests and therapies for gout been evaluated? Curr Opin Rheumatol 1999;11:441–445.
31. Agudelo CA, Weinberger A, Schumacher HR, et al. Definitive diagnosis of gout by identification of urate crystals in asymptomatic metatarsophalangeal joints. Arthritis Rheum 1979;22:559–560.
32. Logan JA, Morrison E, McGill PE. Serum uric acid in acute gout. Ann Rheum Dis 1997;56:696–697.
33. Wallace SL, Robinson H, Masi AT, et al. Preliminary criteria for the classification of the acute arthritis of primary gout. Arthritis Rheum 1977;20:895–900.
34. Zhang W, Doherty M, Pascual E, et al. EULAR evidence based recommendations for gout. Part I. Diagnosis. Report of a task force of the Standing Committee for International Clinical Studies Including Therapeutics (ESCISIT). Ann Rheum Dis 2006;65:1301–1311.
35. Yu T. Nephrolithiasis in patients with gout. Postgrad Med 1978;63:164–170.
36. Klineberg JR. Role of the kidneys in the pathogenesis of gout. Postgrad Med 1978;63:145–150.
37. Zhang W, Doherty M, Bardin T, et al. EULAR evidence based recommendations for gout. Part II. Management. Report of a task force of the EULAR Standing Committee for International Clinical Studies Including Therapeutics (ESCISIT). Ann Rheum Dis 2006;65:1312–1324.
38. Hawkey CJ, Karrasch JA, Szczepanski L, et al. Omeprazole compared with misoprostol for ulcers associated with nonsteroidal anti-inflammatory drugs. Omeprazole versus Misoprostol for NSAID-induced Ulcer Management (OMNIUM) Study Group. N Engl J Med 1998;338:727–734.
39. Yeomans ND, Tulassay Z, Juhasz L, et al. A comparison of omeprazole with ranitidine for ulcers associated with nonsteroidal anti-inflammatory drugs. Acid Suppression Trial: Ranitidine versus Omeprazole for NSAID-associated Ulcer Treatment (ASTRONAUT) Study Group. N Engl J Med 1998;338:719–726.
40. Roberts WN, Liang MH, Stern SH. Colchicine in acute gout. Reassessment of risks and benefits. JAMA 1987;257:1920–1922.
41. Ahern MJ, Reid C, Gordon TP, et al. Does colchicine work? The results of the first controlled study in acute gout. Aust N Z J Med 1987;17:301–304.
42. Rollot F, Pajot O, Chauvelot-Moachon L, et al. Acute colchicine intoxication during clarithromycin administration. Ann Pharmacother 2004;38:2074–2077.
43. Dogukan A, Oymak FS, Taskapan H, et al. Acute fatal colchicine intoxication in a patient on continuous ambulatory peritoneal dialysis (CAPD). Possible role of clarithromycin administration. Clin Nephrol 2001;55:181–182.
44. Hung IF, Wu AK, Cheng VC, et al. Fatal interaction between clarithromycin and colchicine in patients with renal insufficiency: A retrospective study. Clin Infect Dis 2005;41:291–300.
45. Cheng VC, Ho PL, Yuen KY. Two probable cases of serious drug interaction between clarithromycin and colchicine. South Med J 2005;98:811–813.
46. Bonnel RA, Villalba ML, Karwoski CB, Beitz J. Deaths associated with inappropriate intravenous colchicine administration. J Emerg Med 2002;22:385–387.
47. Wallace SL, Singer JZ. Systemic toxicity associated with the intravenous administration of colchicine—Guidelines for use. J Rheumatol 1988;15:495–499.
48. Schlesinger N, Schumacher HR. Gout: Can management be improved? Curr Opin Rheumatol 2001;13:240–246.
49. Siegel LB, Alloway JA, Nashel DJ. Comparison of adrenocorticotropic hormone and triamcinolone acetonide in the treatment of acute gouty arthritis. J Rheumatol 1994;21:1325–1327.
50. Axelrod D, Preston S. Comparison of parenteral adrenocorticotropic hormone with oral indomethacin in the treatment of acute gout. Arthritis Rheum 1988;31:803–805.
51. Taylor CT, Brooks NC, Kelley KW. Corticotropin for acute management of gout. Ann Pharmacother 2001;35:365–368.
52. Ritter J, Kerr LD, Valeriano-Marcet J, Spiera H. ACTH revisited: Effective treatment for acute crystal induced synovitis in patients with multiple medical problems. J Rheumatol 1994;21:696–699.
53. Schlesinger N. Management of acute and chronic gouty arthritis: Present state-of-the-art. Drugs 2004;64:2399–2416.
54. Davis JC. A practical approach to gout: Current management of an "old" disease. Postgrad Med 1999;106:115–123.

55. Kramer HJ, Choi HK, Atkinson K, et al. The association between gout and nephrolithiasis in men: The Health Professionals' Follow-Up Study. Kidney Int 2003;64:1022–1026.
56. Schlesinger N, Detry MA, Holland BK, et al. Local ice therapy during bouts of acute gouty arthritis. J Rheumatol 2002;29:331–334.
57. Dessein PH, Shipton EA, Stanwix AE, et al. Beneficial effects of weight loss associated with moderate calorie/carbohydrate restriction, and increased proportional intake of protein and unsaturated fat on serum urate and lipoprotein levels in gout: A pilot study. Ann Rheum Dis 2000;59:539–543.
58. Riese RJ, Sakhaee K. Uric acid nephrolithiasis: Pathogenesis and treatment. J Urol 1992;148:765–771.
59. Pak CY, Sakhaee K, Fuller C. Successful management of uric acid nephrolithiasis with potassium citrate. Kidney Int 1986;30:422–428.
60. Ferraz MB, O'Brien B. A cost effectiveness analysis of urate lowering drugs in nontophaceous recurrent gouty arthritis. J Rheumatol 1995;22:908–914.
61. Dincer HE, Dincer AP, Levinson DJ. Asymptomatic hyperuricemia: To treat or not to treat. Cleve Clin J Med 2002;69:594–602.
62. Shoji A, Yamanaka H, Kamatani N. A retrospective study of the relationship between serum urate level and recurrent attacks of gouty arthritis: Evidence for reduction of recurrent gouty arthritis with antihyperuricemic therapy. Arthritis Rheum 2004;51:321–325.
63. Li-Yu J, Clayburne G, Sieck M, et al. Treatment of chronic gout. Can we determine when urate stores are depleted enough to prevent attacks of gout? J Rheumatol 2001;28:577–580.
64. Bull PW, Scott JT. Intermittent control of hyperuricemia in the treatment of gout. J Rheumatol 1989;16:1246–1248.
65. Riedel AA, Nelson M, Joseph-Ridge N, et al. Compliance with allopurinol therapy among managed care enrollees with gout: A retrospective analysis of administrative claims. J Rheumatol 2004;31:1575–1581.
66. Hande KR, Noone RM, Stone WJ. Severe allopurinol toxicity. Description and guidelines for prevention in patients with renal insufficiency. Am J Med 1984;76:47–56.
67. Vazquez-Mellado J, Morales EM, Pacheco-Tena C, Burgos-Vargas R. Relation between adverse events associated with allopurinol and renal function in patients with gout. Ann Rheum Dis 2001;60:981–983.
68. Fam AG. Difficult gout and new approaches for control of hyperuricemia in the allopurinol-allergic patient. Curr Rheumatol Rep 2001;3:29–35.
69. Fam AG, Dunne SM, Iazzetta J, Paton TW. Efficacy and safety of desensitization to allopurinol following cutaneous reactions. Arthritis Rheum 2001;44:231–238.
70. Harris M, Bryant LR, Danaher P, Alloway J. Effect of low dose daily aspirin on serum urate levels and urinary excretion in patients receiving probenecid for gouty arthritis. J Rheumatol 2000;27:2873–2876.
71. Becker MA, Schumacher HR, Wortmann RL, et al. Febuxostat compared with allopurinol in patients with hyperuricemia and gout. N Engl J Med 2005;353:2450–2461.
72. de la Serna G, Cadarso C. Fenofibrate decreases plasma fibrinogen, improves lipid profile, and reduces uricemia. Clin Pharmacol Ther 1999;66:166–172.
73. Feher MD, Hepburn AL, Hogarth MB, et al. Fenofibrate enhances urate reduction in men treated with allopurinol for hyperuricaemia and gout. Rheumatology 2003;42:321–325.
74. Hepburn AL, Kaye SA, Feher MD. Long-term remission from gout associated with fenofibrate therapy. Clin Rheumatol 2003;22:73–76.
75. Hepburn AL, Kaye SA, Feher MD. Fenofibrate: A new treatment for hyperuricaemia and gout? Ann Rheum Dis 2001;60:984–986.
76. Wurzner G, Gerster JC, Chiolero A, et al. Comparative effects of losartan and irbesartan on serum uric acid in hypertensive patients with hyperuricaemia and gout. J Hypertens 2001;19:1855–1860.
77. Shahinfar S, Simpson RL, Carides AD, et al. Safety of losartan in hypertensive patients with thiazide-induced hyperuricemia. Kidney Int 1999;56:1879–1885.
78. Abbott RD, Brand FN, Kannel WB, et al. Gout and coronary heart disease: The Framingham Study. J Clin Epidemiol 1988;41:237–242.
79. Freedman DS, Williamson DF, Gunter EW, et al. Relation of serum uric acid to mortality and ischemic heart disease. The NHANES I Epidemiologic Follow-up Study. Am J Epidemiol 1995;141:637–644.
80. Langford HG, Blaufox MD, Borhani NO, et al. Is thiazide-produced uric acid elevation harmful? Analysis of data from the Hypertension Detection and Follow-up Program. Arch Intern Med 1987;147:645–649.
81. Bengtsson C, Lapidus L, Stendahl C, Waldenstrom J. Hyperuricaemia and risk of cardiovascular disease and overall death. A 12-year follow-up of participants in the population study of women in Gothenburg, Sweden. Acta Med Scand 1988;224:549–555.
82. Gutman AB. The past four decades of progress in the knowledge of gout, with an assessment of the present status. Arthritis Rheum 1973;16:431–445.
83. Mikuls TR, MacLean CH, Olivieri J, et al. Quality of care indicators for gout management. Arthritis Rheum 2004;50:937–943.

SECTION 13
OPHTHALMIC AND OTOLARYNGOLOGIC DISORDERS

CHAPTER 97

Glaucoma

RICHARD G. FISCELLA, TIMOTHY S. LESAR, AND DEEPAK P. EDWARD

KEY CONCEPTS

1. Primary open-angle glaucoma (POAG) or ocular hypertension (ocular hypertension) is more prevalent than closed- or narrow-angle glaucoma.
2. In any form of glaucoma, reduction of intraocular pressure (IOP) is essential.
3. IOP is a very important risk factor for glaucoma, but the most important considerations are progression of glaucomatous changes in the back of the eye (optic disk and nerve fiber layer) and visual field changes when diagnosing and monitoring for POAG or ocular hypertension.
4. Optic nerve changes often occur before visual field changes are exhibited.
5. Recent studies demonstrate that reduction in IOP prevents progression or even onset of glaucoma.
6. Newer medications simplify treatment regimens for patients. Prostaglandin analogs are considered the most potent topical medications for reducing IOP and flattening diurnal variations in intraocular pressure.
7. Local adverse events are common with topical glaucoma medications, but patient education and reinforcing adherence are essential to prevent glaucoma progression.

The glaucomas are a group of ocular disorders that lead to an optic neuropathy characterized by changes in the optic nerve head (optic disk) that is associated with loss of visual sensitivity and field. Increased intraocular pressure (IOP), a traditional diagnostic criterion for glaucoma, is thought to play an important role in the pathogenesis of glaucoma, but is no longer a diagnostic criterion for glaucoma.[1–10] Two major types of glaucoma have been identified: open angle and closed angle. Open-angle glaucoma accounts for the great majority of cases. Either type can be a primary inherited disorder, congenital, or secondary to disease, trauma, or drugs, and can lead to serious complications.[11–16] Both primary and secondary glaucomas may be caused by a combination of open-angle and closed-angle mechanisms (Table 97–1).

Learning objectives, review questions, and other resources can be found at **www.pharmacotherapyonline.com.**

BASIC CONCEPTS

AQUEOUS HUMOR DYNAMICS AND INTRAOCULAR PRESSURE

An understanding of IOP and aqueous humor dynamics will assist the reader in understanding the drug therapy of glaucoma.[1,2,17–19]

Aqueous humor is formed in the ciliary body and its epithelium (Figs. 97–1 and 97–2) through both filtration and secretion. Because ultrafiltration depends on pressure gradients, blood pressure and IOP changes influence aqueous humor formation. Osmotic gradients produced by active secretion of sodium and bicarbonate, and possibly other solutes such as ascorbate from the ciliary body epithelial cells into the aqueous humor, result in movement of water from the pool of ciliary stromal ultrafiltrate into the posterior chamber, forming aqueous humor. Carbonic anhydrase (primarily isoenzyme type II), α- and β-adrenergic receptors, and sodium- and potassium-activated adenosine triphosphatases are found on the ciliary epithelium and appear to be involved in this secretion of the solutes sodium and bicarbonate.

Receptor systems controlling aqueous inflow have not been elucidated fully. Pharmacologic studies suggest that β-adrenergic agents increase inflow, whereas α_2-adrenergic blocking, α-adrenergic blocking, β-adrenergic blocking, dopamine-blocking, carbonic, anhydrase-inhibiting, and adenylate cyclase-stimulating agents decrease aqueous inflow. Aqueous humor produced by the ciliary body is secreted into the posterior chamber at a rate of approximately 2 to 3 μL/min. The pressure in the posterior chamber produced by the constant inflow pushes the aqueous humor between the iris and lens and through the pupil into the anterior chamber of the eye (see Fig. 97–2).[1,2,17–22]

Aqueous humor in the anterior chamber leaves the eye by two routes: (a) filtration through the trabecular meshwork (conventional outflow) to the Schlemm canal (80% to 85%) and (b) through the

TABLE 97-1 General Classification of Glaucoma

I. Primary glaucoma
A. Open angle
B. Angle closure
1. With pupillary block
2. Without pupillary block
II. Secondary glaucoma
A. Open angle
1. Pretrabecular
2. Trabecular
3. Posttrabecular
B. Angle closure
1. Without pupillary block
2. With pupillary block
III. Congenital glaucoma

ciliary body and the suprachoroidal space (uveoscleral outflow or unconventional outflow). Cholinergic agents such as pilocarpine increase outflow by physically opening the meshwork pores secondary to ciliary muscle contraction. The uveoscleral outflow of aqueous humor is also increased by prostaglandin analogs, and β- and α_2-adrenergic agonists. Constant inflow of aqueous humor from the ciliary body and resistance to outflow result in an IOP great enough to produce an outflow rate equal to the inflow rate (see Fig. 97–2).

The median IOP measured in large populations is 15.5 ± 2.5 mm Hg; however, the distribution of pressures around the mean is skewed to the right (toward higher readings). IOP is not constant and changes with pulse, blood pressure, forced expiration or coughing, neck compression, and posture. IOP is measured by tonometry: indentation tonometry, applanation tonometry, or a noncontact method using an air pulse. These methods may result in slightly different pressure readings. IOPs consistently greater than 21 mm Hg are found in 5% to 8% of the general population. The incidence increases with age, such that "abnormal" (i.e., >22 mm Hg) IOP is found in 15% of those 70 to 75 years of age. Intermittently high IOP (>40 mm Hg) is found in patients with closed-angle glaucoma (CAG). The increased IOP in all types of glaucoma results from the decreased facility for aqueous humor outflow through the trabecular meshwork. Aqueous humor production in primary open-angle glaucoma (POAG) is normal.[1,2,17–19]

IOP demonstrates considerable circadian variation (often referred to as *diurnal* IOP or the IOP during the daily 24-hour cycle)

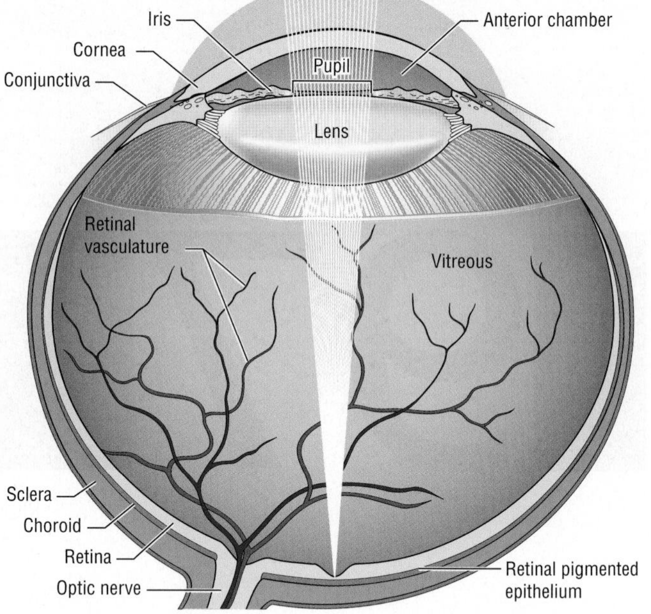

FIGURE 97-1. Anatomy of the eye.

primarily because of changes in the rate of aqueous humor formation. This circadian variation results in a minimum IOP at approximately 6 PM and a maximum IOP at awakening, although some studies suggest that both healthy and glaucoma patients may have their highest IOP at night after falling asleep.[20] Low systemic blood pressure in conjunction with high IOPs (decreased ocular perfusion pressure) at night can result in optic nerve head damage.[20] Generally, the circadian IOP variation is usually less than 3 to 4 mm Hg; however, it may be greater in patients with glaucoma. This circadian variation and the poor relationship of IOP with visual loss make measurement of IOP a poor screening test for glaucoma.

Although increased IOP within any range is associated with a higher risk of glaucomatous damage, it is both an insensitive and nonspecific diagnostic and monitoring tool. Of individuals with IOP between 21 and 30 mm Hg, only 0.5% to 1% per year will develop optic disk changes and visual field loss (i.e., glaucoma) over 5 to 15 years. However, more subtle retinal damage, such as alteration of color vision or decreased contrast sensitivity, occurs in a higher

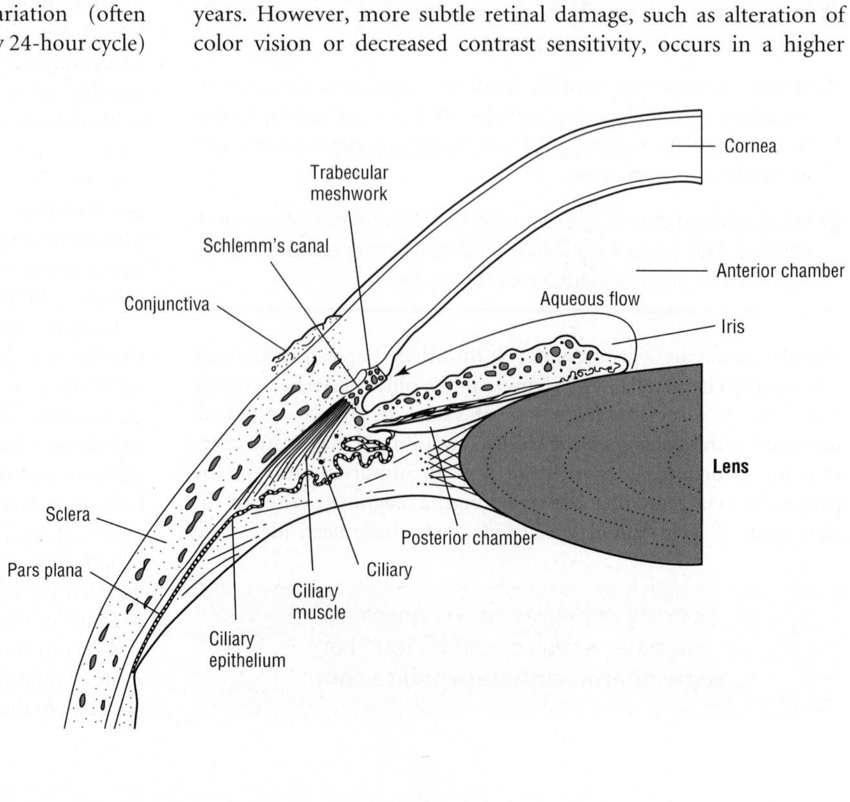

FIGURE 97-2. Anterior chamber of the eye and aqueous humor flow.

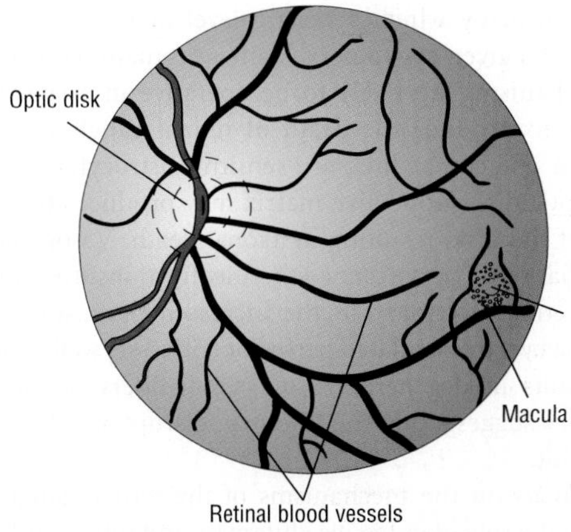

FIGURE 97-3. Normal fundus of the eye and optic disk and cup.

percentage of patients with IOPs greater than 21 mm Hg, and the incidence of visual field defects increases to as high as 28% in individuals with IOPs above 30 mm Hg. For a given abnormal IOP, the incidence of glaucoma increases with age. In patients with preexisting optic nerve damage, the worse the existing damage, the more sensitive the eye is to a given IOP. As many as 20% to 30% of patients with glaucomatous visual field loss have an IOP of less than 21 mm Hg (called *normal-tension glaucoma,* referring to the normal IOP). Thus the absolute IOP is a less-precise predictor of optic nerve damage. More direct measurements of therapeutic outcome, such as optic disk examination and visual-field evaluation, also must be used as monitors of disease progression.[1–7,17–24] Taking the above factors into consideration, glaucoma medications that provide maximal reduction of IOP over 24 hours and have minimal influence on blood pressure may be advantageous in treating glaucoma patients.

OPTIC DISK AND VISUAL FIELDS

The optic disk is the portion of the optic nerve ophthalmoscopically visible as it leaves the eye. It consists of approximately 1 million retinal ganglion nerve cell axons, blood vessels, and supporting connective tissue structures (lamina cribrosa). The small depression within the disk is termed the *cup* (Fig. 97–3). A normal physiologic cup does not extend beyond the optic nerve rim and has a varying diameter of less than one-third to one-half that of the disk (cup-to-disk ratio: 0.33 to 0.5). Table 97–2 lists the common alterations of the optic disk found in glaucoma. These disk changes result from optic nerve axonal degeneration and remodeling of the supporting structures. As the nerve axons die, the cup becomes larger in relation to the whole disk. A loss of retinal nerve fiber layer visibility might be visualized in glaucoma patients with detectable visual field loss. This pattern of changes is consistent with visual field losses and loss of visual sensitivity seen in glaucoma.[1,2,17–24]

Determination of the visual field allows assessment of optic nerve damage and is an important monitoring parameter in treatment. However, visual field changes lag behind optic disk changes, and a loss of 25% to 35% of retinal ganglion cells is usually required before detectable visual field defects are noted. The peripheral visual field is measured using a visual field instrument called a *perimeter.* Characteristic visual field loss occurs in glaucoma (Fig. 97–4; see also Table

TABLE 97-2 Optic Disk and Visual Field Findings

Optic disk
Cup-to-disk ratio >0.5
Progressive increase in cup size
Cup-to-disk ratio asymmetry >0.2
Vertical elongation of the cup
Excavation of the cup
Increased exposure of lamina cribrosa
Pallor of the cup
Splinter hemorrhages
Cupping to edge of disk
Notching of the cup (usually superior or inferior)
Nerve fiber defects
Visual field findings
General peripheral field constriction
Isolated scotomas (blind spots)
Nasal visual field depression ("nasal step")
Enlargement of blind spot
Large arc-like scotomas
Reduced contrast sensitivity
Reduced peripheral acuity
Altered color vision

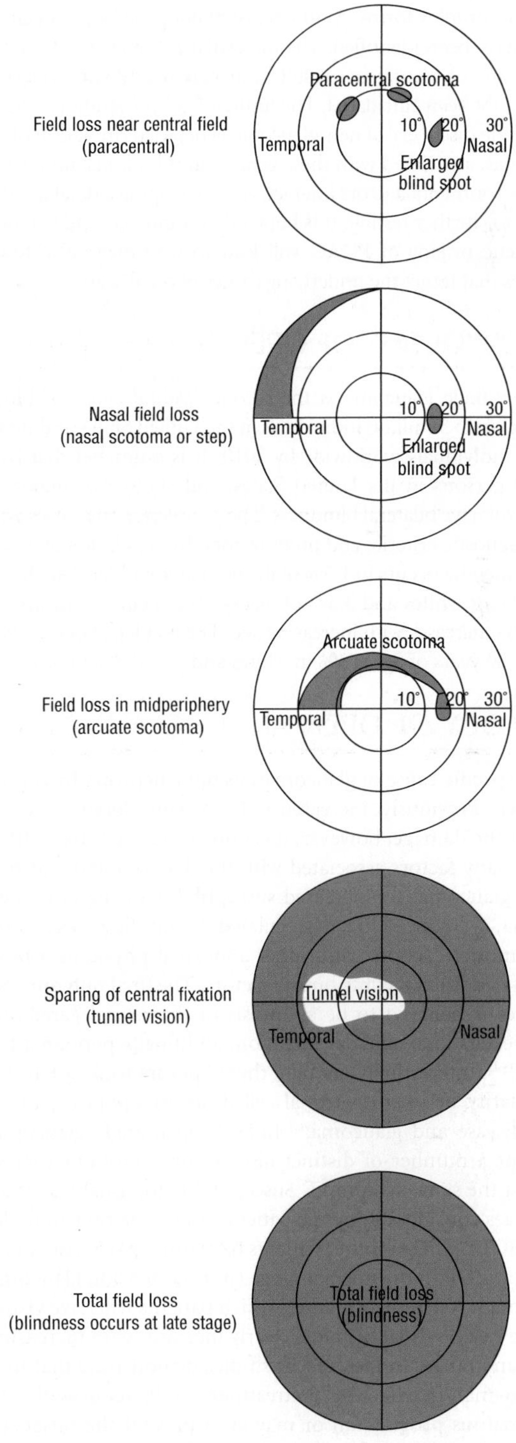

FIGURE 97-4. Schematic of the progression of visual field loss in glaucoma.

97–2), but loss of central visual acuity usually does not occur until late in the disease. Other indicators, such as color vision changes and contrast sensitivity, may allow earlier and more sensitive detection of glaucomatous changes.[1,2]

GENETICS

Glaucoma is often inherited as a complex multifactorial disease, but it can also be inherited as a mendelian autosomal-dominant or autosomal-recessive trait form. The common age-related adult-onset glaucoma, like POAG, although containing heritability of some significance, is more complex and is influenced by environmental factors. Genetic studies have more clearly defined the underlying molecular events responsible for the mendelian forms of the disease. However, the chromosome locations identified may play some factor in the more complex forms. A number of major gene loci associated with POAG have been identified. The molecular mechanism of how mutations in any of these genes result in increased IOP with loss of visual field has not been elucidated. The future of genetic studies in glaucoma will include discovery of new glaucoma genes, determination of clinical phenotypes associated with these genes and mutations, understanding how environmental factors interact, and developing a database that can be used for further testing. It is hoped that improved understanding of the genetic origins of POAG will lead to new diagnostic tools and therapies that target the underlying causes of the disease.[1,2,25,26]

EPIDEMIOLOGY OF OPEN-ANGLE GLAUCOMA

❶ Open-angle glaucoma is the second leading cause of blindness, affecting up to 3 million individuals in the United States and up to 60.5 million individuals worldwide by 2010. It is estimated that by 2010, 135,000 persons in the United States, and about 4.5 million in the world, will have bilateral blindness. The prevalence rate varies with age, race, diagnostic criteria, and other factors. In the United States, open-angle glaucoma occurs in 1.5% of the population older than 30 years of age, 1.3% of whites and 3.5% of blacks. The incidence of open-angle glaucoma increases with increasing age. The incidence of the disease in patients 80 years of age is 3% in whites and 5% to 8% in blacks.

ETIOLOGY OF OPEN-ANGLE GLAUCOMA

❷ The specific cause of glaucomatous optic neuropathy is presently unknown. Previously, increased IOP was considered to be the sole cause of the damage; however, it is now recognized that IOP is only one of many factors associated with the development and progression of glaucoma.[1–10] Increased susceptibility of the optic nerve to ischemia, a reduced or dysregulated blood flow, excitotoxicity, autoimmune reactions, and other abnormal physiologic processes are likely additional contributory factors. The final outcome of these processes is believed to be apoptosis of the retinal ganglion cells, which results in axonal degeneration, and finally permanent loss of vision.[11–16] Interestingly enough, there appears to be a fair amount of similarity between neuronal cell death by apoptosis in Alzheimer's disease and glaucoma.[13] Indeed, open-angle glaucoma may represent a number of distinct diseases or conditions that simply manifest the same symptoms. Susceptibility to visual loss at a given IOP varies considerably; some patients do not demonstrate damage at high IOPs, whereas other patients have progressive visual field loss despite an IOP in the normal range (normal-tension glaucoma).

Although IOP poorly predicts which patients will have visual field loss, the risk of visual field loss clearly increases with increasing IOP within any range. In fact, recent studies demonstrate that lowering IOP, no matter what the pretreatment IOP, reduces the risk of glaucomatous progression or may even prevent the onset to early glaucoma in patients with ocular hypertension.[3–7]

The mechanism by which a certain level of IOP increases the susceptibility of a given eye to nerve damage remains controversial. Multiple mechanisms are likely to be operative in a spectrum of combinations to produce the death of retinal ganglion cells and their axons in glaucoma. Pressure-sensitive astrocytes and other cells in the optic disk supportive matrix may produce changes and remodeling of the disk, resulting in axonal death. Vasogenic theories suggest that optic nerve damage results from insufficient blood flow to the retina secondary to the increased perfusion pressure required in the eye, dysregulated perfusion, or vessel wall abnormalities, and results in degeneration of axonal fibers of the retina. Another theory suggests that the IOP may disrupt axoplasmal flow at the optic disk.

Recently, focus on the mechanisms of the retinal ganglion cell apoptosis and the role of excessive glutamate and nitric oxide found in glaucoma patients has broadened the focus of drug therapy research to include evaluation of agents that act as neuroprotectants.[12–15] Such agents may be particularly useful in patients with normal-pressure glaucoma, in whom pressure-independent factors may play a relatively larger role in disease progression. These agents would target risk factors and underlying pathophysiologic mechanisms of disease other than IOP.[11–16]

PATHOPHYSIOLOGY OF OPEN-ANGLE GLAUCOMA

❸ As stated previously, optic nerve damage in POAG can occur at a wide range of intraocular pressures, and the rate of progression is highly variable. Patients may exhibit pressures in the 20 to 30 mm Hg range for years before any disease progression is noticed in the optic disk or visual fields. That is why open-angle glaucoma is often referred to as the "sneak thief of sight."

CLINICAL PRESENTATION OF GLAUCOMA

General

- Glaucoma can be detected in otherwise asymptomatic patients, or patients can present with characteristic symptoms, especially vision loss. POAG is a chronic, slowly progressive disease found primarily in patients older than 50 years of age, whereas CAG is more typically associated with symptomatic acute episodes.

Symptoms

- POAG: None until substantial visual field loss occurs.
- CAG: Nonsymptomatic or prodromal symptoms (blurred or hazy vision with halos around lights that is caused by a hazy, edematous cornea, and occasionally headache) may be present. Acute episodes produce symptoms associated with a cloudy, edematous cornea, ocular pain or discomfort, nausea, vomiting, abdominal pain, and diaphoresis.

Signs

- POAG: Disk changes and visual field loss (see Table 97–2); IOP can be normal or elevated (>21 mm Hg).
- CAG: Hyperemic conjunctiva, cloudy cornea, shallow anterior chamber, and occasionally an edematous and hyperemic optic disk; IOP is generally elevated markedly (40 to 90 mm Hg) when symptoms are present.

Laboratory Tests

- None

Other Diagnostic Tests

- Emerging tests include optical coherence tomography, retinal nerve fiber analyzers, and confocal scanning laser tomography of the optic nerve.

CLINICAL PRESENTATION OF OPEN-ANGLE GLAUCOMA

POAG is a bilateral, genetically determined disorder constituting 60% to 70% of all glaucomas and 90% to 95% of primary glaucomas (see Clinical Presentation of Glaucoma above). An increased IOP is not required for diagnosis of POAG. Symptoms do not present until substantial visual field constriction occurs. Central visual acuity typically is maintained, even in the late stages of the disease. Even though POAG is a bilateral disease, it may have greater progression and severity in one eye.

❹ Detection and diagnosis involve evaluation of the optic disk and retinal nerve fiber layer, assessment of the visual fields, and measurement of IOP. The presence of characteristic disk changes and visual field loss with or without increased IOP confirms the diagnosis of glaucoma. Typical disk changes and field loss occurring at an IOP of less than 21 mm Hg account for 20% to 30% of patients and are referred to as *normal-tension glaucoma.* Elevated IOP (>21 mm Hg) without disk changes or visual field loss is observed in 5% to 7% of individuals (known as *glaucoma suspects*) and is referred to as *ocular hypertension.* New technologies such as optical coherence tomography, retinal nerve fiber analyzers, or confocal scanning laser tomography of the optic nerve head may allow early identification of signs of glaucomatous retinal changes in ocular hypertensives, thus allowing for earlier initiation of therapy.[1–3,17]

Secondary open-angle glaucoma has many causes, including exfoliation syndrome, pigmentary glaucoma, systemic diseases, trauma, surgery, ocular inflammatory diseases, and medications. A system for classifying secondary glaucomas into pretrabecular, trabecular, and posttrabecular forms has been proposed. This classification allows drug therapy to be chosen on the basis of the pathogenic mechanism involved. In pretrabecular forms, a normal meshwork is covered that does not permit aqueous humor outflow. Trabecular forms of secondary glaucoma result from either an alteration of meshwork or an accumulation of material in the intertrabecular spaces. The posttrabecular forms result primarily from disorders causing increased episcleral venous blood pressure.[1,2,15–17]

PROGNOSIS OF OPEN-ANGLE GLAUCOMA

❺ In most cases of POAG, the overall prognosis is excellent when it is discovered early and treated adequately. Even patients with advanced visual field loss can have continued visual field loss reduced if the IOP is maintained at low enough pressures (often <10 to 12 mm Hg). Progression of visual field loss still occurs in 8% to 20% of patients despite reaching standard therapy IOP goals. However, in untreated patients and in those who fail to achieve target IOP reduction, up to 80% have continued visual field loss. Estimates of progression to bilateral blindness in treated patients range from 4% to 22%. Thus the keys to medical treatment of POAG are an effective, well-tolerated drug regimen, close monitoring of therapy, and adherence. Medications will control IOP successfully in 60% to 80% of patients over a 5-year period. Availability of newer, highly effective, well-tolerated agents may improve the prognosis further.[1,2,5,17–19,23–28]

EPIDEMIOLOGY OF CLOSED-ANGLE GLAUCOMA

The incidence of closed-angle glaucoma varies by ethnic group, with a higher incidence in individuals of Inuit, Chinese, and Asian-Indian descent. Incidence rates of 1% to 4% have been reported in these populations.[1,2]

ETIOLOGY OF CLOSED-ANGLE GLAUCOMA (ANGLE-CLOSURE GLAUCOMA)

Primary CAG accounts for 5% or less of primary glaucomas; however, when CAG occurs, it may need to be treated as an emergency to avoid visual loss. CAG results from mechanical blockage of the (usually normal) trabecular meshwork by the peripheral iris. Partial or complete blockage of the meshwork occurs intermittently, resulting in extreme fluctuations between normal IOP with no symptoms, and very high IOP with symptoms of acute CAG. Between attacks of CAG, the IOP is usually normal unless the patient has concomitant open-angle glaucoma or nonreversible blockage of the meshwork with synechiae ("creeping" angle closure) that develops over time in the narrow-angle eye. Primary CAG occurs in patients with inherited shallow anterior chambers, which produce a narrow angle between the cornea and iris or tight contact between the iris and lens (pupillary block). The presence of a narrow angle is determined mainly by visualization of the angle by gonioscopy. Other tests for CAG involve provocation of an angle-closure–induced IOP increase. These tests, which attempt to produce angle closure through mydriasis (darkroom test or mydriasis test), or gravity (prone test), are rarely performed in the clinical setting.

Two major types of classic, reversible primary CAG have been described: CAG with pupillary block and CAG without pupillary block. CAG with pupillary block results when the iris is in firm contact with the lens. This produces a relative block of aqueous flow through the pupil to the anterior chamber (pupillary block), resulting in a bowing forward of the iris, which blocks the trabecular meshwork. CAG with pupillary block occurs most commonly when the pupil is in middilation. In this position, the combination of pupillary block and relaxed iris allows the greatest bowing of the iris; however, angle closure may occur during miosis or mydriasis.

CAG can occur without significant pupillary block in patients with an abnormality called a *plateau iris.* The ciliary processes in these cases are situated anteriorly, which indent the iris forward and cause closure of the trabecular meshwork, especially during mydriasis. The mydriasis produced by anticholinergic drugs or any other drug results in precipitation of both types of CAG glaucoma, whereas drug-induced miosis may produce pupillary block.

PATHOPHYSIOLOGY OF CLOSED-ANGLE GLAUCOMA

The mechanism of IOP elevation in CAG is clearer than that of POAG. In CAG, a physical blockage of trabecular meshwork is present. In many cases, single or multiple episodes of excessively high IOP (>40 mm Hg) result in optic nerve damage. Very high IOP (>60 mm Hg) may result in permanent loss of visual field within a matter of hours to days.

One type of CAG, known as "creeping" angle closure, occurs in patients with narrow angles in which the iris adheres to the trabecular meshwork and may result in continuously increased IOP in ranges more similar to those of POAG, and the clinical behavior is similar to POAG, with individuals differing in the degree and rapidity of visual loss from any given elevated IOP.[1]

CLINICAL PRESENTATION OF CLOSED-ANGLE GLAUCOMA

Patients with untreated CAG typically experience intermittent nonsymptomatic or prodromal symptoms brought on by precipitating events (see Clinical Presentation of Glaucoma above). Increased IOP during such prodromal episodes is not great enough or long enough to produce the other symptoms of a full-blown

TABLE 97-3 Drugs That May Induce or Potentiate Increased Intraocular Pressure

Open-angle glaucoma
Ophthalmic corticosteroids (high risk)
Systemic corticosteroids
Nasal/inhaled corticosteroids
Fenoldopam
Ophthalmic anticholinergics
Succinylcholine
Vasodilators (low risk)
Cimetidine (low risk)
Closed-angle glaucoma
Topical anticholinergics
Topical sympathomimetics
Systemic anticholinergics
Heterocyclic antidepressants
Low-potency phenothiazines
Antihistamines
Ipratropium
Benzodiazepines (low risk)
Theophylline (low risk)
Vasodilators (low risk)
Systemic sympathomimetics (low risk)
Central nervous system stimulants (low risk)
Serotonin selective reuptake inhibitors
Imipramine
Venlafaxine
Topiramate
Tetracyclines (low risk)
Carbonic anhydrase inhibitors (low risk)
Monoamine oxidase inhibitors (low risk)
Topical cholinergics (low risk)

attack. Such prodromal attacks last 1 to 2 hours, at which time pupillary block is broken by further mydriasis or miosis; or when miosis or mydriasis occurs in patients with plateau iris. The rate at which IOP increases may be a determinant of when full-blown symptoms occur. Visual fields demonstrate generalized constriction or typical glaucomatous defects. In prolonged attacks, total loss of vision may occur if the IOP is high enough. Tonometry reveals IOPs as high as 40 to 90 mm Hg. Patients who have developed adhesions between the iris and meshwork (anterior synechiae) may have chronic IOP elevation with intermittent spikes of high IOP when angle closure occurs.

DRUG-INDUCED GLAUCOMA

A number of medications are associated with increased IOP or carry labeling that cautions against use of the medication in glaucoma patients. The potential for a medication to produce or worsen glaucoma depends on the type of glaucoma and whether or not the patient is treated adequately.[25]

Patients with treated, controlled POAG are at minimal risk of induction of an increase in IOP by systemic medications with anticholinergic properties or vasodilators; however, in patients with untreated glaucoma or uncontrolled POAG, the potential of these medications to increase IOP should be considered. Topical anticholinergic agents used to produce mydriasis may result in an increase in IOP. Potent anticholinergic agents such as atropine or homatropine are most likely to increase IOP. Weaker anticholinergics, such as tropicamide, that produce less cycloplegia are less likely to increase IOP and are favored, along with phenylephrine, when mydriasis is desired in POAG patients. Inhaled, nasal, topical, or systemic glucocorticoids may increase IOP in both normal individuals and patients with POAG.

Patients with POAG appear to be particularly susceptible to glucocorticoid-induced increases in IOP. Glucocorticoids reduce the facility of aqueous humor outflow through the trabecular meshwork. The decreased facility of outflow appears to result from the accumulation of extracellular material blocking the trabecular channels. The potential of a glucocorticoid to increase IOP is related to its antiinflammatory potency and intraocular penetration. Thus patients should be treated with the lowest potency and dose and for the shortest time possible when steroids are indicated.

In patients predisposed to CAG (i.e., narrow anterior chambers), angle closure may be produced by any drug that causes mydriasis (e.g., anticholinergics). A wide range of sulfa compounds cause idiosyncratic reactions that result in anterior choroidal effusions with anterior movement of the iris and lens, resulting in angle closure. The topical use of anticholinergics or sympathomimetic agents most likely will result in angle closure. Systemic and inhaled anticholinergic and sympathomimetic agents also must be used with caution in such patients. As discussed previously, potent miotic agents such as echothiophate may produce angle closure by increasing pupillary block. Table 97–3 lists the drugs associated with potentiation of glaucoma.

TREATMENT

Ocular Hypertension

Treatment of the patient with possible glaucoma (ocular hypertension; i.e., patients with IOP >22 mm Hg) is less controversial than it was in the past, with the recent results of the Ocular Hypertensive Treatment Study (OHTS).[3] The OHTS helped to identify risk factors for treatment. Patients with intraocular pressures higher than 25 mm Hg, vertical cup-to-disk ratio of more than 0.5, and central corneal thickness of less than 555 micrometers are at greater risk for developing glaucoma. Risk factors such as family history of glaucoma, black ethnicity, severe myopia, and patients with only one eye must also be taken into consideration when deciding which individuals need treatment.

Patients without risk factors typically are not treated and are monitored for the development of glaucomatous changes. Patients with significant risk factors usually are treated with a well-tolerated topical agent such as a β-blocking agent, an α_2-agonist (brimonidine), a topical carbonic anhydrase inhibitor (CAI), or a prostaglandin analog, depending on individual patient characteristics. Optimally, therapy is initiated in one eye to assess efficacy and tolerance. Use of second- or third-line agents (e.g., pilocarpine or dipivefrin) when first-line agents fail to reduce IOP depends on the risk-to-benefit assessment of each patient. The cost, inconvenience, and frequent adverse effects of combination therapies, anticholinesterase inhibitors, and oral CAIs result in an unfavorable risk-to-benefit ratio in patients with possible glaucoma.[29]

The goal of therapy is to lower the IOP to a level associated with a decreased risk of optic nerve damage, usually at least a 20%, if not a 25% to 30%, decrease from the baseline IOP. Greater decreases may be required in high-risk patients or those with higher initial IOPs. Drug therapy should be monitored by measurement of IOP, examination of the optic disk, assessment of the visual fields, and evaluation of the patient for drug adverse effects and compliance with therapy. Patients who are unresponsive to or intolerant of a drug should be switched to an alternative agent rather than given an additional drug. Many clinicians prefer to discontinue all medications in patients who fail to respond adequately to simple topical therapy, closely monitor for development of disk changes or visual field loss, and treat again when such changes occur.[1,2,17–19,29]

More recently risk calculators have been suggested as a means of determining who are at greatest risk in developing glaucoma. It is hoped that with future improvement in such calculators, one would be able to tailor treatment to those at greatest risk for developing glaucoma.

TREATMENT

Open-Angle Glaucoma

All patients with elevated IOP and characteristic optic disk changes and/or visual field defects not caused by other factors (i.e., glaucoma by definition) should be treated. Recent findings that 1 in 5 patients with "normal" IOP and glaucomatous retinal nerve findings (i.e., normal-tension glaucoma) do not have progression of visual field loss if left untreated have prompted recommendations to monitor normal-tension glaucoma patients without immediate threat of loss of central vision, and treat only when progression is documented. Some controversy exists as to whether the initial therapy of glaucoma should be surgical trabeculectomy (filtering procedure), argon laser trabeculectomy, or medical therapy.[1,2,17,18] Presently, drug therapy remains the most common initial treatment modality. Drug therapy of patients with documented glaucomatous change with either elevated or normal IOP is initiated in a stepwise manner (Fig. 97–5), starting with lower concentrations of a single, well-tolerated topical agent. The goal of therapy is to prevent further visual loss. A "target" IOP is chosen based on a patient baseline IOP and the amount of existing visual field loss. Typically, an initial target IOP reduction of 30% is desired. Greater reductions may be desired in patients with very high baseline IOPs or advanced visual field loss. Patients with normal baseline IOPs (normal-tension glaucoma) may have target IOPs of less than 10 to 12 mm Hg.

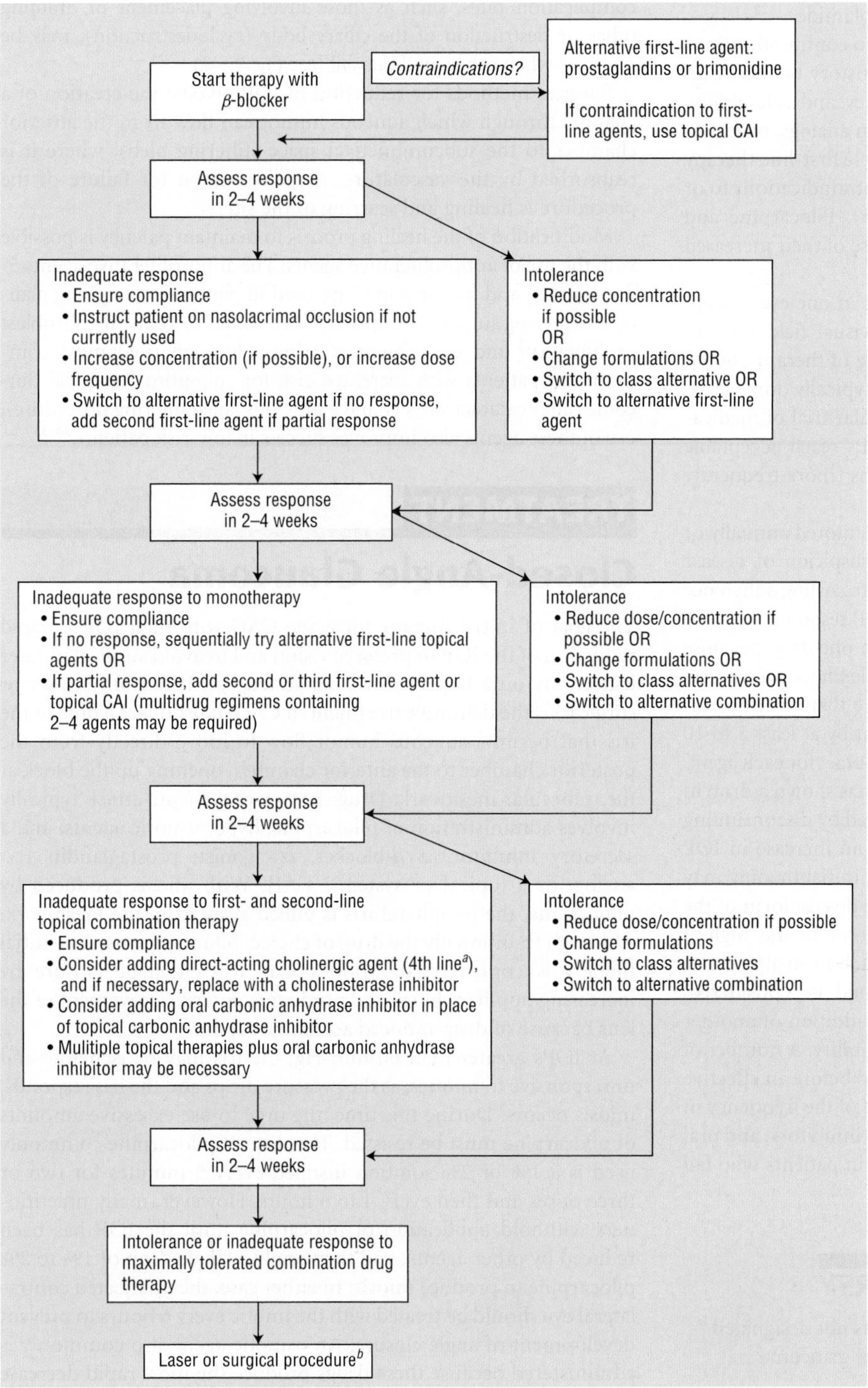

FIGURE 97-5. Algorithm for the pharmacotherapy of open-angle glaucoma. [a]Fourth-line agents not commonly used any longer. [b]Most clinicians believe laser procedure should be performed earlier (e.g., after three-drug maximum, poorly adherent patient). (CAI, carbonic anhydrase inhibitor.)

CLINICAL CONTROVERSY

How much should the IOP be reduced in patients who may have POAG? Although the major clinical trial (OHTS[3]) required a 20% reduction in IOP for patients with ocular hypertension, many clinicians believe a further lowering of IOP may be more beneficial in preventing the progression of ocular hypertension to glaucoma. The American Academy of Ophthalmology Preferred Practice Guidelines suggest 20% to 30% IOP lowering. It remains to be seen if a more aggressive approach earlier in the treatment of the POAG suspect would be more beneficial.

PHARMACOTHERAPEUTIC APPROACH

❻ Medications most commonly used to treat glaucoma are the nonselective β-blockers, the prostaglandin analogs (latanoprost, travoprost, and bimatoprost), brimonidine (an α_2-agonist), and the fixed combination product of timolol and dorzolamide.[21–22]

Before 1996, a β-blocker was used provided no contraindications existed, because this class of drugs has a long history of successful use, providing a combination of clinical efficacy and tolerability. The newer agents, in particular the prostaglandin analogs, brimonidine, and topical CAIs, are also considered suitable first-line therapy or alternative initial therapy in patients with contraindications to or other concerns with β-blockers (see Fig. 97–5). Pilocarpine and dipivefrin are used as third-line therapies because of their increased frequency of adverse effects or reduced efficacy.

Therapy optimally is started as a single agent in one eye (except in patients with very high IOP or advanced visual field loss) to evaluate drug efficacy and tolerance. Monitoring of therapy should be individualized: Initial response to therapy is typically done 4 to 6 weeks after the medication is started. A monocular trial of medication is recommended when possible. Once IOPs reach acceptable levels, the IOP is monitored every 3 to 4 months (more frequently after any change in drug therapy).

Visual fields and disk changes are typically monitored annually or earlier if the glaucoma is unstable or there is suspicion of disease worsening. Patients should always be questioned regarding adherence to and tolerance of prescribed therapy. Initial IOP response does not predict long-term IOP control. Using more than one drop per dose does not improve response, but increases the likelihood of adverse effects and the cost of therapy. When using more than one medication, separation of drop instillation of each agent by at least 5 to 10 minutes is suggested to provide optimal ocular contact for each agent.

The value of an agent with which the patient has shown a drop in IOP following an initial response can be measured by discontinuing the medication completely and determining if an increase in IOP occurs. Patients responding to but intolerant of initial therapy may be switched to another drug or to an alternative dosage form of the same medication. For patients failing to respond to the highest tolerated concentrations of an initial drug, a switch to an alternative agent after 1 day of concurrent therapy should be considered. Alternatively, if only a partial response occurs, addition of another topical drug to be used in combination is a possibility. A number of drugs or drug combinations may need to be tried before an effective and well-tolerated regimen is identified. Because of the frequency of adverse effects, carbachol, topical cholinesterase inhibitors, and oral CAIs are considered last-line agents to be used in patients who fail less-toxic combination topical therapy.

CLINICAL CONTROVERSY

The American Academy of Ophthalmology has not designated any agent as the drug of choice for initiation of glaucoma treatment. In recent years, many clinicians have used the prostaglandin analogs because they are dosed once daily and achieve the best pressure reduction. However, others believe that even though the β-blockers are less potent in reducing IOP, they should still be used as initial agents because they are dosed once or twice daily and are available as generic products, and thus are more cost-effective.

NONPHARMACOLOGIC THERAPY: LASER AND SURGICAL PROCEDURES

When drug therapy fails, is not tolerated, or is excessively complicated, surgical procedures such as laser trabeculoplasty (argon or selective) or a surgical trabeculectomy (filtering procedure) may be performed to improve outflow. Laser trabeculoplasty is usually an intermediate step between drug therapy and trabeculectomy. Procedures with higher complication rates, such as those involving placement of draining tubes or destruction of the ciliary body (cyclodestruction), may be required when other methods fail (see Fig. 97–2).[1,2,25]

Surgical methods for reduction of IOP involve the creation of a channel through which aqueous humor can flow from the anterior chamber to the subconjunctival space (filtering bleb), where it is reabsorbed by the vasculature. A major reason for failure of the procedure is healing and scarring of the site.

Modification of the healing process to maintain patency is possible with the use of antiproliferative agents. The antiproliferative agents 5-fluorouracil and mitomycin C are used in patients undergoing glaucoma-filtering surgery to improve success rates by reducing fibroblast proliferation and consequent scarring. Although used most commonly in patients with increased risk for suboptimal surgical outcome (after cataract surgery and a previous failed filtering procedure), use of these agents also improves success in low-risk patients.[30–33]

TREATMENT

Closed-Angle Glaucoma

The goal of initial therapy for acute CAG with high IOP is rapid reduction of the IOP to preserve vision and to avoid surgical or laser iridectomy on a hypertensive, congested eye. Iridectomy (laser or surgical) is the definitive treatment of CAG; it produces a hole in the iris that permits aqueous humor flow to move directly from the posterior chamber to the anterior chamber, opening up the block at the trabecular meshwork. Drug therapy of an acute attack typically involves administration of pilocarpine, hyperosmotic agents, and a secretory inhibitor (a β-blocker, α_2-agonist, prostaglandin $F_2\alpha$ analog, or a topical or systemic CAI). With miosis produced by pilocarpine, the peripheral iris is pulled away from the meshwork. Although traditionally the drug of choice, pilocarpine used as initial therapy is controversial. Miotics may worsen angle closure by increasing pupillary block and producing anterior movement of the lens because of drug-induced accommodation.

At IOPs greater than 60 mm Hg, the iris may be ischemic and unresponsive to miotics; as the pressure drops and the iris responds, miosis occurs. During this time, the urge to use excessive amounts of pilocarpine must be resisted. The dose of pilocarpine commonly used is a 1% or 2% solution instilled every 5 minutes for two or three doses and then every 4 to 6 hours. However, many practitioners withhold application of pilocarpine until the IOP has been reduced by other agents, and then apply a single drop of 1% to 2% pilocarpine to produce miosis. In either case, the unaffected contralateral eye should be treated with the miotic every 6 hours to prevent development of angle closure. An osmotic agent also commonly is administered because these drugs produce the most rapid decrease in IOP. Oral glycerin 1 to 2 g/kg can be used if an oral agent is tolerated; if not, intravenous mannitol 1 to 2 g/kg should be used. Osmotic agents reduce IOP by withdrawing water from the eye secondary to the osmotic gradient between the blood and the eyes. These drugs are among the first-line agents in the short-term treatment of CAG or other forms of acute very high IOP elevations. Topical corticosteroids often are used to reduce the ocular inflammation and reduce the development of synechiae in CAG eyes. In classic CAG, once the IOP is controlled, pilocarpine may be given every 6 hours until iridectomy is performed. Patients failing therapy altogether will require an emergency iridectomy.

Peripheral iridectomy essentially "cures" primary CAG without significant synechiae. Long-term drug therapy is not used unless IOP remains high because of the presence of synechiae blocking the trabecular meshwork or concurrent POAG. In such cases, the pharmacotherapeutic approach is essentially identical to that for the POAG patient, or laser or surgical procedures are performed.[1,2]

PHARMACOLOGIC AGENTS USED IN GLAUCOMA

β-BLOCKING DRUGS

The topical β-blocking agents are one of the most commonly used antiglaucoma medications (Table 97–4). β-Blockers lower IOP by

TABLE 97-4 Topical Drugs Used in the Treatment of Open-Angle Glaucoma

Drug	Pharmacologic Properties	Common Brand Names	Dose Form	Strength (%)	Usual Dose[a]	Mechanism of Action
β-Adrenergic blocking agents						
Betaxolol	Relative β_1-selective	Generic	Solution	0.5	1 drop twice a day	All reduce aqueous production of ciliary body
		Betoptic-S	Suspension	0.25	1 drop twice a day	
Carteolol	Nonselective, intrinsic sympathomimetic activity	Generic	Solution	1	1 drop twice a day	
Levobunolol	Nonselective	Betagan	Solution	0.25, 0.5	1 drop twice a day	
Metipranolol	Nonselective	OptiPranolol	Solution	0.3	1 drop twice a day	
Timolol	Nonselective	Timoptic, Betimol, Istalol	Solution	0.25, 0.5	1 drop every day–one to two times a day	
		Timoptic-XE	Gelling solution	0.25, 0.5	1 drop every day[a]	
Nonspecific adrenergic agonists						
Dipivefrin	Prodrug	Propine	Solution	0.1	1 drop twice a day	Increased aqueous humor outflow
α_2-Adrenergic agonists						
Apraclonidine	Specific α_2-agonists	Iopidine	Solution	0.5, 1	1 drop two to three times a day	Both reduce aqueous humor production; brimonidine known to also increase uveoscleral outflow
Brimonidine		Alphagan P	Solution	0.15, 0.1	1 drop two to three times a day	
Cholinergic agonists direct acting						
Carbachol	Irreversible	Carboptic, Isopto Carbachol	Solution	1.5, 3	1 drop two to three times a day	All increase aqueous humor outflow through trabecular meshwork
Pilocarpine	Irreversible	Isopto Carpine, Pilocar	Solution	0.25, 0.5, 1, 2, 4, 6, 8, 10	1 drop two to three times a day 1 drop four times a day	
		Pilopine HS	Gel	4	Every 24 h at bedtime	
Cholinesterase inhibitors						
Echothiophate		Phospholine Iodide	Solution	0.125	Once or twice a day	
Carbonic anhydrase inhibitors						
Topical						
Brinzolamide	Carbonic anhydrase type II inhibition	Azopt	Suspension	1	Two to three times a day	All reduce aqueous humor production of ciliary body
Dorzolamide		Trusopt	Solution	2	Two to three times a day	
Systemic						
Acetazolamide		Generic	Tablet	125 mg, 250 mg	125–250 mg two to four times a day	
			Injection	500 mg/vial	250–500 mg	
		Diamox Sequels	Capsule	500 mg	500 mg twice a day	
Methazolamide		Generic	Tablet	25 mg, 50 mg	25–50 mg two to three times a day	
Prostaglandin analogs						
Latanoprost	Prostaglandin $F_{2\alpha}$ analog	Xalatan	Solution	0.005	1 drop every night	Increases aqueous uveoscleral outflow and to a lesser extent trabecular outflow
Bimatoprost	Prostamide analog	Lumigan	Solution	0.03	1 drop every night	
Travoprost		Travatan, Travatan Z	Solution	0.004	1 drop every night	
Combinations						
Timolol-dorzolamide		Cosopt	Solution	Timolol 0.5% dorzolamide 2%	1 drop twice daily	
Timolol-brimonidine		Combigan	Solution	Timolol 0.5% brimonide 0.2%	1 drop twice daily	

[a]Use of nasolacrimal occlusion will increase number of patients successfully treated with longer dosage intervals.

20% to 30% with a minimum of local ocular adverse effects. These are commonly one of the agents of first choice in treating POAG if no contraindications exist.[1,2,17–19,34–36]

The β-blocking agents produce ocular hypotensive effects by decreasing the production of aqueous humor by the ciliary body without producing substantial effects on aqueous humor outflow facility. The mechanism by which β-blockers decrease aqueous humor inflow remains controversial, but it is most frequently attributed to β_2-adrenergic receptor blockade in the ciliary body.

Five ophthalmic β-blockers are presently available: timolol, levobunolol, metipranolol, carteolol, and betaxolol. Timolol, levobunolol, and metipranolol are nonspecific β-blocking agents, whereas betaxolol is a relatively β_1-selective agent. Carteolol is a nonspecific blocker with intrinsic sympathomimetic activity. Despite differences in potency, selectivity, lipophilicity, and intrinsic sympathomimetic activity, the five agents reduce IOP to a similar degree, although betaxolol has been reported to produce somewhat less lowering of IOP than timolol and levobunolol. Levobunolol may be more effective than timolol and betaxolol in reducing postcataract surgery IOP increases. Levobunolol solution is more effective in controlling IOP than other agents when given as aqueous solutions on a once-daily schedule (up to 70% of patients). Timolol in the form of a gel-forming solution (Timoptic-XE) provides equivalent IOP control with once-daily administration when compared with the same concentration of the aqueous solution administered twice daily. The choice of a specific β-blocking agent generally is based on differences in adverse effect potential, individual patient response, and cost. Long-term treatment with topical β-blockers results in tachyphylaxis in 20% to 25% of patients. The mean IOP reduction from baseline may be smaller in patients receiving topical β-blockers with concurrent systemic β-blockers.[29]

Local adverse effects with β-blockers usually are tolerable, although stinging on application occurs commonly, particularly with betaxolol solution (less with betaxolol suspension) and metipranolol. Other local effects include dry eyes, corneal anesthesia, blepharitis, blurred vision, and, rarely, conjunctivitis, uveitis, and keratitis. Some local reactions may be a result of preservatives used in the commercially available products. Switching from one agent to another or switching the type of formulation may improve tolerance in patients experiencing local adverse effects.

Systemic effects are the most important adverse effects of β-blockers. Drug absorbed systematically may produce decreased heart rate, reduced blood pressure, negative inotropic effects, conduction defects, bronchospasm, central nervous system effects, and alteration of serum lipids, and may block the symptoms of hypoglycemia. The β_1-specific agents betaxolol and possibly carteolol (as a consequence of intrinsic sympathomimetic activity) are less likely to produce the systemic adverse effects caused by β-adrenergic blockade, such as the cardiac effects and bronchospasm, but a real risk still exists. The use of timolol as a gel-forming liquid or betaxolol as a suspension allows for administration of less drug per day, and therefore reduces the chance for systemic adverse effects compared with the aqueous solutions.

Because of their systemic adverse effects, all ophthalmic β-blockers should be used with caution in patients with pulmonary diseases, sinus bradycardia, second- or third-degree heart block, congestive heart failure, atherosclerosis, diabetes, and myasthenia gravis, as well as in patients receiving oral β-blocker therapy. Use of nasolacrimal occlusion (NLO; see Patient Education below for description) technique during administration reduces the risk or severity of systemic adverse effects, as well as optimizes response. Overall, β-adrenergic blocking agents are well tolerated by most patients, and most potential problems can be avoided by appropriate patient evaluation, drug choice, and monitoring of drug therapy.

In patients failing or having an inadequate response to single-drug therapy with a β-blocking agent, the addition of a CAI, parasympathomimetic agent, prostaglandin analog, or an α_2-adrenergic receptor agonist usually will result in additional IOP reduction. Epinephrine or dipivefrin added to a β-blocking agent (particularly nonspecific β-blockers) usually results in only minimal additional IOP reduction.[1–3,17–19,29]

α_2-ADRENERGIC AGONISTS

Brimonidine and the less lipid-soluble and less receptor-selective apraclonidine are α_2-adrenergic agonists structurally similar to clonidine. Apraclonidine is indicated and brimonidine is effective for prevention or control of postoperative or postlaser treatment increases in IOP. Brimonidine is considered a first-line or adjunctive agent in the therapy of POAG, and apraclonidine is seen as a second-line or adjunctive therapy. Use of apraclonidine has fallen dramatically because of a high incidence of loss of control of IOP (tachyphylaxis) and a more severe and prevalent ocular allergy rate.

α_2-Agonists reduce IOP by decreasing the rate of aqueous humor production (some increase in uveoscleral outflow also occurs with brimonidine). The drugs reduce IOP by 18% to 27% at peak (2 to 5 hours) and by 10% at 8 to 12 hours. Comparative trials demonstrate a reduction in IOP similar to that obtained with 0.5% timolol. Use of brimonidine 0.2% every 8 to 12 hours appears to provide maximum IOP-lowering effects in long-term use. Use of NLO (see Patient Education, below) may improve response and allow the longer dosing frequency (i.e., every 12 hours). Combinations of α_2-agonists with β-blockers, prostaglandin analogs, or CAIs produce additional IOP reduction.

An allergic-type reaction characterized by lid edema, eye discomfort, foreign-object sensation, itching, and hyperemia occurs in approximately 30% of patients with apraclonidine. Brimonidine produces this adverse effect in up to 8% of patients. This reaction commonly necessitates drug discontinuation. Systemic adverse effects with brimonidine include dizziness, fatigue, somnolence, dry mouth, and possibly a slight reduction in blood pressure and pulse. α_2-Agonists should be used with caution in patients with cardiovascular diseases, renal compromise, cerebrovascular disease, and diabetes, as well as in those taking antihypertensives and other cardiovascular drugs, monoamine oxidase inhibitors, and tricyclic antidepressants.

Brimonidine is also contraindicated in infants because of apneic spells and hypotensive reactions. In terms of overall efficacy and tolerability, brimonidine approximates that achieved with β-blockers.[1,2,17–19,29]

Brimonidine-purite 0.15% or 0.1% is a formulation of brimonidine in a lower concentration than the original product, that contains a less-toxic preservative than the most commonly employed benzalkonium chloride. The newer formulations are as effective as the original because the more neutral pH of brimonidine-purite (0.15% pH 7.2; 0.1% pH 7.7) allows for higher concentrations of brimonidine in the aqueous humor with a similar reduction in IOP and a reduced incidence of ocular allergy.[29]

The combination product timolol 0.5%/brimonidine 0.2% (Combigan) may provide additional IOP lowering than either agent alone. A new treatment option, this product is marketed in solution that is dosed twice daily.

CLINICAL CONTROVERSY

Many animal trials demonstrate that brimonidine has excellent neuroprotective properties.[12–15] Some clinicians believe that one of the major advantages of using brimonidine lies in its potential neuroprotective properties. However, neuroprotection has not been demonstrated in human trials.

PROSTAGLANDIN ANALOGS

The prostaglandin analogs, including latanoprost, travoprost, and bimatoprost, reduce IOP by increasing the uveoscleral and, to a lesser extent, trabecular outflow of aqueous humor. Some differences in receptor sites and mechanisms of action may exist between the two prostaglandins (latanoprost and travoprost), the prostamide (bimatoprost). Bimatoprost may be slightly more effective in lowering IOP, getting a larger percentage of patients to lower IOPs, and in patients unresponsive to latanoprost.[29,37–39]

Reduction in IOP with once-daily doses of prostaglandin $F_2\alpha$ analogs (a 25% to 35% reduction) is often greater than that seen with timolol 0.5% twice daily. In addition, nocturnal control of IOP is improved compared with timolol. Interestingly, administration of prostaglandin $F_2\alpha$ analogs twice daily may reduce the IOP comparably to once-daily dosing. The drugs are administered at nighttime, although they are probably as effective if given in the morning.

Prostaglandin analogs are well tolerated and produce fewer systemic adverse effects than timolol. Local ocular tolerance generally is good, but ocular reactions such as punctate corneal erosions and conjunctival hyperemia do occur. Local intolerance occurs in 10% to 25% of patients with these agents.

With prostaglandin analogs, altered iris pigmentation occurs in 15% to 30% of patients, particularly those with mixed-color irises (blue-brown, green-brown, blue-gray-brown, or yellow-brown eyes), which become more brown in color over 3 to 12 months. The change in iris pigmentation will often appear within 2 years, and long-term consequences of this pigment change appear to be mostly cosmetic but irreversible upon discontinuation. Hypertrichosis is fairly common and reverses upon discontinuation of the drug. Hyperpigmentation around the lids and lashes has also been reported and appears to reverse upon discontinuation.

These agents are associated with uveitis, and caution is recommended in patients with ocular inflammatory conditions. Cystoid macular edema also has been reported. Cases of worsening of herpetic keratitis have been reported.

Prostaglandin analogs can be used in combination with other antiglaucoma agents for additional IOP control because of their unique mechanism of action. Given their excellent efficacy and side-effect profile, prostaglandin analogs provide effective monotherapy or adjunctive therapy in patients who are not responding to or tolerating other agents. Many glaucoma experts have advocated the use of prostaglandin analogs as first-line therapy in POAG. Long-term studies of these agents are ongoing, but they appear to be safe, efficacious, and well tolerated in glaucoma therapy.[17–19,29,37,38]

CARBONIC ANHYDRASE INHIBITORS

Topical Agents

CAIs reduce IOP by decreasing ciliary body aqueous humor secretion. CAIs appear to inhibit aqueous production by blocking active secretion of sodium and bicarbonate ions from the ciliary body to the aqueous humor.[1,2,29] Topical CAIs such as dorzolamide and brinzolamide are well tolerated and are indicated for monotherapy or adjunctive therapy of open-angle glaucoma and ocular hypertension. Relatively specific inhibitors of carbonic anhydrase enzyme II such as dorzolamide and brinzolamide reduce IOP by 15% to 26%.

Topical CAIs generally are well tolerated. Local adverse effects include transient burning and stinging, ocular discomfort and transient blurred vision, tearing, and, rarely, conjunctivitis, lid reactions, and photophobia. A superficial punctate keratitis occurs in 10% to 15% of patients. Brinzolamide produces more blurry vision but is less stinging than dorzolamide. Systemic adverse effects are unusual despite the accumulation of drug in red blood cells. Because of their favorable adverse-effect profile, topical CAIs provide a useful alternative agent for monotherapy or adjunctive therapy in patients with inadequate response to or who are unable to use other agents. The drugs may add additional IOP reduction in patients using other single or multiple topical agents. The usual dose of a topical CAI is 1 drop every 8 to 12 hours. Administration every 12 hours produces somewhat less IOP reduction than administration every 8 hours. Use of NLO should optimize response to CAI given at any interval.[1,2,17–19,29,34,36] The combination product timolol 0.5% and dorzolamide 2% (Cosopt) is dosed twice daily and produces equivalent IOP lowering to each product dosed separately.

Systemic Agents

Systemic CAIs are indicated in patients failing to respond to or tolerate maximum topical therapy. Systemic and topical CAIs should not be used in combination because no data exist concerning improved IOP reduction, and the risk for systemic adverse effects is increased. Oral CAIs reduce aqueous humor inflow by 40% to 60% and IOP by 25% to 40%. The available systemic CAIs (see Table 97–4) produce equivalent IOP reduction but differ in potency, adverse effects, dosage forms, and duration of action. Despite their excellent effects on elevated IOP of any etiology, the systemic CAIs frequently produce intolerable adverse effects. As a result, CAIs are considered third-line agents in the treatment of POAG and often used for short-term administration to lower IOP.

On average, only 30% to 60% of patients are able to tolerate oral CAI therapy for prolonged periods. Intolerance to CAI therapy results most commonly from a symptom complex attributable to systemic acidosis and including malaise, fatigue, anorexia, nausea, weight loss, altered taste, depression, and decreased libido. Other adverse effects include renal calculi, increased uric acid, blood dyscrasias, diuresis, and myopia. Elderly patients do not tolerate CAIs as well as younger patients. The available CAIs produce the same spectrum of adverse effects; however, the drugs differ in the frequency and severity of the adverse effects listed.

CAIs should be used with caution in patients with sulfa allergies (all CAIs, topical or systemic, contain sulfonamide moieties), sickle cell disease, respiratory acidosis, pulmonary disorders, renal calculi, electrolyte imbalance, hepatic disease, renal disease, diabetes mellitus, or Addison's disease. Concurrent use of a CAI and a diuretic may rapidly produce hypokalemia. High-dose salicylate therapy may increase the acidosis produced by CAIs, whereas the acidosis produced by CAIs may increase the toxicity of salicylates.[1,2,17–19,21,29,34,35]

PARASYMPATHOMIMETIC AGENTS

The parasympathomimetic (cholinergic) agents reduce IOP by increasing aqueous humor trabecular outflow. The increase in outflow is a result of physically pulling open the trabecular meshwork secondary to ciliary muscle contraction, thereby reducing resistance to outflow. These agents may reduce uveoscleral outflow. Cholinergics agents work well to decrease IOP, but their use as primary or even adjunctive agents in the treatment of glaucoma has decreased significantly because of local ocular adverse effects and/or frequent dosing requirements.

Pilocarpine, the parasympathomimetic agent of choice in POAG, is available as an ophthalmic solution, an ocular insert, and a hydrophilic polymer gel (see Table 97–4). Pilocarpine produces similar (20% to 30%) reductions in IOP as those seen with β-blocking agents. Pilocarpine in POAG or "glaucoma suspects" is initiated as 0.5% or 1% solution, 1 drop three to four times daily. The use of NLO improves response and reduces the need for an every-6-hour dosing frequency. The use of 1 drop of 2% pilocarpine every 6 to 12 hours and NLO provides optimal response in many patients. Both drug concentration and frequency may be increased if IOP reduction is inadequate. Patients with darkly pigmented eyes frequently require higher concentrations of pilocarpine than do patients with lightly pigmented eyes. Concentrations of pilocarpine above 4% rarely improve IOP control in patients, other than those patients with darkly pigmented eyes.

Pilocarpine 4% gel (Pilopine HS) once daily is equivalent to treatment with pilocarpine solution 4% four times daily or timolol 0.5% twice daily. When using every-24-hour dosing of pilocarpine gel, the adequacy of IOP control late in the dosing interval should be confirmed. Ocular adverse effects of pilocarpine include miosis, which decreases night vision and vision in patients with central cataracts. Visual field constriction may be seen secondary to miosis and should be considered when evaluating visual field changes in a glaucoma patient. Pilocarpine ciliary muscle contraction produces accommodative spasm, particularly in young patients still able to accommodate (prepresbyopic). Pilocarpine also may produce frontal headache, brow ache, periorbital pain, eyelid twitching, and conjunctival irritation or injection early in therapy, which tends to decrease in severity over 3 to 5 weeks of continued therapy.

Cholinergics produce a breakdown of the blood–aqueous humor barrier and may result in a worsening of an ocular inflammatory reaction or condition. Systemic cholinergic adverse effects of pilocarpine—such as diaphoresis, nausea, vomiting, diarrhea, cramping, urinary frequency, bronchospasm, and heart block—are rare but may be seen in patients who are using products with high pilocarpine concentrations (6% to 8%), or in those patients who are using such products overzealously in treatment of acute-angle closure. Other adverse effects associated with direct-acting miotics include retinal tears or detachment, allergic reaction, permanent miosis, cataracts, precipitation of CAG, and, rarely, miotic cysts of the pupillary margin.

Carbachol is a potent direct-acting miotic agent; its duration of action is longer than that of pilocarpine (8 to 10 hours) because of resistance to hydrolysis by cholinesterases. This drug also may act as a weak inhibitor of cholinesterase. Patients with an inadequate response to or intolerance of pilocarpine as a result of ocular irritation or allergy frequently do well on carbachol. The ocular and systemic adverse effects of carbachol are similar to but more frequent, constant, and severe than those of pilocarpine.[1,2,17–19,29,34,35] Clinical use of carbachol is limited and may not be commercially available in the near future.

The cholinesterase inhibitors used most commonly in the treatment of POAG are the long-acting, relatively irreversible agents demecarium and echothiophate (limited commercial availability; see Table 97–4). These agents are potent inhibitors of pseudocholinesterase, but they also inhibit true cholinesterase. Because of the serious ocular and systemic toxic effects of these agents, the cholinesterase inhibitors are reserved primarily for patients who are either not responding to or are intolerant of other therapy. Because of their cataractogenic properties, most ophthalmologists use these agents only in patients without lenses (aphakia) and in patients with artificial lenses (pseudophakia). The ocular and periocular parasympathomimetic adverse effects are more common and more severe than with pilocarpine or carbachol.

In addition to the parasympathomimetic effects, the cholinesterase inhibitors may produce severe fibrinous iritis (particularly with the irreversible inhibitors), synechiae, iris cysts, conjunctival thickening, occlusion of the nasolacrimal ducts, and cataracts. The inhibition of systemic pseudocholinesterase by these agents decreases the rate of succinylcholine hydrolysis, resulting in prolonged muscle paralysis. Cholinesterase inhibitors should be discontinued at least 2 weeks before procedures in which succinylcholine is used.

The role of cholinesterase inhibitors in glaucoma is limited by the frequency and potential toxicity of these agents. In phakic patients, cholinesterase inhibitors should be administered only if intolerance or failure results with other antiglaucoma medications. Cholinesterase inhibitors have been shown to provide additional IOP-lowering effects when used with β-blockers, CAIs, and sympathomimetic (adrenergic) agents. As with all agents for glaucoma, therapy should be initiated with lower concentrations of these agents. A once-daily administration frequency should be used in most patients unless very high IOP is present.

Use of NLO likely improves response and reduces systemic adverse effects and should be performed by all patients administering cholinesterase inhibitors. These agents should be used with caution in patients with asthma, retinal detachments, narrow angles, bradycardia, hypotension, heart failure, Down's syndrome, epilepsy, parkinsonism, peptic ulcer, and ocular inflammation, as well as in those receiving cholinesterase inhibitor therapy for myasthenia gravis or exposure to carbamate or organophosphate insecticides and pesticides.[1,2,17–19,29,34,35]

EPINEPHRINE AND DIPIVEFRIN

The mechanism of action by which epinephrine lowers IOP has not been fully elucidated; however, a β_2-receptor–mediated increase in outflow facility through the trabecular meshwork and the uveoscleral route appears to be the primary mechanism. Compared with β-blockers or miotics, epinephrine and dipivefrin reduce IOP less. With the advent of the better tolerated and more efficacious agents to treat glaucoma, the clinical use of epinephrines has decreased dramatically.

Epinephrine is not commercially available anymore. Use of the prodrug of epinephrine, dipivefrin, allows use of lower concentrations secondary to improved intraocular absorption (10- to 15-fold higher). The 0.1% dipivefrin produces equivalent IOP reduction to 1% to 2% epinephrine. Consequently, dipivefrin may be tolerated by patients who are unable to tolerate epinephrine solutions, and it is often chosen over other epinephrine products when this class of drugs is indicated.

A factor limiting the usefulness of epinephrine was the high frequency of local ocular adverse effects. Tearing, burning, ocular discomfort, brow ache, conjunctival hyperemia, punctate keratopathy, allergic blepharoconjunctivitis, rare loss of eyelashes, stenosis of the nasolacrimal duct, and blurred vision may occur. Prolonged use (>1 year) may result in deposition of pigment (adrenochrome) in the conjunctiva and cornea. Pigment also may deposit in soft contact lenses, turning them black. These adverse effects occur less frequently with dipivefrin. Epinephrine may produce mydriasis (particularly when combined with a β-blocker) and may precipitate acute CAG in patients with narrow anterior chambers. A transient increase in IOP may occur with initial therapy, particularly in patients not using other antiglaucoma medications. A relative contraindication to the use of dipivefrin is aphakia (i.e., after cataract removal) or lens dislocation because of the development of swelling of the macular portion of the retina. The edema is dose dependent and disappears with drug discontinuation.

Systemic adverse effects of epinephrine include headache, faintness, increased blood pressure, tachycardia, arrhythmias, tremor, pallor, anxiety, and increased perspiration. Epinephrine should be used with caution in patients with cardiovascular diseases, cerebrovascular diseases, aphakia, CAG, hyperthyroidism, and diabetes mellitus, as well as in patients undergoing anesthesia with halogenated hydrocarbon anesthetics. Using NLO with epinephrine and dipivefrin will improve therapeutic response and reduce the risk of systemic adverse effects.[1,2,17–19,29,34,35]

FUTURE DRUG THERAPIES

It is hoped that new agents, improved formulations, and novel approaches to the reduction of IOP and other methods of prevention of glaucomatous visual field loss will provide more effective and better-tolerated therapies. Agents that are neuroprotective and act through mechanisms other than IOP reduction are likely to be part of glaucoma therapy in the future.[13–15,40]

EVALUATION OF THERAPEUTIC OUTCOMES

The ultimate goal of drug therapy in the patient with glaucoma is to preserve visual function through reduction of IOP to a level at which no further optic nerve damage occurs. Because of the poor relationship between IOP and optic nerve damage, no specific target IOP exists. Indeed, drugs used to treat glaucoma may act in part to halt visual field loss through mechanisms separate from or in addition to IOP reduction, such as improvements in retinal or choroidal blood flow. Often a 25% to 30% reduction is desired, but greater reductions (40% to 50%) may be desired in patients with initially high IOPs. For patients with glaucoma, an IOP of less than 21 mm Hg generally is desired, with progressively lower target pressures needed for greater levels of glaucomatous damage. Even lower IOPs (possibly even below 10 mm Hg) are required in patients with very advanced disease, those showing continued damage at higher IOPs, and those with normal-tension glaucoma and pretreatment pressures in the low to middle teens. The IOP considered acceptable for a patient is often a balance of desired IOP and acceptable treatment-related toxicity and patient quality of life.

PATIENT EDUCATION

❼ An important consideration in patients failing to respond to drug therapy is adherence. Poor adherence or nonadherence occurs in 25% to 60% of glaucoma patients.

A large percentage of patients also fail to use topical ophthalmic drugs correctly. Patients should be taught the following procedure:

1. Wash and dry the hands; shake the bottle if it contains a suspension.
2. With a forefinger, pull down the outer portion of the lower eyelid to form a "pocket" to receive the drop.
3. Grasp the dropper bottle between the thumb and fingers with the hand braced against the cheek or nose and the head held upward.
4. Place the dropper over the eye while looking at the tip of the bottle; then look up and place a single drop in the eye.
5. The lids should be closed (but not squeezed or rubbed) for 1 to 3 minutes after instillation. This increases the ocular availability of the drug.
6. Recap bottle and store as instructed.

Note that many patients are physically unable to administer their own eyedrops without assistance. NLO also should be used to improve ocular bioavailability and reduce systemic absorption.[1,2,17–19,29,34,35] The patient induces NLO for 1 to 3 minutes by closing the eyes and placing the index finger over the nasolacrimal drainage system in the inner corner of the eye. This maneuver, as well as eyelid closure itself, decreases nasolacrimal drainage of drug, thereby decreasing the amount of drug available for systemic absorption by the nasopharyngeal mucosa. The use of NLO may improve drug response significantly, reduce adverse effects, and allow less frequent dosing intervals and the use of lower drug concentrations.

Use of more than 1 drop per dose increases costs, does not improve response significantly, and may increase adverse effects. When two drugs are to be administered, instillations should be separated by at least 3 to 5 minutes (preferably 10 minutes) to prevent the drug administered first from being washed out. The patient should be taught not to touch the dropper bottle tip with eye, hands, or any surface.

Adherence to glaucoma therapy commonly is inadequate, and it always should be considered as a possible cause of drug therapy failure. Assessment of adherence by healthcare providers generally is poor, so all patients should be encouraged continually to administer prescribed therapy diligently as instructed. To improve adherence, the patient, family, and care providers should be fully informed of the expectations of therapy and the need to continue therapy despite a lack of symptoms. Possible adverse effects of the medication and ways to reduce them should be discussed. Adherence will be improved by good communication, close monitoring, and use of well-tolerated and convenient drug regimens.[1,2,17–19,29]

CONCLUSIONS

The glaucomas are a group of primary and secondary diseases, the management of which presents a considerable challenge to the clinician. Successful therapy requires rational use of antiglaucoma medications and patient adherence to the selected regimen, combined with conscientious monitoring for adverse effects and disease progression. The reward for successful therapy is considerable—the maintenance of vision. The overview of the clinical findings, pathology, and drug therapy presented in this chapter provides the clinician with the fundamentals necessary to understand and treat glaucoma.

ABBREVIATIONS

CAG: closed-angle glaucoma

CAI: carbonic anhydrase inhibitor

IOP: intraocular pressure

NLO: nasolacrimal occlusion

OHTS: Ocular Hypertensive Treatment Study

POAG: primary open-angle glaucoma

REFERENCES

1. Coleman AL. Glaucoma. Lancet 1999;354:1803–1810.
2. Infield DA, O'Shea J. Glaucoma: Diagnosis and management. Postgrad Med J 1998;74:709–715.
3. Kass MA, Heuer DK, Higginbotham EJ, et al. The ocular hypertension treatment study: A randomized trial determines that topical ocular hypotensive medication delays or prevents the onset of primary open-angle glaucoma. Arch Ophthalmol 2002;120:701–713, discussion 829–830.
4. Leske MC, Heijl A, Hussein M, et al. Factors for glaucoma progression and the effect of treatment: The early manifest glaucoma trial. Arch Ophthalmol 2003;121:48–56.
5. Van Veldhuisen PC, Schwartz AL, Gaasterland DE, et al. The advanced glaucoma intervention study (AGIS): 7. The relationship between control of intraocular pressure and visual field deterioration. Am J Ophthalmol 2000;130:429–440.
6. Janz NK, Wren PA, Lichter PR, et al. Quality of life in newly diagnosed glaucoma patients: The collaborative initial glaucoma treatment study. Ophthalmology 2001;108:887–897.
7. Collaborative Normal-Tension Glaucoma Study Group. Comparison of glaucomatous progression between untreated patients with normal-tension glaucoma and patients with therapeutically reduced intraocular pressures. Am J Ophthalmol 1998;126:487–497.
8. Khaw PT, Cordiero MF. Towards better treatment of glaucoma. BMJ 2000;320:1619–1620.
9. Weinreb RN, Khaw PT. Primary open-angle glaucoma. Lancet 2004;363:1711–1720.
10. Tsai JC, Kanner EM. Current and emerging medical therapies for glaucoma. Expert Opin Emerg Drugs, 2005;10:109–118.
11. Chung HS, Harris A, Evans DW, et al. Vascular aspects in the pathophysiology of glaucomatous optic neuropathy. Surv Ophthalmol 1999;43(Suppl 1):S43–S50.

12. Levin LA. Retinal ganglion cells and neuroprotection for glaucoma. Surv Ophthalmol 2003;48(Suppl 1):S21–S24.
13. Tatton W, Chen D, Chalmers-Redman R, et al. Hypothesis for a common basis for neuroprotection in glaucoma and Alzheimer's disease: Anti-apoptosis by α-2-adrengeric receptor activation. Surv Ophthalmol 2003;48(Suppl 1):S25–S37.
14. Levin LA. Extrapolation of animal models of optic nerve injury to clinical trial design. J Glaucoma 2004;13:1–5.
15. Nickells, RW. From ocular hypertension to ganglion cell death: A theoretical sequence of events leading to glaucoma. Can J Ophthalmol 2007;42:278–287.
16. Yu DY, Su EN, Cringle SJ, et al. Systemic and ocular vascular roles of the antiglaucoma agents β-adrenergic antagonists and Ca^{2+} entry blockers. Surv Ophthalmol 1999;43(Suppl 1):S214–S222.
17. Alward WL. Medical management of glaucoma. N Engl J Med 1998;339:1298–1307.
18. King A, Migdal C. Clinical management of glaucoma. J R Soc Med 2000;93:175–177.
19. Hoyng PF, van Beek LM. Pharmacological therapy for glaucoma: A review. Drugs 2000;59:411–434.
20. Wax MB, Camras CB, Fiscella RG, et al. Emerging perspectives in glaucoma: Optimizing 24-hour control of intraocular pressure. Am J Ophthalmol 2002;133:S1–S10.
21. Kooner KS. New agents in glaucoma therapy. Int Ophthalmol Clin 1999;39:1–15.
22. Kaufman PL, Gabelt B, Tian B, Liu X. Advances in glaucoma diagnosis and therapy for the next millennium: New drugs for trabecular and uveoscleral outflow. Semin Ophthalmol 1999;14:130–143.
23. Ocular Hypertension Treatment Study Group; European Glaucoma Prevention Study Group; Gordon MO, Torri V, Miglior S, Beiser JA, Floriani I, Miller JP, Gao F, Adamsons I, Poli D, D'Agostino RB, Kass MA. Validated prediction model for the development of primary open-angle glaucoma in individuals with ocular hypertension. Ophthalmology 2007;114(1):10–19.
24. Kamal D, Hitchings R. Normal-tension glaucoma: A practical approach. Br J Ophthalmol 1998;82:835–840.
25. Triptahi RC, Tripathi BJ, Haggerty C. Drug-induced glaucomas. Drug Saf 2003;26:749–767.
26. Wiggs JL. Genetic etiologies of glaucoma. Arch Ophthalmol, 2007;125:30–37.
27. Hattenhaurr MG, Johnson DH, Ing HH. The probability of blindness from open angle glaucoma. Ophthalmology 1998;105:2099–2104.
28. Quigley HA, Broman AT. The number of people with glaucoma worldwide in 2010 and 2020. Br J Ophthalmol 2006;90:262–267.
29. Cantor L. Achieving low target pressures with today's glaucoma medications. Surv Ophthalmol 2003;48(Suppl 1):S8–S16.
30. Cooper R. Surgical management of the glaucomas. Aust N Z J Ophthalmol 1999;27:352.
31. Mearza AA, Aslanides IM. Uses and complications of mitomycin C in ophthalmology. Expert Opin Drug Saf 2007;6:27–32.
32. Donohue EK, Cioffi GA. Glaucoma surgery: Are there new perspectives in perioperative pharmacology? Curr Opin Ophthalmol 1999;10:93–98.
33. Loon SC, Chew PT. A major review of antimetabolites in glaucoma therapy. Ophthalmologica 1999;213:234–245.
34. Schuman JS. Antiglaucoma medications: A review of safety and tolerability issues related to their use. Clin Ther 2000;22:167–208.
35. Kanner E, Tsai JC. Glaucoma medications. Use and safety in the elderly population. Drugs Aging 2006;23:321–332.
36. Stewart WC, Garrison PM. β-Blocker-induced complications and patients with glaucoma. Arch Intern Med 1998;158:221–226.
37. Noecker R, Dirks M, Choplin N. A six-month randomized clinical trial comparing the IOP lowering efficacy of bimatoprost and latanoprost in patients with ocular hypertension or glaucoma. Am J Ophthalmol 2003;135:55–63.
38. van der Valk R, Webers CA, Schouten JSAG, et al. Intraocular pressure-lowering effects of all commonly used glaucoma drugs. A meta-analysis of randomized clinical trials. Ophthalmology 2005;112:1177–1185.
39. Gandolfi SA, Cimino L. Effect of bimatoprost on patients with primary open-angle glaucoma or ocular hypertension who are nonresponders to latanoprost. Ophthalmology 2003;110:609–614.
40. Naskar R, Vorwerk CK, Dreyer EB. Saving the nerve from glaucoma: Memantine to caspases. Semin Ophthalmol 1999;14:152–158.

CHAPTER 98

Allergic Rhinitis

J. RUSSELL MAY AND PHILIP H. SMITH

KEY CONCEPTS

1. Allergic rhinitis is a common disease. Treatment is justified in most cases because of the potential for complications.
2. Because an immediate immune response to allergens results in release of inflammatory mediators that cause allergic rhinitis symptoms, patients must understand the rationale for the proper timing and administration of prophylactic regimens.
3. Proven therapies include avoidance of allergens and pharmacologic management with antihistamines, topical and systemic decongestants, topical steroids, cromolyn sodium, and immunotherapy.
4. Immunotherapy can be highly successful, offering long-term benefits, but expense, potential risks, and a major time commitment makes proper patient selection critical.

Allergic rhinitis involves inflammation of the nasal mucous membrane. In a sensitized individual, allergic rhinitis occurs when inhaled allergenic materials contact mucous membranes and elicit a specific response mediated by immunoglobulin E (IgE). This acute response involves the release of inflammatory mediators and is characterized by sneezing, nasal itching, and watery rhinorrhea, often associated with nasal congestion. Itching of the throat, eyes, and ears frequently accompanies allergic rhinitis.

Allergic rhinitis may be regarded as seasonal allergic rhinitis, commonly known as hay fever, or perennial allergic rhinitis (increasingly called "intermittent" and "persistent"). Seasonal rhinitis occurs in response to specific allergens usually present at predictable times of the year, during plants' blooming seasons (typically the spring or fall). Seasonal allergens include pollen from trees, grasses, and weeds. Perennial allergic rhinitis is a year-round disease caused by nonseasonal allergens, such as house-dust mites, animal dander, and molds, or multiple allergic sensitivities. It typically results in more subtle, chronic symptoms. Many patients have a combination of these two types of allergic rhinitis, with symptoms year-round and seasonal exacerbations. About one-third to one-half of sufferers have recognizable seasonal disease with the remainder having perennial or a combination of both.[1]

EPIDEMIOLOGY AND ETIOLOGY

(1) Allergic rhinitis is one of the most common medical disorders found in humans. Prevalence in the United States is estimated between 8.8% and 16%, with some believing the percentage to be higher.[2,3] It ranks as the sixth most prevalent chronic illness in the United States.[1] Patients are limited in their ability to carry out normal daily functions; higher levels of general fatigue, mental fatigue, anxiety, and depressive disorders are seen.[4,5]

In addition, the impact of allergic rhinitis goes well beyond these central nervous system issues. Allergic rhinitis is associated with several other serious medical conditions, including asthma, chronic rhinosinusitis, otitis media, nasal polyposis, respiratory infections, and orthodontic malocclusions.

Learning objectives, review questions, and other resources can be found at **www.pharmacotherapyonline.com.**

PREDISPOSING FACTORS

The development of allergic rhinitis is determined by genetics, allergen exposure, and the presence of other risk factors. A family history of allergic rhinitis, atopic dermatitis, or asthma suggests that rhinitis is allergic. The risk of developing allergic disease is approximately 50% for children with one atopic parent and 66% for those with two allergic parents.[3]

Allergen exposure is another necessary factor. For allergic rhinitis to occur, an individual must be exposed over time to a protein that elicits the allergic response in that individual. Many potential sufferers never develop symptoms because they do not come into contact with the allergen that would produce symptoms in them.

Evidence suggests microbial exposure in the first years of life could help prevent allergic disease by stimulating a nonatopic immune response.[6] Farm children are exposed to higher concentrations of endotoxin, derived from cell walls of gram-negative bacteria, in stables and in dust around the farmhouse. Consumption of nonpasteurized farm milk may cause further exposure. This concept has led to the idea that allergic disease could be prevented by proactively increasing exposure to harmless bacteria early in life (see Alternative Treatment Options below). This could explain why positive skin tests indicating allergen sensitization have been observed more frequently in people in higher socioeconomic classes and in people who live in suburban areas.[7]

Other predisposing factors include an elevated serum IgE (>100 international units/mL) before the age of 6 years, eczema, and heavy exposure to secondhand cigarette smoke.[8]

ALLERGENS

Allergens that produce seasonal rhinitis include protein components of airborne pollen grains, often enzymes, from a variety of trees, grasses, and weeds. Ragweed and grass pollen are the most common offenders in the United States; however, this varies with the geographic region. In general, tree pollens cause symptoms in the spring, grass pollens cause symptoms in the late spring and summer, and weed pollens are the culprits from late summer to early fall. Patients who are hypersensitive to all three may have overlapping problem periods, and may be described as having perennial rhinitis, when they are actually experiencing prolonged seasonal rhinitis. For this reason and the fact that most patients with seasonal problems are sensitive to at least some of the perennial allergens, many allergists are less often distinguishing between the two types of allergic rhinitis. To complicate matters further, the antigenic components of many grasses—including fescue, Kentucky bluegrass, orchard, redtop, and timothy—are similar, resulting in cross-allergenicity. By contrast, most trees that produce many of the offending airborne pollens produce antigenically distinct pollens. These trees include ash, beech, birch, cedar, hickory, maple, oak, poplar, and sycamore. Flowering plants that depend on insect pollination do not cause allergic rhinitis.

Mold spores are also important, but less common allergens. Various spores are present year-round; however, mold growth on decaying vegetation increases seasonally. Just walking through uncut fields or raking leaves can increase exposure. Thus mold spores can be responsible for both perennial and seasonal allergies.

Indoor allergens are always present. Most important among these are house-dust mite fecal proteins, animal dander, cockroaches, and certain mold species. Dust mite levels are on the rise, possibly as a result of the construction of energy-efficient homes and offices with reduced ventilation and increased humidity, use of wall-to-wall carpeting, and the popularity of cool water detergents and cold-water washing.[3]

PATHOPHYSIOLOGY

Knowledge of nasal physiology aids in the understanding of allergic rhinitis. The nose performs three "air conditioning" functions to prepare incoming gases and their contents for the lungs. During the fraction of a second that air is in the nose, it is heated, humidified, and cleaned. The cleaning process plays a role in the development of allergic rhinitis. As the air passes through the nose, the turbulence throws particulate matter against a mucous blanket. The rhythmic movements of the nasal cilia cause the mucous blanket to move posteriorly at approximately 9 mm/min, where it is eventually swallowed; thus trapped foreign particles are removed via the gastrointestinal tract and do not reach the lungs.

The vascular tissue in the nose is erectile. Stimulation of sympathetic fibers causes vasoconstriction, reduction in erectile tissue size, and airway widening. Parasympathetic stimulation causes vasodilation, an increase in erectile tissue size, and airway narrowing.

Located in the nasal mucosa are the mast cells, which participate in the regulation of nasal patency by releasing such mediators as histamine. These are described below.

IMMUNE RESPONSE TO ALLERGENS

❷ Allergic reactions in the nose are mediated by antigen-antibody responses, during which allergens interact with specific IgE molecules bound to nasal mast cells and basophils. In allergic people, these cells are increased in both number and reactivity. During inhalation, airborne allergens enter the nose and are processed by lymphocytes, which produce antigen-specific IgE, thereby sensitizing genetically predisposed hosts to those agents. Upon nasal reexposure, IgE bound to mast cells interacts with airborne allergen, triggering release of inflammatory mediators (Fig. 98–1).[9]

Both immediate and late-phase reactions are observed after allergen exposure. The immediate reaction occurs within seconds to minutes, resulting in the rapid release of preformed mediators and newly generated mediators from the arachidonic acid cascade as the mast cell membrane is disturbed (Table 98–1). These mediators of immediate hypersensitivity include histamine, leukotrienes C_4, D_4, E_4, prostaglandin D_2, tryptase, and kinins.[9] In addition, the mast cell has been found to be a source of several cytokines that probably are relevant to the chronicity of the mucosal inflammation that characterizes allergic rhinitis.[10] Sensory nerve stimulation produces itching, and sneezing occurs via reflex stimulation of efferent vagal pathways. Neuropeptides substance P and calcitonin gene-related peptide from nonadrenergic, noncholinergic nerves affect vascular engorgement directly and via modulation of sympathetic tone. Histamine produces rhinorrhea, itching, sneezing, and obstruction, with the obstruction only partially blocked by H_1- or H_2-blocking agents.[11] Nasal obstruction is also caused by kinins, prostaglandin D_2, and leukotrienes C_4/D_4. Kinins, when directly administered, produce pain rather than itching.[12] These inflammatory mediators also produce vasodilation, increased vascular permeability, and production of nasal secretions.[13]

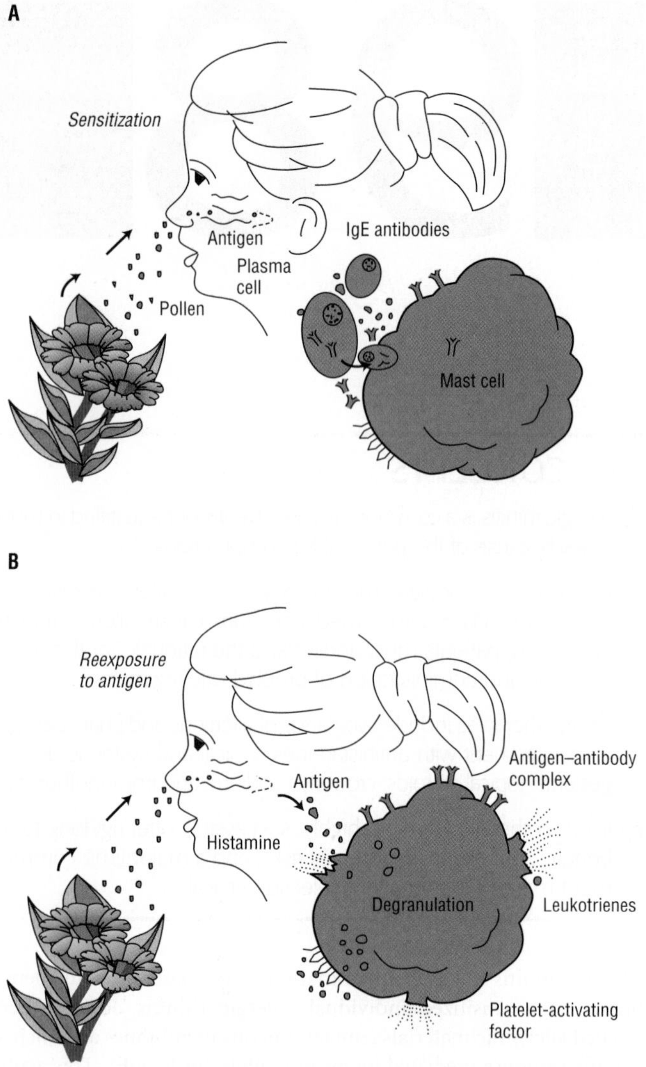

FIGURE 98-1. Allergen sensitization and the allergic response. *A.* Exposure to antigen stimulates IgE production and sensitization of mast cells with antigen-specific IgE antibodies. *B.* Subsequent exposure to the same antigen produces an allergic reaction when mast cell mediators are released.

Four to 8 hours after the initial exposure to an allergen, a late-phase reaction occurs in 50% of allergic rhinitis patients.[14] This response, thought to be caused by cytokines released primarily by mast cells and thymus-derived helper lymphocytes, is characterized by profound infiltration and activation of migrating cells. This inflammatory response likely is responsible for the persistent, chronic symptoms of allergic rhinitis, including nasal congestion. The inflamed mucosa becomes hyperresponsive, a state characterized by exacerbation of nasal reactions to nonspecific or irritant triggers. In this state, the patient also reacts to increasingly lower amounts of the same allergen.[15]

TABLE 98-1 Mast Cell Mediators

Mediator	Effect
Preformed and rapidly released	
Histamine	Stimulates irritant receptors
	Pruritus
	Vascular permeability
	Mucosal permeability
	Smooth muscle contraction
Neutrophil chemotactic factor	Influx of inflammatory cells
Eosinophil chemotactic factor	Influx of inflammatory cells
Kinins	Vascular permeability
N-α-tosyl L-arginine methyl esterase	Vascular permeability
Newly generated	
Leukotrienes	Smooth muscle contraction
	Vascular permeability
	Mucus secretion
	Chemotaxis
	Neutrophil chemotaxis
Thromboxanes	Smooth muscle spasm
Platelet-activating factor	Mucus secretion
	Airway permeability
	Chemotaxis
	Vascular permeability
Granule matrix contents	
Heparin	Antiinflammatory
Tryptase	Protein hydrolysis
Kallikrein	Protein hydrolysis

CLINICAL PRESENTATION

SYMPTOMS AND DIAGNOSIS

The patient with allergic rhinitis typically complains of clear rhinorrhea, paroxysms of sneezing, nasal congestion, postnasal drip, and pruritic eyes, ears, nose, or palate. Symptoms of allergic conjunctivitis are associated more frequently with seasonal than perennial allergic rhinitis, because a majority of the perennial allergens, such as dust mites and molds, are indoors, where air velocity is too low for substantial deposition of allergenic particles on the conjunctivae. However, with heavy exposure from animal or mold allergens, allergic conjunctivitis can be pronounced.

Symptoms secondary to the late-phase reaction, predominantly nasal congestion, begin 3 to 5 hours after antigen exposure and peak at 12 to 24 hours. Subsequent symptoms, both allergic and irritant, are elicited more easily because of the priming effect. For instance, a ragweed-sensitive patient, when exposed to ragweed pollen out of season, responds with modest symptoms and may be very tolerant of irritants such as air pollution or tobacco smoke. During the ragweed season, however, when the nasal mucosa is already inflamed, exposure to small doses of pollen or to irritants to which the patient is usually tolerant elicits a response clinically indistinguishable from the patient's allergy.

Allergic rhinitis is distinguished from other causes of rhinitis by a thorough history, physical examination, and certain diagnostic tests. The medical history consists of a careful description of symptoms, environmental factors and exposures, results of previous therapy, use of other medications, previous nasal injuries, previous nasal or sinus surgery, family history, and the presence of other medical problems and medications. Historical identification of specific causative allergens may be difficult. For example, a reaction induced by mowing the lawn may not be caused by grass pollens, but by the disturbance of various weeds, molds, or other plants in the lawn. With perennial allergic rhinitis, the cause–effect and temporal relationships are less clear, making the diagnosis more difficult, especially with such covert allergens as house-dust mites and molds.

In children, physical examination may reveal allergic shiners, a transverse nasal crease caused by repeated rubbing of the nose, and adenoidal breathing. Pale, bluish, edematous nasal turbinates coated with thin, clear secretions are characteristic of a purely allergic reaction. Tearing, conjunctival injection and edema, and periorbital swelling may be present. Physical findings are generally less clear-cut in adults.

Nasal scrapings will provide a representative sample of cells infiltrating the nasal mucosa and can be helpful in supporting the diagnosis.[16] Microscopic examination of the nasal smear from an allergic individual typically will show numerous eosinophils. The blood eosinophil count may be elevated in allergic rhinitis, but it is nonspecific and has limited usefulness.[17]

Allergy testing can help determine whether a patient's rhinitis is caused by an allergic response to allergens. Immediate-type hypersensitivity skin tests are used for the diagnosis of allergic rhinitis. These include skin tests performed by the percutaneous route, where the diluted allergen is pricked or scratched into the skin surface, or by the intradermal route, where a small volume (0.01 to 0.05 mL) of diluted allergen is injected between the layers of skin. Percutaneous tests are more commonly performed and are safer and more generally accepted, with intradermal tests reserved for patients requiring confirmation in special circumstances.

In percutaneous testing, a positive control (histamine) and a negative control are essential for correct interpretation. After 15 minutes of the application of the allergen, the site is examined for a positive reaction (defined as a wheal-and-flare reaction). Because correct testing is done with extremely minute doses, undetectable by nonsensitized individuals, this reaction is evidence of the presence of mast cell-bound IgE specific to the allergen tested. Many, but not all, common allergens are available as standardized allergenic extracts.

Antihistamines and a few other medications interfere with the wheal-and-flare reaction. First-generation antihistamines should be stopped 3 to 5 days before testing, and second-generation, nonsedating antihistamines should be stopped for 10 days.[18] Medications with antihistamine properties (e.g., sympathomimetic agents, phenothiazines, and tricyclic antidepressants) and H_2-receptor antagonists (e.g., cimetidine, ranitidine, and famotidine) should be discontinued before skin testing.

The radioallergosorbent test (RAST) was the first commonly used method for detecting IgE antibodies in the blood that are specific for a given allergen. Several other quantitative assays that include a reference curve calculated against standardized IgE are available.[19] These tests are highly specific but less sensitive than percutaneous tests.

COMPLICATIONS

❶ Not only is allergic rhinitis aggravating, it also frequently leads to further complications, particularly if the patient does not receive adequate treatment. Symptoms of untreated rhinitis may lead to disturbed sleep, chronic malaise, fatigue, and poor work or school performance. Patients often are plagued by loss of smell or taste, with sinusitis or polyps underlying many cases of allergy-related hyposmia. Postnasal drip with cough, hoarseness, and even vocal polyps also can be bothersome.

The role of allergic rhinitis in the development of acute otitis media or chronic middle ear effusion is often less clear. Children with allergic rhinitis appear to be at greater risk of these conditions because of nasal obstruction, insufflation of nasal secretions into the middle ear via eustachian tube obstruction, and negative middle ear pressure. Hearing problems in children related to middle ear effusion may lead to delayed development of language in young children or to school problems in older children.

Structural facial and dental problems can result from chronic allergic rhinitis.[20,21] The chronic edema and venous stasis may contribute to the development of a high-arched, V-shaped palate. Mouth breathing caused by nasal obstruction can be responsible for dental malocclusion and orthodontic problems. Constant upward rubbing of the nose (allergic salute) can cause a transverse crease across the lower nose; nasal congestion often leads to venous pooling and dark circles under the eyes known as *allergic shiners*.

Allergic rhinitis is clearly a risk factor for asthma. As many as 78% of asthma patients have nasal symptoms, whereas approximately 38% of allergic rhinitis patients have asthma.[3] Asthma is more common in those with perennial than seasonal allergic rhinitis, and it is less likely to be "outgrown" when associated with allergic rhinitis.[22]

Recurrent and chronic sinusitis are relatively common complications of allergic rhinitis. The structure of the mucus blanket breaks down, with decreased water production by serous glands, leaving hair cells trapped in the thicker mucus layer. This greatly reduces the clearance of trapped bacteria and offers ideal breeding grounds for the bacteria. Nasal polyps are less common but nonetheless bothersome; they require specific therapy but may improve with management of the underlying allergic state. Epistaxis also can be a problem; it is related to mucosal hyperemia and inflammation.

TREATMENT

Allergic Rhinitis

DESIRED OUTCOME

The therapeutic goal for patients with allergic rhinitis is to minimize or prevent symptoms. This goal should be accomplished with no or minimal adverse medication effects and reasonable medication expenses. The patient should be able to maintain a normal lifestyle, including participating in outdoor activities, yard work, and playing with pets as desired.

GENERAL APPROACH TO TREATMENT

❸ Once the causative allergens and the specific symptoms are identified, management consists of three possible approaches: (a) allergen avoidance, (b) pharmacotherapy for prevention or treatment of symptoms, and (c) specific immunotherapy. The pharmacotherapy for symptoms approach includes several options that are based on patient-specific information (Table 98–2). Figure 98–2 depicts an algorithm for treatment options.

AVOIDANCE

Avoidance of offending allergens is the most direct method of preventing allergic rhinitis, but it is often the most difficult to accomplish, especially for perennial allergens. Mold growth can be reduced by maintaining household humidity below 50% and removing obvious growth with bleach or disinfectant. Patients sensitive to animals will benefit most by removing pets from the home; however, most animal lovers are reluctant to comply with this approach. Cats may be more of a problem than dogs. Cat allergen is so prevalent and persistent in the air that up to 25% of cat-free houses contain detectable cat allergen.[23] Washing cats weekly may reduce allergens but studies are inconclusive.[24] Some dogs display more profuse antigens than do others; clinically, a sensitized person may tolerate one animal better than another.

Efforts to eliminate dust mites should be rigorous, particularly in the bedroom. Exposure to dust mites can be reduced by encasing mattresses and pillows with impermeable covers and washing bed linens in hot water. Washable area rugs are preferable to wall-to-wall carpeting. Acaricide treatment of carpets denatures the dust mite allergen, but must be done repeatedly, resulting in inconvenience and expense. Atopic infants who are exposed to high levels of dust mites are at increased risk for developing asthma.[25] Environmental control of these allergens may be helpful in forestalling further rhinitis and preventing later asthma.

Older central air-filtration systems for houses were expensive and minimally effective. High-efficiency particulate air (HEPA) filters have minimal effect on the dust mite allergens because these allergens are heavy and heavily charged electrically and are not typically floating in the air in the first place. These filters are effective in removing lightweight airborne particulates, including pollens, mold spores, and cat allergen, thus reducing allergic respiratory symptoms.[26]

Patients with seasonal allergic rhinitis should keep windows closed and minimize time spent outdoors during pollen seasons. Immediate hair washing and change of clothes are recommended upon returning indoors. Use of fans that direct outside air into the house should be avoided. Filter masks can be worn while gardening or mowing the lawn. Table 98–3 summarizes recommendations for environmental control.

The few clinical trials on the effectiveness of avoidance measures are inconclusive.[24] These measures are intended to be a part of a comprehensive treatment strategy that will likely include pharmacotherapy and in selected cases, immunotherapy.

PHARMACOLOGIC THERAPY

First-line therapeutic modalities for treating allergic rhinitis are directed at relief of symptoms (see Table 98–2). Antihistamines and decongestants (both oral and topical) generally are used first in treating allergic rhinitis with medications. Several options in these two categories are available without a prescription, but patients will

TABLE 98-2 Pharmacotherapeutic Options for Allergic Rhinitis

Medication Class	Symptoms Controlled	Comments
Antihistamines		
Systemic	Sneezing, rhinorrhea, itching, conjunctivitis	For seasonal allergic rhinitis, begin treatment before allergen exposure. Nonsedating agents should be tried first. If ineffective or too expensive for the patient, the older agents may be used. For perennial allergic rhinitis, use an intranasal steroid as an alternative to or in combination with systemic antihistamines.
Ophthalmic	Conjunctivitis	Logical addition to nasal steroids if ocular symptoms are present.
Intranasal	Sneezing, rhinorrhea, nasal pruritus	Option for seasonal allergic rhinitis. Warn patients of potential drowsiness.
Decongestants		
Systemic	Nasal congestion	Only needed when nasal congestion is present.
Topical	Nasal congestion	Only needed when nasal congestion is present. Do not exceed 3–5 days.
Intranasal corticosteroids	Sneezing, rhinorrhea, itching, nasal congestion	For seasonal allergic rhinitis, an option when congestion is present. Must begin therapy before allergen exposure. Excellent choice for perennial rhinitis.
Mast cell stabilizers	See comments	Prevents symptoms; therefore, for seasonal allergic rhinitis, use before offending allergen's season starts. For perennial rhinitis, improvement may not be seen for up to 1 month.
Intranasal anticholinergics	Rhinorrhea	Reserve for use when above therapies fail or cannot be tolerated.

Note: Level of evidence for each of these treatment options is Level I: strong evidence from at least one published systematic review of multiple, well-designed, randomized clinical trials.

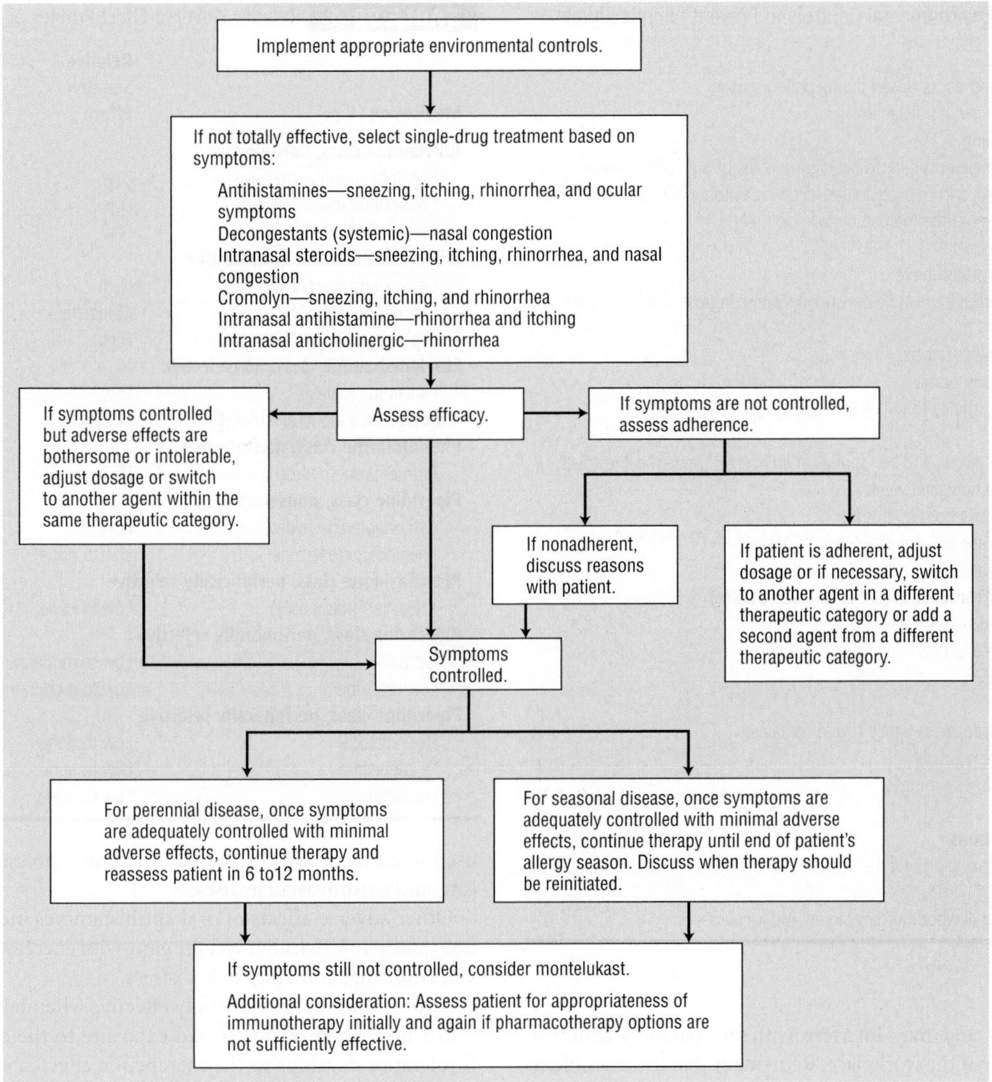

FIGURE 98-2. Treatment algorithm for allergic rhinitis.

need sound advice to make appropriate choices. Knowledge of pathophysiology and the inflammatory state has led to prophylactic therapy for more severe disease using agents such as cromolyn and topical steroids. However, in attempting to assess the evidence supporting any particular therapy, clinicians have difficulty interpreting the medical literature for a variety of reasons, including lack of uniformity in the research methodologies, inappropriate drug controls, and failure to identify types of rhinitis in study subjects (perennial versus seasonal and allergic versus nonallergic).

Antihistamines

Histamine (H_1)-receptor antagonists are competitive antagonists to histamine. They bind to H_1 receptors without activating them, preventing histamine binding and action. Newer antihistamines may also affect components of the inflammatory response such as histamine release, generation of adhesion molecules, and influx of inflammatory cells. Although it was once thought that the older antihistamines had no antiinflammatory action, some were shown to have these effects as early as the 1950s.[27] Antihistamines are available in oral, ophthalmic, and intranasal dosage forms.

The oral antihistamines are the most commonly used and can be divided into two major categories: nonselective (first generation) and peripherally selective (second generation). Nonselective agents are commonly referred to as *sedating antihistamines*, and peripherally selective agents are referred to as *nonsedating antihistamines*. These generalizing terms can be misleading. Individual agents should be judged on their specific characteristics because variation within these broad categories exists. Also, the nonsedating claim is only valid when the newer agents are used at recommended doses.[28] This is of particular concern as some of these antihistamines are now available without a prescription. The mechanism for sedation is not well understood, but its central effect depends on the drugs' ability to cross the blood–brain barrier. Most older antihistamines are lipid-soluble and cross this barrier easily. The peripherally selective agents have little or no central or autonomic nervous system effects. Table 98–4 lists common antihistamines, their chemical classifications, their relative potential for causing sedation, and their relative anticholinergic effects.

Antihistamines are much more effective in preventing the actions of histamines than in reversing these actions once they have taken place. Reversal of symptoms is largely caused by the anticholinergic properties of these drugs. This activity is responsible for the drying effect of antihistamines, which reduces the problem of nasal, salivary, and lacrimal gland hypersecretion. Antihistamines antagonize increased capillary permeability, wheal-and-flare formation, and itching.

In general, the antihistamines are well absorbed, have large volumes of distribution, and are metabolized by the liver. Serum half-lives vary considerably between patients. Also, the therapeutic effects of these agents are more prolonged than might be predicted by their half-lives.

Drowsiness is usually the chief complaint of patients who take antihistamines. It can interfere with a patient's ability to drive a car or

TABLE 98-3 Environmental Controls to Prevent Allergic Rhinitis

Pollens
- Keep windows and doors closed during pollen season
- Avoid fans that draw in outside air
- Use air conditioning
- If possible, eliminate outside activities during times of high pollen counts
- Shower, shampoo, and change clothes following outdoor activity
- Use a vented dryer rather than an outside clothesline

Molds
- Use similar controls as above
- Avoid walking through uncut fields, working with compost or dry soil, and raking leaves
- Clean indoor moldy surfaces
- Fix all water leaks in home
- Reduce indoor humidity to <50% if possible

House-dust mites
- Encase mattress, pillow, and box springs in an allergen-impermeable cover
- Wash bedding in hot water weekly
- Remove stuffed toys from bedroom
- Minimize carpet use and upholstered furniture
- Reduce indoor humidity to <50% if possible

Animal allergens (if removal of pet is not acceptable)
- Keep pet out of patient's bedroom
- Isolate pet from carpet and upholstered furniture
- Wash pet weekly

Cockroaches
- Keep food and garbage in tightly closed containers
- Take out garbage regularly
- Clean up dirty dishes promptly
- Use roach traps

Other recommendations
- Do not allow smoking around the patient, in the patient's house, or in the family car
- Minimize the use of wood-burning stoves and fireplaces

Adapted from reference 3.

TABLE 98-4 Relative Adverse-Effect Profiles of Antihistamines

Medication	Relative Sedative Effect	Relative Anticholinergic Effect
Alkylamine class, nonselective		
Brompheniramine maleate	Low	Moderate
Chlorpheniramine maleate	Low	Moderate
Dexchlorpheniramine maleate	Low	Moderate
Ethanolamine class, nonselective		
Carbinoxamine maleate	High	High
Clemastine fumarate	Moderate	High
Diphenhydramine hydrochloride	High	High
Ethylenediamine class, nonselective		
Pyrilamine maleate	Low	Low to none
Tripelennamine hydrochloride	Moderate	Low to none
Phenothiazine class, nonselective		
Promethazine hydrochloride	High	High
Piperidine class, nonselective		
Cyproheptadine hydrochloride	Low	Moderate
Phenindamine tartrate	Low to none	Moderate
Phthalazinone class, peripherally selective		
Azelastine (nasal only)	Low to none	Low to none
Piperazine class, peripherally selective		
Cetirizine	Low to moderate	Low to none
Levocetirizine	Low to moderate	Low to none
Piperidine class, peripherally selective		
Desloratadine	Low to none	Low to none
Fexofenadine	Low to none	Low to none
Loratadine	Low to none	Low to none

operate machinery and may interfere with the patient's ability to function adequately at the workplace. Remember that these problems can also be a reflection of the disease itself. For this reason, many recommend the use of peripherally selective agents as first-line treatment for any patient who is at high risk for the development of adverse events. This includes patients with renal or hepatic impairment, those with small weights (for whom adult doses may provide larger-than-recommended doses on a milligram-per-kilogram basis), patients with preexisting central nervous system or cardiac disorders, patients who require higher doses, and patients who have shown a tendency to overuse nonprescription or prescription medications.[27]

The sedative effects of antihistamines can be useful in patients who suffer from sleeplessness caused by the symptoms of allergic rhinitis. In these patients, a bedtime dose may prove beneficial. However, they may cause residual daytime sedation, decreased alertness, and performance impairment.[24]

The logic of preferentially using the newer agents is not clear cut. A recent meta-analysis of performance-impairment trials did not show a clear and consistent distinction between diphenhydramine and the peripherally selective agents.[29] Another study showed that tolerance to sedation secondary to diphenhydramine developed by day 4 of treatment, becoming indistinguishable from placebo,[30] but sedation must be distinguished from impairment, as the two are not equivalent.

Anticholinergic (drying) effects contribute to the agents' therapeutic efficacy, but they also cause most adverse effects. Dry mouth, difficulty in voiding urine, constipation, and potential cardiovascular effects may be troublesome. Keep in mind that the differences may be small. Patients with a predisposition to urinary retention (e.g., older men and those on concurrent anticholinergic therapy) should use antihistamines with caution. Caution also should be used in patients with increased intraocular pressure, hyperthyroidism, and cardiovascular disease.

Other adverse effects of oral antihistamines include loss of appetite (and paradoxically, weight gain with increased appetite), nausea, vomiting, and epigastric distress.

Antihistamines are only fully effective when taken approximately 1 to 2 hours before anticipated exposure to the offending allergen. If tolerance develops to the therapeutic effect, a change to an agent in a different chemical class is usually effective.

Patients should be counseled about the proper use of antihistamines. Adverse effects, especially drowsiness, should be emphasized. Patients should be warned against taking other central nervous system depressants, including the use of alcohol. Patients should be told not to take a double dose when a dose is missed. Taking the antihistamine with meals or at least a full glass of water will help prevent gastrointestinal adverse effects such as nausea, vomiting, and epigastric distress. Patients should check with their healthcare professional and read labels before taking nonprescription medications. Many cold products and sleep aids contain antihistamines. Patients should be instructed not to use more than one antihistamine at a time. Table 98–5 lists the recommended dosages of the commonly used agents with their prescription status.

Many patients respond to and tolerate the older agents quite well. Because many of the older agents are available generically, they are much less expensive. Patient cost for many of the older nonprescription agents is less than $5 for a 30-day supply, compared with more than $20 for some of the nonprescription selective agents, and more than $70 dollars for the selective prescription-only products. Although cost is a concern, patient safety should be the first consideration. Interestingly, the most frequently recommended nonprescription antihistamine to adults by pharmacists was diphenhydramine.[32] This may be because of diphenhydramine's use as a sleep aid. With the heavy promotion of competing brands of nonprescription loratadine, this ranking may soon change. Loratadine in combination with pseudoephedrine did show up in the same survey as the top pharmacists' pick in the "adult multisymptom allergy" category.

TABLE 98-5 Oral Dosages of Commonly Used Oral Antihistamines and Decongestants

Medication	Availability	Dosage and Interval[a]	
		Adults	***Children***
Nonselective (first-generation) antihistamines			
Chlorpheniramine maleate, plain[b]	OTC	4 mg every 6 h	6–12 y: 2 mg every 6 h 2–5 y: 1 mg every 6 h
Chlorpheniramine maleate, sustained-release	OTC	8–12 mg daily at bedtime or 8–12 mg every 8 h	6–12 y: 8 mg at bedtime <6 y: Not recommended
Clemastine fumarate[b]	OTC	1.34 mg every 8 h	6–12 y: 0.67 mg every 12 h
Diphenhydramine hydrochloride[b]	OTC	25–50 mg every 8 h	5 mg/kg per day divided every 8 h (up to 25 mg per dose)
Peripherally selective (second-generation) antihistamines			
Loratadine[b]	OTC	10 mg once daily	6–12 y: 10 mg once daily 2–5 y: 5 mg once daily
Fexofenadine	Rx	60 mg twice daily or 180 mg once daily	6–11 y: 30 mg twice daily
Cetirizine[b]	OTC	5–10 mg once daily	>6 y: 5 mg once daily Infants 6–11 mo[c]
Levocetirizine	Rx	5 mg every evening	6–11 y: 2.5 mg every evening
Oral decongestants			
Pseudoephedrine, plain[b]	OTC[e]	60 mg every 4–6 h	6–12 y: 30 mg every 4–6 h 2–5 y: 15 mg every 4–6 h
Pseudoephedrine, sustained-release[d]	OTC[e]	120 mg every 12 h	Not recommended
Phenylephrine[f]	OTC	10–20 mg every 4 h	6–12 y: 10 mg every 4 h 2–6 y: 0.25% drops, 1 mL every 4 h

OTC, nonprescription; Rx, prescription.
[a]Dosage adjustment may be needed in renal/hepatic dysfunction. Refer to manufacturers' prescribing information.
[b]Available in liquid form.
[c]0.25 mg/kg orally demonstrated to be safe.[31]
[d]Controlled-release product available: 240 mg once daily (60-mg immediate-release with 180-mg controlled-release).
[e]See text regarding nonprescription requirements.
[f]Phenylephrine has replaced pseudoephrine in many nonprescription antihistamine–decongestant combination products. Read product labels carefully.

For seasonal allergic rhinitis, an intranasal antihistamine, azelastine, is available. Azelastine has been used successfully in patients who did not respond to loratadine.[33] Using the nasal route offers an alternative to switching to another oral antihistamine. Patient satisfaction has been varied because while the product produces rapid symptom relief, patients complain of drying effects, headache, and diminished effectiveness over time. Patients should be warned of the medication's potential to produce drowsiness, as its systemic availability is approximately 40%.[34]

Allergic conjunctivitis, often associated with allergic rhinitis, can be treated with an ophthalmic antihistamine such as levocabastine. Because systemic antihistamines usually are also effective for allergic conjunctivitis, levocabastine is a logical addition to nasal steroids when ocular symptoms occur, and is an acceptable approach in patients whose only symptoms involve the eyes or to add for those whose symptoms persist on oral treatment.

CLINICAL CONTROVERSY

Although many clinicians strongly prefer a peripherally selective agent as the first antihistamine choice, economic considerations still result in the first-line choice of the less expensive and more sedating products by some prescription plans and clinicians.

Decongestants

Topical and systemic decongestants are sympathomimetic agents that act on adrenergic receptors in the nasal mucosa, producing vasoconstriction. Decongestants shrink swollen mucosa and improve ventilation. When nasal congestion is part of the clinical picture, decongestants work well in combination with antihistamines.

■ TOPICAL DECONGESTANTS

Topical decongestants are applied directly to swollen nasal mucosa via drops or sprays. Table 98–6 lists the common topical decongestants and their durations of action. The use of these agents results in little or no systemic absorption.

Because these agents are extremely effective and are available to patients without a prescription, they are widely used. However, prolonged use of these agents (for more than 3 to 5 days) can result in a condition known as *rhinitis medicamentosa*, or *rebound vasodilation*, with even more severe congestion. Patients who develop this condition use increasingly more spray more often with less response. Although the methods used to treat this "addiction" have not been studied formally, several are used commonly. Abrupt cessation works, but it is difficult because of rebound congestion that may leave the patient congested for several days or weeks. Sleeping may become difficult. Nasal steroids have been used successfully, but they take several days to work. Weaning the patient off topical decongestants can be accomplished by decreasing the dosing frequency or the concentration over several weeks. Combining the weaning process with nasal steroids may prove useful. Ultimately, the success of any plan depends on the patient's resolve and clear understanding of the importance of stopping the drug to end the problem.

Other adverse effects of topical decongestants include burning, stinging, sneezing, and dryness of the nasal mucosa.

Patients should be counseled on the use of topical decongestants to prevent rhinitis medicamentosa. Patients should be instructed to

TABLE 98-6 Duration of Action of Topical Decongestants

Medication	Duration (h)
Short acting	
Phenylephrine hydrochloride	Up to 4
Intermediate acting	
Naphazoline hydrochloride	4–6
Tetrahydrozoline hydrochloride	
Long acting	
Oxymetazoline hydrochloride	Up to 12
Xylometazoline hydrochloride	

use as small a dose as possible as infrequently as possible and only when absolutely necessary (e.g., at bedtime to aid in falling asleep). Duration of therapy always should be limited to 3 to 5 days.

Systemic Decongestants

Oral decongestants are not as effective on an immediate basis as the topical agents, but their effects sometimes last longer and they cause less local irritation. Also, rhinitis medicamentosa is not a problem with oral agents. The most commonly used agent is pseudoephedrine. Table 98–5 lists the usual doses for the regular and sustained-release versions. The use of phenylephrine is increasing as a result of new regulations related to pseudoephedrine described below.

Concerns of safety have greatly limited the systemic decongestant options. Recently, new legal requirements for the sale of pseudoephedrine were put into place to combat the misuse of the drug as a component in making methamphetamine. Pseudoephedrine must now be sold behind the counter and the monthly amount a patient can purchase is limited. Until this new requirement, pseudoephedrine was the most frequently used systemic decongestant and it was considered the safest. Doses of 180 mg have been shown to produce no measurable change in blood pressure or heart rate.[35] In higher doses (210 to 240 mg), pseudoephedrine has raised both blood pressure and heart rate.[36] Pseudoephedrine can cause mild central nervous system stimulation, even at therapeutic doses. Stroke, related to use of oral decongestants such as pseudoephedrine, can occur in patients with hypertension and/or vasospasm.[37] Although stroke complications seem to be associated with higher-than-recommended doses, there is also a stroke risk when these agents are taken properly. Severe hypertensive reactions can occur when pseudoephedrine is given concomitantly with monoamine oxidase inhibitors.[38] Hypertensive patients should, unless absolutely necessary, avoid systemic decongestants.

Combination Products

Numerous products combine an antihistamine with a decongestant. The combination is rational because of the different mechanisms of action. Both nonselective and peripherally selective antihistamines are available in such combinations. As mentioned previously, patients should read labels to avoid therapeutic duplication. Consideration should be given to whether the patient is always congested before recommending these combinations.

■ NASAL STEROIDS

Nasal steroids are an excellent choice for treating perennial rhinitis, and can be useful in seasonal rhinitis, especially if begun in advance of symptoms. Nasal steroids appear to be effective with minimal adverse effects. Some believe that nasal steroids should be recommended as initial therapy over antihistamines because of their high level of efficacy when used properly and along with avoidance of allergens.[39] Multiple mechanisms are involved with the effects of nasal steroids on the nasal mucosa: reducing inflammation by reducing mediator release, suppressing neutrophil chemotaxis, reducing intracellular edema, causing mild vasoconstriction, and inhibiting mast cell-mediated late-phase reactions.[40] Table 98–7 lists the available nasal steroids and their usual doses.

Topical steroids produce only minor adverse effects, most commonly sneezing, stinging, headache, and epistaxis. Despite concerns about safety of systemic steroids, nasal steroids have been found to have no significant association with hypothalamic–pituitary axis suppression, cataract formation, glaucoma, or bone mineral density changes in the doses used for allergic rhinitis. Growth suppression remains a question with some evidence showing that nasal steroids with higher bioavailability (e.g., beclomethasone) may have a greater growth suppression effect than less bioavailable agents.[41] These findings require more study. Most likely, all currently available nasal steroids are safe in the majority of patients and their clinical benefits outweigh any small growth suppressive effect. Other concerns include local infections with *Candida albicans*, which occur rarely.

TABLE 98-7 Dosage of Nasal Steroids

Medication	Dosage and Interval
Beclomethasone dipropionate, monohydrate	>12 y: 1–2 inhalations (42–84 mcg) twice daily in each nostril 6–12 y: 1 inhalation per nostril (42 mcg) twice daily to start
Budesonide	>6 y: 2 sprays (64 mcg) per nostril in am and pm or 4 sprays per nostril in am (maximum: 256 mcg)
Flunisolide	Adults: 2 sprays (50 mcg) per nostril twice daily (maximum: 400 mcg) Children: 1 spray per nostril three times a day
Fluticasone	Adults: 2 sprays (100 mcg) per nostril once daily; after a few days decrease to 1 spray per nostril Children >4 y and adolescents: 1 spray per nostril once daily (maximum: 200 mcg/day)
Mometasone furoate	>12 y: 2 sprays (100 mcg) per nostril once daily
Triamcinolone acetonide	>12 y: 2 sprays (110 mcg) per nostril once daily (maximum: 440 mcg/day)

The therapeutic benefits of topical steroids are not immediate and they are not decongestants. Patients need to understand this to ensure cooperation and continuation of therapy. Some patients notice improvement in a few days, but peak responses may not be observed for 2 to 3 weeks. Once a response is achieved the dosage may be reduced. Blocked nasal passages should be cleared with a decongestant or saline irrigation before administration to ensure adequate penetration of the spray. Patients should be advised to avoid sneezing or blowing their noses for at least 10 minutes after administration. Topical steroids should not be used in patients with nasal septum ulcers or recent nasal surgery or trauma.

One additional benefit of nasal steroids in treating allergic rhinitis in individuals with asthma and upper airway conditions is that they may confer some protection against exacerbations of asthma, leading to fewer emergency room visits. The overall relative risk for an emergency visit among asthma patients who received intranasal steroids was 0.7.[42] No effect was seen in patients receiving antihistamines.

■ OTHER INHALANT MEDICATIONS

Cromolyn sodium and ipratropium bromide offer two additional approaches for treating allergic rhinitis. Cromolyn sodium is a mast cell stabilizer. Increased interest in this product has resulted from it becoming available without a prescription. Ipratropium bromide is an anticholinergic agent useful in perennial allergic rhinitis.

Cromolyn sodium nasal spray is used for the symptomatic prevention and treatment of allergic rhinitis. It curtails antigen-triggered mast cell degranulation and release of the mediators of allergic reactions, including histamine. Cromolyn sodium has no direct antihistaminic, anticholinergic, or antiinflammatory properties. Similarly to topical steroids, the most common adverse effects—sneezing and nasal stinging—result from local irritation. The dose in adults and children at least 2 years of age is one spray in each nostril three to four times per day at regular intervals every 4 to 6 hours. Cromolyn sodium must cover the entire nasal lining; therefore patients should be instructed to clear nasal passages before administration. Inhaling gently through the nose during administration aids in this process. Dosing must be repeated at 6-hour intervals to maintain the effect.

For seasonal rhinitis, treatment with cromolyn sodium should be initiated just before the usual start of the offending allergen's season and continued throughout the season. In perennial rhinitis, the effects may not be seen for 2 to 4 weeks; therefore antihistamines or decongestants may be needed during this initial phase of therapy. As cromolyn sodium begins to work, the need for these medications should decrease.

Ipratropium nasal spray is an anticholinergic agent that exhibits antisecretory properties when applied locally. It provides symptomatic relief of rhinorrhea associated with allergic and other forms of chronic rhinitis. The 0.03% solution is given as two sprays (42 mcg) two to three times daily. The optimal dose should be determined based on the specific patient's symptoms and response. Adverse effects are mild, with the most common being headache, nosebleeds, and nasal dryness.

IMMUNOTHERAPY

❹ The first report of the successful use of grass pollen extract injections to treat allergic rhinitis was published in 1911 by Noon.[43] The therapy was first called *desensitization*; however, this did not seem appropriate because skin reactivity sometimes remained. The name was later changed to *hyposensitization*. Although this term is still used today, *immunotherapy* is used more commonly and is less confusing.

Immunotherapy is the slow, gradual process of injecting increasing doses of antigens responsible for eliciting allergic symptoms into a patient with the hope of inducing tolerance to the allergen when natural exposure occurs. Several mechanisms have been proposed to explain the beneficial effects of immunotherapy, including: induction of IgG blocking antibodies, reduction in specific IgE (long-term), reduced recruitment of effector cells, altered T-cell cytokine balance (a shift from T-helper type 1 to T-helper type 2), T-cell anergy, and induction of regulatory T cells.[44]

Immunotherapy is expensive, has significant potential risks, and requires a major time commitment from the patient. For these reasons, it should be considered only in a select group of patients. Candidates for immunotherapy should have significant symptoms unsuccessfully controlled by avoidance and pharmacotherapy, or stand to achieve more benefit in other significant ways, such as with asthma. Immunotherapy may postpone the onset of asthma or possibly even prevent it.[45] Patients who are unable to tolerate the adverse effects of properly managed drug therapy also should be considered. Patients must be committed to the necessary regular office visits required to complete this course of therapy over several years.

The effectiveness of immunotherapy for seasonal allergic rhinitis appears to be better than that seen with perennial rhinitis, in part because it is more difficult to determine which allergen is responsible for perennial symptoms, and it is more often due to multiple sensitizations. Effectiveness has been shown in a number of clinical studies using a variety of pollen extracts, even in patients with severe disease resistant to pharmacotherapy.[44] Specific immunotherapy for house-dust mites has had good results in appropriately selected patients, while several studies have described marked improvement in patients with allergy to cats. Data indicate that in some patients 3 years of immunotherapy may be sufficient to give lasting benefit.[46] However, many require longer treatment.

The selection of antigens should be based on patient history and skin test results. Numerous regimens for administration of selected allergens have been suggested. In the beginning, very dilute solutions are given initially one to two times per week. The concentration is increased until the maximum tolerated dose is achieved. This maintenance dose is continued every 2 to 6 weeks, depending on clinical response. In light of the present understanding of the immunologic results of immunotherapy, it should be given year-round rather than seasonally.

Adverse reactions can occur with immunotherapy and range from mild to life-threatening. Among the most common are mild local reactions, consisting of induration and swelling at the site of the injection. These may be immediate or delayed. Other more serious reactions (e.g., generalized urticaria, bronchospasm, laryngospasm, and vascular collapse) occur rarely; deaths can result from anaphylactic reactions. Severe reactions are treated with epinephrine as well as other modalities recommended for anaphylaxis. Because of this potential risk, immunotherapy must not be given without adequate direct observation in a medical facility.

Several patient types have been identified as poor candidates for immunotherapy, including patients with any medical condition that would compromise the ability to tolerate an anaphylactic-type reaction, patients with impaired immune systems, and patients with a history of nonadherence to therapy.[47]

TABLE 98-8 Dosage Regimens for Montelukast in Treatment of Allergic Rhinitis

Age	Dosage[a]
Adults and adolescents >15 years	One 10-mg tablet daily
Children 6–14 years	One 5-mg chewable tablet daily
Children 2–5 years	One 4-mg chewable tablet or oral granule packet daily

[a]The timing of drug administration can be individualized. If the patient has combined asthma and seasonal allergic rhinitis, the dose should be given in the evening.

ALTERNATIVE TREATMENT OPTIONS

Montelukast is the first leukotriene receptor antagonist that has received approved labeling for the treatment of seasonal allergic rhinitis. Leukotriene receptor antagonists inhibit the cysteinyl leukotriene receptor. The cysteinyl leukotrienes are among the inflammatory mediators released from mast cells. Montelukast is effective alone or in combination with an antihistamine.[48] Table 98–8 lists dosage regimens. Although this class represents a therapeutic alternative, studies published to date show them to be no more effective than peripherally selective antihistamines and less effective than intranasal steroids, but when combined with antihistamines, more effective than the antihistamine alone.[49]

CLINICAL CONTROVERSY

The exact role of montelukast in treating allergic rhinitis remains to be defined. Although expensive, it may be advantageous in men with significant prostatic hypertrophy who cannot tolerate antihistamines and in patients who have difficulty stopping antihistamines a week before skin testing.

The development of monoclonal antibodies directed against the binding site of IgE provides an additional way to treat allergic respiratory diseases. Omalizumab, a recombinant humanized anti-IgE monoclonal antibody, is the first to show efficacy in allergic rhinitis.[50] The actual mechanism of how this agent is thought to work is quite complex.[51] Anti-IgE antibodies bind to the site on the IgE molecule that recognizes the IgE receptor, thereby preventing the IgE molecule from binding to mast cells or basophils. The half-life of IgE antibodies on the mast cell surface is about 6 weeks, and as the antibodies turn over, they become available for binding to anti-IgE antibodies. Thus by giving repeated doses of omalizumab, the number of IgE antibodies on the mast cell surface can be significantly reduced over time. These new IgE molecules are not eliminated, but remain in circulation as small immune complexes. IgE receptor numbers on basophils and mast cells may be decreased as a result of down regulation. Because of the extremely expensive nature of this therapy, omalizumab's role strictly limited to severe allergic asthma.

CLINICAL CONTROVERSY

Omalizumab may offer significant long-term benefits to allergic rhinitis patients, but it may prove to be too expensive to gain widespread acceptance.

As mentioned earlier in this chapter, microbial exposure in the early years of life could help prevent allergic disease by favoring a nonatopic immune response.[6] This concept was further studied by administering *Lactobacillus rhamnosus* prenatally to mothers who had at least one first-degree relative or partner with atopic disease (eczema, allergic rhinitis, or asthma) and postnatally for 6 months to their infants.[52] However, their use may be limited to treatment or prevention of childhood eczema as available evidence shows little benefit in allergic airway diseases.[53]

Other avenues for treating allergic rhinitis include Chinese herbal medicine and acupuncture. Although study designs and the small number of patients included have been questioned, these treatments deserve further study.[54]

PHARMACOECONOMIC CONSIDERATIONS

The economic impact of allergic rhinitis is enormous. The direct costs have grown significantly over the past few years because of the increasing use of peripherally selective antihistamines and nasal steroids. The most recent detailed review estimated expenditures of $3.4 billion annually in the United States, with the majority of this cost attributed to prescription medications and outpatient visits.[55] Of prescribed medications, 51% were peripherally selective antihistamines, 25% intranasal steroids, and 5% were older antihistamines. A total of 58% of patients received one or more agents. The mean prescription medication expenditure was $103 per patient for those on Medicaid, $155 for patients with private insurance, and $69 for patients with no insurance. Indirect costs related to missed school or workdays and loss of productivity may approach the amount for the direct costs.[56] These figures do not include expenditures for nonprescription medications. With various brands and generic equivalents of nonprescription nonsedating products being heavily marketed to consumers, one would guess that usage of these agents would greatly increase. Direct-to-consumer advertising for prescription-only allergic rhinitis treatment options has also increased significantly. How this will affect the prescription market is unknown.

The most cost-effective choice of treatment for allergic rhinitis is an individualized decision. Seasonal allergic rhinitis patients who see improvement and can tolerate nonprescription and/or generic antihistamines will experience the least impact on out-of-pocket medical and drug expenses. If these are ineffective, the economic picture becomes more complicated. Choices should follow the logical path based on symptoms, tolerance, and efficacy, as described earlier in this chapter. Knowledge of an individual patient's drug coverage or lack of drug coverage may drive drug choices.

EVALUATION OF THERAPEUTIC OUTCOMES

With allergic rhinitis, the major outcomes issues include the effect of the disease on a patient's life, the efficacy and tolerability of treatment, and patient satisfaction. Consideration must be given to how the condition is affecting the patient's job or school performance, family and social interactions, and other aspects of quality of life. The drug therapy should prevent or minimize symptoms with minimal or no adverse effects. The patient should not have difficulty obtaining needed medication for financial or other reasons. Patients should be questioned about their satisfaction with the management of their allergic rhinitis. The management should result in minimal disruption to their lives.

Both the Medical Outcomes Study 36-Item Short Form Health Survey and the Rhinoconjunctivitis Quality of Life Questionnaire have been used to evaluate outcomes of treatment for seasonal and perennial allergic rhinitis.[57–59] These tools go beyond measuring improvement in symptoms and include such items as sleep quality, nonallergic symptoms (e.g., fatigue, poor concentration, and others), emotions, and participation in a variety of activities. How well each of the current treatment modalities performs and how they compare in improving patient outcomes remain to be determined.

Clinicians caring for allergic rhinitis patients should develop a comprehensive pharmaceutical care plan that addresses several areas. Discuss and agree on therapeutic end points for allergic rhinitis, including the patient's acceptable level of symptom relief, onset of symptom relief expectations, and seasonal starts and stops. Discuss adverse drug reaction self-monitoring and prevention based on treatment selection. Assess patient attitude toward adherence to and persistence with oral, ocular, intranasal, or immunologic therapies. Ensure proper matching of treatment to symptoms and intervene with the prescriber if necessary. Conduct seasonal or annual review with patient.

The therapeutic goal for all patients with allergic rhinitis is to minimize or prevent symptoms. Evaluation of success is accomplished primarily through the discussions with the patient, in whom both relief of symptoms and tolerance of drug therapy must be discussed.

CONCLUSIONS

Allergic rhinitis is a common disease with symptoms ranging from mild to severe. If avoidance measures are unsuccessful, it should be treated to improve quality of life and prevent long-term complications. Timing of treating is essential. Treatment regimens should be individualized based on patient symptoms and response.

ABBREVIATION

IgE: immunoglobulin E

REFERENCES

1. McCrory DC, Williams JW, Dolor RJ, et al. Management of Allergic Rhinitis in the Working-Age Population. Evidence Report/Technology Assessment No. 67. Prepared by Duke Evidence-based Practice Center under Contract No. 290–97–0014. Washington, DC: Agency for Healthcare Research and Quality, 2003.
2. Plaut M, Valentine MD. Allergic rhinitis. N Engl J Med 2005;353:1934–1944.
3. The American Academy of Allergy, Asthma, and Immunology Inc. The Allergy Report. *http://www.aaaai.org/ar/*.
4. Marshall PS, O'Hara C, Steinberg P. Effects of seasonal allergic rhinitis on fatigue levels and mood. Psychosom Med 2002;64:684–691.
5. Sauder A, Kovacs M. Anxiety symptoms in allergic patients: Identification and risk factors. Psychosom Med 2003;65:816–823.
6. Riedler J, Braun-Fahrlander C, Eder W, et al. Exposure to farming early in life and development of asthma and allergy: A cross-sectional survey. Lancet 2001;358:1129–1133.
7. Crimi P, Boidi M, Minale P, et al. Differences in prevalence of allergic sensitization in urban and rural school children. Ann Allergy Asthma Immunol 1999;83:252–256.
8. Skoner DP. Allergic rhinitis: Definition, epidemiology, pathophysiology, detection, and diagnosis. J Allergy Clin Immunol 2001;8:S2–S8.
9. Wilson SJ, Shute JK, Holgate ST, et al. Localization of interleukin (IL)-4 but not 5 to human mast cell secretory granules by immunoelectron microscopy. Clin Exp Allergy 2000;30:493–500.
10. Riccio AAM, Tosco MA, Cosentino C, et al. Cytokine pattern in allergic and non-allergic chronic rhinosinusitis in asthmatic children. Clin Exp Allergy 2002;32:422–426.
11. Wood-Baker R, Lau L, Howarth PH. Histamine and the nasal vasculature: The influence of H1 and H2-histamine receptor antagonism. Clin Otolaryngol 1996;21:348–352.
12. Howarth PH. Mediators of nasal blockage in allergic rhinitis. Allergy 1997;52(40 Suppl):12–18.

13. Howarth PH. Leukotrienes in rhinitis. Am J Respir Crit Care Med 2000;161(2 Pt 2):S133–S136.
14. Clark RR, Baroody FM. What drives the symptoms of allergic rhinitis? J Respir Dis 1998;19:S6–S15.
15. Gerth van Wijk R. Perennial allergic rhinitis and nasal hyperreactivity. Am J Rhinol 1998;12:33–35.
16. Klaewsongkram J, Ruxrungtham K, Wannakrairot P, et al. Eosinophil count in nasal mucosa is more suitable than the number of ICAM-1-positive nasal epithelial cells to evaluate the severity of house dust mite-sensitive allergic rhinitis: A clinical correlation study. Int Arch Allergy Immunol 2003;132:68–75.
17. Braunstahl GJ, Fokkens WJ, Overbeek SE, et al. Mucosal and systemic inflammatory changes in allergic rhinitis and asthma: A comparison between upper and lower airways. Clin Exp Allergy 2003;33:579–587.
18. Lasley MV, Shapiro GG. Testing for allergy. Pediatr Rev 2000;21:39–43.
19. Li JT. Allergy testing. Am Fam Physician 2002;66:621–626.
20. Trask G, Shapiro G, Shapiro P. The effects of perennial allergic rhinitis on dental and skeletal development: A comparison of sibling pairs. Am J Orthod Dentofacial Orthop 1987;92:286–293.
21. Shapiro G, Shapiro P. Nasal airway obstruction and facial development. Clin Rev Allergy 1984;2:225–236.
22. Verdiani P, Di CS, Baronti A. Different prevalence and degree of nonspecific bronchial hyperreactivity between seasonal and perennial rhinitis. J Allergy Clin Immunol 1990;86:576–582.
23. Ferguson BJ. Allergic rhinitis: Recognizing signs, symptoms and triggering allergens. Postgrad Med 1997;101:110–116.
24. Rosenwasser LJ. Treatment of allergic rhinitis. Am J Med 2002;113:17S–24S.
25. Sporik S, Holgate S, Platts-Mills T. Exposure to house dust mite allergen and the development of asthma in childhood: A prospective study. N Engl J Med 1990;323:502.
26. Reisman R, Mauriello P, Davis G, et al. A double-blind study of the effectiveness of a high efficiency particulate air (HEPA) filter in the treatment of patients with perennial allergic rhinitis and asthma. J Allergy Clin Immunol 1990;85:1050–1057.
27. Casale TB, Blaiss MS, Gelfand E, et al. First do no harm: Managing antihistamine impairment in patients with allergic rhinitis. J Allergy Clin Immunol 2003;111:S835–S842.
28. Sansgiry SS, Shringarpure GS. Springtime confusion: Are consumers getting the right information on how to treat seasonal allergies? J Allergy Clin Immunol 2003;112:627–628.
29. Bender BG, Berning S, Dudden R, et al. Sedation and performance impairment of diphenhydramine and second-generation antihistamines: A meta-analysis. J Allergy Clin Immunol 2003;111:770–776.
30. Richardson GS, Roehrs TA, Rosenthal L, et al. Tolerance to daytime sedative effects of H1 antihistamines. J Clin Psychopharmacol 2002;22:511–515.
31. Simons FE, Silas P, Portnoy JM, et al. Safety of cetirizine in infants 6 to 11 months of age: A randomized, double-blind, placebo-controlled study. J Allergy Clin Immunol 2003;111:1244–1248.
32. 2003 Survey Pharmacist Survey of OTC Products. Pharm Today 2003(October Supplement):22–26.
33. Berger WE, White MV. Efficacy of azelastine nasal spray in patients with an unsatisfactory response to loratadine. Ann Allergy Asthma Immunol 2003;91:205–211.
34. Astelin. Product information. Cranbury, NJ: Wallace Laboratories, 1997.
35. Empey DE, Young GA, Letley E, et al. Dose response study of the nasal decongestant and cardiovascular effects of pseudoephedrine. Br J Clin Pharmacol 1980;9:351–358.
36. Drew CDM, Knight GT, Hughes DTD, et al. Comparison of the effects of D-()-ephedrine and L-(+)-pseudoephedrine on the cardiovascular and respiratory systems in man. Br J Clin Pharmacol 1978;6:221–225.
37. Cantu C, Arauz A, Murilla-Bonilla LM, et al. Stroke associated with sympathomimetics contained in over-the-counter cough and cold drugs. Stroke 2003;34:1667–1673.
38. Facts and Comparisons 4.0 Online Version. St. Louis: Wolters Kluwer, 2006.
39. Weiner JM, Abramson MJ, Puy RM. Intranasal corticosteroids versus oral H1 receptor antagonists in allergic disease: Systematic review of randomized controlled trials. BMJ 1998;317:1624–1629.
40. Quintiliani R. Hypersensitivity and adverse reactions associated with the use of newer intranasal corticosteroids for allergic rhinitis. Curr Ther Res 1996;57:478–488.
41. Mehle ME. Are nasal steroids safe? Curr Opin Otolaryngol Head Neck Surg 2003;11:201–205.
42. Adams RJ, Fuhlbrigge AL, Finkelstein JA, Weiss ST. Intranasal steroids and the risk of emergency department visits for asthma. J Allergy Clin Immunol 2002;109:636–642.
43. Noon L. Prophylactic inoculation against hay fever. Lancet 1911;1:1572–1573.
44. Frew AJ. Immunotherapy of allergic disease. J Allergy Clin Immunol 2003;111:S712–S719.
45. Moller C, Dreborg S, Ferdousi HA, et al. Pollen immunotherapy reduces the development of asthma in children with seasonal rhinoconjunctivitis (the PAT-study). J Allergy Clin Immunol 2002;109:251–256.
46. Durham SR, Walker SM, Varga EM, et al. Long-term clinical efficacy of grass pollen immunotherapy. N Engl J Med 1999;341:468–475.
47. Li JT, Lockey RF, Bernstein IL, et al. Allergen immunotherapy: A practice parameter. Ann Allergy Asthma Immunol 2003;90:1–40.
48. Meltzer EO, Malmstrom K, Lu S, et al. Concomitant montelukast and loratadine as treatment for seasonal allergic rhinitis: A randomized placebo controlled clinical trial. J Allergy Clin Immunol 2000;105:917–922.
49. Rodrigo GT, Yanez A. The role of antileukotriene therapy in seasonal allergic rhinitis: A systematic review randomized trials. Ann Allergy Asthma Immunol 2006;96:779–786.
50. Casale TB, Condemi J, LaForce C, et al. Effect of omalizumab on symptoms of seasonal allergic rhinitis. JAMA 2001;286:2956–2967.
51. Frew AJ. Anti-IgE and asthma. Ann Allergy Asthma Immunol 2003;91:117–118.
52. Kalliomaki M, Salminen S, Arvilommi H, et al. Probiotics in primary prevention of atopic disease: A randomized placebo-controlled trial. Lancet 2001;357:1076–1079.
53. Boyle RJ, Tang ML The role of probiotics in the management of allergic disease. Clin Exp Allergy 2006;36:568–576.
54. Xue CC, Li CG, Hugel HM, et al. Does acupuncture or Chinese herbal medicine have a role in the treatment of allergic rhinitis. Curr Opin Allergy Clin Immunol 2006;6:175–179.
55. Law AW, Reed SD, Sundy JS, Schulman KA. Direct costs of allergic rhinitis in the United States: Estimates from the 1996 medical expenditure survey. J Allergy Clin Immunol 2003;111:296–300.
56. Rossoff LJ, Stempel DA, Alam R, et al. The health and economic impact of allergic rhinitis. Am J Manage Care 1997;3:S8–S18.
57. Bousquet J, Duchateau J, Pignat JC, et al. Improvement of quality of life by treatment with cetirizine in patients with perennial allergic rhinitis as determined by a French version of the SF-36 questionnaire. J Allergy Clin Immunol 1996;98:309–316.
58. Meltzer EO, Nathan RA, Selner JC, Storms W. Quality of life and rhinitic symptoms: Results of a nationwide survey with the SF-36 and RQLQ questionnaires. J Allergy Clin Immunol 1997;99:S815–S819.
59. Harvey RP, Comer C, Sanders B, et al. Model for outcomes assessment of antihistamine use for seasonal allergic rhinitis. J Allergy Clin Immunol 1996;97:1233–1241.

SECTION 14
DERMATOLOGIC DISORDERS

CHAPTER 99
Dermatologic Drug Reactions and Self-Treatable Skin Disorders

NINA H. CHEIGH

KEY CONCEPTS

1. Pharmacists are often expected to offer advice regarding skin, hair, and nail conditions. Proper assessment includes not only identification of the condition, but also to identification of patients who need further referral.
2. In attempting to make a proper assessment, the healthcare professional must assess factors such as patient age, hormonal status, subjective complaints, and history, as well as examine the lesions.
3. Dermatitis is one of the most common reasons why patients seek advice. Symptomatic control, as well as identification of the offending agent, is typically the mainstay of therapy.
4. Goals of treating seborrheic dermatitis include loosening and removing scales, preventing yeast colonization, controlling any secondary infections, and reducing itching and erythema.
5. Maculopapular eruptions are the most common manifestation of drug-induced skin reactions. Lesions tend to resemble those of measles, often involving the trunk or pressure areas, and are frequently symmetrical.
6. A fixed-drug reaction appears as a round or oval pigmented lesion and typically reappears with a rechallenge within 30 minutes to 8 hours.
7. Sun- or hormonal-induced hyperpigmentation can be treated with skin bleaching agents such as hydroquinone or kojic acid.
8. Lesions that have the following: asymmetry, border irregularity, changes in color, and changes in diameter should be further evaluated by a dermatologist for possible melanoma.

As the largest organ of the body, the skin, also known as the integumentary system, is the site of a vast number of pathologic conditions.

Learning objectives, review questions, and other resources can be found at **www.pharmacotherapyonline.com.**

Patients present with insults to and infections of the skin in a variety of primary care settings ranging from community pharmacies to the emergency department, requesting evaluation of and advice about skin lesions.

In a survey of patients about the sources of advice they use for skin conditions, pharmacists ranked second just behind physicians. Interestingly, the advice sought seemed to depend on the nature of the condition, in that patients sought more pharmacists for advice on conditions such as dermatitis, psoriasis, skin cancer, and acne.[1] To properly assess a patient, pharmacists and other primary care providers must not only understand clinical presentations of common skin disorders, but also be able to quickly identify patients who may need referral for further evaluation by a physician.

1 In this chapter, skin disorders that are self-treatable and dermatologic reactions to medications are presented from the primary care perspective of a pharmacist or other healthcare professional who primarily recommends nonprescription therapies or refers patients to prescribers or physician specialists. Skin infections are mentioned here but discussed in detail in Chap. 114.

SKIN STRUCTURE AND FUNCTION

The skin has many important functions. Its three layers—the epidermis, dermis, and hypodermis (subcutaneous tissue)—provide a barrier, prevent dehydration, and protect from external injury or microorganisms, maintain body temperature, and even express emotions through dilation or constriction of blood vessels. The dermal layer contains most of the structural components of skin, such as mast cells, fibroblasts, collagen, elastic fibers, sweat glands, sebaceous glands, pigment-producing melanin cells, and vasculature.

The hair and nails are considered appendages of the skin. Hair, comprising keratinized epithelial cells, is protein bound and grows in cycles. Scalp hair grows at a rate of approximately 35 mm/day, but this can be affected by various medications and hormones. The nails, also comprising keratinized cells, have different anatomic components. The nail plate is the main part of the nail, and is highly adherent to the nail bed, which grows underneath. Generally, toenails tend to grow at a much slower rate than fingernails. Several factors affect the growth of the nails, including genetics, age, and weather.[2]

PATIENT ASSESSMENT

❷ Before a treat-or-refer recommendation can be made, the pharmacist or other healthcare professional must make a reasoned assessment of the problem and make a presumptive diagnosis (or at least rule out some of the many skin disorders). Several factors play into this decision, including patient age and hormonal status, patient complaint and history, and lesion assessment.

AGE AND HORMONAL STATUS

A primary factor to consider in evaluation is the age of the patient. Changes in the anatomy and physiology of skin and its appendages relate closely to patient age and for women, hormonal status.

Geriatric Considerations

In addition to wrinkling and dryness, expected age-related skin changes include an increase in uneven pigmentation and thinning of the protective layers, thus predisposing the skin to external injuries. Langerhans cells are reduced by 50% in number, reducing natural immunity to skin cancers. The vascularity of the skin declines, and thus older patients tend to look pale (pallor), feel cold to the touch, and develop certain conditions such as psoriasis, seborrhea, pemphigoid, and candidiasis. Changes in the skin appendages can also occur in the elderly, such as thinning, graying, and balding of the scalp. Women can develop facial hair as a result of the reduction of estrogen. The thickness of the nails is reduced, and nails change in color.

Pediatric Considerations

Certain dermatologic conditions, such as atopic dermatitis, are most likely to occur in children. Also, the rate and amount of absorption of medications through the skin are higher in children. Infants may not be able to safely metabolize or excrete medications because of immaturity of their hepatic and renal systems. They also have immature sebaceous gland activity, and thus present frequently with seborrheic dermatitis on the scalp, also known as "cradle cap."

In adolescence, hair appears in new places: the face in boys, and the pubic and other areas in both boys and girls. Sweating and sebaceous gland activity is greater, thus resulting in increased body odor and skin conditions such as acne (see Chap. 100).

Hormone-Related Considerations

Variations in progesterone and estrogen can result in dermatologic disorders as women go through changes and events of their lives.

Menopausal women tend to develop brown hyperpigmentation, or melasma. Women who are on hormone-replacement therapy or oral contraceptives also develop these nonspecific brown discolorations on their skin.

Pregnant women develop many changes, including hyperpigmentation of the areola and genitalia. These women can also develop melasma, commonly known as the "mask of pregnancy." Most pregnant women develop stretch marks, or striae gravidarum around the abdomen, thighs, breasts, and buttocks. They can also develop disorders such as pruritic urticarial papules and plaques of pregnancy, referred to by clinicians as its acronym, PUPPS. Women who are pregnant also typically notice changes in their hair, whether it be thinner or thicker, straighter or curlier.

SUBJECTIVE QUESTIONING

In addition to clues offered by patient age and special conditions such as pregnancy, several key questions can provide insights into the patient's skin disorder or injury. Getting an accurate history and other information from the patient is critical for ensuring optimal treatment and avoiding undue complications.

Interview

When interviewing the patient, the healthcare professional should make note of the interaction. Questions that are helpful in assessment include the following:

- *Are you having other symptoms—difficulty breathing, fever, or nausea/vomiting?* When patients present with a rash or skin lesion, the first thought should be any potential anaphylaxis or angioedema. Many medications can be responsible for these reactions, and these must be ruled out. If a patient has a severe reaction, with difficulty breathing, the patient may require immediate or even emergent referral to an emergency care facility to obtain proper care. Epinephrine, intravenous corticosteroids, or oral prednisone may be needed immediately.
- *Where did the problem first appear? Where are you affected? Did it spread?* Asking where the skin lesions are is of importance, as most likely, the entire skin is not visible to the healthcare professional, and the source of the infection may be covered. For example, although the arms and legs can demonstrate a rash, it would be pertinent to determine if the trunk is also affected, leading to more of a systemic cause, as opposed to an unaffected trunk, which would likely indicate a nonsystemic cause.
- *If not visible, what do the lesions look like?* The patient can be asked whether the lesion is painful or itching, and can thus can be assessed for any infection requiring immediate treatment. For example, if the area is oozing, erythematous, and warm to the touch, it is most likely infected. Alternatively, if the lesion is not painful and no other symptoms are present, other conditions are likely present. The lesions, if appropriate, can be assessed by the pharmacist for color, texture, size, and temperature. Also, it is important to note any symmetrical differences (e.g., present on only one side of the body).
- *How long have the lesions been present?* Some patients present after having had a skin condition for quite sometime without seeking any advice. This information is also helpful if to the lesions' appearance was after the start of a certain suspected medication.
- *Have the lesions changed in size, shape, color, or consistency?* This question is important in determining any changes that might have occurred with the condition. Most importantly, this question enables evaluation of the patient's melanoma risk. Typically, any skin lesion that changes in these elements should be further examined by a physician.
- *What do you think the problem may be?* Many patients have some thought as to what the source of their problem may be. It is helpful to ask this question, and get their opinion and observation.
- *Obtain general medical/allergy history.* After questioning the patient, a pharmacist or other healthcare professional may be able to rule out recently started drugs or new diseases as causes of the patient's reaction.

LESION ASSESSMENT

If appropriate and acceptable to the patient, the healthcare professional should make a quick visual assessment of the skin lesions. The skin surface should be examined, preferably in natural light. As proper diagnosis is based on pattern recognition, the pharmacist or other health professional must understand and demonstrate com-

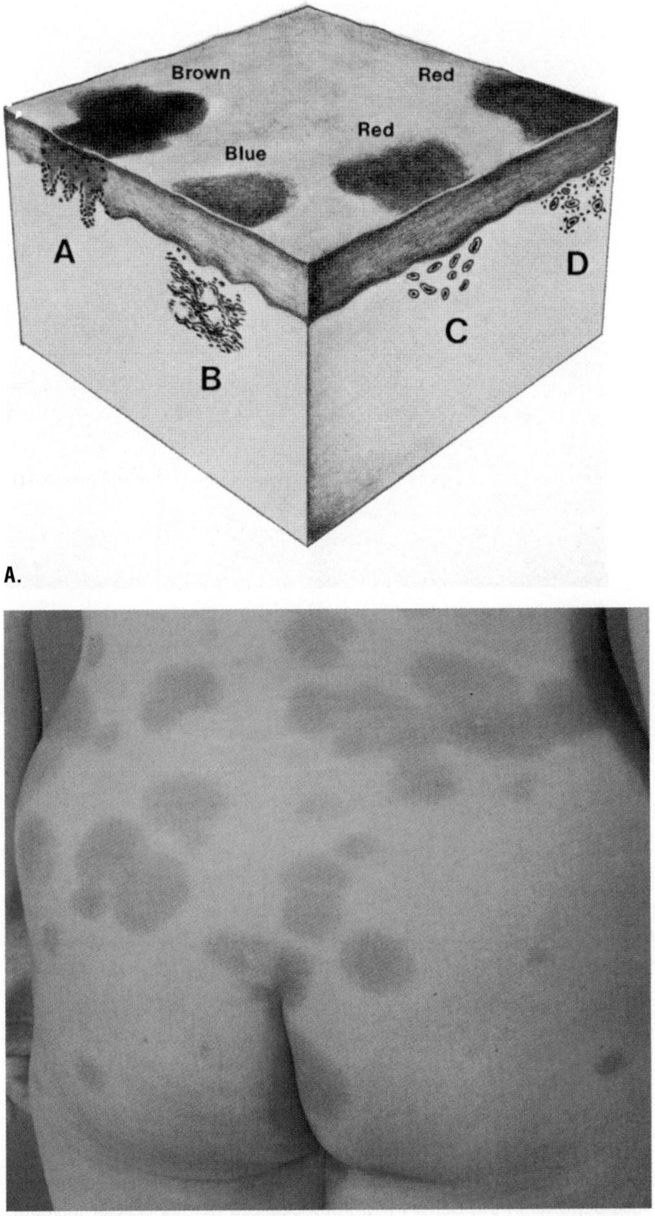

A.

B.

FIGURE 99-1. Macules are circumscribed, flat lesions of any shape or size that differ from surrounding skin because of their color. *A.* Macules may be the result of hyperpigmentation (*A*), hypopigmentation, dermal pigmentation (*B*), vascular abnormalities, capillary dilation (erythema) (*C*), or purpura (*D*). *B.* The clinical appearance of a drug reaction that has produced an eruption consisting of multiple, well-defined red macules of varying size that blanch upon pressure (diascopy) and are thus a result of inflammatory vasodilation. *(Reprinted with permission from Stewart MI, Bernhard JD, Cropley TG, Fitzpatrick TB. The structure of skin lesions and fundamentals of diagnosis. In: Freedberg IM, Eisen AZ, Wolff K, et al., eds. Fitzpatrick's Dermatology in General Medicine, 6th ed. New York: McGraw-Hill, 2003:18.)*

petence in assessing the lesion (Figs. 99–1 through 99–6).[3] In addition, when referral is needed, the pharmacist or other healthcare professional should describe lesions to dermatologists or other physicians in a consistent manner.

Site Distribution and Arrangement

Note the area involved (e.g., face, trunk, arms, legs) and number of lesions present (single or multiple). Identifying the arrangement of the lesions is helpful, such as stating that the lesions are linear (in a line), grouped, annular (limited to one lesion), or serpiginous (resembling a snake). Symmetry or asymmetry should be noted; in skin cancer, lesions are typically asymmetrical.

Surface Texture

Unless the lesions are oozing or appear to be infectious (see Fig. 99–6B), they should be palpated with caution. Palpation helps the healthcare professional determine whether the lesion is smooth or rough, firm or soft, or scaly or crusting.

Type of Lesions

The size of lesions should be measured. Typically, lesions are demarcated as being less than or greater than 0.5 cm in diameter. A *macule* (see Fig. 99–1A) or a papule (see Fig. 99–2A) is typically 1 cm or less in diameter, while the term *patch* is sometimes used for larger flat macules (see Fig. 99–1B).

Border

Poorly circumscribed lesions are those for which it is hard to tell where the "normal" skin begins and ends (see Fig. 99–3B), whereas well-defined lesions have clearer demarcations between healthy skin and lesions (see Fig. 99–4B).

Lesions and Skin Color

Lesions should be examined for variations from the patient's predominant skin color. Increased pigmentation (brownish color), loss of pigmentation, redness (erythema), pallor, cyanosis, and yellowing should be noted. Color can be very indicative of an underlying systemic diseases. For example, anemia and reduced blood flow can result in decreased skin redness. Cyanosis can indicate reduced heart blood flow or lung disease. Jaundice can suggest liver disease.

Other Features

An assessment of the nails, hair, and mucous membranes should also be performed as needed and appropriate.

Once the healthcare professional identifies the specific questions to ask and can provide a reasonable description of the lesion, referral or appropriate therapies can be recommended. As there are hundreds of varieties of dermatologic disorders, this chapter focuses on the common conditions most frequently encountered by the pharmacist and other primary care professionals, with an emphasis on skin disorders that are often treated with nonprescription medications, and on drug-induced skin disorders. Infectious skin conditions are discussed in detail in Chap. 114.

SKIN DISORDERS

DERMATITIS

The term *dermatitis* is a general word denoting an inflammatory, erythematous rash. Many types of dermatitis have been described, with the most common ones being atopic dermatitis (see Chap. 102 for a complete discussion) and contact dermatitis. Although atopic dermatitis can occur at any age, it is most common in infants and children; consequently, age can be a critical identifier in distinguishing between atopic and contact dermatitis. Atopic dermatitis is also frequently associated with elevated immunoglobulin E levels and family history of atopic disease such as dermatitis, allergic rhinitis, and asthma.[4]

Contact Dermatitis

Contact dermatitis is an acute (Fig. 99–7) or chronic (Fig. 99–8) inflammatory skin condition that results from contact of a triggering

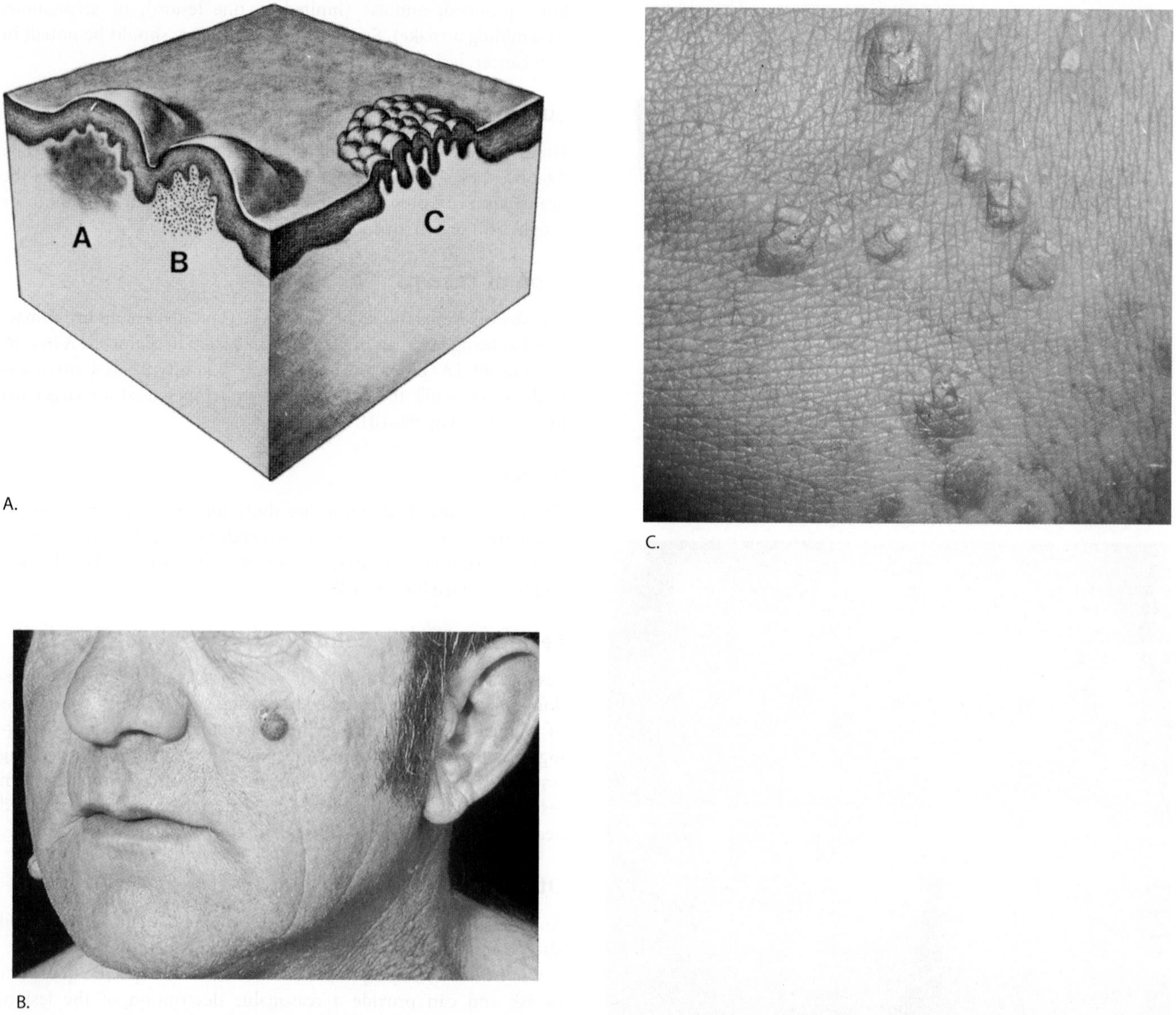

FIGURE 99-2. Papules are small, solid, elevated lesions that are usually less than 1 cm in diameter. The major portion of a papule projects above the plane of the surrounding skin. *A.* Papules may result, for example, from metabolic deposits in the dermis (*A*), from localized dermal cellular infiltrates (*B*), and from localized hyperplasia of cellular elements in the dermis and epidermis (*C*). Papules with scaling are referred to as papulosquamous lesions, as in psoriasis (see Chap. 101). *B.* Clinical examples of papules. The examples are two well-defined and dome-shaped papules of firm consistency and brownish color, which are dermal melanocytic nevi. *C.* Multiple, well-defined, and coalescing papules of varying size are seen. Their violaceous color, glistening surface, and flat tops are characteristic of lichen planus. *(Reprinted with permission from Stewart MI, Bernhard JD, Cropley TG, Fitzpatrick TB. The structure of skin lesions and fundamentals of diagnosis. In: Freedberg IM, Eisen AZ, Wolff K, et al., eds. Fitzpatrick's Dermatology in General Medicine, 6th ed. New York: McGraw-Hill, 2003:18.)*

factor with the skin. Typically, contact dermatitis can be further divided into two major subgroups, allergic or irritant, depending on whether the cause is an antigen (allergen) or irritant, such as an organic substance. Irritant contact dermatitis accounts for 80% of cases of contact dermatitis. In allergies, the antigenic substance triggers the Langerhans cells, and their immunologic responses produce the allergic skin reaction, sometimes several days later. Irritant contact dermatitis is more likely to be the result of a reaction within a few hours of exposure. Although symptoms of either type of contact dermatitis (erythematous vesicles with pruritus) are generally similar, the allergic type can result in more serious erosions or oozing pustules. Table 99–1 lists common offending agents for contact dermatitis.[5]

❸ When patients present with symptoms of contact dermatitis, pharmacists and other primary care providers should initially ask key questions about exposure to potentially offending substances. Initial treatment of contact dermatitis should always focus on identification and removal of the offending agent. When this is not possible, the patient should be advised to avoid exposure to those agents considered most likely responsible.

TABLE 99-1 Common Allergens Producing Contact Dermatitis Among People in the United States

Fragrances	Lanolin (wool)
Flavorings	Neomycin sulfate
Rubber	Nickel (jewelry)
Metals	Paraben mix
Adhesives	Thimerosal
Glues	Urushiol (resin found in poison ivy, oak, sumac)
Plastics	
Formaldehyde (clothing, nail polish)	Preservatives

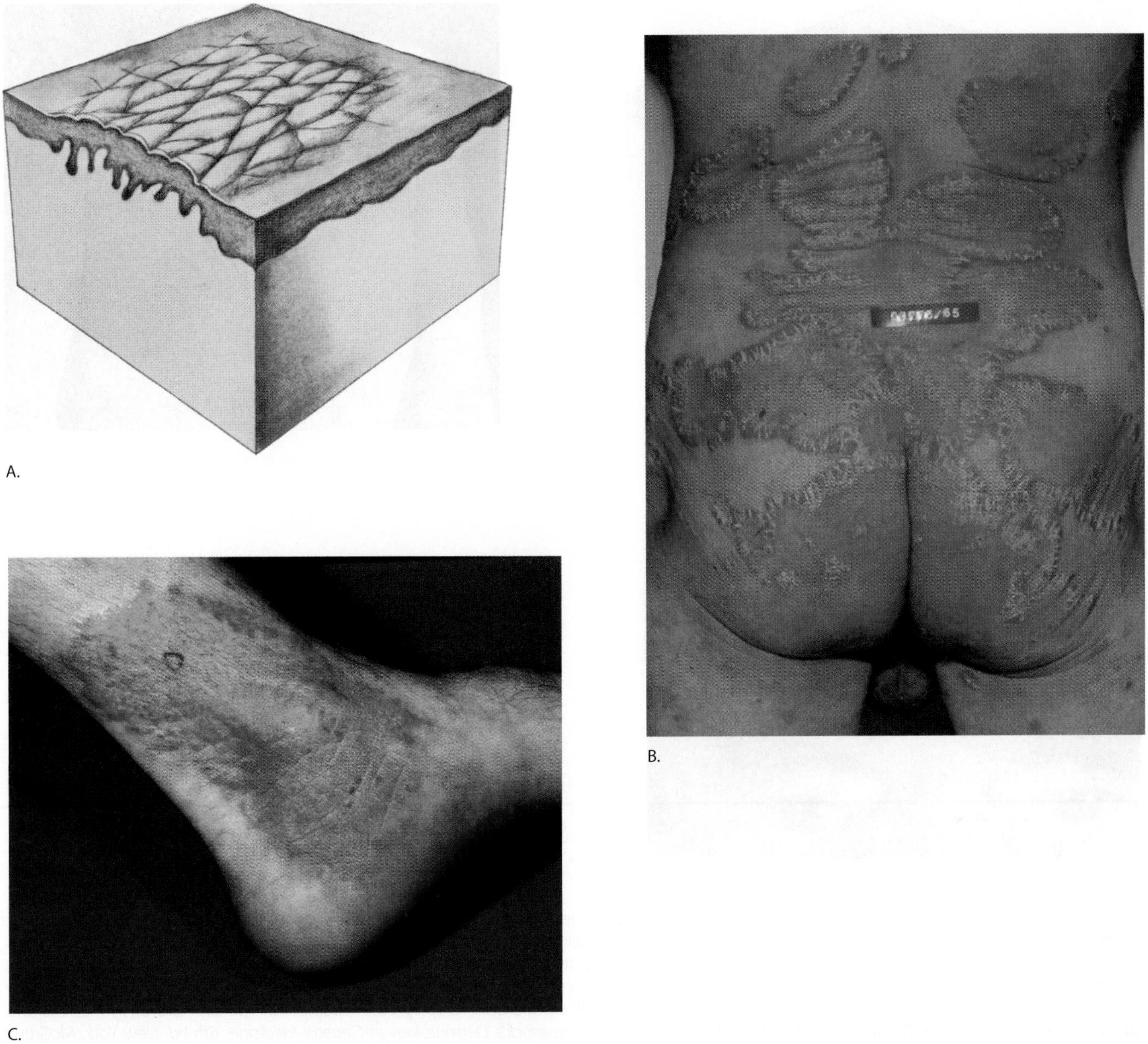

FIGURE 99-3. *A.* Plaque is a mesa-like elevation that occupies a relatively large surface area in comparison with its height above the skin surface. *B.* Well-defined, reddish, scaling plaques can coalesce to cover large areas of the back and buttocks, with some regression in the center as is common in psoriasis (see Chap. 101). *C.* Lichenification, a thickening of the skin and accentuation of skin, can result from repeated rubbings. It develops frequently in patients with atopy, and also occurs in eczematous dermatitis or other conditions associated with pruritus. Lesions of lichenification are not as well defined as most plaques and often show signs of scratching, such as in excoriations and crusts. *(Reprinted with permission from Stewart MI, Bernhard JD, Cropley TG, Fitzpatrick TB. The structure of skin lesions and fundamentals of diagnosis. In: Freedberg IM, Eisen AZ, Wolff K, et al., eds. Fitzpatrick's Dermatology in General Medicine, 6th ed. New York: McGraw-Hill, 2003:18.)*

The second goal of treatment is the relief of symptoms. Products that relieve itching, rehydrate the skin, and decrease weeping of the lesions will provide some immediate relief. The dosage form of topical preparations is determined by the stage of inflammation. In the acute stage, wet dressings are preferred because ointments and creams further irritate the tissue. Astringents such as aluminum acetate, Burrow solution, or witch hazel decrease weeping from lesions, "dry out" the skin, and provide relief from itching. These agents are applied as wet dressings and should not be used for more than 7 days.

For chronic dermatitis, lubricants, emollients, or moisturizers should be applied after bathing. Soap-free (or mild) cleansers and products containing colloidal oatmeal also contribute to alleviating itch and soothing the skin. If the patient's reaction does not subside within a few days, or further spread occurs, the patient should be referred for prescriber or specialist followup and for prescription therapy with stronger topical corticosteroids and possibly oral corticosteroid bursts.

Seborrheic Dermatitis

The prevalence of seborrheic dermatitis peaks during infancy, and then again during the fourth to seventh decades of life, affecting 3% to 5% of adults in the United States. In infants, seborrheic dermatitis is commonly referred to as "cradle cap." Typically, this condition occurs around the areas of skin rich in sebaceous follicles, such as the face (Fig. 99–9), ears, scalp, and upper trunk (Fig. 99–10), although

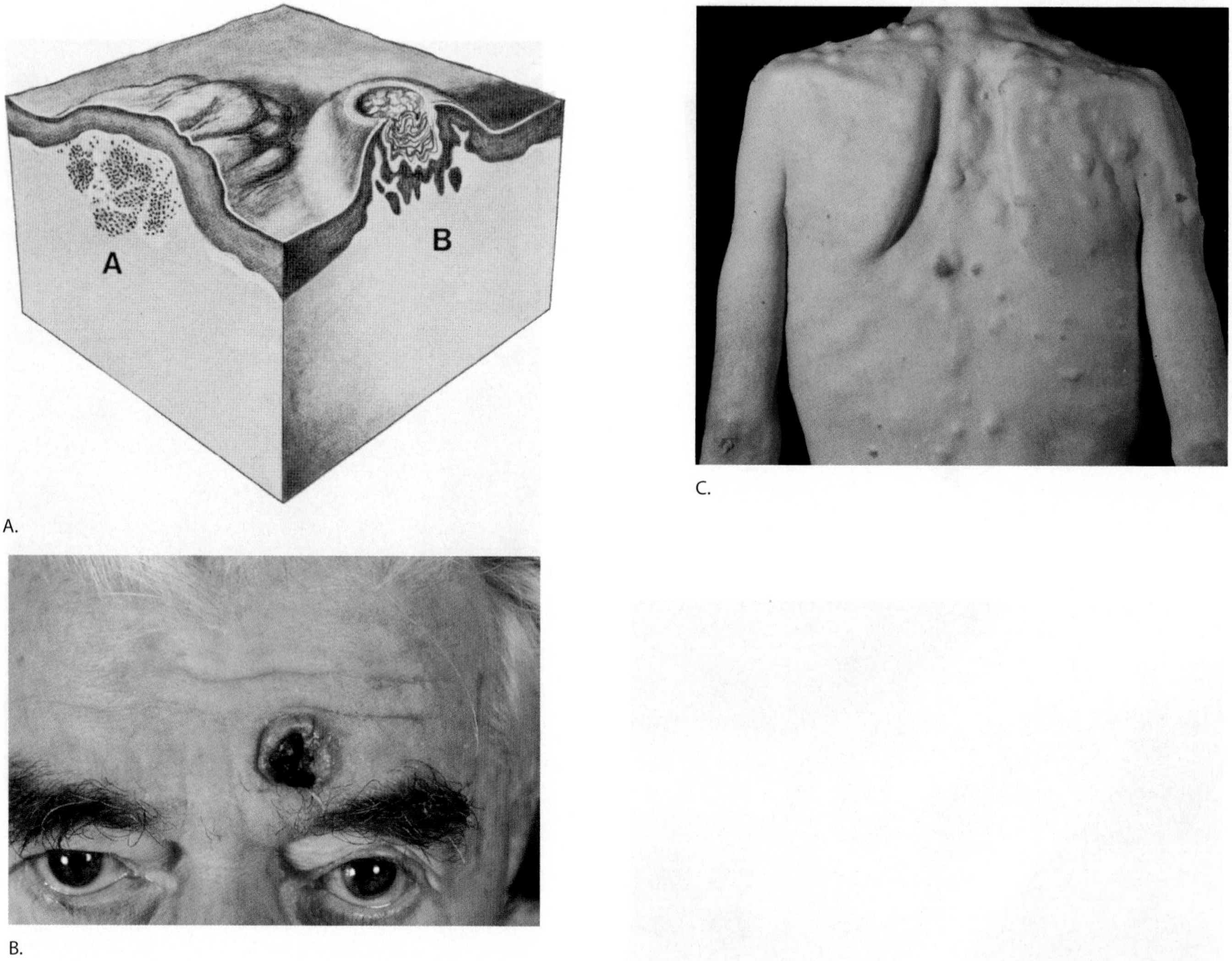

FIGURE 99-4. Nodules are palpable, solid, round or ellipsoidal lesions. Depth of involvement and/or substantive palpability rather than diameter differentiates a nodule from a papule. *A.* Nodules may be located in the epidermis (*B*) or extend into the dermis or subcutaneous tissue (*A*). *B.* This photograph shows a well-defined, firm nodule with a smooth and glistening surface through which telangiectasia (dilated capillaries) can be seen; there is central crusting indicating tissue breakdown and thus incipient ulceration (nodular basal cell carcinoma). *C.* Multiple nodules of varying size can be seen (melanoma metastases). *(Reprinted with permission from Stewart MI, Bernhard JD, Cropley TG, Fitzpatrick TB. The structure of skin lesions and fundamentals of diagnosis. In: Freedberg IM, Eisen AZ, Wolff K, et al., eds. Fitzpatrick's Dermatology in General Medicine, 6th ed. New York: McGraw-Hill, 2003:18.)*

it is not classified as a disease of the sebaceous glands per se.[6] Little is known about its etiology, although factors such as hormone levels, fungal infections (often caused by *Malassezia furfur*), and various nutritional deficits can be associated with the condition. Adult and adolescent seborrheic dermatitis usually starts as mild, greasy scaling of the scalp with erythema and possible scaling of the nasolabial folds. It typically appears oily and occurs in areas of increased sebaceous glad activity (nose, eyebrows, beard area). Adults may develop seborrheic dermatitis on the chest that can appear as small, reddish-brown papules with greasy scales. Infants can have scalp ("cradle cap"), forehead, and ear involvement that typically look like white to yellow scales. Generalized seborrheic dermatitis is uncommon in healthy children, so those who have this should be evaluated for immunodeficiences.[7]

Therapy of seborrheic dermatitis has four major goals: to loosen and remove scales, prevent yeast colonization, control any secondary infections, and reduce itching and erythema. ❹ Interestingly, the disease typically seems to improve with warmer weather and worsens when the air is colder.

Many topical agents are used to manage seborrheic dermatitis. Depending on what area of the body is affected, the pharmacist or other healthcare professional can assist in selection of proper vehicles (i.e., solutions or shampoos for scalp). Adults with seborrheic dermatitis of the scalp can be treated with twice daily topical corticosteroids. This is often used in conjunction with a shampoo containing selenium sulfide, coal tar, or salicylic acid to help loosen the scales. Topical calcineurin inhibitors such as tacrolimus ointment and pimecrolimus cream have fungicidal and antiinflammatory properties and can be used for the scalp or face.[8,9]

Diaper Dermatitis

Diaper dermatitis, or diaper rash, is an acute, inflammatory dermatitis of the buttocks, genital, and perineum region. Commonly seen in infants in diapers, this condition resulting in erythematous patches, erosion of skin, vesicles, and ulcerations can be seen in adults who might wear diapers for incontinence. This reaction is a

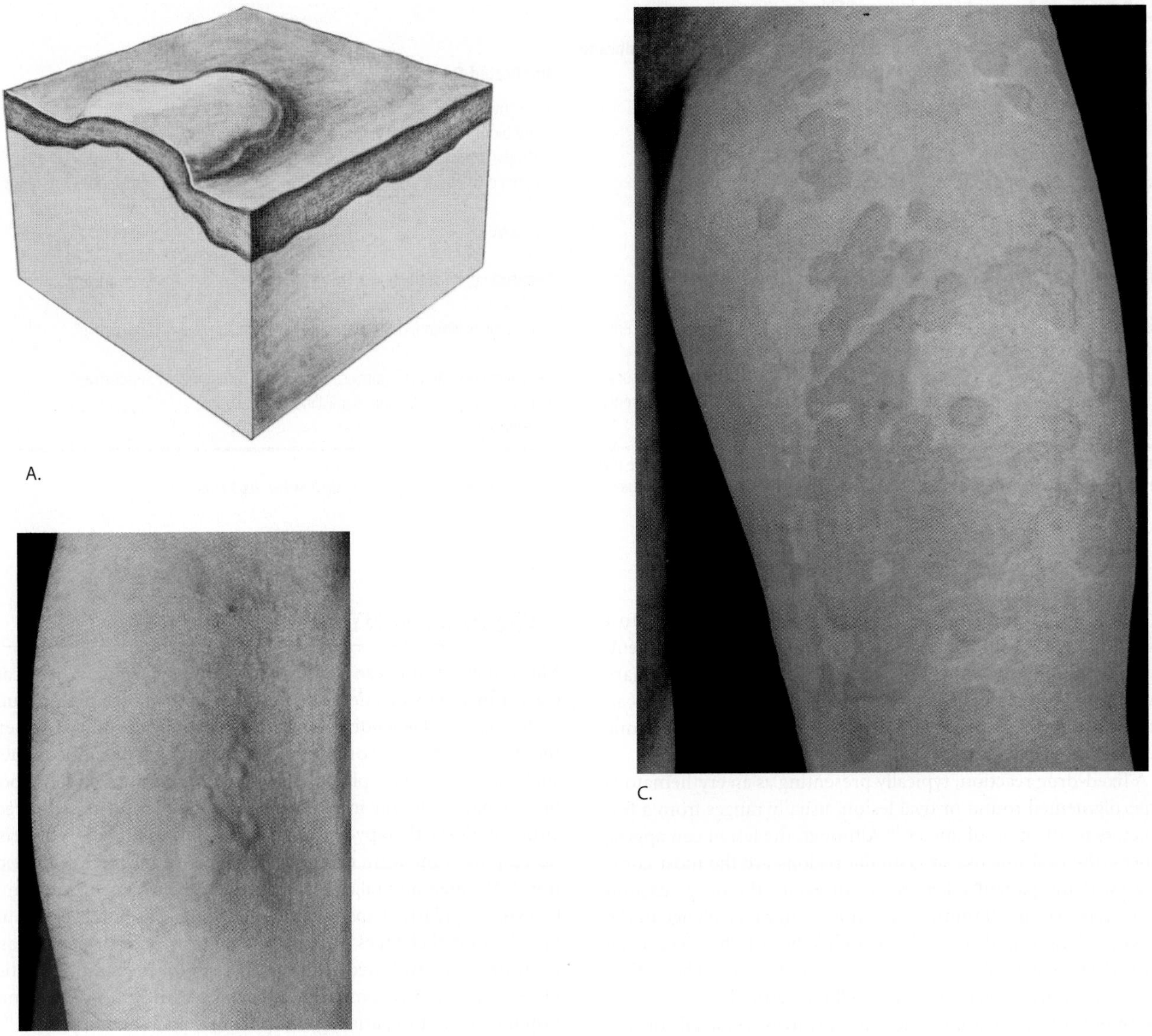

FIGURE 99-5. *A.* Wheals are rounded or flat-topped papules or plaques that are characteristically evanescent, disappearing within hours. An eruption consisting of wheals is termed urticaria and usually itches. *B.* Wheals may be tiny papules 3 to 4 mm in diameter, as in cholinergic urticaria. *C.* Alternatively, wheals may present as large, coalescing plaques, as in allergic reactions to penicillin, other drug, or alimentary allergens. *(Reprinted with permission from Stewart MI, Bernhard JD, Cropley TG, Fitzpatrick TB. The structure of skin lesions and fundamentals of diagnosis. In: Freedberg IM, Eisen AZ, Wolff K, et al., eds. Fitzpatrick's Dermatology in General Medicine, 6th ed. New York: McGraw-Hill, 2003:18.)*

type of contact dermatitis, as it results from direct fecal and moisture contact to the skin in an occlusive environment.

Treatment of diaper dermatitis includes frequent diaper changes and keeping the area dry. Lukewarm water and mild soap can be used to cleanse the area thoroughly, which is then allowed to dry. Occlusive agents—such as zinc oxide, titanium dioxide, petrolatum, or any combination of these—should be generously applied to the area before the diaper is applied.

DRUG-INDUCED SKIN DISORDERS

Approximately 2% to 3% of hospitalized patients experience an adverse cutaneous drug reaction, with a higher incidence in older individuals. Almost every commonly used drug has been implicated in producing local and/or systemic drug reactions (Table 99–2). Typically, these reactions are unpredictable, ranging from mild, self-limiting episodes to more severe, life-threatening ones. Some reactions are nonallergic, but drug-induced skin reactions tend to be immunologic in origin and relate to hypersensitivity.

Pharmacists and other primary care providers should develop an organized and thorough approach to evaluation of patients with potential drug-induced skin disorders. This process begins with a comprehensive drug history, including episodes of previous drug allergies, and is based on an understanding the mechanisms involved in drug reactions.

CUTANEOUS DRUG REACTIONS

Maculopapular eruptions are the most common manifestation of drug-induced skin reactions. Lesions tend to resemble those of measles, often involving the trunk or pressure areas, and are frequently symmetrical. ❺ These eruptions are classified as either early, appearing within a few hours to 3 days after ingestion of the

TABLE 99-2 Types of Drug-Induced Skin Eruptions

Clinical Presentation	Pattern and Distribution of Skin Lesions	Mucous Membrane Involvement	Implicated Drugs	Treatment
Erythema multiforme	Target lesions, limbs	Absent	Anticonvulsants (including lamotrigine), sulfonamide antibiotics, allopurinol, nonsteroidal antiinflammatory drugs, dapsone	Supportive[a]
Stevens-Johnson syndrome	Atypical targets, widespread	Present	As above	Intravenous immunoglobulins, cyclosporine
Toxic epidermal necrolysis	Epidermal necrosis with skin detachment	Present	As above	Supportive[a]
Pseudoporphyria	Skin fragility, blister formation in photodistribution	Absent	Tetracycline, furosemide, naproxen	Supportive[a]
Linger immunoglobulin A disease	Bullous dermatosis	Present or absent	Vancomycin, lithium, diclofenac, piroxicam, amiodarone	Supportive[a]
Pemphigus	Flaccid bullae, chest	Present or absent	Penicillamine, captopril, piroxicam, penicillin, rifampin	Supportive[a]
Bullous pemphigoid	Tense bullae, widespread	Present or absent	Furosemide, penicillamine, penicillins, sulfasalazine, captopril	Supportive[a]

[a]Supportive care includes administration of systemic glucocorticoids until all symptoms of active disease disappear.

Reprinted with permission from Freedberg IM, Eisen AZ, Wolff K, et al., eds. Fitzpatrick's Dermatology in General Medicine, 6th ed. New York: McGraw-Hill, 2003:1199.

drug, or late, appearing up to 9 days after the exposure. Most reactions disappear within a few days after discontinuing the agent, and thus symptomatic control of the affected area is the primary intervention. Topical corticosteroids and oral antihistamines can relieve pruritus. In severe eruptions, a short course of systemic corticosteroids may be warranted.

❻ A fixed-drug reaction, typically presenting as an erythematous or hyperpigmented round or oval lesion, usually ranges from a few millimeters to 20 cm in diameter.[10] Although the lesion can appear anywhere, the oral mucosa or genitalia regions are the most common sites. If the patient takes the agent again, the drug reaction tends to recur within 30 minutes to 8 hours after rechallenge in the exact same location; this is highly indicative of the fixed-drug reaction (lesions may also occur in other locations).[11] The pathogenesis of fixed drug reactions is not well understood.

Treatment of fixed-drug reactions involves removal of the offending agent. Rechallenge should be avoided when possible. Other therapeutic measures include the use of corticosteroids, antihistamines to relieve itch, and perhaps cool water compresses to the affected area.[11]

Sun-induced drug eruptions tend to appear similar to a sunburn, and present with erythema, papules, edema, and sometimes vesicle formations. They also appear in areas that tend to be most susceptible to sunlight, such as the ears, nose, cheeks, forearms, and hands. Photosensitivity is subdivided into phototoxicity, which is defined as a nonimmunologic reaction, and photoallergic reaction, which involves an immunologic mechanism and is far less common.[12] Common medications associated with photosensitivity reactions include fluoroquinolones, nonsteroidal antiinflammatory drugs, phenothiazines, antihistamines, estrogens, progestins, sulfonamides, sulfonylureas, thiazide diuretics, and tricyclic antidepressants.[2] Typically, patients can achieve symptom resolution by discontinuing the medication.

Patients with photosensitivity reactions should be treated much as a burn victim would be. Management of the "burn" is of primary importance. Some patients benefit from topical corticosteroids and oral antihistamines, but these are relatively ineffective. Systemic corticosteroids, typically with oral prednisone at 1 mg/kg per day tapered over 3 weeks, is more effective for these patients. Pharmacists and other healthcare professionals should provide proper sunscreen use counseling and recommend a protective product that covers ultraviolet A and B rays.[13]

HYPERPIGMENTATION

Many medications can cause changes in skin color. These can be caused by the medication or by disturbances in melanin production or formation. Depending on the medication, the site of hyperpigmentation can vary. For example, patients receiving anticonvulsants such as phenytoin, phenobarbital, and carbamazepine report a brown patchy lesion in sun-exposed areas.[10] Patients who receive anticonvulsant therapy for longer than 1 year are at a 10% risk of developing some form of hyperpigmentation related to the medication.[14] Women on oral contraceptives frequently report melasma, or brown, irregularly shaped macules on the cheeks, forehead, or upper lip. Hormonal changes in estrogen and progesterone, as well as sun exposure, are attributed with the increase in melanin deposition.[15] Other medications commonly associated with skin hyperpigmentation include antimalarial agents, phenothiazines, tetracyclines,[16] and amiodarone (Fig. 99–11).[17]

Patients with drug-induced hyperpigmentation can use skin-bleaching creams and/or cosmetic agents that help to even out skin tone. Many such products have been marketed. Hydroquinone or kojic acid are most commonly found in cosmetic agents to aid in bleaching the darkened area of skin. ❼ Many times, these agents are formulated in conjunction with α-hydroxy acids, which help to slowly slough off the outermost layer of skin. Those patients who are using bleaching creams absolutely must use sunscreen, as areas being treated with these creams tend to be even more sun-sensitive.

SKIN CANCERS

Actinic keratoses (AKs) are abnormal keratinocytes that develop in response to prolonged exposure to ultraviolet radiation. These lesions can develop into squamous cell or basal cell carcinomas, and the presence of suspicious lesions is one of the top reasons that patients seek medical attention for dermatologic disorders.

AK usually presents as a small (2- to 6-mm), erythematous papule that feels flat, rough, or scaly when palpated (Fig. 99–12). It tends to be found in chronically sun-exposed areas, such as the top of the hands, head, neck, and forearms. Patients with AKs are frequently elderly and have fair skin, light-colored eyes, freckles, and a history of significant sun exposure and sunburning easily. Because AKs are likely caused by

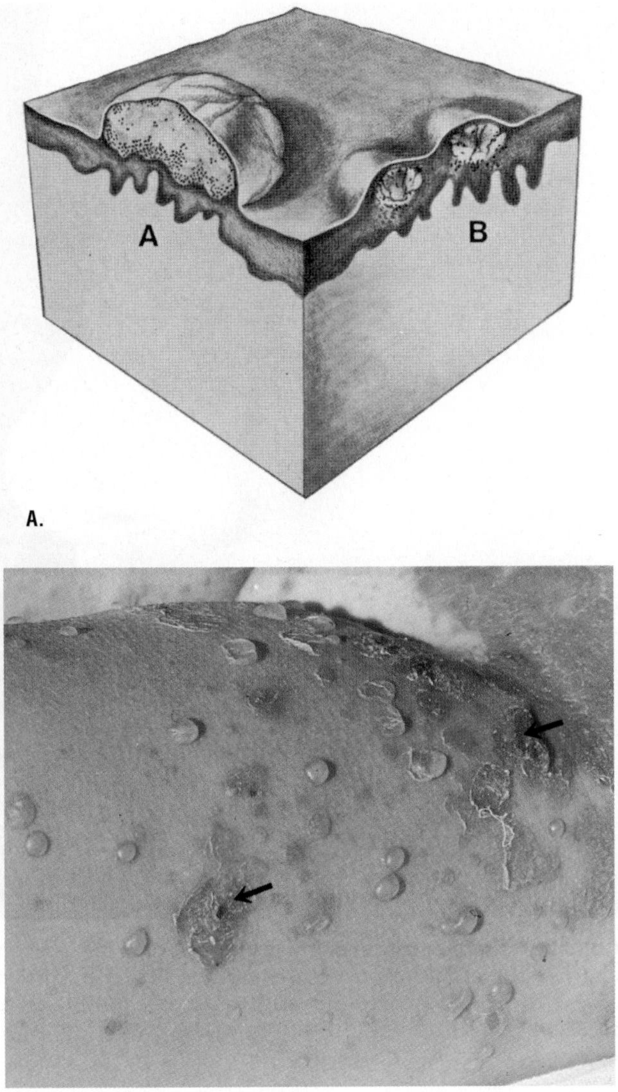

A.

B.

FIGURE 99-6. Vesicles and bullae are the technical terms for blisters. Vesicles are circumscribed lesions that contain fluids, while bullae are vesicles that are larger than 0.5 cm in diameter. *A.* Subcorneal vesicles (*A*) result from fluid accumulation just below the stratum corneum, whereas spongiotic vesicles (*B*) result from intercellular edema. *B.* Multiple translucent subcorneal vesicles are extremely fragile, collapse easily, and thus lead to crusting (*arrows*). These lesions are staphylococcal impetigo. *(Reprinted with permission from Stewart MI, Bernhard JD, Cropley TG, Fitzpatrick TB. The structure of skin lesions and fundamentals of diagnosis. In: Freedberg IM, Eisen AZ, Wolff K, et al., eds. Fitzpatrick's Dermatology in General Medicine, 6th ed. New York: McGraw-Hill, 2003:18.)*

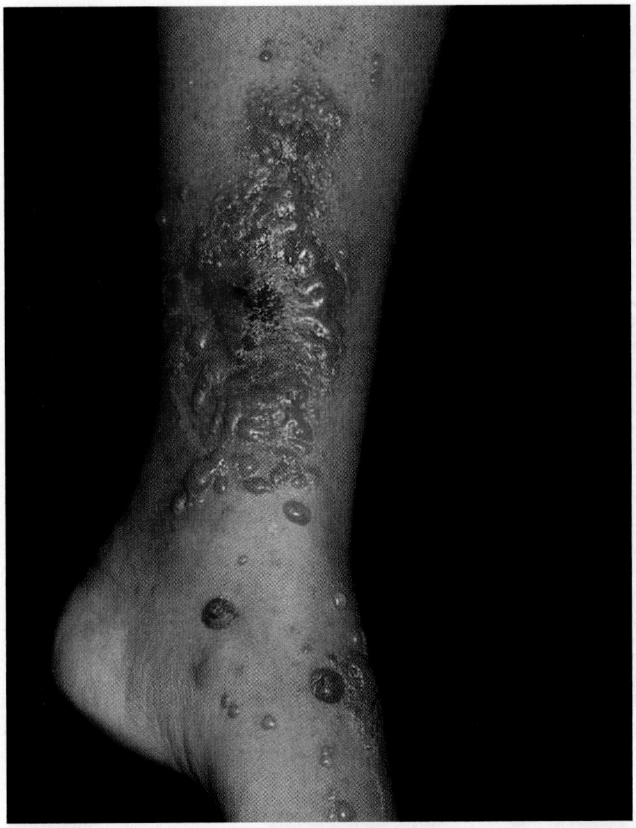

FIGURE 99-7. Acute dermatitis caused by poison ivy. Note the linear arrangement of lesions typical of phytodermatitis acquired by inadvertent contact with the plant. The severe vesiculobullous reaction is typical for urushiol, an oily poisonous irritant found in *Toxicodendron* spp. *(Reprinted with permission from Belsito DV. Allergic contact dermatitis. In: Freedberg IM et al., eds. Fitzpatrick's Dermatology in General Medicine, 6th ed. New York: McGraw-Hill, 2003:1167.)*

ultraviolet radiation, sun-preventive measures, particularly in childhood, are of utmost importance.[18] Most commonly, AKs are treated with liquid nitrogen, which will remove the affected AK. Another frequently used therapy is topical 5-fluorouracil. Patients who are prescribed topical 5-fluorouracil should be properly counseled, as significant erythema, erosion, crusting, and even ulceration normally occur during treatment.

Squamous cell carcinoma (SCC) is a cutaneous malignancy, with estimates of approximately 200,000 cases in the United States in 2001. SCC seems to be more common in advanced age, and twice as common in men than in women. Because of their susceptibility to the negative effects of long-term sun exposure, patients of Celtic ancestry and those with blue/green eyes, red hair, and fair complexion are at the greatest risk of developing SCC.[19] Other risk factors include precursor lesions, such as AKs, long-term immunosuppression, and ultraviolet radiation. SCC can appear in many areas, but mainly occurs in sun-exposed areas such as the head, neck, and dorsal aspect of the hands. Most SCCs appear as a firm, flesh-colored, or erythematous papule or plaque (Fig. 99–13). Some resemble an ulcer. Treatment for SCC is determined by the tumor risk for metastasis, but commonly involves some form of surgical excision.

Basal cell carcinoma is the most common cancer in humans, with an estimated 900,000 cases per year in the United States.[19] Basal cell carcinomas can occur anywhere on the body, but they appear most commonly on the head and neck, usually as a nodular, pigmented lesion (Fig. 99–14). Treatment varies depending on the histology of the lesion, but frequently requires Mohs micrographic surgery, surgical excision, and possible use of topical agents. Topical imiquimod is approved by the U.S. Food and Drug Administration for treating basal cell carcinoma of areas other than the face, and this agent resulted in some clearances in a phase II study.[20] Topical 5-fluorouracil has also been used, but needs further evaluation to warrant routine use.

❽ The risk of malignant melanoma is increasing, with a prediction that prevalence could reach 1 in 50 by 2010.[21] Most frequently, melanoma occurs on the back and extremities of white males and females, whereas in Asians and blacks, it tends to appear on mucous membranes and soles and palms. Risk factors include skin type, sun exposure and response to the sun (i.e., ability to tan), family history, and changing moles. Exposure to environmental radiation or chronic

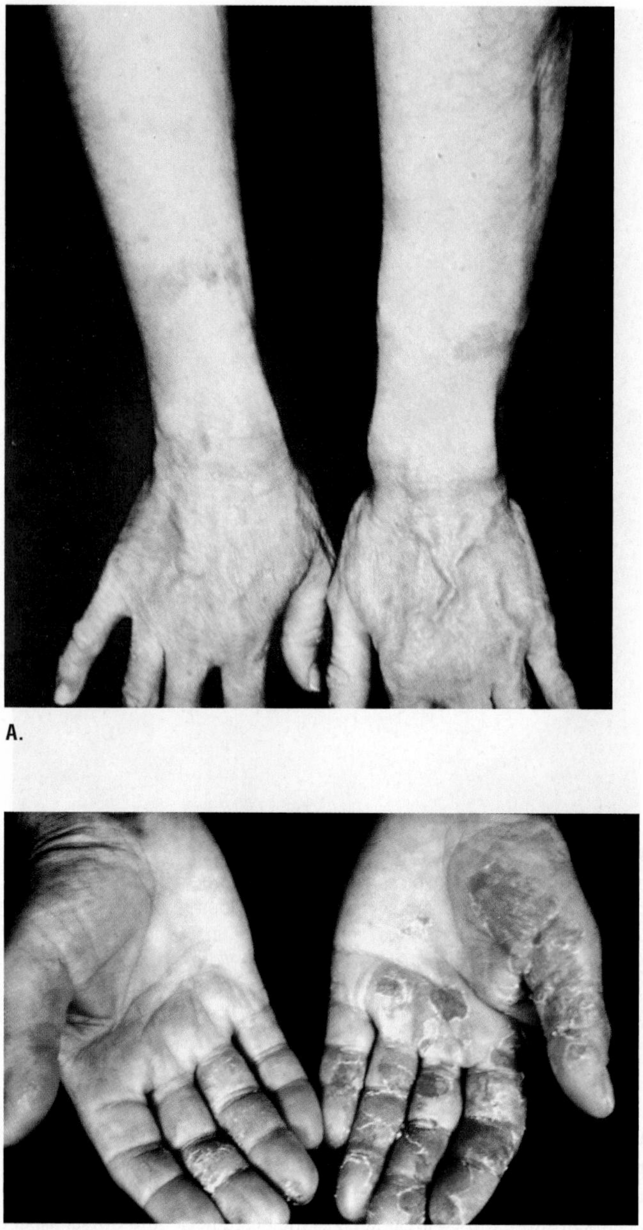

A.

B.

FIGURE 99-8. *A.* This patient has allergic chronic dermatitis involving the dorsal aspects of the hands and the distal forearms. but with minimal involvement of the palms. In this case, contact dermatitis is secondary to use of thiuram present in rubber gloves, prescribed for treatment of an irritant hand dermatitis. *B.* This patient, a florist, has allergic contact dermatitis as a consequence of exposure to tuliposide A, the allergen in Peruvian lilies (*Alstroemeria* spp.). Note the more prominent involvement of the palms of the dominant hand. *(Reprinted with permission from Belsito DV. Allergic contact dermatitis. In: Freedberg IM et al., eds. Fitzpatrick's Dermatology in General Medicine, 6th ed. New York: McGraw-Hill, 2003:1167.)*

immunosuppression can lead to an increased incidence of SCCs.[22] The presence of any nonhealing lesion should raise the suspicion of skin cancer. In addition to assessing these risk factors, pharmacists can play a key role in examining the questionable lesion(s) and by assessing the lesion's asymmetry, border, color, diameter, and history, as when a mole has changed and led to the lesion (Fig. 99–15). Patients who fit these criteria should be further evaluated by a dermatologist.

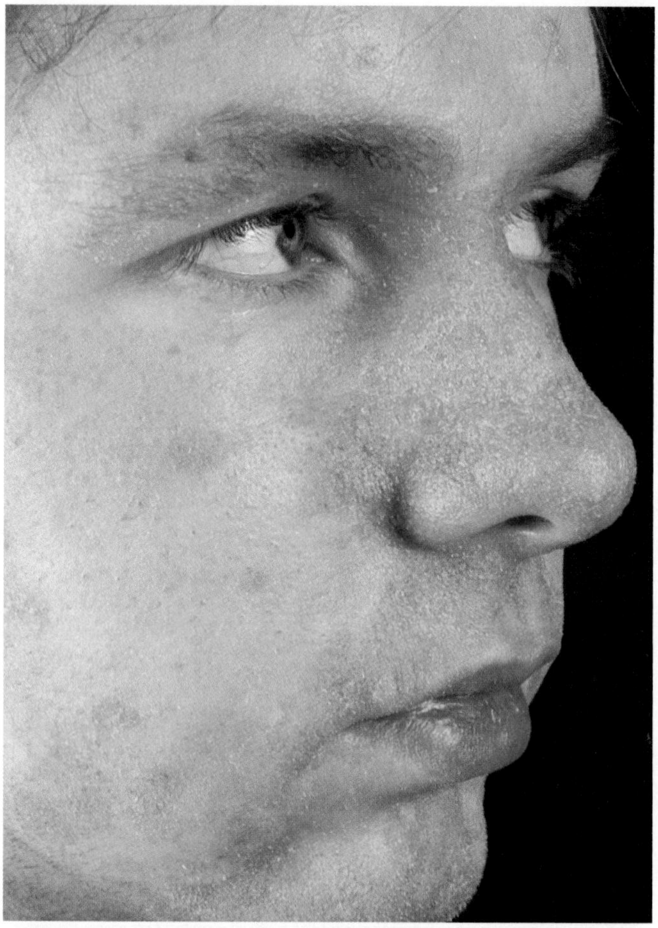

FIGURE 99-9. Seborrheic dermatitis with involvement of the nasolabial folds, cheeks, eyebrows, and nose. *(Reprinted with permission from Plewig G, Jansen T. Seborrheic dermatitis. In: Freedberg IM, Eisen AZ, Wolff K, et al., eds. Fitzpatrick's Dermatology in General Medicine, 6th ed. New York: McGraw-Hill, 2003:1199.)*

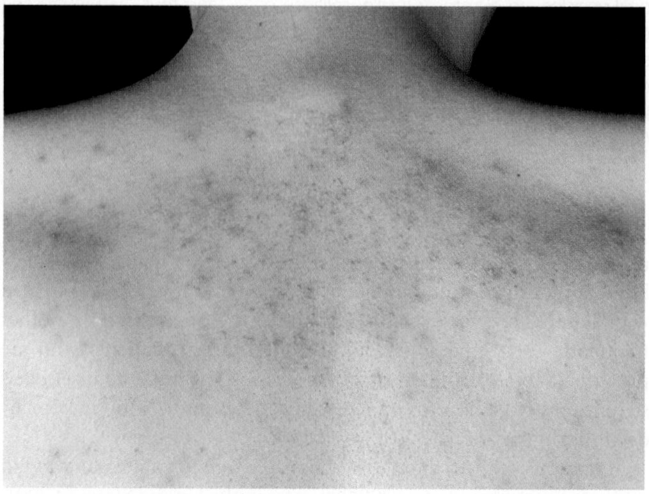

FIGURE 99-10. Seborrheic dermatitis of the upper back. *(Reprinted with permission from Plewig G, Jansen T. Seborrheic dermatitis. In: Freedberg IM, Eisen AZ, Wolff K, et al., eds. Fitzpatrick's Dermatology in General Medicine, 6th ed. New York: McGraw-Hill, 2003:1199.)*

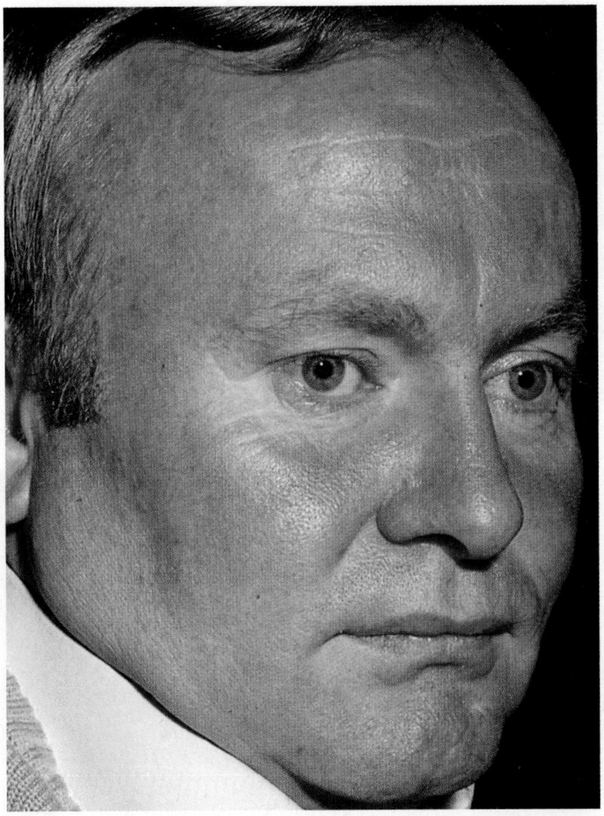

FIGURE 99-11. This patient exhibits a striking amiodarone-induced, late-gray pigmentation of the face. The blue color (ceruloderma) is caused by deposition of a brown pigment in the dermis, contained in macrophages, and endothelial cells. *(Reprinted with permission from Ortonne J-P, Bahadoran P, Fitzpatrick TB, et al. Hypomelanoses and hypermelanoses. In: Freedberg IM, Eisen AZ, Wolff K, et al., eds. Fitzpatrick's Dermatology in General Medicine, 6th ed. New York: McGraw-Hill, 2003:876.)*

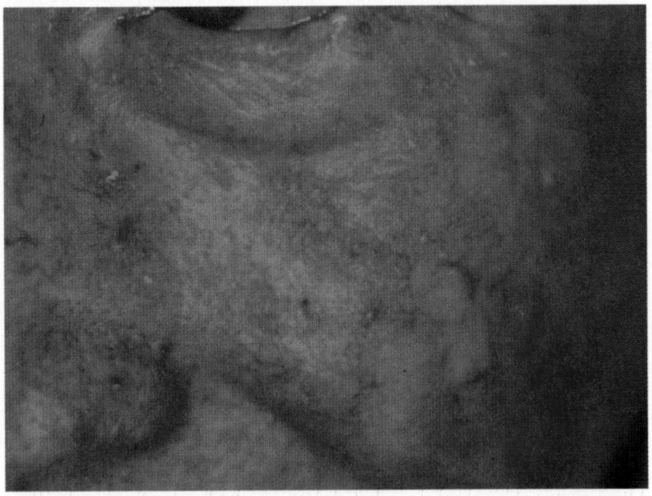

FIGURE 99-12. Severe solar damage of the face revealing both telangiectasias and actinic keratoses at different stages in development, including the flat, pink macules and hyperkeratotic papules. *(Reprinted with permission from Duncan KO, Leffell DJ. Epithelial precancerous lesions. In: Freedberg IM, Eisen AZ, Wolff K, et al., eds. Fitzpatrick's Dermatology in General Medicine, 6th ed. New York: McGraw-Hill, 2003:722.)*

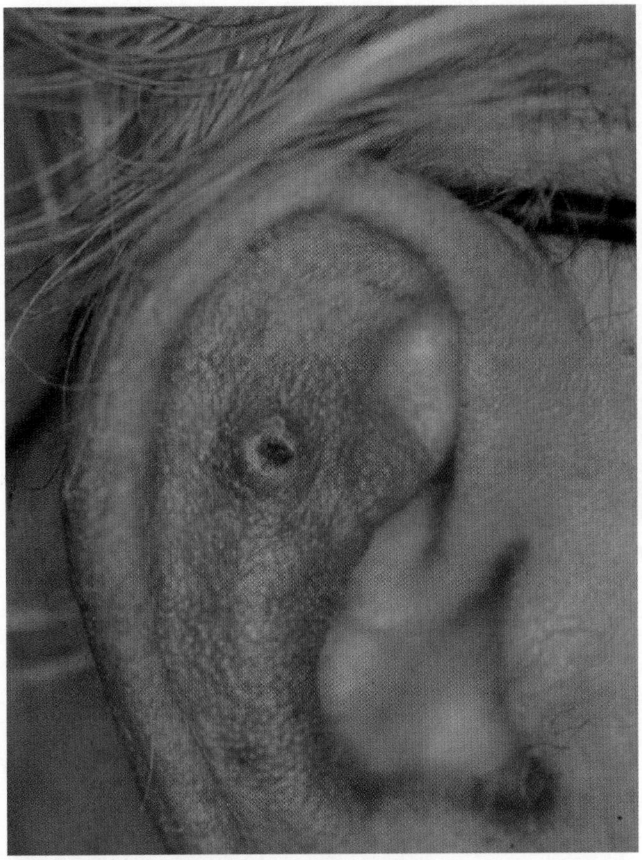

FIGURE 99-13. This case of squamous cell carcinoma must be differentiated in diagnosis from chondrodermatitis nodularis helicis, which, unlike the carcinoma, is painful. *(Reprinted with permission from Grossman D, Leffell DJ. Squamous cell carcinoma. In: Freedberg IM, Eisen AZ, Wolff K, et al., eds. Fitzpatrick's Dermatology in General Medicine, 6th ed. New York: McGraw-Hill, 2003:738.)*

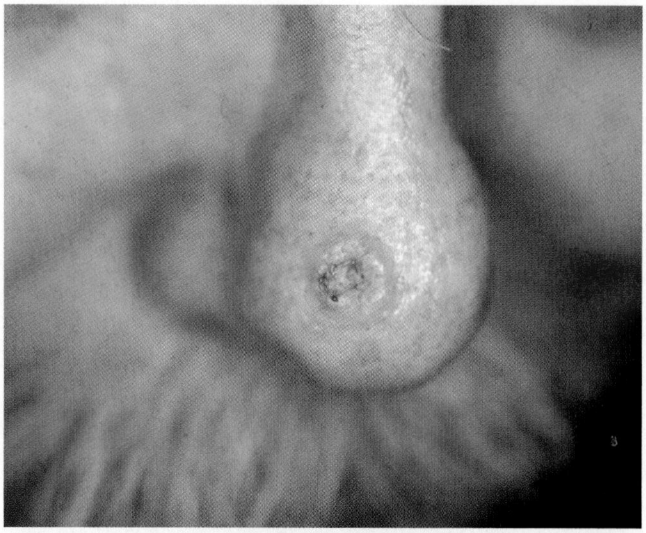

A.

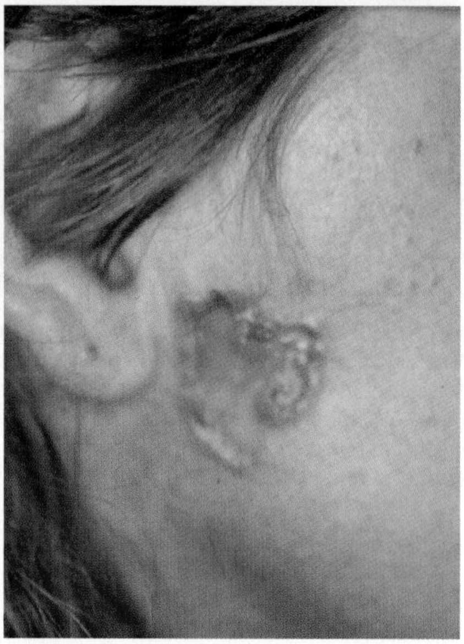

B.

FIGURE 99-14. *A.* Basal cell carcinoma, nodular type. *B.* An ulcerated nodular basal cell carcinoma. *(Reprinted with permission from Carucci JA, Leffell DJ. Basal cell carcinoma. In: Freedberg IM, Eisen AZ, Wolff K, et al., eds. Fitzpatrick's Dermatology in General Medicine, 6th ed. New York: McGraw-Hill, 2003:749.)*

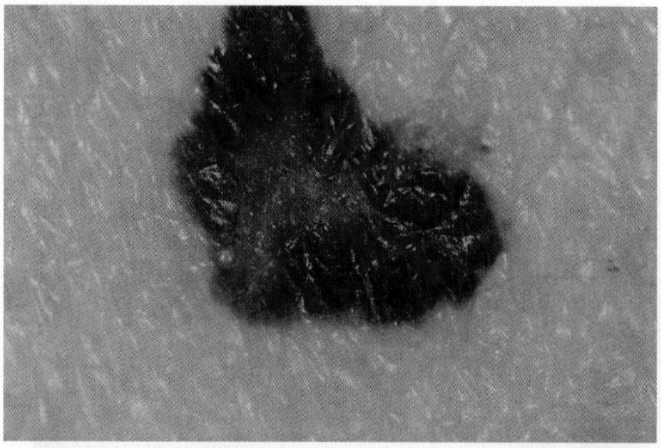

A.

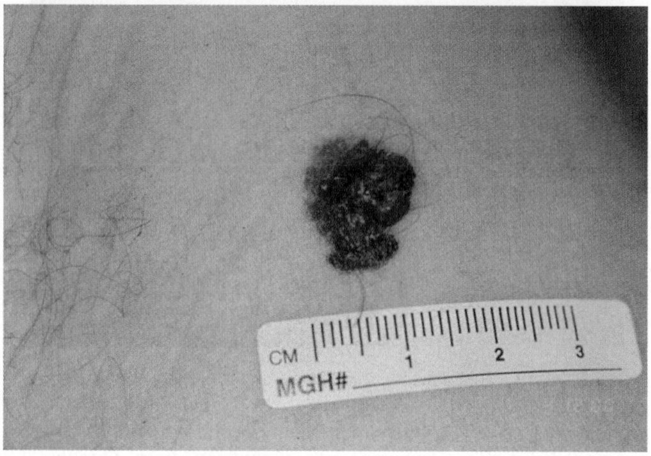

B.

FIGURE 99-15. These two superficial spreading melanomas illustrate the ABCDs of melanoma. *A*, asymmetry. The lesions are not symmetrical and often have irregular borders. *B*, border. Note the highly irregular, uneven, and notched border. *C*, color. The color is variegated with different shades of brown, black, and tan. *D*, diameter. The diameter is usually (but not always) more than 6 mm in melanomas. *(Reprinted with permission from Langley RGB, Barnhill RL, Mihm MC Jr, et al. Neoplasms: Cutaneous melanoma. In: Freedberg IM, Eisen AZ, Wolff K, et al., eds. Fitzpatrick's Dermatology in General Medicine, 6th ed. New York: McGraw-Hill, 2003:925.)*

ABBREVIATIONS

AKs: actinic keratoses

SCC: squamous cell carcinoma

REFERENCES

1. Kilkenny M, Stathakis V, Jolley D, et al. Maryborough skin health survey: Prevalence and sources of advice for skin conditions. Australas J Dermatol 1998;39:235–237.
2. DeSimone II EM. Skin, Hair and nails. In: Jones RM, Rospond RM, eds. Patient Assessment in Pharmacy Practice. Baltimore, MD: Lippincott Williams & Wilkins, 2003:102–128.
3. Ashton RE. Teaching non-dermatologists to examine the skin: A review of the literature and some recommendations. Br J Dermatol 1995;132:221–225.
4. Leung DYM, Eichenfield LF, Boguniewicz M. Atopic dermatitis (atopic eczema). In: Freedberg IM, Eisen AZ, Wolff K, et al., eds. Dermatology in General Medicine, 6th ed. New York: McGraw-Hill; 2003:1180–1194.
5. Belsito DV. Allergic contact dermatitis. In: Freedberg IM, Eisen AZ, Wolff K, et al., eds. Dermatology in General Medicine, 6th ed. New York: McGraw-Hill, 2003:1164–1180.
6. Burton JL, Pye PJ. Seborrhea is not a feature of seborrheic dermatitis. Br Med J 1983;286:1169.
7. Schwartz RA, Janusq CA, Janniger CK. Seborrheic dermatitis: An overview. Am Fam Physician 2006;74:125–130.
8. Meshkinpour A, Sun J, Weinstein G. An open pilot study using tacrolimus ointment in the treatment of seborrheic dermatitis. J Am Acad Dermatol 2003;49:145–147.
9. Rigopoulos D, Ioannides D, Kalogeronitros D, et al. Pimecrolimus 1% cream versus betamethasone 17-valerate 0.1% cream in the treatment of seborrheic dermatitis: A randomized open-label clinical trial. Br J Dermatol 2004;151(5):1071–1075.
10. Bruinsma W. A Guide to Drug Eruptions, 6th ed. Oosthuizen, Netherlands: DeZwaluw, 1995.
11. Korkij, W. Soltani K. Fixed drug eruption. Arch Dermatol 1984; 120:520–524.

12. Garnis-Jones S. Dermatologic side effects of psychopharmacologic agents. Dermatol Clin 1996;14:503–507.
13. Mammen L, Schmidt CP. Photosensitivity reactions: A case report involving NSAIDs. Am Fam Physician 1995;52:575–578.
14. Moller H. Pigmentary disturbances due to drugs. Acta Derm Venereol 1966;46:423–431.
15. Jelinek JE. Cutaneous side effects of oral contraceptives. Arch Dermatol 1970;101:181–186.
16. Granstein RD, Sober AJ. Drug and heavy metal-induced hyperpigmentation. J Am Acad Dermatol 1981;5:1–18.
17. Trimble JW, Mendelson DS, Fetter BF, et al. Cutaneous pigmentation secondary to amiodarone therapy. Arch Dermatol 1983;119:914–918.
18. Salasche S. Epidemiology of actinic keratoses and squamous cell carcinoma. J Am Acad Dermatol 200;42:S4.
19. Miller DL, Weinstock MA. Nonmelanoma skin cancer in the United States: Incidence. J Am Acad Dermatol 1994;30:774.
20. Marks R, Gebauer K, Shumack S, et al. Imiquimod 5% cream in the treatment of superficial basal cell carcinoma: Results of a multicenter 6-week dose-response trial. J Am Acad Dermatol 2001;44:807–813.
21. Rigel DS. Melanoma update, 2001. Skin Cancer Found J 2001;19:13.
22. Lindelof B, Sigurgeirsson B, Gabel H, et al. Incidence of skin cancer in 5356 patients following organ transplantation. Br J Dermatol 2000;143:513.

CHAPTER 100 Acne Vulgaris

DENNIS P. WEST, AMY LOYD, KIMBERLY A. BAUER, LEE E. WEST, LAURA SCUDERI, AND GIUSEPPE MICALI

KEY CONCEPTS

1. In the United States, acne vulgaris is the most common skin disorder, affecting up to 50 million people.
2. Four primary factors are identified as being involved in the formation of acne lesions: increased sebum production, sloughing of keratinocytes, bacterial growth, and inflammation.
3. Acne vulgaris is a disease of the pilosebaceous unit (i.e., the sebaceous glands and adjacent hair follicle).
4. Several types of lesions present at the same time in various stages of development, including noninflammatory and inflammatory lesions, scars, and residual hyperpigmentation.
5. Most therapeutic interventions function primarily to prevent the formation of new acne lesions and have minimal impact on existing lesions.
6. Because most treatments for acne reduce or prevent new eruptions, they can take up to 8 weeks for visible results.
7. *Mild acne* usually is managed with topical retinoids alone or with topical antimicrobials, salicylic acid, or azelaic acid. *Moderate acne* can be managed with topical retinoids in combination with oral antibiotics, and if indicated, benzoyl peroxide. *Severe acne* is often managed with oral isotretinoin.
8. Minocycline has more adverse effects than the other tetracyclines.
9. Acne is a common, chronic inflammatory disorder of the pilosebaceous unit in which a microcomedo develops as the initial condition. The most common form of acne is acne vulgaris. Other variants of acne are neonatal acne, adult acne, acne cosmetica, and acne mechanica. These descriptors refer to age of onset or causative factors.

Localization of acne vulgaris on the facial area, especially in an adolescent population, significantly impacts self-esteem. Although acne is self-limiting, it can persist for years and can result in disfigurement and scarring.[1] Acne can also be associated with anxiety, depression, and higher-than-average unemployment rates.[2] As the emotional impact of acne is not always easy to assess clinically, it is important for the healthcare professional to educate patients on causes of acne, discussing treatment regimens, and counseling on proper medication use.[3]

Learning objectives, review questions, and other resources can be found at **www.pharmacotherapyonline.com.**

EPIDEMIOLOGY

❶ In the United States, acne vulgaris is the most common skin disorder, affecting up to 50 million people.[4] Acne vulgaris affects approximately 80% of the population between the ages of 11 and 30 years,[5] with no gender, race, or ethnicity prevalence.[6]

Acne age of onset varies but usually begins at puberty. A form of acne called *adult acne* can first occur after the mid-20s, affecting females more than males, and with lesions generally distributed in the lower facial area around the mouth, chin, and jaw line.[7]

ETIOLOGY

❷ Four primary factors are identified as being involved in the formation of acne lesions: increased sebum production, sloughing of keratinocytes, bacterial growth, and inflammation.[5,8,9]

INCREASED SEBUM PRODUCTION

Androgen stimulation is enhanced at puberty and sebaceous glands actively produce sebum. Testosterone, the predominant androgen, and its metabolites along with androstenedione, dehydroepiandrosterone, and dehydroepiandrosterone sulfate, are all increased in acne and apparently capable of enhancing sebaceous gland activity. Anatomic sites for acne tend to be more metabolically active in converting androgens to dihydrotestosterone.

Androgenic activity drives sebum production in the sebaceous glands; however, most acne patients do not have an endocrine abnormality. Acne-affected pilosebaceous units apparently have a hyperresponsiveness to circulating androgens.[5] Increased sebum production per se is not necessarily responsible for acne but can rather be viewed as an underlying factor.

SLOUGHING OF KERATINOCYTES

A primary factor in the development of acne is the process of follicular keratinization. Sloughing of keratinocytes within the hair follicle is a normal process, but in acne, follicular keratinization more readily involves keratinocyte clumping and subsequent plugging of the hair follicle pore. Increased sloughing of keratinocytes correlates with comedo formation and can be related to influences such as local cytokine modulation, a decrease in sebaceous linoleic acid, and androgen stimulation.[5] Abnormal follicular keratinization can be a primary event, or can be a secondary response to irritation or other factors.

BACTERIAL GROWTH AND COLONIZATION

The mix of "trapped" keratinocytes and sebum provide an environment for the normally occurring bacteria *Propionibacterium acnes* to

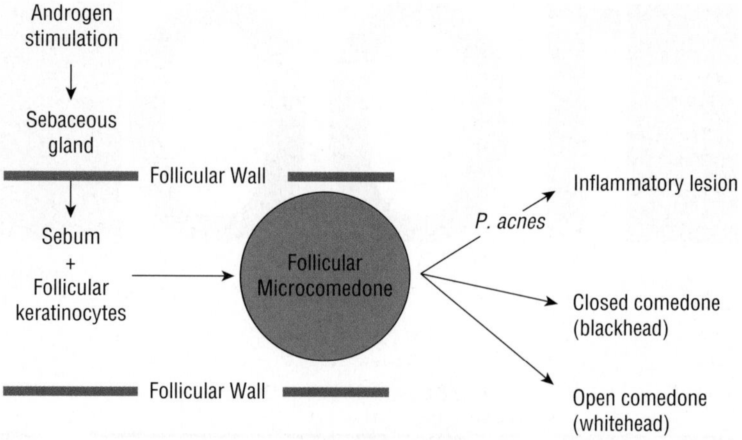

FIGURE 100-1. Principal influence in the formation of acne lesions. *(P. acnes, Propionibacterium acnes.)*

flourish.[10] Although *P. acnes,* a partial anaerobe, resides in the follicle as normal flora, it triggers immune responses such that titers of antibodies to *P. acnes* are higher in patients with severe acne than in non-acne control subjects.

INFLAMMATION AND IMMUNE RESPONSE

Inflammation can be a consequence of increased sebum production, keratinocyte sloughing, and bacterial growth. Also, *P. acnes* can trigger inflammatory acne lesions by producing biologically active mediators and promoting proinflammatory cytokine release.[11]

PATHOPHYSIOLOGY

❸ Acne vulgaris is a disease of the pilosebaceous unit (i.e., the sebaceous gland and adjacent hair follicle). Sebaceous glands, predominant on the face, chest, and upper back, respond to androgen stimulation. These glands provide sebum to the follicular canal and eventually to the skin surface through the follicular opening (the pore). Follicular canal contents include keratinocytes, *P. acnes*, and free fatty acids.

Formation of the primary lesion, the comedo, can be thought of as a plugging of the pilosebaceous follicle. In acne, the follicular canal widens and an increase in cell production can be seen. Sebum mixes with excess loose cells in the follicular canal to form a keratinous plug. The resulting lesion appears as a "blackhead," or open comedo. The brown or black color is not a result of dirt accumulation, but that of melanin (pigment). Inflammation or trauma to the follicle can lead to formation of a "whitehead," or closed comedo. If the follicular wall is damaged or ruptured, the contents of the follicle can extrude into dermis and present clinically as a pustule. Closed comedones are of clinical importance as they can become larger, inflammatory lesions secondary to local *P. acnes* activity (Fig. 100–1).[5,12] Acne lesions can take months to heal completely, and fibrosis associated with healing can lead to permanent scarring.[13]

CLINICAL PRESENTATION OF ACNE VULGARIS

❹ Acne lesions typically occur on the face, back, upper chest, and shoulder area. Severity of the disease varies from a mild comedonal form to severe inflammatory necrotic acne.[14] Acne vulgaris is described as mild, moderate, or severe, depending on the type and severity of lesions present. See Table 100–1 for descriptions of mild, moderate, and severe acne.

Symptoms

- Generally, the diagnosis of acne vulgaris consists of findings that include a mixture of lesions of acne (e.g., comedones, pustules, papules, nodules, and cysts) on the face, back, or chest. Although there is no precise definition for acne, many practitioners consider the presence of 5 to 10 comedones to be diagnostic.

Signs

- There can be more than one morphologic type of lesion present (see Table 100–1), in various stages of development, including noninflammatory and inflammatory lesions, scars, and residual hyperpigmentation.[14]

Noninflammatory Lesions

- An open comedo or blackhead is a plug of sebum, keratinocytes, and microorganisms blocking a *dilated* hair follicle opening, whereas a closed comedone or whitehead is a similar plug blocking a *closed* hair follicle opening to the surface of the skin.

Inflammatory Lesions

- A papule is a well-defined, elevated, palpable, distinct area of skin generally less than 1 cm in diameter involving the epidermis and/or dermis. Papules may not have a change in skin color, but are always raised and can have variable textures.
- A pustule is an elevated, distinct, superficial cavity filled with purulent fluid, typically surrounding a hair follicle.
- A nodule is an elevated, firm, distinct, palpable, round or oval lesion up to 1 cm in diameter that occurs in the dermis and/or hypodermis.

TABLE 100-1 Predominance of Acne Lesion Type by Acne Severity

		Typical Frequency of Lesion Type					
Acne Severity	**Predominant Lesions**	***Closed Comedones***	***Open Comedones***	***Papules***	***Pustules***	***Nodules***	***Scarring***
Mild	Noninflammatory lesions (open and closed comedones)	Few to numerous	Few to numerous	Possible	Possible	None	None
Moderate	Inflammatory papules and pustules with some noninflammatory lesions	Few to numerous	Few to numerous	Numerous	Numerous	Few	Possible
Severe	Inflammatory lesions and scarring with some noninflammatory lesions	Few to numerous	Few to numerous	Extensive	Extensive	Extensive	Extensive

Scars

- Permanent scars can occur as a result of inflammatory acne lesions.

Residual Hyperpigmentation

- Inflammatory acne lesions can trigger noticeable hyperpigmentation that can persist weeks to months after resolution of the lesion.[15]

Laboratory Tests

- There are no laboratory tests to diagnose acne vulgaris.[16] Diagnosis is based on clinical signs. Other dermatologic conditions, such as folliculitis, acne rosacea, and other various acneiform disorders, sometimes can be confused with acne vulgaris.[17]

TREATMENT

Acne Vulgaris

5 Most therapeutic interventions function primarily to prevent the formation of new acne lesions and have minimal impact on existing lesions. Among the factors that can affect acne are genetics, climate, diet, environment, stress, and physical activity.

Stress seems to aggravate, but not induce, acne.[18] In response to stress, immunoreactive nerve fibers can stimulate sebaceous gland activity and provoke inflammatory reactions via mast cells.[19]

The ingestion of iodine can exacerbate acne or induce acneiform lesions.[8] Dietary factors in acne are controversial.

CLINICAL CONTROVERSY

An observational study has concluded that the incidence of acne in Western and non-Western societies is greatly different and suggests that it is not because of genetic influence alone, but most likely occurs because of differences in diet. These authors thought that a non-Westernized diet, representing a substantially low glycemic index, influenced a dramatically lower incidence of acne.[4] It is disputed whether this conclusion is accurate, as acne is influenced by multiple factors, and there are no data to support an effect of glycemic index on acne.[20,21] Whether proven or not, some clinicians feel that diet is a factor in skin conditions, including acne, and needs to be further addressed.[22]

GENERAL APPROACH TO TREATMENT

6 Severity, lesion types, scarring, and skin discoloration, as well as previous treatment history, helps to determine a treatment approach to acne vulgaris (see Table 100–1).[5,9,23,24] Most treatments reduce or prevent new eruptions and can take up to 8 weeks to produce visible results. During the first few weeks of therapy, acne can appear to worsen as existing acne lesions can resolve more rapidly. Patients must understand the need to continue therapy for optimal outcome.

7 Patient education with emphasis on goals, realistic expectations, and dangers of overtreatment is important to optimize therapeutic outcomes. Treatment regimens are targeted to types of lesions and acne severity.[5,14] Mild acne usually is managed with topical retinoids alone or with topical antimicrobials, salicylic acid, or azelaic acid. Moderate acne can be managed with topical retinoids in combination with oral antibiotics, and if indicated, benzoyl peroxide.[24] Severe acne is often managed with oral isotretinoin.

Initial treatment is aimed at reducing lesion count and will vary in duration from a few months to a few years, depending on severity and response to treatment. Once control is achieved, chronic indefinite treatment can be required. Therapy with both topical and systemic antibiotics should be for the minimum duration necessary to achieve control of acne, to minimize the likelihood of resistance.[5,23,24]

Topical treatment forms include creams, lotions, solutions, gels, and disposable wipes. Responses to different formulations can be dependent on skin type and individual preferences:

- Oily to normal skin types can tolerate gels, solutions, and lotions.
- Normal skin can tolerate gels, solutions, lotions, and creams.
- Normal to dry skin can tolerate lotions and creams.

Ointments are not typically included in topical acne therapy because of their occlusive nature and possible induction of acne cosmetica.

Systemic treatment is required in patients with moderate to severe acne, especially when acne scarring is a possibility.[25]

Antibiotics such as tetracyclines and macrolides are the agents of choice for papulopustular acne. In severe papulopustular and nodulocystic/conglobate acne, oral isotretinoin is the treatment of choice. Hormonal therapy represents an alternative effective regimen in female patients.

NONPHARMACOLOGIC THERAPY

Scrubbing the skin with abrasive scrubs or excessive face washing does not necessarily open or cleanse pores. Follicular plugging originates too deeply to be affected by superficial epidermal scrubbing, which often leads to skin irritation.

Because surface cleansing with soap and water primarily affects sebum and bacteria on the surface of the skin and has minimal impact within the follicle, cleansing has a relatively small impact on the treatment of acne.

To avoid skin irritation and dryness during some acne therapies, it is important to use gentle, nondrying cleansing agents.

PHARMACOLOGIC THERAPY

Recently, worldwide consensus statements regarding management and treatment of acne have been widely distributed to improve and optimize outcomes. See Table 100–2 for highlights of consensus statements from the Global Alliance to Improve Outcomes in Acne.[5] In addition, Table 100–3 shows the American Academy of Dermatology evidence basis for acne vulgaris treatment.[16] Figure 100–2 provides acne treatment algorithms based on acne severity. See Table 100–4 for the mechanism of action of selected acne treatments.

Topical Agents: First-Line Therapies

Benzoyl Peroxide Superficial inflammatory acne is typically treated with benzoyl peroxide (BPO), a nonantibiotic antibacterial agent that is rapidly bacteriostatic and possibly bactericidal against *P. acnes*.[26] Its antibacterial mechanism of action is uncertain, although BPO is decomposed on the skin by cysteine, liberating free oxygen radicals that oxidize bacterial proteins.[27] BPO increases the sloughing rate of epithelial cells, loosens the follicular plug structure, and thus possesses some degree of comedolytic activity. An advantage to using topical BPO is that *P. acnes* resistance is not known to develop.[5,24]

BPO is available in soaps, lotions, creams, washes, and gels, in concentrations ranging from 1% to 10%;[5] 10% concentrations are not significantly more efficacious and can be more irritating. Gel formulations have better stability and are usually most potent, whereas lotions, creams, and soaps are weaker. Gels are usually based on alcohol, propylene glycol, or water; the alcohol-based preparations generally cause more dryness and irritation. The addition of a 10% urea to the vehicle is theorized to increase skin moisturization because of its humectant properties as well as to enhance the efficacy of BPO.[28] Fair or moist skin usually is more sensitive to irritation from BPO; thus patients should be advised to

TABLE 100-2 Treatment Guidelines for Acne Vulgaris

Therapy	Recommendations
Topical retinoids	• Should be primary treatment for most forms of acne vulgaris • Use early for best results • Should be applied to the entire affected area • Combine with antimicrobial therapy when inflammatory lesions are present • Essential part of maintenance therapy
Hormonal therapy	Excellent choice for women who also need oral contraceptives for gynecologic reasons • Use early in female patients with moderate to severe acne or with symptoms of seborrhea, acne, hirsutism, or alopecia • Useful as part of combination therapy in women with or without endocrine abnormalities • Sometimes used in women with late-onset acne
Oral isotretinoin	*Indications:* • Severe nodulocystic acne • Severe acne variants • Inflammatory acne with scarring after conventional therapy has failed • Moderate to severe acne, especially frequently relapsing cases • Acne with severe psychological distress *Typical dose:* • 0.5–1.0 mg/kg daily in two divided doses, with cumulative dose of 120–150 mg/kg per treatment course (4–6 months) • A lower dose (<0.5 mg/kg) can be used but is associated with a higher relapse rate • Patient counseling is critical
Combination therapy	• Should be used when inflammatory lesions are present • Speeds clearing and provides greater resolution of both inflammatory lesions and comedones • Topical retinoid should be started at the initiation of antimicrobial therapy • Antibiotic should be discontinued when inflammatory lesions resolve adequately • If this is not possible, then switch to a combination agent with benzoyl peroxide plus an antibiotic • Continue use of topical retinoid to maintain remission of new acne lesions when antibiotic therapy is discontinued

Recommendations from Gollnick et al.[5]

apply medication to dry skin (at least 30 minutes after washing) to decrease irritation. Cleansing dosage forms (washes) that contain anti-acne ingredients such as α-hydroxy acids, BPO, or salicylic acid are available. BPO cleansers can be considered for adolescent boys, both to enhance compliance and to cover large skin areas such as the chest and back.[5]

Dryness and irritation from a primary irritant such as BPO can limit therapy in some patients; allergic contact dermatitis has also been reported.[29]

To limit irritation and increase patient tolerance of BPO, one can initiate therapy with a low-potency formulation (2.5%), and increase either strength (5% to 10%) or application frequency (every other day, each day, and then twice a day). To minimize irritation potential, BPO should be applied to cool, clean, dry skin, no more frequently than twice daily. Use should be discontinued if excessive irritation or allergy occurs. One disadvantage is that BPO can bleach or discolor some fabrics (clothing, bed linen, or towels). Tolerability and effectiveness are enhanced when used in combination with other agents such as topical retinoids, clindamycin, and erythromycin.[5,24,26,30,31]

Retinoids Topical retinoids—tretinoin, adapalene, tazarotene, and in some countries, topical isotretinoin, motretinide, retinaldehyde, and retinoyl-β-glucuronide[5]—can be used as first-line therapy for mild to moderate inflammatory acne and comedonal acne. They can also be viewed by some as preferred agents for maintenance therapy to minimize antibiotic use in acne therapy.[5] To optimize efficacy in moderate inflammatory acne, topical retinoids should be combined with topical antibiotics or BPO.[24,32]

TABLE 100-3 American Academy of Dermatology Evidence Basis for Acne Vulgaris Treatment

Therapy	Therapeutic Approach	Strength of Recommendation	Level of Evidence
Topical	Retinoids	A	I
	Benzoyl peroxide	A	I
	Antibiotics	A	I
	Other agents	A	I
Systemic antibiotics	Tetracyclines	A	I
	Macrolides	A	I
	Trimethoprim-sulfamethoxazole	A	I
Hormonal agents	Contraceptive agents	A	I
	Spironolactone	B	II
	Antiandrogens	B	II
	Oral corticosteroids	B	II
Systemic isotretinoin	Isotretinoin	A	I
Miscellaneous therapy	Intralesional steroids	C	III
	Chemical peels	C	III
	Comedo removal	C	III
Complementary	Herbal agents	B	II
	Psychological approaches	C	III
	Hypnosis/biofeedback	B	II

Strength of recommendation: A, recommendation based on consistent and good-quality patient-oriented evidence; B, recommendation based on inconsistent or limited quality patient-oriented evidence; C, recommendation based on consensus, opinion, or case studies.
Level of evidence: I, good quality patient-oriented evidence; II, limited quality patient-oriented evidence; III, other evidence including consensus guidelines, extrapolations from bench research, opinion, or case studies.
Data from Strauss et al.[16]

Tretinoin Tretinoin, a topical vitamin A analogue, is a comedolytic agent that increases cell turnover in the follicular wall and decreases cohesiveness of cells, leading to extrusion of existing comedones and inhibition of the formation of new comedones,[27] and can reduce the number of inflammatory acne lesions.[24] Tretinoin significantly decreases the number of cell layers in the stratum corneum from approximately 14 to approximately 5.[27]

In a typical 12-week study of tretinoin, the reduction of lesion counts ranged from 32% to 81% for noninflammatory lesions, and 17% to 71% for inflammatory lesions (22% to 83% for the total lesion count).[24]

Tretinoin is available as 0.05% solution (most irritating); 0.01% and 0.025% gels; and 0.025%, 0.05%, and 0.1% creams (least irritating).[5] Treatment initiation with 0.025% cream usually is recommended for mild acne in patients with easily irritated and nonoily skin, 0.01% gel for moderate acne in easily irritated skin with oily complexion, and 0.025% gel for moderate acne with nonsensitive and oily skin. A "flare" of acne can appear suddenly after initiation of treatment, followed by clinical clearing in approximately 8 to 12 weeks.[27]

Once control is established, therapy should be continued at the lowest effective concentration and at the maximum effective interval sufficient to minimize acne exacerbations.

Concomitant use of an antibacterial agent with tretinoin can decrease keratinization, inhibit *P. acnes*, and decrease inflammation. In addition, both BPO and tretinoin have shown additive or synergistic effects in the treatment of inflammatory acne.[33] A regimen of BPO each morning and tretinoin at bedtime can enhance efficacy and be less irritating than either agent used alone.[33] By slowly increasing application frequency from every other day, to daily, and then twice daily, tolerance to tretinoin can be increased. Increased sensitivity to sun exposure, wind, cold, and other irritants can also be evident in patients using tretinoin.

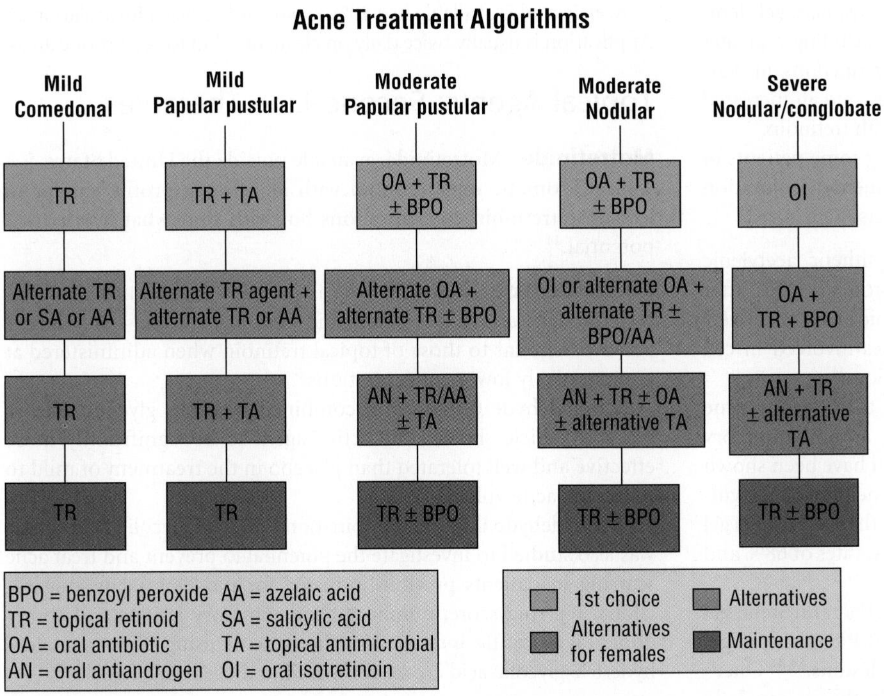

FIGURE 100-2. Algorithms for acne treatment.

Two reformulations of tretinoin include a porous bead (0.01% gel) (microspheres) and liquid polymer (0.025% cream and 0.025% gel). These are designed to be less irritating than standard vehicles for tretinoin and to release tretinoin in a sustained controlled manner.[34] In a topical gel formulation containing polyolprepolymer-2, tretinoin penetration is significantly reduced while epidermal deposition is enhanced, compared with a commercially available gel preparation at the same concentration. Polyolprepolymer-2 is designed to promote retention of drug molecules on the skin surface and in the upper layers of the skin.[34]

A microsponge delivery system represents another formulation approach consisting of macroporous beads 10 to 15 micrometers in diameter that are loaded with tretinoin. Gradual release of active ingredient after topical application depends on mechanical rubbing, temperature, pH, and other factors.[35] Tretinoin 0.1% gel microsponge, tretinoin 0.025% gel, tazarotene 0.1% gel, and adapalene 0.1% gel all showed equivalent facial tolerability in a split-face study.[35] In another variation, a formulation of liposomally encapsulated tretinoin showed somewhat better tolerance than gel dosage forms, yet demonstrated equivalent efficacy.[36]

Adverse reactions to tretinoin—such as skin irritation, erythema, and peeling—vary depending on individual skin type and dosage form used. Allergic contact dermatitis is rare and much less common than with BPO. Teratogenicity risk with topical retinoids remains controversial.

CLINICAL CONTROVERSY

During treatment with topical tretinoin, plasma tretinoin concentrations are typically less than endogenous levels, and apparently do not affect endogenous levels of tretinoin or its metabolites or alter plasma vitamin A levels. However, controversy continues with regard to teratogenicity and embryotoxicity risk-to-benefit issues in the use of topical retinoids during pregnancy.[24,37]

Adapalene Adapalene, a third-generation retinoid,[5] is a retinoid-mimetic compound (a naphthoic acid derivative), available as 0.1% gel, cream, alcoholic solution, and pledgets. Recently, a new 0.3% gel formulation of adapalene has been developed.[38] Adapalene has selective affinity for retinoic acid receptor (RAR) subtypes RAR-β and RAR-γ found in the epidermis,[39] and has comedolytic, keratolytic, and antiinflammatory activity.[9,40,41] Vehicle-controlled and comparative studies have demonstrated the usefulness of adapalene in treatment of acne.[40,41,42]

Adapalene is indicated for mild to moderate acne vulgaris. Adapalene 0.1% gel can be used as an alternative to tretinoin 0.025% gel to achieve better tolerability in some patients.[39,42] Adapalene coadministered with a topical or oral antibiotic represents a rational therapy for moderate forms of acne.[9]

TABLE 100-4 Mechanism of Action of Selected Pharmacotherapeutic Agents in Acne

Treatment	Antimicrobial	Antiinflammatory	Decreased Sebum Production	Keratolytic/Comedolytic
Adapalene	+	++	–	+++
Antibacterial oral agents	+++	++	–	+
Antibacterial topical agents	+++	+	–	+
Azelaic acid	++	+	–	++
Benzoyl peroxide	+++	++	–	+
Oral isotretinoin	++	++	+++	+++
Oral contraceptives	–	–	+++	++
Salicylic acid	–	–	–	+
Spironolactone	–	++	++	–
Topical retinoids	–	+	–	+++

–, No activity; +, low activity; ++, moderate activity; +++, high activity.

In a double-blind 12-week study, tretinoin microsphere gel demonstrated faster onset of action than adapalene, including a greater reduction in comedone counts at week 4. Yet reductions in acne lesions at 12 weeks were similar with the two drugs, and an increased incidence of dryness and peeling was associated with tretinoin.[43]

Adapalene can also be an alternative in treating some patients of color as it produces less skin irritation and subsequent discoloration than the first-generation topical tretinoin products.[9]

Tazarotene Tazarotene, a prodrug and a synthetic acetylenic retinoid, is converted to its active form, tazarotenic acid, after topical application. This new-generation retinoid also selectively binds to RARs and can alter expression of genes involved in cell proliferation, cell differentiation, and inflammation.[44]

Tazarotene is used in the treatment of mild to moderate acne vulgaris and has comedolytic, keratolytic, and antiinflammatory action. Tazarotene 0.1% and 0.05% gel and cream have been shown to be more effective than vehicle in the treatment of acne vulgaris.[45,46] The 0.1% gel was slightly more effective than the 0.05% gel in decreasing lesion counts, with treatment success rates of 68% and 51% of patients, respectively.[6]

Clinical studies have shown that once-daily 0.1% tazarotene gel is more effective than 0.025% tretinoin gel and 0.1% tretinoin gel microsphere in reducing noninflammatory acne lesions.[44,47] Once-daily 0.1% tazarotene gel is also more effective than once-daily adapalene 0.1% gel in reducing both noninflammatory and inflammatory acne lesions.[44,48,49] However, the occurrence of perilesional irritation can limit the use of tazarotene.[48] Once-daily short contact applications significantly reduced irritation potential, yet maintained therapeutic equivalency to standard application regimens.[50] Also, when alternate-day therapy with tazarotene 0.1% gel was compared with once-daily adapalene 0.1% gel therapy, there were no clinically significant differences in improvement or tolerability.[51]

Both 0.1% and 0.05% concentrations had acceptable tolerability profiles, with no serious adverse events.[46] Dose-related local adverse effects include erythema, pruritus, stinging, and burning.[52]

Erythromycin Erythromycin in topical form in concentrations of 1% to 4% with or without the addition of zinc is effective against inflammatory acne. Zinc combination products possibly enhance penetration of erythromycin into the pilosebaceous unit.[53]

Combinations of erythromycin and BPO have shown greater efficacy in treating acne than a combination of erythromycin and tretinoin.[32] Development of *P. acnes* resistance to erythromycin can be reduced by combination therapy with BPO.

Topical erythromycin, usually applied twice daily, is formulated as a gel, lotion, solution, and disposable pad. Reduction of the percentage of free fatty acids in sebum has been noted with the use of topical erythromycin.[53]

Clindamycin Topical clindamycin inhibits *P. acnes* and provides comedolytic as well as antiinflammatory activity.[54] It is available in gel, lotion, solution, foam and disposable pad formulations, and is usually applied twice daily.[49] Combination with BPO increases efficacy.[55] Although rare, diarrhea and pseudomembranous colitis can occur secondary to topical clindamycin.[56]

Azelaic Acid Azelaic acid has a dicarboxylic acid structure that confers antibacterial, antiinflammatory, and comedolytic activity.[54] Azelaic acid is useful for treating mild to moderate acne in patients who do not tolerate BPO. It is useful in treating postinflammatory hyperpigmentation as it also has skin-lightening properties.[57]

Azelaic acid has no likelihood of bacterial resistance, systemic adverse effects, or photosensitivity reactions. Although uncommon, adverse effects, usually transient, include burning, pruritus, stinging, and tingling.[5,24]

Azelaic acid is available in a 20% cream and 15% gel formulations.[58] Application is usually twice daily on clean, dry skin to acne prone areas.

Topical Agents: Second-Line Therapies

Motretinide Motretinide, available outside the United States, is a topical aromatic ester retinoid with an efficacy profile similar to low-dose tretinoin concentrations but with somewhat less irritant potential.[24]

Retinaldehyde Retinaldehyde is biotransformed into all-*trans*-retinoic acid and induces biologic effects including comedolytic activity[59] similar to those of topical tretinoin when administered at comparatively lower concentrations.[5]

Retinaldehyde 0.1% cream combined with 6% glycolic acid vs placebo vehicle showed the active agent to be significantly more effective and well tolerated than placebo in the treatment of mild to moderate acne vulgaris.[60]

Retinaldehyde 0.1% in combination with 6% glycolic acid cream was also studied to investigate the potential to prevent and treat acne scarring in patients previously treated for moderate acne vulgaris. Global scarring score, number of inflammatory lesions and comedones significantly improved in the patients using 0.1% retinaldehyde/6% glycolic acid cream compared to those using vehicle.[59,61]

Retinoyl-β-Glucuronide Retinoyl-β-glucuronide is a naturally occurring, biologically active metabolite of vitamin A. It is a retinoid that possesses the biologic activity of all-trans-retinoic acid but with fewer adverse effects. Topically applied retinoyl-β-glucuronide is safe and effective for treatment of mild forms of acne.[62]

Isotretinoin Isotretinoin is available outside the United States as a gel formulation; it does not significantly alter sebum secretion as does oral isotretinoin. Used topically, the effectiveness of isotretinoin is similar to that of other topical retinoids, but it causes somewhat less skin irritation.[20] It reduces noninflammatory lesions from 46% to 78% and inflammatory lesions from 24% to 55% after 12 to 14 weeks of treatment.[24]

Keratolytic Agents In addition to keratolytic activity, salicylic acid, sulfur, and resorcinol are mildly antibacterial.

Salicylic acid has comedolytic and antiinflammatory action.[23] Also known as β-hydroxy acid, it is deemed a more effective comedolytic than most α-hydroxy acids.[10] In addition, it increases penetration of other substances, and in low concentrations is bacteriostatic and fungistatic.[24]

Although evidence for efficacy in the treatment of acne is conflicting, each agent has been classified as safe and effective by the FDA. Some combinations of these agents can be considered synergistic (e.g., sulfur and resorcinol, salicylic acid, BPO). Keratolytic products, in the concentration allowed, can be less irritating than BPO and tretinoin; however, they are not considered as effective comedolytic agents, as are BPO and tretinoin.

Disadvantages of these agents include the odor created by hydrogen sulfide on reaction of sulfur with the skin, the brown scale from use of resorcinol, and the possibility of salicylism from repeated and widespread use of sufficient concentrations of salicylic acid on highly permeable (inflamed and/or abraded) skin.[56]

Corticosteroids Topical corticosteroids can be applied in very selected patients with very inflammatory acne for short periods of time. They may play a role in reducing flare-up reactions in severe conglobate acne and for reduction of granuloma pyogenicum–like lesions under systemic isotretinoin treatment.[24]

Chemical Peeling Light chemical peels can be useful in some acne patients to reduce superficial scarring and hyperpigmentation.[63] Chemical peeling targets the interfollicular epidermis.[24]

Some currently available substances for chemical peeling include: α-hydroxy acids (glycolic acid), salicylic acid, and trichloroacetic acid.[63] Salicylic acid is lipid soluble and can penetrate into sebum-laden follicles more readily than water-soluble α-hydroxy acids. Salicylic acid can also have some ability to reduce the inflammatory component of acne.[5,23] Patients with sensitive skin types usually tolerate salicylic acid peels.[64]

Dapsone Topical dapsone has both antibacterial and antiinflammatory properties. Topical dapsone 5% gel is FDA approved for use in the treatment of acne in patients older than 12 years of age.[65]

Systemic Agents: First-Line Therapy—Severe Nodular/Conglobata

Isotretinoin As an oral retinoid, isotretinoin is the most effective sebosuppressive agent that affects all of the etiologic factors involved in inflammatory acne, including induction of atrophy of the sebaceous gland with decreased sebum production and change in sebum composition, inhibition of *P. acnes* growth within follicles, inhibition of inflammation, and altered patterns of keratinization within follicles (decreased size and increased differentiation).[66] These characteristics make it the treatment of choice in severe nodulocystic acne.[16,67] It can be used in patients who have failed conventional treatment, those who have scarring acne, those who have chronic relapsing acne, and those who have acne with severe psychological distress.[16,68]

Adverse effects from orally administered isotretinoin are numerous, frequent, and often dose related.[69] Approximately 90% of patients receiving isotretinoin therapy suffer from mucocutaneous effects. Drying of the mucosa of the mouth, nose, and eyes is the most common problem, with relatively rare involvement of the genito-anal mucosa. Cheilitis and skin desquamation occurs in more than 80% of patients. Less frequently, the conjunctiva and nasal mucosa are affected. Table 100–5 shows selected responses to some of the adverse effects of oral isotretinoin.

Disturbances in lipid metabolism also can occur, resulting in transitory increase of blood values for cholesterol and triglycerides.[68] Liver function and serum lipids should initially be monitored, typically at baseline and at weeks 4 and 8.[70] Serious adverse effects of isotretinoin therapy include: increased creatine phosphokinase and blood glucose, as well as photosensitivity, pseudotumor cerebri, excess granulation tissue, hepatomegaly with abnormal liver function tests, bone abnormalities, arthralgias, muscle stiffness, and headaches.[71]

TABLE 100-5 Principal Adverse Effects of Oral Isotretinoin

Adverse Effect	Recommendations for prevention
Teratogenicity	Contraindicated during pregnancy
Depression	Patient monitoring and counseling; antidepressants
Dryness	
Mouth	Sugar-free candy, lozenges, or gum
Eyes	Eyedrops; avoid contact lenses if possible during treatment course
Nose	Lubricant
Skin	Nondrying gentle skin cleansers; noncomedolytic moisturizers
Lips	Lip moisturizer with sunscreen
Muscle and joint pain	Nonsteroidal antiinflammatory drugs
Alopecia	Reversible when drug discontinued or dose decreased
Hypertriglyceridemia	Reversible when drug discontinued or dose decreased
Acne flare at start of therapy	Continue therapy
Photosensitivity	Use sunscreens (moisturizing), protective clothing, and sun avoidance

Hyperlipidemia, diabetes mellitus, and severe osteoporosis are relative contraindications for oral isotretinoin. The drug can very occasionally produce significant mood changes, depression, and other significant psychiatric adverse effects. Although relationship to drug therapy is controversial, current recommendations are that patients be counseled about and screened for depression during therapy.[72]

Oral isotretinoin is a potent teratogen and therefore all patients must participate in the iPLEDGE program, which requires pregnancy tests and assurances by prescribers and pharmacists that they will follow certain procedures, in order to receive oral isotretinoin treatment. It is mandatory for all prescribers, patients, pharmacies, drug wholesalers, and manufacturers in the United States to register and comply with the iPLEDGE program.[16]

Isotretinoin dosing guidelines range from 0.5 to 1 mg/kg per day, but the cumulative dose taken by patients during a treatment course can be the major factor influencing long-term outcome. Optimal results generally have occurred when cumulative doses have attained a range of 120 to 150 mg/kg.[16] One study using dosages of 0.3 to 0.4 mg/kg per day over 6 months found that lower doses over a longer period of time are effective in the treatment of moderate acne with a lower incidence of severe mucocutaneous side effects and laboratory abnormalities.[73]

Although a 5-month course of therapy is sufficient for most patients, it has been observed that an initial dose of 1 mg/kg per day for 3 months, then reduced to 0.5 mg/kg per day, and if possible, to 0.2 mg/kg per day for 3 to 9 additional months can optimize the therapeutic outcome.[25] Generally, after 2 to 4 weeks of treatment, a 50% reduction in pustules can be expected. Pustules clear more rapidly than papules or nodules. Improvement continues during the posttreatment period. In female patients contraception is required because of teratogenicity, recommended to begin 1 month before therapy, continuing during the entire period of treatment, and for up to 3 months after discontinuation of isotretinoin.[69]

Although costs of therapy with isotretinoin are greater in the first year, isotretinoin can be more cost effective than long-term antibiotic treatment.[74]

Systemic Agents: First-Line Therapy—Moderate Papular Pustular/Nodular

Macrolide Antibiotics The macrolide antibiotics (erythromycin, azithromycin, and clindamycin) exhibit antiinflammatory properties in patients with acne.

Erythromycin can be used for patients who require systemic antibiotics but cannot tolerate tetracyclines, or who acquire bacterial strains resistant to tetracyclines.[75,76] The dosage is usually 1 g/day with meals to minimize gastrointestinal intolerance. Zinc combination products possibly enhance penetration of erythromycin into the pilosebaceous unit.[53] The efficacy of erythromycin is similar to tetracycline, but it induces higher rates of bacterial resistance.[75,76] Development of erythromycin resistance by *P. acnes* can be reduced by combination therapy with BPO.

Azithromycin, an azalide antibiotic and derivative of erythromycin, is a safe and effective alternate treatment of moderate to severe inflammatory acne. With a half-life of 68 hours, it can be intermittently dosed three times a week.[77] One study comparing 100 mg doxycycline daily in addition to topical 0.05% tretinoin cream to 500 mg azithromycin once a day for four days per month along with 0.05% topical tretinoin for a total of 12 weeks found that the monthly dose of azithromycin was as effective as daily doxycycline.[78] Adherence is high with this regimen, and phototoxicity and resistance have not been reported.[77]

Although clindamycin is very effective in the treatment of acne, it is seldom used for long-term therapy because of the possible induction of pseudomembranous colitis.[79]

Tetracyclines The tetracyclines are effective in reducing *P. acnes*.[79] In addition to their antibacterial effects, they reduce the amount of keratin in sebaceous follicles and have antiinflammatory properties inhibiting chemotaxis, phagocytosis, complement activation (by the alternate pathway), and cell-mediated immunity.[80,81] Tetracyclines also appear to have an affinity for inflammatory cells and bacteria, resulting in higher drug concentration in areas of inflamed skin.

The recent discovery that tetracyclines have biologic actions affecting inflammation, proteolysis, angiogenesis, apoptosis, metal chelation, ionophoresis, and bone metabolism has led to the development of chemically modified tetracyclines, also known as inhibitors of multiple proteases and cytokines. These are tetracyclines modified by the removal of the dimethylamino group at carbon 4. This eliminates its antibiotic properties and enhances antiinflammatory properties.[81] Incyclinide, one chemically modified tetracycline, is in initial trials for acne.

Adverse reactions involving the gastrointestinal tract can occur with the tetracyclines. Drawbacks to the use of tetracyclines include hepatotoxicity and predisposition to superinfections (vaginal candidiasis), and very rarely benign intracranial hypertension. All tetracyclines are photosensitizing, and a sun protection plan should be used. Also, these agents should not be used in children younger than 10 years of age or in pregnant women because the risk of tooth discoloration when used in children and inhibition of skeletal growth in the developing fetus and child. Emergence of resistant strains of *P. acnes*,[75] adverse events, and adherence issues associated with long-term systemic tetracycline use have led to new treatment approaches.

Moreover, adverse effects of tetracyclines include resistant bacteria, folliculitis, candidiasis, gastrointestinal upset, and phototoxic effects. Tetracyclines must not be combined with systemic retinoids because of the increased probability for development of intracranial hypertension. Tetracycline is used in the treatment of moderate to severe acne vulgaris. It is the least expensive of the tetracyclines and therefore often prescribed for initial therapy.[27] A common initial approach includes tetracycline 1 g daily (500 mg twice daily), 1 hour before meals; after 1 or 2 months, when marked improvement of inflammatory lesions is observed, the dose can be decreased to 500 mg every day, for another 1 or 2 months.[75] Drawbacks to the use of tetracycline include also a drug–food interaction with dairy products.

Doxycycline is commonly used in the treatment of moderate to severe acne vulgaris. It is more effective and produces less resistance than tetracycline. The initial dosage is usually 100 or 200 mg daily, followed after improvement by 50 mg/day as a maintenance dose; it can be taken with food even though it is more effective when taken 30 minutes before meals. Subantimicrobial-dose doxycycline (20 mg) has been investigated in a double-blind, placebo-controlled trial in the treatment of moderate facial acne. Positive outcomes were achieved with no development of resistant organisms or change in normal skin flora.[82,83] Adverse effects include resistant bacteria, folliculitis, candidiasis, gastrointestinal upset, and phototoxic effects such as photoonycholysis.[84]

Minocycline is another commonly prescribed oral antibiotic used in the treatment of moderate to severe acne vulgaris. It is more effective than tetracycline because of greater lipid solubility and enhanced penetration into tissue and sebaceous follicles.[26] It is dosed similarly to doxycycline (100 mg/day or 50 mg twice daily) and on an indefinite basis in selected patients.

Of the tetracyclines, minocycline has the most reported adverse effects.[79] Neither tetracycline nor doxycycline contains an amino acid side chain found in minocycline that has potential to form a reactive metabolite. Perhaps related to this, in addition to usual tetracycline adverse effects, minocycline can cause hypersensitivity syndromes, serum sickness–like illness discoloration of skin, nail, and bone; hepatitis, nephritis, vestibular toxicity, drug-induced lupus erythematosus, intracranial hypertension, pseudotumor cerebri,[85] systemic eosinophilia,[79] severe fever,[86] depersonalization symptoms,[87] and cutaneous hyperpigmentation of at least four distinct types:[88]

1. Blue-black pigmentation confined to sites of scarring or inflammation on the face
2. Blue-gray circumscribed pigmentation of normal skin of the lower legs and forearms
3. Diffuse muddy brown pigmentation of normal skin accentuated in sun-exposed areas
4. Circumscribed blue-gray pigmentation within acne scars confined to the back

Systemic Agents: Second-Line Therapy Cotrimoxazole Cotrimoxazole (trimethoprim-sulfamethoxazole) or trimethoprim alone can be used for treating patients who do not tolerate tetracycline and erythromycin or in cases of resistance to these antibiotics.[26] The adult dosage is usually 800 mg sulfamethoxazole and 160 mg trimethoprim twice daily.

Hormonal Therapy Hormonal therapy is useful in treating acne in women with elevated or normal serum androgens. It can also be warranted for female patients with severe seborrhea, clinically apparent androgenic alopecia, seborrhea/acne/hirsutism/alopecia syndrome, late-onset acne, and with proven ovarian or adrenal hyperandrogenism.[89]

Hormonal therapy is absolutely contraindicated in women who want to become pregnant because of the risk of sexual organ malformation in a developing fetus.[25]

Antiandrogens, or androgen-receptor blockers, should be avoided during pregnancy.[5] Both cyproterone (not available in the United States) and spironolactone should be used for acne only in women, because they lead to feminization in men.[90]

Cyproterone Acetate Cyproterone acetate (CPA) (although not available in the United States) is the most widely used antiandrogen compound. It is a progestational agent that blocks the androgen receptors and also inhibits synthesis of adrenal androgens. In Europe and Canada, CPA is widely used in women for the treatment of acne, with or without signs of hyperandrogenism, and as an oral contraceptive formulation (CPA 2 mg with ethinyl estradiol 35 mcg or 50 mcg).[91]

Adverse effects include menstrual abnormalities, breast tenderness and enlargement, nausea and vomiting, fluid retention, leg edema, headache, and melasma.

Chlormadinone Acetate Chlormadinone acetate (2 mg), alone or in combination with 50 mcg ethinyl estradiol or 50 mcg mestranol in a contraceptive pill, is available in several European countries and is slightly less efficacious than CPA.[92]

Spironolactone Spironolactone, an antiandrogen and inhibitor of 5α-reductase, reduces sebum production and improves acne at dosages of 50 to 200 mg twice daily in patients with acne resistant to conventional therapy.[89] Most commonly, it is used in countries where other antiandrogen drugs are not available.

Adverse effects are dose dependent and can be lessened by initiating therapy with doses as low as 25 mg/day. They include potential hyperkalemia, irregular menses, breast tenderness, headache, and fatigue.[23]

Drospirenone Drospirenone, a derivative of spironolactone, has been introduced in Europe as another antiandrogen agent that is a useful alternative in some patients.[91]

Flutamide Flutamide, a drug approved for treatment of prostate cancer, blocks the androgen receptor. It is used in combination with oral contraceptives in seborrhea and acne therapy for females.[90] The dose is usually 250 to 500 mg twice daily over 6 months.

Flutamide use is limited because of reports of fatal hepatitis requiring monitoring of liver function during therapy.[90] Pregnancy must be avoided because of the risk of feminization of a male fetus.[5]

Estrogens Estrogens are indicated in female patients with clinical evidence of hyperandrogenism. They suppress the ovarian production of androgens. In addition, they can decrease acne by directly opposing the effects of androgens locally within the sebaceous gland and regulating genes that negatively influence sebaceous gland growth or lipid production.[93]

Estrogens are of limited use because the dose of estrogen required for suppression of sebum production is greater than that required to suppress ovulation. Response to 0.035 to 0.050 mcg of ethinyl estradiol or its esters occurs in some women, but higher doses are often required.[93] Breast examinations and Pap smears can be recommended in women receiving long-term estrogen therapy; other serious adverse effects such as clotting and hypertension are possible but very rare in young healthy females.

The mechanism of action of estrogens in acne can include: a direct effect within the sebaceous gland opposing the effects of androgens, inhibition of androgen production by gonadal tissue via a negative feedback loop on pituitary gonadotrophin release, and regulation of genes that influence sebaceous gland growth or lipid production.

Oral Contraceptives Oral contraceptives containing two agents, an estrogen and a progestin, are used as an alternate treatment for moderate acne in women. Estrogen-containing contraceptive agents that are currently approved for the treatment of acne are norgestimate with ethinyl estradiol and norethindrone acetate with ethinyl estradiol.[16]

Oral contraceptives decrease free testosterone levels by increasing sex hormone–binding globulin, which binds circulating testosterone causing it to be biologically inactive. They also inhibit the ovarian production of androgens by suppressing ovulation. This overall antiandrogen effect leads to a decrease in sebum production.[94]

Common adverse effects of oral contraceptives include nausea and vomiting, breast tenderness, headache, spotting and breakthrough bleeding, edema of the venous system of the lower extremities, decreased libido, increased appetite, and weight gain. A transient flare of inflammatory acne can also accompany the initiation of therapy. The most serious adverse effect of oral contraceptives, thromboembolism, has been greatly reduced by the use of lowered doses of estrogens.[89]

Gonadotropin-Releasing Hormone Agonists Gonadotropin-releasing hormone agonists (buserelin, nafarelin, and leuprolide), available as injectable drugs or nasal spray, suppress the production of ovarian androgens and are reported to have some efficacy in acne. However, by reducing estrogen, they can produce menopausal symptoms (headache and bone loss). They have not been demonstrated to be safe and effective for treatment of acne.[89]

Corticosteroids Low-dose corticosteroids (prednisone, prednisolone, or dexamethasone) are indicated in patients with adrenal hyperandrogenism or acne fulminans.

Dapsone Oral dapsone, a sulfone, has been used for treatment of acne conglobata (a rare condition that is highly inflammatory; onset usually occurs in adults) and acne inversa (chronic lesions in the axillary and groin areas).[95]

Nicotinamide Topical 2% nicotinamide can be effective in reducing sebum excretion rate in some individuals.[96]

Oral nicotinamide in combination with oral zinc, copper and folic acid is noted to have both antiinflammatory and antibacterial activity and has undergone clinical studies for the treatment of acne vulgaris. This combination tablet can be an effective therapy for the treatment of acne vulgaris when used alone or with topical therapies.[97]

PHARMACOECONOMIC CONSIDERATIONS

Although costs of therapy with oral isotretinoin are greater than with other therapeutic choices in the first year, this option can be more cost-effective than long-term antibiotic treatment in severe acne.[74]

EVALUATION OF THERAPEUTIC OUTCOMES

See Tables 100–6 through 100–10 for prototypical examples of pharmaceutical care plans in the evaluation of therapeutic outcomes for each grade of acne severity.

TABLE 100-6 Typical Pharmaceutical Care Plan for Mild Comedonal Acne

Mild Comedonal Acne	Baseline	2 wk	1 mo	2 mo	3 mo	4 mo	5 mo	6 mo	9 mo	12 mo	Every 12 mo
First choice											
TR	PA PT		PA		PA			PA		PA	PA
Alternatives											
Alternate TR, SA, or AA	PA		PA		PA			PA		PA	PA
Alternatives for females											
TR	PA		PA		PA			PA		PA	PA
Maintenance											
TR											PA

AA, azelaic acid; blank, N/A; PA, physical assessment; PT, pregnancy test; SA, salicylic acid; TR, topical retinoid.

TABLE 100-7 Typical Pharmaceutical Care Plan for Mild Papular Pustular Acne

Mild Papular Pustular Acne	Baseline	2 wk	1 mo	2 mo	3 mo	4 mo	5 mo	6 mo	9 mo	12 mo	Every 12 mo
First choice											
TR + TA	PA PT		PA		PA			PA		PA	PA
Alternatives											
Alternate TA agent + alternate TR or AA	PA PT		PA		PA			PA		PA	PA
Alternatives for females											
TR + TA	PA PT		PA		PA			PA		PA	PA
Maintenance											
TR											PA

AA, azelaic acid; blank, N/A; PA, physical assessment; PT, pregnancy test; TA, topical antimicrobial; TR, topical retinoid.

TABLE 100-8 Typical Pharmaceutical Care Plan for Moderate Papular Pustular Acne

Papular Pustular Acne	Baseline	2 wk	1 mo	2 mo	3 mo	4 mo	5 mo	6 mo	9 mo	12 mo	Every 12 mo
First choice											
OA + TR ± BPO	PA PT lab		PA		PA lab			PA	PA	PA lab	PA lab
Alternatives											
Alternate OA + alternate TR ± BPO	PA PT lab		PA		PA lab			PA	PA	PA lab	PA lab
Alternatives for females											
AN + TR/AA ± TA	PA PT lab		PA		PA lab			PA		PA lab	PA lab
Maintenance											
TR ± BPO											PA lab

AA, azelaic acid; AN, oral antiandrogen; blank, N/A; BPO, benzoyl peroxide; lab, complete blood count, chemical screen, urinalysis; OA, oral antibiotic; PA, physical assessment; PT, pregnancy test; TA, topical antimicrobial; TR, topical retinoid.

TABLE 100-9 Typical Pharmaceutical Care Plan for Moderate Nodular Acne

Moderate Nodular Acne	Baseline	2 wk	1 mo	2 mo	3 mo	4 mo	5 mo	6 mo	9 mo	12 mo	Every 12 mo
First choice											
OA + TR ± BPO	PA PT lab		PA		PA lab			PA	PA	PA lab	PA lab
Alternatives											
OI or alternate OA + alternate TR ± BPO/AA	PA PT lab SLA	PA PT lab SLA	PA PT lab SLA	PA PT	PA PT lab SLA	PA PT	PA PT	PA PT lab SLA			
Alternatives for females											
AN + TR ± OA ± alternate TA	PA PT lab		PA lab		PA lab			PA		PA lab	PA lab
Maintenance											
TR ± BPO± OA											PA lab

AA, azelaic acid; AN, oral antiandrogen; blank, N/A; BPO, benzoyl peroxide; lab, complete blood count, chemical screen, urinalysis; OA, oral antibiotic; OI, oral isotretinoin; PA, physical assessment; PT, pregnancy test; SLA, serum lipid analysis; TA, topical antimicrobial; TR, topical retinoid.

TABLE 100-10 Typical Pharmaceutical Care Plan for Severe Nodular/Conglobata Acne

Severe Nodular Acne	Baseline	2 wk	1 mo	2 mo	3 mo	4 mo	5 mo	6 mo	9 mo	12 mo	Every 12 mo
First choice											
OI	PA PT lab SLA	PA PT lab SLA	PA PT lab SLA	PA PT	PA PT lab SLA	PA PT	PA PT	PA PT lab SLA			
Alternatives											
OA + TR + BPO	PA PT lab		PA lab		PA lab			PA	PA	PA lab	PA lab
Alternatives for females											
AN + TR ± alternate TA	PA PT lab		PA lab		PA lab			PA		PA lab	PA lab
Maintenance											
TR ± BPO											PA

AN, oral antiandrogen; blank, N/A; BPO, benzoyl peroxide; lab, complete blood count, chemical screen, urinalysis; OA, oral antibiotic; OI, oral isotretinoin; PA, physical assessment; PT, pregnancy test; SLA, serum lipid analysis; TA, topical antimicrobial; TR, topical retinoid.

ABBREVIATIONS

BPO: benzoyl peroxide

CPA: cyproterone acetate

RAR: retinoic acid receptor

REFERENCES

1. Goodman GJ, Baron JA. Postacne scarring—A quantitative global scarring grading system. J Cosmet Dermatol 2006;5(1):48–52.
2. Hanna S, Sharma J, Klotz J. Acne vulgaris: More than skin deep. Dermatol Online J 2003;9(3):8.
3. Dreno B. Assessing quality of life in patients with acne vulgaris: Implications for treatment. Am J Clin Dermatol 2006;7(2):99–106.
4. Cordain L, Lindeberg S, Hurtado M, et al. Acne vulgaris: A disease of Western civilization. Arch Dermatol 2002;138(12):1584–1590.
5. Gollnick H, Cunliffe W, Berson D, et al. Management of acne: A report from a Global Alliance to Improve Outcomes in Acne. J Am Acad Dermatol 2003;49(1 Suppl):S1–37.
6. Berson DS, Chalker DK, Harper JC, et al. Current concepts in the treatment of acne: Report from a clinical roundtable. Cutis 2003;72(1 Suppl):5–13.
7. Williams C, Layton AM. Persistent acne in women: Implications for the patient and for therapy. Am J Clin Dermatol 2006;7(5):281–290.
8. Hunter JAA, Savin JA, Dahl MV. Sebaceous and sweat gland disorders. In: Clinical Dermatology, 3rd ed. Malden, MA: Blackwell Science, 2002:148–161.
9. Leyden JJ. A review of the use of combination therapies for the treatment of acne vulgaris. J Am Acad Dermatol 2003;49(3 Suppl):S200–210.
10. Baumann L. Acne. In: Cosmetic Dermatology. New York: McGraw-Hill, 2002:55–61.
11. Burkhart CN, Burkhart CG. Microbiology's principle of biofilms as a major factor in the pathogenesis of acne vulgaris. Int J Dermatol 2003;42(12):925–927.
12. Cunliffe WJ, Holland DB, Jeremy A. Comedone formation: Etiology, clinical presentation, and treatment. Clin Dermatol 2004;22(5):367–374.
13. Holland DB, Jeremy AH, Roberts SG, et al. Inflammation in acne scarring: A comparison of the responses in lesions from patients prone and not prone to scar. Br J Dermatol 2004;150(1):72–81.
14. Katsambas AD, Stefanaki C, Cunliffe WJ. Guidelines for treating acne. Clin Dermatol 2004;22(5):439–444.
15. Callender VD. Considerations for treating acne in ethnic skin. Cutis 2005;76(2 Suppl):19–23.
16. Strauss JS, Krowchuk DP, Leyden JJ, et al. Guidelines of care for acne vulgaris management. J Am Acad Dermatol 2007;56(4):651–663.
17. Webster GF. Acne vulgaris and rosacea: Evaluation and management. Clin Cornerstone 2001;4(1):15–22.
18. Chiu A, Chon SY, Kimball AB. The response of skin disease to stress: Changes in the severity of acne vulgaris as affected by examination stress. Arch Dermatol 2003;139(7):897–900.
19. Toyoda M, Morohashi M. New aspects in acne inflammation. Dermatology 2003;206(1):17–23.
20. Thiboutot DM, Strauss JS. Diet and acne revisited. Arch Dermatol 2002;138(12):1591–1592.
21. Bershad S. The unwelcome return of the acne diet. Arch Dermatol 2003;139(7):940–941.
22. Treloar V. Diet and acne redux. Arch Dermatol 2003;139(7):941.
23. Longshore SJ, Hollandsworth K. Acne vulgaris: One treatment does not fit all. Cleve Clin J Med 2003;70(8):670, 2–4.
24. Gollnick HP, Krautheim A. Topical treatment in acne: Current status and future aspects. Dermatology 2003;206(1):29–36.
25. Zouboulis CC, Piquero-Martin J. Update and future of systemic acne treatment. Dermatology 2003;206(1):37–53.
26. Tan HH. Antibacterial therapy for acne: A guide to selection and use of systemic agents. Am J Clin Dermatol 2003;4(5):307–14.
27. Arndt K, Bowers, KE. Acne. In: Manual of Dermatologic Therapeutics, 6th ed. Philadelphia: Lippincott Williams & Wilkins, 2002:3–20.
28. Gold MH. A multicenter efficacy and tolerability evaluation of benzoyl peroxide in a 10% urea vehicle for the treatment of acne vulgaris. J Drugs Dermatol 2006;5(5):442–445.
29. Shwereb C, Lowenstein EJ. Delayed type hypersensitivity to benzoyl peroxide. J Drugs Dermatol 2004;3(2):197–199.
30. Rodriguez D, Davis MW. The BEST study: Results according to prior treatment. Cutis 2003;71(2 Suppl):27–34.
31. Fagundes DS, Fraser JM, Klauda HC. New therapy update—A unique combination formulation in the treatment of inflammatory acne. Cutis 2003;72(1 Suppl):16–9.
32. Gupta AK, Lynde CW, Kunynetz RA, et al. A randomized, double-blind, multicenter, parallel group study to compare relative efficacies of the topical gels 3% erythromycin/5% benzoyl peroxide and 0.025% tretinoin/erythromycin 4% in the treatment of moderate acne vulgaris of the face. J Cutan Med Surg 2003;7(1):31–37.
33. Shalita AR, Rafal ES, Anderson DN, et al. Compared efficacy and safety of tretinoin 0.1% microsphere gel alone and in combination with benzoyl peroxide 6% cleanser for the treatment of acne vulgaris. Cutis 2003;72(2):167–172.
34. Del Rosso JQ. The role of the vehicle in combination acne therapy. Cutis 2005;76(2 Suppl):15–18.
35. Leyden J, Grove GL. Randomized facial tolerability studies comparing gel formulations of retinoids used to treat acne vulgaris. Cutis 2001;67(6 Suppl):17–27.
36. Patel VB, Misra A, Marfatia YS. Clinical assessment of the combination therapy with liposomal gels of tretinoin and benzoyl peroxide in acne. AAPS PharmSciTech 2001;2(3):E-TN4.
37. Nau H. Teratogenicity of isotretinoin revisited: Species variation and the role of all-trans-retinoic acid. J Am Acad Dermatol 2001;45(5):S183–187.
38. Thiboutot D, Pariser DM, Egan N, et al. Adapalene gel 0.3% for the treatment of acne vulgaris: a multicenter, randomized, double-blind, controlled, phase III trial. J Am Acad Dermatol 2006;54(2):242–250.
39. Waugh J, Noble S, Scott LJ. Adapalene: A review of its use in the treatment of acne vulgaris. Drugs 2004;64(13):1465–1478.
40. Thiboutot DM, Gollnick HP. Treatment considerations for inflammatory acne: Clinical evidence for adapalene 0.1% in combination therapies. J Drugs Dermatol 2006;5(8):785–794.
41. Millikan LE. Adapalene: An update on newer comparative studies between the various retinoids. Int J Dermatol 2000;39(10):784–788.
42. Wolf JE. An update of recent clinical trials examining adapalene and acne. J Eur Acad Dermatol Venereol 2001;15(Suppl 3):23–29.
43. Nyirady J, Grossman RM, Nighland M, et al. A comparative trial of two retinoids commonly used in the treatment of acne vulgaris. J Dermatolog Treat 2001;12(3):149–157.
44. Chivot M. Retinoid therapy for acne. A comparative review. Am J Clin Dermatol 2005;6(1):13–19.
45. Phillips TJ. An update on the safety and efficacy of topical retinoids. Cutis 2005;75(2 Suppl):14–22.
46. Shalita AR, Berson DS, Thiboutot DM, et al. Effects of tazarotene 0.1 % cream in the treatment of facial acne vulgaris: Pooled results from two multicenter, double-blind, randomized, vehicle-controlled, parallel-group trials. Clin Ther 2004;26(11):1865–1873.
47. Webster GF, Berson D, Stein LF, et al. Efficacy and tolerability of once-daily tazarotene 0.1% gel versus once-daily tretinoin 0.025% gel in the treatment of facial acne vulgaris: A randomized trial. Cutis 2001;67(6 Suppl):4–9.
48. Thielitz A, Krautheim A, Gollnick H. Update in retinoid therapy of acne. Dermatol Ther 2006;19(5):272–279.
49. Shalita AR, Myers JA, Krochmal L, Yaroshinsky A. The safety and efficacy of clindamycin phosphate foam 1% versus clindamycin phosphate topical gel 1% for the treatment of acne vulgaris. J Drugs Dermatol 2005;4(1):48–56.
50. Bershad S, Kranjac Singer G, Parente JE, et al. Successful treatment of acne vulgaris using a new method: Results of a randomized vehicle-controlled trial of short-contact therapy with 0.1% tazarotene gel. Arch Dermatol 2002;138(4):481–489.
51. Leyden J, Lowe N, Kakita L, Draelos Z. Comparison of treatment of acne vulgaris with alternate-day applications of tazarotene 0.1% gel and once-daily applications of adapalene 0.1% gel: A randomized trial. Cutis 2001;67(6 Suppl):10–16.
52. Guenther LC. Optimizing treatment with topical tazarotene. Am J Clin Dermatol 2003;4(3):197–202.
53. Tan HH. Topical antibacterial treatments for acne vulgaris: Comparative review and guide to selection. Am J Clin Dermatol 2004;5(2):79–84.

54. Gollnick H. Current concepts of the pathogenesis of acne: Implications for drug treatment. Drugs 2003;63(15):1579–1596.
55. Bikowski JB. Clinical experience results with clindamycin 1% benzoyl peroxide 5% gel (Duac) as monotherapy and in combination. J Drugs Dermatol 2005;4(2):164–171.
56. Akhavan A, Bershad S. Topical acne drugs: Review of clinical properties, systemic exposure, and safety. Am J Clin Dermatol 2003;4(7):473–492.
57. Fleischer AB, Jr. The evolution of azelaic acid. Cutis 2006;77(2 Suppl):4–6.
58. Gollnick HP, Graupe K, Zaumseil RP. [Azelaic acid 15% gel in the treatment of acne vulgaris. Combined results of two double-blind clinical comparative studies]. J Dtsch Dermatol Ges 2004;2(10):841–847.
59. Katsambas AD. RALGA (Diacneal), a retinaldehyde and glycolic acid association and postinflammatory hyperpigmentation in acne—A review. Dermatology 2005;210(Suppl 1):39–45.
60. Poli F, Ribet V, Lauze C, et al. Efficacy and safety of 0.1% retinaldehyde/ 6% glycolic acid (Diacneal) for mild to moderate acne vulgaris. A multicentre, double-blind, randomized, vehicle-controlled trial. Dermatology 2005;210(Suppl 1):14–21.
61. Dreno B, Katsambas A, Pelfini C, et al. Combined 0.1% retinaldehyde/ 6% glycolic acid cream in prophylaxis and treatment of acne scarring. Dermatology 2007;214(3):260–267.
62. Barua AB, Sidell N. Retinoyl beta-glucuronide: A biologically active interesting retinoid. J Nutr 2004;134(1):286S-289S.
63. Monheit GD. Chemical peels. Skin Therapy Lett 2004;9(2):6–11.
64. Lee HS, Kim IH. Salicylic acid peels for the treatment of acne vulgaris in Asian patients. Dermatol Surg 2003;29(12):1196–1199.
65. Draelos ZD, Carter E, Maloney JM, et al. Two randomized studies demonstrate the efficacy and safety of dapsone gel, 5% for the treatment of acne vulgaris. J Am Acad Dermatol 2007;56(3):439 e1–10.
66. Zaenglein A, Thiboutot DM. Acne vulgaris. In: Bolognia J, Jorizzo JL, Rapini RP, ed. Dermatology. London: Mosby, 2003:531–544.
67. Goulden V. Guidelines for the management of acne vulgaris in adolescents. Paediatr Drugs 2003;5(5):301–313.
68. Cooper AJ. Treatment of acne with isotretinoin: Recommendations based on Australian experience. Australas J Dermatol 2003;44(2):97–105.
69. Charakida A, Mouser PE, Chu AC. Safety and side effects of the acne drug, oral isotretinoin. Expert Opin Drug Saf 2004;3(2):119–129.
70. Altman RS, Altman LJ, Altman JS. A proposed set of new guidelines for routine blood tests during isotretinoin therapy for acne vulgaris. Dermatology 2002;204(3):232–235.
71. Kunynetz RA. A review of systemic retinoid therapy for acne and related conditions. Skin Therapy Lett 2004;9(3):1–4.
72. Hersom K, Neary MP, Levaux HP, et al. Isotretinoin and antidepressant pharmacotherapy: A prescription sequence symmetry analysis. J Am Acad Dermatol 2003;49(3):424–32.
73. Amichai B, Shemer A, Grunwald MH. Low-dose isotretinoin in the treatment of acne vulgaris. J Am Acad Dermatol 2006;54(4):644–646.
74. Doshi A. The cost of clear skin: Balancing the social and safety costs of iPLEDGE with the efficacy of Accutane (isotretinoin). Seton Hall Law Rev 2007;37(2):625–660.
75. Ross JI, Snelling AM, Carnegie E, et al. Antibiotic-resistant acne: Lessons from Europe. Br J Dermatol 2003;148(3):467–478.
76. Eady EA, Gloor M, Leyden JJ. Propionibacterium acnes resistance: A worldwide problem. Dermatology 2003;206(1):54–56.
77. Fernandez-Obregon AC. Azithromycin for the treatment of acne. Int J Dermatol 2000;39(1):45–50.
78. Parsad D, Pandhi R, Nagpal R, Negi KS. Azithromycin monthly pulse vs daily doxycycline in the treatment of acne vulgaris. J Dermatol 2001;28(1):1–4.
79. Ochsendorf F. Systemic antibiotic therapy of acne vulgaris. J Dtsch Dermatol Ges 2006;4(10):828–841.
80. Sadick NS. Antibiotics: unapproved uses or indications. Clin Dermatol 2000;18(1):11–6.
81. Sapadin AN, Fleischmajer R. Tetracyclines: Nonantibiotic properties and their clinical implications. J Am Acad Dermatol 2006;54(2):258–265.
82. Bikowski JB. Subantimicrobial dose doxycycline for acne and rosacea. Skinmed 2003;2(4):234–245.
83. Skidmore R, Kovach R, Walker C, et al. Effects of subantimicrobial-dose doxycycline in the treatment of moderate acne. Arch Dermatol 2003;139(4):459–464.
84. Carroll LA, Laumann AE. Doxycycline-induced photo-onycholysis. J Drugs Dermatol 2003;2(6):662–663.
85. Smith K, Leyden JJ. Safety of doxycycline and minocycline: A systematic review. Clin Ther 2005;27(9):1329–1342.
86. Grim SA, Romanelli F, Jennings PR, Ofotokun I. Late-onset drug fever associated with minocycline: Case report and review of the literature. Pharmacotherapy 2003;23(12):1659–1662.
87. Cohen PR. Medication-associated depersonalization symptoms: Report of transient depersonalization symptoms induced by minocycline. South Med J 2004;97(1):70–73.
88. Mouton RW, Jordaan HF, Schneider JW. A new type of minocycline-induced cutaneous hyperpigmentation. Clin Exp Dermatol 2004;29(1):8–14.
89. Thiboutot D, Chen W. Update and future of hormonal therapy in acne. Dermatology 2003;206(1):57–67.
90. Shaw JC. Hormonal therapies in acne. Expert Opin Pharmacother 2002;3(7):865–874.
91. van Vloten WA, van Haselen CW, van Zuuren EJ, et al. The effect of two combined oral contraceptives containing either drospirenone or cyproterone acetate on acne and seborrhea. Cutis 2002;69(4 Suppl):2–15.
92. Worret I, Arp W, Zahradnik HP, et al. Acne resolution rates: Results of a single-blind, randomized, controlled, parallel phase III trial with EE/CMA (Belara) and EE/LNG (Microgyn). Dermatology 2001;203(1):38–44.
93. Thiboutot D. Acne: Hormonal concepts and therapy. Clin Dermatol 2004;22(5):419–28.
94. Harper JC. Hormonal therapy for acne using oral contraceptive pills. Semin Cutan Med Surg 2005;24(2):103–106.
95. Kaminsky A. Less common methods to treat acne. Dermatology 2003;206(1):68–73.
96. Draelos ZD, Matsubara A, Smiles K. The effect of 2% niacinamide on facial sebum production. J Cosmet Laser Ther 2006;8(2):96–101.
97. Niren NM, Torok HM. The Nicomide Improvement in Clinical Outcomes Study (NICOS): Results of an 8-week trial. Cutis 2006;77(1 Suppl):17–28.

CHAPTER 101 Psoriasis

DENNIS P. WEST, AMY LOYD, LEE E. WEST, KIMBERLY A. BAUER, MARIA LETIZIA MUSUMECI, AND GIUSEPPE MICALI

KEY CONCEPTS

1. Exogenous trigger factors such as climate, stress, alcohol, smoking, infection, trauma, and drugs can aggravate psoriasis.
2. As a result of pathogenic T-cell production and activation, psoriatic epidermal cells proliferate at a rate sevenfold faster than normal epidermal cells.
3. In general, psoriatic lesions are characterized by sharply demarcated, erythematous papules and plaques often covered with silver-white scales.
4. Goals of treatment are usually directed at skin normalization: reduction or clearing of erythema, papules, and plaques, as well as scales.
5. A variety of topical (corticosteroids, anthralin, and vitamin D analogues) and systemic (acitretin, cyclosporine, tacrolimus, methotrexate, mycophenolate mofetil, sulfasalazine, 6-thioguanine, and hydroxyurea) pharmacotherapeutic agents can be used for treating psoriasis, with treatment determined by the severity of a patient's condition and the probability of controlling long-term symptoms with minimal adverse effects. Biologic agents (infliximab, etanercept, alefacept, adalimumab or efalizumab) and photochemotherapy with oral methoxypsoralen and ultraviolet A light (PUVA) or ultraviolet B light can provide additional options, especially for patients with severe or refractory cases.
6. Combination, rotational, and sequential therapy is commonly used in the treatment of psoriasis to achieve a response, increase effectiveness of treatment, or enable lowering of doses of individual agents.

Psoriasis is a common chronic inflammatory skin disorder characterized by recurrent exacerbations and remissions of thickened, erythematous, and scaling plaques. The clinical appearance of psoriasis can be cosmetically disfiguring, and the disease can be physically and emotionally debilitating, especially for patients with severe disease.

EPIDEMIOLOGY

Psoriasis is universal in occurrence and affects nearly 7 million Americans with approximately 14 million physician visits over the 12-year period from 1990 to 2001.[1] The disorder occurs in all racial groups but is most prevalent in whites. It is equally common in males and females. Two peaks of age of onset have been described: The greatest incidence is between 20 and 30 years, and a smaller peak occurs between 50 and 60 years of age[2]; however, the age of onset is widely variable from infancy to old age. Although rarely life-threatening, psoriasis has an adverse physical and emotional impact on quality of life.[3,4]

Learning objectives, review questions, and other resources can be found at **www.pharmacotherapyonline.com.**

ETIOLOGY

Psoriasis is a complex and multifactorial disease that is apparently associated with interaction between environmental factors (exogenous or endogenous antigens) and a specific genetic background. Environmental factors involved in disease development are not completely known or understood.[5]

ENVIRONMENTAL FACTORS

Factors such as climate, stress, alcohol, smoking, infection, trauma, and drugs can aggravate psoriasis. Warm seasons and sunlight reportedly improve psoriasis in 80% of patients, whereas 90% report worsening in cold weather. In addition, stress worsens psoriasis in up to 40% of patients; however, the exact role stress plays in exacerbation of psoriasis is uncertain. Alcohol seems to have a greater influence on the progression of psoriasis in men, and the association between smoking and psoriasis seems to be stronger in women.[6]

Infection has been identified retrospectively as a common precipitating factor in psoriasis.[7] Approximately 25% of patients have initial onset of the disease after clinically documented infections, and more than one-half have exacerbations within 3 weeks after an upper respiratory infection. A variant known as guttate (small drop-like plaques) psoriasis is often associated with infections of group A β-hemolytic streptococci.[7]

Psoriatic lesions can develop at the site of injury on normal-appearing skin (Koebner response). This response can be induced by a variety of trauma that includes rubbing, venipuncture, bites, surgery, and mechanical pressure. The mechanism for a Koebner response is unknown, is not unique to psoriasis, and yet occurs in a majority of psoriatic patients. Duration of time between injury and lesion development can vary from a day to several weeks.

Lithium carbonate, β-adrenergic blocking agents, some antimalarial agents, nonsteroidal antiinflammatory drugs, and tetracyclines are among the most commonly reported drugs to exacerbate psoriasis or to trigger psoriasiform lesions.[8]

GENETIC FACTORS

There is a significant genetic component in psoriasis, but the exact mode of inheritance is uncertain.[9] Most patients with psoriasis have at least one immediate relative with the disorder.[10] Monozygotic twins have a higher concordance for psoriasis than dizygotic twins. Some studies have implied that the development and severity of psoriasis is influenced by gender of the contributing parent. However, recent linkage analysis indicates that the susceptibility genes likely play an important role in the pathogenesis of early onset psoriasis with no predilection for gender.[11]

A number of genetic loci have been identified by genome-wide linkage scans and several loci have been replicated: *PSORS1* on chromosome 6p, within the major histocompatibility complex, *PSORS2* on chromosome 17q, PSORS3 in the SLC12A8 gene, and PSORS4 on chromosome 1q. PSORS4 is likely to be involved in terminal differentiation of keratinocytes. Several other loci have been identified; however they are not always replicated in other pedigrees. The most consistently identified loci *PSORS1* accounts for an estimated 30% to 50% of the genetic contribution to psoriasis.[12]

Studies of histocompatibility antigens in psoriatic patients indicate statistically significant associations on the B, C, and D loci, more specifically, human leukocyte antigen (HLA) B13, HLA-B17, and HLA-B37.[2]

A significant association also occurs with HLA-Cw6, where the relative likelihood for developing psoriasis is 9 to 15 times normal.[2] Moreover, evidence exists for an "early onset" psoriasis susceptibility locus at 9q33-9q34.[11] Identification of multiple loci for psoriasis susceptibility indicates that psoriasis is a genetically heterogeneous disease with different genetic causes, and a strong candidate gene for sequencing remains to be identified.

PATHOPHYSIOLOGY

IMMUNOLOGIC MECHANISMS

Recently, attention has been directed to cell-mediated immune mechanisms in psoriasis. A central role for activated T cells has been demonstrated by response to drugs that block T-cell activation, migration, or cytokine secretion in psoriasis.[13]

Cutaneous inflammatory T-cell–mediated immune activation requires two T-cell signals that are mediated via cell–cell interactions by surface proteins and by antigen-presenting cells (APCs) such as dendritic cells or macrophages.

The "first signal" is the interaction of the T-cell receptor with antigen presented by the APC.

The "second signal," also called *costimulation*, is mediated through various surface interactions. Both signals are essential for initial activation of T cells in psoriasis.[14]

Once T cells are activated, they migrate from lymph nodes and the circulation into skin. In psoriatic lesions, T cells migrate into the epidermis, whereas T cells are not normally located in the epidermis of normal skin. Specific cell-surface proteins on T cells and vascular endothelium including selectins, integrins, and other adhesion molecules mediate this movement. For example, the mechanism of cellular interaction between lymphocyte function-associated antigen-1 (LFA-1) on T cells and intercellular adhesion molecule-1 on endothelial cells is the basis for development of one of the biologic agents, alefacept. Once in the skin, activated T cells secrete various cytokines that induce the pathologic changes of psoriasis.[15] Cytokines are proteins secreted by immune cells that bind to very specific receptors on the cell surface, influencing keratinocytes and other cells to produce pathologic changes characteristic of psoriasis.

The cytokine profile in psoriasis is known as a T-helper cell type 1 (TH_1) response; this subset of T cells produces primarily interferon-γ (INF-γ), tumor necrosis factor-α (TNF-α), and interleukin (IL)-2.[16] Other local cells, including keratinocytes, dendritic cells, and local neutrophils, are induced to produce other cytokines, including TNF-α, IL-23, IL-20,[12] transforming growth factor-α (TGF-α), TGF-β, amphiregulin, IL-1, IL-6, and IL-8,[16] which are believed to be important in the pathophysiology of psoriasis. All of these cytokines are important in the pathophysiologic development of psoriasis CSTL, and represent possible targets of biologic therapies.

TABLE 101-1 Chemical Mediators of Inflammation in Psoriasis (CMI)

CMI	Cell Type	Outcome
GM-CSF	T cells	↑ mononuclear cells, ↑ neutrophils
INF-γ	T cells	↑ E selectin, ↑ ICAM, ↓ IL-4, ↑ keratinocytes, ↑ MHC I and II, ↑ VCAM, ↓ TH_2
IL-2	T cells	↑ macrophages, ↑ TH_1 cells
IL-3	T cells	↑ dendritic cells, ↑ macrophages
IL-8	Keratinocytes, neutrophils	↑ vascular response
IL-12	APC	↑ TH_1 cells
IP-10	Keratinocytes	↑ leukocyte adhesion
MIG	Keratinocytes	↑ leukocyte adhesion
RANTES	Keratinocytes	↑ IL-12
TNF-α	Keratinocytes, macrophages, T cells	↑ E selectin, ↑ ICAM, ↑ TH_1 cells, ↑ VCAM
VEGF	Keratinocytes, T cells	↑ angiogenesis

APC, antigen-presenting cell; GM-CSF, granulocyte-macrophage colony-stimulating factor; ICAM, intercellular adhesion molecule; INF, interferon; IL, interleukin; IP, inflammatory protein; MHC, major histocompatibility complex; MIG, monokine induced by interferon-γ; RANTES, regulated on activation, normal T-cell expressed and secreted; TNF, tumor necrosis factor; TH_1, T-helper cell type 1; TH_2, T-helped cell type 2; VCAM, vascular cell adhesion molecule; VEGF, vascular endothelial growth factor.
Data from Mehlis S, Gordon KB. From laboratory to clinic: Rationale for biologic therapy. Dermatol Clin 2004;22(4):371–377, vii–viii.

Cytokines and chemokines with a currently recognized potential role in psoriasis include the following (Table 101–1): granulocyte-macrophage colony-stimulating factor; regulated on activation, normal T-cell expressed and secreted (RANTES; causes keratinocyte proliferation); epidermal growth factor and monokine induced by interferon-γ(MIG; increases neutrophil migration); IL-8 and inducible protein-10 (increases differentiation of TH_1 cells); IL-12 and macrophage inflammatory protein-3α (MIP-3α; produces angiogenesis); IL-1 and thymus and activation-regulated chemokine (TARC; produces epidermal hyperplasia); IL-6 (increases other chemokine release); INF-γ(increases upregulation of adhesion molecules on endothelial cells); TNF-α; and vascular endothelial growth factor (VEGF).

DEFECTS IN THE EPIDERMAL CELL CYCLE

As a result of pathogenic T-cell production and activation, psoriatic epidermal cells proliferate at a rate sevenfold faster than normal epidermal cells. The germinative cell population increases in psoriatic skin, and duration of the epidermal cell cycle is nearly eight times faster than normal skin.[17] Lesion-free skin in psoriatic patients generally is considered to be involved because epidermal proliferation is elevated in apparently normal skin of psoriatic patients.

CLINICAL PRESENTATION OF PSORIASIS

General

- Although psoriasis is a nonmalignant, hyperproliferative epidermal cell disorder, it results in accumulated, immature, excessively thickened skin that is manifested as plaques.

Symptoms

- Psoriatic lesions are relatively asymptomatic; however, pruritus is a complaint in about 25% of patients. Severe, widespread psoriasis can involve symptomatology similar to that of exfoliative dermatitis, which can include fever and chills. Psoriatic arthritis is a distinct clinical entity in which both psoriatic lesions and inflammatory arthritis-like symptoms occur. Classically, distal interphalangeal joints and adjacent nails are involved, but knees, elbows, wrists and ankles also can be involved.

Signs

- In general, psoriatic lesions are characterized by sharply demarcated, erythematous papules and plaques often covered with silver-white scales. Initial lesions are usually small papules that enlarge over time and coalesce into plaques, sometimes as serpiginous or geographic forms. If the covering scale is removed, a salmon-pink to erythematous lesion is exposed, perhaps with punctate bleeding from prominent dermal capillaries (Auspitz sign).
- Psoriatic lesions vary in appearance depending on the anatomic site and the variant of psoriasis. The most common type of psoriasis is psoriasis vulgaris. Scalp involvement can vary from diffuse scaling on an erythematous scalp to thickened plaques with exudation, microabscesses and fissures. Trunk, back, arm, and leg lesions can appear as generalized, scattered, discrete, guttate (resembling drops or spots), or large plaques. Palms, soles, face, and genitalia can be commonly involved. Affected nails often are pitted with subungual keratotic material. Yellowing under the nail plate also can be seen.

Laboratory Tests

- Skin biopsy of lesional skin is useful in confirming the diagnosis.

Other Diagnostic Tests

- None

TREATMENT

Psoriasis

Goals of treatment of psoriasis are directed at skin normalization: reduction or clearing of erythema, papules, and plaques, as well as scales. Reduction or clearing of skin signs as a treatment objective leads to normalized cosmesis and improvement in quality of life. A goal of therapy is to achieve resolution of lesions, but partial clearing is sometimes acceptable when using regimens with decreased toxicity and increased patient acceptability.

The psoriasis area and severity index (PASI) serves as a uniform method to determine the extent of body surface area affected, along with the degree of erythema, induration, and scaling. Mild psoriasis is considered to have a PASI score of less than 12, moderate involvement is PASI 12 to 18, and severe psoriasis is PASI greater than 18.

Another method to determine disease activity is the Physician Global Assessment (PGA), which summarizes erythema, induration, scaling and extent of plaques relative to baseline assessment. Although the PASI and PGA are commonly used, they fail to measure quality of life and patient well-being. The National Psoriasis Foundation Psoriasis Score (NPF-PS) was developed in response to these limitations by incorporating quality of life and patient's perception of well-being as well as induration, extent of involvement, physician's static global assessment and pruritus.

The results of a comparison study of disease measurement systems showed that NPF-PS strongly correlated with PASI and PGA but better reflected patient perception.[18]

As a new class of agents, the biologic agents were required to demonstrate a PASI 75% decrease for approval by the Food and Drug Administration (FDA). No prior nonbiologic agents were required to meet such a high standard to be approved.

GENERAL APPROACH TO TREATMENT

Although the exact cause of psoriasis is unknown, in a majority of patients, pharmacotherapy is usually effective in establishing good clinical control. Psoriasis can be a lifelong relapsing and remitting disease, so therapy should be selected with careful consideration of long-term adverse effects. Major points for consideration include the extent and site of disease involvement, the patient's age, and concurrent associated diseases.

Keratolytics

Keratolytic agents are used to remove scale, smooth the skin, and decrease hyperkeratosis. The mechanism of action of salicylic acid, one of the most commonly used keratolytics, is disruption in corneocyte-to-corneocyte cohesion in the abnormal horny layer of psoriatic skin. For this reason, salicylic acid is especially useful at anatomic sites where thick scales are present.

When applied to large, inflamed areas of skin, salicylic acid can induce salicylism, with symptoms of nausea, vomiting, tinnitus, and hyperventilation. Salicylate poisoning in small children is potentially more serious than in older people because they are at higher risk of developing metabolic acidosis. Fatal cases of percutaneous salicylate intoxication have been reported in children and adults.

The keratolytic effect of salicylic acid enhances penetration and efficacy of some other topical agents such as corticosteroids.[5]

Salicylic acid, as a gel or lotion, is usually applied two to three times a day in concentrations of 2% to 10%.

NONPHARMACOLOGIC THERAPY

Emollients

Emollients are frequently used during therapy-free periods to minimize skin dryness that can lead to early recurrence. These agents hydrate stratum corneum and minimize cutaneous transepidermal water loss (evaporation). Hydration causes the stratum corneum to swell and flattens the surface contour. Emollients effective as moisturizers decrease binding forces within the horny layer, enhance desquamation, and eliminate scaling. Emollients also can increase pliability of the skin, have antipruritic activity, and possess mild vasoconstrictor activity.

As lotions, creams, or ointments, emollients often need to be applied several times per day (about four times per day) to achieve a beneficial response. Adverse effects of emollients include folliculitis and allergic or irritant contact dermatitis.

Balneotherapy

Balneotherapy (and climatotherapy) is a therapeutic approach that consists of bathing in waters containing certain salts, often combined with natural exposure to the sun. Certain areas around the world have been targeted as excellent places to receive balneotherapy (or climatotherapy); the Dead Sea is salt filled, located below sea level, and capable of enhancing exposure to a natural ultraviolet A (UVA) light source. The Kangal hot spring in Turkey and the Blue Lagoon in Iceland are also notable salt-containing waters. The salts in these waters are a mixture of salts that reduce activated T cells in skin and are remittive for psoriasis. Reduction in serum manganese and lithium levels is significant after bathing with Dead Sea salt, an effect believed to be related to effectiveness of the salts.[19]

PHARMACOLOGIC THERAPY

Topical treatments for mild to moderate psoriasis include corticosteroids, vitamin D analogues, tazarotene, and others. The systemic treatments for moderate to severe psoriasis include biologic agents, cyclosporine, acitretin, and others. See Tables 101–2 and 101–3 for topical and systemic psoriasis treatment regimens and adverse effects.

Various pharmacotherapeutic approaches to psoriasis management include combinations of topical and systemic agents.

TABLE 101-2 Selected Topical Psoriasis Treatment Regimens and Adverse Effects

Therapy	Regimen	Selected Adverse Effects
Emollients	Approximately 4 times per day	Folliculitis, allergic or irritant contact dermatitis
Salicylic acid	2–3 times per day	Irritation, salicylism with symptoms of nausea, vomiting, tinnitus, or hyperventilation
Coal tar	Apply in the evening, allowing to remain through the night	Irritation, photoreactions, unpleasant odor, staining skin and clothing
Corticosteroids	2–4 times per day	Local tissue atrophy, degeneration, and striae; epidermal thinning; acneiform eruptions; bacterial or fungal skin infections; glucocorticoid systemic effects
Calcipotriene	1–2 times/day, no more than 100 g/wk	Burning and stinging (10% of patients), irritant contact dermatitis
Anthralin	Usually applied in the evening, allowed to remain overnight; short-contact regimens can also be used	Stains skin and clothing; irritation
Tazarotene	1 time per day, usually in the evening	Pruritus, burning, stinging, and erythema

Topical Therapy: First-Line Agents

Corticosteroids Topical corticosteroids are the most widely used agents for the treatment of psoriasis in the United States. They are often used to decrease erythema, scaling, and pruritus. Topical vasoconstricting potencies of corticosteroids are ranked by the Stoughton-Cornell classification in seven classes (Table 101–4). Class I corticosteroids, very high-potency, include products such as clobetasol propionate, halobetasol propionate, and betamethasone dipropionate (optimized vehicle).[20]

High-potency agents are used primarily as alternatives to systemic adrenocorticoid therapy when local therapy is feasible. Examples of conditions for which very-high-potency products are used include thick, chronic psoriatic plaques. They should be used for finite periods of time (as short as possible) and on relatively small body surface areas.

Class VII corticosteroids are agents with the lowest level of vasoconstricting potency (e.g., hydrocortisone 1%). They have a weak antiinflammatory effect and are safest for long-term application. These products are also the safest products for use on the face and intertriginous areas, in infants and young children, and with occlusion when necessary and appropriate.

Intermediate classes include products with a medium-potency ranking and are used in moderate inflammatory dermatoses. Medium-potency preparations can be used on the face and intertriginous areas for limited periods of time.[20]

The mechanism of action of corticosteroids in psoriasis is not fully understood.[21] Topical corticosteroids appear to inhibit phos-

TABLE 101-3 Selected Systemic Psoriasis Treatment Regimens and Adverse Effects

Therapy	Regimen	Selected Adverse Effects
Acitretin	25–50 mg/day until lesions have resolved	Hypervitaminosis A (dry lips/cheilitis, dry mouth, dry nose, dry eyes/conjunctivitis, dry skin, pruritus, scaling, and hair loss), hepatotoxicity, skeletal changes, hypercholesterolemia, hypertriglyceridemia
Adalimumab	40 mg subcutaneously once weekly or every other week	Rhinitis, injection site reactions, upper respiratory infections, flu-like symptoms, nausea, headache; can increase opportunistic infections, malignancy, neurologic demyelinating diseases
Alefacept	15 mg intramuscularly once weekly	Pharyngitis, influenza-like symptoms, chills, dizziness, nausea, headache, injection site pain and inflammation, and nonspecific infection; opportunistic infections and malignancy are rare
Cyclosporine	2.5–4 mg/kg per day in two divided doses; can increase to 5 mg/kg per day in 1 month if no response	Nephrotoxicity, malignancies, hypertension, hypomagnesemia, hyperkaliemia, alterations in liver function tests, elevations of serum lipids, gastrointestinal intolerance, paresthesias, hypertrichosis, gingival hyperplasia
Etanercept	50 mg subcutaneously twice a week	Local reaction at the injection site (20% of patients); respiratory tract and gastrointestinal infections, abdominal pain, nausea and vomiting, headaches, rash; serious infections (including tuberculosis) and malignancies are rare
Efalizumab	1 mg/kg subcutaneously once weekly	Headache, nausea, chills, nonspecific infection, pain, fever, and asthenia; no evidence drug causes organ toxicity, serious infection, or malignancy
Infliximab	5 or 10 mg/kg for three intravenous infusions at weeks 0, 2, and 6	Headaches, fever, chills, fatigue, diarrhea, pharyngitis, upper respiratory and urinary tract infections; hypersensitivity reactions (urticaria, dyspnea, hypotension); lymphoproliferative disorders
Hydroxyurea	1 g/day; can increase to 2 g/day	Bone marrow toxicity with leukopenia or thrombocytopenia, cutaneous reactions, leg ulcers, megaloblastic anemia
Methotrexate	7.5–15 mg per week, increased incrementally by 2.5 mg every 2 to 4 weeks until response; maximal doses are approximately 25 mg/wk	Anemia, leukopenia, thrombocytopenia, hepatotoxicity, gastrointestinal upset, nausea, vomiting, mucosal ulceration, stomatitis, malaise, headaches, pulmonary toxicity
Mycophenolate mofetil	500 mg 4 times a day, up to maximum of 4 g/day	Gastrointestinal toxicity (diarrhea, nausea, vomiting), hematologic effects (anemia, neutropenia, thrombocytopenia), viral and bacterial infections; lymphoproliferative disease or lymphoma can occur
Sulfasalazine	3–4 g/day for 8 weeks	Gastrointestinal upset
Tacrolimus	0.05 mg/kg daily, with increases to 0.10 mg/kg daily at 3 weeks and to 0.15 mg/kg daily at 6 weeks, depending on results	Nephrotoxicity, immunosuppression, gastrointestinal upset, diarrhea, nausea, paresthesias, hypertension, tremor, insomnia
Tazarotene	4.5 mg daily	Cheilitis, dry skin, headache, arthralgia, myalgia, back pain; no evidence of drug causing hyperlipidemia, hypercholesterolemia, abnormal liver function tests, desquamation, eye dryness, or alopecia
6-Thioguanine	80 mg twice weekly, increased by 20 mg every 2–4 weeks; maximum dose 160 mg three times per week	Bone marrow suppression; gastrointestinal complications including nausea and diarrhea; elevation of liver function tests

TABLE 101-4 Selected Topical Corticosteroids and Vasoconstricting Potency

Corticosteroids	Dosage Forms	Strength (%)	Vasoconstricting Potency Ranking[a]
Alclometasone dipropionate	Cream	0.05	VI
	Ointment	0.05	V
Amcinonide	Lotion, ointment	0.1	II
	Cream	0.1	III
Beclomethasone dipropionate	Cream, lotion, ointment	0.025	–
Betamethasone benzoate	Cream, gel	0.025	III
	Ointment	0.025	IV
Betamethasone dipropionate	Cream AF (optimized vehicle)	0.05	I
	Cream	0.05	III
	Gel, lotion, ointment (optimized vehicle)	0.05	I
	Lotion	0.05	V
	Ointment	0.05	II
	Topical aerosol	0.1	–
Betamethasone valerate	Cream	0.01, 0.05, 0.1	V
	Lotion, ointment	0.05, 0.1	III
	Foam	0.12	IV
Clobetasol propionate	Cream, ointment, solution, foam	0.05	I
Clobetasol butyrate	Cream, ointment	0.05	–
Clocortolone pivalate	Cream	0.1	–
Desonide	Cream, lotion, ointment	0.05	VI
Desoximetasone	Cream	0.05	II
	Cream, ointment	0.25	II
	Gel	0.05	II
Dexamethasone	Gel	0.1	VII
	Topical aerosol	0.01, 0.04	VII
Dexamethasone sodium phosphate	Cream	0.1	VII
Diflorasone diacetate	Cream	0.05	III
	Ointment	0.05	II
	Ointment (optimized vehicle)	0.05	II
Diflucortolone valerate	Cream, ointment	0.1	–
Flumethasone pivalate	Cream, ointment	0.03	–
Fluocinolone acetonide	Cream	0.01	VI
	Cream	0.025	V
	Cream	0.2	–
	Ointment	0.025	IV
	Solution	0.01	VI
Fluocinonide	Gel, cream, ointment	0.05	II
	Solution	0.05	II
Flurandrenolide	Cream, ointment	0.0125	–
	Ointment	0.05	IV
	Cream, lotion	0.05	V
	Tape	4 mcg/cm^2	I
Fluticasone propionate	Cream	0.05	IV
	Ointment	0.05	III
Halcinonide	Cream	0.025, 0.1	II
	Ointment	0.1	III
	Solution	0.1	–
Halobetasol propionate	Cream, ointment	0.05	I
Hydrocortisone	Cream, lotion, ointment	All strengths	VII
Hydrocortisone acetate	Cream, lotion, ointment	All strengths	VII
Hydrocortisone butyrate	Cream	0.1	V
	Ointment	0.1	V
Hydrocortisone valerate	Cream	0.2	V
	Ointment	0.2	IV
Methylprednisolone acetate	Cream, ointment	0.25	VII
	Ointment	1	VII
Mometasone furoate	Cream	0.1	IV
	Lotion, ointment	0.1	II
Triamcinolone acetonide	Cream, ointment	0.1	IV
	Cream, lotion, ointment	0.025	–
	Cream (Aristocort)	0.1	VI
	Cream (Kenalog)	0.1	IV
	Lotion	0.1	V
	Ointment (Aristocort, Kenalog)	0.1	III
	Cream, ointment	0.5	III
	Topical aerosol	0.015	–

[a]Vasoconstricting potency ranking is I (highest) to VII (lowest); denotes unreported vasoconstricting potency ranking.

pholipase A, and to thus reduce levels of arachidonic acid, prostaglandins, and leukotrienes in skin. Moreover, steroid receptors have been identified in skin, with synthesis and mitosis of DNA in epidermal cells being inhibited by topical corticosteroids as demonstrated by decreased epidermal proliferation.[22]

Topical corticosteroid adverse reactions are not uncommon. Local tissue atrophy, epidermal and dermal degeneration, and striae are manifestations of corticosteroid effect on collagen synthesis and fibroblast growth. If detected early, atrophy and striae can be reversible on drug discontinuation, but in numerous cases of prolonged therapy with high-potency agents, these atrophic changes can be long lasting. Thinning of the epidermis can result in visibly distended capillaries (telangiectasias) and purpura. Acneiform eruptions and masking of symptoms of bacterial or fungal skin infections also have been reported with topical corticosteroid use.[23]

Systemic consequences of topical corticosteroid use include risk of suppression of the hypothalamic-pituitary-adrenal axis, hyperglycemia, and development of cushingoid features. Avoidance of prolonged therapy with very-high-potency agents minimizes the risk of these adverse effects. Tachyphylaxis and rebound flare of psoriasis after abrupt cessation of topical corticosteroid therapy can also occur. With proper monitoring, topical corticosteroids are a safe and effective adjunctive approach to psoriasis treatment.[23]

Topical corticosteroids are available in ointments, creams, lotions, gels, sprays, shampoos, and mousses. An ointment is considered the most clinically effective dosage form in psoriasis treatment because it consists of an oily phase that is occlusive and conveys a hydrating effect. Because of the lipophilicity of ointments, penetration of corticosteroid into dermis is enhanced, resulting in increased vasoconstriction.

Ointments are not suitable for use in areas such as the axilla, groin, or other intertriginous areas where maceration and folliculitis can develop secondary to the occlusive effect. Creams—typically emulsified products with an aqueous phase—are preferred by some patients as more cosmetically desirable. They can be used in intertriginous areas even though their lower oil content makes them more drying than ointments.

Topical corticosteroids are usually applied 2 to 4 times daily during long-term therapy.

Vitamin D Analogues Vitamin D, important in cellular and systemic calcium metabolism, also inhibits keratinocyte differentiation and proliferation, suggesting a role in the treatment of hyperkeratotic skin disease. Vitamin D and its analogues provide antiinflammatory benefits by inducing a shift toward TH_2 cytokine expression, with a decrease in IL-2, IL-6, IL-8, INF-γ, and granulocyte-macrophage colony-stimulating factor.[24] Moreover, it induces inhibition of nuclear factor kappa B (NF-κB) protein in lymphocytes and nuclear factor of activated T cells leading to a reduced transcription of IL-2.[24]

However, use of vitamin D has been limited by its propensity to cause hypercalcemia. This has driven the development of analogues of vitamin D with less effect on calcium homeostasis. Calcipotriene binds to vitamin D receptors as does vitamin D, but it is 100 times less active on systemic calcium metabolism because of its rapid local metabolism.[25] Its long-term effect on altered calcium homeostasis is unknown. On average, improvement is seen within 2 weeks of treatment with calcipotriene, with approximately 70% of patients demonstrating marked improvement after 8 weeks of therapy. Adverse effects of calcipotriene include lesional and perilesional irritation, occurring in approximately 10% of treated patients and consisting of mild burning and stinging. Irritant contact dermatitis is reported to occur more commonly on the face. Calcipotriene, available in a 0.005% concentration as a cream, ointment, and solution, is generally applied one to two times per day (no more than 100 g/wk).

Although calcitriol (1,25-dihydroxyvitamin D_3) is not yet available in the United States, it is used in the treatment of mild to moderate plaque psoriasis. As demonstrated in several open-label or randomized, double-blind, controlled trials, calcitriol is effective in improving or clearing psoriatic plaques. A 0.03% formulation showed clearance or considerable improvement in 89% of patients.[26]

Tacalcitol (1α, 24-dihydroxyvitamin D_3) is a biologically active hormone derived from vitamin D. In a study of 157 patients with chronic plaque psoriasis, tacalcitol ointment applied once daily during a 6-month treatment period decreased mean PASI score by 67% and body area affected from 13.3% to 8.8%. Reported adverse effects of tacalcitol are limited to local, transient, mild irritation.[27]

Tazarotene Tazarotene, a synthetic retinoid, is a prodrug that exerts its pharmacologic activity when hydrolyzed to its active metabolite, tazarotenic acid. Like other topical retinoids, it modulates keratinocyte proliferation and differentiation.[28]

Based on the results of clinical trials, tazarotene is effective for the treatment of mild to moderate plaque psoriasis. These trials have demonstrated treatment success, defined as greater than 50% improvement of psoriasis from baseline including reduction of plaque elevation, scaling, and erythema, for both the gel and cream formulations.[28]

Predominant treatment-related adverse effects are mild to moderate pruritus, burning, stinging, or erythema. These local reactions have been shown to be dose- and frequency-related.[28] Tazarotene is often used in combination with topical corticosteroids to decrease the incidence of local adverse events and to increase efficacy.[10] Application of the gel to eczematous skin or to more than 20% of body surface area is not recommended because this can lead to extensive systemic absorption.

Tazarotene is available as a 0.05 or 0.1% gel and cream, and is applied once a day, usually in the evening.

Topical Therapy: Second-Line Agents

Coal Tar The use of tar as coal tar, shale tar, or wood tar has a long history in antipsoriatic therapy. In recent years, wood and shale tars have fallen out of use because they demonstrate relatively less efficacy than coal tar. Coal tar contains numerous hydrocarbon compounds formed from distillation of bituminous coal.

Although the mechanism of action is not fully understood, coal tar, when applied to normal skin, stimulates transient epidermal hyperplasia followed by a cytostatic effect with epidermal thinning. There is evidence that ultraviolet B (UVB) light–activated topical coal tar forms photo adducts with epidermal DNA, thereby inhibiting DNA synthesis. This downregulated epidermal proliferation rate approaches a normal rate of proliferation and leads to reduction in plaque elevation.[29]

Coal tar treatment is a burdensome, time-consuming treatment with disadvantages that include local irritation, unpleasant odor, staining of skin and clothing, and increased sensitivity to ultraviolet (UV) light, including the sun. The risk of carcinogenicity is low; however, there are cases indicating a higher rate of nonmelanoma skin cancers in patients chronically exposed to tar and UV light.[30]

Coal tar preparations of 2% to 5% tar are available in lotions, creams, shampoos, ointments, gels, and solutions. It also can be used in bath water. It is generally applied in the evening and allowed to remain in skin contact through the night.

Anthralin Anthralin, an anthrone derivative of chrysarobin, was introduced under the name dithranol in Great Britain decades ago. Chronic plaque-type and guttate psoriasis respond better than other variants to anthralin treatment. Topical anthralin, particularly with UV light, is long established as an effective approach to the treatment of psoriasis.[31]

Anthralin possesses antiproliferative activity on human keratinocytes, inhibiting DNA synthesis by intercalation between DNA strands.[32] It induces NF-κB in murine keratinocytes. Because NF-κB is involved in the transcription of proinflammatory cytokines such as IL-6, IL-8, and TNF-α, these findings can be helpful in explaining the irritant properties of anthralin. Other hypotheses support the role of anthralin-generated free radicals in producing both antipsoriatic effects and irritation.

The patient must apply anthralin products only to affected areas of skin because contact with uninvolved skin can result in excessive and unwanted irritation and staining. Skin staining usually disappears within 1 to 2 weeks of discontinuation. Staining of affected plaques is a positive response sign because cell turnover has been slowed enough to take up the stain.

Inflammation, irritation, and staining of skin and clothing (via oxidation and binding to keratins) are often therapy-limiting effects.

Fortunately, anthralin exerts its clinical effects at low cellular concentrations; classic anthralin therapy starts with low concentrations (0.1% to 0.25%) and gradually proceeds to higher concentrations (0.5% to 1%). Short-contact anthralin therapy regimens are alternative modes of application with decreased local adverse effects. Liposomal-based anthralin 0.5% gel can also be used for short contact therapy (10–20 minutes) and can noticeably reduce staining of skin and irritation.[31]

Anthralin traditionally was formulated in stiff paste bases to provide adherence to plaques. Subsequently, cream and ointment formulations have been developed that are more cosmetically appealing and appear to be equivalent in efficacy. Usually it is applied in the evening and allowed to remain overnight.

Topical Calcineurin Inhibitors (TCIs) Pimecrolimus and tacrolimus are calcineurin inhibitors capable of exerting a local immunomodulating effect that can serve to normalize hyperproliferation of epidermis. As topical agents, tacrolimus and pimecrolimus are approved for the treatment of atopic dermatitis; however, regulatory approval regarding the efficacy of these agents in psoriasis is yet to be completed. The benefit in using these agents, as opposed to topical corticosteroids, is that these immunomodulators do not cause skin atrophy. Although pivotal trials are not yet published regarding the efficacy of pimecrolimus and tacrolimus in the treatment of plaque-type psoriasis, clinical studies have shown efficacy on facial and intertriginous psoriasis.[33]

Although not commercially available in the United States, sirolimus is an immunosuppressive drug similar in structure to tacrolimus, however it does not inhibit calcineurin. Sirolimus inhibits a central kinase that transduces signals from the IL-2 receptor. By blocking this receptor, sirolimus inhibits T-cell stimulation by IL-2.[34] Clinical studies have demonstrated that topical sirolimus sufficiently crosses the stratum corneum/epidermis and is therefore effective in psoriasis.[35]

Systemic Therapy: First-Line Agents

Biologic Therapy The field of biologic therapy is expanding rapidly as a result of advances in recombinant DNA technology, microbiology, and immunology. In dermatology, biologic therapies—primarily immunomodulating agents designed to alter immune responses—are the basis for treatment of cutaneous diseases such as psoriasis and atopic dermatitis. These agents, produced in vitro through recombinant DNA technology, fall into three categories: (1) recombinant human cytokines, (2) humanized monoclonal antibodies, and (3) molecular receptors that can bind target molecules.

The biologic agents currently FDA approved for the treatment of moderate to severe psoriasis are infliximab, etanercept, alefacept, and efalizumab. One agent, adalimumab, is currently FDA approved for the treatment of psoriatic arthritis but not yet approved for psoriasis.

CLINICAL CONTROVERSY

Although some authors seem to successfully argue the advantages of remittive therapy in a potentially lifelong disorder,[36] others hypothesize the notion that biologic agents are excessively costly and that less expensive alternatives need development.[37] Although difficult to assess, and not established for all agents, given careful oversight, patient quality of life can be improved with an acceptable risk-to-benefit ratio, and improved cost effectiveness can be attained if remittive therapy is accomplished with some biologic agent.[38]

In psoriasis, biologic agents typically act through one or more of the following mechanisms: (1) elimination of activated T cells, (2) inhibition of T-cell activation, (3) interference with T-cell trafficking to the skin, (4) neutralization of the effects of TH_1-type cytokines, and (5) induction of immune deviation by introducing TH_2-type cytokines.[39]

Tumor Necrosis Factor Inhibitors

Infliximab Infliximab is a chimeric monoclonal antibody (immunoglobulin G_1; IgG_1) directed against TNF-α. It binds with high affinity to the soluble and transmembranous forms of TNF-α and inhibits binding of TNF-α with its receptors. TNF-α is believed to play an important role in the pathogenesis of psoriasis. Increased amounts of TNF-α have been found in psoriatic lesions. The proposed mechanism of action of TNF-α includes stimulation of synthesis of numerous cytokines and induction of the expression of intracellular adhesion molecules on endothelial cells and keratinocytes.[40]

Infliximab has been used for treatment of rheumatoid arthritis and Crohn disease for years. Recently, the FDA expanded the indications for infliximab to include psoriatic arthritis, and now also adults with chronic severe plaque psoriasis.

One double-blind, randomized, placebo-controlled clinical trial studied the effectiveness and safety of infliximab in patients with moderate to severe psoriasis. A good response was seen in 82% and 91% of patients treated with infliximab 5 mg/kg or 10 mg/kg, respectively. Median time to response for all patients receiving infliximab was 4 weeks. The investigators concluded that patients treated with infliximab had a high degree of clinical improvement with rapid response rate, similar to that observed with cyclosporine therapy.[41]

The most common adverse effects of infliximab are headaches, fever, chills, fatigue, diarrhea, pharyngitis, upper respiratory and urinary tract infections, and hypersensitivity reactions (urticaria, dyspnea, and hypotension). Infliximab has been also associated with infections and lymphoproliferative disorders. It is not associated with end-organ toxicity, and blood counts, liver enzyme levels, kidney function, and complement values can be expected to remain normal during treatment. This gives it a major advantage over other systemic psoriasis treatments.

Infliximab is administered in three doses at weeks 0, 2, and 6, of 5 mg/kg or 10 mg/kg by slow intravenous infusion.[41]

Etanercept Etanercept, another TNF-α blocker, is a genetically engineered fusion protein that combines the extracellular domain of the TNF-α receptor with the crystallizable fragment (Fc) region of human IgG_1. Etanercept binds free and membrane-bound TNF-α, competitively interfering with the interaction of TNF-α with cell-bound receptors and inhibits the effects of this cytokine on target cells. Unlike the chimeric infliximab, etanercept is fully humanized, thereby minimizing the risk of immunogenicity.[42]

Etanercept has been approved in several countries, including the United States, for subcutaneous treatment of rheumatoid arthritis, psoriatic arthritis, and more recently psoriasis. Safety and efficacy of etanercept for psoriatic arthritis and psoriasis were demonstrated in a 12-week randomized, double-blind, placebo-controlled trial of twice-weekly subcutaneous injections of etanercept 25 mg. The median reduction in PASI in the treatment group was 46%, compared with 8.7% in the placebo group.[43] During phase III trials etanercept was evaluated at 3 different doses: low (25 mg per week), medium (25 mg twice weekly), and high (50 mg given twice weekly). After 12 weeks of treatment a 75% reduction in PASI score was achieved by 4% of subjects given placebo, 14% of subjects given low-dose, 34% of the subjects given medium-dose, and 49% of the subjects given the high-dose. These results were statistically significant for all three doses when compared to the placebo group. The subjects continued to improve with further treatment and at 24 weeks 25%, 44%, and 59% of the low, medium, and high-dose subjects, respectively, achieved a 75% reduction in PASI score.[44]

Adverse effects of etanercept include a local reaction at the injection site (20% of patients), respiratory tract and gastrointestinal infections, abdominal pain, nausea and vomiting, headaches, and rash. Serious infections (including tuberculosis) and malignancies have rarely been observed.

Etanercept is usually given in doses up to 50 mg subcutaneously twice a week.

Adalimumab Adalimumab is a human IgG_1 monoclonal TNF-α antibody. The binding of adalimumab results in the inactivation of the proinflammatory cytokine TNF-α. It is currently approved for the treatment of rheumatoid arthritis and psoriatic arthritis and is undergoing trials for psoriasis.

In a series of nine patients adalimumab was found to be effective for psoriasis refractory to other treatments including infliximab and etanercept. Adalimumab was dosed at 40 mg every 14 days administered subcutaneously as monotherapy, and after 12 weeks 56% of patients showed a 75% reduction in PASI score. There was continued improvement after 20 weeks.[45]

In a multicenter, randomized, placebo-controlled trial, the efficacy and safety of two dosages of adalimumab (40 mg every other week or weekly) versus placebo were assessed for 12 weeks in the treatment of moderate to severe plaque psoriasis with a 48-week extension trial. At 12 weeks 53% of the subjects that received 40 mg every other week and 80% of the subjects that received 40 mg per week had a reduction of 75% or more in the PASI score. Also, these responses were sustained for those who continued treatment for 60 weeks.[46]

Adalimumab has a favorable safety profile. The most common adverse events were rhinitis, upper respiratory tract infections, nausea, flu-like syndrome, headache, and injection site reactions. In clinical trials for rheumatoid arthritis, anti-adalimumab antibodies were seen in 12% of subjects receiving adalimumab as monotherapy. Theoretically adalimumab should be less immunogenic than the chimeric antibody infliximab.[47]

There is concern that adalimumab can be associated with malignancy, in particular lymphoma, infections, such as tuberculosis, histoplasmosis, pneumococcus, and listeria; adverse neurologic effects including the potential role in causing demyelinating disease.[13]

Adalimumab is given as a dose of 40 mg every other week or every week.

CLINICAL CONTROVERSY

It has been reported that treatment with adalimumab, infliximab and etanercept leads to non-neutralizing antibody production, the long-term significance of which is unknown. Some clinicians believe that antibody production can be related to a lack of efficacy, although others believe that antibody production and efficacy are unrelated. Further, adalimumab as a "fully humanized" product would be expected to produce less antibody production.

Although 12% of subjects in a trial of adalimumab tested positive for adalimumab antibodies, efficacy and pattern or frequency of adverse events did not correlate with production, or lack of production, of antibodies to adalimumab.[48]

In an adalimumab cohort study, anti-adalimumab antibodies were detected in 17% of subjects. Significantly more nonresponders had anti-adalimumab antibodies than responders (34% vs. 5%), and subjects with anti-adalimumab antibodies had less clinical improvement of disease. On follow-up, subjects with anti-adalimumab antibodies also had lower serum adalimumab concentrations than those without anti-adalimumab antibodies.[49]

In a further adalimumab study, 87% of subjects showed antibodies to adalimumab. Five of seven subjects with adverse drug reactions and all subjects with lack of efficacy were associated with antibody formation. Adalimumab, in spite of its "fully humanized" status, apparently also has immunogenic potential.[50]

Thirteen percent of subjects were positive for anti-infliximab antibodies after the first 2 intravenous infusions. With subsequent infusions, more subjects became antibody positive (44% at 6 months), correlating with diminished trough levels of infliximab. These authors concluded that the development of anti-infliximab antibodies is associated with increased risk of infusion reaction and treatment failure.[51]

Immunogenicity of etanercept has also been studied with once-weekly dosing. Antibodies to etanercept are likely to be non-neutralizing and occur in approximately 5% of patients.[52]

T-Cell Activation Inhibitors

Alefacept Alefacept is a dimeric fusion protein that combines the first extracellular domain of human LFA-3 with the Fc portion of human IgG_1. The LFA-3 segment of alefacept binds specifically to the cluster of differentiation 2 (CD2) on T cells to prevent costimulatory signals delivered by LFA-3 and thereby inhibits cutaneous T-cell activation and proliferation. Alefacept also induces selective apoptosis of memory-effector T cells and produces a dose-dependent decrease in circulating total lymphocytes.[10,53]

Alefacept is approved for treatment of moderate to severe plaque psoriasis and is also effective for the treatment of psoriatic arthritis.[54] Significant clinical response is achieved after approximately 3 months of therapy, and improvements are relatively long lasting.

Alefacept is well tolerated, and its safety profile is equivalent to that of placebo. The most common adverse events are mild and include pharyngitis, influenza-like symptoms, chills, dizziness, nausea, headache, injection site pain and inflammation, and nonspecific infection; the frequency of these effects is low. Also, the drug produces no increase in the rate of opportunistic infections or malignancies.[55] Weekly visits to a physician's office for drug administration and CD4 T-cell monitoring are required, and not all patients respond to treatment.

Alefacept is administered by intramuscular injection in once-weekly doses of 15 mg for 12 weeks.

Efalizumab Efalizumab is a humanized monoclonal antibody (IgG_1) against CD11-α integrin. CD11-α/CD18 comprise subunits of LFA-1, a T-cell surface molecule important in T-cell activation, T-cell migration into skin, and cytotoxic T-cell function.[56]

Clinical studies with efalizumab have shown efficacy with few adverse effects. In an open-label, multicenter, dose-escalating study of repeated intravenous infusions of efalizumab over 7 weeks in 39 subjects with moderate to severe psoriasis, the individuals who were exposed to the optimum dose (1 mg/kg weekly) showed a mean decrease in PASI of 47%.[57]

In a phase III multicenter trial subjects received efalizumab subcutaneously at 1.0 or 2.0 mg/kg/week or placebo for 12 weeks. Twenty-two percent of the subjects that received 1 mg/kg/week and

28% of the subjects that received 2 mg/kg/week had an improvement of 75% or more in the PASI. Also, 77% of those subjects who improved 75% or more at the initial 12-week treatment period maintained improvement through week 24.[58]

The most frequent adverse effects of efalizumab are mild to moderate influenza-like complaints such as headache, nausea, chills, nonspecific infection, pain, fever, and asthenia.[59] There have been cases of exacerbations of psoriasis on discontinuation of the drug, leading to the suggestion that patients might need to continue treatment with this drug to maintain suppression of their disease. However, there have been no significant increases in malignant disease, opportunistic infections, signs of immunosuppression, hepatotoxicity, or nephrotoxicity.[13]

The usual dose is 1 mg/kg subcutaneously once weekly.

Systemic Therapy: Second-Line Agents

Acitretin Acitretin, an oral retinoid, is the active metabolite of etretinate and has demonstrated clinical effects similar to etretinate but with fewer adverse effects.[60] Acitretin is indicated for the treatment of severe psoriasis, including erythrodermic and generalized pustular types but is more useful as an adjunct in the treatment of plaque psoriasis. In contrast to the fast-acting cyclosporine and methotrexate, acitretin resolves psoriatic lesions more slowly.

Acitretin has a shorter half-life than etretinate. Its mechanism of action is not completely understood; it might achieve benefits by acting on retinoid receptors in the keratinocyte nucleus to correct abnormal cell differentiation.

Acitretin has shown good results when combined with other psoriatic therapies, including PUVA and UVB and topical calcipotriol. [28] The combination of acitretin and PUVA is highly effective and provides faster and more complete clearance, as well as allowing a decrease in the doses of both agents, thereby limiting the risk of adverse effects.[60]

Adverse effects are dose dependent. They include hypervitaminosis A (i.e., dry lips/cheilitis, dry mouth, dry nose, dry eyes/conjunctivitis, dry skin, pruritus, scaling, and hair loss), hepatotoxicity, skeletal changes, hypercholesterolemia, and hypertriglyceridemia. To counteract hyperlipidemic effects, gemfibrozil has been studied for concomitant use with acitretin. In addition, acitretin is a known teratogen and thus is contraindicated in females who are pregnant or who plan pregnancy within the 3 years following drug discontinuation.[28]

Absorption is enhanced when taken with food. Concurrent ingestion of alcohol converts acitretin to etretinate, which has a longer half-life. Therefore, alcohol must not be ingested by female patients during treatment with acitretin and for 2 months following treatment.

An initial recommended dose of acitretin is 25 to 50 mg once daily, with therapy continued until lesions have resolved. A dosage of 50 mg/day is typically required for plaque psoriasis, and even at this relatively high dose, acitretin is only moderately effective. It is better tolerated when taken in conjunction with a meal.

Cyclosporine An effective immunosuppressive agent that inhibits the first phase of T-cell activation, cyclosporine is used in the treatment of both cutaneous and arthritic manifestations of severe psoriasis.[61] It also inhibits the release of inflammatory mediators from mast cells, basophils, and polymorphonuclear cells.[62]

A meta-analysis of 579 patients with severe psoriasis treated with either 2.5 or 5 mg/kg per day of cyclosporine for 10 to 12 weeks found that the PASI decreased by 70% and 72%, respectively.[63] An oral microemulsion formulation of cyclosporine has shown a better pharmacokinetic profile, resulting in a more consistent and predictable rate of absorption than the original formulation.[5]

The major concerns with the use of cyclosporine are nephrotoxicity, hypertension, and potential risk of malignancy. Published studies have demonstrated interstitial fibrosis and renal tubular atrophy on kidney biopsy specimens in patients treated for more than 2 years with cyclosporine. To decrease the risk of nephrotoxicity, the dose of cyclosporine should be kept below 5 mg/kg per day, and if serum creatinine levels increase by more than 30% the dose of cyclosporine should be decreased or discontinued. In addition, use for more than 2 years of cumulative treatment can increase the risk of malignancy, including skin cancers (non-melanoma) and lymphoproliferative disorders. One study has suggested that cyclosporine renders malignancies more aggressive.[60] Other complications include hypomagnesemia, hyperkalemia, decreased liver function, elevation of serum lipids, gastrointestinal intolerance, paresthesias, hypertrichosis, and gingival hyperplasia.[62,64]

Before initiating therapy with cyclosporine, patients should have the following laboratory tests done: electrolyte panel, renal panel (calcium, phosphate, magnesium, blood urea nitrogen, and two baseline measurements of serum creatinine), uric acid, liver function tests, triglycerides and complete blood count, as well as an accurate baseline blood pressure.

Serum creatinine should be monitored every 2 weeks for the first 3 months, then once a month for the duration of treatment.[64]

See Chap. 92 on solid organ transplantation for a discussion of drug interactions involving cyclosporine.

The typical dose of cyclosporine is usually between 2.5 and 5 mg/kg per day.

Tacrolimus Tacrolimus is a macrolide immunosuppressive agent indicated for the prevention of organ transplant rejection and can be useful as an alternative treatment in severe recalcitrant psoriasis. Tacrolimus, like cyclosporine, inhibits T-cell activation.[10]

Adverse effects include diarrhea, nausea, paresthesias, hypertension, tremor, and insomnia. Other toxicities with topical tacrolimus—including renal insufficiency and immunosuppression—have been rarely reported.[65]

See Chap. 92 on solid organ transplantation for a discussion of drug interactions involving tacrolimus.

Although not FDA approved in recalcitrant plaque-type psoriasis, patients have received tacrolimus at oral doses of 0.05 mg/kg per day (increased up to 0.15 mg/kg per day as needed).[66]

Pimecrolimus Pimecrolimus is a macrolide immunosuppressive agent that inhibits both TH_1 and TH_2 cytokines as well as inhibits degranulation of mast cells. Although it is currently not commercially available in the United States, it is being studied for treatment of moderate to severe psoriasis. A multicenter 12-week clinical trial demonstrated a dose-dependent reduction in psoriasis severity when oral pimecrolimus was given at dosages of 10 mg, 20 mg, 30 mg, or placebo twice daily. Responses at 20 mg and 30 mg doses were statistically significant ($P < 0.001$). The drug is well tolerated, and it is not expected to produce major organ toxicities. The most common adverse event reported is a transient feeling of warmth.[67]

Methotrexate Methotrexate, a common antimetabolite, was introduced several decades ago for the treatment of psoriasis and remains an effective therapeutic approach for psoriasis. It is a synthetic analogue of folic acid that acts as a competitive inhibitor of the enzyme dihydrofolate reductase and is responsible for the conversion of dihydrofolate to tetrahydrofolate. Tetrahydrofolate is an essential cofactor for the synthesis of thymidylate and purine nucleotides required for DNA and RNA synthesis.[65]

Methotrexate inhibits replication and function of T and B cells and suppresses secretion of various cytokines such as IL-1, INF-γ, and TNF-α. It also suppresses epidermal cell division. Methotrexate is indicated in patients with moderate to severe psoriasis.[65]

Methotrexate is particularly beneficial for patients with psoriatic arthritis. It is also indicated for patients that are refractory to topical or UV therapy.[60] Methotrexate should be avoided in patients with active infections because of its immunosuppressive activity.[68]

Methotrexate is associated with nausea and vomiting as well as mucosal ulceration, stomatitis, malaise, headaches, macrocytic anemia, and pulmonary toxicity. Nausea and macrocytic anemia can be ameliorated by administering oral folic acid in doses of 1 to 5 mg/day.

Bone marrow toxicity that leads to leukopenia, anemia, and thrombocytopenia has been shown to be induced by methotrexate. A serious long-term adverse effect is hepatotoxicity. Consequently, methotrexate should typically be avoided in patients with liver disease. Risk factors for hepatotoxicity include a history of excessive alcohol consumption, hepatitis, persistent elevated liver function tests, and family history of inheritable liver disease.[65]

Malignant lymphomas have been reported in several patients treated with methotrexate.

In some cases, lymphomas regressed when methotrexate was discontinued, suggesting a causal relationship. A large cohort study indicated that patients with psoriasis are at increased risk for developing lymphoma. However, the cause of this increased rate of lymphoma is unknown and could be attributed to psoriasis severity, the treatment, or an interaction between these risk factors.[69] Methotrexate is contraindicated in pregnant women because it is teratogenic.[65]

The starting methotrexate dose is 7.5 to 15 mg per week, and this is increased incrementally by 2.5 mg every 2 to 4 weeks until a response is evident. Maximal doses are typically approximately 25 mg per week. It can be administered orally, subcutaneously, or intramuscularly. During treatment complete blood count, renal function, and liver panel should be checked monthly. Methotrexate is renally excreted and should therefore not be administered to patients with impairment of kidney function.[65]

Drug interactions can potentiate methotrexate toxicity. For example nonsteroidal antiinflammatory drugs can reduce renal clearance of methotrexate, resulting in toxic levels.[70] Leucovorin (folinic acid) can be given (20 mg every 6 hours) when there is evidence of methotrexate toxicity. Table 101–5 lists selected drugs that interact with, and increase toxicity of, methotrexate.

Mycophenolate Mofetil Mycophenolate mofetil, a semisynthetic morpholinoester of mycophenolic acid, initially was used to prevent acute rejection after renal and cardiac transplantation, but it is now used as part of combination therapy in moderate to severe psoriasis and other autoimmune dermatoses. It reversibly blocks de-novo synthesis of guanine nucleotides required for DNA and RNA synthesis. The drug has been shown to have a specific lymphocyte antiproliferative effect.[71]

Although not FDA approved for this indication, oral mycophenolate mofetil appears effective in the treatment of moderate to severe plaque-type psoriasis; however, additional clinical trials will be necessary to demonstrate efficacy and safety.[65] Future therapy can also include topical mycophenolic acid, which is not commercially available.[72] Commonly reported adverse effects of mycophenolate mofetil include gastrointestinal toxicity (diarrhea, nausea, and vomiting), hematologic effects (anemia, neutropenia, and thrombocytopenia), and an increased incidence of viral and bacterial infections. Lymphoproliferative disease or lymphoma has developed in up to 1% of patients who received mycophenolic acid with other immunosuppressive agents increased up to 4 g/day.

See Chap. 92 on solid organ transplantation for a discussion of drug interactions involving mycophenolate mofetil.

Mycophenolate mofetil is usually given 500 mg 4 times a day, up to a maximum of 4 g/day.

TABLE 101-5 Selected Drugs That Can Increase the Toxicity of Methotrexate

Mechanism	Drug
Additive or synergistic toxicity	Ethanol
	Pyrimethamine
	Trimethoprim-sulfamethoxazole
Decreased renal elimination of methotrexate	Aminoglycosides
	Cephalothin
	Colchicines
	Cyclosporine
	Nonsteroidal antiinflammatory drugs (naproxen and ibuprofen)
	Penicillins
	Phenylbutazone
	Probenecid
	Salicylates
	Sulfonamides
Displacement of methotrexate from protein binding	Barbiturates
	Phenytoin
	Probenecid
	Retinoids
	Salicylates
	Sulfonamides
	Sulfonylureas
	Tetracycline
Hepatotoxicity	Ethanol
	Retinoids
Intracellular accumulation of methotrexate	Dipyridamole

Sulfasalazine Sulfasalazine, commonly used in the treatment of inflammatory bowel disease and rheumatoid arthritis, is selectively used as an alternative treatment, particularly in patients with concurrent psoriatic arthritis. Sulfasalazine is an antiinflammatory agent that inhibits 5-lipoxygenase. When used as a single agent in the treatment of psoriasis, it is not as effective as is therapy with methotrexate, PUVA, or acitretin. One possible advantage of sulfasalazine therapy compared with other systemic treatments is its relatively high margin of safety.

See Chap. 94 on rheumatoid arthritis for a discussion of drug interactions involving sulfasalazine. The usual dose of oral sulfasalazine is 3 to 4 g/day for 8 weeks.[10]

6-Thioguanine A purine analog that acts as an antimetabolite in the S-phase of cell division, 6-thioguanine is approved for treatment of leukemia but has been used as an alternative treatment for psoriasis for decades when conventional therapies have failed.[73] It appears to be less hepatotoxic than methotrexate and therefore may be more useful in treating hepatically compromised patients with severe psoriasis.

Adverse effects of 6-thioguanine include bone marrow suppression, gastrointestinal complications including nausea and diarrhea, and elevation of liver function tests.

The typical dose of 6-thioguanine is 80 mg twice weekly, increased by 20 mg every 2 to 4 weeks. Its maximum dose is considered to be 160 mg three times a week.

See Chap. 130 on cancer treatment and chemotherapy for a discussion of drug interactions involving 6-thioguanine.

Hydroxyurea Hydroxyurea inactivates the enzyme ribonucleotide reductase, inhibiting cell synthesis in the S-phase of the DNA cycle. An antimetabolite that is primarily used to treat hematologic malignancies, it has been used for the treatment of psoriasis for more than three decades.[60] It is selectively used, particularly in those with liver disease who would be at risk of adverse effects with other antipsoriatic agents. However, hydroxyurea is less effective than methotrexate.[10]

Adverse effects of hydroxyurea are bone marrow toxicity with leukopenia or thrombocytopenia, cutaneous reactions, leg ulcers, and megaloblastic anemia.

See Chap. 130 on cancer treatment and chemotherapy for a discussion of drug interactions involving hydroxyurea.

The typical dose of hydroxyurea is 1 g/day, with gradual increase to 2 g/day as needed as tolerated. Improvement is gradual, usually seen after 4 weeks of therapy.[10]

Tazarotene Tazarotene is a receptor selective retinoid. The oral dosage form is not yet FDA approved. Oral retinoids have been successfully used in the treatment of psoriasis, however, their use is limited because of systemic adverse effects and teratogenicity.

Phase III trials demonstrate that oral tazarotene given 4.5 mg daily is effective for the treatment of moderate to severe psoriasis. Safety and tolerability data suggest that tazarotene may have an improved profile compared to established retinoids. Also, tazarotene does not significantly increase triglycerides, cholesterol, liver function tests, desquamation, eye dryness, or alopecia. However, there are no head-to-head trials with the currently approved oral retinoid, acitretin, therefore it remains unclear whether tazarotene is any safer or more effective. The major limitation with the use of oral tazarotene is embryotoxicity and teratogenicity.[74]

COMBINATION, ROTATIONAL, AND SEQUENTIAL THERAPY

Frequently, monotherapy with a systemic agent does not provide optimal outcomes. Combination therapy of systemic agents with other modalities can enhance therapeutic benefit. In addition, the dose of each pharmacotherapeutic agent can be reduced if used in combination, and this can result in lower toxicity.[60]

Combinations can include:

- Acitretin + UVB light
- Acitretin + PUVA (UVA combined with psoralen, usually methoxsalen)
- Methotrexate + UVB light
- PUVA + UVB light
- Methotrexate + cyclosporine

In addition to combination therapy, biologic agents can also be used in rotational therapy. Patients can receive a biologic regimen for a limited period of time and can be then switched to a nonbiologic regimen, continuing on a rotational basis. One objective of rotational therapy is to minimize cumulative drug toxicity.

Sequential therapy is another treatment strategy designed to optimize therapeutic outcome. It involves rapid clearing of psoriasis with aggressive therapy by an agent such as cyclosporine, followed by a transitional period in which a safer long-term drug such as acitretin is introduced at maximal dosing. Subsequently, a maintenance period with acitretin in lower doses, or if necessary, acitretin in combination with UVB or PUVA, can be continued.[75] Topical sequential therapy can involve the use of a class I corticosteroid (very high potency) and calcipotriene in three different phases to attain rapid clearing of psoriatic lesions while minimizing side effects.[76]

Combination or rotational therapies with biologic agents can also be clinically useful.[25]

Possible pharmacotherapeutic approaches to the treatment of psoriasis are shown in the treatment algorithm (Fig. 101–1).

Phototherapy

Ultraviolet B Light Therapy and PUVA Therapy UVB light (290 to 320 nm) continues to be an important phototherapeutic intervention for psoriasis.

Exposure to UV light by natural sunlight has been used to treat psoriasis for centuries. At the beginning of the 20th-century patients were treated with topical, occlusive coal tar all day and night, removing the tar just before exposure to a hot quartz mercury vapor lamp (Goeckerman therapy).[10] Subsequent development of various forms of UVB phototherapy has led to the use of more precise wavelengths within the UVB range to achieve an optimal therapeutic benefit for psoriasis.

The most effective wavelength of UVB for treatment of psoriasis is 310 to 315 nm, and this has led to the development of a UVB *narrowband* (NB) light source, in which 83% of the UVB emission is at 310 to 313 nm.[77] Numerous clinical trials have demonstrated efficacy of NB-UVB for the treatment of plaque-type psoriasis.[78]

Numerous topical and systemic psoriatic therapies (discussed individually below) are used adjunctively to hasten and improve the response to UVB phototherapy. Emollients enhance efficacy of UVB and can be applied to the skin just before treatments for this purpose.[20] Several studies showed an advantage to combining short-contact anthralin with UVB.[20] The addition of calcipotriene or topical retinoids also improved results compared to UVB alone. However, topical application should be after or at least 2 hours before UVB therapy because phototherapy can inactivate the topical product.[79] UVB phototherapy has also produced more effective results when added to systemic psoriatic treatments, such as methotrexate and retinoids.[79]

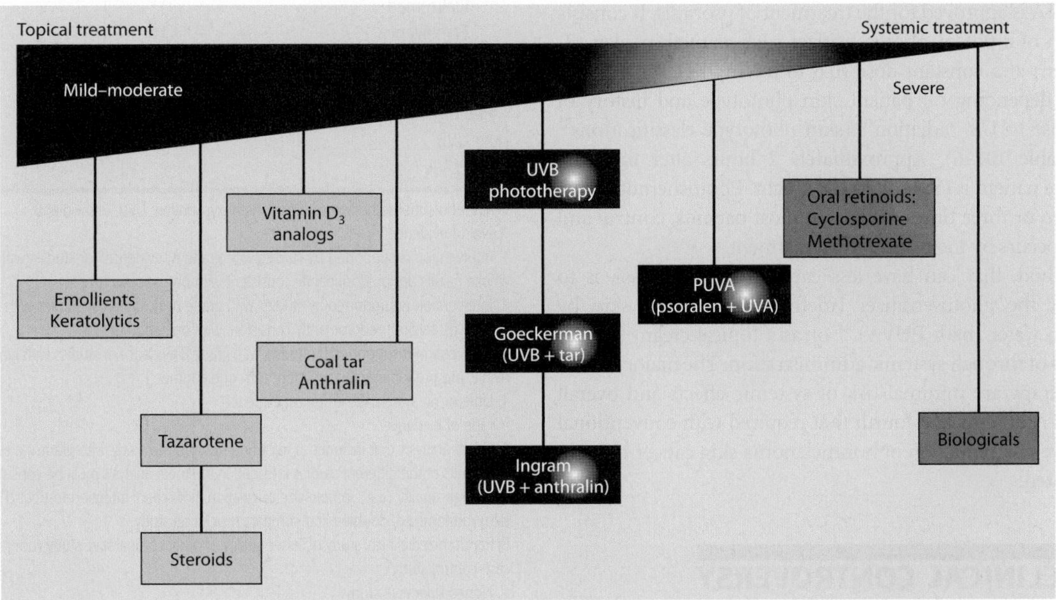

FIGURE 101-1. Psoriasis treatment spectrum. (PUVA, photochemotherapy with oral methoxypsoralen using ultraviolet A light; UVA, ultraviolet A light; UVB, ultraviolet B light.)

TABLE 101-6 Light-Reactive Skin Types

Fitzpatrick Phototypes		I	II	III		IV	V		VI
	Lightest skin								Darkest skin
Cesarini phototypes	0	I	II	IIIa		IIIb	IV	V	VI

Data from Guinot C, Malvy DJ, Latreille J, et al. Sun-reactive Skin Type in 4912 French adults participating in the SU.VI.MAX study. Photochem Photobiol 2005;81(4):934–940.

PUVA is a photochemotherapeutic approach to treatment of psoriasis. Although burdensome, photochemotherapy is an important treatment consideration for patients with moderate to severe psoriasis, when time needed to treat and risk factors are balanced with potential benefit.

The mechanism of action of both UVB and PUVA in treating psoriasis is thought to be immunomodulatory. Although the mechanism of action is not fully understood, UVB and PUVA have antiproliferative, antiinflammatory, and immunosuppressive effects. Phototherapy with UVB also induces T-cell apoptosis.[80] Candidates for PUVA therapy usually have moderate to severe, incapacitating psoriasis unresponsive to conventional topical and systemic therapies.

A randomized double-blind study compared PUVA with NB-UVB for the treatment of chronic plaque psoriasis in 88 subjects. In those with skin phototypes I through IV, PUVA was significantly more effective than NB-UVB (84% vs. 65%; $P = 0.02$). The median number of treatments to clearance was significantly lower in the PUVA group (17.0 vs. 28.5; $P < 0.001$). Six months after the cessation of therapy, 68% of PUVA-treated subjects and 35% of NB-UVB–treated subjects were still in remission. This study indicates that PUVA achieves clearance in more subjects with fewer treatment sessions and results in longer remissions than NB-UVB.[81]

Adverse effects from oral methoxsalen include nausea, dizziness, and headache. Long-term adverse effects from combined psoralen (methoxsalen) and UV light include actinic skin damage, solar elastosis, dry and wrinkled skin, and hyperpigmentation or hypopigmentation. An increased risk of skin cancers, both squamous cell carcinoma and melanoma, exists after PUVA therapy, and is correlated with the cumulative UVA exposure.[82] Although the proportion of patients with malignant melanoma has remained small, an increase in malignant melanoma has been observed in patients who received more than 250 PUVA sessions.

Oral methoxsalen is usually dosed with milk or food to minimize risk of nausea and gastrointestinal upset.

Systemic PUVA is approved for the treatment of psoriasis. It consists of oral ingestion of a potent photosensitizer such as methoxsalen (8-methoxypsoralen) at a constant dose (0.6 to 0.8 mg/kg) and variable doses of UVA, depending on patient skin phototype and history of previous response to UV radiation[10] (skin phototype classifications[83] are listed in Table 101–6). Approximately 2 hours after ingesting methoxsalen, the patient is exposed to UVA light. Photochemotherapy is performed two or three times a week. In most patients, control and partial clearing occurs by the twenty-fifth treatment.

Another method, that can have less carcinogenic potential, is to topically deliver the photosensitizer (methoxsalen) to the skin by addition to bath water (bath PUVA),[84] or as a topical cream (PUVA cream)[85] instead of through systemic administration. The major advantages of this therapy are minimal risk of systemic effects and overall reduction of UVA dose to one-fourth that required with conventional PUVA. A relative risk reduction of nonmelanoma skin cancer has also been demonstrated.

CLINICAL CONTROVERSY

Although PUVA is apparently not responsible for increased incidence of internal malignancy,[86] the risk-to-benefit considerations with regard to melanoma and nonmelanoma skin cancers indicate an increased risk for melanoma,[82] or at least the risk cannot be ruled out,[87] and also an increased incidence of nonmelanoma skin cancers in association with PUVA.[88] One study demonstrated a dose-dependent increased risk for genital tumors in men treated with PUVA, specifically, a 53-fold increased risk for invasive penile and scrotal squamous cell carcinoma.[89]

Excimer Laser Phototherapy

Lasers have been used for the treatment of psoriasis with variable results. Most laser therapy has been ineffective, whereas the excimer laser, which generates a high-energy 308-nm UVB wavelength is effective at clearing psoriasis and inducing moderately prolonged remissions.[90,91] Unfortunately, this approach to therapy is limited to treatment of individual, isolated plaques. The excimer laser has some advantages over traditional NBUVB phototherapy, including

TABLE 101-7 Evidence Basis for Selected Pharmacotherapeutic Approaches to the Treatment of Psoriasis

Pharmacotherapy	Level of Evidence[a]
Topical	
Calcineurin inhibitors	4
Coal tar	4
Corticosteroids	1
Anthralin	1
Tazarotene	2
Vitamin D analogs	1
Systemic	
Acitretin	3
Cyclosporine	1
Methotrexate	3
Biologics	
Efalizumab	1
Etanercept	1
Infliximab	1
Adalimumab	1
Phototherapy	
UVB	2
PUVA	2

PUVA, photochemotherapy with oral methoxypsoralen; UVB, ultraviolet B.

[a]Level of evidence:

1. Intervention is supported by studies with grade A_1 evidence[b] or studies with grade A2 evidence whose results are predominantly consistent with one another.
2. Intervention is supported by studies with grade A_2 evidence or studies with grade B evidence whose results are predominantly consistent with one another.
3. Intervention is supported by studies with grade B evidence or studies with grade C evidence whose results are predominantly consistent with one another.
4. Little or no systematic empirical evidence.

[b]Grade of evidence

A_1, Meta-analysis that includes at least one randomized study with grade A2 evidence. In addition, the results of the different studies included in the meta-analysis must be consistent with one another.

A_2, A high-quality (e.g., sample-size calculation, flow chart, intention-to-treat (ITT) analysis, sufficient size) randomized, double-blind comparative clinical study.

B, Randomized clinical study of lesser quality or other comparative study (nonrandomized, cohort, or case-control study).

C, Noncomparative study.

D, Expert opinion.

Data from Nast A, Kopp I, Augustin M, et al. German evidence-based guidelines for the treatment of Psoriasis vulgaris (short verision). Arch Dermatol Res 2007;299(3):111–138.

the capability to successfully treat psoriatic plaques with fewer treatments and with a smaller UV radiation dose. Moreover, it may have a lower risk of carcinogenicity and photoaging.[91,92]

PHARMACOECONOMIC CONSIDERATIONS

Outpatient costs for a patient with mild to moderate psoriasis can run as high as $4,000 per patient per year. Psoriasis is a chronic disease with patients either requiring treatment or being in remission. Patients with severe psoriasis can be disabled. A patient with early onset of psoriasis can require treatment for more than 50 years.

By effectively controlling psoriasis, costs to patients, lost work days, and health plan costs can be reduced. However, relatively high treatment failure rates are reported for traditional therapies in place before the advent of biologic agent therapies.[93] This unmet need will be examined with further placement of biologic agents as established treatment options for moderate to severe psoriasis.

EVALUATION OF THERAPEUTIC OUTCOMES

See Tables 101–2 and 101–3 for pharmaceutical regiments and adverse effects and Fig. 101–1 for treatment algorithm based on severity of psoriasis. Table 101–7 provides evidence basis for selected pharmacotherapeutic approaches to the treatment of psoriasis.[94] An additional evidence-based review compared the equivalent percent reduction in PASI 75% score after 3 months treatment for most pharmacotherapeutic approaches to psoriasis. Of note, in descending order of efficacy: tar + light > cyclosporine > infliximab > PUVA > methotrexate > adalimumab > acitretin > etanercept > efalizumab > alefacept.[95] Although this evidence-based ranking is reported by the authors to be a rough (and not necessarily accurate) attempt to assess peer-reviewed publications, it presents an interesting perspective to consider when determining first-line versus second-line therapy.

ABBREVIATIONS

APC: antigen-presenting cell

CD2: cluster of differentiation 2

CD4: cluster of differentiation 4

CD28: cluster of differentiation 28

Fc: fragment, crystallizable (of immunoglobulin)

HLA: human leukocyte antigen

INF-γ: interferon-γ

IgG_1: immunoglobulin G_1

IL-2: interleukin-2

IL-4: interleukin-4

IL-8: interleukin-8

IL-10: interleukin-10

LFA-1: lymphocyte function-associated antigen-1

LFA-3: lymphocyte function-associated antigen-3

LFA-3/TIP: recombinantly engineered LFA-3/Ig G1 human fusion protein

MIG: monokine induced by interferon-γ

MIP-3α: macrophage inflammatory protein-3α

NBUVB: narrowband ultraviolet B

NF-κB: nuclear factor kappa B

NPF-PS: National Psoriasis Foundation Psoriasis Score

PASI: psoriasis area and severity index

PGA: Physician Global Assessment

PUVA: photochemotherapy with oral methoxypsoralen and ultraviolet A light

RANTES: regulated on activation, normal T-cell expressed and secreted

TARC: thymus- and activation-regulated chemokine

TCI: topical calcineurin inhibitor

TH_1: T-helper cell type 1

TH_2: T-helper cells type 2

TNF-α: tumor necrosis factor-α

UVA: ultraviolet A

UVB: ultraviolet B

VEGF: vascular endothelial growth factor

REFERENCES

1. Pearce DJ, Stealey KH, Balkrishnan R, et al. Psoriasis treatment in the United States at the end of the 20th century. Int J Dermatol 2006; 45(4):370–374.
2. Bowcock AM, Barker JN. Genetics of psoriasis: The potential impact on new therapies. J Am Acad Dermatol 2003;49(2 Suppl):S51–S56.
3. Krueger G, Koo J, Lebwohl M, et al. The impact of psoriasis on quality of life: Results of a 1998 National Psoriasis Foundation patient-membership survey. Arch Dermatol 2001;137(3):280–284.
4. Weiss SC, Kimball AB, Liewehr DJ, et al. Quantifying the harmful effect of psoriasis on health-related quality of life. J Am Acad Dermatol 2002;47(4):512–518.
5. Koo J, Lee E, Lee CS, Lebwohl M. Psoriasis. J Am Acad Dermatol 2004;50(4):613–622.
6. Higgins E. Alcohol, smoking and psoriasis. Clin Exp Dermatol 2000;25 (2):107–110.
7. Rasmussen JE. The relationship between infection with group A beta hemolytic streptococci and the development of psoriasis. Pediatr Infect Dis J 2000;19(2):153–154.
8. Tsankov N, Angelova I, Kazandjieva J. Drug-induced psoriasis. Recognition and management. Am J Clin Dermatol 2000;1(3):159–165.
9. Elder JT, Nair RP, Henseler T, et al. The genetics of psoriasis 2001: The odyssey continues. Arch Dermatol 2001;137(11):1447–1454.
10. Mendonca CO, Burden AD. Current concepts in psoriasis and its treatment. Pharmacol Ther 2003;99(2):133–147.
11. Sun LD, Li W, Yang S, et al. Evidence for a novel psoriasis susceptibility locus at 9q33–9q34 in Chinese Hans. J Invest Dermatol 2007;127(5):1140–1144.
12. Liu Y, Krueger JG, Bowcock AM. Psoriasis: genetic associations and immune system changes. Genes Immun 2007;8(1):1–12.
13. Saini R, Tutrone WD, Weinberg JM. Advances in therapy for psoriasis: An overview of infliximab, etanercept, efalizumab, alefacept, adalimumab, tazarotene, and pimecrolimus. Curr Pharm Des 2005;11(2):273–280.
14. Mehlis SL, Gordon KB. The immunology of psoriasis and biologic immunotherapy. J Am Acad Dermatol 2003;49(2 Suppl):S44–S50.
15. Lowes MA, Bowcock AM, Krueger JG. Pathogenesis and therapy of psoriasis. Nature 2007;445(7130):866–873.
16. Krueger G, Ellis CN. Psoriasis—Recent advances in understanding its pathogenesis and treatment. J Am Acad Dermatol 2005;53(1 Suppl 1):S94–S100.
17. Mehlis S, Gordon KB. From laboratory to clinic: Rationale for biologic therapy. Dermatol Clin 2004;22(4):371–377, vii–viii.
18. Gottlieb AB, Chaudhari U, Baker DG, et al. The National Psoriasis Foundation Psoriasis Score (NPF-PS) system versus the Psoriasis Area Severity Index (PASI) and Physician's Global Assessment (PGA): A comparison. J Drugs Dermatol 2003;2(3):260–266.
19. Hodak E, Gottlieb AB, Segal T, et al. Climatotherapy at the Dead Sea is a remittive therapy for psoriasis: Combined effects on epidermal and immunologic activation. J Am Acad Dermatol 2003;49(3):451–457.

20. Lebwohl M, Ali S. Treatment of psoriasis. Part 1. Topical therapy and phototherapy. J Am Acad Dermatol 2001;45(4):487–498; quiz 499–502.
21. Travis L, Weinberg JM. Medical backgrounder: Psoriasis. Drugs Today (Barc) 2002;38(12):847–865.
22. Lange K, Kleuser B, Gysler A, et al. Cutaneous inflammation and proliferation in vitro: Differential effects and mode of action of topical glucocorticoids. Skin Pharmacol Appl Skin Physiol 2000;13(2):93–103.
23. Hengge UR, Ruzicka T, Schwartz RA, Cork MJ. Adverse effects of topical glucocorticosteroids. J Am Acad Dermatol 2006;54(1):1–15; quiz 16–18.
24. Norris DA. Mechanisms of action of topical therapies and the rationale for combination therapy. J Am Acad Dermatol 2005;53(1 Suppl 1):S17–S25.
25. Lebwohl M. A clinician's paradigm in the treatment of psoriasis. J Am Acad Dermatol 2005;53(1 Suppl 1):S59–S69.
26. Langner A, Stapor W, Ambroziak M. Efficacy and tolerance of topical calcitriol 3 μg(-1) in psoriasis treatment: A review of our experience in Poland. Br J Dermatol 2001;144(Suppl 58):11–16.
27. Lambert J, Trompke C. Tacalcitol ointment for long-term control of chronic plaque psoriasis in dermatological practice. Dermatology 2002;204(4):321–324.
28. van de Kerkhof PCM. Update on retinoid therapy of psoriasis in: An update on the use of retinoids in dermatology. Dermatol Ther 2006;19(5):252–263.
29. Thami GP, Sarkar R. Coal tar: Past, present and future. Clin Exp Dermatol 2002;27(2):99–103.
30. Vlajinac HD, Adanja BJ, Lazar ZF, et al. Risk factors for basal cell carcinoma. Acta Oncol 2000;39(5):611–616.
31. Saraswat A, Agarwal R, Katare OP, et al. A randomized, double-blind, vehicle-controlled study of a novel liposomal dithranol formulation in psoriasis. J Dermatolog Treat 2007;18(1):40–45.
32. Farkas A, Kemeny L, Szony BJ, et al. Dithranol upregulates IL-10 receptors on the cultured human keratinocyte cell line HaCaT. Inflamm Res 2001;50(1):44–49.
33. de Prost Y. New topical immunological treatments for psoriasis. J Eur Acad Dermatol Venereol 2006;20(Suppl 2):80–82.
34. Reynolds NJ, Al-Daraji WI. Calcineurin inhibitors and sirolimus: mechanisms of action and applications in dermatology. Clin Exp Dermatol 2002;27(7):555–561.
35. Ormerod AD, Shah SA, Copeland P, et al. Treatment of psoriasis with topical sirolimus: Preclinical development and a randomized, double-blind trial. Br J Dermatol 2005;152(4):758–764.
36. Rich SJ. Considerations for assessing the cost of biologic agents in the treatment of psoriasis. J Manag Care Pharm 2004;10(3 Suppl B):S38–S41.
37. Elias AN. Anti-thyroid thioureylenes in the treatment of psoriasis. Med Hypotheses 2004;62(3):431–437.
38. Pearce DJ, Nelson AA, Fleischer AB, et al. The cost-effectiveness and cost of treatment failures associated with systemic psoriasis therapies. J Dermatolog Treat 2006;17(1):29–37.
39. Singri P, West DP, Gordon KB. Biologic therapy for psoriasis: the new therapeutic frontier. Arch Dermatol 2002;138(5):657–663.
40. Gottlieb AB. Infliximab for psoriasis. J Am Acad Dermatol 2003;49(2 Suppl):S112–S117.
41. Chaudhari U, Romano P, Mulcahy LD, et al. Efficacy and safety of infliximab monotherapy for plaque-type psoriasis: A randomised trial. Lancet 2001;357(9271):1842–1847.
42. Sobell JM, Hallas SJ. Systemic therapies for psoriasis: Understanding current and newly emerging therapies. Semin Cutan Med Surg 2003;22(3):187–195.
43. Mease PJ, Goffe BS, Metz J, et al. Etanercept in the treatment of psoriatic arthritis and psoriasis: A randomised trial. Lancet 2000;356(9227):385–390.
44. Leonardi CL, Powers JL, Matheson RT, et al. Etanercept as monotherapy in patients with psoriasis. N Engl J Med 2003;349(21):2014–2022.
45. Pitarch G, Sanchez-Carazo JL, Mahiques L, et al. Treatment of psoriasis with adalimumab. Clin Exp Dermatol 2007;32(1):18–22.
46. Gordon KB, Langley RG, Leonardi C, et al. Clinical response to adalimumab treatment in patients with moderate to severe psoriasis: Double-blind, randomized controlled trial and open-label extension study. J Am Acad Dermatol 2006;55(4):598–606.
47. Wilsmann-Theis D, Martin S, Reber M, et al. Biologicals dramatic advances in the treatment of psoriasis. Curr Pharm Des 2006;12(8):989–999.
48. van de Putte LB, Atkins C, Malaise M, et al. Efficacy and safety of adalimumab as monotherapy in patients with rheumatoid arthritis for whom previous disease modifying antirheumatic drug treatment has failed. Ann Rheum Dis 2004;63(5):508–516.
49. Bartelds GM, Wijbrandts CA, Nurmohamed MT, et al. Clinical response to adalimumab: The relationship with anti-adalimumab antibodies and serum adalimumab concentrations in rheumatoid arthritis. Ann Rheum Dis 2007.
50. Bender NK, Heilig CE, Droll B, et al. Immunogenicity, efficacy and adverse events of adalimumab in RA patients. Rheumatol Int 2007; 27(3):269–274.
51. Bendtzen K, Geborek P, Svenson M, et al. Individualized monitoring of drug bioavailability and immunogenicity in rheumatoid arthritis patients treated with the tumor necrosis factor alpha inhibitor infliximab. Arthritis Rheum 2006;54(12):3782–3789.
52. Dore RK, Mathews S, Schechtman J, et al. The immunogenicity, safety, and efficacy of etanercept liquid administered once weekly in patients with rheumatoid arthritis. Clin Exp Rheumatol 2007;25(1):40–46.
53. Krueger GG, Ellis CN. Alefacept therapy produces remission for patients with chronic plaque psoriasis. Br J Dermatol 2003;148(4):784–788.
54. Kraan MC, van Kuijk AW, Dinant HJ, et al. Alefacept treatment in psoriatic arthritis: Reduction of the effector T cell population in peripheral blood and synovial tissue is associated with improvement of clinical signs of arthritis. Arthritis Rheum 2002;46(10):2776–2784.
55. Ellis CN, Krueger GG. Treatment of chronic plaque psoriasis by selective targeting of memory effector T lymphocytes. N Engl J Med 2001;345(4):248–255.
56. Leonardi CL. Efalizumab: An overview. J Am Acad Dermatol 2003;49(2 Suppl):S98–S104.
57. Gottlieb AB, Krueger JG, Wittkowski K, et al. Psoriasis as a model for T-cell-mediated disease: Immunobiologic and clinical effects of treatment with multiple doses of efalizumab, an anti-CD11a antibody. Arch Dermatol 2002;138(5):591–600.
58. Lebwohl M, Tyring SK, Hamilton TK, et al. A novel targeted T-cell modulator, efalizumab, for plaque psoriasis. N Engl J Med 2003; 349(21):2004–2013.
59. Kanitakis J, Butnaru AC, Claudy A. Novel biological immunotherapies for psoriasis. Expert Opin Investig Drugs 2003;12(7):1111–1121.
60. Lebwohl M, Ali S. Treatment of psoriasis. Part 2. Systemic therapies. J Am Acad Dermatol 2001;45(5):649–661; quiz 662–664.
61. Gordon KB, Ruderman EM. The treatment of psoriasis and psoriatic arthritis: an interdisciplinary approach. J Am Acad Dermatol 2006;54(3 Suppl 2):S85–S91.
62. Ho VC. The use of ciclosporin in psoriasis: a clinical review. Br J Dermatol 2004;150(Suppl 67):1–10.
63. Faerber L, Braeutigam M, Weidinger G, et al. Cyclosporine in severe psoriasis. Results of a meta-analysis in 579 patients. Am J Clin Dermatol 2001;2(1):41–47.
64. Feldman SR, Garton R. Cyclosporin in psoriasis: How? J Eur Acad Dermatol Venereol 2004;18(3):250–253.
65. Yamauchi PS, Rizk D, Kormeili T, et al. Current systemic therapies for psoriasis: Where are we now? J Am Acad Dermatol 2003;49(2 Suppl):S66–S77.
66. Skaehill PA. Tacrolimus in dermatologic disorders. Ann Pharmacother 2001;35(5):582–588.
67. Gottlieb AB, Griffiths CE, Ho VC, et al. Oral pimecrolimus in the treatment of moderate to severe chronic plaque-type psoriasis: A double-blind, multicentre, randomized, dose-finding trial. Br J Dermatol 2005;152(6):1219–1227.
68. Saporito FC, Menter MA. Methotrexate and psoriasis in the era of new biologic agents. J Am Acad Dermatol 2004;50(2):301–309.
69. Gelfand JM, Berlin J, Van Voorhees A, Margolis DJ. Lymphoma rates are low but increased in patients with psoriasis: results from a population-based cohort study in the United Kingdom. Arch Dermatol 2003;139(11):1425–1429.
70. Kremer JM. Toward a better understanding of methotrexate. Arthritis Rheum 2004;50(5):1370–1382.
71. Geilen CC, Arnold M, Orfanos CE. Mycophenolate mofetil as a systemic antipsoriatic agent: Positive experience in 11 patients. Br J Dermatol 2001;144(3):583–586.
72. Mydlarski PR. Mycophenolate mofetil: A dermatologic perspective. Skin Therapy Lett 2005;10(3):1–6.

73. Mason C, Krueger GG. Thioguanine for refractory psoriasis: A 4-year experience. J Am Acad Dermatol 2001;44(1):67–72.
74. Weindl G, Roeder A, Schafer-Korting M, et al. Receptor-selective retinoids for psoriasis: Focus on tazarotene. Am J Clin Dermatol 2006;7(2):85–97.
75. Short MW, Vaughan TK. Sequential therapy using cyclosporine and acitretin for treatment of total body psoriasis. Cutis 2004;74(3):185–188.
76. Koo JY. New developments in topical sequential therapy for psoriasis. Skin Therapy Lett 2005;10(9):1–4.
77. Langan SM, Heerey A, Barry M, Barnes L. Cost analysis of narrowband UVB phototherapy in psoriasis. J Am Acad Dermatol 2004;50(4):623–626.
78. Bandow GD, Koo JY. Narrow-band ultraviolet B radiation: A review of the current literature. Int J Dermatol 2004;43(8):555–561.
79. Zanolli M. Phototherapy arsenal in the treatment of psoriasis. Dermatol Clin 2004;22(4):397–406, viii.
80. Naldi L, Griffiths CE. Traditional therapies in the management of moderate to severe chronic plaque psoriasis: An assessment of the benefits and risks. Br J Dermatol 2005;152(4):597–615.
81. Yones SS, Palmer RA, Garibaldinos TT, Hawk JL. Randomized double-blind trial of the treatment of chronic plaque psoriasis: efficacy of psoralen-UV-A therapy vs. narrowband UV-B therapy. Arch Dermatol 2006;142(7):836–842.
82. Stern RS. The risk of melanoma in association with long-term exposure to PUVA. J Am Acad Dermatol 2001;44(5):755–761.
83. Guinot C, Malvy DJ, Latreille J, et al. Sun-reactive skin type in 4912 French adults participating in the SU.VI.MAX study. Photochem Photobiol 2005;81(4):934–940.
84. Vongthongsri R, Konschitzky R, Seeber A, et al. Randomized, double-blind comparison of 1 mg/L versus 5 mg/L methoxsalen bath-PUVA therapy for chronic plaque-type psoriasis. J Am Acad Dermatol 2006;55(4):627–631.
85. Pozo-Roman T, Gonzalez-Lopez A, Velasco-Vaquero ME, Nunez-Cabezon M. Psoralen cream plus ultraviolet A photochemotherapy (PUVA cream): Our experience. J Eur Acad Dermatol Venereol 2006;20(2):136–142.
86. Gach JE, Madrigal AM, Hutton JL, Charles-Holmes R. Retrospective analysis of the occurrence of internal malignancy in patients treated with PUVA between 1986 and 1999 in South Warwickshire. Clin Exp Dermatol 2004;29(2):154–155.
87. Wang SQ, Setlow R, Berwick M, et al. Ultraviolet A and melanoma: A review. J Am Acad Dermatol 2001;44(5):837–846.
88. Nijsten TE, Stern RS. The increased risk of skin cancer is persistent after discontinuation of psoralen + ultraviolet A. A cohort study. J Invest Dermatol 2003;121(2):252–258.
89. Stern RS, Bagheri S, Nichols K. The persistent risk of genital tumors among men treated with psoralen plus ultraviolet A (PUVA) for psoriasis. J Am Acad Dermatol 2002;47(1):33–39.
90. Asawanonda P, Anderson RR, Chang Y, Taylor CR. 308-nm excimer laser for the treatment of psoriasis: a dose-response study. Arch Dermatol 2000;136(5):619–624.
91. Taibjee SM, Cheung ST, Laube S, Lanigan SW. Controlled study of excimer and pulsed dye lasers in the treatment of psoriasis. Br J Dermatol 2005;153(5):960–966.
92. Spann CT, Barbagallo J, Weinberg JM. A review of the 308-nm excimer laser in the treatment of psoriasis. Cutis 2001;68(5):351–352.
93. Feldman SR, Evans C, Russell MW. Systemic treatment for moderate to severe psoriasis: estimates of failure rates and direct medical costs in a north-eastern US managed care plan. J Dermatolog Treat 2005;16(1):37–42.
94. Nast A, Kopp I, Augustin M, et al. German evidence-based guidelines for the treatment of Psoriasis vulgaris (short version). Arch Dermatol Res 2007;299(3):111–138.
95. Leon A, Nguyen A, Letsinger J, Koo J. An attempt to formulate an evidence-based strategy in the management of moderate-to-severe psoriasis: a review of the efficacy and safety of biologics and prebiologic options. Expert Opin Pharmacother 2007;8(5):617–632.

CHAPTER 102

Atopic Dermatitis

NINA H. CHEIGH

KEY CONCEPTS

1. Atopic dermatitis is increasing in prevalence by a two- to threefold increase, particularly in industrialized countries; with an association with other immunoglobulin E (IgE)-mediated diseases such as allergic rhinitis and asthma.
2. Typically starting in infancy, atopic dermatitis can present at any age, although the clinical presentation can differ at varying ages.
3. Infants typically have face, trunk, and neck involvement whereas older children and adults present in the antecubital and popliteal fossa, hands, and face.
4. Patients with atopic dermatitis are extremely susceptible to potential allergens causing irritations: aeroallergens (dander, grass, mold, pollen), food (eggs, peanuts, soy, milk), detergents and soaps, and chemicals, varying humidities, temperature, and emotional stress.
5. Most patients with atopic dermatitis have elevated serum IgE levels, as well as eosinophilia. But, pathogenesis involves this along with a complex process including lymphocytes, macrophages, and mast cells.
6. Control of flare-ups includes identification and elimination of trigger allergens, as well as maintaining skin patency.
7. Topical corticosteroids and emollients are the mainstay for treatment of atopic dermatitis.
8. Topical immunomodulators, tacrolimus and pimecrolimus applied topically, have demonstrated a new option for patients with mild to severe cases of atopic dermatitis.
9. In severe, refractory cases, atopic dermatitis can be treated with ultraviolet (UV) radiation, oral corticosteroids, cyclosporine, azathioprine, methotrexate, and interferon-γ.

Atopic dermatitis, a common pervasive inflammatory skin condition, is notorious for creating a vicious cycle of itching and scratching. Chronic, relapsing, itchy and inflamed skin is the trademark symptom of atopic dermatitis (or atopic eczema).[1] This highly itchy skin, described as an itch so unbearable that patients often find that they must scratch until it is replaced by pain, naturally results in scratching. Although the term *atopy* is widely accepted throughout clinical medicine to describe a person's susceptibility to hay fever, asthma, and atopic dermatitis, there is no precise definition or marker of atopy.[2] Certainly there is an association among these chronic conditions, as some 80% of children with AD eventually develop allergic rhinitis or asthma, or have some family history of either.[3,4]

Learning objectives, review questions, and other resources can be found at **www.pharmacotherapyonline.com.**

The significant increase in prevalence of atopic dermatitis has been well documented over a wide variety of age groups and geographic locations. Levels of air pollution, industrialization and urbanization, dietary modifications, and higher socioeconomic class are some of the factors that have been attributed to the increase in prevalence. Although approximately one half of the cases are diagnosed by the first year of life, atopic dermatitis typically results in a longer-term condition, as one third of these patients have some form of atopic dermatitis into adulthood.[5] Prevalence in school-aged children is approaching 17%.[6] Those with severe symptoms and early onset have a greater likelihood for a more pervasive course of disease.

Many times, atopic dermatitis is not perceived as a major illness and is frequently dismissed as a minor skin condition. However, studies have demonstrated considerable financial, emotional, and social impact on families of those with moderate–severe atopic dermatitis.[7] An Australian study reported results of significantly more stress in taking care of a child with moderate–severe atopic dermatitis than that of a child with insulin-dependent diabetes.[8] Disturbed or lack of sleep has also been reported.[9] In the United States, atopic dermatitis represents some 4% of emergency room visits. The health systems of all countries are burdened with the heavy economic load of direct and indirect costs of treatment and social morbidity.[10]

ETIOLOGY

Over the past few decades, there have been significant contributions to researching the cause of this condition. Even so, there is no absolute known cause, as this seems to be a disease of complicated genetic, environmental, and immunologic mechanisms. There is a notable strong hereditary component with atopic dermatitis, such as if one parent has an atopic condition, there is a 60% likelihood that the child will be atopic. If both parents are afflicted, it is possible that the child will have an 80% chance of developing an atopic condition.[11] It is also known that there is a stronger influence of paternal atopic dermatitis and asthma as opposed to maternal history. Most patients with atopic dermatitis are found to have elevated eosinophils and serum IgE levels, which supports that 80% of children with atopic dermatitis eventually develop some sort of allergic rhinitis or asthma.

It seems almost every immunocyte, including Langerhans cells, monocytes, macrophages, lymphocytes, mast cells, and keratinocytes, have demonstrated some abnormality in atopic dermatitis.[12]

PATHOPHYSIOLOGY AND CLINICAL PRESENTATION

Intense itching (pruritus) and skin reactivity are the hallmarks of atopic dermatitis, and it is characterized by episodic flares. Atopic flares are classified as mild, moderate, or severe depending on the degree and severity of those symptoms. Typically, there are three different types of skin lesions associated with atopic dermatitis: acute, subacute and chronic.[13] The acute rash results in lesions that are intensely pruritic, erythematous papules and vesicles over erythematous skin. These itchy lesions are subsequently associated with scratching that results in excoriations and exudates. Subacute lesions are typically thicker, paler, scaly, erythematous, and excoriated plaques. Chronic lesions are characterized by thickened plaques, accentuated skin markings (lichenification), and fibrotic papules. Most patients exhibit all three lesion types. At all phases, the atopic skin usually has a dry luster to the skin.[1]

Atopic dermatitis commonly involves the extensor surfaces of the extremities, trunk, face, scalp, and neck.[14] Although infantile eczema commonly subsides in severity, it often causes the adult to develop a tendency for inflammatory, erythematous, pruritic reactions when exposed to irritants. When atopic dermatitis presents in older children or adults, the lesions are present in the flexural areas of the antecubital and popliteal fossa. Atopic skin is associated with xerosis, which is recognized as a fine scaling, noninflamed skin involving large areas of the body. Atopic skin has a genetic decreased ability for keratinocytes to bind water, thus giving patients with atopic dermatitis dry skin, despite the weather.[15] The atopic epidermis not only triggers pruritus, but also results in an abnormal protective layer, predisposing irritation from allergens.

DIAGNOSIS

Hanifin and colleagues published the first major and minor diagnostic criteria for atopic dermatitis in 1980.[13] These diagnostic criteria include the presence of pruritus, with three of more of the following:

1. History of flexural dermatitis of the face in children younger than 10 years of age
2. History of asthma or allergic rhinitis in the child or first-degree relative
3. History of generalized xerosis (dry skin) within past year
4. Visible flexural eczema
5. Onset of rash younger than 2 years of age

If diagnosis of atopic dermatitis cannot be made, the presenting symptoms can be indicative of a wide array of other conditions and differential diagnoses, and thus referral to a specialist is warranted.[16] It should be noted that these are working criteria to aid the clinician in proper diagnoses. Although elevated IgE and peripheral eosinophilia are most likely found in atopic dermatitis, there is no one single laboratory test that is used to reliably diagnose atopic dermatitis, as some patients do not present with such abnormalities.[16] Skin prick tests or enzyme-linked immunosorbent assay (ELISA) tests can be used to aid in identification and exclusion of allergic triggers but are not specific or sensitive enough to be diagnostic.

Not only is there a lack of absolute diagnoses or laboratory tests, there also remains a lack of standardization in objective severity scales for the disease. Of the systems available, the Severity Scoring of Atopic Dermatitis (SCORAD) index, adapted by the European Task Force on Atopic Dermatitis[17] was the most often used but also demonstrated interobserver variation. As such, it was concluded that there is no overall consensus of an objective severity scale, and that further research is warranted.[18]

ALLERGEN TRIGGERS

Immunological triggers that contribute to atopic dermatitis development include food allergens and aeroallergens. Serum IgE levels are elevated in most patients with atopic dermatitis. A variety of allergens cause approximately 85% of atopic dermatitis patients to demonstrate an immediately positive skin test of serum IgE antibody.[1] It is important to note, however, that atopic dermatitis is not a purely IgE-type of condition, as this would indicate an immediate hypersensitivity mast-cell mechanism. There is evidence that T-helper type 2 (TH_2) cells are found in atopic individuals, and play an important role in the condition.[19] Studies have demonstrated flaring of atopic dermatitis on exposure to various aeroallergens such as horse dander, grass, and ragweed pollen.[1] Although it is difficult to avoid variation in the performance and evaluation of these types of tests, it is established that patch tests with allergens can result in eczematous reactions.[3] The most common household aeroallergens include dust mites, cat dander, and molds. Dust mites, which are a particularly commonly encountered allergen, were reported in more than 45% of American homes in a concentration that exceeded levels needed for sensitization.[19] Even so, there are many simple steps to aid in reducing the amount of dust mites in homes.

Food allergy is also a contributing factor to atopic dermatitis, and generally, the more severe the atopic dermatitis and younger the patient, the more likely food allergy is the culprit to the symptoms.[20] Egg, milk, peanut, soy, and wheat are noted to account for almost 90% of food allergy in children with atopic dermatitis.[21] Even so, it seems that almost a third of the children with atopic dermatitis and food allergies will "outgrow" the allergy over 1 to 3 years.[22] But given this, it is essential that patients (parents) are properly instructed on how to read labels for "hidden sources" of allergenic foods. It is recommended that patients be rechallenged at certain times to determine if the food allergy is truly outgrown.[22]

Question remains as to whether breast-feeding helps prevent allergy, but for obvious reasons, this cannot be ethically studied. Human breast milk is the most hypoallergenic substance to nourish infants, but there lacks evidence that either prolonged breast-feeding or manipulations of a mother's diet during lactation protects in the development of atopic dermatitis in infants with family history of atopy.[23] In infants with a strong family history, thus posing them as high risk, there may be a decrease in atopic dermatitis during the first 4 years of life by prolonged breast-feeding (4–6 months), and introduction of solid foods at a later development time (4 months of age).[24] Exclusive breast-feeding during the first 3 months of life has also been associated with a lower incidence of atopic dermatitis in childhood.[25]

In stressful situations, where the patient is frustrated or embarrassed, there is an increased likelihood of itching, sweating, and scratching.[1] Although stress itself does not cause atopic dermatitis per se, it can exacerbate the condition.[26] Stress management, relaxation, and behavioral modification can be important.

Knowing that atopic patients are more susceptible to irritants, it is important to identify and eliminate common irritants. Soaps, detergents, abrasive clothing, smoke, and exposure to extremes in temperature and humidity can be aggravating factors. Although UV light can be beneficial to some patients, sunscreens should be used to avoid sunburns, but care should be used in selection as many chemical sunscreens can cause contact dermatitis. In addition, as modernization and "Westernization" occurs, people spend the majority of their time in modern buildings with reduced ventilation. This has resulted in an increased load of chemical vapors and gasses, and indoor house dust mites and mold.[24]

COMPLICATIONS

Atopic skin also has a predisposition for increased microbial organisms, namely *Staphylococcus aureus*, which is found in more than 90% of atopic dermatitis skin lesions.[13] Bacteria can secrete toxins, which bind to a high number of T cells and can lead to erythroderma and acute inflammatory processes of the skin. Although short courses of antistaphylococcal antibiotics or topical therapy is appropriate, colonization with resistant organisms is possible.[6] Patients with atopic dermatitis are also more prone to herpes simplex infections than in the general population.[27] Patients respond well to oral antiviral therapy with acyclovir or valacyclovir. But it is important for the clinician to maintain therapy of the atopic dermatitis lesions while treating the herpes infection.[6] In addition, fungal pathogens, particularly *Malassezia furfur* or *Pityrosporum ovale,* have been identified. Antifungals such as ketoconazole and itraconazole seem to work well as there is additional antiinflammatory effect as well.[6]

Patients with atopic dermatitis can also present with eyelid dermatitis, nipple dermatitis, and cheilitis of the lips. Eyelid dermatitis and chronic blepharitis are commonly associated with atopic dermatitis and can result in visual impairment from corneal scarring. Other ocular complications include atopic keratoconjunctivitis, vernal conjunctivitis, and keratoconus.[1]

TREATMENT

Atopic Dermatitis

Currently, there is no 100% cure for atopic dermatitis. As such, this condition requires a management plan, including identification and avoidance of external triggers, maintenance of skin patency, and various therapeutic options for symptomatic relief. Therapy should be individualized, and a multipronged approach should be initiated. Reduction of symptoms, prevention of recurrent flares, and attempting to modify the course of the disease, while minimizing exposure to potential toxicity of the drugs is the long-term management indicated for atopic dermatitis (Fig. 102–1).

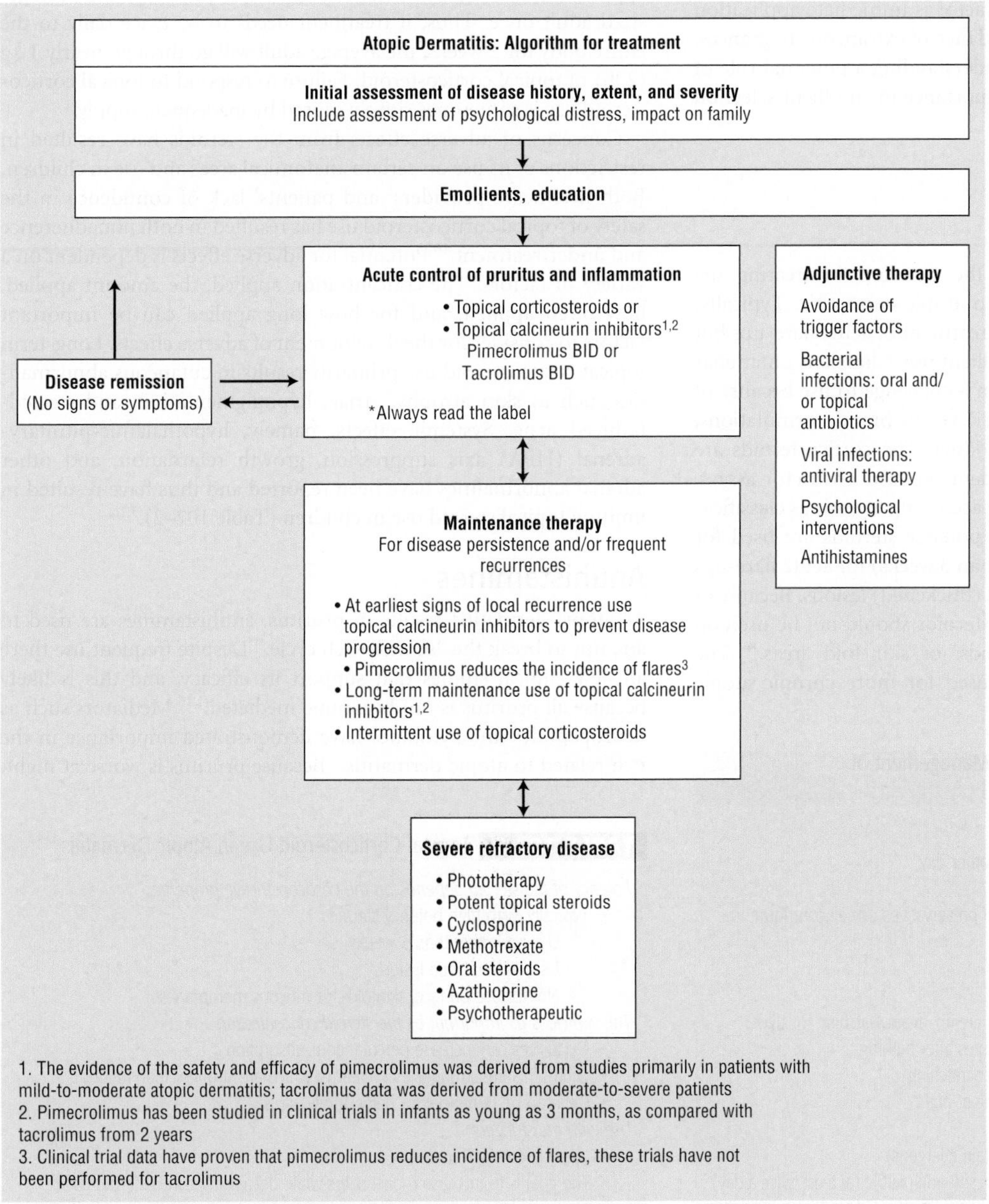

FIGURE 102-1. Treatment of atopic dermatitis. (bid, twice daily.)

NONPHARMACOLOGIC

Given that patients with atopic dermatitis are more susceptible to irritants than normal individuals, it is important to identify possible aggravating factors that can trigger a flare-up. Recommendations can include avoiding extraneous perfumed or dyed soaps and detergents, using a second rinse cycle for laundry, avoiding extremes of temperature fluctuations, and otherwise being cognizant of potential allergens. Sunscreens should be used in patients with atopic dermatitis, but judicious use of nonchemical agents (physical sunscreens such as titanium or zinc-oxide containing products) are probably less likely to cause further irritation or contact dermatitis.[1]

The epidermis of atopic skin has been shown to have a reduced capability of holding moisture. This inherent dry skin is also exacerbated by external changes including weather changes and other allergen exposures. Thus, the importance of maintaining proper skin patency cannot be overstressed, as slight irritations to atopic skin can result in microfissures, which act as a portal of entry for various pathogens.[16] Simple, nonpharmacologic and preventive measure should be recommended for all patients with atopic dermatitis. Skin hydration is a key component to atopic disease management. Lotions can worsen xerosis whereas thick creams (e.g., Cetaphil, Eucerin) or ointments (e.g., Aquaphor, petroleum jelly) are better at protecting against dryness. Although there is some controversy with showering versus bathing, the most important factor is immediate application of the emollient after cleansing. Avoidance of extraneous fragrances, dyes, and preservatives, as well as understanding a potential role of excipient contact allergy is also of importance in emollient selection (Table 102–1).

PHARMACOLOGIC

Topical Corticosteroids

Topical corticosteroids have been the standard in treating the inflammation and pruritus related to atopic dermatitis. Typically, they are used in short-term reactive treatment of acute flare-ups but must still be supplemented with emollient use. Clinicians unfamiliar with topical corticosteroids find them a challenge to use because of the numerous types, strengths, generic versus brand, formulations, and when and where to use the product. The corticosteroids are ranked according to potency dependent on vasoconstrictor assays. Various drug references will list these according to various classifications. Most commonly, the highest potency steroids are used for short periods of time (generally less than 3 weeks) for acute flare-ups of atopic dermatitis, or for lichenified (thickened) lesions. Because of their potential adverse effects, these steroids should not be used on the face, mucous membranes, eyelids, or skin-fold areas.[16] The moderate-strength steroids can be used for more chronic atopic dermatitis, typically on the trunk or extremities. Low potency steroids are typically used in children.

The vehicle in which the steroid is based is also of importance. As in emollients, the ointments are far better at occluding the epidermis, and thus results in enhanced percutaneous absorption of the corticosteroid compared to the same strength cream. This can be a better choice for a lichenified lesion, or if an acute flare-up is being treated as the enhanced occlusion will result in better absorption.[16] Other methods of occlusion, such as use of Saran wrap, tight-fitting clothes, or diapers can also increase the absorption significantly.[28] This may or may not give the desired effect that the clinician expects, and thus he or she should be aware of this potential. The vehicle can also be chosen based on the area of the body. For example, if application should occur in hairy areas such as scalp or beard, a solution or gel can be more aesthetically pleasing. These are important considerations when recommending a corticosteroid, or when counseling a patient on its appropriate use.

Typically, most corticosteroids are applied once to multiple times daily although there is no clear benefit with more than a once daily application.[29] Should the steroid be used in conjunction with other topical agents, including moisturizers, it is important that the corticosteroid be applied first, rubbed in well, followed by the other product. In dispensing a corticosteroid, a good rule of thumb would be that approximately 30 gm of cream or ointment can cover the average-sized adult once. Thus, if treatment needs to be twice daily to the entire body for 2 weeks, the average adult will go through nearly 1 kg (2 lb) of topical corticosteroid. Failure to respond to topical corticosteroid use is sometimes simply caused by inadequate supply.[1]

Concerns of adverse effects from the steroids have resulted in restrictions of its use on certain anatomical areas and use in children. Both healthcare providers' and patients' lack of confidence in the safety of topical corticosteroid use has resulted in both nonadherence and undertreatment.[16] Potential for adverse effects is dependent on a variety of factors. The concentration applied, the amount applied, how often applied, and for how long applied can be important factors to consider for the development of adverse effects. Long-term topical corticosteroid use primarily results in cutaneous abnormalities such as skin atrophy, striae, hypopigmentation, and steroid-induced acne. Systemic effects, namely, hypothalamic-pituitary-adrenal (HPA) axis suppression, growth retardation, and other adrenal abnormalities have been reported and thus have resulted in limiting topical steroid use in children (Table 102–2).[5,16]

Antihistamines

As atopic dermatitis results in pruritus, antihistamines are used to attempt to break the "scratch–itch cycle." Despite frequent use there are few clinical studies that support its efficacy, and this is likely because all pruritus is not histamine mediated.[1,16] Mediators such as neuropeptides and cytokines have demonstrated importance in the itch related to atopic dermatitis.[6] Because pruritus is worse at night,

TABLE 102-1 Nonpharmacologic Management of Atopic Dermatitis

- Identify and eliminate potential allergens
- Reduce frequency of bathing; bathe every other day
- Use tepid water in baths
- Avoid irritating soaps (dyes, fragrances, and preservatives can all contribute to further exacerbations)
- Avoid washcloths or irritating scrubs
- Air dry skin and gently pat dry
- Apply emollient (preferably an ointment or cream, again watching for dyes, fragrances, and preservatives) within 3 minutes after bathing
- Keep fingernails short and clean to prevent scratching
- Consider cotton gloves to prevent scratching at night
- Use cotton sheets and pajamas
- Avoid harsh laundry detergents (some contain allergens)
- Moisturize as often as necessary to keep skin soft and pliable (at least twice a day)

TABLE 102-2 Topical Corticosteroid Use in Atopic Dermatitis

Potency of the steroid depends on the vasoconstrictive properties
- Typically, with high-potency steroids:
  - Use no longer than 3 weeks
  - Use on thickened lesions
  - Not for use on face, skinfolds, or mucous membranes

The vehicle is as important as the steroid concentration
- Occlusives can increase percutaneous absorption
- Ointments are stronger than creams, which are stronger than lotions
- Gels can be beneficial for hairy or oily areas

Use with moisturizers
- Apply corticosteroid first
- The goal is to increase moisturizers while decreasing corticosteroid use

the sedating antihistamines (i.e., hydroxyzine or diphenhydramine), can offer an advantage by facilitating sleep, whereas the newer nonsedating antihistamines have shown variable results. A tricyclic antidepressant, doxepin, which inhibits both H_1 and H_2 receptors, has also been used in doses of 10 to 75 mg at night, and up to 75 mg twice daily in adults. This can be beneficial in those atopic patients who have some depression as well.[1,16,30] Topical antihistamines, such as doxepin 5% cream or diphenhydramine cream, also have demonstrated neutral results but are generally not recommended because of high cutaneous sensitization from its excipient ingredients.[6,16]

Topical Immunomodulators

Topical calcineurin inhibitors, such as tacrolimus and pimecrolimus, offer a more long-term option, as they can be used on all body locations for prolonged periods without fear of corticosteroid-induced adverse effects. As skin atrophy is a main concern for long-term use of topical corticosteroids, the atrophogenic potential of tacrolimus and pimecrolimus were evaluated in healthy volunteers. Data indicate the potential for longer term use without fear of skin atrophy.[31,32] These agents form a complex that results in inhibition of calcineurin, which normally initiates T-cell activation. Through inhibition, the complex subdues the inflammatory component of atopic dermatitis.[33] Although both of the structures are similar, topical pimecrolimus has been shown to be more lipophilic than topical tacrolimus, thus resulting in reduced cutaneous penetration.[33,34]

A number of studies have demonstrated the short-term and long-term effectiveness of topical tacrolimus 0.03% and 0.1% ointment in atopic dermatitis for children and adults.[33] When used twice daily, the patients reported a significant reduction in pruritus, clearance of lesions, and otherwise increased quality of life. Current FDA approvals indicate the 0.03% or 0.1% ointment for moderate to severe atopic dermatitis in adults, and 0.03% ointment for atopic dermatitis in children aged 2 to 15 years.[33] Topical tacrolimus is indicated for second-line therapy for short-term and noncontinuous therapy of moderate–severe atopic dermatitis who have failed other therapies. Several studies in children and adults have demonstrated reduction of frequency of atopic dermatitis flares and symptoms by tacrolimus ointment.[35–40] A head to head comparison found comparable efficacy of tacrolimus 0.1% ointment to topical hydrocortisone butyrate 0.1%, a midpotency corticosteroid.[41]

The safety of topical tacrolimus has been evaluated with the most common complaints being transient itching or burning at the site of application. Although there are no data to support this, many clinicians recommend pretreatment with topical corticosteroids to wave off the tacrolimus induced burning and erythema. There are systemic adverse effects of tacrolimus that have been well documented but have not been observed in patients using the topical ointment for atopic dermatitis.[42] Patients who receive long-term systemic immunosuppressants are prone to developing actinic keratoses, viral warts, and nonmelanoma skin cancers. The FDA issued a black box warning for long-term use of tacrolimus and pimecrolimus acknowledging that there is no direct causal evidence of skin cancers and the use of topical calcineurin inhibitors. Long-term studies are in progress.[43]

Topical pimecrolimus 1% cream has also been demonstrated to be safe and effective in long-term atopic dermatitis.[33] Multicenter, randomized, double-blind trials in infants and children found that flare-ups were prevented, as well as a reduction in disease severity overall.[44] Even those who did require the steroids for flare-ups, it was found that the duration of steroid use was significantly shorter, which support using pimecrolimus as a first-line therapy.[45,46] Pharmacokinetic studies have evaluated the systemic concentration of pimecrolimus absorbed in children. These studies conclude that pimecrolimus is well tolerated locally, and systemic effects were not seen.[47]

Although no comparable data exist, it appears that tacrolimus can be more effective in clearing severe cases of atopic dermatitis than pimecrolimus.[33] There are no direct comparative data as of yet, but there seems to be increased transient local burning with topical tacrolimus, possibly because of a higher immunosuppressant activity. A recent 2-year study of infants who were treated with pimecrolimus 1% cream at the first signs and symptoms of atopic dermatitis flares found progressive reduction in pimecrolimus use, supporting early intervention.[48] Corticosteroids and pimecrolimus cream were evaluated in infants and children 3 months to 11 years of age with mild to severe atopic dermatitis. Pimecrolimus was applied at the first signs of flare, and if the dermatitis was not controlled, a mid-potency steroid was applied in replacement of the evening cream. This was the first study to evaluate efficacy and safety of combined use, and it found that this was an effective steroid-sparing option to treating atopic dermatitis (Table 102–3).[49]

TABLE 102-3 Topical Immunomodulator Use in Atopic Dermatitis

- Tacrolimus (Protopic) 0.1% ointment: for moderate to severe AD in adults not responding adequately to other therapies
- Tacrolimus 0.03% ointment: for moderate to severe AD in children older than 2 years of age
- Pimecrolimus (Elidel) 1% cream: for mild to moderate AD in children and adults (it has been studied in infants as young as 3 months of age)
  - Apply twice daily
  - Can be used for longer term
  - Can result in reduction in flare-ups

AD, atopic dermatitis.

Tar Preparations

Coal tar preparations demonstrated antipruritic and antiinflammatory properties on the skin.[1] Coal tar has been used in combination with topical corticosteroids, as an adjunct to reduce the strength of a corticosteroid, and in conjunction with UV light therapies. These preparations are available as crude coal tar (1%–3%), or liquor carbonis detergens (LCD) (5%–20%). At times, coal tar can be compounded by pharmacists into various concentrations, or even in conjunction with topical corticosteroids. Coal tar preparations should not be used on acute oozing lesions, as this would result in stinging and irritation.[50] The strong odor and staining of clothing is typically a limiting factor to its use. Thus, patients can be instructed to use the product at bedtime and rinse it off in the morning. In addition, folliculitis and photosensitivity have also been reported.

■ REFRACTORY THERAPIES

Wet Dressings and Occlusion

Cool wet dressings or total body wraps placed directly onto the skin can be effective in relieving itch, particularly at night. Wet wraps used in conjunction with topical corticosteroids can be used for acute flares, or those with chronic, lichenified lesions.[50] Skin maceration, fissures, and subsequent infections can occur, and thus these occlusive dressings should be limited to severe, chronic lesions. Tepid compresses applied to skin for 20 minutes four to six times daily can aid in drying out the oozing lesions.

Ultraviolet Light

Ultraviolet light can have phototherapeutic benefits to patients with severe atopic dermatitis. Although natural sunlight can be a source, ensuring that the sunlight is not associated with high heat or humidity (which can exacerbate the condition further) is difficult. Thus, short-wave ultraviolet B (UVB) therapies can be useful as adjunctive therapy in chronic, recalcitrant atopic dermatitis.[51] At times, higher intensity ultraviolet A (UVA) therapy has been therapeutic in acute exacerbations, and the mechanism indicates that eosinophils and epidermal Langerhans cells may be targets for high-intensity UVA.[52] Photochemotherapy with oral methoxypsoralen therapy followed by UVA (PUVA) can be indicated in severe, widespread atopic dermatitis, particularly in corticosteroid failure.[53] Adverse effects, such as erythema and pigmentation, to premature photoaging and cutaneous malignancies are possible, and thus caution should be used in determining the risks versus benefit.

■ SYSTEMIC IMMUNOSUPPRESSANTS

If aggressive topical therapy, or phototherapy fail to control atopic dermatitis symptoms, the systemic immunosuppressant agents can play a role. Given that atopic dermatitis is a T-cell mediated disease with involvement from Langerhans cells, eosinophils, and mast cells, it is logical to consider the use of immunosuppressant agents. However, because of the possible adverse effects associated with these agents, judicious use of systemic immunosuppressants in severe, recalcitrant, or widespread disease is warranted.[54]

Systemic Corticosteroids

Oral corticosteroids, such as prednisone, can be indicated in the treatment of severe chronic atopic dermatitis.[1,6] Typically, a short course (e.g., prednisone 40–60 mg/day for 3–4 days, then 20–30 mg/day for 3–4 days) can be used to control a severe flare. Proper tapering is necessary, as its misuse has resulted in dramatic improvement of symptoms followed by a significant rebound flare on discontinuation of the medication.[16] Long-term use can cause the known adverse effects of systemic corticosteroids, such as hypertension, growth and developmental issues, or cushingoid features. Thus, use of the agents, particularly in children, should be limited to rare, severe conditions.[54] Concomitant and proper use of intensified skin care, particularly of topical corticosteroid and emollient use during the therapy is also of utmost importance.

Cyclosporine

Although cyclosporine is currently approved by the FDA for use in psoriasis, it has been effective in treating many skin diseases.[54] Similar to systemic corticosteroids, rebound flare-ups of atopic dermatitis are possible with cyclosporine use. Oral cyclosporine can be used on a short-term basis for severe, recalcitrant disease in adults at a dose of 5 mg/kg/day.[54,55] Children with recalcitrant disease can be started at a lower dose of 3 mg/kg/day, with caution. Tolerability in children is good, and most common adverse effects are limited to abdominal pain and headaches.[56] In one study of adults, 150 mg/day was effective compared to 300 mg/day in the short term with better renal tolerance.[57] Short courses of 5 mg/kg/day for 12 weeks also have been successful in treating atopic dermatitis.[58] Adverse effects, such as renal toxicity, have been shown to be mild and reversible in a long-term multicenter study evaluating safety for cyclosporine use in adults.[56] Even so, appropriate monitoring parameters, namely electrolytes, renal function, complete blood counts, fasting lipid profiles, and uric acid levels, should be measured at the baseline and reviewed. Cyclosporine also has a large propensity for drug–drug interactions, and careful monitoring is required.

Azathioprine

Azathioprine, a purine analog, is another systemic immunosuppressant that can be helpful in severe atopic dermatitis. The main disadvantage as compared to cyclosporine is its delayed onset of action of 4 to 6 weeks. Most of the reports of azathioprine use has been in uncontrolled, open, and retrospective trials. Thus, it is difficult to determine a dosing regimen, as no consistent regimen was evaluated. Despite the numerous adverse effects including myelosuppression, hepatotoxicity, gastrointestinal disturbances, among others, there is evidence that azathioprine can be helpful in reduction of atopic dermatitis disease activity.[54]

Antimetabolites

Mycophenolate mofetil (MMF), an immunosuppressant used in organ transplant, has demonstrated clearing of atopic dermatitis resistant to other therapies in short-term, open-label studies.[1] As dose finding and well-controlled studies are not available for MMF use in atopic dermatitis, it should be used with caution, and discontinued if the patient does not respond within 4 to 8 weeks of therapy.[1,54]

Methotrexate, an antimetabolite, is a folic acid antagonist primarily used as an antineoplastic agent and in the treatment of psoriasis. Although there are no controlled studies examining its use specifically for atopic dermatitis, there is anecdotal evidence on its effectiveness at a dosage of 2.5 mg per day given four times a week.[1,54] Because of its myelosuppressive effects, patients' hematologic parameters should be closely monitored. Other adverse effects can include hepatotoxicity, pulmonary toxicity, and gastrointestinal toxicity. Folic acid supplementation should also be instituted.

Interferon-γ

Interferon-γ, which is a known inhibitor of TH_2 cells, was considered a logical choice in suppressing the IgE responses in atopic dermatitis. Several multicenter, double-blind, placebo-controlled trials have demonstrated clinical improvement with its use in atopic dermatitis.[1,54] Interferon injections are expensive and can be associated with flulike symptoms such as fever, chills, headache, myalgia, arthralgia, nausea, vomiting, and diarrhea. Further controlled studies are warranted before its routine use for atopic dermatitis patients.

CLINICAL CONTROVERSY

Atopic dermatitis and contact dermatitis (both the irritant and allergic types) are eczematous diseases with similar pathologies. Although atopic dermatitis, unlike contact dermatitis, maintains an important genetic component, there is now evidence that these diseases may be more related to each other. Consensus currently is that atopic and acute contact dermatitis are both immune mediated, and atopic dermatitis increases one's susceptibility to irritant contact dermatitis. More investigations are needed, but understanding the possible links between atopic dermatitis and contact dermatitis can aid clinicians in understanding the pathophysiology, diagnosis, and treatment of patients who are ailing from these diseases.[59]

EVALUATION OF THERAPEUTIC OUTCOMES

The overall goal for managing patients with atopic dermatitis is to control the condition by preventing flare-ups and overall produce a better quality of life without complications. It is important for a patient with atopic dermatitis to consult with a healthcare practitioner in helping to identify and eliminate trigger factors and allergens and to communicate regarding nonpharmacologic management of the disease. All patients with atopic dermatitis should be counseled on the importance of emollient use and other measures for proper skin care.

Depending on the severity of the disease, some patients might warrant a need for low strength topical corticosteroids for maintenance use.

CONCLUSIONS

Management should include controlling "flare-ups," allergen avoidance, proper bathing and skin hydration, and control of humidity. Currently, topical corticosteroids remain as the mainstay for treatment of flare-ups associated with atopic dermatitis. But, a recent study showed that 73% of patients worried about using topical corticosteroids for fear of adverse effects. Twenty-four percent were concerned enough that they were nonadherent with the corticosteroid use.[60]

ABBREVIATIONS

ELISA: enzyme-linked immunoabsorbent assay

HLA: hypothalamic-pituitary-adrenal

IgE: immunoglobulin E

LCD: liquor carbonis detergens

MMF: mycophenolate mofetil

PUVA: photochemotherapy with oral methoxypsoralen therapy followed by UVA

SCORAD: Severity Scoring of Atopic Dermatitis

TH_2: T-helper cell type 2

UV: ultraviolet

UVA: ultraviolet A

UVB: ultraviolet B

REFERENCES

1. Leung DYM, Eichenfield LF, Boguniewicz M. Atopic dermatitis (atopic eczema). In: Freeberg IM, Eisen AZ, et al., eds. Dermatology in General Medicine, 6th ed. New York: McGraw-Hill, 2003:1464–1480.
2. Rocken M, Schallreuther K, et al. What exactly is atopy? Exp Dermatol 1998;7:97–104.
3. Leung DYM. Atopic dermatitis: New insights and opportunities for therapeutic intervention. J Allergy Clin Immunol 2000;105(5):860–876.
4. Bleiker TO, Shahidullah H, et al. The prevalence and incidence of atopic dermatitis in a birth cohort: The importance of a family history of atopy. Arch Dermatol 2000;136(2):274–275.
5. The International Study of Asthma and Allergies in Childhood (ISAAC) Steering Committee. International consensus conference on atopic dermatitis II (ICCAD II): Clinical update and current treatment strategies. Br J Dermatol 2003;148(Suppl 63):3–10.
6. Boguniewicz M, Schmid-Grendelmeier P, Leung DYM. Atopic dermatitis. J Allergy Clin Immunol 2006;118:40–43.
7. Kemp AS. Atopic eczema: Its social and financial costs. J Paediatr Child Health 1999;35(3):229–231.
8. Su JC, Kemp AS, et al. Atopic eczema: Its impact on the family and financial cost. Arch Dis Child 1997;76:159–162.
9. Reid P, Lewis-Jones MS. Sleep difficulties and their management in preschoolers with atopic eczema. Clin Exp Dermatol 1995;20:38–41.
10. Lapidus CS, Schwarz DF, et al. Atopic dermatitis in children: Who cares? Who pays? J Am Acad Dermatol 1993;28:699–703.
11. Uehara M. Kimura C. Descendant family history of atopic dermatitis. Acta Derm Venereol 1993;73:62–63.
12. Kang K. Stevens SR. Pathophysiology of atopic dermatitis. Clin Dermatol 2003;21:116–121.
13. Hanifin JM, Rajka G. Diagnostic features of atopic dermatitis. Acta Derm Venereol 1980;92:44–47.
14. Leung DYM. Pathogenesis of atopic dermatitis. J Allergy Clin Immunol 1999;104(3 Pt 2):S99-S108.
15. Werner Y, Lindberg M. Transepidermal water loss in dry and clinically normal skin in patients with atopic dermatitis. Acta Derm Venereol 1985;65:102–105.
16. Leung DY, Hanifin JM, et al. (Work Group on Atopic Dermatitis) Disease management of atopic dermatitis: a practice parameter. Ann Allergy Asthma Immunol 1997;79:197–209.
17. European Task Force on Atopic Dermatitis. Severity scoring of atopic dermatitis: the SCORAD index. Dermatology 1993;186:23–31.
18. Charman, C, Williams HC. Outcome measures of disease severity in atopic eczema. Arch Dermatol 2000;136(6):763–769.
19. Beltrani VS. The role of house dust mites and other aeroallergens in atopic dermatitis. Clin Dermatol 2003;21:177–182.
20. Guillet G, Guillet MH. Natural history of sensitizations in atopic dermatitis. Arch Dermatol 1992;128:187–192.
21. Sampson HA. The evaluation and management of food allergy in atopic dermatitis. Clin Dermatol 2003;21:183–192.
22. Sampson HA, Scanlon SM. Natural history of food hypersensitivity in children with atopic dermatitis. J Pediatr 1989;115:23–27.
23. Charman, C. Clinical evidence: Atopic eczema. BMJ 1999;318(7198):1600–1604.
24. Halken S, Host A. The lessons of noninterventional and interventional prospective studies on the development of atopic disease during childhood. Allergy 2000;55(9):793–802.
25. Gdalevich M, Mimouni D, David M, et al. Breastfeeding and the onset of AD in childhood: A systematic review and meta-analysis of prospective studies. J Am Acad Dermatol 2001;45:520.
26. Ginsburg IH, et al. Role of emotional factors in adults with dermatitis. Int J Dermatol 1993;32:656.
27. Leyden JJ, Baker DA. Localized herpes simplex infections in atopic dermatitis. Arch Dermatol 1979;115:311–312.
28. Drake LA, Dinehart SM, et al. Guidelines of care for the use of topical glucocorticosteroids. J Am Acad Dermatol 1996;35:615–619.
29. Green C, Colquitt JL, Kirby J, et al. Topical corticosteroids for atopic eczema: Clinical and cost effectiveness of once-daily versus more frequent use. Br J Dermatol 2005;152:130.
30. Klein PA, Clark RAF. An evidence-based review of the efficacy of antihistamines in relieving pruritus in atopic dermatitis. Arch Dermatol 1999;135(12):1522–1525.
31. Queille-Roussel C, Paul C, Duteil L, et al. The new topical azomycin derivative SDZ ASM 981 does not induce sin atrophy when applied to normal skin for 4 weeks: A randomized, double-blind controlled study. Br J Dermatol 2001;144:507–513.
32. Reitamo S, Rissanen C, Paul C, et al. Tacrolimus ointment does not affect collage synthesis: Results of a single-center randomized trial. J Invest Dermatol 1998;111:396–398.
33. Tomi NS, Luger TA. The treatment of atopic dermatitis with topical immunomodulators. Clin Dermatol 2003;21:215–224.
34. Stuetz A. Grassberger M. Meingassner JG. Pimecrolimus (Elidel, SDZ ASM 981): Preclinical pharmacological profile and skin selectivity. Semin Cutan Med Surg 2001;20:233–241.
35. Kapp A, Allen Br, Reitamo S. Atopic dermatitis management with tacrolimus ointment (Protopic). J Dermatolog Treat 2003;14:15–16.
36. Hanifin JM, Ling MR, Langley R, et al. Tacrolimus ointment for the treatment of atopic dermatitis in adult patients: Part I, efficacy. J Am Acad Dermatol 2001;44:S28–S30.
37. Paller A, Eichenfield LF, Leung DY, et al. A 12-week study of tacrolimus ointment for the treatment of atopic dermatitis in pediatric patients. J Am Acad Dermatol 2001;44:S47–S57.
38. Kang S, Lucky AW, Pariser D, et al. Long-term safety and efficacy of tacrolimus ointment for the treatment of atopic dermatitis in children. J Am Acad Dermatol 2001;44:S58–S64.
39. Chapman MS, Schachner LA, Breneman D, et al. Tacrolimus ointment 0.03% shows efficacy and safety in pediatric and adult patients with mild to moderate atopic dermatitis. J Am Acad Dermatol 2005;53:S177–S185.
40. Boguniewicz M, Fiedler VC, Raimer S, et al. A randomized, vehicle-controlled trial of tacrolimus ointment for treatment of atopic dermatitis in children: Pediatric tacrolimus study group. J allergy Clin Immunol 1998;102(4 Pt 1):637–644.
41. Reitamo S, Rustin M, Ruzicka T, et al. Efficacy and safety of tacrolimus ointment compared with that of hydrocortisone butyrate ointment in adult patients with atopic dermatitis. J Allergy Clin Immunol 2002;109:547–555.
42. Plosker GL, Foster RH. Tacrolimus: A further update of its pharmacology and therapeutic use in the management of organ transplantation. Drugs 2000;59:323–389.
43. Fonacier L, Sengel J, Charlesworth EN, et al. Report of the topical calcineurin inhibitors task force of the American College of Allergy, Asthma and Immunology and the American Academy of Allergy, Asthma and Immunology. J Allergy Clin Immunol 2005;115:1249–1253.
44. Kapp A, Papp K. Bingham A, et al. Long-term management of atopic dermatitis in infants with topical pimecrolimus, a nonsteroid anti-inflammatory drug. J Allergy Clin Immunol 2002;10:277–284.

45. Wahn U, Bos JD, Goodfield M, et al. Efficacy and safety of pimecrolimus cream in the long-term management of atopic dermatitis in children. Pediatrics 2002;110(Pt1):e2.
46. Boguniewicz M. Treatment options and new therapeutic approaches in atopic dermatitis. Dermatol Nurs 2003;8(Suppl):12–18.
47. Harper J, Green A, Scott G, et al. First experience of topical SDZ ASM 981 in children with atopic dermatitis. Br J Dermatol 2001;144:781–787.
48. Papp KA, Weifel T, Folster-Holst R, et al. Long-term control of atopic dermatitis with pimecrolimus cream 1% in infants and young children: A two year study. J Am Acad Dermatol 2005;52:2406.
49. Siegfried E, Korman N, Moline C, et al. Safety and efficacy of early intervention with pimecrolimus cream 1% combined with corticosteroids for major flares in infants and children with atopic dermatitis. J Dermatolog Treat 2006;17:143–150.
50. Raimer SS. Managing pediatric atopic dermatitis. Clin Pediatr (Phila) 2000;39(1):1–14.
51. George SA, et al. Narrow band (TL-O1) UVB phototherapy for chronic severe adult atopic dermatitis. Br J Dermatol 1993;128:49.
52. Krutmann J, et al. High-dose UVA1 phototherapy: a novel and highly effective approach for the treatment of acute exacerbation of atopic dermatitis. Acta Derm Venereol Suppl (Stockh)1992;176:120.
53. Morison WL, et al. Oral psoralen photochemotherapy of atopic eczema. Br J Dermatol 1978;98:25.
54. Akhavan A, Rudikoff D. The treatment of atopic dermatitis with systemic immunosuppressive agents. Clin Dermatol 2003;21:225–240.
55. Sowden JM, Berth-Jones J, Ross JS, et al. Double-blind, controlled, crossover study of cyclosporin in adults with severe refractory atopic dermatitis. Lancet 1991;338:137–140.
56. Berth-Jones J, Finlay AY, Zaki I, et al. Cyclosporine in severe childhood atopic dermatitis: A multicenter study. J Am Acad Dermatol 1996;34:1016–1021.
57. Czech W, Brautigam M, Weidnjer G, et al. A body-weight-independent dosing regimen of cyclosporine microemulsion is effective in severe atopic dermatitis and improves the quality of life. J Am Acad Dermatol 2000;42:653.
58. Harper JI, Ahmed I, Barclay G, et al. Cyclosporin for severe childhood atopic dermatitis: Short course versus continuous therapy. Br J Dermatol 2000;152:57.
59. Akhavan A, Cohen SR. The relationship between atopic dermatitis and contact dermatitis. Clin Dermatol 2003;21:158–162.
60. Charman CR, Morris AD, Williams HC. Topical corticosteroids phobia in patients with atopic eczema. Br J Dermatol 200;142(5):931–936.

SECTION 15
HEMATOLOGIC DISORDERS

CHAPTER 103

Hematopoiesis

WILLIAM P. PETROS AND MICHAEL CRAIG

KEY CONCEPTS

1. Leukocytes are subdivided into specific cell types that have important functional differences.
2. All hematopoietic cells are thought to be generated from one common type of cell (stem cell).
3. Blood concentrations of some hematopoietic cell types may not be reflective of total body content.
4. Cytokines such as colony-stimulating factors are important regulators of hematopoiesis.
5. The kinetics of hematopoietic cells vary with cell type, maturity, pathophysiology, and external stimuli.
6. Both the number of cells and other cofactors determine the clinical consequences of neutropenia or anemia.

Hematopoiesis is defined as the formation and maturation of blood cells and their derivatives. This process is important to a wide array of physiologic functions such as hemostasis, immunity, and oxygen delivery. There is a tremendous daily turnover rate of cells in this system, with more than 6 billion cells produced per kilogram of body weight every 24 hours.[1] These accelerated processes result in vastly exaggerated and rapid responses to the slightest perturbation.

In humans, hematopoiesis takes place primarily in the bone marrow. Hematopoietic cells were among the first to be evaluated for their biologic function and pattern of maturation, and identification of the protein molecules (cytokines) that regulate this system has yielded an extraordinary amount of information regarding its control. The process of continual hematopoietic cell production is complicated, involving interactions between immature cells, the surrounding microenvironment, and cytokines.

Learning objectives, review questions, and other resources can be found at **www.pharmacotherapyonline.com.**

HEMATOPOIETIC SYSTEM

The hematopoietic system consists of three primary cell components: leukocytes, platelets, and erythrocytes. The first group encompasses a functionally diverse group of cells that includes neutrophils, eosinophils, basophils, monocytes/macrophages, lymphocytes, and plasma cells. Typical concentrations of mature hematopoietic cells found in the peripheral blood of adults are shown in Table 103–1.

LEUKOCYTES

Neutrophils (Segs and Bands)

1 The major functions of neutrophils (also known as polymorphonuclear leukocytes) are to prevent pathogenic microorganism invasion and to localize and kill these microorganisms if they do invade the body. These effects are mediated by a series of events, including migration to the site (chemotaxis), recognition/attachment to the invader, phagocytosis, lysosomal fusion, degranulation, and local generation of oxidants (respiratory burst) and degrading enzymes (Fig. 103–1).[2] A neutrophil is attracted to the site of infection by chemotactic factors. Once migration to the site has occurred, the neutrophil ingests the opsonized microorganism. Opsonization is the process whereby antibody and complement coat the microorganism, allowing for increased neutrophil recognition. Following ingestion or phagocytosis, the cytoplasmic granules within the neutrophil fuse with the phagosome or phagocytosed microorganism, thereby initiating degranulation and release of enzymes. These degrading enzymes kill the microorganism through oxygen reduction. Secretion of these enzymes can also result in localized host tissue injury. The actions of cytokines such as granulocyte colony-stimulating factor (G-CSF) and granulocyte-macrophage colony-stimulating factor (GM-CSF) may intensify neutrophil activity.[3]

Eosinophils

Although eosinophils are less efficient than neutrophils, they elicit similar effector functions. Eosinophil activity is directed primarily against large invaders, such as helminths and other parasites that cannot be phagocytized. During an allergic reaction, activated mast cells secrete chemicals that attract and stimulate eosinophils, which in turn produce substances that neutralize or degrade the reaction

TABLE 103-1 Average (Normal Range) Adult Blood Cell Concentration

White cell count (cells/mm^3)		7,800 (4,400–11,300)
Red cell count ($\times 10^6/mm^3$)	Male	5.21 (4.52–5.90)
	Female	4.60 (4.10–5.10)
Hemoglobin[a] (g/dL)	Male	15.7 (14.0–17.5)
	Female	13.8 (12.3–15.3)
Hematocrit	Male	0.46 (0.42–0.50)
	Female	0.40 (0.36–0.45)
Mean corpuscular volume (fL/red cell)		88.0 (80.0–96.1)
Platelet count (cells/mm^3)		311,000 (172,000–450,000)

[a]Can be 0.5–1.0 g/dL lower in black patients.

products of mast cells. Unfortunately, the eosinophil constituents can also damage normal tissue and cause secondary histamine release. High concentrations of eosinophils for prolonged periods can result in damage to the cardiac and central nervous systems, with possible pulmonary and dermatologic involvement.[4]

Basophils and Mast Cells

Through a massive release of their granule contents on stimulation, basophils and mast cells function as mediators of inflammatory processes. The released chemicals include heparin, histamine, and other substances. The mediator can be vasoactive, bronchoconstrictive, and/or chemotactic (attractive) for eosinophils.[5,6]

Monocytes/Macrophages

Derived from the granulocyte-monocyte colony-forming unit, monocytes are peripheral cells in transit from the bone marrow to tissues. Once in the tissues, under the influence of local factors, monocytes become macrophages. Macrophages exist in the liver (Kupffer cells), spleen, lymph nodes, microglial (CNS) cells, skin (Langerhans cells), and bone (osteoclasts).

Monocytes and macrophages perform a variety of functions, including initiation of immune responses for recognition by lymphocytes, regulation of immune response intensity, phagocytosis of foreign invaders, tumor cytotoxicity, degradation of cellular debris, and secretion of peptide molecules called *monokines* (a subclassification of cytokines).[7] Examples of monokines include interferons, tumor necrosis factor, and interleukin-1 (IL-1). Monokines and other cytokines regulate the activity of these cells.

Lymphocytes

The primary functions of lymphocytes are to control and be the effector cells for the immune system. Many of these cells also are important synthetic sites for various cytokines. Lymphocytes can be functionally divided into cells that display cell-mediated immunity (T cells) and those that are responsible for humoral immunity (B cells) (Table 103–2). Several different T-cell subtypes are found in peripheral blood. These include the cytotoxic suppressor T cells (CD8), which attack intracellular pathogens and regulate the size and duration of the immune response, as well as helper T-cells (CD4). The latter cells are responsible for delayed hypersensitivity, stimulation of B-cell differentiation (maturation), and antibody production, in addition to regulation of inflammatory reactions. B lymphocytes ultimately become plasma cells, which produce immunoglobulin specific for an antigen attached to the cell's surface.

Null cells are a separate subset of lymphocytes that lack surface markers of B or T origin. These cells, also referred to as large granular

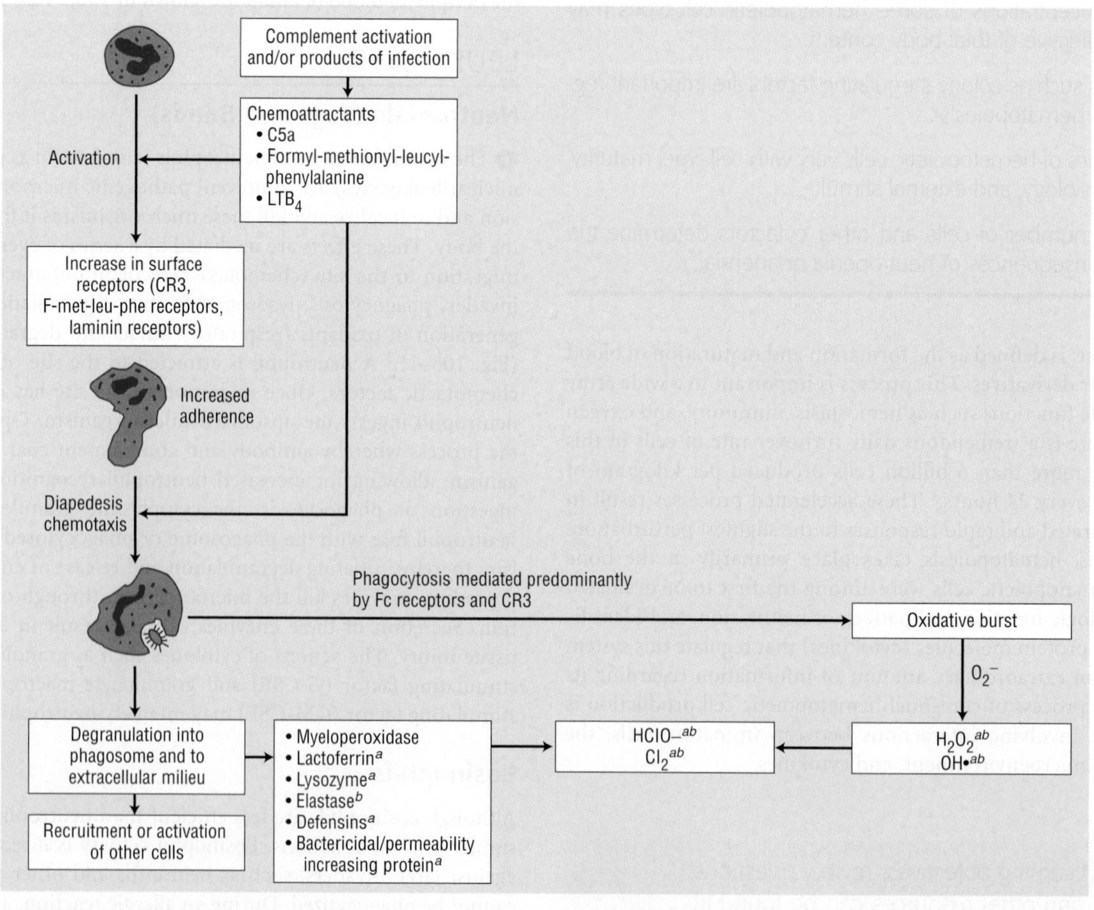

FIGURE 103-1. Neutrophil responses to infection or inflammation. [a]Microbicidal. [b]Damage to host tissues. (CR3, complement receptor type 3; C5a, complement 5a; Fc, crystallizable fragment of immunoglobulin; H_2O_2, hydrogen peroxide; LTB_4, leukotriene B4; O_2, oxygen.)

TABLE 103-2 Lymphocyte-Mediated Immune Function

Cellular immunity (T cells)
1. Provides resistance against intracellular pathogens such as viruses, protozoa, fungi, and bacteria
2. Mediates allogeneic transplant rejection and graft-versus-host disease
3. Responsible for contact dermatitis
4. Mediates adoptive immunotherapy
Humoral immunity (B cells)
1. Serves as major component of allergic reactions and other autoimmune diseases
2. Aids in eradication of encapsulated bacteria
3. Inactivates circulating toxins
4. Can play role in antitumor reactions

lymphocytes, are thought to perform functions such as direct cytotoxicity to foreign entities, and they act either alone (natural killer cells) or in concert with immunoglobulin (antibody-dependent cellular cytotoxicity).[8,9] (Further details regarding lymphocytes are found in Chap. 89.)

PLATELETS

There are several mechanisms by which platelets (thrombocytes) interact to facilitate blood coagulation. These include localization of the thrombus and provision of a specific receptor site for clotting factors, as well as the necessary phospholipid surface for the conversion of prothrombin to thrombin, and protection of thrombin from antithrombin. The process begins with a vascular injury that causes platelets to adhere to the exposed collagen fibers of the damaged wall as blood flows out. These events require the presence of other plasma proteins, namely von Willebrand factor. Platelets then aggregate through a process that is calcium dependent. Following aggregation, various platelet mediators are released (thromboxane, serotonin, and platelet factor V), resulting in the formation of an irreversible platelet aggregate with subsequent formation of a stable fibrin cross-linked clot.[10,11]

ERYTHROCYTES

The primary function of the erythrocyte is to carry oxygen from the lungs to the peripheral tissues. Its optimal design enables efficient oxygen transport via the hemoglobin molecule. The general metabolic state of the patient and local factors control oxygen release.

Some drugs selectively accumulate in erythrocytes, resulting in substantial differences when comparing blood to plasma drug concentrations. In a few instances, enzymes found in erythrocytes (e.g., aldehyde dehydrogenase) can impact on the systemic metabolism of drugs.

HEMATOPOIETIC STRUCTURE AND COMPARTMENTS

Embryonic development of hematopoietic tissue occurs in the yolk sac mesenchyme, with fetal transition occurring in the liver and spleen. Very immature hematopoietic cells can also appear in umbilical cord blood, but not many are evident in the peripheral blood of adults.[12] The ultimate location of immature hematopoietic cells is in the bone marrow. The average adult has approximately 1.7 L of bone marrow, which provides an optimal environment for the development and proliferation of hematopoietic cells.

The hematopoietic bone marrow is located primarily in the central portion of the pelvis, ribs, vertebrae, skull, and femoral and humeral epiphyses. The anatomic structure of the bone marrow is characterized by the central venous marrow sinus, which is linked by coarse vascular sinusoids that intertwine a reticulin mesh where the cells are suspended. Thus hematopoiesis occurs in the extravascular marrow spaces, which also contain endothelial cells, fibroblasts, macrophages, and adipocytes, collectively termed *bone marrow stroma*.[13] Stromal cells are thought to be important hematopoietic components, providing growth factors, collagen, and cell-adhesion proteins.[14] When these cells are combined with accessory cells (lymphocytes/monocytes) and cytokines, the mixture is referred to as the *hematopoietic microenvironment*.

Egress of more mature cells from the bone marrow occurs through the endothelial cell barrier. Release of cells such as neutrophils can be stimulated by complement, steroids, or endotoxin. Immature (progenitor) cells that can ultimately become any one of the blood cellular components can be mobilized from the bone marrow into peripheral blood by the administration of a cytotoxic chemotherapy drug (e.g., cyclophosphamide)[15] or a colony-stimulating factor (G-CSF or GM-CSF).[16] This process is commonly referred to as *priming* the bone marrow for peripheral blood progenitor or stem cell transplantation (see Chap. 142).

❷ The least mature hematopoietic cell, accounting for only a small fraction of a percentage of bone marrow cells, is referred to as the *stem cell*. Because these cells have the unique potential to ultimately become any of the mature hematopoietic cells, they are termed *pluripotent*. Importantly, they have self-renewal capacity (Fig. 103–2).[17] Extensive research has been conducted describing the morphologic and immunologic characteristics indicative of the earliest stem cell, but investigators have yet to arrive at a consensus model. Only a small percentage of these cells are likely to be dividing at any one time, and thus most are dormant in the cell cycle.

Stem cell renewal and differentiation occur within the bone marrow under the influence of the marrow microenvironment. The stromal compartment is divided into mesenchymal stem cells (producing osteoblasts, adiposities and fibroblasts); hematopoietic monocytes-macrophages/osteoclasts; and endothelial-like cells. All of these stromal cells are necessary to support stem cell proliferation and division by providing anchorage for adhesion and secreting various hematopoietic growth factors necessary for differentiation. The characteristics of the local microenvironment (cellular matrix and growth factor concentrations) influence the differentiation of a particular hematopoietic lineage, favoring it over another.

The next step in hematopoietic cell differentiation is thought to be represented by committed pluripotent stem cells that can still differentiate into any cell line (red blood cells [RBCs], white blood cells [WBCs], and platelets); however, they have a limited capacity for self-renewal (see Fig. 103–2).

Cells that differentiate can proceed to either myeloid or lymphoid cell precursors (oligopotent progenitors). These cells can ultimately become B or T lymphocytes in the case of lymphoid cells. Myeloid progenitors can become granulocytes, erythrocytes, monocytes, or megakaryocytes, as displayed in Fig. 103–2. Nomenclature for immature hematopoietic cells often uses terms developed during in-vitro experiments of cell proliferation. Thus the term *burst-forming unit* (BFU) or *colony-forming unit* (CFU) is added to the suffix of the cell lines ultimately produced by the specific cell.

Leukocytes found in the peripheral blood can generally be classified into neutrophils (the most frequently occurring blood leukocyte, subdivided into the more mature segs and less mature bands), lymphocytes, monocytes, eosinophils, basophils, and the tissue derivative of basophils, mast cells. Immature neutrophils such as metamyelocytes are rarely seen in peripheral blood. Strictly speaking, the group of cells referred to as granulocytes includes neutrophils, eosinophils, and basophils, although common use tends to include only the neutrophils. The terminally differentiated leukocytes, which are usually not seen in blood, include the macrophage or histiocyte (derived from monocytes) and plasma cells (derived from B lymphocytes).

❸ Most of the body's neutrophils and neutrophilic precursors reside in the bone marrow (approximately 9 billion cells) in contrast

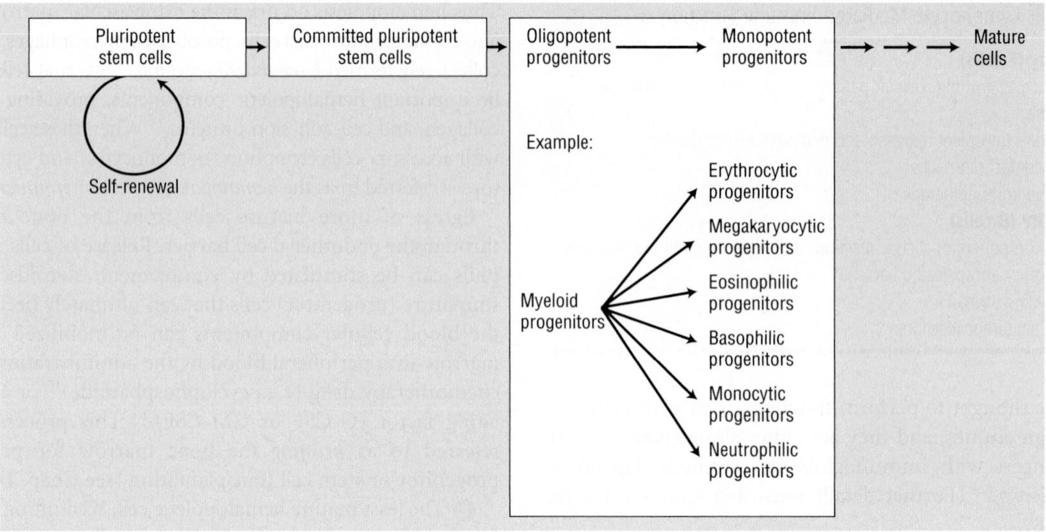

FIGURE 103-2. Rudimentary model of hematopoiesis, displaying the basic steps a cell may take from its inception as a stem cell in the bone marrow, through stages in which it can become multiple (oligopotent) or only one specific (monopotent) type of mature blood cell.

to the circulation (approximately 700 million). Similarly, only 1% of the eosinophils in the body are found in peripheral blood, whereas the skin, lungs, and gastrointestinal tract are the preferred sites of residence.[4] There is no marrow reserve pool of monocytes. Neutrophil development in the bone marrow begins with the stem cell and proceeds through intermediate precursors, such as the myeloblast, promyelocyte, myelocyte, and metamyelocyte.

Only a small fraction of the total body pool of lymphocytes resides in the blood. Immature T cells are evident in the circulation on their way to full maturation in the thymus. Mature B lymphocytes express surface immunoglobulin, which functions as an antigen receptor. Most of these cells migrate from the bone marrow to areas such as the lymph nodes (dense collections of lymphocytes, plasma cells, and macrophages that are supplied by postcapillary venules and drained by a system of efferent lymphatics) and spleen, where antigenic stimulation results in specific immunoglobulin production.[13] Approximately 75% of blood lymphocytes are T cells; 15% null cells, and 10% B cells. Various antigens expressed on the surface of leukocytes, depending on the degree of cell maturity and function, are termed clusters of differentiation (CD).

Progenitor cells that give rise to platelets are referred to as colony-forming unit megakaryocytes. Megakaryocytes account for only 0.05% to 0.02% of marrow cells. Morphologic changes in both the cytoplasm and nucleus accompany the maturation of megakaryocytes. Therefore, at differing stages of maturation, it is possible to see granules, organelles, and increasing segmentation of the nucleus. Cells in this lineage progress through three stages of development: commitment, proliferation, and differentiation, similar to that of leukocytes.[18,19] Receptors for the cytokine thrombopoietin are expressed on both megakaryocytes and platelets, as well as hematopoietic stem cells.

The term *erythron* has been used to describe collectively the erythropoietic cellular pathway, composed of all cells involved in erythropoiesis, starting with the earliest committed erythroid progenitor and ending with the mature circulating RBC. The earliest cell committed to the erythroid lineage is known as a burst-forming unit erythroid (BFU-E). Through in-vitro culture systems, one BFU-E can proliferate into several hundred progeny. These cells are followed in differentiation by the colony-forming unit erythroid (CFU-E) cell, and subsequently by the nucleated normoblast and the immediate RBC precursor, the circulating anuclear reticulocyte as outlined in Fig. 103–3. The remaining RNA is typically lost from the RBC within 2 days of its appearance in the peripheral blood; thus the mature cell does not synthesize new proteins such as enzymes.[20]

The erythrocyte precursor cell types display a continuum of changes in shape, hemoglobin concentration, Rh antigen, and erythropoietin (EPO) receptor expression with maturity. However, mature erythrocytes express significantly lower EPO receptor density than do proerythroblasts.[21]

Neonatal RBCs contain primarily fetal hemoglobin. Adult hemoglobin, 85% of which is synthesized in the erythropoietic marrow,

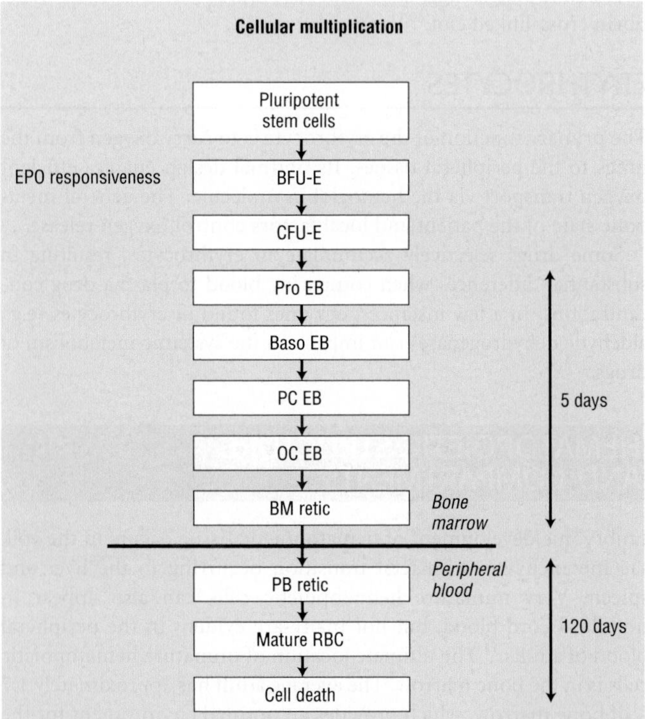

FIGURE 103-3. Proposed differentiation pattern of cells into mature erythrocytes with identification of various immature cell types. In addition, the cells that may be stimulated by the cytokine erythropoietin (EPO) are identified. (BM, bone marrow; BFU, burst-forming unit; CFU, colony-forming unit; E, erythroid; EB, erythroblast; OC, orthochromatophilic; PB, peripheral blood; PC, polychromatophilic; RBC, red blood cell; retic, reticulocyte.)

replaces the fetal hemoglobin within a few months. Heme-synthesizing cells must have mitochondria; therefore its synthesis cannot occur in the mature erythrocyte. Genetic alterations in hemoglobin structure can dramatically alter the stability or solubility of the hemoglobin and also cell confirmation. The characteristic biconcave-disk shape of the normal RBC is approximately 8 × 2 micrometers. Pathologic alterations in plasma lipids can affect the outer phospholipid membrane of the RBC, thus changing the cell's shape and survival. Blood types are characterized by the antigenic structure of the external surface of the cell membrane. The interactions of antibodies with RBC surface antigens affect the membrane function, integrity, and phagocytosis of the cells.

REGULATION OF CELL PROLIFERATION AND DIFFERENTIATION

The generic model of cell maturation presented in Fig. 103–2 includes a population of stem cells, thought to be capable of self-renewal, which provides the initial cell (committed progenitor) for subsequent maturation, differentiation (i.e., commitment to a cell line), and expansion into all blood cell types. This is followed by an initial differentiation step when a cell is produced (oligopotent progenitor) that will ultimately become one of only several mature blood cell types. Finally, monopotent progenitors are noted in which differentiation is restricted to one cell type. The latter cells then undergo a series of maturation steps, ultimately resulting in a mature cell.

STEM CELLS

4 The action of a stem cell in self-renewing rather than differentiating, and the selection of lineage by a multipotential progenitor cell during the differentiation process is thought to be a chain of stochastic (random) events. Conversely, the survival and proliferation of the subsequent progenitor cells are thought to be regulated (positively and negatively) by the group of cytokines referred to as hematopoietic growth factors (colony-stimulating factors, hematopoietins, or hematopoietic cytokines).[22] Receptors for a variety of hematopoietic growth factors are present on the surface of stem cells, which agrees with in vitro studies demonstrating stimulatory activity for cytokines such as stem cell factor (SCF), IL-1, IL-6, G-CSF, IL-10, IL-11, IL-12, IL-13, thrombopoietin, basic fibroblast growth factor, and leukemia inhibitory factor, when present in combinations. The function of hematopoietic growth factors ultimately results in regulating intracellular transcription factors, which are the driving force behind determination of the ultimate cell lineage. Whether or not the therapeutic use of a hematopoietic growth factor that is thought to act primarily on more mature cells will exhaust (deplete) the stem-cell pool over the course of multiple cycles of therapy is under active debate and study.[23] Proposed "cascades" of hematopoiesis are represented in Figs. 103–3 through 103–6. Inserted within some figures are the suspected sites in the process where hematopoietic growth factors are thought to interact by promoting the production, proliferation, and survival of hematopoietic cells. These schema are simple representations of a system of complex interactions between stimulatory and inhibitory cytokines that may not be adequately described by the in-vitro models used thus far to define them. (Details regarding the clinical pharmacology of individual hematopoietic growth factors are presented in Chap. 130.)

Immature bone marrow precursor cells such as the myeloblast (first recognizable cell of granulocytic differentiation), promyelocyte, myelocyte, and erythroblast are thought to be capable of replication. This is in contrast to most mature hematopoietic cells, which are incapable of division. Exceptions to the latter statement include monocytes, macrophages, and tissue mast cells. Evaluation of reasons for a change in hematopoietic cellular concentration over time must be conducted with a thorough knowledge of the mechanisms of both cellular production and destruction.

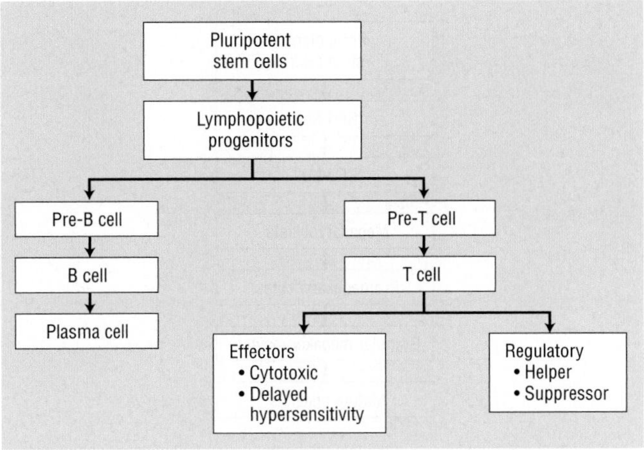

FIGURE 103-4. Pattern of lymphocyte maturation and differentiation into T and B cells. The plasma cell is a factory for antibodies, whereas the T cells have both effector and regulatory functions on the immune system.

NEUTROPHILS

Blood neutrophils are in constant exchange with an equal number of *marginated* cells. The latter are adhered to the walls of vessels in the peripheral blood, liver, lungs, and spleen. Therefore, demargination or the opposite, increased adhesion, can dramatically change the peripheral neutrophil concentration, even though cell production remains constant. A variety of stimuli can result in demargination, including infection, exercise, epinephrine, corticosteroids, and sickle cell anemia.[24] Conversely, transient neutropenia can

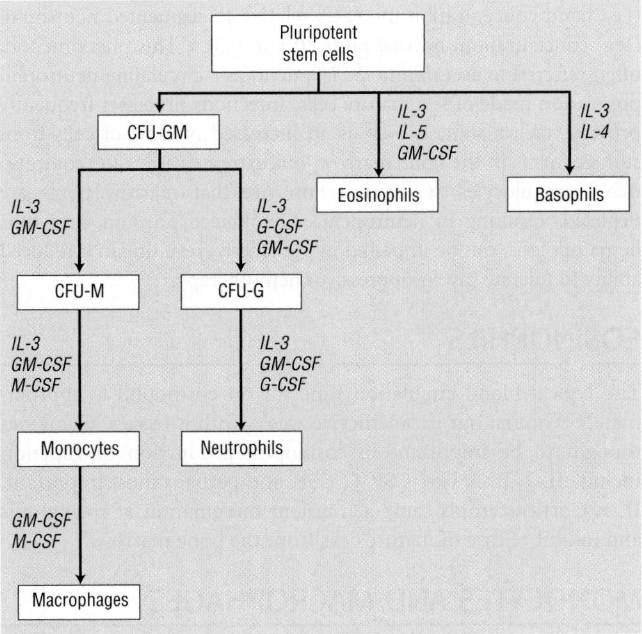

FIGURE 103-5. Maturation of precursor cells into granulocytes and macrophages, including some intermediate precursor cells (CFU-GM, -G, and -M). The hematopoietic growth factors that affect the more terminal (mature) pathways are also shown. (Hematopoietic growth factors that regulate immature cell types are not displayed.) (CFU, colony-forming unit; CSF, colony-stimulating factor; G, granulocyte; GM-CSF, granulocyte-macrophage colony-stimulating factor; IL, interleukin; M, monocyte.)

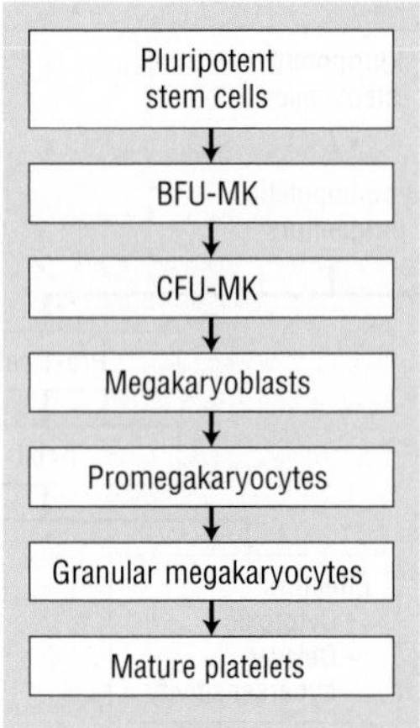

FIGURE 103-6. Maturation steps of megakaryocyte precursors prior to becoming mature platelets. (BFU, burst-forming unit; CFU, colony-forming unit; MK, megakaryocyte.)

occur through stimulation of margination by conditions such as malaria, some viral infections, and onset of hemodialysis.[25]

Normally, it takes 14 days for neutrophil production and differentiation in the bone marrow. It is believed that G-CSF, GM-CSF, and IL-3 are important regulatory molecules of neutrophil production (see Fig. 103–5). A healthy adult will produce approximately 1.6 billion neutrophils per kilogram body weight per day.[26] As blood neutrophils are totally replaced at least twice in each 24-hour period, the average circulation time for any one cell is approximately 6 to 12 hours. Most of this removal is thought to be for effector functions in the tissues and not simply an elimination process.

❺ The total number of noncirculating (i.e., storage) neutrophils is more than 15 times the number in blood. Absolute storage cell numbers are subject to alteration by prior exposure to chemotherapy or deficiency in cofactors required for their synthesis (e.g., folate). When conditions call for an acute increase in blood neutrophils, the pattern of cells thus changes to one more similar to that in the marrow (i.e., band concentration increases relative to segmented neutrophil (seg) concentration; normal ratio <0.1 to 0.3).[27] This phenomenon, often referred to as a *shift to the left*, denotes a circulating neutrophil population made of less mature cells. Infectious processes frequently provoke such a shift, as well as an increased outflow of cells from storage forms in the bone marrow, but extreme cases can require so many granulocytes at the infection site that marrow pools are depleted, resulting in neutropenia. Cytokine expression, and thus hematopoiesis, can be impaired in the elderly, resulting in a reduced ability to tolerate myelosuppressive chemotherapy.[28]

EOSINOPHILS

The typical blood circulation time for an eosinophil is approximately 6 hours, but it can survive weeks within tissues. Cytokines thought to be important in eosinophil production or function include IL-1, IL-3, GM-CSF, G-CSF, and perhaps most important, IL-5. Corticosteroids cause a transient margination of eosinophils and inhibit release of mature cells from the bone marrow.[4]

MONOCYTES AND MACROPHAGES

Both macrophages and T lymphocytes secrete cytokines that stimulate monocytopoiesis.[29] Examples of cytokines that act on relatively mature monocytes include macrophage colony-stimulating factor (M-CSF) and GM-CSF. Blood monocytes have a shorter marrow transit time than neutrophils (6 vs. 13 days, respectively), and there is no monocyte reserve in the marrow.[27] The peripheral blood turnover of these cells is much slower (circulation half-life, 3 days) than for neutrophils; similarly, tissue macrophages are thought to be very long-lived. Macrophages may be able to produce their own progeny as well as attract additional monocytes for differentiation in the local environment.

LYMPHOCYTES

Immature T cells produced in the bone marrow ultimately migrate to the thymus, where they both expand and mature into immunologically competent cells (see Fig. 103–4). A variety of cytokines, including IL-2, IL-4, and IL-7, facilitate lymphopoiesis, whereas others such as transforming growth factor-β may decelerate this process.[30] T lymphocytes are probably the longest lived hematopoietic cell, as there is experimental evidence that the life span of some is more than 10 years.

The term *lymphokine* is used to describe cytokines secreted by T cells. Lymphokines such as IL-2 are important in both activation and proliferation of the immune response, whereas monokines are also important regulators of lymphocyte development. T and B lymphocytes have important interactions with each other in both lymphocyte development and activation, which seem necessary for immunocompetence. There is some evidence for age-associated reductions in circulating helper and suppressor T cells and B cells.[31]

PLATELETS

Thrombopoiesis is the term used to describe the process of platelet production. The bone marrow manufactures 40,000 platelets/mL of blood each day. Proliferation and differentiation of platelet precursors are thought to be primarily influenced by cytokines such as IL-6, IL-11, leukemia inhibitory factor, and perhaps most specifically, by thrombopoietin (Fig. 103–6).[32,33] Other hematopoietins that may act in concert, producing synergistic effects include IL-3, IL-1, GM-CSF, EPO, and SCF.[34] The platelet survival time is a clinical test that can estimate the rate of platelet turnover.[35] In healthy individuals, this time is 9.5 ± 0.6 days.[36]

ERYTHROCYTES

The normal life span of a RBC is approximately 100 to 120 days, with a circulating cell turnover rate of 1% per day. Thus a typical adult produces approximately 200 billion reticulocytes every day. Conditions such as anemia or hypoxemia primarily stimulate the tubular interstitial cells of the renal cortex to produce EPO by interaction with the renal oxygen sensor. The degree of elevation in blood EPO concentrations is dependent on the severity of anemia or hypoxemia. This in turn recruits RBC precursors and shortens the normal time for differentiation if adequate cofactors such as iron, folate, and vitamin B_{12} are present. Although the overall time for differentiation is shortened (as is the duration of time that a reticulocyte spends in the marrow), the RBC's blood maturation time is lengthened. The increase in EPO concentrations is relatively quick (within hours), but the effects on marrow transpire over several days. The ultimate increase in RBC mass occurs at an even slower pace, generally over weeks to months (see Fig. 103–3). Multiple other endogenous cytokines are also thought to play a role in either stimulating or inhibiting erythropoiesis by acting on the early progenitors. These include GM-CSF, G-CSF, IL-1, IL-3, IL-6, IL-9, SCF, and some stromal proteins.[21]

Adequate production of RBCs for a degree of anemia is best assessed by evaluation of the number of circulating reticulocytes. Although the normal range is approximately 0.4% to 1.7% of the RBCs, this percentage would obviously be higher in anemic patients with adequate productive capacity. The calculation of a corrected reticulocyte count involves multiplying the percentage of circulating

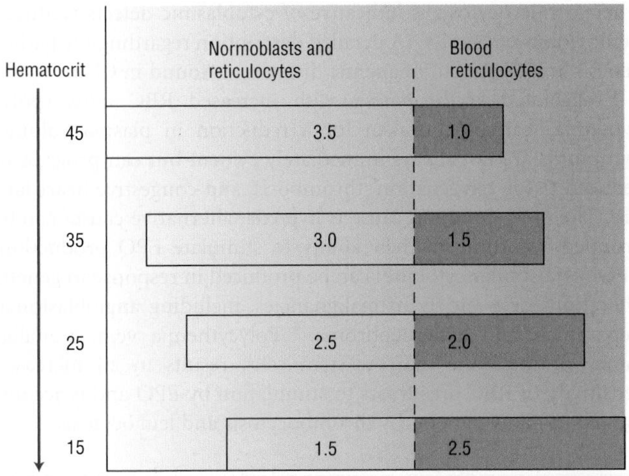

FIGURE 103-7. Correction of hematocrit with the marrow and blood reticulocyte maturation times. With a hematocrit of 45, the blood reticulocytes circulate for 1 day, whereas reduction in hematocrit to 15 results in a 2.5-day circulation time. The numbers found under the blood reticulocyte concentrations can be used as a correction factor in evaluation of reticulocyte concentrations. *(From Hillman et al.[37])*

reticulocytes by the hemoglobin concentration and dividing the result by the normal hemoglobin level expected for a healthy patient with similar characteristics. Additional correction accounts for the increased life span of reticulocytes in the peripheral blood, depending directly on the patient's degree of anemia. Figure 103–7 displays correction factors that can be used to accommodate these changes.[37]

Direct assessment of erythropoiesis in the bone marrow can be performed by estimating the myeloid-to-erythroid cell ratio from a marrow aspirate. The range of the normal adult ratio is 3:1 to 5:1, but changes in erythroid or myeloid production can obviously influence the ratio. RBCs lose flexibility with age and eventually undergo lysis or are phagocytized and removed by the monocyte-macrophage system (primarily via the spleen). Accelerated red cell destruction can be grossly quantitated by determining increases in plasma concentrations of bilirubin and lactate dehydrogenase.[37]

Although clinical laboratories measure RBC concentrations with excellent accuracy, the most useful tool for assessment of the blood's oxygen-carrying capacity is the hemoglobin concentration because of the variability in RBC size. The average RBC and hemoglobin concentrations in healthy adult male and female patients are approximately 5.21 and $4.60 \times 10^6/mm^3$, respectively; and 15.7 and 13.8 g/dL, respectively. Variations in normal concentrations will also be evident, depending on age, menstruation status, race, environmental factors, and pregnancy.[38]

DISEASE-ASSOCIATED HEMATOPOIETIC CHANGES

NEUTROPHILS

❻ The usual definition of neutropenia is an absolute neutrophil count below 1,800 cells/mm^3 in white patients, 1,400 cells/mm^3 in black patients, and 1,500 cells/mm^3 for children 1 month to 10 years old. Clinical manifestations of neutropenia (i.e., infection) are not typically evident without other cofactors until the concentration decreases below 1,000 cells/mm^3.[39] Accompanying factors that can influence the risk of infection for a particular patient include skin and mucous membrane integrity; vascular tissue supply; nutritional status; and lymphopenia, monopenia, or hypogammaglobulinemia. Persistent agranulocytosis (<500 cells/mm^3 or no measurable neutrophils) is almost uniformly fatal without the use of supportive antibiotics.

Disorders resulting in defective granulopoiesis can be subdivided into those that result in marrow aplasia or diseases that replace the normal neutrophilic component (see Chap. 107 for drug-induced neutropenia). Diseases associated with granulopoietic suppression include viral infection, tuberculosis, anorexia, autoimmune diseases (e.g., systemic lupus erythematosus), Felty syndrome (rheumatoid arthritis, splenomegaly, and leukopenia), aplastic anemia, myelodysplastic syndromes, and leukemias.[39,40] A congenital form of severely defective neutrophil production (Kostmann syndrome) has been described that is possibly a result of defective regulation of the late-acting hemopoietin G-CSF.[41] Patients with the rare disorder of cyclic neutropenia display periodic wide fluctuations in the WBCs at approximately 3-week intervals that last for 3 to 6 days. Other forms of chronic neutropenias can occur with adequate marrow stores and can be relatively benign in symptomatology.

Neutrophilia is typically defined as an absolute neutrophil count greater than 7,500 cells/mm^3 of blood and is sometimes referred to as a leukemoid reaction, if extreme.[24] Acute neutrophilia can be a result of emotional or physical stimuli (e.g., exercise, seizures, labor, pain, or temperature changes), infections, inflammation or tissue necrosis, or drugs or toxins (e.g., CSFs, epinephrine, corticosteroids, lithium, vaccines, or endotoxin). Chronic causes of increased neutrophilia include persistent infections, inflammation, malignancies, drugs, metabolic or endocrine disorders, cigarette smoking, hereditary or congenital abnormalities, and myeloproliferative diseases such as polycythemia vera.[24]

EOSINOPHILS

Eosinophilia (absolute count greater than 700 cells/mm^3) can result from neoplastic processes, parasitic or fungal infections, gastrointestinal disorders, malignancies, dermatitis, granulomatous disorders (e.g., sarcoidosis or Wegener granulomatosis), or collagen-vascular diseases in addition to the more typical cause, allergic reactions.[42] One mechanism that may be common to several of these etiologic factors is antigenic stimulation of T cells, which produces a cytokine (IL-5) that mediates eosinophil proliferation.[43] Infections can cause eosinopenia; however, its significance is not thought to be of concern in that setting.

BASOPHILS

Basophilia occurs frequently in patients with myeloproliferative disorders and in association with inflammatory reactions and diseases. Viral infections, iron deficiency, or lung cancer can sometimes increase basophil counts. Mastocytosis is usually evident only on analysis of tissue or bone marrow mast cells. Causes include hypersensitivity reactions, malignancy, osteoporosis, and chronic liver or renal disease.

MONOCYTES

Monocytosis (>800 cells/mm^3 of blood) occurs with some infections (e.g., tuberculosis, histoplasmosis, toxoplasmosis, bacterial endocarditis, and salmonellosis), collagen vascular diseases (rheumatoid arthritis and systematic lupus erythematosus), gastrointestinal disorders (ulcerative colitis and alcoholic liver disease), leukemias, and up to 60% of nonhematologic malignancies, whereas abnormally low monocyte concentrations occur in patients with hairy cell leukemia or aplastic anemia.[44]

LYMPHOCYTES

Significant reductions in lymphocyte concentration (<1,000 cells/mm^3 of blood) can be evident without apparent cause or in a variety of diseases, including acute inflammatory disorders, severe uremia, immune deficiency diseases such as systemic lupus erythematosus, chronic infections such as tuberculosis or human immunodeficiency virus (HIV) infection, malignancies, and connective tissue diseases.[45] Lymphocytosis (>4,000 cells/mm^3) can occur with mononucleosis, pertussis, measles, or chickenpox, and in lymphoid malignancies. A progressive increase in mature lymphocytes can be indicative of chronic lymphocytic leukemia. Increased levels of atypical lymphocytes can occur in patients with infections (e.g., mononucleosis, hepatitis, or cytomegalovirus), allergic reactions, or lymphomas.[46]

PLATELETS

Both qualitative and quantitative platelet disorders have important pathophysiologic consequences. Thrombocytopenia, defined as a platelet count less than 150,000 cells/mm^3, can result from a defect in production, increased sequestration, or accelerated destruction.[47]

Certain stimuli can damage the marrow by reducing the number of megakaryocytes available. Drugs, chemicals, radiation, and infection are among the potential causes of marrow injury. Diseases that produce general bone marrow failure or those that invade the bone marrow can result in thrombocytopenia. Examples of the latter include cancers such as leukemia, lymphoma, myelofibrosis, myelodysplasia, and metastatic solid tumors (breast and prostate cancer), and infections such as those caused by mycobacteria. Suboptimal platelet production can also result from defects in maturation seen with vitamin B_{12} and/or folate deficiency or in congenital syndromes.[48] Alteration in platelet distribution can also result in thrombocytopenia. Splenomegaly is the most frequent cause of increased platelet sequestration.

Idiopathic thrombocytopenic purpura (ITP) is associated with accelerated destruction of platelets and is a common cause of thrombocytopenia. Antiplatelet antibodies combine with platelets in ITP, thus sensitizing them to removal by the immune system. Accelerated platelet destruction can also occur in patients with connective tissue disorders. Approximately 14% of patients with systemic lupus erythematosus experience thrombocytopenia similar to ITP.

Most patients with essential thrombocythemia (450,000 to >1,000,000 cells/mm^3) are initially asymptomatic and diagnosed by the laboratory finding. The high platelet concentration is thought secondary to enhanced destruction. Patients can experience thromboembolic episodes and hemorrhage. The mechanisms mediating these effects are not well understood, but they are observed more frequent in the elderly or in those with platelet concentrations >1,000,000 cells/mm^3.

ERYTHROCYTES

Anemia has been typically defined by data reported from the World Health Organization as follows: men with hemoglobin <13 gm/dL or women with values of <12 gm/dL. The clinical accuracy of these values have been recently challenged.[49] Commonly encountered factors which can significantly impact on what one would consider a "normal" hemoglobin concentration include: race, age, home altitude, and smoking status.

Suboptimal erythropoiesis can be classified by changes in the size of RBCs noted on examination of the peripheral blood. Because the excretory and endocrine functions of the kidney usually mirror each other, renal dysfunction can lead to anemia by reduction in EPO production, resulting in a normochromic, normocytic pattern. Other causes of insufficient erythropoiesis include replacement of bone marrow by fibrosis, solid tumors, or leukemia, as well as defects in erythroid maturation. Relative deficiencies in the cofactors required for heme-RBC synthesis such as iron, folate, and vitamin B_{12} can also be important contributors. Structurally, RBC macrocytosis denotes defects in the maturation of the nucleus, whereas microcytosis is indicative of cytoplasmic defects (reduced hemoglobin synthesis). (A detailed description regarding the pathogenesis and treatment of anemic disorders is found in Chap. 104.)

Exaggerated erythropoiesis with increased RBC mass (polycythemia) can be mistaken for a reduction in plasma volume. Symptoms are not always immediately evident but can progress to reduced tissue oxygenation, thrombosis, and congestive heart failure. The most common cause is hypoxia; alternative causes can be grouped according to their ability to stimulate EPO production. EPO (or a similar cytokine) can be produced in response to genetic alterations or a variety of malignancies, including angioblastoma, hepatomas, and hypernephroma.[50] Polycythemia vera, a malignancy of the bone marrow stem cells, results in an increased sensitivity of RBC precursors to stimulation by EPO and is accompanied in many patients by thrombocytosis and leukocytosis.

CLINICAL USES OF HEMATOPOIETIC CELLS

HEMATOPOIETIC STEM CELL TRANSPLANTATION

High-dose chemotherapy with or without irradiation is beneficial in the treatment of a number of malignant diseases (see Chap. 142). The dose of chemotherapy that can be administered, however, is limited by hematopoietic toxicity that can result in prolonged periods of pancytopenia with the attendant risks of serious infection and bleeding. The infusion (transplantation) of hematopoietic stem cells following the high-dose therapy can overcome this hematopoietic toxicity, resulting in subsequent repopulation of the bone marrow and recovery of hematopoiesis. Hematopoietic stem cell transplantation (HSCT) involves the collection of hematopoietic stem cells from the donor, administration of intensive doses of chemotherapy (with or without irradiation) to the recipient, and infusion of the donor stem cells to the recipient. If the donor and recipient are the same individual (i.e., the patient serves as his or her own donor), the procedure is termed *autologous* HSCT. If the stem cells come from another individual, the procedure is termed *allogeneic* HSCT. Most allogeneic donors are human leukocyte antigen (HLA)-matched siblings, but the use of alternative donors such as HLA-matched unrelated donors or umbilical cord blood cells is increasing.

Allogeneic transplantation is complicated by the immune recognition of host tissues by donor T lymphocytes, resulting in a syndrome called graft-versus-host disease (GVHD). Because immune recognition of tumor cells also occurs (graft-versus-tumor effect), the relapse rates associated with allogeneic transplants are lower than those associated with autologous transplants for similar disease stages. Allogeneic transplantation is commonly used for diseases primarily involving the bone marrow, such as acute and chronic leukemias, aplastic anemia, thalassemia, and severe combined immunodeficiency syndrome.

Autologous transplantation is commonly used in non-Hodgkin lymphoma, Hodgkin lymphoma, multiple myeloma, and a relatively small subset of patients with solid tumors. A number of laboratory techniques are evolving to allow the bone marrow harvested for autologous transplantation to expand in the laboratory prior to infusion and to cleanse the marrow of potential malignant cell contamination.

Small numbers of hematopoietic progenitor (stem) cells capable of reconstituting hematopoiesis circulate in the blood under normal circumstances.[51] Commonly referred to as peripheral blood progenitor cells (PBPCs), these circulating progenitor cells increase in number during recovery from myelosuppressive chemotherapy or after treatment with cytokines such as G-CSF or GM-CSF.[16,52] These cells can be collected by a process called leukapheresis and stored for intravenous reinfusion following high-dose chemotherapy. Intravenous reinfusion is feasible because cell "homing" is facilitated through cytokines, chemokines, adhesion molecules, and integrins. Hematopoietic recovery is generally more rapid following rescue with PBPCs as compared with rescue with bone marrow. Potential tumor cell contamination can also be less with PBPC transplants. The use of PBPCs has essentially replaced the use of autologous and allogeneic bone marrow.

Cytokine-mobilized PBPC transplants from allogeneic donors have been shown to result in more rapid white cell and platelet engraftment and shorter hospital stays than bone marrow transplants.[53] The incidence of acute GVHD is not increased, but there is a significant increase in the incidence of chronic GVHD with PBPC transplants. Relapse rates and overall survival rates are similar with the use of allogeneic PBPC or bone marrow.

Only approximately one-third of patients who would otherwise be eligible for allogeneic bone marrow transplantation (BMT) have HLA-matched related donors. One alternative is the use of closely HLA-matched, unrelated donor marrow. The National Marrow Donor Program (NMDP) is a registry of volunteer marrow donors. By coordinating the activities of a network of donor, collection, and transplant centers, the NMDP facilitates the identification of potential donors and the procurement of marrow. Unrelated donor marrow transplants are associated with an increased risk of GVHD as compared to related donor transplants, but recent advances in tissue typing and donor matching and GVHD prophylaxis have resulted in comparable overall survival rates for many diseases.

Grafts of PBPCs from unrelated donors are also increasingly used for transplantation. The cells are collected by leukapheresis after mobilization of PBPCs by giving the donor G-CSF. This spares the donor from potential complications related to general or spinal anesthesia and pain associated with bone marrow harvest. Unrelated PBPC transplants are associated with more rapid engraftment as compared to unrelated BMT, with no increase in GVHD or relapse rates.[54]

Many patients do not have HLA-matched family members or unrelated donors in the marrow registries. An alternative for these patients is the use of human umbilical cord blood, which contains hematopoietic stem cells capable of reconstituting bone marrow function following high-dose chemotherapy.[55] An almost unlimited number of cord blood donors is potentially available, because the cord and its associated blood are commonly discarded following delivery. There are cord blood banks in which cord blood cells are HLA-typed, cryopreserved, and made available for transplantation for appropriate recipients. The majority of early cord blood progenitor cell transplantations were performed in children because of the relatively small number of cells available from a cord blood unit, although the number of cord blood transplantations performed in adults is increasing.[56] A major problem with cord blood transplants is a more prolonged period of neutropenia (often greater than 1 month.) This leads to additional infectious complications and associated morbidity. Laboratory methods to expand the number of progenitor cells in cord blood units are under investigation. Cord blood transplants are thought to lead to less GVHD than transplants from matched unrelated donors with similar degrees of matching, and they might prove to be an important source of progenitor cells for transplantation in the near future.

The application of allogeneic transplantation has been limited to younger patients without comorbid conditions secondary to the toxicity of the myeloablative preparative regimen and the allogeneic bone marrow or PBPC graft. Recently, a number of centers have reported successful allogeneic engraftment following nonmyeloablative, immunosuppressive conditioning regimens.[57,58] The goal of this approach is to establish donor hematopoiesis and a graft-versus-tumor effect while minimizing toxicity. These transplants can be offered to older patients and to patients with diminished end-organ function. This approach has also been used for patients with disorders that might be responsive to immune-based therapy, such as renal cell carcinoma.

ADOPTIVE IMMUNOTHERAPY

Experiments involving the administration of immune system cells for the purpose of cancer treatment (adoptive immunotherapy) have been conducted for well over a decade; however, the clinical benefit has only recently been substantiated. As described earlier, nonspecific, total depletion of donor T cells following high-dose chemotherapy and stem-cell reinfusion produces fewer graft-versus-host effects, but attenuated anticancer responses. However, it has been shown that careful attention to the T-cell dose and timing of infusion can maximize the potential for beneficial immunologic responses and minimize graft-versus-host effects. It has been found that the administration of allogeneic donor lymphocyte infusions to patients with leukemia relapse following myeloablative stem cell transplantation has anticancer efficacy in diseases such as chronic myelogenous leukemia (65% complete response), acute nonlymphocytic leukemia, or myelodysplastic syndrome (25% complete response).[59] Some of these remissions have prolonged durability. Similar strategies have been used in nonmyeloablative stem cell transplantation. The complications of donor lymphocyte infusions include the obvious risk of GVHD, but the condition does not develop in all patients who have clinical benefit. This mode of therapy can also result in marrow aplasia for approximately 20% of patients, but it is self-limiting or treatable with G-CSF in most cases.

TRANSFUSION AND BLOOD PRODUCT SUPPORT

Advances in blood banking and transfusion support have been critical to the improved outcome of therapy for patients with hematologic and malignant diseases. Platelet transfusions are indicated for the prevention and treatment of bleeding. In general, prophylactic platelet transfusions are not indicated for platelet counts above 10,000 cells/mm^3 unless the patient is febrile or actively bleeding. Platelets are available as pooled random donor concentrates obtained from RBC donations (six to eight donors per transfusion) or single-donor platelets collected by apheresis.

Administration of multiple platelet transfusions increases the risk of developing a platelet-refractory state termed *alloimmunization*. This effect is thought to be an immune-mediated reaction to HLA antigens on donor platelets or WBC contaminants. A common method of identifying such patients is evaluation of platelet counts within an hour of transfusion. For example, a 1-m^2 person should obtain an increase in platelet concentration between 7,000 and 11,000 cells/mm^3 for each unit of platelet concentrate administered (in the absence of other risk factors such as infection, splenomegaly, etc.). The diagnosis can be confirmed by in-vitro demonstration of platelet antibodies. The use of leukocyte filters prior to storage of donated platelets or ultraviolet (UV) irradiation of the product has been shown to decrease the development of alloimmunization and refractoriness to platelet transfusions. Leukocyte filters also decrease the risk of transmission of cytomegalovirus and febrile transfusion reactions. Treatment of alloimmunized patients often entails use of platelets obtained from single donors (to lessen exposure to HLA), or use of HLA-compatible or platelet cross-match–compatible donors. Unfortunately, such approaches are not always effective and additional therapies (plasma exchange or intravenous immunoglobulin) have been added with some limited success.

Packed RBC transfusions are indicated to keep hemoglobin levels above 7 to 8 g/dL to maintain adequate oxygen-carrying capacity. Each unit of packed RBCs should increase the hemoglobin level by approximately 1 g/dL unless active blood loss is evident. RBCs should also be filtered to reduce the risk of nonhemolytic, febrile transfusion reactions. Patients who are candidates for HSCT should receive blood products that have been irradiated with 2,500 cGy to prevent transfusion-associated GVHD.

Fresh frozen plasma (within 6 hours of collection) contains the components of the coagulation system and is indicated for the replacement of deficient coagulation factors II, V, VII, X, XI, and XIII. A unit of fresh frozen plasma has a volume of about 250 mL. Factor VIII and IX deficiencies are treated with specific factor concentrates. Fresh frozen plasma is also used for the rapid reversal of warfarin anticoagulation and in the treatment of disseminated intravascular coagulation. Thrombotic thrombocytopenic purpura is treated by means of therapeutic plasma exchange with fresh frozen plasma as the replacement fluid. Frequent, but inappropriate indications for fresh frozen plasma include: immunodeficiency, burns, wound healing, and volume expansion. Cryoprecipitate, which contains factor VIII, von Willebrand factor, and fibrinogen, is indicated for the treatment of von Willebrand disease that does not respond to desmopressin acetate and for fibrinogen replacement (see Chap. 105).

INTRAVENOUS IMMUNOGLOBULIN

Pharmaceutical products containing immunoglobulin for intravenous use in humans are pooled from blood collection in more than 1,000 donors for each lot of drug. The high number of donors provides a wide diversity in the capability of the antibodies to react with antigenic targets. Products are similar in content of each immunoglobulin G (IgG) subclass, but the titers against specific antigens vary between manufacturers (as do other pharmaceutical characteristics, such as osmolarity).

CLINICAL CONTROVERSIES

Intravenous immunoglobulin products vary by the number of donors used to produce the product, titers for specific antigens, and methods used for purification. Products are often marketed and selected based on these criteria; however, the clinical relevance of each is unclear.

The IV administration of immunoglobulin has been used in a variety of hematologic disorders, but for most of these situations, it is still considered experimental or indicated only when other therapeutic options have been exhausted. Patients with deficient immunoglobulin production (e.g., agammaglobulinemia or hypogammaglobulinemia) or function (e.g., chronic lymphocytic leukemia, multiple myeloma, and children with HIV) can benefit from this therapy, with the goal of increasing the IgG level such that there is less chance for bacterial infection (>500 mg/dL). This approach has other pharmacologic properties as well, including blockade of crystallizable fragment (Fc) of immunoglobulin receptors, modification of complement activation, and modulation of the immune response by anti-idiotypic antibodies.[60] It is also beneficial for patients with ITP who are at high bleeding risk or need higher platelet counts prior to surgery.[61,62] Posttransplant prophylaxis (approximately 3 months) with Ig given IV is also sometimes used in patients receiving allogeneic HSCT for prevention of bacterial sepsis and acute GVHD. The IV treatment with Ig can benefit patients whose platelet counts do not increase substantially despite transfusions, owing to the formation of alloantibodies.

A number of immunoglobulin products are available that provide more specific immunity toward selected antigens. These pharmaceuticals are generated from individuals who have been exposed to the antigen and thus developed antibody "titers" more specific to the infectious agent. Products include antithymocyte globulin, botulism immunoglobulin, cytomegalovirus immunoglobulin, hepatitis B immunoglobulin, rabies immunoglobulin, respiratory syncytial virus immunoglobulin, tetanus immunoglobulin, Rh(D) immunoglobulin, and varicella-zoster immunoglobulin.

ABBREVIATIONS

BFU: burst-forming unit
BFU-E: burst-forming unit erythroid
BMT: bone marrow transplantation
CD: cluster of differentiation
CFU: colony-forming unit
CFU-E: colony-forming unit erythroid
CSF: colony-stimulating factor
EPO: erythropoietin
Fc: crystallizable fragment
G-CSF: granulocyte colony-stimulating factor
GM-CSF: granulocyte-macrophage colony-stimulating factor
GVHD: graft-versus-host disease
HIV: human immunodeficiency virus
HLA: human leukocyte antigen
HSCT: hematopoietic stem cell transplantation
IL: interleukin
ITP: idiopathic thrombocytopenic purpura
M-CSF: macrophage colony-stimulating factor
NMDP: National Marrow Donor Program
PBPC: peripheral blood progenitor cell
RBC: red blood cell
SCF: stem cell factor
Seg: segmented neutrophil
UV: ultraviolet
WBC: white blood cells

REFERENCES

1. Abboud EN, Lichtman MA. Structure of the marrow and the hematopoietic microenvironment. In: Beutler E, Lichtman MA, Coller BS, et al., eds. Williams Hematology, 6th ed. New York: McGraw-Hill, 2001:29.
2. Lehrer RI, Ganz T, Selsted ME, et al. Neutrophils in human diseases. N Engl J Med 1987;317:687–694.
3. Lieschke GJ, Burgess AW. Granulocyte colony-stimulating factor and granulocyte-macrophage colony-stimulating factor. N Engl J Med 1992; 327:28–35.
4. Weller PF. The immunobiology of eosinophils. N Engl J Med 1991; 324:1110–1118.
5. Kitamura Y, Kasugai T, Arizono N, Matsuda H. Development of mast cells and basophils: Processes and regulation mechanisms. Am J Med Sci 1993;306:185–191.
6. Bainton DF. Morphology of neutrophils, eosinophils and basophils. In: Beutler E, Lichtman MA, Coller BS, et al., eds. Williams Hematology, 6th ed. New York: McGraw-Hill, 2001:729.
7. Johnston RB. Monocytes and macrophages. N Engl J Med 1988;318:747–752.

8. Kipps TJ. Functions of B lymphocytes and plasma cells in immunoglobulin production. In: Beutler E, Lichtman MA, Coller BS, et al., eds. Williams Hematology, 6th ed. New York: McGraw-Hill, 2001:937.
9. Kipps TJ. Functions of T lymphocytes: T-cell receptors for antigen. In: Beutler E, Lichtman MA, Coller BS, et al., eds. Williams Hematology, 6th ed. New York: McGraw-Hill, 2001:949.
10. Thompson AR, Harker LA. Manual of Hemostasis and Thrombosis, 3rd ed. Philadelphia, PA: FA Davis, 1983:47.
11. Mustard JF, Packham MA, Kinlough-Rathbone RL. Platelets, blood flow, and the vessel wall. Circulation 1990;81(Suppl 1):I40–I41.
12. Gordon MY. Physiological mechanisms in BMT and haematopoiesis—revisited. Bone Marrow Transplant 1993;11:193–197.
13. Verfaillie CM. Anatomy and physiology of hematopoiesis. In: Hoffman R, Benz EJ, Shattil SJ, et al., eds. Hematology—Basic Principles and Practice. New York: Churchill Livingstone, 2000:139.
14. Greenberger J. The hematopoietic microenvironment. Crit Rev Oncol Hematol 1991;11:65–84.
15. To LB, Shepperd KM, Haylock DN, et al. Single high doses of cyclophosphamide enable the collection of high numbers of hematopoietic stem cells from the peripheral blood. Exp Hematol 1990;18: 442–447.
16. Peters WP, Rosner G, Ross M, et al. Comparative effects of granulocyte-macrophage colony-stimulating factor (GM-CSF) and granulocyte colony-stimulating (G-CSF) factor on priming peripheral blood progenitor cells for use with autologous bone marrow after high-dose chemotherapy. Blood 1993;81:1709–1719.
17. Spangrude GJ, Heimfeld S, Wessman IL. Purification and characterization of mouse hematopoietic stem cells. Science 1988;241:58–62.
18. Williams N, Levine RF. The origin, development, and regulation of megakaryocytes. Br J Haematol 1982;52:173–180.
19. Hoffman R. Regulation of megakaryocytopoiesis. Blood 1989;74:1196–1212.
20. Papayannopoulou T, Abkowitz J, D'Andrea A. Biology of erythropoiesis, erythroid differentiation, and maturation. In: Hoffman R, Benz EJ, Shattil SJ, et al., eds. Hematology—Basic Principles and Practice. New York: Churchill Livingstone, 2000:202.
21. McGuire MJ, Spivak JL. Erythropoiesis. In: Anderson KC, Ness PM, eds. Scientific Basis of Transfusion Medicine—Implications for Clinical Practice. Philadelphia, PA: WB Saunders, 1994:1.
22. Ogawa M. Differentiation and proliferation of hematopoietic stem cells. Blood 1993;81:2844–2853.
23. Moore MAS. Does stem cell exhaustion result from combining hematopoietic growth factors with chemotherapy? If so, how do we prevent it? Blood 1992;80:3–7.
24. Dale DC. Neutrophilia and neutrophilia. In: Beutler E, Lichtman MA, Coller BS, et al., eds. Williams Hematology, 6th ed. New York: McGraw-Hill, 2001:823.
25. Coates T, Baehner R. Leukocytosis and leukopenia. In: Hoffman R, Benz EJ, Shattil SJ, et al., eds. Hematology—Basic Principles and Practice. New York: Churchill Livingstone, 1991:552.
26. Gabrilove J. Granulopoiesis. In: Anderson KC, Ness PM, eds. Scientific Basis of Transfusion Medicine—Implications for Clinical Practice. Philadelphia, PA: WB Saunders, 1994:17.
27. Rosenthal DS. Hematologic manifestations of infectious disease. In: Hoffman R, Benz EJ, Shattil SJ, et al., eds. Hematology—Basic Principles and Practice. New York: Churchill Livingstone, 1991:2420.
28. Rothstein G. Hematopoiesis in the aged: A model of hematopoietic dysregulation? Blood 1993;82:2601–2604.
29. Bagby GC, Heinrich MC. Growth factors, cytokines, and the control of hematopoiesis. In: Hoffman R, Benz EJ, Shattil SJ, et al., eds. Hematology—Basic Principles and Practice. New York: Churchill Livingstone, 2001:154.
30. Jordan SC. Cytokines and lymphocytes. In: Kunkel SL, Remick DG, eds. Cytokines in Health and Disease. New York: Marcel Dekker, 1992:309.
31. Yamashiki M, Nishimura A, Kosaka Y, James SP. Two-color analysis of peripheral lymphocyte surface antigens in inherently healthy adults. J Clin Lab Anal 1994;8:22–26.
32. Du XX, Williams DA. Interleukin-11: A multifunctional growth factor derived from the hematopoietic microenvironment. Blood 1994;83: 2023–2030.
33. Metcalf D. Thrombopoietin—At last. Nature 1994;369:519–520.
34. Gordon MS, Hoffman R. Growth factors affecting human thrombocytopoiesis: Potential agents for the treatment of thrombocytopenia. Blood 1992;80:302–307.
35. Shulman NR, Jordan JV Jr. Platelet kinetics. In: Colman RW, Hirsh J, Marder VJ, Saltzman EW, eds. Hemostasis and Thrombosis. Basic Principles and Clinical Practice, 2nd ed. Philadelphia, PA: JP Lippincott, 1987:341–351.
36. Harker LA, Finch CA. Thrombokinetics in man. J Clin Invest 1969;48:963–974.
37. Hillman RS, Finch CA. Red Cell Manual. Philadelphia, PA: FA Davis, 1996:59.
38. Glassman AB. Anemia: Diagnosis and clinical considerations. In: Harmening DM, ed. Clinical Hematology and Fundamentals of Hemostasis, 2nd ed. Philadelphia, PA: FA Davis, 1992:54.
39. Lichtman MA. Classification and clinical manifestations of neutrophil disorders. In: Beutler E, Lichtman MA, Coller BS, et al., eds. Williams Hematology, 6th ed. New York: McGraw-Hill, 2001:817.
40. Malech HL, Gallin JI. Neutrophils in human disease. N Engl J Med 1987;317:687–694.
41. Dong F, Hoefsloot LH, Schelen AM, et al. Identification of a nonsense mutation in the G-CSF receptor in severe congenital neutropenia. Proc Natl Acad Sci U S A 1994;91:4480–4484.
42. Wardlaw AJ, Kay AB. Eosinophils and their disorders. In: Beutler E, Lichtman MA, Coller BS, et al., eds. Williams Hematology, 6th ed. New York: McGraw-Hill, 2001:785.
43. Sanderson CJ. Interleukin-5 eosinophils and disease. Blood 1992;79:3101–3109.
44. Lichtman MA. Classification and clinical manifestations of disorders of monocytes and macrophages. In: Beutler E, Lichtman MA, Coller BS, et al., eds. Williams Hematology, 6th ed. New York: McGraw-Hill, 2001:877.
45. Williams WJ. Lymphocytosis and lymphocytopenia. In: Beutler E, Lichtman MA, Coller BS, et al., eds. Williams Hematology, 6th ed. New York: McGraw-Hill, 2001:969.
46. Gay JC, Athens JW. Variations of leukocytes in disease. In: Lee GR, Foerster J, Lukens J, et al., eds. Wintrobe's Clinical Hematology, 10th ed. Baltimore, MD: Williams & Wilkins, 1999:1836.
47. Rutherford CJ, Frenkel EP. Thrombocytopenia: Issues in diagnosis and therapy. Med Clin North Am 1994;78:555–575.
48. Seligsohn U, Coller BS. Classification, clinical manifestations, and evaluation of disorders of hemostasis. In: Beutler E, Lichtman MA, Coller BS, et al., eds. Williams Hematology, 6th ed. New York: McGraw-Hill, 2001:1471.
49. Beutler E & Waalen J. The definition of anemia: What is the lower limit of normal of the blood hemoglobin concentration? Blood 2006;107:1747–1750.
50. Tabbara IA. Erythropoietin biology and clinical applications. Arch Intern Med 1993;153:298–304.
51. Kessinger A, Armitage JO, Landmark JD, et al. Autologous peripheral hematopoietic stem cell transplantation restores hematopoietic function following marrow ablative therapy. Blood 1988;71:723–727.
52. To LB, Shepperd KM, Haylock DN, et al. Single high doses of cyclophosphamide enable the collection of high numbers of hematopoietic cells from the peripheral blood. Exp Hematol 1990;18:442–447.
53. Champlin RE, Schmitz N, Horowitz MM, et al. Blood stem cells compared with bone marrow as a source of hematopoietic cells for allogeneic transplantation. Blood 2000;95:3702–3709.
54. Ringden O, Remberger M, Runde V, et al. Peripheral blood stem cell transplantation from unrelated donors: A comparison with marrow transplantation. Blood 1999;94:455–464.
55. Auerbach AD, Liu Q, Ghosh R, et al. Prenatal identification of potential donors for umbilical cord blood transplantation for Fanconi anemia. Transfusion 1990;30:682–687.
56. Ballen KK. New trends in umbilical cord blood transplantation. Blood 2005;105:3786–3792.
57. Slavin S, Nagler A, Naparstek E, et al. Nonmyeloablative stem cell transplantation and cell therapy as an alternative to conventional bone marrow transplantation with lethal cytoreduction for the treatment of malignant and nonmalignant hematologic diseases. Blood 1998;91: 756–763.
58. Khouri IF, Keating M, Korbing M, et al. Transplant-lite: Induction of graft-versus-malignancy using fludarabine-based nonablative chemo-

therapy and allogeneic blood progenitor-cell transplantation as treatment for lymphoid malignancies. J Clin Oncol 1999;16:2817–2824.

59. Baron F, Beguin Y. Adoptive immunotherapy with donor lymphocyte infusions after allogeneic HPC transplantation. Transfusion 2000; 40:468–476.
60. Otten A, Bossuyt PMM, Vermeulen M, Brand A. Intravenous immunoglobulin treatment in hematological diseases. Eur J Haematol 1998; 60:73–85.
61. George JN, Woolf SH, Gary E, et al. Idiopathic thrombocytopenic purpura: A practice guideline developed by explicit methods for the American Society of Hematology. Blood 1996;88:3–40.
62. Beck CE, Nathan PC, Parkin PC, et al. Corticosteroids versus intravenous immune globulin for the treatment of acute immune thrombocytopenic purpura in children: A systemic review and meta-analysis of randomized controlled trials. J Pediatr 2005;147: 521–527.

CHAPTER 104

Anemias

BEATA INECK, BARBARA J. MASON, AND WILLIAM LYONS

KEY CONCEPTS

1. Anemias are a group of diseases characterized by a decrease in either the hemoglobin (Hb) or the volume of red blood cells (RBCs), which results in decreased oxygen-carrying capacity of the blood.

2. Anemias are generally a sign of underlying pathology; therefore, determining the cause of the anemia is important. Possible consequences of chronic anemia include reduced quality-of-life, decreased survival, and increased risk of cardiac complications, neurologic dysfunction, and surgical complications. Awareness of anemia, its detection, investigation, and management must be raised.

3. Patients with acute-onset anemias are most likely to present with tachycardia, lightheadedness, and dyspnea. Patients with chronic anemia often present with weakness, fatigue, headache, vertigo, faintness, and pallor.

4. Iron-deficiency anemia (IDA) is characterized by decreased levels of ferritin (most sensitive marker) and serum iron, as well as decreased transferrin saturation; Hb and hematocrit (Hct) decline later. Total iron-binding capacity (TIBC) is increased. RBC morphology includes hypochromia and microcytosis. Most patients with IDA are adequately treated with oral ferrous (Fe^{2+}) sulfate therapy, although parenteral iron therapy is necessary in selected patient populations.

5. Vitamin B_{12} deficiency, a macrocytic anemia, can be due to inadequate intake, decreased absorption, or inadequate utilization. Anemia caused by a lack of intrinsic factor, resulting in decreased vitamin B_{12} absorption, is called *pernicious anemia.* Vitamin B_{12} levels and the reticulocyte count usually are low. Neurologic symptoms are often present and can become irreversible if the vitamin B_{12} deficiency is not treated promptly. Oral or parenteral therapy can be used for replacement therapy.

6. Folic acid deficiency, a macrocytic anemia, results from inadequate intake, decreased absorption, hyperutilization, or inadequate utilization. Treatment consists of oral administration of folic acid, even in patients with absorption problems. Adequate folic acid intake is essential in women of childbearing age to decrease the risk of neural tube defects in their children.

7. Anemia of chronic disease is a diagnosis of exclusion. It results from chronic inflammation, infection, or malignancy and can occur as early as 1 to 2 months after the onset of these processes. The serum iron level usually is decreased, but in contrast to IDA, the serum ferritin concentration is normal or increased and TIBC is normal or decreased. Treatment is aimed at correcting the underlying pathology.

8. Anemia is a common complication in critically ill patients and is almost universally found in this patient population. Contributing factors include sepsis, frequent blood samples, surgical blood loss, immune-mediated functional iron deficiency, decreased erythropoietin (EPO) production, reduced RBC life span, and active bleeding. Low serum iron, TIBC, and low iron/TIBC ratio result. Serum ferritin is normal to high. Whether exogenous EPO improves clinical outcomes in critically ill patients is not clear.

9. Anemia is one of the most prevalent clinical problems observed in the elderly, although it is not an inevitable outcome of aging. Anemia is associated with an increased risk of hospitalization and mortality, reduced quality of life, and decreased physical functioning. Patients with iron deficiency may have concurrent folic acid or vitamin B_{12} deficiency.

10. IDA is a leading cause of infant morbidity and mortality. The age of the child can yield some clues to the etiology of the anemia. Age- and sex-adjusted norms must be used in the interpretation of laboratory results in pediatric patients. Primary prevention of IDA is the goal. A therapeutic trial of oral iron is the standard of care. EPO can be used for treatment of anemia of prematurity.

11. Hemolytic anemia results in decreased survival time of RBCs secondary to destruction in the spleen or circulation. Hemolytic anemias usually are normocytic and normochromic, with increased levels of reticulocytes, lactate dehydrogenase, and indirect bilirubin. Treatment is directed toward correcting or controlling the underlying pathology.

Learning objectives, review questions, and other resources can be found at **www.pharmacotherapyonline.com.**

According to the World Health Organization, as many as four to five billion people (66%–80% of the world's population) may be iron deficient, and two billion people (30% of the world's population) are anemic. Anemia defined as hemoglobin (Hb) <13 g/dL in men or <12 g/dL in women (as recommended by the World Health Organization) occurs in approximately 3.5 million Americans based on self-reported data from the National Center for Health Statistics. It is estimated that millions of people are unaware they have anemia, making it one of the most underdiagnosed conditions in the United States. The prevalence of iron-deficiency anemia has been stable in the last decade since the mid-1990s in the United States, with the highest rate in minority and poor children.[1] The highest prevalence is seen in women, African Americans, the elderly, and low-income persons. Laboratory data from the third National Health and Nutrition Examination Survey (NHANES) reports anemia prevalence is 5.7% in infants, 5.9% in teenage girls, 5.8% in young women, and 4.4% in elderly men.[2] The estimated prevalence of anemia in the surgical population is as high as 75%.[3] Obesity surgery is increasingly common. Depending on the type of bariatric procedure, nutritional deficiency may be an issue. Gastric bypass may result in calcium, folate, vitamin B_{12}, and iron deficiencies. Prevalence data are confounded by the lack of a standardized definition of anemia. Because no screening guidelines for anemia in the elderly exist, the prevalence may be even higher than suspected. The United States Preventive Services Task Force (USPSTF) guidelines for asymptomatic pregnant women recommend routine screening for iron-deficiency anemia (IDA).

The importance of anemia often is overlooked and undertreated. Evidence suggests that anemia is not an innocent bystander; it can affect both length and quality of life. Retrospective observational studies in hemodialysis patients and heart failure patients suggest that anemia is an independent risk factor for mortality.[4] In addition, anemia significantly influences morbidity, as shown in patients with end-stage renal disease, chronic kidney disease, and heart failure.[5] Quality-of-life data in anemic patients are primarily based on studies in cancer patients.[6] Anemia is associated with psychomotor and cognitive abnormalities in children. Similarly, among adults, anemia is associated with cognitive dysfunction in patients with renal failure, those with cancer, and among community-dwelling elders.[7] During pregnancy, anemia has been associated with increased risk for low birth weights, preterm delivery, and perinatal mortality.[8,9] Maternal IDA may be associated with postpartum depression and poor performance by offspring on mental and psychomotor tests. The effect of treatment on patient outcomes must be the focus of research on each specific type of anemia. Global goals of treatment in anemic patients are to alleviate signs and symptoms, correct the underlying etiology, and prevent recurrence of anemia.

❶ Anemias are a group of diseases characterized by a decrease in either Hb or red blood cells (RBCs), resulting in reduced oxygen-carrying capacity of the blood. Anemias can result from inadequate RBC production, increased RBC destruction, or blood loss. They can be a manifestation of a host of systemic disorders, such as infection, chronic renal disease, or malignancy. Because anemias are often a sign of underlying pathology, rapid diagnosis of the cause is essential.

❷ Anemias can be classified on the basis of the morphology of the RBCs, etiology, or pathophysiology (see Table 104–1 for examples). This chapter focuses on IDA, anemia of chronic disease (ACD), and anemias associated with vitamin B_{12} and folic acid deficiency. Characteristic changes in the size of RBCs seen in erythrocyte indices can be the first step in the morphologic classification and understanding of the anemia.

TABLE 104-1 Classification Systems for Anemias

- I. Morphology
  - Macrocytic anemias
    - Megaloblastic anemias
      - Vitamin B_{12} deficiency
      - Folic acid deficiency anemia
  - Microcytic hypochromic anemias
    - Iron-deficiency anemia
    - Genetic anomaly
      - Sickle cell anemia
      - Thalassemia
      - Other hemoglobinopathies (abnormal hemoglobins)
  - Normocytic anemias
    - Recent blood loss
    - Hemolysis
    - Bone marrow failure
    - Anemia of chronic disease
  - Renal failure
  - Endocrine disorders
  - Myelodysplastic anemias
- II. Etiology
  - Deficiency
    - Iron
    - Vitamin B_{12}
    - Folic acid
    - Pyridoxine
  - Central, caused by impaired bone marrow function
    - Anemia of chronic disease
    - Anemia of the elderly
    - Malignant bone marrow disorders
  - Peripheral
    - Bleeding (hemorrhage)
    - Hemolysis (hemolytic anemias)
- III. Pathophysiology
  - Excessive blood loss
    - Recent hemorrhage
    - Trauma
    - Peptic ulcer
    - Gastritis
    - Hemorrhoids
  - Chronic hemorrhage
    - Vaginal bleeding
    - Peptic ulcer
    - Intestinal parasites
    - Aspirin and other nonsteroidal anti-inflammatory agents
  - Excessive RBC destruction
    - Extracorpuscular (outside the cell) factors
      - RBC antibodies
      - Drugs
      - Physical trauma to RBC (artificial valves)
      - Excessive sequestration in the spleen
    - Intracorpuscular factors
      - Heredity
      - Disorders of hemoglobin synthesis
  - Inadequate production of mature RBCs
    - Deficiency of nutrients (B_{12}, folic acid, iron, protein)
    - Deficiency of erythroblasts
      - Aplastic anemia
      - Isolated (often transient) erythroblastopenia
      - Folic acid antagonists
      - Antibodies
    - Conditions with infiltration of bone marrow
      - Lymphoma
      - Leukemia
      - Myelofibrosis
      - Carcinoma
    - Endocrine abnormalities
      - Hypothyroidism
      - Adrenal insufficiency
      - Pituitary insufficiency
    - Chronic renal disease
    - Chronic inflammatory disease
      - Granulomatous diseases
      - Collagen vascular diseases
    - Hepatic disease

RBC, red blood cell.

Anemias are classified by RBC size as macrocytic, normocytic, or microcytic. Vitamin B_{12} deficiency and folic acid deficiency both are macrocytic anemias. An example of a microcytic anemia is iron deficiency, whereas a normocytic anemia may be associated with recent blood loss or chronic disease. More than one anemia and etiology can occur concurrently. Inclusion of the underlying cause of the anemia makes diagnostic terminology easier to understand (e.g., microcytic anemia secondary to iron deficiency).

Microcytic anemias are pathogenically a result of a quantitative deficiency in Hb synthesis, usually due to iron deficiency or impaired iron utilization. As a result, erythrocytes containing insufficient Hb are formed. Microcytosis and hypochromia are the morphologic abnormalities that provide evidence of impaired Hb synthesis. Macrocytic anemias can be divided into megaloblastic and nonmegaloblastic anemias. The type of macrocytic anemia can be distinguished microscopically by peripheral blood smear examination. Megaloblasts are distinctive cells that express a biochemical abnormality of retarded DNA synthesis, resulting in unbalanced cell growth. Megaloblastic anemias affect all hematopoietic cell lines. The most common cause of megaloblastic anemia is vitamin B_{12} and/or folate deficiency. Nonmegaloblastic anemias do not have a common pathogenic mechanism and may be macrocytic or normocytic. This type of macrocytic anemia may be due to etiologies such as liver disease, hypothyroidism, hemolytic anemia, and alcoholism. Hemolytic anemias often are macrocytic, resulting in increased reticulocyte counts, and reticulocytes are larger on average than more mature red cells.

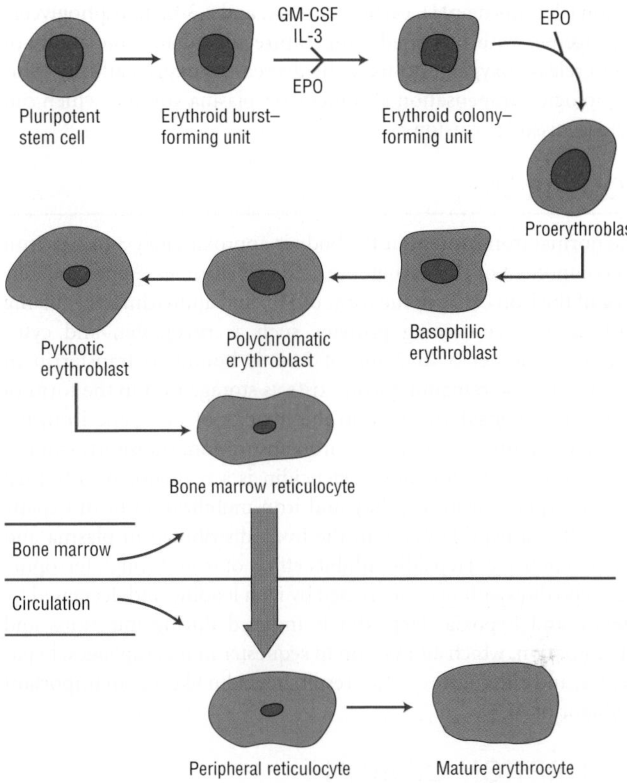

FIGURE 104-1. Erythrocyte maturation sequence. (EPO, erythropoietin; GM-CSF, granulocyte-macrophage colony-stimulating factor; IL-3, interleukin-3.)

MATURATION AND DEVELOPMENT OF RED BLOOD CELLS

In adults, RBCs are formed in the marrow of the vertebrae, ribs, sternum, clavicle, pelvic (iliac) crest, and proximal epiphyses of the long bones. In children, most bone marrow space is hematopoietically active to meet increased RBC requirements.

In normal RBC formation, a pluripotent stem cell yields an erythroid burst-forming unit. Erythropoietin (EPO) and cytokines such as interleukin-3 and granulocyte–macrophage colony-stimulating factor stimulate this cell to form an erythroid colony-forming unit in the marrow. The erythroid colony-forming unit is very sensitive to EPO and produces proerythroblasts. Subsequent divisions yield basophilic erythroblasts, polychromatic erythroblasts, pyknotic erythroblasts, reticulocytes, and finally erythrocytes. During this process, the nucleus becomes smaller with each division, finally disappearing in the normal erythrocyte (Fig. 104–1). Hb and iron are incorporated into the gradually maturing RBC, which eventually is released from the marrow into the circulating blood as a reticulocyte. The maturation process usually takes approximately 1 week. The reticulocyte loses its nucleus and becomes an erythrocyte within several days. The circulating erythrocyte is a nonnucleated, nondividing cell. More than 90% of the protein content of the erythrocyte consists of the oxygen-carrying molecule Hb. Erythrocytes compose 40% to 50% of the total blood volume and have a normal survival time of 120 days.

STIMULATION OF ERYTHROPOIESIS

The hormone EPO, 90% of which is produced by the kidneys, initiates and stimulates the production of RBCs. Erythropoiesis is regulated by a feedback loop. The main mechanism of action of EPO is preventing apoptosis, or programmed cell death, of erythroid precursor cells and allowing their proliferation and subsequent maturation. A decrease in tissue oxygen concentration signals the kidneys to increase the production and release of EPO into the plasma, which (a) stimulates stem cells to differentiate into proerythroblasts, (b) increases the rate of mitosis, (c) increases the release of reticulocytes from the marrow, and (d) induces Hb formation. Under normal circumstances, the RBC mass is kept at an almost constant level by EPO matching new erythrocyte production to the natural rate of loss of RBCs. Accelerated Hb synthesis makes possible achievement of the critical Hb concentration necessary for RBCs to mature more rapidly. A feedback mechanism stops further RBC nucleic acid synthesis, causing an earlier release of reticulocytes. Early appearance of large quantities of reticulocytes in the peripheral circulation (reticulocytosis) is an indication of increased RBC production.

SYNTHESIS OF HEMOGLOBIN

Hb consists of a protein component with two α- and two β–chains. Each chain is linked to a heme group consisting of a porphyrin ring structure with an iron atom chelated at its center, which is capable of binding oxygen. The initial step in the synthesis of heme from the substrate succinyl CoA and glycine requires the presence of pyridoxine phosphate (vitamin B_6) as a catalyst. Following its synthesis in the cytoplasmic mitochondria of the RBC, heme diffuses into the extramitochondrial space, combines with the completed α- and β-chains, and forms Hb.

Under normal conditions, the body produces approximately 6.25 g of Hb daily. If the bone marrow functions at maximal capacity, the normal RBC survival time of 120 days can decrease to 18 to 20 days before an anemia develops. When hemolytic destruction of RBCs exceeds marrow production capacity and anemia develops, the Hb value decreases to a steady-state level at which production is equal to destruction. Hb values in these hemolytic anemias, such as sickle cell anemia (see Chap. 106), will remain stable unless other factors further shorten the RBC life span.

The affinity of Hb for oxygen is influenced by three intracellular components and by temperature. Increasing hydrogen ion concentration (decreasing pH), carbon dioxide, and 2,3-bisphosphoglycerate, together with increased temperature, all enhance the ability of Hb to release oxygen into tissue by decreasing oxygen affinity. This physiologic compensation also increases plasma volume, which can increase tissue perfusion.

BODY IRON

The normal iron content of the body is approximately 3 to 4 g. Iron is a component of Hb, myoglobin, and cytochromes. Approximately 2.5 g of the iron exists in the form of Hb, and approximately 400 mg exists as iron-containing proteins such as myoglobin and cytochromes. Another 3 to 7 mg of iron is bound to transferrin in plasma, and the remaining iron exists as storage iron in the form of ferritin or hemosiderin. Due to the toxicity of inorganic iron, the body has an intricate system for iron absorption, transport, storage, assimilation, and elimination. Hepcidin is a regulator of intestinal iron absorption, iron recycling and iron mobilization from hepatic stores. It is a peptide made in the liver, distributed in plasma and excreted in urine. Hepcidin inhibits efflux of iron through ferroportin. Hepcidin synthesis is increased by iron loading and decreased by anemia and hypoxia. Hepcidin is induced during infections and inflammation, which allows iron to sequester in macrophages, hepatocytes, and enterocytes.[10] As a result, hepcidin likely is an important mediator of ACD.

ABSORPTION OF IRON

Iron is best absorbed in its ferrous (Fe^{2+}) form. The normal daily western diet contains approximately 12 to 15 mg of iron, mainly in the ferric (Fe^{3+}) nonabsorbed form. After iron is ionized by stomach acid and then reduced to the Fe^{2+} state, it is absorbed primarily in the duodenum, and to a smaller extent in the jejunum, via intestinal mucosal cell uptake. Subsequently, it is transferred across the cell into the plasma. Iron absorption is not directly correlated to iron intake. As physiologic iron levels decrease, gastrointestinal absorption of iron increases.

The daily recommended dietary allowance for iron is 8 mg in adult males and postmenopausal females, and 18 mg in menstruating females. Children require more iron because of growth-related increases in blood volume, and pregnant women have an increased iron demand brought about by fetal development. Iron overload does not occur, however, because only the amount of iron lost per day is absorbed. The amount of iron absorbed from food depends on the body stores, the rate of RBC production, the type of iron provided in the diet, and the presence of any substances that may enhance or inhibit iron absorption.

Heme iron, which is found in meat, fish, and poultry, is approximately three times more absorbable than the nonheme iron found in vegetables, fruits, dried beans, nuts, grain products, and dietary supplements. Forty percent of iron from animal sources is in the heme form. Heme and nonheme iron are absorbed by different receptors on the intestinal mucosa. The iron contents of some foods high in iron are listed in Table 104–2. Gastric acid and other dietary components such as ascorbic acid increase the absorption of nonheme iron. Dietary components that form insoluble complexes with iron (phytates, tannates, and phosphates) decrease absorption. Phytates, a natural component of grains, brans, and some vegetables, can form poorly absorbed complexes and partially explain the increased prevalence of IDA in poorer countries, where grains and vegetables compose a disproportionate amount of the normal diet, with the more readily absorbable heme iron lacking in the diet. Polyphenols bind the iron and decrease nonheme iron absorption when large amounts of tea or coffee are consumed with a meal. Although the mechanism is unknown, calcium inhibits absorption of both heme and nonheme iron. Epidemiologic studies show a correlation between milk intake and prevalence of iron deficiency. Finally, because gastric acid improves iron absorption, patients who have undergone a gastrectomy or have achlorhydria have decreased iron absorption.[11]

TABLE 104-2 Good Sources of Iron

Food	Serving Size	Amount (mg)
Total cereal	1 cup	18
Grape-Nuts cereal	1 cup	18
Instant Cream of Wheat	1 cup	8.2
Instant plain oatmeal	1 cup	6.7
Wheat germ	1 oz.	2.6
Broccoli	1 medium stalk	2.1
Baked potato	1 medium	2.7
Raw tofu	1/2 cup	4
Lentils	1/2 cup	3.3
Beef chuck	3 ounces	3.2

INCORPORATION OF IRON INTO HEME

The specific plasma transport protein transferrin delivers iron to the bone marrow for incorporation into the Hb molecule. Transferrin enters cells by binding to transferrin receptors, which circulate and then attach to cells needing iron. Conversely, there are fewer transferrin receptors on the surface of cells that do not need iron, thus preventing iron-replete cells from receiving excess iron.[12]

Circulating transferrin normally is approximately 30% saturated with iron. Transferrin delivers extra iron to other body storage sites, such as the liver, marrow, and spleen, for later use. This iron is stored within macrophages as ferritin or hemosiderin. Ferritin consists of a Fe^{3+} hydroxyphosphate core surrounded by a protein shell called *apoferritin.* Hemosiderin can be described as compacted ferritin molecules with an even greater iron/protein shell ratio. Physiologically it is a more stable, but less available, form of storage iron.

NORMAL DESTRUCTION OF RED BLOOD CELLS

Phagocytic breakdown destroys older blood cells, primarily in the spleen, but also in the marrow (Fig. 104–2). Amino acids from the globin chains return to an amino acid pool; heme oxygenase acts on the porphyrin heme structure to form biliverdin and to release its iron. Iron returns to the iron pool to be reused, although biliverdin is further catabolized to bilirubin. The bilirubin is released into the plasma, where it binds to albumin and is transported to the liver for glucuronide conjugation and excretion via bile. If the liver is unable to perform the conjugation, as occurs with intrinsic liver disease or oversaturation of conjugation enzymes by excessive cell hemolysis, the result is an elevated indirect (unconjugated) bilirubin. If the biliary excretion pathway for the already conjugated bilirubin is obstructed, an elevated direct bilirubin results. Comparison of direct and indirect bilirubin values helps to determine if the defect in bilirubin clearance occurs before or after bilirubin enters the liver. The Hb in RBCs, which is destroyed by intravascular hemolysis, becomes attached to haptoglobin and is carried back to the marrow for processing in the normal manner.

DIAGNOSIS OF ANEMIA

GENERAL PRESENTATION

History, physical examination and laboratory testing are used in the evaluation of anemia. The workup determines if the patient is

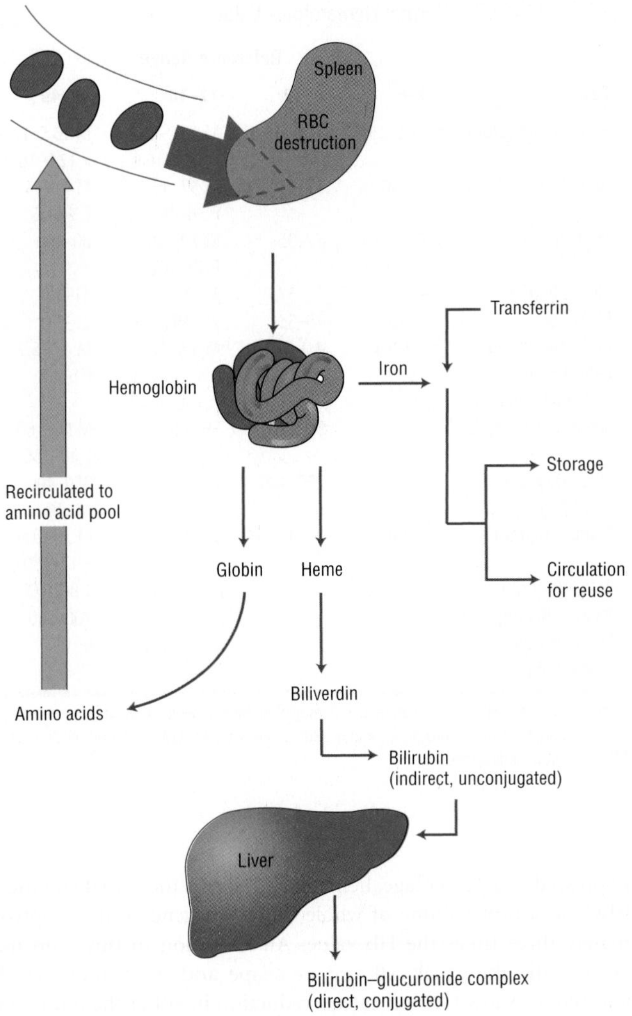

FIGURE 104-2. Destruction of red blood cells (RBCs).

bleeding and investigates potential causes of the anemia, such as increased RBC destruction, bone marrow suppression, or iron deficiency. Occupation, social habits, travel history, and diet all can be important in identifying causes of anemia. Additionally, information about concurrent nonhematologic disease states and a drug ingestion history are essential when evaluating the cause of the anemia (see Chap. 107). History of blood transfusions, liver disease, peptic ulcers, gastrointestinal tract malignancies, and exposure to toxic chemicals also should be obtained.

Because anemias are a sign of disease, clinical presentation may relate to the underlying pathology. Presenting signs and symptoms of anemias depend on the rate of development and the age of the patient, as well as the cardiovascular status of the patient. Severity of symptoms does not always correlate with the degree of anemia. If the myocardium is healthy and the anemia evolves slowly, the combined effects of the shift in the oxygen dissociation curve and increased cardiac output may allow acclimatization at very low Hb concentrations. Mild anemia often is associated with no clinical symptoms and often is found incidentally upon obtaining a complete blood count (CBC) for other reasons. The signs and symptoms in elderly patients with anemia may be attributed to their age or concomitant disease states. Levels of Hb tolerated by younger persons may not be tolerated by the elderly. Patients with cardiac or pulmonary disease may be less tolerant of mild anemia. Premature infants with anemia may be asymptomatic or have tachycardia, poor weight gain, increased supplemental oxygen needs, or increased episodes of apnea or bradycardia.

CLINICAL PRESENTATION OF ANEMIA

General

- Patients may be asymptomatic or have vague complaints
- Patients with vitamin B_{12} deficiency may develop neurologic consequences
- In ACD, signs and symptoms of the underlying disorder often overshadow those of the anemia

Symptoms

- Decreased exercise tolerance
- Fatigue
- Dizziness
- Irritability
- Weakness
- Palpitations
- Vertigo
- Shortness of breath
- Chest pain
- Neurologic symptoms in vitamin B_{12} deficiency

Signs

- Tachycardia
- Pale appearance (most prominent in conjunctivae)
- Decreased mental acuity
- Increased intensity of some cardiac valvular murmurs
- Diminished vibratory sense or gait abnormality in vitamin B_{12} deficiency

Laboratory Tests

- Hb, hematocrit (Hct), and RBC indices may remain normal early in the disease and then decrease as the anemia progresses
- Serum iron is low in IDA and ACD
- Ferritin levels are low in IDA and normal to increased in ACD
- TIBC is high in IDA and is low or normal in ACD
- Mean corpuscular volume is elevated in vitamin B_{12} deficiency and folate deficiency
- Vitamin B_{12} and folate levels are low in their respective types of anemia
- Homocysteine is elevated in vitamin B_{12} deficiency and folate deficiency
- Methylmalonic acid is elevated in vitamin B_{12} deficiency

Other Diagnostic Tests

- Schilling test may help uncover intrinsic factor deficiency
- Bone marrow testing with iron staining can indicate low iron levels in IDA and adequate stores in ACD

❸ Anemia of rapid onset is most likely to present with cardiorespiratory symptoms such as tachycardia, palpitations, angina, hypotension, lightheadedness, and breathlessness due to decreased oxygen delivery to tissues or hypovolemia in those with acute bleeding. With severe intravascular blood volume loss, peripheral vasoconstriction and central vasodilation preserve blood flow to vital organs. Systemic small-vessel dilation eventually increases tissue oxygenation. Vascular compensation results in decreased systemic vascular resistance, increased cardiac output, and tachycardia. With acute hemolysis and reduced RBC mass, some decrease in blood volume, but not in plasma volume, is seen.

If onset is more chronic, presenting symptoms may include fatigue, weakness, headache, symptoms of heart failure, vertigo, faintness, sensitivity to cold, pallor, and loss of skin tone. Traditional signs of anemia, such as pallor, have limited sensitivity and specificity and may be misinterpreted. With chronic bleeding, there is time for equilibration with extravascular space, and total blood volume remains normal.

Possible manifestations of IDA include glossal pain, smooth tongue, reduced salivary flow, pica (compulsive eating of nonfood items), and pagophagia (compulsive eating of ice). These symptoms are not likely to appear until the Hb concentration falls to a level of 9 g/dL or below.

Clinically, patients with vitamin B_{12} deficiency may be pale and mildly icteric, and they may develop gastric mucosal atrophy. Neurologic findings in vitamin B_{12} deficiency, which often precede hematologic findings, may be partly due to impairment of conversion of homocysteine to methionine, as methionine is necessary for production of choline and choline-containing phospholipids. Neurologic effects of vitamin B_{12} deficiency may occur even in the absence of anemia. Early neurologic findings include numbness and paresthesias, then peripheral neuropathy, ataxia, diminished vibratory sense, decreased proprioception, and imbalance, as demyelination of the dorsal columns and corticospinal tract develop. Vision changes may result from optic nerve involvement. Psychiatric findings include irritability, personality changes, memory impairment, dementia, depression, and, infrequently, psychosis. Other reported symptoms include glossitis, muscle weakness, dysphagia, and anorexia. Pernicious anemia is associated with increased risk of gastric cancer.

Symptoms associated with folate deficiency are similar to those seen in patients with vitamin B_{12} deficiency, with the absence of neurologic symptoms. Although the symptoms of anemia will improve with folate replacement and a partial hematologic response will occur, the neurologic manifestations of vitamin B_{12} deficiency will not be reversed with folic acid replacement therapy and consequently may progress or become irreversible if not treated.

LABORATORY EVALUATION

The initial evaluation of anemia involves a CBC (including RBC indices), reticulocyte index, and examination of a stool sample for occult blood. The results of the preliminary evaluation determine the need for other studies, such as examination of a peripheral blood smear. Based on laboratory test results, anemia can be categorized into three functional defects:

1. RBC production failure (hypoproliferative)
2. Cell maturation ineffectiveness
3. Increase in RBC destruction

Table 104–3 lists normal hematologic values, although these values may differ in certain populations, such as individuals living at high altitudes and endurance athletes.

Fig. 104–3 shows a broad, general algorithm for the diagnosis of anemias based on laboratory data. There are many exceptions and additions to this algorithm, but it can serve as a guide to the typical presentation of common types and causes of anemia. The algorithm is less useful in the presence of more than one cause of anemia.

Hemoglobin

Values given for Hb represent the amount of Hb per volume of whole blood. The higher values seen in males are due to stimulation of RBC production by androgenic steroids, whereas the lower values in females are due to decrease in Hb as a result of blood loss during menstruation. The Hb level can be used as a very rough estimate of the oxygen-carrying capacity of blood. Hb levels may be diminished because of a decreased quantity of Hb per RBC or because of a decrease in the actual number of RBCs. In pregnancy, Hb may not reflect red cell mass changes.

TABLE 104-3 Normal Hematologic Values

	Reference Range			
Test	**2–6**	**6–12**	**12–18**	**18–49**
Hemoglobin (g/dL)	11.5–15.5	11.5–15.5	M 13.0–16.0 F 12.0–16.0	M 13.5–17.5 F 12.0–16.0
Hematocrit (%)	34–40	35–45	M 37–49 F 36–46	M 41–53 F 36–46
MCV (fL)	75–87	77–95	M 78–98 F 78–102	80–100
MCHC (%)	–	31–37	31–37	31–37
MCH (pg)	24–30	25–33	25–35	26–34
RBC (million/mm^3)	3.9–5.3	4.0–5.2	M 4.5–5.3	M 4.5–5.9
Reticulocyte count, absolute (%)				0.5–1.5
Serum iron (mcg/dL)		50–120	50–120	M 50–160 F 40–150
TIBC (mcg/dL)	250–400	250–400	250–400	250–400
RDW (%)				11–16
Ferritin (ng/mL)	7–140	7–140	7–140	M 15–200 F 12–150
Folate (ng/mL)				1.8–16.0[a]
Vitamin B_{12} (pg/mL)				100–900[a]
Erythropoietin (mU/mL)				0–19

F, female; M, male; MCH, mean corpuscular hemoglobin; MCHC, mean corpuscular hemoglobin concentration; MCV, mean corpuscular volume; RBC, red blood cell; RDW, red blood cell distribution; TIBC, total iron-binding capacity.
[a]Varies by assay method.

Hematocrit

Expressed as a percentage, hematocrit (Hct) is the actual volume of RBCs in a unit volume of whole blood. In general, it is approximately three times the Hb value. An alteration in this ratio may occur with abnormal cell size or shape and often indicates the pathology. A low Hct indicates a reduction in either the number or the size of RBCs or an increase in plasma volume.

Red Blood Cell Count

The RBC count is an indirect estimate of the Hb content of the blood; it is an actual count of RBCs per unit of blood.

Red Blood Cell Indices

Wintrobe indices describe the size and Hb content of the RBCs and are calculated from the Hb, Hct, and RBC count. RBC indices, such as mean corpuscular volume (MCV) and mean corpuscular Hb (MCH), are single mean values that do not express the variation that can occur in cells.

Mean Corpuscular Volume (Hct/RBC Count) MCV represents the average volume of RBCs. It may reflect changes in MCH, but it can be confounded. Cells are considered *macrocytic* if they are larger than normal, *microcytic* if they are smaller than normal, and *normocytic* if their size falls within normal limits. Folic acid and vitamin B_{12} deficiency anemias yield macrocytic morphology, whereas iron deficiency and thalassemia are examples of microcytic anemias. MCV is falsely elevated in the presence of cold agglutinins and hyperglycemia. When IDA (decreased MCV) is accompanied by folate deficiency (increased MCV), failure to understand that the MCV represents an average RBC size creates the potential for overlooking the real cause of the anemia.

Mean Corpuscular Hemoglobin (Hb/RBC Count) MCH is defined as the percent volume of Hb in an RBC. It reflects the adequacy of iron supply to developing erythron. Two morphologic changes, microcytosis and hypochromia, can reduce MCH. A

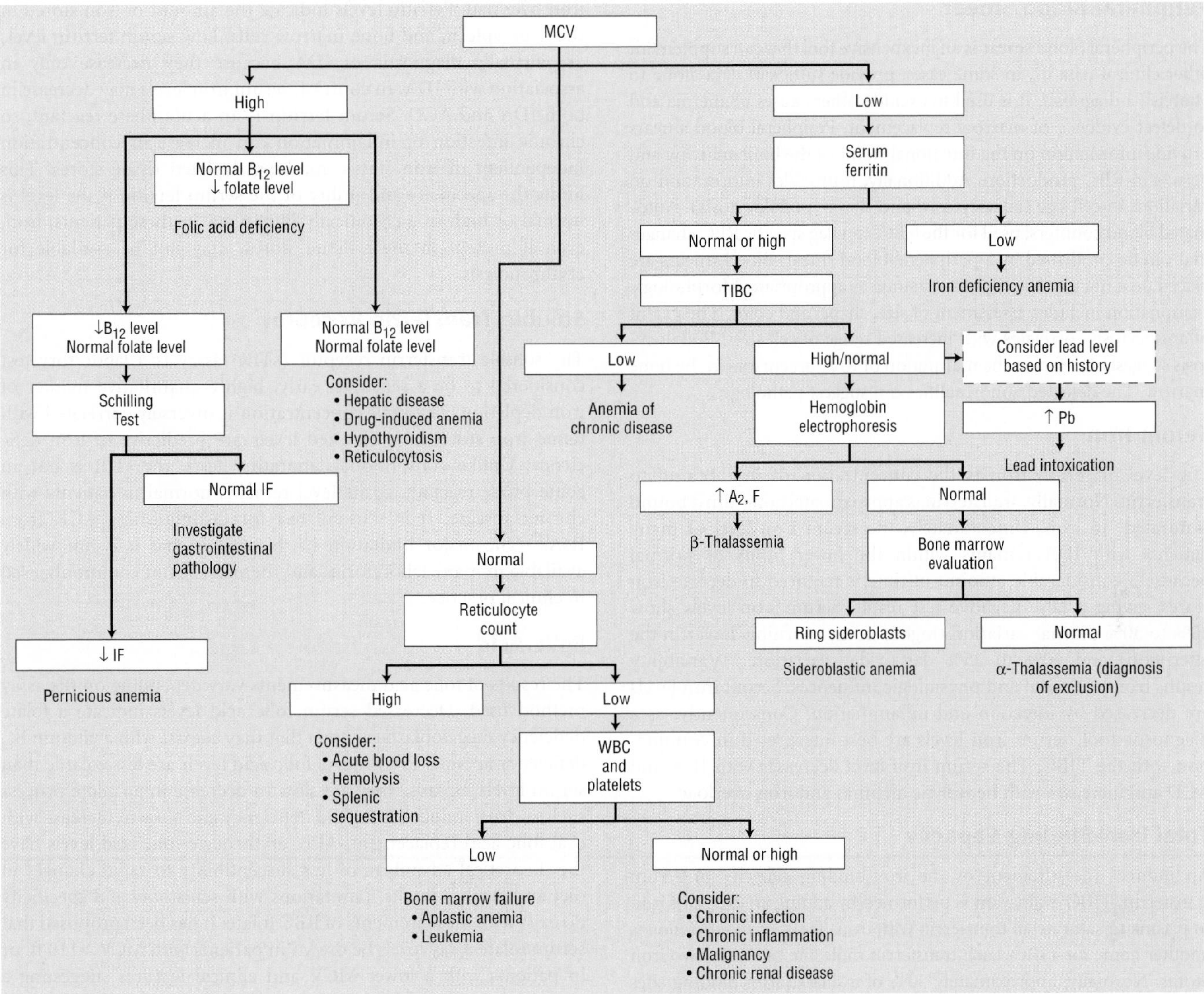

FIGURE 104-3. General algorithm for diagnosis of anemias. (↑, increased; ↓, decreased; A_2, hemoglobin A_2; F, hemoglobin F; IF, intrinsic factor; MCV, mean corpuscular volume; Pb, lead; TIBC, total iron-binding capacity; WBC, white blood cells.)

microcytic cell contains less Hb because it is a smaller cell, whereas a hypochromic cell has a low MCH because of the decreased amount of Hb present in a normocytic cell. Cells can be both microcytic and hypochromic, as seen with IDA, and the MCH alone cannot distinguish between microcytosis and hypochromia. The most common cause of an elevated MCH is macrocytosis (e.g., vitamin B_{12} or folate deficiency).

Mean Corpuscular Hemoglobin Concentration (Hb/Hct)

The weight of Hb per volume of cells is the mean corpuscular Hb concentration (MCHC). Because MCHC is independent of cell size, it is more useful than MCH in distinguishing between microcytosis and hypochromia. A low MCHC always indicates hypochromia; a microcyte with a normal Hb concentration will have a low MCH but a normal MCHC. A decreased MCHC is seen most often in association with IDA.

Total Reticulocyte Count

Although an indirect assessment, the total reticulocyte count is an indication of new RBC production. It measures how quickly immature RBCs (reticulocytes) are produced by bone marrow and released into the blood. Reticulocytes circulate in the blood approximately 2 days before maturing into RBCs. In a normal situation, 1% of RBCs are replaced daily, representing a reticulocyte count of 1%. The reticulocyte count in normocytic anemia can differentiate hypoproliferative marrow from a compensatory marrow response to an anemia. A lack of reticulocytosis in anemia indicates impaired RBC production. Examples include iron deficiency, B_{12} deficiency, ACD, malnutrition, renal insufficiency, and malignancy. A high reticulocyte count may be seen in acute blood loss or hemolysis. Occasionally, a patient's Hct decreases while the absolute number of reticulocytes remains the same, resulting in a falsely elevated reticulocyte percentage. Multiplying the reticulocyte percentage by the patient's Hct and then dividing the product by an average normal Hct (for men or women) produces a corrected percentage of reticulocytes (see Chap. 103). When the reticulocyte count is >2.5%, hemolysis may be present.

Red Blood Cell Distribution Width

The higher the red blood cell distribution width (RDW), the more variable the size of the RBCs. The RDW increases in early IDA because of the release of large, immature, nucleated RBCs to compensate for the anemia, but this change is not specific for IDA. The RDW also can be helpful in the diagnosis of a mixed anemia. A patient can have a normal MCV yet have a wide RDW. This finding indicates the presence of microcytes and macrocytes, which would yield a "normal" average RBC size. Use of RDW to distinguish IDA from ACD is not recommended.

Peripheral Blood Smear

The peripheral blood smear is an inexpensive tool that can supplement other clinical data or, in some cases, provide sufficient data alone to establish a diagnosis. It is used to exclude other causes of anemia and to detect evidence of marrow replacement. Peripheral blood smears provide information on the functional status of the bone marrow and defects in RBC production. Additionally, it provides information on variations in cell size (anisocytosis) and shape (poikilocytosis). Automated blood counters, used for the CBC, can flag specific RBC changes that can be confirmed by a peripheral blood smear. Blood smears are placed on a microscope slide and stained as appropriate. Morphologic examination includes assessment of size, shape, and color. The extent of anisocytosis correlates with increased range of cell sizes. Poikilocytosis suggests a defect in the maturation of RBC precursors in the bone marrow. The detected abnormalities can suggest pathology.

Serum Iron

The level of serum iron is the concentration of iron bound to transferrin. Normally, transferrin is approximately one-third bound (saturated) to iron. Unfortunately, the serum iron level of many patients with IDA remains within the lower limits of normal because a considerable amount of time is required to deplete iron stores, giving a false-negative test result. Serum iron levels show 20% to 30% diurnal variation (higher in the morning, lower in the afternoon) and 20% to 25% day-to-day variation.[13] Variability results from technical and physiologic influences. Serum iron levels are decreased by infection and inflammation. Consequently, as a diagnostic tool, serum iron levels are best interpreted in conjunction with the TIBC. The serum iron level decreases with IDA and ACD and increases with hemolytic anemias and iron overload.

Total Iron-Binding Capacity

An indirect measurement of the iron-binding capacity of serum transferrin, TIBC evaluation is performed by adding an excess of iron to plasma to saturate all transferrin with iron. *Transferrin saturation* is another name for TIBC. Each transferrin molecule can carry two iron atoms. Normally, approximately 30% of available iron binding sites are filled. With this laboratory test, all binding sites are filled to measure TIBC. The excess (unbound) iron is then removed and the serum iron concentration determined. Unlike the serum iron level, the TIBC does not fluctuate over hours or days. TIBC usually is higher than normal when body iron stores are low. The finding of a low serum iron level and a high TIBC indicates IDA. The TIBC is actually a measurement of protein serum transferrin, which can be affected by a variety of factors. Patients with infection, malignancy, inflammation, liver disease, and uremia may have a decreased TIBC and a decreased serum iron level, which are consistent with the diagnosis of ACD. Oral contraceptive use and pregnancy can increase TIBC because serum transferrin production is increased with a variety of other proteins.

Percentage Transferrin Saturation

The ratio of serum iron level to TIBC indicates transferrin saturation. It reflects the extent to which iron-binding sites are vacant on transferrin and indicates the amount of iron readily available for erythropoiesis. It is expressed as a percentage, as described in the following formula: Transferrin saturation = (Serum iron/TIBC) $\times$ 100.

Transferrin normally is 20% to 50% saturated with iron. In IDA, transferrin saturation of 15% or lower is commonly seen. Transferrin saturation is a less sensitive and specific marker of iron deficiency than are ferritin levels.

Serum Ferritin

The concentration of ferritin (storage iron) is proportional to total iron stores and therefore is the best indicator of iron deficiency or iron overload. Ferritin levels indicate the amount of iron stored in the liver, spleen, and bone marrow cells. Low serum ferritin levels are virtually diagnostic of IDA because they decrease only in association with IDA. In contrast, serum iron levels may decrease in both IDA and ACD. Serum ferritin is an acute phase reactant, so chronic infection or inflammation can increase its concentration independent of iron status, masking depleted tissue stores. This limits the specificity and utility of the serum ferritin if the level is normal or high in a chronically ill patient. In these patients, iron, even if present in these tissue stores, may not be available for erythropoiesis.

Soluble Transferrin Receptor

The soluble transferrin receptor (sTfR) assay is a laboratory test considered to be a sensitive, early, highly quantitative marker of iron depletion. The sTfR concentration is inversely correlated with tissue iron stores, and elevated levels are predictive of iron deficiency. Unlike conventional laboratory tests, the sTfR is not an acute phase reactant, so its level remains normal in patients with chronic disease. It is a useful test for distinguishing ACD from IDA.[14] The major limitation of this test is that it is not widely available in many laboratories and therefore is not commonly used in clinical practice.

Folic Acid

The results of folic acid measurements vary depending on the assay method used. Decreased serum folic acid levels indicate a folate deficiency megaloblastic anemia that may coexist with a vitamin B_{12} deficiency anemia. Erythrocyte folic acid levels are less volatile than serum levels, because they are slow to decrease in an acute process such as drug-induced folic acid deficiency and slow to increase with oral folic acid replacement. Also, erythrocyte folic acid levels have the theoretical advantage of less susceptibility to rapid changes in diet and alcohol intake. Limitations with sensitivity and specificity do exist with measurements of RBC folate. It has been proposed that serum folate assay levels be drawn in patients with MCV >110 fL or in patients with a lower MCV and clinical features suggesting a macrocytic anemia. If the serum folate concentration is normal in a patient with suspected folate deficiency, then the red cell folate level should be measured.[15]

Vitamin B_{12}

Low levels of vitamin B_{12} (cyanocobalamin) indicate vitamin B_{12} deficiency. However, a deficiency may exist prior to the recognition of low serum levels, as serum values are maintained at the expense of vitamin B_{12} tissue stores. Because vitamin B_{12} deficiency and folate deficiency may overlap, serum levels of both vitamins should be determined. Vitamin B_{12} levels may be falsely low with folate deficiency, pregnancy, and use of oral contraceptives.[16]

Schilling Test

The purpose of the rarely used Schilling urinary excretion test is to diagnose vitamin B_{12} deficiency anemia caused by a B_{12} absorption defect resulting from a lack of intrinsic factor (pernicious anemia). The patient initially receives an oral dose of radiolabeled vitamin B_{12}. Two hours later, the patient receives a large intramuscular dose of nonlabeled vitamin B_{12} to saturate plasma transport proteins. Any excess vitamin B_{12} that is not taken up by the transport proteins or stored in the liver is excreted in the urine. A 24-hour urine collection then is measured for radioactivity. If production of gastrointestinal intrinsic factor is sufficient, the radiolabeled B_{12} will be absorbed initially, displaced by the injected B_{12}, and excreted in the urine.

If oral absorption is impaired, stage 2 of the test is conducted 5 to 7 days later. The second stage of the Schilling test differentiates inadequate secretion of intrinsic factor by the stomach from an abnormality in absorption by the ileum. Generally, the finding of abnormal results for stage 1 followed by a normal result in stage 2 is consistent with pernicious anemia. If the results in part 2 still are low, then the third stage of the test is conducted to determine whether the cause of the deficiency is bacterial overgrowth or ileal disease.

Homocysteine

Vitamin B_{12} and folate both are required for conversion of homocysteine to methionine. Increased serum homocysteine may suggest vitamin B_{12} or folate deficiency. Homocysteine levels also can be elevated in patients with vitamin B_6 deficiency, renal failure, hypothyroidism, or a genetic defect in cystathionine β-synthase.[17] Additionally, elevated levels have been caused by medications, including nicotinic acid, theophylline, methotrexate, and L-dopa.

Methylmalonic Acid

A vitamin B_{12} coenzyme is needed to convert methylmalonyl coenzyme A to succinyl coenzyme A. Patients with vitamin B_{12} deficiency may have increased concentrations of serum methylmalonic acid (MMA), which is a more specific marker for vitamin B_{12} deficiency compared to homocysteine. MMA levels are not elevated in folate deficiency because folate does not participate in MMA metabolism. Levels of both MMA and homocysteine usually are elevated prior to the development of hematologic abnormalities and reductions in serum vitamin B_{12} levels.[16] MMA levels must be interpreted cautiously in patients with renal disease and hypovolemia because the levels may be elevated due to decreased urinary excretion.

Coombs Test

Antiglobulin tests, also called *Coombs tests,* indicate hemolytic anemia caused by an immune response. A direct Coombs test detects antibodies bound to erythrocytes, whereas an indirect Coombs test measures antibodies present in the serum. A positive finding on a direct Coombs test usually is indicative of antibody-mediated hemolysis.

Erythropoietin Levels

Healthy individuals require 10 to 30 milliunits/mL of EPO to maintain normal Hb and Hct concentrations. Endogenous EPO levels can increase 100- to 1,000-fold during hypoxia or anemia, but this marked increase does not occur in patients with significant renal disease, patients receiving chemotherapy, and patients with acquired immunodeficiency syndrome (AIDS), especially those taking zidovudine. These patients will have an EPO response that is insufficient to correct their anemia.

SPECIFIC ANEMIAS

IRON-DEFICIENCY ANEMIA

Epidemiology

Iron deficiency is the most common nutritional deficiency in developing and developed countries. More than 500 million people worldwide are estimated to have IDA.[2] Data from NHANES III indicates 1% to 2% of adult in the United States have IDA.[18] Prevalence data vary because screening uses a simple Hb test, arbitrary normals are used, and selection of samples in population surveys tends to lead to errors. The normal ranges for Hb and Hct are so wide that a patient may lose up to 15% of RBC mass and still have a Hct within the normal range.

Etiology

Iron deficiency results from prolonged negative iron balance or failure to meet increased physiologic iron need. The onset of iron deficiency depends on an individual's initial iron stores and balance between iron absorption and loss. Multiple etiologic factors usually are involved. Certain groups at higher risk for iron deficiency include children younger than 2 years, adolescent girls, pregnant females, and elderly older than 65 years.

In less industrialized nations, the risks for developing IDA are largely related to dietary factors. Diets limited in meat or fresh fruits and vegetables or diets high in substances that form complexes with iron may result in IDA. Malabsorptive syndromes also may cause IDA. Situations that increase the demand for iron are frequent blood donations, participation in endurance sports, menstruation, pregnancy and lactation, infancy, and adolescence. Iron deficiency in pregnant women is so common that the Centers for Disease Control and Prevention (CDC) guidelines recommend initiation of low-dose iron supplements (30 mg/day) at the woman's first prenatal visit for primary prevention of IDA. At diagnosis, the cause of IDA must be considered a consequence of blood loss until proven otherwise. More than 50% of adults with IDA have some form of gastrointestinal bleeding. Blood loss may occur as a result of many disorders, including trauma, hemorrhoids, peptic ulcers, gastritis, gastrointestinal malignancies, arteriovenous malformations, diverticular disease, copious menstrual flow, nosebleeds, and postpartum bleeding. Occult blood loss from a single gastrointestinal lesion has been shown to be a frequent cause of "idiopathic" IDA.[19]

The possibility of multifactorial causes must always be considered. Medication history, specifically regarding recent or past use of iron or hematinics, alcohol, corticosteroids, aspirin, and nonsteroidal antiinflammatory drugs, is a vital part of the history. Other possible causes of hypochromic microcytic anemia include ACD, thalassemia, sideroblastic anemia, and heavy metal (mostly lead) poisoning (Fig. 104–3). Patients with IDA commonly undergo upper and/or lower endoscopy in an attempt to identify a bleeding gastrointestinal lesion. Patients with a medical history significant for IDA should be periodically reevaluated for iron deficiency.

Pathophysiology

Iron is vital to the function of all cells. It is a critical element in iron-containing enzymes such as the mitochondrial cytochrome system. Without iron, cells lose their capacity for electron transport and energy metabolism. Because iron is a cofactor for oxidative metabolism, dopamine and DNA synthesis, and free radical function in neutrophils, IDA can be associated with abnormal neurotransmitter function and altered immunologic and inflammatory defenses. The balance of iron metabolism is designed to conserve iron for reutilization. The margin between the amount of iron available for absorption and the body's iron requirement is narrow for growing infants and female adults, which explains why IDA prevalence is highest in these populations. Risk of iron deficiency is related to levels of iron loss, iron intake, iron absorption, and physiologic demands. Iron deficiency usually is the result of a long period of negative iron balance. Manifestations of iron deficiency occur in three stages: prelatent, latent, and IDA. *Prelatent* iron deficiency refers to a reduction in iron stores without reduced serum iron levels and can be assessed with serum ferritin measurement. In this first stage, iron stores can be depleted without causing anemia. The stores allow iron to be utilized when there is an increased need for Hb synthesis. Once stores are depleted, there still is adequate iron from daily RBC turnover for Hb synthesis. Further iron losses would make the patient vulnerable to anemia development. *Latent* iron deficiency occurs when iron stores are depleted, but Hb is above the lower limit of normal for the population but may be reduced for a given patient. This can be determined by serial CBC measurements. Findings include reduced transferrin saturation and increased TIBC. *IDA* occurs when the Hb falls to less than normal values. Deficiency progresses to the classic hypochromia and microcytosis of iron-deficient erythropoiesis.

Another classification of iron deficiency is in accordance with clinical state: iron-store depletion, iron-deficient erythropoiesis, or IDA. The mildest form, iron-store depletion, occurs when there is an increase in formal physiologic demands, which occurs in rapid growth in infancy or adolescence, menstruation, or with an inadequate diet. Limited RBC production and iron-deficient erythropoiesis can occur with blood loss or malabsorption, which can progress to IDA. Iron-store depletion and iron-deficient erythropoiesis may not be associated with any distinctive clinical findings.

Laboratory Findings

❹ Abnormal laboratory findings in patients with IDA generally include low serum iron and ferritin levels and high TIBC. The first apparent sign of iron deficiency is the increased RDW, although the finding is not specific to IDA. In the early stages of IDA, RBC size is not changed. Low ferritin concentration is the earliest and most sensitive indicator of iron deficiency. However, ferritin may not correlate with iron stores in the bone marrow because renal or hepatic disease, malignancies, infection, or inflammatory processes may increase ferritin values.[20] Hb, Hct, and RBC indices usually remain normal.

In the later stages of IDA, Hb and Hct fall below normal values, and a microcytic hypochromic anemia develops. Microcytosis may precede hypochromia, as erythropoiesis is programmed to maintain normal Hb concentration in deference to cell size. As a result, even slightly abnormal Hb and Hct levels may indicate significant depletion of iron stores and should not be ignored. In terms of RBC indices, MCV reduction occurs earlier in iron-deficient hematopoiesis than does reduction in Hb concentration.

Transferrin saturation (i.e., serum iron level divided by the TIBC) is useful for assessing IDA. Low values likely indicate IDA, although low serum transferrin saturation values also may be present in inflammatory disorders. Fortunately, the TIBC usually helps to differentiate the diagnosis in these patients: TIBC >400 mcg/dL suggests IDA, whereas values <200 mcg/dL usually represent inflammatory disease. With continued progression of IDA, anisocytosis occurs and poikilocytosis develops, as seen on peripheral blood smear and indicated by increased RDW. In rare cases, a bone marrow examination is indicated to assess bone marrow iron stores. Bone marrow examination reveals absent iron stores in IDA. Documentation of decreased hemosiderin can confirm the diagnosis of IDA. In microcytic anemias due to all other causes, iron stores are detectable. Serum transferrin receptor can be used to diagnose iron-store depletion and defects in iron delivery to the marrow. Commercial assays are available but are not well standardized. An elevated serum transferrin receptor level would be expected in IDA and a normal level in ACD.

TREATMENT

Iron-Deficiency Anemia

The severity and cause of IDA determines the approach to treatment.[21] Treatment is focused on replenishing iron stores. Because iron deficiency can be an early sign of other illnesses, treatment of the underlying disease may aid in the correction of iron deficiency. The USPSTF has concluded that evidence is insufficient to recommend for or against routine iron supplementation for nonanemic pregnant women.

■ DIETARY SUPPLEMENTATION AND THERAPEUTIC IRON PREPARATIONS

Treatment of IDA usually consists of dietary supplementation and administration of therapeutic iron preparations. Iron is poorly absorbed from vegetables, grain products, dairy products, and eggs; it is best absorbed from meat, fish, and poultry. Beverages have been shown to affect iron absorption. Meat, orange juice, and other ascorbic acid–rich foods should be included with meals, whereas milk and tea should be consumed in moderation between meals. In most cases of IDA, oral administration of iron therapy with soluble Fe^{2+} iron salts is appropriate.

CLINICAL CONTROVERSY

Daily Fe^{2+} sulfate is not tolerated by all patients and can be difficult to administer in populations of developing nations. Weekly rather than daily supplements have been used, with conflicting efficacy results. The weekly approach follows the natural pattern of mucosal cell iron turnover.

Fe^{2+} sulfate, succinate, lactate, fumarate, glycine sulfate, glutamate, and gluconate are absorbed similarly. The addition of copper, cobalt, molybdenum, or other minerals or hematinics provides no advantage but adds expense. The carbonyl iron may be advantageous because of lower risk for death in cases of accidental overdose. Iron is best absorbed in the reduced Fe^{2+} form, with maximal absorption occurring in the duodenum, primarily due to the acidic medium of the stomach. The presence of mucopolysaccharide chelator substances prevents the iron from precipitating and maintains the iron in a soluble form. In the alkaline environment of the small intestines, iron tends to form insoluble complexes that are unavailable for absorption. Slow-release or sustained-release iron preparations do not undergo sufficient dissolution until they reach the small intestines, which significantly reduces iron absorption and can attenuate the hematinic effects. This is especially true when enteric-coated preparations are used in achlorhydric patients. The dose of iron replacement therapy depends on the patient's ability to tolerate the administered iron. Tolerance of iron salts improves with a small initial dose and gradual escalation to the full dose. In patients with IDA, the general recommendation is administration of approximately 200 mg of elemental iron daily, usually in two or three divided doses to maximize tolerability. However, if patients cannot tolerate this daily dose of elemental iron, smaller amounts of elemental iron (e.g., single 325-mg tablet of Fe^{2+} sulfate) usually is sufficient to replace iron stores, albeit at a slower rate. Table 104–4 lists the percentage of elemental iron of commonly available iron salts. The percentage of iron absorbed decreases progressively as the dose increases, although the absolute amount absorbed increases. Iron preferably is administered at least 1 hour before meals because food interferes with iron absorption. Many patients must take iron with food because they experience nausea and diarrhea when iron is administered on an empty stomach.

Adverse reactions to therapeutic doses of iron are primarily gastrointestinal in nature and consist of a dark discoloration of feces, constipation or diarrhea, nausea, and vomiting. Gastrointestinal side effects usually are dose-related and are similar among iron salts when equivalent amounts of elemental iron are administered. Administration of smaller amounts of iron with each dose may minimize these adverse effects. Histamine$_2$ blockers or proton pump inhibitors that reduce gastric acidity may impair iron absorption. Table 104–5 lists drug interactions with iron. Failure to develop at least some mild gastrointestinal symptoms may suggest nonadherence. If these side effects become intolerable, the total daily dose can be decreased to 110 to 120 mg of elemental iron, or

TABLE 104-4 Oral Iron Products

Salt	Elemental Iron Percentage	Elemental Iron Provided
Ferrous sulfate	20%	60–65 mg/324–325 mg tablet 18 mg iron/5 mL syrup 44 mg iron/5 mL elixir 15 mg iron/0.6 mL drop
Ferrous sulfate (exsiccated)	30%	65 mg/200 mg tablet 60 mg/187 mg tablet 50 mg/160 mg tablet
Ferrous gluconate	12%	36 mg/325 mg tablet 27 mg/240 mg tablet
Ferrous fumarate	33%	33 mg/100 mg tablet 63–66 mg/200 mg tablet 106 mg/324–325 mg tablet 15 mg/0.6 mL drop 33 mg/5 mL suspension
Polysaccharide iron complex	100%	150 mg capsule 50 mg tablet 100 mg/5 mL elixir
Carbonyl iron	100%	50 mg caplet

the dose can be taken with meals. It should be noted, however, that administration of iron with meals reduces the amount of iron absorbed by more than half.

Failure to respond to appropriate treatment regimens necessitates reevaluation of the patient's condition. Occasionally a "therapeutic trial of iron" approach will be used to confirm a presumptive diagnosis of IDA. Common causes of treatment failure include poor patient adherence, inability to absorb iron, incorrect diagnosis, continued bleeding, or a concurrent condition that impairs full reticulocyte response. Even when iron deficiency is present, response may be impaired when a coexisting cause for anemia exists. Rarely a patient is not able to absorb iron, most often due to previous gastrectomy or celiac disease. Malabsorption can be ruled out by the iron test, in which plasma iron levels are determined at half-hour intervals for 2 hours following the administration of 50 mg of elemental iron as liquid Fe^{2+} sulfate. If plasma iron levels increase by >50 mcg/dl during this time, absorption is satisfactory. Regardless of the form of oral therapy used, treatment should continue for 3 to 6 months after the anemia is resolved to allow for repletion of iron stores and to prevent relapse.

TABLE 104-5 Iron Salt–Drug Interactions

Drugs That Decrease Iron Absorption	Object Drugs Affected by Iron
Al-, Mg-, and Ca^{+2}-containing antacids	Levodopa ↓ (chelates with iron)
Tetracycline and doxycycline	Methyldopa ↓ (decreases efficacy of methyldopa)
$Histamine_2$ antagonists	Levothyroxine ↓ (decreased efficacy of levothyroxine)
Proton pump inhibitors	Penicillamine ↓ (chelates with iron)
Cholestyramine	Fluoroquinolones ↓ (forms ferric ion–quinolone complex)
	Tetracycline and doxycycline ↓ (when administered within 2 hours of iron salt)
	Mycophenolate ↓ (decreases absorption)

PARENTERAL IRON THERAPY

When evidence of iron malabsorption or intolerance to orally administered iron is seen or long-term nonadherence is suspected, parenteral iron therapy may be warranted. Patients with significant blood loss who refuse transfusions and cannot take oral iron therapy also may require parenteral iron therapy. Parenteral iron does not lead to a quicker hematologic response than that of oral iron. The ideal parenteral iron supplement would be safe, efficacious, and convenient and would maintain consistent patient outcomes. Three different parenteral iron preparations currently available in the United States are iron dextran, sodium ferric gluconate, and iron sucrose (Table 104–6). They differ in their molecular size, degradation kinetics, bioavailability, and side-effect profiles. Although toxicity profiles of these agents differ, clinical studies indicate that each is efficacious. Most of the recent research on intravenous iron has been performed in hemodialysis patients. Dextran parenteral preparations have been associated with death due to anaphylactic reactions. These reactions may be related to immune reactions to the iron–carbohydrate or iron–dextran complex. Another theory for the anaphylaxis is the high-molecular-weight dextran component, which may be antigenic even when not complexed to iron. The safety profile of iron is largely assessed by spontaneous reports to the Food and Drug Administration (FDA) and retrospective and open-label prospective studies. Results of these studies suggest that Fe^{3+} gluconate and iron sucrose are safer than iron dextran.[22] The concern with parenteral iron is that iron may be released too quickly and overload the ability

TABLE 104-6 Comparison of Parenteral Iron Preparations

	Sodium Ferric Gluconate	Iron Dextran	Iron Sucrose
Amount of elemental iron	62.5 mg iron/5 mL	50 mg iron/mL	20 mg iron/mL
Molecular weight	Ferrlecit: 289,000–444,000 daltons	InFeD: 165,000 daltons DexFerrum: 267,000 daltons	Venofer: 34,000–60,000 daltons
Composition	Ferric oxide hydrate bonded to sucrose chelates with gluconate in a molar rate of 2 iron molecules to 1 gluconate molecule	Complex of ferric hydroxide and dextran	Complex of polynuclear iron hydroxide in sucrose
Preservative	Benzyl alcohol 9 mg/5 mL 20% (975 mg in 62.5 mg iron)	None	None
Indication	Treatment of iron-deficiency anemia in patients undergoing chronic hemodialysis who are receiving supplemental erythropoietin therapy	Treatment of patients with documented iron deficiency in whom oral therapy is unsatisfactory or impossible	Treatment of iron-deficiency anemia in patients undergoing chronic hemodialysis who are receiving supplemental epoetin alfa therapy
Warning	No black box warning; hypersensitivity reactions	Black box warning: anaphylactic-type reactions	Black box warning: anaphylactic-type reactions
IM injection	No	Yes	No
Usual dose	125 mg (10 mL) diluted in 100 mL normal saline, infused over 60 minutes; also can be administered as a slow IV injection (rate of 12.5 mg/min).	100 mg undiluted at a rate not to exceed 50 mg (1 mL) per min	100 mg into the dialysis line at a rate of 1 mL (20 mg of iron) undiluted solution per minute
Treatment	8 doses × 125 mg = 1,000 mg	10 doses × 100 mg = 1,000 mg	Up to 10 doses × 100 mg = 1,000 mg
Common adverse effects	Cramps, nausea and vomiting, flushing, hypotension, rash, pruritus	Pain and brown staining at injection site, flushing, hypotension, fever, chills, myalgia, anaphylaxis	Leg cramps, hypotension

of transferrin to bind it, leading to free iron reactions that can interfere with neutrophil function.

Iron dextran, a complex of Fe^{3+} hydroxide and the carbohydrate dextran, contains 50 mg of iron per milliliter and can be given via the intramuscular or intravenous route. Different brands of iron dextran are available and differ in their molecular weight. They are not interchangeable.

Iron dextran must be processed by macrophages for the iron to be biologically available. The absorption and metabolism vary with the route and amount of drug given. Absorption of an intramuscular dose of iron dextran occurs in two phases. During the first 72 hours, iron dextran is absorbed primarily through the lymphatics into the left superior vena cava. A smaller amount is absorbed directly through the intramuscular capillary network into the blood. A second, slower phase involves uptake of the iron–dextran complex by macrophages, with subsequent transport through the lymphatics into the blood. The macrophages phagocytize the iron–dextran complex and cleave the dextran moiety, which makes free iron available to the body as circulating iron, transferrin-bound iron, or storage iron (ferritin and hemosiderin). Iron dextran can remain within these cells for many months. Approximately 60% of an intramuscular dose of iron dextran is absorbed after 3 days, and up to 90% is absorbed within 3 weeks. The remainder is absorbed slowly over several months or longer.

When intravenous iron dextran is given, the iron is taken up immediately by the mononuclear phagocytic system. Small-to-intermediate intravenous doses can be cleared from the plasma within 3 days of administration. In contrast, larger intravenous doses of iron dextran are processed by the mononuclear phagocytic system at a constant rate of 10 to 20 mg/h and result in high plasma concentrations of iron dextran for as long as 3 weeks.

The iron dextran package insert carries a black box warning regarding the risk of anaphylaxis and a test dose is required before administration of the repletion dose. Methods of intravenous administration include multiple slow injections of undiluted iron dextran solution or an infusion of a diluted preparation. This latter method often is referred to as *total dose infusion.* The intramuscular administration of iron dextran should take place via Z-tract injection technique (a technique for handling intramuscular injections of irritating substances with minimal tracking of the medication through surrounding tissues) to minimize staining of the skin. Because each intramuscular dose is limited to 2 mL (100 mg of iron), multiple injections often are required. Daily intramuscular doses should not exceed 25 mg in patients weighing less than 5 kg, 50 mg in patients weighing less than 10 kg, and 100 mg in all other patients. Problems with intramuscular administration include patient discomfort, unpredictable delivery, sterile abscesses, tissue necrosis, and atrophy. In addition, up to 30% of an administered dose remains physiologically unavailable. For these reasons, the intravenous route is the preferred parenteral route of administration.

Equations for calculating the appropriate dose of parenteral iron in patients with IDA or anemia secondary to blood loss are listed in Table 104–7. Doses given by intravenous administration should not exceed 50 mg of iron per minute (1 mL/min). It is suggested that all patients considered for an iron dextran injection receive a test dose of 25 mg intramuscularly or intravenously, or a 5- to 10-minute infusion of the diluted solution. Patients then should be observed for more than 1 hour for untoward reactions. An anaphylaxis-like reaction generally responds to intravenous epinephrine, diphenhydramine, and corticosteroids. If the test dose is tolerated, patients receiving total dose infusions can undergo infusion of the remaining solution during the next 2 to 6 hours.

Total replacement doses of intravenous iron dextran have been given as a single dose, diluted in 250 to 1,000 mL normal saline or 5% dextrose in water and infused over 4 to 6 hours. A test dose still is required. The ability to give a total dose infusion is a benefit of iron dextran over the other parenteral iron products. Iron dextran is best utilized when smaller frequent doses of sodium ferric gluconate or iron sucrose are impractical, as with peritoneal dialysis.

TABLE 104-7 Equations for Calculating Doses of Parenteral Iron

In patients with iron deficiency anemia:
Adults + children >15 kg
Dose (mL) = 0.0442 (Desired Hb – Observed Hb) × LBW + (0.26 × LBW)
LBW males = 50 kg + (2.3 × inches over 5 ft)
LBW females = 45.5 kg + (2.3 × inches over 5 ft)
Children 5–15 kg
Dose (mL) = 0.0442 (Desired Hb – Observed Hb) × W + (0.26 × W)
In patients with anemia secondary to blood loss (hemorrhagic diathesis or long-term dialysis):
mg of iron = blood loss × hematocrit,
where blood loss is in milliliters and hematocrit is expressed as a decimal fraction.

Hb, hemoglobin; LBW, lean body weight; mL, milliliter; W, weight.

Patients who receive total dose infusions are at higher risk for adverse reactions, such as arthralgias, myalgias, flushing, malaise, and fever. Other adverse reactions of iron dextran include staining of the skin, pain at the injection site, allergic reactions, and rarely anaphylaxis. Patients most likely to experience adverse effects with iron dextran include individuals with a history of allergies, asthma, or inflammatory diseases. Patients with preexisting immune-mediated diseases, such as active rheumatoid arthritis or systemic lupus erythematosus, are considered at high risk for adverse reactions because of their hyperreactive immune response capabilities.

Sodium ferric gluconate is a complex of iron bound to one gluconate and four sucrose molecules in a repeating pattern. Its molecular weight is 289,000 to 440,000 daltons. Sodium ferric gluconate is available in an aqueous solution. No direct transfer of iron from the Fe^{3+} gluconate to the transferrin occurs. The complex is taken up quickly by the mononuclear phagocytic system and has a half-life of approximately 1 hour in the bloodstream. It is supplied in 5-mL ampules containing 62.5 mg of elemental iron. It has been available in Europe since 1959 and was introduced for use in the United States in 1999. It is FDA-indicated for iron supplementation in hemodialysis patients. The difference in the time of availability between Europe and the United States makes difficult the comparison of allergy and anaphylaxis reports for sodium ferric gluconate complex and iron dextran. Sodium ferric gluconate appears to produce fewer anaphylactic reactions than does iron dextran. According to the package insert, a test dose of sodium ferric gluconate is not required. If given, a test dose is administered as 2 mL (25 mg of elemental iron) in 50 mL normal saline intravenously over 60 minutes. Although sodium ferric gluconate can be administered undiluted as a slow intravenous injection (up to 12.5 mg/min), it is most commonly administered as 10 mL (125 mg of elemental iron) in 100 mL normal saline intravenously over 1 hour. Most hemodialysis patients require a minimum total of 1 g of elemental iron over eight dialysis sessions to replete their stores. Side effects of sodium ferric gluconate include cramps, nausea, vomiting, flushing, hypotension, intense upper gastric pain, rash, and pruritus.

Iron sucrose is a polynuclear iron (III) hydroxide in sucrose complex with a molecular weight of approximately 34,000 to 60,000 daltons. It is available in 5-mL single-dose vials. Each vial contains 100 mg (20 mg/mL) of iron sucrose. Following intravenous administration of iron sucrose, the iron is released directly from the circulating iron sucrose to the transferrin and is taken up by the mononuclear phagocytic system and metabolized. The half-life is approximately 6 hours, with a volume of distribution similar to that of iron dextran. For adults undergoing hemodialysis, iron sucrose is administered as an intravenous dose of 100 mg one to three times per week to a total dose of 1,000 mg in 10 doses. It can be given directly into the dialysis line by slow intravenous injection (20 mg iron [1 mL] per minute) or via infusion without the requirement for a test dose. For infusion, it must be diluted in normal saline (maximum 100 mL) immediately prior to use and infused over a minimum of 15 minutes. Iron sucrose injection should not be administered concomitantly with oral iron preparations because it will reduce the absorption of oral iron. Adverse effects include leg cramps and hypotension. Iron sucrose has been shown to be well tolerated but has less-than-expected efficacy at maintaining Hb >11 g/dL and transferrin saturation >25%.[23] Approximately 50% of patients studied had serum ferritin levels >1,100 ng/mL, which suggests iron overload. The reduced hematologic response and development of high serum ferritin levels may be due to oversaturation of transferrin and release of free iron. Varying doses of iron sucrose may not produce these results. Overall, iron sucrose has been shown to be safe and efficacious.

■ TRANSFUSIONS

Another form of treatment involves blood transfusions. The decision to manage anemia with blood transfusions is based on the evaluation of risks and benefits. Transfusion of allogeneic blood is indicated in acute situations of blood loss when hemodynamic support is needed. Blood transfusion in chronic anemia can elevate Hb concentration in the short term but does not address the underlying disorder. In critically ill patients, the risk of infection, length of stay, and economic cost increase with each unit of transfused packed RBCs.[24] Once Hct decreases to <30%, the oxygen-carrying capacity in patients with coronary disease is dangerously compromised, and ischemia can occur. Tachycardia, angina, ischemic patterns on electrocardiogram, cerebrovascular insufficiency, postural hypotension, and prerenal azotemia may suggest that transfusions should be provided to maintain the Hct >30%. An exception to this treatment option is patients who have developed low Hct values over extended time periods. These patients often demonstrate cardiac compromise after transfusion despite Hct levels in the 20% range. These patients should receive iron therapy, followed by transfusion only if necessary. Guidelines for transfusion in perisurgical anemias suggest 6 to 8 g/dL of Hb as a threshold for treatment, with no benefit at levels >10 g/dL.[25]

Evaluation of Therapeutic Outcomes

A positive response to a trial of oral iron therapy results in a modest reticulocytosis in 5 to 7 days, with an increase in Hb at a rate of approximately 2 to 4 g/dL every 3 weeks until Hb is normalized. As the Hb level approaches normal, the rate of increase slows progressively. A Hb response of <2 g/dL over a 3-week period warrants further evaluation. If the patient does not develop reticulocytosis, reevaluation of the diagnosis or iron replacement therapy is necessary.

Iron therapy should continue for a period sufficient for complete restoration of iron stores. Serum ferritin concentrations should return to the normal range prior to discontinuation of iron. The time interval required to accomplish this goal varies, although at least 3 to 6 months of therapy usually is warranted. Patients with negative iron balances caused by bleeding may require iron replacement therapy for only 1 month after correction of the underlying lesion, whereas patients with recurrent negative balances may require long-term treatment with as little as 30 to 60 mg of elemental iron daily.

When large amounts of parenteral iron are administered, by either total dose infusion or multiple intramuscular or intravenous doses, the patient's iron status should be closely monitored. For patients intolerant of iron dextran, ferric gluconate and iron sucrose are alternatives. Cost, number of infusions, impact on need to transfuse, and concurrent EPO supplementation affect the choice of parenteral iron products. Patients receiving regular intravenous iron should be monitored for clinical or laboratory evidence of iron toxicity or overload. Iron overload may be indicated by abnormal hepatic function tests, serum ferritin >800 ng/mL, or transferrin saturation >50%. Serum ferritin and transferrin saturation should be measured in the first week after doses of 100 to 200 mg and 2 weeks after larger intravenous iron doses. Hb and Hct should be measured weekly, and serum iron and ferritin levels should be measured at least monthly. Serum iron values can be obtained reliably 48 hours after intravenous dosing.

MEGALOBLASTIC ANEMIAS

Macrocytic anemias are divided into megaloblastic and nonmegaloblastic anemias. Macrocytosis, as seen in megaloblastic anemias, is caused by abnormal DNA metabolism resulting from vitamin B_{12} or folate deficiency. It also can be caused by administration of various drugs, such as hydroxyurea, zidovudine, cytosine arabinoside, methotrexate, azathioprine, 6-mercaptopurine, and cladribine.

In vitamin B_{12} or folate deficiency anemia, megaloblastosis results from interference with folic acid– and vitamin B_{12}–interdependent nucleic acid synthesis in the immature erythrocyte. The rate of RNA and cytoplasm production exceeds the rate of DNA production. The maturation process is retarded, resulting in immature large RBCs (macrocytosis). RNA and DNA synthesis depend on a series of reactions catalyzed by vitamin B_{12} and folic acid because of their role in the conversion of uridine to thymidine. As shown in Fig. 104–4, dietary folates are absorbed in this process and converted to 5-methyl-tetrahydrofolate (A), which then is converted via a B_{12}-dependent reaction (B) to tetrahydrofolate (C). After gaining a carbon, tetrahydrofolate is converted to 5,10-methyl-tetrahydrofolate (D), a folate cofactor used by thymidylate synthetase (E) in the biosynthesis of nucleic acids. The 5,10-methyl-tetrahydrofolate cofactor is converted to dihydrofolate (F) during biosynthesis. Dihydrofolate reductase normally reduces dihydrofolate back to tetrahydrofolate (C), which can again pick up a carbon and be recycled to produce more 5,10-methyl-tetrahydrofolate (D).

Although vitamin B_{12} deficiency and folate deficiency are common causes of macrocytosis, other possible causes must be considered if these deficiencies are not found. Other causes of macrocytosis include (a) a shift to immature or stressed RBCs as seen in reticulocytosis, aplastic anemia, and pure RBC aplasia; (b) a primary bone marrow disorder such as myelodysplastic syndromes, congenital dyserythropoietic anemias, and large granular lymphocyte leukemia; (c) lipid abnormalities as seen with liver disease,

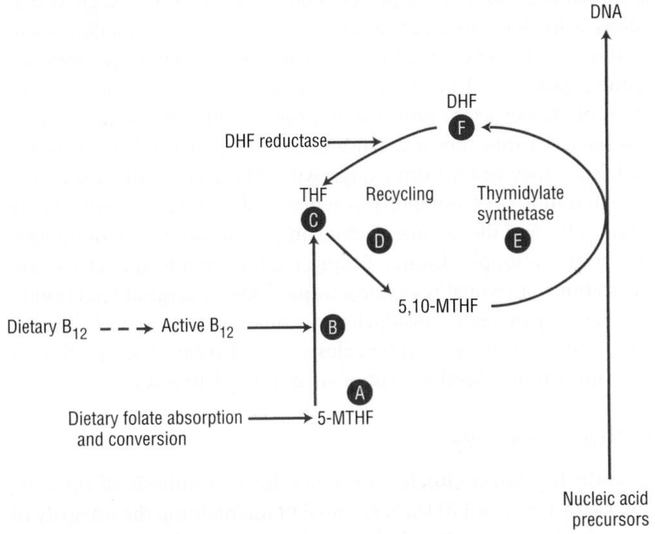

FIGURE 104-4. Drug-induced megaloblastosis. (DHF, dihydrofolate; 5-MTHF, 5-methyl-tetrahydrofolate; 5,10-MTHF, 5,10-methyl-tetrahydrofolate THF; THF, tetrahydrofolate.)

hypothyroidism, or hyperlipidemia; and (d) unknown mechanisms resulting from alcohol abuse and multiple myeloma. Macrocytosis is the most typical morphologic abnormality associated with excessive alcohol consumption. Even with adequate folate and vitamin B_{12} levels and the absence of liver disease, patients may present with an alcohol-induced macrocytosis. Cessation of alcohol ingestion results in resolution of the macrocytosis within a couple of months.

VITAMIN B_{12} DEFICIENCY ANEMIA

Epidemiology

The prevalence of pernicious anemia in the United States has been estimated at 151 per 100,000 and is slightly more common in women.[26] However, this figure may be underestimated because of the aging population and universal use of gastric acid–suppressing agents, which may inhibit the release of cobalamin from food. Older adults in the United States have a high prevalence (up to 15%) of elevated MMA levels and associated low or low–normal vitamin B_{12} levels, likely due to atrophic gastritis and malabsorption of food-bound vitamin B_{12}.[26]

Etiology

❺ The three major causes of vitamin B_{12} deficiency are inadequate intake, malabsorption syndromes, and inadequate utilization. Inadequate dietary consumption of vitamin B_{12} is rare. It usually occurs only in patients who are strict vegans and their breast-fed infants, chronic alcoholics, and elderly patients who consume a "tea and toast" diet because of financial limitations or poor dentition. Decreased vitamin B_{12} absorption is seen in patients with pernicious anemia, which is caused by the absence of intrinsic factor due to autoimmune destruction of the gastric parietal cells, atrophy of the gastric mucosa, or stomach surgery. It is most commonly seen in Europeans of northern descent and in African Americans; it is rarely diagnosed in patients younger than 35 years. Patients with pernicious anemia are prone to gastric polyps and have an increased incidence of stomach cancer. The most frequent cause of low serum B_{12} levels is cobalamin malabsorption, which results in the inability of vitamin B_{12} to be cleaved and released from proteins in food because of inadequate gastric acid production.[27] Conditions leading to this phenomenon include subtotal gastrectomy, atrophic gastritis resulting in decreased acid pepsin production, and prolonged use of acid suppression therapy. In these individuals, supplemental cobalamin is well absorbed because it is not protein bound. Some experts suggest that adults older than 50 years consume vitamin B_{12} in the crystalline form to meet the recommended dietary allowance as this form does not require gastric acid or enzymes for digestion.[28] Additionally, treatment of *Helicobacter pylori* may improve vitamin B_{12} status because this bacterial infection is a cause of chronic gastritis.[29] Vitamin B_{12} deficiency may result from overgrowth of bacteria in the bowel that use vitamin B_{12} or from injury or removal of ileal receptor sites where vitamin B_{12} and the intrinsic factor complex are absorbed. Blind loop syndrome, Whipple disease, Zollinger-Ellison syndrome, tapeworm infestations, intestinal resections, tropical sprue, surgical resection of the ileus, pancreatic insufficiency, inflammatory bowel disease, advanced liver disease, tuberculosis, and Crohn disease all may contribute to the development of vitamin B_{12} deficiency.[30]

Pathophysiology

Vitamin B_{12} works closely with folate in the synthesis of building blocks for DNA and RNA, is essential in maintaining the integrity of the neurologic system, and plays a role in fatty acid biosynthesis and energy production. It is a water-soluble vitamin obtained exogenously by ingestion of meat, fish, poultry, dairy products, and fortified cereals. Body stores range from 2 to 5 mg, of which approximately half is in the liver. The recommended daily allowance is 2 mcg in adults and 2.6 mcg in pregnant or breast-feeding women. The average western diet provides 5 to 7 mcg of vitamin B_{12} daily, of which 1 to 5 mcg is absorbed. Vitamin B_{12} deficiency takes several years to develop following vitamin deprivation because of efficient enterohepatic circulation of the vitamin.

Once dietary cobalamin enters the stomach, pepsin and hydrochloric acid release the cobalamin from animal proteins. The free cobalamin then binds to R-protein, which is released from parietal and salivary cells. In the duodenum, the cobalamin bound to R-protein is joined by cobalamin–R-protein complexes that have been secreted in the bile. Pancreatic enzymes degrade both biliary and dietary cobalamin–R-protein complexes, releasing free cobalamin. The cobalamin then binds with intrinsic factor that serves as a cell-directed carrier protein similar to transferrin for iron. This complex attaches to mucosal cell receptors (cubilin) in the distal ileum, the intrinsic factor is discarded, and the cobalamin is bound to transport proteins (transcobalamin I, II, and III). The cobalamin bound to transcobalamin II is secreted into the circulation and is taken up by the liver, bone marrow, and other cells via endocytosis. The cobalamin then is converted into its two coenzyme forms (methylcobalamin and adenosylcobalamin). Consequently, most circulating cobalamin is bound to transcobalamin I and transcobalamin III. However, an alternate pathway for vitamin B_{12} absorption independent of intrinsic factor or an intact terminal ileum accounts for a small amount of vitamin B_{12} absorption.[30] This alternate pathway involves passive diffusion and accounts for approximately 1% absorption of the ingested vitamin B_{12}.

Laboratory Findings

In macrocytic anemias, MCV usually is elevated to 110 to 140 fL, but some patients deficient in vitamin B_{12} may have a normal MCV. Mild leukopenia and thrombocytopenia are often present because abnormal DNA synthesis can affect all blood cells. Advanced cases of vitamin B_{12} deficiency may result in pancytopenia. A peripheral blood smear demonstrates macrocytosis accompanied by hypersegmented polymorphonuclear leukocytes (one of the earliest and most specific indications of this disease), oval macrocytes, anisocytosis, and poikilocytosis. Serum lactate dehydrogenase and indirect bilirubin levels may be elevated as a result of hemolysis or ineffective erythropoiesis. Other laboratory findings include a low reticulocyte count, low serum vitamin B_{12} level (<150 pg/mL), and low Hct. Bone marrow biopsy will reveal marked erythroid hyperplasia and megaloblastic changes in the cells of erythroid lineage.

In the early stages of vitamin B_{12} deficiency, classic signs and symptoms of megaloblastic anemia may not be evident, and serum levels of vitamin B_{12} may be within normal limits. Therefore, measurement of MMA and homocysteine is useful because these parameters are often the first to change. Because MMA and homocysteine are involved in enzymatic reactions that depend on vitamin B_{12}, a deficiency in vitamin B_{12} leads to accumulation of serum MMA and homocysteine. Elevations in MMA are more specific for vitamin B_{12} deficiency, whereas elevated homocysteine can be indicative of either vitamin B_{12} or folic acid deficiency but offers greater specificity for folate plasma levels. Low levels of vitamin B_{12} result in hyperhomocysteinemia, which some studies have reported to be an independent risk factor for cerebrovascular, peripheral vascular, coronary, and venous thromboembolic disease.[31]

CLINICAL CONTROVERSY

Hyperhomocysteinemia may be linked to dementia and Alzheimer's disease. Controversy exists whether supplementation with vitamin B_{12} or folate for reducing homocysteine levels would have a beneficial effect on cognition.

Blood levels should be drawn in all patients with suspected vitamin B_{12} deficiency. Vitamin B_{12} values <150 pg/mL in patients with macrocytosis, hypersegmented polymorphonuclear leukocytes, peripheral neuropathy, or dementia are suggestive of B_{12} deficiency. Approximately one third of patients with pernicious anemia do not demonstrate macrocytosis if their condition is complicated by iron deficiency, thalassemia, or a predominant neurologic involvement.

Vitamin B_{12} values of 200 to 300 pg/mL are suggestive of depletion, and patients should undergo repeated testing in 1 to 3 months. A Schilling test may be performed to diagnose pernicious anemia, but the usefulness of this test is questionable and rarely alters the clinical management of the vitamin B_{12} deficiency. The Schilling test was once performed to determine whether replacement of vitamin B_{12} should occur via an oral or parenteral route, but evidence now shows that oral replacement is as efficacious as parenteral supplementation because of the vitamin B_{12} absorption pathway independent of intrinsic factor. Other limitations to the Schilling test include its complicated protocol, the need for a 24-hour urine collection, certification issues, difficulty in obtaining radiolabeled vitamin B_{12}, and difficulty in interpreting results in patients with renal insufficiency.[30]

Other potentially useful tests include antibody testing and serum gastrin levels. Positive anti–intrinsic factor antibodies may be present in approximately half of patients with pernicious anemia but is highly specific for the disease.[16] In addition, an estimated 85% of patients have anti–parietal cell antibodies, but this test is not specific because 3% to 10% of healthy patients have these antibodies.[16] When evaluating low serum vitamin B_{12} levels, other causes besides dietary deprivation and malabsorption should be ruled out. For example, levels may be falsely low in patients receiving antibiotics, anticonvulsants, cytotoxic agents, oral contraceptives, and high-dose vitamin C.

TABLE 104-8 Good Sources of Vitamin B_{12}

Food	Serving Size	Amount (mcg)
Beef liver, cooked	3 oz	60
Breakfast cereal, fortified (100%)	3/4 cup	6
Rainbow trout, cooked	3 oz	5.3
Sockeye salmon, cooked	3 oz	4.9
Beef, cooked	3 oz	2.1
Breakfast cereal, fortified (25%)	3/4 cup	1.5
Haddock, cooked	3 oz	1.2
Clams, breaded and fried	3/4 cup	1.1
Oysters, breaded and fried	6 pieces	1
Tuna, canned in water	3 oz	0.9
Milk	1 cup	0.9
Yogurt	8 oz	0.9

TREATMENT

Vitamin B_{12} Deficiency Anemia

The goals of treatment for vitamin B_{12} deficiency include reversal of hematologic manifestations, replacement of body stores, and prevention or resolution of neurologic manifestations. Early treatment is of paramount importance because neurologic damage may be irreversible if the deficiency is not detected and corrected within months. Permanent disabilities may range from mild paresthesias and numbness to memory loss and outright psychosis. In addition to replacement therapy, any underlying etiology that is treatable, such as bacterial overgrowth, should be remedied. In the rare cases of nutritional deficiency, oral or parenteral administration of vitamin B_{12} is beneficial. Patients should be counseled on the types of foods high in vitamin B_{12} content (Table 104–8). Oral administration of vitamin B_{12} also can be used effectively to treat pernicious anemia or cobalamin deficiency due to ileal resection but in much larger doses than those used to treat other causes of vitamin B_{12} deficiency. Oral replacement therapy can be used because of the aforementioned alternate pathway of absorption, independent of intrinsic factor. Daily oral doses (1–2 mg) of vitamin B_{12} is as effective as intramuscular administration in achieving hematologic and neurologic responses.[32] If vitamin B_{12} levels are marginally low and either MMA or both MMA and homocysteine levels are elevated, administration of 1 mg of oral vitamin B_{12} daily should be strongly considered.[33] Timed-release preparations of oral cobalamin should be avoided.[34] Nonprescription 1-mg cobalamin tablets are available. The only contraindications to oral replacement therapy are the inability to take medications orally, diarrhea, and vomiting. A commonly used initial parenteral vitamin B_{12} regimen consists of daily injections of 1,000 mcg of cyanocobalamin for 1 week to saturate vitamin B_{12} stores in the body and resolve clinical manifestations of the deficiency. Thereafter, it can be given weekly for 1 month and monthly thereafter for maintenance. Vitamin B_{12} also can be effectively administered parenterally in 2- to 3-month increments.[35] Hydroxocobalamin is a less popular formulation of parenteral vitamin B_{12}. Its low utilization rate may be due to the occasional development of antibodies to the hydroxocobalamin–transcobalamin II complex. Parenteral therapy is preferred for patients exhibiting neurologic symptoms until resolution of symptoms and hematologic indices because the most rapid-acting therapy is necessary.[36] When patients are converted from the parenteral to the oral form of cobalamin, 1 mg of oral cobalamin daily can be initiated on the due date of the next injection.

In addition to the oral and parenteral forms, vitamin B_{12} is available as a nasal spray for patients in remission following intramuscular vitamin B_{12} therapy who have no nervous system involvement. The nasal spray is administered once weekly. Intranasal administration should be avoided in patients with nasal diseases or those receiving medications intranasally in the same nostril. Patients should not administer the spray 1 hour before or after ingestion of hot foods or beverages, which can impair cobalamin absorption. The efficacy of the nasal spray formulation has not been well studied, and it should be used for maintenance therapy only after hematologic parameters have normalized.

Potential adverse effects with vitamin B_{12} replacement therapy are rare. Uncommon side effects include hyperuricemia and hypokalemia due to marked increase in potassium utilization during production of new hematopoietic cells. Rebound thrombocytosis may precipitate thrombotic events. Another side effect of vitamin B_{12} therapy is fluid retention, which is more likely to occur in patients with compromised cardiovascular status because of an expansion in intravascular volume secondary to the sudden increase in production of RBCs. Rare cases of anaphylaxis with parenteral administration of cobalamin have been reported.

Evaluation of Therapeutic Outcomes

Most patients respond rapidly to vitamin B_{12} therapy. The patient will experience an improvement in strength and well-being within a few days. If glossitis is present, improvement is seen within 24 hours. Bone marrow becomes normoblastic after 24 hours but is not evident in the plasma for another 7 days. Reticulocytosis is evident in 2 to 5 days and peaks around day 7. Hb begins to rise after the first week, and leukocyte and platelet counts normalize after approximately 7 days. Hypersegmented neutrophils persist for approximately 2 weeks. A CBC count and serum cobalamin level usually are drawn 1 to 2 months after initiation of therapy and 3 to 6 months thereafter for surveillance monitoring. Homocysteine and MMA levels should be repeated 2 to 3 months after initiation of replacement therapy to evaluate for normalization of levels, although levels begin to decrease in 1 to 2 weeks. Neuropsychiatric signs and symptoms can be reversible if treated early. If permanent neurologic damage has resulted, progression should cease with replacement therapy. Slow response to therapy or failure to observe normalization of laboratory results may suggest the presence of an additional abnormality such as iron deficiency, thalassemia trait, infection, malignancy, or misdiagnosis.

FOLIC ACID DEFICIENCY ANEMIA

Epidemiology

Folic acid deficiency is one of the most common vitamin deficiencies occurring in the United States, largely as a result of its association with excessive alcohol intake and pregnancy.

Etiology

❻ Major causes of folic acid deficiency include inadequate intake, decreased absorption, hyperutilization, and inadequate utilization. Because folic acid deficiency is associated with poor eating habits, it is common in elderly patients, teenagers whose diets consist of "junk food," alcoholics, food faddists, the poverty stricken, and those who are chronically ill or in demented states. Folic acid absorption may decrease in patients who have malabsorption syndromes or those who have received certain drugs. In alcoholics with poor dietary habits, alcohol interferes with folic acid absorption, interferes with folic acid utilization at the cellular level, and decreases hepatic stores of folic acid.

Hyperutilization of folic acid may occur when the rate of cellular division is increased, as seen in pregnant women; patients with hemolytic anemia, myelofibrosis, malignancy, chronic inflammatory disorders such as Crohn disease, rheumatoid arthritis, or psoriasis; patients undergoing long-term dialysis; burn patients; and in adolescents and infants during their growth spurts. This hyperutilization eventually can lead to anemia, particularly when the daily intake of folate is borderline, resulting in inadequate replacement of folate stores.

Several drugs have been reported to cause a folic acid deficiency megaloblastic anemia. Some drugs (e.g., azathioprine, 6-mercaptopurine, 5-fluorouracil, hydroxyurea, and zidovudine) directly inhibit DNA synthesis. Other drugs are folate antagonists; the most toxic is methotrexate (other examples include pentamidine, trimethoprim, and triamterene). A number of drugs (e.g., phenytoin, phenobarbital and primidone) antagonize folate via poorly understood mechanisms but are thought to reduce vitamin absorption by the intestine (see Chap. 107). Because folic acid doses as low as 1 mg/day may affect serum phenytoin levels, routine folic acid supplementation is not generally recommended. The decline in phenytoin concentration usually is evidenced within the first 10 days and may decrease phenytoin levels by 15% to 50%.[37]

Pathophysiology

Folic acid is a water-soluble vitamin readily destroyed by cooking or processing. It is necessary for the production of nucleic acids, proteins, amino acids, purines, and thymine, and hence DNA and RNA. It acts as a methyl donor to form methylcobalamin, which is used in the remethylation of homocysteine to methionine. Because humans are unable to synthesize sufficient folate to meet total daily requirements, they depend on dietary sources. Major dietary sources of folate include fresh, green, leafy vegetables, citrus fruits, yeast, mushrooms, dairy products, and animal organs such as liver and kidney. Most folate in food is present in the polyglutamate form, which must be broken down into the monoglutamate form prior to absorption in the small intestine. Once absorbed, dietary folate must be converted to the active form tetrahydrofolate through a cobalamin-dependent reaction. In 1997 the U.S. government mandated the fortification of grain products with folic acid in an attempt to increase the dietary intake of folate by 100 mcg of folate daily per person. This amount of supplementation was chosen to decrease the incidence of neural tube defects without masking occult vitamin B_{12} deficiency. As a result of grain product fortification, neural tube defect frequency has decreased by 25% to 30%.[38] Even though body demands for folate are high because of high rates of RBC synthesis and turnover, the minimum daily requirement is 50 to 100 mcg. In the general population, the recommended daily allowance for folate is 400 mcg in nonpregnant females, 600 mcg for pregnant females, and 500 mcg for lactating females.[39] Because the body stores approximately 5 to 10 mg of folate, primarily in the liver, cessation of dietary folate intake can result in megaloblastosis within 4 to 5 months. Folate is distributed to the other tissues primarily via enterohepatic recirculation. The methylated form of folate is reabsorbed from the bile into the serum. As folate enters the tissues, including erythrocytes, it endures for the remaining life span of the cell.

Laboratory Findings

It is of paramount importance to rule out vitamin B_{12} deficiency when folate deficiency is suspected. Laboratory changes associated with folate deficiency are similar to those seen in vitamin B_{12} deficiency, except vitamin B_{12} levels are normal. Serum folate levels decrease to less than 3 ng/mL within a few days of reduced dietary folate intake. The RBC folate level (<150 ng/mL) also declines, and levels remain constant throughout the life span of the erythrocyte. An estimated 60% of patients with pernicious anemia have falsely low RBC folate levels, probably because of the cobalamin requirement for normal transfer of methyl-tetrahydrofolate from plasma to cells.[16] Additionally, if serum or erythrocyte folate levels are borderline, serum homocysteine usually is increased with a folic acid deficiency. If serum MMA levels also are elevated, vitamin B_{12} deficiency must be ruled out given that folate does not participate in MMA metabolism.

TREATMENT

Folic Acid Deficiency Anemia

Therapy for folic acid deficiency consists of administration of exogenous folic acid to induce hematologic remission, replace body stores, and resolve signs and symptoms. In most cases, 1 mg daily is sufficient to replace stores, except in cases of deficiency due to malabsorption, in which case doses of 1 to 5 mg daily may be necessary. Parenteral folic acid is available but rarely necessary. Synthetic folic acid is almost completely absorbed by the gastrointestinal tract and is converted to tetrahydrofolate without cobalamin. Therapy should continue for approximately 4 months if the underlying cause of the deficiency can be identified and corrected to allow for clearance of all folate-deficient RBCs from the circulation. Long-term folate administration may be necessary in chronic conditions associated with increased folate requirements. Patients with a folic acid deficiency should be placed on diets containing foods high in folate (Table 104–9). Low-dose folate therapy (500 mcg daily) can be administered when anticonvulsant drugs produce a megaloblastic anemia so that discontinuation of anticonvulsant therapy may not be necessary. Adverse effects have not been reported with folic acid doses used for replacement therapy. It is considered nontoxic at high doses and is rapidly excreted in the urine.

Although megaloblastic anemia during pregnancy is rare, the most common cause is folate deficiency. The condition usually manifests as an underweight premature infant and suboptimal health of the mother. Periconceptional folic acid supplementation is recommended to decrease the occurrence and recurrence of neural tube defects, specifically anencephaly and spina bifida. Folic acid

TABLE 104-9 Good Sources of Folate

Food	Serving	Amount (mcg)
Chicken liver	3.5 oz	770
Cereal	1/2 to 1 1/2 cups	100–400
Lentils, cooked	1/2 cup	180
Chickpeas	1/2 cup	141
Asparagus	1/2 cup	132
Spinach, cooked	1/2 cup	131
Black beans	1/2 cup	128
Pasta	2 oz	100–120
Kidney beans	1/2 cup	115
Lima beans	1/2 cup	78
White rice, cooked	3/4 cup	60
Tomato juice	1 cup	48
Brussels sprouts	1/2 cup	47
Orange	1 medium	47

supplementation at a dose of 400 mcg daily is recommended in low-risk women. Women who have previously given birth to offspring with neural tube defects or those with a family history of neural tube defects should ingest 4 mg daily of folic acid.[37,38,40] Periconceptual use of a multivitamin containing folic acid is associated with a decreased incidence of congenital heart defects and possibly of orofacial clefts.[41] Higher levels of folic acid supplementation should not be attained via ingestion of excess multivitamins because of the risk for vitamin A toxicity.[40] It is essential that women in their childbearing years maintain adequate folic acid intake.

Evaluation of Therapeutic Outcomes

Symptomatic improvement, as evidenced by increased alertness, appetite, and cooperation, often occurs early during the course of treatment. Reticulocytosis occurs within 2 to 3 days and peaks within 5 to 8 days after beginning therapy. Hct begins to rise within 2 weeks and should reach normal levels within 2 months. MCV initially increases because of an increase in reticulocytes but gradually decreases to normal.

ANEMIA OF CHRONIC DISEASE

Epidemiology

❼ ACD is one of the most common forms of anemia seen clinically, particularly among the elderly. It is especially important in the differential diagnosis of iron deficiency. Because ACD, as the name implies, is associated with other prominent disease states, the usual signs and symptoms are often overlooked. The diagnosis of ACD usually is one of exclusion, with particular emphasis on the possibility of IDA as the primary anemia or as a coexistent anemia with ACD because of chronic disease–associated conditions (e.g., gastrointestinal blood loss from aspirin, other nonsteroidal antiinflammatory drugs, or steroids) or malignancy-associated bleeding. ACD is often observed in patients with diseases that last longer than 1 to 2 months, although it can occur in conditions with a fairly rapid onset of several weeks, such as pneumonia. It can coexist with anemia of chronic kidney disease, chemotherapy-induced anemia, and AIDS-related anemia. Anemia is the most common hematologic abnormality associated with human immunodeficiency virus (HIV), and the yearly incidence of developing anemia increases with disease progression.[42] Anemia occurs commonly in patients with heart failure. A 1-g/dL decrease in Hb was independently associated with significantly increased mortality risk in several studies of the heart failure population.[43] The degree of anemia in ACD is generally associated with the severity of underlying disease. Table 104–10 lists common diseases associated with ACD.

TABLE 104-10 Diseases Causing Anemia of Chronic Disease

Common causes
Chronic infections
Tuberculosis
Other chronic lung infections (e.g., lung abscess, bronchiectasis)
Human immunodeficiency virus
Subacute bacterial endocarditis
Osteomyelitis
Chronic urinary tract infections
Chronic inflammation
Rheumatoid arthritis
Systemic lupus erythematosus
Inflammatory bowel disease
Inflammatory osteoarthritis
Gout
Other (collagen vascular) diseases
Chronic inflammatory liver diseases
Malignancies
Carcinoma
Lymphoma
Leukemia
Multiple myeloma
Less common causes
Alcoholic liver disease
Congestive heart failure
Thrombophlebitis
Chronic obstructive pulmonary disease
Ischemic heart disease

Etiology

ACD is a response to stimulation of the cellular immune system by various underlying disease processes. ACD commonly develops in AIDS patients, especially those with opportunistic infections or malnutrition, and is associated with increased morbidity and mortality. In patients with HIV, anemia is a predictor of progression to AIDS and is independently associated with an increased risk of death.[44] The etiology of anemia in patients with HIV is complex. HIV infects hematopoietic cells, which can lead to abnormal hematopoiesis and bone marrow suppression. In addition, the drugs used to treat AIDS and associated illness can cause bone marrow suppression.

Pathophysiology

ACD is a hypoproliferative anemia that traditionally has been associated with infectious or inflammatory processes, tissue injury, and conditions associated with release of proinflammatory cytokines. Alternative names include anemia of inflammation and cytokine-mediated anemia. The pathogenesis of ACD is multifactorial and is characterized by a blunted EPO response to anemia, impaired proliferation of erythroid progenitor cells, and disturbance of iron homeostasis. Increased iron uptake and retention occur within cells of the mononuclear phagocytic system. The RBCs have a shortened life span, and the bone marrow's capacity to respond to EPO is inadequate to maintain normal Hb concentration. The cause of this defect is uncertain but appears to involve blocked release of iron from cells in the bone marrow. Iron availability to erythroid progenitor cells then is limited. Various cytokines, such as interleukin-1, interferon-γ, and tumor necrosis factor released during these illnesses may inhibit the production or action of EPO or the production of RBCs.[45] Hepcidin may decrease duodenal absorption of iron and block release of iron from macrophages.[46]

Laboratory Findings

No definitive test can confirm the diagnosis of ACD, and the diagnosis is often overlooked. The practitioner should maintain a

TABLE 104-11 Laboratory Value Differences Between Anemia of Chronic Disease and Iron-Deficiency Anemia

	Anemia of Chronic Disease	Iron-Deficiency Anemia	Both
Iron	↓	↓	↓
Transferrin	↓or nl	↓	↓
Transferrin saturation	↓	↓	↓
Ferritin	↑or nl	↓	↓or nl
Soluble transferrin receptor	nl	↑	↑or nl

nl, normal limits.

high index of suspicion in any patient with a chronic inflammatory or neoplastic disease. ACD may coexist with IDA and folic acid deficiency because many patients with these conditions have poor dietary intake or gastrointestinal blood loss. Examination of the bone marrow reveals an abundance of iron, suggesting that the release mechanism for iron is the central defect. Patients with ACD usually have a decreased serum iron level, but unlike patients with IDA, their serum ferritin level is normal or increased and their TIBC decreased. Transferrin saturation is decreased. ACD usually is normocytic and normochromic with mildly depressed Hb. With ACD, hypochromia usually precedes microcytosis, with the opposite finding in IDA. Patients with concurrent ACD and IDA usually have microcytes and a more severe anemia. Erythrocyte survival may be reduced in patients with ACD, but a compensatory erythropoietic response usually does not occur. A low reticulocyte count indicates underproduction of red cells (Table 104–11).

TREATMENT

Anemia of Chronic Disease

Treatment of ACD is somewhat less specific than treatment of other anemias. Guidelines exist for management of anemia in patients with cancer or chronic kidney disease (see Chaps. 130 and 47). Although the goals of therapy should include treating the underlying disorder and correcting reversible causes of anemia, accomplishment of these goals may not totally reverse hematologic and physiologic abnormalities. Iron is effective only if iron deficiency is present. During inflammation, oral or parenteral iron therapy is ineffective. Absorption is poor because of downregulation of ferroportin and iron diversion mediated by cytokines.[45] Because iron is a required nutrient for proliferating microorganisms, supplementation may increase the risk of infections. Parenteral iron may have a role for patients unresponsive to erythropoietic agents.

RBC transfusions are effective but should be limited to situations in which oxygen transport is inadequate due to concomitant medical problems. The transfusion threshold varies from 8 to 10 g/dL based on factors such as cost, convenience, and risk of complications. Risks may include transmission of bloodborne infections, development of autoantibodies, transfusion reactions, and iron overload. Assessment of the symptomatic state should always be considered before blood products are administered.

Erythropoietic agents have been used to stimulate erythropoiesis in patients with ACD as a relative EPO deficiency exists for the degree of anemia. Two agents are available: recombinant epoetin alfa and recombinant darbepoetin alfa. Although both agents share the same mechanism of action, darbepoetin alfa has a longer half-life and can be administered less frequently. FDA-approved uses for these agents include patients with cancer receiving chemotherapy, patients with chronic kidney disease, and patients with HIV receiving myelosuppressive therapy. These agents are sometimes used to treat ACD, currently not an FDA-approved indication. Patients with chronic disease may have a relatively impaired response to epoetin alfa. The dosage of epoetin alfa is 50 to 100 units per kilogram three times per week. The dosage can be increased to 150 units per kilogram per dose if no increase in Hb concentration occurs after 6 to 8 weeks. Response to EPO varies depending on dose and cause of the anemia. EPO treatment is effective when the marrow has an adequate supply of iron, cobalamin, and folic acid. Whether EPO levels are a useful predictor of response is controversial.

EPO therapy usually is well tolerated. Iron deficiency can occur in patients treated with EPO, so close monitoring of iron levels is necessary. Oral iron supplementation should be given if transferrin saturation drops below 20% or the serum ferritin level drops below 100 ng/mL. Some patients develop "functional" iron deficiency, in which the iron stores are normal but the supply of iron to the erythroid marrow is less than necessary to support the demand for RBC production. Therefore, many practitioners routinely supplement EPO therapy with oral iron therapy. The hypertension commonly seen in patients with end-stage renal disease treated with EPO is far less common in AIDS patients. Potential toxicities of exogenous EPO administration include increases in blood pressure, nausea, headache, fever, bone pain, and fatigue. Other adverse effects include seizures, thrombotic events, and allergic reactions such as rashes and local reactions at the injection site.

Evaluation of Therapeutic Outcomes

One of the earliest responses to increased endogenous or exogenous EPO is an increase in blood reticulocyte count, which usually occurs in the first few days. Baseline iron status should be checked before and during treatment, as many patients receiving EPO require supplemental iron therapy. The optimal form and schedule of iron supplementation are not known. Hb levels should be checked 4 weeks after therapy initiation and then every 2 to 4 weeks thereafter. A fall in Hb during EPO therapy generally indicates a need for iron supplementation. Baseline and periodic monitoring of iron, TIBC, transferrin saturation, or ferritin levels may be useful in maximizing iron repletion and limiting the need for epoetin. Patients who do not respond to 8 weeks of optimal dosage should not continue taking EPO. Target Hb levels should be 11 to 12 g/dL. Cost is an issue with EPO therapy, so drug expense must be weighed against the effects on transfusions and hospitalizations.

ANEMIA OF CRITICAL ILLNESS

Epidemiology

❽ Anemia is a common complication in critically ill patients and is found almost universally in this patient population.[47] Approximately 95% of patients have less than normal Hb levels by their third day in the intensive care unit (ICU).[48]

Etiology

Factors that may contribute to anemia in critically ill patients include sepsis, taking of frequent blood samples, hemodilution, surgical blood loss, immune-mediated functional iron deficiency, decreased production of endogenous EPO, reduced RBC life span, and active bleeding, especially in the gastrointestinal tract. More commonly, a combination of these factors exists. Additional comorbid factors include coagulopathies and nutritional deficits such as malnourishment and altered absorption of vitamins and minerals, including iron, vitamin B_{12}, and folate.[49] Deleterious effects of anemia includes increased risk of cardiac-related morbidity and mortality, especially in patients with known cardiovascular disease. Continued tissue hypoxia can result in cerebral ischemia, myocardial ischemia, multiple organ deterioration, lactic acidosis, and death. Consequences of anemia in critically ill patients may be enhanced because of the increased metabolic demands of critical illness. Weaning anemic patients from mechanical ventilation may be more difficult.[50]

Pathophysiology

In anemia of critical illness, the mechanism for RBC replenishment and homeostasis is altered. The effect of various inflammatory cytokines on EPO may partly explain anemia of critical illness because inflammatory cytokines are associated with a blunted erythropoietic response.[51] Inflammatory cytokines appear to directly inhibit RBC production and stimulate iron-binding proteins that sequester iron and limit RBC production.[51] Increased nitric oxide production may alter iron metabolism; it inhibits erythroid amino-levulinic acid, decreases iron consumption, and decreases ferrochelatase activity, resulting in diminished oxygen transport by Hb and myoglobin.

Laboratory Findings

Anemia of critical illness is similar to ACD. Diminished Hb concentration is the most telling sign of anemia in the critically ill patient if hydration status is considered. MCV will assist in determining the cause of the anemia. Laboratory findings frequently seen in anemia of critical illness are low serum iron, TIBC, and iron/TIBC ratio. Transferrin saturation usually is less than 20% in anemia of critical illness due to functional iron deficiency. Serum ferritin is normal to high, as seen with ACD, and EPO levels usually are slightly decreased despite the presence of anemia, with minimal reticulocyte response.[47,51] These findings differs from those in patients with IDA, who generally have elevated EPO concentrations in response to a low Hct.

TREATMENT

Anemia of Critical Illness

Patients with anemia of critical illness require the necessary substrates of iron, folic acid, and vitamin B_{12} for RBC production. Because iron stores usually are insufficient to meet physiologic demands, administration of supplemental iron is necessary to support erythropoiesis. Parenteral iron is generally preferred in this population because patients often are undergoing enteral therapy or because of concerns regarding inadequate iron absorption. The disadvantage of parenteral therapy is the theoretical risk of infection.[52]

CLINICAL CONTROVERSY

The low iron concentrations in critically ill patients may be a defense mechanism, as microbes require iron for sustenance. Therefore, diminished iron levels may inhibit bacterial growth. Further investigation of supplementation with iron is warranted.

Pharmacologic doses of EPO have been used to treat the anemia of critical illness. Few randomized controlled trials have evaluated the role of EPO in critically ill patients, and the results of these trials have not consistently shown a decrease in transfusion requirements in EPO-treated patients.[51] The EPO dose is not firmly established, but a recommended dose is 40,000 units given subcutaneously once weekly for up to four total doses. Patients with a length of stay in the ICU longer than 1 week are most likely to benefit.[53] Further investigation is necessary to determine the effectiveness and the cost effectiveness of EPO in critically ill patients.[48] Use of darbepoetin for treatment of anemia of critical illness has not been examined.

Many critically ill patients receive RBC transfusions despite the inherent risks associated with transfusions. Stored RBCs may not function as well as endogenous blood. Although RBC transfusions may increase oxygen delivery to tissues, cellular oxygen may not increase.[54] Transfusion practices in ICUs vary, and clinicians use different Hb concentrations as thresholds for administering transfusions. Study results suggest that RBC transfusions may decrease the likelihood of survival in some subgroups of critically ill patients.[55] Decisions to use transfusions must consider the risks, including transmission of infections; volume overload, especially in patients with renal or heart failure; iron overload; and immune-mediated reactions such as febrile reactions, hemolysis, and anaphylaxis. The clinician also must consider administrative, logistic, and economic factors, including the shortage of blood supplies.

Evaluation of Therapeutic Outcomes

Goals of therapy include maintenance of adequate tissue oxygenation and perfusion, immediate correction of severe anemia, and prevention and minimization of blood loss. The role of monitoring RBCs, Hb, Hct, EPO levels, and reticulocyte counts remains to be determined. Outcomes used in EPO studies are transfusion requirements and transfusion independence. Morbidity, mortality, and length of stay also are assessed. Clinicians should monitor predose hematocrit values and withhold therapy in patients with Hct exceeding 38% to decrease unnecessary doses of EPO and cost. Iron levels should be monitored to ensure that adequate amounts of iron are present to support an optimal erythropoietic response to epoetin alfa.

ANEMIA IN THE ELDERLY

Epidemiology

❾ One of the most common clinical problems observed in the elderly is anemia. Anemia is a prevalent and increasing problem in the elderly, with approximately 20% of people 85 years and older affected.[56] Elderly patients with the highest incidence of anemia are those who are hospitalized, followed by residents of nursing homes and institutions, with an estimated rate of 31% to 40%.[57] The lowest incidence is seen in elderly patients who are community dwellers. Although the incidence of anemia is high in the elderly, anemia should not be regarded as an inevitable outcome of aging because an underlying cause can be identified in approximately two thirds of patients. Undiagnosed and untreated anemia can have severe ramifications. Anemia has been significantly associated with adverse outcomes, including all-cause hospitalization, hospitalization secondary to cardiovascular disease, and all-cause mortality.[58] Anemia is an independent predictor of death and major clinical adverse events in elderly patients with stable symptomatic coronary artery disease.[59] Anemia can cause neurologic and cognitive complications and can adversely influence quality-of-life and physical performance in the elderly.[60] Anemia may be an indication of serious diseases such as gastrointestinal cancer.

Pathophysiology

Aging is associated with a progressive reduction in hematopoietic reserve, which makes individuals more susceptible to developing anemia in times of hematopoietic stress.[61] Dysregulation of proinflammatory cytokines, most notably interleukin-6, may inhibit EPO production or interact with EPO receptors.[62] Although Hb levels may remain normal, the diminished marrow reserve leaves the elderly patient more susceptible to other causes of anemia. Renal insufficiency, which also is common in elderly patients, may reduce the ability of the kidneys to produce EPO. Patients often have a normal creatinine level but a diminished glomerular filtration rate. It has been suggested that a deficiency in endogenous EPO develops when the glomerular filtration rate falls below 50% of the normal range. Myelodysplasia is the cause of unexplained anemia in 20% of elderly individuals, whereas 30–50% are presumed to have multiple causes for their anemia.

Etiology

In the acute care setting, the top three causes of anemia in the elderly are chronic disease (35%), unexplained cause (17%), and iron deficiency (15%), whereas in community-based outpatient clinics, the most common causes are unexplained (36%), infection (23%), and chronic disease (17%).[63] Risk factors for the development of anemia in the elderly include race and ethnicity. The highest prevalence is seen in elderly blacks, those with serum albumin and serum creatinine abnormalities, and in patients with recent hospitalization or placement in an institution.[57]

Anemia in the elderly usually is hyporegenerative and represents an inability of the aging hematopoietic system to replace the peripheral blood loss or respond to marrow insults. Unexplained causes may be due to inadequate diagnostic evaluation or absolute or relative EPO deficiency. Absolute deficiency may be associated with renal insufficiency, whereas relative deficiency may be due to the body's inability to provide adequate response to declining Hb levels.[63]

Another common problem in the elderly is vitamin B_{12} deficiency. The most common causes of clinically overt vitamin B_{12} deficiency are food/cobalamin malabsorption (more than 60% of cases), pernicious anemia (15%–20% of cases), insufficient dietary intake, and malabsorption.[64] Patients, especially the elderly, with elevated serum MMA in the presence of borderline or even normal cobalamin levels may develop neuropsychiatric abnormalities. Treatment with cyanocobalamin may prevent further deterioration and result in improvement.

One often overlooked major factor that may contribute to anemia in the older population is nutritional status. Cross-sectional studies demonstrate a high prevalence of anemia and other nutritional deficiencies in low socioeconomic populations. Therefore, nutritional deficiencies that are not severe enough to affect the hematopoietic system in the younger population may contribute to anemia in the elderly. Edentulous or infirm elderly who may be too ill to prepare their meals are at risk for nutritional folate deficiency. Risk factors for inadequate folate intake in the elderly include low energy intake, inadequate consumption of fortified cereals, and failure to take a vitamin/mineral supplement.[65] However, unlike cobalamin levels, folate levels often increase rather than decline with age. High folic acid intake can occur if the elderly patient regularly uses a supplement and consumes fortified cereals.[65,66]

Other common anemias in the elderly include IDA and ACD. Iron malabsorption may occur after total gastrectomy. Bleeding with resultant iron deficiency in the elderly may be due to carcinoma, ulcer, atrophic gastritis, drug-induced gastritis, postmenopausal vaginal bleeding, or bleeding hemorrhoids. Elderly women have a much lower incidence of IDA compared to younger, menstruating women. Until proven otherwise, iron deficiency in the elderly should be considered a sign of chronic blood loss. ACD is more common in the elderly, as diseases that contribute to ACD such as cancer, infection, and rheumatoid arthritis are more prevalent in this population.

Laboratory Findings

Elderly males may have lower Hb levels, but whether this condition is secondary to physiologic reasons or increased prevalence of anemia is not known. Low levels may be due to decreased androgen secretion in men or age-related changes in stem cells. For practical purposes, it is best to use usual adult reference values for laboratory tests in the elderly and realize that some mild anemias may go unexplained.

Anemia in elderly persons usually is normocytic and mild, with Hb values ranging between 10 and 12 g/dL in most anemic patients.[56] A CBC, including a peripheral blood smear and reticulocyte count, should be performed in any elderly patient with symptoms that may be related to anemia. Patients also should be evaluated for signs of renal or hepatic failure and gastrointestinal or genitourinary blood loss. If the reticulocyte count is adequate, blood loss or RBC destruction should be suspected. A low count indicates decreased RBC production, so RBC indices should be evaluated. If MCV is >100 fL, further testing should be performed to evaluate for possible vitamin B_{12} or folate deficiency. A vitamin B_{12} deficiency may be present even when plasma levels of vitamin B_{12} are within the normal range, but elevated MMA levels will detect the deficiency. A refractory macrocytic anemia in the elderly should raise suspicion of a myelodysplastic or leukemic syndrome. If MCV is <100 fL, further studies should be performed to determine if IDA or ACD is a possible cause.

With IDA, abnormal laboratory values are similar to those found in patients with microcytic anemia. However, serum iron and TIBC decrease with age, so the transferrin saturation ratio is less useful in the elderly. MCVs and mean cell Hb concentrations may appear normal even in the presence of IDA, as patients may have concurrent vitamin B_{12} or folate deficiency anemias.

TREATMENT

Anemia in the Elderly

Depending on the cause of the anemia, treatment in the elderly is the same as that described for each type of anemia discussed in this chapter. With IDA it is essential to treat the underlying cause, if known (i.e., bleeding), and administer iron supplementation. Lower doses of iron supplementation are often recommended in the elderly (e.g., 325 mg of ferrous sulfate once daily) to decrease the incidence of gastrointestinal adverse effects, which can lead to considerable morbidity and poor adherence. Vitamin B_{12} deficiency is treated with parenteral or oral vitamin B_{12} supplementation; folic acid deficiency is treated with folic acid, generally at a dose of 1 mg daily. A meta-analysis showed that folic acid supplementation did not reduce the risk of cardiovascular disease or all-cause mortality in patients with a history of vascular disease.[67] The goal of treatment of ACD is resolution of the underlying cause, although treating the underlying chronic illness in elderly patients can be difficult. Results of several uncontrolled studies suggest that weekly EPO doses ranging from 9,000 to 20,000 units may be beneficial in elderly patients with ACD.[60] The medical and economic implications of anemia correction remain to be defined for ACD or undefined anemia.

Evaluation of Therapeutic Outcomes

Reticulocytosis usually starts within 1 week of oral supplementation with iron. If the reticulocyte count rises but the anemia does not improve, inadequate absorption of iron or continued blood loss should be suspected. Iron malabsorption due to atrophic or *Helicobacter pylori*-associated gastritis or celiac disease is not uncommon.[68] As with any form of anemia, symptomatic improvement should be evident shortly after starting therapy, and Hb/Hct should begin to rise within a few weeks of initiating therapy.

ANEMIA IN PEDIATRIC POPULATIONS

Epidemiology

⓾ IDA is a leading cause of infant morbidity and mortality around the world.[69] In the United States, the prevalence of IDA among children is declining as a result of improved iron supplementation.[2] Data from NHANES III indicated that 9% of children ages 12 to 36 months in the United States had iron deficiency and 3% had IDA.[70,71] Lack of a normal Hb at birth directly affects nonstorage iron and increases the risk of IDA in the first 3 to 6 months of life. Another study reports that as many as 20% of children in the United States and 80% of children in developing countries will have anemia before age 18 years.[9] Children who are African American or Hispanic have a higher incidence of anemia.[72] Requirements for iron absorption peak during puberty. In infants and children, 30% of daily iron needs must be met by dietary sources, compared to 5% in adults. An anemia of prematurity can occur 3 to 12 weeks after birth in infants younger than 32 weeks' gestation and spontaneously resolves by 3 to 6 months. The prevalence of vitamin B_{12} deficiency has been identified as 1 in 1,255 for levels <100 pg/mL and 1 in 200 for levels of <200 pg/mL, with the lowest levels in non-Hispanic whites.[73]

Pathophysiology

In contrast to anemias in adults, which tend to be manifestations of a broader underlying pathology, anemias in the pediatric population are more often due to a primary hematologic abnormality. The amount of iron present at birth depends on gestational length and weight. Erythropoiesis normally decreases after birth. A concurrent decrease in EPO production results in a physiologic anemia at 2 to 9 weeks of age. Iron stores are mostly depleted by age 6 months, although the blood volume doubles from 4 to 12 months.

Etiology

The age of the child can yield some clues regarding the etiology of the anemia. The optimal amount of nutritional iron and folate required varies among individuals based on life cycle stages. Two peak periods place children at risk of developing IDA. The first peak period occurs during late infancy and early childhood, when children undergo rapid body growth, have low levels of dietary iron, and exhaust stores accumulated during gestation. The second peak period occurs during adolescence, which is associated with rapid growth, poor diets, and onset of menses in girls. Some studies suggest that overweight children are at significantly higher risk for IDA. Proposed factors include genetic influences; physical inactivity, leading to decreased myoglobin breakdown and lower amounts of released iron into the blood; and inadequate diet with limited intake of iron-rich foods.[74]

Conditions in the newborn period that can lead to IDA include prematurity, administration of EPO for anemia of prematurity, and insufficient dietary intake. Premature infants are at increased risk for IDA because of their smaller total blood volume, increased blood loss through phlebotomy, and poor gastrointestinal absorption. Blood loss and hemolysis are other common causes of anemia in neonates. However, iron deficiency can occur only after the birth weight has doubled in premature infants.[9] Factors leading to unbalanced iron metabolism in infants include insufficient iron intake, decreased absorption, early introduction of cow's milk, intolerance of cow's milk, medications, and malabsorption. Dietary deficiency of iron in the first 6 to 12 months of life is less common today because of the increased use of iron supplementation during breastfeeding and use of iron-fortified formulas. Iron deficiency becomes more common when children change to regular diets.

Anorexia associated with infection can lead to decreased ingestion of iron-containing foods. Infection also can decrease erythropoiesis. When screening for iron deficiency in young children, a careful dietary history can help identify children at risk. Dietary deficiency has been defined as one or more of the following: fewer than five servings each of meat, grains, vegetables, and fruit per week; more than 16 oz of milk per day; or daily intake of fatty snacks, sweets, or more than 16 oz of soft drinks. High iron needs and the tendency to eat fewer iron-containing foods contribute to the etiology of iron deficiency during adolescence.

Other causes of microcytic anemia include thalassemia, lead poisoning, and sideroblastic anemia. Use of homeopathic or herbal medications and exposure to paint or certain cooking materials may place children at risk for lead exposure. Normocytic anemias in children include infection with human parvovirus B19 and glucose-6-phosphate dehydrogenase (G6PD) deficiency. Macrocytic anemias are caused by deficiencies in vitamin B_{12} and folate, chronic liver disease, hypothyroidism, and myelodysplastic disorders. Folic acid deficiency usually is due to inadequate dietary intake, but human milk and cow's milk provide adequate sources. Folic acid deficiency may be seen in infants and children who primarily consume goat's milk or health food milk alternatives, or in children with insufficient intake of green leafy vegetables. Vitamin B_{12} deficiency due to nutritional reasons is rare but may occur due to a congenital pernicious anemia.

Laboratory Findings

When evaluating laboratory values in pediatric patients, the clinician must use age- and sex-adjusted norms. It is important to know that many blood samples are capillary samples, such as heel or fingersticks, which may have slightly different results than venous samples.

The USPSTF has concluded that evidence is insufficient to recommend for or against routine screening for IDA in asymptomatic children aged 6 to 12 months. The Hb is a sensitive test for iron deficiency, but it has a low specificity in childhood anemias. If an abnormality is found, a CBC should be ordered to evaluate MCV and determine whether the anemia is microcytic, normocytic, or macrocytic. A peripheral blood smear and reticulocyte count also may be helpful. The peripheral blood smear can indicate the etiology based on RBC morphology, and the reticulocyte count helps differentiate between decreased RBC production and increased RBC destruction. Other laboratory tests include serum iron, ferritin, TIBC, and transferrin saturation. Mild hereditary anemias may produce a mild hypochromic microcytic anemia that can be confused with IDAs. The RDW may be high with iron deficiency and is more likely to be normal with thalassemia. Laboratory features of anemia of prematurity include normocytic normochromic cells, low reticulocyte count, low serum EPO concentrations, and decreased RBC precursors in bone marrow. Laboratory diagnosis of vitamin B_{12} deficiency in children is similar to that of adults and includes a CBC, measurement of vitamin B_{12}, and MMA and homocysteine levels. Serum or erythrocyte folate levels also should be measured if a folic acid deficiency anemia is suspected.

TREATMENT

Anemia in Pediatric Populations

Primary prevention of IDA in infants, children, and adolescents is the most appropriate goal because delays in mental and motor development are potentially irreversible. In 2006, the USPSTF published revised recommendations to screen and supplement iron deficiency in the United States, focusing on children and pregnant women.[75] The USPSTF recommends routine iron supplementation for asymptomatic children aged 6 to 12 months who are at increased risk for IDA. Fair evidence was found that iron supplementation (e.g., iron-fortified formula or iron supplements) may improve neurodevelopmental outcomes in children at risk for IDA and poor evidence for children 6 to 12 months of age not at risk for IDA.

Interventions likely to prevent anemia include diverse foods with bioavailable forms of iron, food fortification for infants and children, and individual supplementation. Routine screening for iron deficiency in nonpregnant adolescents is recommended only for those with risk factors, which include significant physical activity (especially in adolescent female athletes), vegetarian diets, malnutrition, low body weight, chronic illness, or history of heavy menstrual blood loss.

Anemia of prematurity is frequently treated with RBC transfusions, with wide variations in transfusion practices among neonatal ICUs. Reasons for use include improved oxygen delivery, intravascular volume, reduced fatigue during feeding, and improved growth. EPO may be used to treat anemia of prematurity, but it is important to note that EPO pharmacokinetics differ depending on the developmental age of the infant. Use of EPO is controversial because it has not been shown to clearly reduce transfusion requirements. Other questions regarding use of EPO in anemia of prematurity remain unanswered. Which infants respond best to EPO, and what is the long-term benefit (if any) of decreasing transfusions? What is the role of supplemental parenteral iron and nutritional supplementation? Premature infants fed human milk need 2 mg/kg of iron supplementation daily. Infants on full enteral feedings treated with EPO need iron supplements in doses of 6 mg/kg/day.

For infants aged 9 to 12 months with a mild microcytic anemia, the most cost-effective treatment is a therapeutic trial of iron. Fe^{2+} sulfate at a dose of 3 mg/kg of elemental iron once or twice daily between meals for 4 weeks is recommended. In children who respond, iron should be continued for 2 to 3 months to replace storage iron pools, along with dietary intervention and patient education. If the anemia recurs, the workup should include determination of sources of occult blood loss. Higher doses of oral iron (6 mg/kg/day of elemental iron divided into two or three daily doses) are administered to older children. Parenteral iron therapy has a limited role and is rarely necessary. For nonresponders, a serum ferritin level can be drawn.

For the macrocytic anemias in children, folate can be administered in a dose of 1 to 3 mg daily. However, vitamin B_{12} deficiency due to congenital pernicious anemia requires lifelong vitamin B_{12} supplementation. Dose and frequency should be titrated according to clinical response and laboratory values. No data regarding the use of oral vitamin B_{12} supplementation in children are available.

Evaluation of Therapeutic Outcomes

Therapeutic outcomes are assessed in children by monitoring Hb, Hct, and RBC indices 6 to 8 weeks after initiation of iron therapy. In premature infants, Hb or Hct should be monitored weekly. Reticulocyte counts should be checked 4 to 6 weeks after birth. Reticulocyte count, Hct, and absolute neutrophil counts are measured before and 1 to 2 weeks after starting EPO treatment. EPO should be held for an absolute neutrophil count of less than 1,000 cells/mm^3. Serum ferritin levels may be helpful in infants who do not respond to therapy. EPO use in premature infants is not associated with the side effects frequently seen in adults.

HEMOLYTIC ANEMIA

Pathophysiology

⓫ Hemolytic anemia results from decreased survival time of RBCs secondary to destruction in the spleen or circulation. The severity of hemolytic anemia varies with the mechanism. Hemolysis may be mild, chronic, and compensated, or acute, severe, and life-threatening.

The normal 120-day life span of a RBC comes from its inherent flexibility in passing through the microvasculature and spleen without disruption of the cell membrane or sequestration and phagocytosis by the mononuclear phagocytic system. Hemolysis, as defined by an RBC life span of less than 120 days, results from one of three primary defects that are intrinsic or extrinsic in origin: (a) membrane defects, (b) alterations in Hb solubility or stability, and (c) changes in intracellular metabolic processes. Intrinsic defects are intracorpuscular changes and often are genetically determined. Extrinsic defects, or extracorpuscular changes, usually are the cause of acquired hemolytic anemia. Acquired disorders result mainly from a direct effect on the membrane and less often from alterations in Hb or metabolism. Table 104–12 lists examples of the different classes of hemolytic anemias.

TABLE 104-12 Common Classes of Hemolytic Anemias

Intrinsic (intracorpuscular; usually genetically inherited)
Membrane defect
Spherocytosis and elliptocytosis
Hemoglobin defect
Sickle cell anemia
Thalassemia syndrome
Metabolic defect
Glucose-6-phosphate dehydrogenase (G6PD) deficiency
Many other enzyme deficiencies
Extrinsic
Membrane defect
Autoimmune hemolytic anemias
Oxidants, may cause unstable hemoglobin to clump

Causes of hemolytic anemia in younger patients differ from causes in elderly patients. Most younger patients exhibit congenital disease, whereas older patients most often experience autoimmune hemolytic anemia. A positive Coombs test is diagnostic in the latter group.

Alterations in Hb solubility or stability, as seen with sickle cell anemia and the thalassemias, cause cell deformations leading to hemolysis (see Chap. 106).

Finally, alterations in cell metabolism (enzymopathies) lead to hemolytic disease by changing cell dimensions and Hb solubility.

The two major metabolic pathways necessary for normal RBC metabolism are the hexose monophosphate shunt pathway, with its associated enzyme systems, and the Embden-Myerhof pathway of anaerobic glycolysis. The former is responsible primarily for maintaining Hb in the reduced state and thus preventing the formation of methemoglobin, whereas the latter metabolizes glucose to lactic acid, which leads to adenosine triphosphate formation.

The most common metabolic abnormality resulting in a hemolytic syndrome is G6PD deficiency in the hexose monophosphate shunt pathway (see Chap. 107). Hb is oxidized to methemoglobin and then to sulfhemoglobin. Heinz bodies of denatured Hb form, resulting in damage to the RBC membrane. Hemolysis results from the action of the spleen and the mononuclear phagocytic system, which normally removes damaged cells. The disease more typically occurs in whites of Mediterranean descent upon exposure to oxidant drugs (e.g., sulfamethoxazole and dapsone) and chemicals or with infection.

Some drugs and ingested toxins (e.g., nitrofurantoin, cancer chemotherapy agents, phenazopyridine, sulfones, amyl nitrate, mothballs, paraquat, and hydrogen peroxide) can cause direct oxidative damage to erythrocytes (see Chap. 107).

Laboratory Findings

Hemolytic anemias tend to be normocytic and normochromic. An increased reticulocyte count is evidence of an attempt to maintain RBC mass. A peripheral blood smear may reveal sickle cells, target cells, spherocytes, elliptocytes, and fragmented RBCs. Decreased haptoglobin is seen, caused by increased Hb–haptoglobin complex formation. Lactate dehydrogenase level often is elevated secondary to release from RBCs, but this enzyme is very nonspecific. Hemoglobinuria may result, and an increase in indirect bilirubin often occurs.

TREATMENT

Hemolytic Anemia

Therapy for hemolytic anemia consists of managing the underlying cause of the anemia. Patients with G6PD deficiency should avoid use of precipitating oxidant medications and chemicals. No specific therapy compensates for this enzyme deficiency. Steroids and other immunosuppressive agents have been used for management of autoimmune hemolytic anemias. A splenectomy is sometimes indicated in an attempt to reduce RBC destruction.

ANEMIAS CAUSED BY ABNORMAL HEMOGLOBIN SYNTHESIS

A defect in Hb synthesis or acquired defects in erythroid precursor cell metabolism may cause changes in iron incorporation, producing a cell with an excess of nonheme iron within the cytoplasm. These cells, called *sideroblasts,* cause sideroblastic anemia, which usually is microcytic. Sideroblastic anemia can be congenital (hereditary, sex-linked in males) or acquired. The acquired forms can be either primary or secondary to drugs, toxins (e.g., lead or alcohol), or other disease states. Reduced copper content of the blood, known as *hypocupremia,* has long been associated with sideroblastosis. Excess zinc intake causes sideroblastic anemia by binding preferentially to copper, impairing copper absorption, and leading to hypocupremia. Primary acquired sideroblastic anemia usually is classified as myelodysplastic syndrome and may eventually transform into acute myeloblastic leukemia.

Other hereditary defects in heme synthesis can lead to overproduction of heme precursors resulting in porphyria. The most common form, acute intermittent porphyria (AIP), results from a hereditary (autosomal dominant) partial deficiency in the enzyme uroporphyrinogen I synthetase, which is responsible for converting porphobilinogen to uroporphyrinogen. This deficiency inhibits the normal feedback mechanism of porphyrin synthesis, leading to excess production of the heme intermediate pigments uroporphyrin I and coproporphyrin I. The diagnosis of AIP is confirmed by detection of abnormal amounts of these products in urine and feces.

AIP is characterized by neuropsychiatric, neuromuscular, and autonomic dysfunction and intense abdominal pain. In the liver, this enzyme deficiency results in the increased inducibility of abnormal heme intermediates by certain drugs. Drugs and agents known to induce hepatic cytochrome P450 enzymes or to increase hepatic heme turnover are theoretically capable of precipitating porphyria. Barbiturates, estrogens, alcohol, and heavy metals (e.g., lead) have been documented to induce porphyria in genetically susceptible people.[76–78]

Genetic expression of an abnormal amino acid substitution in either the α- or β-globin chains can lead to a variety of hemoglobinopathies causing hemolytic diseases, such as sickle cell anemia and thalassemia (see Chap. 106).[79] Four genes control α-chain production, and two genes regulate β-chain production. Thalassemias result when these genes are defective. If three or four α-genes or both β-genes are not functioning properly, a major thalassemia, which is often incompatible with life, develops. Fortunately, thalassemia minor (trait) is more common. The trait results from deficiencies in one or two α-genes or one β-gene. For example, if α-genes are affected, normal β-chains accumulate in the cell and damage the membrane. This cell is prematurely cleared from the circulation, exacerbating the anemia. Surviving cells have inadequate Hb and are microcytic and hypochromic. Hemolysis and ineffective erythropoiesis cause the anemia.

The thalassemias are widely disseminated throughout parts of Africa, the Mediterranean region, the Middle East, the Indian subcontinent, and southeast Asia, but occur sporadically in all racial groups. Specifically, β-thalassemia is well recognized in persons of Greek and Italian descent; whereas the α-thalassemic syndromes have an increased prevalence in African American, American Indian, and Asian groups. It frequently is asymptomatic. Transfusion therapy allows for normal growth and suppresses ineffective erythropoiesis. Iron supplementation is not needed unless the patient has excessive blood loss and confirmed iron deficiency. It is important to distinguish thalassemia from IDA to avoid inappropriate iron therapy, as the excess iron may be deleterious and lead to possible organ damage. Iron overload causes most of the mortality and morbidity associated with thalassemia. Chelation therapy with deferoxamine is used but has limitations such as painful parenteral administration and cost. New oral iron chelators such as deferasirox are under development. Although both are microcytic, MCV tends to be much lower with thalassemia than with IDA. Target cells may be seen on the peripheral blood smear in patients with thalassemia. Finally, in contrast to patients with IDA, patients with thalassemia have normal or increased ferritin levels.. Hundreds of these abnormal Hb diseases exist and are best diagnosed by Hb electrophoresis.

PHARMACOECONOMIC CONSIDERATIONS

Anemia has an independent impact on many clinical, functional, and economic indicators, and evidence suggests that treatment can improve patient outcomes. The implications of treating anemia are becoming increasingly recognized, especially in the elderly. The cost of the complications associated with anemia in the elderly is considerable because anemia has been associated with an increased risk of falls, dementia, depression, and general functional disability that increases the demand for long-term care services.[80] However, the causal link between anemia and the costs of these diseases is not known. Studies show that treatment of anemia in elderly patients with renal failure and heart failure is beneficial.[80] More research is needed to assess the costs and benefits of therapies in individuals and in groups, especially when treatment of mild anemia is considered.[81]

Although the direct medical costs of anemia are unknown, the direct costs of drug treatment must be weighed against the indirect costs associated with anemia.[82] The costs of laboratory tests used to diagnose anemia, the role of screening for anemia, and the prevention of anemia are components that must be considered in the pharmacoeconomic analysis. Anemia practice guidelines within medical subspecialties must consider cost as they are developed. Additionally, the frequency of blood transfusions must be considered because it impacts cost and therapeutic decision making in patients.

For IDA, intravenous iron is costly but has superior bioavailability compared with oral preparations. In some individuals, the bioavailability advantage of parenteral iron over oral iron can be the difference in achieving a successful outcome. The benefits of using combination oral iron products designed to enhance absorption probably are not warranted.

With regard to vitamin B_{12} deficiency, the cost of oral cyanocobalamin tablets and intramuscular injections is inexpensive. However, the parenteral route has significant additional costs, including the cost of a physician or nurse's visit for the injection or the cost of a home health visit. Additionally, many elderly patients may have difficulties attending extra clinic appointments because of transportation difficulties. A 90-day supply of nonprescription 1-mg oral tablets can be purchased for approximately $5. The disadvantage of the nasal spray is its cost compared to the oral or parenteral route, with a 2-month supply costing approximately $75.

For ACD, EPO is generally effective and safe, but it is expensive. The cost of intravenous iron is low compared with the cost of EPO. Because most patients with ACD are not symptomatic, they may feel no improvement with therapy. Symptom severity should be considered in the decision to use EPO. Transfusion use for treatment of ACD as an alternative to EPO must consider cost, convenience, and risk of complications.

Formal economic evaluation of treatment approaches for anemia of critical illness are generally lacking. Doses used for anemia of critical illness have been 40,000 units weekly, with a cost of approximately $570. The cost of one unit of packed RBCs is $191 to $391 per dose based on factors such as donor recruitment and qualification; blood collection, processing, and screening; blood destruction, donor notification, and tracking; blood inventory, storage, and transport; and transfusion-related costs. Two or three doses of EPO are needed to avoid one RBC transfusion. Future studies may need to assess the cost per unit of RBC saved, which differs among institutions. Other pharmacoeconomic factors for consideration include morbidity and mortality of transfusion reactions, related infections, potential for medical errors, and availability of RBCs as a resource. Length of ICU stay, total hospital stay, and length of time on mechanical ventilation are other key factors.

ABBREVIATIONS

ACD: anemia of chronic disease
AIDS: acquired immunodeficiency syndrome
AIP: acute intermittent porphyria
CBC: complete blood count
CDC: Centers for Disease Control and Prevention
EPO: erythropoietin
Fe^{2+}: ferrous iron
Fe^{3+}: ferric iron
G6PD: glucose-6-phosphate dehydrogenase
Hb: hemoglobin
Hct: hematocrit
HIV: human immunodeficiency virus
IDA: iron-deficiency anemia
MCH: mean corpuscular hemoglobin
MCHC: mean corpuscular hemoglobin concentration
MCV: mean corpuscular volume
MMA: methylmalonic acid
NHANES: National Health and Nutrition Examination Survey
RBC: red blood cell
RDW: red blood cell distribution width
TIBC: total iron-binding capacity
USPSTF: U.S. Preventive Services Task Force

REFERENCES

1. Lozoff B, Georgieff MK. Iron deficiency and brain development. Semin Pediatr Neurol 2006;13:158–165.
2. Gleason G. Iron deficiency anemia finally reaches the global stage of public health. Nutr Clin Care 2002;5:217–219.
3. Shander A, Knight K, Thurer R, et al. Prevalence and outcomes of anemia in surgery: A systematic review of the literature. Am J Med 2004;116(Suppl 7A):58S–69S.
4. Nissenson A. Anemia not just an innocent bystander. Arch Intern Med 2003;163:1400–1404.
5. Mozaffarian D. Anemia predicts mortality in severe heart failure: The prospective randomized amlodipine survival evaluation (PRAISE). J Am Coll Cardiol 2003;41:1933–1939.
6. Bottomley A, Thomas R, Van SK, et al. Human recombinant erythropoietin and quality of life: A wonder drug or something to wonder about? Lancet Oncol 2002;3:1145–1153.
7. Chaves PHM, Carlson MC, et al. Association between mild anemia and executive function impairment in community-dwelling older women: The Women's Health and Aging Study II. J Am Geriatr Soc 2006;54:1429–1435.
8. Gran Ham-McGregor S, Ani C. A review of studies on the effect of iron deficiency on cognitive development in children. J Nutr 2001;131:649S–668S.
9. Irwin JJ, Kirchner JT. Anemia in children. Am Fam Physician 2001;64:1379–1386.
10. Ganz T. Hepcidin—A regulator of intestinal iron absorption and iron recycling by macrophages. Best Pract Res Clin Haematol 2005;18:171–182.
11. Hershko C, Ianculovich M, Souroujon M. A hematologist's view of unexplained iron deficiency anemia in males: Impact of Helicobacter pylori eradication. Blood Cells Mol Dis 2007;38:45–53.
12. Wians FH, Urban JE, Keffer JH, Kroft SH. Discriminating between iron deficiency anemia and anemia of chronic disease using traditional indices of iron status vs. transferrin receptor concentration. Am J Clin Pathol 2001;115:112–118.
13. Andrews NC. Iron metabolism and absorption. Rev Clin Exp Hematol 2000;4:283–301.
14. Baillie FJ, Morrison AE, Fergus I. Soluble transferrin receptor: A discriminating assay for iron deficiency. Clin Lab Haematol 2003;25:353–357.
15. Galloway M, Rushworth L. Red cell or serum folate? Results from the National Pathology Alliance benchmarking review. J Clin Pathol 2003;56:924–926.
16. Snow CF. Laboratory diagnosis of vitamin B_{12} and folate deficiency. Arch Intern Med 1999;159:1289–1298.
17. Dharmarajan TS, Norkus EP. Approaches to vitamin B_{12} deficiency. Early treatment may prevent devastating complications. Postgrad Med 2001;110:99–105.
18. Institute of Medicine. Dietary Reference Intakes (DRI) for Vitamin A, Vitamin K, Arsenic, Boron, Chromium, Copper, Iodine, Iron, Manganese, Molybdenum, Nickel, Silicon, Vanadium, and Zinc. Washington, DC: National Academy Press, 2002:18–19.
19. Annibale B, Chistolin A, D'Ambra G, et al. Gastrointestinal causes of refractory iron deficiency anemia in patients without gastrointestinal symptoms. Am J Med 2001;111:439–445.
20. Tefferi A. Anemia in adults: A contemporary approach to diagnosis. Mayo Clin Proc 2003;78:1274–1280.
21. Guha K. Investigating iron status in microcytic anaemia: Causes and management of iron deficient anaemia. BMJ 2006;333:972.
22. Faich G, Strobos J. Sodium Fe^{3+} gluconate complex in sucrose: Safer IV iron therapy than iron dextrans. Am J Kidney Dis 1999;33:464–470.
23. Chandler G, Harchowal J, Macdougall IC. Intravenous iron sucrose: Establishing a safe dose. Am J Kidney Dis 2001;38:988–991.
24. Houblers JG, et al. Transfusion of red cells is associated with increased incidence of bacterial infection after colorectal surgery: A prospective study. Transfusion 1997;37:126–134.
25. Goodnough LT, Brecher ME, Kamter MH, Aubuchon JP. Transfusion medicine, part 1; blood transfusions. N Engl J Med 1999;340:438–444.
26. Stabler SP, Allen RH. Vitamin B_{12} deficiency as a worldwide problem. Annu Rev Nutr 2004;24:299–326.
27. Wickramasinghe SN. Diagnosis of megaloblastic anaemias. Blood Rev 2006;20:299–318.
28. Park S, Johnson MA. What is an adequate dose of oral vitamin B_{12} in older people with poor vitamin B_{12} status? Nutr Rev 2006;64:373–378.
29. Kaptan K, Beyan C, Ural AU, et al. *Helicobacter pylori*—Is it a novel causative agent in vitamin B_{12} deficiency? Arch Intern Med 2000;160:1349–1353.
30. Oh RC, Brown DL. Vitamin B_{12} deficiency. Am Fam Physician 2003;67:979–986, 993–994.
31. Aronow WS. Homocysteine. The association with atherosclerotic vascular disease in older persons. Geriatrics 2003;58:22–28.
32. Vidal-Alaball J, Butler CC, Cannings-John R, et al. Oral vitamin B_{12} versus intramuscular vitamin B_{12} for vitamin B_{12} deficiency. Cochrane Database Syst Rev 2005;3:CD004655.
33. Cravens DD, Nashelsky J, Oh RC. How do we evaluate a marginally low B_{12} level? J Fam Pract 2007;56:62–63.
34. Solomon LR. Oral vitamin B_{12} therapy: A cautionary note. Blood 2004;103:2863.
35. Hvas AM, Nexo E. Diagnosis and treatment of vitamin B_{12} deficiency—An update. Haematologica 2006;91:1506–1512.
36. Lane LA, Rojas-Fernandez. Treatment of vitamin B_{12}-deficiency anemia: Oral versus parenteral therapy. Ann Pharmacother 2002;36:1268–1272.
37. Yerby MS. Clinical care of pregnant women with epilepsy: Neural tube defects and folic acid supplementation. Epilepsia 2003;44(Suppl 3): 33–40.

38. Pitkin RM. Folate and neural tube defects. Am J Clin Nutr 2007;85:285S–288S.
39. Institute of Medicine. Food and Nutrition Board. Dietary Reference Intakes: Thiamin, Riboflavin, Niacin, Vitamin B_6 Folate, Vitamin B_{12} Pantothenic Acid, Biotin, and Choline. Washington, DC: National Academy Press, 1998.
40. American College of Obstetricians and Gynecologists (ACOG). Neural Tube Defects. ACOG Practice Bulletin No. 44. Washington, DC: American College of Obstetricians and Gynecologists, 2003.
41. Bailey LB, Berry RJ. Folic acid supplementation and the occurrence of congenital heart defects, orofacial clefts, multiple births, and miscarriage. Am J Clin Nutr 2005;81(Suppl):1213S–7S.
42. Volberding P. Consensus statement: Anemia in HIV infection—current trends, treatment options, and practice strategies. Anemia in HIV Working Group. Clin Ther 2000;22:1004–1020.
43. Tang Y, Katz S. Anemia in Chronic Heart Failure. Circulation 2006;113:2454–2461.
44. Belperio PS, Rhew DC. Prevalence and outcomes of anemia in individuals with human immunodeficiency virus: A systemic review of the literature. Am J Med 2004;116:27S–43S.
45. Weiss GW, Goodnough LT. Anemia of chronic disease. N Engl J Med 2005;352:1011–1023.
46. Laftah AH, Ramesh B, Simpson RJ, et al. Effect of hepcidin on intestinal iron absorption in mice. Blood 2004:103:3940–3944.
47. Corwin HL, Gettinger A, Pearl RG, et al. The CRIT Study: Anemia and blood transfusion in the critically ill—Current clinical practice in the United States. Crit Care Med 2004;32:39–52.
48. Stubbs JR. Alternatives to blood product transfusion in the critically ill: Erythropoietin. Crit Care Med 2006;34(Suppl.):S160–S169.
49. Rodriguez RM, Corwin HL, Gettinger A, et al. Nutritional deficiencies and blunted erythropoietin response as cause of anemia of critical illness. J Crit Care 2001;16:36.
50. Silver MR. Anemia in the long-term ventilator-dependent patient with respiratory failure. Chest 2005;128(Suppl):568S–575S.
51. Rudis M, Jacobi J, Hassan E, et al. Managing anemia in the critically ill patient. Pharmacotherapy 2004;24:229–247.
52. Patruta SL, Horl WH. Iron and infection. Kidney Int 1999;55(Suppl 69):S125–S130.
53. Corwin HL, Eckardt KU. Erythropoietin in the critically ill: What is the evidence? Nephrol Dial Transplant 2005;20:2605–2608.
54. Hébert PC, Wells G, Martin C, et al. Do blood transfusions improve outcomes related to mechanical ventilation? Chest 2001;119:1850–1857.
55. Vincent JL, Piagnerelli M. Transfusion in the intensive care unit. Cit Care Med 2006;34(Suppl.):S96–S101.
56. Guralnik JM, Eisenstaedt RS, Ferrucci L, et al. Prevalence of anemia in person 65 years and older in the United States: Evidence for a high rate of unexplained anemia. Blood 2004;104:2263–2268.
57. Carmel R. Anemia and aging: An overview of clinical, diagnostic, and biological issues. Blood Rev 2001;15:9–18.
58. Culleton BF, Manns BJ, Zhang J, et al. Impact of anemia on hospitalization and mortality in older adults. Blood 2006;107:3841–3846.
59. Muzzarelli S, Pfisterer M, TIME Investigators. Anemia as independent predictor of major events in elderly patients with chronic angina. Am Heart J 2006;152:991–996.
60. Woodman R, Ferrucci L, Guralnik J. Anemia in older adults. Curr Opin Hematol 2005;12:123–128.
61. Balducci L, Hardy CL, Lyman GH. Hematopoietic growth factors in the older cancer patient. Curr Opin Hematol 2001;8:170–187.
62. Eisenstaedt R, Penninx BW, Woodman RC. Anemia in the elderly: Current understanding and emerging concepts. Blood Rev 2006;20:213–226.
63. Balducci L. Epidemiology of anemia in the elderly: Information on diagnostic evaluation. J Am Geriatr Soc 2003;51(Suppl):S2–S9.
64. Andres E, Loukili N, Noel E, et al. Vitamin B_{12} (cobalamin) deficiency in elderly patients. CMAJ 2004;171:251–259.
65. Mulligan JE, Greene GW, Caldwell M. Sources of folate and serum folate levels in older adults. J Am Diet Assoc 2007;107:495–499.
66. Ford ES, Bowman BA. Serum and red blood cell folate concentrations, race, and education: Findings from the third National Health and Nutrition Examination Survey. Am J Clin Nutr 1999;69:476–481.
67. Bazzano LA, Reynolds K, Holder KN, et al. Effect of folic acid supplementation on risk of cardiovascular diseases: A meta-analysis of randomized controlled trials. JAMA 2006;296;2720–2726.
68. Annibale B, Capurso G, Chistolini A, et al. Gastrointestinal causes of refractory iron deficiency anemia in patients without gastrointestinal symptoms. Am J Med 2001;111:439–445.
69. Milman N. Iron prophylaxis in pregnancy—General or individual and in which dose? Ann Hematol 2006;85:821–828.
70. Recommendations to prevent and control iron deficiency in the United States. Morb Mortal Wkly Rep 1998;47:1–36.
71. Moy RJ. Prevalence, consequences and prevention of childhood nutritional iron. Clin Lab Haematol 2006;28:291–298.
72. Coyer S. Anemia: Diagnosis and management. J Pediatr Health Care 2005;19:380–385.
73. Wright JD, Bialostosky K, Gunter EW, et al. Blood folate and vitamin B_{12}: United States, 1988–94. Vital Health Stat 1998;11:1–78.
74. Nead KG, Halterman JS, Kaczorowski JM, et al. Overweight children and adolescents: A risk group for iron deficiency. Pediatrics 2004;114:104–108.
75. U.S. Preventive Services Task Force (USPSTF). Screening for Iron Deficiency Anemia—Including Iron Supplementation for Children and Pregnant Women. Rockville, MD: Agency for Healthcare Research and Quality (AHRQ), 2006.
76. Hryhorczuk DO, Hogan MM. Variegate porphyria and heavy metal poisoning from ingestion of moonshine. South Med J 1983;76:1027–1031.
77. McKenzie AW, Acharya U. Oestrogen-induced familial porphyria. Br J Dermatol 1975;92:707–709.
78. Doss M, Baumann H, Sixel F. Alcohol in acute porphyria. Lancet 1982;1:1307.
79. Morris CR, Singer ST, Walters MC. Clinical hemoglobinopathies: Iron, lungs and new blood. Curr Opin Hematol 2006;13:407–418.
80. Robinson B. Cost of anemia in the elderly. J Am Geriatr Soc 2003;51(Suppl):S14–S17.
81. Cogswell M, Kettel-Khan L, Ramakrishnan V. Iron supplement use among women in the United States: Science, policy and practice. J Nutr 2003;133(Suppl):1974S–1977S.
82. Tice JA, Ross E, Coxson PG, et al. Cost-effectiveness of vitamin therapy to lower plasma homocysteine levels for the prevention of coronary heart disease. JAMA 2001;286:936–943.

CHAPTER 105 Coagulation Disorders

BETSY BICKERT AND CHAR WITMER

KEY CONCEPTS

1. Hemophilia is an inherited bleeding disorder resulting from a congenital deficiency in factor VIII or IX.
2. The goal of therapy for hemophilia is to prevent bleeding episodes and their long-term complications and to arrest bleeding when it occurs.
3. Recombinant factor concentrates usually are first-line treatment of hemophilia because they have the lowest risk of infection.
4. The goal of therapy for von Willebrand disease is to increase von Willebrand factor and factor VIII levels to prevent bleeding during surgery or arrest bleeding when it occurs.
5. Factor VIII concentrates that contain von Willebrand factor are the agents of choice for treatment of type 3 von Willebrand disease and some type 2 von Willebrand disease, and for serious bleeding in type 1 von Willebrand disease.
6. Desmopressin acetate often is effective for treatment of type 1 von Willebrand disease. It also may be effective for treatment of some forms of type 2 von Willebrand disease.
7. The optimal approach for patients with disseminated intravascular coagulation remains to be determined. The goal of treatment is to diagnose and treat the underlying cause.
8. Prophylactic use of phytonadione can effectively prevent vitamin K–dependent bleeding in newborns.

Coagulation disorders result from a decreased number of platelets, decreased function of platelets, coagulation factor deficiency, or enhanced fibrinolytic activity. A series of complex actions and reactions of procoagulant and anticoagulant events regulate blood flow. Maintenance of blood flow involves the interplay of four major components: (a) the vessel wall, (b) platelets, (c) the coagulation system, and (d) the fibrinolytic system.

The traditional view of the coagulation cascade consisted of intrinsic, extrinsic, and common pathways where coagulation proteins directed and controlled coagulation. Coagulation could be initiated via either the intrinsic or the extrinsic pathway (Fig. 105–1). The extrinsic pathway is initiated by exposure of tissue during trauma. The intrinsic pathway is initiated when circulating factor XII comes in contact with the subendothelial membrane. These two pathways converge at the activation of factor X, forming the common pathway. Although the historical model in Fig. 105–1 shows the basic dependency of the various coagulation factors, it does not reflect the interactions with platelets and the endothelium. Thus, it has been replaced by the cell-based model that more accurately describes these interactions (Fig. 105–2). This is known as the *tissue factor pathway* because it recognizes the central role of tissue factor in coagulation.

Learning objectives, review questions, and other resources can be found at **www.pharmacotherapyonline.com.**

REGULATION OF HEMOSTASIS

COAGULATION FACTORS

Twelve plasma proteins are considered coagulation factors (Table 105–1). The coagulation factors can be divided into three groups on the basis of biochemical properties. These groups include vitamin K–dependent factors (II, VII, IX, and X), contact activation factors (XI and XII, prekallikrein, high-molecular-weight kininogen), and thrombin-sensitive factors (V, VIII, XIII, and fibrinogen).

Coagulation factors circulate as inactive precursors (zymogens). Coagulation of blood entails a cascading series of proteolytic reactions. At each step, a clotting factor undergoes limited proteolysis and becomes an active protease (designated by a lowercase "a," as in Xa). These coagulation factors play key roles in the coagulation pathway.

VESSEL WALL AND PLATELETS

Blood vessel walls and activated platelets play central roles in primary hemostasis. Damage to a vessel wall initiates vasoconstriction and the exposure of collagen and tissue factor to blood. This exposure initiates coagulation via the tissue factor pathway.

Platelet function in response to vascular injury includes four phases: (a) adhesion, (b) secretion, (c) aggregation, and (d) elaboration of procoagulant activity. Release of von Willebrand factor from activated platelets and fibrinogen from the endothelium causes adhesion of platelets at the site. Platelets release granular contents, such as adenosine diphosphate and thromboxane A_2, which lead to platelet aggregation. A platelet plug is formed that occludes the blood vessel lesion. Activated coagulation factors are generated at the site of bleeding on the activated platelets to form fibrin and stabilize the platelet plug. Factor XIIIa cross-links the fibrin and stabilizes the fibrin clot.[1]

Unbound factors IIa, IXa, Xa, XIa, and XIIa are inactivated by antithrombin when they migrate to the endothelial cell surface. Heparin and heparin-like substances present on the surface of endothelial cells enhance the inhibitory capacity of antithrombin.[1] Thrombomodulin binds thrombin and activates protein C. Activated protein C and its cofactor, protein S, are vitamin K–dependent proteins that inactivate factor Va and VIIIa on the endothelial cell surface. These interactions localize the clotting to the site of injury and prevent clotting in the intact vascular system.

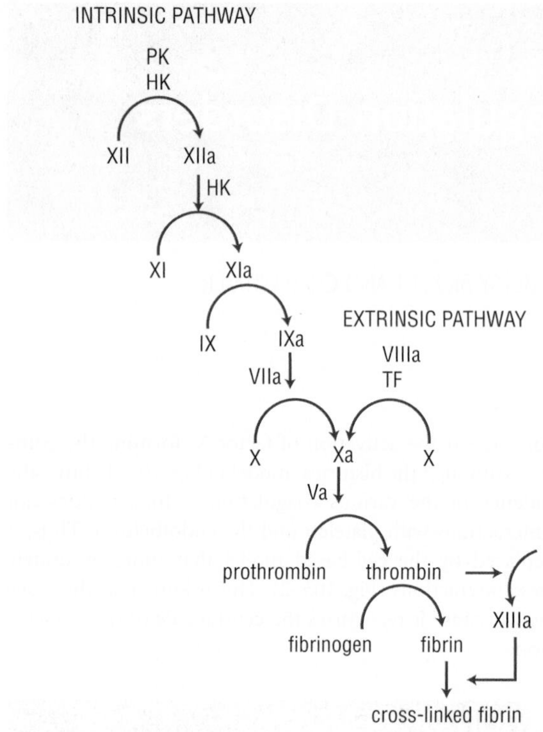

FIGURE 105-1. Cascade model of coagulation demonstrates activation via the intrinsic or extrinsic pathway. This model shows successive activation of coagulation factors proceeding from the top to the bottom where thrombin and fibrin are generated. (HK, high-molecular-weight kininogen; PK, prekallikrein; TF, tissue factor.) *(Reproduced from Roberts HR, Monroe DM, Hoffman M. Molecular biology and biochemistry of the coagulation factors and pathways of hemostasis. In: Beutler E, Coller BS, Lichtman MA, Kipps TJ, Seligsohn U, eds. Williams Hematology, 6th ed. New York: McGraw-Hill, 2001: 1409–1434.)*

TISSUE FACTOR PATHWAY

Tissue factor is a membrane protein found in organs and surrounding the vasculature. Tissue factor is exposed to blood as a consequence of vessel wall damage or inflammatory cytokine release from vascular cells or monocytes.[2] Coagulation is initiated when factor

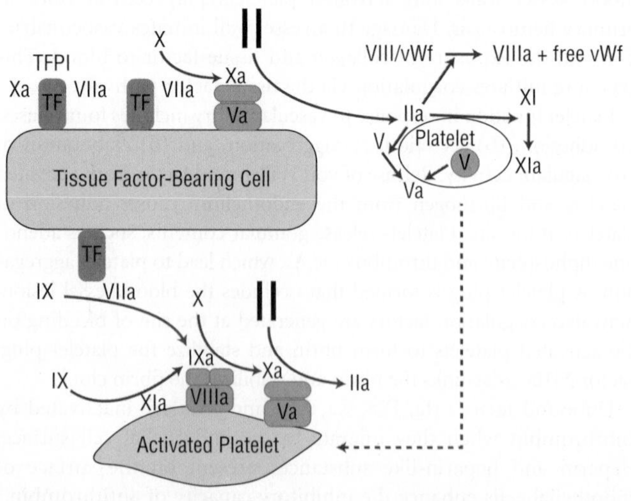

FIGURE 105-2. Cell-based model of hemostasis. (TF, tissue factor; TFPI, tissue factor pathway inhibitor; vWf, von Willebrand factor.) *(Reproduced from Roberts HR, Monroe DM, Hoffman M. Molecular biology and biochemistry of the coagulation factors and pathways of hemostasis. In: Beutler E, Coller BS, Lichtman MA, Kipps TJ, Seligsohn U, eds. Williams Hematology, 6th ed. New York: McGraw-Hill, 2001: 1409–1434.)*

TABLE 105-1 Blood Coagulation Factors

Factor[a]	Synonym	Biologic Half-life (h)	Blood Product Source
I	Fibrinogen	100–150	Cryoprecipitate (200–300 mg/bag)
II	Prothrombin	50–80	FFP, PCC
V	Proaccelerin	12–36	FFP
VII	Proconvertin	4–6	Recombinant VIIa, FFP, PCC
VIII	Antihemophilic factor	12–15	FFP, factor concentrates, cryoprecipitate
IX	Christmas factor	18–30	FFP, PCC, factor concentrates
X	Stuart-Power factor	25–60	FFP, PCC
XI	Plasma thromboplastin antecedent	40–80	FFP
XII	Hageman factor	50–70	Not associated with bleeding diathesis
XIII	Fibrin-stabilizing factor	150	FFP, cryoprecipitate, factor concentrate
VWF	von Willebrand factor	8–12	FFP, cryoprecipitate, factor concentrate

[a]Coagulation factors are numbered with roman numerals in order of their discovery. The most common synonyms are listed. Factor III (tissue factor) and factor IV (calcium ions) have been omitted. There is no factor VI.
FFP, fresh-frozen plasma; PCC, prothrombin complex concentrate.

VIIa binds to exposed or expressed tissue factor (Fig. 105–2). The factor VIIa–tissue factor complex activates factors IX and X.[2] Activated platelets form complexes with factor IXa–factor VIIIa (tenase) and factor Xa-factor Va (prothrombinase). Tenase activates factor X, and prothrombinase converts prothrombin to thrombin. Thrombin activates platelets and catalyzes the conversion of fibrinogen to fibrin. Thrombin also amplifies coagulation by activating factors V, VIII, and XI.

FIBRINOLYSIS

The coagulation system regulates fibrin clot formation, whereas the fibrinolytic system dissolves the polymerized clot and restores blood flow. As a regulatory mechanism for maintaining blood flow, the fibrinolytic system removes fibrin deposits and prevents formation of unnecessary fibrin clots. It also contributes to localized repair of damaged endothelium.

Plasminogen is the primary compound of the fibrinolytic enzyme system. Plasminogen activators (tissue plasminogen activator and urokinase plasminogen activator) are released in response to thrombin, venous stasis, physical exercise, and ischemia.[3] Activators convert plasminogen to plasmin in the presence of fibrin. Plasmin enzymatically digests fibrin, dissolves the clot, and releases a number of fibrin degradation products (FDPs). The interaction among plasminogen activators, plasminogen, and fibrin restricts the fibrinolytic activity to the site of the clot. Plasminogen activator inhibitor type 1 (PAI-1) blocks the plasminogen activators, whereas antiplasmin directly inhibits circulating plasmin to prevent systemic fibrinolysis.[3]

SIMPLE LABORATORY TESTS

The diagnosis of coagulation disorders can be established from a detailed clinical history, physical examination, and laboratory test results. The most common screening tests include prothrombin time (PT), activated partial thromboplastin time (aPTT), thrombin time, platelet count, and bleeding time.[1] The results of these standard laboratory procedures can distinguish bleeding disorders caused by defects in the intrinsic, extrinsic, and common coagulation pathways (Fig. 105–1) or alterations in the number of functioning platelets. Specific assays of individual coagulation factors and

TABLE 105-2 Laboratory Procedures

Procedure	Identifies	Cause of Prolonged Value	Clinical Manifestations
Bleeding time	Platelet number and function	Acquired platelet disorders (uremia) Vasculitis Connective tissue disorder Thrombocytopenia Inherited qualitative platelet defects Antiplatelet drugs von Willebrand disease Factor V or XI deficiency Afibrinogenemia, dysfibrinogenemia	Bleeding from the gums Easy bruising Bleeding following surgery or tooth extraction Epistaxis Menorrhagia
Prothrombin time (PT)	Factors I, II, V, VII, X	Newborn Vitamin K deficiency Inherited factor deficiencies[a] Warfarin Liver disease Lupus anticoagulant Afibrinogenemia	Bleeding following surgery, trauma, etc. Easy bruising
Activated partial thromboplastin time (aPTT)	Factors I, II, V, VIII, IX, X	Inherited factor deficiencies[a] Lupus anticoagulant Heparin therapy Liver disease Afibrinogenemia	Joint and muscle bleeding Bleeding after surgery, trauma, etc.
	HMWK, prekallikrein Factor XII		No bleeding manifestations Increased incidence of thrombotic disease possible with factor XII deficiency
	Factor XI		Variable bleeding tendency Bleeding following surgery, trauma, etc.
Thrombin time (TT)	Fibrinogen Inhibitors of fibrin aggregation	Afibrinogenemia, dysfibrinogenemia Heparin therapy	Lifelong hemorrhagic disease

[a]Bleeding manifestations dependent on factor levels.
HMWK, high-molecular-weight kininogen.

platelet function tests can be performed after abnormalities are identified by initial screening tests. The following is a brief review of widely available tests (summarized in Table 105–2).

Bleeding Time and Platelet Function Analyzer

Bleeding time assesses platelet and capillary function. Bleeding time reflects the time to cessation of bleeding following a standardized skin cut. This technique is patient and operator dependent. In the past 15 years has come increased recognition that the bleeding time has a number of disadvantages when applied as a screening test, resulting in the decreased popularity of this test.[4] The bleeding time is insensitive to mild platelet defects and does not consistently predict a bleeding tendency.[4] The platelet function analyzer (PFA-100) is an in vitro screen for platelet function and has been found to be superior to the in vivo bleeding time.[4] The PFA-100 also has limitations; it is not diagnostic, and abnormal values require further evaluation. Patients with an abnormal bleeding time but a normal platelet count are arbitrarily designated as having qualitative abnormalities of platelet function. A prolonged bleeding time can be caused by incorrect performance of the test, thrombocytopenia, platelet dysfunction, von Willebrand disease, use of antiplatelet drugs (i.e., aspirin), renal failure (uremia), fibrinogen disorders, abnormal blood vessels, or collagen disorders.

Prothrombin Time

PT assesses the activity of the vitamin K–dependent proteins (factors II, VII, IX, and X, and proteins C and S) and the common pathway proteins (factors V and X).[5] PT reflects the time required for fibrin strands to appear after the addition of tissue thromboplastin to the patient's plasma. Thus, PT provides evidence about the current synthetic capacity of the liver, the adequacy of vitamin K absorption, and the inhibition of clotting factor synthesis by warfarin. PT is expressed as an international normalized ratio that normalizes values, which is needed because of the variability of test reagents.[6]

Activated Partial Thromboplastin Time

aPTT measures the activity of the intrinsic system and common pathway (factors II, V, VIII, IX, X, XI, and XII, high-molecular-weight kininogen, prekallikrein, and fibrinogen). aPTT reflects the time required for a fibrin clot to form after a partial thromboplastin, calcium, and an activating agent are added to the patient's plasma. aPTT is widely used for monitoring heparin therapy.

Thrombin Time

The thrombin time measures the conversion of fibrinogen to fibrin and is affected by quantitative or qualitative abnormalities of fibrinogen, the presence of thrombin inhibitors, and fibrinogen degradation products. The thrombin time measures the time required for the formation and appearance of the fibrin clot after thrombin is added to plasma. It can be used to monitor the effect of systemic fibrinolytic therapy and can be modified for monitoring heparin therapy.

CONGENITAL COAGULATION DISORDERS

HEMOPHILIA

❶ Hemophilia is a bleeding disorder that results from a congenital deficiency in a plasma coagulation protein. Hemophilia A (classic hemophilia) is caused by a deficiency of factor VIII, whereas hemophilia B (Christmas disease) is caused by a deficiency of factor IX. The incidence of hemophilia A is approximately 1 in 5,000 male births.[7–9] Hemophilia B occurs less commonly, with only one fourth the incidence of hemophilia A.[7–9] There are no significant racial differences in the incidence of hemophilia.

Approximately one-third of patients with severe hemophilia have a negative family history, presumably representing a spontaneous mutation. Both hemophilia A and hemophilia B are recessive X-linked diseases, that is, the defective gene is located on the X chromosome. The disease usually affects only males; females are carriers. Affected males have the abnormal allele on their X chromosome and no matching allele on their Y chromosome, but their sons would be normal (assuming the mother is not a carrier) and their daughters would be obligatory carriers. Female carriers have one normal allele and therefore do not usually have a bleeding tendency. Sons of a female carrier and a normal male have a 50% chance of having hemophilia, whereas daughters have a 50% chance of being carriers. Thus, there is a "skipped generation" mode of inheritance in which the female carriers, who are the children of patients with hemophilia, do not express the disease but can pass it on to the next male generation.

Hemophilia has been observed in a small number of females. It can occur if both factor VIII and IX genes are defective,[10,11] if a female patient has only one X chromosome, as in Turner syndrome,[12] or if the normal X chromosome is excessively inactivated through a process called *lyonization*.[12]

In 1984, researchers isolated and cloned the human factor VIII gene.[13,14] It is a large gene, consisting of 186 kilobases (kb).[14,15] More than 900 unique mutations in the factor VIII gene, including point mutations, deletions, and insertions, have been reported (*http://europium.csc.mrc.ac.uk*). Deletions and nonsense mutations are often associated with the more severe forms of factor VIII deficiency because no functional factor VIII is produced. In 1993, researchers identified an inversion in the factor VIII gene at intron 22 that accounts for approximately 45% of severe hemophilia A gene abnormalities.[16] That discovery has greatly simplified carrier detection and prenatal diagnosis in families with this gene mutation. A more recently discovered inversion mutation involving intron 1 of the factor VIII gene accounts for an additional 5% of severe hemophilia mutations.[17]

The factor IX gene, cloned and sequenced in 1982,[18] consists of only 34 kb and thus is significantly smaller than the factor VIII gene.[13,15] Unlike the factor VIII gene in patients with severe hemophilia A, the factor IX gene in patients with hemophilia B has no predominant mutation. Direct gene mutation analysis is simpler in hemophilia B because of the smaller gene size, and to date more than 900 different mutations have been reported (*http://kcl.ac.uk/ip/petergreen/haemBdatabase.html*). Most of these mutations are single base pair substitutions. Approximately 3% of factor IX gene mutations are deletions or complex rearrangements, and the presence of these mutations is associated with a severe phenotype.[14]

Hemophilia B Leiden is a rare variant in which factor IX levels initially are low but rise at puberty. This phenotype results from a mutation in the promoter region of the gene that apparently is ameliorated by the action of testosterone.[14,19,20] Identification of this genotype is clinically important because it confers a better prognosis.

Clinical Presentation

The characteristic bleeding manifestations of hemophilia include palpable ecchymoses, bleeding into joint spaces (hemarthroses), muscle hemorrhages, and excessive bleeding after surgery or trauma. The severity of clinical bleeding generally correlates with the degree of deficiency of factor VIII or factor IX. Factor VIII and factor IX activity levels usually are measured in units per milliliter, with 1 unit/mL representing 100% of the factor found in 1 mL of normal plasma. Normal plasma levels range from 0.5 to 1.5 units/mL.[5] Patients with less than 0.01 units/mL (1%) of either factor are classified as having severe hemophilia, those with 0.01 to 0.05 units/mL (1%–5%) are moderate, and those with greater than 0.05 units/mL (5%) have mild hemophilia (Table 105–3). Patients with severe disease experience frequent spontaneous hemorrhages and joint space bleeding, whereas those with moderate disease have excessive bleeding following mild trauma and rarely experience spontaneous hemarthroses. Patients with mild hemophilia may have so few symptoms that their condition is undiagnosed for many years, and they usually have excessive bleeding only after significant trauma or surgery. Occasionally those with severe disease (less than 1% factor activity) may not display a severe phenotype; conversely, some with milder forms of the disease may have more severe bleeding symptomatology. Patients with hemophilia usually present with clinical manifestations after age 1 year, when they begin to walk and increase their risk of bleeding.

TABLE 105-3 Laboratory and Clinical Manifestations of Hemophilia

	Severe (<0.01 units/mL)	Moderate (0.01–0.05 units/mL)	Mild (>0.05 units/mL)
Age at diagnosis	≤1 year	1–2 years	2 years–adult
Neonatal symptoms			
PCB	Usually	Usually	Rarely
ICH	Occasionally	Uncommonly	Rarely
Muscle/joint hemorrhage	Spontaneous	Minor trauma	Minor trauma
CNS hemorrhage	High risk	Moderate risk	Rare
Postsurgical hemorrhage (without prophylaxis)	Frank bleeding, severe	Wound bleeding, common	Wound bleeding
Oral hemorrhage following trauma, tooth extraction	Usually	Common	Common

Normal range of factor VIII/IX activity level is 0.5–1.5 units/mL (50%–150%). 1 unit/mL corresponds to 100% of the factor found in 1 mL of normal plasma.
CNS, central nervous system; ICH, intracranial hemorrhage; PCB, postcircumcisional bleeding.

CLINICAL PRESENTATION OF HEMOPHILIA

Signs and Symptoms

- Ecchymoses (palpable)
- Hemarthrosis (especially knee, ankle, and elbow)
- Joint pain
- Joint swelling and erythema
- Decreased range of motion
- Muscle hemorrhage
- Swelling
- Pain with motion of affected muscle
- Signs of nerve compression
- Potential life-threatening blood loss, especially with thigh bleeding
- Oral bleeding with dental extractions or trauma
- Hematuria
- Intracranial hemorrhage (spontaneous or following trauma)
- Excessive bleeding with surgery

Laboratory Testing

- Prolonged aPTT
- Decreased factor VIII or factor IX level
- Normal PT
- Normal platelet count
- Normal von Willebrand factor antigen and activity
- Normal bleeding time

Diagnosis

The diagnosis of hemophilia should be considered in any male with unusual bleeding. A family history of bleeding is helpful in the diagnosis but is absent in up to one third of patients.[21] Brothers of patients with hemophilia should be screened; sisters should undergo carrier testing.

Advances in molecular genetic analysis have greatly improved the accuracy of carrier status evaluation. Thus, female relatives of patients with hemophilia who are at risk of being carriers for the disorder should be tested. Additionally, the appropriate factor level should be measured in female carriers to identify those with levels less than 0.3 units/mL (30%) who themselves might be at risk for bleeding.

Patients with severe hemophilia A should be tested for the common factor VIII gene inversions. If the patient has this mutation, family members should undergo testing to determine if they also have the mutation and thus are carriers. In patients with hemophilia A who lack the inversion mutation, other methods for determining the carrier status of their family members are available.[22,23] Techniques for determining carrier status in families with hemophilia B are similar, although no predominant mutation like the factor VIII inversion has been found. The smaller size of the factor IX gene facilitates direct DNA mutational analysis.[23]

Hemophilia can be diagnosed prenatally by chorionic villus sampling in gestational weeks 10 to 11 or by amniocentesis after 15 weeks' gestation.[15,22] Fetal blood can be sampled and assayed directly for factor VIII levels by 18 to 20 weeks' gestation.[15,22] This procedure is less useful for diagnosing factor IX deficiency because factor IX levels are physiologically low in fetuses and infants.

TREATMENT

Hemophilia

The comprehensive care of hemophilia requires a multidisciplinary approach. The patient is best managed in specialized centers with trained personnel and appropriate laboratory, radiologic, and pharmaceutical services. The healthcare team includes hematologists, orthopedic surgeons, nurses, physical therapists, dentists, genetic counselors, psychologists, pharmacists, case managers, and social workers.

Patients with hemophilia should receive routine immunizations, including immunization against hepatitis B. Hepatitis A vaccine is also recommended for patients with hemophilia because of the risk (albeit small) of transmitting the causative agent through factor concentrates.[24] Use of a small-gauge needle can prevent excessive bleeding. Some healthcare providers advocate subcutaneous rather than intramuscular immunizations to decrease the risk of hematoma formation.

A few special considerations apply to the perinatal care of male infants of hemophilia carriers. Intracranial or extracranial hemorrhage has been estimated to occur in 1% to 4% of newborns with hemophilia.[25] Vacuum extraction and forceps delivery increase the risk of cranial bleeding. Elective cesarean section has not prevented intracranial bleeding. There is no clear consensus on the optimal mode of delivery or the use of prophylactic factor replacement in male infants of hemophilia carriers.[25] Circumcision should be postponed until a diagnosis of hemophilia is excluded. Factor levels can be assayed from cord blood samples or from peripheral venipuncture. Arterial puncture should be avoided because of the risk of hematoma formation. If an infant has hemophilia, many clinicians recommend a screening head ultrasound to rule out an intracranial hemorrhage prior to discharge from the nursery.

❷ Intravenous factor replacement therapy for treatment or prevention of bleeding is the mainstay of treatment of hemophilia. Families usually learn how to treat patients receiving factor concentrate at home. Parents may learn to infuse factor for younger children, and older children and adult patients may learn self-administration. Home healthcare nursing support may be helpful, particularly for the youngest patients in whom venous access may be difficult. Administration of factor at home is more convenient for families and allows for earlier treatment of acute bleeding episodes. However, serious bleeding episodes always require medical evaluation.

HISTORY OF HEMOPHILIA TREATMENT

Therapy for hemophilia has undergone dramatic advances over the past few decades. Fifty years ago, administration of fresh-frozen plasma was the only available treatment. The introduction of cryoprecipitate in the early 1960s allowed more specific therapy for hemophilia A.[14] Intermediate-purity factor VIII and IX concentrates became available in the 1970s.[14] Plasma-derived factor concentrates are made from the donations of thousands of people. Contamination of plasma pools with hepatitis B, hepatitis C, and the human immunodeficiency virus (HIV) during the late 1970s and early 1980s resulted in transmission to most patients with severe hemophilia. Since the mid-1980s, plasma-derived concentrates have been manufactured with a variety of virus-inactivating techniques, including dry heat, pasteurization, and treatment with chemicals (e.g., solvent detergent mixtures).[14] Since 1986, no transmission of HIV through factor concentrates to patients with hemophilia in the United States has been reported.[14] Protein purification, introduced in the 1990s, produced high-purity concentrates with increased amounts of factor VIII or factor IX relative to the product's total protein content. Recombinant factor VIII and then factor IX also became available.[14] The first-generation recombinant factor VIII products utilize human and animal proteins in culture and add human albumin as a protein stablilizer.[14] Second-generation recombinant factor VIII concentrates removed albumin as a protein stabilizer, and third-generation products lack human and animal proteins in the culture media.[26] Gene therapy for treatment of hemophilia is now in the early stages of clinical trials.

HEMOPHILIA A

Table 105–4 summarizes the factor VIII products currently available in the United States. Most patients are treated with high-purity products. In general, products that have the lowest risk of transmitting infectious disease should be used. Thus, recombinant products, when available, are generally used rather than plasma-derived products.

Recombinant Factor VIII

❸ Derived from cultured Chinese hamster ovary cells or baby hamster kidney cells transfected with the human factor VIII gene,[14] recombinant factor VIII is produced with recombinant DNA technology. Because it is not derived from blood donations, the risk of transmitting infections through administration of recombinant factor VIII is low. For this reason, recombinant products are generally favored over plasma-derived products. There still is a small risk of viral infection of the cell lines used to produce the clotting factor.[27] Furthermore, human and/or animal proteins are utilized in the production process of some recombinant products.[26] Therefore, these products have a theoretical risk of transmitting infection, although hepatitis and HIV infection have never been reported with their use.[14] The presence of parvovirus B19 DNA has been reported in recombinant factor VIII products.[28] First-generation recombinant factor VIII products contain human albumin as a stabilizing protein.[14] Second-generation recombinant factor VIII products add sucrose instead of human albumin as a stabilizer, but human albumin is utilized in the culture process. One second-generation product (ReFacto) has deletion of the B domain of the factor VIII gene, yielding a smaller protein product.[29] This B domain does not appear to be necessary for coagulation function. Third-generation recombinant factor VIII products contain no human protein in either the culture or in the stabilization processes.[26]

Clinical trials have demonstrated that recombinant factor VIII products are comparable in effectiveness to plasma-derived products.[29] The risk of patients with severe hemophilia A developing an

reported side effects include mild headaches, increased heart rate, and decreased blood pressure. Thrombosis is a rare complication associated with desmopressin.[36] Because of its antidiuretic effects, desmopressin has the potential to cause water retention, which may lead to severe hyponatremia. This may be a particular problem in children younger than 2 years, in whom hyponatremic seizures have been reported.[36] Therefore, desmopressin should be used with caution in this age group.[34,35] Patients with congestive heart failure may be at increased risk for developing hyponatremia with use of desmopressin.[34] Mild fluid restriction and monitoring of urine output are recommended with desmopressin administration.[36]

Antifibrinolytic therapy inhibits clot lysis and therefore is a useful adjunctive therapy for treatment of hemophilia. These antifibrinolytic agents are particularly beneficial for treatment of oral bleeding because of the high concentration of fibrinolytic enzymes present in saliva. Two antifibrinolytics are aminocaproic acid and tranexamic acid. Aminocaproic acid is given at a dosage of 100 mg/kg (maximum 6 g) every 6 hours and can be administered orally or intravenously.[15] The dosage of tranexamic acid is 25 mg/kg (maximum 1.5 g) orally every 8 hours or 10 mg/kg (maximum 1 g) intravenously every 8 hours.[15]

■ HEMOPHILIA B

Therapeutic options for hemophilia B have improved greatly over the past several years, first with the development of monoclonal antibody–purified plasma-derived products and then with the licensure of recombinant factor IX. Products currently available in the United States for treatment of hemophilia B are listed in Table 105–4.

Recombinant Factor IX

First marketed in the United States in 1999,[14] recombinant factor IX is produced in Chinese hamster ovary cells transfected with the factor IX gene. Blood and plasma products are not used to produce recombinant factor IX or to stabilize the final product; thus, recombinant factor IX has an excellent viral safety profile.[14] Clinical trials have shown the product to be safe and efficacious in the treatment of acute bleeding episodes and in the management of bleeding associated with surgical procedures.[14,37,38] Although the half-life of recombinant factor IX is similar to that of the plasma-derived products, recovery is approximately 30% lower.[37,39] As a result, doses of recombinant factor IX concentrate must be higher than those of plasma-derived products to achieve equivalent plasma levels. Because individual pharmacokinetics may vary, recovery and survival studies should be performed to determine optimal treatment.[37–39] Recombinant factor IX is often considered the treatment of choice for hemophilia B.

Plasma-Derived Factor IX Products

High-purity factor IX plasma concentrates have been available in the United States since the early 1990s.[14] These products are derived from plasma through biochemical purification and monoclonal immunoaffinity techniques. Other viral inactivation measures, such as solvent detergent or chemical treatment, are also used.

Before the high-purity products were approved for use, hemophilia B patients were treated with factor IX concentrates that also contained other vitamin K–dependent proteins (factors II, VII, and X), known as prothrombin complex concentrates (PCCs). These products contain small amounts of activated factors generated during processing, and their use has been associated with thrombotic complications, including deep-vein thrombosis, pulmonary embolism, myocardial infarction, and disseminated intravascular coagulation (DIC).[14,40] The risk of such complications is highest in patients who are receiving high or repeated doses of PCCs, in those who have hepatic disease (the liver removes the activated factors from circulation), in neonates, and in patients who have experienced crush injuries or who are undergoing major surgery.[14,40] Concomitant use of PCCs and antifibrinolytics should be avoided because of the risk for thrombosis.

Because of the lower purity of PCCs and their thrombogenic potential, these products are not first-line treatment of hemophilia B, although they still are used for treatment of patients with hemophilia A or B who have developed inhibitory antibodies against factor VIII or factor IX, respectively. High-purity factor IX concentrates have excellent efficacy in the treatment of bleeding episodes and in the control of bleeding associated with surgical procedures.[41] Their viral safety profile has been reported to be excellent,[41] and the risk of thromboembolic complications is low.

Factor IX Concentrate Replacement

Factor IX is a relatively small protein. Unlike factor VIII, it is not limited to the intravascular space; it also passes into the extravascular compartment.[31] This results in a volume of distribution that is about twice that of factor VIII. In general, for plasma-derived factor IX concentrates, each unit of factor IX infused per kilogram of body weight yields a 1% rise in the plasma level of factor IX (range 0.67%–1.28%).[31] The following equation can be used to calculate the initial dose:

Plasma-derived factor IX (units) = (Desired level – Baseline level) × (Weight [in kilograms]).

As with the similar calculation for factor VIII dosing, the baseline level term can be omitted from the formula. Because recovery of recombinant factor IX is lower than that of the plasma-derived products, the following adjustment is made:

Pediatric dosing:

Recombinant factor IX (units) = (Desired level – Baseline level) × 1.4 × (Weight [in kilograms]).

Adult dosing:

Recombinant factor IX (units) = (Desired level – Baseline level) × 1.2 × (Weight [in kilograms]).

A recovery study to determine optimal dosing is recommended for patients who receive recombinant factor IX because of the wide interpatient variability in pharmacokinetics.

Because the half-life of factor IX is approximately 24 hours, dosing can be less frequent than with factor VIII. Table 105–5 provides general guidelines for dosing factor IX, based on the site and severity of the bleeding episode. As with factor VIII replacement therapy, individual pharmacokinetics may vary, and monitoring the patient's factor IX levels helps optimize therapy.

Prophylactic Replacement Therapy

Traditionally, factor concentrates for hemophilia patients have been given on demand, as the bleeding episode occurs. However, recurrent joint bleeding can damage the joint and lead to development of severe physical disability. Thus, it would be preferable to prevent bleeding episodes and avoid the resultant damage. Known as *prophylactic factor replacement therapy,* this approach entails regular infusion of concentrate to maintain the deficient factor at a minimum of 0.01 units/mL (1%).

In effect, prophylactic replacement therapy converts severe hemophilia into a milder form of the disease. The rationale for this approach is that patients with moderate hemophilia rarely experience spontaneous hemarthroses, and they have a much lower incidence of chronic arthropathy. Patients with hemophilia A usually require 25 to 40 units of factor VIII per kilogram of body weight, given every other day or three times per week.[15] For hemophilia B, the usual dosage is 40 to 100 units/kg of factor IX given twice weekly instead of three times weekly because of the longer half-life of factor IX.[42]

Primary prophylaxis is regular replacement therapy started at a young age (usually before age 2 years), prior to the onset of joint bleeding.[43,44] The results of primary prophylaxis have been very promising. In the Swedish experience, children who began prophylaxis at age 1 to 2 years experienced almost no bleeding episodes and had normal joint examinations and radiographs over a 5-year period.[14,45] Secondary prophylaxis begins after significant joint bleeding has already occurred. It is associated with a significant reduction in the number of joint bleeding episodes and a better clinical and orthopedic outcome.[46,47] However, radiographic evidence of joint disease rarely improves and often progresses despite the institution of secondary prophylaxis.[14,45] Therefore, it may not be possible to avoid chronic arthropathy when prophylaxis is initiated after significant joint bleeding has already occurred; this supports a need for earlier intervention.

CLINICAL CONTROVERSY

Hemophilia patients may receive prophylactic factor concentrate therapy to prevent or decrease bleeding episodes, or they may receive on-demand factor concentrate therapy in response to a bleeding episode. In addition, prophylaxis may be primary on secondary. Controversy exists over whether the benefits of prophylaxis justify the cost, appropriate time to initiate prophylaxis, and appropriate dosing for prophylaxis.

Prophylactic replacement therapy now is in widespread use in Europe. In 2001 the Medical and Scientific Advisory Council of the National Hemophilia Foundation of the United States recommended primary prophylaxis (prior to onset of frequent bleeding) beginning at age 1 to 2 years for children with severe hemophilia. This therapeutic approach has many challenges and has not been widely accepted in the United States. Many institutions continue to use secondary prophylaxis, in which prophylaxis is started after a pattern of bleeding has been established. Several disadvantages are associated with a primary prophylactic regimen. Perhaps most important is the high cost of prophylactic replacement therapy. Factor requirements are estimated to be twofold to threefold higher with prophylactic regimens than with treatment on demand.[45,48] Use of individual pharmacokinetics to titrate dosage may help to lessen costs.[48] Other issues to consider are the inconvenience to families and possible difficulties with compliance. Central venous lines may be necessary for frequent administration of factor concentrates, particularly in children younger than 5 years, who are at the age targeted for initiation of primary prophylaxis regimens. Potential complications of central venous access include surgical risks, infection, and catheter-related deep-vein thrombosis.[49,50] Catheter-related sepsis has been reported to occur in up to 50% of patients with hemophilia who have central lines.[49] Catheter-related infectious complications appear to be more common in hemophilia patients who have developed inhibitory antibodies.[50] Finally, there are concerns that routine use of primary prophylaxis may overtreat some patients with severe hemophilia who do not have a severe clinical phenotype. Prospective randomized studies and more formal cost-effectiveness analyses are needed to determine the relative benefits and optimal timing of prophylactic factor replacement therapy.

■ TREATMENT OF INHIBITORS IN HEMOPHILIA

Neutralizing antibodies to factor VIII and IX, known as *inhibitors,* develop in a subset of patients with hemophilia, challenging the management of these patients. The development of inhibitors is the most serious complication of factor replacement therapy. The reported incidence of inhibitor development varies considerably, depending on the population studied, the study design, the method of detection, and the frequency and duration of testing. In one systematic review, the overall prevalence of inhibitors in unselected patients with hemophilia was 5% to 7%.[30] The prevalence among patients with severe hemophilia was approximately 12% to 13%, which is higher than for unselected patients.[30] The reported cumulative incidence of inhibitors in hemophilia B is much lower, occurring in only 1% to 4% of patients.[51]

Most inhibitors develop in childhood, often after relatively few exposure days (median 9–12 days).[51] Patients with severe hemophilia are much more likely to develop inhibitors than those with milder forms of the disease.[30] It is possible that the low levels of factor produced in patients with mild and moderate hemophilia induce immune tolerance in these individuals. In contrast, factor levels are undetectable in patients with severe hemophilia, and infused factor VIII, regarded as a foreign protein, may provoke an antibody response. The rate of inhibitor formation varies even among patients with identical mutations, which suggests that host factors modify the risk. One possibility is that human leukocyte antigen (HLA) genotype may influence the risk of inhibitor formation, but studies have been inconclusive.[52]

Inhibitors usually are immunoglobulins of the immunoglobulin G subclass that are directed against the factor coagulant portion of the complex. The presence of an inhibitor is suspected when a decreased clinical response to factor replacement is observed. It may be discovered incidentally on routine laboratory screening. Inhibitors are measured with the Bethesda assay, and titers are reported in Bethesda units (BU). One BU is the amount of inhibitor needed to inactivate half of the factor VIII or factor IX in a mixture of inhibitor-containing plasma and pooled normal plasma.[14] Patients with inhibitors to factor VIII or factor IX are divided into two groups: low responders, who have low levels of inhibitors (<5 BU/mL) and generally have little or no rise in antibody titers after exposure to the factor; and high responders (>5 BU/mL), who have higher inhibitor levels and develop an increase in antibody titer after exposure (anamnestic response).[53]

Therapy for patients with inhibitors involves treatment of acute bleeding episodes and treatment directed at eradicating the inhibitor. The inhibitor titer, the site and magnitude of bleeding, and the patient's past response to therapy determine the approach to treatment. For patients with a low inhibitor titer, administration of high doses of the specific factor often can control bleeding episodes. Two to three times the usual replacement dose and more frequent dosing intervals often are necessary to overcome the antibody. Factor level monitoring and clinical assessments help to evaluate the adequacy of treatment. Additional supportive measures, such as immobilization and administration of antifibrinolytic agents, should be used, where appropriate.

In the presence of a high-titer inhibitor, it may be impossible to administer enough factor VIII or factor IX to neutralize the antibody and achieve a hemostatic plasma level. Therefore, in these patients treatment of bleeding episodes consists of use of agents that bypass the factor to which the antibody is directed. These include PCCs, activated PCCs, and recombinant activated factor VII.

PCCs contain the vitamin K–dependent factors II, VII, IX, and X. Small quantities of activated factors VII and IX are present in these products. Activated PCCs (aPCCs) contain greater quantities of the activated factors.[54] The usual dosage is 50 to 100 units/kg administered every 12 to 24 hours, depending on the severity of the bleeding episode.[30] The maximum dose should not exceed 200 units/kg/day. Use of PCCs and aPCCs, when not restricted to one or two doses, is effective in obtaining hemostasis in approximately 80% of bleeding episodes in patients with inhibitors, and aPCCs appear to be more effective than PCCs. As previously mentioned, there is a risk of serious thrombotic complications, including pulmonary emboli, deep-vein thrombosis, and myocardial infarction associated with use of PCCs and aPCCs.[54] Additionally, because these products contain trace amounts of factor VIII and larger amounts of factor IX, they can stimulate an anamnestic response in patients with hemophilia A and, more commonly, in those with hemophilia B.[54] Other minor side effects include dizziness, nausea, hives, flushing, and headaches.[54] Patients with factor IX inhibitors occasionally develop severe allergic reactions in response to infusion of factor IX–containing products, so these patients should be monitored closely.[55]

Recombinant factor VIIa, a newer bypassing agent, is thought to be hemostatically active only at the site of tissue injury where tissue factor is present; thus, the risk of systemic thrombotic events associated with this agent is minimal.[56] Additionally, because recombinant VIIa is not a plasma-derived product, both viral transmission and anamnestic responses to factor VIII or factor IX are unlikely.[54] The initial dose for bleeding episodes ranges from 35 to 120 mcg/kg.[54] Doses of 70 mcg/kg or higher are more effective, and often a dose of 90 to 120 mcg/kg is used for treatment of patients with hemophilia and inhibitors.[54,57] A drawback is the product's short half-life, which necessitates dosing every 2 hours. Continuous infusion of recombinant factor VIIa, which may be more convenient and cost effective, has been successful, although studies are limited. Recombinant factor VIIa appears to be efficacious in controlling bleeding episodes and managing hemophilia during surgical procedures.[54] Patients treated with bypassing agents must be monitored clinically because no laboratory test directly measures the effectiveness of treatment.

Porcine factor VIII is an alternative therapeutic option for patients who have hemophilia A and inhibitors. In general, porcine factor VIII is most useful when the inhibitor titer is less than 50 BU.[31] The recommended initial dose is 50 to 100 units/kg for those with inhibitor titers less than 50 BU.[31] The rationale is that porcine factor VIII is enough like human factor VIII to participate in the coagulation cascade, yet most factor VIII inhibitors have absent or only weak neutralizing activity against nonhuman factor VIII. However, cross-reactivity with porcine factor VIII does occur, and a high titer of antibody against porcine factor VIII can develop. Although the rise in antibody titer with porcine factor VIII is generally lower than that seen with administration of human factor VIII, anamnestic rises in inhibitor titers to both porcine and human factor VIII may occur and can limit future use.[54] Other potential side effects include severe allergic reactions and thrombocytopenia.[54] Porcine factor VIII is no longer commercially available in the United States, but can be obtained for us in specific patients. Because of these limitations, porcine factor VIII usually is indicated only after the patient has not responded to recombinant factor VIIa and PCC or when the patient has severe hemorrhages.[54] An advantage to porcine factor VIII is that treatment response can be monitored with factor VIII levels.

The ideal therapy for patients with hemophilia and inhibitors is eradication of the inhibitor so that future treatment with factor VIII or factor IX concentrates is possible. Immune tolerance therapy, which involves the regular infusion of high doses of the factor to which the antibody is directed, may accomplish this eradication. A variety of different dosing regimens, ranging from 25 units/kg every other day to more than 200 units/kg every day, have been used. Some treatment protocols include adjunctive immunomodulatory therapy, such as administration of cyclophosphamide, prednisone, and intravenous immune globulin.[58] The overall success rate is 50% to 70% and is higher in patients with low inhibitor titers and in those with recent development of inhibitor.[52] Weeks to years of therapy may be required to eradicate the antibody. Unfortunately, immune tolerance therapy is costly, time-consuming, and often requires placement of a central venous catheter.[59,60] Once achieved, however, immune tolerance facilitates the management of bleeding episodes with specific factor replacement therapy. Rituximab, an anti-CD20 monoclonal antibody has been used with some success in a few patients with acquired factor VIII inhibitors.[61] The mechanism of action involves the rapid depletion of circulating B cells, which produce antibodies, including the anti–factor VIII antibody. Use of rituximab in patients with hemophilia and inhibitors has yet to be tested in large numbers of patients.

Figure 105–3 summarizes the therapeutic options in the management of hemophilia A patients with inhibitors. The same algorithm can be applied to the management of hemophilia B patients, except that factor IX should be substituted for factor VIII. Use of porcine factor VIII is not indicated for inhibitors in hemophilia B.

■ GENE THERAPY IN HEMOPHILIA

Use of gene therapy for hemophilia A and B is currently under investigation. A number of different viral and nonviral vectors have been used to transfer the recombinant factor gene to human cells, such as liver and muscle cells.[62,63] Even low levels of factor expression through gene therapy should reduce bleeding episodes in patients with severe hemophilia, a rationale for gene therapy similar to that for prophylactic factor replacement. Furthermore, given the broad range of physiologically normal factor levels, very tight regulation of gene expression is not necessary. The safety and efficacy of this approach to treatment remain to be determined. Potential benefits to gene therapy include patient convenience, viral safety, and decreased cost. Possible drawbacks to gene therapy include a risk of inhibitor formation, tumorigenesis related to integration of the viral vector, possible germ-line transmission, and concerns about long-term gene expression.[62,63]

■ PAIN MANAGEMENT IN HEMOPHILIA

Pain, both acute and chronic, can be a common occurrence in patients with hemophilia. The likely cause of acute pain is bleeding, and control of the bleeding episode should ease the pain. Chronic pain may be the result of permanent joint changes. Surgical intervention may help to alleviate the pain, as may an intensive physical therapy program.[64] Intraarticular administration of dexamethasone also may be useful.[65] Acetaminophen can be used, although narcotic analgesia may be required for more severe pain. Nonsteroidal antiinflammatory drugs impair platelet function and may increase the risk of bleeding in patients with hemophilia, although these drugs have been used for the management of chronic arthropathy. Cyclooxygenase-2 inhibitors have less antiplatelet activity and may be an option for pain management.

■ SURGERY IN HEMOPHILIA

In the patient with hemophilia undergoing a surgical procedure, the goal of treatment is maintaining factor levels of at least 0.5 to 0.7 units/mL (50%–70%) during surgery and in the postoperative period in order to prevent excessive bleeding. Intermittent dosing or continuous infusion factor replacement may accomplish this goal. Before surgery, factor concentrate usually is infused to obtain a plasma level of 1 unit/mL (100%).[66] Replacement therapy is continued to maintain plasma levels greater than 0.5 units/mL (50%) for 5 to 7 days or longer, depending on the type of surgery. Preoperative evaluation for elective procedures should include measurement of an inhibitor titer and assessment of the recovery and half-life of infused factor in the patient. Elective surgery should not proceed unless therapeutic plasma levels can be obtained.

Evaluation of Therapeutic Outcomes

The main goal in the treatment of hemophilia is controlling and preventing bleeding episodes and their long-term sequelae, such as chronic arthropathies. Pharmacologic and nonpharmacologic inter-

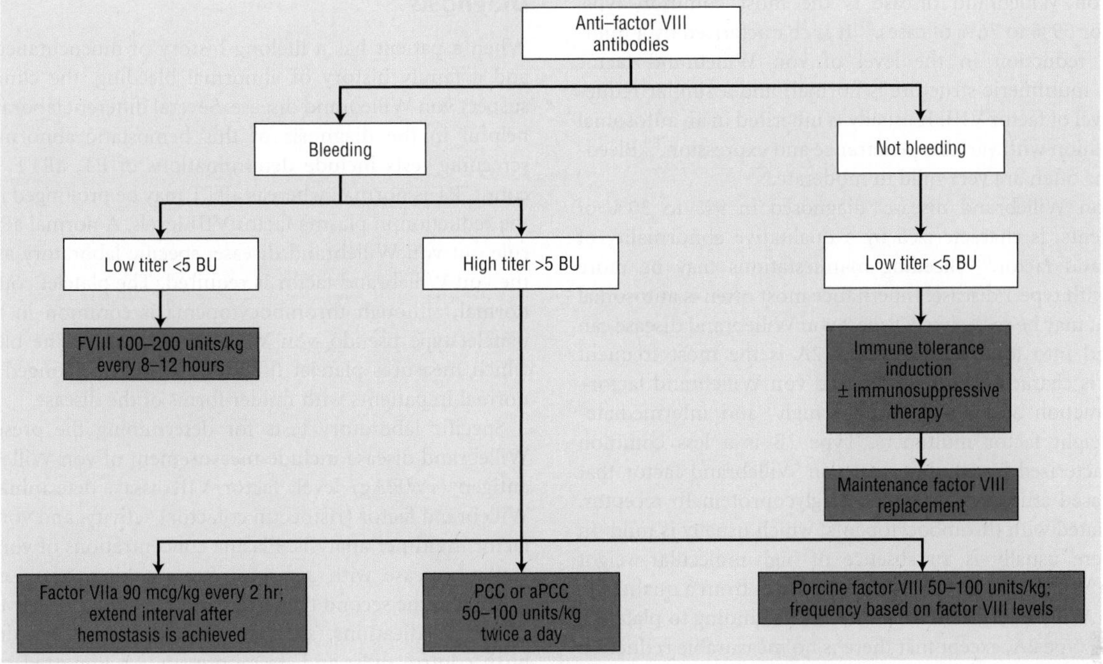

FIGURE 105-3. Treatment algorithm for the management of patients with hemophilia A and factor VIII antibodies. (aPCC, activated prothrombin complex concentrate; BU, Bethesda unit; PCC, prothrombin complex concentrate.)

ventions should be aimed at achieving this goal. Treatment response can be monitored through clinical parameters, such as cessation of bleeding and resolution of symptoms. Determination of plasma factor levels also may be helpful, particularly for severe bleeding episodes. Home therapy for administration of factor concentrates is common among these patients because this approach can lead to earlier treatment and more independence for the patient. Diaries in which the patient documents symptoms, the dose of factor replacement, adjuvant therapies used, and treatment response can help the caregiver evaluate the success of home therapy. Monitoring the number and type of bleeding episodes and measuring trough plasma factor levels makes it possible to evaluate the adequacy of prophylactic regimens. Physical examination with evaluation of joint range of motion and radiographs of target joints indicates the long-term success of preventing and treating arthropathies.

Clinicians should check for the development of inhibitors, especially in patients with severe disease and exposure to factor concentrates, at least yearly and with any suspicion of poor treatment response. The development of inhibitors challenges the management and control of bleeding episodes. A full understanding of the clinical situation and the titer of the inhibitor are mandatory to address all treatment options for each patient. Because no laboratory test measures the effectiveness of therapy in this scenario, close clinical monitoring for worsening or resolution of symptoms is essential for optimizing the outcome.

VON WILLEBRAND DISEASE

The most common congenital bleeding disorder, von Willebrand disease, has a prevalence of 1% to 2%.[67] von Willebrand disease refers to a family of disorders caused by a quantitative and/or qualitative defect of von Willebrand factor, a glycoprotein that plays a role in both platelet aggregation and coagulation. Unlike hemophilia, von Willebrand disease has an autosomal inheritance pattern, resulting in an equal frequency of disease in males and females.

The gene for von Willebrand factor is located on chromosome 12 and is 178 kb in length.[67] Transcription and translation produce a large primary product that subsequently undergoes complex modifications, resulting in von Willebrand factor multimers of various sizes with molecular weights ranging from 500 to 20,000 kDa.[67] Von Willebrand factor is synthesized in endothelial cells, where it is either stored in Weibel-Palade bodies or secreted constitutively. It also is synthesized in megakaryocytes and stored in α-granules, from which it is released following platelet activation.[67]

Von Willebrand factor is important for both primary and secondary hemostasis. In response to vascular injury, it promotes platelet adhesion by interacting with the glycoprotein Ib receptor on platelets.[67,68] It can facilitate platelet aggregation by binding to the platelet glycoprotein IIb/IIIa receptor, although fibrinogen is the main ligand for this receptor.[67,68] The highest-molecular-weight von Willebrand factor multimers appear to be the most important in platelet adhesion because their large surface area contains numerous binding sites for various ligands and receptors. An additional function of von Willebrand factor is that it is the carrier molecule for circulating factor VIII, protecting it from premature degradation and removal.[67] A deficiency of von Willebrand factor reduces the half-life of factor VIII and decreases plasma factor VIII levels. Therefore, von Willebrand factor plays a dual role in hemostasis, affecting both platelet function and coagulation.

Classification of von Willebrand Disease

von Willebrand disease consists of a heterogeneous group of disorders that can be classified into three major subtypes (Table 105–6). Types 1 and 3 are associated with quantitative defects in von Willebrand factor; type 2 mutations refer to functional abnormalities in von Willebrand factor. Determination of the disease subtype is important because it influences treatment.

TABLE 105-6 von Willebrand Disease

von Willebrand factor (vWF)
Large multimeric glycoprotein that is necessary for normal platelet adhesion, normal bleeding time, and stabilizing factor VIII.

von Willebrand factor antigen (vWF:Ag)
Antigenic determinant(s) on vWF measured by immunoassays; usually low in types 1 and 2; virtually absent in type 3.

Ristocetin cofactor activity
Functional assay of vWF activity based on platelet aggregation with ristocetin. Reduced by the same degree as vWF:Ag in types 1 and 3, but to a greater extent in type 2 disease (except 2B).

Type 1 von Willebrand disease is the most common type, accounting for 59% to 76% of cases.[67] It is characterized by a mild-to-moderate reduction in the level of von Willebrand factor (although its multimeric structure is normal) and a similar reduction in the level of factor VIII. It usually is inherited in an autosomal dominant fashion with variable penetrance and expression.[69] Bleeding symptoms often are very mild to moderate.[67]

Type 2 von Willebrand disease, diagnosed in 9% to 30% of affected patients, is characterized by a qualitative abnormality of von Willebrand factor.[67] Bleeding manifestations may be more severe than with type 1 disease. Inheritance most often is autosomal dominant but may be recessive.[69] Type 2 von Willebrand disease can be subdivided into four variants. Type 2A is the most frequent subtype and is characterized by a reduced von Willebrand factor–platelet interaction and an absence of high- and intermediate-molecular-weight factor multimers. Type 2B is a less common variant characterized by an abnormal von Willebrand factor that has an increased affinity for the platelet glycoprotein Ib receptor. This is associated with thrombocytopenia, which usually is mild. In addition, there usually is an absence of high-molecular-weight forms of von Willebrand factor.[69] Type 2M arises from a qualitative defect in von Willebrand factor that impairs its binding to platelets; it is similar to type 2A, except that there is no measurable reduction in the high-molecular-weight multimers.[69] Finally, type 2N von Willebrand disease (Normandy) is a rare form of the disease in which von Willebrand factor has a markedly reduced affinity for factor VIII. This leads to a moderate-to-severe reduction of factor VIII plasma levels with normal von Willebrand factor levels.[69]

Type 3 von Willebrand disease refers to a severe quantitative variant of the disease in which von Willebrand factor is nearly undetectable and factor VIII levels are very low. It often is inherited in an autosomal recessive fashion.[67] The clinical phenotype is severe, reflecting major deficits in primary hemostasis and coagulation. There also is a platelet-type pseudo–von Willebrand disease in which von Willebrand factor is normal but a defect in the platelet glycoprotein Ib receptor causes an increased affinity for normal von Willebrand factor.[67] As a result, platelet-type pseudo–von Willebrand disease is phenotypically similar to type 2B disease but should be distinguished from it because the treatment is different.

Acquired von Willebrand disease is a rare bleeding disorder that is similar to the congenital form of the disease. It has been reported primarily in association with autoimmune disorders, such as systemic lupus erythematosus, lymphoproliferative disorders, myeloproliferative disorders, hypothyroidism, and certain neoplastic diseases such as Wilms tumor and lymphoma.[67,70] It has been reported in situations of high shear stress, such as aortic stenosis. Certain medications have been associated with acquired von Willebrand disease, including valproic acid, griseofulvin, hydroxyethyl starch, and ciprofloxacin.[70] Bleeding manifestations vary from mild to severe, and the condition often resolves with treatment of the underlying disease. Various mechanisms have been proposed, including autoantibodies to von Willebrand factor resulting in rapid removal from the plasma, adsorption to tumor cells or activated platelets, increased proteolysis, or mechanical destruction.[70]

CLINICAL PRESENTATION OF VON WILLEBRAND DISEASE

- Clinical manifestations are variable; some patients are asymptomatic
- Mucocutaneous bleeding: epistaxis, gingival bleeding with minor manipulation, menorrhagia
- Easy bruising
- Postoperative bleeding

Diagnosis

When a patient has a lifelong history of mucocutaneous bleeding and a family history of abnormal bleeding, the clinician should suspect von Willebrand disease. Several different laboratory tests are helpful in the diagnosis of this hemostatic abnormality. Initial screening tests include determinations of PT, aPTT, and platelet count. PT is normal, whereas aPTT may be prolonged in relation to the reduction in plasma factor VIII levels. A normal aPTT does not rule out von Willebrand disease; specific laboratory assessment of the von Willebrand factor is required. The platelet count usually is normal, although thrombocytopenia is common in type 2B and platelet-type pseudo–von Willebrand disease. The bleeding time, which measures platelet function, often is prolonged but may be normal in patients with milder forms of the disease.

Specific laboratory tests for determining the presence of von Willebrand disease include measurement of von Willebrand factor antigen (vWF:Ag) level, factor VIII assay, determination of von Willebrand factor (ristocetin cofactor) activity, and von Willebrand factor multimer analysis. Plasma concentrations of von Willebrand factor increase with age, cigarette smoking, exercise, pregnancy starting in the second trimester, and infection, as well as with use of certain medications, such as corticosteroids, high-dose estrogen birth control pills, and desmopressin.[71,72] Repeated test measurements may be necessary to make the diagnosis because of physiologic variations in plasma levels.

Electroimmunoassay, immunoradiometric assay, or enzyme-linked immunosorbent assay can be used to quantify vWF:Ag.[67] Because vWF:Ag levels are known to vary with different ABO blood types,[73] interpretation requires reference to values specific for the patient's blood type. The vWF:Ag level usually is low in types 1 and 2 von Willebrand disease and virtually absent in type 3 disease. Factor VIII levels are normal or mildly decreased in patients with type 1 or 2 disease and very low (<10%) in those with type 3 disease.[67] Ristocetin, an antibiotic that causes platelet aggregation in the presence of functional von Willebrand factor, is used to measure von Willebrand factor activity. The assay is performed by mixing platelet-free patient plasma, normal formalin-fixed platelets, and ristocetin and then quantitating the extent of platelet agglutination. Ristocetin cofactor activity usually is reduced in parallel to vWF:Ag levels in types 1 and 3 disease and decreased to a greater extent than vWF:Ag in type 2 disease (except type 2B).[69] Ristocetin-induced platelet agglutination is useful for further distinguishing type 2B disease, as a low concentration of ristocetin induces excessive aggregation in type 2B disease.

Von Willebrand factor multimers can be analyzed by separating them by size on an agarose gel. All multimer sizes are present in type 1 disease, whereas reduced levels of intermediate- and high-molecular-weight multimers are characteristic of type 2 disease. Type 3 patients lack all types of von Willebrand factor multimers. A summary of the laboratory findings in the various types of von Willebrand disease is provided in Table 105–6.

TREATMENT

von Willebrand Disease

❹ The specific type of von Willebrand disease, as well as the location and severity of bleeding, determines the approach to treatment. Local measures, including pressure, ice, and topical thrombin, often can control superficial bleeding. Systemic treatment is used for bleeding that cannot be controlled in this manner and for prevention of bleeding with surgery. The goal of systemic therapy is correction of platelet adhesion and coagulation defects by stimulating the release of endogenous von Willebrand factor or by

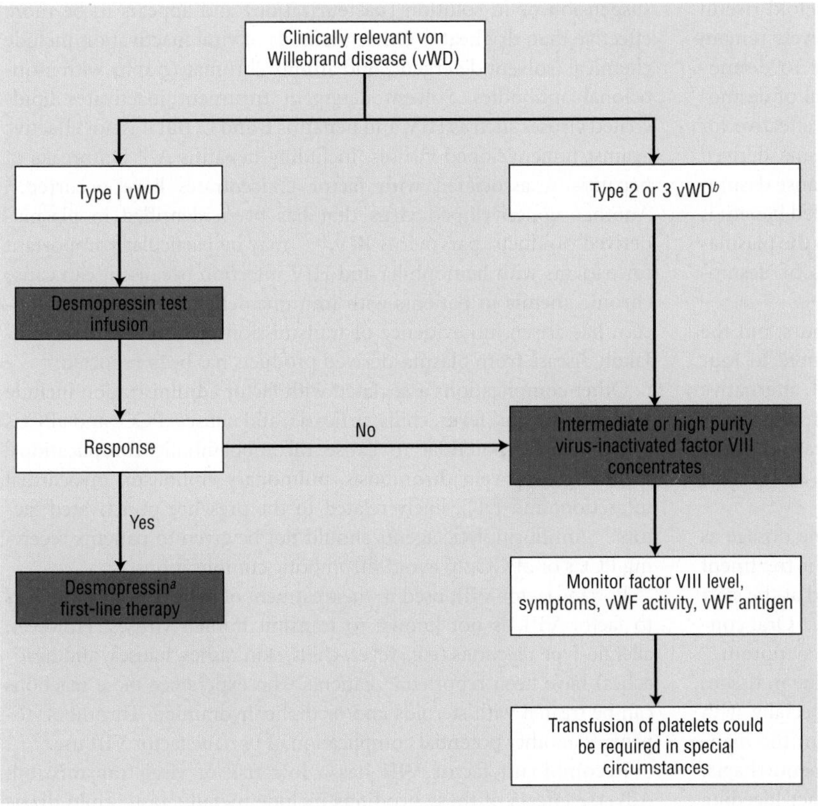

FIGURE 105-4. Guidelines for treatment of von Willebrand disease. [a]Use factor VIII concentrate for life-threatening bleeding. [b]Some patients with type 2 or 3 von Willebrand disease may respond to desmopressin.

administering products that contain von Willebrand factor and factor VIII. General guidelines for treatment of von Willebrand disease are shown in Fig. 105–4.

■ REPLACEMENT THERAPY

❺ The treatment of choice for patients with types 2B, 2M, and 3 von Willebrand disease and for patients with type 1 or 2A von Willebrand disease who are unresponsive to desmopressin is replacement therapy with plasma-derived von Willebrand factor–containing products.[66] Several virus-inactivated, intermediate- or high-purity factor VIII concentrates contain sufficient amounts of functional von Willebrand factor.[66] Ultrahigh-purity (monoclonal antibody-derived) plasma-derived products and recombinant factor VIII products contain only negligible amounts of von Willebrand factor and are inadequate for treatment of von Willebrand disease. A very high-purity plasma-derived von Willebrand factor concentrate and a recombinant von Willebrand factor product are currently in clinical trials.[68] Because these von Willebrand factor concentrates do not contain appreciable factor VIII, concomitant administration of a factor VIII–containing product may be necessary for patients with severe disease and low levels of factor VIII.[68] Cryoprecipitate contains approximately 80 to 100 units of von Willebrand factor per unit (5–10 times more von Willebrand factor and factor VIII than fresh-frozen plasma), and in the past it was the mainstay of therapy for von Willebrand disease.[67] However, because cryoprecipitate is not virally inactivated, it is seldom used as first-line treatment. General guidelines for the dosing of replacement therapy in patients with von Willebrand disease unresponsive to desmopressin are provided in Table 105–7.

■ OTHER PHARMACOLOGIC THERAPY

❻ Desmopressin stimulates the endothelial cell release of von Willebrand factor and factor VIII.[66] It is effective for patients with von Willebrand disease who have adequate endogenous stores of functional von Willebrand factor. This group includes most patients with type 1 disease and some patients with type 2A disease. Conversely, desmopressin is not appropriate for patients with type 3 disease, who lack stores of von Willebrand factor.

CLINICAL CONTROVERSY

Some hematologists find desmopressin beneficial in treating patients with type 2B von Willebrand disease, whereas others believe it may exacerbate thrombocytopenia.

Desmopressin usually is not recommended for treatment of type 2B disease because the release of additional abnormal von Willebrand factor may exacerbate thrombocytopenia.[67] However, desmopressin has been reported to be beneficial in some patients with type 2B disease.[67] If desmopressin is used for treatment of type 2B disease, close monitoring is necessary.

The dose of desmopressin used for treatment of von Willebrand disease is identical to that used for treatment of mild factor VIII deficiency, 0.3 mcg/kg diluted in 30 to 50 mL of normal saline and given intravenously over 15 to 30 minutes.[66] In general, patients with von Willebrand disease have a better response to desmopressin than

TABLE 105-7 Replacement Therapy in von Willebrand Disease[a]

Condition	Therapy
Major surgery	Maintain factor VIII level ≥50% for 1 week Prolonged treatment in type 3 patients (>7 days)
Minor surgery	Maintain factor VIII level ≥50% for 1–3 days Maintain factor VIII level >20%–30% for an additional 4–7 days
Dental extraction	Single infusion to achieve factor VIII level >50% Desmopressin prior to procedure for type I
Spontaneous or post-traumatic bleeding	Usually single infusion of 20–40 units/kg

[a]The yield of factor VIII after first infusion is similar to that observed in hemophilia A (about 2% increment over baseline amount for every 1 unit/kg of factor VIII infused).

those with hemophilia, with an average threefold to fivefold rise in von Willebrand factor and factor VIII levels.[67] These levels remain elevated for approximately 6 to 8 hours. The response to desmopressin in a given patient usually is consistent, and a trial of desmopressin should establish if the medication likely will be effective for the individual. Desmopressin is preferable to use of plasma-derived products for patients who have an adequate response because desmopressin does not carry a risk of viral transmission. An added benefit is the substantially lower cost of desmopressin compared to the plasma-derived products. (For a discussion of the side effects of desmopressin, see Treatment of Hemophilia A above.)

Desmopressin can be administered every 12 to 24 hours, but the response diminishes with repeated treatment.[68] After three to four doses, desmopressin often is no longer effective, and alternative replacement therapy may be necessary if prolonged treatment is required. Laboratory monitoring, including vWF:Ag measurements, factor VIII assays, ristocetin cofactor activity assessments, and clinical examinations, will determine the adequacy of treatment.

Intranasal administration of desmopressin, at the same dosage as that used for mild factor VIII deficiency, can be useful for treatment of mild bleeding episodes. One or two doses administered at the start of menses may be helpful in controlling menorrhagia.[68,74] Oral contraceptives may also be very effective in controlling this symptom.[68] Inhibitors of the fibrinolytic system may be of special value in tissues rich in plasminogen activators, such as the mouth, especially with tooth extractions.[67] Antifibrinolytic agents can be used in the management of epistaxis, gastrointestinal bleeding, and menorrhagia. However, these agents should be avoided in urinary tract bleeding because of the risk of thrombosis and obstruction.[66]

OTHER CONGENITAL FACTOR DEFICIENCIES

In addition to deficiencies in factors VIII and IX, congenital deficiencies in fibrinogen, in factors II, V, VII, X, XI, and XIII, and in combinations of factor deficiencies have been reported.[75] Contact factor abnormalities, including deficiencies in factor XII, high-molecular-weight kininogen, and prekallikrein, prolong the aPTT but do not lead to any bleeding diathesis. Identification of these disorders is important so that inappropriate treatment is not given. The only contact factor deficiency associated with bleeding symptoms is factor XI deficiency. Also known as hemophilia C, this deficiency is particularly common in people of Ashkenazi Jewish descent.[75,76] Bleeding manifestations are variable. Bleeding usually does not occur spontaneously, but excessive bleeding may occur after trauma or surgery. Most other deficiencies are inherited as autosomal recessive disorders and are rare. Some patients with abnormal molecules, such as fibrinogen, may have an increased tendency to develop thromboembolic disease. Most of these deficiencies are treated with fresh-frozen plasma. Newer specific concentrates are becoming available. For example, a factor XIII plasma-derived concentrate is available, and recombinant VIIA is approved for use in patients with congenital VII deficiency. Cryoprecipitate, which is rich in fibrinogen, can be used to treat patients with fibrinogen deficiency or dysfunctional fibrinogen (dysfibrinogenemias).

COMPLICATIONS OF REPLACEMENT THERAPY

Transmission of blood-borne viruses is always a concern when blood and blood-derived products are used. The infection of a large number of hemophiliac patients with hepatitis viruses and HIV during the 1980s prompted the development of virucidal methods to inactivate infectious agents.[8,15] All currently available plasma-derived factor concentrates come from screened donors and undergo viral inactivation procedures in an effort to reduce the risk of viral transmission. Heat treatment, which includes dry and wet heat, is one method of viral inactivation. Wet heat is applied while the concentrate is in suspension or in solution (pasteurization) and appears to be more effective than dry heat.[77] Other methods of viral inactivation include chemical (solvent detergent) and affinity chromatography with monoclonal antibodies. Solvent detergent treatment inactivates lipid-coated viruses such as HIV and hepatitis B and C, but it is not effective against nonenveloped viruses, including hepatitis A.[77] Outbreaks of hepatitis A associated with factor concentrates have occurred.[15] Another nonenveloped virus that has been identified in plasma-derived products, parvovirus B19,[21,77] may be particularly important for patients with hemophilia and HIV infection because it can cause chronic anemia in patients with immune deficiency. Although concern has arisen, no evidence of transmission of variant Creutzfeldt-Jakob disease from plasma-derived products has been reported.[21]

Other complications associated with factor administration include allergic reactions, fever, chills, urticaria, and nausea. PCCs and aPCCs also have the potential to cause thromboembolic complications, including deep-vein thrombosis, pulmonary embolism, myocardial infarction, and DIC, likely related to the presence of activated factors.[14] Antifibrinolytic agents should not be given to patients receiving PCCs or aPCCs to avoid thrombotic complications.

Porcine factor VIII, used in the treatment of patients with inhibitors to factor VIII, is not known to transmit human viruses. However, allergic-type reactions (e.g., fever, chills, skin rashes, nausea, and headaches) have been reported.[54] Patients who experience these reactions can be treated with steroids and/or diphenhydramine. Thrombocytopenia is another potential complication of porcine factor VIII use.[54]

Recombinant factor VIII has a low risk of viral transmission. Adverse effects of these products include metallic taste, mild dizziness, mild rash, burning at the infusion site, and a small drop in blood pressure.[78]

PHARMACOECONOMIC CONSIDERATIONS

Treatment of severe hemophilia often is expensive, with a substantial portion of the cost related to the expense of factor concentrates.[59] The highly purified plasma-derived products and recombinant factor concentrates are considerably more expensive than the low- and intermediate-purity products. However, the viral safety of recombinant products must be weighed against the added cost. Recombinant products are often used, particularly for children with hemophilia. With the more widespread use of prophylactic factor replacement regimens to prevent chronic arthropathy, factor usage and cost of treatment have greatly increased over that for on-demand therapy.[14] The positive impact on patient lifestyle must be weighed against the drawbacks of cost, the potential need for permanent venous access, and patient compliance. Finally, the use of immune tolerance therapy is associated with extremely high factor usage and cost, but with the potential benefit of eradicating an inhibitor a life-threatening complication of hemophilia. A formal economic analysis has suggested that this therapy may be cost-effective over the patient's lifetime.[59]

Optimal management of von Willebrand disease starts with adequate identification of the patient's disease type. Desmopressin is considerably less expensive than plasma-derived factor VIII concentrates.[67] It should be the treatment of choice for all patients responsive to the test dose because of its viral safety, reduced cost, and ease of administration.

ACQUIRED COAGULATION DISORDERS

DISSEMINATED INTRAVASCULAR COAGULATION

Systemic activation of coagulation that results from DIC leads to clot formation in the microvasculature, often with compensatory bleeding

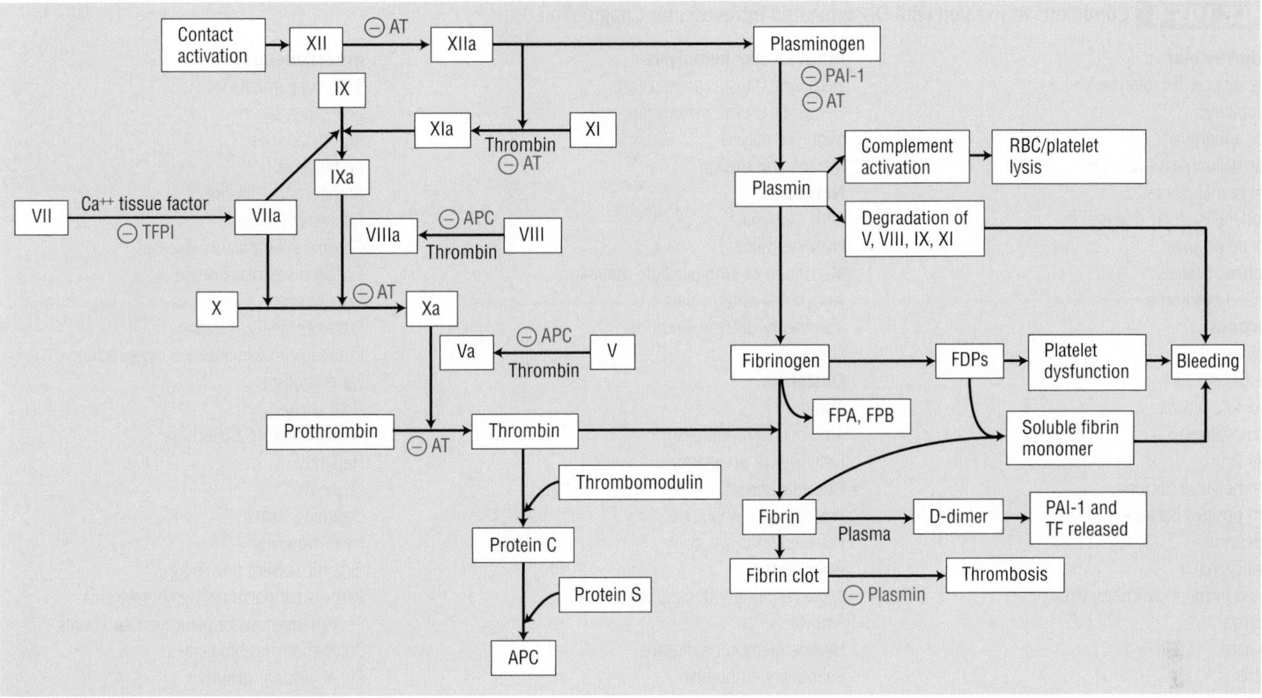

FIGURE 105-5. Pathophysiology of disseminated intravascular coagulation. (APC, activated protein C; AT, antithrombin; FDP, fibrin degradation product; FPA, fibrinopeptide A; FPB, fibrinopeptide B; PAI-1, plasminogen activator inhibitor type 1; RBC, red blood cell; TFPI, tissue factor pathway inhibitor.)

owing to biodegradation of coagulation factors and platelets. Although the causes for DIC can be diverse, the pathophysiology leading to DIC is the same once the triggering event occurs (Fig. 105–5). An overwhelming insult leads to the formation of thrombin and plasmin beyond the control of the regulatory systems. Once formed, thrombin leads to the cleavage of fibrinopeptide A and B from fibrinogen, leaving a fibrin monomer. The monomer polymerizes into a clot, leading to microvascular and macrovascular thrombosis while consuming platelets by trapping them in the clots. Thrombosis ultimately decreases blood flow to multiple organs, leading to organ damage. Plasmin cleaves fibrinogen into fibrin(ogen) degradation products, which can combine with the fibrin monomer before polymerization. This forms a soluble fibrin monomer that impairs hemostasis and leads to hemorrhage. Some of the FDPs may adhere to platelets, causing platelet dysfunction that may contribute to clinically significant hemorrhage. In addition, plasmin is a proteolytic enzyme that can degrade factors V, VIII, IX, and XI and other plasma proteins. Circulation of plasmin can activate the complement system, leading to red blood cell and platelet lysis. The activated complement system also increases vascular permeability that can cause hypotension and shock.[79]

Complicating this process is an intricate web of feedback systems. Thrombin induces activation of factors V and XI, while it also activates protein C that inhibits the activation of the same. Antithrombin is a serine protease that mediates the antithrombotic effect of heparin. It also inhibits the activation of thrombin, plasmin, and factors IXa, Xa, XIa, and XIIa.[80] Acute DIC is characterized by rapid and extensive depletion of coagulation factors and inhibitors and excessive fibrinolysis in an attempt to compensate for microvascular clotting. Normally, a balanced dynamic process of clotting and fibrinolysis operates to prevent organ dysfunction, bleeding, or clotting. In acute DIC, excessive intravascular coagulation overcomes the normal inhibitory processes. In subacute or chronic DIC, the balance between depletion and synthesis of coagulation factors in the circulation may make the diagnosis difficult, because patients may be asymptomatic, bleeding, and/or forming thromboses.

In summary, bleeding problems observed during DIC can be the result of consumption of coagulation factors during clotting, depletion or dysfunction of platelets, interference in fibrin formation by FDPs, and lysis of clots by plasmin. Thrombosis occurs in parallel with the bleeding process, and the extent of microvascular obstruction will determine the degree of organ damage.

CLINICAL PRESENTATION OF DISSEMINATED INTRAVASCULAR COAGULATION

General

- Underlying illness (Table 105–8)

Signs and Symptoms

- Bleeding, thrombosis, or both
- Petechiae and purpura
- Peripheral cyanosis
- Hemorrhagic bullae

Laboratory Tests

- Elevated D-dimer
- Decreased antithrombin
- Decreased fibrinogen
- Thrombocytopenia
- Decreased proteins C and S
- Increased fibrinopeptides A and B
- Elevated prothrombin fragments 1 and 2
- Evidence of end-organ dysfunction or failure

Laboratory Diagnosis

The basis for a diagnosis of DIC is a combination of laboratory test results in the setting of a known causative clinical disorder.[79,81–82] The relative importance of any particular laboratory test is controversial. Routine tests of blood coagulation, including PT and aPTT,

TABLE 105-8 Conditions Associated with Disseminated Intravascular Coagulation

Cardiovascular	**Intravascular hemolysis**	**Miscellaneous**
Acute myocardial infarction	Hemolytic transfusion reaction	Acid–base imbalance
Angiopathy	Hemolytic uremic syndrome	Acute liver failure
Aortic aneurysm	Minor hemolysis	Amphetamines
Aortic balloon assist devices	Massive transfusion	Anaphylaxis
Giant hemangiomas	**Newborn**	Autoimmune diseases
Peripheral vascular disease	Birth asphyxia	Cholestasis
Postcardiac arrest	Hypothermia	Chronic inflammatory diseases
Prosthetic devices	Meconium or amniotic fluid aspiration	Collagen vascular disease
Raynaud syndrome	Necrotizing enterocolitis	Craniotomy
Infectious	Respiratory distress syndrome	Extracorporeal circulation
Arbovirus	Shock	Extracorporeal membrane oxygenation
Aspergillus	**Obstetrics**	Fat embolism
Candida albicans	Abortion	Heat stroke
Cytomegalovirus	Amniotic fluid embolism	Hemorrhagic telangiectasia
Ebola virus	Fatty liver of pregnancy	Hepatitis
Gram-negative bacteria	Placental abruption	Leukemia
Gram-positive bacteria	Preeclampsia/eclampsia	Lightning strikes
Herpesvirus	Retained fetus syndrome	Near drowning
Histoplasma	**Pulmonary**	Organic solvent poisoning
Human immunodeficiency virus	Acute respiratory distress syndrome	Paroxysmal nocturnal hemoglobinuria
Influenza	Empyema	Peritoneovenous or pleurovenous shunts
Kala-azar	Hyaline membrane disease	Polycythemia rubra vera
Malaria	Pulmonary embolism	Renal vascular disorders
Mycobacteria	Pulmonary infarction	Severe anoxia
Mycoplasma	**Tissue injury**	Snake bite
Paramyxoviruses	Burns	Solid tumors
Rocky Mountain spotted fever	Crush injuries	Transplant rejection
Rubella	Extensive surgery	
Typhoid	Head trauma	
Varicella	Multiple trauma	
Variola		

are unreliable and of minimal use. PT and aPTT are prolonged in 50% to 60% of cases, but they may be decreased or normal.[79,82] The thrombin time usually is prolonged because of the absolute decrease in fibrinogen as well as the presence of FDPs, which inhibit the conversion of fibrinogen to fibrin.[79]

Liver disease may cause decreased synthesis of coagulation factors, and the subsequent abnormal laboratory results can be difficult to differentiate from DIC. Increased levels of FDPs are not specific to DIC, but elevated levels occur in 85% to 100% of patients with DIC.[79] Because FDPs are metabolized in the liver and excreted by the kidney, organ damage may increase the level of FDPs. However, an increased FDP level may help to identify compensated DIC, as it may be the only abnormal laboratory result. D-Dimer is formed when plasmin digests cross-linked fibrin; thus, the level of D-dimer is a more specific measure of FDPs.

Fibrinogen levels are an acute phase reactant, and a low level indicates DIC with only 28% sensitivity.[81] Platelet counts usually are decreased in patients with DIC. Fifty percent of patients have schistocytes (red blood cell fragments) in fulminant DIC.[79] Unfortunately, these findings also may be evident in patients with severe liver disease with hypersplenism. Depressed levels of antithrombin, protein C, and protein S are seen in most patients. Severe initial decreases in antithrombin levels occur in septic DIC. Activity levels below 50% to 60% correlate with poor outcome.[80]

Thrombin cleaves fibrinopeptides A and B from fibrinogen, so the levels of fibrinopeptides A and B should be elevated in patients with DIC. Initial studies have shown a good correlation between an elevated level of fibrinopeptide A and DIC, but other inflammatory conditions such as systemic lupus erythematosus, infections, and thrombosis also may result in elevated levels, thus decreasing the specificity of this test. Elevated prothrombin 1 and 2 levels indicate factor Xa generation and are a reliable DIC marker, indicating procoagulant activation.[79]

Factor VIII and V levels should be decreased in DIC, but results of these tests may be quite variable because of systemic activation of the coagulation system. In clinical practice, serial results yielding a declining platelet count associated with an elevated D-dimer level along with depressed antithrombin and fibrinogen levels indicate a diagnosis of DIC.[81,82] In lieu of molecular markers, measurements of prolonged PT or aPTT in conjunction with platelet count and fibrinogen are commonly used.

TREATMENT

Disseminated Intravascular Coagulation

❼ If unrecognized and left untreated, DIC may lead to death as a result of hemorrhage or thrombosis. However, there is some controversy regarding optimal treatment because of the different mechanisms and clinical manifestations that can occur with DIC. Even so, there is a consensus that the most important step in therapy for DIC is treatment of the underlying disease.[79,81] In a pregnant woman with placental abruption or retained placenta in whom the disease is self-limited, delivery of the fetus with the products of conception usually returns hemostasis to normal. In patients who have overwhelming sepsis or shock, antibiotics and treatment of hypotension are the mainstays of therapy. In patients who are receiving maximum treatment for the underlying condition but in whom the process is worsening or in whom bleeding develops, additional treatments may be used.

The efficacy of fresh-frozen plasma or platelet transfusions has not been proven in randomized clinical trials but is rational for patients who are bleeding or require invasive procedures.[81] Fresh-frozen plasma replaces clotting factors, fibrinogen, protein S, protein C, and antithrombin. If hypofibrinogenemia is severe, cryoprecipitate may be useful as a concentrated source of fibrinogen. Although it has been argued that replacement of coagulation factors may worsen the situation, in practice this does not appear to make the situation worse, and it frequently improves hemostasis.

Trials of antithrombin concentrate in the treatment of DIC from various causes show some beneficial effect on improving DIC score, decreasing duration of DIC, or improving end-organ function.[80,81] A large multicenter, randomized controlled trial showed no significant decrease in mortality when used in septic patients. A subset analysis suggests antithrombin may be useful in the absence of heparin.[83] In addition to variable efficacy, antithrombin is an expensive product with only intermittent availability. Therefore, restricting its use to patients at high risk for morbidity and mortality should be considered.

CLINICAL CONTROVERSY

Heparin use in patients with disseminated intravascular coagulation may prevent the formation of new blood clots. The most common complication of heparin therapy is bleeding, so some clinicians find the risk too high to justify heparin use.

Anticoagulation in patients with DIC is controversial. The main pathogenic factor of DIC is considered to be the generation of intravascular thrombin. Interference of thrombin activity by an agent such as heparin appears to be a logical therapeutic step. The main advantage of heparin is that it can prevent further thrombosis and consumption of hemostatic factors, but it has no effect on an already established microthrombus within the vasculature. Because the major complication of heparin therapy is bleeding, some experts argue against heparin use in patients with an existing bleeding disorder. Although case reports have shown improvement in individual patients, heparin has not been shown to reduce morbidity or mortality in controlled clinical trials. Heparin rarely restores the coagulopathy to normal, although both the deficiency of coagulation factors and the thrombocytopenia may improve. If the patient does not respond to the replacement of coagulation factors, the addition of heparin may improve the coagulopathy by forming the heparin–antithrombin complex to inhibit thrombin.

Heparin is given subcutaneously or as a continuous IV infusion. The dosage of heparin for DIC is controversial, ranging anywhere from full-dose to low-dose heparin.[81] Full-dose heparin in adults requires administration of 5,000 units as an IV bolus, followed by a continuous infusion at 1,000 units per hour or according to a weight-based heparin dosing regimen. Some experts advocate low-dose heparin, such as an infusion of 500 units per hour in adults, and adjusting the dose based on clinical and laboratory data. Low-dose heparin given subcutaneously has been used with success. Monitoring of heparin therapy is difficult because the aPTT often is elevated before initiation of heparin therapy, so following D-dimer and fibrinogen levels is best.

Anticoagulation is contraindicated in patients with life-threatening or serious bleeding (e.g., intracranial, retroperitoneal, or pericardial). Patients with symptomatic thromboemboli, extensive fibrin deposition, persistent coagulation abnormalities despite replacement of hemostatic factors, solid tumors, or chronic DIC may benefit from heparin therapy.[81,84] Historically, an infusion of low-dose heparin at 7.5 units/kg/h has been used in patients with acute promyelocytic leukemia, along with administration of platelets, fresh-frozen plasma, and cryoprecipitate.[84] Patients with solid tumors who are symptomatic from a thrombosis should receive an infusion of heparin 15 units/kg/h. Once asymptomatic, heparin can be administered subcutaneously.

In two uncontrolled trials, patients tolerated the use of low-molecular-weight heparin well, and this approach showed a possible beneficial outcome.[79] A randomized, double-blind study compared the efficacy of dalteparin with that of low-dose heparin. Dalteparin was more effective at improving bleeding symptoms, but no difference in mortality was observed.[79]

Antifibrinolytics, such as aminocaproic acid, have been used in patients in whom excessive fibrinolysis was the dominant clinical picture.[79] Because aminocaproic acid can increase fibrin deposition, many experts believe that it usually is contraindicated. In patients with chronic liver disease who manifest dominant fibrinolysis, attempts to inhibit the fibrinolytic system have generally been unsuccessful. Patients with acute promyelocytic leukemia may benefit from an antifibrinolytic, as hyperfibrinolysis is the dominant clinical feature of their condition.[79]

Critically ill patients may develop vitamin K deficiency. In addition, patients with DIC may consume vitamin K and may require supplementation to replenish stores. Other possible treatment may include use of protein C concentrate, lepirudin, anti–tissue factor antibody, tifacogin (recombinant tissue factor pathway inhibitor), or thrombin inhibitors such as dermatan sulfate, anti–plasminogen activator inhibitor type 1, and dithiocarbamates.[79,85]

Activated protein C modulates coagulation (Fig. 105–5). Activation of protein C may be impaired during sepsis. Drotrecogin alfa (activated protein C) administration resulted in an absolute reduction in mortality of 6.1% from severe sepsis without undue bleeding in carefully chosen adult patients.[86] Strategies for use in adults have been developed to target appropriate patients.[87] The pediatric trials closed prematurely. Patients must be carefully chosen to minimize bleeding complications and optimize benefits.

Evaluation of Therapeutic Outcomes

The management of DIC is surrounded by controversy, and the optimal approach to these patients is still to be determined. Diagnosis and treatment of the underlying disease should be the goal in all cases. Determination of the dominant process (i.e., hemorrhage vs. thrombosis) can help focus the treatment approach but often is impossible, so clinicians institute replacement therapy of the deficient clotting factors and attempt to control the clotting problems with agents such as heparin.

Risk versus benefit, as well as any contraindications, should be considered at the start of any given therapy for each patient. Monitoring therapy for DIC with laboratory tests can be difficult because the underlying process can cause a variety of laboratory abnormalities. For example, monitoring the effect of heparin by using the aPTT can be a complex task, especially when the patient has an abnormal baseline aPTT. In this case, monitoring fibrinogen and D-dimer levels may be more useful in detecting any need to adjust therapy. In addition, it is important to combine laboratory parameters with clinical assessment to make rational treatment adjustments. Aggressive hemodynamic stabilization and other supportive measures to prevent organ failure also are important in the overall management and prognosis of patients with DIC.

VITAMIN K DEFICIENCY

Vitamin K is a cofactor for activation of factors II, VII, IX, and X.[88] Vitamin K is required for γ-carboxylation of these clotting factors. Without vitamin K, these factors cannot bind calcium or bind to negatively charge phospholipids membranes and thus remain inactive precursors. Vitamin K also is necessary for the active forms of proteins C and S, which inhibit factor Va and VIIIa. In most clinical situations, vitamin K deficiency causes a bleeding diathesis as a result of marked deficiency of factors II, VII, IX, and X.

Vitamin K is a fat-soluble vitamin. Vitamin K_1, phytonadione, is found in green vegetables. Bacteria in the large intestine produce vitamin K_2, the menaquinones, which require bile salts to be solubilized and absorbed.[88]

Hemorrhagic Disease of the Newborn

Newborns are deficient in vitamin K at birth, as transplacental passage is insignificant.[89] The level may continue to fall during the neonatal period because the infant's gut has not had sufficient time to undergo bacterial colonization, so the infant lacks hepatic stores. Breast milk contains a low content of vitamin K in comparison to infant formulas; therefore, breast-fed infants are more vulnerable to developing vitamin K deficiency. In addition, the plasma concentrations of the vitamin K–dependent factors are physiologically low in infants.[90] Vitamin K deficiency in neonates can cause intracranial hemorrhage and bleeding from the umbilical cord or the gastrointestinal tract.[89]

Bleeding within 24 hours of birth, early vitamin K–dependent bleeding, usually is the result of maternal ingestion of anticonvulsants, warfarin, rifampin, or isoniazid. Classic vitamin K–dependent bleeding usually appears during the first week of life and results from the lack of prophylactic vitamin K administration at birth. Risk factors for late vitamin K–dependent bleeding, which occurs at 2 to 12 weeks, include cholestatic liver disease, cystic fibrosis, α_1-antitrypsin deficiency, exclusive breast-feeding, and failure to give adequate vitamin K at birth.[89] Use of oral vitamin K at birth is associated with a higher incidence of late vitamin K–dependent bleeding. It has been suggested that the intramuscular route of administration allows the vitamin K to act as a depot preparation and may explain the lower rate of late vitamin K–dependent bleeding with this route.[89]

The levels of vitamin K–dependent coagulation factors are low at birth. Without adequate vitamin K, these levels may fall even further. In this situation, PT and aPTT are prolonged, but the thrombin time, fibrinogen level, and platelet count are normal. Most infants achieve adult levels by age 3 months if intramuscular phytonadione was given at birth.[89]

❽ In the United States, infants usually receive 1 mg of phytonadione intramuscularly at birth for prophylaxis. Most infants build up vitamin K_1 and K_2 stores in the liver during the first month of life. The speed of repletion depends on the amount of milk or formula received. Oral supplementation results in late vitamin K–dependent bleeding if vitamin K is not given daily for 3 months, which risks noncompliance. Controversy has arisen over whether the high plasma vitamin K levels achieved with intramuscular injection lead to an increased incidence of childhood cancer. This risk has not been substantiated, and the benefits of widespread use outweigh the minimal risk.[90] Fresh-frozen plasma is used to treat life-threatening hemorrhages.

Malabsorption

Patients may become deficient in vitamin K as a result of poor nutrition or malabsorption. A careful dietary history is important in this regard. Broad-spectrum antibiotics may sterilize the large intestine and prevent vitamin K_2 production.

Vitamin K absorption depends on both bile acids and pancreatic enzymes to create micelles. Malabsorption resulting from diseases of the small intestine or pancreas, such as cystic fibrosis, Crohn disease, ulcerative colitis, cholestatic liver disease, celiac disease, amyloidosis, Whipple disease, and short-bowel syndrome, may cause abnormal development in children, weight loss, muscle wasting, steatorrhea, vitamin deficiencies, and anemia. Significant malabsorption can occur even without the symptoms of diarrhea or steatorrhea.

TREATMENT

Vitamin K Deficiency

Phytonadione is used to treat vitamin K deficiency. The dose, frequency, and duration of vitamin K administration depend on the severity of the deficiency and the patient's response. Vitamin K can be administered orally, intramuscularly, subcutaneously, or intravenously. After an oral dose of vitamin K_1, blood coagulation factors increase within 6 to 12 hours. When vitamin K_1 is administered parenterally, PT may take 12 to 24 hours to normalize, although improvement usually occurs within 1 to 2 hours. Failure of vitamin K_1 to correct PT after 48 hours should raise suspicion about the etiology of the coagulation abnormality (e.g., liver disease).

The appropriate route of administration depends on the severity and the cause of the vitamin K deficiency. For instance, in patients with severe hypoprothrombinemia, it is best to avoid the intramuscular route because of the risk of hematoma formation. Because of the rare anaphylactic reaction associated with intravenous administration, this route often is restricted to patients who are thrombocytopenic or unable to absorb the drug via the gastrointestinal tract.[91] Vitamin K can be administered subcutaneously to patients without intravenous access. Patients with life-threatening bleeding should receive fresh-frozen plasma as a source of vitamin K–dependent factors to ensure immediate correction.

Patients with malabsorption or obstructive jaundice may require parenteral administration of vitamin K. Phytonadione 10 mg weekly usually is sufficient in adults. Patients on long-term total parenteral nutrition should receive daily supplementation.

COAGULOPATHY AND LIVER DISEASE

Bleeding disorders can be associated with acute or chronic liver disease. The degree of coagulopathy correlates with the degree of hepatocellular disease. The liver synthesizes the blood coagulation factors and inhibitors of coagulation (e.g., antithrombin and proteins C and S). All clotting factors except factor VIII are decreased in liver failure.[92] The ability of the liver to clear activated clotting factors and their degradation products is reduced with liver failure.[92] Primary fibrinolysis occurs due to decreased levels of the inhibitors of plasmin activation.[92] Platelet count and function are decreased in patients with liver disease. The development of DIC may worsen the coagulopathy.

PT, aPTT, and thrombin time are useful in screening for a deficiency of liver-dependent factors. PT is sensitive to deficiencies in the vitamin K–dependent factors. aPTT helps to determine deficiencies in factor IX and other factors. Thrombin time can help to detect hypofibrinogenemia, dysfibrinogenemia, and the presence of FDPs that interfere with fibrin polymerization. Defects in polymerization may occur before severe hypofibrinogenemia and may be an indication of the degree of liver dysfunction. The level of D-dimer should be normal unless DIC is present.

Factor V is synthesized by hepatic cells but is not dependent on vitamin K. Therefore, it may be useful in distinguishing vitamin K deficiency from liver disease. Deficiency of antithrombin occurs with severe hepatocellular disease and may contribute to the development of DIC. In acute hepatic failure, the level of plasminogen may be low, reflecting decreased synthesis or increased catabolism associated with DIC. The level of factor VIII usually is normal or elevated in liver disease but is decreased in DIC.

TREATMENT

Coagulopathy and Liver Disease

Treatment of the coagulopathy associated with liver disease is recommended for overt bleeding or for correction of coagulation parameters (e.g., PT and aPTT) prior to an invasive procedure. Major bleeding may occur with normal coagulation parameters secondary to esophageal varices or peptic ulcer disease. To ensure that vitamin K deficiency is not contributing to the abnormalities, adults may receive 10 mg of vitamin K for one or more days.

When a patient bleeds in association with a coagulopathy, replacement therapy with platelets and fresh-frozen plasma may decrease bleeding. Fresh-frozen plasma supplies all of the missing coagulation factors, but fluid overload may be a serious problem. If fluid overload becomes an issue, plasma exchange may be considered. If the patient has ascites, the half-life of many of these factors is decreased, and correcting the coagulopathy is difficult. PCCs can be given, but they may increase the risk of intravascular coagulation and cause DIC if not already present. In general, use of these concentrates is not recommended. Only when administration of fresh-frozen plasma does not correct the coagulopathy and the patient continues to have serious bleeding should PCCs be considered.

The use of heparin and antifibrinolytic drugs is controversial. Administration of aminocaproic acid may be successful, especially with mucosal bleeding. Heparin has not been demonstrated to improve survival in patients with acute liver failure and may exacerbate bleeding. Antithrombin concentrates have been evaluated in fulminant liver failure. They had no benefit on mortality, clinical complications, or coagulation laboratory findings. Desmopressin may decrease the bleeding time in patients with liver failure.[92] Administration of recombinant factor VIIa has successfully corrected coagulation parameters and stopped bleeding in patients with liver disease.[93]

ABBREVIATIONS

aPCC: activated prothrombin complex concentrate
aPTT: activated partial thromboplastin time
BU: Bethesda unit
DIC: disseminated intravascular coagulation
FDP: fibrin degradation product
HIV: human immunodeficiency virus
PAI-1: plasminogen activator inhibitor type 1
PCC: prothrombin complex concentrate
PT: prothrombin time
vWF:Ag: von Willebrand factor antigen

REFERENCES

1. Dahlback B. Blood coagulation. Lancet 2000;355:1627–1632.
2. Tilley R, Mackman N. Tissue factor in hemostasis and thrombosis. Semin Thromb Hemost 2006;32:5–10.
3. Wiman B. The fibrinolytic enzyme system. Basic principles and links to venous and arterial thrombosis. Hematol Oncol Clin North Am 2000;14:325–338.
4. Harrison P. The role of PFA-100 testing in the investigation and management of haemostatic defects in children and adults. Br J Haematol 2005;130:3–10.
5. Colman R, Hirsh J, Marder V, Clowes A, George J, eds. Hemostasis and Thrombosis Basic Principles and Clinical Practice, 4th ed. Philadelphia: Lippincott Williams & Wilkins, 2001;787–816.
6. Adcock DM, Duff S. Enhanced standardization of the International Normalized Ratio through the use of plasma calibrants: A concise review. Blood Coagul Fibrinolysis 2000;11:583–590.
7. Mannucci PM, Tuddenham EG. The hemophilias—From royal genes to gene therapy. N Engl J Med 2001;344:1773–1779.
8. Pruthi RK. Hemophilia: A practical approach to genetic testing. Mayo Clin Proc 2005;80:1485–1499.
9. Soucie JM, Evatt B, Jackson D. Occurrence of hemophilia in the United States. The Hemophilia Surveillance System Project Investigators. Am J Hematol 1998;59:288–294.
10. David D, Morais S, Ventura C, Campos M. Female haemophiliac homozygous for the factor VIII intron 22 inversion mutation, with transcriptional inactivation of one of the factor VIII alleles. Haemophilia 2003;9:125–130.
11. Shetty S, Ghosh K, Mohanty D. Hemophilia B in a female. Acta Haematol 2001;106:115–117.
12. Espinos C, Lorenzo JI, Casana P, Martinez F, Aznar JA. Haemophilia B in a female caused by skewed inactivation of the normal X-chromosome. Haematologica 2000;85:1092–1095.
13. Bowen DJ. Haemophilia A and haemophilia B: Molecular insights. Mol Pathol 2002;55:127–144.
14. Lee C, Berntorp EE, Hoots WK, eds. Textbook of Hemophilia. Malden, MA: Blackwell Publishing, 2005.
15. Dunn AL, Abshire TC. Recent advances in the management of the child who has hemophilia. Hematol Oncol Clin North Am 2004;18:1249–1276.
16. Lakich D, Kazazian HH Jr, Antonarakis SE, Gitschier J. Inversions disrupting the factor VIII gene are a common cause of severe haemophilia A. Nat Genet 1993;5:236–241.
17. Bagnall RD, Waseem N, Green PM, Giannelli F. Recurrent inversion breaking intron 1 of the factor VIII gene is a frequent cause of severe hemophilia A. Blood 2002;99:168–174.
18. Kurachi K, Davie EW. Isolation and characterization of a cDNA coding for human factor IX. Proc Natl Acad Sci U S A 1982;79:6461–6464.
19. Crossley M, Ludwig M, Stowell KM, De Vos P, Olek K, Brownlee GG. Recovery from hemophilia B Leyden: An androgen-responsive element in the factor IX promoter. Science 1992;257:377–379.
20. Reitsma PH, Bertina RM, Ploos van Amstel JK, Riemens A, Briet E. The putative factor IX gene promoter in hemophilia B Leyden. Blood 1988;72:1074–1076.
21. Bolton-Maggs PH, Pasi KJ. Haemophilias A and B. Lancet 2003;361:1801–1809.
22. Ljung R, Tedgard U. Genetic counseling of hemophilia carriers. Semin Thromb Hemost 2003;29:31–36.
23. Peyvandi F, Jayandharan G, Chandy M, et al. Genetic diagnosis of haemophilia and other inherited bleeding disorders. Haemophilia 2006;12(Suppl 3):82–89.
24. Richardson LC, Evatt BL. Risk of hepatitis A virus infection in persons with hemophilia receiving plasma-derived products. Transfus Med Rev 2000;14:64–73.
25. Kulkarni R, Lusher J. Perinatal management of newborns with haemophilia. Br J Haematol 2001;112:264–274.
26. Guidelines on the selection and use of therapeutic products to treat haemophilia and other hereditary bleeding disorders. Haemophilia 2003;9:1–23.
27. Minor PD. Are recombinant products really infection risk free? Haemophilia 2001;7:114–116.
28. Soucie JM, Siwak EB, Hooper WC, Evatt BL, Hollinger FB. Human parvovirus B19 in young male patients with hemophilia A: Associations with treatment product exposure and joint range-of-motion limitation. Transfusion 2004;44:1179–1185.
29. Lusher JM. First and second generation recombinant factor VIII concentrates in previously untreated patients: Recovery, safety, efficacy, and inhibitor development. Semin Thromb Hemost 2002;28:273–276.
30. Wight J, Paisley S. The epidemiology of inhibitors in haemophilia A: A systematic review. Haemophilia 2003;9:418–435.
31. Shord SS, Lindley CM. Coagulation products and their uses. Am J Health Syst Pharm 2000;57:1403–1417.
32. Batorova A, Martinowitz U. Continuous infusion of coagulation factors. Haemophilia 2002;8:170–177.
33. Schulman S. Continuous infusion. Haemophilia 2003;9:368–375.
34. Lethagen S. Desmopressin in mild hemophilia A: Indications, limitations, efficacy, and safety. Semin Thromb Hemost 2003;29:101–106.
35. Revel-Vilk S, Blanchette VS, Sparling C, Stain AM, Carcao MD. DDAVP challenge tests in boys with mild/moderate haemophilia A. Br J Haematol 2002;117:947–951.
36. Villar A, Jimenez-Yuste V, Quintana M, Hernandez-Navarro F. The use of haemostatic drugs in haemophilia: Desmopressin and antifibrinolytic agents. Haemophilia 2002;8:189–193.
37. Roth DA, Kessler CM, Pasi KJ, Rup B, Courter SG, Tubridy KL. Human recombinant factor IX. Safety and efficacy studies in hemophilia B patients previously treated with plasma-derived factor IX concentrates. Blood 2001;98:3600–3606.
38. Shapiro AD, Di Paola J, Cohen A, et al. The safety and efficacy of recombinant human blood coagulation factor IX in previously untreated patients with severe or moderately severe hemophilia B. Blood 2005;105:518–525.

39. Poon MC, Lillicrap D, Hensman C, Card R, Scully MF. Recombinant factor IX recovery and inhibitor safety: A Canadian post-licensure surveillance study. Thromb Haemost 2002;87:431–435.
40. Luu H, Ewenstein B. FEIBA safety profile in multiple modes of clinical and home-therapy application. Haemophilia 2004;10(Suppl 2):10–16.
41. Shapiro AD, Ragni MV, Lusher JM, et al. Safety and efficacy of monoclonal antibody purified factor IX concentrate in previously untreated patients with hemophilia B. Thromb Haemost 1996;75:30–35.
42. Bjorkman S. Prophylactic dosing of factor VIII and factor IX from a clinical pharmacokinetic perspective. Haemophilia 2003;9(Suppl 1):101–108.
43. Berntorp E, Astermark J, Bjorkman S, et al. Consensus perspectives on prophylactic therapy for haemophilia: Summary statement. Haemophilia 2003;9(Suppl 1):1–4.
44. Petrini P. How to start prophylaxis. Haemophilia 2003;9 (Suppl 1):83–85.
45. van den Berg HM, Fischer K. Prophylaxis for severe hemophilia: Experience from Europe and the United States. Semin Thromb Hemost 2003;29:49–54.
46. Astermark J. When to start and when to stop primary prophylaxis in patients with severe haemophilia. Haemophilia 2003;9(Suppl 1):32–36.
47. Panicker J, Warrier I, Thomas R, Lusher JM. The overall effectiveness of prophylaxis in severe haemophilia. Haemophilia 2003;9:272–278.
48. Fischer K, Van Den Berg M. Prophylaxis for severe haemophilia: Clinical and economical issues. Haemophilia 2003;9:376–381.
49. Bollard CM, Teague LR, Berry EW, Ockelford PA. The use of central venous catheters (portacaths) in children with haemophilia. Haemophilia 2000;6:66–70.
50. Ljung R. Central venous lines in haemophilia. Haemophilia 2003;9(Suppl 1):88–92.
51. Key NS. Inhibitors in congenital coagulation disorders. Br J Haematol 2004;127:379–391.
52. Wight J, Paisley S, Knight C. Immune tolerance induction in patients with haemophilia A with inhibitors: A systematic review. Haemophilia 2003;9:436–463.
53. White GC 2nd, Rosendaal F, Aledort LM, Lusher JM, Rothschild C, Ingerslev J. Definitions in hemophilia. Recommendation of the scientific subcommittee on factor VIII and factor IX of the scientific and standardization committee of the International Society on Thrombosis and Haemostasis. Thromb Haemost 2001;85:560.
54. Lloyd Jones M, Wight J, Paisley S, Knight C. Control of bleeding in patients with haemophilia A with inhibitors: A systematic review. Haemophilia 2003;9:464–520.
55. Shibata M, Shima M, Misu H, Okimoto Y, Giddings JC, Yoshioka A. Management of haemophilia B inhibitor patients with anaphylactic reactions to FIX concentrates. Haemophilia 2003;9:269–271.
56. Hedner U. Mechanism of action of factor VIIa in the treatment of coagulopathies. Semin Thromb Hemost 2006;32(Suppl 1):77–85.
57. von Depka M. Managing acute bleeds in the patient with haemophilia and inhibitors: Options, efficacy and safety. Haemophilia 2005;11(Suppl 1):18–23.
58. Paisley S, Wight J, Currie E, Knight C. The management of inhibitors in haemophilia A. Introduction and systematic review of current practice. Haemophilia 2003;9:405–417.
59. Colowick AB, Bohn RL, Avorn J, Ewenstein BM. Immune tolerance induction in hemophilia patients with inhibitors: Costly can be cheaper. Blood 2000;96:1698–1702.
60. Gringeri A, Mantovani LG, Scalone L, Mannucci PM. Cost of care and quality of life for patients with hemophilia complicated by inhibitors: The COCIS Study Group. Blood 2003;102:2358–2363.
61. Wiestner A, Cho HJ, Asch AS, et al. Rituximab in the treatment of acquired factor VIII inhibitors. Blood 2002;100:3426–3428.
62. Walsh CE. Gene therapy progress and prospects: Gene therapy for the hemophilias. Gene Ther 2003;10:999–1003.
63. White GC 2nd. Gene therapy in hemophilia: Clinical trials update. Thromb Haemost 2001;86:172–177.
64. Dunn AL. Management and prevention of recurrent hemarthrosis in patients with hemophilia. Curr Opin Hematol 2005;12:390–394.
65. Fernandez-Palazzi F, Caviglia HA, Salazar JR, Lopez J, Aoun R. Intraarticular dexamethasone in advanced chronic synovitis in hemophilia. Clin Orthop Relat Res 1997;343:25–29.
66. Kasper CK. Protocols for the treatment of haemophilia and von Willebrand disease. Haemophilia 2000;6(Suppl 1):84–93.
67. Federici AB, Castaman G, Mannucci PM. Guidelines for the diagnosis and management of von Willebrand disease in Italy. Haemophilia 2002;8:607–621.
68. Batlle J, Noya MS, Giangrande P, Lopez-Fernandez MF. Advances in the therapy of von Willebrand disease. Haemophilia 2002;8:301–307.
69. Federici AB, Mannucci PM. Advances in the genetics and treatment of von Willebrand disease. Curr Opin Pediatr 2002;14:23–33.
70. Mohri H. Acquired von Willebrand syndrome: Features and management. Am J Hematol 2006;81:616–623.
71. Kouides PA. Aspects of the laboratory identification of von Willebrand disease in women. Semin Thromb Hemost 2006;32:480–484.
72. Sadler JE, Mannucci PM, Berntorp E, et al. Impact, diagnosis and treatment of von Willebrand disease. Thromb Haemost 2000;84:160–174.
73. Gill JC, Endres-Brooks J, Bauer PJ, Marks WJ Jr, Montgomery RR. The effect of ABO blood group on the diagnosis of von Willebrand disease. Blood 1987;69:1691–1695.
74. Mannucci PM. Treatment of von Willebrand's Disease. N Engl J Med 2004;351:683–694.
75. Peyvandi F, Duga S, Akhavan S, Mannucci PM. Rare coagulation deficiencies. Haemophilia 2002;8:308–321.
76. Bolton-Maggs PH. Factor XI deficiency and its management. Haemophilia 2000;6(Suppl 1):100–109.
77. Kasper CK. Concentrate safety and efficacy. Haemophilia 2002;8:161–165.
78. Bray GL, Gomperts ED, Courter S, et al. A multicenter study of recombinant factor VIII (Recombinate): Safety, efficacy, and inhibitor risk in previously untreated patients with hemophilia A. The Recombinate Study Group. Blood 1994;83:2428–2435.
79. Bick RL. Disseminated intravascular coagulation current concepts of etiology, pathophysiology, diagnosis, and treatment. Hematol Oncol Clin North Am 2003;17:149–176.
80. Bucur SZ, Levy JH, Despotis GJ, Spiess BD, Hillyer CD. Uses of antithrombin III concentrate in congenital and acquired deficiency states. Transfusion 1998;38:481–498.
81. Warren BL, Eid A, Singer P, et al. Caring for the critically ill patient. High-dose antithrombin III in severe sepsis: A randomized controlled trial. JAMA 2001;286:1869–1878.
82. Levi M. Disseminated intravascular coagulation: What's new? Crit Care Clin 2005;21:449–467.
83. Toh CH, Downey C. Back to the future: Testing in disseminated intravascular coagulation. Blood Coagul Fibrinolysis 2005;16:535–542.
84. Arkel YS. Thrombosis and cancer. Semin Oncol 2000;27:362–374.
85. Pernerstorfer T, Hollenstein U, Hansen JB, et al. Lepirudin blunts endotoxin-induced coagulation activation. Blood 2000;95:1729–1734.
86. Bernard GR, Vincent JL, Laterre PF, et al. Efficacy and safety of recombinant human activated protein C for severe sepsis. N Engl J Med 2001;344:699–709.
87. Cohen H, Welage LS. Strategies to optimize drotrecogin alfa (activated) use: Guidelines and therapeutic controversies. Pharmacotherapy 2002;22(12 Pt 2):223S–235S.
88. Vermeer C, Schurgers LJ. A comprehensive review of vitamin K and vitamin K antagonists. Hematol Oncol Clin North Am 2000;14:339–353.
89. Tandoi F, Mosca F, Agosti M. Vitamin K prophylaxis: Leaving the old route for the new one? Acta Paediatr Suppl 2005;94:125–128.
90. Ross JA, Davies SM. Vitamin K prophylaxis and childhood cancer. Med Pediatr Oncol 2000;34:434–437.
91. Riegert-Johnson DL, Volcheck GW. The incidence of anaphylaxis following intravenous phytonadione (vitamin K1): A 5-year retrospective review. Ann Allergy Asthma Immunol 2002;89:400–406.
92. Lisman T, Leebeek FW, de Groot PG. Haemostatic abnormalities in patients with liver disease. J Hepatol 2002;37:280–287.
93. Caldwell SH, Chang C, Macik BG. Recombinant activated factor VII (rFVIIa) as a hemostatic agent in liver disease: A break from convention in need of controlled trials. Hepatology 2004;39:592–598.

CHAPTER 106 Sickle Cell Disease

C.Y. JENNIFER CHAN AND REGINALD MOORE

KEY CONCEPTS

1. Sickle cell disease is an inherited disorder caused by a defect in the gene for hemoglobin. Patients can have one defective gene (sickle cell trait) or two defective genes (sickle cell disease).
2. Although sickle cell disease usually occurs in persons of African ancestry, other ethnic groups can be affected. Different mutation variants can result in variation in clinical manifestations.
3. Sickle cell disease involves multiple organ systems. Usual clinical signs and symptoms include anemia, pain crisis, hepatosplenomegaly, and pulmonary diseases. Sickle cell disease can be identified by routine neonatal screening programs. Early diagnosis allows early comprehensive care.
4. Patients with sickle cell disease are at risk for infection. Prophylaxis against pneumococcal infection reduces death during childhood.
5. Hydroxyurea has been shown to decrease the incidence of painful crises, but patients treated with hydroxyurea should be carefully monitored.
6. Neurologic complications caused by vasoocclusion can lead to stroke. Chronic transfusion therapy programs have been shown to be beneficial in decreasing the occurrence of stroke in children with sickle cell disease.
7. Patients with fever greater than 38.5°C (101.3°F) should be evaluated and appropriate antibiotics should include coverage for encapsulated organisms, especially pneumococcal.
8. Pain episodes can usually be managed at home. Hospitalized patients usually require parenteral analgesics. Analgesic options include opioids, nonsteroidal antiinflammatory agents, and acetaminophen. The patient characteristics and the severity of the crisis should determine the choice of agent and regimen.

❶ Sickle cell syndromes, which can be divided into sickle cell disease (SCD) and sickle cell trait (SCT), are a group of hereditary disorders characterized by the presence of sickle cell hemoglobin (HbS) in red blood cells. SCT is the heterozygous inheritance of one normal cell and one sickle cell hemoglobin (HbAS) gene. Individuals with SCT are usually asymptomatic. SCD can be of homozygous or compounded heterozygous inheritance. Homozygous HbS (HbSS) is called sickle cell anemia (SCA); heterozygous inheritance of HbS compounded with another mutation results in sickle cell hemoglobin C (HbSC), sickle cell β-thalassemia (HbSβ^+-thal and HbSβ^0-thal), and some other rare phenotypes.

Learning objectives, review questions, and other resources can be found at **www.pharmacotherapyonline.com.**

This complex disorder was first described in the literature by Herrick in 1910. Since that discovery was made, much progress has been made in identifying the molecular and functional defects and understanding the relationship between genotypes and clinical severity of the disease.[1,2]

SCD is a chronic illness with significant burden for family and society.[3] Frequent crisis episodes can interrupt schooling and result in employment difficulties. Acute complications of the disease can be unpredictable, rapidly progressive, and life-threatening. Later in life, chronic organ damage can develop. Because of the complexity and seriousness of the illness, it is essential that comprehensive care is available and that all providers involved have a good understanding of the disease and its management options.[4]

EPIDEMIOLOGY

More than 50,000 Americans have sickle cell disease, and approximately 2,000 infants with SCD are identified each year in the United States. In addition, for every 1 infant with SCD, approximately 50 infants are identified as carriers. The most common SCD genotype is HbSS (~45%), followed by HbSC (~25%), HbSβ^+-thal (~8%), and HbSβ^0-thal (~2%). Other variants account for less than 1% of patients.[5,6]

Sickle cell gene mutation offers partial protection against serious malarial infection. Abnormal red blood cells (RBCs) are less easily parasitized by *Plasmodium falciparum* than normal RBCs. Consequently, persons with heterozygous sickle cell gene (i.e., SCT) have a selective advantage in regions (tropical areas) where malaria is endemic. The incidence of the sickle cell gene in a population correlates with the historical incidence of malaria.

❷ SCD is most common in people with African heritage, with a frequency of approximately 1 in 400 for SCD and 8% for SCT in African Americans. The prevalence is higher in Africa, where an estimated 120,000 babies are born with SCD each year. The prevalence rate of SCT in Africa varies across regions, with a higher rate in western, central, and eastern Africa (10% to 30%) but lower rates in northern and southern Africa (0% to 5%). Hemoglobin C (HbC) appears primarily in the inhabitants of western and northern Africa or in descendants of people from this area. Approximately 2% to 3% of African Americans carry the HbC gene (HbC-trait).[5–8]

Other areas with sickle cell mutation are the Arabian Peninsula, the Indian subcontinent, and the Mediterranean region. HbS has been reported in up to 25% in certain Middle Eastern populations and greater than 30% in Greece and Cyprus. Genetic analysis shows that the mutation found in Arabic patients is different from those of African descent. Sickle cell gene mutation variants have been associated with different geographic locations and may be responsible for variations in clinical manifestations. In Africa, the variants are

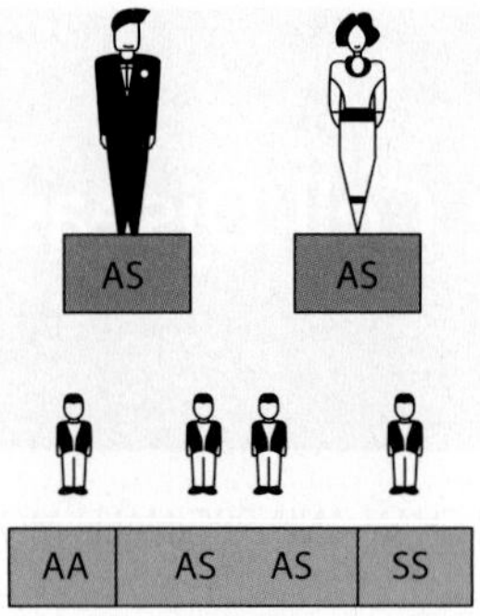

FIGURE 106-1. Sickle cell gene inheritance scheme for both parents with sickle cell trait (SCT). Possibilities with each pregnancy: 25% normal (AA); 50% SCT (AS); 25% sickle cell anemia (SS). (A, normal hemoglobin; S, sickle cell hemoglobin.)

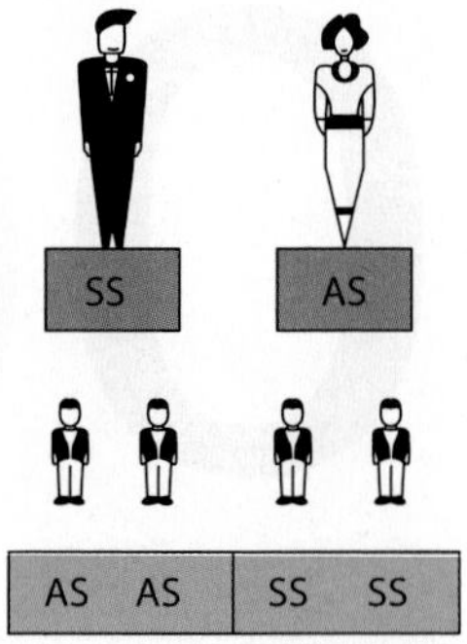

FIGURE 106-3. Sickle cell gene inheritance scheme for one parent with sickle cell trait (SCT) and one parent with sickle cell anemia (SCA). Possibilities with each pregnancy: 50% SCA (SS); 50% SCT (AS). (A, normal hemoglobin; S, sickle cell hemoglobin.)

Senegal (Atlantic West Africa), Benin (Central West Africa), Bantu (Central African Republic), and Cameroon. Arab-Indian haplotype is seen in certain areas of Saudi Arabia and India.[1,7–9] Although there are a number of other haplotypes seen around the world, the major types include Saudi Arabian and Cameroon. Both of these types usually follow milder courses of illness.[2,7,9–10]

ETIOLOGY

Normal hemoglobin (hemoglobin A [HbA]) is composed of two α chains and two β chains ($\alpha_2\beta_2$). The biochemical defect that leads to the development of HbS involves the substitution of valine for glutamic acid as the sixth amino acid in the β-polypeptide chain. Another type of abnormal hemoglobin, hemoglobin C (HbC), is produced by the substitution of lysine for glutamic acid as the sixth amino acid in the β-chain. Structurally, the α-chains of HbS, HbA, and HbC are identical. Therefore, it is the chemical differences in the β-chain that account for sickling and its related sequelae.[1,2,7]

SCA is a form of SCD in which the patient has inherited both genes that code for formation of HbS, one from each parent (HbSS). Figures 106–1, 106–2, 106–3, and 106–4 show the probability of inheritance with each pregnancy for the offspring of parents with HbA, SCT, and SCA. If both parents are carriers, the offspring will have a 25% risk of having SCD and 50% risk of being a carrier (see Fig. 106–1). β-Thalassemia can be found in conjunction with HbS. Because patients with HbSS and HbSβ^0-thal do not have normal β-globulin production, they usually have a more severe course than those with HbSC and HbSβ^+-thal. As discussed earlier, several haplotypes characterize the sickle cell gene, resulting in different clinical and hematologic courses. Included among these types are the three most commonly found in the United States: the Bantu haplotype, characterized by severe disease; the Senegal haplotype, characterized by mild disease; and the Benin haplotype, characterized by a course intermediate to that of the other two haplotypes.

PATHOPHYSIOLOGY

To understand the pathophysiology of SCD, one must understand the normal physiology of RBC production. Normal adult RBCs contain 33 to 35 g/dL hemoglobin, predominantly HbA (96%). Other forms of hemoglobin are HbA_2 (2% to 3%) and fetal hemoglobin (less than 2%). Fetal hemoglobin (HbF) is present predominantly in fetal RBCs. Instead of β chains in HbA or HbS, HbF contains two γ chains ($\alpha_2\gamma_2$). The switch from production of γ chains to β chains occurs shortly before birth. A few red cell clones remain to produce HbF postnatally. Increased production of HbF is seen under severe erythroid stress, such as anemia, hematopoietic stem cell transplantation, or chemotherapy. Both water and hemoglobin content in the RBCs determine the mean corpuscular hemoglobin concentration (MCHC). Passive diffusion and active transport regulate intracellular cation and volume contents, which determine the intracellular viscosity of RBC. Normal RBCs are biconcave shape and able to deform to squeeze through capillaries. As RBCs age, MCHC increases, deformability decreases, and the cells are removed by the mononuclear phagocytic system.[7,12]

In the pathogenesis of SCD, three known problems are primarily responsible for various clinical manifestations: impaired circulation, destruction of RBCs, and stasis of blood flow. These three problems probably relate directly to two major disturbances involving RBCs: polymerization and membrane damage (Fig. 106–5).

The solubility of HbS and HbA are the same when oxygenated. Because of increased hydrophobicity as a result of valine substituting

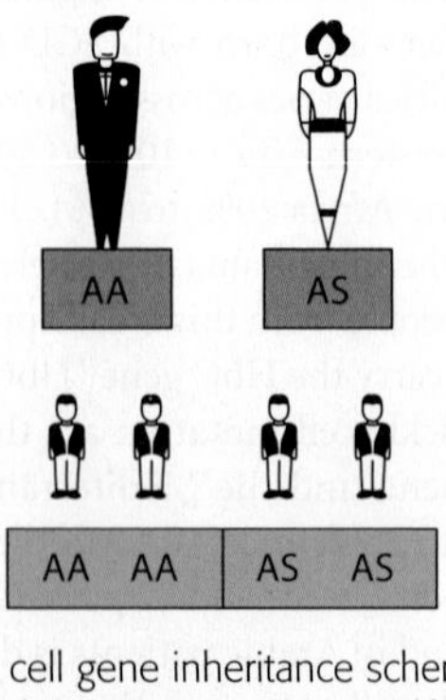

FIGURE 106-2. Sickle cell gene inheritance scheme for one parent with sickle cell trait (SCT) and one parent with no sickle cell gene. Possibilities with each pregnancy: 50% normal (AA); 50% SCT (AS). (A, normal hemoglobin; S, sickle cell hemoglobin.)

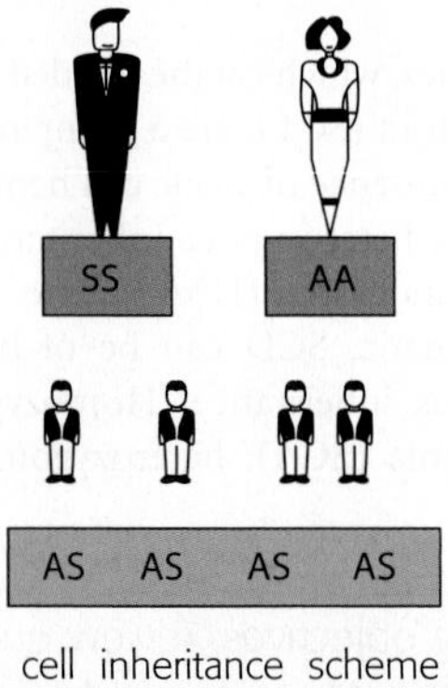

FIGURE 106-4. Sickle cell inheritance scheme for 1 parent without sickle cell gene and 1 parent with sickle cell anemia (SCA). Possibilities with each pregnancy: 100% SCT (AS). (A, normal hemoglobin; S, sickle cell hemoglobin.)

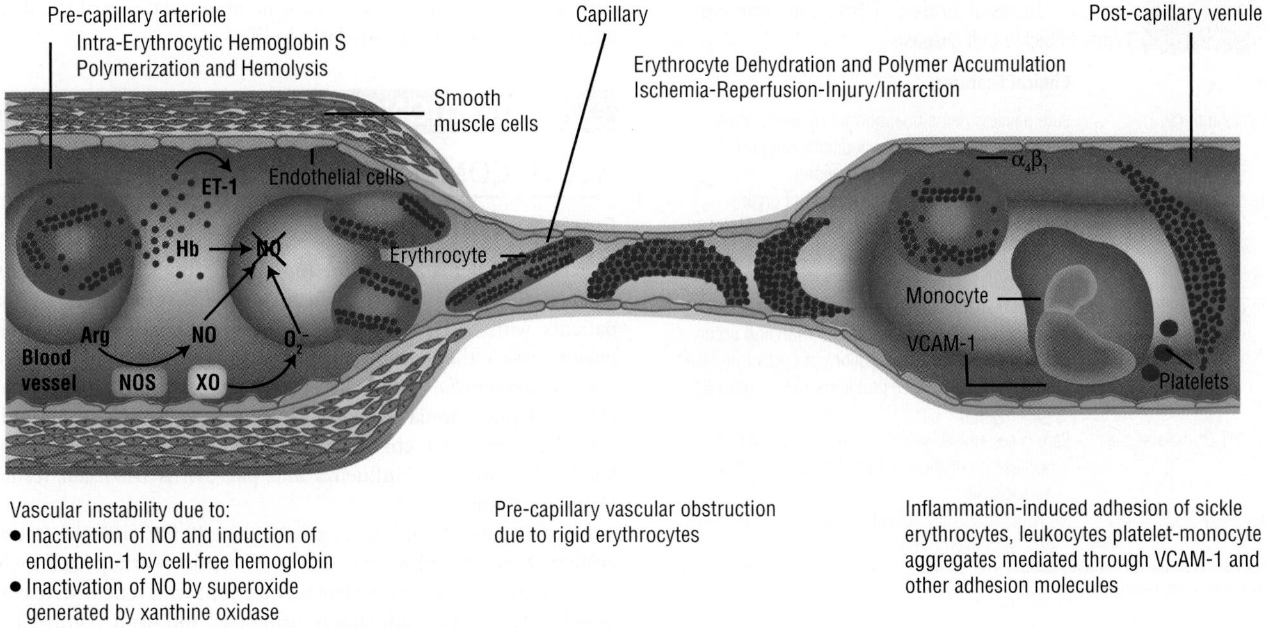

FIGURE 106-5. Pathophysiology of sickle cell disease. (Arg, arginine; ET-1, endothelin-1; Hb, hemoglobin; NO, nitric oxide; NOS, nitrous oxide synthase; VCAM-1, vascular cell adhesion molecule 1; XO, xanthine oxidase.) *(From Kato GJ, Gladwin MT. Sickle cell disease. In: Hall JB, Schmidt GA, Wood LDH. Principles of Critical Care, 3rd ed. New York: McGraw-Hill, 2005:1658.)*

glutamic acid, solubility of deoxygenated HbS is reduced to 17 g/dL. Saturation of deoxy-HbS leads to intermolecular binding and formation of thin bundles of fibers, which initially are unstable, but increased binding of deoxy-HbS eventually results in cross-linking fibers and stable polymers. This process is influenced by MCHC, temperature, intracellular pH, and the amount of HbS. Polymerization allows deoxygenated hemoglobin molecules to exist as a semisolid gel that protrudes into the cell membrane, leading to distortion of RBCs (sickled shape) and loss of deformability. The presence of sickled RBCs increases blood viscosity and encourages sludging in the capillaries and small venous vessels. Such obstructive events lead to local tissue hypoxia, which tends to accentuate the pathologic process.

When reoxygenated, polymers within the RBCs are lost, and the RBCs eventually return to normal shape. This process contributes to the vasoocclusive manifestation in that HbS is able to squeeze into microvasculature when oxygenated, but becomes sickled when deoxygenated. This cycle of sickling and unsickling results in damage to the cell membrane, loss of membrane flexibility, and rearrangement of surface phospholipids. Membrane damage also alters ion transport, resulting in potassium and water loss, which can lead to a dehydrated state that enhances the formation of sickled forms. After continual repetitions of the process, the RBC membrane develops into a more rigid form, irreversibly sickled cell (ISC). Unlike the reversible sickle cells, which have normal morphology when oxygenated, ISCs are elongated cells and remain sickled when oxygenated. More rigid membranes of HbS-containing RBC retard their flow, particularly through the microcirculation. In addition, sickled RBCs tend to adhere to vascular endothelial cells, which further increase polymerization and obstruction.

Intermolecular binding and polymer formation are reduced by HbF and to a lesser degree by HbA_2. RBCs that contain HbF sickle less readily than cells without. ISCs, not surprisingly, have a low HbF level. Increased levels of HbF, as in the case of the Saudi Arabian genotype, result in more benign forms of SCD. The amount of HbF and HbA_2 in relation to HbS influences clinical manifestations and accounts for the variability in severity among different SCD genotypes.

Intravascular destruction of sickle cells can occur at an accelerated rate. The stresses of circulation, and repetitive sickle–unsickle cycles are likely to lead to cell fragmentation. Damage to the cell membrane promotes cell recognition by macrophages. Rigid ISCs are easily trapped, resulting in short circulatory survival and chronic hemolysis. The typical sickled cell survives for approximately 10 to 20 days, whereas the life span of a normal RBC is 100 to 120 days.

In addition to sickling, other factors are also responsible for the clinical manifestations associated with SCD. Obstruction of blood flow to the spleen by sickle cells can result in functional asplenia, defined as the loss of splenic function with an intact spleen. These patients can also have deficient opsonization. Impaired splenic function increases susceptibility to infection by encapsulated organisms, particularly pneumococcal disease. Coagulation abnormalities in SCD can be the result of continuous activation of the hemostatic system or disorganization of the membrane layer.[7–9,12–14]

CLINICAL PRESENTATION

❸ SCD is usually identified by routine neonatal screening programs. The sensitivity and specificity of screening methods, most commonly by isoelectric focusing, are excellent. For infants with a positive screening result, confirmation testing should be performed prior to 2 months of age. Even with universal screening, infants with SCD are sometimes not identified at birth because of extreme prematurity, prior blood transfusion, inability to contact family, or clerical errors.[4]

SCD involves multiple organ systems, and its clinical manifestations vary greatly between and among genotypes (Table 106–1). Persons with SCT are usually asymptomatic and are not considered to have clinical disease. However, some clinical signs and symptoms can occur, and patients should be cautious when participating in exercise under extreme conditions, such as high altitude or military training. Sickling of RBCs in the renal medulla can result in loss of ability to maximally concentrate urine. Patients with such impairment can be at risk of dehydration during periods in which the body normally conserves water. Microscopic hematuria has been observed, and gross hematuria can occur after heavy exercise. An increased incidence of urinary tract infection in women, especially during pregnancy, has been reported.[1,5,7]

The feature presentations of SCD are hemolytic anemia and vasoocclusion. In patients who are homozygous for HbS, anemia usually appears from 4 to 6 months after birth. The delay in presenta-

TABLE 106-1 Clinical Features of Sickle Cell Trait and Common Types of Sickle Cell Disease

Type	Clinical Features
Sickle cell trait (SCT)	Rare painless hematuria; normal Hb level; heavy exercise under extreme conditions can provoke gross hematuria and complications
Sickle cell anemia (SCA)	Pain crises, microvascular disruption of organs (spleen, liver, bone marrow, kidney, brain, and lung), gallstone, priapism, leg ulcers; anemia (Hb 7–10 g/dL)
Sickle cell hemoglobin C	Painless hematuria and rare aseptic necrosis of bone; vasoocclusive crises are less common and occur later in life; other complications are ocular disease and pregnancy-related problems; mild anemia (Hb 10–12 g/dL)
Sickle cell β^+-thalassemia	Rare crises; milder severity than sickle cell disease because production of HbA; Hb 10–14 g/dL with microcytosis
Sickle cell β^0-thalassemia	No HbA production; severity similar to SCA; Hb 7–10 g/dL with microcytosis

HbA, hemoglobin; Hb, hemoglobin.

tion is because during those months, HbF in the infant's RBC is gradually replaced by HbS, which typically leads to attacks of pain frequently accompanied by fever. Pneumonia and splenomegaly are also common findings. Infants can also present with pain and swelling of the hands and feet, commonly referred to as *hand-and-foot syndrome* or *dactylitis*.[1,4,5,7]

The usual clinical signs and symptoms associated with SCA include chronic anemia; fever and pallor; arthralgia; scleral icterus; abdominal pain; weakness; anorexia; fatigue; enlargement of the liver, spleen, and heart; and hematuria. Laboratory findings include low hemoglobin level and increased reticulocyte, platelet, and white blood cell (WBC) counts. The peripheral blood smear demonstrates sickle cell forms.

Presentation of patients with HbSC disease is less severe than that of SCA and is characterized primarily by mild anemia (hemoglobin levels above 9 g/dL), infrequent episodes of pain, persistence of splenomegaly into adult life, and excessive target cells in the peripheral blood smear. In patients with heterozygous HbS and β-thalassemia gene, severity of disease depends on the thalassemia gene involved.[1,5,7]

Patients with SCD experience delayed growth and sexual maturation. Both height and weight are usually below average, and the poor growth cannot be explained by nutritional factors alone. Fertility problems tend to occur more often, and some menstrual abnormalities are more common in female SCD patients than in normal women. Other typical physical characteristics include a protuberant abdomen with exaggerated lumbar lordosis, usually an asthenic appearance with rather long extremities and tapered fingers, and frequently a barrel-shaped chest.[1,4,5,7]

The previously high mortality rate of early childhood has been reduced for patients with SCD with availability of public health programs and comprehensive care.[4] The median survival rate is estimated to be 42 years for males and 48 years for females for HbA, and 60 years for males and 68 years for females for HbSC.[5] Predictors for severe disease in children who are less than 10 years of age include dactylitis before 1 year of age, an average hemoglobin level less than 7 g/dL in the second year of life, and WBC count greater than 13,700 cells/mm^3 in the absence of infection. Early acute chest syndrome during first 3 years of life is a predictor for recurrent episodes throughout childhood. Children with concomitant SCD and asthma have increased episodes of acute chest syndrome and stroke. Risk factors for early death in adults with SCD include acute complications such as pain crisis, anemic events, acute chest syndrome, renal failure, and pulmonary disease.[3,5,15–19] Today, with longer survival for SCD, chronic manifestations of the disease contribute to the morbidity later in life.

COMPLICATIONS

ACUTE COMPLICATIONS

Fever and Infection

Functional asplenia and failure to make antibodies against encapsulated organisms contribute to the high risk of overwhelming sepsis in patients with SCD. The most common pathogen is *Streptococcus pneumoniae*. Other encapsulated organisms are *Haemophilus influenzae* and *Salmonella*, and the latter has been known to cause osteomyelitis and pneumonia in SCD. *Mycoplasma pneumoniae* should be considered in older children with infiltrates on chest radiograph. Viral infections (e.g., influenza and parvovirus B19) can result in severe morbidity.[1,5,20,21]

All SCD patients with fever greater than 38.5°C (101.3°F) must be evaluated to determine the extent of sepsis; workup can include physical examination, complete blood count with reticulocyte count, blood culture, chest radiograph, urinalysis, and urine culture. Lumbar puncture may be needed, especially in young children and toxic-looking children. A low threshold for empiric therapy compared to that in the general population is recommended.[1,5,7,10]

Neurologic

Neurologic abnormalities can occur in both adults and children. Vasoocclusive processes occasionally lead to cerebrovascular occlusion that manifests itself as the signs and symptoms of stroke, such as drowsiness, paralysis, transitory or permanent blindness, aphasia, visual disturbances, spinal cord infarction, and convulsions. Behavioral and performance changes in patients with asymptomatic infarction. The cumulative risk of cerebral infract in HbSS is 11% by age 20 years and 24% by age 45 years with a recurrence rate as high as 70% in 3 years. Some patients recover rapidly and completely, although others are left with permanent neurologic deficits. Evaluation of acute events include computed tomography (CT) scan and magnetic resonance imaging (MRI), magnetic resonance angiography (MRA) for asymptomatic infarction and transcranial Doppler (TCD) ultrasound to detect abnormal velocity and identify high-risk patients. In addition, electroencephalograph (EEG) can be used if there is a history of seizure. Some patients who have SCA with no prior history of stroke have been found to have changes on MRI of the brain consistent with infarction or ischemia. These "silent infarcts" have been reported to occur in up to 22% of HbSS patients and can be associated with increased risk of stroke and decreased neurocognitive functions.[1,13,22–25]

Acute Chest Syndrome

Acute chest syndrome is the leading cause of death among patients with SCD. It is characterized by a new pulmonary infiltrate associated with one or more other symptoms (such as cough, dyspnea, tachypnea, chest pain, fever, wheezing, and new onset hypoxia), and an equivocal response to antibiotic therapy. As many as one-half of patients with SCD experience at least one episode of acute chest syndrome. Pulmonary infarcts often involve the lower lobes of the lungs and are a frequent cause of pleural effusions. Pneumonia occurs most often in the middle and upper lobes. These pulmonary manifestations must be recognized early and managed aggressively because the patient can rapidly progress to pulmonary failure and death.[26–31]

Priapism

Sickling in the sinusoids of the penis can cause priapism, a sustained painful erection that can last several hours or days. Impotence has

TABLE 106-2 Sickle Cell Crisis

Vasoocclusive pain crisis[a]
Clinical features: Acute painful infarction without changes in Hb; almost all patients with SCA will have episodes of acute pain. Recurrent acute crises result in bone, joint, and organ damage and chronic pain. Vasoocclusive crisis most commonly involves the bones, liver, spleen, brain, lungs, and penis. Acute long bone pains can be accompanied by signs of inflammation, making it difficult to differentiate from osteomyelitis. Abdominal involvement can resemble a surgical abdomen. Precipitating factors include infection, extreme weather conditions, dehydration, and stresses.
Signs and symptoms: Deep throbbing pain; local tenderness, erythema, and swelling can be seen. Fever and leukocytosis are common. Dactylitis usually occurs in young infants. Jaundice and increased transaminases present if liver is involved.
Evaluation: Frequent physical examination, CBC, reticulocyte, and urinalysis; based on symptomatology, the following can be needed: needle aspiration to rule out osteomyelitis, abdominal studies (radiograph, computed tomography scan, etc.), liver function tests, bilirubin, culture, and chest radiograph.
Aplastic crisis[b]
Clinical features: Acute decrease in Hb with decreased reticulocyte count (usually less than 1%); transient suppression of RBC production in response to bacterial or viral infection, most common being parvovirus B19
Signs and symptoms: Headache, fatigue, dyspnea, pallor, and tachycardia; can also present with fever, upper respiratory or gastrointestinal infection symptoms.
Evaluation: CBC, reticulocyte count, radiograph, cultures (blood, urine, and throat), evaluation of viral infection (e.g., parvovirus titers)
Acute splenic sequestration crisis[c]
Clinical features: Acute exacerbation of anemia due to sequestration of large blood volume by the spleen. More commonly seen in patients with functioning spleens (e.g., infants and adults with HbSC disease); onset often is associated with viral or bacterial infections; recurrences are common and can be fatal.
Signs and symptoms: Sudden onset of fatigue, dyspnea, and distended abdomen; rapid decrease in Hb and HCT with elevated reticulocyte count, abdominal pain, splenomegaly, vomiting, hypotension, and shock
Evaluation: Close monitoring of vital signs, spleen size, and oxygen saturation, CBC, reticulocyte, and cultures

CBC, complete blood count; HbSC, sickle cell hemoglobin C; Hb, hemoglobin; HCT, hematocrit; RBC, red blood cell; SCA, sickle cell anemia.
[a]From Fixler and Styles,[1] National Institutes of Health,[5] Stuart and Nagel,[7] and Hebbel et al.[12]
[b]From Fixler and Styles,[1] National Institutes of Health,[5] Stuart and Nagel,[7] and Kellermayer et al.[32]
[c]From Fixler and Styles,[1] National Institutes of Health,[5] and Stuart and Nagel.[7]

been reported after repeated episodes. Recurrent and severe priapism is a predictor for other end-organ damage. ASPEN (*a*ssociation of *s*ickle cell disease, *p*riapism, *e*xchange transfusion, and *n*eurologic events) syndrome has occurred in some patients with priapism 1 to 11 days after partial exchange transfusion. This syndrome can range from headaches and seizures to obtundation requiring ventilation.[1,5,7]

Sickle Cell Crisis

Chronic hemolytic anemia in the SCD patient is periodically interrupted by crises, particularly in childhood (see Table 106–2). Patients with HbSS disease experience crises more often than do patients with HbSC disease or some other variants. Although fever, infections, dehydration, hypoxia, acidosis, and sudden temperature alterations can precipitate crises, multiple factors often contribute to development of a crisis.

Vasoocclusive Pain Crisis The most common type of crisis is the vasoocclusive crisis, which is usually characterized by pain affecting the involved areas, without changes in hemoglobin. Laboratory changes that can be seen include leukocytosis, increased fibrinogen levels, and decreased serum pH and bicarbonate level. Dactylitis (hand-and-foot syndrome) occurs in infancy and early childhood and is characterized by redness and swelling of the dorsal aspects of the hands, feet, fingers, and toes. The episodes are painful but usually do not result in permanent damage.[1,5,7,12]

Aplastic Crisis Aplastic crisis is characterized by a decrease in the reticulocyte count and a rapidly developing severe anemia. The bone marrow is hypoplastic. There can be associated pain. The crisis is typically caused by a viral infection, particularly parvovirus B19.[1,5,7,32]

Splenic Sequestration Crisis This is a sudden massive enlargement of the spleen resulting from the sequestration of blood from the mononuclear phagocytic system. There is a dramatic fall in hematocrit and hemoglobin concentrations, with no evidence of marrow failure or accelerated hemolysis. The trapping of the sickled RBCs by the spleen also leads to a decrease in circulating blood volume, which can result in hypotension and shock. The condition is most often seen in infants and children, as their spleens are intact. These crises can cause sudden death in young children. Repeated infarctions lead to autosplenectomy as the disease progresses; therefore, the incidence declines as adolescence approaches.[1,5,7]

CHRONIC COMPLICATIONS

SCD manifests in a variety of chronic problems involving multiple organs. Pulmonary hypertension has been reported to be a risk factor for death in adult patients with SCD.[16,33] Headache is a symptom associated with acute neurologic events, and pseudotumor cerebri presenting with severe headache and blurred vision has also been reported.[34] Destructive bone and joint problems are common. Aseptic necrosis, particularly of the femoral or humeral heads, causes permanent damage and disability. Patients with SCD also have an increased incidence of osteomyelitis; the organism most often responsible is *Salmonella*. In addition to necrosis of joints, chronic leg ulcers can become a difficult skeletal problem. The inner aspect of the lower leg just above the ankle is the site most often affected. Ulcers are often seen after trauma or infection and are usually slow to heal.[1,5,7]

Ocular problems seen in patients with SCD include transient monocular blindness, visual field defects from retinal hemorrhage, retinal detachment, vitreous hemorrhage, venous microaneurysms, and neovascularization. The incidence of proliferative retinopathy in SCD patients varies from 5% to 10%. Vasoocclusion in the eye can occur as early as 20 months of age, and clinically detectable retinal diseases usually occur during adolescence and early adulthood. Despite the less systemic manifestations, patients with HbSC develop serious retinal complications more often and earlier. Annual examination with retinal evaluation is recommended for patients with SCD to prevent blindness from retinopathy and other complications.[5,35,36]

Cholelithiasis is a common occurrence in the SCD patient. It is the result of the chronic hemolysis that results in increased bilirubin production, leading to biliary sludge and/or stone formation. The risk of gallstones increases with age, with 14% younger than age 10 years and 50% by age 22 years. Cholecystitis, exemplified by pain in the right iliac fossa, can be confused with abdominal pain crisis.[1,5,37]

As with any anemia, cardiovascular abnormalities, including cardiac enlargement and various murmurs, can occur in patients with SCD. Patients complain of various degrees of exertional dyspnea, tachycardia, and palpitation owing to the decreased oxygen-carrying capacity of the blood. Acute myocardial infraction has also been reported in children with SCD[5,38,39]

Renal complications include hematuria, tubular acidosis, proteinuria and hyposthenuria (inability to concentrate urine maximally). Enuresis, as a result of increased urine production, is a common complaint. Death from renal disease is unusual among younger patients but does occur among older patients with SCD.[1,5,40]

Depression can be more common than in the general population; especially in patients with unstable disease.[41] Reduction of cognitive function has been reported even in children with no evidence of cerebral infarction.[42] Delay in growth and sexual development are seen in patients with SCD. Adults with SCD have decreased fertility. Finally, pregnancy introduces an increased risk for the mother with SCD and for the fetus. Some patients can experience increased frequency of pain crisis during pregnancy. The anemia of SCD can lead to intrauterine growth retardation. Preterm labor and premature delivery are common occurrences in mothers with SCD, and the risk of spontaneous abortion is increased. The incidence of preeclampsia is also higher when compared to mothers who do not have SCD.[1,5,7,11]

TREATMENT

Sickle Cell Disease

Patients with SCD require lifelong multidisciplinary care. All patients with SCD should receive regularly scheduled comprehensive medical evaluations. The goal of comprehensive care is to reduce hospitalizations, complications, and mortality. Because of the complexity of the disease, a multidisciplinary team is needed to provide medical care, education, counseling, and psychosocial support. Appropriate comprehensive care can have a positive impact on both longevity and general quality of life. This care includes the use of traditional prophylactic and general symptomatic supportive care and the use of newer, more specific therapies aimed at altering hematologic capacity and function.[1,5,7,10,11]

Treatment for patients with SCD involves the use of general measures to meet the unique demands for increased erythropoiesis. Additional interventions can be aimed at preventing or treating complications of the disease. When crises occur, the type and severity of the crisis determine the appropriate therapeutic plan.

■ HEALTH MAINTENANCE

Immunizations

Administration of routine immunizations as recommended by the American Academy of Pediatrics is crucial. In addition to the routine immunizations, SCD patients 6 months and older should receive influenza vaccine annually. Meningococcal vaccine is also recommended for patients older than 2 years of age undergoing splenectomy.[43–45]

Patients with SCD have impaired splenic function, which increases their susceptibility to infection by encapsulated organisms, particularly pneumococci. Prior to the routine use of penicillin prophylaxis and the development of pneumococcal vaccines, invasive pneumococcal disease was 20- to 100-fold more common in children with SCD than in healthy children. Even with these interventions, some groups of children with SCD continue to have a high rate of invasive pneumococcal infections.[20,43]

❹ Two different pneumococcal vaccines are available. The 7-valent pneumococcal conjugate vaccine (PCV7; Prevnar) induces good antibody responses in infants. Immunization with the PCV7 is recommended for all children younger than 24 months of age. Infants should receive the first dose between 6 weeks and 6 months. Two additional doses should be given at 2-month intervals, followed by a fourth dose at age 12 to 15 months. The 23-valent pneumococcal polysaccharide vaccine (PPV 23; Pneumovax 23) is not recommended for use in children younger than 2 years of age because of poor antibody response. To cover for different serotypes, the immunization schedule for children with SCD should include both pneumococcal vaccines. PPV 23 should be given at 2 years of age or older, administered about 2 months after the last dose of the PCV7. An additional dose of the PPV 23 administered 3 to 5 years later should be considered. The recommended immunization schedule and catch-up schedule for PCV7 and PPV 23 are presented in Table 106–3.[44,46] In addition to pneumococcal disease, the risk of meningococcal disease can also be higher in SCD, and routine vaccination is recommended.[45]

TABLE 106-3 Pneumococcal Immunization for Children with Sickle Cell Disease

	Recommended Schedule
Previously unvaccinated	
Age 2–6 months	**PCV7 (Prevnar):** 3 doses 6–8 wk apart; then 1 dose at 12–15 months
Age 7–11 months	**PCV7 (Prevnar):** 2 doses 6–8 wk apart; then 1 dose at 12–15 months
Age ≥12–23 months	**PCV7 (Prevnar):** 2 doses 6–8 wk apart
Age 24–59 months	**PCV7 (Prevnar):** 2 doses 6–8 wk apart **PPV 23 (Pneumovax):** 2 doses; first dose at least 6–8 wk after last PCV7 dose; second dose 3–5 years after the first PPV 23 dose
Age 5 years or older	**PCV7 (Prevnar):** 1 dose **PPV 23 (Pneumovax):** 2 doses; first dose at least 6–8 wk after last PCV7 dose; second dose 3–5 years (for those age 10 years or younger) or more than 5 years (for those age 10 years or older) after the first PPV 23 dose
Previously vaccinated	
Age 12–23 months, incomplete PCV7 series	**PCV7 (Prevnar):** 2 doses 6–8 wk apart
Age 24–59 months, received four doses of PCV7	**PPV 23 (Pneumovax):** 2 doses; first dose at least 6–8 wk after last PCV7 dose; second dose 3–5 years after the first PPV 23 dose
Age 24–59 months, three doses PCV7 given before 24 months of age	**PCV7 (Prevnar):** 1 dose **PPV 23 (Pneumovax):** 2 doses; first dose at least 6–8 wk after last PCV7 dose; second dose 3–5 y after the first PPV 23 dose
Age 24–59 months, 1 dose PPV 23 given	**PCV7 (Prevnar):** 2 doses 6–8 wk apart; first dose at least 8 wk after PPV 23 dose **PPV 23 (Pneumovax):** second dose 3–5 years after first PPV 23
Age 5 years or older, received PPV 23	**PCV7 (Prevnar):** 1 dose 6–8 wk after PPV 23 **If only received 1 dose of PPV 23 (Pneumovax):** Second dose 6–8 wk after PCV7 *and* 3–5 years (for those age 10 years or less) or more than 5 years (for those age 10 years or older) after the first PPV 23 dose

PCV7, 7-valent pneumococcal conjugated vaccine; PPV 23, 23-valent pneumococcal polysaccharide vaccine.
From Advisory Committee on Immunization Practices[44] and Sickle Cell Disease Care Consortium.[46]

Penicillin

❹ Penicillin prophylaxis until at least 5 years of age is recommended in children with SCD, even if they have been immunized with PCV7 as prophylaxis against pneumococcal infections. Prophylactic treatment should begin at 2 months of age or earlier. An effective regimen that reduces the risk of pneumococcal infections by 84% is penicillin V potassium at a dosage of 125 mg orally twice daily until the age of 3 years, followed by 250 mg twice daily until the age of 5 years. An alternate regimen is benzathine penicillin, 600,000 units given intramuscularly every 4 weeks for children age 6 months to 6 years, and 1.2 million units every 4 weeks for those over 6 years of age for whom continued therapy is warranted. Patients who are allergic to penicillin can be given erythromycin 20 mg/kg per day twice daily. Penicillin prophylaxis is not routinely given in older children, based on a study demonstrating no benefit over placebo beyond the age of 5 years. However, continuation of oral pneumococcal prophylaxis should be evaluated on a case-by-case basis, especially in patients with a history of invasive pneumococcal infection or surgical splenectomy.[1,5,7,43,44,46,47]

CLINICAL CONTROVERSY

The need for routine penicillin prophylaxis is controversial in HbSβ^+-thal patients because these patients have less severe disease.

Folic Acid

Patients with SCD have an increased demand for folic acid because of accelerated erythropoiesis. Megaloblastic changes have been reported, but the actual prevalence of megaloblastic anemia in patients with SCD is unknown. Conflicting data on serum folate levels have been reported. In children and adolescents, one study reported normal folate stores in SCD patients without receiving supplemental folic acid, and another study reported that 15% of patients had low folate levels despite daily supplementation. Conversion of homocysteine (Hcy) to methionine depends on folate, and vitamins B_6 and B_{12}. Plasma homocysteine level has been used as a marker for folate and vitamins B_6 and B_{12} status, and increased homocysteine levels have been associated with endothelial damage in pediatric SCD patients. In general, folic acid supplementation at a dose of 1 mg/day is recommended in adult patients, women who are contemplating pregnancy, and patients of all ages with chronic hemolysis. Daily supplementation with folic acid (1 mg), vitamin B_{12} (6 mcg) and vitamin B_6 (6 mg) has also been suggested for patients with increased homocysteine levels to reduce risk of endothelial damage[5,7,48–50]

■ FETAL HEMOGLOBIN INDUCERS

HbF has a direct effect on polymer formation. Increases in HbF levels significantly correlate with decreased RBC sickling and RBC adhesion. Epidemiologic studies show a relationship between HbF concentration and severity of the disease. Patients with low HbF levels have more frequent crises and higher mortality. Based on these observations, HbF induction has become a treatment modality for patients with SCD.[6,13]

Hydroxyurea

Hydroxyurea, a chemotherapeutic agent, increases HbF levels by stimulating the production of HbF. It also increases in the number of HbF-containing reticulocytes and intracellular HbF. Its antineoplastic activity is related to inhibition of DNA synthesis by blocking the conversion of ribonucleoside to deoxyribonucleotides. The exact mechanism on HbF production is unknown, but it alters RBC differentiation toward macrocytosis and HbF production as part of the erythropoietic response to cytoreduction in the bone marrow. In addition, hydroxyurea increases nitric oxide (NO) levels, which provides the rationale for the development of NO as a treatment modality for SCD.[51–54] Hydroxyurea also reduces neutrophils and monocytes, has antioxidant properties, alters RBC membrane properties, increases RBC deformability by increasing intracellular water content, and decreases RBC adhesion to endothelium.[5,51–53]

Hydroxyurea can prevent painful crises and is FDA-approved for adult patients based on a double-blind, placebo-controlled study called the Multicenter Study of Hydroxyurea in Sickle Cell Anemia (MSH). In that study of 299 adults with moderate-to-severe SCD, hydroxyurea significantly reduced the frequency of painful episodes, incidence of acute chest syndrome, need for blood transfusions, and number of hospitalizations.[51] The average number of crises was 44% lower in those who received hydroxyurea, declining from 4.5 to 2.5 crises per year. The incidence of severe crises, defined as those requiring hospitalization, was also lower, with a median rate of 2.4 severe crises per year in the placebo group versus one severe crisis per year in the hydroxyurea group. The risk of acute chest syndrome was also significantly reduced in patients receiving hydroxyurea. Of the 152 patients in the hydroxyurea group, 25 (16%) developed acute chest syndrome, as compared with 51 (35%) of the 147 patients in the placebo group. Blood transfusion requirements were decreased by 34% in the hydroxyurea group. The study was terminated early after interim analyses revealed the significant benefits. The incidence of death, stroke, and hepatic sequestration in the hydroxyurea and placebo groups was not significantly different during the 29-month evaluation period. However, the followup study of 233 of the 299 patients showed a 40% reduction in mortality with hydroxyurea over a 9-year period.[55] It is not clear whether the beneficial results can be extrapolated to patients with milder disease, such as HbSC.

Hydroxyurea is also used in selected children and adolescents with SCD, although its use is not FDA-approved in this patient population. Studies in pediatric patients (Pediatric Hydroxyurea in Sickle Cell Anemia) showed similar benefits as in adults with no adverse effects on growth and development. In addition, patients treated with 4 years of hydroxyurea therapy had possible delayed progression of organ dysfunction, such as splenic function. The results of another study, Pediatric Hydroxyurea Phase III Clinical Trial (BABY HUG), supported by the National Heart, Lung and Blood Institute will be available in the next few years to evaluate if hydroxyurea therapy is effective in prevention of chronic end-organ damage in young children with SCA.[5,51,52,56–59]

The most common side effect of hydroxyurea is bone marrow suppression. In the MSH trial, 14 of 152 patients in the hydroxyurea group and 6 of 147 patients in the placebo group required permanent discontinuation of treatment because of medical reasons. Temporary discontinuation of therapy occurred in almost all patients because of bone marrow suppression, which usually recovered within 2 weeks.[51] Alteration of magnesium levels, an cofactor in cation transport, has been reported in children.[60] Long-term side effects of hydroxyurea therapy in patients with SCD are not fully known. Myelodysplasia, acute leukemia, and chronic opportunistic infection associated with T-lymphocyte abnormalities have been reported.[7,46,59] In the 9-year followup study, 3 of 233 patients treated with hydroxyurea have developed cancer.[55] However, only 23 of those patients received therapy for more than 8 years, a duration that had been associated with an increased risk of acute leukemia.[61] Although no increased risk of cancer has been associated with hydroxyurea use of 2 to 15 years, a pilot study reported acquired DNA mutations in children.[51] Longer followup is needed to determine its carcinogenic or leukemogenic effects. Teratogenicity is another concern, as high-dose hydroxyurea has been shown to be teratogenic in animals. Normal pregnancies resulting in no birth defects have been reported in at least 15 women receiving hydroxyurea.[7,46]

Clinical indications for hydroxyurea use include frequent painful episodes, severe symptomatic anemia, a history of acute chest syndrome, or other severe vasoocclusive complications.[7,46] It is not clear whether hydroxyurea prevents organ damage or reverses previous damage. Splenic regeneration, however, has been reported in adult patients who received the agent. Hydroxyurea does not appear to prevent neurologic complications but can preserve cognitive performance. Hydroxyurea does not prevent strokes, but when given with a transfusion program, it can play an important role in preventing recurrent strokes and reducing iron overload from transfusion.[62] As discussed previously, hydroxyurea has been shown to decrease mortality in adult sickle cell patients in a 9-year followup study.[33,55]

Hydroxyurea is available in 200-, 300-, 400-, and 500-mg capsules. For children who are unable to swallow capsules, liquid preparations (100 mg/mL) can be prepared extemporaneously. The starting dose for hydroxyurea is 10 to 15 mg/kg per day as a single daily dose (Fig. 106–6). The dosage can be increased after 8 to 12 weeks if the patient can tolerate the adverse effects and blood counts are stable. Hydroxyurea dosage should be individualized based on response and toxicity. In general, 3 to 6 months of daily administration are required before improvement is observed. Medication adherence can be an issue.

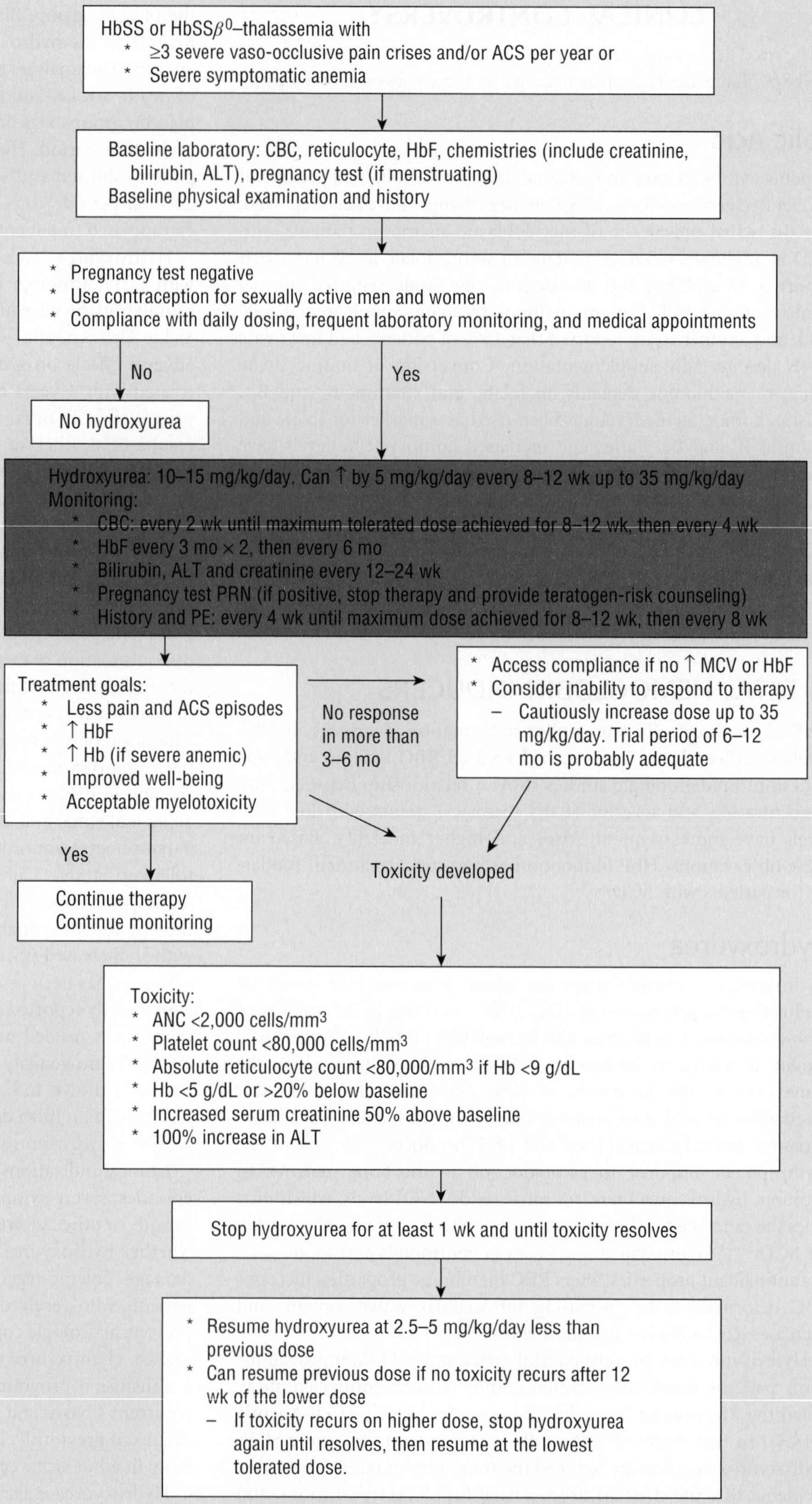
HbSS or HbSSβ0–thalassemia with
* ≥3 severe vaso-occlusive pain crises and/or ACS per year or
* Severe symptomatic anemia
Baseline laboratory: CBC, reticulocyte, HbF, chemistries (include creatinine, bilirubin, ALT), pregnancy test (if menstruating)
Baseline physical examination and history
* Pregnancy test negative
* Use contraception for sexually active men and women
* Compliance with daily dosing, frequent laboratory monitoring, and medical appointments
No
Yes
No hydroxyurea
Hydroxyurea: 10–15 mg/kg/day. Can ↑ by 5 mg/kg/day every 8–12 wk up to 35 mg/kg/day
Monitoring:
* CBC: every 2 wk until maximum tolerated dose achieved for 8–12 wk, then every 4 wk
* HbF every 3 mo × 2, then every 6 mo
* Bilirubin, ALT and creatinine every 12–24 wk
* Pregnancy test PRN (if positive, stop therapy and provide teratogen-risk counseling)
* History and PE: every 4 wk until maximum dose achieved for 8–12 wk, then every 8 wk
Treatment goals:
* Less pain and ACS episodes
* ↑ HbF
* ↑ Hb (if severe anemic)
* Improved well-being
* Acceptable myelotoxicity
No response in more than 3–6 mo
* Access compliance if no ↑ MCV or HbF
* Consider inability to respond to therapy
– Cautiously increase dose up to 35 mg/kg/day. Trial period of 6–12 mo is probably adequate
Yes
Continue therapy
Continue monitoring
Toxicity developed
Toxicity:
* ANC <2,000 cells/mm3
* Platelet count <80,000 cells/mm3
* Absolute reticulocyte count <80,000/mm3 if Hb <9 g/dL
* Hb <5 g/dL or >20% below baseline
* Increased serum creatinine 50% above baseline
* 100% increase in ALT
Stop hydroxyurea for at least 1 wk and until toxicity resolves
* Resume hydroxyurea at 2.5–5 mg/kg/day less than previous dose
* Can resume previous dose if no toxicity recurs after 12 wk of the lower dose
– If toxicity recurs on higher dose, stop hydroxyurea again until resolves, then resume at the lowest tolerated dose.

FIGURE 106-6. Hydroxyurea use in sickle cell disease. (ACS, acute chest syndrome; ALT, alanine aminotransferase; ANC, absolute neutrophil count; CBC, complete blood cell count; HbF, fetal hemoglobin; Hb, hemoglobin; HbSS, homozygous sickle cell hemoglobin; HBSSβ^0, sickle cell β^0-thalassemia; MCV, mean corpuscular volume; PE, physical examination; PRN, as needed; RBC, red blood cell.) *(From Stuart et al.,[7] Sickle Cell Disease Care Consortium,[46] and Halsey and Roberts.[51])*

Since the mean corpuscular volume (MCV) generally increases as the level of HbF increases, monitoring the MCV is an inexpensive and convenient method of monitoring response. With close monitoring, hydroxyurea can be increased by 5 mg/kg per day up to 35 mg/kg per day, the maximal prescribed dose in the MSH study.[7,46,51]

❺ Patients receiving hydroxyurea should be closely monitored for toxicity. Blood counts should be checked every 2 weeks during dose titration and every 4 to 6 weeks thereafter. Treatment should be interrupted if hematologic indices fall below the following values: absolute neutrophil count, 2,000 cells/mm^3; platelet count, 80,000 cells/mm^3; hemoglobin, 5 g/dL; or reticulocytes, 80,000 cells/mm^3 if the hemoglobin concentration is less than 9 g/dL. Other laboratory abnormalities warranting temporary discontinuation of therapy are a 50% increase in serum creatinine and a 100% increase in transaminase. After recovery has occurred, treatment should be resumed at a dose that is 2.5 to 5 mg/kg per day lower than the dose associated with toxicity. If no toxicity occurs after 12 weeks with the lower dose, the dose can be increased by 2.5 to 5 mg/kg per day. A given dose that twice produces a toxic hematologic response should not be tried again. Failure to see an increase in the MCV with hydroxyurea therapy can indicate that the marrow is unable to respond, the hydroxyurea dose is inadequate, or the patient is noncompliant.[7,46,51]

Butyrate

Butyrate, a naturally occurring fatty acid, increases HbF by altering gene expression, which leads to increased γ-globin chain production. Unlike hydroxyurea, butyrate does not appear to be cytotoxic.

Butyrate has been studied in small number of adult patients. Initial trials with continuous infusion butyrate showed an increase in not only HbF, but also in total hemoglobin and in the number of cells containing HbF. However, a sustained effect or an associated clinical benefit has not been observed. A later study with arginine butyrate in a pulse regimen reported a sustained increase in HbF and reduction of hospitalized days in a small number of adult patients. In that study, adult patients received a 4-day course of arginine butyrate, followed by a 10- to 24-day drug-free period before the administration of the next dose. Arginine butyrate was given at a daily dose of 250 to 500 mg/kg over 6 to 12 hours. Although the results are encouraging, the need for intravenous administration can limit widespread use of the regimen.[63]

Oral sodium phenylbutyrate has been used for years in young children with urea cycle disorders. At high doses, side effects include transient fluid retention, rashes, and unusual body odor. Increased HbF levels were seen in patients with SCA who received both high-dose (15 to 20 g/day) and low-dose (1 to 11 g/day) regimens. In the study of low-dose sodium phenylbutyrate, increased HbF was seen within 5 weeks but may not be sustained. The studies of butyrate involved a small number of patients. More clinical trials are needed to determine the optimal dosage and regimen.[5,63]

5-Aza-2'-Deoxycytidine (Decitabine)

5-A'zacytidine and 5-aza-2'-deoxycytidine (decitabine) induce HbF by inhibiting methylation of DNA, thus preventing the switch from γ- to β-globin production. Compared with 5-azacytidine, decitabine has a more favorable safety profile and is a more potent methylation inhibitor. Virtually abandoned in the past because of concerns regarding the cytotoxicity of 5-azacytidine, decitabine has been studied in a small number of patients with SCD who did not respond to hydroxyurea. In one study of eight patients who were resistant or intolerant to hydroxyurea, 5-aza-2'-deoxycytidine was given at a dose of 0.2 mg/kg one to three times a week subcutaneously. An increase in HbF was seen in all patients. In addition, reduction of adhesion was reported in the RBC adhesion study. The only significant toxicity observed was neutropenia. This agent may have a role in treating patients who fail to respond to hydroxyurea.[5,64]

Combinations of Hemoglobin F Inducers

Erythropoietin therapy has been used in only a limited number of patients with SCD, and the clinical results have been inconsistent; therefore, its routine use in these patients cannot be recommended. When used in combination with hydroxyurea, erythropoietin increases HbF levels to a greater extent than hydroxyurea alone. This suggests that there may be a role for addition of erythropoietin therapy in patients who do not respond to hydroxyurea alone, although more studies are needed. Other proposed combinations are hydroxyurea combined with either phenylbutyrate or clotrimazole, based on their different mechanisms of action.[7,52,57,63]

■ CLOTRIMAZOLE

Clotrimazole, an antifungal agent, decreases cell density by blocking cation transport channels in the erythrocyte membrane. The decrease seen, however, is less than that demonstrated with hydroxyurea therapy. It is unclear whether this agent will be clinically useful in the treatment of SCA.[52] Its analog, ICA-17043, is more specific for potassium efflux and is currently undergoing clinical trials for vasoocclusive event reduction.[65]

■ CHRONIC TRANSFUSION THERAPY

Transfusions play an important role in the management of SCD. In acute illness, transfusions can be life-saving and will be discussed in a later section (see Chronic Transfusion Therapy). Maintenance transfusion programs are used to prevent serious complications of SCD. The primary indication for chronic transfusion is stroke prevention and amelioration of other organ damage. Transfusion can be done by simple or exchange transfusions. Exchange transfusion is associated with higher cost but has the advantage of limiting volume, and minimizing hyperviscosity and iron overload.[66]

❻ In children who had a stroke, chronic transfusions are successful in reducing stroke recurrence from approximately 50% to approximately 10% over 3 years. As the initial stroke in SCD can be devastating, transfusions are usually to prevent the initial stroke. In one trial, prophylactic transfusions significantly reduced the incidence of first stroke over a 2-year period in children 2 to 16 years of age with abnormal TCD ultrasonography. Stroke occurrence rate was reduced from 16% in patients receiving usual care to 2% in those who received prophylactic transfusions.[66–68]

Chronic transfusions can also reduce the risk of vasoocclusive pain and acute chest syndrome, and prevent or delay progression of organ damage. They can also reverse preexisting organ dysfunction and improve quality of life, energy levels, exercise tolerance, growth, and sexual development. Selected patients in whom chronic transfusion should be considered are patients with transient ischemic attack, abnormal TCD, severe or recurrent acute chest syndrome, debilitating pain, splenic sequestration, recurrent priapism, chronic organ failure, intractable leg ulcers, severe chronic anemia with cardiac failure, and complicated pregnancies.[5,46,66]

The goal of transfusions is to achieve and maintain an HbS concentration of less than 30% of total hemoglobin. Transfusions are usually given every 3 to 4 weeks, but the frequency of transfusion is adjusted to maintain the desired HbS levels. After 4 years of therapy without development of complications, many clinicians give transfusions less frequently and allow the HbS concentration to increase to 50% of total hemoglobin.[4,5,46,66] The optimal duration of chronic primary prophylactic transfusion therapy is not clear, but discontinuation of transfusions has been associated with a 50% recurrence rate within 12 months and abnormal blood flow velocity in children. For secondary prevention, current recommendations are to continue transfusion for at least 5 years if there has been no neurologic event and imaging studies have been normalized or until age 18 years. A pilot study suggests that hydroxyurea should be started prior to discontinuation of transfusion for secondary stroke prevention.[5,66–71]

Although the benefits of transfusion therapy are clear in some clinical situations, its role in other situations such as priapism and leg ulcer remains controversial.[66] The risks of transfusion therapy must be weighed against possible benefits. The risks associated with transfusion therapy include alloimmunization (sensitization to the blood received), hyperviscosity, viral transmission, volume overload, iron overload, and transfusion reactions. Alloimmunization occurs in 18% to 36% of SCD patients who receive blood transfusions. The use of leukocyte-reduced RBC transfusions or human leukocyte antigen (HLA)-matched units in chronically transfused patients can reduce the risk of alloimmunization. Transfusion-related infections also remain a concern. All patients should be immunized with hepatitis A and B vaccines. Presently, hepatitis C is considered the most serious risk associated with transfusion therapy, with an infection rate of approximately 1 in every 100,000 transfusions. The risk of contracting acquired immune deficiency syndrome (AIDS) from blood transfusions, although still of concern, has decreased with routine blood screening. Iron overload is another complication of transfusions, and patients should be counseled to avoid excess dietary iron. Abnormal liver biopsy results showing mild to moderate inflammation or fibrosis have been reported. Chelation therapy with deferoxamine should be considered after more than 1 year of chronic transfusions or when serum ferritin is greater than 1,500 to 2,000 ng/mL.[5,7,46,66] Deferoxamine has been associated with oto- and ocular toxicity and growth failure. Therefore, patients receiving chelation therapy should have yearly ophthalmologic and auditory examinations. Deferasirox, a new oral chelator, has shown effectiveness in management of iron overload in SCD. It has an advantage of being available as an oral dosage form.[46,66,72,73]

Unique to the population with SCD is a constellation of features that can occur in response to blood transfusion; this is often referred to as the sickle cell hemolytic transfusion reaction syndrome. This syndrome includes manifestations of an acute or delayed transfusion reaction caused by alloimmunization. Delayed reaction can occur 2 to 20 days after transfusion. During the hemolytic reaction, the patient develops symptoms suggestive of a pain crisis, or symptoms worsen if the patient is already in crisis. The patient can also develop an anemia posttransfusion that is more severe than previously observed because of the rapid decline in hemoglobin and hematocrit, accompanied by a suppressed erythropoiesis. Reticulocytopenia is often seen in delayed hemolytic transfusion reactions. Alloantibodies and autoantibodies that formed as a result of past transfusions can serve as a trigger, causing a return of symptoms in the postrecovery period. Subsequent transfusions can further worsen the clinical situation because of the presence of autoimmune antibodies. Life-threatening events can be treated with steroids and intravenous immunoglobulin. Erythropoietin has been used in patients with reticulocytopenia. Recovery, as evidenced by reticulocytosis with a gradual increase in the hemoglobin level, may occur only after further transfusions are withheld. Although some patients tolerate further transfusions after recovery, others experience a recurrence of the hemolytic transfusion reaction.[3,5,13,46,66,74]

■ ALLOGENEIC HEMATOPOIETIC STEM CELL TRANSPLANTATION

Allogeneic hematopoietic stem cell transplantation (HSCT) is currently the only therapy that can cure patients with SCD.[75–77] A report of a multicenter trial of allogeneic HSCT in 50 patients with SCD showed a 94% survival rate and 84% event-free survival. All of the patients in the study were younger than 16 years of age, had symptomatic SCD, and had an HLA-identical sibling donor. Two patients died from chronic graft-versus-host disease, and one died of intracranial hemorrhage. Of the 47 surviving patients, 5 experienced graft rejection and recurrent SCD. These rejections occurred a median of 5.1 months after transplantation.[75–77] Pretransplant use of hydroxyurea has been associated with a lower incidence of rejection or failure of engraftment in a study of children with severe SCD.[78]

The best candidates for allogeneic HSCT are SCD patients who are younger than 16 years of age; have severe complications such as refractory pain, stroke, or recurrent acute chest syndrome; and have an HLA-matched donor. Although allogeneic HSCT in young children before organ damage and alloimmunization occur can be associated with an increased success rate, disease progression is unpredictable, making it difficult to determine the optimal time for transplantation. The risks associated with allogeneic HSCT must be carefully considered, as the transplant-related mortality rate is approximately 5% to 10%, and graft rejection is approximately 10%. The risk of acute or extensive chronic graft-versus-host disease ranges from 6% to more than 50% in various studies. Other risks associated with allogeneic HSCT include secondary malignancies. Neurologic events, such as intracranial hemorrhage and seizures during transplant were seen more frequently in patients with a history of stroke. In addition, transmission of chronic myeloid leukemia has been reported in a sickle cell patient who received a peripheral blood stem cell transplant. Efforts to decrease the posttransplant risk of seizures or intracranial bleeding include prophylactic anticonvulsant therapy, aggressive platelet support, and stringent patient selection.[5,75–79]

Experience with unrelated HLA-matched or related HLA-mismatched donor transplants is very limited. Studies in thalassemia patients do not support the use of these alternate donors at this time. Umbilical cord blood is another donor source. Its advantages include a lower incidence of severe graft-versus-host disease and the potential of using umbilical cord blood from unrelated donors, but such advantages are balanced by longer duration for engraftment and a higher rate of graft rejection.[5,75–79]

TREATMENT OF COMPLICATIONS

■ GENERAL MANAGEMENT

Parents and older children should be educated on the signs and symptoms of complications and conditions that require urgent evaluation. During acute illness, patients should be evaluated promptly, as deterioration can occur rapidly. It is essential to maintain a balanced fluid status because dehydration and fluid overload can worsen complications associated with SCD. Oxygen saturation by pulse oximetry should be maintained at least 92% or at baseline. New or increasing supplemental oxygen requirements should be investigated.[5,7,46]

■ EPISODIC TRANSFUSIONS FOR ACUTE COMPLICATIONS

Indications for RBC transfusions include (1) acute exacerbation of baseline anemia, such as aplastic crisis if the anemia is severe, hepatic or splenic sequestration, or severe hemolysis; (2) severe vasoocclusive episodes, such as acute chest syndrome, stroke, or acute multi-organ failure; and (3) preparation for procedures that require the use of general anesthesia or ionic contrast. Other patients in whom transfusions can be useful include patients with complicated obstetric problems, refractory leg ulcers, or refractory and protracted painful episodes or severe priapism. Transfusion can be done by simple transfusion or partial exchange transfusion. If simple transfusion is used, volume overload leading to congestive heart failure can occur if anemia is corrected too rapidly in patients with severe anemia. In addition, increases in hemoglobin levels to greater than 10 to 11 g/dL can cause hyperviscosity and should be avoided.[5,46,66]

■ INFECTION AND FEVER

Patients with SCD should be evaluated as soon as possible for any fever greater than 38.5°C (101.3°F). Criteria for hospitalization include an infant younger than 1 year old, history of previous bacteremia or sepsis, temperature greater than 40°C (104°F), WBC greater than 30,000 cells/mm^3 or less than 5,000 cells/mm^3 and/or platelets less than 100,000 cells/mm^3, and evidence of other acute complications or toxic appearance. Outpatient management can be considered in older nontoxic children with reliable family caregivers. Antibiotic choice should provide adequate coverage for encapsulated organisms.

❼ Ceftriaxone should be used for outpatient management because it provides coverage for 24 hours. If admitted, cefotaxime can also be used. For patients with cephalosporin allergy, clindamycin can be used. Vancomycin should be considered for acutely ill children or if staphylococcus is suspected. A macrolide antibiotic should be added if mycoplasma pneumonia is suspected. Penicillin prophylaxis should be discontinued while receiving broad-spectrum antibiotics. Acetaminophen or ibuprofen can be used for fever control. Increased fluid requirements can be needed because of dehydration and/or increased insensible loss.[1,4,5,7,46]

CEREBROVASCULAR ACCIDENTS

Patients with acute neurologic events must be hospitalized and monitored closely. Physical and neurologic examination should be performed every 2 hours. Acute treatment for children should include exchange transfusion or simple transfusion to maintain hemoglobin at approximately 10 g/dL and HbS less than 30%, anticonvulsants for patients with a seizure history, and therapy for increased intracranial pressure if needed. Chronic transfusion therapy should be initiated for children with ischemic stroke as discussed above. In adults presenting with ischemic stroke, thrombolytic therapy should be considered if it is less than 3 hours since the onset of symptoms.[1,4,5,7,24,46,67]

ACUTE CHEST SYNDROME

Patients with acute chest syndrome should use incentive spirometry frequently (e.g., at least every 2 hours while awake) to reduce atelectasis development. In addition, proper management of pain is important. The goal is to provide relief while avoiding analgesic-induced hypoventilation. Appropriate fluid therapy is important as overhydration can cause pulmonary edema and exacerbate respiratory distress. Early use of broad-spectrum antibiotics, including a macrolide or quinolone, is also recommended. Studies indicate that infection is common with acute chest syndrome, and can involve gram-positive, gram-negative, or atypical bacteria. Oxygen therapy is indicated for all patients who are hypoxic or in acute distress. In a patient with a history of reactive airway disease or wheezing on examination, a trial of bronchodilators is appropriate. Transfusions are often used in the treatment of acute lung disease.[5,7,30,31,80]

Steroids can decrease inflammation and endothelial cell adhesion. Glucocorticoids can decrease the duration of hospitalization, transfusions, and need for other supportive care but can increase the readmission rate for SCA-related complications. Another promising therapy is the use of NO. NO inhalation relaxes and dilates blood vessels. Its hematologic effects include inhibition of platelet aggregation and reduction in the polymerization tendency of HbS. Marked improvement of pulmonary status and cardiac output has been reported in a patient with acute chest syndrome. Both inhaled NO and oral L-arginine, the precursor of NO, are being evaluated for management of acute chest syndrome.[30,31,80]

PRIAPISM

Stuttering priapism, episodes that last a few minutes to 2 hours, resolve spontaneously. Prolonged episodes lasting more than 2 to 3 hours require prompt medical attention. The initial goals of treatment are to provide appropriate analgesic therapy, reduce anxiety, produce detumescence, and preserve testicular function and fertility. Treatment given within 4 to 6 hours can usually reduce erection. Aggressive hydration and adequate pain control should be initiated. Use of ice packs is not recommended. Heat (hot water bottles, hot packs, or sitz baths) can provide comfort without precipitating pain crisis. Although transfusions have been given to these patients, the efficacy of this therapeutic intervention has not been established.[1,5,81,82]

Clinicians have used both vasoconstrictors and vasodilators in the treatment of priapism. Vasoconstrictors, such as diluted phenylephrine (10 microgram/mL) or epinephrine (1:1,000,000), are thought to work by forcing blood out of the corpus cavernosum into the venous return. In one uncontrolled open-label study, aspiration followed by intrapenile irrigation with epinephrine was effective and well tolerated. In that study, blood was first aspirated from the corpus cavernosum, and then the area was irrigated with a 1:1,000,000 solution of epinephrine. The priapism resolved in 37 of the 39 occasions. A followup study reported that 3 out of 20 patients required a repeat procedure within 24 hours. The therapy was well tolerated with no serious immediate or long-term side effects but on two occasions, a small intrapenile hematoma formed after treatment.[82]

Vasodilators, such as terbutaline and hydralazine, relax the smooth muscle of the vasculature. This relaxation allows oxygenated arterial blood to enter the corpus cavernosum, which displaces or washes out the damaged sickle cells that are stagnant in the corpus cavernosum. Terbutaline has been used to treat priapism, but it has not been formally studied in patients with SCA. In one case report, a single oral sildenafil dose at onset of priapism aborted episodes. Surgical interventions used in severe refractory priapism have included a variety of shunt procedures. These surgical procedures have been successful in some cases, but they have a high failure rate and potential serious complications, which include impotence, skin sloughing, cellulitis, and urethral fistulas.[5,7,82]

Modalities to prevent priapism are limited and not well studied. Pseudoephedrine (30 or 60 mg/day given orally at bedtime) and leuprolide, a gonadotropin-releasing hormone, have been used to decrease the number of recurrent episodes of priapism. Hydroxyurea therapy can also be useful. Finally, low-doses of an antiandrogen, bicalutamide, have been used in two patients with SCD and one patient with spinal cord injury for treatment of recurrent and refractory priapism without major side effects.[5,7,46,82,83] The role of RBC transfusion in preventing priapism remains unclear.[66,82]

CLINICAL CONTROVERSY

Some clinicians transfuse patients to maintain an HbS level less than 30% to prevent recurrent priapism. Duration of such regimens should be limited to 6 to 12 months.

MANAGEMENT OF CRISES

Aplastic Crisis

Treatment of aplastic crisis is primarily supportive, and most patients recover spontaneously. The patient can need blood transfusions if the anemia is severe or symptomatic. Reticulocyte count helps to determine if there is red cell production and the need for transfusions. The most common cause for aplastic crisis is acute infection with human parvovirus B19. As parvovirus is contagious, infected patients should be placed in isolation. In addition, contact with pregnant healthcare providers should be avoided because parvovirus infection during the midtrimester of pregnancy can result in hydrops fetalis and stillbirth.[4,5,7,46]

Sequestration Crisis

Splenic sequestration crisis is a major cause of mortality in young patients with SCD. The sequestration of RBCs in the spleen can result in a rapid drop of hematocrit, leading to hypovolemia, shock, and death. Immediate treatment is RBC transfusion to correct hypovolemia. Broad-spectrum antibiotic therapy, which includes coverage for pneumococci and *H. influenzae,* can also be beneficial because infection can precipitate crises.[4,5,7,46]

Recurrent episodes occur in approximately one-half of patients and are associated with increased mortality. Options for management of recurrence include observation, chronic transfusion, and splenectomy. Adults are often observed because they tend to have milder episodes. Increased risk of invasive infection after splenectomy is a concern in young children. Chronic transfusions delay splenectomy and temporarily restore splenic function, but it is associated with its own risks. Splenectomy is probably indicated, even after a single sequestration crisis, if that event is life-threatening. Splenectomy should be considered after repetitive episodes, even if they are less serious. For children younger than 2 years of age, chronic blood transfusions are recommended to prevent sequestration and delay splenectomy until the age of 2 years, when the risk of postsplenectomy septicemia is less. Finally, splenectomy should also be considered for patients with chronic hypersplenism.[1,4,5,7,46]

Vasoocclusive Pain Crisis

Hydration and analgesia are the mainstays of treatment for vasoocclusive (painful) crises (Table 106–4). Patients with mild pain crisis can be treated as outpatients with rest, increased fluid intake, warm compresses, and oral analgesics. Hospitalization is necessary for moderate to severe crisis. As infection can precipitate crises, an infectious etiology should be ruled out and appropriate empiric therapy should be initiated in patients who have fever or are critically ill. In anemic patients, transfusion to maintain the hemoglobin level at baseline can be needed. Fluid replacement given intravenously or orally at 1.5 times the maintenance requirement is recommended. Close monitoring of fluid status is essential as aggressive hydration, particularly with sodium-containing fluids, can lead to volume overload, acute chest syndrome, and heart failure.[4,5,7,46]

The frequency and severity of acute pain episodes associated with SCD are variable, and pain should be assessed, and analgesic therapy should be tailored for each patient. Several pain assessment tools are available and should be used to quantify the degree of pain. Unfortunately, they have not been validated for sickle cell pain. The healthcare provider should choose one tool appropriate for age and use it routinely to assess pain. Other useful information to guide choice of analgesics should include previous effective agents and their dosages, response to therapy and previous clinical course, and duration of pain crisis.[84–85]

❽ Aggressive therapy that relieves pain and enables the patient to attain maximum functional ability should be initiated in patients with pain crisis. Treatment of mild-to-moderate pain should include the use of nonsteroidal antiinflammatory drugs (NSAIDs) or acetaminophen, unless there are contraindications to their use. Ketorolac is the only injectable NSAID available and is useful for patients requiring intravenous therapy. Because of concerns about gastrointestinal bleeding, it is recommended to limit the duration of therapy to 5 days or less. When acetaminophen is used, it is important to review the total dose of acetaminophen administered in patients who may also be receiving the agent for fever or another acetaminophen-containing product for pain. If mild-to-moderate pain persists, an opioid should be added. Effective combination therapy, such as an NSAID combined with an opioid, can enhance analgesic efficacy while decreasing side effects.[7,84–86]

Severe pain should be treated aggressively until the pain is tolerable. Commonly used opioids include morphine, hydromorphone, fentanyl, and methadone. The weak opioids, codeine and hydrocodone, are used to manage mild-to-moderate pain. Meperidine has no advantages as an analgesic. Its duration of action is short compared to the half-life of the metabolite, normeperidine. The accumulation of normeperidine can cause central nervous system side effects, ranging from dysphoria to seizures. Therefore, meperidine should be avoided if possible and used only for a very brief duration in patients who are allergic or intolerant to other opioids.[7,84–86]

TABLE 106-4 Management of Acute Pain of Sickle Cell Disease

Principles
• Treat underlying precipitating factors
• Avoid delays in analgesia administration
• Use pain scale to assess severity
• Choice of initial analgesic should be based on previous pain crisis pattern, history of response, current status, and other medical conditions
• Schedule pain medication; avoid as-needed dosing
• Provide rescue dose for breakthrough pain
• If adequate pain relief can be achieved with one or two doses of morphine, consider outpatient management with a weak opioid; otherwise hospitalization is needed for parenteral analgesics
• Frequently assess to evaluate pain severity and side effects; titrate dose as needed
• Treating adverse effects of opioids is part of pain management
• Consider nonpharmacologic intervention (e.g., relaxation techniques, guided imagery, deep breathing)
• Transition to oral analgesics as the patient improves; choose an oral agent based on previous history, anticipated duration, and ability to swallow tablets; if sustained-release products are used, a product with a rapid onset is also needed for breakthrough pain
Analgesic regimens
Mild-to-moderate pain: nonopioid ± weak opioid
Moderate-to-severe pain: weak opioid or low dose of a strong opioid ± nonopioid
Severe pain: strong opioid + nonopioid
Weak opioid
Acetaminophen with codeine
Dose based on codeine–children: 1 mg/kg per dose every 6 hours; adult: 30 to 60 mg/dose
Hydrocodone + acetaminophen
Dose based on hydrocodone–children: 0.2 mg/kg per dose every 6 hours; adults: 5 to 10 mg/dose
Nonopioid
Oral antiinflammatory agents
Use with caution in patients with renal failure (dehydration) and bleeding
Ibuprofen–children: 10 mg/kg every 6 to 8 hours; adult: 200 to 400 mg/dose
Naproxen: 5 mg/kg every 12 hours; adult 250 to 500 mg/dose
Intravenous antiinflammatory agents:
Ketorolac: 0.5 mg/kg up to 30 mg/dose every 6 hours
Strong opioid
Morphine: 0.1 to 0.15 mg/kg per dose every 3 to 4 hours for children; 5 to 10 mg/dose for adults
Continuous infusion: 0.04 to 0.05 mg/kg per hour; titrate to effect
Hydromorphone: 0.015 mg/kg per dose every 3 to 4 hours for children; 1.5 to 2 mg/dose for adults
Continuous infusion: 0.004 mg/kg per hour; titrate to effect
Patient-controlled analgesics:
Morphine: 0.01 to 0.03 mg/kg per hours basal; demand 0.01 to 0.03 mg/kg every 6 to 10 min; 4-hour lock out 0.4 to 0.6 mg/kg
Hydromorphone: 0.003 to 0.005 mg/kg per hour basal; demand 0.03 to 0.05 mg/kg every 6–10 minutes; 4 hour lock out 0.06 to 0.08 mg/kg
Rescue therapy:
For breakthrough, give 1/4 to 1/2 of the scheduled dose as bolus every 1 to 2 hour; assess amount of rescue dose used in 8 to 12 hours and readjust scheduled dose or infusion rate as needed
Other adjunct therapy:
Hydration, heating pads, relaxation, and distraction
Stool softener and/or stimulants for constipation
Antihistamine for itching
Antiemetics for nausea or vomiting

From Jacob et al.,[84] Stinson and Naser,[85] Dumaplin,[86] and Elander et al.[87]

Both prior history and current assessment should be considered in the management of pain crisis. For patients whose typical crisis improves in a short time, preparations with a short duration of action are appropriate. For patients whose crises require many days to resolve, sustained-release preparations combined with a short-acting product for breakthrough pain are more appropriate. If the patient has been on long-term opioid therapy at home, tolerance can develop. In these cases, the pain of acute crises can be treated with a different potent opioid or a larger dose of the same medication.

Intravenous administration provides a rapid onset of action and therefore is preferred for severe pain. Intramuscular injections should be avoided. Children might actually deny pain because of fear of injections. Analgesics should be titrated to pain relief. In patients with continuous pain, the analgesic should be given as a scheduled dose or continuous infusion. Continuous infusion has the advantage of less fluctuation of blood levels between dosing intervals. As-needed dosing is only appropriate for breakthrough pain. Patient-controlled analgesia (PCA) is commonly used. When used properly, PCA allows patients to have control over pain therapy and minimizes the lag time between perception of pain and administration of analgesics. The transdermal fentanyl patch has also been used successfully, but its role in sickle cell pain crisis is unclear because of its long time of onset of pain relief (12 to 16 hours) and fixed dosage form, which makes it difficult to titrate the dose. Other alternative pain management techniques such as physical therapy and relaxation therapy can be helpful as adjunct therapy.[7,84–86]

The most common cause of suboptimal pain control in children with SCA is the suspicion of addiction. This obstacle is especially common in adolescents. In one study, 53% of emergency physicians believed that 20% of SCD patients are addicted to analgesics. Elander and associates interviewed 51 SCD patients and used symptoms described in the *Diagnostic and Statistical Manual of Mental Disorders, Fourth Edition* to assess substance dependence. They reported that when pain-related symptoms are included, 31% met criteria for substance dependence, but when symptoms are restricted to those that are not pain related, only 2% met the criteria for substance dependence. Another barrier for effective pain control is the difference in perception between patients, family, and healthcare providers. Patients with SCD often suffer from chronic pain, and they may cope with the pain by being inactive. Patients who have inadequate pain control can exhibit anxiety and drug-seeking behavior for fear of pain. Tolerance to narcotics can also be misinterpreted as drug addiction by healthcare providers and families. Aggressive pain control, frequent monitoring of pain during crises, and tapering medication according to response are factors that minimize physical dependence.[84–89]

Poloxamer 188 (Flocor), a highly purified poloxamer, is an agent currently being evaluated under orphan drug status for the management of vasoocclusive pain crisis in SCD. It acts as a surfactant and normalizes the RBC to its nonadhesive state. In addition, it enhances blood flow in ischemic areas by blocking RBC aggregation. The antiadhesive and hemorheologic properties result in improved blood flow, increased oxygen delivery, and decreased cell injury. A phase III clinical study conducted in adults and children aged 8 to 65 years old with vasoocclusive crises reported more rapid resolution in those treated with poloxamer 188. Patients younger than 15 years and those who were receiving hydroxyurea therapy were two groups that appeared to have the most beneficial effect.[90]

Intracellular adhesion of RBCs contributes to vasoocclusion in SCD. Agents that can alter adhesion molecules on RBCs can potentially reduce or ameliorate clinical manifestation of SCD. Omega-3 fatty acids are important components of cell membrane and organelles and may be important for erythrocyte integrity and play a role in reducing hemolysis. In addition, omega-3 fatty acids have antiadhesion activity by modulating adhesive molecules in membrane. Reduction of disease severity has been reported in clinical trials.[91]

PHARMACOECONOMIC CONSIDERATIONS

Patients with SCD incur considerable healthcare costs. Pharmacoeconomic considerations should include newborn screening, cost of managing acute and chronic complications, and the economic impact of new treatment modalities. Early penicillin prophylaxis prevents pneumococcal sepsis in infants. Newborn screening targeted at African Americans has been shown to be cost-effective. Whether it is cost-effective to screen all infants depends on the prevalence of high-risk infants in the area. The estimated annual cost through universal screening programs ranged from $1,402 in Mississippi to $304,215 in Vermont per case identified. In general, universal screening identifies more infants with disease, prevents more deaths, and can provide for a certain degree of cost-effectiveness because targeted screening might not detect all infants with the disease.[8,92]

Hospitalization is an important societal financial burden. A 1996 national estimate reported the average cost per hospitalization to be $6,300, which totals a cost of $475 million per year. Studies conducted in various regions have shown that a small number of patients consume a disproportionate amount of care as a result of severe illness, and most of the total cost is related to hospitalizations. Patients who are not being followed in settings that provide comprehensive medical care tend to acquire higher costs for emergency room and hospital visits. Another study examining relationships between socioeconomic factors and geographic distribution in Alabama reported that use of comprehensive care was lower for those living in rural areas. Using a mathematical model and data available from studies, researchers estimated lifetime costs for SCA and other hemoglobinopathies to be $83,200 for patients with early diagnoses and $78,400 for late diagnosis.[3,8,93,94]

Newer therapies, diagnostic methods such as TCD, and chronic transfusions further increase cost. Using the data from the MSH trial, Moore and colleagues estimated that the average annual cost for medical care was lower in the hydroxyurea group as compared with the placebo group ($12,160 vs. $22,020). Hospitalization because of pain crisis accounted for the highest cost in both groups and a saving of more than 5,000 per patient per year of medical costs can be achieved if every eligible patient was to receive the agent.[94] However, this cost-saving was not demonstrated in one analysis performed in Maryland.[95] Allogeneic HSCT can potentially cure the disease, and if successful can reduce long-term costs, but it requires a high up-front cost. The new therapies, although expensive, might reduce visits to emergency departments and inpatient hospitalizations, improving the cost-effectiveness of those therapies over a patient's lifetime.[7]

EVALUATION OF THERAPEUTIC OUTCOMES

SCD is a complex disorder that requires multidisciplinary comprehensive care. All patients should be medically evaluated regularly to establish baseline, monitor changes, and provide education appropriate for age. For infants younger than 1 year old, medical evaluations every 2 to 4 months are needed. Beyond 1 year of age, evaluation can be extended to every 6 to 12 months with modifications depending on severity of the illness.[46]

It is important to establish baseline laboratory values and imaging studies. Routine laboratory evaluation includes complete blood cell counts and reticulocyte counts every 3 months up to 2 years of age, then every 6 months; HbF level should be taken every 6 months until 2 years of age, then annually. Evaluation of renal, hepatobiliary, and pulmonary function should be done annually. TCD screening is recommended to start at age 2 years, then annually. Ophthalmologic examination to screen for retinopathy is recommended at around age 10 years. In patients with recurrent acute chest syndrome, pulmonary function tests should be done to establish baseline values and identify declines in lung function.

It is essential that prophylactic immunizations and antibiotics are given. When infections do occur, appropriate antibiotic therapy should be initiated, and the patient should be monitored for laboratory and clinical improvement. The efficacy of hydroxyurea can best be assessed in terms of the decrease in number, severity, and duration of sickle cell pain crises. HbF concentrations or MCV values can also provide some indication of the patient's response to therapy. When painful crises do occur, the effectiveness of analgesics can be measured by subjective assessments made by the patient, family, and healthcare practitioners. The success of poststroke blood transfusions can be measured by clinical progression or the occurrence of subsequent strokes.

CONCLUSIONS

The goals of the general management of SCA are to decrease the number of sickle cell crises, decrease the complications arising from the disease, and improve the overall quality of the patient's life. The general care of SCA patients still includes early penicillin prophylaxis and appropriate immunization. HbF inducers such as hydroxyurea can decrease the frequency and severity of painful episodes. Continued studies of other possible agents and treatment modalities that can reduce crises or reverse organ damage are warranted.

ABBREVIATIONS

ASPEN syndrome: association of sickle cell disease, priapism, exchange transfusion, and neurologic events

HbAS: one normal (hemoglobin A) and one sickle cell hemoglobin (hemoglobin S) geneHbC: Hemoglobin C

HbF: fetal hemoglobin

HbSβ^{+}-thal, HbSβ^{0}-thal: hemoglobin sickle cell β^{+}-thalassemia and hemoglobin sickle cell β^{0}-thalassemia

HbSC: sickle cell hemoglobin C

HbSS: homozygous sickle cell hemoglobin (hemoglobin S)

HbS: sickle cell hemoglobin

HLA: human leukocyte antigen

HSCT: hematopoietic stem cell transplantation

ISC: irreversibly sickled cell

MCHC: mean corpuscular hemoglobin concentration

MCV: mean corpuscular volume

MSH: Multicenter Study of Hydroxyurea in Sickle Cell Anemia

NO: nitric oxide

NSAID: nonsteroidal antiinflammatory drug

PCA: patient-controlled analgesia

PCV7: 7-valent pneumococcal conjugate vaccine

PPV 23: 23-valent pneumococcal polysaccharide vaccine

RBC: red blood cell

SCA: sickle cell anemia

SCD: sickle cell disease

SCT: sickle cell trait

TCD: transcranial Doppler

WBC: white blood cell

REFERENCES

1. Fixler J, Styles L. Sickle cell disease. Pediatr Clin North Am 2002;49:1193–1210.
2. Eaton WA. Linus Pauling and sickle cell disease. Biophys Chem 2003;100:109–116.
3. Nietert PJ, Silverstein MD, Abboud MR. Sickle cell anaemia epidemiology and cost of illness. Pharmacoeconomics 2002;20:357–366.
4. Ad Hoc Writing Committee, American Academy of Pediatrics. Health supervision for children with sickle cell disease. Pediatrics 2002;109:526–535.
5. National Institutes of Health, Division of Blood Diseases and Resources, Public Health Service. The Management of Sickle Cell Disease. Bethesda, MD: U.S. Department of Health and Human Services, June 2002:1–88. NIH publication 02–2117.
6. Ashley-Koch A, Yang Q, Olney RS. Sickle hemoglobin (HbS) allele and sickle cell disease: A huge review. Am J Epidemiol 2000;151:839–844.
7. Stuart MJ, Nagel RL. Sickle-cell disease. Lancet 2004;364:1343–1360.
8. Miller St, Sleeper LA, Pegelow CH, et al. Reduction of adverse outcomes in children with sickle cell disease. N Engl J Med 2000;342:83–89.
9. Steensma DP, Hoyer JD, Fairbanks VF. Hereditary red blood cell disorders in Middle Eastern patients. Mayo Clin Proc 2001;76:285–293.
10. Agrawal MB. Advances in management of sickle cell disease. Indian J Pediatr 2003;70:649–654.
11. Wilson KE, Krishnamurti L, Kamat D. Management of sickle cell disease in primary care. Clin Pediatr 2003;42:753–761.
12. Hebbel RP, Osarogiagbon R, Kaul D. The endothelial biology of sickle cell disease: Inflammation and a chronic vasculopathy. Microcirculation 2004;11:129–151.
13. Ballas SK, Mohandas N. Sickle red cell microheology and sickle blood rheology. Microcirculation 2004;11:209–225.
14. Parise LV, Telen MJ. Erythrocyte adhesion in sickle cell disease. Curr Hematol Rep 2003;2:102–108.
15. Quinn CT, Rogers ZR, Buchanan GR. Survival of children with sickle cell disease. Blood 2004;103:4023–4027.
16. Darbari DS, Kple-Faget P, Kwagyan J, et al. Circumstances of death in adult sickle cell disease patients. Am J Hematol 2006;81:858–863.
17. Prasad R, Hasan S, Castro O, et al. Long-term outcomes in patients with sickle cell disease and frequent vaso-occlusive crises. Am J Med Sci 2003;325:107–109.
18. Quinn CT, Shull EP, Ahmad N, et al. Prognostic significance of early vaso-occlusive complications in children with sickle cell anemia. Blood 2006;109:40–45.
19. Nordness ME, Lynn J, Zacharisen MC, et al. Asthma is a risk factor for acute chest syndrome and cerebral vascular accidents in children with sickle cell disease. Clin Molecular Allergy 2005;3:2–6.
20. Hord J, Byrd R, Stowe L, et al. *Streptococcus pneumoniae* sepsis and meningitis during the penicillin prophylaxis era in children with sickle cell disease. J Pediatr Hematol Oncol 2002;24:470–472.
21. Smithy-Whitley K, Zhao H, Hodinka RL, et al. The epidemiology of human parvovirus B 19 in children with sickle cell disease. Blood 2004;103:422–427.
22. Pegelow CH, Mackoin EA, Moser FG, et al. Longitudinal changes in brain magnetic resonance imaging findings in children with sickle cell disease. Blood 2002;15:3014–3018.
23. Kral MC, Brown RT, Nietert PJ, et al. Transcranial Doppler ultrasonography and neurocognitive functioning in children with sickle cell disease. Pediatrics 2003;112:324–331.
24. Wong W, Powars DR. Overt and incomplete (silent) cerebral infarction in sickle cell anemia: diagnosis and management. Hematol Oncol Clin North Am 2005:839–855.
25. Prengler M, Pavlakis SG, Boyd S, et al. Sickle cell disease: Ischemia and seizures. Ann Neurology 2005;58:290–302.
26. Dean D, Neumayr L, Kelly DM, et al. *Chlamydia pneumoniae* and acute chest syndrome in patients with sickle cell disease. J Pediatr Hematol Oncol 2003;25:46–55.
27. Siddiqui AK, Ahmed S. Pulmonary manifestations of sickle cell disease. Postgrad Med J 2003;79:384–390.
28. Sylvester KP, Patey RA, Milligan P, et al. Impact of acute chest syndrome on lung function of children with sickle cell disease. J Pediatr 2006:149:17–22.
29. Neumayr L, Lennette E, Kelly D, et al. Mycoplasma disease and acute chest syndrome in sickle cell disease. Pediatrics 2003;112:87–95.
30. Vichinsky E. Novel therapeutic approaches in sickle cell disease: Understanding the pathophysiology and treatment of pulmonary injury in sickle cell disease. Hematology (Am Soc Hematol Educ Program) 2002;16–22.
31. Johnson CS. The acute chest syndrome. Hematol Oncol Clin North Am 2005;198;857–879.
32. Kellermayer R, Faden H, Grossi M. Clinical presentation of parvovirus B19 infection in children with aplastic crisis. Pediatr Infect Dis J 2003;22:1100–1101.
33. Gladwin MT, Sachdev V, Jison ML, et al. Pulmonary hypertension as a risk factor for death in patients with sickle cell disease. N Engl J Med 2004;350:886–895.

34. Henry M, Driscoll CM, Miller M, et al. Pseudotumor cerebri in children with sickle cell disease: a case series. Pediatrics 2004;113:e265–e269.
35. Hasan S, Elbedawi M, Castro O, et al. Central retinal vein occlusion in sickle cell disease. South Med J 2004;97:202–204.
36. Babalola OE, Wambebe CO. When should children and young adults with sickle cell disease be referred for eye assessment? Afr J Med Med Sci 2001;30:261–263.
37. Suell MN, Horton TM, Dishop MK, et al. Outcomes for children with gallbladder abnormalities and sickle cell disease. J Pediatr 2004;145:617–621.
38. de Montalembert M, Maunoury C, Acar P, et al. Myocardial ischaemia in children with sickle cell disease. Arch Dis Child 2004;89:359–362.
39. Assanasen C, Quinton RA, Buchanan GR. Acute myocardial infraction in sickle cell anemia. J Pediatr Hematol/Oncol 2003;25:978–981.
40. Simsek B, Bayazit AK, Ergin M, et al. Renal amyloidosis in a child with sickle cell anemia. Pediatr Nephrol 2006;21:877–879.
41. Hassan SP, Hashmi S, Alhassen M, et al. Depression in sickle cell disease. J Natl Med Assoc 2003;95:533–537.
42. Schatz J, Finke RL, Kellett JM, Kramer JH. Cognitive functioning in children with sickle cell disease: A meta-analysis. J Pediatr Psychol 2002;27:739–748.
43. Adamkiewicz TV, Sarnaik S, Buchanan GR, et al. Invasive pneumococcal infections in children with sickle cell disease in the era of penicillin prophylaxis antibiotic resistance and 23-valent pneumococcal polysaccharide vaccination. J Pediatr 2003;143:438–444.
44. Advisory Committee on Immunization Practices, CDC. Preventing pneumococcal disease among infants and young children. MMWR Morb Mortal Wkly Rep 2000;49:1–38.
45. Advisory Committee on Immunization Practices, CDC. Prevention and control of meningococcal disease. MMWR Morb Mortal Wkly Rep 2005;54:7:1–21.
46. Sickle Cell Disease Care Consortium. Sickle Cell Disease in Children and Adolescents: Diagnosis, Guidelines for Comprehensive Care, and Care Paths and Protocols for Management of Acute and Chronic Complications. 2001, *http://www.tdh.texas.gov/newborn/sedona02.htm.*
47. Falletta JM, Woods RM, Verter JI, et al. Discontinuing penicillin prophylaxis in children with sickle cell anemia. J Pediatr 1995;127:685–690.
48. Kennedy TS, Fung EB, Kawchak DA, et al. Red blood cell folate and serum vitamin B12 status in children with sickle cell disease. J Pediatr Hematol Oncol 2001;23:165–169.
49. Lowenthal EA, Mayo MS, Cornwell PE, et al. Homocysteine elevation in sickle cell disease. J Am Coll Nutr 2000;19:608–612.
50. van der Dijs, Fokkema MR, Dijck-Brouwer DA, et al. Optimization of folic acid, vitamin B12 and vitamin B6 supplements in pediatric patients with sickle cell disease. Am J Hematol 2002;69:239–246.
51. Halsey C, Roberts IA. The role of hydroxyurea in sickle cell disease. Br J Haematol 2003;120:177–186.
52. Nathan DG. Search for improved therapy of sickle cell anemia. J Pediatr Hematol Oncol 2002;24:700–703.
53. Cokic VP, Smith RD, Beleslin-Cokic BB, et al. Hydroxyurea induces fetal hemoglobin by the nitric oxide-dependent activation of soluble guanylyl cyclase. J Clin Invest 2003;111:231–239.
54. Gladwin MT, Schechter AN. Nitric oxide therapy in sickle cell disease. Semin Hematol 2001;38:333–342.
55. Steinberg MH, Bartin F, Castro O, et al. Effect of hydroxyurea on mortality and morbidity in adult sickle cell anemia. Risks and benefits up to 9 years of treatment. JAMA 2003;289:1645–1651.
56. Hankins JS, Ware RE, Rogers ZR, et al. Long-term hydroxyurea therapy for infants with sickle cell anemia: the HUSOFT extension study. Blood 2005;106:2269–2275.
57. Little JA, McGowan VR, Kato Gj, et al. Combination erythropoietin-hydroxyurea therapy in sickle cell disease: Experience from National Institute of Health and a literature review. Haematologica 2006;91:1076–1083.
58. National Heart, Lung, and Blood Institute (NHLBI). Pediatric Hydroxyurea in Sickle Cell Anemia (BABY HUG). Study Details. 2006, *http://www.clinicaltrials.gov.*
59. Zimmerman SA, Schultz WH, Davis JS, et al. Sustained long-term hematological efficacy of hydroxyurea at maximal tolerated dose in children with sickle cell disease. Blood 2004;103:2039–2045.
60. Altura RA, Want WC, Wynn L, et al. Hydroxyurea therapy associated with declining serum levels of magnesium in children with sickle cell anemia. J Pediatr 2002;140:565–569.
61. Wilson S. Acute leukemia in a patient with sickle cell anemia treated with hydroxyurea (letter). Ann Intern Med 2000;133:925–926.
62. Ware RE, Zimmerman SA, Sylvestre PB, et al. Prevention of secondary stroke and resolution of transfusional iron overload in children with sickle cell anemia using hydroxyurea and phlebotomy. J Pediatr 2004;145:346–352.
63. Resar LMS, Segal JB, Fitzpatric LK, et al. Induction of fetal hemoglobin synthesis in children with sickle cell anemia on low-dose oral sodium phenylbutyrate therapy. J Pediatr Hematol Oncol 2002;24:737–741.
64. Saunthararajah Y, Hillery CA, Lavelle D, et al. Effects of 5-aza-2′-deoxycytidine on fetal hemoglobin levels, red cell adhesion and hematopoietic differentiation in patients with sickle cell disease. Blood 2003;102:3865–3870.
65. Ataga KI, Orringer EP, Styles L, et al. Dose-escalation study of ICA-17043 in patients with sickle cell disease. Pharmacotherapy 2006;26: 1557–1564.
66. Wanko SO, Telen MJ. Transfusion management in sickle cell disease. Hematol Oncol Clin North Am 2005;19:803–826.
67. Switzer J, Hess DC, Nichols FT, et al. Pathophysiology and treatment of stroke in sickle cell disease: present and future. Lancet Neurol 2006;5:501–512.
68. Hillery CA, Panepinto JA. Pathophysiology of stroke in sickle cell disease. Microcirculation 2004;11:195–208.
69. Adams RJ, Brambilla D. Discontinuing prophylactic transfusions used to prevent stroke in sickle cell disease. N Engl J Med 2005;29:2769–2978.
70. Ware RE, Zimmerman SA, Sylvestre PB, et al. Prevention of secondary stroke and resolution of transfusional iron overload in children with sickle cell anemia using hydroxyurea and phlebotomy. J Pediatr 2004:145:346–352.
71. Lee MT, Piomelli S, Granger S, et al. Stroke prevention trial in sickle cell anemia (STOP) extended follow-up and final results. Blood 2006:108:847–852.
72. Vichinsky E, Onyekwere O, Porter J, et al. A randomized comparison of deferasirox versus deferoxamine for the treatment of transfusion iron overload in sickle cell disease. Br J Haematol 2007;136:501–508.
73. Stumpf JL. Deferasirox. Am J Health Syst Pharm 2007;64:6006–6016.
74. Win N, Yeghen T, Needs M, et al. Use of intravenous immunoglobulin and intravenous methylprednisolone in hyperhaemolysis syndrome in sickle cell disease. Hematol 2004;9:433–436.
75. Adamkiewicz TV, Mehta PS, Boyer MW, et al. Transplantation of unrelated placental blood cells in children with high-risk sickle cell disease. Bone Marrow Transplant 2004;34:405–411.
76. Atkins RC, Walters MC. Haematopoietic cell transplantation in the treatment of sickle cell disease. Expert Opin Biol Ther 2003;3:1215–1224.
77. Horan JT, Liesveld JL, Fenton P, et al. Hematopoietic stem cell transplantation for multiply transfused patients with sickle cell disease and thalassemia after low-dose total body irradiation, fludarabine and rabbit anti-thymocyte globulin. Bone Marrow Transplant 2005;35: 171–177.
78. Brachet C, Azzi N, Demulder A, et al. Hydroxyurea treatment for sickle cell disease: Impact on haematopoietic stem cell transplantation's outcome. Bone Marrow Transplant 2004;33:779–803.
79. Walters MC. Novel therapeutic approaches in sickle cell disease: Stem cell transplantation for sickle cell disease: How and when to intervene? Hematology (Am Soc Hematol Educ Program) 2002;22–29.
80. Knight-Madden J, Hambleton I. Inhaled bronchodilators for acute chest syndrome in people with sickle cell disease. Cochrane Database Syst Rev 2003;3:CD003733.
81. Li M, Fogarty J, Whitney KD, Stone P. Repeated testicular infarction in a patient with sickle cell disease: A possible mechanism for testicular failure. Urology 2003;62:551.
82. Rogers ZR. Priapism in sickle cell disease. Hematol Oncol Clin North Am 2005;19:917–928.
83. Dahm P, Rao DS, Donatucci CF. Antiandrogens in the treatment of priapism, case report. Urology 2002;59:138.
84. Jacob E, Miaskowski C, Savedra M, et al. Management of vaso-occlusive pain in children with sickle cell disease. J Pediatr Hematol Oncol 2003;25:307–311.
85. Stinson J, Naser B. Pain management in children with sickle cell disease. Paediatr Drugs 2003;5:229–238.

86. Dumaplin CA. Avoiding admission for afebrile pediatric sickle cell pain: Pain management methods. J Pediatr Health Care 2006;20:115–122.
87. Elander J, Lusher J, Bevan D, et al. Pain management and symptoms of substance dependence among patients with sickle cell disease. Soc Sci Med 2003;7:1683–1696.
88. Labbe E, Herbert D, Haynes J. Physicians' attitude and practices in sickle cell disease pain management. J Palliat Care 2005;21:246–251.
89. Elander J, Lusher, J, Bevan D, et al. Understanding the causes of problematic pain management in sickle cell disease: Evidence that pseudoaddiction plays a more important role than genuine analgesic dependence. J Pain Symptom Manage 2004;27:156–169.
90. Gibbs WJ, Hagemann TM. Purified poloxamer 188 for sickle cell vaso-occlusive crisis. Ann Pharmacother 2004;38:320–324.
91. Okpala IE. New therapies for sickle cell disease. Hematol Oncol Clin North Am 2005;19:975–987.
92. Panepinto JA, Magid D, Rewers MJ, Lane PA. Universal versus targeted screening of infants for sickle cell disease: A cost effectiveness analysis. J Pediatr 2000;136:201–208.
93. Telfair J, Haque A, Etienne M, et al. Rural/urban difference in access to and utilization of services among people in Alabama with sickle cell disease. Public Health Rep 2003;118:27–36.
94. Moore RD, Charache S, Errin ML, et al. Cost-effectiveness of hydroxyurea in sickle cell anemia. Am J Hematol 2000;64:26–31.
95. Lanzkron S, Haywood C, Segal JB, et al. Hospitalization rates and costs of care of patients with sickle-cell anemia in the state of Maryland in the era of hydroxyurea. Am J Hematol 2006;81:927–932.

CHAPTER 107 Drug-Induced Hematologic Disorders

DALE H. WHITBY AND THOMAS E. JOHNS

KEY CONCEPTS

1. The most common drug-induced hematologic disorders include aplastic anemia, agranulocytosis, megaloblastic anemia, hemolytic anemia, and thrombocytopenia.
2. Drug-induced hematologic disorders are generally rare adverse effects associated with drug therapy.
3. Reporting during postmarketing surveillance of a drug is usually the method by which the incidence of rare adverse drug reactions is established.
4. Because drug-induced blood disorders are potentially dangerous, rechallenging a patient with a suspected agent in an attempt to confirm a diagnosis may not be ethical.
5. The mechanisms of drug-induced hematologic disorders are the result of direct toxicity or an immune reaction.
6. The primary treatment of drug-induced hematologic disorders is removal of the drug in question and symptomatic support of the patient.
7. Frequent laboratory monitoring may be warranted for agents commonly demonstrating severe hematologic reactions.

(1) Hematologic disorders have long been a potential risk of modern pharmacotherapy. Granulocytopenia (agranulocytosis) was reported in association with one of medicine's early therapeutic agents, sulfanilamide, in 1938.[1] Some agents cause predictable hematologic disease (e.g., antineoplastics), but others induce idiosyncratic reactions not directly related to the drugs' pharmacology. The most common drug-induced hematologic disorders include aplastic anemia, agranulocytosis, megaloblastic anemia, hemolytic anemia, and thrombocytopenia.

(2) The incidence of idiosyncratic drug-induced hematologic disorders varies depending on the condition and the associated drug. Few epidemiologic studies have evaluated the actual incidence of these adverse reactions, but these reactions appear to be rare. A report from the Netherlands estimated the incidence of drug-associated agranulocytosis as 1.6 to 2.5 cases per million inhabitants per year.[2] Similar results were reported in epidemiologic studies conducted in Thailand and Brazil.[3,4] However, the incidence of drug-induced thrombocytopenia is more frequent, with some reports suggesting that as many as 5% of patients who receive heparin develop heparin-induced thrombocytopenia.[5]

Although drug-induced hematologic disorders are less common than other types of adverse reactions, they are important because they are associated with significant morbidity and mortality. An epidemiologic study conducted in the United States estimated that 4,490 deaths in 1984 were attributable to blood dyscrasias from all causes. Aplastic anemia was the leading cause of death, followed by thrombocytopenia, agranulocytosis, and hemolytic anemia.[6] Like most other adverse drug reactions, drug-induced hematologic disorders are more common in the elderly than in the young; the risk of death also appears to be greater with increasing age. The risk of agranulocytosis has been reported to be higher in women than in men.[4]

(3) Because of the seriousness of drug-induced hematologic disorders, it is necessary to track the development of these disorders to predict their occurrence and to estimate their incidence. Reporting during postmarketing surveillance of a drug is the most common method of establishing the incidence of adverse drug reactions. The MedWatch program supported by the Food and Drug Administration is one such program.[7] Many facilities have similar drug-reporting programs to follow adverse drug reaction trends and to determine whether an association between a drug and an adverse drug reaction is causal or coincidental. In the case of drug-induced hematologic disorders, these programs can enable practitioners to confirm that an adverse event is indeed the result of drug therapy rather than one of many other potential causes; general guidelines are readily available.[8,9]

(4) Because drug-induced blood disorders are potentially dangerous, rechallenging a patient with a suspected agent in an attempt to confirm a diagnosis may not be ethical. In-vitro studies with the offending agent and cells or plasma from the patient's blood can be performed to determine causality.[10] These methods are often expensive, however, and require facilities and expertise that are not generally available. Therefore, it is extremely important that practitioners be able to clinically evaluate suspect drugs quickly and to interrupt therapy when necessary.

Throughout the past decades, lists of drugs that have been associated with adverse events have been developed to help clinicians identify possible causes. Unfortunately, these lists are comprehensive and include commonly used drugs, making it difficult to determine the cause of any abnormality. Furthermore, the absence of a drug from such a list should not discourage the investigation and reporting of an agent associated with an adverse event. It is imperative that clinicians use a rational approach to determine causality and identify the agents associated with a reaction. The clinician should focus on the issue, perform a rigorous investigation, develop appropriate criteria, use objective criteria to grade the response, and complete a quantitative summary. A systematic approach to evaluate the information available in the literature also helps the clinician to focus and intervene in the cause of the disorder.

A common tool employed by clinicians to rate the likelihood of causality in adverse drug reaction (ADR) investigations is an ADR probability scale (algorithm). One such scale was developed and tested by Naranjo and colleagues.[11] This tool provides a series of scored questions that lead an investigator to the likelihood that an ADR was caused by the suspected medication. Depending on the aggregate score, the causality is rated as *doubtful, possible, probable*, or *definite*. The scale gives the most weight to the temporal relationship of the reaction with relation to administration of the drug, observations following a rechallenge of the suspected medication, and alternate explanations for the ADR. As mentioned above, it is often unethical to rechallenge patients who experience severe hematologic toxicities. Thus without a rechallenge it is difficult to achieve a causality rating of *definite* with such an algorithm.

In determining the likelihood that an observed reaction is caused by a particular medication, clinicians should review the medical literature for past reports supporting the observation. Using an evidence-based approach such as that proposed by Sackett,[12] the investigator assigns greater weight to prospective study designs such as clinical trials or cohort studies than to case reports or expert opinion. This will provide a framework for the investigator's confidence in published literature describing ADRs.

In this chapter, we use both methods described to review and present published information on hematologic drug toxicities. When only case reports were available, the Naranjo algorithm was applied to the cases (if not already used). *Definite* and those rated as *probable* when only a lack of rechallenge prevented a rating of *definite* were included in the lists. An evidence-based approach was incorporated through a review of the medical literature for prospective and retrospective studies of the adverse reactions and medications of interest. Drugs significantly associated with an adverse reaction of interest through studies were also deemed to have a causal relationship to the reaction.

The understanding of drug-induced hematologic disorders requires a basic understanding of hematopoiesis (see Chap. 103 on hematopoiesis). The pluripotential hematopoietic stem cells in the bone marrow, which have the ability to self-reproduce, maintain the blood. These pluripotential hematopoietic stem cells further differentiate to intermediate precursor cells, which are also called *progenitor cells* or *colony-forming cells*. Committed to a particular cell line, these intermediate stem cells differentiate into colonies of each type of blood cell in response to specific colony-stimulating factors (Fig. 107–1).

Drug-induced hematologic disorders can affect any cell line, including white blood cells (WBCs), red blood cells (RBCs), and platelets. When a drug causes decreases in all three cell lines accompanied by a hypoplastic bone marrow, the result is drug-induced aplastic anemia. The decrease in WBC count alone by a medication is drug-induced agranulocytosis. Drugs can affect RBCs by causing a number of different anemias, including drug-induced immune hemolytic anemia, drug-induced oxidative hemolytic anemia, or drug-induced megaloblastic anemia. A drug-induced decrease in platelet count is drug-induced thrombocytopenia.

DRUG-INDUCED APLASTIC ANEMIA

Aplastic anemia is a rare, serious disease of unclear etiology. It was first described by Ehrlich in 1888 following an episode of failed hematopoiesis identified during the autopsy of a pregnant woman.[13] Since that first report, numerous cases of aplastic anemia have been described, but the true incidence of the disease remains uncertain. Best estimates report an incidence of two to seven cases per million inhabitants.[14–16] Interestingly, the incidence of aplastic anemia is different in different regions, which suggests an environmental component to the etiology of this condition.[14,15,17] There is also debate regarding the peak age at

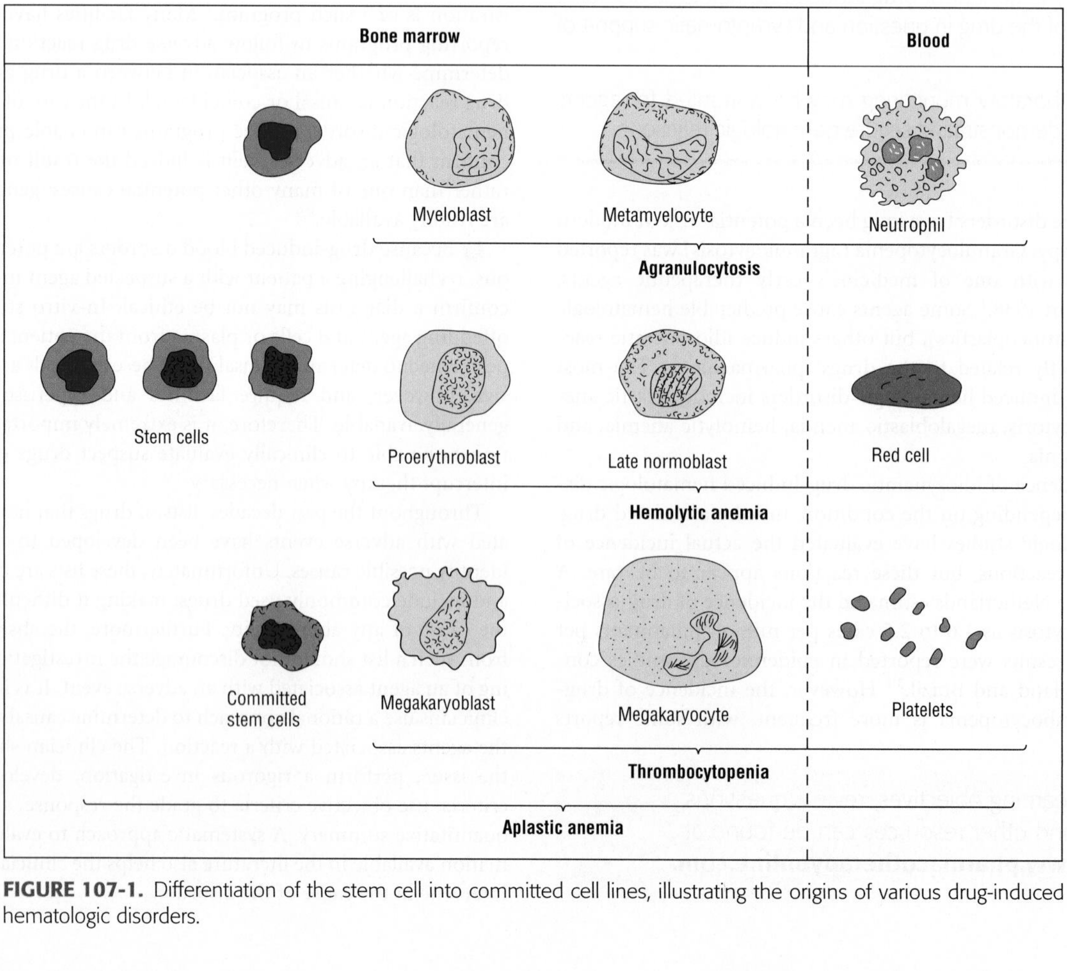

FIGURE 107-1. Differentiation of the stem cell into committed cell lines, illustrating the origins of various drug-induced hematologic disorders.

which aplastic anemia is most common. Some authors have reported a peak incidence in patients younger than 30 years of age, although others report the highest incidence in those older than 60 years of age.[14,17–19] When the results of all studies are considered, the young and elderly appear to be at increased risk for the development of aplastic anemia.

Aplastic anemia can be broken down into two very broad categories—inherited and acquired. Although this chapter will focus on one specific type of acquired aplastic anemia, it is important to be aware of inherited disorders of bone marrow failure because they can be misdiagnosed as acquired.[18] Inherited types of bone marrow failure typically present in the first decade of life, are often associated with physical anomalies (e.g., short stature and café-au-lait spots), and rarely respond to immunosuppressive therapies.[18] Acquired aplastic anemia accounts for the large majority of cases, and as with many other autoimmune disorders, genetic factors may predispose some patients to acquire aplastic anemia.[20,21] A number of variables can incite immune destruction of the bone marrow; the most common are drugs, insecticides, benzene and other chemical exposure, viruses, and radiation. It has been estimated that 25% to 40% of aplastic anemia cases are related to one of these external factors.[22] However, in the large majority of modern cases, a definitive causative agent cannot be identified.[18,23]

Aplastic anemia is characterized by pancytopenia (presence of anemia, neutropenia, and thrombocytopenia) with a hypocellular bone marrow and no gross evidence of increased peripheral blood cell destruction.[24] A diagnosis of aplastic anemia can be made by the presence of two of the following criteria: a WBC count of 3,500 cells/mm^3 or less, a platelet count of 55,000 cells/mm^3 or less, or a hemoglobin value of 10 g/dL or less with a reticulocyte count of 30,000 cells/mm^3 or less.[25] However, all of these blood counts do not decrease at the same rate.

Once diagnosed, acquired aplastic anemia can be classified as nonsevere, severe, or very severe based on the degree of bone marrow cellularity and peripheral neutrophil, platelet, and reticulocyte counts. Severe aplastic anemia is defined by at least two of the following three peripheral blood findings: neutrophil count of less than 500 cells/mm^3, platelet count of less than 20,000 cells/mm^3, and anemia with a corrected reticulocyte index of less than 1%.[26,27] The prognosis is poor if the neutrophil count declines to less than 200 cells/mm^3.[3,32,28] A bone marrow aspirate and biopsy are required to exclude other causes of pancytopenia, including neoplastic infiltration or significant myelofibrosis.[29] There must also be no history of iatrogenic exposure to cytotoxic chemotherapy that is known to cause transient bone marrow suppression or to intensive radiation.

Aplastic anemia is considered the most serious drug-induced blood dyscrasia because of the associated high mortality rate as compared to other blood dyscrasias.[26,30] The onset of drug-induced aplastic anemia is variable and insidious. Symptoms have been reported to appear from days to months after initiation of the offending drug, with the average being approximately 6.5 weeks.[28] In some instances, symptoms appear after the drug has been discontinued. Neutropenia typically presents first, followed by thrombocytopenia and finally, because of the longer life span of the RBCs, anemia evolves slowly.[31] Clinical features of drug-induced aplastic anemia depend on the degree to which each cell line is suppressed, similar to idiopathic disease. Symptoms of anemia include pallor, fatigue and weakness, whereas fever, chills, pharyngitis, or other signs of infection can characterize neutropenia. Thrombocytopenia, often the initial clue to diagnosis, is manifest by easy bruisability, petechiae, and bleeding.

❺ The cause of drug-induced aplastic anemia is damage to the pluripotential hematopoietic stem cells before their differentiation to committed stem cells. This damage effectively reduces the normal levels of circulating erythrocytes, neutrophils, and platelets. Three mechanisms have been proposed as causes of damage to the pluripotential hematopoietic stem cells.[32] The first is direct, dose-dependent drug toxicity. This type of injury leads to transient marrow failure secondary to direct suppression of proliferating cell lines, and hematopoietic suppression continues with dose escalation. Most often caused by chemotherapy or radiotherapy, this injury is frequently iatrogenic. The second mechanism is idiosyncratic and may operate through toxic metabolites of the parent drug. Furthermore, individual variations in the pharmacokinetics of the suspected drug, genetic polymorphisms altering metabolism or a hypersensitivity of the stem cells to the destructive effects of the implicated drug may increase the potential for toxicity. The third mechanism is a drug- or metabolite-induced immune reaction specific to the stem-cell population, and it is this mechanism that has received much attention over the past few decades. Currently, it is believed that most cases of aplastic anemia are immune mediated.[16] It is proposed that exposure to an inciting antigen (drug), activates cells and cytokines of the immune system, leading to the death of stem cells.[32] Table 107–1 lists drugs that have been associated with drug-induced aplastic anemia.

The antineoplastic agents exemplify the dose-dependent mechanism for the development of aplastic anemia. Many of these agents have the ability to suppress one or more cell lines in a reversible manner. The degree of suppression and the cell line involved depend on the nature of the particular drug and its potential for inhibiting marrow proliferation. Chloramphenicol, an antimicrobial agent, also causes a bone marrow depression that is dose-dependent and reversible.[33]

Idiosyncratic drug-induced aplastic anemia secondary to direct toxicity can be characterized by dose independence, a latent period prior to the onset of anemia, and continued marrow injury following

TABLE 107-1 Drugs Associated with Aplastic Anemias

Observational study evidence
Carbamazepine
Furosemide
Gold salts
Mebendazole
Methimazole
NSAIDs
Oxyphenbutazone
Penicillamine
Phenobarbital
Phenothiazines
Phenytoin
Propylthiouracil
Sulfonamides
Thiazides
Tocainide
Case report evidence (*probable* or *definite* causality rating)
Acetazolamide
Aspirin
Captopril
Chloramphenicol
Chloroquine
Chlorothiazide
Chlorpromazine
Dapsone
Felbamate
Interferon alfa
Lisinopril
Lithium
Nizatidine
Pentoxifylline
Quinidine
Sulindac
Ticlopidine

NSAID, nonsteroidal antiinflammatory drug.

drug discontinuation.[34] Chloramphenicol, already known to cause a dose-dependent reaction, is the prototype drug for the idiosyncratic mechanism, with an estimated incidence of 1 case per 20,000 patients treated;[28] however, the overall prevalence has fallen with decreased use of this agent.[34] The idiosyncratic mechanism is believed to result from abnormal metabolism of chloramphenicol. The nitrobenzene ring on chloramphenicol is thought to be reduced to form a nitroso group on the chloramphenicol molecule.[33] The nitroso group may then interact with DNA in the stem cell, causing damage to the chromosomes, and eventually cell death. Other investigators have hypothesized that bacteria from the gastrointestinal tract may metabolize chloramphenicol to marrow-toxic metabolites.[35] There appears to be no relationship between the dose-dependent and idiosyncratic reactions seen with chloramphenicol.

Other drugs thought to induce aplastic anemia through toxic metabolites include phenytoin and carbamazepine. Investigators have theorized that metabolites of phenytoin and carbamazepine bind covalently to macromolecules in the cell and then cause cell death either by exerting a direct toxic effect on the stem cell or by causing the death of lymphocytes involved in regulating hematopoiesis.[36]

Of the three potential mechanisms, the most common cause of drug-induced aplastic anemia is the development of an immune reaction. Early laboratory studies showed that removal of T lymphocytes from patients with aplastic anemia improved in-vitro colony formation.[37] Furthermore, overproduction of cytokines (e.g., tumor necrosis factor and interferon-γ) from activated T lymphocytes appears to be responsible for hematopoietic failure, as well as for the initiation of apoptosis.[16,38] The observation of improved hematopoiesis in aplastic anemia patients who receive a conditioning regimen with antithymocyte globulin and cyclophosphamide prior to allogeneic hematopoietic stem cell transplantation (HSCT) supports this hypothesis.[39] After the initiation of immunosuppressive therapy, bone marrow concentrations of interferon-γ decreased whereas all cell lines improved.[40]

Additional support for an immunologic basis as a mechanism of aplastic anemia comes from a prospective, randomized, placebo-controlled trial evaluating the efficacy of antilymphocyte globulin and methylprednisolone, with or without cyclosporine, in patients with severe aplastic anemia.[41] The primary response variable was an improvement in blood counts (i.e., platelets, erythrocytes, and leukocytes) at 3 months. Patients receiving therapy with antilymphocyte globulin, methylprednisolone, and cyclosporine had a response rate of 65% versus a response rate of 39% in the group not receiving cyclosporine. The favorable response rate from this study, using immunosuppressant drugs, supports the overall hypothesis of an immune-based mechanism for aplastic anemia. One can also conclude that the degree of immunosuppression is related to a better response rate.

Genetic predisposition can also influence the development of drug-induced aplastic anemia. Studies in animals and a case report of chloramphenicol-induced aplastic anemia in identical twins suggest a genetic predisposition to the development of drug-induced aplastic anemia.[28,33] Furthermore, pharmacogenetic research that focuses on patients who may be slow or normal metabolizers of drugs can increase the clinician's ability to predict the development of aplastic anemia. Initial case-control studies have not had the statistical power necessary to identify a significant difference between controls and cases, but continued research may establish the role of altered metabolism in patients with aplastic anemia.[42]

TREATMENT

Drug-Induced Aplastic Anemia

Because of the high mortality rate associated with severe and very severe aplastic anemia, it is imperative that drug-induced aplastic anemia be diagnosed quickly and therapy initiated immediately. Treatment should be based on the degree of cytopenia, and the goals of therapy are to improve peripheral blood counts, which limits the requirement for transfusions and minimizes the risk for opportunistic infections.

❻ As with all cases of drug-induced hematologic disorders, the first step is to remove the suspected offending agent. Early withdrawal of the drug can allow for reversal of the aplastic anemia.[28] The next step is to provide adequate supportive care, including appropriate antimicrobial therapy for the treatment of infection and transfusion support with erythrocytes and platelets. Appropriate supportive care is essential because the major causes of mortality in patients with aplastic anemia are bacterial or fungal infections and bleeding. Current treatment guidelines for aplastic anemia do not include chemoprophylaxis, except in patients undergoing allogeneic HSCT. Therefore, fever of unknown origin should be initially managed with broad-spectrum antibiotics.

The clinical course of aplastic anemia is variable. The condition can progress to severe or very severe disease in some patients, although it can remain relatively stable or even resolve in others.[16] The treatment of moderate disease ranges from no clinical intervention to immunosuppressive regimens, and treatment should be based on the degree of cytopenias.[16,18]

For patients with disease requiring treatment, the two major treatment options for patients with drug-induced aplastic anemia are allogeneic HSCT and immunosuppressive therapy. Most experts consider allogeneic HSCT the treatment of choice for young patients who have human leukocyte antigen (HLA)-matched sibling donors.[18] Most patients are cured after HSCT, and the 5-year survival of patients following a matched sibling donor transplant has been reported to be 77% for adults and up to 80% to 90% in children.[16,43] Despite these promising results, relatively few patients are eligible for HSCT because less than 30% of patients have a matched sibling donor.[18] For those patients who do not have a matched sibling donor, mismatched related and matched unrelated donor transplants may be an option, but the prognosis is less optimistic. In one recent study reporting the results of 318 mismatched related or matched unrelated donor transplants for aplastic anemia, the 5-year survival rate ranged from 30% to 49%.[44] The highest mortality rate was seen in older patients and those with poorer clinical status at the time of transplantation. Complications for HSCT, such as graft-versus-host disease (GVHD) and graft rejection, require all patients to be closely monitored for an extended period of time.

An alternative to allogeneic HSCT is immunosuppressive therapy, which tends to be first-line therapy for older patients and those who are not candidates for HSCT. The current standard regimen against which new therapies are measured is combination therapy with antithymocyte globulin (ATG) and cyclosporine.[45] ATG is composed of polyclonal immunoglobulin G (IgG) against human T-lymphocytes derived from either horses or rabbits, and it has been a standard component of immunosuppressive therapy for aplastic anemia for many years. Monotherapy may achieve response rates of 40% to 70%, and long-term survival rates are similar to those receiving allogeneic HSCT.[46] Most of these studies used horse-derived ATG, and one recent trial showed a lower response rate in patients whose regimen contained rabbit-derived ATG versus those who received horse-derived ATG.[47] More data are needed to determine the role of rabbit-derived ATG in the treatment of aplastic anemia. Recommended dosing of antithymocyte globulin (horse-derived) has varied from 40 mg/kg per day for 4 days to 10 to 20 mg/kg per day for 8 to 14 days. Shorter, more intense regimens are preferred, as they are associated with fewer adverse events (i.e., serum sickness).[16]

Cyclosporine plays a key role in immunosuppressant therapy for aplastic anemia. Although cyclosporine monotherapy has been used in moderate cases of aplastic anemia, it is more often used in combination with ATG. The addition of cyclosporine to ATG therapy has been shown to increase response rate, improve failure-free survival, and reduce the number of immunosuppressive courses needed.[45,47] Cyclosporine inhibits interleukin-2 production and release and subsequent activation of resting T cells. Cyclosporine dosing has varied from 4 to 6 mg/kg per day to 10 to 12 mg/kg per day, with the most frequently reported initial dose of 5 mg/kg per day in two divided doses. Cyclosporine doses are titrated to a target blood concentration that can be patient- and institution-specific but is usually in the range of 200 to 400 ng/mL. Although it does not provide a cure for the disease, immunosuppressive therapy with regimens that include ATG and cyclosporine provides a response rate between 60% and 80% with a 5-year survival rate similar to allogeneic HSCT.[18]

Corticosteroids are sometimes added to ATG-based immunosuppression. Although the addition of corticosteroids does not clearly improve the efficacy of regimens that include ATG and cyclosporine, they are still commonly used today because they reduce adverse reactions to the ATG portion of the therapy. For this reason, some practitioners currently use abbreviated courses (e.g., 2 weeks). Several dosing regimens of methylprednisolone or prednisolone have been used including 1 mg/kg per day for 2 to 4 weeks or a tapered therapy using higher doses (e.g., 2 mg/kg/day) during the initial weeks of therapy followed by lower doses. Despite the abbreviated regimen used, all patients receiving immunosuppressive therapy must be monitored for long-term complications including infection, relapse, and conversion to other stem-cell disorders (e.g., myelodysplastic syndrome, acute myelogenous leukemia, and paroxysmal nocturnal hemoglobinuria).

In an effort to improve outcomes, several other agents have also been investigated in the treatment of aplastic anemia. The additive benefits of other immunosuppressive agents such as mycophenolate, cyclophosphamide, and sirolimus have been evaluated.[16] However, they have not been shown to be superior to the combination of ATG and cyclosporine, and their place in therapy is not defined. Granulocyte colony-stimulating factor (G-CSF),[48] granulocyte-macrophage colony-stimulating factor (GM-CSF),[47] and erythropoietin,[47] have also been investigated in the supportive care of aplastic anemia. Results of these trials have varied. Some patients have had a faster neutrophil recovery, whereas others showed no difference in hematopoietic recovery. No improvement in survival has been observed.[18,47,48] If long-term bone-marrow suppression continues after initial treatment with optimal immunosuppression, the only viable available option is allogeneic HSCT.

CLINICAL CONTROVERSY

HSCT has long been the established treatment of drug-induced aplastic anemia. More recently, immunosuppressive regimens combining antithymocyte globulin, glucocorticoids, and cyclosporine are gaining favor. The usefulness of each treatment modality is limited by various factors. Clinical data suggest that there is no difference in survival achieved with the two treatments among patients followed for 6 years. Parity between the treatments will necessitate that clinicians individualize treatment decisions, while considering risk factors, economics, and quality of life.

DRUG-INDUCED AGRANULOCYTOSIS

Agranulocytosis is defined as a reduction in the number of mature myeloid cells in the blood (granulocytes and immature granulocytes [bands]) to a total count of 500 cells/mm^3 or less. It occurs most commonly in females and the elderly (i.e. >60 years of age),[49] with an estimated annual incidence of 1.1 to 12 cases per million population.[15,50] The overall mortality rate of agranulocytosis is estimated to be 3.5% to 16%, and that rate is highest among the elderly and patients with renal failure, bacteremia, or shock at the time of diagnosis.[15,50] Of those cases reported since 1990, approximately 5% to 6% have resulted in fatal outcomes.[51] Symptoms of agranulocytosis include sore throat, fever, malaise, weakness, chills, and other signs and symptoms of infection. These symptoms can appear rapidly, within days to weeks after the initiation of the offending drug. The median duration of exposure prior to the development of agranulocytosis ranges from 19 to 60 days for most drugs associated with this adverse event, but the time to onset is greater than 1 month for most of these agents.[51] Drug-induced agranulocytosis will usually resolve over time with supportive care and management of infection. Time to neutrophil recovery typically has been reported to range from 4 to 24 days.[51] Table 107–2 provides a list of medications that have been associated with drug-induced agranulocytosis.

The cause of drug-induced agranulocytosis is not fully understood, and several mechanisms have been proposed. Initially, it was thought that drugs affected only the mature granulocytes, causing a *maturation arrest*. However, more recent studies have demonstrated that drugs may have either a direct toxic effect or an antibody-mediated effect on the bone marrow, neutrophils, or stem cells. Several immune-mediated mechanisms have been proposed.[49]

The first type of immune-mediated mechanism involves the drug or drug metabolite, antibodies, and neutrophils. This mechanism involves drug adsorption on the membrane of the neutrophil. The drug-membrane complex then acts as a hapten to stimulate antibody formation. The antibodies produced bind to the drug-membrane complex, causing WBC destruction through complement activation and removal by the phagocytic system (Fig. 107–2). This hapten-type reaction is often seen when drugs, such as the penicillin derivatives, are given in large doses. Continuous presence of the drug is required for the destruction of neutrophils in this type of reaction.

The second mechanism of immune-mediated agranulocytosis is called the *innocent bystander phenomenon*. In this reaction, the drug combines with a drug-specific antibody. The complex is nonspecifically adsorbed to the neutrophil membrane, resulting in complement activation. The activated complement then destroys the cell (Fig. 107–3). Quinidine has been associated with this type of reaction. Functioning in a manner somewhat similar to that of the second mechanism, the third mechanism of immune response involves a protein carrier that combines with the drug and then attaches to the cell membrane. This in turn causes antibody formation. The antibodies bind to the drug protein carrier–membrane complex and activate complement. The cells are then cleared by the phagocytic system (Fig. 107–4).

In addition, there are several other immune-mediated mechanisms that have been identified. The production of autoantibodies to a *spoiled membrane* is a mechanism in which the offending drug alters the neutrophil membrane. This alteration induces the formation of autoantibodies (antibodies that attach directly to the neutrophil), which causes cellular destruction by the phagocytic system. High concentrations of β-lactam antibiotics, carbamazepine, and valproic acid have been associated with inhibition of colony-forming units of granulocytes and macrophages. Finally, drug-induced apoptosis and direct toxicity for pluripotent or bipotent hematopoietic progenitor stem cells have also been associated with clozapine and ticlopidine respectively.[49]

In the case of penicillin-induced agranulocytosis, the patient can often begin taking penicillin again, at a lower dosage, after the neutropenia has resolved without any relapse of drug-induced agranulocytosis.[52] Because of the rapid onset of symptoms and the dose-related phenomenon, a second mechanism could possibly be involved with penicillin-induced agranulocytosis. That mechanism involves an accumulation of drug to toxic concentrations in hyper-

TABLE 107-2 Drugs Associated with Agranulocytosis

Observational Study Evidence	Case Report Evidence (*probable* or *definite* causality rating)	
β-Lactam antibiotics	Acetaminophen	Levodopa
Carbamazepine	Acetazolamide	Meprobamate
Carbimazole	Ampicillin	Methazolamide
Clomipramine	Captopril	Methyldopa
Digoxin	Carbenicillin	Metronidazole
Dipyridamole	Cefotaxime	Nafcillin
Ganciclovir	Cefuroxime	NSAIDs
Glyburide	Chloramphenicol	Olanzapine
Gold salts	Chlorpromazine	Oxacillin
Imipenem-cilastatin	Chlorpropamide	Penicillamine
Indomethacin	Chlorpheniramine	Penicillin G
Macrolide antibiotics	Clindamycin	Pentazocine
Methimazole	Clozapine	Phenytoin
Mirtazapine	Colchicine	Primidone
Phenobarbital	Doxepin	Procainamide
Phenothiazines	Dapsone	Propylthiouracil
Prednisone	Desipramine	Pyrimethamine
Propranolol	Ethacrynic acid	Quinidine
Spironolactone	Ethosuximide	Quinine
Sulfonamides	Flucytosine	Rifampin
Sulfonylureas	Gentamicin	Streptomycin
Ticlopidine	Griseofulvin	Terbinafine
Valproic acid	Hydralazine	Ticarcillin
Zidovudine	Hydroxychloroquine	Tocainide
	Imipenem-cilastatin	Tolbutamide
	Imipramine	Vancomycin
	Lamotrigine	

NSAID, nonsteroidal antiinflammatory drug.

sensitive individuals. Researchers have shown with in-vitro cell cultures that penicillin derivatives in high concentrations inhibit the growth of myeloid colony-forming units in patients recovering from drug-induced agranulocytosis.[53] Penicillin derivatives, therefore, may suppress WBCs by several mechanisms.

Antithyroid medications, such as propylthiouracil and methimazole, have been reported to cause agranulocytosis. The current incidence of this adverse effect is unknown, but early publications report agranulocytosis in approximately 0.3% to 0.6% of patients.[54] In two more recent reports, antithyroid medications accounted for 7% to 23% of drug-induced agranulocytosis cases investigated.[55,56] The mechanism by which antithyroid agents cause agranulocytosis is unknown, but antineutrophil cytoplasmic antibodies have been identified.[57] In a study by Cooper and coworkers,[54] agranulocytosis occurred more frequently in older patients (>40 years old), and it appeared within 2 months after the initiation of therapy. The investigators also reported a possible dose-response relationship with methimazole.[54] For patients receiving less than 30 mg/day of methimazole, no agranulocytosis occurred, but in patients receiving higher doses, neutropenia was evident. No dose-response relationship has been observed with conventional doses of propylthiouracil. However, another study demonstrated no relationship between age or dose and the incidence of thionamide-induced agranulocytosis.[58]

Ticlopidine is an antiplatelet agent indicated for the treatment of cerebrovascular disease and the prevention of reocclusion associated with stent placement. It produces neutropenia in approximately 2.4% of patients and agranulocytosis in 0.8%,[59] possibly by inhibiting hematopoietic progenitor stem cells.[49] Patient factors that can be associated with the development of agranulocytosis include poor bone marrow reserve and age. Agranulocytosis most commonly occurs within 1 to 3 months from the initiation of ticlopidine. Removal of the drug is the best treatment option with counts usually returning to normal within 2 to 4 weeks.

The phenothiazine class of drugs is known to cause drug-induced agranulocytosis by the innocent bystander mechanism. The onset of phenothiazine-induced agranulocytosis is approximately 2 to 15

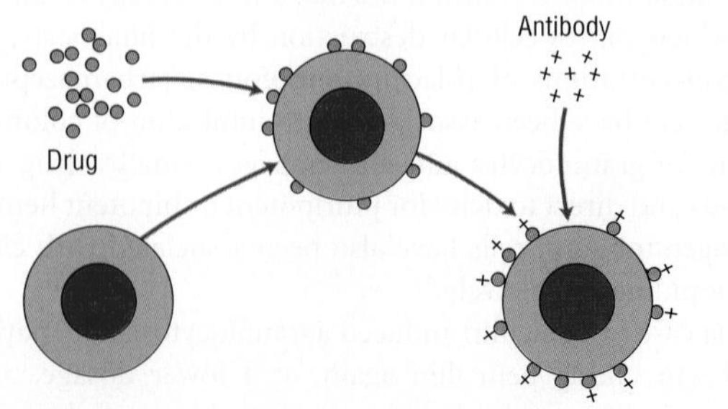

FIGURE 107-2. Drug adsorption mechanism. The drug binds to the membrane of the blood cell. Antibodies are formed to the drug–membrane complex (hapten). The antibodies then attach to the complex, and cell toxicity occurs. *(Reproduced with permission from Petz LD. Drug-induced autoimmune hemolytic anaemia. Transfus Med Rev Oct 1993;7:242–254.)*

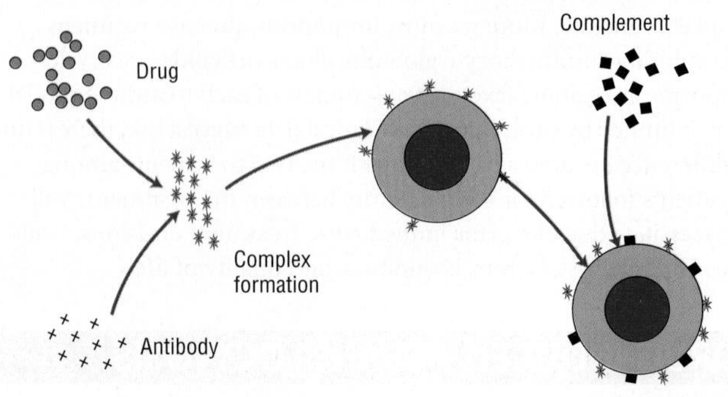

FIGURE 107-3. Innocent bystander mechanism. The drug induces antibody formation. The antibodies and drug form a complex in the serum, and the complex nonspecifically binds to the cell membrane. Complement is activated, and the cell is lysed. *(Reproduced with permission from Petz LD. Drug-induced haemolytic anaemia. Ballieres Clin Haematol 1980;91:455–482.)*

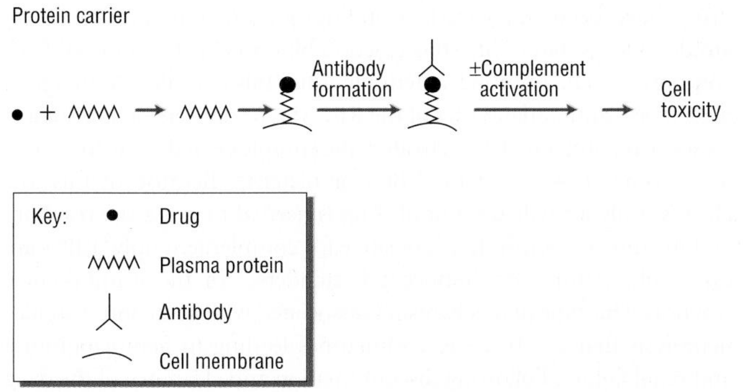

FIGURE 107-4. Protein carrier mechanism. The drug combines with a plasma protein. The complex then attaches to the cell membrane, and antibody formation is stimulated. Antibodies later attach to the complex and activate complement. The cell is then lysed by the complement. *(Reproduced with permission from Young GA, Vincent PC. Drug-induced agranulocytosis. Clin Haematol 1980 Oct;9:483–504.)*

weeks after the initiation of therapy, with a peak onset between 3 and 4 weeks.[60,61] The mechanism by which phenothiazines cause drug-induced agranulocytosis has been studied primarily with chlorpromazine,[62] which is thought to affect cells in the cell cycle phase that manufactures enzymes needed for DNA synthesis (G_1 phase), or the phase in which cells are resting and not committed to cell division (G_0 phase).[62] The antipsychotic agents are known to precipitate proteins and may coprecipitate polynucleotides so they can no longer participate in nucleic acid synthesis. Chlorpromazine also increases the loss of macromolecules from the intracellular pools that are essential for cellular replication.[62] When the bone marrow from a patient with phenothiazine-induced agranulocytosis is examined, it initially appears to have no cellularity (aplastic), but over time it becomes hyperplastic. It is believed that toxic effects of the phenothiazines are not seen in all patients taking the medications because most patients have enough bone marrow reserve to overcome the toxic effects.[62]

Clozapine, an antipsychotic agent, is associated with a significantly higher risk of agranulocytosis as compared to other antipsychotic medications and has received much attention over recent years.[63] The annual incidence of clozapine-induced agranulocytosis in the United States is reported to be 1.3% and can occur at any time during treatment, although the risk is highest at around 3 months after initiation.[64] Because of the frequency and seriousness of clozapine-induced agranulocytosis and because of its reversible nature if detected early in therapy, clozapine is currently only available through a limited distribution program which requires strict WBC count monitoring.[64] In-vitro studies have suggested that the formation of a nitrenium ion unstable metabolite may be responsible for clozapine-induced agranulocytosis.[49] The resulting oxidative stress caused by this metabolite may cause cytotoxicity or an immune reaction.[65]

TREATMENT

Drug-Induced Agranulocytosis

The primary treatment of drug-induced agranulocytosis is the removal of the offending drug. Following discontinuation of the drug, most cases of neutropenia resolve over time, and only symptomatic treatment (e.g., antimicrobials for infections) and appropriate vigilant hygiene practices are necessary. Sargramostim (GM-CSF) and filgrastim (G-CSF) have been shown to shorten the duration of neutropenia, length of antibiotic therapy, and hospital length of stay.[50] Although the use of both agents has been reported in the literature, a commonly reported regimen is G-CSF 300 mcg/day via subcutaneous injection. The only prospective, randomized trial to date did not confirm the benefit of these growth factors.[66] However, some experts have questioned the validity of these results based on the small sample size ($n = 24$) and the lower than standard dose of filgrastim used (i.e., 100–200 mcg/day). One systematic review found that patients with a neutrophil nadir less than 100 cells/mm^3 had a higher rate of infections and fatal complications as compared to those with a higher nadir.[51] Therefore, some clinicians recommend the use of growth factors in patients with a neutrophil nadir less than 100 cells/mm^3, regardless of the presence of infection.

DRUG-INDUCED HEMOLYTIC ANEMIA

Following their release from the bone marrow, normal RBCs survive for approximately 120 days before they are removed by phagocytic cells of the spleen and liver. The process of premature RBC destruction is referred to as hemolysis, which can occur either because of defective RBCs or abnormal changes in the intravascular environment. Drugs can promote hemolysis by both processes.

The causes of drug-induced hemolytic anemia can be divided into two categories: immune or metabolic. Those in the first category may operate much like the process that leads to immune-mediated agranulocytosis, or they can suppress regulator cells, which can lead to the production of autoantibodies. The second category involves the induction of hemolysis by metabolic abnormalities in the RBCs.

Patients with drug-induced hemolytic anemia can present with signs of intravascular or extravascular hemolysis. Intravascular hemolysis, the lysis of RBCs in the circulation, can result from trauma, complement fixation to the RBC, or exogenous toxic factors. Extravascular hemolysis refers to the ingestion of RBCs by macrophages in the spleen and liver, a process that requires the presence of surface abnormalities on RBCs, such as bound immunoglobulin.[67]

The onset of drug-induced hemolytic anemia is variable and depends on the drug and mechanism of the hemolysis. Symptoms of hemolytic anemia can include fatigue, malaise, pallor, and shortness of breath. Table 107–3 provides a list of drugs that have been associated with drug-induced immune hemolytic anemia.

DRUG-INDUCED IMMUNE HEMOLYTIC ANEMIA

In immune hemolytic anemia, IgG and/or immunoglobulin M (IgM) bind to antigens on the surface of RBCs and initiate their destruction through the complement and mononuclear phagocytic systems.[68] Depending on the antigenic stimulus, immune hemolytic anemia is either classified as autoimmune, alloimmune, or drug-induced.[68] Drug-induced antibodies may recognize the host's intrinsic RBC antigens or RBCs bound to drug. If the antibodies react against RBC-bound drug, then the drug must be present to induce hemolysis.[68]

A laboratory test called the direct Coombs test (or direct antiglobulin test [DAT]), which identifies foreign immunoglobulins either in the patient's serum or on the RBCs themselves, is the best means to diagnose drug-induced immune hemolytic anemia. The Coombs test begins with the antiglobulin serum, which is produced by injecting rabbits with preparations of human complement, crystallizable fragment (of immunoglobulin) (Fc), or immunoglobulins. The rabbits produce antibodies that are foreign to human immunoglobulins and complement. The direct Coombs test involves combining the patient's RBCs with the antiglobulin serum. If the patient's RBCs are coated with antibody or complement (as a result of a drug-induced process), the antibodies in the serum (produced by the rabbit) will attach to the Fc regions of the autoimmune globulins on two separate RBCs, creating a lattice formation called agglutination.[69] This agglutination is considered positive for the presence of IgG or complement on the cell surfaces.

TABLE 107-3 Drugs Associated with Hemolytic Anemia

Observational study evidence
Phenobarbital
Phenytoin
Case report evidence (*probable* or *definite* causality rating)
Acetaminophen
Angiotensin-converting enzyme inhibitors
β-Lactam antibiotics
Cephalosporins
Ciprofloxacin
Clavulanate
Erythromycin
Hydrochlorothiazide
Indinavir
Interferon alfa
Ketoconazole
Lansoprazole
Levodopa
Levofloxacin
Methyldopa
Minocycline
NSAIDs
Omeprazole
p-Aminosalicylic acid
Phenazopyridine
Probenecid
Procainamide
Quinidine
Rifabutin
Rifampin
Streptomycin
Sulbactam
Sulfonamides
Sulfonylureas
Tacrolimus
Tazobactam
Teicoplanin
Tolbutamide
Tolmetin
Triamterene

NSAID, nonsteroidal antiinflammatory drug.

An indirect Coombs test can identify antibodies in a patient's serum. This test is performed by combining the patient's serum with normal RBCs, then subjecting them to the direct Coombs test. Antibodies that have attached to the normal RBCs will be identified. This process is important in blood bank procedures.

The mechanisms that have been proposed to explain how drugs can induce immune hemolytic anemia are similar to the mechanisms that produce drug-induced agranulocytosis. The first mechanism is the adsorption of the drug to the RBC membrane to form a hapten, and subsequently, an antibody. The antibody attaches to the drug without direct interaction with the erythrocyte. The extravascular anemia that follows is usually caused by IgG, and generally complement is not activated. The anemia usually develops gradually over 7 to 10 days and reverses over a couple of weeks after the offending drug is discontinued. The direct Coombs test may remain positive for several weeks. The penicillin and cephalosporin derivatives given in high doses are primarily associated with this type of immune reaction.[70] Other drugs that have been reported to cause drug-induced immune hemolytic anemia by this process include minocycline, tolbutamide, and semisynthetic penicillins.[70] Streptomycin is also associated with this type of reaction and is associated with activation of the complement system.[71]

Like drug-induced agranulocytosis, immune hemolytic anemia has been associated with the formation of immune complexes in a reaction formally known as the *innocent bystander phenomenon*. Quinidine and phenacetin are the prototype drugs of this reaction, but many other drugs have been implicated, including quinine and several sulfonamides. Drugs that induce this reaction bind weakly to a normal RBC component. The immune system identifies this complex as foreign, a *neoantigen*, and initiates lysis of the RBC via the complement system.[68] As soon as complement is activated, the complex can detach and move on to other RBCs, and to WBCs or platelets. Because of this low affinity, only a small amount of drug is needed to cause the reaction, and the direct Coombs test is positive for complement only. RBCs are essentially victims, or "innocent bystanders," of the immunologic reaction. This type of mechanism is associated with acute intravascular hemolysis that can be severe, sometimes leading to hemoglobinuria and renal failure. Following discontinuation and clearance of the drug from the circulation, the direct Coombs test will become negative.

The third mechanism is drug-induced autoimmune hemolytic anemia. The first drug implicated in this type of hemolytic anemia was methyldopa.[72] Like some other drugs, methyldopa is known to induce true autoantibodies to RBCs; the antibodies can be identified without the presence of the offending drug or its metabolites. Approximately 10% to 20% of patients receiving methyldopa will develop a positive Coombs test, usually within 6 to 12 months of initiating therapy.[73] However, less than 1% of these patients experience hemolysis, and hemolysis can develop from 4 to 6 months to more than 2 years after the start of therapy. After the withdrawal of the drug, results of the Coombs test can remain positive for many months.[71] The mechanism by which methyldopa induces antibody production is not completely known, but there are two main hypotheses.[72] The first suggests that methyldopa or its metabolites acts on the immune system and impairs immune tolerance. An alternative hypothesis suggests that the offending drug may bind to immature RBCs, altering the membrane antigens and inducing autoantibodies.

It is not known why only some patients develop autoantibodies, and why only some of the patients who have autoantibodies develop hemolytic disease. In an effort to explain why patients have a positive result from a Coombs test and no hemolysis, Kelton demonstrated that methyldopa impairs the ability of these patients to remove antibody-sensitized cells.[74] In Coombs-positive patients receiving methyldopa, patients with impairment of the mononuclear phagocytic system could not clear the RBCs coated with autoantibodies from their bloodstream, and therefore hemolysis did not occur. Patients with hemolysis had no impairment of the mononuclear phagocytic system. Procainamide has also been reported to cause a positive result on the indirect Coombs test and hemolytic anemia.[75] Other drugs that have been reported to cause autoimmune hemolytic anemia include levodopa, mefenamic acid, and diclofenac.[76]

DRUG-INDUCED OXIDATIVE HEMOLYTIC ANEMIA

A hereditary condition, drug-induced oxidative hemolytic anemia, most often accompanies a glucose-6-phosphate dehydrogenase (G6PD) enzyme deficiency, but it can occur because of other enzyme defects (reduced nicotinamide adenine dinucleotide phosphate [NADPH] methemoglobin reductase or reduced glutathione peroxidase). A G6PD deficiency is a disorder of the hexose monophosphate shunt, which is responsible for producing NADPH in RBCs, which in turn keeps glutathione in a reduced state. Reduced glutathione is a substrate for glutathione peroxidase, an enzyme that removes peroxide from RBCs, thus protecting them from oxidative stress.[77] Without reduced glutathione, oxidative drugs can oxidize the sulfhydryl groups of hemoglobin, removing them prematurely from the circulation (i.e., causing hemolysis).

A G6PD deficiency is the most common of all enzyme defects, affecting millions of people. Because the G6PD gene is located on the X chromosome, the disorder is therefore inherited through a sex-linked mode. Both homozygotes and heterozygotes can be symptomatic, but

TABLE 107-4 Drugs Associated with Oxidative Hemolytic Anemia

Observational study evidence
Dapsone
Case report evidence (*probable* or *definite* causality rating)
Ascorbic acid
Metformin
Methylene blue
Nalidixic acid
Nitrofurantoin
Phenazopyridine
Primaquine
Sulfacetamide
Sulfamethoxazole
Sulfanilamide

homozygotes tend to have the most severe cases.[78] There are many G6PD variants, but the most common types occur in American and African blacks (approximately 10%), people from Mediterranean areas (e.g., Greeks, Sardinians, and Khurdic and Sephardic Jews), and Asians.[78]

The degree of hemolysis depends on the severity of the enzyme deficiency and the amount of oxidative stress. However, the dose required for hemolysis to occur is often less than prescribed quantities of the suspected drug.[71,77] Although severe hemolysis is rare, any drug that places oxidative stress on RBCs can cause drug-induced oxidative hemolytic anemia. One case of drug-induced oxidative hemolytic anemia has been reported in a child when dapsone (an oxidizing agent) was transferred through the breast milk of the mother, who was taking the drug.[79] For a list of agents associated with drug-induced oxidative hemolytic anemia, refer to Table 107–4.

TREATMENT

Drug-Induced Hemolytic Anemia

■ DRUG-INDUCED IMMUNE HEMOLYTIC ANEMIA

The severity of drug-induced immune hemolytic anemia depends on the rate of hemolysis. Hemolytic anemia caused by drugs through the hapten/adsorption and autoimmune mechanisms tend to be slower in onset and mild to moderate in severity. Conversely, hemolysis prompted through the neoantigen mechanism (innocent bystander) phenomenon can have a sudden onset, lead to severe hemolysis, and result in renal failure. The treatment of drug-induced immune hemolytic anemia includes the removal of the offending agent and supportive care. In severe cases, glucocorticoids can be helpful,[68] but some practitioners have questioned their efficacy.[76] Other agents such as the chimeric anti-CD20 monoclonal antibody rituximab and immunoglobulin treatments have been used, but their role is yet to be clearly defined.[80,81]

■ DRUG-INDUCED OXIDATIVE HEMOLYTIC ANEMIA

Removal of the offending drug is the primary treatment for drug-induced oxidative hemolytic anemia. No other therapy is usually necessary, as most cases of drug-induced oxidative hemolytic anemia are mild in severity. Patients with these enzyme deficiencies should be advised to avoid medications capable of inducing the hemolysis.

DRUG-INDUCED MEGALOBLASTIC ANEMIA

In drug-induced megaloblastic anemia, the development of RBC precursors called megaloblasts in the bone marrow is abnormal. Deficiencies in either vitamin B_{12} or folate are responsible for the impaired proliferation and maturation of hematopoietic cells, resulting in cell arrest and subsequent sequestration. Examination of peripheral blood shows an increase in the mean corpuscular hemoglobin concentration. These megaloblastic changes are caused by the direct or indirect effects of the drug on DNA synthesis. Some patients can have a normal-appearing cell line, and the diagnosis must be made by measurement of vitamin B_{12} and folate concentrations. The abnormality can be seen in any portion of the replication process, including DNA assembly, base precursor metabolism, or RNA synthesis.[82]

TABLE 107-5 Drugs Associated with Megaloblastic Anemia

Case report evidence (*probable* or *definite* causality rating)
Azathioprine
Chloramphenicol
Colchicine
Cotrimoxazole
Cyclophosphamide
Cytarabine
5-Fluorodeoxyuridine
5-Fluorouracil
Hydroxyurea
6-Mercaptopurine
Methotrexate
Oral contraceptives
p-Aminosalicylate
Phenobarbital
Phenytoin
Primidone
Pyrimethamine
Sulfasalazine
Tetracycline
Vinblastine

Because of their pharmacologic action on DNA replication, the antimetabolite class of chemotherapeutic agents is most frequently associated with drug-induced megaloblastic anemia. Methotrexate, an irreversible inhibitor of dihydrofolate reductase, causes megaloblastic anemia in 3% to 9% of patients.[83] Dihydrofolate reductase is an enzyme responsible for generating tetrahydrofolate, an essential factor in making deoxythymidine triphosphate, which is necessary for DNA synthesis. Other drugs such as cotrimoxazole, phenytoin, or the barbiturates have also been implicated in megaloblastic anemia. Cotrimoxazole, for example, has been reported to cause drug-induced megaloblastic anemia with both low and high doses,[84,85] particularly in patients with a partial vitamin B_{12} or folate deficiency.[82] Because the drug's affinity for human dihydrofolate reductase is low, patients with adequate stores of these vitamins are at low risk of developing drug-induced megaloblastic anemia. It has been postulated that phenytoin, primidone, and phenobarbital cause drug-induced megaloblastic anemia by either inhibiting folate absorption or by increasing folate catabolism. In both instances, the patient develops a relative deficiency of folate. Table 107–5 provides a list of drugs that have been suggested as causative factors in drug-induced megaloblastic anemia.

TREATMENT

Drug-Induced Megaloblastic Anemia

When drug-induced megaloblastic anemia is related to chemotherapy, no real therapeutic option is available, and the anemia becomes an accepted side effect of therapy. If drug-induced megaloblastic anemia results from cotrimoxazole, a trial course of folinic acid, 5 to 10 mg up to four times a day, can correct the anemia.[84,85] Folic acid supplementation of 1 mg every day often corrects the drug-induced megaloblastic anemia produced by either phenytoin or phenobarbital, but some clinicians suggest that folic acid supplementation can decrease the effectiveness of the antiepileptic medications.[86]

DRUG-INDUCED THROMBOCYTOPENIA

Thrombocytopenia is usually defined as a platelet count below 100,000 cells/mm^3 or >50% reduction from baseline values. Thrombocytopenia can be caused by numerous conditions such as blood loss, infection, diffuse intravascular coagulation, and the use of some medications. The annual incidence of drug-induced thrombocytopenia is approximately 10 cases per 1,000,000 population (excluding those cases associated with heparin).[87] Although numerous epidemiologic studies have been reported, none of them have identified patient-specific risk factors, other than exposure to certain classes of medications, that increase the risk for the development of drug-induced thrombocytopenia.[87]

Several mechanisms have been proposed for the development of drug-induced thrombocytopenia: direct toxicity reactions, hapten-type immune reactions, platelet-reactive autoantibodies, and drug-dependent antibodies. Direct toxicity reactions, as often associated with chemotherapeutic agents, result in suppressed thrombopoiesis and produce a decrease in the number of megakaryocytes in the bone marrow. In contrast, immune reactions result in an increased peripheral destruction of platelets and an increased number of megakaryocytes. Early symptoms of drug-induced thrombocytopenia include increased bruising, petechiae, ecchymoses, and epistaxis. Bleeding from mucous membranes and severe purpura can appear later in the disorder. A list of medications associated with drug-induced thrombocytopenia can be found in Table 107–6.

Most of the drugs that induce thrombocytopenia by their toxic effects are cancer chemotherapy agents, but organic solvents, pesticides, drugs that influence folic acid metabolism, and inamrinone (formally named amrinone) have also been implicated. Although orally administered inamrinone has been reported to cause thrombocytopenia in up to 18.6% of patients,[88] only the intravenous formulation is currently commercially available in the United States. Some studies suggest that this toxic effect might be caused by the metabolite of inamrinone, instead of the parent drug.[89] Regardless of the cause, inamrinone use has been largely replaced by other phosphodiesterase-3 inhibitors that are not associated with the same high risk of side effects.

Drug-induced thrombocytopenia usually develops through an immunologic mechanism. The agents most commonly implicated are quinine, quinidine, gold salts, sulfonamide antibiotics, rifampin, glycoprotein IIb/IIIa (GPIIb/IIIa) receptor antagonists, and heparin.[87] Studies of these agents have helped to elucidate the mechanisms of drug-induced immune thrombocytopenia. In hapten-type reactions, the offending drug binds to certain platelet glycoproteins. Antibodies are generated that bind to these drug-bound glycoprotein epitopes. After the binding of drug-dependent antibodies to the platelet surface, lysis occurs through complement activation or through clearance from the circulation by macrophages.[90] Hapten-mediated immune thrombocytopenia usually occurs at least 7 days after the initiation of the drug, although it can occur much sooner if the exposure is actually a reexposure to a previously administered drug. The recovery period, once the suspected drug is discontinued, is often short in duration with a median recovery time within 1 week.[91] A recently published study suggests that vancomycin-induced thrombocytopenia is related to drug-dependent antibodies,[92] and although relatively rare, penicillins and cephalosporins can cause thrombocytopenia through this mechanism.[87]

Gold compounds and procainamide appear to induce thrombocytopenia through the platelet-specific autoantibody type reaction.[87] In this type of reaction, a drug induces the production of autoantibodies that bind to platelet membranes and cause destruction, but the causative drug does not have to be present for the reaction to occur. In contrast, the drug-dependent antibody reaction requires the presence of the drug to allow antibody binding. Although several mechanisms of drug-induced thrombocytopenia have been proposed, it is often not possible to determine the

TABLE 107-6 Drugs Associated with Thrombocytopenia

Observational study evidence	Diazoxide	Morphine
Carbamazepine	Diclofenac	Nalidixic acid
Phenobarbital	Diethylstilbestrol	Naphazoline
Phenytoin	Digoxin	Naproxen
Valproic acid	Ethambutol	Nitroglycerin
Case report evidence (*probable* or *definite* causality rating)	Felbamate	Octreotide
Abciximab	Fluconazole	Oxacillin
Acetaminophen	Gold salts	p-Aminosalicylic acid
Acyclovir	Haloperidol	Penicillamine
Albendazole	Heparin	Pentoxifylline
Aminoglutethimide	Hydrochlorothiazide	Piperacillin
Aminosalicylic acid	Ibuprofen	Primidone
Amiodarone	Inamrinone	Procainamide
Amphotericin B	Indinavir	Pyrazinamide
Ampicillin	Indomethacin	Quinidine
Aspirin	Interferon alfa	Quinine
Atorvastatin	Isoniazid	Ranitidine
Captopril	Isotretinoin	Recombinant hepatitis B vaccine
Chlorothiazide	Itraconazole	Rifampin
Chlorpromazine	Levamisole	Simvastatin
Chlorpropamide	Linezolid	Sirolimus
Cimetidine	Lithium	Sulfasalazine
Ciprofloxacin	Low-molecular-weight heparins	Sulfonamides
Clarithromycin	Measles, mumps, and rubella vaccine	Sulindac
Clopidogrel	Meclofenamate	Tamoxifen
Danazol	Mesalamine	Tolmetin
Deferoxamine	Methyldopa	Trimethoprim
Diazepam	Minoxidil	Vancomycin

mechanism for an individual drug or patient and more than one mechanism can be responsible for the condition.

Approximately 1% of patients who receive the GPIIb/IIIa receptor antagonist abciximab develop acute thrombocytopenia, and that rate increases to approximately 4% after a second exposure.[93] Three GPIIb/IIIa receptor antagonists are currently marketed in the United Sates, abciximab, eptifibatide, and tirofiban, and all three agents have been associated with thrombocytopenia. The pathogenesis of GPIIb/IIIa-induced thrombocytopenia remains unclear, and one of the unique aspects is the varying presentations. Some patients develop a precipitous drop in platelets within hours of their first exposure to the medication, which can be associated with fever, dyspnea, hypotension, and even anaphylaxis in some cases.[93,94] Several authors have proposed a nonimmune mechanism for this type of drug-induced thrombocytopenia because of the acute nature of the platelet drop.[93] In addition to the acute thrombocytopenia that can occur with GPIIb/IIIa receptor antagonists, delayed thrombocytopenia has also been reported, which suggests an immune-based reaction.[64,95] Although the exact mechanism is unknown, growing evidence suggests that the binding of GPIIb/IIIa receptor antagonists to the GPIIb/IIIa receptors can induce the expression of ligand-induced binding sites.[93] These new binding sites may then react with antibodies, leading to an increased clearance of platelets.[96,97]

Because GPIIb/IIIa receptor antagonists are coadministered with heparin, it is important to distinguish between GPIIb/IIIa receptor antagonist-induced and heparin-induced thrombocytopenia. A heparin-induced platelet aggregation study can help to determine the offending agent.

CLINICAL CONTROVERSY

Profound thrombocytopenia (i.e., platelet count less than 20,000 cells/mm^3) has been reported with the GPIIb/IIIa receptor antagonists. Before this effect was fully appreciated, many clinicians attributed this event to heparin. The current challenge for clinicians is to distinguish between GPIIb/IIIa receptor antagonist-induced and heparin-induced thrombocytopenia, so that the patient's adverse event is documented properly. Thrombocytopenia associated with GPIIb/IIIa receptor antagonists can present with a nadir of platelet counts of 1,000 to 4,000 cells/mm^3 occurring from 2 to 31 hours following bolus infusion, which is much sooner than the 5 to 10 days observed with initial heparin exposure. However, reexposure to heparin can produce profound thrombocytopenia within hours. The ubiquity of heparin use for flushing catheters makes it difficult to determine previous exposure in many cases. Clinicians can choose from several types of assays to aid in the diagnosis of heparin-induced thrombocytopenia, including platelet activation assays, platelet aggregation studies, and enzyme-linked immunosorbent assay methods, each with varying sensitivity, specificity, and availability.

Pseudothrombocytopenia, defined as in-vitro platelet aggregation in blood anticoagulated with ethylenediamine tetraacetic acid (EDTA), is clinically insignificant, but it must also be differentiated from thrombocytopenia induced by GPIIb/IIIa receptor antagonists. In this case, microscopic examination of a peripheral blood smear, along with repeated platelet counts in citrate-anticoagulated blood samples, makes the distinction possible.[93]

Probably the most recognized, complex type of drug-induced thrombocytopenia is that associated with heparin. At least two types of heparin-induced thrombocytopenia (HIT) have been identified. The most common, type I, occurs in approximately 10% to 20% of patients treated with heparin.[98] It is a mild, reversible, nonimmune-mediated reaction that usually occurs within the first 2 days of therapy.[5] The platelet count slowly returns to baseline following an initial decline, despite continued heparin therapy. HIT type I is usually an asymptomatic condition and is thought to be related to platelet aggregation.[5]

HIT type II is less common but more severe and can be associated with more complications. Approximately 1 to 5% of patients receiving unfractionated heparin and up to 0.8% of patients receiving low-molecular-weight heparin (LMWH) can develop HIT.[5,98] Patients typically present with a low platelet count (e.g., below 150,000 cells/mm^3) or a 50% or more decrease in platelet count from baseline and thrombosis can occur.[99] The platelet count generally begins to decline 5 to 10 days after the start of heparin therapy. However, this decline can occur within hours of receiving heparin if the patient has recently received heparin (i.e., within 100 days).[99] Thrombocytopenia and thrombosis can develop with low-dose heparin,[100] heparin-coated catheters,[101] or even heparin flushes. Certain patient populations have a higher risk for developing HIT than others; patients who have had recent, major surgery are one of the highest risk groups.[98] The next highest risk groups include patients receiving heparin for thrombosis prophylaxis following peripheral vascular surgery, cardiac surgery, and orthopedic surgery.[102] A lower incidence in seen in medical, obstetric, and pediatric patients, especially those receiving LMWH instead of unfractionated heparin.[98] The most recent practice guidelines by the American College of Chest Physicians recommend varying degrees of platelet monitoring based on the relative risk of developing HIT.[103]

HIT is caused by the development of antibodies against platelet factor-4 (PF-4) and heparin complexes[99] (Fig. 107–5). Low-molecular-weight heparins bind less well to PF-4 than unfractionated heparin, and therefore antibody formation is less common. However, there is cross-reactivity between antibodies developed by patients receiving unfractionated heparin and LMWH, and LMWH should therefore not be used in patients with HIT.[98] Once the antibodies bind to the complexes, platelet activation and aggregation occur, with subsequent release of more circulating PF-4 to interact with heparin. In addition, procoagulant microparticles are also released that increase the risk of thrombosis.[98] Thrombosis is one of the major complications of HIT and can occur in up to 20% to 50% of patients with HIT.[99] In fact, thrombosis is the precipitating factor that leads the clinician to diagnose HIT in many patients. This high risk of thrombosis continues for days to weeks after heparin discontinuation and platelet recovery, and continued anticoagulation with an alternative agent is essential during this time period.[99] Other less frequent manifestations of HIT include heparin-induced skin necrosis and venous gangrene of the limbs.[98,99] The diagnosis of HIT is frequently a clinical one, supported by laboratory testing. Several types of assays are available to aid in the diagnosis of HIT, including platelet activation assays, platelet aggregation studies, and enzyme-linked immunosorbent assay methods, each with varying sensitivities and specificities.[5]

TREATMENT

Drug-Induced Thrombocytopenia

The primary treatment of drug-induced thrombocytopenia is removal of the offending drug and symptomatic treatment of the patient. The use of corticosteroid therapy in the treatment of drug-induced thrombocytopenia is controversial, although some authors recommend it in severe symptomatic cases.[104]

In the case of HIT, the main goal of management is to reduce the risk of thrombosis or reduce thrombosis-associated complications in patients who have already developed a clot. All forms of heparin must be discontinued, including heparin flushes, and alternative

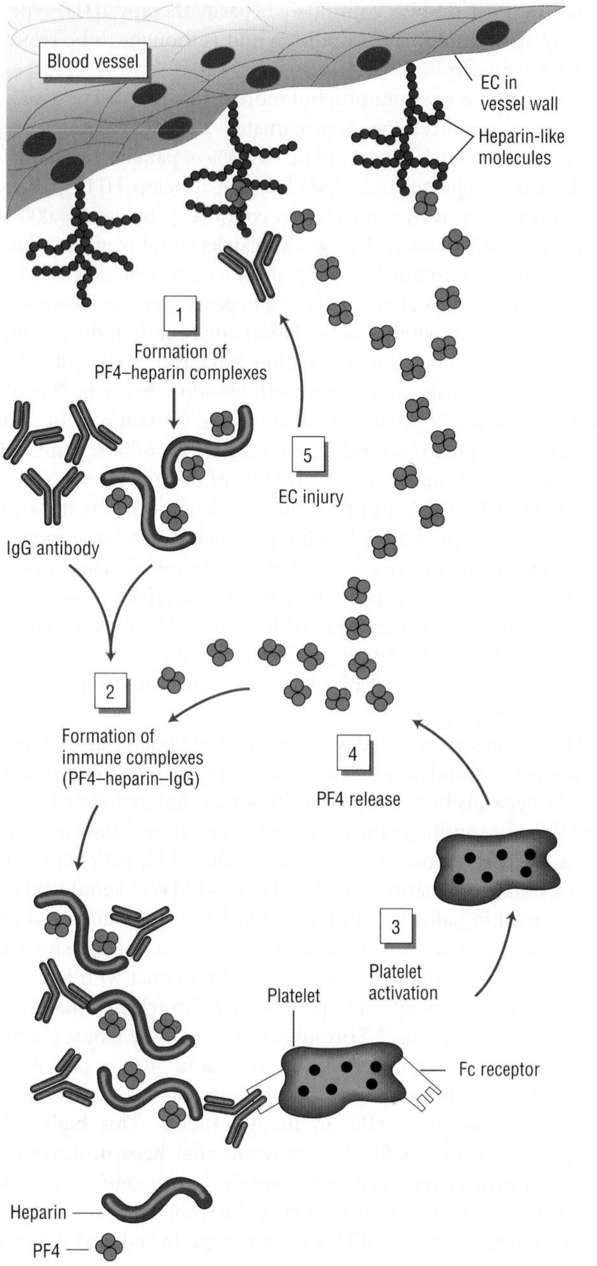

FIGURE 107-5. Proposed explanation for the presence of both thrombocytopenia and thrombosis in heparin-sensitive patients who are treated with heparin. Injected heparin reacts with platelet factor-4 (PF-4), which is normally present on the surface of endothelial cells (ECs) or released in small quantities from circulating platelets, to form PF-4–heparin complexes *(1)*. Specific immunoglobulin G (IgG) antibodies react with these conjugates to form immune complexes *(2)* that bind to crystallizable fragment (Fc) receptors on circulating platelets. Fc-mediated platelet activation *(3)* releases PF-4 from α-granules in platelets *(4)*. Newly released PF-4 binds to additional heparin, and the antibody forms more immune complexes, establishing a cycle of platelet activation. PF-4 released in excess of the amount that can be neutralized by available heparin binds to heparin-like molecules (glycosaminoglycans) on the surface of ECs to provide targets for antibody binding. This process leads to immune-mediated EC injury *(5)* and heightens the risk of thrombosis and disseminated intravascular coagulation. *(Reproduced with permission from Aster RH. Heparin-induced thrombocytopenia and thrombosis. N Engl J Med 1995;332:1374–1376. Copyright ©1995 Massachusetts Medical Society. All rights reserved.)*

anticoagulation must begin immediately.[105] The direct thrombin inhibitors are the alternative anticoagulants most commonly used in current practice. Three direct thrombin inhibitors are currently available: lepirudin, argatroban, and bivalirudin. Lepirudin, the first drug that was approved for the treatment of HIT, is a recombinant analogue of hirudin, a natural anticoagulant found in leeches. Lepirudin is renally eliminated and requires dosage adjustment in those patients with kidney dysfunction. It is also important to note that antibodies to lepirudin develop in approximately 30% of patients who receive this agent for the first time, and it is therefore recommended that patients receive only one treatment course of lepirudin.[99] Argatroban is another intravenous thrombin inhibitor indicated for the management of HIT. But unlike lepirudin, argatroban is metabolized in the liver and can be used in patients with end-stage renal disease. However, dosage adjustment is needed for patients with significant hepatic impairment. The most recently approved direct thrombin inhibitor is bivalirudin. It is similar to lepirudin in that is parenteral bivalent analog of hirudin. It requires dosage adjustment only in severe renal failure. These agents should also be considered for the treatment of patients who have acute HIT without thrombosis because of the increased risk of thrombosis occurring in these patients. Because of the increased risk of venous limb gangrene, warfarin should not be used alone to treat acute HIT complicated by deep vein thrombosis.[103]

SUMMARY

❻ Drug-induced hematologic disorders are rare but potentially life-threatening conditions. Clinicians should be cognizant of medications with the potential of causing hematologic disorders and educate patients to recognize the symptoms associated with such events. Frequent laboratory monitoring of patients taking medications associated with severe hematologic events can facilitate diagnosis and treatment. Identifying the etiology of the event and documenting the causative agents can serve to prevent a recurrence secondary to the use of a related medication. Reporting these events to national adverse event reporting services and in the peer-reviewed medical literature can serve to improve the understanding of the prevalence and risk factors for this disorder.

ABBREVIATIONS

ADR: adverse drug reaction

ATG: antithymocyte globulin

DAT: direct antiglobulin test

EDTA: ethylenediamine tetraacetic acid

Fc: crystallizable fragment (of immunoglobulin)

G6PD: glucose-6-phosphate dehydrogenase

G-CSF: granulocyte colony-stimulating factor

GM-CSF: granulocyte-macrophage colony-stimulating factor

GPIIb/IIIa: glycoprotein IIb/IIIa

GVHD: graft-versus-host disease

HIT: heparin-induced thrombocytopenia

HLA: human leukocyte antigen

HSCT: hematopoietic stem cell transplantation

IgG: immunoglobulin G

IgM: immunoglobulin M

LMWH: low-molecular-weight heparin

NADPH: reduced nicotinamide adenine dinucleotide phosphate

PF-4: platelet factor-4

RBC: red blood cell

WBC: white blood cell

REFERENCES

1. Johnston FD. Granulocytopenia following the administration of sulfanilamide compounds. Lancet 1938;2:1004–1047.
2. van der Klauw MM, Goudsmit R, Halie MR, et al. A population-based case-cohort study of drug-associated agranulocytosis. Arch Intern Med 1999;159:369–374.
3. Maluf EM, Pasquini R, Eluf JN, et al. Aplastic anemia in Brazil: incidence and risk factors. Am J Hematol 2002;71:268–274.
4. Shapiro S, Issaragrisil S, Kaufman DW, et al. Agranulocytosis in Bangkok, Thailand: a predominantly drug-induced disease with an unusually low incidence. Aplastic Anemia Study Group. Am J Trop Med Hyg 1999;60:573–577.
5. Franchini M. Heparin-induced thrombocytopenia: an update. Thromb J [serial on the Internet] 2005 [cited 2006 Dec 12];3(14):[about 5 p.] Available from: *http://www.thrombosisjournal.com/content/3/1/14*
6. Hine LK, Gerstman BB, Wise RP, et al. Mortality resulting from blood dyscrasias in the United States, 1984. Am J Med 1990;88:151–153.
7. Kessler DA. Introducing MEDWatch. A new approach to reporting medication and device adverse effects and product problems. JAMA 1993;269:2765–2768.
8. ASHP guidelines on adverse drug reaction monitoring and reporting. American Society of Hospital Pharmacy. Am J Health Syst Pharm 1995;52:417–419.
9. Rieder MJ. In vivo and in vitro testing for adverse drug reactions. Pediatr Clin North Am 1997;44:93–111.
10. Parent-Massin DM, Sensebe L, Leglise MC, et al. Relevance of in vitro studies of drug-induced agranulocytosis. Report of 14 cases. Drug Saf 1993;9:463–469.
11. Naranjo CA, Busto U, Sellers EM, et al. A method for estimating the probability of adverse drug reactions. Clin Pharmacol Ther 1981;30:239–245.
12. Sackett D. Clinical Epidemiology: A basic science for clinical medicine, 2nd ed. Boston: Little Brown, 1991:xiii, 370, plates 1.
13. Ehrlich P. Ueber einem Fall von Anamie mit Berner-kungen uber regenerative Veranderungen des Knochenmarks. Charite-Annalen 1888;13:301–309.
14. Issaragrisil S, Kaufman DW, Anderson T, et al. The epidemiology of aplastic anemia in Thailand. Blood 2006;107:1299–1307.
15. Kaufman DW, Kelly JP, Issaragrisil S, et al. Relative incidence of agranulocytosis and aplastic anemia. Am J Hematol 2006;81:65–67.
16. Young NS, Calado RT, Scheinberg P. Current concepts in the pathophysiology and treatment of aplastic anemia. Blood 2006;108:2509–2519.
17. Issaragrisil S, Leaverton PE, Chansung K, et al. Regional patterns in the incidence of aplastic anemia in Thailand. The Aplastic Anemia Study Group. Am J Hematol 1999;61:164–168.
18. Brodsky RA, Jones RJ. Aplastic anaemia. Lancet 2005;365:1647–1656.
19. Gale RP, Champlin RE, Feig SA, et al. Aplastic anemia: biology and treatment. Ann Intern Med 1981;95:477–494.
20. Nimer SD, Ireland P, Meshkinpour A, et al. An increased HLA DR2 frequency is seen in aplastic anemia patients. Blood 1994;84:923–927.
21. Poonkuzhali B, Shaji RV, Salamun DE, et al. Cytochrome P4501A1 and glutathione S transferase gene polymorphisms in patients with aplastic anemia in India. Acta Haematol 2005;114:127–132.
22. Kaufman DW, Kelly JP, Levy M, et al. The drug etiology of agranulocytosis and aplastic anemia, 1st ed. New York: Oxford University Press, 1991.
23. Gewirtz AM, Hoffman R. Current considerations of the etiology of aplastic anemia. Crit Rev Oncol Hematol 1985;4:1–30.
24. Council for International Organizations of Medical Sciences. Standardization of definitions and criteria of assessment of adverse drug reactions: Drug-induced cytopenia. Int J Clin Pharmacol Ther Toxicol 1991;29:75–81.
25. Heimpel H. Epidemiology and etiology of aplastic anemia. In: Schrezenmeier H, ed. Aplastic anemia: pathophysiology and treatment. Cambridge, UK: Cambridge University Press, 2000:97–116.
26. The International Agranulocytosis and Aplastic Anemia Study Group. Risks of agranulocytosis and aplastic anemia. A first report of their relation to drug use with special reference to analgesics. JAMA 1986;256:1749–1757.
27. Camitta BM, Thomas ED, Nathan DG, et al. A prospective study of androgens and bone marrow transplantation for treatment of severe aplastic anemia. Blood 1979;53:504–514.
28. Shadduck R. Aplastic anemia. In: Williams W, ed. Hematology. New York: McGraw-Hill, 1995:238–251.
29. Vincent PC. In vitro evidence of drug action in aplastic anemia. Blut 1984;49:3–12.
30. Howard SC, Naidu PE, Hu XJ, et al. Natural history of moderate aplastic anemia in children. Pediatr Blood Cancer 2004;43:545–551.
31. Vandendries ER, Drews RE. Drug-associated disease: hematologic dysfunction. Crit Care Clin 2006;22:347–355, viii.
32. Young NS, Maciejewski J. The pathophysiology of acquired aplastic anemia. N Engl J Med 1997;336:1365–1372.
33. Yunis AA, Miller AM, Salem Z, et al. Chloramphenicol toxicity: pathogenetic mechanisms and the role of the p-NO2 in aplastic anemia. Clin Toxicol 1980;17:359–373.
34. Malkin D, Koren G, Saunders EF. Drug-induced aplastic anemia: pathogenesis and clinical aspects. Am J Pediatr Hematol Oncol 1990;12:402–410.
35. Jimenez JJ, Arimura GK, Abou-Khalil WH, et al. Chloramphenicol-induced bone marrow injury: possible role of bacterial metabolites of chloramphenicol. Blood 1987;70:1180–1185.
36. Gerson WT, Fine DG, Spielberg SP, et al. Anticonvulsant-induced aplastic anemia: increased susceptibility to toxic drug metabolites in vitro. Blood 1983;61:889–893.
37. Kagan WA, Ascensao JA, Pahwa RN, et al. Aplastic anemia: Presence in human bone marrow of cells that suppress myelopoiesis. Proc Natl Acad Sci USA 1976;73:2890–2894.
38. Selleri C, Sato T, Anderson S, et al. Interferon-gamma and tumor necrosis factor-alpha suppress both early and late stages of hematopoiesis and induce programmed cell death. J Cell Physiol 1995;165:538–546.
39. Mathe G, Amiel JL, Schwarzenberg L, et al. Bone marrow graft in man after conditioning by antilymphocytic serum. Br Med J 1970;2:131–136.
40. Platanias L, Gascon P, Bielory L, et al. Lymphocyte phenotype and lymphokines following anti-thymocyte globulin therapy in patients with aplastic anaemia. Br J Haematol 1987;66:437–443.
41. Frickhofen N, Kaltwasser JP, Schrezenmeier H, et al. Treatment of aplastic anemia with antilymphocyte globulin and methylprednisolone with or without cyclosporine. The German Aplastic Anemia Study Group. N Engl J Med 1991;324:1297–1304.
42. Marsh JC, Chowdry J, Parry-Jones N, et al. Study of the association between cytochromes P450 2D6 and 2E1 genotypes and the risk of drug and chemical induced idiosyncratic aplastic anaemia. Br J Haematol 1999;104:266–270.
43. Horowitz MM. Current status of allogeneic bone marrow transplantation in acquired aplastic anemia. Semin Hematol 2000;37:30–42.
44. Passweg JR, Perez WS, Eapen M, et al. Bone marrow transplants from mismatched related and unrelated donors for severe aplastic anemia. Bone Marrow Transplant 2006;37:641–649.
45. Frickhofen N, Heimpel H, Kaltwasser JP, et al. Antithymocyte globulin with or without cyclosporin A. 11-year follow-up of a randomized trial comparing treatments of aplastic anemia. Blood 2003;101:1236–1242.
46. Bacigalupo A, Brand R, Oneto R, et al. Treatment of acquired severe aplastic anemia: bone marrow transplantation compared with immunosuppressive therapy—The European Group for Blood and Marrow Transplantation Experience. Semin Hematol 2000;37:69–80.
47. Zheng Y, Liu Y, Chu Y. Immunosuppressive therapy for acquired severe aplastic anemia (SAA): a prospective comparison of four different regimens. Exp Hematol 2006;34:826–831.
48. Gluckman E, Rokicka-Milewska R, Hann I, et al. Results and follow-up of a phase III randomized study of recombinant human-granulocyte stimulating factor as support for immunosuppressive therapy in patients with severe aplastic anaemia. Br J Haematol 2002;119:1075–1082.
49. Bhatt V, Saleem A. Review: Drug-induced neutropenia—pathophysiology, clinical features, and management. Ann Clin Lab Sci 2004;34:131–137.
50. Andres E, Noel E, Kurtz JE, et al. Life-threatening idiosyncratic drug-induced agranulocytosis in elderly patients. Drugs Aging 2004;21:427–435.
51. Andersohn F, Konzen C, Garbe E. Systematic review: agranulocytosis induced by nonchemotherapy drugs. Ann Intern Med 2007;146:657–665.
52. Neftel K, Muller M, Hauser S, et al. More on penicillin-induced leukopenia. N Engl J Med 1983;308:901–902.
53. Neftel KA, Hauser SP, Muller MR. Inhibition of granulopoiesis in vivo and in vitro by beta-lactam antibiotics. J Infect Dis 1985;152:90–98.

54. Cooper DS, Goldminz D, Levin AA, et al. Agranulocytosis associated with antithyroid drugs. Effects of patient age and drug dose. Ann Intern Med 1983;98:26–29.
55. Andres E, Maloisel F, Kurtz JE, et al. Modern management of non-chemotherapy drug-induced agranulocytosis: a monocentric cohort study of 90 cases and review of the literature. Eur J Intern Med [serial on the Internet] 2002 [cited 2006 Dec 17];13:[about 4 p.]. Available from: *http://www.ispub.com/journals/ijim.htm*
56. Ibanez L, Vidal X, Ballarin E, et al. Population-based drug-induced agranulocytosis. Arch Intern Med 2005;165:869–874.
57. Akamizu T, Ozaki S, Hiratani H, et al. Drug-induced neutropenia associated with anti-neutrophil cytoplasmic antibodies (ANCA): possible involvement of complement in granulocyte cytotoxicity. Clin Exp Immunol 2002;127:92–98.
58. Werner MC, Romaldini JH, Bromberg N, et al. Adverse effects related to thionamide drugs and their dose regimen. Am J Med Sci 1989;297:216–219.
59. Ticlid (ticlopidine). Prescribing information. 2001, *http://www.roche-usa.com/products/ticlid/pi.pdf.*
60. Young GA, Vincent PC. Drug-induced agranulocytosis. Clin Haematol 1980;9483–504.
61. Stubner S, Grohmann R, Engel R, et al. Blood dyscrasias induced by psychotropic drugs. Pharmacopsychiatry 2004;37 (Suppl 1):S70–S78.
62. Pisciotta V. Drug-induced agranulocytosis. Drugs 1978;15:132–143.
63. Schulte PF. Risk of clozapine-associated agranulocytosis and mandatory white blood cell monitoring. Ann Pharmacother 2006;40:683–688.
64. Bosco A, Kidson-Gerber G, Dunkley S. Delayed tirofiban-induced thrombocytopenia: two case reports. J Thromb Haemost 2005;3:1109–1110.
65. Fischer V, Haar JA, Greiner L, et al. Possible role of free radical formation in clozapine (Clozaril)-induced agranulocytosis. Mol Pharmacol 1991;40:846–853.
66. Fukata S, Kuma K, Sugawara M. Granulocyte colony-stimulating factor (G-CSF) does not improve recovery from antithyroid drug-induced agranulocytosis: A prospective study. Thyroid 1999;9:29–31.
67. Tabbara IA. Hemolytic anemias. Diagnosis and management. Med Clin North Am 1992;76:649–668.
68. Gehrs BC, Friedberg RC. Autoimmune hemolytic anemia. Am J Hematol 2002;69:258–271.
69. McKenzie S. Hemolytic anemias due to extrinsic factors. In: Balado D, et al., ed. Textbook of Hematology. Baltimore: Williams & Wilkins, 1996;1233–1263.
70. Thomas A. Autoimmune hemolytic anemias. In: Lee R, et al., eds. Wintrobe's Clinical Hematology. Baltimore: Williams & Wilkins, 1999:1233–1263.
71. Jandl J. Immunohemolytic anemias. In: Strangis J, ed. Textbook of Hematology. Boston: Little Brown, 1996:421–518.
72. Dacie SJ. The immune haemolytic anaemias: a century of exciting progress in understanding. Br J Haematol 2001;114:770–785.
73. Aldomet (methyldopa). Prescribing Information. 1998, *http://www.merck.com/product/usa/pi_circulars/a/aldomet/aldomet_pi.pdf.*
74. Kelton JG. Impaired reticuloendothelial function in patients treated with methyldopa. N Engl J Med 1985;313:596–600.
75. Kleinman S, Nelson R, Smith L, et al. Positive direct antiglobulin tests and immune hemolytic anemia in patients receiving procainamide. N Engl J Med 1984;311:809–812.
76. Packman C, Leddy J. Drug-related immune hemolytic anemia. In: Williams W, et al., eds. Hematology. New York: McGraw-Hill, 1995:691–697.
77. Beutler E. G6PD deficiency. Blood 1994;84:3613–3636.
78. Frank JE. Diagnosis and management of G6PD deficiency. Am Fam Physician 2005;72:1277–1282.
79. Sanders SW, Zone JJ, Foltz RL, et al. Hemolytic anemia induced by dapsone transmitted through breast milk. Ann Intern Med 1982;96:465–466.
80. Ahrens N, Kingreen D, Seltsam A, et al. Treatment of refractory autoimmune haemolytic anaemia with anti-CD20 (rituximab). Br J Haematol 2001;114:244–245.
81. Flores G, Cunningham-Rundles C, Newland AC, et al. Efficacy of intravenous immunoglobulin in the treatment of autoimmune hemolytic anemia: results in 73 patients. Am J Hematol 1993;44: 237–242.
82. Scott JM, Weir DG. Drug-induced megaloblastic change. Clin Haematol 1980;9:587–606.
83. Weinblatt ME. Toxicity of low dose methotrexate in rheumatoid arthritis. J Rheumatol 1985; 12 (Suppl 12):35–39.
84. Kobrinsky NL, Ramsay NK. Acute megaloblastic anemia induced by high-dose trimethoprim-sulfamethoxazole. Ann Intern Med 1981; 94:780–781.
85. Magee F, O'Sullivan H, McCann SR. Megaloblastosis and low-dose trimethoprim-sulfamethoxazole. Ann Intern Med 1981;95:657.
86. Rivey MP, Schottelius DD, Berg MJ. Phenytoin-folic acid: a review. Drug Intell Clin Pharm 1984;18:292–301.
87. van den Bemt PM, Meyboom RH, Egberts AC. Drug-induced immune thrombocytopenia. Drug Saf 2004;27:1243–1252.
88. Ansell J, Tiarks C, McCue J, et al. Amrinone-induced thrombocytopenia. Arch Intern Med 1984;144:949–952.
89. Sadiq A, Tamura N, Yoshida M, et al. Possible contribution of acetylamrinone and its enhancing effects on platelet aggregation under shear stress conditions in the onset of thrombocytopenia in patients treated with amrinone. Thromb Res 2003;111:357–361.
90. Aster RH. Drug-induced immune thrombocytopenia: an overview of pathogenesis. Semin Hematol 1999;36(Suppl 1):2–6.
91. George JN, Raskob GE, Shah SR, et al. Drug-induced thrombocytopenia: a systematic review of published case reports. Ann Intern Med 1998;129:886–890.
92. Von Drygalski A, Curtis BR, Bougie DW, et al. Vancomycin-induced immune thrombocytopenia. N Engl J Med 2007;356:904–910.
93. Aster RH. Immune thrombocytopenia caused by glycoprotein IIb/IIIa inhibitors. Chest 2005;127(Suppl):53S–59S.
94. Iakovou Y, Manginas A, Melissari E, et al. Acute profound thrombocytopenia associated with anaphylactic reaction after abciximab therapy during percutaneous coronary angioplasty. Cardiology 2001;95:215–216.
95. Onitilo AA. Delayed profound thrombocytopenia associated with eptifibatide. Am J Hematol 2006;81:984.
96. Cines DB. Glycoprotein IIb/IIIa antagonists: potential induction and detection of drug-dependent antiplatelet antibodies. Am Heart J 1998;135(Pt 2 Su):S152–S159.
97. Jubelirer SJ, Koenig BA, Bates MC. Acute profound thrombocytopenia following C7E3 Fab (Abciximab) therapy: Case reports, review of the literature and implications for therapy. Am J Hematol 1999;61:205–208.
98. Menajovsky LB. Heparin-induced thrombocytopenia: clinical manifestations and management strategies. Am J Med 2005;118(Suppl 8A):21S–30S.
99. Arepally GM, Ortel TL. Clinical practice. Heparin-induced thrombocytopenia. N Engl J Med 2006;355:809–817.
100. Girolami B, Prandoni P, Stefani PM, et al. The incidence of heparin-induced thrombocytopenia in hospitalized medical patients treated with subcutaneous unfractionated heparin: a prospective cohort study. Blood 2003;101:2955–2959.
101. Laster JL, Nichols WK, Silver D. Thrombocytopenia associated with heparin-coated catheters in patients with heparin-associated antiplatelet antibodies. Arch Intern Med 1989;149:2285–2287.
102. Lindhoff-Last E, Wenning B, Stein M, et al. Risk factors and long-term follow-up of patients with the immune type of heparin-induced thrombocytopenia. Clin Appl Thromb Hemost 2002;8:347–352.
103. Warkentin TE, Greinacher A. Heparin-induced thrombocytopenia: recognition, treatment, and prevention: the Seventh ACCP Conference on Antithrombotic and Thrombolytic Therapy. Chest 2004;126(Suppl):311S–337S.
104. Pedersen-Bjergaard U, Andersen M, Hansen PB. Drug-induced thrombocytopenia: clinical data on 309 cases and the effect of corticosteroid therapy. Eur J Clin Pharmacol 1997;52:183–189.
105. Dager WE, Dougherty JA, Nguyen PH, et al. Heparin-induced thrombocytopenia: treatment options and special considerations. Pharmacotherapy 2007;27:564–587.

SECTION 16
INFECTIOUS DISEASES

CHAPTER 108

Laboratory Tests to Direct Antimicrobial Pharmacotherapy

MICHAEL J. RYBAK AND JEFFREY R. AESCHLIMANN

KEY CONCEPTS

1. Familiarity with normal host flora and typical pathogens will help to determine whether a patient is truly infected or merely colonized.
2. Direct examination of tissue and body fluids by Gram stain provides simple and rapid information about the potential pathogen.
3. Isolation of the offending organism by culture assists in the diagnosis of infection and allows for more definitive directed treatment.
4. The development of molecular testing systems has improved our ability to diagnose infection and determine the antimicrobial susceptibilities for numerous fastidious or slow-growing pathogens, such as mycobacteria and viruses.
5. Although highly standardized, in-vitro antimicrobial susceptibility testing has limitations and often cannot truly mimic the conditions found at the site of an infection. This can cause discordance between in-vitro susceptibility results and in-vivo response to therapy.
6. The laboratory evaluation of antimicrobial activity is an important component of the pharmacotherapeutic management of infectious diseases.
7. Antimicrobial pharmacodynamics have become a crucial consideration for the clinician during the selection of both empirical and pathogen-directed therapy in the current era of antimicrobial resistance.
8. When used appropriately, rapid automated susceptibility test systems appear to improve therapeutic outcomes of patients with infection, especially when they are linked with other clinical information systems.
9. Laboratory tests such as minimal bactericidal concentration tests, timed-kill tests, post-antibiotic-effect tests, and antimicrobial combination testing are important for the clinician to understand because they help to determine an antimicrobial's pharmacodynamic properties.
10. Routine monitoring of serum concentrations is currently used for a select few antimicrobials (e.g., aminoglycosides, chloramphenicol, and vancomycin) in an attempt to minimize toxicity and maximize efficacy.
11. Appropriate timing for the collection of serum samples when measuring antimicrobial serum concentrations is crucial to ensure that proper data are generated on the pharmacokinetics of antimicrobials.
12. The monitoring of serum concentrations of aminoglycosides and the use of extended-interval doses of aminoglycosides can help to maximize the probability of therapeutic success and minimize the probability of aminoglycoside-related toxicity.
13. Vancomycin serum concentration monitoring should be routinely done to ensure adequate serum concentrations, minimize toxicity, and avoid the potential for resistance.
14. Optimization of antimicrobial pharmacodynamic parameters such as the ratio of the peak serum concentration to minimum inhibitory concentration or the time that the serum concentration remains above the minimum inhibitory concentration can improve infection treatment outcomes.

Learning objectives, review questions, and other resources can be found at **www.pharmacotherapyonline.com.**

Appropriate antimicrobial pharmacotherapy for a given infectious disease requires knowledge of the infecting pathogen, host characteristics, and the drug's expected activity against the pathogen. The most fundamental aspect of therapy starts with an appropriate diagnosis. A vast array of laboratory tests is available to assist the clinician in verifying the presence of infection and for monitoring the response to therapy. Although useful, these tests are subject to interpretation and cannot be substituted for sound clinical judgment. Organism susceptibility to the administered antimicrobials is key to determining the outcome from a patient's therapy. Host characteristics, however, such as immune status, infection-site location, and body-organ function, play a significant role in selecting the most appropriate antimicrobial for a given individual.[1] This chapter reviews the routine laboratory tests that are used to assist in the diagnosis and treatment of infection.

LABORATORY TESTS CONFIRMING THE PRESENCE OF INFECTION

NONSPECIFIC TESTS

Many tests are used by clinicians to determine whether a patient has an infection. Although no single test can prove that a patient is infected, when used in combination with clinical findings, tests are helpful to establish the diagnosis of infection. Because many tests are nonspecific, there are often factors other than infection that can cause a test to be reported as positive when no infection exists. Therefore, the importance of careful interpretation and sound clinical judgment cannot be overemphasized. This chapter reviews the commonly employed tests and their interpretation and application for the diagnosis and management of infection.

White Blood Cell Count and Differential

❶ Understanding the role of the white blood cell (WBC) in fighting infection is important in the diagnosis of infection, the selection of drug therapy, and the monitoring of patient progress. The major role of the WBC is to defend the body against invading organisms such as bacteria, viruses, and fungi. The normal range of the WBC is 4,500 to 10,000 cells/mm^3. WBCs usually are elevated in response to infection. The WBC count can become elevated in response to a number of noninfectious causes, including stress, inflammatory conditions such as rheumatoid arthritis, and leukemia or in response to certain drugs (e.g., corticosteroids).

WBCs are divided into two groups: the granulocytes, which have prominent cytoplasmic granules, and the agranulocytes, which lack granules. Polymorphonuclear (PMN) granulocytes are made up of neutrophils, basophils, and eosinophils. The two other classes of WBCs are the monocytes and lymphocytes. Neutrophils are the most common type of WBCs in the blood, comprising approximately 70% of the total WBC count. In response to infection, they leave the bloodstream and enter the tissue to interact with and phagocytize offending pathogens. Mature neutrophils sometimes are referred to as *segs* because of their segmented nucleus, which usually consists of two to five lobes. Immature neutrophils lack this segmented feature and are referred to as *bands.* During an acute infection, immature neutrophils, such as bands (single-lobed nucleus), are released from the bone marrow into the bloodstream at an increased rate, and the percentage of bands (usually 5%) can increase in relationship to mature cells. The change in the ratio of mature to immature cells is often referred to as a *shift to the left* because of the way the cells were counted by hand with a microscope and charted from immature to mature cells.

Leukocytosis is a normal host defense to infection and is an important adjunct to antimicrobial therapy. Unfortunately, bacterial infection is a common complication of neutropenia from cancer chemotherapy. These patients are incapable of increasing their WBCs in response to infection. In fact, susceptibility to infection in these patients is highly dependent on their WBC status. Patients with neutrophil counts of less than 500 cells/mm^3 are at high risk for the development of bacterial or fungal infections. The absence of leukocytosis also occurs in the elderly and in severe cases of sepsis.[2,3]

Lymphocytes comprise 15% to 40% of all WBCs and are of central importance to the immune system. Two functional types of lymphocytes are the T cell, which is involved in cell-mediated immunity, and the B cell, which produces antibodies involved in humoral immunity. Lymphocytosis frequently is associated with acute viral infections such as Epstein-Barr virus infection (mononucleosis) and Cytomegalovirus (CMV) infection and rarely with unusual bacterial infections (i.e., *Brucella* species infections).

T lymphocytes are characterized on the basis of function (type 1 or type 2) and on the basis of surface antigen. Most type 1 and type 2 T cells carry a T4 (CD4) marker that recognizes class II major histocompatibility complex (MHC) antigens, and most cytoxic T cells carry a T8 (CD8) marker that recognizes class I MHC antigens. A severe deficiency of CD4 cells is associated with human immunodeficiency virus (HIV) infection.[4] Malignancies also can adversely affect cellular immunity. Patients with Hodgkin's disease and other types of lymphoma exhibit defective cell-mediated immunity that predisposes them to a variety of infections, notably fungal diseases and infections by the *Listeria* species. Drug treatment with cytotoxic chemotherapy and corticosteroids also can have profound deleterious effects on cell-mediated immunity.[5] Defects in cell-mediated immune function can be demonstrated by a variety of simple laboratory tests, including quantification of lymphocytes on a routine complete blood cell count and skin testing for anergy. A more detailed investigation includes quantitative measurements of CD4+ and CD8+ cells. Monocytosis is correlated less frequently with acute bacterial infection, although its presence has been associated with the response of certain infections (e.g., tuberculosis) to chemotherapy. Eosinophilia can result from parasitic infection.[6] Figure 108–1 describes a number of cell types and their biologic function.

Other Tests

Some nonspecific laboratory tests are useful to support the diagnosis of infection. The inflammatory process initiated by an infection sets

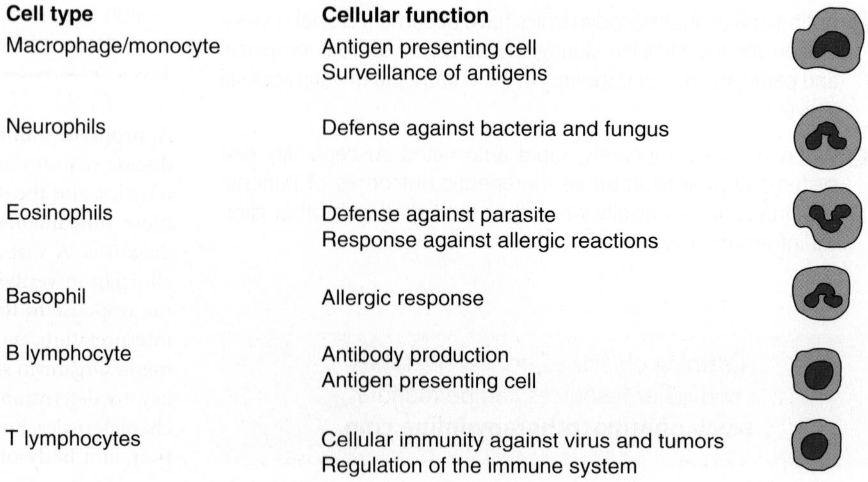

Cell type
Cellular function
Macrophage/monocyte
Antigen presenting cell
Surveillance of antigens
Neurophils
Defense against bacteria and fungus
Eosinophils
Defense against parasite
Response against allergic reactions
Basophil
Allergic response
B lymphocyte
Antibody production
Antigen presenting cell
T lymphocytes
Cellular immunity against virus and tumors
Regulation of the immune system

FIGURE 108-1. Various cell types and their biologic functions.

up a complex host response. Activation of complements, such as C3a and C5a, initiates inflammation and sets off a cascade of changes and the subsequent release of mediators, all of which can be measured and monitored. Serum complement concentrations, particularly C3, usually are consumed as part of the host defense mechanism and subsequently are reduced during the early stages of an acute infectious process.[7] Acute-phase reactants, such as the erythrocyte sedimentation rate (ESR) and the C-reactive protein concentration, are elevated in the presence of an inflammatory process but do not confirm the presence of infection because they are often elevated in noninfectious conditions, such as collagen-vascular diseases and arthritis. Large elevations in ESR are associated with infections such as endocarditis, osteomyelitis, and intraabdominal infections.[8,9]

Changes in endothelial membranes and the presence of a foreign pathogen and its endotoxins cause certain cytokines, such as interleukin 1 (IL-1), IL-6, and IL-8 and tumor necrosis factor-α (TNF-α), to be produced by macrophages or lymphocytes. Fluctuations in cytokine levels occur during the course of an infection, which can be useful in staging and monitoring the response to therapy. Although abnormally high levels of TNF have been associated with a variety of noninfectious causes, spiked elevations in TNF are found in patients with serious infections, such as sepsis. Studies of the relationship of circulating mediators to patient outcome have determined the value of endotoxin and cytokine measurements in patients with sepsis. Although the combination of elevations in endotoxin and individual cytokines has correlated well with the mortality rate, measurement of IL-6 was by far the best individual cytokine that predicted patient outcome.[9] There is a significant relationship between monocyte human leukocyte antigen (HLA)-DR expression and the risk of mortality in patients with community-acquired severe infections.[10] Understanding the balance between these proinflammatory and antiinflammatory processes likely will lead to interventions that can have a direct impact on the outcome of patients with sepsis.[11]

LABORATORY IDENTIFICATION OF PATHOGENS

COLONIZATION VERSUS INFECTION

❷ Pathogens are organisms that are capable of damaging host tissues and that elicit specific host responses and symptoms that are consistent with an infectious process. These organisms are transferred from patient to patient, vector to patient (animals, insects, and so on), environment to patient (e.g., hospital settings) or are derived from the patient's own flora. Conversely, the human body contains a vast variety of microorganisms that colonize body systems and make up the so-called *normal* flora. These organisms occur naturally in the tissues of the host and provide some benefits, including defense by occupying space, competing for essential nutrients, stimulating cross-protective antibodies, and suppressing the growth of potentially pathogenic bacteria and fungi (Table 108–1).

Organisms that comprise the normal flora can become pathogenic when host defenses become impaired or if they are translocated to other body sites during trauma. The identification of an organism that is considered to be normal flora in a wound or otherwise sterile body cavity or fluid often becomes a dilemma for the clinician in deciding whether or not a patient is infected and whether or not the patient requires treatment. Such is the case with *Staphylococcus epidermidis* when it is identified in the blood of a hospitalized patient. *S. epidermidis* is considered normal skin flora and commonly colonizes intravenous catheters. In these conditions, identification of the organism must be taken in light of the patient circumstances (signs and symptoms, laboratory indices supporting infection) and the probability of the organism being responsible for the infection. Often the simple removal of the catheter can eliminate the organism from the bloodstream, thereby preventing misdiagnosis and unnecessary application of antimicrobials.[12]

DIRECT EXAMINATION

❸ Direct examination of tissue or body fluids believed to be infected can provide simple, rapid information to the clinician. Microscopic examination of wet-mount specimen preparations can provide valuable information regarding potential pathogens. Applications of this procedure with or without staining preparations include direct examination of sputum, bronchial aspirates, scrapings of mucosal lesions, and urinary sediment. The Gram stain is one of the first identification tests run on a specimen brought to the laboratory. For this procedure, crystal violet is applied as the primary stain, with iodine added to enhance the staining process and to form a crystal violet–iodine complex. Alcohol decolorization is the next step in the procedure. Gram-negative cells are decolorized by the addition of alcohol, and they take in a red color when counterstained by safranin. Gram-positive cells are not decolorized by alcohol and retain the crystal violet color and appear purple. Gram staining in conjunction with microscopic examination can provide a presumptive diagnosis and some indication of the organism's characteristics (gram-positive, gram-negative, gram-variable, bacillus, or cocci). This is extremely useful information for the selection of empirical antibiotic therapy.

Gram stains are performed routinely on cerebrospinal fluid (CSF) in cases of suspected meningitis, on urethral smears for venereal diseases, and on abscess or effusion specimens. They are helpful in identifying organisms that may not grow on culture and which otherwise would be missed. Although Gram stains of sputum are performed routinely when respiratory tract infections are suspected, there is controversy regarding the usefulness of this test because the sputum is often contaminated with mixed or normal flora. The predominance of one particular organism, the overall number of organisms present, the amount of PMN granulocyte present, and the presence or absence of a significant amount of squamous epithelial cells (<10 per low-power field) can improve the significance of the sputum Gram stain specimen. Figure 108–2 lists some common infecting pathogens grouped according to Gram stain and other characteristics.

Other staining techniques are used to identify pathogens such as those that are best identified microscopically because of their poor growth characteristics in the laboratory setting. The best examples

TABLE 108-1 Examples of Normal Bacterial Flora

	Gram-Positive		Gram-Negative		
	Cocci	***Rods***	***Cocci***	***Rods***	***Other***
Skin	*Staphylococcus* spp. (e.g., *S. epidermidis*), *Streptococcus* spp.	*Corynebacterium* spp., *Propionibacterium* spp.		Enteric bacilli (some sites), *Acinetobacter* spp. (Coccobacilli)	
Oropharynx	Streptococci–viridans group Micrococcus	*Corynebacterium* spp.	Neisseria	*Haemophilus* spp.	Spirochetes
Gastrointenstinal tract	*Enterococcus* spp., *Peptostreptococcus* spp.	*Lactobacillus, Clostridium*		*Bacteroides* spp., Enteric bacilli (*E. coli, Klebsiella* spp.)	
Genital tract	*Streptococcus* spp., *Staphylococcus* spp.	*Lactobacillus, Corynebacterium* spp.		Enterobacteriaceae, *Prevotella* spp.	*Mycoplasma*

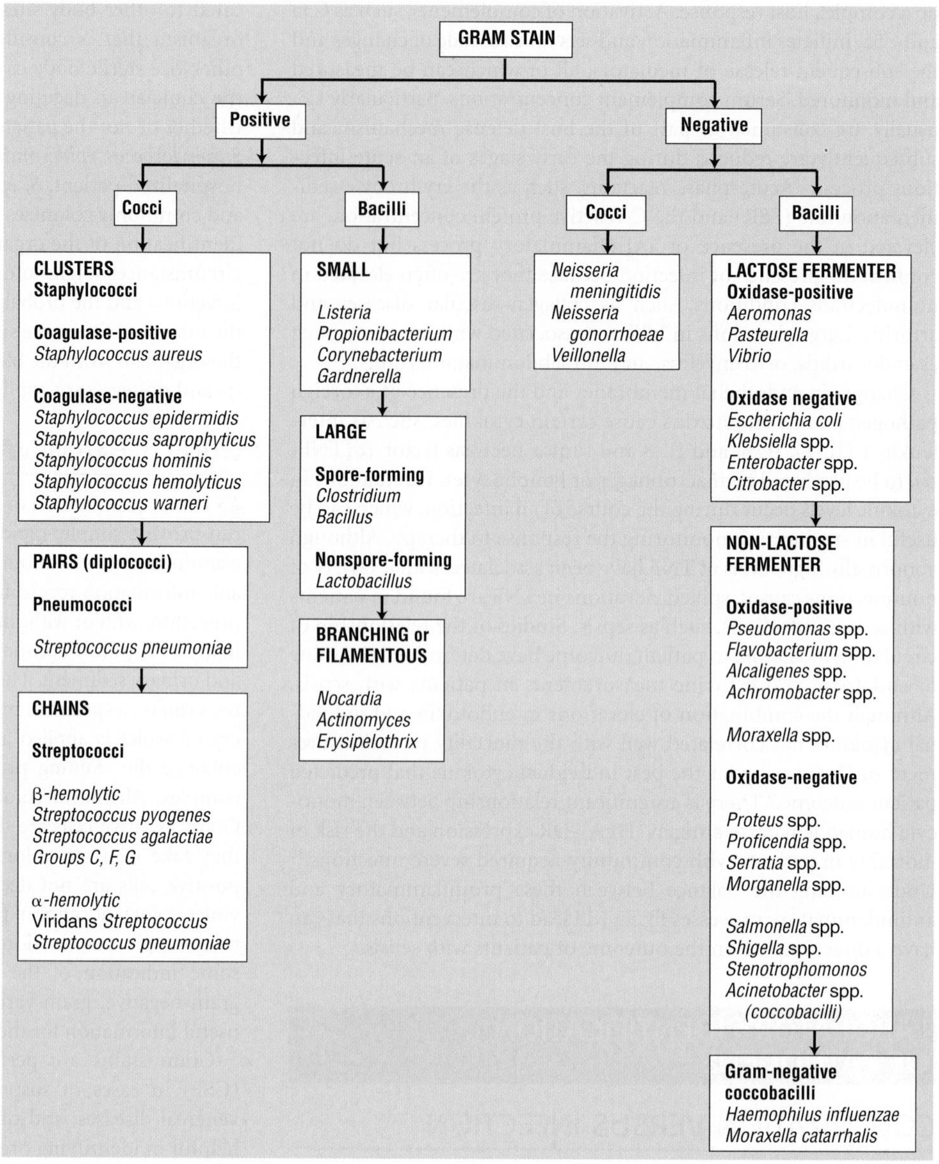

FIGURE 108-2. Important bacterial pathogens classified according to Gram stain and morphologic characteristic.

of these are the Ziehl-Neelsen stain for acid-fast bacilli, which is used for the identification of mycobacteria, and the India ink, potassium hydroxide (KOH), and Giemsa stains, which are useful for detecting certain fungi.[13]

CULTURES

❹ Isolation of the etiologic agent by culture is the most definitive method available for the diagnosis and eventual treatment of infection. Although suspicion of a specific pathogen or group of pathogens is helpful to the laboratory for the selection of a specific cultivating medium, the more common procedure for the laboratory is to screen for the presence of any potential pathogen. After receipt of a clinical specimen, the laboratory will inoculate the specimen in a variety of artificial media. Some culture media are designed to differentiate various organisms on the basis of biochemical characteristics or to select specific organisms on the basis of resistance to certain antimicrobials. Other media are employed commonly for the isolation of more fastidious organisms, such as *Listeria, Legionella, Mycobacterium,* or *Chlamydia.* Cultures for viruses are more difficult to perform and are undertaken primarily by larger institutions or outside laboratories because of the technical expense and time involved in processing samples.

When a culture is obtained, careful attention must be paid to ensuring that specimens are collected and transported appropriately to the laboratory. Every effort should be made to avoid contamination with normal flora and to ensure that the specimen is placed in the appropriate transport medium. Culture specimens should be transported to the laboratory as soon as possible because organisms can perish from prolonged exposure to air or drying. This is especially important for swab specimen preparations. Transport media may not be ideal for all organisms. Specimens that contain fastidious organisms or anaerobes require special transport media and should be forwarded immediately to the laboratory for processing. Finally, the source of the specimen should be clearly recorded and forwarded along with the culture to the laboratory. This process will aid the laboratory in differentiating true pathogens from the expected normal flora, and it will help in the selection of the appropriate culture media. Detection of microorganisms in the bloodstream by standard culturing techniques is difficult because of the inherently low yield of organisms diluted by blood, humoral factors with bactericidal activity, and the potential of antimicrobial pretreatment affecting organism growth. Newer automated systems employing the use of medium-containing culture bottles and innovative organism-detection techniques have improved this situation. Most blood collection bottles dilute the blood specimen 1:10 with growth medium to neutralize the bactericidal properties of blood and antimicrobials. The addition of a polyanionic anticoagulant abolishes the effect of complement and antiphagocytic activity in the specimen. Some laboratories also add β-lactamase to their blood collection bottles. Antibiotic-binding resin bottles, such as BACTEC 16B, are also commercially available. Rapid detection of bacteria or fungi within a few hours of specimen collection is now possible by the use of automated culturing systems, such as BACTEC (Becton Dickinson Diagnostic Instruments, Sparks, MD), that use bottles of growth medium containing a fluorescent sensor to monitor culture bottles for the presence of carbon dioxide (CO_2) every 10 minutes as a by-product of microorganism growth. Computers monitoring the system alert laboratory personnel of positive culture results by both audible and visual alarms. Once detected, a battery of testing can be performed rapidly that shortens the reporting time and that enables clinicians to obtain preliminary information about the organism.[13,14] The initial identity of the organism can be determined by a variety of testing procedures. General schemes differentiate organisms into primary groups, such as gram-positive and gram-negative bacteria. This can be accomplished by simple Gram staining, as described previously, by evaluating organism growth patterns on selective media, and by testing for the presence or absence of specific enzymes and chemical characteristics, such as hemolytic and fermentation properties. For example, non–lactose-fermenting gram-negative bacilli that are oxidase-positive can suggest *Pseudomonas aeruginosa* as opposed to a variety of other potential gram-negative organisms. This preliminary information, which is readily obtainable from the laboratory, can greatly assist the clinician in choosing the appropriate empirical therapy. Definitive identification of organisms requires more complex testing procedures and devices that can further differentiate the organism on the basis of specific fermentation and biochemical reactive properties. Commercially available automated systems can inoculate the test organism into a series of panels containing a variety of test media, sugars, and other reagents. The system can then photometrically determine the results and compare the findings to a library of organism characteristics to produce a definitive identification.[14] Viral agents can be detected by direct observation of inoculated culture cells for cytopathic effects or by detection of antigens after incubation by immunofluorescent methods. The culture method is most useful for organisms such as CMV or herpes simplex virus because these viral agents are rapidly propagated in culture cells, making them easily detected.[15]

DIAGNOSIS OF INFECTION USING IMMUNOLOGIC AND MOLECULAR METHODS

ANTIBODY AND ANTIGEN DETECTION

❺ The use of immunologic methods for the diagnosis and monitoring of human host immune response to infection has become an indispensable laboratory tool. This is especially important in the detection of microorganisms, such as bacteria, fungi, and viruses, that otherwise would elude detection or severely delay results from conventional culturing techniques. These methods have the advantage of a rapid turnaround time and an acceptable level of sensitivity and specificity. Some tests (e.g., identification of group A streptococci) are simple to use, can be performed conveniently in the physician's office, and often can be used to decide whether antibiotics should be administered for a suspected upper respiratory infection.

The primary immunologic methods involve the detection and quantification of antibodies directed against a specific pathogen or its components (i.e., surface proteins of HIV, such as p24 antigen). The commercial availability of specific monoclonal antibodies in a variety of testing formats has led to an increased use of these methods for direct pathogen detection. Although pathogen antigenic proteins can be increased and, therefore, detected easily during acute infection, detection of past or asymptomatic infection can be difficult because of undetectable levels of antigen and, therefore, low antibody titers. Continued advancement in test sensitivity (the capability to detect a true-positive state) and specificity (the capability to detect a negative state), as well as the use of amplification techniques, likely will improve these tests in the near future.

Antibody or antigen detection can be accomplished by a variety of techniques, including immunofluorescence, which has been used routinely for the detection of CMV, respiratory syncytial virus, varicella-zoster virus, *Treponema pallidum* (syphilis), *Borrelia burgdorferi* (Lyme disease), and *Chlamydia trachomatis.* Latex agglutination is useful for detecting meningococcal capsular antigens in CSF of patients suspected of having bacterial meningitis and as an aid in the diagnosis of *Legionella pneumophila.* Enzyme-linked immunosorbent assay (ELISA) is a commonly employed method for detecting HIV, herpes simplex virus, respiratory syncytial virus, pneumococcal serum antibody, *Neisseria gonorrhoeae,* and *Haemophilus pylori.*[15]

MOLECULAR TECHNIQUES FOR THE DETECTION OF MICROORGANISMS

Hybridization DNA Probes

Highly sensitive and specific molecular methods are now available for the rapid detection and identification of a variety of pathogens. The two primary molecular techniques used commonly are nucleic acid hybridization, which involves the binding of a specific DNA or RNA probe to its target, and DNA amplification schemes. Probe-based methods require the extraction of DNA or RNA from a clinical specimen (i.e., body fluid, tissue, or WBC) or directly from a microorganism culture. The extract is then tested for the presence of pathogen DNA or RNA using a probe that contains a specific oligonucleic acid–based sequence for the organism. For example, a probe with a sequence of ACTGTT would bind to the complementary organism nucleic acid sequence of TGACAA. Because the probe is labeled with a signal-emitting molecule (i.e., radiolabeled, colorimetric, or chemoluminescent), a match would be detected. The primary means for detection involves the use of separation of the organism DNA into specific fragments (gel electrophoresis), transfer and fixation of the mixture to specialized paper or nylon membranes (Southern or Northern blotting), the mixing of the DNA fragments with the labeled probe (hybridization), and transfer to radiographic or photographic film for processing. These techniques have been used for many years and are fairly standardized methods for the detection of a variety of organisms. Hybridization probes are useful for a variety of diagnostic and clinical applications, including the direct examination of organisms in tissue, which enables the evaluation and documentation of organism infestation, location, distribution, and host response. The use of hybridization probes is particularly helpful for the detection of slow-growing organisms such as *Mycobacterium tuberculosis, N. gonorrhoeae,* and certain species of fungi. This technique is also used to document the presence or absence of antimicrobial-resistant genes in a cell culture and to track the spread of resistant microorganisms in hospital and outpatient settings. Although employed widely, the use of hybridization probes is often limited by their lack of sensitivity. Probe amplification methods are available that improve the sensitivity of these assays. The principle of these probe-amplification schemes is to boost the probe's signal-emitting molecule to make it more easily detected. The most advanced signal-amplification system available is the branched DNA (bDNA) probe system (Chiron Corp., Emeryville, CA). This system uses multiple probes and multiple signal-emitting molecules (reporters). The target-binding probe contains two hybridization regions. One region is complementary to the target, and the other region is capable of binding with the bDNA amplification multimer. The amplification multimer binds multiple reporter molecules (as many as 3,000), which provides a significant boost in the probe's signal. Branched DNA probe systems are being developed for rapid detection of hepatitis B and C, HIV-1, and CMV. Because of the system's high specificity and quantitative ability, bDNA probe assays can be useful for therapeutic monitoring, such as in the case of monitoring the response to antiretroviral therapy in acquired immunodeficiency syndrome (AIDS).[16,17]

Nucleic Acid Amplification Methods

Nucleic acid amplification methods are now considered a standard laboratory tool. They have had a tremendous impact on the diagnosis and treatment of infectious diseases. These highly sensitive methods have the capability to detect and quantitate minute amounts of target nucleic acid in a rapid manner. The polymerase chain reaction (PCR) is based on the capability of a DNA polymerase to copy and elongate a targeted strand of DNA. This is accomplished by the use of short oligonucleotide primers (20 to 25 nucleotides long) that correspond to the DNA targeted to be expanded. After an excess of primers and heat-stable DNA polymerases are added to the targeted DNA mixture, the targeted DNA is denatured and separated by a process of cycling hot and cool temperatures. The heat-stable DNA polymerase elongates the primers on the two separate strands of DNA, thereby generating two new strands of targeted DNA. The process of cycling typically is repeated 20 to 35 times. Each cycle doubles the amount of DNA originally present at the start of the cycle, thereby exponentially increasing the overall number of DNA copies. In theory, more than 1 million copies of the original DNA can be generated from as few as 20 cycles. Although this amplification technique is very sensitive and has tremendous application potential, it is not without problems. The powerful amplification procedure can yield false-positive results when samples are contaminated by nucleic acid left over from previously amplified DNA. Other problems include primer artifact formation and nonspecific hybridization of primers to DNA samples. Several modifications to the original PCR technology have been made over the years to improve the sensitivity and application potential for PCR, including the use of multiple sets of amplification primers, multiplex PCR, PCR amplification of RNA by converting targeted RNA with reverse transcriptase to complementary DNA templates (which are then suitable for DNA amplification by traditional PCR techniques), and real-time quantitative PCR. The cost-benefit ratio of PCR as compared with traditional microbiologic methods must be evaluated. Molecular amplification schemes such as PCR have become routine in situations in which rapid turnaround time is essential to improve patient diagnosis and outcome, for example, real-time universal screening for acute HIV infection and routine testing and monitoring of patients receiving treatment for HIV infection, and the isolation and detection of fastidious or slow-growing organisms such as *M. tuberculosis, B. burgdorferi,* and *Helicobacter pylori.* Another potential application for this technology is the early detection of multidrug-resistant organisms. Amplification of resistant gene markers would aid in rapid selection of the most appropriate therapy in the treatment of organisms in which days or weeks traditionally are required for culturing and determining basic susceptibility. Examples fitting this description include the rapid detection of isoniazid and rifampin gene markers for *M. tuberculosis,* early detection of the *mec* gene responsible for methicillin resistance in *Staphylococcus aureus,* and identification of resistant genes responsible for production of β-lactamase capable of destroying specific cephalosporins and multidrug resistant *H. pylori.*[17–20]

EVALUATION OF ANTIMICROBIAL ACTIVITY AND DETERMINATION OF ANTIMICROBIAL PHARMACODYNAMICS

❻ The laboratory evaluation of antimicrobial activity is an important component of the pharmacotherapeutic management of infectious diseases. The integration of this activity with various pharmacokinetic properties of the antimicrobial agent determines the ❼ drug's pharmacodynamic characteristics. Antimicrobial pharmacodynamics have become a crucial consideration for the clinician for selecting both empirical and pathogen-directed therapy, formulary decision-making, developing antimicrobial streamlining programs, and for intravenous-to-oral antimicrobial switch protocols.

❺ Most antimicrobial susceptibility testing methods that are used in the clinical laboratory are well characterized and have been standardized by the Clinical and Laboratory Standards Institute (CLSI). However, controversies exist about which test methods provide the most useful information, how to report these results, and how to apply them to the treatment of patients.[21] Nevertheless, there are many investigations that show that the general antimicrobial susceptibility or resistance profile of an infecting organism correlates with clinical and/or microbiologic responses to therapy.

Most of the standardized and well-accepted test methods evaluate the susceptibility of aerobic, nonfastidious bacteria. However, substantial progress has been made to develop sensitive, specific, reproducible, and clinically useful susceptibility tests for anaerobic bacteria, yeasts, mycobacteria, and viruses. Continued advances in technology should further improve test methods and the rapidity with which the results can be applied to the management of patients. Although these newer systems are often very expensive, the increased quality and decreased overall costs of patient care can determine their cost-effectiveness.

QUANTITATIVE ANTIMICROBIAL SUSCEPTIBILITY TESTING

MINIMAL INHIBITORY CONCENTRATIONS

The *minimal inhibitory concentration* (MIC) is defined as the lowest antimicrobial concentration that prevents visible growth of an organism after approximately 24 hours of incubation in a specified growth medium. The MIC quantitatively determines in-vitro antibacterial activity. Classically, MICs were determined through the macrotube dilution method, which uses liquid growth medium (broth), doubling serial dilutions of antimicrobials in test tubes, and a standard inoculum of bacteria (approximately 10^5 colony-forming units [CFU]/mL). The tubes (up to 10 mL) were incubated at approximately 35°C (95°F) for 18 to 24 hours and then examined for visible bacterial growth (Fig. 108–3). Because macrodilution MIC testing is laborious and supply-intensive, it is not used often in the contemporary clinical microbiology laboratory. However, one advantage of this method is that it tests a large inoculum of bacteria—a factor that can improve the detection of small numbers of resistant subpopulations or document the presence of inducible resistance.[22]

The use of 96-well microtiter plates substantially reduces the amount of growth medium and preparation time needed for broth-dilution MIC testing in the clinical laboratory. Volumes of 100 to 200 microliters (mcL) or less of medium are used, and multichannel pipets and/or automated systems allow efficient preparation of numerous tests (Fig. 108–4). The microdilution MIC test method is currently the most commonly-used susceptibility test method in the clinical microbiology laboratory. Although microdilution MIC testing is a vast improvement over macrodilution MIC testing, it still has important shortcomings. These include both limitations in the

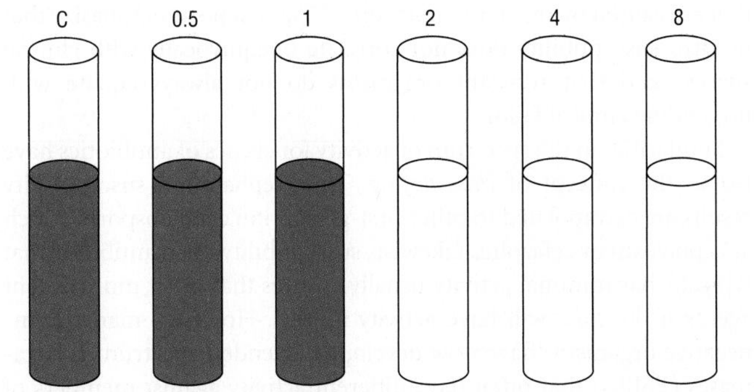

FIGURE 108-3. Macrotube minimal inhibitory concentration (MIC) determination. The growth control *(C)*, 0.5 mg/L, and 1 mg/L tubes are visibly turbid, indicating bacterial growth. The MIC is read as the first clear test tube (2 mg/L).

numbers and various types of antimicrobials to use in the test (especially with premade or premanufactured trays) and a limited ability to detect some forms of antimicrobial resistance (e.g., β-lactamases in gram-negative bacteria).[23]

The MIC also can be determined using solid agar growth medium. For the agar dilution MICs, the test antimicrobial is added to the molten agar at the desired concentration just prior to its solidification. After the agar has hardened, suspensions of test bacteria are applied to the agar. As with broth MICs, the agar dilution MIC is defined as the lowest concentration that prevents the visible growth of the organism after an overnight incubation period. The primary advantages of the agar dilution MICs are the ability to test many bacteria on the same agar plate and the flexibility to choose specific antimicrobials. These advantages often are outweighed by the need to prepare agar plates manually and the instability of the antimicrobial in the agar as compared with commercially prepared microtiter MIC trays. Although agar dilution MIC once was considered the standard susceptibility test for many bacteria and for certain slow-growing organisms such as *M. tuberculosis*, its use has declined in most clinical laboratories with the advent of more rapidly performed and less cumbersome susceptibility testing methods (e.g., microtiter MICs, PCR, radiometric, and/or fluorometric tests).

LIMITATIONS AND PROBLEMS WITH MIC TESTING

Some of the limitations and problems of MIC testing are academic in nature, whereas others can have important implications for the clinician's everyday management of patients with serious infections. For example, because the MIC only represents the concentration of antimicrobial that is needed to inhibit visual growth of the most resistant cells within the tested bacterial population, there can be small numbers of cells present within the large numbers of cells within the infection that are more antimicrobial-resistant than the MIC would indicate. Use of the antimicrobial then could select these more resistant subpopulations, resulting in poor clinical response. This phenomenon can be observed with intermediate vancomycin resistance in *S. aureus*, as well as in strains of gram-negative bacteria such as the *Enterobacteriaceae* species that produce both plasmid-borne and chromosomal β-lactamases.[23,24]

❽ Many other factors also can influence the in-vitro MIC value obtained and its subsequent application to the in-vivo situation. The bacterial growth medium used and cation content can affect the activity of many drugs significantly. For example, aminoglycosides are more active against *P. aeruginosa* in a medium supplemented with physiologic concentrations of magnesium and calcium (CLSI standardized method) than in a medium without these cations. MIC values of antibiotics that are highly bound to plasma proteins are significantly higher when the test medium contains human serum. As testing of these drugs in a serum-supplemented medium has not gained widespread acceptance, their in-vivo activity can be overestimated by in-vitro MIC test results. Fortunately, the standardized guidelines for testing and quality assurance procedures proposed by the CLSI attempt to minimize the impact of these problems and are followed by most clinical and research laboratories.[25] However, when a patient infected with an apparently susceptible organism fails therapy, it is important for the clinician to consider these potential confounding factors as possibly being related to the observed failure. In such situations, consideration of antimicrobial pharmacokinetics and pharmacodynamics also often can help to better predict therapeutic response as compared with organism susceptibility alone.

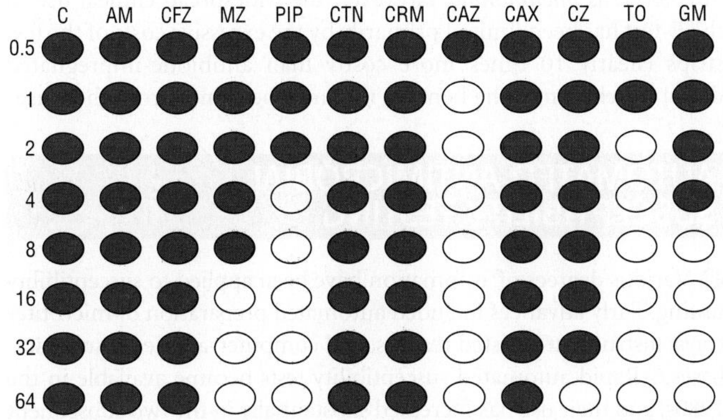

FIGURE 108-4. A prepared microtiter minimal inhibitory concentration (MIC) panel represents antibiotics tested commonly against gram-negative pathogens. This tray indicates that the organism is resistant to ampicillin (AM), cefazolin (CFZ), cefotetan (CTN), cefuroxime (CRM), ceftriaxone (CAX), and gentamicin (GM). The isolate is susceptible to mezlocillin (MZ), piperacillin (PIP), ceftazidime (CAZ), and tobramycin (TO). The isolate would be considered intermediately susceptible to ceftizoxime (CZ).

QUALITATIVE ANTIMICROBIAL SUSCEPTIBILITY TEST METHODS

DISK DIFFUSION ASSAY

The disk diffusion assay method for susceptibility testing (Bauer-Kirby method) was developed in the 1960s by Bauer and coworkers as a way to reduce the labor needed for tube dilution susceptibility testing.[26] It still remains one of the more common susceptibility test methods used in the clinical microbiology laboratory owing to its high degree of standardization, reliability, flexibility, low cost, and simplicity of test interpretation. Up to 12 user-selected antibiotic-impregnated disks are placed on an agar plate previously streaked with a standard suspension of bacteria (1–2 × 10^8 CFU/mL). The drug contained in the disk diffuses in a concentration gradient out into the agar. The plate is incubated (18 to 24 hours at 35°C), and visual bacterial growth occurs only in areas in which the drug concentrations are below those required for growth inhibition. The diameters of the zones of inhibition are measured via calipers or automated scanners and are compared with standard zone size ranges that determine susceptibility, intermediate susceptibility, or resistance to the antimicrobials that were tested (Fig. 108–5). Although factors such as agar composition, incubation temperature, bacterial inoculum, and antibiotic paper disk composition can influence results, the standards for testing conditions and interpretive zone sizes are well defined by the CLSI.

QUALITATIVE VERSUS QUANTITATIVE SUSCEPTIBILITY TESTING OF MICROORGANISMS

Quantitative MIC data often are reported to the clinician qualitatively by deeming an organism "susceptible," "intermediate or

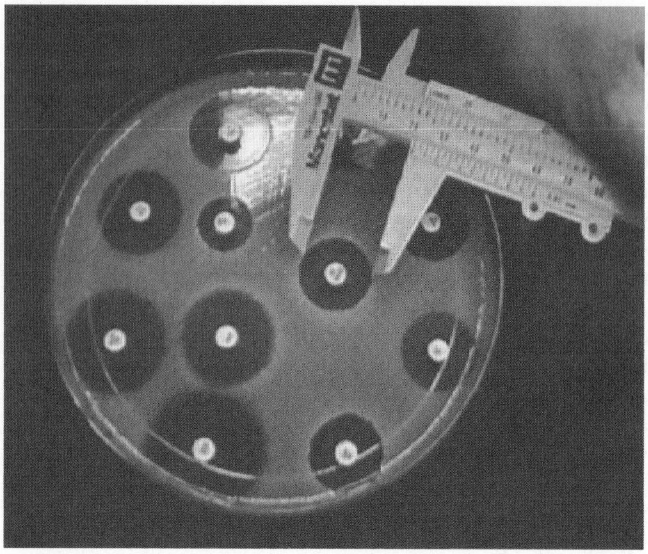

FIGURE 108-5. Disk diffusion susceptibility test. Antibiotic-impregnated disks are placed on the surface of a plate previously inoculated with the test organism. The plate is incubated for 18 hours, and the subsequent zones of inhibition are measured. The zone size correlates with the sensitivity of the organism. The larger the zone, the more sensitive is the organism to the specific antibiotic. On the basis of predetermined zone breakpoints, organisms can be classified as susceptible, resistant, or intermediately susceptible to the antibiotic. *(Photograph courtesy of the Anti-Infective Research Laboratory, Wayne State University, Detroit, Michigan.)*

indeterminate" or "moderately susceptible," or "resistant" to a given antimicrobial agent. Many factors are considered to determine these qualitative susceptibility classifications, including pharmacokinetic properties, the distribution of MICs for the organisms, and the clinical and bacteriologic responses observed for the antimicrobial against strains of bacteria with various MIC values This simplification makes the susceptibility data easily interpretable by non–infectious-disease clinicians. Pathogens classified as susceptible to an antibiotic are those with the lowest MICs, and they are the most likely to be eradicated during therapy of infections using typical drug doses. Conversely, resistant organisms are bacteria with significantly higher MICs that, when treated with the antimicrobial, will result in a less-than-optimal clinical response, even at the highest doses. The indeterminate classification exists when the number of strains with MICs in the given range is too small to derive robust conclusions on susceptibility or resistance to the antimicrobial. Responses to therapy for organisms that are moderately susceptible/intermediately susceptible/indeterminate can be variable. These organisms can respond to treatment with maximal doses of the antimicrobial or can respond when the drug is known to be concentrated at the site of infection (e.g., urinary tract infections treated by drugs excreted by the kidneys).

There are concerns that the "user friendly" susceptible/resistant classification system can oversimplify the decision-making process for treating infections. For example, a critically ill patient may not respond to the antimicrobial therapy of a susceptible organism at the usual doses. If serum concentrations or concentrations at the site of infection could be assayed (not practically done), one might discover suboptimal concentrations as a result of inadequate tissue perfusion. Likewise, a patient with severe vascular insufficiency and a diabetic foot infection may fail a course of therapy with normal doses of an antimicrobial and a susceptible organism because of inadequate drug delivery. Additionally, some investigators have shown that different outcomes can be achieved for "susceptible" organisms with different MIC values[27] and also that substantial (although not clinically acceptable) clinical and/or microbiologic cure rates can occur for infections that are caused by resistant organisms.[28] These reports emphasize that in-vitro susceptibility does not correlate unequivocally with clinical success and that resistant organisms do not always equate with impending clinical failure.

Similarities in the spectrum of activity for classes of antibiotics have led to the concept of *class testing.* Thus cephalothin susceptibility results are extrapolated to other first-generation cephalosporins, such as cephalexin or cefazolin. Likewise, susceptibility to an antibiotic that typically has minimal activity usually ensures that other more potent agents in its class will have activity as well. However, many gram-negative organisms have now developed extended-spectrum β-lactamases (ESBLs) that often have different activity against members of the same drug class. These developments significantly limit the utility of class testing to reduce susceptibility testing workload.

CLINICAL CONTROVERSY

Some clinicians believe that the MICs of all antimicrobials for which susceptibility testing was performed should be reported to allow for proper selection of the best antimicrobial for a given infection in a patient. However, other clinicians argue that the additional information can be misapplied or that the nonselective reporting of all antimicrobial susceptibility data will result in the increased use of more costly broad-spectrum antimicrobials.

OTHER SUSCEPTIBILITY TESTS

EPSILOMETER TEST

8 The Epsilometer test (Etest; AB Biodisk, Solna, Sweden) combines the benefits of quantitative MIC test methods with the ease of agar diffusion testing. The E-test is a plastic strip impregnated with a known, prefixed concentration gradient of antibiotic that is placed on an agar plate streaked with a suspension of known bacterial inoculum. The drug instantly diffuses from the plastic strip to form an effective concentration gradient within the agar. After overnight incubation, elliptical zones of inhibition are formed; the point where the bottom of the ellipse crosses the plastic strip is correlated with an MIC value printed on the strip (Fig. 108–6). Many investigators have analyzed the E-test's correlation with standard susceptibility methods and assessed its potential clinical use. In general, values obtained with E-test methods are comparable with or even more consistent and accurate than standard methods. In fact, the E-test method is the recommended method for susceptibility testing of *Streptococcus pneumoniae.* However, the widespread clinical use of the E-test has been limited primarily by the excessive costs of the test strips (nearly 10 times more costly than antibiotic-impregnated disks) in relation to the benefits that may be gained from their use.

AUTOMATED ANTIMICROBIAL SUSCEPTIBILITY TESTING

8 Various degrees of automation have been applied to susceptibility testing. Early advances included automated preparation of microtiter trays, instrument-assisted readers, and computer-assisted result databases.[29] Rapid automated susceptibility tests became available in the 1980s, and their use has increased substantially in the two subsequent decades. These systems often incorporate microprocessors, robotics, and microcomputers to rapidly identify organisms and produce susceptibility test results in as few as 3 hours.

There are two rapid automated susceptibility test systems in common use in clinical microbiology laboratories. The Vitek system (bioMerieux Vitek, Hazelwood, MO) uses small plastic reagent "cards" that contain 30 or 45 wells for the testing of various antimi-

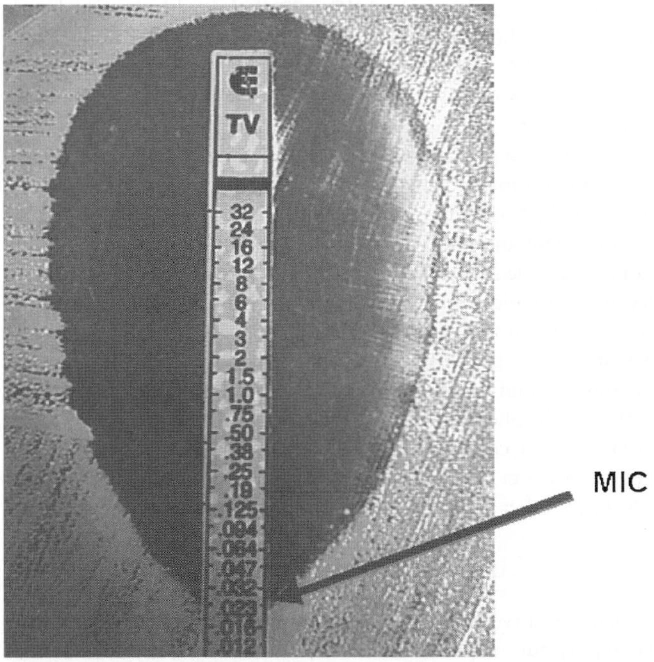

FIGURE 108-6. Photograph of E-test susceptibility strip. The minimal inhibitory concentration (MIC) is determined from the point where the zone of inhibition intersects with the numerical scale. *(Photograph courtesy of the Anti-Infective Research Laboratory, Wayne State University, Detroit, Michigan.)*

crobials or indicator chemicals. Bacterial test suspensions (25 mcL total, providing 1×10^5 CFU/well) enter the wells by capillary diffusion, and growth is monitored automatically via photometric assessment of turbidity every hour for up to 15 hours. When the growth control reaches a specified turbidity level, growth curves for all wells are calculated and compared with the growth control curve for slope normalization. Computerized linear regression and the use of best-fit line coefficients produce an algorithm-derived MIC. The clinical laboratory can control the result output that is generated (qualitative susceptibility, quantitative susceptibility, or both).

The Microscan Walkaway system (Dade Microscan, West Sacramento, CA) is a rapid test system that uses fluorogenic substrate hydrolysis as an indicator of bacterial growth. This system uses standard microdilution test trays and a computer-controlled incubator and reader unit that can perform robotic manipulations, such as reagent addition and tray rotation, to allow for spectrophotometric or fluorometric growth assessments. Bacterial inocula (approximately 6×10^4 CFU/well for gram-negative organisms and approximately 10^5 CFU/well for gram-positive organisms are added to the wells), and growth is detected by the production of fluorophores from hydrolysis of amidomethylcoumarin or methylumbelliferyl fluorogenic substrates. Although this method is a more sensitive assessment of growth as compared with turbidity, its indirect nature allows for the possibility of bacterial growth without hydrolysis of the fluorophores; this occurrence is rare, however. As with the Vitek system, growth curves are generated, and algorithms applied for the determination of MICs; output is via computer or video display.

❽ The results obtained from both systems are comparable. Both the Vitek and Walkaway systems also contain information management systems that allow for the storage and rapid retrieval of susceptibility data. Both systems are also capable of producing chartable patient data reports, antibiograms, and epidemiologic reports. Importantly, these systems can be interfaced with other clinical information systems, such as the pharmacy, infection control, or other laboratory data systems, which can help to improve clinical outcomes.[30]

ADVANCES IN SUSCEPTIBILITY TESTING FOR MYCOBACTERIA, FUNGI, AND VIRUSES

Impressive advances have been made in the past decade in the areas of mycobacterial, fungal, and viral susceptibility testing. The use of radiometric techniques, such as the BACTEC TB460 system (Becton Dickinson Biosciences, Sparks, MD), has revolutionized the analysis of antimicrobial susceptibility for *M. tuberculosis* and other slow-growing mycobacteria.[31] Radiometric susceptibility testing involves the incubation of *M. tuberculosis* in liquid medium containing carbon-14 (^{14}C)-labeled growth substrate. As organisms grow, respiration causes the release of ^{14}C, which is then detected. The growth indices for antimicrobial-containing bottles are compared with those of a control bottle with the calculation of an MIC. Use of this method, when coupled with the rapid processing of samples, can reduce the time to susceptibility result generation to approximately 1 week. A newer mycobacterial susceptibility testing method (the BACTEC Mycobacteria Growth Indicator Tube [MGIT 960], Becton Dickinson Diagnostic Instruments, Sparks, MD) that is fully automated and that employs detection of fluorescence related to growth also has been developed; it produces results in a similar time frame and with similar reliability as the radiometric method.[32] Primary advantages of this system are its automation, the elimination of radioactivity, and the elimination of needle use. Although the slower agar proportion susceptibility method (generating results in approximately 1 month) is still considered the reference standard for mycobacterial susceptibility testing by the CLSI, the group now recommends the use of a rapid susceptibility testing method to ensure that the Centers for Disease Control and Prevention (CDC) guidelines for reporting susceptibility results for *M. tuberculosis* infections within 28 days of specimen receipt in the laboratory can be met.[33] In the future, the use of molecular probes for mycobacterial resistance genes most likely will become a more important component of mycobacterial susceptibility determinations, especially in light of the increasing problems with antimicrobial resistance.[34]

There has been a substantial increase in the prevalence of fungal infections in the past two decades. An increase in the development and use of newer antifungal agents has followed. Historically, antifungal susceptibility testing was imprecise and fraught with many inconsistencies. However, pioneering research in the past decade has resulted in the development of CLSI guidelines for the antifungal susceptibility testing methods of both yeasts and filamentous fungi (molds).[35,36] Use of these techniques can result in greater than 90% inter- and intralaboratory reproducibility. Although routine antifungal testing of every isolate is not generally necessary for most clinical microbiology laboratories, periodic batch testing for antibiograms and surveillance of resistance and/or antifungal testing of patients with such infections as cryptococcal meningitis or oropharyngeal candidiasis refractory to therapy are warranted.

DETECTION OF RESISTANCE FACTORS

There are a number of methods in use that directly detect the production of antimicrobial resistance in pathogens. β-Lactamase production can be detected rapidly and easily in the clinical laboratory with the use of nitrocephin disks. Nitrocephin is a chromogenic cephalosporin derivative that changes color on hydrolysis by β-lactamase. Colonies from a growing bacterial culture can be touched to a disk, with β-lactamase production noted within a few minutes. Although rapid and reliable, this method is limited to the assessment of strains of staphylococci, enterococci, *H. influenzae, Moraxella catarrhalis,* and *N. gonorrhoeae.* The nitrocephin disk also cannot detect β-lactam resistance caused by altered penicillin-binding proteins or by some of the newer ESBLs. The use of PCR or DNA probes for detection of β-lactamases improves sensitivity/specificity but is still limited to the research setting. In the years to come, these molecular biologic techniques should become more refined and more prominent in the clinical microbiology laboratory.

PCR has now become a standard method to quantify the replication of the HIV and hepatitis viruses in infected patients (the *viral load,* described as copies per milliliter).[37] Similar methods are used to determine the presence of genetic mutations in the HIV that are associated with increased resistance to one or more of the many antiretroviral medications available for clinical use. The use of these genotyping methods as an aid to select an optimized antiretroviral regimen has been correlated with an improved clinical response to therapy, as well as with a more potent reduction in the viral load.[37]

The detection of methicillin resistance in *Staphylococcus* (methicillin-resistant *S. aureus* [MRSA]) is crucial to ensure appropriate therapy. Methicillin resistance is the result of the *mecA* gene, which encodes for an altered penicillin-binding protein (penicillin-binding protein 2a) that has a low binding affinity for β-lactams. It is particularly difficult to detect this resistance, although, because of the heterogeneous expression of the phenotype—it is common for only 1 in 10^{4-6} tested cells to express methicillin resistance (even though all cells may have the genetic ability to do so). Screening via oxacillin disks or by oxacillin-containing agar (6 mcg/mL) was once considered the gold standard for resistance detection prior to the development of PCR and DNA probes that were specific for *mecA.* The *mecA* PCR test is available for clinical use, is 99% sensitive and specific, and allows for the rapid (within 6 hours) determination of the presence of methicillin resistance. Although the *mecA* PCR test has been available for many years, many laboratories do not use it commonly because of its high cost relative to other screening methods with acceptable sensitivity/specificity. For example, the presence of MRSA in a nasal swab or a blood culture sample can now be determined directly and rapidly within 24 hours using chromogenic technology (CHROMagar MRSA). This technology uses chromogenic substrates and a cephalosporin; MRSA strains will grow in the presence of cephalosporins such as cefoxitin and will produce mauve-colored colonies resulting from hydrolysis of the chromogenic substrates. The sensitivity and specificity for this test is as high as 97% and 99%, respectively.[38,39] In addition, fluorescence in situ hybridization (FISH) is a novel technique that uses peptide nucleic acid probes to target ribosomal RNA (rRNA) to rapidly identify both bacteria and yeasts in culture. Peptide nucleic acid probes that specifically target 16S rRNA of *S. aureus* have now been developed for rapid and specific identification of *S. aureus* directly from blood cultures that are Gram-stain positive for gram-positive cocci. The assay has 100% sensitivity and 96% specificity.[40]

The detection of decreased vancomycin susceptibility in gram-positive organisms has become more important with the increased prevalence of both vancomycin-resistant Enterococcus (VRE) and vancomycin-intermediate-resistant and vancomycin-resistant *S. aureus* (VISA and VRSA). The vancomycin agar screening method (Brain-Heart Infusion agar containing 6 mcg/mL of vancomycin) is an inexpensive and reliable way to detect vancomycin resistance for both of these problem pathogens.[24] With this test, the growth of any colonies from a sample of the test organism (10^5–10^6 CFU) after 24 hours of incubation indicates the presence of decreased vancomycin susceptibility (VISA) or vancomycin resistance (VRE, VRSA) within the test strain. Most MIC test methods used in the clinical laboratory that incorporate at least a 16-hour incubation period also appear to reliably detect strains of VRE, VISA, and VRSA.

SPECIAL IN-VITRO TESTS OF ANTIMICROBIAL ACTIVITY

MINIMAL BACTERICIDAL CONCENTRATION

9 In certain infections (e.g., meningitis and endocarditis), the bactericidal (killing) activity may be more predictive of a favorable infection outcome than the MIC.[41] The minimal bactericidal concentration (MBC) can be performed in conjunction with the broth microtiter MIC test by taking aliquots of broth from microtiter wells that demonstrate no visible growth and plating the samples onto antibiotic-free agar plates for subsequent incubation. The MBC is defined as the lowest concentration of drug that kills 99.9% of the total initially viable cells (representing a 3 $\log_{10}$ CFU/mL or greater reduction in the starting inoculum).

For certain antibiotic classes such as the aminoglycosides and the quinolones, the MIC often approximates the MBC. However, for β-lactam antibiotics and glycopeptides, the MBC can exceed the MIC substantially, resulting in an overestimation of in-vivo bactericidal activity. When the MBC exceeds the MIC by 32-fold or more, an organism is said to be *tolerant* to the antimicrobial's killing activity. Although the phenomenon of tolerance has been documented for β-lactams and glycopeptides against certain staphylococci, streptococci, and enterococci, its impact on the outcome of infections caused by organisms other than those just mentioned appears to be limited.

TIMED-KILL CURVE TESTS

Timed-kill curve tests are not performed routinely in the clinical laboratory but can provide important additional data on the effects of an antimicrobial on bacteria. For timed-kill curve tests, a standard inoculum of bacteria (10^6 CFU/mL) is placed in a test tube containing liquid growth medium with or without desired test concentrations of antimicrobial. Samples are removed periodically to determine the number of living cells at the given time points. The viable cell counts are plotted versus time to construct the timed-kill profile of the antimicrobial. The tested concentration of antimicrobial is considered to be bactericidal if it causes at least a 3 $\log_{10}$ CFU/mL reduction in viable inoculum. Comparisons of the relative rates of bacterial killing also can be performed in timed-kill curve experiments. Additionally, the presence of concentration-dependent killing activity (where killing increases with increasing drug concentrations above the MIC) versus concentration-independent killing activity can be determined from a timed-kill curve experiment. An example of results from a timed-kill curve experiment is depicted in Fig. 108–7. These data can help to predict the best way to administer an antimicrobial to maximize activity. For example, lower-dose, more frequent (or continuous) infusions would be preferable for concentration-independent antibiotics, while higher-dose intermittent administrations would maximize activity for concentration-dependent antibiotics.

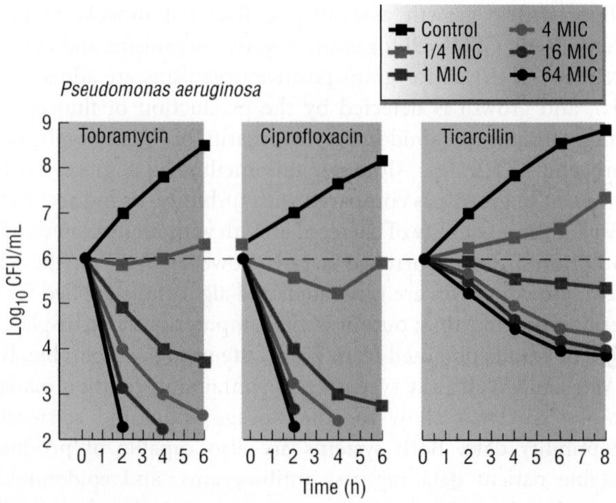

FIGURE 108-7. Killing curve depicting the effect of concentration on antibiotic bactericidal activity. (CFU, colony-forming unit; MIC, minimal inhibitory concentration [0.25–64 times the MIC; the organism tested was *P. aeruginosa* ATCC 27853]). *(From Pape et al.[39])*

POSTANTIBIOTIC EFFECT

The *postantibiotic effect* (PAE) is defined as the persistent suppression of an organism's growth after a brief exposure to an antibiotic.[42] A PAE experiment is performed by exposing a fixed inoculum of organism to a set concentration of antibiotic (typically some multiple of the MIC) (Fig. 108–8). The antibiotic is then removed either by inactivation (e.g., inactivation by a β-lactamase or binding the antibiotic to a resin) or by filtration/centrifugation of the mixture. The cells are resuspended in antibiotic-free growth medium, and samples are removed frequently (every 0.5 to 2 hours) to determine resumption of normal growth. The PAE is quantified as the difference in time that it takes the organism exposed to the antibiotic to demonstrate a 10-fold increase in viable cells per milliliter as compared with a separate culture of organism not subjected to the antibiotic. A PAE equal to or greater than 1 hour has been demonstrated for most antibiotics against gram-positive bacteria. As a general rule, antibiotics that inhibit DNA or protein synthesis (e.g., quinolones and aminoglycosides) demonstrate significant PAEs against gram-negative organisms. An exception to this rule are the carbapenem cell wall synthesis inhibitors (e.g., ertapenem, imipenem, and meropenem), which demonstrate PAEs against selected strains of gram-negative organisms. The primary clinical application of the PAE is to allow for less frequent administration of antimicrobials while still maintaining adequate antibacterial activity (e.g., extended-interval aminoglycoside administration).[42]

ANTIMICROBIAL COMBINATION EFFECT TEST

Antimicrobial combination therapy is used frequently to treat serious infections. Combination therapy can be used prior to knowing the pathogen or antibiotic susceptibility for the treatment of infections in neutropenic patients and in patients with enterococcal endocarditis or bacteremia, sepsis, or pneumonia caused by *P. aeruginosa*. In these cases, it is important to know whether the combination will have beneficial (or detrimental) effects on the overall antibacterial activity of the regimen. For example, the combination can result in activity that is significantly greater than the sum of activity of either agent alone (i.e., synergy). Conversely, the combination can result in activity that is worse than either agent alone (i.e., antagonism). Combination activity that is neither synergistic nor antagonistic is said to be *indifferent* or *additive*.[43]

Two methods are used to determine the expected effects of combination antibiotic therapy. For the most part, both methods are not used commonly in the clinical microbiology laboratory owing to the substantial labor involved with these tests and the lack of strong correlation with clinical outcome in the majority of infections. The first method is the microtiter fractional inhibitory concentration (FIC, or "checkerboard" method). The FIC is performed in a similar manner to the microtiter broth MIC except that two antibiotics are tested in the same microtiter plate. Twofold serial dilutions of one antibiotic are made in one direction on the plate (e.g., from right to left), whereas dilutions of the second antibiotic are made from the other direction on the same plate (e.g., from top to bottom). This method produces all possible combinations of twofold concentrations for the two drugs being tested. An inoculum of test bacteria is added to all wells, and the results are read in a similar manner as the MIC test. The FIC is expressed mathematically by calculation of the FIC index. The FIC index is calculated as

$$\text{FIC index} = \frac{A}{\text{MIC}_A} + \frac{B}{\text{MIC}_B}$$

where *A* or *B* is the lowest concentration of the drug that is inhibitory in the presence of the second drug, and the MIC is the minimal inhibitory concentration of each drug tested alone. Synergism is defined as an FIC index of 0.5 or less, indifference is defined as an FIC index of between 0.6 and 4.0, and antagonism is defined as an FIC index of greater than 4.0.[44] The microtiter FIC methods have been adapted to allow the use of E-test antibiotic-susceptibility test strips.[45] In this method, two antibiotic E-test strips are crossed at the individual MIC of each antibiotic; an extension of the zone of inhibition beyond that from either antibiotic alone is considered additive or synergistic activity, and an FIC index can be calculated in a similar manner as the microtiter method.

The second most common method to determine the effects of antibiotic combinations is an adaptation of timed-kill curve tests. Two antibiotics are added to the same test tube at fixed concentration fractions of the MIC for each drug, and killing is quantified. With this method, synergism is defined as a 100-fold decrease in viable organisms at 24 hours for the combination as compared with the most potent antibiotic tested alone. Antagonism is defined as a 100-fold or greater increase in viable organism count[44] (Fig. 108–9). It is important to note that although antagonism has been demonstrated for several combinations in vitro (e.g., penicillin plus tetracycline, chloramphenicol and an aminoglycoside, fluoroquinolones and rifampin), antagonism in vivo has been demonstrated only infrequently.

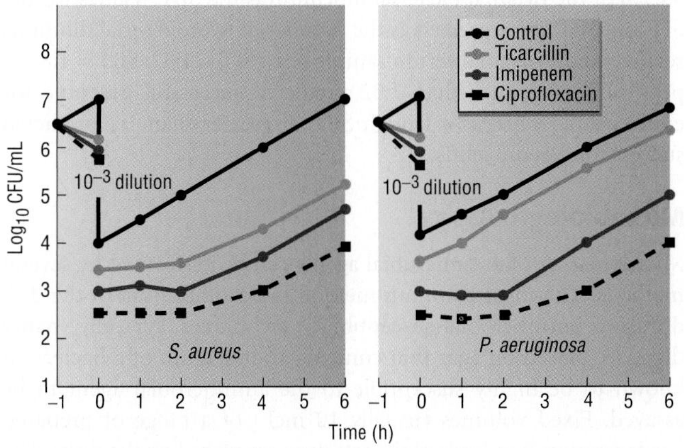

FIGURE 108-8. Postantibiotic effect. In this experiment, fixed inocula of *Staphylococcus aureus* and *Pseudomonas aeruginosa* are exposed to ticarcillin, imipenem, and ciprofloxacin at a set concentration of four times the MIC. The organism and the antibiotic are then diluted 1,000-fold to a point where the antibiotic concentration is far below the MIC of the organism. Growth suppression of *S. aureus* following exposure to the three drugs (postantibiotic effect [PAE]) occurs for approximately 2 hours. Growth suppression of *P. aeruginosa,* however, is only demonstrated for imipenem and ciprofloxacin. The β-lactam ticarcillin has no effect on the growth of *P. aeruginosa*. (CFU, colony-forming unit; MIC, minimal inhibitory concentration.) *(From Oliveria et al.[40])*

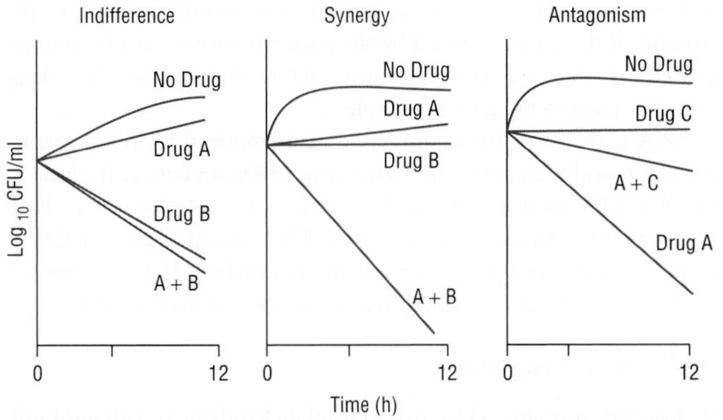

FIGURE 108-9. Timed-kill curve illustrating indifference, synergy, and antagonism. (CFU, colony-forming unit.)

Although the methods for testing the effects of antimicrobial combinations are well described, the results from these tests have not been adequately studied in the context of infection outcome. There is little debate that the combination of a β-lactam antibiotic and an aminoglycoside is required for successful treatment of enterococcal endocarditis. For enterococci, susceptibility to high concentrations of aminoglycosides (e.g., gentamicin, 500 mg/mL) is evaluated in the clinical laboratory because it correlates closely with synergy when the drug is combined with β-lactam antibiotics.

The concept of combination therapy is not universally accepted for the treatment of other infections. There is ongoing debate as to whether the combination of a broad-spectrum β-lactam and an aminoglycoside is needed (versus the β-lactam alone) for the therapy of such infections as gram-negative bloodstream infections or infections in neutropenic patients.[46] In individual studies, combination therapy has resulted in improved outcomes in patients with severe illness and in patients with *P. aeruginosa* bloodstream infections, but pooled meta-analyses have disputed these results.[46]

LABORATORY MONITORING OF ANTIMICROBIAL THERAPY

⑩ The clinician should have an understanding of in-vivo antimicrobial agent disposition to select the most appropriate therapy for a given infection and to help monitor for clinical or bacteriologic efficacy. Serum concentration monitoring is the most common method used to attempt to maximize efficacy and minimize toxicity of antimicrobials. Because most antimicrobials are well tolerated at their usual doses, only a select few agents (e.g., aminoglycosides, chloramphenicol, and vancomycin) are monitored routinely in the current clinical environment. There are a number of direct and indirect methods that are used to quantify the concentration of antimicrobial in an experimental sample.

METHODS OF ANTIMICROBIAL CONCENTRATION DETERMINATION IN CLINICAL SAMPLES

Fluorescence-Polarization Immunoassay

The fluorescence-polarization immunoassay (FPIA) technique involves the application of the principles of fluorescence when molecules are exposed to light. A fluorescein-labeled drug and antibody that is directed against the drug are added in constant amounts to samples with unknown drug concentrations and to concentration standards. When the fluorescein-labeled drug complexes with the antibody, a quantifiable change in the fluorescence polarization occurs. When a sample containing non–fluorescein-labeled drug (i.e., a patient's serum sample) is mixed with the standard mixture, competition for antibody binding occurs. Comparison of the change caused by the patient's sample to the changes caused by standard concentrations determines the specific drug concentration in the patient sample.

FPIA is the most commonly used assay method for the determination of aminoglycoside and vancomycin serum concentrations in the clinical laboratory setting. Advantages of this technique include its automation through the use of the TDx system (Abbott Laboratories, North Chicago, IL). Disadvantages include the expenses for reagents and the cost for the purchase of the automated system.

Radioimmunoassay

Radioimmunoassay (RIA) uses a radiolabeled drug and an antibody directed against the specific drug to determine the concentration contained in an unknown sample. The theory behind the assay is similar to FPIA because radiolabeled antibiotic and unlabeled antibiotic (in the patient's serum sample) are equilibrated with the antibody. The amount of free radiolabeled drug is measured and compared with the values obtained with standard concentrations of the radiolabeled drug alone to determine the concentration in the patient sample. Although RIA has good sensitivity and specificity, its main disadvantage compared with FPIA is the expense and hassle of handling and disposal of the radioactive waste generated during the test.

High-Pressure Liquid Chromatography

High-performance liquid chromatography (HPLC) permits the separation of different molecular species by passing a mobile solvent phase over a stationary phase. Drugs with a polarity similar to that of the stationary phase are retained for a time on the chromatographic column and then released after various retention times. Detection can be accomplished via fluorescence, electrochemical, or radiometric methods. The detector signal is proportional to the amount of molecules present. Standard curves are generated from known concentrations of the drug (usually recorded as peak area or peak height). Advantages of HPLC include a rapid turnaround time, precision, and an ability to detect the test drug in the presence of its metabolites and/or other drugs. Disadvantages include the high cost of HPLC instruments and the expertise required to perform the assays. These disadvantages usually relegate HPLC drug assay to the experimental and/or research settings.

Serum Inhibitory/Bactericidal Titers

Serum inhibitory titers (SITs) and serum bactericidal titers (SBTs) sometimes are used to monitor the antimicrobial therapy of certain serious infections (e.g., osteomyelitis and endocarditis). SITs and SBTs for antimicrobials are determined in a similar standardized manner as microdilution MICs and MBCs, but dilutions of the patient's serum are used instead of known concentrations of antimicrobial.[47] Patient serum can be collected near the expected peak, midpoint, and/or trough concentration(s) of the antimicrobial dose. The SIT is the highest twofold dilution of the serum sample that inhibits the visible growth of the patient's infecting organism, whereas the SBT is defined as the highest dilution of serum that kills 99.9% of the original bacterial inoculum is the SBT. Values for the SIT and SBT are expressed as the number of twofold serial dilutions relative to the original serum sample (e.g., SIT = 1:32, SBT = 1:8). A peak SBT of greater than 1:32 predicted successful outcome for endocarditis, whereas a trough SBT of greater than 1:2 predicted success for osteomyelitis.[48,49]

Microbiologic Assay

Microbioassay of antimicrobial agents can be performed by several methods. The most common method is a modification of the disk diffusion antimicrobial-susceptibility technique. Typically, paper disks are placed on agar that contains an inoculum of a bacterium known to be highly susceptible to the antimicrobial agent to be assayed. Fixed volumes (usually 10 mcL) of a range of prepared concentration standards of the test drug are placed on the disks. The zones of growth inhibition are measured and plotted versus the drug concentration to generate a standard curve. Zone sizes from samples containing the unknown concentrations of the test drug are measured, and the concentrations are determined from the plotted curve; the drug concentration in unknown samples is determined from the standard curve generated from the known concentrations of the drug. The advantages of this method include its relative ease of performance and the minimal cost for equipment. The disadvantages of this method include interference from other antibiotics that can be present in the unknown sample, a lack of sensitivity/

specificity for certain antimicrobials, and a slow turnaround time (usually 24 to 48 hours) for generation of results.

TIMING OF COLLECTION OF SERUM SAMPLES

⓫ Peak and/or trough concentrations are monitored routinely for only a select few antimicrobials (e.g., aminoglycosides and vancomycin) during the contemporary management of infections. It is crucial for the healthcare team to ensure that the antimicrobial's administration time and serum sample time(s) are meticulously recorded because even small errors in recording these (e.g., 1 hour) can have a substantial impact on the calculation of pharmacokinetics for antibiotics such as the aminoglycosides, which have relatively short elimination half-lives.

Samples ideally should be obtained after steady state is achieved (usually defined as the passage of at least 3 to 4 anticipated half-lives), but in certain situations, this may not be possible (e.g., critically ill patients with fluctuations in drug elimination owing to fluctuating hemodynamics, kidney function, and/or liver function). Generally, the timing of the peak serum sample collection is usually more critical than the trough concentration because adequate time must elapse to allow for completion of the distribution phase and to avoid underestimating the drug's volume of distribution.

SPECIFIC AGENTS

The aminoglycosides (i.e., amikacin, gentamicin, and tobramycin) and vancomycin remain the most common agents for which serum concentrations are monitored. A summary of the recommendations for serum concentration monitoring of these agents is shown in Table 108–2.

Aminoglycosides

⓬ There are many studies that have linked serum aminoglycoside concentrations with clinical response and with the occurrence of nephrotoxicity. One of the classic investigations into the relationship between serum aminoglycoside activity and clinical outcome revealed that peak serum concentrations of at least 5 mcg/mL for gentamicin and tobramycin and at least 20 mcg/mL for amikacin were associated with a lower prevalence of clinical failure rates during the treatment of gram-negative bacteremia.[50] Although earlier studies suggested that trough concentrations exceeding 2 to 4 mcg/mL for gentamicin and tobramycin and 10 mcg/mL for amikacin predisposed patients to nephrotoxicity, more recent investigations indicate that the development of aminoglycoside-related ototoxicity and nephrotoxicity is more complex and also is associated with the total exposure to the aminoglycoside (as measured by the AUC) and/or the total duration of aminoglycoside therapy.[51] The specific recommended serum peak and trough concentrations for the various aminoglycosides are described in Table 108–2.

Newer regimens of once-daily or extended-interval aminoglycoside administration have gained widespread acceptance for use in the clinical setting. These regimens exploit the pharmacodynamic properties of these agents (i.e., concentration-dependent bacterial killing and a substantial PAE) to maximize activity while also attempting to minimize drug nephrotoxicity by reducing the total aminoglycoside exposure time for the patient's kidneys. The doses employed for extended-interval treatment typically range from 5 to 7 mg/kg of lean body weight (administered every 24 to 48 hours), with the dose and/or interval adjusted based on renal function or observed mid-dose serum concentrations.[52] Many prospective studies have been performed to evaluate the safety and efficacy of once-daily aminoglycoside dosing, and most have revealed similar rates of efficacy and toxicity, or trends toward improved efficacy and reduced toxicity for once-daily dosage regimens as compared with traditional (thrice daily) regimens.

Traditional methods of aminoglycoside serum concentration monitoring (evaluating peak and trough serum concentrations) cannot be applied to extended-interval dosing because the serum concentrations 24 hours after a dose ideally should be undetectable. A mid-interval serum sample can be taken approximately 6 to 12 hours after the dose to allow for use of first-order pharmacokinetic equations.

CLINICAL CONTROVERSY

Although some clinicians believe that the clinical data are sufficient to support widespread use of once-daily aminoglycoside dosing without determination of individualized patient pharmacokinetics, other clinicians believe that the data from investigations on once-daily aminoglycosides are incomplete and that patients still should receive individualized pharmacokinetic assessments and dosage adjustments.

TABLE 108-2 Suggested Therapeutic Serum Concentrations for Selected Antimicrobial Agents

Drug	Sample	Target Concentrations (mg/L)	Comments
Gentamicin, Tobramycin (Traditional dosage regimens)	Peak (1 hour after the start of a 15- to 45-minute infusion)	<5	Urinary tract infections
		>5	Bacteremia
		>6	Bacterial pneumonia
		>12	Endocarditis caused by *Pseudomonas aeruginosa*
	Trough	<2–3	High trough concentrations are most likely a result of and not a cause of nephrotoxicity
Amikacin	Peak	>15	Urinary tract infections
		>20	Bacteremia
		>24	Bacterial pneumonia, other serious infections
	Trough	>9–10	See comments regarding trough gentamicin/ tobramycin concentrations
Single daily dosage regimens[49]			
Gentamicin Netilmicin Tobramycin	8-hour postdose (*mid-dose*)	1.5–6	Concentrations above this range associated with nephrotoxicity in one study with netilmicin
Vancomycin	Peak (1–2 hours after a 60-minute infusion)	20–50	Recommendations should be considered tentative, as definitive data are not available
	Trough	15-20	Recent data suggest this higher trough range in pneumonia due to low lung penetration and increasing vancomycin MICs/MBCs[52,53]

MIC, minimal inhibitor concentration; MBC, minimal bactericidal concentration.
Data from Weinstein et al.,[49] Nicalau et al.,[52] and Rybak.[53]

Vancomycin

⑬ Although vancomycin appears to possess a time-dependent killing profile, the area under the concentration-time curve to MIC ratio (AUC/MIC) appears to be the most likely parameter predicting efficacy as demonstrated by animal and limited human data.[53] Although intravenous vancomycin has been associated with oto- and nephrotoxicity in humans, most of these reports occurred with older, impure formulations of the drug, with extremely high concentrations uncommon with contemporary dosing regimens, or when vancomycin was combined with known nephrotoxic agents. Indeed, continuous infusions of vancomycin that resulted in constant serum vancomycin concentrations of 20 to 25 mcg/mL caused no substantial nephrotoxicity when compared with intermittent regimens that targeted the "accepted" serum trough concentration range.[54]

Because vancomycin appears to possess a time-dependent killing-activity profile, it has been recommended that vancomycin concentrations remain above the organism's MIC during the entire dosing interval. Most methods of empirical vancomycin dosing result in peak concentrations of between 20 and 50 mcg/mL and trough concentrations of between 5 and 15 mcg/mL. A number of weight-based dosage regimens and/or nomogram-based dosage methods can be used to minimize monitoring of serum concentrations for the vast majority of patients. However, recent data suggest that higher vancomycin trough concentrations are now needed because of its poor penetration into the lung tissue, combined with the trend toward increased prevalence of strains of staphylococci with higher MICs and/or MBCs. Recent guidelines for the treatment of hospital- and ventilator-associated pneumonia reflect these trends, as troughs of 15 to 20 mg/L are recommended.[55,56]

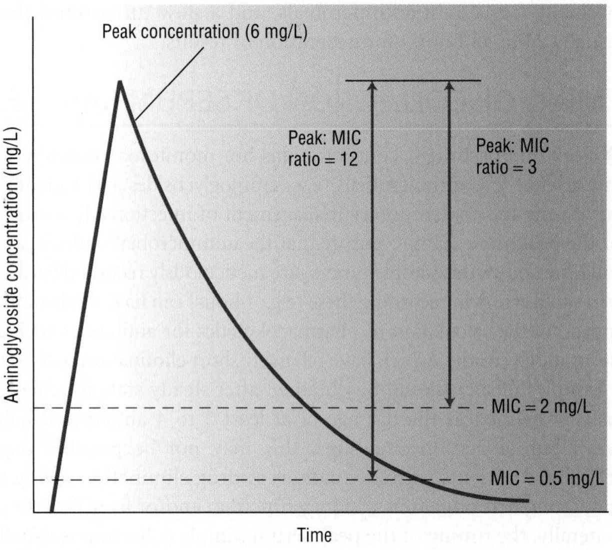

FIGURE 108-10. Illustration of the concept of peak concentration to the minimal inhibitory concentration (MIC) ratio for aminoglycosides. The MIC for the given organism to gentamicin is 2 mg/L, whereas the tobramycin MIC is 0.5 mg/L. Administration of gentamicin would result in a suboptimal peak:MIC ratio (<10), which could increase the chances for development of resistance or an inadequate response. Administration of tobramycin would result in a peak:MIC ratio of 12, which should improve efficacy. Note that modification of the gentamicin regimen to produce peak serum concentrations of 20 mg/L or more (as commonly done with once-daily administration) also would result in a peak:MIC ratio of 10 or greater.

INTEGRATING ORGANISM SUSCEPTIBILITY WITH SERUM CONCENTRATION DATA TO IMPROVE ANTIMICROBIAL THERAPY

❼ ⑭ We have advanced our understanding substantially of the importance of considering both antimicrobial pharmacokinetics and organism susceptibility when selecting therapy for the treatment of infections. Antimicrobial regimens should be selected and/or designed to maximize the probability that bacterial killing is optimized and that the probability of resistance is minimized. For example, the activity of antimicrobials such as the fluoroquinolones and the aminoglycosides can be maximized if the ratio of the peak serum concentration to the organism MIC (peak-to-MIC ratio) is greater than or equal to 10.[57] Similarly, the probability of clinical and/or microbiologic infection cure can be maximized if a fluoroquinolone is chosen that achieves an area under the curve (AUC)-to-MIC ratio of 100 to 125 or greater for gram-negative bacteria (e.g., *P. aeruginosa*) and 30 to 40 or greater for gram-positive bacteria (e.g., *S. pneumoniae*).[58,59] The clinical application of these principles to aminoglycoside dosage regimen optimization is depicted in Fig. 108–10. Although the maintenance of concentrations above the infecting organism's MIC (the time above the MIC) best predicts the clinical efficacy of the β-lactam antimicrobials, the AUC-to-MIC ratio also appears to be a strong predictor for treatment outcome for certain organisms and in certain clinical situations (e.g., vancomycin for staphylococcal infections).[53,60]

Most of the data on optimization of antimicrobial pharmacodynamics have been generated in in-vitro models of infection, in animal models of infection, within the context of controlled clinical trials, or through mathematical modeling of small data sets. However, research continues to emerge on the best ways to apply these valuable data to the everyday management of patients in the clinical setting. The recognition of the importance of antimicrobial pharmacodynamics already has resulted in the expansion of serum concentration monitoring for select antimicrobials (e.g., antiretroviral agents, antifungal agents), suggested revisions of breakpoint values that define antimicrobial susceptibility and/or resistance, development of nomograms or computer programs that can suggest optimal drugs and doses for a given infection, and/or the development of newer antimicrobial agents that minimize the probability of suboptimal pharmacodynamics. These developments present exciting opportunities for healthcare providers to improve the outcomes of patients with infections in a variety of different healthcare settings.

ABBREVIATIONS

AIDS: acquired immunodeficiency syndrome

AUC: area under the curve

bDNA: branched DNA

CDC: Centers for Disease Control and Prevention

CLSI: Clinical and Laboratory Standards Institute

CFU: colony-forming unit

CMV: cytomegalovirus

ELISA: enzyme-linked immunosorbent assay

ESBL: extended-spectrum β-lactamase

ESR: erythrocyte sedimentation rate

FIC: fractional inhibitory concentration

FISH: fluorescence in situ hybridization

FPIA: fluorescence polarization immunoassay

HIV: human immunodeficiency virus

HPLC: high-performance liquid chromatography

KOH: potassium hydroxide

MBC: minimum bactericidal concentration

MHC: major histocompatibility complex

MIC: minimum inhibitory concentration
PAE: postantibiotic effect
PCR: polymerase chain reaction
PMN: polymorphonuclear leukocyte
RIA: radioimmunoassay
SBT: serum bactericidal titer
SIT: serum inhibitory titer
TNF: tumor necrosis factor
VISA: vancomycin-intermediate *S. aureus*
VRE: vancomycin-resistant enterococci
VRSA: vancomycin-resistant *S. aureus*

REFERENCES

1. Reese RE, Betts RF. Principles of Antibiotic Use. In: Betts RF, Chapman SW, Penn RL, eds. A Practical Approach to Infectious Diseases, 5th ed. Philadelphia: Lippincott Williams & Wilkins, 2003:969–988.
2. Andro V, Cainelli F. Infections in patients with cancer undergoing chemotherapy: Aetiology, prevention, and treatment. Lancet Oncol 2003;595–604.
3. Crawford J, Dale DC, Lyman GH. Chemotherapy-induced neutropenia: Risks, consequences, and new directions for its management. Cancer 2003;100:228–237.
4. Day CL, Walker BD. Progress in defining CD4 helper cell responses in chronic viral infections. J Exp Med 2003;198:1773–1777.
5. Smith JM, Nemeth TL, McDonald RA. Current immunosuppressive agents: Efficacy, side effects and utilization. Pediatr Clin North Am 2003;6:1283–1300.
6. Penn RL, Betts RF. Lower respiratory tract infections (including tuberculosis). In: Betts RF, Chapman SW, Penn RL, eds. A Practical Approach to Infectious Diseases, 5th ed. Philadelphia: Lippincott Williams & Wilkins, 2003:295–371.
7. Lannergard A, Larsson A, Kragsbjerg P, Friman G. Correlation between serum amyloid A protein and C-reactive protein in infectious diseases. Scand J Clin Lab Invest 2003;4:267–272.
8. Priest DH, Peakcock JE Jr. Hematogenous vertebral osteomyelitis due to Staphylococcus aureus in the adult: Clinical features and therapeutic outcomes. South Med J 2005;98:854–862.
9. Cavaillon JM, Adib-Conquy M, Fitting C, et al. Cytokine cascade in sepsis. Scand J Infect Dis 2003;35:535–544.
10. Lekkou A, Karakantza M, Mouzaki A, et al. Cytokine production and monocyte HLH-DR expression as predictors of outcome for patients with community-acquired severe infections. Clin Diagn Lab Immunol 2004;11:161–167.
11. Dorman NJ. Sepsis. In: Betts RF, Chapman SW, and Penn RL, eds. A Practical Approach to Infectious Diseases, 5th ed. Philadelphia: Lippincott Williams & Wilkins, 2003:19–66.
12. Safdar N, Kluger DM, Maki DG. A review of risk factors for catheter-related bloodstream infection caused by percutaneously inserted, non-cuffed central venous catheters: Implications for preventive strategies. Medicine 2002;86:466–479.
13. Graman PS, Menegus MA. Microbiology laboratory tests In: Betts RF, Chapman SW, Penn RL, eds. A Practical Approach to Infectious Diseases, 5th ed. Philadelphia: Lippincott Williams & Wilkins, 2003:929–956.
14. O'Hara CM, Weinstein MP, Miller JM. Manual and automated systems for detection and identification of microorganisms. In: Murry PR, Baron EJ, Jorgensen JH, et al., eds. Manual of Clinical Microbiology, 8th ed. Washington, DC: ASM Press, 2003:185–207.
15. Constantine NT, Lana DP. Immunoassays for the diagnosis of infectious diseases. In: Murray PR, Baron EJ, Jorgensen JH, et al., eds. Manual of Clinical Microbiology, 8th ed. Washington, ASM Press, 2003:218–256.
16. Gill VJ, Fedorko DP, Witebsky FG. The clinician and the microbiology laboratory. In: Mandell GL, Bennet JE., Dolin R, eds. Principles and Practice of Infectious Diseases, 6th ed. New York: Churchill-Livingstone, 2005:203–241.
17. Nolte FS, Caliendo AM. Molecular detection and identification of microorganisms. In: Murry PR, Baron EJ, Jorgensen JH, et al., eds. Manual of Clinical Microbiology, 8th ed. Washington, ASM Press, 2003:234–256.
18. Pilcher CD, McPherson JD, Leone PA, et al. Real-time, universal screening for acute HIV infection in a routine HIV counseling and testing population. JAMA 2002;288:216–221.
19. Bryant P, Venter D, Robins-Browne R, Curtis N. Chips with everything: DNA microarrays in infectious diseases. Lancet Infect Dis 2004;4:100–111.
20. Owen RJ. Molecular testing for antibiotic resistance in *Helicobacter pylori.* Gut 2002;50:285–289.
21. Varaldo PE. Antimicrobial resistance and susceptibility testing: An evergreen topic. J Antimicrob Chemother 2002;50:1–4.
22. Jorgensen JH, Ferraro MJ. Antimicrobial susceptibility testing: Special needs for fastidious organisms and difficult-to-detect resistance mechanisms. Clin Infect Dis 2000:30:799–808.
23. Pfaller MA, Segreti J. Overview of the epidemiological profile and laboratory detection of extended-spectrum beta-lactamases. Clin Infect Dis 2006;42(Suppl 4):S153–163.
24. Appelbaum PC. The emergence of vancomycin-intermediate and vancomycin-resistant Staphylococcus aureus. Clin Microbiol Infect 2006;12(Suppl 1):16–23.
25. Clinical and Laboratory Standards Institute (CLSI). Methods for Antimicrobial Susceptibility Tests for Bacteria that Grow Aerobically; Approved Standard, 7th ed. CLSI document M7-A7. Wayne, PA: Clinical and Laboratory Standards Institute.
26. Bauer AW, Kirby MM, Sherris JC, et al. Antibiotic susceptibility testing by a standardized, single-disk method. Am J Clin Pathol 1966;45:493–496.
27. Hidayat LK, Hsu DI, Quist R, Shriner KA, Wong-Beringer A. High-dose vancomycin therapy for methicillin-resistant Staphylococcus aureus infections: Efficacy and toxicity. Arch Intern Med 2006;166:2138–2144.
28. Craig WA. Does the dose matter? Clin Infect Dis 2001;33(Suppl 3):S233–237.
29. Jorgensen JH, Ferraro MJ. Antimicrobial susceptibility testing: General principles and contemporary practices. Clin Infect Dis 1998;26:973–980.
30. Pestotnik SL. Expert clinical decision support systems to enhance antimicrobial stewardship programs: Insights from the Society of Infectious Diseases Pharmacists. Pharmacotherapy 2005;25:1116–1125.
31. Woods GL. Susceptibility testing for mycobacteria. Clin Infect Dis 2000;31:1209–1215.
32. Ardito F, Posteraro B, Sanguinetti M, et al. Evaluation of BACTEC Mycobacteria Growth Indicator Tube (MGIT 960) automated system for drug susceptibility testing of *Mycobacterium tuberculosis.* J Clin Microbiol 2001;38:4440–4444.
33. Clinical and Laboratory Standards Institute (CLSI). Susceptibility Testing for Mycobacteria, Nocardiae, and Other Aerobic Actinomycetes—Approved Standard. CLSI Document M24-A. Wayne, PA: Clinical and Laboratory Standards Institute, 2003.
34. Garcie de Viedma D. Rapid detection of resistance in *Mycobacterium tuberculosis*: A review discussing molecular approaches. Clin Microbiol Infect 2003;9:349–359.
35. Clinical and Laboratory Standards Institute (CLSI). Reference Method for Broth Dilution Antifungal Susceptibility Testing of Yeasts; Approved Standard, 2nd ed. CLSI Document M27-A2. Wayne, PA: Clinical and Laboratory Standards Institute, 2002.
36. Clinical and Laboratory Standards Institute (CLSI). Reference Method for Broth Dilution Antifungal Susceptibility Testing of Filamentous Fungi—Approved Standard. CLSI Document M38-A. Wayne, PA: Clinical and Laboratory Standards Institute, 2002.
37. Dybul M, Fauci AS, Bartlett JG, et al. Guidelines for using antiretroviral agents among HIV-infected adults and adolescents: Recommendations of the Panel on Clinical Practices for Treatment of HIV. MMWR 2002;51:1–56.
38. Flayhart D, Hindler JF., Bruckner DA, et al. Multicenter evaluation of BBL CHROMagar MRSA medium for direct detection of methicillin-resistant *Staphylococcus aureus* from surveillance cultures of the anterior nares. J Clin Microbiol 2005;43:5336–5340.
39. Pape J, Waldlin J, Nackamkin I. Use of BBL CHROMagar MRSA medium for identification of methicillin-resistant *Staphylococcus*

aureus directly from blood cultures. J Clin Microbiol 2006;44:2575–2576.
40. Oliveria K, Procop GW, Wilson D, et al. Rapid identification of *Staphylococcus aureus* directly from blood cultures by fluorescence in situ hybridization with peptide nucleic acid probes. J Clin Microbiol 2002;40;247–251.
41. Voorn GP, Kuyvenhoven J, Goessens WHF, et al. Role of tolerance in treatment and prophylaxis of experimental *Staphylococcus aureus* endocarditis with vancomycin, teicoplanin, and daptomycin. Antimicrob Agents Chemother 1994;38:487–493.
42. Craig WA, Gudmundsson S. Postantibiotic effect. In: Lorian V, ed. Antibiotics in Laboratory Medicine, 5th ed. Baltimore, MD: Williams & Wilkins, 2005:296–329.
43. Rybak MJ, McGrath BJ. Combination antimicrobial therapy for bacterial infections: Guidelines for the clinician. Drugs 1996;52:390–405.
44. Elipoulos G, Moellering RC Jr. Antimicrobial combinations. In; Lorian V, ed. Antibiotics in Laboratory Medicine, 4th ed. Baltimore, MD: Williams & Wilkins, 1996:330–397.
45. White RL, Burgess DS, Manduru M, Bosso JA. Comparison of three different in vitro methods of detecting synergy: Time-kill, checkerboard, and E test. Antimicrob Agents Chemother 1996;40:1914–1918.
46. Paul M, Silbiger I, Grozinsky S, Soares-Weiser K, Leibovici L. Beta lactam antibiotic monotherapy versus beta lactam-aminoglycoside antibiotic combination therapy for sepsis. Cochrane Database Syst Rev 2006:CD003344.
47. Clinical and Laboratory Standards Institute (CLSI). Methodology for the Serum Bactericidal Test; Approved Guideline. NCCLS Document M21-A. Wayne, PA: Clinical and Laboratory Standards Institute, 1999.
48. Weinstein MP, Stratton CW, Acklery A, et al. Multicenter collaborative evaluation of a standardized serum bactericidal test as a prognostic indicator in infective endocarditis. Am J Med 1985;78:262–269.
49. Weinstein MP, Stratton CW, Hawley HB, et al. Multicenter collaborative evaluation of a standardized serum bactericidal test as a predictor of therapeutic efficacy in acute and chronic osteomyelitis. Am J Med 1987;83:218–222.
50. Moore RD, Smith CR, Lietman PS. The association of aminoglycoside plasma levels with mortality in patients with gram-negative bacteremia. J Infect Dis 1984;149:443–448.
51. Rybak MJ, Abate BJ, Kang SL, Ruffing MJ, Lerner SA, Drusano GL. Prospective evaluation of the effect of an aminoglycoside dosing regimen on rates of observed nephrotoxicity and ototoxicity. Antimicrob Agents Chemother 1999;43:1549–1555.
52. Nicolau DP, Freeman CD, Belliveau PP, et al. Experience with a once-daily aminoglycoside program administered to 2,184 adult patients. Antimicrob Agents Chemother 1995;39:650–655.
53. Rybak MJ. The pharmacokinetic and pharmacodynamic properties of vancomycin. Clin Infect Dis 2006;42(Suppl 1):S35–39.
54. Wysocki M, Delatour F, Faurisson F, et al. Continuous versus intermittent infusion of vancomycin in severe staphylococcal infections: Prospective, multicenter randomized study. Antimicrob Agents Chemother, 2001;45:2460–2467.
55. Guidelines for the management of adults with hospital-acquired, ventilator-associated, and healthcare-associated pneumonia. Am J Respir Crit Care Med 2005;171:388–416.
56. Jones RN. Microbiological features of vancomycin in the 21st century: minimum inhibitory concentration creep, bactericidal/static activity, and applied breakpoints to predict clinical outcomes or detect resistant strains. Clin Infect Dis 2006;42(Suppl 1):S13–24.
57. Preston S, Drusano G, Berman A, et al. Pharmacodynamics of levofloxacin: A new paradigm for early clinical trials. JAMA 1998;279:125–129.
58. Forrest A, Nix DE, Ballow CH, et al. Pharmacodynamics of intravenous ciprofloxacin in seriously ill patients. Antimicrob Agents Chemother 1993;37:1073–1081.
59. Ambrose P, Grasela, D, Grasela T, et al. Pharmacodynamics of fluoroquinolones against *Streptococcus pneumoniae* in patients with community-acquired respiratory tract infections. Antimicrob Agents Chemother 2001;45:2793–2797.
60. Moise PA, Forrest A, Bhavnani SM, et al. Area under the inhibitory curve and a pneumonia scoring system for predicting outcomes of vancomycin therapy for respiratory infections by *Staphylococcus aureus*. Am J Health Syst Pharm 2000;57:S4–9.

CHAPTER 109

Antimicrobial Regimen Selection

DAVID S. BURGESS

KEY CONCEPTS

1. Every attempt should be made to obtain specimens for culture and sensitivity testing prior to initiating antibiotics.

2. Empirical antibiotic therapy should be based on knowledge of likely pathogens for the site of infection, information from patient history (e.g., recent hospitalizations, work-related exposure, travel, and pets), and local susceptibility.

3. Patients with delayed dermatologic reactions to penicillin generally can receive cephalosporins. Patients with type I hypersensitivity reactions (anaphylaxis) to penicillins should not receive cephalosporins or carbapenems (alternatives include aztreonam, quinolones, sulfa drugs, or vancomycin based on type of coverage indicated).

4. Estimated renal function should be calculated for every patient who is to receive antibiotics and the antibiotic dose interval adjusted accordingly. Hepatic function should be considered for drugs eliminated through the hepatobiliary system, such as clindamycin, erythromycin, and metronidazole.

5. All concomitant drugs and nutritional supplements should be reviewed when an antibiotic is added to a patient's therapy.

6. Combination antibiotic therapy may be indicated for polymicrobial infections (abdominal, gynecologic infections), to produce synergistic killing (β-lactam plus aminoglycoside versus *Pseudomonas aeruginosa*), or to prevent the emergence of resistance.

7. All patients receiving antibiotics should be monitored for resolution of infectious signs and symptoms (e.g., decreasing temperature and white blood cell [WBC] count) and adverse drug events.

8. Antibiotic agents with the narrowest effective spectrum of activity are preferred. Antibiotic route of administration should be evaluated daily, and conversion from intravenous to oral therapy should be attempted as signs of infection improve for patients with functioning gastrointestinal tracts (general exceptions are endocarditis and central nervous system infections).

9. Patients not responding to an appropriate antibiotic treatment in 2 to 3 days should be reevaluated to ensure (a) the correct diagnosis, (b) that therapeutic drug concentrations are being achieved, (c) that the patient is not immunosuppressed, (d) that the patient does not have isolated infection (i.e., abscess, foreign body), or (e) that resistance has not developed.

Learning objectives, review questions, and other resources can be found at **www.pharmacotherapyonline.com.**

Choosing an antimicrobial agent to treat an infection is far more complicated than matching a drug to a known or suspected pathogen.[1,2] Most clinicians generally follow a systematic approach to select an antimicrobial regimen (Table 109–1). Problems arise when this systematic approach is replaced by prescribing broad-spectrum therapy to cover as many organisms as possible. Consequences of not using the systematic approach include the use of more expensive and potentially more toxic agents, which can, in turn, lead to widespread resistance and difficult-to-treat superinfections. Another abuse of antimicrobial agents is administration when they are not needed. An example of this is prescribing antibacterials for self-limited clinical conditions that are most likely viral in origin (i.e., the common cold).

Initial selection of antimicrobial therapy is nearly always empirical, which is the initiation of antimicrobials sometimes prior to documentation of the presence of infection and before the offending organism is identified. Infectious diseases generally are acute, and a delay in antimicrobial therapy can result in serious morbidity or even mortality. Thus empirical antimicrobial therapy selection is based on information gathered from the patient's history and physical examination and results of Gram stains or of rapidly performed tests on specimens from the infected site. This information, combined with knowledge of the most likely offending organism(s) and an institution's local susceptibility patterns, should result in a rational selection of antibiotics to treat the patient.

This chapter introduces a systematic approach to the selection of antimicrobial therapeutic regimens.

TABLE 109-1 Systematic Approach for Selection of Antimicrobials

Confirm the presence of infection
Careful history and physical
Signs and symptoms
Predisposing factors
Identification of the pathogen (see Chap. 108)
Collection of infected material
Stains
Serologies
Culture and sensitivity
Selection of presumptive therapy considering every infected site
Host factors
Drug factors
Monitor therapeutic response
Clinical assessment
Laboratory tests
Assessment of therapeutic failure

CONFIRMING THE PRESENCE OF INFECTION

FEVER

The presence of a temperature greater than the expected 37°C (98.6°F) "normal" body temperature is considered a hallmark of infectious diseases. Body temperature is controlled by the hypothalamus. In addition, the circadian rhythm, a built-in temperature cycle, is also operational. The daily temperature rhythm can vary for each individual. In a healthy person, the internal thermostat is set between the morning low temperature and the afternoon peak as controlled by the circadian rhythm. During fever, the hypothalamus is reset at a higher temperature level.

Fever is defined as a controlled elevation of body temperature above the normal range. The average normal body temperature range taken orally is 36.7 to 37°C (98.0 to 98.6°F). Body temperatures obtained rectally generally are 0.6° (1°F) higher and axillary temperatures are 0.6°C (1°F) lower than oral temperatures, respectively. Skin temperatures are also less than the oral temperature but can vary depending on the specific measurement method. Fever can be a manifestation of disease states other than infection. Collagen-vascular (autoimmune) disorders and several malignancies can have fever as a manifestation. Fever of unknown or undetermined origin is a diagnostic dilemma and is reviewed extensively elsewhere.[3]

Many drugs have been identified as causes of fever.[4] *Drug-induced fever* is defined as persistent fever in the absence of infection or other underlying condition. The fever must coincide temporally with the administration of the offending agent and disappear promptly on its withdrawal, after which the temperature remains normal. Possible mechanisms of drug-induced fever are either a hypersensitivity reaction or development of antigen-antibody complexes that result in the stimulation of macrophages and the release of interleukin 1 (IL-1). Although this is not a common drug effect (accounting for no more than 5% of all drug reactions), it should be suspected when obvious reasons for fever are not present. Almost any medication can produce fever, but β-lactam antibiotics, anticonvulsants, allopurinol, hydralazine, nitrofurantoin, sulfonamides, phenothiazines, and methyldopa appear to be responsible more often than others.[4]

Noninfectious etiologies of fever can be referred to as "false-positives." Although these certainly can confuse the clinician, even more troublesome are false-negatives: the absence of fever in a patient with signs and symptoms consistent with an infectious disease. Careful questioning of the patient or family is vital to assess the ingestion of any medication that can mask fever (e.g., aspirin, acetaminophen, nonsteroidal antiinflammatory agents, and corticosteroids). The use of antipyretics should be discouraged during the treatment of infection unless absolutely necessary because they can mask a poor therapeutic response. Moreover, elevated body temperature, unless very high (>40.5°C [105°F]), is not harmful and may be beneficial.

SIGNS AND SYMPTOMS

White Blood Cell Count

Most infections result in elevated WBC counts (leukocytosis) because of the increased production and mobilization of granulocytes (neutrophils, basophils, and eosinophils), lymphocytes, or both to ingest and destroy invading microbes. The generally accepted range of normal values for WBC counts is between 4,000 and 10,000 cells/mm^3. Values above or below this range hold important prognostic and diagnostic value.

Bacterial infections are associated with elevated granulocyte counts, often with immature forms (band neutrophils) seen in peripheral blood smears. Mature neutrophils are also referred to as *segmented neutrophils* or *polymorphonuclear* (PMN) *leukocytes*. The presence of immature forms (left shift) is an indication of an increased bone marrow response to the infection. With infection, peripheral WBC counts can be very high, but they are rarely higher than 30,000 to 40,000 cells/mm^3. Because leukocytosis indicates the normal host response to infection, low leukocyte counts after the onset of infection indicate an abnormal response and generally are associated with a poor prognosis.

The most common granulocyte defect is neutropenia, a decrease in absolute numbers of circulating neutrophils. A thorough description of the consequences of neutropenia is given in Chap. 120. Lymphocytosis, even with normal or slightly elevated total WBC counts, generally is associated with tuberculosis and viral or fungal infections. Increases in monocytes can be associated with tuberculosis or lymphoma, and increases in eosinophils can be associated with allergic reactions to drugs or infections caused by metazoa. Many types of infections can be accompanied by a completely normal WBC count and differential.

Local Signs

The classic signs of pain and inflammation can manifest as swelling, erythema, tenderness, and purulent drainage. Unfortunately, these are only visible if the infection is superficial or in a bone or joint. The manifestations of inflammation in deep-seated infections (e.g., meningitis, pneumonia, endocarditis, and urinary tract infection) must be ascertained by examining tissues or fluids. For example, the presence of neutrophils in spinal fluid, lung secretions (sputum), or urine is highly suggestive of a bacterial infection.

Symptoms referable to an organ system must be sought out carefully because not only do they help in establishing the presence of infection, but they also aid in narrowing the list of potential pathogens. For example, a febrile patient with complaints of flank pain and dysuria can well have pyelonephritis. In this situation, enteric gram-negative bacilli, especially *Escherichia coli,* are the predominant pathogens. If a febrile patient has no symptoms suggestive of an organ system but only constitutional complaints, the list of possible infectious diseases is lengthy.[3] A febrile individual with cough and sputum production probably has a pulmonary infection. What is not so evident, however, is the etiologic organism in this situation, because it can be caused by bacteria, mycobacteria, viruses, chlamydia, or mycoplasmas.[5] In this situation, attention to the patient's history and background disease states is important. Even more important is a careful examination of the infected material (in this case sputum) to ascertain the identity of the pathogen.

IDENTIFICATION OF THE PATHOGEN

MICROBIOLOGY ISSUES

❶ Infected body materials must be sampled, if at all possible or practical, before institution of any antimicrobial therapy for two reasons. First, a Gram stain of the material might reveal bacteria, or an acid-fast stain might detect mycobacteria or actinomycetes. Second, a delay in obtaining infected fluids or tissues until after antimicrobial therapy is started might result in false-negative culture results or alterations in the cellular and chemical composition of infected fluids. This is particularly true in patients with urinary tract infections, meningitis, and septic arthritis.[6]

Blood cultures usually should be performed in the acutely ill febrile patient. Blood culture collection should coincide with sharp elevations in temperature, suggesting the possibility of microorganisms or microbial antigens in the bloodstream. Ideally, blood should be obtained from peripheral sites as two sets (one set consists of an aerobic bottle and one set an anaerobic bottle) from two different sites approximately 1 hour apart. In selected infections, bacteremia is qualitatively continuous (e.g., endocarditis), so cultures can be obtained at any time.[7]

In addition to the infected materials produced by the patient (e.g., blood, sputum, urine, stool, and wound or sinus drainage), other less accessible fluids or tissues must be obtained based on localized signs or symptoms (e.g., spinal fluid in meningitis and joint fluid in arthritis). Abscesses and cellulitic areas also should be aspirated.

INTERPRETING RESULTS

After a positive Gram stain, culture results, or both are obtained, the clinician must be cautious in determining whether the organism recovered is a true pathogen, a contaminant, or a part of the normally expected flora (see Chap. 108). This latter consideration is especially problematic with cultures obtained from the skin, oropharynx, nose, ears, eyes, throat, and perineum. These surfaces are heavily colonized with a wide variety of bacteria, some of which can be pathogenic in certain settings. For example, coagulase-negative staphylococci are found in cultures of all the aforementioned sites yet are seldom regarded as pathogens unless recovered from blood, venous access catheters, or prosthetic devices.

Importantly, cultures of specimens from purportedly infected sites that are obtained by sampling from or through one of these contaminated areas might contain significant numbers of the normal flora. In the case of urine cultures, the urinalysis should be used in combination with culture results to assess the presence of WBCs, nitrite, and leukocyte esterase to help confirm infection and rule out colonization.

Particularly problematic are expectorated sputum specimens that must be evaluated carefully by determination of the presence of squamous epithelial cells and leukocytes.[5] A predominance of epithelial cells in sputum specimens reduces the likelihood that recovered bacteria are pathogenic, especially when multiple types of organisms are seen on Gram stain. In contrast, the discovery of leukocytes in large numbers with one predominant type of organism is a more reliable indicator of a valid collection. In general, however, sputum evaluation has poor sensitivity and specificity as a diagnostic test.[5]

Caution also must be used in the evaluation of positive culture results from normally sterile sites (e.g., blood, cerebrospinal fluid, or joint fluid). The recovery of bacteria normally found on the skin in large quantities (e.g., coagulase-negative staphylococci or diphtheroids) from one of these sites can be a result of contamination of the specimen rather than a true infection. These organisms can be pathogenic in certain settings.

Gram-staining techniques, culture methods, and serologic identification, as well as susceptibility testing, are discussed in detail in Chap. 108. Emphasis must be placed on the proper collection and handling of specimens and careful assessment of Gram stain or other test results in guiding the clinician toward appropriate selection of initial antimicrobial therapy.[8]

SELECTION OF PRESUMPTIVE THERAPY

❷ To select rational antimicrobial therapy for a given clinical situation, a variety of factors must be considered. These include the severity and acuity of the disease, host factors, factors related to the drugs used, and the necessity for using multiple agents. In addition, there are generally accepted drugs of choice for the treatment of most pathogens (see Appendix 109–1).

Drugs of choice are compiled from a variety of sources and are intended as guidelines rather than as specific rules for antimicrobial use. These choices are influenced by local antimicrobial susceptibility data rather than information published by other institutions or national compilations. Each institution should publish an annual summary of antibiotic susceptibilities (antibiogram) for organisms cultured from patients. Antibiograms contain both the number of nonduplicate isolates for common species and the percentage susceptible to the antibiotics tested. To further guide empirical antibiotic therapy, some hospitals publish unit-specific antibiograms in unique patient care areas, such as intensive care units or burn units.

Susceptibility of bacteria can differ substantially among hospitals within a community. For example, the prevalence of hospital-acquired methicillin-resistant *Staphylococcus aureus* (HA-MRSA) in some centers is quite high, whereas in other centers the problem might be nonexistent. This particular situation will influence the selection of therapy for possible *S. aureus* infection, where the clinician must choose either a β-lactam or vancomycin. The problem of differing susceptibilities is limited not only to gram-positive bacteria but also to gram-negative organisms, and all drug classes are affected.

Empirical therapy is directed at organisms that are known to cause the infection in question. These organisms for different sites of infection are discussed in Chap. 110 to 129. To define the most likely infecting organisms, a careful history and physical examination must be performed. The place where the infection was acquired should be determined, for example, the home (community-acquired), nursing home environment, or hospital-acquired (nosocomial). Nursing home patients can be exposed to potentially more resistant organisms because they are often surrounded by ill patients who are receiving antibiotics. Other important questions to ask infected patients regarding the history of the present illness include the following:

1. Are any other people sick at home, especially children?
2. Are any unusual pets kept in the home such as pigeons?
3. Where are you employed (i.e., are you exposed to contaminated meat or infectious biohazards)?
4. Has there been any recent travel, for example, to endemic areas of fungal infections or developing countries?

HOST FACTORS

Several host factors should be considered when evaluating a patient for antimicrobial therapy. The most important factors are drug allergies, age, pregnancy, genetic or metabolic abnormalities, renal and hepatic function, site of infection, concomitant drug therapy, and underlying disease states.

Allergy

❸ Allergy to an antimicrobial agent generally precludes its use. Careful assessment of allergy histories must be performed because many patients confuse common adverse drug effects (i.e., gastrointestinal disturbance) with true allergic reactions.[9] Among the most commonly cited antimicrobial allergies are those to penicillin, penicillin-related compounds, or both. In the absence of complete penicillin skin testing capabilities, a rule of thumb for giving cephalosporins or carbapenems to patients allergic to penicillin is to avoid giving them to patients who give a good history for immediate or accelerated reactions (e.g., anaphylaxis, laryngospasm) and to give them under close supervision in patients with a history of delayed reactions, such as a rash.[10] If gram-negative infection is suspected or documented, therapy with a monobactam may be appropriate because cross-reactivity with other β-lactams is virtually nil.

Age

The patient's age is an important factor both in trying to identify the likely etiologic agent and in assessing the patient's ability to eliminate the drug(s) to be used. The best example of an age determinant of organisms is in bacterial meningitis, where the pathogens differ as the patient grows from the neonatal period through infancy and childhood and into adulthood.[6]

In the case of the neonate, hepatic and liver functions are not well developed. The use of chloramphenicol can lead to shock and cardiovascular collapse (gray baby syndrome) caused by the inability of the newborn's liver to metabolize and detoxify the drug.[4] Serum concentrations of chloramphenicol must be monitored to ensure that concentrations of the drug do not exceed 20 to 25 mcg/mL. Neonates (especially when premature) can develop kernicterus when given sulfonamides. This results from displacement of bilirubin from serum albumin.[4] Additional special drug considerations for pediatric patients include low frequency of adverse effects and compliance-enhancing features (e.g., absorption not affected by food, once- to twice-daily dosing, and good taste).[11]

The major physiologic change in persons older than 65 years of age is a decline in the number of functioning nephrons that, in turn, results in decreased renal function.[12] This is usually manifested by an increased incidence of side effects caused by antimicrobials that are eliminated renally. For example, renal toxicity caused by aminoglycosides may be apparent much sooner during therapy than in younger patients.

Pregnancy

During pregnancy, not only is the fetus at risk for drug teratogenicity (see Chap. 81), but also the pharmacokinetic disposition of certain drugs can be altered.[13] Penicillins, cephalosporins, and aminoglycosides are cleared from the peripheral circulation more rapidly during pregnancy. This is probably a result of marked increases in intravascular volume, glomerular filtration rate, and hepatic and metabolic activities. The net result is that maternal serum antimicrobial concentrations can be as much as 50% lower during this period than in the nonpregnant state. Increased dosages of certain compounds might be necessary to achieve therapeutic levels during late pregnancy.

Metabolic Abnormalities

Inherited or acquired metabolic abnormalities will influence the therapy of infectious diseases in a variety of ways. For example, patients with impaired peripheral vascular flow may not absorb drugs given by intramuscular injection. In addition, certain metabolic states can predispose patients to enhanced drug toxicity. For example, patients who are phenotypically slow acetylators of isoniazid are at greater risk for peripheral neuropathy.[14] Patients with severe deficiency of glucose-6-phosphate dehydrogenase can develop significant hemolysis when exposed to such drugs as sulfonamides, nitrofurantoin, nalidixic acid, antimalarials, dapsone, and perhaps, chloramphenicol.[4] Although mild deficiencies are found in African Americans, the more severe forms of the disease generally are confined to persons of eastern Mediterranean origin.

Organ Dysfunction

❹ Patients with diminished renal or hepatic function or both will accumulate certain drugs unless the dosage is adjusted.[15,16] Recommendations for dosing antibiotics in patients with liver dysfunction are not as formalized as guidelines for patients with renal dysfunction. Antibiotics that should be adjusted in severe liver disease include clindamycin, erythromycin, metronidazole, and rifampin. Significant accumulation can occur when both liver dysfunction and renal dysfunction are present for these drugs: cefotaxime, nafcillin, piperacillin, and sulfamethoxazole.

Concomitant Drugs

❺ Any concomitant therapy that the patient is receiving can influence the drug selection, dose, and monitoring. For example, administration of isoniazid to a patient who is also receiving phenytoin can result in phenytoin toxicity secondary to inhibition of phenytoin metabolism by isoniazid. Furthermore, drugs that possess similar adverse-effect profiles can increase the risk for effects, for example, two drugs that cause nephrotoxicity or neutropenia. A detailed review of drug interactions is beyond the scope of this chapter, but an excellent textbook on this subject is available.[17] Lists of potentially severe drug-drug interactions are provided in Table 109–2.

Concomitant Disease States

Concomitant disease states can influence the selection of therapy. Certain diseases will predispose patients to a particular infectious disease or will alter the type of infecting organism. For example, patients with diabetes mellitus and the resulting peripheral vascular disease often develop infections of the lower extremity soft tissue. Moreover, the alterations in peripheral blood flow associated with the disease and perhaps altered immunity make such infections more difficult to treat than in nondiabetics. Patients with chronic lung disease or cystic fibrosis develop frequent pulmonary infections that can be caused by somewhat different microorganisms than are found in otherwise normal hosts.

Patients with immunosuppressive diseases, such as malignancies or acquired immunologic deficiencies, are highly predisposed to infections, and the types of organisms can be vastly different from what would be expected (see Chap. 126). For example, patients undergoing chemotherapy for acute forms of leukemia often are profoundly granulocytopenic and are predisposed to infections caused by bacteria and fungi.[18] Patients with the acquired immunodeficiency syndrome (AIDS) often become infected with an enormous variety of organisms (see Chap. 129).[19]

Many factors predisposing to infection are related to disruption of the host's integumentary barriers. For example, trauma, burns, and iatrogenic wounds induced in surgery can lead to a substantial risk of infection depending on the severity and location of the injury or disruption. For a complete discussion of the various risks involved in surgical procedures, see Chap. 127.

DRUG FACTORS

Pharmacokinetic and Pharmacodynamic Considerations

Integration of both pharmacokinetic and pharmacodynamic properties of an agent is important when choosing antimicrobial therapy to ensure efficacy and to prevent resistance.[20] Early researchers relied solely on pharmacokinetic properties such as the area under the (drug concentration) curve (AUC), maximum observed concentration (peak), and drug half-life to optimize therapy. Pharmacodynamics is the study of the relationship between drug concentration and the effects on the microorganism (see Chap. 108). Researchers now realize the important relationship between both pharmacokinetic and microbiologic parameters that has resulted in new measurements such as AUC:minimal inhibitory concentration (MIC) ratio, peak:MIC ratio, and time (T) the concentration is above MIC ($T >$ MIC).[21,22]

Aminoglycosides exhibit concentration-dependent bactericidal effects.[20–22] An example of the integration of pharmacokinetics and microbiological activity is the use of high-dose, once-daily aminoglycosides. For these regimens, the drug is given as a single large daily dose to maximize the peak:MIC ratio. Aminoglycosides also possess a postantibiotic effect (persistent suppression of organism growth after concentrations decrease below the MIC) that appears to contribute to the success of high-dose, once-daily administration.[20] Fluoroquinolones exhibit concentration-dependent killing activity, but optimal killing appears to be characterized by the AUC:MIC ratio.[20–23]

TABLE 109-2 Major Drug Interactions with Antimicrobials

Antimicrobial	Other Agent(s)	Mechanism of Action/Effect	Clinical Management
Aminoglycosides	Neuromuscular blocking agents	Additive adverse effects	Avoid
	Nephrotoxins (N) or ototoxins (O) (e.g., amphotericin B (N) cisplatin (N/O), cyclosporine (N), furosemide (O), NSAIDs (N), radio contrast (N), vancomycin (N)	Additive adverse effects	Monitor aminoglycoside SDC and renal function
Amphotericin B	Nephrotoxins (e.g., aminoglycosides, cidofovir, cyclosporine, foscarnet, pentamidine)	Additive adverse effects	Monitor renal function
Azoles	See Chap. 125		
Chloramphenicol	Phenytoin, tolbutamide, ethanol	Decreased metabolism of other agents	Monitor phenytoin SDC, blood glucose
Foscarnet	Pentamidine IV	Increased risk of severe nephrotoxicity/hypocalcemia	Monitor renal function/serum calcium
Isoniazid	Carbamazepine, phenytoin	Decreased metabolism of other agents (nausea, vomiting, nystagmus, ataxia)	Monitor drug SDC
Macrolides/azalides	Digoxin	Decreased digoxin bioavailability and metabolism	Monitor digoxin SDC; avoid if possible
	Theophylline	Decreased metabolism of theophylline	Monitor theophylline SDC
Metronidazole	Ethanol (drugs containing ethanol)	Disulfiram-like reaction	Avoid
Penicillins and cephalosporins	Probenecid, aspirin	Blocked excretion of β-lactams	Use if prolonged high concentration of β-lactam desirable
Ciprofloxacin/norfloxacin	Theophylline	Decreased metabolism of theophylline	Monitor theophylline
Quinolones	Class Ia and III Antiarrhythmics	Increased Q-T interval	Avoid
	Multivalent cations (antacids, iron, sucralfate, zinc, vitamins, dairy, citric acid) didanosine	Decreased absorption of quinolone	Separate by 2 hours
Rifampin	Azoles, cyclosporine, methadone propranolol, PIs, oral contraceptives, tacrolimus, warfarin	Increased metabolism of other agent	Avoid if possible
Sulfonamides	Sulfonylureas, phenytoin, warfarin	Decreased metabolism of other agent	Monitor blood glucose, SDC, PT
Tetracyclines	Antacids, iron, calcium, sucralfate	Decreased absorption of tetracycline	Separate by 2 hours
	Digoxin	Decreased digoxin bioavailability and metabolism	Monitor digoxin SDC; avoid if possible

PI, protease inhibitor; PT, prothrombin time; SDC, serum drug concentrations.
Azalides: azithromycin; Azoles: fluconazole, itraconazole, ketoconazole, and voriconazole; Macrolides: erythromycin, clarithromycin; Protease inhibitors: amprenavir, indinavir, lopinavir/ritonavir, nelfinavir, ritonavir, and saquinavir; Quinolones: ciprofloxacin, gatifloxacin, levofloxacin, moxifloxacin.

β-Lactams display time-dependent bactericidal effects. Killing activity is enhanced only marginally if drug concentration exceeds the MIC. Therefore, the important pharmacodynamic relationship for these antimicrobials is the duration that drug concentrations exceed the MIC ($T >$ MIC). Effective dosing regimens require serum drug concentrations to exceed the MIC for at least 40% to 50% of the dosing interval.[20–23] Frequent small doses or a continuous infusion of β-lactams appears to be correlated with positive outcomes.

The ability of bacteriostatic antimicrobial agents to eradicate infections is reliant on host immune function and a postantibiotic effect. Examples include clindamycin, macrolides, ketolides, and tetracyclines.[20–23]

Tissue Penetration

The importance of tissue penetration varies with site of infection. Some of the difficulties in interpreting data include a lack of correlation with clinical outcomes and poor understanding of whether the antimicrobial agents are present in a biologically active form. An example of the former problem is the recognized efficacy of drugs with low biliary fluid concentrations in the treatment of cholecystitis, cholangitis, or both and the absence of the enhanced efficacy of drugs whose primary route of elimination is biliary excretion of active drug. An example of the latter difficulty is with penetration to deep infections, such as abscesses, where various factors such as acid pH, WBC products, and various enzymes can inactivate even high concentrations of certain drugs.

The central nervous system (CNS) is one body site where antimicrobial penetration is relatively well defined, and correlations with clinical outcomes are established.[6,24] Cerebrospinal fluid (CSF) concentrations of antimicrobial agents necessary to cure bacterial meningitis have been defined, and drugs that do not reach significant concentrations in the CSF should either be avoided or instilled directly, if feasible.

Caution must be exercised when selecting an antimicrobial agent for clinical use on the basis of tissue or fluid penetration. Body fluids where drug concentration data are clinically relevant include CSF, urine, synovial fluid, and peritoneal fluid. Apart from these areas, more attention should be paid to clinical efficacy, antimicrobial spectrum, toxicity, and cost than to comparative data on penetration into a given body site.

The proper route of administration for an antimicrobial depends on the site of infection. Parenteral therapy is warranted when patients are being treated for febrile neutropenia or deep-seated infections such as meningitis, endocarditis, and osteomyelitis. Severe pneumonia often is treated initially with intravenous antibiotics and switched to oral therapy as clinical improvement is evident.[5,25] Patients treated in the ambulatory setting for upper respiratory tract infections (e.g., pharyngitis, bronchitis, sinusitis, and otitis media), lower respiratory tract infections, skin and soft tissue infections, uncomplicated urinary tract infections, and selected sexually transmitted diseases can receive oral therapy.

Drug Toxicity

It is incumbent on health professionals to avoid toxic drugs whenever possible. Antibiotics associated with CNS toxicities, usually when not dose-adjusted for renal function, include penicillins, cephalosporins, quinolones, and imipenem. Hematologic toxicities generally are manifested with prolonged use of nafcillin (neutropenia), piperacillin (platelet dysfunction), cefotetan (hypoprothrombinemia), chloramphenicol (bone marrow suppression, both idiosyncratic and dose-related toxicity), and trimethoprim (megaloblastic anemia). Reversible nephrotoxicity classically is associated with aminoglycosides and vancomycin. Reversible ototoxicity can occur with aminoglycosides or erythromycin. In the outpatient setting, patients must be counseled regarding photosensitivity with azithromycin, quinolones, tetracyclines, pyrazinamide, sulfamethoxazole, and trimethoprim. Lastly, all antibiotics have been implicated in causing diarrhea and colitis secondary to *Clostridium difficile*[26] (see Chap. 38).

Aside from consideration of drug toxicity, some antimicrobial use requires more intensive risk-benefit analysis. An example of this is the decision to use isoniazid prophylactically to prevent tuberculosis. Because the hepatotoxicity of isoniazid increases in frequency with age, older persons (>45 years of age) who are candidates for isoniazid prophylaxis (positive skin test) must have additional risk factors for tuberculosis to balance the potential toxic effects. These include evidence of recent skin-test conversion, immunosuppression, or previous gastrectomy. Older patients without additional risk factors are more likely to suffer toxicity from isoniazid than derive benefit from its use.[27]

Cost

The costs of drug therapy are increasing dramatically, especially as new products, derived from biotechnology, are introduced. Greater attention is being paid to the pharmacoeconomics of drug therapy, where patient outcomes are valued, and the costs to arrive at those outcomes are estimated. Understanding the true cost of antimicrobial therapy is more important than ever. The total cost of antimicrobial therapy includes much more than just the acquisition cost of the drugs.[28]

Many ancillary costs and factors affect the true cost of therapy. These include factors such as storage, preparation, distribution, and administration, as well as all the costs incurred from monitoring for adverse effects and factors such as length of hospitalization, readmissions, and all directly provided healthcare goods and services. More difficult to value but equally as important are indirect costs such as patient quality-of-life issues. Pharmacoeconomic and outcomes analyses are becoming more widely applied and used in order to derive values such as cost-benefit ratios and the cost-effectiveness of various products as compared with other products. A detailed review of pharmacoeconomic analyses is beyond the scope of this chapter, but excellent reviews of the subject are available.[29] A great deal more research in this area is needed, and multidisciplinary, collaborative efforts with the involvement of pharmacy, medicine, nursing, and microbiology are essential.

Many oral antimicrobials have been approved, including cephalosporins, linezolid, and fluoroquinolones, that can be used in place of more expensive parenteral therapy. These agents offer extended-spectrum killing activity, increased tissue penetration, and excellent safety and pharmacokinetic profiles. When oral therapy is being considered, the choice between convenient once-a-day expensive agents versus multiple-dose inexpensive agents arises. It is easy to calculate the difference in acquisition cost; however, the overall cost between agents is more difficult to determine. Factors to weigh include safety, effectiveness, tolerability, patient compliance, and potential drug-drug interactions. In some instances, more expensive agents can be warranted to avoid adverse outcomes.

COMBINATION ANTIMICROBIAL THERAPY

❻ In selecting a drug regimen for a given patient, consideration must be given to the necessity of using more than one drug. Combinations of antimicrobials generally are used to broaden the spectrum of coverage for empirical therapy, achieve synergistic activity against the infecting organism, and prevent the emergence of resistance.

Broadening the Spectrum of Coverage

Increasing the coverage of antimicrobial therapy generally is necessary in mixed infections where multiple organisms are likely to be present. This is the case in intraabdominal and female pelvic infections, in which a variety of aerobic and anaerobic bacteria can produce disease.[30] Traditionally, a combination of a drug active against aerobic gram-negative bacilli, such as an aminoglycoside, and a drug active against anaerobic bacteria, such as metronidazole or clindamycin, is selected. Newer compounds, which possess good activity against both these types of organisms, such as the β-lactam/β-lactamase inhibitor combinations, carbapenems or glycylcyclines, might be adequate to replace the combination and thereby reduce the cost of therapy. The other clinical situation in which an increased spectrum of activity is desirable is with nosocomial infections.[25]

Synergism

The achievement of synergistic antimicrobial activity is advantageous for infections caused by enteric gram-negative bacilli in immunosuppressed patients. Laboratory tests to identify synergy between antibiotic combinations are described in Chap. 108. Traditionally, combinations of aminoglycosides and β-lactams have been used because these drugs together generally act synergistically against a wide variety of bacteria. However, the data supporting superior efficacy of synergistic over nonsynergistic combinations are weak. At best, it would appear that synergistic combinations produce better results in certain infections caused by *P. aeruginosa and Enterococcus* species.[31,32]

The most obvious example of the use of synergy is the treatment of enterococcal endocarditis. The causative organism is usually only inhibited by penicillins, but it is killed rapidly by the addition of streptomycin or gentamicin to a penicillin.[31] The need for bactericidal activity in the treatment of endocarditis underscores the need for these synergistic combinations.

Preventing Resistance

The use of combinations to prevent the emergence of resistance is applied widely but not often realized. The only circumstance where this has been clearly effective is in the treatment of tuberculosis. The prevalence of resistance to a first-line drug such as isoniazid or rifampin in a population of organisms may be as high as 1 in 10^6 to 10^8. Because the bacterial load in a patient with active tuberculosis often exceeds this, two drugs are given to reduce the likelihood of encountering resistance to less than 1 in 10.[27] There is ample evidence from in-vitro data and experimental bacterial infections that combinations of drugs with different mechanisms are effective in the prevention of the emergence of resistance. Data from clinical trials, however, are either conflicting or do not convincingly support this concept.[33]

Disadvantages of Combination Therapy

Although there are potentially beneficial effects from combining drugs, there also are potential disadvantages, including increased cost, greater risk of drug toxicity such as nephrotoxicity such as aminoglycosides, amphotericin, and possibly vancomycin, and superinfection with even more resistant bacteria.[32.33]

The combination of two or more antibiotics can result in antagonistic effects. Clinically, the effect of antagonism may be evident when one drug induces β-lactamase production and another drug is β-lactamase unstable. Cefoxitin and imipenem are examples of drugs capable of inducing β-lactamases and may result in more rapid inactivation of penicillins when used together.

MONITORING THERAPEUTIC RESPONSE

❼ After antimicrobial therapy has been instituted, the patient must be monitored carefully for a therapeutic response. Culture and sensitivity reports from specimens sent to the microbiology laboratory must be reviewed and the therapy changed accordingly. Use of agents with the narrowest spectrum of activity against identified pathogens is recommended. If anaerobes are suspected, even if they are not identified, anaerobic therapy should be continued.

Patient monitoring should include many of the same parameters used to diagnose the infection. The WBC count and temperature should start to normalize. Physical complaints from the patient also should diminish (i.e., decreased pain, shortness of breath, cough, or sputum production). Appetite should improve. Radiologic improvement can lag behind clinical improvement. Determinations of serum (or other fluid) levels of antimicrobials can be useful in ensuring outcome, preventing toxicity, or both. There are only a few antimicrobials that require serum concentration monitoring and then only in selected situations. These include the aminoglycosides, flucytosine, and chloramphenicol. Achievement of adequate aminoglycoside concentrations within the first few days of therapy of gram-negative infection has been correlated with better therapeutic outcome.[34]

Changes in the volume of distribution can have a significant impact on the efficacy, safety, or both of therapy. An unexpectedly low volume of distribution (such as in the dehydrated patient) will result in higher, potentially toxic drug concentrations, whereas a larger-than-expected volume of distribution (such as in patients with edema or ascites) will result in low, potentially subtherapeutic concentrations. The most effective methods use measured serum concentrations of the drugs rather than estimations from renal function tests to assess true drug clearance from the body.

❽ As patients improve clinically, the route of administration should be reevaluated. Streamlining therapy from parenteral to oral (switch therapy) has become an accepted practice for many infections.[5] Criteria that should be present to justify a switch to oral therapy include (1) overall clinical improvement, (2) lack of fever for 8 to 24 hours, (3) decreased WBC count, and (4) a functioning gastrointestinal tract. Drugs that exhibit excellent oral bioavailability when compared with intravenous formulations include ciprofloxacin, clindamycin, doxycycline, levofloxacin, metronidazole, moxifloxacin, linezolid, and trimethoprim-sulfamethoxazole.

FAILURE OF ANTIMICROBIAL THERAPY

❾ A variety of factors may be responsible for an apparent lack of response to therapy. Patients who fail to respond over 2 to 3 days require a thorough reevaluation. It is possible that the disease is not infectious or is nonbacterial in origin, or there is an undetected pathogen in a polymicrobial infection. Other factors include those directly related to drug selection, the host, or the pathogen. Laboratory error in identification, susceptibility testing, or both (presence of inoculum effect or resistant subpopulations) is a rare cause of antimicrobial failure.

Failures Caused by Drug Selection

Factors related directly to the drug selection include an inappropriate drug selection or dosage or route of administration. Malabsorption of a drug product because of gastrointestinal (GI) disease, such as a short-bowel syndrome, or a drug interaction, such as complexation of fluoroquinolones with multivalent cations resulting in reduced absorption, can lead to potentially subtherapeutic serum concentrations. Accelerated drug elimination is also possible. This can occur in patients with cystic fibrosis or during pregnancy, when more rapid clearance or larger volumes of distribution can result in low serum concentrations, particularly for aminoglycosides. A common cause of failure of therapy is poor penetration into the site of infection. This is especially true for sites such as the CNS, eye, and prostate gland. Drug failure also can result from drugs that are highly protein bound or that are chemically inactivated at the site of infection.

Failures Caused by Host Factors

Host defenses must be considered when evaluating a patient who is not responding to antimicrobial therapy. Patients who are immunosuppressed (e.g., granulocytopenia from chemotherapy or AIDS) may respond poorly to therapy because their defenses are inadequate to eradicate the infection despite seemingly adequate drug regimens. A good example is the poor response of infection in granulocytopenic patients that is seen when their WBC counts remain low during therapy. This contrasts with a much better response when granulocyte counts increase during therapy.

Other host factors are related to the need for surgical drainage of abscesses or removal of foreign bodies, necrotic tissue, or both. If these situations are not corrected, they result in persistent infection and, occasionally, bacteremia despite adequate antimicrobial therapy.

Failures Caused by Microorganisms

Factors related to the pathogen include the development of drug resistance during therapy.[35] *Primary resistance* refers to the intrinsic resistance of the pathogens producing the infection. Several infections are more likely to result in drug resistance because of drug inaccessibility (e.g., pneumonia, endocarditis, abdominal and deep-seated skin and soft tissue infections). It has become increasingly obvious that despite the development and introduction of new antimicrobial agents, bacterial resistance has continued to increase both within and across different bacterial genera.

Organisms in which resistance has increased most dramatically include enterococci, pneumococci, and *Mycobacterium tuberculosis.* Enterococci have been isolated with multiple resistance patterns. They may be resistant to β-lactams (by virtue of β-lactamase production, altered penicillin-binding proteins [PBPs], or both), vancomycin (via alterations in peptidoglycan synthesis), and high levels of aminoglycosides (via enzymatic degradation).

Pneumococci resistant to penicillins, certain cephalosporins, and macrolides are increasingly common. These organisms generally are susceptible to vancomycin, the new fluoroquinolones, and cefotaxime or ceftriaxone. *M. tuberculosis* resistant to one or more first-line antitubercular agents (e.g., isoniazid, rifampin, ethambutol, streptomycin, and pyrazinamide) have increased in frequency as well. This has been observed principally in populations of prison inmates and patients with AIDS.

The increase in resistance among these organisms is believed to be a result of continued overuse of antimicrobials in the community, as well as in hospitals, and the increasing prevalence of immunosuppressed patients receiving long-term suppressive antimicrobials for the prevention of infections. These resistance patterns are regionally variable, and susceptibility patterns in the community (or hospital) should be monitored closely to promote rational antimicrobial selection.[36]

Antimicrobial agents such as linezolid, daptomycin, and tigecycline have been targeted at resistant gram-positive bacteria. Several other drugs currently in development also have enhanced activity against these bacteria.

The emergence of resistance during antimicrobial therapy is reported most frequently in pulmonary or other deep-seated infections caused by *P. aeruginosa.* This occurs in 20% to 30% of cases and with all the available antibacterial agents, including imipenem. This organism and a group of enteric gram-negative bacilli (*Enterobacter aerogenes, Enterobacter cloacae, Citrobacter freundii, Serratia marcescens,* and a few others) can produce a β-lactamase that is capable of hydrolyzing broad-spectrum cephalosporins and, to a lesser extent, penicillins.[35,36] These enzymes are categorized as Bush group I, and their genetic code is found on the chromosome. Resistant mutants of these aforementioned organisms that produce large quantities of these enzymes can be present within an infection and can be responsible for the emergence of resistance during therapy. The mutants occur at a frequency of 1 in 10^6 to 1 in 10^8 bacteria, the numbers of bacteria commonly encountered in clinical infections.[36] Because only 10^4 to 10^5 bacteria are tested for susceptibility in the microbiology laboratory, however, this potential resistance may not be detected.

Treatment of an infection caused by *Enterobacter, Citrobacter, Serratia,* or *P. aeruginosa* with a third-generation cephalosporin or aztreonam may produce an initial clinical response by eradicating all the susceptible bacteria in the population. Within a few days, however, the highly resistant subpopulations have a selective advantage and can overgrow the infection site to produce a relapse.[35,36] These bacteria usually retain susceptibility to aminoglycosides, carbapenems, and fluoroquinolones but are resistant to all other β-lactams. Host defenses are extremely important in this scenario. Debilitated patients with pulmonary infections, abscesses, or osteomyelitis are at high risk for drug failure. In these situations, a combination regimen to prevent the emergence of resistance or the use of carbapenem or a fluoroquinolone may be warranted for empirical therapy.

ANTIMICROBIAL USE MANAGEMENT

ANTIBIOTIC FORMULARY

Institutions must decide which antibiotics to include on their formularies. The actual decision to have a formulary remains controversial; however, restricting choices does encourage familiarity with a core of antibiotics for residents and attending physicians.[37] Open formularies allow the empirical use of any commercially available antibiotics, with recommended guidelines for changes when culture and sensitivity results are finalized. Many institutions have organized an antibiotic subcommittee to the pharmacy and therapeutics committee that meets to discuss trends in resistance and review new agents. The subcommittee is generally a multidisciplinary group including representation from microbiology, infection control, pharmacy, and physicians from several disciplines, including infectious disease. The actual implementation of the guidelines and restrictions recommended by such groups requires the cooperation of the entire medical staff. Education is vital to the success of the antibiotic formulary.[38]

ANTIMICROBIAL CYCLING

An interesting topic in formulary management that continues to gain interest and scientific research is *antimicrobial cycling.* Antimicrobial cycling is a predetermined change in an antimicrobial recommendation for empirical therapy of a specific infection at a predetermined time. It also has been called *rotation of antimicrobials.* This strategy should not be confused with *antimicrobial switch therapy,* which involves changes in the route of administration of antimicrobial therapy (i.e., intravenous to oral).

Antimicrobial cycling is employed as a mechanism to reduce or prevent antimicrobial resistance. *Proactive cycling* is a planned switch to preempt resistance at a predetermined point or series of points with a predetermined schedule. *Reactive cycling* is a response to high or unacceptable resistance and is often a one-time switch. Most programs incorporate aspects of both types of cycling. Cycling implies returning to the original drug after other choices have been used. Rotation implies several planned changes.

Antimicrobial cycling is based on the assumptions that the resistance problem is (1) caused by the overuse of a particular agent or class of agents and (2) that discontinuation of the particular agent or class of agents will restore susceptibility. These assumptions correlate best with nosocomial gram-negative organisms that can rapidly develop resistance. Theoretically, antimicrobial agents should be sequenced in such an order that mechanisms of resistance do not overlap (i.e., changing drug classes).[39,40] However, to date there has been insufficient evidence to clearly demonstrate the usefulness of antibiotic cycling.

KEEPING CURRENT

Attention must be paid to the literature on antimicrobials to assist in the selection of therapy. The results from prospective, controlled, randomized clinical trials should be evaluated whenever possible when considering appropriate antimicrobial therapy. Results from prelicensing open trials offer only limited information that can be useful in this regard because patients in these trials generally are not seriously ill and are not infected with multiple resistant bacteria and other confounding factors found in most clinical situations are excluded by virtue of the study design. Therefore, comparative data in more seriously ill patients are essential for the appropriate application of new agents.

Postmarketing trials are also important because results can demonstrate superiority of one regimen over another, either in efficacy, safety, or cost-effectiveness. Appropriate antimicrobial therapy can change as new organisms are discovered, susceptibility patterns change, new drugs become available, and new clinical trial results are published. Classical thinking in the treatment of infectious diseases will continue to change and evolve to maintain antimicrobial efficacy. Optimal use of modern antimicrobials is just beginning to be defined.

ABBREVIATIONS

AUC: area under the curve

IL: interleukin

MIC: minimal inhibitory concentration

PBP: penicillin-binding protein

PMN: polymorphonuclear leukocytes

WBC: white blood cell

REFERENCES

1. Hessen TM, Kaye D. Principles of selection and use of antibacterial agents: In vitro activity and pharmacology. Infect Dis Clin North Am 2000;14:265–279.
2. Slama TG, Amin A, Brunton SA, et al. A clinician's guide to the appropriate and accurate use of antibiotics: The Council for Appropriate and Rational Antibiotic Therapy (CARAT) criteria. Am J Med 2005;118(7A):1S–6S.
3. Mackowiak PA, Durach DT. Fever of unknown origin. In: Mandell GL, Bennett JE, Dolin R, eds. Mandell, Douglas and Bennett's Principles and Practice of Infectious Diseases, 6th ed. New York: Churchill-Livingstone, 2005:718–729.
4. Cunha BA. Antibiotic side effects. Med Clin North Am 2001;85:149–185.
5. Mandell LA, Wunderink RG, Anzueto A, et al. Infectious Diseases Society of America/American Thoracic Society Consensus Guidelines on the management of community-acquired pneumonia in adults. Clin Infect Dis 2007;44:S27–S72.
6. Tunkel AR, Hartman BJ, Kaplan SL, et al. Practice guidelines for the management of bacterial meningitis. Clin Infect Dis 2004;39:1267–1284.
7. Baddour LM, Wilson WR, Bayer AS, et al. Infective Endocarditis. Diagnosis, Antimicrobial Therapy, and Management of Complications: A Statement for Healthcare Professionals from the Committee on Rheumatic Fever, Endocarditis, and Kawasaki Disease, Council on Cardiovascular Disease in the Young, and the Councils on Clinical Cardiology, Stroke, and Cardiovascular Surgery and Anesthesia, American Heart Association. Circulation 2005;111:e394-e434.

8. Thomson RB Jr, Miller JM. Specimen collection, transport, and processing: Bacteriology. In: Murray PR, Baroon EJ, Jorgensen JH, et al. eds. Manual of Clinical Microbiology, 8th ed. Washington, DC: ASM Press, 2003:286–330.
9. Park MA, Li JTC. Diagnosis and management of penicillin allergy. Mayo Clin Proc 2005;80:405–410.
10. Kelkar PS, Li JTC. Cephalosporin allergy. N Engl J Med 2001;345:804–809.
11. San Joaquin VH, Stull TL. Antibacterial agents in pediatrics. Infect Dis Clin North Am 2000;14:341–355.
12. Stalam M, Kaye D. Antibiotic agents in the elderly. Infect Dis Clin North Am 2000;14:357–369.
13. Anderson GD. Pregnancy-induced changes in pharmacokinetics. Clin Pharmacokinetic 2005;44:989–1008.
14. Weinshilboum R. Inheritance and drug response. N Engl J Med 2003;348:529–537.
15. Livornese LL, Slavin D, Benz RL, et al. Use of antibacterial agents in renal failure. Infect Dis Clin North Am 2000;14:371–389.
16. Tschida SJ, Vance-Bryan K, Zaske DE. Anti-infective agents in hepatic disease. Med Clin North Am 1995;79:895–917.
17. Piscitelli SC, Rodvold KA. Drug Interactions in Infectious Diseases, 2nd ed. Totowa, NJ: Humana Press, 2005.
18. Hughes WT, Armstrong D, Bodey GP, et al. 2002 Guidelines for the use of antimicrobial agents in neutropenic patients with cancer. Clin Infect Dis 2002;34:730–751.
19. Treating Opportunistic Infections among HIV-Exposed and Infected Children. Recommendations from CDC, the National Institutes of Health, and the Infectious Diseases Society of America. MMWR Recomm Rep 2004;53(RR-12):1–63.
20. Levison ME. Pharmacodynamics of antibacterial agents. Infect Dis Clin North Am 2004;18:451–465.
21. Owens RC Jr, Ambrose PG, Nightingale. Antibiotic Optimization: Concepts and Strategies in Clinical Practice, 1st ed. New York: Marcel Dekker, 2005.
22. Nightingale Ch, Murakawa T, Ambrose PG. Antimicrobial Pharmacodynamics in Theory and Clinical Practice, 1st ed. New York: Marcel Dekker, 2002.
23. McKinnon PS, Davis SL. Pharmacokinetic and pharmacodynamic issues in the treatment of bacterial infectious diseases. Eur J Clin Microbiol Infect Dis 2004;23:271–288.
24. Sinner SW, Tunkel AR. Antimicrobial agents in the treatment of bacterial meningitis. Infect Dis Clin North Am 2004;18:581–602.
25. American Thoracic Society (ATS), Infectious Diseases Society of America (IDSA). Official ATS and IDSA statement: Guidelines for the management of adults with hospital-acquired, ventilator-associated, and healthcare-associated pneumonia Am J Respir Crit Care Med 2005;171:388–416.
26. Starr J. *Clostridium difficile* associated diarrhoea: Diagnosis and treatment. BMJ 2005;331:498–501.
27. Recommendations from the American Thoracic Society, Centers for Disease Control and Prevention, and Infectious Diseases Society of America. Controlling Tuberculosis in the United States. MMWR Recomm Rep 2005;54(RR-12):1–81.
28. McNabb J, Quintiliani R, Nicolau DP, et al. Cost-effectiveness in the use of antibiotics. Curr Clin Top Infect Dis 2002;20:24–42.
29. Scott RD 2d, Solomon SL, McGowan JE Jr. Applying economic principles to health care. Emerg Infect Dis 2001;7:282–285.
30. Solomkin JS, Mazuski JE, Baron EJ, et al. Guidelines for the selection of anti-infective agents for complicated intra-abdominal infections. Clin Infect Dis 2003;37:997–1005.
31. Murray BE. Vancomycin-resistant enterococcal infections. N Engl J Med 2000;342:710–721.
32. Bliziotis IA, Samonis G, Vardakas KZ, et al. Effect of aminoglycoside and β-lactam combination therapy versus β-lactam monotherapy on the emergence of antimicrobial resistance: A meta-analysis of randomized, controlled trials. Antimicrob Agents Chemother 2005;41:149–158.
33. Safdar N, Handelsman J, Maki DG. Does combination antimicrobial therapy reduce mortality in gram-negative bacteraemia? A meta-analysis. Lancet Infect Dis 2004;4:519–527.
34. Turnidge J. Pharmacodynamics and dosing of aminoglycosides. Infect Dis Clin N Am 2003;17:503–528.
35. Kaye KS, Fraimiw HS, Abrutyn E. Pathogens resistant to antimicrobial agents: Epidemiology, molecular mechanisms, and clinical management. Infect Dis Clin North Am 2000;14:293–319.
36. Shlaes DM, Gerding DN, John JF Jr, et al. Society for Healthcare Epidemiology of America and Infectious Diseases Society of America Joint Committee on the Prevention of Antimicrobial Resistance: Guidelines for the prevention of antimicrobial resistance in hospitals. Infect Control Hosp Epidemiol 1997;18:275–291.
37. Polk RE. Antimicrobial formularies: Can they minimize antimicrobial resistance. Am J Health Syst Pharm 2003;60(Suppl 1):S16–S19.
38. Fishman N. Antimicrobial stewardship. Am J Med 2006:119(6A):S53-S61.
39. McGowan JE Jr. Strategies for study of the role of cycling on antimicrobial use and resistance. Infect Control Hosp Epidemiol 2000;21:S36–43.
40. van Loon HJ, Vriens MR, Fluit AC, et al. Antibiotic rotation and development of gram-negative antibiotic resistance. Am J Respir Crit Care Med 2005;171:480–487.

Appendix 109-1

Drugs of Choice, First Choice, Alternative(s)

GRAM-POSITIVE COCCI

Enterococcus faecalis (generally not as resistant to antibiotics as *Enterococcus faecium*)
Serious infection (endocarditis, meningitis, pyelonephritis with bacteremia)
Ampicillin (or penicillin G) + (gentamicin or streptomycin)
Vancomycin + (gentamicin or streptomycin), linezolid, daptomycin, tigecycline
Urinary tract infection (UTI)
Ampicillin, amoxicillin
Fosfomycin or nitrofurantoin
E. faecium (generally more resistant to antibiotics than *E. faecalis*)
Recommend consultation with infectious disease specialist.
Linezolid, quinupristin/dalfopristin, daptomycin, tigecycline
Staphylococcus aureus/Staphylococcus epidermidis
Methicillin (oxacillin)-sensitive
PRP[a]
FGC,[b,c] trimethoprim-sulfamethoxazole, clindamycin,[d] ampicillin-sulbactam, or amoxicillin-clavulanate
Methicillin (oxacillin)–resistant
Vancomycin ± (gentamicin or rifampin)
Trimethoprim-sulfamethoxazole, doxycycline[e] or clindamycin[d], Linezolid, quinupristin-dalfopristin, daptomycin, or tigecycline
Streptococcus (groups A, B, C, G, and *Streptococcus bovis*)
Penicillin G[f] or V[g] or ampicillin
FGC,[b,c] erythromycin, azithromycin, clarithromycin,[h]
Streptococcus pneumoniae
Penicillin-sensitive (MIC <0.1 mcg/mL)
Penicillin G or V or ampicillin
Erythromycin, FGC,[b,c] doxycycline, azithromycin, clarithromycin[h]
Penicillin intermediate (MIC 0.1–1.0 mcg/mL)
High-dose penicillin (12 million units/day for adults) or ceftriaxone[c] or cefotaxime[c]
Levofloxacin,[i] moxifloxacin,[i] gemifloxacin,[i] telithromycin, or vancomycin
Penicillin-resistant (MIC ≥1.0 mcg/mL)
Recommend consultation with infectious disease specialist.
Vancomycin ± rifampin
Per sensitivities: TGC,[c,j] telithromycin, levofloxacin,[i] moxifloxacin,[i] or gemifloxacin[i]
Streptococcus, viridans group
Penicillin G ± gentamicin[k]
TGC,[c,j] erythromycin, azithromycin, clarithromycin,[h] or vancomycin ± gentamicin

GRAM-NEGATIVE COCCI

Moraxella (Branhamella) catarrhalis
Amoxicillin-clavulanate, ampicillin-sulbactam
Trimethoprim-sulfamethoxazole, erythromycin, azithromycin, clarithromycin,[h] doxycycline,[e] SGC,[c,l] TGC,[c,j] or TGC PO[c,m]
Neisseria gonorrhoeae (also give concomitant treatment for *Chlamydia trachomatis*)
Disseminated gonococcal infection
Ceftriaxone[c] or cefotaxime[c]
Oral followup: Cefpodoxime,[c] ciprofloxacin,[i] or levofloxacin [i]
Uncomplicated infection
Ceftriaxone[c] or cefotaxime,[c] or cefpodoxime[c]
Ciprofloxacin[i] or levofloxacin[i]
Neisseria meningitides
Penicillin G
TGC[c,j]

GRAM-POSITIVE BACILLI

Clostridium perfringens
Penicillin G ± clindamycin
Metronidazole, clindamycin, doxycycline,[e] cefazolin,[c] imipenem,[n] meropenem,[n] or ertapenem[n]
Clostridium difficile
Oral metronidazole
Oral vancomycin

GRAM-NEGATIVE BACILLI

Acinetobacter spp.
Imipenem or meropenem ± aminoglycoside[o] (amikacin usually most effective)
Ciprofloxacin,[i] ampicillin-sulbactam, colistin, or tigecycline
Bacteroides fragilis (and others)
Metronidazole
BLIC,[p] clindamycin, cephamycins,[c,q] or carbapenem[n]
Enterobacter spp.
Imipenem, meropenem, ertapenem, or cefepime ± aminoglycoside[p]
Ciprofloxacin,[i] levofloxacin,[i] piperacillin-tazobactam, ticarcillin-clavulanate, or tigecycline
Escherichia coli
Meningitis
TGC[c,j] or meropenem
Systemic infection
TGC[c,j]
Ampicillin-sulbactam, FGC,[b,c] BL/BLI,[p] fluoroquinolone,[i,n,r] imipenem,[n] meropenem[n]
Urinary tract infection
Most oral agents: check sensitivities
Ampicillin, amoxicillin-clavulanate, doxycyline,[e] or cephalexin[c]
Aminoglycoside,[p] FGC[b,c] nitrofurantoin, fluoroquinolone[i,n,r]
Gardnerella vaginalis
Metronidazole
Clindamycin
Haemophilus influenzae
Meningitis
Cefotaxime[c] or ceftriaxone[c]
Meropenem[n] or chloramphenicol[s]
Other infections
BLIC,[p] or if β-lactamase-negative, ampicillin or amoxicillin
Trimethoprim-sulfamethoxazole, cefuroxime,[c] azithromycin, clarithromycin,[h] or fluoroquinolone[i,n,r]

Klebsiella pneumoniae
TGC[e,k] (if UTI only: aminoglycoside[p])
Cefuroxime,[e] fluoroquinolone,[b,r] BLIC,[g] imipenem,[o] meropenem,[o] or ertapenem

Legionella spp.
Erythromycin ± rifampin or fluoroquinolone[i,r]
Trimethoprim-sulfamethoxazole, clarithromycin,[h] azithromycin, or doxycycline[e]

Pasteurella multocida
Penicillin G, ampicillin, amoxicillin
Doxycycline,[e] BLIC,[p] trimethoprim-sulfamethoxazole or ceftriaxone[c,j]

Proteus mirabilis
Ampicillin
Trimethoprim-sulfamethoxazole, most antibiotics except PRP[a]

Proteus (indole-positive) (including *Providencia rettgeri, Morganella morganii,* and *Proteus vulgaris*)
TGC[c,h] or fluoroquinolone[f,r]
BLIC,[p] aztreonam,[t] imipenem,[n] or TGC PO[c,m]

Providencia stuartii
TGC[c,j] or fluoroquinolone[i,r]
Trimethoprim-sulfamethoxazole, aztreonam,[t] imipenem,[n] meropenem,[n] or ertapenem

Pseudomonas aeruginosa
Cefepime,[c] ceftazidime,[c] piperacillin-tazobactam, or ticarcillin-clavulanate plus aminoglycoside[o]
Ciprofloxacin,[i] levofloxacin,[i] aztreonam,[t] imipenem,[n] meropenem,[n] or colistin
UTI only: aminoglycoside[o]
Ciprofloxacin,[i] levofloxacin[i]

Salmonella typhi
Ciprofloxacin,[i] levofloxacin,[i] ceftriaxone,[c] or cefotaxime[c]
Trimethoprim-sulfamethoxazole

Serratia marcescens
Piperacillin-tazobactam, ticarcillin-clavulanate, or TGC[c,j] ± gentamicin
Trimethoprim-sulfamethoxazole, ciprofloxacin,[i] levofloxacin,[i] aztreonam,[t] imipenem,[n] meropenem,[n] or ertapenem

Stenotrophomonas (Xanthomonas) maltophilia
Trimethoprim-sulfamethoxazole
Generally very resistant to all antimicrobials; check sensitivities to ceftazidime,[e] ticarcillin-clavulanate, doxycycline,[e] and minocycline[e]

MISCELLANEOUS MICROORGANISMS

Chlamydia pneumoniae
Doxycycline[e]
Erythromycin, azithromycin, clarithromycin,[h] telithromycin or fluoroquinolone[f,r]

C. trachomatis
Doxycycline[e] or azithromycin
Levofloxacin[i] or ofloxacin[i]

Mycoplasma pneumoniae
Erythromycin, azithromycin, clarithromycin[h]
Doxycycline[e] or fluoroquinolone[f,r]

SPIROCHETES

Treponema pallidum
Neurosyphilis
Penicillin G
Ceftriaxone[c]
Primary or secondary
Benzathine penicillin G
Doxycycline[e] or ceftriaxone[c]

Borrelia burgdorferi (choice depends on stage of disease)
Ceftriaxone[c] or cefuroxime axetil,[c] doxycycline,[e] amoxicillin
High-dose penicillin, cefotaxime,[c] or azithromycin

BLIC, β-lactamase inhibitor combination; BL/BLI, β-lactamase/β-lactamase inhibitor; FGC, first-generation cephalosporin; MIC, minimal inhibitory concentration; PO, orally; PRP, penicillinase-resistant penicillin; SGC, second-generation cephalosporin; TGC, third-generation cephalosporin.
[a]Penicillinase-resistant penicillin: nafcillin or oxacillin.
[b]First-generation cephalosporins—IV: cefazolin; PO: cephalexin, cephradine, or cefadroxil.
[c]Some penicillin-allergic patients may react to cephalosporins.
[d]Not reliably bactericidal; should not be used for endocarditis.
[e]Not for use in pregnant patients or children younger than 8 years old.
[f]Either aqueous penicillin G or benzathine penicillin G (pharyngitis only).
[g]Only for soft tissue infections or upper respiratory infections (pharyngitis, otitis media).
[h]Do not use in pregnant patients.
[i]Not for use in pregnant patients or children younger than 18 years old.
[j]Third-generation cephalosporins—IV: cefotaxime, ceftriaxone.
[k]Gentamicin should be added if tolerance or moderately susceptible (MIC >0.1 g/mL) organisms are encountered; streptomycin is used but can be more toxic.
[l]Second-generation cephalosporins—IV: cefuroxime; PO: cefaclor, cefditoren, cefprozil, cefuroxime axetil, and loracarbef.
[m]Third-generation cephalosporins—PO: cefdinir, cefixime, cefetamet, cefpodoxime proxetil, and ceftibuten.
[n]Reserve for serious infection.
[o]Aminoglycosides: gentamicin, tobramycin, and amikacin; use per sensitivities.
[p]β-Lactamase inhibitor combination—IV: ampicillin-sulbactam, piperacillin-tazobactam, ticarcillin-clavulanate; PO: amoxicillin-clavulanate.
[q]Cefoxitin
[r]IV/PO: ciprofloxacin, levofloxacin, and moxifloxacin.
[s]Reserve for serious infection when less toxic drugs are not effective.
[t]Generally reserved for patients with hypersensitivity reactions to penicillin.

CHAPTER 110

Central Nervous System Infections

ISAAC F. MITROPOULOS, ELIZABETH D. HERMSEN, JEREMY A. SCHAFER, AND JOHN C. ROTSCHAFER

KEY CONCEPTS

1. The three most likely pathogens of bacterial meningitis in the United States are *Streptococcus pneumoniae, Neisseria meningitidis,* and *Haemophilus influenzae.* Routine vaccination is having a dramatic effect on the incidence of these pathogens causing infection.

2. In cases of meningitis, initial findings can include (a) *presenting signs and symptoms:* fever, headache, and nuchal rigidity (classic triad), Brudzinski or Kernig sign, and altered mental status, and (b) *abnormal cerebrospinal fluid (CSF) chemistries:* elevated white blood cell count (>100 cells/mm^3), elevated protein (>50 mg/dL), and decreased glucose levels (<40 mg/dL).

3. Two main microbiologic tests that should be obtained include a Gram stain of the CSF and CSF cultures.

4. Three primary goals of treatment in meningitis are (a) *eradication* of infection, (b) *amelioration* of signs and symptoms, and (c) *prevention* of development of neurologic sequelae, such as seizures, deafness, coma, and death.

5. When selecting antibiotics, the clinician must consider the antibiotic concentration at the site of infection as well as the spectrum of antibacterial activity. Empirical choices should be based on age and predisposing conditions. (a) *Ceftriaxone* or *cefotaxime* and *vancomycin* are reasonable initial choices for empirical coverage of community-acquired meningitis in adult patients. (b) *Listeria monocytogenes* is a common pathogen in infants and elderly; therefore, *ampicillin* should be added empirically to antimicrobial coverage.

6. Empirical coverage with an appropriate antibiotic should be started as soon as possible when clinical suspicion of meningitis exists. If lumbar puncture is to be delayed (even by 30–60 minutes) or if the patient is to undergo neuroimaging, the first dose of an antibiotic *should not* be withheld. Changes in CSF after initiation of antibiotics usually take 12 to 24 hours.

7. In contrast to treatment of other infectious diseases, antibiotic dosages for treatment of meningitis should be maximized to optimize central nervous system penetration.

8. The duration of antibiotic treatment for meningitis is not standardized; however, the duration of antibiotic therapy generally is based on the causative organism and the individual case and may range from 7 to 21 days.

9. Close contacts and relatives of the index case should be assessed for appropriate prophylaxis, particularly with *N. meningitidis* and *H. influenzae* meningitis.

10. Steroid treatment includes dexamethasone 0.15 mg/kg per dose given four times daily for 4 days in infants and children older than 2 months with proven or strongly suspected bacterial meningitis. Steroids should be given *prior* to antibiotics.

Learning objectives, review questions, and other resources can be found at **www.pharmacotherapyonline.com.**

Central nervous system (CNS) infections are caused by various pathogens, including bacteria, viruses, fungi, and parasites. Infections are the result of hematogenous spread from a primary infection site, seeding from a parameningeal focus, reactivation from a latent site, trauma, or congenital defects in the CNS. Newer diagnostic techniques have enabled more rapid and definitive diagnoses, thus diminishing the number of unknown "aseptic meningitis" diagnoses and improving targeted therapy. Bacteria resistant to multiple antibiotics present new challenges in the management of meningitis. This chapter presents the etiologies, pathophysiology, therapy, and prophylaxis of these infections, with concentration on bacterial meningitis.

EPIDEMIOLOGY

Approximately 1.2 million cases of acute bacterial meningitis, excluding epidemics, occur every year around the world, resulting in 135,000 deaths.[1] Overall mortality rates for patients with meningitis range from 2% to 30% depending on the causative microorganism, approaching 20% in most cases of bacterial meningitis.[2] Neurologic sequelae frequently associated with meningitis include seizures, sensorineural hearing loss, and hydrocephalus. Risk for development of neurologic sequelae depends on the infecting organism, with pneumococcal meningitis associated with the highest risk.[3] Generally, 30% to 50% of patients who survive meningitis may develop neurologic disabilities.[4,5] Despite the availability of antimicrobial therapy against the most common CNS pathogens, CNS infections continue to have significant morbidity and mortality.

Two findings have the potential for great epidemiologic impact on bacterial meningitis. First, both passive and active exposure to cigarette smoke were shown to be risk factors for bacterial meningitis, especially meningococcal disease.[6] Second, children with cochlear implants that include a positioner are at increased risk for bacterial meningitis, specifically pneumococcal meningitis. The incidence of meningitis due to *Streptococcus pneumoniae* in children with cochlear implants was more than 30 times the incidence in a similar cohort of the U.S. population without implants.[7]

ETIOLOGY

❶ CNS infections are caused by a variety of microorganisms. Historically, CNS infections were primarily community acquired; however, an increasing number now are nosocomial.[8] *Haemophilus influenzae* was the most commonly identified cause of bacterial meningitis (45%), followed by *S. pneumoniae* (18%) and *Neisseria meningitidis* (14%). However, in 1995, approximately 5 years after introduction of the *H. influenzae* type b conjugate (Hib) vaccine, *S. pneumoniae* became the most commonly identified cause of bacterial meningitis (47%), followed by *N. meningitidis* (25%), *Listeria monocytogenes* (8%), and *H. influenzae* (7%).

The incidence of invasive *H. influenzae* infections has decreased by more than 90% since the introduction of the Hib vaccine.[9] Mass immunization with the Hib vaccine also has resulted in alterations in the age distribution of bacterial meningitis. Whereas in 1986 the median age was 15 months, by 1995 that age increased to 25 years. Accordingly, the proportion of cases in those 18 years and older increased from 20.8% to 51.5%.[9] However, many developing countries have not adopted the Hib vaccine as part of the standard vaccines offered to children because of cost. Thus, approximately 350,000 to 700,000 children die each year worldwide due to invasive *H. influenzae* infections.[1]

Following the release of the heptavalent protein–polysaccharide conjugate vaccine, the rate of invasive pneumococcal disease dropped from 24.3 cases per 100,000 people in 1999 to 17.3 per 100,000 in 2001. The largest impact was in children younger than 2 years, in whom a nearly 70% decline in infection rate was reported as a result of implementation of the routine childhood vaccination schedule. Among children younger than 5 years, the rates of pneumococcal meningitis were reduced nearly 60% from 10.3 cases per 100,000 to 4.2 cases during the same time period. Interestingly, the effect carried into the adult population as well, with significant reduction in invasive pneumococcal disease across all age groups.[10] Both the Hib and pneumococcal vaccines are of limited availability in developing countries, where cost often is prohibitive.

ANATOMY AND PHYSIOLOGY OF THE CENTRAL NERVOUS SYSTEM

MENINGES

The skull and vertebrae protect the CNS from blunt or penetrating trauma (Fig. 110–1). The brain is suspended in these structures by cerebrospinal fluid (CSF) and is surrounded by the meninges. The meninges are made up of three separate membranes: dura mater, arachnoid, and pia mater.[11] *Dura mater,* or *pachymeninges,* lies directly beneath and is adherent to the skull. The other two membranes are referred to collectively as *leptomeninges. Pia mater* lies directly over brain tissue. Arachnoid, the middle layer, lies between the dura mater and the pia mater. The *subarachnoid space,* located between the arachnoid and the pia mater, is the conduit for CSF. By definition, *meningitis* refers to inflammation of the subarachnoid space or spinal fluid, whereas *encephalitis* is an inflammation of the brain itself. Because infectious microorganisms frequently are an underlying cause of these inflammatory processes, the terms *meningitis* and *encephalitis* frequently are used to denote an infectious process. The decision regarding the diagnosis of meningoencephalitis depends on radiographic, laboratory, and clinical information but refers to inflammation of both tissue and fluid.

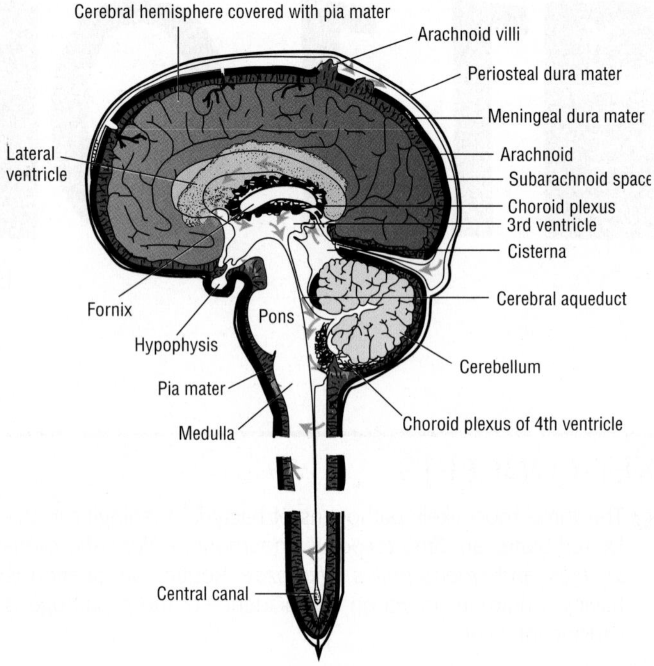

FIGURE 110-1. Diagram of the central nervous system.

CEREBROSPINAL FLUID

Approximately 85% of the CSF is produced within the third, fourth, and lateral ventricles by the choroid plexus (Fig. 110–1). CSF volume in the CNS is related to patient age. Infants have approximately 40 to 60 mL of CSF, older children have 60 to 100 mL, and adults have 110 to 160 mL. Normally, CSF is produced at the rate of approximately 500 mL/day and flows unidirectionally downward through the spinal cord. The CSF is removed by the arachnoid villi and vertebral venous plexus located in the spinal cord and does not recommunicate with the point of production.[11]

The CSF normally is clear, with a protein content <50 mg/dL, glucose concentration approximately 50% to 66% of the simultaneous peripheral serum glucose concentration, and pH approximately 7.4. It typically contains fewer than five white blood cells (WBCs) per cubic millimeter, all of which should be lymphocytes (Table 110–1). As meninges become inflamed, the constituency of the CSF changes, and these changes can be used diagnostically as markers of infection.

TABLE 110-1 Mean Values of Components of Normal and Abnormal Cerebrospinal Fluid

Type	Normal	Bacterial	Viral	Fungal	Tuberculosis
WBC (cells/mm^3)	<5	1,000–5,000	100–1,000	40–400	100–500
Differential (%)	>90[a]	≥80 PMNs	50[b,c]	>50[b]	>80[b,c]
Protein (mg/dL)	<50	100–500	30–150	40–150	≤40–150
Glucose (mg/dL)	50–66% simultaneous serum value	<40 (<60% simultaneous serum value)	<30–70	<30–70	<30–70

[a]Monocytes.
[b]Lymphocytes.
[c]Initial cerebrospinal fluid; while blood cell (WBC) count may reveal a predominance of polymorphonuclear neutrophils (PMNs).
From Schuchat et al.[9] and Bennett et al.[92]

BLOOD–BRAIN BARRIER/BLOOD–CEREBRAL SPINAL FLUID BARRIER

Natural barriers to the exchange of drugs and endogenous compounds among the blood, brain, and CSF are the blood–brain barrier and the blood–CSF barrier (Fig. 110–2). The blood–brain barrier consists of tightly joined capillary endothelial cells. Drug entry into brain tissue is accomplished by direct passage through the capillary endothelial cells and further penetration of the glial cells that envelop the capillary structure.[11]

Passage of drugs into the CSF is controlled by the blood–CSF barrier. This barrier is created by ependymal cells of the choroid plexus, which function as an active transport system similar to the renal tubular epithelial cells. The inflammatory process associated with meningitis inhibits the active transport system of the choroid plexus.[12] As in the active transport system in the kidney, secretion of substances out of the choroid plexus can be inhibited by administration of probenecid.[11]

PATHOPHYSIOLOGY OF CENTRAL NERVOUS SYSTEM INFECTION

The development of bacterial meningitis occurs following bacterial invasion of the host and CNS, bacterial multiplication with subsequent inflammation of the CNS, specifically the subarachnoid space and the ventricular space, pathophysiologic alterations owing to progressive inflammation, and the resulting neuronal damage.[13] The critical first step in the acquisition of acute bacterial meningitis is nasopharyngeal colonization of the host. Immunoglobulins (Igs) such as secretory IgA are found in high concentrations within nasopharyngeal secretions and work to inhibit bacterial colonization. However, the mucus barrier is deteriorated by IgA proteases secreted by the bacteria, which then extend pili that allow adherence to the host cell surface receptors.[14] Bacterial pathogens attach themselves to nasopharyngeal epithelial cells and are phagocytized into the host's bloodstream. After accessing the patient's bloodstream, bacteria must overcome the host's defense mechanisms.[1] Commonly, CNS bacterial pathogens produce an extensive polysaccharide capsule resistant to neutrophil phagocytosis and complement opsonization. *H. influenzae, Escherichia coli,* and *N. meningitidis* strains lacking polysaccharide capsules are unable to cause meningitis. Capsular polysaccharides activate the alternate complement pathway, which promotes phagocytosis and clearance of infecting pathogens. Patients unable to activate the alternative complement pathway, such as patients with asplenic and sickle cell, are predisposed to bacterial infections caused by encapsulated microorganisms and therefore are at risk for meningitis.

Although the exact site and mechanism of bacterial invasion into the CNS are unknown, studies suggest that invasion into the subarachnoid space occurs by continuous exposure of the CNS to large bacterial inocula. Bacteremia with inoculum densities of at least 10^3 colony-forming units per milliliter appears to be essential for subarachnoid space invasion.[5] Although several sites of bacterial invasion have been theorized, the most plausible sites are the choroid plexus and/or the cerebral microvasculature. Successful translocation of *E. coli* across the blood–brain barrier requires a high bacterial inoculum, *E. coli* binding to and invading the brain microvascular endothelial cells through specific ligand-receptor interactions, host cytoskeletal reorganization, and activation of various signaling pathways.[5] Host defense mechanisms within the subarachnoid space are inadequate to combat bacterial pathogens; therefore, bacteria replicate freely within the CSF until either overgrowth occurs or an effective antibiotic regimen is administered that terminates the process.

The effects of meningitis, namely, inflammation within the subarachnoid space and the ensuing neurologic damage, are not a direct result of the pathogens themselves. The neurologic sequelae occur due to activation of the host's inflammatory pathways, which is induced by the pathogens or their products.[2] Bacterial cell death can cause the release of cell wall components, such as lipopolysaccharide, lipid A (endotoxin), lipoteichoic acid, teichoic acid, and peptidoglycan, depending on whether the pathogen is gram-positive or gram-negative (Fig. 110–3). These cell wall components cause capillary endothelial cells and CNS macrophages to release cytokines (interleukin 1 [IL-1], tumor necrosis factor [TNF]) and other inflammatory mediators

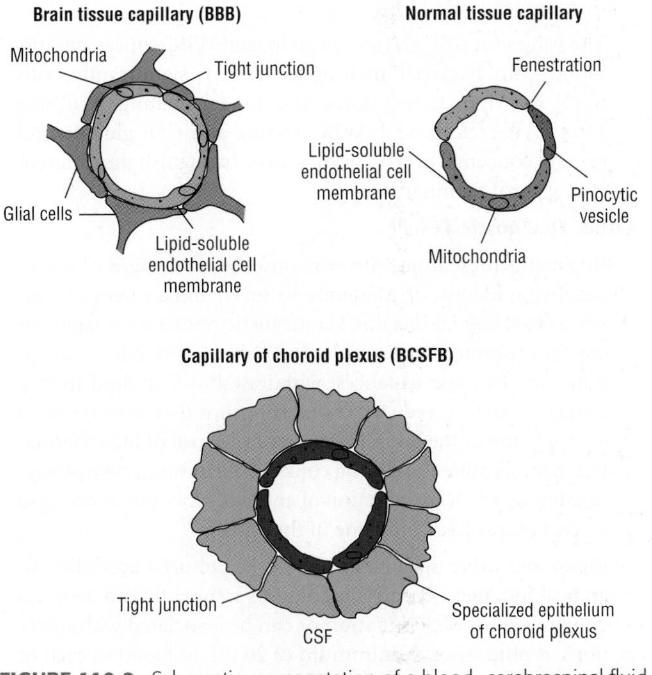

FIGURE 110-2. Schematic representation of a blood–cerebrospinal fluid barrier capillary, brain tissue capillary, and normal tissue capillary *(below)*.

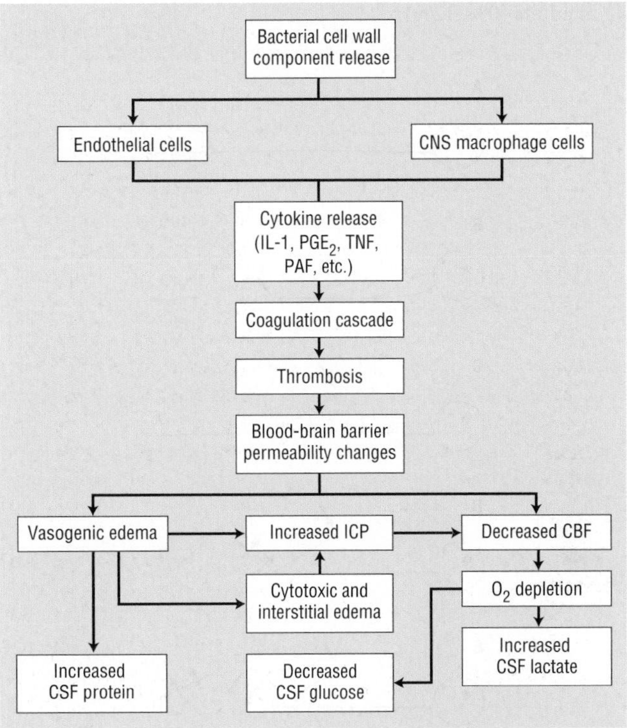

FIGURE 110-3. Hypothetical schema of pathophysiologic events that occur during bacterial meningitis. (CBF, cerebral blood flow; CSF, cerebrospinal fluid; ICP, intracranial pressure; IL-1, interleukin 1; PAF, platelet-activating factor; PGE_2, prostaglandin E_2; TNF, tumor necrosis factor.)

(IL-6, IL-8, platelet-activating factor [PAF], nitric oxide, arachidonic acid metabolites [e.g., prostaglandin and prostacyclin], macrophage-derived proteins). Proteolytic products and toxic oxygen radicals are released from the capillary endothelium, causing an alteration in the permeability of the blood–brain barrier. PAF activates the coagulation cascade, and arachidonic acid metabolites stimulate vasodilation. These events propagate other sequential events that lead to cerebral edema, elevated intracranial pressure (ICP), CSF pleocytosis, decreased cerebral blood flow, cerebral ischemia, and death.[2]

CLINICAL PRESENTATION AND DIAGNOSIS

CLINICAL PRESENTATION OF ACUTE MENINGITIS

General

- Clinical presentation varies with age; generally, the younger the patient, the more atypical and the less pronounced is the clinical picture.
- Up to 50% of patients may receive antibiotics before a diagnosis of meningitis is made, delaying presentation to the hospital. Prior antibiotic therapy may cause the Gram stain and CSF culture to be negative, but antibiotic therapy rarely affects CSF protein or glucose.[15]

Signs and Symptoms

- ❷ Classic signs and symptoms include fever, nuchal rigidity, and altered mental status (the classic triad), chills, vomiting, photophobia, and severe headache. Kernig and Brudzinski signs may be present but are poorly sensitive and frequently are absent in children[15,16] (Figs. 110–4 and 110–5).
- Other signs and symptoms include irritability, delirium, drowsiness, lethargy, and coma.
- Clinical signs and symptoms in young children also may include bulging fontanelle, apneas, purpuric rash, and convulsions.[15]
- Seizures occur more commonly in children (20%–30%) than in adults (0%–12%).[17]

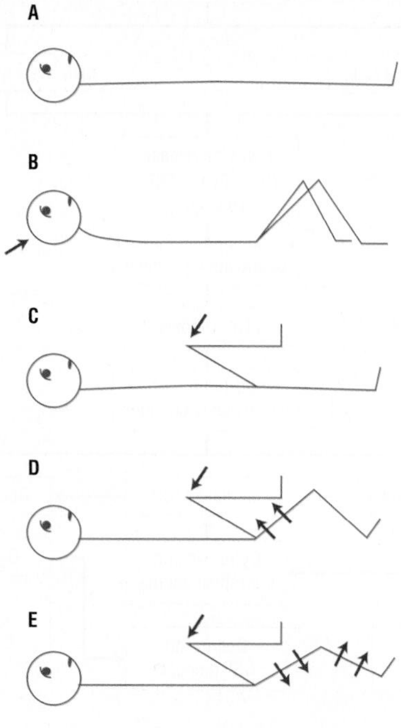

FIGURE 110-4. *A, B.* Brudzinski neck signs. Hip and knee flexion occur as a result of flexion of the neck *(B)*. *C–E.* Brudzinski leg signs. *C.* Patient's leg is flexed by examiner *(arrow)*. *D.* Contralateral leg begins to flex–identical contralateral sign *(arrows)*. *E.* Contralateral leg now begins to extend spontaneously, resembling a little kick *(arrows)*.

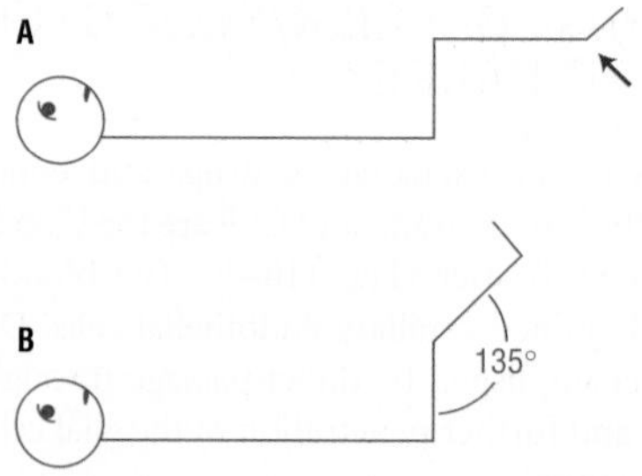

FIGURE 110-5. Kernig sign. *A.* Knees are raised to form a 90-degree angle relative to the trunk, and the examiner attempts to extend the knees. *B.* Once the knee angle reaches approximately 135 degrees, contracture or extensor spasm occurs.

Differential Signs and Symptoms[2]

- Purpuric and petechial skin lesions typically indicate meningococcal involvement, although the lesions may be present with *H. influenzae* meningitis. Rashes rarely occur with pneumococcal meningitis.
- Waterhouse-Friderichsen syndrome, a rapid eruption of multiple hemorrhagic lesions associated with a shock-like state, is associated with meningococcal meningitis.
- *H. influenza* meningitis and meningococcal meningitis both can cause involvement of the joints during the illness.
- A history of head trauma with or without skull fracture or presence of a chronically draining ear is associated with pneumococcal involvement.

Laboratory Tests

- Several tubes of CSF are collected via lumbar puncture for chemistry, microbiologic, and hematologic tests. Theoretically, the first tube has a higher likelihood of being contaminated with both blood and bacteria during the puncture, although in practice the total volume is more important than the tube cultured. CSF should not be refrigerated or stored on ice.[18]
- Analysis of CSF chemistries typically includes measurement of glucose and total protein concentrations. An elevated CSF protein ≥100 mg/dL and CSF glucose concentration <50% of the simultaneously obtained peripheral value suggest bacterial meningitis (Table 110–1).
- The values for CSF glucose, protein, and WBC concentrations found with bacterial meningitis overlap significantly with those for viral, tuberculous, and fungal meningitis (Table 110–1). Therefore, CSF WBC counts and CSF glucose and protein concentrations cannot always distinguish the different etiologies of meningitis.

Other Diagnostic Tests[18]

- In patients presenting with new-onset seizures, signs of space-occupying lesions, or moderate-to-severe impairment of consciousness, cranial imaging via magnetic resonance imaging or cranial computed tomography (CT) should precede a lumbar puncture. In these instances, withdrawal of CSF fluid from a lumbar puncture reduces counterpressure that may result in compression of the brain from above with risk of brain herniation complicating the clinical course.[19,20] However, neuroimaging should not delay initiation of antibiotic therapy, as doing so can result in a poor outcome in this disease.[21]
- Blood and other specimens should be cultured according to clinical judgment because meningitis frequently can arise via hematogenous dissemination or can be associated with infections at other sites. A minimum of 20 mL of blood in each of two to three separate cultures per each 24-hour period is necessary for detection of most bacteremias.

- ❸ Gram stain and culture of the CSF are the most important laboratory tests performed for bacterial meningitis. The Gram stain continues to be the most rapid and accurate method of presumptively diagnosing acute bacterial meningitis. When performed before antibiotic therapy is initiated, Gram stain is both rapid and sensitive and can confirm the diagnosis of bacterial meningitis in 75% to 90% of cases. The sensitivity of the Gram stain decreases to 40% to 60% in patients who received prior antibiotic therapy. Culture is required to differentiate the various bacterial etiologies.
- Polymerase chain reaction (PCR) techniques can be used to diagnose meningitis caused by *N. meningitidis, S. pneumoniae,* and Hib. PCR is considered to be highly sensitive and specific, but use of this powerful diagnostic approach is limited because of expense and availability.
- Latex fixation, latex coagglutination, and enzyme immunoassay tests provide for rapid identification of several bacterial causes of meningitis, including *S. pneumoniae, N. meningitidis,* and Hib.[13] Rapid-identification latex tests work by bringing potential capsular antigens of the pathogen causing meningitis in contact with a specific antibody, causing an antigen–antibody reaction. This capsular antigen–antibody reaction can be observed visually and quickly without waiting for culture results. The rapid antigen tests should be used in situations where in which the Gram stain is negative.[17] The sensitivity and specificity of latex fixation and coagglutination tests can vary with the manufacturer of the antibody, density of the antigen present in the CSF, and pathogen being tested.
- Diagnosis of tuberculosis meningitis uses acid-fast staining, culture, and PCR of the CSF.
- PCR testing of the CSF is the preferred method for diagnosing most viral meningitis infections.
- The standard diagnostic tests for fungal meningitis include culture, direct microscopic examination of stained and unstained specimens of CSF, antigen detection of cryptococcal or histoplasmal antigens, and antibody assay of serum and/or CSF.

TREATMENT

Central Nervous System Infections

DESIRED OUTCOME

Supportive care, particularly early in the course of treatment, is critically important. Administration of fluids, electrolytes, antipyretics, analgesics, and other supportive measures is indicated for patients presenting with acute bacterial meningitis. Although supportive care is important initially, appropriate antibiotic therapy (empirical or definitive) should be started as soon as possible. ❹ Understanding antibiotic selection and the issues surrounding antibiotic penetration will assist in meeting the goals of treatment, which include eradication of infection with amelioration of signs and symptoms and prevention of neurologic sequelae, such as seizures, deafness, coma, and death.

APPROACH TO TREATMENT

This section discusses issues surrounding the approach to treatment, such as antibiotic penetration within the CNS, duration of antibiotic therapy, and use of adjunctive corticosteroids. Until a pathogen is identified, prompt empirical antibiotic coverage often is needed. ❺ Based on the patient's profile (i.e., allergies, age, and

TABLE 110-2 Most Likely and Empirical Therapy for Bacterial Meningitis by Age Group

Age Commonly Affected	Most Likely Organisms	Empirical Therapy	Risk Factors for All Age Groups
Newborn–1 month	Group B *Streptococcus* Gram-negative enterics[a] *Listeria monocytogenes*	Ampicillin plus cefotaxime or ceftriaxone or aminoglycoside	Respiratory tract infection Otitis media Mastoiditis Head trauma Alcoholism High-dose steroids
1 month–4 years	*S. pneumoniae* *N. meningitidis* *H. influenzae*	Vancomycin[b] and cefotaxime or ceftriaxone	Splenectomy Sickle cell disease Immunoglobulin deficiency
5–29 years	*N. meningitidis* *S. pneumoniae* *H. influenzae*	Vancomycin[b] and cefotaxime or ceftriaxone	Immunosuppression
30–60 years	*S. pneumoniae* *N. meningitidis*	Vancomycin[b] and cefotaxime or ceftriaxone	
>60 years	*S. pneumoniae* Gram-negative enterics *L. monocytogenes*	Vancomycin[b] plus ampicillin plus cefotaxime or ceftriaxone	

[a]*Escherichia coli, Klebsiella* species, *Enterobacter* species common.
[b]Vancomycin use should be based on local incidence of penicillin-resistant *S. pneumoniae* and until cefotaxime or ceftriaxone minimum inhibitory concentration results are available.

tion, and spectrum of activity, appropriate recommendations can be made, and therapy should last at least 48 to 72 hours or until the diagnosis of ❻ bacterial meningitis can be ruled out (Tables 110–2 and 110–3). The first dose of antibiotics should not be withheld even if lumbar puncture is to be delayed or neuroimaging is to be performed. Changes in the CSF after antibiotic administration usually take 12 to 24 hours. Continued therapy should be based on the assessment of clinical improvement, cultures, and susceptibility testing results. Once a pathogen is identified, antibiotic therapy should be tailored to the specific pathogen (Tables 110–4 and 110–5). Throughout the course of treatment, efficacy parameters (e.g., signs and symptoms, microbiologic findings, and CSF examination) should be followed to evaluate the success of meeting the desired outcomes.

Several factors influence the transfer of antibiotic from capillary blood into the CNS, including inflammation of the meninges, which increases antibiotic penetration through damage to tight junctions between capillary endothelial cells and decreases the activity of an energy-dependent efflux pump in the choroid plexus responsible for movement of penicillins, and, to a much lesser extent, fluoroquinolones and aminoglycosides (Table 110–3). Antibiotics having low molecular weights are passed more easily through biologic barriers than are compounds of higher molecular weight. Only antibiotics that are nonionized at physiologic or pathologic pH are capable of diffusion. Highly lipid-soluble compounds penetrate more readily than are water-soluble compounds. Antibiotics not extensively protein bound in the serum provide a larger free fraction of drug capable of passing into the CSF. Passage of large, polar antibiotics into the CSF may be assisted, however, by a carrier transport system. ❼ Unlike the treatment of many other infections, antibiotic dosages in the treatment of CNS infections must be maximized to optimize penetration to the site of infection.

Problems of CSF penetration may be overcome by direct instillation of antibiotics intrathecally, intracisternally, or intraventricularly (Table 110–6). However, advantages of direct instillation must be weighed against the risks of invasive CNS procedures. Intrathecal administration of antibiotics is unlikely to produce therapeutic

TABLE 110-3 Penetration of Antimicrobial Agents into the Cerebrospinal Fluid

Therapeutic levels in CSF with or without inflammation	
Chloramphenicol	Pyrazinamide
Cycloserine	Rifampin
Ethionamide	Sulfonamides
Isoniazid	Trimethoprim
Metronidazole	
Therapeutic levels in CSF with inflammation of meninges	
Acyclovir	Ganciclovir
Ampicillin ± sulbactam	Imipenem
Aztreonam	Levofloxacin
Carbenicillin	Linezolid
Cefotaxime	Meropenem
Ceftazidime	Mezlocillin
Ceftizoxime	Moxifloxacin
Ceftriaxone	Nafcillin
Cefuroxime	Ofloxacin
Ciprofloxacin	Penicillin G
Colistin	Piperacillin
Daptomycin	Pyrimethamine
Ethambutol	Quinupristin/dalfopristin
Fluconazole	Ticarcillin ± clavulanic acid
Flucytosine	Vancomycin
Foscarnet	Vidarabine
Nontherapeutic levels in CSF with or without inflammation	
Aminoglycosides	Cephalosporins (second-generation)[a]
Amphotericin B	Clindamycin[b]
Cefoperazone	Itraconazole[c]
Cephalosporins (first-generation)	Ketoconazole

CSF, cerebrospinal fluid.
[a]Cefuroxime is an exception.
[b]Achieves therapeutic brain tissue concentrations.
[c]Achieves therapeutic concentrations for *Cryptococcus neoformans* therapy.

concentrations in the ventricles, possibly because of the unidirectional flow of CSF.[22] Although intraventricular administration from a therapeutic standpoint may be preferred over intrathecal administration, the former requires neurosurgical placement of a subcutaneous reservoir. Intraventricular delivery may be necessary when bacteria that require treatment with aminoglycosides, such as *L. monocytogenes*, *Pseudomonas aeruginosa* or enterococci, are isolated. In a review of antibiotic-induced endotoxin release, children receiving both parenteral antibiotics and intrathecal gentamicin had higher CSF endotoxin levels, higher CSF IL-1β levels, and higher mortality than did children receiving only parenteral antibiotics. Interestingly, the differences were attributed to direct CSF administration of gentamicin, which generally is thought to blunt the endotoxin release caused by β-lactam antibiotics.[23]

8 Although the length of treatment for bacterial meningitis generally is based on the causative organism, there is no universally accepted standard (Table 110–4). Meningitis caused by *S. pneumoniae* has been treated successfully with 10 to 14 days of antibiotic therapy. Meningitis caused by *N. meningitidis* usually can be treated with a 7-day course of antibiotics. In contrast, a longer duration (≥21 days) has been recommended for patients infected with *L. monocytogenes* (A-III, see guidelines in Table 110–4). Therapy should be individualized, and some patients may require longer courses.

CAUSATIVE AGENTS

Neisseria meningitidis (Meningococcus)

N. meningitidis is the leading cause of bacterial meningitis in children and young adults in the United States.[24] The source of infection usually is an asymptomatic carrier. Most cases occur in the winter or spring when viral meningitis is relatively uncommon. Five serogroups of *N. meningitidis* (A, B, C, Y, and W-135) are primarily

TABLE 110-4 Antimicrobial Agents of First Choice and Alternative Choice for Treatment of Meningitis Caused by Gram-Positive and Gram-Negative Microorganisms

Organism	Antibiotic of First Choice	Alternative Antibiotics	Recommended Duration of Therapy
Gram-positive			
Streptococcus pneumoniae			10–14 days
Penicillin susceptible	Penicillin G or ampicillin (A-III)	Cefotaxime (A-III), ceftriaxone (A-III), chloramphenicol (A-III)	
Penicillin intermediate	Cefotaxime or ceftriaxone (A-III)	Cefepime (B-II), meropenem (B-II), moxifloxacin (B-II), linezolid (C-III)	
Penicillin resistant	Vancomycin[a] plus cefotaxime or ceftriaxone (A-III)	Cefepime (B-II), meropenem (B-II), moxifloxacin (B-II), linezolid (C-III)	
Group B *Streptococcus*	Penicillin G or ampicillin ± gentamicin[a] (A-III)	Cefotaxime (B-III), ceftriaxone (B-III), chloramphenicol (B-III)	14–21 days
Staphylococcus aureus			14–21 days[e]
Methicillin susceptible	Nafcillin or oxacillin (A-III)	Vancomycin[a] (A-III), meropenem (B-III)	
Methicillin resistant	Vancomycin[a] (A-III)	Trimethoprim-sulfamethoxazole (A-III), linezolid (B-III)	
Staphylococcus epidermidis	Vancomycin[a] (A-III)	Linezolid (B-III)	14–21 days[e]
Listeria monocytogenes	Penicillin G or ampicillin ± gentamicin[a] (A-III)	Trimethoprim-sulfamethoxazole (A-III), meropenem (B-III)	≥21 days
Gram-negative			
Neisseria meningitis			7 days
Penicillin susceptible	Penicillin G or ampicillin (A-III)	Cefotaxime (A-III), ceftriaxone (A-III), chloramphenicol (A-III)	
Penicillin resistant	Cefotaxime or ceftriaxone (A-III)	Chloramphenicol (A-III), meropenem (A-III), fluoroquinolone (A-III)	
Haemophilus influenzae			7 days
β-Lactamase negative	Ampicillin (A-III)	Cefotaxime (A-III), ceftriaxone (A-III), chloramphenicol (A-III), cefepime (A-III), fluoroquinolone (A-III)	
β-Lactamase positive	Cefotaxime or ceftriaxone (A-I)	Cefepime (A-I), fluoroquinolone (A-III), chloramphenicol (A-III)	
Enterobacteriaceae[d]	Cefotaxime or ceftriaxone (A-II)	Cefepime (A-III), fluoroquinolone (A-III), meropenem (A-III), aztreonam (A-III)	21 days
Pseudomonas aeruginosa	Cefepime or ceftazidime (A-II) ± tobramycin[a,b] (A-III)	Ciprofloxacin (A-III), meropenem (A-III), piperacillin plus tobramycin[a,b] (A-III), colistin sulfomethate[a,c] (B-III), aztreonam (A-III)	21 days

Strength of recommendation: A, good evidence to support a recommendation for use; should always be offered; B, moderate evidence to support a recommendation for use; should generally be offered.
Quality of evidence: I, evidence from ≥1 properly randomized, controlled trial; II, evidence from ≤1 well-designed clinical trial, without randomization; from cohort or case-controlled analytic studies (preferably from >1 center) or from multiple time-series; III, evidence from opinions of respected authorities, based on clinical experience, descriptive studies, or reports of expert committees
[a]Monitor drug levels in serum.
[b]Direct central nervous system administration may be added; see Table 110–6 for dosage.
[c]Should be reserved for multidrug-resistant pseudomonal or *Acinetobacter* infections for which all other therapeutic options have been exhausted.
[d]Includes *Escherichia coli* and *Klebsiella* species.
[e]Based on clinical experience; no clear recommendations.

TABLE 110-5 Dosing of Antimicrobial Agents by Age Group

Antimicrobial Agent	Infants and Children	Adults
Antibacterials		
Ampicillin	75 mg/kg every 6 h	2 g every 4 h
Aztreonam		2 g every 6–8 h
Cefepime	50 mg/kg every 8h	2 g every 8 h
Cefotaxime	75 mg/kg every 6–8 h	2 g every 4–6 h
Ceftazidime	50 mg/kg every 8 h	2 g every 8 h
Ceftriaxone	100 mg/kg once daily	2 g every 12–24 h
Chloramphenicol	25 mg/kg every 6 h	1–1.5g every 6 h
Ciprofloxacin	10 mg/kg every 8 h	400 mg every 8–12 h
Colistin[a,c]	5 mg/kg once daily	5 mg/kg once daily
Gentamicin[a,b]	2.5 mg/kg every 8 h	2 mg/kg every 8 h
Linezolid	10 mg/kg every 8 h	600 mg every 12 h
Meropenem	40 mg/kg every 8 h	2 mg every 8 h
Moxifloxacin		400 mg once daily
Oxacillin/nafcillin	50 mg/kg every 6 h	2 mg every 4 h
Penicillin G	0.05 million units /kg every 4–6 h	4 million units every 4h
Piperacillin	50 mg/kg every 4–6 h	3 g every 4–6 h
Tobramycin[a,b]	2.5 mg/kg every 8 h	2 mg/kg every 8 h
Trimethoprim-sulfamethoxazole[d]	5 mg/kg every 6–12 h	5 mg/kg every 6–12 h
Vancomycin[a]	15 mg/kg every 6 h	15 mg/kg every 8–12 h
Antimycobacterials		
Isoniazide	10–15 mg/kg once daily	5 mg/kg once daily
Rifampin	10–20 mg/kg once daily	600 mg once daily
Pyrazinamide	15–30 mg/kg once daily	15–30 mg/kg once daily
Ethambutol	15–25 mg/kg once daily	15–25 mg/kg once daily
Antifungals		
Amphotericin B		0.7–1 mg/kg once daily
Lipid amphotericin B		4 mg/kg once daily
Flucytosine		25 mg/kg every 6 h
Fluconazole		400-800 mg once daily
Voriconazole		6 mg/kg every 12 h × 2 doses, then 4 mg/kg every 12 h
Antivirals		
Acyclovir	20 mg/kg every 8 h	10 mg/kg every 8 h
Foscarnet		60 mg/kg every 8–12 h

[a]Monitor drug levels in serum.
[b]Direct central nervous system administration may be added; see Table 110-6 for dosage.
[c]Should be reserved for multidrug-resistant pseudomonal or *Acinetobacter* infections for which all other therapeutic options have been exhausted.
[d]Dosing based on trimethoprim component.
[e]Supplemental pyridoxine hydrochloride (vitamin B_6) 50 mg/day is recommended.

TABLE 110-6 Intraventricular and Intrathecal Antibiotic Dosage Recommendation

Antibiotic	Dose (mg)	Expected CSF Concentration[a] (mg/L)	Reference
Ampicillin	10–50	60–300	104–106
Methicillin	25–100	160–600	104–106
Nafcillin	75	500	105
Cephalothin	25–100	160–600	104–106
Chloramphenicol	25–100	160–600	104, 106, 107
Gentamicin	1–10	6–60	104–108
Quinupristin/dalfopristin	1–2	7–13	109
Tobramycin	1–10	6–60	108
Vancomycin	5	30	110–112
Amphotericin B	0.05–0.25 mg/day to 0.05–1 mg 1–3 times weekly	–	113

[a]Assumes adult cerebrospinal fluid (CSF) volume = 150 mL.

responsible. Clusters of meningococcal disease, defined as two or more cases of the same serogroup that are closer in time and space than expected for the population or group under observation, generally are associated with schools.[25] Although some of these clusters have been due to serogroup B, the majority have been due to serogroup C. Serogroup A, which is associated with meningococcal outbreaks in Africa and Asia, is a rare cause of disease in the United States.[26] Serogroup Y, which frequently is associated with pneumonia, is emerging as an important cause of invasive meningococcal disease in select areas.[27,28] Overall, *N. meningitidis* accounts for 25% of all meningitis cases and 60% of cases in persons aged 2 to 18 years, and it carries a case-fatality rate of approximately 10%.[9,27]

Initially, patients are colonized and, at some point, develop a bacteremia, which most likely occurs prior to hospital admission. Meningitis occurs after the bacteria seeds into the meninges, which can occur in 50% of cases of meningococcal disease.[29] After the acute phase of meningitis has resolved, a unique immune reaction occurs that distinguishes meningococcal meningitis from other bacterial causes. The patient develops a characteristic immunologic reaction of fever, arthritis (usually involving large joints), and pericarditis approximately 10 to 14 days after the onset of disease and despite successful treatment.[30] At this time, examination of the synovial fluid will reveal a large number of polymorphonuclear cells, elevated protein concentrations, normal glucose concentrations, and sterile cultures. The reaction may last 1 week or longer, and no additional antibiotic therapy is required. However, patients may benefit from nonsteroidal antiinflammatory drugs and supportive care.[30]

Seizures and coma are uncommon with meningococcal meningitis. However, patients may behave aggressively and often are maniacal. Patients may develop deafness and transiently impaired ocular movements. Deafness unilaterally or, more commonly, bilaterally may develop early or late in the disease course.[30] Hearing loss secondary to sensory nerve damage (sensorineural hearing) usually is permanent, whereas conductive hearing impairment, such as damage to the tympanic membrane, often is reversible.

The presence of petechiae may be the primary clue that the underlying pathogen is *N. meningitidis*. Approximately 50% of patients with meningococcal meningitis have purpuric lesions, petechiae, or both. Patients may have an obvious or subclinical picture of disseminated intravascular coagulation, which may progress to infarction of the adrenal glands and renal cortex and cause widespread thrombosis.

Aggressive, early intervention with high-dose intravenous crystalline penicillin G (50,000 units/kg every 4 hours) usually is recommended for treatment of *N. meningitidis* meningitis. Chloramphenicol is bactericidal for *N. meningitidis* and can be used in place of penicillin G. However, chloramphenicol has unpredictable metabolism in young infants and several drug–drug interactions and is used rarely in developed countries.[2] Several third-generation cephalosporins (e.g., cefotaxime, ceftriaxone, ceftazidime, ceftizoxime) have indications for treatment of meningitis and are acceptable alternatives to penicillin G (Table 110–5). Meropenem and fluoroquinolones are suitable alternatives for treatment of penicillin-nonsusceptible meningococci (A-III).

Cases of meningitis caused by relatively (minimum inhibitory concentration [MIC] 0.1–1 mg/L) and highly (MIC ≥256 mg/L) penicillin-resistant meningococci have been reported. Prevalence varies geographically, ranging from 0.4% to 42.6%.[31] Isolated cases of treatment failure with penicillin have been reported.[32,33] Completely resistant strains produce β-lactamase, whereas relatively resistant strains have an alteration of penicillin-binding proteins. Given the emergence of β-lactamase–producing strains of meningococci, more practitioners are prescribing third-generation cephalosporins (cefotaxime or ceftriaxone) instead of penicillin, which long has been considered the drug of choice for meningococcal meningitis.[34]

N. meningitidis is spread by direct person-to-person close contact, including respiratory droplets and pharyngeal secretions.[29] Close contacts of patients contracting *N. meningitidis* meningitis are at an increased risk for developing meningitis. Close contacts include daycare center contacts, members of the household, or anyone who has been exposed to respiratory or oral secretions through activities such as coughing, sneezing, or kissing. Household contacts of people who have sporadic disease are estimated to have an incidence of meningococcal meningitis that is 500 to 800 times greater than that of the overall population.[29] Secondary cases of meningitis usually develop within the first week following exposure but may take up to 60 days after contact with the index case.[35] Young children are at the greatest risk for contracting *N. meningitidis;* however, persons of all ages are at risk, especially close contacts exposed via household, daycare, or military contact.

❾ Prophylaxis of close contacts should be started only after consultation with the local health department. In general, rifampin is given as prophylaxis for 2 days.[26] The adult dose is 600 mg every 12 hours, whereas children 1 month and older should receive 10 mg/kg every 12 hours, and children younger than 1 month should receive 5 mg/kg every 12 hours (A-III). Intramuscular ceftriaxone (250 mg in adults, 125 mg in children younger than 12 years) and oral ciprofloxacin (500 mg in adults and children older than 12 years) are alternatives to rifampin (A-III).[15] Further discussion of who should receive prophylaxis is beyond the scope of this chapter; interested readers can refer to the recommendations of the U.S. Centers for Disease Control and Prevention (CDC) for that information.[36]

Streptococcus pneumoniae (Pneumococcus or Diplococcus)

S. pneumoniae is the leading cause of meningitis in adults. Moreover, *S. pneumoniae* is the most common cause of bacterial meningitis in children younger than 2 years, accounting for four to six cases per 100,000 of this population, and is the second most common cause in children older than 2 years.[37] Case-fatality rates in children are highest with this organism and approach 20%. Approximately 50% of cases are secondary infections resulting from primary infections of parameningeal foci, such as the ear or paranasal sinuses. Pneumonia, endocarditis, CSF leak secondary to head trauma, splenectomy, alcoholism, sickle cell disease, and bone marrow transplantation may predispose the patient to the development of pneumococcal meningitis.

Neurologic complications, such as coma and seizures, are common with pneumococcal meningitis. Children with pneumococcal meningitis have lower mortality rates (4%–17%) compared with adults (20%–30%), but children who survive have a high rate of neurologic sequelae (29%–56%).[38,39] Risk factors for recurrent pneumococcal meningitis include traumatic tears of the dura, fracture of the cribriform plate or paranasal sinuses, nasal meningoceles, repeated episodes of otitis media, basilar skull fractures, and CSF leaks. The prognosis of pneumococcal meningitis depends on a variety of factors, including the number of WBCs in the CSF, number of WBCs in the periphery, CSF glucose concentration, CSF protein concentration, serum sodium concentration, and presence of a comatose state and/or shock.[40]

Treatment with intravenous crystalline penicillin G (50,000 units/kg every 4 hours) in adult patients with a penicillin-susceptible isolate and normal renal function usually results in a favorable outcome. However, the frequency of penicillin-resistant pneumococcal strains (MIC ≥2 mg/L) in the United States increased from 14% in 1994 to 25% in 1997 and continues to rise.[34] Based on these resistance patterns and the fact that sufficient CSF concentrations of penicillin are difficult to achieve with standard intravenous doses, penicillin should not be used as empirical therapy if *S. pneumoniae* is a suspected pathogen. Furthermore, appropriate Clinical Laboratory Standards Institute (CLSI)–approved testing of all CSF isolates for penicillin resistance is recommended. Ceftriaxone and cefotaxime have served as alternatives to penicillin in the treatment of penicillin intermediate- and high-resistant pneumococci. Of note, treatment failures with third-generation cephalosporins in the management of penicillin-resistant pneumococci have been reported.[34] Therapeutic approaches to cephalosporin-resistant pneumococcus include the addition of vancomycin and rifampin, which have demonstrated synergistic activity with ceftriaxone. However, no data from controlled clinical trials supporting the use of rifampin are available. Therefore, the combination of vancomycin and ceftriaxone has been suggested as empirical treatment until the results of antimicrobial susceptibility testing are available.[2,34] Some investigators have suggested that the addition of vancomycin to the initial empirical regimen may not be necessary because the prevalence of β-lactam–resistant pneumococci has been reduced greatly as a result of the pneumococcal vaccines.[2]

Ceftriaxone and vancomycin are the agents of choice for treatment of presumed pneumococcal meningitis empirically until the susceptibility is known. Penicillin can be used for drug-susceptible isolates with MIC ≤0.06 mg/L, but for intermediate isolates, ceftriaxone is used, and for highly drug resistant isolates, a combination of ceftriaxone and vancomycin should be used. Vancomycin should not be used as monotherapy.[34] In severe cases, therapeutic drug monitoring of the CSF and possibly even direct antibiotic instillation may be necessary.

Reports of the isolation of pneumococcal strains exhibiting tolerance to vancomycin are of great concern, but the clinical significance is unknown.[41,42] Based on concern about the limited therapeutic options for penicillin- and cephalosporin-resistant pneumococcal meningitis, newer agents have been evaluated. Meropenem is approved by the Food and Drug Administration (FDA) for treatment of bacterial meningitis in children aged 3 months and older and has shown similar clinical and microbiologic efficacy to cefotaxime or ceftriaxone. Meropenem currently is recommended as an alternative to a third-generation cephalosporin in penicillin-nonsusceptible isolates (B-II). Some concern is warranted with use of imipenem for CNS infections because of the possibility of drug-induced seizures, especially if the dose is not adjusted for renal function. Of note, seizures may be caused by the meningitis itself or by imipenem, and the cause is difficult to differentiate. The newer fluoroquinolones are another therapeutic option as a result of favorable activity against multidrug-resistant pneumococci and good penetration into the CSF.[43] However, clinical data regarding fluoroquinolone treatment of pneumococcal meningitis are limited mainly to animal models. Comparative, controlled clinical efficacy trials in patients with meningitis will be necessary before routine use of the fluoroquinolones is viable. Interestingly, some of the newer fluoroquinolones act synergistically with vancomycin and β-lactam antibiotics against penicillin-resistant pneumococcal meningitis in an animal model, but this claim has not been substantiated in humans.[34,44,45]

Linezolid and daptomycin have emerged as therapeutic options for treatment of multidrug-resistant gram-positive infections. Linezolid in combination with ceftriaxone has been used to treat a limited number of cases of pneumococcal meningitis with outcomes similar to standard treatment.[46] Penetration of daptomycin in the CSF was approximately 6% following a 15 mg/kg bolus and achieved maximum concentration approximately 4 hours after the dose in a rabbit meningitis model. The 15 mg/kg dose produces similar serum concentrations in rabbits as the 6 mg/kg dose in humans. In this study, daptomycin was able to clear both the penicillin-resistant and the quinolone-resistant pneumococci from the CSF more rapidly than the standard regimen of vancomycin and ceftriaxone.[47] However, limited data are available, and use of these agents cannot be recommended for treatment of pneumococcal meningitis.

CLINICAL CONTROVERSY

Some investigators believe that use of vancomycin for empirical treatment of pneumococcal meningitis is no longer necessary because the widespread use of pneumococcal vaccines has greatly reduced the prevalence of β-lactam–resistant pneumococci. However, because the infecting organism is rarely known initially, most clinicians still use the combination of a third-generation cephalosporin and vancomycin for empirical treatment.

Pneumococcal vaccines help reduce the risk of invasive pneumococcal disease. Virtually all serotypes of *S. pneumoniae* exhibiting intermediate or complete resistance to penicillin are found in the 23-serotype pneumococcal polysaccharide vaccine. However, in 1997, surveillance data indicated that only 30% of people 65 years and older had been immunized against pneumococcal disease.[48] Therefore, the CDC issued stronger recommendations for use of the pneumococcal polysaccharide vaccine, calling for vaccination of the following high-risk groups: persons older than 65 years; persons aged 2 to 64 years who have a chronic illness, who live in high-risk environments (e.g., Alaskan Natives and residents of long-term care facilities), and who lack a functioning spleen (e.g., sickle cell disease and splenectomy); and immunocompromised persons older than 2 years, including those with human immunodeficiency virus (HIV) infection. Additionally, the question of whether or not college students living in dormitories, a possible high-risk environment, should be vaccinated remains debatable. Unfortunately, variability in the host's ability to mount an immune response to the vaccine limits its usefulness for penicillin-resistant pneumococci in children younger than 2 years and in immunocompromised adults.

In 2000, a heptavalent pneumococcal conjugate vaccine (Prevnar) was approved for use in children aged 2 months and older. Use of the vaccine has reduced invasive pneumococcal infections, including sepsis and meningitis, by more than 90%.[49] Moreover, the vaccine is safe and effective in low-birth-weight and preterm infants.[50,51] Widespread vaccination is expected to have a significant impact on the prevalence of pneumococcal meningitis, including infection caused by antibiotic-resistant strains. A cohort study of 3.8 million healthy infants projected that vaccination would prevent more than 12,000 cases of invasive disease for each U.S. birth cohort, resulting in substantial decreases in morbidity and mortality as well as possible cost savings.[52] According to current recommendations, all healthy infants younger than 2 years should be immunized with the heptavalent vaccine at 2, 4, 6, and 12 to 15 months. The recommendations are extended to include Alaskan Native, Native American, and African American children between the ages of 2 and 5 years. In 2003, the CDC issued a recommendation that all persons with cochlear implants receive age-appropriate vaccination with the pneumococcal conjugate vaccine, pneumococcal polysaccharide vaccine, or both.[53]

Haemophilus influenzae

Historically, *H. influenzae* was the most common cause of meningitis in children aged 6 months to 3 years. Since the introduction of effective vaccines, however, the incidence of *H. influenzae* type B disease in the United States has declined dramatically. Widespread vaccination of infants and children has decreased the incidence of bacterial meningitis due to *H. influenzae* in children between the ages of 1 month and 5 years by 87%, resulting in a 55% decline in all cases of bacterial meningitis.[14] Worldwide, in countries that have adopted universal immunization, the incidence of bacterial meningitis caused by *H. influenzae* type b has decreased more than 99%.[2] In children older than 3 years and in adults, meningitis caused by *H. influenzae* may indicate a parameningeal focus of infection such as middle ear infection, paranasal sinus infection, or CSF leakage. Spread of the organism occurs through direct spread from infected sinuses, draining of these areas via the veins, or bacteremia originating from the local focus of infection.[54]

In the past, ampicillin and chloramphenicol were the drugs of choice to treat pediatric meningitis. However, because approximately 30% to 40% of *H. influenzae* now are ampicillin resistant, many clinicians prescribe a third-generation cephalosporin until sensitivities are available. If the organism is found to be sensitive to ampicillin, the patient can be switched to ampicillin and the third-generation cephalosporin discontinued. Most clinicians regard third-generation cephalosporins as the drugs of choice for meningitis caused by *H. influenzae* (A-1). Third-generation cephalosporins (cefotaxime and ceftriaxone) are active against β-lactamase–producing and non–β-lactamase–producing strains of *H. influenzae,* are relatively free of toxicity, and do not require serum concentration monitoring. Cefepime (A-I) and fluoroquinolones (A-III) are suitable alternatives regardless of β-lactamase activity.

Secondary cases resulting from close contact with an index case occur within 30 days of the onset of disease. Close contacts, which include household members, individuals sharing sleeping quarters, daycare attendees, nursing home residents, and crowded, confined populations, may be at 200 to 1,000 times the risk of the general population for acquiring *H. influenzae* meningitis. The risk of acquiring *H. influenzae* meningitis is low without intimate contact with the index patient's respiratory secretions.[55]

❾ The aim of prophylaxis is to protect close contacts from the index case by eliminating nasopharyngeal and oropharyngeal carriage of *H. influenzae.* Invasive disease should be reported to the local public health department and the CDC. Prophylaxis of close contacts should be started only after consultation with the local health department. In general, children should receive rifampin 20 mg/kg/day (maximum 600 mg) and adults 600 mg/day in one dose for 4 days. Any unvaccinated children between the ages of 12 and 48 months should receive one dose of the vaccine, whereas those between the ages of 2 and 11 months should be given three doses of the vaccine.[15] Individuals fully vaccinated are not recommended to receive prophylaxis.[26] Further discussion of who should receive prophylaxis is beyond the scope of this chapter; interested readers can refer to the recommendations of the American Academy of Pediatrics for that information.[56]

Vaccination includes a series of doses and usually is started in children at age 2 months. The diphtheria, tetanus toxoids, acellular pertussis–*H. influenzae* type B (DTaP–Hib) combination vaccine also is available as a booster following the Hib series. In addition to pediatric immunization, the vaccine should be considered in patients older than 5 years with the following underlying conditions: sickle cell disease, asplenia, and immunocompromising diseases (see Chap. 128 for further information on dosing and administration).

Listeria monocytogenes

L. monocytogenes is a gram-positive diphtheroid-like organism responsible for 8% of all reported cases of meningitis. This disease primarily affects neonates, alcoholics, immunocompromised adults, and the elderly. *Listeria* infections in healthy individuals are extremely rare. *L. monocytogenes* is implicated in 20% of meningitis cases in patients older than 60 years and carries a case-fatality rate of approximately 15%.[9]

Transmission usually involves colonization of the patient's gastrointestinal (GI) tract with the organisms, which then penetrate the gut lumen. Coleslaw, unpasteurized milk, Mexican-style soft cheese, ready-to-eat foods, and raw beef and poultry all have been identified as sources of this food-borne pathogen.[26] If a sufficient cell-mediated immune response (T lymphocytes, macrophages) is not produced, bacteremia, meningitis, meningoencephalitis, or cerebritis may develop. Infection of the CNS may be diffuse or localized, possibly involving the cerebral hemispheres, thalamus, and brainstem. In immunocompromised hosts, approximately 75% of *L. monocytogenes* infections result in transmission into the CNS.[57]

Incidence of *L. monocytogenes* meningitis tends to peak in the summer and early fall. As with gram-negative meningitis, presentation may be subtle and insidious, and clinical suspicion should prompt lumbar puncture. *L. monocytogenes* produces primarily a mononuclear CSF response.[57] One common laboratory error seen with *L. monocytogenes* is a tendency to misidentify the organism on Gram stain as a diphtheroid, streptococcus, or poorly staining gram-negative rod.

Treatment of *L. monocytogenes* meningitis with penicillin G or ampicillin may result in only a bacteriostatic effect and possible persistence of infection. Usually the combination of penicillin G or ampicillin with an aminoglycoside results in a bactericidal effect. Patients should be treated for 2 to 3 weeks after defervescence (A-III).[15] Combination therapy usually is given for at least 10 days, with the remaining course of therapy completed with penicillin G or ampicillin alone. Trimethoprim-sulfamethoxazole may be an effective alternative because adequate CSF penetration is achieved (A-III). Chloramphenicol and vancomycin both possess in vitro activity against *Listeria*, but they are not recommended for use in meningitis caused by *L. monocytogenes* because of unacceptably high failure rates.[34]

Gram-Negative Meningitis

During the last several years, the incidence of gram-negative bacillary meningitis, excluding *H. influenzae,* has been increasing in both children and adults. Enteric gram-negative organisms are the fourth leading cause of meningitis, with only *S. pneumoniae, H. influenzae,* and *N. meningitidis* having higher incidences.

Several factors predispose patients to the development of gram-negative meningitis: congenital defects involving the CNS, accidental cranial trauma, neurosurgery, use of antimicrobial agents with exclusive gram-positive activity preoperatively in neurosurgery, any form of communication between the skin and subarachnoid space (e.g., dermal sinus), diabetes, malignancy, urinary tract infection in neonates, cirrhosis, parameningeal infection, spinal anesthesia, advanced age, immunosuppression, and hospitalization in general.

Elderly debilitated patients are at increased risk for gram-negative meningitis but typically lack the classic signs and symptoms of the disease. Nuchal rigidity may be difficult to detect secondary to cervical arthritis. Presence of a low-grade fever and changes in mental status without other obvious cause should prompt consideration of meningitis and a lumbar puncture. Neonates also are at risk for gram-negative meningitis with *E. coli* and *Klebsiella pneumoniae,* which are responsible for 60% to 70% of cases.

Optimal antimicrobial therapies for gram-negative bacillary meningitis have not been fully defined. Therapy for gram-negative meningitis is complex because of the variety of organisms that can infect the CNS. Treatment of meningitis due to *P. aeruginosa* remains a unique problem because antibiotics showing good antibacterial activity against *P. aeruginosa,* such as antipseudomonal penicillins and aminoglycosides, penetrate the CSF poorly. Furthermore, many isolates of *P. aeruginosa* are resistant to multiple, if not all, commonly used agents, and this trend in resistance is increasing. Initially, cases of *P. aeruginosa* meningitis should be treated with an extended-spectrum β-lactam such as ceftazidime or cefepime (A-II), or alternatively piperacillin ± tazobactam, or meropenem plus an aminoglycoside, usually tobramycin.[2] Because aminoglycosides penetrate the CSF poorly, they are included predominantly to aid in the treatment of extracerebral infections. If multidrug-resistant *Pseudomonas* is suspected initially, intraventricular administration of aminoglycoside should be considered along with intravenous administration. Preservative-free forms of gentamicin and tobramycin are available and should be used for direct administration into the CSF. Intraventricular aminoglycoside dosages should be adjusted to the estimated CSF volume (0.03 mg tobramycin or gentamicin per milliliter of CSF and 0.1 mg amikacin per milliliter of CSF every 24 hours). Because CSF flows unidirectionally with gravity, intraventricular aminoglycoside administration is more likely to produce therapeutic concentrations throughout the CSF than will intrathecal administration. Although intraventricular administration of aminoglycosides is considered for treatment of *P. aeruginosa* meningitis, this method produced higher mortality in a sample of infants treated for gram-negative bacillary meningitis.[22] Thus, intraventricular administration of aminoglycosides to infants is not recommended routinely. Ventricular levels of aminoglycoside should be monitored every 2 or 3 days, just prior to the next intraventricular dose, and should approximate 2 to 10 mg/L. Interpretation of drug levels may be difficult because determinations often are contaminated with residual aminoglycoside from the preceding dose.

One patient exhibited favorable effects of high-dose intravenous ciprofloxacin (400 mg every 8 hours) plus intravenous ceftazidime for treatment of pseudomonal meningitis.[58] However, this information must be evaluated in a controlled clinical trial before use of high-dose ciprofloxacin can be recommended.

Multidrug-resistant *Pseudomonas* and *Acinetobacter* infections are of concern to clinicians because of the limited therapeutic options available for treatment. This concern has led to the reemergence of the use of older antibiotics, such as colistin. Colistin can be used, both intravenously and intrathecally, for treatment of multidrug-resistant *Pseudomonas* or *Acinetobacter* CNS infections.[59–61] Furthermore, there is synergistic activity with the combination of colistin and ceftazidime against multidrug-resistant *P. aeruginosa*.[62] Use of colistin should be reserved for only the most severe cases.

Other gram-negative organisms causing meningitis, excluding *P. aeruginosa* and *Acinetobacter* species, most likely can be treated with a third or fourth-generation cephalosporin, such as cefotaxime, ceftriaxone, ceftazidime, or cefepime. However, ceftazidime, may not be the best choice of empirical antibiotic for situations where the offending organism is not known initially because CSF antibiotic concentrations more than 10 times the minimal bactericidal concentration may not be produced reliably for gram-positive organisms. In adults, daily doses of 8 to 12 g/day of third-generation cephalosporins (ceftriaxone 2 g twice daily) should produce CSF concentrations of 5 to 20 mg/L. Ceftriaxone is not recommended for use in the neonatal period because of the potential for displacement of bilirubin from albumin-binding sites.[2] in this situation, cefotaxime should be used in place of ceftriaxone.

Trimethoprim-sulfamethoxazole is useful in the management of the Enterobacteriaceae family and may be useful in the management of *L. monocytogenes*.[2,8] One advantage of trimethoprim-sulfamethoxazole is that its penetration into the CSF does not depend on meningeal inflammation. However, trimethoprim-sulfamethoxazole is not bactericidal. Trimethoprim-sulfamethoxazole produces CSF levels of 1.9 to 5.7 mg/L for the former and 20 to 63 mg/L for the latter when given parenterally in doses of trimethoprim 10 mg/kg/day and sulfamethoxazole 50 mg/kg/day.

Fluoroquinolones have good penetration into the CSF and are effective in animal models of both gram-negative and gram-positive meningitis. However, data on the efficacy of fluoroquinolones in clinical practice are limited. Ciprofloxacin is recommended as an alternative for treatment of *E. coli* and other *Enterobacteriaceae* as well as *Pseudomonas aeruginosa* (A-III). Cefepime and meropenem are other therapeutic options for treatment of gram-negative bacterial meningitis, as is aztreonam (A-III).[2,34]

CSF cultures may remain positive for at least several days with a regimen that eventually will be curative. Therapeutic efficacy can be monitored through bacterial colony counts every 2 or 3 days, which should decrease progressively over the period of therapy. Therapy for gram-negative meningitis should be continued for a minimum of 21 days from the start of treatment.[15]

Bacillus anthracis

B. anthracis is a large, endospore-forming, aerobic, gram-positive bacteria capable of producing infection via the cutaneous, pulmonary, or GI routes. Cases of meningitis following both cutaneous and inhalational infection have been reported. Prior to the bioterrorism-related outbreak of 11 inhalational and 12 suspected or confirmed cases of cutaneous anthrax in 2001, only 18 sporadic cases had occurred in the United States in the 20th century, with the last occurrence in 1976.[63] However, since the terrorist attack on the United States on September 11, 2001, heightened awareness of biologic warfare agents, including *B. anthracis*, has percolated throughout the United States.

The major neurologic complication of anthrax infection is fulminant, rapidly fatal hemorrhagic meningoencephalitis. The inhalational form of anthrax seems to be a potent inducer of neurologic symptoms, and death usually occurs within 1 week in those with neurologic complications.[63] Neurologic manifestations may be the initial symptoms leading to the diagnosis of anthrax. An index case of fatal inhalational anthrax from bioterrorism developed acute fever, emesis, disorientation, and confusion. A head CT scan showed no abnormalities, but spinal tap revealed cloudy CSF, low CSF glucose concentration, high CSF protein concentration, increased leukocytes in the CSF, and large gram-positive bacilli in chains. Shortly thereafter, the patient developed a generalized seizure and died on the third hospital day.[64]

Consistent findings in the CSF of anthrax meningitis cases include a low CSF glucose level, marked infiltration of WBCs into the CSF, and presence of gram-positive bacilli in chains. High suspicion of anthrax meningitis is warranted in the additional presence of grossly visible blood or elevated red blood cell counts in the CSF with hemorrhagic changes on a CT scan. Molecular advances can aid in the rapid diagnosis of *B. anthracis* infections. Rapid PCR techniques, such as the Light Cycler (Roche Applied Science, Indianapolis, IN), can provide molecular confirmation of the presence of anthrax within 1 hour.[63] Extreme caution is warranted for diagnosis without the use of molecular techniques because *B. anthracis* can be confused easily with *B. cereus*, which is found commonly in soil and often considered a contaminant if identified.

B. anthracis typically is susceptible to penicillin, amoxicillin, erythromycin, doxycycline, ciprofloxacin, and chloramphenicol. The bioterrorism-related strain was susceptible to the fluoroquinolones, rifampin, tetracycline, vancomycin, imipenem, meropenem, chloramphenicol, clindamycin, and the aminoglycosides. However, the strain was resistant to third-generation cephalosporins and trimethoprim-sulfamethoxazole. Ciprofloxacin or doxycycline plus one or two of the aforementioned antibiotics is the currently recommended regimen for treatment of inhalational anthrax, but doxycycline is not recommended for treatment of anthrax meningitis because of poor CNS penetration and recent in vitro resistance.[63]

Dexamethasone as Adjunctive Treatment of Meningitis

In addition to antibiotics, dexamethasone has become a commonly used therapy for treatment of meningitis. Corticosteroids inhibit the production of TNF and IL-1, which both are potent proinflammatory cytokines. A series of clinical studies assessing the efficacy of corticosteroid therapy for the initial treatment of bacterial meningitis has reported conflicting results.[65–69] A fundamental problem with corticosteroid investigations is that the majority of patients in the trials had *H. influenzae* meningitis. Although *H. influenzae* was the most commonly identified causative pathogen responsible for bacterial meningitis in the United States in 1986, the incidence of *H. influenzae* meningitis has decreased dramatically because of the introduction of polysaccharide conjugate vaccines. Additionally, the majority of studies examining dexamethasone use for pneumococcal meningitis were conducted before the widespread problem of penicillin-resistant pneumococcus had emerged or were conducted in parts of the world where penicillin resistance was minimal. Whether or not steroids are beneficial for treatment of meningitis caused by penicillin-resistant *S. pneumoniae, N. meningitidis,* and group B streptococci is unclear at this time.

The findings of several studies have shown significant improvement in markers of active infection, such as CSF levels of proinflammatory cytokines, as well as CSF protein, glucose, and lactate concentrations, after corticosteroid administration as adjunctive treatment.[14] Trials consistently detected a significantly lower incidence of neurologic sequelae commonly associated with bacterial meningitis with corticosteroid use. In trials that measured inflammatory mediators, lower levels of TNF, PAF, or IL-1 were detected in patients treated with dexamethasone.[65,66,69]

The majority of clinical trials on the use of adjunctive dexamethasone in bacterial meningitis has involved children. A retrospective analysis of pediatric patients with pneumococcal meningitis and one unblinded, noncontrolled trial suggested that adjunctive steroids may decrease the neurologic sequelae and mortality associated with *S. pneumoniae* meningitis.[65,70] A meta-analysis suggests that, with the possible exception of hearing loss, dexamethasone does not protect against neurologic sequelae.[71] The protective effect of dexamethasone was observed to be strongest in patients with meningitis due to *H. influenzae.*

⑩ The American Academy of Pediatrics suggests that dexamethasone be considered for infants and children aged 2 months and older with pneumococcal meningitis (C-II) and given to those with *H. influenzae* meningitis.[56,72] The recommended intravenous dose is 0.15 mg/kg every 6 hours for 4 days. Alternatively, prospective, randomized, double-blinded studies have found dexamethasone 0.15 mg/kg every 6 hours for 2 days or dexamethasone 0.4 mg/kg every 12 hours for 2 days to be equally effective and potentially less toxic.[69,73] Dexamethasone should be administered prior to or with the first antibiotic dose and not after antibiotics already have been started (A-I).[14] Additionally, serum hemoglobin and stool guaiac should be monitored for evidence of GI bleeding.[66,68,70,73] Dexamethasone should not be given to neonates or any infant younger than 6 weeks.[14,22] Use of dexamethasone interferes with the interpretation of clinical response to treatment. For example, corticosteroid use interferes with resolution of fever. Thus, all infants and children are recommended to undergo a repeat lumbar puncture 24 to 48 hours after treatment to verify CSF sterilization.[14]

Data supporting the use of corticosteroids in adults with meningitis are scarce. A prospective, randomized, double-blinded multicenter study evaluated the use of adjuvant therapy plus dexamethasone compared with adjuvant therapy plus placebo in adults with acute bacterial meningitis.[74] Early treatment with dexamethasone improved clinical outcome in adults with bacterial meningitis, reducing the risk of both unfavorable outcome and death. However, the study did not show a beneficial effect of dexamethasone on neurologic sequelae, including hearing loss. Furthermore, a meta-analysis of five trials[75] involving 623 adults with acute bacterial meningitis described a significant reduction in mortality in patients treated with steroids and antibiotics compared to those treated with antibiotics alone. There was no significant reduction in neurologic sequelae, but this could have been limited by the sample size, as two of the five trials did not investigate neurologic complications. The safety and adverse events were similar between those who received steroids and those who did not.[75]

If pneumococcal meningitis is suspected or proven, it is recommended that adults receive dexamethasone 0.15 mg/kg every 6 hours for 2 to 4 days, with the first dose administered 10 to 20 minutes prior to first dose of antibiotics. Patient outcome likely will not improve if dexamethasone is given after the first dose of antibiotic and therefore should be avoided (A-I). Because ascertaining the responsible pathogen on presentation often is difficult, some clinicians recommend initiating dexamethasone in all adult patients presenting with meningitis (B-III).

Routine use of dexamethasone in meningitis is not without controversy. A potential concern is that adjunctive dexamethasone therapy might reduce the penetration of antibiotics into the CSF by inhibiting meningeal inflammation. In experimental models of meningitis, steroids decreased the CSF concentrations of ampicillin, rifampin, vancomycin, and gentamicin.[69,76] Ceftriaxone and vancomycin penetration into CSF was unaffected by concurrent dexamethasone administration in pediatric patients.[77,78]

CLINICAL CONTROVERSY

Some clinicians believe that dexamethasone should be initiated in all patients older than 2 months with bacterial meningitis and continued for the recommended 2 to 4 days regardless of bacterial etiology. However, others believe corticosteroids have limited proven benefit in the treatment of nonpneumococcal meningitis and recommend stopping dexamethasone if another bacterial pathogen is identified.

Mycobacterium tuberculosis

M. tuberculosis is the primary cause of tuberculous meningitis. Tuberculous meningitis is associated with significant morbidity and mortality and is difficult to diagnose in a timely manner. The most life-threatening form of extrapulmonary tuberculosis is tuberculous meningitis.[79] The epidemiology of tuberculous meningitis as a cause of extrapulmonary tuberculosis has changed. Between 1997 and 1990, an average of 193 cases of tuberculous meningitis was reported to the CDC, representing 4.7% of extrapulmonary cases. The number of cases reported in 1990 was 284, or 6.2% of extrapulmonary cases. This change most likely is secondary to HIV/acquired immune deficiency syndrome (AIDS) and rising rates among minority adults leading to increased tuberculosis in their children.[80] The incidence of tuberculosis in general has increased 15% since 1985, and the increase is more substantial in children than in adults.[79]

The most useful clue to the diagnosis of tuberculous meningitis is the presence of inflammation of the CSF in an individual who is at epidemiologic risk for tuberculosis. Although up to 40% of patients may present with evidence of pulmonary involvement with hilar adenopathy, tuberculous meningitis still may exist in the absence of disease in the lung or extrapulmonary sites. The tuberculin skin test (purified protein derivative) is negative in 5% to 50% of cases.[81]

On initial examination, CSF usually contains 100 to 1,000 WBCs/mm^3, which may be 75% to 80% polymorphonuclear cells. Over time, the pattern of WBCs in the CSF will shift to lymphocytes and monocytes (Table 110–1). CSF glucose concentration initially may be normal but gradually decreases as the disease progresses.[81,82] Protein concentration within the CSF may be normal or elevated, with high protein levels shown to correlate with advanced disease.[81–83] CSF cultures often are positive for *M. tuberculosis* even if the patient is asymptomatic.

One potentially useful diagnostic sign unique to tuberculous meningitis is paralysis of cranial nerve VI, which initially is unilateral and then progresses to bilateral.[30] Initial acid-fast bacilli smears are approximately 37% sensitive and as high as 87% sensitive following subsequent smears. Sensitivity of the acid-fast bacilli smear is enhanced by examination of multiple CSF specimens collected on consecutive days. Cultures of CSF are positive in 45% to 90% of cases depending on the quantity of CSF used in the culture, pathogen density, and experience of the laboratory in culturing *M. tuberculosis*. Some clinicians obtain fluid from the base of the brain or the ventricles in an attempt to increase the yield. Positive culture results may take up to 8 weeks, providing little help with the initial diagnosis.[81,82] Several systems using rapid broth culture (Organon Teknika MB/BacT, Organon Teknika, Durham, NC; ESP system, Trek Diagnostic Systems, Inc., Westlake, OH; and Bactec 9000 TB series or Bactec 460, Becton Dickinson Diagnostic Instruments, Sparks, MD) have considerably shortened the time to detection and are able to detect organisms in less than 3 weeks.[18] Nucleic acid amplification products, such as Amplicor (Roche) and MTD (Gen-Probe), allow for direct identification of *M. tuberculosis* within 48 hours and yield higher sensitivity than a smear.

The incidence of multidrug-resistant strains of *M. tuberculosis* has increased, necessitating the use of at least three antitubercular agents for treatment of active pulmonary disease. The CDC recommends an initial regimen of four drugs for empirical treatment of *M. tuberculosis*.[84] This regimen consists of isoniazid, rifampin, pyrazinamide, and ethambutol 15 to 20 mg/kg/day (maximum 1.6 g/day) for the first 2 months, generally followed by isoniazid plus rifampin for the remaining duration of therapy. The recommended therapy for HIV-positive individuals is the same as for immunocompetent patients, although rifabutin may be considered in place of other rifamycins in an effort to minimize drug interactions with protease inhibitors and nonnucleoside reverse transcriptase inhibitors. Therapy in HIV-negative and HIV-positive patients should be individualized based on susceptibility patterns and guidelines from the CDC and the American Thoracic Society, which are updated frequently and available on the Internet (*www.cdc.gov/nchstp/tb/pubs/mmwrhtml/maj_guide.htm*). Patients with *M. tuberculosis* meningitis should be treated with multiple-drug therapy for 9 months or longer, and patients with rifampin-resistant strains should receive 18 to 24 months of therapy.

Isoniazid, the mainstay in virtually any regimen for treatment of *M. tuberculosis*, penetrates the CSF with or without meningeal inflammation and achieves concentrations more than 30 times the MIC of *M. tuberculosis* (MIC 0.05–0.2 mg/L).[57,81,82] Rifampin's penetration of CSF approximates only 20% of serum concentrations in the presence of meningeal inflammation. *M. tuberculosis* typically is so exquisitely sensitive to rifampin that the low penetration ratio is of little clinical significance.[81,82,85] However, the incidence of *M. tuberculosis* resistance to rifampin has increased, necessitating empirical multiple-antibiotic regimens.

Pyrazinamide is a small molecule that penetrates the CSF well in the presence or absence of meningeal inflammation. Streptomycin, an aminoglycoside, penetrates the CSF poorly, even in the presence of meningeal inflammation. The incidence of resistance to streptomycin is increasing, and this drug should not be recommended unless susceptibility is known. Ethambutol is a weak antitubercular agent that reaches the CSF in moderate concentrations. Use of ethambutol is also limited by a high incidence of dose-related optic neuritis. Ethionamide and cycloserine are two other agents that sometimes are used to treat tuberculous meningitis. Both of these agents penetrate the CSF well in the absence of meningeal inflammation.[81,82]

The usual dose of isoniazid in children is 10 to 15 mg/kg/day (maximum 300 mg/day); adults usually receive 5 mg/kg/day or a daily dose of 300 mg.[84] Supplemental doses of pyridoxine hydrochloride (vitamin B_6) 50 mg/day are recommended to prevent the peripheral neuropathy associated with isoniazid administration.[81,82] Concurrent administration of rifampin is recommended at doses of 10 to 20 mg/kg/day (maximum 600 mg/day) for children and 600 mg/day for adults. The addition of pyrazinamide (children and adults 15–30 mg/kg/day; maximum 2 g/day in both) to the regimen of isoniazid and rifampin is recommended.[84] Duration of concomitant pyrazinamide therapy generally should be limited to 2 months to avoid hepatotoxicity.

The role of steroids in the management of tuberculous meningitis remains unclear. Administration of oral prednisone 60 to 80 mg/day or 0.2 mg/kg/day of intravenous dexamethasone for adults and prednisone 1 to 2 mg/kg/day for children, tapered over 4 to 8 weeks, has been used in clinical practice. Corticosteroids improve neurologic sequelae and survival in adults and decrease mortality, long-term neurologic complications, and permanent sequelae in children. Concerns regarding the use of steroids include possible interference with CSF chemistry studies and decreased penetration of antitubercular agents because of a decrease in inflammation. Despite the controversy, the trend toward an improved outcome generally supports their use for tuberculous meningitis.[86,87]

Tuberculous meningitis has a mortality rate of 10% to 50% despite early diagnosis and treatment.[81,82,88] The level of patient consciousness at the start of therapy is the most useful prognostic indicator. Patients who are comatose at the beginning of therapy have a mortality rate of approximately 75%.[82] Other negative prognostic factors include old age, poor nutrition, evidence of miliary disease, high initial CSF protein concentrations, presence of hydrocephalus, and evidence of elevated ICP.[82] Between 10% and 30% of patients surviving the disease have physical or mental sequelae, including deafness, vertigo, and short-term memory loss.[81,82]

Cryptococcus neoformans

Cryptococcal meningitis is the most common form of fungal CNS infection in the United States and is a major cause of morbidity and mortality in immunosuppressed patients. In the United States, 85% of cases occur in HIV-infected patients. *C. neoformans* is a soil fungus acquired by inhalation of spores from the environment leading to a pneumonia that usually is asymptomatic. Most patients present initially with disseminated disease, especially meningoencephalitis. The incubation period in AIDS patients may be very short, as opposed to a relatively normal host, in whom the incubation period may be very long.

Symptoms of cryptococcal meningitis are insidious and may be present for varying periods, depending on the host involved, before the definitive diagnosis is made. Fever and a history of headaches are the most common symptoms, although altered mentation and evidence of focal neurologic deficits may be present. Examination of the CSF usually reveals small numbers of WBCs (<150/mm^3), which are primarily lymphocytes (Table 110–1). Diagnosis is based on the presence of a positive CSF, blood, sputum, or urine culture for *C. neoformans*. CSF cultures are positive in more than 90% of cases. Organisms may be seen by microscope when stained with India ink and are more likely to be seen in AIDS patients compared with other hosts. An additional rapid test helpful in diagnosis is latex agglutination, which detects the presence of cryptococcal antigens.[89] Latex agglutination is positive in more than 90% of culture-positive cases. A cryptococcal antigen test can be used to follow the prognosis of non-AIDS patients, but cryptococcal antigen titers do not correlate well with treatment efficacy in AIDS patients.[90] A cryptococcal antigen detection test must be considered in any patient presenting initially with meningitis. Risk factors predictive of a poor outcome include lethargy at presentation, high CSF cryptococcal antigen titer, and low CSF WBC count.[91]

Despite poor penetration into the CSF, amphotericin B has long been the drug of choice for treatment of acute *C. neoformans* meningitis. Amphotericin B 0.5 to 1 mg/kg/day combined with flucytosine 100 mg/kg/day is more effective than amphotericin alone, with successful outcomes in 75% of non-AIDS patients and 50% in AIDS patients.[92] Unfortunately, flucytosine often is poorly tolerated in the AIDS population, causing bone marrow suppression and GI distress. Amphotericin B alone, although less effective, has been used in AIDS patients with preexisting granulocytopenia.[92,93] Because of the high acute mortality rate of up to 40% and a relapse rate of 50% in AIDS patients receiving therapy, many new agents and regimens are being investigated in this population.[91] A small, noncomparative open study evaluating the safety and efficacy of liposomal amphotericin B (AmBisome) found the product to be well tolerated and moderately effective.[94] A second study found high-dose liposomal amphotericin B (4 mg/kg) to clear CSF cultures more rapidly relative to standard amphotericin B, although clinical efficacy was not significantly different.[95]

Azole therapy is the most studied alternative regimen for treatment of *C. neoformans* meningitis in AIDS patients. Fluconazole at doses of 200 mg/day was compared with amphotericin B alone (0.4 mg/kg/day), with no significant difference in overall mortality between groups. However, patients receiving fluconazole had a higher 2-week mortality rate and time to CSF conversion.[96] High-dose fluconazole therapy (800 mg/day) as salvage therapy was attempted in eight AIDS patients who had not responded to antifungal therapy, but success was limited.[97] A randomized trial in Thailand compared amphotericin B (0.7 mg/kg/day), amphotericin B plus flucytosine (100 mg/kg/day), amphotericin B plus fluconazole (400 mg/day) and triple therapy with amphotericin B, flucytosine, and fluconazole daily for treatment of HIV-associated cryptococcal meningitis. The addition of fluconazole to the standard therapy of amphotericin B plus flucytosine resulted in less fungicidal activity against *C. neoformans* than the current standard of amphotericin B plus flucytosine.[98] Itraconazole 200 mg orally twice daily was less effective than amphotericin B plus flucytosine in a small nonblinded study.[99] Voriconazole has demonstrated good in vitro activity against *C. neoformans*; however, no comparative data suggest an improvement over fluconazole.[100] Posaconazole has demonstrated clinical activity against cryptococcal and other fungal infections of the CNS in patients with refractory disease or who are otherwise intolerant to standard antifungal agents. Posaconazole at oral doses of 800 mg/day divided appeared well tolerated.[101] More data are needed to determine the role new azole antifungal agents will play in treatment of cryptococcal meningitis.

Patients with AIDS often require lifelong maintenance or suppressive therapy because of high relapse rates following acute therapy for *C. neoformans*. A large multicenter, controlled trial compared fluconazole (200 mg/day) and amphotericin B (1 mg/kg/wk) in the prevention of relapse.[102] Two percent of patients receiving fluconazole versus 18% of patients receiving amphotericin B relapsed. In addition, the amphotericin B group had significantly more frequent bacterial infections, bacteremias, and drug-related toxicity.[102] Fluconazole is superior to itraconazole in the prevention of relapse.[103] Current guidelines for patients with AIDS-associated cryptococcal meningitis recommend 2 weeks of therapy with a combination of amphotericin B 0.7–1 mg/kg/day and flucytosine 100 mg/kg/day. This is often referred to as the *induction phase* and is followed by 8 weeks of fluconazole 400 mg/day as part of the *consolidation phase*. Therapy should be continued thereafter with fluconazole 200 mg/day until immune reconstitution occurs. Guidelines for prevention of opportunistic infections in HIV-infected persons are updated frequently and can be found at *www.aidsinfo.nih.gov*.

Viral Encephalitis

The epidemiology of viral encephalitis in the United States has changed dramatically since the mid-1960s because of the introduction of large-scale polio and mumps immunization programs. In the United States, the incidence of mumps decreased 98% between 1967 and 1985. Worldwide, mumps remains a causative agent of viral encephalitis in countries with low vaccination rates. Poliomyelitis, once a significant cause of encephalitis, now is confined to only a few less developed countries and soon likely will be eradicated as an infectious agent.

Nonpolio enteroviruses such as coxsackievirus A and B, echoviruses, and enterovirus 70 and 71 cause approximately 85% of all viral encephalitis cases.[104,105] The remaining 10% to 15% of viral encephalitis cases are caused by a variety of pathogens, such as arboviruses, adenoviruses, influenzae virus A and B, rotavirus, corona virus, cytomegalovirus, varicella-zoster, herpes simplex virus, Epstein-Barr virus, and lymphocytic choriomeningitis.[18,104] In the past, the St. Louis and LaCrosse viruses have been the most common cause of arbovirus encephalitis.[18] However, in 2002, the largest arboviral meningoencephalitis epidemic in the western hemisphere was caused by the West Nile virus, accounting for 4,156 human cases of West Nile disease in 44 states and the District of Columbia.[106] To date, nearly 20,000 cases of West Nile disease and almost 800 deaths have been reported in the United States since surveillance began in 1999.[107]

Viral encephalitis is acquired primarily by hematogenous spread or, alternatively, by neuronal spread of the causative pathogen. After entry into the host, viral replication occurs, resulting in dissemination through the reticuloendothelial system or vasculature. Infection of the capillary endothelial cells and choroid plexus may provide a conduit for CNS infections. Viruses such as polio, herpes, and varicella-zoster virus also may gain access to the CNS by axonal retrograde transmission from peripheral nerve endings.[108] Once a virus gains access to the CNS, the course of infection depends on the virulence of the particular virus and the host immune response. Host response to aseptic CNS infections is mediated by a complex cascade of inflammatory cytokines in a manner similar to purulent meningitis. In contrast with purulent meningitis, host response to viral encephalitis is mediated primarily through cytotoxic T lymphocytes. Although TNF is a prominent mediator in purulent bacterial meningitis, TNF concentrations are not increased in viral encephalitis, whereas increases in concentrations of IL-1 and interferon (INF) and INF- occur. TNF concentrations have been suggested as a diagnostic tool for differentiating between bacterial meningitis and viral encephalitis.[109] Although cytokine assays are available for investigational use, they are not used routinely in the clinical diagnosis of viral encephalitis.

The clinical syndrome associated with viral encephalitis generally is independent of viral etiology and may vary depending on the patient's age. Common signs in adults include headache, mild fever (<40°C), nuchal rigidity, malaise, drowsiness, nausea, vomiting, and photophobia. Only fever and irritability may be evident in the infant, and meningitis must be ruled out as a cause of fever when no other localized findings are observed in a child. Symptoms generally last 1 to 2 weeks, and specific manifestations outside the meninges can occur depending on the viral etiology.

Laboratory examination of the CSF usually reveals a pleocytosis with 100 to 1,000 WBCs/mm^3, which are primarily lymphocytic; however, 20% to 75% of patients with viral encephalitis may have a predominance of polymorphonuclear cells on initial examination of the CSF, especially in enteroviral meningitis.[92] On repeat lumbar puncture, 90% of patients initially presenting with a predominance of neutrophils experience a shift to a predominance of mononuclear cells. Other laboratory findings include normal to mildly elevated protein concentrations and normal or mildly reduced glucose concentrations (Table 110–1).[104]

Historically, pathogens responsible for viral encephalitis were not identified.[110] Poor laboratory recovery of viral pathogens and limited treatment options for viral encephalitis made the need for specific identification of pathogens of questionable value. Advances in diagnostic laboratory techniques and the potential for decreased costs associated with longer duration of hospitalization for patients with unconfirmed viral encephalitis have led to a reevaluation of the need for confirmatory pathogen diagnosis.[111] When clinical signs warrant pathogen identification, appropriate laboratory diagnostic techniques, including PCR, should be undertaken. Molecular methods are preferred to conventional laboratory tests for diagnosis of viral encephalitis because of the ability to detect a specific virus in 30% to 70% of cases as compared with the 14% to 24% sensitivity of viral culture.[18]

Although there are numerous pathogenic causes of viral encephalitis, much of the clinical presentation, diagnosis, and treatment are similar. The most commonly isolated viral etiologies are described here.

Commonly, the incidence of enteroviral encephalitis peaks in late summer and continues into early fall. Enteroviruses are transmitted in the host via the fecal–oral route. Clinical presentation of enteroviral infection frequently is nonspecific and characterized by fever, nausea, vomiting, and malaise; GI symptoms may not be present. Following a prodrome of 1 to 2 days, headache, photophobia, and neck stiffness develop. Diagnosis can be confirmed by cell culture from the CSF, where the incidence of successful isolation has ranged from 40% to 80%.[109] In addition, enterovirus can be isolated from throat swabs (60%) and stool cultures (80%), but they are not necessarily diagnostic because the virus is shed in the stool for 1 to 2 weeks following infection.[110] Conversely, an enterovirus-specific reverse-transcription PCR test can provide prompt results within 24 hours, with sensitivity and specificity of 100%.[112] Treatment of enteroviral encephalitis consists of supportive care, fluids, antipyretics, and analgesics. Generally, disease progression is self-limiting, and the patient recovers fully without long-term neurologic complications.

Both herpes simplex virus type 1 (HSV-1) and herpes simplex virus type 2 (HSV-2) have been associated with infections of the CNS. HSV-1 is associated with encephalitis in adults, whereas HSV-2 is associated predominantly with encephalitis in newborns.[105] An HSV infection of the CNS most likely is spread via retrograde movement from the dorsal root ganglion. Sexually active adults acquire herpes simplex meningitis during or after an attack of genital or rectal herpes. Although HSV-2 frequently can be cultured from CSF, HSV-1 cannot. As such, PCR may be more useful than culture in detecting infection with HSV; diagnosis usually is made by PCR, culture, or a fourfold rise in complement-fixing antibody to the virus. Establishing the correct diagnosis as early as possible is paramount because mortality rates range between 50% and 85% without treatment, and, unlike other viral encephalitides, specific and effective therapy is available. As a result, empirical therapy of suspected HSV encephalitis is necessary while awaiting results of laboratory tests. Additionally, a clinical decision to treat may be needed regardless of test results.

Acyclovir is the drug of choice for herpes simplex encephalitis. In patients with normal renal function, acyclovir usually is administered 10 mg/kg intravenously every 8 hours for 2 to 3 weeks.[105] Herpes virus resistance to acyclovir has been reported with increasing incidence, particularly from immunocompromised patients with prior or chronic exposures to acyclovir.[113] The alternative treatment of acyclovir-resistant herpes simplex virus is foscarnet.[105] The major toxicity of foscarnet is renal impairment, and doses must be individualized for renal function.[114] The dose for patients with normal renal function is 40 mg/kg infused over 1 hour every 8 to 12 hours for 2 to 3 weeks. Ensuring adequate hydration is imperative. Patients receiving foscarnet should be monitored for seizures related to alterations in plasma electrolyte levels.

Historically, the four most important arboviral pathogens in the United States were the St. Louis virus, the La Crosse virus, and the eastern and western equine viruses. However, West Nile virus has been recognized as an emerging pathogen and has been implicated in an epidemic occurring in the United States since 1999. Transmission occurs through the bites of mosquitoes. Typically, an incubation period of 2 to 14 days precedes the onset of clinical symptoms. Infection of the brain tissue results in fever, headache, paralysis, and coma. Although many patients have a benign presentation, symptomatic cases are associated with a higher degree of mortality. Mortality rates of 50% to 75% have been reported for eastern equine virus, whereas mortality rates for western equine and St. Louis viruses are 3% to 4% and 10% to 20%, respectively.[105,108] Treatment is supportive, including treatment of seizures and increased ICP. In the majority of cases, the disease is self-limiting.[108]

Because of the recent epidemic in the United States, a separate discussion of the West Nile virus is warranted. Although West Nile virus is transmitted primarily by mosquitoes, transmission of the virus via blood products, organ transplantation, transplacental transfer, and breast milk has been documented.[106] Similar to the other arboviruses, the incubation period for West Nile virus ranges from 3 days to 2 weeks. West Nile virus infection is asymptomatic in most adults or causes a mild flu-like syndrome characterized by fever, malaise, myalgia, and lymphadenopathy. Typically, less than 1% of patients develop neurologic disease, and approximately two thirds have encephalitis, with the remainder having meningitis without encephalitis.[14] Many patients develop a maculopapular, erythematous rash, which is more common in children than in adults and is uncommon in other forms of viral encephalitis.[14] Other neurologic manifestations include fever, nausea, vomiting, headache, altered mental status, movement disorders, and/or a syndrome much like poliomyelitis.[14,115,116] The primary risk factor for this manifestation seems to be advanced age. The poliomyelitis syndrome is characterized by an early prodromic phase of fevers and weakness followed by the sudden onset of flaccid paralysis. Among patients hospitalized with West Nile virus, the mortality rate is approximately 10% to 15%, whereas patients with encephalitis and weakness have a mortality rate of 30%.[14] CSF examination of West Nile virus encephalitis typically shows pleocytosis and a slightly elevated CSF protein concentration.[14] Several diagnostic methods have been developed for West Nile virus, including a PCR assay and an enzyme-linked immunosorbent assay (ELISA). However, serologic tests (ELISA) can cross-react with other flaviviruses, causing a false-positive result. Moreover, the IgM antibodies for West Nile virus can persist for up to 1 year, leading to confusion regarding whether the infection is an acute or previous infection.[14] Ribavirin has shown inhibitory effects on the West Nile virus in neural tissue cultures, but this has not been studied in controlled trials.

HIV encephalitis is the most common CNS complication associated with AIDS. Patients frequently may complain of headache, photophobia, or stiff neck at the time of presumed seroconversion. As the disease progresses, however, neurologic symptoms are reported frequently secondary to other opportunistic infections. Diagnosis of viral encephalitis is difficult because mental status and neurologic examinations are not sensitive enough to detect early changes. Direct evidence of HIV encephalitis can be obtained through CSF culture, p24 antigen testing, or qualitative or quantitative PCR for HIV RNA. Diagnostic workup of other potential copathogens, such as HSV, *Toxoplasma gondii, M. tuberculosis, Aspergillus* species, and *Cryptococcus,* also should be performed (see Chap. 126 for a complete discussion of infectious complications in HIV-positive individuals.)

EVALUATION OF THERAPEUTIC OUTCOMES

SIGNS AND SYMPTOMS

Because of the potential for rapid deterioration associated with meningitis, signs and symptoms of fever, headache, meningismus (e.g., nuchal rigidity, Brudzinski sign, Kernig sign), vital signs, and signs of cerebral dysfunction should be evaluated every 4 hours for the initial 3 days and daily thereafter. The Glasgow Coma Scale should be used in severely ill patients. Trends in improvement and resolution rather than single evaluations in time are more important in monitoring the signs and symptoms of meningitis.

MICROBIOLOGIC FINDINGS

CSF and blood samples for Gram stain, cultures, and sensitivity testing should be taken prior to starting antibiotic therapy. If lumbar puncture is delayed, however, antibiotics should be started. Although the CSF cultures may be negative, antibiotic therapy rarely interferes with the protein and/or glucose concentrations in the CSF.[15] Furthermore, if the laboratory is made aware of the antibiotic therapy, steps can be taken to diminish the effects of the antibiotic during the detection process.[18] Gram stain results can be obtained immediately and can guide empirical antibiotic treatment. Identification of the organism can be made within 24 hours, and sensitivities should be available within 48 hours. Repeat cultures should be performed to help determine if sterilization is achieved. A second tube of blood should be taken to allow for latex agglutination tests of antigens to common meningeal pathogens (*H. influenzae, S. pneumoniae, N. meningitidis, E. coli,* group B streptococcus) if the Gram stain has not been helpful.

CEREBRAL SPINAL FLUID EXAMINATION

In bacterial meningitis, the CSF WBC count usually is >1,000 cells/mm^3, CSF protein concentration is elevated, and CSF glucose concentration (hypoglycorrhachia) often is low (<50 mg/dL or 50%–60% of a simultaneous blood glucose value). In contrast, viral encephalitis results in relatively normal CSF protein and glucose levels and typically does not result in >90% polymorphonuclear neutrophils in the CSF (Table 110–1).

ABBREVIATIONS

AIDS: acquired immunodeficiency syndrome

CDC: Centers for Disease Control and Prevention

CNS: central nervous system

CSF: cerebrospinal fluid

CT: computed tomography

FDA: Food and Drug Administration

GI: gastrointestinal

Hib: *Haemophilus influenzae* type b

HIV: human immunodeficiency virus

ICP: intracranial pressure

IL: interleukin

INF: interferon

MIC: minimum inhibitory concentration

PAF: platelet-activating factor

PCR: polymerase chain reaction

TNF: tumor necrosis factor

WBC: white blood cell

REFERENCES

1. Scheld WM, Koedel U, Nathan B, et al. Pathophysiology of bacterial meningitis: Mechanism(s) of neuronal injury. J Infect Dis 2002;186(Suppl 2):S225–S33.
2. Saez-Llorens X, McCracken GH Jr. Bacterial meningitis in children. Lancet 2003;361:2139–2148.

3. van de Beek D, de Gans J, Spanjaard L, et al. Clinical features and prognostic factors in adults with bacterial meningitis. N Engl J Med 2004;351:1849–1859.
4. Meli DN, Christen S, Leib SL, et al. Current concepts in the pathogenesis of meningitis caused by Streptococcus pneumoniae. Curr Opin Infect Dis 2002;15:253–257.
5. Kim KS. Pathogenesis of bacterial meningitis: From bacteraemia to neuronal injury. Nat Rev Neurosci 2003;4:376–385.
6. Gold R. Epidemiology of bacterial meningitis. Infect Dis Clin North Am 1999;13:515–525.
7. Reefhuis J, Honein MA, Whitney CG, et al. Risk of bacterial meningitis in children with cochlear implants. N Engl J Med 2003;349:435–445.
8. Parodi S, Lechner A, Osih R, et al. Nosocomial Enterobacter meningitis: Risk factors, management, and treatment outcomes. Clin Infect Dis 2003;37:159–166.
9. Schuchat A, Robinson K, Wenger JD, et al. Bacterial meningitis in the United States in 1995. Active Surveillance Team. N Engl J Med 1997;337:970–976.
10. Whitney CG, Farley MM, Hadler J, et al. Decline in invasive pneumococcal disease after the introduction of protein-polysaccharide conjugate vaccine. N Engl J Med 2003;348:1737–1746.
11. Greenlee J. Anatomic considerations in central nervous system infections. In: GL Mandell; JE Bennett; R Dolin, eds. Principles and Practice of Infectious Diseases, 4th ed. New York: Churchill Livingstone, 1995:821–831.
12. Spector R, Lorenzo AV. Inhibition of penicillin transport from the cerebrospinal fluid after intracisternal inoculation of bacteria. J Clin Invest 1974;54:316–325.
13. Leib SL, Tauber MG. Pathogenesis of bacterial meningitis. Infect Dis Clin North Am 1999;13:527–548.
14. Bonthius DJ, Karacay B. Meningitis and encephalitis in children: An update. Neurol Clin North Am 2002;20:1013–1038.
15. Bashir HE, Laundy M, Booy R. Diagnosis and treatment of bacterial meningitis. Arch Dis Child 2003;88:615–620.
16. Thomas KE, Hasbun R, Jekel J, et al. The diagnostic accuracy of Kernig's sign, Brudzinski's sign, and nuchal rigidity in adults with suspected meningitis. Clin Infect Dis 2002;35:46–52.
17. Kaplan SL. Clinical presentations, diagnosis, and prognostic factors of bacterial meningitis. Infect Dis Clin North Am 1999;13:579–593.
18. Thomson RB, Bertram H. Laboratory diagnosis of central nervous system infections. Infect Dis Clin North Am 2001;15:1047–1071.
19. van Crevel H, Hijdra A, de Gans J. Lumbar puncture and the risk of herniation: When should we first perform CT? J Neurol 2002;249:129–137.
20. Hasbun R, Abrahams J, Jekel J, et al. Computed tomography of the head before lumbar puncture in adults with suspected meningitis. N Engl J Med 2001;345:1727–1733.
21. Proulx N, Frechette D, Toye B, et al. Delays in the administration of antibiotics are associated with mortality from adult acute bacterial meningitis. QJM 2005;98:291–298.
22. Heath PT, Yusoff NK, Baker CJ. Neonatal meningitis. Arch Dis Child Fetal Neonatal Ed 2003;88:F173–F178.
23. Prins JM, van Deventer SJ, Kuijper EJ, et al. Clinical relevance of antibiotic-induced endotoxin release. Antimicrob Agents Chemother 1994;38:1211–1218.
24. Shepard CW, Rosenstein NE, Fischer M. Neonatal meningococcal disease in the United States, 1990 to 1999. Pediatr Infect Dis J 2003;22:418–422.
25. Gold R. Epidemiology of bacterial meningitis. Infect Dis Clin North Am 1999;13:515–525.
26. Spach DH, Jackson LA. Bacterial meningitis. Neurol Clin 1999;17:711–735.
27. Moura AS, Mendez AP, Layton M, et al. Epidemiology of meningococcal disease, New York City, 1989–2000. Emerg Infect Dis 2003;9:355–361.
28. Rosenstein NE, Perkins BA, Stephens DS, et al. The changing epidemiology of meningococcal disease in the United States. J Infect Dis 1999;180:1894–1901.
29. Kelleher JA, Raebel MA. Meningococcal vaccine use in college students. Ann Pharmacother 2002;36:1776–1784.
30. Weinstein L. Bacterial meningitis. Specific etiologic diagnosis on the basis of distinctive epidemiologic, pathogenetic, and clinical features. Med Clin North Am 1985;69:219–229.
31. Klugman KP, Madhi SA. Emergence of drug resistance. Impact on bacterial meningitis. Infect Dis Clin North Am 1999;13:637–646.
32. Glodani LZ. Inducement of Neisseria meningitidis resistance to ampicillin and penicillin in a patient with meningococcemia treated with high doses of ampicillin. Clin Infect Dis 1998;26:772.
33. Casado-Flores J, Osona B, Domingo P, et al. Meningococcal meningitis during penicillin therapy for meningococcemia. Clin Infect Dis 1997;25:1479.
34. Chowdhury MH, Tunkel AR. Antibacterial agents in infections of the central nervous system. Infect Dis Clin North Am 2000;14:391–407.
35. Schwartz B. Chemoprophylaxis for bacterial infections: Principles of and application to meningococcal infections. Rev Infect Dis 1991;13(Suppl 2):S170–S173.
36. Anonymous. Prevention and control of meningococcal disease. Recommendations of the Advisory Committee on Immunization Practices (ACIP). MMWR Morb Mortal Weekly Rep 2000;49(RR-7):1–10.
37. Kaplan SL. Management of pneumococcal meningitis. Pediatr Infect Dis J 2002;21:589–591.
38. Aronin SI. Current pharmacotherapy of pneumococcal meningitis. Expert Opin Pharmacother 2002;3:121–129.
39. Kastanbauer S, Pfister HW. Pneumococcal meningitis in adults. Brain 2003;126:1015–1025.
40. Kaplan SL. Clinical presentations, diagnosis, and prognostic factors of bacterial meningitis. Infect Dis Clin North Am 1999;13:579–593.
41. Mitchell L, Tuomanen E. Vancomycin-tolerant Streptococcus pneumoniae and its clinical significance. Pediatr Infect Dis J 2001;20:531–533.
42. Novak R, Henriques B, Charpentier E, et al. Emergence of vancomycin tolerance in Streptococcus pneumoniae. Nature 1999;399:590–593.
43. Ross GH, Wright DH, Ibrahim KH, et al. Use of fluoroquinolones in central nervous system infections. J Infect Dis Pharmacother 2001;4:47–72.
44. Cottagnoud P, Tauber MG. Fluoroquinolones in the treatment of meningitis. Curr Infect Dis Rep 2003;5:329–336.
45. Kuhn F, Cottagnoud M, Acosta F, et al. Cefotaxime acts synergistically with levofloxacin in experimental meningitis due to penicillin-resistant pneumococci and prevents selection of levofloxacin-resistant mutants in vitro. Antimicrob Agents Chemother 2003;47:2487–2491.
46. Faella F, Pagliano P, Fusco U, et al. Combined treatment with ceftriaxone and linezolid of pneumococcal meningitis: A case series including penicillin-resistant strains. Clin Microbiol Infect 2006;12:391–394.
47. Cottagnoud P, Pfister M, Acosta F, et al. Daptomycin is highly efficacious against penicillin-resistant and penicillin- and quinolone-resistant pneumococci in experimental meningitis. Antimicrob Agents Chemother 2004;48:3928–3933.
48. CDC. Prevention of pneumococcal disease: Recommendations of the advisory committee on immunization practices. MMWR Recomm Rep 1997;46(RR-08):1–24.
49. Black S, Shinefield H, Fireman B, et al. Efficacy, safety and immunogenicity of heptavalent pneumococcal conjugate vaccine in children. Northern California Kaiser Permanente Vaccine Study Center Group. Pediatr Infect Dis J 2000;19:187–195.
50. Shinefield H, Black S, Ray P, et al. Efficacy, immunogenicity and safety of heptavalent pneumococcal conjugate vaccine in low birth weight and preterm infants. Pediatr Infect Dis J 2002;21:182–186.
51. Black S, Shinefield H. Safety and efficacy of the seven-valent pneumococcal conjugate vaccine: Evidence from Northern California. Eur J Pediatr 2002;161(Suppl 2):S127–S131.
52. Lieu TA, Ray GT, Black SB, et al. Projected cost-effectiveness of pneumococcal conjugate vaccination of healthy infants and young children. JAMA 2000;283:1460–1468.
53. CDC. Pneumococcal vaccination for cochlear implant candidates and recipients: Updated recommendations of the Advisory Committee on Immunization Practices. MMWR Morb Mortal Wkly Rep 2003;52: 739–740.
54. Tang LM, Chen ST, Wu YR. Haemophilus influenzae meningitis in adults. Diagn Microbiol Infect Dis 1998;32:27–32.
55. Lieberman JM, Greenberg DP, Ward JI. Prevention of bacterial meningitis. Vaccines and chemoprophylaxis. Infect Dis Clin North Am 1990;4:703–729.
56. Pediatrics AA. Haemophilus influenzae infections. In: LK Pickering, ed. 2000 Red Book: Report of the Committee on Infectious Diseases,

25 ed. Elk Grove Village, IL: American Academy of Pediatrics, 2000:262–272.

57. Rubin RH, Hooper DC. Central nervous system infection in the compromised host. Med Clin North Am 1985;69:281–296.
58. Lipman J, Allworth A, Wallis SC. Cerebrospinal fluid penetration of high doses of intravenous ciprofloxacin in meningitis. Clin Infect Dis 2000;31:1131–1133.
59. Levin AS, Barone AA, Penco J, et al. Intravenous colistin therapy for nosocomial infections caused by multidrug-resistant Pseudomonas aeruginosa and Acinetobacter baumannii. Clin Infect Dis 1999;28:1008–1011.
60. Jimenez-Mejias ME, Pichardo-Guerrero C, Marquez-Rivas FJ, et al. Cerebrospinal fluid penetration and pharmacokinetic/pharmacodynamic parameters of intravenously administered colistin in a case of multidrug-resistant Acinetobacter baumannii meningitis. Eur J Clin Microbiol Infect Dis 2002;21:212–214.
61. Vasen W, Desmery P, Ilutovich S, et al. Intrathecal use of colistin. J Clin Microbiol 2000;38:3523.
62. Gunderson BW, Ibrahim KH, Hovde LB, et al. Synergistic activity of colistin and ceftazidime against multiantibiotic-resistant Pseudomonas aeruginosa in an in vitro pharmacodynamic model. Antimicrob Agents Chemother 2003;47:905–909.
63. Meyer MA. Neurologic complications of anthrax. Arch Neurol 2003;60:483–488.
64. Bush LM, Abrams BH, Beall A, et al. Index case of fatal inhalational anthrax due to bioterrorism in the United States. N Engl J Med 2001;345:1607–1610.
65. Girgis NI, Farid Z, Mikhail IA, et al. Dexamethasone treatment for bacterial meningitis in children and adults. Pediatr Infect Dis J 1989;8:848–851.
66. Lebel MH, Freij BJ, Syrogiannopoulos GA, et al. Dexamethasone therapy for bacterial meningitis. Results of two double-blind, placebo-controlled trials. N Engl J Med 1988;319:964–971.
67. Lebel MH, Hoyt MJ, Waagner DC, et al. Magnetic resonance imaging and dexamethasone therapy for bacterial meningitis. Am J Dis Child 1989;143:301–306.
68. Odio CM, Faingezicht I, Paris M, et al. The beneficial effects of early dexamethasone administration in infants and children with bacterial meningitis. N Engl J Med 1991;324:1525–1531.
69. Schaad UB, Lips U, Gnehm HE, et al. Dexamethasone therapy for bacterial meningitis in children. Swiss Meningitis Study Group. Lancet 1993;342:457–461.
70. Kennedy WA, Hoyt MJ, McCracken GH Jr. The role of corticosteroid therapy in children with pneumococcal meningitis. Am J Dis Child 1991;145:1374–1378.
71. McIntyre PB, Berkey CS, King SM, et al. Dexamethasone as adjunctive therapy in bacterial meningitis. A meta-analysis of randomized clinical trials since 1988. JAMA 1997;278:925–931.
72. Pediatrics AAo. Pneumococcal infections. In: LK Pickering, ed. 2000 Red Book: Report of the Committee on Infectious Diseases, 25 ed. Elk Grove Village, IL: American Academy of Pediatrics, 2000:452–460.
73. Syrogiannopoulos GA, Lourida AN, Theodoridou MC, et al. Dexamethasone therapy for bacterial meningitis in children: 2- versus 4-day regimen. J Infect Dis 1994;169:853–858.
74. De Gans J, Van De Beek D. Dexamethasone in adults with bacterial meningitis. N Engl J Med 2002;347:1549–1556.
75. van de Beek D, de Gans J, McIntyre P, et al. Steroids in adults with acute bacterial meningitis: A systematic review. Lancet Infect Dis 2004;4:139–143.
76. Paris MM, Hickey SM, Uscher MI, et al. Effect of dexamethasone on therapy of experimental penicillin- and cephalosporin-resistant pneumococcal meningitis. Antimicrob Agents Chemother 1994;38:1320–1324.
77. Klugman KP, Friedland IR, Bradley JS. Bactericidal activity against cephalosporin-resistant Streptococcus pneumoniae in cerebrospinal fluid of children with acute bacterial meningitis. Antimicrob Agents Chemother 1995;39:1988–1992.
78. Gaillard JL, Abadie V, Cheron G, et al. Concentrations of ceftriaxone in cerebrospinal fluid of children with meningitis receiving dexamethasone therapy. Antimicrob Agents Chemother 1994;38:1209–1210.
79. Tung YR, Lai MC, Lui CC, et al. Tuberculous meningitis in infancy. Pediatr Neurol 2002;27:262–266.
80. Iseman MD. Extrapulmonary tuberculosis in adults. In: A Clinician's Guide to Tuberculosis. Philadelphia: Lippincott Williams & Wilkins, 2000:145–197.
81. Leonard JM, Des Prez RM. Tuberculous meningitis. Infect Dis Clin North Am 1990;4:769–787.
82. Holdiness MR. Management of tuberculosis meningitis. Drugs 1990;39:224–233.
83. Kent SJ, Crowe SM, Yung A, et al. Tuberculous meningitis: A 30-year review. Clin Infect Dis 1993;17:987–994.
84. CDC. Treatment of tuberculosis. MMWR Recomm Rep 2003;52(RR-11):1–77.
85. Ellard GA, Humphries MJ, Allen BW. Cerebrospinal fluid drug concentrations and the treatment of tuberculous meningitis. Annu Rev Resp Dis 1993;148:650–655.
86. Byrd T, Zinser P. Tuberculosis meningitis. Curr Treat Options Neurol 2001;3:427–432.
87. Waecker NJ. Tuberculosis meningitis in children. Curr Treat Options Neurol 2002;4:249–257.
88. Alzeer AH, FitzGerald JM. Corticosteroids and tuberculosis: Risks and use as adjunct therapy. Tubercle Lung Dis 1993;74:6–11.
89. Sugar AM, Stern JJ, Dupont B. Overview: Treatment of cryptococcal meningitis. Rev Infect Dis 1990;12(Suppl 3):S338–S348.
90. Powderly WG, Cloud GA, Dismukes WE, et al. Measurement of cryptococcal antigen in serum and cerebrospinal fluid: Value in the management of AIDS-associated cryptococcal meningitis. Clin Infect Dis 1994;18:789–792.
91. Powderly WG, Saag MS, Cloud GA, et al. A controlled trial of fluconazole or amphotericin B to prevent relapse of cryptococcal meningitis in patients with the acquired immunodeficiency syndrome. The NIAID AIDS Clinical Trials Group and Mycoses Study Group. N Engl J Med 1992;326:793–798.
92. Bennett JE, Dismukes WE, Duma RJ, et al. A comparison of amphotericin B alone and combined with flucytosine in the treatment of cryptococcal meningitis. N Engl J Med 1979;301:126–131.
93. Chuck SL, Sande MA. Infections with Cryptococcus neoformans in the acquired immunodeficiency syndrome. N Engl J Med 1989;321:794–799.
94. Coker RJ, Viviani M, Gazzard BG, et al. Treatment of cryptococcosis with liposomal amphotericin B (AmBisome) in 23 patients with AIDS. AIDS 1993;7:829–835.
95. Leenders AC, Reiss P, Portegies P, et al. Liposomal amphotericin B (AmBisome) compared with amphotericin B both followed by oral fluconazole in the treatment of AIDS-associated cryptococcal meningitis. AIDS 1997;11:1463–1471.
96. Saag MS, Powderly WG, Cloud GA, et al. Comparison of amphotericin B with fluconazole in the treatment of acute AIDS-associated cryptococcal meningitis. The NIAID Mycoses Study Group and the AIDS Clinical Trials Group. N Engl J Med 1992;326:83–89.
97. Berry AJ, Rinaldi MG, Graybill JR. Use of high-dose fluconazole as salvage therapy for cryptococcal meningitis in patients with AIDS. Antimicrob Agents Chemother 1992;36:690–692.
98. Brouwer AE, Rajanuwong A, Chierakul W, et al. Combination antifungal therapies for HIV-associated cryptococcal meningitis: A randomised trial. Lancet 2004;363:1764–1767.
99. de Gans J, Portegies P, Tiessens G, et al. Itraconazole compared with amphotericin B plus flucytosine in AIDS patients with cryptococcal meningitis. AIDS 1992;6:185–190.
100. Pfaller MA, Messer SA, Boyken L, et al. Global trends in the antifungal susceptibility of Cryptococcus neoformans (1990 to 2004). J Clin Microbiol 2005;43:2163–2167.
101. Pitisuttithum P, Negroni R, Graybill JR, et al. Activity of posaconazole in the treatment of central nervous system fungal infections. J Antimicrob Chemother 2005;56:745–755.
102. Powderly WG. Therapy for cryptococcal meningitis in patients with AIDS. Clin Infect Dis 1992;14(Suppl 1):S54–S59.
103. Saag MS, Cloud GA, Graybill JR, et al. A comparison of itraconazole versus fluconazole as maintenance therapy of AIDS-associated cryptococcal meningitis. Clin Infect Dis 1999;28:291–296.
104. Maxson S, Jacobs RF. Viral meningitis. Tips to rapidly diagnose treatable causes. Postgrad Med 1993;93:153–156, 1599–160, 163–166.
105. Roos KL. Encephalitis. Neurol Clin 1999;17:813–833.
106. CDC. Epidemic/epizootic West Nile Virus in the United States: Guidelines for surveillance, prevention, and control. Fort Collins, CO:

National Center for Infectious Diseases, Division of Vector-Borne Infectious Diseases, 2003.
107. CDC. Summary of West Nile Virus Activity, United States 2005. Fort Collins, CO: National Center for Infectious Diseases, Division of Vector-Borne Infectious Diseases, 2005.
108. Rubeiz H, Roos RP. Viral meningitis and encephalitis. Semin Neurol 1992;12:165–177.
109. Glimaker M. Enteroviral meningitis. Diagnostic methods and aspects on the distinction from bacterial meningitis. Scand J Infect Dis Suppl 1992;85:1–64.
110. Overall JC Jr. Is it bacterial or viral? Laboratory differentiation. Pediatr Rev 1993;14:251–261.
111. Dalton M, Newton RW. Aseptic meningitis. Dev Med Child Neurol 1991;33:446–451.
112. Sawyer MH, Holland D, Aintablian N, et al. Diagnosis of enteroviral central nervous system infection by polymerase chain reaction during a large community outbreak. Pediatr Infect Dis J 1994;13:177–182.
113. Gateley A, Gander RM, Johnson PC, et al. Herpes simplex virus type 2 meningoencephalitis resistant to acyclovir in a patient with AIDS. J Infect Dis 1990;161:711–715.
114. Astra USA I. Package insert: Foscavir injection.
115. Kelley TW, Prayson RA, Ruiz AI, et al. The neuropathology of West Nile virus meningoencephalitis. Am J Clin Pathol 2003;119:749–753.
116. Sejvar JJ, Haddad MB, Tierney BC, et al. Neurologic manifestations and outcome of West Nile virus infection. JAMA 2003;290:511–515.

CHAPTER 111

Lower Respiratory Tract Infections

MARK L. GLOVER AND MICHAEL D. REED

KEY CONCEPTS

1. Respiratory infections remain the major cause of morbidity from acute illness in the United States and likely represent the most common reasons why patients seek medical attention.

2. The majority of pulmonary infections follow colonization of the upper respiratory tract with potential pathogens, whereas microbes less commonly gain access to the lungs via the blood from an extrapulmonary source or by inhalation of infected aerosol particles. The competency of a patient's immune status is an important factor influencing the susceptibility to infection, etiologic cause, and disease severity.

3. An appropriate treatment regimen for the patient with uncomplicated lower respiratory tract infection usually can be established by patient history, physical examination, chest radiograph, and properly collected sputum for culture interpreted in light of current knowledge of the most common lung pathogens and their antibiotic susceptibility patterns within the community.

4. Acute bronchitis is caused most commonly by respiratory viruses and almost always is self-limiting. Therapy targets associated symptoms, such as lethargy, malaise, or fever (ibuprofen or acetaminophen), and fluids for rehydration. Routine use of antibiotics should be avoided.

5. Chronic bronchitis is caused by several interacting factors, including inhalation of noxious agents (most prominent are cigarette smoke and exposure to occupational dusts, fumes, and environmental pollution) and host factors including genetic factors and bacterial (and possibly viral) infections. The hallmark of this disease is a chronic cough, excessive sputum production, and expectoration with persistent presence of microorganisms in the patient's sputum.

6. Treatment of acute exacerbations of chronic bronchitis includes attempts to mobilize and enhance sputum expectoration (chest physiotherapy, humidification of inspired air), oxygen if needed, aerosolized bronchodilators (albuterol) in select patients with demonstrated benefit, and antibiotics.

7. Respiratory syncytial virus is the most common cause of acute bronchiolitis, an infection that mostly affects infants during their first year of life. In the well infant, bronchiolitis usually is a self-limiting viral illness, whereas in the child with underlying respiratory disease, cardiac disease, or both, the child may develop severe respiratory compromise (failure) necessitating in-hospital treatment, such as rehydration, oxygen, and, in select patients, bronchodilators, ribavirin aerosol, or both.

8. The most prominent pathogen causing community-acquired pneumonia in otherwise healthy adults is *Streptococcus pneumoniae*, whereas the most common pathogens causing hospital-acquired pneumonia (including nursing home residents) are *Staphylococcus aureus* and gram-negative aerobic bacilli. Anaerobic bacteria are the most common etiologic agents in pneumonia that follows aspiration of gastric or oropharyngeal contents.

9. Treatment of community-acquired pneumonia may consist of humidified oxygen for hypoxemia, bronchodilators (albuterol) when bronchospasm is present, rehydration fluids, and chest physiotherapy for marked accumulation of retained respiratory secretions. Antibiotic regimens should be selected based on presumed causative pathogens and pulmonary distribution characteristics and should be adjusted to provide optimal activity against pathogens identified by culture (sputum or blood).

10. Treatment of nosocomial pneumonia requires aggressive therapy with careful consideration of the dominance and susceptibility patterns of the pathogens present within the institution. The epidemiology of these common pathogens should be evaluated on a regular basis in order to identify changing resistance patterns and subsequent alternation of treatment guidelines.

Learning objectives, review questions, and other resources can be found at **www.pharmacotherapyonline.com.**

(1) Respiratory tract infections remain the major cause of morbidity from acute illness in the United States and most likely represent the single most common reason patients seek medical attention. This chapter focuses on bacterial and viral infections involving the lower respiratory tract, which includes the tracheobronchial tree and lung parenchyma.

(2) The respiratory tract has an elaborate system of host defenses, including humoral immunity, cellular immunity, and anatomic mechanisms.[1] When functioning properly, the host defenses of the respiratory tract are markedly effective in protecting against pathogen invasion and removing potentially infectious agents from the lungs. For the most part, infections in the lower respiratory tract occur only when these defense mechanisms are impaired, as in cases of dysgammaglobulinemia or compromised ciliary function, such as that caused by the chronic inflammation accompanying cigarette smoking. In addition, local defenses may be overwhelmed when a particularly virulent microorganism or excessive inoculum invades lung parenchyma. The majority of pulmonary infections follow colonization of the upper respiratory tract with potential pathogens, which, after achieving sufficiently high concentrations, gain access to the lung via aspiration of oropharyngeal secretions. Less commonly, microbes enter the lung via the blood from an extrapulmonary source or by

inhalation of infected aerosolized particles. The specific type of pulmonary infection caused by an invading microorganism is determined by a variety of host factors, including age, anatomic features of the airway, and specific characteristics of the infecting agent.

The most common infections involving the lower respiratory tract are bronchitis, bronchiolitis, and pneumonia. Lower respiratory tract infections in children and adults most commonly result from either viral or bacterial invasion of lung parenchyma. The diagnosis of viral infections rests primarily on the recognition of a characteristic constellation of clinical signs and symptoms. Because treatment is largely supportive, only occasionally does the diagnosis require laboratory confirmation; this is achieved through serologic tests or identification of the organism by culture or antigen detection in respiratory secretions.[2] New laboratory techniques using polymerase chain reaction and genetic "fingerprinting" technology have emerged as a means to identify specific pathogens rapidly and accurately.[3]

In contrast, because bacterial pneumonia usually necessitates expedient, effective, and specific antibiotic therapy, its management depends, in large part, on isolation of the etiologic agent by culture from lung tissue or secretions.[4,5] The pharynx is colonized with many organisms that can cause pneumonia; therefore, culture of expectorated sputum can be misleading unless the specimen is examined to ensure that it has originated from the lower respiratory tract. The Gram stain provides the easiest method for distinguishing lower from upper respiratory tract secretions; moreover, through determination of the shape and color of the bacteria, the Gram stain frequently narrows the microbiologic differential diagnosis sufficiently to allow accurate initial therapy. Scanned under low-power microscopy, Gram-stained expectorated upper respiratory tract secretions contain many irregularly shaped epithelial cells with little evidence of inflammation. In contrast, a lower-tract specimen from a patient with bacterial pneumonia usually contains multiple neutrophils per high-powered field and a single or predominant bacterial species. Culture of specimens confirmed to originate from the lower tract by Gram stain provides valuable diagnostic information in the majority of patients with bacterial pneumonia. In addition, pneumonia promotes the release of inflammatory mediators and acute phase proteins such as C-reactive protein, which is significantly elevated in serum in the presence of respiratory tract infections.[6]

❸ An appropriate treatment regimen for the patient with an uncomplicated lower respiratory tract infection usually can be established by history, physical examination, chest radiograph, and properly collected sputum cultures interpreted in light of the most common lung pathogens and their antibiotic susceptibility patterns within the community.[2,4,5,7,8] More sophisticated or invasive diagnostic methods (e.g., computed tomography, bronchoscopy, and lung biopsy)[9,10] should be reserved for very ill patients who are unable to expectorate sputum or who are not responding to empirical therapy or for pulmonary infections occurring in immunocompromised patients.

BRONCHITIS

Bronchitis and bronchiolitis are inflammatory conditions of the large and small elements, respectively, of the tracheobronchial tree. The inflammatory process does not extend to the alveoli. Bronchitis frequently is classified as acute or chronic. Acute bronchitis occurs in individuals of all ages, whereas chronic bronchitis primarily affects adults. Bronchiolitis is a disease of infancy.

ACUTE BRONCHITIS

Epidemiology and Etiology

Acute bronchitis occurs most commonly during the winter months, following a pattern similar to those of other acute respiratory tract infections. Cold, damp climates and the presence of high concentrations of irritating substances (e.g., air pollution, cigarette smoke) may precipitate attacks.

❹ Respiratory viruses are by far the most common infectious agents associated with acute bronchitis.[11] The common cold viruses (rhinovirus and coronavirus) and lower respiratory tract pathogens (influenza virus and adenovirus) account for the majority of cases. In children, similar pathogens are observed, with the addition of the parainfluenza viruses. Although the true incidence remains to be defined, *Mycoplasma pneumoniae* appears to be a frequent cause of acute bronchitis. Additionally, *Chlamydia pneumoniae*[12] and *Bordetella pertussis*[13] (agent responsible for whooping cough) have been associated with acute respiratory tract infections. Although a variety of bacteria, including *Streptococcus pneumoniae, Streptococcus* species, *Staphylococcus* species, and *Haemophilus* species, may be isolated from throat or sputum culture, these organisms probably represent contamination by normal flora of the upper respiratory tract rather than true pathogens. Although a primary bacterial etiology for acute bronchitis appears rare, secondary bacterial infection may be involved.

Pathogenesis

❹ Because acute bronchitis is primarily a self-limiting illness and rarely a cause of death, few data describing the pathology are available. In general, infection of the trachea and bronchi yields hyperemic and edematous mucous membranes with an increase in bronchial secretions. Destruction of respiratory epithelium can range from mild to extensive and may affect bronchial mucociliary function. In addition, the increase in bronchial secretions, which can become thick and tenacious, further impairs mucociliary activity. The probability of permanent damage to the airways as a result of acute bronchitis remains unclear; however, epidemiologic evaluations support the belief that recurrent acute respiratory infections may be associated with increased airway hyperreactivity and possibly the pathogenesis of asthma or chronic obstructive pulmonary disease (COPD).

Clinical Presentation

Acute bronchitis usually begins as an upper respiratory infection with nonspecific complaints (Table 111–1).[11,14] Cough is the hallmark of acute bronchitis and occurs early. The onset of cough may be insidious or abrupt, and the symptoms persist despite resolution of nasal or nasopharyngeal complaints. Frequently, the cough initially is nonproductive but then progresses, yielding mucopurulent sputum. In older children and adults, the sputum is raised and expectorated; in the young child, sputum often is swallowed and can result in gagging and vomiting. Substantial discomfort may result from the coughing. Dyspnea, cyanosis, or signs of airway obstruction are observed rarely unless the patient has underlying pulmonary disease, such as emphysema or COPD. Fever, when present, rarely exceeds 39°C (102.2°F) and appears most commonly with adenovirus, influenza virus, and *M. pneumoniae* infections. The diagnosis

TABLE 111-1 Clinical Presentation of Acute Bronchitis

Signs and symptoms
Cough persisting >5 days to weeks
Coryza, sore throat, malaise, headache
Fever rarely >39°C
Physical examination
Rhonchi or coarse, moist, bilateral rales
Purulent sputum in ~50% of patients
Chest radiograph
Normal

typically is made on the basis of a characteristic history and physical examination. Bacterial cultures of expectorated sputum generally are of limited use because of the inability to avoid normal nasopharyngeal flora by the sampling technique. In routine cases, viral cultures are unnecessary and frequently unavailable. Viral antigen detection tests, developed to identify respiratory viral antigens from nasal secretions rapidly, can be obtained in many hospital laboratories and in some practice settings when a specific diagnosis is necessary for clinical or epidemiologic reasons. Cultures or serologic diagnosis of *M. pneumoniae* and culture or direct fluorescent antibody detection for *B. pertussis* should be obtained in prolonged or severe cases when epidemiologic considerations would suggest their involvement.

TREATMENT

Acute Bronchitis

■ DESIRED OUTCOME

In the absence of a complicating bacterial superinfection, acute bronchitis almost always is self-limiting. The goals of therapy are to provide comfort to the patient and, in the unusually severe case, to treat associated dehydration and respiratory compromise.[11]

■ GENERAL APPROACH TO TREATMENT

❹ Treatment of acute bronchitis is symptomatic and supportive in nature. Reassurance and antipyretics frequently are all that are needed. Bed rest for comfort may be instituted as desired. Patients should be encouraged to drink fluids to prevent dehydration and possibly to decrease the viscosity of respiratory secretions. Mist therapy (use of a vaporizer) may promote the thinning and loosening of respiratory secretions.

■ PHARMACOLOGIC THERAPY

Mild analgesic–antipyretic therapy often is helpful in relieving the associated lethargy, malaise, and fever. Aspirin or acetaminophen (650 mg in adults or 10–15 mg/kg per dose in children; maximum daily pediatric dose 60 mg/kg; maximum daily adult dose 4 g) or ibuprofen (200–800 mg in adults or 10 mg/kg per dose in children; maximum daily pediatric dose 40 mg/kg; maximum daily adult dose 3.2 g) should be administered every 4 to 6 hours. In children, aspirin should be avoided and acetaminophen used as the preferred agent because of the possible association between aspirin use and the development of Reye syndrome.[15]

Use of ibuprofen as an antipyretic has increased. The drug's antipyretic efficacy appears identical to that of aspirin or acetaminophen, although its duration of antipyretic effect may be slightly longer (e.g., 3–4 hours for aspirin and acetaminophen versus 5–6 hours for ibuprofen). Caution should be exercised in the administration of ibuprofen in patients younger than 3 months, elderly patients, and individuals with poor renal function. Aspirin and ibuprofen inhibit prostaglandin synthesis and may adversely influence renal function in these predisposed patient populations.

Patients suffering from acute bronchitis frequently medicate themselves with nonprescription cough and cold remedies containing various combinations of antihistamines, sympathomimetics, and antitussives despite the lack of definitive evidence supporting their effectiveness. In fact, the tendency of these agents to dehydrate bronchial secretions could aggravate and prolong the recovery process. Although not recommended for routine use, persistent, mild cough, which may be bothersome, can be treated with dextromethorphan; more severe coughs may require intermittent codeine or other similar agents.[14] In severe cases, the cough may be persistent enough to disrupt sleep, and use of a mild sedative–hypnotic, concomitantly with a cough suppressant, may be desirable. However, antitussives should be used cautiously when the cough is productive. The primary or supplemental use of expectorants is questionable because their clinical effectiveness has not been well established.

Routine use of antibiotics for treatment of acute bronchitis should be discouraged.[11] In previously healthy patients who exhibit persistent fever or respiratory symptoms for more than 4 to 6 days or in predisposed patients (e.g., elderly, immunocompromised), the possibility of a concurrent bacterial infection should be suspected. When possible, antibiotic therapy should be directed toward anticipated respiratory pathogen(s) (i.e., *S. pneumoniae*). *M. pneumoniae*, if suspected by history, by finding of cold hemagglutinins in serum (immunoglobulin M antibodies) with titers >1:32, or if confirmed by culture or serology, can be treated with azithromycin. Alternatively and empirically, a fluoroquinolone antibiotic with activity against these suspected pathogens (e.g., levofloxacin) can be used. During known epidemics involving the influenza A virus, amantadine or rimantadine may be effective in minimizing associated symptoms if administered early in the course of the disease.[16] Also, the neuraminidase inhibitors (e.g., zanamivir and oseltamivir) are active against both influenza A and B viral infections and may reduce the severity and duration of the influenza episode if administered promptly during the onset of the viral infection (see Chap. 114).[17,18] Unfortunately, the incidence of influenzae virus resistance to available antiviral drugs is increasing.[19]

CHRONIC BRONCHITIS

Epidemiology and Etiology

Chronic bronchitis is a nonspecific disease that primarily affects adults. Between 10% and 25% of the adult population 40 years of age and older suffer from chronic bronchitis, resulting in substantial healthcare dollar expenditures and lost wages. This disease is so common that acute bronchitis and acute exacerbations of chronic bronchitis result in approximately 16 million physician visits per year in the United States. Similar to acute bronchitis, cold, damp climates and elevated airborne concentrations of irritating substances may favor this disease. Chronic bronchitis occurs more commonly in men than in women.[20,21]

❺ Chronic bronchitis is a result of several contributing factors; the most prominent include cigarette smoking, exposure to occupational dusts, fumes, and environmental pollution; and host factors (e.g., genetic factors and bacterial [and possibly viral] infections). The contribution of each of these factors and of others (either alone or in combination) to chronic bronchitis is unknown. Cigarette smoke is a well-known airway irritant and is believed to be the predominant factor in the etiology of chronic bronchitis. Studies of lungs from smoking and nonsmoking individuals clearly have demonstrated a substantial increase in the number of alveolar macrophages, as well as the presence of bronchial inflammation, in individuals who smoke cigarettes. Although the majority of patients who suffer from chronic bronchitis have a positive smoking history, no history of smoking can be identified in as many as 10% of patients. These findings suggest that additional airway irritants, either alone or more probably in combination, are responsible for the pathogenesis of chronic bronchitis. It appears from candidate gene association studies that a genetic basis for some COPD phenotypes will be described in the near future.[22] In addition, the influence of recurrent respiratory tract infections during childhood or young adult life on the later development of chronic bronchitis remains obscure. Recurrent respiratory infections may predispose individuals to the development of chronic bronchitis[23]; however, whether these recurrent respiratory tract infections are a result of unrecognized anatomic abnormalities of the airways or impaired pulmonary defense mechanisms is unclear.

Chronic bronchitis is a disease of the bronchi that is manifested by cough and excessive sputum expectoration that occurs on most days of the week for a minimum of 3 consecutive months per year for at least 2 consecutive years that is unrelated to other pulmonary or cardiac disease. Numerous consensus statements and published authoritative guidelines define chronic bronchitis and emphysema as the two main components of chronic obstructive pulmonary (lung) disease (COPD/COLD).[20,21,24] The NHLBI/WHO Global Initiative for Chronic Obstruction Lung Disease (GOLD)[21] guidelines document does not distinguish these two diagnosis (e.g., emphysema or chronic bronchitis) in the definition of COPD, but it does define COPD as a disease characterized by airflow obstruction that is not fully reversible and progressive.[20] The GOLD guidelines provide a COPD classification scoring system according to severity that can be very helpful in staging patients for intensity of therapy and prognosis.[21] Unfortunately, differences in definitions between authoritative organizations[20,21,24] may cause confusion in the assignment of patients in clinical trials and thus to assessment and applications of study results to clinical care.

Pathogenesis

Chronic inhalation of an irritating noxious substance compromises the normal secretory and mucociliary function of bronchial mucosa. Bronchial biopsy specimens in bronchitic patients underscore the importance of proinflammatory cytokines (e.g., interleukins 1, 6, and 8, and tumor necrosis factor-α) in the pathogenesis and propagation of the observed inflammatory changes. In chronic bronchitis, the bronchial wall is thickened, and the number of mucus-secreting goblet cells on the surface epithelium of both larger and smaller bronchi is increased markedly. In contrast, goblet cells generally are absent from the smaller bronchi of normal individuals. In addition to the increased number of goblet cells, hypertrophy of the mucous glands and dilation of the mucous gland ducts are observed. As a result of these changes, chronic bronchitics have substantially more mucus in their peripheral airways, further impairing normal lung defenses. This increased quantity of tenacious secretions within the bronchial tree frequently causes mucous plugging of the smaller airways. Accompanying these changes are squamous cell metaplasia of the surface epithelium, edema, and increased vascularity of the basement membrane of larger airways and variable chronic inflammatory cell infiltration. Continued progression of this pathology can result in residual scarring of small bronchi and peribronchial fibrosis augmenting airway obstruction and weakening of bronchial walls.

Clinical Presentation

5 The hallmark of chronic bronchitis is a cough that may range from a mild "smoker's cough" to severe, incessant coughing productive of purulent sputum. Coughing may be precipitated by multiple stimuli, including simple, normal conversation. Expectoration of the largest quantity of sputum usually occurs on arising in the morning, although many patients expectorate sputum throughout the day. The expectorated sputum usually is tenacious and can vary in color from white to yellow–green. Patients with chronic bronchitis often expectorate as much as 100 mL/day more than normal. As a result, many patients complain of a frequent bad taste in their mouth and of halitosis.

The diagnosis of chronic bronchitis is based primarily on clinical assessment and history. Any patient who reports coughing sputum on most days for at least 3 consecutive months each year for 2 consecutive years presumptively has chronic bronchitis.[20] The diagnosis of chronic bronchitis is made only when the possibilities of bronchiectasis, cardiac failure, cystic fibrosis, and lung carcinoma have been effectively excluded. In an attempt to be more specific in the diagnosis, some investigators have added the criteria of lost wages for 3 or more weeks. In addition, many clinicians attempt to subdivide their patients based on severity of disease to guide therapeutic interventions. As noted earlier, GOLD has published a COPD classification system that many clinicians find useful (Table 111–2). The importance of accurate classification for grouping patients of similar disease involvement cannot be overemphasized with respect to assessing publications outlining treatment strategies for these patients.[25] The typical clinical presentation of chronic bronchitis is listed in Table 111–3.

In more advanced stages of chronic bronchitis, physical findings associated with cor pulmonale, including cardiac enlargement, hepatomegaly, and edema of the lower extremities, are observed. In general, chronic bronchitics tend to maintain at least normal body weight and commonly are obese. Radiographic studies are of limited value either in the diagnosis or followup of a patient. The microscopic and laboratory assessments of sputum are considered important components in the overall evaluation of patients with chronic bronchitis. A fresh sputum specimen obtained as an early-morning sample is preferred. Comparison of the cellular constituents of chronic bronchitic sputum with those of normal sputum can provide insight into the degree of activity of the disease processes. An increased number of polymorphonuclear granulocytes often suggests continual

TABLE 111-2 Useful Clinical Classification System for Patients with Chronic Bronchitis and Initial Treatment Options

Baseline Status	Criteria or Risk Factors	Usual Pathogens	Initial Treatment Options
Class I			
Acute tracheobronchitis	No underlying structural disease	Usually a virus	1. None unless symptoms persist 2. Amoxicillin; amoxicillin–clavulanate; a macrolide/azalide if bacterial infection is suspected/documented
Class II			
Chronic bronchitis	FEV_1 >50% predicted value, increased sputum volume and purulence	*Haemophilus influenzae* (usually nontypeable), *Haemophilus* species, *Moraxella catarrhalis*, *Streptococcus pneumoniae* (β-lactam resistance possible)	1. Same as Class I, no. 2, or a fluoroquinolone if prevalence of H. influenzae resistance to amoxicillin is >20% 2. Fluoroquinolone, amoxicillin–clavulanate, azithromycin, tetracycline, or trimethoprim–sulfamethoxazole
Class III			
Chronic bronchitis with complications	FEV_1 <50% predicted value, increased sputum volume and purulence, advanced age, at least four flares per year, or significant comorbidity	Same as class II; also *E. coli*, *Klebsiella*, *Enterobacter* species, *Pseudomonas aeruginosa* (β-lactam resistance common)	1. Fluoroquinolone 2. Extended spectrum cephalosporin, amoxicillin–clavulanate, or azithromycin
Class IV			
Chronic bronchial infection	Same as for class III plus yearlong production of purulent sputum	Same as class III	1. Oral or parenteral fluoroquinolone, carbapenem, or extended spectrum cephalosporin

Carbapenem: imipenem–cilastatin; meropenem; extended-spectrum cephalosporin; ceftazidime, cefepime; fluoroquinolone; ciprofloxacin, levofloxacin, moxifloxacin; tetracycline, tetracycline HCl, doxycycline; 1, preferred therapy; 2, alternative treatment options.

TABLE 111-3 Clinical Presentation of Chronic Bronchitis

Signs and symptoms
Cyanosis (advanced disease)
Obesity
Physical examination
Chest auscultation usually reveals inspiratory and expiratory rales, rhonchi, and mild wheezing with an expiratory phase that is frequently prolonged; hyperresonance on percussion with obliteration of the area of cardiac dullness
Normal vesicular breathing sounds are diminished
Clubbing of digits (advanced disease)
Chest radiograph
Increase in anteroposterior diameter of the thoracic cage (observed as a barrel chest)
Depressed diaphragm with limited mobility
Laboratory tests
Erythrocytosis (advanced disease)
Pulmonary function tests
Decreased vital capacity
Prolonged expiratory flow

bronchial irritation, whereas an increased number of eosinophils suggests an allergic component that should be further investigated. Gram staining of the sputum often reveals a mixture of both gram-positive and gram-negative bacteria, reflecting normal oropharyngeal flora and chronic tracheal colonization (in order of frequency) by nontypeable *Haemophilus influenzae, S. pneumoniae,* and *Moraxella catarrhalis.* Table 111–4 lists the most common bacterial isolates identified from sputum culture in patients experiencing an acute exacerbation of chronic bronchitis. In patients with more severe airflow disease (e.g., forced expiratory volume in the first second of expiration [FEV_1] <40%), enteric gram-negative bacilli, *Escherichia coli, Klebsiella, Enterobacter,* and *Pseudomonas aeruginosa* may be significant pathogens during acute exacerbations.[26]

TABLE 111-4 Common Bacterial Pathogens Isolated from Sputum of Patients with Acute Exacerbation of Chronic Bronchitis

Pathogen	Percent of Cultures
Haemophilus influenzae[a]	45
Moraxella catarrhalis[a]	30
Streptococcus pneumoniae[b]	20
Escherichia coli, Enterobacter species, *Klebsiella, Pseudomonas aeruginosa*	5

[a]Often β-lactamase positive; vast majority are nontypeable strains.
[b]As many as 25% of strains may have intermediate or high resistance to penicillin.

TREATMENT

Chronic Bronchitis

■ DESIRED OUTCOME

The goals of therapy for chronic bronchitis are twofold: to reduce the severity of chronic symptoms and to ameliorate acute exacerbations and achieve prolonged infection-free intervals.

■ GENERAL APPROACH TO TREATMENT

The approach to treatment of chronic bronchitis is multifactorial. First and foremost, attempts must be made to reduce the patient's exposure to known bronchial irritants (e.g., smoking, workplace pollution). A complete occupational and environmental history for determination of exposure to noxious, irritating gases, as well as preference toward cigarette smoking, must be assessed. Often easier discussed than accomplished, honest, yet reasonable attempts should be made with the patient to reduce or eliminate completely the number of cigarettes smoked daily and to reduce exposure to secondhand smoke. In an organized, coordinated, smoking cessation program, including counseling and hypnotherapy, the adjunctive use of nicotine substitutes (e.g., nicotine gum or patch) may promote the reduction or complete withdrawal from cigarette smoking. Often just as difficult is modification of exposure to irritating substances within the home and workplace.

❻ Measures to provide pulmonary toilet can be instituted. During acute pulmonary exacerbations of the disease, the patient's ability to mobilize and expectorate sputum may be reduced dramatically. In these instances, attempts at postural drainage techniques, with instruction, active participation, or both from a respiratory therapist, may assist in promoting clearance of pulmonary secretions. In addition, humidification of inspired air may promote the hydration (liquefaction) of tenacious secretions, allowing for more productive removal. Use of mucolytic aerosols, such as *N*-acetylcysteine and DNAse, is of questionable therapeutic value, particularly considering their propensity to induce bronchospasm (*N*-acetylcysteine) and their excessive cost. A Cochrane meta-analysis of mucolytic therapy in subjects with chronic bronchitis or COPD found that treatment with mucolytics was associated with a small reduction in acute exacerbations and a reduction in total number of days of disability. The clinical benefit may be greater in chronic bronchitics/COPD patients who have frequent or prolonged exacerbations or in those who are repeatedly admitted to hospitals with acute exacerbations. Mucolytics may have the greatest benefit in patients with moderate or severe COPD who are not receiving inhaled corticosteroids.[27] Although limited data are available, chronic use of oral or aerosolized bronchodilators may be of benefit by increasing mucociliary and cough clearance. In patients with moderate-to-severe COPD, twice-daily inhaled salmeterol/fluticasone propionate 50/250 or 50/500 micrograms for 24–52 weeks improves FEV_1 significantly more than does salmeterol or fluticasone monotherapy and results in clinically significant improvements in health-related quality of life.[28] Furthermore, patients may benefit from inhaled corticosteroids; patients with severe disease (FEV_1 <50%) with a history of frequent exacerbations should receive chronic inhaled corticosteroid therapy. Use of systemic corticosteroid therapy (oral or IV) in patients with an acute exacerbation significantly reduces treatment failures and the need for additional medical treatment.[29] Finally, in the face of an acute exacerbation, a trial of antibiotics directed against the most likely underlying pathogens should be initiated.

■ PHARMACOLOGIC THERAPY

For patients who consistently demonstrate clinical limitation in airflow, a therapeutic challenge of β_2-agonist bronchodilators (e.g., as albuterol aerosol) should be considered. Pulmonary function tests can be performed before and after β_2-agonist aerosol administration for more objective determination of a patient's propensity to benefit from supplemental aerosol therapy. However, this laboratory assessment, often performed at times of better health, may not accurately predict a patient's potential benefit from β_2-agonists during acute exacerbations of chronic bronchitis. Nevertheless, sufficient published experience supports the use of inhalation therapy with short-acting β_2-agonist in patients with chronic bronchitis to improve pulmonary function and exercise tolerance and to reduce the sense of breathlessness.[20] As noted earlier, chronic inhalation of the salmeterol/fluticasone combination has been associated with improved pulmonary function and quality of life.

Published experience with inhaled anticholinergic drugs, including ipratropium and tiotropium, is limited. In stable patients, long-term inhalation of ipratropium has been associated with a decreased frequency of cough, less severe coughing, and a decrease in the volume of expectorated sputum. Once-daily tiotropium inhalation was associated with significant bronchodilation and dyspnea relief compared to placebo but had no significant effect on the incidence or severity of cough.[20] Although chronic theophylline administration has been used extensively in the past, this therapy is being used with decreasing frequency in favor of aerosolized β_2-receptor agonists.

Use of antimicrobials for treatment of chronic bronchitis is controversial. Numerous comparative evaluations, including placebo-controlled studies of antibiotic administration with acute and chronic treatment of chronic bronchitics, have suggested definite clinical benefit, whereas other similar studies have not.[26] The antibiotics selected most frequently possess variable in-vitro activity against the common sputum isolates *H. influenzae, S. pneumoniae, M. catarrhalis,* and *M. pneumoniae.* In general, these conflicting results appear independent of the antibiotic used or the regimen compared. The wide disparity that exists in the results from these studies, combined with the difficulties in recognition and lack of standardized diagnostic criteria for acute exacerbations of chronic bronchitis, serves as the basis for the enormous controversy surrounding the use of antibiotics in this condition.[30] A review of 14 double-blinded randomized clinical trials compared fluoroquinolones to more standard antibiotic regimens (e.g., macrolides, azalides, oral cephalosporins, and the combination drug amoxicillin–clavulanate).[26] As expected, no statistically significant differences were observed between treatment arms. However, in a small subset of studies (n = 4), the sputum culture became negative in a significantly higher number of fluoroquinolone-treated patients. Other studies showed an increase in the interval between acute exacerbations in patients who received fluoroquinolone therapy. An additional advantage of fluoroquinolone therapy is the short course (e.g., 5 days) and once-daily dosing compared to other antibiotic regimens.

The increasing resistance of the common bacterial pathogens to first-line agents further complicates antibiotic selection. As many as 30% to 40% of *H. influenzae* and 95% of *M. catarrhalis* isolates produce β-lactamases. Moreover, up to 30% of *S. pneumoniae* isolates demonstrate resistance to penicillin (minimum inhibitory concentration [MIC] = 0.1–2 mg/L), with approximately 14% of isolates being highly resistant (MIC >2 mg/L). In addition, concern regarding *S. pneumoniae* resistance is increasing, given the incidence of macrolide resistance approximating 20%. Despite these changes in bacterial susceptibility, the current recommendation is to initiate therapy with first-line agents in less severely affected patients.

Regardless of the antibiotic selected, careful attention to predetermined outcome measures should be monitored closely in each patient to determine the success or failure of the therapeutic intervention. Oral antibiotics with broader antibacterial spectra (e.g., amoxicillin–clavulanate, fluoroquinolones, or azalides) that possess more potent in-vitro activity against sputum isolates are increasingly becoming first-line antibiotics as initial therapy for treatment of acute exacerbations of chronic bronchitis.[26]

An important clinical outcome variable directing drug selection and criteria for beginning antibiotics in individual patients is the infection-free period when chronic bronchitics are off antibiotics. The actual length of the infection-free time period and the change in the number of physician office visits and hospital admissions with a particular antibiotic regimen are extremely important to identify, whenever possible, for each patient. The antibiotic regimen that results in the longest infection-free period defines the "regimen of choice" for specific patients for future acute exacerbations of their disease.

Antibiotics should be selected that are effective against responsible pathogens, demonstrate the least risk of drug interactions, and can be administered in a manner that promotes compliance. Antibiotics commonly used for treatment of these patients and their respective adult starting doses are listed in Table 111–5. Doses of antibiotics should be adjusted as needed to the desired clinical effect and the lowest incidence of acceptable side effects. A frequently used clinical strategy to enhance the duration of symptom-free periods incorporates higher-dose antibiotic regimens using the upper limit of the recommended daily antibiotic dose for a period of 5 to 7 days.

TABLE 111-5 Oral Antibiotics Commonly Used for the Treatment of Acute Respiratory Exacerbations in Chronic Bronchitis

Antibiotic	Usual Adult Dose (g)	Dose Schedule (doses/day)
Preferred drugs		
Ampicillin	0.25–0.5	4
Amoxicillin	0.5–0.875	3–2
Amoxicillin–clavulanate	0.5–0.875	3–2
Ciprofloxacin	0.5–0.75	2
Levofloxacin	0.5–0.75	1
Moxifloxacin	0.4	1
Doxycycline	0.1	2
Minocycline	0.1	2
Tetracycline HCl	0.5	4
Trimethoprim-sulfamethoxazole[a]	1 DS	2
Supplemental drugs		
Azithromycin	0.25–0.5	1
Erythromycin	0.5	4
Clarithromycin	0.25–0.5	2
Cephalexin	0.5	4

[a]DS, double-strength tablet (160-mg trimethoprim/800-mg sulfamethoxazole).

In the patient whose history suggests recurrent exacerbations of disease that might be attributable to specific events (e.g., seasonal or related to the winter months), a trial of prophylactic antibiotics might be beneficial. If no clinical improvement is noted over an appropriate time period (2–3 months per year for 2–3 years), further attempts at prophylactic therapy can be discontinued. Similarly, patient-specific antibiotic trials can be performed in individuals experiencing acute exacerbations, focusing on attaining the maximum infection-free period. Although less than desirable, this method of clinical assessment may distinguish patients who will benefit from prophylactic antibiotic therapy from those who will not.

BRONCHIOLITIS

EPIDEMIOLOGY AND ETIOLOGY

❼ Bronchiolitis is an acute viral infection of the lower respiratory tract that affects approximately 50% of children during the first year of life and 100% by age 3 years. The occurrence of bronchiolitis peaks during the winter months and persists through early spring. Bronchiolitis remains the major reason for hospital admission during the first year of life. The incidence of bronchiolitis appears to be more common in males than in females.[31,32]

Respiratory syncytial virus (RSV) is the most common cause of bronchiolitis, accounting for up to 70% of all cases. During epidemic periods, the incidence of RSV-induced bronchiolitis can exceed 80% of cases. Parainfluenza viruses type 3 (10%–15%), type 1 (5%–10%), and type 2 (1%–5%) are the second most common pathogens, constituting as a group nearly 25% of cases. Bacteria serve as secondary pathogens in a minority of cases.[31,33]

CLINICAL PRESENTATION

A prodrome suggesting an upper respiratory tract infection, usually lasting from 2 to 8 days, precedes the onset of clinical symptoms (Table 111–6). As a result of limited oral intake because of coughing combined with fever, vomiting, and diarrhea, infants frequently are dehydrated. The increased work of breathing and tachypnea most

TABLE 111-6 Clinical Presentation of Bronchiolitis

Signs and symptoms
Prodrome with irritability, restlessness, and mild fever
Cough and coryza
Vomiting, diarrhea, noisy breathing, and increased respiratory rate as symptoms progress
Labored breathing with retractions of the chest wall, nasal flaring, and grunting
Physical examination
Tachycardia and respiratory rate of 40–80 per minute in hospitalized infants
Wheezing and inspiratory rales
Mild conjunctivitis in one third of patients
Otitis media in 5%–10% of patients
Laboratory tests
Peripheral white blood cell count normal or slightly elevated
Abnormal arterial blood gases (hypoxemia and, rarely, hypercarbia)

likely further increases fluid loss. In most cases, this clinical picture persists between 3 and 7 days. Although the hospital course of bronchiolitic children often is variable, substantial clinical improvement usually is observed within the first 2 days, with gradual improvement and complete resolution requiring 4 to 8 weeks.

The diagnosis of bronchiolitis is based primarily on history and clinical findings. It is important for the clinician to attempt to differentiate between bronchiolitis and a host of other clinical entities affecting infants, which may produce a similar picture of dyspnea and wheezing. Asthma, congestive heart failure, anatomic airway abnormalities, cystic fibrosis, foreign bodies, and gastroesophageal reflux are the primary disease entities that may present with wheezing on physical examination in children. Isolation of a viral pathogen in the respiratory secretions of a wheezing child establishes a presumptive diagnosis of infectious bronchiolitis. However, the ability to identify specific viral pathogens often is hindered by the limited availability of special virology laboratories. In addition, in the elderly and in immunocompromised patients, antigen detection lacks adequate sensitivity, and patients frequently seek medical care after the acute stage of the infection, thus compromising the ability of the available tests to diagnose RSV. However, the proliferation of commercial enzyme-linked immunosorbent assays and fluorescent antibody staining techniques of nasopharyngeal secretions has increased the ability to identify viral antigens within several hours.[31] Identification of RSV by polymerase chain reaction should be available routinely from most clinical laboratories, but its relevance to the clinical management of bronchiolitis remains obscure.

Multiple clinical laboratory determinations have been used to assist in the management of cases of bronchiolitis. Roentgenographic evaluation of the chest in children with bronchiolitis yields variable findings but may help to distinguish this illness from other entities characterized by wheezing. In children requiring hospitalization, abnormalities in blood gas tensions are frequent and appear to relate to disease severity. Hypoxemia is common and increases the respiratory drive, whereas hypercarbia is seen in only the most severe cases. Despite the presence of moderate degrees of hypoxemia, clinical cyanosis is unusual.

TREATMENT

Bronchiolitis

DESIRED OUTCOME

❼ In the well infant, bronchiolitis usually is a self-limiting illness, and reassurance and antipyretics usually are all that are necessary while waiting for resolution of the underlying viral infection. In-hospital support is necessary for the child suffering from respiratory failure or dehydration; underlying cardiac and pulmonary diseases potentiate these conditions.

GENERAL APPROACH TO TREATMENT

❼ Almost all otherwise healthy babies with bronchiolitis can be followed as outpatients. Such infants are treated for fever, provided generous amounts of oral fluids, and observed closely for evidence of respiratory deterioration.[34] In severely affected children, the mainstays of therapy for bronchiolitis are oxygen therapy and intravenous fluids. In a subset of patients, aerosolized bronchodilators may have a role. In selected infants, particularly those with underlying pulmonary disease, cardiac disease, or both, therapy with the antiviral agent ribavirin can be considered.[35]

PHARMACOLOGIC THERAPY

❼ Aerosolized β_2-adrenergic therapy appears to offer little benefit for the majority of patients and may even be detrimental.[33] However, this therapy may offer some benefit to the child with a predisposition toward bronchospasm. In addition, although clinical trials have demonstrated varied results, nebulized epinephrine seems to be more efficacious than salbutamol in hospitalized patients with bronchiolitis.[36,37] In such patients, bronchodilator therapy may be offered initially but should not be pursued in the absence of a clear-cut clinical benefit. Similarly, controlled trials of corticosteroids have failed to reveal any therapeutic benefit (or harmful effect) when administered to bronchiolitic infants.[33] As a result, the routine use of systemically administered corticosteroids is discouraged. Although placing children with bronchiolitis in mist tents has been common practice, no data have documented the effectiveness of this practice.

CLINICAL CONTROVERSY

Because bacteria are not primary pathogens in the etiology of bronchiolitis, antibiotics should not be administered routinely. Despite this, many clinicians frequently administer antibiotics while awaiting culture results because the clinical and radiographic findings in bronchiolitis often are suggestive of possible bacterial pneumonia.

Ribavirin may offer benefit to a subset of infants with bronchiolitis. Although ribavirin, a synthetic nucleoside, possesses in-vitro antiviral properties against a variety of RNA and DNA viruses, including influenza A, influenza B, parainfluenza, and adenovirus,[33] it is approved only in aerosolized form against RSV. Use of the drug requires special equipment (small-particle aerosol generator) and specially trained personnel for administration via oxygen hood or mist tent. Special care must be taken to avoid drug particle deposition and the resulting clogging of respiratory tubing and valves in mechanical ventilators.

Among hospital admissions for RSV infection, ribavirin therapy failed to decrease length of hospital stay, number of days in the intensive care unit, or number of days receiving mechanical ventilation. Consequently, the American Academy of Pediatrics has modified its recommendation for the use of ribavirin from "should be used" to "may be considered."[33] In light of this and because of the requirement for special aerosolization equipment and the cost of the drug itself, most experts recommend reserving use of ribavirin for severely ill patients, especially those with chronic lung disease (particularly bronchopulmonary dysplasia), congenital heart disease, prematurity, and immunodeficiency (especially severe combined immunodeficiency and human immunodeficiency virus [HIV] infection). Ribavirin also can be considered in otherwise healthy patients with severe distress because of RSV infection.

In infants with underlying pulmonary or cardiovascular disease, prophylaxis against RSV may be warranted. When administered monthly during the RSV season, both RSV immune globulin[38] and palivizumab[39,40] (a monoclonal antibody for RSV) may decrease the number of RSV episodes and the need for hospitalization. Between the two, palivizumab appears to be preferred, given its ease of administration, lack of administration-related adverse effects, and noninterference with select immunizations.

PNEUMONIA

EPIDEMIOLOGY

Pneumonia is the most common infectious cause of death in the United States, where approximately three million cases are diagnosed annually at a cost of more than $20 billion to the healthcare system.[41,42] Pneumonia occurs throughout the year, with the relative prevalence of disease resulting from different etiologic agents varying with the seasons. It occurs in persons of all ages, although the clinical manifestations are most severe in the very young, the elderly, and the chronically ill.

PATHOGENESIS

Microorganisms gain access to the lower respiratory tract by three routes. They may be inhaled as aerosolized particles, or they may enter the lung via the bloodstream from an extrapulmonary site of infection; however, aspiration of oropharyngeal contents, a common occurrence in both healthy and ill persons during sleep, is the major mechanism by which pulmonary pathogens gain access to the normally sterile lower airways and alveoli. When pulmonary defense mechanisms are functioning optimally, aspirated microorganisms are cleared from the region before infection can become established; however, aspiration of potential pathogens from the oropharynx can result in pneumonia if lung defenses are impaired.[1] Factors that promote aspiration, such as altered sensorium and neuromuscular disease, may result in an increase in the size of the inoculum delivered to the lower respiratory tract, thereby overwhelming local defense mechanisms. Lung infections with viruses suppress the antibacterial activity of the lung by impairing alveolar macrophage function and mucociliary clearance, thus setting the stage for secondary bacterial pneumonia. Mucociliary transport is also depressed by ethanol and narcotics and by obstruction of a bronchus by mucus, tumor, or extrinsic compression. All these factors can severely impair pulmonary clearance of aspirated bacteria.

❽ The most prominent pathogen causing community-acquired pneumonia in otherwise healthy adults is *S. pneumoniae* (pneumococcus) and accounts for up to 75% of all acute cases. Other common pathogens include *M. pneumoniae, Legionella, C. pneumoniae, H. influenzae,* and a variety of viruses including influenza.[41,42] Community-acquired pneumonias caused by *Staphylococcus aureus* and gram-negative rods are observed primarily in the elderly, especially those residing in nursing homes, and in association with alcoholism and other debilitating conditions. The term *atypical* may be applied to pneumonia to indicate that the pneumonia may be caused by an atypical pathogen. Although this older terminology is slowly fading, atypical pneumonia or atypical pathogens refers to pneumonia (e.g., bilateral lobar pneumonia with a negative Gram stain of sputum) caused by *M. pneumoniae, C. pneumoniae,* or *Legionella.*[43]

Gram-negative aerobic bacilli and *S. aureus* are the leading causative agents in hospital-acquired pneumonia.[44] Anaerobic bacteria are the most common etiologic agents in pneumonia that follows the gross aspiration of gastric or oropharyngeal contents.[45]

Pneumonia in infants and children is caused by a wider range of microorganisms, and, unlike the situation in adults, nonbacterial pathogens predominate. Most pneumonias occurring in the pediatric age group are caused by viruses, especially RSV, parainfluenza, and adenovirus.[33] *M. pneumoniae* is an important pathogen in older children. Beyond the neonatal period, pneumococcus is the major bacterial pathogen in childhood pneumonia, followed by group A *Streptococcus* and *S. aureus. H. influenzae* type b, once a major childhood pathogen, has become an infrequent cause of pneumonia since the introduction of active vaccination against this organism in the late 1980s.

CLINICAL PRESENTATION

Bacterial Pneumonia

Bacterial pneumonia is caused most commonly by gram-positive streptococci and staphylococci and gram-negative organisms that normally inhabit the gastrointestinal tract (enterics) and soil and water (nonenterics). In addition, *Legionella,* itself a weakly staining gram-negative nonenteric organism, accounts for a small percentage of community- and hospital-acquired bacterial pneumonia, although the true incidence may be underreported.[46] Finally, *Mycobacterium tuberculosis,* an acid-fast staining bacillus, has reemerged as an important cause of pneumonia in urban centers throughout the United States.[47]

A wide array of gram-positive and gram-negative organisms can cause pneumonia, but they usually present a similar clinical appearance (Table 111–7). Pneumococcus, *Staphylococcus,* the enteric gram-negative rods, and occasionally other organisms may produce local irritation or destruction of blood vessels leading to rust-colored sputum or hemoptysis. Pleural effusions, both sterile and empyematous, may be associated with many of these entities, as evidenced by distant breath sounds and a wide area of dulled percussion. The chest radiograph and sputum examination and culture are the most useful diagnostic tests for gram-positive and gram-negative bacterial pneumonia. Typically, the chest radiograph reveals a dense lobar or segmental infiltrate. However, patchy consolidation may be seen occasionally with virtually all these pathogens. Occasionally, pneumonia resulting from hematogenous spread of the organisms results in a diffuse, alveolar pattern on chest radiograph. Gram stain of the expectorated sputum demonstrates many polymorphonuclear cells per high-powered field in the presence of a predominant organism, which is reflected as heavy growth of a single species on culture. Other laboratory tests are less sensitive or specific. Blood cultures may be helpful in identifying the offending organism but are positive in only a minority of patients. The complete blood count usually reflects a leukocytosis with a predominance of polymorphonuclear cells; in some instances, particularly with pneumococcus, elevation of the white blood cell (WBC) count may be pronounced. Normal or

TABLE 111-7 Clinical Presentation of Pneumonia

Signs and symptoms
Abrupt onset of fever, chills, dyspnea, and productive cough
Rust-colored sputum or hemoptysis
Pleuritic chest pain
Physical examination
Tachypnea and tachycardia
Dullness to percussion
Increased tactile fremitus, whisper pectoriloquy, and egophony
Chest wall retractions and grunting respirations
Diminished breath sounds over affected area
Inspiratory crackles during lung expansion
Chest radiograph
Dense lobar or segmental infiltrate
Laboratory tests
Leukocytosis with predominance of polymorphonuclear cells
Low oxygen saturation on arterial blood gas or pulse oximetry

mildly elevated WBC counts, however, do not exclude bacterial pneumonic disease. The patient also may be hypoxic, as reflected by low oxygen saturation on arterial blood gas or pulse oximetry.

Although the clinical appearance of gram-positive and gram-negative pneumonias is similar, epidemiologic and clinical clues render one more likely than the other.

Gram-Positive Bacteria

8 Pneumococcus is the most common community-acquired bacterial pneumonia, accounting for up to 76% of cases.[42] It is particularly prevalent and severe in patients with splenic dysfunction, diabetes mellitus, chronic cardiopulmonary or renal disease, or HIV infection. *S. aureus* pneumonia occurs in both the community and hospital settings.[48] Community-acquired disease with *S. aureus* is identified most frequently in young infants, patients with early cystic fibrosis, and those recovering from an antecedent respiratory viral infection. *S. aureus* is a prominent cause of nosocomial pneumonia and may result from hematogenous spread from a distant source. In both settings, it is characteristically severe and accompanied by the formation of pneumatoceles (air-containing cavities within the lung). Group B *Streptococcus,* although rare in adults, is the most common cause of bacterial pneumonia among neonates, in whom it typically causes a clinical and radiographic picture nearly indistinguishable from hyaline membrane disease.[49] Group A *Streptococcus* is an uncommon cause of community-acquired pneumonia and frequently occurs after a viral respiratory tract infection. Only occasionally is it associated with streptococcal pharyngitis. The organism is pyogenic, and the presentation can be severe.

Enteric Gram-Negative Bacteria

Community-acquired enteric gram-negative pneumonia is identified most frequently among patients with chronic illness, especially alcoholism and diabetes mellitus. The enteric gram-negative bacteria are leading causes of nosocomial pneumonia because the upper respiratory tract becomes rapidly colonized with gram-negative organisms after hospitalization, particularly among critically ill patients and those receiving antibiotics.[50] Outbreaks of nosocomial disease may be caused occasionally by contaminated respiratory therapy equipment. *Klebsiella pneumoniae* is the most frequently encountered pathogen among the gram-negative enteric bacteria, although the relative prominence of these organisms varies among hospitals. The gram-negative bacilli are associated with high mortality, sometimes exceeding 50%; their potential to produce significant morbidity and mortality has been enhanced by the emergence of highly antibiotic-resistant organisms in some hospital settings.[51]

Nonenteric Gram-Negative Bacteria

The most prominent nonenteric gram-negative rods associated with pneumonia include *Pseudomonas, Haemophilus,* and *Moraxella.* Like the enteric gram-negative organisms, *P. aeruginosa* is a frequent cause of hospital-acquired pneumonia and is particularly prominent among neutropenic and burn patients.[51] In addition, cystic fibrosis patients suffer from chronic, multilobar infections with *P. aeruginosa* as well as other *Pseudomonas* species; these infections are punctuated with acute exacerbations.[52] *H. influenzae* type b historically has been a prominent pathogen in childhood pneumonia. However, the incidence of all invasive disease due to this organism in the pediatric age group has dropped dramatically since the introduction of the conjugated *Haemophilus* vaccines in the late 1980s. However, two different clinical presentations of *H. influenzae* pneumonia still are seen in adults. The most common by far is the bronchopneumonia form, which develops most frequently in patients with underlying chronic lung disease and is believed to represent, in most patients, an exacerbation of chronic bronchitis. In the second form of *H. influenzae* pneumonia, segmental or lobar involvement predominates. The course of this illness is more acute, with sudden onset of cough, fever, and pleuritic chest pain. Finally, *M. catarrhalis,* an important cause of otitis media and sinusitis, is an increasingly important cause of lower respiratory tract infections in immunoincompetent and hospitalized patients.

Legionella pneumophila

Of the several *Legionella* species known to cause pneumonia in humans, *Legionella pneumophila* is by far the most important, accounting for 2% to 15% of all community-acquired pneumonias in North America and Europe.[46] *Legionella* is a water and soil organism and most probably is transmitted by inhalation of aerosols containing the organism or by microaspiration of contaminated water. Outbreaks of illness caused by *L. pneumophila* have been linked to excavation sites and to contaminated water from air conditioners and showers. Person-to-person transmission has not been demonstrated. In addition to epidemics, *L. pneumophila* causes sporadic illness that peaks in summer and fall. Individuals who are male, middle-aged or older, immunocompromised, chronic bronchitics, or cigarette smokers are at increased risk.

Infection with *L. pneumophila* is characterized by multisystem involvement, including rapidly progressive pneumonia. It has a gradual onset, with prominent constitutional symptoms (e.g., malaise, lethargy, weakness, anorexia) occurring early in the course of the illness. A dry, nonproductive cough is present initially and becomes productive of mucoid or purulent sputum over several days. Fevers exceeding 40°C (104°F) develop in more than half of patients, typically are unremitting, and are associated with a relative bradycardia. Pleuritic chest pain and progressive dyspnea may be seen. Extrapulmonary symptoms, particularly diarrhea, nausea, and vomiting, remain evident throughout the course of the illness. Myalgias and arthralgias also occur. Substantial changes in the patient's mental status, often out of proportion to the degree of fever, are seen in approximately one fourth of patients. Obtundation, hallucinations, grand mal seizures, and focal neurologic findings are also associated with this illness. Chest roentgenograms initially reveal patchy alveolar infiltrates that may be bilateral. Progression to lobar or multilobar consolidation is frequent, as are small pleural effusions.

Laboratory findings include leukocytosis with a predominance of mature and immature granulocytes in 50% to 75% of patients. Urinalysis may reveal proteinuria, hematuria, and casts; liver function tests may be abnormal. Hyponatremia and hypophosphatemia have been reported frequently. Because *L. pneumophila* stains poorly with commonly used stains, routine microscopic examination of sputum is of little diagnostic value. Although it exhibits slow growth and has highly selective growth requirements, *L. pneumophila* has been isolated successfully from tissue using a specialized medium. Direct fluorescent antibody examination of respiratory tract secretions, lung tissue, or pleural fluid is the most rapid means of establishing the diagnosis. The sensitivity of this method approaches 70% for sputum and 90% for lung tissue, and diagnostic specificity is high for both. Commercially available urine antigen tests have been developed for *L. pneumophila.* These tests are 70% sensitive and remain positive for weeks, even after effective antibiotics have been started. Because these diagnostic tests are unavailable in many clinical laboratories, the diagnosis of Legionnaires' disease often is presumptive and based on a suggestive clinical presentation.

Anaerobic Pneumonia

8 Anaerobic pneumonitis is most likely to occur in individuals predisposed to aspiration by impaired consciousness and may be

more prevalent in those with periodontal disease or dysphagia. Bronchogenic carcinoma is an associated underlying condition. A variety of gram-positive and gram-negative anaerobic bacteria indigenous to the upper airway may cause pneumonitis when large quantities of oropharyngeal secretions are aspirated into the lower airways. The organisms most frequently implicated are *Peptostreptococcus* species, *Fusobacteria, Bacteroides melaninogenicus, Bacteroides fragilis,* and *Peptococcus* species; polymicrobial infections with anaerobes and aerobes, such as *S. aureus, S. pneumoniae,* and gram-negative bacilli, are common.[45]

The course of illness typically is indolent, with cough, low-grade fever, and weight loss, although an acute presentation may occur. Rigors are notably absent, and bacteremia is rare. Putrid sputum, when present, is highly suggestive of the diagnosis. Chest radiographs reveal infiltrates typically located in dependent lung segments, and lung abscesses develop in 20% of patients 1 to 2 weeks into the course of the illness.

Tuberculosis

The acid-fast bacillus *M. tuberculosis* causes tuberculosis. After years of steady decline, the number of cases of pneumonia caused by *M. tuberculosis* in the United States began to increase in the middle to late 1980s. The new epidemic was a consequence of an increased incidence among prison inmates, intravenous drug abusers, immigrants, and, most prominently, HIV-infected patients.[53] It is most prominent in urban neighborhoods afflicted with crowded conditions and poor access to healthcare. Unlike previous eras in which tuberculosis was seen most frequently in elderly men, infection currently is identified in increasing numbers of young minority adults. As mentioned, the resurgence of tuberculosis is at least partially related to coinfection with HIV; HIV-infected patients are more likely to develop symptomatic disease with its associated fits of coughing than are their immunocompetent counterparts, and this enables further spread of infection. Other groups prone to tuberculosis include the homeless and patients in chronic care facilities and homes for the elderly. Fortunately, since 1992, the incidence of tuberculosis in the United States has declined, reaching a record low. However, the incidence of tuberculosis worldwide continues to increase. Both the sustained worldwide increase in tuberculosis and the reemergence of tuberculosis in the United States are important reasons for the development of multiple-drug resistance, that is, mycobacteria that are resistant to two or more of the first-line antituberculosis drugs. Infection caused by these organisms is poorly responsive to alternative therapy and is associated with mortality rates exceeding 50% (see Chap. 116).

Tuberculosis is spread from person to person by inhalation of droplet nuclei generated by vigorous coughing. Most patients who become infected with *M. tuberculosis* remain asymptomatic despite lifelong infection and have a normal chest radiograph. Infection in these patients is detected only through routine skin testing. Less frequently, particularly in those with poor immunity, the infection cannot be contained by local macrophages, and the tuberculous burden grows sufficiently to cause clinical manifestations.

Adult disease (from adolescence onward) begins with constitutional complaints, followed by a prominent chronic, troublesome cough productive of mucopurulent material. The infection initially appears in the lung apices with little or no hilar adenopathy and, in advanced disease, results in lung necrosis, producing a cavity containing enormous numbers of organisms. With sufficient cough, the cavitary contents are mobilized and aspirated into other areas of the lung, where additional cavities may be formed.

In contrast, pediatric tuberculosis commonly is associated with little cough even in the presence of extensive pulmonary infection. Instead, the child presents with a subacute course of poor appetite, weight loss, lethargy, fever, and sweats. Chest radiograph reveals a widened mediastinum representing enlarged hilar lymph nodes reacting to the tuberculin inoculum. In progressive cases, the nodes impinge on or erode through a large bronchus, resulting in a dense consolidation of the segment distal to the lesion. Cavitary disease is uncommon.

Nonbacterial Pneumonia

Viruses, *Mycoplasma* species, *Chlamydia* species, and fungi are recognized causes of pneumonia syndromes in all age groups. The designation *atypical pneumonia,* distinct from the typical bacterial pneumonia seen most commonly in adults, has been used to describe the illness caused by many of these agents.[54]

Mycoplasma Pneumonia

Taxonomically, the mycoplasmas are included in their own class labeled Mollicutes. Although their small size and filterability are similar to viruses, the structure of their ribosomal RNA indicates that they have evolved from bacteria, and, unlike any virus, they contain cytoplasm and can replicate in an extracellular environment. They are distinguished from eubacteria by their low genetic content. In addition, the mycoplasmas lack a cell wall and are surrounded instead by a lipid membrane.[55]

M. pneumoniae causes human disease throughout the year, with a slightly increased incidence in fall and early winter. During the summer months when other causes of pneumonia are less common, *M. pneumoniae* is responsible for a greater proportion of cases. Both infection and disease from *M. pneumoniae* are common, with two thirds of children ages 2 to 5 years and 97% of persons older than 17 years having detectable serum antibody to the organism. Overall, *M. pneumoniae* is responsible for approximately 20% of pneumonia cases, although in enclosed populations, such as military recruits and college dormitory residents, it may cause more than 50%. Infection is spread by close person-to-person contact, and the incubation period is 2 to 3 weeks. *M. pneumoniae* infections are unusual in children younger than 5 years and show a peak incidence in older children and young adults. Only 3% to 10% of persons infected with *M. pneumoniae* develop pneumonia, with the majority of respiratory tract involvement manifested as pharyngitis and tracheobronchitis. Asymptomatic infection is common.

M. pneumoniae presents with a gradual onset of fever, headache, and malaise, with the appearance 3 to 5 days after the onset of illness of a persistent, hacking cough that initially is nonproductive. Sore throat, ear pain, and rhinorrhea often are present. Chills are seen only occasionally, and pleuritic pain is uncommon. Lung findings generally are limited to rales and rhonchi; findings of consolidation are rare. Nonpulmonary manifestations are extremely common and include nausea, vomiting, diarrhea, myalgias, arthralgias, polyarticular arthritis, skin rashes, myocarditis and pericarditis, hemolytic anemia, meningoencephalitis, cranial neuropathies, and Guillain-Barré syndrome. Systemic symptoms generally clear in 1 to 2 weeks, whereas respiratory symptoms may persist for up to 4 weeks. Although the course of mycoplasmal pneumonia usually is benign and self-limited, severe respiratory disease may develop in patients with sickle cell disease, agammaglobulinemia, and COPD.[55]

Radiographic findings generally are more impressive than the patient's physical findings and include patchy or interstitial infiltrates, which are seen most commonly in the lower lobes. Small unilateral, transient pleural effusions are common, but large effusions and empyema are rare. Roentgenographic abnormalities resolve slowly, and 4 to 6 weeks may be required for complete resolution.

Sputum Gram stain may reveal mononuclear or polymorphonuclear leukocytes, with no predominant organism. Although *M. pneumoniae* can be cultured from respiratory secretions using specialized medium, its growth is slow, and 2 to 3 weeks may be necessary for culture identification. Indirect evidence of infection by *M. pneumoniae* is the presence of elevated levels of serum cold hemagglutinins. These immunoglobulin M antibodies develop in approximately half of patients with mycoplasmal pneumonia and can be elevated in other illnesses, especially viral infection. A definitive diagnosis also can be made by demonstrating a fourfold or greater rise in serum antibodies to *M. pneumoniae.* However, because this test also requires 2 to 4 weeks for results, the diagnosis of mycoplasmal pneumonia during the acute phase of the illness must be based on the characteristic history, appropriate clinical setting, and typical physical findings.

Chlamydia Pneumonia

C. pneumoniae, formally designated the *TWAR agent,* after the laboratory designations for the first two isolates, is a relatively recently identified pathogen antigenically similar to *Chlamydia psittaci. C. pneumoniae* infection is ubiquitous worldwide, but only a small percentage of infections result in clinically apparent pneumonia. Conversely, approximately 5% to 15% of pneumonia is associated with this pathogen.[56] Primary-infection *Chlamydia* pneumonia typically occurs in young adults and is characterized by mild respiratory symptoms with a gradual onset. Constitutional manifestations, particularly fever and headache, are common. The radiographic findings are nonspecific and usually consist of multilobular interstitial infiltrates. Immunity is incomplete, and reinfection with *C. pneumoniae* is common, particularly among the elderly. Definitive diagnosis of *C. pneumoniae*–associated pneumonia depends on identification of the organism in sputum. Culture of this organism is difficult, and commercially available antigen detection systems are insensitive.

Viral Pneumonia

Viruses are an uncommon cause of pneumonia in adults, except in the immunosuppressed.[3] Influenza virus, usually type A, is the most common cause of pneumonia in the adult civilian population[56]; adenoviruses cause most cases in military trainees. In contrast, viruses are by far the most common agents producing pneumonia in infants and young children, with RSV, parainfluenza, and adenovirus producing most cases.[31]

All viral respiratory tract infections occur more commonly in the winter, and rapid person-to-person spread through susceptible populations is typical. Underlying cardiac or pulmonary disease predisposes to an increased incidence and severity of viral lower respiratory tract infection, especially with influenza virus in adults and RSV in children. Radiographic findings are nonspecific and include bronchial wall thickening and perihilar and diffuse interstitial infiltrates. Pleural effusions may be seen, especially in adenovirus and parainfluenza pneumonia.

The clinical pictures produced by respiratory viruses are sufficiently variable and overlap to such a degree that an etiologic diagnosis cannot be made confidently based on clinical grounds alone. Although virus isolation in tissue culture is possible, a period of 7 or more days often is required for virus identification; thus, this method usually cannot be used for definitive diagnosis during the acute phase of illness. Serologic tests for virus-specific antibodies are used often in the diagnosis of viral infections. The diagnostic fourfold rise in titer between acute and convalescent phase sera may require 2 to 3 weeks to develop. Same-day diagnosis of viral infections now is possible through the use of indirect immunofluorescence tests on exfoliated cells from the respiratory tract. The immunofluorescence technique frequently uses a battery of monoclonal antibodies, including those against influenza A and B, RSV, parainfluenza, and adenovirus, to provide rapid diagnosis of a range of viral infections.[3]

PNEUMONIA IN SPECIAL CLINICAL CIRCUMSTANCES

Pneumonia in the HIV-Infected Patient

HIV infects and destroys helper T lymphocytes bearing the CD4 surface molecule; these cells are critical for orchestrating a wide variety of immunologic responses. Their depletion consequently results in dysfunction of both cell-mediated and humoral immunity. As a result, a broad range of pathogens can cause pneumonia in HIV infection (Table 111–8).[57–59] The HIV-infected patient may be afflicted with pneumonia multiple times in his or her lifetime, particularly in the advanced stages of the disease, and a given episode may be caused by more than one species.

The clinical presentation of pneumonia in HIV-infected persons frequently is not helpful in distinguishing one pathogen from another. The pneumonia usually is subacute in onset and consists of fever, nonproductive cough, and dyspnea. Radiographically, most of these entities produce a multilobular or diffuse pattern. Some practitioners initially treat the HIV-infected patient with pneumonia empirically, covering the most common entities (bacteria and *Pneumocystis carinii*). However, given the wide array of possible pathogens, more frequently a specific microbiologic diagnosis is aggressively pursued early in the patient's course through sputum induction or bronchoalveolar lavage to allow a rational choice of an antimicrobial regimen. The diagnosis and treatment of HIV-infected patients with pulmonary disease is discussed in detail in Chap. 129.

Pneumonia in the Neutropenic Host

Neutropenia in the cancer patient is a common complication of aggressive chemotherapy but occasionally results from the cancer itself. The risk of infection in the cytopenic patient is increased significantly

TABLE 111-8 Pulmonary Complications of Human Immunodeficiency Virus Infection

Infections
Viruses
Cytomegalovirus
Herpes simplex virus
Varicella-zoster virus
Respiratory syncytial virus and other common respiratory pathogens (parainfluenza virus, adenovirus)
Measles virus
Bacteria
Pyogenic organisms (especially *Streptococcus pneumoniae, Haemophilus influenzae*; in late disease, *Staphylococcus aureus* and gram-negative organisms)
Mycobacterium tuberculosis
Mycobacterium avium complex and other nontuberculous mycobacteria
Fungi
Histoplasma capsulatum
Coccidioides immitis
Cryptococcus neoformans
Candida species
Aspergillus species
Parasites
Pneumocystis carinii
Toxoplasma gondii
Cryptosporidia
Strongyloides stercoralis
Malignancies
Kaposi sarcoma
Non-Hodgkin's lymphoma
Smooth muscle tumors
Lymphocytic interstitial pneumonitis
Nonspecific interstitial pneumonitis
Drug-induced pneumonitis

From Viscoli et al.[61]

when the absolute neutrophil count falls below 500 cells/mm^3 and the neutropenia persists for more than 7 days.[60–62] In many patients, the duration of chemotherapy-induced cytopenia can be reduced by judicious application of colony-stimulating factors.[63,64]

The organisms that cause pneumonia in the cytopenic cancer patient include a broad range of bacteria and fungi.[60] The most prominent among these are gram-positive bacteria (staphylococci and streptococci); others include enteric and nonenteric (particularly *Pseudomonas*) gram-negative rods as well as the fungi (*Candida, Aspergillus*). The chest radiograph may reveal the lobar pattern typical of bacterial infection in the normal host, or it may exhibit a diffuse pattern. Sometimes the pneumonia remains invisible by chest radiograph until the neutropenia resolves. Noninfectious entities that may cause pulmonary symptoms include toxicity from radiation or chemotherapy or infiltration of the lung parenchyma by the tumor itself.

Nosocomial Pneumonia

After the urinary tract and the bloodstream, the lungs are the most frequent site of infection acquired in the hospital. Nosocomial pneumonia is seen most commonly in critically ill patients.[65,66] Factors that predispose patients to the development of nosocomial pneumonia include the severity of illness, duration of hospitalization, supine positioning, witnessed aspiration, coma, acute respiratory distress syndrome, patient transport, and prior antibiotic exposure.[67] The strongest predisposing factor, however, is mechanical ventilation (intubation), which bypasses the natural airway defenses against the migration of upper respiratory tract organisms into the lower tract. This situation is exacerbated by the wide use of H_2-receptor blocking agents in the intensive care unit, which increases the pH of gastric secretions and may promote the proliferation of microorganisms in the upper gastrointestinal tract. Subclinical microaspirations are events that occur routinely in intubated patients and result in the inoculation of bacteria-contaminated gastric contents into the lung and a higher incidence of nosocomial pneumonia. Ventilator-associated pneumonia can be diagnosed accurately by any one of multiple standard criteria, including histopathologic examination of lung tissue obtained by open-lung biopsy, rapid cavitation of a pulmonary infiltrate in the absence of cancer or tuberculosis, positive pleural fluid culture, and same species with an identical antibiogram for a pathogen(s) isolated from blood and respiratory secretions without another identifiable source of bacteremia.[8]

The organisms most commonly associated with nosocomial pneumonia are *S. aureus* and enteric (e.g., *Klebsiella* or *E. coli*) and nonenteric (e.g., *Pseudomonas*) gram-negative bacilli, organisms that colonize the pharynx of the hospitalized, critically ill patient. The diagnosis of nosocomial pneumonia usually is established by the presence of a new infiltrate on chest radiograph, fever, worsening respiratory status, and the appearance of thick, neutrophil-laden respiratory secretions. In actuality, the diagnosis often is difficult to make in the intensively ill patient with underlying lung pathology that itself can be associated with an abnormal changing radiograph, as occurs with congestive heart failure or chronic lung disease. Broad-spectrum antibiotics frequently are started empirically even in equivocal circumstances, with bronchoscopy reserved for poorly responsive patients.[51]

Severe Acute Respiratory Syndrome

In November 2002, an extremely contagious atypical pneumonia manifested in China that since has been termed *severe acute respiratory syndrome* (SARS).[68] The etiology of SARS is an enveloped RNA virus, a coronavirus, referred to as SARS-CoV. The virus is transmitted primarily via large-droplet spread; however, surface contamination and airborne and fecal spread are possible. Signs and symptoms associated with SARS include high fever, myalgias, headache, diarrhea, and a dry nonproductive cough. Respiratory symptoms may progress to shortness of breath and hypoxemia, necessitating the need for intubation and mechanical ventilation. Diagnostic tests for patients suspected of contracting SARS should include chest x-ray film, blood cultures, sputum cultures and Gram stain, pulse oximetry, and identification of other potential pathogens, including influenza A and B, *Legionella,* and RSV. For unclear reasons, SARS appears to be less severe in pediatric patients.

Avian Influenza (Bird Flu)

All influenza viruses may be present in aquatic birds, with the H5N1 subtype being extremely pathogenic and fatal to fowl.[69,70] The first known cases of humans infected with this subtype occurred in Hong Kong in 1997, with six deaths among 18 infected patients. Signs and symptoms typical of the H5N1 virus are those common to other subtypes and include conjunctivitis, fever, rhinitis, and pharyngitis. However, pneumonia, respiratory distress syndrome, lymphopenia, and clotting abnormalities tend to occur rapidly in patients infected with this highly virulent subtype. Laboratory tests used to detect the H5N1 virus include immunoassays and reverse-transcription polymerase chain reactions.

TREATMENT

Pneumonia

■ DESIRED OUTCOME

Eradication of the offending organism through selection of the appropriate antibiotic and complete clinical cure are the goals of therapy for bacterial pneumonia. Therapy should minimize associated morbidity, including one or both of the following: reversible or irreversible disease and drug-induced organ toxicity (e.g., renal, lung, or hepatic dysfunction). Most cases of viral pneumonia are self-limiting, although therapy of influenza pneumonia with specific antiviral agents (amantadine or rimantadine) may hasten recovery. All efforts should focus on the design of the most cost-effective approach to therapy. Whenever possible, the oral (versus parenteral) route for drug administration should be selected, encouraging outpatient management rather than hospitalization.

■ GENERAL APPROACH TO TREATMENT

❾ The first priority in assessing the patient with pneumonia is to evaluate the adequacy of respiratory function and to determine the presence of signs of systemic illness, specifically dehydration or sepsis with resulting circulatory collapse. Oxygen or, in severe cases, mechanical ventilation and fluid resuscitation should be provided as necessary. Further supportive care of the patient with pneumonia includes humidified oxygen for hypoxemia, administration of bronchodilators (albuterol) when bronchospasm is present, and chest physiotherapy with postural drainage if evidence of retained secretions is seen. Additional therapeutic adjuncts include adequate hydration (intravenously if necessary), optimal nutritional support, and control of fever. Appropriate sputum samples may be obtained to determine the microbiologic etiology. Rehydration should be provided to replace losses that may have occurred as a result of fever, poor intake, and/or associated vomiting. Selection of an appropriate antimicrobial must be made based on the patient's probable or documented microbiology, distribution in the respiratory tract, side effects, and cost.

■ PHARMACOLOGIC THERAPY

Antibiotic Concentrations

Antibiotic concentrations in respiratory secretions in excess of the pathogen MIC are necessary for successful treatment of pulmonary infections.[71] The concept of a blood–bronchus barrier, analogous but dissimilar to the blood–brain barrier, has been used to assess the characteristics of drug penetration into pulmonary secretions. The ability of a drug to penetrate respiratory secretions depends on multiple physicochemical factors, including molecular size, lipid solubility, and degree of ionization at serum and biologic fluid pH and extent of protein binding. Studies performed in animals and cystic fibrosis patients suggest that larger molecular size favors the accumulation of drugs in bronchial secretions. This finding contrasts with data on drug penetration of other physiologic compartments, such as the cerebrospinal fluid, and may be a result of the trapping of lower-molecular-weight compounds in mucin pores. Nevertheless, the rate at which a drug may accumulate in certain respiratory secretions appears to remain an important factor relative to the drug's clinical efficacy in treating pulmonary infections. The un-ionized form of a drug and lipid solubility also appear to favor drug penetration. Of note, the pH of the infected bronchi often is more acidic than that of normal tissue and blood.

Fewer data are available for assessing the influence of drug protein binding on the rate and amount of respiratory secretion penetration. Clearly, it is the free antibiotic fraction reaching the infected site capable of binding to the bacterial cell target that is responsible for antibacterial activity. Given that the degree of protein binding influences a drug's ability to traverse membranes, a similar relationship would be expected within the lung. However, focusing on the absolute amount of an antibiotic bound to plasma/tissue proteins without accounting for the drug's overall antibacterial potency is errant. To completely assess an antibiotic's therapeutic potential in the treatment of pneumonia or any infectious process, it is prudent to assess the antibiotic's integrated pharmacokinetic–pharmacodynamic characteristics (e.g., bacterial killing may be concentration dependent or time dependent) that account for the drug's degree of binding to serum proteins, tissue distribution, and in-vitro potency. Thus, simply focusing on a drug's degree of protein binding is an errant, overly simplistic approach that does not account for the drug's inherent antibacterial activity or distribution characteristics.

These concepts relating to antibiotic activity and overall drug penetration of respiratory secretions have supported the clinical practice of administering certain antibiotics (aminoglycosides) to achieve high peak serum concentrations on the assumption that higher (and possibly more effective) biologic fluid concentrations of the drug will be achieved. The aminoglycosides are large polar molecules that diffuse poorly into tissue and respiratory secretions; however, with increasing concentrations obtained with once-daily dosing, increased target-tissue concentrations would be expected with increasing individual doses. Substantial clinical experience supports this practice for treating pulmonary infections with certain antibiotics (e.g., concentration-dependent antimicrobials), although more data are needed to describe the relationships between these variables and clinical response.

CLINICAL CONTROVERSY

Prior to the availability of newer β-lactam and fluoroquinolone antibiotics possessing consistently potent activity against multiple gram-negative pathogens, some investigators promoted the administration of antibiotics by direct endotracheal instillation. This method of drug administration attempts to provide increased topical concentrations of antibiotics that do not appear to penetrate respiratory secretions effectively while reducing the likelihood of systemic toxicity. In addition, greater local concentrations of antibiotics, particularly of the polymyxins and aminoglycosides, are believed to overcome partially the substantial decrease in antibiotic bioactivity observed when these agents interact with the purulent material present in infectious foci. Despite these potential theoretical advantages, the role of antibiotic aerosols or direct endotracheal instillation in clinical practice remains controversial.[71]

Sputum is frequently assessed as possibly representing the pharmacodynamic interface for pulmonary infections. Sputum is only one of many pulmonary fluids and secretions, and it may serve as a reservoir for pathogen growth. These beliefs have led many investigators to assess antibiotic concentrations in sputum, frequently describing sputum drug concentrations as a ratio of serum to sputum drug concentration. Although sputum drug concentrations provide some insight into the characteristics of drug penetration of respiratory secretions, caution should be exercised in the interpretation of these data. Data describing sputum drug concentrations often are difficult to interpret because of differences in analytic techniques, method of sputum sampling, and random nature of sampling times relative to drug dose. Moreover, representation of sputum drug concentrations as a ratio of serum drug concentration can be misleading and most probably should be described relative to absolute drug concentration or apparent area under the drug concentration versus time curve in sputum. To more accurately describe the distribution characteristics of antimicrobial agents in sputum, research studies should be designed to allow sequential repeated sputum sampling over a dosage interval under both first-dose and steady-state conditions. Thus, until greater sophistication is achieved in our understanding of the relationships between antibiotic concentrations in specific anatomic sites, plasma (blood)-based integrated pharmacokinetic–pharmacodynamic correlates should be used for antibiotic and dose selection.

Selection of Antimicrobial Agents

Treatment of bacterial pneumonia, like the treatment of most infectious diseases, initially involves the empirical use of a relatively broad-spectrum antibiotic that is effective against probable pathogens after appropriate cultures and specimens for laboratory evaluation have been obtained.[56] Therapy should be narrowed to cover specific pathogens after the results of cultures are known. Multiple factors that help to define the potential pathogens involved include patient age, previous and current medication history, underlying disease(s), major organ function, and present clinical status. These factors must be evaluated to select an appropriate and effective empirical antibiotic regimen as well as the most appropriate route for drug administration (oral or parenteral). For a more detailed discussion on the principles of antibiotic selection, see Chap. 109.

Numerous antibiotics are available, and the majority are effective in the treatment of bacterial pneumonia. Superiority of one antibiotic over another when both demonstrate similar in-vitro activity and tissue distribution characteristics is difficult to define. Our opinions on appropriate empirical choices for the treatment of bacterial pneumonias relative to a patient's underlying disease are listed in Table 111–9 for adults and Table 111–10 for children. A complete listing of antimicrobial agents for specific pathogens is beyond the scope of this chapter and is presented in Chap. 108.

Table 111–11 lists dosages for the treatment of bacterial pneumonia. The list of commercially available antimicrobial agents with documented bacterial and clinical effectiveness in the treatment of pneumonia appears endless. The large number of expensive drugs mandates critical evaluation for formulary selection and clinical use. Similarities of in-vitro activity, resistance to bacterial-inactivating enzymes, and overall effectiveness often make rational therapeutic decisions difficult and even appear random. However, some general principles can be applied to guide rational antibiotic choice, including direct comparison of the antibiotic's likely attainment of the defined pharmacokinetic–pharmacodynamic target correlate for specific bacterial species within the infected site. For treatment of bacterial pneumonia with concentration-independent antimicrobials (e.g., β-lactams and carbapenems), a plasma drug concentration exceeding the pathogen MIC for more than 50% of the dosing interval correlates with bacteriologic cure. For concentration-depen-

TABLE 111-9 Empirical Antimicrobial Therapy for Pneumonia in Adults[a]

Clinical Setting	Usual Pathogen(s)	Presumptive Therapy
Previously healthy, ambulatory patient	Pneumococcus, *Mycoplasma pneumoniae*	Macrolide/azalide,[b] tetracycline[c]
Elderly	Pneumococcus, gram-negative bacilli (e.g., *Klebsiella pneumoniae*); *Staphylococcus aureus, Haemophilus influenzae*	Piperacillin–tazobactam, cephalosporin,[d] carbapenem[e]
Chronic bronchitis	Pneumococcus, *H. influenzae, M. catarrhalis*	Amoxicillin, tetracycline,[c] trimethoprim–sulfamethoxazole, cefuroxime, amoxicillin–clavulanate, macrolide/azalide,[b] fluoroquinolone
Alcoholism	Pneumococcus, *K. pneumoniae, S. aureus, H. influenzae*, possibly mouth anaerobes	Ticarcillin–clavulanate, piperacillin–tazobactam, plus aminoglycoside; carbapenem,[e] fluoroquinolone[f]
Aspiration		
Community	Mouth anaerobes	Penicillin or clindamycin
Hospital/residential care	Mouth anaerobes, *S. aureus*, gram-negative enterics	Clindamycin, ticarcillin–clavulanate, piperacillin–tazobactam, plus aminoglycoside
Nosocomial pneumonia	Gram-negative bacilli (e.g., *K. pneumoniae, Enterobacter* species, *Pseudomonas aeruginosa*), *S. aureus*	Piperacillin-tazobactam, carbapenem,[e] or extended spectrum cephalosporin[g] plus aminoglycoside; fluoroquinolone[f]

[a]See section on treatment of bacterial pneumonia.
[b]Macrolide/azalide: erythromycin, clarithromycin, azithromycin.
[c]Tetracycline: tetracycline HCl, doxycycline.
[d]Cephalosporin: cefuroxime, ceftriaxone, cefotaxime.
[e]Carbapenem: imipenem-cilastatin, meropenem.
[f]Fluoroquinolone: ciprofloxacin, gatifloxacin, or levofloxacin.
[g]Extended-spectrum cephalosporin: ceftazidime, cefepime.

dent antimicrobials (e.g., aminoglycosides and fluoroquinolones), a peak drug concentration to pathogen MIC ratio >8 to 10 or ratio of pathogen MIC to antibiotic area under the curve >25 to 40 for gram-positive pathogens and >100 for gram-negative pathogens correlates with bacteriologic cure. An understanding and application of these inherent drug characteristics appears to be of the utmost importance for the selection of an optimal therapeutic regimen. Thus, whenever possible, identification of the causative pathogen and expected/defined antibiotic activity (e.g., MIC) is of paramount importance to the selection/design of the optimal antibiotic regimen.

Community-Acquired Pneumonia

Tables 111–12 and 111–13 provide evidence-based guidelines for the treatment of community-acquired pneumonia.[72] The bacterial causes are relatively constant, even across geographic areas and patient populations. Unfortunately, pathogen resistance to standard antimicrobials is increasing (e.g., penicillin-resistant pneumococci), necessitating careful attention by the clinician to local and regional bacterial susceptibility patterns.[73] Thus, whenever possible, initial therapy should be based on presumed antibacterial susceptibility and consist of older, less-expensive agents, with newer and more

TABLE 111-10 Empirical Antimicrobial Therapy for Pneumonia in Pediatric Patients[a]

Age	Usual Pathogen(s)	Presumptive Therapy
1 month	Group B streptococcus, *Haemophilus influenzae* (nontypeable), *Escherichia coli, Staphylococcus aureus, Listeria*, CMV, RSV, adenovirus	Ampicillin–sulbactam, cephalosporin[b] carbapenem[c] Ribavirin for RSV
1–3 months	*Chlamydia*, possibly *Ureaplasma*, CMV, *Pneumocystis carinii* (afebrile pneumonia syndrome)	Macrolide/azalide,[d] trimethoprim-sulfamethoxazole
	RSV	Ribavirin
	Pneumococcus, *S. aureus*	Semisynthetic penicillin[e] or cephalosporin[f]
3 months–6 years	Pneumococcus, *H. influenzae*, RSV, adenovirus, parainfluenza	Amoxicillin or cephalosporin[f] Ampicillin–sulbactam, amoxicillin–clavulanate Ribavirin for RSV
>6 years	Pneumococcus, *Mycoplasma pneumoniae*, adenovirus	Macrolide/azalide[d] cephalosporin,[f] amoxicillin–clavulanate

CMV, cytomegalovirus; RSV, respiratory syncytial virus.
[a]See section on treatment of bacterial pneumonia.
[b]Third-generation cephalosporin: ceftriaxone, cefotaxime, cefepime. Note that cephalosporins are not active against *Listeria*.
[c]Carbapenem: imipenem–cilastatin, meropenem.
[d]Macrolide/azalide: erythromycin, clarithromycin/azithromycin.
[e]Semisynthetic penicillin: nafcillin, oxacillin.
[f]Second-generation cephalosporin: cefuroxime, cefprozil.
See text for details regarding ribavirin treatment for RSV infection.

TABLE 111-11 Antibiotic Doses for Treatment of Bacterial Pneumonia

		Daily Antibiotic Dose	
Antibiotic Class	Antibiotic	*Pediatric (mg/kg/day)*	*Adult (total dose/day)*
Macrolide	Clarithromycin	15	0.5–1 g
	Erythromycin	30–50	1–2 g
Azalide	Azithromycin	10 mg/kg × 1 day, then 5 mg/kg/day × 4 days	500 mg day 1, then 250 mg/day × 4 days
Tetracycline[a]	Tetracycline HCl	25–50	1–2 g
	Oxytetracycline	15–25	0.25–0.3 g
Penicillin	Ampicillin	100–200	2–6 g
	Amoxicillin/amoxicillin–clavulanate[b]	40–90	0.75–1 g
	Piperacillin–tazobactam	200–300	12 g
	Ampicillin–sulbactam	100–200	4–8 g
Extended-spectrum cephalosporins	Ceftriaxone	50–75	1–2 g
	Ceftazidime	150	2–6 g
	Cefepime	100–150	2–4 g
Fluoroquinolones	Gatifloxacin[c]	10–20	0.4 g
	Levofloxacin	10–15	0.5–0.75 g
	Ciprofloxacin	20–30	0.5–1.5 g
Aminoglycosides	Gentamicin	7.5	3–6 mg/kg
	Tobramycin	7.5	3–6 mg/kg

Doses can be increased for more severe disease and may require modification in patients with organ dysfunction.
[a]Tetracyclines are rarely used in pediatric patients, particularly in those younger than 8 years because of tetracycline-induced permanent tooth discoloration.
[b]Higher-dose amoxicillin, amoxicillin–clavulanate (e.g., 90 mg/kg/day) is used for penicillin-resistant *S. pneumoniae*.
[c]Fluoroquinolones are avoided in pediatric patients because of the potential for cartilage damage; however, their use in pediatrics is emerging. Doses shown are extrapolated from adults and require further study.

TABLE 111-12 Evidence-Based Guidelines for Management of Community-Acquired Pneumonia in Immunocompetent Adults

Recommendation	Recommendation Grade[a]
Preferred parenteral agents for treatment of pneumococcal pneumonia for strains with reduced susceptibility to penicillin are cefotaxime or ceftriaxone.	B-III
For susceptible strains, amoxicillin is the preferred antibiotic for oral treatment of pneumococcal pneumonia.	B-II
Recommended initial therapy for a hospitalized patient consists of a β-lactam plus macrolide combination or a respiratory fluoroquinolone alone.	A-I
For an intensive care patient and in the absence of a *Pseudomonas* infection, a combination of a β-lactam plus either a macrolide or a respiratory fluoroquinolone should be prescribed.	B-III
For an intensive care patient and in the presence of a penicillin-resistant isolate, cefotaxime, ceftriaxone, or a respiratory fluoroquinolone or other agent indicated by in-vitro testing may be prescribed.	A-III
For hospitalized patients, the preferred treatment for Legionnaires' disease is azithromycin or a fluoroquinolone.	B-II
For nonhospitalized patients, Legionnaires' disease may be treated with erythromycin, doxycycline, azithromycin, clarithromycin, or a fluoroquinolone.	A-II
Amantadine, rimantadine, oseltamivir, or zanamivir is effective for early (within 48 hours of appearance of symptoms) treatment of influenza A and oseltamivir and zanamivir for influenza B.	B-I

[a]Quality of evidence: I, evidence from at least one properly randomized, controlled trial; II, evidence from at least one well-designed clinical trial without randomization, from cohort or case-controlled analytic studies (preferably from more than one center), or from multiple time-series studies or dramatic results from uncontrolled experiments; III, evidence from opinions of respected authorities based on clinical experience, descriptive studies, or reports of expert committees. Strength of recommendation: A, good evidence to support a recommendation for use; B, moderate evidence to support a recommendation for use.

expensive antibiotics reserved for unresponsive illness or special circumstances. Indiscriminate use of recently introduced agents increases healthcare costs and, in some instances (e.g., widespread use of fluoroquinolones), induces resistance among a significant percentage of community-acquired organisms.[74,75] It must be emphasized, however, that the rapidly evolving epidemiology of bacterial resistance, including the increasing emergence of penicillin-resistant pneumococcus in many areas of the United States and Europe,[76] forces the clinician to be vigilant and knowledgeable about antibiotic sensitivity patterns in each community. Indiscriminate use of antimicrobials for treatment of pneumonia has contributed to the problem of antimicrobial resistance, underscoring the need for defining the optimal antibiotic regimen for each patient.[74]

❾ Evidence-based empirical therapy differs among outpatients, hospitalized patients, and hospitalized patients admitted to an intensive care unit (Table 111–13).[72,77,78] Antimicrobial therapy should be initiated in hospitalized patients with acute pneumonia within 8 hours of admission because an increase in mortality has been demonstrated when therapy was delayed beyond 8 hours of admission.

Nosocomial Pneumonia

❿ Antibiotic selection within the hospital environment demands greater care because of constant changes in antibiotic resistance patterns in-vitro and in-vivo. Ironically, some β-lactam antibiotics, which were developed to treat multiple-antibiotic–resistant hospital-acquired organisms, can themselves induce broad-spectrum bacterial β-lactamases and thereby lead to even greater problems with resistance.[79] These facts underscore the importance of regularly documenting the epidemiology of pathogens and infectious diseases within a specific

TABLE 111-13 Initial Evidence-Based Empirical Therapy for Suspected Bacterial Community-Acquired Pneumonia

Clinical Setting	Empirical Therapy
Outpatient	
Previously healthy	
No recent antibiotic therapy	A macrolide[a] or doxycycline
Recent antibiotic therapy[b]	A respiratory fluoroquinolone[c] alone, an advanced macrolide[d] plus high-dose amoxicillin, or an advanced macrolide plus high-dose amoxicillin–clavulanate
Comorbidities (chronic obstructive pulmonary disease, diabetes, renal or congestive heart failure, malignancy)	
No recent antibiotic therapy	An advanced macrolide[d] or a respiratory fluoroquinolone
Recent antibiotic therapy[b]	A respiratory fluoroquinolone[c] alone or an advanced macrolide plus a β-lactam[e]
Suspected aspiration with infection	Amoxicillin–clavulanate or clindamycin
Influenza with bacterial superinfection	A β-lactam[e] or a respiratory fluoroquinolone
Inpatient	
Medical ward	
No recent antibiotic therapy[b]	A respiratory fluoroquinolone alone or an advanced macrolide plus a β-lactam[f]
Recent antibiotic therapy[b]	An advanced macrolide plus a β-lactam or a respiratory fluoroquinolone alone (regimen selected will depend on nature of recent antibiotic therapy)
Intensive Care Unit (ICU)	
Pseudomonas infection is not an issue	A β-lactam[f] plus either an advanced macrolide or a respiratory fluoroquinolone
Pseudomonas infection is not an issue but patient has a β-lactam allergy	A respiratory fluoroquinolone, with or without clindamycin
Pseudomonas infection is an issue[g]	Either (a) an antipseudomonal agent[h] plus ciprofloxacin, or (b) an antipseudomonal agent plus an aminoglycoside plus a respiratory fluoroquinolone or a macrolide
Pseudomonas infection is an issue but the patient has a β-lactam allergy	Either (a) aztreonam plus levofloxacin or (b) aztreonam plus moxifloxacin or gatifloxacin, with or without an aminoglycoside

[a]Erythromycin, azithromycin, or clarithromycin.
[b]The patient was given a course of antibiotic(s) for treatment of any infection within the past 3 months, excluding the current episode of infection. Such treatment is a risk factor for drug-resistant *Streptococcus pneumoniae* and possibly for infection with gram-negative bacilli. Depending on the class of antibiotics recently given, one or another of the suggested options may be selected. Recent use of a fluoroquinolone should dictate selection of a nonfluoroquinolone regimen, and vice versa.
[c]Moxifloxacin, gatifloxacin, levofloxacin, or gemifloxacin (oral).
[d]Azithromycin or clarithromycin.
[e]High-dose amoxicillin, high-dose amoxicillin-clavulanate, cefpodoxime, cefprozil, or cefuroxime.
[f]Cefotaxime, ceftriaxone, ampicillin–sulbactam, or ertapenem; ertapenem was recently approved for such use (in once-daily parenteral treatment) but little experience is available.
[g]The antipseudomonal agents chosen reflect this concern. Risk factors for *Pseudomonas* infection include severe structural lung disease (e.g., bronchiectasis), and recent antibiotic therapy or stay in hospital (especially in the ICU). For patients with CAP in the ICU, coverage for *S. pneumoniae* and *Legionella* species must always be assured. Piperacillin–tazobactam, imipenem, meropenem, and cefepime are excellent β-lactams and are adequate for most *S. pneumoniae* and *Haemophilus influenzae* infections. They may be preferred when there is concern for relatively unusual CAP pathogens, such as *Pseudomonas aeruginosa*, *Klebsiella* species, and other gram-negative bacteria.
[h]Piperacillin, piperacillin–tazobactam, imipenem, meropenem, or cefepime.
Data from Mandell LA, Wunderink RG, Anzueto A, et al. Infectious Diseases Society of America/American Thoracic Society consensus guidelines on the management of community-acquired pneumonia in adults. Clin Infect Dis 2007;44:S27–S72.

practice or institution. As a result, an antimicrobial agent for a specific infectious disease favored in one practice site may not be the most desirable selection in another site despite similarities in size and patient profile. Strict and careful control and, possibly, rotation of empirical antibiotics in the hospital environment may help to limit the emergence of resistant organisms. Newer antibiotics developed for treatment of resistant, hospital-acquired pathogens are costly, so their use must be moderated to some extent in an era where capitated hospital costs and mandated budget cuts will not tolerate careless antibiotic use.

Severe Acute Respiratory Syndrome

Treatment of SARS involves primarily supportive care and procedures to prevent transmission to others.[68] Owing to the uncertainty associated with the diagnosis of SARS, empirical therapy with broad-spectrum antibiotics should be used. To date, fluoroquinolones (e.g., moxifloxacin, levofloxacin) or macrolides/azalides (e.g., erythromycin, clarithromycin, azithromycin) typically have been used. Although its efficacy is unproven, ribavirin also has been used to treat patients. Owing to the potential benefit of corticosteroids in the presence of progressive pulmonary disease, methylprednisolone has been used in doses ranging from 80 to 500 mg/day.

Avian Influenza

Treatment of avian influenza is primarily supportive, with the majority of patients requiring aggressive oxygen therapy and intensive care monitoring.[69,70] Due to observed resistance with amantadine, the neuraminidase inhibitors are the recommended treatment of avian influenza, with oseltamivir being the preferred agent. For optimal efficacy, treatment should be initiated within 48 hours of the first sign of infection. Of note, there is concern regarding oseltamivir, with a resistant A/H5N1 isolate identified in Vietnam.[70]

■ FLUOROQUINOLONE ANTIBIOTICS

The in-vitro spectrum of antibacterial activity of systemically absorbed fluoroquinolone antibiotics (e.g., ciprofloxacin, levofloxacin, moxifloxacin, gatifloxacin) suggests that these drugs have an important role in the treatment of bacterial infections of the lower respiratory tract. Numerous clinical studies describe the efficacy of these drugs for treatment of purulent bronchitis, acute exacerbations of chronic bronchitis, pneumonia, and cystic fibrosis.[80] However, the widespread use of earlier analogs (ciprofloxacin) by primary care physicians has led to pathogen resistance and treatment failures, including, perhaps most important, isolates of *S. pneumoniae.* Although newer fluoroquinolones are more active than older agents against common respiratory tract pathogens, this experience renders difficult the recommendation of their indiscriminate use for routine community-acquired pneumonia. Nevertheless, these drugs may be effective alternative agents for treatment of community-acquired pneumonia or for the initial treatment of nosocomial pneumonia in hospitalized patients and patients residing in extended-care facilities. The availability of newer analogs with broad spectra of antibacterial activity, including *S. pneumoniae* (e.g., gatifloxacin), further enhances the desirability of a fluoroquinolone as a first-line agent, expanding the therapeutic armamentarium for both community-acquired and nosocomially acquired pneumonia.

At present, fluoroquinolone use in pediatric patients remains restricted and limited because of possible fluoroquinolone-induced destructive lesions of growing cartilage, primarily of the weight-bearing joints. These fluoroquinolone-associated arthritic lesions were determined in animals following large doses but have not been reflected in the human experience. The need for fluoroquinolones for treatment of selected infections arising in pediatric patients continues, and their continued safety in these patients has served as the foundation for ongoing controlled clinical efficacy and safety trials in pediatric patients.

■ MACROLIDE/AZALIDE ANTIBIOTICS

Among the more recently introduced classes of oral antibiotics, the newer macrolide/azalide antibiotics (clarithromycin–azithromycin) possess excellent activity against most *S. pneumoniae* and *Mycoplasma* organisms. They appear to offer viable alternatives to erythromycin, particularly in patients who are intolerant of erythromycin analogs (e.g., patients with gastrointestinal upset) and, with azithromycin, in patients who are taking medications that may result in a clinically significant drug–drug interaction (e.g., erythromycin with carbamazepine or theophylline). Azithromycin offers the added advantage of once-daily dosing and short-course therapy because of the drug's extensive tissue distribution characteristics and prolonged elimination half-life.

PREVENTION

Prevention of some cases of pneumonia is possible through the use of vaccines and medications against selected infectious agents. Polyvalent polysaccharide vaccines are available for two of the leading causes of bacterial pneumonia, pneumococcus and *H. influenzae* type b. In addition, evidence-based guidelines for preventing health-care-associated pneumonia have been published (Table 111–14)[81] (see Chap. 114 for a full discussion of prevention of influenza and Chap. 128).

EVALUATION OF THERAPEUTIC OUTCOMES

After therapy has been instituted, appropriate clinical parameters should be monitored to ensure the efficacy and safety of the therapeutic regimen. In patients with bacterial infections of the upper or lower respiratory tract, the time to resolution of initial presenting symptoms and the lack of appearance of new associated symptomatology are important to determine. In patients with community-acquired pneumonia or pneumonia from any source of mild-to-moderate clinical severity, the time to resolution of cough, decreasing sputum production, and fever, as well as other constitutional symptoms of malaise, nausea, vomiting, and lethargy, should be noted. If the patient requires supplemental oxygen therapy, the amount and need should be assessed regularly. A gradual and persistent improvement in the resolution of these symptoms and

TABLE 111-14 Evidenced-Based Guidelines for Preventing Health-Care Associated Pneumonia

Recommendation	Recommendation Grade[a]
For nebulizers, use aerosolized medications in single-dose vials. If multidose medication vials are used, follow manufacturers' instructions for handling, storing, and dispensing the medications.	1B
Pneumococcal vaccination is recommended for patients at high risk for severe pneumococcal infections.	1A
Unless contraindicated, administer a macrolide to any person who has had close contact with persons having pertussis.	1B
In acute-care settings, offer vaccine to inpatients and outpatients at high risk for complications from influenza beginning in September and throughout the influenza season.	1A
Unless contraindicated, provide prophylactic treatment to all patients without influenza illness in the involved unit with amantadine, rimantadine, or oseltamivir for a minimum of 2 weeks or until approximately 1 week after the end of the outbreak.	1A
Unless contraindicated, patients with influenza should receive amantadine, rimantadine, oseltamivir, or zanamivir within 48 hours of the onset of symptoms.	1A

[a]Category IA, strongly recommended for implementation and strongly supported by well-designed experimental, clinical, or epidemiologic studies; category IB, strongly recommended for implementation and supported by certain clinical or epidemiologic studies and by strong theoretical rationale.

therapies should be observed. Initial resolution should be observed within the first 2 days and progression to complete resolution within 5 to 7 days but usually no more than 10 days. In patients with nosocomial pneumonia, substantial underlying diseases, or both, additional parameters can be followed, including the magnitude and character of the peripheral blood WBC count, chest radiograph, and blood gas determinations. Similar to patients with less severe disease, some resolution of symptoms should be observed within 2 days of instituting antibiotic therapy. If no resolution of symptoms is observed within 2 days of starting seemingly appropriate antibiotic therapy or if the patient's clinical status is deteriorating, the appropriateness of initial antibiotic therapy should be critically reassessed. The patient should be evaluated carefully for deterioration of underlying concurrent disease(s). Additionally, the caregiver should consider the possibility of changing the initial antibiotic therapy to expand antimicrobial coverage not included in the original regimen (e.g., *Mycoplasma, Legionella,* and anaerobes). Furthermore, the need for antifungal therapy (amphotericin B) should be considered. Some resolution of symptoms should be observed within 2 days of starting proper antibiotic therapy, with complete resolution expected within 10 to 14 days.

ABBREVIATIONS

COPD: chronic obstructive pulmonary disease

MIC: minimum inhibitory concentration

RSV: respiratory syncytial virus

SARS: severe acute respiratory syndrome

REFERENCES

1. Mason CM, Nelson S. Pulmonary host defenses and factors predisposing to lung infection. Clin Chest Med 2005;26:11–17.
2. Zaas AK, Alexander BD. New developments in the diagnosis and treatment of infections in lung transplant recipients. Respir Care Clin N Am 2004;10:531–547.
3. Yip TTC, Chan JW, Cho WCS, et al. Protein chip array profiling analysis in patients with severe acute respiratory syndrome identified serum amyloid a protein as a biomarker potentially useful in monitoring the extent of pneumonia. Clin Chem 2005;51:47–55.
4. Don M, Fasoli L, Paldanius M, et al. Aetiology of community-acquired pneumonia: Serological results of a paediatric survey. Scand J Infect Dis 2005;37:806–812.
5. Koulenti D, Rello J. Hospital-acquired pneumonia in the 21st century: A review of existing treatment options and their impact on patient care. Expert Opin Pharmacother 2006;7:1555–1569.
6. Almirall J, Bolibar I, Toran P, et al. Contribution of C-reactive protein to the diagnosis and assessment of severity of community-acquired pneumonia. Chest 2004;125:1335–1342.
7. Howard LSGE, Sillis M, Pasteur MC, et al. Microbiological profile of community-acquired pneumonia in adults over the last 20 years. J Infect 2005;50:107–113.
8. Porzecanski I, Bowton DL. Diagnosis and treatment of ventilator-associated pneumonia. Chest 2006:130:597–604.
9. Trotman-Dickenson B. Radiology in the intensive care unit (part 1). J Intensive Care Med 2003;18:198–210.
10. Donnelly LF. Imaging in immunocompetent children who have pneumonia. Radiol Clin North Am 2005;43:253–265.
11. Wenzel RP, Fowler AA III. Clinical practice. Acute bronchitis. N Engl J Med 2006;355:2125–2130.
12. Tsai MH, Huang YC, Chen CJ, et al. Chlamydial pneumonia in children requiring hospitalization: Effect of mixed infection on clinical outcome. J Microbiol Immunol Infect 2005;38:117–122.
13. Crowcroft NS, Pebody RG. Recent developments in pertussis. Lancet 2006;367:1926–1936.
14. Braman SS. Chronic cough due to acute bronchitis: ACCP evidence-based clinical practice guidelines. Chest 2006;129:95S–103S.
15. Bhutta AT, Savell VH, Schexnayder SM. Reye's syndrome: Down but not out. South Med J 2003;96:43–45.
16. Committee on Infectious Diseases. American Academy of Pediatrics. Reduction of the influenza burden in children. Pediatrics 2002;110:1246–1252.
17. Jefferson TO, Demicheli V, Di Pietrantonj C. Neuraminidase inhibitors for preventing and treating influenza in healthy adults. Cochrane Database Syst Rev 2006;3:CD001265.
18. Cooper NJ, Sutton AJ, Abrams KR, et al. Effectiveness of neuraminidase inhibitors in treatment and prevention of influenza A and B. Systemic review and meta-analyses of randomised controlled trials. BMJ 2003;326:1235–1240.
19. Regoes RR, Bonhoeffer S. Emergence of drug-resistant influenza virus: Population dynamical considerations. Science 2006;312:389–391.
20. Braman SS. Chronic cough due to chronic bronchitis: ACCP evidence-based clinical practice guidelines. Chest 2006;129:104S–115S.
21. Pauwels RA, Buist AS, Calvery PM, et al., Global strategy for the diagnosis, management, and prevention of chronic obstructive pulmonary disease. NHLBI/WHO Global Initiative for Chronic Obstruction Lung Disease (GOLD) workshop summary. Am J Respir Crit Care Med 2001;163:1256–1276.
22. Molfino NA. Genetics of COPD. Chest 2004;125:1929–1940.
23. Holtzman MJ, Tyner JW, Kim EY, et al. Acute and chronic airway responses to viral infection: Implications for asthma and chronic obstructive pulmonary disease. Proc Am Thorac Soc 2005;2:132–140.
24. Pierson DJ. Clinical practice guidelines for chronic obstructive pulmonary disease: A review and comparison of current resources. Respir Care 2006;51:277–288.
25. Wilson R, Jones P, Schaberg T. Antibiotic treatment and factors influencing short and long term outcomes of acute exacerbations of chronic bronchitis. Thorax 2006;61:337–342.
26. Mensa J, Trilla A. Should patients with acute exacerbation of chronic bronchitis be treated with antibiotics? Advantages of the use of fluoroquinolones. Clin Microbiol Infect 2006;12(Suppl 3):42–54.
27. Poole PJ, Black PN. Mucolytic agents for chronic bronchitis or chronic obstructive pulmonary disease. Cochrane Database Syst Rev 2006;3:CD001287.
28. Fenton C, Keating GM. Inhaled salmeterol/fluticasone propionate: A review of its use in chronic obstructive pulmonary disease. Drugs 2004;64:1975–1996.
29. Wood-Baker RR, Gibson PG, Hannay M. Systemic corticosteroids for acute exacerbations of chronic obstructive pulmonary disease. Cochrane Database Syst Rev 2005;1:CD001288.
30. Miravitlles M. No more equivalence trials for anitbiotics in exacerbations of COPD, please. Chest. 2004;124:811–813.
31. Hall CB. Respiratory syncytial virus and parainfluenza virus. N Engl J Med 2001;344:1917–1928.
32. Mejias A, Chavez-Bueno S, Jafri HS, et al. Respiratory syncytial virus infections: Old challenges and new opportunities. Pediatr Infect Dis J 2005;24:S189–S197.
33. King VJ, Viswanathan M, Bordley WC, et al. Pharmacologic treatment of bronchiolitis in infants and children: A systematic review. Arch Pediatr Adolesc Med 2004;158:127–137.
34. Panitch HB. Respiratory syncytial virus bronchiolitis: Supportive care and therapies designed to overcome airway obstruction. Pediatr Infect Dis J 2003;22:S83–S88.
35. Kimpen JLL. Management of respiratory syncytial virus infection. Curr Opin Infect Dis 2001;14:323–328.
36. Bertrand P, Aranibar H, Castro E, et al. Efficacy of nebulized epinephrine versus salbutamol in hospitalized infants with bronchiolitis. Pediatr Pulmonol 2001;31:284–288.
37. Langley JM, Smith MB, LeBlanc JC, et al. Racemic epinephrine compared to salbutamol in hospitalized young children with bronchiolitis; a randomized controlled clinical trial (ISRCTN46561076). BMC Pediatr 2005;5:1–7.
38. Prais D, Danino D, Schonfeld T, et al. Impact of palivizumab on admission to ICU for respiratory syncytial virus bronchiolitis. Chest 2005;128:2765–2771.
39. Feltes TF, Cabalka AK, Meissner HC, et al. Palivizumab prophylaxis reduces hospitalizations due to respiratory syncytial virus in young

children with hemodynamically significant congenital heart disease. J Pediatr 2003;143:532–540.
40. Pedraz C, Carbonell-Estrany X, Figueras-Aloy J, et al. Effect of palivizumab prophylaxis in decreasing respiratory syncytial virus hospitalizations in premature infants. Pediatr Infect Dis J 2003;22:823–827.
41. File Jr. TM, Garau J, Blasi F, et al. Guidelines for empiric antimicrobial prescribing in community-acquired pneumonia. Chest 2004;125:1888–1901.
42. Reimer LG. Community-acquired bacterial pneumonias. Semin Respir Infect 2000;15:95–100.
43. Shefet D, Robenshtok E, Paul M, et al. Empirical atypical coverage for inpatients with community-acquired pneumonia: Systematic review of randomized controlled trials. Arch Intern Med 2005;165:1992–2000.
44. Lynch III JP. Hospital-acquired pneumonia: Risk factors, microbiology, and treatment. Chest 2001;119:373S–384S.
45. Levison ME. Anaerobic pleuropulmonary infection. Curr Opin Infect Dis 2001;14:187–191.
46. Roig J, Sabria M, Pedro-Botet ML. *Legionella* spp.: Community acquired and nosocomial infections. Curr Opin Infect Dis 2003;16:145–151.
47. Martin G, Lazarus A. Epidemiology and diagnosis of tuberculosis. Postgrad Med 2000;108:42–54.
48. Cunha BA. Nosocomial pneumonia: Diagnostic and therapeutic considerations. Med Clin North Am 2001;85:79–114.
49. Gibbs RS, Schrag S, Schuchat A. Perinatal infections due to group B streptococci. Obstet Gynecol 2004;104:1062–1076.
50. Lim WS, Macfarlane JT. Hospital acquired pneumonia. Clin Med 2001;1:180–184.
51. Fiel S. Guidelines and critical pathways for severe hospital-acquired pneumonia. Chest 2001;119:412S–418S.
52. Starner TD, McCray PB Jr. Pathogenesis of early lung disease in cystic fibrosis: A window of opportunity to eradicate bacteria. Ann Intern Med 2005;143:816–822.
53. Nahid P, Daley CL. Prevention of tuberculosis in HIV-infected patients. Curr Opin Infect Dis 2006;19:189–193.
54. Plouffe JF. Importance of typical pathogens of community acquired pneumonia. Clin Infect Dis 2000;31(Suppl 2):S35–S39.
55. Hammerschlag MR. Mycoplasma pneumoniae infections. Curr Opin Infect Dis 2001;14:181–186.
56. Bartlett JG, Dowell SF, Mandell LA, et al. Practice guidelines for the management of community-acquired pneumonia in adults. Clin Infect Dis 2000;31:347–382.
57. Ashley EA, Johnson MA, Lipman MC. Human immunodeficiency virus and respiratory infection. Curr Opin Pulm Med 2000;6:240–245.
58. Afessa B, Green B. Bacterial pneumonia in hospitalized patients with HIV infection: The pulmonary complications, ICU support, and prognostic factors of hospitalized patients with HIV (PIP) study. Chest 2000;117:1017–1022.
59. Feldman C. Pneumonia associated with HIV infection. Curr Opin Infect Dis 2005;18:165–170.
60. Hughes WT, Armstrong D, Bodey GP, et al. 2002 guidelines for the use of antimicrobial agents in neutropenic patients with cancer. Clin Infect Dis 2002;34:730–751.
61. Viscoli C, Varnier O, Machetti M. Infections in patients with febrile neutropenia: Epidemiology, microbiology, and risk stratification. Clin Infect Dis 2005;40:S240–S245.
62. Viscoli C, Castagnola E. Treatment of febrile neutropenia: What is new? Curr Opin Infect Dis 2002;15:377–382.
63. Smith TJ, Khatcheressian J, Lyman GH, et al. 2006 update of recommendations for the use of white blood cell growth factors: An evidence-based clinical practice guideline. J Clin Oncolol 2006;24:3187–3205.
64. Gruson D, Hilbert G, Vargas F, et al. Impact of colony-stimulating factor therapy on clinical outcome and frequency rate of nosocomial infections in intensive care unit neutropenic patients. Crit Care Med 2000;28:3155–3160.
65. Mehta RM, Niederman MS. Nosocomial pneumonia. Curr Opin Infect Dis 2002;15:387–394.
66. Rello J. Pneumonia in the intensive care unit. Crit Care Med 2003;31:2544–2551.
67. Kollef MH. Prevention of hospital-associated pneumonia and ventilator-associated pneumonia. Crit Care Med 2004;32:1396–1405.
68. Sampathkumar P, Temesgen Z, Smith TF, et al. SARS. Epidemiology, clinical presentation, management, and infection control measures. Mayo Clin Proc 2003;78:882–890.
69. Liu JP. Avian influenza—a pandemic waiting to happen? J Microbiol Immunol Infect 2006;39:4–10.
70. Wong SSY, Yuen KY. Avian influenza virus infections in humans. Chest 2006;129:156–168.
71. Smaldone GC, Palmer LB. Aerosolized antibiotics: Current and future. Respir Care 2000;45:667–675.
72. Mandell LA, Wunderink RG, Anzueto A, et al. Infectious Diseases Society of America/American Thoracic Society consensus guidelines on the management of community-acquired pneumonia in adults. Clin Infect Dis 2007;44:S27–S72.
73. Heffelfinger JD, Dowell SF, Jorgensen JH. Management of community-acquired pneumonia in the era of pneumococcal resistance: A report from the Drug-Resistant *Streptococcus pneumoniae* Therapeutic Working Group. Arch Intern Med 2000;160:1399–1408.
74. Low DE. Antimicrobial drug use and resistance among respiratory pathogens in the community. Clin Infect Dis 2001;33(Suppl):S206–S213.
75. Collignon P, Turnidge JD. Antibiotic resistance in *Streptococcus pneumoniae.* Med J Aust 2000;173(Suppl):S58–S64.
76. Steinke D, Davey P. Association between antibiotic resistance and community prescribing: A critical review of bias and confounding in published studies. Clin Infect Dis 2001;33(Suppl):S193–S205.
77. Mandell LA, Bartlett JG, Dowell SF, et al. Update of practice guidelines for the management of community-acquired pneumonia in immunocompetent adults. Clin Infect Dis 2003;37:1405–1433.
78. Cunha BA. Empiric therapy of community-acquired pneumonia. Chest 2004;125:1913–1919.
79. Owens RC Jr, Rice L. Hospital-based strategies for combating resistance. Clin Infect Dis 2006;42:S173–S181.
80. Aminimanizani A, Beringer P, Jelliffe R. Comparative pharmacokinetics and pharmacodynamics of the newer fluoroquinolone antibacterials. Clin Pharmacokinet 2001;40:169–187.
81. Tablan OC, Anderson LJ, Besser R, Bridges C, et al. Guidelines for preventing health-care–associated pneumonia 2003: Recommendations of CDC and the Healthcare Infection Control Practices Advisory Committee. MMWR Recomm Rep 2004;26;53(RR-3):1–36.

CHAPTER 112

Upper Respiratory Tract Infections

YASMIN KHALIQ, SARAH FORGIE, AND GEORGE ZHANEL

KEY CONCEPTS

1. Most nonspecific upper respiratory tract infections have a viral, not bacterial, etiology and tend to resolve spontaneously.
2. Each time antibiotics are administered for an upper respiratory tract infection, the recipient is at increased risk of selection and carriage of resistant organisms that can be passed to others. This can lead to future antibiotic failure.
3. Amoxicillin is the drug of choice for acute otitis media. High-dose amoxicillin (80 to 90 mg/kg/day) is recommended as it is not always known if the patient is at high risk for a penicillin-resistant pneumococcal infection.
4. Vaccination against influenza and pneumococcus may decrease the risk of acute otitis media, especially in those with recurrent episodes.
5. Viral and bacterial sinusitis are difficult to differentiate because their clinical presentations are similar. Viral infections, however, tend to resolve by 7 to 10 days. Persistence of symptoms beyond this time or worsening of symptoms likely indicates a bacterial infection.
6. Amoxicillin is first-line treatment for acute bacterial sinusitis. As there is no difference in clinical outcome among antibiotics, the advantages of amoxicillin include proven efficacy and safety, a relatively narrow antibacterial spectrum that minimizes emergence of resistance, good tolerability, and low cost.
7. Viruses cause the majority of acute pharyngitis cases. Of all the bacterial causes, group A β-hemolytic *Streptococcus* (*S. pyogenes*) is the most common and it is the only commonly occurring form of acute pharyngitis for which antimicrobial therapy is indicated.
8. Antimicrobial treatment of pharyngitis should be limited to those who have clinical and epidemiologic features of group A streptococcal pharyngitis with a positive laboratory test. Penicillin is the drug of choice; amoxicillin can be used for children because of its better taste.

Upper respiratory tract infections include otitis media, sinusitis, pharyngitis, laryngitis (croup), rhinitis, and epiglottitis. These infections are responsible for the majority of antibiotics prescribed in ambulatory practice and the cost is significant.[1] In 1998, for example, the estimated cost of otitis media was $3 to $4 billion in the United States, and $600 million in Canada.[2]

Learning objectives, review questions, and other resources can be found at **www.pharmacotherapyonline.com.**

❶ Most nonspecific upper respiratory tract infections have a viral, not bacterial, etiology and tend to resolve spontaneously.[3,4] Strategies for limiting unnecessary antibiotic use have been developed[1,3,5] in an effort to address the problem of increased bacterial resistance that is associated with antibiotic use. This is particularly important for *Streptococcus pneumoniae,* the leading bacterial cause of meningitis, pneumonia, otitis media, and sinusitis.[1] In Canada, an average of 15 deaths per year caused by *S. pneumoniae* are reported in children younger than 5 years of age.[6]

This chapter focuses primarily on otitis media, sinusitis, and pharyngitis because these infectious entities are frequently bacterial in origin, and appropriate antibiotic treatment can minimize morbidity and potentially prevent complications.

OTITIS MEDIA

Otitis media is an inflammation of the middle ear. The diagnosis of acute otitis media includes signs and symptoms of infection of the middle ear, such as otalgia, fever, and irritability, as well as the presence of fluid in the middle ear.[7–11] In otitis media with effusion, middle ear fluid is present, but signs and symptoms of infection are absent. Otitis media is most common in infants and children, 75% of whom have had at least one episode by the age of 1 year.[12] Table 112–1 lists the risk factors for otitis media. Risk factors for bacterial otitis media caused by resistant pathogens include (a) day-care attendance, (b) recent antibiotic exposure, (c) age younger than 2 years, and (d) frequent bouts of otitis media.[13]

PATHOPHYSIOLOGY

Acute bacterial otitis media usually follows a viral upper respiratory tract infection that causes eustachian tube dysfunction and mucosal swelling in the middle ear.[12,13] Bacteria that colonize the nasopharynx thus enter the middle ear and are not cleared properly by the mucociliary system.[7] In the presence of effusion, the bacteria proliferate and cause infection.[7,13] Children tend to be more susceptible to otitis media than adults because the anatomy of their eustachian tube is shorter and more horizontal, facilitating bacterial entry into the middle ear.[13]

MICROBIOLOGY

S. pneumoniae is the most common bacterial cause of acute otitis media, with an incidence of 20% to 35%.[6,8,14] Nontypeable *Haemophilus influenzae* and *Moraxella catarrhalis* are each responsible for 20% to 30% and 20% of cases, respectively. Bacterial organisms that have been associated less frequently with otitis media include *Staphy-*

TABLE 112-1 Risk Factors for Otitis Media

Winter season/outbreaks of respiratory syncytial or influenza virus
Attendance at day care centers
Lack of breast-feeding in infants
Aboriginal or Inuit origin
Early age of first diagnosis
Nasopharyngeal colonization with middle ear pathogens
Genetic predisposition
Siblings in the home
Lower socioeconomic status
Exposure to tobacco smoke
Use of a pacifier
Male gender
Immunodeficiency
Allergy
Urban population

From Faden et al.,[12] and Hoberman et al.[13]

lococcus aureus, *Streptococcus pyogenes*, and gram-negative bacilli such as *Pseudomonas aeruginosa*.[13] In 20% to 30% of cases, no bacterial pathogen is found, and in up to 44%, a viral etiology is found with or without concomitant bacteria.[7]

Bacterial Resistance

Bacterial resistance to antimicrobial therapy for acute otitis media is of growing concern, particularly in view of the increasing levels of drug-resistant *S. pneumoniae*. Data from the United States (1999–2000) indicate that 8.3% to 34.2% of all *S. pneumoniae* isolates are penicillin-nonsusceptible (minimum inhibitory concentration [MIC] = 0.12 to 1 mcg/mL), that 12.2% to 21.5% are highly penicillin-resistant (MIC ≥2 mcg/mL), and that these rates are highly variable depending on the region of the country.[15,16] International data collected from Europe, Latin America, and North America between 1999 and 2003 indicate penicillin nonsusceptibility rates of 28.6, 28.7, and 33%, respectively. High-level resistance was reported as 14.7, 12.7, and 15.9% respectively.[17] Canadian data from isolates collected between 1997 and 2005 indicate that 16.1% to 25.3% of *S. pneumoniae* isolates are penicillin-nonsusceptible.[17] High-level penicillin resistance fluctuated between 2.3% and 9.7% over this time period, with a rate of 7.4% in 2006. Macrolide and fluoroquinolone resistance have been steadily increasing over 1997 to 2006, from 7.5% to 17.2%, and 0.6% to 7.3%, respectively.[18] Multidrug resistance in the United States is reported as 12.2% to 22.4% of *S. pneumoniae* isolates.[15,16] Multidrug resistance is defined as concomitant resistance to at least three different antibiotic classes. Therefore, antibiotic resistance rates with other β-lactams (penicillins other than penicillin, as well as cephalosporins), macrolides (azithromycin and clarithromycin), clindamycin, trimethoprim-sulfamethoxazole, tetracyclines, and fluoroquinolones also must be considered. In otitis media, non–β-lactam antibiotic treatment is mostly considered when penicillin-allergic patients are treated or when treatment failure occurs.

S. pneumoniae resistance to amoxicillin with clavulanate is reported to range from 0.3% to 1% in Canada, and up to 14% in the United States.[16,17] The second-generation cephalosporins that have been found most active are cefuroxime and cefprozil, followed by cefixime and cefaclor, with resistance rates of 6% to 12% in Canada and approximately 25% to 30% in the United States.[15,16,18] The approximate rates of resistance for individual agents are clarithromycin (8% to 26%), trimethoprim-sulfamethoxazole (16% to 30%), doxycycline (3% to 8%), and levofloxacin (0.5% to 2.5%).[16,17]

β-Lactamase-producing *H. influenzae* and *M. catarrhalis* are found in 23% to 35% and up to 100% of infected patients, respectively.[16,19,20] Susceptibilities, however, vary by geographic region. Although these organisms tend to cause infection that is more likely to resolve spontaneously as compared with *S. pneumoniae*, they are still pathogens that must be accounted for, particularly in treatment failures.

TABLE 112-2 Clinical Presentation of Acute Bacterial Otitis Media

General
The acute onset of signs and symptoms of middle ear infection following cold symptoms of runny nose, nasal congestion, or cough
Signs and symptoms
Pain that can be severe (more than 75% of patients)
Children may be irritable, tug on the involved ear, and have difficulty sleeping
Fever is present in less than 25% of patients and, when present, occurs more often in younger children
Examination shows a discolored (gray), thickened, bulging eardrum
Pneumatic otoscopy or tympanometry demonstrates an immobile eardrum; 50% of cases are bilateral
Draining middle ear fluid occurs (less than 3% of patients) that usually reveals a bacterial etiology
Laboratory tests
Gram stain, culture, and sensitivities of draining fluid or aspirated fluid if tympanocentesis is performed

Data from Hendley JO: Otitis media. N Engl J Med 2002; 347:1169–1174.

❷ Each time antibiotics are administered for an upper respiratory tract infection, the recipient is at increased risk of selection and carriage of resistant organisms that can be passed to others. This can lead to future antibiotic failure. Without antibiotic therapy, however, acute otitis media secondary to *S. pneumoniae* is less likely to resolve spontaneously than that from other causes. *S. pneumoniae* is increasingly resistant to penicillin, and penicillin-resistant *S. pneumoniae* is more likely to be resistant to multiple antibiotics.[14,15,18]

CLINICAL PRESENTATION AND DIAGNOSIS

Acute otitis media presents as an acute onset of symptoms such as fever, otalgia, irritability, and tugging on the ear, accompanied by signs such as a gray, bulging, nonmotile tympanic membrane. Bacterial otitis media often follows a viral upper respiratory tract infection, and the child will experience symptoms of runny nose, nasal congestion, or cough (Table 112–2).

Resolution of the symptoms of acute otitis media occurs over 1 week. Pain and fever tend to resolve after 2 to 3 days, with most children becoming asymptomatic at 7 days. Over a period of 1 week, changes in the eardrum normalize, and the pus becomes serous fluid. Air–fluid levels are apparent behind the eardrum, at which point the stage is now referred to as *otitis media with effusion*. This does not represent ongoing infection, nor are additional antibiotics required.[12] Otitis media with effusion also can occur de novo and is thought to be a result of respiratory viruses. The diagnosis of acute otitis media and otitis media with effusion are easily confused, and careful attention to history, signs, and symptoms as well as results from pneumatic otoscopy are important. Otitis media with effusion usually occurs in spring or autumn, not winter, and may be a result of allergens or viruses common at these times. It also differs from acute otitis media in that pain is not present, nor a bulging eardrum. Effusions resolve slowly. At 3 months, 90% have disappeared.[10,12] Younger children and those with a history of recurrent infections have a further delay in resolution.[7,12] Complications of otitis media are infrequent but include mastoiditis, bacteremia, meningitis, and auditory sequelae with potential for speech and language impairment.[21,22]

TREATMENT

Acute Otitis Media

■ DESIRED OUTCOME

The goals of treatment of acute otitis media are the reduction in signs and symptoms, eradication of the infection, and prevention of complications. Avoidance of unnecessary antibiotic prescribing is another goal in view of the increasing problem of *S. pneumoniae* resistance.

■ GENERAL APPROACH TO TREATMENT

The management of acute otitis media is not without controversy. For example, a systematic review of studies demonstrated that antimicrobial therapy provides resolution of symptoms in approximately 95% of patients,[23] whereas approximately 80% of placebo-treated patients also have a resolution of symptoms.[23,24] Based on the theory that many of these studies likely included children with viral otitis leading to the small benefit of antimicrobials,[23–25] antimicrobial treatment is still considered an appropriate management strategy in *correctly diagnosed* bacterial acute otitis media.[9,14]

■ NONPHARMACOLOGIC THERAPY

Acetaminophen or a nonsteroidal antiinflammatory drug (NSAID) such as ibuprofen should be offered early to relieve pain and malaise in acute otitis media regardless of the use of antibiotics.[11] Decongestants, antihistamines, topical corticosteroids, and expectorants have not been proven effective for acute otitis media,[10,26] and side effects associated with these treatments may be unpleasant.

Surgical insertion of tympanostomy tubes (T tubes) is an effective method for the prevention of recurrent otitis media. These small tubes are placed through the inferior portion of the tympanic membrane under general anesthesia and aerate the middle ear. Children with recurrent otitis who have more than three episodes in 6 months or four or more episodes (one of which is recent) in a year should be considered for T-tube placement.

■ PHARMACOLOGIC THERAPY

Delayed Antimicrobial Therapy

It is difficult to identify who will benefit from antimicrobial therapy, but it is likely that in children viral otitis media will resolve without antibiotics, whereas children with bacterial otitis media will require antimicrobials. With or without treatment, approximately 60% of children who have acute otitis media become symptom-free within 24 hours.[27] Antibiotic use reduces the duration of symptoms (including pain and crying) by about 1 day.[28] Delayed treatment decreases antibiotic use to approximately 30%, decreases side effects, and minimizes bacterial resistance.[29,30]

Patients who are eligible for delayed therapy are children ages 6 months to 2 years, if symptoms are not severe.[11] Children in this age range with severe symptoms, and those younger than 6 months old, should receive antibiotic therapy. Delayed treatment is not advisable in children who have severe symptoms, those with recent antimicrobial exposure, or when underlying conditions exist, because these patients are at increased risk of invasive disease and resistant bacterial infections. If delayed therapy is tried, use of appropriate pain medication, such as oral ibuprofen or acetaminophen, is strongly advised. It is also important that the parent be aware of the symptoms of deterioration, and has easy access to followup.[9,11] If no improvement is noted in 48 to 72 hours, antibiotics should be started. In children ages 6 months to 2 years, some clinicians recommend reevaluation in 24 hours.[29]

Immediate symptom improvement, and prevention of mastoiditis and meningitis are reasons to prescribe immediate antibiotic treatment for acute otitis media. The rates of mastoiditis in the Netherlands, Norway, and Denmark, countries that use delayed therapy, and those in Canada, the United States, Australia, and the United Kingdom (immediate antibiotic use) are similar, although about 1,600 fewer children per 100,000 experienced antibiotic side effects in the former.[30] Given the interest in reducing overprescription and minimizing bacterial resistance, North American countries are now suggesting this wait-and-see approach in certain situations as an alternative.[31]

Antimicrobial Therapy

Acute otitis media must be distinguished from otitis media with effusion. Antimicrobials are indicated only in the former unless the effusion persists beyond 3 months in otitis media with effusion. Middle ear effusion in acute otitis media tends to continue after antimicrobial therapy is completed but does not require retreatment.

Studies have not demonstrated any one antimicrobial agent to be superior in the treatment of acute uncomplicated otitis media.[23]

❸ Amoxicillin is the drug of choice for acute otitis media. High-dose amoxicillin (80 to 90 mg/kg per day) is recommended as it is not always known if a patient is at risk for a penicillin-resistant pneumococcal infection.[9,11] Amoxicillin has the best pharmacodynamic profile (time above the MIC_{90} in the middle ear fluid for more than 40% of the dosing interval) against drug-resistant *S. pneumoniae* of all available oral agents. In addition, amoxicillin has a long record of safety, possesses a narrow spectrum, and is inexpensive.[9] Higher middle ear fluid concentrations of amoxicillin as a result of higher dosing overcome most drug-resistant *S. pneumoniae* even with its increased MIC.[33] Its excellent efficacy against *S. pneumoniae* outweighs the issue of β-lactamase–producing *H. influenzae* and *M. catarrhalis*, against which amoxicillin may not be effective. This is because *H. influenzae* and *M. catarrhalis* are both more likely than *S. pneumoniae* to lead to a spontaneous resolution of the infection. In patients with moderate-severe illness (severe otalgia, and temperature >39°C [102.2°F]), amoxicillin-clavulanate is recommended. Table 112–3 lists treatment recommendations for acute otitis media.

If treatment failure occurs with amoxicillin, an agent should be chosen with activity against β-lactamase–producing *H. influenzae* and *M. catarrhalis,* as well as drug-resistant *S. pneumoniae.*[13,20] High-dose amoxicillin-clavulanate is recommended. Other choices include cefuroxime, cefdinir, cefpodoxime, cefprozil, and intramuscular ceftriaxone.[11,14] Second-generation cephalosporins, while β-lactamase stable, are expensive, have an increased incidence of side effects, and may increase selective pressure for resistant bacteria. Furthermore, most

TABLE 112-3 Acute Otitis Media Treatment Recommendations

First Line	Penicillin Allergy	Treatment Failure
Amoxicillin high dose 80–90 mg/kg/day divided twice daily	Non–type I: Cefdinir 14 mg/kg/day once or twice daily Cefuroxime 30 mg/kg/day divided twice daily Cefpodoxime 10 mg/kg/day once daily Cefprozil 30 mg/kg/day divided twice daily	Amoxicillin-clavulanate[a]
	Type I: Azithromycin 10 mg/kg/day 1, then 5 mg/kg/day for days 2–5 Clarithromycin 15 mg/kg/day divided twice daily	Ceftriaxone 50 mg/kg/day IM/IV for 3 days
If severe symptoms (severe otalgia and temperature above 39°C [102.2°F]) Amoxicillin-clavulanate[a]		Alternatives: Clindamycin 30–40 mg/kg/day in 3 divided doses Tympanocentesis

[a]Amoxicillin component 80–90 mg/kg/day divided twice daily; clavulanate component 6.4 mg/kg/day. Amoxicillin-clavulanate 90:6.4 or 14:1 ratio is available in the United States; 7:1 ratio is available in Canada (use amoxicillin 45 mg/kg for one dose, amoxicillin 45 mg/kg with clavulanate 6.4 mg/kg for second dose).
From Forgie et al.,[9] and American Academy of Pediatrics.[11]

cephalosporins do not achieve adequate middle ear fluid concentrations against drug-resistant *S. pneumoniae* for the desired duration over the dosing interval. Use of trimethoprim-sulfamethoxazole and erythromycin-sulfisoxazole are discouraged because of high rates of resistance.[9,11] Intramuscular ceftriaxone is the only agent other than amoxicillin that achieves middle ear fluid concentrations above the MIC for more than 40% of the dosing interval.[20] Although single doses have been used, daily doses for 3 days are recommended to optimize clinical outcomes.[11,13,14] Ceftriaxone should be reserved for severe and unresponsive infections or for patients in whom oral medication is inappropriate because of vomiting, diarrhea, or possible nonadherence. Ceftriaxone is an expensive agent, and the intramuscular injections are painful. The drug can be given intravenously, but the risk-to-benefit ratio of starting an intravenous line must also be examined. Tympanocentesis also can be considered for treatment failure or persistent acute otitis media. It has a therapeutic effect of relieving pain and pressure and can be used to collect fluid to identify the causative agent. This procedure, however, is not frequently performed in practice in Canada.[13] Clindamycin may also be considered at this point for coverage of documented penicillin-resistant *S. pneumoniae*.[9,11,14] Patients with penicillin allergy can be treated with several alternative antibiotics. If the reaction is not type I hypersensitivity, cefdinir, cefpodoxime, or cefuroxime can be used.[11] If the reaction is type I, a macrolide such as azithromycin or clarithromycin may be used. If *S. pneumoniae* is documented, clindamycin is an alternative. However, the incidence of resistance is much higher with these agents,[9,13] and of these agents, only clindamycin is recommended by the Centers for Disease Control and Prevention (CDC) and American Academy of Pediatrics guidelines.[11,14] Table 112–4 lists evidence-based principles guiding management of otitis media.

Short Courses of Therapy

A meta-analysis of 32 trials[32] reported no difference in effect (cure rates) after short (<7 days) and usual durations (≥7 days) of antibiotic therapy in children. The advantages of short-term therapy are an increased likelihood the patient will adhere to the full course of treatment, decreased side effects and cost, and decreased bacterial-selective pressure for both the individual and the community. However, the data has limitations, including inadequate study sample sizes, lack of use of standardized diagnostic criteria, and subtherapeutic doses. Short treatment courses in children younger than 2 years of age are not recommended.[33] In children at least 6 years old who have mild to moderate acute otitis media, a 5- to 7-day course may be used.[11]

TABLE 112-4 Evidence-Based Principles for the Treatment of Acute Otitis Media

Recommendations	Rating
Properly diagnosed acute otitis media should be treated with antibiotics.	AI
Delayed therapy (observation) may be an option in nonsevere cases.	BI
Antimicrobial resistance should be considered before choosing an antibiotic.	AII-1
High-dose amoxicillin (80–90 mg/kg/day) is first line for uncomplicated infection.	AI-II-2
Short-course therapy may be considered in some instances.	AI
Ten-day courses are recommended for children older than age 2 years and in recurrent otitis media, or otitis media with perforated tympanic membrane.	AI-AIII
When episodes of acute otitis media are frequent, preventive measures are recommended, including handwashing, and limiting exposure to daycare, pacifiers, and second-hand smoke.	BII-III
Influenza vaccine is recommended in children with chronic medical conditions.	AII
Pneumococcal conjugate vaccine is recommended for children ages 2 months to 2 years, and in those with high-risk conditions and older than age 2.	AI

Rating system:
Strength: A, good evidence; B, fair evidence; C, conflicting evidence; D, evidence against; I, insufficient evidence.
Level of evidence: I, randomized controlled trials; II-1, controlled trials not randomized; II-2, cohort or case control studies; II-3, dramatic results from uncontrolled experiments; III, expert opinion.
From Forgie et al.[9]

CLINICAL CONTROVERSY

Some guidelines suggest that children between 2 and 5 years of age should not receive short-course therapy for acute otitis media. Others suggest there is adequate data unless it is a case of recurrent otitis media or the otitis media is accompanied by a perforated tympanic membrane.[9,11]

EVALUATION OF THERAPEUTIC OUTCOMES

Treatment failure is a lack of clinical improvement after 3 days in the signs and symptoms of infection, including pain, fever, and redness/bulging of the tympanic membrane. Early reevaluation of the eardrum when signs and symptoms are improving can be misleading because effusions persist. Immediate reevaluation is appropriate if hearing loss results from persistent middle ear effusions following infection.[10]

Antibiotic Prophylaxis of Recurrent Infections

Recurrent otitis media is defined as at least three episodes in 6 months or at least four episodes in 12 months. Recurrent infections are of concern because patients younger than 3 years of age are at high risk for hearing loss and language and learning disabilities.[21] Data from studies generally do not favor prophylaxis. A meta-analysis demonstrated that prophylaxis prevents one infection each time one child is treated for 9 months.[35] Of further concern is antibiotic resistance. Treatment can be delayed until the onset of symptoms of an upper respiratory tract infection (viral symptoms), or antibiotic prophylaxis can be limited to 6 months duration during the winter months. T-tube placement, adenoidectomy, and tonsillectomy may be of value in children with recurrent treatment failure.

Vaccination

❹ Vaccination against influenza and pneumococcus may decrease the risk of acute otitis media, especially in individuals with recurrent episodes. Immunization with the influenza vaccine is associated with up to a 36% reduction in the incidence of acute otitis media infection.[36] Others have described a benefit during the influenza season.[12,37] The influenza vaccine can be administered to any healthy person without contraindications, especially individuals with chronic disease who are at least 6 months of age.[6,14,25]

A conjugate pneumococcal vaccine that is indicated in infants and children provides a 6% reduction in the frequency of acute otitis media and a 20% reduction in the need for placement of T tubes.[38] Also, vaccine use has demonstrated an 8% decrease in office visits, as well as a 10% to 26% decrease in otitis media episodes in children who experienced 3 to 10 infections per year.[39] Pneumococcal conjugate vaccine is recommended for all children ages 2 to 23 months; it is also recommended for those 24 to 59 months of age who are at high risk of invasive disease.[6,40] Previously unvaccinated children who are older than 1 year of age and who have had recurrent otitis media infections do not benefit from later vaccination.[41]

SINUSITIS

Sinusitis is an inflammation and/or infection of the paranasal sinus mucosa.[42–44] The term *rhinosinusitis* is used by some specialists because sinusitis typically also involves the nasal mucosa.[42,44] Even though the majority of these infections are viral in origin, antimicrobials are prescribed frequently. It is thus important to differentiate between viral and bacterial sinusitis to aid in optimizing treatment decisions.

❺ Viral sinusitis and bacterial sinusitis are difficult to differentiate because their clinical presentations are similar. Viral infections, however, tend to resolve by 7 to 10 days. Persistence of symptoms beyond this time or worsening of symptoms likely indicates a bacterial infection.[43] Acute bacterial sinusitis lasts less than 30 days with complete resolution of symptoms, whereas chronic sinusitis is defined as episodes of inflammation lasting more than 3 months with persistence of respiratory symptoms.[42,47]

Bacterial sinusitis is overdiagnosed by family physicians and thus antibiotics are overprescribed.[42,46] No one clinical finding can accurately diagnose this disease as compared to the gold standard, sinus aspiration (>10^5 organisms/mL).[42] Table 112–5 illustrates the signs and symptoms that best predict a diagnosis of bacterial sinusitis. Between 5% and 13% of viral upper respiratory tract infections in children are complicated by bacterial sinusitis, whereas only 0.5% to 2% of viral upper respiratory tract infections in adults are complicated by sinusitis.[42–44,47] Other factors that can be associated with sinus disease include allergic inflammation, systemic diseases, trauma, environmental exposures, and anatomic abnormalities.[44,46,47] Complications include osteitis, orbital cellulitis, meningitis, and brain abscess, but are extremely rare.[43]

PATHOPHYSIOLOGY

Similar to acute otitis media, acute bacterial sinusitis usually is preceded by a viral respiratory tract infection that causes mucosal inflammation.[42,43,47] This can lead to obstruction of the sinus ostia—the pathways that drain the sinuses. Mucosal secretions become trapped, local defenses are impaired, and bacteria from adjacent surfaces begin to proliferate. The pathogenesis of chronic sinusitis has not been well studied. Whether it is caused by more persistent pathogens or there is a subtle defect in the host's immune function, some patients develop chronic symptoms after their acute infection.[44,48,49]

MICROBIOLOGY

Viruses are responsible for most cases of acute sinusitis; however, when symptoms are persistent (≥7 days) or severe, bacteria may be a primary cause or the cause of secondary infection.[42] Acute sinusitis that is bacterial in origin is caused most often by the same bacteria implicated in acute otitis media: *S. pneumoniae* and *H. influenzae*.[1,44,45,50] These organisms are responsible for approximately 70% of bacterial causes of acute sinusitis in both adults and children.[45] *M. catarrhalis* is also frequently implicated in children (approximately 25%).[45,47] *S. pyogenes, S. aureus,* fungi, and anaerobes are associated less frequently with acute sinusitis.[42,45] Issues of bacterial resistance are similar to those found with otitis media and are further addressed in that section of this chapter.

TABLE 112-5 Clinical Presentation and Diagnosis of Bacterial Sinusitis

General
A nonspecific upper respiratory tract infection that persists beyond 7 to 14 days
Signs and symptoms
Acute
Adults
Nasal discharge/congestion
Maxillary tooth pain, facial or sinus pain that may radiate (unilateral in particular) as well as deterioration after initial improvement
Severe or persistent (beyond 7 days) signs and symptoms are most likely bacterial and should be treated with antimicrobials
Children
Nasal discharge and cough for greater than 10 to 14 days or severe signs and symptoms such as temperature above 39°C (102.2°F) or facial swelling or pain are indications for antimicrobial therapy
Chronic
Symptoms are similar to acute sinusitis but more nonspecific
Rhinorrhea is associated with acute exacerbations
Chronic unproductive cough, laryngitis, and headache may occur
Chronic/recurrent infections occur three to four times a year and are unresponsive to steam and decongestants

Compiled from Hickner et al.,[42] Piccirillo,[43] ref. 44, Scheid et al.,[46] and ref. 47.

TREATMENT

Sinusitis

DESIRED OUTCOME

The goals of treatment of acute sinusitis are the reduction in signs and symptoms, achieving and maintaining patency of the ostia, limiting antimicrobial treatment to those who may benefit, eradicating bacterial infection with appropriate antimicrobial therapy, minimizing the duration of illness, preventing complications, and preventing progression from acute disease to chronic disease.[45,47,48]

GENERAL APPROACH TO TREATMENT

Approximately 65% of patients with acute sinusitis will recover spontaneously (these are likely patients with viral sinusitis).[44,45] When the decision to treat with antimicrobials thus is made, the choice must be effective and safe, and cost must be considered. Tables 112–6 and 112–7 provide the evidence-based principles for acute bacterial sinusitis in children and adults.

CLINICAL CONTROVERSY

Is antimicrobial treatment warranted in bacterial sinusitis? Because most studies have not used sinus aspiration to diagnose bacterial sinusitis, it is likely that patients with viral infections have diluted the results of studies of antimicrobial therapy. It is recommended that patients with mild acute sinusitis be given decongestants and reassurance, whereas those with moderate disease for 7 days or more, and those with severe disease, be given antimicrobial therapy.

PHARMACOLOGIC THERAPY

Data regarding supportive therapy are limited, but such therapy may be useful in reducing symptoms in some patients.[46] Nasal deconges-

TABLE 112-6 Evidence-Based Principles for Acute Bacterial Sinusitis in Children

Recommendation	Rating
The diagnosis of acute bacterial sinusitis is based on clinical criteria in children who present with upper respiratory symptoms that are either persistent or severe.	Strong–limited scientific data
Imaging studies are not necessary to confirm a diagnosis of clinical sinusitis in children ≤6 years of age.	Strong–limited scientific data
Antibiotics are recommended for the management of acute bacterial sinusitis to achieve more rapid clinical cure.	Strong–good evidence
No recommendations are made for adjuvant therapies or antibiotic prophylaxis.	Controversial and limited data

Rating: Strong recommendations are based on high-quality scientific evidence or when such was unavailable, strong expert panel consensus from a subcommittee of the American Academy of Pediatrics, the Agency for Healthcare Research and Quality, the New England Medical Center for Evidence Based Practice, and colleagues from family practice and otolaryngology organizations.
Data from American Academy of Pediatrics. Pediatrics 2001;108:798–808.

TABLE 112-7 Evidence-Based Principles on Acute Bacterial Sinusitis in Adults

Recommendations	Rating
Most cases of acute rhinosinusitis diagnosed in ambulatory care are caused by uncomplicated viral upper respiratory tract infections.	A
Bacterial and viral rhinosinusitis are difficult to differentiate on clinical grounds.	B
Sinus radiography is not recommended for diagnosis in routine cases.	B
Acute rhinosinusitis resolves without antibiotic therapy in most cases.	A

Rating: A indicates randomized controlled trials with little or no heterogeneity; *B* indicates randomized controlled trials with some heterogeneity or a well-designed cohort study; *C* indicates case series or poor cohort studies; *D* indicates expert opinion.
Data from Hickner JM, Bartlett JG, Besser RE, et al. Ann Intern Med 2001;134:498–505.

TABLE 112-8 Approach to Treatment of Acute Bacterial Sinusitis

Uncomplicated Sinusitis	Amoxicillin
Uncomplicated sinusitis, penicillin-allergic patient	*Non–immediate-type hypersensitivity*: β-lactamase–stable cephalosporin *Immediate-type hypersensitivity:* Clarithromycin or azithromycin or trimethoprim-sulfamethoxazole or doxycycline or respiratory fluoroquinolone
Treatment failure or prior antibiotic therapy in past 4 to 6 weeks	High-dose amoxicillin with clavulanate or β-lactamase–stable cephalosporin Second choice: respiratory fluoroquinolone
High suspicion of penicillin-resistant *Streptococcus pneumoniae*	High-dose amoxicillin or clindamycin Second choice: respiratory fluoroquinolone

Compiled from ref. 44, ref. 45, and ref. 47.

tant sprays that reduce inflammation by vasoconstriction, such as phenylephrine and oxymetazoline, are used often in sinusitis.[42,44] Use should be limited to the recommended duration of the product to prevent rebound congestion. Oral decongestants also may aid in nasal/sinus patency. Irrigation of the nasal cavity with saline and steam inhalation may be used to increase mucosal moisture, and mucolytics (e.g., guaifenesin) may be used to decrease the viscosity of nasal secretions.[42,44]

Antihistamines should not be used for acute bacterial sinusitis in view of their anticholinergic effects that can dry mucosa and disturb clearance of mucosal secretions.[46] Second-generation antihistamines may play a role in chronic sinusitis where allergy is a component. Glucocorticoids intranasally may decrease inflammation causing headache, nasal congestion, and facial pain;[51] however, there is little data in acute sinusitis.

Antimicrobial Therapy

Two meta-analyses[44,52] have demonstrated that antimicrobial therapy is superior to placebo in reducing or eliminating symptoms in acute sinusitis, with a reduction in clinical failure of 25% to 30% reported. Results from individual randomized controlled trials are conflicting, and are confounded by flaws in methodology. Of two randomized, controlled, double-blind studies,[50,53] one demonstrated that amoxicillin provided no benefit over placebo, while the other demonstrated that amoxicillin or penicillin were more effective than placebo. Although neither study used sinus aspiration for diagnosis, the study that showed no benefit with antibiotic treatment used radiography for diagnosis of sinusitis, and duration of illness was not specified. Viral infection thus was likely present in a number of patients, underestimating the value of antimicrobial therapy. The second study[50] demonstrated the effectiveness of penicillin and amoxicillin in patients with at least 7 days of illness and findings of sinusitis on computed tomography (CT). CT is considered more specific for diagnosis than radiography.[46] With more rigorous inclusion criteria and better diagnostic tools, more patients with bacterial sinusitis were likely included.

No difference between cure rates, clinical improvement, or relapse rates was noted between different antibiotics according to one meta-analysis.[52] Another report suggests that amoxicillin-clavulanate was 41% more effective in reducing clinical failure than cephalosporins when used within 10 to 25 days; however, by 45 days, the difference disappeared.[44] There was no difference noted when other antibiotic classes were compared, but there is a lack of studies comparing older, less expensive antibiotics with newer, more costly agents.

❻ Amoxicillin is first-line treatment for acute bacterial sinusitis. Because there is no difference in clinical outcome among antibiotics, the advantages of amoxicillin include proven efficacy and safety, a relatively narrow antibacterial spectrum that minimizes emergence of resistance, good tolerability, and low cost. Most consensus reports and reviews consider amoxicillin as first-line treatment for acute bacterial sinusitis (Table 112–8). It is cost-effective in acute uncomplicated disease, and initial use of newer broad-spectrum agents is not justified.[44,47,54,55] If a patient is penicillin-allergic, trimethoprim-sulfamethoxazole, doxycycline, azithromycin, or clarithromycin may be used. There is concern, however, regarding increasing resistance to trimethoprim-sulfamethoxazole and macrolides,[45] as well as the high failure rate of all these agents. In adults, a respiratory fluoroquinolone such as levofloxacin or gatifloxacin is an alternative in the penicillin-allergic patient. Use of fluoroquinolones also should be restricted, if possible, to those who have recently received antibiotics, those with severe disease, and those with drug-resistant *S. pneumoniae.*[45,56] Furthermore, gatifloxacin should no longer be used because of well-documented hypoglycemia and hyperglycemia. If the penicillin allergy is not a true immunoglobulin (Ig) E-mediated reaction (e.g., hives or anaphylaxis), a second-generation cephalosporin is initially recommended (e.g., cefprozil, cefuroxime, or cefpodoxime).[47,57]

If drug-resistant *S. pneumoniae* is highly suspected (daycare attendance, recent antibiotic use, age younger than 2 years), high-dose amoxicillin should be given. Some recommend clindamycin, but it is important to note that this drug is not active against *H. influenzae* and *M. catarrhalis.*[47]

In the case of treatment failure with amoxicillin (i.e., no improvement in symptoms 72 hours after starting therapy) or in patients who have received antimicrobial therapy in the prior 4 to 6 weeks, limitations of initial treatment coverage must be considered.[45] Improved coverage of *H. influenzae* and *M. catarrhalis* with either high-dose amoxicillin plus clavulanate or a β-lactamase–stable cephalosporin that covers *S. pneumoniae* (e.g., cefprozil, cefuroxime, or cefpodoxime) is an option.[45,47] Other alternatives include cefdinir, azithromycin, clarithromycin, and trimethoprim-sulfamethoxazole.[46,47] Clinical cure rates are similar among antimicrobial agents,[54,55] although local-area resistance rates also must be considered, as well as increasing resistance of *S. pneumoniae, H. influenzae,* and *M. catarrhalis* to trimethoprim-sulfamethoxazole, and of *S. pneumoniae* to macrolides. Respiratory fluoroquinolones have also been recommended, as well as ceftriaxone and telithromycin. Combination therapy is recommended in the otolaryngology guidelines in cases of treatment failure.[45] Examples include high-dose amoxicillin or clindamycin with cefixime or rifampin. However, there is no clinical evidence of the safety and efficacy of these combinations at this time. Table 112–9 lists dosing guidelines for these drugs.

Duration of therapy for treatment of sinusitis is not well established. Most trials have used 10- to 14-day antimicrobial courses, although some trials also have investigated courses as short as 3 days.[58] In one placebo-controlled comparison of 3- versus 10-day treatment with trimethoprim-sulfamethoxazole and a decongestant, a similar number in each group were cured or improved at 14 days. Since the publication of this study, however, rates of *S. pneumoniae* resistant to trimethoprim-sulfamethoxazole have increased dramatically. Furthermore, extrapolation of these results to other antimicro-

TABLE 112-9 Dosing Guidelines for Acute Bacterial Sinusitis

Drug	Adult Dosage	Pediatric Dosage
Amoxicillin	500 mg three times daily	Low dose: 40–50 mg/kg/day divided in three doses
	High dose: 1 g three times daily	High dose: 80–100 mg/kg/day divided in three doses
Amoxicillin-clavulanate	500/125 mg three times daily	40–50 mg/kg/day divided in three doses
	High dose: 2 g/125 mg twice daily	High dose: can add 40–50 mg/kg/day amoxicillin
Cefuroxime	250–500 mg twice daily	15 mg/kg/day divided in two doses
Cefaclor	250–500 mg three times daily	20 mg/kg/day divided in three doses
Cefixime	200–400 mg twice daily	8 mg/kg/day in one dose or divided in two doses
Cefdinir	600 mg daily or divided in two doses	14 mg/kg/day in one dose or divided in two doses
Cefpodoxime	200 mg twice daily	10 mg/kg/day in two divided doses (max: 400 mg daily)
Cefprozil	250–500 mg twice daily	15–30 mg/kg/day divided in two doses
Doxycycline	100 mg every 12 hours	–
Trimethoprim-sulfamethoxazole	160/800 mg every 12 hours	6–8 mg/kg/day trimethoprim, 30–40 mg/kg/day sulfamethoxazole divided in two doses
Clindamycin	150–450 mg every 6 hours	30–40 mg/kg/day divided in three doses
Clarithromycin	250–500 mg twice daily	15 mg/kg/day divided in two doses
Azithromycin	500 mg day 1, then 250 mg/day x days 2–5	10 mg/kg day 1, then 5 mg/kg/day x days 2–5
Levofloxacin	500 mg daily	–
Telithromycin	800 mg daily for 5 days	–
Ceftriaxone	1 g daily	50–75 mg/kg/day divided every 12–24 hours

Compiled from Piccirillo,[43] Scheid and Hamm,[46] and ref. 47.

bials is inappropriate. Recently, a 3-day course of azithromycin was approved for use in sinusitis in both Canada and the United States. A randomized double-blind study demonstrated that azithromycin 500 mg daily for 3 or 5 days was as effective as amoxicillin-clavulanate over 10 days.[57] Furthermore, a new extended-release single-dose preparation of azithromycin was recently approved in the United States. However, data supporting these short regimens are limited and new guidelines express concern over macrolide-resistant *S. pneumoniae*.[45] The current recommendations are 10 to 14 days of antimicrobial therapy or at least 7 days after signs and symptoms are under control.[43,45]

EVALUATION OF THERAPEUTIC OUTCOMES

Antimicrobial therapy reduces the median duration of illness from 17 to 9 days (amoxicillin) or 11 days (penicillin).[50] A patient with persistence or worsening of symptoms 72 hours after initiating antimicrobial therapy may be considered a treatment failure.[45] Referral to a specialist should be considered for patients who have not responded to first- or second-line therapy; for those with severe, recurrent, and chronic disease; and for patients who are at risk for complications. Surgery may be considered in more complicated patients.

PHARYNGITIS

Pharyngitis is an acute infection of the oropharynx or nasopharynx.[59] It is the reason for 1% to 2% of all outpatient visits.[60] While viral causes are most common, group A β-hemolytic *Streptococcus*, or *S. pyogenes*, is the primary bacterial cause and is the focus of this section.[59,61] In the pediatric population, group A *Streptococcus*, or "strep throat," causes 15% to 30% of cases of pharyngitis. In adults, it is the cause of 5% to 15% of all symptomatic episodes of pharyngitis.[59–62]

MICROBIOLOGY

❼ Viruses cause the majority of acute pharyngitis cases. Specific etiologic agents include rhinovirus (20%), coronavirus (≥5%), adenovirus (5%), herpes simplex (4%), influenza virus (2%), parainfluenza virus (2%), and Epstein-Barr virus (<1%).[49,59,61] A bacterial etiology for acute pharyngitis is far less likely. Of all the bacterial causes, group A *Streptococcus* is the most common (10% to 30% of persons of all ages with pharyngitis[49]), and it is the only commonly occurring form of acute pharyngitis for which antimicrobial therapy is indicated.[59]

Other, less-common causes of acute pharyngitis include groups C and G *Streptococcus, Corynebacterium diphtheriae, Neisseria gonorrhoeae, Mycoplasma pneumoniae, Arcanobacterium haemolyticum, Yersinia enterocolitica,* and *Chlamydia pneumoniae.* Treatment options for these organisms are not addressed in this chapter.[59,61]

PATHOPHYSIOLOGY

The mechanism by which group A *Streptococcus* causes pharyngitis is not well defined.[49] Asymptomatic pharyngeal carriers of the organism may have an alteration in host immunity (e.g., a breach in the pharyngeal mucosa) and the bacteria of the oropharynx, allowing colonization to become infection. Pathogenic factors associated with the organism itself also may play a role. These include pyrogenic toxins, hemolysins, streptokinase, and proteinase.

CLINICAL PRESENTATION

Group A streptococcal pharyngitis is difficult to differentiate from viral pharyngitis based on history and clinical findings. However, although all age groups are susceptible, epidemiologic data show that certain groups are at higher risk. Children ages 5 to 15 years old are most susceptible; parents of school-age children and those who work with children are also at increased risk. Pharyngitis in a child younger than 3 years of age is rarely caused by group A *Streptococcus.*[59,61]

Seasonal outbreaks occur, and the occurrence of group A streptococcal pharyngitis is highest in winter and early spring.[59,63] The incubation period is 2 to 5 days, and the illness often occurs in clusters.[60,63] Spread occurs via direct contact (usually from hands) with droplets of saliva or nasal secretions, and transmission is thus worse in institutions, schools, families, and areas of crowding.[62,64] Untreated, patients with streptococcal pharyngitis are infectious during the acute illness and for another week thereafter.[65] Effective antimicrobial therapy reduces the infectious period to about 24 hours. Table 112–10 gives clinical presentation and diagnosis of pharyngitis.

Nonsuppurative complications such as acute rheumatic fever, acute glomerulonephritis, and reactive arthritis may occur, as well as suppurative complications, such as peritonsillar abscess, retropharyngeal abscess, cervical lymphadenitis, mastoiditis, otitis media, sinusitis, and necrotizing fasciitis.

Acute rheumatic fever is rarely seen in developed countries. Acute rheumatic fever secondary to group A streptococcal infection was a cause of concern in the 1950s and was the major reason for penicillin therapy, but the annual incidence of this disease today is extremely rare (≤1 case, per 1 million population). Some risk however, does remain; outbreaks have been reported in the United States as recently as the late 1980s and early 1990s. Furthermore, acute rheumatic fever is widespread in developing countries (e.g., it is estimated that there are 50,000 cases of acute rheumatic fever per year in India).

TABLE 112-10 Clinical Presentation and Diagnosis of Group A Streptococcal Pharyngitis

General
A sore throat of sudden onset that is mostly self-limited
Fever and constitutional symptoms resolving in about 3 to 5 days
Clinical signs and symptoms are similar for viral causes as well as nonstreptococcal bacterial causes
Signs and symptoms
Sore throat
Pain on swallowing
Fever
Headache, nausea, vomiting, and abdominal pain (especially children)
Erythema/inflammation of the tonsils and pharynx with or without patchy exudates
Enlarged, tender lymph nodes
Red swollen uvula, petechiae on the soft palate, and a scarlatiniform rash
Several symptoms that are not suggestive of group A *Streptococcus* are cough, conjunctivitis, coryza, and diarrhea
Laboratory tests
Throat swab and culture or rapid antigen detection testing

Compiled from Mandell et al.,[49] Bisno et al.,[59] Snow et al.,[60] Bisno,[61] Cooper et al.,[62] American Academy of Pediatrics,[63] Schwartz et al.,[66] and Hayes and Williamson.[67]

DIAGNOSIS

For a patient presenting with pharyngitis, the most important clinical decision that needs to be made is whether or not the pharyngitis is caused by group A *Streptococcus.* Diagnosis is essential because it directs management.

Clinical scoring systems such as the Centor criteria[67] or modifications[68] have been advocated for diagnosis in adults as a way to overcome the lack of sensitivity and specificity of clinician judgment and to avoid laboratory testing of all patients.[60,62] Table 112–11 lists the modified Centor criteria. However, concern exists that use of these criteria alone leads to overprescribing.[59,61,70] Guidelines from the Infectious Disease Society of America, the American Academy of Pediatrics, and the American Heart Association suggest that testing be done in all patients with signs and symptoms of pharyngitis. Only those with a positive test for group A *Streptococcus* require antibiotic treatment.[59,63,70] Recent studies suggest that limiting testing to patients who meet two or more Centor criteria will minimize overtesting.[68,70] The simplest approach is likely bedside testing with culture confirmation in cases of negative results. This ensures those with disease are not missed.

It is important to note that laboratory testing should not be used without consideration of clinical criteria. This is because a positive test does not necessarily indicate disease. A positive test may indicate carriage (not active infection) with group A *Streptococcus.*

TABLE 112-11 Modified Centor Criteria for Clinical Prediction of Group A Streptococcal Pharyngitis

Criteria	Points
Temperature >38°C (100.4°F)	1
Absence of cough	1
Swollen tender anterior cervical nodes	1
Tonsillar swelling or exudate	1
Age	
3–14 years	1
15–44 years	0
45 years or older	−1
Score	Risk of streptococcal infection
≤0	1%–2.5%
1	5%–10%
2	11%–17%
3	28%–35%
≥4	51%–53%

The original Centor score applies to adults only. This modified version allows for age.
Data from McIsaac WJ, Kellner JD, Aufricht P, et al. JAMA 2004;291:1587–1595.

TABLE 112-12 Evidence-Based Principles for Diagnosis of Group A *Streptococcus*

Recommendations	Level
Selective use of diagnostic testing in only those with clinical features suggestive of group A *Streptococcus* will increase the proportion of positive tests as well as results of those truly infected, not carriers.	A-II
Clinical diagnosis cannot be made with certainty even by the most experienced clinician; bacteriologic confirmation is required.	A-II
Throat culture remains the diagnostic standard with a sensitivity of 90%–95% for detection of group A *Streptococcus* if done correctly.	A-II
Rapid identification and treatment of patients with disease can reduce transmission, allow patients to return to work or school earlier, and reduce the acute morbidity of the disease.	A-II
The majority of rapid antigen-detection tests available have a specificity >95% (minimizes overprescription to those without disease), and a sensitivity of 80%–90%, compared to culture.	A-II
Early initiation of antimicrobial therapy results in faster resolution of signs and symptoms. Delays in therapy (if awaiting cultures) can be made safely for up to 9 days after symptom onset and still prevent major complications such as rheumatic fever.	A-I

Rating:
Strength of recommendation–A to E
Evidence to support use: A, good; B, moderate; C, poor
Evidence against use: D, moderate; E, good
Quality of evidence–I, II, or III
I: at least 1 randomized controlled trial
II: at least 1 well-designed clinical trial, not randomized, or a cohort or case-controlled analytical study, or from multiple time series, or from dramatic results of an uncontrolled trial
III: opinions of respected authorities
Data from Bisno AL, Gerber MA, Gwaltney JM, et al. Clin Infect Dis 2002;35:113–125.

The incidence of carriage in children is 5% to 20%; it is considerably lower in adults.[63] Table 112–12 lists the evidence-based principles for diagnosis of group A *Streptococcus.* There are several options to test for group A streptococcal pharyngitis. A throat swab can be sent for culture or used for the rapid antigen-detection test (RADT). Cultures are the "gold standard" but require 24 to 48 hours for results.[61] The RADT is more practical in that it provides results quickly, it can be performed at the bedside, and it is less expensive than culture. Cultures are recommended for children, adolescents, parents, and schoolteachers with negative RADTs, as well as in situations of outbreak or to monitor resistance.[62,63,66] Delaying therapy while awaiting culture results does not affect the risk of complications (although some argue that symptomatic benefit is postponed, and contagion remains), and patients must be educated as to the value of waiting given the low false-negative rate of RADT.

TREATMENT

Pharyngitis

DESIRED OUTCOME

The goals of treatment of pharyngitis are to improve clinical signs and symptoms, minimize adverse drug reactions, prevent transmission to close contacts, and prevent acute rheumatic fever and suppurative complications, such as peritonsillar abscess, cervical lymphadenitis, and mastoiditis.[59,60]

GENERAL APPROACH TO TREATMENT

Antimicrobial therapy should be limited to those who have clinical and epidemiologic features of group A streptococcal pharyngitis with a positive laboratory test. Empiric therapy is not recommended. Antimicrobial overuse in those without disease and underuse in those with disease is well documented.[59,70]

TABLE 112-13 Dosing Guidelines for Pharyngitis

Drug	Adult Dosage	Pediatric Dosage	Duration
Penicillin VK	250 mg three or four times daily or 500 mg twice daily	50 mg/kg/day divided in three doses	10 days
Penicillin benzathine	1.2 million units intramuscularly	0.6 million units for weight <27 kg (50,000 units/kg)	One dose
Penicillin G procaine and benzathine mixture	Not recommended in adolescents and adults	1.2 million units (benzathine 0.9 million units, procaine 0.3 million units)	One dose
Amoxicillin	500 mg three times daily	40–50 mg/kg/day divided in three doses	10 days
Erythromycin			10 days
Estolate	20–40 mg/kg/day divided two to four times daily (max: 1 g/day)	Same as adults	
Stearate	1 g daily divided two to four times daily (adolescents, adults)	–	
Ethylsuccinate	40 mg/kg/day divided two to four times daily (max: 1 g/day)	Same as adults	
Cephalexin	250–500 mg orally four times daily	25–50 mg/kg/day divided in four doses	10 days

Compiled from Bisno et al.,[59] Bisno,[61] and American Academy of Pediatrics.[63]

PHARMACOLOGIC THERAPY

Because pain is often the primary reason for visiting a physician, emphasis on analgesics such as acetaminophen and NSAIDs to aid in pain relief is strongly recommended.[71] However, acetaminophen is a better option because there is some concern that NSAIDs may increase the risk for necrotizing fasciitis/toxic shock syndrome. Toxic shock syndrome has been linked to group A streptococcal pharyngitis. Either systemic or topical analgesics can be used, as well as antipyretics and other supportive care, including rest, fluids, lozenges, and saltwater gargles. Symptoms may resolve 1 to 2 days sooner with such interventions.[60–62]

Antimicrobial Therapy

Antimicrobial therapy decreases the duration of signs and symptoms by 1 to 2 days.[60,72] Therapy also decreases the severity of symptoms when initiated within 2 to 3 days of onset in patients with proven group A *Streptococcus*. Microbiologic eradication will occur in 48 to 72 hours, which aids in decreasing transmission.[60]

❽ Antimicrobial treatment of pharyngitis should be limited to those who have clinical and epidemiologic features of group A streptococcal pharyngitis with a positive laboratory test. Penicillin is the drug of choice (Table 112–13).[59,60] It has the narrowest spectrum of activity, and it is effective, safe, and inexpensive.

The only controlled studies that have demonstrated that antimicrobial therapy prevents rheumatic fever following group A streptococcal pharyngitis were done with procaine penicillin, which was later replaced with benzathine penicillin.[73,74] Penicillin given by other routes is assumed to be equally efficacious. The ability of other antibiotics to eradicate group A *Streptococcus* has led to extrapolation that these agents also will prevent rheumatic fever.[62] Amoxicillin can be used in children because the suspension has a better taste than that of penicillin.[59,64] Gastrointestinal side effects and rash, however, are more common.

In patients who are allergic to penicillin, a macrolide such as erythromycin or a first-generation cephalosporin such as cephalexin (if the reaction is non–IgE-mediated hypersensitivity) can be used.[59] Newer macrolides such as azithromycin and clarithromycin are equally effective as erythromycin and cause fewer gastrointestinal adverse effects. Second-generation cephalosporins, such as cefuroxime and cefprozil, or third-generation cephalosporins, such as cefpodoxime and cefdinir, which are β-lactamase–stable, have been advocated for clinical failures with penicillin. In cases of documented macrolide resistance (owing to low-level macrolide resistance—erythromycin MIC 1 to 8 mcg/mL—because of expression of the *mefA/E* gene leading to efflux of macrolide out of the bacterial cell), clindamycin is an alternative. The new ketolides, such as telithromycin, may also have a role to play, especially in regions with a high prevalence of macrolide-resistant strains. If patients are unable to take oral medications, intramuscular benzathine penicillin can be given, although it is painful and is no longer available in Canada.[59] Amoxicillin-clavulanate or clindamycin may be considered for recurrent episodes of pharyngitis to maximize bacterial eradication in potential carriers and to counter copathogens that produce β-lactamases.[59,63,66] Tables 112–13 and 112–14 outline dosing for acute and recurrent episodes of pharyngitis.

To date, no resistance of group A *Streptococcus* to penicillin has been reported in clinical isolates.[59,60,63,75,80] Macrolide resistance is low (>5%) and is not widespread.[75–81] There has been a report of an outbreak of macrolide-resistant group A streptococcal pharyngitis in the United States and increasing rates in New York City.[80] Internationally, higher rates have also been reported,[81] and as usage of macrolides increases, these rates will continue to rise. There is concern that if macrolide use continues to increase, macrolide resistance rates also will increase.[77,78] Consequently, use of newer macrolides as first-line therapy is discouraged in febrile patients with upper respiratory tract infections. Group A *Streptococcus* resistance rates to tetracyclines and sulfonamides are high; consequently, use of these agents is no longer recommended.[59]

The duration of therapy for group A streptococcal pharyngitis is 10 days to maximize bacterial eradication.[59] Short-course therapy has been advocated to help overcome compliance issues that lead to bacteriologic failure.[82] A 6-day course of amoxicillin shows promising results; in addition, recent studies with newer broad-spectrum agents (e.g., azithromycin, cefuroxime, cefprozil, cefdinir, cefixime, cefpodoxime, and telithromycin) have demonstrated durations of 5 days to be effective.

CLINICAL CONTROVERSY

Although some clinicians propose short courses of treatment for pharyngitis, confounding factors from these studies, such as lack of strict entry criteria or differentiation between new or failed infections, limit the widespread application of short antibiotic courses at this time.[59] As well, newer agents that have been studied in this fashion are more expensive and may be more likely to lead to resistance in light of their broad spectra of activity.[61]

TABLE 112-14 Antibiotics and Dosing for Recurrent Episodes of Pharyngitis

Drug	Adult Dosage	Pediatric Dosage
Clindamycin	600 mg orally divided in two to four doses	20 mg/kg/day in three divided doses (max: 1.8 g/day)
Amoxicillin-clavulanate	500 mg twice daily	40 mg/kg/day in three divided doses
Penicillin benzathine	1.2 million units intramuscularly for one dose	0.6 million units for weight <27 kg (50,000 units/kg)
Penicillin benzathine with rifampin	As above Rifampin 20 mg/kg/day orally in two divided doses during last 4 days of treatment with penicillin	As above Rifampin dose same as adults

CLINICAL CONTROVERSY

Once-daily amoxicillin given at a dose of 750 mg is as effective as penicillin 250 mg three times daily (duration 10 days each) in children ages 4 to 18 years with group A streptococcal pharyngitis.[83] This dosing regimen has not yet been endorsed by expert panels but may gain support in the future if the results are reproducible.[59,60,62]

Overprescribing is a large concern that requires consideration. Antibiotics are prescribed in 73% of patients who visit their physician with a complaint of sore throat.[84] This is well above the incidence of group A *Streptococcus.* For those who receive antibiotics, 68% of prescriptions are described as being nonrecommended treatments, for example, extended-spectrum macrolides (e.g., azithromycin and clarithromycin) or fluoroquinolones (e.g., ciprofloxacin, gatifloxacin, levofloxacin, and moxifloxacin). Cost and resistance are factors that should discourage this practice.

EVALUATION OF THERAPEUTIC OUTCOMES/CONTACT CASES

Most cases of pharyngitis are self-limited; however, antimicrobial therapy will hasten resolution when given early to proven cases of group A *Streptococcus.*[59] Symptoms generally resolve by 3 to 4 days even without therapy.[61] Children should be kept home from daycare or school until afebrile and for the first 24 hours after antimicrobial treatment is initiated, after which time transmission is unlikely.[62–64]

Followup testing generally is not necessary for index cases or in asymptomatic contacts of the index patient.[59,61,63] Symptomatic contacts may be treated without cultures.[64] In epidemics or in cases of severe infection, followup testing may be prudent. The incidence of invasive group A streptococcal infection in household contacts is rare, and routine chemoprophylaxis is not recommended by the CDC,[86] although testing is advocated and guides management.[59,63] Twenty-five percent of household contacts are carriers, but treatment would only be required in persons with signs and symptoms of disease or contacts of severe or resistant disease.[59]

ABBREVIATIONS

MIC: minimal inhibitory concentration

MIC_{90}: minimal inhibitory concentration for 90% of isolates

NSAID: nonsteroidal antiinflammatory drug

RADT: rapid antigen-detection test

REFERENCES

1. Snow V, Mottur-Pilson C, Gonzales R, for the American College of Physicians-American Society of Internal Medicine. Principles of appropriate antibiotic use for treatment of nonspecific upper respiratory tract infections in adults. Ann Intern Med 2001;134:487–489.
2. Elden LM, Coyte PC. Socioeconomic impact of otitis media in North America. J Otolaryngol 1998;27(Suppl 2):9–16.
3. Gonzales R, Bartlett JG, Besser RE, et al. Principles of appropriate antibiotic use for treatment of nonspecific upper respiratory tract infections in adults: Background. Ann Intern Med 2001;134:490–494.
4. Turnidge J. Responsible prescribing for upper respiratory tract infections. Drugs 2001;61:2065–2077.
5. Gonzales R, Bartlett JG, Besser RE, et al. Principles of appropriate antibiotic use for treatment of acute respiratory tract infections in adults: Background, specific aims, and methods. Ann Intern Med 2001;134:479–486.
6. Canadian Medial Association. Canadian Immunization Guide, 6th ed. Ottawa: Health Canada, 2002. *http://dsp-psd.pwgsc.gc.ca/Collection/H49-8-2002E.pdf*
7. Hendley JO. Otitis media. N Engl J Med 2002;347:1169–1174.
8. Dowell SF, Marcy SM, Phillips WR, et al. Otitis media: Principles of judicious use of antimicrobial agents. Pediatrics 1998;101(Suppl):165–171.
9. Forgie S, Zhanel GG, and the Canadian Pediatric Society (CIDS). Canadian guidelines on the treatment of acute otitis media. Pediatr Child Health 2006 (in press).
10. American Academy of Pediatrics. Managing otitis media with effusion: Practice guideline. Pediatrics 1994;94:766–773.
11. American Academy of Pediatrics and American Academy of Family Physicians. Diagnosis and management of acute otitis media. Pediatrics 2004;113(5):1451–1465.
12. Faden H, Duffy L, Boeve M. Otitis media: Back to the basics. Pediatr Infect Dis J 1998;17:1103–1113.
13. Hoberman S, Marchant CD, Kaplan SL, et al. Treatment of acute otitis media consensus recommendations. Clin Pediatr 2002;41:373–390.
14. Dowell SF, Butler JC, Giebink GS, et al. Acute otitis media: Management and surveillance in an era of pneumococcal resistance. A report from the Drug-Resistant *Streptococcus pneumoniae* Therapeutic Working Group. Pediatr Infect Dis J 1999;18:1–9.
15. Doern GV, Heilmann KP, Huynh HK, et al. Antimicrobial resistance among clinical isolates of *Streptococcus pneumoniae* in the United States during 1999–2000 including a comparison of resistance rates since 1994–1995. Antimicrob Agents Chemother 2001;45:1721–1729.
16. Thornsberry C, Sahm DF, Kelly LJ, et al. Regional trends in antimicrobial resistance among clinical isolates of *Streptococcus pneumoniae, Haemophilus influenzae*, and *Moraxella catarrhalis* in the United States: Results from the TRUST surveillance program, 1999–2000. Clin Infect Dis 2002;34(Suppl 1):S4–S16.
17. Johnson DM, Stilwell MG, Fritsche TR, et al. Emergence of multidrug-resistant Streptococcus pneumoniae: report from the SENTRY Antimicrobial Surveillance Program (1999–2003). Diagn Microbiol Infect Dis. 2006;56:69–74.
18. Hoban DJ, Weshnoweski B, Vashisht R, et al. Incidence of penicillin, doxycycline, macrolide, trimethoprim-sulfamethoxazole and fluoroquinolone resistance in 12,045 Streptococcus pneumonia (SPN) in Canada 1997–2006 [Abstract] 47th Annual Interscience Conference on Antimicrobial Agents and Chemotherapy, Chicago, Illinois, 2007.
19. Zhanel GG, Palatnick L, Nichol KA, et al. Five-year incidence of antimicrobial resistance in respiratory tract isolates of *Haemophilus influenzae* and *Moraxella catarrhalis*: Results of the Canadian Respiratory Organism Susceptibility Study (CROSS), 1997–2002. Antimicrob Agents Chemother 2003;47:1875–1881.
20. McCracken GH. Prescribing antimicrobial agents for treatment of acute otitis media. Pediatr Infect Dis J 1999;18:1141–1146.
21. Luotonen M, Uhari M, Aitola L, et al. Recurrent otitis media during infancy and linguistic skills at the age of nine years. Pediatr Infect Dis J 1996;15:854–858.
22. Teele DW, Klein JO, Chase C, et al. Otitis media in infancy and intellectual ability, school achievement, speech, and language at age 7 years. J Infect Dis 1990;162:685–694.
23. Rosenfeld RM, Vertrees JE, Carr J, et al. Clinical efficacy of antimicrobial drugs for acute otitis media: Metaanalysis of 5400 children from thirty-three randomized trials. J Pediatr 1994;124:355–367.
24. Takata GS, Chan LS, Morphew T, et al. Evidence assessment of the accuracy of methods of diagnosing middle ear effusion in children with otitis media with effusion. Pediatrics 2003;112:1379–1387.
25. Glasziou PP, Del Mar CB, Sanders SL, et al. Antibiotics for acute otitis media in children. Cochrane Database Syst Rev 2004;(1):CD000219.
26. Flynn CA, Griffin G, Tudiver F. Decongestants and antihistamines for acute otitis media in children. Cochrane Database Syst Rev 2002;(1):D001727.
27. Del Mar CB, Glasziou P, Hayem M. Are antibiotics indicated as initial treatment for children with acute otitis media? A meta analysis. BMJ 1997;314:1526–1528.
28. Little P, Gould C, Williamson I, et al. Pragmatic randomised, controlled trial of two prescribing strategies for childhood acute otitis media. BMJ 2001;322:336–342.
29. Froom J, Culpepper L, Jacobs M, et al. Antimicrobials for acute otitis media? A review from the international primary care network. BMJ 1997;315:98–102.

30. van Zuijlen DA, Schilder AG, van Balen FA. National differences in incidence of acute mastoiditis: Relationship to prescribing patterns of antibiotics for acute otitis media? Pediatr Infect Dis J 2001;20:140–144.
31. Spiro DM, Tay K-Y, Arnold DH, et al. Wait-and-see prescription for the treatment of acute otitis media. JAMA 2006;296:1235–1241.
32. Kozyrskyj AL, Hildes-Ripstein GE, Longstaffe SEA, et al. Short courses of antibiotics for acute otitis media. Cochrane Database Syst Rev 2000;(2):CD001095.
33. Cohen R, Levy C, Boucherat M, et al. A multicentre, randomized, double-blind trial of 5 versus 10 days of antibiotic therapy for acute otitis media in young children. J Pediatr 1998;133:634–639.
34. Seikel K, Shelton S, McCracken G. Middle ear fluid concentrations of amoxicillin after large dosages in children with acute otitis media. Pediatr Infect Dis J 1997;16:710–711.
35. Williams RL, Chalmers TC, Stange KC, et al. Use of antibiotics in preventing recurrent otitis media and in treating otitis media with effusion: A meta-analytic attempt to resolve the brouhaha. JAMA 1993;270:1344–1351.
36. Heikkinen T, Ruuskanen O, Waris M, et al. Influenza vaccination in the prevention of acute otitis media in children. Am J Dis Child 1991;145:445–448.
37. Clements DA, Langdon L, Bland C, et al. Influenza A vaccine decreases the incidence of otitis media in 6- to 30-month-old children in day care. Arch Pediatr Adolesc Med 1995;149:1113–1117.
38. Eskola J, Kilpi T, Palmu A, et al. Efficacy of a pneumococcal conjugate vaccine against acute otitis media. N Engl J Med 2001;344:403–409.
39. Fireman B, Black SB, Shinefield HR, et al. Impact of the pneumococcal conjugate vaccine on otitis media. Pediatr Infect Dis J 2003;22:10–15.
40. Recommendations of the Advisory Committee on Immunization Practices (ACIP) Advisory Committee on Immunization Practices. Preventing pneumococcal disease among infants and young children. MMWR 2000;43(RR-09):1–38.
41. Vennhoven R, Bogaert D, Uiterwaal C, et al. Effect of conjugate pneumococcal vaccine followed by polysaccharide pneumococcal vaccine on recurrent acute otitis media: A randomised study. Lancet 2003;361:2189–2195.
42. Hickner JM, Bartlett JG, Besser RE, et al. Principles of appropriate antibiotic use for acute rhinosinusitis in adults: Background. Ann Intern Med 2001;134:498–505.
43. Piccirillo JF. Acute bacterial sinusitis. N Engl J Med 2004;351:902–910.
44. Update on Acute Bacterial Rhinosinusitis. Summary, Evidence Report/Technology Assessment: June 2005. Rockville, MD: Agency for Health Care Policy and Research, 2005, *http://www.ahrq.gov/clinic/epcsums/rhinoupsum.htm*.
45. Sinus and Allergy Health Partnership. Executive summary: Antimicrobial treatment guidelines for acute bacterial rhinosinusitis. Otolaryngol Head Neck Surg Suppl 2004;130(1):S1–S45.
46. Scheid DC, Hamm RM. Acute bacterial sinusitis in adults: Part II. Treatment. Am Fam Phys 2004;70:1697–1704, 1711–1712.
47. American Academy of Pediatrics. Clinical practice guidelines: Management of sinusitis. Pediatrics 2001;108:798–808.
48. Wald E. Microbiology of acute and chronic sinusitis. In: Lusk RP, ed. Pediatric Sinusitis. New York: Raven Press, 1992:43–47.
49. Mandell GL, Bennett JE, Dolin R, eds. Principles and Practice of Infectious Diseases, 6th ed. New York: Churchill-Livingstone, 2005.
50. Lindbaek M, Hjortdahl P, Johnsen ULH. Randomised, double-blind, placebo-controlled trial of penicillin V and amoxicillin in treatment of acute sinus infections. BMJ 1996;313:325–329.
51. Meltzer EO, Bachert C, Staudinger H. Treating acute rhinosinusitis: Comparing efficacy and safety of mometasone furoate nasal spray, amoxicillin, and placebo. J Allergy Clin Immunol 2005;116:1289–1295.
52. Williams JW Jr, Aguilar C, Cornell J, et al. Antibiotics for acute maxillary sinusitis. Cochrane Database Syst Rev 2003;(2):CD000243.
53. van Buchem FL, Knottnerus JA, Schrijnemaekers VJJ, et al. Primary-care-based randomised, placebo-controlled trial of antibiotic treatment in acute maxillary sinusitis. Lancet 1997;349:683–687.
54. Piccirillo JF, Mager DE, Frisse ME, et al. Impact of first-line vs second-line antibiotics for the treatment of acute uncomplicated sinusitis. JAMA 2001;286:1849–1856.
55. de Bock GH, Dekker FW, Stolk J, et al. Antimicrobial treatment in acute maxillary sinusitis: A meta-analysis. J Clin Epidemiol 1997;50:881–890.
56. Azithromycin extended release (Zmax) for sinusitis and pneumonia. Med Lett Drugs Ther 2005;47(1218):78–80.
57. Henry DC, Riffer E, Sokol WN, et al. Randomized double-blind study comparing 3- and 6-day regimens of azithromycin with a 10-day amoxicillin-clavulanate regimen for treatment of acute bacterial sinusitis. Antimicrob Agents Chemother 2003;47:2770–2774.
58. Williams JW Jr, Holleman DR Jr, Samsa GP, et al. Randomized controlled trial of 3 vs 10 days of trimethoprim-sulfamethoxazole for acute maxillary sinusitis. JAMA 1995;273:1015–1021.
59 Bisno AL, Gerber MA, Gwaltney JM, et al. Practice guidelines for the diagnosis and management of group A streptococcal pharyngitis (IDSA guidelines). Clin Infect Dis 2002;35:113–125.
60. Snow V, Mottur-Pilson C, Cooper RJ, et al. Principles of appropriate antibiotic use for acute pharyngitis in adults. Clinical practice guideline, part I. Ann Intern Med 2001;134:506–508.
61. Bisno A. Acute pharyngitis. N Engl J Med 2001;344:205–211.
62. Cooper RJ, Hoffman JR, Bartlett JG, et al. Principles of appropriate antibiotic use for acute pharyngitis in adults: Background. Clinical practice guideline, part II (endorsed by the Centers for Disease Control, American Academy of Family Physicians, and the American College of Physicians-American Society of Internal Medicine). Ann Intern Med 2001;134:509–517.
63. American Academy of Pediatrics. Group A streptococcal infections. In: Pickering LK, ed. Red Book 2003: Report of the Committee on Infectious Diseases, 26th ed. Elk Grove Village, IL: American Academy of Pediatrics, 2003:526–536.
64. Hayes CS, Williamson HW. Management of group A β-hemolytic streptococcal pharyngitis. Am Fam Phys 2001;63:1557–1565.
65. Vincent MT, Celestin N, Hussain AN. Pharyngitis. Am Fam Physicians 2004;69:1465–1470.
66 Schwartz B, Marcy M, Phillips WR, et al. Pharyngitis: Principles of judicious use of antimicrobial agents. Pediatrics 1998;101;171–174.
67. Centor RM, Witherspoon JM, Dalton HP, et al. The diagnosis of strep throat in adults in the emergency room. Med Decis Making 1981;1:239–246.
68 McIsaac WJ, Kellner JD, Aufricht P, et al. Empirical validation of guidelines for the management of pharyngitis in children and adults. JAMA 2004;291:1587–1595.
69. Dajani A, Taubert K, Ferrieri P, et al. Treatment of acute streptococcal pharyngitis and prevention of rheumatic fever: A statement for health professionals. Committee on Rheumatic Fever, Endocarditis, and Kawasaki Disease of the Council on Cardiovascular Disease in the Young, the American Heart Association. Pediatrics 1995;96:758–764.
70. Humair JP, Revaz SA, Bovier P, et al. Management of acute pharyngitis in adults: Reliability of rapid streptococcal tests and clinical findings. Arch Intern Med 2006;166:640–644.
71. Dickinson JA. Acute pharyngitis [letter]. N Engl J Med 2001;344:1479–1480.
72. Del Mar CB, Glasziou PP, Spinks AB. Antibiotics for sore throat. Cochrane Rev 2000;2.
73. Chamovitz R, Catanzaro FJ, Stetson CA, et al. Prevention of rheumatic fever by treatment of previous streptococcal infections. N Engl J Med 1954;251:466–471.
74. Denny FW, Wannamaker LW, Brink WR, et al. Prevention of rheumatic fever. JAMA 1950;143:151–153.
75. Kaplan EL, Johnson DR, del Rosario MC, et al. Susceptibility of group A β-hemolytic streptococci to thirteen antibiotics: Examination of 301 strains isolated in the United States between 1994 and 1997. Pediatr Infect Dis J 1999;18:1069–1072.
76. de Azavedo JCS, Yeung RH, Bast DJ, et al. Prevalence and mechanisms of macrolide resistance in clinical isolates of group A streptococci from Ontario, Canada. Antimicrob Agents Chemother 1999;43:2144–2147.
77. Martin JM, Green M, Barbadora KA, et al. Erythromycin-resistant group A streptococcus in schoolchildren in Pittsburgh. N Engl J Med 2002;346:1200–1206.
78. Seppala H, Klaukka T, Vuopio-Varkila J, et al. The effect of changes in the consumption of macrolide antibiotics on erythromycin resistance in group A streptococci in Finland. N Engl J Med 1997;337:441–446.
79. Littauer P, Caugant DA, Sangvik M, et al. Macrolide-resistant *Streptococcus pyogenes* in Norway: Population structure and resistance determinants. Antimicrob Agents Chemother 2006;50:1896–1899.

80. Lin K, Tierno PM, Komisar A. Increasing antibiotic resistance of streptococcus species in New York City. Laryngoscope 2004;114:1147–1150.
81. Grivea IN, Al-Lahham A, Katopodis GD, et al. Resistance to erythromycin and telithromycin in *Streptococcus pyogenes* isolates obtained between 1999 and 2002 from Greek children with tonsillopharyngitis: Phenotypic and genotypic analysis. Antimicrob Agents Chemother 2006:50:256–261.
82. Guay DRP. Short-course antimicrobial therapy of respiratory tract infections. Drugs 2003;63:2169–2184.
83. Feder HMJ, Gerber MA, Randolph MF, et al. Once daily therapy for streptococcal pharyngitis with amoxicillin. Pediatrics 1999;103:47–51.
84. Linder JA, Stafford RS. Antibiotic treatment of adults with sore throat by community primary care physicians: A national survey, 1989–1999. JAMA 2001;286:1181–1186.
85. Robinson KA, Rothrock G, Phan Q, et al. Risk for severe group A streptococcal disease among patients' household contacts. Emerg Infect Dis 2003;9:443–447.

CHAPTER 113

Influenza

ELIZABETH D. HERMSEN AND MARK E. RUPP

KEY CONCEPTS

1. Influenza is a viral illness associated with high mortality and high hospitalization rates among persons younger than age 65 years. The aging of the population is contributing to an increased disease burden in the United States.
2. Seasonal influenza epidemics are the result of viral antigenic drift, which is why the influenza vaccine is changed on a yearly basis. Antigenic drift forms the foundation of the recommendation for annual influenza vaccination.
3. The acquisition of a new hemagglutinin and/or neuraminidase by the influenza virus is called *antigenic shift*, which results in a novel influenza virus that has the potential to cause a pandemic.
4. The primary route of influenza transmission is person-to-person via inhalation of respiratory droplets, and transmission can occur for as long as the infected person is shedding virus from the respiratory tract.
5. Clinical diagnosis of influenza is difficult. Classic signs and symptoms include abrupt onset of fever, muscle pain, headache, malaise, nonproductive cough, sore throat, and rhinitis. These signs and symptoms usually resolve within 1 week of presentation.
6. In the United States, the primary mechanism of influenza prevention is annual vaccination. Vaccination not only prevents influenza illness and influenza-related hospitalizations and deaths, but also may decrease healthcare resource use and the overall cost to society.
7. The trivalent influenza vaccine (TIV) and the live-attenuated influenza vaccine (LAIV) are the two commercially available vaccines for prevention of influenza. Both vaccines contain an influenza A (H3N2), influenza A (H1N1), and influenza B virus, which are initially grown in hens' eggs.
8. Antiviral drugs for prophylaxis of influenza should be considered adjuncts to vaccine and are not replacements for annual vaccination.
9. The sooner the antivirals are started after the onset of illness, the more effective they are.
10. Oseltamivir and zanamivir, neuraminidase inhibitors that have activity against both influenza A and influenza B viruses, are the agents of choice for treatment of influenza. They are most effective if started within 48 hours of the onset of illness.

Learning objectives, review questions, and other resources can be found at **www.pharmacotherapyonline.com.**

Influenza causes significant morbidity and mortality, particularly among young children and the elderly. Seasonal influenza epidemics result in 25 to 50 million influenza cases, approximately 200,000 hospitalizations, and more than 30,000 deaths each year in the United States. Globally, influenza causes nearly 500,000 deaths each year. Overall, more people die of influenza than of any other vaccine-preventable illness. Significant societal consequences associated with influenza include visits to physicians' offices and emergency departments and days lost from school and/or work. The societal costs associated with influenza are more than $37 billion in the United States alone.[1]

Vaccination is the primary mechanism of prevention of influenza in the United States. The antiviral armamentarium for treatment and prophylaxis of influenza is limited, which further emphasizes the importance of prevention with vaccination and appropriate use of infection control measures during outbreaks. Research toward the development of novel antivirals and vaccines is needed for effective control of seasonal epidemics and for pandemic preparedness.

ETIOLOGY AND EPIDEMIOLOGY

Influenza infection can occur at any time during the year with the highest rates of influenza-associated illness during the winter months. The highest rate of infection occurs in children, but the highest rates of severe illness, hospitalization, and death occur among those older than age 65 years, young children (younger than 2 years old), and those who have underlying medical conditions, including pregnancy and cardiopulmonary disorders, that increase their risk of complications from influenza. (1) The seasonal influenza epidemics from 1979 through 2000 resulted in an average of 226,000 hospitalizations per year with more than 63% of the hospitalizations occurring in those older than age 65 years.[2] More than 90% of influenza-related deaths occur in those older than age 65 years.[3,4] Thus the aging of the population is contributing to an increased disease burden. Deaths associated with influenza often result from secondary bacterial pneumonia, primary viral pneumonia, and/or exacerbation of underlying comorbidities.

INFLUENZA VIRUSES A, B, AND C

Influenza virus types A, B, and C are members of the Orthomyxoviridae family and affect many species, including humans, pigs, horses, and birds. Influenza A and B viruses are the two types that cause disease in humans. Influenza A viruses are responsible for the regular, seasonal epidemics of the flu, whereas influenza B viruses are typically associated with sporadic outbreaks, particularly among residents of long-term care facilities. Influenza A viruses are further categorized into different subtypes based on changes in two surface antigens—hemagglutinin and neuraminidase. Influenza B viruses are not categorized into subtypes.

Hemagglutinin and Neuraminidase

Hemagglutinin allows the influenza virus to enter host cells by attaching to sialic acid receptors and is the major antigen to which antibodies are directed upon exposure.[5] Neuraminidase allows the release of new viral particles from host cells by catalyzing the cleavage of linkages to sialic acid.[5]

Sixteen hemagglutinin subtypes (H1 to H16) and nine neuraminidase subtypes (N1 to N9) of influenza A have been isolated from birds. However, the only influenza A subtypes that have circulated among humans since the 1918 pandemic (see Pandemics and Antigenic Shift below) are H1 to H3 and N1 and N2.[5] The primary subtypes of influenza A that have been circulating among humans for the last three decades are H3N2 and H1N1.

EPIDEMICS AND ANTIGENIC DRIFT

❷ Immunity to influenza virus occurs as a result of the development of antibody directed at the surface antigens, particularly hemagglutinin. However, immunity to one influenza subtype does not offer protection against other subtypes or types of influenza. Moreover, immunity to one antigenic variant of a subtype of influenza may not confer protection against other antigenic variants. Antigenic variants are created by point mutations in the surface antigens of a particular subtype, resulting in small changes in the hemagglutinin and/or neuraminidase molecules, which is called *antigenic drift*. Antigenic drift is the basis for seasonal epidemics of influenza, the reason for changes in the annual influenza vaccine, and the rationale behind the recommendation for annual vaccination.

PANDEMICS AND ANTIGENIC SHIFT

Immunity to one subtype of influenza does not confer protection against other subtypes or types. ❸ Antigenic shift occurs when the influenza virus acquires a new hemagglutinin and/or neuraminidase via genetic reassortment rather than point mutations.[5] Most likely, the genetic reassortment occurs when an animal that supports the growth of multiple subtypes of influenza, such as a pig, is concurrently infected with two subtypes of the influenza virus. Conversely, antigenic shift may occur directly from avian strains that have gained competency in the human host. Antigenic shift results in the emergence of a novel influenza virus and carries the potential of causing a pandemic. However, novelty alone is insufficient cause for an influenza pandemic; the virus must be able to replicate in humans, spread person-to-person, and affect a susceptible population.[5]

Spanish Flu of 1918

The influenza pandemic of 1918 was the most significant infectious disease outbreak known to man, causing approximately 40 to 50 million deaths in a year, with more than 500,000 deaths occurring in the United States.[5–8] Although the reports of the first illnesses associated with this pandemic occurred in Spain, there is no evidence that the virus associated with this pandemic actually originated there, indicating a misnomer. The pandemic occurred almost concurrently in Europe, Asia, and North America.[7]

The 1918 pandemic was caused by a particularly virulent influenza A H1N1 virus, which was entirely of avian origin.[9–11] In contrast to the other pandemics of the 20th century, the 1918 pandemic resulted in an unusual mortality pattern. The mortality peaked for those younger than age 4 years, those between the ages of 25 and 35 years, and those older than 65 years of age, which resulted in a W-shaped mortality curve, as opposed to the U- or J-shaped curve typically associated with influenza.[3,8] Over half of the deaths occurred in persons ages 20 to 40 years. The death toll associated with this pandemic culminated in an almost 10-year drop in the life expectancy of the population at the time.[8]

Asian Flu of 1957

The Asian flu pandemic began when a new H2 subtype of influenza A surfaced in Hunan province in China in 1957.[12] The virus appears to have formed from coinfection with an avian H2N2 virus and a human H1N1 virus in a common host, possibly a pig or a human.[13] The H2N2 virus quickly spread to Japan, South America, the United States, New Zealand, and Europe, resulting in approximately 4 million deaths worldwide, with 70,000 deaths occurring in the United States.[7,8,12] Unlike the Spanish flu of 1918, the mortality curve for the Asian flu pandemic was U- or J-shaped, with infants and elderly being most affected.[7]

Hong Kong Flu of 1968

The H2N2 virus of the Asian flu circulated in the human population until 1968, when a new H3 subtype emerged in China and Hong Kong[12] following genetic reassortment with the H2N2 virus.[7,12] The H3N2 virus quickly spread to the United States and later to Europe. This pandemic caused more than 30,000 deaths in the United States and approximately 2 million deaths worldwide.[7,8,12] The lower morbidity and mortality associated with the Hong Kong flu may be explained by previous exposure of the population to the N2 subtype.[14] Similar to the Asian flu of 1957, the mortality curve for the Hong Kong flu pandemic was U- or J-shaped, primarily affecting infants and elderly.

Avian Influenza

Influenza viruses are in circulation in southern China during all months of the year.[5] Given this fact and the close proximity of dense populations of people, pigs, and wild and domestic birds, this area proves ideal for the development of new influenza viruses via genetic reassortment (antigenic shift), as demonstrated by the pandemics of 1957 and 1968 and, most recently, the emergence of what is known as avian influenza.[5]

The first report of human infection with the avian H5N1 virus occurred in 1997 in Hong Kong in a 3-year-old who had a direct link with chickens and later died.[15] This was followed by 18 confirmed cases and 6 deaths.[16] The virus reemerged in 2003 as an antigenically and genetically different virus that has spread widely through wild and domestic bird populations in Asia, Africa, and Europe as well as infecting humans in 10 countries: China, Vietnam, Thailand, Indonesia, Cambodia, Turkey, Iraq, Azerbaijan, Djibouti, and Egypt.[7] As of November 13, 2006, 258 cases and 153 deaths caused by H5N1 infection have been reported.[17] The current overall case fatality is 59.3%, with 20 years being the median age at death for the first 152 cases.

In contrast to the animal-to-human transmission of the 1997 epidemic, occasional human-to-human transmission has been suggested during the recent outbreaks associated with the H5N1 virus,[18,19] although no cases of transmission via aerosolization have been identified.[20] Clinical presentation includes high fever and influenza-like illness, and watery diarrhea without blood may occur up to 1 week prior to respiratory symptoms.[20] Almost all patients have clinically apparent pneumonia. Progression to death, most commonly as a consequence of respiratory failure, occurs a mean of 9 to 10 days after the onset of illness.[20] The neuraminidase inhibitors, oseltamivir and zanamivir, have activity against the H5N1 virus, although higher doses may be needed. Oseltamivir resistance has been detected in several patients infected with the H5N1 virus who were treated with oseltamivir.[20] Amantadine and rimantadine are ineffective against H5N1, and no H5N1 vaccines are currently licensed, although several are under investigation.

The potential for H5N1 to cause a pandemic is of concern as it could spread more quickly than pandemics of the past because of the mobility of people in today's world. International travel has increased 73% since 1990, with 763 million people crossing international borders in 2004.[21] A severe pandemic, like that of 1918, could cause more than 9 million hospitalizations and more than 1.9 million deaths, whereas a moderate pandemic, like those of 1957 and 1968, could result in more than 800,000 hospitalizations and more than 200,000 deaths in the United States alone.[7]

Pandemic Preparedness

This chapter is not meant to provide an exhaustive review of the biology of influenza or pandemic preparedness. This topic is rapidly changing and interested readers are referred to the following websites: *www.pandemicflu.gov* and *www.who.int/csr/disease/avian_influenza/en/*.

The United States Department of Health and Human Services released a *Pandemic Influenza Plan* focusing on surveillance, vaccine development and production, antivirals, communications, and preparedness on the state and local levels.[22] The current goal for the national antiviral drug stockpile is 81 million courses of therapy, with 6 million to contain the initial outbreak and 75 million to treat 25% of the population in the United States.[23–25] The estimated illness attack rate during a pandemic in the United States is 30%, which means that the planned antiviral drug stockpile would not be enough to treat all those infected.[7] The current goal for the national vaccine stockpile is 20 million courses of prepandemic vaccine with the ability to dramatically increase vaccine production during a pandemic resulting in 300 million doses within 4 to 6 months.[23] Furthermore, a population previously unexposed to the pandemic subtype would likely require at least two doses of an inactivated vaccine to induce immunity, which presents challenges in prevention and control during a pandemic.[25] A vital component of pandemic preparedness is forethought—plans must be established for how to effectively triage large numbers of ill patients, prioritize and/or ration vaccine and antivirals, and communicate with the public through mass media during a period of severe labor shortage (a result of stress and illness amongst healthcare workers) and supply shortfall (a result of societal and economic disruption).

PATHOGENESIS

❹ The route of influenza transmission is person-to-person via inhalation of respiratory droplets, which can occur when an infected person coughs or sneezes.[26,27] Transmission may also occur if a person touches an object contaminated with respiratory secretions and then touches their mucus membranes. The incubation period for influenza ranges between 1 and 4 days, with an average incubation of 2 days.[28] Transmission can occur for as long as the infected person is shedding virus from the respiratory tract. Adults are considered infectious from the day before their symptoms begin through the fifth day after the onset of illness, while children can be infectious for longer than 10 days after the onset of illness.[29] Viral shedding can persist for weeks to months in severely immunocompromised people.[30]

The pathogenesis of influenza in humans is not well understood. The severity of the infection is determined by the balance between viral replication and the host immune response.[5] Severe illness is likely a result of both a lack of ability of host defense mechanisms to inhibit viral replication and an overproduction of cytokines leading to tissue damage in the host.[31]

CLINICAL PRESENTATION AND DIAGNOSIS OF INFLUENZA

General

- The clinical diagnosis of influenza can be difficult because the presentation is similar to a number of other respiratory illnesses. The sensitivity of clinical diagnosis ranges from 38% for children to 77% for adults and largely depends on the relative prevalence of influenza and other respiratory viruses circulating in a community.[32]
- The clinical course and outcome are affected by age, immunocompetence, viral characteristics, smoking, comorbidities, pregnancy, and the degree of preexisting immunity.
- Complications of influenza may include exacerbation of underlying comorbidities, primary viral pneumonia, secondary bacterial pneumonia or other respiratory illnesses (e.g., sinusitis, bronchitis, otitis), encephalopathy, transverse myelitis, myositis, myocarditis, pericarditis, and Reye syndrome.

Signs and Symptoms

- ❺ Classic signs and symptoms of influenza include rapid onset of fever, myalgia, headache, malaise, nonproductive cough, sore throat, and rhinitis.
- Nausea, vomiting, and otitis media are also commonly reported in children.[33]
- Signs and symptoms typically resolve in approximately 3 to 7 days, although cough and malaise may persist for more than 2 weeks.
- Primary viral pneumonia, occurring predominantly in pregnant women and in those with underlying cardiovascular disease, usually begins with fever and dry cough, which changes to a productive cough of bloody sputum. This rapidly progresses to dyspnea, hypoxemia, and cyanosis with radiologic evidence of bilateral interstitial infiltrates.[34]
- Secondary bacterial pneumonia is usually seen in individuals with underlying pulmonary disorders and presents during the early stages of defervescence from the influenza infection. These patients usually present with fever, productive cough, and radiologic evidence of consolidation.[34]

Laboratory Tests

- Complete blood count and chemistry panels should be obtained to assess the overall status of the patient.
- The gold standard for diagnosis of influenza is viral culture, which can provide information on the specific strain and subtype. Viral culture has a high sensitivity but can take as long as a week to develop, limiting the clinical relevancy of the results.
- Tests such as the rapid antigen and point-of-care (POC) tests, direct fluorescence antibody (DFA) test, and the reverse-transcription polymerase chain reaction (RT-PCR) assay may be used for rapid detection of virus.

Other Diagnostic Tests

- Cultures of potential sites of infection should be obtained if co-infection, superinfection, or secondary infection is suspected.
- Chest radiograph should be obtained if pneumonia is suspected.

Rapid Tests

- Rapid tests have allowed for prompt diagnosis and initiation of antiviral therapy and decreased inappropriate use of antibiotics. Rapid antigen or POC tests use enzyme immunoassay technology to provide results within 1 hour of specimen collection. Appropriate specimens for collection, in decreasing order of sensitivity, are nasopharyngeal aspirates, nasopharyngeal swabs/washes, and throat swabs.[32] POC tests allow for differentiation of influenza viruses A and B, with sensitivity and specificity ranging from 57% to 90% and 65% to 99%, respectively.[32] In general, use of POC tests is contraindicated in those who have had symptoms for longer than 3 days, and results may be confounded following recent immunization with live-attenuated influenza vaccine.[32]
- DFA testing requires more technical expertise and infrastructure than POC tests. The advantages of DFA are increased sensitivity over POC tests and simultaneous detection of other respiratory viruses, such as respiratory syncytial virus and adenovirus.[32] DFA provides results between 1 and 4 hours after specimen collection and may serve as a confirmatory assay for a POC test.
- RT-PCR assay is a nucleic acid amplification test and is the most sensitive, specific, and versatile diagnostic test for influenza.[32] RT-PCR is replacing viral isolation as the reference standard and can determine the type, subtype, and strain of influenza. Results are provided within 4 to 6 hours of specimen collection.

PREVENTION

The best means to decrease the morbidity and mortality associated with influenza is to prevent infection through vaccination. Appropriate infection control measures, such as hand hygiene, basic respiratory etiquette (cover your cough, throw tissues away), and contact avoidance, are also important in preventing the spread of influenza. Additionally, chemoprophylaxis is useful in certain situations.

VACCINATION

❻ The primary means of influenza prevention employed in the United States is annual vaccination. Vaccination can help prevent hospitalization and death among those at high risk, decrease influenza-like illness, decrease visits to physicians' offices and emergency rooms, decrease otitis media in children, and prevent school and/or work absenteeism. Annual vaccination is recommended for those at high risk for complications and severe disease, such as[29]

- Children between 6 and 59 months old.
- Pregnant women.
- People older than age 50 years.
- Children between 6 months and 18 years old who are receiving long-term aspirin therapy, placing them at risk for Reye syndrome following influenza.
- People of any age with chronic pulmonary or cardiovascular disorders, including asthma but not including hypertension.
- People of any age who have required regular medical followup or hospitalization in the prior year because of chronic metabolic diseases, including diabetes, renal dysfunction, hemoglobinopathies, or immunodeficiency, including medication-induced immunosuppression and human immunodeficiency virus (HIV).

TABLE 113-1 Influenza Vaccination Rates and Goals by Patient Population

Patient Population	Vaccination Coverage	Vaccination Coverage National Goal (2000/2010)
Children ages 6–23 months	18%[a]	N/A
Persons ages 18–49 years with high-risk conditions	26%[a]	60%/60%
Persons ages 50–64 years	36%[a]	60%/60%
Persons ages 50–64 years with high-risk conditions	46%[a]	60%/60%
Persons ages >65 years	65%[a]	60%/90%
Nursing home residents	83%[b]	80%/90%
Pregnant women without other high-risk conditions	13%[a]	N/A
Healthcare workers	42%[a]	N/A

N/A, not applicable; no goals established.
[a]2004 data.
[b]1998 data.
From Smith et al.[29]

- People of any age who have any condition that may compromise respiratory function or increase the risk of aspiration (e.g., cognitive dysfunction, spinal cord injuries, or epilepsy).
- Residents of long-term care facilities.

Vaccination is also recommended for those who live with and/or care for people who are at high risk, including household contacts and healthcare workers.

The ideal time for vaccination is during October or November to allow for the development and maintenance of immunity during the peak of the influenza season. Table 113–1 lists the vaccination coverage rates and goals for various patient populations.

❼ The two vaccines currently available for prevention of influenza are the trivalent influenza vaccine (TIV) and the live-attenuated influenza vaccine (LAIV). Both vaccines contain an influenza A (H3N2), influenza A (H1N1), and influenza B virus; the specific strains included in the vaccine each year change based on antigenic drift. The viruses used for both vaccines are initially grown in embryonated hens' eggs, which explains the contraindication for vaccination of persons with a severe allergic reaction to eggs.

Trivalent Influenza Vaccine

❼ TIV is FDA-approved for use in people over 6 months of age, regardless of their immune status. Of note, several commercial products are available and are approved for different age groups (Table 113–2). TIV is administered intramuscularly and is made with killed viruses, meaning it cannot cause signs and symptoms of influenza-like illness (Table 113–3). Age and immune status can affect the efficacy of TIV as can the similarity of the vaccine to the viruses in circulation.

In children between 6 and 24 months of age, a 2-year randomized study of TIV exhibited 89% seroconversion and efficacy of 66% in year 1 and 7% in year 2 versus culture-confirmed influenza.[35] In children between 1 and 15 years of age, the efficacy of TIV was 91.4% and 77.3% against culture-confirmed influenza A H1N1 and H3N2, respectively. Two doses of TIV are important for children under the age of 9 years, supporting the rationale for the recommendation of a booster dose of TIV at least 1 month after the initial dose in children between 6 months and 9 years of age (see Table 113–2).[29]

TIV is also effective in adult populations under and older than the age of 65 years. A double-blind, randomized, controlled trial evaluating TIV in healthy adults younger than the age of 65 years demonstrated an efficacy of 50% against serologically confirmed influenza during a season in which the vaccine and the circulating viruses were not well-matched and an efficacy of 86% during a season in which the

TABLE 113-2 Approved Influenza Vaccines for Different Age Groups—United States, 2006–2007 Season

Vaccine	Trade Name	Manufacturer	Dose/Presentation	Thimerosal Mercury Content (mcg Hg/0.5 mL dose)	Age Group	Number of Doses
TIV	Fluzone	Sanofi Pasteur	0.25 mL prefilled syringe	0	6–35 mo	1 or 2[a]
			0.5 mL prefilled syringe	0	≥36 mo	1 or 2[a]
			0.5 mL vial	0	≥36 mo	1 or 2[a]
			5 mL multidose vial	25	≥6 mo	1 or 2[a]
TIV	Fluvirin	Novartis Vaccine	0.5 mL prefilled syringe	<1	≥4 y	1 or 2[a]
			5 mL multidose vial	24.5	≥4 y	1 or 2[a]
TIV	Fluarix	GlaxoSmithKline	0.5 mL prefilled syringe	<1.25	≥18 y	1
LAIV	FluMist	MedImmune	0.5 mL sprayer	0	5–49 y	1 or 2[b]

LAIV, live-attenuated influenza vaccine; TIV, trivalent influenza vaccine.
[a]Two doses administered at least 1 month apart are recommended for children ages 6 months to less than 9 years who are receiving influenza vaccine for the first time.
[b]Two doses administered at least 6 weeks apart are recommended for children ages 5 to 9 years who are receiving influenza vaccine for the first time.
From Smith et al.[29]

vaccine and the circulating viruses were well-matched.[36] These findings were corroborated by a large Cochrane Database System review, which found that TIV had an efficacy of 70% in healthy adults younger than 65 years of age, regardless of virus and vaccine concordance.[37] Vaccination of those younger than 65 years old during seasons when the virus and vaccine are well-matched results in decreased work absenteeism and healthcare resource use.[36,37]

Adults older than the age of 65 years benefit from influenza vaccination, including prevention of complications and decreased risk of influenza-related hospitalization and death. However, people in this population may not generate a strong antibody response to the vaccine and may remain susceptible to infection. In patients older than the age of 60 years who do not reside in a long-term care facility, TIV efficacy was 58% against influenza illness.[29] Although the efficacy against influenza illness for those living in long-term care facilities is between 30% and 40%, the vaccine is 50% to 60% effective in preventing influenza-related hospitalization or pneumonia and 80% effective in preventing influenza-related death.[29]

The most frequent adverse effect associated with TIV is soreness at the injection site that lasts for less than 48 hours. TIV may cause fever and malaise in those who have not previously been exposed to the viral antigens in the vaccine.[29] Allergic-type reactions (hives, systemic anaphylaxis) rarely occur after influenza vaccination and are likely a result of a reaction to residual egg protein in the vaccine.

The 1976 swine influenza vaccine was linked to a rise in the incidence of Guillain-Barré syndrome (GBS), and this has propagated the belief that TIV may cause GBS.[29] However, there is insufficient evidence to establish causality. Although several studies have failed to establish a relationship between influenza vaccination and increased frequency of GBS, two studies have demonstrated a small but significant increase in GBS following influenza vaccination.[38,39] Therefore, vaccination should be avoided in persons who are not at high risk for influenza complications and who have experienced GBS within 6 weeks of receiving a previous influenza vaccine.[29] The potential benefits of influenza vaccination in terms of prevention of severe illness, hospitalization, and mortality significantly outweigh the risks of GBS, and vaccination is recommended for all groups previously discussed.

The multidose vials and a few of the single-dose preparations of TIV contain trace to small amounts of a preservative, thimerosal, which is a mercury-containing compound (see Table 113–2). Some individuals are concerned about thimerosal exposure, particularly among children, because of the unfounded belief that thimerosal exposure is linked to the development of autism. No scientifically persuasive evidence exists to suggest harm from thimerosal exposure from a vaccine. Conversely, accumulating evidence reports the lack of harm from such exposure.[40–42] Thus, similar to GBS, the potential benefits of influenza vaccination in terms of prevention of severe illness, hospitalization, and mortality significantly outweigh the theoretical risk associated with thimerosal exposure, and vaccination is recommended for all groups previously discussed. However, to maximize the public health benefit and placate concerned individuals, thimerosal-free vaccine is available (see Table 113–2).

Live-Attenuated Influenza Vaccine

7 LAIV is made with live, attenuated viruses and is approved for intranasal administration in healthy people between 5 and 49 years of age (see Table 113–3). Advantages of LAIV include its ease of administration, intranasal rather than intramuscular administration, and the potential induction of broad mucosal and systemic immune response.[29] The mucosal response occurs at the site of viral entry and may prevent infection before viral replication occurs.[43] LAIV is more expensive than TIV and is approved for use in a more limited population.

Controlled studies support the use of LAIV in healthy people between the ages of 5 and 49 years. Although LAIV is FDA-approved for children who are at least 5 years old, a double-blind, placebo-controlled trial demonstrated efficacy of 93% against culture-confirmed influenza in children as young as 15 months (range: 15 to 71 months).[44] Moreover, those receiving vaccine had 30% fewer episodes of acute otitis media, suggesting a decrease in healthcare resource use.[44] LAIV is only approved for children over the age of 5 years in part because of data showing an increase in asthma or reactive airway disease in those younger than 5 years old.[45,46] However, in children ages 6 to 71 months there was a 52.7% reduction in culture-confirmed influenza in those who received LAIV compared to those who received TIV, and there was no difference between groups in the incidence of wheezing after vaccination.[47]

Although LAIV is FDA approved for adults younger than the age of 49 years, LAIV is effective in healthy adults between 18 and 64 years old.[48,49] Vaccination reduced the number of severe febrile illnesses by 18.8% and febrile upper respiratory tract illnesses by 23.6%.[48] Additionally, vaccination led to fewer days of illness, fewer days lost from

TABLE 113-3 Comparison of Trivalent (TIV) and Live-Attenuated Influenza Vaccine (LAIV)

Characteristic	TIV	LAIV
Age groups approved for use	>6 months	5 to 49 years
Immune status requirements	Immunocompetent or immunocompromised	Immunocompetent
Viral properties	Inactivated (killed) influenza A (H3N2), A (H1N1), and B viruses	Live-attenuated influenza A (H3N2), A (H1N1), and B viruses
Route of administration	Intramuscular	Intranasal
Immune system response	High serum IgG antibody response	Lower IgG response and high serum IgA mucosal response

TABLE 113-4 Recommended Daily Dosage of Influenza Antiviral Medications for Treatment and Prophylaxis–United States

	Age Group (y)				
Antiviral Agent	*1–6*	*7–9*	*10–12*	*13–64*	*At Least 65*
Zanamivir					
Treatment	N/A	10 mg twice daily	10 mg twice daily	10 mg twice daily	10 mg twice daily
Prophylaxis	Ages 1–4, N/A	Ages 5–9, 10 mg once daily	10 mg once daily	10 mg once daily	10 mg once daily
Oseltamivir					
Treatment[a]	According to weight[b]	According to weight[b]	According to weight[b]	75 mg twice daily	75 mg twice daily
Prophylaxis[a]	According to weight[c]	According to weight[c]	According to weight[c]	75 mg once daily	75 mg once daily

N/A, not applicable.
[a]Dose reduction recommended in those with creatinine clearance less than 30 mL/min.
[b]Treatment dosing of oseltamivir for children weighing ≤15 kg is 30 mg twice daily; for those >15 kg to 23 kg, the dose is 45 mg twice daily; for those weighing >23 kg to 40 kg, the dose is 60 mg twice daily; and for those >40 kg, the dose is 75 mg twice daily.
[c]The prophylactic dosing of oseltamivir for children weighing ≤15 kg is 30 mg once daily; for those >15 kg to 23 kg, the dose is 45 mg once daily; for those weighing >23 kg up to 40 kg, the dose is 60 mg once daily; and for those >40 kg, the dose is 75 mg once daily.
From Smith et al.[29]

work, fewer visits to healthcare providers, and decreased use of prescription antibiotics and nonprescription medications.[48]

The adverse effects typically associated with LAIV administration include runny nose, congestion, sore throat, and headache. Because LAIV contains live, attenuated viruses, viral shedding may occur for several days following vaccination with LAIV, although this should not be equated with person-to-person transmission.[29] Additionally, because LAIV contains live-attenuated viruses, which carry a theoretical infection risk, LAIV should not be given to immunosuppressed patients or given by healthcare workers who are severely immunocompromised. Moreover, for the reasons discussed in the TIV section, LAIV should not be administered to persons with a history of GBS or hypersensitivity to eggs.

CLINICAL CONTROVERSY

LAIV is not recommended in several populations, including people younger than 5 or older than 50 years and pregnant women, largely because the vaccine has not been studied extensively in these populations. However, many clinicians believe the use of LAIV in these populations is acceptable.

POSTEXPOSURE PROPHYLAXIS

8 Antiviral drugs available for prophylaxis of influenza should be considered adjuncts but are not replacements for annual vaccination. The two classes of antiviral drugs available for influenza prophylaxis are the adamantanes and the neuraminidase inhibitors. The adamantanes, amantadine and rimantadine, are currently not recommended for prophylaxis or treatment in the United States because 92% of the circulating influenza A viruses are resistant to these agents.[29] Both of the neuraminidase inhibitors, oseltamivir and zanamivir, are effective prophylactic agents against influenza in terms of preventing laboratory-confirmed influenza when used for seasonal prophylaxis (67% and 85% effective for zanamivir and oseltamivir, respectively) and preventing influenza illness among persons exposed to a household contact who was diagnosed with influenza (79% to 81% and 68% to 89% effective for zanamivir and oseltamivir, respectively).[50–52] Additionally, oseltamivir was 92% effective against influenza and also reduced associated complications when used as seasonal prophylaxis among immunized, institutionalized, elderly patients.[53] Oseltamivir is approved for prophylaxis in those older than the age of 1 year, and zanamivir is approved for prophylaxis in those older than the age of 5 years. Table 113–4 gives dosing recommendations.

In those patients who did not receive the influenza vaccination and are receiving an antiviral drug for prevention of disease during the influenza season, the medication should optimally be taken for the entire duration of influenza activity in the community. The use of prophylaxis requires clinical judgment and depends on a variety of factors, but prophylaxis should be considered during influenza season for the following groups of patients:

- Persons at high risk of serious illness and/or complications who cannot be vaccinated.
- Persons at high risk of serious illness and/or complications who are vaccinated after influenza activity has begun in their community since the development of sufficient antibody titers after vaccination takes approximately 2 weeks.
- Unvaccinated persons who have frequent contact with those at high risk.
- Persons who may have an inadequate response to vaccination (e.g., advanced HIV disease).
- Long-term care facility residents, regardless of vaccination status, when an outbreak has occurred in the institution.
- Unvaccinated household contacts of someone who was diagnosed with influenza.

LAIV should not be administered until 48 hours after influenza antiviral therapy has stopped, and influenza antiviral drugs should not be administered for 2 weeks after the administration of LAIV because the antiviral drugs inhibit influenza virus replication.[29] No contraindication exists for concomitant use of TIV and influenza antiviral drugs.

SPECIAL POPULATIONS

Pregnant women and immunocompromised hosts are special populations at increased risk of influenza complications and are also populations in whom careful consideration must be given in regard to prevention strategies.

Pregnant Women

Pregnant women, regardless of trimester, should receive annual influenza vaccination with TIV but not with LAIV. No studies have demonstrated an increased incidence of adverse effects in mothers or their infants related or potentially related to TIV, but no such data exist for LAIV.[54] TIV is also safe for breast-feeding mothers. No data exist for LAIV and breast-feeding, but caution is warranted because of the potential for viral shedding.[29] In those who are not vaccinated or those who develop disease, limited treatment options exist. The adamantanes and neuraminidase inhibitors are not recommended during pregnancy because of concerns regarding the effects of the drugs on the fetus.

Immunocompromised Hosts

Immunocompromised hosts should receive annual influenza vaccination with TIV but not LAIV. TIV was 100% effective against laboratory-confirmed influenza in HIV-positive patients with no significant effect on viral load or CD4 cell count.[55] However, antibody titers may not be as high as in immunocompetent individuals and are not improved with a second dose of vaccine.[56] Similarly, antibody titers may not be as high in solid-organ transplant patients as in immunocompetent persons, but conversely, antibody titers were increased significantly after a second dose of TIV in adult liver transplant patients.[57] Although this suggests a potential benefit from a two-dose regimen, such a regimen is not currently recommended for solid-organ transplant recipients.

Large, clinical trials evaluating the use of influenza antivirals for prophylaxis are lacking in immunocompromised hosts. Viral shedding occurs for prolonged periods in this population and may promote the development of antiviral resistance, which has already been documented with oseltamivir in HIV-positive patients.[58,59]

TREATMENT

Influenza

When prevention efforts fail or are not used, clinicians must turn to the agents available for treatment of influenza. Currently, the antiviral treatment options are limited, particularly in the face of high resistance to the adamantanes.

■ GOALS OF THERAPY

The four primary goals of therapy of influenza are as follows:

1. Control symptoms;
2. Prevent complications;
3. Decrease work and/or school absenteeism;
4. Prevent the spread of infection.

■ GENERAL APPROACH TO TREATMENT

In the era of pandemic preparedness and increasing resistance, early and definitive diagnosis of influenza is crucial. ❾ The currently available antiviral drugs are most effective if started within 48 hours of the onset of illness. Moreover, the sooner the antiviral drugs are started after the onset of illness, the more effective they are. Antiviral drugs shorten the duration of illness and provide symptom control. Adjunct agents, such as acetaminophen for fever or an antihistamine for rhinitis, may be used concomitantly with the antiviral drugs.

■ NONPHARMACOLOGIC THERAPY

Patients suffering from influenza should get adequate sleep and maintain a low level of activity. They should stay home from work and/or school in order to rest and prevent the spread of infection. Appropriate fluid intake should be maintained. Cough/throat lozenges, warm tea, or soup may help with symptom control (cough, sore throat).

■ PHARMACOLOGIC THERAPY

The two classes of antiviral drugs available for treatment of influenza are the same as those available for prophylaxis and include the adamantanes, amantadine and rimantadine, and the neuraminidase inhibitors, oseltamivir and zanamivir. Because of widespread resistance to the adamantanes among influenza A viruses in the United States, amantadine and rimantadine are not recommended for treatment of influenza until susceptibility can be reestablished. A limited discussion of these two agents can be found below, but the focus will be on the two available agents of choice, oseltamivir and zanamivir.

Amantadine/Rimantadine

Amantadine and rimantadine are adamantanes that have activity against influenza A only. The adamantanes block the M2 ion channel, which is specific to influenza A viruses, and inhibit viral uncoating. Rapid emergence of resistance is a problem with these agents because cross-resistance is conferred by a single point mutation.[29] Ninety-two percent of the circulating influenza A viruses are resistant to the adamantanes, which is why these agents are not currently recommended for treatment or prophylaxis of influenza in the United States.[29]

Oseltamivir/Zanamivir

❿ Oseltamivir and zanamivir are neuraminidase inhibitors that have activity against both influenza A and influenza B viruses. Without neuraminidase, release of the virus from infected cells is impaired, and thus, viral replication is decreased. When administered within 48 hours of the onset of illness, oseltamivir and zanamivir may reduce the duration of illness by approximately one day versus placebo.[29] In a pivotal trial, oseltamivir reduced the time to return to normal health in adults by 1.9 days and the time to return to normal activity by 2.8 days.[60] These reductions have a significant effect on not only the quality of life for the patient but also the societal costs associated with influenza. ❾ Of note, the benefits of treatment are highly dependent on the timing of the initiation of treatment, with the ideal initiation period being within 12 hours of illness onset.[61]

Oseltamivir treatment in adults and adolescents with documented influenza illness resulted in a 26.7% reduction in overall antibiotic use, a 55% reduction in lower respiratory tract complications (bronchitis, pneumonia), and a 59% reduction in hospitalizations.[62] Zanamivir treatment in adults and adolescents with influenza-like illness resulted in a 28% reduction in antibiotic use and a 40% reduction in lower respiratory tract complications.[63] The data in these studies largely come from healthy individuals rather than those at highest risk for complications associated with influenza. The impact of appropriate treatment in high-risk populations may be even greater than that which has been documented to date.

Oseltamivir is approved for treatment in those older than the age of 1 year, while zanamivir is approved for treatment in those older than the age of 7 years. The recommended dosages vary by agent and age (see Table 113–4), and the recommended duration of treatment for both agents is 5 days.

Resistance to the neuraminidase inhibitors has been documented but remains rare, and transmission of resistant viruses has not been documented to date.[29] Moreover, cross-resistance between the neuraminidase inhibitors has not been reported. A small study of oseltamivir treatment in Japanese children demonstrated a high frequency of resistant viruses (18%),[64] but this was likely caused by suboptimal dosing of oseltamivir in these children.[51]

The FDA has received 103 reports, occurring between August 29, 2005 and July 6, 2006, of delirium, hallucinations, and self-injury in pediatric patients (mostly from Japan) following treatment with oseltamivir.[65] Although a causal relationship has not been established, the label for oseltamivir has been updated to include neuropsychiatric events as a precaution.[66]

CLINICAL CONTROVERSY

Some clinicians debate the cost-benefit of the use of diagnostic tests for influenza as well as treatment of influenza in otherwise healthy individuals who are likely to experience resolution without treatment. This controversy is compounded by the fact that the diagnostic tests and the benefits associated with treatment of influenza are highest early in the disease process, and many patients present after this time period.

SPECIAL POPULATIONS

Inadequate data exist regarding the use of antiinfluenza medications in special populations, such as immunocompromised hosts. Furthermore, no clinical studies have been conducted evaluating the safety and efficacy of the adamantanes or the neuraminidase inhibitors during pregnancy, and all of the drugs are Pregnancy Category C. The adamantanes are embryotoxic and teratogenic in rats, and limited case reports of adverse fetal outcomes following amantadine use in humans have been published. No such data exist for the neuraminidase inhibitors. Both the adamantanes and the neuraminidase inhibitors are excreted in breast milk and should be avoided by mothers who are breast-feeding their infants. More studies are needed in these populations who are at high risk for serious disease and complications from influenza.

EVALUATION OF THERAPEUTIC OUTCOMES

Patients should be monitored daily for resolution of signs and symptoms associated with influenza, such as fever, myalgia, headache, malaise, nonproductive cough, sore throat, and rhinitis. These signs and symptoms will typically resolve within approximately 1 week. If the patient continues to exhibit signs and symptoms of illness beyond 10 days or a worsening of symptoms after 7 days, a physician visit is warranted as this may be an indication of a secondary bacterial infection. Ideally, antiviral therapy should not be started until influenza is confirmed via the laboratory. However, therapy should be initiated within 48 hours of illness onset, emphasizing the need for rapid diagnosis. Repeat diagnostic tests to demonstrate clearance of the virus are not necessary.

CONCLUSIONS

Influenza is associated with significant morbidity and mortality and substantial burden to society in terms of both direct and indirect costs. Prevention of influenza by vaccination may yield significant benefit to society in terms of reductions in influenza-related complications, decreased work/school absenteeism, reductions in hospitalizations and deaths, and general cost savings. Two highly effective influenza vaccines are currently available in the United States, yet influenza remains the leading cause of vaccine-preventable mortality. This underscores the need for targeted efforts toward populations at high risk for serious disease and complications as well as the need for more vaccines, particularly for certain populations (e.g., those younger than 6 months old, those with hypersensitivity to eggs).

Four antiviral drugs are available for treatment and prophylaxis of influenza. Thus, the antiinfluenza antiviral armamentarium is limited and has been further reduced by the significant resistance to the adamantanes in recent years. Importantly, these agents are not a replacement for vaccination but rather an adjunct. Although the neuraminidase inhibitors remain useful as agents for treatment and prophylaxis of influenza, information on the use of these agents in special populations, such as immunocompromised hosts and pregnant women, is limited. The best mechanism to decrease the morbidity, mortality, and societal burden associated with influenza remains prevention of the disease through annual vaccination.

ABBREVIATIONS

DFA: direct fluorescent antibody

FDA: Food and Drug Administration

GBS: Guillain-Barré syndrome

HIV: human immunodeficiency virus

LAIV: live-attenuated influenza vaccine

POC: point of care

RT-PCR: reverse-transcription polymerase chain reaction

TIV: trivalent influenza vaccine

REFERENCES

1. American Lung Association. Trends in Pneumonia and Influenza Morbidity and Mortality. American Lung Association. New York. Research and Scientific Affairs Epidemiology and Statistics Unit, 2004.
2. Thompson WW, Shay DK, Weintraub E, et al. Influenza-associated hospitalizations in the United States. JAMA 2004;292(11):1333–1340.
3. Simonsen L, Clarke MJ, Schonberger LB, et al. Pandemic versus epidemic influenza mortality: A pattern of changing age distribution. J Infect Dis 1998;178(1):53–60.
4. Thompson WW, Shay DK, Weintraub E, et al. Mortality associated with influenza and respiratory syncytial virus in the United States. JAMA 2003;289(2):179–186.
5. Nicholson KG, Wood JM, Zambon M. Influenza. Lancet 2003; 362(9397):1733–1745.
6. Barry JM. The site of origin of the 1918 influenza pandemic and its public health implications. J Transl Med 2004;2(1):3.
7. Monto AS, Comanor L, Shay DK, Thompson WW. Epidemiology of pandemic influenza: Use of surveillance and modeling for pandemic preparedness. J Infect Dis 2006;194(Suppl 2):S92–S97.
8. Palese P. Influenza: Old and new threats. Nat Med 2004;10(12 Suppl):S82–S87.
9. Taubenberger JK, Morens DM. 1918 influenza: The mother of all pandemics. Emerg Infect Dis 2006;12(1):15–22.
10. Kash JC, Basler CF, Garcia-Sastre A, et al. Global host immune response: Pathogenesis and transcriptional profiling of type A influenza viruses expressing the hemagglutinin and neuraminidase genes from the 1918 pandemic virus. J Virol 2004;78(17):9499–9511.
11. Tumpey TM, Garcia-Sastre A, Taubenberger JK, et al. Pathogenicity and immunogenicity of influenza viruses with genes from the 1918 pandemic virus. Proc Natl Acad Sci U S A 2004;101(9):3166–3171.
12. Oxford JS. Influenza a pandemics of the 20th century with special reference to 1918: Virology, pathology and epidemiology. Rev Med Virol 2000;10(2):119–133.
13. Belshe RB. The origins of pandemic influenza—lessons from the 1918 virus. N Engl J Med 2005;353(21):2209–2211.
14. Lipatov AS, Govorkova EA, Webby RJ, et al. Influenza: Emergence and control. J Virol 2004;78(17):8951–8959.
15. Yuen KY, Chan PK, Peiris M, et al. Clinical features and rapid viral diagnosis of human disease associated with avian influenza A H5N1 virus. Lancet 1998;351(9101):467–471.
16. Mounts AW, Kwong H, Izurieta HS, et al. Case-control study of risk factors for avian influenza A (H5N1) disease, Hong Kong, 1997. J Infect Dis 1999;180(2):505–508.
17. Anonymous. Epidemic and Pandemic Alert and Response: Avian Influenza. *http://www.who.int/csr/disease/avian_influenza/en/index.html.* Nov 13, 2006.
18. Tran TH, Nguyen TL, Nguyen TD, et al. Avian influenza A (H5N1) in 10 patients in Vietnam. N Engl J Med 2004;350(12):1179–1188.
19. Ungchusak K, Auewarakul P, Dowell SF, et al. Probable person-to-person transmission of avian influenza A (H5N1). N Engl J Med 2005;352(4):333–340.
20. Beigel JH, Farrar J, Han AM, et al. Avian influenza A (H5N1) infection in humans. N Engl J Med 2005;353(13):1374–1385.
21. Hill DR. The burden of illness in international travelers. N Engl J Med 2006;354(2):115–117.
22. U.S. Department of Health and Human Services. HHS Pandemic Influenza Plan. *http://www.hhs.gov/pandemicflu/plan/.* Nov 2005.
23. Fauci AS. Seasonal and pandemic influenza preparedness: Science and countermeasures. J Infect Dis 2006;194(Suppl 2):S73–S76.
24. U.S. Department of Health and Human Services. HHS Buys More Antiviral Medication for the Strategic National Stockpile. *http://www.hhs.gov/news/press/2006pres/20060322.html.* March 22, 2006.

25. Nichol KL, Treanor JJ. Vaccines for seasonal and pandemic influenza. J Infect Dis 2006;194(Suppl 2):S111–S118.
26. Bridges CB, Kuehnert MJ, Hall CB. Transmission of influenza: Implications for control in health care settings. Clin Infect Dis 2003;37(8):1094–1101.
27. Salgado CD, Farr BM, Hall KK, Hayden FG. Influenza in the acute hospital setting. Lancet Infect Dis 2002;2(3):145–155.
28. Cox NJ, Subbarao K. Influenza. Lancet 1999;354(9186):1277–1282.
29. Smith NM, Bresee JS, Shay DK, et al. Prevention and control of influenza: Recommendations of the Advisory Committee on Immunization Practices (ACIP). MMWR Recomm Rep 2006;55(RR-10):1–42.
30. Boivin G, Goyette N, Bernatchez H. Prolonged excretion of amantadine-resistant influenza A virus quasi species after cessation of antiviral therapy in an immunocompromised patient. Clin Infect Dis 2002; 34(5):E23–E25.
31. Cheung CY, Poon LL, Lau AS, et al. Induction of proinflammatory cytokines in human macrophages by influenza A (H5N1) viruses: A mechanism for the unusual severity of human disease? Lancet 2002;360(9348):1831–1837.
32. Petric M, Comanor L, Petti CA. Role of the laboratory in diagnosis of influenza during seasonal epidemics and potential pandemics. J Infect Dis 2006;194(Suppl 2):S98–S110.
33. Neuzil KM, Zhu Y, Griffin MR, et al. Burden of interpandemic influenza in children younger than 5 years: A 25-year prospective study. J Infect Dis 2002;185(2):147–152.
34. Newton DW, Treanor JJ, Menegus MA. Clinical and laboratory diagnosis of influenza virus infections. Am J Manag Care 2000;6(5 Suppl):S265–S275.
35. Hoberman A, Greenberg DP, Paradise JL, et al. Effectiveness of inactivated influenza vaccine in preventing acute otitis media in young children: A randomized controlled trial. JAMA 2003;290(12):1608–1616.
36. Bridges CB, Thompson WW, Meltzer MI, et al. Effectiveness and cost-benefit of influenza vaccination of healthy working adults: A randomized controlled trial. JAMA 2000;284(13):1655–1663.
37. Demicheli V, Rivetti D, Deeks JJ, Jefferson TO. Vaccines for preventing influenza in healthy adults. Cochrane Database Syst Rev 2004;(3):CD001269.
38. Juurlink DN, Stukel TA, Kwong J, et al. Guillain-Barré syndrome after influenza vaccination in adults: A population-based study. Arch Intern Med 2006;166(20):2217–2221.
39. Lasky T, Terracciano GJ, Magder L, et al. The Guillain-Barré syndrome and the 1992–1993 and 1993–1994 influenza vaccines. N Engl J Med 1998;339(25):1797–1802.
40. Summary of the joint statement on thimerosal in vaccines. American Academy of Family Physicians, American Academy of Pediatrics, Advisory Committee on Immunization Practices, Public Health Service. MMWR Morb Mortal Wkly Rep 2000;49(27):622, 631.
41. McCormick MC. The autism "epidemic": Impressions from the perspective of immunization safety review. Ambul Pediatr 2003;3(3):119–120.
42. Verstraeten T, Davis RL, DeStefano F, et al. Safety of thimerosal-containing vaccines: A two-phased study of computerized health maintenance organization databases. Pediatrics 2003;112(5):1039–1048.
43. Boyce TG, Poland GA. Promises and challenges of live-attenuated intranasal influenza vaccines across the age spectrum: A review. Biomed Pharmacother 2000;54(4):210–218.
44. Belshe RB, Mendelman PM, Treanor J, et al. The efficacy of live attenuated, cold-adapted, trivalent, intranasal influenzavirus vaccine in children. N Engl J Med 1998;338(20):1405–1412.
45. Belshe RB, Nichol KL, Black SB, et al. Safety, efficacy, and effectiveness of live, attenuated, cold-adapted influenza vaccine in an indicated population aged 5–49 years. Clin Infect Dis 2004;39(7):920–927.
46. Bergen R, Black S, Shinefield H, et al. Safety of cold-adapted live attenuated influenza vaccine in a large cohort of children and adolescents. Pediatr Infect Dis J 2004;23(2):138–144.
47. Ashkenazi S, Vertruyen A, Aristegui J, et al. Superior relative efficacy of live attenuated influenza vaccine compared with inactivated influenza vaccine in young children with recurrent respiratory tract infections. Pediatr Infect Dis J 2006;25(10):870–879.
48. Nichol KL, Mendelman PM, Mallon KP, et al. Effectiveness of live, attenuated intranasal influenza virus vaccine in healthy, working adults: A randomized controlled trial. JAMA 1999;282(2):137–144.
49. Treanor JJ, Kotloff K, Betts RF, et al. Evaluation of trivalent, live, cold-adapted (CAIV-T) and inactivated (TIV) influenza vaccines in prevention of virus infection and illness following challenge of adults with wild-type influenza A (H1N1), A (H3N2), and B viruses. Vaccine 1999;18(9–10):899–906.
50. Hayden FG, Atmar RL, Schilling M, et al. Use of the selective oral neuraminidase inhibitor oseltamivir to prevent influenza. N Engl J Med 1999;341(18):1336–1343.
51. Hayden FG, Pavia AT. Antiviral management of seasonal and pandemic influenza. J Infect Dis 2006;194(Suppl 2):S119–S126.
52. Monto AS, Pichichero ME, Blanckenberg SJ, et al. Zanamivir prophylaxis: An effective strategy for the prevention of influenza types A and B within households. J Infect Dis 2002;186(11):1582–1588.
53. Peters PH Jr, Gravenstein S, Norwood P, et al. Long-term use of oseltamivir for the prophylaxis of influenza in a vaccinated frail older population. J Am Geriatr Soc 2001;49(8):1025–1031.
54. Englund JA. Maternal immunization with inactivated influenza vaccine: Rationale and experience. Vaccine 2003;21(24):3460–3464.
55. Tasker SA, Treanor JJ, Paxton WB, Wallace MR. Efficacy of influenza vaccination in HIV-infected persons. A randomized, double-blind, placebo-controlled trial. Ann Intern Med 1999;131(6):430–433.
56. Kroon FP, van Dissel JT, de Jong JC, et al. Antibody response after influenza vaccination in HIV-infected individuals: A consecutive 3-year study. Vaccine 2000;18(26):3040–3049.
57. Soesman NM, Rimmelzwaan GF, Nieuwkoop NJ, et al. Efficacy of influenza vaccination in adult liver transplant recipients. J Med Virol 2000;61(1):85–93.
58. Ison MG, Gubareva LV, Atmar RL, et al. Recovery of drug-resistant influenza virus from immunocompromised patients: A case series. J Infect Dis 2006;193(6):760–764.
59. Whitley RJ, Monto AS. Prevention and treatment of influenza in high-risk groups: Children, pregnant women, immunocompromised hosts, and nursing home residents. J Infect Dis 2006;194(Suppl 2):S133–S138.
60. Treanor JJ, Hayden FG, Vrooman PS, et al. Efficacy and safety of the oral neuraminidase inhibitor oseltamivir in treating acute influenza: A randomized controlled trial. US Oral Neuraminidase Study Group. JAMA 2000;283(8):1016–1024.
61. Aoki FY, Macleod MD, Paggiaro P, et al. Early administration of oral oseltamivir increases the benefits of influenza treatment. J Antimicrob Chemother 2003;51(1):123–129.
62. Kaiser L, Wat C, Mills T, et al. Impact of oseltamivir treatment on influenza-related lower respiratory tract complications and hospitalizations. Arch Intern Med 2003;163(14):1667–1672.
63. Kaiser L, Keene ON, Hammond JM, et al. Impact of zanamivir on antibiotic use for respiratory events following acute influenza in adolescents and adults. Arch Intern Med 2000;160(21):3234–3240.
64. Kiso M, Mitamura K, Sakai-Tagawa Y, et al. Resistant influenza A viruses in children treated with oseltamivir: Descriptive study. Lancet 2004;364(9436):759–765.
65. Bridges A. FDA. Tamiflu patients need monitoring. Washington, DC: Associated Press, November 14, 2006.
66. Tamiflu product information. Roche Laboratories Inc. *http://www.rocheusa.com/products/tamiflu/pi.pdf*. July 2007.

CHAPTER 114 Skin and Soft-Tissue Infections

DOUGLAS N. FISH, SUSAN L. PENDLAND, AND LARRY H. DANZIGER

KEY CONCEPTS

1. Folliculitis, furuncles (boils), and carbuncles begin around hair follicles and are caused most often by *Staphylococcus aureus*. Folliculitis and small furuncles are generally treated with warm, moist heat to promote drainage; large furuncles and carbuncles require incision and drainage. A penicillinase-resistant penicillin such as dicloxacillin is commonly used for extensive or serious infections (e.g., fever).

2. Erysipelas, a superficial skin infection with extensive lymphatic involvement, is caused by *Streptococcus pyogenes*. The treatment of choice is penicillin, administered orally or parenterally, depending on the severity of the infection.

3. Impetigo is a superficial skin infection that occurs most commonly in children. It is characterized by fluid-filled vesicles that develop rapidly into pus-filled blisters that rupture to form golden-yellow crusts. Effective therapy includes penicillinase-resistant penicillins (dicloxacillin), first-generation cephalosporins (cephalexin), and topical mupirocin. *S. aureus* is the primary cause of impetigo, with infections caused by community-associated methicillin-resistant *S. aureus* (CA-MRSA) emerging in recent years.

4. Lymphangitis, an infection of the subcutaneous lymphatic channels, is generally caused by *S. pyogenes*. Acute lymphangitis is characterized by the rapid development of fine, red, linear streaks extending from the initial infection site toward the regional lymph nodes, which are usually enlarged and tender. Penicillin is the drug of choice.

5. Cellulitis is an infection of the epidermis, dermis, and superficial fascia most commonly caused by *S. pyogenes* and *S. aureus*. Lesions generally are hot, painful, and erythematous, with nonelevated, poorly defined margins. Treatment generally consists of a penicillinase-resistant penicillin (dicloxacillin) or first-generation cephalosporin (cephalexin) for 5 to 10 days. Trimethoprim-sulfamethoxazole should be considered for treatment of suspected staphylococcal infections in areas with a high prevalence of CA-MRSA.

6. Necrotizing fasciitis is a rare but life-threatening infection of subcutaneous tissue that results in progressive destruction of superficial fascia and subcutaneous fat. Early and aggressive surgical debridement is an essential part of therapy for treatment of necrotizing fasciitis. Infections caused by *S. pyogenes* or *Clostridium* species should be treated with the combination of penicillin and clindamycin.

7. Diabetic foot infections are managed with a comprehensive treatment approach that includes both proper wound care and antimicrobial therapy. Antimicrobial regimens for diabetic foot infections should include broad-spectrum coverage of staphylococci, streptococci, enteric gram-negative bacilli, and anaerobes. Outpatient therapy with oral antimicrobials should be used whenever possible.

8. Prevention is the single most important aspect in the management of pressure sores. After a sore develops, successful local care includes a comprehensive approach consisting of relief of pressure, proper cleaning (debridement), disinfection, and appropriate antimicrobial therapy if an infection is present. Good wound care is crucial to successful management.

9. All bite wounds (either animal or human) should be irrigated thoroughly with large volumes of sterile normal saline, and the injured area should be immobilized and elevated. Depending on the severity of the bite wound, amoxicillin-clavulanic acid or ampicillin-sulbactam are often used for treatment of animal bites because of their coverage of *Pasteurella multocida*, *S. aureus*, and anaerobes typically present in the oral flora of dogs and cats.

10. Although antimicrobial prophylaxis of dog or cat bites is not recommended routinely, patients with human bite injuries should be given prophylactic antimicrobial therapy for 3 to 5 days. Infected wounds, particularly clenched-fist injuries, should be treated for 7 to 14 days with ampicillin-sulbactam, cefoxitin, or other combination that has activity against *Eikenella corrodens*, *S. aureus*, and β-lactamase–producing anaerobes.

Learning objectives, review questions, and other resources can be found at **www.pharmacotherapyonline.com.**

The skin serves as a barrier between humans and their environment and therefore functions as a primary defense mechanism against infections. The skin consists of the epidermis, the dermis, and subcutaneous fat. The epidermis is the outermost, nonvascular layer of the skin. It varies in thickness from approximately 0.1 mm on most areas of the body to a maximum of 1.5 mm on the soles of the feet. Although extremely thin, the epidermis is composed of several layers. The innermost layer consists of continuously dividing cells. The outer layers are renewed as cells are gradually pushed outward. As the cells approach the surface, they become flattened, lose their nuclei, and are filled with keratin. The outermost layer, the stratum corneum, is composed of flattened, cornified, nonnucleated cells. The dermis is the layer of skin directly beneath the epidermis. It consists of connective tissue and contains blood vessels and lymphatics, sensory nerve endings, sweat and sebaceous glands, hair follicles, and smooth muscle fibers. Beneath the dermis is a layer of loose connective tissue containing primarily fat cells. This subcutaneous fat layer is of variable thickness over the body. Beneath the subcutaneous fat lies the fascia, which separates the skin from underlying muscle. It is generally divided into superficial fascia, which is located immediately beneath the skin, and deep fascia, which forms sheaths for muscles.

Skin and soft-tissue infections (SSTIs) may involve any or all layers of the skin, fascia, and muscle. They also may spread far from the initial site of infection and lead to more severe complications, such as endocarditis, gram-negative sepsis, or streptococcal glomerulonephritis. Sometimes the treatment of SSTIs may necessitate both medical and surgical management. This chapter presents details of the pathogenesis and management of some of the most common infections involving the skin and soft tissues. The first part of the chapter discusses a variety of SSTIs that range in severity from superficial to life-threatening. The remainder of the chapter discusses diabetic foot infections, pressure sores, and human and animal bites.

EPIDEMIOLOGY

A number of classification schemes have been developed to describe SSTIs. Bacterial infections of the skin can be classified as primary or secondary (Table 114–1). Primary bacterial infections usually involve areas of previously healthy skin and typically are caused by a single pathogen. In contrast, secondary infections occur in areas of previously damaged skin and are frequently polymicrobic. SSTIs are also classified as complicated or uncomplicated. Infections are considered complicated when they involve deeper skin structures (e.g., fascia, muscle layers), require significant surgical intervention, or occur in patients with compromised immune function (e.g., diabetes mellitus, human immunodeficiency virus [HIV] infection).[1]

The classification system developed by Eron divides SSTIs into four classes based on severity of signs and symptoms, as well as the presence and stability of any comorbidities.[2] The classification was used to develop an algorithm to help with admission and treatment decisions. Class 1 includes patients who are afebrile and otherwise healthy. These patients generally can be managed on an outpatient basis with topical or oral antimicrobials. Class 2 includes patients who are febrile and ill-appearing but who have no unstable comorbid conditions. Some class 2 patients may be treated with oral antimicrobials, but most are likely to require some parenteral therapy, either as an outpatient or with short-term hospitalization. Patients having a toxic appearance, unstable comorbidity, or a limb-threatening infection are grouped into class 3. Class 4 includes patients with sepsis syndrome or another life-threatening infection, such as necrotizing fasciitis. Patients in classes 3 and 4 require hospitalization and parenteral antimicrobial therapy initially but may be candidates for oral or outpatient parenteral therapy once their condition has stabilized. Patients in class 4 also generally require some type of surgical intervention.

TABLE 114-1 Bacterial Classification of Important Skin and Soft-Tissue Infections

Primary infections	
Erysipelas	Group A streptococci
Impetigo	*Staphylococcus aureus*, group A streptococci
Lymphangitis	Group A streptococci; occasionally *S. aureus*
Cellulitis	Group A streptococci, *S. aureus*; occasionally other gram-positive cocci, gram-negative bacilli, and/or anaerobes
Necrotizing fasciitis	
Type I	Anaerobes (*Bacteroides* spp., *Peptostreptococcus* spp.) and facultative bacteria (streptococci, Enterobacteriaceae)
Type II	Group A streptococci
Secondary infections	
Diabetic foot infections	*S. aureus*, streptococci, Enterobacteriaceae, *Bacteroides* spp., *Peptostreptococcus* spp., *Pseudomonas aeruginosa*
Pressure sores	*S. aureus*, streptococci, Enterobacteriaceae, *Bacteroides* spp., *Peptostreptococcus* spp., *Pseudomonas aeruginosa*
Bite wounds	
Animal	*Pasteurella multocida*, *S. aureus*, streptococci, *Bacteroides* spp.
Human	*Eikenella corrodens*, *S. aureus*, streptococci, *Corynebacterium* spp., *Bacteroides* spp., *Peptostreptococcus* spp.
Burn wounds	*Pseudomonas aeruginosa*, Enterobacteriaceae, *S. aureus*, streptoccocci

SSTIs are among the most common infections seen in both community and hospital settings.[3] However, data on the exact incidence of SSTIs are lacking. Most infections are believed to be mild and therefore are treated in an outpatient setting, making it difficult to quantify community-acquired SSTIs. One description of office visits among health plan members listed cellulitis and impetigo as the primary diagnosis for 2.2% and 0.3% of patients, respectively.[4] According to the most recent Healthcare Cost and Utilization Project Nationwide Inpatient Sample, SSTIs are the 28th most common diagnosis of patients in community hospitals.[5] Soft-tissue infections were the leading cause of admissions for medical or surgical treatment in a large academic medical center.[3] Approximately 0.1% of the adult population in the United States required hospitalization for SSTIs in 1995.[2]

Although the exact incidence of SSTIs is unknown, the frequency of infections caused by invasive group A streptococci and drug-resistant gram-positive cocci has been increasing.[1] Group A streptococci (*Streptococcus pyogenes*) are among the most common etiologic agents of SSTIs. Although they may be found in many mild, superficial skin infections, they are also responsible for life-threatening cases of necrotizing fasciitis.[1] A dramatic increase in necrotizing fasciitis caused by *S. pyogenes* is a major concern because of the high morbidity and mortality associated with these infections.

Another worrisome trend is the increased in vitro resistance reported for many gram-positive bacteria.[1] While the high incidence of nosocomial methicillin-resistant *Staphylococcus aureus* (MRSA) has been a major concern for the past decade,[6–8] the recent emergence of community-associated MRSA (CA-MRSA) is even more problematic.[9–16] CA-MRSA strains have been isolated from patients lacking typical risk factors (e.g., prior hospitalization, long-term care facility) and are generally susceptible to non–β-lactam antibiotics (trimethoprim-sulfamethoxazole, doxycycline, clindamycin).[9,11,13] They also differ genetically from nosocomial strains of MRSA with methicillin resistance carried on the type IV staphylococcal chromosomal cassette *mec* (SCC*mec*) element of the *mecA* gene. CA-MRSA strains often harbor genes for Panton-Valentine leukocidin, a cytotoxin responsible for leukocyte destruction and tissue necrosis. In contrast, nosocomial strains usually lack genes for Panton-Valentine leukocidin and are associated with SCC*mec* alleles I to III.[10,11,16] Clinicians should suspect CA-MRSA in geographic areas with a high prevalence of these strains, or in recurrent or persistent infections that are not responding to appropriate β-lactam therapy. In addition to the emergence of CA-MRSA, treatment choices for SSTIs have been further complicated by the increased incidence of macrolide-resistant strains of *Staphylococcus aureus* and *S. pyogenes*.[1,8,11]

ETIOLOGY

The majority of SSTIs are caused by gram-positive organisms present on the skin surface.[1] Gram-positive bacteria (coagulase-negative staphylococci, diphtheroids) are the predominant flora of the skin, with gram-negative organisms (*Escherichia coli* and other

TABLE 114-2 Predominant Microorganisms of Normal Skin

Bacteria
Gram-positive
Coagulase-negative staphylococci
Micrococci (*Micrococcus luteus*)
Corynebacterium species (diphtheroids)
Propionibacterium species
Gram-negative
Acinetobacter species
Fungi
Malassezia species
Candida species

Enterobacteriaceae) being relatively uncommon[17] (Table 114–2). *S. aureus*, as well as a variety of gram-negative bacteria, can be found in moist intertriginous areas (e.g., axilla, groin, and toe webs) of the body. *Acinetobacter* species have been cultured from these moister areas in 25% of the population.[17] *S. aureus* also inhabits the anterior nares of approximately 30% of healthy individuals.[17] Colonization, whether transient or permanent, provides a nidus for infection should the integrity of the epidermis be compromised.

S. aureus and *S. pyogenes* account for the majority of community-acquired SSTIs.[1] Data from the most recent SENTRY Antimicrobial Surveillance Program showed *S. aureus* to be the most common cause (45%) of SSTIs in hospitalized patients.[6,7] Also of note in this study was the 36% incidence of methicillin resistance among strains of *S. aureus*. Other common nosocomial pathogens included *Pseudomonas aeruginosa* (11%), enterococci (9%), and *E. coli* (7%).[6,7]

PATHOPHYSIOLOGY

The skin and subcutaneous tissues normally are extremely resistant to infection but may become susceptible under certain conditions. Even when high concentrations of bacteria are applied topically or injected into the soft tissue, resulting infections are rare.[17] Several host factors act together to confer protection against skin infections. Because the surface of the skin is relatively dry and has a pH of approximately 5.6, it is not conducive to bacterial growth.[17] Continuous renewal of the epidermal layer results in the shedding of keratocytes, as well as skin bacteria. In addition, sebaceous secretions are hydrolyzed to form free fatty acids that strongly inhibit the growth of many bacteria and fungi.[4] The conditions that may predispose a patient to the development of skin infections include (a) a high concentration of bacteria ($>10^5$ microorganisms), (b) excessive moisture of the skin, (c) inadequate blood supply, (d) availability of bacterial nutrients, and (e) damage to the corneal layer allowing for bacterial penetration.[4,17]

The majority of SSTIs result from the disruption of normal host defenses by processes such as skin puncture, abrasion, or underlying diseases (e.g., diabetes). The nature and severity of the infection depend on both the type of microorganism present and the site of inoculation.

FOLLICULITIS, FURUNCLES, AND CARBUNCLES

❶ Folliculitis is inflammation of the hair follicle and can be caused by physical injury, chemical irritation, or infection.[4] Infection occurring at the base of the eyelid is referred to as a stye. While folliculitis is a superficial infection with pus present only in the dermis, furuncles and carbuncles occur when a follicular infection extends from around the hair shaft to involve the deeper areas of the skin. A furuncle, commonly known as an *abscess* or *boil*, is a walled-off mass of purulent material arising from a hair follicle.[4] The lesions are called *carbuncles* when they coalesce and extend to the subcutaneous tissue. This aggregate of infected hair follicles forms deep masses that generally open and drain through multiple sinus tracts.[4] *S. aureus* is the most common cause of folliculitis, furuncles, and carbuncles. Inadequate chlorine levels in whirlpools, hot tubs, and swimming pools have been responsible for outbreaks of folliculitis caused by *P. aeruginosa*.[18] Outbreaks of furunculosis caused by *S. aureus* and CA-MRSA have been reported in settings involving close contact (such as with families, prisons), especially when skin injury was common (such as with sports). In addition, some individuals experience repeated attacks of furunculosis. The major predisposing factor in this population is the presence of *S. aureus* in the anterior nares.[11]

CLINICAL PRESENTATION

Folliculitis

- Pruritic, erythematous papules typically appear within 48 hours (range: 6 to 72 hours) of exposure to large numbers of organisms.
- Papules evolve into pustules that generally heal in several days.
- Systemic signs such as fever and malaise are uncommon, although they have been reported in cases caused by *P. aeruginosa*.

Furuncles

- Furuncles can occur anywhere on hairy skin but generally develop in areas subject to friction and perspiration.
- Furuncles are discrete lesions, whether occurring as singular or multiple nodules.
- The lesion starts as a firm, tender, red nodule that becomes painful and fluctuant.
- Lesions often drain spontaneously.
- Lesions caused by CA-MRSA often have necrotic centers characteristic of "spider bites."

Carbuncles

- Carbuncles are broad, swollen, erythematous, deep, and painful follicular masses.
- Carbuncles commonly develop on the back of the neck and are more likely to occur in patients with diabetes.
- Unlike folliculitis and furuncles, carbuncles are commonly associated with fever, chills, and malaise.
- Bacteremia with secondary spread to other tissues is common.

TREATMENT

Folliculitis, Furuncles, and Carbuncles

Table 114–3 summarizes evidence-based treatment recommendations from recently published clinical guidelines for SSTIs.[11,19] Treatment of folliculitis generally requires only local measures, such as warm moist compresses or topical therapy (e.g., clindamycin, erythromycin, mupirocin, or benzoyl peroxide).[20] Topical agents generally are applied two to four times daily for 7 days. Small furuncles generally can be treated with moist heat, which promotes localization and drainage of pus.[20] Large and/or multiple furuncles and carbuncles require incision and drainage.[20] Systemic antibiotics are generally not necessary unless accompanied by fever or extensive cellulitis.[11] For more severe infections, treatment generally consists of a penicillinase-resistant penicillin or a first-generation cephalosporin for 5 to 10 days (refer to Table 114–4 for adult and pediatric doses). An alternative agent for penicillin-allergic patients is clindamycin. For individuals with nasal

TABLE 114-3 Evidence-Based Recommendations for Treatment of Skin and Soft-Tissue Infections

Recommendations	Recommendation Grade
Folliculitis, furuncles, carbuncles	
Folliculitis and small furuncles can be treated with moist heat; large furuncles and carbuncles require incision and drainage. Antimicrobial therapy is unnecessary unless extensive lesions or fever are present.	E-III
Erysipelas	
Most infections are caused by *Streptococcus pyogenes*. Penicillin (oral or intravenous depending on clinical severity) is the drug of choice.	A-I
If *Staphylococcus aureus* is suspected, a penicillinase-resistant penicillin or first-generation cephalosporin should be used.	A-I
Impetigo	
S. aureus accounts for the majority of infections; consequently, a penicillin-resistant penicillin or first-generation cephalosporin is recommended.	A-I
Topical therapy with mupirocin is equivalent to oral therapy.	A-I
Cellulitis	
Mild-moderate infections can generally be treated with oral agents (dicloxacillin, cephalexin, clindamycin) unless resistance is high in the community.	A-I
Serious infections should be treated intravenously with a penicillinase-resistant penicillin (nafcillin) or first-generation cephalosporin (cefazolin). Patients with penicillin allergies should be treated with vancomycin or clindamycin.	A-I
Vancomycin, linezolid, and daptomycin should be used to treat serious infections caused by methicillin-resistant *S. aureus*.	A-I
Necrotizing fasciitis	
Early and aggressive surgical debridement of all necrotic tissue is essential.	A-III
Necrotizing fasciitis caused by *S. pyogenes* should be treated with the combination of clindamycin and penicillin.	A-II
Clostridial gas gangrene (myonecrosis) should be treated with clindamycin and penicillin.	B-III
Diabetic foot infections	
Many mild to moderate infections can be treated with oral agents that possess high bioavailability.	A-II
All severe infections should be treated with intravenous therapy. After initial response, step-down therapy to oral agents can be used.	C-III
Broad-spectrum antimicrobial therapy is not generally required, except for some severe cases.	B-III
Definitive therapy should be based on results of appropriately collected cultures and sensitivities, as well as clinical response to empiric antimicrobial agents.	C-III
Optimal wound care, in additional to appropriate antimicrobial therapy, is essential for wound healing.	A-1
Animal bites	
Many bite wounds can be treated on an outpatient basis with amoxicillin-clavulanic acid.	B-II
Serious infections requiring intravenous antimicrobial therapy can be treated with a β-lactam/β-lactamase inhibitor combination or second-generation cephalosporin with activity against anaerobes (cefoxitin).	B-II
Penicillinase-resistant penicillins, first-generation cephalosporins, macrolides, and clindamycin should not be used for treatment because of their poor activity against *Pasteurella multocida*.	D-III
Human bites	
Antimicrobial therapy should provide coverage against *Eikenella corrodens*, *S. aureus*, and β-lactamase producing anaerobes.	B-III

Strength of recommendation: A, good evidence for use; B, moderate evidence for use; C, poor evidence for use, optional; D, moderate evidence to support not using; E, good evidence to support not using.
Quality of evidence: I, evidence from ≥1 properly randomized, controlled trials; II, evidence from ≥1 well-designed clinical trials without randomization, case-controlled analytic studies, multiple time series, or dramatic results from uncontrolled experiments; III, evidence from expert opinion, clinical experience, descriptive studies, or reports of expert committees.

colonization, application of mupirocin ointment twice daily in the anterior nares for the first 5 days of each month decreases recurrent furunculosis by almost half.[11] In addition, a single oral daily dose of clindamycin 150 mg for 3 months reduced recurrent infections caused by susceptible strains of *S. aureus* by approximately 80%.[11]

EVALUATION OF THERAPEUTIC OUTCOMES

Many follicular infections resolve spontaneously without medical or surgical intervention. Lesions should be incised if they do not respond to a few days of moist heat and nonprescription topical agents. Following drainage, most lesions begin to heal within several days without antimicrobial therapy. Any patient who is unresponsive to several days of therapy with a penicillinase-resistant penicillin or first-generation cephalosporin should have a culture and sensitivity performed because of the increasing frequency of CA-MRSA.

ERYSIPELAS

❷ Erysipelas is an infection of the more superficial layers of the skin and cutaneous lymphatics.[21] The intense red color and burning pain associated with this skin infection led to the common name of St. Anthony's fire. The infection is almost always caused by β-hemolytic streptococci, with the organisms gaining access via small breaks in the skin. Group A streptococci (*S. pyogenes*) are responsible for most infections.[11,22] Infections are more common in infants, young children, the elderly, and patients with nephrotic syndrome.[20] Erysipelas also commonly occurs in areas of preexisting lymphatic obstruction or edema.[20] Diagnosis is made on the basis of the characteristic lesion.

CLINICAL PRESENTATION

General

- The lower extremities are the most common sites for erysipelas.

Symptoms

- Patients often experience flu-like symptoms (fever, malaise) prior to the appearance of the lesion.
- The infected area is described as painful or as a burning pain.

Signs

- The lesion is bright red and edematous, often with lymphatic streaking.
- Temperature is often mildly elevated.
- The clinical presentation differs from cellulitis in that the lesion has clearly demarcated raised margins.

TABLE 114-4 Recommended Drugs and Dosing Regimens for Outpatient Treatment of Mild–Moderate Skin and Soft-Tissue Infections

Infection	Oral Adult Dose	Oral Pediatric Dose
Folliculitis	None; warm saline compresses usually sufficient	
Furuncles and carbuncles	Dicloxacillin 250–500 mg every 6 h	Dicloxacillin 25–50 mg/kg in four divided doses
	Cephalexin 250–500 mg every 6 h	Cephalexin 25–50 mg/kg in four divided doses
	Clindamycin 300–600 mg every 6–8 h[a]	Clindamycin 10–30 mg/kg/day in three to four divided doses[a]
Erysipelas	Procaine penicillin G 600,000 units intramuscularly every 12 h	Penicillin VK 25,000–90,000 units/kg in four divided doses
	Penicillin VK 250–500 mg every 6 h	Clindamycin 10–30 mg/kg in three to four doses[a]
	Clindamycin 150–300 mg every 6–8 h[a]	Erythromycin 30–50 mg/kg in four divided doses[a]
	Erythromycin 250–500 mg every 6 h[a]	
Impetigo	Dicloxacillin 250–500 mg every 6 h	Dicloxacillin 25–50 mg/kg in four divided doses
	Cephalexin 250–500 mg every 6 h	Cephalexin 25–50 mg/kg in two to four divided doses
	Cefadroxil 500 mg every 12 h	Cefadroxil 30 mg/kg in two divided doses
	Clindamycin 150–300 mg every 6–8 h[a]	Clindamycin 10–30 mg/kg/day in three to four divided doses[a]
	Mupirocin ointment every 8 h[a]	Mupirocin ointment every 8 h[a]
Lymphangitis	Initial intravenous therapy, followed by penicillin VK 250–500 mg every 6 h	Initial intravenous therapy, followed by penicillin VK 25,000–90,000 units/kg in four divided doses
	Clindamycin 150–300 mg every 6–8 h[a]	Clindamycin 10–30 mg/kg/day in three to four divided doses[a]
Diabetic foot infections	Amoxicillin-clavulanic acid 875 mg/125 mg every 12 h	
	Fluoroquinolone (levofloxacin 750 mg every 24 or moxifloxacin 400 mg every 24 h) + metronidazole 250–500 mg every 8 h or clindamycin 300–600 mg every 6–8 h[a]	
Animal bite	Amoxicillin-clavulanic acid 875 mg/125 mg every 12 h	Amoxicillin-clavulanic acid 40 mg/kg (of the amoxicillin component) in two divided doses
	Doxycycline 100–200 mg every 12 h[a]	
	Dicloxacillin 250–500 mg every 6 h + penicillin VK 250–500 mg every 6 h	Dicloxacillin 25–50 mg/kg in four divided doses + penicillin VK 40,000–90,000 units/kg in four divided doses
	Cefuroxime axetil 500 mg every 12 h + metronidazole 250–500 mg every 8 h or clindamycin 300–600 mg every 6–8 h	Cefuroxime axetil 20–30 mg/kg in two divided doses + metronidazole 30 mg/kg in three to four divided doses or clindamycin 10–30 mg/kg/day in three to four divided doses
	Fluoroquinolone (levofloxacin 500–750 mg every 24 h or moxifloxacin 400 mg every 24 h) or clindamycin 300-600 mg every 6–8 h[a]	Trimethoprim-sulfamethoxazole 4–6 mg/kg (of the trimethoprim component) every 12 h + metronidazole 30 mg/kg in three to four divided doses or clindamycin 10–30 mg/kg/day in three to four divided doses[a]
	Erythromycin 500 mg every 6 h + metronidazole 250–500 mg every 8 h or clindamycin 300–600 mg every 6–8 h[a]	Erythromycin 30–50 mg/kg in four divided doses + every 12 h + metronidazole 30 mg/kg in three to four divided doses or clindamycin 10–30 mg/kg/day in three to four divided doses[a]
Human bite	Amoxicillin-clavulanic acid 875 mg/125 mg every 12 h	Amoxicillin-clavulanic acid 40 mg/kg (of the amoxicillin component) in two divided doses
	Doxycycline 100–200 mg every 12 h[a]	
	Dicloxacillin 250–500 mg every 6 h + penicillin VK 250–500 mg every 6 h	Dicloxacillin 25–50 mg/kg in four divided doses + penicillin VK 40,000–90,000 units/kg in four divided doses
	Cefuroxime axetil 500 mg every 12 h metronidazole 250–500 mg every 8 h or clindamycin 300–600 mg every 6–8 h	Cefuroxime axetil 20–30 mg/kg in two divided doses + metronidazole 30 mg/kg in three to four divided doses or clindamycin 10–30 mg/kg/day in three to four divided doses
	Fluoroquinolone (levofloxacin 500–750 mg every 24 h or moxifloxacin 400 mg every 24 h) + metronidazole 250–500 mg every 8 h or clindamycin 300–600 mg every 6–8 h[a]	Trimethoprim-sulfamethoxazole 4–6 mg/kg (of the trimethoprim component) every 12 h + metronidazole 30 mg/kg in three to four divided doses or clindamycin 10–30 mg/kg/day in 3–4 divided doses[a]

[a]Recommended for patients with penicillin allergy.

Laboratory Tests

- The causative organism usually cannot be cultured from the surface skin but sometimes may be aspirated from the edge of the advancing lesion.
- Cultures may be considered in more severe cases or those with atypical clinical findings such as fluid-filled blisters.

Other Diagnostic Tests

- A complete blood count is often performed because leukocytosis is common.
- C-reactive protein is also generally elevated.

TREATMENT

Erysipelas

The goal of treatment of erysipelas is rapid eradication of the infection. Mild to moderate cases of erysipelas are treated with intramuscular procaine penicillin G or penicillin VK for 7 to 10 days (see Table 114–4).[20,23] Penicillin-allergic patients can be treated with clindamycin or erythromycin. For more serious infections, the patient should be hospitalized and aqueous penicillin G 2 to 8 million units daily administered intravenously.[20,21] Marked improvement usually is seen within 48 hours, and the patient often may be switched to oral penicillin to complete the course of therapy. One randomized, double-blind, placebo-controlled study showed that the median time for cure, intravenous antibiotics, and hospital stay was reduced in patients receiving prednisolone in addition to antibiotics.[22] Further studies are needed, however, before corticosteroids can be recommended for routine use.[11]

EVALUATION OF THERAPEUTIC OUTCOMES

Erysipelas generally responds quickly to appropriate antimicrobial therapy. Temperature and white blood count should return to normal within 48 to 72 hours. Erythema, edema, and pain also should resolve gradually.

IMPETIGO

❸ Impetigo is a superficial skin infection that is seen most commonly in children.[24] The infection is generally classified as bullous or nonbullous based on clinical presentation.[4] Impetigo is most common during hot, humid weather, which facilitates microbial colonization of the skin.[20] Minor trauma, such as scratches or insect bites, allows entry of organisms into the superficial layers of skin, and infection ensues.[20] Impetigo is highly communicable and readily spreads through close contact, especially among siblings and children in daycare centers and schools.[20,21]

Most cases of impetigo were caused by *S. pyogenes*, but recently *S. aureus*, either alone or in combination with *S. pyogenes*, has emerged as the principal cause of impetigo.[24] The bullous form is caused by strains of *S. aureus* capable of producing exfoliative toxins.[24] The bullous form most frequently affects neonates and accounts for approximately 10% of all cases of impetigo.[20,24]

CLINICAL PRESENTATION

General

- Exposed skin, especially the face, is the most common site for impetigo.

Symptoms

- Pruritus is common, and scratching of the lesions may further spread infection through excoriation of the skin.
- Other systemic signs of infection are minimal.
- Weakness, fever, and diarrhea sometimes are seen with bullous impetigo.

Signs

- Nonbullous impetigo manifests initially as small, fluid-filled vesicles.
- These lesions rapidly develop into pus-filled blisters that rupture readily.
- Purulent discharge from the lesions dries to form golden-yellow crusts that are characteristic of impetigo.
- In the bullous form of impetigo, the lesions begin as vesicles and turn into bullae containing clear yellow fluid.
- Bullae soon rupture, forming thin, light brown crusts.
- Regional lymph nodes may be enlarged.

Laboratory Tests

- Cultures should be collected.
- Crusted tops of lesions should be raised so that purulent material at the base of the lesion can be cultured.
- Cultures should not be collected from open, draining skin pustules because they may be colonized with staphylococci and other normal skin flora.

Other Diagnostic Tests

- A complete blood count is often performed because leukocytosis is common.

TREATMENT

Impetigo

Although impetigo may resolve spontaneously, antimicrobial treatment is indicated to relieve symptoms, prevent formation of new lesions, and prevent complications, such as cellulitis. Penicillinase-resistant penicillins are preferred for treatment because of the increased incidence of infections caused by *S. aureus*.[11] First-generation cephalosporins are also commonly used. Penicillin, administered as a single intramuscular dose of benzathine penicillin G (300,000 to 600,000 units in children, 1.2 million units in adults) or as oral penicillin VK, is effective for infections known to be caused by *S. pyogenes*. Penicillin-allergic patients can be treated with clindamycin. The duration of therapy is 7 to 10 days. Topical therapy with mupirocin ointment (applied three times daily for 7 days) is as effective as erythromycin.[11] Although erythromycin has long been a mainstay of therapy for impetigo and other SSTIs, increased macrolide resistance in both *S. aureus* and *S. pyogenes* may limit its future usefulness.[11] With proper treatment, healing of skin lesions generally is rapid and occurs without residual scarring. Removal of crusts by soaking in soap and warm water also may be helpful in providing symptomatic relief.[20,23]

EVALUATION OF THERAPEUTIC OUTCOMES

Clinical response should be seen within 7 days of initiating antimicrobial therapy for impetigo. Treatment failures could be a result of noncompliance or antimicrobial resistance. A followup culture of exudates should be collected for culture and sensitivity, with treatment modified accordingly.[24]

LYMPHANGITIS

❹ Acute lymphangitis is an inflammation involving the subcutaneous lymphatic channels. Lymphangitis usually occurs secondary to puncture wounds, infected blisters, or other skin lesions. Most infections are caused by *S. pyogenes*.[23,25]

CLINICAL PRESENTATION

General

- Lymphadenitis (acute or chronic inflammation of the lymph nodes) also may occur when microorganisms reach the lymph nodes and elicit an inflammatory response.

Symptoms

- Systemic manifestations of infection (i.e., fever, chills, malaise, and headache) often develop rapidly before any sign of infection is evident at the initial site of inoculation or even after the initial lesion has subsided.
- Systemic symptoms often are more profound than would be expected based on examination of the cutaneous lesion.

Signs

- Identification of a peripheral lesion associated with proximal red linear streaks directed toward the regional lymph nodes is diagnostic of acute lymphangitis.
- Lymph nodes usually are enlarged and tender.
- Peripheral edema of the involved extremity often is present.
- Thrombophlebitis and acute lymphangitis in the lower extremities may be confused because both are associated with red linear streaking and tender areas; however, in thrombophlebitis, no portal of entry is identifiable.

Laboratory Tests

- Cultures of the affected lesions often yield negative results because the infection resides within the lymphatic channels.
- Offending pathogens often can be identified by Gram stain of the initial lesion if done early in the course of the disease.

Other Diagnostic Tests

- A complete blood count frequently is performed because leukocytosis is common.

TREATMENT

Lymphangitis

The goal of therapy for lymphangitis is rapid eradication of infection and prevention of further systemic complications. Penicillin is the antibiotic of choice. Because these infections are potentially serious and rapidly progressive, initial treatment should be with intravenous penicillin G 1 to 2 million units every 4 to 6 hours. Parenteral treatment should be continued for 48 to 72 hours, followed by oral penicillin VK for a total of 10 days.[23,25] Nondrug therapy includes immobilization and elevation of the affected extremity and warm-water soaks every 2 to 4 hours.[23] For penicillin-allergic patients, clindamycin may be used.

EVALUATION OF THERAPEUTIC OUTCOMES

Lymphangitis usually responds rapidly to appropriate therapy; signs and symptoms often are decreased markedly or absent within 24 hours of starting antibiotics.

CELLULITIS

❺ Cellulitis is an acute, infectious process that represents a serious type of SSTI. Cellulitis initially affects the epidermis and dermis and may spread subsequently within the superficial fascia. Cellulitis is considered a serious disease because of the propensity of the infection to spread through lymphatic tissue and to the bloodstream. *S. pyogenes* and *S. aureus* are the most frequent etiologic agents. However, many bacteria have been implicated in various types of cellulitis (see Table 114–1). The rising incidence of infections caused by MRSA is a major concern in both the community and hospital settings.[6,7,9–16]

Injection-drug users are predisposed to a number of infectious complications, including abscess formation and cellulitis at the site of injection.[26] These SSTIs are located most frequently on the upper extremities and often are polymicrobic in nature.[27] Infecting organisms are believed to originate from the skin and/or oropharynx, as well as from contaminated needles, syringes, and diluents.[27] *S. aureus* is the most common pathogen isolated from these infections. The incidence of MRSA is also rising in SSTIs in injection-drug users.[28] Anaerobic bacteria, especially oropharyngeal anaerobes, are also found commonly, particularly in polymicrobic infections.[27] Outbreaks caused by *Clostridium* species have been reported recently in injection-drug users, particularly as a consequence of injection of contaminated black-tar heroin.[29,30]

Acute cellulitis with mixed aerobic and anaerobic flora generally occurs in diabetics, where the skin is adjacent to some site of trauma, at sites of surgical incisions to the abdomen or perineum, or where host defenses have been otherwise compromised (vascular insufficiency). In older patients, cellulitis of the lower extremities also may be complicated by thrombophlebitis. Other complications of cellulitis include local abscess, osteomyelitis, and septic arthritis.[11,23]

CLINICAL PRESENTATION

General

- There is usually a history of an antecedent wound from a minor trauma, abrasion, ulcer, or surgery.
- Because these infections occur often in patients with alterations in host defense mechanisms, poor nutrition, or both, systemic findings such as hypotension, dehydration, and altered mental status are common.

Symptoms

- Patients often experience fever, chills, or malaise and complain that the affected area feels hot and painful.

Signs

- Cellulitis is characterized by erythema and edema of the skin.
- Lesions, which may be extensive, are nonelevated and have poorly defined margins.
- Affected areas generally are warm to touch.
- Inflammation generally is present with little or no necrosis or suppuration of soft tissue.
- Tender lymphadenopathy associated with lymphatic involvement is common.

Laboratory Tests

- Cultures should be collected when possible.
- A Gram stain of fluid obtained by injection and aspiration of 0.5 mL of saline (using a small 22-gauge needle) into the advancing edge of the lesion may aid the microbiologic diagnosis but often yields negative results.
- Diagnosis usually is made on clinical grounds, that is, the appearance of the lesion.

Other Diagnostic Tests

- A complete blood count frequently is performed because leukocytosis is common.
- Because bacteremia may be present in as many as 30% of cases of cellulitis, blood cultures may be useful for diagnosis in some patients.

TREATMENT

Cellulitis

The goal of therapy of acute bacterial cellulitis is rapid eradication of the infection and prevention of further complications. Antimicrobial therapy of bacterial cellulitis is directed against the type of bacteria either documented or suspected to be present based on the clinical presentation. Local care of cellulitis includes elevation and immobilization of the involved area to decrease swelling. Cool sterile saline dressings may decrease pain and can be followed later with moist heat to aid in localization of the cellulitis. Surgical intervention (incision and drainage) as a mode of therapy is rarely indicated in the treatment of uncomplicated cellulitis. The use of inappropriate antibiotic therapy for cellulitis is associated with significantly higher risk of clinical treatment failures.[31] Therefore, in the selection of antibiotics for treatment of cellulitis, particular attention must be paid to patients with risk factors for more atypical or resistant bacterial pathogens (e.g., gram-negative bacteria, anaerobes, MRSA).

Because staphylococcal and streptococcal cellulitis are indistinguishable clinically,[21] administration of a penicillinase-resistant penicillin (nafcillin or oxacillin) or first-generation cephalosporin (cefazolin) is recommended until a definitive diagnosis, by skin or blood cultures, can be made (Table 114–5).[2,11,20,23] Mild to moderate infections not associated with systemic symptoms may be treated orally with dicloxacillin or cephalexin. Other oral cephalosporins, such as cefadroxil, cefaclor, cefprozil, cefpodoxime proxetil, and cefdinir, are also effective in the treatment of cellulitis but are considerably more expensive.[23,32] If documented to be a mild cellulitis secondary to streptococci, oral penicillin VK or intramuscular procaine penicillin may be administered. More severe infections, either staphylococcal or streptococcal, should be treated initially with intravenous antibiotic regimens. Ceftriaxone 50 to

TABLE 114-5 Initial Treatment Regimens for Cellulitis Caused by Various Pathogens

Antibiotic	Adult Dose and Route	Pediatric Dose and Route
Staphylococcal or unknown gram-positive infection		
Mild infection	Dicloxacillin 0.25–0.5 g orally every 6 h[a,b]	Dicloxacillin 25–50 mg/kg/day orally in four divided doses[a,b]
Moderate–severe infection	Nafcillin or oxacillin 1–2 g IV every 4–6 h[a,b]	Nafcillin or oxacillin 150–200 mg/kg/day (not to exceed 12 g/24 h) IV in four to six equally divided doses[a,b]
Streptococcal (documented)		
Mild infection	Penicillin VK 0.5 g orally every 6 h[a] or procaine penicillin G 600,000 units IM every 8–12 h[a]	Penicillin VK 125–250 mg orally every 6–8 h, or procaine penicillin G 25,000–50,000 units/kg (not to exceed 600,000 units) IM every 8–12 h[a]
Moderate–severe infection	Aqueous penicillin G 1–2 million units IV every 4–6 h[a,c]	Aqueous penicillin G 100,000–200,000 units/kg/day IV in four divided doses[a]
Gram-negative bacilli		
Mild infection	Cefaclor 0.5 g orally every 8 h[d] or cefuroxime axetil 0.5 g orally every 12 h[d]	Cefaclor 20–40 mg/kg/day (not to exceed 1 g) orally in three divided doses or cefuroxime axetil 0.125–0.25 g (tablets) orally every 12 h
Moderate–severe infection	Aminoglycoside[e] or IV cephalosporin (first- or second-generation depending on severity of infection or susceptibility pattern)[d]	Aminoglycoside[e] or intravenous cephalosporin (first- or second-generation depending on severity of infection or susceptibility pattern)
Polymicrobic infection without anaerobes		
	Aminoglycoside[e] + penicillin G 1–2 million units every 4–6 h or a semisynthetic penicillin (nafcillin 1–2 g every 4–6 h) depending on isolation of staphylococci or streptococci[b]	Aminoglycoside[e] + penicillin G 100,000–200,000 units/kg/day IV in four divided doses or a semisynthetic penicillin (nafcillin 150–200 mg/kg/day [not to exceed 12 g/24 h] IV in four to six equally divided doses) depending on isolation of staphylococci or streptococci[b]
Polymicrobic infection with anaerobes		
Mild infection	Amoxicillin/clavulanate 0.875 g orally every 12 h or A fluoroquinolone (ciprofloxacin 0.4 g orally every 12 h or levofloxacin 0.5–0.75 g orally every 24 h) plus clindamycin 0.3–0.6 g orally every 8 h or metronidazole 0.5 g orally every 8 h	Amoxicillin/clavulanic acid 20 mg/kg/day orally in three divided doses
Moderate–severe infection	Aminoglycoside[e,f] + clindamycin 0.6–0.9 g IV every 8 h or metronidazole 0.5 g IV every 8 h or Monotherapy with second- or third-generation cephalosporin (cefoxitin 1–2 g IV every 6 h or ceftizoxime 1–2 g IV every 8 h) or Monotherapy with imipenem 0.5 g IV every 6–8 h, meropenem 1 g IV every 8 h, ertapenem 1 g IV every 24 h, extended-spectrum penicillins with a β-lactamase inhibitor (piperacillin/tazobactam 4.5 g IV every 6 h), or tigecycline 100 mg IV as loading dose, then 50 mg IV every 12 h	Aminoglycoside[e] plus clindamycin 15 mg/kg/day IV in three divided doses or metronidazole 30–50 mg/kg/day IV in three divided doses

IM, intramuscularly; IV, intravenous.
[a]For penicillin-allergic patients, use clindamycin 150–300 mg orally every 6–8 h (pediatric dosing: 10–30 mg/kg/day in three to four divided doses).
[b]For methicillin-resistant staphylococci, use vancomycin 0.5–1 g every 6–12 h (pediatric dosing 40 mg/kg/day in divided doses) with dosage adjustments made for renal dysfunction.
[c]For type II necrotizing fasciitis, use clindamycin 0.6–0.9 g IV every 8 h (in children, clindamycin 15 mg/kg/day IV in 3 divided doses).
[d]For penicillin-allergic adults, use a fluoroquinolone (ciprofloxacin 0.5–0.75 g orally every 12 h or 0.4 g IV every 12 h; levofloxacin 0.5–0.75 g orally or IV every 24 h; or moxifloxacin 0.4 g orally or IV every 24 h).
[e]Gentamicin or tobramycin, 2 mg/kg loading dose, then maintenance dose as determined by serum concentrations.
[f]A fluoroquinolone or aztreonam 1 g IV every 6 h may be used in place of the aminoglycoside in patients with severe renal dysfunction or other relative contraindications to aminoglycoside use.

100 mg/kg as a single daily dose is efficacious in the treatment of cellulitis in pediatric patients.[33] The usual duration of therapy for cellulitis is 5 to 10 days.[11,20,23]

In penicillin-allergic patients, oral or parenteral clindamycin may be used.[1,2] Alternatively, a first-generation cephalosporin may be used cautiously for patients who have not experienced immediate or anaphylactic penicillin reactions and are negative for a penicillin skin test. In severe cases in which cephalosporins cannot be used because of suspected and/or documented methicillin-resistant staphylococci or severe β-lactam allergies, vancomycin should be administered.[2,11]

Although the most optimal treatment for CA-MRSA infections is not known, initial therapy with trimethoprim-sulfamethoxazole appears to be effective in most cases and should be considered in geographic areas in which CA-MRSA infections are commonly encountered.[9,13,14] Hospital-acquired strains of MRSA tend to be more antibiotic resistant and vancomycin is a more appropriate choice for initial treatment of patients in whom hospital-acquired MRSA is a suspected or documented pathogen. Alternative agents for infections with resistant gram-positive bacteria such as MRSA and vancomycin-resistant enterococci include linezolid, quinupristin-dalfopristin, daptomycin, and tigecycline.[1,2,34–40] The excellent activity of these drugs against resistant gram-positive pathogens and significantly higher cost make them most appropriate for treatment of complicated or refractory infections, or those caused by multidrug-resistant pathogens, rather than as initial therapy. The availability of orally administered linezolid may provide a cost-effective "step-down" option for many patients with more complicated infections and/or those patients who require initial hospitalization as an alternative to prolonged treatment with parenteral agents.[41] Tigecycline may be considered in complicated infections, particularly those in which the presence of mixed gram-negative and/or anaerobic pathogens is suspected or documented alongside resistant gram-positive bacteria.[39,40]

CLINICAL CONTROVERSY

Because of the recent emergence and increasing prevalence of CA-MRSA, clinicians are now debating whether current treatment guidelines for empiric antimicrobial therapy of SSTIs should change.[42,43] Although numerous studies have documented the rise in infections caused by CA-MRSA,[9–16] none have reported poor clinical outcomes even though the majority of patients were treated with β-lactam antibiotics.[42] Trimethoprim-sulfamethoxazole has excellent in vitro activity against CA-MRSA, but no clinical trials have been published that correlate susceptibility data with clinical outcomes. Another concern is the lack of activity of trimethoprim-sulfamethoxazole against *S. pyogenes*, another organism commonly isolated in SSTIs. The combination of trimethoprim-sulfamethoxazole and a β-lactam antibiotic has been suggested when empiric therapy is needed for coverage of both organisms.[42,43] Clindamycin has activity against both organisms, but with the high incidence of macrolide resistance, there is concern of inducible clindamycin resistance during therapy.[13] Of note, most skin abscesses, even those caused by MRSA, can be cured with adequate drainage without the need for antimicrobials.[42,43]

The carbapenems (i.e., imipenem, meropenem, and ertapenem) and the β-lactam–β-lactamase inhibitor combination antibiotics (ampicillin-sulbactam, ticarcillin-clavulanic acid, and piperacillin-tazobactam) also appear to be equivalent to standard therapies in adults.[1,44–47] The greater cost of these newer agents without increased efficacy compared with other reliable regimens, however, makes them less desirable.

For cellulitis caused by gram-negative bacilli or a mixture of microorganisms, immediate antimicrobial chemotherapy, as determined by Gram stain, is essential (see Table 114–5). Surgical excision of necrotic tissue and drainage also may be appropriate. Gram-negative cellulitis may be treated appropriately with an aminoglycoside or first- or second-generation cephalosporin. If gram-positive aerobic bacteria are also present, penicillin G or a penicillinase-resistant penicillin should be added to the regimen. Ceftazidime and the fluoroquinolones are effective in the treatment of cellulitis caused by both gram-negative and gram-positive bacteria.[1,48]

Because some infections may be polymicrobic in nature, antibiotic therapy may need to be broadened to include agents with good activity against anaerobic bacteria. Many different treatment regimens are possible depending on the bacteriology of the lesion (see Table 114–5). Usually an aminoglycoside combined with an anti-anaerobic cephalosporin, extended-spectrum penicillin, or clindamycin is used. Second- or third-generation cephalosporins have been suggested as single-agent therapy in certain instances.[1,2,11] Monotherapy with a β-lactam plus β-lactamase inhibitor combination antibiotic or a carbapenem also may be appropriate in seriously ill patients.[1,44–47] Therapy should be 10 to 14 days in duration.

CLINICAL CONTROVERSY

Oral fluoroquinolones have demonstrated efficacy similar to parenteral cephalosporins in the treatment of soft-tissue infections caused by gram-positive organisms.[1,48–50] Caution is warranted when treating SSTIs with ciprofloxacin owing to the unreliable activity of this agent against streptococci.[1] Lower eradication rates of streptococci also have been reported with moxifloxacin when compared with cephalexin in the treatment of uncomplicated SSTIs.[49] Levofloxacin and moxifloxacin are effective for both uncomplicated and complicated SSTIs.[1,46,49–51] The use of fluoroquinolones is of concern, however, because of increasing reports of resistance among both gram-positive and gram-negative bacteria.[52,53] Sensitivity testing is recommended when a fluoroquinolone is to be used. Also, fluoroquinolones are not approved for use in children because of toxicity concerns.

Because gram-negative and mixed aerobic-anaerobic cellulitis can progress quickly to serious tissue invasion, therapeutic intervention should be immediate. If treated early, a rapid response can be seen. Unfortunately, because these infections often occur in patients with compromised immune defenses, they may still progress, even with therapeutic intervention. If the infectious process is secondary to a systemic cause (e.g., diabetes), the treatment course often is prolonged and may be associated with high morbidity and mortality.

Infections in injection-drug users generally are treated similarly to those in other types of patients.[27] It is important that blood cultures be obtained because 25% to 35% of patients may be bacteremic.[27,54] Also, patients should be assessed for the presence of abscesses; incision, drainage, and culture of these lesions are of extreme importance.[20] Initial antimicrobial therapy while awaiting culture results of abscesses should include coverage for anaerobic organisms, in addition to *S. aureus* and streptococci.[27] In areas where MRSA is prevalent, treatment with vancomycin plus metronidazole is preferred.[27]

EVALUATION OF THERAPEUTIC OUTCOMES

If treated promptly with appropriate antibiotics, the majority of patients with cellulitis are cured rapidly. Culture and sensitivity results should be evaluated carefully both for the adequacy of culture material and the presence of resistant organisms. Additional high-quality samples for culture may be needed for microbiologic analysis. Failure to respond to therapy also may be indicative of an underlying local or systemic problem or a misdiagnosis.

NECROTIZING SOFT-TISSUE INFECTIONS

Necrotizing soft-tissue infections consist of a group of highly lethal infections that require early and aggressive surgical debridement in addition to appropriate antibiotics and intensive supportive care.[55,56] A number of different descriptive terms have been used to classify necrotizing infections. These have been based on factors such as predisposing conditions, onset of symptoms, pain, skin appearance, etiologic agent, gas production, muscle involvement, and systemic toxicity. While many of the necrotizing soft-tissue infections have been designated as unique infectious processes, they all share similar pathophysiologies, clinical features, and treatment approaches.[55,56] The major clinical entities of necrotizing infections are *necrotizing fasciitis* and *clostridial myonecrosis* (gas gangrene).[55]

❻ Necrotizing fasciitis is a rare but very severe infection of the subcutaneous tissue that may be caused by aerobic and/or anaerobic bacteria and results in progressive destruction of the superficial fascia and subcutaneous fat. It is generally characterized as one of two different types based on bacterial etiology. Type I necrotizing fasciitis generally occurs after trauma and surgery and involves a mixture of anaerobes (*Bacteroides, Peptostreptococcus*) and facultative bacteria (streptococci and members of Enterobacteriaceae) that act synergistically to cause destruction of fat and fascia. Type I necrotizing fasciitis is also being reported more commonly among injection-drug users.[56,57] In type I infections, the skin may be spared, and the speed at which the infection spreads is somewhat slower than type II. Necrotizing fasciitis affecting the male genitalia has been termed *Fournier gangrene.* Type II necrotizing fasciitis is caused by virulent strains of *S. pyogenes* and is more commonly referred to as *streptococcal gangrene.* This type of infection has received considerable attention in recent years because of reports of "flesh-eating bacteria" by the lay press. Unlike previous reports of streptococcal gangrene that affected older individuals with underlying diseases, recent reports have occurred primarily in young, previously healthy adults following some type of minor trauma. It differs from the polymicrobial type I infections in its clinical presentation. Type II infections have rapidly extending necrosis of subcutaneous tissues and skin, gangrene, severe local pain, and systemic toxicity.[21] Type II infections are also highly associated with an early onset of shock and organ failure and are present in approximately half the cases of streptococcal toxic shock-like syndrome.[21]

Clostridial myonecrosis is a necrotizing infection that involves the skeletal muscle. Gas production and muscle necrosis are prominent features of this infection, which readily explains why this infection is commonly referred to as *gas gangrene*.[55,56] The infection advances rapidly, often over a matter of a few hours.[55] Most infections occur after surgery or trauma, with *Clostridium perfringens* identified as the most common etiologic agent. Recently, outbreaks have been reported in injection-drug users who injected contaminated coal-tar heroin.[30,33]

CLINICAL PRESENTATION

General

- These infections may occur in almost any anatomic location but most frequently involve the abdomen, the perineum, and the lower extremities.
- Patients often have predisposing factors such as diabetes mellitus, local trauma or infection, or recent surgery.

Symptoms

- Systemic symptoms generally are marked (e.g., fever, chills, and leukocytosis) and may include shock and organ failure, especially in patients with type II infections.
- In general, pain in the affected area and systemic toxicity are more pronounced than would be expected with cellulitis.

Signs

- At the beginning of an infection, it may be difficult to differentiate between necrotizing fasciitis and cellulitis.
- Like cellulitis, the affected area is initially hot, swollen, and erythematous without sharp margins.
- The affected area is often shiny, exquisitely tender, and painful.
- Diffuse swelling of the area is followed by the appearance of bullae filled with clear fluid.
- The infectious process progresses rapidly, with the skin taking on a maroon or violaceous color after several days.
- Without appropriate intervention, the infection will evolve rapidly into a frank cutaneous gangrene, sometimes with myonecrosis (involvement of skin and muscle).
- Because of the aggressive nature and high mortality (20% to 50%) associated with these infections, a rapid diagnosis is critical.

Laboratory Tests

- Although computed tomography and magnetic resonance imaging studies can distinguish these infections, the best and most rapid diagnosis of necrotizing infections is obtained via surgical exploration.
- Intraoperative samples should be collected for culture and sensitivity, as well as for histologic examination.
- Unlike necrotizing fasciitis, clostridial myonecrosis shows little inflammation on histologic examination.

Other Diagnostic Tests

- Because marked systemic symptoms are seen commonly in necrotizing infections, blood samples should be collected for complete blood count and chemistry profile, as well as for bacterial culture.

TREATMENT

Necrotizing Soft-Tissue Infections

After the diagnosis is made, immediate and aggressive surgical debridement of all necrotic tissue is essential.[55,56] Patients often require further surgical intervention following initial debridement to ensure that all necrotic tissue has been removed.[2,11] Broad-spectrum antibiotics should be administered, with coverage against streptococci, Enterobacteriaceae, and anaerobes. A number of antibiotic regimens have been used successfully to treat necrotizing soft-tissue infections; these are generally similar to those used for severe polymicrobic cellulitis involving anaerobes (see Table 114–5). Other combination antibiotic regimens that may be used prior to obtaining bacteriologic data include ampicillin with gentamicin and clindamycin (or metronidazole); ampicillin-sulbactam with gentamicin; and imipenem with metronidazole.[20]

Antibiotic therapy can be modified after Gram stain and culture reports are available. If a diagnosis of type II necrotizing fasciitis is established, the broad-spectrum empirical therapy should be replaced with the combination of penicillin and clindamycin.[21] Although *S. pyogenes* remains susceptible to penicillin, clindamycin is more effective.[21] A number of factors have been postulated to explain the higher efficacy of clindamycin, including the mechanism of action (inhibition of protein synthesis), which is not affected by the size of the inoculum or the stage of bacterial growth.[21] In addition, clindamycin has immunomodulatory properties that may account for the higher efficacy.[21] The combination of penicillin and clindamycin is also recommended for treatment of clostridial myonecrosis.[11,55,56] Hyperbaric oxygen also may be of some benefit for clostridial myonecrosis.[55,58]

EVALUATION OF THERAPEUTIC OUTCOMES

Because of the high mortality associated with necrotizing infections, rapid and complete debridement of all devitalized and necrotic tissue is essential. Surgical debridement, coupled with appropriate antimicrobial therapy and typical supportive measures for management of shock and organ failure, should stabilize the patient. Vital signs and laboratory tests should be monitored carefully for signs of resolution of the infection. Change in antimicrobial therapy or additional surgical debridement may be needed in patients who do not show signs of improvement.

DIABETIC FOOT INFECTIONS

Three major types of foot infections are seen in diabetic patients: deep abscesses, cellulitis of the dorsum, and mal perforans ulcers.[59] Most deep abscesses involve the central plantar space (arch) and are caused by minor penetrating trauma or by an extension of infection of a nail or web space of the toes. Skin infections of the dorsal area generally arise from infections in the toes that are related to routine care of the nails, nail beds, and calluses of the toes. Mal perforans ulcer is a chronic ulcer of the sole of the foot. The ulcer develops on thickened, hardened calluses over the first or fifth metatarsal. Mal perforans ulcers are associated with neuropathy, which is responsible for the misalignment of the weight-bearing bones of the foot.[59] Osteomyelitis is one of the most serious complications of foot problems in diabetic patients and may occur in 30% to 40% of infections.[19,59,60]

EPIDEMIOLOGY

Disorders of the foot are among the most common complications of diabetes, accounting for as many as 20% of all hospitalizations in diabetic patients at an annual cost of $200 to $350 million.[61] The cost of treating a patient with a diabetic foot ulcer has been estimated at $14,000 to $18,000 each year.[62,63] Approximately 25% of diabetic patients experience significant soft-tissue infection at some time during the course of their lifetime. Approximately 55,000 lower-extremity amputations, often sequelae of uncontrolled infection, are performed each year on diabetic patients; this represents 50% of all nontraumatic amputations in the United States.[61] Between 10% and 20% of diabetics will undergo additional surgery or amputation of a second limb within 12 months of the initial amputation.[64] By 5 years, this increases to 25% to 50%, with death reported in as much as two-thirds of patients.[64]

ETIOLOGY

Diabetic foot infections begin with local bacterial invasion and typically involve a number of different bacterial pathogens.[64] The infections are polymicrobic in nature, with an average of 2.3 to 5.8 isolates per culture (Table 114–6).[19,64–66] Staphylococci (especially *S. aureus*) and streptococci are the most common pathogens, although gram-negative bacilli and/or anaerobes occur in approximately 50% of cases.[19,64–66] Common gram-negative bacilli isolated include *E. coli*, *Klebsiella* spp., *Proteus* spp., and *P. aeruginosa*. *Bacteroides fragilis* and *Peptostreptococcus* spp. are among the most common anaerobes isolated.

The optimum technique for obtaining culture material from ulcerated lesions is still debated.[59] Routine swab cultures of ulcerative lesions are difficult to interpret because of organisms that colonize the surface of the wounds. Cultures of material from sinus tracts are also unreliable. The correlation between these superficial cultures and true deep cultures (via biopsy or needle aspiration of drainage or abscess fluid) is often poor, particularly in chronic lesions.[19,65] Therefore, cultures and sensitivity tests should be done with specimens obtained from a deep culture whenever possible. Before the wound is cultured, it should be scrubbed vigorously with saline-moistened sterile gauze to remove any overlying necrotic debris.[67] Cultures then can be obtained from the wound base, preferably from expressed pus.[67] Specimens obtained from curettage of the base of the ulcer correlate best with results from deep-tissue or bone biopsies.[67]

TABLE 114-6 Bacterial Isolates from Foot Infections in Diabetic Patients

Organisms	Percentage of Isolates
Aerobes	63%–75%
Gram-positive	42%–64%
Staphylococcus aureus	15%–20%
Streptococcus spp.	6%–12%
Enterococcus spp.	7%–20%
Coagulase-negative staphylococci	6%–10%
Other gram-positive aerobes	0%–12%
Gram-negative	16%–18%
Proteus spp.	5%–6%
Enterobacter spp.	1%–2%
Escherichia coli	3%–5%
Klebsiella spp.	1%–2%
Pseudomonas aeruginosa	1%–3%
Other gram-negative bacilli	3%–8%
Anaerobes	25%–40%
Peptostreptococcus spp.	8%–12%
Bacteroides fragilis group	4%–7%
Other *Bacteroides* spp.	3%–6%
Clostridium spp.	0%–2%
Other anaerobes	7%–10%

Compiled from Pellizzer et al.,[65] and Lipsky et al.[66]

PATHOPHYSIOLOGY

Three key factors are involved in the development of diabetic foot problems: (a) neuropathy, (b) angiopathy and ischemia, and (c) immunologic defects. Any of these disorders can occur in isolation; however, they frequently occur together.

Neuropathic changes to the autonomic nervous system as a consequence of diabetes may affect the motor nerve supply of small intrinsic muscles of the foot, resulting in muscular imbalance, abnormal stresses on tissues and bone, and repetitive injuries.[68] Diminished sensory perception causes an absence of pain and unawareness of minor injuries and ulceration. Also, the sympathetic nerve supply may be damaged and can result in an absence of sweating; this leads to dry cracked skin, which can become secondarily infected.[19,64]

Atherosclerosis is more common, appears at a younger age, and progresses more rapidly in the diabetic than in the nondiabetic. Diabetics may have problems with both small vessels (microangiopathy) and large vessels (macroangiopathy) that can result in varying degrees of ischemia, ultimately leading to skin breakdown and infection.

Diabetic patients typically have normal humoral immunity, normal levels of immunoglobulins, and normal antibody responses. Patients with diabetes, however, have impaired phagocytosis and intracellular microbicidal function as compared with nondiabetics; this may be related to angiopathy and low tissue levels of oxygen.[19,64,68] These defects in cell-mediated immunity make patients with diabetes more susceptible to certain types of infection and impair the patients' ability to heal wounds adequately.[68]

CLINICAL PRESENTATION

General

- Infections are often much more extensive than they appear initially.

Symptoms

- Patients with peripheral neuropathy often do not experience pain but seek medical care for swelling or erythema in the foot.

Signs

- Clinical signs of infection in the diabetic foot may not be present secondary to the angiopathy and neuropathy.
- When present, lesions vary in size and clinical features (e.g., erythema, edema, warmth, presence of pus, draining sinuses, pain, and tenderness).
- A foul-smelling odor suggests the presence of anaerobic organisms.
- Temperature may be mildly elevated or normal.

Laboratory Tests

- Specimens for culture and sensitivities should be collected.
- If possible, deep intraoperative samples should be obtained during surgical debridement.
- Because of the complex microbiology of these infections, wounds must be cultured for both aerobic and anaerobic organisms.

Other Diagnostic Tests

- The presence of osteomyelitis also must be assessed via radiograph, bone scan, or both, as appropriate.

TREATMENT

Diabetic Foot Infections

7 The goal of therapy of diabetic foot infections is preservation of as much normal limb function as possible while preventing additional infectious complications. Up to 90% of these infections can be treated successfully with a comprehensive treatment approach that includes both wound care and antimicrobial therapy.[19] After carefully assessing the extent of the lesion and obtaining necessary cultures, necrotic tissue must be thoroughly debrided, with wound drainage and amputation as required. Wounds must be kept clean and dressings changed frequently (two to three times daily). Because of the relationship between hyperglycemia and immune system defects, glycemic control must be maximized to ensure optimal wound healing. In addition, the patient's activities should be restricted initially to bedrest for leg elevation and control of edema, if present. Adequate pressure relief from a foot wound (i.e., off-loading) is crucial to the healing process.[19,69] Finally, appropriate antimicrobials must be initiated.[19,60,61,67,68] However, the optimal antimicrobial therapy for diabetic foot infections has yet to be defined.

The majority of mild, uncomplicated infections can be managed successfully on an outpatient basis with oral antimicrobials and good wound care. Many different agents have been studied, including cefaclor, cephalexin, fluoroquinolones, clindamycin, and amoxicillin-clavulanic acid, and provide clinical cure rates of 60% to 85%.[19,60,68] However, significant failure rates and/or relapse rates have been reported with the use of oral agents. In addition, the development of resistance was problematic in some infections involving *P. aeruginosa* and staphylococci.[70] Many clinicians consider amoxicillin-clavulanic acid to be the preferred agent because of its broad spectrum of activity, which includes staphylococci, streptococci, enterococci, and many Enterobacteriaceae and anaerobes.[19,67,68] However, this agent does not have activity against *P. aeruginosa.* Fluoroquinolones, which provide coverage against *P. aeruginosa,* have been studied extensively as monotherapy, but they, perhaps, are most appropriately used in combination with metronidazole or clindamycin to provide anaerobic activity.[2,19] Oral antimicrobials should be used cautiously in serious infections, especially those complicated by osteomyelitis, extensive ulceration, areas of necrosis, or a combination of these.

Initial therapy for patients requiring hospitalization for moderate to severe infections is similar to that for polymicrobic cellulitis with anaerobes (see Table 114–5). Monotherapy with broad-spectrum parenteral antimicrobials, along with appropriate medical or surgical management, or both, is often effective in treating these infections, including those in which osteomyelitis is present.[66,71,72] Monotherapy is particularly attractive because of the potential advantages of convenience, cost, and avoidance of toxicities. Microbiologic and clinical cure rates ranging from 60% to 90% may be expected from any of these agents; selection of a specific regimen is determined primarily by cost. In penicillin-allergic patients, metronidazole or clindamycin plus either a fluoroquinolone, aztreonam, or possibly a third-generation cephalosporin is appropriate.[2,19,60,68] Vancomycin also is used frequently in severe infections because of its excellent activity against gram-positive pathogens. With the increased incidence of MRSA, linezolid, quinupristin-dalfopristin, daptomycin, and tigecycline are alternatives for treatment of these resistant organisms.[1,2,34–40] Tigecycline may be particularly useful in this setting because of its activity against gram-negative aerobes and anaerobic bacteria, thus allowing it to be used as monotherapy for the treatment of mixed infections. Because these patients already may have some degree of diabetic nephropathy that may place them at higher risk of nephrotoxicity, strong recommendations have been made for the avoidance of aminoglycoside antibiotics unless no alternative agents are available.[19] When an aminoglycoside is used, care must be taken to avoid further compromising renal function. All antibiotic regimes should be adjusted as necessary for renal dysfunction.

Empirical therapy that is totally comprehensive in its coverage of all possible pathogens is not necessary unless the infection is life-threatening.[19,66,71,72] No differences have been reported in the efficacy of ampicillin-sulbactam versus imipenem-cilastatin for treatment of limb-threatening diabetic foot infections despite the higher incidence of potential pathogens resistant to the ampicillin-sulbactam regimen.[71] Other studies demonstrate good clinical efficacy despite the presence of pathogens such as MRSA and *Pseudomonas,* which were resistant to the antibiotics used.[47,66] These studies highlight the importance of good wound care as part of a comprehensive treatment approach.

Mild to moderate infections can be treated with oral agents that are highly bioavailable. Duration of therapy is usually 7 to 14 days, although some infections may require an additional 1 to 2 weeks of therapy. More severe infections require initial parenteral therapy. Duration of therapy for most moderate to severe infections ranges from 2 to 4 weeks.[19] In cases of underlying osteomyelitis, treatment should continue for 6 to 12 weeks.[19,60,68] After healing of the infection has occurred, a well-designed program for prevention of further infections should be instituted.

EVALUATION OF THERAPEUTIC OUTCOMES

Therapy should be reevaluated carefully after 48 to 72 hours to assess favorable response. Change in therapy (or route of administration, if oral) should be considered if clinical improvement is not observed at this time. For optimal results, drug therapy should be appropriately modified according to information from deep-tissue culture and the clinical condition of the patient. Infections in diabetic patients often require extended courses of therapy because of impaired host immunity and poor wound healing.

PRESSURE SORES

The terms *decubitus ulcer, bed sore,* and *pressure sore* are used interchangeably. The decubitus ulcer and the bed sore are types of pressure sores. The term *decubitus ulcer* is derived from the Latin word *decumbere,* meaning "lying down." Pressure sores, however, can develop regardless of a patient's position.

Numerous systems for classification of pressure sores have been described. The two most frequently used systems are those of Shea[73] and the 1989 National Pressure Ulcer Advisory Panel.[74] These classification systems define the various stages of progression through which a pressure sore may pass (Table 114–7).

TABLE 114-7 Pressure Sore Classification

Stage 1	Pressure sore is generally reversible, is limited to the epidermis, and resembles an abrasion. It is best described as an irregularly shaped area of soft-tissue swelling with induration and heat.
Stage 2	A stage 2 sore also may be reversible; it extends through the dermis to the subcutaneous fat along with extensive undermining.
Stage 3[a]	In this instance, the sore or ulcer extends further into subcutaneous fat along with extensive undermining.
Stage 4[a]	The sore or ulcer is characterized by penetration into deep fascia involving both muscle and bone.

[a]Stages 3 and 4 lesions are unlikely to resolve on their own and often require surgical intervention.

From Shea[73] and National Pressure Ulcer Advisory Panel.[74]

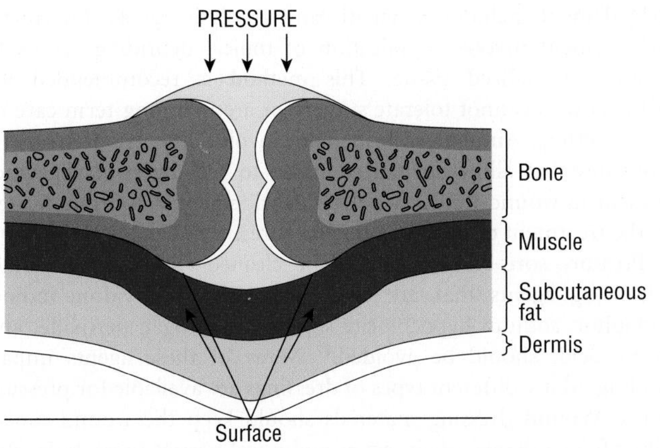

FIGURE 114-1. Distribution of forces involved with sore formation in a conical fashion.

Complications of pressure sores are not uncommon and may be life-threatening. Infection is one of the most serious and most frequently encountered complications of pressure ulcers. Bacterial colonization must be differentiated from true bacterial infection. Although most pressure sore wounds are colonized, the majority of these eventually heal.[75] When the tissue is infected, there is bacterial invasion of previously healthy tissue. Without treatment, an initial small, localized area of ulceration can progress rapidly to 5 to 6 cm within days. The visible ulcer is just a small portion of the actual wound; up to 70% of the total wound is below the skin. A pressure-gradient phenomenon is created by which the wound takes on a conical nature; the smallest point is at the skin surface, and the largest portion of the defect is at the base of the ulcer (Fig. 114–1).

EPIDEMIOLOGY

Pressure sores are seen most frequently in chronically debilitated persons, the elderly, and persons with serious spinal cord injury. Generally, patients who are at risk for pressure sores are elderly or chronically ill young patients who are immobilized, either in bed or a wheelchair, and who may have altered mental status and/or incontinence.

ETIOLOGY

Similar to diabetic foot infections, a large variety of aerobic gram-positive and gram-negative organisms, as well as anaerobes, frequently are isolated from wound cultures.[76] Curettage of the ulcer base after debridement provides more reliable culture information than does needle aspiration.[75] Biopsy specimens give the most reliable data but may not be practical to obtain. Deep-tissue cultures from different sites may give different results. Cultures collected from pressure ulcers reveal polymicrobial growth. A culture collected by swab is likely to identify surface bacteria colonizing the wound rather than to diagnose the infection.[75,76]

PATHOPHYSIOLOGY

Many factors are thought to predispose patients to the formation of pressure sores: paralysis, paresis, immobilization, malnutrition, anemia, infection, and advanced age. Four factors thought to be most critical to their formation are pressure, shearing forces, friction, and moisture; however, there is still debate as to the exact pathophysiology of pressure sore formation.

Pressure is the essential element in the formation of pressure sores. The areas of highest pressure are generated most often over the bony prominences. Studies show that when the pressure is relieved intermittently within a 2-hour period, only minimal changes occur in soft-tissue and skin structures.[75] Therefore, both the degree of pressure and the length of time that the pressure is applied are important.

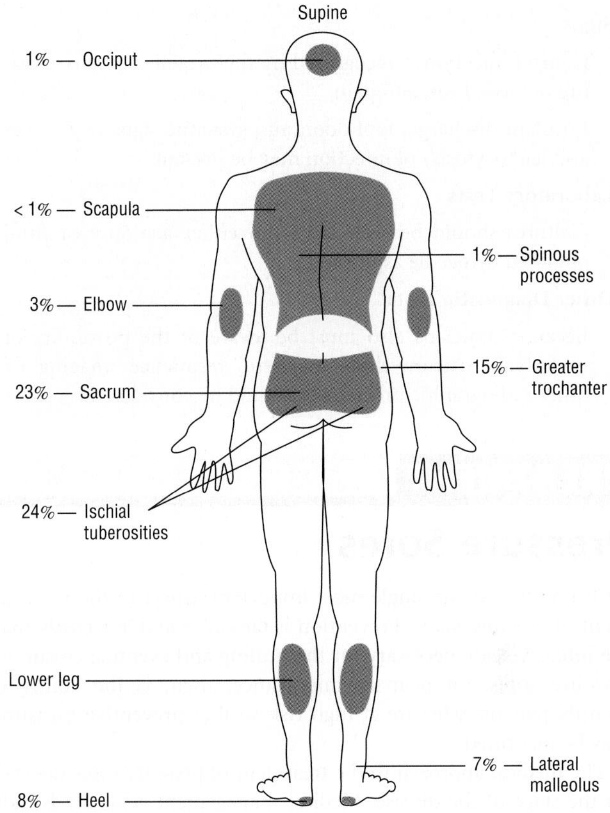

FIGURE 114-2. Supine view of areas where pressure sore formation tends to occur.

Shearing forces are caused by the sliding of adjacent parallel surfaces of soft tissues in an unequal fashion. This situation can occur when the head of a bed is raised, causing the upper torso to slide downward, transmitting pressure to the sacrum and other areas. This effect results in occlusion or distortion of vessels, leading to compromise of the dermis. At the same time, sitting and gravity create shearing forces; the posterior sacral skin area can become fixed secondary to friction with the bed. The effects of friction and shearing forces combine, resulting in transmission of force to the deep portion of the superficial fascia and leading to further damage of soft tissue structures.

Compounding the problems of shearing and friction forces are the macerating effects of excessive moisture in the local environment, resulting from incontinence and perspiration. This factor is of critical importance because when combined with the other forces, it increases the risk of pressure sore formation fivefold.[75]

CLINICAL PRESENTATION

General

- Pressure sores can occur anywhere on the body.
- However, more than 95% of all pressure sores are located on the lower part of the body (65% in the region of the pelvis and 3.4% on the lower extremities; Fig. 114–2).
- The most common sites on the lower portion of the body are the sacral and coccygeal areas, ischial tuberosities, and greater trochanter.

Symptoms

- Patients with pressure sores commonly have other medical problems that may mask the typical signs and symptoms of infection.

Signs

- Clinical infection is recognized by the presence of surrounding redness, heat, and pain.
- Purulent discharge, foul odor, and systemic signs (e.g., fever and leukocytosis) of infection may be present.

Laboratory Tests

- Cultures should be collected from either a biopsy or fluid obtained by needle aspiration.

Other Diagnostic Tests

- Because clinicians also must be aware of the possibility of underlying osteomyelitis, magnetic resonance imaging or other radiographic procedures should be considered.

TREATMENT

Pressure Sores

8 Prevention is the single most important aspect in the management of pressure sores. Prevention is far easier and less costly than the intensive care necessary for the healing and eventual closure of pressure sores. Of primary importance, then, is the ability to identify patients who are at high risk so that preventive measures may be instituted.

The medical approach to the treatment of pressure sores depends on the stage of the disease. Medical management generally is indicated for lesions that are of moderate size and relatively shallow depth (stage 1 or 2 lesions) and are not located over a bony prominence. Depending on their location and severity, from 30% to 80% of these ulcers will heal without an operation. Surgical intervention is almost always necessary for ulcers that extend through superficial fascia or into bone (stage 3 and 4 lesions).

The goal of therapy is to clean and decontaminate the ulcer to promote wound healing by permitting the formation of healthy granulation tissue or to prepare the wound for an operative procedure. The main factors to be considered for successful topical therapy (local care) are (a) relief of pressure, (b) debridement of necrotic tissue as needed, (c) wound cleansing, (d) dressing selection, and (e) prevention, diagnosis, and treatment of infection.[77]

Friction and shearing forces can be minimized with proper positioning. Skin care and prevention of soilage are important, with the intent being to keep the surface relatively free of moisture. Patients with problems of incontinence should be cleaned frequently, and efforts should be made to keep the involved areas dry. Natural sheepskin is believed to be useful in minimizing the effects of moisture, shearing forces, and friction. Relief of pressure is probably the single most important factor in preventing pressure sore formation. Relief for a period of only 5 minutes once every 2 hours is believed to give protection against pressure sore formation.[74,76,77]

The goals of debridement and cleansing measures are removal of devitalized tissue and reduction of bacterial contamination, which can slow granulation time and, therefore, impede healing. Debridement can be accomplished by surgical, mechanical, or chemical means. Surgical debridement rapidly removes necrotic material from the wound and is recommended for urgent situations (e.g., cellulitis and sepsis).[77] Mechanical debridement generally involves wet-to-dry dressing changes. Saline-soaked gauze is applied to the wound; after drying, the gauze is removed and with it any adherent necrotic tissue. Other effective mechanical therapies include hydrotherapy (use of the whirlpool [Hubbard tank] to remove necrotic tissue and debris), wound irrigation, and dextranomers (beads placed in the wound to absorb exudate and bacteria). Chemical debridement includes enzymatic and autolytic agents. Enzymatic debridement involves application of topical debriding agents to remove devitalized tissue. This method is recommended for patients who cannot tolerate surgery or are in a long-term care or home setting. Autolytic debridement involves the use of synthetic dressings that allow devitalized tissue to self-digest via enzymes present in wound fluids. Autolytic debridement is contraindicated in the treatment of infected pressure sores.

Pressure sore wounds should be cleaned with normal saline. Cleansing agents that are cytotoxic, such as povidone-iodine, iodophor, sodium hypochlorite solution, hydrogen peroxide, and acetic acid, should be avoided.[77] Many of these agents impair healing. Many different types of dressings are available for pressure sores. Wound dressing materials should keep the wound moist, allow free exchange of air, act as a physical barrier to bacteria, and prevent physical damage. Controlled studies of the various types of wound dressings have shown no significant differences in healing outcomes.[77] Occlusive dressings should be avoided if infection is present.[74–77] If occlusive dressings are used, any infection should be controlled or the dressing frequency increased.

Systemic treatment (see Table 114–5) of an infected pressure ulcer should be guided by results from appropriately collected cultures. Systemic antibiotics generally are reserved for treatment of bacteremia, sepsis, cellulitis, or osteomyelitis.[74–77] However, a 2-week trial of topical antibiotics (silver sulfadiazine or triple antibiotic) is recommended for a clean ulcer that is not healing or is producing a moderate amount of exudate despite appropriate care.[74]

Other nonpharmacologic approaches to shortening the healing time have included the use of hyperbaric oxygenation, hydrotherapy, high-frequency/high-intensity sound waves, and electrotherapy.[75,78] Electrical stimulation is the only adjunctive therapy that is effective.[75,78]

EVALUATION OF THERAPEUTIC OUTCOMES

With appropriate wound care and antimicrobial therapy, infected pressure sores can heal. A reduction in erythema, warmth, pain, and other signs and symptoms should be seen in 48 to 72 hours.

BITE WOUNDS

Approximately half the population in the United States will be bitten by either an animal or another human sometime during their lifetimes.[79] Bite wounds have a substantial potential for infectious complications. If left untreated, complications such as soft tissue infection and osteomyelitis may occur, possibly requiring extensive débridement or amputation.

ANIMAL BITES

Epidemiology

Dog bites account for approximately 80% of all animal bite wounds requiring medical attention. Data from U.S. emergency departments reported 368,245 visits for new dog bite-related injuries in 2001.[80] Based on the data gathered in this study, approximately 1,000 new dog bite injuries are seen in emergency departments every day. Approximately one-half of dog bites occur in individuals younger than 20 years of age, usually males (55%). More than 70% of bites are to the extremities. Facial bites are also seen, particularly in children younger than 5 years of age. Up to 65% of bite wounds in young children involve the head and neck, and can be a lethal event because of blood loss. From 1979 through 1994, 279 deaths were the result of attacks by dogs.[81]

Patients at greatest risk of acquiring an infection after a bite have had a puncture wound (usually the hand), have not sought medical attention within 12 hours of the injury, and are older than 50 years of age.[82,83]

Cat bites, with an estimated incidence of 5% to 15% of all animal bites, are the second most common cause of animal bite wounds in the United States.[82] Bites and scratches occur most commonly on the upper extremities, with most injuries reported in women.[79] Infection rates, estimated at 30% to 50%, are more than double those seen with dog bites.[79,82,83]

Etiology

Infections from dog bite wounds are caused predominantly by mouth flora from the animal.[84–86] Most infections are polymicrobial, with approximately five bacterial isolates per culture.[84] *Pasteurella multocida* is the most frequent isolate. Other common aerobes include streptococci, staphylococci, *Moraxella,* and *Neisseria.* The most common anaerobes are *Fusobacterium, Bacteroides, Porphyromonas,* and *Prevotella.*[84] Wound-site cultures in both infected and noninfected patients have similar bacteria present, with aerobic organisms isolated from 74% to 90% and anaerobic organisms isolated from 41% to 49% of patients.[79,82,84]

Infections arising from cat bites or scratches are frequently (75%) caused by *P. multocida,* which has been isolated in the oropharynx of 50% to 70% of healthy cats.[82,86] Mixed aerobic and anaerobic infections have been reported in 63% of cat bite wounds, whereas approximately one-third of cultures grow aerobes only.[84] Both tularemia (*Pasteurella tularensis*) and rabies also have been transmitted by cat bites.[79,82,84]

Pathophysiology

The potential for infection from an animal bite is great owing to the pressure that can be exerted during the bite and the vast number of potential pathogens that make up the normal oral flora.[85] Cats' teeth are slender and extremely sharp. Their teeth easily penetrate into bones and joints, resulting in a higher incidence of septic arthritis and osteomyelitis.[79,82] Although a dog's teeth may not be as sharp, they can exert a pressure of 200 to 450 lb/in^2 and therefore result in a serious crush injury with much devitalized tissue.[85] Known human pathogens such as *S. aureus, P. multocida,* and anaerobes are among the more than 64 species of bacteria that are harbored in the average dog mouth.[85] In addition, the polymicrobic (aerobic and anaerobic) nature of animal bites provides a synergistic relationship, thus making an infection harder to eradicate.[85]

CLINICAL PRESENTATION

General

- Health care providers see two distinct groups of patients seeking medical attention for dog bites.
- The first group presents within 12 hours of the injury; these patients require general wound care, repair of tear wounds, or rabies and/or tetanus treatment. The second group of patients presents more than 12 hours after the injury has occurred; these patients usually have clinical signs of infection and seek medical attention for infection-related complaints.

Symptoms

- Patients seek medical care for infection-related complaints (i.e., pain, purulent discharge, and swelling).

Signs

- Patients with infected dog bite wounds generally present with a localized cellulitis and pain at the site of injury.
- Cellulitis usually spreads proximally from the initial site of injury, and a gray malodorous discharge may be encountered.
- If *P. multocida* is present, a rapidly progressing cellulitis is observed, with pain and swelling developing within 24 (70%) to 48 (90%) hours of initial injury.
- Fever is uncommon.
- Fewer than 20% of patients have a concomitant adenopathy or lymphangitis.

Laboratory Tests

- Samples for bacterial cultures (aerobic and anaerobic) should be obtained.
- Wounds seen less than 8 hours or more than 24 hours after injury that show no signs of infection may not need to be cultured.

Other Diagnostic Tests

- A roentgenogram of the affected part should be considered when infection is documented in proximity to a bone or joint.

TREATMENT

Dog and Cat Bites

Table 114–4 lists the recommended drugs and dosing regimens for animal bite wounds.

Cultures obtained from early, noninfected bite wounds are not of great value in predicting the subsequent development of infection. Documentation of the mechanism of injury is important; if possible, an immunization history of the animal should be obtained. It is also important for the patient's tetanus immune status to be determined.

Wounds should be irrigated thoroughly with a copious volume (>150 mL) of sterile normal saline. Proper irrigation reduces the bacterial count in the wound. Antibiotic or iodine solutions do not offer any advantage over saline and actually may increase tissue irritation. Several management techniques used in the treatment of bite wounds remain controversial, including the extent and type of debridement,[82,87,88] suturing wounds within 8 hours of the injury,[11] and indications for the use of antibiotics.

The role of prophylactic antimicrobial therapy for the early, noninfected bite wound remains controversial.[82,86,89,90] Unfortunately, suggestions concerning the use of prophylactic antibiotics are based on minimal data because few clinical trials have been performed. Most reports are of retrospective studies or observations of complicated cases. A systematic review of eight randomized trials of bite wounds (caused by both animals and humans) evaluated the use of antibiotics for the prevention of infectious complications and concluded that antibiotics did not significantly reduce the risk of infection in patients with dog or cat bites, but that wounds involving the hands may benefit from antimicrobial prophylaxis.[90] However, this review also concluded that additional studies are required to support these conclusions.[90]

Controlled studies have not shown benefits definitively with prophylactic antibiotics for noninfected bites. Because up to 20% of bite wounds may become infected, a 3- to 5-day course of antimicrobial therapy generally is recommended.[11,79,82,86] This is especially important for patients at greater risk for infection (patients older than 50 years of age and those with puncture wounds and wounds to the hands, and those who are immunocompromised).[86,89] Treatment should be directed at the typical aerobic and anaerobic oral flora of dogs, as well as at potential pathogens from the skin flora of the bite victim. The length of antimicrobial therapy depends on the severity of the injury/infection.[11,82]

CLINICAL CONTROVERSY

To date, there is no single, universally agreed-on treatment regimen for bite wounds. Penicillin provides excellent coverage for *P. multocida* but not for *S. aureus* and most of the other staphylococci that are commonly isolated from bite wounds. Although penicillinase-resistant penicillins, first-generation cephalosporins, erythromycin, and clindamycin have excellent activity against staphylococci, these agents are not active against most strains of *P. multocida.*

Amoxicillin-clavulanic acid is commonly recommended for oral outpatient therapy.[11,82,86,91] Alternative oral agents include doxycycline or the combination of penicillin VK and dicloxacillin. Trimethoprim-sulfamethoxazole and fluoroquinolones have activity against *P. multocida* and are recommended as alternatives for patients who are allergic to penicillins.[11,82,91] However, these agents should not be used in children and/or pregnant women; trimethoprim-sulfamethoxazole also should be avoided during pregnancy. Macrolides or azalides may be considered as alternatives in growing children or pregnant women.[11,82,87] If erythromycin or similar-class agent is selected, bacterial sensitivities should be obtained and clinical response monitored carefully because most strains of *P. multocida* are resistant. Cefuroxime is another viable alternative for patients with mild penicillin allergies. Many of these alternative agents will likely require an additional agent (metronidazole, clindamycin) with activity against anaerobes. Failure to provide adequate initial treatment of bite wounds results in treatment failures and increased need for hospitalization for administration of parenteral antibiotics.[92]

Treatment options for patients requiring intravenous therapy include β-lactam–β-lactamase inhibitor combinations (ampicillin-sulbactam, piperacillin-tazobactam), second-generation cephalosporins with antianaerobic activity (cefoxitin), and carbapenems.[11,79,82,86,91]

In addition to irrigation and antibiotics, when indicated, the injured area should be immobilized and elevated. Clinical failures due to edema have occurred despite appropriate antibiotic therapy.[82] Therefore, it is important to stress to patients that the affected area should be elevated for several days or until edema has resolved.

Tetanus does not occur commonly after dog bites; however, it is possible. If the immunization history of a patient with anything other than a clean, minor wound is unknown, tetanus-diphtheria (TD) toxoids should be administered (0.5 mL intramuscularly).[93] Both TD toxoids and tetanus immune globulin (250 units intramuscularly) should be administered to patients who have never been immunized.[86,94]

Because the rabies virus can be transmitted via saliva, rabies may be a potential complication of a bite. When the symptoms of rabies develop after a bite, the prognosis for survival is poor. Roughly 3% of rabies cases documented in animals were in dogs (the most frequent vectors are skunks, raccoons, and bats).[95]

After a patient has been exposed to rabies, the treatment objectives consist of thorough irrigation of the wound, tetanus prophylaxis, antibiotic prophylaxis, if indicated, and immunization. Prompt, thorough irrigation of the wound with soap or iodine solution may reduce the development of rabies.[95] Postexposure prophylaxis immunization against rabies consists of the administration of both passive antibody and vaccine.[94,95] The vaccine is administered as a series of five 1-mL intramuscular injections given on days 0, 3, 7, 14, and 28, beginning on the day of exposure or as soon as possible afterward. Rabies hyperimmune globulin is administered at a dose of 40 international units/kg; as much of the total dose as possible should be infiltrated into and around the wound, with the remainder being injected intramuscularly at a site different from that of the vaccine.[94] The only exceptions to administration of hyperimmune globulin are patients who were immunized previously and who have the appropriate degree of documented rabies antibody titers. However, even individuals who have been fully vaccinated should receive two doses of vaccine on days 0 and 3 after actual rabies exposure.[94,95]

The management of cat bites is similar to that discussed for dog bites. Cat scratches typically involve the same organisms as bites and should be treated accordingly.

Evaluation of Therapeutic Outcomes

Bite victims treated on an outpatient basis with oral antimicrobials should be followed up within 24 hours either by phone or office visit.[11] Hospitalization or change to intravenous therapy should be considered if the infection has progressed. For hospitalized patients with no improvement in signs and symptoms following 24 hours of appropriate therapy, then surgical debridement may be needed.

HUMAN BITES

Epidemiology

Human bites are the third most frequent type of bite. Infected human bites can occur as bites from the teeth or from blows to the mouth (clenched-fist injuries). Human bites generally are more serious than animal bites and carry a higher likelihood of infection than do most animal bites. Infectious complications occur in 10% to 50% of patients with human bites.[82,96,97]

Self-inflicted bites most commonly occur on the lips or around the fingernails (from sucking or biting the nails). Bites by others can occur to any part of the body, but most often involve the hands. Bites to the hand are most serious and become infected more frequently. The clenched-fist injury is a traumatic laceration caused by one person hitting another in the mouth and is a very serious bite wound. The areas most commonly affected by this injury are the third and fourth metacarpophalangeal joints.

Etiology

Infections caused by these injuries are similar and are caused most often by the normal oral flora, which include both aerobic and anaerobic microorganisms. *Streptococcus* spp. (especially *Streptococcus anginosus*) are the most common isolates, followed by *Staphylococcus* spp. (predominately *S. aureus*).[98] *Eikenella corrodens* is isolated from human bite wounds approximately 30% of the time.[82,98] Anaerobic microorganisms have been isolated in approximately 40% of human bites and 55% of clenched-fist injuries. Common anaerobes recovered from human bite infections include *Fusobacterium*, *Prevotella*, *Porphyromonas*, and *Peptostreptococcus* species.[98]

Pathophysiology

Human bites generally are more serious and more prone to infection than animal bites, particularly clenched-fist injuries.[85] While the force of a punch may sever a tendon or nerve or break a bone, it most often causes a breach in the capsule of the metacarpophalangeal joint, leading to direct inoculation of bacteria into the joint or bone.[82] When the hand is relaxed, the tendons carry bacteria into deeper spaces of the hand, resulting in more extensive infection.[82]

CLINICAL PRESENTATION

General

- Most clenched-fist injuries are already infected by the time patients seek medical care, and most require hospitalization.

Symptoms

- Patients with infected bites to the hand may develop a painful, throbbing, swollen extremity.

- Wounds often have a purulent discharge, and the patient complains of a decreased range of motion.

Signs

- Signs of infection include erythema, swelling, and clear or pussy discharge.
- Adjacent lymph nodes may be enlarged.
- In clenched-fist injuries, edema may limit the ability of tendons to glide in their sheaths, thereby limiting a joint's range of motion.

Laboratory Tests

- Samples for bacterial cultures (aerobic and anaerobic) should be collected as per animal bites.
- In severe infections, a peripheral leukocytosis of 15,000 to 30,000 cells/mm^3 may be seen; therefore, the white blood count should be monitored for resolution of infection.

Other Diagnostic Tests

- If damage to a bone or joint is suspected, radiographic evaluation should be undertaken.

TREATMENT

Human Bites

Table 114–4 lists the recommended drugs and dosing regimens for human bite wounds.

❾ Management of bite wounds consists of aggressive irrigation and topical wound cleansing. Surgical debridement and immobilization of the affected area is often required. Prophylactic antimicrobial agents should be given as soon as possible to all patients, regardless of the appearance of the wound, unless it can be documented that the wound does not involve hands, feet, or joints and penetrates no deeper than the epidermis.[11,83] Patients with clenched-fist injuries should be seen by a specialist in hand care to evaluate for penetration into the synovium, joint capsule, and bone.[11,82] Primary closure for human bites generally is not recommended. Tetanus toxoid and antitoxin may be indicated. Because transmission of viruses (HIV, herpes, hepatitides B and C) is a possibility with human bites, information about the biter is important. Although the possibility of acquiring HIV through bites is believed to be unlikely, the presence of the virus in the saliva makes disease transmission possible. If the biter is HIV-positive, the victim should have a baseline blood specimen drawn to determine preexposure HIV status and then be retested in 3 months and 6 months.[97] The bite wound should be irrigated thoroughly and vigorously with a virucidal agent such as povidone-iodine.[79,82] Bite victims exposed to blood-tainted saliva should be offered antiretroviral chemoprophylaxis.

❿ Patients with human bite injuries should receive prophylactic antibiotic therapy for 3 to 5 days.[99] First-generation cephalosporins, macrolides, clindamycin, and aminoglycosides are not recommended because the sensitivity of these agents to *E. corrodens* is variable.[79,82,89] Amoxicillin-clavulanic acid (500 mg every 8 hours) is commonly recommended. Alternatives for penicillin-allergic patients include fluoroquinolones or trimethoprim-sulfamethoxazole in combination with clindamycin or metronidazole.[11,79,82,89]

Hospitalization for minor wounds is unnecessary if surgical repair of vital structures has not been performed. Patients suffering serious injuries or clenched-fist injuries should be started on intravenous antibiotics. Recommended agents include cefoxitin (1 g every 6 to 8 hours), ampicillin-sulbactam (1.5 to 3 g every 6 hours), or ertapenem (1 g every 24 hours).[11,91] Therapeutic failures have been documented when either first-generation cephalosporins or penicillinase-resistant penicillins have been used alone, most likely because of their poor and variable activity against *E. corrodens.* Therapy should be continued from 7 to 14 days.[99]

Evaluation of Therapeutic Outcomes

Evaluation of treatment should follow the same general guidelines as discussed for animal bite wounds. Complications with clenched-fist injuries are common and may result in residual joint stiffness and loss of function. Physical therapy can be needed to improve these complications.

ABBREVIATIONS

HIV: human immunodeficiency virus

MRSA: methicillin-resistant *Staphylococcus aureus*

CA-MRSA: community-associated methicillin-resistant *S. aureus*

SSTI: skin and soft-tissue infection

TD: tetanus-diphtheria

REFERENCES

1. Fung HB, Chang JY, Kuczynski S. A practical guide to the treatment of complicated skin and soft tissue infections. Drugs 2003;63:1459–1480.
2. Eron LJ, Lipsky BA, Low DE, et al. Managing skin and soft tissue infections: Expert panel recommendations on key decision points. J Antimicrob Chemother 2003;59;52(Suppl S1):i3–i17.
3. Centers for Disease Control and Prevention. Soft tissue infections among injection drug users: San Francisco, California—1996–2000. MMWR Morb Mort Wkly Rep 2001;50:381–384.
4. Stulberg DL, Penrod MA, Blatny RA. Common bacterial skin infections. Am Fam Physician 2002;66:119–124.
5. Elixhauser A, Steiner CA. Most Common Diagnoses and Procedures in U.S. Community Hospitals, 1996: Summary. HCUP Research Note. Rockville, MD: Agency for Health Care Policy and Research, 1996. Available at *http://www.ahrq.gov/data/hcup/commdx/commdx.htm.*
6. Rennie RP, Jones RN, Mutnick AH, and the SENTRY Program Study Group (North America). Occurrence and antimicrobial susceptibility patterns of pathogens isolated from skin and soft tissue infections: Report from the SENTRY Antimicrobial Surveillance Program (United States and Canada, 2000). Diagn Microbiol Infect Dis 2003;45:287–293.
7. Moet GJ, Jones RN, Biedenbach DJ, Stilwell MG, Fritsche TR. Contemporary causes of skin and soft tissue infections in North America, Latin America, and Europe: Report from the SENTRY Antimicrobial Surveillance Program (1998–2004). Diagn Microbiol Infect Dis 2007;57:7–13.
8. Wilson MA. Skin and soft-tissue infections: Impact of resistant gram-positive bacteria. Am J Surg 2003;186(Suppl 5A):35S–41S.
9. Eady EA, Cove JH. Staphylococcal resistance revisited: Community-acquired methicillin-resistant *Staphylococcus aureus*—An emerging problem for the management of skin and soft tissue infections. Curr Opin Infect Dis 2003;16:103–124.
10. Diep BA, Sensabaugh GF, Somboona NS, et al. Widespread skin and soft-tissue infections due to two methicillin-resistant *Staphylococcus aureus* strains harboring the genes for Panton-Valentine leucocidin. J Clin Microbiol 2004;42:2080–2084.
11. Stevens DL, Bisno AL, Chambers HF, et al. Practice guidelines for the diagnosis and management of skin and soft-tissue infections. Clin Infect Dis 2005;41:1373–1406.
12. Frazee BW, Lynn J, Charlebois ED, Lambert L, Lowery D, Perdreau-Remington F. High prevalence of methicillin-resistant *Staphylococcus aureus* in emergency department skin and soft tissue infections. Ann Emerg Med 2005;45:311–320.
13. Moran GJ, Amil RN, Abrahamian FM, Talan DA. Methicillin-resistant *Staphylococcus aureus* in community-acquired skin infections. Emerg Infect Dis 2005;11:928–930.
14. Moran GJ, Krishnadasan A, Gorwitz RJ, et al. Methicillin-resistant *S. aureus* infections among patients in the emergency department. N Eng J Med 2006;355:666–674.

15. King MD, Humphrey BJ, Wang YF, et al. Emergence of community-acquired methicillin-resistant *Staphylococcus aureus* USA 300 clone as the predominant cause of skin and soft-tissue infections. Ann Intern Med 2006;144:309–317.
16. Tenover FC, McDougal LK, Goering RV, et al. Characterization of a strain of community-associated methicillin-resistant *Staphylococcus aureus* widely disseminated in the United States. J Clin Microbiol 2006;44:108–118.
17. Granato PA. Pathogenic and indigenous microorganisms of humans. In: Murray PR, Baron EJ, Jorgensen JH, et al., eds. Manual of Clinical Microbiology, 8th ed. Washington, DC: ASM Press, 2003:44–54.
18. Centers for Disease Control and Prevention. *Pseudomonas* dermatitis/folliculitis associated with pools and hot tubs: Colorado and Maine, 1999–2000. MMWR 2000;49:1087–1091.
19. Lipsky BA, Berendt AR, Deery HG, et al. Diagnosis and treatment of diabetic foot infections. Clin Infect Dis 2004;39:885–910.
20. Swartz MN, Pasternak MS. Cellulitis and subcutaneous tissue infections. In: Mandell GL, Bennett JE, Dolin R, eds. Principles and Practice of Infectious Diseases, 6th ed. New York: Churchill-Livingstone, 2000:1172–1193.
21. Bisno AL, Stevens DL. Streptococcal infections of skin and soft tissues. N Engl J Med 1996;334:240–245.
22. Bergkvist P, Sjobeck K. Antibiotic and prednisolone therapy of erysipelas: A randomized, double-blind, placebo-controlled study. Scand J Infect Dis 1997;29:377–382.
23. Sadick NS. Current aspects of bacterial infections of the skin. Dermatol Clin 1997;15:341–349.
24. Brown J, Shriner DL, Schwartz RA, Janniger CK. Impetigo: An update. Int J Dermatol 2003;42:251–255.
25. Pasternak MS, Swartz MN. Lymphadenitis and lymphangitis. In: Mandell GL, Bennett JE, Dolin R, eds. Principles and Practice of Infectious Diseases, 6th ed. New York: Churchill-Livingstone, 2006:1204–1214.
26. Binswanger IA, Kral AH, Bluthenthal RN, et al. High prevalence of abscesses and cellulitis among community-recruited injection drug users in San Francisco. Clin Infect Dis 2000;30:579–581.
27. Ebright JR, Pieper B. Skin and soft tissue infections in injection drug users. Infect Dis Clin North Am 2002;16:697–712.
28. Bassetti S, Battegav M. *Staphylococcus aureus* infections in injection drug users: Risk factors and prevention strategies. Infection 2004;32:163–169.
29. Kimura AC, Higa JI, Levin RM, Simpson G, Vargas Y, Vugla DJ. Outbreak of necrotizing fasciitis due to *Clostridium sordellii* among black-tar heroin users. Clin Infect Dis 2004;38:e87–e91.
30. Brett MM, Hood J, Brazier JS, Duerden BI, Hahne SJ. Soft tissue infections caused by spore-forming bacteria in injecting drug users in the United Kingdom. Epidemiol Infect 2005;133:575–582.
31. Falagas ME, Barefoot L, Griffith J, et al. Risk factors leading to clinical failure in the treatment of intra-abdominal or skin/soft tissue infections. *Eur J Clin Microbiol Infect Dis* 1996;15:913–921.
32. Tack KJ, Littlejohn TW, Mailloux G, et al. Cefdinir versus cephalexin for the treatment of skin and skin-structure infections. The Cefdinir Adult Skin Infection Study Group. Clin Ther 1998;20:244–256.
33. Ladhani S, Garbash M. Staphylococcal skin infections in children: Rational drug therapy recommendations. Paediatr Drugs 2005;7:77–102.
34. Stevens DL, Herr D, Lampiris H, et al. Linezolid versus vancomycin for the treatment of methicillin-resistant *Staphylococcus aureus* infections. Clin Infect Dis 2002;34:1481–1490.
35. Stevens DL, Smith LG, Bruss JB, et al. Randomized comparison of linezolid (PNU-100766) versus oxacillin-dicloxacillin for treatment of complicated skin and soft tissue infections. Antimicrob Agents Chemother 2000;44:3408–3413.
36. Nichols RL, Graham DR, Barriere SL, et al. Treatment of hospitalized patients with complicated gram-positive skin and skin structure infections: Two randomized, multicentre studies of quinupristin/dalfopristin versus cefazolin, oxacillin or vancomycin. Synercid Skin and Skin Structure Infection Group. J Antimicrob Chemother 1999;44:263–273.
37. Tedesco KL, Rybak MJ. Daptomycin. Pharmacotherapy 2004;24:41–57.
38. Arbeit RD, Maki D, Tally FP, et al. The safety and efficacy of daptomycin for the treatment of complicated skin and skin-structure infections. Clin Infect Dis 2004;38:1673–1681.
39. Breedt J, Teras J, Gardovskis J, et al. Safety and efficacy of tigecycline in treatment of skin and skin structure infections: Results of a double-blind phase 3 comparison study with vancomycin-aztreonam. Antimicrob Agents Chemother 2005;49:4658–4666.
40. Wilcox MH. Efficacy of tigecycline in complicated skin and skin structure infections and complicated intra-abdominal infections. J Chemother 2005;17(Suppl 1):23–29.
41. McKinnon PS, Sorensen SV, Liu LZ, Itani KM. Impact of linezolid on economic outcomes and determinants of cost in a clinical trial evaluating patients with MRSA complicated skin and soft-tissue infections. Ann Pharmacother 2006;40:1017–1023.
42. Moran GJ, Talan DA. Community-associated methicillin-resistant *Staphylococcus aureus*: Is it in your community and should it change practice? Ann Emerg Med 2005;45:321–322.
43. Grayson LG. The treatment triangle for staphylococcal infections. N Engl J Med 2006;355:724–727.
44. Grayson ML, Gibbons GW, Habershaw GM, et al. Use of ampicillin/sulbactam versus imipenem/cilastatin in the treatment of limb-threatening foot infections in diabetic patients. Clin Infect Dis 1994;18:683–693.
45. Graham DR, Lucasti C, Malafaia O, et al. Ertapenem once daily versus piperacillin-tazobactam four times per day for treatment of complicated skin and skin-structure infections in adults: Results of a prospective, randomized, double-blind multicenter study. Clin Infect Dis 2002;34:1460–1468.
46. Graham DR, Talan DA, Nichols RL, et al. Once-daily, high-dose levofloxacin versus ticarcillin-clavulanate alone or followed by amoxicillin-clavulanate for complicated skin and skin-structure infections: A randomized, open-label trial. Clin Infect Dis 2002;35:381–389.
47. Fabian TC, File TM Jr, Embil JM, et al. Meropenem versus imipenem-cilastatin for the treatment of hospitalized patients with complicated skin and skin structure infections: Results of a multicenter, randomized, double-blind comparative study. Surg Infect 2005;6:269–282.
48. Gentry LO. Therapy with newer oral β-lactam and quinolone agents for infections of the skin and skin structures: A review. Clin Infect Dis 1992;14:285–297.
49. Parish LC, Routh HB, Miskin B, et al. Moxifloxacin versus cephalexin in the treatment of uncomplicated skin infections. Int J Clin Pract 2000;54:497–503.
50. Nichols RL, Smith JW, Gentry LO, et al. Multicenter randomized study comparing levofloxacin and ciprofloxacin for uncomplicated skin and skin structure infections. South Med J 1997;90:1193–1200.
51. Giordano P, Song J, Pertel P, et al. Sequential intravenous/oral moxifloxacin versus intravenous piperacillin-tazobactam followed by oral amoxicillin-clavulanate for the treatment of complicated skin and skin structure infection. Int J Antimicrob Agents 2005;26:357–365.
52. Zervos MJ, Hershberger E, Nicolau DP, et al. Relationship between fluoroquinolone use and changes in susceptibility to fluoroquinolones of selected pathogens in 10 United States teaching hospitals, 1991–2000. Clin Infect Dis 2003;37:1643–1648.
53. Neuhauser MM, Weinstein RA, Rydman R, et al. Antibiotic resistance among gram-negative bacilli in US intensive care units. Implications for fluoroquinolone use. JAMA 2003;289:885–888.
54. Crane L, Levine D, Aervos M, et al. Bacteremia in narcotic addicts at Detroit Medical Center: Microbiology, epidemiology, risk factors, and empiric therapy. Rev Infect Dis 1986;8:364–373.
55. Urschel JD. Necrotizing soft tissue infections. Postgrad Med J 1999;75:645–649.
56. Vinh DC, Embil JM. Rapidly progressive soft tissue infections. Lancet Infect Dis 2005;5:501–513.
57. Chen JL, Fullerton KE, Flynn NM. Necrotizing fasciitis associated with injection drug use. Clin Infect Dis 2001;33:6–15.
58. Jallali N, Withey S, Butler PE. Hyperbaric oxygen as adjuvant therapy in the management of necrotizing fasciitis. Am J Med 2005;189:462–466.
59. Gentry LO. Diagnosis and management of the diabetic foot ulcer. J Antimicrob Chemother 1993;32(Suppl A):77–89.
60. Smith AJ, Daniels T, Bohnen JMA. Soft tissue infections and the diabetic foot. Am J Surg 1996;172(Suppl 6A):7S–12S.
61. Levin ME. Foot lesions in patients with diabetes mellitus. Endocrinol Metab Clin North Am 1996;25:447–462.
62. Ramsey SD, Newton K, Blough D, et al. Incidence, outcomes, and cost of foot ulcers in patients with diabetes. Diabetes Care 1999;22:382–387.
63. Tennvall GR, Apelqvist J, Eneroth M. Costs of deep foot infections in patients with diabetes mellitus. Pharmacoeconomics 2000;18:225–238.

64. Slovenkai MP. Foot problems in diabetes. Med Clin North Am 1998;82:949–971.
65. Pellizzer G, Strazzabosco M, Presi S, et al. Deep tissue biopsy vs. superficial swab culture monitoring in the microbiological assessment of limb-threatening diabetic foot infection. Diabet Med 2001;18:822–827.
66. Lipsky BA, Armstrong DG, Citron DM, et al. Ertapenem versus piperacillin/tazobactam for diabetic foot infections (SIDESTEP): Prospective, randomized, controlled, double-blinded, multicentre trial. Lancet 2005;366:1695–1703.
67. Shea KW. Antimicrobial therapy for diabetic foot infections. Postgrad Med 1999;106:85–94.
68. West NJ. Systemic antimicrobial treatment of foot infections in diabetic patients. Am J Health Syst Pharm 1995;52:1199–1207.
69. Armstrong DG, Lavery LA, Nixon BP, Boulton AJ. It's not what you put on, but what you take off; techniques for debriding and off-loading the diabetic foot wound. Clin Infect Dis 2004;39(Suppl 2):S92–S99.
70. Eron LJ, Harvey L, Hixon DL, et al. Ciprofloxacin therapy of infections caused by *Pseudomonas aeruginosa* and other resistant bacteria. Antimicrob Agents Chemother 1985;28:308–310.
71. Grayson ML, Gibbons GW, Habershaw GM, et al. Use of ampicillin-sulbactam versus imipenem-cilastatin in the treatment of limb-threatening foot infections in diabetic patients. Clin Infect Dis 1994;18:683–693.
72. Lipsky BA, Baker PD, Landon GC, et al. Antibiotic therapy for diabetic foot infections: Comparison of two parenteral-to-oral regimens. Clin Infect Dis 1997;24:643–648.
73. Shea JD. Pressure sores: Classification and management. Clin Orthop 1975;112:89–100.
74. National Pressure Ulcer Advisory Panel. Pressure ulcers: Incidence, economics, risk. Consensus Development Conference Statement. Decubitus 1989;2:24–29.
75. Kanj LF, Wilking SVB, Phillips TJ. Pressure ulcers. J Am Acad Dermatol 1998;38:517–536.
76. Garcia AD, Thomas DR. Assessment and management of chronic pressure ulcers in the elderly. Med Clin North Am 2006;90:925–944.
77. Cervo FA, Cruz AC, Posillico JA. Pressure ulcers: Analysis of guidelines for treatment and management. Geriatrics 2000;55:55–60.
78. Cuddigan J, Frantz RA. Pressure ulcer research: Pressure ulcer treatment. A monograph from the National Pressure Ulcer Advisory Panel. Adv Wound Care 1998;2:294–300.
79. Smith PF, Meadowcraft AM, May DB. Treating mammalian bite wounds. J Clin Pharm Ther 2000;25:85–99.
80. Centers for Disease Control and Prevention. Nonfatal dog bite-related injuries treated in hospital emergency departments—United States, 2001. MMWR 2003;52:605–610.
81. Anonymous. Dog bite related fatalities—United States, 1995–1996. MMWR 1997;46:463–467.
82. Brook, I. Management of human and animal bite wounds: An overview. Adv Skin Wound Care 2005;18:197–203.
83. Broder J, Jerrard D, Olshaker J, Witting M. Low risk of infection in selected human bites treated without antibiotics. Am J Emerg Med 2004;22:10–13.
84. Talan DA, Citron DM, Abrahamian FM, et al. Bacteriologic analysis of infected dog and cat bites. N Engl J Med 1999;340:85–92.
85. Brook I. Microbiology and management of human and animal bite wound infections. Prim Care 2003;30:1–11.
86. Goldstein EJC. Bites. In: Mandell GL, Bennett JE, Dolin R, eds. Principles and Practice of Infectious Diseases, 6th ed. New York: Churchill-Livingstone, 2005:3552–3556.
87. Benson LS, Edwards SL, Schiff AP, et al. Dog and cat bites to the hand: Treatment and cost assessment. J Hand Surg 2006;31:468–473.
88. Stefanopoulos PK, Tarantzopoulou AD. Facial bite wounds: Management update. Int J Oral Maxillofac Surg 2005;34:464–472.
89. Taplitz RA. Managing bite wounds. Currently recommended antibiotics for treatment and prophylaxis. Postgrad Med 2004;116:49–52, 55–56.
90. Medeiros I, Saconato H. Antibiotic prophylaxis for mammalian bites. Cochrane Database Syst Rev 2001;2:CD001738.
91. Goldstein EJ, Citron DM, Merriam CV, et al. Comparative in vitro activity of ertapenem and 11 other antimicrobial agents against aerobic and anaerobic pathogens isolated from skin and soft tissue animal and human bite wound infections. J Antimicrob Chemother 2001;48:641–651.
92. Holm M, Tarnvik A. Hospitalization due to *Pasteurella multocida*-infected animal bite wounds: Correlation with inadequate primary antibiotic medication. Scand J Infect Dis 2000;32:181–183.
93. Centers for Disease Control and Prevention. Diphtheria, tetanus, and pertussis: Recommendations for vaccine use and other preventive measures: Recommendations of the Immunization Practices Advisory Committee (ACIP). MMWR 1991:40(RR-10):1–28.
94. Orenstein WA, Wharton M, Bart KJ, Hinman AR. Immunization. In: Mandell GL, Bennett JE, Dolin R, eds. Principles and Practice of Infectious Diseases, 6th ed. New York: Churchill-Livingstone, 2005:3557–3588.
95. Rupprecht CE, Gibbons RV. Prophylaxis against rabies. N Engl J Med 2004;351:2626–2635.
96. Stierman KL, Lloyd KM, De Luca-Pytell DM, et al. Treatment and outcome of human bites in the head and neck. Otolaryngol Head Neck Surg 2003;128:795–801.
97. Bunzli WF, Wright DH, Hoang AD, et al. Current management of human bites. Pharmacotherapy 1998;18:227–234.
98. Talan DA, Abrahamian FM, Moran PM, et al. Clinical presentation and bacteriologic analysis of infected human bites in patients presenting to emergency departments. Clin Infect Dis 2003;37:1481–1489.
99. Talan D. Infectious disease issues in the emergency department. Clin Infect Dis 1996;23:1–14.

CHAPTER 115 Infective Endocarditis

MICHAEL A. CROUCH AND ANGIE VEVERKA

KEY CONCEPTS

1. Infective endocarditis is an uncommon infection usually occurring in persons with preexisting cardiac valvular abnormalities (e.g., prosthetic heart valves) or with other specific risk factors (e.g., intravenous drug abuse).
2. Three groups of organisms cause a majority of infective endocarditis cases: streptococci, staphylococci, and enterococci.
3. The clinical presentation of infective endocarditis is highly variable and nonspecific, although a fever and murmur usually are present. Classic peripheral manifestations (Osler nodes) may or may not occur.
4. The diagnosis of infective endocarditis requires the integration of clinical, laboratory, and echocardiographic findings. The two major diagnostic criteria are bacteremia and echocardiographic changes (e.g., valvular vegetation).
5. Treatment of infective endocarditis involves isolation of the infecting pathogen and determination of antimicrobial susceptibilities, followed by high-dose, parenteral, bactericidal antibiotics for an extended period.
6. Surgical replacement of the infected heart valve is an important adjunct to endocarditis treatment in certain situations (e.g., patients with acute heart failure).
7. *β*-Lactam antibiotics, such as penicillin G (or ceftriaxone), nafcillin, and ampicillin, remain the drugs of choice for streptococcal, staphylococcal, and enterococcal endocarditis, respectively.
8. Aminoglycosides are essential to obtain a synergistic bactericidal effect in the treatment of enterococcal endocarditis. Adjunctive aminoglycosides also may decrease the emergence of resistant organisms (e.g., prosthetic valve endocarditis caused by coagulase-negative staphylococci) and hasten the pace of clinical and microbiologic response (e.g., some streptococcal and staphylococcal infections).
9. Vancomycin is reserved for patients with immediate *β*-lactam allergies and the treatment of resistant organisms.
10. Antimicrobial prophylaxis is used as an attempt to prevent infective endocarditis in patients who are at the highest risk (such as persons with prosthetic heart valves) before a bacteremia-causing procedure (e.g., dental extraction).

Learning objectives, review questions, and other resources can be found at **www.pharmacotherapyonline.com.**

Endocarditis is an inflammation of the endocardium, the membrane lining the chambers of the heart and covering the cusps of the heart valves.[1,2] More commonly, *endocarditis* refers to infection of the heart valves by various microorganisms. Although it typically affects native valves, it also may involve nonvalvular areas or implanted mechanical devices (e.g., mechanical heart valves). Bacteria primarily cause endocarditis, but fungi and other atypical microorganisms can lead to the disease; hence, the more encompassing term *infective endocarditis* is preferred.

Endocarditis is often referred to as acute or subacute depending on the pace and severity of the clinical presentation. The acute, fulminating form is associated with high fevers and systemic toxicity. Virulent bacteria, such as *Staphylococcus aureus,* frequently cause this syndrome, and if untreated, death may occur within days to weeks. On the other hand, subacute infective endocarditis is more indolent and it is caused by less-invasive organisms, such as viridans streptococci, usually occurring in preexisting valvular heart disease. Although infective endocarditis is often referred to as acute or subacute, it is best classified based on the etiologic organism, the anatomic site of infection, and pathogenic risk factors.[2] Infection also may follow surgical insertion of a prosthetic heart valve, resulting in prosthetic-valve endocarditis (PVE).[3]

EPIDEMIOLOGY AND ETIOLOGY

Infective endocarditis is an uncommon, but not rare, infection affecting about 10,000 to 20,000 persons annually in the United States. The infection accounts for approximately 1 in every 1,000 hospital admissions.[1] Yet, the incidence of infective endocarditis may be increasing, and it is now the fourth leading cause of infectious disease syndromes that are life-threatening, after urosepsis, pneumonia, and intraabdominal sepsis.[4] The mean male-to-female ratio is 1.7:1. Overall, most cases occur in individuals older than 50 years of age, and it is uncommon in children.[1,2] PVE accounts for 10% to 30% of cases of infective endocarditis.[5] As the population ages, and as valve replacement surgery becomes more common, the mean age of patients with infective endocarditis increases. However, those with a history of intravenous drug abuse (IVDA) are also at high risk of infective endocarditis. Other conditions associated with a higher incidence of infective endocarditis include diabetes, long-term hemodialysis, and poor dental hygeine.[6,7]

❶ Most persons with infective endocarditis have risk factors, such as preexisting cardiac valvular abnormalities. Many types of structural heart disease result in turbulent blood flow that increases the risk for infective endocarditis. A predisposing risk factor, however, may be absent in up to 25% of cases. Some of the more important risk factors include[6]:

- Presence of a prosthetic valve (highest risk)
- Previous endocarditis (highest risk)

- Complex cyanotic congenital heart disease (e.g., single-ventricle states)
- Surgically constructed systemic pulmonary shunts or conduits
- Acquired valvular dysfunction (e.g., rheumatic heart disease)
- Hypertrophic cardiomyopathy
- Mitral valve prolapse with regurgitation
- IVDA

In the past, rheumatic heart disease was a prevalent risk factor for infective endocarditis, but the incidence of this disease continues to decline. The risk of infective endocarditis in persons with mitral valve prolapse and regurgitation is small; however, because the condition is prevalent, it is an important contributor to the overall number of infective endocarditis cases.[6,7] Prosthetic valve endocarditis occurs in 1% to 3% of patients undergoing valve replacement surgery in the first postoperative year.[3,5,8]

❷ Nearly every organism causing human disease has been reported to cause infective endocarditis, but three groups of organisms result in a majority of cases: streptococci, staphylococci, and enterococci (Table 115–1).[1,5] The incidence of staphylococci, particularly *S. aureus,* continues to increase, and recent case series document staphylococci have surpassed viridans streptococci as the leading cause of infective endocarditis.[6,8,9] In general, streptococci cause infective endocarditis in patients with underlying cardiac abnormalities, such as mitral valve prolapse or rheumatic heart disease. Staphylococci (*S. aureus* and coagulase-negative staphylococci) are the most common cause of PVE within the first year after valve surgery, and *S. aureus* is common in those with a history of IVDA. Although polymicrobial infective endocarditis is uncommon, it is encountered most often in association with IVDA.[5,6,7] Enterococcal endocarditis tends to follow genitourinary manipulations (older men) or obstetric procedures (younger women).[5] There are many exceptions to the preceding generalizations; thus, isolation of the causative pathogen and determination of its antimicrobial susceptibilities offer the best chance for successful therapy.

The mitral and aortic valves are affected most commonly in cases involving a single valve. Subacute endocarditis tends to involve the mitral valve, whereas acute disease often involves the aortic valve. Up to 35% of cases involve concomitant infections of both the aortic and the mitral valves. Infection of the tricuspid valve is less common, with a majority of these cases occurring in patients with a history of IVDA. It is rare for the pulmonary valve to be infected.[1,2]

PATHOPHYSIOLOGY

The development of infective endocarditis via hematogenous spread, the most common route, requires the sequential occurrence of several factors. These components are complex and not fully elucidated.[1,2,5]

- *The endothelial surface of the heart is damaged.* This injury occurs with turbulent blood flow associated with the valvular lesions previously described.
- *Platelet and fibrin deposition occurs on the abnormal epithelial surface.* These platelet-fibrin deposits are referred to as *nonbacterial thrombotic endocarditis.*
- *Bacteremia gives organisms access to and results in colonization of the endocardial surface.* Bacteremia is the result of trauma to a mucosal surface with a high concentration of resident bacteria, such as the oral cavity and gastrointestinal tract. Transient bacteremia commonly follows certain dental, gastrointestinal, urologic, and gynecologic procedures. Staphylococci, viridans streptococci, and enterococci are most likely to adhere to nonbacterial thrombotic endocarditis, probably because of production of specific adherence factors, such as dextran by some oral streptococci and glycocalyx for staphylococci.[2,8,86] Gram-negative bacteria rarely adhere to heart valves and are uncommon causes of infective endocarditis.
- *After colonization of the endothelial surface, a "vegetation" of fibrin, platelets, and bacteria forms.* The protective cover of fibrin and platelets allows unimpeded bacterial growth to concentrations as high as 10^9 to 10^{10} organisms per gram of tissue.

TABLE 115-1 Etiologic Organisms in Infective Endocarditis

Agent	Percentage of Cases (%)
Streptococci	60–80
Viridans streptococci	30–40
Other streptococci	15–25
Staphylococci	20–35
Coagulase positive	10–27
Coagulase negative	1–3
Enterococci	5–18
Gram-negative aerobic bacilli	1.5–13
Fungi	2–4
Miscellaneous bacteria	<5
Mixed infections	1–2
"Culture negative"	<5–24

Adapted from Fowler G, Scheld WM, Bayer AJ. Endocarditis and intravascular infection. In Mandell GL, Bennett JE, Dolin R, eds., Principles and Practice of Infectious Diseases, 6th Ed. New York: Churchill-Livingstone, 2005, 975–1022.

The pathogenesis of early PVE differs from the infective endocarditis acquired by the hematogenous route because surgery may directly inoculate the valve with bacteria from the patient's skin or operating room personnel. The recently placed nonendothelialized valve is more susceptible to bacterial colonization than are native valves. Bacteria also may colonize the new valve from contaminated bypass pumps, cannulas, and pacemakers, or from a nosocomial bacteremia subsequent to an intravascular catheter.[3,10] The mechanism of bacterial colonization and pathogenesis in late PVE is similar to native-valve endocarditis.[3]

The vegetations seen in infective endocarditis may be single or multiple and vary in size from a few millimeters to centimeters. Bacteria within the vegetation grow slowly and are protected from antibiotics and host defenses. The adverse effects of infective endocarditis and the resulting lesions can be far-reaching and include (a) local perivalvular damage, (b) embolization of septic fragments with potential hematogenous seeding of remote sites, and (c) formation of antibody complexes.[1,2,5]

Formation of vegetations may destroy valvular tissue, and continued destruction can lead to acute heart failure via perforation of the valve leaflet, rupture of the chordae tendineae or papillary muscle, or in patients with PVE, valve dehiscence. Occasionally, valvular stenosis may occur. Abscesses can develop in the valve ring or in myocardial tissue itself. Even with resolution of the process, fibrosis of tissue with some residual dysfunction is possible.

Vegetations may be friable, and fragments may be released downstream. These infected particles, termed *septic emboli,* can result in organ abscess or infarction. Septic emboli from right-sided endocarditis commonly lodge in the lungs, causing pulmonary abscesses. Emboli from left-sided vegetations commonly affect organs with high blood flow, such as the kidneys, spleen, and brain.[1,2,5]

Circulating immune complexes consisting of antigen, antibody, and complement may deposit in organs, producing local inflammation and damage (e.g., glomerulonephritis in the kidneys). Other potential pathologic changes that result from immune-complex deposition or septic emboli include the development of "mycotic" aneurysms (although the aneurysm is usually bacterial in origin, not fungal), cerebral infarction, splenic infarction and abscess, and skin manifestations such as petechiae, Osler nodes, and Janeway lesions.[1,2,5]

CLINICAL PRESENTATION

3 The clinical presentation of infective endocarditis is highly variable and nonspecific. Fever is the most common finding and is often accompanied by other vague symptoms (Table 115–2). Fever may be relatively low grade, particularly in subacute cases. Heart murmurs are found in a majority of patients, most often preexisting, with some documented as new or changing. Infective endocarditis usually begins insidiously and worsens gradually. Patients may present with nonspecific findings, such as fever, chills, weakness, dyspnea, night sweats, weight loss, or malaise. In contrast, patients with acute disease, such as those with a history of IVDA and *S. aureus* infective endocarditis, may appear with classic signs of sepsis.

Splenomegaly is a frequent finding in patients with prolonged endocarditis. Other important clinical signs especially prevalent in subacute illness may include the following peripheral manifestations ("stigmata") of endocarditis[1,2,6]:

- *Osler nodes*—Purplish or erythematous subcutaneous papules or nodules on the pads of the fingers and toes. These lesions are 2 to 15 mm in size and are painful and tender. These nodes are not specific for infective endocarditis and may be the result of embolism, immunologic phenomena, or both.
- *Janeway lesions*—Hemorrhagic, painless plaques on the palms of the hands or soles of the feet. These lesions are believed to be embolic in origin.
- *Splinter hemorrhages*—Thin, linear hemorrhages found under the nail beds of the fingers or toes. These lesions are not specific for infective endocarditis and more commonly are the result of traumatic injuries. Distal lesions are more likely the result of trauma, whereas proximal lesions tend to be associated with infective endocarditis.
- *Petechiae*—Small (usually 1 to 2 mm in diameter), erythematous, painless, hemorrhagic lesions. These lesions appear anywhere on the skin but more frequently on the anterior trunk, buccal mucosa and palate, and conjunctivae. Petechiae are nonblanching and resolve after a few days.
- *Clubbing of the fingers*—Proliferative changes in the soft tissues about the terminal phalanges observed in long-standing endocarditis.
- *Roth spots*—Retinal infarct with central pallor and surrounding hemorrhage.
- *Emboli*—Embolic phenomena occur in up to one-third of cases and may result in significant complications. Left-sided endocarditis can result in renal artery emboli causing flank pain with hematuria, splenic artery emboli causing abdominal pain, and cerebral emboli, which may result in hemiplegia or alteration in mental status. Right-sided endocarditis may result in pulmonary emboli, causing pleuritic pain with hemoptysis.

Patients with infective endocarditis typically have laboratory abnormalities; however, none of these changes is specific for the disease.[6] Anemia (normocytic, normochromic), leukocytosis, and thrombocytopenia may be present. The white blood cell count is often normal or only slightly elevated, sometimes with a mild left shift. Acute bacterial endocarditis, however, may present with an elevated white blood cell count, consistent with a fulminant infection. The erythrocyte sedimentation rate is elevated in 90% to 100% of patients, and the level of C-reactive protein also may be elevated.[1,6] Often the urinary analysis is abnormal, with proteinuria and microscopic hematuria occurring in approximately 50% of individuals.

TABLE 115-2 Clinical Presentation of Infective Endocarditis

General	The clinical presentation of infective endocarditis is highly variable and nonspecific.
Symptoms	The patient may complain of fever, chills, weakness, dyspnea, night sweats, weight loss, and/or malaise.
Signs	Fever is common, as is a heart murmur (sometimes new or changing). The patient may or may not have embolic phenomenon, splenomegaly, or skin manifestations (e.g., Osler nodes, Janeway lesions).
Laboratory tests	The patient's white blood cell count may be normal or only slightly elevated. Nonspecific findings include anemia (normocytic, normochromic), thrombocytopenia, an elevated erythrocyte sedimentation rate or C-reactive protein, and altered urinary analysis (proteinuria/microscopic hematuria). The hallmark laboratory finding is continuous bacteremia; three sets of blood cultures should be collected over 24 hours.
Other diagnostic tests	An electrocardiogram, chest radiograph, and echocardiogram are commonly performed. Echocardiography to determine the presence of valvular vegetations plays a key role in the diagnosis of infective endocarditis; it should be performed in all suspected cases.

The hallmark of infective endocarditis is a continuous bacteremia caused by bacteria shedding from the vegetation into the bloodstream; more than 95% of patients with infective endocarditis have positive blood cultures.[1,2] Three sets of blood cultures, each from separate venipuncture sites, should be collected over 24 hours, and antibiotics should be withheld until adequate blood cultures are obtained. On the other hand, if a patient has a toxic appearance, several blood cultures should be collected promptly, followed by immediate empirical antimicrobial treatment. The blood cultures in patients who have received previous antibiotics should be monitored more closely because pathogen growth may be suppressed.[1,2] "Culture negative" endocarditis describes a patient in whom a clinical diagnosis of infective endocarditis is likely but blood cultures do not yield a pathogen.[11] This condition is often the consequence of previous antibiotic therapy, improperly collected blood cultures, or unusual organisms.[9] When blood cultures from patients suspected of having infective endocarditis show no growth after 48 to 72 hours, the laboratory should be advised and cultures held for up to a month to detect growth of fastidious organisms.[1,2]

An electrocardiogram, chest radiograph, and echocardiogram are performed in patients suspected of endocarditis. The electrocardiogram rarely shows important diagnostic findings but may reveal heart block, suggesting extension of the infection. The chest radiograph may provide more diagnostic information, especially in a patient with right-sided endocarditis. Septic pulmonary emboli may occur, leading to multiple lung foci. The echocardiogram is the most important test and should be performed in all patients suspected of this infection.

Echocardiography plays an important role in the diagnosis and management of infective endocarditis.[9] The chosen approach, transthoracic echocardiography (TTE) or transesophageal echocardiography (TEE), depends on the clinical setting. The TEE technique is more sensitive for detecting vegetations (90% to 100%) as compared with TTE (58% to 63%), and TEE maintains good specificity (85% to 95%).[2,5,9] TTE appears reasonable in the evaluation of children or adults in whom the clinical suspicion of infective endocarditis is relatively low.[9,12] TEE is preferred in high-risk patients such as those with prosthetic heart valves, many congenital heart diseases, previous endocarditis, new murmur, heart failure, or other stigmata of endocarditis.[9,13,14] The lack of vegetation on echocardiogram does not exclude infection even if the transesophageal approach is used. Conversely, the test may reveal an unsuspected large vegetation, extension of the disease into surrounding tissue, valvular defects, abscess formation, cordial rupture, or an intracardiac fistula. Thus, in addition to helping in the diagnosis of infective endocarditis, the echocardiogram allows the physician to evaluate hemodynamic stability and the need for urgent surgical intervention; it also provides a rough estimate of the likelihood of embolism.[9,15,16]

DIAGNOSIS

❹ The signs and symptoms of infective endocarditis are not specific, and the diagnosis is often unclear. The identification of infective endocarditis requires the integration of clinical, laboratory, and echocardiographic findings. The Duke diagnostic criteria include major and minor variables (Table 115–3).[17,18] Based on the number of major and minor criteria that are fulfilled, patients suspected of infective endocarditis are categorized into three separate groups: definite infective endocarditis, possible infective endocarditis, or infective endocarditis rejected.[18]

TABLE 115-3 Diagnosis of Infective Endocarditis According to the Modified Duke Criteria

Major Criteria
Blood culture positive for infective endocarditis
Typical microorganisms consistent with infective endocarditis from two separate blood cultures:
Viridans streptococci, *Streptococcus bovis*, HACEK group, *Staphylococcus aureus*; or
Community-acquired enterococci, in the absence of a primary focus; or
Microorganisms consistent with infective endocarditis from persistently positive blood cultures, defined as follows:
At least two positive cultures of blood samples drawn greater than 12 h apart; or
All of three or a majority of four or more separate cultures of blood (with first and last sample drawn at least 1 h apart)
Single positive blood culture for *Coxiella burnetii* or antiphase I immunoglobulin G antibody titer greater than 1:800
Evidence of endocardial involvement
Echocardiogram positive for infective endocarditis (transesophageal echocardiography recommended in patients with prosthetic valves, rated at least "possible infective endocarditis" by clinical criteria, or complicated infective endocarditis [paravalvular abscess]; transthoracic echocardiography as first test in other patients), defined as follows:
Oscillating intracardiac mass on valve or supporting structures, in the path of regurgitant jets, or on implanted material in the absence of an alternative anatomic explanation; or
Abscess; or
New partial dehiscence of prosthetic valve
New valvular regurgitation (worsening or changing of preexisting murmur not sufficient)
Minor Criteria
Predisposition, predisposing heart condition or injection drug use
Fever, temperature greater than 38°C (100.4°F)
Vascular phenomena, major arterial emboli, septic pulmonary infarcts, mycotic aneurysm, intracranial hemorrhage, conjunctival hemorrhages, and Janeway lesions
Immunologic phenomena: glomerulonephritis, Osler nodes, Roth spots, and rheumatoid factor
Microbiologic evidence: positive blood culture but does not meet a major criterion as noted above or serologic evidence of active infection with organism consistent with infective endocarditis
Echocardiographic minor criteria eliminated

HACEK, *Haemophilus* species (*H. parainfluenzae, H. aphrophilus, H. paraphrophilus*), *Actinobacillus actinomycetemcomitans, Cardiobacterium hominis, Eikenella corrodens*, and *Kingella kingae*.
Note: Cases are defined clinically as definite if they fulfill two major criteria, one major criterion plus three minor criteria, or five minor criteria; cases are defined as possible if they fulfill one major and one minor criterion or three minor criteria; cases are rejected if there is a firm alternate diagnosis explaining evidence of infective endocarditis; resolution of infective endocarditis syndrome with antibiotic therapy for less than 4 days; or no pathologic evidence of infective endocarditis at surgery or autopsy, with antibiotic therapy for less than 4 days; or does not meet criteria for possible infective endocarditis, as above.
Adapted from Durack et al.,[17] and Li et al.[18]

PROGNOSIS

The outcome for endocarditis is improved with rapid diagnosis, appropriate treatment (i.e., antimicrobial therapy, surgery, or both), and prompt recognition of complications should they arise. Factors associated with increased mortality include (a) heart failure, (b) culture-negative endocarditis, (c) endocarditis caused by resistant organisms such as fungi or gram-negative bacteria, (d) left-sided endocarditis caused by *S. aureus,* and (e) prosthetic-valve endocarditis.[1,6,19] The presence of heart failure has the greatest negative impact on the short-term prognosis.[9] For native-valve infective endocarditis, mortality rates range from 20% to 25%; lower rates occur with viridans streptococci (4% to 16%), and higher rates occur with left-sided infective endocarditis caused by enterococci (15% to 25%) and staphylococci (25% to 47%). Even higher rates of mortality are seen with unusually encountered organisms (e.g., mortality greater than 50% for *Pseudomonas aeruginosa*). The mortality rate for right-side infective endocarditis associated with IVDA is generally low (e.g., 10%).[6] For those who relapse after treatment for infective endocarditis, most will do so within the first 2 months after discontinuation of antimicrobials. Relapse rates for viridans streptococcus are generally low (2%), whereas relapse is more likely in those with enterococcal infection (8% to 20%) and PVE (10% to 15%).[6] After appropriate treatment and recovery, the risk of morbidity and mortality following infective endocarditis persist for years, although it gradually declines annually. Morbidity remains elevated because of a greater likelihood of recurrent infective endocarditis, heart failure, and embolism or, if a valve is replaced, the risk of anticoagulation, valve thrombosis, or additional valve surgery.[20]

TREATMENT

Infective Endocarditis

■ DESIRED OUTCOMES

The desired outcomes for treatment and prophylaxis of infective endocarditis are to

- Relieve the signs and symptoms of the disease.
- Decrease morbidity and mortality associated with the infection.
- Eradicate the causative organism with minimal drug exposure.
- Provide cost-effective antimicrobial therapy determined by the likely or identified pathogen, drug susceptibilities, hepatic and renal function, drug allergies, and anticipated drug toxicities.
- Prevent infective endocarditis from occurring or recurring in high-risk patients with appropriate prophylactic antimicrobials.

■ GENERAL APPROACH TO TREATMENT

❺ The most important approach in the treatment of infective endocarditis is isolation of the infecting pathogen and determination of antimicrobial susceptibilities, followed by high-dose, parenteral, bactericidal antibiotics for an extended period.[1,2] Identification of susceptibilities is crucial given the escalating level of antibiotic resistance to commonly encountered pathogens. Treatment usually is started in the hospital, but in selected patients it is often completed in the outpatient setting so long as defervescence has occurred and followup blood cultures show no growth.[6] Large doses of parenteral antimicrobials usually are necessary to achieve bactericidal concentrations within vegetations. An extended duration of therapy is required, even for susceptible pathogens, because microorganisms are enclosed within valvular vegetations and fibrin deposits. These barriers impair host defenses and protect microbes from phagocytic cells. In addition, high bacterial concentrations within vegetations may result in an inoculum effect that further resists killing (see Chap. 108 for additional discussion). Many bacteria are not actively dividing, further limiting the rate of bacterial death. For most patients, 4 to 6 weeks of therapy is required.[5,7]

NONPHARMACOLOGIC THERAPY

❻ Surgery is an important adjunct in the management of endocarditis. In most surgical cases, valvectomy and valve replacement are performed to remove infected tissue and to restore hemodynamic function. Echocardiographic features that suggest the need for surgery include persistent vegetation or an increase in vegetation size after prolonged antibiotic treatment, valve dysfunction, or perivalvular extension (e.g., abscess).[9] Surgery also may be considered in cases of PVE endocarditis caused by resistant organisms (e.g., fungi or gram-negative bacteria), or if there is persistent bacteremia or other evidence of failure despite appropriate antimicrobial therapy.[3,5,21] The major indications for surgical intervention in the past have been heart failure in left-sided infective endocarditis and persistent infection in right-sided infective endocarditis.[1]

PHARMACOLOGIC THERAPY

Specific treatment recommendations from the American Heart Association (AHA) provide guidance for the management of infective endocarditis and these were updated in 2005,[9] with slight modification.[22] A new aspect of the revised guidelines is the use of the AHA evidence-based scoring system where recommendations are given a classification as well as level of evidence. Class I recommendations are conditions for which there is evidence, general agreement, or both that a given procedure or treatment is useful and effective. Class II recommendations are conditions for which there is conflicting evidence, a divergence of opinion, or both about the usefulness/efficacy of a procedure or treatment (IIa implies the weight of evidence/opinion is in favor of usefulness/efficacy whereas IIb implies usefulness/efficacy is less-well established by evidence/opinion). Class III recommendations are conditions for which there is evidence, general agreement, or both that the procedure/treatment is not useful/effective and in some cases may be harmful. Level of evidence is listed as A (data derived from multiple randomized clinical trials), B (data derived from a single randomized trial or nonrandomized studies), and C (consensus opinion of experts).

❼ *β*-Lactam antibiotics, such as penicillin G (or ceftriaxone), nafcillin, and ampicillin, remain the drugs of choice for streptococcal, staphylococcal, and enterococcal endocarditis, respectively. Tables 115–4 through 115–11 summarize these recommendations, which are discussed in more detail in the following sections. Because these guidelines focus on common causes of endocarditis, readers are referred to other references for more in-depth discussion of unusually encountered organisms.[4,9]

❽ For some pathogens, such as enterococci, the use of synergistic antimicrobial combinations (including an aminoglycoside) is essential to obtain a bactericidal effect. Combination antibiotics also may decrease the emergence of resistant organisms during treatment (e.g., PVE caused by coagulase-negative staphylococci) and hasten the pace of clinical and microbiologic response (e.g., some streptococcal and staphylococcal infections). Occasionally, combination treatment will result in a shorter treatment course.

TABLE 115-4 Therapy of Native Valve Endocarditis Caused by Highly Penicillin-Susceptible Viridans Group Streptococci and *Streptococcus bovis*

Regimen	Dosage[a] and Route	Duration (wk)	Strength of Recommendation	Comments
Aqueous crystalline penicillin G sodium	12–18 million units/24 h IV either continuously or in four or six equally divided doses	4	I A	Preferred in most patients older than age 65 years or patients with impairment of 8th cranial nerve function or renal function
or				
Ceftriaxone sodium	2 g/24 h IV/IM in one dose *Pediatric dose*[b]: penicillin 200,000 units/kg per 24 h IV in four to six equally divided doses; ceftriaxone 100 mg/kg per 24 h IV/IM in 1 dose	4	I A	
Aqueous crystalline penicillin G sodium	12–18 million units/24 h IV either continuously or in six equally divided doses	2	I B	2-wk regimen not intended for patients with known cardiac or extracardiac abscess or for those with creatinine clearance of less than 20 mL/min, impaired 8th cranial nerve function, or *Abiotrophia, Granulicatella*, or *Gemella* spp. infection; gentamicin dosage should be adjusted to achieve peak serum concentration of 3–4 mcg/mL and trough serum concentration of less than 1 mcg/mL when three divided doses are used (second option to single daily dose)
or				
Ceftriaxone sodium	2 g/24 h IV/IM in 1 dose	2	I B	
plus				
Gentamicin sulfate[c]	3 mg/kg per 24 h IV/IM in 1 dose *Pediatric dose*: penicillin 200,000 units/kg per 24 h IV in four to six equally divided doses; ceftriaxone 100 mg/kg per 24 h IV/IM in 1 dose; gentamicin 3 mg/kg per 24 h IV/IM in 1 dose or 3 equally divided doses[d]	2		
Vancomycin hydrochloride[e]	30 mg/kg per 24 h IV in two equally divided doses not to exceed 2 g/24 h unless concentrations are inappropriately low *Pediatric dose*: 40 mg/kg per 24 h IV in two to three equally divided doses	4	I B	Vancomycin therapy recommended only for patients unable to tolerate penicillin or ceftriaxone; vancomycin dosage should be adjusted to obtain peak (1 h after infusion completed) serum concentration of 30–45 mcg/mL and a trough concentration range of 10–15 mcg/mL

Minimum inhibitory concentration less than 0.12 mcg/mL.
[a]Dosages recommended are for patients with normal renal function.
[b]Pediatric dose should not exceed that of a normal adult.
[c]Other potentially nephrotoxic drugs (e.g., nonsteroidal antiinflammatory drugs) should be used with caution in patients receiving gentamicin therapy.
[d]Data for once-daily dosing of aminoglycosides for children exist, but no data for treatment of infective endocarditis exist.
[e]Vancomycin dosages should be infused during course of at least 1 h to reduce risk of histamine-release "red man" syndrome.
From Baddour LM, Wilson WR, Bayer AS, et al. Infective endocarditis diagnosis, antimicrobial therapy, and management of complications. Circulation 2005;111:e394–e433, with permission. Copyright 2005, American Medical Association. Modified based on reference 22.

TABLE 115-5 Therapy of Native Valve Endocarditis Caused by Strains of Viridans Group Streptococci and *Streptococcus bovis* Relatively Resistant to Penicillin

Regimen	Dosage[a] and Route	Duration (wk)	Strength of Recommendation	Comments
Aqueous crystalline penicillin G sodium	24 million units/24 h IV either continuously or in four to six equally divided doses	4	I B	Patients with endocarditis caused by penicillin-resistant (MIC greater than 0.5 mcg/mL) strains should be treated with regimen recommended for enterococcal endocarditis (see Table 115-9)
or				
Ceftriaxone sodium	2 g/24 h IV/IM in one dose	4	I B	
plus				
Gentamicin sulfate[b]	3 mg/kg per 24 h IM/IV in one dose *Pediatric dose*[c]: penicillin 300,000 units/24 h IV in four to six equally divided doses; ceftriaxone 100 mg/kg per 24 h IV/IM in one dose; gentamicin 3 mg/kg per 24 h IV/IM in one dose or three equally divided doses	2		Although it is preferred that gentamicin (3 mg/kg) be given as a single daily dose to adult patients, as a second option, gentamicin can be administered daily in three equally divided doses
Vancomycin hydrochloride[c]	30 mg/kg per 24 h IV in two equally divided doses not to exceed 2 g/24 h unless serum concentrations are inappropriately low *Pediatric dose*: 40 mg/kg 24 h in two or three equally divided doses	4	I B	Vancomycin[d] therapy recommended only for patients unable to tolerate penicillin or ceftriaxone therapy

Minimum inhibitory concentration (MIC) greater than 0.12 mcg/mL to less than or equal to 0.5 mcg/mL.
[a]Dosages recommended are for patients with normal renal function.
[b]See Table 115-4 for appropriate dosage of gentamicin.
[c]Pediatric dose should not exceed that of a normal adult.
[d]See Table 115-4 for appropriate dosage of vancomycin.
From Baddour LM, Wilson WR, Bayer AS, et al. Infective endocarditis diagnosis, antimicrobial therapy, and management of complications. Circulation 2005;111:e394–e433, with permission. Copyright 2005, American Medical Association. Modified based on reference 22.

TABLE 115-6 Therapy for Endocarditis of Prosthetic Valves or Other Prosthetic Material Caused by Viridans Group Streptococci and *Streptococcus bovis*

Regimen	Dosage[a] and Route	Duration (wk)	Strength of Recommendation	Comments
Penicillin-susceptible strain (minimum inhibitory concentration ≤0.12 mcg/mL)				
Aqueous crystalline penicillin G sodium	24 million units/24 h IV either continuously or in four to six equally divided doses	6	I B	Penicillin or ceftriaxone together with gentamicin has not demonstrated superior cure rates compared with monotherapy with penicillin or ceftriaxone for patients with highly susceptible strain; gentamicin therapy should not be administered to patients with creatinine clearance of less than 30 mL/min
or				
Ceftriaxone sodium	2 g/24 h IV/IM in one dose	6	I B	
with or without				
Gentamicin sulfate[b]	3 mg/kg per 24 h IM/IV in one dose *Pediatric dose*[c]: penicillin 300,000 units/24 h IV in four to six equally divided doses; ceftriaxone 100 mg/kg per 24 h IV/IM in one dose; gentamicin 3 mg/kg per 24 h IV/IM in one dose or three equally divided doses	2		
Vancomycin hydrochloride[d]	30 mg/kg per 24 h IV in two equally divided doses *Pediatric dose*: 40 mg/kg 24 h in two or three equally divided doses	6	I B	Vancomycin therapy recommended only for patients unable to tolerate penicillin or ceftriaxone therapy
Penicillin relatively or fully resistant strain (minimum inhibitory concentration >0.12 mcg/mL)				
Aqueous crystalline penicillin sodium	24 million units/24 h IV either continuously or in four to six equally divided doses	6	I B	
or				
Ceftriaxone	2 g/24 h IV/IM in one dose	6	I B	
plus				
Gentamicin sulfate	3 mg/kg per 24 h IV/IM in one dose *Pediatric dose*: penicillin 300,000 units/kg per 24 h IV in four to six equally divided doses	6		
Vancomycin hydrochloride	30 mg/kg per 24 h IV in two equally divided doses *Pediatric dose*: 40 mg/kg per 24 h IV in two or three equally divided doses	6	I B	Vancomycin therapy recommended only for patients unable to tolerate penicillin or ceftriaxone therapy

[a]Dosages recommended are for patients with normal renal function.
[b]See Table 115-4 for appropriate dosage of gentamicin.
[c]Pediatric dose should not exceed that of a normal adult.
[d]See text and Table 115-4 for appropriate dosage of vancomycin.
From Baddour LM, Wilson WR, Bayer AS, et al. Infective endocarditis diagnosis, antimicrobial therapy, and management of complications. Circulation 2005;111:e394–e433, with permission. Copyright 2005, American Medical Association.

TABLE 115-7 Therapy for Endocarditis Caused by Staphylococci in the Absence of Prosthetic Materials

Regimen	Dosage[a] and Route	Duration	Strength of Recommendation	Comments
Oxacillin-susceptible strains				
Nafcillin or oxacillin[b] ***with***	12 g/24 h IV in four to six equally divided doses	6 wk	I A	For complicated right-sided infective endocarditis and for left-sided infective endocarditis; for uncomplicated right-sided infective endocarditis, 2 wk (see text)
Optional addition of gentamicin sulfate[c]	3 mg/kg per 24 h IV/IM in two or three equally divided doses	3–5 days		Clinical benefit of aminoglycosides has not been established
For penicillin-allergic (nonanaphylactoid type) patients:				Consider skin testing for oxacillin-susceptible staphylococci and questionable history of immediate-type hypersensitivity to penicillin
Cefazolin ***with***	6 g/24 h IV in three equally divided doses	6 wk	I B	Cephalosporins should be avoided in patients with anaphylactoid-type hypersensitivity to β-lactams; vancomycin should be used in these cases[d]
Optional addition of gentamicin sulfate	3 mg/kg per 24 h IV/IM in two or three equally divided doses *Pediatric dose*: cefazolin 100 mg/kg per 24 h IV in three equally divided doses; gentamicin 3 mg/kg per 24 h IV/IM in three equally divided doses	3–5 days		Clinical benefit of aminoglycosides has not been established
Oxacillin-resistant strains				
Vancomycin[e]	30 mg/kg per 24 h IV in two equally divided doses *Pediatric dose*: 40 mg/kg per 24 h IV in two or three equally divided doses	6 wk	I B	Adjust vancomycin dosage to achieve 1-h serum concentration of 30–45 mcg/mL and trough concentration of 10–15 mcg/mL

[a]Dosages recommended are for patients with normal renal function.
[b]Penicillin G 24 million units/24 h IV in four to six equally divided doses may be used in place of nafcillin or oxacillin if strain is penicillin susceptible (minimum inhibitory concentration ≤0.1 mcg/mL) and does not produce β-lactamase.
[c]Gentamicin should be administered in close temporal proximity to vancomycin, nafcillin, or oxacillin dosing. See Table 115–4 for appropriate dosage of gentamicin.
[d]Pediatric dose should not exceed that of a normal adult.
[e]For specific dosing adjustment and issues concerning vancomycin, see Table 115–4 footnotes.
From Baddour LM, Wilson WR, Bayer AS, et al. Infective endocarditis diagnosis, antimicrobial therapy, and management of complications. Circulation 2005;111:e394–e433, with permission. Copyright 2005, American Medical Association. Modified based on reference 22.

TABLE 115-8 Therapy for Prosthetic Valve Endocarditis Caused by Staphylococci

Regimen	Dosage[a] and Route	Duration (wk)	Strength of Recommendation	Comments
Oxacillin-susceptible strains				
Nafcillin or oxacillin ***plus***	12 g/24 h IV in four to six equally divided doses	≥6	I B	Penicillin G 24 million units/24 h IV in four to six equally divided doses may be used in place of nafcillin or oxacillin if strain is penicillin susceptible (minimum inhibitory concentration ≤0.1 mcg/mL) and does not produce β-lactamase; vancomycin should be used in patients with immediate-type hypersensitivity reactions to beta-lactam antibiotics (see Table 115–4 for dosing guidelines); cefazolin may be substituted for nafcillin or oxacillin in patients with non–immediate-type hypersensitivity reactions to penicillins
Rifampin ***plus***	900 mg per 24 h IV/orally in three equally divided doses	≥6		
Gentamicin[b]	3 mg/kg per 24 h IV/IM in two or three equally divided doses *Pediatric dose*[c]: nafcillin or oxacillin 200 mg/kg per 24 h IV in four to six equally divided doses; rifampin 20 mg/kg per 24 h IV/orally in three equally divided doses; gentamicin 3 mg/kg per 24 h IV/IM in three equally divided doses	2		
Oxacillin-resistant strains				
Vancomycin ***plus***	30 mg/kg 24 h in two equally divided doses	≥6	I B	Adjust vancomycin to achieve 1-h serum concentration of 30–45 mcg/mL and trough concentration of 10–15 mcg/mL
Rifampin ***plus***	900 mg/24 h IV/orally in three equally divided doses	≥6		
Gentamicin	3 mg/kg per 24 h IV/IM in two or three equally divided doses *Pediatric dose*: vancomycin 40 mg/kg per 24 h IV in two or three equally divided doses; rifampin 20 mg/kg per 24 h IV/orally in three equally divided doses (up to adult dose); gentamicin 3 mg/kg per 24 h IV or IM in three equally divided doses	2		

[a]Dosages recommended are for patients with normal renal function.
[b]Gentamicin should be administered in close proximity to vancomycin, nafcillin, or oxacillin dosing. See Table 115–4 for appropriate dosage of gentamicin.
[c]Pediatric dose should not exceed that of a normal adult.
From Baddour LM, Wilson WR, Bayer AS, et al. Infective endocarditis diagnosis, antimicrobial therapy, and management of complications. Circulation 2005;111:e394–e433, with permission. Copyright 2005, American Medical Association. Modified based on reference 22.

TABLE 115-9 Therapy for Native Valve or Prosthetic Valve Enterococcal Endocarditis Caused by Strains Susceptible to Penicillin, Gentamicin, and Vancomycin

Regimen	Dosage[a] and Route	Duration (wk)	Strength of Recommendation	Comments
Ampicillin sodium	12 g/24 h IV in six equally divided doses	4–6	I A	Native valve: 4-wk therapy recommended for patients with symptoms of illness less than 3 mo;
or				
Aqueous crystalline penicillin G sodium	18–30 million units/24 h IV either continuously or in six equally divided doses	4–6	I A	6-wk therapy recommended for patients with symptoms greater than 3 mo
plus				Prosthetic valve or other prosthetic cardiac material: minimum of 6 wk of therapy recommended
Gentamicin sulfate[b]	3 mg/kg per 24 h IV/IM in three equally divided doses	4–6		
Vancomycin hydrochloride[d]	30 mg/kg per 24h IV in 2 equally divided doses	6	I B	Vancomycin therapy recommended only for patients unable to tolerate penicillin or ampicillin
plus				
Gentamicin sulfate	3 mg/kg per 24 h IV/IM in three equally divided doses *Pediatric dose*[c]: vancomycin 40 mg/kg per 24 h IV in two or three equally divided doses; gentamicin 3 mg/kg per 24 h IV/IM in three equally divided doses	6		6 wk of vancomycin therapy recommended because of decreased activity against enterococci

[a]Dosages recommended are for patients with normal renal function.
[b]Dosage of gentamicin should be adjusted to achieve peak serum concentration of 3–4 mcg/mL and a trough concentration of less than 1 mcg/mL. See Table 115–4 for appropriate dosage of gentamicin.
[c]Pediatric dose should not exceed that of a normal adult.
[d]See text and Table 115–4 for appropriate dosing of vancomycin.
From Baddour LM, Wilson WR, Bayer AS, et al. Infective endocarditis diagnosis, antimicrobial therapy, and management of complications. Circulation 2005;111:e394–e433, with permission. Copyright 2005, American Medical Association. Modified based on reference 22.

CLINICAL CONTROVERSY

In the past, the AHA guidelines recommended traditional aminoglycoside dosing (three times daily) whenever clinicians use these antibiotics. Extended-interval dosing (once-daily administration) is an intriguing dosing strategy, but data only support this approach for the treatment of streptococcal infective endocarditis.

■ STREPTOCOCCAL ENDOCARDITIS

Streptococci are a common cause of infective endocarditis, with most isolates being viridans streptococci. *Viridans streptococci* refer to a large number of different species, such as *Streptococcus sanguinis, Streptococcus oralis, Streptococcus salivarius, Streptococcus mutans,* and *Gemella morbillorum.*[9] These bacteria are common inhabitants of the human mouth and gingiva, and they are especially common causes of endocarditis involving native valves.[1,23] During dental surgery, and even when brushing the teeth, these organisms can cause a transient bacteremia. In susceptible individuals, this may result in infective endocarditis. Streptococcal endocarditis is usually subacute, and the response to medical treatment is good. *Streptococcus bovis* is not a viridans streptococcus, but it is included in this group because it is penicillin sensitive and requires the same treatment as viridans streptococci. *S. bovis* is a nonenterococcal group D *Streptococcus* that resides in the gastrointestinal tract. Infective endocarditis caused by this organism is often associated with a gastrointestinal pathology, especially colon carcinoma. Endocarditis caused by *Streptococcus pneumoniae, Streptococcus pyogenes,* and groups B, C, and G streptococci are uncommon, and their treatment is not well defined.[1]

Antimicrobial regimens for viridans streptococci are well studied, and in uncomplicated cases, response rates as high as 98% can be expected. Viridans streptococci are penicillin-susceptible, although some are more susceptible than others. Most are exquisitely sensitive

TABLE 115-10 Therapy for Both Native and Prosthetic Valve Endocarditis Caused by HACEK[a] Microorganisms

Regimen	Dosage and Route	Duration (wk)	Strength of Recommendation	Comments
Ceftriaxone[b] sodium	2 g/24 h IV/IM in one dose	4	I B	Cefotaxime or another third- or fourth-generation cephalosporin may be substituted
or				
Ampicillin-sulbactam[c]	12 g/24 h IV in four equally divided doses	4	IIa B	
or				
Ciprofloxacin[c,d]	1,000 mg/24 h orally or 800 mg/24 h IV in two equally divided doses *Pediatric dose*[e]: Ceftriaxone 100 mg/kg per 24 h IV/IM once daily; ampicillin-sulbactam 300 mg/kg per 24 h IV divided into four or six equally divided doses; ciprofloxacin 20–30 mg/kg per 24 h IV/orally in two equally divided doses	4	IIb C	Fluoroquinolone therapy recommended only for patients unable to tolerate cephalosporin and ampicillin therapy; levofloxacin, gatifloxacin, or moxifloxacin may be substituted; fluoroquinolones generally not recommended for patients younger than 18 y old Prosthetic valve: patients with endocarditis involving prosthetic cardiac valve or other prosthetic cardiac material should be treated for 6 wk

[a]*Haemophilus parainfluenzae, H. aphrophilus, Actinobacillus actinomycetemcomitans, Cardiobacterium hominis, Eikenella corrodens,* and *Kingella kingae.*
[b]Patients should be informed that IM injection of ceftriaxone is painful.
[c]Dosage recommended for patients with normal renal function.
[d]Fluoroquinolones are highly active in vitro against HACEK microorganisms. Published data on use of fluoroquinolone therapy for endocarditis caused by HACEK are minimal.
[e]Pediatric dose should not exceed that of a normal adult.
From Baddour LM, Wilson WR, Bayer AS, et al. Infective endocarditis diagnosis, antimicrobial therapy, and management of complications. Circulation 2005;111:e394–e433, with permission. Copyright 2005, American Medical Association.

TABLE 115-11 Therapy for Culture-Negative Endocarditis Including *Bartonella* Endocarditis

Regimen	Dosage[a] and Route	Duration (wk)	Strength of Recommendation	Comments
Native valve				
Ampicillin-sulbactam	12 g/24 h IV in four equally divided doses	4–6	IIb C	Patients with culture-negative endocarditis should be treated with consultation with an infectious diseases specialist
plus				
Gentamicin sulfate[b]	3 mg/kg per 24 h IV/IM in three equally divided doses	4–6		
Vancomycin[c]	30 mg/kg per 24 h IV in 2 equally divided doses	4–6	IIb C	Vancomycin recommended only for patients unable to tolerate penicillins
plus				
Gentamicin sulfate	3 mg/kg per 24 h IV/IM in three equally divided doses	4–6		
plus				
Ciprofloxacin	1,000 mg/24 h orally or 800 mg/24 h IV in two equally divided doses	4–6		
	Pediatric dose[d]: ampicillin-sulbactam 300 mg/kg per 24 h IV in four to six equally divided doses; gentamicin 3 mg/kg per 24 h IV/IM in three equally divided doses; vancomycin 40 mg/kg per 24 h in two or three equally divided doses; ciprofloxacin 20–30 mg/kg per 24 h IV/orally in two equally divided doses			
Prosthetic valve (early, <1 y)				
Vancomycin	30 mg/kg per 24 h IV in two equally divided doses	6	IIb C	
plus				
Gentamicin sulfate	3 mg/kg per 24 h IV/IM in three equally divided doses	2		
plus				
Cefepime	6 g/24 h IV in three equally divided doses	6		
plus				
Rifampin	900 mg/24 h orally/IV in three equally divided doses	6		
	Pediatric dose: vancomycin 40 mg/kg per 24 h IV in two or three equally divided doses; gentamicin 3 mg/kg per 24 h IV/IM in three equally divided doses; cefepime 150 mg/kg per 24 h IV in three equally divided doses; rifampin 20 mg/kg per 24 h orally/IV in three equally divided doses			
Prosthetic valve (late, >1 y)		6	IIb C	Same regimens as listed above for native valve endocarditis with the addition of rifampin
Suspected *Bartonella*, culture negative				
Ceftriaxone sodium	2 g/24 h IV/IM in one dose	6	IIa B	Patients with *Bartonella* endocarditis should be treated in consultation with an infectious diseases specialist
plus				
Gentamicin sulfate	3 mg/kg per 24 h IV/IM in three equally divided doses	2		
with/without				
Doxycycline	200 mg per 24 h IV/orally in two equally divided doses	6		
Documented *Bartonella*, culture positive				
Doxycycline	200 mg/24 h IV or orally in two equally divided doses	6	IIa B	If gentamicin cannot be given, then replace with rifampin, 600 mg/24 h orally/IV in two equally divided doses
plus				
Gentamicin sulfate	3 mg/kg per 24 h IV/IM in three equally divided doses	2		
	Pediatric dose: ceftriaxone 100 mg/kg per 24 h IV/IM once daily; gentamicin 3 mg/kg per 24 h IV/IM in three equally divided doses; doxycycline 2–4 mg/kg per 24 h IV/orally in two equally divided doses; rifampin 20 mg/kg per 24 h orally/IV in two equally divided doses			

[a]Dosages recommended are for patients with normal renal function.
[b]See text and Table 115–4 for appropriate dosing of gentamicin.
[c]See Table 115–4 for appropriate dosing of vancomycin.
[d]Pediatric dose should not exceed that of a normal adult.
From Baddour LM, Wilson WR, Bayer AS, et al. Infective endocarditis diagnosis, antimicrobial therapy, and management of complications. Circulation 2005;111:e394–e433, with permission. Copyright 2005, American Medical Association. Modified based on reference 22.

to penicillin G and have minimal inhibitory concentrations (MICs) of less than 0.12 mcg/mL.[9,23] Approximately 10% to 20% are moderately susceptible (MIC 0.12 to 0.5 mcg/mL). This difference in in vitro susceptibility led to recommendations that the MIC be determined for all viridans streptococci and that the results be used to guide therapy. Some streptococci are deemed tolerant to the killing effects of penicillin, where the minimal bactericidal concentration (MBC) exceeds the MIC by 32 times. A tolerant organism is inhibited but not killed by an antibiotic normally considered bactericidal.[24] Bactericidal activity is required for successful treatment of infective endocarditis; therefore, infections with a tolerant organism may relapse after treatment. Despite some animal studies of endocarditis suggesting that tolerant strains do not respond as readily to β-lactam therapy as nontolerant ones, this phenomenon is primarily a laboratory finding with little clinical significance.[9,25] Treatment for tolerant strains is identical to that for nontolerant organisms, and measurement of the MBC is not recommended.[9]

An assortment of regimens can be used to treat uncomplicated, native-valve endocarditis caused by fully susceptible viridans streptococci (Table 115–4). Two single-drug regimens consist of high-dose parenteral penicillin G or ceftriaxone for 4 weeks. If a shorter course of therapy is desired, the guidelines suggest high-dose parenteral penicillin G plus an aminoglycoside.[9] When used in select patients, this combination is as effective as 4 weeks of penicillin alone. Although streptomycin was listed in previous guidelines, gentamicin is the preferred aminoglycoside because serum drug concentrations are obtained easily, clinicians are more familiar with its use, and the few strains of streptococci resistant to the effects of streptomycin-penicillin remain susceptible to gentamicin-penicillin. Other aminoglycosides are not recommended.

The decision of which regimen to use depends on the perceived risk versus benefit. For example, a 2-week course of gentamicin in an elderly patient with renal impairment may be associated with ototoxicity, worsening renal function, or both. Furthermore, the 2-week regimen is not recommended for patients with known extracardiac infection. On the other hand, a 4-week course of penicillin alone generally entails greater expense, especially if the patient remains in the hospital. Monotherapy with once-daily ceftriaxone offers ease of administration, facilitates home health care treatment, and may be cost-effective.[9,26]

The British Society for Antimicrobial Chemotherapy guidelines suggest that all of the following conditions be present to consider a 2-week treatment regimen for penicillin-sensitive streptococcal endocarditis:[27]

- Penicillin-sensitive viridans streptococcus or *S. bovis* (penicillin MIC <0.1 mcg/mL)
- No cardiovascular risk factors such as heart failure, aortic insufficiency, or conduction abnormalities
- No evidence of thromboembolic disease
- Native-valve infection
- No vegetation of greater than 5 mm diameter on echocardiogram
- Clinical response within 7 days (the temperature should return to normal, the patient should feel well, and the patient's appetite should return to normal)

❾ When a patient has a history of an immediate-type hypersensitivity to penicillin, vancomycin is chosen for infective endocarditis caused by viridans streptococci. When vancomycin is used, the addition of gentamicin is not recommended.[9] Most patients who report a penicillin allergy have a negative penicillin skin test and consequently are at low risk of anaphylaxis.[28] The published experience with penicillin is more extensive than with alternative regimens; consequently, a thorough allergy history must be obtained before a second-line therapy is administered.

In patients with complicated infections (e.g., extracardiac foci) or when the streptococcus has an MIC of 0.12 to less than or equal to 0.5 mcg/mL, combination therapy with an aminoglycoside and penicillin (higher dose) or ceftriaxone for the first 2 weeks is recommended, followed by penicillin or ceftriaxone alone for an additional 2 weeks (Table 115–5).[9] Some viridans streptococci have biologic characteristics that complicate diagnosis and treatment, previously referred to as nutritionally variant streptococci. *Abiotrophia defectiva* and *Granulicatella* species have nutritional deficiencies that hinder growth in routine culture media.[2,9] These organisms require special broth supplemented with pyridoxal hydrochloride or cysteine. For patients infected with nutritionally variant streptococci or when the *Streptococcus* has an MIC of more than 0.5 mcg/mL, treatment should follow the enterococcal endocarditis treatment guidelines.[9]

The rationale for combination therapy of penicillin-susceptible viridans streptococci is that enhanced activity against these organisms usually is observed when cell wall active agents are combined with aminoglycosides in vitro.[25] Combined treatment results in quicker sterilization of vegetations in animal models of endocarditis and probably explains the high response rates observed in patients treated for a total of 2 weeks.[9] The combined treatment, however, is not superior to penicillin alone. Some authors question the need for combination therapy in relatively resistant streptococci, emphasizing that few human data suggest that patients with endocarditis caused by these organisms respond less well to penicillin alone.[29]

In patients with endocarditis of prosthetic valves or other prosthetic material caused by viridans streptococci and *S. bovis*, choices of treatment are similar to those without prosthetic material (e.g., penicillin or ceftriaxone); however, treatment courses are extended to 6 weeks (Table 115–6). In fact, if the organism is relatively resistant, gentamicin is recommended for 6 weeks.

Whether or not extended-interval aminoglycoside dosing has a role in infective endocarditis continues to be debated. At this time, data support extended-interval dosing for the treatment of streptococcal infective endocarditis, and as compared with three times-daily dosing this approach may have greater efficacy.[30–33] One study specifically evaluated the combination of ceftriaxone (2 g daily) with gentamicin (3 mg/kg daily) for 2 weeks compared with ceftriaxone (2 g daily) alone for 4 weeks for penicillin-sensitive streptococci. Both regimens were safe and effective with similar clinical cure rates at 3 months following treatment.[34]

■ STAPHYLOCOCCAL ENDOCARDITIS

Endocarditis caused by staphylococci has become more prevalent, mainly because of increased IVDA, more frequent use of peripheral and central venous catheters, and increased frequency of valve-replacement surgery.[35,36] *S. aureus* is the most common organism causing infective endocarditis among those with IVDA and persons with venous catheters. Coagulase-negative staphylococci (usually *Staphylococcus epidermidis*) are prominent causes of PVE.

Staphylococcal endocarditis is not a homogeneous disease; appropriate management requires consideration of several questions: Is the organism methicillin resistant? Should combination therapy be used? Is the infection on a native or prosthetic valve? Does the patient have a history of IVDA? Is the infection on the left or right side of the heart? Another consideration in staphylococcal endocarditis is that some organisms may exhibit tolerance to antibiotics. Similar to streptococci, however, the concern for tolerance among staphylococci should not affect antibiotic selection.[9]

Any patient who develops staphylococcal bacteremia is at risk for endocarditis. Many investigators have attempted to develop criteria that identify the bacteremic patient likely to have infective endocarditis.[36] In the past, patients were considered to be at high risk for infective endocarditis if *S. aureus* bacteremia was community acquired versus hospital acquired.[17] However, more recent evidence has resulted in nosocomial *S. aureus* bacteremia being considered as a major criterion for development of infective endocarditis.[18] In hospitalized patients with *S. aureus* bacteremia and an identified focus of infection, such as a vascular catheter, the risk of concomitant infective endocarditis is low, and treatment of the bacteremia can be reduced to 2 weeks. This approach applies only if the patient does not have a prosthetic valve or additional clinical evidence for endocarditis.[35,36] Additionally, the following parameters predict higher risk of infective endocarditis in patients with *S. aureus* bacteremia: (a) the absence of a primary site of infection, (b) metastatic signs of infection, and (c) valvular vegetations detected by echocardiography.[1,4]

The recommended therapy for patients with left-sided, native-valve infective endocarditis caused by methicillin-sensitive *S. aureus* (MSSA) is 6 weeks of nafcillin or oxacillin, often combined with a short course of gentamicin (Table 115–7). Four weeks of monotherapy with nafcillin or oxacillin may be sufficient for uncomplicated infections (no perivalvular abscess or septic metastatic complications). From in vitro studies, the combination of an aminoglycoside and penicillinase-resistant penicillin or vancomycin enhances the activity of these drugs for MSSA. In animal models of endocarditis, combinations of penicillin with an aminoglycoside eradicate organisms from vegetations more rapidly than penicillins alone.[35] In human studies, the addition of an aminoglycoside to nafcillin hastens the resolution of fever and bacteremia, but it does not affect survival or relapse rates and can increase renal toxicity.[37] Traditional twice or three times-daily dosing of aminoglycosides is recommended when administered for staphylococcal infective endocarditis, albeit initial data have evaluated gentamicin given once a day.[38]

If a patient has a mild, delayed allergy to penicillin, first-generation cephalosporins (such as cefazolin) are effective alternatives, but they should be avoided in patients with a history of immediate-type hypersensitivity reactions to penicillins (see Table 115–7). The potential for a true immediate-type allergy should be assessed carefully. A penicillin skin test should be conducted before giving antibiotic treatment to any patient with infective endocarditis caused by MSSA if there is a questionable penicillin allergy.[39] ⑨ In a patient with a positive skin test or a history of immediate hypersensitivity to penicillin, vancomycin is chosen. Vancomycin, however, kills *S. aureus* slowly and is regarded as inferior to penicillinase-resistant penicillins for MSSA.[36] Alternatively, patients with immediate-type hypersensitivity reactions to penicillin who fail to respond to vancomycin therapy should be considered for penicillin desensitization.[9] Generally, antibiotic therapy should be continued for 6 weeks. Unfortunately, left-sided infective endocarditis caused by *S. aureus* continues to have a poor prognosis, with a mortality rate of 25% to 47%.[6] For reasons discussed in the following section, those with infective endocarditis associated with IVDA have a more favorable response to therapy.

During the past decade, greater numbers of staphylococci became resistant to penicillinase-resistant penicillins (e.g., methicillin). ⑨ Vancomycin is used in this situation because most methicillin-resistant *S. aureus* (MRSA) and coagulase-negative staphylococci are susceptible to it (see Table 115–7). Reports of *S. aureus* strains resistant to vancomycin are emerging.[40] This is concerning as there are currently no standard treatment regimens to treat *S. aureus* infective endocarditis if the strain is resistant to both methicillin and vancomycin. There is emerging literature documenting success with daptomycin or linezolid in these patients.[41–44] The presence or lack of a prosthetic heart valve in patients with a methicillin-resistant organism guides therapy and determines whether vancomycin should be used alone or, if a prosthetic valve is present, whether combination therapy is necessary (Table 115–8).[3,9]

Staphylococcus Endocarditis: Intravenous Drug Abuser

Infective endocarditis in those with IVDA is frequently (60% to 70%) caused by *S. aureus,* although other organisms may be common in certain geographic locations.[45] In this setting, the tricuspid valve is frequently infected, resulting in right-sided infective endocarditis. Most patients have no history of valve abnormalities, are usually otherwise healthy, and have a good response to medical treatment. Nonetheless, surgery may be required.

An uncomplicated, left-sided MSSA endocarditis may be treated sufficiently with 4 weeks of monotherapy with penicillinase-resistant penicillin.[9] In the intravenous drug abuser, however, the clinical response with right-sided MSSA endocarditis is usually excellent. These patients may be treated effectively (clinical and microbiologic cure exceeding 85%) with a 2-week course of nafcillin or oxacillin plus an aminoglycoside.[45–51] Short-course vancomycin, in place of nafcillin or oxacillin, appears ineffective.[49] Another trial suggested that a 2-week regimen of a penicillinase-resistant penicillin alone, without the addition of an aminoglycoside, is as effective as combined therapy in MSSA tricuspid valve endocarditis.[52] Although these data suggest that an aminoglycoside is unnecessary for short-course treatment in the intravenous drug abuser with right-sided infective endocarditis, most clinicians are uncomfortable with monotherapy and choose combination treatment so long as there are no reasons to avoid an aminoglycoside. Short-course therapy should not be used in left-sided endocarditis, and it is inappropriate in patients with underlying acquired immunodeficiency syndrome, renal failure, meningitis or substantial pulmonary complications, such as lung abscess from right-sided infective endocarditis.[9]

An intriguing therapeutic approach for staphylococcal endocarditis in those with IVDA is oral treatment. Preliminary data suggest that short-course intravenous treatment (primarily nafcillin; mean: 16 days) followed by oral treatment (dicloxacillin or oxacillin; mean: 26 days) might be effective for tricuspid valve MSSA endocarditis.[53] The positive results of this trial can be explained by the duration of intravenous antibiotics (>2 weeks), which may be a sufficient treatment course. Yet, two other studies that predominantly used oral therapy (ciprofloxacin and rifampin) found this approach to be effective (cure rates exceeding 90%) in addicts with uncomplicated right-sided endocarditis caused by MSSA.[54,55] At this time, concerns with resistance (e.g., ciprofloxacin) and limited published data preclude routine use of oral antibacterial regimens for the treatment of infective endocarditis in the intravenous drug abuser.[9]

Staphylococcal Endocarditis: Prosthetic Valves

PVE accounts for approximately 15% of all infective endocarditis cases.[56] An episode of PVE occurring within 2 months of surgery strongly suggests that the cause is staphylococci implanted during the procedure.[3] Yet the risk of staphylococcal endocarditis remains elevated for up to 12 months after valve replacement. Because this type of infective endocarditis is typically a nosocomial infection, methicillin-resistant organisms are common, and vancomycin is the cornerstone of therapy. Combination antimicrobials are recommended because of the high morbidity and mortality associated with PVE and its refractoriness to therapy.[3,9] Although the addition of rifampin to a penicillinase-resistant penicillin or vancomycin does not result in predictable bacterial synergism, rifampin may have unique activity against staphylococcal infection that involves prosthetic material, where its addition results in a higher microbiologic cure rate.[2] Combination therapy also decreases the emergence of resistance to rifampin, which frequently occurs when it is used alone. For methicillin-resistant staphylococci (both MRSA and coagulase-negative staphylococci), vancomycin is recommended with rifampin for 6 weeks or more (see Table 115–8). An aminoglycoside is added for the first 2 weeks if the organism is aminoglycoside-susceptible. For MSSA, a penicillinase-resistant penicillin is administered in place of vancomycin. PVE responds poorly to medical treatment and has a higher mortality compared with native-valve endocarditis. Valve dehiscence and incompetence can result in acute heart failure, and surgery is often a component of treatment.[3,9]

Twelve months or more after valve replacement the likely organism for PVE parallels that of native-valve endocarditis. As with native-valve endocarditis, antimicrobial therapy should be based on the identified organism and in vitro susceptibility. If an organism is identified other than staphylococci, the treatment regimen should be guided by susceptibilities and should be at least 6 weeks in duration.[3,9] Additionally, a concomitant aminoglycoside is recommended if streptococci or enterococci are identified. Once-daily aminoglycoside regimens have not been adequately evaluated in PVE and are not recommended.[3]

The use of anticoagulation is controversial in PVE. In general, those who require anticoagulation for a prosthetic valve should continue the anticoagulant cautiously during endocarditis therapy, unless a contraindication to therapy exists. It is recommended to hold all anticoagulation for at least 2 weeks in patients with *S. aureus* PVE if a recent CNS embolic event has occurred.[9]

CLINICAL CONTROVERSY

Oral antibiotics for the treatment of infective endocarditis have been assessed primarily in those with IVDA. Although treating infective endocarditis with oral antibiotics would decrease adverse events associated with prolonged use of intravenous catheters, the paucity of data preclude this being a routine treatment. Oral rifampin is used as part of combination therapy in PVE caused by staphylococci. The AHA guidelines recently added ciprofloxacin orally as an option for treatment of infective endocarditis caused by the HACEK group of organisms.

■ ENTEROCOCCAL ENDOCARDITIS

Enterococci are normal inhabitants of the human gastrointestinal tract and, occasionally, of the anterior urethra. These organisms are usually of low virulence but can become pathogens in predisposed patients following genitourinary manipulations (older men) or obstetric procedures (younger women).[2] Historically, enterococci were considered group D streptococci, but they have been reclassified into the genus *Enterococcus (E. faecalis* and *E. faecium). E. faecalis* is the most common clinical isolate (approximately 90%) of the two species. Enterococci cause 5% to 18% of endocarditis cases, but they are more resistant to therapy than staphylococci and streptococci. Enterococci are noteworthy for these reasons: (a) no single antibiotic is bactericidal, (b) MICs to penicillin are relatively high (1 to 25 mcg/mL), (c) intrinsic resistance occurs to all cephalosporins and relative resistance occurs to aminoglycosides (e.g., "low-level" aminoglycoside resistance), (d) combinations of a cell wall active agent such as a penicillin or vancomycin and an aminoglycoside are necessary for killing, and (e) resistance to all available drugs is increasing.[1,9]

Monotherapy with penicillin for infective endocarditis caused by enterococci results in relapse rates of 50% to 80%. When used alone, penicillins are only bacteriostatic against enterococci, and combination therapy is always recommended for susceptible strains.[9] The relapse rate following penicillin-gentamicin therapy for susceptible strains is less than 15%.[16] The killing of enterococci by the bactericidal combination of an aminoglycoside and a penicillin is the best clinical example of antibiotic synergy. Because the aminoglycoside cannot penetrate the bacterial cell in the absence of the penicillin, enterococci usually will appear to be resistant to aminoglycosides by routine susceptibility testing (low-level resistance). However, in the presence of an agent that disrupts the cell wall such as penicillin, the aminoglycoside can gain entry, attach to bacterial ribosomes, and cause rapid cell death. An aminoglycoside-vancomycin combination is also synergistic against enterococci and is appropriate therapy for the penicillin-allergic patient.[57]

Enterococcal endocarditis ordinarily requires 4 to 6 weeks of ampicillin or high-dose penicillin G plus an aminoglycoside for cure (Table 115–9). Ampicillin has greater in vitro activity than penicillin G, although there are no clinical data to document differences in efficacy. A 6-week course is recommended for patients with symptoms lasting longer than 3 months and those with PVE. Streptomycin has been the most extensively studied aminoglycoside, but gentamicin is presently favored. Because of resistance, other aminoglycosides, such as tobramycin and amikacin, cannot be substituted routinely. In the treatment of enterococcal endocarditis, relatively low serum concentrations of aminoglycosides appear adequate for successful therapy, such as a gentamicin peak concentration of approximately 3 to 4 mcg/mL.[9,58] Treatment of enterococcal endocarditis does not have the high success rate seen with infective endocarditis caused by viridans streptococci presumably because the organism is more resistant to killing.

Although some data support the use of extended-interval aminoglycoside dosing for other types of endocarditis (i.e., streptococci), the data are more vague regarding this strategy in enterococcal infective endocarditis.[59] Even though some studies suggest that extended-interval aminoglycoside dosing and short-interval (traditional) dosing are clinically equivalent,[60–62] discordant studies imply otherwise.[63,64] The paucity of human data precludes routine use of extended-interval aminoglycoside dosing in this setting and the guidelines recommend three-times daily dosing.[9]

Resistance among enterococci to penicillins and aminoglycosides is increasing.[9] Enterococci that exhibit high-level resistance to streptomycin (MIC >2000 mcg/mL) are not synergistically killed by penicillin and streptomycin because the aminoglycoside either no longer binds to the ribosome or is inactivated by an aminoglycoside-modifying enzyme, streptomycin adenylase. Because enterococci will appear resistant to aminoglycosides on routine susceptibility testing, the only way to distinguish high-level from low-level resistance is by performing special susceptibility tests using 500 to 2,000 mcg/mL of the aminoglycoside. High-level streptomycin-resistant enterococci occur with a frequency approaching 60%, and high-level resistance to gentamicin is now found in 10% to 50% of isolates. Although most gentamicin-resistant enterococci are resistant to all aminoglycosides (including amikacin), 30% to 50% remain susceptible to streptomycin.[1,5] High-level gentamicin resistance is mediated by a bifunctional aminoglycoside-modifying enzyme, 6-acetyltransferase/2-phosphotransferase, and most strains also possess streptomycin adenylase. These organisms do not commonly cause infective endocarditis; data on appropriate therapy are sparse, and therapeutic options are few. Case reports indicate that some patients will respond to high doses of ampicillin, as observed in the early trials of penicillin monotherapy.[65]

In addition to isolates with high-level aminoglycoside resistance, β-lactamase–producing enterococci (especially *E. faecium*) have been reported.[66] If these organisms are discovered, use of vancomycin or ampicillin-sulbactam in combination with gentamicin should be considered. Vancomycin-resistant enterococci are reported increasingly, primarily with *E. faecium.* Vancomycin resistance occurs when the bacterium replaces the normal vancomycin target with a peptidoglycan precursor that does not bind vancomycin.[67] Because of the difficulty of treating multidrug-resistant enterococci, surgery and replacement of the infected cardiac valve may be the only cure.

HACEK Group

Fastidious gram-negative bacteria from the HACEK group account for up to 10% of native valve, community-acquired infective endocarditis.[9] Frequently, these types of infective endocarditis present as subacute illnesses with large vegetations and emboli.[68] These oropharyngeal organisms typically are slow growing and should be considered as possible causes of "culture negative" endocarditis. In the past, high-dose ampicillin with gentamicin for 4 weeks was an acceptable treatment regimen for HACEK endocarditis, but β-lactamase–producing organisms are occurring more often; hence, HACEK organisms should be considered resistant to ampicillin alone. Numerous treatments are reasonable for the treatment of HACEK infective endocarditis, including ceftriaxone and ampicillin-sulbactam; the newest addition to the guidelines is oral ciprofloxacin for selected patients (Table 115–10).[9] Treatment is usually for 4 weeks, but it should be extended to 6 weeks in PVE caused by one of these organisms.

LESS-COMMON TYPES OF INFECTIVE ENDOCARDITIS

Atypical Microorganisms

Endocarditis caused by organisms such as *Bartonella; Coxiella burnetii; Brucella, Candida,* and *Aspergillus* spp.; *Legionella*; and gram-negative bacilli (e.g., *Pseudomonas*) is relatively uncommon. Medical therapy for infective endocarditis caused by these organisms is usually unsuccessful.[6,9] Consultation with an infectious disease expert is warranted when these microorganisms are identified.

In addition to *Pseudomonas* spp., other gram-negative bacilli that have been implicated include *Salmonella* spp., *Escherichia coli, Citrobacter* spp., *Klebsiella-Enterobacter* spp., *Serratia marcescens, Proteus* spp., and *Providencia* spp.[1] Generally, these infections have a poor prognosis, with mortality rates as high as 60% to 80%.[19] Cardiac surgery in concert with extended course antibacterial therapy is the recommended course (Class IIa; Level of Evidence: B) for most patient with gram-negative bacillary infective endocarditis. Readers are referred to the AHA guidelines for more extensive review of *Pseudomonas* spp. infective endocarditis and unusual gram-negative bacteria treatment regimens.[9]

Fungi cause between 2% and 4% of endocarditis cases; most patients with fungal endocarditis have undergone recent cardiovascular surgery, are intravenous drug abusers, have received prolonged treatment with intravenous catheters or antibiotics, or are immunocompromised.[1,2,69] *Candida* spp. and *Aspergillus* spp. are the most commonly involved, and the mortality rate is high (greater than 80%) for these reasons: (a) large, bulky vegetations that often form, (b) systemic septic embolization that may occur, (c) the tendency for fungi to invade the myocardium, (d) poor penetration of vegetations by antifungals, (e) the low toxic-to-therapeutic ratio of agents such as amphotericin B, and (f) the lack of consistent fungicidal activity of available antifungal agents.[1,70] When fungal infective endocarditis is identified, the combined medical–surgical approach is recommended. Because these infections occur infrequently, scant clinical data are available to make solid treatment recommendations; however, the use of antifungal agents alone has been globally unsuccessful. Amphotericin B has been the mainstay pharmacologic approach. The availability of newer antifungal agents challenges this historical approach, although clinical trial data are lacking.[9]

C. burnetii (Q fever) was recently recovered from blood cultures, but infection is more likely to be identified via serologic tests. It is a common cause of infective endocarditis in certain areas of the world where goat, cattle, and sheep farming are widespread. The most favorable therapy for Q fever is unknown but may include doxycycline with trimethoprim-sulfamethoxazole, rifampin, or fluoroquinalones.[4] *Brucella* are facultative intracellular gram-negative bacilli. Humans are infected by this organism after ingesting infected unpasteurized milk or undercooked meat, inhalation of infectious aerosols, or contact with infected tissues. This type of infective endocarditis is more common in veterinarians and livestock handlers. Cure requires valve replacement and antimicrobial agents including doxycycline with streptomycin or gentamicin or doxycycline with trimethoprim-sulfamethoxazole or rifampin for an extended period (8 weeks to months).[4]

Culture-Negative Endocarditis

Sterile blood cultures are reported in 5% to 20% of patients with infective endocarditis if strict diagnostic criteria are used.[1,6,71] This type of infective endocarditis may occur as a result of unidentified subacute right-sided infective endocarditis, previous antibiotic therapy, slow-growing fastidious organisms, nonbacterial etiologies (e.g., fungi), and improperly collected blood cultures. When blood cultures from patients suspected of infective endocarditis show no growth after 48 to 72 hours, the laboratory should be advised and cultures held for up to a month to detect growth of fastidious organisms.[9]

The AHA guidelines provide general recommendations for culture-negative infective endocarditis (Table 115–11), although clinicians should individualize therapy, as necessary. Selection of treatment can be difficult, balancing the need to cover all likely organisms against potential toxic drug effects (e.g., aminoglycosides). Antimicrobial selection should be in consultation with an infectious diseases specialist. Irrespective of the chosen treatment, extended antimicrobial therapy is required. The preceding empirical approaches for culture-negative infective endocarditis highlight the need for proper collection and monitoring of blood cultures and an extensive medication history.

PHARMACOECONOMIC CONSIDERATIONS

Infective endocarditis remains an uncommon disease, but the cost of treatment can be substantial. In the past, the long duration of hospitalization required to administer intravenous antimicrobials was the major expense. In selected cases, abbreviated and/or outpatient, and perhaps oral antimicrobial therapy may appreciably reduce the cost of care.

Shorter-course antimicrobial regimens are advocated when possible. For instance, in exquisitely sensitive streptococcal endocarditis (MICs less than 0.12 mcg/mL), a 2-week regimen of high-dose parenteral penicillin G or ceftriaxone in combination with an aminoglycoside is as effective as 4 weeks of penicillin alone.[9] Uncomplicated right-sided MSSA endocarditis in the intravenous drug abuser may be treated with a 2-week course. Treatment with nafcillin or oxacillin in combination with an aminoglycoside appears to be cost-effective.

The initiation of outpatient parenteral antibiotics should be considered early in the treatment of infective endocarditis, after the patient is stable clinically and responds favorably to initial antibiotics. Outpatient treatment is safe and cost-effective in select situations.[72] Patients considered for home therapy must be hemodynamically stable, compliant with therapy, have careful medical monitoring, understand the potential complications of the disease, and have immediate access to medical care. Advances in technology allow for the outpatient administration of complex antibiotic regimens that significantly reduce the cost of therapy. Simple regimens, such as single daily doses of ceftriaxone for streptococcal infective endocarditis, are particularly attractive. Although endocarditis is common in those with a history of IVDA and home healthcare would substantially reduce the cost of treatment, many clinicians are uncomfortable with outpatient intravenous therapy because central venous access is required. Sudden cardiac decompensation in an outpatient setting is also of concern.[9]

EVALUATION OF THERAPEUTIC OUTCOMES

The evaluation of patients treated for infective endocarditis includes assessment of disease signs and symptoms, blood cultures, microbiologic tests, serum drug concentrations, and other tests that evaluate organ function.

SIGNS AND SYMPTOMS

Fever usually subsides within 1 week of initiating therapy.[1,2] Persistence of fever may indicate ineffective antimicrobial therapy, emboli, infections of intravascular catheters, or drug reactions. In some patients, low-grade fever may persist even with appropriate antimicrobial therapy. With defervescence, the patient should begin to feel better, and other symptoms, such as lethargy or weakness, should subside. Echocardiography should be performed when antibiotic therapy has been completed to determine new baseline cardiac function (i.e., ventricular size and function). A TTE is usually sufficient.

BLOOD CULTURES

Blood cultures should be negative within a few days, although microbiologic response to vancomycin may be slower.[1,2] If bacteria continue to be isolated from blood beyond the first few days of therapy, it may indicate that the antimicrobials are inactive against the pathogen or that the doses are not producing adequate concentrations at the site of infection. After the initiation of therapy, blood cultures should be rechecked until negative. During the remainder of therapy, frequent blood culturing is not necessary. Additional blood cultures should be rechecked after successful treatment (e.g., once or twice within the 8 weeks after treatment) to ensure cure.

MICROBIOLOGIC TESTS

For all isolates from blood cultures, MICs should be determined; MBCs are no longer recommended.[9] The agent currently being used should be tested, as well as alternatives that may be required if intolerance, allergy, or resistance occurs. Occasionally, it is useful to determine whether synergy exists for antimicrobial combinations, although synergistic regimens usually can be predicted from the literature. Chapter 108 summarizes the methods for in vitro determinations of synergy.

Serum bactericidal titers (SBTs; also called *Schlichter tests*) have been used in the past in association with a number of infectious diseases. The SBT is the greatest dilution of a patient's serum sample that is obtained while receiving antimicrobial treatment that kills greater than 99.9% of an inoculum of the infecting pathogen in vitro over 18 to 24 hours.

Although specific SBTs have been evaluated in endocarditis, at present, SBTs have little value in monitoring treatment of common types of infective endocarditis and should not be recommended routinely.[9,73,74] This test may be useful when the causative organisms are only moderately susceptible to antimicrobials, when less-well-established regimens are used, or when response to therapy is suboptimal and dosage escalation is being considered.

SERUM DRUG CONCENTRATIONS

Of the agents used commonly for infective endocarditis, measurement of serum drug concentrations is routinely available for aminoglycosides (except streptomycin) and vancomycin. Few data, however, support attaining any specific serum concentrations in patients with infective endocarditis. In general, serum concentrations of the antimicrobial should exceed the MBC of the organisms. Aminoglycoside concentrations rarely exceed the MBC for certain organisms, such as streptococci and enterococci, and concentrations have not been correlated with response, such as aminoglycosides and vancomycin for staphylococci.[74,75]

When aminoglycosides are administered for infective endocarditis caused by gram-positive cocci with a traditional three times-daily regimen, peak serum concentrations are recommended to be on the low side of the traditional ranges (3 to 4 mcg/mL for gentamicin). If extended-interval dosing is used, which is only recommended in streptococcal infective endocarditis, the most appropriate method of monitoring has not been determined. When vancomycin is administered, the most recent treatment guidelines recommend serum drug monitoring.[9] Although the guidelines recommend that clinicians obtain a peak serum concentrations when using vancomycin, measuring peak concentrations has limited applicability. The primary goal of serum vancomycin monitoring clinically is to ensure adequate trough concentrations are achieved.

PREVENTION

⑩ Antimicrobial prophylaxis is used as an attempt to prevent infective endocarditis in patients who are at the highest risk.[76,77] The use of antimicrobials for this purpose requires consideration of (a) cardiac conditions associated with endocarditis, (b) procedures causing bacteremia, (c) organisms likely to cause endocarditis, and (d) pharmacokinetics, spectrum, cost, adverse effects, and ease of administration of available antimicrobial agents. The objective of prophylaxis is to diminish the likelihood of infective endocarditis in high-risk individuals from procedures that result in bacteremia. Although there are no prospective, controlled human trials demonstrating that prophylaxis in high-risk individuals protects against the development of endocarditis during bacteremia-induced procedures, animal studies suggest possible benefit.[76] Many causes of infective endocarditis, however, appear not to be secondary to an invasive procedure. Bacteremia as a consequence of daily activities in fact may be the major culprit, and the value of antibiotic prophylaxis before bacteremia-causing procedures has been questioned.[78] Retrospective human studies, though, support that a reduction of endocarditis occurs in selected patients following dental surgery where prophylaxis is employed.[79] The common practice of using antimicrobial therapy in this setting remains controversial. The mechanism of a beneficial effect in humans is unclear, but antibiotics may decrease the number of bacteria at the surgical site, kill bacteria after they are introduced into the blood, and prevent adhesion of bacteria to the valve. Prophylaxis does not reduce the frequency of bacteremia immediately following tooth extraction as compared with a control group, suggesting that a reduction in adhesion or effects after the bacteria adhere to the endocardium are more likely mechanisms.[80,81] Other studies have further questioned the benefit of antibiotic prophylaxis.[82]

CLINICAL CONTROVERSY

The common practice of administering antibiotics to high-risk individuals before a bacteremia-causing procedure is controversial. Despite limited data supporting this approach and the fact that 100% compliance with AHA preventative guidelines would have only a modest benefit, the use of single-dose antibiotics for the prevention of endocarditis remains a standard of care.

TABLE 115-12 Cardiac Conditions Associated with the Highest Risk of Adverse Outcome from Endocarditis for Which Prophylaxis with Dental Procedures Is Recommended

Prosthetic cardiac valves
Previous infective endocarditis
Congenital heart disease (CHD)[a]
Unrepaired cyanotic CHD, including palliative shunts and conduits
Completely repaired congenital heart defect with prosthetic material or device, whether placed by surgery or by catheter intervention, during the first 6 months after the procedure[b]
Repaired CHD with residual defects at the site or adjacent to the site of a prosthetic patch or prosthetic device (which inhibit endothelialization)
Cardiac transplantation recipients who develop cardiac valvulopathy

[a]Except for the conditions listed above, antibiotic prophylaxis is no longer recommended for any other form of CHD.

[b]Prophylaxis is recommended because endothelialization of prosthetic material occurs within 6 months after the procedure.

From Wilson W, Taubert KA, Gewitz M, et al. Prevention of infective endocarditis. Circulation 2007:116:1736–1754 with permission. Copyright 2007, American Medical Association.

TABLE 115-13 Dental Procedures for Which Endocarditis Prophylaxis is Recommended for Patients in Table 115–12

All dental procedures that involve manipulation of gingival tissue or the periapical region of teeth or perforation of the oral mucosa[a]

[a]The following procedures and events do not need prophylaxis: routine anesthetic injections through noninfected tissue, taking dental radiographs, placement of removable prosthodontic or orthodontic appliances, adjustment of orthodontic appliances, placement of orthodontic brackets, shedding of deciduous teeth, and bleeding from trauma to the lips or oral mucosa.

From Wilson W, Taubert KA, Gewitz M, et al. Prevention of infective endocarditis. Circulation 2007:116:1736–1754 with permission. Copyright 2007, American Medical Association.

Regardless of the controversy about whether prophylactic antibiotics should be used, infective endocarditis prophylaxis is recommended in selected situations, specifically dental procedures, in those with underlying high-risk cardiac conditions. Recently the American Heart Association released new guidelines that better define who should and should not receive infective endocarditis prophylaxis.[83] This update is timely as data show overuse of infective endocarditis prophylaxis occurs in low-risk patients, and underuse occurs in those at greater risk.[84]

Key points of this report are that (a) only a small number of cases of infective endocarditis might be prevented with antibiotic prophylaxis for dental procedures, even if 100% effective; (b) infective endocarditis prophylaxis for dental procedures should be recommended only for patients with underlying cardiac conditions associated with the highest risk; (c) in those with high-risk underlying cardiac conditions, prophylaxis is recommended for all dental procedures involving manipulation of gingival tissue or the periapical region of teeth or perforation of the oral mucosa; (d) prophylaxis is not recommended based solely on an increased lifetime risk of acquisition of infective endocarditis; and (e) administration of antibiotics solely to prevent endocarditis is not recommended for patients who undergo a genitourinary or gastrointestinal tract procedure.

To determine whether a patient should receive prophylactic antibiotics, one needs to assess the patient's risk (Table 115–12) and if they are undergoing a procedure resulting in bacteremia (Table 115–13). When antibiotic prophylaxis is appropriate a single 2-g dose of amoxicillin is recommended for adult patients at risk, given 30 to 60 minutes before undergoing procedures associated with bacteremia (Table 115–14). Because the duration of antimicrobial prophylaxis appears to be relatively short, these guidelines do not advocate a second oral dose of amoxicillin, which was recommended previously. Alternative prophylaxis regimens for patients allergic to penicillins or those unable to take oral medications are also provided.

TABLE 115-14 Antibiotic Regimens for a Dental Procedure

		Regimen: Single Dose 30 to 60 Min Before Procedure	
Situation	**Agent**	***Adult***	***Children***
Oral	Amoxicillin	2 g	50 mg/kg
Unable to take oral medication	Ampicillin	2 g IM or IV	50 mg/kg IM or IV
	or		
	Cefazolin or ceftriazone	1 g IM or IV	50 mg/kg IM or IV
Allergic to penicillins or ampicillin–oral	Cephalexin[a,b]	2 g	50 mg/kg
	or		
	Clindamycin	600 mg	20 mg/kg
	or		
	Azithromycin or clarithromycin	500 mg	15 mg/kg
Allergic to penicillins or ampicillin and unable to take oral medication	Cefazolin or ceftriaxone[b]	1 g IM or IV	50 mg/kg IM or IV
	or		
	Clindamycin	600 mg IM or IV	20 mg/kg IM or IV

[a]Or other first- or second-generation oral cephalosporin in equivalent adult or pediatric dosage.
[b]Cephalosporins should not be used in an individual with a history of anaphylaxis, angioedema, or urticaria with penicillins or ampicillin.

From Wilson W, Taubert KA, Gewitz M, et al. Prevention of infective endocarditis. Circulation 2007:116:1736–1754 with permission. Copyright 2007, American Medical Association.

ABBREVIATIONS

AHA: American Heart Association

HACEK: The group of bacteria including *Haemophilus parainfluenzae, Haemophilus aphrophilus, Actinobacillus actinomycetemcomitans, Cardiobacterium hominis, Eikenella corrodens,* and *Kingella kingae*

IVDA: intravenous drug abuse

MBC: minimal bactericidal concentration

MIC: minimal inhibitor concentration

MRSA: methicillin-resistant *Staphylococcus aureus*

MSSA: methicillin-sensitive *Staphylococcus aureus*

PVE: prosthetic valve endocarditis

SBT: serum bactericidal titers

TEE: transesophageal echocardiogram

TTE: transthoracic echocardiogram

REFERENCES

1. Fowler VG, Scheld WM, Bayer AS. Endocarditis and intravascular infections. In: Mandell GL, Bennett JE, Dolin R, eds. Principles and Practice of Infectious Diseases, 6th ed. New York: Churchill-Livingstone, 2005:975–1022.
2. Karchmer AW. Infective endocarditis. In: Zipes DP, Libby P, Bonow RO, Braunwald E, eds. Braunwald's Heart Disease: A Textbook of Cardiovascular Medicine, 7th ed. Philadelphia: WB Saunders, 2005:1633–1658.
3. Baddour LM, Wilson SR. Infections of prosthetic valves and other cardiovascular devices. In: Mandell GL, Bennett JE, Dolin R, eds. Principles and Practice of Infectious Diseases, 6th ed. New York: Churchill-Livingstone, 2005:1022–1044.
4. Bayer AS, Bolger AF, Taubert KA, et al. Diagnosis and management of infective endocarditis and its complications. Circulation 1998;98:2936–2948.
5. Bashore TM, Cabell C, Fowler V. Update on Infective Endocarditis. Curr Probl Cardiol 2006;31:274–352.
6. Mylonakis E, Calderwood SB. Infective endocarditis in adults. N Engl J Med 2001;345:1318–1320.
7. Moreillon P, Que Y. Infective endocarditis. Lancet 2004;363:139–149.
8. Winston LG, Bolger AF. Modern epidemiology, prophylaxis, and diagnosis and therapy for infective endocarditis. Curr Cardiol Rep 2006;8:102–108.
9. Baddour LM, Wilson WR, Bayer AS, et al. Infective endocarditic: Diagnosis, antimicrobial therapy, and management of complications: A statement for healthcare professionals from the Committee on Rheumatic Fever, Endocarditis, and Kawasaki Disease, Council on Cardiovascular Disease in the Young, and the Councils on Clinical Cardiology, Stroke, and Cardiovascular Surgery and Anesthesia, American Heart Association: endorsed by the Infectious Diseases Society of America. Circulation 2005;111:e394-e433.
10. Guoello JP, Asfar P, Brenet O. Nosocomial endocarditis in the intensive care unit: An analysis of 22 cases. Crit Care Med 2000;28:377–382.
11. Werner M, Andersson R, Olaison L. A clinical study of culture-negative endocarditis. Medicine (Baltimore) 2003;82:263–273.
12. Cheitlin MD, Armstrong WF, Aurigemma GP, et al. AHA/ACC/ASE 2003 Guideline Update for the Clinical Application of Echocardiogra-

phy. A Report of the American College of Cardiology/American Heart Association Task Force on Practice Guidelines, 2003. *www.acc.org/clinical/guidelines/echo/index/pdf.*
13. Sachdev M, Peterson GE, Jollis JG. Imaging techniques for diagnosis of infective endocarditis. Cardiol Clin 2003;21:185–195.
14. Kupferwasser LI, Darius H, Muller AM, et al. Diagnosis of culture-negative endocarditis: The role of the Duke criteria and the impact of transesophageal echocardiography. Am Heart J 2001;142:146–152.
15. Mugge A. Echocardiographic detection of cardiac valve vegetations and prognostic implications. Infect Dis Clin North Am 1993;7:877–898.
16. Flachskampf FA, Daniel WG. Role of transoesophageal echocardiography in infective endocarditis. Heart 2000;84:3–4.
17. Durack DT, Lukes AS, Bright DK. New criteria for diagnosis of infective endocarditis: Utilization of specific echocardiographic findings. Am J Med 1994;96:200–209.
18. Li JS, Sexton DJ, Mick N, et al. Proposed modifications to the Duke criteria for the diagnosis of infective endocarditis. Clin Infect Dis 2000;30:633–638.
19. Gold MJ. Cure rates and long-term prognosis. In: Kaye D, ed. Infective Endocarditis, 2d ed. New York: Raven Press, 1992:455–464.
20. Pokorski RJ. Long-term survival of patients with infective endocarditis. J Insur Med 1998;30:76–87.
21. Ferguson E, Reardon MJ, Letsou GV. The surgical management of bacterial valvular endocarditis. Curr Opin Cardiol 2000;15:82–85.
22. Anonymous. Correction: Infective endocarditic: Diagnosis, antimicrobial therapy, and management of complications: A statement for healthcare professionals from the Committee on Rheumatic Fever, Endocarditis, and Kawasaki Disease, Council on Cardiovascular Disease in the Young, and the Councils on Clinical Cardiology, Stroke, and Cardiovascular Surgery and Anesthesia, American Heart Association: Endorsed by the Infectious Diseases Society of America. Circulation 2005;112:2374.
23. Hoen B. Special issues in the management of infective endocarditis caused by gram-positive cocci. Infect Dis Clin North Am 2002;16:437–452.
24. Levison ME. In vitro assays. In: Kaye D, ed. Infectious Endocarditis, 2d ed. New York: Raven Press, 1992:151–167.
25. Baldassarre JS, Kaye D. Principles and overview of antibiotic therapy. In: Kaye D, ed. Infectious Endocarditis, 2d ed. New York: Raven Press, 1992:169–190.
26. Francioli PB. Ceftriaxone and outpatient treatment of infective endocarditis. Infect Dis Clin North Am 1993;7:97–116.
27. Shanson DC. New guidelines for the antibiotic treatment of streptococcal, enterococcal and staphylococcal endocarditis. J Antimicrob Chemother 1998;42:292–296.
28. Weiss ME, Adkinson NF. Beta-lactam allergy. In: Mandell GL, Bennett JE, Dolin R, eds. Principles and Practice of Infectious Diseases, 6th ed. New York: Churchill-Livingstone, 2005:318–325.
29. DiNubile MJ. Treatment of endocarditis caused by relatively resistant nonenterococcal streptococci: Is penicillin enough? Rev Infect Dis 1990;12:112–115.
30. Blatter M, Fluckiger U, Entenza J, et al. Simulated human serum profiles of one daily dose of ceftriaxone plus netilmicin in treatment of experimental streptococcal endocarditis. Antimicrob Agents Chemother 1993;37:1971–1976.
31. Francioli PB, Glauser MP. Synergistic activity of ceftriaxone combined with netilmicin administered once daily for treatment of experimental streptococcal endocarditis. Antimicrob Agents Chemother 1993;37:207–212.
32. Gavalda J, Pahissa A, Almirante B, et al. Effect of gentamicin dosing interval on therapy of viridans streptococcal experimental endocarditis with gentamicin plus penicillin. Antimicrob Agents Chemother 1995;39:2098–2103.
33. Francioli P, Ruch W, Stamboulian D, et al. Treatment of streptococcal endocarditis with a single daily dose of ceftriaxone and netilmicin for 14 days: A prospective multicenter study. Clin Infect Dis 1995;21:1406–1410.
34. Sexton DJ, Tenenbaum MJ, Wilson WR, et al. Ceftriaxone once daily for 4 weeks compared to ceftriaxone plus gentamicin once daily for 2 weeks for treatment of penicillin-susceptible streptococcal endocarditis. Clin Infect Dis 1998;27:1470–1474.
35. Karchmer A. Staphylococcal endocarditis. In: Kaye D, ed. Infectious Endocarditis, 2d ed. New York: Raven Press, 1992:225–249.
36. Petti CA, Fowler VG. *Staphylococcus aureus* bacteremia and endocarditis. Cardiol Clin 2003;21:219–233.
37. Korzeniowski O, Sande MA. The National Collaborative Endocarditis Study Group: Combination antimicrobial therapy for *Staphylococcus aureus* endocarditis in patients addicted to parenteral drugs and in nonaddicts. Ann Intern Med 1982;97:496–503.
38. Gavalda J, Lopez P, Martin T, et al. Efficacy of ceftriaxone and gentamicin given once a day using human-like pharmacokinetics in treatment of experimental staphylococcal endocarditis. Antimicrob Agents Chemother 2002;46:378–384.
39. Dodek P, Phillip P. Questionable history of immediate-type hypersensitivity to penicillin in staphylococcal endocarditis: Treatment based on skin test results versus empirical alternative treatment—A decision analysis. Clin Infect Dis 1999;29:1251–1256.
40. Fridkin SK, Hageman J, McDougal LK, et al. Vancomycin-Intermediate *Staphylococcus aureus* Epidemiology Study Group. Epidemiological and microbiological characterization of infections caused by *Staphylococcus aureus* with reduced susceptibility to vancomycin, United States, 1997–2001. Clin Infect Dis 2003;36:429–439.
41. Woods CW, Cheng AC, Fowler VG, et al. Endocarditis caused by *Staphylococcus aureus* with reduced susceptibility to vancomycin. Clin Infect Dis 2004;38:1188–1191.
42. Howden BP, Ward PB, Charles PGP, et al. Treatment outcomes for serious infections causes by methicillin-resistant *Staphylococcus aureus* with reduced vancomycin susceptibility. Clin Infect Dis 2004;38:521–528.
43. Segreti JA, Crank CW, Finney MS. Daptomycin for the treatment of gram-positive bacteremia and infective endocarditis: A retrospective case series of 31 patients. Pharmacotherapy 2006;26:347–352.
44. Fowler VG, Boucher HW, Corey GR, et al. Daptomycin versus standard therapy for bacteremia and endocarditis caused by *Staphylococcus aureus.* N Engl J Med 2006;355:653–665.
45. Miro JM, del Rio A, Mestres CA. Infective endocarditis and cardiac surgery in intravenous drug abusers and HIV-1 infected patients. Cardiol Clin 2003;21:167–184.
46. Chambers HF. Short-course combination and oral therapies of *Staphylococcus aureus* endocarditis. Med Clin North Am 1993;7:69–80.
47. DiNubile MJ. Abbreviated therapy for right-sided *Staphylococcus aureus* endocarditis in injection drug users: The time has come? Eur J Clin Microbiol Infect Dis 1994;13:533–534.
48. DiNubile MJ. Short-course antibiotic therapy for right-sided *Staphylococcus aureus* endocarditis in injection drug users. Ann Intern Med 1994;121:873–876.
49. Chambers HF, Miller T, Newman MD. Right-sided endocarditis in intravenous drug abusers: Two-week combination therapy. Ann Intern Med 1988;109:619–624.
50. Espinosa FJ, Valdes M, Martin-Luengo M, et al. Right sided endocarditis caused by *Staphylococcus aureus* in parenteral drug addicts: Evaluation of a combined therapeutic scheme for 2 weeks versus conventional treatment. Enferm Infect Microbiol Clin 1993;11:235–240.
51. Torres-Tortosa M, de Cueto M, Vergara A, et al. Prospective evaluation of a two-week course of intravenous antibiotics in intravenous drug addicts with infective endocarditis. Eur J Clin Microbiol Infect Dis 1994;13:559–564.
52. Ribera E, Gomez-Jimenez J, Cortes E, et al. Effectiveness of cloxacillin with and without gentamicin in short-term therapy for right-sided *Staphylococcus aureus* endocarditis: A randomized, controlled trial. Ann Intern Med 1996;125:969–974.
53. Parker RH, Fossieck BE. Intravenous followed by oral antimicrobial therapy for staphylococcal endocarditis. Ann Intern Med 1980;93:832–834.
54. Dworkin RJ, Lee BL, Sande MA, Chambers HF. Treatment of right-sided *Staphylococcus aureus* endocarditis in intravenous drug abusers with ciprofloxacin and rifampin. Lancet 1989;2:1071–1073.
55. Heldman AW, Hartert TV, Ray SC, et al. Oral antibiotic treatment of right-sided staphylococcal endocarditis in injection drug users: Prospective, randomized comparison with parenteral therapy. Am J Med 1996;101:68–76.
56. Berlin JA, Abrutyn E, Strom BL, et al. Incidence of infective endocarditis in the Delaware Valley, 1988–1990. Am J Cardiol 1995;76:933–936.
57. Murray BE. The life and times of the enterococcus. Clin Microbiol Rev 1990;3:46–65.

58. Wilson WR, Wilkowske CJ, Wright AJ, et al. Treatment of streptomycin-susceptible and streptomycin resistant enterococcal endocarditis. Ann Intern Med 1984;100:816–823.
59. Tam VH, Preston SL, Briceland LL. Once-daily aminoglycosides in the treatment of gram-positive endocarditis. Ann Pharmacother 1999;33:600–606.
60. Houlihan HH, Stokes DP, Rybak MJ. Pharmacodynamics of vancomycin and ampicillin alone and in combination with gentamicin once daily or thrice daily against *Enterococcus faecalis* in an in vitro infection model. J Antimicrob Chemother 2000;46:79–86.
61. Gavalda J, Cardona PJ, Almirante B, et al. Treatment of experimental endocarditis due to *Enterococcus faecalis* using profiles of ampicillin in human serum. Antimicrob Agents Chemother 1996;40:173–178.
62. Schwank S, Blaser J. Once versus thrice-daily netilmicin combined with amoxicillin, penicillin, or vancomycin against *Enterococcus faecalis* in a pharmacodynamic in vitro model. Antimicrob Agents Chemother 1996;40:2258–2261.
63. Fantin B, Carbon C. Importance of the aminoglycoside dosing regimen in the penicillin-netilmicin combination for treatment of *Enterococcus faecalis*–induced experimental endocarditis. Antimicrob Agents Chemother 1990;34:2387–2391.
64. Marangos MN, Nicolau DP, Quintiliani R, Nightingale CH. Influence of gentamicin dosing interval on the efficacy of penicillin-containing regimens in experimental *Enterococcus faecalis* endocarditis. J Antimicrob Chemother 1997;39:519–522.
65. Lipman ML, Silva J. Endocarditis due to *Streptococcus faecalis* with high-level resistance to gentamicin. Rev Infect Dis 1989;11:325–328.
66. Wells VD, Wong ES, Murray BE, et al. Infections due to beta-lactamase-producing, high-level gentamicin-resistant *Enterococcus faecalis.* Ann Intern Med 1992;116:285–292.
67. Tailor SA, Bailey EM, Rybak MJ. *Enterococcus*: An emerging pathogen. Ann Pharmacother 1993;27:1231–1242.
68. Hessen MT, Abrutyn E. Gram-negative bacterial endocarditis. In: Kaye D, ed. Infective Endocarditis, 2d ed. New York: Raven Press, 1992:251–264.
69. Moyer DV, Edwards JE. Fungal endocarditis. In: Kaye D, ed. Infective Endocarditis, 2d ed. New York: Raven Press, 1992:299–312.
70. Pierrotti LC, Baddour LM. Fungal endocarditis, 1995–2000. Chest 2002;122:302–310.
71. Werner M, Andersson R, Olaison L, et al. A clinical study of culture-negative endocarditis. Medicine (Baltimore) 2003;82:263–273.
72. Rehm SJ. Outpatient intravenous antibiotic therapy for endocarditis. Infect Dis Clin North Am 1998;12:879–901.
73. Tunkel AR, Scheld WM. Experimental models of endocarditis. In: Kaye D, ed. Infectious Endocarditis, 2d ed. New York: Raven Press, 1992:37–56.
74. Weinstein MP, Stratton CW, Ackley A, et al. Multicenter collaborative evaluation of a standardized serum bactericidal test as a prognostic indicator in infective endocarditis. Am J Med 1985;78:262–269.
75. McCormack JP, Jewesson PJ. A critical reevaluation of the "therapeutic range" of aminoglycosides. Clin Infect Dis 1992;14:320–339.
76. Dajani AS, Taubert KA, Wilson W, et al. Prevention of bacterial endocarditis: Recommendations by the American Heart Association. JAMA 1997;277:1794–1801.
77. Ramsdale DR, Turner-Stokes L on behalf of the Advisory Group of the British Cardiac Society Clinical Practice Committee and the RCP Clinical Effectiveness and Evaluation Unit. Prophylaxis and treatment of infective endocarditis in adults: A concise guide. Clin Med 2004;4:545–550.
78. Roberts GJ. Dentist are innocent! "Everyday" bacteremia is real culprit: A review and assessment of the evidence that dental surgical procedures are a principal cause of bacterial endocarditis. Pediatr Cardiol 1999;20:317–325.
79. Greenman RL, Bisno AL. Prevention of bacterial endocarditis. In: Kaye D, ed. Infective Endocarditis, 2d ed. New York: Raven Press, 1992:465–481.
80. Hall G, Hedstrom SA, Heimdahl A, Nord CE. Prophylactic administration of penicillins for endocarditis does not reduce the incidence of postextraction bacteremia. Clin Infect Dis 1993;17:188–194.
81. Van der Meer JT, Van Wijk W, Thompson J, et al. Efficacy of antibiotic prophylaxis for prevention of native-valve endocarditis. Lancet 1992;339:135–139.
82. Strom BL, Abrutym E, Berlin JA, et al. Risk factors for infective endocarditis: Oral hygiene and nondental exposures. Circulation 2000;102:2842–2848.
83. Wilson, W, Taubert KA, Gewitz M, et al. Prevention of infective endocarditis. Circulation 2007:116:1736–1754.
84. Seto TB, Kwiat D, Taira DA, et al. Physicians' recommendations to patients for use of antibiotic prophylaxis to prevent endocarditis. JAMA 2000;284:68–71.

CHAPTER 116

Tuberculosis

CHARLES A. PELOQUIN

KEY CONCEPTS

1. Tuberculosis (TB) is the most prevalent communicable infectious disease on earth; it remains out of control in many developing nations. These nations require medical and financial assistance from developed nations in order to control the spread of TB globally.

2. In the United States, TB disproportionately affects ethnic minorities as compared with whites, reflecting greater ongoing transmission in ethnic minority communities. Additional TB surveillance and preventive treatment are required within these communities.

3. Coinfection with human immunodeficiency virus (HIV) and TB accelerates the progression of both diseases, thus requiring rapid diagnosis and treatment of both diseases.

4. Mycobacteria are slow-growing organisms; in the laboratory, they require special stains, special growth media, and long periods of incubation to isolate and identify.

5. TB can produce atypical signs and symptoms in infants, the elderly, and immunocompromised hosts, and it can progress rapidly in these patients.

6. Latent TB infection (LTBI) can lead to reactivation disease years after the primary infection occurred.

7. The patient suspected of having active TB disease must be isolated until the diagnosis is confirmed and the patient is no longer contagious. Often, isolation takes place in specialized "negative-pressure" hospital rooms to prevent the spread of TB.

8. Isoniazid and rifampin are the two most important TB drugs; organisms resistant to both these drugs (multidrug-resistant TB [MDR-TB]) are much more difficult to treat.

9. Never add a single drug to a failing regimen!

10. Directly observed treatment should be used whenever possible to reduce treatment failures and the selection of drug-resistant isolates.

(1) Tuberculosis (TB) remains a leading infectious killer globally. TB is caused by *Mycobacterium tuberculosis*, which can produce either a silent, latent infection or a progressive, active disease.[1] Left untreated or improperly treated, TB causes progressive tissue destruction and, eventually, death. Because of renewed public health efforts, TB rates in the United States continue to decline. In contrast, TB remains out of control in many developing countries—to the point that one-third of the world's population currently is infected.[1] Approximately 1 person dies of TB in India each minute (*Times of India*, August 29, 2003). Given increasing drug resistance, it is critical that a major effort be made to control TB before the most effective drugs are lost permanently.

M. tuberculosis preferentially infects humans, and the closely related *Mycobacterium bovis* causes a similar disease in cattle and other livestock. Although uncommon today, humans frequently developed TB by drinking milk contaminated with *M. bovis*—a threat that spurred the development of pasteurization. Today, airborne *M. tuberculosis* is the main threat to humans.

Evidence of TB has been found in ancient human remains, and ancient texts describe it.[1–3] TB commonly was known as "consumption" because of the pronounced weight loss that it caused.[1] Other common names included "wasting disease" and the "white plague." As the term *plague* implies, TB had a profound impact on human history, most notably in Europe. (*Note:* The "black plague," or bubonic plague, is a separate disease caused by *Yersinia pestis.*)

TB rates generally have risen with increasing urbanization and overcrowding because it is easier for an airborne disease to spread when people are packed closely together.[3] Hence TB became a significant pathogen in Europe during the Middle Ages and peaked during the Industrial Revolution, when it caused approximately 25% of all deaths in Europe and in the United States.[1–3] This dire threat led to the rise of public health departments and to procedures such as the isolation of infected patients. Thus TB was directly responsible for many of the healthcare practices that we take for granted today. Unfortunately, in developing nations, some of these practices are not widely available, and TB continues to rage unabated.

EPIDEMIOLOGY

Globally, roughly 2 billion people are infected by *M. tuberculosis*, and roughly 2 to 3 million people die from active TB each year despite the fact that it is curable.[1,2,4] In the United States, about 13 million people are latently infected with *M. tuberculosis*, meaning that they are not currently sick but that they could fall ill with TB at any time. The United States had 14,093 new cases of active TB in 2005 and about 1,500 deaths.[5] (For detailed data analysis, visit the Centers for Disease Control and Prevention [CDC] website at *www.cdc.gov/nchstp/tb.*) The annual incidence of TB in the United States declined by approximately 5% per year from 1953 to 1983[6] (Fig. 116–1). In 1984, this decline slowed, and then the incidence of TB rose from 1988 to 1992, reaching 10.5 cases per 100,000 population. Since 1992, more effective infection control practices and treatment protocols have reduced TB rates to 4.8 per 100,000 population as of 2005.[5] Despite this good news, the eradication of TB from the United States remains very

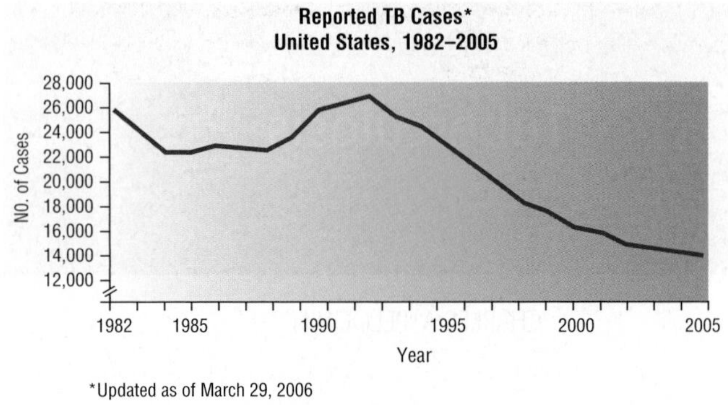

FIGURE 116-1. Reported tuberculosis cases in the United States, 1982–2005.

difficult. One reason is that we continue to import new cases from countries where TB remains out of control.[4,5]

RISK FACTORS FOR INFECTION

Location and Place of Birth

TB can infect anyone, but the risk is not evenly distributed across the U.S. population. The major points of entry into the United States have the most TB cases. Seven states (California, Florida, Georgia, Illinois, New Jersey, New York, and Texas) reported more than 400 cases each for 2005; combined, these seven states accounted for 59.7% (8,414 cases) of the national total.[5] Within these states, TB is most prevalent in large urban areas.[4]

The TB rate among foreign-born persons was 8.7 times that of U.S.-born persons in 2005.[5] The percentage of foreign-born TB patients in the United States has increased annually since 1986, reaching 54% in 2005.[5] More than half (56.0%) of the foreign-born cases in 2005 were reported in persons from Mexico (1,930), the Philippines (826), Vietnam (576), India (563), and China (389).[5] Therefore, healthcare workers must "think TB" when caring for patients from these countries who experience symptoms such as cough, fever, and weight loss.

Close contacts of pulmonary TB patients are most likely to become infected.[2–4] These include family members, coworkers, or coresidents in places such as prisons, shelters, or nursing homes. The more prolonged the contact, the greater is the risk, with infection rates as high as 30%.[5,6] Although many circumstances exist, TB patients frequently have limited access to healthcare, live in crowded conditions, or are homeless.[2,4] Many patients have histories of alcohol abuse or illicit drug use, and many are coinfected with hepatitis B or human immunodeficiency virus (HIV). These concurrent social and health problems make treating some TB patients particularly difficult.

Race, Ethnicity, Age, and Gender

❷ In the United States, TB disproportionately affects ethnic minorities. Hispanics, blacks, and Asians had TB rates 7.3, 8.3, and 19.6 times higher than whites in 2005.[5] Hispanics accounted for 28.4% of all TB cases, followed by blacks at 27.9%.[5] Asians and Pacific Islanders accounted for 22.5%, whereas non-Hispanic whites accounted for only 21.2% of the new TB cases.[5]

TB is most common among people 25 to 44 years of age (35% of all U.S. cases in 2002), followed by those 45 to 64 years of age (28%) and 65 years of age and older (21%).[6] TB is more common in older whites and Asians compared with younger people from these groups. This reflects reactivation of latent infection acquired many years earlier when TB was very common. Older blacks and Hispanics also have more TB than younger individuals, but the differences by age are not as pronounced.[6] This reflects a greater recent transmission among younger blacks and Hispanics compared with younger whites and Asians. Until the age of 15 years, TB rates are similar for males and females, but after that, the male predominance increases with each decade of life.[6]

Coinfection with Human Immunodeficiency Virus (HIV)

❸ HIV is the most important risk factor for active TB, especially among people 25 to 44 years of age.[2,4,6,7] TB and HIV seem to act synergistically within patients and across populations, making each disease worse than it might otherwise be. *Roughly 10% of U.S. TB patients are coinfected with HIV, and roughly 20% of TB patients ages 25 to 44 years are coinfected.*[5,6] HIV coinfection may not increase the risk of acquiring *M. tuberculosis* infection, but it does increase the likelihood of progression to active disease.[1,7] Furthermore, TB and HIV patients share a number of behavioral risk factors that contribute to the high rates of coinfection.[2,8,9]

RISK FACTORS FOR DISEASE

Once infected with *M. tuberculosis*, a person's lifetime risk of active TB is approximately 10%.[2,4,7] The greatest risk for active disease occurs during the first 2 years after infection. Children younger than 2 years of age and adults older than 65 years of age have two to five times greater risk for active disease compared with other age groups. Patients with underlying immune suppression (e.g., renal failure, cancer, and immunosuppressive drug treatment) have 4 to 16 times greater risk than other patients. Finally, HIV-infected patients with *M. tuberculosis* infection are 100 times more likely to develop active TB than normal hosts.[4,10] HIV-infected patients have an annual risk of active TB of approximately 10%, rather than a lifetime risk at that rate. Therefore, all patients with HIV infection should be screened for tuberculous infection, and those known to be infected with *M. tuberculosis* should be tested for HIV infection.

ETIOLOGY

M. tuberculosis is a slender bacillus with a waxy outer layer.[2,7] It is 1 to 4 microns in length, and under the microscope, it is either straight or slightly curved in shape.[1,11,12] It does not stain well with Gram stain, so the Ziehl-Neelsen stain or the fluorochrome stain must be used instead.[1,2,7] After Ziehl-Neelsen staining with carbol-fuchsin, mycobacteria retain the red color despite acid–alcohol washes. Hence they are called *acid-fast bacilli.*[11] After staining, microscopic examination ("smear") detects about 8,000 to 10,000 organisms per milliliter of specimen, so a patient can be "smear negative" but still grow *M. tuberculosis* on culture. Microscopic examination also cannot determine which of the 100+ mycobacterial species is present or whether the organisms in the original samples were alive or dead.[1,11,12] On smear, they are all dead. On culture, *M. tuberculosis* grows slowly, doubling about every 20 hours. This is very slow compared with gram-positive and gram-negative bacteria, which double about every 30 minutes.

Among the mycobacteria, only *M. tuberculosis* is a frequent human pathogen. Some nontuberculous mycobacteria such as *Mycobacterium kansasii, Mycobacterium fortuitum*, and *Mycobacterium avium* complex (MAC) cause infections in patients with other medical problems, especially the acquired immunodeficiency syndrome (AIDS). Chapter 129 discusses the treatment of these infections.

CULTURE AND SUSCEPTIBILITY TESTING

❹ Direct susceptibility testing involves inoculating specialized media with organisms taken directly from a concentrated, smear-positive specimen.[1,11,12] This approach produces susceptibility results in 2 to 3 weeks. Indirect susceptibility testing involves inoculating the test media with organisms obtained from a pure culture of the organisms, which can take several more weeks. The most common agar method, known as the *proportion method,* uses the ratio of colony counts on drug-containing agar to that on drug-free agar.[1,12] In the United States, the critical proportion for resistance is 1%. That means that if a drug-containing plate shows only 2% of the growth seen on a drug-free plate, some of the organisms from the specimen were resistant to that drug. Therefore, it is likely that many of the organisms in the patient also are resistant to that drug, and it should not be used to treat that patient.

The proportion method's limitations include many weeks to obtain results, drug degradation during the incubation, and a qualitative result (susceptible or resistant). The BACTEC system (Becton-Dickinson, Sparks, MD) uses liquid medium (7H12 broth) and detects live mycobacteria based on the release of radiolabeled CO_2.[11] Advantages of the BACTEC system include reduced incubation time (as few as 9 to 14 days), reduced drug loss in the medium, and when multiple concentrations are tested, a truly quantitative end point (minimal inhibitory concentration [MIC]).[1,11,12] Newer, nonradiometric rapid methods such as the MGIT system are now being used by some laboratories.[13]

Rapid-identification tests are now available.[13] Nucleic acid probes such as the AccuProbe (Gen-Probe, San Diego, CA) use DNA probes to identify the presence of complementary rRNA (ribosomal ribonucleic acid) for several mycobacterial species.[7,11,14] DNA fingerprinting using restriction-fragment-length polymorphism analysis has been used to identify clusters of cases.[1,11,14] Amplification of the genetic material can be achieved through polymerase chain reaction (Roche Molecular Systems, Branchburg, NJ), the amplified *M. tuberculosis* direct (MTD) test (Gen-Probe, San Diego, CA), and strand-displacement amplification (SDA; Becton-Dickinson, Sparks, MD).[11,15] Thin-layer chromatography, high-performance liquid chromatography for mycolic acid identification, and gas chromatography for short-chain fatty acids (methyl esters) have been used to speciate mycobacterial isolates.[1,11,14] Other tests are designed to detect common genetic changes associated with drug resistance, such as changes in the *katG* gene associated with isoniazid resistance and the *rpoB* gene associated with rifampin resistance.[7,16–18] These tests offer clinicians a chance to know rapidly what organism they are treating and what drugs might be good initial choices.

TRANSMISSION

M. tuberculosis is transmitted from person-to-person by coughing or sneezing.[2,7,13] This produces "droplet nuclei" that are dispersed in the air. Each droplet nuclei contains one to three organisms. Riley and colleagues showed that air circulated from a hospital TB ward could cause disease in guinea pigs.[19] When this air was filtered or treated with ultraviolet radiation, the animals were not infected. Approximately 30% of individuals who experience prolonged contact with an infectious TB patient will become infected.

A person with cavitary, pulmonary TB and a cough may infect roughly one person per month until that person is treated effectively, although this number can vary significantly. A person with the uncommon laryngeal form of TB can spread organisms even when talking, so the transmission rates can be very high. HIV-infected patients acquire the organisms through the lungs just like normal hosts, but their weakened immune system puts them at very high risk for active disease.[2,4,7,13]

PATHOPHYSIOLOGY

IMMUNE RESPONSE

Good T-lymphocyte responses are essential to controlling *M. tuberculosis* infections.[2,7,20,21] In the mouse model, two different T-cell responses—the T-helper type 1 (TH_1) response and the T-helper type 2 (TH_2) response—have been described. The TH_1 response is the preferred response to TB, and the TH_2 response, including the potentially subversive influence of interleukin (IL) 4, is undesirable.[2,20,21] Some workers have argued that this dichotomy is clearer in the mouse model, and in many humans, the T-cell response may be classified as TH_0 (elements of both TH_1 and TH_2).[20] In either case, T-lymphocytes activate macrophages that, in turn, engulf and kill mycobacteria. T lymphocytes also destroy immature macrophages that harbor *M. tuberculosis* but are unable to kill the invaders.[20,21] CD4+ cells are the primary T cells involved, with contributions by $\gamma\delta$ T cells and CD8+ T cells.[20] CD4+ T cells produce interferon γ (INF-γ) and other cytokines, including IL-2 and IL-10, that coordinate the immune response to TB.[20] Because CD4+ cells are depleted in HIV-infected patients, these patients are unable to mount an adequate defense to TB.[20,21]

Although B-cell responses and antibody production can be demonstrated in TB-infected mammals, these humoral responses do not appear to contribute much to the control of TB within the host.[2,7,20] T cells are responding to certain mycobacterial antigens, but the key antigen(s) invoking the immune response have not been identified.[20] Tumor necrosis factor-α (TNF-α) and INF-γ are important cytokines involved in coordinating the host's cell-mediated response. Rheumatoid arthritis patients treated with TNF-α inhibitors (infliximab) have high rates of reactivation TB.[22] Therefore, patients known to be deficient in the activity of TNF-α or INF-γ should be screened for TB infection and offered appropriate treatment.

M. tuberculosis has several ways of evading or resisting the host immune response.[20,21] In particular, *M. tuberculosis* can inhibit the fusion of lysosomes to phagosomes inside macrophages. This prevents the destructive enzymes found in the lysosomes from getting to the bacilli captured in the phagosomes. This stay of execution allows time for *M. tuberculosis* to escape into the cytoplasm. Virulent *M. tuberculosis* are able to multiply in the macrophage cytoplasm, thus perpetuating their spread. Finally, lipoarabinomannan, the principal structural polysaccharide of the mycobacterial cell wall, inhibits the host immune response.[20,21] Lipoarabinomannan induces immunosuppressive cytokines, thus blocking macrophage activation; additionally, lipoarabinomannan scavenges O_2, thus preventing attack by superoxide anions, hydrogen peroxide, singlet oxygen, and hydroxyl radicals.[20,21] These survival mechanisms make *M. tuberculosis* a particularly difficult organism to control. Any defects in the host immune system make it likely that *M. tuberculosis* will not be controlled and that active disease will ensue.

PRIMARY INFECTION

Primary infection usually results from inhaling airborne particles that contain *M. tuberculosis.*[2,7,21] These particles, called *droplet nuclei,* contain one to three bacilli and are small enough (1 to 5 mm) to reach the alveolar surface. Ingestion (swallowing) and inoculation (puncture wound) are other rare pathways to acquire *M. tuberculosis* infection.[21]

The progression to clinical disease depends on three factors: (a) the number of *M. tuberculosis* organisms inhaled (infecting dose), (b) the virulence of these organisms, and (c) the host's cell-mediated immune response.[2,5,7,13,21,23] At the alveolar surface, the bacilli that were delivered by the droplet nuclei are ingested by pulmonary macrophages.[21] If these macrophages inhibit or kill the bacilli, infection is aborted.[21] If the macrophages cannot do this, the organisms continue to multiply. The macrophages eventually rupture, releasing many bacilli, and these mycobacteria are then phagocytized by other macrophages. This cycle continues over several weeks until the host is able to mount a more coordinated response.[21] During this early phase of infection, *M. tuberculosis* multiplies logarithmically.[21]

Some of the intracellular organisms are transported by the macrophages to regional lymph nodes in the hilar, mediastinal, and retroperitoneal areas. The cycle of phagocytosis and cell rupture continues. During lymph node involvement, the mycobacteria may be held in check. More frequently, *M. tuberculosis* spreads throughout the body through the bloodstream.[2,7,21] When this intravascular dissemination occurs, *M. tuberculosis* can infect any tissue or organ in the body. Most commonly, *M. tuberculosis* infects the posterior apical region of the lungs. This may be so because of the high oxygen content, and it may be because of a less-vigorous immune response in this area.

After about 3 weeks of infection, T lymphocytes are presented with *M. tuberculosis* antigens. These T cells become activated and begin to secrete INF-γ and the other cytokines noted earlier. The processes described in the immune response section earlier then begin to occur. First, T-lymphocytes stimulate macrophages to become bactericidal.[21] Large numbers of activated microbicidal macrophages surround the solid caseous (cheese-like) tuberculous foci (the necrotic area of infection).[21] This process of creating activated microbicidal macrophages is known as *cell-mediated immunity*.[21]

At the same time that cell-mediated immunity occurs, delayed-type hypersensitivity also develops through the activation and multiplication of T lymphocytes. Delayed-type hypersensitivity refers to the cytotoxic immune process that kills nonactivated immature macrophages that are permitting intracellular bacillary replication.[21] These immature macrophages are killed when the T-lymphocytes initiate Fas-mediated apoptosis (programmed cell death).[21] The bacilli released from the immature macrophages then are killed by the activated macrophages.[21]

By this time (>3 weeks), macrophages have begun to form granulomas to contain the organisms. In a typical tuberculous granuloma, activated macrophages accumulate around a caseous lesion and prevent its further extension.[21] At this point, the infection is largely under control, and bacillary replication falls off dramatically. Depending on the inflammatory response, tissue necrosis and calcification of the infection site plus the regional lymph nodes may occur.

Over 1 to 3 months, activated lymphocytes reach an adequate number, and tissue hypersensitivity results. This is shown by a positive tuberculin skin test. Any remaining mycobacteria are believed to reside primarily within granulomas or within macrophages that have avoided detection and lysis, although some residual bacilli have been found in various types of cells.[2,7,20]

Approximately 90% of infected patients have no further clinical manifestations. Most patients only show a positive skin test (70%), whereas some also have radiographic evidence of stable granulomas (approximately 20%). This radiodense area on chest radiograph is called a *Ghon complex*. Approximately 5% of patients (usually children, the elderly, and the immunocompromised) experience "progressive primary" disease that occurs before skin test conversion.[24,25] This presents as a progressive pneumonia, usually in the lower lobes. Disease frequently spreads, leading to meningitis and other severe forms of TB.[24,25] Because of this risk of severe disease, very young, elderly, and immunocompromised patients, including those with HIV, should be evaluated and treated for latent or active TB.

REACTIVATION DISEASE

❻ Roughly 10% of infected patients develop reactivation disease at some point in their lives. Nearly half of these cases occur within 2 years of infection.[2,7,13] In the United States, most cases of TB are believed to result from reactivation. Reinfection is uncommon in the United States because of the low rate of exposure and because previously sensitized individuals possess some degree of immunity to reinfection.[2,21] Exceptions include patients coinfected with HIV who live in areas of higher exposure to *M. tuberculosis*.

The apices of the lungs are the most common sites for reactivation (85% of cases).[2] This reflects the fact that *M. tuberculosis* prefers areas with high oxygen content and possibly because the immune response may not be as effective in this region.[2,21] For reasons that are not entirely known (waning cellular immunity, loss of specific T-cell clones, blocking antibody), organisms within granulomas emerge and begin multiplying extracellularly.[24] The inflammatory response produces caseating granulomas, which eventually will liquefy and spread locally, leading to the formation of a hole (cavity) in the lungs.

The immune response contributes to the severity of the lung damage. There is targeted killing of immature macrophages that are allowing mycobacterial multiplication (delayed-type hypersensitivity).[20,21] In addition, there is "innocent bystander" killing of host cells and locally thrombosed blood vessels.[21] The killing of mycobacteria, macrophages, and neutrophils that have entered the battle releases cytokines and lysozymes into the infectious foci. This toxic mixture can be too much for the surrounding alveoli and airway cells, causing regional necrosis and structural collapse.[2,21] These unstable foci liquefy, spreading the infection to neighboring areas of the lung, creating a cavity. Some of this necrotic material is coughed out, producing droplet nuclei. Bacterial counts in the cavities can be as high as 10^8 per milliliter of cavitary fluid. Partial healing may result from fibrosis, but these lesions remain unstable and may continue to expand.[2,21] If left untreated, pulmonary TB continues to destroy the lungs, resulting in hypoxia, respiratory acidosis, and eventually death.

EXTRAPULMONARY AND MILIARY TUBERCULOSIS

Caseating granulomas at extrapulmonary sites can undergo liquefaction, releasing tubercle bacilli and causing symptomatic disease.[2,7] Extrapulmonary TB without concurrent pulmonary disease is uncommon in normal hosts but more common in HIV-infected patients. Because of these unusual presentations, the diagnosis of TB is difficult and often delayed in immunocompromised hosts.[2,4,7] Lymphatic and pleural diseases are the most common forms of extrapulmonary TB, followed by bone, joint, genitourinary, meningeal, and other forms.[2,7] Left untreated, these forms will spread to other organs and may result in death.

Occasionally, a massive inoculum of organisms enters the bloodstream, causing a widely disseminated form of the disease known as *miliary TB*. It is named for the millet seed appearance of the small granulomas seen on chest radiographs, and it can be rapidly fatal.[20] Miliary TB is a medical emergency requiring immediate treatment.

INFLUENCE OF HIV INFECTION ON PATHOGENESIS

❸ HIV infection is the largest risk factor for active TB.[2,7,20] As CD4+ lymphocytes multiply in response to the mycobacterial infection, HIV multiplies within these cells and selectively destroys them. In turn, the TB-fighting lymphocytes are depleted.[20] This vicious cycle puts HIV-infected patients at 100 times the risk of active TB compared with HIV-negative people.[25] In addition, the combination of HIV infection and certain social behaviors increases the risk of newly acquired TB. In selected areas of the United States, up to 50% of new TB cases are the result of recent infection, particularly among HIV-infected individuals.[26–28]

As mycobacteria spread throughout the body, HIV replication accelerates in lymphocytes and macrophages. This leads to progression of HIV disease.[20,29] HIV-infected patients who are infected with TB deteriorate more rapidly unless they receive antimycobacterial chemotherapy.[30,31] Most clinicians elect to begin TB treatment first, and once this is under control, begin HIV treatment as well. Starting both treatments at the same time can lead to paradoxical worsening of the TB.[13,32] This appears to result from a reinvigorated inflammatory response to TB. Because TB can be very dangerous in HIV-positive patients, they should be screened for tuberculous infection or disease soon after they are shown to be HIV-positive.[2,4,7,20]

CLINICAL PRESENTATION

The classical presentation of TB is shown below. The onset of TB may be gradual, and the diagnosis may not be considered until a chest radiograph is performed. Unfortunately, many patients do not seek medical attention until more dramatic symptoms, such as frank hemoptysis, occur. At this point, patients typically have large cavitary lesions in the lungs. These cavities are loaded with *M. tuberculosis*. Expectoration or swallowing of infected sputum may spread the disease to other areas of the body.[1,2,7,23] Physical examination is nonspecific but suggestive of progressive pulmonary disease.

CLINICAL PRESENTATION OF TUBERCULOSIS

Signs and Symptoms

- Patients typically present with weight loss, fatigue, a productive cough, fever, and night sweats[1,2,7,23]
- Frank hemoptysis

Physical Examination

- Dullness to chest percussion, rales, and increased vocal fremitus are observed frequently on auscultation

Laboratory Tests

- Moderate elevations in the white blood cell (WBC) count with a lymphocyte predominance

Chest Radiograph

- Patchy or nodular infiltrates in the apical areas of the upper lobes or the superior segment of the lower lobes[2,7,23]
- Cavitation that may show air-fluid levels as the infection progresses

❺ Patients coinfected with HIV may have atypical presentations.[1,2,7,23,33] As their CD4+ counts decline, HIV-positive patients are less likely to have positive skin tests, cavitary lesions, or fever. Pulmonary radiographic findings may be minimal or absent. HIV-positive patients have a higher incidence of extrapulmonary TB and are more likely to present with progressive primary disease. Because their symptoms are not specific to TB, a thorough workup for TB is essential.[2,7,20,23]

Extrapulmonary TB typically presents as a slowly progressive decline in organ function.[2,7,23] Patients may have low-grade fever and other constitutional symptoms. Patients with genitourinary TB may present with sterile pyuria and hematuria. Lymphadenitis often involves the cervical and supraclavicular nodes and may appear as a neck mass with spontaneous drainage. Tuberculous arthritis and osteomyelitis occur most commonly in the elderly and usually affect the lower spine and weight-bearing joints. TB of the spine is known as *Pott's disease*.[2] Abnormal behavior, headaches, or convulsions suggest tuberculous meningitis. Involvement of the peritoneum, pericardium, larynx, and adrenal glands also occurs.[2,7,23]

THE ELDERLY

❺ TB in the elderly is easily confused with other respiratory diseases. Many clinical findings are muted or absent altogether. Compared with younger patients, TB in the elderly is far less likely to present with positive skin tests, fevers, night sweats, sputum production, or hemoptysis.[2,23,34,35] Weight loss may occur but is nonspecific. In contrast, mental status changes are twice as common in the elderly, and mortality is six times higher.[2,23,34] TB is a preventable cause of death in the elderly that should not be overlooked.

CHILDREN

❺ TB in children, especially those younger than 12 years of age, may present as a typical bacterial pneumonia and is called *progressive primary TB*.[23–25] Clinical disease often begins 1 to 2 months after exposure and precedes skin-test positivity. Unlike adults, pulmonary TB in children often involves the lower and middle lobes.[23–25] Dissemination to the lymph nodes, gastrointestinal and genitourinary tracts, bone marrow, and meninges is fairly common. Because of delays in recruitment of cellular immunity, cavitary disease is infrequent, and the number of organisms present typically is smaller than in an adult. Because cavitary lesions are uncommon, children do not spread TB readily. However, TB can be rapidly fatal in a child, and it requires prompt chemotherapy.

DIAGNOSIS

SKIN TESTING

The key to stopping the spread of TB is early identification of infected individuals.[1,2,7,23] Table 116–1 lists the populations most likely to benefit from skin testing (column 1 patients are at highest risk for TB, followed by those in column 2). Members of these high-risk groups should be tested for TB infection and educated about the disease.

The Mantoux test is the preferred TB skin test. It uses tuberculin purified protein derivative (PPD), and unlike the Heaf or tine test, the Mantoux test is quantitative. The standard 5-tuberculin-unit PPD dose is placed intracutaneously on the volar aspect of the forearm with a 26- or 27-gauge needle.[2,23,30] This injection should produce a small, raised, blanched wheal. An experienced professional should read the test in 48 to 72 hours. The area of induration (the "bump") is the important end point, not the area of redness. Table 116–1 lists the criteria for interpretation.[1,2,7,23,30] The CDC does not recommend the routine use of anergy panels.[30,36] Aplisol and Tubersol 5-tuberculin-unit products are available commercially, but because of more predictable results, Tubersol appears to be the preferred product.

The "booster effect" occurs in patients who do not respond to an initial skin test but show a positive reaction if retested about a week later.[23,36] Patients with past *M. tuberculosis* infection and some patients with past immunization with bacillus Calmetté-Guerin (BCG) vaccine or past infection with other mycobacteria may "boost" with a second skin test. Individuals who require periodic skin testing, such as healthcare workers, should receive a two-stage test initially.[23,36,37] Once they are shown to be skin-test–negative, any positive skin test later shows recent infection, and this requires treatment.

The PPD skin test is an imperfect diagnostic tool. Up to 20% of patients with active TB are falsely skin-test–negative, presumably because their immune systems are overwhelmed.[20,36] False-positive results are more common in low-risk patients and those recently vaccinated with BCG. Despite BCG vaccination, one should not ignore a positive PPD result. These patients require careful evaluation for active disease, and they may be offered preventive treatment because many come from areas where TB infection is common.

The QuantiFERON-TB Gold test measures the release of INF-γin whole blood.[38] For latently infected persons, INF-γ is released in response to in vitro stimulation by PPD, whereas no release occurs in blood samples taken from uninfected persons. This test can provide a diagnosis of latent TB infection within hours, instead of the 2 to 3 days required for the traditional PPD skin test. Also, QuantiFERON-TB testing does not require a return visit by the patient to the clinic for reading of the PPD skin test, making it more convenient for the patient. Ongoing research seeks to find a diagnostic test that will confirm TB infection within minutes, allowing for immediate treatment decisions while the patient is still in the

TABLE 116-1 Criteria for Tuberculin Positivity by Risk Group

Reaction 5 mm of Induration	Reaction ≥10 mm of Induration	Reaction ≥15 mm of Induration
Human immunodeficiency virus (HIV)-positive persons Recent contacts of tuberculosis (TB) case patients Fibrotic changes on chest radiograph consistent with prior TB	Recent immigrants (i.e., within the last 5 y) from high-prevalence countries Injection-drug users Residents and employees[a] of the following high-risk congregate settings: prisons and jails; nursing homes and other long-term care facilities for the elderly; hospitals and other healthcare facilities; residential facilities for patients with acquired immunodeficiency syndrome (AIDS); homeless shelters	Persons with no risk factors for TB
Patients with organ transplants and other immunosuppressed patients (receiving the equivalent of ≥15 mg/day of prednisone for 1 mo or more)[b]	Mycobacteriology laboratory personnel Persons with the following clinical conditions that place them at high risk: silicosis; diabetes mellitus; chronic renal failure; some hematologic disorders (e.g., leukemias and lymphomas); other specific malignancies (e.g., carcinoma of the head or neck and lung); weight loss of ≥10% of ideal body weight; gastrectomy; jejunoileal bypass Children younger than 4 y of age or infants, children, and adolescents exposed to adults at high risk	

[a]For persons who are otherwise at low risk and who are tested at the start of employment, a reaction of ≥15 mm induration is considered positive.
[b]Risk of TB in patients treated with corticosteroids increases with higher dose and longer duration.
Adapted from Centers for Disease Control and Prevention. Screening for tuberculosis and tuberculosis infection in high-risk populations: recommendations of the Advisory Council for the Elimination of Tuberculosis. MMWR 1995;44(RR-11):19–34.

clinic. Another related test, T-SPOT.TB, is available in Europe, and is undergoing review by the FDA here in the United States.[39]

ADDITIONAL TESTS

When active TB is suspected, attempts should be made to isolate *M. tuberculosis* from the site of infection.[2,7,23,36] Sputum collected in the morning usually has the highest yield.[2,11,23] Daily sputum collection over 3 consecutive days is recommended.

For patients unable to expectorate, sputum induction with aerosolized hypertonic saline may produce a diagnostic sample. Bronchoscopy, or aspiration of gastric fluid via a nasogastric tube, may be attempted in selected patients.[23] For patients with suspected extrapulmonary TB, samples of draining fluid, biopsies of the infected site, or both may be attempted. Blood cultures are positive occasionally, especially in AIDS patients.[23,33,40]

TREATMENT

Tuberculosis

DESIRED OUTCOMES

The desired outcomes for the treatment of tuberculosis are

1. Rapid identification of a new TB case
2. Initiation of specific antituberculosis treatment
3. Prompt resolution of the signs and symptoms of disease
4. Achievement of a noninfectious state in the patient, thus ending isolation
5. Adherence to the treatment regimen by the patient
6. Cure of the patient as quickly as possible (generally at least 6 months of treatment)

It is also important that patients with active disease are isolated to prevent spread of the disease and that appropriate samples for smears and cultures are collected. Secondary goals are identification of the index case that infected the patient, identification of all persons infected by both the index case and the new case of TB ("contact investigation"), and completion of appropriate treatments for those individuals.

GENERAL APPROACHES TO TREATMENT

Drug treatment is the cornerstone of TB management.[2,7,13,41] Monotherapy can be used only for infected patients who do not have active TB (latent infection, as shown by a positive skin test). Once active disease is present, a minimum of two drugs, and generally three or four drugs, must be used simultaneously.[2,7,13,41] The duration of treatment depends on the condition of the host, extent of disease, presence of drug resistance, and tolerance of medications. The shortest duration of treatment generally is 6 months, and 2 to 3 years of treatment may be necessary for cases of multidrug-resistant TB (MDR-TB).[2,7,13,41] Because the duration of treatment is so long, and because many patients feel better after a few weeks of treatment, careful followup is required. Directly observed therapy by a healthcare worker is a cost-effective way to ensure completion of treatment.[2,7,13,41–43]

PRINCIPLES FOR TREATING LATENT INFECTION AND FOR TREATING DISEASE

Asymptomatic patients with tuberculous infection have a bacillary load of about 10^3 organisms, compared with 10^{11} organisms in a patient with cavitary pulmonary TB.[2,7,44] As the number of organisms increases, the likelihood of naturally occurring drug-resistant mutants also increases. Naturally occurring mutants are found at rates of 1 in 10^6 to 1 in 10^8 organisms for the antituberculosis drugs.[2,41,44] When treating asymptomatic latent infection with isoniazid monotherapy, the risk of selecting out isoniazid-resistant organisms is low. The isoniazid mutation rate is about 1 in 10^6, but only about 10^3 organisms are present in the body. In contrast, the risk of selecting out isoniazid-resistant organisms is unacceptably high in patients with cavitary TB. One can prevent selection of these resistant mutants by adding more drugs because the rates for resistance mutations to multiple drugs are additive functions of the individual rates. For example, only 1 in 10^{13} organisms would be naturally resistant to both isoniazid (1 in 10^6) and rifampin (1 in 10^7).[2,41,44] It is unlikely that such rare organisms are present in a previously untreated patient.

Combination chemotherapy is required for treating active TB disease. The patient should receive at least two drugs to which the isolate is susceptible, and generally four drugs are given at the outset of treatment. Rifampin and isoniazid are the best drugs for preventing drug resistance, followed by ethambutol, streptomycin, and pyrazinamide.[2,7,41,44,45]

Three subpopulations of mycobacteria are proposed to exist within the body, and each appears to respond to certain drugs.[2,41,44] Most numerous are the extracellular, rapidly dividing bacteria, often found within cavities (about 10^7 to 10^9 organisms). These are killed most readily by isoniazid, followed by rifampin, streptomycin, and the other drugs. A second group resides within caseating granulomas (possibly 10^5 to 10^7 organisms). These organisms appear to be in a semidormant state, with occasional bursts of metabolic activity. Pyrazinamide, through its conversion within *M. tuberculosis* to pyrazinoic acid, appears most active against these organisms. Rifampin and isoniazid also may be active against this subpopulation. The third subset is the intracellular mycobacteria present within macrophages (10^4 to 10^6). Rifampin, isoniazid, and the quinolones appear to be most active against intracellular *M. tuberculosis*. While this appears to explain what happens during the treatment of TB, there is no practical way to quantitate these populations within a given patient.

NONPHARMACOLOGIC THERAPY

7 Nonpharmacologic interventions aim to (a) prevent the spread of TB, (b) find where TB has already spread using contact investigation, and (c) replenish the weakened (consumptive) patient to a state of normal weight and well-being. The first two items are performed by public health departments. Clinicians involved in the treatment of TB should verify that the local health department has been notified of all new cases of TB.

Workers in hospitals and other institutions must prevent the spread of TB within their facilities.[2,4,13,30] All such workers should learn and follow each institution's infection control guidelines. This includes using personal protective equipment, including properly fitted respirators, and closing doors to "negative pressure" rooms. These hospital isolation rooms draw air in from surrounding areas rather than blowing air (and *M. tuberculosis*) into these surrounding areas. The air from the isolation room may be treated with ultraviolet lights and then vented safely outside. However, these isolation rooms work properly only if the door is closed.

Debilitated TB patients may require therapy for other medical problems, including substance abuse and HIV infection, and some may need nutritional support. Therefore, clinicians involved in substance abuse rehabilitation and nutritional support services should be familiar with the needs of TB patients.

Surgery may be needed to remove destroyed lung tissue, space-occupying infected lesions (*tuberculomas*), and certain extrapulmonary lesions.[2,13,41] Vaccines against TB include BCG and *M. vaccae*.[41] However, these vaccines are of limited value, and neither can prevent infection by *M. tuberculosis*. BCG (discussed below) may prevent extreme forms of TB in infants, whereas *Mycobacterium vaccae* cannot be recommended.[41,46]

PHARMACOLOGIC THERAPY

Treating Latent Infection

Isoniazid is the preferred drug for treating latent TB infection.[2,7,13,41] Generally, isoniazid alone is given for 9 months. The treatment of latent TB infection (LTBI) reduces a person's lifetime risk of active TB from approximately 10% to approximately 1%. Because TB is spread easily through the air, each case prevented also prevents a second wave of cases that each prevented case would have produced. Historically, the treatment of LTBI has been called *prophylaxis, chemoprophylaxis*, or *preventive treatment*. By any name, it is one of the primary mechanisms for reducing TB in the United States. Table 116–2 lists the LTBI treatment options.

Because young children, the elderly, and HIV-positive patients are at greater risk of active disease once infected with *M. tuberculosis*, they require careful evaluation. Once active TB is ruled out, they should receive treatment for latent infection.[2,22,23,41]

The keys to successful treatment of LTBI are (a) infection by an isoniazid-susceptible isolate, (b) adherence to the 9-month regimen, and (c) no exogenous reinfection.[2] Isoniazid adult doses are usually 300 mg daily (5 to 10 mg/kg of body weight)[55] (see Table 116–2). Lower doses are less effective.[2,52] Isoniazid should be given on an empty stomach, and antacids should be avoided within 2 hours of dosing. When adherence is an issue, twice-weekly isoniazid (900 mg in an adult) can be given using directly observed treatment. Nine months of treatment is recommended, but 6 months still provides considerable benefit.

Rifampin 600 mg daily for 4 months can be used when isoniazid resistance is suspected or when the patient cannot tolerate isoniazid.[2,25,51,52] Rifabutin 300 mg daily might be substituted for rifampin for patients at high risk of drug interactions. The combination of pyrazinamide plus rifampin is no longer recommended because of higher than expected rates of hepatotoxicity. When resistance to isoniazid and rifampin is suspected in the isolate causing infection, there is no regimen proved to be effective.[2,41] Regimens that *might* be effective include ethambutol plus levofloxacin, but data regarding efficacy are lacking.

For recent skin-test converters of all ages, the risk of active TB outweighs the risk for drug toxicity.[30,41] Pregnant women, alcoholics, and patients with poor diets who are treated with isoniazid should receive pyridoxine (vitamin B_6) 10 to 50 mg daily to reduce the incidence of central nervous system (CNS) effects or peripheral neu-

TABLE 116-2 Recommended Drug Regimens for Treatment of Latent Tuberculosis (TB) Infection in Adults

Drug	Interval and Duration	Comments	Rating[a] (Evidence)[b] HIV–	HIV+
Isoniazid	Daily for 9 mo[c,d]	In human immunodeficiency virus (HIV)-infected patients, isoniazid may be administered concurrently with nucleoside reverse transcriptase inhibitors (NRTIs), protease inhibitors, or nonnucleoside reverse transcriptase inhibitors (NNRTIs)	A (II)	A (II)
	Twice weekly for 9 mo[c,d]	Directly observed therapy (DOT) must be used with twice-weekly dosing	B (II)	B (II)
Isoniazid	Daily for 6 mo[d]	Not indicated for HIV-infected persons, those with fibrotic lesions on chest radiographs, or children	B (I)	C (I)
	Twice weekly for 6 mo[d]	DOT must be used with twice-weekly dosing	B (II)	C (I)
Rifampin	Daily for 4 mo	For persons who are contacts of patients with isoniazid-resistant, rifampin-susceptible TB who cannot tolerate pyrazinamide	B (II)	B (III)

[a]Strength of recommendation: A, preferred; B, acceptable alternative; C, offer when A and B cannot be given.

[b]Quality of evidence: I, randomized clinical trial data; II, data from clinical trials that are not randomized or were conducted in other populations; III, expert opinion.

[c]Recommended regimen for children younger than 18 years of age.

[d]Recommended regimen for pregnant women. Some experts would use rifampin and pyrazinamide for 2 months as an alternative regimen in HIV-infected pregnant women, although pyrazinamide should be avoided during the first trimester.

Adapted from Centers for Disease Control and Prevention. Targeted tuberculin testing and treatment of latent tuberculosis infection. MMWR 2000;49(RR-6):31.

ropathies. All patients who receive treatment of LTBI should be monitored monthly for adverse drug reactions and for possible progression to active TB.

Treating Active Disease

(8) The treatment of active TB requires the use of multiple drugs. There are two primary antituberculosis drugs, isoniazid and rifampin, with the rest of the drugs having specific roles.[41,44,45] Isoniazid and rifampin should be used together whenever possible. Typically, *M. tuberculosis* is either very susceptible or very resistant to a given drug. This contrasts with *M. avium*, where moderately resistant organisms are a frequent occurrence. Theoretically, MIC results could be used to guide dosing in the treatment of moderately resistant *M. tuberculosis*, but this remains to be studied prospectively.[2,13,41]

Drug-susceptibility testing should be done on the initial isolate for all patients with active TB. These data should guide the selection of drugs over the course of treatment.[2,7,13,41] However, some patients are unable to provide a suitable specimen for laboratory testing. If susceptibility data are not available for a given patient, the drug-susceptibility data for the suspected source case or regional susceptibility data should be used.[2,41]

Drug resistance should be expected in patients presenting for the retreatment of TB. These patients require retesting of drug susceptibility using freshly collected specimens. It is imperative to learn what drugs the patient received and for how long the patient received them.[2,13,41] A treatment history, often called a "drug-o-gram," shows the start and stop dates of all antimycobacterial drugs on a horizontal bar graph.[2,41] A "drug-o-gram" should be constructed for all retreatment patients.

(10) The standard TB treatment regimen is isoniazid, rifampin, pyrazinamide, and ethambutol for 2 months, followed by isoniazid and rifampin for 4 months, for a total of 6 months of treatment.[2,13,41] If susceptibility to isoniazid, rifampin, and pyrazinamide is shown, ethambutol can be stopped at any time. Without pyrazinamide, a total of 9 months of isoniazid and rifampin treatment is required. Table 116–3 shows the recommended treatment regimens. When intermittent therapy is used, directly observed treatment is essential. Doses missed during an intermittent TB regimen decrease its efficacy and increase the relapse rate. Note that Table 116–3 shows recommendations that differ for HIV-negative and HIV-positive patients. HIV-positive patients should not receive highly intermittent regimens. In general, regimens given daily five times each week or three times weekly can be used for HIV-positive patients. Less-frequent dosing is associated with higher failure and relapse rates and the selection of rifampin-resistant organisms.[41]

CLINICAL CONTROVERSY

The recommended duration of treatment often is the same for HIV-negative and HIV-positive patients. However, some clinicians believe that therapy should be extended for patients with weakened immune systems. These clinicians treat HIV-positive patients with drug-susceptible TB for 9 months rather than the usual 6 months.

TABLE 116-3 Drug Regimens for Culture-Positive Pulmonary Tuberculosis Caused by Drug-Susceptible Organisms

Initial Phase			Continuation Phase				Rating[a] (Evidence)[b]	
Regimen	***Drugs***	***Interval and Doses[c] (Minimal Duration)***	***Regimen***	***Drugs***	***Interval and Doses[c,d] (Minimal Duration)***	***Range of Total Doses (Minimal Duration)***	***HIV–***	***HIV+***
1	Isoniazid, rifampin, pyrazinamide, ethambutol	Seven days per week for 56 doses (8 wk) or 5 days/wk for 40 doses (8 wk)[c]	1a	Isoniazid/ rifampin	Seven days per week for 126 doses (18 wk) or 5 days/wk for 90 doses (18 wk)[c]	182–130 (26 wk)	A (I)	A (II)
			1b	Isoniazid/ rifampin	Twice weekly for 36 doses (18 wk)	92–76 (26 wk)	A (I)	A (II)[f]
			1c[g]	Isoniazid/ rifapentine	Once weekly for 18 doses (18 wk)	74–58 (26 wk)	B (I)	E (I)
2	Isoniazid, rifampin, pyrazinamide, ethambutol	Seven days per week for 14 doses (2 wk), then twice weekly for 12 doses (6 wk) or 5 days/wk for 10 doses (2 wk)[e] then twice weekly for 12 doses (6 wk)	2a	Isoniazid/ rifampin	Twice weekly for 36 doses (18 wk)	62–58 (26 wk)	A (II)	B (II)[f]
			2b[g]	Isoniazid/ rifapentine	Once weekly for 18 doses (18 wk)	44–40 (26 wk)	B (I)	E (I)
3	Isoniazid, rifampin, pyrazinamide, ethambutol	Three times weekly for 24 doses (8 wk)	3a	Isoniazid/ rifampin	Three times weekly for 54 doses (18 wk)	78 (26 wk)	B (I)	B (II)
4	Isoniazid, rifampin, ethambutol	Seven days per week for 56 doses (8 wk) or 5 days/wk for 40 doses (8 wk)[c]	4a	Isoniazid/ rifampin	Seven days per week for 217 doses (31 wk) or 5 days/wk for 155 doses (31 wk)[e]	273–195 (39 wk)	C (I)	C (II)
			4b	Isoniazid/ rifampin	Twice weekly for 62 doses (31 wk)	118–102 (39 wk)	C (I)	C (II)

[a]Ratings: A, preferred; B, acceptable alternative; C, offer when A and B cannot be given; E, should never be given.
[b]Evidence ratings: I, randomized clinical trial; II, data from clinical trials that were not randomized or were conducted in other populations; III, expert opinion.
[c]When directly observed therapy is used, drugs may be given 5 days per week and the necessary number of doses adjusted accordingly. Although there are no studies that compare five with seven daily doses, extensive experience indicates this would be an effective practice.
[d]Patients with cavitation on initial chest radiograph and positive cultures at completion of 2 months of therapy should receive a 7-month (31-week; either 217 doses [daily] or 62 doses [twice weekly]) continuation phase.
[e]Five-day-a-week administration is always given by directly observed therapy. Rating for 5 day per week regimens is A (III).
[f]Not recommended for HIV-infected patients with CD4+ cell counts <100 cells/μL.
[g]Options 1c and 2b should be used only in HIV-negative patients who have negative sputum smears at the time of completion of 2 months of therapy and who do not have cavitation on initial chest radiograph (see text). For patients started on this regimen and found to have a positive culture from the 2-month specimen, treatment should be extended an extra 3 months.
From Centers for Disease Control and Prevention. Treatment of tuberculosis. MMWR 2003;52 (RR-11).

When a patient's sputum smears convert to a negative, the risk of the patient infecting others is greatly reduced, but it is not zero.[2,21,41] Such patients can be removed from respiratory isolation, but they must be careful not to cough on others and should meet with others only in well-ventilated places. Smear-negative patients still may be culture-positive, so they still can transmit TB to others.

Patients who are slow to respond clinically, those who remain culture-positive at 2 months of treatment, those with cavitary lesions on chest radiograph, and perhaps HIV-positive patients should be treated for a total of 9 months and for at least 6 months from the time that they convert to smear and culture negativity.[2,7,13,41] Some authors recommend therapeutic drug monitoring for such patients.[2,41,45,47] When isoniazid and rifampin cannot be used, treatment durations become 2 years or more regardless of immune status.[2,13,41,45]

Adjustments to the regimen should be made once the susceptibility data are available.[2,13,41] If the organism is drug-resistant, careful consideration of the remaining therapeutic options must be made. Two or more drugs with in vitro activity against the patient's isolate and that the patient has not received previously should be added to the regimen, as needed.[2,13,41] TB specialists should be consulted regarding cases of drug-resistant TB.[2,13,41]

❾ There is no standard regimen for MDR-TB.[2,13,41] Each patient's exposure history, previous treatment history (including toxicity and adherence issues), and current susceptibility data must be considered simultaneously. *It is critical to avoid monotherapy, and it is critical to avoid adding a single drug to a failing regimen.*[2,13,41] Adding one drug at a time leads to the sequential selection of drug resistance until there are no drugs left. The treatment of MDR-TB should be managed by TB specialists. It may take several months for a patient with MDR-TB to become culture-negative because the drugs used lack the potency of isoniazid and rifampin.[2,44,45] Consequently, prolonged respiratory isolation may be required.

Drug resistance should be suspected in the following situations:

- Patients who have received prior therapy for TB
- Patients from areas with a high prevalence of resistance (New York City, Mexico, Southeast Asia, the Baltic countries, and the former Soviet states)
- Patients who are homeless, institutionalized, intravenous drug abusers, or infected with HIV
- Patients who still have acid-fast bacilli-positive sputum smears after 1 to 2 months of therapy
- Patients who still have positive cultures after 2 to 4 months of therapy
- Patients who fail treatment or relapse after treatment
- Patients known to be exposed to MDR-TB cases

The patients just listed should be considered infected with drug-resistant TB until proved otherwise. Empirical therapy with four or more drugs may be needed for acutely ill patients.[2,13,41] These regimens may be altered when the susceptibility pattern becomes known. If the index case is known, then the same effective regimen should be employed for the new case. Again, MDR-TB cases should be referred to specialists. A new term in use, "XDR-TB," refers to "extensively drug-resistant TB." Such organisms are resistant to at least isoniazid, rifampin, a fluoroquinolone and one second-line injectable drug (amikacin, capreomycin, or kanamycin).[48]

Special Populations

Tuberculous Meningitis and Extrapulmonary Disease

Patients with CNS tuberculosis usually are treated for longer periods (9 to 12 months instead of 6 months) (Table 116–4).[2,13,41] In general, isoniazid, pyrazinamide, ethionamide, and cycloserine penetrate the cerebrospinal fluid readily, but rifampin, ethambutol, and streptomycin have variable CNS penetration.[49] Of the quinolones, levofloxacin may be preferred based on current data. Extrapulmonary TB of the soft tissues can be treated with conventional regimens.[2,13,41] TB of the bone typically is treated for 9 months, occasionally with surgical debridement.[2,13,41]

Children TB in children may be treated with regimens similar to those used in adults, although some physicians still prefer to extend treatment to 9 months.[2,13,23,24,41,50,51] Pediatric doses of isoniazid and rifampin on a milligram-per-kilogram basis are higher than those used in adults (Table 116–5).[41]

Pregnancy Women with TB should be cautioned against becoming pregnant because the disease poses a risk to the fetus and to the mother. If already pregnant, the usual treatment is isoniazid, rifampin, and ethambutol for 9 months.[41] Isoniazid or ethambutol are relatively safe for use in pregnant women.[2,41,49–51] B vitamins are particularly important during pregnancy and should be provided to women being treated for TB. Rifampin is associated rarely with birth defects, including limb reduction and CNS lesions.[49] In general, rifampin is used in pregnant women with TB. Pyrazinamide has not been studied in large numbers of pregnant women, but anecdotal data suggest that it may be safe.[41]

Streptomycin use during pregnancy may lead to hearing loss in the newborn, including complete deafness. Streptomycin and the other aminoglycosides must be reserved for critical situations where alternatives do not exist.[2,41] Although the polypeptide capreomycin has not been studied, it probably carries the same risks.

Ethionamide may cause premature delivery and congenital deformities when used during pregnancy.[41,49] Mongolism also has been reported with ethionamide, so it cannot be recommended in this setting. *p*-Aminosalicylic acid has been used safely in pregnancy, but specific data are lacking.[41,49] Cycloserine is known to cross the placenta, but the effects on the developing fetus are not known. Therefore, cycloserine generally cannot be recommended during pregnancy.[49]

TABLE 116-4 Evidence-Based[a] Guidelines for the Treatment of Extrapulmonary Tuberculosis and Adjunctive Use of Corticosteriods[b]

Site	Length of Therapy (mo)	Rating (Duration)	Corticosteroids[c]	Rating (Corticosteroids)
Lymph node	6	A (I)	Not recommended	D (III)
Bone and joint	6–9	A (I)	Not recommended	D (III)
Pleural disease	6	A (II)	Not recommended	D (I)
Pericarditis	6	A (II)	Strongly recommended	A (I)
CNS tuberculosis including meningitis	9–12	B (II)	Strongly recommended	A (I)
Disseminated disease	6	A (II)	Not recommended	D (III)
Genitourinary	6	A (II)	Not recommended	D (III)
Peritoneal	6	A (II)	Not recommended	D (III)

[a]For rating system, see Table 116–3.
[b]Duration of therapy for extrapulmonary tuberculosis caused by drug-resistant organisms is not known.
[c]Corticosteroid preparations vary among studies.

TABLE 116-5 Doses[a] of Antituberculosis Drugs for Adults and Children[b]

Drug	Preparation	Adults/Children	Doses: *Daily*	*1×/wk*	*2×/wk*	*3×/wk*
First-line drugs						
Isoniazid	Tablets (50 mg, 100 mg, 300 mg); elixir (50 mg/5 mL); aqueous solution (100 mg/mL) for intravenous or intramuscular injection	Adults (max)	5 mg/kg (300 mg)	15 mg/kg (900 mg)	15 mg/kg (900 mg)	15 mg/kg (900 mg)
		Children (max)	10–15 mg/kg (300 mg)	–	20–30 mg/kg (900 mg)	–
Rifampin	Capsule (150 mg, 300 mg); powder may be suspended for oral administration; aqueous solution for intravenous injection	Adults[c] (max)	10 mg/kg (600 mg)	–	10 mg/kg (600 mg)	10 mg/kg (600 mg)
		Children (max)	10–20 mg/kg (600 mg)	–	10–20 mg/kg (600 mg)	–
Rifabutin	Capsule (150 mg)	Adults[c] (max)	5 mg/kg (300 mg)	–	5 mg/kg (300 mg)	5 mg/kg (300 mg)
		Children	Appropriate dosing for children is unknown	Appropriate dosing for children is unknown	Appropriate dosing for children is unknown	Appropriate dosing for children is unknown
Rifapentine	Tablet (150 mg, film coated)	Adults	–	10 mg/kg (continuation phase) (600 mg usual adult dose)	–	–
		Children	The drug is not approved for use in children	The drug is not approved for use in children	The drug is not approved for use in children	The drug is not approved for use in children
Pyrazinamide	Tablet (500 mg, scored)	Adults	1,000 mg (40–55 kg)	–	2,000 mg (40–55 kg)	1,500 mg (40–55 kg)
			1,500 mg (56–75 kg)	–	3,000 mg (56–75 kg)	2,500 mg (56–75 kg)
			2,000 mg (76–90 kg)[k]	–	4,000 mg (76–90 kg)[k]	3,000 mg (76–90 kg)[k]
		Children (max)	15–30 mg/kg (2 g)	–	50 mg/kg (2 g)	–
Ethambutol	Tablet (100 mg, 400 mg)	Adults	800 mg (40–55 kg)	–	2,000 mg (40–55 kg)	1,200 mg (40–55 kg)
			1,200 mg (56–75 kg)	–	2,800 mg (56–75 kg)	2,000 mg (56–75 kg)
			1,600 mg (76–90 kg)[k]	–	4,000 mg (76–90 kg)[k]	2,400 mg (76–90 kg)[k]
		Children[d] (max)	15–20 mg/kg daily (1 g)	–	50 mg/kg (2.5 g)	–
Second-line drugs						
Cycloserine	Capsule (250 mg)	Adults (max)	10–15 mg/kg/day (1 g in two doses), usually 500–750 mg/day in two doses[e]	There are no data to support intermittent administration	There are no data to support intermittent administration	There are no data to support intermittent administration
		Children (max)	10–15 mg/kg/day (1 g/day)	–	–	–
Ethionamide	Tablet (250 mg)	Adults[f] (max)	15–20 mg/kg/day (1 g/day), usually 500–750 mg/day in a single daily dose or two divided doses[f]	There are no data to support intermittent administration	There are no data to support intermittent administration	There are no data to support intermittent administration
		Children (max)	15–20 mg/kg/day (1 g/day)	There are no data to support intermittent administration	There are no data to support intermittent administration	There are no data to support intermittent administration
Streptomycin	Aqueous solution (1-g vials) for intravenous or intramuscular administration	Adults (max)	g	g	g	g
		Children (max)	20–40 mg/kg/day (1 g)	–	20 mg/kg	–
Amikacin-kanamycin	Aqueous solution (500-mg and 1-g vials) for intravenous or intramuscular administration	Adults (max)	g	g	g	g
		Children (max)	15–30 mg/kg/day (1 g) intravenous or intramuscular as a single daily dose	–	15–30 mg/kg	–
Capreomycin	Aqueous solution (1-g vials) for intravenous or intramuscular administration	Adults (max)	g	g	g	g
		Children (max)	15–30 mg/kg/day (1 g) as a single daily dose	–	15–30 mg/kg	–
p-Aminosalicylic acid (PAS)	Granules (4-g packets) can be mixed with food; tablets (500 mg) are still available in some countries, but not in the United States; a solution for intravenous administration is available in Europe	Adults	8–12 g/day in two or three doses	There are no data to support intermittent administration	There are no data to support intermittent administration	There are no data to support intermittent administration
		Children (max)	200–300 mg/kg/day in two to four divided doses (10 g)	There are no data to support intermittent administration	There are no data to support intermittent administration	There are no data to support intermittent administration
Levofloxacin	Tablets (250 mg, 500 mg, 750 mg); aqueous solution (500-mg vials) for intravenous injection	Adults	500–1,000 mg daily	There are no data to support intermittent administration	There are no data to support intermittent administration	There are no data to support intermittent administration
		Children	h	h	h	h

(continued)

TABLE 116-5 Doses[a] of Antituberculosis Drugs for Adults and Children[b] (continued)

Drug	Preparation	Adults/Children	Doses: Daily	1×/wk	2×/wk	3×/wk
Moxifloxacin	Tablets (400 mg); aqueous solution (400 mg/250 mL) for intravenous injection	Adults	400 mg daily	There are no data to support intermittent administration	There are no data to support intermittent administration	There are no data to support intermittent administration
		Children	i	i	i	i
Gatifloxacin	Tablets (400 mg); aqueous solution (200 mg/20 mL; 400 mg/40 mL) for intravenous injection	Adults	400 mg daily	There are no data to support intermittent administration	There are no data to support intermittent administration	There are no data to support intermittent administration
		Children	j	j	j	j

[a] Dose per weight is based on ideal body weight. Children weighing more than 40 kg should be dosed as adults.
[b] For purposes of this document adult dosing begins at age 15 years.
[c] Dose may need to be adjusted when there is concomitant use of protease inhibitors or nonnucleoside reverse transcriptase inhibitors.
[d] The drug can likely be used safely in older children but should be used with caution in children less than 5 years of age, in whom visual acuity cannot be monitored. In younger children, ethambutol at the dose of 15 mg/kg per day can be used if there is suspected or proven resistance to isoniazid or rifampin.
[e] It should be noted that, although this is the dose recommended generally, most clinicians with experience using cycloserine indicate that it is unusual for patients to be able to tolerate this amount. Serum concentration measurements are often useful in determining the optimal dose for a given patient.
[f] The single daily dose can be given at bedtime or with the main meal.
[g] Dose: 15 mg/kg per day (1 g), and 10 mg/kg in persons older than 59 years of age (750 mg). Usual dose: 750–1,000 mg administered intramuscularly or intravenously, given as a single dose 5–7 days/week and reduced to two or three times per week after the first 2–4 months or after culture conversion, depending on the efficacy of the other drugs in the regimen.
[h] The long-term (more than several weeks) use of levofloxacin in children and adolescents has not been approved because of concerns about effects on bone and cartilage growth. However, most experts agree that the drug should be considered for children with tuberculosis caused by organisms resistant to both isoniazid and rifampin. The optimal dose is not known.
[i] The long-term (more than several weeks) use of moxifloxacin in children and adolescents has not been approved because of concerns about effects on bone and cartilage growth. The optimal dose is not known.
[j] The long-term (more than several weeks) use of gatifloxacin in children and adolescents has not been approved because of concerns about effects on bone and cartilage growth. The optimal dose is not known.
[k] Maximum dose regardless of weight.

Ciprofloxacin, levofloxacin, moxifloxacin, and the other quinolones are associated with permanent damage to cartilage in the weight-bearing joints of immature animals, especially dogs and rabbits.[41,49] Although these drugs have not been shown to frequently cause joint problems in humans, other antituberculosis agents should be used during pregnancy.

Pregnant women with LTBI are not at the same level of risk compared with those with active disease. Therapy with isoniazid for LTBI may be delayed until after pregnancy or, if recent skin-test conversion has occurred, started during the second trimester of pregnancy.[41,49–51] Although most antituberculosis drugs are excreted in breast milk, the amount of drug received by the infant through nursing is insufficient to cause toxicity. Quinolones should be avoided in nursing mothers, if possible.

HIV Infection Patients with AIDS and other immunocompromised hosts may be managed with chemotherapeutic regimens similar to those used in immunocompetent individuals, although treatment is often extended to 9 months (see Table 116–3).[2,13,41] The precise duration to recommend remains a matter of debate. Highly intermittent regimens (twice or once weekly) are not recommended for HIV-positive TB patients. Prognosis has been particularly poor for HIV-infected patients infected with MDR-TB. Differentiation must be made between infection with *M. tuberculosis* and nontuberculous mycobacteria, such as MAC, because the drugs used are different. While awaiting laboratory results, the patient can be treated empirically for TB if there is any doubt about the causative organism. Some patients with AIDS malabsorb their oral medications; this is discussed under Therapeutic Drug Monitoring below.[2,41,45,47] The major issue of drug interactions is discussed further below under Rifampin.

Renal Failure In nearly all patients, isoniazid and rifampin do not require dose modification in renal failure. They are eliminated primarily by the liver.[45,49,52] In the unlikely event that peripheral neuropathies develop, the frequency of isoniazid dosing may be reduced. Pyrazinamide and ethambutol typically require a reduction in dosing frequency from daily to three times weekly (Table 116–6).[41,52]

TABLE 116-6 Dosing Recommendations for Adult Patients with Reduced Renal Function and for Adult Patients Receiving Hemodialysis

Drug	Change in Frequency?	Recommended Dose and Frequency for Patients with Creatinine Clearance <30 mL/min or for Patients Receiving Hemodialysis
Isoniazid	No change	300 mg once daily, or 900 mg three times per week
Rifampin	No change	600 mg once daily, or 600 mg three times per week
Pyrazinamide	Yes	25–35 mg/kg per dose three times per week (not daily)
Ethambutol	Yes	15–25 mg/kg per dose three times per week (not daily)
Levofloxacin	Yes	750–1,000 mg per dose three times per week (not daily)
Cycloserine	Yes	250 mg once daily, or 500 mg/dose three times per week[a]
Ethionamide	No change	250–500 mg/dose daily
p-Aminosalicylic acid	No change	4 g/dose, twice daily
Streptomycin	Yes	12–15 mg/kg per dose two or three times per week (not daily)
Capreomycin	Yes	12–15 mg/kg per dose two or three times per week (not daily)
Kanamycin	Yes	12–15 mg/kg per dose two or three times per week (not daily)
Amikacin	Yes	12–15 mg/kg per dose two or three times per week (not daily)

Standard doses are given unless there is intolerance.
The medications should be given after hemodialysis on the day of hemodialysis.
Monitoring of serum drug concentrations should be considered to ensure adequate drug absorption, without excessive accumulation, and to assist in avoiding toxicity.
Data currently are not available for patients receiving peritoneal dialysis. Until data become available, begin with doses recommended for patients receiving hemodialysis and verify adequacy of dosing, using serum concentration monitoring.
[a] The appropriateness of 250-mg daily doses has not been established. There should be careful monitoring for evidence of neurotoxicity.

Renally cleared TB drugs include the aminoglycosides (amikacin, kanamycin, and streptomycin), capreomycin, ethambutol, cycloserine, and levofloxacin.[41,49,52,53] Dosing intervals need to be extended for these drugs (see Table 116–6). Ciprofloxacin and moxifloxacin are approximately 50% cleared by the kidneys but may not require a change in dose from once daily, as used for TB. The metabolites of isoniazid, pyrazinamide, and *p*-aminosalicylic acid are cleared primarily by the kidneys. The role of these metabolites in causing toxicity is unknown, so their accumulation in renal failure may carry some risk.

Ethionamide and its sulfoxide metabolite are hepatically cleared, so dosing is unchanged.[41,53] *p*-Aminosalicylic acid is converted largely to metabolites prior to renal elimination; these metabolites may accumulate in renal failure.[53] For patients on hemodialysis, the usual 12-hour dosing interval for *p*-aminosalicylic acid granules seems to be safe. Dialysis will remove the metabolites. Serum concentration monitoring must be performed for cycloserine to avoid dose-related toxicities in renal failure patients.[45,47,53]

Hepatic Failure Antituberculosis drugs that rely on hepatic clearance for most of their elimination include isoniazid, rifampin, pyrazinamide, ethionamide, and *p*-aminosalicylic acid.[49] Ciprofloxacin and moxifloxacin are approximately 50% cleared by the liver. Elevations of serum transaminase concentrations generally are not correlated with the residual capacity of the liver to metabolize drugs, so these markers cannot be used as guides for drug dosing. Furthermore, isoniazid, rifampin, pyrazinamide, and, to a lesser degree, ethionamide, *p*-aminosalicylic acid, and, rarely, ethambutol may cause hepatotoxicity.[41,45,49] For some patients with drug-susceptible TB, a "liver-sparing" regimen of streptomycin, levofloxacin, and ethambutol may be used, at least temporarily.[41,45,49] Because this regimen requires 18 or more months of treatment to be successful, patients usually are switched to isoniazid- and rifampin-containing regimens as soon as they are able.

Morbid Obesity Data are not available for dosing the TB drugs in patients with morbid obesity.[49] Relatively hydrophilic drugs (isoniazid, pyrazinamide, the aminoglycosides, capreomycin, ethambutol, *p*-aminosalicylic acid, and cycloserine) can be dosed initially based on ideal body weight. Very low or very high serum concentrations can be avoided by checking the serum concentrations.

The TB Drugs

The interested reader is referred to several other publications for more detailed information regarding these drugs.[2,12,41,44,45,47,49,54–56] Note that although the American Thoracic Society (ATS)/CDC guidelines recommend "maximum" doses, I disagree with this approach to therapy (see Table 116–5).[41] In my view, the "maximum" dose for a given patient is the dose that produces the desired response with an acceptable level of toxicity.[45,47] This can only be determined on a case-by-case basis. Artificially capping doses may deprive patients of needed drug.

Primary Antituberculosis Drugs ***Isoniazid.*** Isoniazid is one of the two most important TB drugs. It is highly specific for mycobacteria, with a MIC against *M. tuberculosis* of 0.01 to 0.25 mcg/mL. Most nontuberculous mycobacteria such as *M. avium* are resistant to isoniazid, although *M. kansasii* and *Mycobacterium xenopi* are susceptible. The most common mechanisms of resistance result from mutations in the *katG* or *inhA* genes.

Isoniazid is readily absorbed from the gastrointestinal tract and from intramuscular injection sites. It also can be given as a short intravenous infusion over 5 minutes if diluted in about 20 mL of normal saline.[57] Isoniazid should be given on an empty stomach whenever possible.[58] *N*-acetyltransferase 2 forms the principal metabolite acetylisoniazid, which lacks antimycobacterial activity. The rate at which humans acetylate isoniazid is determined genetically; slow acetylation is an autosomal recessive trait and reflects a relative lack of *N*-acetyltransferase 2. Fast acetylators have isoniazid half-lives of less than 2 hours. Approximately 50% of whites and blacks and 80% to 90% of Asians and Eskimos are rapid acetylators. Slow acetylators have isoniazid half-lives of 3 to 4 hours and may be at an increased risk of neurotoxicity. The association of acetylator status and risk of hepatotoxicity, however, appears to be weak.[59] Poor absorption and rapid clearance of isoniazid in patients receiving highly intermittent therapy are associated with poor clinical outcomes.[60,61]

Transient elevations of the serum transaminases occur in 12% to 15% of patients receiving isoniazid and usually occur within the first 8 to 12 weeks of therapy.[41] Overt hepatotoxicity, however, occurs in only 1% of cases. Risk factors for hepatotoxicity include patient age, preexisting liver disease, excessive alcohol intake, pregnancy, and the postpartum state. Isoniazid also may result in neurotoxicity, most frequently presenting as peripheral neuropathy or, in overdose, as seizures and coma. Patients with pyridoxine deficiency, such as pregnant women, alcoholics, children, and the malnourished, are at increased risk. Isoniazid may inhibit the metabolism of phenytoin, carbamazepine, primidone, and warfarin.[45] Patients who are being treated with these agents should be monitored closely, and appropriate dose adjustments should be made when necessary.

Rifampin. The introduction of rifampin into routine use during the 1970s allowed for true short-course treatment of TB (6 to 9 months).[2,13,41] Without rifampin, treatment is generally 18 months or longer. Drug resistance to rifampin is an ominous prognostic factor because it is frequently associated with isoniazid resistance and leaves the patient with few good therapeutic options. Clinicians *must* take care to protect susceptibility to rifampin by carefully treating their patients. Rifampin shows bactericidal activity against *M. tuberculosis* and several other mycobacterial species, including *M. bovis* and *M. kansasii.*[62] Other nontuberculous mycobacteria, including MAC, show variable susceptibility to rifampin. Rifampin also is active against a broad array of other bacteria. Alteration of the target site on RNA polymerase, primarily through changes in the *rpoB* gene, leads to most forms of rifampin resistance.[41,62]

Rifampin usually is given orally, but it also can be given as a 30-minute intravenous infusion.[54,62] Oral doses are best given on an empty stomach.[63] Patients with AIDS, diabetes, and other gastrointestinal problems appear to have difficulty absorbing rifampin after oral doses, and this has been associated with therapeutic failures in some cases.[45,47,61] Rifampin is metabolized to 25-desacetylrifampin, which retains most of rifampin's activity; most of rifampin and its metabolite are cleared in the bile. Rifampin generally is given at 600 mg daily or intermittently, although this dose does not take full advantage of rifampin's concentration-dependent killing.[45,47] Higher doses should be tested in humans within the context of clinical trials.

CLINICAL CONTROVERSY

Rifampin shows concentration-dependent killing. Larger doses produce higher concentrations that more effectively kill bacteria and mycobacteria. High-dose rifampin fell out of favor because high doses given once or twice weekly caused flu-like symptoms. However, high doses (900 to 1,200 mg and possibly higher) can be given safely daily. Studies should be performed in humans with TB to take full advantage of rifampin's potent activity.

Elevations in hepatic enzymes have been attributed to rifampin in 10% to 15% of patients, with overt hepatotoxicity occurring in less than 1%.[41,62] More frequent adverse effects of rifampin include rash, fever, and gastrointestinal distress. Allergic reactions to rifampin have been reported and occur more frequently with intermittent rifampin doses 900 mg or more twice weekly. These reactions may

TABLE 116-7 Clinically Significant Drug–Drug Interactions Involving the Rifamycins

Drug Class	Drugs Whose Concentrations Are Substantially Decreased by Rifamycins (References)	Comments
Antiinfectives	HIV-1 protease inhibitors (saquinavir, indinavir, nelfinavir, amprenavir, ritonavir, lopinavir-ritonavir)	Can be used with rifabutin. Ritonavir, 400–600 mg twice daily, probably can be used with rifampin. The combination of saquinavir and ritonavir can also be used with rifampin.
	Nonnucleoside reverse transcriptase inhibitors (delavirdine, nevirapine, efavirenz)	Delavirdine should not be used with any rifamycin. Doses of nevirapine and efavirenz need to be increased if given with rifampin; no dose increase needed if given with rifabutin.
	Macrolide antibiotics (clarithromycin, erythromycin)	Azithromycin has no significant interaction with rifamycins.
	Doxycycline	May require use of a drug other than doxycycline.
	Azole antifungal agents (ketoconazole, itraconazole, voriconazole)	Itraconazole, ketoconazole, and voriconazole concentrations may be subtherapeutic with any of the rifamycins. Fluconazole can be used with rifamycins, but the dose of fluconazole may have to be increased.
	Atovaquone	Consider alternate form of *Pneumocystis carinii* treatment or prophylaxis.
	Chloramphenicol	Consider an alternative antibiotic.
	Mefloquine	Consider alternate form of malaria prophylaxis.
Hormone therapy	Ethinylestradilol, norethindrone	Women of reproductive potential on oral contraceptives should be advised to add a barrier method of contraception when taking a rifamycin.
	Tamoxifen	May require alternate therapy or use of a nonrifamycin-containing regimen.
	Levothyroxine	Monitoring of serum thyroid-stimulating hormone recommended; may require increased dose of levothyroxine.
Narcotics	Methadone	Rifampin and rifapentine use may require methadone dose increase; rifabutin infrequently causes methadone withdrawal.
Anticoagulants	Warfarin	Monitor prothrombin time; may require two- to threefold dose increase.
Immunosuppressive agents	Cyclosporine, tacrolimus	Rifabutin may allow concomitant use of cyclosporine and a rifamycin; monitoring of cyclosporine serum concentrations may assist with dosing.
	Corticosteroids	Monitor clinically; may require two- to threefold increase in corticosteroid dose.
Anticonvulsants	Phenytoin, lamotrigine	Therapeutic drug monitoring recommended; may require anticonvulsant dose increase.
Cardiovascular agents	Verapamil, nifedipine, diltiazem (a similar interaction is also predicted for felodipine and nisoldipine)	Clinical monitoring recommended; may require change to an alternate cardiovascular agent.
	Propranolol, metoprolol	Clinical monitoring recommended; may require dose increase or change to an alternate cardiovascular drug.
	Enalapril, losartan	Monitor clinically; may require a dose increase or use of an alternate cardiovascular drug.
	Digoxin (among patients with renal insufficiency), digitoxin	Therapeutic drug monitoring recommended; may require digoxin or digitoxin dose increase.
	Quinidine	Therapeutic drug monitoring recommended; may require quinidine dose increase.
	Mexiletine, tocainide, propafenone	Clinical monitoring recommended; may require change to an alternate cardiovascular drug.
Bronchodilators	Theophylline	Therapeutic drug monitoring recommended; may require theophylline dose increase.
Sulfonylurea hypoglycemics	Tolbutamide, chlorpropamide, glyburide, glimepiride, repaglinide	Monitor blood glucose; may require dose increase or change to an alternate hypoglycemic drug.
Hypolipidemics	Simvastatin, fluvastatin	Monitor hypolipidemic effect; may require use of an alternate hypolipidemic drug.
Psychotropic drugs	Nortriptyline	Therapeutic drug monitoring recommended; may require dose increase or change to alternate psychotropic drug.
	Haloperidol, quetiapine	Monitor clinically; may require a dose increase or use of an alternate psychotropic drug.
	Benzodiazepines (e.g., diazepam, triazolam), zolpidem, buspirone	Monitor clinically; may require a dose increase or use of an alternate psychotropic drug.

take the form of a flu-like syndrome with development of fever, chills, headache, arthralgias, and, rarely, hypotension and shock.[41,55] Alternatively, hemolytic anemia or acute renal failure may occur, requiring permanent discontinuation.

Rifampin's potent induction of hepatic enzymes, especially cytochrome P450 3A4, may enhance the elimination of many other drugs, most notably the protease inhibitors used to treat HIV (Table 116–7). HIV-positive patients may benefit from the use of rifabutin instead of rifampin (see below).[41,64–67] Also, women who use oral contraceptives must use another form of contraception during therapy because increased clearance of the hormones may lead to unexpected pregnancies. Patient records should be reviewed for potential drug interactions before dispensing rifampin.[54] Rifampin may turn urine and other secretions orange-red and may permanently stain some types of contact lenses.

Other Rifamycins. Rifabutin is used for disseminated *M. avium* infection in AIDS patients and is quite active against *M. tuberculosis*. Most rifampin-resistant organisms are resistant to rifabutin. Because rifabutin is a less-potent enzyme inducer than rifampin, it may be used in patients who are receiving protease inhibitors.[41,64–67] For HIV-positive patients, the ATS/CDC recommends regimens with three or more doses of the TB drugs per week (see Table 116–3). Rifapentine is a long-acting rifamycin that can be used once weekly in the continuation phase of treatment (after the first 2 months) in carefully selected HIV-negative patients. Rifapentine is approximately 85% as potent an enzyme inducer as rifampin, so similar drug interactions are likely.[41,64–67]

Pyrazinamide. Adding pyrazinamide to the first 2 months of treatment with isoniazid and rifampin shortens the duration to 6 months for most patients.[2,41] It is usually well absorbed and displays a fairly long half-life.[68,69] The most common toxicities of pyrazinamide are gastrointestinal distress, arthralgias, and elevations in the serum uric acid concentrations.[41,55] Most patients do not experience true gout. Hepatotoxicity is the major limiting adverse effect and is dose-related when pyrazinamide is given daily.

A fixed-combination product (Rifater, Aventis) of rifampin 120 mg, isoniazid 50 mg, and pyrazinamide 300 mg is designed to prevent drug resistance by keeping the self-medicating patient from using only one drug at a time. If the patient is receiving directly observed treatment, there is no particular advantage to this product. The typical dose of Rifater will be five to six tablets daily. When pyrazinamide is discontinued after 2 months of treatment, the combination product Rifamate (isoniazid 150 mg and rifampin 300 mg) can be substituted.

Ethambutol. Ethambutol replaced *p*-aminosalicylic acid as a first-line agent in the 1960s because it was better tolerated by patients.[2,41] Ethambutol is used as a fourth drug for TB while awaiting susceptibility data.[41] If the organism is susceptible to isoniazid, rifampin, and pyrazinamide, ethambutol can be stopped. Ethambutol is active against most mycobacteria, including *M. tuberculosis* and *M. avium*, but it is generally bacteriostatic.

Ethambutol should not be given with antacids.[70] In patients with renal failure, the ethambutol dose should be reduced to three times per week.[52,71] Retrobulbar neuritis is the major adverse effect. Patients may complain of a change in visual acuity, the inability to see the color green, or both. They should be monitored monthly while on the drug using Snellen wall charts for visual acuity and Ishihara red-green color discrimination cards.[41,54,55]

Second-Line Antituberculosis Drugs ***Streptomycin.*** Streptomycin is one of three aminoglycoside antibiotics (along with amikacin and kanamycin) that are active against mycobacteria. Streptomycin is quite active against MAC and several other mycobacteria, enterococci, *Brucella*, *Yersinia*, and various other bacteria. Although labeled only for intramuscular dosing, streptomycin can be given safely as intravenous infusions (100 mL of dextrose 5% water or normal saline) over 30 minutes, similar to the other aminoglycosides.[72] Streptomycin, like other aminoglycosides, is renally cleared by glomerular filtration and must be given less often in patients with renal dysfunction.[41,45,54]

Streptomycin occasionally causes nephrotoxicity, although it tends to be mild and reversible. It also is capable of causing ototoxicity (vestibular and cochlear), which may become permanent with continued use.[41,55] Older patients and those receiving long durations of treatment are most likely to experience hearing loss, whereas vestibular toxicity is highly unpredictable.

Resistance to amikacin and kanamycin is frequently linked but independent of resistance to streptomycin and independent of resistance to capreomycin. Therefore, susceptibility tests should guide the selection of these injectable drugs.

p-Aminosalicylic Acid. In the United States, only the enteric-coated, sustained-release granule form (Paser) is available.[73–75] Gastrointestinal disturbances are the most common adverse effects from *p*-aminosalicylic acid. Diarrhea is usually self-limited, with symptoms improving after the first 1 to 2 weeks of therapy. Occasionally, a few doses of an opioid will resolve the problem. It is also important to tell the patient that the empty granules will appear in the stool. Although FDA approved for three daily doses, pharmacokinetic data support twice-daily dosing.[74]

Various types of malabsorption, including steatorrhea, were reported with previous dosage forms of *p*-aminosalicylic acid. Hypersensitivity may occur and, rarely, severe hepatitis. *p*-Aminosalicylic acid is known to produce goiter, with or without myxedema, that seems to occur more frequently with concomitant ethionamide therapy.

Cycloserine. Cycloserine is only used to treat MDR-TB. It is well absorbed orally and is best taken on an empty stomach.[76] It is cleared primarily through the kidneys by glomerular filtration and requires dosage reduction in renal failure. Cycloserine can produce dose-related CNS toxicity, including lethargy, confusion, or unusual behavior. Seizures, although reported, are exceedingly rare.[2,41,54] Therapy is improved by maintaining 2-hour postdose serum concentrations between 20 and 35 mcg/mL.[45,47] Most patients reach a maximum dose of 750 mg daily, divided unevenly into two doses. This can be achieved by starting with 250 mg daily for 2 days, followed by 250-mg increments over 2-day intervals. This dose of cycloserine can be maintained if the patient complains of only occasional mild CNS effects, such as difficulty concentrating. Serum concentrations can be checked 1 to 2 weeks into therapy. The addition of pyridoxine 50 mg daily may improve patient tolerance of cycloserine.

Ethionamide. Ethionamide shares structural features with two other antimycobacterial agents, isoniazid and, more distantly, thiacetazone, a drug not used in the United States. Prothionamide, the *n*-propyl derivative of ethionamide, is used in Europe. Ethionamide is only active against organisms of the genus *Mycobacterium*, and it should be considered primarily bacteriostatic because it is difficult to achieve serum concentrations that would be bactericidal.[41,45,47]

Gastrointestinal toxicity is the dose-limiting adverse effect. The drug should be introduced gradually in 250-mg increments, as described earlier for cycloserine. Rarely will a patient tolerate more than 1,000 mg daily in divided oral doses. Ethionamide may be administered with a light snack or prior to bedtime to minimize gastrointestinal intolerance. Food does not affect absorption significantly.[77] Little ethionamide is recovered in the urine, so doses remain the same in renal failure. Ethionamide may cause goiter, with or without hypothyroidism (especially when given with *p*-aminosalicylic acid), gynecomastia, alopecia, impotence, menorrhagia, photodermatitis, and acne. The management of diabetes also may be more difficult in patients receiving ethionamide. Because of these problems, ethionamide is only used when absolutely necessary.

Clofazimine. Clofazimine is a drug with good activity against *Mycobacterium leprae* and weak activity against *M. tuberculosis* and *M. avium*. It is used in doses of 100 to 200 mg daily in advanced cases of MDR-TB or MAC, especially when therapeutic options are limited.[41,45] The drug has a terminal elimination half-life that is weeks long. Gastrointestinal distress and skin discoloration are the most important adverse reactions. Although uncommon, severe gastrointestinal pain may occur because of deposition of clofazimine crystals within the intestines; this may require surgical correction.

Thiacetazone. Thiacetazone is a weak agent used rarely in parts of the developing world because of its low cost. Skin reactions, including rash and Stevens-Johnson's syndrome, may occur. Thiacetazone must be discontinued permanently as soon as a rash appears. Similar to trimethoprim-sulfamethoxazole, the incidence of skin reactions is much higher in AIDS patients.[78]

Quinolones. Levofloxacin, ciprofloxacin, and moxifloxacin are sometimes used to treat MDR-TB. Moxifloxacin also is being studied as a possible replacement for certain first line agents.[2,13,41,45,79] Quinolones are useful because most are available in oral and intravenous dosage forms, so they can be used in critically ill patients.

β-Lactam and β-Lactamase Inhibitor Combinations. The *β*-lactams have limited activity against mycobacteria because of *β*-lactamases and because *β*-lactams fail to enter macrophages.[41,45,80] Cefoxitin, a *β*-lactamase–stable cephalosporin, has useful activity against rapidly growing mycobacteria, such as *M. fortuitum* and *Mycobacterium chelonae*. Combinations of *β*-lactam with *β*-lactamase inhibitors have been used in salvage regimens for TB patients with no other options, but are not used routinely to treat TB.

Macrolides/Azalides. The macrolide clarithromycin and azalide azithromycin represent substantial advances in the treatment of MAC but demonstrate limited activity against *M. tuberculosis* and are not used frequently for TB.[2,13,41,45]

New Drugs and Delivery Systems. The nitroimidazopyran PA 824, which is chemically related to metronidazole and tinidazole, has activity against *M. tuberculosis* in vitro.[81,82] This class, along with the oxazolidinones, may produce useful agents for TB. Linezolid has been used in a few patients with TB.[96] Long-term use of linezolid requires careful monitoring of hematologic indices for potential anemia and thrombocytopenia. Although not proved conclusively, it may be possible to reduce the incidences of these toxicities by giving linezolid 600 mg daily for the slow-growing *M. tuberculosis* rather than the usual twice-daily dose used for gram-positive organisms. Chemical modification of existing compounds, such as pyrazinamide, may produce new TB drugs. Finally, continuing research on the construction of the mycobacterial cell wall and intracellular pathways may lead to agents with unique activity against this genus.

Liposomes have been investigated as delivery systems for various agents against mycobacteria, including isoniazid, rifampin, and the aminoglycosides. Liposomes also could be used to deliver β-lactams or other agents that generally are excluded from macrophages. By changing the pharmacokinetic profile of such agents, their use in the treatment of mycobacterial infections could be enhanced greatly. Currently, no such product is licensed for use against TB.

Corticosteroids. Adjunctive therapy with corticosteroids may be of benefit in some patients with tuberculous meningitis or pericarditis to relieve inflammation and pressure (see Table 116–4).[2,41] They should be avoided in most other circumstances because they detract from the immune response to TB.

Bacille Calmette-Guérin Vaccine. The BCG vaccine is an attenuated, hybridized strain of *M. bovis*. It was developed in 1921 and is used as a prophylactic vaccine against TB. Administration of BCG vaccine is compulsory in many developing countries and is officially recommended in many others. Vaccination with BCG produces a subclinical infection resulting in sensitization of T lymphocytes and cross-immunity to *M. tuberculosis*, as well as cutaneous hypersensitivity and, in many cases, a positive tuberculin skin test.

In the published clinical trials, several different BCG preparations were used, and the efficacy of these vaccinations ranged from negative 56% (some patients did worse with the vaccine) to positive 80%.[2,41] Trials within the United States and Puerto Rico have shown efficacy rates of 6% to 29%. The primary benefit of BCG vaccination appears to be the prevention of severe forms of TB in children. Data from the BCG trials show that the incidence of tuberculous meningitis and miliary TB is 52% to 100% lower and that the incidence of pulmonary TB is 2% to 80% lower in vaccinated children younger than 15 years of age than it was in unvaccinated controls.

Unfortunately, BCG does not appear to be very reliable in preventing disease by *M. tuberculosis* in other segments of the population. Side effects occur in 1% to 10% of vaccinated persons and usually include severe or prolonged ulceration at the vaccination site, lymphadenitis, and lupus vulgaris. It is recommended that pregnant women and patients with impaired immune systems, including those with HIV infection, avoid vaccination. The World Health Organization has recommended, however, that in populations where the risk of TB is high, HIV-infected infants who are asymptomatic should receive BCG vaccine at birth or as soon as possible thereafter. Because BCG infection has occurred in AIDS patients given the vaccine, individuals with symptomatic HIV infection should not be vaccinated.[2,41]

In the United States, BCG vaccination is recommended only for uninfected children who are at unavoidable risk of exposure to TB and for whom other methods of prevention and control have failed or are not feasible.[2,41] Its use is very limited.

PHARMACOECONOMIC CONSIDERATIONS

The World Health Organization and the World Bank agree that the control of TB is one of the most cost-effective health interventions any nation can pursue. Early identification of TB cases and the effective use of isoniazid, rifampin, and pyrazinamide (plus ethambutol) while the isolate is still drug-susceptible always should be the primary goals of public health departments. Contact investigation and treatment of those infected but without disease are important secondary goals to reduce the number of future cases.

Patients who complete all their treatment for drug-susceptible TB have cure rates over 95%. Noncompliance (nonadherence), drug resistance, extrapulmonary disease, and concomitant disease states reduce the overall effectiveness of chemotherapy of TB to approximately 75%.

The treatment of TB is not particularly expensive, especially if hospitalization is not required.[83] Furthermore, TB is quite curable. Because the various TB drugs each have a role to play in the treatment of TB or MDR-TB, all the antituberculosis drugs approved by the Food and Drug Administration should be on institutional formularies. Centers that see little MDR-TB need not keep stocks of the second-line drugs, provided that they are readily available should the need arise. Because the treatment of MDR-TB is difficult, and because missteps are potentially disastrous, such patients should be referred to centers experienced in the management of MDR-TB.[2,41,84,85]

EVALUATION OF THERAPEUTIC OUTCOMES

MONITORING OF THE PHARMACEUTICAL CARE PLAN

The most serious problem with TB therapy is patient nonadherence to the prescribed regimens.[86,87] Unfortunately, there is no reliable way to identify such patients a priori. In the study by Brudney and Dobkin,[86] 89% of the patients were noncompliant with therapy. It is critical to the control of TB that such adherence rates be improved dramatically. The most effective way to achieve this end is with directly observed treatment.[2,13,41] Despite criticisms that it will cost more money, it is far cheaper in the long run to prevent the further spread of disease with directly observed treatment than to track down and treat additional cases of TB continuously.

The homeless and other underprivileged individuals are assumed to constitute the group of patients considered "unreliable," and directly observed treatment should be reserved for them; it is also assumed that "responsible" patients cared for by private physicians may be treated with daily, unsupervised therapy. A study conducted in Baltimore, however, compared outcomes (sputum culture conversion to negative at 3 months) in patients with pulmonary TB who were treated by private physicians with outcomes in patients treated via directly observed treatment in a city-run clinic. Surprisingly, 3-month culture conversion occurred in only 40% of the private-care patients, compared with 90% in the city clinic-care patients.[88] Clearly, expansion of the use of directly observed treatment to nearly all patients with TB may be of benefit.

For patients who are acid-fast bacilli smear positive, they should have sputum samples sent for acid-fast bacilli stains every 1 to 2 weeks until two consecutive smears are negative. This provides early evidence of a response to treatment.[41] Once on maintenance therapy, sputum cultures can be performed monthly until two consecutive cultures are negative, which generally occurs over 2 to 3 months. If sputum cultures continue to be positive after 2 months, drug susceptibility testing should be repeated, and serum concentrations of the drugs should be checked.

Serum chemistries, including blood urea nitrogen, creatinine, aspartate transaminase, and alanine transaminase, and a complete blood count with platelets should be performed at baseline and periodically thereafter, depending on the presence of other factors that may increase the likelihood of toxicity (e.g., advanced age, alcohol abuse, pregnancy).[2,41] Hepatotoxicity should be suspected in patients whose transaminases exceed five times the upper limit of normal or whose total bilirubin concentration exceeds 3 mg/dL and in patients with symptoms such as nausea, vomiting, or jaundice. At this point, the offending agent(s) should be discontinued. Sequential reintroduction of the drugs with frequent testing of liver enzymes is often successful in identifying the offending agent; other agents may be continued. Alternative agents should be selected as needed. Audiometric testing should be performed at baseline and monthly in patients who must receive streptomycin for more than 1 to 2 months. Vision testing (Snellen visual acuity charts and Ishihara color discrimination plates) should be performed on all patients who receive ethambutol. All patients diagnosed with TB should be tested for HIV infection.

THERAPEUTIC DRUG MONITORING

Therapeutic drug monitoring (TDM) or applied pharmacokinetics is the use of serum drug concentrations to optimize therapy.[41,45,47,88,89] Non-AIDS patients with drug-susceptible TB generally do well, and TDM generally should be used if they are failing appropriate directly observed treatment (no clinical improvement after 2 to 4 weeks or smear-positive after 4 to 6 weeks). On the other hand, patients with AIDS, diabetes, cystic fibrosis, and various gastrointestinal disorders often fail to absorb these drugs properly and are candidates for TDM. Also, patients with hepatic or renal disease should be monitored, given their potential for overdoses.

In the treatment of MDR-TB, the differences between the maximum serum concentration (C_{max}) and the minimal inhibitory concentration (MIC) for the second-line agents are much smaller that with isoniazid and rifampin. Therefore, alterations in the absorption of these drugs can have significant impact on the outcome of therapy.[45,47] Although the optimal serum concentrations for TB are not known, target serum peak concentrations have been proposed.[45,47] Blood samples collected at 2 and 6 hours after a dose have been used with some success, although they may not be the optimal sampling times for all the drugs. Long-half-life drugs (e.g., pyrazinamide and cycloserine) can be sampled at 2 and 10 hours if an estimate of the half-life is desired. Finally, TDM of the TB and HIV drugs is perhaps the most logical way to untangle the complex drug interactions that take place (see Table 116–7).[91]

CLINICAL CONTROVERSY

Some TB centers employ TDM for many of their patients at the outset of treatment in order to identify drug-delivery problems early. Other centers wait to see how the patient responds and perform TDM only if problems arise. An argument can be made for either approach. The latter can save money, but delays in effective treatment can affect the patient's outcome adversely. Most otherwise healthy TB patients will absorb their drugs adequately. Patients who are critically ill or who have MDR-TB can benefit from early TDM.

CONCLUSIONS

Good patient adherence to treatment regimens is the cornerstone to effective antimycobacterial chemotherapy. Pharmacists should monitor TB therapy with particular interest in drug-drug interactions, drug malabsorption, and avoiding the error of adding a single drug to a failing regimen. They should educate patients on the importance of continuing their chemotherapy despite symptomatic improvement. Pharmacists should become part of a multidisciplinary team (with nurses, physicians, social workers) devoted to successful chemotherapy of TB patients and their families.

ABBREVIATIONS

ATS: American Thoracic Society
BCG: bacillus Calmette-Guérin
CDC: Centers for Disease Control and Prevention
INF: interferon
IL: interleukin
LTBI: latent tuberculosis infection
MAC: *Mycobacterium avium* complex
MDR: multidrug resistance
MIC: minimal inhibitory concentration
PPD: purified protein derivative
TB: tuberculosis
TDM: therapeutic drug monitoring
TH: T-helper cell
TNF: tumor necrosis factor

REFERENCES

1. World Health Organization Report on the Global Tuberculosis Epidemic. Geneva: WHO, 1998.
2. Iseman MD. A Clinician's Guide to Tuberculosis. Philadelphia: Lippincott Williams & Wilkins, 2000.
3. Stead WW. The origin and erratic global spread of tuberculosis. Clin Chest Med 1997;18:65–77.
4. McCray E, Weinbaum CM, Braden CR, Onorato IM. The epidemiology of tuberculosis in the United States. Clin Chest Med 1997;18:99–113.
5. Centers for Disease Control and Prevention. Trends in tuberculosis morbidity—United States, 2005. MMWR 2006:55;305–308.
6. Centers for Disease Control and Prevention. Tuberculosis in the United States, 2002. Atlanta, GA: CDC, September 2005.
7. Haas DW. *Mycobacterium tuberculosis.* In: Mandell GL, Bennett JE, Dolin R, eds. Principles and Practice of Infectious Diseases, 5th ed. New York: Churchill-Livingstone, 2000:2576–2607.
8. Small PM, Shafer RW, Hopewell PC, et al. Exogenous reinfection with multidrug-resistant *Mycobacterium tuberculosis* in patients with advanced HIV infection. N Engl J Med 1993;328:1137–1144.
9. Beck-Sague C, Dooley SW, Hutton MD, et al. Hospital outbreak of multidrug-resistant *Mycobacterium tuberculosis* infections: Factors in transmission to staff and HIV-infected patients. JAMA 1992;268:1280–1286.
10. Centers for Disease Control and Prevention. Meeting the challenge of multidrug-resistant tuberculosis: Summary of a conference. MMWR 1992;41:51–71.
11. Heifets L. Mycobacteriology laboratory. Clin Chest Med 1997;18:35–53.
12. Heifets LB. Drug susceptibility tests in the management of chemotherapy of tuberculosis. In: Heifets LB, ed. Drug Susceptibility in the Chemotherapy of Mycobacterial Infections. Boca Raton, FL: CRC Press, 1991:89–122.
13. Daley CL, Chambers HF. *Mycobacterium tuberculosis* complex. In: Yu VL, Weber R, Raoult D, eds. Antimicrobial Therapy and Vaccines, Vol I. Microbes, 2d ed. New York: Apple Trees Productions, 2002:841–865.
14. Roberts GD, Böttger EC, Stockman L. Methods for the rapid identification of mycobacterial species. Clin Lab Med 1996;16:603–615.
15. Sandin RL. Polymerase chain reaction and other amplification techniques in mycobacteriology. Clin Lab Med 1996;16:617–639.
16. Blanchard JS. Molecular mechanisms of drug resistance in *Mycobacterium tuberculosis.* Annu Rev Biochem 1996;65:215–239.
17. Somoskovi A, Parsons LM, Salfinger M. The molecular basis of resistance to isoniazid, rifampin, and pyrazinamide in *Mycobacterium tuberculosis.* Respir Res 2001;2:164–168.
18. Marin M, Garcia de Viedma D, Ruiz-Serrano MJ, Bouza E. Rapid direct detection of multiple rifampin and isoniazid resistance mutations in Mycobacterium tuberculosis in respiratory samples by real-time PCR. Antimicrob Agents Chemother 2004;48:4293–4300.
19. Riley RL, Mills CC, Nyka W, et al. Aerial dissemination of pulmonary tuberculosis: A two-year study of contagion in a tuberculosis ward. Am J Hygiene 1959;70:185–196.
20. Daniel TM, Boom WH, Ellner JJ. Immunology of tuberculosis. In: Reichman LB, Hershfield ES, eds. Tuberculosis: A Comprehensive International Approach, 2d ed. New York: Marcel Dekker, 2000:157–185.

21. Piessens WF, Nardell EA. Pathogenesis of tuberculosis. In: Reichman LB, Hershfield ES, eds. Tuberculosis: A Comprehensive International Approach, 2d ed. New York: Marcel Dekker, 2000:241–260.
22. Long, R, Gardam, M. Tumour necrosis factor-α inhibitors and the reactivation of latent tuberculosis infection. CMAJ 2003;168:1153–1156.
23. American Thoracic Society/Centers for Disease Control and Prevention. Diagnostic standards and classification of tuberculosis in adults and children. Am J Respir Crit Care Med 2000;161:1376–1395.
24. Peloquin CA, Berning SE. Tuberculosis and multi-drug resistant tuberculosis in children. Pediatr Nurs 1995;21:566–572.
25. Correa AG. Unique aspects of tuberculosis in the pediatric population. Clin Chest Med 1997;18:89–98.
26. Alland D, Kalkut GE, Moss AR, et al. Transmission of tuberculosis in New York City: An analysis of DNA fingerprinting and conventional epidemiologic methods. N Engl J Med 1994;330:1710–1716.
27. Small PM, Hopewell PC, Singh SP, et al. The epidemiology of tuberculosis in San Francisco: A population-based study using conventional and molecular methods. N Engl J Med 1994;330:1703–1709.
28. Daley CL, Small PM, Schecter GF, et al. An outbreak of tuberculosis with accelerated progression among persons infected with the human immunodeficiency virus: An analysis using restricted-fragment-length polymorphisms. N Engl J Med 1992;326:231–235.
29. Wallis RS, Vjecha M, Amir-Tahmasseb M, et al. Influence of tuberculosis on human immunodeficiency virus (HIV-1): Enhanced cytokine expression and elevated β_2-microglobulin in HIV-1–associated tuberculosis. J Infect Dis 1993;167:43–48.
30. American Thoracic Society/Centers for Disease Control and Prevention. Targeted tuberculin skin testing and treatment of latent tuberculosis infection. Am J Respir Crit Care Med 2000;161:S221–S247.
31. Pape JW, Jean SS, Ho JL, et al. Effect of isoniazid prophylaxis on incidence of active tuberculosis and progression of HIV infection. Lancet 1993;342:268–272.
32. Narita M, Ashkin D, Hollender ES, Pitchenik AE. Paradoxical worsening of tuberculosis following antiretroviral therapy in patients with AIDS. Am J Respir Crit Care Med 1998;158:157–161.
33. Barnes PF, Bloch AB, Davidson PT, Snider DE. Tuberculosis in patients with human immunodeficiency virus infection. N Engl J Med 1991;324:1644–1650.
34. Alvarez S, Shell C, Berk SL. Pulmonary tuberculosis in elderly men. Am J Med 1987;82:602–606.
35. Umeki S. Comparison of younger and elderly patients with pulmonary tuberculosis. Respiration 1989;55:75–83.
36. Centers for Disease Control and Prevention. Anergy skin testing and preventive therapy for HIV-infected persons: Revised recommendations. MMWR 1997;46:1–10.
37. Rosenberg T, Manfreda J, Hershfield ES. Two-step tuberculin testing in staff and residents of a nursing home. Am Rev Resp Dis 1993;148:1537–1540.
38. Centers for Disease Control and Prevention. Guidelines for using the QuantiFERON-TB test for diagnosing latent *Mycobacterium tuberculosis* infection. MMWR 2002;51:1–5.
39. Barnes PF. Weighing gold or counting spots. Am J Respir Crit Care Med 2006;174:731–735.
40. Bouza E, Diaz-Lopez MD, Moreno S, et al. *Mycobacterium tuberculosis* bacteremia in patients with and without human immunodeficiency virus infection. Arch Intern Med 1993;153:496–500.
41. American Thoracic Society/Centers for Disease Control/Infectious Disease Society of America. Treatment of tuberculosis. Am J Respir Crit Care Med 2003;167:603–662.
42. Fujiwara PI, Larkin C, Frieden TR. Directly observed therapy in New York City. Clin Chest Med 1997;18:135–148.
43. Weis SE. Universal directly observed therapy. Clin Chest Med 1997;18:155–163.
44. Mitchison DA. Basic mechanisms of chemotherapy. Chest 1979;1994;76(Suppl):771–781.
45. Peloquin CA. Pharmacological issues in the treatment of tuberculosis. Ann N Y Acad Sci 2001;953:157–164.
46. Fourie PB, Ellner JJ, Johnson JL. Whither *Mycobacterium vaccae*—encore. Lancet 2002;360:1032–1033.
47. Peloquin CA. Therapeutic drug monitoring in the treatment of tuberculosis. Drugs 2002;62:2169–2183.
48. Lawn SD, Wilkinson R. Extensively drug resistant tuberculosis. BMJ 2006;333;559–560.
49. Peloquin CA. Antituberculosis drugs: Pharmacokinetics. In: Heifets LB, ed. Drug Susceptibility in the Chemotherapy of Mycobacterial Infections. Boca Raton, FL: CRC Press, 1991:59–88.
50. Hamadeh MA, Glassroth J. Tuberculosis and pregnancy. Chest 1992;101:1114–1120.
51. Vallejo JG, Starke JR. Tuberculosis and pregnancy. Clin Chest Med 1992;13:693–707.
52. Malone RS, Fish DN, Spiegel DM, et al. The effect of hemodialysis on isoniazid, rifampin, pyrazinamide, and ethambutol. Am J Respir Crit Care Med 1999;159:1580–1584.
53. Malone RS, Fish DN, Spiegel DM, et al. The effect of hemodialysis on cycloserine, ethionamide, *para*-aminosalicylate, and clofazimine. Chest 1999;116:984–990.
54. McEvoy GK, ed. AHFS Drug Information. Bethesda, MD: American Society of Health-Systems Pharmacists, 2003.
55. Girling DJ. Adverse effects of antituberculous drugs. Drugs 1982;23:56–74.
56. Holdiness MR. Clinical pharmacokinetics of the antituberculosis drugs. Clin Pharmacokinet 1984;9:511–544.
57. Crabbe SJ. Drug infosearch—intravenous isoniazid. P&T 1990;15:1483–1484.
58. Peloquin CA, Namdar R, Dodge AA, Nix DE. Pharmacokinetics of isoniazid under fasting conditions, with food, and with antacids. Intl J Tuberc Lung Dis 1999;3:703–710.
59. Berning SE, Peloquin CA. Antimycobacterial agents: Isoniazid. In: Yu VL, Merigan TC, Barriere S, White NJ, eds. Antimicrobial Chemotherapy and Vaccines. Baltimore: Williams & Wilkins, 1998:654–663.
60. Weiner M, Burman W, Vernon A, et al. Low isoniazid concentration associated with outcome of tuberculosis treatment with once-weekly isoniazid and rifapentine. Am J Respir Crit Care Med 2003;167:1341–1347.
61. Weiner M, Benator D, Burman W, et al. Association between acquired rifamycin resistance and the pharmacokinetics of rifabutin and isoniazid among patients with HIV and tuberculosis. Clin Infect Dis 2005;40:1481–1491.
62. Morris AB, Kanyok TP, Scott J, et al. Rifamycins. In: Yu VL, Merigan TC, Barriere S, White NJ, eds. Antimicrobial Chemotherapy and Vaccines. Baltimore: Williams & Wilkins, 1998:901–963.
63. Peloquin CA, Namdar R, Singleton MD, Nix DE. Pharmacokinetics of rifampin under fasting conditions, with food, and with antacids. Chest 1999;115:12–18.
64. Centers for Disease Control and Prevention. Prevention and treatment of tuberculosis among patients infected with human immunodeficiency virus: Principles of therapy and revised recommendations. MMWR 1998;47:1–58.
65. Centers for Disease Control and Prevention. Updated guidelines for the use of rifabutin or rifampin for the treatment and prevention of tuberculosis among HIV-infected patients taking protease inhibitors on nonnucleoside reverse transcriptase inhibitors. MMWR 2000;49:185–189.
66. Burman WJ, Gallicano K, Peloquin CA. Therapeutic implications of drug interactions in the treatment of HIV-related tuberculosis. Clin Infect Dis 1999;28:419–430.
67. Burman WJ, Gallicano K, Peloquin CA. Comparative pharmacokinetics and pharmacodynamics of the rifamycin antibiotics. Clin Pharmacokinet 2001:40:327–341.
68. Peloquin CA, Jaresko GS, Yong CL, et al. Population pharmacokinetic modeling of isoniazid, rifampin, and pyrazinamide. Antimicrob Agents Chemother 1997;41:2670–2679.
69. Peloquin CA, Bulpitt AE, Jaresko GS, et al. Pharmacokinetics of pyrazinamide under fasting conditions, with food, and with antacids. Pharmacotherapy 1998;18:1205–1211.
70. Peloquin CA, Bulpitt AE, Jaresko GS, et al. Pharmacokinetics of ethambutol under fasting conditions, with food, and with antacids. Antimicrob Agents Chemother 1999;43:568–572.
71. Summers KK, Hardin TC. Treatment of tuberculosis in hemodialysis patients. J Infect Dis Pharmacother 1996;2:37–55.
72. Peloquin CA, Berning SE. Comment: Intravenous streptomycin. Ann Pharmacother 1993;27:1546–1547.
73. Peloquin CA, Henshaw TL, Huitt GA, et al. Pharmacokinetic evaluation of *p*-aminosalicylic acid granules. Pharmacotherapy 1994;14:40–46 (and correction: Pharmacotherapy 1994;14:2).
74. Peloquin CA, Berning SE, Huitt GA, et al. Once-daily and twice-daily dosing of *p*-aminosalicylic acid (PAS) granules. Am J Respir Crit Care Med 1999;159:932–934.

75. Peloquin CA, Zhu M, Adam RD, et al. Pharmacokinetics of *p*-aminosalicylate under fasting conditions, with orange juice, food, and antacids. Ann Pharmacother 2001;35:1332–1338.
76. Zhu M, Nix DE, Adam RD, et al. Pharmacokinetics of cycloserine under fasting conditions, with orange juice, food, and antacids. Pharmacotherapy 2001;21:891–897.
77. Zhu M, Namdar R, Stambaugh JJ, et al. Population pharmacokinetics of ethionamide in patients with tuberculosis. Tuberculosis 2002;82:91–96.
78. Elliott AM, Foster SD. Thiacetazone: Time to call a halt? Tuber Lung Dis 1996;77:27–29.
79. Burman WJ, Goldberg S, Johnson JL, et al. Moxifloxacin versus ethambutol in the first 2 months of treatment for pulmonary tuberculosis. Am J Respir Crit Care Med, 2006;174:331–338.
80. Zhang Y, Steingrube VA, Wallace RJ. Beta-lactamase inhibitors and the inducibility of the beta-lactamase of *Mycobacterium tuberculosis*. Am Rev Respir Dis 1992;145:657–660.
81. Stover CK, Warrener P, VanDevanter DR, et al. A small-molecule nitroimidazopyran drug candidate for the treatment of tuberculosis. Nature 2000;405:962–966.
82. Nuermberger E, Rosenthal I, Tyagi S, Williams KN, Almeida D, Peloquin CA, Bishai WR, Grosset JH. Combination chemotherapy with the nitroimidazopyran PA-824 and first-line drugs in the murine model of tuberculosis. Antomicrob Agents Chemother 2006;50:2621–2625.
83. Reves R, Burman W, Dalton C, et al. A cost-effectiveness analysis of directly-observed therapy versus self-administered therapy for treatment of tuberculosis. Am J Respir Crit Care Med 1997;155(Suppl):A33.
84. Goble M, Iseman MD, Madsen LA, et al. Treatment of 171 patients with pulmonary tuberculosis resistant to isoniazid and rifampin. N Engl J Med 1993;328:527–532.
85. Iseman MD. Treatment of multidrug-resistant tuberculosis. N Engl J Med 1993;329:784–791.
86. Brudney K, Dobkin J. Resurgent tuberculosis in New York City: Human immunodeficiency virus, homelessness, and the decline of tuberculosis control programs. Am Rev Respir Dis 1991;144:745–749.
87. Mahmoudi A, Iseman MD. Pitfalls in the care of patients with tuberculosis: Common errors and their association with the acquisition of drug resistance. JAMA 1993;270:65–68.
88. Chaulk CP, Friedman M, Dunning R. Modeling the epidemiology and economics of directly observed therapy in Baltimore. Int J Tuberc Lung Dis 2000;4:201–207.
89. Tappero JW, Bradford WZ, Agerton TB, et al. Serum concentrations of antimycobacterial drugs in patients with pulmonary tuberculosis in Botswana. Clin Infect Dis 2005;41:461–469.
90. Perlman DC, Segal Y, Rosenkranz S, et al. The clinical pharmacokinetics of rifampin and ethambutol in HIV-infected persons with tuberculosis. Clin Infect Dis 2005;41:1638–1647.
91. Peloquin CA. Agents for tuberculosis. In: Piscitelli SC, Rodvold KA, eds. Drug Interactions in Infectious Diseases. Totowa, NJ: Humana Press, 2001:109–120.

CHAPTER 117

Gastrointestinal Infections and Enterotoxigenic Poisonings

STEVEN MARTIN AND ROSE JUNG

KEY CONCEPTS

1. The etiology of infectious diarrhea includes bacteria, viruses, and protozoans. Viral infections are the leading cause of diarrhea in the world.
2. Fluid and electrolyte replacement is the cornerstone of therapy. Oral rehydration therapy is preferred in most cases of mild and moderate diarrhea. The necessary components of oral replacement therapy are glucose, sodium, potassium, chloride, and water.
3. Antimicrobial therapy often is not indicated for enteritis because many cases are mild and self-limited or are viral in nature.
4. Diarrheal illness can be prevented by following simple rules of personal hygiene and safe food preparation.
5. The most common pathogens for traveler's diarrhea include enterotoxigenic *Escherichia coli*, *Shigella*, *Campylobacter*, *Salmonella*, and viruses.
6. Patient education and prevention strategies are important in preventing and treating traveler's diarrhea. Prophylaxis with antibiotics is not recommended in most situations.
7. Common pathogens responsible for food poisoning include *Staphylococcus, Salmonella, Shigella,* and *Clostridium.*

Gastrointestinal (GI) infections encompass a wide variety of syndromes from mild gastroenteritis to life-threatening systemic infections. Dehydration from GI infections is the second leading cause of morbidity and mortality worldwide, especially in infants and children younger than 5 years of age. From 1992 to 2000, the median incidence of diarrhea for all children younger than 5 years of age was 3.2 episodes per child per year. The incidence of diarrhea was higher in younger children, with 4.8 episodes per child per year among children ages 6 to 11 months in comparison with 1.4 episodes per child per year for 4-year-olds. Younger children also had a higher risk for death from acute dehydrating diarrhea. For children younger than 1 year of age and those ages 1 to 4 years, the median mortality rates were 8.5 and 3.8 per 1,000 children per year, respectively.[1] Although this was a decrease from 13.6 per 1,000 children per year during 1955–1979 and 5.6 per 1,000 children per year during 1980 to 1989, diarrhea remains a major health problem in children, especially in those younger than 1 year of age.[2,3]

Although outbreaks of infectious diarrhea and deaths in the United States are not as prevalent, the economic burden of GI infections still remains high. The estimates by the Centers for Disease Control and Prevention (CDC) suggest that 211 million episodes of acute gastroenteritis occur each year in the United States, resulting in more than 900,000 hospitalizations and more than 6,000 deaths.[4] In contrast to the developing world where the risk of death is highest among young children, in the United States most of those who die of diarrheal illness are elderly. According the National Center for Health Statistics, during 1979 to 1987, 51% of deaths caused by diarrheal illness were among patients older than 74 years of age, and 27% were among 55- to 74-year-olds, while 11% were in those younger than 5 years.[5] Similarly, a study of the McDonnell-Douglas Health Information System database revealed that 25% of all hospitalizations and 85% of all mortality associated with diarrhea involved the elderly (≥60 years old).[6] In addition to children and elderly, other groups at risk for GI infections include travelers and campers, immunocompromised patients such as those with acquired immunodeficiency syndrome (AIDS), patients in chronic care facilities, and military personnel assigned overseas.

Fortunately, diarrheal mortality has declined substantially in the past two decades, especially among children younger than 1 year of age. Interventions for diarrheal disease such as breast-feeding, better weaning practices, improved sanitation, and higher use of oral rehydration therapy are responsible for the decrease in case-fatality rates. Although reassuring, diarrhea still accounts for 1.6 to 2.5 million deaths annually.[1] To achieve further declines in mortality, a more complex approach needs to be adopted that includes distinguishing acute watery diarrhea from dysentery and persistent diarrhea and providing appropriate case management for each syndrome.

(1) A variety of pathogens are responsible for acute infectious diarrhea. Viruses are suspected to be the most common cause of gastroenteritis, especially in children. However, bacterial species are the most commonly identified cause of infectious diarrhea in the United States. This chapter focuses on the bacterial and viral etiologies of GI infections such as *Vibrio cholerae, Escherichia coli, Salmonella, Shigella, Campylobacter jejuni*, rotaviruses, noroviruses, astrovirus, and enteric adenovirus. Clinical presentation, diagnosis, treatment and prevention strategies are discussed in general terms initially for all GI infections and further elaborated in regards to specific etiologies in subsequent sections.

Learning objectives, review questions, and other resources can be found at **www.pharmacotherapyonline.com.**

CLINICAL PRESENTATION AND DIAGNOSIS

Appropriate management of moderate to severe cases requires an organism-specific diagnosis and thus, stool cultures are often ordered. Unfortunately, the yield of such cultures is very low. Unlike cultures of sterile sites, normal feces contain many enteric pathogens and differential and selective media are required to isolate pathogenic bacteria from among those that are nonpathogenic. A routine stool culture will screen for presence of *C. jejuni*, *Salmonella* species, and *Shigella* species. Although other pathogens such as *Yersinia enterocolitica* and *Vibrio* species may also be detected, the yield of positive cultures for nonroutine organisms is increased if requested specifically based on clinical suspicion of likely etiologies.

Current guidelines recommend selective approaches to identify patients who are likely to have positive cultures and those who would benefit from organism-specific diagnosis in order to improve the usefulness of stool cultures.[7] A careful history and physical examination are crucial in providing clues to the likely etiology. Fecal testing is recommended in patients with a recent use of antibiotics, daycare center attendance, hospitalization, or illness accompanied by fever, bloody stools, systemic illness, or dehydration if they have community-acquired diarrheal illnesses lasting for more than 1 day. For community-acquired or traveler's diarrhea, stool samples should be sent for culture of *Salmonella, Shigella, Campylobacter,* and *E. coli* O157:H7.

A careful history may further point to other etiologic agents. Bloody diarrhea may indicate enterohemorrhagic *E. coli*. Outbreaks should prompt consideration of *Staphylococcus aureus, Bacillus cereus, Clostridium perfringens, Vibrio, Salmonella, Campylobacter, Shigella,* or *E. coli* infection. Ingestion of inadequately cooked seafood should increase suspicions for infections with *Vibrio* or noroviruses. Use of antibiotics predisposes patients to cytotoxigenic *Clostridium difficile*. Travel to tropical areas increases the chances of developing enterotoxigenic *E. coli*, viral (norovirus or rotavirus), and parasitic infections (*Giardia, Entamoeba, Strongyloides,* and *Cryptosporidium*).

In hospitalized patients, fecal testing for routine bacterial pathogens or ova and parasites is not recommended for diarrhea that occurs 3 days after the start of hospitalization owing to low yield. Instead, 15% to 20% of cases are caused by *C. difficile*, thus the stool specimen should be tested for *C. difficile* toxin(s), especially in those who are exposed to antimicrobial therapy or chemotherapy. Stool culture is recommended, however, in persons 65 years of age and older with comorbid diseases, neutropenia, or human immunodeficiency virus (HIV) infection. In immunocompromised hosts, a wide range of viral, bacterial, and parasitic agents should be tested. Microscopic examination for fecal polymorphonuclear cells or a simple immunoassay for the neutrophil marker lactoferrin can further provide evidence of an inflammatory process and increase the yield of culture for invasive pathogens in patients presenting with fever or bloody stool.

TREATMENT

Diarrhea

GENERAL APPROACHES TO MANAGEMENT

Rehydration Therapy

❷ Initial assessment of fluid loss is essential for rehydration and should include acute weight loss as it is the most reliable means of determining the extent of water loss. However, if accurate baseline weight is not available, clinical signs are helpful in determining approximate deficits (Table 117–1). Physical assessment generally is more reliable in young children and infants than in adults.[8]

❷ Fluid replacement is the cornerstone of therapy for diarrhea regardless of etiology. Oral rehydration therapy (ORT) reverses dehydration in nearly all patients with mild to moderate diarrhea; treatment failure with ORT is infrequent (3% to 6%).[9] ORT offers the advantages of being inexpensive and noninvasive and does not require hospitalization for administration. In those who are able to take oral fluids, ORT is superior to administration of intravenous (IV) fluids. Moreover, thirst drives use of ORT and provides a safeguard against overhydration.

The American Academy of Pediatrics recommends rehydration with an electrolyte-concentrated rehydration phase followed by a maintenance phase using dilute electrolyte solutions and larger volumes (see Table 117–1).[10] The necessary components of glucose-based ORT include glucose, sodium, potassium, chloride, and water (Table 117–2). Glucose-based ORT takes advantage of glucose-coupled sodium transport in the small bowel. Glucose enhances sodium and subsequently water transport across intestinal walls. In children with vomiting and diarrhea, ORT may be given as 5 mL every 2 to 3 minutes in a teaspoon or oral syringe. Nasogastric administration of ORT is an alternative method of administration in a child with persistent vomiting. After starting rehydration therapy, patients should be observed for a reversal of the signs of dehydration, increased stool consistency, and decreased stool frequency.

TABLE 117-1 Clinical Assessment of Degree of Dehydration in Children Based on Percentage of Body Weight Loss[a]

Variable	Mild: 3%–5%	Moderate: 6%–9%	Severe: ≥10%
Blood pressure	Normal	Normal	Normal to reduced
Quality of pulses	Normal	Normal or slightly decreased	Moderately decreased
Heart rate	Normal	Increased	Increased (bradycardia in severe cases)
Skin turgor	Normal	Decreased	Decreased
Fontanelle	Normal	Sunken	Sunken
Mucous membranes	Slightly dry	Dry	Dry
Eyes	Normal	Sunken orbits/decreased tears	Deeply sunken orbits/decreased tears
Extremities	Warm, normal capillary refill	Delayed capillary refill	Cool, mottled
Mental status	Normal	Normal to listless	Normal to lethargic or comatose
Urine output	Slightly decreased	<1 mL/kg/h	<1 mL/kg/h
Thirst	Slightly increased	Moderately increased	Very thirsty or too lethargic to indicate
Fluid replacement	ORT 50 mL/kg over 2–4 h	ORT 100 mL/kg over 2–4 h	Ringer lactate 40 mL/kg in 15–30 min, then 20–40 mL/kg if skin turgor, alertness, and pulse have not returned to normal or
	Replace ongoing losses with low-sodium ORT (40–60 mEq/L Na+) at 10 mL/kg per stool or emesis	Replace ongoing losses with low-sodium ORT (40–60 mEq/L Na^+) at 10 mL/kg per stool or emesis	Ringer lactate or NS 20 mL/kg, repeat if necessary, and then replace water and electrolyte deficits over 1–2 days Followed by ORT 100 mL/kg over 4 h. Replace ongoing losses with low-sodium ORT (40–60 mEq/L Na^+) at 10 mL/kg per stool or emesis

ORT, oral rehydration therapy.
[a]Percentages vary among authors for each dehydration category; hemodynamic and perfusion status is most important; when unsure of category, therapy for more severe category is recommended.
Data from American Academy of Pediatrics[10] and Holliday et al.[12]

TABLE 117-2 Comparison of Common Solutions Used in Oral Rehydration and Maintenance

Product	Na (mEq/L)	K (mEq/L)	Base (mEq/L)	Carbohydrate (mmol/L)	Osmolality (mOsm/L)
Naturalyte (unlimited beverage)	45	20	48	140	265
Pediatric electrolyte (NutraMax)	45	20	30	140	250
Pedialyte (Ross)	45	20	30	140	250
Infalyte (formerly Ricelyte; Mead Johnson)	50	25	30	70	200
Rehydralyte (Ross)	75	20	30	140	310
WHO/UNICEF oral rehydration salts	90	20	30	111	310
Cola[a]	2	0	13	700	750
Apple juice[a]	5	32	0	690	730
Chicken broth[a]	250	8	0	0	500
Sports beverage[a]	20	3	3	255	330

[a]These solutions should be avoided.
From American Academy of Pediatrics.[10]

Maintenance rehydration requires sodium concentrations of 40 to 60 mEq/L, compared to 50 to 90 mEq/L for initial rehydration. ORT solutions with high sodium content may be alternated with water if a low-sodium fluid is not available. The maintenance phase should provide 100 to 150 mL/kg per day plus additional replacement for stool losses. Clear fluids, such as soda, apple juice, broth, and Gatorade should be avoided in both the rehydration and maintenance phase of dehydration. Those solutions are hyperosmolar and may draw free water into the gut lumen and cause hypernatremia. In addition, high glucose concentrations may produce an osmotic diarrhea (see Table 117–2).

Glucose-based ORT primarily prevents dehydration without much influence on the duration of diarrhea or stool volume; low-osmolarity ORT solutions (rice- or cereal-based), however, reduce the diarrhea stool number, volume, and frequency, as well as the duration of diarrhea, and the replacement volume requirements.[11] The efficacy of rice-based ORT solutions may be a result, in part, of their hypotonicity, which promotes intestinal water absorption. Also, slow rice hydrolysis allows some rice (glucose) absorption to take place before hydrolysis occurs. Starch and simple proteins provide more cotransport molecules with a lower intraluminal osmotic load, thus increasing fluid and electrolyte uptake by enterocytes and reducing stool losses. Therefore, a larger carbohydrate load can be given with rice solutions, resulting in a greater nutritional advantage.

If ORT does not improve the fluid status and the patient continues to produce frequent, large-volume watery stools, close supervision with medical support is warranted. Weight loss of 9% to 10% is considered severe and requires IV fluid replacement with Ringer lactate or normal saline. Intravenous fluid therapy is also indicated in patients with uncontrolled vomiting, the presence of a paralytic ileus, stool output greater than 10 mL/kg per hour, shock, or loss of consciousness. Rapid IV rehydration is preferred over more prolonged deficit-replacement regimens for restoring extracellular fluids and electrolytes because it more effectively reestablishes gastrointestinal and renal perfusion.[12] Table 117–1 summarizes fluid-replacement guidelines for each dehydration category.

Early refeeding as tolerated is recommended.[13] The American Academy of Pediatrics guidelines recommend age-appropriate diet resumption as soon as dehydration is corrected.[10] Breast milk, lactose-free soy formula, and cow's-milk-based formulas often can be continued.[8,13] Early initiation of feeding has shortened the course of diarrhea. In a study of severely malnourished children younger than 5 years of age with diarrhea, using a standardized protocol of slower oral rehydration, immediate feeding, and intensive management of complications resulted in a significant reduction of mortality as compared with standard therapy. Initially, easily digested foods, such as bananas, applesauce, and cereal, may be added. Foods high in fiber, sodium, and sugar should be avoided. Lactase deficiency may be exacerbated among known lactase-deficient patients and may persist up to 10 days.

Antimicrobial Therapy

The indiscriminate use of antimicrobial therapy in GI infections produces increases in antimicrobial resistance, side effects of antimicrobial agents, and the threat of superinfections owing to eradication of normal flora. Increasing fluoroquinolone resistance in *Campylobacter* and multidrug resistance in *Salmonella* species worldwide reinforce the importance of judicious use of antibiotics and prudent infection control measures.[14,15] Furthermore, it stresses the need to take local susceptibility patterns into account in the selection of initial choice of antimicrobial regimen.

❸ Antibiotics are not essential in the treatment of most mild diarrheas, and empirical therapy for acute GI infections may result in courses of unnecessary antibiotics. However, appropriate antibiotic therapy shortens the duration of illness and reduces morbidity in some bacterial (cholera, enterotoxigenic *E. coli*, shigellosis, campylobacteriosis, yersiniosis) infections and can be lifesaving in invasive infections (*C. difficile*, salmonellosis). Antibiotic treatment also reduces the duration and shedding of organisms in infections with susceptible *Shigella* species and possibly in infection with susceptible *Campylobacter* species.[16] Table 117–3 summarizes antibiotic recommendations, and further details in the treatment of specific infections are discussed in appropriate sections.

It is also important to note that outcomes of some bacterial diarrheal illnesses may be worsened by the use of antibiotics. Antibiotic treatment may prolong asymptomatic carriage of *Salmonella*.[17] In patients infected with *E. coli* O157, use of an antimicrobial agent may worsen the risk of hemolytic uremic syndrome (HUS), which is defined by the triad of acute renal failure, thrombocytopenia, and microangiopathic hemolytic anemia, by increasing the production of shiga-like toxin.[18]

Antimotility Agents

Antiperistaltic drugs such as diphenoxylate and loperamide offer symptomatic relief in patients with mild diarrhea. However, these agents are contraindicated in most toxin-mediated diarrheal illnesses (enterohemorrhagic *E. coli*, pseudomembranous colitis, shigellosis) and thus should be avoided in patients with high fever and bloody diarrhea. Slowing of fecal transit time is thought to result in extended toxin-associated damage.

PREVENTION OF GASTROINTESTINAL INFECTIONS

❹ Public health measures of improved water supply and sanitation facilities and the quality control of commercial products are important for the control of the majority of enteric infections. In addition, many diarrheal diseases can be prevented by following simple rules of personal hygiene and safe food preparation. Handwashing with soap is instrumental in preventing the spread of illness and should

TABLE 117-3 Recommendations for Antibiotic Therapy

Pathogen	First-Line Agents	Alternative Agents
Enterotoxigenic (cholera-like) diarrhea		
Vibrio cholerae O1 or O139	Doxycycline 300 mg oral single dose; tetracycline 500 mg orally four times daily × 3 days; or trimethoprim-sulfamethoxazole DS tablet twice daily × 3 days; norfloxacin 400 mg orally twice daily × 3 days; or ciprofloxacin 500 mg orally twice daily × 3 days or 1 g orally single dose	Chloramphenicol 50 mg/kg IV every 6 hours, erythromycin 250–500 mg orally every 6–8 hours, and furazolidone
Enterotoxigenic *Escherichia coli*	Norfloxacin 400 mg or ciprofloxacin 500 mg orally twice daily × 3 days	Trimethoprim-sulfamethoxazole DS tablet every 12 hours
Clostridium difficile	Metronidazole 250 mg four times daily to 500 mg three times daily × 10 days	Vancomycin 125 mg orally four times daily × 10 days; bacitracin 20,000–25,000 units four times daily × 7–10 days
Invasive (dysentery-like) diarrhea		
Shigella species[a]	Trimethoprim-sulfamethoxazole DS twice daily × 3–5 days	Ofloxacin 300 mg, norfloxacin 400 mg, or ciprofloxacin 500 mg twice daily × 3 days, or nalidixic acid 1 g/day × 5 days; azithromycin 500 mg orally × 1, then 250 mg orally daily × 4 days
Salmonella		
Nontyphoidal[a]	Trimethoprim-sulfamethoxazole DS twice daily; ofloxacin 300 mg, norfloxacin 400 mg, or ciprofloxacin 500 mg twice daily × 5 days; or ceftriaxone 2 g IV daily or cefotaxime 2 g IV three times daily × 5 days	Azithromycin 1,000 mg orally × 1 day, followed by 500 mg orally once daily × 6 days
Enteric fever	Ciprofloxacin 500 mg orally twice daily × 3–14 days (ofloxacin and pefloxacin equally efficacious)	Azithromycin 1,000 mg orally × 1 day, followed by 500 mg daily × 5 days; or cefixime, cefotaxime, and cefuroxime; or chloramphenicol 500 mg four times daily orally or IV × 14 days
Campylobacter[a]	Erythromycin 500 mg orally twice daily × 5 days; azithromycin 1,000 mg orally × 1 day, followed by 500 mg daily or clarithromycin 500 mg orally twice daily	Ciprofloxacin 500 mg or norfloxacin 400 mg orally twice daily × 5 days
Yersinia species[a]	A combination therapy with doxycycline, aminoglycosides, trimethoprim-sulfamethoxazole, or fluoroquinolones	
Traveler's diarrhea		
Prophylaxis[a]	Norfloxacin 400 mg or ciprofloxacin 500 mg orally daily (in Asia, Africa, and South America); trimethoprim-sulfamethoxazole DS tablet orally daily (in Mexico)	Rifaximin 200 mg one to three times daily × 2 weeks
Treatment	Norfloxacin 400 mg or ciprofloxacin 500 mg orally twice daily × 3 days, or trimethoprim-sulfamethoxazole DS tablet orally twice daily × 3 days (in Mexico), or azithromycin 500 mg orally once daily × 3 days (only in areas of high prevalence of quinolone-resistant *Campylobacter* species, such as Thailand)	Rifaximin 200 mg three times a day or 400 mg twice a day × 3 days

[a]For high-risk patients only. See the preceding text for the high-risk patients in each infection.

be emphasized for caregivers and persons with diarrheal illnesses. Safe food handling and preparation practices can significantly decrease the incidence of certain types of enteric infections.

Reporting suspected outbreaks and cases of notifiable illness to local health authorities is vital in investigation of threats of enteric infection arising from increasingly global and industrialized food supplies. The reporting of specific infectious diseases to the appropriate public health authorities is the cornerstone of public health surveillance, outbreak detection, and prevention and control efforts.

Vaccines are used to boost specific immune processes directed against the bacteria themselves or against adherence appendages, cytotoxins, or enterotoxins. Unfortunately, there are only a few vaccines available for prevention of gastroenteritis. Currently available vaccines for typhoid fever are the parenteral Vi capsular polysaccharide vaccine and the oral live-attenuated Ty21a vaccine.[19] Both vaccines have efficacy of 50% to 80%.[31] A new rotavirus vaccine, RotaTeq, licensed in 2006, is intended for infants ages 6 weeks through 32 weeks. The three-dose regimen's efficacy is 74%.[20]

PATIENT ASSESSMENT

Appropriate followup care of patients with acute diarrhea is based on successful restoration of fluid losses. The clinical signs and symptoms (see Table 117–1) that led to the diagnosis also can indicate adequate rehydration and should be assessed frequently. Because oral rehydration therapy is now preferred, routine laboratory testing often is unnecessary. Electrolytes should be measured in those receiving parenteral fluids, when oral replacement fails, or when signs of hypernatremia or hypokalemia are present. Followup stool samples to ensure complete evacuation of the infecting pathogen may be necessary only in patients who are at high risk to initiate or contribute to a community outbreak. All patients should be monitored for complications associated with the infecting pathogen, resolution of the diarrhea, and adverse reactions to the pharmacologic agents used. One panel suggests prompt discharge of hospitalized children when rehydration is achieved, IV fluids have not been required, oral intake equals or exceeds losses, or adequate family education and medical followup are ensured. For most patients, discharge can occur in 16 to 24 hours.

BACTERIAL INFECTIONS

Bacterial agents are important causes of GI infections, and syndromes caused by these pathogens are better understood than viral gastroenteritis. For a simple generalization, the bacterial pathogens presented in this section are divided into either those that cause watery (enterotoxigenic) diarrhea or those that cause dysentery (invasive diarrhea). Watery diarrhea is usually self-limiting, whereas those who present with dysenteric symptoms, such as fever, tenesmus, and blood and/or pus in the stool, require close monitoring and intensive follow-up. Table 117–4 lists the clinical signs and symptoms of these two broad categories.

TABLE 117-4 Acute Infectious Diarrhea Clinical Syndromes: Watery vs. Dysenteric

	Watery	Dysenteric
Percentage of patients	90	5–10
Stools		
Appearance	Watery	Bloody
Volume	Increased: ++/+++	Increased: +/++
Number per day	<10	>10
Reducing substances	0 to +++	0
pH	5.0–7.5	6.0–7.5
Occult blood	Negative	Positive
Fecal polymorphonuclear cells	Absent or few	Many
Mechanisms	Toxins Reduced absorption	Mucosal invasion
Complications		
Dehydration	Could be severe	Mild
Others	Acidosis, shock, electrolyte imbalance	Tenesmus, rectal prolapse, seizures
Etiology	Rotaviruses Enterotoxigenic *Escherichia coli* *Vibrio cholerae*	*Shigella* spp. *Campylobacter* spp. *Salmonella enteritidis*

From Guerrant et al.[7] *and Armon et al.*[8]

ENTEROTOXIGENIC (CHOLERA-LIKE) DIARRHEA

Cholera (*Vibrio cholerae*)

Epidemiology Cholera has been endemic in the Ganges delta, West Bengal, Bangladesh, and southern Asia (including Southeast Asia) since at least 1817.[21] A 1994 outbreak of a multidrug-resistant strain of cholera among Rwandan refugees resulted in more than 20,000 deaths. Cholera epidemics in 1991 and 1998 caused more than 1 million deaths in Latin America. As international travel has increased, cholera has also been reported in all major regions of the United States. However, the incidence, 1 case per 1 million persons, is extremely low.[22]

V. cholerae O1 is the most common serogroup associated with epidemics and pandemics. Within this serogroup, there are two biotypes, classic and El Tor.[21] In 1992, a new serogroup, *V. cholerae* O139 Bengal, appeared in India and spread rapidly through Southeast Asia. Four mechanisms for transmission have been proposed, including animal reservoirs, chronic carriers, asymptomatic or mild disease victims, and water reservoirs.

A relatively large inoculum of 10^3 to 10^6 organisms is required for infection if water is the vehicle and 10^2 to 10^4 if the vehicle is food. Approximately half the people infected with *V. cholerae* O1 are symptomatic, whereas only 1% to 5% of those infected with *V. cholerae* O139 manifest symptoms. The hallmark of cholera is the production of watery diarrhea, and severe dehydration may develop within a few hours, causing death within 24 hours. An estimated 25% to 50% of cases are fatal if left untreated. The prevention of cholera transmission depends on the provision of clean drinking water and public sanitation, which is difficult in impoverished developing countries.[21]

Pathogenesis *V. cholerae* is a gram-negative bacillus sharing similar characteristics with the family Enterobacteriaceae. Most pathology of cholera results from an enterotoxin (cholera toxin) produced by the bacteria.[21] Conditions that reduce gastric acidity, such as the use of antacids, histamine receptor blockers, or proton pump inhibitors or infections with *Helicobacter pylori,* increase the risk for clinical disease. Cholera toxin stimulates adenylate cyclase, which increases intracellular cyclic adenosine monophosphate (cAMP) and results in inhibition of sodium and chloride absorption by microvilli and promotes the secretion of chloride and water by crypt cells. The toxin likely acts along the entire intestinal tract, but most fluid loss occurs in the duodenum.[23] The net effect of the cholera toxin is isotonic fluid secretion (primarily in the small intestine) that exceeds the absorptive capacity of the intestinal tract (primarily the colon). This results in the production of watery diarrhea with electrolyte concentrations similar to that of plasma.

Clinical Presentation The average incubation period for *V. cholerae* infection is 1 to 3 days.[23] The clinical presentation can vary from asymptomatic to life-threatening dehydration owing to watery diarrhea. Patients may lose up to 1 L of isotonic fluid every hour. The onset of diarrhea is abrupt and is followed rapidly or sometimes preceded by vomiting. Fever occurs in less than 5% of patients, and the physical examination correlates well with the severity of dehydration. In some cases, fluid accumulates within the intestinal lumen causing abdominal distension and ileus and may cause intravascular depletion without diarrhea. In the most severe state, this disease can progress to death in 2 to 4 hours if not treated.

Laboratory abnormalities, such as increased packed red blood cell volume and total protein, magnesium, and calcium levels, are a result of hemoconcentration. Hypoglycemia, seizures, fever, and mental alterations are seen more often in children, perhaps as a reflection of the greater degree of dehydration and electrolyte losses observed with diarrhea in children.[21,23] Other complications include metabolic acidosis, prerenal azotemia, iatrogenic water intoxication from overhydration, and aspiration pneumonia. Children, the elderly, and pregnant women are at an increased risk of complications caused by cholera.

TREATMENT

Cholera

Regardless of the serotypes, the primary goal of therapy is restoration of fluid and electrolyte losses caused by watery diarrhea. ORT is the preferred method of rehydration, and several studies showed reduction in fluid requirements by 32% to 35% when rice-based instead of glucose-based ORT solutions are used (50 to 80 g rice instead of 20 g glucose/L).[24] In patients who cannot tolerate ORT, IV Ringer lactate solution can be used. Normal saline is not recommended because it does not correct metabolic acidosis. After rehydration, maintenance fluid is given based on accurate recording of intake and output volumes.

Antibiotics shorten the duration of diarrhea, decrease fluid loss, and shorten the duration of the carrier state.[23] There appears to be substantial mobility in genetic elements encoding antibiotic resistance in *V. cholerae*, and the drug resistance patterns may change between outbreaks. For example, O139 strains isolated during 1992 and 1993 showed a trend toward increased resistance to trimethoprim-sulfamethoxazole, but those isolated in India during 1996 and 1997 showed susceptibility to the same agent.[23] A single dose of doxycycline is the preferred agent, especially in endemic areas, although it has been associated with prolonged fecal excretion of bacteria. In children younger than 7 years of age, trimethoprim-sulfamethoxazole, erythromycin, and furazolidone are preferred. In pregnant women, erythromycin or furazolidone can be used. In areas of high tetracycline resistance, fluoroquinolones such as ciprofloxacin are effective. Ciprofloxacin has been studied more extensively than other fluoroquinolones.[25]

The manufacture of the only licensed whole-cell cholera vaccine in the United States has been discontinued. Two oral vaccines are available in other countries.[23] Dukoral consists of killed *V. cholerae* organisms and the cholera B subunit, and Orochol is an avirulent mutant of *V. cholerae* strain CVD103HgR. Both vaccines are effective in field trials and volunteer studies, but their cost-effectiveness in endemic settings is uncertain. The World Health Organization does not require vaccination for international travel to or from endemic areas because the series of two injections is effective in only 50% of people and immunity wanes in 6 months or less.

Escherichia coli

Diarrheagenic *E. coli* is differentiated into several distinct categories based on pathogenic features of diarrheal disease: enterotoxigenic *E. coli* (ETEC), enteroinvasive *E. coli* (EIEC), enteropathogenic *E. coli* (EPEC), enteroaggregative *E. coli* (EAEC), and enterohemorrhagic *E. coli* (EHEC).[26] The most common diarrheagenic *E. coli* infection is caused by ETEC manifested by watery (enterotoxigenic) diarrhea. Dysentery is caused by EHEC. In this section, commonly known categories of diarrheagenic *E. coli* that cause watery diarrhea are discussed separately from EHEC that cause bloody diarrhea.[26]

Epidemiology ETEC occurs most commonly, and accounts for about half of all cases of *E. coli* diarrhea. There are an estimated 79,420 cases in the United States each year.[26,27] ETEC is the most common cause of traveler's diarrhea and a common cause of food- and water-associated outbreaks. Infections with EIEC and EPEC are primarily a disease of children in developing countries. EAEC strains are implicated in persistent diarrhea (≥14 days) in HIV-infected patients.

Recognized as a common and potentially deadly cause of infectious diarrhea, EHEC is believed to be the major etiologic factor responsible for the development of hemorrhagic colitis and HUS.[28] The CDC estimates the annual disease burden of *E. coli* O157:H7 in the United States to be more than 20,000 infections and as many as 250 deaths, but the failure of many clinical laboratories to screen for this organism greatly complicates any estimates. In the United States, serotype O157:H7 causes 50% to 80% of all EHEC infections, but in the southern hemisphere, such as Argentina, Australia, Chile, and South Africa, non-O157:H7 serotypes are often more important.[28] Transmission usually occurs via food and water, and outbreaks have been associated with undercooked ground beef and feces-contaminated vegetables.[28]

Pathogenesis *E. coli* is a gram-negative bacillus commonly found in the human GI tract as well as in intestines of healthy cattle, deer, goats, and sheep. Enterotoxigenic *E. coli* are capable of producing either or both plasmid-mediated enterotoxins: heat-labile toxin and heat-stable toxin.[29] A cholera-like toxin, heat-labile toxin has two subunits (A and B) that have similar antigenic properties and action on the gut mucosa. The net effect is luminal accumulation of electrolytes that draws water into the intestine, and production of a cholera-like secretory diarrhea. Heat-stable toxin is nonantigenic and produces watery diarrhea by acting on the small intestine.[28]

The mode of pathogenesis of the non-ETEC varieties is less-well understood. The hallmark histopathologic lesions of EPEC infections is the effacing of microvilli and intimate adherence between the bacterium and the epithelial cell membrane throughout the intestine. These attaching and effacing lesions disrupt the integrity of the intestinal epithelium, leading to diarrhea. EAEC adheres to intestinal mucosal cells by mucus production and deposition of bacteria in a bacterium–mucus biofilm. This persistent colonization of EAEC potentially leads to cytotoxic damage of intestinal cells, resulting in persistent diarrhea. EIEC closely resembles *Shigella* species and penetrates the intestinal mucosa; predominantly the lining of the large intestine. The resulting histological damage is inflammation and mucosal ulceration which are characteristic of bacillary dystentery.[26]

The pathogenicity of EHEC is related to the production of shiga-like toxins, so named because of their resemblance to the shiga toxin of *Shigella dysenteriae*.[28] The cytotoxic effect of shiga-like toxins disrupts the mucosal integrity of the large intestine causing diarrhea. In addition, the toxin is able to pass through the intestinal epithelium to reach the endothelial cells lining small blood vessels that supply the gut, kidney, and other viscera, causing the myriad metabolic events that eventually lead to HUS.

Clinical Presentation Nausea and watery stools, with or without abdominal cramping, are characteristic of the disease caused by ETEC.[26] Usually there is no blood or pus in the stool. Signs and symptoms depend directly on the extent of fluid loss, which in most cases is subclinical. Most ETEC diarrhea is typically abrupt in onset and resolves within 24 to 48 hours without complication. Common symptoms of EPEC infection include acute onset of profuse watery diarrhea, vomiting, and low-grade fever. The clinical features of EAEC diarrhea are characterized as persistent, watery, mucoid, secretory diarrhea with low-grade fever and little or no vomiting. EIEC infection presents most commonly as watery diarrhea, which can be indistinguishable from the secretory diarrhea seen with ETEC. However, in a minority of cases, patients experience the dysentery syndrome, manifested as blood, mucus, and leukocytes in the stool with tenesmus and fever.

Symptoms from EHEC infection can be severe, with as many as 11 to 12 bloody stools per day.[29] Initially EHEC infections typically manifest as cramping abdominal pain, abdominal distension, and watery diarrhea. Nausea occurs in about two-thirds of patients, and vomiting occurs in less than half. The white blood cell count is elevated and accompanied by a left shift, but patients often remain afebrile. Within 1 to 2 days the diarrhea becomes bloody with increased abdominal pain. The illnesses typically resolves in 1 week; however in approximately 2% to 7% of cases, particularly in children younger than 5 years of age and the elderly, the disease causes a complication termed HUS. This syndrome is defined by a triad of hemolytic anemia, thrombocytopenia, and renal failure. Death may occur rarely, usually as a result of HUS.[28]

TREATMENT

Escherichia coli Diarrhea

The cornerstone of management of all diarrheagenic *E. coli* infection is to prevent dehydration by correcting fluid and electrolyte imbalances. ORT is often lifesaving in infants and children.[27] Although antimicrobial prophylaxis with doxycycline, trimethoprim-sulfamethoxazole, or a fluoroquinolone is effective in preventing ETEC diarrhea, the growing problem of antibiotic resistance and the possibility of adverse effects from antimicrobial agents deter recommendations of prophylaxis. Instead, experts recommend avoiding risk factors while traveling. In addition, if significant disease occurs, bismuth subsalicylate and loperamide are effective in decreasing the severity of ETEC diarrhea, and empirical antibiotics shorten the duration of the disease.[30] Fluoroquinolones (e.g., ciprofloxacin, norfloxacin, and ofloxacin) are the most commonly recommended agents owing to increasing antimicrobial resistance among other drug classes.

CLINICAL CONTROVERSY

Loperamide should not be used in patients with fever or dysentery because antimotility agents are contraindicated in the management of diarrhea caused by EHEC. There is evidence that the use of such agents can increase the risk for development of HUS, possibly by delaying intestinal clearance of the organism and thereby increasing toxin absorption.

The use of antibiotics remains controversial in EHEC infection.[31] Their use may be harmful because of lysis of bacteria leading to increased release of toxin and alteration of normal intracolonic bacterial flora, thereby increasing the systemic absorption of the toxin. Treatment of EHEC infection is primarily limited to supportive care, which may include dialysis, hemofiltration, transfusion of packed erythrocytes, platelet infusions, and other interventions as indicated clinically.[29] Severe disease may cause chronic kidney failure and require renal transplant.

Pseudomembranous Colitis (*Clostridium difficile*)

Epidemiology Pseudomembranous colitis (PMC) was first reported in 1893 and was associated with antibiotic therapy in 1955. Although described in the preantibiotic era, the incidence increasingly has been associated with antibiotic administration. *C. difficile* is thought to be the cause in 10% to 20% of patients experiencing antibiotic-associated diarrhea, in 50% to 75% of those with antibiotic-associated colitis, and in greater than 90% of those with antibiotic-associated PMC.[32] It is also the most common cause of nosocomial diarrhea, infecting 16% to 20% of inpatients, one-third of whom are symptomatic.[33]

The incidence of intestinal colonization is variable, ranging from 30% to 70% in infants to 3% to 5% in healthy adults.[32] The relationship between the colonized state and active disease is poorly understood. Many people are colonized with the bacteria yet do not go on to develop PMC. It occurs most often in high-risk groups, such as the elderly, debilitated patients, cancer patients, surgical patients, patients receiving antibiotics, patients with nasogastric tubes, and patients who frequently use laxatives.[33] PMC is associated with use of broad-spectrum antimicrobials, including clindamycin, ampicillin, and third-generation cephalosporins.[32] Other agents that have been implicated, albeit at a lower incidence rate, include aminoglycosides, erythromycin, fluoroquinolones, trimethoprim-sulfamethoxazole, and, surprisingly, vancomycin and metronidazole, two of the most commonly used antimicrobials for treatment of *C. difficile*.[32]

Pathogenesis *C. difficile* is a gram-positive spore-forming anaerobic bacillus and causes a toxin-mediated disease. Once antibiotics disrupt normal colonic flora and colonization of *C. difficile* occurs, two toxins (A and B) are released to mediate diarrhea and colitis. This toxin production is essential in disease manifestation. Toxin A is the major pathogenic factor and has been characterized as an enterotoxin that causes intestinal fluid secretion, mucosal injury, and inflammation through actin disaggregation, intracellular calcium release, and damage to neurons. Toxin B is a nonenterotoxic cytotoxin that causes depolymerization of filamentous actin and mediates more potent damage to human colonic mucosa than toxin A. Initially, raised white and yellowish plaques form, and the surrounding mucosa may be inflamed. With progression of disease, these pseudomembranous plaques become enlarged and scatted over the colorectal mucosa.[34]

Clinical Presentation *C. difficile* infection may cause a spectrum of disease from mild antibiotic-associated diarrhea to pseudomembranous entercolitis.[34] In colitis without pseudomembrane formation, patients present with malaise, abdominal pain, nausea, anorexia, watery diarrhea, low-grade fever, and leukocytosis. PMC is characterized by more severe illness, with severe abdominal pain, perfuse diarrhea, high fever, marked leukocytosis, and classic pseudomembrane formation evident with sigmoidoscopic examination. Symptoms can start a few days after the start of antibiotic therapy or several weeks after antibiotics have been discontinued.

C. difficile infection should be suspected in patients experiencing diarrhea with a recent history of antibiotic use (within the previous 2 months) or in those whose diarrhea began 72 hours after hospitalization. Diagnosis can be established by detection of toxin A or B, stool culture for *C. difficile,* or endoscopy. If the stool sample is negative, a second analysis is recommended because the testing sensitivity may be increased with repeat testing. Endoscopy should be reserved for situations where rapid diagnosis is needed, ileus is present, a stool is not available, or other colonic diseases are in the differential diagnosis.[35]

TREATMENT

Pseudomembranous Colitis

Initial therapy should include discontinuation of the offending agent with a change to an alternative antibiotic if possible.[32] Fluid and electrolyte replacement therapy is necessary. Although diarrhea will resolve in 15% to 23% of patients without therapy, most patients require antibiotics. Both vancomycin and metronidazole are effective, but metronidazole 250 mg orally four times daily is the drug of choice.[32] It is similar to vancomycin in time to resolution of diarrhea, incidence of side effects, and relapse rates. However, it is less expensive than vancomycin, and the concern for vancomycin resistance promotes metronidazole use.

Oral vancomycin 125 mg four times daily is second-line therapy. Its use is appropriate in the following situations: the patient has not responded to oral metronidazole; the organism is resistant to metronidazole; the patient is allergic or intolerant to metronidazole; treatment includes ethanol-containing solutions; the patient is either pregnant or younger than 10 years of age; the patient is critically ill because of *C. difficile* diarrhea or colitis; and there is evidence suggesting that the diarrhea is caused by *S. aureus.*[32] The duration of diarrhea is reduced to 3 versus 4.6 days with metronidazole. Vancomycin must be administered orally because IV vancomycin does not achieve gut lumen concentrations high enough for effective bacterial elimination.

Bacitracin is third-line treatment. In resolving symptoms, 80,000 units of bacitracin orally daily is as effective as vancomycin but is not as effective in eradicating the organism. Bacitracin's poor taste, which reduces patient adherence, limits its use.[35] Teicoplanin and fusidic acid have been effective in resolving symptoms and eradicating the organism.[35]

Relapse after antibiotic treatment occurs in approximately 20% to 25% of patients and does not appear to be influenced by the choice of initial therapy, dose of drug used, or duration of treatment.[32] Recurrences occur because of the persistence of the spore forms of *C. difficile* that are not killed by antibiotic therapy or reinfection by a new strain. Recurrences usually occur 3 to 21 days after antibiotics are stopped. Retreatment with metronidazole or vancomycin at the previous dose for 10 to 14 days generally is successful. The addition of rifampin to vancomycin also has been effective.[32]

CLINICAL CONTROVERSY

Some investigators have found prophylaxis with competing, nonpathogenic organisms such as *Lactobacillus* spp. or *Saccharomyces* spp. to be helpful in preventing relapse in small numbers of patients.[36] It is thought that these organisms help to restore the natural flora in the gut and make patients more resistant to colonization by *C. difficile.*

Vancomycin has been used in combination with anion-exchange resins dosed to avoid drug-resin binding, and this has been used successfully in a small number of cases.[35] Cholestyramine 4 g orally three to four times daily and colestipol 5 g orally twice daily have been used as alternatives to antibiotics in mild cases.

Drugs that inhibit peristalsis, such as diphenoxylate, are contraindicated in PMC.[32] Slowing of fecal transit time is thought to result in extended toxin-associated damage. Strict handwashing and contact precautions are imperative measures in preventing the spread of the organism. *C. difficile* can be cultured in rooms of infected individuals up to 40 days after discharge.[35]

INVASIVE (DYSENTERY-LIKE) DIARRHEA

Bacillary Dysentery (Shigellosis)

Epidemiology Approximately 450,000 cases of shigellosis occur in the United States and 165 million cases occur in the world annually, resulting in more than 1 million deaths worldwide each year.[37] Shigellosis is primarily a disease of children, with the highest incidence in children between the ages of 6 months and 5 years. Only a third of all cases occur in adults. Most cases result from fecal–oral transmission. A few well-documented food- and water-associated outbreaks have been reported. Peak incidence in the United States is in late summer.

The shigellae have worldwide distribution, with regional differences in prevalence of subgroups responsible for disease. Four species most often associated with disease are *S. dysenteriae* type I, *Shigella flexneri, Shigella boydii,* and *Shigella sonnei.*[37] In the United States, the common causes of shigellosis are *S. sonnei* and *S. flexneri.* Cases caused by other shigellae are successfully acquired during travel to developing countries. Because of overuse of antibiotics in human and animal feed, Southeast Asia and India have higher levels of resistance. Poor sanitation, poor personal hygiene, inadequate water supply, malnutrition, and increased population density are associated with an increased risk of *Shigella* gastroenteritis epidemics, even in developed countries.

Pathogenesis The shigellae are gram-negative bacilli belonging to the family Enterobacteriaceae. Ingestion of as few as 10 to 200 viable organisms of the *Shigella* species causes disease in healthy adults, explaining the ease with which the disease is transmitted from person to person.[38] The bacteria multiply and spread within the submucosa of the small bowel, but they rarely extend beyond the mucosa. Penetration of the mucosa is conferred genetically by large "invasion plasmids" and results in distortion of the crypts, death to intestinal epithelium, causing focal ulceration, sloughing of mucosal cells, bloody mucoid exudate into the gut lumen, and submucosal accumulation of inflammatory cells with microabscess formation.[39] Microabscesses eventually may coalesce, forming larger abscesses. Infection frequently involves the entire colon. In addition to the virulence characteristics of invasiveness, *S. dysenteriae* type 1 and, to lesser degree, *S. flexneri* and *S. sonnei* produce a cytotoxin, or shiga toxin, the pathogenic role of which is unclear, although it is thought to damage endothelial cells of the lamina propria, resulting in microangiopathic changes that can progress to HUS.[40]

Clinical Presentation Initial signs and symptoms include abdominal pain, cramping, and fever followed by frequent watery stools.[41] Within a few days, patients experience a decrease in fever, severe abdominal pain, and tenderness prior to the development of bloody diarrhea and other signs of dysentery (see Table 117–4). Stools are often greenish in color and contain leukocytes. Fluid and electrolyte losses may be significant, particularly in infants and elderly patients. In the early stages of the disease, stool cultures are positive. A rapid diagnostic test kit that uses DNA amplification by the polymerase chain reaction is also available.

If left untreated, bacillary dysentery usually lasts about 1 week (range: 1 to 30 days). Complications are unusual but may include severe dehydration, generalized seizures, septicemia, toxic megacolon, perforated colon, arthritis, protein-losing enteropathy, and HUS. Mortality is rare, but it may be more likely with *S. dysenteriae* type I. Less than 3% of persons who are infected with *S. flexneri* will later develop Reiter syndrome, characterized by pains in the joints, irritation of the eyes, and painful urination. This can lead to chronic arthritis.[42]

TREATMENT

Bacillary Dysentery (Shigellosis)

Shigellosis is usually a self-limiting disease. Most patients recover in 4 to 7 days, although 10% may experience a recurrence. Oral fluid and electrolyte replacement is the foundation of treatment (dysentery is not generally associated with significant fluid loss). However, intravenous fluid replacement therapy may be necessary, especially in children and the elderly.

Owing to the self-limiting nature of the illness and rapid development of antimicrobial resistance on completion of therapy, antibiotic treatment is reserved for the elderly and infirm, those who are immunocompromised, children in daycare centers, malnourished children, and healthcare workers. Antibiotics shorten the period of fecal shedding and attenuate the clinical illness. The choice of agent depends on location (see Table 117–3). For infections acquired in the United States, the agent of choice is trimethoprim-sulfamethoxazole (only 4% resistance). For infections acquired outside the United States, the agents of choice are ciprofloxacin, norfloxacin, and azithromycin.[16]

Antimotility agents such as diphenoxylate are not recommended because they can worsen bacillary dysentery and could be involved in the development of toxic dilatation of the colon. Oral vaccines currently in development contain attenuated strains of *Shigella* and provide protection against shigellosis in human challenges.[43]

Salmonellosis

Epidemiology *Salmonella* species are gram-negative bacilli belonging to the family Enterobacteriaceae. As a result of DNA hybridization experiments, the classification and nomenclature of *Salmonella* spp. have been changing, causing much confusion.[44] Owing to a high degree of DNA similarity, all important *Salmonella* isolates have been classified into a single species, *Salmonella enterica,* with approximately 2,500 different serotypes. Because various serotypes were known formally as species, it has been acceptable to refer to serotypes as species. For example *S. enterica* serotype Typhi is commonly referred to as *Salmonella typhi.*

Specific *Salmonella* serotypes produce characteristic human disease.[45] *S. enterica* serotypes Typhimurium or Enteritidis causes gastroenteritis, whereas serotypes Typhi or Paratyphi causes enteric fever. Clinical manifestations produced by *Salmonella* serotypes commonly include acute gastroenteritis (enterocolitis), bacteremia, extraintestinal localized infection, enteric fever (typhoid and paratyphoid fever), and a chronic carrier state.

In the United States, approximately 1.4 million cases of salmonellosis, 16,000 hospitalizations, and 600 deaths occur annually.[4] There is decreasing incidence in rates of salmonellosis in the United States, which is believed to be a result of improved food-handling practices and water treatment. Salmonellosis is a disease primarily of infants, children, and adolescents. Children younger than 5 years of age account for approximately 25% of all diagnosed cases.[17] Conditions that may predispose to infection include those which decrease gastric acidity, antibiotic use, malnutrition, and immunodeficiency states. Contaminated food or water has been implicated in the majority of cases. Direct fecal–oral transmission occurs less frequently but is particularly important in children. Foods most often implicated in human salmonellosis are poultry, poultry products, beef, pork, and dairy products. Pets, particularly reptiles, are a common source of infection.

Pathogenesis The incubation period, symptoms, and disease severity depend on the amount of organism ingested. The inoculum necessary for infection is estimated to less than 1,000 organisms, and this infectious dose is lowered in patients with achlorhydria (gastric pH >4.0). If the organisms survive the gastric acid barrier, mucosal invasion of the small intestine begins.[46] After penetration, microorganisms translocate to the intestinal lymphoid follicles and the draining mesenteric lymph nodes, in addition to the reticuloendothelial cells of the liver and spleen. Thereafter, the ability of organisms to survive and multiply within the mononuclear phagocytic cells of the lymphoid follicles, liver, and spleen plays an instrumental role in the pathogenesis. In the asymptomatic phase, the organisms are sequestered intracellularly. Once the critical number of organisms has been reached, bacteria are released into the bloodstream, and the symptoms of enteric fever are manifested. This dissemination of organisms via bloodstream also causes secondary infection in the liver, spleen, bone marrow, gallbladder, and Peyer patches of the terminal ileum. After several weeks of infection, recruitment of mononuclear cells and lymphocytes induced by *Salmonella* is thought to be responsible for necrosis of Peyer patches and the abdominal pain observed in enteric fever.[46]

The mechanism by which nontyphoidal salmonellae cause enterocolitis is less-well understood. Although a number of enterotoxins have been described in salmonellae, their role remains illusive.[47] Some salmonellae, such as *S. enterica* serotype Choleraesuis, which is the most invasive, are frequently associated with bacteremia and metastatic localization, whereas others seldom cause disease. Enterocolitis often is characterized by massive neutrophil infiltration into both the large and small bowel mucosa. The serotypes that are responsible for human illness cause intestinal epithelial cells to secrete interleukin 8, a potent neutrophil chemotactic factor. Degranulation and release of toxic substances by neutrophils may contribute to inflammation and result in tissue damage, fluid secretion, or leakage across the intestinal mucosa.

Clinical Presentation ***Enterocolitis.*** Most patients experience symptoms within 72 hours of ingestion of contaminated food or water.[47] Patients often complain of nausea and vomiting followed by abdominal cramps, headache, fever, and diarrhea, although the actual presentation is quite variable. Some patients do not have increased stool frequency, whereas others have more than 1 stool per hour. Stools generally are loose and may be mucoid or bloody (dysentery-like) or both. Febrile episodes usually range between 37.7°C and 38.8°C (100°F and 102°F) but may be higher. Some evidence suggests that fever of 40°C (104°F) or higher is associated with shorter bacterial excretion.[48] Diarrhea and fever usually resolve spontaneously within 1 to 5 days but may last 2 weeks.

Stool cultures inevitably yield the causative organism if obtained early (i.e., in patients hospitalized less than 3 days).[7] Recovery of organisms continues to decrease with time so that by 3 to 4 weeks, only 5% to 15% of adult patients are passing *Salmonella.* Infants and children tend to pass bacteria for longer periods than adults. Some patients may continue to shed *Salmonella* for a year or longer. These "chronic carrier" states are rare for serotypes other than Typhi.[46]

Bacteremia. Salmonellae can produce bacteremia without classic enterocolitis or enteric fever. Bacteremia rarely occurs in older adults, but it can occur in up to 40% of infants.[49] It is also reported more frequently in persons with severe underlying illness or immunosuppression, including AIDS. The clinical syndrome is characterized by persistent bacteremia and prolonged intermittent fever with chills. Stool cultures frequently are negative. This clinical syndrome is most frequent with serotype Choleraesuis infections (50%). Leukocyte counts are often within the normal range.

Localized Infections. Localized infections develop in 5% to 10% of patients with bacteremia.[47] Extraluminal infection or abscess formation or both can occur at any site. They may follow any of the other syndromes, or they may be the primary presentation. Metastatic infections involve bone, cysts, heart, kidney, liver, lungs, pericardium, spleen, and tumors. The clinical presentation usually is determined by the organ systems involved. Polymorphonuclear leukocyte counts often are elevated.

Enteric Fever (Typhoid and Paratyphoid). Enteric fever caused by serotype Typhi is called typhoid fever.[46] If caused by any other serotype, it is referred to as paratyphoid fever. The clinical presentations of typhoid fever and paratyphoid fever generally are indistinguishable, although paratyphoid fever tends to be less severe than typhoid fever. The incubation period can range from 10 to 14 days. The onset of symptoms is gradual. Nonspecific symptoms of fever, dull headache, malaise, anorexia, and myalgia are most common. Initially, fever tends to be remittent, but it progresses gradually over the first week to temperatures that are often sustained higher than 40°C (104°F). Other frequently encountered symptoms include chills, nausea, vomiting, cough, weakness, and sore throat. Symptoms subside slowly within 4 weeks.

Physical examination generally reveals an acutely ill patient. An erythematous maculopapular rash known as *rose spots* appears primarily on the abdomen in 15% to 50% of patients. The abdomen also may be tender, particularly in the lower quadrants. Hepatomegaly, splenomegaly, or both also may be present in 50% of the cases, and cervical lymph nodes may be enlarged.

A normochromic anemia may develop rapidly without evidence of GI blood loss, although intestinal bleeding may be contributory. Leukopenia may be reflective of a relative decrease in polymorphonuclear leukocytes. White blood cell counts may range from 1,200 to 20,000 cells/mm^3. As many as one-third of the patients have elevated levels of the liver enzymes glutamic-oxaloacetic transaminase and alkaline phosphatase in serum. Approximately 80% of patients have positive blood cultures. Bacteremia persists in about a third of cases for several weeks if not treated. Intestinal perforation, intestinal hemorrhage, thrombophlebitis, toxemia with circulatory collapse, encephalopathy, and pneumonia all contribute to a fatality rate of 1% to 2%. Without treatment, mortality may be 10%.[46]

TREATMENT

Salmonellosis

■ ENTEROCOLITIS

Fluid and electrolyte replacement is the primary mode of treatment. Most patients respond well to ORT (self-limited illness).[47] Antimotility drugs should be avoided because they increase the risk of mucosal invasion and complications. Antibiotic therapy is not indicated in healthy adults. Antibiotics have no effect on the duration of fever or diarrhea, and their frequent use increases the likelihood of resistance and the duration of fecal shedding. Antibiotics should be used in (a) neonates or infants younger than 6 months of age because young children have an increased risk of complicated infection, (b) patients with primary or secondary immunodeficiency such as AIDS or chemotherapy patients, (c) severely symptomatic patients with fever and bloody diarrhea, and (d) patients after splenectomy.[47] Susceptibility testing is recommended because many drug-resistant strains of *Salmonella* have emerged. Recommended antibiotics include the fluoroquinolones, trimethoprim-sulfamethoxazole, ampicillin, and third-generation cephalosporins. If susceptibility results are not available, a fluoroquinolone or third-generation cephalosporins should be instituted owing to resistance with trimethoprim-sulfamethoxazole and ampicillin. Azithromycin and aztreonam also have been studied and may be used as alternative agents.

■ BACTEREMIA AND LOCALIZED INFECTIONS

Owing to increasing resistance, empirical therapy for life-threatening bacteremia or focal infections following nontyphoidal *Salmonella* infection should include both a third-generation cephalosporin (such as ceftriaxone 2 g IV daily) and a fluoroquinolone (ciprofloxacin 500 mg orally twice daily) until the susceptibilities are known.[49] The duration of antibiotic therapy is dictated by the site of infection. Bacteremia without endovascular infection should be treated for 7 to 14 days. In documented or suspected endovascular infection, 6 weeks of intravenous therapy with ampicillin or ceftriaxone is recommended. Chloramphenicol is no longer recommended in patients with endovascular infection owing to high rates of failure.

■ ENTERIC FEVER (TYPHOID AND PARATYPHOID)

Antibiotic choice is dictated by susceptibility testing.[46] Fluoroquinolones are the drugs of choice for the treatment of enteric fever.[50] A short course of 3 to 5 days is effective in uncomplicated enteric fever, but a minimum of 10 days is recommended in severe cases. In patients who are infected with fluoroquinolone-susceptible *S. enterica* serotype Typhi, the average time for defervescence is less than 4 days, and the cure rates exceed 96%, with fewer than 2% of treated patients having persistent fecal carriage or relapse. Unfortunately, fluoroquinolone resistance is increasing in some areas, and these strains are also often multidrug-resistant, limiting the choice of antibiotics. Among patients with fluoroquinolone-resistant *S. enterica* serotype Typhi infection, fluoroquinolones still can be used but at the maximal possible dose for a minimum of 10 to 14 days. These patients should be monitored carefully to determine whether they are excreting the organism in their feces. High-dose fluoroquinolone regimens have been successful in 90% to 95% of patients with multidrug-resistant infection.[51] However, the average time to defervescence is 7 days, and the rate of fecal carriage during convalescence can be as high as 20%.

The third-generation cephalosporins (e.g., ceftriaxone, cefixime, cefotaxime, and cefoperazone) and azithromycin are also effective drugs for typhoid. Chloramphenicol, amoxicillin, and trimethoprim-sulfamethoxazole remain appropriate for the treatment of typhoid fever in areas of the world where the bacterium is still fully susceptible to these drugs and where the fluoroquinolones are not available or affordable.[46] Although fluoroquinolones are not recommended in children, the pediatric use of ciprofloxacin in areas where multidrug-resistant *S. typhi* occurs is acceptable. In pregnant women, the β-lactam antibiotics are safe, and there are some case reports to support fluoroquinolone use.

Adults and children with severe enteric fever characterized by delirium, obtundation, stupor, coma, or shock benefit from prompt administration of dexamethasone 1 mg/kg every 6 hours for 24 to 48 hours.[52] Two vaccines against *S. typhi* are licensed in the United States: an orally administered vaccine (Ty21a, Vivotif Berna) and a parenteral polysaccharide vaccine (ViCPS, Typhim Vi).[19] The efficacy of these vaccines ranges from 42% to 77%, and immunity persists for 3 to 5 years. The Ty21a and Vi vaccines are recommended for travelers to areas of endemic disease and those in high-risk groups, including household contacts of *S. typhi* carriers, laboratory technicians with repeated exposure, and sanitation workers in endemic areas. Because the Ty21a vaccine is a live-attenuated vaccine, it should not be administered to immunocompromised persons, patients taking antibiotics, or patients with gastroenteritis.

■ "CHRONIC CARRIERS" OF *SALMONELLA*

"Chronic carriers" of *Salmonella* usually have negative stool cultures at 12 weeks after the onset of illness, but some may have continued positive stool cultures at 6 to 12 months. Chronic fecal shedding of *Salmonella* has been associated with chronic biliary infection and cholelithiasis. To alleviate the chronic carrier state, the drug of choice is norfloxacin 400 mg orally twice daily for 28 days. In addition, amoxicillin and trimethoprim-sulfamethoxazole are effective in eradicating the bacteria in greater than 80% of cases after 6 weeks of therapy.[17] Chronic carriers should take preventative measures (i.e., antibiotics and hygiene) so that they do not serve as reservoirs of infection to the community.

Campylobacteriosis

Epidemiology The *Campylobacter* spp. are flagellated, curved, gram-negative rods that are thought to be one of the most common bacterial causes of diarrheal illnesses worldwide. Although there are 14 different species, *C. jejuni* is the species responsible for more than 99% of *Campylobacter*-associated gastroenteritis.[53] In the United States, the incidence of *Campylobacter* infection decreased 26% from 1996 to 1999. However, surveillance studies indicate that *Campylobacter* spp. remain the most commonly isolated enteric pathogen, detected two to seven times more frequently than *Salmonella* or *Shigella.*[53] Currently, the CDC estimates that 2.4 million persons are affected each year in the United States, involving almost 1% of the entire population.

In developed countries, the peak incidence of *Campylobacter* infections occurs in children younger than 1 year of age and in young adults 15 to 44 years of age. The incidence is also higher in males than in females, although the reason for this is unknown. Patients with AIDS are particularly susceptible; the incidence in AIDS patients is 40 times that of the general population.[53] Most reported cases occur during the summer months, beginning in May and peaking in August. In tropical developing countries, *Campylobacter* infections are common among children younger than 2 years of age, and asymptomatic infections of children and adults are more common than those seen in industrialized nations. This decrease in the case-to-infection ratio suggests that previous exposure confers immunity to the infecting strain.

The transmission of infection occurs primarily by ingestion of contaminated food or water. Although *Campylobacter* spp. have varied reservoirs, such as livestock, dogs, cats, and birds, the consumption of chicken is the major vector of infections in industrialized nations.[54] Poultry products are nearly always contaminated with *Campylobacter* spp. during the slaughtering process, and it is estimated that 1 drop of chicken juice may contain 500 infectious organisms. Although public education emphasizes safe handling and cooking of chicken, it is easy to see how simple errors may result in human illness.

Pathogenesis *Campylobacter* spp. are labile in acidic environments, much like *Salmonella.* Therefore, an inoculum of approximately 800 organisms is required to initiate infection. Conditions in the upper small intestine are favorable for multiplication. Flagella-mediated adherence and tissue invasion by bacteria have been demonstrated in the jejunum, ileum, and colon. Infection results in an acute inflammatory enteritis. *C. jejuni* can produce an enterotoxin or cytotoxin.[55] Both cytotoxins and enterotoxins may be produced in many strains. Symptom manifestation depends on immunity. Patients infected with *Campylobacter* develop specific immunoglobulin (Ig) G, IgM, and IgA antibodies in serum and IgA antibodies in intestinal secretions. Volunteer studies indicate that immunity does protect against illness.

Clinical Presentation The average incubation period of *Campylobacter* is 2 to 4 days.[53] The most common presenting symptoms include diarrhea, abdominal pain, and fever. Nausea, vomiting, headache, myalgia, and malaise also may occur. Bowel movements may be numerous, bloody (dysentery-like), and foul smelling, and range from loose to watery. Cramping and abdominal pain usually are relieved by defecation. In 75% of cases, leukocytes and red blood cells are detected in the stool samples. Peripheral leukocytosis also may be present. The disease usually is self-limited to about 1 week, but it may persist for several weeks in 10% to 20% of patients. The case-fatality rate is 0.05 per 1,000 infections.

Complications, including pseudoappendicitis, pancreatitis, gastrointestinal hemorrhage, thrombophlebitis, abscess, septicemia, peritonitis, empyema, urinary tract infection, and cholecystitis, are uncommon, but occur more frequently in those who are immunocompromised. *C. jejuni* has been associated with Guillain-Barré syndrome (GBS), but the relationship is not well understood.[56] *C. jejuni* infections are a common trigger of GBS, accounting for approximately 30% of GBS cases, but the risk of developing GBS after *C. jejuni* infection appears to be low (<1 case of GBS per 1,000 *C. jejuni* infections). A reactive arthritis may develop several weeks after infection in persons with the HLA-B27 histocompatibility antigens.[42] Diagnosis is made by stool culture, but the bacteria sometimes are identifiable with Gram stain or carbol-fuchsin stain.

TREATMENT

Campylobacteriosis

The primary treatment of campylobacteriosis is oral fluid and electrolyte replacement.[53] Most people recover from this self-limiting disease in 4 to 7 days. Antibiotics are *not* useful unless started within 4 days of the start of the illness because they do not shorten the duration or severity of diarrhea but only shorten the duration of bacterial excretion. However, antibiotics are warranted in patients who present with high fevers, severe bloody diarrhea, prolonged illnesses (>1 week), pregnancy, and immunocompromised states, including HIV infection (see Table 117–3).

C. jejuni is susceptible to a wide variety of antimicrobial agents.[53] Fluoroquinolone resistance has increased to 10% to 13% in the United States (41% to 88% in Europe and Asia) in recent years, and may be a result of the use of quinolone antibiotics in poultry feed and their frequent use overseas in treating enteric infections. Erythromycin is considered the drug of choice owing to its low cost, high efficacy, safety profile, and ease of administration. Newer macrolides such as clarithromycin and azithromycin are equally effective. Tetracycline, chloramphenicol, clindamycin, and aminoglycosides may be effective.[53] Antimotility agents such as loperamide are contraindicated because slowing fecal transit time may extend the duration of infection and increase toxin mucosal invasion.

Yersiniosis

Yersinia spp. are non-lactose-fermenting gram-negative coccobacilli that are widely distributed in nature. The genus *Yersinia* includes six species known to cause disease in humans. *Y. enterocolitica* and, to lesser extent, *Yersinia pseudotuberculosis* are most likely associated with intestinal infection, but overall, both are a relatively infrequent cause of diarrhea and abdominal pain. More than 50 serotypes of *Y. enterocolitica* exist; of these, serotypes 0:3, 0:8, and 0:9 are associated most frequently with enterocolitis.[57] Infections are reported commonly from northern Europe, and the peak incidence occurs during the winter months.

Children are most likely to experience illness with *Y. enterocolitica* infection.[58] Transmission of infection occurs frequently by ingestion of contaminated food or water. The organisms have been isolated from a variety of food sources, including pigs and raw goat and cow milk. Refrigeration does not deter the development of adherence and invasive virulence factors.

Y. enterocolitica invade the intestinal epithelium and penetrate the intestinal mucosa.[59] An inoculum of 10^9 organisms may be required for infection. Most strains produce an enterotoxin, but the role of toxin production in causing diarrhea is not well established. However, this infection causes mucosal ulcerations in the terminal ileum, necrotic lesions in Peyer patches, and enlargement of mesenteric lymph nodes.

Clinical Presentation These bacteria cause a wide spectrum of clinical syndromes.[58] Most patients with *Y. enterocolitica* infection present with enterocolitis that is mild and self-limiting. Symptoms include vomiting, abdominal pain, diarrhea, and fever; up to 60% of patients will have blood-streaked stools. Diarrhea resolves after 1 to 3 weeks, but bacteria excretion may continue for up to 3 months after diarrhea subsides. Most patients with this type of infection are younger than 5 years of age. In older children and adolescents, mesenteric adenitis and/or terminal ileitis with fever, right lower quadrant pain, and leukocytosis are common. Mesenteric adenitis, which is difficult to distinguish from acute appendicitis, is also seen in patients infected with *Y. pseudotuberculosis*.

Approximately 10% to 30% of adult patients develop a reactive arthritis 1 to 2 weeks after recovery from enteritis. This arthritis, involving the knees, ankles, toes, fingers, and wrists, usually resolves in 1 to 4 months but may persist in approximately 10% of patients.[42] This complication is more common in persons with the HLA-B27 antigen. Other postinfection complications include erythema nodosum, exudative pharyngitis, pneumonia, empyema, and lung abscess. Although rare, *Y. enterocolitica* bacteremia has been reported in patients with diabetes mellitus, severe anemia, hemochromatosis, cirrhosis, and malignancy. Other groups at risk include the elderly and those who received frequent red blood cell transfusions (iron overload).[60] These patients are at increased risk for hepatic or splenic abscesses, peritonitis, septic arthritis, osteomyelitis, wound infections, meningitis, and endocarditis.

TREATMENT

Yersiniosis

Oral fluid and electrolyte replacement is an important initial approach. Owing to the self-limiting nature of the illness, antibiotics may not alter the time to resolution of the diarrhea or the rate of bacteriologic cure. Antibiotics should be used in high-risk patients who develop bacteremia (i.e., infants younger than 3 months of age and patients with cirrhosis or iron overload) or in patients with bone and joint infections.[58]

Drugs of choice are not yet identified. Fluoroquinolones alone or in combination with third-generation cephalosporins or aminoglycosides may be effective for *Yersinia* bacteremia or for those with bone and joint infections.[58] Other antibiotics effective in vitro are chloramphenicol, tetracyclines, and trimethoprim-sulfamethoxazole. Agents frequently resistant to *Yersinia* are penicillin G, ampicillin, and first-generation cephalosporins.

ACUTE VIRAL GASTROENTERITIS

Acute viral gastroenteritis was unknown until the 1970s. Viruses are now recognized as the leading cause of diarrhea in the world, although in many cases an exact pathogen cannot be determined. In Asia, Africa, and Latin America, viral gastroenteritis accounts for an estimated 3 to 5 billion cases and is associated with 5 to 10 million deaths.[82] Viruses that cause gastroenteritis include rotavirus, calicivirus, enteric adenovirus, and astrovirus. Other viruses, such as toroviruses, coronaviruses, picobirnaviruses, and pestiviruses, are being identified increasingly as causative agents of diarrhea.

ROTAVIRUSES

Epidemiology

Rotavirus is the most common cause of diarrhea in infants and children worldwide, and 1 million people die annually from the infection. In the United States, approximately 3.5 million cases of diarrhea, 500,000 physician visits, 50,000 hospitalizations, and 20 deaths occur each year in children younger than 5 years of age.[62] Serologic surveys show that nearly all children are infected by age 5 years, but dehydrating diarrhea occurs primarily among young children ages 3 to 35 months during their initial infection.[63] Thereafter, they are shielded from severity of subsequent infection. In fact, after the initial infection with rotavirus, 40% of children are protected against subsequent infection, 75% are protected against subsequent gastroenteritis, and up to 88% are protected against severe gastroenteritis. Unfortunately, both immunocompromised children and adults are at increased risk for severe, prolonged, and even fatal rotavirus gastroenteritis. The fecal–oral route is thought to be the most common mode of transmission. In the United States, rotavirus infection rates peak from November to May each year.

Pathogenesis

Rotaviruses are double-stranded, wheel-shaped, RNA viruses. The outermost layer contain two structural viral proteins. The protease-cleaved protein (P protein) VP4 and the glycoprotein (G protein) VP7 define the serotype of the virus and are the basis for vaccine development. Once ingested, these strains cause diarrhea by inducing changes in transepithelial fluid balance, malabsorption as a consequence of destruction of epithelial lining of intestine, and vacular damage and ischemia of villi. Changes to the villi include shortening of villus height, crypt hyperplasia, and mononuclear cell infiltration of the lamina propria.[64]

Clinical Presentation

The incubation period of rotavirus infection is typically 1 to 3 days.[65] Clinical manifestations vary from asymptomatic (which is common in adults) to severe nausea, vomiting, and diarrhea with dehydration. Because the first infection tends to be the most severe, dehydration and electrolyte disturbances occur more frequently in children. The symptoms begin abruptly, with vomiting often preceding the onset of diarrhea. Fever is present in a third of patients. Other signs and symptoms include respiratory symptoms, irritability, lethargy, pharyngeal erythema, rhinitis, red tympanic membranes, and palpable cervical lymph nodes. These gastrointestinal symptoms resolve in 3 to 7 days.

Laboratory findings reflect the degree of vomiting, diarrhea, or both. Transient rises in liver enzymes may be seen in 60% of children hospitalized for rotavirus diarrhea. The white blood cell count is usually normal. Stools rarely contain blood or leukocytes. Rotavirus detection in stool samples is possible with an enzyme immunoassay and a latex agglutination assay, both of which are available commercially.

TREATMENT

Rotavirus Infection

Oral fluid and electrolyte replacement is the cornerstone of treatment.[66] Oral *Lactobacillus* therapy may reduce the duration of diarrhea and of viral excretion. There is no role for antibiotics in acute infection. Bismuth subsalicylate, although shown to decrease the duration of diarrhea and stool output, is not recommended for routine use because of the self-limiting nature of the disease and the risk of bismuth subsalicylate overdose. Antimotility agents are not recommended because they do not decrease the duration or volume of diarrhea.

The first vaccine (RotaShield) to prevent rotavirus infection was licensed for use in the United States in 1998, but it was withdrawn after 1 year because of an increased rate of idiopathic intussusception.[67] Postlicensure surveillance found that the risk for intussusception was the highest within 3 to 14 days after receipt of the first dose, which was estimated to be 1 case per 10,000 vaccine recipients.[68] There was also a suggestion that the risk was age-dependent, and possibly infants younger than 3 months were in less danger than older ones.

In 2006, a live, oral vaccine (RotaTeq) received its licensure in United States. This is a pentavalent vaccine that contains five reassortant rotaviruses.[20] Because these viral strains are derived by inserting the gene encoding capsid protein from G1, G2, G3, or G4 human rotavirus strain into a bovine rotavirus backbone, they contain segmented genome from different parents and are referred to as *reassortant rotaviruses*. Four reassortant rotavirus express one of the outer capsid proteins, G types (G1 to G4), and the fifth expresses the attachment protein, P1A. Therefore, this vaccine provides protection against the serotypes G1, G2, G3, and G4 when administered as a three-dose series to infants between the ages of 6 and 32 weeks. After completion of a three-dose regimen, the vaccine offered protection against any rotavirus infection of 74% and severe gastroenteritis of 98%.[68] This oral vaccine decreased office visits because of rotavirus infection by 86%, emergency department visits by 94%, and hospitalizations by 96%. Moreover, the vaccinated children showed similar cases of intussusception as nonvaccinated children (six cases versus five cases; adjusted relative risk of 1.6; confidence interval [CI] = 0.4 to 6.4). Other serious side effects, including deaths, were similar among vaccine and placebo recipients. There were small but significantly greater rates of vomiting, diarrhea, nasopharyngitis, otitis media, and bronchospasm among vaccine recipients. Concurrent administration of this rotavirus vaccine did not diminish the immune responses of other vaccines, diphtheria, tetanus toxoids, and acellular pertussis (DTaP), *Haemophilus influenzae* type b vaccine, inactivated poliovirus vaccine, hepatitis B vaccine, and pneumococcal conjugate vaccine.

Another rotavirus vaccine, RotaRix, has completed clinical trials and received licensure in many Latin America countries. A trial of this monovalent vaccine, based on an attenuated human rotavirus strain of P1A G1 specificity, in approximately 60,000 infants, has shown a clinical efficacy of 85% against severe rotavirus disease, and no increase in intussusception among vaccine recipients.[69]

CALICIVIRUSES

The human caliciviruses are assigned to two genera, Norovirus and Sapovirus, responsible for gastroenteritis. The Norovirus causes illness in all age groups, whereas Sapovirus causes illness mainly in children.[70] Although the relative importance of these viruses as causes of GI infections is unknown, Noroviruses are important causes of outbreaks. The Norwalk virus was the first of norovirus to be described in 1972 in Norwalk, Ohio.

As with most viruses, the epidemiology of the norovirus is not well understood. The disease commonly affects children and adults, but it is not often associated with disease in neonates and preschool children.[80] Outbreaks occur throughout the year and have been documented in families, healthcare systems, cruise ships, and college dormitories. Noroviruses are often spread from person to person. Other vectors of transmission include contaminated water supplies, fecal–oral spread, and food-borne outbreaks. Almost any food that has come in contact with contaminated water can serve as a vehicle for an outbreak. A major source of food-borne gastroenteritis is contamination of shellfish beds from raw sewage dumped into the water supply.

The pathophysiology of this disease is similar to that caused by the rotavirus. Human volunteer studies show histopathologic changes in the jejunum within 24 hours of viral challenge, and clinical manifestations appear within 48 hours.[70] The exact mechanisms of virus-induced vomiting or diarrhea are unknown. Brush-border enzyme activity may be decreased, resulting in lactose intolerance, but it generally returns to preinfection levels within 2 weeks. Virus shedding in the stool can occur over the first 24 to 48 hours after illness.

Gastroenteritis caused by norovirus is characterized by sudden onset of abdominal cramps with nausea, vomiting, or both.[71] Although adults frequently experience nonbloody diarrhea, and children experience vomiting more often than diarrhea. Other complaints are myalgia, headache, and malaise, which are accompanied by fever in approximately 50% of patients. Signs and symptoms generally last 12 to 48 hours.[71]

The disease is generally self-limiting. Oral fluid and electrolyte replacement should be used, if necessary.[71] A norovirus vaccine produced via expression of viral antigens in plants is under investigation, but the clinical availability of such a product is several years in the future.

ASTROVIRUSES

Astroviruses increasingly are being recognized as important causes of gastroenteritis. Astroviral illness is often reported in children younger than 3 years of age, but it also been described in adults and elderly.[72] Astroviruses have been detected in the stools of children, as well as in patients with immunodeficiency conditions such as HIV infection or bone marrow transplantation. Transmission is suspected to occur via the fecal–oral route. Outbreaks have been reported in schools, daycare settings, and pediatric wards. The pathogenesis of astroviral infection is believed to be similar to that noted for rotavirus. The clinical presentation consists of diarrhea, headache, malaise, nausea, and to lesser extent, vomiting. These symptoms appear to be similar to those observed with rotavirus but milder. The incubation period is estimated to be 3 to 4 days, and the disease is usually self-limiting within 5 days. Maintenance of adequate hydration and electrolyte balance is the only therapeutic issue. The duration of viral shedding may be as long as 35 days.[73]

ENTERIC ADENOVIRUS

Adenovirus is an icosahedral virus previously associated with respiratory, ocular, and genitourinary infections; however, serotypes 40 and 41 are GI pathogens. The peak incidence is in children younger than 2 years of age, and infections occur year-round. Transmission is primarily person to person and fecal–oral, and viral shedding from the gut may occur for extended periods. The incubation time is 8 to 10 days. Diarrhea and vomiting often last 1 to 2 weeks. Low-grade fever and respiratory symptoms are also common.[74] The diagnosis can be made by enzyme immunoassay that identifies serotypes.

OTHER POTENTIAL VIRAL PATHOGENS

Although less-commonly associated with severe GI disease, pestivirus, torovirus, and coronavirus-like particles have been recovered from diarrheal stools. In HIV-infected patients, the presence of diarrhea is associated with virus in 35% of stool specimens. Astrovirus, picobirnavirus, calicivirus, and adenovirus appear to be the most commonly isolated viral pathogens.[75] Table 117–5 presents specific characteristics of these agents.

TRAVELER'S DIARRHEA

Traveler's diarrhea describes the clinical syndrome manifested by malaise, anorexia, and abdominal cramps followed by the sudden onset of diarrhea that incapacitates many travelers.[76] Traveler's diarrhea interferes with planned activities or work in 30% of those affected, accounting for unknown but substantial direct and indirect lost dollars because of decreased productivity.[77] In particular, an increased risk lies with North Americans and northern Europeans traveling to Latin America, southern Europe, Africa, and Asia. The highest risk is observed with patients with immunocompromised conditions, achlorhydria, or inflammatory bowel disease, and people taking diuretics, digoxin, lithium, or insulin (because of the need for appropriate hydration). Overall, an estimated 20% to 50% of people traveling to high-risk areas will develop the illness.

❺ The onset of symptoms usually occurs during the first week of travel but can occur anytime during the visit or after returning home.[76] Traveler's diarrhea is caused by contaminated food or water. Foods at high risk for contamination include raw or undercooked meat and seafood and raw fruits and vegetables. Tap water, ice, and unpasteurized milk and dairy products are also associated with increased risk. The most common pathogens are bacterial in nature and include ETEC (20% to 72%), *Shigella* (3% to 25%), *Campylobacter* (3% to 17%), and *Salmonella* (3% to 7%).[76] Viruses (0% to 30%) are also potential causes, as are parasites, although they are rare during short-term travels, accounting for less than 5% of cases. The severity of the syndrome is determined by the number of stools per day and the presence or absence of cramping, nausea, and vomiting. Mild diarrhea is defined as 1 to 4 loose stools per day that are associated with abdominal cramps lasting less than 14 days. Moderate diarrhea indicates more than 4 loose stools daily associated with dehydration and severe diarrhea is defined as presence of fever or blood in stools. Traveler's diarrhea is rarely life-threatening and in most cases, symptoms resolve in 1 to 2 days without treatment. Travelers to high-risk areas should pack a kit that includes a thermometer, loperamide, 3 days of antibiotics (see Prevention below), oral rehydration solution salts, and a water purification method.[78]

TABLE 117-5 Agents Responsible for Acute Viral Gastroenteritis and Diarrhea

Virus	Peak Age of Onset	Time of Year	Duration	Mode of Transmission	Symptoms
Rotavirus	6 mo–2 y	October to April	3–8 days	Fecal–oral, water, food	Vomiting, diarrhea, fever, abdominal pain, lactose intolerance
Enteric adenovirus	<2 y	Year-round	7–9 days	Fecal–oral	Diarrhea, respiratory symptoms, vomiting, fever
Calicivirus	3 mo–6 y	Peak in winter	4 days	Fecal–oral, water, shellfish	Vomiting, diarrhea
Astrovirus	<7 y	Winter	1–4 days	Fecal–oral, water, shellfish	Vomiting, diarrhea, fever, abdominal pain
Pestivirus	<2 y	NR	3 days	NR	Mild
Coronavirus-like particles	<2 y	Fall and early winter	7 days	NR	Respiratory disease
Enterovirus	NR	NR	NR	NR	Mild diarrhea, secondary organ damage
Norwalk	>5 y	Variable	12–24 h	Fecal–oral, food, aerosol	Nausea, vomiting, diarrhea, abdominal cramps, headache, fever, chills, myalgia

NR, not reported.

From Wilhelmi et al.,[61] Koopmans et al.,[70] Bresee et al,[71] and Taterka et al.[74]

PREVENTION

❻ Patient education in avoiding high-risk food and beverages is the best method for minimizing the risk. High-risk foods and beverages include moist foods served at room temperature, fruit that cannot be peeled, milk from a questionable source, hot sauces on the table, tap water, unsealed bottle water, iced drinks, and food from a street vendor. Slogans such as "Peel it, boil it, cook it, or forget it" remind travelers to avoid contaminated food and to use water purification or reliable bottled beverages.[78] These measures can decrease the risk to less than 15%, even in endemic areas.

Bismuth subsalicylate 524 mg (2 tablets, caplets, tablespoonfuls) orally four times daily for up to 3 weeks is a commonly recommended prophylactic regimen.[79] Bismuth subsalicylate may inhibit enterotoxin activity and prevent diarrhea. Persons taking this regimen should be informed of adverse events, including temporary black discoloration of tongue and stools, and, rarely, tinnitus.

Although efficacy of prophylactic antibiotics have been documented, their uses are discouraged owing to the increased risk of selection of drug-resistant organisms, side effects of antibiotics (e.g., photosensitivity), and possible acquisition of more severe infections. Prophylactic antibiotics (see Table 117–3) are recommended only in high-risk individuals or in situations in which short-term illness could ruin the purpose of the trip, such as a military mission.[76]

A nonabsorbed oral rifamycin, rifaximin, has activity against enteric pathogens and may have a role in prevention of traveler's diarrhea. A randomized, double-blind trial of rifaximin 200 mg once, twice, or three times daily with meals for 2 weeks resulted in equal protection of 72% with each of the three dosing regimens compared to placebo.[80] Notably, rifaximin did not alter colonic flora and coliform or enterococcal antimicrobial susceptibility patterns. Consequently, chemoprophylaxis with rifaximin may be beneficial in high-risk individuals with underlying medical conditions or those on tight schedules where short-term illness could ruin the purpose of the trip. Rifaximin has a tolerability and safety profile comparable to that of placebo.

TREATMENT

Traveler's Diarrhea

Fluid and electrolyte replacement should be initiated at the onset of diarrhea. (ORT generally is not required in otherwise healthy individuals; flavored mineral water offers a good source of sodium and glucose.[76]) For symptom relief, loperamide (preferred because of its quicker onset and longer duration of relief relative to bismuth) should be taken (4 mg orally initially and then 2 mg with each subsequent loose stool to a maximum of 16 mg/day in patients without bloody diarrhea and discontinued if symptoms persist for more than 48 hours). Other symptomatic therapy includes bismuth subsalicylate 525 mg every 30 minutes up to 8 doses.

Antibiotics (see Table 117–3) are recommended in addition to loperamide in travelers who develop three or more loose stools in an 8-hour period, especially with nausea, vomiting, abdominal cramps, fever, or blood in stools. Currently, the drug of choice is a fluoroquinolone usually given for 3 to 5 days.[76] In clinical trials, 3 days of antibiotic therapy is as effective as 5 days, and some studies indicate that single-dose treatment may be effective in most cases.[81,82] In pregnant women and children younger than 16 years of age, a combination of trimethoprim-sulfamethoxazole and erythromycin has been suggested. Macrolides are the drugs of choices only in areas of high prevalence of *Campylobacter* species resistant to quinolones, such as Thailand.

Rifaximin was as effective as a 3-day course of ciprofloxacin in shortening the duration of diarrhea in noninvasive traveler's diarrhea.[83] However, rifaximin was not as effective in patients with fever and bloody diarrhea and in those with invasive pathogens. Therefore, rifaximin 200 mg three times a day for 3 days has been approved for the treatment of traveler's diarrhea caused by noninvasive strains of *E. coli*. A dosage of 400 mg two times per day for 3 days has also been shown to be effective.[84]

FOOD POISONING

❼ Food poisoning results from the ingestion of food containing pathogenic microorganisms, preformed toxins that were produced by microorganisms, or other toxic compounds. In the United States, food-borne disease causes approximately 76 million illnesses, 325,000 hospitalizations, and 5,200 deaths each year.[4] Food-borne transmission may account for up to 35% of acute gastroenteritis cases caused by unknown agents. A number of bacteria can cause food poisoning (Table 117–6). Common bacterial (*Campylobacter, Salmonella, Shigella, E. coli, Yersinia, Vibrio*) and viral (Norovirus) causes of GI infections were discussed in the preceding sections. Other common food-borne pathogens that cause gastroenteritis include *S. aureus, Bacillus cereus, C. perfringens,* and *Clostridium botulinum*. Unfortunately, sporadic illnesses caused by these agents are not reportable through passive or active systems, and thus it is difficult to determine their disease burden.

Because food-borne disease can appear as sporadic cases or outbreaks, the diagnosis should be suspected whenever two or more people present with acute gastrointestinal or neurologic manifestations after sharing a meal within the previous 72 hours. Important clues about etiologic agents can be gathered from demographic information (age, gender, etc.), the clinical syndrome, incubation period, medical history, type of foods consumed, seasonality, and geographic location of the outbreak.

Staphylococcal food poisoning results from the ingestion of food contaminated by an enterotoxin produced by certain strains of *S. aureus* growing within the food.[85] Enterotoxin production generally results from leaving foods at room temperature, allowing the staphylococci to grow. Symptoms are rapid in onset, generally occurring within 1 to 6 hours of ingestion of preformed toxin-containing foods. The condition is characterized by nausea and vomiting (75%), although abdominal cramps and diarrhea also may be present. Symptoms resolve in less than 12 hours. ORT should be provided in severe cases, but antibiotics are not indicated.

B. cereus causes two different types of clinical syndromes.[86] The first one is characterized by a short incubation period with vomiting, abdominal cramps, and to a lesser extent, diarrhea within 1 to 6 hours of ingestion of contaminated food. This syndrome is caused by a preformed heat-stable toxin. Similar to staphylococcal food poisoning, illnesses caused by *B. cereus* usually last less than 12 hours. The second syndrome has a longer incubation period (8 to 16 hours) and is caused by toxins produced in vivo after the ingestion of contaminated food. In this syndrome, patients experience diarrhea, abdominal cramps, and less frequently, vomiting. The heat-labile enterotoxin produced in this syndrome activates intestinal adenylate cyclase and causes intestinal fluid secretion. This illness usually resolves within 24 hours, but symptom durations of several days to weeks also have been observed.

Food-borne *C. perfringens* infection may present as two distinct syndromes.[87] Type A organisms are seen in Western nations and result in a 24-hour illness characterized by watery diarrhea and epigastric pain. Symptoms generally resolve within 24 hours. This enterotoxin-related syndrome damages the brush borders of epithelial cells at the villus tips to cause a noninflammatory diarrhea. Type C organisms can be found in undercooked pork and occur in underdeveloped tropical regions. Type C organisms can produce a toxin-related syndrome called *enteritis necroticans,* which is a coag-

TABLE 117-6 Food Poisonings

Organism	Time to Symptoms (h)	Principal Foods	Peak Incidence (U.S.)	Principal Mechanism of Pathophysiology	Duration	Treatment
Staphylococcus aureus	1–6	Salad, pastries, ham, poultry	Summer	Preformed toxins A–E (heat stable)	12 h	Supportive
Bacillus cereus	1–6	Meats, vegetables, fried rice	None	Preformed toxin	12 h	Supportive
	8–16			Toxin production (in vivo)	24 h	Supportive
Clostridium perfringens (type A)	6–24	Meats, poultry	Fall, winter, spring	Toxin production (in vivo)	24 h	Supportive
Vibrio parahaemolyticus	16–72	Shellfish	Spring, summer, fall	Toxin production and tissue invasion	2–7 days	Supportive
Salmonella spp.	16–48	Beef, poultry, water, eggs, dairy products	Summer	Tissue invasion	2–7 days	Supportive
Shigella spp.	16–48	Salad, water	Summer	Tissue invasion	2–7 days	Supportive
EPEC	16–48	Water	None	Tissue invasion	2–7 days	Supportive
Campylobacter	16–48	Poultry, dairy products, clams, water	Spring, summer	Tissue invasion	2–7 days	Supportive
ETEC	16–72	Water	None	Toxin production (in vivo)	1–7 days	Supportive
Vibrio cholerae	16–72	Water		Toxin production (in vivo)	2–12 days	Supportive, antibiotics
Yersinia enterocolitica	16–48	Dairy products		Toxin production and/or tissue invasion	1–30 days	Supportive
Clostridium botulinum	12–72	Canned fruits, vegetables, meats, honey	None	Preformed toxins A, B, and E (children and adults) Toxin production (in vivo) (infants)		Supportive (including mechanically assisted ventilation), trivalent antitoxin

EPEC, enteropathogenic *E. coli*; ETEC, enterotoxigenic *E. coli*.

ulative transmural necrosis of the intestinal wall. This syndrome can result in intestinal perforation leading to sepsis and mortality in approximately 40% of victims.

Food-borne botulism results from the ingestion of food contaminated with preformed toxins or toxin-producing spores from *C. botulinum. C. botulinum* poisoning is relatively rare; only 110 cases are reported per year in the United States. Botulism is almost always associated with improper preparation or storage of food. Seven distinct toxins (A to G) have been described. The toxins, which are produced by the bacteria and released on lysis, are the most potent biologic or chemical toxins known to humans. The toxin prevents the release of acetylcholine at the peripheral cholinergic nerve terminal. Toxin activity has prompted the use of minute locally injected doses to treat select spastic disorders, such as blepharospasm, hemifacial spasm, and certain dystonias.[88]

Food-borne botulism is suspected when patients present with acute GI symptoms concurrently or just prior to the onset of a symmetric descending paralysis without sensory or central nervous system involvement. Symptoms usually begin 18 to 24 hours after ingestion and progress over days to weeks. Other symptoms can include blurred vision, photophobia (90%), dysphagia (76%), generalized weakness (58%), nausea and vomiting (56%), and dysphonia (55%). Diagnosis is made by culturing *C. botulinum* from the stool.[89] Guillain-Barré syndrome associated with *C. jejuni* infection has been a common differential diagnosis in patients who present with these symptoms. The difference lies in the onset of neurologic symptoms, which typically occur 1 to 3 weeks after the onset of *C. jejuni* infection, and the condition usually is manifested by an ascending paralysis in *C. jejuni*-associated Guillain-Barré syndrome.[56]

Treatment consists primarily of respiratory support and use of botulinum antitoxin.[90] Respiratory failure may occur prior to involvement of other upper muscle groups. If evaluation is performed within several hours of ingestion, gastric lavage or induction of vomiting is suggested. Cathartics and enemas also can be used to remove residual toxin from the bowel, but they are contraindicated in cases of ileus. Although the effectiveness of antitoxins is unknown, patients diagnosed with botulism should receive botulinum antitoxin. Botulinum antitoxin is a concentrated preparation of equine globulins obtained from horses immunized with toxins A, B, and E. Because trivalent antitoxin is equine in origin, patients should be tested for hypersensitivity before receiving the product intravenously. Other agents used experimentally as adjunctive therapy are guanidine, which antagonizes the effect of botulinum toxin at the neuromuscular junction, and 4-aminopyridine, which increases acetylcholine release.[91] Newer and more effective methods of treatment and prevention are under development, including a botulinum toxin vaccine consisting of nontoxic botulinum fragments. Prevention always should be stressed. Botulinum toxins are heat labile and readily destroyed by 10 minutes of boiling. All home-canned foods should be processed according to directions and boiled, not just warmed, prior to consumption.

In food-borne illnesses, the cornerstone of therapy remains supportive care. ORT is preferred in replenishing and maintaining fluid and electrolyte balance, and intravenous fluid therapy should be reserved for those who are severely ill and cannot tolerate oral therapy. Antiemetics and antiperistaltic agents offer symptomatic relief, but the latter should not be given in patients who present with high fever, bloody diarrhea, or fecal leukocytes. Antimicrobial therapy is not effective in the management of *S. aureus, C. perfringens*, or *B. cereus* food poisonings. In developed countries, many of the food-borne illness can be prevented with proper food selection, preparation, and storage. However, in developing countries, sanitation and clean water supply are larger concerns.

ABBREVIATIONS

AIDS: acquired immunodeficiency syndrome

CDC: Centers for Disease Control and Prevention

EAEC: enteroaggregative *Escherichia coli*

EHEC: enterohemorrhagic *Escherichia coli*

EIEC: enteroinvasive *Escherichia coli*

EPEC: enteropathogenic *Escherichia coli*

ETEC: enterotoxigenic *Escherichia coli*

GBS: Guillain-Barré syndrome

HUS: hemolytic-uremic syndrome

ORT: oral rehydration solution

REFERENCES

1. Kosek M, Bern C, Guerrant RL. The global burden of diarrhoeal disease, as estimated from studies published between 1992 and 2000. Bull World Health Organ 2003;81:197–204.
2. Snyder JD, Merson MH. The magnitude of the global problem of acute diarrhoeal disease: A review of active surveillance data. Bull World Health Organ 1982;60:604–613.
3. Bern C, Martines J, de Zoysa I, et al. The magnitude of the global problem of diarrhoeal disease: A ten-year update. Bull World Health Organ 1992;70:705–714.
4. Lew JF, Glass RI, Gangarosa RE, et al. Diarrheal deaths in the United States, 1979 through 1987: A special problem for the elderly. JAMA 1991;265:3280–3284.
5. Ganarosa RE, Glass RI, Lew JF, et al. Hospitalizations involving gastroenteritis in the United States, 1985: The special burden of the disease among the elderly. Am J Epidemiol 1992;135:281–290.
6. Mead PS, Slutsker L, Dietz V, et al. Food-related illness and death in the United States. Emerg Infect Dis 1999;5:607–625.
7. Guerrant RL, Van Gilder T, Steiner TS, et al. Practice guidelines for the management of infectious diarrhea. Clin Infect Dis 2001;32:331–350.
8. Armon K, Stephenson T, MacFaul R, et al. An evidence and consensus based guideline for acute diarrhoea management. Arch Dis Child 2001;85:132–142.
9. Gavin N, Merrick N, Davidson B. Efficacy of glucose-based oral rehydration therapy. Pediatrics 1996;98:45–51.
10. American Academy of Pediatrics. Practice parameter: The management of acute gastroenteritis in young children. Pediatrics 1996;97:424–435.
11. Gore SM, Fontaine O, Pierce MF. Impact of rice-based oral rehydration solution on stool output and duration of diarrhoea: Meta-analysis of 13 clinical trials. BMJ 1992;304:287–291.
12. Holliday MA, Friedman AL, Wassner SJ. Extracellular fluid restoration in dehydration: A critique of rapid versus slow. Pediatr Nephrol 1999;13:292–297.
13. Sandhu BK. Rationale for early feeding in childhood gastroenteritis. J Pediatr Gastroenterol Nutr 2001;33:S13–S16.
14. Hoge CW, Gambel JM, Srijan A, et al. Trends in antibiotic resistance among diarrheal pathogens isolated in Thailand over 15 years. Clin Infect Dis 1998;26:341–345.
15. Parry CM. Antimicrobial drug resistance in *Salmonella enterica*. Curr Opin Infect Dis 2003;16:467–472.
16. Khan WA, Seas C, Dhar U, et al. Treatment of shigellosis: V. Comparison of azithromycin and ciprofloxacin. A double-blind, randomized, controlled trial. Ann Intern Med 1997;126:697–703.
17. Graham SM. Salmonellosis in children in developing and developed countries and population. Curr Opin Infect Dis 2002;15:507–512.
18. Carter AO, Borczyk AA, Carlson JAK, et al. A severe outbreak of *Escherichia coli* O157:H7–associated hemorrhagic colitis in a nursing home N Engl J Med, 1987;317:1496–1500.
19. Centers for Disease Control and Prevention. Typhoid immunization: Recommendations for the Immunization Practice Advisory Committee (ACIP). MMWR 1990;39:1–5.
20. Centers for Disease Control and Prevention. Prevention of rotavirus gastroenteritis among infants and children: Recommendation of the Advisory Committee on Immunization Practices (ACIP). MMWR 2006;55:1–14.
21. Faruque SM, Albert MJ, Mekalanos JJ. Epidemiology, genetics, and ecology of toxigenic *Vibrio cholerae*. Microbiol Mol Bio Rev 1998;64:1301–1314.
22. Chang MH, Glynn MK, Groseclose SL. Endemic, notifiable bioterrorism-related diseases, United States, 1992–1999. Emerg Infect Dis 2003;9:556–564.
23. Sack DA, Sack RB, Nair GB, et al. Cholera. Lancet 2004;363:223–233.
24. Molla A, Sarker S, Hossain M, et al. Rice-power electrolyte solution as oral-therapy in diarrhea due to *Vibrio cholerae* and *Escherichia coli*. Lancet 1982;1:1317–1319.
25. Khan WA, Bennish ML, Seas C, et al. Randomized, controlled comparison of single-dose ciprofloxacin and doxycycline for cholera caused by *Vibrio cholerae* 01 or O139. Lancet 1996;348:296–300.
26. Nataro JP, Kaper JB. Diarrheagenic *Escherichia coli*. Clin Microbiol Rev 1998;11:142–201.
27. Robins-Browne RM, Hartland EL. *Escherichia coli* as a cause of diarrhea. J Gastroenterol Hepatol 2002;17:467–475.
28. Slutsker L, Ries AA, Greene KD, et al. *Escherichia coli* O157:H7 diarrhea in the United States: Clinical and epidemiologic features. Ann Intern Med 1997;126:505–513.
29. Karch H, Bielaszewask M, Bitzan M, et al. Epidemiology and diagnosis of shiga toxin–producing *Escherichia coli* infections. Diagn Microbiol Infect Dis 1999;34:229–243.
30. Ericsson CD, DuPont HL, Mathewson JJ, et al. Treatment of traveler's diarrhea with sulfamethoxazole and trimethoprim and loperamide. JAMA 1990;263:257.
31. Wong CS, Jelacic S, Habeeb RL, et al. The risk of the hemolytic-uremic syndrome after antibiotic treatment of *Escherichia coli* O157:H7 infections. N Engl J Med 2000;342:1930–1936.
32. Bartlett JG. Antibiotic-associated diarrhea. N Engl J Med 2002;346:334–339.
33. Al-Eidan FA, McElnay JC, Scott MG, et al. Clostridium difficile-associated diarrhea in hospitalized patients. J Clin Pharm Ther 2000;25:101–109.
34. Hurley BW, Nguyen CC. The spectrum of pseudomembranous enterocolitis and antibiotic-associated diarrhea. Arch Intern Med 2002;162:2177–2184.
35. Feteky R. Guidelines for the diagnosis and management of *Clostridium difficile*–associated diarrhea and colitis. Am J Gastroenterol 1997;92:739–750.
36. Elmer GW, Surawicz CM, McFarland LV. Biotherapeutic agents: A neglected modality for the treatment and prevention of selected intestinal and vaginal infections. JAMA 1996;275:870–876.
37. Kotloff KL, Winickoff B, Ivanoff JD, et al. Global burden of *Shigella* infections: Implications for vaccine development and implementation. Bull World Health Organ 1999;77:651–656.
38. DuPont HL, Levine MM, Hornick RB, et al. Inoculum size in shigellosis and implications for expected mode of transmission. J Infect Dis 1989;159:1126–1128.
39. Fernandez MI, Sansonetti PJ. *Shigella* interaction with intestinal epithelial cells determines the innate immune response in shigellosis. Int J Med Microbiol 2003;293:55–67.
40. Keusch GT, Jacewicz M. The pathogenesis of shigella diarrhea: VI. Toxin and antitoxin in *Shigella flexneri* and *Shigella sonnei* infections in humans. J Infect Dis 1977;135:552–556.
41. Lopez EL, Prado-Jimenez V, O'Ryan-Gallardo M. Shigella and shiga toxin-producing *Escherichia coli* causing bloody diarrhea in Latin America. Infect Dis Clin North Am 2000;14:41–65.
42. Hill Gaston JS, Lillicrap MS. Arthritis associated with enteric infection. Best Pract Res Clin Rheumatol, 2003;17:219–239.
43. Katz DE, Coster TS, Wolf MK, et al. Two studies evaluating the safety and immunogenicity of a live, attenuated *Shigella flexneri* 2a vaccine (SC602) and excretion of vaccine organisms in North American volunteers. Infect Immun 2004;72:923–930.
44. Brenner F, Villar R, Angulo F, et al. *Salmonella* nomenclature. J Clin Microbiol 2000;38:2465–2467.
45. Olsen SJ, Bishop R, Brenner FW, et al. The changing epidemiology of *Salmonella*: Trends in serotypes isolated from humans in the United States, 1987–1997. J Infect Dis 2001;183:753–761.
46. Parry CM, Hien TT, Dougan G, et al. Typhoid fever. N Engl J Med 2002;347:1770–1782.
47. Hohmann EL. Nontyphoidal salmonellosis. Clin Infect Dis 2001;32:263–269.
48. El-Radhi AS, Rostila T, Vesikari T. Association of high fever and short bacterial excretion after salmonellosis. Arch Dis Child 1992;67:531–532.
49. Stutman HR. *Salmonella, Shigella,* and *Campylobacter:* Common bacterial causes of infectious diarrhea. Pediatr Ann 1994;23:538–543.
50. Hosek G, Leschinsky D, Irons S, Safranek TJ. Multidrug-resistant *Salmonella* serotype typhimurium—United States, 1996. JAMA 1997;277:1513.
51. Wain J, Hoa NT, Chinh NT, et al. Quinolone-resistant *Salmonella typhi* in Viet Nam: Molecular basis of resistance and clinical response to treatment. Clin Infect Dis 1997;25:1404–1410.
52. Hogan DE. The emergency department approach to diarrhea. Emerg Med Clin North Am 1996;14:673–694.
53. llos BM. *Campylobacter jejuni* infections: Update on emerging issues and trends. Clin Infect Dis 2001;32:1201–1206.

54. Harris NV, Weiss NS, Nolan CM. The role of poultry and meats in the etiology of *Campylobacter jejuni* enteritis. Am J Public Health 1986;76:407–410.
55. Wallis MR. The pathogenesis of *Campylobacter jejuni*. Br J Biomed Sci 1994;51:57–64.
56. Allos BM. Association between *Campylobacter* infection and Guillain-Barré syndrome. J Infect Dis 1997;(Suppl 2):S125–S128.
57. Hoogkamp-Korstanje JAA, de Koning J, Samsom JP. Incidence of human infection with *Yersinia enterocolitica* serotypes O3, O8, and O9 and the use of indirect immunofluorescence in diagnosis. J Infect Dis 1986;153:138–141.
58. Marks MI, Pai CH, LaFleur L, et al. *Yersinia enterocolitica* gastroenteritis: A prospective study of clinical, bacteriologic, and epidemiologic features. J Pediatr 1980;96:26–31.
59. San Joaquin VH. *Aeromonas, Yersinia,* and miscellaneous bacterial enteropathogens. Pediatr Ann 1994;23:544–548.
60. Haverly RM, Harrison CR, Dougherty TH. *Yersinia enterocolitica* bacteremia associated with red blood cell transfusion. Arch Pathol Lab Med 1996;120:499–500.
61. Wilhelmi I, Roman E, Sanchez-Fauquier A. Viruses causing gastroenteritis. Clin Microbiol Infect 2003;9:247–262.
62. Charles MD, Holman RC, Curns At, et al. Hospitalizations associated with rotavirus gastroenteritis in the United States, 1993–2002. Pediatr Infect Dis J 2006;25:489–493.
63. Lundgren O, Svensson L. Pathogenesis of rotavirus diarrhea. Microb Infect 2001;3:1145–1156.
64. Parashar UD, Holman RC, Clarke MJ, et al. Hospitalizations associated with rotavirus diarrhea in the United States, 1993 through 1995: Surveillance based on the new ICD-9-CM rotavirus-specific diagnostic code. J Infect Dis 1998;177:13–17.
65. Centers for Disease Control and Prevention (CDC). Outbreak of severe rotavirus gastroenteritis among children—Jamaica, 2003. MMWR 2003;52:1103–1105.
66. Centers for Disease Control and Prevention. Withdrawal of rotavirus vaccine recommendations. MMWR 1999;48:1007.
67. Peter G, Myers MG. Intussusception, rotavirus, and oral vaccines: Summary of a workshop. Pediatrics 2002:54:1–67.
68. Vesikari T, Matson DO, Dennehy P, et al. Safety and efficacy of a pentavalent human-bovine (WC3) reassortant rotavirus vaccine. N Engl J Med 2006;354:23–33.
69. Ruiz-Palacios GM, Perez-Schael I, Velazquez FR, et al. Safety and efficacy of an attenuated vaccine against severe rotavirus gastroenteritis. N Engl J Med 2006;354:11–22.
70. Koopmans M, von Bonsdorff CH, Vinje J, et al. Food-borne viruses. FEMS Microbiol Rev 2002;26:187–205.
71. Bresee JS, Widdowson MA, Monroe SS, et al. Food-borne viral gastroenteritis: Challenges and opportunities. Clin Infect Dis 2002;35:748–753.
72. Oishi I, Yamazaki K, Kimoto T, et al. A large outbreak of acute gastroenteritis associated with astrovirus among students and teachers in Osaka, Japan. J Infect Dis 1994;170:439–443.
73. Walter JE, Mitchell DK. Astrovirus infection in children. Curr Opin Infect Dis 2003;16:247–253.
74. Taterka JA, Cuff CF, Rubin DH. Viral gastrointestinal infections. Gastroenterol Clin North Am 1992;21:303–329.
75. Grohmann GS, Glass RI, Pereira HG, et al. Enteric viruses and diarrhea in HIV-infected patients. N Engl J Med 1993;329:14–20.
76. Shlim DR. Update in traveler's diarrhea. Infect Dis Clin North Am 2005;19:137–148.
77. von Sonnenburg F, Tornieporth N, Waiyaki P, et al. Risk and aetiology of diarrhea at various tourist destinations. Lancet 2000;356:133–134.
78. Centers for Disease Control and Prevention. Health Information for International Travel 1999–2000. Atlanta, GA: Department of Health and Human Services (also *www.cdc.gov/travel/diarrhea.htm*).
79. Ericsson CD. Nonantimicrobial agents in the prevention and treatment of traveler's diarrhea. Clin Infect Dis 2005;41:S557–S563.
80. DuPont HL, Jiang ZD, Okhuysen PC, et al. A randomized, double-blind, placebo-controlled trial of rifaximin to prevent travelers' diarrhea. Ann Intern Med 2005;142:805–812.
81. DuPont HL, Ericsson CD, Mathewson JJ, et al. Five versus three days of ofloxacin therapy for traveler's diarrhea: A placebo-controlled study. Antimicrob Agents Chemother 1992;36:87–91.
82. Adachi JA, Ericsson CD, Jiang ZD, et al. Azithromycin found to be comparable to levofloxacin for the treatment of US travelers with acute diarrhea acquired in Mexico. Clin Infect Dis 2003;37:1165–1171.
83. Taylor DN, Bourgeois AL, Ericsson CD, et al. A randomized, double-blind, multicenter study of rifaximin compared with placebo and with ciprofloxacin in the treatment of travelers' diarrhea. Am J Trop Med Hyg 2006;74:1060–1066.
84. DuPont HL, Jiang ZD, Ericsson CD, et al. Rifaximin versus ciprofloxacin for the treatment of traveler's diarrhea: A randomized, double-blind clinical trial. Clin Infect Dis 2001;33:1807–1815.
85. Le Loir Y, Baron F, Gautier M. *Staphylococcus aureus* and food poisoning. Genet Mol Res 2003;2:63–76.
86. Schoeni JL, Wong AC. Bacillus cereus food poisoning and its toxins. J Food Prot 2005;68:636–648.
87. Hatheway CL. Toxigenic clostridia. Clin Microbiol Rev 1990;3:66–98.
88. Roblot P, Roblot F, Fauchere JL, et al. Retrospective study of 108 cases of botulism in Poitiers, France. J Med Microbiol 1994;40:379–384.
89. Linstrom M, Korkeala H. Laboratory diagnostics of botulism. Clin Microb Rev 2006;19:298–314.
90. Shapiro RL, Hatheway C, Swerdlow DL. Botulism in the United States: A clinical and epidemiologic review. Ann Intern Med 1998;129:221–228.
91. Middlebrook JL. Protection strategies against botulinum toxin. Adv Exper Med Biol 1995;383:93–98.

CHAPTER 118 Intraabdominal Infections

JOSEPH T. DIPIRO AND THOMAS R. HOWDIESHELL

KEY CONCEPTS

1. Most intraabdominal infections are "secondary" infections that are polymicrobic and are caused by a defect in the gastrointestinal tract that must be treated by surgical drainage, resection, and/or repair.
2. Primary peritonitis generally is caused by a single organism (*Staphylococcus aureus* in patients undergoing chronic ambulatory peritoneal dialysis [CAPD] or *Escherichia coli* in patients with cirrhosis).
3. Secondary intraabdominal infections usually are caused by a mixture of bacteria including enteric gram-negative bacilli and anaerobes, which enhances the pathogenic potential of the bacteria.
4. For peritonitis, early and aggressive intravenous fluid resuscitation and electrolyte replacement therapy are essential. A common cause of early death is hypovolemic shock caused by inadequate intravascular volume and tissue perfusion.
5. Cultures of secondary intraabdominal infection sites generally are not useful for directing antimicrobial therapy. Treatment generally is initiated on a "presumptive" or empirical basis.
6. Antimicrobial regimens for secondary intraabdominal infections should include coverage for enteric gram-negative bacilli and anaerobes. Antimicrobials that may be used for the treatment of secondary intraabdominal infections include (a) a β-lactam–β-lactamase inhibitor combination (such as piperacillin-tazobactam), (b) a carbapenem (imipenem or meropenem), (c) quinolone (ciprofloxacin) plus metronidazole, or an aminoglycoside (gentamicin) plus clindamycin (or metronidazole).
7. Treatment of primary peritonitis for CAPD patients should include an antistaphylococcal antimicrobial such as a first-generation cephalosporin (cefazolin) or vancomycin (usually given by the intraperitoneal route).
8. The duration of antimicrobial treatment should be for a total of 5 to 7 days for most secondary intraabdominal infections.
9. Patients treated for intraabdominal infections should be assessed for the occurrence of drug-related adverse effects, particularly hypersensitivity reactions (β-lactam antimicrobials), diarrhea (most agents), fungal infections (most agents), and nephrotoxicity (aminoglycosides).

Learning objectives, review questions, and other resources can be found at **www.pharmacotherapyonline.com.**

Intraabdominal infections are those contained within the peritoneal cavity or retroperitoneal space. The peritoneal cavity extends from the undersurface of the diaphragm to the floor of the pelvis and contains the stomach, small bowel, large bowel, liver, gallbladder, and spleen. The duodenum, pancreas, kidneys, adrenal glands, great vessels (aorta and vena cava), and most mesenteric vascular structures reside in the retroperitoneum. Intraabdominal infections may be generalized or localized. They may be contained within visceral structures, such as the liver, gallbladder, spleen, pancreas, kidney, or female reproductive organs. Two general types of intraabdominal infection are discussed throughout this chapter: peritonitis and abscess. *Peritonitis* is defined as the acute inflammatory response of the peritoneal lining to microorganisms, chemicals, irradiation, or foreign-body injury. This chapter deals only with peritonitis of infectious origin.

An *abscess* is a purulent collection of fluid separated from surrounding tissue by a wall consisting of inflammatory cells and adjacent organs. It usually contains necrotic debris, bacteria, and inflammatory cells. These processes differ considerably in presentation and approach to treatment.

EPIDEMIOLOGY

Peritonitis may be classified as primary, secondary, or tertiary.[1–3] Primary peritonitis, also called *spontaneous bacterial peritonitis,* is an infection of the peritoneal cavity without an evident source in the abdomen. Bacteria may be transported from the bloodstream to the peritoneal cavity, where the inflammatory process begins. In secondary peritonitis, a focal disease process is evident within the abdomen. Secondary peritonitis may involve perforation of the gastrointestinal (GI) tract (possibly because of ulceration, ischemia, or obstruction), postoperative peritonitis, or posttraumatic peritonitis (blunt or penetrating trauma). Tertiary peritonitis occurs in critically ill patients and is infection that persists or recurs at least 48 hours after apparently adequate management of primary or secondary peritonitis.

❶ Primary peritonitis develops in up to 10 to 30% of patients with alcoholic cirrhosis.[4] Patients undergoing chronic ambulatory peritoneal dialysis (CAPD) average one episode of peritonitis every 2 years.[5] Epidemiologic data for secondary and tertiary intraabdominal infections are limited. Secondary peritonitis may be caused by perforation of a peptic ulcer; traumatic perforation of the stomach, small or large bowel, uterus, or urinary bladder; appendicitis; pancreatitis; diverticulitis; bowel infarction; inflammatory bowel disease, cholecystitis; operative contamination of the peritoneum; or diseases of the female genital tract, such as septic abortion, postoperative uterine infection, endometritis, and salpingitis. Appendicitis is one of the most common causes of intraabdominal infection. In 1998, 278,000 appendectomies were performed in the United States for suspected appendicitis.[6]

TABLE 118-1 Primary Bacterial Peritonitis

Primary bacterial peritonitis		
	Peritoneal dialysis	
	Cirrhosis with ascites	
	Nephrotic syndrome	
Secondary bacterial peritonitis		
	Miscellaneous causes	
		Diverticulitis
		Appendicitis
		Inflammatory bowel diseases
		Salpingitis
		Biliary tract infections
		Necrotizing pancreatitis
	Neoplasms	
		Intestinal obstruction
		Perforation
	Mechanical gastrointestinal problems	
		Any cause of small bowel obstruction (adhesions, hernia)
	Vascular causes	
		Mesenteric arterial or venous occlusion (atrial fibrillation)
		Mesenteric ischemia without occlusion
	Trauma	
		Blunt abdominal trauma with rupture of intestine
		Penetrating abdominal trauma
	Iatrogenic intestinal perforation (endoscopy)	
	Intraoperative events	
	Peritoneal contamination during abdominal operation	
	Leakage from gastrointestinal anastomosis	

ETIOLOGY

Primary peritonitis in adults occurs most commonly in association with alcoholic cirrhosis, especially in its end stage, or with ascites caused by postnecrotic cirrhosis, chronic active hepatitis, acute viral hepatitis, congestive heart failure, malignancy, systemic lupus erythematosus, or nephritic syndrome. It also may result from the use of a peritoneal catheter for dialysis or central nervous system ventriculoperitoneal shunting for hydrocephalus. Rarely, primary peritonitis occurs without apparent underlying disease.

Table 118–1 summarizes many of the potential causes of bacterial peritonitis. Causes include inflammatory processes of the GI tract or abdominal organs, bowel obstruction, vascular occlusions that may lead to gangrene of the intestines, and neoplasia that may cause intestinal perforation or obstruction. Other possible causes include those resulting from traumatic injuries or postoperative infections.

Abscesses are the result of chronic inflammation and may occur without preceding generalized peritonitis. They may be located within one of the spaces of the peritoneal cavity or within one of the visceral organs, and may range from a few milliliters to a liter or more in volume. These collections often have a fibrinous capsule and may take from a few weeks to years to form.

The causes of intraabdominal abscess overlap those of peritonitis and, in fact, may occur sequentially or simultaneously. Appendicitis is the most frequent cause of abscess. Other potential causes of intraabdominal abscess include pancreatitis, diverticulitis, lesions of the biliary tract, genitourinary tract infections, perforating tumors in the abdomen, trauma, and leaking intestinal anastomoses. In addition, pelvic inflammatory disease in women may lead to tuboovarian abscess. For some diseases, such as appendicitis and diverticulitis, abscesses occur more frequently than generalized peritonitis.

MICROFLORA OF THE GASTROINTESTINAL TRACT AND FEMALE GENITAL TRACT

A full appreciation of intraabdominal infection requires an understanding of the normal microflora within the GI tract. There are striking differences in bacterial species and concentrations of flora within the various segments of the GI tract (Table 118–2), and this bacterial environment usually determines the severity of infectious processes in the abdomen. Generally, the low gastric pH eradicates bacteria that enter the stomach. With achlorhydria, bacterial counts may rise to 10^5 to 10^7 organisms/mL. The normally low bacterial count also may increase by 1,000- or 10,000-fold with gastric outlet obstruction, hemorrhage, gastric cancer, and in patients receiving histamine 2 (H_2)-receptor antagonists, proton pump inhibitors, or antacids.

The biliary tract (gallbladder and bile ducts) is sterile in most healthy individuals, but in people older than 70 years or age, those with acute cholecystitis, jaundice, or common bile duct stones, it is likely to be colonized by aerobic gram-negative bacilli (particularly *Escherichia coli* and *Klebsiella* spp.) and enterococci.[7] Patients with biliary tract bacterial colonization are at greater risk of intraabdominal infection.

In the distal ileum, bacterial counts of aerobes and anaerobes are quite high. In the colon, there may be 500 to 600 different types of bacteria in stool, with concentrations often reaching 10^{11} organisms/mL and anaerobic bacteria outnumbering aerobic bacteria by more than 1,000 to 1.[2] In fact, up to 50% of the dry mass of stool is bacteria. Fortunately, most colonic bacteria are not pathogens because they cannot survive in environments outside the colon. Perforation of the colon results in the release of large numbers of anaerobic and aerobic bacteria into the peritoneum. The colonic flora generally are consistent unless broad-spectrum antimicrobials have been used, in which case there are increases in *Candida* or gram-negative bacteria.

The lower female genital tract generally is colonized by a large number of aerobic and anaerobic bacteria. Anaerobes may number 10^9 organisms per milliliter and often include lactobacilli, eubacteria, clostridia, anaerobic streptococci, and, less frequently, *Bacteroides fragilis.* Aerobic bacteria most often are streptococci and *Staphylococcus epidermidis,* and these may number 10^8 organisms per milliliter.

PATHOPHYSIOLOGY

Intraabdominal infection results from bacterial entry into the peritoneal or retroperitoneal spaces or from bacterial collections within intraabdominal organs. In primary peritonitis, bacteria may enter

TABLE 118-2 Usual Microflora of the Gastrointestinal Tract

Site	Commonly Found Bacteria	Approximate Concentration (Log No. Organisms/mL) Aerobes	Anaerobes
Stomach[a]	*Streptococcus, Lactobacillus*	10–100	Rare
Biliary tract	Normally sterile (*Escherichia coli, Klebsiella*, or enterococci in some patients)	0	0
Proximal small bowel	*Streptococcus* (including enterococci), *E. coli, Klebsiella, Lactobacillus,* diphtheroids	100	Few
Distal ileum	*E. coli, Klebsiella, Enterobacter*, enterococci, *Bacteroides fragilis, Clostridium,* peptostreptococci	10^4–10^6	10^5–10^7
Colon	*Bacteroides* spp., peptostreptococci, *Clostridium, E. coli, Klebsiella,* enterococci, *Enterobacter*, and many others	10^5–10^8	10^9–10^{11}

[a]With achlorhydria, H_2-antagonist therapy, gastric cancer, or gastric outlet obstruction, bacterial counts may rise to 10^5/mL.

the abdomen via the bloodstream or the lymphatic system by transmigration through the bowel wall, through an indwelling peritoneal dialysis catheter, or via the fallopian tubes in females. Hematogenous bacterial spread (through the bloodstream) occurs more frequently with tuberculosis peritonitis or peritonitis associated with cirrhotic ascites. When peritonitis results from peritoneal dialysis, skin surface flora are introduced via the peritoneal catheter. In secondary peritonitis, bacteria most often enter the peritoneum or retroperitoneum as a result of perforation of the GI or female genital tracts caused by diseases or traumatic injuries. Also, peritonitis or abscess may result from contamination of the peritoneum during a surgical procedure or following anastomotic leak.

The physiologic characteristics of the peritoneal cavity determine the nature of the response to infection or inflammation within it.[1] The peritoneum is lined by a highly permeable serous membrane with a surface area approximately that of skin. The peritoneal cavity is lubricated with less than 100 mL of sterile, clear yellow fluid, normally with fewer than 300 cells/mm^3, a specific gravity below 1.016, and protein content below 3 g/dL. These conditions change drastically with peritoneal infection or inflammation, as described below.

After bacteria are introduced into the peritoneal cavity, there is an immediate response to contain the insult. Humoral and cellular defenses respond first; then the omentum adheres to the affected area. A limited bacterial inoculum is handled rapidly by defense mechanisms, including complement activation. Under certain conditions, the bacterial insult is not contained, and bacteria disseminate throughout the peritoneal cavity, resulting in peritonitis. This is more likely to occur in the presence of a foreign body, hematoma, dead tissue, a large bacterial inoculum, continuing bacterial contamination, and contamination involving a mixture of synergistic organisms. Protein-calorie malnutrition, antecedent steroid therapy, and diabetes mellitus also may contribute to the formation of an intraabdominal abscess.

When bacteria become dispersed throughout the peritoneum, the inflammatory process involves most of the peritoneal lining. There is an outpouring into the peritoneum of fluid containing leukocytes, fibrin, and other proteins that form exudates on the inflamed peritoneal surfaces and begin to form adhesions between peritoneal structures. This process, combined with a paralysis of the intestines (ileus), may result in confinement of the contamination to one or more locations within the peritoneum. Fluid also begins to collect in the bowel lumen and wall, and distension may result.

The fluid and protein shift into the abdomen (called *third-spacing*) may be so dramatic that circulating blood volume is decreased, which causes decreased cardiac output and hypovolemic shock. Accompanying fever, vomiting, or diarrhea may worsen the fluid imbalance. A reflex sympathetic response, manifested by sweating, tachycardia, and vasoconstriction, may be evident. With an inflamed peritoneum, bacteria and endotoxins are absorbed easily into the bloodstream (translocation), and this may result in septic shock.[1] Other foreign substances present in the peritoneal cavity potentiate peritonitis. These adjuvants, notably feces, dead tissues, barium, mucus, bile, and blood, have detrimental effects on host defense mechanisms, particularly on bacterial phagocytosis.

Many of the manifestations of intraabdominal infections, particularly peritonitis, result from cytokine activity. Inflammatory cytokines, such as tumor necrosis factor-α (TNF-α), interleukin (IL) 1, IL-6, IL-8, and interferon γ(INF-γ), are produced by macrophages and neutrophils in response to bacteria and bacterial products or in response to tissue injury resulting from the surgical incision.[1,8] These cytokines produce wide-ranging effects on the vascular endothelium of organs, particularly the liver, lungs, kidneys, and heart. With uncontrolled activation of these mediators, sepsis may result (see Chap. 123).[9]

Peritonitis may result in death because of the effects on major organ systems. Fluid shifts and endotoxin may result in hypovolemic and septic shock. Hypoalbuminemia may result from protein loss into the peritoneum exacerbating intravascular volume loss. Pulmonary function may be compromised by the inflamed peritoneum producing splinting (muscle rigidity caused by pain) that inhibits adequate diaphragmatic movement leading to atelectasis and pneumonia. Increased lung vascular permeability and resulting shunting of blood may induce onset of the respiratory distress syndrome and associated hypoxemia and hypercarbia. With fluid loss, hypotension, endotoxemia, and renal and hepatic perfusion may be compromised, and acute renal and hepatic failure are potential threats.

If peritoneal contamination is localized but bacterial elimination is incomplete, an abscess results. This collection of necrotic tissue, bacteria, and white blood cells may be at single or multiple sites and may be within one of the spaces of the peritoneal cavity or in one of the visceral organs. The location of the abscess often is related to the site of primary disease. For example, abscesses resulting from appendicitis tend to appear in the right lower quadrant or the pelvis; those resulting from diverticulitis tend to appear in the left lower quadrant or pelvis.

An abscess begins by the combined action of inflammatory cells (such as neutrophils), bacteria, fibrin, and other inflammatory mediators. Bacteria may release heparinases that cause local thrombosis and tissue necrosis or fibrinolysins, collagenases, or other enzymes that allow extension of the process into surrounding tissues. Neutrophils gathered in the abscess cavity die in 3 to 5 days, releasing lysosomal enzymes that liquefy the core of the abscess. A mature abscess may have a fibrinous capsule that isolates bacteria and the liquid core from antimicrobials and immunologic defenses.

Within the abscess, the oxygen tension is low, and anaerobic bacteria thrive, and thus the size of the abscess may increase because it is hypertonic, resulting in an additional influx of fluid. Hypertonicity promotes the formation of bacterial L forms, which are resistant to antimicrobial agents that disrupt cell walls. Abscess formation may continue and mature for long periods of time and may not be readily evident to either patient or physician. In some instances, the abscess may resolve spontaneously, and infrequently, it may erode into adjacent organs or rupture and cause diffuse peritonitis. If the abscess erodes through the skin, it may result in an enterocutaneous fistula, connecting bowel to skin, or in a draining sinus tract.

The overall outcome from an intraabdominal infection depends on five key factors: inoculum size, virulence of the contaminating organisms, the presence of adjuvants within the peritoneal cavity that facilitate infection, the adequacy of host defenses, and the adequacy of initial treatment.[10]

MICROBIOLOGY OF INTRAABDOMINAL INFECTION

❷ Primary bacterial peritonitis often is caused by a single organism. In children, the pathogen is usually group A *Streptococcus*, *E. coli*, *Streptococcus pneumoniae*, or *Bacteroides* species.[11] When peritonitis occurs in association with cirrhotic ascites, *E. coli* is isolated most frequently. Other potential pathogens are: *Haemophilus pneumoniae*, *Klebsiella*, *Pseudomonas*, anaerobes, and *S. pneumoniae*.[12] Occasionally, primary peritonitis may be caused by *Mycobacterium tuberculosis*. Peritonitis in patients undergoing peritoneal dialysis is caused most often by common skin organisms, such as *S. epidermidis*, *Staphylococcus aureus*, streptococci, and diphtheroids. Occasionally, aerobic gram-negative bacilli may cause infections, particularly in patients undergoing dialysis during hospitalization. Mortality from primary peritonitis caused by gram-negative bacteria is much greater than that from gram-positive bacteria.[13]

❸ Because of the diverse bacteria present in the GI tract, secondary intraabdominal infections often are polymicrobial.[2] The mean number of different bacterial species isolated from infected intraabdominal

TABLE 118-3 Pathogens Isolated from Patients with Secondary Peritonitis

Gram-negative bacteria	
Escherichia coli	32%–61%
Enterobacter	8%–26%
Klebsiella	6%–26%
Proteus	4%–23%
Gram-positive bacteria	
Enterococci	18%–24%
Streptococci	6%–55%
Staphylococci	6%–16%
Anaerobic bacteria	
Bacteroides	25%–80%
Clostridium	5%–18%
Fungi	2%–5%

Data from Marshall JC, Innes M. Intensive care unit management of intraabdominal infection. Crit Care Med 2003;31:2228–2237.

sites ranged from 2.9 to 3.7, including an average of 1.3 to 1.6 aerobes and 1.7 to 2.1 anaerobes.[14,15] With proper anaerobic specimen collection, anaerobic organisms are isolated in most patients. In one report of patients with gangrenous and perforated appendicitis, an average of 10.2 different organisms was isolated from each patient, including 2.7 aerobes and 7.5 anaerobes.[16] Purely aerobic or anaerobic infections are uncommon, as are infections caused by fungi. Table 118–3 gives the frequencies with which specific bacteria were isolated from patients with peritonitis.[17] *E. coli, Streptococcus* spp., and *Bacteroides* spp. were isolated most often from the infection site, as well as from blood cultures. In patients diagnosed with severe infections, the pattern of bacterial isolates may change and commonly includes *Candida,* enterococci, Enterobacteriaceae, and *S. epidermidis.*

Visceral organ abscesses differ in character from the typical intraabdominal abscess. Hepatic abscesses may be polymicrobial (involving *E. coli* and anaerobes) or occasionally may be caused by amoeba. Pancreatic abscesses are often polymicrobial, involving enteric bacteria that ascend through the biliary system. Splenic abscesses usually result from hematogenous dissemination of bacteria, such as *S. aureus,* streptococci, and occasionally, *Salmonella* or anaerobic organisms. Pelvic inflammatory disease is associated initially with *Neisseria gonorrhoeae* or *Chlamydia trachomatis.* However, tuboovarian abscesses usually are polymicrobial, having a mix of gram-positive and gram-negative aerobes and anaerobes.

BACTERIAL SYNERGISM

The size of the bacterial inoculum and the number and types of bacterial species present in intraabdominal infections influence patient outcome. The combination of aerobic and anaerobic organisms appears to increase the severity of infection greatly. In animal studies, combinations of aerobic and anaerobic bacteria were much more lethal than infections caused by aerobes or anaerobes alone.

Facultative bacteria may provide an environment conducive to the growth of anaerobic bacteria.[2] Although many bacteria isolated in mixed infections are nonpathogenic by themselves, their presence may be essential for the pathogenicity of the bacterial mixture.[4] The role of facultative bacteria in mixed infections can include (a) promotion of an appropriate environment for anaerobic growth through oxygen consumption, (b) production of nutrients necessary for anaerobes, and (c) production of extracellular enzymes that promote tissue invasion by anaerobes.

Rat models of intraabdominal infection demonstrate that uncontrolled infection with an implanted mix of aerobes and anaerobes leads to a two-stage (biphasic) infectious process. There is an early peritonitis phase with a high mortality rate and isolation of *E. coli* from blood and a late abscess formation phase in all survivors with isolation of anaerobes such as *B. fragilis* and *Fusobacterium varium.* These experiments and others support the concept that aerobic enteric organisms and anaerobes are pathogens in intraabdominal infection. Aerobic bacteria, particularly *E. coli,* appear responsible for the early mortality from peritonitis, whereas anaerobic bacteria are major pathogens in abscesses, with *B. fragilis* predominating.[17]

Enterococcus can be isolated from many intraabdominal infections in humans, but its role as a pathogen is not clear. Enterococcal infection occurs more commonly in postoperative peritonitis, in the presence of specific risk factors indicating failure of the host's defenses (immunocompromised patients), or with the use of broad-spectrum antibiotics.[18,19]

CLINICAL PRESENTATION

Intraabdominal infections have a wide spectrum of clinical features often depending on the specific disease process, the location and magnitude of bacterial contamination, and concurrent host factors. Peritonitis usually is recognized easily, but intraabdominal abscess often may continue for considerable periods of time, either going unrecognized or being attributed to an unrelated disease process. Patients with primary and secondary peritonitis present quite differently (Table 118–4).[1]

Primary peritonitis can develop over a period of days to weeks and usually is a more indolent process than secondary peritonitis.

TABLE 118-4 Clinical Presentation of Peritonitis

Primary Peritonitis

General

The patient may not be in acute distress, particularly with peritoneal dialysis.

Signs and symptoms

The patient may complain of nausea, vomiting (sometimes with diarrhea), and abdominal tenderness.
- Temperature may be only mildly elevated or not elevated in patients undergoing peritoneal dialysis.
- Bowel sounds are hypoactive.
- The cirrhotic patient may have worsening encephalopathy.
- Cloudy dialysate fluid with peritoneal dialysis.

Laboratory tests

The patient's white blood cell (WBC) count may be only mildly elevated.
- Ascitic fluid usually contains greater than 300 leukocytes/mm^3, and bacteria may be evident on Gram stain of a centrifuged specimen.
- In 60% to 80% of patients with cirrhotic ascites, the Gram stain is negative.

Other diagnostic tests

Culture of peritoneal dialysate or ascitic fluid should be positive.

Secondary Peritonitis

Signs and symptoms

Generalized abdominal pain.
- Tachypnea.
- Tachycardia.
- Nausea and vomiting.
- Temperature normal initially then increasing to 37.7°C to 38.8°C (100°F to 102°F) within the first few hours and may continue to rise for the next several hours.
- Hypotension and shock if volume is not restored.
- Decreased urine output due to dehydration.

Physical examination

Voluntary abdominal guarding changing to involuntary guarding and a "board-like abdomen."
- Abdominal tenderness and distension.
- Faint bowel sounds that cease over time.

Laboratory tests

Leukocytosis (15,000–20,000 WBC/mm^3, with neutrophils predominating and an elevated percentage of immature neutrophils (bands).
- Elevated hematocrit and blood urea nitrogen because of dehydration.
- Patient progresses from early alkalosis because of hyperventilation and vomiting to acidosis and lactic acidemia.

Other diagnostic tests

Abdominal radiographs may be useful because free air in the abdomen (indicating intestinal perforation) or distension of the small or large bowel is often evident.

The first sign of peritonitis may be a cloudy dialysate in patients undergoing peritoneal dialysis or worsening encephalopathy in a cirrhotic patient.

The patient with generalized bacterial peritonitis presents most often in acute distress. The patient lies still, usually on his or her back, possibly with hips slightly flexed. Any movement of the patient, including rocking the bed or breathing, worsens the generalized abdominal pain.

If peritonitis continues untreated, the patient may experience hypovolemic shock from third-space fluid loss into the peritoneum, bowel wall, and lumen. This may be accompanied by sepsis because the inflamed peritoneum absorbs bacteria and toxins into mesenteric blood vessels and lymph nodes, initiating production of inflammatory cytokines. Hypovolemic shock is the major factor contributing to mortality in the early stage of peritonitis.

Intraabdominal abscess may pose a difficult diagnostic challenge because the symptoms are neither specific nor dramatic. The patient may complain of abdominal pain or discomfort, but these symptoms are not reliable. Fever usually is present; often it is low grade, but it may be high, with a spiking pattern. The patient may have a paralytic ileus and abdominal distension. The abdominal examination is unreliable; tenderness and pain may be present, and a mass may be palpated.

Peritonitis may result from an abscess that ruptures, spreading bacteria and toxins throughout the peritoneum. In other patients, the entry of bacterial toxins into the systemic circulation from the abscess may lead to sepsis and progressive multisystem organ failure (e.g., renal, hepatic, pulmonary, or cardiovascular).

Laboratory studies generally are not helpful in the diagnosis of intraabdominal abscess, although most patients will have leukocytosis. Some patients may have positive blood cultures, whereas others, particularly diabetics, may have hyperglycemia. The finding of *Bacteroides* or any two enteric bacteria in the bloodstream is often indicative of an intraabdominal infectious process.

Radiographic methods are used to make the diagnosis of an intraabdominal abscess. Plain radiographs may show air–fluid levels or a shift of normal intraabdominal contents by the abscess mass. GI contrast studies also may demonstrate this displacement of abdominal structures. Both these modalities provide indirect evidence of abscess presence but are not generally helpful in precisely locating the abscess.

Ultrasound is a frequent first diagnostic method used when an intraabdominal abscess is suspected. The procedure may be done at the bedside, which is particularly helpful in the patient in the intensive care unit.

Computed tomography (CT) scanning frequently is used to evaluate the abdomen for the presence of an abscess and is the imaging modality of greatest value. An oral radiocontrast agent should be given to allow differentiation of the abscess from the bowel. Intravenous radiocontrast material will be taken up preferentially in the wall of the abscess, creating a unique radiographic appearance, so-called rim enhancement.

Magnetic resonance imaging is used infrequently to locate an intraabdominal abscess, particularly in the retroperitoneum, but this modality offers no significant advantage when compared with CT scanning.

Radioactive isotope imaging with ^{67}Ga citrate-, ^{99m}Tc-, or ^{111}In-labeled leukocytes also may be used.[20] These studies require long preparation and image acquisition and are not used routinely unless CT scanning fails to demonstrate a suspected abscess.

Intraabdominal infection caused by disease processes at specific sites often produces characteristic manifestations that are helpful in diagnosis. For example, a patient with diverticulitis may exhibit stabbing left-lower-quadrant abdominal pain and constipation. Fever and leukocytosis frequently are present, and a tender mass sometimes is palpable. With appendicitis, the findings may be inconsistent, but many patients have a sudden onset of periumbilical or epigastric pain that usually is colicky and later shifts to the right lower quadrant. The location of pain may vary because the appendix can be in many locations (e.g., retrocecal or pelvic) in the abdomen. A mass may be palpable on abdominal, pelvic, or rectal examination. The patient's temperature generally is mildly elevated early and then increases. If perforation and peritonitis occur, findings would include diffuse abdominal pain, rigidity, and sustained fever. More often, however, appendiceal perforation results in a local abscess.

TREATMENT

Intraabdominal Infections

■ DESIRED OUTCOME

The primary goals of treatment are correction of the intraabdominal disease processes or injuries that have caused infection and the drainage of purulent collections (abscesses). A secondary objective is to achieve a resolution of infection without major organ system complications (pulmonary, hepatic, cardiovascular, or renal failure) or adverse drug effects. Ideally, the patient should be discharged from the hospital with full function for self-care and routine daily activities.

■ GENERAL APPROACH TO TREATMENT

The treatment of intraabdominal infection most often requires hospitalization and the coordinated use of three major modalities: (a) prompt drainage of the infected site, (b) hemodynamic resuscitation and support of vital functions, and (c) early administration of appropriate antimicrobial therapy to treat infection not eradicated by surgery.[2]

Antimicrobials are an important adjunct to drainage procedures in the treatment of secondary intraabdominal infections; however, the use of antimicrobial agents without surgical intervention usually is inadequate. For most cases of primary peritonitis, drainage procedures may not be required, and antimicrobial agents become the mainstay of therapy.

❹ In the early phase of serious intraabdominal infections, attention should be given to the maintenance of organ system functions. With generalized peritonitis, large volumes of intravenous (IV) fluids are required to restore vascular volume, to improve cardiovascular function, and to maintain adequate tissue perfusion and oxygenation. Adequate urine output should be maintained to ensure adequate resuscitation and proper renal function. Respiratory function can be assisted by a variety of methods, including oxygen therapy, pulmonary physiotherapy, and ventilatory support in severely ill patients. Often the critically ill patient with intraabdominal infection will require intensive care management, particularly if there is cardiovascular or respiratory instability. Also, isolation procedures may be required if the infectious process poses a threat to other hospitalized patients.

An additional important component of therapy is nutrition. Intraabdominal infections often directly involve the GI tract or disrupt its function (paralytic ileus). The return of GI motility may take days, weeks, and occasionally, months. In the interim, enteral or parenteral nutrition as indicated facilitates improved immune function and wound healing to ensure recovery.

■ NONPHARMACOLOGIC TREATMENT

Drainage Procedures

Primary peritonitis is treated with antimicrobials and rarely requires drainage. Secondary peritonitis requires surgical correction of the underlying pathology. The drainage of the purulent material is the critical component of management of an intraabdominal abscess. Without adequate drainage of the abscess, antimicrobial therapy and fluid resuscitation can be expected to fail.

Secondary peritonitis is treated surgically and this is often called *source control*, which refers to all the physical measures undertaken to eradicate the focus of infection.[2] At the time of laparotomy (surgical opening and exploration of the abdomen) attempts are made to correct the cause of the peritonitis. This may include patching a perforated ulcer with omentum, removal of a segment of perforated colon, or excision of a portion of gangrenous small intestine. The goal of all these procedures is to repair or remove the inflamed or gangrenous viscus and to prevent further bacterial contamination. The presence of active inflammation increases the difficulty of the surgical procedure, which results in a higher morbidity and mortality rate than if the same procedures were performed in an elective setting without inflammation.

The presence of active inflammation may make it technically impossible to perform the definitive surgical procedure. In this situation, attempts are made to provide drainage of the infected or gangrenous structures. If an intraabdominal abscess, separate from any intraabdominal organ, is discovered during an exploratory laparotomy, it may be debrided, excised, or drained. If the intraabdominal abscess involves an abdominal structure, then a resection of part or all of that organ may be required. An example of this situation is an abscess associated with diverticular disease of the colon. Management may include drainage of the abscess and resection of the involved colon. All foreign material, necrotic tissue, feces, blood, or pus should be removed from the operative field, and the peritoneum should be copiously irrigated with 0.9% sodium chloride to decrease the concentrations of bacteria or other noxious substances.

After an abscess is located, it must be drained. This may be performed surgically or using percutaneous, image-guided techniques.[21] Typically, image-guided techniques are done using ultrasonography or CT scanning. The management of an intraabdominal abscess with percutaneous catheter drainage may be sufficient to resolve the infection. Some patients may require a subsequent procedure to treat the underlying gastrointestinal conditions; however, a significant advantage is obtained by first draining the abscess percutaneously. This allows the surgical procedure to be performed on a patient who is no longer suffering the systemic manifestations of uncontrolled infection. Drainage techniques may be performed using endoscopy or laparoscopy. These minimal-access techniques may offer advantages when compared with traditional surgery but probably will be used less often than radiologically assisted percutaneous drainage techniques.

The most valuable microbiologic information may be obtained at the time of percutaneous or operative abscess drainage. If pus or fluid is found that is believed to be infected, it is best to aspirate 2 to 3 mL into a syringe, remove any air, and tightly cap the syringe. The specimen should be taken promptly to the microbiology laboratory, where a Gram stain should be performed immediately and cultures prepared for identification of aerobic and anaerobic bacteria. If no fluid is available for collection, culture swab devices may be applied to the infected area; however, anaerobic organisms often are not isolated from swabs.

Fluid Therapy

❹ Aggressive fluid repletion and management are required for successful treatment of intraabdominal infections. Fluid therapy is instituted for the purposes of achieving or maintaining proper intravascular volume to ensure adequate cardiac output, tissue perfusion, and correction of acidosis. Loss of fluid through vomiting, diarrhea, or a nasogastric suction contributes to dehydration. Intravascular volume can be assessed by blood pressure and heart rate but more accurately by measurement of central venous pressure, pulmonary capillary wedge pressure, or urinary output. When a contracted vascular volume is accompanied by hemorrhage, the initial hematocrit may be normal, but if there is no associated hemorrhage, the hematocrit usually is elevated as an indication of hemoconcentration. Urine output should be monitored continuously in severely ill patients by use of a urinary bladder catheter, quantitated hourly, and should equal or exceed 0.5 mL/kg of body weight per hour.

In patients with peritonitis, hypovolemia often is accompanied by acidosis, so a reasonable IV fluid would be lactated Ringer solution, which contains the bicarbonate precursor lactate, as well as sodium, chloride, potassium, and calcium. In the initial hour of treatment, large volumes of solution may be required to restore intravascular volume. Thereafter, fluids may be required at a rate of 1 L/h. Maintenance fluids should be instituted (after intravascular volume is restored) with 0.9% sodium chloride and potassium chloride (20 mEq/L) or 5% dextrose and 0.45% sodium chloride with potassium chloride (20 mEq/L). The administration rate should be based on estimated daily fluid loss through urine and nasogastric suction, including 0.5 to 1.0 L for insensible fluid loss. Potassium would not be included routinely if the patient is hyperkalemic or has renal insufficiency.

In patients with significant blood loss, blood transfusion may be indicated. This is generally in the form of packed red blood cells. The criteria for blood transfusion are controversial, but a hematocrit of 25% generally is accepted. In the individual patient, the decision is often determined by the overall clinical status and the ability of the patient to compensate for the reduction in oxygen-carrying capacity associated with an acute anemia. Additional blood component therapy with fresh-frozen plasma or platelets is also based on the needs of the individual patient. Aggressive fluid therapy often must be continued in the postoperative period because fluid will continue to sequester in the peritoneal cavity, bowel wall, and lumen.

■ PHARMACOLOGIC TREATMENT

Antimicrobial Therapy

The goals of antimicrobial therapy are (a) to control bacteremia and prevent the establishment of metastatic foci of infection, (b) to reduce suppurative complications after bacterial contamination, and (c) to prevent local spread of existing infection. After suppuration has occurred (e.g., an abscess has formed), a cure by antibiotic therapy alone is very difficult to achieve; antimicrobials may serve to improve the results with surgery.

❺ An empirical antimicrobial regimen should be started as soon as the presence of intraabdominal infection is suspected. Therefore, antibiotics usually are initiated before identification of the infecting organisms is complete. Therapy must be initiated based on the likely pathogens. Predominant pathogens, as discussed in the preceding section, vary depending on the site of intraabdominal infection and the underlying disease process. Table 118–5 lists the likely pathogens against which antimicrobial agents should be directed.

Antimicrobial Experience Many studies have been conducted evaluating or comparing the effectiveness of antimicrobials for the treatment of intraabdominal infections. Substantial differences in patient outcomes from treatment with a variety of agents generally have not been demonstrated.[22]

Important findings from over 20 years of clinical trials regarding selection of antimicrobials for intraabdominal infections are the following:

- Antimicrobial regimens should cover a broad spectrum of aerobic and anaerobic bacteria from the gastrointestinal tract.
- Single-agent regimens (such as antianaerobic cephalosporins, extended-spectrum penicillins with β-lactamase inhibitors, and carbapenems) are as effective as combinations of ami-

TABLE 118-5 Likely Intraabdominal Pathogens

Type of Infection	Aerobes	Anaerobes
Primary bacterial peritonitis		
Children (spontaneous)	Group A *Streptococcus, Escherichia coli*, pneumococci	–
Cirrhosis	*E. coli, Klebsiella*, pneumococci (many others)	–
Peritoneal dialysis	*Staphylococcus, Streptococcus*	–
Secondary bacterial peritonitis		
Gastroduodenal	*Streptococcus, E. coli*	–
Biliary tract	*E. coli, Klebsiella*, enterococci	*Clostridium* or *Bacteroides* (infrequent)
Small or large bowel	*E. coli, Klebsiella* spp., *Proteus* spp.	*Bacteroides fragilis* and other *Bacteroides, Clostridium*
Appendicitis	*E. coli, Pseudomonas*	*Bacteroides* spp.
Abscesses	*E. coli, Klebsiella*, enterococci	*B. fragilis* and other *Bacteroides, Clostridium*, anaerobic cocci
Liver	*E. coli, Klebsiella*, enterococci staphylococci, amoeba	*Bacteroides* (infrequent)
Spleen	*Staphylococcus, Streptococcus*	

noglycosides with antianaerobic agents. This is also true for antimicrobial treatment of acute bacterial contamination from penetrating abdominal trauma.[23,24]

- Clindamycin and metronidazole appear to be equivalent in efficacy when combined with agents effective against aerobic gram-negative bacilli (gentamicin or aztreonam).
- For most patients, antimicrobial treatment can be completed orally with amoxicillin-clavulanate or the combination of ciprofloxacin and metronidazole.
- Five to 7 days of antimicrobial treatment is sufficient for most intraabdominal infections of mild to moderate severity.

Intraabdominal infection presents in many different ways and with a wide spectrum of severity. The regimen employed and duration of treatment depend on the specific clinical circumstances (i.e., the nature of the underlying disease process and the condition of the patient). Compromised patients require more aggressive therapies than do otherwise healthy patients who experience the same intraabdominal infection.

Recommendations ❻ For most intraabdominal infections, the antimicrobial regimen should be effective against both aerobic and anaerobic bacteria.[25] Although it is impossible to provide antimicrobial activity against every possible pathogen, agents with activity against enteric gram-negative bacilli such as *E. coli* and *Klebsiella*, and anaerobes such as *B. fragilis* and *Clostridium* spp. should be administered. If most of the organisms can be eliminated through drainage or antimicrobials, the synergistic effect may be removed, and the patient's defenses may be able to resolve the remaining infection.

Table 118–6 presents the recommended agents for treatment of community-acquired and complicated intraabdominal infections from the Infectious Diseases Society of America and the Surgical Infection Society.[25–27] These recommendations were formulated using an evidence-based approach. Table 118–7 lists additional evidence-based recommendations. Most community-acquired infections are "mild to moderate," whereas healthcare-associated infections tend to be more severe and difficult to treat. Table 118–8 presents guidelines for treatment and alternative regimens for specific

TABLE 118-6 Recommended Agents for the Treatment of Community-Acquired Complicated Intraabdominal Infections

Agents Recommended for Mild to Moderate Infections	Agents Recommended for High-Severity Infections
β-Lactamase inhibitor combinations	
Ampicillin-sulbactam	Piperacillin-tazobactam
Ticarcillin-clavulanate	
Carbapenems	
Ertapenem	Imipenem/cilastatin Meropenem
Combination regimens	
Cefazolin or cefuroxime plus metronidazole	Third- or fourth-generation cephalosporins (cefotaxime, ceftriaxone, ceftizoxime, ceftazidime, cefepime) plus metronidazole
Ciprofloxacin, levofloxacin, moxifloxacin, or gatifloxacin in combination with metronidazole	Ciprofloxacin in combination with metronidazole Aztreonam plus metronidazole

From Solomkin et al.,[25] and Mazuski et al.[26,27]

situations. These are general guidelines; there are many factors that cannot be incorporated into such a table.

Most patients with severe intraabdominal infection, generalized peritonitis, or sepsis should be placed on a β-lactam–β-lactamase inhibitor combination or carbapenem such as imipenem, ertapenem, or meropenem. Combinations of an aminoglycoside with an antianaerobic agent, such as clindamycin or metronidazole, may be used, but such combinations are considered to be obsolete. Gentamicin is the aminoglycoside of choice based on its lower cost. Other aminoglycosides, such as tobramycin or amikacin have no advantage in intraabdominal infection and generally are not drugs of first choice. Aztreonam may be used as an alternative to an aminoglycoside to avoid potential nephrotoxicity.

The dosage for aminoglycosides should be determined initially based on the patient's weight and renal function. Dosage adjustment should be performed by applying pharmacokinetic principles and by using peak and trough serum drug levels. Unless relatively resistant bacteria are suspected, a gentamicin or tobramycin peak concentration of 5 to 6 mcg/mL usually is effective. To achieve these serum concentrations, gentamicin or tobramycin dosage may range from 1 to 3 mg/kg per dose given as often as every 6 hours or as infrequently as every 48 hours if the patient has renal failure. Because aminoglycosides have concentration-dependent killing and a relatively long postantibiotic effect for aerobic gram-negative bacilli, once-daily administration (5 to 7 mg/kg) is a reasonable alternative and appears to be equivalent to multiple daily dosing.

When used for intraabdominal infection, aminoglycosides should be combined with agents that are effective against the majority of *B. fragilis*. Clindamycin or metronidazole is the agent of first choice, but others, such as antianaerobic cephalosporins (e.g., cefoxitin, cefotetan, or ceftizoxime), piperacillin, mezlocillin, and combinations of extended-spectrum penicillins with β-lactamase inhibitors, would be suitable alternatives. Clindamycin should be administered intravenously in a dosage of 600 or 900 mg every 8 hours. Patients receiving multiple broad-spectrum antimicrobial agents who are immunocompromised should receive an oral antifungal agent (nystatin) for prevention of fungal overgrowth in the mouth and GI tract. The benefits of systemic antifungal prophylaxis (with fluconazole) have not been established for intraabdominal infection and should not be used routinely.

With intraabdominal contamination from the upper GI tract (perforation of a peptic ulcer or biliary tract disease), *B. fragilis* is an uncommon pathogen, and other agents therefore may be substituted for clindamycin or metronidazole. Alternatives include ampicillin, penicillin, or first-generation cephalosporins.

TABLE 118-7 Evidence-Based Recommendations for Treatment of Complicated Intraabdominal Infections

	Grade of Recommendation[a]
Acute contamination as a result of trauma	
Bowel injuries caused by penetrating, blunt, or iatrogenic trauma that are repaired within 12 h and intraoperative contamination of the operative field by enteric contents under other circumstances should be treated with antibiotics ≤24 h.	A-1
Acute appendicitis	
Acute appendicitis without evidence of gangrene, perforation, abscess, or peritonitis requires only prophylactic administration of inexpensive regimens active against facultative and obligate anaerobes.	A-1
Community-acquired infections	
Antibiotics used for empirical treatment of community-acquired intraabdominal infections should be active against empiric gram-negative aerobic and facultative bacilli and β-lactam–susceptible gram-positive cocci.	A-1
For patients with mild-to-moderate community-acquired infections, agents that have a narrower spectrum of activity, such as ampicillin-sulbactam, cefazolin, or cefuroxime-metronidazole, ticarcillin-clavulanate, and ertapenem are preferable to more-costly agents that have broader coverage against gram-negative organisms and/or greater risk of toxicity.	A-1
Anaerobic coverage	A-1
Coverage against obligate anaerobic bacilli should be provided for distal small-bowel and colon-derived infections and for more-proximal gastrointestinal perforations when obstruction is present.	
Nosocomial infections	
Agents used to treat nosocomial infections in the intensive care unit (e.g., expanded gram-negative bacterial spectrum) should not be routinely used to treat community-acquired infections.	B-2
If a patient with diagnosed infection has previously been treated with an antibiotic, that patient should be treated as if he or she has had a healthcare-associated (nosocomial) infection.	B-3
Aminoglycosides	
Aminoglycosides are not recommended for routine use in community-acquired intraabdominal infections.	A-1
Oral completion therapy	
Completion of the antimicrobial course with oral forms of a quinolone plus metronidazole,	A-1
or with amoxicillin-clavulanic acid is acceptable for patients who are able to tolerate an oral diet.	B-3
Suspected fungal infection	
Antiinfective therapy for *Candida* should be withheld until the infecting species is identified.	C-3
Enterococcal infection	
Routine coverage against *Enterococcus* is not necessary for patients with community-acquired intraabdominal infections.	A-1

[a]Strength of recommendations: A, B, C = good, moderate, and poor evidence to support recommendation, respectively. Quality of evidence: 1 = Evidence from >1 properly randomized, controlled trial. 2 = Evidence from >1 well-designed clinical trial with randomization, from cohort or case-controlled analytic studies; from multiple time series, or from dramatic results from uncontrolled experiments. 3 = Evidence from opinions of respected authorities, based on clinical experience, descriptive studies, or reports of expert communities.

From Solomkin et al.,[25] and Mazuski et al.[26,27]

CLINICAL CONTROVERSY

Enterococci often are isolated from intraabdominal infections, and many antimicrobials are ineffective against enterococci (such as cephalosporins and fluoroquinolones). Regimens without activity against enterococci (gentamicin with clindamycin or cephalosporins) generally are effective in treating intraabdominal infections; however, there are numerous reports of enterococcal superinfection in immunocompromised patients, particularly after broad-spectrum antimicrobial use. The Infectious Disease Society of America guidelines state that "Routine coverage against enterococcus is not necessary for patients with community-acquired intraabdominal infections. Antimicrobial therapy for enterococci (e.g., ampicillin, penicillin, or vancomycin) should be given when enterococci are recovered from patients with "healthcare-associated infections."

The failure of host defenses may be a critical factor in the pathogenicity of enterococci. In immunocompromised patients or patients with valvular heart disease or a prosthetic heart valve, there is justification to provide specific antimicrobial activity against enterococci. Ampicillin or other penicillins that are active against enterococci (e.g., penicillin, piperacillin, and mezlocillin) should be used in patients at high risk, patients with persistent or recurrent intraabdominal infection, or patients who are immunosuppressed, such as after organ transplantation. Ampicillin remains the drug of choice for this indication because it is most active in vitro against enterococcus and is relatively inexpensive. Vancomycin is active against most enterococci; however, resistance is increasing, and this agent should be reserved for established infections when first-line therapies cannot be used.

❼ Intraperitoneal administration of antibiotics is preferred over IV therapy in the treatment of peritonitis that occurs in patients undergoing CAPD. The International Society of Peritoneal Dialysis revised its guidelines for the diagnosis and pharmacotherapy of peritoneal dialysis-associated infections.[28] The guidelines provide dosing recommendations for intermittent and continuous therapy based on the modality of dialysis (CAPD or automated peritoneal dialysis) and the extent of the patient's residual renal function.

Antimicrobial agents effective against both gram-positive and gram-negative organisms should be used for initial intraperitoneal empiric therapy for peritonitis in peritoneal dialysis patients. The most important factors to take into consideration for initial antimicrobial selection are the dialysis center's and the patient's history of infecting organisms and their sensitivities. The use of cefazolin (loading dose [LD] 500 mg/L; maintenance dose [MD] 125 mg/L) plus ceftazidime (LD 500 mg/L; MD 125 mg/L) or cefepime (LD 500 mg/L; MD 125 mg/L) or an aminoglycoside (gentamicin-tobramycin LD 8 mg/L; MD 4 mg/L) is suitable for initial empiric therapy; if patients are allergic to cephalosporin antibiotics, vancomycin (LD 1,000 mg/L; MD 25 mg/L) or an aminoglycoside should be substituted. Another option is monotherapy with imipenem-cilastin (LD 500 mg/L; MD 200 mg/L) or cefepime. Antimicrobial doses should empirically be increased by 25% in patients with residual renal function (more than 100 mL/day urine output).[28] Antimicrobial therapy should be continued for at least 1 week after the dialysate fluid is clear and for a total of at least 14 days. The reader is referred to these guidelines for additional information.[28]

After acute bacterial contamination, such as with abdominal trauma where GI contents spill into the peritoneum, combination antimicrobial regimens are not required. If the patient is seen soon after injury (within 2 hours) and surgical measures are instituted promptly, antianaerobic cephalosporins (such as cefoxitin or cefotetan) or extended-spectrum penicillins are effective in preventing most infectious complications. Antimicrobials should be administered as soon as possible after injury.

For appendicitis, the antimicrobial regimen used should depend on the appearance of the appendix at the time of operation, which may be normal, inflamed, gangrenous, or perforated. Because the condition of the appendix is unknown preoperatively, it is advisable

TABLE 118-8 Guidelines for Initial Antimicrobial Agents for Intraabdominal Infections

	Primary Agents	Alternatives
Primary bacterial peritonitis		
Cirrhosis	Cefotaxime	1. Add clindamycin or metronidazole if anaerobes are suspected 2. Other third-generation cephalosporins, extended-spectrum penicillins, aztreonam, and imipenem as alternatives 3. Aminoglycoside with antipseudomonal penicillin
Peritoneal dialysis	Initial empiric regimens Cefazolin or cephalothin plus ceftazidime or cefepime	1. An aminoglycoside may be used in place of ceftazidime or cefepime 2. Imipenem/cilastatin or cefepime may be used alone 3. Quinolones may be used in place of ceftazidime or cefepime if local susceptibilities allow
	1. *Staphylococcus*: penicillinase-resistant penicillin or first-generation cephalosporin	1. Alternative for methicillin resistant staphylococci is vancomycin 2. For vancomycin-resistant *Staphylococcus aureus*, linezolid, daptomycin, or quinupristin-dalfopristin must be used.
	2. *Streptococcus or Enterococcus*: ampicillin	1. An aminoglycoside may be added for enterococcal peritonitis 2. Linezolid or quinupristin-dalfopristin should be used to treat vancomycin-resistant enterococcus not susceptible to ampicillin.
	3. Aerobic gram-negative bacilli: ceftazidime or cefepime 4. *Pseudomonas aeruginosa*: two agents with differing mechanisms of actions, such as an oral quinolone plus ceftazidime, cefepime, tobramycin, or piperacillin	1. The regimen should be based on in vitro sensitivity tests
Secondary bacterial peritonitis		
Perforated peptic ulcer	First-generation cephalosporins	1. Antianaerobic cephalosporins[a] 2. Possibly add aminoglycoside if patient condition is poor 3. Aminoglycoside with clindamycin or metronidazole; add ampicillin if patient is immunocompromised or if biliary tract origin of infection
Other	Imipenem-cilastatin, meropenem, ertapenem, or extended-spectrum penicillins with β-lactamase inhibitor	1. Ciprofloxacin with metronidazole 2. Aztreonam with clindamycin or metronidazole 3. Antianaerobic cephalosporins[a]
Abscess		
General	Imipenem-cilastatin, meropenem, ertapenem, or extended-spectrum penicillins with β-lactamase inhibitor	1. Aztreonam with clindamycin or metronidazole 2. Ciprofloxacin with metronidazole 3. Aminoglycoside with clindamycin or metronidazole;
Liver	As above but add a first-generation cephalosporin	Use metronidazole if amoebic liver abscess is suspected
Spleen	Aminoglycoside plus penicillinase-resistant penicillin	Alternatives for penicillinase-resistant penicillin are first-generation cephalosporins or vancomycin
Appendicitis		
Normal or inflamed	Antianaerobic cephalosporins[a] (discontinued immediately postoperation)	1. Ampicillin-sulbactam
Gangrenous or perforated	Imipenem-cilastatin, meropenem, ertapenem, antianaerobic cephalosporins, or extended-spectrum penicillins with β-lactamase inhibitor	1. Aztreonam with clindamycin or metronidazole 2. Ciprofloxacin with metronidazole 3. Aminoglycoside with clindamycin or metronidazole
Acute cholecystitis	First-generation cephalosporin	Aminoglycoside plus ampicillin if severe infection
Cholangitis	Aminoglycoside with ampicillin with or without clindamycin or metronidazole	Use vancomycin instead of ampicillin if patient is allergic to penicillin
Acute contamination from abdominal trauma	Antianaerobic cephalosporins[a] or ampicillin-sulbactam	1. A carbapenem 2. Ciprofloxacin plus metronidazole
Pelvic inflammatory disease	Cefotetan or cefoxitin with doxycycline	1. Clindamycin with gentamicin 2. Ampicillin-sulbactam with doxycycline 3. Ciprofloxacin with doxycycline and metronidazole

[a]Cefoxitin, cefotetan, and ceftizoxime.

to begin antimicrobial agents before the appendectomy is performed. Reasonable regimens would be antianaerobic cephalosporins or, if the patient is seriously ill, a carbapenem or β-lactam–β-lactamase inhibitor combination. If, at operation, the appendix is normal or inflamed, postoperative antimicrobials are not required. If the appendix is gangrenous or perforated, a treatment course of 5 to 7 days with the agents listed in Table 118–8 is appropriate.

8 The necessary duration of treatment for intraabdominal infections is not clearly defined. Acute intraabdominal contamination, such as after a traumatic injury, may be treated with a very short course (24 hours).[29] For established infections (i.e., peritonitis or intraabdominal abscess), an antimicrobial course limited to 5 to 7 days is justified. This allows eradication of bacteria remaining in the peritoneum after a surgical procedure that may enter the peritoneum through healing suture lines. Under certain conditions, therapy for longer than 7 days would be justified (e.g., if the patient remains febrile or is in poor general condition, when relatively resistant bacteria are isolated, or when a focus of infection in the abdomen may still be present). For some abscesses, such as pyogenic liver abscess, antimicrobials may be required for a month or longer.

Intraperitoneal irrigation of antimicrobial agents for treatment of intraabdominal infection has been studied often with conflicting results.[30] Intraoperative antimicrobial irrigation does not improve patient outcomes in comparison with copious intraoperative irrigation with normal saline. Possibly the most important aspect of peritoneal irrigation is the dilutional effect on bacteria and adjuvants that promotes infection (intestinal contents and hemoglobin). Most systemically administered antimicrobials easily cross the peritoneal membrane so that peritoneal fluid concentrations are similar to serum. Confined areas, such as an abscess, can be expected to attain much lower antimicrobial concentrations.

EVALUATION OF THERAPEUTIC OUTCOMES

Whichever antimicrobial regimen is chosen, the patient should be reassessed continually to determine the success or failure of therapies. The clinician should recognize that there are many reasons for poor patient outcome with intraabdominal infection; improper antimicrobial administration is only one. The patient may be immunocompromised, which decreases the likelihood of successful outcome with any regimen. It is impossible for antimicrobials to compensate for a nonfunctioning immune system. There may be surgical reasons for poor patient outcome. Failure to identify all intraabdominal foci of infection or leaks from a GI anastomosis may cause continued intraabdominal infection. Even when intraabdominal infection is controlled, accompanying organ system failure, most often renal or respiratory, may lead to patient demise.

The outcome from intraabdominal infection is not determined solely by what transpires in the abdomen. Unsatisfactory outcomes in patients with intraabdominal infections may result from complications that arise in other organ systems. Infectious complications commonly associated with mortality after intraabdominal infection are urinary tract infections and pneumonia.[31] A high APACHE (Acute Physiology and Chronic Health Evaluation) II score, low serum albumin concentration, and high New York Heart Association cardiac function status were significantly and independently associated with increased mortality from intraabdominal infection.[32]

❾ Once antimicrobials are initiated and the other important therapies described earlier are used, most patients should show improvement within 2 to 3 days. Usually, temperature will return to near normal, vital signs should stabilize, and the patient should not appear in distress, with the exception of recognized discomfort and pain from incisions, drains, and nasogastric tube. At 24 to 48 hours, aerobic bacterial culture results should return. If a suspected pathogen is not sensitive to the antimicrobial agents being given, the regimen should be changed if the patient has not shown sufficient improvement. If the isolated pathogen is extremely sensitive to one antimicrobial and the patient is progressing well, concurrent antimicrobial therapy often may be discontinued.

CLINICAL CONTROVERSY

❺ Although some investigators suggest that routine culturing of patients with community-acquired intraabdominal infections contributes little to their management,[33] other investigators suggest that antimicrobial therapy should be based on susceptibility of the bacteria collected from the operative site because this correlates with clinical outcome.[34]

With anaerobic culturing techniques and the slow growth of these organisms, anaerobes often are not identified until 4 to 7 days after culture, and sensitivity information is difficult to obtain. For this reason, there are usually few data with which to alter the antianaerobic component of the antimicrobial regimen. A report indicating that anaerobes were not isolated should not be the sole justification for discontinuing antianaerobic drugs because anaerobic bacteria that were present in the infectious process may not have been transported properly to the microbiology laboratory, or other problems may have led to cell death in vitro.

Reasons for antimicrobial failure may not always be apparent. Even when antimicrobial susceptibility tests indicate that an organism is susceptible in vitro to the antimicrobial agent, therapeutic failures may occur. Possibly there is poor penetration of the antimicrobial agent into the focus of infection, or bacterial resistance may develop after initiation of antimicrobial therapy. Also, it is possible that an antimicrobial regimen may encourage the development of infection by organisms not susceptible to the regimen being used. Superinfection in patients being treated for intraabdominal infection can be caused by *Candida;* however, enterococci or opportunistic gram-negative bacilli such as *Pseudomonas* or *Serratia* may be involved.

Treatment regimens for intraabdominal infection can be judged as successful if the patient recovers from the infection without recurrent peritonitis or intraabdominal abscess and without the need for additional antimicrobials. A regimen can be considered unsuccessful if a significant adverse drug reaction occurs, reoperation or percutaneous drainage is necessary, or patient improvement is delayed beyond 1 or 2 weeks.

ABBREVIATIONS

CAPD: chronic ambulatory peritoneal dialysis

CT: computed tomography

IL: interleukin

LD: loading dose

MD: maintenance dose

REFERENCES

1. Ordonez CA, Puyana JC. Management of peritonitis in the critically ill patient. Surg Clin North Am 2006;86:1323–1349.
2. Marshall JC. Intra-abdominal infections. Microbes Infect 2004;6:1015–1025.
3. Marshall JC, Innes M. Intensive care unit management of intraabdominal infection. Crit Care Med 2003;31:2228–2237.
4. Mowat C, Stanley AJ. Spontaneous bacterial peritonitis—Diagnosis, treatment, and prevention. Aliment Pharmacol Ther 2001;15:1851–1859.
5. Vas S, Oreopoulos DG. Infections in patients undergoing peritoneal dialysis. Infect Dis Clin North Am 2001;15:743–774.
6. Hall MJ, Popovic JR. 1998 Summary: National Hospital Discharge Survey, Number 316. Washington, DC: National Center for Health Statistics, 2000.
7. Toloza EM, Wilson SE. Cholecystitis and cholangitis. In: Fry DE, ed. Surgical Infections. Boston: Little, Brown, 1995:254–263.
8. Schein M, Wittman DH, Holzheimer R, et al. Hypothesis: Compartmentalization of cytokines in intraabdominal infection. Surgery 1996;119:694–700.
9. Riche FC, Cholley BP, Panis YH, et al. Inflammatory cytokine response in patients with septic shock secondary to generalized peritonitis. Crit Care Med 2000;28:433–437.
10. Malangoni MA. Contributions to the management of intraabdominal infection. Am J Surg 2005;190:255–259.
11. Thompson AE, Marshall JC, Opal SM. Intraabdominal infections in infants and children: descriptions and definitions. Pediatr Crit Care Med 2005;6:S30–S35.
12. Johnson DH, Cuhna BA. Infections in cirrhosis. Infect Dis Clin North Am 2001;15:363–371.
13. Troidle L, Gordon-Brennan N, Kliger A, Finkelstein F. Differing outcomes of gram-positive and gram-negative peritonitis. Am J Kidney Dis 1998;32:623–628.
14. Brook I, Frazier EH. Aerobic and anaerobic microbiology of retroperitoneal abscesses. Clin Infect Dis 1998;26:938–941.
15. Bennion RS, Baron EJ, Thompson JE, et al. The bacteriology of gangrenous and perforated appendicitis—Revisited. Ann Surg 1990;211:165–171.
16. Sawyer RG, Rosenlof LK, Adams RB, et al. Peritonitis into the 1990s: Changing pathogens and changing strategies in the critically ill. Am Surg 1992;58:82–87.
17. Onderdonk AB, Bartlett JG, Louie T, et al. Microbial synergy in experimental intraabdominal abscess. Infect Immun 1997;13:22–26.

18. Donskey CJ, Chowdhry TK, Hecker MT, et al. Effect of antibiotic therapy on the density of vancomycin-resistant enterococci in the stool of colonized patients. Ann Surg 2000;343:1925–1932.
19. Sitges-Serra A, Lopez MJ, Girvent M, et al. Postoperative enterococcal infection after treatment of complicated intraabdominal sepsis. Br J Surg 2002;89:361–367.
20. Youssef IM, Milardovic R, Perone RWM, Heiba SI, Abdel-Dayem HM. Importance of 99mTc-sulfur colloid liver-spleen scans performed before 111indium labeled leukocyte imaging for localization of abdominal infection. Clin Nucl Med 2005;30:87–90.
21. Jaffe TA, Nelson RC, Delong DM, Paulson EK. Practice patterns in percutaneous image-guided intraabdominal abscess drainage: survey of academic and private practice centers. Radiology 2004;233:750–756.
22. Wong PF, Gilliam AD, Kumar S, et al. Antibiotic regimens for secondary peritonitis of gastrointestinal origin in adults. Cochrane Database Syst Rev 2007;2;CD 004539.
23. Hooker KD, DiPiro JT, Wynn JJ. Aminoglycoside combinations versus single β-lactams for penetrating abdominal trauma: A meta analysis. J Trauma 1991;31:1155–1160.
24. Solomkin JS, Dellinger EP, Christou NV, et al. Results of a multicenter trial comparing imipenem/cilastatin to tobramycin/clindamycin for intraabdominal infections. Ann Surg 1990;212:581–591.
25. Solomkin JS, Mazuski JE, Baron EJ, et al. Guidelines for the selection of anti-infective agents for complicated intraabdominal infections. Clin Infect Dis 2003;37:997–1005.
26. Mazuski JE, Sawyer RG, Nathens AB, et al. The Surgical Infection Society guidelines on antimicrobial therapy for intraabdominal infections: An executive summary. Surg Infect (Larchmt) 2002;3: 161–174.
27. Mazuski JE, Sawyer RG, Nathens AB, et al. The Surgical Infection Society guidelines on antimicrobial therapy for intraabdominal infections: Evidence for recommendations. Surg Infect (Larchmt) 2002;3:175–234.
28. Piraino B, Bailie GR, Bernardini J, et al. Peritoneal dialysis related infections: 2005, update. Perit Dial Int 2005;25:107–131.
29. Bozorgzadeh A, Pizzi WF, Barie PS, et al. The duration of antibiotic administration in predicting abdominal trauma. Am J Surg 1999;172:125–135.
30. Schein M, Gecelter G, Freinkel W, et al. Peritoneal lavage in abdominal sepsis: A controlled clinical study. Arch Surg 1990;125:1132–1135.
31. Merlino JI, Yowler CJ, Malangoni MA. Nosocomial infections adversely affect the outcomes of patients with serious intraabdominal infections. Surg Infect (Larchmt) 2004;5:21–27.
32. Christou NV, Barie PS, Dellinger EP, et al. Surgical infection society intraabdominal infection study. Arch Surg 1993;128:193–199.
33. Dougherty SH. Antimicrobial culture and susceptibility testing has little value for routine management of secondary bacterial peritonitis. Clin Infect Dis 1997;25(Suppl 2):S258–S261.
34. Nathens AB. Relevance and utility of peritoneal cultures in patients with peritonitis. Surg Infect (Larchmt) 2001;2:153–160.

CHAPTER 119

Parasitic Diseases

J. V. ANANDAN

KEY CONCEPTS

1. Parasites normally inflict some degree of injury to the host, the extent of which depends on such factors as parasite load, nutritional status, and immunologic competence of the host.
2. All symptomatic adults and children older than 8 years of age with giardiasis should be treated with metronidazole 250 mg three times daily for 5 to 7 days.
3. Intestinal amebiasis is diagnosed by demonstrating *Entamoeba histolytica* cysts or trophozoites (may contain ingested erythrocytes) in fresh stool or from a specimen obtained by sigmoidoscopy. Three stool samples obtained 24 hours apart will produce a 60% to 90% yield for *E. histolytica.*
4. The drug of choice for enterobiasis, hookworm, and ascariasis is mebendazole, and the agent of choice for strongyloidiasis is albendazole.
5. The primary reasons for deaths as a result of malaria are failure to take chemoprophylaxis, inappropriate chemoprophylaxis, delay in seeking medical care, and misdiagnosis.
6. In adults (including pregnant women) traveling from a nonendemic to an endemic area, the chemoprophylaxis for all species of plasmodia is chloroquine phosphate 300 mg (base) once weekly beginning 1 week prior to departure and continuing for 4 weeks after leaving an endemic area. In an uncomplicated attack of malaria (for all plasmodia except chloroquine-resistant *Plasmodium falciparum*), the recommended regimen is chloroquine 600 mg (base) initially, followed by 300 mg (base) 6 hours later, and then 300 mg (base) daily for 2 days.
7. Because falciparum malaria is associated with serious complications, including pulmonary edema, hypoglycemia, jaundice, renal failure, confusion, delirium, seizures, coma, and death, careful monitoring of fluid status and hemodynamic parameters is mandatory.
8. In chronic trypanosomiasis (Chagas' disease), patients present with cardiomyopathy and heart failure.
9. The resistance of lice to permethrin is increasing, and 0.5% malathion is an effective alternative.
10. The treatment of choice for scabies is 5% permethrin cream; oral ivermectin is an alternative therapy.

Learning objectives, review questions, and other resources can be found at **www.pharmacotherapyonline.com.**

Parasitic diseases are receiving increasing attention from clinicians in the United States because of the high frequency of travel, deployment of personnel for humanitarian and military missions (e.g., Peace Corps volunteers), inflow of immigrants from a wider geographic distribution, and the presence of immunosuppressed populations (e.g., acquired immune deficiency syndrome [AIDS] and transplant patients). Migrant farm workers who work and live in substandard hygienic conditions, the large and growing Central and South American immigrant population, and other poorly medically screened immigrants from Asia represent significant sources of parasitic infections in the United States.[1–9] Clinicians need to have a heightened awareness of parasitic diseases and how to treat them. Clinical signs and symptoms, together with the patient's travel history, should be used with other diagnostic aids in the identification of parasitic diseases. Parasitic infections caused by pathogenic protozoa or helminths affect more than 3 billion people worldwide and impose tremendous health and economic burdens on developing countries.[9]

This chapter discusses the major parasitic diseases, including protozoan diseases (giardiasis, amebiasis, malaria, and Chagas' disease), helminthic infections (ascariasis, enterobiasis, hookworm, strongyloidiasis, and cestodiasis), and ectoparasitic infestations (head and body lice). Emphasis is placed on diseases seen more frequently in the United States. World distribution of parasites depends on the presence of suitable hosts, habitats, and environmental conditions.[9] A human parasite that does not use an intermediate host is likely to be found in any inhabited region of the world as long as the environmental conditions are suitable. *Ascaris* (roundworm) and *Trichuris* (whipworm) require carelessness of habits for transfer and require time outside the body, where they are exposed to heat and dryness, to reach the infective stage. The distribution of the hookworm is more limited because the free-living forms are unprotected by resistant shells or cysts. African trypanosomiasis never occurs outside the range of the tsetse fly; malaria never occurs beyond the range of the infective *Anopheles* mosquito; and schistosomiasis never occurs in the absence of a specific water snail. The prevalence of clonorchiasis (Chinese liver fluke) is an example of the impact of both environmental and geographic factors. Clonorchiasis requires the simultaneous presence of not only humans, specific snail species, and certain fish, but also unsanitary conditions that make the eggs accessible to the snails, an association of the snail and fish, and the established local habit of eating raw fish. The ability of some parasites to infect hosts other than humans may perpetuate an infection even when human habits preclude the possibility of more than occasional access to the human body. In North America, the broad tapeworm (*Diphyllobothrium latum*) would perish if it were not that dogs and other carnivores, such as the brown bear, serve as reservoir hosts.

HOST–PARASITE RELATIONSHIP

Symbiosis is the association of two species for the purpose of obtaining food for either one or the other. *Parasitism* is a symbiotic relationship in which one species, the host, is injured through the activities of the other. Through evolution, parasites have made specific morphologic adaptations. Adaptation to the host has taken a number of forms: loss of locomotor organelles in the protozoan *Sporozoa;* partial and complete lack of digestive systems in the trematodes and cestodes, respectively; elaboration of proteolytic enzymes to penetrate the host intestinal mucosa by *Entamoeba histolytica;* the cercariae of the blood fluke that penetrate the skin of the host by elaborate enzymes; and, finally, the ability to infect an intermediate host to increase reproductive capacity, as seen among the cestodes and trematodes.[9]

❶ Parasites normally inflict some degree of injury to the host, the extent of which depends on such factors as parasite load, nutritional status, and immunologic competence of the host. *Entamoeba coli* is considered commensal because it subsists on the bacterial flora of the gut and does not cause any harm to the host. Unlike *Entamoeba coli, Fasciolopsis buski,* the giant intestinal fluke, can produce severe local damage to the intestinal wall. *Ascaris,* the roundworm, can perforate the bowel wall, cause intestinal obstruction, and invade the appendix and bile duct. Malarial parasites destroy red cells by multiplying inside them. *D. latum,* or the broad fish tapeworm, removes vitamin B_{12} from the gastrointestinal tract (GI) tract, resulting in megaloblastic anemia.[9]

PROTOZOAN DISEASES

GIARDIASIS

Epidemiology and Etiology

Giardia lamblia (also known as *Giardia intestinalis* or *Giardia duodenalis*), an enteric protozoan, is the most common intestinal parasite responsible for diarrheal syndromes throughout the world.[10–12,14] *Giardia* is the most frequently identified intestinal parasite in the United States, with a prevalence rate of 15% in some areas. *G. lamblia* has been identified as the first enteric pathogen seen in children in developing countries, with prevalence rates between 15% and 30%.[12]

There are two stages in the life cycle of *G. lamblia*: the trophozoite and the cyst. *G. lamblia,* which is found in the small intestine, the gallbladder, and biliary drainage, is a pear-shaped trophozoite with four pairs of flagella. Two nuclei lie in the area of the sucking disk, giving the protozoan a characteristic face-like image.

The distribution of giardiasis is worldwide. Children seem to be affected more frequently than adults. Children in daycare centers may infect parents and other family members.[12] In less-developed countries, fecal contamination of the environment and lack of potable water, education, and housing continue to be risk factors for giardiasis among children.

Pathology

Giardiasis results from ingestion of *G. lamblia* cysts in fecally contaminated water or food. The protozoan excysts under the stimulus of low gastric pH to release the trophozoite.[12] Colonization and multiplication of the trophozoite lead to mucosal invasion, localized edema, and flattening of the villi, resulting in malabsorption states in the host.[10–16]

Lactose intolerance precipitated by giardiasis can persist even after eradication of the protozoan. Achlorhydria, hypogammaglobulinemia, or deficiency in secretory immunoglobulin A (IgA) are predispositions for giardiasis.[10,12,14] Table 119–1 describes the clinical presentation of giardiasis.

TABLE 119-1 Clinical Presentation of Giardiasis

Acute onset
Diarrhea, cramp-like abdominal pain, bloating, and flatulence[10–12]
Malaise, anorexia, nausea, and belching[12]
Chronic
Diarrhea: foul-smelling, copious, light-colored, fatty stools; weight loss
Periods of diarrhea alternating with constipation
Steatorrhea, lactose intolerance, vitamin B_{12}, and fat-soluble vitamin deficiencies[12–16]

Diagnosis of giardiasis is made by examination of fresh stool or a preserved specimen during the acute diarrheal phase. Fresh stool specimens may show the trophozoites, whereas preserved specimens usually yield the cysts. If both the stool examination and string test prove unsuccessful, it may be necessary to attempt duodenal aspiration and biopsy to confirm the diagnosis; this may be more important in AIDS patients and in patients with hypogammaglobulinemia.[10,12] Most clinicians advocate a clinical trial of the standard therapy before undertaking invasive diagnostic tests. Detection of the trophozoites or cysts in fecal samples by enzyme-linked immunosorbent assay (ELISA) or immunofluorescence or identification of the *Giardia* antigen by counterimmunoelectrophoresis are alternative ways for diagnosis of giardiasis.[9,10,12]

TREATMENT

Giardiasis

■ DESIRED OUTCOME

To reduce morbidity and to avoid complications in patients identified with prolonged diarrhea and malabsorption and who have a recent history of travel to an endemic area, rapid identification by ova and parasite examination or by antigen detection test should be used to institute appropriate therapy.

■ PHARMACOLOGIC THERAPY

❷ All symptomatic adults and children older than 8 years of age should be treated with metronidazole 250 mg three times daily for 5 to 7 days. The alternative drugs include furazolidone 100 mg four times or paromomycin 25 to 30 mg/kg per day in divided doses daily for 1 week.[11–14] Paromomycin 25 to 30 mg/kg per day in three doses for 7 days is a safe agent in pregnancy.[11,12] The pediatric dose for metronidazole is 15 mg/kg per day three times daily for 5 to 7 days.[13] Furazolidone suspension 6 mg/kg per day in four doses for 7 to 10 days and nitazoxanide (Alinia) suspension 100 to 200 mg every 12 hours for 3 days are alternative drugs for children.[12,13] Quinacrine, which was the drug of choice in giardiasis, has been discontinued by the manufacturer but is obtained in the United States from a specialized pharmacy (see Appendix 119–1). Albendazole 400 mg daily for 5 days has been cited to produce cure rates of 97% and as being equivalent to metronidazole in children. However, other investigators have disputed the efficacy of this agent.[11]

Evaluation of Therapeutic Outcomes

Patients with symptomatic giardiasis, positive stool samples, or the detection of *Giardia* antigen by counterimmunoelectrophoresis or ELISA should be treated with metronidazole for 5 to 7 days. Metronidazole produces cure rates of between 85% and 95%.[11,12] Diarrhea will stop within a few days, although in some patients it may take 1 to 2 weeks. Cyst excretion will cease within days; however, intestinal dysfunction (manifested as increased transit time) and radiologic changes (irregular thickening of the folds in the upper small intestine) may take a few months to resolve.[10] Patients who fail initial therapy with metronidazole should receive a second course of therapy. Nitazoxanide (500 mg twice daily for 3 days) is effective in patients who are not responding to metronidazole.[12] Pregnant patients can receive paromomycin 25 to 30 mg/kg per day in divided doses for 7 days. Metronidazole has been used in the second and third trimesters of pregnancy.[12]

Giardiasis can be prevented by good personal hygiene and by caution in food and drink consumption.

AMEBIASIS

Epidemiology and Etiology

Because of its worldwide distribution and serious gastrointestinal manifestations, amebiasis is one of the most important parasitic diseases of humans.[9,18–21] The major causative organism in amebiasis is *E. histolytica,* which inhabits the colon and must be differentiated from the *Entamoeba dispar,* which is associated with an asymptomatic carrier state and is considered nonpathogenic. Although *E. histolytica* and *E. dispar* are indistinguishable morphologically, recent research using monoclonal antibodies has been able to separate the two.[20,21] Invasive amebiasis is almost exclusively the result of *E. histolytica* infection. Approximately 50 million cases of invasive disease result each year worldwide, leading to an excess of 100,000 deaths.[19,21] In the United States, the incidence of amebiasis is estimated at approximately 4% in the general population.[21] The highest incidence is found in institutionalized mentally retarded patients, sexually active homosexuals, patients with AIDS, the Native American population, and new immigrants from endemic areas (e.g., Mexico, India, West and South Africa, and portions of Central and South America).[19,21]

Pathology

E. histolytica invades mucosal cells of colonic epithelium, producing the classic flask-shaped ulcer in the submucosa.[19–23] The trophozoite has a cytolethal effect on cells through a toxin. If the trophozoite gets into the portal circulation, it will be carried to the liver, where it produces abscess and periportal fibrosis.[19–23] Amebic ulcerations can affect the colon, perineum, and genitalia, and abscesses may occur in the lung and brain.[20,21,24]

Clinical Presentation

The most frequent clinical manifestations of the disease are gastrointestinal (Table 119–2).

Liver abscesses can spread to the lungs and pleura.[20,21] Pericardial infections, although rare, may be associated with extension of the amebic abscess from the left lobe of the liver. Erosion of liver abscesses also present as peritonitis.[19–22]

❸ Review of the patient's history and recent travel should be strongly emphasized. Intestinal amebiasis is diagnosed by demonstrating *E. histolytica* cysts or trophozoites (may contain ingested erythrocytes) in fresh stool or from a specimen obtained by sigmoidoscopy. Three stool samples obtained 24 hours apart will produce a 60% to 90% yield for *E. histolytica.* Microscopy may not differentiate between the pathogenic *E. histolytica* and the nonpathogenic *E. dispar* in stools. Sensitive techniques are available to detect *E. histolytica* in stool, including ELISA and antigen detection.[19–21] Endoscopy with scraping or biopsy may provide more definitive diagnosis where stool examinations do not provide adequate evidence.[19,21]

When amebic liver abscess is suspected from initial physical examination and history, confirmatory diagnostic procedures will include serology and liver scans (using isotopes by ultrasound or computed tomography) or magnetic resonance imaging.[20,21] Leukocytosis (>10,000/mm^3) and an elevated alkaline phosphatase concentration (>75%) are common findings. In rare instances, needle aspiration of the hepatic abscess may be attempted using ultrasound guidance.[20–22]

TABLE 119-2 Most Common Manifestations of Amebiasis

Intestinal disease
Vague abdominal discomfort, malaise to severe abdominal cramps, flatulence, bloody diarrhea (heme-positive in 100% of cases) with mucus[19–21]
Eosinophilia is usually absent, although moderate leukocytosis is not unusual[20,21]
Amebic liver abscess
High fever, significant leukocytosis with left shift, elevated alkaline phosphatase, and liver tenderness on palpation[20–22]
Right-upper-quadrant pain, hepatomegaly, and liver tenderness, with referred pain to the left or right shoulder
Erosion of liver abscesses also present as peritonitis[19–21]

TREATMENT

Amebiasis

■ DESIRED OUTCOME

In amebiasis, the goals of therapy are initially to eradicate the parasite by use of specific amebicides and then to render supportive therapy.

■ TREATMENT REGIMENS

A number of different regimens have been suggested depending on the category of amebiasis: asymptomatic cyst passers, intestinal amebiasis, and amebic liver abscess.[13,19–22] Electrolyte replacement, antibiotic therapy, and nutritional support are essential adjunctive treatment modalities. Large hepatic abscess or amebic pericarditis may require needle aspiration, percutaneous catheter drainage, or, rarely, surgery before drug therapy.[20–22] Most regimens require a combination of drugs administered concurrently or sequentially.[19,21]

A careful history should be taken when one of the differential diagnoses is ulcerative colitis because corticosteroid administration has the potential to unmask amebiasis and produce toxic megacolon.[22]

■ PHARMACOLOGIC THERAPY

Metronidazole (Flagyl), dehydroemetine, and chloroquine (Aralen) are tissue-acting agents, whereas iodoquinol (Yodoxin), diloxanide furoate (Furamide), and paromomycin (Humatin) are luminal amebicides. A systemic agent may be so well absorbed that only small amounts of the drug stay in the bowel, which might prove ineffective as a luminal agent.[20–22] A luminal-acting agent, on the other hand, may be too poorly absorbed to be effective in the tissue. In the asymptomatic cyst passer, it is necessary to eradicate the causative agent from the lumen to prevent intestinal amebiasis or the development of amebic liver abscess. Drug effectiveness must be monitored by stool examination, that is, from one to three negative specimens from 1 to 3 months after treatment.

Asymptomatic cyst passers and patients with mild intestinal amebiasis should receive one of the following luminal agents: paromomycin 25 to 30 mg/kg per day three times daily for 7 days, iodoquinol 650 mg three times daily for 20 days, or diloxanide furoate 500 mg three times daily for 10 days. These regimens have cure rates of between 84% and 96%.[21] Diloxanide furoate is available only from Ponorama Compounding Pharmacy [6744 Balboa Blvd., Van Nuys, CA 91406; (800)-247-9767].[13] The pediatric dose for paromomycin is the same as in adults, whereas the dose of iodoquinol is 30 to 40 mg/kg per day in three doses for 20 days, and the dose of diloxanide furoate is 20 mg/kg per day in three doses for 10 days.[13] Paromomycin is the preferred luminal agent in pregnant patients.[13,21]

Patients with severe intestinal disease or liver abscess should receive metronidazole 750 mg three times daily for 10 days, followed by a course of one of the luminal agents indicated earlier.[13,20–21] Tinidazole 800 mg three times daily for 5 days has been suggested for amebic liver abscess.[22] In the pediatric patient, the dose of oral metronidazole is 50 mg/kg per day in divided doses to be followed by a luminal agent.[13] Patients who are too ill to take oral metronidazole should receive the drug in equivalent doses by the intravenous route.[21]

Evaluation of Therapeutic Outcomes

Followup in patients with amebiasis should include repeat stool examination, serology, colonoscopy (for colitis), or computed tomography (CT) (for liver abscess) between days 5 and 7, at the end of the course of therapy, and a month after the end of therapy.[19,21] Most patients with either intestinal amebiasis or colitis will respond in 3 to 5 days with amelioration of symptoms. Patients with liver abscesses may take from 7 to 10 days to respond; patients not responding during this period may require aspiration of abscesses or exploratory laparotomy. Serial liver scans have demonstrated healing of liver abscesses over 4 to 8 months after adequate therapy.

Sanitation and Preventive Measures

Travelers and tourists visiting an epidemic area should avoid local tap water, ice, salads, and unpeeled fruits. Water can be disinfected by the use of iodine (tincture of iodine or commercial sources: Potable Aqua tablet, Wisconsin Pharmacal, or Globaline, Wallace & Trernain) or a strong chlorine (laundry bleach) solution, but boiled water is probably the safest. An alternative or additional measure may be to carry a portable water purifier (such as Safewater, Durango, CO; *www.outgear.com*). Because food handlers in Asia and Latin America may be a source of amebiasis, travelers should avoid eating at food stalls and open markets.

HELMINTHIC DISEASES

Most intestinal helminthic infections may not be associated with clearly defined manifestation of disease, but they can cause significant pathology.[9,25–33] One factor that determines the pathogenicity of helminths is their population density. Light infections may be fairly well tolerated, whereas high populations of intestinal helminths can result in predictable disease presentations. In the United States, these infections are seen most frequently in recent immigrants from Southeast Asia, the Caribbean, Mexico, and Central America.[1,2,8,26,27] Other populations that have a high risk of infestation include institutionalized patients (both young and elderly), preschool children in daycare centers, residents of Indian reservations, and homosexual individuals. Certain conditions and drugs (fever, corticosteroids, and anesthesia) can cause atypical localization of worms.[34–38] Immunocompromised hosts can be overwhelmed by some helminthic infections, such as strongyloidiasis.[34]

NEMATODES

Hookworm Disease

This is an infection of the small intestine caused by either *Ancylostoma duodenale* or *Necator americanus. N. americanus* is found in the southeastern United States, where the temperature and humidity provide the proper environment. *Ancylostoma* is seen rarely in the United States.[25,27]

The life cycles of both species of hookworm are similar. The adult worms live in the small intestine attached to the mucosa. The females liberate eggs, which are eliminated in the feces and develop into larvae. Infective larva enter the host in contaminated food or water or penetrate the skin, where a papular eruption with localized edema and erythema can result.

TABLE 119-3 Clinical Presentations of Nematode Infections and Cysticercosis

Hookworm[27]
Mild epigastric pain and tenderness, headache, fatigue, anemia, hypoproteinemia, and cutaneous larva migrans
Ascariasis[26]
Abdominal pain, right-upper-quadrant pain, biliary coli, cholangitis, pancreatitis, and abdominal obstruction
Enterobiasis[25]
Mild abdominal discomfort and perianal itch
Strongyloidiasis[34,35,37]
Gastrointestinal: abdominal pain, bloating, nausea, constipation, and small obstruction
Cardiopulmonary: cough, wheezing, pleural effusion, chest pain, and dyspnea
Dermatologic/hematologic: pruritic linear streaks of lower thighs and buttocks and eosinophilia
Central nervous system: headache, altered mental status, and meningitis
Cysticercosis[41,42,45]
Abdominal pain, nausea, diarrhea, painless nodules on arms, chest and legs, and myalgia
Neurocysticercosis: headache, intracranial hypertension, hydrocephalus, and seizures

In the small intestine, where the adult worm lives attached to the mucosa, injury is usually caused by mechanical and lytic destruction of tissue. The loss of blood can lead to anemia and hypoproteinemia (Table 119–3).[26–29]

Stool should be examined for eggs and the rhabditiform larvae. Eosinophilia (30% to 60%) may be present in patients during early infection.

TREATMENT

Hookworm Disease

❹ Mebendazole (Vermox), an oral synthetic benzimidazole, is the agent of first choice. It is also effective against ascariasis, enterobiasis, trichuriasis, and hookworm.[13,25,26] The adult dose for treatment of hookworm infestation is 100 mg twice daily for 3 days. Pediatric patients older than 2 years of age should receive the same dose as adults.[13] Albendazole is an alternative agent.[13]

Ascariasis

Ascariasis is caused by the giant roundworm *Ascaris lumbricoides.* Female worms range from 20 to 35 cm in length. The worm is found worldwide but more commonly in areas where sanitation is poor. In the United States, endemic areas include southeastern parts of the Appalachian range and the Gulf Coast states.

Clinical Manifestations During migration of the larvae through the lungs, patients can present with pneumonitis, fever, cough, eosinophilia, and pulmonary infiltrates.[9,25,26] Other symptoms of ascariasis include abdominal discomfort, abdominal obstruction, vomiting, and appendicitis (see Table 119–3).[9,25,31,32] Diagnosis is made by demonstrating the characteristic egg in the stool.

TREATMENT

Ascariasis

In both adults and pediatric patients older than 2 years of age, the treatment for ascariasis is mebendazole (Vermox) 100 mg twice daily for 3 days.[13] An alternative drug for ascariasis is albendazole 400 mg as a single dose.[13]

Enterobiasis

Enterobiasis, or pinworm infection, is caused by *Enterobius vermicularis.* The pinworm is a small, thread-like, spindle-shaped worm about 1 cm in length. It is the most widely distributed helminthic infection in the world. There are estimated to be 42 million cases in the United States.[25] The majority of those infected are children.

The most common problem with enterobiasis is cutaneous irritation in the perianal region, made by the migrating females or the presence of eggs. However, there are reports of other complications, including appendicitis and intestinal perforation.[33] The intense pruritus and scratching can cause dermatitis and secondary bacterial infections. In children, the itching can cause loss of sleep and restlessness (see Table 119–3).

The most effective method of diagnosing pinworm infections is by the use of perianal swab using adhesive Scotch tape. The Scotch tape, which is applied to the perianal region with a tongue depressor, is examined microscopically for eggs.[9,25]

TREATMENT

Enterobiasis

The common agents for treatment include pyrantel pamoate, mebendazole, or albendazole (Albenza). The dose of pyrantel pamoate is 11 mg/kg (maximum 1 g) as a single dose that can be repeated in 2 weeks. The dose of mebendazole for adults and children older than 2 years of age is 100 mg as a single dose; this may be repeated in 2 weeks.[13,25] The dose of albendazole for adults and children older than 2 years of age is 400 mg, and should be repeated in 2 weeks.[25] Following treatment, all bedding and underclothes should be sterilized by steaming or washing in the hot water cycle of a regular washing machine; this will eradicate the eggs. Bathroom rugs and toilet accessories also should be cleaned in a similar way.

Strongyloidiasis

Strongyloidiasis is caused by *Strongyloides stercoralis*, which has a worldwide distribution and is predominantly prevalent in South America (Brazil and Columbia) and in Southeast Asia. Strongyloidiasis is primarily seen among institutionalized populations (mental homes, mentally disabled children's homes) and immunocompromised individuals (patients with human immunodeficiency virus [HIV], AIDS, and hematologic malignancies).[8,34–38] The worm is usually found in the upper intestine where the eggs are deposited and hatch to form the rhabditiform larvae. The rhabditiform larvae (male and female) migrate to the bowel where they may be excreted in the feces. If excreted in the feces, the larvae can evolve into either one of two forms after copulation: (a) free-living noninfectious rhabditiform larvae or (b) infectious filariform larvae. The filariform larvae can penetrate host skin, travel to the lungs via the bronchi and glottis and make their way to the small intestine. At times, the filariform larvae may not pass out in the feces but instead migrate to the lungs and produce progeny, a process called autoinfection. This can result in hyperinfection (i.e., increased number of larvae in intestine, lungs and other internal organs), especially in immunocompromised hosts.[34–36]

Symptoms with acute infection may appear with localized pruritic rash but heavy infestations can produce eosinophilia (10% to 15%), diarrhea, abdominal pain and intestinal obstruction (see Table 119–3).[37–39] Administration of corticosteroids or other immunosuppressive drugs to an infected individual can result in hyperinfections and disseminated strongyloidiasis. Diagnosis of strongyloidiasis is made by identification of the rhabditiform larvae in stool, sputum, duodenal fluid, and cerebrospinal fluid, by small bowel biopsy specimens, or by antigen testing (ELISA assay).[34,37]

TREATMENT

Strongyloidiasis

❹ The drug of choice for strongyloidiasis is oral ivermectin 200 mcg/kg/day for 2 days and the alternative is albendazole 400 mg twice daily for 7 days.[13,34,39,40] In a patient with hyperinfection or disseminated strongyloidiasis, immunosuppressive drugs should be discontinued and treatment initiated with ivermectin 200 mcg/kg/day until all symptoms are resolved (duration: 5 to 14 days). Patients should be tested periodically to ensure the elimination of the larvae. Individuals from endemic areas, who are candidates for organ transplantation, must be screened for *S. stercoralis.*

Taenia solium: Cysticercosis and Neurocysticercosis

Tapeworm infection caused by *Taenia solium* is a result of ingestion of poorly cooked pork that contains the larvae or cysticercus.[41,42] Cysticercus, when released from the contaminated meat by host digestive juices, matures into the adult tapeworm and attaches to the host jejunum. Cysticercosis is a systemic disease caused by the larva of *T. solium* (oncosphere) and is usually acquired by ingestion of eggs in contaminated food or by autoinfection.[41–46] The larvae can penetrate the bowel and migrate through the bloodstream to infect different organs including the central nervous system (neurocysticercosis). The larvae matures in about 8 weeks and remain as a semitransparent, oval-shaped, fluid-filled bladder in tissues. In the United States, the highest incidence of cysticercosis has been reported in immigrants from Mexico.[2,43,44] Cysticercosis in most tissues may not produce major symptoms and usually manifest as subcutaneous nodules, primarily in the arms, legs, and chest. However, penetration of the larval stage (cysticercus) into the central nervous system can produce hydrocephalus, intracranial hypertension, stroke, and seizure activity. Epileptic seizures (50% to 80%) may be the presenting symptoms in patients with neurocysticercosis (see Table 119–3).[42,45] Clinical presentation, primarily seizure history, together with radiographic demonstration (CT and magnetic resonance imaging) of the cysticercus within the bladder or calcified cysts in the central nervous system, is diagnostic for neurocysticercosis. Serologic diagnosis is made by the use of an enzyme-linked immunoelectrotransfer blot assay, which is considered highly sensitive and specific for cysticercosis.[41,42,45,46]

TREATMENT

Neurocysticercosis

CLINICAL CONTROVERSY

❹ Cysticercosis (excluding neurocysticercosis) is normally not treated. The management for neurocysticercosis remains controversial but may include surgery, anticonvulsants (neurocysticercosis-induced seizures), and antihelminthic therapy.[2,41,42,45,47] Antihelminthic therapy, if one decides this is an option, is albendazole 400 mg twice daily for 8 to 30 days.[13] However, the dose and duration of therapy with albendazole is not clearly defined.[42,47] The pediatric dose of albendazole is 15 mg/kg (maximum: 800 mg) in two divided doses for 8 to 30 days. The doses for both adults and pediatric subjects may be repeated if necessary. Praziquantel is an alternative therapy.[13]

Evaluation of Therapeutic Outcome

Morbidity and disease with intestinal nematodes are related to the intensity of infection or worm burden; subjects with transient exposure have less-severe disease. The major adverse effects of intestinal nematodes are malnutrition, fatigue, and diminished work capacity. Treatment with antihelmintic agents results in complete eradication and significant change in the well-being of patients. Unlike other nematode infections, strongyloidiasis can perpetuate itself by autoinfection, and in the immunosuppressed host, the filariform larvae can invade various organs (e.g., lungs, central nervous system, and the like) to produce disseminated infection that can be fatal.[9,34–38]

The most serious complication of cysticercosis is invasion of the central nervous system which results in neurocysticercosis. Neurocysticercosis can cause obstructive hydrocephalus, strokes and seizures; antihelminthic treatment for these conditions remains controversial.[2,42,45,47]

MALARIA

❺ Malaria represents the most devastating disease in terms of human suffering and economics. It affects the largest number of people (between 300 and 500 million new infections are reported annually) in the world, and between 1 to 2 million deaths worldwide.[3,5,48–50] In the United States, deaths from malaria are preventable. The primary reasons for deaths are failure to take chemoprophylaxis, inappropriate chemoprophylaxis, delay in seeking medical care, and misdiagnosis.[3,4,7,50]

EPIDEMIOLOGY

The exact geographic distribution of the various species is not well documented; it is reported that *Plasmodium vivax* is more prevalent in India, Pakistan, Bangladesh, Sri Lanka, and Central America, whereas *Plasmodium falciparum* is predominant in Africa, Haiti, Dominican Republic, the Amazon region of South America, and New Guinea. Most of the infections with *Plasmodium ovale* occur in Africa, and the distribution of *Plasmodium malariae* is considered worldwide.[7,49]

In the United States, most cases of malaria are reported in immigrants from endemic areas and in American travelers. Blood transfusion also has been cited as a cause of malarial infection.[48,51]

ETIOLOGY

Malaria is transmitted by the bite of an infected *Anopheles* mosquito that introduces the sporozoites (tissue parasites) of the plasmodia (*P. falciparum, P. vivax, P. malariae,* and *P. ovale*) into the bloodstream. The asexual reproduction stage develops in humans, whereas the sexual stage occurs in the mosquito.[9,48,49] The sporozoites invade parenchymal hepatocytes, multiply in stages referred to as *exoerythrocytic stages,* and become hepatic vegetative forms or schizonts. Schizonts rupture to release daughter cells, or merozoites, that then infect erythrocytes.

P. falciparum and *P. malariae* remain in the primary exoerythrocytic stage in the liver for about 4 weeks before invading erythrocytes, whereas *P. vivax* and *P. ovale* can exist in the liver in the latent exoerythrocytic form for extended periods, and, therefore, infected subjects can experience relapses. The merozoites that invade the erythrocytes develop sequentially into ring forms, trophozoites, schizonts, and finally, merozoites, which can invade other erythrocytes or can develop into gametocytes, which undergo the sexual stage in the *Anopheles* vector. Because erythrocytic forms never reinvade the liver without developing into sporozoites in the vector, malaria infections from transfusion never result in the exoerythrocytic, or "liver," form.[9,49] *P. falciparum* can result in high levels of parasitemia because of its ability to invade erythrocytes of all ages, unlike *P. vivax* and *P. ovale,* which only invade young cells.[48,49]

TABLE 119-4 Clinical Presentation of Malaria

Initial presentation
Nonspecific fever, chills, rigors, diaphoresis, malaise, vomiting[15,49]
Orthostatic hypotension
Electrolyte abnormalities
Erythrocytic phase
Prodrome: headache, anorexia, malaise, fatigue, myalgia
Nonspecific complaints such as abdominal pain, diarrhea, chest pain, and arthralgia
Paroxysm: high fever, chills, and rigor[2,3,9,49,54,55]
Cold phase: severe pallor, cyanosis of the lips and cutis anserina ("goose flesh")[9,49,55]
Hot phase: fever between 40.5°C (104.9°F) and 41°C (105.8°F).
Sweating phase:
Follows hot phase by 2–6 hours
Fever resolves
Marked fatigue and drowsiness, warm, dry skin, tachycardia, cough, severe headache, nausea, vomiting, abdominal pain, diarrhea, and delirium
Lactic acidosis and hypoglycemia (with falciparum malaria)[48,49,54,55]
Anemia
Splenomegaly
***P. falciparum* infections**
Hypoglycemia, acute renal failure, pulmonary edema, severe anemia, thrombocytopenia, high-output heart failure, cerebral congestion, seizures and coma, and adult respiratory syndrome[49,54,55]

PATHOLOGY

The erythrocytic phase causes extensive hemolysis, which results in anemia and splenomegaly. The most serious complications usually are associated with *P. falciparum* infections.[48–50,52–59] Infants and children younger than 5 years of age and nonimmune pregnant women are at high risk for severe complications from falciparum malaria.[52–55] The complications associated with falciparum malaria are primarily a result of the high parasitemia and the ability of the parasites to sequester in capillaries and postcapillary vessels of organs such as the brain and the kidney. It has been postulated that tissue hypoxia from anemia, together with *P. falciparum*-parasitized red blood cell adherence to endothelial cells in capillaries, contributes to extensive vascular disease and severe metabolic effects.[52,53] *P. malariae* is implicated in immune-mediated glomerulonephritis and nephrotic syndrome (Table 119–4).[49,52]

To ensure a positive diagnosis, blood smears should be obtained every 12 to 24 hours for 3 consecutive days.[9,48,52] The presence of parasites in the blood 3 to 5 days after initiation of therapy suggests drug resistance. Recent advances for detecting malaria parasite have included DNA or RNA probes by polymerase chain reaction (PCR) and rapid dipstick tests (*Para*Sight F, Becton-Dickinson, Cockeysville, MD) and OptiMAL.[48,49,52,60] The dipstick is reported to have a sensitivity of 88% and a specificity of 97%; however, microscopy is still considered the optimal test.

TREATMENT

Malaria

■ DESIRED OUTCOME

The primary goal in the management of malaria is the rapid diagnosis of the *Plasmodia* spp. by blood smears (repeated every 12 hours for 3 days) so as to initiate timely antimalarial therapy to eradicate the infection within 48 to 72 hours and to avoid complications such as hypoglycemia, pulmonary edema, and renal failure that are responsible for increased mortality in malaria.

■ PHARMACOLOGIC THERAPY

❻ In adults (including pregnant women), the chemoprophylaxis for all species of *Plasmodium* is chloroquine phosphate 300 mg (base) once weekly beginning 1 week prior to departure and continued for 4 weeks after leaving an endemic area.[3,13,48,49,52,61–63] The pediatric dose of chloroquine phosphate is 5 mg (base) per kilogram of body weight (maximum: 300 mg). When departing an area endemic for *P. vivax* or *P. ovale,* primaquine phosphate 30 mg (base) daily for 14 days beginning the last 2 weeks of chloroquine prophylaxis should be added to the regimen. The pediatric dose of primaquine is 0.6 mg (base) per kilogram of body weight per day for 14 days. The pediatric doses of chloroquine can be calculated based on body weight, and the tablets can be pulverized and placed in gelatin capsules. Parents can be instructed to suspend the dose in food, simple syrup, chocolate milk, or drink.[13,61]

In areas where chloroquine-resistant *P. falciparum* strains exist, travelers should receive mefloquine (Lariam) for prophylaxis. The adult dose of mefloquine is 250 mg once weekly beginning 1 week prior to departure and continuing for the full period of exposure, followed by 250 mg for 4 weeks after last exposure.[13,48,49] The pediatric dose of mefloquine for prophylaxis is based on body weight:

Body Weight (kg)	Dose
15 to 19 kg	5 mg/kg
15 to 19 kg	one-quarter tablet
20 to 30 kg	one-half tablet
31 to 45 kg	three-quarters tablet
>45 kg	1 tablet

In travelers who are at immediate risk for drug-resistant falciparum malaria, a loading dose of mefloquine may be considered. Mefloquine is administered at 250 mg daily for 3 days before travel, followed by 250 mg once weekly while in the endemic area and continued for 4 weeks after last exposure.[13,48,49] Patients may experience neuropsychiatric reactions from mefloquine and may need to be monitored closely.[13,62–64]

CLINICAL CONTROVERSY

Because there remains public concern with mefloquine therapy, primarily about its neuropsychiatric effects,[63] an alternative regimen for chemoprophylaxis is the combination of atovaquone and proguanil (Malarone): 1 tablet daily beginning 1 to 2 days prior to travel and continuing for the duration of stay and 1 week after leaving the area.[13,62] Daily primaquine 30 mg (base) also has been recommended for prophylaxis for both *P. vivax* and *P. falciparum* malaria.[13]

An alternative regimen for prophylaxis in chloroquine-resistant areas for those who cannot tolerate mefloquine or Malarone, is to take doxycycline 100 mg daily starting 1 to 2 days prior to departure, during the exposure period, and continuing for 4 weeks after leaving the endemic area.[13] Children older than 8 years of age should receive 2 mg/kg per day (up to 100 mg) of doxycycline. Doxycycline is contraindicated in children younger than 8 years of age, in pregnant women, and during breast-feeding.[13,49,63,65]

In an uncomplicated attack of malaria (for all plasmodia except chloroquine-resistant *P. falciparum*), the recommended regimen is chloroquine 600 mg (base) initially, followed by 300 mg (base) 6 hours later, and then 300 mg (base) daily for 2 days. In severe illness or when oral therapy is not tolerated or parenteral quinine is not available, quinidine gluconate 10 mg/kg as a loading dose (maximum 600 mg) in 250 mL normal saline should be administered slowly over 1 to 2 hours, followed by continuous infusion of 0.02 mg/kg per minute until oral therapy can be started.[13,48,49] In patients who have received either quinine or mefloquine, the loading dose of quinidine should be omitted. Oral quinine (650 mg every 8 hours) together with doxycycline 100 mg twice daily should follow the intravenous dose of quinidine to complete a total of 7 days of therapy.[13,48] The pediatric dose of intravenous quinidine gluconate is the same as the dose for adults.[13] The pediatric dose of quinine is 30 mg/kg per day in three divided doses for 7 days. Children younger than age 8 years and pregnant women should get clindamycin 20 mg/kg/day in divided doses for 7 days instead of doxycycline.[13,49]

In *P. falciparum* (chloroquine-resistant) infections, a dose of 750 mg mefloquine followed by 500 mg 12 hours later is recommended. The pediatric dose of mefloquine is 15 mg/kg (<45 kg) followed by 10 mg/kg 8 to 12 hours later.[13] Intravenous quinidine gluconate followed by oral quinine plus doxycycline to complete a total of 7 days of therapy should follow in a severe illness, as already indicated.[13,49] An alternative oral treatment for chloroquine-resistant *P. falciparum* infection in adults, especially in those with a history of seizures or psychiatric disorders, is the combination of atovaquone 250 mg and proguanil 100 mg (Malarone) (4 tablets daily for 3 days).[13,48,49] The intravenous quinidine regimen requires close monitoring of the electrocardiogram and other vital signs (e.g., hypotension, QT interval prolongation, and hypoglycemia).[13,49,55]

❼ Because falciparum malaria is associated with serious complications, including pulmonary edema, hypoglycemia, jaundice, renal failure, confusion, delirium, seizures, coma, and death, careful monitoring of fluid status and hemodynamic parameters is mandatory.[48,49,55] Exchange transfusion that may be required in patients with *P. falciparum* malaria in whom parasitemia is 5% to 15% remains a questionable modality.[13,58] Either hemofiltration or hemodiafiltration is indicated in renal failure.[55]

Malarial infection does not produce immunity in patients, and active research has been initiated to develop a malaria vaccine.[66–68] A vaccine that blocks the entry of sporozoites into the liver cells will prevent malaria at this stage. However, immunity to sporozoites does not protect the host against parasites in the erythrocytic cycle. Infective sporozoites of *P. falciparum* are covered by a polypeptide, circumsporozoite protein. Isolation and identification of the gene encoding for this circumsporozoite protein have led to the development of a monoclonal antibody by recombinant DNA technology; *P. falciparum* sporozoite vaccine is now under investigation.[68]

EVALUATION OF THERAPEUTIC OUTCOMES

When advising potential travelers on prophylaxis for malaria, be aware of the incidence of chloroquine-resistant *P. falciparum* malaria and the countries where this is prevalent.[13,62,63] Detailed recommendations for prevention of malaria may be obtained by checking the World Wide Web (e.g., *www.cdc.gov/travel/* or *www2.cdc.gov/mmwr/*)[63,69] or by calling the Centers for Disease Control and Prevention (CDC) (see Appendix 119–1). A number of newer drugs are under active study and include the water-soluble artesunate and the oil-soluble artemether and combinations with other agents.[7,13,49,62,63,70–73,75]

Acute *P. falciparum* malaria resistant to chloroquine should be treated with intravenous quinidine. These patients should have a central venous catheter to follow fluid status, and the electrocardiogram should be monitored closely. Hypoglycemia that is associated with *P. falciparum* should be checked and corrected with dextrose infusions.[48,49,55] Quinidine infusion should be slowed temporarily or stopped if electrocardiogram shows a QT interval of greater than 0.6 seconds, an increase in the QRS complex to greater than 50%, or hypotension unresponsive to fluid challenge results. The suggested quinidine levels should be maintained at 3 to 7 mg/L.[49] Blood smears should be checked every 12 hours until parasitemia is less than 1%. Resolution of fever should take place between 36 and 48 hours after initiation of the intravenous quinidine therapy and the blood should be clear of parasites in 5 days.[48,49,52] If parenteral therapy is required for more than 48 hours, the dose of quinidine be lowered by half.[13]

Travelers to endemic areas for malaria should be advised to remain in well-screened areas, to wear clothes that cover most of the body, and to sleep in mosquito nets.[4,7,71,74] It is prudent to carry the insect repellent DEET (N,N,diethyl-metatol) or Picaridin (Cutter Advanced) insect spray for use in mosquito-infested areas. Readers are urged to check publications from the CDC for the list of countries where chloroquine-resistant *P. falciparum* exist.[13,63]

AMERICAN TRYPANOSOMIASIS

ETIOLOGY

Two distinct forms of the genus *Trypanosoma* occur in humans. One is associated with African trypanosomiasis (sleeping sickness) and the other with American trypanosomiasis (Chagas' disease).[76–79] *Trypanosoma brucei gambiense* and *Trypanosoma brucei rhodesiense* are the causative organisms for the East African and West African trypanosomiasis, respectively. *T. brucei rhodesiense* causes the acute disease and is the more virulent of the two species. Both East and West African trypanosomiasis are transmitted by various species of tsetse fly belonging to the genus *Glossina*. Further discussion of this subject will focus on American trypanosomiasis.

Trypanosoma cruzi is the agent that causes American trypanosomiasis. American trypanosomiasis is transmitted by a number of species of a reduviid bug (*Triatoma infestans, Rhodnius prolixus*) that live in wall cracks of houses in rural areas of North, Central, and South America. The reduviid bug is infected by sucking blood from animals (e.g., opossums, dogs, and cats) or humans infected with circulating trypomastigotes (Table 119–5).

8 In chronic trypanosomiasis, patients present with cardiomyopathy and heart failure. Electrocardiograms are usually abnormal, demonstrating extrasystoles, first-degree heart block, right bundle-branch block, and other serious conduction disturbances.[77–79] Degeneration of the autonomic ganglia in the smooth muscle of the esophagus and colon leads to uncoordinated peristalsis. The end result has been reported to be "megasyndromes" of affected organs.[78–79] Penetration of central nervous system results in meningoencephalitis, strokes, seizures, and focal paralysis.[78–80]

A history to verify the possible exposure to *T. cruzi* should be an important initial diagnostic workup. Recovery of *T. cruzi* is definitive, but this is not always possible, especially in chronic disease. Positive serologic tests using indirect immunofluorescent antibody test and ELISA (Chagas' EIA, Abbott Labs) may be diagnostic for the disease. The only serologic test available in United States is Chagas' Kit (Hemagen Diagnostics, Inc., Columbia, MD).[78] A PCR test has been used to diagnosis *T. cruzi*.[81] Specimens may be sent to the CDC for testing. All candidates from an endemic area for Chagas' disease who are candidates for transplantation should be tested for *T. cruzi*.[82]

TABLE 119-5 Clinical Presentation of South American Trypanosomiasis

Acute
Unilateral orbital edema ("Romana sign")[76,78,79]
Granuloma or "chagoma"
Fever, hepatosplenomegaly, and lymphadenopathy
Chronic
Cardiac: cardiomyopathy and heart failure
ECG: first-degree heart block, right bundle-branch block, and arrhythmias[77,78]
Gastrointestinal: enlargement of esophagus and colon ("mega" syndrome)[76,78]
Central nervous system: meningoencephalitis, strokes, seizures, and focal paralysis[78–80]

TREATMENT

American Trypanosomiasis

■ DESIRED OUTCOME

The primary goal of drug therapy in trypanosomiasis is to reduce the duration and severity of the illness and to decrease mortality.

■ PHARMACOLOGIC THERAPY

The drugs that have been used to treat *T. cruzi* infections include nifurtimox (Lampit, Bayer 2502) and benznidazole (Rochagan).[13,78,79,83,84] Oral nifurtimox is available from the CDC, whereas benznidazole is only available in Brazil. Neither of these agents are optimal therapy and there is ongoing search for newer agents.[76,78] The adult dose of nifurtimox is 8 to 10 mg/kg per day in divided doses for 120 days. Because pediatric patients tolerate the drug better than adults, the dose for children aged 1 to 10 years is 15 to 20 mg/kg per day, and for children aged 11 to 16 years it is 12.5 to 15 mg/kg per day in divided doses.[13,84] Symptomatic treatment for heart failure includes digitalis and diuretics; the gastrointestinal complications, however, may require surgical revisions and reconstruction.[78,79]

EVALUATION OF THERAPEUTIC OUTCOMES

American trypanosomiasis (Chagas' disease), which is endemic in all Latin American countries, can be transmitted congenitally, by blood transfusion, and by organ transplantation.[78,79] Treatment with nifurtimox of the acute phase (i.e., fever, malaise, edema of face, generalized lymphadenopathy, and hepatosplenomegaly) produces between 10% and 30% cure rates.[78] Treatment of chronic infection with nifurtimox is not recommended. It is essential to identify *T. cruzi*-infected patients by serology and to monitor the cardiovascular status of these patients by electrocardiogram periodically. The congestive failure of cardiomyopathic Chagas' disease is treated the same way as cardiomyopathies from other causes.[76,78]

ECTOPARASITES

A parasite that lives on the outside the body of the host is called an *ectoparasite*. Approximately 6 to 12 million people become infested with pediculosis yearly in the United States.[85] Pediculosis usually is associated with poor personal hygiene, and infections are passed from person to person through social and sexual contact. The three types of human lice belong to two genera: *Pediculus*, including the head and body lice, and *Phthirus*, with only one species, the crab louse.[9,85,86] The human louse is detectable to the human naked eye and measures approximately 2 to 3 mm in length.

LICE

The two species that belong to this group include *Pediculus humanus capitis* (head louse) and *Pediculus humanus corporis* (body louse). Female lice deposit eggs on the hair. The eggs (or nits) remain firmly attached to the hair, and in about 10 days, the lice hatch to form nymphs, which mature in 2 weeks. Using both their piercing mouth parts and a pumping device, the larva and adults feed on the blood of the host. The body louse and head louse are essentially identical, although they live on different parts of the body. Unlike the head louse, which lives on the hair, the body louse is more frequently found on clothing of the infected host.

Pubic or crab lice are found on the hairs around the genitals, although they can occur in other areas of the body (e.g., eyelashes, beards, and axillae). Patients usually complain of severe pruritus from papular lesions produced by the bite of the louse. Hypersensitivity to foreign material injected by the lice can produce macular swellings and occasionally can lead to secondary bacterial infections.[85]

TREATMENT

Lice

The goal of therapy is to eradicate the causative organisms and provide symptomatic relief to patients. The agent of choice for all three infections (body, head, and crab lice) is 1% permethrin (Nix).[85–90] Permethrin is a derivative of the flowers of the plant *Chrysanthemum cinerariifolium.* The term *pyrethrin* is usually applied to several esters of chrysanthemic acid and pyrethric acid. Permethrin has both pediculicidal and ovicidal activity against *P. humanus* var. *capitis.* The cure rate is reported to be in the range of 85% to 95%.[85] Individuals who have a history of ragweed or chrysanthemum allergy should use this compound with caution. The side effects reported with permethrin products include itching, burning, stinging, and tingling.[90] Permethrin 1% is applied to the scalp after the hair has been dried following a shampooing. The scalp should be saturated with permethrin liquid, and a towel should be wrapped around the scalp to allow the application to stay on for 10 minutes. The hair then should be rinsed thoroughly. A cream rinse of permethrin 1% (Nix-Creme Rinse) is also available. To ensure complete eradication, especially of newly hatched lice, it may be necessary to repeat the application.

❾ Recent reports suggest increasing lice resistance to permethrin 1%.[87–89] An alternative preparation for lice is 0.5% malathion (Ovide), which is very effective.[13,85] To ensure complete eradication of lice infestation, the malathion application should be left on the scalp for about 90 minutes.[90] For the relief of pruritus, a soothing lotion of calamine liniment or lotion with 0.1% menthol may be used. Other members of the family or sexual partners also should be treated. All bedding and clothes should be sterilized by boiling or washing in the hot water cycle of the washing machine to avoid reinfections. Seams of clothes should be examined to verify that all organisms are eradicated. An ocular lubricant (e.g., Lacri-Lube S.O.P.) applied twice daily may be used to remove crab louse infection of the eyelids.

SCABIES

Scabies is caused by the itch mite *Sarcoptes scabiei,* which affects both humans and animals. Mange in domestic animals is caused by the same organism. Infection usually affects the interdigital and popliteal folds, axillary folds, the umbilicus, and the scrotum.[91–93]

Clinical Presentation

Patients will complain of severe itching and an inability to sleep and may have excoriations in the interdigital web spaces, wrists, elbows, buttocks, groin, and scalp. Excoriations may lead to secondary bacterial infections. The diagnosis is made by looking for burrows formed by the mite and taking skin scrapings, which will demonstrate the mite on a wet mount.

TREATMENT

Scabies

Because these infections cause a great deal of discomfort and distress to patients and families, the goals of therapy are to eradicate the infestations rapidly, to institute symptomatic treatment, and to provide counseling and reassurance. The treatment of choice is permethrin 5% (Elimite) cream.[13,91–93] To initiate the treatment, the skin should be scrubbed thoroughly in a warm soapy bath using a soft brush to remove all scabs. The lotion is then applied to the whole body, avoiding the face, mucous membranes, and eyes. The application should be left on for 8 to 14 hours before bathing. A single application eradicates 97% of scabies in subjects.[91] All close contacts should be checked and treated appropriately.

Other agents used to treat scabies include topical crotamiton 10% (Eurax) and oral ivermectin (Stromectol) 200 mcg/kg as a single dose which may be repeated in 2 weeks.[13,93] Crotamiton and oral ivermectin may be used in patients who have hypersensitivity to permethrin preparations. Topical corticosteroids and antihistamines may be used to decrease pruritus.

❿ Permethrin (1% and 5%) for pediculosis and scabies respectively, is the preferred agent and remains the safest agent, especially in infants and children.[85,93] One application of permethrin is consistently effective in eradicating more than 90% of all infections. However, pruritus may persist for 2 to 4 weeks because of the remnants of mite parts in the skin. Ivermectin is an alternative therapy for scabies.

ABBREVIATIONS

AIDS: acquired immunodeficiency syndrome

ELISA: enzyme-linked immunosorbent assay

PCR: polymerase chain reaction

REFERENCES

1. Garg PK, Perry S, Dorn M, Hardcastle L, Parsonnet J. Risk of intestinal helminth and protozoan infection in a refugee population. Am J Trop Med Hyg 2005;73:386–391.
2. White AC, Atmar RL. Infections in Hispanic immigrants. Clin Infect Dis 2002;34:1627–1632.
3. Bledsoe GH. Malaria Primer for Clinicians in the United States. South Med J 2005;98:1197–1204.
4. Dardick K. Educating travelers about malaria: Dealing with resistance and patient noncompliance. Cleve Clin J Med 2000;69:469–479.
5. Malaria Surveillance—United States, 2004. MMWR 2006;55(SS-04):1–19.
6. Beigel Y, Greenberg Z, Ostfeld I. Letting the patient off the hook. N Engl J Med 2000;342:1658–1661.
7. Franco-Paredes C, Santos-Preciado JI. Problem pathogens: Prevention of malaria in travelers. Lancet Infect Dis 2006;6:139–149.
8. Nuesch R, Zimmerli L, Stockli R, Gyr N, Hatz CFR. Imported strongyloidosis: A longitudinal analysis of 31 cases. J Travel Med 2005;29:80–84.
9. John DT, Petri WA Jr. Markell and Voge's Medical Parasitology, 9th ed. Philadelphia: WB Saunders, 2006.
10. Farthing MJG, Cevellos AM, Kelly P. Intestinal protozoa. The Mastigophora (flagellates): *Giardia intestinalis.* In: Cook GC, Zumla A, eds. Mansons Topical Diseases, 21st ed. London: WB Saunders, 2003:1387–1396.
11. Gardner TB, Hill DR. Treatment of giardiasis. Clin Microbiol Rev 2001;14:14–128.
12. Hill DR. *Giardia lamblia.* In: Mandell GL, Bennett JE, Dolin R, eds. Principles and Practice of Infectious Diseases, 6th ed. New York: Elsevier Churchill-Livingstone, 2005:3198–3205.
13. Abramowicz M. (Editor). Drugs for parasitic infections. In: Handbook of Antimicrobial Therapy, 17th ed. New Rochelle, NY: Medical Letter, 2005:179–193.
14. Lebwohl B, Deckelbaum RJ, Green PHR. Giardiasis. Gastrointest Endosc 2003;57:906–913.
15. Walkowiak J, Krawczynski M, Herzig KH. Giardiasis aggravates malabsorption in cystic fibrosis. Scand J Gastroenterol 2004;39:607–608.
16. Sorell L, Garrote JA, Galvan JA, Velazco C, Endrosa CR, Arranz E. Celiac disease diagnosis in patients with giardiasis: High value of antitransglutaminase antibodies. Am J Gastroenterol 2004;99:1330–1332.
17. Nitazoxanide (Alinia): A new antiprotozoal agent. Med Lett 2003;45:29–31.

18. Hung C-C, Deng H-Y, Hsiao W-H, et al. Invasive amebiasis as an emerging parasite disease in patients with human immunodeficiency virus type 1 infection in Taiwan. JAMA 2005;165:409–415.
19. Farthing MJG. Intestinal protozoa. *Entamoeba histolytica*. In: Cook GC, Zumla A, eds. Mansons Tropical Diseases, 21st ed. London: WB Saunders, 2003:1373–1386.
20. Haque R, Huston CD, Hughes M, et al. Amebiasis. N Engl J Med 2003;348:1565–1573.
21. Ravdin J, Stauffer WM. *Entamoeba histolytica* (amebiasis). In: Mandell GL, Bennett JA, Dolin R, eds. Principles and Practice of Infectious Diseases, 6th ed. New York: Elsevier Churchill-Livingstone, 2005:3097–3111.
22. Hughes MA, Petri WA Jr. Amebic liver abscess. Infect Dis Clin North Am 2000;14:565–581.
23. Katz DE, Taylor DN. Parasitic infections of the gastrointestinal tract. Gastroenterol Clin North Am 2001;30:797–815.
24. Ozdogan M, Baykal A, Aran O. Amebic perforation of the colon: Rare and frequently fatal complication. World J Surg 2004;28:926–929.
25. Maguire JH. Intestinal nematodes (Roundworms). In: Mandell GL, Bennett JE, Dolin R, eds. Principles and Practice of Infectious Diseases, 6th ed. New York: Elsevier Churchill-Livingstone, 2005:3260–3267.
26. Bethony J, Brooker S, Albonico M, et al. Soil-transmitted helminth infection: Ascariasis, trichuriasis, and hookworm. Lancet 2006;367:1521–1532.
27. Hotez PJ, Brooker S, Bethony JM, et al. Hookworm Infection. N Engl J Med 2004;357:799–807.
28. Gabriella AF, Ramsan M, Naumann C, et al. Soil-transmitted helminths and haemoglobin status among Afghan children in World Food Programme Assisted Schools. J Helminthol 2005;79:381–384.
29. Larocque R, Casapia M, Gotuzzo E, Gyorkos TW. Relationship between intensity of soil-transmitted helminth infections and anemia in pregnancy. Am J Trop Med Hyg 2005;73:783–789.
30. Sahoo PK, Satapathy AK, Michael E, Ravindran B. Concomitant parasitism: Bancroftian filariasis and intestinal helminths and response to albendazole. Am J Trop Med Hyg 2005;73:877–880.
31. Malik AH, Saima BD, Wani MY. Management of hepatobiliary and pancreatic ascariasis in children of endemic area. Pediatr Surg Int 2006;22:164–168.
32. Huratado RM, Sahani DV, Kradin RL. Case records of the Massachusetts General Hospital. Case 9–2006. A 35-year-old woman with recurrent upper-quadrant pain. N Engl J Med 2006;354:1295–1303.
33. Petro M, Iavu K, Minocha A. Unusual endoscopic and microscopic view of *Enterobius vermicularis*: A case report with review of the literature. Southern Med J 2005;98:927–929.
34. Keiser PB, Nutman TB. *Strongyloides stercoralis* in the immunocompromised population. Clin Microbiol Rev 2004;17:208–217.
35. Lim S, Katz K, Krajden S, Fuksa M, Keystone JS, Kain KC. Complicated and fatal *Strongyloides* infection in Canadians: Risk factors, diagnosis and management. CMAJ 2004;171:479–484.
36. Schaeffer MW, Buell JF, Gupta M, et al. *Strongyloides* hyperinfection syndrome after heart transplantation: Case report and review of literature. J Heart Lung Transplant 2004;23:905–911.
37. Concho R, Harrington W, Rogers AI. Intestinal strongyloidiasis: Recognition, management, and determinants of outcome. Clin Gastroenterol 2005;39:203–211.
38. Newberry AM, Williams DN, Stauffer WM, et al. *Strongyloides* hyperinfection presenting as acute respiratory failure and gram-negative sepsis. Chest 2005;128:3681–3684.
39. Satoh M, Kokaze A. Treatment strategies in controlling strongyloidiasis. Expert Opin Pharmacother 2004;5:2293–2301.
40. Muennig P, Pallin D, Challah C, Khan K. The cost-effectiveness of ivermectin vs albendazole in the presumptive treatment of strongyloidiasis in immigrants to the United States. Epidemiol Infect 2004;132:1055–1063.
41. King CH. Cestodes (Tapeworms). In: Mandell GL, Dolin R, Bennett JE, eds. Principles and Practice of Infectious Diseases, 6th ed. New York: Elsevier Churchill-Livingstone, 2005:3285–3293.
42. Garcia HH, Gonzalez AE, Evans CAW, Gilman RH. *Taenia solium* cysticercosis. Lancet 2003;361:547–556.
43. Del La Garza Y, Graviss EA, Daver NG, et al. Epidemiology of neurocysticercosis in Houston, Texas. Am J Trop Med Hyg 2005;73:766–770.
44. Townes JM, Hoffmann CJ, Kohn MA. Neurocysticercosis in Oregon, 1995–2000. Emerg Infect Dis 2004;10:508–510.
45. Dua T, Aneja S. Neurocysticercosis: Management issues. Indian Pediat 2006:43:227–235.
46. Garcia HH, Del Brutto OH, Nash TE, White AC Jr, Tsang VCW, Gilman RH. New concepts in the diagnosis and management of neurocysticercosis (*Taenia solium*). Am J Trop Med Hyg 2005;72:3–9.
47. Gongora-Rivera F, Soto-Hernandez JL, Esquivel DG, et al. Albendazole trial at 15 or 30 mg/kg/day for subarachnoid and intraventricular cysticercosis. Neurology 2006;66:436–438.
48. Fairhurst RM, Wellems TE. *Plasmodium* species (Malaria). In: Mandell GL, Dolin R, Bennett JE, eds. Principles and Practice of Infectious Diseases, 6th ed. New York: Elsevier Churchill-Livingstone, 2005:3121–3144.
49. White NJ, Breman JG. Malaria and babesiosis: Diseases caused by red blood cell parasites. In: Kasper DL, Fauci AS, Longo DL, et al. eds. Harrison's Principles of Internal Medicine, 16th ed. New York: McGraw-Hill, 2005:1218–1233.
50. Newman RD, Parise ME, Barber AM, Steketee RW. Malaria-related deaths among travelers, 1963–2001. Ann Intern Med 2004;141:547–555.
51. Kitchen AD, Chiodini PL. Malaria and blood transfusion. Vox Sang 2006;90:77–84.
52. White NJ. Malaria. In: Cook GC, Zumla A, eds. Manson's Tropical Diseases, 21st ed. London: WB Saunders, 2003:1205–1295.
53. Idro R, Carter JA, Fegan G, Neville BG, Newton CR. Risk factors for persisting neurological and cognitive impairment following cerebral malaria. Arch Dis Child 2006;91:142–148.
54. Idro R, Jenkins NE, Newton Newton CRJC. Pathogenesis, clinical features, and neurological outcome of cerebral malaria. Lancet Neurol 2005;4:827–840.
55. Pasvol G. Management of severe malaria: Interventions and controversies. Infect Dis Clin North Am 2005;19:211–240.
56. Eiam-Ong S. Malarial nephropathy. Semin Nephrol 2003;23:21–33.
57. Murphy SC, Breman JG. Gaps in childhood malaria burden in Africa: Cerebral malaria, neurological sequelae, anemia, respiratory distress, hypoglycemia, and complications of pregnancy. Am J Trop Med Hyg 2001;64:57–67.
58. Riddle MS, Jackson JL, Sanders JW, Blazes DL. Exchange transfusion as an adjunct therapy in severe *Plasmodium falciparum* malaria: A meta-analysis. Clin Infect Dis 2002;34:1192–1198.
59. Taylor WRJ, White NJ. Malaria and the lung. Clin Chest Med 2002;23:457–468.
60. Singh N, Saxena A. Usefulness of a rapid on-site *Plasmodium falciparum* diagnosis (Paracheck PF) in forest migrants and among the indigenous population at the site of their occupational activities in central India. Am J Trop Med Hyg 2005;72:26–29.
61. Magill AJ. The prevention of malaria. Prim Care Clin Off Pract 2002;29:815–842.
62. Shanks GD, Kain KC, Keystone JS. Malaria chemoprophylaxis in the age of drug resistance: II. Drugs that may be available in the future. Clin Infect Dis 2001;33:381–385.
63. Shanks GD, Edstein MD. Modern malaria chemoprophylaxis. Drugs 2005;65:2091–2110.
64. Taylor WRJ, White NJ. Antimalarial drug toxicity. Drugs Safety 2004;27:25–61.
65. Tako EA, Zhou A, Lohoue J, et al. Risk factors for placental malaria and its effect on pregnancy outcome in Yaounde, Cameroon. Am J Trop Med Hyg 2005;72:236–242.
66. Hoffman SL, Subramanian GM, Collins FH, Venter JC. *Plasmodium*, human and *Anopheles* genomics and malaria. Nature 2002:415:702–709.
67. Ballou WR, Arevalo-Herrera M, Carucci D, et al. Update on the clinical development of candidate malaria vaccines. Am J Trop Med Hyg 2004;71:239–247.
68. Alonso P, Sacarlal J, Aponte JJ, et al. Efficacy of the RTS,S/ASO2A vaccine against *Plasmodium* infection and disease in young African children: Randomized controlled trial. Lancet 2004;364:1411–1420.
69. Angus BJ. Malaria on the World Wide Web. Clin Infect Dis 2001;33:651–661.
70. Rathore D, McCutchan TF, Sullivan M, Kumar S. Antimalarial drugs: Current status and new developments. Expert Opin Investig Drugs 2006;14:871–883.
71. Chen LH, Keystone JS. New strategies for the prevention of malaria in travelers. Infect Dis Clin North Am 2005;19:185–210.
72. Davis TME, Karunajeewa HA, Ilett KF. Artemisin-based combination therapies for uncomplicated malaria. Med J Aust 2005;182:181–185.

73. Price RN, Uhlemann A-C, van Vugt M, et al. Molecular and Pharmacological determinants of the therapeutic response to Artemether-Lumefantrine in multi-resistant *Plasmodium falciparum* malaria. Clin Infect Dis 2006;42:1570–1577.
74. Fradin MS, Day JF. Comparative efficacy of insect repellents against mosquito bites. N Engl J Med 2002;347:13–18.
75. Rosenthal PJ. Antiprotozoal drugs. In: Katzung BG, ed. Basic and Clinical Pharmacology, 9th ed. New York: Lange Medical Books/McGraw-Hill, 2004:864–885.
76. Barrett MP, Burchmore RJS, Stich A, et al. The trypanosomiasis. Lancet 2003;362:1469–1480.
77. Rassi A Jr, Rassi A, Little WC. Chagas' heart disease. Clin Cardiol 2000;23:883–889.
78. Kirchhoff LV. *Trypanosoma* species (American trypanosomiasis, Chagas' disease): Biology of trypanosomes. In: Mandell GL, Bennett JE, Dolin R, eds. Principles and Practice of Infectious Diseases, 6th ed. New York: Elsevier Churchill-Livingstone, 2005:3156–3164.
79. Miles MA. American trypanosomiasis (Chagas' Disease). In: Cook GC, Zumla A, eds. Manson's Tropical Diseases, 21st ed. London: WB Saunders, 2003:1325–1337.
80. Carod-Artal FJ, Vargas AP, Melo M, Horan TA. American trypanosomiasis (Chagas' disease): An unrecognized cause of stroke. J Neurol Neurosurg Psychiatry 2003;74:516–518.
81. Schijman AG, Vigliano CA, Viotti RJ, et al. *Trypanosoma cruzi* DNA in cardiac lesions of Argentine patients with end-stage chronic Chagas' heart disease. Am J Trop Med Hyg 2004;70:210–220.
82. Chagas' disease after organ transplantation—United States 2001. MMWR 2002;51:210–212.
83. Viotti R, Vigliano C, Lococo B, et al. Long-term cardiac outcomes of treating chronic Chagas' disease with benznidazole versus no treatment. A nonrandomized trial. Ann Intern Med 2006;144:724–734.
84. Rosenthal PJ, Goldsmith RS. Clinical pharmacology of the antihelmintic drugs. In: Katzung BG, ed. Basic and Clinical Pharmacology, 9th ed. New York: Lange Medical Books/McGraw-Hill, 2004:886–897.
85. Mathieu ME, Wilson BB. Lice (pediculosis). In: Mandell GL, Bennett JR, Dolin R, eds. Principles and Practice of Infectious Diseases, 6th ed. New York: Elsevier Churchill-Livingstone, 2005:3302–3304.
86. Roberts RJ. Head lice. N Engl J Med 2002;346:1645–1650.
87. Yoon KS, Gao J-R, Taplin D, et al. Permethrin-resistant human head lice, *Pediculus capitis,* and their treatment. Arch Dermatol 2003;139:994–1000.
88. Burkhart CG. Relationship of treatment-resistant head lice to the safety and efficacy of pediculicides. Mayo Clin Proc 2004;79:661–666.
89. Meinking TL, Clineschmidt CM, Chen C, et al. An observer blinded study of 10% permethrin creme rinse with and without adjunctive combing in patients with head lice. J Pediatr 2002;141:665–670.
90. Jones KN, English JC III. Review of common therapeutic options in the United States for the treatment of pediculosis capitis. Clin Infect Dis 2003;36:1355–1361.
91. Wendel K, Rompalo A. Scabies and pediculosis pubis. Clin Infect Dis 2002;35(Suppl 2):S146–S151.
92. Johnson G, Sladden M. Scabies: Diagnosis and treatment. BMJ 2005;331:619–622.
93. Chosidow O. Scabies. N Engl J Med 2006;354:1718–1727.

Appendix 119-1 Antiparasitic Drugs

Drug	Indications	Side Effects	Comments	References
Albendazole 200 mg tablet (Albenza)	Giardiasis Ascariasis, Neurocysticercosis	GI: abdominal pain, nausea, diarrhea, increase in liver function enzymes	Not recommended in children <2 years old	9, 13, 37, 39, 42, 46, 47
Atovaquone 250 mg *plus* proguanil 100 mg (Malarone)[a]	Prevention and treatment of *Plasmodium falciparum* malaria	Abdominal pain, nausea, vomiting and headache		9,13, 48, 49, 52, 61, 62, 64, 65, 75
Chloroquine phosphate (Aralen, Nivaquine) 250- and 500-mg tablets; 50 mg/mL (as HCl); 5-mL ampule	Malaria	GI: nausea, vomiting, diarrhea CNS: Dizziness, headache, blurring of vision, confusion, fatigue Derm: Pruritus	Administer oral dose after meals IV route: recommend ECG monitoring *Contraindication*: patients with psoriasis or porphyria	9, 13, 48, 49, 52, 61, 62, 64, 75
Diloxanide furoate[b] (Furamide) 500-mg tablet	Amebiasis	GI: nausea, flatulence Derm: pruritus		9, 13, 19, 20, 21, 23, 75
Furazolidone (Furoxone) 100-mg tablet Suspension: 50 mg/5 mL	Giardiasis Alternative to metronidazole	GI: Nausea, vomiting Hypersensitivity: hypotension, fever, arthralgia, urticaria Other: headache	Disulfiram-like reaction with alcohol; avoid in G6PD deficiency; may cause hemolysis; chances color of urine to brown	9–14
Iodoquinol (Yodoxin) 210-mg tablet	Amebiasis	GI: abdominal pain, diarrhea Derm: rash	May interfere with thyroid function test *Contraindication*: patients with iodine intolerance	9, 13, 19–23, 75
Ivermectin (Stromectol) 6-mg tablet	Strongyloidiasis Pediculosis Scabies	Dizziness, somnolence, tremor, vertigo, pruritus, abdominal pain	Should be taken with a full glass of water	9, 13, 34, 37, 39, 92
Mebendazole (Vermox) 100-mg chewable tablet	Ascariasis, trichuriasis, hookworm, pinworm	GI: abdominal pain, diarrhea CNS: headache, dizziness Other: pyrexia, neutropenia	Drug should be taken with meals *Contraindication*: pregnancy *Drug interaction*: can increase serum levels of theophylline	9, 13, 25, 26, 84
Mefloquine (Lariam) 250-mg tablet	*P. falciparum* malaria	Incidence 17% GI: nausea, vomiting, abdominal pain, diarrhea Card: sinus bradycardia CNS: vertigo, dizziness, confusion, hallucinations, psychosis, convulsions Derm: itching, skin rash	Patients given doses in excess of 12 mg/kg should be monitored carefully because the side effects are dose related	9, 13, 48–50, 52, 55, 61, 62, 65, 75
Metronidazole (Flagyl) Oral: 250-mg, 500-mg tablets	Amebiasis Giardiasis	GI: nausea, anorexia, vomiting, diarrhea, abdominal cramping, glossitis, metallic taste CNS: dizziness, vertigo, headache, paresthesia	Avoid alcohol; alcohol ingestion will cause the disulfiram reaction: abdominal distress, vomiting, hypotension *Contraindication*: First trimester of pregnancy	9, 11–14, 19–21
Nifurtimox[c] (Lampit, Bayer 2502)	South American trypanosomiasis	GI: anorexia, nausea CNS: peripheral neuritis, psychosis Hemat: hemolysis in G6PD deficiency patients	Monitor pulmonary function and hematologic parameters	9, 13, 75, 76, 78, 79
Nitazoxanide (Alinia) 100-mg/5-mL suspension	Cryptosporidiosis Giardiasis	Abdominal pain, diarrhea, vomiting, and headache	Rarely may produce yellow sclerae	12, 13, 17
Primaquine phosphate 26.3-mg tablet	Malaria (*P. vivax*) (*P. ovale*)	GI: nausea, abdominal pain CNS: mental depression	In G6PD deficiency can cause hemolysis	9, 13, 48, 49, 52, 55, 62
Pyrimethamine 25 mg *plus* sulfadoxine 500 mg (Fansidar)	*P. falciparum*-resistant malaria	GI: nausea, abdominal pain, stomatitis, headache, and glossitis Hemat: agranulocytosis, aplastic anemia, leukopenia, megaloblastic anemia, hemolytic anemia, hemolysis in with G6PD deficiency	Combination was recently reported to cause the Stevens-Johnson syndrome; patients should be advised to call their physician/pharmacist if a skin rash or other reaction is seen	9, 13, 48, 49, 75
Quinacrine 100 mg[d]	Giardiasis	GI: nausea, anorexia, vomiting Headache, toxic psychosis, hepatitis, and aplastic anemia	Avoid in pregnancy, psychosis, and psoriasis	9, 12, 13
Quinidine gluconate 500 mg base/mL; 10 mL	Acute malaria	GI: nausea, vomiting, diarrhea Card: hypotension, widening of QRS and QT on ECG, heart block	Administration of IV quinidine requires close monitoring; should normally monitor ECG and all vital signs	9, 13, 48, 49, 52, 55
Quinine sulfate 325-mg and 650-mg tablets	Acute malaria	Cinchonism: flushing, dizziness, nausea, vomiting, diarrhea (levels over 10 mcg/mL) Card: hypotension, widening of QRS complex Hemat: hemolysis, leukopenia, thrombocytopenia	When drug is administered IV, it should be administered by slow infusion (600 mg over 8 h); dose monitoring of vitals and ECG *Avoid use*: IM administration	9, 13, 48, 49, 52, 55

Card, cardiologic; Derm, dermatologic; ECG, elecetrocardiogram; G6PD, glucose-6-phosphate dehydrogenase; Hemat, hematologic.

[a]Atovaquone 62.5 mg/proguanil 25 mg (Malarone), pediatric dosage strength.

[b]Investigational drugs obtained from Ponorama Compounding Pharmacy, 6744 Balboa Blvd, Van Nuys, CA 91406 (800–247–9767).

[c]Investigational drug obtained from the Centers for Disease Control and Prevention, Parasitic Disease Service, Atlanta, GA 30333 (707–488–7760–business hours: 8:00 AM to 4:30 PM EST; 404–639–2888–nights, weekends, or holidays, for emergency calls only).

[d]Available from Ponorama Compounding Pharmacy.

CHAPTER 120 Urinary Tract Infections and Prostatitis

ELIZABETH A. COYLE AND RANDALL A. PRINCE

KEY CONCEPTS

1. Urinary tract infections (UTIs) are classified as uncomplicated and complicated. *Uncomplicated* refers to an infection in an otherwise healthy female who lacks structural or functional abnormalities of the urinary tract. Most often complicated infections are associated with a predisposing lesion of the urinary tract; however, the term may be used to refer to all other infections, except for those in the otherwise healthy adult female.

2. Recurrent UTIs are considered either reinfections or relapses. Reinfection usually happens more than 2 weeks after the last UTI, and is treated as a new uncomplicated UTI. Relapse usually happens within 2 weeks of the original infection and is a relapse of the original infection either because of unsuccessful treatment of the original infection, a resistant organism, or anatomical abnormalities.

3. Eighty-five percent of uncomplicated urinary tract infections are caused by *Escherichia coli,* and the remainder are caused primarily by *Staphylococcus saprophyticus, Proteus* spp., and *Klebsiella* spp. Complicated infections are more frequently associated with gram-negative organisms and *Enterococcus faecalis.*

4. Symptoms of lower urinary tract infections include dysuria, urgency, frequency, nocturia, and suprapubic heaviness, whereas upper urinary tract infections involve more systemic symptoms such as fever, nausea, vomiting, and flank pain.

5. Significant bacteriuria traditionally has been defined as bacterial counts of greater than 100,000 (10^5)/mL of urine. Many clinicians, however, have challenged this as too general a statement. Indeed, significant bacteriuria in patients with symptoms of a urinary tract infection may be defined as greater than 10^2 organisms per milliliter.

6. The goals of treatment of urinary tract infections are to prevent or treat systemic consequences of infections, eradicate the invading organism(s), and prevent the recurrence of infection.

7. Uncomplicated urinary tract infections can be managed most effectively with short-course (3 days) therapy with either trimethoprim-sulfamethoxazole or a fluoroquinolone. Complicated infections require longer treatment periods (2 weeks) usually with one of these agents.

8. In choosing appropriate antibiotic therapy, practitioners need to be cognizant of antibiotic resistance patterns, particularly to *E. coli*. Trimethoprim-sulfamethoxazole has demonstrated diminished activity against *E. coli* in some areas of the country, with reported resistance up to 20%.

9. Acute bacterial prostatitis can be managed with many agents that have activity against the causative organism. Chronic prostatitis requires an agent that is not only active against the causative organism but also concentrates in the prostatic secretions. Therapy with trimethoprim-sulfamethoxazole or a fluoroquinolone is preferred for 4 to 6 weeks.

Learning objectives, review questions, and other resources can be found at **www.pharmacotherapyonline.com.**

Infections of the urinary tract represent a wide variety of syndromes, including urethritis, cystitis, prostatitis, and pyelonephritis. Urinary tract infections (UTIs) are the most commonly occurring bacterial infections and account for 8 million patient visits annually.[1–3] Approximately 1 in 3 females will have had a urinary tract infection by age 24 years.[2] Infections in men occur much less frequently until the age of 65 years, at which point the incidence rates in men and women are similar.

A UTI is defined as the presence of microorganisms in the urinary tract that cannot be accounted for by contamination. The organisms present have the potential to invade the tissues of the urinary tract and adjacent structures. Infection may be limited to the growth of bacteria in the urine, which frequently may not produce symptoms. A UTI can present as several syndromes associated with an inflammatory response to microbial invasion and can range from asymptomatic bacteriuria to pyelonephritis with bacteremia or sepsis.

UTIs are classified by several methods. Typically, they have been described by anatomic site of involvement. Lower tract infections include cystitis (bladder), urethritis (urethra), prostatitis (prostrate gland), and epididymitis. Pyelonephritis is an infection involving the kidneys and represents upper tract infection.

1 Also, UTIs are designated as uncomplicated or complicated. Uncomplicated infections occur in individuals who lack structural or functional abnormalities of the urinary tract that interfere with the normal flow of urine or voiding mechanism. These infections occur in females of childbearing age (15 to 45 years) who are otherwise normal, healthy individuals. Infections in males generally are not classified as uncomplicated because these infections are rare and most often represent a structural or neurologic abnormality.

Complicated UTIs are the result of a predisposing lesion of the urinary tract, such as a congenital abnormality or distortion of the urinary tract, a stone, indwelling catheter, prostatic hypertrophy, obstruction, or neurologic deficit that interferes with the normal flow of urine and urinary tract defenses. Complicated infections occur in both genders and frequently involve the upper and lower urinary tract.

Recurrent UTIs in healthy nonpregnant women, three or more UTIs occurring within 1 year, are a common problem. They are

TABLE 120-1 Diagnostic Criteria for Significant Abacteriuria

$\geq 10^2$ CFU coliforms/mL or $\geq 10^5$ CFU noncoliforms/mL in a symptomatic female
$\geq 10^3$ CFU bacteria/mL in a symptomatic male
$\geq 10^5$ CFU bacteria/mL in asymptomatic individuals on two consecutive specimens
Any growth of bacteria on suprapubic catheterization in a symptomatic patient
$\geq 10^2$ CFU bacteria/mL in a catheterized patient

CFU, colony-forming unit.

characterized by multiple symptomatic infections with asymptomatic periods occurring between each episode and may be either reinfections or relapses. Reinfections are caused by a different organism than originally isolated and account for the majority of recurrent UTIs. Relapses are the development of repeated infections with the same initial organism and usually indicate a persistent infectious source.

Asymptomatic bacteriuria is a common finding, particularly among those 65 years of age and older, when there is significant bacteriuria ($>10^5$ bacteria/mL of urine) in the absence of symptoms. Symptomatic abacteriuria or acute urethral syndrome consists of symptoms of frequency and dysuria in the absence of significant bacteriuria. This syndrome is commonly associated with *Chlamydia* infections.

Significant abacteriuria is a term used to distinguish the presence of microorganisms that represent true infection versus contamination of the urine as it passes through the distal urethra prior to collection. Historically, bacterial counts equal to or greater than 100,000 organisms/mL of urine in a "clean-catch" specimen were judged to indicate true infection.[4,5] Counts of less than 100,000 organisms/mL of urine, however, may represent true infection in certain situations, for example, with concurrent antibacterial drug administration, rapid urine flow, low urinary pH, or upper tract obstruction.[5] Table 120–1 lists the clinical definitions of significant bacteriuria, which are dependent on the clinical setting and the method of specimen collection.[5] These criteria allow for more appropriate specificity and sensitivity in documenting infection under differing clinical circumstances.

EPIDEMIOLOGY

The prevalence of UTIs varies with age and gender. In newborns and infants up to 6 months of age, the prevalence of abacteriuria is approximately 1% and is more common in boys. Most of these infections are associated with structural or functional abnormalities of the urinary tract and have been correlated with noncircumcision.[6] Between the ages of 1 and 6 years, UTIs occur more frequently in females. The prevalence of abacteriuria in females and males of this age group is 7% and 2%, respectively.[6] Infections occurring in preschool boys usually are associated with congenital abnormalities of the urinary tract. These infections are difficult to recognize because of the age of the patient, but they often are symptomatic. In addition, the majority of renal damage associated with UTI develops at this age.[7]

Through grade school and before puberty, the prevalence of UTI is approximately 1%, with 5% of females reported to have significant bacteriuria prior to leaving high school. This percentage increases dramatically to 1% to 4% after puberty in nonpregnant females primarily as a result of sexual activity. Approximately 1 in 5 women will suffer a symptomatic UTI at some point in their lives. Many women have recurrent infections, with a significant proportion of these women having a history of childhood infections. In contrast, the prevalence of bacteriuria in adult men is very low (<0.1%).[8]

In the elderly, the ratio of bacteriuria in women and men is dramatically altered and is approximately equal in persons older than age 65 years.[9] The overall incidence of UTI increases substantially in this population, with the majority of infections being asymptomatic. The rate of infection increases further for elderly persons who are residing in nursing homes, particularly those who are hospitalized frequently. The increase is probably the result of a number of factors, including obstruction from prostatic hypertrophy in males, poor bladder emptying as a result of prolapse in females, fecal incontinence in demented patients, neuromuscular disease, including strokes, and increased urinary instrumentation (catheterization).

ETIOLOGY

❸ The bacteria causing UTIs usually originate from bowel flora of the host. Although virtually every organism is associated with UTIs, certain organisms predominate as a result of specific virulence factors. The most common cause of uncomplicated UTIs is *Escherichia coli,* which accounts for 85% of community-acquired infections. Additional causative organisms in uncomplicated infections include *Staphylococcus saprophyticus* (5% to 15%), *Klebsiella pneumoniae, Proteus* spp., *Pseudomonas aeruginosa,* and *Enterococcus* spp. (5% to 10%).[10] Because *Staphylococcus epidermidis* is frequently isolated from the urinary tract, it should be considered initially a contaminant. Repeat cultures should be performed to help confirm the organism as a real pathogen.

Organisms isolated from individuals with complicated infections are more varied and generally are more resistant than those found in uncomplicated infections. *E. coli* is a frequently isolated pathogen, but it accounts for less than 50% of infections. Other frequently isolated organisms include *Proteus* spp., *K. pneumoniae, Enterobacter* spp., *P. aeruginosa,* staphylococci, and enterococci. Enterococci represent the second most frequently isolated organisms in hospitalized patients.[10] In part, this finding may be related to the extensive use of third-generation cephalosporin antibiotics, which are not active against the enterococci. Vancomycin-resistant *Enterococcus faecalis* and *Enterococcus faecium* (vancomycin-resistant enterococci) have become more widespread, especially in patients with long-term hospitalizations or underlying malignancies. Vancomycin-resistant enterococci are major therapeutic and infection control issues because the organisms are susceptible to few antimicrobials.[10,11]

Staphylococcus aureus infections may arise from the urinary tract, but they are more commonly a result of bacteremia producing metastatic abscesses in the kidney. *Candida* spp. are common causes of UTI in the critically ill and chronically catheterized patient.

Most UTIs are caused by a single organism; however, in patients with stones, indwelling urinary catheters, or chronic renal abscesses, multiple organisms may be isolated. Depending on the clinical situation, the recovery of multiple organisms may represent contamination, and a repeat evaluation should be done.

PATHOPHYSIOLOGY

ROUTE OF INFECTION

In general, organisms gain entry into the urinary tract via three routes: the ascending, hematogenous (descending), and lymphatic pathways. The female urethra usually is colonized by bacteria believed to originate from the fecal flora. The short length of the female urethra and its proximity to the perirectal area make colonization of the urethra likely. Other factors that promote urethral colonization include the use of spermicides and diaphragms as methods of contraception.[2] Although there is evidence in females that bladder infections follow colonization of the urethra, the mode of ascent of the microorganisms is incompletely understood. Massage of the female urethra and sexual intercourse allow bacteria to reach the bladder.[12] Once bacteria have reached the bladder, the organisms quickly multiply and can ascend the ureters to the kidneys. This sequence of events is more likely to occur if vesicoureteral reflux (reflux of urine into the ureters and kidneys while voiding) is present. That UTIs are more common in females than in males because of the anatomic differences in location and length of the urethra tends to support the ascending route of infections as the primary acquisition route.

Infection of the kidney by hematogenous spread of microorganisms usually occurs as the result of dissemination of organisms from a distant primary infection in the body. Infections via the descending route are uncommon and involve a relatively small number of invasive pathogens. Bacteremia caused by *S. aureus* may produce renal abscesses. Additional organisms include *Candida* spp., *Mycobacterium tuberculosis, Salmonella* spp., and enterococci. Of particular interest, it is difficult to produce experimental pyelonephritis by intravenously administering common gram-negative organisms such as *E. coli* and *P. aeruginosa.* Overall, less than 5% of documented UTIs result from hematogenous spread of microorganisms.

There appears to be little evidence supporting a significant role for renal lymphatics in the pathogenesis of UTIs. There are lymphatic communications between the bowel and kidney, as well as between the bladder and kidney. There is no evidence, however, that microorganisms are transferred to the kidney via this route.

After bacteria reach the urinary tract, three factors determine the development of infection: the size of the inoculum, the virulence of the microorganism, and the competency of the natural host defense mechanisms. Most UTIs reflect a failure in host defense mechanisms.

HOST DEFENSE MECHANISMS

The normal urinary tract generally is resistant to invasion by bacteria and is efficient in rapidly eliminating microorganisms that reach the bladder. The urine under normal circumstances is capable of inhibiting and killing microorganisms. The factors thought to be responsible include a low pH, extremes in osmolality, high urea concentration, and high organic acid concentration. Bacterial growth is further inhibited in males by the addition of prostatic secretions.[13,14]

The introduction of bacteria into the bladder stimulates micturition, with increased diuresis and efficient emptying of the bladder. These factors are critical in preventing the initiation and maintenance of bladder infections. Patients who are unable to void urine completely are at greater risk of developing UTIs and frequently have recurrent infections. Also, patients with even small residual amounts of urine in their bladder respond less favorably to treatment than patients who are able to empty their bladders completely.[15]

An important virulence factor of bacteria is their ability to adhere to urinary epithelial cells, resulting in colonization of the urinary tract, bladder infections, and pyelonephritis. Various factors that act as antiadherence mechanisms are present in the bladder, preventing bacterial colonization and infection. The epithelial cells of the bladder are coated with a urinary mucus or slime called *glycosaminoglycan.* This thin layer of surface mucopolysaccharide is hydrophilic and strongly negatively charged. When bound to the uroepithelium, it attracts water molecules and forms a layer between the bladder and urine. The antiadherence characteristics of the glycosaminoglycan layer are nonspecific, and when the layer is removed by dilute acid solutions, rapid bacterial adherence results.[16]

In addition, the Tamm-Horsfall protein is a glycoprotein produced by the ascending limb of Henle and distal tubule that is secreted into the urine and contains mannose residues. These mannose residues bind *E. coli* that contain small surface-projecting organellae on their surfaces called *pili* or *fimbriae.* Type 1 fimbriae are mannose sensitive, and this interaction prevents the bacteria from binding to similar receptors present on the mucosal surface of the bladder. Other factors that possibly prevent adherence of bacteria include immunoglobulins (Ig) G and A. Investigators have documented both systemic and local kidney immunoglobulin synthesis in upper tract infections. The role of immunoglobulins in preventing bladder infection is less clear. Patients with reduced urinary levels of secretory IgA are, however, at increased risk of infections of the urinary tract.

After bacteria actually have invaded the bladder mucosa, an inflammatory response is stimulated with the mobilization of polymorphonuclear leukocytes (PMNs) and resulting phagocytosis. PMNs are primarily responsible for limiting the tissue invasion and controlling the spread of infection in the bladder and kidney. They do not play a role in preventing bladder colonization or infections and actually contribute to renal tissue damage.

Other host factors that may play a role in the prevention of UTIs are the presence of *Lactobacillus* in the vaginal flora and circulating estrogen levels. In premenopausal women, circulating estrogen supports the vaginal tract growth of lactobacilli, which produce lactic acid to help maintain a low vaginal pH, thereby preventing *E. coli* vaginal colonization. Spermicide use, β-lactam antimicrobials use, lower estrogen levels, intercourse with a new partner, and douching can lead to decreases in lactobacilli colonization.[17,18]

BACTERIAL VIRULENCE FACTORS

Pathogenic organisms have differing degrees of pathogenicity (virulence), which play a role in the development and severity of infection. Bacteria that adhere to the epithelium of the urinary tract are associated with colonization and infection. The mechanism of adhesion of gram-negative bacteria, particularly *E. coli,* is related to bacterial fimbriae that are rigid, hair-like appendages of the cell wall.[19] These fimbriae adhere to specific glycolipid components on epithelial cells. The most common type of fimbriae is type 1, which binds to mannose residues present in glycoproteins. Glycosaminoglycan and Tamm-Horsfall protein are rich in mannose residues that readily trap those organisms that contain type 1 fimbriae, which are then washed out of the bladder.[20] Other fimbriae are mannose resistant and are associated more frequently with pyelonephritis, such as P fimbriae, which bind avidly to specific glycolipid receptors on uroepithelial cells. These bacteria are resistant to washout or removal by glycosaminoglycan and are able to multiply and invade tissue, especially the kidney. In addition, PMNs, as well as secretory IgA antibodies, contain receptors for type 1 fimbriae, which facilitates phagocytosis, but they lack receptors for P fimbriae.

Other virulence factors include the production of hemolysin and aerobactin.[21] Hemolysin is a cytotoxic protein produced by bacteria that lyses a wide range of cells, including erythrocytes, PMNs, and monocytes. *E. coli* and other gram-negative bacteria require iron for aerobic metabolism and multiplication. Aerobactin facilitates the binding and uptake of iron by *E. coli;* however, the significance of this property in the pathogenesis of UTIs remains unknown.

PREDISPOSING FACTORS TO INFECTION

The normal urinary tract typically is resistant to infection and colonization by pathogenic bacteria. In patients with underlying structural abnormalities of the urinary tract, the typical host defenses previously discussed usually are lacking. There are several known abnormalities of the urinary tract system that interfere with its natural defense mechanisms, the most important of which is obstruction. Obstruction can inhibit the normal flow of urine, disrupting the natural flushing and voiding effect in removing bacteria from the bladder and resulting in incomplete emptying. Common conditions that result in residual urine volumes include prostatic hypertrophy, urethral strictures, calculi, tumors, bladder diverticula, and drugs such as anticholinergic agents. Additional causes of incomplete bladder emptying include neurologic malfunctions associated with stroke, diabetes, spinal cord injuries, tabes dorsalis, and other neuropathies.

Vesicoureteral reflux represents a condition in which urine is forced up the ureters to the kidneys. Urinary reflux is associated not only with an increased incidence of UTIs and pyelonephritis but also with renal damage.[15] Reflux may be the result of a congenital abnormality or, more commonly, bladder overdistension from obstruction.

TABLE 120-2 Clinical Presentation of Urinary Tract Infections in Adults

Signs and symptoms	
	Lower UTI: dysuria, urgency, frequency, nocturia, suprapubic heaviness
	Gross hematuria
	Upper UTI: flank pain, fever, nausea, vomiting, malaise
Physical examination	
	Upper UTI: costovertebral tenderness
Laboratory tests	
	Bacteriuria
	Pyuria (white blood cell count >10/mm^3)
	Nitrite-positive urine (with nitrite reducers)
	Leukocyte esterase-positive urine
	Antibody-coated bacteria (upper UTI)

UTI, urinary tract infection.

Other risk factors include urinary catheterization, mechanical instrumentation, pregnancy, and the use of spermicides and diaphragms.

CLINICAL PRESENTATION

❹ The presenting signs and symptoms of UTIs in adults are recognized easily (Table 120–2). Women frequently will report gross hematuria. Systemic symptoms, including fever, typically are absent in this setting. Unfortunately, large numbers of patients with significant bacteriuria are asymptomatic. These patients may be normal, healthy patients, elderly patients, children, pregnant patients, and patients with indwelling catheters. It is important to note that attempts at differentiating upper tract from lower tract infections on the basis of symptoms alone are not reliable.

Elderly patients frequently do not experience specific urinary symptoms, but they will present with altered mental status, change in eating habits, or gastrointestinal symptoms. In addition, patients with indwelling catheters or neurologic disorders commonly will not have lower tract symptoms, whereas flank pain and fever may be recognized. Many of the aforementioned patients, however, frequently will develop upper tract infections with bacteremia and no or minimal urinary tract symptoms.

Symptoms alone are unreliable for the diagnosis of bacterial UTIs. The key to the diagnosis of UTI is the ability to demonstrate significant numbers of microorganisms in an appropriate urine specimen to distinguish contamination from infection. The type and extent of laboratory examination required depend on the clinical situation.

URINE COLLECTION

Examination of the urine is the cornerstone of laboratory evaluation for UTIs. There are three acceptable methods of urine collection. The first is the *midstream clean-catch method.* After cleaning the urethral opening area in both men and women, 20 to 30 mL of urine is voided and discarded. The next part of the urine flow is collected and should be processed immediately (refrigerated as soon as possible). Specimens that are allowed to sit at room temperature for several hours may result in falsely elevated bacterial counts. The midstream clean catch is the preferred method for the routine collection of urine for culture. When a routine urine specimen cannot be collected or contamination occurs, alternative collection techniques must be used.

The two acceptable alternative methods include catheterization and suprapubic bladder aspiration. Catheterization may be necessary for patients who are uncooperative or who are unable to void urine. If catheterization is performed carefully with aseptic technique, the method yields reliable results. Note, however, that introduction of bacteria into the bladder may result, and the procedure is associated with infection in 1% to 2% of patients. Suprapubic bladder aspiration involves inserting a needle directly into the bladder and aspirating the urine. This procedure bypasses the contaminating organisms present in the urethra, and any bacteria found using this technique generally are considered to represent significant bacteriuria. Suprapubic aspiration is a safe and painless procedure that is most useful in newborns, infants, paraplegics, seriously ill patients, and others in whom infection is suspected and routine procedures have provided confusing or equivocal results.

BACTERIAL COUNT

❺ The diagnosis of UTI is based on the isolation of significant numbers of bacteria from a urine specimen. Microscopic examination of a urine sample is an easy-to-perform and reliable method for the presumptive diagnosis of bacteriuria. The examination may be performed by preparing a Gram stain of unspun or centrifuged urine. The presence of at least one organism per oil-immersion field in a properly collected uncentrifuged specimen correlates well with more than 100,000 bacteria/mL of urine. For detecting smaller numbers of organisms, a centrifuged specimen is more sensitive. Such examinations detect more than 10^5 bacteria/mL with a sensitivity of greater than 90% and a specificity of greater than 70%.[22] Counts of less than 30,000/mL, however, usually are not recognized reliably by these methods.[23]

PYURIA, HEMATURIA, AND PROTEINURIA

Microscopic examination of the urine for leukocytes is also used to determine the presence of pyuria. The presence of pyuria in a symptomatic patient correlates with significant bacteriuria.[24] Pyuria is defined as a white blood cell (WBC) count of greater than 10 WBC/mm^3 of urine. A count of 5 to 10 WBC/mm^3 is accepted as the upper limit of normal. It should be emphasized that pyuria is nonspecific and signifies only the presence of inflammation and not necessarily infection. Thus patients with pyuria may or may not have infection. Sterile pyuria has long been associated with urinary tuberculosis, as well as chlamydial and fungal urinary infections.

Hematuria, microscopic or gross, is frequently present in patients with UTI but is nonspecific. Hematuria may indicate the presence of other disorders, such as renal calculi, tumors, or glomerulonephritis. Proteinuria is found commonly in the presence of infection.

CHEMISTRY

Several biochemical tests have been developed for screening urine for the presence of bacteria. A common dipstick test detects the presence of nitrite in the urine, which is formed by bacteria that reduce nitrate normally present in the urine. False-positive tests are uncommon. False-negative tests are more common and frequently are caused by the presence of gram-positive organisms or *P. aeruginosa* that do not reduce nitrate.[25] Other causes of false tests include low urinary pH, frequent voiding, and dilute urine.

The leukocyte esterase dipstick test is a rapid screening test for detecting the presence of pyuria. Leukocytes esterase is found in primary neutrophil granules and indicates the presence of WBCs. The leukocyte esterase test is a sensitive and highly specific test for detecting more than 10 WBC/mm^3 of urine. When the leukocyte esterase test is used with the nitrite test, the range of reported sensitivity and specificity is 45.5% to 100% and 60% to 98%, respectively, for the detection of bacteriuria.[26,27] These tests can be useful in the outpatient evaluation of uncomplicated UTIs. However, urine culture is still the "gold standard" test in determining the presence of UTIs.

CULTURE

The most reliable method of diagnosing UTI is by quantitative urine culture. Urine in the bladder is normally sterile, making it statistically possible to differentiate contamination of the urine from infection by quantifying the number of bacteria present in a urine sample. This criterion is based on a properly collected midstream clean-catch urine specimen. Patients with infection usually have greater than 10^5 bacteria/mL of urine. It should be emphasized that as many as one-third of women with symptomatic infection have less than 10^5 bacteria/mL. A significant portion of patients with UTIs, either symptomatic or asymptomatic, also have less than 10^5 bacteria/mL of urine.

Several laboratory methods are used to quantify bacteria present in the urine. The most accurate method is the pour-plate technique. This method is unsuitable for a high-volume laboratory because it is expensive and time-consuming. The streak-plate method is an alternative that involves using a calibrated-loop technique to streak a fixed amount of urine on an agar plate. This method is used most commonly in diagnostic laboratories because it is simple to perform and less costly.

After identification and quantification are complete, the next step is to determine the susceptibility of the organism. There are several methods by which bacterial susceptibility testing may be performed. Knowledge of bacterial susceptibility and achievable urine concentration of the antibiotics puts the clinician in a better position to select an appropriate agent for treatment.

Infection Site

Several methods have been evaluated to determine the location of infection within the urinary system and differentiate upper tract from lower tract involvement. The most direct method is a ureteral catheterization procedure as described by Stamey and colleagues.[28] The method involves the passage of a catheter into the bladder and then into each ureter, where quantitative cultures are obtained. History and physical examination were of little value in predicting the site of infection. Although this method provides direct quantitative evidence for UTI, it is invasive, technically difficult, and expensive. The Fairley bladder washout technique is a modification of the Stamey procedure that involves Foley catheterization only.[29] After the catheter is passed into the bladder, bladder samples are obtained, and the bladder is washed out, with culture samples taken at 10, 20, and 30 minutes. The procedure shows that up to 50% of patients have renal involvement regardless of signs and symptoms. Other investigators found 10% to 20% of tests to be equivocal.[29]

Noninvasive methods of localization may be more acceptable for routine use; however, they have limited clinical value. Patients with pyelonephritis can have abnormalities in urinary concentrating ability. The use of concentrating ability for localization of UTIs, however, is associated with high false-positive and false-negative responses and is not useful clinically.[25] The antibody-coated bacteria test is an immunofluorescent method that detects bacteria coated with Ig in freshly voided urine, indicating upper urinary tract infection. The sensitivity and specificity of this test to localize the site of infection are reported to average 88% and 76%, respectively.[30] Because of the high incidence of false-positive and false-negative results, antibody-coated bacteria testing is not used routinely in the management of UTIs.

Virtually all patients with uncomplicated lower tract infections can be cured with a short course of antibiotic therapy, and this assumption sometimes can be used to distinguish between patients with lower and upper tract infections. Patients who do not respond or who relapse do so because of upper tract involvement. It is rarely necessary to localize the site of infection to direct the clinical management of such patients.

TREATMENT

DESIRED OUTCOME

❻ The goals of UTI treatments are (a) to prevent or to treat systemic consequences of infection, (b) to eradicate the invading organism(s), and (c) to prevent the recurrence of infection.

MANAGEMENT

The management of a patient with a UTI includes initial evaluation, selection of an antibacterial agent and duration of therapy, and followup evaluation. The initial selection of an antimicrobial agent for the treatment of UTI is based primarily on the severity of the presenting signs and symptoms, the site of infection, and whether the infection is determined to be uncomplicated or complicated. Other considerations include antibiotic susceptibility, side-effect potential, cost, and the comparative inconvenience of different therapies.

Various pharmacologic factors may affect the action of antibacterial agents. Certainly the ability of the agent to achieve appropriate concentrations in the urine is of utmost importance. Factors that affect the rate and extent of excretion through the kidney include the patient's glomerular filtration rate and whether or not the agent is actively secreted. Filtration depends on the molecular size and degree of protein binding of the agent. Agents such as sulfonamides, tetracyclines, and aminoglycosides enter the urine via filtration. As the glomerular filtration rate is reduced, the amount of drug that enters the urine is reduced. Most β-lactam agents and quinolones are filtered and are actively secreted into the urine. For this reason, these agents achieve high urinary concentrations despite unfavorable protein-binding characteristics or the presence of renal dysfunction.

The ability to eradicate bacteria from the urine is related directly to the sensitivity of the microorganism and the achievable concentrations of the antimicrobial agent in the urine. Unfortunately, most susceptibility testing is directed at achievable concentrations in the blood. There is a poor correlation between achievable blood levels of antimicrobial agents and the eradication of bacteria from the urine.[31] In the treatment of lower tract infections, plasma concentrations of antibacterial agents may not be important, but achieving appropriate plasma concentrations appears critical in patients with bacteremia and renal abscesses.

A number of nonspecific therapies have been advocated in the treatment and prevention of UTIs. Fluid hydration has been used to produce rapid dilution of bacteria and removal of infected urine by increased voiding. A critical factor appears to be the amount of residual volume remaining after voiding. As little as 10 mL of residual urine can alter the eradication of infection significantly.[15] Paradoxically, increased diuresis also may promote susceptibility to infection by diluting the normal antibacterial properties of the urine. Often in clinical practice the concentrations of antimicrobial agents in the urine are so high that dilution has little effect on efficacy.

The antibacterial activity of the urine is related to the low pH, which is the result of high concentrations of various organic acids. Large volumes of cranberry juice increase the antibacterial activity of the urine and prevent the development of UTIs.[2,32] Apparently, the fructose and other unknown substances (condensed tannins) in cranberry juice act to interfere with adherence mechanisms of some pathogens, thereby preventing infection. Acidification of the urine by cranberry juice does not appear to play a significant role. The use of other agents (ascorbic acid) to acidify the urine to hinder bacterial growth does not achieve significant acidification. Consequently, attempts to acidify urine with systemic agents are not recommended. *Lactobacillus* probiotics also may aid in the prevention of female UTIs by decreasing the vaginal pH, thereby decreasing *E. coli* colonization.[18] In postmenopausal women, estrogen replacement may be of help in the prevention of recurrent UTIs. After 1 month of topical estrogen replacement, decreases in vaginal *Lactobacillus,* as well as decreases in and pH and *E. coli* colonization, have been found.[17]

CLINICAL CONTROVERSY

The role of nonantibiotic alternatives such as cranberry juice and estrogens in the treatment and/or prevention of urinary tract infections has long been discussed. Possible clinical benefits with cranberry juice in sexually active adult women with recurrent UTI have been suggested. However, the consistency of study results has varied, as have the types of cranberry products tested, leading to inconclusive evidence.[32] In a randomized, double-blind, placebo-controlled study, postmenopausal women receiving topical estriol vaginal cream had significantly fewer UTIs than did those receiving placebo.[17] More thorough studies on the overall effectiveness of cranberry juice or estrogen replacement needs to be performed before a uniform opinion of the role of these agent in UTIs can be resolved.

Urinary analgesics such as phenazopyridine hydrochloride are used frequently by many clinicians.[2] If the pain or dysuria present in a UTI is a consequence of infection, then urinary analgesics have little clinical role because most patients' symptoms respond quite rapidly to appropriate antibacterial therapy. Urinary analgesics also may mask signs and symptoms of UTIs not responding to antimicrobial therapy.

■ PHARMACOLOGIC THERAPY

Ideally, the antimicrobial agent chosen should be well tolerated, well absorbed, achieve high urinary concentrations, and have a spectrum of activity limited to the known or suspected pathogen(s). Table 120–3 lists the most common agents used in the treatment of UTIs along with comments concerning their general use. Table 120–4 presents an overview of various therapeutic options for outpatient therapy of UTI. Table 120–5 describes empirical treatment regimens for selected clinical situations.

❽ The therapeutic management of UTIs is best accomplished by first categorizing the type of infection: acute uncomplicated cystitis, symptomatic abacteriuria, asymptomatic bacteriuria, complicated UTIs, recurrent infections, or prostatitis. In choosing the appropriate antibiotic therapy, it is important to be aware of the increasing resistance of *E. coli* and other pathogens to many antimicrobials. Resistance to *E. coli* is as high as 30% for amoxicillin and cephalosporins.[33,34] Overall, most *E. coli* remain susceptible to trimethoprim-sulfamethoxazole, although resistance as high as 22% has been reported in various places.[35] However, resistant infections still may be treated successfully with trimethoprim-sulfamethoxazole, most likely owing to its high urinary concentrations. Current or recent antibiotic exposure is the most significant risk factor associated with *E. coli* resistance.[35–39] Although resistance to the fluoroquinolones remains low, there is an increasing incidence of fluoroquinolone-resistant *E. coli,* with many of these isolates being multidrug resistant.[36] Antibiotic therapy should be determined based on the geographic resistance patterns of the prescriber, as well as the patient's recent history of antibiotic exposure.

■ ACUTE UNCOMPLICATED CYSTITIS

Acute uncomplicated cystitis is the most common form of UTI. These infections typically occur in women of childbearing age and often are related to sexual activity. Although the presence of dysuria, frequency, urgency, and suprapubic discomfort frequently is associated with lower tract infection, a significant number of patients have upper tract involvement as well.[40] Because these infections are predominantly caused by *E. coli,* antimicrobial therapy initially should be directed against this organism. Other common causes include *S. saprophyticus* and, occasionally, *K. pneumoniae* and *Proteus mirabilis.* Because the causative organisms and their susceptibility generally are known, many clinicians advocate a cost-effective approach to management. This approach includes a urinalysis and initiation of empirical therapy without a urine culture (Fig. 120–1).[1] Therefore, geographic pathogen and susceptibility patterns are directed by cultures drawn in cases of complicated cystitis and not necessarily the actual pathogens causing uncomplicated UTIs.

The goal of treatment for uncomplicated cystitis is to eradicate the causative organism and to reduce the incidence of recurrence caused by relapse or reinfection. The ability to reduce the chance of recurrence depends on the agent's efficacy in eradicating the uropathogenic bacteria from the vaginal and gastrointestinal reservoir. In the past, conventional therapy consisted of an effective oral antibiotic administered for 7 to 14 days. It is now apparent, however, that acute cystitis is a superficial mucosal infection that can be eradicated with much shorter courses of therapy (3 days). Advantages of short-course therapy include increased compliance, fewer side effects, decreased cost, and less potential for the development of resistance.

CLINICAL CONTROVERSY

Single-dose therapy is used frequently, although it can be associated with lower cure rates and increased reoccurrence compared with longer therapies.[1,41,42] Clinicians should not assume that all antimicrobial agents are effective as single-dose therapies. Trimethoprim-sulfamethoxazole or the fluoroquinolones are most efficacious as single-dose therapies. Fosfomycin given once daily also has been used, although other therapies appear superior.[1,43] The efficacy of these agents probably is related to observations that *E. coli* causing community-acquired UTIs are increasingly resistant to ampicillin, amoxicillin, and sulfonamides. In addition, oral *β*-lactam antibiotics are eliminated more rapidly and do not achieve high renal tissue concentrations compared with trimethoprim-sulfamethoxazole and are less successful in eradicating uropathogens from the vaginal and gastrointestinal reservoirs.

❼ Three-day courses of trimethoprim-sulfamethoxazole or a fluoroquinolone (e.g., ciprofloxacin, levofloxacin, or norfloxacin) are superior to single-dose therapies.[42,44–46] The fluoroquinolone moxifloxacin is not recommended for use in UTIs owing to the inadequate urinary concentrations.[47] The use of amoxicillin and sulfonamides is not recommended because of the high incidence of resistant *E. coli.* For most adult females, short-course therapy is the treatment of choice for uncomplicated lower UTIs. Short-course therapy is inappropriate for patients who have had previous infections caused by resistant bacteria, for male patients, and for patients with complicated UTIs. If symptoms do not respond or recur, a urine culture should be obtained and conventional therapy with a suitable agent instituted.[1]

■ SYMPTOMATIC ABACTERIURIA

Symptomatic abacteriuria or acute urethral syndrome represents a clinical syndrome in which females present with dysuria and pyuria, but the urine culture reveals less than 10^5 bacteria/mL of urine. Acute urethral syndrome is estimated to account for more than half the complaints of dysuria seen in the community today. These women most likely are infected with small numbers of coliform bacteria, including *E. coli, Staphylococcus* spp., or *Chlamydia trachomatis.* Additional causes include *Neisseria gonorrhoeae, Gardnerella vaginalis,* and *Ureaplasma urealyticum.*

TABLE 120-3 Commonly Used Antimicrobial Agents in the Treatment of Urinary Tract Infections

Agent	Comments
Oral therapy	
Sulfonamides	These agents generally have been replaced by more agents due to resistance.
Trimethoprim-sulfamethoxazole	This combination is highly effective against most aerobic enteric bacteria except *Pseudomonas aeruginosa*. High urinary tract tissue levels and urine levels are achieved, which may be important in complicated infection treatment. Also effective as prophylaxis for recurrent infections.
Penicillins Ampicillin Amoxicillin-clavulanic acid	Ampicillin is the standard penicillin that has broad-spectrum activity. Increasing *Escherichia coli* resistance has limited amoxicillin use in acute cystitis. Drug of choice for enterococci sensitive to penicillin. Amoxicillin-clavulanate is preferred for resistance problems.
Cephalosporins Cephalexin Cefaclor Cefadroxil Cefuroxime Cefixime Cefprozil Cefpodoxime	There are no major advantages of these agents over other agents in the tratment of UTIs, and they are more expensive. They may be useful in cases of resistance to amoxicillin and trimethoprim–sulfamethoxazole. These agents are not active against enterococci.
Tetracyclines Tetracycline Doxycycline Minocycline	These agents have been effective for initial episodes of urinary tract infections; however, resistance drops rapidly, and their use is limited. These agents also lead to candidal overgrowth. They are useful primarily for chlamydial infections.
Fluoroquinolones Ciprofloxacin Norfloxacin Levofloxacin	The newer quinolones have a greater spectrum of activity, including *P. aeruginosa*. These agents are effective for pyelonephritis and prostatitis. Avoid in pregnancy and children. Moxifloxacin should not be used owing to inadequate urinary concentrations.
Nitrofurantoin	This agent is effective as both a therapeutic and prophylactic agent in patients with recurrent UTIs. Main advantage is the lack of resistance even after long courses of therapy. Adverse effects may limit use (GI intolerance, neuropathies, pulmonary reactions).
Azithromycin	Single-dose therapy for chlamydial infections.
Fosfomycin	Single-dose therapy for uncomplicated infections.
Parenteral therapy	
Aminoglycosides Gentamicin Tobramycin Amikacin	Gentamicin and tobramycin are equally effective; gentamicin is less expensive. Tobramycin has better pseudomonal activity, which may be important in serious systemic infections. Amikacin generally is reserved for multiresistant bacteria.
Penicillins Ampicillin Ampicillin-sulbactam Ticarcillin-clavulanate Piperacillin-tazobactam	These agents generally are equally effective for susceptible bacteria. The extended-spectrum penicillins are more active against *P. aeruginosa* and enterococci and often are preferred over cephalosporins. They are very useful in renally impaired patients or when an aminoglycoside is to be avoided.
Cephalosporins, first-, second-, and third-generation	Second- and third-generation cephalosporins have a broad spectrum of activity against gram-negative bacteria but are not active against enterococci and have limited activity against *P. aeruginosa*. Ceftazidime and cefepime are active against *P. aeruginosa.* They are useful for nosocomial infections and urosepsis due to susceptible pathogens.
Carbapenems/Monobactams	These agents have broad spectrum of activity, including gram-positive, gram-negative, and anaerobic bacteria.
Imipenem-cilastatin Meropenem Ertapenem	Imipenem and meropenem are active against *P. aeruginosa* and enterococci, but ertapenem is not. All may be associated with candidal superinfections.
Aztreonam	A monobactam that is only active against gram-negative bacteria, including some strains of *P. aeruginosa.* Generally useful for nosocomial infections when aminoglycosides are to be avoided and in penicillin-sensitive patients.
Fluoroquinolones Ciprofloxacin Levofloxacin	These agents have broad-spectrum activity against both gram-negative and gram-positive bacteria. They provide urine and high-tissue concentrations and are actively secreted in reduced renal function.

Most patients presenting with pyuria will, in fact, have infection that requires treatment. Single-dose or short-course therapy with trimethoprim-sulfamethoxazole has been used effectively, and prolonged courses of therapy are not necessary for most patients. If single-dose or short-course therapy is ineffective, a culture should be obtained. If the patient reports recent sexual activity, therapy for *C. trachomatis* should be considered. Chlamydial treatment should consist of 1 g azithromycin or doxycycline 100 mg twice daily for 7 days. Often, concomitant treatment of all sexual partners is required to cure chlamydial infections and prevent reacquisition (see Chap. 121).

ASYMPTOMATIC BACTERIURIA

Asymptomatic bacteriuria is the finding of two consecutive urine cultures with more than 10^5 organisms/mL of the same organism in the absence of urinary symptoms. Most patients with asymptomatic bacteriuria are elderly and female. Pregnant women frequently presents with asymptomatic bacteriuria. Although this group of patients typically responds to treatment, relapse and reinfection are very common, and chronic asymptomatic bacteriuria is difficult to eradicate.

TABLE 120-4 Overview of Outpatient Antimicrobial Therapy for Lower Tract Infections in Adults

Indications	Antibiotic	Dose[a]	Interval	Duration
Lower tract infections	Trimethoprim-sulfamethoxazole	2 DS tablets	Single dose	1 day
Uncomplicated		1 DS tablet	Twice a day	3 days
	Ciprofloxacin	250 mg	Twice a day	3 days
	Norfloxacin	400 mg	Twice a day	3 days
	Levofloxacin	250 mg	Once a day	3 days
	Amoxicillin	6 × 500 mg	Single dose	1 day
		500 mg	Twice a day	3 days
	Amoxicillin-clavulanate	500 mg	Every 8 hours	3 days
	Trimethoprim	100 mg	Twice a day	3 days
	Nitrofurantoin	100 mg	Every 6 hours	3 days
	Fosfomycin	3 g	Single dose	1 day
Complicated	Trimethoprim-sulfamethoxazole	1 DS tablet	Twice a day	7–10 days
	Trimethoprim	100 mg	Twice a day	7–10 days
	Norfloxacin	400 mg	Twice a day	7–10 days
	Ciprofloxacin	250–500 mg	Twice a day	7–10 days
	Levofloxacin	250 mg	Once a day	7–10 days
	Amoxicillin-clavulanate	500 mg	Every 8 hours	7–10 days
Recurrent infections	Nitrofurantoin	50 mg	Once a day	6 months
	Trimethoprim	100 mg	Once a day	6 months
	Trimethoprim-sulfamethoxazole	1/2 SS tablet	Once a day	6 months
Acute urethral syndrome	Trimethoprim-sulfamethoxazole	1 DS tablet	Twice a day	3 days
Failure of trimethoprim-sulfamethoxazole	Azithromycin	1 g	Single dose	
	Doxycycline	100 mg	Twice a day	7 days
Acute pyelonephritis	Trimethoprim-sulfamethoxazole	1 DS tablet	Twice a day	14 days
	Ciprofloxacin	500 mg	Twice a day	14 days
	Levofloxacin	250 mg	Once a day	14 days
	Amoxicillin-clavulanate	500 mg	Every 8 hours	14 days

DS, double strength; SS, single strength.
[a]Dosing intervals for normal renal function.

The management of asymptomatic bacteriuria depends on the age of the patient and whether or not the patient is pregnant. In children, because of a greater risk of developing renal scarring and long-standing renal damage, treatment should consist of conventional courses of therapy as that for symptomatic infection. The greatest risk of renal damage occurs during the first 5 years of life.[48] In the nonpregnant female, therapy is controversial; however, treatment has little effect on the natural course of infections. Two groups characterize asymptomatic bacteriuria in the elderly: those with persistent bacteriuria and those with intermittent bacteriuria.

Several studies in hospitalized elderly subjects, however, have not found antimicrobial therapy to be efficacious for aberteruria.[49–51] A number of questions remain unanswered, for example: What is the effect of eradication of bacteriuria on life expectancy? What are the

TABLE 120-5 Evidence-Based Empirical Treatment of Urinary Tract Infections and Prostatitis

Diagnosis	Pathogens	Treatment Recommendation	Comments
Acute uncomplicated cystitis	*Escherichia coli* *Staphylococcus saprophyticus*	1. Trimethoprim-sulfamethoxazole × 3 days (A, I)[a] 2. Fluoroquinolone × 3 days (A, II)[a] 3. Nitrofurantion × 7 days (B, I)[a] 4. β-lactams × 3 days (E, III)[a]	Short-course therapy more effective than single dose β-Lactams as a group are not as effective in acute cystitis then trimethoprim/sulfamethoxazole or the fluoroquinolones[a]
Pregnancy	As above	1. Amoxicillin-clavulanate × 7 days 2. Cephalosporin × 7 days 3. Trimethoprim-sulfamethoxazole × 7 days	Avoid trimethoprim-sulfamethoxazole during third trimester
Acute pyelonephritis			
Uncomplicated	*E. coli*	1. Quinolone × 14 days (A, II)[a] 2. Trimethoprim-sulfamethoxazole (if susceptible) × 14 days (B, II)[a]	Can be managed as outpatient
	Gram-positive bacteria	1. Amoxicillin or amoxicillin-clavulanic acid × 14 days (B, III)[a]	
Complicated	*E. coli* *Proteus mirabilis* *Klebisella pneumoniae* *Pseudomonas aeruginosa* *Enterococcus faecalis*	1. Quinolone × 14 days (B, III)[a] 2. Extended-spectrum penicillin plus aminoglycoside (B, III)[a]	Severity of illness will determine duration of IV therapy; culture results should direct therapy Oral therapy may complete 14 days of therapy
Prostatitis	*E. coli* *K. pneumoniae* *Proteus* spp. *P. aeruginosa*	1. Trimethoprim-sulfamethoxazole × 4–6 weeks 2. Quinolone × 4–6 weeks	Acute prostatitis may require IV therapy initially Chronic prostatitis may require longer treatment periods or surgery

[a]Strength of recommendations: A, good evidence for; B, moderate evidence for; C, poor evidence for and against; D, moderate against; E, good evidence against. Quality of evidence: I, at least one proper randomized, controlled study; II, one well-designed clinical trial; III, evidence from opinions, clinical experience, and expert committees.
Data from Warren JW, Abrutyn E, Hebel JR, et al. Surviving sepsis campaign guidelines for management of severe sepsis and septic shock. Crit Care Med 2004;32:858–873.

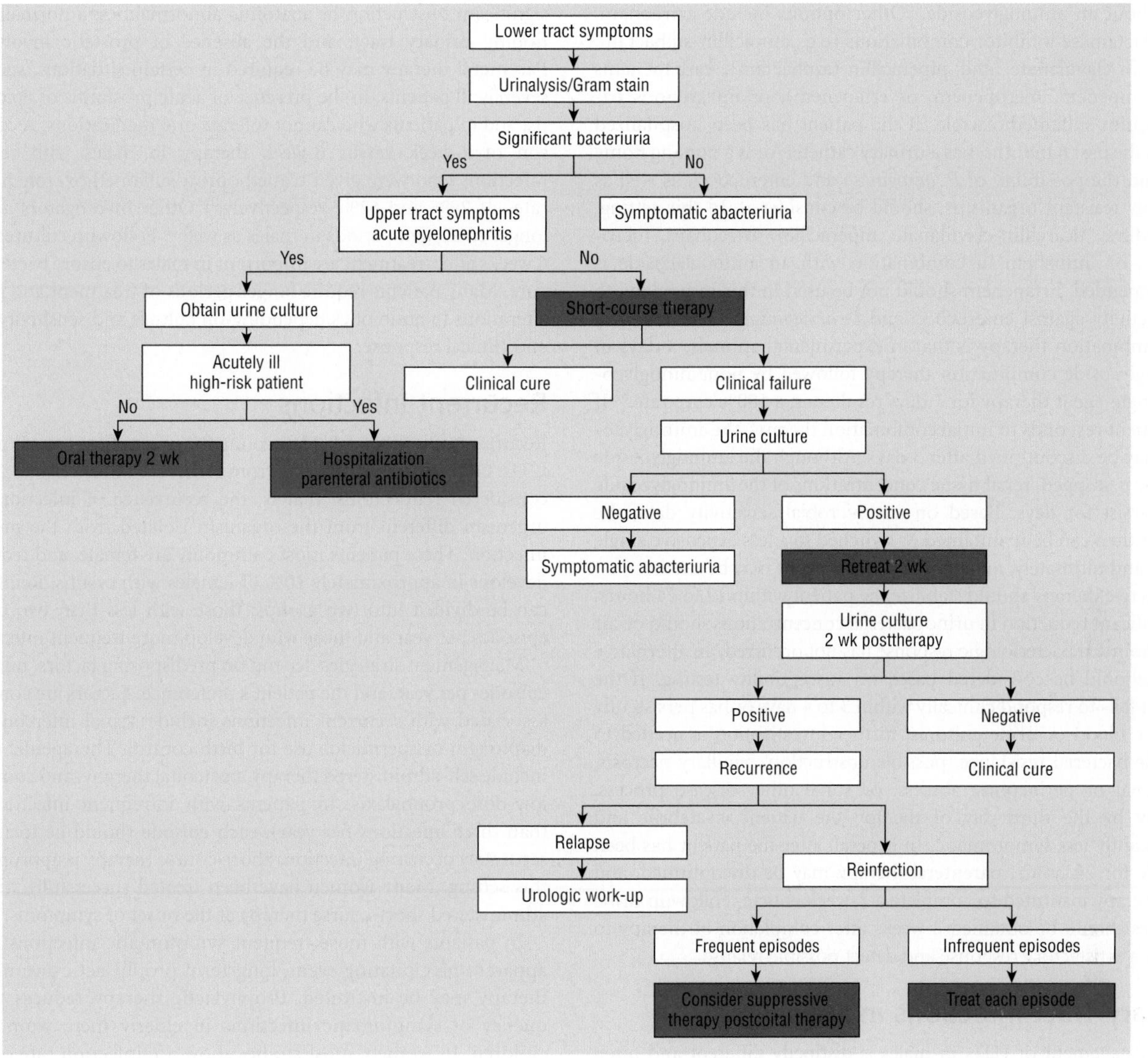

FIGURE 120-1. Management of UTIs in females.

cost-effectiveness and risk-to-benefit ratio of therapy? What is the effect on morbidity. Certainly, with the information available and the high adverse reaction rate in the elderly, vigorous treatment and screening programs cannot be advocated.

■ COMPLICATED URINARY TRACT INFECTIONS

Acute Pyelonephritis

The presentation of high-grade fever (>38.3°C [100.9°F]) and severe flank pain should be treated as acute pyelonephritis, warranting aggressive management. Severely ill patients with pyelonephritis should be hospitalized and intravenous antimicrobials administered initially (see Table 120–5). However, milder cases may be managed with orally administered antibiotics in an outpatient setting. Symptoms of nausea, vomiting, and dehydration may require hospitalization.

At the time of presentation, a Gram stain of the urine should be performed, along with a urinalysis, culture, and sensitivity tests. The Gram stain should indicate the morphology of the infecting organism(s) and help to direct the selection of an appropriate antibiotic. However, the precise identity and susceptibility of the infecting organism(s) will be unknown initially, warranting empirical therapy. The goals of treatment include the achievement of therapeutic concentrations of an antimicrobial agent in the bloodstream and urinary tract to which the invading organism is susceptible and sufficient therapy to eradicate residual infection in the tissues of the urinary tract.

In the mildly to moderately symptomatic patient in whom oral therapy is considered, an effective agent should be administered for at least a 2-week period, although use of highly active agents for 7 to 10 days may be sufficient.[1,52] Oral antibiotics that are highly active against the probable pathogens and that are sufficiently bioavailable are preferred. Although the sulfonamides and ampicillin or amoxicillin have been the primary choices for the treatment of gram-negative bacillary infections, they are no longer considered reliable agents for UTIs;[38] reports of increasing resistance to *E. coli* have tempered their use. In addition, treatment with trimethoprim-sulfamethoxazole (one double-strength tablet twice daily) for 2 weeks was superior to ampicillin, despite the organism being susceptible to both agents.[1,53] Agents such as trimethoprim-sulfamethoxazole and the fluoroquinolones are the agents of choice. If a Gram stain reveals gram-positive cocci, *Streptococcus faecalis* should be considered and treatment directed against this potential pathogen (ampicillin). Close followup of outpatient treatment is mandatory to ensure success.

In the seriously ill patient, parenteral therapy should be administered initially. Therapy should provide a broad spectrum of coverage and should be directed toward bacteremia or sepsis, if present. A number of antibiotic regimens have been used as empirical therapy, including an intravenous fluoroquinolone, an aminoglycoside with or without ampicillin, and extended-spectrum cephalosporins with or without an aminoglycoside.[1] Other options include aztreonam, the β-lactamase inhibitor combinations (e.g., ampicillin-sulbactam, ticarcillin-clavulanate, and piperacillin-tazobactam), carbapenems (e.g., imipenem, meropenem, or ertapenem), or intravenous trimethoprim-sulfamethoxazole. If the patient has been hospitalized within the past 6 months, has a urinary catheter, or is a nursing home resident, the possibility of *P. aeruginosa* and enterococci, as well as multiply resistant organisms, should be considered. In this setting, ceftazidime, ticarcillin-clavulanate, piperacillin, aztreonam, meropenem, or imipenem in combination with an aminoglycoside is recommended. Ertapenem should not be used in this case owing to its inactivity against enterococci and *P. aeruginosa*.[54] The rationale for combination therapy is that in experimental animals, 3 days of aminoglycoside combination therapy followed by nonaminoglycoside single-agent therapy for 7 days resulted in a 100% cure rate.[52] If the patient responds to initial combination therapy, the aminoglycoside may be discontinued after 3 days. Although the aminoglycoside therapy is stopped, renal tissue concentrations of the aminoglycoside will persist for days. Based on antimicrobial sensitivity data, the patient then can be maintained or switched to a less expensive single agent, and ultimately, an appropriate oral agent may be used.

Effective therapy should stabilize the patient within 12 to 24 hours. A significant reduction in urine bacterial concentrations should occur in 48 hours. If bacteriologic response has not occurred, an alternative agent should be considered based on susceptibility testing. If the patient fails to respond clinically within 3 to 4 days or has persistently positive blood or urine cultures, further investigation is needed to exclude bacterial resistance, possible obstruction, papillary necrosis, intrarenal or perinephric abscess, or some other disease process. Usually by the third day of therapy the patient is afebrile and significantly less symptomatic. In general, after the patient has been afebrile for 24 hours, parenteral therapy may be discontinued, and oral therapy instituted to complete a 2-week course. Followup urine cultures should be obtained 2 weeks after completion of therapy to ensure a satisfactory response and detect possible relapse.

Urinary Tract Infections in Males

The management of UTIs in males is distinctly different and often more difficult than in females. Infections in male patients are considered to be complicated because endogenous bacteria in the presence of functional or structural abnormalities that disrupt the normal defense mechanisms of the urinary tract cause them. The incidence of infections in males younger than 60 years of age is much less than the incidence in females. During the adult years, the occurrence of infection can be related directly to some manipulation of the urinary tract. The most common causes are instrumentation of the urinary tract, catheterization, and renal and urinary stones. Uncomplicated infections are rare, but they may occur in young males as a result of homosexual activity, noncircumcision, and having sex with partners who are colonized with uropathogenic bacteria. As the patient ages, the most common cause of infection is related to bladder outlet obstruction because of prostatic hypertrophy. In addition, the prostate gland may become infected and provide a nidus for recurrent infection in males.

The conventional view is that therapy in males requires prolonged treatment (Fig. 120–2). A urine culture should be obtained before treatment because the cause of infection in men is not as predictable as in women. Single-dose or short-course therapy is not recommended in males. Considerably fewer data are available comparing various antimicrobial agents in males as compared with females. If gram-negative bacteria are presumed, trimethoprim-sulfamethoxazole or the quinolone antimicrobials should be considered because these agents achieve high renal tissue, urine, and prostatic concentrations.[14]

Initial therapy should be for 10 to 14 days. Factors associated with treatment success are isolation of a single organism, the absence of significant obstruction or anatomic abnormalities, a normally functioning urinary tract, and the absence of prostatic involvement. Parenteral therapy may be required in certain situations, such as in severely ill patients, in the presence of acute prostatitis or epididymitis, and in patients who cannot tolerate oral medications. A comparison of 2-week versus 6-week therapy in males with recurrent infections who were given trimethoprim-sulfamethoxazole had cure rates of 29% and 62%, respectively.[55] Other investigators advocate longer treatment periods in males as well.[56] Followup cultures at 4 to 6 weeks after treatment are important in males to ensure bacteriologic cure. Many patients require longer periods of treatment and possible alterations in antibiotics depending on culture and sensitivity results and clinical response.

Recurrent Infections

Recurrent episodes of UTI account for a significant portion of all UTIs. Of the patients suffering from recurrent infections, 80% can be considered reinfections, that is, the recurrence of infection by an organism different from the organism isolated from the preceding infection. These patients most commonly are female, and recurrence develops in approximately 20% of females with cystitis. Reinfections can be divided into two groups: those with less than two or three episodes per year and those who develop more frequent infections.

Management strategies depend on predisposing factors, number of episodes per year, and the patient's preference. Factors are commonly associated with recurrent infections include sexual intercourse and diaphragm or spermicide use for birth control. Therapeutic options include self-administered therapy, postcoital therapy, and continuous low-dose prophylaxis. In patients with infrequent infections (less than three infections per year), each episode should be treated as a separately occurring infection. Short-course therapy is appropriate in this setting. Many women have been treated successfully with self-administered short-course therapy at the onset of symptoms.[57]

In patients with more frequent symptomatic infections and no apparent precipitating event, long-term prophylactic antimicrobial therapy may be instituted. Prophylactic therapy reduces the frequency of symptomatic infections in elderly men, women, and children. In women, most studies show a reinfection rate of 2 to 3 per patient-year reduced to 0.1 to 0.2 per patient-year with treatment.[58] Before prophylaxis is initiated, patients should be treated conventionally with an appropriate agent. Trimethoprim-sulfamethoxazole (one-half of a single-strength tablet), trimethoprim (100 mg daily), a fluoroquinolone (levofloxacin 500 mg daily) and nitrofurantoin (50 or 100 mg daily) all reduce the rate of reinfection as single-agent therapy.[58] Full-dose therapy with these agents is unnecessary, and single daily doses can be used. Therapy generally is prescribed for a period of 6 months, during which time urine cultures are followed monthly. If symptomatic episodes develop, the patient should receive a full course of therapy with an effective agent and should be restarted on prophylactic therapy.

In women who experience symptomatic reinfections in association with sexual activity, voiding after intercourse may help to prevent infection. Also, single-dose prophylactic therapy with trimethoprim-sulfamethoxazole taken after intercourse reduces the incidence of recurrent infection significantly.[59]

In postmenopausal women with recurrent infections, the lack of estrogen results in changes in the bacterial flora of the vagina, resulting in increased colonization with uropathogenic *E. coli*. Topically administered estrogen cream reduces the incidence of infections in this population.[17]

The remaining 20% of recurrent UTIs are relapses, that is, persistence of infection with the same organism after therapy for an isolated UTI. The recurrence of symptomatic or asymptomatic bacteriuria after therapy usually indicates that the patient has renal involvement, a structural abnormality of the urinary tract, or chronic bacterial

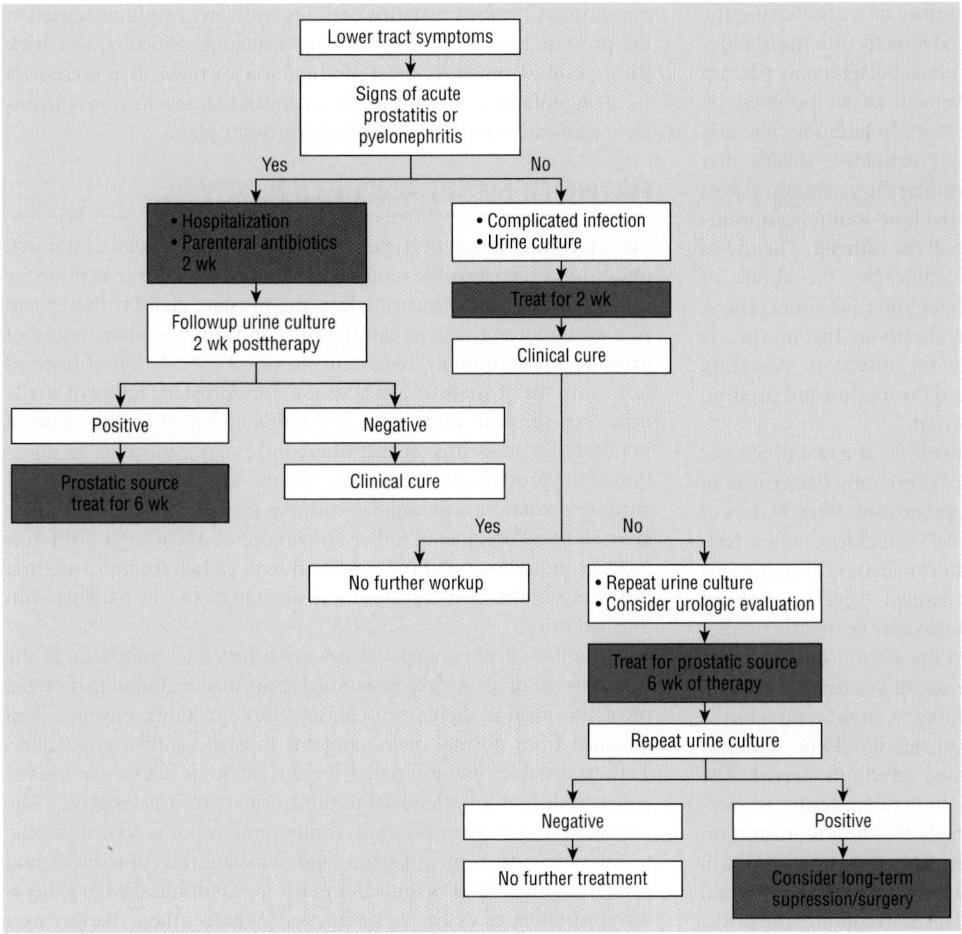

FIGURE 120-2. Management of UTIs in male.

prostatitis. In the absence of structural abnormalities, relapse often is related to renal infection and requires a long duration of treatment. Women who relapse after short-course therapy should receive a 2-week course of therapy. In patients who relapse after 2 weeks of therapy, therapy should be continued for another 2 to 4 weeks. If relapse occurs after 6 weeks of therapy, urologic evaluation should be performed, and any obstructive lesion should be corrected. If this is not possible, therapy for 6 months or longer may be considered. Asymptomatic adults who have no evidence of urinary obstruction should not receive long-term therapy.

In males, relapse usually indicates bacterial prostatitis, the most common cause of persistent bacteriuria. Although many agents have been used for long-term therapy of relapses, trimethoprim-sulfamethoxazole and the fluoroquinolones appear to be highly effective.

■ SPECIAL CONDITIONS

UTIs in Pregnancy

During pregnancy, significant physiologic changes occur to the entire urinary tract that dramatically alter the prevalence of UTIs and pyelonephritis. Severe dilation of the renal pelvis and ureters, decreased ureteral peristalsis, and reduced bladder tone occur during pregnancy.[60] These changes result in urinary stasis and reduced defenses against reflux of bacteria to the kidneys. In addition, increased urine content of amino acids, vitamins, and nutrients encourages bacterial growth. All these factors increase the incidence of bacteriuria, resulting in symptomatic infections, especially during the third trimester.

Asymptomatic bacteriuria occurs in 4% to 7% of pregnant patients. Of these, 20% to 40% will develop acute symptomatic pyelonephritis during pregnancy. If untreated, asymptomatic bacteriuria has the potential to cause significant adverse effects, including prematurity, low birth weight, and stillbirth.[61,62] Because pyelonephritis is associated with significant adverse events during pregnancy, routine screening tests for bacteriuria should be performed at the initial prenatal visit and again at 28 weeks' gestation. In patients with significant bacteriuria, symptomatic or asymptomatic, treatment is recommended so as to avoid possible complications. Organisms associated with bacteriuria are the same as those seen in uncomplicated UTIs, with *E. coli* isolated most frequently.

Therapy should consist of an agent administered for 7 days that has a relatively low adverse-effect potential and is safe for the mother and baby. The administration of a sulfonamide, amoxicillin, amoxicillin-clavulanate, cephalexin, or nitrofurantoin is effective in 70% to 80% of patients. Tetracyclines should be avoided because of teratogenic effects, and sulfonamides should not be administered during the third trimester because of the possible development of kernicterus and hyperbilirubinemia. In addition, the available fluoroquinolones should not be given because of their potential to inhibit cartilage and bone development in the newborn. A followup urine culture 1 to 2 weeks after completing therapy and then monthly until gestation is complete is recommended.

Catheterized Patients

The use of an indwelling catheter frequently is associated with infection of the urinary tract and represents the most common cause of hospital-acquired infection. The incidence of catheter-associated infection is related to a variety of factors, including method and duration of catheterization, the catheter system (open or closed), the care of the system, the susceptibility of the patient, and the technique of the healthcare personnel inserting the catheter. The incidence of infection from a single catheterization in a healthy ambulatory patient is 1%.[63]

Bacteria may enter the bladder in a number of ways. During the catheterization, bacteria may be introduced directly into the bladder from the urethra. Once the catheter is in place, bacteria may pass up the lumen of the catheter via the movement of air bubbles, by motility of the bacteria, or by capillary action. In addition, bacteria may reach the bladder from around the exudative sheath that surrounds the catheter in the urethra. Cleaning the periurethral area thoroughly and applying an antiseptic (povidone-iodine) can minimize infection occurring during insertion of the catheter. The use of closed drainage systems has reduced significantly the ability of bacteria to pass up the lumen of the catheter and cause infection. A bacterium passing around the catheter sheath in the urethra is probably the most important pathway for infection. Avoiding manipulation of the catheter and trauma to the urethra and urethral meatus can minimize this path of acquisition.

Patients with indwelling catheters acquire UTIs at a rate of 5% per day.[63–65] The closed systems are capable of preventing bacteriuria in most patients for up to 10 days with appropriate care. After 30 days of catheterization, however, there is a 78% to 95% incidence of bacteriuria despite use of a closed system.[63,66] Unfortunately, UTI symptoms in catheterized patient are not clearly defined. Fever, peripheral leukocytosis, and urinary signs and symptoms may be of little predictive value.[64,65] When bacteriuria occurs in the asymptomatic, short-term catheterized patient (<30 days), the use of systemic antibiotics should be withheld and the catheter removed as soon as possible. If the patient becomes symptomatic, the catheter should be removed and treatment as described for complicated infections started. The optimal duration of therapy is unknown. In the long-term catheterized patient (>30 days), bacteriuria is inevitable.[63] The administration of systemic antibiotics active against the infecting organism will sterilize the urine; however, reinfection occurs rapidly in more than 50% of patients. In addition, resistant organisms recolonize the urine. Symptomatic patients must be treated because they are at risk of developing pyelonephritis and bacteremia. Bacteria adhere to the catheter and to produce a biofilm consisting of bacterial glycocalyces, Tamm-Horsfall protein, as well as apatite and struvite salts, that act to protect the bacteria from antibiotics.[65] Recatheterization with a new, sterile unit should be performed in those symptomatic patients if the existing catheter has been in place for more than 2 weeks.

Various methods have been proposed to prevent the development of bacteriuria and infection in the patient with an indwelling catheter (see Table 120–5). The success of these methods depends on the type of catheter and the length of time it is in place. The use of constant bladder irrigation with antiseptic or antibacterial solutions reduces the incidence of infection in those with open drainage systems, but this approach has no advantage in those with closed systems. The use of prophylactic systemic antibiotics in patients with short-term catheterization reduces the incidence of infection over the first 4 to 7 days.[64,66] In long-term catheterized patients, however, antibiotics only postpone the development of bacteriuria and lead to the emergence of resistant organisms.

PROSTATITIS

Bacterial prostatitis is an inflammation of the prostate gland and surrounding tissue as a result of infection. It is classified as either acute or chronic. By definition, pathogenic bacteria and significant inflammatory cells must be present in prostatic secretions and urine to make the diagnosis of bacterial prostatitis. Prostatitis occurs rarely in young males, but it is commonly associated with recurrent infections in persons older than 30 years of age. As many as 50% of all males develop some form of prostatitis at some period in their life.[67,68] The acute form typically is an acute infectious disease characterized by a sudden onset of fever, tenderness, and urinary and constitutional symptoms. Chronic prostatitis presents with few symptoms related to the prostate but rather symptoms of urinating difficulty, low back pain, perineal pressure, or a combination of these. It represents a recurring infection with the same organism that results from incomplete eradication of bacteria from the prostate gland.

PATHOGENESIS AND ETIOLOGY

The exact mechanism of bacterial infection of the prostate is not well understood. The possible routes of infection are the same as those for UTIs. Reflux of infected urine into the prostate gland is thought to play an important role in causing infection. Intraprostatic reflux of urine occurs commonly and results in direct inoculation of infected urine into the prostate.[67,68] In addition, intraprostatic reflux of sterile urine can result in a chemical prostatitis and may be the cause of nonbacterial prostatitis. Sexual intercourse may contribute to infection of the prostate gland because prostatic secretions from men with chronic prostatitis and vaginal cultures from their sexual partners grew identical organisms. Other known causes of bacterial prostatitis include indwelling urethral and condom catheterization, urethral instrumentation, and transurethral prostatectomy in patients with infected urine.

A number of physiologic factors are believed to contribute to the development of prostatitis. Functional abnormalities found in bacterial prostatitis include altered prostate secretory functions. Prostatic fluid obtained from normal males contains prostatic antibacterial factor. This heat-stable, low-molecular-weight cation is a zinc-complexed polypeptide that is bactericidal to most urinary tract pathogens.[69] The antibacterial activity of prostatic antibacterial factor is related directly to the zinc content of prostatic fluid. Prostate fluid zinc levels and prostatic antibacterial factor activity also appear diminished in patients with prostatitis, as well as in the elderly.[69] Whether these changes are a cause or effect of prostatitis remains to be determined.

The pH of prostatic secretions in patients with prostatitis is altered.[70] Normal prostatic secretions have a pH in the range of 6.6 to 7.6. With increasing age, the pH tends to become more alkaline. In patients with inflammation of the prostate, prostatic secretions may have an alkaline pH in the range of 7 to 9. These changes suggest a generalized secretory dysfunction of the prostate that not only can affect the pathogenesis of prostatitis but also can influence the mode of therapy.

Gram-negative enteric organisms are the most frequent pathogens in acute bacterial prostatitis.[67,68] *E. coli* is the predominant organism, occurring in 75% of cases. Other gram-negative organisms frequently isolated include *K. pneumoniae, P. mirabilis,* and less frequently, *P. aeruginosa, Enterobacter* spp., and *Serratia* spp. Occasionally, cases of gonococcal and staphylococcal prostatitis occur, but they are infrequent.

E. coli most commonly causes chronic bacterial prostatitis, with other gram-negative organisms isolated less frequently. The importance of gram-positive organisms in chronic bacterial prostatitis remains controversial. *S. epidermidis, S. aureus,* and diphtheroids have been isolated in some studies.

CLINICAL PRESENTATION

Acute bacterial prostatitis presents as other acute infections (Table 120–6). Massage of the prostate will express a purulent discharge that will readily grow the pathogenic organism. Prostatic massage is contraindicated in acute bacterial prostatitis, however, because of the risk of inducing bacteremia and associated local pain. The diagnosis of acute bacterial prostatitis can be made from the patient's clinical presentation and the presence of significant bacteriuria. As with other UTIs, the infecting organism can be isolated from a midstream specimen.

TABLE 120-6 Clinical Presentation of Bacterial Prostatitis

Signs and symptoms	
	Acute bacterial prostatitis: high fever, chills, malaise, myalgia, localized pain (perineal, rectal, sacrococcygeal), frequency, urgency, dysuria, nocturia, and retention
	Chronic bacterial prostatitis: voiding difficulties (frequency, urgency, dysuria), low back pain, and perineal and suprapubic discomfort
Physical examination	
	Acute bacterial prostatitis: swollen, tender, tense, or indurated gland
	Chronic bacterial prostatitis: boggy, indurated (enlarged) prostate in most patients
Laboratory tests	
	Bacteriuria
	Bacteria in expressed prostatic secretions

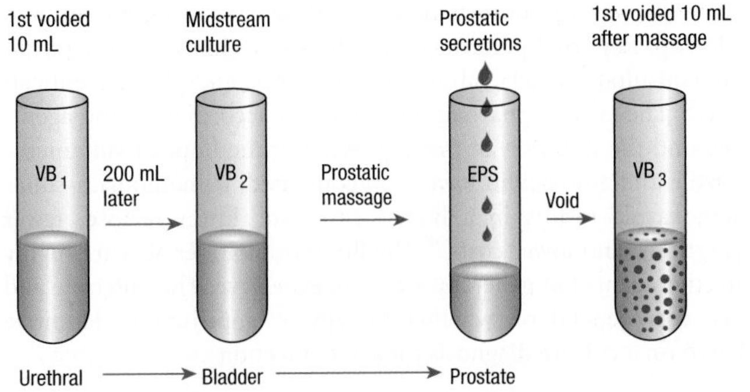

FIGURE 120-3. Segmented cultures of the lower tract in men. (EPS, expressed prostatic secretions; VB_1, voiding bladder 1; VB_2, voiding bladder 2; VB_3, voiding bladder 3.)

In contrast, chronic bacterial prostatitis is more difficult to diagnose and treat. Chronic bacterial prostatitis typically is characterized by recurrent UTIs with the same pathogen and is the most common cause of recurrent UTI in males. The patient's clinical presentation can vary widely (see Table 120–6). Many adults, however, are asymptomatic.

Because physical examination of the prostate is often normal, urinary tract localization studies are critical to the diagnosis of chronic bacterial prostatitis. The method of quantitative localization culture, as described by Meares and Stamey,[71] remains the diagnostic standard (Fig. 120–3). The method compares the bacterial growth in sequential urine and prostatic fluid cultures obtained during micturition. The first 10 mL of voided urine is collected (voiding bladder 1, or VB_1) and constitutes urethral urine. After approximately 200 mL of urine has been voided, a 10-mL midstream sample is collected (VB_2). This specimen represents bladder urine. After the patient voids, the prostate is massaged, and expressed prostatic secretions (EPS) are collected. After prostatic massage, the patient voids again, and 10 mL of urine is collected (VB_3).

The diagnosis of bacterial prostatitis is made when the number of bacteria in EPS is 10 times that of the urethral sample (VB_1) and midstream sample (VB_2). If no EPS is available, the urine sample following massage (VB_3) should contain a bacterial count 10-fold greater than that of VB_1 or VB_2. If significant bacteriuria is present, ampicillin, cephalexin, or nitrofurantoin should be given for 2 to 3 days to sterilize the urine prior to performing the localization study.

TREATMENT

❾ The goals in the management of bacterial prostatitis are, in general, the same as those for UTIs. Acute bacterial prostatitis responds well to appropriate antimicrobial therapy that is directed at the most commonly isolated organisms. Prostatic penetration of antimicrobials occurs because the acute inflammatory reaction alters the cellular membrane barrier between the bloodstream and the prostate. Most patients can be managed with oral antimicrobial agents, such as trimethoprim-sulfamethoxazole and the fluoroquinolones (e.g., ciprofloxacin, levofloxacin) (see Table 120–5). Other effective agents in this setting include cephalosporins, and β-lactam–β-lactamase combinations. Although intravenous therapy is rarely necessary for total treatment, intravenous to oral sequential therapy with trimethoprim-sulfamethoxazole or the fluoroquinolones is appropriate. The conversion to an oral antibiotic can be considered after the patient is afebrile for 48 hours or after 3 to 5 days of intravenous therapy. The total course of antibiotic therapy should be 4 weeks in order to reduce the risk of development of chronic prostatitis. Therapy may be prolonged with chronic prostatitis (6 to 12 weeks). Long-term suppressive therapy also may be initiated for recurrent infections, such as three times weekly ciprofloxacin, trimethoprim-sulfamethoxazole regular-strength tablet daily, or nitrofurantoin 100 mg daily.[72]

Chronic bacterial prostatitis often presents a more vexing situation because cures are obtained rarely. Despite high serum concentrations of antibacterial drugs in excess of the minimal inhibitory concentrations of the infecting organisms, bacteria persist in prostatic fluid. Most likely the failure to eradicate sensitive bacteria is caused by the inability of antibiotics to reach sufficient concentrations in the prostatic fluid and cross the prostatic epithelium.

Several factors that determine antibiotic diffusion into prostatic secretions were delineated from the canine model. Lipid solubility is a major determinant in the ability of drugs to diffuse from plasma across epithelial membranes. The degree of ionization in plasma also affects the diffusion of drugs. Only unionized molecules can cross the lipid barrier of prostatic cells, and the drug's pK_a (negative logarithm of acid ionization constant) directly determines the fraction of unchanged drug.

The pH gradient across the membrane has an influence on tissue penetration as well. A pH gradient of at least 1 pH unit between separate compartments allows for ion trapping. As the unionized drug crosses the epithelial barrier into prostatic fluid, it becomes ionized, allowing less drug to diffuse back across the lipid barrier. In early studies with the canine model, the prostatic pH was reported to be acidic (6.4).[70] More recent studies in humans, however, have reported that the pH of prostatic secretions from an inflamed prostate is actually basic (8.1 to 8.3).[70]

The choice of antibiotics in chronic bacterial prostatitis should include agents that are capable of reaching therapeutic concentrations in the prostatic fluid and which possess the spectrum of activity to be effective. Agents that achieve therapeutic prostatic concentrations include trimethoprim and the fluoroquinolones. Sulfamethoxazole penetrates poorly and probably contributes very little to trimethoprim. The fluoroquinolones appear to provide the best therapeutic options in the management of chronic bacterial prostatitis. Trimethoprim-sulfamethoxazole is also effective. Therapy should be continued for 4 to 6 weeks initially. Longer treatment periods may be necessary in some cases. If therapy fails with these regimens, chronic suppressive therapy may be used or surgery considered.

PHARMACOECONOMIC CONSIDERATIONS

The cost-effective management of UTIs requires knowledge of its pathogenesis and causative organisms associated with the various clinical syndromes described in this chapter. The costs associated with managing a UTI include direct costs, such a laboratory tests, medication, and healthcare visits. The indirect costs include lost work time and general quality-of-life issues such as disease or therapy adverse effects.

Direct costs are those associated with diagnosis, treatment, and followup. Reported percentages for these costs in cystitis are physician consultation 23%, laboratory costs 64%, and pharmaceuticals 13%.[73] The cost of pharmaceuticals varies according to the agents used and the duration of therapy. When trimethoprim-sulfamethoxazole and amoxicillin have been compared, trimethoprim-sulfamethoxazole results in a higher cure rate, lower relapse, fewer symptoms, and lower costs.[74] The fluoroquinolones also are highly effective agents but generally are more expensive. The outcome and total cost depend on whether therapy is empirical or definitive (based on a culture diagnosis for acute infection).

ABBREVIATIONS

EPS: expressed prostatic secretions

PMN: polymorphonuclear leukocyte

UTI: urinary tract infection

WBC: white blood cell

REFERENCES

1. Warren JW, Abrutyn E, Hebel JR, et al. Guidelines for antimicrobial treatment of uncomplicated acute bacterial cystitis and acute pyelonephritis. Clin Infect Dis 1999;29:745–758.
2. Fihn SD. Acute uncomplicated urinary tract infection in women. N Engl J Med 2003;349:259–266.
3. Foxman B. Epidemiology of urinary tract infections: Incidence, morbidity, and economic considerations. Am J Med 2002;113(Suppl 1A): 5S–13S.
4. Bent S, Nallamothu BK, Simel DL, Fihn SD, Saint S. Does this woman have an acute, uncomplicated urinary tract infection? JAMA 2002; 287(20):2701–2710.
5. Platt R. Quantitative definition of bacteriuria. Am J Med 1983;75:44–52.
6. Alper BS, Curry SH. Urinary tract infection in children. Am Fam Physician 2005;72(12):2483–2488.
7. Smellie JM. Reflections of thirty years of treating children with urinary tract infections. J Urol 1991;146:665–668.
8. Sobel JD, Kaye D. Urinary tract infections. In: Mandell GL, Bennett JE, Dolin R, eds. Principles and Practice of Infectious Diseases, 6th ed. New York: Churchill-Livingstone, 2005:906–926.
9. Shortliffe LM, McCue JD. Urinary tract infections at the age extremes: Pediatrics and geriatrics. Am J Med 2002;113(Suppl 1A):55S–66S.
10. Gordon KA, Jones RN, et al. Susceptibility patterns of orally administered antimicrobials among urinary tract infections pathogens from hospitalized patients in North America: Comparison report to Europe and Latin America. Results from the SENTRY Antimicrobial Surveillance Program (2000). Diagn Microbiol Infect Dis 2003;45:295–301.
11. Wong AH, Wnzel RP, Edmond MB. Epidemiology of bacteriuria caused by vancomycin-resistant enterococci: A retrospective study. Am J Infect Control 2000;28:277–281.
12. Stamatiou C, Bovis C, Panaguopoulos P, Petrakos G, Economou A, Lycoudt A. Sex-induced cystitis—Patient burden and other epidemiological features. Clin Exp Obstet Gynecol 2005;32(13):180–182.
13. Stamey TA, Fair WR, Timothy MM, et al. Antibacterial nature of prostatic fluid. Nature 1968;218:444–447.
14. Lipsky BA. Prostatitis and urinary tract infection in men: What's new; what's true? Am J Med 1999;106:327–334.
15. Shand DG, Nimmon CC, O'Grady F, et al. Relation between residual urine volume and response to treatment of urinary infection. Lancet 1970;1:1305–1306.
16. Parsons CL, Schrom SH, Hanno P, et al. Bladder surface mucin: Examination of possible mechanisms for its antibacterial effect. Invest Urol 1978;6:196–200.
17. Raz R, Stamm WE. A controlled trial of intravaginal estriol in postmenopausal women with recurrent urinary tract infections. N Engl J Med 1993;329:753–756.
18. Gupta K, Stapleton AE, Hooton TM, et al. Inverse association of H_2O_2-producing lactobacilli and vaginal *Escherichia coli* colonization in women with recurrent urinary tract infections. J Infect Dis 1998;178:446–450.
19. Ronald A. The etiology of urinary tract infections: Traditional and emerging pathogens. Am J Med 2002;113(1A):14S–19S.
20. Orskov I, Ferencz A, Orskov F. Tamm-Horsfall protein or uromucoid is the normal urinary slime that traps type-1 fimbriated *Escherichia coli.* Lancet 1980;1:887.
21. Measley RE, Levison ME. Host defense mechanisms in the pathogenesis of urinary tract infection. Med Clin North Am 1991;75:275–286.
22. Jenkins RD, Fenn JP, Matsen JM. Review of urine microscopy for bacteriuria. JAMA 1986;255:3397–3403.
23. Pezzlo M. Detection of urinary tract infections by rapid methods. Clin Microbiol Rev 1988;2:268–280.
24. Stamm WE. Measurement of pyuria and its relation to bacteriuria. Am J Med 1983;75(Suppl 1):53–58.
25. Pappas PG. Laboratory in the diagnosis and management of urinary tract infections. Med Clin North Am 1991;75:313–325.
26. St John A, Boyd JC, Lowes AJ, Price CP. The use of urinary dipstick tests to exclude urinary tract infection: A systematic review of the literature. Am J Clin Pathol 2006;126(3):428–436.
27. VanNostrand JD, Junkins AD, Bartholdi RK. Poor predictive ability of urinalysis and microscopic examination to detect urinary tract infection. Am J Clin Pathol 2000;113:709–713.
28. Stamey TA, Govan DE, Palmer JM. The localization and treatment of urinary tract infections: The role of bactericidal urine levels as opposed to serum levels. Medicine (Baltimore) 1965;44:1–36.
29. Fairley KF, Bond AG, Brown RB, et al. Simple test to determine the site of urinary tract infection. Lancet 1967;2:427–428.
30. Thomas VC, Forland M. Antibody-coated bacteria in urinary tract infection. Kidney Int 1982;21:1–7.
31. Stamey TA, Fair WR, Timothy MM, et al. Serum versus urinary antimicrobial concentrations in cure of urinary tract infections. N Engl J Med 1974;291:1159–1163.
32. Raz R, Chazan B, Dan M. Cranberry juice and urinary tract infections. Clin Infect Dis 2004;38:1413–1419.
33. Gupta K. Addressing antibiotic resistance. Am J Med 2002;113(1A):295–345.
34. Kahlmeter G. The ECO-SENS Project: A prospective, multinational, multicenter, epidemiological survey of the prevalence and antimicrobial susceptibility of urinary tract pathogens-interim report. J Antimicrob Chemother 2000;46(Suppl S1):15–22.
35. Steinke DT, Seaton RA, Phillips G, et al. Factors associated with trimethoprim-resistant bacteria isolated from urine samples. J Antimicrob Chemother 1999;43:841–843.
36. Goettsch W, VanPelt W, Naglekerke N, et al. Increasing resistance to fluoroquinolones in *Escherichia coli* from urinary tract infections in the Netherlands. J Antimicrob Chemother 2000;46:223–228.
37. Karlowsky JA, Hoban DJ, DeCarby MR, Laing NM, Zhanel GG. Fluoroquinolone-resistant urinary isolates of *Escherichia coli* from outpatients are frequently multi-drug resistant: Results from the North American urinary tract infection collaborative. Antimicrob Agents Chemother 2006;50:2251–2254.
38. Gupta K, Hooton TM, and Stamm WE. Increasing antimicrobial resistance and the management of uncomplicated community-acquired urinary tract infections. Ann Intern Med 2001;135:41–50.
39. Gupta K, Sahm DF, Mayfield D, Stamm WE. Antimicrobial resistance among uropathogens that cause community-acquired urinary tract infections in women: A nationwide analysis. Clin Infect Dis 2001;33:89–94.
40. Fihn SD. Acute uncomplicated urinary tract infections in women. N Engl J Med 2003;349(3):259–266.
41. Stamm WE, Hooton TM. Management of urinary tract infections in adults. N Engl J Med 1993;329:1328–1334.
42. Tice AD. Short course therapy of acute cystitis: A brief review of therapeutic strategies. J Antimicrob Chemother 1999;43(Suppl A):85–93.
43. Stein GE. Comparison of single-dose fosfomycin and a 7-day course of nitrofurantoin in female patients with uncomplicated urinary tract infections. Clin Ther 1999;21:1864–1872.
44. Cox CE, Marbury TC, Pittman WG, et al. A randomized, double-blind, multicenter comparison of gatifloxacin versus ciprofloxacin in the treatment of complicated urinary tract infection and pyelonephritis. Clin Ther 2002;24:223–236.

45. Irvani A, Klimberg I, Briefer C, et al. A trial comparing low-dose, short-course ciprofloxacin and standard 7-day therapy with co-trimoxazole or nitrofurantoin in the treatment of uncomplicated urinary tract infections. J Antimicrob Chemother 1999;43(Suppl A):67–75.
46. McCarty JM, Richard G, Huck W, et al. A randomized trial of short-course ciprofloxacin, ofloxacin, or trimethoprim-sulfamethoxazole for treatment of acute urinary tract infections in women. Am J Med 1999;106:292–299.
47. Stass H, Kubitza D. Pharmacokinetics and elimination of moxifloxacin after oral and intravenous administration in man. J Antimicrob Chemother 1999;43(Suppl B):83–90.
48. Chang SL, Shortliffe LD. Pediatric urinary tract infections. Pediatr Clin North Am 2006;53(3):379–400.
49. Nicolle LE, Bradley S, Colgan R, Rice JC, Schaeffer A, Hooton TM. Infectious Disease Society of America guidelines for diagnosis and treatment of asymptomatic bacteruria in adults. Clin Infect Dis 2005;40:643–654.
50. Nicolle LE. Urinary tract infection in long-term-care facility residents. Clin Infect Dis 2000;31:757–761.
51. Nicolle LE, Bjornson J, Harding GKM, et al. Bacteriuria in elderly institutionalized men. N Engl J Med 1983;309:1420–1425.
52. Melekos MD, Naber KG. Complicated urinary tract infections. Int J Antimicrob Agents 2000;15:247–256.
53. Katchman EA, Milo G, Paul M, Christiaens T, Baerheim A, Leibovici L. Three days vs longer duration of antibiotic treatment for cystitis in women: A systemic review and meta-analysis. Am J Med 2005;118(11):1196–1207.
54. Curran MP, Simpson D, Perry CM. Ertapenem, a review of its use in the management of bacterial infections. Drugs 2003;63:1855–1878.
55. Gleckman R, Crowley M, Natsios GA. Therapy of recurrent invasive urinary tract infection in men. N Engl J Med 1979;301:878–880.
56. Lipsky GA. Urinary tract infections in men: Epidemiology, pathophysiology, diagnosis, and treatment. Ann Intern Med 1989;110:138–150.
57. Wong ES, McKevitt M, Running K, et al. Management of recurrent urinary tract infections with patient-administered single-dose therapy. Ann Intern Med 1985;102:302–307.
58. Hooton TM. Recurrent urinary tract infection in women. Int J Antimicrob Agents 2001;17:259–268.
59. Stapleton A, Latham RH, Johnson C, et al. Post-coital antimicrobial prophylaxis for recurrent urinary tract infection. JAMA 1990;264:703–706.
60. Macejko AM, Shaeffer AJ. Asymptomatic bacteruria and symptomatic urinary tract infections during pregnancy. Urol Clin North Am 2007;34(1):35–42.
61. Christensen B. Which antibiotics are appropriate for treating bacteriuria in pregnancy. J Antimicrob Chemother 2000;46(Suppl S1):29–34.
62. McDermott S, Daguise V, Mann H, Szwejbka L, Callaghan W. Perinatal risk for mortality and mental retardation associated with maternal urinary tract infections. J Fam Pract 2001;50:433–437.
63. Trautner BW, Darouiche RO. Catheter-associated infections: Pathogenesis affects prevention. Arch Intern Med 2004;164(8):842–850.
64. Tambyah PA, Maki DG. Catheter-associated urinary tract infection is rarely symptomatic. Arch Intern Med 2000;160:678–682.
65. Ohkawa M, Sugata T, Sawaki M, et al. Bacterial and crystal adherence to the surfaces of indwelling urethral catheters. J Urol 1990;143:717–721.
66. Johnson JR, Duskowski MA, Wilt TJ. Systemic review: Antimicrobial urinary catheters prevent catheter-associated urinary tract infections in hospital patients. Arch Intern Med 2006;144(2):116–126.
67. Schaefer AJ. Urinary tract infection in men: State of the art. Infection 1994;22(Suppl 1):S19–S21.
68. Drieger JN, Nyberg L, Nickel JC. NIH consensus definition and classification of prostatitis. JAMA 1999;282:236–237.
69. Fair WR, Couch J, Wehner M. Prostatic antibacterial factor: Identity and significance. Urology 1976;7:169–177.
70. Pfau A, Perlberg S, Shapiro A. The pH of prostatic fluid in health and disease: Implications of treatment in chronic bacterial prostatitis. J Urol 1978;119:384–387.
71. Meares EM. Prostatitis. Med Clin North Am 1991;75:405–424.
72. Wagenlehner FM, Naber KG. Current challenges in the treatment of complicated urinary tract infections and prostatitis. Clin Microbiol Infect 2006;12(Suppl 3):67–80.
73. Patton JP, Nash DB, Abrutyn E. Urinary tract infection: Economic considerations. Med Clin North Am 1991;75:495–513.
74. MacDonald TM, Collins D, McGilchrist MM, et al. The utilization and economic evaluation of antibiotics prescribed in primary care. J Antimicrob Chemother 1995;35:191–204.

CHAPTER 121 Sexually Transmitted Diseases

LEROY C. KNODEL

KEY CONCEPTS

1. All recommended treatment regimens for gonorrhea include antibiotic therapy directed against *Chlamydia* species because of the high prevalence of coexisting infections, unless chlamydia has been ruled out.

2. Parenteral penicillin is the treatment of choice for all syphilis infections. For patients who are penicillin-allergic, few well-studied alternative agents are available, and all are oral medications that require 2 to 4 weeks of therapy to be effective. Patient compliance and thus efficacy are a concern when alternative regimens must be used.

3. Chlamydia genital tract infections represent the most frequently reported communicable disease in the United States. In females, these infections are frequently asymptomatic or minimally symptomatic and, if left untreated, are associated with the development of pelvic inflammatory disease and attendant complications such as ectopic pregnancy and infertility. As a result, all sexually active females, females aged 20 to 25 years, and sexually active women with multiple sexual partners should be screened annually for this infection.

4. Oral acyclovir, famciclovir, and valacyclovir are effective in reducing viral shedding, duration of symptoms, and time to healing of first-episode genital herpes infections, with maximal benefits seen when therapy is initiated at the earliest stages of infection. Depending on the severity of recurrent infections, which generally tend to be of shorter duration and produce less severe symptoms, symptomatic benefits may not be as obvious.

5. Metronidazole and tinidazole are the only agents currently approved in the United States to treat trichomoniasis. Although a single 2-g dose of either agent is widely used for compliance and other reasons, the alternative 7-day metronidazole regimen may be a better choice if sexual partners of treated individuals cannot be treated concurrently.

The spectrum of sexually transmitted diseases (STDs) has broadened from the classic venereal diseases—gonorrhea, syphilis, chancroid, lymphogranuloma venereum, and granuloma inguinale—to include a variety of pathogens known to be spread by sexual contact (Table 121–1). Because of the large number of infected individuals, the diversity of clinical manifestations, the changing drug-susceptibility patterns of some pathogens, and the high frequency of multiple STDs occurring simultaneously in infected individuals, the diagnosis and management of patients with STDs are much more complex today than they were even a decade ago.[1–4]

Despite a higher reported incidence of most major STDs in men, the complications of STDs generally are more frequent and severe in women. In particular, serious effects on maternal and infant health during pregnancy are well documented.[4] Damage to reproductive organs, increased risk of cancer, complications associated with pregnancy, and transmission of disease to the fetus or newborn are associated with several STDs. As a result of the physiologic, psychosocial, and economic consequences of STDs, and because of the increasing prevalence of some viral STDs, such as human immunodeficiency virus (HIV) and genital herpes, for which curative therapy is not available, there is continuing research into STDs and the primary prevention of these diseases.[2–5]

With the exception of HIV infection, which is reviewed in detail in Chap. 129, the most frequently occurring STDs in the United States are discussed in this chapter. For other less common STDs, only recommended treatment regimens are presented. The most current information on the epidemiology, diagnosis, and treatment of STDs provided by the Centers for Disease Control and Prevention (CDC) can be obtained at the CDC website (*www.cdc.gov*).

Numerous interrelated factors contribute to the epidemic nature of STDs. Sociocultural, demographic, and economic factors, together with patterns of sexual behavior, host susceptibility to infection, changing properties of the causative pathogens, disease transmission by asymptomatic individuals, and environmental factors, are important determinants of the frequency and distribution of STDs in the United States and worldwide.

Age is one of the most important demographic determinants of STD incidence. Overall, two-thirds of STD cases each year occur in persons in their teens and twenties, the peak years of sexual activity. With increasing age, the incidence of most STDs decreases exponentially. In sexually active teenagers, STD rates are highest in the youngest, suggesting that physiologic differences may contribute to increased susceptibility.[2–5]

Age-specific rates of STDs are higher in men than in women; however, reported rates may not represent true gender differences but rather may reflect greater ease of detection in men. In recent years, the ratio of male-to-female cases for most STDs has declined, possibly reflecting improvements in the diagnosis of STDs in asymptomatic women or changes in female sexual behavior following the availability of improved methods of contraception. Although some racial disparity exists for rates of STD infection, it is possible that this is a reflection of socioeconomic differences.[2–5]

The single greatest risk factor for contracting STDs is the number of sexual partners. As the number of sexual partners increases, the risk of being exposed to someone infected with an STD increases. Sexual

TABLE 121-1 Sexually Transmitted Diseases

Disease	Associated Pathogens
Bacterial	
Gonorrhea	*Neisseria gonorrhoeae*
Syphilis	*Treponema pallidum*
Chancroid	*Haemophilus ducreyi*
Granuloma inguinale	*Calymmatobacterium granulomatis*
Enteric disease	*Salmonella* spp., *Shigella* spp., *Campylobacter* fetus
Campylobacter infection	*Campylobacter jejuni*
Bacterial vaginosis	*Gardnerella vaginalis, Mycoplasma hominis, Bacteroides* spp., *Mobiluncus* spp.
Group B streptococcal infections	Group B *Streptococcus*
Chlamydial	
Nongonococcal urethritis	*Chlamydia trachomatis*
Lymphogranuloma venereum	*Chlamydia trachomatis*, type L
Viral	
Acquired immune-deficiency syndrome (AIDS)	Human immunodeficiency virus
Herpes genitalis	Herpes simplex virus, types I and II
Viral hepatitis	Hepatitis A, B, C, and D viruses
Condylomata acuminata	Human papillomavirus
Molluscum contagiosum	Poxvirus
Cytomegalovirus infection	Cytomegalovirus
Mycoplasmal	
Nongonococcal urethritis	*Ureaplasma urealyticum*
Protozoal	
Trichomoniasis	*Trichomonas vaginalis*
Amebiasis	*Entamoeba histolytica*
Giardiasis	*Giardia lamblia*
Fungal	
Vaginal candidiasis	*Candida albicans*
Parasitic	
Scabies	*Sarcoptes scabiei*
Pediculosis pubis	*Phthirus pubis*
Enterobiasis	*Enterobius vermicularis*

preference also plays a major role in the transmission of STDs. For all major STDs, rates are disproportionately greater in men who have sex with men (MSM) than in heterosexuals. Also, a number of less common STDs, including several caused by enteric protozoans and bacterial pathogens, occur primarily in MSM. The major risk factors for MSM appear to be related to the greater number of sexual partners and the practice of unprotected anal-genital, oral-genital, and oral-anal intercourse. In addition, prostitution and illicit drug use are associated with a higher incidence of most STDs.[1–4]

Some of the most serious sequelae of STDs are associated with congenital or perinatal infections. Most neonatal infections are acquired at birth, after infant passage through an infected cervix or vagina. Neonatal *Chlamydia trachomatis, Neisseria gonorrhoeae,* and herpes simplex virus (HSV) infections are associated with this type of spread. For pregnant women with syphilis, infection is usually transmitted transplacentally, producing a congenital infection. Depending on the organism, neonatal infections can manifest in a variety of ways, produce significant morbidity, and in some cases result in infant death.[1–4]

Other than complete abstinence, the most effective way to prevent STD transmission is by maintaining a mutually monogamous sexual relationship between uninfected partners. Short of this, use of barrier contraceptive methods, such as the male and female condoms, diaphragm, cervical cap, vaginal sponges, and vaginal spermicides alone or in combination, provides varying degrees of protection from a number of STDs. When used correctly and consistently, male latex condoms with or without spermicide are more effective than natural skin condoms in protecting against STD transmission, including HIV, gonorrhea, chlamydia, trichomoniasis, HSV, and human papillomavirus (HPV). When lubrication is desired with latex condoms, water-based products, such as K-Y jelly, are recommended because oil-based agents (e.g., petroleum jelly) can weaken latex condoms and reduce their effectiveness. For latex-allergic individuals, other synthetic condoms (e.g., polyurethane) appear to possess efficacy against STD transmission similar to latex condoms. The female condom is a lubricated polyurethane sheath with a diaphragm-like ring on each end that can be used as a protective device for women with male sexual partners who do not desire to use a condom. Limited data suggest that the female condom blocks penetration of viruses, including HIV; for nonviral STDs, the female condom provides STD protection similar to the male condom.[1,3,5,6] At one time, use of nonoxynol-9, a vaginal spermicide with cytolytic activity, was advocated to reduce the transmissibility of several STDs. This was based in large part on in-vitro and animal data. However, nonoxynol-9 does not significantly reduce the risk of transmission of common STDs but actually can increase the risk of HIV transmission in some users. Frequent use of nonoxynol-9 damages vaginal, cervical, and rectal epithelium, leading to increased transmissibility of HIV and possibly other STDs. Diaphragms may protect against cervical gonorrheal, chlamydial, and trichomonal infections.[1,6–8]

The varied spectrum of clinical syndromes produced by common STDs is determined not only by the etiologic pathogen(s) but also by differences in male and female anatomy and reproductive physiology. For a number of STDs, the signs and symptoms overlap sufficiently to prevent accurate diagnosis without microbiologic confirmation. Frequently, symptoms are minimal or absent despite the presence of infection. Table 121–2 lists common clinical syndromes associated with STDs.[1–3]

GONORRHEA

EPIDEMIOLOGY AND ETIOLOGY

N. gonorrhoeae is a gram-negative diplococcus estimated to cause up to 600,000 infections per year in the United States.[1] Of even greater concern are the substantial number of infections that remain undiagnosed and unreported.[1,9] Humans are the only known natural host of this intracellular parasite. Because of its rapid incubation period and the large number of infected individuals with asymptomatic disease, gonorrhea is difficult to control.[1,10–15]

Although the risk of a female acquiring a cervical infection after a single episode of vaginal intercourse with an infected male partner is high and increases with multiple exposures, the risk of transmission from an infected female to an uninfected male is not as great following a single act of coitus. No data are available on the risk of transmission after other types of sexual contact.[10–12]

PATHOPHYSIOLOGY

On contact with a mucosal surface lined by columnar, cuboidal, or noncornified squamous epithelial cells, the gonococci attach to cell membranes by means of surface pili and are then pinocytosed. The virulence of the organism is mediated primarily by the presence of pili and other outer membrane proteins. After mucosal damage is established, polymorphonuclear (PMN) leukocytes invade the tissue, submucosal abscesses form, and purulent exudates are secreted.[10,11]

CLINICAL PRESENTATION

Individuals infected with gonorrhea can be symptomatic or asymptomatic, have complicated or uncomplicated infections, and have infections involving several anatomic sites. Interestingly, most of the symptomatic patients who are not treated become asymptomatic within 6 months, with only a few becoming asymptomatic carriers of

TABLE 121-2 Selected Syndromes Associated with Common Sexually Transmitted Pathogens

Syndrome	Commonly Implicated Pathogens	Common Clinical Manifestations[a]
Urethritis	*Chlamydia trachomatis*, herpes simplex virus, *Neisseria gonorrhoeae, Trichomonas vaginalis, Ureaplasma urealyticum*	Urethral discharge, dysuria
Epididymitis	*C. trachomatis, N. gonorrhoeae*	Scrotal pain, inguinal pain, flank pain, urethral discharge
Cervicitis/vulvovaginitis	*C. trachomatis, Gardnerella vaginalis*, herpes simplex virus, human papillomavirus, *N. gonorrhoeae, T. vaginalis*	Abnormal vaginal discharge, vulvar itching/irritation, dysuria, dyspareunia
Genital ulcers (painful)	*Haemophilus ducreyi*, herpes simplex virus	Usually multiple vesicular/pustular (herpes) or papular/pustular (*H. ducreyi*) lesions that can coalesce; painful, tender lymphadenopathy[b]
Genital ulcers (painless)	*Treponema pallidum*	Usually single papular lesion
Genital/anal warts	Human papillomavirus	Multiple lesions ranging in size from small papular warts to large exophytic condylomas
Pharyngitis	*C. trachomatis* (?), herpes simplex virus, *N. gonorrhoeae*	Symptoms of acute pharyngitis, cervical lymphadenopathy, fever[c]
Proctitis	*C. trachomatis*, herpes simplex virus, *N. gonorrhoeae, T. pallidum*	Constipation, anorectal discomfort, tenesmus, mucopurulent rectal discharge
Salpingitis	*C. trachomatis, N. gonorrhoeae*	Lower abdominal pain, purulent cervical or vaginal discharge, adnexal swelling, fever[d]

[a]For some syndromes, clinical manifestations can be minimal or absent.
[b]Recurrent herpes infection can manifest as a single lesion.
[c]Most cases of pharyngeal gonococcal infection are asymptomatic.
[d]Salpingitis increases the risk of subsequent ectopic pregnancy and infertility.

the disease.[10–12] The most common clinical features of gonococcal infections are presented in Table 121–3.

Complications associated with untreated gonorrhea appear more pronounced in women, likely a result of a high percentage who experience signs and symptoms that are nonspecific and minimally symptomatic. As a result, many women do not seek treatment until after the development of serious complications, such as pelvic inflammatory disease (PID). Approximately 15% of women with gonorrhea develop PID. Left untreated, PID can be an indirect cause of infertility and ectopic pregnancies. In 0.5% to 3.0% of patients with gonorrhea, the gonococci invade the bloodstream and produce disseminated disease. Disseminated gonococcal infection (DGI) is three times more common in women than in men. The usual clinical manifestations of DGI are tender necrotic skin lesions, tenosynovitis, and monarticular arthritis.[1,10–13]

DIAGNOSIS

Diagnosis of gonococcal infections can be made by Gram-stained smears, culture, or methods based on the detection of cellular components of the gonococcus (e.g., enzymes, antigens, DNA, or lipopolysaccharide) in clinical specimens. Various stains have been used to identify gonococci microscopically, with the Gram stain the most widely used in clinical practice. Gram-stained smears are positive for gonococci when gram-negative diplococci of typical kidney bean morphology are identified within PMN leukocytes.[1,10–13] In the presence of equivocal smears (extracellular gonococcal forms that can be nonpathogenic, commensal Neisseria, or gram-negative diplococci of atypical morphology), culture is mandatory. In urethral smears from men with symptomatic urethritis, the smear is highly sensitive and specific, and is considered diagnostic for infection. Because of their low sensitivity, Gram-stained smears are not recommended in the diagnosis of endocervical, rectal, cutaneous, and asymptomatic male urethral infections. Because of the presence of nonpathogenic Neisseria in the pharynx, the Gram stain is not useful in the diagnosis of pharyngeal infection.[1,10,11,14]

Although no longer considered the most sensitive of diagnostic tests for gonorrhea, culture is considered the test of choice because of its high specificity in medicolegal situations (e.g., suspected abuse, rape); in diagnosing anorectal, pharyngeal, and conjunctival infections; and in screening populations with a low prevalence. Anatomic sites to be cultured depend on the individual's sexual preferences and body areas exposed. In women, because the urethra and other sites are rarely the sole locus of infection, cervical cultures produce the highest yield and frequently are performed in conjunction with rectal cultures. Urethral cultures are recommended in women who have had hysterectomies and heterosexual men.[1,10–14]

Because technical constraints and cost preclude the use of culture techniques in many office settings and clinics, alternative methods of diagnosis have been developed, including enzyme immunoassay, DNA probe techniques, and nucleic acid amplification techniques

TABLE 121-3 Presentation of Gonorrhea Infections

	Males	Females
General	Incubation period 1–14 days Symptom onset in 2–8 days	Incubation period 1–14 days Symptom onset in 10 days
Site of infection	Most common–urethra Others–rectum (usually caused by rectal intercourse in MSM), oropharynx, eye	Most common–endocervical canal Others–urethra, rectum (usually caused by perineal contamination), oropharynx, eye
Symptoms	Can be asymptomatic or minimally symptomatic Urethral infection–dysuria and urinary frequency Anorectal infection–asymptomatic to severe rectal pain Pharyngeal infection–asymptomatic to mild pharyngitis	Can be asymptomatic or minimally symptomatic Endocervical infection–usually asymptomatic or mildly symptomatic Urethral infection–dysuria, urinary frequency Anorectal and pharyngeal infection–symptoms same as for men
Signs	Purulent urethral or rectal discharge can be scant to profuse Anorectal–pruritus, mucopurulent discharge, bleeding	Abnormal vaginal discharge or uterine bleeding; purulent urethral or rectal discharge can be scant to profuse
Complications	Rare (epididymitis, prostatitis, inguinal lymphadenopathy, urethral stricture) Disseminated gonorrhea	Pelvic inflammatory disease and associated complications (i.e., ectopic pregnancy, infertility) Disseminated gonorrhea (three times more common than in men)

MSM, men who have sex with men.

(NAATs). With the exception of Gram stain for symptomatic gonococcal urethritis, these tests offer increased sensitivity and/or specificity over both Gram stain and culture.[10,16] Additionally, many of these tests can provide a more rapid means of diagnosis than culture. Of particular clinical importance is the high sensitivity of NAATs for detecting *N. gonorrhoeae* using noninvasive specimens (e.g., self-collected urine specimens, vaginal swabs). This technology is also being used to concurrently test for *C. trachomatis* using a single specimen. However, a major drawback of NAATs is their inability to provide resistance data on isolated gonococcal strains.[1,14,16]

TREATMENT

Gonorrhea

❶ All gonorrhea treatment regimens recommended by the CDC consist of various oral or parenteral cephalosporins and fluoroquinolones given as a single dose[1] (Table 121–4). These regimens have documented efficacy in the treatment of urethral, cervical, rectal, and pharyngeal infections. Coexisting chlamydial infection, which is documented in up to 50% of women and 20% of men with gonorrhea, constitutes the major cause of postgonococcal urethritis, cervicitis, and salpingitis in patients treated for gonorrhea for whom concurrent chlamydial infection has not been ruled out.[1,15,17] As a result, concomitant treatment with doxycycline or azithromycin is recommended in all patients treated for gonorrhea. Although none of the single-dose regimens recommended for gonorrhea in the CDC guidelines is effective against chlamydia, azithromycin (2 g) as a single dose is highly effective in eradicating both gonorrhea and chlamydia.

CLINICAL CONTROVERSY

Some clinicians advocate that a single 2-g dose of azithromycin should be the treatment of choice for gonorrhea because it is also effective in eradicating concomitant chlamydial infection. However, azithromycin therapy is associated with a greater incidence of gastrointestinal side effects and is much more expensive than other recommended first-line therapies.

TABLE 121-4 Treatment of Gonorrhea

Type of Infection	Recommended Regimens[a]	Alternative Regimens[b]
Uncomplicated infections of the cervix, urethra, and rectum in adults[c,d]	Ceftriaxone 125 mg IM once,[e,f] or cefixime 400 mg PO once,[f,g] or ciprofloxacin 500 mg PO once,[e] or ofloxacin 400 mg PO once,[e] or levofloxacin 250 mg PO once *plus* A treatment regimen for presumptive *C. trachomatis* coinfection if chlamydial infection has not been ruled out (see Table 121–8)	Spectinomycin 2 g IM once, or ceftizoxime 500 mg IM once, or cefotaxime 500 mg IM once, or cefoxitin 2 g IM once with probenecid 1 g PO once, or gatifloxacin 400 mg PO once, or lomefloxacin 400 mg PO once, or norfloxacin 800 mg PO once *plus* A treatment regimen for presumptive *C. trachomatis* coinfection if chlamydial infection has not been ruled out (see Table 121–8)
Gonococcal infections in pregnancy	Ceftriaxone 125 mg IM once,[h,i] or Cefixime 400 mg PO once *plus* A recommended treatment regimen for presumptive *C. trachomatis* infection during pregnancy,[i] if chlamydial infection has not been ruled out (see Table 121–8)	Spectinomycin 2 g IM once, or ceftizoxime 500 mg IM once, or cefotaxime 500 mg IM once, or cefoxitin 2 g IM once with probenecid 1 g PO once *plus* a recommended treatment regimen for presumptive *C. trachomatis* infection during pregnancy,[i] if chlamydial infection has not been ruled out (see Table 121–8)
Disseminated gonococcal infection in adults (>45 kg)[i,j,k,l]	Ceftriaxone 1 g IM or IV every 24 hours[l]	Cefotaxime 1 g IV every 8 hours[l] or ceftizoxime 1 g IV every 8 hours,[l] or ciprofloxacin 400 mg IV every 12 hours,[f,l] or ofloxacin 400 mg IV every 12 hours,[f,l] or levofloxacin 250 mg IV every 24 hours,[f,l] or spectinomycin 2 g IM every 12 hours[l]
Uncomplicated infections of the cervix, urethra, and rectum in children (<45 kg)	Ceftriaxone 125 mg IM once[m]	Spectinomycin 40 mg/kg IM once (not to exceed 2 g)
Gonococcal conjunctivitis in adults	Ceftriaxone 1 g IM once[n]	
Ophthalmia neonatorum	Ceftriaxone 25–50 mg/kg IV or IM once (not to exceed 125 mg)	
Infants born to mothers with gonococcal infection (prophylaxis)	Erythromycin (0.5%) ophthalmic ointment in a single application[o]; or Tetracycline (1%) ophthalmic ointment in a single application[o]	

CDC, Centers for Disease Control and Prevention; *C. trachomatis, Chlamydia trachomatis*; MSM, men who have sex with men; PO, orally.

[a]Recommendations are those of the CDC.

[b]A number of other antimicrobials have demonstrated efficacy in treating uncomplicated gonorrhea but are not included in the CDC guidelines.

[c]Treatment failures are usually caused by reinfection and necessitate patient education and sex-partner referral; additional treatment regimens for gonorrhea and chlamydia infections should be administered. Epididymitis should be treated for 10 days (see Table 121–8).

[d]Patients allergic to β-lactams should receive a quinolone. Persons unable to tolerate a β-lactam (penicillin or cephalosporin) or a quinolone should receive spectinomycin.

[e]Also recommended for the treatment of uncomplicated infections of the pharynx in combination with a treatment regimen for presumptive *C. trachomatis* infection, if chlamydial infection has not been ruled out.

[f]Fluoroquinolones are *not* recommended for treating infections in MSM or infections acquired in Hawaii, California, or other parts of the world where high-level resistance to fluoroquinolones is reported, or in heterosexuals with a history of recent foreign travel (including exposure from a partner with a history of recent foreign travel).

[g]In July 2002, Wyeth Pharmaceutical discontinued manufacturing cefixime; at the time of publication, Lupin, Ltd, which has FDA approval to market cefixime, had marketed only a suspension formulation of the drug and not the 400-mg tablet dosage form.

[h]Another recommended IM or PO cephalosporin also can be used.

[i]The fluoroquinolones, doxycycline, and erythromycin ethylsuccinate are contraindicated during pregnancy.

[j]Patients treated with one of the recommended regimens should be treated with doxycycline or azithromycin for possible coexistent chlamydial infection.

[k]Patients with gonococcal meningitis should be treated for 10 to 14 days and those with endocarditis for at least 4 weeks with ceftriaxone 1–2 g IV every 12 hours.

[l]All treatment regimens should be continued for 24–48 hours after improvement begins; at this time therapy can be switched to one of the following oral regimens to complete a 7-day course of treatment: cefixime 400 mg PO twice daily, or ciprofloxacin 500 mg PO twice daily, or ofloxacin 400 mg PO twice daily, or levofloxacin 500 mg PO once daily; ciprofloxacin, ofloxacin, and levofloxacin are not recommended for treating infections in MSM or infections acquired in Hawaii, California, or other parts of the world where high-level resistance to fluoroquinolones is reported, or in heterosexuals with a history of recent foreign travel (including exposure from a partner with a history of recent foreign travel).

[m]Patients with bacteremia or arthritis should receive ceftriaxone 50 mg/kg (maximum 1 g) IM or IV once daily for 7 days.

[n]A single lavage of the infected eye should be considered.

[o]Efficacy in preventing chlamydial ophthalmia is unclear.

Ceftriaxone, the only parenteral agent included in CDC recommended first-line agents for the treatment of gonorrhea, is administered intramuscularly (IM) as a single 125-mg dose, and in comparison with recommended oral antibiotics, it is an expensive alternative.[1,14–17,18,19]

Although oral therapy offers a promising alternative to the expense and pain associated with parenteral therapy, it may not be preferred for all cases of gonorrhea. Of the regimens of choice, only ceftriaxone is effective in eradicating both gonorrhea and incubating syphilis. Because the overall incidence of concomitant infection with both gonorrhea and syphilis appears low in most areas, selection of ceftriaxone based on this criterion should be considered only in areas in which the incidence of syphilis infection is high.[1,13,18,19] Resistance to the broad-spectrum cephalosporins recommended for the treatment of gonorrhea has not been reported. However, because of the increasing prevalence of quinolone-resistant *N. gonorrhoeae* (QRNG) throughout most parts of the world and in some parts of the United States (i.e., Hawaii and California), fluoroquinolones are no longer recommended for treating infections acquired in these locations. Similarly, fluoroquinolones are no longer recommended as first-line therapy in MSM because of increasing resistance in this population.[1,19] Ofloxacin is useful in eradicating both *N. gonorrhoeae* and *C. trachomatis;* however, different dosage regimens are required for each pathogen, and it is unknown whether the lower, multiple-dose daily regimen used in chlamydial infections is effective in eradicating gonorrheal infections.[1,18,19] Spectinomycin is still the preferred alternative for patients unable to tolerate the recommended cephalosporin or fluoroquinolone regimens. Although some resistance to spectinomycin is reported, its limited use appears to have prevented widespread resistance from developing. Unlike ceftriaxone and the fluoroquinolones, spectinomycin has only limited efficacy in treating pharyngeal infections.

Pregnant women infected with *N. gonorrhoeae* should be treated with either a cephalosporin or spectinomycin because fluoroquinolones are contraindicated. For presumed or diagnosed concurrent *C. trachomatis* infection, either azithromycin or amoxicillin is the preferred treatment.[1,10,11,18,19]

Ceftriaxone is the recommended therapy for DGI, gonococcal meningitis, endocarditis, and any type of gonococcal infection in children. In cases of DGI, patients should be hospitalized and treated initially with one of the recommended parenteral antibiotics (see Table 121–4). Although marked improvement is usually noted within 48 hours of initiating therapy, treatment should be continued as an outpatient with one of the recommended oral antibiotics to complete at least 7 days of antibiotic therapy.[1,18,19] Children and pregnant or lactating women should not receive fluoroquinolones because of the concern for bone and joint disorders. In MSM with DGI, ceftriaxone is preferred because of its efficacy in treating coexisting rectal, pharyngeal, and urethral infections QRNG infections.[1,10,18]

Gonococcal ophthalmia is highly contagious in adults and neonates and requires IM ceftriaxone therapy. Single-dose therapy is adequate for gonococcal conjunctivitis, although some physicians recommend continuing therapy until cultures are negative at 48 to 72 hours. Topical antibiotics are not sufficiently effective when used alone for ocular infections and are not necessary with appropriate systemic therapy. Infants with either type of ophthalmologic infection should be evaluated for signs of DGI.[1,10,18–20]

Treatment of gonorrhea during pregnancy is essential to prevent ophthalmia neonatorum. Gonococcal infection in newborns results primarily from passage through an infected birth canal, but it also can be transmitted in utero. Ophthalmia neonatorum is the most common ophthalmic infection in newborns (1.6% to 12%), although membranes of the vagina, pharynx, or rectum also can become colonized. Conjunctival involvement usually develops within 7 days of delivery and is characterized by intense, bilateral conjunctival inflammation with chemosis. If not treated promptly, corneal ulceration and blindness can develop. Because the law in most states requires neonatal prophylaxis with topical ocular antimicrobials, gonococcal ophthalmia neonatorum is rare in the United States. The CDC recommends that either tetracycline (1%) ophthalmic ointment or erythromycin (0.5%) ophthalmic ointment be instilled in each conjunctival sac immediately postpartum.[1,10–13,18–20]

EVALUATION OF THERAPEUTIC OUTCOMES

Although some clinicians recommend obtaining followup cultures at least 3 days after treatment, combination gonorrhea and chlamydial therapy rarely results in treatment failures, and routine followup of patients treated with a regimen included in the CDC guidelines is not recommended. Persistence of symptoms following any treatment requires culture of the site(s) of gonorrheal infection, as well as susceptibility testing if gonococci are isolated. In most cases, the presence of gonococci indicates reinfection rather than treatment failure and reflects the need for improved patient education and sex partner referral. Persistence of symptoms also can be caused by other infectious causes, such as *C. trachomatis.*[1,18,19]

SYPHILIS

EPIDEMIOLOGY AND ETIOLOGY

Although the actual number of reported cases is still relatively low (8,724 in 2005), the incidence of primary and secondary syphilis has increased in the United States by more than 40% since 2001.[9] In addition to being highly contagious, syphilis is of major concern because, if left untreated, it can progress to a chronic systemic disease that can be fatal or seriously disabling.[21–27]

Syphilis usually is acquired by sexual contact with infected mucous membranes or cutaneous lesions, although on rare occasions it can be acquired by nonsexual personal contact, accidental inoculation, or blood transfusion. The causative organism of syphilis is *Treponema pallidum,* a spirochete. The risk of acquiring syphilis from an infected individual after a single sexual encounter is approximately 50% to 60%. After sexual contact, the organism penetrates the intact mucous membrane or a break in the cornified epithelium, and spirochetemia occurs.[21,24,25]

Evidence of a strong association between syphilis and HIV infection has been noted. Although complex and incompletely understood, it appears that syphilis, similar to other sexually transmitted genital ulcer diseases, can increase the risk of acquiring HIV in exposed individuals. Also, immunologic defects in HIV-infected individuals can produce an atypical serologic response to syphilis. In particular, the possibility of delayed seroreactivity, markedly elevated serologic titers, and increased false-positive results could complicate the diagnosis, as well as assessment of treatment efficacy, in HIV-positive individuals infected with syphilis. Furthermore, anecdotal evidence suggests that compromised immune function can result in an accelerated progression of syphilis, particularly to neurosyphilis, requiring more aggressive antibiotic therapy in comparison with an immunocompetent host. As a result of this association, the CDC recommends that all patients diagnosed with syphilis be tested for HIV infection.[1,22–24,26,27]

CLINICAL PRESENTATION

The clinical presentation of syphilis is varied with progression through multiple stages possible in untreated or inadequately treated patients (Table 121–5).

Primary Syphilis

The primary stage, characterized by the appearance of a chancre on cutaneous or mucocutaneous tissue exposed to the organism, is

TABLE 121-5 Presentation of Syphilis Infections

General	
Primary	Incubation period 10–90 days (mean 21 days)
Secondary	Develops 2–8 weeks after initial infection in untreated or inadequately treated individuals
Latent	Develops 4–10 weeks after secondary stage in untreated or inadequately treated individuals
Tertiary	Develops in approximately 30% of untreated or inadequately treated individuals 10–30 years after initial infection
Site of infection	
Primary	External genitalia, perianal region, mouth, and throat
Secondary	Multisystem involvement secondary to hematogenous and lymphatic spread
Latent	Potentially multisystem involvement (dormant)
Tertiary	CNS, heart, eyes, bones, and joints
Signs and symptoms	
Primary	Single, painless, indurated lesion (chancre) that erodes, ulcerates, and eventually heals (typical); regional lymphadenopathy is common; multiple, painful, purulent lesions possible but uncommon
Secondary	Pruritic or nonpruritic rash, mucocutaneous lesions, flulike symptoms, lymphadenopathy
Latent	Asymptomatic
Tertiary	Cardiovascular syphilis (aortitis or aortic insufficiency), neurosyphilis (meningitis, general paresis, dementia, tabes dorsalis, eighth cranial nerve deafness, blindness), gummatous lesions involving any organ or tissue

highly infectious. Even without treatment, chancres persist only for 1 to 8 weeks before healing spontaneously. Because syphilitic chancres can be confused with other infectious etiologies, appropriate diagnostic testing is important.[21–24,26,27]

Secondary Syphilis

The secondary stage of syphilis is characterized by a variety of mucocutaneous eruptions resulting from widespread hematogenous and lymphatic spread of *T. pallidum*. Skin lesions can be either generalized or localized to a small portion of the body and, with the exception of follicular lesions, are nonpruritic. Generalized lymphadenopathy also is seen in the majority of patients, as are nonspecific symptoms such as mild and transitory malaise, fever, pharyngitis, headache, anorexia, and arthralgia. If untreated, secondary syphilis disappears in 4 to 10 weeks; however, lesions can recur at any time within 4 years.[12,21–27]

Latent Syphilis

By definition, persons with a positive serologic test for syphilis but with no other evidence of disease have latent syphilis. Latent syphilis is further divided into early and late latency. During early latency, the patient is considered potentially infectious because of the 25% risk of spontaneous mucocutaneous relapse. The U.S. Public Health Service defines early latency as 1 year from the onset of infection, although other investigators propose a longer interval, such as 2 to 4 years. With the exception of pregnancy in which the mother can pass the disease to the fetus, late latency is considered noninfectious, although the patient remains a host.[1,21–27]

Most untreated patients with late latent syphilis have no further sequelae; however, approximately 25% to 30% progress either to neurosyphilis or to late syphilis with clinical manifestations other than neurosyphilis. Treatment of all patients with latent syphilis is essential because there is no way to predict which patients will have progression of their disease.[21–27]

Tertiary Syphilis and Neurosyphilis

If left untreated, syphilis can slowly produce an inflammatory reaction in virtually any organ in the body. Manifestations of this disease progression were referred to previously as *tertiary syphilis*.[24] These clinical manifestations now are differentiated into two subgroups based on the presence or absence of central nervous system (CNS) involvement: neurosyphilis or tertiary syphilis (i.e., gumma and cardiovascular syphilis).[1,21–27]

Currently, the term *neurosyphilis* encompasses any patient with cerebrospinal fluid (CSF) abnormalities consistent with CNS infection.[1,21,24,27] Approximately 40% of patients with primary or secondary syphilis exhibit such abnormalities, although most remain asymptomatic. Persistence of CSF abnormalities into late latency is associated with a greater risk of progression to symptomatic neurosyphilis. Although data are conflicting, some investigators suggest that HIV-infected patients are at greater risk of developing symptomatic neurosyphilis than patients with intact immune systems.[1,22,25]

Rarely seen, the most common manifestations of disease progression from late latency are benign gumma formation and cardiovascular syphilis. The gumma, a nonspecific granulomatous lesion, is the classic lesion of late syphilis and develops in 50% of patients with disease progression. These chronic, destructive lesions characteristically infiltrate the skin, bone, soft tissue, and liver but can be found in any organ or tissue. Gummas of critical organs, such as the heart or brain, can be fatal.[1,21,24–28]

Congenital Syphilis

In pregnant women with syphilis, *T. pallidum* can cross the placenta at any time during pregnancy. The risk of fetal infection is greatest in pregnant women with primary and secondary syphilis and declines in pregnant women with late disease. Transmission of syphilis during pregnancy occurs primarily transplacentally and can result in fetal death, prematurity, or congenital syphilis. Symptoms can be seen during the first months of life (early congenital syphilis) or later in childhood or adolescence (late congenital syphilis). Manifestations of early congenital syphilis resemble those of secondary syphilis, whereas those of late congenital syphilis correspond to the tertiary stage in adults.[21–25]

DIAGNOSIS

Because *T. pallidum* is difficult to culture in vitro, diagnosis is based primarily on microscopic examination of serous material from a suspected syphilitic lesion or on results from serologic testing. In primary syphilis, diagnosis is established by the presence of *T. pallidum* on dark-field microscopic examination of material from cutaneous lesions and enlarged lymph nodes in patients with secondary syphilis. In incubating syphilis, confirmation frequently is by dark-field microscopic examination because serologic tests can be unreactive early in the disease. Another method of direct microscopic examination, the direct fluorescent antibody (test) for *T. pallidum* (DFA-TP), which uses monoclonal or polyclonal antibodies specific for *T. pallidum*, has greater specificity and sensitivity than does dark-field examination, and does not require the immediate examination of fresh specimens.[12,24–28]

Serologic tests are the mainstay in the diagnosis of syphilis and traditionally are categorized as nontreponemal or treponemal. Common nontreponemal tests include the Venereal Disease Research Laboratory (VDRL) slide test, rapid plasma reagin (RPR) card test, unheated serum reagin (USR) test, and the toluidine red unheated serum test (TRUST). Nontreponemal tests, which are inexpensive and easily performed, rely on the detection of treponemal antibodies directed against an alcoholic solution of cardiolipin, lecithin, and cholesterol contained in these tests. A positive nontreponemal test can indicate the presence of any stage of syphilis or congenital syphilis, although incubating syphilis and very early primary syphilis produce a negative reaction; however, because they are nonspecific tests, false-positive reactions occur, making them inappropriate to confirm the diagnosis alone. Transiently false-positive results can be seen in patients with acute febrile illnesses, after immunizations, and during pregnancy. Chronic false-positive results are commonly associated with heroin addiction, aging, chronic infections, autoimmune diseases, and malignant disease. In some cases, false-positive reactions are familial and are related to abnormal serum globulin levels.[23–28]

Nontreponemal tests are used primarily as screening tests; however, because *T. pallidum* antibody titers also can be quantitated by testing serial dilutions of the patient's serum for reactivity, they are useful in following the progression of the disease, recovery after therapy, and possible reinfection. Because antibody titers vary to some extent between tests, it is important that sequential serologic testing be performed using the same method each time. In patients treated successfully for primary and secondary syphilis, nontreponemal tests almost always will return to seronegativity. If these tests are going to return to negative in patients with early latent syphilis, they will do so within the first 4 years after adequate therapy; patients with disease of longer duration usually remain seropositive for life. In addition to their use in serologic testing, nontreponemal tests often are used on CSF to diagnose neurosyphilis.[23–28]

In some patients with secondary syphilis, a prozone phenomenon occurs that produces a negative VDRL test despite the presence of high reaginic antibody titers. This is corrected by diluting the patient's serum prior to testing.[26,27] For HIV-positive individuals with syphilis, the reactivity of nontreponemal tests can vary depending on the stage of the HIV infection. In the early stages, reaginic titers higher than in non–HIV-infected patients have been seen, resulting in the prozone phenomenon. During the later stages of HIV infection, however, when immune function deteriorates to a greater extent, serologic responses can be reduced or delayed. As a result, the diagnosis of syphilis in HIV-infected individuals can be more difficult.[1,24–28]

In diagnosing all stages of syphilis, treponemal tests are more sensitive than nontreponemal tests. Because these tests are technically more demanding and are more expensive, they are used primarily as confirmatory rather than as screening tests. The fluorescent treponemal antibody absorption (FTA-ABS) test is the most frequently used treponemal test. The FTA-ABS test uses the *T. pallidum* antigen to detect specific antibodies to treponemal organisms. The FTA-ABS test becomes positive earlier than nontreponemal tests in primary syphilis. After adequate antibiotic therapy for any stage of syphilis, the FTA-ABS test usually remains reactive for life and therefore is not useful in assessing serologic response to therapy, relapse, or reinfection. In suspected neurosyphilis when the CSF is negative with nontreponemal tests, FTA-ABS testing of the CSF is recommended to confirm these results. Although less specific than the VDRL test for CSF involvement, the FTA-ABS test appears to be highly sensitive.

Other serologic tests that are specific for the *Treponema pallidum* antibody are the *T. pallidum* hemagglutination assay (TPHA), microhemagglutination assay for antibodies to *T. pallidum* (MHA-TP), and the *T. pallidum* particle agglutination assay (TPPA). Recently, several enzyme immunoassays for *T. pallidum* have become available and are gaining wide use as confirmatory tests. Polymerase chain reaction (PCR)-based tests also are being investigated, particularly in situations in which serologic testing has poor sensitivity and specificity (e.g., congenital syphilis, early primary syphilis, and neurosyphilis). Additionally, multiplex PCR tests that can identify the presence of *T. pallidum,* herpes simplex virus type 1 (HSV-1) and herpes simplex virus type 1 (HSV-2), and *Haemophilus ducreyi* from genital ulcer specimens are under study.[23,24,26–28]

TREATMENT

Syphilis

Table 121–6 presents the CDC's treatment recommendations.[1] Parenteral penicillin G is the treatment of choice for all stages of syphilis. Because *T. pallidum* multiplies slowly, single doses of short- or intermediate-acting penicillins do not provide the prolonged, low-level exposure to penicillin required for eradication of the treponeme. As a result, benzathine penicillin G is the only penicillin effective for single-dose therapy.[1,12,22–29]

The recommended treatment for syphilis of less than 1 year's duration is benzathine penicillin G 2.4 million units as a single dose. Although the relapse rate for this regimen is less than 3%, some investigators advocate that 2.4 million units be administered once a week for 2 consecutive weeks. In patients with syphilis of longer than 1 year's duration and normal CSF examination, benzathine penicillin G is administered weekly for three successive doses. Although not specifically recommended by the CDC, this three-dose regimen is used by some experts to treat HIV-infected patients with syphilis of less than 1 year's duration based on data suggesting a greater risk of treatment failure with single-dose therapy.[1,24,25,29]

CLINICAL CONTROVERSY

Some experts even prefer to treat all patients with syphilis of less than 1 year's duration with the three-dose regimen because single-dose therapy is not consistently effective in eradicating treponemes from the CSF; this is of primary concern in patients with undiagnosed CSF involvement, such as HIV-infected individuals.

Patients with abnormal CSF findings should be treated as having neurosyphilis. Preferred regimens for neurosyphilis provide treatment over 10 to 14 days with parenteral penicillin G administered every 4 hours. Benzathine penicillin G alone in standard weekly doses and procaine penicillin G in doses under 2.4 million units do not consistently provide treponemicidal levels in the CSF and have resulted in treatment failures.[1,24–29] Because *T. pallidum* resistance to penicillin has not emerged, the primary need for alternative drugs in treating syphilis is for penicillin-allergic patients.[1,24,25,29]

❷ Alternative regimens recommended for penicillin-allergic patients are doxycycline 100 mg orally twice daily or tetracycline 500 mg orally four times daily for 2 to 4 weeks depending on the duration of syphilis infection.[1,24,25,29] These regimens should be used only in cases of documented penicillin allergy, and given concerns regarding patient compliance with these regimens, followup serologic testing is of particular importance.[1,23,24]

Other antibiotics used successfully in treating syphilis include various β-lactam antibiotics; however, none offers significant advantages over benzathine penicillin G. Even though ceftriaxone is considered effective in eradicating incubating syphilis when given as a single 125-mg dose, higher doses and more frequent administration (e.g., 1,000 mg daily for 8 to 10 days) appear necessary for more advanced syphilis, and treatment failures are reported in HIV-infected patients. Although data indicate that azithromycin 2 g as a single dose produces good results in patients with early syphilis, treatment failures and resistance to azithromycin are reported.[1,21,24,25,29]

For pregnant patients, penicillin is the treatment of choice at the dosage recommended for that particular stage of syphilis. To ensure treatment success and prevent transmission to the fetus, some experts advocate an additional IM dose of benzathine penicillin G 2.4 million units 1 week after completion of the recommended regimen. In women allergic to penicillin, safe and effective alternatives are not available; therefore, skin testing should be performed to confirm a penicillin allergy. It is recommended that women with positive skin tests undergo penicillin desensitization and receive the appropriate treatment regimen for their stage of disease.[1,24,25]

Most patients treated for primary and secondary syphilis experience the Jarisch-Herxheimer reaction after treatment. This benign, self-limiting reaction is characterized by flulike symptoms, such as transient headache, fever, chills, malaise, arthralgia, myalgia, tachy-

TABLE 121-6 Drug Therapy and Followup of Syphilis

Stage/Type of Syphilis	Recommended Regimens[a,b]	Followup Serology
Primary, secondary, or early latent syphilis (<1 year's duration)	Benzathine penicillin G 2.4 million units IM in a single dose[c]	Quantitative nontreponemal tests at 6 and 12 months for primary and secondary syphilis; at 6, 12, and 24 months for early latent syphilis[d]
Late latent syphilis (>1 year's duration) or latent syphilis of unknown duration	Benzathine penicillin G 2.4 million units IM once a week for 3 successive weeks (7.2 million units total)	Quantitative nontreponemal tests at 6, 12, and 24 months[e]
Neurosyphilis	Aqueous crystalline penicillin G 18–24 million units IV (3–4 million units every 4 hours or by continuous infusion) for 10–14 days[f] *or* Aqueous procaine penicillin G 2.4 million units IM daily plus probenecid 500 mg PO four times daily, both for 10–14 days[f]	CSF examination every 6 months until the cell count is normal; if it has not decreased at 6 months or is not normal by 2 years, retreatment should be considered
Congenital syphilis (infants with proven or highly probable disease)	Aqueous crystalline penicillin G 50,000 units/kg IV every 12 hours during the first 7 days of life and every 8 hours thereafter for a total of 10 days *or* Procaine penicillin G 50,000 units/kg IM daily for 10 days	Serologic followup only recommended if antimicrobials other than penicillin are used
Penicillin-allergic patients[g]		
Primary, secondary, or early latent syphilis	Doxycycline 100 mg PO two times daily for 14 days[g,h] *or* Tetracycline 500 mg PO four times daily for 14 days[h] *or* Ceftriaxone 1 g IM or IV daily for 8–10 days	Same as for non–penicillin-allergic patients
Late latent syphilis (>1 year's duration) or syphilis of unknown duration	Doxycycline 100 mg PO twice a day for 28 days[h,i] *or* Tetracycline 500 mg PO four times daily for 28 days[h,i]	Same as for non–penicillin-allergic patients

CDC, Centers for Disease Control and Prevention; CSF, cerebrospinal fluid; PO, orally.
[a]Recommendations are those of the CDC.
[b]The CDC recommends that all patients diagnosed with syphilis be tested for HIV infection.
[c]Some experts recommend multiple doses of benzathine penicillin G or other supplemental antibiotics in addition to benzathine penicillin G in HIV-infected patients with primary or secondary syphilis; HIV-infected patients with early latent syphilis should be treated with the recommended regimen for latent syphilis of more than 1 year's duration.
[d]More frequent followup (i.e., 3, 6, 9, 12, and 24 months) recommended for HIV-infected patients.
[e]More frequent followup (i.e., 6, 12, 18, and 24 months) recommended for HIV-infected patients.
[f]Some experts administer benzathine penicillin G 2.4 million units IM once per week for up to 3 weeks after completion of the neurosyphilis regimens to provide a total duration of therapy comparable to that used for late syphilis in the absence of neurosyphilis.
[g]For nonpregnant patients; pregnant patients should be treated with penicillin after desensitization.
[h]Pregnant patients allergic to penicillin should be desensitized and treated with penicillin.
[i]Limited data suggest that ceftriaxone my be effective, although the optimal dosage and treatment duration are unclear.

pnea, peripheral vasodilation, and aggravation of syphilitic lesions. The exact mechanism of the reaction is unknown, although proposed etiologies, including immunologic mechanisms and release of endotoxin or other toxic treponemal products, are not substantiated. The Jarisch-Herxheimer reaction is independent of the drug and dose used and should not be confused with penicillin allergy. It usually begins within 2 to 4 hours of initiating therapy, peaks at 8 hours, and is complete within 12 to 24 hours. Most reactions can be managed symptomatically with analgesics, antipyretics, and rest. Steroids and antihistamines have been administered prior to initiation of syphilitic therapy but are of limited value.[1,23–26]

EVALUATION OF THERAPEUTIC OUTCOMES

Table 121–6 lists the CDC recommendations for serologic followup of patients treated for syphilis.[1] Quantitative nontreponemal tests should be performed at 6 and 12 months in all patients treated for primary and secondary syphilis and at 6, 12, and 24 months for early and late latent disease. The CDC recommends more frequent monitoring of HIV-infected individuals (i.e., 3, 6, 9, 12, and 24 months after therapy). In general, the time to reach seronegativity is proportional to the duration of the disease. Table 121–6 also includes specific testing recommendations for other stages of syphilis. Despite adequate therapy, some patients can remain seropositive based on nontreponemal test results. In these cases, stabilization of low antibody titers is indicative of adequate therapy. For women treated during pregnancy, monthly quantitative nontreponemal tests are recommended in those at high risk of reinfection.[1,23–26]

CHLAMYDIA TRACHOMATIS

EPIDEMIOLOGY AND ETIOLOGY

Based on CDC data, the number of reported cases of chlamydia infection, the most frequently reported infectious disease in the United States, has doubled in the past 10 years.[1,7] Although this most likely is a result of improved screening and detection, it can also represent a true increase in the infection rate. Chlamydial infections represent the most common cause of nongonococcal urethritis (NGU), accounting for as much as 50% of such infections.[1,30,31]

PATHOPHYSIOLOGY

C. trachomatis is an obligate intracellular parasite that shares properties of both viruses and bacteria. Like viruses, chlamydiae require cellular material from host cells for replication; however, unlike viruses, chlamydiae maintain their cellular identity throughout development. Although *C. trachomatis* lacks a cell-wall peptidoglycan, its major outer membrane is similar to gram-negative bacteria. At least 18 serovars (subspecies) of *C. trachomatis* exist, of which only the lymphogranuloma venereum strains produce potentially invasive infections. The remaining serovars are involved primarily with superficial infection of epithelial cells.[31–33]

The risk of transmissibility of chlamydia after exposure is unknown but is believed to be less than that following exposure to *N. gonorrhoeae*.[1,31–33] Coinfection with chlamydia occurs in a substantial number of individuals with gonorrhea and all individuals diagnosed with *N. gonorrhoeae* should be assumed also to have *C. trachomatis* present, if chlamydial infection has not been ruled out.[1,15,16,34] Of major concern is that chlamydial infections are associated with a significantly increased risk of acquiring HIV infection.[33] In addition to genital infections, ocular infections in adults owing to autoinoculation and infants owing to vaginal delivery through an infected birth canal are reported. Pharyngeal and rectal infections can develop secondary to orogenital or receptive anal intercourse, respectively, with an infected individual.[1,30–36]

CLINICAL PRESENTATION

In comparison with gonorrhea, chlamydial genital tract infections are more frequently asymptomatic, and when present, symptoms tend to be less noticeable. Urethral discharge usually is less profuse and more mucoid or watery than the urethral discharge associated with gonorrhea.[30–34] Table 121–7 summarizes the usual clinical presentation of chlamydial infections.

Similar to gonorrhea, chlamydia can be transmitted to an infant during contact with infected cervicovaginal secretions. Nearly two-thirds of infants acquire chlamydial infection after endocervical exposure, with the primary morbidity associated with seeding of the infant's eyes, nasopharynx, rectum, or vagina. In exposed infants, neonatal conjunctivitis develops in as many as 50%, and pneumonia develops in up to 16%. Inclusion conjunctivitis in newborns is usually self-limited, but it can result in scarring and micropannus of the cornea. Interstitial pneumonitis occurring secondary to carriage in the nasopharynx typically is mild, but it can be severe and require hospitalization.[1,28,30–34]

DIAGNOSIS

❸ Because of the high rate of asymptomatic disease and the high prevalence of chlamydial infection in sexually active adolescent females, females aged 20 to 25 years, and sexually active women with multiple sex partners, the CDC recommends routine annual screening in these individuals. Laboratory confirmation of chlamydial infection is important because of the relative lack of specificity of symptoms when present.[1,32]

TABLE 121-7 Presentation of *Chlamydia* Infections

	Males	Females
General	Incubation period–35 days Symptom onset–7–21 days	Incubation period–7–35 days Usual symptom onset–7–21 days
Site of infection	Most common–urethra Others–rectum (receptive anal intercourse), oropharynx, eye	Most common–endocervical canal Others–urethra, rectum (usually caused by perineal contamination), oropharynx, eye
Symptoms	More than 50% of urethral and rectal infections are asymptomatic Urethral infection–mild dysuria, discharge Pharyngeal infection–asymptomatic to mild pharyngitis	More than 66% of cervical infections are asymptomatic Urethral infection–usually subclinical; dysuria and frequency uncommon Rectal and pharyngeal infection–symptoms same as for men
Signs	Scant to profuse, mucoid to purulent urethral or rectal discharge Rectal infection–pain, discharge, bleeding	Abnormal vaginal discharge or uterine bleeding, purulent urethral or rectal discharge can be scant to profuse
Complications	Epididymitis, Reiter syndrome (rare)	Pelvic inflammatory disease and associated complications (i.e., ectopic pregnancy, infertility) Reiter syndrome (rare)

Cell culture is the reference standard against which all other diagnostic tests are measured. Because chlamydiae are obligate intracellular parasites, specimens for culture must be obtained from endocervical (women) or urethral (men) epithelial cell scrapings rather than from urine or urethral discharges. Although tissue culture techniques have close to 100% specificity, the sensitivity is reported to be as low as 70% in part because of problems of improper specimen collection, transport, or processing. Because of the technical demands, expense, and length of time until results are available (3 to 7 days), culture is not used widely for diagnostic purposes today. However, culture remains the diagnostic standard in medicolegal cases such as sexual assault and child abuse because of its high specificity and ability to detect only viable organisms.[14,28,32,34,37–39]

Tests that detect chlamydial antigens and nucleic acid provide more rapid results, are technically less demanding to perform, are less costly, and in some situations have greater sensitivity than culture. Commonly used nonculture tests for detection of *C. trachomatis* are the enzyme immunosorbent assay (EIA), DNA hybridization probe, and NAATs.[14,28,32,34,37–39]

Most commercially available tests used to detect *C. trachomatis* use EIA techniques that detect chlamydial lipopolysaccharide (LPS) antigen. Some EIA methods, however, are not specific for *C. trachomatis,* and false-positive results are reported with other *chlamydia* species, as well as with some gram-negative bacteria. The sensitivity and specificity of the test are generally lower when urine specimens are used.[14,28,32,34,37–40]

Rapid office tests that employ EIA technology for diagnosing chlamydial infections are widely available, and most provide results in 30 minutes. These tests generally are much less sensitive and specific than laboratory-performed EIA, and they are subject to a high false-positive rate because of the cross-reactivity of LPS from other microorganisms. As a result, a positive rapid office test should only be considered presumptive, and test results should be confirmed by a laboratory-based method.[14,38–40]

Of all the advances in the diagnosis of *C. trachomatis* infections, the most important has been the development of NAATs, which can detect small amounts of chlamydial DNA. These tests are highly sensitive and specific for detecting infection in urogenital and anal specimens and in urine. Use of self-collected vaginal or anal specimens or first-void urine samples offers greater patient acceptability, particularly when used to screen asymptomatic individuals. A further advantage of tests that can screen urine for the presence of infection is that up to 30% of women are reported to have urethral infection only, which would be missed using a test on endocervical samples. Because of their ability to detect as little as a single gene copy in a specimen, nucleic acid residues that persist following successful antibiotic therapy of a chlamydial infection can result in a false-positive test for several weeks following eradication of the organism.[14,32–41]

TREATMENT

Chlamydia

A number of antimicrobials, including tetracyclines, macrolides, azithromycin, and some fluoroquinolones, display good in-vitro and in-vivo activity against *C. trachomatis.* In most clinical trials, cure rates exceeding 90% are reported for these agents. All these antimicrobials also appear to have good efficacy against *Ureaplasma urealyticum,* the second most common cause of NGU.[30–33]

Azithromycin 1 g orally as a single dose and doxycycline 100 mg orally twice daily for 7 days are the regimens of choice for the treatment of uncomplicated chlamydial infections[1] (Table 121–8). Because of its prolonged serum and tissue half-life, azithromycin is the only single-dose therapy that is effective in treating *C. trachomatis.* Of the fluoroquinolones, ofloxacin and levofloxacin are

TABLE 121-8 Treatment of Chlamydial Infections

Infection	Recommended Regimens[a]	Alternative Regimen
Uncomplicated urethral, endocervical, or rectal infection in adults	Azithromycin 1 g PO once, or doxycycline 100 mg PO twice daily for 7 days	Ofloxacin 300 mg PO twice daily for 7 days, or levofloxacin 500 mg PO once daily for 7 days, or erythromycin base 500 mg PO four times daily for 7 days, or erythromycin ethyl succinate 800 mg PO four times daily for 7 days
Urogenital infections during pregnancy	Azithromycin 1 g PO as a single dose or amoxicillin 500 mg PO three times daily for 7 days	Erythromycin base 500 mg PO four times daily for 7 days, or erythromycin base 250 mg PO four times daily for 14 days, or erythromycin ethyl succinate 800 mg PO four times daily for 7 days (or 400 mg PO four times daily for 14 days)
Conjunctivitis of the newborn or pneumonia in infants	Erythromycin base 50 mg/kg/day PO in four divided doses for 14 days[b]	

CDC, Centers for Disease Control and Prevention; PO, orally.
[a]Recommendations are those of the CDC.
[b]Topical therapy alone is inadequate and is unnecessary when systemic therapy is administered.

included in the CDC recommendations, but neither appears to offer an advantage over other first-line or alternative therapies. Although ciprofloxacin and some other fluoroquinolones have activity against *C. trachomatis* and *U. urealyticum*, high dosages have not consistently eradicated chlamydial infections.[1,34–37,41,42]

For pregnant women with chlamydial urogenital infections, treatment can reduce the risk of pregnancy complications and transmission to the newborn significantly. Because the use of tetracyclines and fluoroquinolones is contraindicated during pregnancy, azithromycin and amoxicillin are the recommended drug treatments (see Table 121–8). When compliance with a multiday regimen is a concern, azithromycin is the preferred treatment in women, regardless of pregnancy status. It is recommended that posttreatment cultures be obtained for pregnant patients treated for chlamydial infections to ensure eradication of the infection.[1,35–37] Persons treated for chlamydia should abstain from sexual intercourse for 7 days following the initiation of treatment.[1,34–37,41,42]

C. trachomatis transmission during perinatal exposure can result in infections of the eye, oropharynx, lungs, urogenital tract, and rectum of the neonate or infant. Despite their efficacy in preventing gonococcal ophthalmia, topical erythromycin ointment (0.5%), tetracycline ointment (1%), and silver nitrate solution (1%) appear less effective in preventing chlamydial ophthalmia. Additionally, topical therapy has no effect on nasal carriage or colonization of other parts of the infant's body, so the potential for other infections, including pneumonia, remains. Because of the high percentage of treatment failures, topical therapy is not recommended to treat ophthalmia caused by *C. tracho matis*. Instead, an oral erythromycin regimen is recommended.[1,31–33,36]

EVALUATION OF THERAPEUTIC OUTCOMES

Treatment of chlamydial infections with the recommended regimens is highly effective; therefore, posttreatment laboratory testing is not recommended routinely unless symptoms persist or there are other specific concerns (e.g., pregnancy).[1,34–37] Posttreatment tests should not be performed for at least 3 weeks following completion of therapy.[1] When posttreatment tests are positive, they usually represent noncompliance, failure to treat sexual partners, or laboratory error rather than inadequate therapy or resistance to therapy. Infants with pneumonitis should receive followup testing because erythromycin is only 80% effective, and a second course of therapy can be necessary.[1,30–34,36]

GENITAL HERPES

EPIDEMIOLOGY AND ETIOLOGY

Genital herpes infections represent the most common cause of genital ulceration seen in the United States. More than 50 million Americans have genital herpes, and this number is increasing by at least 500,000 each year.[1,7,43–48] Because of its morbidity, recurrent nature, and potential for complications, as well as its ability to be transmitted asymptomatically, genital herpes is of major public health importance.[45–54] Similar to syphilis and other STDs, the presence of genital herpes lesions is associated with an increased risk of acquiring HIV following exposure.[1,46,47,52]

PATHOPHYSIOLOGY

Herpes comes from the Greek word meaning "to creep" and is used to describe two distinct but antigenically related serotypes of herpes simplex virus. HSV-1 is associated most commonly with oropharyngeal disease, and HSV-2 is associated most closely with genital disease; however, each virus is capable of causing clinically indistinguishable infections in both anatomic areas.[46,47,50,54]

Humans are the sole known reservoir for HSV. Infection is transmitted via inoculation of virus from infected secretions onto mucosal surfaces (e.g., urethra, oropharynx, cervix, and conjunctivae) or through abraded skin. Evidence that the virus survives for a limited time on environmental surfaces suggests the possibility of fomitic transfer as a nonvenereal route of transmission.[46,48–50]

The cycle of HSV infection occurs in five stages: primary mucocutaneous infection, infection of the ganglia, establishment of latency, reactivation, and recurrent infection. After viral inoculation, HSV infection is associated with cytoplasmic granulation, ballooning degeneration of cells, and production of mononucleated giant cells. Initially, the cellular response is predominantly polymorphonuclear, followed by a lymphocytic response. Replication occurs with viral spread to contiguous cells and peripheral sensory nerves. Latency then is established in sensory or autonomic nerve root ganglia. Latency appears to be lifelong, interrupted only by reactivation of the viral infection. It is unclear what factors are important in maintaining latency, but immune responses and emotional and physical stresses appear important in reactivating latent virus.[46,48]

CLINICAL PRESENTATION

The signs and symptoms of genital herpes infection are influenced by many factors, including previous exposure to HSV, viral type, and host factors such as age and site of infection. Because a high percentage of initial and recurrent infections are asymptomatic, and because viral shedding can occur in the absence of apparent lesions or symptoms, identification and education of individuals with genital herpes are essential in controlling its transmission.[46,53,55] A summary of the clinical presentation of genital herpes is provided in Table 121–9.

Complications

Complications from genital herpes infections result from both genital spread and autoinoculation of the virus and occur most commonly with primary first episodes. Lesions at extragenital sites, such as the eye, rectum, pharynx, and fingers, are not uncommon. CNS involvement is seen occasionally and can take several forms,

TABLE 121-9 Presentation of Genital Herpes Infections

General	Incubation period 2–14 days (mean–4 days)
	Can be caused by either HSV-1 or HSV-2
Classification of infection	
First-episode primary	Initial genital infection in individuals lacking antibody to either HSV-1 or HSV-2
First-episode nonprimary	Initial genital infection in individuals with clinical or serologic evidence of prior HSV (usually HSV-1) infection
Recurrent	Appearance of genital lesions at some time following healing of first-episode infection
Signs and symptoms	
First-episode infections	Most primary infections are asymptomatic or minimally symptomatic
	Multiple painful pustular or ulcerative lesions on external genitalia developing over a period of 7–10 days; lesions heal in 2–4 weeks (mean 21 days)
	Flulike symptoms (e.g., fever, headache, malaise) during first few days after appearance of lesions
	Others–local itching, pain or discomfort; vaginal or urethral discharge, tender inguinal adenopathy, paresthesias, urinary retention
	Severity of symptoms greater in females than in males
	Symptoms are less severe (e.g., fewer lesions, more rapid lesion healing, fewer or milder systemic symptoms) with nonprimary infections
	Symptoms more severe and prolonged in the immunocompromised
	On average viral shedding lasts approximately 11–12 days for primary infections and 7 days for nonprimary infections
Recurrent	Prodrome seen in approximately 50% of patients prior to appearance of recurrent lesions; mild burning, itching, or tingling are typical prodromal symptoms
	Compared to primary infections, recurrent infections associated with (1) fewer lesions that are more localized, (2) shorter duration of active infection (lesions heal within 7 days), and (3) milder symptoms
	Severity of symptoms greater in females than in males
	Symptoms more severe and prolonged in the immunocompromised
	On average viral shedding lasts approximately 4 days
	Asymptomatic viral shedding is more frequent during the first year after infection with HSV
Therapeutic implications of HSV-1 versus HSV-2 genital infection	Primary infections caused by HSV-1 and HSV-2 virtually indistinguishable
	Recurrent infections and subclinical viral shedding are less frequent with HSV-1
	Recurrent infections with HSV-2 tend to be more severe
Complications	Secondary infection of lesions; extragenital infection because of autoinoculation; disseminated infection (primarily in immunocompromised patients); meningitis or encephalitis; neonatal transmission

HSV-1, herpes simplex virus type 1; HSV-2, herpes simplex virus type 2.

including an aseptic meningitis, transverse myelitis, or sacral radiculopathy syndrome.[47,50,51,54]

A major concern is the effect of genital herpes on neonates exposed during pregnancy. Neonatal herpes is associated with a high mortality and significant morbidity. It is transmitted to the newborn primarily through exposure to HSV in the birth canal but, in rare cases, also is transmitted transplacentally. The risk of transmission during birth appears much greater for first-episode primary infections than for recurrent infections. Neonatal herpes infection has a case-fatality rate of approximately 50%, with a large proportion of surviving infants experiencing significant morbidity, including permanent neurologic damage.[49–51]

DIAGNOSIS

Confirmation of a genital herpes infection can be made only with laboratory testing. Tissue culture is the most specific (100%) and sensitive method (80% to 90%) of confirming the diagnosis of first-episode genital herpes; however, culture is relatively insensitive in detecting HSV in ulcers in the latter stages of healing and in recurrent infections, as a result, in part, of reduced viral load. Viral culture is expensive and time-consuming, and improper collection or transport of specimens can result in false-negative results. In most situations, HSV isolation on tissue culture takes 48 to 96 hours. Following isolation, it is recommended that typing of the virus be performed because of prognostic implications (HSV-1 is associated with a lower rate of asymptomatic and symptomatic recurrence).[28,54–57] In instances in which rapid detection is necessary, such as an impending birth, other detection methods can be more useful. Amplified culture techniques that combine cell culture for 24 hours and subsequent staining for HSV antigen have sensitivities and specificities only slightly less than those of culture.[28,47,49,50,52–57]

Several serologic tests capable of distinguishing HSV-1 and HSV-2 antibodies are available. These tests detect antibodies to type-specific HSV-1 and HSV-2 proteins gG-1 and gG-2, respectively. Whereas antibody formation begins immediately following a primary herpes infection, complete seroconversion (i.e., complete antibody development) can take several months. Until the full expression of all antigenic determinants of HSV-1 and HSV-2 occurs, these tests are not useful in differentiating HSV-1 and HSV-2 infection.[48,53,54,57] Older antibody detection tests, some of which are still marketed, are unable to distinguish between HSV-1 and HSV-2 owing to the considerable cross-reactivity between the two serotypes. Given the high prevalence of HSV-1 antibody in the adult population, accurate interpretation of positive results is not possible.[28,46,54]

In recent years, PCR assays that detect HSV DNA and can differentiate HSV-1 and HSV-2 infections have become increasingly available. These assays are more sensitive than culture and are considered the diagnostic test of choice for suspected CNS infections (i.e., HSV encephalitis and HSV meningitis). Although PCR assays are not used widely in diagnosing genital ulcer disease at this time, some data suggest that they also may prove useful in diagnosing asymptomatic viral shedding.[52,55–57]

Although the diagnosis of genital herpes can be confirmed only by laboratory tests, less stringent diagnostic criteria (e.g., characteristic physical findings or clinical history) frequently are used in clinical practice. A presumptive diagnosis of genital herpes commonly is made based on the presence of dark-field-negative, vesicular, or ulcerative genital lesions. A prior history of similar lesions or recent sexual contact with an individual with similar lesions also is useful in making the diagnosis. Other STDs, including chancroid, lymphogranuloma venereum, and granuloma inguinale, and causes such as trauma, allergic reactions, and bacterial or fungal infections are considered in the differential diagnosis.[48,55–57]

TREATMENT

Genital Herpes

The most achievable goals in the management of genital herpes are to relieve symptoms and to shorten the clinical course, to prevent complications and recurrences, and to decrease disease transmission. Although research has focused primarily on the treatment of active infection and suppression of recurrences, increasing emphasis is being placed on various approaches, including immunotherapy that might provide protection from disease transmission or possibly eliminate established latency.[46–48,55]

Palliative and supportive measures are the cornerstone of therapy for patients with genital herpes. Pain and discomfort usually respond to warm saline baths or the use of analgesics, antipyretics, or antipruritics; good genital hygiene can prevent the development of bacterial superinfection.

❹ Specific chemotherapeutic approaches to treating genital herpes include antiviral compounds, topical surfactants, photodynamic dyes, immune modulators, vaccines, and interferons. Few of these have undergone extensive evaluation, however, and only the antiviral agents have demonstrated any consistent clinical efficacy. The most recent CDC recommendations for the treatment of genital herpes include the antiviral agents acyclovir, valacyclovir, and famciclovir[1] (Table 121–10). The overall efficacy of these agents in treating genital HSV infection appears comparable, although patient compliance can be improved with regimens requiring less frequent dosing.[1,42–52,58]

TABLE 121-10 Treatment of Genital Herpes

Type of Infection	Recommended Regimens[a,b]	Alternative Regimen
First clinical episode of genital herpes[c]	Acyclovir 400 mg PO three times daily for 7–10 days,[d] *or* Acyclovir 200 mg PO five times daily for 7–10 days,[d] *or* Famciclovir 250 mg PO three times daily for 7–10 days,[d] *or* Valacyclovir 1 g PO twice daily for 7–10 days[d]	Acyclovir 5–10 mg/kg IV every 8 hours for 2–7 days or until clinical improvement occurs, followed by oral therapy to complete at least 10 days of total therapy[e]
Recurrent infection		
Episodic therapy	Acyclovir 400 mg PO three times daily for 5 days,[g] *or* Acyclovir 800 mg PO twice daily for 5 days,[g] *or* Acyclovir 800 mg PO three times daily for 2 days,[g] *or* Famciclovir 125 mg PO twice daily for 5 days,[g] *or* Valacyclovir 500 mg PO twice daily for 3–5 days,[g] *or* Valacyclovir 1 g PO once daily for 5 days[g]	
Suppressive therapy	Acyclovir 400 mg PO twice daily, *or* Famciclovir 250 mg PO twice daily, *or* Valacyclovir 500 mg or 1,000 mg PO once daily[h]	

CDC, Centers for Disease Control and Prevention; HIV, human immunodeficiency virus; PO, orally.
[a]Recommendations are those of the CDC.
[b]HIV-infected patients can require more aggressive therapy.
[c]Primary or nonprimary first episode.
[d]Treatment duration can be extended if healing is incomplete after 10 days.
[e]Only for patients with severe symptoms or complications that necessitate hospitalization.
[f]Recommendations based on studies using this dosage regimen rather than the lower dosage regimens recommended for first clinical episodes of genital herpes. It is not clear whether lower dosage regimens would have comparable efficacy. Famciclovir and valacyclovir are probably also effective for proctitis and oral infection, but clinical experience is limited.
[g]Requires initiation of therapy within 24 hours of lesion onset or during the prodrome that precedes some outbreaks.
[h]Valacyclovir 500 mg appears less effective than valacyclovir 1,000 mg in patients with approximately 10 recurrences per year.

FIRST-EPISODE INFECTIONS

Oral formulations of acyclovir, famciclovir, and valacyclovir have demonstrated efficacy in reducing viral shedding, duration of symptoms, and time to healing of first-episode genital herpes infections, with maximal benefits seen when therapy is initiated at the earliest stages of infection.[1,44–48,52,58–61] Table 121–10 lists the recommended acyclovir, famciclovir, and valacyclovir oral regimens for first-episode infections. In immunocompromised patients or those with severe symptoms or complications necessitating hospitalization, parenteral acyclovir can be beneficial; however, the IV regimen has been associated with renal, gastrointestinal, bone marrow, and CNS toxicity, particularly in patients with renal dysfunction receiving high doses. No antiviral regimen is known to prevent latency or alter the subsequent frequency and severity of recurrences in humans.[1,42–52,61–64]

RECURRENT INFECTIONS

CLINICAL CONTROVERSY

The role of antiviral agents in the treatment of most recurrent genital herpes episodes is controversial. Because signs and symptoms of recurrent infections generally are milder and of shorter duration than those of first-episode infections in immunocompetent hosts, demonstration of clinically important therapeutic benefits is difficult. However, as episodic, asymptomatic viral shedding is common in HSV-2 infection, suppressive therapy in combination with use of condoms provides some protection to uninfected sexual partners.

There are two approaches to management of recurrent episodes: episodic or chronic suppressive therapy.[1,47,50,51,55,56,61–64] Episodic therapy is initiated early during the course of the recurrence, preferably at the onset of prodromal symptoms but no more than 24 hours after the appearance of lesions. In most patients, appreciable effects on symptomatology are not seen. Patients with prolonged episodes of recurrent infection or severe symptomatology are most likely to benefit from episodic therapy. Table 121–10 lists the recommended acyclovir, famciclovir, and valacyclovir suppressive regimens. Because of the relative mildness and brevity of recurrent infections, parenteral administration of acyclovir usually is not justifiable.[32,47,51,55,56]

Suppressive therapy with recommended antivirals reduces the frequency and severity of recurrences in 70% to 80% of patients experiencing frequent recurrences. Asymptomatic viral shedding is markedly reduced in patients receiving suppressive therapy; however, the extent to which this decreases disease transmission to sexual partners remains to be determined. Despite antiviral suppressive therapy, low-level virus shedding still occurs. Because the frequency of recurrences tends to diminish over time, periodic "drug holidays" are advocated to assess changes in the underlying recurrence rate and determine if continued suppressive therapy is warranted. In patients experiencing 10 recurrences or more each year, the valacyclovir 500 mg regimen can be less effective than the other recommended regimens.[1,46,55,56,61–64]

Resistant HSV isolates have been identified in some patients experiencing breakthrough recurrences while taking acyclovir. Although there is concern about the development of resistant strains with suppressive therapy, clinical trials have found no evidence of cumulative toxicity or significant resistance in patients treated continuously with the recommended antivirals.[44,46,47,50,56,58,60,61]

SELECTED POPULATIONS

Immunocompromised patients are at greatest risk for severe and recurrent HSV infections. Acyclovir, valacyclovir, and famciclovir have been used to prevent reactivation of infection in patients seropositive for HSV who undergo transplantation procedures or induction chemotherapy for acute leukemia. Immunocompromised individuals, such as patients with acquired immune deficiency syndrome (AIDS), who fail treatment or prophylaxis with recommended antiviral doses frequently demonstrate improved response with higher doses. If resistance is suspected or confirmed with recommended first-line antivirals, foscarnet is usually effective. However, its use is associated with a greater risk of serious adverse effects.[45,51,52,56] Lesional application of an extemporaneous compounded cidofovir (1%) gel or trifluridine ophthalmic solution appears to offer some benefits also.[1,43]

The safety of acyclovir, famciclovir, and valacyclovir during pregnancy is not established, although considerable experience with acyclovir in pregnant patients has produced no evidence of teratogenic effects. Because of the high maternal and infant morbidity associated with first-episode primary genital infections or severe recurrent infections at or near term, many clinicians advocate the use of systemic acyclovir as the standard of care in such cases; however, the effectiveness of such therapy is unknown. The use of acyclovir to suppress recurrent episodes near term is more controversial primarily because of the lack of data demonstrating significant benefits in this situation.[32,50,55,56,59–61]

With the increasing prevalence of genital herpes worldwide, the potential exists for widespread use and misuse of acyclovir, valacyclovir, and famciclovir, resulting in development of resistant HSV isolates. In-vitro resistance to these three agents usually is mediated by alterations in viral thymidine kinase; most resistant isolates are either thymidine kinase–deficient or have altered thymidine kinase. The incidence and clinical implications of HSV resistance require further study particularly with respect to immunocompromised hosts, in whom resistance can develop with greater frequency and be of greater clinical importance. Unlike acyclovir, valacyclovir, and famciclovir, foscarnet does not require the presence of thymidine kinase to be effective.[47,50,52,55,56]

Numerous agents for the prophylaxis and treatment of genital herpes infections are being studied. Neither topical nor systemic interferons have demonstrated consistent beneficial effects in genital HSV infections; however, a reduction in pain and time of healing of lesions has been reported with an interferon preparation incorporated into a gel containing nonoxynol-9. Other treatments under investigation include cidofovir and immune modulators such as imiquimod and resiquimod.[47,53,56] Agents that can eliminate ganglionic latency and prevent recurrent HSV infections are not expected to be available in the near future. Development of vaccines capable of protecting against HSV infection has proved challenging given the relative lack of protection offered by humoral and cell-mediated immunity in preventing naturally occurring recurrent infections. Safety concerns with live attenuated virus vaccines resulted in research focused primarily on recombinant protein vaccines that have exhibited relatively poor immunogenicity. In recent years, investigations using replication-defective HSV mutants that are not pathogenic, as well as DNA vaccines that foster host cell uptake of foreign DNA that encodes for an antigenic viral protein, have shown some promise in animal models. Use of heterologous vaccines (bacillus Calmette-Guérin and influenza vaccines) to stimulate the immune system in patients with recurrent genital herpes has proved of no significant benefit.[47,55,62–64]

EVALUATION OF THERAPEUTIC OUTCOMES

Available antiviral compounds are of greatest benefit in patients experiencing first-episode primary infections, immunocompromised patients, and patients with frequent or severe recurrent infections. Antivirals, however, are palliative and not curative, and patients receiving these agents should be monitored closely for adverse drug effects. CDC guidelines suggest that discontinuation of suppressive therapy after 1 year should be considered to assess for possible changes in the patient's intrinsic pattern of recurrence. In many patients, decreases in recurrence rates and the severity of symptoms occur over time. However, some clinicians prefer to continue suppressive therapy indefinitely because it significantly reduces asymptomatic viral shedding, a potential benefit in reducing the risk of disease transmission to uninfected sexual partners.[1,47,48,61]

TRICHOMONIASIS

EPIDEMIOLOGY AND ETIOLOGY

Trichomonas vaginalis, a flagellated, motile protozoan is responsible for 3 to 5 million cases of trichomoniasis annually in the United States.[65–68] Humans are host to two other *Trichomonas* species, *Trichomonas tenax* and *Trichomonas hominis,* but *T. vaginalis* is the only species thought to be pathogenic. Although infection by nonsexual contact is reported, it is rare. Contamination of inanimate objects and spread of infection via communal bathing or contact with infected bath or toilet articles is possible because *T. vaginalis* can survive for several hours on moist surfaces.[65–73] Neonatal infections also represent another possible nonvenereal route of disease transmission.[67–71,73,74]

Coinfection with other STDs is not unusual in patients diagnosed with trichomoniasis. Women infected with *T. vaginalis* are three times more likely to have gonorrhea than those who do not have trichomoniasis; approximately 20% of men with gonococcal urethritis also have trichomoniasis.[67,68] In patients treated appropriately for genital *C. trachomatis* or *U. urealyticum* infection, persistent urethritis can result from coexisting trichomonal infection.[1,70,71] Although not well documented, it is proposed that the inflammatory response produced by trichomoniasis may increase the risk of acquiring HIV.[66,68,70,74,75]

PATHOPHYSIOLOGY

Trichomonads typically can be isolated from the vagina, urethra, and paraurethral ducts and glands in the majority of infected women. Infrequently, they are recovered from the endocervix. Extragenital sites are epidemiologically important because infection can persist and result in reinfection of the vagina if local therapy alone is used.[68,71,72] This may account for the higher relapse rates reported for local versus systemic therapy.[71,72,75] After attachment to the vaginal or urethral mucosa, trichomonads usually elicit an inflammatory response that manifests as a discharge containing large numbers of PMN leukocytes.[68–72]

CLINICAL PRESENTATION

Trichomonal infections are reported more commonly in women than in men. In part this might be because of the smaller number of organisms found in the male urethra making detection more difficult, greater disease transmission rates from males to females, and the nature of male infections, which have a high spontaneous cure rate even in the absence of treatment.[66,67,70–72,75] The typical clinical presentation of trichomoniasis in males and females is presented in Table 121–11.

DIAGNOSIS

T. vaginalis produces nonspecific symptoms also consistent with bacterial vaginosis; as a result, laboratory diagnosis is required. Because *T. vaginalis* requires a pH range of 4.9 to 7.5 for survival, a vaginal discharge pH of greater than 5.0 usually indicates the pres-

TABLE 121-11 Presentation of *Trichomonas* Infections

	Males	Females
General	Incubation period 3–28 days Organism can be detectable within 48 hours after exposure to infected partner	Incubation period 3–28 days
Site of infection	Most common—urethra Others—rectum (usually caused by rectal intercourse in MSM), oropharynx, eye	Most common—endocervical canal Others—urethra, rectum (usually caused by perineal contamination), oropharynx, eye
Symptoms	Can be asymptomatic (more common in males than females) or minimally symptomatic Urethral discharge (clear to mucopurulent) Dysuria, pruritus	Can be asymptomatic or minimally symptomatic Scant to copious, typically malodorous vaginal discharge (50–75%) and pruritus (worse during menses) Dysuria, dyspareunia
Signs	Urethral discharge	Vaginal discharge Vaginal pH 4.5–6 Inflammation/erythema of vulva, vagina, and/or cervix Urethritis
Complications	Epididymitis and chronic prostatitis (uncommon) Male infertility (decreased sperm motility and viability)	Pelvic inflammatory disease and associated complications (i.e., ectopic pregnancy, infertility) Premature labor, premature rupture of membranes, and low-birth-weight infants (risk of neonatal infections is low) Cervical neoplasia

MSM, men who have sex with men.

ence of either *T. vaginalis* or *Gardnerella vaginalis,* a common cause of bacterial vaginosis. The simplest and most reliable means of diagnosis is a wet-mount examination of the vaginal discharge.[28,67,70–72,75] Trichomoniasis is confirmed if characteristic pear-shaped, flagellating organisms are observed. The wet mount is only about 60% to 80% sensitive in detecting the presence of trichomonads, with lower sensitivities reported in men and in women with low-grade, subacute, or chronic infections.[68–70,72,74]

Although the presence of trichomonads may be reported on a Papanicolaou (Pap) smear, the sensitivity of this cytologic technique is less than for wet mount and also is associated with a number of false-positive results. Stained smears of cervical specimens have been used in diagnosis, but they are less sensitive and more time-consuming than the wet mount and therefore are not recommended. Culture techniques for trichomonads are highly specific and more sensitive than the wet mount, but they are not useful in rapid diagnosis because up to 48 hours or longer is necessary for growth. Cultures can be necessary, however, to confirm the diagnosis in the absence of a positive wet mount or to determine antimicrobial susceptibility in intractable cases.[1,28,67–72,74,75]

Newer diagnostic tests such as monoclonal antibody or DNA probe techniques, as well as PCR tests that can detect small amounts of trichomonal DNA, have been developed. These office-based tests are highly sensitive and specific for detecting infection in both vaginal specimens. Such tests could replace more traditional diagnostic tests in the future.[66,68,71,72]

In males, demonstration of trichomonads in urethral specimens or urine sediment by wet mount is difficult, and diagnosis depends largely on culture. Specimens from males should be taken prior to first voiding because the small number of trichomonads in males may be reduced by micturition.[28,70–72,74,75]

TREATMENT

Trichomoniasis

Recommended and alternative treatment regimens for *T. vaginalis* include either metronidazole or tinidazole, both of which produce high cure rates in these infections. In only a few cases have *T. vaginalis* isolates been resistant to standard metronidazole or tinidazole doses. In these instances, longer courses of therapy or doses higher than those recommended routinely as initial therapy usually produce a cure.[1,67,68,70–76]

Table 121–12 provides treatment recommendations for trichomonas infections.[1] The standard therapy for trichomoniasis is either metronidazole or tinidazole 2 g orally as a single dose; cure rates are comparable with the recommended alternative regimen of metronidazole 500 mg twice daily for 7 days. When sexual partners are treated simultaneously, cure rates greater than 95% are reported. If sexual partners are not treated concurrently, cure rates are somewhat lower. In limited clinical testing, single metronidazole doses of less than 1.5 g are associated with high failure rates.[1,65,67,68,70–77]

Advantages of single-dose therapy over the multidose alternative regimen include better patient compliance, lower total dose, lower cost, and shorter exposure of the patient's gastrointestinal and urogenital anaerobic bacterial flora to the drug. As a result of the latter, the likelihood of developing pseudomembranous colitis or symptomatic candidal vulvovaginitis is decreased.[68,69,71,76,77] Because high doses of metronidazole have mutagenic effects in bacteria and oncogenic effects in mice, a reduced time of exposure in humans can be beneficial. There is no conclusive evidence for either of these effects in humans after short-term therapy with recommended doses.[69,71,75,76] Gastrointestinal complaints (e.g., anorexia, nausea, vomiting, and diarrhea) are more common with the single 2-g dose of either metronidazole or tinidazole, occurring in 5% to 10% of treated patients. Some patients also complain of a bitter metallic taste in the mouth with metronidazole. Patients intolerant of the single 2-g dose because of gastrointestinal adverse effects usually tolerate the alternative metronidazole multidose regimen.[68–73,74,76]

❺ To achieve maximal cure rates and prevent relapse with either metronidazole or tinidazole as a single 2-g dose, simultaneous treatment of infected sexual partners is necessary. In women treated with the alternative 7-day course, however, relapse rates are not

TABLE 121-12 Treatment of Trichomoniasis

Type	Recommended Regimen[a]	Alternative Regimen
Symptomatic and asymptomatic infections	Metronidazole 2 g PO in a single dose[b] *or* Tinidazole 2 g PO in a single dose	Metronidazole 500 mg PO 2 times daily for 7 days[c] *or* Tinidazole 2 g PO in a single dose[d]
Treatment in pregnancy	Metronidazole 2 g PO in a single dose[e]	

CDC, Centers for Disease Control and Prevention; PO, orally.

[a]Recommendations are those of the CDC.

[b]Treatment failures should be treated with metronidazole 500 mg PO twice daily for 7 days. Persistent failures should be managed in consultation with an expert. Metronidazole or tinidazole 2 g PO daily for 5 days has been effective in patients infected with *Trichomonas vaginalis* strains mildly resistant to metronidazole, but experience is limited; higher doses also have been used.

[c]Metronidazole labeling approved by the FDA does not include this regimen. Dosage regimens for treatment of trichomoniasis included in the product labeling are the single 2 g dose; 250 mg three times daily for 7 days; and 375 mg twice daily for 7 days. The 250 mg and 375 mg dosage regimens are currently not included in the CDC recommendations.

[d]For treatment failures with metronidazole 2 g as a single dose.

[e]Metronidazole is pregnancy category B and tinidazole is pregnancy category C; both drugs are contraindicated in the first trimester of pregnancy. Some clinicians recommend deferring metronidazole treatment in asymptomatic pregnant women until after 37 weeks gestation.

appreciably different regardless of whether or not sexual partners are treated. It is speculated that in men, spontaneous resolution of trichomonal infection or a reduction in the number of trichomonads below the inoculum necessary to transmit disease may occur during the 7 days of a female's therapy. In patients who fail to respond to an initial course of metronidazole therapy, a second course of therapy with metronidazole 500 mg twice daily for 7 days or a single 2-g dose of tinidazole is recommended. Patients refractory to a second course of treatment usually respond to a regimen using higher dosages of either agent (i.e., 2 to 4 g daily for 5 days). Good response rates also are reported for metronidazole 2 to 3 g orally plus either a single 500-mg tablet administered intravaginally or intravaginal metronidazole gel (0.75%) for 7 to 14 days.[65,67,68,70–77] Topical vaginal therapy alone is associated with low cure rates because infections involving the urethra or periurethral glands are unaffected and can serve as the source of reinfection.[67] Use of intravenous metronidazole can be warranted for rare cases of intolerance to oral medication or infections resistant to high-dose oral metronidazole. Sexual partners of all patients who require retreatment also should be treated or retreated because the majority of apparent treatment failures appear to be caused by reinfection or noncompliance.[65,67,68,70–77]

Concerns regarding the use of metronidazole in women who are pregnant or breast-feeding have been raised. Because metronidazole is secreted in breast milk, it is recommended that breast-feeding be interrupted for 12 to 24 hours after maternal ingestion of a single 2-g dose.[1,70,74–77] Metronidazole (pregnancy category B) and tinidazole (pregnancy category C) are contraindicated during the first trimester of pregnancy based on Food and Drug Administration (FDA)–approved labeling. Although some experts recommend avoiding use of either agent throughout pregnancy, others advocate the use of metronidazole during any stage of pregnancy because of the potential adverse pregnancy outcomes associated with trichomoniasis.[1,70,74,75,78] Currently no consensus exists on whether or how to treat trichomonas infections in pregnant women.

Various local therapies for trichomoniasis have been proposed, particularly for pregnant patients. Clotrimazole vaginal suppositories, 100 mg at bedtime for 1 to 2 weeks, relieve symptoms in many women and produce cure rates of 50% or greater.[68,72–74,76] An alternative therapy is gentle douching with either a diluted solution of vinegar or a 1% zinc sulfate solution until symptoms improve and then less frequently thereafter. This therapy generally provides some symptomatic improvement but few cures. Although once recommended, povidone-iodine douches should be avoided during pregnancy because of the risk of fetal thyroid suppression.[70,71,74,75]

Several other nitroimidazole antibiotics related to metronidazole and tinidazole (e.g., nimorazole, ornidazole, and carnidazole) are being investigated worldwide for the treatment of trichomoniasis. Unfortunately, none of these agents differs significantly from metronidazole or tinidazole in terms of efficacy (i.e., cross-resistance is high) or toxicity against metronidazole-susceptible strains of *T. vaginalis*.[69–71,74,77]

EVALUATION OF THERAPEUTIC OUTCOMES

Followup is considered unnecessary in patients who become asymptomatic after treatment with recommended therapy. When patients remain symptomatic, it is important to determine if reinfection has occurred. In these cases, a repeat course of therapy, as well as identification and treatment or retreatment of infected sexual partners, is recommended. In situations in which reinfection can be excluded, a relative resistance to metronidazole or tinidazole should be assumed, and an alternative regimen should be prescribed. Culture and sensitivity are warranted for infections unresponsive to alternative regimens.

HUMAN PAPILLOMAVIRUS AND OTHER STDS

Several STDs other than those just discussed occur with varying frequency in the United States and throughout the world. Although an in-depth discussion of these diseases is beyond the scope of this chapter, Table 121–13 lists recommended treatment regimens.[1] Of notable importance among these other STDs, however, is genital HPV infection, the most common viral STD in the United States. More than 100 HPV types have been characterized by genomic makeup, with approximately 30 types associated with genital tract lesions.[79–81] Of these, types 6 and 11 are associated most commonly with the development of low-grade dysplasia manifested as exophytic genital warts. In most individuals, genital infection with HPV is subclinical, and patients with visible acuminate warts represent less than 1% of all infected individuals. When present, genital warts can be large and multifocal, producing variable degrees of discomfort. Based on HPV DNA detection methods, most warts will regress spontaneously within 1 to 2 years of their initial appearance. However, reinfection is common in young, sexually active populations.[1,80,81]

Infection with several HPV types, particularly HPV-16 and HPV-18, is considered the major risk factor for the development of cervical neoplasia, the second most common cancer in women worldwide. Although epidemiologic, virologic, and clinical data strongly support this association, HPV infection alone is insufficient to cause cervical cancer development because only a small percentage of infected women develop the disease. It appears that the interplay of host immune defenses, genetic factors, and infection with HPV types containing a more aggressive variant all contribute to the risk of developing cervical neoplasia.[78–81]

The Pap smear is the most cost-effective and frequently used diagnostic test for HPV. It can detect abnormal cytology in patients with clinical manifestations and those with subclinical disease (i.e., no overt condylomata) but not latent HPV infection. Visual inspection of genital surfaces under magnification can assist in making the diagnosis. Various tests for detecting HPV DNA also are available, and unlike the Pap smear do not require subjective interpretation of the results. Currently HPV DNA testing is only approved in women with abnormal Pap smears or women older than 30 years of age. However, use of HPV DNA testing as a routine screening test in lieu of Pap smears is expected in the near future. In women identified to have high-risk HPV infections by these tests, followup cytology would be performed.[78–81]

No consensus exists on the best approach to treating patients with genital HPV infection, particularly because most cases appear to be transient with spontaneous regression of lesions. A number of treatments are recommended (see Table 121–13), but none is clearly superior to the others. Treatment generally is directed toward patients with manifestations of genital warts, with the goal of removing or destroying these lesions and grossly infected surrounding tissue. Because such treatment neither stops viral expression in surrounding tissue nor eliminates viral latency, recurrence of lesions is not uncommon.[78–81]

A quadrivalent HPV vaccine (Gardasil®) is marketed for females between the ages of 9 and 26 years. The vaccine provides protection against cervical cancer caused by HPV-16 and HPV-18 (which account for up to 70% of cervical cancers) and genital warts caused by HPV-6 and HPV-11 (which account for up to 90% of genital warts).[82] Questions regarding use in males, and how long immunity from the 3-dose regimen persists remain to be answered. At least one other HPV vaccine is in final stages of clinical testing and expected to be marketed in the near future.[83]

CONCLUSIONS

More than 20 different diseases have been identified for which sexual transmission is epidemiologically important. For most STDs,

TABLE 121-13 Treatment Regimens for Miscellaneous Sexually Transmitted Diseases

Infection	Recommended Regimen[a]	Alternative Regimen
Chancroid *(Haemophilus ducreyi)*	Azithromycin 1 g PO in a single dose, *or* Ceftriaxone 250 mg IM in a single dose, *or* Ciprofloxacin 500 mg PO twice daily for 3 days,[b] *or* Erythromycin base 500 mg PO four times daily for 7 days	
Lymphogranuloma venereum	Doxycycline 100 mg PO twice daily for 21 days[c]	Erythromycin base 500 mg PO four times daily for 21 days
Human Papillomavirus (HPV) Infection:		
External genital warts	*Provider-Administered Therapies:* Cryotherapy (e.g., liquid nitrogen or cryoprobe), *or* Podophyllin resin 10–25% in compound tincture of benzoin applied to lesions; repeat weekly if necessary,[d,e] *or* Trichloroacetic acid (TCA) 80–90% *or* bichloracetic acid (BCA) 80–90% applied to warts; repeat weekly if necessary, *or* Surgical removal (tangential scissor excision, tangential shave excision, curettage, or electrosurgery) *Patient-Applied Therapies:* Podofilox 0.5% solution or gel applied twice daily for 3 days, followed by 4 days of no therapy; cycle is repeated as necessary for up to four cycles,[e] or Imiquimod 5% cream applied at bedtime three times weekly for up to 16 weeks[e]	Intralesional interferon or laser surgery
Human Papillomavirus Infection:		
Vaginal and anal warts	Cryotherapy with liquid nitrogen, or TCA or BCA 80–90% as for external HPV warts; repeat weekly as necessary[f] Surgical removal (*not* for vaginal or urethral meatus warts)	
Urethral meatus warts	Cryotherapy with liquid nitrogen, or podophyllin resin 10–25% in compound tincture of benzoin applied at weekly intervals[e,g]	

[a]Recommendations are those of the Centers for Disease Control and Prevention (CDC).
[b]Ciprofloxacin is contraindicated for pregnant and lactating women and for persons aged <18 years.
[c]Azithromycin 1 g PO once weekly for 3 weeks can be effective.
[d]Some experts recommended washing podophyllin off after 1–4 hours to minimize local irritation.
[e]Safety during pregnancy is not established.
[f]Surgical removal of anal warts is also a recommended treatment.
[g]Some specialists recommend the use of podofilox and imiquimod for treating distal meatal warts.

curative drug therapies are available; however, therapeutic approaches to viral STDs, such as genital herpes, provide only palliation and suppression of symptoms. Technologic advances in laboratory medicine have resulted in improved and more rapid diagnostic capabilities for many STDs. These advances are of particular importance for individuals with undiagnosed, asymptomatic disease who comprise a vast reservoir for continued disease transmission. Sexually active persons can reduce their risk of transmitting or acquiring an STD by avoidance of unsafe sexual practices, maintaining a mutually monogamous sexual relationship, or proper use of physical barriers during intercourse. In the future, vaccines providing protection from common STDs may have a significant effect on reducing the incidence of these infections.

ABBREVIATIONS

AIDS: acquired immune deficiency syndrome
CDC: Centers for Disease Control and Prevention
CSF: cerebrospinal fluid
DFA-TP: direct fluorescent-antibody test
DGI: disseminated gonorrhea infection
EIA: enzyme immunoassay
FDA: Food and Drug Administration
FTA-ABS: fluorescent treponemal antibody absorption
HIV: human immunodeficiency virus
HPV: human papillomavirus
HSV: herpes simplex virus
HSV-1: herpes simplex virus type 1
HSV-2: herpes simplex virus type 2
LPS: lipopolysaccharide
MHA-TP: microhemagglutination assay for antibodies to *T. pallidum*
MSM: men who have sex with men
NAATs: nucleic acid amplification tests
NGU: nongonococcal urethritis
Pap: papanicolaou
PCR: polymerase chain reaction
PID: pelvic inflammatory disease
PMN: polymorphonuclear
QRNG: quinolone-resistant *N. gonorrhoeae*
RPR: rapid plasma reagin
STD: sexually transmitted disease
TPHA: *T. pallidum* hemagglutination assay
TPPA: *T. pallidum* particle agglutination assay
TRUST: toluidine red unheated serum test
USR: unheated serum reagin
VDRL: Venereal Disease Research Laboratory

REFERENCES

1. Centers for Disease Control and Prevention. Workowski KA, Berman SM. Sexually transmitted diseases treatment guidelines 2006. MMWR Recomm Rep 2006;21;55(RR 11):1–94.
2. Holmes KK. Sexually transmitted diseases: Overview and clinical approach. In: Kasper DL, Fauci AS, Longo DL, et al., eds. Harrison's Principles of Internal Medicine, 16th ed. New York: McGraw-Hill, 2005:762–774.

3. Braverman PK. Sexually transmitted diseases in adolescents. Med Clin North Am 2000;84:869–889.
4. Sulak PJ. Sexually transmitted diseases. Semin Reprod Med 2003;21:399–413.
5. Rietmeijer CA, McMillan A. Some aspects of the prevention of sexually transmissible infections. In: McMillan A, Young H, Ogilvie MM, Scott GR, eds. Clinical Practice in Sexually Transmissible Infections. London: WB Saunders, 2002:11–28.
6. Gilliam ML, Derman RJ. Barrier methods of contraception. Obstet Gynecol Clin North Am 2000;27:841–858.
7. Roddy RE, Zekeng L, Ryan KA, et al. Effect of nonoxynol-9 gel on urogenital gonorrhea and chlamydial infection: A randomized, controlled trial. JAMA 2002;287:1117–1122.
8. Stone A. Microbicides: A new approach to preventing HIV and other sexually transmitted infections. Nat Rev Drug Discov 2002;1:977–985.
9. Centers for Disease Control. Jajosky RA, Hall PA, Adams DA, et al. Summary of notifiable diseases—United States, 2004. MMWR 2006;53(53):1–79.
10. Ram S, Rice PA. Gonococcal infections. In: Kasper DL, Fauci AS, Longo DL, et al., eds. Harrison's Principles of Internal Medicine, 16th ed. New York: McGraw-Hill, 2005:855–861.
11. Handsfield HH, Sparling PF. *Neisseria gonorrhoeae.* In: Mandell GL, Bennett JE, Dolin R, eds. Principles and Practice of Infectious Diseases, 6th ed. New York: Churchill Livingstone, 2005:2514–2529.
12. Emmert DH, Kirchner JT. Sexually transmitted diseases in women: Gonorrhea and syphilis. Postgrad Med 2000;107:181–197.
13. Marrazzo JM. Infections due to *Neisseria.* In: Federman DD, Dale DC, eds. WebMD Scientific American Medicine. New York: WebMD Corporation, 2004; *http://online.statref.com/document.aspx?fxid=48&docid=1019.*
14. Johnson RE, Newhall WI, Papp JR, et al. Screening tests to detect *Chlamydia trachomatis* and *Neisseria gonorrhoeae* infections—2002. MMWR 2002;51(RR 15):1–39.
15. Lyss SB, Kamb ML, Peterman TA, et al. *Chlamydia trachomatis* among patients infected with and treated for *Neisseria gonorrhoeae* in sexually transmitted disease clinics in the United States. Ann Intern Med 2003;139:178–185.
16. Gaydos CA. Nucleic acid amplification tests for gonorrhea and Chlamydia: Practice and applications. Infect Dis Clin North Am 2005;19:367–386.
17. Dicker LW, Mosure DJ, Berman SM, et al. Gonorrhea prevalence and coinfection with chlamydia in women in the United States, 2000. Sex Transm Dis 2003;30:472–476.
18. Fox KK, Cohen MS. Gonococcal, chlamydial, and mycoplasma urethritis. In: Cohen J, Powderly WG, Berkley SF, et al., eds. Infectious Diseases, 2nd ed. St. Louis: Mosby, 2004:795–805.
19. Young H, McMillan A. Gonorrhea. In: McMillan A, Young H, Ogilvie MM, Scott GR, eds. Clinical Practice in Sexually Transmissible Infections. London: WB Saunders, 2002:313–356.
20. Woods CR. Gonococcal infections in neonates and young children. Semin Pediatr Infect Dis 2005;16:258–270.
21. LaFond RE, Lukehart SA. Biological basis for syphilis. Clin Microbiol Rev 2006;19:29–49.
22. Golden MR, Marra CM, Holmes KK. Update on syphilis: Resurgence of an old problem. JAMA 2003;290:1510–1514.
23. Lukehart SA. Syphilis. In: Kasper DL, Fauci AS, Longo DL, et al., eds. Harrison's Principles of Internal Medicine, 16th ed. New York: McGraw-Hill, 2005:977–984.
24. Young H, McMillan A. Syphilis and the endemic treponematoses. In: McMillan A, Young H, Ogilvie MM, Scott GR, eds. Clinical Practice in Sexually Transmissible Infections. London: WB WB Saunders, 2002:395–456.
25. Kinghorn GR. Syphilis. In: Cohen J, Powderly WG, Berkley SF, et al., eds. Infectious Diseases, 2nd ed. St Louis: Mosby, 2004:807–816.
26. Zeltser R, Kurban AK. Syphilis. Clin Dermatol 2004;22:461–468.
27. Goh BT. Syphilis in adults. Sex Transm Infect 2005;81:448–452.
28. Hall CS, Klausner JD. Diagnostic tests for common STDs and HSV-2. MLO Med Lab Obs 2004;36:10–16.
29. Pao D, Goh BT, Bingham JS. Management issues in syphilis. Drugs 2002;61:1447–1461.
30. Kirchner JT, Emmert DH. Sexually transmitted diseases in women: *Chlamydia trachomatis* and herpes simplex infections. Postgrad Med 2000:107:55–58, 61–65.
31. Stamm WE, Jones RB, Batteiger BE. *Chlamydia trachomatis* (trachoma, perinatal infections, lymphogranuloma venereum, and other genital infections). In: Mandell GL, Bennett JE, Dolin R, eds. Principles and Practice of Infectious Diseases, 6th ed. New York: Churchill Livingstone, 2005:2239–2255.
32. Stamm WE. Chlamydial infections. In: Kasper DL, Fauci AS, Longo DL, et al., eds. Harrison's Principles of Internal Medicine, 16th ed. New York: McGraw-Hill, 2005:1011–1018.
33. Fox KK, Cohen MS. Gonococcal, chlamydial and *Mycoplasma* urethritis. In: Cohen J, Powderly WG, Berkley SF, et al., eds. Infectious Diseases, 2nd ed. St Louis: Mosby, 2004:795–805.
34. McMillan A, Ballard RC. Non-specific genital tract infection and chlamydial infection, including lymphogranuloma venereum. In: McMillan A, Young H, Ogilvie MM, Scott GR, eds. Clinical Practice in Sexually Transmissible Infections. London: WB Saunders, 2002:281–312.
35. Geisler WM. Approaches to the management of uncomplicated genital *Chlamydia trachomatis* infections. Expert Rev Anti Infect Ther 2004;2:771–785.
36. Zar HJ. Neonatal chlamydial infections: Prevention and treatment. Paediatr Drugs 2005;7:103–110.
37. Peipert JF. Genital chlamydial infections. N Engl J Med 2003;349:2424–2430.
38. Hollblad-Fadiman K, Goldman SM. American College of Preventive Medicine practice policy statement: Screening for *Chlamydia trachomatis.* Am J Prev Med 2003;24:287–292.
39. Ostergaard L. Microbiological aspects of the diagnosis of *Chlamydia trachomatis.* Best Pract Res Clin Obstet Gynaecol 2002;16:789–799.
40. Watson EJ, Templeton A, Russell I, et al. The accuracy and efficacy of screening tests for *Chlamydia trachomatis*: A systematic review. J Med Microbiol 2002:51:1021–1031.
41. Guaschino S, Ricci G. How, and how efficiently, can we treat *Chlamydia trachomatis* infections in women? Best Pract Res Clin Obstet Gynaecol 2002:16:875–888.
42. Anonymous. Drugs for sexually transmitted infections. Treat Guidel Med Lett 2004;2:67–74.
43. McMillan A, Ogilvie MM. Herpes simplex virus infection. In: McMillan A, Young H, Ogilvie MM, Scott GR, eds. Clinical Practice in Sexually Transmissible Infections. London: WB Saunders, 2002:107–144.
44. Corey L. Herpes simplex virus. In: Mandell GL, Bennett JE, Dolin R, eds. Principles and Practice of Infectious Diseases, 6th ed. New York: Churchill Livingstone, 2005:1762–1780.
45. Marques AR, Straus SE. Herpes simplex type 2 infections: An update. Dis Mon 2000;46:325–359.
46. Kimberlin DW, Rouse DJ. Genital herpes. N Engl J Med 2004;350:1970–1977.
47. Goade D. Genital herpes. In: Cohen J, Powderly WG, Berkley SF, et al., eds. Infectious Diseases, 2nd ed. St. Louis: Mosby, 2004:817–826.
48. Corey L. Herpes simplex viruses. In: Kasper DL, Fauci AS, Longo DL, et al., eds. Harrison's Principles of Internal Medicine, 16th ed. New York: McGraw-Hill, 2005:1035–1041.
49. Dwyer DE, Cunningham AL. Herpes simplex and varicella-zoster virus infections. Med J Aust 2002;177:267–273.
50. Whitley RJ, Roizman B. Herpes simplex virus infections. Lancet 2001;357:1513–1518.
51. Simmons A. Clinical manifestations and treatment considerations of herpes simplex virus infection. J Infect Dis 2002;186(Suppl 1):S71–S77.
52. Beauman JG. Genital herpes: A review. Am Fam Physician 2005;72:1527–1534.
53. Leung DT, Sacks SL. Current recommendations for the treatment of genital herpes. Drugs 2000;60:1329–1352.
54. Geers TA, Isada CM. Update on antiviral therapy for genital herpes infection. Cleve Clin J Med 2000;67:567–573.
55. Wald A, Ashley-Morrow R. Serological testing for herpes simplex virus (HSV)-1 and HSV-2 infection. Clin Infect Dis 2002;35(Suppl 2): S173–S182.
56. Wald A. Testing for genital herpes: How, who, and why. Curr Clin Top Infect Dis 2002;22:166–180.
57. Scoular A. Using the evidence base on genital herpes: Optimising the use of diagnostic tests and information provision. Sex Transm Infect 2002;78:160–165.
58. Patel R. Progress in meeting today's demands in genital herpes: An overview of current management. J Infect Dis 2002;186(Suppl 1):S47–S56.

59. Hill J, Roberts S. Herpes simplex virus in pregnancy: New concepts in prevention and management. Clin Perinatol 2005;32:657–670.
60. Corey L. Challenges in genital herpes simplex virus management. J Infect Dis 2002;186(Suppl 1):S29–S33.
61. Mills J, Mindel A. Genital herpes simplex infections: Some therapeutic dilemmas. Sex Transm Dis 2003;30:232–233.
62. Stanberry LR. Clinical trials of prophylactic and therapeutic herpes simplex virus vaccines. Herpes 2004;11(Suppl 3):161A–169A.
63. Snoeck R, De Clercq E. New treatments for genital herpes. Curr Opin Infect Dis 2002;15:49–55.
64. Miller RL, Tomai MA, Harrison CJ, Bernstein DI. Immunomodulation as a treatment strategy for genital herpes: Review of the evidence. Int Immunopharmacol 2002;2:443–451.
65. Weller PF. Protozoal intestinal infections and trichomoniasis. In: Kasper DL, Fauci AS, Longo DL, et al., eds. Harrison's Principles of Internal Medicine, 16th ed. New York: McGraw-Hill, 2005:1248–1252.
66. Soper D. Trichomoniasis: Under control or undercontrolled? Am J Obstet Gynecol 2004;190:281–290.
67. Sobel JD. Vaginitis, vulvitis, cervicitis and cutaneous vulval lesions. In: Cohen J, Powderly WG, Berkley SF, et al., eds. Infectious Diseases, 2nd ed. St. Louis: Mosby, 2004:683–691.
68. McMillan A. Vaginal infections and vulvodynia. In: McMillan A, Young H, Ogilvie MM, Scott GR, eds. Clinical Practice in Sexually Transmissible Infections. London: WB Saunders, 2002:473–516.
69. Martin DH, Rein MF. *Trichomonas vaginalis.* In: Mandell GL, Bennett JE, Dolin R, eds. Principles and Practice of Infectious Diseases, 6th ed. New York: Churchill Livingstone, 2005:3205–3209.
70. Schwebke JR, Burgess D. Trichomoniasis. Clin Microbiol Rev 2004;17:794–803.
71. Schwebke JR. Update on trichomoniasis. Sex Transm Infect 2002;78:378–379.
72. Say PJ, Jacyntho C. Difficult-to-manage vaginitis. Clin Obstet Gynecol 2005;48:753–768.
73. Faro S. Vaginitis: Differential Diagnosis and Management. Boca Raton, FL: Parthenon Publishing, 2004:67–92.
74. Eckert LO. Acute vulvovaginitis. N Engl J Med 2006;355:1244–1252.
75. Sobel JD. What's new in bacterial vaginosis and trichomoniasis. Infect Dis Clin North Am 2005;19:387–406.
76. Forna F, Gülmezoglu AM. Interventions for treating trichomoniasis in women. Cochrane Database Syst Rev 2003;2:CD000218. DOI. 10.1002/14651858.
77. Cudmore SL, Delgaty KL, Hayward-McClelland SF, et al. Treatment of infections caused by metronidazole-resistant *Trichomonas vaginalis.* Clin Microbiol Rev 2004;17:783–793.
78. Gunter J. Genital and perianal warts: New treatment opportunities for human papillomavirus infection. Am J Obstet Gynecol 2003;189(Suppl 3):S3–S11.
79. Lacey CJ. Therapy for genital human papillomavirus-related disease. J Clin Virol 2005;32 (Suppl 1):S82–S90.
80. Eiley DJ, Douglas J, Beutner K, et al. External genital warts: Diagnosis, treatment, and prevention. Clin Infect Dis 2002;35(Suppl 2):S210–S224.
81. Zanotii KM, Belinson J. Update on the diagnosis and treatment of human papillomavirus infection. Cleve Clin J Med 2002;69:948–961.
82. Anon. A human papillomavirus vaccine. Med Lett Drugs Ther 2006;48:65–66.
83. Partridge JM, Koutsky LA. Genital human papillomavirus infection in men. Lancet Infect Dis 2006;6:21–31.

CHAPTER 122 Bone and Joint Infections

EDWARD P. ARMSTRONG AND ALLAN D. FRIEDMAN

KEY CONCEPTS

1. The most common cause of osteomyelitis (particularly that acquired by hematogenous spread) and infectious arthritis is *Staphylococcus aureus.*

2. Culture and susceptibility information are essential as a guide for antimicrobial treatment of osteomyelitis and infectious arthritis.

3. Joint aspiration and examination of synovial fluid are extremely important to evaluate the possibility of infectious arthritis.

4. The most important treatment modality of acute osteomyelitis is the administration of appropriate antibiotics in adequate doses for a sufficient length of time.

5. Antibiotics generally are given in high doses so that adequate antimicrobial concentrations are reached within infected bone and joints.

6. The standard duration of antimicrobial treatment for osteomyelitis is 4 to 6 weeks.

7. Oral antimicrobial therapy can be used for osteomyelitis to complete a parenteral regimen in children who have had a good clinical response to intravenous antibiotics and in adults without diabetes mellitus or peripheral vascular disease when the organism is susceptible to the oral antimicrobial, a suitable oral agent is available, and compliance is ensured.

8. The three most important therapeutic maneuvers in the management of infectious arthritis are appropriate antibiotics, joint drainage, and joint rest.

Bone and joint infections are comprised of two disease processes known, respectively, as *osteomyelitis* and *septic* or *infectious arthritis.* As such, they are unique and separate infectious entities with different signs and symptoms and infecting organisms. Despite advances in therapy, however, these infections continue to cause significant morbidity from residual damage and chronic recurring infections. Emphasis on initiating antibiotic therapy as soon as possible is important in reducing long-term complications.

Learning objectives, review questions,
and other resources can be found at
www.pharmacotherapyonline.com.

EPIDEMIOLOGY

Osteomyelitis generally is an uncommon disease. One classic publication reported that 247 patients had osteomyelitis in a prominent American teaching hospital during a 4-year period.[1] Acute osteomyelitis has an estimated annual incidence of 0.4 per 1,000 children.[2] Osteomyelitis caused by contiguous spread, including postoperative, direct puncture, and that associated with adjacent soft tissue infections, comprises 47% of infections. Hematogenous osteomyelitis comprises 19% of infections, and osteomyelitis occurring in patients with significant peripheral vascular disease comprises 34% of infections. A review of osteomyelitis cases based on duration of disease shows that acute disease constitutes 56% of patients and that chronic osteomyelitis, defined as having a previous hospitalization for the same infection, constitutes 44% of patients.

Infectious or septic arthritis is an inflammatory reaction within the joint space. Distinct from osteomyelitis, septic arthritis is a more common disease and is known to be one of the most common causes of new cases of arthritis. One study identified 22 patients with culture-proven septic arthritis at a tertiary teaching hospital over 10 years.[3] Another hospital reported 15 cases of neonatal septic arthritis of the hip in a 3-year period.[4] Overall, the yearly incidence of bacterial arthritis varies from 2 to 10 per 100,000 inhabitants.[5]

ETIOLOGY

OSTEOMYELITIS

The most common method of classifying osteomyelitis is based on the route in which the infecting organism reaches the bone. Infection that results from spread through the bloodstream is termed *hematogenous osteomyelitis.* When the organism reaches the bone from an adjoining soft tissue infection, it is termed *contiguous osteomyelitis.* Osteomyelitis that results from direct inoculation, such as from trauma, puncture wounds, or surgery, generally is also classified under the contiguous osteomyelitis category. Patients with peripheral vascular disease are at risk for the development of osteomyelitis, and these patients often are separated into a third distinct category because of their unique management features.

Osteomyelitis also can be classified based on the duration of the disease. Acute osteomyelitis describes infections of recent onset, usually several days to 1 week, whereas chronic infections are those of a longer duration. Some authors describe chronic infections as those with symptoms for more than 1 month before therapy, whereas other authors define chronic infections as relapse of an initial infection. Yet a third system sometimes used to classify osteomyelitis is based on the anatomic location of the infection (medullary or superficial) and the physiologic status of the patient (otherwise healthy, systemic immunologic compromise, local immu-

TABLE 122-1 Types of Osteomyelitis, Age Distribution, Common Sites, and Risk Factors

Type of Osteomyelitis	Typical Age (y)	Site(s) Involved	Risk Factors
Hematogenous	Less than 1	Long bones and joints	Prematurity, umbilical catheter or venous cutdown, respiratory distress syndrome, perinatal asphyxia
	1–20	Long bones (femur, tibia, humerus)	Infection (pharyngitis, cellulitis, respiratory infections), trauma, sickle cell disease, puncture wounds to feet
	Older than 50	Vertebrae	Diabetes mellitus, blunt trauma to spine, urinary tract infection
Contiguous	Older than 50	Femur, tibia, mandible	Hip fractures, open fractures
Vascular insufficiency	Older than 50	Feet, toes	Diabetes mellitus, peripheral vascular disease, pressure sores

nologic compromise).[6,7] This classification system can be useful when comparing patients among different studies and attempting to categorize the severity of infection.

INFECTIOUS ARTHRITIS

Infectious arthritis can occur from many different types of microorganisms. Most infecting organisms are known to produce an infection in a single joint, termed *monarticular infections;* however, infections also can involve two or more joints.[8] As with osteomyelitis, joint infections also can be classified according to the mechanisms by which the infecting organism reaches the joint. Infectious arthritis can result from the spread of an adjacent bone infection, direct contamination of the joint space, or hematogenous dissemination. Hematogenous spread of the disease comprises the majority of infections; spread from osteomyelitis and direct inoculation is much less frequent.[9] Infectious arthritis occurs most commonly in patients older than age 16; however, approximately one-fourth of cases occur in children 15 years of age or younger.[10]

PATHOPHYSIOLOGY

HEMATOGENOUS OSTEOMYELITIS

Hematogenous osteomyelitis is described classically as a disease of children because most cases occur in patients younger than 16 years of age.[7] Table 122–1 summarizes the primary characteristics of osteomyelitis. Less commonly, these infections occur in adults. One exception, vertebral osteomyelitis, involves the vertebrae and occurs most frequently in patients older than 50 years of age.

Unique features of the anatomy and physiology of some bones appear to predispose them to become infected.[11] The vascular structure within the long bones appears to predispose the bone for hematogenous infections to begin within the metaphyses (Fig. 122–1). The nutrient arteries of the long bones divide within the medullary canal of the bone into small arterioles. These end in hairpin turns near the growth plate and flow into veins, of much wider diameter, that drain the medullary cavity.[1] An infection in hematogenous disease is initiated within the bend of the arterioles. There is considerable slowing of blood flow passing through the hairpin turns within the arterioles and then into the wider venous structures. This sludging of blood flow allows bacteria present within the bloodstream to settle and initiate an inflammatory response. In addition to these structural features, there also appears to be less active phagocytosis within the metaphysis. After the bacteria settle in the bone, avascular necrosis can occur from occlusion of the nutrient vessels and release of bacterial enzymes.

In addition to these anatomic and functional features, there is some evidence that trauma is associated with developing an infection in specific bones. Children who develop hematogenous osteomyelitis may report some type of trauma as an etiologic event. Animal data also indicate that traumatized bone is more likely to become infected than normal bone.

Once the infection is initiated, exudate begins to form within the bone, which produces increased pressure. The age of the patient largely determines the next stage in the pathophysiology. In children older than 12 to 18 months, the infection that started in the metaphysis of a long bone is prevented from spreading into the joint because of the growth plate; however, the exudate often expands laterally through the thin outer cortex of the bone and raises the loose periosteum. The periosteum is thick and not easily broken, and the resulting pus usually remains subperiosteal. If there is significant periosteal damage, a soft-tissue abscess can develop. Impairment of blood flow to the outer portion of the cortical bone can occur, producing dead bone that separates from healthy bone, termed *sequestra.* The elevated periosteum remains viable because its blood supply, derived from the overlying muscle, is unaffected. The raised periosteum will continue to produce bone; however, this new bone is now separated from the cortex because the periosteum has been raised from the infection. This new bone is termed *involucrum.*

In adults, the periosteum is tightly bound, and the cortex is thick. These anatomic features generally cause the infections to remain intramedullary. As expected, subperiosteal abscess formations are less common in this population. The infection can spread to adjacent bone structures through the Haversian and Volkmann canals. Chronic osteomyelitis is more likely to occur if large segments of bone become avascular and necrotic.

Neonatal patients also have unique characteristics. In these patients, there are blood vessels that spread through the cortex of the metaphyses and up into the epiphyses. This enables an infection that started within the metaphyseal area to spread easily to involve the epiphyses and then into the joint. Therefore, in infants, not only can the infection spread to involve the periosteum and the shaft as in children, but the infection also can spread to involve the joint.[12]

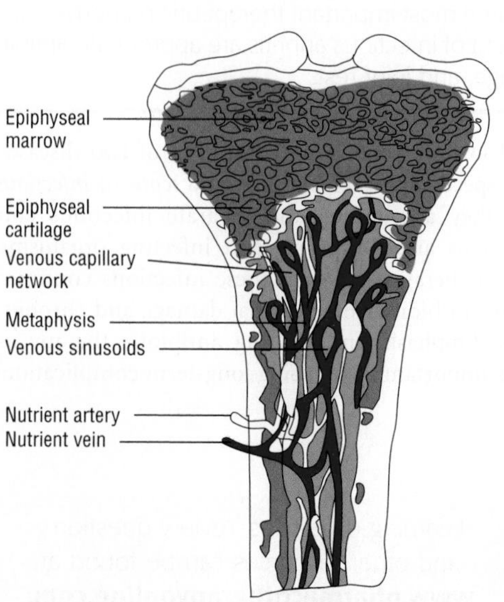

FIGURE 122-1. Cross-section of normal bone.

Hematogenous osteomyelitis also is known to have a predilection for certain bones. The specific bones most likely to be involved also depend on the age of the patient. Children most commonly develop infections within the femur, tibia, humerus, and fibula.[12] Vertebral infections are more common in patients older than 50 years of age. Neonatal infections commonly involve multiple bones.

❶ The bacteriology of hematogenous osteomyelitis is unique compared with osteomyelitis caused by other routes of infection. A single organism is responsible for the vast majority of hematogenous infections. *Staphylococcus aureus* is isolated most frequently with hematogenous infections in children. In immunocompetent children who have been fully vaccinated with the *Haemophilus influenzae* type b vaccine, this is now an uncommon pathogen causing bone and joint infections.[13] However, neonatal osteomyelitis has a wider spectrum of infecting organisms.[14] The three most common etiologic agents are *S. aureus,* group B streptococcus, and *Escherichia coli.* The infections from *S. aureus* and *E. coli* have been linked to complications occurring during pregnancy or delivery, and they are involved most frequently in multiple-bone infections.

Vertebral osteomyelitis has several unique features. Vertebral osteomyelitis occurs most commonly in adults 50 to 60 years of age. The lumbar and thoracic regions are the locations of most infections. Hematogenous infections are most likely to develop in the vascular areas near the subchondral plate region of the vertebral body. Staphylococci cause approximately 60% of these infections; however, gram-negative organisms now play a significant role. It is presumed that these gram-negative organisms, particularly *E. coli,* most likely originate within the urinary tract. *E. coli* vertebral infections have been associated with urinary tract infections, positive urine cultures, and bacteremias. *Mycobacterium tuberculosis* also is known to cause infections in the spine. Skin and respiratory tract infections are other foci of infections known to lead to vertebral infections.

A unique category of osteomyelitis patients consists of individuals with a history of intravenous drug abuse. More than 50% of the osteomyelitis infections in this group of patients are found in the vertebral column. Less than 20% of infections are located in either the sternoarticular or pelvic girdle. Infections are much less frequent within the extremities. An unusual feature of osteomyelitis in the intravenous drug-abusing population is the spectrum of organisms. Gram-negative organisms are responsible for 88% of infections. *Pseudomonas aeruginosa,* either singly or in combination with other organisms, is cultured in 78% of all infections. *Klebsiella, Enterobacter,* and *Serratia* species also can be found but less commonly. In addition, staphylococcal and streptococcal organisms can be cultured.

Patients with sickle cell anemia and related hemoglobinopathies have a much higher rate of infection with *Salmonella* species as compared with other populations. *Salmonella* species are responsible for two-thirds of the infections in these patients. Bowel infarctions from the sickle cell disease can facilitate salmonellae entry into the bloodstream from the colon and spread hematogenously to the bone. Osteomyelitis in patients with sickle cell disease may occur in any bone, but it is observed to be most common in the medullary cavity of long or tubular bones. Because of the difficulty in separating bone pain during a sickle cell crisis from that of an infection, osteomyelitis can be relatively advanced in these patients when the diagnosis is made. Although salmonellae are cultured most frequently, staphylococci and other gram-negative organisms also can be isolated.

CONTIGUOUS-SPREAD OSTEOMYELITIS

This category of osteomyelitis includes infections caused by direct entrance of organisms from a source outside the body or progressive spread of an infection from tissue adjacent to the bone. Penetrating wounds (e.g., trauma), open fractures, and various invasive orthopedic procedures can result in direct inoculation of organisms into the bone. Infections also can occur secondary to pressure ulcers.[15] More than 80% of cases of postoperative osteomyelitis are known to occur following open reductions of fractures. Specifically, these infections occur most commonly after internal fixation of a hip fracture or femoral or tibial shaft fracture.

Osteomyelitis secondary to an adjoining soft tissue infection comprises another very important group of contiguous infections and most often involves the fingers and toes. Less commonly, infections can spread from infected teeth to involve the mandible or occur secondary to sinus infections by spreading through the mucosal lining of the sinuses into the vascular system surrounding the bone.

In contrast to hematogenous osteomyelitis, which occurs most commonly in children, contiguous-spread osteomyelitis occurs most commonly in patients older than age 50. Most likely this is so because important predisposing factors, such as hip fractures, are more common in this age group.

Contiguous-spread disease has several important differences compared with hematogenous osteomyelitis. Although *S. aureus* is still the most common organism isolated, infections with multiple organisms, including gram-negative bacilli, occur frequently. *Pseudomonas aeruginosa,* streptococcus, *E. coli, Staphylococcus epidermidis,* and anaerobes all can be isolated. One important exception to this wide range of organisms is puncture wounds of the feet. There is a strong correlation between puncture wounds of the feet and gram-negative osteomyelitis (often classified as *osteochondritis*), especially infections caused by *P. aeruginosa.*[16]

Patients with osteomyelitis in association with severe vascular insufficiency are extremely difficult to manage.[17,18] As anticipated, most of these patients have diabetes mellitus or severe atherosclerosis, and they develop their infections from contiguous-spread mechanisms. Generally, these patients are between the ages of 50 and 70 years when they develop osteomyelitis. Frequently, patients with vascular disease develop osteomyelitis in their toes and fingers, and there is usually an adjacent area of infection, such as cellulitis or dermal ulcers.

Another important characteristic of osteomyelitis in association with vascular insufficiency is the spectrum of infecting organisms. Infections in these patients almost always include multiple organisms. The mixed-flora infections often include staphylococcus and streptococcus or the combination of staphylococcus, streptococcus, and Enterobacteriaceae. Enterococci and anaerobic organisms also can be seen.

Anaerobic organisms also play a role in osteomyelitis. When anaerobes are grown from cultures, they usually are found in association with other organisms, including aerobic bacteria. The two most common predisposing factors in patients who have anaerobic osteomyelitis are previous fractures and diabetes mellitus. The anaerobic infections in association with diabetes mellitus almost always occur within the feet. *Bacteroides fragilis* and *Bacteroides melaninogenicus* comprise the majority of anaerobic isolates.

INFECTIOUS ARTHRITIS

Distinct from osteomyelitis, infectious arthritis usually is acquired by hematogenous spread.[8] The synovial tissue is highly vascular and does not have a basement membrane, so organisms in the blood can easily reach the synovial fluid. Table 122–2 summarizes the characteristics of acute infectious arthritis. Some organisms, such as *Neisseria gonorrhoeae,* are especially likely to infect a joint during bacteremia. In addition, organisms also can gain access to the joint from a deep-penetrating wound, an intraarticular steroid injection, arthroscopy, prosthetic joint surgery, and contiguous osteomyelitis expansion into the joint.[3]

TABLE 122-2 Characteristics of Acute Infectious Arthritis

Feature	Finding
Peak incidence	Children younger than 16 years Adults older than 50 years
Clinical findings	Fever of 38–40°C (100.4–104°F) in children; painful swollen joint in the absence of trauma Physical examination: Effusion, restriction of joint motion, tenderness, and warmth of joint
Most commonly affected joints	Knee, hip, ankle, elbow, wrist, and shoulder
Laboratory findings:	
Erythrocyte sedimentation rate	Elevated in 90% of cases
White blood cell count	Elevated in 30–60% of cases
Left shift	Seen in two-thirds of patients
Blood culture	Positive in 40% of cases
Needle aspiration of joint	Gram-stain diagnostic in 30–50% of cases. Synovial fluid cultures are positive in 60–80% of cases. Synovial fluid differential reveals 90% polymorphonuclear leukocytes. Synovial fluid glucose decreased relative to serum glucose. Lactic acid levels elevated in nongonococcal infectious arthritis but not in gonococcal infectious arthritis

The risk factors associated with adult infectious arthritis (more than one factor may be present) are systemic corticosteroid use, preexisting arthritis, arthrocentesis, distant infection, diabetes mellitus, trauma, and other diseases.

Trauma also appears to be a risk factor in facilitating microorganism entry into the synovial space. One study found that 35% of patients with infectious arthritis had preexisting joint disease.[10] Unlike children, adults often have significant systemic diseases that predispose them to infectious arthritis, such as diabetes mellitus, immunosuppressive states (cancer, liver disease), or preexisting arthritis. Intravenous drug abusers also are prone to develop septic arthritis. Arthritis, joint trauma, and surgery are other important risk factors because chronic inflammation or trauma makes the joint more susceptible to infection.[19] In addition, rheumatoid arthritis patients can be prone to bacterial infection because of an inherent phagocytic defect, as well as concomitant corticosteroid therapy. Hormonal factors appear to play a role in *N. gonorrhoeae* infectious arthritis. Women are more prone to develop disseminated gonococcal infections than men. The second and third trimesters of pregnancy and during menstruation appear to be the times of greatest risk for developing gonococcal bacteremia.

After bacteria gain access to the joint, the organisms begin to multiply and produce a persistent purulent effusion within the joint. If this joint effusion is present beyond 7 days, chronic, and sometimes irreversible, damage can occur. Purulent effusions can promote cartilage destruction by increasing leukocyte enzyme activity. In conjunction with the development of the effusion, almost all patients will develop a hot, swollen, painful joint. The proteolytic enzymes within the effusion and pressure necrosis can lead to cartilage and bone damage.

❶ *Staphylococcus aureus,* the single most common infecting organism, is found in 48% of cases of nongonococcal bacterial arthritis. Streptococcal infections account for 18% of cases, and gram-negative organisms are less common.[10] Overall, *E. coli* is the most common of the gram-negative organisms; however, *P. aeruginosa* is the most frequent organism in intravenous drug abusers. Neonates may have infectious arthritis because of a broad range of organisms, with *S. aureus,* streptococcus, and gram-negative organisms being most common. *Staphylococcus aureus* and streptococcus are the most common pathogens in children younger than 5 years of age. If the child has not been fully vaccinated or is immunocompromised, *H. influenzae* type b may be seen. Within the adult population, *S. aureus* is responsible for the vast majority of nongonococcal infections. The most common cause of bacterial arthritis in adults 18 to 30 years of age is *N. gonorrhoeae,* which are the most common infections in women.[20] Patients with a terminal complement deficiency (C5–C9) are at increased risk of disseminated infections with *Neisseria* species. Although less common, nonbacterial causes of osteomyelitis and septic arthritis include fungi and viruses.[21]

CLINICAL PRESENTATION

The clinical presentation of acute hematogenous osteomyelitis is summarized in Table 122–3. Although neonatal hematogenous osteomyelitis can spread rapidly to involve the joint, often there are few systemic symptoms present. A joint effusion is present in 60% to 70% of neonatal infections. Decreased limb motion and edema over the affected area may be the only signs from which to make a diagnosis. Pyogenic vertebral osteomyelitis produces nonspecific symptoms, such as severe back pain, fever or night sweats, and weight loss. The pain typically is present at rest and increases in severity with movement. Neurologic symptoms can occur if the infection extends and compresses the spinal cord. With contiguous-spread osteomyelitis there is often an area of localized tenderness, warmth, edema, and erythema over the infected site. Patients with significant vascular insufficiency usually have local symptoms, such as pain, swelling, and redness. Less commonly, patients with vascular disease also can have a fever and elevated white blood cell (WBC) count. The presentation of osteomyelitis from surgery or trauma depends on the precipitating cause. If the infection follows surgery or bone trauma, the symptoms usually are noted within 1 month. The most frequent symptom is simply pain in the area of infection. Less commonly, patients also can develop a fever and elevated WBC count.

Patients with nongonococcal bacterial arthritis almost always present with a fever, and 50% of patients have an elevated WBC count (see Table 122–2). The average initial synovial WBC count is 100,000 cells/mm^3 or greater in nongonococcal bacterial disease. The most frequent initial sign of disseminated gonococcal infections is a migratory polyarthralgia. In addition, two-thirds of patients also complain of fever, dermatitis, and tenosynovitis (inflammation of the tendon sheath).

Nongonococcal bacterial arthritis almost always involves only a single joint. The knee is the most commonly involved joint, but infections also can occur in the shoulder, wrist, hip, ankle, interphalangeal joints, and elbow joints. Usually, the initial focus of infection that acted as the source for bacterial or microbial entrance can be identified. Common routes for bacterial entrance include infections of the respiratory tract, skin, and urinary tract. Blood cultures are important in these patients because they can be positive in 50% of patients.

Another type of infectious arthritis occurs following prosthetic joint surgery. With these infections, the erythrocyte sedimentation

TABLE 122-3 Clinical Presentation of Hematogenous Osteomyelitis

Signs and symptoms

Significant tenderness of the affected area, pain, swelling, fever, chills, decreased motion, and malaise

Laboratory tests

Elevated erythrocyte sedimentation rate, C-reactive protein, and white blood cell count

50% of patients will have positive blood cultures

Diagnostic studies

Bone changes observed on radiographs 10–14 days after the onset of infection. Technetium and gallium scans positive as early as 1 day after the onset of infection.

rate usually is elevated, although a leukocytosis often is absent. Infections that result from postoperative contamination usually become apparent within 1 year of surgery.

RADIOLOGIC AND LABORATORY TESTS

The evaluation of a patient who potentially may have osteomyelitis has several unusual aspects. Radiographs of the involved area should be obtained; however, bone changes characteristic of osteomyelitis are not seen for at least 10 to 14 days after the onset of the infection.[22] Radiologists may note soft tissue swelling before any bone changes become obvious. Bone lesions do not appear on roentgenogram films until 10 days after infection because more than 50% of the bone matrix must be removed before the lesions can be detected. As an aide to improve the diagnosis, bone scanning is used commonly.[23]

Despite the seriousness of osteomyelitis, often there are few laboratory abnormalities. The erythrocyte sedimentation rate (ESR), C-reactive protein, and WBC count may be the only laboratory abnormalities.[12] The degree of abnormality of these laboratory findings does not correlate with the disease outcome; however, they are useful for monitoring therapy. C-reactive protein can be elevated because of the presence of inflammation, and it can be substituted for the ESR. C-reactive protein is generally the more sensitive and specific marker of response to therapy and often increases and decreases before the ESR.

When a clinical assessment of osteomyelitis is suspected, it is important to establish a bacteriologic diagnosis by culture of the infected bone. Accurate culture information is especially important as a guide for treatment of osteomyelitis. Bone aspiration is valuable in determining an accurate bacteriologic diagnosis.[24] In addition, performing a bone aspiration determines whether or not there is an abscess present. If an abscess is located, the pus is cultured, and a Gram stain is performed. If an abscess is found, the fluid needs to be drained and cultured. Aspirates of subperiosteal pus or metaphyseal fluid yield a pathogen in 70% of cases. Cultures should be done for both aerobic and anaerobic bacteria. A Gram stain of the aspirate can be useful in initiating empirical antibiotic therapy. This allows a more appropriate choice of antibiotics from the first day of therapy rather than waiting several days while culture results are pending.

If a specimen is obtained from a previously undrained or unopened wound abscess, the pathogen usually can be identified. In chronic osteomyelitis, however, identification can be more difficult. Open wounds and draining sinuses frequently are contaminated with other organisms and thus provide inaccurate culture information.[25] Therefore, because of the inaccuracies with sinus tract cultures, they cannot be relied on to reflect the pathogen. Cultures of loculated pus aspirates in the area of orthopedic devices removed from infected bone can be trusted, however, to identify the infecting organism. The preferable time to obtain culture material in a patient with a chronic draining sinus is at the time of open surgical débridement.

❷ In addition to performing cultures from the involved bone, it also is important to obtain cultures from any site believed to be the source of a bacteremia. Blood cultures should be obtained. Approximately 50% of patients with hematogenous osteomyelitis will have positive blood cultures.

❸ When evaluating the possibility of a patient having infectious arthritis, immediate joint aspiration with subsequent analysis of the synovial fluid is extremely important. The presence of purulent fluid usually indicates the presence of a septic joint. The synovial fluid WBC count is usually 50,000 to 200,000 cells/mm^3 when an infection is present. Approximately half the patients with an infected joint have a low synovial glucose level, usually less than 40 mg/dL. Gram stains of joint fluid demonstrate bacteria in 50% of patients with septic arthritis; however, such stains can be positive in only 25% of patients with gonococcal arthritis infections. Synovial fluid cultures usually are positive in patients with nongonococcal infections. Both blood and joint fluid should be cultured aerobically and anaerobically in a patient suspected of having an infected joint. Blood cultures are positive in one-half of patients with nongonococcal infections but in only 20% of those with gonococcal infections. Pharyngeal, rectal, cervical, or urethral smears and cultures, as well as cultures of cutaneous lesions, should be performed if a disseminated gonococcal infection is considered. As with osteomyelitis, most patients will have an elevated C-reactive protein concentration and ESR. Radiographs of infected joints often reveal distension of the joint capsule with soft tissue swelling in the adjacent space. Magnetic resonance imaging can be helpful in identifying an infected hip. In patients who have developed an infected prosthetic joint, loosening of the prosthesis can be seen radiographically.

TREATMENT

■ DESIRED OUTCOME

The goals of treatment are resolution of the infection and prevention of long-term sequelae. The ultimate outcome of osteomyelitis depends on the acute or chronic nature of the disease and how rapidly appropriate therapy is initiated. Patients with acute osteomyelitis have the best prognosis. Cure rates exceeding 80% can be expected for patients with acute osteomyelitis who have surgery as indicated and receive injectable antibiotics for 4 to 6 weeks.[26] In contrast, patients with chronic osteomyelitis have a much poorer prognosis.[27] Dead bone and other necrotic material from the infection act as a bacterial reservoir and make the infection very difficult to eliminate. Adequate surgical débridement to remove all the dead bone and necrotic material, combined with prolonged administration of antibiotics, provides the best chance to obtain a cure.[28] The inability to remove all the dead bone can allow residual infection and require suppressive antibiotics to control the infection.

In comparison, many patients who develop infectious arthritis recover with no long-term sequelae. Gonococcal arthritis usually resolves rapidly with antibiotics; however, patients with staphylococcal arthritis have a higher incidence of joint damage. Individuals at greatest risk for long-term sequelae are those who have symptoms present for more than 7 days before starting therapy and those with infections occurring within the hip joint and infections caused by gram-negative organisms. Common long-term residual effects following infectious arthritis are limited joint motion and persistent pain. Shortening of the affected extremity is another well-known complication. More than half the children who subsequently developed residual joint damage were believed normal at the time of hospital discharge.

■ GENERAL APPROACH TO TREATMENT

❹ Following completion of the steps needed to determine the infecting organism, the most important treatment modality of acute osteomyelitis is the administration of appropriate antibiotics in adequate doses for a sufficient length of time. It is important to stress that early antibiotic therapy can mitigate the need for surgery.[29] A delay in treatment can allow bone necrosis to occur and make eradication of the infection much more difficult. In these patients, recurrent exacerbations of the infection can result if all necrotic tissue is not removed surgically and all microorganisms eliminated. Adjunctive treatment with hyperbaric oxygen or antibiotic-impregnated implants during surgery also has been used.[30–32]

If a patient with hematogenous osteomyelitis does not respond by having a decrease in fever, local swelling, redness, and pain following the initiation of adequate antibiotic therapy, the patient should undergo surgical débridement of the infected area. It is important to emphasize the priority of starting antibiotics immediately after the cultures have been obtained. No treatment failures have been reported when injectable antibiotics were started within 48 hours of the onset of symptoms in children with osteomyelitis.

■ PHARMACOLOGIC THERAPY

Antibiotic Bone Concentration

❺ Antibiotics used in the management of acute osteomyelitis generally are given in high doses (adjusted for weight, renal function, hepatic function, or both) so that adequate antimicrobial concentrations are reached within the infected bone and joint. Between 8 and 12 g/day of a penicillinase-resistant penicillin (nafcillin or oxacillin), ampicillin, or cephalosporin or a similar large dose of another parenteral antibiotic is used in the initial management of adults with osteomyelitis. These dosing recommendations, however, are empirical; the relationship between a specific dose of a given antibiotic and its resulting concentration within the infected bone is largely unknown.[33] Semisynthetic penicillins, cephalosporins, clindamycin, and the aminoglycosides can be detected in bone homogenates soon after their administration.

CLINICAL CONTROVERSY

Some clinicians recommend coverage empirically for methicillin-resistant *Staphylococcus aureus* (MRSA) when staphylococcal infection is suspected. Others believe that culture results and sensitivity testing or lack of response to routine staphylococcal antibiotics should trigger use of antibiotics directed against MRSA. The frequency of MRSA in a community may help govern which approach is used.

Duration of Antibiotic Therapy

❻ The specific duration of antibiotic therapy needed in the management of osteomyelitis is usually 4 to 6 weeks.[34] Failure rates approaching 20% have been observed in children treated with injectable antibiotics for 3 weeks or less. Thus, with the data indicating a minimum of 3 weeks of antibiotic therapy, the standard treatment for osteomyelitis has been parenteral antibiotics for 4 to 6 weeks.[35–37] Although these data were determined in children, this duration-of-therapy recommendation is also used in adults. A trial assessing ceftriaxone 2 g intravenously once daily for at least 6 weeks for *S. aureus* osteomyelitis achieved a cure rate of 77%.[38] The failures in this study were in patients with infected necrotic bone or infected hardware (wires, plates, screws, and rods) that could not be removed.

A modification of this recommendation has been used in some patients. Children receiving an appropriate oral antibiotic regimen and adults receiving an oral fluoroquinolone antibiotic, such as ciprofloxacin, for a duration of 6 weeks have been treated successfully. Monitoring the patient's clinical signs and symptoms and the C-reactive protein level or ESR is an important parameter to assess therapy. If signs or symptoms are still present at 6 weeks, therapy should be extended. In contrast, children who have had a puncture wound of the foot resulting in *P. aeruginosa* osteochondritis and who have had surgical débridement of infected material can be treated with parenteral antibiotics for 10 days.[39]

Oral Antibiotic Therapy

❼ One of the most significant changes in the management of osteomyelitis is the use of oral antibiotics to complete therapy.[40] Criteria for the use of oral outpatient antibiotic therapy for osteomyelitis include all of the following:

- Confirmed osteomyelitis
- Initial clinical response to parenteral antibiotics
- Suitable oral agent available
- Compliance ensured

Suitable candidates are children with good clinical response to intravenous therapy and adults without diabetes mellitus or peripheral vascular disease.

Two primary populations have benefited from oral treatment. Children responding to initial parenteral therapy may be excellent candidates to receive followup oral therapy with an agent such as dicloxacillin, cephalexin, or amoxicillin depending on their culture and sensitivity results.[41] Although more controversial, the other population to benefit from oral therapy is adults with an infecting organism sensitive to a fluoroquinolone.[42] These two populations now no longer routinely require expensive and complicated courses of long-term parenteral antibiotics.

The use of oral antibiotics is well studied in children. Several studies documenting the effectiveness of oral therapy used injectable antibiotics initially and then switched to oral antibiotics when there was a decrease in the signs of inflammation and the ESR or when the patient was afebrile for 3 days.[41] If pus was obtained on the initial needle aspirate, or if a reduction in fever, local swelling, and tenderness did not occur despite adequate rest, immobilization, and intensive antibiotic therapy, the patients underwent surgical drainage.

The patients enrolled in oral antibiotic trials generally had disease of recent onset, identification of a specific infecting organism, enforced compliance, and surgery as indicated. In patients who meet these criteria, oral antibiotics appear to offer a great advantage in the treatment of osteomyelitis. Patients not meeting these criteria are more likely to develop chronic osteomyelitis with resulting recurrent exacerbations of the infection if oral therapy is attempted. A systematic literature review in acute hematogenous osteomyelitis compared studies using less than 7 days of intravenous therapy plus oral antibiotics versus patients who received more than one week of intravenous antibiotics plus oral therapy. The analysis found no difference between groups, with cure rates at least 95%.[43]

Ciprofloxacin is effective in the treatment of osteomyelitis caused by gram-negative strains, such as *Enterobacter cloacae* and *Serratia marcescens*.[44] Many strains of streptococci are relatively resistant. Its activity against gram-negative bacilli allows patients to be treated orally and avoids the potential toxic complications of 4 to 6 weeks of aminoglycoside therapy. Ciprofloxacin and other fluoroquinolones also have demonstrated effectiveness in the treatment of chronic osteomyelitis along with adequate surgical débridement.[45,46] Another benefit with this agent is that it can be administered on an every-12-hour schedule. An important limitation of this antibiotic class, however, is that fluoroquinolones should not be used in children younger than 16 to 18 years of age or in pregnant women because of the potential to cause cartilage damage. Other limitations of ciprofloxacin are that it has poor coverage against anaerobic organisms and staphylococci and that *P. aeruginosa* can develop resistance.[47] Newer fluoroquinolones have additional gram-positive activity; however, additional well-controlled clinical trials are needed to determine most appropriately their role in the treatment of osteomyelitis.[48,49]

CLINICAL CONTROVERSY

Some clinicians believe that oral fluoroquinolones should be preferred treatments for osteomyelitis, whereas others believe that there have been inadequate studies to date to determine their comparative clinical effectiveness.

Concern has been raised about staphylococci resistance to fluoroquinolones. Methicillin-resistant *S. aureus* infections do not respond

TABLE 122-4 Empirical Treatment of Osteomyelitis

Patient Subtype	Likely Infecting Organism	Antibiotic[a]	Recommendation Grades[b]
Newborn	*Staphylococcus aureus*, streptococci, *Escherichia coli*	Nafcillin or oxacillin 50–150 mg/kg/day IV plus cefotaxime 100–200 mg/kg/day IV	B-3
Children 5 years of age or younger	1. If vaccinated for *Haemophilus influenzae* type b: *S. aureus* or streptococci	1. Nafcillin 150 mg/kg/day IV or cefazolin 100 mg/kg/day IV	B-3
	2. If not vaccinated against *H. influenzae* type b	2. Cefuroxime 150 mg/kg/day IV	B-3
Children older than 5 years of age	*S. aureus*	Nafcillin 150 mg/kg/day IV or cefazolin 100 mg/kg/day IV	A-3
Adults	*S. aureus*	Nafcillin 2 g IV every 4 hours or cefazolin 2 g IV every 8 hours	A-3
Intravenous drug abusers	*Pseudomonas*	Ciprofloxacin 750 mg PO twice daily or ceftazidime 2 g IV every 8 hours plus tobramycin 5 mg/kg/day IV	B-3
Postoperative or posttrauma patients	Gram-positive and gram-negative organisms	Nafcillin 2 g IV every 4 hours plus ceftazidime 2 g IV every 8 hours or ticarcillin-clavulanate 3.1 g IV every 4 hours	B-3
Patients with vascular insufficiency	Gram-positive and gram-negative organisms	Nafcillin 2 g IV every 4 hours or cefazolin 2 g IV every 8 hours plus ceftazidime 2 g IV every 8 hours	B-3
	If anaerobes suspected	Cefotetan 2 g IV every 12 hours or clindamycin 900 mg IV every 8 hours plus ceftazidime 2 g IV every 8 hours	C-3

PO, orally.

[a]Dosage should be adjusted for some agents in patients with renal and/or hepatic dysfunction.

[b]Strength of recommendations: A, B, C = good, moderate, and poor evidence to support recommendation, respectively. Quality of evidence: 1 = Evidence from more than one properly randomized, controlled trial. 2 = Evidence from more than one well-designed clinical trial with randomization, from cohort or case-controlled analytic studies or multiple time series; or dramatic results from uncontrolled experiments. 3 = Evidence from opinions of respected authorities, based on clinical experience, descriptive studies, or reports of expert communities.

well to ciprofloxacin; however, resistance also can be troublesome for methicillin-sensitive strains. It is now recommended that when ciprofloxacin is to be used to treat osteomyelitis with mixed etiologies that include *S. aureus,* it should be combined with an antistaphylococcal drug such as dicloxacillin, cephalexin, or clindamycin.

Antibiotic Selection

A critical component in the management of osteomyelitis is the selection of appropriate antibiotics. Empirical therapy must be selected on the basis of the most likely infecting organism while the results of culture and sensitivity data are pending. Table 122–4 summarizes empirical therapy recommendations. It is difficult to make evidence-based recommendations on the treatment of these infections as very little high quality clinical evidence exists. Experimental evidence, case series, and published expert opinion are used to suggested preferred treatment options.[29,48] Dosages expressed in terms of milligrams per kilograms per day generally are given in divided doses every 6 to 8 hours (three to four times a day).

Because *S. aureus,* streptococci, and *E. coli* are the most common infecting organisms in newborns, an intravenous dosage of 150 mg/kg per day (given in four divided doses) of oxacillin or nafcillin plus cefotaxime 150 mg/kg per day (given in three to four divided doses) is appropriate. For children 5 years of age or younger, *S. aureus* and streptococci are the most common infecting organisms. Appropriate therapy in this age group is nafcillin or oxacillin 150 mg/kg per day intravenously or cefazolin 100 mg/kg per day. If the patient is immunocompromised or has not been fully vaccinated, empirical therapy is needed to also cover *H. influenzae* type b. In this setting, intravenous cefuroxime 150 mg/kg per day is appropriate empirical therapy. For children older than 5 years, *S. aureus* is the most likely infecting organism, and either nafcillin 150 to 200 mg/kg per day intravenously or cefazolin 100 mg/kg per day intravenously is recommended. If patients are allergic to penicillins or cephalosporins or are infected with MRSA, vancomycin, clindamycin, or linezolid can be used.[50] Children with culture-negative osteomyelitis can be managed as presumed staphylococcal disease with excellent long-term results.[51] Children with osteomyelitis usually can be treated successfully with 4 weeks of parenteral therapy or parenteral followed by oral therapy.

CLINICAL CONTROVERSY

Some clinicians believe that empirical therapy of osteomyelitis and septic arthritis in a child younger than 5 years of age no longer requires *H. influenzae* type b coverage, whereas others are concerned about children not being fully vaccinated and desire to use an antibiotic with activity against this organism.

An oral regimen can be an alternative to the previous recommendation in many cases of osteomyelitis in children. Children who have undergone surgery, if needed, and have had a good clinical response to intravenous therapy may be candidates for the alternate oral antibiotic regimen. Parenteral antibiotic therapy should be initiated and continued until there has been a resolution in the erythema, swelling, and tenderness and until the patient is afebrile. Dicloxacillin, cloxacillin, and cephalexin (100 mg/kg per day) are effective oral agents. Patients should be monitored with periodic WBC counts, C-reactive protein (or ESR) determinations, and radiographic findings. When oral antibiotics are used, the total duration of oral and injectable therapy is usually at least 4 to 6 weeks. As stated previously, because of the risk of cartilage damage, fluoroquinolones should not be used in children. Hematogenous osteomyelitis in adults is caused most frequently by *S. aureus* and thus is treated appropriately with 8 to 12 g/day of a penicillinase-resistant penicillin such as nafcillin. A similar dose of a first-generation cephalosporin (e.g., cefazolin), clindamycin 2.4 g/day, or vancomycin 2 g/day (with normal renal function) can be used in individuals allergic to penicillin; however, if the infection is located within the vertebrae, *E. coli* must be considered, and thus, depending on the culture and sensitivity data, a switch to a cephalosporin may be needed.[52] After institution of appropriate antibiotic therapy, the antimicrobial agent should be continued for at least 4 to 6 weeks total (parenteral plus oral).

Special Populations Osteomyelitis in a patient with a hemoglobinopathy, such as sickle cell anemia, is commonly caused by either *Salmonella* or *S. aureus.* Thus empirical antibiotics of first choice are ceftriaxone or cefotaxime. Alternatives are chloramphenicol and ciprofloxacin (in adults).

Bone infections in patients with a history of intravenous drug abuse require coverage for gram-negative organisms; therefore, empirical treatment with ceftazidime 2 g intravenously every 8 hours plus an aminoglycoside is indicated. If compliance can be ensured, these patients are excellent candidates to receive oral ciprofloxacin 750 mg twice daily. Antibiotic therapy in these patients should be continued for at least 4 to 6 weeks.

As discussed previously, several microorganisms can cause bone infections that occur after surgery or from contiguous spread of an adjacent soft tissue infection. *S. aureus* is the single most common organism, but multiple organisms can be involved. To provide the required broad-spectrum coverage, nafcillin 2 g intravenously every 4 hours plus ceftazidime 2 g intravenously every 8 hours should be used as initial therapy. An alternative single agent is ticarcillin–clavulanate potassium 3.1 g intravenously every 4 hours; however, there is less experience with this agent. Other broad-spectrum alternatives can be cefepime and imipenem. The antibiotic regimen can require modification after culture and sensitivity information is evaluated. Based on the culture and sensitivity data, ciprofloxacin can be an appropriate oral alternative for these patients. Frequently, the antibiotics must be continued for 6 weeks to obtain a cure, and surgery often is required to remove any infected or devitalized tissue.

Patients with established vascular insufficiency who subsequently develop osteomyelitis are extremely difficult to manage.[6] Impaired blood flow to the extremities impedes the healing process, possibly requiring vascular bypass surgery.[53] Infections in these patients involve a wide range of organisms, including *S. aureus, Streptococcus,* anaerobes, and gram-negative organisms. Broad-spectrum therapy with a penicillinase-resistant penicillin in combination with ceftazidime is the preferred initial therapy. If anaerobes are suspected, an antianaerobic cephalosporin (e.g., cefoxitin) or clindamycin plus ceftazidime can be substituted. Ampicillin may need to be added to the regimen to provide coverage against enterococci. Despite aggressive antibiotic therapy along with surgical débridement, these patients continue to have very low cure rates. Amputation of the involved area may be required to obtain a cure of the infection.[54]

Home Antibiotic Therapy Because the management of bone and joint infections frequently requires prolonged parenteral antibiotics, newer antibiotic regimens are being evaluated.[55] Administration of antibiotics in the home environment and the use of antibiotics with extended elimination half-lives are being studied.[56] Although acute osteomyelitis is one of the more common infectious diseases that can be treated with home intravenous antibiotics, not all patients are acceptable candidates for home administration.[57] Patients must be screened to include only those who are receiving a stable treatment program, those who are interested and are motivated in participating, and those who have good venous access, as well as those who have support from family members or neighbors and have home facilities for storage and refrigeration.[58] Patients with adequate vascular access may be able to use a peripheral intravenous catheter; however, a central intravenous catheter may be required if venous access difficulties occur. Certain exclusion criteria also must be considered. Complications of other preexisting diseases, such as diabetic retinopathy, intention tremor, disabling inflammation or degenerative joint disease, coagulopathies, or various neurologic disorders can prevent individuals from receiving home antibiotics. A history of alcoholism or of intravenous drug abuse also are important exclusion criteria. Patients who are fluent in only a foreign language and patients who are illiterate or hard of hearing may have to be excluded if a qualified guardian is unavailable. In addition to meeting these initial screening criteria, patients must complete a thorough training program successfully before hospital discharge. Aseptic technique, proper catheter care, and correct administration techniques must be documented. Once a patient is receiving therapy in the home environment, continued monitoring of their antimicrobial therapy is important. It is vital to ensure compliance with the antimicrobial regimen.

In addition, the specific antibiotic regimen characteristics must be considered when evaluating a patient for home antibiotics.[59] Some important features are microbiologic culture and sensitivity data, the number of required daily antimicrobial doses, antibiotic stability data, and requirements for unique monitoring for the specific antimicrobial regimen, such as serum creatinine and peak and trough concentration measurements with aminoglycosides. Although an organism can be sensitive to several antimicrobial agents, one antibiotic can provide practical benefits over other agents. Patients who have an infecting organism that is sensitive to one of the longer-acting (less frequently dosed) cephalosporins and is resistant to less expensive agents (cefazolin) may benefit from the newer antibiotics. It is important, however, to monitor for the development of resistant strains and superinfections.

Infectious Arthritis ❽ The three most important therapeutic maneuvers in the management of infectious arthritis are appropriate antibiotics, joint drainage, and joint rest.[60] Smears of the synovial fluid can be useful to select appropriate antibiotic therapy initially.[61] If bacteria are not observed on the Gram stain in a patient who has a purulent joint effusion, antibiotics still should be initiated because of the high risk of an infection being present.[62] A delay in initiating antibiotics significantly increases the likelihood for long-term complications.

The specific antibiotic selected depends on the most likely infecting organism. In infants younger than 1 month of age, the infecting organisms vary widely, and empirical therapy thus must provide broad-spectrum coverage. A penicillinase-resistant penicillin such as nafcillin or oxacillin plus an aminoglycoside is appropriate. Children younger than 5 years of age who have been immunized for *H. influenzae* type b should receive nafcillin, oxacillin, or cefazolin.

In children older than 5 years of age and in adults, initial therapy with a penicillinase-resistant penicillin is appropriate to provide the necessary coverage against *S. aureus.* Therapy should be changed to clindamycin, vancomycin, or linezolid if the *S. aureus* is resistant to methicillin. Preliminary data indicate that children with infectious arthritis can be converted to oral therapy after initial intravenous therapy.[63,64] As with osteomyelitis, intravenous drug abusers require coverage for *P. aeruginosa,* and therefore, combination therapy with an aminoglycoside is needed. The antibiotics selected usually are administered parenterally. Antibiotics administered by this route achieve sufficient concentrations within the synovial fluid, and thus intraarticular antibiotic injections are unnecessary. Although studies to define clearly the appropriate length of therapy have not been conducted, 2 to 3 weeks of antibiotic therapy generally is adequate in nongonococcal infections. Joint fluid cultures usually are no longer positive after 7 days of antibiotics.

Disseminated gonococcal infections often respond quickly to antibiotics.[65] Ceftriaxone 1 g/day for 7 to 10 days is the treatment of choice. After culture and sensitivity results are available and the organism is determined to be sensitive, therapy can be switched on the fourth day to oral amoxicillin or to doxycycline or tetracycline to complete the 7- to 10-day course. Clinical resolution of signs and symptoms usually is rapid.

Closed-needle aspiration is recommended for all infected joints except the hip. Joint drainage can be repeated daily for 5 to 7 days until effusions no longer reaccumulate. Open drainage is required in hip infections because closed-needle aspiration is difficult and inadequate. During the initial phase of the infection, weight bearing, such as walking, on the joint should be avoided. Passive range-of-motion exercises should be initiated when the pain begins to subside to maintain joint mobility.[66] Approximately one-third of patients with bacterial arthritis have a poor joint outcome, such as severe functional deterioration.[67] Poor joint outcomes are associated with older patients, those with preexisting joint disease, and patients with an infected joint containing synthetic material. Treatment guidelines are useful with septic arthritis of the hip.[68]

PHARMACOECONOMIC CONSIDERATIONS

Cost and outcome issues are important in osteomyelitis and infectious arthritis. If long-term sequelae develop, such as impaired joint motion or draining sinus tracts, or if amputation is required, patient quality of life can be significantly diminished. Cost and quality-of-life issues have clearly played a major role in evaluating other treatment alternatives (oral therapy or home antibiotic treatment) rather than requiring patients to remain hospitalized to receive 4 to 6 weeks of parenteral antibiotics.[69] One study compared a series of decision analytic models to provide estimates of the costs and outcomes of different regimens.[70] Another study used a Markov model to compare different treatments in non–insulin-dependent diabetes mellitus patients who had foot infections and suspected osteomyelitis.[71] This study found that a 10-week course of culture-guided oral antibiotics after surgical débridement may be as effective as and less costly than other treatment approaches, such as immediate amputation.

EVALUATION OF THERAPEUTIC OUTCOMES

Patients with bone and joint infections must be monitored closely. Table 122–5 summarizes a pharmaceutical care monitoring protocol. An assessment of a therapy's success or failure is based on the patient's clinical findings and laboratory values. The clinical signs of inflammation, such as swelling, tenderness, pain, redness, and fever, should resolve with appropriate therapy. Initially, the clinical signs are assessed daily until improvement and then periodically thereafter. Elevations in WBC count also should decline gradually. The ESR usually is determined weekly. Elevations in the C-reactive protein or ESR may not return to normal for several weeks of therapy. The WBC count usually is obtained once or twice per week until it returns to the normal range. If by the end of the 4- to 6-week antibiotic course the clinical findings of osteomyelitis are no longer present and the C-reactive protein or ESR is within normal limits, the patient can be considered a clinical cure. Patients can relapse, however, after initially appearing to be cured. No relapse for 1 year generally is considered a complete cure.

If a patient fails to resolve the clinical signs and symptoms of inflammation after appropriate empirical antibiotics, surgical débridement may be needed. In addition, the patient might have a resistant infecting organism or an atypical infecting organism that can require a modification of the antibiotic therapy. It is especially important to note the infecting organism and its sensitivity pattern.

TABLE 122-5 Monitoring Protocol

Parameter	Frequency	Notes
Culture and sensitivity	At initiation of treatment	
White blood cell count	One time per week until within normal range	
C-reactive protein or erythrocyte sedimentation rate	Weekly	May not decrease to normal range until several weeks of therapy
Clinical signs of inflammation (redness, pain, swelling, tenderness, fever)	Daily during initiation of therapy	
Compliance of outpatient therapy	Reinforce before starting oral therapy and with each healthcare visit	Compliance is critical if treatment is to be successful

Followup cultures at subsequent débridements can be useful to assess the antibiotic therapy.

Despite apparently adequate surgery and antibiotics, some patients can fail therapy and have recurrent relapses in their infection. This scenario is more common in the population with chronic osteomyelitis. These patients can require long-term oral antibiotics to keep the infection under control.

ABBREVIATIONS

ESR: erythrocyte sedimentation rate

MRSA: methicillin-resistant *Staphylococcus aureus*

WBC: white blood cell

REFERENCES

1. Waldvogel FA, Medoff G, Swartz MN. Osteomyelitis: A review of clinical features, therapeutic considerations and unusual aspects. N Engl J Med 1970;282:198–206, 260–266, 316–322.
2. Van den Bruel A, Bartholomeeusen S, Aertgeerts B, Truyers C, Buntinx F. Serious infections in children: An incidence study in family practice. BMC Family Practice 2006;7:23.
3. Uthman I, Bizri AR. Clinical features of septic arthritis at a tertiary teaching hospital in Lebanon. Clin Rheumatol 2003;22:359–360.
4. Deshpande SS, Taral N, Modi N, Singrakhia M. Changing epidemiology of neonatal septic arthritis. J Orthop Surg (Hong Kong) 2004;12:10–13.
5. Garcia-De La Torre I. Advances in the management of septic arthritis. Rheum Dis Clin North Am 2003;29:61–75.
6. Gutierrez K. Bone and joint infections in children. Pediatr Clin North Am 2005;52:779–794.
7. Berendt T, Byren I. Bone and joint infection. Clin Med 2004;4:510–518.
8. Smith JW, Chalupa P, Shabaz HM. Infectious arthritis: Clinical features, laboratory findings and treatment. Clin Microbial Infect 2006;12:309–314.
9. Shetty AK, Avinash K, Gedalia A. Management of septic arthritis. Indian J Pediatr 2004;71:819–824.
10. Levine M, Siegel LB. A swollen joint: Why all the fuss? Am J Ther 2003;10:219–224.
11. McCarthy JJ, Dormans JP, Kozin SH, Pizzutillo PD. Musculoskeletal infections in children: Basic treatment principles and recent advancements. Instr Course Lect 2005;54:515–528.
12. Offiah AC. Acute osteomyelitis, septic arthritis and discitis: Differences between neonates and older children. Eur J Radiol 2006;DOI:10.1016/J.EJRAD 2006.07.016.
13. Goergens ED, McEvoy A, Watson M, Barrett IR. Acute osteomyelitis and septic arthritis in children. J Paediatr Child Health 2005;41:59–62.
14. Aroojis AJ, Johari AN. Epiphyseal separations after neonatal osteomyelitis and septic arthritis. J Pediatr Orthop 2000;20:544–549.
15. Hirshberg J, Rees RS, Marchant B, Dean S. Osteomyelitis related to pressure ulcers: The cost of neglect. Adv Skin Wound Care 2000;13:25–29.
16. Waagner DC. Musculoskeletal infections in adolescents. Adolescent Med State Art Rev 2000;11:375–400.
17. Ansari MA, Shukla VK. Foot infections. Int J Low Extrem Wounds 2005;4:74–87.
18. Brem H, Sheehan P, Boulton AJ. Protocol for treatment of diabetic foot ulcers. Am J Surg 2004;187:1S–10S.
19. Gupta MN, Sturrock RD, Field M. A prospective 2-year study of 75 patients with adult-onset septic arthritis. Rheumatology 2001;40:24–30.
20. Rice PA. Gonococcal arthritis (disseminated gonococcal infection). Infect Dis Clin North Am 2005;19:853–861.
21. Kohli R, Hadley S. Fungal arthritis and osteomyelitis. Infect Dis Clin North Am 2005;19:831–851.
22. Song KM, Sloboda JF. Acute hematogenous osteomyelitis in children. J Am Acad Orthop Surg 2001;9:166–175.
23. Delcourt A, Huglo D, Prangere T, et al. Comparison between Leukoscan (Sulesomab) and Gallium-67 for the diagnosis of osteomyelitis in the diabetic foot. Diabetes Metab 2005;31:125–133.

24. Khatri G, Wagner DK, Sohnle PG. Effect of bone biopsy in guiding antimicrobial therapy for osteomyelitis complicating open wounds. Am J Med Sci 2001;321:367–371.
25. Zuluaga AF, Galvis W, Jaimes F, Vesga O. Lack of microbiological concordance between bone and non-bone specimens in chronic osteomyelitis: An observational study. BMC Infect Dis 2002;2:8–17.
26. Ezra E, Cohen N, Segev E, et al. Primary subacute epiphyseal osteomyelitis: Role of conservative treatment. J Pediatr Orthop 2002;22:333–337.
27. Ray PS, Simonis RB. Management of acute and chronic osteomyelitis. Hosp Med 2002;63:401–407.
28. Reinehr T, Burk G, Michel E, Andler W. Chronic osteomyelitis in childhood: Is surgery always indicated? Infection 2000;28:282–286.
29. Davis JS. Management of bone and joint infections due to *Staphylococcus aureus*. Internal Med J 2005;35:S79-S96.
30. Wang J, Li F, Calhoun JH, Mader JT. The role and effectiveness of adjunctive hyperbaric oxygen therapy in the management of musculoskeletal disorders. J Postgrad Med 2002;48:226–231.
31. Gitelis S, Brebach GT. The treatment of chronic osteomyelitis with a biodegradable antibiotic-impregnated implant. J Orthop Surg (Hong Kong) 2002;10:53–60.
32. Strauss MB, Bryant B. Hyperbaric oxygen. Orthopedics 2002;25:303–310.
33. Khatri G, Wagner DK, Sohnle PG. Effect of bone biopsy in guiding antimicrobial therapy for osteomyelitis complicating open wounds. Am J Med Science 2001;321:367–371.
34. Lazzarini L, Lipsky BA, Mader JT. Antibiotic treatment of osteomyelitis: what have we learned from 30 years of clinical trials? Int J Infect Dis 2005;9:127–138.
35. Le Saux N, Howard A, Barrowman NJ, et al. Shorter courses of parenteral antibiotic therapy do not appear to influence response rates for children with acute hematogenous osteomyelitis: A systematic review. BMC Infect Dis 2002;2:16–24.
36. Vinod MB, Matussek J, Curtis N, et al. Duration of antibiotics in children with osteomyelitis and septic arthritis. J Paediatr Child Health 2002;38:363–367.
37. Jaberi FM, Shahcheraghi GH, Ahadzadeh M. Short-term intravenous antibiotic treatment of acute hematogenous bone and joint infection in children: A prospective, randomized trial. J Pediatr Orthop 2002;22:317–320.
38. Guglielmo BJ, Luber AD, Paletta D, Jacobs RA. Ceftriaxone therapy for staphylococcal osteomyelitis: A review. Clin Infect Dis 2000;30:205–207.
39. Bradley JS, Nelson JD. 2002–2003 Nelson's Pocket Book of Pediatric Antimicrobial Therapy, 15th ed. Philadelphia, PA: Lippincott Williams & Wilkins, 2002:24.
40. Steer AC, Carapetis JR. Acute hematogenous osteomyelitis in children: Recognition and management. Paediatr Drugs 2004;6:333–346.
41. Darville T, Jacobs RF. Management of acute hematogenous osteomyelitis in children. Pediatr Infect Dis J 2004;23:255–257.
42. Greenberg RN, Newman MT, Shariaty S, Pectol RW. Ciprofloxacin, lomefloxacin, or levofloxacin as treatment for chronic osteomyelitis. Antimicrob Agents Chemother 2000;44:164–166.
43. Le Saux N, Howard A, Barrowman NJ, et al. Shorter courses of parenteral antibiotic therapy do not appear to influence response rates for children with acute hematogenous osteomyelitis: A systematic review. BMC Infect Dis 2002;2:16.
44. Shuford JA, Steckelberg JM. Role of oral antimicrobial therapy in the management of osteomyelitis. Curr Opin Infect Diseas 2003;16:515–519.
45. Greenberg RN, Newman MT, Shariaty S, Pectol RW. Ciprofloxacin, lomefloxacin, or levofloxacin as treatment for chronic osteomyelitis. Antimicrob Agents Chemother 2000;44:164–166.
46. Grady RW. Systemic quinolone antibiotics in children: A review of the use and safety. Expert Opin Drug Saf 2005;4:623–630.
47. Greenberg RN, Newman MT, Shariaty S, Pectol RW. Ciprofloxacin, lomefloxacin, or levofloxacin as treatment for chronic osteomyelitis. Antimicrob Agents Chemother 2000;44:164–166.
48. Stengel D, Bauwens K, Sehouli J, et al. Systematic review and meta-analysis of antibiotic therapy for bone and joint infections. Lancet Infect Dis 2001;1:175–188.
49. Andriole VT. The quinolones: Past, present, and future. Clin Infect Dis 2005;41(Suppl 2):S113–S119.
50. Till M, Wixson RL, Pertel PE. Linezolid treatment for osteomyelitis due to vancomycin-resistant *Enterococcus faecium*. Clin Infect Dis 2002;34:1412–1414.
51. Floyed RL, Steele RW. Culture-negative osteomyelitis. Pediatr Infect Dis J 2003;22:731–735.
52. Jones ME, Karlowsky JA, Draghi DC, et al. Antibiotic susceptibility of bacteria most commonly isolated from bone related infections: The role of cephalosporins in antimicrobial therapy. Int J Antimicrob Agents 2004;23:240–246.
53. Brem H, Sheehan P, Boulton AJ. Protocol for treatment of diabetic foot ulcers. Am J Surg 2004;187:1S-10S.
54. Aksoy DY, Gurlek A, Cetinkaya Y, et al. Change in the amputation profile in diabetic foot in a tertiary reference center: Efficacy of team working. Exp Clin Endocrinol Diabetes 2004;112:526–530.
55. Tice A. The use of outpatient parenteral antimicrobial therapy in the management of osteomyelitis: Data from the outpatient parenteral antimicrobial therapy outcomes registries. Chemotherapy 2001;47(Suppl 1):5–16.
56. Bernard L, Hajj E, Pron B, et al. Outpatient parenteral antimicrobial therapy (OPAT) for the treatment of osteomyelitis: Evaluation of efficacy, tolerance and cost. J Clin Pharm Ther 2001;26:445–451.
57. Tice AD, Hoaglund PA, Shoultz DA. Outcomes of osteomyelitis among patients treated with outpatient parenteral antimicrobial therapy. Am J Med 2003;114:723–728.
58. Gomez M, Maraqa N, Alvarez A, Rathore M. Complications of outpatient parenteral antibiotic therapy in childhood. Pediatr Infect Dis J 2001;20:541–543.
59. Tice AD, Hoaglund PA, Shoultz DA. Outcomes of osteomyelitis among patients treated with outpatient parenteral antimicrobial therapy. Am J Med 2003;114:723–728.
60. Cimmino MA. Recognition and management of bacterial arthritis. Drugs 1997;54:50–60.
61. Ross JJ. Septic arthritis. Infect Dis Clin North Am 2005;19:799–817.
62. De Boeck H. Osteomyelitis and septic arthritis in children. Acta Orthop Belg 2005;71:505–515.
63. Nade S. Septic arthritis. Best Pract Res Clin Rheumatol 2003;17:183–200.
64. Kim HKW, Alman B, Cole WG. A shortened course of parenteral antibiotic therapy in the management of acute septic arthritis of the hip. J Pediatr Orthop 2000;20:44–47.
65. Bardin T. Gonococcal arthritis. Best Pract Res Clin Rheumatol 2003;17:201–208.
66. Mathews CJ, Coakley G. Acute hot joint. Br J Hosp Med 2006;67:232–234.
67. Shirtliff ME, Mader JT. Acute septic arthritis. Clin Microbiol Rev 2002;15:527–544.
68. Kocher MS, Mandiga R, Murphy JM, et al. A clinical practice guideline for treatment of septic arthritis in children: Efficacy in improving process of care and effect on outcome of septic arthritis of the hip. J Bone Joint Surg Am 2003;85A:994–999.
69. Bernard L, El-Hajj PB, Lotthe A, et al. Outpatient parenteral antimicrobial therapy (OPAT) for the treatment of osteomyelitis: Evaluation of efficacy, tolerance and cost. J Clin Pharmacol Ther 2001;26:445–451.
70. Tavakoli M, Davey P, Clift BA, Davies HT. Diagnosis and management of osteomyelitis: Decision analytic and pharmacoeconomic considerations. Pharmacoeconomics 1999;16:627–647.
71. Eckman MH, Greenfield S, Mackey WC, et al. Foot infections in diabetic patients: Decision and cost-effectiveness. JAMA 1995;273:712–720.

CHAPTER 123 Sepsis and Septic Shock

S. LENA KANG-BIRKEN AND JOSEPH T. DIPIRO

KEY CONCEPTS

1. The spectrum of microorganisms associated with sepsis has changed from predominantly gram-negative bacteria in the late 1970s and 1980s to gram-positive bacteria as the major pathogens since 1987.
2. The incidence of fungal infections has increased threefold from 1979 to 2000, and despite the recent addition of several potent antifungal agents, mortality ranges from 41% to 71%.
3. Sepsis represents a complex pathophysiology, characterized by the activation of multiple overlapping and interacting cascades leading to systemic inflammation, a procoagulant state, and decreased fibrinolysis.
4. Mortality rates with sepsis are higher for patients with preexisting disease, intensive care unit (ICU) care and multiple organ failure.
5. Prompt, aggressive initiation of broad-spectrum, parenteral antibiotic therapy is required because of the high incidence of complications and mortality.
6. Significant fluid leaks from the vasculature occur with sepsis and initial fluid resuscitation with large volumes of fluid is required. There is no clinical outcome difference between colloids and crystalloids.
7. Norepinephrine is generally the preferred vasopressor to correct hypotension in septic shock over dopamine. Low-dose dopamine does not maintain or improve renal function.
8. Early goal-directed therapy of sepsis consisting of a hemodynamic monitoring with a central venous catheter, volume resuscitation, inotropic therapy, and red blood cell transfusions, demonstrated a significant clinical outcome benefit with a 16% absolute reduction in 28-day mortality.
9. Intensive insulin therapy maintaining the blood glucose level <150 mg per deciliter should be initiated to reduce the morbidity and mortality rates among critically ill patients without the increased risk of hypoglycemia.
10. Low-dose hydrocortisone therapy in patients with severe septic shock demonstrated a significant shock reversal and reduction of mortality rate in patients with relative adrenal insufficiency.
11. Recombinant human activated protein C, which has both anti-inflammatory and anticoagulant properties, was associated with a 6.1% reduction in 28-day all cause mortality in comparison to placebo.

Learning objectives, review questions, and other resources can be found at **www.pharmacotherapyonline.com.**

Sepsis represents a significant burden to the national health care system. In 2000, sepsis affected approximately 660,000 people, an increase of 8.7 % per year since 1979.[1] More than one-half of the patients were admitted to the ICU with a mean length of stay of 15.7 days.[2] The total number of deaths increased from 21.9 per 100,000 population in 1979 to 43.9 per 100,000 populations in 2000.[1] With the annual cost of approximately $16.7 billion, there remains a vital need for clinicians to comprehend the pathophysiology and to appreciate the management options available for acutely ill patients with sepsis or septic shock.[2]

DEFINITIONS

In 1992, a joint committee of the American College of Chest Physicians and the Society of Critical Care Medicine standardized the terminology related to sepsis for several reasons: (a) widespread confusion with the use of these terms; (b) the need to provide a flexible classification scheme for patient identification; (c) identification of an earlier therapeutic intervention; (d) standardization of research protocols.[3]

The criteria for the new terms provide specific physiologic variables that can be used to categorize a patient as having bacteremia, systemic inflammatory response syndrome (SIRS), sepsis, severe sepsis, septic shock, or multiple-organ dysfunction syndrome (MODS), suggesting an important continuum of progressive physiologic decline (Table 123–1). Introduction of the term SIRS reflects the knowledge that a physiologically similar systemic inflammatory response can be seen even in the absence of identifiable infection (Fig. 123–1).[4] Severe sepsis refers to patients with an acute organ dysfunction such as acute renal failure or respiratory failure. These patients have a mortality rate of approximately 40%.[5] Septic shock refers to sepsis patients with arterial hypotension that is refractory to adequate fluid resuscitation, thus requiring vasopressor administration. These patients usually require intensive care and ultimately die in 50% to 80% of cases.[2,5] It is important to note that progression from sepsis to MODS can occur in the absence of an intervening period of septic shock.

At the most recent consensus conference, the definitions were revised to include additional criteria for the diagnosis of SIRS and sepsis.[6] A new staging system was developed to facilitate a more accurate staging of sepsis disease and the associated risks and prognosis. However, extensive testing and further refinement is needed before clinical application.

INFECTION SITES AND PATHOGENS

The leading primary sites of microbiologically documented infections that led to sepsis were the respiratory tract (21%–68%), intraabdom-

TABLE 123-1 Definitions Related to Sepsis

Condition	Definition
Bacteremia (fungemia)	Presence of viable bacteria (fungi) in the bloodstream
Infection	Inflammatory response to invasion of normally sterile host tissue by the microorganisms
Systemic inflammatory response syndrome (SIRS)	Systemic inflammatory response to a variety of clinical insults that can be infectious or noninfectious etiology. The response is manifested by two or more of the following conditions: T >38°C (100.4°F) or <36°C (96.8°F); HR > 90 beats/min; RR > 20 breaths/min or Pa_{CO_2} <32 torr; WBC >12,000 cells/mm^3, <4,000 cells/mm^3, or >10% immature (band) forms; positive fluid balance (>20 mL/kg over 24 h); hyperglycemia; plasma C-reactive protein/procalcitonin >2 SD above normal value; arterial hypotension; cardiac index >3.5 L/min; arterial hypoxemia; acute oliguria; creatinine increase >0.5 mg/dL; coagulation abnormalities; ileus, platelets <100,000 mcL; bilirubin >4 mg/dL; hyperlactatemia; decreased capillary refill
Sepsis	The SIRS secondary to infection
Severe sepsis	Sepsis associated with organ dysfunction, hypoperfusion, or hypotension. Hypoperfusion and perfusion abnormalities can include, but are not limited to, lactic acidosis, oliguria, or acute alteration in mental status.
Septic shock	Sepsis with persistent hypotension despite fluid resuscitation, along with the presence of perfusion abnormalities. Patients who are on inotropic or vasopressor agents may not be hypotensive at the time perfusion abnormalities are measured.
Multiple-organ dysfunction syndrome (MODS)	Presence of altered organ function requiring intervention to maintain homeostasis

HR, heart rate; Pa_{CO_2}, arterial carbon dioxide tension; RR, respiratory rate; SD, standard deviation; T, temperature; WBC, white blood cell.

inal space (14%–22%), and urinary tract (14%–18%).[5,7–9] Although almost any microorganism can be associated with sepsis and septic shock, the most common etiologic pathogens are gram-positive bacteria (40% of patients), followed by gram-negative bacteria (38%) and fungi (17%).[5] Certain viruses and rickettsiae can produce a similar syndrome.

GRAM-POSITIVE BACTERIAL SEPSIS

❶ Since 1987, gram-positive organisms are the predominant pathogens in sepsis and septic shock, accounting for approximately 40% to 50% of all cases.[1] They are commonly caused by *Staphylococcus aureus, Streptococcus pneumoniae,* coagulase-negative staphylococci, and *Enterococcus* species. *Streptococcus pyogenes* and viridans streptococci are less commonly involved.[5,8–10]

S. pneumoniae sepsis is associated with an overall mortality rate of more than 25%. Factors related to a higher mortality include shock, respiratory insufficiency, preexisting renal failure, and the presence of a rapidly fatal underlying disease. *Staphylococcus epidermidis* is most often related to infected intravascular devices, such as artificial heart valves and stents and the use of intravenous and intraarterial catheters. The rates of nosocomial enterococcal bacteremia and associated sepsis are also increasing. Enterococci are isolated most commonly in blood cultures following a prolonged hospitalization and treatment with broad-spectrum cephalosporins.

GRAM-NEGATIVE BACTERIAL SEPSIS

A greater proportion of patients with gram-negative bacteremia develop clinical sepsis, and gram-negative bacteria are also more likely to produce septic shock in comparison to gram-positive organisms, 50% versus 25%, respectively.[8,11] Gram-negative sepsis also results in a higher mortality rate compared with sepsis from any other groups of organisms.[11–13] The major factor associated with the outcome of gram-negative sepsis appears to be the severity of any underlying condition. Patients with rapidly fatal conditions, such as acute leukemia, aplastic anemia, and >70% of the body's surface burn injury, have a significantly worse prognosis than do those patients with nonfatal underlying conditions, such as diabetes mellitus or chronic renal insufficiency.[1,2,11]

Escherichia coli and *Pseudomonas aeruginosa* are the most commonly isolated gram-negative microorganisms in sepsis.[5,7–11] Other common gram-negative pathogens include *Klebsiella* species, *Serratia* species, *Enterobacter* species, and *Proteus* species *P. aeruginosa,* although not considered a predominant endogenous flora, is found widely in the environment and is the most frequent cause of sepsis fatality. In a European study evaluating sepsis occurring in acutely ill patients, *P. aeruginosa* was isolated from 14% of all cultures.[5]

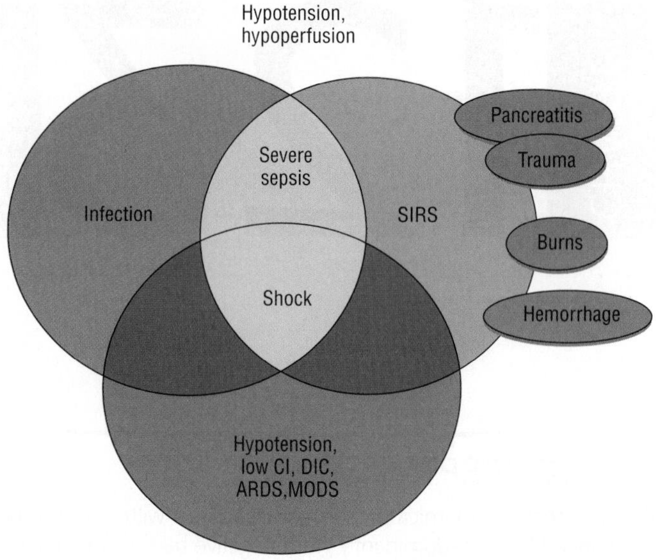

FIGURE 123-1. Relationship of infection, systemic inflammatory response syndrome (SIRS), sepsis, severe sepsis, and septic shock.

ANAEROBIC AND MISCELLANEOUS BACTERIAL SEPSIS

Anaerobes are usually considered low-risk organisms for the development of sepsis. If present, anaerobes are often found together with other pathogenic bacteria that are commonly found in sepsis. Epidemiology reports suggested that polymicrobial infections accounted for 5% to 39% of sepsis.[1,5,7–9] Mortality rates associated with polymicrobial infections are similar to sepsis caused by a single organism. Although some clinicians believe the particular combination of organisms present in polymicrobial sepsis can provide clues to the source of infection, no clear source for the infection can be identified in up to 25% of cases. Other less common pathogens include meningococcus, gonococcus, rickettsia, chlamydia, and spirochetes.

FUNGAL SEPSIS

❷ The rate of fungal infections increased more than 200% from 1979 to 2000.[1] *Candida* species are common causes of fungal sepsis in hospitalized patients. Although *Candida albicans* remains the most dominant species, non-*albicans Candida* species, particularly *Candida glabrata, Candida parapsilosis, Candida tropicalis,* and *Candida krusei,* have gradually emerged from 24% in the 1980s to 46% during 1997 to 2000.[12,13] Other fungi identified as causes of sepsis include Cryptococcus, Coccidioides, Fusarium, and Aspergillus. Risk factors for fungal infection include abdominal surgery, poorly controlled diabetes mellitus, prolonged granulocytopenia, broad-spectrum antibiotic treatment, corticosteroid treatment, prolonged hospitalization, central venous catheter, total parenteral nutrition, hematologic malignancy, and chronic, indwelling bladder (Foley) catheter.

Mortality ranges from 41% to 71% in patients with fungemia.[14] *Candida* species, the fourth most common bloodstream pathogens in all recent U.S. studies of nosocomial bloodstream infections, are associated with the highest mortality (40%) of all bloodstream pathogens. Hematologic diseases, neutropenia, and a higher number of positive blood cultures were associated with poor outcome irrespective of patient's gender, age, or days of antifungal drug treatment.

PATHOPHYSIOLOGY

The pathophysiologic sequelae resulting from the interaction between the invading pathogen and the human host are diverse and complex. Proinflammatory mediators that contribute to eradication of invading microorganisms are produced, and antiinflammatory mediators control this response. The inflammatory response leads to damage to host tissue and the antiinflammatory response causes leukocytes to activate. Once the balance to control the local inflammatory process to eradicate the invading pathogens is lost, systemic inflammatory response occurs, converting the infection to sepsis, severe sepsis, or septic shock.[15]

CELLULAR COMPONENTS FOR INITIATING THE INFLAMMATORY PROCESS

The pathophysiologic focus of gram-negative sepsis has been on the lipopolysaccharide component of the bacterial cell wall. Commonly referred to as endotoxin, this substance is unique to the outer membrane of the gram-negative cell wall, and is generally released with bacterial lysis. Lipid A, the innermost region of the lipopolysaccharide, is highly immunoreactive and is considered responsible for most of the toxic effects observed with gram-negative sepsis. Although lipid A can affect tissues directly, its predominant effect is to activate macrophages and trigger inflammatory cascades critical in the progression to sepsis and septic shock.[15] Endotoxin forms a complex with a protein called a *lipopolysaccharide-binding protein,* which then engages the CD14 receptor on the surface of a macrophage. Subsequently, cytokine mediators are activated and released.

In gram-positive sepsis, the exotoxin peptidoglycan appears to exhibit proinflammatory activity. Peptidoglycan comprises up to 40% of gram-positive cell mass, and is exposed on the cell wall surface. Although it competes with lipid A for similar binding sites on CD14, the potency of peptidoglycan is less than that of endotoxin.[15] However, an important feature of gram-positive bacteria is the production of potent exotoxins, some of which have been associated with septic shock.[16] Toxic shock syndromes have been reported with *S. aureus* producing toxic shock syndrome toxin-1 and *S. pyogenes* producing pyrogenic exotoxins.

PRO- AND ANTIINFLAMMATORY MEDIATORS

Sepsis involves activation of inflammatory pathways, and a complex interaction between proinflammatory and antiinflammatory mediators plays a major role in the pathogenesis of sepsis. The key proinflammatory mediators include tumor necrosis factor-α (TNF-α), interleukin-1 (IL-1), and interleukin-6 (IL-6), which are released by activated macrophages.[15,17–19] Other mediators that may be important for the pathogenesis of sepsis include interleukin-8 (IL-8), platelet-activating factor (PAF), leukotrienes, and thromboxane A_2.

The TNF-α is considered the primary mediator of sepsis.[17,19] Although the TNF-α levels can be increased in patients with a variety of diseases and in many healthy people, there is a correlation of TNF-α levels with the severity of sepsis. The TNF-α level is highly elevated very early in the inflammatory response in most patients with sepsis.[20] In meningococcemia, increased morbidity and mortality are associated with high plasma concentrations of TNF-α. The TNF-α release leads to activation of other cytokines (IL-1 and IL-6) associated with cellular damage.[18] In addition, TNF-α stimulates the release of cyclooxygenase-derived arachidonic acid metabolites (thromboxane A_2 and prostaglandins) that contribute to vascular endothelial damage. TNF-α also causes endothelial cells to express adhesion molecules, facilitating influx of granulocytes.

Although IL-1 levels have been inconsistently associated with sepsis, IL-6 is a more consistent predictor of sepsis as it remains elevated for a longer period of time than does TNF-α.[18] The highest circulating levels of IL-6 have been associated with severity and mortality.[21,22] A high level of IL-8 can be detected in blood during sepsis, and it appears to be related to sepsis severity and mortality.[17,23]

The significant antiinflammatory mediators include interleukin-1 receptor antagonist (IL-1RA), interleukin-4 (IL-4), and interleukin-10 (IL-10).[15,17–19] These antiinflammatory cytokines inhibit the production of the proinflammatory cytokines and down regulate some inflammatory cells. All antiinflammatory cytokines are produced in large amounts in sepsis. Levels of IL-10 and IL-1RA are higher in septic shock than in sepsis and higher levels are found among nonsurviving patients than in survivors.[17]

The net effect of a given mediator can vary depending on the state of activation of the target cell, the presence of other mediators near the target cell, and the ability of the target cell to release mediators that can augment or inhibit the primary mediator. As Fig. 123–2 illustrates, when there is a systemic spillover of excessive proinflammatory mediators, the patient presents with SIRS and possibly

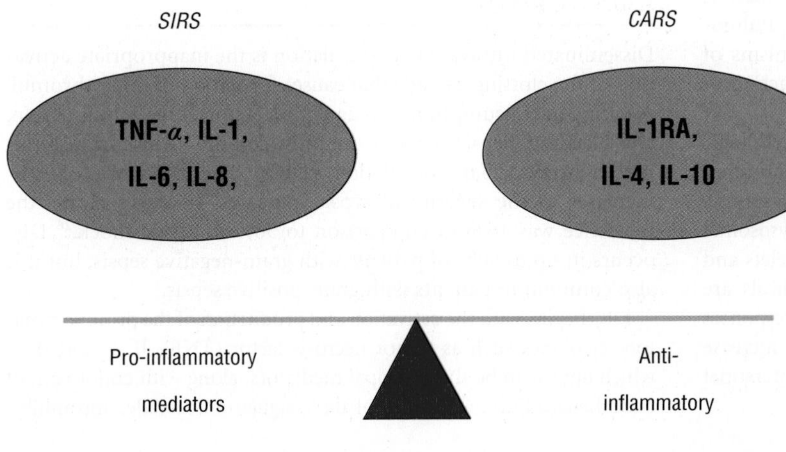

FIGURE 123-2. The balance between pro- and antiinflammatory mediators. (CARS, compensatory antiinflammatory response syndrome; IL, interleukin; IL-1RA, interleukin-1 receptor antagonist; SIRS, systemic inflammatory response syndrome; TNF-α, tumor necrosis factor-α.)

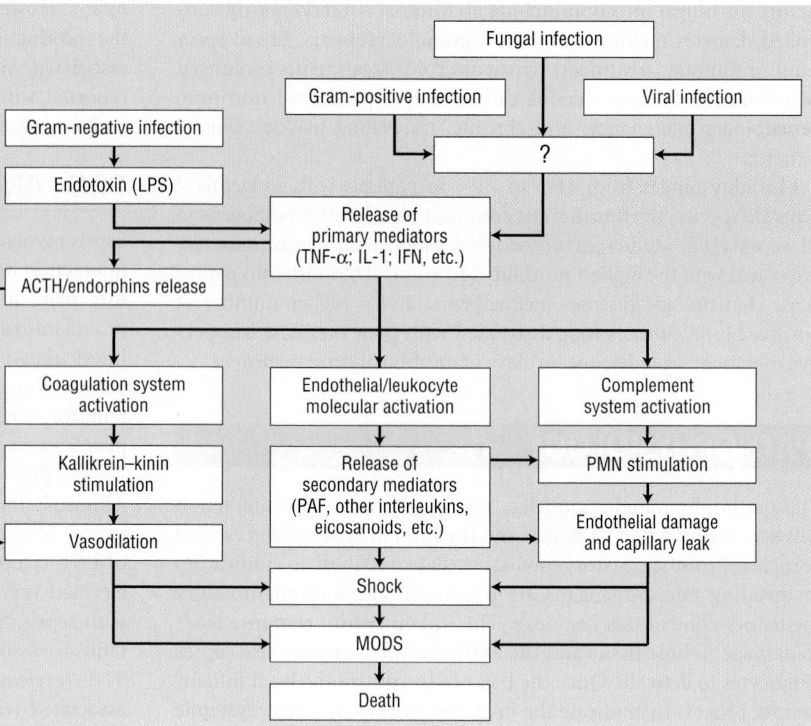

FIGURE 123-3. Cascades of sepsis. (ACTH, adrenocorticotropic hormone.)

MODS. Shortly after this initial phase, counterregulatory pathways become activated, and there is a systemic spillover of excessive antiinflammatory mediators, representing a compensatory anti-inflammatory response syndrome (CARS). The balance between pro- and antiinflammatory mechanisms determines the degree of inflammation, ranging from local antibacterial activity to systemic tissue toxicity or organ failure.[15]

CASCADE OF SEPSIS

❸ The cascade leading to development of sepsis is complex and multifactorial, involving various mediators and cell lines (Fig. 123–3).[15–17,19] Through the actions of the mediators, a variety of cells become activated, initiating detrimental cascades. Initially, macrophages become activated and produce inflammatory cytokines. These cytokines then influence a wide range of cells, including endothelial cells, lymphocytes, hepatocytes, neutrophils, and platelets. Endothelial cells that respond to and produce a variety of cytokines mediate a primary mechanism of injury with sepsis. When injured, endothelial cells allow circulating cells such as granulocytes and plasma constituents to enter inflamed tissues, which can result in organ damage.

The microcirculation is affected by sepsis-induced inflammation.[24] The arterioles become less responsive to either vasoconstrictors or vasodilators. The capillaries are less perfused, and there is neutrophil infiltration and protein leakage into the venules. Pulmonary dysfunction can result from the destructive mechanisms of neutrophils that are attracted to lung tissue through the action of mainly IL-8.

Activation of complement in sepsis leads to pathophysiologic consequences including generation of anaphylactic toxins and other substances that augment or exaggerate the inflammatory response. Stimulation of leukocyte chemotaxis, phagocytosis with lysosomal enzyme release, increased aggregation and adhesion of platelets and neutrophils, and the production of toxic superoxide radicals are attributed, in part, to complement activation. Among these responses are the release of histamine from mast cells and the resultant increase in capillary permeability and the "third-spacing" of fluid in interstitial spaces.

The inflammatory process in sepsis is also directly linked to the coagulation system. Proinflammatory mechanisms that promote sepsis are also procoagulant and antifibrinolytic, whereas fibrinolytic mechanisms can be antiinflammatory. A key endogenous substance involved in inflammation of sepsis is activated protein C, which enhances fibrinolysis and inhibits inflammation. Levels of protein C are reduced in patients with sepsis.[25]

COMPLICATIONS

The majority of patients with severe sepsis have dysfunction of two organs and the three most frequent organ dysfunctions were respiratory, circulatory, and renal.[9] Shock is the most ominous complication associated with sepsis, and mortality occurs in approximately one-half of the patients with septic shock. Severe hypotension appears to be caused, in part, by the release of vasoactive peptides, such as bradykinin and serotonin, and by endothelial cell damage leading to the extravasation of fluids into interstitial spaces. Septic shock is associated with several complications including disseminated intravascular coagulation, acute respiratory distress syndrome, and multiple organ failure.

DISSEMINATED INTRAVASCULAR COAGULATION

Disseminated intravascular coagulation is the inappropriate activation of the clotting cascade that causes formation of microthrombi, resulting in consumption of coagulation factors, organ dysfunction, and bleeding. Sepsis remains the most common cause of disseminated intravascular coagulation (DIC). The incidence of DIC increases as the severity of sepsis increases. In sepsis alone, the incidence was 16% in comparison to 38% in septic shock.[26] DIC occurs in up to 50% of patients with gram-negative sepsis, but it is also common in patients with gram-positive sepsis.

DIC begins with the activation and production of the proinflammatory cytokines such as tumor necrosis factor (TNF), IL-1, and IL-6, which appear to be the principal mediators, along with endotoxin, of endothelial injury, activation of the coagulation cascade, and inhibition of fibrinolysis. The combination of excessive fibrin formation, inhibited fibrin removal from a depressed fibrinolytic system, and endothelial injury results in microvascular thrombosis and DIC.[26]

Complications of DIC vary and depend on the target organ affected and severity of the coagulopathy. DIC can produce acute renal failure, hemorrhagic necrosis of the gastrointestinal mucosa, liver failure, acute pancreatitis, acute respiratory distress syndrome, and pulmonary failure. Furthermore, as the procoagulant state appears to be the key in the pathogenesis of MODS, coagulation dysfunction and MODS often coexist in sepsis.

ACUTE RESPIRATORY DISTRESS SYNDROME

Pulmonary dysfunction usually precedes dysfunction in other organs, and it can even initiate the development of SIRS with resultant MODS. Activated neutrophils and platelets adhere to the pulmonary capillary endothelium, initiating multiple inflammatory cascades with a release of a variety of toxic substances. There is diffuse pulmonary endothelial cell injury, increased capillary permeability, and alveolar epithelial cell injury.[27] Consequently, interstitial pulmonary edema occurs that gradually progresses to alveolar flooding and collapse. The end result is loss of functional alveolar volume, impaired pulmonary compliance, and profound hypoxemia.

A large body of basic and preclinical evidence has implicated abnormalities of pathways of fibrin turnover in the pathogenesis of acute inflammation and fibrotic repair.[28,29] Coagulation is locally upregulated in the injured lung, whereas fibrinolytic activity is depressed. These abnormalities occur concurrently and favor alveolar fibrin deposition. Preliminary data indicate that anticoagulant interventions that block the extrinsic coagulation pathway can protect against the development of pulmonary fibrin deposition as well as lung dysfunction and acute inflammation.[29] Overall, fibrin deposition in the injured lung as well as abnormalities of coagulation and fibrinolysis are integral to the pathogenesis of acute respiratory distress syndrome (ARDS).

HEMODYNAMIC EFFECTS

The hallmark of the hemodynamic effect of sepsis is the hyperdynamic state characterized by high cardiac output and an abnormally low systemic vascular resistance (SVR).[30] TNF-α and endotoxin directly depress cardiovascular function. Endotoxin depresses left ventricular function independent of changes in left ventricular volume or vascular resistance.

Persistent hypotension raises concern for the balance of oxygen delivery (DO_2) to the tissues and oxygen consumption (VO_2) by the tissues.[27,30] Sepsis results in a distributive shock characterized by inappropriately increased blood flow to selected tissues at the expense of other tissues, which is independent of specific tissue oxygen needs. This perfusion defect is accentuated by an increased precapillary atrioventricular shunt. If perfusion decreases, oxygen extraction increases, and the arteriovenous oxygen gradient widens. Cellular DO_2 is decreased, but VO_2 remains unaffected. When increased oxygen demand occurs without increased blood flow, the increased VO_2 is compensated by increased oxygen extraction. If perfusion decreases sufficiently in the face of high metabolic demands, then the reserve DO_2 can be exceeded, and tissue ischemia results. Significant tissue ischemia leads to organ dysfunction and failure. Therefore, systemic DO_2 relative to VO_2 should be optimized by increasing oxygen delivery or decreasing oxygen consumption in a hypermetabolic patient.

ACUTE RENAL FAILURE

Renal dysfunction such as acute oliguric or anuric renal failure occurs in approximately one quarter of the patients, and in the event of severe sepsis and MODS, renal dysfunction is potentially lethal with a mortality of 50% to 90%.[2,27] Without normal urine output, fluid overload in extravascular space including the lungs develops, leading to impairment of pulmonary gas exchange and severe hypoxemia. Consequently, compromised oxygen delivery would exacerbate peripheral ischemia and organ damage.[31] Adequate renal perfusion and a trial of loop diuretics should be initiated promptly in oliguric or anuric patients with MODS. In addition, renal replacement therapy such as continuous hemofiltration or intermittent hemodialysis should be used to facilitate volume and electrolytes.[32,33]

CLINICAL PRESENTATION

Table 123–2 lists some of the common clinical features of sepsis, although a number of these findings are not limited to infectious processes. The initial clinical presentation can be referred to as signs and symptoms of early sepsis, and they typically include fever, chills, and change in mental status. Hypothermia can occur with a systemic infection, and this is often associated with a poor prognosis.[3,6] In patients with sepsis caused by gram-negative bacilli, hyperventilation can occur even before fever and chills, and it can lead to respiratory alkalosis as the earliest metabolic change.

Progression of uncontrolled sepsis leads to clinical evidence of organ system dysfunction as represented by the signs and symptoms attributed to late sepsis. With the exception of rapidly progressing cases as in meningococcemia, *P. aeruginosa*, or *Aeromonas* infection, the onset of shock is slow and usually follows a period of several hours of hemodynamic instability. Oliguria often follows hypotension. Increased glycolysis with impaired clearance of the resulting lactate by the liver and kidneys and tissue hypoxia because of hypoperfusion result in elevated lactate levels, contributing to metabolic acidosis. Altered glucose metabolism, including impaired gluconeogenesis and excessive insulin release, is evidenced by either hyperglycemia or hypoglycemia. The distinction between early and late sepsis is arbitrary, and it is recognized that sepsis represents a spectrum of clinical findings.

PROGNOSIS

❹ As the patient progresses from SIRS to sepsis to severe sepsis to septic shock, mortality increases in a stepwise fashion. Mortality rates are higher for patients with advanced age, preexisting disease including chronic obstructive pulmonary disease, neoplasm, and human immunodeficiency virus (HIV) disease, ICU care, more organ failure, positive blood cultures, and *Pseudomonas* species infection.[5,9] Mortality increased with age from 10% in children to 38.4% in those ≥85

TABLE 123-2 Signs and Symptoms Associated with Sepsis

Early Sepsis	Late Sepsis
Fever or hypothermia	Lactic acidosis
Rigors, chills	Oliguria
Tachycardia	Leukopenia
Tachypnea	DIC
Nausea, vomiting	Myocardial depression
Hyperglycemia	Pulmonary edema
Myalgias	Hypotension (shock)
Lethargy, malaise	Hypoglycemia
Proteinuria	Azotemia
Hypoxia	Thrombocytopenia
Leukocytosis	ARDS
Hyperbilirubinemia	Gastrointestinal hemorrhage
	Coma

ARDS, acute respiratory distress syndrome; DIC, disseminated intravascular coagulation.

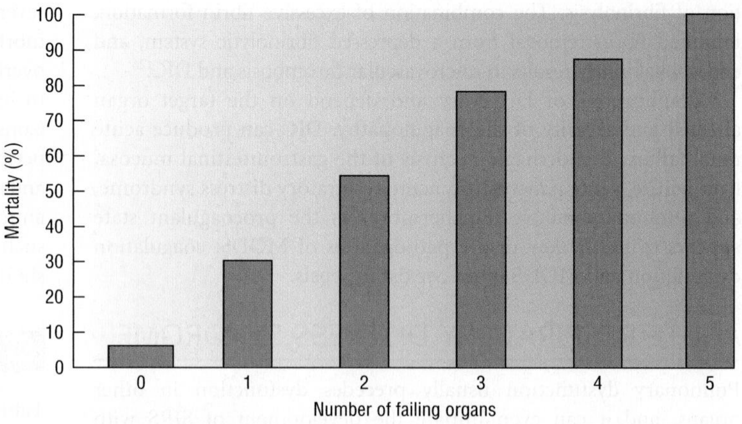

FIGURE 123-4. Mortality related to the number of failing organs.

years.[2] ICU admission was required in 51.1% of the patients with severe sepsis and of those patients, mortality was reported in 34.1%.[2] Mortality from severe sepsis and MODS is most closely related to the number of dysfunctioning organs. As the number of failing organs increased from two to five, mortality increased from 54% to 100% (Fig. 123–4).[27] Duration of organ dysfunction can also affect the overall mortality rate.

An elevated lactate concentration of >4 mmol/L in the presence of the SIRS significantly increases intensive care unit admission rates, and persistent elevations in lactate for more than 24 hours are associated with a mortality rate as high as 89%.[34] Inversely, patients with higher lactate clearance after 6 hours of emergency department intervention have improved outcome compared with those lower lactate clearance. There was an approximately 11% decrease likelihood of mortality for each 10% increase in lactate clearance.[34]

TREATMENT

In 2003, a surviving sepsis campaign guideline for management of severe sepsis and septic shock was developed as an international effort to increase awareness and improve outcome in severe sepsis.[35] The primary goals of therapy for patients with sepsis include (a) timely diagnosis and identification of pathogen; (b) rapid elimination of the source of infection medically and/or surgically; (c) early initiation of aggressive antimicrobial therapy; (d) interruption of pathogenic sequence leading to septic shock; (e) avoidance of organ failure. Supportive care such as stress ulcer prophylaxis and nutritional support is important to prevent complications during the stay in the intensive care unit. Table 123–3 describes the summary of the surviving sepsis campaign treatment recommendations.

■ DIAGNOSIS AND IDENTIFICATION OF PATHOGEN

The presence of clinical features suggesting sepsis should prompt further evaluation of the patient. In addition to obtaining a careful history of any underlying conditions and recent travel, injury, animal exposure, infection or use of antibiotics, a complete physical examination should be performed to determine the source of the infection.

A collection of specimens should be sent for culture prior to initiating any antimicrobial therapy. Generally, at least two sets of blood samples from a peripheral vein and through a vascular access device should be obtained for aerobic and anaerobic culture. In critically ill septic patients, two or three sets of blood cultures should be collected without temporal separation between the sets.[36] With suspected catheter-related infection, a pair of blood cultures obtained through the catheter hub and a peripheral site should be obtained simultaneously.[36] In severe community-acquired pneumonia, blood

TABLE 123-3 Evidence-Based Treatment Recommendations for Sepsis and Septic Shock

Recommendations	Recommendation Grades[a]
Antibiotic therapy	
Use a broad initial empirical antibiotic regimen against all likely pathogens	D
There is no evidence of higher efficacy with combination therapy	E
Fluid therapy	
Immediate initial resuscitation of a patient in severe sepsis or sepsis-induced tissue hypoperfusion should be instituted to achieve central venous pressure 8–12 mm Hg, mean arterial pressure ≥65 mm Hg, urine output ≥0.5 mL/kg/h, central venous or mixed venous oxygen saturation ≥70%	B
There is no clinical outcome difference between colloids and crystalloids	C
Vasopressors	
The advantages of norepinephrine and dopamine over epinephrine (potential tachycardia, possibly disadvantageous effects on splanchnic circulation) and phenylephrine (decrease in stroke volume) are not supported by the literature.	D
There is no support of low doses of dopamine to maintain or improve renal function	B
Inotropic therapy	
Dobutamine as the first-choice inotrope to increase cardiac output combined with norepinephrine in the presence of low blood pressure is not supported in the literature.	E
Glucose control	
There is minimal support for maintaining blood glucose <150 mg/dL to improve survival	D
Steroids	
The value of intravenous hydrocortisone 200–300 mg/day for 7 days in three or four divided doses in patients with septic shock is not clear.	C
The use of fludrocortisone 50 mcg orally per day is not supported	E
Drotrecogin	
Drotrecogin is effective in patients at high risk of death (Acute Physiology and Chronic Health Evaluation II >25, sepsis-induced multiple organ failure, septic shock, or sepsis-induced acute respiratory distress syndrome)	B
Deep vein thrombosis prophylaxis	
Either low-dose unfractionated heparin or low-molecular weight heparin are effective in preventing deep vein thrombosis	A
Stress ulcer prophylaxis	
H_2 receptor inhibitors are more efficacious than sucralfate	A

[a]Grading of recommendations: A, B, C, D, E = at least two level I investigations, one level I investigation, level II investigations, at least one level III investigation, and level IV or V evidence to support recommendation, respectively. Quality of evidence: I = Large, randomized trials with clear-cut results; low risk of false-positive (alpha) error or false-negative (beta) error. II = Small, randomized trials with uncertain results; moderate-to-high risk of false-positive and/or false-negative error. III = Nonrandomized, contemporaneous controls. IV = Nonrandomized, historical controls and expert opinion. V = Case series, uncontrolled studies, and expert opinion.

Data from Dellinger RP, Carlet JM, Masur H, et al. Surviving sepsis campaign guidelines for management of severe sepsis and septic shock. Crit Care Med 2004;32:858–873.

cultures and respiratory secretions must be obtained. Urinary antigen detection of *Legionella* serogroup 1 is recommended during outbreaks. To document a soft tissue infection, a Gram stain and bacterial culture of any obvious wound exudates should be performed. A needle aspiration of a closed infection such as cellulitis or abscess may be needed for stain and bacterial culture. In abdominal infections, fluid collections identified by imaging studies should be aspirated for Gram stains and aerobic and anaerobic cultures.[36] A lumbar puncture is indicated in case of mental alteration, severe headache, or a seizure, assuming there are no focal cranial lesions identified by computed tomography scan. Further tests can be indicated to assess any systemic organ dysfunction caused by severe sepsis. The laboratory tests should include hemoglobin, white blood cell count with differential, platelet count, complete chemistry profile, coagulation parameters, serum lactate, and arterial blood gases.

ELIMINATION OF SOURCE OF INFECTION

After the source of infection is identified, prompt efforts to remove or to eliminate the source should be initiated.[37] With an infected intravascular catheter, the catheter should be removed and cultured. Urinary tract catheters should be removed if association with sepsis is suspected. Suspicion of soft tissue (cellulitis or wound infection) or bone involvement should lead to aggressive débridement of the affected area. Evidence of an abscess or sepsis associated with any intraabdominal pathology should prompt surgical intervention.

ANTIMICROBIAL THERAPY

(5) Aggressive, early antimicrobial therapy is critical in the management of septic patients because of high incidence of complications and mortality. Because of the inherent problems associated with the timely identification of the infecting organism or organisms, empiric antimicrobial regimens are usually started initially. Selection of empiric regimen should be based on the suspected site of infection, the most likely pathogens, acquisition of the organism from the community or hospital, the patient's immune status, and the antibiotic susceptibility and resistance profile for the institution. All patients should be treated initially with parenteral antibiotics for optimal drug concentrations within the first hour of recognition of severe sepsis after appropriate cultures have been taken.[35] Empiric therapy for an immunocompromised patient should be broad enough to cover likely pathogens and penetrate into the presumed infection site.[35] Once the pathogen and its susceptibility pattern are known, antimicrobial regimen should be modified accordingly.

Pathophysiologic changes have been reported in sepsis. These changes can affect drug distribution and different dosing regimens are required in critically ill patients with sepsis.[38] Initially high creatinine clearance can be seen in patients with normal serum creatinine because of increased renal preload. Volume of distribution can increase because of leaky capillaries and/or altered protein binding. Consequently, some antimicrobial agents including aminoglycosides, β-lactams and carbapenems, and vancomycin can achieve lower peak serum concentrations. However, as sepsis progresses, organ perfusion decreases because of significant myocardial depression and leads to multiple organ dysfunction. Consequently, clearance of antimicrobial agents is decreased, prolonging the elimination half-life and accumulation of metabolites.

Selection of Antimicrobial Agents

In a study evaluating 904 patients with microbiologically confirmed severe sepsis or septic shock, appropriate initial antimicrobial therapy was an important determinant of survival.[7] The 28-day mortality was 24% in patients who received appropriate initial antimicrobial treatment versus 39% in those who received inappropriate initial treatment. The overall incidence of inappropriate antibiotics treatment ranged from 14.5% to 52.8% among critically ill adult patients.[8,39]

Table 123–4 lists antimicrobial regimens that can be used empirically based on the possible source of infection. In the nonneutropenic patient with urinary tract infection, fluoroquinolones are generally recommended. In case of increased risk of *P. aeruginosa* in sepsis or hospital-acquired infections, an antipseudomonal antibiotic, such as ceftazidime is recommended.[40] *S. pneumoniae* is the most common cause of community-acquired pneumonia, and it accounts for approximately 60% of all deaths. The rising incidence of penicillin-resistant *S. pneumoniae* requires empiric use of newer "respiratory" fluoroquinolones. Newer fluoroquinolones, such as levofloxacin, moxifloxacin, and gemifloxacin can be used as monotherapy as they offer excellent coverage against penicillin-resistant pneumococci and aerobic gram-negative bacteria, as well as atypical pathogens including *Legionella pneumophila, Mycoplasma pneumoniae,* and *Chlamydia pneumoniae.*[41,42] Clarithromycin and azithromycin, are very effective against atypical pathogens and better tolerated than erythromycin.

In nosocomial pneumonia, enteric gram-negative bacteria such as *Enterobacter* and *Klebsiella* species and *P. aeruginosa* are the major pathogens in addition to *S. aureus.* If *P. aeruginosa* infection is suspected, a short course of aminoglycoside (5 days) should be added to antipseudomonal penicillin or third- or fourth-generation cephalosporin because of the high mortality rate associated with *Pseudomonas* infection.[39,43] When an aminoglycoside is undesirable, an antipseudomonal fluoroquinolone such as ciprofloxacin or levofloxacin can be used instead. In case of pneumonia caused by methicillin-resistant *S. aureus*, linezolid may be preferred over vancomycin because of the poor penetration of vancomycin into the lungs as well as worldwide emergence of glycopeptide-intermediately resistant *S. aureus.*[44,45]

Secondary peritonitis as a consequence of perforation of the gastrointestinal tract is usually polymicrobial involving enteric aerobes and anaerobes, and as many as five organisms are isolated per patient.

TABLE 123-4 Empiric Antimicrobial Regimens in Sepsis

Infection (Site or Type)	Antimicrobial Regimen: ***Community-Acquired***	***Hospital-Acquired***	
Urinary tract	Ciprofloxacin or levofloxacin	Ciprofloxacin, levofloxacin or ceftazidime, ceftriaxone	± gentamicin
Respiratory tract	Newer fluoroquinolone[a] or ceftriaxone + clarithromycin/azithromycin	Piperacillin, ceftazidime, or cefepime	+ gentamicin or ciprofloxacin
Intraabdominal	β-Lactamase inhibitor combo[b] or ciprofloxacin + metronidazole	Piperacillin/tazobactam or carbapenem	
Skin/soft tissue	Vancomycin or linezolid or daptomycin	β-Lactamase inhibitor combo[b] or clindamycin plus ciprofloxacin or carbapenem	
Catheter-related		Vancomycin	
Unknown		Piperacillin or ceftazidime/cefepime or imipenem/meropenem	+ gentamicin ± vancomycin

[a]Levofloxacin, moxifloxacin, gemifloxacin.
[b]Ampicillin/sulbactam, ticarcillin/clavulanic acid, piperacillin/tazobactam.

In addition to surgical intervention, broad-spectrum antibiotics such as β-lactamase inhibitor combination agents (piperacillin/tazobactam or ticarcillin/clavulanate) are appropriate in intraabdominal infections.[46] Carbapenems such as imipenem and meropenem are indicated in treatment of resistant pathogens including Enterobacteriaceae and *P. aeruginosa* in critically ill patients.[47] Differences between the two drugs are subtle. Imipenem generally exhibits more potent in-vitro activity against gram-positive bacteria and meropenem against gram-negative rods, but the clinical difference has not been observed. Meropenem has been initially described as better tolerated than imipenem, but recent reports on seizure rates for the two carbapenem are similar.[47,48] Metronidazole is preferred in infections caused by anaerobes as it remains active against >99% of anaerobes including *Bacteroides*, *Prevotella*, and *Porphyromonas* species.[49]

In skin and skin-structure infections, there is a concern over a growing resistance to macrolide among *S. pyogenes*. The Centers for Disease Control and Prevention reported the national surveillance data demonstrating increase in macrolide resistance from 4% to 5% in 1996 through 1998 to 8% to 9% in 1999 through 2001. However, 99.5% of strains remained susceptible to clindamycin, and 100% were susceptible to penicillin.[50] In the case of *S. aureus*, the empiric agents effective against methicillin-resistant *S. aureus* (MRSA) should be initiated because of the high prevalence of community-associated MRSA strains.[50,51] Vancomycin, daptomycin, and linezolid have comparable clinical efficacy and safety data for complicated skin and skin-structure infections caused by MRSA.[52,53]

The antimicrobial regimen should be reassessed after 48 to 72 hours based on the microbiological and clinical data. A narrow-spectrum antibiotic should be used to prevent development of resistant organisms, to reduce toxicity, and to reduce costs. Although there is no evidence that combination therapy is more effective than monotherapy, some experts prefer combination therapy for patients with *Pseudomonas* infections and for neutropenic patients with severe sepsis or septic shock.[35]

In addition to selecting the most appropriate antimicrobial agents, a clinician must ensure effective antibiotic usage such as proper dosing, interval administration, optimal duration of treatment, monitoring of drug levels when appropriate, and avoidance of unwanted drug interactions. Lack of adherence to these requirements can lead to suboptimal or excessive tissue concentrations that can promote antibiotic resistance, toxicity, and inadequate efficacy despite appropriate antibiotic selection.

CLINICAL CONTROVERSY

The rationale of antibiotic combination therapy for severe infections includes broadening the antibacterial spectrum, exertion of additive or synergistic effects, and possible reduction of emergence of resistant bacteria or superinfection. Earlier studies have evaluated combinations such as a β-lactam and an aminoglycoside.[54,55] However, superiority of the combination therapy over single-agent therapy was not demonstrated with the exception of those patients with rapidly declining diseases such as severe sepsis. With the introduction of highly bactericidal, broad-spectrum antibiotics such as piperacillin/tazobactam, ceftazidime, cefepime, and the carbapenems, more studies have compared the efficacy and toxicities of monotherapy against a β-lactam and an aminoglycoside combination regimen during the last two decades.

Monotherapy with a broad-spectrum β-lactam antibiotic is as efficacious and less toxic than a combination of β-lactam and an aminoglycoside as empirical therapy for critically ill patients with severe sepsis or septic shock.[35,54] However, it would be premature to initiate monotherapy for all patients with severe sepsis as standard of care because of limitations in the clinical trials such as small sample sizes (less than 200 patients) and the variability in antimicrobials used.[55,56]

Antifungal Therapy

Candida species are most frequently associated with fungal infections, and the resulting candidemia is frequently associated with sepsis syndrome and a high mortality rate.[12,13,57] Treatment of invasive candidiasis involves amphotericin B–based preparations, the azole antifungal agents, the echinocandin antifungal agents, or combination therapy with fluconazole plus amphotericin B. The choice depends on the clinical status of the patient, fungal species and its susceptibility, the relative drug toxicity, the presence of organ dysfunction that would affect drug clearance, and the patient's prior exposure to antifungal agents.

CLINICAL CONTROVERSY

Three new lipid formulations of amphotericin (amphotericin B lipid complex, amphotericin B cholesteryl sulfate, and liposomal amphotericin B) offer several advantages over amphotericin B deoxycholate.[58] They are less nephrotoxic, allow increased daily dose, have high tissue concentrations in the reticuloendothelial organs such as lungs, liver, and spleen, and have decreased infusion-associated side effects. However, superior clinical efficacy over the conventional amphotericin B or between the lipid formulations has not clearly been established in comparative clinical trials. Higher cost and the lack of overall benefit of using a lipid formulation have led to placing the lipid-associated preparations as primarily for patients who are intolerant of or have an infection refractory to the deoxycholate preparation.[59] However, recent data reported association of amphotericin B–induced nephrotoxicity with increased mortality, up to 6.6-fold, suggesting the usage of a lipid formulation initially for those patients at high risk of being intolerant.[57,60]

Fluconazole is less toxic and easier to administer than amphotericin B. However, fluconazole resistance among *C. albicans* has been well described among HIV-infected individuals and is increasing in immunocompetent adults.[57] *Candida glabrata* often has reduced susceptibility to fluconazole. Itraconazole exhibits a similar activity profile as fluconazole, and is well known to be active against mucosal forms of candidiasis. However, formal clinical trials using intravenous itraconazole are not available for invasive candidiasis. Voriconazole appears to be active against *Candida* species including fluconazole-resistant isolates. A recently completed worldwide study will aid in analyzing voriconazole for the indication of treatment of serious invasive, fluconazole-resistant *Candida* infections including *C. krusei*.[57,61]

Caspofungin, the first echinocandin antifungal agent appears to be potent against all *Candida* species including *C. glabrata, C. krusei,* and *Candida lusitaniae,* and *Aspergillus* species. Intravenous caspofungin was equally effective but better tolerated than amphotericin B deoxycholate for invasive candidiasis.[62] Recently, two more echinocandin antifungal agents, micafungin and anidulafungin, were approved. Open label trials evaluating the efficacy of micafungin for patients with invasive candidiasis demonstrated approximately 85% clinical response rate.[63,64] In an open-label dose, dose-ranging study evaluating anidulafungin, higher success rates were observed in the groups of 100 mg and 150 mg (85% and 83%, respectively), compared to the 50 mg group (72%).[65]

In general, suspected systemic mycotic infection leading to sepsis in neutropenic and critically ill patients should be empirically treated with parenteral amphotericin B or caspofungin especially if the patient is clinically unstable because of its greater activity against fluconazole-resistant *Candida* species and non-*albicans* species including *C. glabrata* and *C. krusei*.[57,66] To date, there is no data on the efficacy of voriconazole compared with that of echinocandins in the management of invasive candidiasis.

Inadequate antimicrobial treatment is an independent determinant of hospital mortality, and fungal bloodstream infections are associated with the highest rates of inappropriate initial treatment. Empirical fluconazole therapy for suspected nosocomial blood stream infections can be appropriate for hospitalized patients at high risk for fungal infections including those receiving total parenteral nutrition, with bowel perforation, or with persistent or new signs and symptoms of infections despite receiving broad-spectrum antibacterial therapy. Of the patients with candidemia, mortality rates were lowest for patients who began empirical fluconazole therapy on day 0 (15%) and highest for patients who began on day 3 or later (41%).[67] Although prompt empirical fluconazole therapy significantly impacts mortality of the hospitalized patients with candidemia, it can increase overprescribing of antifungal agents for patients without candidemia. Rapid diagnostic tests or identification of unique risk factors for bloodstream infections caused by *Candida* species are needed.

Duration of Therapy

The average duration of antimicrobial therapy in the normal host with sepsis is 7 to 10 days and fungal infections can require 10 to14 days.[7,35,43,57] However, the duration can vary depending on the site of the infection, as well as the overall response to therapy. After the patient is hemodynamically stable, has been afebrile for 48 to 72 hours, has a normalizing white blood cell (WBC) count, and is able to take oral medications, then a "step-down" from parenteral to oral antibiotics can be considered for the remaining duration of therapy. Treatment can continue considerably longer if the infection is persistent. In a neutropenic patient, therapy is usually continued until the patient is no longer neutropenic and has been afebrile for at least 72 hours.

■ HEMODYNAMIC SUPPORT

A high cardiac output and a low systemic vascular resistance characterize septic shock. Patients can have hypotension as a result of low systemic vascular resistance and abnormal distribution of blood flow in the microcirculation, resulting in compromised tissue perfusion. Because approximately half of patients with septic shock die of multiple organ system failure, they should be monitored carefully and aggressive hemodynamic support should be initiated.

Hemodynamics change rapidly in sepsis, and noninvasive evaluation can give inaccurate assessment of filling pressures and cardiac output, requiring a right-sided heart catheter in an intensive care unit.[68] Hemodynamic support can be divided into three main categories: fluid therapy, vasopressor therapy, and inotropic therapy.

Fluid Therapy

❻ Septic patients have enormous fluid requirements as a result of peripheral vasodilation and capillary leakage.[68] Rapid fluid resuscitation is the best initial therapeutic intervention for treatment of hypotension in sepsis. In approximately 50% of septic patients who initially present with hypotension, fluids alone will reverse hypotension and restore hemodynamic stability. The goal of fluid therapy is to maximize cardiac output by increasing the left ventricular preload, which will ultimately restore tissue perfusion.[68] Fluid administration should be titrated to clinical endpoints such as heart rate, urine output, blood pressure, and mental status. An increased serum lactate, a by-product of cellular anaerobic metabolism, should normalize as the tissue perfusion improves.

Isotonic crystalloids, such as 0.9% sodium chloride (normal saline) or lactated Ringer solution are commonly used for fluid resuscitation. A patient in septic shock typically requires up to 10 L of crystalloid solution during the first 24-hour period. These solutions distribute into the extracellular compartment. Approximately 25% of the infused volume of crystalloid remains in the intravascular space, whereas the balance distributes to extravascular spaces. Although this could impair diffusion of oxygen to tissues, clinical impact is unproven.

The most commonly used colloids are 5% albumin, naturally occurring plasma protein and 6% hetastarch, a synthetic colloid formulation. These solutions offer more rapid restoration of intravascular volume because they produce greater intravascular volume expansion per quantity of volume infused. Colloids produce less peripheral edema than crystalloid, but there is no significant clinical impact. The use of colloid solutions and blood products can be particularly important if there is significant blood loss associated with sepsis or if the patient had severe preexisting anemia.

Meta-analysis of clinical studies comparing crystalloid and colloid resuscitation indicated no clinical outcome differences.[69] The Saline versus Albumin Fluid Evaluation (SAFE) trial found no difference in 28-day mortality rate in critically ill patients (21.1% with saline versus 20.9% with albumin).[70] Although crystalloid solutions require two to four times more volume than colloids, they are generally recommended for fluid resuscitation because of the lower cost. However, colloids can be preferred especially when the serum albumin is less than 2.0 g/dL.

The major complications with fluid resuscitation are pulmonary and systemic edema. Aggressive volume expansion can cause increase in pulmonary capillary pressure leading to an increase in lung water and associated hypoxemia. There is no significant difference in the incidence of pulmonary edema between the crystalloid and colloid solutions.

Vasopressor and Inotropic Therapy

When fluid resuscitation alone provides inadequate arterial pressure and organ perfusion, vasopressors and inotropic agents should be initiated. Inotropic agents such as dopamine and dobutamine have been effective in improving cardiac output. Vasopressors should be considered when a systolic blood pressure is less than 90 mm Hg or mean arterial pressure (MAP) is lower than 60 to 65 mm Hg after adequate left ventricular preload and inotrope therapy. Although inotropes and vasopressors are effective in life-threatening hypotension and in improving cardiac index, there are significant complications such as tachycardia and myocardial ischemia and infarction as a result of change in myocardial oxygen consumption in patients with coexisting coronary disease. Thus, a catecholamine infusion should be titrated gradually to restore MAP without impairing stroke volume.

❼ Agents commonly considered for vasopressor or inotropic support include dopamine, dobutamine, norepinephrine, phenylephrine, and epinephrine (Table 123–5).[71–73] Recently, norepinephrine should generally be considered to be the first choice vasopressor after failure to restore adequate blood pressure and organ perfusion with appropriate fluid resuscitation. Norepinephrine is a potent α-adrenergic agent with less pronounced β-adrenergic activity, and it increases mean arterial pressure because of its vasoconstrictive effects on peripheral vascular beds. Doses of 0.01 to 3 mcg/kg/min can reliably increase blood pressure with little changes in heart rate or cardiac index. Norepinephrine is a more potent agent than dopamine in refractory septic shock. Despite the earlier concern of decreased renal blood flow associated with norepinephrine, data in humans and animals demonstrate a norepinephrine-induced renal blood flow as well as urine and cardiac output.[71,74] Norepinephrine resulted in greater increases in arterial blood pressure in comparison

TABLE 123-5 Receptor Activity of Cardiovascular Agents Commonly Used in Septic Shock

Agent	α_1	α_2	β_1	β_2	Dopaminergic
Dopamine	++/+++	?	++++	++	++++
Dobutamine	+	+	++++	++	0
Norepinephrine	+++	+++	+++	+/++	0
Phenylephrine	++/+++	+	?	0	0
Epinephrine	++++	++++	++++	+++	0

α_1, α_1-adrenergic receptor; α_2, α_2-adrenergic receptor; β_1, β_1-adrenergic receptor; β_2, β_2-adrenergic receptor; 0, no activity; ++++, maximal activity; ?, unknown activity.

to patients with septic shock who were treated with dopamine (93% with norepinephrine versus 31% with dopamine).[75] Norepinephrine was also associated with higher rate of survival comparison to dopamine and epinephrine.[73,76]

Dopamine, an α- and β-adrenergic agent with dopaminergic activity, appears to increase MAP and cardiac output, primarily because of an increase in stroke volume and heart rate. Doses of >5 mcg/kg/min exhibit α and β activity and are frequently used to support blood pressure and to improve cardiac function such as increase in cardiac index (CI). Because of combined vasopressor and inotropic effects, dopamine can be more useful in patients with hypotension and compromised systolic function, but it can cause more tachycardia and can be more arrhythmogenic.[35,76,77] A large randomized trial and a meta-analysis demonstrated low-dose dopamine (1 to 5 mcg/kg/min) does not maintain renal perfusion.[74,78]

Dobutamine is a β-adrenergic inotropic agent that many clinicians consider to be the preferred drug for improvement of cardiac output and oxygen delivery, particularly in early sepsis before significant peripheral vasodilation has occurred. Doses of 2 to 20 mcg/kg/min increases the CI, ranging from 20% to 66%. However, heart rate often increases significantly.[68] Dobutamine should be considered in severely septic patients with adequate filling pressures and blood pressure but low CI. A vasopressor such as norepinephrine and an inotrope such as dobutamine can be used to maintain both mean arterial pressure and cardiac output.

Phenylephrine, a selective α_1-agonist, has a rapid onset, short duration, and primary vascular effects, and it is least likely to produce tachycardia. The limited available information suggests that it can increase blood pressure modestly in fluid-resuscitated patients, and it does not appear to impair cardiac or renal function. Phenylephrine appears useful when tachycardia limits the usage of other vasopressors.[68,71]

Epinephrine, a nonspecific α- and β-adrenergic agonist, is capable of increasing CI and producing significant peripheral vasoconstriction in doses of 0.1 to 0.5 mcg/kg/min. However, because of its undesirable effects, including a propensity to increase lactate level and to impair blood flow to the splanchnic system, it should be reserved for patients who fail to respond to traditional therapies for increasing or maintaining blood pressure.[68,76]

During hypotension, endogenous vasopressin levels increase and maintain arterial blood pressure as vasopressin is a direct vasoconstrictor without inotropic or chronotropic effects. However, there is a vasopressin deficiency in septic shock most likely caused by inadequate production. Low doses of vasopressin (0.01–0.04 units/min) produce a significant increase in mean arterial pressure in septic shock, leading to the discontinuation of other vasopressors.[71,79] Doses higher than 0.04 units/min have been associated with myocardial ischemia, significant decreases in cardiac output, and cardiac arrest.[79,80] Although it can be beneficial to those patients requiring high-dose vasopressors, routine usage is not currently recommended because of lack of large, randomized, prospective clinical trials.[35,71,80]

In summary, for the septic patient with clinical signs of shock and significant hypotension unresponsive to aggressive fluid therapy, norepinephrine is the preferred agent for increasing the blood pressure. Epinephrine should be considered for refractory hypotension. Dopamine and epinephrine are more likely to induce or exacerbate tachycardia than norepinephrine and phenylephrine. In a septic patient with low cardiac index after adequate fluid therapy and an adequate MAP, dobutamine is the first-line agent. Alternatively, dopamine in moderate doses (5–10 mcg/kg/min) can also be used as an initial agent because of its selective effect on increasing cardiac output with its minimal effect on the systemic vascular resistance.

EARLY GOAL-DIRECTED THERAPY

8 Initial resuscitation of a patient in severe sepsis or sepsis-induced tissue hypoperfusion should begin as soon as the syndrome is recognized. A randomized, controlled trial evaluated the timing of the goal-directed therapy involving adjustments of cardiac preload, afterload, and contractility to balance oxygen delivery with demand prior to admission to the ICU.[81] The goals during the first 6 hours included central venous pressure of 8 to 12 mm Hg, mean arterial pressure of ≥65 mm Hg, urine output of ≥0.5 mL/kg/h, and a central venous or mixed venous oxygen saturation of ≥70%. During the first 6 hours of resuscitation, the early goal-directed therapy group had a central venous catheter placed and received more fluid than with traditional therapy (5 versus 3.5 L), dobutamine therapy to a maximum of 20 mcg/kg/min, and red blood cell transfusions. The 28-day mortality rate was 30% in the early goal-directed therapy group, in comparison to 46.5% in the traditional therapy group consisting of fluid resuscitation, followed by vasopressor therapy if required. Increased oxygen delivery from the red blood cell transfusions to achieve a hematocrit of ≥30% in the early goal-directed therapy group appeared to be the primary difference between the two groups. One institution evaluated the impact of 6-hour sepsis care bundle and found the compliance rate to be 52%.[82] The noncompliant group had a more than twofold increase in hospital mortality in comparison to the compliant group (49% vs. 23%).

ADJUNCTIVE THERAPIES

ARDS and hypoxia are common in septic patients, even in septic patients without pulmonary infection. Oxygen therapy is indicated to maintain oxygen saturation greater than 90%, and with progressive pulmonary insufficiency, the patient can require assisted ventilation.

9 Hyperglycemia is frequently associated with sepsis, and it is usually quite refractory to exogenous insulin. Intensive insulin therapy, maintaining blood glucose level at 80 to 110 mg per deciliter resulted in lower morbidity and mortality among critically ill patients in comparison to those with blood glucose level at 180 to 200 mg per deciliter.[83,84] However, hypoglycemia was reported in 40% of patients. Post hoc data analysis suggested achieving a goal of <150 mg/dL also improved outcome, and this goal is likely to reduce the risk of hypoglycemia.[85] Insulin therapy also reduced the rate of death from multiple-organ failure among patients with sepsis, regardless of presence of diabetes prior to sepsis.

10 The corticosteroids have been the subject of much controversy in the management of septic patients.[86–88] Although routine use of

corticosteroids for the treatment of sepsis is not recommended, it appears to have a role in severe septic shock. A multi-center, randomized, controlled trial demonstrated a significant shock reversal and decrease in mortality (absolute reduction 10%) in patients with severe septic shock.[89] Fludrocortisone 50 mcg orally and hydrocortisone 200 to 300 mg/day, for 7 days in three or four divided doses or by continuous infusion were used in patients with adrenal insufficiency, requiring high-dose or increasing vasopressor therapy within the first 8 hours of septic shock[89]. There was no benefit for those patients without adrenal insufficiency. Higher doses of hydrocortisone (<300 mg daily) were ineffective or harmful.[35] Subsequent *post hoc* analysis of this trial addressed the efficacy and safety of low doses of corticosteroids in septic shock-associated early ARDS.[90] More favorable outcomes were achieved only in septic shock-associated early ARDS nonresponders. Of the 129 nonresponders, the mortality rates between the placebo and the steroid group were 75% and 53%. There was no significant difference between groups in responders.

Deep vein thrombosis prophylaxis with either low-dose unfractionated heparin or low-molecular weight heparin should be initiated in general ICU patients including those with severe sepsis and septic shock.[35] Similarly, stress ulcer prophylaxis should be initiated in all patients with severe sepsis and septic shock.[35] Proton pump inhibitors and H_2 receptor antagonists are equivalent in their ability to increase gastric pH.

IMMUNOTHERAPY

A variety of strategies have been used to reverse or control the inflammatory process initiated during sepsis.[91] Despite the initial enthusiasm in immunotherapeutic interventions for sepsis, overall results have been generally disappointing with the exception of recombinant human activated protein C (rhAPC; drotrecogin alfa), an endogenous anticoagulant with antiinflammatory properties.

⓫ Recombinant human activated protein C, the first antiinflammatory agent to be approved for sepsis, promotes fibrinolysis and associated antiinflammatory mechanisms. The Recombinant Human Activated Protein C Worldwide Evaluation in Severe Sepsis (PROWESS) trial studied the effects of 96 hours of continuous infusion of recombinant activated protein C.[25] All-cause mortality at 28 days was significantly reduced from 30.8% with placebo to 24.7% in those receiving rhAPC. However, a major risk associated with rhAPC is hemorrhage. Serious bleeding including intracranial hemorrhage and a life-threatening bleeding episode occurred in 3.5% of patients in comparison to 2% of patients in the placebo group. Regardless, activated protein C appears to have a significant role in the treatment of septic shock. Currently, activated protein C is recommended in patients at high risk of death including Acute Physiology and Chronic Health Evaluation (APACHE) II score ≥25, sepsis-induced multiple organ failure, septic shock, or sepsis-induced ARDS and with no absolute contraindication related to bleeding risk. Cost-benefit analysis studies support for activated protein C therapy especially for the patients with APACHE II scores greater than 25.[25,92,93]

The debate regarding certain aspects of the study design, patient selection, and safety continues.[94,95] Activated protein C may be underused in patients aged 75 years and older, possibly because of incidence of bleeding, high drug cost, and clinician's tendency to treat elderly patients less aggressively.[96] Sub-analysis of the PROWESS trial demonstrated significant absolute risk reductions in 28-day and inhospital mortality among patients aged ≥75 years (15.5% and 15.6%, respectively) in comparison to the placebo group.[97] There was no significant difference between the activated protein C treated group and the placebo group with respect to the incidences of serious bleeding (3.9% versus 2.2%). A multicenter trial evaluated the efficacy of activated protein C for adults who had severe sepsis and a low risk of death defined by an APACHE score <25 or single organ failure.[98] There was no significant difference between the placebo and the treatment group in 28-day mortality (17.0% versus 18.5%, respectively). The incidence of serious bleeding was higher in the treatment group than in the placebo group (3.9% versus 2.2%). Consequently, activated protein C should not be used in patients with severe sepsis at low risk for death.

ABBREVIATIONS

APACHE: Acute Physiology and Chronic Health Evaluation

ARDS: acute respiratory distress syndrome

CARS: compensatory antiinflammatory response syndrome

CI: cardiac index

DIC: disseminated intravascular coagulation

DO_2: oxygen delivery to tissues

HIV: human immunodeficiency virus

ICU: intensive care unit

IL: interleukin

IL-1RA: interleukin-1 receptor antagonist

MAP: mean arterial pressure

MODS: multiple-organ dysfunction syndrome

MRSA: methicillin-resistant *Staphylococcus aureus*

PAF: platelet-activating factor

PROWESS: Recombinant Human Activated Protein C Worldwide Evaluation in Severe Sepsis (trial)

rhAPC: recombinant human activated protein C

SAFE: Saline versus Albumin Fluid Evaluation (trial)

SIRS: systemic inflammatory response syndrome

SVR: systemic vascular resistance

TNF: tumor necrosis factor

VO_2: oxygen consumption

WBC: white blood cell

REFERENCES

1. Martin GS, Mannino DM, Eaton S, Moss M. The epidemiology of sepsis in the United States from 1979 through 2000. N Engl J Med 2003;348:1546–1554.
2. Angus DC, Linde-Zwirble WT, Lidicker J, et al. Epidemiology of severe sepsis in the United States: Analysis of incidence, outcome, and associated costs of care. Crit Care Med 2001;29:1303–1310.
3. American College of Chest Physicians/Society of Critical Care Medicine Consensus Conference. Definitions for sepsis and organ failure and guidelines for the use of innovative therapies in sepsis. Crit Care Med 1992;20:864–874.
4. Robertson CM Coopersmith CM. The systemic inflammatory response syndrome. Microbes Infect 2006;8:1382–1389.
5. Vincent JL, Sakr Y, Sprung CL, et al. Sepsis in European intensive care units: Results of the SOAP study. Crit Care Med 2006;34:344–353.
6. Levy MM, Fink MP, Marshall JC, et al. 2001 SCCM/ESICM/ACCP/ATS/SIS International Sepsis Definitions Conference. Crit Care Med 2003;31:1250–1256.
7. Harbarth S, Garbino J, Pugin J, et al. Inappropriate initial therapy and its effect on survival in a clinical trial of immunomodulating therapy for severe sepsis. Am J Med 2003;115:529–535.
8. Valles J, Rello J, Ochagavia A, et al. Community-acquired bloodstream infection in critically ill adult patients. Chest 2003;123:1615–1624.
9. Guidet B, Aegerter P, Gauzit R, et al. Incidence and impact of organ dysfunctions associated with sepsis. Chest 2005;127:942–951.

10. Garnacho-Montero J, Garcia-Garmendia JL, Barrero-Almodovar A, et al. Impact of adequate empirical antibiotic therapy on the outcome of patients admitted to the intensive care unit with sepsis. Crit Care Med 2003;31:2742–2751.
11. Laupland KB, Kirkpatrick AW, Church DL, et al. Intensive-care-unit-acquired bloodstream infections in a regional critically ill population. J Hosp Infect 2004;58:137–145.
12. Pfaller MA, Diekema DJ, Jones RN, et al. Trends in antifungal susceptibility of *Candida* spp. isolated from pediatric and adult patients with bloodstream infection: SENTRY Antimicrobial surveillance program, 1997 to 2000. J Clin Microbiol 2002;40:852–856.
13. Bodey GP, Mardani M, Hanna HA, et al. The epidemiology of *Candida glabrata* and *Candida albicans* fungemia in immunocompromised patients with cancer. Am J Med 2002;112:380–385.
14. Costa SF, Marinho I, Araujo EA, et al. Nosocomial fungaemia: A 2-year prospective study. J Hosp Infect 2000;45:69–72.
15. Annane D, Bellissant E, Cavaillon JM. Septic shock. Lancet 2005;365:63–78.
16. Cohen J. The immunopathogenesis of sepsis. Nature 2002;420:885–891.
17. Cavaillon JM, Adib-Conquy M, Fitting C, et al. Cytokine cascade in sepsis. Scand J Infect Dis 2003;35:535–544.
18. Marie C, Muret J, Fitting C, et al. Interleukin-1 receptor antagonist production during infectious and noninfectious systemic inflammatory response syndrome. Crit Care Med 2000;28:2277–2282.
19. Kim PK, Deutschman CS. Inflammatory responses and mediators. Surg Clin North Am 2000;80:885–894.
20. Heper Y, Akalin EH, Mistik R, et al. Evaluation of serum C-reactive protein, procalcitonin, tumor necrosis factor alpha, and interleukin-10 levels as diagnostic and prognostic parameters in patients with community-acquired sepsis, severe sepsis, and septic shock. Eur J Clin Microbiol Infect Dis 2006;25:481–491.
21. Steinmetz HT, Herbertz A, Bertram M, Diehl V. Increase in interleukin-6 serum level preceding fever in granulocytopenia and correlation with death from sepsis. J Infect Dis 1995;171:225–228.
22. O'Malley K, Moldawer LL. Interleukin-6: Still crazy after all these years. Crit Care Med 2006;34:2690–2691.
23. Lin KJ, Lin J, Hanasawa K, et al. Interleukin-8 as a predictor of the severity of bacteremia and infectious disease. Shock 2000;14:95–100.
24. Lush CW, Kvietys PR. Microvascular dysfunction in sepsis. Microcirculation 2000;7:83–101.
25. Bernard GR, Vincert JL, Laterre PF, et al. Efficacy and safety of recombinant human activated protein C for severe sepsis. N Engl J Med 2001;344:699–709.
26. Nimah M, Brill RJ. Coagulation dysfunction in sepsis and multiple organ failure. Crit Care Clin 2003;19:441–458.
27. Awad SS. State-of-the-art therapy for severe sepsis and multisystem organ failure. Am J Surg 2003;186:23S-30S.
28. Bastarache JA, Ware LB, Bernard GR. The role of the coagulation cascade in the continuum of sepsis and acute lung injury and acute respiratory distress syndrome. Semin Respir Crit Care Med 2006;27:365–376.
29. Idell S. Adult respiratory distress syndrome: Do selective anticoagulants help? Am J Respir Med 2002;1:383–91.
30. Young JD. The heart and circulation in severe sepsis. Br J Anaesth 2004;93:114–120.
31. Wan L, Bellomo R, Di Giantomasso D, et al. The pathogenesis of septic acute renal failure. Curr Opin Crit Care 2003;9:496–502.
32. Mehta RL, McDonald B, Gabbai FB, et al. A randomized clinical trial of continuous versus intermittent dialysis for acute renal failure. Kidney Int 2001;60:1154–12163.
33. Kellum J, Angus DC, Johnson JP, et al. Continuous versus intermittent renal replacement therapy: A meta-analysis. Intensive Care Med 2002;28:29–37.
34. Nguyen HB, Rivers EP, Knoblich BP, et al. Early lactate clearance is associated with improved outcome in severe sepsis and septic shock. Crit Care Med 2004;32:1637–1642.
35. Dellinger RP, Carlet JM, Masur H, et al. Surviving sepsis campaign guidelines for management of severe sepsis and septic shock. Crit Care Med 2004;32:858–873.
36. Cohen J, Brun-Buisson C, Torres A, Jorgensen J. Diagnosis of infection in sepsis: An evidence-based review. Crit Care Med 2004:32:S466–S494.
37. Jimenez MF, Marshall JC. Source control in the management of sepsis. Intensive Care Med 2001;27:S49–S62.
38. Roberts JA, Lipman J. Antibacterial dosing in intensive care. Clin Pharmacokinet 2006;45:755–773.
39. Kang CI, Kim SH, Park WB, et al. Bloodstream infections caused by antibiotic-resistant gram-negative bacilli: Risk factors for mortality and impact of inappropriate initial antimicrobial therapy on outcome. Antimicrob Agents Chemother 2005;49:760–766.
40. Liu H, Mulholland G. Appropriate antibiotic treatment of genitourinary infections in hospitalized patients. Am J Med 2005;118:14S–20S.
41. Carratala J, Martin-Herrero JE, Mykietiuk A, et al. Clinical experience in the management of community-acquired pneumonia: Lessons from the use of fluoroquinolones. Clin Microbiol Infect 2006;12(S3):2–11.
42. Mandell LA, Bartlett JG, Dowell SF, et al. Update of practice guidelines for the management of community-acquired pneumonia in immunocompetent adults. Clin Infect Dis 2003;37:1405–1433.
43. American Thoracic Society Documents. Guidelines for the management of adults with hospital-acquired, ventilator-associated, and healthcare-associated pneumonia. Am J Respir Crit Care Med 2005;171:388–416.
44. Wunderink RG, Rello J, Cammarata SK, et al. Linezolid vs vancomycin. Analysis of two double-blind studies of patients with methicillin-resistant *Staphylococcus aureus* nosocomial pneumonia. Chest 2003; 124:1789–1797.
45. Mullins CD, Kuznik A, Shaya FT, et al. Cost-effectiveness analysis of linezolid compared with vancomycin for the treatment of nosocomial pneumonia caused by methicillin-resistant *Staphylococcus aureus*. Clin Ther 2006;28:1184–1198.
46. Solomkin JS, Mazuski JE, Baron EJ, et al. Guidelines for the selection of anti-infective agents for complicated intra-abdominal infections. Clin Infect Dis 2003;37:997–1005.
47. Verwaest C. Meropenem versus imipenem/cilastatin as empirical monotherapy for serious bacterial infections in the intensive care unit. Clin Microbiol Infect 2000;6:294–302.
48. Novelli A, Adembri C, Livi P, et al. Pharmacokinetic evaluation of meropenem and imipenem in critically ill patients with sepsis. Clin Pharmacokinet 2005;44:539–549.
49. Falagas ME, Siakavellas E. Bacteroides, prevotella, and porphyromonas species: A review of antibiotic resistance and therapeutic options. Int J Antimicrob Agents 2000;15:1–9.
50. Stevens BL, Bisno AL, Chambers HF, et al. Practice guidelines for the diagnosis and management of skin and soft-tissue infections. Clin Infect Dis 2005;41:1373–1406.
51. Sabol KE, Schevarria KL, Lewis JS. Community-associated methicillin-resistant *Staphylococcus aureus*: New bug, old drugs. Ann Pharmacother 2006;40:1125–1133.
52. Arbeit RD, Maki D, Tally FP, et al. The safety and efficacy of daptomycin for the treatment of complicated skin and skin-structure infections. Clin Infect Dis 2004;38:1673–1681.
53. Sharpe JN, Shively EH, Polk HC. Clinical and economic outcomes of oral linezolid versus intravenous vancomycin in the treatment of MRSA-complicated, lower-extremity skin and soft-tissue infections caused by methicillin-resistant *Staphylococcus aureus*. Am J Surg 2005;189:425–428.
54. Paul M, Benuri-Silbiger I, Soares-Weiser K, et al. β-Lactam monotherapy versus β-lactam-aminoglycoside combination therapy for sepsis in immunocompetent patients: Systematic review and meta-analysis of randomized trials. BMJ 2004;328:668–681.
55. Safdar N, Handelsman, Maki D. Does combination antimicrobial therapy reduce mortality in gram-negative bacteraemia? A meta-analysis. Lancet Infect Dis 2004;4:519–527.
56. Paul M, Leibovici L. Combination antibiotic therapy for *Pseudomonas aeruginosa* bacteraemia. Lancet Infect Dis 2005;5:192–194.
57. Pappas PG, Rex JH, Sobel JD, et al. Guidelines for treatment of candidiasis. Infectious Diseases Society of America. Clin Infect Dis 2004;38:161–189.
58. Robinson RF, Nahata MC. A comparative review of conventional and lipid formulations of amphotericin B. J Clin Pharm Ther 1999;24:249–257.
59. Cagnoni PJ, Walsh TJ, Prendergast MM, et al. Pharmacoeconomic analysis of liposomal amphotericin B versus conventional amphotericin B in the empirical treatment of persistently febrile neutropenic patients. J Clin Oncol 2000;18:2476–2483.
60. DW, Su L, Yu DT, et al. Mortality and costs of acute renal failure associated with amphotericin-B therapy. Clin Infect Dis 2001;32:686–693.

61. Kullberg BJ, Sobel JD, Ruhnke M, et al. Voriconazole versus a regimen of amphotericin B followed by fluconazole for candidemia in non-neutropenic patients: A randomized non-inferiority trial. Lancet 2005;366:1435–1442.
62. Mora-Duarte J, Betts R, Rotstein R, et al. Comparison of caspofungin and amphotericin B for invasive candidiasis. N Engl J Med 2002;347:2020–2029.
63. Ostrosky-Zeichner L, Kontoyiannia D, Raffalli J, et al. International, open-label, noncomparative, clinical trial of micafungin alone and in combination for treatment of newly diagnosed and refractory candidemia. Eur J Clin Microbiol Infect Dis 2005;24:654–661.
64. Kohno S, Masaoka T, Yamaguchi H, et al. A multicenter, open-label clinical study of micafungin (FK-463) in the treatment of deep-seated mycosis in Japan. Scand J Infect Dis 2004;36:372–379.
65. Krause DS, Reinhardt J, Vazquez JA, et al. Phase 2 randomized, dose-ranging study evaluating the safety and efficacy of anidulafungin in invasive candidiasis and candidemia. Antimicrob Agents Chemother 2004;38:2021–2024.
66. Spanakis EK, Aperis G, Mylonakis E. New agents for the treatment of fungal infections: Clinical efficacy and gaps in coverage. Clin Infect Dis 2006;43:1060–1068.
67. Garey KW, Rege M, Pai MP, et al. Time to initiation of fluconazole therapy impacts mortality in patients with candidemia: A multi-institutional study. Clin Infect Dis 2006;43:25–31.
68. Hollenberg SM, Ahrens TS, Annane D, et al. Practice parameters for hemodynamic support of sepsis in adult patients: 2004 Update. Crit Care Med 2004;32:1928–1948.
69. Choi PTL, Yip G, Quinonez LG, et al. Crystalloids versus colloids in fluid resuscitation: Systemic review. Crit Care Med 1999;27:200–210.
70. Finfer S, Bellomo R, Boyce N, et al. A comparison of albumin and saline for fluid resuscitation in the intensive care unit. N Engl J Med 2004;350:2247–2256.
71. Dellinger RP. Cardiovascular management of septic shock. Crit Care Med 2003;31:946–955.
72. Beale RJ, Hollenberg SM, Vincent JL, Parrillo JE. Vasopressor and inotropic support in septic shock: An evidence-based review. Crit Care Med 2004;32:S455–S465.
73. Martin C, Viviand X, Leone M, Thirion X. Effect of norepinephrine on the outcome of septic shock. Crit Care Med 2000;28:2758–2765.
74. Kellum J, Decker J. Use of dopamine in acute renal failure: A meta-analysis. Crit Care Med 2001;29:1526–1531.
75. Levy MM, Macias WL, Vincent JL, et al. Early changes in organ function predict eventual survival in severe sepsis. Crit Care Med 2005;33:2194–2201.
76. De Backer D, Creteur J, Silva E, et al. Effects of dopamine, norepinephrine, and epinephrine on the splanchnic circulation in septic shock: Which is best? Crit Care Med 2003;31:1659–1667.
77. Sakr Y, Reinhart K, Vincent JL, et al. Dose dopamine administration in shock influence outcome? Results of the sepsis occurrence in acutely ill patients (SOAP) study. Crit Care Med 2006;34:589–597.
78. Bellomo R, Chapman M, Finfer S, et al. Low-dose dopamine in patients with early renal dysfunction: A placebo-controlled randomized trial. Australian and New Zealand Intensive Care Society (ANZICS) Clinical Trials Group. Lancet 2000;356:2139–2143.
79. Klinzing S, Simon M, Reinhart K, et al. High-dose vasopressin is not superior to norepinephrine in septic shock. Crit Care Med 2003;31:2646–2650.
80. Russell JA. Vasopressin in septic shock: Clinical equipoise mandates a time for restraint. Crit Care Med 2003;31:2707–2708.
81. Rivers E, Nguyen B, Havstad S, et al. Early goal-directed therapy in the treatment of severe sepsis and septic shock. N Engl J Med 2001;345:1368–1377.
82. Gao F, Melody T, Daniels D, et al. The impact of compliance with 6-hour and 24-hour sepsis bundles on hospital mortality in patients with severe sepsis: A prospective observational study. Crit Care 2005;9:R764–770.
83. Van Den Berghe G, Wouters P, Weekers F, et al. Intensive insulin therapy in critically ill patients. N Engl J Med 2001;345:1359–1367.
84. Pittas AG, Siegel RD, Lau J. Insulin therapy for critically ill hospitalized patients: A meta-analysis of randomized controlled trials. Arch Intern Med 2004;164:2005–2011.
85. Finney SJ, Zekveld C, Elia A, et al. Glucose control and mortality in critically ill patients. JAMA 2003;290:2041–2047.
86. Sessler CN. Steroids for septic shock back from the dead? (Con). Chest 2003;123:482S–489S.
87. Balk RA. Steroids for septic shock back from the dead? (Pro). Chest 2003;123:490S–499S.
88. Annane D, Dellissant E, Bollaert PE, et al. Corticosteroids for severe sepsis and septic shock: A systematic review and meta-analysis. BMJ 2004;329:480.
89. Annane D, Sebille V, Charpentier C, et al. Effects of treatment with low-dose hydrocortisone and fludrocortisone on mortality in patients with septic shock. JAMA 2002;288:862–871.
90. Annane D, Sebille Veronique, Bellisssant E, et al. Effect of low doses of corticosteroids in septic shock patients with or without early acute respiratory distress syndrome. Crit Care Med 2006;34:22–30.
91. Nasraway SA. The problems and challenges of immunotherapy in sepsis. Chest 2003;123:451S–459S.
92. Manns BJ, Lee H, Doig CJ, et al. An economic evaluation of activated protein C treatment for severe sepsis. N Engl J Med 2002;347:993–1000.
93. Angus DC, Linde-Zwirble WT, Clermont G, et al. Cost-effectiveness of drotrecogin alfa (activated) in the treatment of severe sepsis. Crit Care Med 2003;31:1–11.
94. Bernard GR. Drotrecogin alfa (activated) recombinant human activated protein C for the treatment of severe sepsis. Crit Care Med 2003;31:S85–S93.
95. Eichacker RQ, Natanson C. Recombinant human activated protein C in sepsis: Inconsistent trial results, an unclear mechanism of action, and safety concerns resulted in labeling restrictions and the need for phase IV trials. Crit Care Med 2003:31:S94–S96.
96. Alexander SL, Ernst FR. Use of drotrecogin alfa (activated) in older patients with severe sepsis. Pharmacotherapy 2006;26:533–538.
97. Ely EW, Angus DC, Williams MD, et al. Drotrecogin alfa (activated) treatment of older patients with severe sepsis. Clin Infect Dis 2003;37:187–195.
98. Abraham E, Laterre PF, Garg R, et al. Drotrecogin alfa (activated) for adults with severe sepsis and a low risk of death. N Engl J Med 2005;353:1332–1341.

CHAPTER 124

Superficial Fungal Infections

THOMAS E. R. BROWN AND THOMAS W. F. CHIN

KEY CONCEPTS

1. Vulvovaginal candidiasis (VVC) can be classified as uncomplicated or complicated. This classification is useful in determining appropriate pharmacotherapy.
2. *Candida albicans* is the major pathogen responsible for VVC. The number of cases of non-*albicans* species appears to be increasing.
3. Signs and symptoms of VVC are not pathognomonic, and reliable diagnosis must be made with laboratory tests.
4. *Candida albicans* is the predominant species causing all forms of mucosal candidiasis. Important host and exogenous risk factors have been identified that predispose an individual to the development of mucosal candidiasis. In oropharyngeal and esophageal candidiasis, the key risk factor is impaired host immune system.
5. A topical agent is the first choice for treating oropharyngeal candidiasis, whereas systemic therapy can be used in patients not responding to an adequate trial of topical treatment or unable to tolerate topical agents and in those at high risk for systemic candidiasis. Fluconazole and itraconazole solution are the most effective azole agents.
6. In esophageal candidiasis, topical agents are not of proven benefit; fluconazole or itraconazole solution is the first choice.
7. Patients with human immunodeficiency virus (HIV) infection must be on concurrent optimal antiretroviral therapy, which is important for the prevention of recurrent and refractory candidiasis.
8. Primary or secondary prophylaxis of fungal infection is not recommended routinely for HIV-infected patients; use of secondary prophylaxis should be individualized for each patient.
9. Topical agents are first-line agents for fungal skin infections. Oral therapy is preferred for the treatment of extensive or severe infection or those of tinea capitis or onychomycosis.
10. Oral agents, in particular terbinafine and itraconazole, are first-line treatment for toenail and fingernail onychomycosis.

Superficial mycoses are among the most common infections in the world and the second most common vaginal infections in North America. Mucocutaneous candidiasis can occur in three forms, oropharyngeal, esophageal, and vulvovaginal disease, with oropharyngeal and vulvovaginal disease being the most common forms. These infections were reported in humans as far back as 1839. Over the last 15 to 20 years, the occurrence rates of some fungal infections have increased dramatically. The prevalence of fungal skin infections varies throughout different parts of the world from the most common causes of skin infections in the tropics to relatively rare disorders in the United States. This chapter reviews the pharmacotherapy of vulvovaginal candidiasis, oropharyngeal and esophageal candidiasis, and common dermatophyte infections.

Learning objectives, review questions, and other resources can be found at **www.pharmacotherapyonline.com.**

VULVOVAGINAL CANDIDIASIS

❶ *Vulvovaginal candidiasis* (VVC) refers to infections in individuals with or without symptoms who have positive vaginal cultures for *Candida* species. Depending on episodic frequency, VVC can be classified as either sporadic or recurrent.[1] This classification is essential to understanding the pathophysiology, as well as the pharmacotherapy, of VVC. Furthermore, VVC may be defined as *uncomplicated,* which refers to sporadic infections that are susceptible to all forms of antifungal therapy regardless of the duration of treatment, or *complicated,* in which consideration of factors affecting the host, microorganism, and pharmacotherapy all have an essential role in successful treatment.[1] Complicated VVC includes recurrent VVC, severe disease, non-*albicans* candidiasis, and abnormal host factors, including diabetes mellitus, immunosuppression, and pregnancy.[1]

EPIDEMIOLOGY

Minimal information on the incidence and prevalence of VVC exists. Healthcare workers are not required to report cases of VVC; therefore, estimates are derived from self-reported histories. Epidemiologic data are limited because VVC usually is diagnosed without microscopy and/or cultures, and antifungal nonprescription preparations are available for self-treatment.[1] By 25 years of age, approximately 50% of college women will have had at least one episode of VVC.[1] It is rare before menarche and increases dramatically at approximately 20 years of age, with the peak incidence between 30 and 40 years of age. It is associated with the initial act of sexual intercourse. As many as 75% of women experience one bout of symptomatic VVC in their lifetime. Between 40% and 50% of women who experience one episode of VVC experience a second episode, and 5% experience recurrent VVC.[2,3] Black women appear to be at higher risk of developing VVC as compared with whites (62.8% versus 55%, respectively).[4] The incidence after menopause remains unknown.

PATHOPHYSIOLOGY

❷ *Candida albicans* is the major pathogen responsible for VVC, accounting for 80% to 92% of symptomatic episodes. The remainder are caused by non-*albicans* species, with *Candida glabrata* dominating.[5] The number of cases of non-*albicans* candidiasis appears to be increasing, possibly related to the use of nonprescription vaginal antifungal preparations and short-course therapy and/or the increased use of long-term maintenance therapy in preventing recurrent infections.[1]

Candida species can act as commensal members of the vaginal flora. Asymptomatic colonization with *Candida* species has been found in 10% to 20% of reproductive-aged women.[5,6] *Candida* organisms are dimorphic; blastospores are believed to be responsible for colonization (transmission and spread), whereas germinated *Candida* forms are associated with tissue invasion and symptomatic infections.[7] To colonize the vagina, *Candida* species must be able to attach to the mucosa. The attachment process is complex. Not only are candidal surface structures important for attachment, but appropriate receptors for attachment must be present in the epithelial tissue. Not all women have the same range of receptors, which may explain variation in colonization.[6] Changes in the host's vaginal environment or response are necessary to induce a symptomatic infection. Unfortunately, in most cases of symptomatic VVC, no precipitating factor can be identified.[7]

RISK FACTORS

Several factors predispose a woman to VVC. VVC is not considered to be a sexually transmitted disease, although sexual factors can be important. There is a dramatic increase in the frequency of VVC when women become sexually active. In addition, oral–genital contact can increase the risk.[1] However, current guidelines do not recommend the treatment of asymptomatic partners.[5] Contraceptive agents, including the diaphragm with spermicide, the contraceptive sponge, and the intrauterine device, increase the risk of VVC. Oral contraceptive users demonstrated increased risk of candidiasis; however, these reports were with the higher-dose oral contraceptive pills, and the risk may not be as great with the lower-estrogen-dose oral contraceptives.[8]

Antibiotic use can increase the risk of VVC, but it is only significant in a small number of women. The mechanism by which antibiotics can increase the risk of VVC is unknown; colonization, however, is a prerequisite.[1] Diet (excess refined carbohydrate), douching, and tight-fitting clothing often are listed as important risk factors; however, no association has been established between these factors and increased risk of VVC.[1]

CLINICAL PRESENTATION

❸ The clinical presentation of VVC is given in Table 124–1.[1,5] These signs and symptoms are not pathognomonic, and a reliable diagnosis cannot be made without laboratory tests. Self-diagnosis has a sensitivity of 35% and a specificity of 89% and a positive predictive value of 62%.[4] More than 50% of women who had self-diagnosed VVC did not have yeast as the causative agent.[9] This limits the value of self-diagnosis and the success of self-treatment. The American College of Obstetricians and Gynecologists (ACOG) recommend that whenever possible women requesting treatment for VVC should be examined and evaluated. They only recommend self-diagnosis in compliant women with multiple confirmed prior cases of VVC who report the same symptoms. They further recommend that if these individuals fail to improve on a short course of therapy, they be evaluated for a further diagnosis.[10] Therefore in most instances the diagnosis should be based on both clinical presentation and investigations, including vaginal pH, saline microscopy, and 10% potassium hydroxide (KOH) microscopy. The vaginal pH remains normal in VVC, and microscopic investigations should detect blastospores or pseudohyphae. *Candida* cultures usually are not required in the diagnosis of uncomplicated VVC; however, they are recommended when an individual presents with classic signs and symptoms of VVC, has a normal vaginal pH, but microscopy is inconclusive or recurrence is suspected.[5]

TABLE 124-1 Clinical Presentation of Vulvovaginal Candidiasis

General	Often involves both the vulva and the vagina
Symptoms	Intense vulvar itching, soreness, irritation, burning on urination, and dyspareunia
Signs	Erythema, fissuring, curdy "cheese"-like discharge, satellite lesions, edema
Laboratory tests	Vaginal pH—normal, saline and 10% KOH microscopy—blastospores or pseudohyphae
Other diagnostic tests	*Candida* cultures not recommended unless classic signs and symptoms with normal vaginal pH and microscopy is inconclusive or recurrence is suspected

KOH, potassium hydroxide.

TREATMENT

Vulvovaginal Candidiasis

GOALS OF THERAPY

The goal of therapy is complete resolution of symptoms in patients who have symptomatic VVC. Test of cure is not necessary if symptoms resolve.[5] Antimycotic agents used in the treatment of VVC do not meet the definition of being fungicidal agents because of their slower killing rate. At the end of therapy, the number of viable organisms drops below the detectable range. However, by 6 weeks after a course of therapy, 25% to 40% of women will have positive yeast cultures and remain asymptomatic.[1] Asymptomatic colonization with *Candida* species does not require therapy.

GENERAL APPROACHES TO TREATMENT

The approach to therapy is to remove or improve any predisposing factors if they can be identified. A pharmacologic agent should have limited local and systemic side effects, a high cure rate, and easy administration. Additionally, it would be advantageous to use a therapy that is able to resolve symptoms within 24 hours, that has broad antimycotic activity (to cover increasing rates on non-*albicans Candida* species), that prevents recurrence, and that can be used over a shortened period of time such as 1 to 3 days.

Avoid harsh soaps and perfumes that can cause or worsen vulvar irritation. Keep the genital area clean and dry by avoiding constrictive clothing and frequent or prolonged exposure to hot tub use.[3] Douching is not recommended for either prevention or treatments.[10] Cool baths can soothe the skin.[3] Daily ingestion of 240 mL yogurt containing *Lactobacillus acidophilus* decreased colonization and symptomatic infections of VVC in women with recurrent infections.[11]

PHARMACOLOGIC TREATMENTS

Uncomplicated Vulvovaginal Candidiasis

Cure rates for uncomplicated VVC are between 80% and 95% with topical or oral azoles and between 70% and 90% with nystatin preparations. Table 124–2 lists available topical and oral preparations for the treatment of uncomplicated VVC. There are many topical nonprescription preparations for the treatment of VVC. No significant differences in in-vitro activity or clinical efficacy exist between the topical azole agents.[1,3,5,10] The selection of a topical azole should be based primarily on an individual patient's preference as to product formulation. Some topical products can cause vaginal burning, stinging, or irritation; conversely, the vehicle used

TABLE 124-2 Treatment for Uncomplicated Vulvovaginal Candidiasis

Active Ingredient	Preparation	Regimen
Over-the-counter/topical vaginal products		
Butoconazole	2% cream	one applicator × 3 days
Clotrimazole	1% cream	one applicator × 1 day
	100-mg tablet	one 100 mg tablet × 7 days
	2% cream	one applicator × 1 day
	200-mg tablet	one 200 mg tablet × 3 days
	10% cream	one applicator × 1 day
	500-mg tablet	one 500 mg tablet × 1 day
Miconazole[a]	2% cream	one applicator × 1 day
	100-mg suppository	one 100 mg suppository × 7 days
	200-mg suppository	one 200 mg suppository × 3 days
	1200-mg ovule	one ovule × 1 day
Ticonazole	2% cream	one applicator × 3 days
	6.5% cream	one applicator × 1 day
Prescription/topical		
Nystatin	100,000-unit tablet	one tablet × 14 days
Terconazole	0.4% cream	one applicator × 7 days
	0.8% cream	one applicator × 3 days
Oral products		
Fluconazole	150 mg	one tablet × 1 day

[a]The U.S. Food and Drug Administration warns of possible increase in anticoagulant effects of warfarin with concomitant use.

in topical creams or gels can provide initial symptomatic relief.[1] Of note, most topical preparations can decrease the efficacy of latex condoms and diaphragms.

Oral azoles have been used in the treatment of VVC. Patients prefer oral therapy because of its convenience.[12] Oral and topical therapy are therapeutically equivalent.[1] A Cochrane review of 17 trials analyzing oral versus topical antifungal use concluded that there were no differences between the routes in short-term and long-term clinical and mycologic cure rates.[13]

In the treatment of uncomplicated VVC, the duration of therapy is not critical. Cure rates with different lengths of treatment have not demonstrated that one therapy is significantly better.[12,13,14] Shorter-duration therapies (e.g., clotrimazole 1-day therapy) consist of higher concentrations of azoles that maintain the local therapeutic effect for up to 72 hours and allow for resolution of signs and symptoms.[15] A review of 14 trials that examined 1-day treatments showed less than 7% difference in short-term cure rates or improvement between any two treatments in any two studies and no significant differences in short- or long-term clinical cure rates among 1-day regimens.[14] Table 124–2 lists the therapeutic options for the treatment of uncomplicated VVC.

Complicated Vulvovaginal Candidiasis

Complicated VVC occurs in patients who are immunocompromised or have uncontrolled diabetes mellitus.[1] These individuals need a more aggressive treatment plan.[10] Current recommendations are to lengthen therapy to 10 to 14 days regardless of the route of administration.[10] Therapeutic options include those listed in Table 124–2; however, regimens should be continued for 10 to 14 days. A study of oral fluconazole therapy in women with complicated VVC demonstrated that cure rates increased from 67% with single dose therapy to 80% when the 150 mg dose of fluconazole was repeated 72 hours after the initial dose.[16]

VVC during pregnancy also can be considered complicated because consideration of host factors such as hormonal changes that can affect normal flora are essential in selecting therapeutic regimens. Topical agents are considered to be safe throughout pregnancy Oral agents are contraindicated in pregnancy because of the concern for fetal complications. A prospective assessment of pregnancy outcomes in 226 women exposed to fluconazole in the first trimester did not indicate increased risk of congenital abnormalities or other adverse outcomes.[17] The median dose of fluconazole was 200 mg, with 46.5% of the cohort receiving a single dose of fluconazole 150 mg.[18] However, ACOG recommends avoiding oral therapy as larger doses of fluconazole have been linked to birth defects.[18] They recommend a topical imidazole therapy for 7 days.[10]

Recurrent Vulvovaginal Candidiasis

Recurrent vulvovaginal candidiasis (RVVC) is defined as having more than four episodes of VVC within a 12-month period.[1,5] Fewer than 5% of women develop RVVC, and its pathogenesis is poorly understood. A proper diagnosis should be obtained to rule out other infections or nonmycotic contact dermatitis. Recurrent VVC is best treated in two stages: an initial intensive stage followed by prolonged antifungal therapy to achieve mycologic remission. This was demonstrated in a randomized controlled trial in which women were assigned to receive 150 mg fluconazole daily for 10 days followed by 6 months of either fluconazole 150 mg weekly or placebo. Ninety percent of women receiving both active treatments were symptom free for the 6 months following initial treatment (during the weekly fluconazole therapy), and there were 50% fewer symptomatic episodes in the 6 months following weekly suppressive therapy.[19]

Antifungal Resistant Vulvovaginal Candidiasis

Resistance to azole antifungals should be considered in individuals who have persistently positive yeast cultures and fail to respond to therapy despite adherence to prescribed regimens.[1] These infections can be treated with boric acid or 5-flucytosine.[20,21] Boric acid is administered as a 600-mg intravaginal capsule daily for 14 days of induction therapy, followed by a maintenance regimen of one capsule intravaginally twice weekly. Boric acid should not be administered orally as it is toxic. 5-Flucytosine cream is administered vaginally, 1,000 mg inserted nightly for 7 days.

PHARMACOECONOMIC CONSIDERATIONS

Costs from VVC can be related to direct costs of medical visits and self-treatment as well as indirect costs nonmedical expenses; time loss from work, costs of travel and time required in obtaining treatment. There are an estimated 6 million visits to healthcare providers each ear, resulting in more than $1 billion spent annually on these medical visits and self treatment.[22]

EVALUATION OF THERAPEUTIC OUTCOMES

Treatment of VVC will be considered to have positive outcomes if the symptoms of VVC are resolved within 24 to 48 hours and no adverse medication events are experienced. Self-assessment of symptom relief is appropriate for most cases of VVC. If symptoms remain unresolved or recur, then further testing and treatment can be required.

CLINICAL CONTROVERSY

Self-diagnosis of VVC is unreliable, however, the availability of nonprescription antifungal agents encourages self-diagnosis and self-treatment for the majority of women. Therefore women who self-treat should be monitored to ensure that the infection clears within a few days, or they need to see a physician for an accurate diagnosis.

OROPHARYNGEAL AND ESOPHAGEAL CANDIDIASIS

Oropharyngeal candidiasis (OPC) refers to an infection of the oral mucosa, and it is usually referred to informally as *thrush. Candida* is the predominant fungi responsible for the majority of oral fungal infections, and *C. albicans* is the principal species causing the infection, commonly referred to as *candidiasis* (the proper but less commonly used term being *candidosis*). The infection may extend into the esophagus, causing esophageal candidiasis.

MICROBIOLOGY AND EPIDEMIOLOGY

Candida species are normal inhabitants of the human gastrointestinal tract. They can be isolated from the oral cavity in up to 65% of healthy adults without producing any signs or symptoms. [23] This is referred to as *asymptomatic colonization.* The incidence of candidal carriage is increased under immunocompromised conditions, and the organism is capable of rapid conversion to a pathogen causing symptomatic mucosal infections. In HIV-infected individuals, asymptomatic colonization approaches 76%.[24] *C. albicans* is the predominant colonizing *Candida* species (70% to 80%), but any of the non-*albicans Candida* species can be colonizers. Colonization rates are influenced by the severity and nature of the underlying medical illness and the duration of hospitalization, as well as age (highest in infants younger than 18 months of age and in adults older than 60 years of age). A variety of host and exogenous factors (Table 124–3) can lead to the transformation of asymptomatic colonization to symptomatic disease such as oropharyngeal and esophageal candidiasis. *C. albicans* is the most common species causing all forms of mucosal candidiasis in humans. Less frequently non-*albicans Candida* species can be pathogenic and cause disease. These include *C. glabrata, Candida tropicalis, Candida krusei, Candida guilliermondi, Candida parapsilosis,* and others.[25,26] *Candida krusei*, although relatively uncommon, generally is recovered from mucosal surfaces of neutropenic patients with hematologic malignancies.[25] Another species, *Candida dubliniesis,* has been identified in both HIV-infected and noninfected patients, and may cause approximately 15% of infections previously ascribed to *C. albicans.*[25] In patients with cancer, non-*albicans Candida* species account for almost half of all *Candida* infections.

Oropharyngeal candidiasis is the most common opportunistic infection in patients with HIV disease, and it may be the first clinical manifestation of the HIV infection in the majority of untreated patients. OPC occurs in 50% to 90% of HIV-infected patients at some point during the progressive course of the disease to acquired immune deficiency syndrome (AIDS),[23,24,26] although significant reductions in the incidence have been observed after the introduction of highly active antiretroviral therapy (HAART). The incidence of OPC increases as the level of immunity decreases, especially when the CD4 T-cell counts are between 500 and 200 cells/mm^3 and is further increased when the CD4 T-cell counts drop below 200 cells/mm^3.[23] Oropharyngeal candidiasis is considered one of the earliest indicators of HIV infection and is a relatively reliable indirect marker of disease progression. Regardless of the CD4 T-cell count, OPC is predictive for the development of AIDS-related illnesses if left untreated.[23,26] In non-HIV diseases, such as cancer, the incidence of OPC varies depending on the type of malignant neoplastic disease, level of immune suppres-

TABLE 124-3 Risk Factors for Development of Oropharyngeal and/or Esophageal Candidiasis

Local Factors	**Potential Mechanisms**
Use of steroids and antibiotics	Suppression of cellular immunity and inhibition of phagocytosis by steroids, including chronic use of inhaled and topical steroids. Alteration of endogenous oral flora by broad-spectrum antibiotics, especially when used with steroids, creates a milieu for proliferation of *Candida* species because of reduced environmental and nutritional competition.
Dentures	Enhanced adherence of *Candida* species to acrylic material of dentures, reduced saliva flow under surfaces of denture fittings, improperly fitted dentures, or poor oral hygiene; these provide a milieu conducive to survival of microorganisms.
Xerostomia caused by drugs (e.g., tricyclic antidepressants, phenothiazine) and chemotherapy, radiotherapy to head-neck and various diseases, e.g., Sjögren's syndrome, HIV, cancer of head-neck, bone marrow transplant recipients	Reduced dilutional and cleansing effect caused by low secretion rate and low pH in saliva. Saliva and mucosa secretions have defense factors, such as lactoferrin, sialoperoxidase, lsozyme, histidine-rich polypeptide, secretory IgA antibodies, specific anti-*Candida* antibodies that help prevent adhesion and overgrowth of *Candida* species.
Smoking	
Disruption of oral mucosa caused by chemotherapy and radiotherapy, ulcers, endotracheal intubation trauma, and burns	Oral mucositis induced by radiation and breaks in physical barrier of oral epithelium, which is protective against invasion by microorganisms; altered rate of mucosa regeneration by cancer chemotherapy, which increases vulnerability to infection.
Systemic Factors	**Potential Mechanisms**
Drugs (cytotoxic agents, corticosteroids, immunosuppressants after organ transplant), omeprazole, environmental chemicals (benzene, pesticides)	Reduced immunity because of drug-induced neutropenia or cell-mediated immunity. Potent inhibition of gastric acid by proton pump inhibitors (PPI) can facilitate growth of *Candida* species; PPI also can inhibit cytotoxic effect of lymphocytes and reduce salivary secretion.
Neonates or elderly	Immature immune system of neonates who usually acquire infection during birth to a mother with vaginal candidiasis or from exposure to infected bottle nipples or to skin of adult care giver. Elderly–Unclear if this is the direct effect of age per se or contribution from dentures or underlying comorbidity.
HIV infection/AIDS	Depletion of CD4 T-lymphocytes especially below 200–300 cells/mm^3; anti-*Candida* protective mechanism of T-lymphocytes at a mucosal level is unclear but can be caused by altered cytokines, especially γ-interferon that inhibit transformation of *Candida* blastoconidia to the more invasive hyphal phase.
Diabetes	Higher than normal numbers of *Candida albicans* cultured from saliva of diabetic patients. Can be related to the elevated glucose levels and reduced chemotactic factor in saliva, altered neutrophil function, and reduced saliva volume and flow.
Malignancies (e.g., leukemia, head-neck cancer)	Use of intensive radiotherapy and chemotherapy can disrupt oral mucosa and also cause xerostomia; also prolonged use of broad-spectrum antibiotics in neutropenic patients can alter the normal oral flora. Because of the prolonged neutropenia, the principal immune defect, seen especially in leukemic patients, the initial oropharyngeal candidiasis can become systemic or invasive.
Nutritional deficiencies (e.g., iron, folate, vitamins B_1, B_2, B_6, B_{12}, and C)	Can be related to dietary restriction or GI absorption problems. Deficiencies can serve to enhance the pathogenic potential of the candida inhabitants, alter host defense mechanisms, or change epithelial barrier integrity.

AIDs, aquired immune deficiency syndrome; GI, gastrointestinal; HIV, human immunodeficiency virus; IgA, immunoglobulin A.

sion, and type and duration of treatment, but it is less common than in HIV-infected patients. OPC was initially reported in approximately 25% of patients with solid tumors, and up to 60% in those with hematologic malignancies or bone marrow transplant recipients.[27] Current rates of OPC have decreased significantly in these patients because of widespread use of antifungal prophylaxis.

Oropharyngeal candidiasis can predispose patients to develop more invasive disease, including esophageal candidiasis.[26] The esophagus is the second most common site of gastrointestinal candidiasis. The prevalence of esophageal candidiasis has increased mainly because of AIDS, as well as the increased numbers of other severely immunocompromised patients, especially those with hematologic malignancies.[25] Esophageal candidiasis is the first opportunistic infection in 3% to 10% of HIV-infected patients and is the second most common AIDS-defining disease after *Pneumocystis jiroveci* pneumonia.[26] The mean incidence of esophageal candidiasis among HIV-infected patients is less than OPC, and ranges from 15% to 20%.[26] The risk of esophageal candidiasis is increased in HIV-infected patients when the CD4 T-cell count has dropped below 100 to 200 cells/mm^3, and in those with OPC.[28,29] However the absence of OPC does not necessarily exclude the possibility of esophageal disease. Like OPC, the presence of esophageal candidiasis can help predict HIV disease progression and prognosis. [26] The incidence of esophageal candidiasis in non–HIV-infected immunocompromised patients is not well established. *Candida albicans* is also the most common cause of esophageal candidiasis, accounting for approximately 80% of cases, with the rest being caused by non-*albicans* species.[25,26]

The epidemiology of mucosal candidiasis has been affected by two factors. The introduction of HAART appears to have resulted in a significant decline in the incidence of OPC and esophageal candidiasis.[23,24] This is postulated to be caused both by enhanced immune responsiveness as well as by direct action on the organism by HAART.[24] The widespread use of the azole agents has led to a decline in the prevalence of mucosal candidiasis while leading to the emergence of refractory infections that have become difficult to treat.

PATHOGENESIS AND HOST DEFENSES

There appear to be several levels of immune defense against the development of OPC in HIV-infected persons, and they involve both systemic and local immunity. The primary line of host defense against *C. albicans* is cell-mediated immunity (CMI) at the mucosal surfaces, which is mediated by CD4 T-cells.[23] The efficacy of the CD4 T-cells is reduced when the number of cells drops below a protective threshold, and protection against infection becomes dependent on secondary or local immune mechanisms.[23,24] When the number of CD4 T-cells drops too low, recruitment of these cells to the oral cavity is impaired. The CD4 T-cell count has been considered as the hallmark predictor for development of OPC. However HIV viral load may have a stronger association with OPC than CD4 cell number.[30] This requires further confirmation by larger cohort studies. The possibility that HIV plays a strong role in susceptibility to infection is supported clinically by the fact that OPC is more common in HIV-infected persons than in those with similar immunosuppression, such as lymphoma and bone marrow transplant. When the primary line of defense fails, the secondary host defenses become crucial. These include the CD8 T-cells, salivary cytokines and other innate immune cells, such as the neutrophils, macrophages and epithelial cells (with anti-*Candida* activity). Deficiencies or dysfunction in any of these can result in susceptibility to OPC. The problem with the CD8 T-cells is caused more by a dysfunction of the micro-environment, specifically reduction in the E-cadherin adhesion molecule that promotes migration of the cells through mucosal tissues.[24] The role of humoral immunity by antibodies as a protective mechanism is unclear and controversial. The changeover of the role of *Candida* species from commensal to pathogenic in the human host usually occurs when break-down in these host defenses occurs. The pathogenesis of OPC is still not completely understood. It is important to develop a better understanding of the pathogenesis and role of host defenses, including the mechanism of CD8 T-cell activity, reduced adhesion molecules, and whether other cofactors, such as HIV viral load, HAART, and intravenous drug use play a role. Immunotherapeutic modalities can then be developed to eliminate the susceptibility factors and significantly reduce OPC in the at-risk populations.

Significant differences exist in the virulence among *Candida* species in mucosal candidiasis. One virulence factor is the ability of the organism to adapt and survive in response to changes in the host environment.[25] The genes required for virulence are regulated in response to the environmental signals indigenous to the host environment (e.g., temperature, pH, osmotic pressure, iron and calcium ion concentrations, oxygenation, carbon and nitrogen availability). The ability of *C. albicans* to undergo reversible morphologic transition between the budding pseudohyphal and the more invasive hyphal growth forms is also a determinant of virulence, and genes are recognized to play a role.[25] Other virulence factors include adhesive ability of *C. albicans* to epithelial cells and proteins and ability to invade host cells by means of phospholipase and proteinase enzymes.

RISK FACTORS

❹ Several host and exogenous factors contribute to the ability of *Candida* species to cause infection (see Table 124–3). Local and systemic factors, as well as characteristics of the organism itself, can increase the susceptibility of an individual to *Candida* infections.[23,25,27] Endocrine disorders besides diabetes mellitus, such as hypothyroidism, hypoparathyroidism, and hypoadrenalism, also can predispose patients to *Candida* species overgrowth. Patients with primary immune deficiencies such as lymphocytic abnormalities, phagocytic dysfunction, immunoglobulin A (IgA) deficiency, viral-induced immune paralysis, and severe congenital immunodeficiencies are also at risk for oropharyngeal candidiasis as well as disseminated candidiasis. Oral mucosal disease, such as lichen planus, can be preexistent causes of candidiasis. Smoking has been suggested as a predisposing risk factor. In many cases, multiple concurrent predisposing factors to candidiasis can exist; for example, xerostomia with mucositis and a break in the epithelial surface or immunosuppression, such as might occur in a leukemic patient receiving radiation and chemotherapy. The severity and extent of *Candida* infections increase with the number and severity of predisposing risk factors.

CLINICAL PRESENTATION AND DIAGNOSIS

Oropharyngeal candidiasis can manifest in several major forms (Table 124–4).[23,25,27] The clinical signs and symptoms of OPC and the locations of the lesions can be quite diverse (Table 124–5). A presumptive diagnosis of OPC usually is made by the characteristic appearance on the oral mucosa, with resolution of signs and symptoms after antifungal therapy. Pseudomembranous candidiasis, commonly known as *oral thrush,* is the classic and most common form seen in immunosuppressed and immunocompetent hosts. Erythematous and hyperplastic candidiasis and angular cheilitis occur less commonly in the HIV-infected population. Dysphagia, odynophagia, and retrosternal chest pain are common complaints of esophageal candidiasis which is usually, but not always, accompanied by the presence of OPC. Clinical symptomatology, along with a therapeutic trial of antifungal, can provide a reliable presumptive diagnosis of esophageal candidiasis. If antifungal therapy does not lead to resolution, more invasive tests such as upper gastrointestinal endoscopy can be undertaken.

TABLE 124-4 Clinical Classification of Oropharyngeal Candidiasis

Types	Population at Risk	Clinical Signs and Appearance
Pseudomembranous (thrush)	Neonates, patients with HIV or cancer, debilitated elderly, patients on broad-spectrum antibiotics or steroid inhalers, patients with dry mouth from various causes, smokers	Classic "cottage cheese" appearance, yellowish-white, soft plaques (or milk-curds) overlying areas of erythema on the buccal mucosa, tongue, gums and throat; plaques are easily removed by vigorous rubbing but can leave red or bleeding sites when removed; lesions on the tongue dorsum gives it a bald depapillated appearance.
Erythematous (acute atrophic)	Patients with HIV, patients on broad-spectrum antibiotics or steroid inhalers	Sensitive and painful erythematous mucosa with few, if any, white plaques; lesions are generally on dorsal surface of tongue or hard palate, occasionally on soft palate, but any part of mucosa can be involved; appear as flat red patches on the palate or atrophic patches on tongue dorsum with loss of papillae.
Hyperplastic (candidal leukoplakia)	Smokers; uncommon in patients with HIV	Thick white and adherent keratotic plaques commonly seen on the buccal mucosa and lateral border of tongue; can also see on lips and bottom of mouth; plaques cannot be easily scraped off or only partially removed. This condition is distinct from oral hairy leukoplakia, and it can progress to severe dysplasia or malignancy.
Angular cheilitis	Patients with HIV, denture wearers	Painful red, ulcerative, cracking or fissuring lesion at one or both comers of the mouth because of inflammatory reaction; usually lesions are small and rather punctate, but occasionally can extend in a linear fashion from the angles onto the facial skin.
Denture stomatitis (chronic atrophic)	Denture wearers who tend to be elderly and have poor oral hygiene	Red, flat lesions on mucosa beneath the denture and extends to right up to the denture border; more commonly located beneath a maxillary denture, although can be encountered beneath a mandibular denture.

HIV, human immunodeficiency virus.

TABLE 124-5 Clinical Presentation of Oropharyngeal and Esophageal Candidiasis

Oropharyngeal Candidiasis	Esophageal Candidiasis
General The clinical features can be quite diverse (see Table 124–4) **Symptoms** Symptoms are diverse and range from none to sore, painful mouth, burning tongue, metallic taste, and dysphagia and odynophagia with involvement of hypopharynx. **Signs** Signs are variable and can include diffuse erythema and white patches on the surfaces of buccal mucosa, throat, tongue, or gums. Constitutional signs are absent. **Laboratory tests** Scraping of an active lesion for microscopic examination can help confirm the diagnosis (presence of pseudohyphae and budding yeast) but is usually not necessary. Cultures are also not necessary since isolation of *Candida* species does not distinguish between colonization and true infection. Cultures can be taken in patients responding poorly to therapy to determine the infecting species and to predict likely drug resistance.	**General** This usually occurs as an extension of OPC. However, the esophagus can be the only site involved. The distal two-thirds, rather than the proximal one-third, is the most common site. **Symptoms** Typically the symptoms are dysphagia, odynophagia, and retrosternal chest pain but can be asymptomatic in some patients. Although rare, epigastric pain can be the dominant symptom. **Signs** Constitutional signs, including fever, occasionally occur. Physical findings can range from a few to numerous white or beige plaques of variable size. Plaques can be hyperemic or edematous, with ulceration in more severe cases. Most advanced cases can occur with increased mucosal friability and narrowing of lumen. Uncommon complications include perforation and aortic–esophageal fistula formation. **Laboratory tests** The best test is upper GI endoscopy (more useful than barium swallow); helps exclude other causes of esophagitis (e.g., viral, aphthous ulcers). Diagnosis is confirmed by the histologic presence of *Candida* species in biopsy lesions taken during endoscopy. Cultures to look for drug-resistant *Candida* species are warranted in patients who require endoscopy.

GI, gastrointestinal; OPC, oropharyngeal candidiasis.

TREATMENT

Oropharyngeal and Esophogeal Candidiasis

■ DESIRED OUTCOMES

The primary desired outcome in the management of OPC is a clinical cure, that is, elimination of clinical signs and symptoms. Even when the patient is relatively asymptomatic, it is important to treat the initial episode of OPC to avoid progression to more extensive disease. In the most severe cases, the patient's quality of life can be impaired, and this can result in decreased fluid and nutritional intake. Lack of appropriate treatment of OPC can lead to more extensive oral disease, especially in patients who are immunocompromised. The most serious complication of untreated OPC is extension of the infection to esophageal candidiasis. Because esophageal candidiasis is more debilitating, the patient's quality of life is more affected. It is important to initiate appropriate antifungal therapy for both OPC and esophageal candidiasis. Preventing or minimizing the number of future recurrences of both types of candidiasis is an equally important outcome. The approach depends largely on the underlying predisposing conditions. Mycologic cure is not a necessary treatment outcome because it may not be feasible or realistic given that *Candida* species exist commonly as part of the normal mouth flora.

Minimizing toxicities and drug-drug interactions of systemic antifungal agents, as well as maximizing adherence by ensuring that the patient understands directions to take the medication appropriately, is an important secondary outcome of therapy.

■ GENERAL APPROACH TO TREATMENT

The management of *Candida* infections should be individualized for each patient, taking into consideration the underlying immune status, other concurrent mucosal and medical diseases, concomitant medications, and exogenous infectious sources. In HIV-infected patients with inadequately controlled disease, anti-fungal treatment produces only a transient clinical response, and the relapse rates are higher than in other patient populations. These patients usually require frequent courses of anti-fungal treatment. Therefore in patients with HIV disease, treatment with effective HAART is paramount because this would provide the best prophylaxis against recolonization and recurrence of symptoms.[25,27,29]

Whenever feasible, it is desirable to minimize all predisposing factors, such as administration of corticosteroids, chemotherapeutic agents, and antimicrobials, as well as instituting proper oral hygiene and resolving concurrent conditions such as denture stomatitis. Selection of an appropriate antifungal agent for treatment of candidiasis requires consideration of several factors, including the patient's drug adherence, adequate saliva for dissolution of solid topical medications, risk of caries from sucrose- or dextrose-containing preparations, potential drug interactions, coexisting medication conditions (e.g., liver disease can affect certain systemic drugs), location and severity of the infection, and the need for long-term maintenance therapy. Another factor that could affect drug selection is overuse of fluconazole leading to the emergence of fluconazole-resistant species of *C. albicans,* and in some cases to all azoles, and other intrinsically more resistant species such as *C. krusei, C. glabrata,* and *C. tropicalis.*

❺ Topical therapies should be the first choice for milder forms of infections. The efficacy of antifungal agents for OPC varies in different patient populations. Until the polyene antifungal agents became available in the 1950s, gentian violet, an aniline dye, was used commonly to treat oropharyngeal candidiasis. Problems with gentian violet include fungal resistance, skin irritation, and especially the unaesthetic staining of the oral mucosa. Topical agents, such as nystatin and clotrimazole, have been the standard of treatment for uncomplicated OPC and generally are effective for treatment in otherwise healthy adults and infants with no underlying immunodeficiencies. Topical agents are available in an assortment of formulations, including oral rinses (suspension), troches, powder, vaginal tablets, and creams. The two most common types of formulations currently used are the suspension and troches (Table 124–6).

Topical agents require frequent applications because of the short contact time with the oral mucosa; the ideal contact time is 20 to 30 minutes. Sufficient saliva is needed to dissolve clotrimazole troches, and this can be problematic for patients with xerostomia. Also, the rough surface of the tablet can become irritating to the oral soft

TABLE 124-6 Therapeutic Options for Mucosal Candidiasis

Initial Episodes of OPC[a] – Treat for 7–14 days	**Common/Significant Side Effects**
Clotrimazole 10-mg troche: Hold 1 troche in mouth for 15–20 minutes for slow dissolution four to five times times daily. (B-2)	Altered taste, mild nausea, vomiting
Nystatin 100,000 units/mL suspension: 5-mL swish and swallow four times daily. (B-2)	Mild nausea, vomiting, diarrhea
Fluconazole100-mg tablets[b]: 100 mg daily. (A-1)	GI upset, hepatitis not common
Itraconazole 10 mg/mL solution[c]: 200 mg daily. (A-1)	GI upset, not common: hepatotoxicity, CHF, pulmonary edema with long-term use[e]
Posaconazole 40 mg/mL suspension: 100 mg BID on day 1, then 100 mg daily with a full meal. (B-1)	GI upset, fever, headache, increased hepatic transaminases not common
Fluconazole-Refractory OPC–Treat for ≥14 days	**Common/Significant Side Effects**
Itraconazole 10 mg/mL solution: 200–400 mg daily. (A-2)	See above
Voriconazole 200 mg tablets: 200 mg twice daily (>40 kg), taken on empty stomach. (UR)	GI upset, rash, reversible visual disturbance (altered light perception, photopsia, chromatopsia, photophobia), increased hepatic transaminases, hallucinations or confusion
Posaconazole 40 mg/mL suspension: 400 mg twice daily with a full meal. (UR)	See above
Amphotericin B 100 mg/mL suspension[d]: 1–5 mL swish and swallow four to five times daily. (B-2)	Oral: Nausea, vomiting, diarrhea with higher dose.
Amphotericin B deoxycholate 50-mg injection: 0.3–0.7 mg/kg/day infusion. (B-2)	IV: Fever, chills, sweats, nephrotoxicity, electrolyte disturbances, bone marrow suppression
Caspofungin 50 mg IV daily. (UR)	Fever, headache, infusion related-reactions (<5%), e.g., rash, facial swelling, pruritus, and vasodilation, hypokalemia, increased hepatic transaminases, anemia, neutropenia
Esophageal Candidiasis[a]–Treat for 14–21 days	**Common/Significant Side Effects**
Fluconazole 100-mg tablets: 100–400 mg daily. (A-1)	See above
Itraconazole 10 mg/mL solution[c]: 200 mg daily. (A-1)	See above
Voriconazole and caspofungin (A-1): generally reserved for refractory cases	See above
Fluconazole-Refractory EC–Treat for 21–28 days	**Common/Significant Side Effects**
Itraconazole 10 mg/mL solution: 200–400 mg daily. (A-2)	See above
Voriconazole 200 mg tablets: 200 mg twice daily (>40 kg), taken on empty stomach. (A-2)	See above
Caspofungin 50 mg IV daily. (A-2)	See above
Micafungin 150 mg IV daily. (UR)	Similar to caspofungin
Anidulafungin 100 mg IV on day 1, then 50 mg IV daily. (*UR)	Similar to caspofungin
Amphotericin B deoxycholate: 0.3–0.7 mg/kg/day IV, or lipid-based amphotericin 3–5 mg/kg/day IV. (B-2)	See above

BID, twice daily; CHF, congestive heart failure; E, esophageal candidiasis; GI, gastrointestinal; OC, oropharyngeal candidiasis.

[a]Initial episodes of OPC can be adequately treated first with topical agents before resorting to systemic therapy (B-2), but systemic therapy is required for effective treatment of EC. (A-2) Suppressive therapy is generally not recommended (D-3) unless patients have frequent or severe recurrences.

[b]Fluconazole is more effective than ketoconazole (A-1).

[c]Solution is more effective than capsule (A-1); solution is better taken on an empty stomach.

[d]Suspension is not marketed; can be prepared extemporaneously by pharmacy.[44]

[e]See discussion under onychomycosis.

Recommendation Grades:

Strength of recommendation: **A**–Both strong evidence for efficacy and substantial clinical benefit to support recommendation for use. *Should always be offered.* **B**–Moderate evidence for efficacy but only limited clinical benefit, to support recommendation for use. *Should generally be offered.* **C**–Evidence for efficacy is insufficient to support recommendation for or against use; or evidence for efficacy might not outweigh adverse consequences or cost of the treatment under consideration. *Optional.* **D**– Moderate evidence for lack of efficacy or adverse outcome supports a recommendation against use. *Should generally not be offered.*

Quality of evidence: **1**–Evidence from at least one properly designed randomized, controlled trial. **2**–Evidence from at least one well-designed trial without randomization, from cohort or case-controlled analytic studies (preferably from more than one center), or from multiple time-series studies, or dramatic results from uncontrolled experiments. **3**– Evidence from opinions of respected authorities based on clinical experience, descriptive studies, or reports of expert committees. (UR) Evidence currently unrated.

tissue. Troches also contain dextrose, which has cariogenic potential. Nystatin suspension might be a better choice for patients with xerostomia, but it is difficult to maintain adequate contact time with the oral mucosa. Some patients complain of the unpleasant taste of nystatin, which can cause nausea and vomiting, and this is problematic in cancer patients experiencing chemotherapy-induced nausea. The high sucrose content of nystatin suspension is cariogenic in dentate patients, and it should be used with caution in diabetic patients. Topical creams, such as clotrimazole, ketoconazole, miconazole, and nystatin (usually mixed with a steroid), are more appropriate for application three times daily to the corners of the mouth in treating angular cheilitis.[31]

Systemic therapy is necessary in patients with OPC that is refractory to topical treatment, those who cannot tolerate topical agents, and those at high risk for disseminated systemic or invasive candidiasis. Effective treatment of esophageal candidiasis generally requires the use of systemic antifungal agents. However, these agents have the disadvantage of producing more side effects (see Table 124–6) and drug-drug interactions (see Chap. 125). Fluconazole is inexpensive, generally well tolerated, and its absorption is unaffected by food or gastric acidity. Ketoconazole requires gastric acidity for absorption, which can be problematic in AIDS patients with achlorhydria, and hence it is best given with an acidic beverage. It is generally not used today with the availability of more effective triazoles. Itraconazole capsules also have the same absorption problem, and should be taken after a meal. In contrast, itraconazole solution has enhanced absorption, and is best taken in a fasting state; in addition, the solution provides the benefit of both topical effects to the oral mucosa and systemic effects and is beneficial to patients with mucositis or swallowing problems. Whenever possible, it is generally beneficial to limit the use of systemic azole agents to prevent unnecessary drug exposure and to minimize the potential for occurrence of drug-resistant candidiasis, particularly from fluconazole resistance.

When patients become unresponsive to topical agents or fluconazole and itraconazole, alternative agents are available.[28,29,32] These include amphotericin B, and newer triazoles (voriconazole and posaconazole) and echinocandins (caspofungin, micafungin and anidulafungin) (see discussion below).

Oropharyngeal Candidiasis—HIV-Infected Patients

It is appropriate to initiate therapy with topical agents for initial or recurrent episodes of OPC, provided that clinical symptoms are not severe and that there is minimal risk of esophageal involvement.[28,32] Clinical responses with the resolution of signs and symptoms generally occur within 5 to 7 days of starting treatment. Clotrimazole appears to be the most effective topical agent and demonstrates comparable clinical response rates with both fluconazole and itraconazole.[26,29] However, topical therapy is associated with more frequent relapses than with fluconazole.[28,29] This may be of limited clinical significance in patients receiving effective HAART owing to their decreased susceptibility to opportunistic infection. In practice, nystatin suspension is still used frequently in initial episodes of OPC, although it is the least effective agent and is associated with frequent treatment failures and early relapses, especially in patients with advanced HIV disease or neutropenia.[26,29]

Systemic oral azoles should be reserved for use in the more severe episodes of OPC unresponsive to topical agents or in patients with concurrent esophageal involvement.[26,28,29] In clinical practice, fluconazole usually is the systemic azole agent of choice because of its proven efficacy, favorable absorption, safety, and drug-interaction profiles, and it is relatively inexpensive. Fluconazole is superior to ketoconazole and itraconazole capsules.[26,28,29] Itraconazole oral solution with an improved absorption profile compared with the capsule formulation, is as effective as fluconazole with comparable clinical and mycologic response and relapse rates.[26,28,29] However itraconazole carries a higher risk of drug interactions because it is a potent inhibitor of the cytochrome P450 enzymes, and it is associated with more nausea than fluconazole. Posaconazole is a new extended-spectrum triazole with potent in-vitro activity against both *albicans* and non-*albicans Candida* species. It is equivalent to fluconazole in efficacy, safety and tolerability.[33] The role of posaconazole in uncomplicated OPC remains to be defined. Other agents that are also effective include amphotericin B, voriconazole, a triazole, and the echinocandins (caspofungin, micafungin, and anidulafungin). They are better reserved for refractory OPC either because of greater toxicity, more expensive or less convenient to use.

Oropharyngeal Candidiasis—Non–HIV-Infected Patients

This patient population includes patients with hematologic malignancy (e.g., leukemias) or blood and marrow transplantation (BMT) with a long duration of neutropenia and chronic graft-versus-host disease, patients with solid tumors, patients with solid-organ transplants who are receiving immunosuppressive therapy, and patients with diabetes mellitus; as well as patients on prolonged courses of antibiotics or corticosteroids and the debilitated elderly. Factors to consider in deciding whether to use topical or systemic antifungal therapy include the severity and extent of mucosal involvement (oropharyngeal versus esophageal), predisposing risk factors, and risk for dissemination. Patients who develop neutropenia (e.g., leukemic and BMT patients) are usually at high risk for disseminated and invasive fungal disease, and treatment of oral candidiasis is more aggressive. Patients with cell-mediated immune deficits but normal or near-normal granulocyte function and number (e.g., solid tumors, solid-organ transplants, or diabetic patients) are at low risk for dissemination of infection.

Specific antifungal therapy can be unnecessary for asymptomatic patients at relatively low risk for disseminated candidiasis, such as those who are not granulocytopenic or who are expected to have a short duration of granulocytopenia.[34] Many of these infections will clear spontaneously after recovery of the granulocytes or discontinuation of antibiotic and/or immunosuppressive therapy. However, antifungal therapy usually is required for patients who have persistent infection or significant symptoms, usually pain, or who are granulocytopenic with a relatively high risk of fungal dissemination. Topical agents first can be given a therapeutic trial depending on the severity of infection and degree of immunosuppression. Although both nystatin and clotrimazole can be effective in treating OPC, nystatin suspension does not effectively reduce the incidence of either oropharyngeal or systemic *Candida* infections in immunocompromised patients receiving chemotherapy or radiation; its use often is associated with treatment failures and early relapses.[34,35] Clotrimazole appears to more effective in reducing colonization and treating acute episodes in cancer patients who are immunocompromised.

Systemic azole agents are used for treating OPC in patients who have failed or who are unable to take topical therapy.[29,34] The preceding discussion on the relative efficacy of fluconazole, itraconazole, and ketoconazole in HIV-infected patients can be extrapolated to the non–HIV-infected population. Fluconazole 100 to 200 mg daily is used more commonly because of more extensive experience with its use, and it is more effective and has a more favorable absorption and side-effect profile compared with ketoconazole.[26] If the oral route is not feasible for reasons such as severe chemotherapy-induced mucositis, fluconazole can be administered intravenously. In patients unresponsive to azoles, intravenous amphotericin B in relatively low doses of 0.1 to 0.3 mg/kg per day can be tried.[34] Because of the higher risk for dissemination in patients who are severely neutropenic (<0.1 × 10^9 neutrophils/L) or clinically unstable (hypotensive, febrile), some clinicians prefer to initiate therapy with intravenous amphotericin B at 0.6 mg/kg per day, with therapy continued until the neutropenia has resolved.[34]

Topical therapy with clotrimazole or nystatin for 7 days is usually adequate for treating mucocutaneous candidiasis in most solid-organ transplant patients.[36] Use of topical therapy will reduce the number of systemic drugs that these patients receive and hence minimize the risk of drug–drug interactions. Failure to respond to topical agents warrants the use of fluconazole. Low-dose amphotericin B 5 to 10 mg daily for 7 to 10 days is reserved for the unusual cases of treatment failure.

Patients who develop OPC because of prolonged antibiotic use or aerosolized corticosteroids use usually can be managed successfully by discontinuation of the offending agent, and the infection usually will resolve. If there is a strong desire to treat because of discomfort or need to hasten symptom resolution or an inability to stop the offending agent, therapy with a topical agent, either clotrimazole or nystatin, is effective in most cases. The advantage of systemic azoles is the convenience of less frequent dosing. Symptoms usually improve in 3 to 4 days. Infants should be given smaller amounts more frequently (e.g., nystatin 100,000 units every 2 to 3 hours) to ensure better contact time. For denture-related OPC, or candidal stomatitis, effective therapy requires treatment of both the mouth and the dentures to avoid relapse. The dentures must be brushed vigorously and disinfected every night by soaking in antiseptic solution, such as chlorhexidine gluconate 0.25% or a product such as Polident or Efferdent.[27,29] Topical antifungal therapy of the oral cavity is required. Consistent proper oral hygiene and care of the dentures can help prevent relapse.

Esophageal Candidiasis—HIV-Infected Patients

❻ Treatment of esophageal candidiasis has not been as well studied as OPC. Because of the significant morbidity of esophageal candidiasis and the absence of evidence supporting the efficacy of topical antifungals, treatment requires systemic antifungal agents.[28,29,32] Fluconazole is superior to ketoconazole and itraconazole capsules with respect to endoscopic cure and clinical response and usually produces a more rapid onset of action and resolution of symptoms.[26,28,29,32] Fluconazole is as effective as itraconazole solution, with reported response rates of more than 80% to 90%.[29] However itraconazole solution causes more nausea and drug interactions because of inhibition of the cytochrome P450 enzymes. Amphotericin B, voriconazole, and the echinocandins are also effective in esophageal candidiasis, but they are generally reserved for patients with advanced or inadequately controlled HIV disease where the candidiasis tends to recur or becomes refractory to azole therapy.[37–40]

Esophageal Candidiasis—Non–HIV-Infected Patients

As in the case of HIV-infected patients, treatment of esophageal candidiasis requires systemic therapy. Patients can be started on fluconazole 100 to 200 mg/day for 14 to 21 days.[32] However, higher fluconazole doses (up to 400 mg/day) have been suggested for patients with severe symptoms or those who are neutropenic.[34] Itraconazole solution is an effective alternative for those not responding adequately to fluconazole. If the symptoms worsen or fail to respond, intravenous amphotericin B 0.6 mg/kg per day can be used. Intravenous amphotericin B can be considered for initial therapy in neutropenic patients who present with severe symptoms or who are at high risk for dissemination of *Candida* species, such as those receiving other aggressive immunosuppressive therapy (e.g., corticosteroids, total-body irradiation, or antithymocyte globulin) and who have documented evidence of esophageal candidiasis or who have failed an initial empirical trial of oral nonabsorbable agents or systemic azoles.[34] Amphotericin B should be continued until at least the neutropenia resolves. For patients whose symptoms have resolved and who are afebrile and clinically stable, amphotericin B should be discontinued, and the patients should be monitored closely for infection recurrence. In high-risk patients, particularly those with persistent fever and neutropenia, the potential presence of clinically occult, diffuse gastrointestinal or disseminated candidiasis should be considered. Less toxic alternatives or oral agents are now available, such as the echinocandins and voriconazole, and are preferred in patients who are intolerant of amphotericin B deoxycholate or who have preexisting renal impairment.[25,41,42] Their efficacy and safety can be extrapolated from studies in HIV-infected patients as majority of randomized controlled trials have been conducted in HIV-patient population. There is limited data on the clinical efficacy of anidulafungin compared to fluconazole, 95% versus 89% cure rates, respectively, in the non–HIV-infected patients.[43]

Antifungal-Refractory Oral Mucosal Candidiasis

Treatment failure is generally defined as persistence of signs and symptoms of OPC or esophageal candidiasis after an appropriate trial of antifungal therapy.[28] Treatment of refractory oral mucosal candidiasis is frequently unsatisfactory, and clinical response is usually short-lived, with rapid and periodic recurrences. The key risk factors for occurrence of refractory candidiasis are advanced stage of AIDS with low CD4 cell counts (<50 cells/mm^3) and repeated or prolonged courses of various systemic antifungal agents, in particular systemic azoles.[25,29,32] Frequent or prolonged use of fluconazole can be associated with fluconazole-refractory candidiasis because of selection of more resistant non-*albicans* species. An important initial management strategy is to assess and optimize the antiretroviral therapy of the patient with refractory OPC to help improve the immune function. With the widespread use of HAART, fluconazole-refractory OPC is now less commonly encountered. It is also important to identify and rectify potentially correctable causes of clinical failures of mucosal candidiasis, such as poor drug adherence, adequate dosing, reduced drug absorption associated with hypochlorhydria, and drug–drug interactions.

There have been few controlled studies that assess the effectiveness of antifungals. Doubling of the fluconazole dosage to 400 or 800 mg/day can be effective in some patients with infection caused by *Candida* species of intermediate resistance, although the response can be only transient.[25] Fluconazole oral suspension can be beneficial in some patients because of increased salivary concentrations obtained when the suspension is taken with the swish-and-swallow technique.[32] Patients with fluconazole-refractory mucosal candidiasis can be treated with itraconazole oral suspension because it can be effective in between 64% and 80% of patients; however, the benefit is short-lived if chronic suppressive therapy is not maintained.[28,32] Amphotericin B oral suspension is another alternative for azole-refractory patients.[28,32] It has broad spectrum activity against many fungal species and low likelihood of *Candida* species resistance. There are limited data and experience on its use in immunosuppressed patients, and results from small studies have yielded mixed results.[44] Amphotericin B suspension is no longer available commercially in the United States, but it can be prepared extemporaneously by the pharmacy.[44]

Until recently, intravenous amphotericin B deoxycholate has been the alternative for patients with endoscopically proven disease who have failed fluconazole or itraconazole therapy.[25] Patients with severe disease unresponsive to other agents require intravenous amphotericin B 0.3 to 0.7 mg/kg per day for 7 to 10 days to achieve clinical response; higher dose or longer treatment duration can be needed in more severe disease.[25,28,29,32] After response, suppressive therapy with amphotericin B is required to increase disease-free intervals. Patients who fail to respond to amphotericin B and require more than 1 mg/kg per day might be candidates for liposomal amphotericin B preparations because of renal and/or bone marrow toxicities, although at a markedly higher cost. Flucytosine usually is not used as monotherapy because of rapid development of resistance but can be used in combination with an azole or amphotericin B.[25] Less toxic agents that are also effective include voriconazole and the echinocandins.[41–43] Voriconazole, a triazole antifungal available in both oral and intravenous preparations, appears to be as effective as fluconazole for esophageal candidiasis, and it has shown success in treatment of fluconazole-refractory disease.[40] However drawbacks of voriconazole include more side effects and multiple pharmacokinetic drug interactions than fluconazole.[25,42] Caspofungin is the first of the echinocandins to be approved for esophageal candidiasis, and more recently micafungin and anidulafungin have also been approved for this indication. All three echinocandins have similar efficacy and tolerability profile as fluconazole, although higher relapse has been reported with caspofungin and anidulafungin compared to fluconazole.[29,43] Because the echinocandins require intravenous administration and are expensive, they are primarily used in patients who are refractory to the triazoles or have serious triazole-related adverse effects. As a class the echinocandins have a favorable adverse effect profile. They are less toxic than amphotericin B (see Table 124–6), and have lesser impact on the cytochrome P450 enzymes than itraconazole or voriconazole.

Antifungal Prophylaxis

❼ Ensuring that the HIV-infected patient is receiving appropriate antiretroviral therapy to enhance the immune system is perhaps the most important measure in preventing future episodes of mucosal candidiasis (oropharyngeal, esophageal, and vulvovaginal).[29,32] Initial success of treatment often is followed by symptomatic recurrences, especially in patients with advanced or poorly controlled HIV disease. Long-term suppressive therapy with fluconazole is effective in preventing recurrences or new infections of OPC in AIDS and in patients with cancer.[29,32] However the indications for antifungal prophylaxis and the best long-term management strategy still have not been well established. Fluconazole does not provide complete protection, and breakthrough infections can occur.[25] The reduced risk of recurrence of OPC also has not been demonstrated to improve survival. In addition, chronic exposure to azole therapy has been a concern that it might lead to the development of refractory disease or emergence of azole resistance. [29,32] However in a randomized trial of continuous versus episodic fluconazole therapy, continuous therapy did not result in a higher rate of refractory OPC or esophageal disease.[45] ❽ Currently HIV specialists do not recommend primary or secondary prophylaxis for OPC.[28] The rationale includes effectiveness of therapy for acute episodes of OPC, low incidence of serious invasive fungal disease, low mortality associated with mucosal candidiasis, potential for drug interactions, potential for emergence of drug resistance, and the prohibitive long-term cost of prophylaxis.

The decision to use secondary prophylaxis should be individualized for each patient. Secondary prophylaxis can be considered in patients with multiple recurrent episodes of symptomatic OPC, or when the disease is sufficiently severe and affecting the quality of life.[28] Patients with a history of one or more episodes of documented esophageal candidiasis, and CD4 T-cell count still is below 200 cells/mm^3 despite being on HAART are candidates for secondary prophylaxis. Fluconazole 100 mg daily is the usual regimen recommended for OPC and esophageal candidiasis,[28,29,32] although 200 mg three times weekly also appears to be effective.[45] Once-weekly fluconazole (200 mg) is also effective for preventing OPC recurrences in those with less advanced AIDS.[25] Itraconazole solution 200 mg daily is an alternative as suppressive therapy for OPC.[32]

Patients with malignant neoplastic diseases who are receiving irradiation, cytotoxic, and/or immunosuppressive therapy are at high risk for fungal infections in addition to bacterial and viral infections. Prophylaxis of *Candida* infection is controversial, and results of studies have been conflicting and difficult to evaluate. The value of antifungal prophylaxis in these patients needs to be considered in the broader context of not only reducing colonization and the risk of superficial candidiasis but also, more importantly, reducing the risk for invasive candidiasis and improving survival. Management of these infections in this patient population is discussed further in Chap. 126.

EVALUATION OF THERAPEUTIC OUTCOMES

Efficacy end points for oropharyngeal and esophageal candidiasis include rapid relief of symptoms and prevention of complications without early relapse after completion of the course of therapy.[28,32] Sterilization of the oral cavity is not a feasible end point because mycologic eradication is rarely achievable, especially in HIV-positive patients. Symptomatic relief of presenting signs and symptoms (see Table 124–5) generally occurs within 48 to 72 hours of starting therapy, with complete resolution by 7 to 10 days. Patients should be advised about the time course and told to return for reassessment when signs and symptoms recur. It is usually unnecessary for the patient to be reassessed soon after finishing the treatment course. However, HIV patients should be questioned and examined for the occurrence of mucosal candidiasis as part of their regular followup. The frequency of monitoring can be more often in neutropenic patients because of concern for dissemination of candidiasis. During the period of neutropenia, temperature should be monitored daily, as well as signs of dissemination.

Efficacy of the antifungal agent is partly influenced by patient adherence to the medication regimen. Patients must be counseled on proper administration and dosing, in particular for topical agents (Table 124–7).[31] Safety end points include monitoring for occurrence of the relevant drug side effects and drug interactions (Table 124–6). Mild gastrointestinal (GI) intolerance can occur with topical therapy, but serious adverse effects are rare. It is still prudent to monitor for hypersensitivity reactions, with rash and pruritus that might occur

TABLE 124-7 Patient Counseling Tips for Managing Oropharyngeal Candidiasis

1. Clean the oral cavity prior to administering the topical antifungal agent. Daily fluoride rinses can help reduce the risk of caries when using an agent containing sucrose or dextrose.
2. Use the topical antifungal agent after meals as saliva flow and mouth movements can reduce the contact time.
3. Troches should be slowly dissolved in mouth, not chewed or swallowed whole, over 15 to 30 minutes and the saliva swallowed.
4. Suspension should be swished around the mouth in the oral cavity to cover all areas for as long as possible, ideally at least 1 minute, then gargled and swallowed.
5. Remove dentures while medication is being applied to the oral tissues.
6. Use a suspension instead of a troche if xerostomia is present; if a troche is preferred, the patient should rinse or drink water prior to dosing. For xerostomia, suggest nonpharmacologic measures for symptomatic relief, e.g., ice chips, sugarless gum or hard candy, citrus beverages.
7. Dentures should be removed and disinfected overnight using an antiseptic solution (e.g., chlorhexidine 0.12–0.2%). Disinfect oral tissues in addition to dental prosthesis.
8. Complete treatment course even though symptomatic improvement can occur in 48–72 hours.
9. Maintain good oral hygiene. Brush teeth daily (twice daily) and floss, rinse mouth or brush teeth after eating sweets.
10. Stop smoking; avoid alcohol.

From Akpan et al.[31]

with any medication. Gastrointestinal intolerance is more associated with the oral azoles. Hepatotoxicity can occur when azole therapy is prolonged beyond 7 to 10 days or high doses are used. Periodic monitoring of liver enzymes (alanine transaminase, aspartate aminotransferase) should be considered especially if prolonged therapy (more than 21 days) is anticipated. Patients who are receiving intravenous amphotericin B require daily monitoring by the pharmacist.

CLINICAL CONTROVERSY

The optimal strategy for the management of recurrent oral mucosal candidiasis is unclear. Specific criteria for use of secondary prophylaxis are not well defined, and a wide range of approaches can be seen in clinical practice.

CLINICAL CONTROVERSY

Several new antifungal agents, in both the triazole and echinocandin class, are now available in the armamentarium from which to choose to treat oral mucosal candidiasis. Although they have demonstrated efficacy in treatment of oral mucosal candidiasis, their place in therapy remains to be defined. It is not established which specific agent should be used next after failing fluconazole or itraconazole, and where amphotericin fits in the list of therapeutic options. Factors to consider in the selection can include underlying clinical condition, risk for drug interaction, and side-effect profiles.

MYCOTIC INFECTIONS OF THE SKIN, HAIR, AND NAILS

Superficial mycotic infections of the skin are referred to as *dermatophytoses.* They are common infections that usually are caused by dermatophytes classified by genera: *Trichophyton, Epidermophyton,* or *Microsporum.*[46] Dermatophytes have the ability to penetrate keratinous structures of the body. These infections affect both male and female genders and all races. Reservoirs of mycotic infections include humans, animals, and soil.[46] Individuals can develop an infection if they come in contact with a reservoir in addition to having a conducive environment for mycotic growth (i.e., moist conditions).[47] Risk factors for the development of an infection include prolonged exposure to sweaty clothes, failure to bathe regularly, many skin folds, sedentariness, and confinement to bed.[47]

Mycotic infections of the skin have a classic appearance that consists of a central clearing surrounded by an advancing red, scaly, elevated border.[47] Infections of the nail can appear chalky and dull yellow or white and become brittle and crumbly.

Diagnosis usually is based on patient history, as well as the physical examination.[48] Diagnostic tests include direct microscopic examination of a specimen after the addition of potassium hydroxide (KOH) or fungal cultures. The KOH test is quick, inexpensive, and easy to perform, whereas cultures are more expensive and take longer to obtain results. Diagnostic tests are recommended when systemic therapy is likely to be prescribed.[48]

❾ A general approach to treatment of superficial mycotic infections includes keeping the infected area dry and clean and limiting exposure to the infected reservoir. Topical agents generally are considered to be first-line therapy for infections of the skin. Oral therapy is preferred when the infection is extensive or severe or when treating tinea capitis or onychomycosis.[49–51] Table 124–8 lists specific treatments for each mycotic infection. Superficial mycotic infections are categorized by the pattern and site of infection.[46] The most commonly occurring infections in North America are detailed below.

TINEA PEDIS

Tinea pedis is the most common dermatophytoses (affecting approximately 70% of adults). It is better known as "athlete's foot" and occurs in hot weather, with exposure to surface reservoirs (locker room floors), and with use of occlusive footwear.[47] Treatment with topical therapy for 2 to 4 weeks often is adequate for mild infections; however, severe infections or involvement of the nails requires oral therapy[47] (see Table 124–8). Recurrence of infection occurs in up to 70% of individuals. Prolonged treatment with either topical or systemic therapy may be required.[48,49]

TINEA MANUUM

Tinea manuum usually involves the palmar surface of the hands, is unilateral, and can involve the feet. Treatment of this infection is similar to tinea pedis (see Table 124–8). Emollients that contain lactic acid also can be useful.[47]

TINEA CRURIS

Tinea cruris is an infection of the proximal thighs and buttocks.[50] It is referred to as "jock itch" and is more common in males. The scrotum and penis often are spared from infection. Treatment with topical therapy is recommended and should continue for 1 to 2 weeks after symptom resolution. Severe infections can require oral therapy (see Table 124–8). Relief of pruritus and burning can be facilitated by the use of short-term (2 to 3 days) topical steroids (2.5% hydrocortisone).[47]

TINEA CORPORIS

Tinea corporis is an infection the glabrous skin of the trunk and extremities.[50] Therapy is similar to that for tinea pedis, tinea manuum, and tinea cruris (see Table 124–8).

TINEA CAPITIS

Tinea capitis is a mycotic infection involving the scalp, hair follicles, and adjacent skin[51,52] that primarily affects children. Treatment should consist of oral therapy, as well as the cleaning of combs and brushes, which can be contaminated (see Table 124–8). Daily shampooing is recommended for removal of scales. Some children and adults can be asymptomatic carriers, thereby facilitating spread of the infection.[51] Family members who culture positive for tinea tonsurans should be treated with a antifungal shampoo (e.g., ketoconazole, selenium sulfide, or povidone-iodine).[51]

TINEA BARBAE

Tinea barbae affects the hairs and follicles of beards and mustaches.[51] Treatment is similar to that for tinea capitis (see Table 124–8). Removal of the beard or mustache is recommended.[47]

PITYRIASIS VERSICOLOR

Hyperpigmented and hypopigmented scaly patches characterize pityriasis versicolor. These patches are found on the trunk and extremities.[53] It is more common in adults and in areas with tropical ambient temperatures. Topical treatment usually is adequate unless there is extensive involvement, recurrent infections, or failure of topical therapy[53] (see Table 124–8).

CLINICAL CONTROVERSY

Evidence for the treatment of superficial mycotic infections of the skin and hair come from a small number of trials with relatively small numbers of subjects.

TABLE 124-8 Treatment of Mycoses of the Skin, Hair, and Nails

	Topical[a,b]	Oral[c]
Tinea pedis	Butenafine, daily	Fluconazole 150 mg 1 × per wk 1–4 wk
Tinea manuum	Ciclopirox, twice daily	Ketoconazole 200 mg daily × 4 wk
Tinea cruris	Clotrimazole, twice daily	Itraconazole 200–400 mg/day × 1 wk
Tinea corporis	Econazole, daily	Terbinafine 250 mg/day × 2 wk
	Haloprogin, twice daily	
	Ketoconazole cream, daily	
	Miconazole, twice daily	
	Naftifine cream, daily; gel, twice daily	
	Oxiconazole, twice daily	
	Sulconazole, twice daily	
	Terbinafine, twice daily	
	Tolnaftate, twice daily	
	Triacetin cream, solution, three times daily	
	Undecylenic acid, various preparations apply as directed	
Tinea capitis	Shampoo only in conjunction with oral therapy or for treatment	Terbinafine 250 mg/day 4–8 wk
Tinea barbae	of asymptomatic carriers	Ketoconazole 200 mg daily × 4 wk
	Ketoconazole 2 × per wk × 4 wk	Itraconazole 100–200 mg/day × 4–6 wk
	Selenium sulfide daily × 2 wk	Griseofulvin 500 mg/day × 4–6 wk
Pityriasis versicolor	Clotrimazole, twice daily	Ketoconazole 400 mg × 1
	Econazole, daily	
	Haloprogin, twice daily	Fluconazole 400 mg × 1
	Ketoconazole, daily	
	Miconazole, twice daily	Itraconazole 200 mg daily × 3–7 days
	Oxiconazole cream only, twice daily	
	Sulconazole, twice daily	
	Tolnaftate, three times daily	
Onychomycosis	Ciclopirox 8% nail lacquer apply solution at night for up to 48 wk	Terbinafine 250 mg/day × 6 wk (finger), 12 wk (toe)
Fingernail		Itraconazole 200 mg twice daily × 1 wk per month; repeat for total of two pulses (finger), or three pulses (toe)
Toenail		Itraconazole 200 mg daily for 6 weeks (finger), or for 12 weeks (toe)
		Fluconazole 50 mg daily or 300 mg once weekly for ≥6 months (finger), or for 12 months (toe)

[a]Other products are available, including combination products.
[b]Length of therapy depends on mycotic sensitivity and severity of infection.
[c]Only capsule formulation studied; give with food for increased absorption.

ONYCHOMYCOSIS (TINEA UNGUIUM)

Onychomycosis is a fungal infection of the nail apparatus, and it is a common condition that accounts for up to 50% of all nail problems.[54,55] Onychomycosis more commonly affects the toenails, approximately 4 to 19 times more frequently than fingernails.[54] This can be partly because of the slower growth of toenails, three times slower than fingernails, making it easier for fungi to establish infection. The dermatophytes responsible for causing more than 90% of onychomycosis are *Trichophyton rubrum* (71%) and *Trichophyton mentagrophytes* (20%).[54,55] Less common fungi causing onychomycosis are the nondermatophytic molds (2.3 to 11%) and yeasts (5.6%). *Candida albicans* is the most commonly isolated yeast, and typically affect fingernails rather than toenails.[54,56] Risk factors for dermatophytic onychomycosis include increasing age (especially older than 40 years of age), family history and genetic factors, immunodeficiency (such as HIV, renal transplant, immunosuppressive therapy, defective polymorphonuclear chemotaxis), diabetes mellitus, psoriasis, peripheral vascular disease, smoking, prevalence of tinea pedis, frequent nail trauma, and sporting activities such as swimming.[56,57] These risk factors also appear to apply to recurrence of onychomycosis. Mold onychomycosis does not seem to be associated with systemic or local predisposing factors, but there is a risk of systemic dissemination in the immunosuppressed patients.[57] *Candida* onychomycosis seems to always occur in immunosuppressed patients.[57]

Onychomycosis can present in four to five different major clinical forms, of which lateral distal subungual onychomycosis (DSO) is the most common type.[54,57,58] In DSO the nail plate, the nail bed, and in advanced cases, the matrix are all affected, and *T. rubrum* is the most common etiologic cause. The worst case of onychomycosis is progression of the infection to total dystrophic onychomycosis, characterized by almost complete destruction of the nail plate. White superficial onychomycosis is usually caused by *Trichophyton mentagrophytes*, where the infection is localized to the surface of the nail plate. In proximal subungual onychomycosis (PSO), the fungi (usually *T. rubrum*) invade the nail through the proximal nail fold and spreads to the nail plate and matrix. Although PSO is relatively uncommon in the general population, it occurs most frequently in severely immunocompromised patients and is often considered a marker for AIDS.[56,58] Because of the multifactorial etiology of onychomycosis, it is important to differentiate onychomycosis from other causes of nail dystrophies so that the patient receives appropriate therapy and is not subjected to prolonged treatment with unnecessary drugs. Besides clinical history and physical examination, proper diagnosis of onychomycosis can include combination of direct microscopy of scrapings from appropriate nail area to look for fungal hyphae, and fungal cultures, and if necessary histologic examination.[55,59,60]

TREATMENT

Onychomycosis (Tinea Unguium)

■ GENERAL APPROACH

Onychomycosis merits proper treatment because it is a debilitating disease and can exert a negative impact on quality of life (cosmetic and psychosocial effects, pain, discomfort, and decreased ambulation).[55,56,61] Untreated onychomycosis can lead to complications such as cellulitis or reduced mobility, which further compromises peripheral circulation in those with diabetes or peripheral vascular disease; and infected nails can serve as a source for transmission of fungi to other areas of the body, as well as to other people, such as close household contacts or in communal bathing places.[55,56,61,62] The primary end point of treatment is eradication of the organism, with secondary end points being clinical cure or improvement.[55] Assessment of clinical success (cure or improvement) requires followup for several months after the end of treatment because of the slow growth rate of nails, especially toenails.[55,56] Successful eradication of the fungus does not always result in normalization of the nails because they can have been dystrophic prior to infection. This can cause patient dissatisfaction especially if this is not explained before starting treatment.[58] There are several factors that must be taken into account on a patient-by-patient basis to ensure appropriate treatment decisions (Table 124–9). The impact of patient adherence on success of treatment cannot be overemphasized. Patients need to be educated about their disease, expectation from treatment and prevention of recurrence, and various strategies have been suggested to improve treatment success.[60]

In general, onychomycosis of the toenail is more difficult to treat than fingernails, requires longer treatment duration, and is associated with a higher recurrence. The treatment options for onychomycosis include oral and topical therapies, mechanical or chemical nail avulsion, or a combination of these. Mechanical or chemical nail avulsion is used primarily as adjunct to oral therapy in patients with total dystrophic onychomycosis, in whom there is severe onycholysis and extensive nail thickening or longitudinal spikes. This is to enhance penetration of the antifungal agent to the entire nail plate and unit.[55,60,62]

TOPICAL THERAPY

⑩ Conventional topical antifungal products are available as creams, ointments, powders, and solutions. Because these formulations do not penetrate through the nail plate to the nail bed, they are most appropriately used when the nail plate has been removed.[62] Even then cure rates are still low and variable, and are influenced by patient adherence.[56,62] Nail lacquer represents the latest advance in topical formulation. The volatile vehicle, used to deliver the drug, evaporates and leaves an occlusive film with a high drug concentration on the nail surface.[56,62] There are only two marketed nail lacquers, amorolfine 5% and ciclopirox 8% solution (Penlac), the latter being the only one approved in North America for the treatment of mild to moderate onychomycosis caused by *T. rubrum* without lunula involvement.[56,61,62] Ciclopirox, a hydroxypyridine, has a broad spectrum of antifungal activity (dermatophytes, *Candida* spp. and some molds), and requires treatment for 1 year. Although ciclopirox was significantly better than vehicle alone, mycologic cure rate was only 32% with ciclopirox versus 10% for vehicle alone after 48 weeks of treatment; overall treatment cure (mycological cure with 0%–10% involvement of target nail) was 9% versus 0.9% for drug and vehicle, respectively.[56,62] However higher mycologic cure rates of 45% to 65% have been reported in a variety of open-label trials involving 6 to 12 months of treatment.[56] Amorolfine appears to produce higher mycologic and treatment cure rates than ciclopirox.[56,61] Most experts consider topical therapy a feasible option when the infection is superficial involving the nail plate without matrix involvement, such as white superficial onychomycosis, involves a partial area of the nail plate not exceeding 50% (owing to difficulty of applying treatment to the margin of the nail), is limited to a few (three or four) nails, is in the very early stages of DSO when infection is still confined to the distal edge of the nail, or when systemic therapy is contraindicated.[55,56,61] Topical therapy is not associated with systemic adverse effects or drug interactions. Any adverse effect will be localized to the application site, such as mild erythema in the adjacent skin area.

TABLE 124-9 Factors That May Impact Treatment Decisions and Outcomes

- Type and severity of onychomycosis
- Causative organism—dermatophyte versus molds or yeast
- Infection of the finger versus toenail
- Extent of disease—involvement of matrix, one or two lateral edges, number of nails
- Thickness of nail plate
- Other sites of mycotic infection (palms, soles, toe webs)
- Other nail alterations affecting outcome (onycholysis, paronychia, dermatophytoma, etc.)
- Other nail diseases and symptoms
- Age and underlying medical conditions (diabetes, poor perfusion, immunocompromised)
- Drug interactions and adverse effects
- Cost of therapy

Data from Effendy,[54] Gupta,[60] Lecha,[61] Gupta.[62]

SYSTEMIC THERAPY

⑩ Oral antifungal therapy is considered to be more effective than topical for treating onychomycosis. Terbinafine and itraconazole (capsule), the current first-line agents for treatment, have yielded higher efficacy rates using shorter treatment periods (generally 3 months or shorter) for toenail and fingernail onychomycosis compared with the traditional agents, such as griseofulvin and ketoconazole, which are rarely used nowadays. Terbinafine, an allylamine, exerts fungicidal activity and demonstrates the greatest in-vitro activity against dermatophytes compared with the other oral antifungals; it has good activity against nondermatophyte molds and only marginal activity against *Candida* species.[55,62] Like other azoles, itraconazole, is fungistatic, has a broad antifungal spectrum and is very active against dermatophytes, nondermatophytes, and *Candida* species.[55,62] Both agents have lipophilic and keratinophilic properties, which explain their excellent penetration (appearing in the nail plate within days of treatment initiation) and accumulation in the nails, achieving concentrations far exceeding the minimal inhibitory concentration (MIC) of most dermatophytes. Nail terbinafine concentrations are detected within 1 week of starting therapy, whereas itraconazole can be detected 1 (fingernails) to 2 weeks (toenails) after starting therapy.[58] Both drugs are slowly eliminated from the nail, with effective drug concentrations persisting in nails for 30 to 36 weeks after completion of treatment with terbinafine and for 27 weeks with itraconazole.[58] The persistence of drug in the nails explains in part the long-term protection against relapses after the end of treatment and also permit use of intermittent (*pulse*) dosing.

Treatment of toenail onychomycosis requires a 12-week course, whereas a 6-week course generally is adequate for fingernail onychomycosis with either drug.[55,58] In general, cure rates of 80% to 90% for fingernail infection and 70% to 80% for toenail can be expected.[55] Terbinafine is licensed for daily dosing (see Table 124–8).[55,58,63] Although various terbinafine pulse regimens have been evaluated,[62] pulse dosing was less effective than continuous dosing, and it did not provide clear safety advantages.[64,65] Itraconazole pulse therapy is the preferred method over continuous dosing for fingernail infections, and it is licensed as twice-daily dosing for a 1-week cycle per month for 2 consecutive months (i.e., two pulses), or as daily therapy for 6 weeks (see Table 124–8).[58,63] Although itraconazole pulse therapy is not approved by the Food and Drug Administration (FDA), three to four pulses are effective for toenail infections; otherwise, half the dose is taken daily for 3 months (see Table 124–8).[58,63] In addition to lower drug cost, potential advantages of itraconazole pulse therapy compared with continuous therapy include a lower risk of adverse drug effects and improved patient adherence.

Terbinafine is generally considered by most experts as first-line agent for onychomycosis, whereas itraconazole is the alternative. Direct comparative trials generally have shown that terbinafine is more effective than itraconazole either by continuous or pulse dosing.[55,61,62] Mycologic cure rates for terbinafine range from 77% to 100% depending on the study.[61] In a cumulative meta-analysis of randomized controlled trials, mycologic cure rates for terbinafine, itraconazole pulse, itraconazole continuous, fluconazole, and griseofulvin were 76% ± 3%, 63% ± 7%, 59% ± 5%, 60% ± 6% and 48% ± 5%, respectively.[66] An earlier meta-analysis and systematic review also reported that continuous terbinafine was the most effective therapy for toenail onychomycosis.[67,68] In addition, terbinafine was reported to achieve high cure rates in high-risk immunosuppressed patients, such as diabetics, organ transplant recipients, comparable to the immunocompetent population, with no significant adverse effects or drug interactions. It also appears to be effective in HIV patients and nondermatophyte infections.[63,69] A pharmacoeconomic analysis of oral and topical (ciclopirox) therapies showed that from a managed-care perspective, terbinafine was the most cost-effective therapy in terms of highest success rate, lowest relapse rate, and highest number of disease-free days for both fingernail and toenail infections.[70]

Both terbinafine and itraconazole generally are well tolerated. The more common adverse effects reported with terbinafine are gastrointestinal (e.g., diarrhea, dyspepsia, nausea, and abdominal pain), dermatologic (e.g., rash, urticaria, and pruritus), and headache; less common adverse effects include taste disturbances, fatigue, inability to concentrate, and asymptomatic liver enzyme abnormalities.[58,61,63] Terbinafine can cause transient decrease in absolute lymphocyte counts; hence monitoring of complete blood counts can be useful especially in immunocompromised patients.[63] Although uncommon, severe adverse effects have been reported with terbinafine, including erythema multiforme, Stevens-Johnson's syndrome and toxic epidermal necrolysis, pancytopenia, lupus erythematosus, psoriasis, hair loss, and hepatotoxicity. Although the incidence of severe hepatotoxicity is considered rare, the FDA issued a Public Health Advisory in 2001 regarding the association of terbinafine tablets with 16 possible cases of liver failure, including 2 liver transplants and 11 deaths.[71] Terbinafine thus is not recommended for patients with chronic or active liver disease, although hepatotoxicity can occur in patients with no preexisting liver disease or serious underlying medical condition. Prior to initiating terbinafine treatment, it is recommended to obtain appropriate nail specimens for laboratory testing to confirm the diagnosis of onychomycosis. Liver function parameters (serum transaminases) should be assessed at baseline and periodically during treatment with terbinafine.[63,71]

The common adverse effects of itraconazole are similar to those of terbinafine, such as gastrointestinal disturbance, dermatologic disorders, and headache; less common adverse effects include dizziness, fatigue, fever, decreased libido, and asymptomatic liver enzyme abnormalities (1% to 5% with continuous dosing and about 2% with pulse dosing).[58,61,63,72] Although still considered rare, 24 serious cases of liver failure, including transplantation and death, have been reported with the use of itraconazole, resulting in a recent FDA Public Health Advisory warning.[71] Some of these patients did not have preexisting liver disease or serious underlying medical conditions, and some developed within the first week of treatment. It has been suggested to avoid itraconazole in patients with elevated liver enzymes or active liver disease or in those who have experienced other drug-induced liver toxicity. Liver function parameters (serum transaminases) should be assessed prior to and periodically during treatment. However, some experts have suggested that frequent monitoring is not as necessary if pulse therapy is used because symptomatic hepatotoxicity has not been reported with pulse therapy.[72] In addition, there is an FDA warning on the risk of developing congestive heart failure (CHF) associated with the use of itraconazole, possibly related to its potential negative inotropic effect.[58,71] Therefore, itraconazole should not be used in patients with evidence of ventricular dysfunction, such as CHF. Symptomatic assessment for the development of CHF also should be included as part of therapy monitoring. Before a patient is subjected to several months of itraconazole treatment, it is important to confirm the diagnosis of onychomycosis.

In contrast to the azoles, terbinafine does not inhibit the cytochrome P450 (CYP) 3A4 isoenzymes, but it is a potent inhibitor of the CYP2D6 isoenzymes, which are responsible for metabolism of tricyclic antidepressants and other psychotropic drugs.[55,58,63] The most significant drug interactions with terbinafine are decreased clearance of 33% by cimetidine and increased clearance of 100% by rifampin. Other drug interactions of variable clinical significance include tricyclic antidepressants, cyclosporine, caffeine, theophylline, and terfenadine. Itraconazole and its major metabolite can inhibit the CYP3A4 isoenzymes, and result in numerous clinically significant drug interactions where coadministration with several drugs are contraindicated (e.g., alprazolam, midazolam, triazolam, pimozide, lovastatin, simvastatin, cisapride, terfenadine). [55,58,63]

Fluconazole is also active against dermatophytes, *Candida* species, and some nondermatophytes.[58,62] Fluconazole does not have current FDA-approved indication for treatment of onychomycosis. The overall mycologic cure rate of fluconazole is 48%, which is lowest compared to all other oral agents.[66] The most effective dose and treatment duration have not been clearly established, with a variety of dosing regimens used, ranging from 50 mg daily to 300 mg once weekly for 6 to 12 months (see Table 124–8).[58,63] Advantages of fluconazole include a relatively good safety profile, and fewer drug interactions compared to itraconazole.[58,63]

These three oral antifungal agents have superseded the use of griseofulvin and ketoconazole as treatments of choice for onychomycosis.[55,61,62] Griseofulvin has a narrow antifungal spectrum, low clinical efficacy, especially for toenail infections, high relapse rates, and the need for prolonged treatment duration (up to 12 to 18 months for toenails). Use of ketoconazole is also associated with high relapse rates, and the prolonged treatment duration carries an increased risk of hepatotoxicity.

■ TREATMENT RESPONSE AND RECURRENCE

Treatment failures and recurrence rates of infection following initial cure are high, ranging from 20% to 50%.[55,60] Recurrence could be either a relapse (original infection not completely cured) or reinfection (new infection after achieving a cure of the original). Factors associated with poor response to systemic therapy include a compromised immune system (AIDS), reduced blood flow (diabetes, peripheral vascular disease, vasculitis, connective tissue disease, congestive heart failure), coexisting nail disease (psoriasis), nail factors (slow growth, thick nails, severe disease), drug-resistant organisms because of extensive prior drug exposure, and reduced bioavailability (absorption problems, poor compliance, drug interactions).[58,60] To help to improve treatment outcomes and reduce recurrence, patients should be counseled on the importance of proper foot hygiene, for example, wearing breathable footwear and 100% cotton socks with frequent changes, keeping the nails short and clean, keeping the feet dry, protecting the feet in shared bathing areas, treating tinea pedis, and controlling other predisposing medical conditions.[60]

The use of combination therapy (topical–oral or oral–oral agents) can improve cure rates and shorten treatment duration, as this approach provides complementary mechanisms of attack.[60,61] Studies in Europe have reported favorable results achieved with itraconazole or terbinafine combined with amorolfine.[61] To date no specific combination has been approved or endorsed for use. Other novel approaches include giving supplemental therapy and use of boosted therapy.[60,61] The efficacy and role of either approach remains to be defined.

CHAPTER 125

Invasive Fungal Infections

PEGGY L. CARVER

KEY CONCEPTS

1. Systemic mycoses can be caused by pathogenic fungi and include histoplasmosis, coccidioidomycosis, cryptococcosis, blastomycosis, paracoccidioidomycosis, and sporotrichosis, or infections by opportunistic fungi such as *Candida albicans, Aspergillus* species, *Trichosporon, Candida glabrata, Fusarium, Alternaria,* and *Mucor.*

2. The diagnosis of fungal infection generally is accomplished by careful evaluation of clinical symptoms, results of serologic tests, and histopathologic examination and culture of clinical specimens.

3. Histoplasmosis is caused by *Histoplasma capsulatum* and is endemic in parts of the central United States along the Ohio and Mississippi River valleys. Although most patients experience asymptomatic infection, some can experience chronic, disseminated disease.

4. Asymptomatic patients with histoplasmosis are not treated, although non-acquired immune deficiency syndrome (AIDS) patients with evident disease are treated with either oral ketoconazole or intravenous amphotericin B; AIDS patients are treated with amphotericin B and then receive lifelong suppression.

5. Blastomycosis is caused by *Blastomyces dermatitidis* and generally is an asymptomatic, self-limited disease; however, reactivation can lead to chronic disease. Although treatment for self-limited disease is controversial, patients with chronic pulmonary disease or extrapulmonary disease should be treated with ketoconazole, and those with central nervous system (CNS), progressive, or life-threatening disease should receive amphotericin B.

6. Coccidioidomycosis is caused by *Coccidioides immitis* and is endemic in some parts of the southwestern United States. It can cause nonspecific symptoms, acute pneumonia, or chronic pulmonary or disseminated disease. Primary pulmonary disease (unless severe) frequently is not treated, whereas extrapulmonary disease is treated with amphotericin B, and meningitis is treated with fluconazole.

7. Cryptococcosis is caused by *Cryptococcus neoformans* and occurs primarily in immunocompromised patients. Patients with acute meningitis are treated with amphotericin B with flucytosine. Patients infected with human immunodeficiency virus (HIV) often require long-term suppressive therapy with fluconazole or itraconazole.

8. A variety of *Candida* species (including *C. albicans, C. glabrata, Candida tropicalis, and Candida krusei*) can cause diseases such as mucocutaneous, oral, esophageal, vaginal, and hematogenous candidiasis, as well as candiduria. Candidemia can be treated with a variety of antifungal agents; the optimal choice depends on previous patient exposure to antifungal agents, potential drug interactions and toxicities of each agent, and local epidemiology of intensive care unit or hematology-oncology centers.

9. Aspergillosis can be caused by a variety of *Aspergillus* species that can cause superficial infections, pneumonia, allergic bronchopulmonary aspergillosis, or invasive infection. Treatment with amphotericin B or voriconazole generally is instituted but often is not successful. Combination therapy, while widely used, lacks clinical trial data to support its use.

Learning objectives, review questions, and other resources can be found at **www.pharmacotherapyonline.com.**

For many years, fungal infections were classified as either superficial "nuisance diseases," such as athlete's foot or vulvovaginal candidiasis, or as relatively rare infections confined primarily to endemic areas of the country. When invasive fungal infections were encountered, amphotericin B was the only consistently effective, systemically active agent available for the treatment of systemic mycoses. (1) Advances in medical technology, including organ and bone marrow transplantation, cytotoxic chemotherapy, the widespread use of indwelling intravenous (IV) catheters, and the increased use of potent broad-spectrum antimicrobial agents all have contributed to the dramatic increase in the incidence of fungal infections worldwide.

Fungal infections have emerged as a major cause of death among cancer patients and transplant recipients.[1–4] In addition, patients with AIDS experience substantially more frequent and severe forms of cryptococcosis, histoplasmosis, coccidioidomycosis, and mucocutaneous (esophageal, oral, and vulvovaginal) candidiasis.

Problems remain in the diagnosis, prevention, and treatment of fungal infections. Unlike the available diagnostic techniques for most bacterial pathogens, there remains a host of unresolved issues regarding standardization of susceptibility testing methods, in-vitro and in-vivo models of infection, the usefulness of monitoring antifungal plasma concentrations, and the development and identification of resistant pathogens.[1,5,6] The Infectious Diseases Society of America published guidelines for the treatment of many commonly encountered fungal infections. These guidelines provide summaries of the literature and a consensus of expert opinions regarding the treatment of these difficult infections.[6]

MYCOLOGY

Fungi are eukaryotic organisms with a defined nucleus enclosed by a nuclear membrane; a cytoplasmic membrane containing lipids, glycoproteins, and sterols, mitochondria, Golgi apparatus, and ribosomes bound to endoplasmic reticulum; and a cytoskeleton

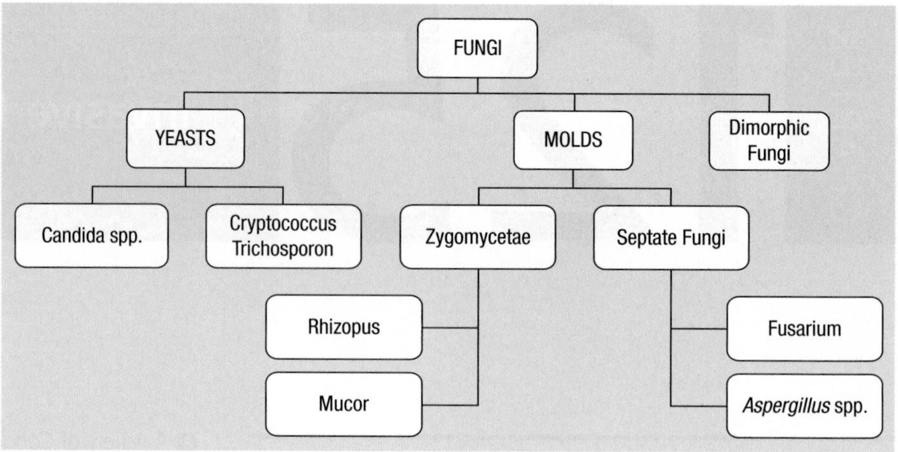

FIGURE 125-1. Morphologically, pathogenic fungi can be grouped as either filamentous molds or unicellular yeasts. *Molds* grow as multicellular branching, threadlike filaments (hyphae) that are either septate (divided by transverse walls) or coenocytic (multinucleate without cross walls).

with microtubules, microfilaments, and intermediate filaments. Fungi have rigid cell walls composed of chitin, cellulose, or both that stain with Gomori methenamine silver or periodic acid–Schiff reagent. Most fungi, except *Candida* species, are too weakly gram-positive to be seen well on Gram's stain. *Cryptococcus neoformans* has a polysaccharide capsule surrounding the cell wall.[6]

Morphologically, pathogenic fungi can be grouped as either filamentous molds or unicellular yeasts (Fig. 125–1). *Molds* grow as multicellular branching, threadlike filaments (hyphae) that are either septate (divided by transverse walls) or coenocytic (multinucleate without cross walls). On agar media, molds grow outward from the point of inoculation by extension of the tips of filaments and then branch repeatedly, interweaving to form fuzzy, matted growths called *mycelia.* Yeasts are oval or spherically shaped unicellular forms that generally produce pasty or mucoid colonies on agar medium similar to those observed with bacterial cultures. Yeasts have rigid cell walls and reproduce by budding, a process in which daughter cells arise from pinching off a portion of the parent cell.

Fungi reproduce by forming spores asexually through mitosis to produce motile sporangiospores or nonmotile conidia (singular, conidium), or they reproduce sexually through meiosis to produce ascospores, basidiospores, oospores, or zygospores. Although terms such as *spore* and *conidia* should no longer be used interchangeably, some newer literature and much of the older medical literature continue to confuse these terms.

Many pathogenic fungi, termed *dimorphic fungi,* exist as either a yeast or a mold, depending on pathogen, site of growth (in the host or in the laboratory setting), and temperature. Usually yeasts are the parasitic form that invades human or animal host tissue, whereas molds are the free-living form found in the environment. For example, *Histoplasma capsulatum* exists as a yeast in humans and as a mold in the laboratory.[1]

SUSCEPTIBILITY TESTING OF ANTIFUNGAL AGENTS

Most laboratories do not routinely perform susceptibility tests on fungal isolates, but standardized methods for performing these tests are being developed and are now available for testing selected yeasts. To date, reference broth macrodilution and microdilution methods have been established for *Candida* and *Cryptococcus* species, whereas the broth microdilution method has been standardized for filamentous fungi. Additionally, minimal inhibitory concentration (MIC) reference ranges for American Type Culture Collection (ATCC) quality control strains have been established against various antifungal agents, as well as interpretive breakpoints for fluconazole, itraconazole, and flucytosine against *Candida* species[5] (Tables 125–1 and 125–2). For further detail, refer to the section outlining treatment of *Candida* infections. Reliable and convincing interpretive breakpoints are not yet available for amphotericin B. The National Committee for Clinical Laboratory Standards (NCCLS) M27-A methodology does not reliably identify amphotericin B–resistant isolates; variations of the methodology using different media appear to enhance detection of resistant isolates.[5,7] It is important that the breakpoints be used following testing with the standardized, reproducible laboratory methodology (NCCLS 27-A) used to develop the test and that they be interpreted in the context of the delivered dose of the antifungal agent.

Because in-vitro correlations with in-vivo outcomes in patients are not yet known, the role of routine susceptibility testing is unknown at this time. Several concerns need to be considered as the use of MIC breakpoints is incorporated into the clinical practice setting: First, MICs are not actual physical measurements; rather, they provide estimates of drug activity. Because the MICs obtained can span greater than three twofold dilutions for the same isolate despite meticulous technique, MICs must be interpreted with caution. Second, host factors contribute greatly to clinical outcome. The same isolate in an immunocompetent patient might not result in the same outcome as in an immunocompromised patient. Thus, in-vitro susceptibility does *not* necessarily equate with in-vivo clinical success, and in-vitro resistance might *not* always correlate with treatment failure. Susceptibility testing occasionally is indicated, for example, in a patient with prolonged fungemia with a presumed susceptible isolate. Because of wide interlaboratory variability in test results, isolates should be tested at specialty laboratories that routinely perform these specialized tests. Susceptibility testing is most helpful in dealing with infections caused by non-*albicans* species of *Candida.*[5,7]

RESISTANCE TO ANTIFUNGAL AGENTS

It is important to distinguish between clinical resistance and microbial resistance. *Clinical resistance* refers to failure of an antifungal agent in the treatment of a fungal infection that arises from factors other than microbial resistance, such as failure of the antifungal agent to reach the site of infection or inability of a patient's immune system to eradicate a fungus whose growth is retarded by an antifungal agent.[8]

Microbial resistance can refer to *primary* or *secondary* resistance, as determined by in-vitro susceptibility testing using standardized methodology. NCCLS resistance breakpoints are based on data relating treatment outcomes and fungal MICs and indicate the MIC at

TABLE 125-1 General Patterns of Susceptibility and Interpretive Breakpoints of *Candida Species*[a]

	Patterns of Susceptibility							
	Azoles				*Echinocandins*			
***Candida* Species**	**Fluconazole**	**Itraconazole**	**Voriconazole**	**Posaconazole**	**Caspofungin**	**Micafungin**	**Anidulafungin**	**Amphotericin B**
C. albicans	+++ S	+++ S	+++ S	S	+++	+++	+++	+++
C. tropicalis	+++ S	+++ S	+++ S	+++ S	+++ S	+++ S	+++ S	+++ S
C. parapsilosis	S	S	S	S	S[d]	S[d]	S[d]	S
C. glabrata	++ S-DD to R[b]	++ S-DD to R[c]	++	S	S	S	S	S-I[e]
C. krusei	R	S-DD to R[c]	S	S	S	S	S	S-I[e]
C. lusitaniae	S	S	S	S	S	S	S	S to R
Interpretive breakpoints								
Sensitive	≤8	≤0.125	≤0.1	NA	NA	NA	NA	NA
S-DD or I	S-DD: 16–32	S-DD: 0.25–0.5	2	NA	NA	NA	NA	NA
R	>32	>0.5	≥4	NA	NA	NA	NA	NA

[a]Except for amphotericin B, interpretations are based on the use of a broth sensitivity test.
[b]Approximately 15% of *C. glabrata* isolates are resistant to fluconazole
[c]Approximately 46% of *C. glabrata* isolates and 31% of *C. krusei* isolates are resistant to itraconazole.
[d]Most isolates of *C. parapsilosis* have reduced susceptibility to echinocandins.
[e]A significant proportion of *C. glabrata* and *C. krusei* isolates have reduced susceptibility to amphotericin B.
[f]Although frank resistance to amphotericin B is not observed in all isolates, it is well described for isolates of *C. lusitaniae*.
For antifungal drugs and pathogens for which susceptibility breakpoints have been established (fluconazole, itraconazole, voriconazole):
S = susceptible; S-DD = susceptible-dose dependent (see text); I = intermediate; R = resistant; NA = not available (has not been established for this antifungal against this pathogen).
For antifungal drugs and pathogens for which susceptibility breakpoints have not been established, an estimate of relative activity:
+++ = reliable activity with occasional resistance
++ = moderate activity but resistance is noted
+ = occasional activity
0 = no meaningful activity
Data from NCCLS,[5] Pappas et al.,[7] and Eschenauer et al.[12]

which clinical responses demonstrate a marked decline.[8] However, they do not serve as absolute predictors of therapeutic success or failure.

Primary, or *intrinsic, resistance* refers to resistance recorded prior to drug exposure in vitro or in vivo. *Secondary*, or *acquired resistance* develops on exposure to an antifungal agent and can be either reversible, owing to transient adaptation, or acquired as a result of one or more genetic alterations. The clinical consequences of antifungal resistance can be observed in treatment failures and in changes in the prevalences of *Candida* species causing disease. The evidence for the emergence of antifungal-resistant yeasts in patients other than those with HIV infection is confounded by the lack of standardized susceptibility testing methods and definitions of resistance. Large-scale surveys of yeasts from blood cultures, tested by standardized methodology, do not yet suggest that antifungal resistance is a significant or growing therapeutic problem.[8]

It is possible for a patient to respond clinically to treatment with an antifungal agent despite resistance to that agent in vitro because the patient's own immune system may eradicate the infection, or the agent may reach the site of infection in high concentrations.[8] Resistance to azole antifungal agents has been studied intensively partly because of the increased number of fluconazole-resistant *Candida* strains isolated from AIDS patients. Resistance can be acquired (i.e., transferred from other organisms or developed dur-

TABLE 125-2 General Patterns of In-Vitro Susceptibility of Non-*Candida* Fungal Pathogens[a]

	Patterns of Susceptibility[a]							
	Azoles				*Echinocandins*			
Pathogen	**Fluconazole**	**Itraconazole**	**Voriconazole**	**Posaconazole**	**Caspofungin**	**Micafungin**	**Anidulafungin**	**Amphotericin B**
Aspergillus								
A. fumigatus	No	Yes	Yes	Yes	Yes	Yes	Yes	Yes
A. flavus	No	Yes	Yes	Yes	Yes	Yes	Yes	Yes
A. terreus	No	Yes	Yes		Yes			No
Fusarium	No	No	Yes (but breakthrough infections are seen)	Conflicting data (species dependent)	No	No	No	Yes but occasional resistance
Scedosporium	No	No	Yes	Yes (apiospermum)	No	No	No	No
Zygomycetes[b]	No	No	No	Yes	No	No	No	Yes
Trichosporon	No	No	Yes	Yes	No	No	No	No
Cryptococcus	Yes	Yes	Yes	Yes	No	No	No	

[a]No = has minimal or no in-vitro activity versus the pathogen; Yes = possesses adequate in-vitro activity versus the pathogen
[b]Includes *Rhizopus, Mucor, Absidia* species.
Data from Eschenauer et al.[12] and Dodds.[78]

ing therapy as a result of exposure to the antifungal agent) or intrinsic (innate lack of susceptibility of the antifungal agent to a pathogen). This issue has been reviewed extensively.

The most exhaustive and definitive accounts of antifungal resistance have been described in *Candida* species, in particular *Candida albicans* and, to a lesser extent, *C. glabrata*, *C. tropicalis*, and *C. krusei*, as well as in a few *Cryptococcus neoformans* isolates.[9–11] There are four different mechanisms that result in azole resistance: (1) mutations or upregulation of *ERG11* (an enzyme involved in the ergosterol biosynthesis pathway), (2) expression of multidrug efflux transport pumps that decrease antifungal drug accumulation within the fungal cell, (3) alteration of the structure or concentration of antifungal drug target proteins, and (4) alteration of membrane sterol proteins (Fig. 125–2). It is beyond the scope of this chapter to provide a complete discussion of the biochemical mechanisms of fungal resistance. Interested readers are referred to several excellent reviews concerning this topic.[8–11] Efflux pumps have been identified in *C. albicans, C. glabrata, C. tropicalis,* and *Candida dubliniensis* and appear to be the most common mechanism of resistance encountered in clinical isolates. It is interesting to note that some of these mechanisms (efflux pumps in particular) appear to be reversible when selective pressure of antifungal agents is withdrawn.

Even though ketoconazole was used widely for the treatment of mucocutaneous candidiasis, resistant strains appeared very rarely. In patients with the uncommon syndrome of chronic mucocutaneous candidiasis, however, the chronic use of ketoconazole was associated with the emergence of ketoconazole-resistant *C. albicans.* Resistance likely developed in this specific population of patients because of two factors: the chronic use of ketoconazole and the inability of patients with this syndrome to eradicate the organism by normal host defense mechanisms. Fluconazole-resistant *C. albicans* have been noted primarily in AIDS patients, usually after CD4 counts are less than 50 cells/mm^3 and after fluconazole has been used chronically for repeated episodes of thrush over months to years. Resistance develops in a stepwise progression in patients who have repeated episodes of thrush with one or several persisting strains of *C. albicans.*

Among hospitalized patients, there is increasing evidence for a shift toward isolation of other resistant species, such as *C. glabrata* and *C. krusei,* that have moderate or high-level resistance to fluconazole. This phenomenon has been especially common among patients in whom fluconazole has been used extensively.[3]

Resistance has not been described widely with itraconazole. This can be partly related to the fact that the drug has been used primarily for the treatment of endemic mycoses and not candidiasis. Even in patients never treated with itraconazole, however, *C. albicans* strains that are resistant to fluconazole also show decreased susceptibility to itraconazole.

The most commonly reported mechanisms of azole resistance among *C. albicans* isolates include reduced permeability of the fungal cell membrane to azoles, alteration in the target fungal enzymes (cytochrome P450) resulting in decreased binding of the azole to the target site, and overproduction of the fungal cytochrome P450 (CYP) enzymes. Studies also suggest the presence of efflux pumps capable of actively pumping azoles from the target pathogen, thereby conferring multidrug resistance to azole antifungals.[8–11]

C. glabrata is intrinsically more resistant than *C. albicans* to ketoconazole. Several strains of *C. glabrata* have been well characterized in terms of the mechanism of ketoconazole resistance. Decreased permeability to azoles has been described, but other strains show enhanced activity of the P450 cell membrane enzymes as well. *C. krusei* is inherently resistant to fluconazole, but it appears to be more susceptible to the other azoles. Decreased uptake of fluconazole into the fungal cell has been noted for several *C. krusei* strains.[8–11]

Although rare, in-vitro intrinsic resistance to amphotericin B is described, mainly in *Candida lusitaniae*, *Candida guilliermondii*, and some molds (*Fusarium* spp. and *Pseudallescheria boydii*).[11] However, it is important to keep in mind that the current in-vitro M27-A methodology discriminates poorly between rates of susceptibility of *Candida* species to amphotericin B. Although the rate of apparent resistance to amphotericin B appears to be quite low, breakthrough bacteremias in patients treated with amphotericin B have been observed. *C. glabrata*, *C. guilliermondii*, *C. krusei*, and *C. lusitaniae* appear to have a higher propensity than other *Candida* species to develop resistance to amphotericin B; this point should be kept in mind when treating patients with infections caused by one of these pathogens.[8] Because polyenes target ergosterol in the membranes of fungal cells, it is not surprising that amphotericin B–resistant strains of *Candida* generally have a marked decrease in ergosterol content compared with amphotericin B–susceptible strains. Resistant isolates of *Cryptococcus neoformans* have been reported to have a mutation in the C8 isomerization step of ergosterol synthesis.[11]

Although spontaneous resistance of *C. albicans* to echinocandins has been documented in vitro, the specific mechanisms of resistance have not been fully elucidated and prospective worldwide surveillance of clinical *Candida* isolates has revealed no evidence of emerging caspofungin resistance.[12]

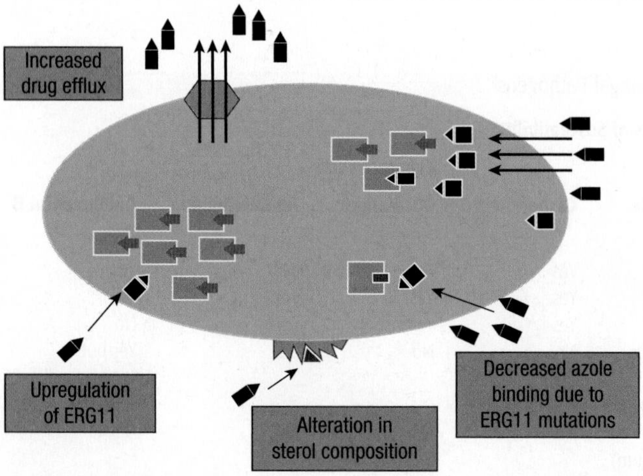

FIGURE 125-2. Mechanisms of azole resistance. Four different mechanisms result in azole resistance: (1) mutations or upregulation of *ERG11*, the target enzyme of azoles, (2) expression of multidrug efflux transport pumps that decrease antifungal drug accumulation within the fungal cell, (3) alteration of the structure or concentration of antifungal drug target proteins, and (4) alteration of membrane sterol proteins.

PATHOGENESIS AND EPIDEMIOLOGY

Systemic mycoses caused by primary or pathogenic fungi include histoplasmosis, coccidioidomycosis, cryptococcosis, blastomycosis, paracoccidioidomycosis, and sporotrichosis. Primary pathogens can cause disease in both healthy and immunocompromised individuals, although disease generally is more severe or disseminated in the immunocompromised host. In contrast, mycoses caused by opportunistic fungi such as *C. albicans, Aspergillus* species, *Trichosporon, Torulopsis (Candida) glabrata, Fusarium, Alternaria,* and *Mucor* generally are found only in the immunocompromised host.[1]

Most fungal infections are acquired as a result of accidental inhalation of airborne conidia. For example, *Histoplasma capsulatum* is found in soil contaminated by bat, chicken, or starling excreta, and *C. neoformans* is associated with pigeon droppings. Although some fungi, including *C. albicans, C. neoformans,* and *Aspergillus* species, are ubiquitous pathogens with worldwide distribution, other fungi have regional distributions associated with specific geographic environments.[1]

Systemic fungal infections are a major cause of morbidity and mortality in the immunocompromised patient. Fungal infections account for 20% to 30% of fatal infections in patients with acute leukemia, 10% to 15% of fatal infections in patients with lymphoma, and 5% of fatal infections in patients with solid tumors. The frequency of fungal infections among transplant recipients ranges from 0% to 20% for kidney and bone marrow transplant recipients to 10% to 35% for heart transplant recipients and 30% to 40% for liver transplant recipients.[4]

Approximately 2% to 4% of all hospitalized patients develop a nosocomial infection. Of these, bacteria comprise the most common etiologic agent.[1] Fungi, however, are becoming increasingly significant nosocomial pathogens. Fungi account for 10% of all bloodstream isolates. *Candida* species (primarily *C. albicans*) are the fourth most commonly isolated bloodstream isolate and account for 78% of all nosocomial fungal infections.[13]

Nosocomially acquired fungal infections can arise from either exogenous or endogenous flora. Endogenous flora can include normal commensal organisms of the skin, gastrointestinal (GI), genitourinary, or respiratory tract. *C. albicans* is found as a normal commensal of the GI tract in 20% to 30% of humans.

A complex interplay of host and pathogen factors influences the acquisition and development of fungal infections. Intact skin or mucosal surfaces serve as primary barriers to infection. Desiccation, epithelial cell turnover, fatty acid content, and low pH of the skin are believed to be important factors in host resistance. Bacterial flora of the skin and mucous membranes compete with fungi for growth. Alterations in the balance of normal flora caused by the use of antibiotics or alterations in nutritional status can allow the proliferation of fungi such as *Candida,* increasing the likelihood of systemic invasion and infection.[1]

The growth of fungi within tissues is restrained by a number of mechanisms. For example, serum has fungistatic activity against *Candida* in part because of transferrins, the human iron-binding proteins that deprive microbes of the iron needed for synthesis of respiratory enzymes. Serum also contains globulins, which cause a nonimmunologic clumping of *Candida,* facilitating their elimination by inflammatory cells.[1]

Tissue reaction in the presence of fungi varies with fungal species, site of proliferation, and duration of infection. Phagocytosis by neutrophils and macrophages is the earliest mechanism that prevents the establishment of fungi. Consequently, patients with decreased neutrophil counts or decreased neutrophil function are at higher risk of infections, particularly infections caused by *Candida* and *Aspergillus* species. Some mycoses are characterized by a low-grade inflammatory response that does not eliminate the fungi. Fungal cells sometimes can persist within macrophages without being killed, perhaps because of resistance to the effects of lysosomal enzymes.[1]

DIAGNOSIS

❷ The diagnosis of invasive fungal infections generally is accomplished by careful evaluation of clinical symptoms, results of serologic tests, and histopathologic examination and culture of clinical specimens. Skin tests generally are not useful diagnostically because they do not distinguish between active and past infection. They remain useful as screening tools and in epidemiologic studies to determine endemic areas. It is beyond the scope of this chapter to discuss the relative merits of each of the immunologic tests used in the diagnosis of invasive fungal infections. Interested readers, however, are referred to several excellent reviews concerning this topic.[14]

TREATMENT

Invasive Mycoses

Strategies for the prevention or treatment of invasive mycoses can be classified broadly as prophylaxis, early empirical therapy, empirical therapy, and secondary prophylaxis or suppression.[1] In patients undergoing cytotoxic chemotherapy, antifungal therapy is directed primarily at the prevention or treatment of infections caused by *Candida* and *Aspergillus* species. Prophylactic therapy with topical, oral, or intravenous antifungal agents is administered prior to and throughout periods of granulocytopenia (absolute neutrophil count <1000 cells/L). The potential benefits of prophylactic therapy must be weighed against the potential risks inherent in each regimen, including safety, efficacy, cost, the prevalence of infection, and the potential consequences (e.g., resistance) of widespread use.

Early empirical therapy is the administration of systemic antifungal agents at the onset of fever and neutropenia. Empirical therapy with systemic antifungal agents is administered to granulocytopenic patients with persistent or recurrent fever despite the administration of appropriate antimicrobial therapy.

Secondary prophylaxis (or suppressive therapy) is the administration of systemic antifungal agents (generally prior to and throughout the period of granulocytopenia) to prevent relapse of a documented invasive fungal infection that was treated during a previous episode of granulocytopenia.

Although these treatment classifications also have been applied to the treatment of fungal infections in AIDS, patients with AIDS rarely acquire systemic infections caused by *Candida* or *Aspergillus* species unless they become granulocytopenic because of disease or drugs. The use of antifungal prophylaxis is much less widely studied in this population, although studies suggest that early antifungal prophylaxis decreases the incidence of invasive cryptococcal disease.[15] Suppressive therapy generally is necessary following acute therapy for histoplasmosis, coccidioidomycosis, and cryptococcosis because of the high rates of relapse when antifungal therapy is discontinued.

■ PROPHYLAXIS OF FUNGAL INFECTION IN THE HIV-INFECTED PATIENT

The use of antifungal prophylaxis to prevent fungal infections in HIV-infected patients has been assessed. Fluconazole prevented cryptococcosis and local *Candida* infections, including esophagitis, in HIV-infected patients, but overall mortality was not improved. Because of the high costs of long-term prophylaxis, improved therapeutic regimens available for treating cryptococcal meningitis, and increasing reports of fluconazole resistance among *Candida* isolates from AIDS patients, many clinicians prefer not to use fluconazole prophylaxis in AIDS patients. For some patients with very low CD4 counts (<50 cells/microliter), however, some clinicians feel that it is cost-effective to use fluconazole prophylaxis (100 to 200 mg daily) to prevent cryptococcosis.

HISTOPLASMOSIS

In humans, histoplasmosis is caused by inhalation of dust-borne microconidia of the dimorphic fungus *H. capsulatum.* Although there exist two dimorphic varieties of *H. capsulatum,* the small-celled (2–5 microns) form (var. *capsulatum*) occurs globally, whereas the large-celled (8–15 microns) form (var. *duboisii*) is confined to the African continent and Madagascar. In tissues stained by conventional techniques, *H. capsulatum* appears as an oval or round, narrow-pore, budding, unencapsulated yeast.[16]

EPIDEMIOLOGY

❸ Although histoplasmosis is found worldwide, certain areas of North and Latin America are recognized as endemic areas; in the United States, most disease is localized along the Ohio and Mississippi River valleys, where more than 90% of residents may be affected. Precise reasons for this endemic distribution pattern are unknown but are thought to include moderate climate, humidity, and soil characteristics. *H. capsulatum* is found in nitrogen-enriched soils, particularly those heavily contaminated by avian or bat guano, which accelerates sporulation. Blackbird or pigeon roosts, chicken coops, and sites frequented by bats, such as caves, attics, or old buildings, serve as "microfoci" of infections. Although birds are not infected because of their high body temperature, bats (mammals) may be infected and can pass yeast forms in their feces, allowing the spread of *H. capsulatum* to new habitats. Air currents carry the spores for great distances, exposing individuals who were unaware of contact with the contaminated site.[16–18]

PATHOPHYSIOLOGY

At ambient temperatures, *H. capsulatum* grows as a mold. The mycelial phase consists of septate branching hyphae with terminal micro- and macroconidia that range in size from 2 to 14 microns in diameter. When soil is disturbed, these conidia become aerosolized and reach the bronchioles or alveoli.[16]

Animal studies demonstrate that within 2 to 3 days after reaching lung tissue, the conidia germinate, releasing yeast forms that begin multiplying by binary fission. During the next 9 to 15 days, organisms are ingested but not destroyed by large numbers of macrophages that are recruited to the infected site, resulting in small infiltrates. Infected macrophages migrate to the mediastinal lymph nodes and other sites within the mononuclear phagocyte system, particularly the spleen and liver. At this time, the onset of specific T-cell immunity in the nonimmune host activates the macrophages, rendering them capable of fungicidal activity. Tissue granulomas form, many of which develop central caseation and necrosis over the next 2 to 4 months. Over a period of several years, these foci become encapsulated and calcified, often with viable yeast trapped within the necrotic tissue.[16,19]

Cellular immunity, as measured by histoplasmin skin-test reactivity, wanes in the absence of occasional reexposure. Although exposure to heavy inocula can overcome these immune mechanisms, resulting in severe disease, reinfection occurs frequently in endemic areas. In the immune individual, the reactions of acquired immunity begin 24 to 48 hours after the appearance of yeast forms, resulting in milder forms of illness and little proliferation of organisms. Although viable organisms can be found within granulomas years after initial infection, the organisms appear to have little ability to proliferate within the fibrous capsules, except in immunocompromised patients.[16,19]

CLINICAL PRESENTATION[15,16,18,19]

General

The outcome of infection with *H. capsulatum* depends on a complex interplay of host, pathogen, and environmental factors. Host factors include the degree of immunosuppression and the presence of immunity (from prior infection). Environmental factors include inoculum size, exposure within an enclosed area, and duration of exposure. Hematogenous dissemination from the lungs to other tissues probably occurs in all infected individuals during the first 2 weeks of infection before specific immunity has developed but is nonprogressive in most cases, which leads to the development of calcified granulomas of the liver and/or spleen. Progressive pulmonary infection is common in patients with underlying centrilobular emphysema.

A number of acute and chronic manifestations of histoplasmosis appear to result from unusual inflammatory or fibrotic responses to the pathogen, including pericarditis and rheumatologic syndromes during the first year after exposure, with chronic mediastinal inflammation or fibrosis, broncholithiasis, and enlarging parenchymal granulomas later in the course of disease.

Acute Pulmonary Histoplasmosis

In the vast majority of patients, low-inoculum exposure to *H. capsulatum* results in mild or asymptomatic pulmonary histoplasmosis. The course of disease generally is benign, and symptoms usually abate within a few weeks of onset. Patients exposed to a higher inoculum during an acute primary infection or reinfection can experience an acute, self-limited illness with flulike pulmonary symptoms, including fever, chills, headache, myalgia, and a nonproductive cough. Patients with diffuse pulmonary histoplasmosis can have diffuse radiographic involvement, become hypoxic, and require ventilatory support. A small percentage of patients present with arthritis, erythema nodosum, pericarditis, or mediastinal granuloma.

Chronic Pulmonary Histoplasmosis

Chronic pulmonary histoplasmosis generally presents as an opportunistic infection imposed on a preexisting structural abnormality, such as lesions resulting from emphysema. Patients demonstrate chronic pulmonary symptoms and apical lung lesions that progress with inflammation, calcified granulomas, and fibrosis. Patients with early, noncavitary disease often recover without treatment. Progression of disease over a period of years, seen in 25% to 30% of patients, is associated with cavitation, bronchopleural fistulas, extension to the other lung, pulmonary insufficiency, and often death.

Disseminated Histoplasmosis

In patients exposed to a large inoculum and in immunocompromised hosts, successful containment of the organism within macrophages may not occur, resulting in a progressive illness characterized by yeast-filled phagocytic cells and an inability to produce granulomas. This disease, termed *disseminated histoplasmosis,* is characterized by persistent parasitization of macrophages. The clinical severity of the diverse forms of disseminated histoplasmosis (Table 125–3) generally parallels the degree of macrophage parasitization observed.

Acute (infantile) disseminated histoplasmosis is characterized by massive involvement of the mononuclear phagocyte system by yeast-engorged macrophages. Classically, this severe type of infection is seen in infants and young children and (rarely) in adults with Hodgkin's disease or other lymphoproliferative disorders. In infants or children, acute disseminated histoplasmosis is characterized by unrelenting fever, anemia, leukopenia or thrombocytopenia, enlargement of the liver, spleen, and visceral lymph nodes, and GI symptoms, particularly nausea, vomiting, and diarrhea. The chest roentgenogram often demonstrates remnants of the initiating acute pulmonary lesion. Untreated disease is uniformly fatal in 1 to 2 months. A less severe "subacute" form of the disease, which occurs in both infants and immunocompetent adults, is characterized by focal destructive lesions in various organs, weight loss, weakness, fever, and malaise. Untreated disease generally is fatal in approximately 10 months.

Most adults with disseminated histoplasmosis demonstrate a mild, chronic form of the disease. Untreated patients often are ill for 10 to 20 years, demonstrating long asymptomatic periods interrupted by relapses of clinical illness characterized primarily by weight loss, weakness, and fatigue. Chronic disseminated histoplasmosis can be seen in patients with lymphoreticular neoplasms (Hodgkin disease) and patients undergoing immunosuppressant chemotherapy for organ transplantation or for rheumatic diseases. Although CNS involvement occurs in 10% to 20% of patients with severe underlying immunosuppressive conditions, focal organ involvement is uncommon. The disease is characterized by the development of focal granulomatous lesions, often with bone marrow involvement resulting in thrombocytopenia, anemia, and leukemia. Fever, hepatosplenomegaly, and GI ulceration are common.

TABLE 125-3 Clinical Manifestations and Therapy of Histoplasmosis

Type of Disease and Common Clinical Manifestations	Approximate Frequency (%)[a]	Therapy/Comments
Nonimmunosuppressed host		
Acute pulmonary histoplasmosis		
Asymptomatic or mild disease	50–99	*Asymptomatic, mild, or symptoms <4 weeks:* No therapy generally required *Symptoms >4 weeks:* Itraconazole 200 mg once daily × 6–12 weeks[b]
Self-limited disease	1–50	*Self-limited disease:* Amphotericin B[c] 0.3–0.5 mg/kg/day × 2–4 weeks (total dose 500 mg) or ketoconazole 400 mg orally daily × 3–6 months can be beneficial in patients with severe hypoxia following inhalation of large inocula Antifungal therapy generally not useful for arthritis or pericarditis; NSAIDs or corticosteroids can be useful in some cases
Mediastinal granulomas	1–50	Most lesions resolve spontaneously; surgery or antifungal therapy with amphotericin B 40–50 mg/day × 2–3 weeks or itraconazole 400 mg/day orally × 6–12 months can be beneficial in some severe cases; mild to moderate disease can be treated with itraconazole for 6–12 months
Severe diffuse pulmonary disease		Amphotericin B 0.7 mg/kg/day, for a total dose of ≤35 mg/kg (or 3 mg/kg/day of one of the lipid preparations) + prednisone 60 mg daily tapered over 2 weeks,[d] followed by itraconazole 200 mg twice daily for 6–12 weeks; in patients who do not require hospitalization, itraconazole 200 mg once or twice daily for 6–12 weeks can be used
Inflammatory/fibrotic disease	0.02	*Fibrosing mediastinitis:* The benefit of antifungal therapy (itraconazole 200 mg twice daily × 3 months) is controversial but should be considered, especially in patients with elevated ESR or CF titers ≥1:32; surgery can be of benefit if disease is detected early; late disease can not respond to therapy *Sarcoid-like:* NSAIDs or corticosteroids can be of benefit for some patients *Pericarditis:* Severe disease: corticosteroids 1 mg/kg/day or pericardial drainage procedure
Chronic pulmonary histoplasmosis	0.05	Antifungal therapy generally recommended for all patients to halt further lung destruction and reduce mortality *Mild–moderate disease:* Itraconazole 200–400 mg PO daily × 6–24 months is the treatment of choice Itraconazole and ketoconazole (200–800 mg/day orally for 1 year) are effective in 74% to 86% of cases, but relapses are common; fluconazole 200–400 mg daily is less effective (64%) than ketoconazole or itraconazole, and relapses are seen in 29% of responders *Severe disease:* Amphotericin B 0.7 mg/kg/day for a minimum total dose of 35 mg/kg is effective in 59% to 100% of cases and should be used in patients who require hospitalization or are unable to take itraconazole because of drug interactions, allergies, failure to absorb drug, or failure to improve clinically after a minimum of 12 weeks of itraconazole therapy
Immunosuppressed host		
Disseminated histoplasmosis	0.02 – 0.05	*Disseminated histoplasmosis:* Untreated mortality 83% to 93%; relapse 5% to 23% in non-AIDS patients; therapy is recommended for all patients
Acute (Infantile)		*Nonimmunosuppressed patients:* Ketoconazole 400 mg/day orally × 6–12 months or amphotericin B 35 mg/kg IV
Subacute		*Immunosuppressed patients (non-AIDS) or endocarditis or CNS disease:* Amphotericin B >35 mg/kg × 3 months followed by fluconazole or itraconazole 200 mg orally twice daily × 12 months
Progressive histoplasmosis (immunocompetent patients and immunosuppressed patients without AIDS)		*Life-threatening disease:* Amphotericin B 0.7–1 mg/kg/day IV for a total dosage of 35 mg/kg over 2–4 months; once the patient is afebrile, able to take oral medications, and no longer requires blood pressure or ventilatory support, therapy can be changed to itraconazole 200 mg orally twice daily for 6–18 months *Non–life-threatening disease:* Itraconazole 200–400 mg orally daily for 6–18 months; fluconazole therapy 400–800 mg daily) should be reserved for patients intolerant to itraconazole, and the development of resistance can lead to relapses
Progressive disease of AIDS	25–50[e]	Amphotericin B 15–30 mg/kg (1–2 g over 4–10 weeks)[f] or itraconazole 200 mg three times daily for 3 days then twice daily for 12 weeks, followed by lifelong suppressive therapy with itraconazole 200–400 mg orally daily. Although patients receiving secondary prophylaxis (chronic maintenance therapy) might be at low risk for recurrence of systemic mycosis when their CD4+ T-lymphocyte counts increase to >100 cells/microliter in response to HAART, the number of patients who have been evaluated is insufficient to warrant a recommendation to discontinue prophylaxis.

AIDS, acquired immunodeficiency syndrome; CF, complement fixation; ESR, erythrocyte sedimentation rate; HAART, highly active antiretroviral therapy; NSAIDs, nonsteroidal anti-nflammatory drugs; PO, orally.
[a]As a percentage of all patients presenting with histoplasmosis.
[b]Itraconazole plasma concentrations should be measured during the second week of therapy to ensure that detectable concentrations have been achieved. If the concentration is below 1 mcg/mL, the dose may be insufficient or drug interactions can be impairing absorption or accelerating metabolism, requiring a change in dosage. If plasma concentrations are greater than 10 mcg/mL, the dosage can be reduced.
[c]Desoxycholate amphotericin B.
[d]Effectiveness of corticosteroids is controversial.
[e]As a percentage of AIDS patients presenting with histoplasmosis as the initial manifestation of their disease.
[f]Liposomal amphotericin B (AmBisome) may be more appropriate for disseminated disease.
Data from Deepe,[16] Wheat et al.,[18] and Wheat and Kauffman.[19]

Histoplasmosis in HIV-Infected Patients

Adult patients with AIDS demonstrate an acute form of disseminated disease that resembles the syndrome seen in infants and children. Progressive disseminated histoplasmosis (PDH) can occur as the direct result of initial infection or because of the reactivation of dormant foci. In endemic areas, 50% of AIDS patients demonstrate PDH as the first manifestation of their disease. PDH is characterized by fever (75% of patients), weight loss, chills, night sweats, enlargement of the spleen, liver, or lymph nodes, and anemia. Pulmonary symptoms occur in only one-third of patients and do not always correlate with the presence of infiltrates on chest roentgenogram. A clinical syndrome resembling septicemia is seen in approximately 25% to 50% of patients.[19]

DIAGNOSIS

Detection of single, yeastlike cells 2 to 5 microns in diameter with narrow-based budding by direct examination or by histologic study of blood smears or tissues should raise strong suspicion of infection with *H. capsulatum* because colonization does not occur as with *Aspergillus* or *Candida* infection. Identification of mycelial isolates from clinical cultures can be made by conversion of the mycelium to the yeast form (requires 3 to 6 weeks) or through a rapid (2-hour) and 100% sensitive DNA probe that recognizes ribosomal DNA. In patients with suspected disseminated or chronic cavitary histoplasmosis, two to three blood, sputum, and bone marrow cultures and stains should be obtained using the lysis centrifugation technique, and the cultures should be held for 14 to 21 days for optimal yield of *H. capsulatum*. In patients with acute self-limited histoplasmosis, extensive testing to verify the diagnosis may not be necessary.

In most patients, serologic evidence remains the primary method in the diagnosis of histoplasmosis. Results obtained from commercially available complement fixation (CF), immunodiffusion (ID), and latex agglutination (LA) antibody tests are used alone or in combination. In general, the use of histoplasmin skin tests is of little value except in epidemiologic studies because histoplasmin reactivity waxes in the absence of occasional reexposure. In addition, histoplasmin skin testing can result in a false increase in the CF titer for mycelial antigen (CF-M) to *H. capsulatum*. A fourfold rise in the CF titer is usually indicative of recent infection, although some patients with severe disease or profound immunosuppression can demonstrate a weaker antibody response.

Because the ID test is not as sensitive as CF, it should be used to assess the importance of weakly reactive results obtained by CF rather than as a screening procedure. Radioimmunoassay (RIA), which measures immunoglobulin M (IgM) and immunoglobulin G (IgG) antibodies against a histoplasmin extract, is the most sensitive test, but it can show a large number of false-positive reactions in patients living in an endemic area.

In the AIDS patient with PDH, the diagnosis is best established by bone marrow biopsy and culture, which yield positive cultures in more than 90% of patients, although blood cultures and histopathologic examination and culture of pulmonary tissue, sputum, skin, and lymph nodes also can be helpful. Detection of *H. capsulatum* polysaccharide antigen (HPA) in urine, blood, or cerebrospinal fluid (CSF) by enzyme-linked immunosorbent assay (ELISA) or by modified RIA offer promising new techniques for the rapid diagnosis of histoplasmosis. The HPA (RIA) levels also have been used successfully to monitor the course of therapy and to detect relapses in patients with AIDS, and the clearance of antigen from serum and urine correlates with clinical efficacy during maintenance therapy with itraconazole.[19]

TREATMENT

Histoplasmosis

■ NON–HIV-INFECTED PATIENT

Table 125–3 summarizes the recommended therapy for the treatment ❹ of histoplasmosis. In general, asymptomatic or mildly ill patients and patients with sarcoid-like disease do not benefit from antifungal therapy. In the vast majority of patients, low-inoculum exposure to *H. capsulatum* results in *mild* or *asymptomatic* pulmonary histoplasmosis. The course of disease generally is benign, and symptoms usually abate within a few weeks of onset. Therapy can be helpful in symptomatic patients whose conditions have not improved during the first month of infection. Fever persisting more than 3 weeks can indicate that the patient is developing progressive disseminated disease, which can be aborted by antifungal therapy. Whether antifungal therapy hastens recovery or prevents complications is unknown because it has never been studied in prospective trials.

Patients with mild, self-limited disease, chronic disseminated disease, or chronic pulmonary histoplasmosis who have no underlying immunosuppression usually can be treated with either oral ketoconazole or IV amphotericin B. The goals of therapy are resolution of clinical abnormalities, prevention of relapse, and eradication of infection whenever possible, although chronic suppression of infection can be adequate in immunosuppressed patients, including those with HIV disease.[18,19]

Patients with arthritis, erythema nodosum, pericarditis, or mediastinal granuloma can require the addition of a 2-week course of corticosteroids to their therapy.[16]

■ HIV-INFECTED PATIENT

In AIDS patients, intensive 12-week primary antifungal therapy (induction and consolidation therapy) is followed by lifelong suppressive (maintenance) therapy with itraconazole. Amphotericin B dosages of 50 mg/day (up to 1 mg/kg per day) should be administered intravenously to a cumulative dose of 15 to 35 mg/kg (1 to 2 g) in patients who require hospitalization. Amphotericin B can be replaced with itraconazole 200 mg orally twice daily when the patient no longer requires hospitalization or intravenous therapy to complete a 12-week total course of induction therapy. In patients who do not require hospitalization, itraconazole therapy for 12 weeks can be used.

Fluconazole 800 mg/day orally as induction, followed by 400 mg/day, was effective in 88% of patients, but relapses occurred in approximately one-third of patients, and in-vitro resistance developed in approximately 50% of patients who relapsed.

In regions experiencing high rates of histoplasmosis (>5 cases/100 patient-years), itraconazole 200 mg/day is recommended as prophylactic therapy in HIV-infected patients. Fluconazole is not an acceptable alternative because of its inferior activity against *H. capsulatum* and its lower efficacy for the treatment of histoplasmosis.[18]

Although patients receiving secondary prophylaxis (chronic maintenance therapy) might be at low risk for recurrence of systemic mycosis when their CD4+ T lymphocyte counts increase to >100 cells/microliter in response to highly active antiretroviral therapy (HAART), the number of patients who have been evaluated is insufficient to warrant a recommendation to discontinue prophylaxis.

EVALUATION OF THERAPEUTIC OUTCOMES

Response to therapy should be measured by resolution of radiologic, serologic, and microbiologic parameters and by improvement in signs and symptoms of infection. Although investigators are limited by the lack of standardized criteria to quantify the extent of infection, degree of immunosuppression, or treatment response, response rates (based on resolution or improvement in presenting signs and symptoms) of greater than 80% have been reported in case series in AIDS patients receiving varied dosages of amphotericin B. Rapid responses are reported, with the resolution of symptoms in 25% and 75% of patients by days 3 and 7 of therapy, respectively.

After the initial course of therapy for histoplasmosis is complete, lifelong suppressive therapy with oral azoles or amphotericin B (1–1.5 mg/kg weekly or biweekly) is recommended because of the frequent recurrence of infection.[20] Relapse rates in AIDS patients not receiving maintenance therapy range from 50% to 90%.[18]

Antigen testing can be useful for monitoring therapy in patients with disseminated histoplasmosis. Antigen concentrations decrease with therapy and increase with relapse. Some investigators recommend that treatment should continue until antigen concentrations revert to negative or less than 4 units. If treatment is discontinued before antigen concentrations in serum and urine revert to negative, patients should be followed closely for relapse, and antigen levels should be monitored every 3 to 6 months until they become negative.[18]

BLASTOMYCOSIS

North American blastomycosis is a systemic fungal infection caused by *Blastomyces dermatitidis,* a dimorphic fungus that infects primarily the lungs. Patients, however, can present with a variety of pulmonary and extrapulmonary clinical manifestations. Pulmonary disease can be acute or chronic and can mimic infection with tuberculosis, pyogenic bacteria, other fungi, or malignancy. Blastomycosis can disseminate to virtually every other body organ, and approximately 40% of patients with blastomycosis present with skin, bone and joint, or genitourinary tract involvement without any evidence of pulmonary disease.[21]

Pulmonary infection probably occurs by inhalation of conidia, which convert to the yeast form in the lung. A vigorous inflammatory response ensues, with neutrophilic recruitment to the lungs followed by the development of cell-mediated immunity and the formation of noncaseating granulomas.

EPIDEMIOLOGY

Blastomycosis was renamed *North American blastomycosis* in 1942, when Conant and Howell named a similar fungus endemic to South America, *Blastomyces braziliensis,* and the disease it caused *South American blastomycosis.* Although the disease is now recognized to be endemic to the southeastern and south central states of the United States (especially those bordering on the Mississippi and Ohio River basins) and the midwestern states and Canadian provinces bordering on the Great Lakes, numerous cases of North American blastomycosis have been diagnosed in Africa, northern parts of South America, India, and Europe. Endemic areas have been defined primarily by analysis of sporadic cases and epidemics or clusters of disease because the lack of a dependable skin or laboratory test makes widescale epidemiologic testing to determine the incidence of infection unfeasible at present.[19,20] Although initial review of sporadic cases suggested that males with outdoor occupations that exposed them to soil were at greatest risk for blastomycosis, there is no sex, age, or occupational predilection for blastomycosis.[19,21]

Although *B. dermatitidis* generally is considered to be a soil inhabitant, attempts to isolate the organism in nature frequently have been unsuccessful. *B. dermatitidis* has been isolated from soil containing decayed vegetation, decomposed wood, and pigeon manure, frequently in association with warm, moist soil of wooded areas that is rich in organic debris.[19,21]

PATHOPHYSIOLOGY AND CLINICAL PRESENTATION[13,19,21]

General

Colonization does not occur with *Blastomyces. Acute pulmonary blastomycosis* generally is an asymptomatic or self-limited disease characterized by fever, shaking chills, and productive, purulent cough, with or without hemoptysis, in immunocompetent individuals. The clinical presentation can be difficult to differentiate from other respiratory infections, including bacterial pneumonia, on the basis of clinical symptoms alone.

Sporadic (nonepidemic) pulmonary blastomycosis can present as a more chronic or subacute disease, with low-grade fever, night sweats, weight loss, and productive cough that resembles tuberculosis rather than bacterial pneumonia. *Chronic pulmonary blastomycosis* is characterized by fever, malaise, weight loss, night sweats, chest pain, and productive cough. Patients often are thought to have tuberculosis and frequently have evidence of disseminated disease that can appear 1 to 3 years after the primary pneumonia has resolved. Reactivation of disease can occur in the lungs or as the focus of new infection in other organs.

In approximately 40% of patients, dissemination is not accompanied by reactivation of pulmonary disease. The most common sites for disseminated disease include the skin and bony skeleton, although less commonly the prostate, oropharyngeal mucosa, and abdominal viscera are involved. CNS disease, while exceedingly uncommon, is associated with the highest mortality rate.

Laboratory and Diagnostic Tests

The simplest and most successful method of diagnosing blastomycosis is by direct microscopic visualization of the large, multinucleated yeast with single, broad-based buds in sputum or other respiratory specimens following digestion of cells and debris with 10% potassium hydroxide. Histopathologic examination of tissue biopsies and culture of secretions also should be used to identify *B. dermatitidis,* although it can require up to 30 days to isolate and identify a small inoculum.

No reliable skin test exists to determine the incidence and prevalence of disease in endemic populations, and reliable serologic diagnosis of blastomycosis has long been hampered by the lack of specific and standardized reagents. Serologic response does not always correlate with clinical improvement, although some investigators have noted that a decline in the number of precipitins or CF titers can offer evidence of a favorable prognosis in patients with established disease.

Acute pulmonary blastomycosis generally is an asymptomatic or self-limited disease characterized by fever, shaking chills, and productive, purulent cough, with or without hemoptysis, in immunocompetent individuals. The clinical presentation can be difficult to differentiate from other respiratory infections, including bacterial pneumonia, on the basis of clinical symptoms alone. Sporadic (nonepidemic) cases of pulmonary blastomycosis can present as a more chronic or subacute disease with low-grade fever, night sweats, weight loss, and productive cough that resembles tuberculosis rather than bacterial pneumonia.

TREATMENT

Blastomycosis

■ NON–HIV-INFECTED PATIENT

❺ In patients with mild pulmonary blastomycosis, the clinical presentation of the patient, the immune competence of the patient, and the toxicity of the antifungal agents are the main determinants of whether or not to administer antifungal therapy. All immunocompromised patients and patients with progressive pulmonary disease or with extrapulmonary disease should be treated (Table 125–4). In the case of disease limited to the lungs, cure might have occurred before the diagnosis is made and without treatment. Regardless of whether or not the patient receives treatment, however, he or she must be followed carefully for many years for evidence of reactivation or progressive disease.[19,21]

Some authors recommend ketoconazole therapy for the treatment of self-limited pulmonary disease, with the hope of preventing late extrapulmonary disease; however, data supporting the efficacy of these regimens are lacking.[19,21] Itraconazole 200 to 400 mg/day demonstrated 90% efficacy as a first-line agent in the treatment of non–life-threatening non-CNS blastomycosis, and for compliant patients who completed at least 2 months of therapy, a success rate of 95% was noted. No therapeutic advantage was noted with the higher (400 mg) dosage as compared with patients treated with 200 mg.

All patients with disseminated blastomycosis, as well as those with extrapulmonary disease, require therapy. Ketoconazole 400 mg/day orally for 6 months cures more than 80% of patients with chronic

TABLE 125-4 Therapy of Blastomycosis

Type of Disease	Preferred Treatment	Comments
Pulmonary[a]		
Life-threatening	Amphotericin B[b] IV 0.7–1 mg/kg/day IV (total dose 1.5–2.5 g)	Patients can be initiated on amphotericin B and changed to oral itraconazole 200–400 mg orally daily once patient is clinically stabilized and a minimum dose of 500 mg of amphotericin B has been administered
Mild to moderate	Itraconazole 200 mg orally twice daily × ≥6 months[c]	*Alternative therapy:* Ketoconazole 400–800 mg orally daily × ≥6 months or fluconazole 400–800 mg orally daily × ≥6 months[d]
		In patients intolerant of azoles or in whom disease progresses during azole therapy: Amphotericin B 0.5–0.7 mg/kg/day IV (total dose 1.5–2.5 g)
Disseminated or extrapulmonary		
CNS	Amphotericin B 0.7–1 mg/kg/day IV (total dose 1.5–2.5 g)	For patients unable to tolerate a full course of amphotericin B, consider lipid formulations of amphotericin B or fluconazole ≥800 mg orally daily
Non-CNS		
Life-threatening	Amphotericin B 0.7–1 mg/kg/day IV (total dose 1.5–2.5 g)	Patients can be initiated on amphotericin B and changed to oral itraconazole 200–400 mg orally daily once stabilized
Mild to moderate	Itraconazole 200–400 mg orally daily × ≥6 months	Ketoconazole 400–800 mg orally daily or fluconazole 400–800 mg orally daily × ≥6 months
		In patients intolerant of azoles or in whom disease progresses during azole therapy: Amphotericin B 0.5–0.7 mg/kg/day IV (total dose 1.5–2.5 g)
		Bone disease: Therapy with azoles should be continued for 12 months
Immunocompromised host (including patients with AIDS, transplants, or receiving chronic glucocorticoid therapy)		
Acute disease	Amphotericin B 0.7–1 mg/kg/day IV (total dose 1.5–2.5 g)	Patients without CNS infection can be switched to itraconazole once clinically stabilized and a minimum dose of 1 g of amphotericin B has been administered; long-term suppressive therapy with an azole is advised
Suppressive therapy	Itraconazole 200–400 mg orally daily	For patients with CNS disease or those intolerant of itraconazole, consider fluconazole 800 mg orally daily

AIDS, acquired immunodeficiency syndrome.
[a]Some patients with acute pulmonary infection can have a spontaneous cure. Patients with progressive pulmonary disease should be treated.
[b]Desoxycholate amphotericin B.
[c]In patients not responding to 400 mg, dosage should be increased by 200 mg increments every 4 weeks to a maximum of 800 mg daily.
[d]Therapy with ketoconazole is associated with relapses, and fluconazole therapy achieves a lower response rate than itraconazole.
Data from Wheat and Kauffman[19] and O'Shaughnessy et al.[21]

pulmonary and nonmeningeal disseminated blastomycosis. Amphotericin B is more efficacious but more toxic and therefore is reserved for noncompliant patients and patients with overwhelming or life-threatening disease, CNS infection, and treatment failures. Cumulative amphotericin B dosages of more than 1 g have resulted in cure without relapse in 70% to 91% of patients with blastomycosis. Relapse rates depend on the total dosage of amphotericin B administered.[19,21] Patients with genitourinary tract disease should be treated initially with 600–800 mg/day of ketoconazole because of the low concentrations of drug achieved in the urine and prostate tissue.

Patients should be monitored carefully for signs of clinical failure, and those who fail or are unable to tolerate itraconazole therapy or who develop CNS disease should be treated with amphotericin B for a total cumulative dose of 1.5 to 2.5 g.[19,21]

Lipid preparations of amphotericin B are effective in animal models of blastomycosis, but they have not been evaluated adequately in humans. Limited clinical experience suggests that these preparations can provide an alternative for patients unable to experience standard therapy with amphotericin B because of toxicity. Surgery has only a limited role in the treatment of blastomycosis.

■ HIV-INFECTED PATIENT

For unclear reasons, blastomycosis is an uncommon opportunistic disease among immunocompromised individuals, including AIDS patients; however, blastomycosis can occur as a late (CD4 lymphocytes <200 cells/mm^3) and frequently fatal complication of HIV infection. In this population, overwhelming disseminated disease with frequent involvement of the CNS is common.[19] Following induction therapy with amphotericin B (total cumulative dose of 1 g), HIV-infected patients should receive chronic suppressive therapy with an oral azole antifungal. Despite its higher cost, itraconazole has become the drug of choice for non–life-threatening histoplasmosis (mild to moderate disease) in HIV-infected patients.[21]

COCCIDIOIDOMYCOSIS

EPIDEMIOLOGY

Coccidioidomycosis is caused by infection with *Coccidioides immitis,* a dimorphic fungus found in the southwestern and western United States, as well as in parts of Mexico and South America. In North America, the endemic regions encompass the semiarid areas of the southwestern United States from California to Texas known as the Lower Sonoran Zone, where there is scant annual rainfall, hot summers, and sandy, alkaline soil. *Coccidioides immitis* grows in the soil as a mold, and mycelia proliferate during the rainy season. During the dry season, resistant arthroconidia form and become airborne when the soil is disturbed.

Although generally considered to be a regional disease, coccidioidomycosis has increased in importance in recent years because of the increased tourism and population in endemic areas, the increased use of immunosuppressive therapy in transplantation and oncology, and the AIDS epidemic. Although there is no racial, hormonal, or immunologic predisposition for acquiring primary disease, these factors affect the risk of subsequent dissemination of disease (Table 125–5).[20]

PATHOPHYSIOLOGY

When individuals come in contact with contaminated soil during ranching, dust storms, or proximity to construction sites or archaeologic excavations, arthroconidia are inhaled into the respiratory tree, where they transform into spherules, which reproduce by cleavage of the cytoplasm to produce endospores. The endospores are released when the spherules reach maturity. Similar to histoplasmosis, an acute inflammatory response in the tissue leads to infiltration of mononuclear cells, ultimately resulting in granuloma formation.[20]

TABLE 125-5 Risk Factors for Severe, Disseminated Infection with Coccidioidomycosis

Race (Filipinos > African-Americans > Native Americans > Hispanics > Asians)
Pregnancy (especially when infection is acquired or reactivated in the second or third trimester)
Compromised cellular immune system, including
AIDS patients
Patients receiving
Corticosteroids
Immunosuppressive agents
Chemotherapy
Male gender
Neonates
Patients with B or AB blood types

AIDS, acquired immune deficiency syndrome.
Data from Galgiani JM, Ampel NM, Blair JE, Catanzaro A, et al. Practice guidelines for the treatment of coccidioidomycoses. Clin Infect Dis 2005;30:658–661.

CLINICAL PRESENTATION OF COCCIDIOIDOMYCOSIS[11,19–22]

Coccidioidomycosis encompasses a spectrum of illnesses ranging from primary uncomplicated respiratory tract infection that resolves spontaneously to progressive pulmonary or disseminated infection. Initial or primary infection with *C. immitis* almost always involves the lungs. Although approximately one-third of the population in endemic areas is infected, the average incidence of symptomatic disease is only approximately 0.43%.

Signs and Symptoms

In *asymptomatic disease* (60% of patients), patients have nonspecific symptoms that are often indistinguishable from ordinary upper respiratory infections, including fever, cough, headache, sore throat, myalgias, and fatigue. A fine, diffuse rash can appear during the first few days of the illness. Primary pneumonia can be the first manifestation of disease, characterized by a productive cough that can be blood-streaked, as well as single or multiple soft or dense homogeneous hilar or basal infiltrates on chest roentgenogram. Chronic, persistent pneumonia or persistent pulmonary coccidioidomycosis (primary disease lasting more than 6 weeks) is complicated by hemoptysis, pulmonary scarring, and the formation of cavities or bronchopleural fistulas.

Necrosis of pulmonary tissue with drainage and cavity formation occurs commonly. Most parenchymal cavities close spontaneously or form dense nodular scar tissue that can become superinfected with bacteria or spherules of *C. immitis.* These patients often have persistent cough, fevers, and weight loss.

Valley fever occurs in approximately 25% of patients and is characterized by erythema nodosum and erythema multiforme of the upper trunk and extremities in association with diffuse joint aches or fever. More commonly, a diffuse, mild erythroderma or maculopapular rash is observed. Patients can have pleuritic chest pain and peripheral eosinophilia.

Disseminated disease occurs in less than 1% of infected patients. The most common sites for dissemination are the skin, lymph nodes, bone, and meninges, although the spleen, liver, kidney, and adrenal gland also can be involved. Occasionally, miliary coccidioidomycosis occurs, with rapid, widespread dissemination, often in concert with positive blood cultures for *C. immitis.* Patients with AIDS frequently present with miliary disease. Coccidioidomycosis in AIDS patients appears to be caused by reactivation of disease in most patients.

CNS infection occurs in approximately 16% of patients with disseminated coccidioidomycosis. Patients can present with meningeal disease without previous symptoms of primary pulmonary infection, although disease usually occurs within 6 months of the primary infection. The signs and symptoms are often subtle and nonspecific, including headache, weakness, changes in mental status (lethargy and confusion), neck stiffness, low-grade fever, weight loss, and occasionally, hydrocephalus. Space-occupying lesions are rare, and the main areas of involvement are the basilar meninges.

DIAGNOSIS

Laboratory Tests

Recovery of *C. immitis* from infected tissues or secretions for direct examination and culture provides an accurate and rapid method of diagnosis. Direct microscopic examination and histopathologic studies of infected tissues will reveal the large, mature endosporulating spherules. Young spherules without endospores can be confused, however, with other fungi. Silver stains of body fluids or tissue biopsies are also helpful.

With chronic, persistent pneumonia, *C. immitis* often can be cultured from the sputum for a period of several years. Chest radiographs usually demonstrate apical fibronodular lesions or slowly progressive cavitation. With CNS infection, analysis of the CSF generally reveals a lymphocytic pleocytosis with elevated protein and a decreased glucose concentration. Although serum usually is positive for coccidioidal CF antibodies, the coccidioidal skin test is often negative.

Other Diagnostic Tests

Most patients develop a positive skin test within 3 weeks of the onset of symptoms. Baseline evaluation of skin test reactivity and serology is essential to assess cell-mediated immunity. Patients who develop early positive skin-test reactivity or whose coccidioidin skin-test reactivity turns from negative to positive during therapy have an improved prognosis compared with patients whose skin-test reactivity develops later or does not change during therapy. Patients with disseminated coccidioidomycosis whose skin tests are persistently negative are more likely to require prolonged therapy, and they are more likely to relapse after completion of therapy.

Antibody production can be used to follow the course of disease because most patients produce antibodies in response to infection with *C. immitis.* Early infection is characterized by the development of the IgM antibody, which peaks within 2 to 3 weeks of infection and then declines rapidly. The IgM antibody can be detected by either tube precipitin or immunodiffusion techniques.

The IgG antibody levels increase between 4 and 12 weeks after infection and decrease slowly over months to years, and IgG can be detected in many body fluids, including serum, CSF, and pleural fluid, by CF and ID techniques. Higher titers (>1:16 or 1:32) occur more frequently with severe disease. Titers can be followed serially to evaluate the efficacy of antifungal therapy.

Radiographic features tend to be quite variable; hilar adenopathy with alveolar infiltrates, tissue excavation of an infiltrate (resulting in a thin-walled cavity), or small pleural effusions are all seen commonly. With chronic persistent pneumonia, chest radiographs usually demonstrate apical fibronodular lesions or slowly progressive cavitation.[21,22]

TREATMENT

Coccidioidomycosis

■ GENERAL GUIDELINES

❻ Therapy for coccidioidomycosis is difficult, and the results are unpredictable. Guidelines are available for treatment of this disease; however, optimal treatment for many forms of this disease still generates debate.[20] The efficacy of antifungal therapy for coccidioidomycosis is often less certain than that for other fungal etiologies, such as blastomycosis, histoplasmosis, or cryptococcus, even when in-vitro susceptibilities and the sites of infections are similar. The refractoriness of coccidioidomycosis can relate to the ability of *C. immitis* spherules to release hundreds of endospores, maximally challenging host defenses.[20,22] Fortunately, only approximately 5% of infected patients require therapy.[22]

■ GOALS OF THERAPY

Desired outcomes of treatment are resolution of signs and symptoms of infection, reduction of serum concentrations of anticoccidioidal antibodies, and return of function of involved organs. It would also be desirable to prevent relapse of illness on discontinuation of therapy, although current therapy is often unable to achieve this goal.

■ SPECIFIC AGENTS USED FOR THE TREATMENT OF COCCIDIOIDOMYCOSIS

Azole antifungals, primarily fluconazole and itraconazole, have replaced amphotericin B as initial therapy for most chronic pulmonary or disseminated infections. Amphotericin B is now usually reserved for patients with respiratory failure because of infection with Coccidioides species, those with rapidly progressive coccidioidal infections, or women during pregnancy. Therapy often ranges from many months to years in duration, and in some patients, lifelong suppressive therapy is needed to prevent relapses. Specific antifungals (and their usual dosages) for the treatment of coccidioidomycosis include intravenous amphotericin B (0.5 to 1.5 mg/kg per day), ketoconazole (400 mg/day orally), intravenous or oral fluconazole (usually 400 to 800 mg/day, although dosages as high as 1200 mg/day have been used without complications), and itraconazole (200 to 300 mg orally twice daily or three times daily, as either capsules or solution).[20,22] If itraconazole is used, measurement of serum concentrations can be helpful to ascertain whether oral bioavailability is adequate.

Amphotericin B generally is preferred as initial therapy in patients with rapidly progressive disease, whereas azoles generally are preferred in patients with subacute or chronic presentations. The lipid formulations of amphotericin B have not been studied extensively in coccidioidal infection but can offer a means of giving more drug with less toxicity. Fluconazole probably is the most frequently used medicine given its tolerability, although high relapse rates have been reported in some studies. Relapse rates with itraconazole therapy can be lower than with fluconazole.[20,22]

The usefulness of newly available antifungal agents of possible benefit for the treatment of refractory coccidioidal infections has not been adequately assessed and are not yet FDA approved for use in this population. Case reports have suggested that voriconazole can be effective in selected patients. Caspofungin has been effective in treating experimental murine coccidioidomycosis, but in-vitro susceptibility of isolates varies widely, and there is only one report regarding its value. Posaconazole was shown to be an effective treatment in a small clinical trial and in patients with refractory infections. Its efficacy relative to other triazole antifungals is unknown.

Combination therapy with members of different classes of antifungal agents has not been evaluated in patients, and there is a hypothetical risk of antagonism. However, some clinicians feel that outcome in severe cases is improved when amphotericin B is combined with an azole antifungal. If the patient improves, the dosage of amphotericin B can be slowly decreased while the dosage of azole is maintained.[20,22]

■ PRIMARY RESPIRATORY INFECTION

Although most patients with symptomatic primary pulmonary disease recover without therapy, management should include followup visits for 1 to 2 years to document resolution of disease or to identify as early as possible evidence of pulmonary or extrapulmonary complications.

CLINICAL CONTROVERSY

Because of the lack of prospective, controlled trials, there is continued disagreement among experts in endemic areas whether patients with coccidioidomycosis should be treated and, if so, which ones and for how long. The excellent tolerability of oral azoles has lowered the threshold for deciding to treat primary infection, and some clinicians treat all primary infections. Rationale for treating a primary self-limiting infection include the ability to lessen the morbidity associated with the acute infection and the possible ability to reduce the development of more serious complications. However, there is currently no evidence that treatment of the primary infection accomplishes either of these goals.[22]

Patients with a large inoculum, severe infection, or concurrent risk factors (e.g., HIV infection, organ transplant, pregnancy, or high doses of corticosteroids) probably should be treated, particularly those with high CF titers, in whom incipient or occult dissemination is likely. Because some racial or ethnic populations have a higher risk of dissemination, some clinicians advocate their inclusion in the high-risk group. Common indicators used to judge the severity of infection include weight loss (>10%), intense night sweats persisting more than 3 weeks, infiltrates involving more than one-half of one lung or portions of both lungs, prominent or persistent hilar adenopathy, CF antibody titers of greater than 1:16, failure to develop dermal sensitivity to coccidial antigens, inability to work, or symptoms that persist for more than 2 months.[20,22]

Commonly prescribed therapies include currently available oral azole antifungals at their recommended doses for courses of therapy ranging from 3 to 6 months.[20,22] In patients with diffuse pneumonia with bilateral reticulonodular or miliary infiltrates, therapy usually is initiated with amphotericin B; several weeks of therapy generally are required to produce clear evidence of improvement. Consolidation therapy with oral azoles can be considered at that time. The total duration of therapy should be at least 1 year, and in patients with underlying immunodeficiency, oral azole therapy should be continued as secondary prophylaxis. Although HIV-infected patients receiving secondary prophylaxis might be at low risk for recurrence of systemic mycosis when their CD4+ T-lymphocyte counts increase to >100 cells/microliter in response to HAART, the number of patients who have been evaluated is insufficient to warrant a recommendation to discontinue prophylaxis.

■ INFECTIONS OF THE PULMONARY CAVITY

Many pulmonary infections that are caused by *C. immitis* are benign in their course and do not require intervention. In the absence of controlled clinical trials, evidence of the benefit of antifungal therapy is lacking, and asymptomatic infections generally are left untreated. Symptomatic patients can benefit from oral azole therapy, although recurrence of symptoms can be seen in some patients once therapy is discontinued. Surgical resection of localized cavities provides resolution of the problem in patients in whom the risks of surgery are not too high.[20,22]

■ EXTRAPULMONARY (DISSEMINATED) DISEASE

Nonmeningeal Disease

Almost all patients with disease located outside the lungs should receive antifungal therapy; therapy usually is initiated with 400 mg/

day of an oral azole. Amphotericin B is an alternative therapy and can be necessary in patients with worsening lesions or with disease in particularly critical locations such as the vertebral column. Approximately 50% to 75% of patients treated with amphotericin B for nonmeningeal disease achieve a sustained remission, and therapy usually is curative in patients with infections localized strictly to skin and soft tissues without extensive abscess formation or tissue damage. The efficacy of local injection into joints or the peritoneum, as well as intraarticular or intradermal administration, remains poorly studied. Amphotericin B appears to be most efficacious when cell-mediated immunity is intact (as evidenced by a positive coccidioidin or spherulin skin test or low CF antibody titer). Controlled trials that document these clinical impressions are lacking, however.[20,22]

Meningeal Disease

Fluconazole has become the drug of choice for the treatment of coccidioidal meningitis. A minimum dose of 400 mg/day orally leads to a clinical response in most patients and obviates the need for intrathecal amphotericin B. Some clinicians will initiate therapy with 800 or 1,000 mg/day, and itraconazole dosages of 400 to 600 mg/day are comparably effective. It is also clear, however, that fluconazole only leads to remission rather than cure of the infections; thus suppressive therapy must be continued for life. Ketoconazole cannot be recommended routinely for the treatment of coccidioidal meningitis because of its poor CNS penetration following oral administration. Patients who do not respond to fluconazole or itraconazole therapy are candidates for intrathecal amphotericin B therapy with or without continuation of azole therapy. The intrathecal dose of amphotericin B ranges from 0.01 to 1.5 mg given at intervals ranging from daily to weekly. Therapy is initiated with a low dosage and is titrated upward as patient tolerance develops.[20,22]

CRYPTOCOCCOSIS

EPIDEMIOLOGY

Cryptococcosis is a noncontagious, systemic mycotic infection caused by the ubiquitous encapsulated soil yeast *Cryptococcus neoformans,* which is found in soil, particularly in pigeon droppings, although disease occurs throughout the world, even in areas where pigeons are absent. Infection is acquired by inhalation of the organism. The incidence of cryptococcosis has risen dramatically in recent years, reflecting the increased numbers of immunocompromised patients, including those with malignancies, diabetes mellitus, chronic renal failure, and organ transplants and those receiving immunosuppressive agents. The AIDS epidemic also has contributed to the increased numbers of patients; cryptococcosis is the fourth most common infectious complication of AIDS and the second most common fungal pathogen.[23]

Although *C. neoformans* produces no toxins and evokes only a minimal inflammatory response in tissue, the polysaccharide capsule appears to allow the organism to resist phagocytosis by the host. The capsular polysaccharide of *C. neoformans* appears to comprise the major virulence factor for this pathogen. Four serotypes of *C. neoformans* (A through D) have been identified; they vary in their polysaccharide content, virulence, geographic foci, and response to antifungal therapy. Serotypes A and D are commonly associated with pigeon droppings and other environmental sites and generally require shorter therapy than do infections caused by serotypes B or C, which have been found only in infected humans and animals. Serotypes B and C appear more resistant to antifungal agents in vitro. Patients with AIDS are almost always infected with serotypes A and D, even in areas endemic for serotypes B and C. There is no particular geographic area of endemic focus for *C. neoformans.*

Cell-mediated immunity appears to play a major role in host defense against infection with *C. neoformans;* 29% to 55% of patients with cryptococcal meningitis have a predisposing condition. Many patients with disseminated cryptococcosis demonstrate defects in cell-mediated immunity. The predilection of *C. neoformans* for the CNS appears to be caused by the lack of immunoglobulins and complement and the excellent growth medium afforded by CSF.[23]

Disease can remain localized in the lungs or can disseminate to other tissues, particularly the CNS, although the skin also can be affected. Hematogenous spread generally occurs in the immunocompromised host, although it also has been seen in individuals with intact immune systems. Cryptococcemia is the most common symptomatic extraneural infection associated with *C. neoformans.* Cryptococcemia can be documented in 5% to 22% of non-AIDS patients, and CNS involvement of *C. neoformans* can be found in 18% to 50% of AIDS patients. Cryptococcal disease is present in 7.5% to 10% of AIDS patients. Therefore, patients with evidence of extraneural cryptococcosis should be evaluated for CNS disease.

CLINICAL PRESENTATION OF CRYPTOCOCCOSIS[11,23,24]

Primary cryptococcosis in humans almost always occurs in the lungs, although the pulmonary focus usually produces a subclinical infection. Symptomatic infections usually are manifested by cough, rales, and shortness of breath that generally resolve spontaneously. In non-AIDS patients, the symptoms of cryptococcal meningitis are nonspecific. Headache, fever, nausea, vomiting, mental status changes, and neck stiffness generally are observed. Less common symptoms include visual disturbances (photophobia and blurred vision), papilledema, seizures, and aphasia. In AIDS patients, fever and headache are common, but meningismus and photophobia are much less common than in non-AIDS patients. Approximately 10% to 12% of AIDS patients have asymptomatic disease, similar to the rate observed in non-AIDS patients.[24]

Laboratory Tests

With cryptococcal meningitis, the CSF opening pressure generally is elevated. There is a CSF pleocytosis (usually lymphocytes), leukocytosis, a decreased glucose concentration, and an elevated CSF protein concentration. There is also a positive cryptococcal antigen (detected by LA). The test is rapid, specific, and extremely sensitive, but false-negative results can occur. False-positive tests can result from cross-reactivity with rheumatoid factor and *Trichosporon beigelli. C. neoformans* can be detected in approximately 60% of patients by India ink smear of CSF, and it can be cultured in more than 96% of patients. Occasionally, large volumes of CSF are required to confirm the diagnosis.

The CSF parameters in patients with AIDS are similar to those seen in non-AIDS patients, with the exception of a decreased inflammatory response to the pathogen, resulting in a strikingly low number of leukocytes in CSF and extraordinarily high cryptococcal antigen titers.

TREATMENT

Cryptococcosis

The choice of treatment for disease caused by *C. neoformans* depends on both the anatomic sites of involvement and the host's immune status.

■ NONIMMUNOCOMPROMISED PATIENTS

For asymptomatic immunocompetent hosts with isolated pulmonary disease and no evidence of CNS disease, careful observation can be warranted; in the case of symptomatic infection, fluconazole or amphotericin B is warranted (Table 125–6). In individuals with non-CNS cryptococcemia, a positive serum cryptococcal antigen titer (>1:8), cutaneous infection, a positive urine culture, or prostatic disease, the clinician must decide whether to follow the regimen for isolated pulmonary disease or the more aggressive regimen for patients with CNS (disseminated) disease.[15]

Prior to the introduction of amphotericin B, cryptococcal meningitis was an almost uniformly fatal disease; approximately 86% of patients died within 1 year. The use of large (1 to 1.5 mg/kg) daily doses of amphotericin B resulted in cure rates of approximately 64%. ❼ When amphotericin B is combined with flucytosine, a smaller dose of amphotericin B can be employed because of the in-vitro and in-vivo synergy between the two antifungal agents. Resis-

TABLE 125-6 Therapy of Cryptococcosis[a,b]

Type of Disease and Common Clinical Manifestations	Therapy/Comments
Nonimmunocompromised host	Comparative trials for amphotericin B[c] versus azoles not available
Isolated pulmonary disease (without evidence of CNS infection)	*Asymptomatic disease:* Drug therapy generally not required; observe carefully or fluconazole 400 mg orally daily × 3–6 months
	Mild to moderate symptoms: Fluconazole 200–400 mg orally daily × 3–6 months;
	Severe disease or inability to take azoles: Amphotericin B 0.4–0.7 mg/kg/day (total dose of 1–2 g)
Cryptococcemia with positive serum antigen titer (>1:8), cutaneous infection, a positive urine culture, or prostatic disease	Clinician must decide whether to follow the pulmonary therapeutic regimen or the CNS (disseminated) regimen
Recurrent or progressive disease not responsive to amphotericin B.	Amphotericin B[d] IV 0.5–0.75 mg/kg/day ± IT amphotericin B 0.5 mg 2–3 times weekly
Isolated pulmonary disease (without evidence of CNS infection)	*Mild to moderate symptoms or asymptomatic with a positive pulmonary specimen:* Fluconazole 200–400 mg orally daily × lifelong
	or
	Itraconazole 200–400 mg orally daily × lifelong
	or
	Fluconazole 400 mg orally daily + flucytosine 100–150 mg/kg/day orally × 10 weeks
	Severe disease: Amphotericin B until symptoms are controlled, followed by fluconazole
CNS disease	
Acute (induction/consolidation therapy) (follow all regimens with suppressive therapy)	Amphotericin B[d] IV 0.7–1 mg/kg/day + flucytosine 100 mg/kg/day orally × ≥2 weeks, then fluconazole 400 mg orally daily × ≥8 weeks[e]
	or
	Amphotericin B[d] IV 0.7–1 mg/kg/day + flucytosine 100 mg/kg/day orally × 6–10 weeks[e]
	or
	Amphotericin B[d] IV 0.7–1 mg/kg/day × 6–10 weeks[e]
	or
	Fluconazole 400–800 mg orally daily × 10–12 weeks
	or
	Itraconazole 400–800 mg orally daily × 10–12 weeks
	or
	Fluconazole 400–800 mg orally daily + flucytosine 100–150 mg/kg/day orally × 6 weeks[e]
	or
	Lipid formulation of amphotericin B IV 3–6 mg/kg/day × 6–10 weeks
	Note: Induction therapy with azoles alone is discouraged.
CNS disease	Amphotericin B[d] IV 0.7–1 mg/kg/day + flucytosine 100 mg/kg/day orally × 2 weeks, followed by fluconazole 400 mg orally daily for a minimum of 10 weeks (in patients intolerant to fluconazole, substitute itraconazole 200–400 mg orally daily)
	or
	Amphotericin B[d] IV 0.7–1 mg/kg/day + 5-flucytosine 100 mg/kg/day orally × 6–10 weeks
	or
	Amphotericin B[d] IV 0.7–1 mg/kg/day × 10 weeks
	Refractory disease: Intrathecal or intraventricular amphotericin B
Immunocompromised patients	
Non-CNS pulmonary and extrapulmonary disease	Same as nonimmunocompromised patients with CNS disease
CNS disease	Amphotericin B[d] IV 0.7–1 mg/kg/day × 2 weeks, followed by fluconazole 400–800 mg orally daily 8–10 weeks, followed by fluconazole 200 mg orally daily × 6–12 months (in patients intolerant to fluconazole, substitute itraconazole 200–400 mg orally daily)
	Refractory disease: Intrathecal or intraventricular amphotericin B
HIV-infected patients	
Suppressive/maintenance therapy	Fluconazole 200–400 mg orally daily × lifelong
	or
	Itraconazole 200 mg orally twice daily × lifelong
	or
	Amphotericin B IV 1 mg/kg 1–3 times weekly × lifelong

HIV, human immunodeficiency virus; IT, intrathecal.
[a]When more than one therapy is listed, they are listed in order of preference.
[b]See text for definitions of induction, consolidation, suppressive/maintenance therapy, and prophylactic therapy.
[c]Deoxycholate amphotericin B.
[d]In patients with significant renal disease, lipid formulations of amphotericin B can be substituted for deoxycholate amphotericin B during the induction.
[e]Or until cerebrospinal fluid (CSF) cultures are negative
Data from Bennett et al.,[23] Francis and Walsh,[24] Powderly et al.,[25] Saag et al.,[26] and van der Horst et al.[27]

tance develops to flucytosine in up to 30% of patients treated with flucytosine alone, limiting its usefulness as monotherapy.[24,25] Combination therapy with amphotericin B and flucytosine will sterilize the CSF within 2 weeks of treatment in 60% to 90% of patients, and most immunocompetent patients will be treated successfully with 6 weeks of combination therapy.[23] However, because of the need for prolonged IV therapy and the potential for renal and hematologic toxicity with this regimen, alternative regimens have been advocated. Despite a lack of clinically controlled trials in this population, amphotericin B induction therapy for 2 weeks, followed by consolidation therapy with fluconazole for an additional 8 to 10 weeks, is frequently recommended based on data extrapolated from studies conducted in HIV-infected patients. Suppressive therapy with fluconazole 200 mg/day for 6 to 12 months after the completion of induction and consolidation therapy is optional.[15,25–27]

Pilot studies evaluating combination therapy with fluconazole plus flucytosine as initial therapy yielded unsatisfactory results, and this approach is discouraged even in "low risk" patients. Ketoconazole has been used successfully in the treatment of cutaneous cryptococcosis, but it is not useful in the treatment of CNS disease, probably because of its poor penetration into the CNS.[15]

Despite low CSF concentrations of amphotericin B (2% to 3% of those observed in plasma), the use of intrathecal amphotericin B is not recommended for the treatment of cryptococcal meningitis except in very ill patients or in patients with recurrent or progressive disease despite aggressive therapy with IV amphotericin B. The dosage of amphotericin B employed is usually 0.5 mg administered through the lumbar, cisternal, or intraventricular (through an Ommaya reservoir) route two or three times weekly. Side effects of intrathecal amphotericin B include arachnoiditis and paresthesias. Intrathecal amphotericin B therapy should be administered in combination with IV amphotericin B.[27]

■ IMMUNOCOMPROMISED PATIENTS

Immunocompromised hosts with isolated pulmonary and extrapulmonary disease without CNS disease should be treated similarly to nonimmunocompromised patients with CNS disease. Immunocompromised patients with CNS infection require more prolonged therapy; treatment regimens are based on those used in the HIV-infected population and follow induction and consolidation therapy with 6 to 12 months of suppressive therapy with fluconazole.[15]

HIV-Infected Patients

There are no controlled clinical trials evaluating the therapy of isolated pulmonary infection; thus the specific treatment of choice is unclear. However, because these patients are at high risk for disseminated infection, antifungal therapy is warranted in all patients. Lifelong therapy with fluconazole is recommended; in patients for whom fluconazole is not an option, itraconazole can be used.

Fluconazole is beneficial for both acute and chronic maintenance therapy for cryptococcal meningitis. Amphotericin B 0.4 to 0.5 mg/kg IV daily was compared with oral fluconazole 200 mg/day. Although the overall 10-week mortality was the same in both groups, the time until the CSF culture became negative was longer, and there were more deaths in the first 2 weeks of therapy in the fluconazole group.[26] In later trials,[27] amphotericin B 0.7 mg/kg IV daily for 2 weeks (with or without oral flucytosine 100 mg/kg per day), followed by consolidation therapy with either itraconazole 400 mg/day orally or fluconazole 400 mg/day orally, led to markedly improved outcomes in comparison with earlier regimens. This study confirmed the benefit of early high-dose (0.7 mg/kg per day) amphotericin B use, the usefulness of flucytosine added to amphotericin B for induction therapy, and the slight superiority of fluconazole over itraconazole for consolidation therapy.

Amphotericin B combined with flucytosine is the initial treatment of choice. In patients who cannot tolerate flucytosine, amphotericin B alone is an acceptable alternative. After the initially successful 2-week induction period, consolidation therapy with fluconazole can be administered for 8 weeks or until CSF cultures are negative. In patients in whom fluconazole cannot be given, itraconazole is an acceptable, albeit less effective, alternative. Combination therapy with fluconazole plus flucytosine is effective; however, it is recommended as an alternative to the preceding therapies because of its potential for toxicity. Lipid formulations of amphotericin B are effective, but the optimal dosage is unknown.[15]

In HIV-infected patients, mortality is highly associated with elevated intracranial pressure (CSF opening pressure >250 mm). At the initiation of antifungal therapy, lumbar drainage should remove enough CSF to reduce the opening pressure by 50%. Patients initially should undergo daily lumbar punctures to maintain CSF opening pressure in the normal range. When the CSF pressure is normal for several days, the procedure can be suspended. Adjunctive steroid treatment is not recommended because therapy has resulted in mixed results and its impact on outcome is unclear. Similarly, neither mannitol nor acetazolamide therapy provides any clear benefit in the management of elevated intracranial pressure.[15]

Suppressive (Maintenance) Therapy for Cryptococcal Meningitis in the HIV-Infected Patient

Relapse of *C. neoformans* meningitis occurs in approximately 50% of AIDS patients after completion of primary therapy. Persistence of asymptomatic urinary *C. neoformans* has been documented in a high percentage of AIDS patients despite seemingly adequate courses of therapy for primary meningeal disease. The prostate appears to act as a sequestered reservoir of infection in these patients, resulting in systemic relapse. Fluconazole is recommended for chronic suppressive therapy of cryptococcal meningitis in AIDS patients. The AIDS Clinical Trials Group's (ACTG) 026 study demonstrated that oral fluconazole 200 mg/day was superior to IV administration of amphotericin B 1 mg/kg weekly in preventing relapse. In addition, the fluconazole-treated group showed a lower incidence of adverse drug reactions and bacterial infections.[27] Randomized comparative trials also demonstrated the superiority of fluconazole versus itraconazole as maintenance therapy. Thus itraconazole should be reserved for patients intolerant to fluconazole. Ketoconazole is not effective as maintenance therapy.

Although the numbers of patients who have been evaluated remain limited, and recurrences can occur, patients are at low risk for recurrence of cryptococcosis when they have successfully completed a course of initial therapy for cryptococcosis, remain asymptomatic with regard to signs and symptoms of cryptococcosis, and have a sustained increase (e.g., >6 months) in their CD4+ T-lymphocyte counts to >100 to 200 cells/microliter and an HIV viral load of fewer than 50 copies/mL.[15,25–28]

EVALUATION OF THERAPEUTIC OUTCOMES

Once the CNS is involved, the usual course is weeks to months of progressive deterioration, with 80% of untreated patients dying within the first year. The prognosis of cryptococcal meningitis depends largely on the underlying predisposing factors of the host. Although cryptococcal antigen is positive in 90% of patients with cryptococcal meningitis, fewer than one-half of the patients with cryptococcal meningitis develop antibody to capsular polysaccharide. Those who produce antibody have a slightly improved prognosis. In contrast, the presence of headache is a favorable symptom presumably because it leads to an earlier diagnosis. A favorable outcome is also associated with a normal mental status on diagnosis and a CSF white blood cell (WBC) count of less than 20 cells/mm^3. A poor outcome is predicted, however, by the presence of one or more underlying diseases (including hematopoietic disorders and AIDS), corticosteroid or immunosuppressive therapy, pretreatment serum cryptococcal antigen titers of 1:32, and posttherapy serum antigen titers of 1:8. In non-AIDS patients, the cryptococcal antigen titer can be followed during therapy to assess response to antifungal therapy. In AIDS patients, decreasing titers are not necessarily predictive of success, and titers rarely become negative at the completion of therapy.

CANDIDA INFECTIONS

Candida species are yeasts that exist primarily as small (4–6 microns), unicellular, thin-walled, ovoid cells that reproduce by budding. On agar medium, they form smooth, white, creamy colonies resembling staphylococci. Although there are more than 150 species of *Candida*, eight species—*C. albicans, C. tropicalis, Candida parapsilosis, C. krusei, Candida stellatoidea, C. guilliermondii, C. lusitaniae,* and *C. glabrata*—are regarded as clinically important pathogens in human disease.[13] Yeast forms, hyphae, and pseudohyphae can be found in clinical specimens.

PATHOPHYSIOLOGY

8 *C. albicans* is a normal commensal of the skin, female genital tract, and entire GI tract of humans. Therefore, the mere presence of hyphae or pseudohyphae in a clinical specimen is insufficient for the diagnosis of invasive disease. The majority of infections with *C. albicans* are acquired endogenously, although human-to-human transmission also can occur. Oral candidiasis in the newborn probably is acquired during passage through the birth canal, and balanitis in the uncircumcised male can be acquired through contact with a female with vaginal candidiasis. Although the term *fungemia* refers to the presence of fungi in the blood, the most commonly isolated organism is *C. albicans.* Candidiasis can cause mucocutaneous or systemic infection, including endocarditis, peritonitis, arthritis, and infection of the CNS. (Mucocutaneous infections caused by *Candida* are discussed in further detail in Chap. 124.)

The role of an intact integument is crucial in the prevention of mucocutaneous or hematogenous candidiasis. After *Candida* invades the dermis or enters the bloodstream, polymorphonuclear (PMN) leukocytes play a major role in the defense of the patient because PMN leukocytes are capable of damaging pseudohyphae and can phagocytize and kill blastoconidia. In addition to neutrophils, lymphocytes, monocytes, macrophages, complement, and eosinophils play a role in the prevention of infection. Adherence of *C. albicans* is important in the pathogenesis of oral candidiasis and subsequent colonization of the GI tract. Because evidence suggests that the GI tract is often the portal of entry for *Candida* in disseminated disease, factors that alter the adherence of *Candida* are crucial in the development of local and systemic infection. *Candida tropicalis* adheres to intravascular catheters at a higher rate than *C. albicans,* a factor that may help to account for the increased incidence of systemic infections caused by this pathogen.

HEMATOGENOUS CANDIDIASIS

EPIDEMIOLOGY

The incidence of fungal infections caused by *Candida* species has increased substantially in the past three decades, and *Candida* infections currently constitute a significant cause of morbidity and mortality among severely ill patients. *Candida* species now constitute the fourth most common cause of bloodstream infections (BSIs) for patients hospitalized in intensive care units (ICUs) in the United States, following coagulase-negative staphylococci, *Staphylococcus aureus*, and enterococci. The Centers for Disease Control and Prevention's (CDC) National Nosocomial Infection Survey implicated fungi as the cause of 8% of nosocomial infections. Although *C. albicans* accounted for approximately 50% of *Candida* species, non-*albicans* species of *Candida,* including *C. glabrata, C. tropicalis, C. krusei,* and *C. parapsilosis,* are increasingly frequent causes of invasive candidal infections.[29–31] *Candida lusitaniae* infections are a cause of breakthrough fungemia in cancer patients; *C. parapsilosis* has emerged as the second most common pathogen, following *C. albicans*, in neonatal ICU patients, where it is often associated with central lines and parenteral nutrition, and fungemias in patients outside the United States, in particular in South America. Fungemia caused by *C. glabrata* is observed more commonly in adults older than 65 years of age.[29,32] The change in species is of concern clinically because certain pathogens, such as *C. krusei* and *C. glabrata*, are intrinsically more resistant to commonly used triazole drugs (see Table 125–1).

PATHOPHYSIOLOGY

Candida generally is acquired via the GI tract, although organisms also can enter the bloodstream via indwelling IV catheters. Immunosuppressed patients, including those with lymphoreticular or hematologic malignancies, diabetes, and immunodeficiency diseases and those receiving immunosuppressive therapy with high-dose corticosteroids, immunosuppressants, antineoplastic agents, or broad-spectrum antimicrobial agents, are at high risk for invasive fungal infections. However, a number of prospective, randomized, controlled trials have validated the efficacy of antifungal prophylaxis and the use of antifungal agents for the treatment of persistently febrile patients with neutropenia who do not respond to antibiotics, and in the prophylaxis of patients undergoing hematopoietic stem cell transplantation (HSCT), in particular in HSCT patients with graft-versus-host disease (GVHD).[33] These efforts have resulted in a reduction in the frequency of bloodstream infections caused by *Candida* species and systemic candidiasis in patients with neutropenia. In fact, most bloodstream infections caused by *Candida* species now occur in patients who have been hospitalized in ICUs, especially adult and neonatal ICUs. Retrospective studies have identified a number of risk factors for candidal bloodstream infections in ICU patients, most of which have been verified in multiple studies, although some remain controversial[34] (Table 125–7). Major risk factors include the use of central venous catheters, total parenteral nutrition, receipt of multiple antibiotics, extensive surgery and burns, renal failure and hemodialysis, mechanical ventilation, and prior fungal colonization. Patients who have undergone surgery (particularly surgery of the GI tract) are increasingly susceptible to disseminated candidal infections.[34,35]

CLINICAL PRESENTATION OF HEMATOGENOUS CANDIDIASIS[11,13]

Dissemination of *C. albicans* can result in infection in single or multiple organs, particularly the kidney, brain, myocardium, skin, eye, bone, and joints. In most patients, multiple micro- and macroabscesses are formed. Infection of the liver and spleen is becoming recognized as a particularly common and difficult-to-treat site of infection that characteristically occurs in patients undergoing chemotherapy for acute leukemia or lymphoma.

Diagnosis

Signs and Symptoms Several distinct presentations of disseminated *C. albicans* have been recognized.[10]

TABLE 125-7 Risk Factors for Invasive Candidiasis

Neutropenia
Lymphoreticular or hematologic malignancies
Diabetes
Immunodeficiency diseases
High-dose corticosteroids
Immunosuppressants
Antineoplastic agents
Central venous catheters
Total parenteral nutrition (TPN)
Receipt of multiple antibiotics
Extensive surgery (particularly surgery of the gastrointestinal tract)
Burns
Renal failure and hemodialysis
Mechanical ventilation
Prior fungal colonization

Data from Fraser et al.[34] and Wey et al.[35]

1. Patients present with the acute onset of fever, tachycardia, tachypnea, and occasionally, chills or hypotension. The clinical presentation generally is indistinguishable from that seen with sepsis of bacterial origin.
2. Patients develop intermittent fevers and are ill only when febrile.
3. Patient manifests progressive deterioration of their condition with or without fever.
4. Hepatosplenic candidiasis often is manifested only as fever while the patient remains neutropenic (<1000 WBCs/mm^3).

Laboratory Tests Although a variety of serologic tests have been proposed for the detection of *Candida* protein antigens, serum antibodies to *Candida*, and antibodies to cell wall components such as mannan, no test has demonstrated reliable accuracy in the clinical setting for the diagnosis of disseminated infection with *Candida*. Only 25% to 45% of neutropenic patients with disseminated candidiasis at autopsy had a positive blood culture with *C. albicans* prior to death. The interpretation of positive surveillance cultures of the skin, mouth, sputum, feces, or urine is hampered by their occurrence as commensal pathogens and in distinguishing colonization from invasive disease.

Until recently, a rapid presumptive identification of *C. albicans* could be made by incubation of the organism in serum; formation of a germ tube (the beginning of hyphae, which arise as perpendicular extensions from the yeast cell, with no constriction at their point of origin) within 1 to 2 hours offered a positive identification of *C. albicans*. Unfortunately, *C. dubliniensis*, a new species of *Candida* that was identified recently as an important cause of mucosal colonization and infection in HIV-infected individuals, also can produce a germ tube. A negative germ tube test does not rule out the possibility of *C. albicans*, but further biochemical tests must be performed to differentiate between other non-*albicans* species.[36]

In patients with hepatosplenic candidiasis, as the WBC count increases to more than 1,000 cells/mm^3, imaging studies can detect the presence of abscess or microabscesses in the liver and spleen, often found with acute suppurative and granulomatous reactions.

A new peptide nucleic acid (PNA) fluorescence in situ hybridization (FISH) method uses fluorescein-labeled PNA probes that targets *C. albicans* 26S rRNA for the identification of *C. albicans* directly from blood culture bottles that test positive and in which yeasts are observed by Gram staining has been developed. The probe is added to smears made directly from the contents of blood culture bottles and is hybridized for 90 minutes, and the smears are subsequently examined by fluorescence microscopy. The test has excellent sensitivity (99%–100%) and specificity (100%) in the direct identification of *C. albicans* from blood cultures.[14]

TREATMENT

Hematogenous Candidiasis

Fraser and colleagues[34] documented the high rate of mortality in nonneutropenic patients with fungal blood cultures. Mortality was highest in patients with sustained positive blood cultures, those who did not receive antifungal therapy, and those infected with non-*albicans* strains of *Candida*. This study clearly documented the importance of early recognition and treatment of positive fungal blood cultures. Prompt initiation of therapy is important: Delays in empiric antifungal treatment greater than 12 hours after obtaining a positive blood sample is associated with greater hospital mortality.[37,38,39] Despite increased awareness of the importance of treating patients with positive blood cultures, mortality associated with candidemia remains high.[40]

Treatment of candidiasis should be guided by knowledge of the infecting species; the clinical status of the patient; when available, the antifungal susceptibility of the infecting isolate; and whether the patient has received antifungal therapy previously (Table 125–8). Therapy should be continued for 2 weeks after the last positive blood culture and resolution of signs and symptoms of infection. All patients should undergo an ophthalmologic examination to exclude the possibility of candidal endophthalmitis.[7] Amphotericin B can be switched to fluconazole (intravenous or oral) for the completion of therapy. Susceptibility testing of the infecting isolate is a useful adjunct to species identification during selection of a therapeutic approach because it can be used to identify isolates that are unlikely to respond to fluconazole or amphotericin B. However, this is not currently available at most institutions.

■ NONIMMUNOCOMPROMISED PATIENT

Prophylaxis

In ICUs, the use of fluconazole for prophylaxis or empirical therapy has increased exponentially in the past decade. However, studies that demonstrated benefit in the prevention of invasive candidal bloodstream infections did so either by using highly selective criteria or by studying patients in an unusually high-risk ICU setting, and the role of antifungal prophylaxis in the surgical ICU remains extremely controversial. Rex and colleagues[7] have suggested that for a study to demonstrate efficacy in clinical trials, the baseline rate of invasive candidiasis must be >10%, and that prophylaxis must result in >fourfold reduction of disease. Although ICU-specific, a >10% rate of invasive candidiasis is generally found only in the setting of high-risk transplant patients (e.g., patients undergoing liver transplantation), or in patients with one or more of the following risk factors by day 3 of their ICU stay: new onset dialysis, receipt of broad-spectrum antibiotics, the presence of diabetes, and in patients receiving parenteral nutrition.[41–43]

Empirical Therapy

Few data are available for assessing the role of fluconazole as empirical therapy for suspected fungemia or for isolates other than *C. albicans*. Because fluconazole has poor activity against *Aspergillus* species and some non-*albicans* strains of *Candida*, many clinicians advocate amphotericin B as the therapy of choice in patients with suspected fungemia. If therapy is given, its use should be limited to patients with (1) *Candida* colonization at multiple sites, (2) multiple other risk factors, and (3) the absence of any other uncorrected causes of fever.[7]

Specific Therapy

Several large randomized studies in nonneutropenic patients have demonstrated that azoles (fluconazole or voriconazole) and deoxy-

TABLE 125-8 Therapy of Invasive Candidiasis

Type of Disease and Common Clinical Manifestations	Therapy/Comments
Prophylaxis of candidemia	
Nonneutropenic patients[a]	Not recommended except for severely ill/high-risk patients in whom fluconazole IV/PO 400 mg daily should be used (see text)
Neutropenic patients[a]	The optimal duration of therapy is unclear but at a minimum should include the period at risk for neutropenia: Fluconazole IV/PO 400 mg daily *or* itraconazole solution 2.5 mg/kg every 12 hours PO *or* micafungin 50 mg (1 mg/kg in patients under 50 kg) intravenously daily
Solid-organ transplantation	
Liver transplantation	*Patients with two or more key risk factors[b]:*
	Amphotericin B IV 10–20 mg daily *or* liposomal amphotericin B (AmBisome) 1 mg/kg/day *or* fluconazole 400 mg orally daily
Empirical antifungal therapy (unknown *Candida* species)	
Suspected disseminated candidiasis in febrile nonneutropenic patients	None recommended; data are lacking defining subsets of patients who are appropriate for therapy (see text)
Febrile neutropenic patients with prolonged fever despite 4–6 days of empirical antibacterial therapy	*Treatment duration:* Until resolution of neutropenia
	Amphotericin B IV 0.5–0.7 mg/kg/day *or* liposomal amphotericin B (AmBisome) IV 3 mg/kg/day *or* itraconazole 200 mg IV every 12 hours × 2 days, then 200 mg/day × 12 days, then 400 mg PO (solution) daily *or* voriconazole 6 mg/kg IV loading dose every 12 hours × 2 doses, then 3 mg/kg every 12 hours (restrict to allogeneic bone marrow transplant and relapsed leukemia patients) *or* fluconazole 400 mg/day IV/PO (restrict to patients with a low risk for invasive aspergillosis or azole-resistant strains of *Candida* in patients with no previous azole exposure or signs and symptoms suggesting aspergillosis)
Treatment of candidemia and acute hematogenously disseminated candidiasis	
Nonimmunocompromised host[c]	*Treatment duration:* 2 weeks after the last positive blood culture and resolution of signs and symptoms of infection
	Remove existing central venous catheters when feasible plus
Candida albicans, Candida tropicalis, Candida parapsilosis	Amphotericin B IV 0.6 mg/kg/day *or* fluconazole IV/PO 6 mg/kg/day *or* an echinocandin[d] *or* amphotericin B IV 0.7 mg/kg/day plus fluconazole IV/PO 800 mg/day
	Patients intolerant or refractory to other therapy[e]:
	Amphotericin B lipid complex IV 5 mg/kg/day
	Liposomal amphotericin B IV 3–5 mg/kg/day
	Amphotericin B colloid dispersion IV 2–6 mg/kg/day
Candida krusei	Amphotericin B IV ≥1 mg/kg/day *or* an echinocandin[d]
Candida lusitaniae	Fluconazole IV/PO 6 mg/kg/day
Candida glabrata	Amphotericin B IV ≥0.7 mg/kg/day *or* fluconazole IV/PO 6–12 mg/kg/day (400–800 mg/day in a 70 kg patient) *or* an echinocandin[d]
Neutropenic host[f]	*Treatment duration:* Until resolution of neutropenia
	Remove existing central venous catheters when feasible plus
	Amphotericin B IV 0.7–1 mg/kg/day (total dosages 0.5–1 g)
	or Patients failing therapy with traditional amphotericin B: Lipid formulation of amphotericin B IV 3–5 mg/kg/day
Chronic disseminated candidiasis (hepatosplenic candidiasis)	*Treatment duration:* Until calcification or resolution of lesions
	Stable patients: Fluconazole IV/PO 6 mg/kg/day
	Acutely ill or refractory patients: Amphotericin B IV 0.6–0.7 mg/kg/day
Urinary candidiasis	*Asymptomatic disease:* Generally no therapy is required
	Symptomatic or high-risk patients[g]: Removal of urinary tract instruments, stents, and Foley catheters, +7–14 days therapy with fluconazole 200 mg orally daily *or* amphotericin B IV 0.3–1 mg/kg/day

PO, orally.

[a]Patients at significant risk for invasive candidiasis include those receiving standard chemotherapy for acute myelogenous leukemia, allogeneic bone marrow transplants, or high-risk autologous bone marrow transplants. However, among these populations, chemotherapy or bone marrow transplant protocols do not all produce equivalent risk, and local experience should be used to determine the relevance of prophylaxis.

[b]Risk factors include retransplantation, creatinine of more than 2 mg/dL, choledochojejunostomy, intraoperative use of 40 units or more of blood products, fungal colonization detected within the first 3 days after transplantation.

[c]Therapy is generally the same for acquired immunodeficiency syndrome (AIDS)/non-AIDS patients except where indicated and should continued for 2 weeks after the last positive blood culture and resolution of signs and symptoms of infection. All patients should receive an ophthalmologic examination. Amphotericin B can be switched to fluconazole (intravenous or oral) for the completion of therapy. Susceptibility testing of the infecting isolate is a useful adjunct to species identification during selection of a therapeutic approach because it can be used to identify isolates that are unlikely to respond to fluconazole or amphotericin B. However, this is not currently available at most institutions.

[d]Echinocandin = caspofungin 70 mg loading dose, then 50 mg IV daily maintenance dose, or micafungin 100 mg daily, or anidulafungin 200 mg loading dose, then 100 mg daily maintenance dose.

[e]Often defined as failure of ≥500 mg amphotericin B, initial renal insufficiency (creatinine ≥2.5 mg/dL or creatinine clearance <25 mL/min), a significant increase in creatinine (to 2.5 mg/dL for adults or 1.5 mg/dL for children), or severe acute administration-related toxicity.

[f]Patients who are neutropenic at the time of developing candidemia should receive a recombinant cytokine (granulocyte colony-stimulating factor or granulocyte-monocyte colony-stimulating factor) that accelerates recovery from neutropenia.

[g]Patients at high risk for dissemination include neutropenic patients, low-birth-weight infants, patients with renal allografts, and patients who will undergo urologic manipulation.

Data from NCCLS,[5] Pappas et al.[7,40]

cholate amphotericin B are similarly effective; however, fewer adverse effects are observed with azole therapy (Table 125–9). Similarly, echinocandins are at least as effective as amphotericin B or fluconazole in (mainly nonneutropenic) adult patients with candidemia with fewer drug-related adverse events. Although the use of combination therapy (high-dose fluconazole plus amphotericin B) was demonstrated recently to be superior to treatment with fluconazole alone, it was associated with a higher rate of nephrotoxicity, and the routine use of combination therapy in this patient population is not yet recommended. Alternatives to fluconazole should be considered when patients have a history of recent exposure to fluconazole or other azoles, when a broader spectrum is desirable (e.g., persistently neutropenic patient), or when non-*albicans* species are isolated during or immediately following azole therapy, and in unstable or severely immunocompromised patients.[44–50]

Neonates with disseminated candidiasis usually are treated with amphotericin B because of its low toxicity in this patient population and because of the lack of experience with other agents in this population; however, micafungin or caspofungin may offer safe, effective alternatives.[7,12,40] Treatment should continue until 2 weeks

TABLE 125-9 Treatment of Candidemia in the Nonneutropenic Host

Year Published	Study Drugs and Dosages	Study Design	Results and Comments
1994	Fluconazole vs. amphotericin B	Randomized, non-blinded, multicenter	Similar outcomes but higher rate of nephrotoxicity in the amphotericin B group
2002	Caspofungin (70 mg IV × 1 loading dose; then 50 mg IV daily) vs. amphotericin B (0.6–0.7 mg/kg/day IV) each antifungal agent was changed to fluconazole after ≥10 days to complete therapy	Randomized, multicenter	Successful outcome was achieved in 73.9% and 61.7% of patients receiving caspofungin and amphotericin B, respectively, but there was a higher rate of nephrotoxicity in the amphotericin B group.
2003	Fluconazole 800 mg/day + placebo vs fluconazole 800 mg/d + amphotericin B 0.7 mg/kg/day	Randomized, blinded, multicenter	The study was confounded by differences in the severity of illness of the two study populations (the fluconazole group had more severe illness). The regimens were comparable and noted a trend toward better response (based principally on more effective bloodstream clearance) in the group receiving combination therapy.
2005	Voriconazole (6 mg/kg IV every 12 hours on day 1; 3 mg/kg every 12 hours IV on days 2 and 3; then 200 mg PO every 12 hours) vs. amphotericin B (≥0.7 mg/kg/day) followed by fluconazole (≥400 mg PO/IV daily)	Randomized, non-blinded, multicenter	Voriconazole was as effective as the regimen of amphotericin B followed by fluconazole in the clearing of blood cultures. Treatment discontinuations cased by all-cause adverse events were more frequent in the voriconazole group, although most discontinuations were caused by non–drug-related events, and there were significantly fewer serious adverse events and cases of renal toxicity than in the amphotericin B/fluconazole group.
2005 (abstract)	Anidulafungin (200 mg loading dose × 1, then 100 mg/day) vs. IV fluconazole (800 mg loading dose × 1, then 400 mg/day)	Randomized, double-blind	A statistically significantly greater response was observed with anidulafungin in the microbiologic intent-to-treat arm at the end of IV therapy, and at the 2-wk and 6-wk followups in patients with APACHE II scores of >20. Survival was improved with anidulafungin.
2005 (abstract)	Micafungin (100 mg/day IV) vs. liposomal amphotericin B (3 mg/kg/day) × 2–4 weeks	Randomized, double-blind	Micafungin treatment was considered effective (clinical plus mycological response) in 89.6% of patients (181:202), compared to 89.5% (170:190) in the amphotericin B group. The amphotericin B group had a significantly higher incidence of side effects, including infusion-related reactions and increases in serum creatinine.
2006 (abstract)	Caspofungin (70 mg IV × 1 loading dose; then 50 mg IV daily) vs. micafungin 100 mg/day vs. micafungin 150 mg/day	Randomized, double-blind	Micafungin was found noninferior to caspofungin. Higher dosages of micafungin (150mg/day vs. 100mg/day) were not more efficacious. The safety profiles for the three treatments were similar.

APACHE, Acute Physiology and Chronic Health Evaluation; PO, orally.

Data from Rex et al.,[44] Mora-Duarte et al.,[46] Rex et al.,[47] Kullberg et al.,[48] Ruhnke et al.,[49] Betts et al.,[50] and Goodman et al.[51]

following the last positive blood culture and resolution of signs and symptoms of infection.

CLINICAL CONTROVERSY

Because *C. glabrata* demonstrates reduced susceptibility in vitro to both fluconazole and amphotericin B, optimal therapy is unclear. Larger doses of fluconazole (800 mg/day in a 70-kg patient) have been used in less critically ill patients or amphotericin B (≥0.7 mg/kg per day). However, observational studies demonstrated no difference in mortality in nonneutropenic patients administered fluconazole versus amphotericin B for bloodstream infections caused by *C. glabrata.*[40] In vitro, echinocandin antifungal agents appear very active, and these agents are widely used, however, their usefulness in vivo has not been adequately assessed in controlled trials.[7,40]

C. krusei infections should be treated with large doses of amphotericin B (≥1 mg/kg per day) or with caspofungin (70-mg IV loading dose, followed by 50 mg/day IV).[7] *C. tropicalis*, and *C. parapsilosis* can be treated with either amphotericin B at 0.6 mg/kg per day or fluconazole at 6 mg/kg per day. Amphotericin B resistance remains relatively rare despite more than 45 years of clinical use, although it has been reported in *C. lusitaniae* (now *Clavispora lusitaniae*) and *C. guilliermondii*. *Candida rugosa* often is considered to be "polyene tolerant," and these isolates are believed to be selected owing to the wide use of amphotericin B.

Among the lipid-associated formulations of amphotericin B, only liposomal amphotericin B (AmBisome) and amphotericin B lipid complex (Abelcet) have been approved for use in proven cases of candidiasis; however, patients with invasive candidiasis also have been treated successfully with amphotericin B colloid dispersion (Amphotec or Amphocil). The lipid-associated formulations are less toxic but as effective as amphotericin B deoxycholate.

CLINICAL CONTROVERSY

Owing to the higher cost and paucity of randomized trials showing the efficacy of lipid-associated formulations of amphotericin B against proven invasive candidiasis, many clinicians limit their first-line use for the treatment of these infections to individuals who are intolerant to, at high risk of intolerance to, or refractory to amphotericin B deoxycholate. However, the data demonstrating up to a 6.6-fold increase in mortality in patients with amphotericin B–induced nephrotoxicity have convinced other clinicians that high-risk patients (e.g., residence in an ICU care or intermediate care unit at the time of initiation of amphotericin B therapy) warrant first-line therapy with these agents.

■ IMMUNOCOMPROMISED PATIENTS

In immunocompromised patients, the presence of candidemia is associated with evidence of disseminated disease in more than 70% of patients and with a 70% to 80% fatality rate. Therapy should include removal of the catheter and administration of systemic antifungal therapy.[7] The optimal agent, dose, and duration of therapy are unclear, and patients must be monitored carefully with serial blood cultures and careful physical examinations, particularly of the retina. Patients who are neutropenic at the time of developing candidemia should receive a recombinant cytokine (granulocyte colony-stimulating factor or granulocyte-monocyte colony-stimulating factor) that accelerates recovery from neutropenia.[7]

Prophylaxis

Recognition of the role of the GI tract in invasive *Candida* infections has led to efforts to decrease infections by prophylactic administration of topical or systemically absorbed antifungal agents in immunocompromised patients. The use of systemically absorbable agents such as azole antifungal agents appears to decrease the risk of invasive fungal infections.[7,51,52]

Fluconazole, given at 400 mg/day from the start of the conditioning regimen until day 75, can reduce the frequency of invasive *Candida* infections and decrease mortality at day 110 in patients undergoing allogeneic bone marrow transplantation.[52,53] In less risk-selected patients with hematologic malignancies who are undergoing remission-induction chemotherapy, both fluconazole (400 mg/day) and itraconazole cyclodextrin (2.5 mg/kg orally twice daily) are effective in preventing systemic infection and death caused by *Candida* species.[54,55] Intravenous caspofungin (50 mg daily) was compared with intravenous itraconazole (200 mg twice daily for 2 days, then 200 mg once daily). Mortality was similar in both groups. Micafungin 50 mg daily was compared to intravenous fluconazole 400 mg daily in patients undergoing HSCT. Significantly fewer patients in the micafungin arm versus the fluconazole arm required empiric antifungal therapy, and mortality was decreased, although not significantly, in the micafungin arm. Based on this limited data, micafungin and caspofungin may provide options for prophylaxis in patients undergoing HSCT. However, more compelling data have been demonstrated with posaconazole.[12] In a double-blinded, multicenter clinical trial of the prophylaxis of invasive fungal infections in patients who had undergone HSCT with GVHD, posaconazole (200 mg every 8 hours), was superior to fluconazole (400 mg daily) in preventing aspergillosis and comparable to fluconazole in preventing other breakthrough invasive fungal infections.[56]

Empirical Therapy for Febrile Neutropenic Patients

Many clinicians advocate early institution of empirical IV amphotericin B in patients with neutropenia and persistent (>5–7 days) fever.[57] However, the potential toxicities (particularly nephrotoxicity) of this agent preclude its routine use in all patients. Suggested criteria for the empirical use of amphotericin B include (1) fever of 5 to 7 days' duration that is unresponsive to antibacterial agents, (2) neutropenia of more than 7 days' duration, (3) no other obvious cause for fever, (4) progressive debilitation, (5) chronic adrenal corticosteroid therapy, and (6) indwelling intravascular catheters. In patients who fail therapy with amphotericin B, lipid formulations of amphotericin B can be used (3–5 mg/kg per day). Comparative trials have indicated that lipid formulations of amphotericin B can be used as alternatives to amphotericin B deoxycholate for empirical therapy. Although they do not appear to be substantially more effective, there is less drug-related toxicity (Table 125–10).[57]

Itraconazole and fluconazole have demonstrated efficacy equivalent to that of deoxycholate amphotericin B in patients with hematologic malignancy (not treated with allogeneic hematopoietic stem cell transplantation).[58–60] However, as fluconazole is not active against filamentous fungi, its use in patients at high risk for these pathogens should be avoided. If itraconazole is used, the intravenous formulation should be used because the bioavailability of the oral formulations (including the solution) is unreliable. Voriconazole and caspofungin were compared with liposomal amphotericin B in large randomized, multicenter trials of empirical antifungal therapy in febrile neutropenic patients. Voriconazole did not fulfill the protocol-defined criteria for noninferiority (a difference in success rates between voriconazole and amphotericin B of no more than 10 percentage points) to liposomal amphotericin; however, it was superior in reducing documented breakthrough infections, infusion-related toxicity, and nephrotoxicity. Patients who received voriconazole had more frequent episodes of transient visual disturbances and hallucinations. Caspofungin demonstrated equivalent efficacy but was superior in the successful treatment of baseline invasive fungal infections.[12,61]

Specific Therapy

Amphotericin B, the azoles, and the echinocandins have roles in the treatment of hematogenous candidiasis, and the choice of therapy is guided by weighing the greater activity of amphotericin B for some non-*albicans* species (e.g., *C. krusei*) against the lower toxicity and ease of administration of fluconazole and the echinocandins.[7]

Most clinicians recommend amphotericin B in total dosages of 0.5 to 1 g administered over approximately 1 to 2 weeks in patients with *Candida* endophthalmitis and in all neutropenic patients with candidemia.[13] Longer courses of therapy can be needed in some patients.[13] Fluconazole and amphotericin B appear similarly effective for the treatment of *C. albicans* bloodstream infections in the neutropenic patient; controlled data, however, are lacking. In patients with uncom-

TABLE 125-10 Comparative Trials for Empiric Therapy in the Febrile Neutropenic Host

Year Published	Study Drugs	Study Design	Results and Comments
1982	Placebo vs. amphotericin B	Randomized	Favored amphotericin B
1989	Placebo vs. amphotericin B	Randomized	Favored amphotericin B
1996	Fluconazole vs. amphotericin B	Randomized	Defervescence: equivalence; safety analysis favored fluconazole
1998	Fluconazole vs. amphotericin B	Randomized	Composite: equivalence; secondary analysis favored fluconazole
2000	Fluconazole vs. amphotericin B	Randomized	Composite: equivalence; safety analysis favored fluconazole
1999	liposomal amphotericin B vs. amphotericin B	Randomized, double blind	Composite: equivalence; secondary analysis favors liposomal amphotericin B
2000	liposomal amphotericin B vs amphotericin B lipid complex	Randomized, double blind	Liposomal amphotericin B had superior safety vs. amphotericin B lipid complex and a similar therapeutic success rate
2001	Itraconazole vs. amphotericin B	Randomized, open label	Composite: equivalence; secondary analysis favors itraconazole
2002	Voriconazole vs. liposomal amphotericin B	Randomized, open label	Composite: equivalence; secondary analysis variable (voriconazole failed to meet criteria for noninferiority). Fewer breakthrough infections with voriconazole.
2004	Caspofungin vs. liposomal amphotericin B	Randomized, double blind	Composite: equivalence; secondary analysis favored caspofungin for treatment of baseline infections
2005 (abstract)	Liposomal amphotericin B loading regimen (10 mg/kg/day ×14 day) vs. standard dosing (3 mg/kg/day)	Randomized, prospective, double blind	Loading regimen did not demonstrate any benefit in overall response or survival and was associated with higher rates of nephrotoxicity and hypokalemia

Data from Boogaerts et al.,[58] Winstan et al.,[59] Marr,[60] Walsh et al.,[61] Cornely et al.,[80] and Walsh et al.[86]

plicated *C. albicans* fungemia who have not received systemic prophylaxis with antifungal azoles, therapy with fluconazole 400 to 800 mg/day IV can be considered.[62] However, in patients who have undergone allogeneic HSCT, the role of fluconazole is becoming more limited because of its widespread use for antifungal prophylaxis. In this setting, particularly if the patient has been treated previously with an azole antifungal agent, the possibility of microbiologic resistance must be considered.[7] Infections with fluconazole-resistant *Candida* species, including *C. glabrata*, *C. krusei*, and fluconazole-resistant *C. albicans*, or with *Aspergillus* species, are more likely.

In patients intolerant to amphotericin B or fluconazole, one of the lipid formulations can be used. In a randomized trial, amphotericin B lipid complex (ABLC) was found to be equivalent to 0.6 to 1 mg/kg per day of amphotericin B, and open-label therapy with amphotericin B colloid dispersion (ABCD) has been successful.

CANDIDURIA

Within the urinary tract, most common lesions are either *Candida* cystitis or hematogenously disseminated renal abscesses. *Candida* cystitis often follows catheterization or therapy with broad-spectrum antimicrobial agents. The diagnosis of *Candida* cystitis can be problematic because of the frequent presence of *Candida* pseudohyphae and yeast cells in urine specimens secondary to urethral colonization. The usefulness of urine colony counts or antibody coating techniques is questionable. The recovery of 10,000 organisms or visualization of both yeast and pseudohyphae from fresh midstream urine or from bladder urine obtained by single catheterization (not indwelling) is suggestive of genitourinary candidiasis. In most patients, the infection is asymptomatic and clears spontaneously without specific antifungal therapy.

Initial therapy of candidal cystitis should focus on removal of urinary catheters whenever possible. Changing the catheter will eliminate candiduria in only 20% of patients, whereas discontinuation will eradicate *Candida* in 40% of patients. Asymptomatic candiduria rarely requires therapy. Therapy should be used in symptomatic patients and in neutropenic patients, as well as in patients with renal allografts and those who will undergo urologic manipulation, because of the risk of dissemination.[63,64]

Fluconazole 200 mg/day for 14 days hastens the time to a negative urine culture as compared with placebo treatment, but 2 weeks after the end of therapy, the frequency of a negative urine culture remains the same with both treatments.[64] Short courses of therapy are not recommended; treatment should include removal of catheters and stents whenever possible plus 7 to 14 days of therapy. Bladder irrigation with amphotericin B (50 mg in 500 mL sterile water instilled twice daily into the bladder via a three-way catheter) is only transiently effective. Minimal quantities (<3%) of amphotericin B are absorbed systemically from the bladder.[17,64]

ROLE OF CATHETER REMOVAL

Although it is common practice in today's standard of care to place indwelling catheters in patients for the administration of medications and parenteral nutrition (PN), catheter-related infections are a common complication. These foreign bodies (especially triple-lumen catheters) double as entry ports for normal skin flora or other nosocomial pathogens, and they provide a readily available site for the binding of pathogens through microbiotic biofilms. Their subsequent role as a source of bloodstream infections is facilitated by frequent use, PN, and the potential for contamination of catheters by medical staff who are colonized with *Candida* species.

Most consensus recommendations urge that, if feasible, initial nonmedical management should include removal of all existing tunneled central venous catheters (CVCs) and implantable devices, particularly in patients with fungemia caused by *C. parapsilosis*, which is very frequently associated with catheters.[7] Arguments against the removal of all catheters in patients with candidemia include the prominent role of the gut as a source for disseminated candidiasis, the significant cost and potential for complications, and the problems that can be encountered in patients with difficult vascular access.[65] However, in an individual patient it is often difficult to determine the relative contribution of gut versus catheter as the primary source of fungemia. The evidence for this recommendation is weakest in cancer patients with severe neutropenia and mucositis (e.g., acute leukemia, stem cell transplant), in whom candidemia is almost always primarily of gut origin, and removal of CVCs is least likely to have an impact on mortality. Nucci and Anaissie[62] have proposed that CVCs be removed in nonneutropenic patients without a short life expectancy who have one of the following criteria: (1) otherwise unexplained hemodynamic instability, (2) lack of clinical improvement of resolution of candidemia after more than 72 hours of an optimal dose of an appropriate antifungal agent, (3) established or at high risk for endocarditis or septic thrombophlebitis, or (4) a pocket infection or cellulitis. In patients with more than one CVC, they recommend removal if one tunneled or implanted CVC is the likely source of infection and the patient meets the preceding criteria.[62]

ASPERGILLOSIS

EPIDEMIOLOGY

Aspergillus is a ubiquitous mold that grows well on a variety of substrates, including soil, water, decaying vegetation, moldy hay or straw, and organic debris. Although more than 300 species of *Aspergillus* have been characterized, three species are most commonly pathogenic: *Aspergillus fumigatus*, *Aspergillus flavus*, and *Aspergillus niger*. The varying degrees of pathogenicity of each species depend on their relative geographic prevalence, conidial size and shape, thermotolerance, and production of mycotoxins. For example, transport of *A. fumigatus* conidia into the lungs is facilitated by their smaller diameter in comparison with *A. flavus* and *A. niger*.

9 The term *aspergillosis* may be broadly defined as a spectrum of diseases attributed to allergy, colonization, or tissue invasion caused by members of the fungal genus *Aspergillus*. A single satisfactory classification system for these disease entities is difficult because different populations of patients can develop the same type of infection. For example, osteomyelitis can result from local trauma or hematogenous dissemination in an immunocompromised host. Colonization in normal hosts can lead to allergic diseases ranging from asthma to allergic bronchopulmonary aspergillosis or, rarely, invasive disease.[66]

PATHOPHYSIOLOGY

Aspergillosis generally is acquired by inhalation of airborne conidia that are small enough (2.5–3 microns) to reach alveoli or the paranasal sinuses. Each conidiophore releases 10^4 conidia that remain suspended for long periods and are viable for months in dry locations. Although some authors advocate monitoring of hospital air for *Aspergillus* conidia, guidelines for interpreting results do not exist. The use of high-efficiency particulate air (HEPA) filters in operating rooms and laminar flow rooms and removal of immunocompromised patients from hospital renovation sites can be helpful in preventing infection in this population. Although the fate of *Aspergillus* conidia in the GI tract has not been closely studied, limited evidence suggests that this route may provide an important portal of entry for disseminated infections in humans.[67]

Superficial Infection

Superficial or locally invasive infections of the ear, skin, or appendages often can be managed with topical antifungal therapy. Skin infections in patients with burn wounds, although uncommon, can progress to deep-tissue invasion despite the use of topical or parenteral antifungal agents. Risk factors for deep infection include extensive thermal injuries, malnutrition, cirrhosis, and previous infection with *Pseudomonas aeruginosa*.[67]

Allergic Bronchopulmonary Aspergillosis

Allergic manifestations of *Aspergillus* range in severity from mild asthma to allergic bronchopulmonary aspergillosis (BPA). BPA, which is almost always caused by *A. fumigatus,* is characterized by severe asthma with wheezing, fever, malaise, weight loss, chest pain, and a cough productive of blood-streaked sputum. Following recurrent episodes of severe asthma, the disease usually progresses to fibrosis and bronchiectasis with granuloma formation. When *Aspergillus* conidia become trapped in the viscous mucus of asthmatic patients, BPA develops. The fungus grows, releasing toxins and antigens. The resulting host sensitization results in a variety of immune reactions. Early in the course of disease, an immunoglobulin E (IgE)-mediated (type I) immune reaction results in bronchospasm, eosinophilia, and immediate skin reactivity. The ensuing fibrosis and pulmonary infiltrates appear to be mediated by circulating or precipitating antibody complexes of IgG antibody, followed by granuloma formation and mononuclear infiltration because of a type IV delayed hypersensitivity reaction. Therapy is aimed at minimizing the quantity of antigenic material released in the tracheobronchial tree. Management of acute asthma attacks minimizes trapping of *Aspergillus* by bronchial secretions, and administration of parenteral corticosteroids clears lung infiltrates.[67] Antifungal therapy generally is not indicated in the management of allergic manifestations of aspergillosis, although some patients have demonstrated a decrease in their corticosteroid dose following therapy with itraconazole. A recent double-blind, randomized, placebo-controlled trial showed that itraconazole 200 mg twice daily for 16 weeks resulted in significant differences in the amelioration of disease, as measured by the reduction in corticosteroid dose and improvement in exercise tolerance and pulmonary function.[66]

Aspergilloma

In the nonimmunocompromised host, *Aspergillus* infections of the sinuses most commonly occur as saprophytic colonization (aspergillomas or "fungus balls") of previously abnormal sinus tissue. An aspergilloma is composed of intertwined *Aspergillus* hyphae matted together with fibrin, mucus, and cellular debris. Infection usually is localized in the maxillary sinus and rarely is associated with local invasion of adjacent bone or brain tissue. Sinus aspergillosis also can present as allergic sinusitis with nasal drainage of brownish mucous plugs. Therapy with corticosteroids and surgery generally is successful. In the immunocompromised host, subacute, chronic, or fulminant invasive disease can be seen, and a combination of antifungal and surgical therapy generally is required.[67,68]

Pulmonary aspergillomas are fungus balls arising in preexisting cavities because of tuberculosis, histoplasmosis, lung tumors, or radiation fibrosis, although occasionally no previous pulmonary disease is present. The diagnosis of aspergilloma generally is made on the basis of chest radiographs, on which aspergillomas appear as a solid rounded mass, sometimes mobile, of water density within a spherical or ovoid cavity and separated from the wall of the cavity by an airspace of variable size and shape. Patients generally experience chest pain, dyspnea, and sputum production. Hemoptysis is observed in 50% to 80% of patients probably because of ulceration of the epithelial lining of the cavity with formation of granulation tissue, and hemoptysis is the cause of death in up to 26% of patients with aspergilloma. A poor prognosis is associated with increasing size or number of aspergillomas, immunosuppression (including corticosteroids), increasing *Aspergillus*-specific titers, underlying sarcoidosis, and HIV infection. Although *Aspergillus* can be cultured in only 50% to 60% of patients, precipitating antibodies are positive in virtually 100% of patients.

Invasive disease occurs rarely, and therapy therefore is controversial. There are no controlled clinical trials with which to guide therapy, and recommendations for treatment have been generated from uncontrolled trials and case reports.[68] Concern regarding the risk of severe hemorrhage has led some clinicians to use aggressive surgical excision of aspergillomas or pulmonary resection in patients with hemoptysis. Complications, including bronchopulmonary fistulas, hemorrhage, empyema, and persistent airspace problems, have led to the recommendation that surgical intervention be reserved for patients with severe (>500 mL/24 h) hemoptysis, however. Bronchial artery embolization (BAE) has been used to occlude the vessel that supplies the bleeding site in patients experiencing hemoptysis. Unfortunately, BAE generally is unsuccessful or only temporarily effective. Collateral circulation eventually develops, supplying blood flow to the affected area, and hemoptysis often recurs; consequently, reembolization is often unsuccessful. BAE should be used as a temporizing procedure in a patient with life-threatening disease who might respond to more definitive therapy if hemoptysis is stabilized. Mild to moderate hemoptysis should be managed conservatively. Although IV amphotericin B generally is not useful in eradicating aspergillomas, inhaled or intracavitary instillation of amphotericin B has been employed successfully in a limited number of patients. Itraconazole has been efficacious in uncontrolled studies; however, the dose and duration of therapy have not been standardized. Hemoptysis generally ceases when the aspergilloma is eradicated.[67,68]

Invasive Aspergillosis

Although exposure to *Aspergillus* conidia is nearly universal, impaired host defenses are required for the development of invasive disease. Phagocytes (neutrophils, monocytes, and macrophages) rather than antibodies or lymphocytes constitute the primary host defense system against invasive disease with aspergillosis. Macrophages prevent germination of conidia and also eradicate conidia, providing the first line of defense against invasive disease. Administration of corticosteroids appears to impair the killing of conidia by macrophages and to impair mobilization of neutrophils. Neutrophils halt hyphal growth and dissemination and kill mycelia, constituting a second line of defense. Prolonged neutropenia appears to be the most important predisposing factor to the development of invasive aspergillosis, accounting for the high frequency of disease in patients with acute leukemia. Complement provides a source of chemotactic factor and facilitates neutrophil damage to hyphae and monocyte killing of conidia. Complement is not necessary for the attachment or ingestion of conidia by human alveolar macrophages.[67,69]

Until recently, aspergillosis was an uncommon fungal infection in patients with AIDS. AIDS patients may be at less risk for aspergillosis than other fungal infections because the primary cellular defect in AIDS patients is in the T-lymphocytes, whereas neutrophils and macrophages constitute the primary lines of defense to infection with aspergillosis. Until recently, aspergillosis was reported as a late complication of disease in AIDS patients with additional risk factors for aspergillosis, such as corticosteroid use, neutropenia, previous *Pneumocystis carinii* or cytomegalovirus pneumonia, marijuana smoking, or the use of broad-spectrum antibiotics. However, approximately 50% of patients with aspergillosis have no classic risk factors. The majority of these patients had CD4 counts of fewer than 50 cells/mm^3. Although some patients diagnosed early in their infection responded to treatment, most patients do not respond to therapy with amphotericin B 0.5 mg/kg per day or itraconazole 200 to 600 mg/day.[70]

Invasive disease with *Aspergillus* can arise de novo or from any of the allergic or colonizing forms of aspergillosis. Predisposing factors to the development of invasive aspergillosis include glucocorticoid therapy, particularly following chronic administration or with higher dosages (30–200 mg/day of prednisone), cytotoxic agents, and recent or concurrent therapy with broad-spectrum antimicrobial agents. Patients with chronic hepatitis, alcoholism, diabetes mellitus, chronic granulomatous disease, leukopenia (<1000 cells/mm^3), leukemia (particularly acute lymphocytic or myelogenous leukemia), lymphoma, and acute rejection of an organ transplant are also at a higher risk of invasive disease. Although rare, invasive aspergillosis has been reported in apparently normal hosts.[67]

CLINICAL PRESENTATION[67,68]

The lung is the most common site of invasive disease. In the immunocompromised host, aspergillosis is characterized by vascular invasion leading to thrombosis, infarction, necrosis of tissue, and dissemination to other tissues and organs in the body. Survival beyond 2 or 3 weeks is uncommon. If bone marrow function returns, cavitation of the pulmonary lesion generally occurs, and the spread of infection can be halted. The progressive nature of the disease and its refractoriness to therapy are, in part, caused by the organism's rapid growth and its tendency to invade blood vessels.

Signs and Symptoms Patients often present with classic signs and symptoms of acute pulmonary embolus: pleuritic chest pain, fever, hemoptysis, and friction rubs. The CNS, liver, spleen, heart, GI tract, pericardium, and other body sites are involved in a substantial minority of cases. In neutropenic patients with *Aspergillus* pneumonia, hyphae invade the walls of bronchi and surrounding parenchyma, resulting in an acute necrotizing, pyogenic pneumonitis. As a result, patients often present with classic signs and symptoms of acute pulmonary embolus: pleuritic chest pain, fever, hemoptysis, and friction rubs.

Diagnosis

The diagnosis of aspergillosis is complicated by the presence of *Aspergillus* as a normal commensal in the human GI tract and respiratory secretions, and establishment of a definitive diagnosis of disease is difficult. Although suggestive of infection, the presence of hyphae in a smear or biopsy specimen is not diagnostic. Demonstration of *Aspergillus* by repeated culture and microscopic examination of tissue provides the most firm diagnosis. The appearance of *Aspergillus* in tissues varies with increasing host resistance from the normal vegetative hyphae found with necrotic tissue and exudate in the alveoli of immunocompromised hosts to the compact, tangled filaments (*granules*) observed in fungal balls. Identification of *Aspergillus* generally is based on the appearance of 2- to 4-micron-wide septate hyphae that are dichotomously branched at 45-degree angles. Sporulation is observed rarely in tissue. Although growth on Sabouraud dextrose or brain-heart infusion agar can be used for primary culture, bronchoscopy or bronchoalveolar lavage cultures are positive in only 40% of histopathologically identified specimens. Blood, CSF, and bone marrow cultures are rarely positive for *Aspergillus.*

Many clinicians treat positive respiratory cultures of *Aspergillus* as a common contaminant and argue that a minimum of two to three positive cultures is necessary before antifungal therapy is indicated. Any positive culture, however, can be indicative of true infection in the immunocompromised host, and the positive predictive value can be as high as 80% to 90% in patients with leukemia or bone marrow transplants.

Diagnostic Tests Galactomannan is a cell-wall polysaccharide specific to *Aspergillus* species that is detectable in serum and other body fluids during invasive aspergillosis (IA). Galactomannan levels, reported as optical density values, can be measured in body fluids by means of a double-sandwich enzyme immunosorbent assay (EIA). The Platelia *Aspergillus* EIA test (Bio-Rad Laboratories) is FDA-approved for use in the diagnosis of invasive aspergillosis in HSCT recipients and in patients with leukemia; its usefulness in solid-organ transplant and pediatric populations need to be established. The use of mold-active antifungals can decrease the sensitivity of the test. In most patients, circulating antigen can be detected at a mean of 8 days before diagnosis by other means. However, false-positive galactomannan assay results have been reported for patients receiving piperacillin-tazobactam and amoxicillin-clavulanate, those with bifidobacteria infections, and in neonates.[14]

The BG test (Fungitell; Associates of Cape Cod) detects (1,3)-β-D glucan (BG) in the serum of patients with symptoms of or medical conditions predisposing to invasive fungal infections and aids in the diagnosis of deep seated mycoses and fungemia. BG is a cell-wall constituent of many pathogenic fungi, including *Aspergillus* and *Candida* species, and is detectable in patients' serum during invasive disease due to these organisms. In addition to patients with IA and candidiasis, BG is also detectable in patients with infections caused by species of *Fusarium, Trichosporon, Saccharomyces,* and *Acremonium,* which are less common but very important fungal pathogens, especially in immunocompromised hosts. Detection of BG in serum uses a chromogenic variant of the limulus amoebocyte lysate assay. Although a positive test result for the presence of BG does not identify the infecting fungus, the practical application of this test includes its use as a screening assay (presumptive marker) for invasive fungal infection to allow the earlier initiation of antifungal therapy. Other tests are necessary for the confirmation and identification of the fungal pathogen.[14]

Late findings on radiographic studies include wedge-shaped pleural-based infiltrates or cavities on chest radiographs. Findings on computed tomographic (CT) scans include the halo sign (an area of low attenuation surrounding a nodular lung lesion) initially (caused by edema or bleeding surrounding an ischemic area) and, later, the crescent sign (an air crescent near the periphery of a lung nodule caused by contraction of infarcted tissue). CT abnormalities are best documented in neutropenic marrow transplant recipients and commonly precede plain chest radiograph abnormalities.

TREATMENT

Invasive Aspergillosis

Therapy for invasive aspergillosis is far from optimal at this time in part because of the difficulties in establishing a diagnosis and in part because of a lack of truly effective antifungal agents. Administration of amphotericin B appears to decrease mortality from more than 90% to approximately 45%. These data, however, are difficult to interpret because many patients were diagnosed postmortem, or amphotericin B therapy was not administered until the patient had very advanced disease. Mortality from pulmonary aspergillosis in bone marrow transplant recipients exceeds 94% regardless of therapy.[67] Although early diagnosis and administration of antifungal therapy can result in higher response rates, correction of underlying immune deficits (in particular, return of neutrophil counts) is of paramount importance in eradication of infection.[68]

Until the diagnosis of aspergillosis can be determined more rapidly and definitively, empirical therapy must be instituted when invasive disease is suspected. In patients at highest risk for invasive disease (acute leukemia and bone marrow transplant recipients), the most important predisposing factors include prolonged severe neutropenia (<100 cell/microliter for more than 1 week), graft rejection, chronic administration of corticosteroids, and tissue damage from preexisting infection. In these patients, antifungal therapy should be instituted in any of these conditions: (1) persistent fever or progressive sinusitis unresponsive to antimicrobial therapy, (2) an eschar over the nose, sinuses, or palate, (3) the presence of characteristic radiographic findings, including wedge-shaped infarcts, nodular densities, and new cavitary lesions, or (4) any clinical manifestation suggestive of orbital or cavernous sinus disease or an acute vascular event associated with fever. Isolation of *Aspergillus* species from nasal or respiratory tract secretions should be considered confirmatory evidence in any of the previously mentioned clinical settings.[67]

■ NON–HIV-INFECTED PATIENT

Prophylaxis

Unfortunately, effective chemoprophylaxis against infections by *Aspergillus* species has not been demonstrated thus far.[7] As noted above in the discussion of prophylaxis for Candida infections in immunocompromised hosts, prophylaxis with azoles or echinocandins can reduce the incidence of fungal infections in select high-risk populations.

Specific Therapy

Even though older azole antifungal agents (miconazole and ketoconazole) possess poor in-vitro activity against *Aspergillus* species, newer triazoles demonstrate improved activity both in vitro and in animal models of infection.[71] Voriconazole has emerged as the drug of choice of most clinicians for primary therapy of most patients with invasive aspergillosis.[72] A randomized trial, which compared voriconazole with amphotericin B (followed by other licensed antifungal therapy) for primary therapy of aspergillosis, noted better responses, improved survival, and fewer severe side effects with voriconazole.[73]

In patients who are unable to tolerate voriconazole, amphotericin B can be used. Because *Aspergillus* is only moderately susceptible to amphotericin B, full doses (1–1.5 mg/kg/day) are generally recommended, with response measured by defervescence and radiographic clearing. To treat microfoci, therapy should be continued after resolution of clinical and radiographic abnormalities until cultures (if they can be obtained) are negative, and reversible underlying predispositions have abated. Clinical response rather than any arbitrary total dose should guide duration of therapy. The optimal dosage or duration of amphotericin B therapy for the treatment of invasive disease is unknown and dependent on the extent of disease, the response to therapy, and the patient's underlying disease(s) and immune status. Unfortunately, the response rate averages only 37% (range, 14% to 83%), and the response to therapy is largely related to the extent of aspergillosis at the time of diagnosis, and host factors, such as resolution of neutropenia and the return of neutrophil function, lessening immunosuppression, and the return of graft function from a bone marrow or organ transplant.

Lipid formulations of amphotericin B can be indicated in patients with impaired renal function, and in those patients who develop nephrotoxicity while receiving deoxycholate amphotericin B. The lipid-based formulations may be preferred as initial therapy in patients with marginal renal function or in patients receiving other nephrotoxic drugs. Although these preparations appear less toxic than standard preparations, only limited data regarding their relative efficacy for invasive aspergillosis are available at this time, as the studies with the lipid preparations have been open-label or with historical conventional amphotericin B controls.[70,74]

Caspofungin was approved by the FDA for use as salvage therapy in patients who are intolerant or who fail therapy with one of the amphotericin B formulations.[12] Caspofungin has in vitro activity against *Aspergillus* species and is indicated for the treatment of invasive aspergillosis in patients who are refractory to or intolerant of other therapies such as conventional amphotericin B, lipid formulations of amphotericin B, and/or itraconazole. Caspofungin has not yet been studied for first-line therapy for patients with aspergillosis. Because of the high risk of mortality from invasive aspergillosis even following treatment with standard therapy such as amphotericin B or itraconazole, caspofungin can offer a new mechanism for salvage therapy for patients with this disease.

The use of adjuvant therapies, such as granulocyte transfusions or recombinant colony-stimulating factors, remains controversial, and controlled trials are lacking at this time. Although some authors advocate combination therapy with azoles, flucytosine, or rifampin plus amphotericin B, controlled clinical studies verifying the efficacy of these combination therapies are lacking.

Secondary Prophylaxis

The use of prophylactic antifungal therapy to prevent primary infection or reactivation of aspergillosis during subsequent courses of chemotherapy is controversial.[18] Studies assessing the utility of IV administration of amphotericin B in low doses (0.1 mg/kg per day) as prophylactic therapy or with higher dosages (0.5–0.6 mg/kg per day) as empirical therapy for invasive fungal infections in patients with granulocytopenia have not included sufficient numbers of patients to enable detection of differences in the number of *Aspergillus* infections.

The prophylactic use of intranasal amphotericin B aerosol sprays (5 or 10 mg/day in three divided doses) appeared beneficial in small studies in human and animal models. A larger randomized trial found, however, that amphotericin B sprays reduced colonization of the nasal mucosal without any reduction in the frequency of invasive pulmonary infections with aspergillosis. Because failure of amphotericin B sprays can be a result of the ability of small airborne conidia to access the alveolar spaces directly and to establish infection, use of aerosolized forms of amphotericin B capable of reaching the alveolar spaces can be required.

In granulocytopenic patients who recover from an episode of invasive aspergillosis, the risk of relapse of aspergillosis during subsequent courses of chemotherapy is greater than 50%. Secondary prophylaxis of aspergillosis with empirical administration of high-dose amphotericin B decreases the risk of relapse. Amphotericin B 1 mg/kg per day is started 24 to 48 hours prior to the start of chemotherapy and continued throughout the period of granulocytopenia. Some investigators recommend the addition of flucytosine (dosed to achieve peak serum concentrations of 30–60 mcg/mL) to the amphotericin B regimen. Although the use of itraconazole (alone or in combination with amphotericin B or flucytosine) can be beneficial in this patient population, little is known regarding its efficacy in this setting. If itraconazole is administered, serum levels should be monitored to assess absorption because poor absorption of drug has been documented in this patient population.[12]

EMERGING PATHOGENS

The increased frequency of fungal pathogens that were once rare is gaining attention from the medical community. Permissive environmental conditions, selective antifungal pressure, and increased numbers of immunosuppressed patients have led to increased numbers of infections caused by the Zygomycetes (e.g., *Mucor*, *Rhizopus* spp., or *Absidia*) or filamentous fungi such as *Scedosporium* or *Fusarium* species. Unfortunately, the early presentation of *Fusarium* and *Scedosporium* infections often mimics that of aspergillosis. On histopathology, *Scedosporium* species resembles *Aspergillus* species with dichotomously branching, septate hyphae and has a tendency for invasion of vascular structures.[75] These pathogens often demonstrate intrinsic resistance to amphotericin B and are associated with high mortality rates.[73] For example, mortality caused by *Scedosporium prolificans*, previously known as *Scedosporium inflatum*, exceeds 85%; *Scedosporium apiospermum* (the asexual state of *P. boydii*), was uniformly fatal in 23 solid-organ transplant recipients with disseminated disease.[75] However, in-vitro data suggest that *S. prolificans* is more sensitive to voriconazole than to amphotericin B or itraconazole.[75] Voriconazole recently received FDA approval for the treatment of serious fungal infections caused by *S. apiospermum* and *Fusarium* species, including *Fusarium solani,* in patients intolerant of or refractory to other therapy.[77] Posaconazole appears promising for the treatment of zygomycoses infections.

ANTIFUNGAL THERAPY

The antifungal armamentarium for the treatment of invasive fungal infections includes (1) inhibitors of the fungal cell membrane, such as polyenes (e.g., amphotericin B) and azole antifungals, (2) inhibitors of DNA (5-flucytosine), and more recently, (3) inhibitors of cell wall biosynthesis (echinocandins).[78]

Antifungal therapy generally uses one or more of these agents depending on the severity of infection and the patients' immune status. Rarely are the agents used in combination. Often therapy is initiated with an intravenous agent such as amphotericin B, and therapy is changed to an oral (azole) regimen as the patient's clinical status improves and oral therapy is tolerated. The most widely used combination therapy consists of flucytosine plus amphotericin B. The role of combination therapy is unclear at this time; controlled trials are lacking, and the possibility of therapeutic antagonism when using azoles in combination with amphotericin B remains debated. Controlled trials are needed to define the role of azoles plus amphotericin B and azoles or amphotericin B plus an echinocandin.

AMPHOTERICIN B

Amphotericin B remains the therapy of choice for many systemic fungal infections despite a lack of controlled clinical trials documenting the optimal dosage, duration of therapy, or relative efficacy of this agent in comparison with newer azole antifungal agents. During pregnancy, amphotericin B remains the treatment of choice for most fungal infections because azole antifungals are teratogenic.[17,79]

The side effects of amphotericin B generally are categorized as acute (infusion related) or long term. Gallis and Drew[17] recently reviewed the side effects and clinical uses of amphotericin B.

LIPID FORMULATIONS OF AMPHOTERICIN B

The use of deoxycholate amphotericin B frequently is associated with the development of induced nephrotoxicity. In an attempt to decrease the incidence of nephrotoxicity, three lipid formulations of amphotericin B have been developed and approved for use in humans: amphotericin B lipid complex (ABLC, Abelcet; Enzon Pharmaceuticals), amphotericin B colloidal dispersion (ABCD, Amphotec; Intermune Pharmaceuticals), and liposomal amphotericin B (AmBisome; Gilead Pharmaceuticals). In these preparations, amphotericin B is incorporated into the phospholipid bilayer membrane rather than in the enclosed aqueous phase.

The various lipid formulations of amphotericin B exhibit markedly different pharmacokinetics; however, the clinical implications of these differences remain unclear. Although larger doses of these preparations are required to achieve similar pharmacologic effects as the deoxycholate form of amphotericin B, the toxicity appears to be much lower.[79] Although the FDA-approved dosages of these agents are 5 mg/kg per day (amphotericin B lipid complex), 3 to 6 mg/kg per day (amphotericin B colloid dispersion), and 3 to 5 mg/kg per day (liposomal amphotericin B), the agents appear generally equipotent. The optimal dose of these compounds for serious *Candida* infections is unknown; however, dosages of 3 to 5 mg/kg per day appear reasonable. Liposomal amphotericin B administered at 3 mg/kg per day was equally as effective but less toxic than a dosage of 10 mg/kg per day as initial therapy for invasive mold infections.[80] The relative efficacy of these agents is unknown; whether differences in pharmacokinetic features result in different outcomes in the treatment of specific types of infections (e.g., CNS infections) is unclear.[7]

Lipid formulations of amphotericin B are indicated for patients intolerant of, refractory to, or at high risk of being intolerant to conventional antifungal therapy.[7,81] Intolerance generally is defined as initial renal insufficiency (creatinine >2.5 mg/ dL or creatinine clearance <25 mL/min), a significant increase in creatinine (to 2.5 mg/dL for adults or 1.5 mg/dL for children), or severe acute administration-related toxicity, whereas refractory infections are defined as therapeutic failure of more than 500 mg amphotericin B.

Only ABLC and liposomal amphotericin B have been approved for use in proven candidiasis. Both in-vivo and clinical studies indicate that these compounds are less toxic but as effective as amphotericin B when used in appropriate dosages. Nevertheless, their higher cost and the paucity of randomized trials in proven invasive candidiasis limit their front-line use in these infections.[81]

CLINICAL CONTROVERSY

Should lipid formulations of amphotericin B be used rather than the traditional deoxycholate formulation? Many clinicians feel that lipid formulations have shown clear superiority in the treatment of aspergillosis and histoplasmosis and are "at least as good" as deoxycholate amphotericin B for the treatment of *Candida*, cryptococcosis, and febrile neutropenia. However, they lack FDA approval for these infections except (in some cases) as salvage therapy and their costs can be prohibitive.[81]

FLUCYTOSINE

Flucytosine (also known as 5-flucytosine) is a fluorinated pyrimidine analogue that is highly water-soluble. Patients with creatinine clearances of less than 40 mL/min should receive 100 to 150 mg/kg daily in four divided doses. The dosage should be reduced by 50% in patients with a creatinine clearance of 25 to 50 mL/min and by 75% in patients with a clearance of 13 to 25 mL/min. Peak serum concentrations (2 hours after an oral dose) should be monitored in all patients (particularly those with a creatinine clearance of less than 10 mL/min) to maintain peak serum concentrations of more than 100 mg/L.[24,25]

Flucytosine generally is associated with very few side effects in patients with normal renal, GI, and hematologic function, although rash, GI discomfort, diarrhea (5% to 10%), and reversible elevations in hepatic enzymes are observed occasionally. In patients with renal dysfunction or concomitant amphotericin B therapy, leukopenia, thrombocytopenia, and (rarely) enterocolitis can occur. Although studies have suggested that little or no conversion of flucytosine to fluorouracil occurs in vitro, serum concentrations of greater than 1,000 ng/mL (therapeutic for the treatment of malignancies) have been documented in some patients. Investigators have theorized that flucytosine may be secreted into the GI tract, deaminated by intestinal bacteria, and reabsorbed as 5-fluorouracil.[24,25]

Flucytosine is used in combination with amphotericin B or fluconazole in the treatment of cryptococcosis or (less commonly) candidiasis. The rapid development of resistance to flucytosine, however, precludes its use as single-agent therapy. Mechanisms for drug resistance can include loss of deaminase and decreased permeability to the drug.[24,25]

ECHINOCANDINS

The echinocandins (caspofungin, micafungin, and anidulafungin) are a new class of antifungal agents that act as concentration-dependent, noncompetitive inhibitors of β(1,3)-D-glucan synthase, an essential component of the cell wall of susceptible filamentous fungi that is absent in mammalian cells.[12]

All echinocandins display linear pharmacokinetics following administration of intravenous dosages, and are degraded primarily by the liver (also in the adrenals and spleen) by hydrolysis and *N*-acetylation. Following initial distribution, echinocandins are taken up by red blood cells (micafungin) and the liver (caspofungin and micafungin) where they undergo slow degradation to mainly inactive metabolites, although two uncommon metabolites of micafungin possess antifungal activity. Degradation products are excreted slowly over many days, primarily through the bile. Among the echinocandins, anidulafungin is unique in being elimination almost exclusively by slow chemical degradation rather than undergoing hepatic metabolism.[12]

Echinocandins are available only as parenteral formulations, are not dialyzable, and do not require dosage adjustment in patients with renal insufficiency. They have minimal CSF penetration, largely because of their high protein binding and large molecular weights, although the clinical relevance of these findings can be disputed, given that several other antifungal agents (amphotericin B and itraconazole) are effective for the treatment of fungal meningitis despite low CSF concentrations.

Adverse effects of echinocandins include histamine release resulting in rash, facial swelling, and itchiness. Limited experience suggests that caspofungin and micafungin are safe to use in pediatric patients; the safety and effectiveness of anidulafungin in pediatric patients has not been established. At the time of FDA approval, there were concerns regarding the safety of caspofungin when combined with cyclosporine. However, three retrospective analyses of the use of caspofungin and cyclosporine in patients do not support a risk of clinically relevant hepatotoxicity.[12]

AZOLE ANTIFUNGAL AGENTS

The introduction of the azole antifungal agents has rapidly expanded the armamentarium of agents useful in the treatment of systemic fungal infections.[9] Adverse effects of azoles include GI disturbances (primarily nausea, vomiting, epigastric pain, and diarrhea), which appear to be more common in patients receiving ketoconazole and the solution formulation of itraconazole. Although cyclodextrin is not absorbed following oral administration, use of the IV formulations of itraconazole and voriconazole is limited to 2 weeks because of concerns for potential nephrotoxicity secondary to accumulation of the cyclodextrin vehicle.[82] Fluconazole is well tolerated; intestinal complaints are the most frequently reported, followed by headaches and rash. Unlike ketoconazole, fluconazole does not inhibit testicular or adrenal steroidogenesis in healthy volunteers or hospitalized patients. Reversible alopecia occurs not infrequently and usually appears after several months of treatment with higher doses of fluconazole. Azoles are potentially teratogenic and should be avoided in pregnant women.[82]

Itraconazole

Itraconazole is triazole antifungal with a broad spectrum of antifungal activity. Despite its marked structural similarity to ketoconazole, itraconazole differs in several important respects. Itraconazole appears to have greater specificity against fungal versus mammalian CYP, resulting in greater potency and a decrease in CYP-mediated side effects. In addition, itraconazole possesses excellent in-vitro activity against *Aspergillus* and *Sporothrix* species.

Like ketoconazole, the capsule formulation of itraconazole depends on the availability of low gastric pH for dissolution and absorption. Administration with food appears to enhance significantly the bioavailability of itraconazole capsules, whereas it decreases the bioavailability of the oral solution. Because itraconazole exhibits pH-dependent dissolution and absorption, absorption of the capsule formulation is impaired in patients receiving antacids or H_2-receptor antagonists and in patients with achlorhydria.[82] Plasma concentrations of itraconazole following a single oral dose (capsules) in HIV-infected patients are approximately 50% lower than concentrations observed in healthy volunteers. The capsule formulation of itraconazole exhibits unpredictable oral bioavailability, particularly in subjects with hypochlorhydria and in patients with enteropathy caused by mucositis or graft-versus-host gut disease. Recently, oral suspension and IV formulations of itraconazole became available; both use cyclodextrin as a solubilizing vehicle to increase the solubility of the drug. The oral bioavailability of the solution is unaffected by alterations in gastric pH or in patients with enteropathy.[7,82]

Fluconazole

Fluconazole is a triazole antifungal agent with markedly different pharmacologic features than other marketed azole antifungals. The small molecular weight, low protein binding, and increased water solubility of fluconazole result in rapid, essentially complete absorption of drug following oral administration. Because fluconazole is excreted primarily (>80%) as unchanged drug in the urine, dosage adjustments are necessary in patients with renal dysfunction.[71]

Voriconazole

The hepatic biotransformation of voriconazole is fairly complex and involves CYP2C19, CYP3A4, and CYP2C9. Two of the CYPs involved in voriconazole metabolism (CYP2C19 and CYP2C9) exhibit genetic polymorphism; variability in the CYP2C19 genotype accounts for approximately 30% of the overall between-subject variability in voriconazole pharmacokinetics. Voriconazole drug interactions are dose-dependent, as they exhibit unpredictable nonlinear pharmacokinetics; thus, drug interactions are more difficult to predict and manage.

The most common side effect of voriconazole is a reversible disturbance of vision (photopsia), which occurs in approximately 30% of patients but rarely leads to discontinuation of the drug. Symptoms tend to occur during the first week of therapy and decrease or disappear despite continued therapy. Patients experience altered color discrimination, blurred vision, the appearance of bright spots and wavy lines, and photophobia. Patients should be cautioned that driving can be hazardous because of the risk of visual disturbances. The visual effects are associated with changes in electroretinogram tracings, which revert to normal when treatment with the drug is stopped; no permanent damage to the retina has been demonstrated.[71]

Posaconazole

Posaconazole has a broad spectrum of antifungal activity, including *Aspergillus* and *Candida* species and zygomycetes. In-vitro studies demonstrate that posaconazole is an inhibitor but not a substrate of hepatic (but not total) CYP3A4, and both a substrate and an inhibitor of P-glycoprotein (Pgp), suggesting that it may exhibit a drug interaction profile similar to other azoles. In addition, posaconazole undergoes glucuronidation by uridine diphosphate (UDP)-glucuronosyltransferase enzymes.[71]

DRUG INTERACTIONS WITH ANTIFUNGAL AGENTS

Drug interactions with azole antifungals generally can be placed into three broad categories: (1) decreases in azole bioavailability because of chelation or secondary to increases in gastric pH, (2) interactions with other CYP–metabolized drugs, and (3) interactions caused by inhibition of Pgp. Drug interactions in the latter two categories can result in increases or decreases in the azole antifungal, in the interacting drug, or in both drugs.

The interaction of azole antifungal agents with other CYP–metabolized drugs is well recognized. The azoles appear to be metabolized almost entirely via the CYP3A4 subfamily. As expected, they interact with other drugs metabolized partly or wholly through this enzyme pathway. In addition, fluconazole and voriconazole use the CYP2C19 pathway. Numerous clinically significant interactions have been documented with azole antifungals and a variety of other drugs. In most cases, the azole interferes with the metabolism of the other CYP–metabolized drug.[71]

The interaction between ketoconazole and cyclosporine has been exploited to reduce drug costs associated with administration of cyclosporine following organ transplantation. Relative to ketoconazole and itraconazole, fluconazole appears to be intermediate in its ability to inhibit human cytochromes P450. The magnitude of fluconazole-induced inhibition of cyclosporine metabolism appears, however, to depend on the dosage of fluconazole.

Predictably, drugs such as rifampin, rifabutin, isoniazid, phenytoin, and carbamazepine, which are known to induce the activity of cytochromes P450, result in increased metabolism of the azole antifungals and can result in therapeutic failures. Increased dosages of azole antifungals can be required in patients receiving these combinations of drugs.

Itraconazole is an inhibitor of intestinal Pgp. Significant increases in digoxin (a Pgp substrate) have been observed in patients receiving both agents concurrently. Interactions with other substrates of Pgp would be expected to occur.

Echinocandins are not inducers of cytochrome P450 enzymes, nor do they interact with Pgp, and are considered poor substrates of CYP3A4. Nevertheless, cyclosporine increases the area under the curve (AUC) of caspofungin by ~35%, and tacrolimus AUC, peak, and 12-hour concentrations are decreased by approximately 20% during concomitant administration with caspofungin. Additionally, when caspofungin was administered concurrently with tacrolimus, tacrolimus levels were reduced by 20% compared to administration with tacrolimus alone. The mechanism for these interactions is not yet known. Rifampin both inhibits (acutely) and induces (after chronic administration) caspofungin metabolism. A dosage increase is recommended in patients receiving other enzyme inducers, such as efavirenz, nevirapine, phenytoin, dexamethasone, and carbamazepine. Although micafungin does not significantly affect the clearance (or AUC) of tacrolimus, it increases the AUC of sirolimus by 21%, and of nifedipine by 18%, and decreases the clearance of cyclosporine by 16%; monitoring of cyclosporine levels during combination therapy with micafungin is recommended. Administration of cyclosporine and anidulafungin revealed only a clinically insignificant 22% increase in the AUC of anidulafungin following 4 days of concomitant cyclosporine therapy, and concurrent administration of rifampin or a variety of other substrates, inhibitors, or inducers of CYP450 with anidulafungin does not affect its clearance.[12]

COMBINATION ANTIFUNGAL THERAPY FOR ASPERGILLOSIS

Based on extensive experience in the management of bacterial and, more recently, retroviral infections, the use of combination agents for synergistic or additive effects is now common practice, particularly for the treatment of invasive aspergillosis. High-dose fluconazole, alone or in combination with amphotericin B, in nonimmunocompromised patients with candidemia demonstrated no antagonism and a trend toward improved success and more rapid clearance of *Candida* from the bloodstream.[47]

CLINICAL CONTROVERSY

Controversy has arisen about whether single-drug therapy or combination therapy (e.g., voriconazole plus and echinocandin or voriconazole plus a lipid formulation of amphotericin B) is optimum therapy. At present, the highest interest concerns combination therapy in the treatment of aspergillosis, given the continued high mortality of these infections.[84] However, in-vitro and animal data have produced conflicting results. Several retrospective studies have suggested an improvement in mortality with combination therapy with two or three antifungal agents, however, prospective, controlled human studies are lacking. Thus there are as yet no firm recommendations regarding the use of such combinations in humans.[12]

PLASMA CONCENTRATION MONITORING OF ANTIFUNGAL AGENTS

Routine monitoring of plasma concentrations of antifungal agents to assess efficacy or toxicity of these agents generally is not available. Correlations between plasma concentrations of antifungal agents and therapeutic outcomes have been poorly studied. Under certain circumstances, serum or plasma concentration monitoring is warranted, for example, in patients susceptible to flucytosine toxicity or to document adequate oral absorption of ketoconazole, itraconazole, or voriconazole in cases of suspected treatment failure, concern about compliance or absorption, or when drug interactions that might reduce the solubility or accelerate the metabolism of azoles are suspected (Table 125–11).

TABLE 125-11 Plasma Concentration Monitoring of Antifungal Agents

	Serum Concentration Monitoring Necessary?	Target Concentration Range	Timing of Sample
Echinocandins	No	NA	NA
Amphotericin B (including lipids)	No	NA	NA
Fluconazole	No	NA	NA
Itraconazole	Yes, to ensure absorption & efficacy	>0.5 mcg/mL	Trough after 7 days therapy
Voriconazole	Yes, (1) metabolism is variable, (2) low concentrations are associated with poor outcome, (3) high concentrations are associated with adverse effects (hepatotoxicity, visual disturbances)	Troughs >1 mcg/mL; concentrations >2.05 mcg/mL have been associated with improved outcomes; the likely therapeutic range is ~2–6 mcg/mL	Trough after 7 days therapy
Posaconazole	? Unclear; perhaps to ensure absorption	>0.25 mcg/mL ?	Trough after 7 days therapy
Flucytosine	Yes–high concentrations are associated with bone marrow suppression	Peak concentration <100 mcg/mL	2-hour post-dose peak

NA, not applicable.
Data from Dodds-Ashley E et al. CID 2006;43:S28–S39 and from Smith et al. AAC 2006;50:1570.

CLINICAL CONTROVERSY

Although "therapeutic" levels have not been defined, some investigators recommend maintenance of serum concentrations of itraconazole (2 to 4 hours after administration) of 1 mcg/mL, measured by bioassay, and voriconazole.[18] Among AIDS patients, those receiving itraconazole dosages of 200 mg once or twice daily achieved median plasma concentrations of 3 or 6 mcg/mL, respectively.[18] Although pharmacokinetic-pharmacodynamic analysis of early clinical trials of voriconazole did not reveal an association between voriconazole concentration and efficacy, they did suggest a trend toward worse outcome in those patients with voriconazole concentrations of <0.5 mcg/mL. This lack of association is likely because the antifungal exposure far exceeded the MICs of most pathogens (MIC_{90}, ≤0.5 mcg/mL). However, in a recent study, favorable responses were observed in 10:10 patients with voriconazole plasma concentrations >2.05 mcg/mL, whereas disease progressed in 44% of patients with concentrations <2.05 mcg/mL.[85]

ABBREVIATIONS

AIDS: acquired immunodeficiency syndrome
ACTG: AIDS Clinical Trials Group
ATCC: American Type Culture Collection
ABCD: amphotericin B colloid dispersion
ABLC: amphotericin B lipid complex
BG: (13)-β-D-Glucan
BPA: bronchopulmonary aspergillosis
BSI: bloodstream infection
CDC: Centers for Disease Control and Prevention
CNS: central nervous system
CVC: central venous catheter
CSF: cerebrospinal fluid
CF-M: CF titer for mycelial antigen
CF: complement fixation
ELISA: enzyme-linked immunosorbent assay
FISH: fluorescence in-situ hybridization
GI: gastrointestinal
GVHD: graft-versus-host disease
HEPA: high-efficiency particulate air
HAART: highly active antiretroviral therapy
HSCT: hematopoietic stem cell transplantation
ID: immunodiffusion
IgM: immunoglobulin M
ICUs: intensive care units
IV: intravenous
LA: latex agglutination
NCCLS: National Committee for Clinical Laboratory Standards
PMN: polymorphonuclear leukocytes
PDH: progressive disseminated histoplasmosis
PN: total parenteral nutrition
PNA: peptide nucleic acid
RIA: radioimmunoassay
WBC: white blood cell

REFERENCES

1. Bennett JE. Introduction to mycoses. In: Mandell GL, Bennett JE, Dolin R, eds. Principles and Practice of Infectious Diseases, 6th ed. Philadelphia, PA: Churchill Livingstone, 2005:2935–2938.
2. Pfaller MA, Jones RN, Messer SA, et al. National surveillance of nosocomial blood stream infection due to *Candida* albicans: Frequency of occurrence and antifungal susceptibility in the SCOPE program. Diagn Microbiol Infect Dis 1998;31:327–332.
3. Pfaller MA, Jones RN, Doern GV, et al. International surveillance of blood stream infections due to *Candida* species in the European SENTRY Program: Species distribution and antifungal susceptibility including the investigational triazole and echinocandin agents. SENTRY Participant Group (Europe). Diagn Microbiol Infect Dis 1999;35:19–25.
4. Singh N. Invasive mycoses in organ transplant recipients: Controversies in prophylaxis and management. J Antimicrob Chemother 2000;45:749–755.
5. National Committee for Clinical Laboratory Standards (NCCLS). Reference method for broth dilution antifungal susceptibility testing of yeasts: Approved Standard. Wayne, PA: NCCLS, 1997. NCCLS document M27-A.
6. Sobel JD. Practice guidelines for the treatment of fungal infections. Clin Infect Dis 2000;30:652.
7. Pappas PG, Rex JH, Walsh TJ, et al. Guidelines for treatment of candidiasis. Clin Infect Dis 2004;38:161–189.
8. Sanglard D, Odds FC. Resistance of *Candida* species to antifungal agents: Molecular mechanisms and clinical consequences. Lancet Infect Dis 2002;2:73185.
9. White TC, Marr KA, Bowden RA. Clinical, cellular, and molecular factors that contribute to antifungal drug resistance. Clin Microbiol Rev 1998;11:382–402.
10. Lupetti A, Danesi R, Campa M, et al. Molecular basis of resistance to azole antifungals. Trends Mol Med 2002;8:76–81.
11. Bille J. Mechanisms and clinical significance of antifungal resistance. Int J Antimicrob Agents 2000;16:331–333.
12. Eschenauer G, DePestel DD, Carver PL. Comparison of Echinocandin Antifungals. Therapeutics and Clinical Risk Management, 2007;3(1):71–97.
13. Edwards JE. *Candida* species. In: Mandell GL, Bennett JE, Dolin R, eds. Principles and Practice of Infectious Diseases, 6th ed. Philadelphia, PA: Churchill Livingstone, 2005:2938–2953.
14. Alexander BD, Pfaller MA. Contemporary tools for the diagnosis and management of invasive mycoses. Clin Infect Dis 2006;2006;43:S15–27.
15. Saag MS, Graybill RJ, Larsen RA, et al. Practice guidelines for the management of cryptococcal disease. Clin Infect Dis 2000;30:710–718.
16. Deepe GS. Histoplasma capsulatum. In: Mandell GL, Bennett JE, Dolin R, eds. Principles and Practice of Infectious Diseases, 6th ed. Philadelphia, PA: Churchill Livingstone, 2005:3012–3026.
17. Gallis HA, Drew RH, Pickard WW. Amphotericin B. 30 years of clinical experience. Rev Infect Dis 1990;12:308–329.
18. Wheat J, Sarosi G, McKinsey D, et al. Practice guidelines for the management of patients with histoplasmosis. Clin Infect Dis 2000;30:688–695.
19. Wheat LJ, Kauffman CA. Histoplasmosis. Infect Dis Clin North Am 2003;17(1):1–19.
20. Galgiani JN, Ampel NM, Blair JE, et al. Practice guidelines for the treatment of coccidioidomycoses. Clin Infect Dis 2005;41:1217–1223.
21. O'Shaughnessy EM, Shea YM, Witebsky FG. Laboratory diagnosis of invasive mycoses. Infect Dis Clin North Am 2003;17(1):135–158.
22. Chiller TM, Galgiani JN, Stevens DA. Coccidioidomycosis. Infect Dis Clin North Am 2003;17:41–57.
23. Bennett JE, Dismukes WE, Duma RJ, et al. A comparison of amphotericin B alone and combined with flucytosine in the treatment of cryptococcal meningitis. N Engl J Med 1979;301:126–131.
24. Francis P, Walsh TJ. Evolving role of flucytosine in immunocompromised patients: New insights into safety, pharmacokinetics, and antifungal therapy. Clin Infect Dis 1992;15:1003–1018.
25. Powderly WG, Saag MS, Cloud GA, et al. A controlled trial of fluconazole or amphotericin B to prevent relapse of cryptococcal meningitis in patients with the acquired immunodeficiency syndrome. N Engl J Med 1992;326:793–798.
26. Saag MS, Powderly WG, Cloud GA, et al. Comparison of amphotericin B with fluconazole in the treatment of acute AIDS-associated crypto-

coccal meningitis: The NIAID Mycoses Study Group and the AIDS Clinical Trials Group. N Engl J Med 1992;326:83–89.
27. van der Horst CM, Saag MS, Cloud GA, et al. Treatment of cryptococcal meningitis associated with the acquired immunodeficiency syndrome. N Engl J Med 1997;37:15–21.
28. Vibhagool A, Sungkanuparph S, Mootsikapun P, et al. Discontinuation of secondary prophylaxis for cryptococcal meningitis in human immunodeficiency virus-infected patients treated with highly active antiretroviral therapy: A prospective, multicenter, randomized study. Clin Infect Dis 2003;36:1329–1331.
29. Minari A, Hachem R, Raad I. *Candida lusitaniae:* A cause of breakthrough fungemia in cancer patients. Clin Infect Dis 2001;32:186–190.
30. Pfaller MA, Jones RN, Doern GV, et al. International surveillance of bloodstream infections due to *Candida* species: Frequency of occurrence and antifungal susceptibilities of isolates collected in 1997 in the United States, Canada, and South America for the SENTRY program. J Clin Microbiol 1998;36:1886–1889.
31. Winston DJ, Chandrasekar PH, Lazarus HM, et al. Fluconazole prophylaxis of fungal infections in patients with acute leukemia: Results of a randomized placebo-controlled, double-blind, multicenter trial. Ann Intern Med 1993;118:495–503.
32. Rangel-Frausto MS, Wiblin T, Blumberg HM, et al. National Epidemiology of Mycoses Survey (NEMIS): Variations in rates of blood stream infections due to *Candida* species in seven surgical intensive care units and six neonatal intensive care units. Clin Infect Dis 1999;29:253–258.
33. Edmond MB, Wallace SE, McClish DK, et al. Nosocomial bloodstream infections in United States hospitals: A three-year analysis. Clin Infect Dis 1999;29:239–244.
34. Fraser VJ, Jones M, Dunkel J, et al. Candidemia in a tertiary care hospital: Epidemiology, risk factors, and predictors of mortality. Clin Infect Dis 1992;15:414–421.
35. Wey SB, Mori M, Pfaller MA, et al. Risk factors for hospital-acquired candidemia: A matched case-control study. Arch Intern Med 1989;149: 2349–2353.
36. Sullivan DJ, Moran GP, Coleman DC. Candida dubliniensis: Ten years on. FEMS Microbiol Lett 2005;253(1):9–17.
37. Morrell M, Fraser VJ, Kollef MH. Delaying the empiric treatment of candida bloodstream infection until positive blood culture results are obtained: A potential risk factor for hospital mortality. Antimicrob Agents Chemother 2005;49:3640–3645.
38. Gudlaugsson O, Gillespie S, Lee K, et al. Attributable mortality of nosocomial candidemia, revisited. Clin Infect Dis 2003;37:1172–1177.
39. Garey KW, Rege M, Pai MP, et al. Time to initiation of fluconazole therapy impacts mortality in patients with candidemia: A multi-institutional study. Clin Infect Dis 2006;43(1):25–31.
40. Pappas, PG, Rex JH, Lee J, et al. A prospective observational study of candidemia: Epidemiology, therapy, and influences on mortality in hospitalized adult and pediatric patients. Clin Infect Dis 2003;37:634–643.
41. Eggimann P, Francioli P, Bille J, et al. Fluconazole prophylaxis prevents intraabdominal candidiasis in high-risk surgical patients. Crit Care Med 1999;27:1066–1072.
42. Rocco TR, Reinert SE, Simms H. Effect of fluconazole administration in critically ill patients. Arch Surg 2000;135:160–165.
43. Sobel JD, Rex JH. Invasive candidiasis: Turning risk into a practical prevention policy? Clin Infect Dis 2001;33:187–190.
44. Rex JH, Bennett JE, Sugar AM, et al. A randomized trial comparing fluconazole with amphotericin B for the treatment of candidemia in patients without neutropenia. N Engl J Med 1994;331:1325–1330.
45. Phillips P, Shafran S, Garber G, et al. Multicenter randomized trial of fluconazole versus amphotericin B for treatment of candidemia in non-neutropenic patients: Canadian candidemia study group. Eur J Clin Microbiol Infect Dis 1997;16:337–345.
46. Mora-Duarte J, Betts R, Rotstein C, et al. Comparison of caspofungin and amphotericin B for invasive candidiasis. N Engl J Med 2002;347:2020–2029.
47. Rex JH, Pappas PG, Karchmer AW, et al. A randomized and blinded multicenter trial of high-dose fluconazole plus placebo versus fluconazole plus amphotericin B as therapy for candidemia and its consequences in nonneutropenic subjects. Clin Infect Dis 2003;36:1221–1228.
48. Kullberg BJ, Sobel JD, Ruhnke M, et al. Voriconazole versus a regimen of amphotericin B followed by fluconazole for candidemia in non-neutropenic patients: A randomised non-inferiority trial. Lancet 2005;366(9495):1435–1442.
49. Ruhnke M, Kuse E, Chetchotisakd P, et al. Comparison of micafungin and liposomal amphotericin B for invasive candidiasis bstract M-722c]. In: Abstracts of the 45th Interscience Conference on Antimicrobial Agents and Chemotherapy. Washington, DC: American Society for Microbiology, 2005.
50. Betts RF, Rotstein C, Talwar D, et al. Comparison of micafungin and caspofungin for candidemia or invasive candidiasis [abstract M-1308a]. In: Abstracts of the 46th Interscience Conference on Antimicrobial Agents and Chemotherapy. San Francisco, CA: American Society for Microbiology, 2006.
51. Goodman JL, Winston DJ, Greenfield RA, et al. A controlled trial of fluconazole to prevent fungal infections in patients undergoing bone marrow transplantation. N Engl J Med 1992;326:845–851.
52. Slavin MA, Osborne B, Adams R, et al. Efficacy and safety of fluconazole prophylaxis for fungal infections after marrow transplantation: A prospective, randomized, double-blind study. J Infect Dis 1995;171:1545–1552.
53. Marr KA, Seidel K, Slavin MA, et al. Prolonged fluconazole prophylaxis is associated with persistent protection against candidiasis-related death in allogeneic marrow transplant recipients: Long-term follow-up of a randomized, placebo-controlled trial. Blood 2000;96:2055–2061.
54. Menichetti F, Del Favero A, Martino P, et al. Itraconazole oral solution as prophylaxis for fungal infections in neutropenic patients with hematologic malignancies: A randomized, placebo-controlled, double-blind, multicenter trial. GIMEMA Infection Program. Gruppo Italiano Malattie Ematologiche dell' Adulto. Clin Infect Dis 1999;28:250–255.
55. Rotstein C, Bow EJ, Laverdiere M, et al. Randomized placebo-controlled trial of fluconazole prophylaxis for neutropenic cancer patients: Benefit based on purpose and intensity of cytotoxic therapy. Clin Infect Dis 1999;28:331–340.
56. Ullmann AJ, Lipton JH, Vesole DH, et al. A multicenter trial of oral posaconazole vs. fluconazole for the prophylaxis of invasive fungal infections in recipients of allogeneic hematopoietic stem cell transplantation with graft-vs.-host disease. Mycoses 2005;48(Suppl 2):26a–27a.
57. Hughes WT, Armstrong D, Bodey GP, et al. 2002 Guidelines for the use of antimicrobial agents in neutropenic patients with cancer. Clin Infect Dis 200215;34:730–51.
58. Boogaerts M, Winston DJ, Bow EJ, et al. Intravenous and oral itraconazole versus intravenous amphotericin B as empirical antifungal therapy for persistent fever in neutropenic patients with cancer who are receiving broad-spectrum antibacterial therapy. Ann Intern Med 2001;135:412–422.
59. Winston DJ, Hathorn JW, Schuster MG, et al. A multicenter, randomized trial of fluconazole versus amphotericin B for empiric antifungal therapy of febrile neutropenic patients with cancer. Am J Med 2000;108:282–289.
60. Marr KA. Empirical antifungal therapy—New options, new tradeoffs. N Engl J Med, 2002;346:278–80.
61. Walsh TJ, Pappas P, Winston DJ, et al. Voriconazole compared with liposomal amphotericin B for empirical antifungal therapy in patients with neutropenia and persistent fever. N Engl J Med 2002;346:225–234.
62. Anaissie EJ, Darouiche RO, Abi-Said D, et al. Management of invasive candidal infections: Results of a prospective, randomized, multicenter study of fluconazole versus amphotericin B and review of the literature. Clin Infect Dis 1996;23:964–972.
63. Kauffman CA, Vazquez JA, Sobel JD, et al. Prospective multicenter surveillance study of funguria in hospitalized patients. Clin Infect Dis 2000;30:14–18.
64. Sobel JD, Kauffman CA, McKinsey D, et al. Candiduria: A randomized, double-blind study of treatment with fluconazole and placebo. Clin Infect Dis 2000;30:19–24.
65. Nucci M, Anaissie E. Should vascular catheters be removed from all patients with candidemia? An evidence-based review. Clin Infect Dis 2002;34:591–599.
66. Stevens DA, Schwartz HJ, Lee JT, et al. A randomized trial of itraconazole in allergic bronchopulmonary aspergillosis. N Engl J Med 2000;342:756–762.
67. Steinbach WJ, Stevens DA. Review of newer antifungal and immunomodulatory strategies for invasive aspergillosis. Clin Infect Dis 2003;37(Suppl 3):S157–187.
68. Stevens DA, Kan VL, Judson MA, et al. Practice guidelines for diseases caused by *Aspergillus.* Clin Infect Dis 2000;30:696–709.

69. Lin SJ, Schranz J, Teutsch SM. Aspergillus case fatality rate: Systematic review of the literature. Clin Infect Dis 2001;32:358–366.
70. Holding KJ, Dworkin MS, Wan PCT, et al. Aspergillosis among people infected with human immunodeficiency virus: Incidence and survival. Clin Infect Dis 2000;31:1253–1257.
71. Saad A, DePestel DD, Carver PL. Factors influencing the magnitude and clinical significance of drug interactions between azole antifungals and select immunosuppressants. Pharmacotherapy 2006;26: 1730–1744.
72. Dismukes, WE. Antifungal therapy: Lessons learned over the past 27 years. Clin Infect Dis 2006;42:1289–96.
73. Herbrecht R, Denning DW, Patterson TF, et al. 2002. Voriconazole versus amphotericin B for primary therapy of invasive aspergillosis. N Engl J Med 347:408–415.
74. Ellis M, Spence D, de Pauw B, et al. An EORTC international multicenter randomized trial (EORTC no. 19923) comparing two dosages of liposomal amphotericin B for treatment of invasive aspergillosis. Clin Infect Dis 1998;27:1406–1412.
75. Castiglioni B, Sutton DA, Rinaldi MG, et al. *Pseudallescheria boydii* (anamorph *Scedosporium apiospermum*) infection in solid organ transplant recipients in a tertiary medical center and review of the literature. Medicine 2002;81:333–348.
76. Lamaris, GA, Chamilos G, Lewis, RE, et al. Scedosporium infection in a tertiary care cancer center: A review of 25 cases from 1989–2006. Clin Infect Dis 2000;43:1580–4.
77. Vfend (voriconazole). Package insert. New York: Pfizer, 2002.
78. Dodds Ashley ES. Treatment options for invasive fungal infections. Pharmacotherapy 2006;26(6 Pt 2):55S–60S.
79. King CT, Rogers PD, Cleary JD, et al. Antifungal therapy during pregnancy. Clin Infect Dis 1998;27:1151–1160.
80. Cornely O, Maertens J, Bresnik M, Herbrecht R. Liposomal amphotericin B (L-AMB) as initial therapy for invasive filamentous fungal infections (IFFI): A randomized, prospective trial of a high loading regimen vs. standard dosing (AmBiLoad trial) [abstract 3222]. In: Program and abstracts of the 47th Annual Meeting of the American Society for Hematology, Atlanta, GA, 2005.
81. Ostrosky-Zeichner L, Marr KA, Rex JH, Cohen SH. Amphotericin B. Time for a new "gold standard." Clin Infect Dis 2003;37:415–425.
82. Stevens DA. Itraconazole in cyclodextrin solution. Pharmacotherapy 1999;19:603–611.
83. Reboli A, Rotstein C, Pappas P, et al. Anidulafungin vs. fluconazole for treatment of candidemia and invasive candidiasis (c/ic) [abstract M-718]. In: Abstracts of the 45th Interscience Conference on Antimicrob Agents Chemother. Washington, DC: American Society for Microbiology, 2005:418.
84. Marr KA, Boeckh M, Carter RA, et al. Combination antifungal therapy for invasive aspergillosis. Clin Infect Dis 2004;39:797–802.
85. Smith J, Safdar N, Knasinski V, et al. Voriconazole therapeutic drug monitoring. Antimicrob Agents Chemother 2006;50(4):1570–1572.
86. Walsh TJ, Teppler H, Donowitz GR, et al. Caspofungin versus liposomal amphotericin B for empirical antifungal therapy in patients with persistent fever and neutropenia. N Engl J Med 2004;351:1391–1402.

CHAPTER 126 Infections in Immunocompromised Patients

DOUGLAS N. FISH

KEY CONCEPTS

1. An *immunocompromised host* is a patient with defects in host defenses that predispose to infection. Risk factors include neutropenia, immune system defects (from disease or immunosuppressive drug therapy), compromise of natural host defenses, environmental contamination, and changes in normal flora of the host.

2. Immunocompromised patients are at high risk for a variety of bacterial, fungal, viral, and protozoal infections. Bacterial infections caused by gram-positive cocci (staphylococci and streptococci) occur most frequently, followed by gram-negative bacterial infections caused by Enterobacteriaceae and *Pseudomonas aeruginosa.* Fungal infections caused by *Candida* and *Aspergillus,* as well as certain viral infections (herpes simplex virus, cytomegalovirus), are also important causes of morbidity and mortality.

3. Risk of infection in neutropenic patients is associated with the severity and duration of neutropenia. Patients with severe neutropenia (absolute neutrophil count [ANC] <500 cells/mm^3) for more than 7 to 10 days are considered to be at high risk for infection.

4. Fever (single oral temperature ≥38.3°C [≥101°F] or temperature ≥38°C [≥100.4°F] for ≥1 hour) is the most important clinical finding in neutropenic patients and usually is the stimulus for further diagnostic workup and initiation of antimicrobial treatment. Infection should be considered as the cause of fever until proved otherwise. Usual signs and symptoms of infection may be altered or absent in neutropenic patients. Appropriate empirical broad-spectrum antimicrobial therapy must be instituted rapidly to prevent excessive morbidity and mortality.

5. Empirical antimicrobial regimens for neutropenic infections should take into account patients' individual risk factors as well as institutional infection and susceptibility patterns. The significant morbidity and mortality associated with gram-negative infections require that initial empirical regimens for treatment of febrile neutropenia have good activity against *P. aeruginosa* and Enterobacteriaceae. Inpatient parenteral regimens most commonly recommended for initial treatment include monotherapy with an antipseudomonal cephalosporin (cefepime or ceftazidime), carbapenem (imipenem or meropenem), or a combination regimen consisting of an antipseudomonal cephalosporin or carbapenem plus an aminoglycoside. Low-risk patients can be treated successfully with oral antibiotics (ciprofloxacin plus amoxicillin-clavulanate), with the treatment setting determined by the patient's clinical status.

6. Neutropenic patients who remain febrile after 3 to 5 days of initial antimicrobial therapy should be reevaluated to determine whether treatment modifications are necessary. Common regimen modifications include the addition of vancomycin (if not already present) and antifungal therapy (amphotericin B or fluconazole). Therapy should be directed at causative organisms, if identified, but broad-spectrum regimens should be maintained during neutropenia.

7. The optimal duration of therapy for febrile neutropenia is controversial. The decision to discontinue antimicrobials is based on resolution of neutropenia, defervescence, culture results, and clinical stability of the patient.

8. Prophylactic antimicrobials are administered to cancer patients expected to experience prolonged neutropenia as well as to both hematopoietic stem cell and solid-organ transplant recipients. Prophylactic regimens may include antibacterial, antifungal, antiviral, or antiprotozoal agents, or a combination of these, selected according to risk of infection with specific pathogens. Optimal prophylactic regimens should take into account individual patient risk for infection and institutional infection and susceptibility patterns.

9. Patients undergoing hematopoietic stem cell transplantation are at extremely high risk for infection because of prolonged neutropenia following intensive chemotherapy with or without irradiation, whereas solid-organ transplant recipients are at high risk because of prolonged administration of immunosuppressive drugs. Fungal *(Aspergillus)* and viral (cytomegalovirus) infections are particularly troublesome in these populations, and prophylactic regimens directed against these pathogens are used commonly. When documented, these infections must be treated aggressively in order to optimize patient outcomes. Nevertheless, mortality rates often are very high despite appropriate and aggressive antimicrobial therapy.

10. Immunocompromised patients must be assessed continuously for evidence of infection and response to antimicrobial therapy. Because a large number of antimicrobials potentially may be used, the occurrence of drug-related adverse effects also must be assessed carefully. Efforts should be directed at designing cost-effective treatment strategies that promote optimal patient outcomes.

Learning objectives, review questions, and other resources can be found at **www.pharmacotherapyonline.com.**

An immunocompromised host is a patient with intrinsic or acquired defects in host defenses that predispose to infection. Advances in modern medicine are creating more immunocompromised hosts than ever before. Historically, many of these patients died of their underlying diseases. Dramatic improvements in survival have been achieved by more aggressive therapy of underlying diseases and improved supportive care. Because aggressive therapy often renders patients profoundly immunosuppressed for long periods, opportunistic infections remain important causes of morbidity and mortality. This chapter focuses on risk factors for infection, common pathogens and infection sites, and prevention and management of suspected or documented infections in cancer patients (including hematopoietic stem cell transplantation [HSCT] patients) and solid-organ transplant recipients. Chapter 129 discusses infectious complications associated with human immunodeficiency virus (HIV) infection.

RISK FACTORS FOR INFECTION/EPIDEMIOLOGY

NEUTROPENIA

❶ ❷ ❸ Neutropenia is defined as an abnormally reduced number of neutrophils circulating in peripheral blood. Although exact definitions of neutropenia often vary, an absolute neutrophil count (ANC) less than 1,000 cells/mm^3 indicates a reduction sufficient to predispose patients to infection.[1] ANC is the sum of the absolute numbers of both mature neutrophils (polymorphonuclear cells [PMNs], also called *polys* or *segs*) and immature neutrophils (*bands*). The absolute number of PMNs and bands is determined by dividing the total percentage of these cells (obtained from the white blood cell [WBC] differential) by 100 and then multiplying the quotient obtained by the total number of WBCs.

The degree or severity of neutropenia, rate of neutrophil decline, and duration of neutropenia are important risk factors for infection.[1–5] All neutropenic patients are considered to be at risk for infection, but those with ANC less than 500 cells/mm^3 are at greater risk than those with ANCs of 500 to 1,000 cells/mm^3. Most treatment guidelines use ANC less than 500 cells/mm^3 as the critical value in making therapeutic decisions regarding the management of suspected or documented infections.[1–5] Risk of infection and death are greatest among patients with less than 100 neutrophils/mm^3.[1,2] In patients with chemotherapy-induced neutropenia, the risk of infection is increased according to the rapidity of ANC decline. Infection risk also increases as the duration of neutropenia increases; patients with severe neutropenia of more than 7 to 10 days' duration are considered to be at especially high risk for serious infections.[3] The duration of chemotherapy-induced neutropenia varies considerably among subsets of cancer patients according to the specific chemotherapeutic agents used and the intensity of treatment. Patients undergoing HSCT may have no detectable granulocytes in peripheral blood for up to 3 to 4 weeks and are at particular risk for severe infections with a variety of pathogens.[6]

Bacteria and fungi commonly cause infections in neutropenic patients. Gram-positive cocci (*Staphylococcus aureus, Staphylococcus epidermidis,* streptococci, and enterococci) have emerged as the most common cause of acute bacterial infections among neutropenic patients. Gram-negative bacilli (*Escherichia coli, Klebsiella pneumoniae, Pseudomonas aeruginosa*) traditionally were the most common causes of bacterial infection and remain frequent pathogens.[4,7,8] Although not now as common as gram-positive bacteria, the incidence of gram-negative infections may again be increasing.[3,8] Gram-negative infections are associated with significant morbidity and mortality, in large part due to increasing antibiotic resistance among these pathogens.[7,8] Patients who are neutropenic for extended periods and who receive broad-spectrum antibiotics are at high risk for fungal infections, usually due to *Candida* or *Aspergillus* spp.[2,3,9] Viral infections, although not as common as bacterial and fungal infections, also may cause severe infection in neutropenic patients.[2,3,5,10] Successful treatment of infections in neutropenic patients depends on resolution of neutropenia.[1–3,5]

Although not readily quantifiable, abnormalities may exist in granulocyte function as well as in cell numbers. Defects in phagocyte function may be caused by underlying disease (e.g., leukemia) or its treatment (e.g., corticosteroids, antineoplastic agents, and radiation).[3,11,12]

IMMUNE SYSTEM DEFECTS

In addition to neutropenia, defects in T-lymphocyte and macrophage function (cell-mediated immunity), B-cell function (humoral immunity), or both predispose patients to infection. Cellular immune dysfunction is the result of underlying disease or immunosuppressive drug therapy; these defects result in a reduced ability of the host to defend against intracellular pathogens. Patients with Hodgkin's disease and transplant patients receiving a wide variety of immunosuppressive drugs, such as cyclosporine, tacrolimus, sirolimus, mycophenolate, corticosteroids, azathioprine, and antineoplastic agents, are at risk for a variety of bacterial, fungal, viral, and protozoal infections (Table 126–1). Although some of these pathogens are associated with asymptomatic or mild disease in normal hosts, they can cause disseminated, life-threatening infections in immunocompromised hosts.

Underlying disease frequently causes defects in humoral immune function. Patients with multiple myeloma and chronic lymphocytic leukemia have progressive hypogammaglobulinemia that results in defective humoral immunity. Splenectomy performed as a part of the staging process for Hodgkin's disease places patients at risk for infectious complications. Disease states with humoral immune dysfunction predispose the patient to serious, life-threatening infection with encapsulated organisms such as *Streptococcus pneumoniae, Haemophilus influenzae,* and *Neisseria meningitidis.*

DESTRUCTION OF PROTECTIVE BARRIERS

Loss of protective barriers is a major factor predisposing immunocompromised patients to infection. Damage to skin and mucous membranes by surgery, venipuncture, intravenous (IV) and urinary catheters, radiation, and chemotherapy disrupts natural host defense systems, leaving patients at high risk for infection. Chemotherapy-induced mucositis may erode mucous membranes of the oropharynx and gastrointestinal (GI) tract and establish a portal for subsequent infection by bacteria, herpes simplex virus (HSV), and *Candida.*[3,13] Medical and surgical procedures, such as transplant surgery, indwelling IV catheter placement, bone marrow aspiration, biopsies, and endoscopy, further damage the integument and predispose patients to infection. Infections resulting from disruption of protective barriers usually are a result of skin flora, such as *S. aureus, S. epidermidis,* and various streptococci.[1,3,5,11,13]

ENVIRONMENTAL CONTAMINATION/ ALTERATION OF MICROBIAL FLORA

Infections in immunocompromised patients are caused by organisms either colonizing the host or acquired from the environment. Microorganisms may be transferred easily from patient to patient on the hands of hospital personnel unless strict infection control guidelines are followed. Contaminated equipment, such as nebulizers or ventilators, and contaminated water supplies have been responsible for outbreaks of *P. aeruginosa* and *Legionella pneumophila* infections, respectively. Foods, such as fruits and green leafy vegetables, which often are colonized with gram-negative bacteria and fungi, are sources of microbial contamination in immunocompromised hosts.[3,14]

TABLE 126-1 Risk Factors and Common Pathogens in Immunocompromised Patients

Risk Factor	Patient Conditions	Common Pathogens
Neutropenia	Acute leukemia Chemotherapy	Bacteria: *Staphylococcus aureus, Staphylococcus epidermidis, Escherichia coli, Klebsiella pneumoniae, Pseudomonas aeruginosa*, streptococci, enterococci Fungi: *Candida, Aspergillus, Zygomycetes* Viruses: Herpes simplex
Impaired cell-mediated immunity	Lymphoma Immunosuppressive therapy (steroids, cyclosporine, chemotherapy)	Bacteria: *Listeria, Nocardia, Legionella*, Mycobacteria Fungi: *Cryptococcus neoformans, Candida, Aspergillus, Histoplasma capsulatum* Viruses: Cytomegalovirus, varicella-zoster, herpes simplex Protozoal: *Pneumocystis jiroveci*
Impaired humoral immunity	Multiple myeloma Chronic lymphocytic leukemia Splenectomy Immunosuppressive therapy (steroids, chemotherapy)	Bacteria: *S. pneumoniae, H. influenzae, N. meningitidis*
Loss of protective skin barriers	Venipuncture, bone marrow aspiration, urinary catheterization, vascular access devices, radiation, biopsies	Bacteria: *S. aureus, S. epidermidis, Bacillus* spp., *Corynebacterium jeikeium* Fungi: *Candida*
Mucous membranes	Respiratory support equipment, endoscopy, chemotherapy, radiation	Bacteria: *S. aureus, S. epidermidis*, streptococci, Enterobacteriaceae, *P. aeruginosa, Bacteroides* spp. Fungi: *Candida* Viruses: Herpes simplex
Surgery	Solid-organ transplantation	Bacteria: *S. aureus, S. epidermidis*, Enterobacteriaceae, *P. aeruginosa, Bacteroides* spp. Fungi: *Candida* Viruses: Herpes simplex
Alteration of normal microbial flora	Antimicrobial therapy Chemotherapy Hospital environment	Bacteria: Enterobacteriaceae, *P. aeruginosa, Legionella, S. aureus, S. epidermidis* Fungi: *Candida, Aspergillus*
Blood products, donor organs	Bone marrow transplantation Solid-organ transplantation	Fungi: *Candida* Viruses: Cytomegalovirus, Epstein-Barr virus, hepatitis B, hepatitis C Protozoal: *Toxoplasma gondii*

Compiled from references 1, 3, 4, 5, 7, 11, 15, 18, 23, 25, 27, and 31.

Most infections in cancer patients are caused by organisms colonizing body sites, such as the skin, oropharynx, and GI tract.[1,3,13,14] Approximately 80% of infecting bacterial pathogens are from the patient's endogenous flora.[1,3] The GI tract is the most common site from which infections in immunocompromised hosts originate. Periodontitis, pharyngitis, esophagitis, colitis, perirectal cellulitis, and bacteremias are caused predominantly by normal flora of the gut; bloodstream infections are thought to arise from microbial translocation across injured GI mucosa.[1,13,14] Normal flora may be significantly disrupted and altered; oropharyngeal flora rapidly change to primarily gram-negative bacilli in hospitalized patients. Many cancer patients may already be colonized with gram-negative bacilli on admission as a result of frequent prior hospitalizations and clinic visits. In hospitalized cancer patients, however, 50% of infections are caused by colonizing organisms acquired after admission.[1,3]

Although hospitalization and severity of illness are risk factors for colonization by gram-negative bacilli, administration of broad-spectrum antimicrobial agents has the greatest impact on flora of immunocompromised hosts. Use of these agents disrupts the delicate balance of GI tract flora and predisposes patients to infection with more virulent pathogens. Antineoplastic drugs (e.g., cyclophosphamide, doxorubicin, and fluorouracil) and acid-suppressive therapy (e.g., H_2-receptor antagonists, proton pump inhibitors, and antacids) also may result in changes in GI flora and possibly predispose patients to infection.[1,3,14]

Numerous factors, such as underlying disease, immunosuppressive drug therapy, and antimicrobial administration, determine the immunocompromised host's risk of developing infection. Several risk factors are present concomitantly in many patients (see Table 126–1).

ETIOLOGY OF INFECTIONS IN NEUTROPENIC CANCER PATIENTS

❷ Infection remains a significant cause of morbidity and mortality in neutropenic cancer patients. More than 50% of febrile neutropenic patients have an established or occult infection.[1,5] Patients with profound neutropenia are at greatest risk for systemic infection, with at least 20% of these individuals developing bacteremia. Areas of impaired or damaged host defenses, such as the oropharynx, lungs, skin, sinuses, and GI tract, are common sites of infection. These local infections may progress to cause systemic infection and bacteremia.[13] Febrile episodes in neutropenic cancer patients can be attributed to microbiologically documented infection in approximately 30% of cases, about half of which are due to bacteremia. Further, infections can be documented clinically (but not microbiologically) in another 30% to 40% of patients, with the remaining 30% of patients manifesting infection only by fever.[3,8,11]

Table 126–1 lists organisms commonly infecting immunocompromised patients. Approximately 45% to 70% of bacteremic episodes in cancer patients are the result of gram-positive organisms compared with less than 30% of episodes documented during the 1970s and 1980s.[1,4,7] This shift is attributed to the frequent use of indwelling central and peripheral IV catheters, frequent use of broad-spectrum antibiotics with excellent gram-negative activity but relatively poor gram-positive coverage, higher rates of mucositis caused by aggressive cancer treatments, and prophylaxis with trimethoprim–sulfamethoxazole or quinolones.[1,4,7,11] *S. aureus* and coagulase-negative staphylococci (especially *S. epidermidis*) are the most common organisms, but *Bacillus* spp. and *Corynebacterium jeikeium* are also important pathogens.[1,5,11] Data from the United States Centers for Disease Control and Prevention's (CDC) National Nosocomial Infection Surveillance System (NNIS) indicate increasing rates of infection due to methicillin-resistant *Staphylococcus aureus* (MRSA) in the hospital setting.[15] Resistance also is being observed in community-acquired staphylococcal infections.[16,17] Viridans streptococci, which may be resistant to β-lactams, also have emerged as important pathogens, particularly in patients with chemotherapy-induced mucositis of the oropharynx.[4,11,18] Enterococci, including vancomycin-resistant strains, also may be problematic in many institutions.[2,7] Bacteremia caused by vancomycin-resistant enterococci (VRE) in neutropenic patients is associated with a mortality rate exceeding 70%.[4,19]

Gram-positive infections do not always cause immediately life-threatening infections and are associated with somewhat lower mortality rates compared with gram-negative infections.[1,11] However, increasing rates of antibiotic resistance have made treatment of gram-positive infections in immunocompromised patients more challenging.[7] MRSA infections are associated with increased morbidity and mortality and hospital costs compared with susceptible organisms.[20] Methicillin resistance among coagulase-negative staphylococci, which may cause 40% to 80% of infections in certain populations, is very common (70%–90% of isolates).[7,21,22] Certain organisms that are intrinsically resistant to vancomycin (e.g., *Lactobacillus*) are increasing in importance.[7] Thus, prevention and timely diagnosis and treatment of gram-positive infections are clearly of great importance in the management of neutropenic cancer patients.

Gram-negative infections remain important causes of morbidity and mortality in immunocompromised cancer patients, but the relative frequency of infection owing to specific pathogens has been shifting among gram-negative infections. *Escherichia coli* and *Klebsiella* spp. remain the most common isolates at many centers. Strains of *Klebsiella* spp. producing plasmid-mediated extended-spectrum β-lactamases that hydrolyze extended-spectrum cephalosporins have emerged and are cause for concern.[1,7] The frequency of infections resulting from other gram-negative organisms, such as *Enterobacter, Serratia,* and *Citrobacter,* has been increasing.[7] *Enterobacter* spp. are important causes of bacteremias; use of broad-spectrum antibiotics, particularly third-generation cephalosporins, is thought to have played a major role in this trend. Infections with *Enterobacter, Serratia,* and *Citrobacter* may be difficult to treat because of the ease of β-lactamase induction and the more frequent development of resistance to multiple antibiotics.[3,7,11]

P. aeruginosa has long been an important pathogen in cancer patients. *P. aeruginosa* infection rates are decreasing in patients with solid tumors but not in patients with hematologic malignancies.[4,7,23] Infections caused by *P. aeruginosa* are associated with significant morbidity and mortality in neutropenic patients, with mortality rates of 33% to 75% reported.[11] The frequency of infection caused by difficult-to-treat organisms such as *Stenotrophomonas maltophilia* and *Burkholderia cepacia* appears to be increasing at many centers, probably because of selective pressures of broad-spectrum antimicrobial use.[4,11] Although the GI tract is a common site of bacterial infection, severe infections caused by anaerobic organisms are relatively infrequent. Anaerobes are found most frequently in mixed infections, such as perirectal cellulitis and mucositis-associated oropharyngeal infections.[11] As with gram-positive organisms, antibiotic resistance among gram-negative organisms has continued to increase at alarming rates and has made appropriate antibiotic selection for treatment of febrile neutropenia more difficult.[1,7,15]

In addition to bacterial infections, neutropenic cancer patients are at risk for invasive fungal infections. Patients with extended periods of profound neutropenia who have been receiving broad-spectrum antibiotics, corticosteroids, or both are at the highest risk for invasive fungal infection. Up to one third of febrile neutropenic patients who do not respond to 1 week of broad-spectrum antibiotic therapy will have a systemic fungal infection.[1] A large international autopsy study revealed that up to 40% of patients with hematologic malignancies had deep fungal infections, many of which were undiagnosed prior to death. Approximately 65% of these infections were the result of *Candida* spp., and another 30% were caused by *Aspergillus* spp.[24]

Candida albicans is the most common fungal pathogen in neutropenic cancer patients.[4,25,26] Other species of *Candida,* such as *C. tropicalis, C. parapsilosis,* and *C. krusei,* are being isolated with increasing frequency. An increase also has been noted in infections caused by *Candida glabrata, Trichosporon* spp., *Fusarium* spp., and *Curvularia*.[25–30] Because *Candida* spp. are normal flora, alteration of body host defenses is an important risk factor for the development of these infections. Oral thrush is the most common clinical manifestation of fungal infection. Mucous membranes damaged from chemotherapy and radiation serve as areas of *Candida* surface colonization and subsequent entry into the bloodstream; disease then may disseminate throughout the body. Organs such as the liver, spleen, kidney, and lungs are commonly involved in disseminated disease.[12,24,26,27] Hepatosplenic candidiasis is a particularly important infection in patients with hematologic malignancies.[3,26] Diagnosis of candidal infections is difficult and often requires invasive tissue sampling.[6] Overall mortality attributed to candidal infections in patients with invasive candidiasis is as high as 38%.[4,26]

Invasive infections caused by *Aspergillus* spp. are a serious complication of neutropenia, with mortality approaching 80% in patients with prolonged neutropenia and/or patients undergoing allogeneic HSCT.[4] These infections are particularly prevalent in patients with hematologic malignancies and in patients undergoing HSCT.[4,26,30] Infections resulting from *Aspergillus* spp. (including *A. fumigatus, A. terreus, A. flavus,* and *A. niger*) usually are acquired via inhalation of airborne spores. After colonizing the lungs, *Aspergillus* invades the lung parenchyma and pulmonary vessels, resulting in hemorrhage, pulmonary infarcts, and a high mortality rate. Invasive pulmonary disease is the dominant manifestation of infection in patients with neutropenia. However, *Aspergillus* spp. also may cause other infections, including sinusitis, cutaneous infection, and disseminated disease involving multiple organs, including the central nervous system (CNS).[31] Prolonged neutropenia is the primary risk factor for invasive pulmonary aspergillosis in neutropenic patients with acute leukemia; use of corticosteroids also may predispose patients to disease.[31] Invasive aspergillosis should be suspected in neutropenic cancer patients colonized with *Aspergillus* (in sputum and/or nasal cultures) who remain persistently febrile despite at least 1 week of broad-spectrum antibiotic therapy.[1,31]

Chemotherapy-induced mucous membrane damage may predispose neutropenic cancer patients to the reactivation of HSV, manifesting as gingivostomatitis or recurrent genital infections. Untreated oropharyngeal HSV infections may spread to involve the esophagus and often coexist with candidal infections. Clinical disease resulting from HSV occurs most often in patients with serologic evidence (e.g., serum antibodies to HSV) of prior infection. Both HSV-seropositive HSCT patients and HSV-seropositive leukemics receiving intensive chemotherapy are at high risk for recurrent HSV disease during periods of immunosuppression.[6]

Pneumocystis jiroveci and *Toxoplasma gondii* are the most common parasitic pathogens found in immunocompromised cancer patients. Patients with hematologic malignancies (i.e., acute lymphocytic leukemia, lymphoma, and Hodgkin's disease) and those receiving high-dose corticosteroids as part of chemotherapy regimens are at the greatest risk of infection.[6] Routine use of trimethoprim–sulfamethoxazole prophylaxis has reduced substantially the incidence of these infections.[1,6]

Because the majority of infecting organisms in cancer patients are from the host's own flora, some centers have used routine surveillance cultures in an attempt to prospectively identify causes of fever and suspected infection. In a typical surveillance culture program, cultures of the nose, mouth, axillae, and perirectal area are performed twice weekly, and culture results are correlated with the clinical status of the patient. Because these cultures are costly and have low diagnostic yield, the utility of surveillance culture programs is believed to be limited.[1] However, surveillance cultures are useful as research tools and in certain clinical situations, including patients with prolonged profound neutropenia and in institutions that have high rates of antimicrobial resistance or have problems with virulent pathogens such as *P. aeruginosa* or *A. flavus.* Surveillance cultures should be limited to the anterior nares for detecting colonization with MRSA, *Aspergillus,* and penicillin-resistant pneumococci and to the rectum for detecting *P. aeruginosa,* multiple-antibiotic-resistant gram-negative rods, and VRE.[1,11]

Knowledge of infection rates and local susceptibility patterns is essential for guiding optimal management of febrile neutropenia. These parameters must be monitored closely because the spectrum of infectious complications is related to multiple factors, including cancer chemotherapy regimens and antimicrobial therapy used for treatment and prophylaxis.

CLINICAL PRESENTATION

❹ The most important clinical finding in the neutropenic cancer patient is fever. Because of the potential for significant morbidity and mortality associated with infection in these patients, fever should be considered to be the result of infection until proved otherwise.[1–3,8] At the appearance of fever, the patient should be evaluated carefully for other signs and symptoms of infection.

CLINICAL PRESENTATION OF FEBRILE NEUTROPENIA[1,3,4,6,10]

General

- Because neutropenic cancer patients are at high risk for serious infections, frequent (at least daily) careful clinical assessments must be performed to search for possible evidence of infection.
- Physical assessment should include examination of all common sites of infection, including mouth/pharynx, nose and sinuses, respiratory tract, GI tract, urinary tract, skin, soft tissues, perineum, and intravascular catheter insertion sites.

Symptoms

- Usual signs and symptoms of infection may be absent or altered in neutropenic patients owing to low numbers of leukocytes and an inability to mount an inflammatory response (e.g., no infiltrate on chest x-ray film, urinary tract infection without pyuria).
- Pain may be present at the infection site(s).

Signs

- Fever in this setting is defined as a single oral temperature ≥38.3°C (≥101°F) in the absence of other causes or temperature ≥38°C (≥100.4°F) for 1 hour or more. Other causes of fever unrelated to infection in this patient population include reactions to blood products, chemotherapeutic agents (and other drugs, including biologics), cell lysis, and underlying malignancy.
- Usual signs of infection may be absent or altered; patients with bacteremia commonly exhibit no signs of infection other than fever.

Laboratory Tests

- Neutropenia (ANC ≤1,000 cells/mm^3).
- Blood cultures (two or more sets, including vascular access devices) for bacteria and fungi; cultures of other suspected infection sites (infection can be documented microbiologically in only about 30% of cases, about half of which are due to bacteremia).
- Other cultures should be obtained as indicated clinically according to the presence of signs or symptoms.
- Recent surveillance cultures (nasal, rectal) should be reviewed, if available.
- Complete blood count and blood chemistries should be obtained frequently to monitor neutropenia, plan supportive care, guide drug dosing, and assess patient's overall status.

Other Diagnostic Tests

- Chest x-ray film
- Aspiration, biopsy of skin lesions
- Other diagnostic tests as indicated clinically on the basis of physical examination and other assessments

TREATMENT

Infections in Cancer Patients

■ FEBRILE EPISODES IN NEUTROPENIC CANCER PATIENTS

❹ ❺ The goals of antimicrobial therapy in neutropenic patients (including HSCT recipients) are (a) to protect the neutropenic patient from early death caused by undiagnosed infection; (b) to prevent breakthrough bacterial, fungal, viral, and protozoal infections during periods of neutropenia; and (c) to treat established infections effectively, all aimed at reducing patient morbidity and mortality and allowing for administration of optimal antineoplastic therapy. All these goals must be achieved at the lowest possible toxicity and cost.

Approach to Treatment

Guidelines for management of febrile episodes and documented infections in neutropenic patients are shown in Fig. 126–1 (from the Infectious Diseases Society of America [IDSA], revised in 2002).[1] Although many controversies remain regarding optimal management of these patients, the IDSA guidelines and those of other expert panels, such as the National Comprehensive Cancer Network (NCCN),[5] offer an evidence-based consensus approach to the management of febrile neutropenia. Selected specific recommendations as discussed in the following sections of this chapter, and their associated evidence-based rankings are summarized in Table 126–2. Updated guidelines from the IDSA are expected in late 2008.

Because fever in the neutropenic cancer patient is considered to be caused by infection until proved otherwise, high-dose broad-spectrum bactericidal, usually parenteral, empirical antibiotic therapy should be initiated at the onset of fever or at the first signs or symptoms of infection. Withholding antibiotic therapy until an organism is isolated results in unacceptably high mortality rates. At least 50% of febrile neutropenic cancer patients have an established or occult infection, and at least 20% of profoundly neutropenic patients (ANC <100 cells/mm^3) experience bacteremia.[1,5] In immunocompromised patients, undiagnosed infection can rapidly disseminate and result in death if left untreated or if treated improperly. Failure to initiate appropriate antibiotic therapy for *P. aeruginosa* bacteremia at the onset of fever in neutropenic cancer patients resulted in mortality rates of 15% and 70% within 12 and 48 hours, respectively.[1] Empirical antibiotic therapy is 70% to 90% effective at reducing early morbidity and mortality.[11] Therapy must be appropriate and initiated promptly. Antimicrobial therapy also should be initiated promptly in afebrile cancer patients with clinical signs and symptoms of infection.

When designing optimal empirical antibiotic regimens, clinicians must consider infection patterns and antimicrobial susceptibility trends in their respective institutions. Patient factors, such as risk for infection, drug allergies and concomitant nephrotoxins, and previous antimicrobial exposure (including prophylaxis), must be considered.[1,5] Assessment of the patient's risk of infection will help determine the appropriate route and setting for antibiotic administration. Patients with neutropenia can be divided into low-, moderate-, and high-risk groups based on the projected duration of neutropenia and

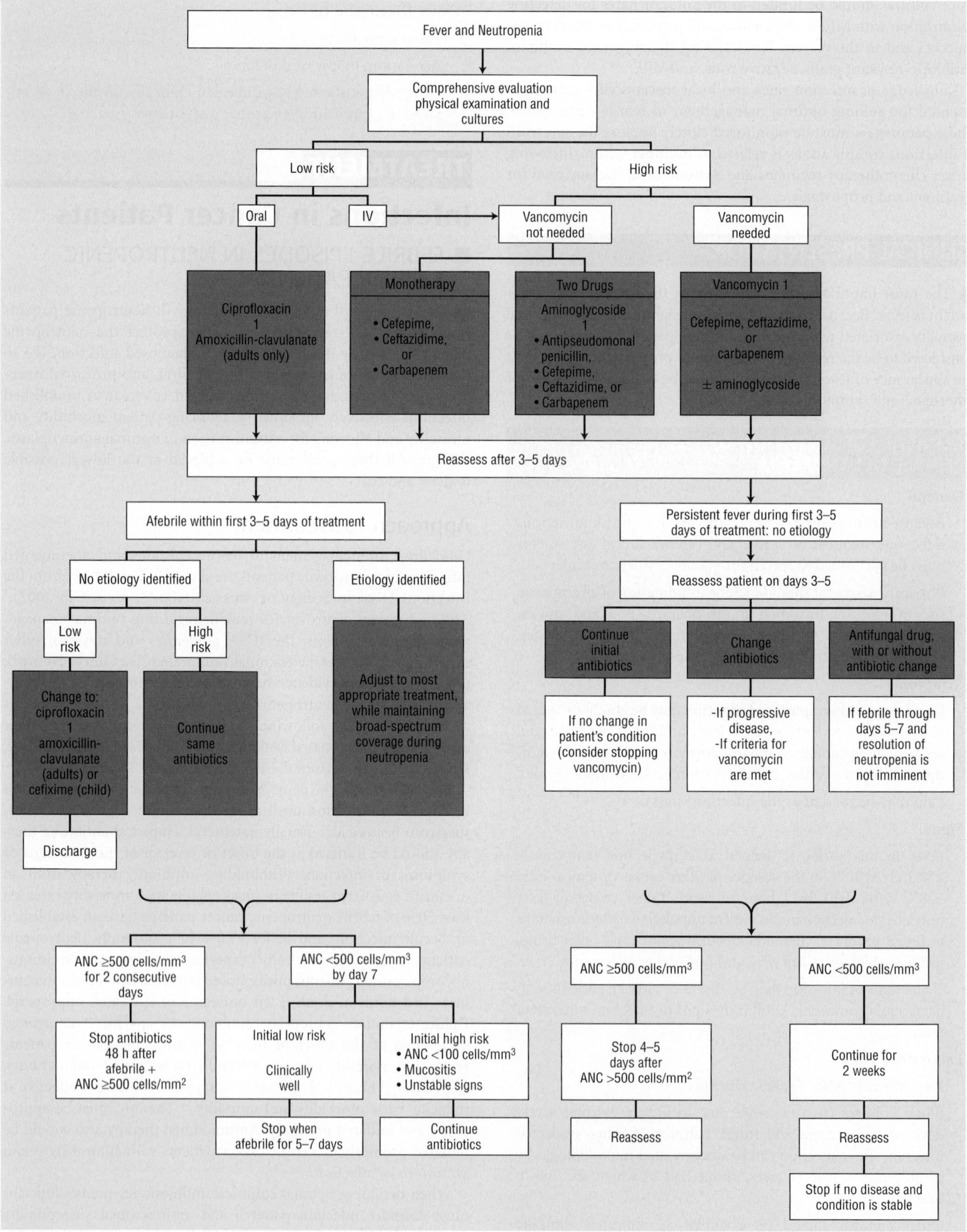

FIGURE 126-1. Management of febrile episodes in neutropenic cancer patients. (ANC, absolute neutrophil count; carbapenem, imipenem–cilastatin, meropenem.) *(Adapted from Hughes WT, Armstrong D, Bodey GP, et al. 2002 guidelines for the use of antimicrobial agents in neutropenic patients with cancer. Clin Infect Dis 2002;34:730–751. ©2002 by the Infectious Diseases Society of America. Used with permission of the University of Chicago Press.)*

TABLE 126-2 Summary of Evidence-Based Recommendations for Management of Febrile Episodes in Neutropenic Patients

Recommendations	Recommendation Grades[a]
Use of oral antibiotics for outpatient management	
Oral antibiotics are feasible for treatment of carefully selected patients at low risk for complications.	A-1
Use of monotherapy	
Monotherapy with appropriate antibiotics is as effective as combination regimens for initial empirical treatment of febrile neutropenic episodes.	A-1
Route of antibiotic administration for initial treatment	
Patients at high risk for serious life-threatening infections must be initially treated with intravenous antibiotics. patients at low risk can be treated with either intravenous or oral drugs (see text for risk stratification criteria).	A-2
Management of patients who become afebrile	
Patients who become afebrile within 3–5 days of beginning initial empirical antibiotic therapy and in whom specific organisms have been identified should be treated for ≥7 days (until cultures are negative and patient has clinically recovered). Low-risk patients in whom no organism is identified can be switched to oral antibiotics if desired, whereas patients originally classified as high risk should continue on intravenous antibiotics.	B-2
Management of patients with persistent fever during first 3–5 days of treatment	
In patients initially receiving monotherapy or a two-drug regimen *not* including vancomycin, addition of vancomycin can be considered if any criteria for use of vancomycin are present (see text for specific criteria).	C-3
In patients *already* receiving vancomycin as part of the initial empirical regimen, withdrawal of vancomycin should be considered in the absence of a documented pathogen requiring continued therapy. Other initial antibiotics can be continued if the disease has not progressed, or switched to oral therapy if the patient was classified as low risk even in the presence of continued fever.	C-3
Management of patients with fever persisting for more than three days after initial treatment	
Reassess patient after 3 days of treatment. If still febrile by day 5, then continue the same antibiotics if clinically stable; change antibiotics if any evidence of disease progression or antibiotic toxicities; or add an antifungal drug if the duration of neutropenia is expected to be more than 5–7 additional days.	B-2
Continuation of antibiotics in afebrile patients with no identified infection	
Antibiotic therapy can be discontinued after 3 days of treatment if patient is afebrile for ≥48 hours and absolute neutrophil count (ANC) is ≥500 cells/mm^3 for 2 consecutive days.	C-3
If patient remains neutropenic, continue intravenous or oral antibiotics.	B-2
Antibiotics should be continued in patients with profound neutropenia (ANC <100 cells/mm^3), mucous membrane lesions of mouth or gastrointestinal tract, unstable vital signs, or other identified risk factors.	C-3
Antibiotics can be stopped after 2 weeks in patients with prolonged neutropenia of unclear continued duration, no identified site of infection, and who can be closely observed.	C-3
Alternatively, antibiotics can be discontinued after 4 days if no infection is documented and the patient shows no response to therapy.	C-3
Granulocyte transfusions	
There are no specific indications for routine use of granulocyte transfusions.	C-2
Colony-stimulating factors	
Colony-stimulating factors are not indicated for routine treatment of neutropenia in either febrile or afebrile patients.	D-2
Antimicrobial prophylaxis in neutropenic patients	
Prophylaxis with trimethoprim-sulfamethoxazole should be administered to all patients at risk for *Pneumocystis jiroveci* pneumonia, regardless of whether they are neutropenic.	A-1
Routine use of prophylactic antifungal agents (i.e., fluconazole, itraconazole) for all patients with neutropenia is not recommended.	D-2

[a]Strength of recommendations: A, B, C = good, moderate, and poor evidence to support recommendation for use, respectively; D = moderate evidence to support a recommendation against use.
Quality of evidence: 1 = evidence from ≥1 properly randomized, controlled trial; 2 = evidence from ≥1 well-designed clinical trial without randomization, from cohort or case-control analytic studies, from multiple time series, or from dramatic results from uncontrolled experiments; 3 = evidence from opinions of respected authorities, based on clinical experience, descriptive studies, or reports of expert committees.

Hughes WT, Armstrong D, Bodey GP, et al. ©2002 guidelines for the use of antimicrobial agents in neutropenic patients with cancer. Clin Infect Dis 2002;34:730–751. © 2002 by the Infectious Disease Society of America. Used with permission of the University of Chicago Press.

other risk factors for serious infection (Table 126–3).[3,4] Patients with neutropenia of short duration (≤7 days) are considered to be at relatively low risk of severe infection. Patients with neutropenia lasting 7 to 14 days are considered to be at moderate risk for severe infection. High-risk patients are those with neutropenia for 14 or more days; these patients are at increased risk for severe infection from bacteria as well as from fungi, viruses, and parasites.

Oral empirical antimicrobial therapy may be appropriate for low-risk patients.[1,5,32] The patient's overall clinical condition and other risk factors for infection determine whether oral therapy is administered on an inpatient or outpatient basis. If therapy is administered on an outpatient basis, the patient must be compliant with treatment and have prompt access to medical care around the clock, should his or her condition worsen. Patients considered at moderate risk of infection should receive at least the first few days of therapy administered parenterally in the hospital setting.[1] High-risk patients generally are treated with hospital-based parenteral therapy for the entire course of their treatment.

The optimal antibiotic regimen for empirical therapy in febrile neutropenic cancer patients remains controversial. Although empirical antimicrobial therapy for febrile neutropenia has been studied extensively for nearly 4 decades, no single regimen can be recommended for all patients. Because of their frequency and relative pathogenicity, *P. aeruginosa* and other gram-negative bacilli and staphylococci remain the primary targets of empirical antimicrobial therapy.[1,11] Although *P. aeruginosa* is documented in fewer than 5% of bloodstream infections in the population of hospitalized patients, adequate antipseudomonal antibiotic coverage still must be included in empirical regimens because of the significant morbidity and mortality associated with this pathogen.[1,11,15,23]

At least four different types of empirical parenteral antibiotic regimens are in use: (a) monotherapy with an antipseudomonal cephalosporin (cefepime or ceftazidime) or antipseudomonal carbapenem (imipenem–cilastatin or meropenem); (b) combination therapy with an aminoglycoside plus an antipseudomonal penicillin (piperacillin–tazobactam or ticarcillin–clavulanate), an antipseudomonal cephalosporin, or an antipseudomonal carbapenem; (c) vancomycin plus an antipseudomonal cephalosporin or antipseudomonal carbapenem, with or without an aminoglycoside; and (d) a fluoroquinolone (ciprofloxacin or levofloxacin) in combination with an antipseudomonal cephalosporin, antipseudomonal carbapenem, aminoglycoside, or vancomycin.[1,3,5,11] Each of these regimens has advantages and disad-

TABLE 126-3 Risk-Based Therapy for Febrile Patients with Neutropenia

Risk Group	Patient Characteristics	Treatment Strategies
High risk	*Neutropenia:* Severe (absolute neutrophil count <100/mm^3) and/or prolonged (≥14 days) *Malignancy/treatment:* Hematologic malignancy or allogeneic HSCT *Comorbidities:* Substantial comorbidity; poor performance status *Clinical status:* Clinical or hemodynamic instability (e.g., shock) and/or complex infection (e.g., pneumonia, bacteremia) *Response to initial therapy:* Slow response	*Therapy/setting:* Broad-spectrum, parenteral (IV) therapy, hospital-based for duration of febrile neutropenia
Moderate risk	*Neutropenia:* Moderate duration (7–14 days) *Malignancy/treatment:* Solid tumor treated with autologous HSCT *Comorbidities:* Minimal medical comorbidity *Clinical status:* Clinically stable *Response to initial therapy:* Favorable (e.g., early defervescence)	*Therapy/setting:* Initial parenteral, hospital-based therapy, followed by early discharge on a parenteral or oral regimen (sequential)
Low risk	*Neutropenia:* Short duration (≤7 days) *Malignancy/treatment:* Solid tumor treated with conventional chemotherapy *Comorbidities:* None *Clinical status:* Clinically stable at onset of fever; no identified focus of infection, or simple infection (e.g., urinary tract infection)	*Therapy/setting:* Broad-spectrum outpatient therapy (parenteral, sequential, or oral) for the entire episode

HSCT, hematopoietic stem cell transplantation.

Compiled from Hughes et al.,[1] Donowitz et al.,[4] Freifeld at al.,[33] Kern et al.,[34] Escalante et al.,[35] Shenep et al.,[36] Giamarellou et al.,[37] and the National Comprehensive Cancer Network, Fever and Neutropenia, Pract. Guidelines Oncol 2002;1.

vantages, which are summarized in Table 126–4. There is no overwhelming evidence that any one of these regimens is superior to the others. The overall response to empirical antibiotic regimens in febrile neutropenic cancer patients is approximately 70% to 90% regardless of whether a pathogen is isolated or which antimicrobial regimen is used.[4,11]

Regardless of initial antibiotic selection, all empirical regimens must be monitored appropriately and revised on the basis of documented infections, susceptibilities of bacterial isolates, development of more defined clinical signs and symptoms of infection, or a combination of these factors. Consensus guidelines recommend three general empirical parenteral antibiotic regimens: monotherapy with an antipseudomonal cephalosporin or carbapenem; two-drug therapy without vancomycin (aminoglycoside plus antipseudomonal penicillin, cephalosporin, or carbapenem); or vancomycin plus one to two other drugs (antipseudomonal cephalosporin or carbapenem, with or without an aminoglycoside; Fig. 126–1).[1,5] However, other alternative regimens also may be appropriate, based on specific patient characteristics.

Prompt initiation of broad-spectrum empirical antibiotic therapy is essential to prevent early morbidity and mortality in febrile neutropenic patients with cancer. Choice of empirical regimens should take into account the patient's risk of infection and clinical status as well as patterns of hospital infections and susceptibility.

TABLE 126-4 Comparative Advantages and Disadvantages of Various Antibiotic Regimens for Empiric Therapy of Febrile Neutropenic Cancer Patients

Regimen	Potential Advantages	Potential Disadvantages
β-Lactam monotherapy (ceftazidime 1–2 g every 8 h, cefepime 1–2 g every 12 h, piperacillin–tazobactam 4.5 g every 6 h, imipenem–cilastatin 0.5 g every 6 h, or meropenem 1 g every 8 h)[a]	Efficacy comparable to combination regimens; decreased drug toxicities; ease of administration; possibly less expensive	Possibly less efficacy in profound neutropenia or prolonged neutropenia; limited gram-positive activity; no potential for additive/synergistic effects; increased selection of resistant organisms; increased colonization and superinfection rates
Antipseudomonal β-lactam plus aminoglycoside (e.g., cefepime 1–2 g every 12 h or ceftazidime 1–2 g every 8 h + gentamicin or tobramycin)[a,b]	Traditional regimen, broad-spectrum coverage; optimal therapy of *Pseudomonas aeruginosa;* rapidly bactericidal; synergistic activity; decreased bacterial resistance; reduction of superinfections	Limited gram-positive activity; potential for nephrotoxicity; need for therapeutic monitoring of aminoglycoside concentrations
Empirical regimens containing vancomycin[c] (ceftazidime 1–2 g every 8 h + vancomycin 0.5–1 g every 6–12 h)[a] ± gentamicin or tobramycin[b]	Early effective therapy of gram-positive infections	No demonstrated benefit of vancomycin empirical therapy vs. addition of vancomycin if needed later; increased risk of selection for vancomycin-resistant enterococci; risk of toxicities; excessive cost; need for therapeutic monitoring of vancomycin concentrations
Empirical regimens containing fluoroquinolones (ciprofloxacin 0.4 g every 8–12 h + ceftazidime 1–2 g every 8 h, aminoglycoside, or vancomycin[c] 0.5–1 g every 6–12 h)[a]	Efficacy similar to other regimens when used in combination therapy; no cross resistance with β-lactams; possibility for oral administration; may be useful in patients with renal impairment in whom aminoglycosides are undesirable	Marginal gram-positive activity; fluoroquinolones not recommended as monotherapy; resistance may develop rapidly
Oral antibiotic regimens (e.g., ciprofloxacin 0.75 g every 12 h or levofloxacin 0.75 g every 24 h + amoxicillin–clavulanate 0.75 g every 12 h or clindamycin 0.6-0.9 g every 8 h)[d]	Efficacy comparable with parenteral therapy in low-risk patients; less expensive; reduced exposure of patients to nosocomial pathogens	Least studied treatment approach; less potent than parenteral antibiotics; requires compliant patient with 24-h access to medical care should clinical instability develop

[a]Dosing guidelines in patients with normal renal function.
[b]Gentamicin or tobramycin 2 mg/kg loading dose, followed by maintenance dose determined by serum concentrations. Choice of specific agent determined according to institutional susceptibilities to individual drugs.
[c]Vancomycin dosing may be guided by serum concentrations.
[d]Clindamycin recommended for patients with β-lactam allergy.
Compiled from references 1, 3, 4, 5, and 11.

β-Lactam Monotherapy

Several β-lactam antibiotics in current use have been evaluated as monotherapy for management of febrile episodes in neutropenic cancer patients, including antipseudomonal cephalosporins (ceftazidime and cefepime), antipseudomonal penicillins (ticarcillin–clavulanic acid and piperacillin–tazobactam), and antipseudomonal carbapenems (imipenem–cilastatin and meropenem).[1,3,5,11] A meta-analysis of 29 randomized clinical trials involving almost 4,800 patients concluded that monotherapy with an antipseudomonal cephalosporin or carbapenem is at least as effective as aminoglycoside-containing combination regimens in the empirical treatment of febrile neutropenia.[38] These results were confirmed in a second meta-analysis of 46 clinical trials involving more than 7,600 patients who revealed no significant differences between monotherapy and combination therapy (β-lactam/aminoglycoside) in rates of survival, treatment response, and bacterial/fungal superinfections but a higher rate of adverse events in patients receiving combination therapy.[39] A third meta-analysis of 33 clinical trials found no overall advantage to the use of combination therapy compared to monotherapy. However, the study found that cefepime monotherapy was associated with a significantly higher risk of mortality compared to the other β-lactams evaluated.[40] Significantly lower response rates for ceftazidime (but not cefepime) monotherapy have been reported in another review of the clinical literature.[41] However, until the results of these conflicting studies can be validated, both ceftazidime and cefepime still are among the monotherapy regimens routinely recommended as appropriate initial therapy of febrile neutropenic patients.[1,10,40,41]

At least six clinical studies have documented the efficacy of piperacillin–tazobactam monotherapy for the empirical treatment of febrile neutropenic patients.[39–41] Although piperacillin–tazobactam has good activity against *P. aeruginosa* and other gram-negative organisms as well as many gram-positive pathogens, the most recent consensus guidelines did not recommend piperacillin–tazobactam as appropriate for monotherapy due to a relative lack of supportive clinical evidence at the time the guidelines were written.[1] This issue likely will be addressed in the next updated version of the IDSA guidelines.

Use of monotherapy has several potential advantages and disadvantages (see Table 126–4). Perhaps the most common concerns are those regarding the selection of resistant strains of organisms, such as *P. aeruginosa, Enterobacter* spp., and *Serratia* spp., through extended-spectrum β-lactamases and type 1 β-lactamases, especially with ceftazidime.[1,5,7] Activity against gram-positive organisms, such as coagulase-negative staphylococci, MRSA, enterococci (including VRE), penicillin-resistant *S. pneumoniae,* and some strains of viridans streptococci is poor with some single β-lactams, but cefepime and antipseudomonal carbapenems have good activity against viridans streptococci and pneumococci.[1] Although ceftazidime has been studied widely and used for treatment of febrile neutropenia, newer agents may be more optimal owing to ceftazidime's susceptibility to β-lactamase induction and lower activity against gram-positive organisms.[1,7,41] Ertapenem, a new carbapenem antibiotic, has excellent activity against many gram-negative organisms but should not be used in the empirical treatment of febrile neutropenia due to its weaker activity against *P. aeruginosa.*

As with all empirical antibiotic regimens, patients receiving monotherapy should be monitored closely for treatment failure, secondary infections, and development of resistance. Use of monotherapy may not be appropriate in institutions with high rates of gram-positive infections or infections caused by relatively resistant gram-negative pathogens such as *P. aeruginosa* and *Enterobacter* spp. Imipenem–cilastatin and meropenem are less susceptible to inducible β-lactamases and often may be used effectively in these institutions. Overall, similar efficacy has been observed with monotherapy with antipseudomonal β-lactams and aminoglycoside combination therapy for treatment of *P. aeruginosa* infections.[23]

Aminoglycoside Plus Antipseudomonal β-Lactam

Regimens consisting of an aminoglycoside plus an antipseudomonal penicillin, antipseudomonal cephalosporin, or antipseudomonal carbapenem traditionally have been the most commonly used for empirical treatment of febrile neutropenia, although many such regimens may lack adequate gram-positive activity (see Table 126–4).[1] This relative lack of activity remains a concern because of the increasing frequency of gram-positive infections. The choice of aminoglycoside and β-lactam for inclusion in empirical regimens should be based on institutional epidemiology and antimicrobial susceptibility patterns. Use of empirical tobramycin or amikacin may be strongly considered because these agents are generally more active than gentamicin against *P. aeruginosa.* However, gentamicin still is an appropriate choice in many institutions based on known susceptibility patterns in those locations. Similar efficacy is observed with an antipseudomonal penicillin, antipseudomonal cephalosporin, or antipseudomonal carbapenem in combination with an aminoglycoside.[1]

Combinations of broad-spectrum β-lactams and aminoglycosides often provide synergistic activity against bacteria commonly infecting neutropenic patients. The exact role of synergy in the outcome of febrile neutropenic patients treated with empirical antibiotic therapy is somewhat controversial, particularly in light of the efficacy of single-drug regimens. Nevertheless, synergistic combinations of antibiotics appear to be beneficial in patients with persistent profound neutropenia. Moreover, administration of antipseudomonal β-lactams in combination with an aminoglycoside may result in a lower rate of drug resistance.[4]

Aminoglycoside toxicity may be a concern in patients receiving these regimens who are already receiving other nephrotoxic drugs, such as cisplatin and cyclosporine. Administration of aminoglycosides in large single daily doses (once-daily dosing) may be as effective, less costly, and no more toxic than conventional dosing methods.[42] A review of randomized, prospective trials of febrile neutropenia failed to find significant differences in either efficacy or toxicity between once-daily dosing and traditional dosing of aminoglycosides.[42] Although once-daily aminoglycoside dosing regimens appear to be safe and effective in these patients, data are not sufficient to recommend once-daily dosing for routine use in this population.[4]

Empirical Regimens Containing Vancomycin

The inclusion of vancomycin in initial empirical therapy of febrile neutropenic cancer patients remains an ongoing debate. This controversy continues because of the increasing incidence of gram-positive infections in this population. One approach is to include vancomycin in the initial empirical antibiotic regimen, thereby providing early effective treatment of possible gram-positive infections. Decreased mortality from penicillin-resistant viridans streptococcal infections has been observed when vancomycin was included in initial therapy.[1,4] A second approach is to withhold vancomycin from initial empirical regimens, later adding the drug if gram-positive organisms are isolated from cultures or if there is no response to initial therapy. Support for both these approaches can be found in the medical literature.[1,5,7,11,43,44] Prospective studies and at least one meta-analysis indicate no advantage to adding vancomycin to initial empirical regimens routinely if vancomycin can be added later as needed.[14,43–45] In addition to increased costs of therapy, it is widely recognized that the selection of VRE is associated with excessive vancomycin use.[46]

Inclusion of vancomycin in initial empirical regimens may be more appropriate today because of higher rates of MRSA infections as well as aggressive chemotherapy regimens causing significant mucosal damage that increases the risk for streptococcal infections. Vancomycin is recommended for inclusion in initial empirical regimens in patients at high risk for gram-positive infection, particularly due to MRSA and coagulase-negative staphylococci (including patients with evidence of infection of central venous catheters and other indwelling lines), high risk for viridans streptococcal infection due to severe mucositis, or pneumonitis in hospitals with high rates of MRSA infections.[1,3,5,7,11,18,46] Rates of β-lactam resistance among viridans streptococci range from 18% to 29%.[5] Empirical vancomycin use may be justified in institutions using empirical or prophylactic antibiotic regimens without good activity against streptococci (e.g., ciprofloxacin) and in patients known to be colonized with MRSA or β-lactam–resistant pneumococci. In patients with preliminary culture results indicating gram-positive infection, empirical vancomycin is appropriate while the susceptibility results are pending. Lastly, empirical use of vancomycin may be recommended in patients with hypotension or other evidence of cardiovascular impairment or sepsis without an identified pathogen.[5,18,46] If empirical vancomycin therapy is initiated and no evidence of gram-positive infection is found after 24 to 48 hours, the drug should be discontinued.[1,4,5] Continuing vancomycin when not warranted results in higher costs, more toxicities, and greater risk of development of VRE.[43]

Vancomycin plus carbapenem regimens may have advantages over vancomycin plus cephalosporin regimens because of lower rates of carbapenem resistance to gram-negative bacilli.[1] Newer antimicrobial agents, such as quinupristin–dalfopristin, linezolid, daptomycin, and dalbavancin, should be reserved for documented infections caused by multiresistant gram-positive pathogens such as VRE. The role of these drugs in the routine treatment of fever in neutropenic patients is undetermined, and linezolid is associated with myelosuppression.[1,5]

CLINICAL CONTROVERSY

Inclusion of vancomycin into empirical antimicrobial regimens for febrile neutropenia remains controversial. Although the incidence of bacterial infections caused by gram-positive pathogens has increased significantly over the past 2 decades, the benefits of adding vancomycin or other agents with specific gram-positive activity to initial treatment regimens have not been conclusively demonstrated.

Fluoroquinolones as a Component of Empirical Regimens

Because the fluoroquinolone antibiotics have broad-spectrum activity (particularly against gram-negative pathogens), rapid bactericidal activity, and favorable pharmacokinetic and toxicity profiles, these agents have been investigated as empirical therapy for febrile neutropenic patients. Ciprofloxacin is the preferred quinolone for use in this clinical setting because of its relatively better activity against *P. aeruginosa* and more extensive evidence-based support for its use.[1,11] Response rates to quinolone-containing combination regimens are comparable to those obtained with the other regimens described previously.[1,4,47,48] Ciprofloxacin is not recommended for monotherapy, however, because of its relatively poor activity against gram-positive pathogens, particularly streptococci, and variable response rates in clinical studies.[1] Quinolones should not be used as empirical therapy in patients who have received quinolones as infection prophylaxis because of the risk of drug resistance.[1,5,11] Rates of fluoroquinolone resistance are increasing, and streptococcal treatment failures are a concern.[49] Although fluoroquinolones are not generally considered first-line empirical therapy, they may be useful as one component of combination regimens in patients with allergies or other contraindications to first-line agents.

Oral Antibiotic Therapy for Management of Febrile Neutropenia

An individual patient's risk of severe infection (influenced by degree/duration of neutropenia and other patient variables) determines appropriate antibiotic therapy and the setting for administration (see Table 126–3 for patient characteristics and levels of infection risk in patients with neutropenia).[1,4,5] Risk stratification is based on several parameters, including duration and degree of neutropenia, type of cancer and its management (including history of HSCT), clinical status, comorbidities, and response to empirical antimicrobial therapy.[1] Because of the excellent spectrum of activity and favorable pharmacokinetics of relatively newer oral antibiotics, particularly the fluoroquinolones, oral antibiotics have a role in the management of selected patients. In patients at low risk for severe or complicated bacterial infection, empirical therapy with broad-spectrum oral antibiotic agents achieves similar patient outcomes as parenteral antibiotics, with response rates of 77% to 95%.[4,32–34] The availability of oral antibiotics with broad-spectrum activity has made possible the treatment of febrile neutropenia in low-risk patients completely in the outpatient setting. Patients with solid tumors undergoing conventional chemotherapy with an expected duration of neutropenia of less than 7 to 10 days and who are clinically stable may be appropriate candidates for oral antibiotic therapy administered on an outpatient basis.[4,3–35] Fluoroquinolones, either as monotherapy or in combination with amoxicillin–clavulanate (or clindamycin for penicillin-allergic patients) for enhanced gram-positive coverage, have been most commonly studied for outpatient therapy in low-risk patients. IDSA and NCCN guidelines recommend oral antibiotic therapy with ciprofloxacin plus amoxicillin–clavulanate in clinically stable low-risk adults (particularly those with recovering neutrophils) with no focus of bacterial infection and no signs of infection other than fever.[1,5] Oral cephalosporins such as cefixime also may be suitable for outpatient treatment.[1] Careful patient selection obviously is required for such management strategies. Important patient characteristics include a history of medication compliance, good caregiver support, and close proximity to medical care in the event of failure to respond to outpatient antibiotic therapy. Benefits of oral therapy on an outpatient basis include increased convenience and quality of life for patients and caregivers and reduced exposure to multidrug-resistant institutional pathogens.[4] Outpatient therapy of low-risk patients now is common practice in most institutions.

In patients at moderate risk for severe bacterial infection, oral antibiotics may play a role in step-down therapy. Carefully selected neutropenic patients may be safely switched from broad-spectrum parenteral therapy to oral antibiotic regimens (e.g., ciprofloxacin plus amoxicillin–clavulanate) with response rates comparable to patients remaining on IV therapy.[11,32,36] Patient selection criteria generally include defervescence within 72 hours of initiation of parenteral therapy, hemodynamic stability, absence of positive cultures or a discernible site of infection, and ability to take oral medications. Many of these patients are able to complete their course of therapy at home.[1,11,36] Changing parenteral antimicrobials to oral regimens in carefully selected patients is now relatively common practice and allows for less expensive hospitalizations and earlier patient discharges.

■ ANTIMICROBIAL THERAPY AFTER INITIATION OF EMPIRICAL THERAPY

6 After initiation of empirical antimicrobial therapy, judicious assessment of febrile neutropenic cancer patients is mandatory to evaluate response, clinical status, laboratory data, and potential need for therapy adjustments. After 72 hours or more of empirical antimicrobial therapy, the clinical status and culture results of febrile neutropenic patients should be reevaluated to determine whether therapeutic modifications are necessary. Additions or modifications to the initial antimicrobial regimen likely will be required for patients with ANC less than 500 cells/mm^3 for more than 1 week. Modifications of antimicrobial therapy should be based on clinical and laboratory data; antibiotic therapy should be optimized based on culture results. However, during periods of neutropenia, patients generally should continue to receive broad-spectrum therapy because of risk of secondary infections or breakthrough bacteremias when antimicrobial coverage is too narrow.[1,4,11]

In patients who become afebrile after 3 to 5 days of therapy with no infection identified, it is generally optimal to continue antibiotic therapy until neutropenia has resolved (ANC ≥500 cells/mm^3). Some clinicians switch therapy from IV antibiotics to an oral regimen (e.g., ciprofloxacin plus amoxicillin-clavulanate) after 2 days of IV therapy in low- to moderate-risk patients who become afebrile and have no evidence of infection. This approach may facilitate earlier hospital discharge. In high-risk patients, the parenteral antibiotic regimen should be continued for at least 7 days.[1,5] However, in afebrile patients with prolonged neutropenia but no signs or symptoms of infection, consideration can be given to discontinuing antibiotic therapy, provided patients can be observed carefully and have ready access to medical care.

The optimal management of patients who remain febrile in the absence of microbiologic or clinical documentation of infection remains highly controversial. The median time to defervescence of febrile neutropenic cancer patients receiving empirical antibiotic therapy is 5 to 7 days.[50] Persistently febrile patients should be evaluated carefully, but modifications generally are not made to initial antimicrobial regimens within the first 5 days of therapy unless there is evidence of clinical deterioration (see Fig. 126–1).[1,4,5] It important to note that the persistence of fever does not necessarily mean failure of a given antimicrobial regimen; up to 25% of neutropenic patients have fever due to noninfectious causes.[8] This is particularly true if patients are otherwise clinically stable. Fever after 3 or more days of antibiotic therapy can be due to a number of causes, including nonbacterial infection, resistant bacterial infection or infection slow to respond to therapy, emergence of a secondary infection, inadequate drug concentrations, drug fever, cell wall–deficient bacteremia, and fever at an avascular site (e.g., catheter infection or abscess).[1,4] Patients with documented infection who are receiving appropriate antimicrobial therapy (based on in vitro susceptibility tests) often remain febrile until resolution of neutropenia occurs. Therefore, the same antibiotic regimen can be continued in patients who remain febrile despite 3 to 5 days of antibiotic therapy but are otherwise clinically stable, especially if neutropenia is expected to resolve within 1 week. However, antibiotic regimens may require modification in patients experiencing toxicities as well as in patients with evidence of progressive disease or documentation of an organism not covered by the initial regimen. When a causative organism is identified, specific therapy directed at the organism should be included; however, patients should continue to receive broad-spectrum therapy while they remain neutropenic.[1,3,4,11] Need for addition of vancomycin should be considered as warranted by clinical and laboratory findings; however, if vancomycin was a component of the initial empirical regimen and the patient still is febrile after 3 days of therapy, discontinuation of vancomycin should be considered to reduce the risk of resistance.

Initiation of Antifungal Therapy

Neutropenic patients who remain febrile despite 5 or more days of broad-spectrum antibiotic therapy are candidates for antifungal therapy. A high percentage of febrile patients who die during prolonged neutropenia have evidence of invasive fungal infection on autopsy, even though many had no evidence of fungal disease before death.[24] Persistence of fever or development of a new fever during broad-spectrum antibiotic therapy may indicate the presence of a fungal infection, most commonly due to *Candida* and *Aspergillus* spp.[11] Blood cultures are positive in fewer than 50% of neutropenic patients with invasive fungal infections.[11,30] The lack of rapid, sensitive diagnostic tests for fungi and the high morbidity and mortality associated with waiting for isolation of fungal organisms justify the empirical addition of antifungal therapy in this clinical setting.[1,11,30] Therefore, empirical antifungal therapy should be initiated after 5 to 7 days of broad-spectrum antibiotic therapy at adequate doses to treat undiagnosed fungal infection and prevent fungal superinfection in high-risk febrile neutropenic patients.[25]

The optimal empirical antifungal regimen is not known. Empirical coverage for both *Candida* spp. and *Aspergillus* should be considered because these organisms are responsible for more than 90% of fungal infections in neutropenic cancer patients.[6] *Aspergillus* is particularly common in patients with hematologic malignancies and in patients undergoing HSCT; therefore, amphotericin B traditionally has been preferred for these patients.[11,24,51] In the setting of febrile neutropenia, lipid-associated amphotericin B products are similar in efficacy to conventional amphotericin B while causing fewer toxicities.[52,53] However, the significantly higher cost and relative lack of experience in comparison with conventional amphotericin B, as well as no clear improvement in efficacy, make their role in the empirical therapy of febrile neutropenia uncertain.[1,11,51–53] Lipid-associated amphotericin B agents may be appropriate in patients with preexisting renal dysfunction, in patients with infusion-related or renal toxicities from conventional amphotericin B therapy, and in patients experiencing treatment failure of suspected/documented fungal infections on conventional amphotericin B therapy.[1,13]

The azole compounds fluconazole, itraconazole, and voriconazole are used in the management of febrile neutropenia. Despite the high rate of amphotericin B toxicities, concerns regarding the emergence of azole-resistant fungi and unclear efficacy advantages relative to other agents have prevented these agents from replacing amphotericin B as the "gold standard" in persistently febrile neutropenic patients.[30,51] However, fluconazole can be a useful alternative to amphotericin B for empirical antifungal use in hospitals in which *Aspergillus* infections and infections due to *C. krusei* and drug-resistant *C. glabrata* are not common.[1] If fluconazole is used as antifungal prophylaxis in cancer patients, it should not be included in empirical antifungal regimens. Itraconazole has similar efficacy as amphotericin B, with fewer toxicities, and availability in both parenteral and oral forms provides a platform for step-down therapy if indicated clinically.[54] Voriconazole has shown efficacy in the treatment of documented invasive fungal infections but may be less desirable for empirical therapy in febrile neutropenic patients due to lack of improved efficacy compared to amphotericin B.[30,51,55] Use of empirical voriconazole should be limited to allogeneic HSCT patients and patients with relapsed leukemia who are at very high risk of invasive *Aspergillus* infections.[25,55]

The echinocandin antifungals (caspofungin, micafungin, and anidulafungin) are attractive agents for treatment of febrile neutropenia because of their broad spectrum of antifungal activity and favorable adverse effect profiles. Caspofungin is as effective as, and also generally better tolerated than, liposomal amphotericin B for empirical treatment of neutropenic patients with persistent fever.[56] Therefore, caspofungin can be considered an alternative agent for use in patients who are intolerant of amphotericin B or in whom severe renal insufficiency makes the use of amphotericin B less desirable.[30,51] Micafungin and anidulafungin have not been well studied for this indication and cannot be recommended for routine use at this time.

As with antibiotic therapy, the optimal duration of antifungal therapy remains controversial. Most clinicians agree that antifungal therapy can be discontinued when neutropenia has resolved in clinically stable patients with no evidence of fungal infection. In neutropenic patients, antifungal therapy generally should be continued for at least 2 weeks in the absence of signs and symptoms of active fungal disease, but many experts advocate continuing therapy until resolution of the neutropenia.[4,25] In neutropenic patients with documented fungal disease, antifungal therapy should be directed at the causative organism, and therapy should be continued for at least 2 weeks and clinical and culture data indicate resolution of the infection. In addition to fungal infections, other causes of persistent fever of unknown origin include resistant bacterial infection, tissue necrosis as a result of underlying tumor, nonbacterial and nonfungal infection (e.g., viral, mycobacterial, or parasitic), and drug or blood product administration. The persistence of fever should not be considered the sole indication for modification of antifungal regimens, assuming that an agent active against *Aspergillus* was initially selected.[30] Treatment recommendations for specific fungal infections are given in Table 126–5.

Initiation of Antiviral Therapy

Febrile neutropenic patients with vesicular or ulcerative skin or mucosal lesions should be evaluated carefully for infection due to HSV or varicella-zoster virus (VZV). Mucosal lesions from viral infections provide a portal of entry for bacteria and fungi during periods of immunosuppression. If viral infection is presumed or documented, neutropenic patients should receive aggressive antiviral therapy to aid healing of primary lesions and prevent disseminated disease. Acyclovir traditionally has been used in this population. However, the newer antivirals valacyclovir and famciclovir have

TABLE 126-5 Infectious Complications after Bone Marrow and Solid Organ Transplantation: Syndromes of Disease and Treatment Guidelines

Pathogen	Syndromes of Disease	Treatment
Bacterial		
Gram-negative aerobic bacilli (Enterobacteriaceae, *Pseudomonas aeruginosa, Haemophilus influenzae)*	Blood, urinary tract, pulmonary, abdomen	*Empiric:* Ceftazidime 1–2 g every 8 h + aminoglycoside,[a,b] cefepime 1–2 g every 12 h + aminoglycoside[a,b]; piperacillin–tazobactam 3.375–4.5 g every 4–6 h; imipenem–cilastatin 0.25–0.5 g every 6 h ± aminoglycoside[a,b] *Definitive:* According to culture and sensitivity results
Gram-positive cocci (*Staphylococcus aureus, Staphylococcus epidermidis, Streptococcus pneumoniae, Enterococcus faecalis*)	Skin, blood, urinary tract, pulmonary, abdomen	*Empiric:* Nafcillin 1–2 g every 4–6 h; vancomycin 0.5–1 g every 6–12 h[c] *Definitive:* According to culture and sensitivity results
Legionella spp.	Pulmonary	Erythromycin 0.5–1 g every 6 h; ciprofloxacin 0.4 g every 8–12 h; levofloxacin 0.75 g every 24 h
Listeria monocytogenes	Central nervous system	Ampicillin 1–2 g every 4–6 h with gentamicin[a]; trimethoprim–sulfamethoxazole 4 mg/kg every 12 h[d]
Nocardia spp.	Skin, pulmonary, central nervous system	Sulfadiazine 1 g every 4–6 h; trimethoprim–sulfamethoxazole 4 mg/kg every 12 h[d]
Fungal		
Candida spp.	Blood, urinary tract, mucous membranes, skin	Clotrimazole 10 mg five times daily; nystatin 100,000 units every 6 h; ketoconazole 200 mg daily; fluconazole 100–800 mg daily; itraconazole 200–400 mg daily; amphotericin B 0.5–0.7 mg/ kg/day ± 5-flucytosine 100–150 mg/kg/day divided every 6 h; caspofungin 50 mg daily[e]; anidulafungin 100 mg daily[e]
Aspergillus spp.	Skin, pulmonary, central nervous system	Amphotericin B 1 mg/kg/day ± 5-flucytosine; itraconazole 200–400 mg daily; lipid-associated amphotericin B 4–5 mg/kg daily[e]; caspofungin 50 mg daily[e]; voriconazole 4 mg/kg every 12 h[e]
Cryptococcus neoformans	Skin, pulmonary, central nervous system	Amphotericin B 0.5 mg/kg/day ± 5-flucytosine; fluconazole 400 mg daily
Zygomycetes (*Mucor*)	Rhinocerebral disease	Amphotericin B 1 mg/kg/day; lipid-associated amphotericin B 4–5 mg/kg daily[e]; posaconazole 200 mg every 8 h[e]
Viral		
Herpes simplex virus	Skin, central nervous system, mucous membranes, pulmonary	Acyclovir 5–10 mg/kg every 8 h; foscarnet 60 mg/kg every 8 h
Cytomegalovirus	Pulmonary, blood, urinary tract, gastrointestinal tract	Ganciclovir 5 mg/kg every 12 h; foscarnet 60 mg/kg every 8 h; hyperimmune globulins 100–500 mg/kg every 1–2 wk
Varicella-zoster virus	Skin, disseminated disease	Acyclovir 10 mg/kg every 8 h; foscarnet 60 mg/kg every 8 h
Epstein-Barr virus	Lymphoproliferative disease	No effective treatment
Papovaviruses (BK, JC)	Skin, central nervous system	No effective treatment
Protozoal/parasitic		
Pneumocystis jiroveci	Pulmonary	Trimethoprim–sulfamethoxazole 15–20 mg/kg/day divided every 6 h[d]; atovaquone 750 mg every 12 h; pentamidine 4 mg/kg daily; dapsone 100 mg daily + trimethoprim 15–20 mg/kg/day divided every 6 h; clindamycin 450–600 mg every 6 h + primaquine 15 mg daily
Toxoplasma gondii	Central nervous system	Pyrimethamine 50–100 mg daily + sulfadiazine 1 g every 4–6 h[f]; pyrimethamine 50–100 mg daily + clindamycin 450–600 mg every 6 h[f]
Strongyloides stercoralis	Pulmonary, central nervous system	Thiabendazole 25 mg/kg every 12 h (maximum 3 g/day)

[a] Gentamicin or tobramycin 2 mg/kg loading dose, followed by maintenance dose determined by serum concentrations. Choice of specific agent determined according to institutional susceptibilities to individual drugs.
[b] For penicillin-allergic adults, use ciprofloxacin 0.4 g every 8–12 h plus an aminoglycoside.
[c] Vancomycin dosing may be guided by serum concentrations.
[d] Based on the trimethoprim component of the combination.
[e] For use in cases refractory to amphotericin B or itraconazole, or in patients with relative contraindications to other agents based on potential for toxicities or potential drug–drug interactions.
[f] Folinic acid (5–10 mg/day) often recommended in conjunction with pyrimethamine-containing regimens for prevention of bone marrow toxicity.

better oral absorption and more convenient dosing schedules. Routine use of antiviral agents in the management of patients without mucosal lesions or other evidence of viral infection generally is not recommended.[1] Treatment recommendations for viral infections are given in Table 126–5.

Duration of Antimicrobial Therapy

❼ The optimal duration of antimicrobial therapy in the neutropenic cancer patient remains controversial. Decisions regarding discontinuation of empirical antimicrobial therapy often are more difficult and complex than those regarding initiation of therapy (see Fig. 126–1). One point on which experts agree, however, is that the most important determinant of the total duration of antibiotic therapy is the patient's ANC.[1,3,5,11] If ANC is ≥500 cells/mm^3 for 2 consecutive days, if the patient is afebrile and clinically stable for 48 to 72 hours or more, and if no pathogen has been isolated, then antibiotics can be discontinued. Some clinicians advocate that patients with ANC less than 500 cells/mm^3 be maintained on antibiotic therapy until resolution of neutropenia, even if they are afebrile. However, prolonged antibiotic use has been associated with superinfections resulting from resistant bacteria and fungi and increases the risk of antibiotic-related toxicities.[11] If low-risk patients are stable clinically but the ANC still is less than 500 cells/mm^3, antibiotics may be discontinued after a total of 5 to 7 afebrile days. However, patients with profound neutropenia (ANC <100 cells/mm^3), mucosal lesions, or unstable vital signs or other risk factors should continue to receive antibiotics until ANC has increased to 500 cells/mm^3 or greater or the patient is stable clinically.

Patients who are persistently neutropenic and febrile but who are stable clinically with no active site of infection often can be discontinued successfully from antimicrobial therapy for at least 2 weeks. However, these patients must be monitored carefully because reinstitution of antibiotics may be necessary.[1,11] An alternative approach is to place these patients on antimicrobial prophylaxis (discussed below in Prophylaxis of Infections in Neutropenic Cancer Patients). Patients with documented infections should receive antimicrobial therapy until the infecting organism is eradicated and signs and symptoms of infection have resolved (at least 10–14 days of therapy).

Consensus guidelines provide useful information regarding the management of febrile episodes in cancer patients with neutropenia.[1,5] However, therapy (including initial empirical regimens, modifications, and duration of treatment) must be individualized based on individual patient parameters and response to therapy.

CLINICAL CONTROVERSY

The optimal time to stop empirical antimicrobial therapy in patients who remain persistently febrile remains a key controversy in the overall management of febrile neutropenia in cancer patients. One unresolved issue is whether the patient's neutropenia must be resolved prior to discontinuing antimicrobial therapy. The patient's individual risk of severe infection (determined by extent and duration of neutropenia as well as other risk factors) helps to guide treatment decisions in this setting.

Colony-Stimulating Factors

Because resolution of neutropenia is the most important determinant of patient outcome from both febrile episodes and documented infections, numerous studies have evaluated hematopoietic colony-stimulating factors (CSFs) (sargramostim [granulocyte-macrophage colony-stimulating factor] and filgrastim [granulocyte colony-stimulating factor]) as adjunct therapy to antimicrobial treatment of febrile neutropenic cancer patients.[57] These studies consistently found that use of CSFs reduces the total duration and severity of chemotherapy-related neutropenia. However, these studies failed to demonstrate consistent benefits of CSFs compared with placebo in relation to important outcomes such as overall survival and disease-free survival, but use of CSFs did result in fewer hospitalizations.[57,58] An expert panel of the American Society of Clinical Oncology (ASCO) has concluded that there is no clear support for routine use of CSFs in uncomplicated fever and neutropenia.[57] The ASCO panel reported that use of CSFs may be useful in patients with ANC ≤500 cells/mm^3, uncontrolled primary disease, pneumonia, invasive fungal infections, multiorgan dysfunction, sepsis syndrome, hypotension, or other factors likely to cause rapid clinical deterioration. However, the panel emphasized that even under these severe circumstances, the benefits of CSF therapy were not substantiated.[57] Clinical judgment must be exercised in determining which patients may benefit from judicious use of these expensive agents. Patients with prolonged neutropenia and documented infections who are not responding to appropriate antimicrobial therapy may benefit from treatment with CSFs.[57]

Direct transfusion of neutrophils has been studied for treatment of febrile neutropenia or opportunistic infections. Routine use of neutrophil transfusions is not supported, but use should be considered in patients with profound prolonged neutropenia with severe documented infections and in whom causative organisms have not been eradicated with appropriate antimicrobial therapy in combination with CSFs.[1,5,59] At present, the use of neutrophil transfusions is considered investigational and is not recommended for routine management of febrile neutropenic patients.[59,60]

PROPHYLAXIS OF INFECTIONS IN NEUTROPENIC CANCER PATIENTS

❽ Owing to the potential morbidity and mortality of infections in neutropenic cancer patients, a number of environmental modifications and prophylactic antimicrobial regimens have been implemented to prevent these complications. The goal of antimicrobial prophylaxis in cancer patients is to decrease the number and severity of systemic infections during prolonged periods of neutropenia. Decisions regarding prophylactic antimicrobials must be made with the realization of associated issues, such as resistance.

General Measures

Because approximately 50% of pathogens infecting neutropenic cancer patients are acquired in the hospital, reducing acquisition of infectious organisms from the environment is a basic component in controlling nosocomial infections.[1,2,5,6] Neutropenic patients should be placed in reverse isolation (isolation to protect patients from contracting infections after exposure to others), with strict adherence to infection control guidelines by hospital personnel.[1,5] Proper meticulous handwashing by hospital personnel is a simple yet very effective infection control measure. To reduce the risk of infection caused by airborne pathogens, such as *Aspergillus* spp., laminar airflow rooms are used at some cancer centers performing HSCT. Laminar airflow rooms work by directing filtered air away from the patient, thus minimizing the risk of infection from airborne or environmental pathogens. Laminar airflow rooms are expensive, and use of these protective environments does not improve overall survival in HSCT recipients.[6]

Bacterial Infections

Combinations of oral nonabsorbable antibiotics, such as gentamicin, nystatin, vancomycin, polymyxin B, and colistin, have been widely studied as a means of reducing colonization of the GI tract with virulent pathogens, such as *P. aeruginosa*, and their translocation into the bloodstream. Although clinical trials have demonstrated that selective intestinal decontamination with oral nonabsorbable antibiotics successfully reduces infections, these regimens are not routinely recommended for prophylaxis because of problems that include unpalatability, high cost, and frequent adverse effects (e.g., nausea, vomiting, diarrhea).[1,2,5,6] Use of nonabsorbable antibiotic regimens has been associated with the development of resistance to aminoglycosides among gram-negative bacilli, rendering the aminoglycosides useless as treatment alternatives for ensuing infections.[1,2] Owing to concerns regarding development of resistance, prophylaxis with aminoglycosides and vancomycin should be avoided.[1,5]

Combining selective decontamination with systemic antimicrobial prophylaxis has been done with oral agents, particularly the fluoroquinolones.[1,2,61] Prospective clinical trials have shown that orally absorbed prophylactic antibiotics, including trimethoprim–sulfamethoxazole and fluoroquinolones, are more effective and better tolerated than nonabsorbable antibiotics.[1,5] Most placebo-controlled studies indicate that trimethoprim–sulfamethoxazole significantly reduces infection rates in cancer patients.[1,5] Although trimethoprim–sulfamethoxazole is effective as prophylaxis against *P. jiroveci,* its lack of activity against *P. aeruginosa* is worrisome, particularly in institutions where pseudomonal infections are frequent.[1] Other concerns with trimethoprim–sulfamethoxazole prophylaxis include selection of resistant organisms, predisposition to development of oral fungal infections, and delay in bone marrow recovery resulting in prolonged neutropenic episodes.[1,5,6]

Numerous studies have shown that oral fluoroquinolones are more effective than placebo, nonabsorbable antibiotics, or trimethoprim–sulfamethoxazole in preventing gram-negative infections in neutropenic cancer patients.[61] Fluoroquinolone prophylaxis during periods of neutropenia decreases the incidence of fever and microbiologically documented gram-negative infections and may decrease the risk of death in these patients.[61] However, there are several potential limitations to their use. In particular, some quinolones (e.g., ciprofloxacin) may lack adequate gram-positive activity. As a result, combination of a quinolone with a second agent providing enhanced gram-positive activity (e.g., rifampin, penicillin, or a macrolide) may be required for effective prophylaxis.[62] Although fluoroquinolone prophylaxis has been associated with the development of resistant gram-negative organisms, a meta-analysis suggests that the risk of infection with resistant pathogens is not significantly increased.[61] This same analysis also found that the risk of colonization or infection with strains resistant to the prophylactic agent is lower with fluoroquinolones than with trimethoprim–sulfamethoxazole. However, patients experiencing breakthrough infection during fluoroquinolone prophylaxis should not be subsequently placed on a fluoroquinolone-containing empirical antibiotic regimen.

Although studies have concluded that the benefits of prophylaxis with fluoroquinolones outweigh the potential risks, antibacterial prophylaxis in general remains controversial due to continued concerns regarding the potential for development of resistant bacteria, high cost, and lack of impact on patient survival.[1,2,5] Therefore, antibacterial prophylaxis is not recommended routinely for all neutropenic patients. Prophylaxis (with trimethoprim–sulfamethoxazole or quinolone plus penicillin) generally is indicated for patients expected to be profoundly neutropenic for more than 1 week, such as HSCT patients.[1,6] Additional risk factors that may provide justification for prophylaxis include mucous membrane or skin lesions, presence of indwelling catheters, need for instrumentation or severe periodontal disease.[1,5] Neutrophil recovery eliminates the need for continued prophylaxis, and recovery may be facilitated by use of CSFs.[57] In contrast to their unclear role in the treatment of febrile neutropenia, CSFs have been formally recommended by the ASCO for prevention of febrile neutropenia in high-risk patients.[57] Patients include those receiving chemotherapy regimens that produce a high rate of febrile neutropenia (>40% incidence) and patients with active tissue infection at the time of chemotherapy, history of febrile neutropenia with previous courses of chemotherapy, or underlying bone marrow compromise.[57]

Fungal Infections

Because neutropenic patients are at risk for mucocutaneous and invasive fungal infections that are difficult to diagnose and treat in this population, antifungal prophylaxis can be considered during high-risk periods at institutions where fungal infections in cancer patients occur frequently.[63] The goal of antifungal prophylaxis is to prevent development of invasive fungal infections during periods of risk, thereby reducing morbidity and mortality. A meta-analysis of antifungal prophylaxis in 38 trials involving more than 7,000 cancer patients reported a decrease in the use of parenteral antifungal therapy, superficial and invasive systemic fungal infections, and fungal infection–related mortality rate.[64] Antifungal prophylaxis in these studies resulted in decreased mortality in patients with prolonged neutropenia and HSCT but no effect on rates of invasive *Aspergillus* infections.

Although the choice of antifungal prophylaxis agents remains controversial, fluconazole prophylaxis (400 mg/day) has been particularly well studied and reduces the incidence of both superficial and systemic fungal infections; it also significantly decreases mortality from fungal infections in patients with leukemia and HSCT recipients.[62–64] However, use of fluconazole prophylaxis has resulted in the emergence of infections caused by *C. krusei* and *C. glabrata,* pathogens that frequently are resistant to fluconazole and other azole-type antifungal agents.[63] Therefore, routine antifungal prophylaxis with oral fluconazole (400 mg/day) or itraconazole oral solution (2.5 mg/kg every 12 hours) is not routinely recommended.[6,25] However, prophylaxis against fungal infection is beneficial in leukemic patients, and the choice of fluconazole, itraconazole, or amphotericin B should be determined by the types of fungal isolates at individual institutions.[25,65] Itraconazole may be more effective than fluconazole for long-term antifungal prophylaxis in allogeneic HSCT recipients; however, itraconazole use was associated with more frequent GI side effects.[66] After initiation, antifungal prophylaxis should be continued until resolution of neutropenia or the need for institution of antifungal therapy for suspected/documented infection.[25]

Itraconazole, low to moderate doses of amphotericin B, intranasal and aerosolized amphotericin B, lipid-associated amphotericin B products, voriconazole, and the echinocandin agents have been investigated for *Aspergillus* prophylaxis in neutropenic patients.[6,67] The new triazole agent posaconazole (200 mg suspension three times daily) was shown to be more effective than either fluconazole 400 mg/day or itraconazole 200 mg twice daily in the prevention of *Aspergillus* and other invasive fungal infections in patients with hematologic malignancies and prolonged neutropenia.[67] However, neither posaconazole nor other interventions are routinely recommended for febrile neutropenic patients at this time.

Other Infections

Use of trimethoprim–sulfamethoxazole in cancer patients at risk for *P. jiroveci* pneumonia has substantially reduced the incidence of this protozoal infection.[1] Antiviral prophylaxis with acyclovir, valacyclovir, or famciclovir is used in most centers to reduce the risk of HSV reactivation in patients with acute leukemia undergoing intensive chemotherapy. Varicella vaccine provides good protection (90%) in leukemic children and may be useful in seronegative adults, although the vaccine has been less well studied in this population.

When considering use of antimicrobial (antibacterial, antifungal, antiprotozoal, and antiviral) prophylaxis in neutropenic patients with cancer, the risks and benefits of prophylaxis must be weighed against issues with development of resistance, toxicities, and other concerns.

PHARMACOECONOMIC CONSIDERATIONS

⑩ As in all areas of modern healthcare, attention has been directed increasingly toward providing cost-effective management of febrile neutropenia in cancer patients. Use of oral and/or outpatient antimicrobial therapy in low-risk patients is an effective, less costly alternative that is preferred by patients.[1,68,69] Potent oral antimicrobials facilitate conversion from IV antibiotics to oral therapy when appropriate. Judicious use of antimicrobials, such as reserving lipid-associated amphotericin B products for patients intolerant to conventional amphotericin B, helps to contain costs. In the situation of febrile neutropenia in a cancer patient, clinicians often are tempted to treat suspected/documented infections extremely aggressively; however, following guidelines such as those published by the IDSA and NCCN helps to assure the most appropriate use of available antimicrobials. Future consequences of antimicrobial overuse, such as resistance and limited treatment options, must be considered when choosing antimicrobial therapy for any indication, including management of febrile neutropenia. Each institution should examine its own infection and susceptibility patterns and use this information to guide empirical treatment decisions while individualizing therapy for each patient.

EVALUATION OF THERAPEUTIC OUTCOMES

⑩ Close monitoring of febrile neutropenic patients, including both clinical and laboratory parameters, is essential for early detection and treatment of infectious complications. Three general therapeutic outcomes have been defined in the setting of febrile neutropenia: (a) success (survival during the febrile episode until resolution of neutropenia by judicious selection of empirical antimicrobial therapy), (b) success with modification (same as 1 but with additions/modifications to empirical therapy), and (c) failure (death during febrile neutropenia).[11] Because many of the drugs that can be used in this setting (e.g., aminoglycosides and amphotericin B) have significant toxicity potential, careful attention must be paid to prevention and management of drug-related adverse effects. Evaluations of the parameters given in the Clinical Presentation are appropriate to help monitor and guide therapy. In addition, the NCCN guidelines for febrile neutropenia provide comprehensive recommendations on clinical/laboratory monitoring parameters, including schedules.[5] The reader is referred to individual chapters within this book for more detailed discussions of monitoring parameters related to specific types of infections (e.g., pneumonia and urinary tract infections).

INFECTIONS IN PATIENTS UNDERGOING HSCT

① Infection remains a major barrier to successful HSCT.[70,71] Numerous advances in HSCT have occurred over the past decade and have resulted in greatly improved patient outcomes. Recipients of HSCT are at enhanced risk for infection because of prolonged periods of neutropenia. In addition, patients receiving allogeneic or matched unrelated donor transplants have immune system insults imposed by prolonged immunosuppressive drug therapy for prevention and treatment of graft-versus-host disease (GVHD). Intensive pretransplant conditioning regimens (high-dose chemotherapy and total-body irradiation), as well as GVHD itself, often disrupt protective barriers, such as mucous membranes, skin, and the GI tract, placing patients at further risk of infection. Patients experiencing failure to engraft have extended periods of profound neutropenia often resulting in death from infectious causes. The Food and Drug Administration (FDA) approved sargramostim for marrow graft failure in both autologous and allogeneic transplants.

ETIOLOGY AND CLINICAL PRESENTATION OF INFECTIONS

② ⑩ The timing with which specific types of infections typically occur following HSCT is shown in Fig. 126–2. Figure 126–2 illustrates the general time course for infections in all types of HSCT, but the relative incidence and importance of specific pathogens vary greatly according to the specific type of HSCT performed. Patients receiving allogeneic transplants are at greatest risk for infection after HSCT and are predisposed to earlier and more severe infections with opportunistic pathogens such as *Aspergillus*. The presence of GVHD also has an impact on the incidence and timing of various infections.

After administration of intensive conditioning regimens to eliminate malignant cells and prevent rejection of donor cells, patients may remain profoundly neutropenic for 3 to 4 weeks. During this preengraftment period, patients are at risk for the same types of infectious complications that occur in other granulocytopenic cancer patients (e.g., bacterial and fungal infections) and should be managed accordingly (see Table 126–1). Table 126–5 lists regimens for treatment of specific infections.

Patients undergoing HSCT are at significant risk for serious bacterial infections.[70–72] The risk of bacterial infection is particularly increased in patients undergoing allogeneic transplantation and those with GVHD. Gram-negative bacteremia occur in approximately 20% of patients, and mortality rates may reach 25%.[72]

Fungal infections, especially those caused by *Candida* and *Aspergillus* spp., are serious and often result in fatal complications associated with HSCT. Fungi remain a serious cause of infection, particularly in allogeneic HSCT recipients, for up to 1 to 2 years following transplantation and may occur in as many as 10% of patients.[70,71,73] Mortality rates associated with invasive aspergillosis infections may be as high as 90%.[74]

In addition to bacterial and fungal infections, HSCT recipients are at risk for serious HSV infections manifesting as severe gingivostomatitis, esophagitis, genital lesions, and, rarely, pneumonia during the first month after transplant.[70,71] Clinical disease is more common in patients with serologic evidence (e.g., serum antibodies) of prior exposure and latent HSV infection pretransplant. Therefore, reactivation of latent disease during periods of immunosuppression is the most common etiology of HSV infection. Without prophylaxis, as many as 80% of HSV-seropositive patients experience mucocutaneous disease after intensive chemotherapy compared with less than 25% of seronegative patients.[71,73] HSV infections often coexist with candidal infection and mucositis secondary to chemotherapy, radiation, or both.[75] Acyclovir-resistant HSV infections occur following HSCT but are not common.[73,76] Painful swallowing associated with these conditions often makes it difficult for patients to take oral medications and maintain adequate nutritional intake. Because of the considerable morbidity associated with reactivation of HSV after transplantation, the HSV serologic status of patients should be determined prior to transplant.

HSCT recipients remain at high risk for infection after bone marrow engraftment has occurred.[70,71] Significant defects in neutrophil function and cell-mediated and humoral immunity, persisting for several months after transplantation, predispose patients to infectious complications. Acute and chronic GVHD also result in prolonged periods of immunosuppression and increased infection rates.

Bone marrow transplant patients are at high risk for cytomegalovirus (CMV) infections during the early postengraftment period. They range in severity from asymptomatic viral shedding (urine, throat, lungs) to life-threatening disseminated disease and interstitial pneumonia.[70,71,73,75]

As with HSV, patients seropositive for CMV before transplantation are at high risk for recurrent disease during periods of immunosuppression; approximately 70% of seropositive patients develop recur-

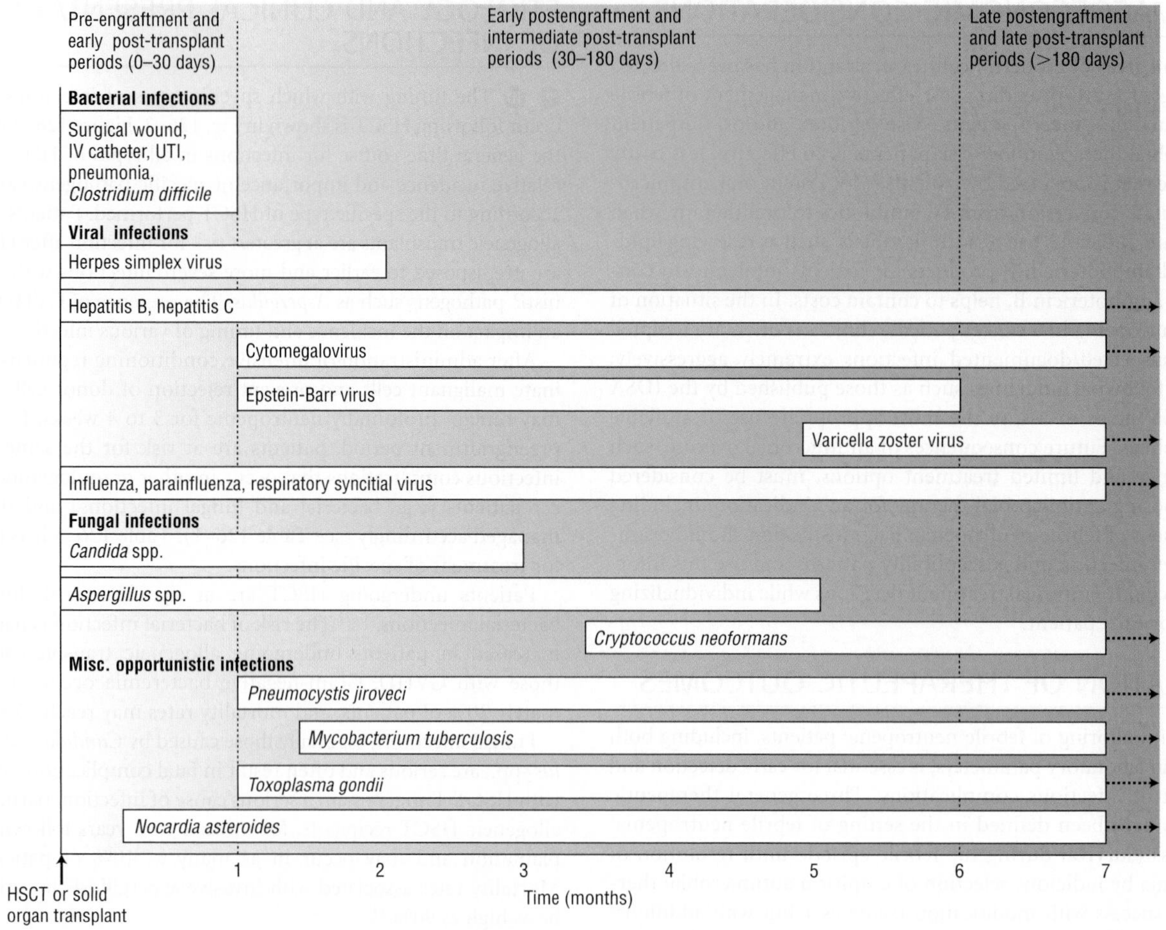

FIGURE 126-2. Timetable for the occurrence of infections in hematopoietic stem cell transplantation HSCT and solid organ-transplant patients. (IV, intravenous; UTI, urinary tract infection.)

rent CMV disease after transplantation compared with only 3% of seronegative patients.[73,75] Other risk factors for CMV disease in HSCT patients include advanced age, human lymphocyte antigen mismatch, total-body irradiation, multiagent conditioning regimens, and presence of GVHD.[71,73] Patients without evidence of latent CMV infection (CMV seronegative) before transplantation may develop primary CMV disease after receiving bone marrow or blood products from CMV-seropositive donors. Although the typical onset of both primary and recurrent CMV infection is 1 to 2 months after transplantation, late-onset infections occurring more than 100 days after transplantation are increasing in frequency.[70–73,75,77] Patients receiving allogeneic transplants are at highest risk for CMV disease.[71,73,75]

The most serious clinical manifestation of CMV disease and the leading cause of infectious death in HSCT recipients is interstitial pneumonia, which is associated with an 85% mortality rate if left untreated.[73] This clinical syndrome manifests as fever, dyspnea, hypoxia, nonproductive cough, and diffuse pulmonary infiltrates. As many as 40% of allogeneic HSCT patients will develop interstitial pneumonia; of the patients with interstitial pneumonia, up to 40% of cases are caused by CMV.[73] Interstitial pneumonia also may result from other infectious (*P. jiroveci,* VZV) and noninfectious causes (pulmonary damage by radiation and chemotherapy).[73]

During the late postengraftment period (beginning approximately 100 days after transplantation), infections remain a major problem in patients suffering from chronic GVHD. Additional immunosuppressive therapy for treatment of GVHD places these patients at added risk for infection. Infections common during the late postengraftment period include those caused by encapsulated bacteria, such as *S. pneumoniae* and *H. influenzae*, and viruses, including CMV and VZV.[70,71,73] Patients not undergoing allogeneic transplantation or suffering from chronic GVHD generally have few infections in this period.

Up to 50% of all patients surviving up to 10 months after transplantation develop an infection caused by VZV.[71,73] Infection with VZV is most common in patients receiving allogeneic transplants with acute or chronic GVHD.[73,75] Both primary (varicella) or recurrent disease (herpes zoster) usually present as skin lesions, most of which remain contained to local areas; however, 30% to 45% of these infections may disseminate to other cutaneous areas or body organs, causing mortality as high as 50%.[73,75]

TREATMENT

Prophylaxis and Management: Infections in Recipients of HSCT

❽ ❾ Goals of antimicrobial drug use in HSCT patients include (a) prevention of bacterial, fungal, viral, and protozoal infections during preengraftment and postengraftment periods and (b) effective treatment of established infections. The overall goal of prophylaxis and treatment of infection in HSCT patients is prevention of infectious morbidity and mortality. These goals must be achieved at the lowest possible toxicity and cost. Prophylactic therapy should be specifically aimed at pathogens known to cause a high incidence of infection within the HSCT population, the specific institution, or both. In addition, prophylactic therapy should be limited to regimens proved to be effective through well-designed clinical trials.

Appropriate immunizations should be a primary consideration in the prevention of infections in HSCT recipients. Immunizations against common bacterial and viral pathogens are timed to avoid periods of severe immunosuppression following HSCT when the protective response to vaccination potentially would be decreased.[6] Current recommendations for immunization of HSCT patients include three doses each of diphtheria-pertussis-tetanus or diphtheria-tetanus, inactivated polio, conjugated *H. influenzae* type b, and hepatitis B vaccines at 12, 14, and 24 months after transplantation. The 23-valent pneumococcal vaccine should be administered at 12 and 24 months after HSCT, and the influenza vaccine should be administered prior to HSCT, resumed at least 6 months after transplantation, and continued for life. Family members, close contacts, and healthcare providers of HSCT patients also should be vaccinated annually against influenza. Finally, the measles-mumps-rubella vaccine should be administered no sooner than 24 months after HSCT when the patient is considered to be immunocompetent. The varicella vaccine is contraindicated for administration to HSCT patients owing to the live-attenuated nature of the product and the risk of VZV infection.[6]

■ BACTERIAL INFECTIONS

Prophylaxis of infections in HSCT patients is similar in many ways to that used in other neutropenic patients. Selective decontamination with oral antimicrobials is used commonly; considerations are the same as those discussed previously in the "Prophylaxis of Infections in Neutropenic Cancer Patients" section. Although some studies have shown decreased rates of bacteremia and other bacterial infections after HSCT, overall mortality rates were not reduced.[6,73] Therefore, routine use of prophylactic antibiotics in HSCT is still controversial. Fluoroquinolones have become the most frequently used agents, often combined with another agent (e.g., macrolides or rifampin), for enhanced gram-positive activity.[6,73] These regimens usually are started either within 72 hours of beginning the chemotherapy conditioning regimens or on the day of hematopoietic stem cell infusion and continued throughout the neutropenic period. Patients who become febrile while receiving prophylaxis should be managed according to general guidelines for febrile neutropenic patients.

Routine use of parenteral vancomycin for prophylactic therapy is not recommended. Prophylaxis with vancomycin has been studied because of the high incidence of gram-positive infections following transplantation. Vancomycin prophylaxis appears to decrease the overall incidence of gram-positive bacterial infections, number of days of empirical antimicrobial therapy, and cost of therapy.[6,73] However, important mortality benefits were not demonstrated consistently, and there are significant concerns regarding the selection of vancomycin-intermediate *S. aureus* and vancomycin-resistant enterococci. Thus, prophylactic vancomycin use is not generally recommended except in institutions with high rates of MRSA infection among HSCT recipients.[6] There currently is no role for linezolid, quinupristin–dalfopristin, or daptomycin except in documented infections caused by VRE.

Antibiotic prophylaxis against bacterial infection is recommended in the late postengraftment period (>100 days after transplantation) in certain high-risk patients, specifically allogeneic transplant recipients with chronic GVHD.[6] Antibiotics should be targeted against encapsulated bacteria such as *S. pneumoniae* and *H. influenzae* and should be selected based on local susceptibility patterns for these organisms. Patients receiving trimethoprim–sulfamethoxazole for prophylaxis of other opportunistic infections may be protected adequately and do not necessarily require an additional antibiotic.[6,73] Prophylaxis should be continued as long as the chronic GVHD is being actively treated.

■ VIRAL INFECTIONS

Prophylaxis of recurrent HSV infection is recommended for all HSV-seropositive patients undergoing HSCT.[6,73] Approximately 0% to 10% of HSV-seropositive patients receiving acyclovir experienced viral shedding, clinical symptoms of viral reactivation, or both compared with 60% to 80% of patients receiving placebo.[6,71] Acyclovir doses recommended for prophylaxis are 250 mg/m^2 (5 mg/kg) IV every 12 hours or 200 mg orally three times daily.[6,73] Intravenous therapy eventually is necessary in most patients because of the development of severe mucositis from conditioning regimens. Oral acyclovir is effective and considerably less expensive in patients who can take oral medications. Valacyclovir in doses of 500–1,000 mg/day have been used, but clinical experience is limited. It is not currently recommended as first-line prophylaxis therapy.[6] Although the duration of antiviral prophylaxis differs among centers, acyclovir usually is started at the time of the conditioning regimen and continued until bone marrow engraftment or resolution of mucositis (approximately 30 days after HSCT).[6] In addition to preventing recurrence of HSV disease, acyclovir prophylaxis may reduce the incidence of CMV reactivation.[6] Patients developing active HSV or VZV infection should be treated with high-dose acyclovir (10 mg/kg IV every 8 hours).

Although high-dose oral acyclovir given for 6 months after transplantation significantly reduces reactivation of VZV infections, routine use of long-term acyclovir is controversial and not generally recommended for this indication.[6,73] Patients who received HSCT within the previous 24 months or those more than 24 months after HSCT who have chronic GVHD or are undergoing immunosuppressive therapy should receive varicella-zoster immunoglobulin 625 units intramuscularly within 48 to 96 hours after close contact with persons with chickenpox or shingles for prevention of VZV-related disease.[6]

Acyclovir-resistant HSV has been reported occasionally in HSCT patients receiving acyclovir prophylaxis. Foscarnet is the drug of choice for treatment of acyclovir-resistant HSV. Foscarnet for HSV prophylaxis has not been well studied.[6,73]

Prevention of CMV disease has been studied extensively in HSCT patients and is a well-accepted indication for prophylaxis because of the high associated infectious morbidity and mortality. If possible, CMV-seronegative patients should receive donor cells and supportive blood products from seronegative donors only; however, CMV-seropositive patients are not at additional risk by receiving blood or donor cells from seropositive donors.[73] Although acyclovir has relatively poor in vitro activity against CMV, a decrease in CMV infection and an improvement in overall survival were reported in HSV- and CMV-seropositive allogeneic HSCT recipients receiving IV acyclovir.[6]

Ganciclovir has been well studied for prophylaxis because of its superior activity against CMV compared with acyclovir.[6] Although administration of prophylactic ganciclovir to CMV-seropositive patients may significantly decrease the occurrence of CMV disease, studies have found no clear survival benefit, and ganciclovir-related bone marrow suppression frequently was problematic. Therefore, ganciclovir prophylaxis is only recommended routinely among allogeneic HSCT recipients for the first 100 days after transplantation.[6,73] The recommended dose of ganciclovir in these patients is 5 mg/kg IV every 12 hours for the first 5 to 7 days, followed by 5 to 6 mg/kg IV once daily five times per week until day 100 after HSCT.[6]

Perhaps a more appropriate role for ganciclovir is early or preemptive therapy, in which ganciclovir is administered at first isolation of CMV from the blood or bronchoalveolar lavage fluid. Detection of CMV can be accomplished by use of either a monoclonal antibody–based test for viral antigens or by detection of viral DNA through polymerase chain reaction (PCR)–based tests. Preemptive therapy was evaluated in several studies. It significantly reduced the occurrence of CMV disease (including CMV pneumonia) and improved survival significantly up to 180 days after transplantation.[73] Because CMV viremia and bronchoalveolar lavage cultures are highly predictive of subsequent CMV disease, preemptive ganciclovir therapy should be considered for autologous HSCT recipients within the first 100 days after transplantation or in allogeneic HSCT recipients at any time after transplantation.[6,73] The dose of ganciclovir for preemptive therapy is the same as that used for prophylaxis. Foscarnet can be used for either prophylaxis or preemptive therapy of CMV disease in patients intolerant of ganciclovir. The recommended foscarnet dose is 60 mg/kg IV every 12 hours for 7 days, followed by 90 to 126 mg/kg IV daily.[78] Oral valganciclovir 900 mg every 12 hours has not been well studied in the setting of HSCT and is not recommended routinely. CSFs are beneficial in this setting, providing benefits similar to those noted in neutropenic patients with acquired immunodeficiency syndrome receiving ganciclovir therapy for CMV retinitis.

Pharmacologic prevention of CMV disease with either intravenous immunoglobulin (IVIG) or CMV hyperimmune globulin (CMVIG) produced variable and inconclusive results.[79] The benefits of immunoglobulins for CMV prophylaxis in HSCT patients have not been demonstrated conclusively, and their use is not currently recommended.[73,79]

Ganciclovir is the drug of choice for treatment of active CMV infection in HSCT patients (see Table 126–5). Foscarnet also may be of benefit for treatment or prevention of infections in HSCT patients and may be used as an alternative to ganciclovir because of its relative lack of bone marrow toxicity. Foscarnet-related nephrotoxicity may be problematic, however, especially in the posttransplant period when patients may be receiving other nephrotoxic agents. Use of cidofovir is limited by the risk of nephrotoxicity, and this agent has not been well studied in HSCT patients.

Numerous single-agent treatments, such as vidarabine, interferon, and ganciclovir, have been used unsuccessfully as treatment for CMV pneumonitis. However, the combination of high-dose IVIG and ganciclovir may decrease the mortality of the syndrome from 85% to only 30% to 50%.[73,79,80] Ganciclovir plus hyperimmune CMVIG also is considered effective for treatment of CMV disease, although this regimen has not been studied as extensively in the HSCT population in a controlled fashion. The potential for ganciclovir-associated bone marrow suppression prior to marrow engraftment and in patients who are just recovering from granulocytopenia remains a concern, especially in patients with unstable renal function. Ganciclovir plus CMVIG is used widely as the treatment regimen of choice for severe or life-threatening CMV disease. Ganciclovir plus IVIG also is used frequently, although CMVIG is replacing IVIG in most institutions.[79,80]

CLINICAL CONTROVERSY

Use of CMVIG for prophylaxis and/or treatment of CMV infections in HSCT and solid-organ transplantation patients is advocated by many clinicians. However, the clinical benefits of this expensive adjunct therapy have not been clearly demonstrated in these patients. Although CMVIG often is recommended in combination with ganciclovir for treatment of CMV pneumonia in transplant patients, its role in other types of infections is not clear.

■ FUNGAL INFECTIONS

Prophylaxis with antifungal agents is efficacious for prevention of mucocutaneous and disseminated candidal infections in high-risk HSCT patients.[6,25,30,67,73,81] Patients specifically recommended for prophylaxis include all allogeneic transplant recipients and autologous recipients who are expected to have prolonged neutropenia, have received intensive conditioning regimens associated with extensive mucositis, or have recently received fludarabine.[6,30,67,73,81] Fluconazole 400 mg IV or orally once daily is the most commonly used regimen; it is started on the day of transplantation and continued until engraftment or resolution of neutropenia.[6,25,73] The variable activity of fluconazole against non-*albicans* species of *Candida* may be problematic in this population, as is lack of activity against *Aspergillus*.[30,67] Prophylaxis with fluconazole (as well as itraconazole), although effectively reducing colonization and infection with yeasts, has not been consistently demonstrated to reduce overall mortality or invasive infections such as aspergillosis in HSCT recipients.[30,67,73,81] Low-dose amphotericin B (0.10–0.25 mg/kg/day) and liposomal amphotericin B (1 mg/kg/day) have occasionally been used in institutions with high rates of *Aspergillus* infection after HSCT.[30,67,81] As with the azoles, amphotericin B prophylaxis has not been clearly demonstrated to reduce either overall or infection-related mortality following HSCT.[25,30,81] Despite the controversies regarding absolute benefits of prophylaxis, fluconazole generally is recommended for most patients undergoing HSCT.[6,30,67,81]

Two newer antifungal agents have shown efficacy in the prevention of fungal infections in patients undergoing HSCT. Micafungin 50 mg IV once daily was demonstrated to be more efficacious than fluconazole in the prevention of early-onset *Candida* infections in patients with neutropenia prior to engraftment. Posaconazole 200 mg suspension three times daily was more effective than fluconazole 400 mg orally once daily in the late prevention of invasive *Aspergillus* and other fungal infections in HSCT patients with GVHD. Although both of these agents show efficacy better than that of fluconazole, their exact roles in preventing fungal infections in high-risk HSCT patients is not known.[30,67,81]

Fluconazole, posaconazole, and other azole antifungals may cause significant elevations in serum cyclosporine concentrations and predispose to cyclosporine toxicities; this interaction should be monitored closely in HSCT patients receiving these agents concurrently.[25]

■ PROTOZOAL INFECTIONS

Pulmonary infection with *P. jiroveci* is a relatively infrequent complication of HSCT. However, mortality rates in this population are approximately 60% and are especially high in patients with GVHD.[6,73] Prophylactic trimethoprim–sulfamethoxazole (one double-strength tablet three times per week or one single-strength tablet daily) is given commonly in this setting. Toxoplasmosis is not a common infection in HSCT patients but is associated with mortality rates of approximately 70%.[82] Toxoplasmosis should be prevented by trimethoprim–sulfamethoxazole prophylaxis.[6,73]

■ USE OF COLONY-STIMULATING FACTORS

Several studies have evaluated the use of filgrastim and sargramostim in HSCT patients in an effort to speed bone marrow recovery, reduce the period of neutropenia, and decrease infectious complications. Although the time to neutrophil recovery was consistently decreased, the studies failed to show significant differences in infection rates, transplant-related mortality, or overall survival. CSFs appear to be safe, but their use in HSCT patients is not formally recommended because of lack of clear benefits.[57]

EVALUATION OF THERAPEUTIC OUTCOMES

⑩ Close monitoring of HSCT patients, including clinical and laboratory data, is essential for early detection and treatment of infectious complications. In addition, because many of the drugs commonly used in this setting (e.g., ganciclovir, amphotericin B, and trimethoprim–sulfamethoxazole) have significant toxicity potential in HSCT patients, careful attention must be paid to prevention and management of drug-related adverse effects. Monitoring parameters related to specific types of infections (e.g., pneumonia and urinary tract infections) should be applied as appropriate.

The reader is referred to other chapters within this book for more specific information.

INFECTIONS IN SOLID-ORGAN TRANSPLANT RECIPIENTS

Since the introduction of cyclosporine in 1980, solid-organ transplantation has become an established mode of treatment for end-stage diseases of the kidney, liver, heart, lungs, and pancreas. Small bowel transplantation is becoming more common. Patient and allograft survival rates greatly exceed those of the past. Reasons for improved survival include continuous improvements in immunosuppressive drug therapy, candidate selection, and transplant surgery techniques and more experience in the management of complications (including infection) in these patients. Major hindrances to successful transplantation and extended long-term survival include problems with allograft dysfunction and rejection and infectious complications. Despite advances in diagnostic techniques and antimicrobial therapy, infection remains an important cause of morbidity and mortality.

RISK FACTORS

❶ Many of the risk factors for infection are present in solid-organ transplant patients (see Table 126–1). The most important risk factor in this population is immunosuppressive drug therapy for prevention and treatment of allograft rejection. Risk of infection depends on specific immunosuppressive drug regimens as well as the intensity (dose) and duration of immunosuppression. Most opportunistic infections in transplant patients occur during the first 6 months after transplantation, when the intensity and total cumulative doses of immunosuppressive therapy are very high.[83,84]

Immunosuppressive drugs, often in escalated doses, are used to treat episodes of graft rejection. Drugs used to treat rejection include immunoglobulins directed against T cells (e.g., antithymocyte globulin), murine monoclonal antibodies (muromonab), antibodies against interleukin-2 receptors (daclizumab and basiliximab), and high-dose IV or oral corticosteroids. Rejection episodes often occur during the posttransplant period when the overall cumulative dose or net state of immunosuppression is highest (2–4 months posttransplant).[83] Therefore, patients already at risk for infection are placed at even higher risk if additional immunosuppressive therapy is needed to treat one or more episodes of graft rejection. Immunosuppressive drug therapy must be evaluated carefully when infections occur because, in many cases, immunosuppression may have to be reduced to allow patients to survive the infectious episode, at the expense of increased risk of graft rejection. Risk of increased infectious complications from immunosuppressive therapy used to treat rejection episodes is determined, at least in part, by the specific therapy used.[83,84]

ETIOLOGY

❷ As with cancer patients, microorganisms infecting solid-organ transplant patients are present before transplantation or are acquired from exogenous sources. All transplant recipients are at risk for mucocutaneous candidiasis from species colonizing body sites. Invasive fungal infection is less common following kidney and pancreas transplantation (5%–15%) but also may occur in 30% to 60% of heart, lung, liver, and small bowel transplant recipients. Rates are highest following liver and small bowel transplantation and are associated with mortality rates up to 60% to 70%.[74,83,85,86] Approximately 50% to 90% of all systemic fungal infections in transplant recipients are caused by *Candida* spp.[74,83,85,86] Abdominal surgery, especially the more complex procedures required for liver and small bowel transplantation, predispose patients to serious fungal disease, most likely as a consequence of entering an area highly colonized with *Candida* spp.[85] Lung and heart transplant recipients are particularly at risk for invasive aspergillosis; these infections may occur in up to 10% of patients.[85] Liver and lung transplant recipients are at high risk for serious gram-negative bacterial infections as a result of the technically difficult surgical procedures.[83]

Organisms present as latent tissue infections may reactivate and cause clinical disease after transplantation with administration of immunosuppressive drug therapy. Disease resulting from infection reactivation has been noted with viral (HSV-1 and HSV-2, CMV, VZV, Epstein-Barr virus), protozoal *(Toxoplasma gondii, P. jiroveci),* and mycobacterial *(Mycobacterium tuberculosis)* pathogens.[87,88] Serologic or immunologic tests are performed prior to transplantation to assess the risk for infection because of reactivation and identify other subclinical infections (e.g., hepatitis B, hepatitis C, *Legionella*). Many patients with reactivated disease have no clinical symptoms; often the only evidence of active infection is a rise in antibody titer from the pretransplant baseline, positive culture, or histologic evidence. Reactivation of latent infection may result in severe life-threatening disease in immunosuppressed hosts.[88]

Exogenous sources of infection in transplant patients include environmental contamination and transmission of microorganisms via transplanted organs and blood products. Environmental sources of infection are similar to those noted in other immunocompromised hosts, such as cancer patients. Airborne pathogens, especially fungi, such as *Aspergillus* and *Cryptococcus neoformans,* may cause infections in transplant patients; this is thought to be a direct cause of increased *Aspergillus* infections among lung transplant patients.[83,85] Transplant patients are at risk for common nosocomial infections and infections occurring as hospital outbreaks *(P. aeruginosa* and *Legionella).* Optimal prevention and management of nosocomial infections in transplant patients require knowledge of the current epidemiology of infections and susceptibility patterns in the institution.

Infections transmitted via donor organs or blood products are major causes of morbidity and mortality in transplant patients and may include HSV, *T. gondii,* and hepatitis B and C. The most important infections transmitted from the donor, however, are caused by CMV. These infections may cause serious disease (e.g., pneumonia, hepatitis, hematologic disorders, and chorioretinitis). They also may predispose patients to other opportunistic infections and contribute to acute and chronic allograft dysfunction or rejection, posttransplant lymphoproliferative disorders, and cardiac complications and atherosclerosis in heart transplant recipients.[83,89] In contrast to reactivation disease, transplant patients contracting primary CMV disease are at increased risk for serious life-threatening infections.[83,90–92] The most important source of primary CMV infection in transplant patients is the donor organ. Efforts are made to avoid transplanting organs from CMV-seropositive donors into CMV-seronegative recipients because of the potentially severe consequences. With the relative scarcity of suitable organs and the rapidity with which transplant decisions often must be made, however, this is not always possible. The consequences of transplanting an organ from a CMV-seropositive donor into an already CMV-seropositive recipient are less clear. Evidence exists that CMV reinfection (as well as reactivation) syndromes may occur in these patients.[83,84,92] In addition to transmission from donor organs, primary CMV disease may be transmitted from seropositive blood products, although this is a much less common mode of transmission. Risk of such transmission increases with the administration of large numbers of blood products.

Organs from donors seropositive for *T. gondii* or HSV generally are not withheld from seronegative patients. Organs from known HIV-infected donors, however, are not used for transplantation.

Asymptomatic HIV-seropositive individuals with $CD4^+$ lymphocyte count greater than 400 cells/mm^3 may be considered for liver, heart, or lung transplantation without prohibitively high risk for acceleration of HIV disease.[91,93] However, this practice is not widespread because of the shortage of donor organs. The impact of protease inhibitors and highly active antiretroviral therapy on long-term outcome of HIV-infected patients following transplantation is not precisely known but is believed to have improved the overall feasibility of transplanting these individuals.[93]

Table 126–5 provides information on microbiology, clinical presentation, and treatment of infections in HSCT and solid-organ transplant recipients. Although opportunistic viral, fungal, and protozoal infections may occur commonly, bacterial infections remain the most frequent infectious complications after transplantation in all allograft recipients.

TIMING OF INFECTIONS AFTER TRANSPLANTATION

Although risk of infection with specific pathogens varies with the type of transplant, the time course of infections is similar in all transplant recipients. The overall risk of infection is greatest during the first 6 months after transplantation, when the greatest number of risk factors are present. Both daily and cumulative doses of immunosuppressive drugs are at high levels, and additional agents may be necessary for treatment of acute rejection episodes.[83,84]

As with HSCT, the overall time course for infections can be divided into three general periods after transplantation (see Fig. 126–2). During the early posttransplant period (within the first month after transplantation), patients are at risk for infections already present and brought forward from the pretransplant period (e.g., hepatitis B); postoperative infections, such as surgical wound and catheter infections; infection resulting from colonized donor organs (pneumonia following lung transplant); and reactivation of HSV.[83,84,88] In the intermediate posttransplant period (2–6 months after transplant), risk is highest for viral infections, including CMV, Epstein-Barr virus, and hepatitis B and C. The combination of these "immunomodulating" viruses plus sustained immunosuppressive therapy leads to a high risk for opportunistic infections with pathogens such as *P. jiroveci, Aspergillus,* and *Nocardia asteroides.*[83–85,88] In the late posttransplant period (>6 months after transplant), patients are at risk for persistent infections (particularly viral) from earlier posttransplant periods, reactivation of VZV and *C. neoformans,* and routine infections affecting the general population.[83] In addition, patients who required additional immunosuppression therapy for acute or chronic rejection are at continued high risk for opportunistic infections *(Aspergillus* and *P. jiroveci).*[83–85] Although Fig. 126–2 illustrates infection patterns common to all solid-organ transplants, the relative incidence and importance of a particular pathogen vary according to the type of transplant.

TYPES OF INFECTIONS AND CLINICAL PRESENTATION

⑩ Transplant patients are at risk for infections occurring at a variety of sites, including skin, surgical wound, urinary tract, lungs, blood, abdomen, and CNS. However, most infections occur at or near the site of the transplanted organ. For example, heart transplant and heart and lung transplant recipients most often are infected within the lungs or thoracic cavity. Urinary tract infections remain an important cause of morbidity in renal transplant patients, especially in the early posttransplant period. Administration of prophylactic antibiotics (e.g., trimethoprim–sulfamethoxazole) to these patients has reduced the incidence and severity of urinary tract infections.[83,84] Serious bacterial and fungal infections originating from the abdomen and GI tract are most common after liver transplantation and are related to variables such as length of surgery and surgical procedures performed. Risk of bacteremia, usually originating from the gut, is highest in liver transplant patients. Renal transplant recipients are at the lowest risk for infections and infectious deaths, whereas patients receiving heart, lung, and liver transplants are at the highest risk for infection-related morbidity and mortality.[83–85]

CLINICAL PRESENTATION OF INFECTIONS IN SOLID-ORGAN TRANSPLANT PATIENTS

General

- Because transplant patients are at high risk for serious infections, frequent (at least daily), careful clinical assessments must be performed to search for evidence of infection.
- Clinical presentation of infection is variable and depends on the type and site of infection, type of transplant, time after transplantation, immune status of the host, and dose and duration of immunosuppressive therapy.
- Primary viral disease usually is more symptomatic and severe than disease caused by reactivation.
- Physical assessment should include examination of all common sites of infection, including mouth/pharynx, nose and sinuses, respiratory tract, GI tract, urinary tract, skin, soft tissues, perineum, and intravascular catheter insertion sites.

Symptoms

- Usual signs and symptoms of infection may be absent or altered in patients receiving intensive immunosuppressive regimens owing to an inability to mount a typical inflammatory response (e.g., no infiltrate on chest x-ray film, urinary tract infection without pyuria).
- Pain may be present at infection site(s).

Signs

- Fever is the single most important clinical sign indicating the presence of infection. Other causes of fever unrelated to infection in this patient population include reactions to blood products, drugs, embolic events, and ischemic injury.
- Usual signs of infection may be absent or altered.
- Signs of allograft dysfunction may be related to infection. Distinguishing fever caused by allograft rejection from that caused by infection often is difficult and frequently requires allograft biopsy.

Laboratory Tests

- Blood cultures (at least two sets, including vascular access devices) for bacteria and fungi; cultures of other suspected or potential infection sites (urine, lungs, surgical wounds, and soft tissue infections).
- Other cultures should be obtained as clinically indicated according to the presence of signs or symptoms.
- Complete blood count and chemistries should be obtained frequently to monitor allograft function, plan supportive care, guide drug dosing, and assess patient's overall status.
- Surveillance cultures for CMV and HSV may be useful during first 3 months after transplantation for early detection of infection.

Other Diagnostic Tests

- Chest x-ray film
- Aspiration, biopsy of skin lesions
- Other diagnostic tests as indicated clinically on the basis of physical examination and other assessments

In contrast to febrile neutropenic patients, the threshold for initiating empirical antimicrobial therapy is higher in febrile transplant patients. Appropriate therapy for the large numbers of pathogens that may cause infections in transplant patients varies greatly from organism to organism (Table 126–5). Therefore, careful attempts at definitive diagnosis of suspected infections must be made. If comprehensive workup reveals no source of infection, careful observation of the febrile transplant patient (rather than empirical therapy) is common practice. Surveillance cultures may be useful during the first 3 months for detecting CMV and HSV infections.[83,85,90,91,94] Management and monitoring of documented infections are similar to that in other types of patients.

Prevention of Infection in Solid-Organ Transplantation

❽ The goals of antimicrobial drug use in solid-organ transplant recipients are (a) prevention of infectious complications in the immediate postoperative period, (b) prevention of late infectious complications associated with prolonged periods of immunosuppression, and (c) effective treatment of established infections in order to prevent graft dysfunction and rejection and decrease patient morbidity and mortality. All of these goals must be achieved at the lowest possible toxicity and cost.

Prevention of infection in the transplant patient can be accomplished in a number of ways. First, risk of environmental contamination should be minimized.[95] Patients should be protected from institutional infectious outbreaks. Transplant patients should receive the pneumococcal vaccine once and the influenza vaccine yearly; however, their immunologic responses to these vaccines may be blunted by immunosuppressive therapy.[83]

Because the most important source of primary CMV disease is an infected donor organ, CMV-seronegative patients should not receive organs or blood products from seropositive donors if possible. A number of pharmacologic strategies have been studied in an attempt to prevent CMV infection. Prophylactic ganciclovir (administered as either 5 mg/kg IV every 12 hours or oral valganciclovir in doses ranging from 900 mg once daily to 1,000 mg three times daily) is effective in reducing the incidence of both primary and reactivated CMV disease in solid-organ transplantation.[78,83,84,89–92] Ganciclovir prophylaxis also may reduce reactivation of CMV disease significantly in seropositive patients receiving antithymocyte globulin or muromonab for treatment of acute rejection.[84,91,92] High-dose oral acyclovir effectively reduces the incidence of CMV infection and disease following renal transplantation. However, acyclovir is less efficacious in high-risk renal transplant patients (donor positive, recipient negative for CMV serum antibodies) and other nonrenal transplant types.[83,84,89,91,92,96] Preemptive ganciclovir (initiated after actual isolation of CMV from blood, urine, bronchoalveolar lavage fluid, or other site) is more effective than acyclovir in preventing both primary and reactivation disease in liver transplant recipients. Preemptive ganciclovir effectively prevents CMV disease in other types of solid-organ transplants as well.[90,91,94] Ganciclovir-related bone marrow suppression is not as problematic in solid-organ transplant recipients as in HSCT patients; most studies report the drug is reasonably well tolerated.[83,91,94,96]

Whether prophylaxis or preemptive therapy is the best approach to preventing CMV disease is controversial.[83,90–92,94] Prophylaxis is effective and easy to administer without the need for careful discrimination among suitable patients. However, universal prophylaxis results in unnecessary exposure of low-risk individuals to adverse effects of drugs, and there are concerns that prolonged exposure may increase the risk of viral resistance to drugs.[90,91,96] Preemptive therapy is effective and results in exposure of fewer patients to drugs. However, this strategy requires the availability and routine use of sensitive and specific diagnostic tests in order to identify high-risk individuals at an early stage of CMV infection. Although currently available PCR-based methods make this latter consideration less of an issue, PCR testing is not available at all centers. Prophylactic therapy should be used primarily in patients at highest risk of disease (i.e., seronegative patients receiving organs from seropositive donors), whereas other lower-risk patients should receive only preemptive therapy.[83,90,91,94] These recommendations are not universally accepted or practiced.

A number of studies have demonstrated the value of CMVIG in decreasing the incidence and severity of CMV disease following kidney, heart, lung, and liver transplantation.[83,90] Although prophylaxis with CMVIG has been strongly recommended for CMV-seronegative transplant recipients receiving organs from seropositive donors, the benefits of CMVIG relative to other therapies (e.g., prophylactic or preemptive ganciclovir) are not well known, and available studies have conflicting results. Whether the combination of CMVIG plus ganciclovir offers advantages over the use of either agent alone, either for primary prophylaxis or for treatment of established CMV disease, in solid-organ transplantation is unclear.[83,90] However, some authorities recommend use of CMVIG in combination with ganciclovir for treatment of severe, life-threatening CMV pneumonitis in solid-organ transplant recipients.[79,80]

Although use of prophylactic acyclovir in HSV-seropositive patients undergoing HSCT is well accepted, prophylaxis in solid-organ transplant recipients remains controversial. Reactivation disease caused by HSV occurs in approximately 25% of HSV-seropositive patients who are not receiving prophylaxis.[83] Oral or genital mucocutaneous disease is the most common presentation, but HSV pneumonitis also is seen occasionally and is associated with a mortality rate of approximately 75%.[83] Acyclovir is used at some centers because of the high incidence of clinical HSV infection, including pneumonias, after transplantation.

Prophylactic antimicrobial agents are of benefit to transplant patients in certain clinical situations. Antibiotic prophylaxis, with agents such as cefazolin started perioperatively and continued for less than 24 hours, is considered to reduce wound infection rates effectively following renal transplantation.[83,95] Although the benefits of perioperative prophylaxis have not been well demonstrated in other types of transplantation procedures, surgical prophylaxis usually is considered mandatory for liver, heart, and lung transplant patients because of the high risk of perioperative bacterial infections.[83,95] Pulmonary infections are particularly common in lung and heart and lung transplant recipients. They often are caused by bacteria colonizing the airways prior to transplantation. Therefore, perioperative antibiotics for lung and heart and lung procedures often are selected based on pretransplant sputum cultures.[83,95] In addition, posttransplant antibiotic prophylaxis is effective in decreasing the number of bacterial infections in renal transplant patients. Prophylactic trimethoprim–sulfamethoxazole traditionally has been used because it is inexpensive and well tolerated; other antibiotics, such as the fluoroquinolones, also have been evaluated.[83] Administration of oral low-dose trimethoprim–sulfamethoxazole (one double-strength tablet daily) for 6 to 12 months for prevention of *P. jiroveci* infection following heart and lung transplantation is common, although the efficacy and optimal duration are somewhat controversial.[83,97] Selective bowel decontamination with nonabsorbable antibiotics in combination with a low-bacterial diet (no fresh fruits and vegetables) effectively reduces oropharyngeal and GI colonization with gram-negative aerobes and *Candida* in liver transplant patients. However, selective bowel contamination is less efficacious when administered for a period of less than 1 week prior to transplantation.[95] Because liver transplantation usually is performed without advance notice as organs become emergently available, the practice of selective bowel decontamination remains controversial and is not recommended routinely.[83,95]

Because immunosuppressed transplant recipients are at risk for mucocutaneous fungal infections, prophylactic oral or topical antifungal agents may be indicated in these patients. Liver transplant patients are clearly at high risk for invasive fungal infections and should receive prophylaxis with fluconazole (400 mg/day).[25,83,85,98] High-dose fluconazole prophylaxis for lung and heart and lung transplant recipients has been suggested, but data supporting this recommendation are lacking.[25,85] Concentrations of immunosuppressant drugs should be monitored closely in transplant patients receiving fluconazole and other azole antifungal agents.

Transplant patients, especially heart and heart and lung recipients, without serologic evidence of prior exposure to *T. gondii* who receive organs from seropositive donors are at high risk for toxoplasmosis.[83] Many of these patients will be receiving trimethoprim–sulfamethoxazole for prophylaxis of *P. jiroveci* infection; this agent will provide effective prophylaxis against *T. gondii* as well as *N. asteroides.* Although prophylaxis is not given routinely at all centers, this therapy may be justified in high-risk patients because of the delays in diagnosis and serious infections associated with toxoplasmosis.[83]

Use of prophylactic isoniazid therapy for transplant patients with evidence of exposure to *M. tuberculosis* (positive purified protein derivative skin test) remains controversial. Risk of reactivation and development of clinical tuberculosis is enhanced with posttransplant immunosuppression. Some clinicians believe, however, that the risk of isoniazid-induced hepatotoxicity, especially in liver transplant recipients in whom the rate of hepatotoxicity has been reported as high as 40%, outweighs the benefits of treatment. High-risk patients who can be considered for isoniazid prophylaxis include those with a positive skin test, those with previously diagnosed tuberculosis who may not have been treated adequately, patients in close contact with individuals with active pulmonary disease, and patients with abnormal chest radiographs consistent with old tuberculosis who have not received prior prophylaxis.[83]

EVALUATION OF THERAPEUTIC OUTCOMES

Close monitoring of transplant recipients, including both clinical and laboratory data, is essential for early detection and treatment of potentially severe opportunistic infections.

ABBREVIATIONS

ANC: absolute neutrophil count

ASCO: American Society for Clinical Oncology

CDC: Centers for Disease Control and Prevention

CMVIG: cytomegalovirus hyperimmune globulin

CSF: colony-stimulating factor

GVHD: graft-versus-host disease

HSCT: hematopoietic stem cell transplantation

HSV: herpes simplex virus

IDSA: Infectious Diseases Society of America

MRSA: methicillin-resistant *Staphylococcus aureus*

NCCN: National Comprehensive Cancer Network

NNIS: National Nosocomial Infection Surveillance

PCR: polymerase chain reaction

PMN: polymorphonuclear leukocyte

VRE: vancomycin-resistant enterococci

VZV: varicella-zoster virus

REFERENCES

1. Hughes WT, Armstrong D, Bodey GP, et al. 2002 guidelines for the use of antimicrobial agents in neutropenic patients with cancer. Clin Infect Dis 2002;34:730–751.
2. Bow EJ. Management of the febrile neutropenic cancer patient: Lessons from 40 years of study. Clin Microbiol Infect 2005;11(Suppl 5):24–29.
3. Viscoli C, Varnier O, Machetti M. Infections in patients with febrile neutropenia: Epidemiology, microbiology, and risk stratification. Clin Infect Dis 2005;40(Suppl 4):S240–S245.
4. Donowitz GR, Maki DG, Crnich CJ, et al. Infections in the neutropenic patient: New views of an old problem. Hematology (Am Soc Hematol Educ Program) 2001;113–139.
5. National Comprehensive Cancer Network. Fever and neutropenia. Pract Guidelines Oncol 2002;1.
6. Sullivan KM, Dykewicz CA, Longworth DL, et al. Preventing opportunistic infections after hematopoietic stem cell transplantation: The Centers for Disease Control and Prevention, Infectious Diseases Society of America, and American Society for Blood and Marrow Transplantation practice guidelines and beyond. Hematology (Am Soc Hematol Educ Program) 2001;392–421.
7. Rolston KVI. Challenges in the treatment of infections caused by Gram-positive and Gram-negative bacteria in patients with cancer and neutropenia. Clin Infect Dis 2005;40(Suppl 4):S246–S252.
8. Toussaint E, Bahel-Ball E, Vekemans M, et al. Causes of fever in cancer patients (prospective study over 477 episodes). Support Care Cancer 2006;14:763–769.
9. Neuburger S, Maschmeyer G. Update on the management of infections in cancer and stem cell transplant patients. Ann Hematol 2006;85:345–356.
10. Hicks KL, Chemaly RF, Kontoyiannis DP. Common community respiratory viruses in patients with cancer: More than just "common colds." Cancer 2003;97:2576–2587.
11. Giamarellou H, Antoniadou A. Infectious complications of febrile leukopenia. Infect Dis Clin North Am 2001;15:457–482.
12. Safdar A. Managing opportunistic infections against the odds of neutropenia. Abstr Hematol Oncol 2003;6:20–26.
13. O'Brien SN, Blijlevens NMA, Mahfouz TH, Anaissie EJ. Infections in patients with hematological cancer: Recent developments. Hematology (Am Soc Hematol Educ Program) 2003;438–472.
14. Pascoe J, Cullen M. The prevention of febrile neutropenia. Curr Opin Hematol 2006;18:325–329.
15. U.S. Department of Public Health and Human Services, Public Health Service. National Nosocomial Infections Surveillance (NNIS) System Report, data summary from January 1992 through June 2004, issued October 2004. Am J Infect Control 2004;32:470–485.
16. Moran GJ, Amil RN, Abrahamian FM, Talan DA. Methicillin-resistant *Staphylococcus aureus* in community-acquired skin infections. Emerg Infect Dis 2005;11:928–930.
17. King MD, Humphrey BJ, Wang YF, et al. Emergence of community-acquired methicillin-resistant *Staphylococcus aureus* USA 300 clone as the predominant cause of skin and soft-tissue infections. Ann Intern Med 2006;144:309–317.
18. Tunkel AR, Sepkowitz KA. Infections caused by viridans streptococci in patients with neutropenia. Clin Infect Dis 2002;34:1524–1529.
19. Avery R, Kalaycio M, Pohlman B, et al. Early vancomycin-resistant enterococcus (VRE) bacteremia after allogeneic bone marrow transplantation is associated with a rapidly deteriorating clinical course. Bone Marrow Transplant 2005;35:497–499.
20. Engemann JJ, Carmeli Y, Cosgrove SE, et al. Adverse clinical and economic outcomes attributable to methicillin resistance among patients with *Staphylococcus aureus* surgical site infection. Clin Infect Dis 2003;36:592–598.
21. Bissinger AL, Einsele H, Hamprecht K, et al. Infectious pulmonary complications after stem cell transplantation or chemotherapy: Diagnostic yield of bronchoalveolar lavage. Diagn Microbiol Infect Dis 2005;52:275–280.
22. Junghanss C, Marr KA, Carter RA, et al. Incidence and outcome of bacterial and fungal infections following nonmyeloablative compared with myeloablative allogeneic hematopoietic stem cell transplantation: A matched case control study. Biol Blood Marrow Transplant 2002;8:512–520.

23. Chatzinikolaou I, Abi-Said D, Bodey, GP, et al. Recent experience with *Pseudomonas aeruginosa* bacteremia in patients with cancer: Retrospective analysis of 245 episodes. Arch Intern Med 2000;160:501–509.
24. Bodey GP, Bueltmann B, Duguid W, et al. Fungal infections in cancer patients: An international autopsy survey. Eur J Clin Microbiol Infect Dis 1992;11:99–109.
25. Pappas PG, Rex JH, Sobel JD, et al. Guidelines for treatment of candidiasis. Clin Infect Dis 2004:38:161–189.
26. Viscoli C, Girmenia C, Marinus A, et al. Candidemia in cancer patients: A prospective, multicenter surveillance study by the Invasive Fungal Infections Group (IFIG) of the European Organization for Research and treatment of Cancer (EORTC). Clin Infect Dis 1999;28:1071–1079.
27. Segal BH, Bow EJ, Menichetti F. Fungal infections in nontransplant patients with hematologic malignancies. Infect Dis Clin North Am 2002;16:935–964.
28. Groll AH, Walsh TJ. Uncommon opportunistic fungi: New nosocomial threats. Clin Microbiol Infect 2001;7(Suppl 2):8–24.
29. Malani A, Hmoud J, Chiu L, et al. *Candida glabrata* fungemia: Experience in a tertiary care center. Clin Infect Dis 2005;41:975–981.
30. Segal BH, Almyroudis NG, Battiwalla M, et al. Prevention and early treatment of invasive fungal infection in patients with cancer and neutropenia and in stem cell transplant recipients in the era of newer broad-spectrum antifungal agents and diagnostic adjuncts. Clin Infect Dis 2007;44:402–409.
31. Stevens DA, Kan VL, Judson MA, et al. Practice guidelines for diseases caused by *Aspergillus*. Clin Infect Dis 2000;30:696–709.
32. Vidal L, Paul M, Ben dor I, et al. Oral versus intravenous antibiotic treatment for febrile neutropenia in cancer patients: A systematic review and meta-analysis of randomized trials. J Antimicrob Chemother 2004;54:29–37.
33. Freifeld A, Marchigiani D, Walsh T, et al. A double-blind comparison of empirical oral and intravenous antibiotic therapy for low-risk febrile patients with neutropenia during cancer chemotherapy. N Engl J Med 1999;341:305–311.
34. Kern WV, Cometta A, DeBock R, et al. Oral versus intravenous empirical antimicrobial therapy for fever in patients with granulocytopenia who are receiving cancer chemotherapy. N Engl J Med 1999;341:312–318.
35. Escalante CP, Rubenstein EB, Rolston KV. Outpatient antibiotic therapy for febrile episodes in low-risk neutropenic patients with cancer. Cancer Invest 1997;15:237–242.
36. Shenep JL, Flynn PM, Baker DK, et al. Oral cefixime is similar to continued intravenous antibiotics in the empirical treatment of febrile neutropenic children with cancer. Clin Infect Dis 2001;32:36–43.
37. Giamarellou H, Bassaris HP, Petrikkos G, et al. Monotherapy with intravenous followed by oral high-dose ciprofloxacin versus combination therapy with ceftazidime plus amikacin as initial empirical therapy for granulocytopenic patients with fever. Antimicrob Agents Chemother 2000;44:3264–3271.
38. Furno P, Bucaneve G, Del Favero A. Monotherapy or aminoglycoside-containing combinations for empirical antibiotic treatment of febrile neutropenic patients: A meta-analysis. Lancet Infect Dis 2002;2:231–242.
39. Paul M, Soares-Weiser K, Grozinsky S, Leibovici L. β-Lactam versus β-lactam-aminoglycoside combination therapy in cancer patients with neutropaenia. Cochrane Database Syst Rev 2003;3:CD003038.
40. Paul M, Yahava D, Fraser A, Leibovici L. Empirical antibiotic monotherapy for febrile neutropenia: Systematic review and meta-analysis of randomized controlled trials. J Antimicrob Chemother 2006;57:176–189.
41. Glasmacher A, von Lilienfeld-Toal M, Schulte S, et al. An evidence-based evaluation of important aspects of empirical antibiotic therapy in febrile neutropenic patients. Clin Microbiol Infect 2005;11(Suppl 5):17–23.
42. Hatala R, Dinh TT, Cook DJ. Single daily dosing of aminoglycosides in immunocompromised adults: A systematic review. Clin Infect Dis 1997;24:810–815.
43. Feld R. Vancomycin as part of initial empirical antibiotic therapy for febrile neutropenia in patients with cancer: Pros and cons. Clin Infect Dis 1999;29:503–507.
44. Paul M, Borok S, Fraser A, et al. Empirical antibiotics against Gram-positive infections for febrile neutropenia: Systematic review and meta-analysis of randomized controlled trials. J Antimicrob Chemother 2005;55:436–444.
45. Cometta A, Kern WV, De Bock R, et al. Vancomycin versus placebo for treating persistent fever in patients with neutropenic cancer receiving piperacillin-tazobactam monotherapy. Clin Infect Dis 2003;37:382–389.
46. Centers for Disease Control and Prevention. Recommendations for preventing the spread of vancomycin resistance: Recommendations of the Hospital Infection Control Practices Advisory Committee (HICPAC). MMWR 1995;44(RR-12):1–13.
47. Antabli BA, Bross P, Siegel RS, et al. Empirical antimicrobial therapy of febrile neutropenic patients undergoing haematopoietic stem cell transplantation. Int J Antimicrob Agents 1999;13:127–130.
48. Peacock JE Jr, Herrington DA, Wade JC, et al. Ciprofloxacin plus piperacillin compared with tobramycin plus piperacillin as empirical therapy in febrile neutropenia patients: A randomized, double-blind trial. Ann Intern Med 2002;137:77–87.
49. Scheld WM. Maintaining fluoroquinolone class efficacy: Review of influencing factors. Emerg Infect Dis, 2003, *http://www.cdc.gov/ncidod/eid/vol9no1/02-0277.htm.*
50. Elting LS, Rubenstein EB, Rolston K, et al. Time to clinical response: An outcome of antibiotic therapy of febrile neutropenia with implications for quality and cost of care. J Clin Oncol 2000;18:3699–3706.
51. Martino R, Viscoli C. Empirical antifungal therapy in patients with neutropenia and persistent of recurrent fever of unknown origin. Br J Haematol 2005;132:138–154.
52. Blau IW, Fauser AA. Review of comparative studies between conventional and liposomal amphotericin B (AmBisome®) in neutropenic patients with fever of unknown origin and patients with systemic mycosis. Mycoses 2000;43:325–332.
53. Walsh TJ, Finberg RW, Arndt C, et al. Liposomal amphotericin B for empirical therapy in patients with persistent fever and neutropenia. N Engl J Med 1999;340:764–771.
54. Boogaerts M, Winston DJ, Bow EJ, et al. Intravenous and oral itraconazole versus intravenous amphotericin B deoxycholate as empirical antifungal therapy for persistent fever in neutropenic patients with cancer who are receiving broad-spectrum antibacterial therapy: A randomized, controlled trial. Ann Intern Med 2001;135:412–422.
55. Walsh TJ, Pappas P, Winston DJ, et al. Voriconazole compared with liposomal amphotericin B for empirical antifungal therapy in patients with neutropenia and persistent fever. N Engl J Med 2002;346:225–234.
56. Walsh TJ, Teppler H, Donowitz GR, et al. Caspofungin versus liposomal amphotericin B for empirical antifungal therapy in patients with persistent fever and neutropenia. N Engl J Med 2004;351:1391–1402.
57. Ozer H, Armitage JO, Bennett CL, et al. 2000 update of recommendations for the use of hematopoietic colony-stimulating factors: Evidence-based, clinical practice guidelines. J Clin Oncolol 2000;18:3558–3585.
58. Clark OA, Lyman G, Castro AA, et al. Colony-stimulating factors for chemotherapy-induced febrile neutropenia. Cochrane Database Syst Rev 2003;3:CD003039.
59. Atallah E, Schiffer CA. Granulocyte transfusion. Curr Opin Hematol 2006;13:45–49.
60. Hubel K, Dale DC, Engert A, Liles WC. Current status of granulocyte (neutrophil) transfusion therapy for infectious diseases. J Infect Dis 2001;183:321–328.
61. Gafter-Gvili A, Paul M, Fraser A, Leibovici L. Effect of quinolone prophylaxis in afebrile neutropenic patients on microbial resistance: Systematic review and meta-analysis. J Antimicrob Chemother 2007;59:5–22.
62. Munoz L, Martino R, Subira M, et al. Intensified prophylaxis of febrile neutropenia with ofloxacin plus rifampin during severe short-duration neutropenia in patients with lymphoma. Leuk Lymphoma 1999;34:585–589.
63. Cornely OA, Ullmann AJ, Karthaus M. Evidence-based assessment of primary antifungal prophylaxis in patients with hematologic malignancies. Blood 2003;101:3365–3372.
64. Bow EJ, Laverdiere M, Lussier N, et al. Antifungal prophylaxis for severely neutropenic chemotherapy recipients: A meta-analysis of randomized-controlled clinical trials. Cancer 2002;94:3230–3246.
65. Rotstein C, Bow EJ, Laverdiere M, et al. Randomized placebo-controlled trial of fluconazole prophylaxis for neutropenic cancer patients: Benefit based on purpose and intensity of cytotoxic therapy. Clin Infect Dis 1999;28:331–340.
66. Winston DJ, Maziarz RT, Chandrasekar PH, et al. Intravenous and oral itraconazole versus intravenous and oral fluconazole for long-

term antifungal prophylaxis in allogeneic hematopoietic stem-cell transplant recipients: A multicenter, randomized trial. Ann Intern Med 2003;138:705–713.
67. Ullmann AJ, Cornely OA. Antifungal prophylaxis for invasive mycoses in high risk patients. Curr Opin Infect Dis 2006;19:571–576.
68. de Lalla F. Antibiotic treatment of febrile episodes in neutropenic cancer patients: Clinical and economic considerations. Drugs 1997;53:789–804.
69. van Tiel FH, Harbers MM, Kessels AG, Schouten HC. Home care versus hospital care of patients with hematological malignancies and chemotherapy-induced cytopenia. Ann Oncol 2005;16:195–205.
70. Gratwohl A, Brand R, Frassoni F, et al. Cause of death after allogeneic hematopoietic stem cell transplantation (HSCT) in early leukemias: An EBMT analysis of lethal infectious complications and changes over calendar time. Bone Marrow Transplant 2005;36:757–769.
71. Afessa B, Peters SG. Major complications following hematopoietic stem cell transplantation. Semin Respir Crit Care Med 2006;27:297–309.
72. Mitchell AE, Derrington P, Turner P, et al. Gram-negative bacteraemia (GNB) after 428 unrelated donor bone marrow transplants (UD-BMT): Risk factors, prophylaxis, therapy, and outcome. Bone Marrow Transplant 2004;33:303–310.
73. Leather HL, Wingard JR. Infections following hematopoietic stem cell transplantation. Infect Dis Clin North Am 2001;15:483–520.
74. Lin S-J, Schranz J, Teutsch SM. Aspergillosis case-fatality rate: Systematic review of the literature. Clin Infect Dis 2001;32:358–366.
75. Ketterer N, Espinouse D, Chomarat M, et al. Infections following peripheral blood progenitor cell transplantation for lymphoproliferative malignancies: Etiology and potential risk factors. Am J Med 1999;106:191–197.
76. Darville JM, Ley BE, Roome AP, et al. Acyclovir-resistant herpes simplex virus infections in a bone marrow transplant population. Bone Marrow Transplant 1998;22:587–589.
77. Nguyen Q, Champlin R, Giralt S, et al. Late cytomegalovirus pneumonia in adult allogeneic blood and marrow transplant recipients. Clin Infect Dis 1999;28:618–623.
78. Razonable RR, Paya CV. Valganciclovir for the prevention and treatment of cytomegalovirus disease in immunocompromised hosts. Expert Rev Anti Infect Ther 2004;2:27–42.
79. Orange JS, Hossny EM, Weiler CR, et al. Use of intravenous immunoglobulin in human disease: A review of evidence by members of the Primary Immunodeficiency Committee of the American Academy of Allergy, Asthma, and Immunology. J Allergy Clin Immunol 2006; 117:S525–S553.
80. Crumpacker CS, Wadhwa S. Cytomegalovirus. In: Mandell GL, Bennett JE, Dolin R, eds. Principles and Practice of Infectious Diseases, 6th ed. New York: Churchill-Livingstone, 2005:1786–1801.
81. Strasfeld L, Weinstock DM. Antifungal prophylaxis among allogeneic hematopoietic stem cell transplant recipients: Current issues and new agents. Expert Rev Anti Infect Ther 2006;4:457–468.
82. Mele A, Paterson PJ, Prentice HG, et al: Toxoplasmosis in bone marrow transplantation: A report of two cases and systematic review of the literature. Bone Marrow Transplant 2002;29:691–698.
83. Simon DM, Levin S. Infectious complications of solid organ transplantations. Infect Dis Clin North Am 2001;15:521–549.
84. Varon NF, Alangaden GJ. Emerging trends in infections among renal transplant recipients. Expert Rev Anti-Infect Ther 2004;2:95–109.
85. Singh N. Fungal infections in the recipients of solid organ transplantation. Infect Dis Clin North Am 2003;17:113–134.
86. Montoya JG, Giraldo LF, Efron B, et al. Infectious complications among 620 consecutive heart transplant recipients at Stanford University Medical Center. Clin Infect Dis 2001;33:629–640.
87. Kotton CN. Zoonoses in solid-organ and hematopoietic stem cell transplant recipients. Clin Infect Dis 2007;44:857–866.
88. Kotton CN, Fishman JA. Viral infection in the renal transplant recipient. J Am Soc Nephrol 2005;16:1758–1774.
89. Pescovitz MD. Benefits of cytomegalovirus prophylaxis in solid organ transplantation. Transplantation 2006;82:S4–S8.
90. Kletzmayr J, Kreuzwieser E, Klauser R. New developments in the management of cytomegalovirus infection and disease after renal transplantation. Curr Opin Urol 2001;11:153–158.
91. Singh N. Preemptive therapy versus universal prophylaxis with ganciclovir for cytomegalovirus in solid organ transplant recipients. Clin Infect Dis 2001;32:742–751.
92. Pereyra F, Rubin RH. Prevention and treatment of cytomegalovirus infection in solid organ transplant recipients. Curr Opin Infect Dis 2004;17:357–361.
93. Roland ME, Adey D, Carlson LL, Terrault NA. Kidney and liver transplantation in HIV-infected patients: Case presentations and review. AIDS Patient Care STDs 2003;17:501–507.
94. Strippoli GFM, Hodson EM, Jones C, Craig JC. Preemptive treatment for cytomegalovirus viremia to prevent cytomegalovirus disease in solid organ transplant recipients. Transplantation 2006;81:139–145.
95. Soave R. Prophylaxis strategies for solid-organ transplantation. Clin Infect Dis 2001;33(Suppl 1):S26–S31.
96. Van der Bij W, Speich R. Management of cytomegalovirus infection and disease after solid-organ transplantation. Clin Infect Dis 2001;33(Suppl 1):S33–S37.
97. Fishman JA. Prevention of infection caused by *Pneumocystis jiroveci* in transplant recipients. Clin Infect Dis 2001;33:1397–1405.
98. Paya CV. Prevention of fungal and hepatitis viral infections in liver transplantation. Clin Infect Dis 2001;33(Suppl 1):S47–S52.

CHAPTER 127

Antimicrobial Prophylaxis in Surgery

SALMAAN KANJI AND JOHN W. DEVLIN

KEY CONCEPTS

1. *Prophylactic* antibiotic therapy differs from *presumptive* and *therapeutic* antibiotic therapy in that the latter two involve treatment regimens for documented or presumed infections, whereas the goal of prophylactic therapy is to prevent infections in high-risk patients or procedures.

2. The risk of a surgical site infection (SSI) is determined from both the type of surgery and patient-specific risk factors; however, most commonly used classification systems account for only procedure-related risk factors.

3. Timing of antimicrobial prophylaxis is of paramount importance. Antibiotics should be administered within 1 hour before surgery to ensure adequate drug levels at the surgical site prior to the initial incision.

4. Antimicrobial agents with short half-lives (e.g., cefazolin) may require intraoperative redosing during long (>3 hours) procedures.

5. The type of surgery, intrinsic patient risk factors, most commonly identified pathogenic organisms, institutional antimicrobial resistance patterns, and cost must be considered when choosing an antimicrobial agent for prophylaxis.

6. Single-dose prophylaxis is appropriate for many types of surgery. First-generation cephalosporins (e.g., cefazolin) are the mainstay for prophylaxis in most surgical procedures because of their spectrum of activity, safety, and cost.

7. Vancomycin as a prophylactic agent should be limited to patients with a documented history of life-threatening β-lactam hypersensitivity or patients in whom the incidence of infections with organisms resistant to cefazolin (e.g., methicillin-resistant *Staphylococcus aureus*) is high enough to justify use.

According to the National Center for Health Statistics, approximately 46 million surgical procedures are performed annually in the United States, the majority of which are done in an outpatient setting.[1] Infection is the most common complication of surgery.[2] Surgical site infections (SSIs) occur in approximately 3% to 6% of patients and prolong hospitalization by an average of 7 days at a direct annual cost of $5 to $10 billion.[3,4] SSIs are the third (14%–16%) most frequent cause of nosocomial infections among hospitalized patients, and the primary (40%) cause of nosocomial infection in surgical patients.[3] Prophylactic administration of antibiotics decreases the risk of infection after many surgical procedures and represents an important component of care for this population.

Learning objectives, review questions, and other resources can be found at **www.pharmacotherapyonline.com.**

Antibiotics administered prior to the contamination of previously sterile tissues or fluids are called *prophylactic* antibiotics. The goal of therapy is to *prevent* an infection from developing. Although eradication of distal (preexisting, unrelated to surgery) infections lowers the risk for subsequent postoperative infections, it does not, per se, constitute a prophylactic regimen. In fact, surgical prophylaxis often is prescribed concurrently under these circumstances because of important antimicrobial spectrum- and timing-related concerns. Both SSIs and infections not directly related to the surgical site (e.g., urinary tract infections, pneumonia) are termed *nosocomial.* Prevention of hospital-acquired infections is a major goal of antibiotic prophylaxis.

1 *Presumptive* antibiotic therapy is administered when an infection is suspected but not yet proven. Clinical scenarios where presumptive therapy is used commonly include acute cholecystitis, open compound fractures, and acute appendicitis of less than 24 hours' duration. In these situations, if signs of perforation or infection are absent during surgery, then routine prophylactic rather than presumptive therapy is warranted. An operative finding of a gangrenous gallbladder or a perforated appendix, however, is suggestive of an established infectious process, and a *therapeutic* antibiotic regimen is required.[3]

According to the Centers for Disease Control and Prevention's (CDC) National Nosocomial Infections Surveillance System (NNIS),[3] SSIs can be categorized as either incisional (e.g., cellulitis of the incision site) or organ/space (e.g., meningitis; Fig. 127–1). Incisional SSIs are subcategorized into superficial (involving only the skin or subcutaneous tissue) and deep (fascial and muscle layers) infections. Organ/space SSIs can involve any anatomic area other than the incision site. For example, a patient who develops bacterial peritonitis after bowel surgery has an organ/space SSI. By definition, SSIs must occur within 30 days of surgery. If a prosthetic implant is involved, a deep incisional or organ/space SSI can be reported up to 1 year from the date of surgery. Although microbiologic testing of surgical drainage material or sites may help to guide care, the specificity of a negative culture is poor and generally does not rule out an SSI.[3]

SSI RISK FACTORS

2 SSI incidence depends on both procedure- and patient-related factors. Traditionally, the risk for SSIs has been stratified by surgical procedure in a classification system developed by the National Research Council (NRC; Table 127–1).[5] The NRC classification system proposes that the risk of an SSI depends on the microbiology of the surgical site, presence of a preexisting infection, likelihood of

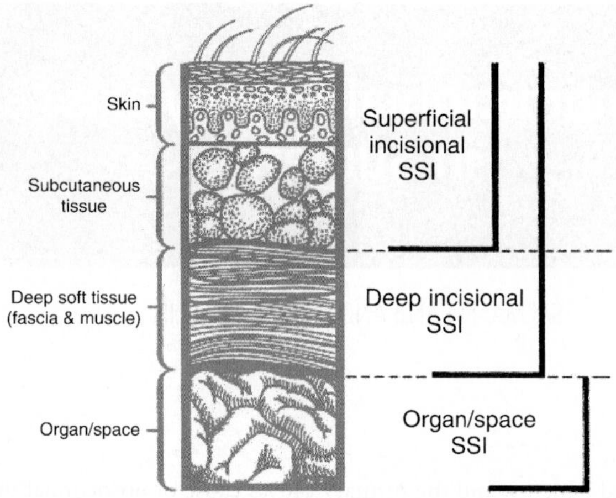

FIGURE 127-1. Cross section of abdominal wall depicting Centers for Disease Control and Prevention classifications of surgical site infections (SSI). *(Reprinted from Am J Infect Control, Vol. 27, Mangram AJ, Horan TC, Pearson ML, et al. Guideline for prevention of surgical site infection. Copyright 1999, with permission from Elsevier. Centers for Disease Control and Prevention (CDC) Hospital Infection Control Practices Advisory Committee, Pages 97–132, Copyright 1999, with permission from the Association for Professionals in Infection Control and Epidemiology.)*

contaminating previously sterile tissue during surgery, and events during and after surgery.[5,6] A patient's NRC procedure classification is the primary determinant of whether antibiotic prophylaxis is warranted. However, because a patient's NRC wound classification is influenced by surgical findings (e.g., gangrenous gallbladder) and perioperative events (e.g., major technique breaks), categorization generally occurs intraoperatively.[7]

INHERENT PATIENT RISK

The NRC classification system does not account for the influence of underlying patient risk factors for SSI development, instead categorizing the risks for SSIs simply based on a specific surgical procedure. Disease states and conditions known to increase SSI risk are listed in Table 127–2. Preexisting distal infections increase SSI rates and should be resolved prior to surgery whenever possible. Diabetic patients have an increased risk for SSIs, especially patients with uncontrolled perioperative blood sugars.[8] Preoperative smoking has been identified as an independent risk factor for SSI because of the deleterious effects of nicotine on wound healing. Preoperative immunosuppression, including corticosteroid use, may increase infection risk. Malnutrition is a well-described risk factor for postoperative complications, including SSI, impaired wound and colonic anastomosis healing, and prolonged hospital stay. Although enteral feeding during the perioperative period can reduce bacterial translocation by maintaining the integrity of the intestinal mucosa, nutritional supplementation does not decrease the incidence of infection.[9]

CLINICAL CONTROVERSY

Several studies have investigated the role of specialized enteral formulas fortified with a variety of immunomodulating micronutrients thought to enhance the immune response and gut function after trauma or surgery. Although many clinicians are exploring the role of supplements such as glutamine, arginine, ω-3 fatty acids, and nucleotides, no study to date has shown a significant reduction in postoperative infection rates using these formulations.

Colonization of the nares with *Staphylococcus aureus* is a well-described SSI risk factor.[3] Although intranasal application of mupirocin ointment reduces the rate of nasal carriage of *S. aureus*, one large, randomized, double-blinded study of 4,030 surgical patients found that prophylactic intranasal mupirocin did not reduce the rate of *S. aureus* SSI, although it did reduce the rate of nosocomial *S. aureus* infections among patients who were *S. aureus* carriers.[10] Other factors shown to increase the risk of SSI are age, length of preoperative hospital stay, and obesity.[3]

IDENTIFYING SSI RISK

Two large epidemiologic studies have objectively quantified SSI risk based on specific patient- and procedure-related factors. The Study on the Efficacy of Nosocomial Infection Control (SENIC) analyzed more than 100,000 surgery cases to identify and validate risk factors for SSI.[11] Abdominal operations, operations lasting longer than 2 hours, contaminated or "dirty" procedures (as per NRC classification), and more than three underlying medical diagnoses each was associated with an increased incidence of SSI. When NRC classification was stratified by number of SENIC risk factors present, SSI incidence varied by as much as a factor of 15 within the same NRC operative category (Table 127–3).[12]

In a subsequent analysis of more than 84,000 surgical cases, the NNIS attempted to simplify and refine the SENIC system by quantifying intrinsic patient risk using the American Society of Anesthesiologists (ASA) preoperative assessment score (Table 127–4).[14,15] An ASA score ≥3 was a strong predictor for the development of an SSI. Other factors associated with increased SSI incidence include contaminated or "dirty" operations (NRC criteria) and surgical proce-

TABLE 127-1 NRC Wound Classification, Risk of SSI, and Indication for Antibiotics

	SSI Rate (%)			
Classification	***Preoperative Antibiotics***	***No Preoperative Antibiotics***	**Criteria**	**Antibiotics**
Clean	5.1	0.8	No acute inflammation or transection of gastrointestinal, oropharyngeal, genitourinary, biliary, or respiratory tracts. Elective case, no technique break.	Not indicated unless high-risk procedure[a]
Clean–contaminated	10.1	1.3	Controlled opening of aforementioned tracts with minimal spillage/minor technique break. Clean procedures performed emergently or with major technique breaks.	Prophylactic antibiotics indicated
Contaminated	21.9	10.2	Acute, nonpurulent inflammation present. Major spillage/technique break during clean–contaminated procedure.	Prophylactic antibiotics indicated
Dirty	N/A	N/A	Obvious preexisting infection present (abscess, pus, or necrotic tissue present).	Therapeutic antibiotics required

NRC, National Research Council; SSI, surgical-site infection.
[a]High-risk procedures include implantation of prosthetic materials and other procedures where surgical site infection is associated with high morbidity (see text).
Adapted from refs. 5 and 11.

TABLE 127-2 Patient and Operation Characteristics That May Influence the Risk of Surgical Site Infection

Patient	Operation
Age	Duration of surgical scrub
Nutritional status	Preoperative skin preparation
Diabetes	Preoperative shaving
Smoking	Duration of operation
Obesity	Antimicrobial prophylaxis
Coexisting infections at distal body sites	Operating room ventilation
Colonization with resistant microorganisms	Sterilization of instruments
Altered immune response	Implantation of prosthetic materials
Length of preoperative stay	Surgical drains
	Surgical technique

Reprinted and adapted from Am J Infect Control, Vol. 27, Mangram AJ, Horan TC, Pearson ML, et al. Guideline for prevention of surgical site infection. Copyright 1999, with permission from Elsevier. Centers for Disease Control and Prevention (CDC) Hospital Infection Control Practices Advisory Committee, Pages 97–132, Copyright 1999, with permission from the Association for Professionals in Infection Control and Epidemiology.

dures lasting longer than average. Similar to the SENIC study, the SSI rate was linked to the number of risk factors present and varied considerably within NRC class. The NNIS basic SSI risk index is composed of the following criteria: ASA score = 3, 4, or 5; wound class; and duration of surgery. Overall, for 34 of the 44 NNIS procedure categories, SSI rates increased proportionally with the number of risk factors present.[13] The SSI rate was generally lower when the procedure was performed done laparoscopically.

Although evidence-based recommendations for antimicrobial prophylaxis during surgery are best established using the results of randomized clinical trials, many studies have small sample sizes and do not stratify patients according to overall SSI risk. Future studies, particularly those involving clean procedures, should be stratified by SSI risk so that the subset of high-risk patients who might benefit the most from prophylaxis is clearly established.

BACTERIOLOGY

The most important consideration when choosing antibiotic prophylaxis is the bacteriology of the surgical site. Organisms involved in an SSI are acquired one of two ways: endogenously (from the patient's own normal flora) or exogenously (from contamination during the surgical procedure). Based on the type and anatomic location of the procedure and the NRC classification (see Table 127–1), resident flora can be predicted and appropriate antibiotic choices made. According to NNIS data, *S. aureus*, coagulase-negative Staphylococci, Enterococci, *Escherichia coli*, and *Pseudomonas aeruginosa* are the pathogens most commonly isolated (Table 127–5).[14] With the widespread use of broad-spectrum antibiotics, however, *Candida* spp. and methicillin-resistant *Staphylococcus aureus* (MRSA) are becoming more prevalent.[14]

Factors affecting the ability of an organism to induce an SSI depend on organism count, organism virulence, and host immunocompetency. Organisms in the commensal flora generally are not pathogenic. These organisms often serve the host as a form of protection against invasive organisms that otherwise would colonize the surgical site. Opportunistic organisms usually are kept in check by normal flora and rarely are problematic unless they are present in large numbers. Loss of normal flora through use of broad-spectrum antibiotics can destabilize homeostasis, allowing pathogenic bacteria to proliferate and infection to occur.[4]

Normal flora translocated to a normally sterile tissue site or fluid during a surgical procedure can become pathogenic. For example, *S. aureus* or *S. epidermidis* may be translocated from the surface of the skin to deeper tissues or *E. coli* from the colon to the peritoneal cavity, bloodstream, or urinary tract. Studies in animals and healthy volunteers have shown bacterial virulence to be an important determinant in the development of secondary infections.[16,17] Whereas more than one million *S. aureus* per square centimeter or gram of tissue are required to produce infection in animals, less than 100,000 *Streptococcus pyogenes* per square centimeter or gram of tissue are required at the same site.[17,18]

Impaired host defense reduces the number of bacteria required to establish an infection. A breach of normal host defenses through surgical intervention (e.g., insertion of a prosthetic device) may enable organisms to cause infection. In addition, the loss of specific immune factors, such as complement activation, tissue-derived inhibitors (e.g., proinflammatory cytokines), cell-mediated response (e.g., T-cell function), and granulocytic or phagocytic function (e.g., neutrophils or macrophages) can greatly increase the risk for SSI development.[19] Vascular occlusive states related to the surgical procedure or those occurring from hypovolemic shock can greatly affect blood flow to the surgical site, thus diminishing host defense mech-

TABLE 127-3 Surgical Site Infection Incidence (%) Stratified by NRC Wound Classification and SENIC Risk Factors

No. of SENIC Risk Factors[a]	Clean	Clean–Contaminated	Contaminated	Dirty
0	1.1	0.6	N/A	N/A
1	3.9	2.8	4.5	6.7
2	8.4	8.4	8.3	10.9
3	15.8	17.7	11.0	18.8
4	N/A	N/A	23.9	27.4

[a]Study on the Efficacy of Nosocomial Infection Control (SENIC) risk factors include abdominal operation, operations lasting >2 hours, contaminated or dirty procedures by National Research Council (NRC) classification, and more than three underlying medical diagnoses.

Gaynes RP, Culver DH, Horan TC, et al. Surgical site infection (SSI) rates in the United States, 1992–1998: The national nosocomial infections surveillance system basic SSI risk index. Clin Infect Dis 2001;33(Suppl 2):S69–S77. Copyright The University of Chicago Press.

TABLE 127-4 American Society of Anesthesiologists Physical Status Classification

Class	Description
1	Normal healthy patient
2	Mild systemic disease
3	Severe systemic disease that is not incapacitating
4	Incapacitating systemic disease that is a constant threat to life
5	Not expected to survive 24 hours with or without operation

Data from Owens WD, Felts JA, Spitznagel EL: ASA physical status classifications: A study of consistency of ratings. Anesthesiology 1978;49:239–243.

TABLE 127-5 Major Pathogens in Surgical Wound Infections

Pathogen	Percent of Infections[a]
Staphylococcus aureus	20
Coagulase-negative staphylococci	14
Enterococci	12
Escherichia coli	8
Pseudomonas aeruginosa	8
Enterobacter spp.	7
Proteus mirabilis	3
Klebsiella pneumoniae	3
Other *Streptococcus* spp.	3
Candida albicans	3
Group D streptococci	2
Other gram-positive aerobes	2
Bacteroides fragilis	2

[a]Data reported by the National Nosocomial Infections Surveillance System from January 1992 through June 2004.

Data from NNIS; adapted from ref. 5.

anisms against microbial invasion. Traumatized tissue, hematomas, and the presence of foreign material also lead to more infections. When a foreign body is introduced during a surgical procedure, fewer than 100 bacterial colony-forming units are required to cause an SSI.[20] Studies examining *S. aureus*–contaminated wound infections on the skin of healthy volunteers demonstrate a 10,000-fold reduction in the number of organisms required to establish a wound infection if sutures are not present.[16]

ANTIMICROBIAL RESISTANCE

Colonization of the host with antibiotic-resistant hospital flora prior to or during surgery may lead to an SSI that is unresponsive to routine antibiotic therapy. The most common cause of nosocomially acquired multiresistant organisms is transmission from hospital personnel.[21] Patients treated with broad-spectrum antibiotic therapy are at increased risk for colonization with hospital flora.

With cephalosporins established as first-line agents for prophylaxis over the past decade, organisms resistant to cephalosporins represent the majority of pathogens causing SSIs. The CDC has reported an alarming increase in the incidence of vancomycin-resistant enterococci (VRE) infections, particularly those with *E. faecium.*[3] Risk factors for VRE colonization include severe concomitant diseases, immunosuppression, admission to the intensive care unit, previous intraabdominal or cardiothoracic surgery, placement of indwelling catheters, and prolonged courses of antimicrobials, ❼ particularly vancomycin.[22,23] In an effort to control the spread of VRE, the CDC has published recommendations that include strict criteria for use of vancomycin as surgical prophylaxis.[23] The guidelines suggest vancomycin substitution for cefazolin as SSI prophylaxis only in cases with a high suspicion of MRSA or in patients with a documented history of a life-threatening allergy to penicillins or cephalosporins. Other limitations to vancomycin use, other than risk of inducing resistant organisms, are the drug's narrow spectrum of activity, its poor penetration into some tissues, and the potential for infusion-related reactions.

The emergence of *S. aureus* displaying intermediate resistance (minimum inhibitory concentration [MIC] ≥8 mcg/mL) further underscores the need to limit routine use of vancomycin for prophylaxis.[24] Methicillin resistance not only limits the options available to treat these infections but is associated with patient mortality twice that of patients with infections caused by methicillin-sensitive *Staphylococcus aureus* (MSSA).[25] Postoperative factors associated with MRSA include discharge to a long-term care facility and duration of postoperative antibiotic treatment >1 day.[26] Although several published guidelines for surgical prophylaxis recommend use of vancomycin for prophylaxis for some operations performed in hospitals with a high rate of infection due to MRSA, there is little guidance on what constitutes a "high rate" of MRSA infection and whether providing prophylaxis with vancomycin alone will result in fewer SSIs.[4]

Although cefazolin remains a mainstay in cardiovascular SSI prophylaxis, its failure has been reported in cases involving MSSA. In a comparison trial between cefamandole and cefazolin, significantly more failures were attributed to cefazolin, even though the primary pathogen was MSSA.[27] However, a similar trial comparing cefazolin and cefuroxime did not show any difference in SSI incidence between the two regimens.[27] It has been proposed that the β-lactamase expressed by some MSSA is capable of hydrolyzing cefazolin more readily than cefuroxime or cefamandole. Although this trend is disturbing, the overall incidence of cefazolin failure remains low, and cefazolin remains the drug of choice for SSI prophylaxis in cardiovascular surgery.[27]

The increase in frequency of fungal infections in surgical patients has drawn concern. In hospitalized patients, the incidence of nosocomial *Candida* infections has approximately doubled from 1992 to 2004.[14,28] Overzealous use of broad-spectrum antibiotics is the most likely cause for this increase. A study of patients undergoing cardiovascular surgery identified sex (female), length of stay in the intensive care unit, and duration of central venous catheterization as risk factors for postoperative *Candida* infections.[29] Although presurgical *Candida* colonization is associated with a higher risk of fungal SSIs, routine preoperative use of prophylactic antifungal agents is not being advocated at this time.[28,30]

SCHEDULING ANTIBIOTIC ADMINISTRATION

❸ ❹ The following principles must be considered when providing antimicrobial surgical prophylaxis: (a) the agents should be delivered to the surgical site prior to the initial incision, and (b) bactericidal antibiotic concentrations should be maintained at the surgical site throughout the surgical procedure. Although animal and human models have demonstrated the efficacy of a single dose of an antibiotic administered just prior to bacterial contamination, long operations often require intraoperative doses of antibiotics to maintain adequate concentrations at the surgical site for the duration of surgery.[31] Antibiotics should be administered with anesthesia just prior to the initial incision. Administration of antibiotics too early may result in concentrations below the MIC toward the end of the operation, and administration too late leaves the patient unprotected at the time of initial incision. In a study examining the timing of antibiotic administration to 2,847 patients receiving prophylaxis, Classen et al.[31] evaluated patients who received prophylaxis early (2–24 hours before surgery), preoperative prophylaxis (0–2 hours prior to surgery), perioperative prophylaxis (up to 3 hours after first incision), and postoperative prophylaxis (>3 hours after first incision). The risk of infection was lowest (0.6%) for patients who received preoperative prophylaxis, moderate (1.4%) for those who received perioperative antibiotics, and greatest for those who received postoperative antibiotics (3.3%) or preoperative antibiotics too early (3.8%). One study that evaluated the effect of vancomycin prophylaxis timing in relationship to SSI in 2,048 cardiac surgery patients found that vancomycin administration between 16 and 60 minutes before the first surgical incision was associated with the lowest incidence of SSI.[32] The risk for an SSI increases dramatically with each hour from the time of initial incision to the time when antibiotics are eventually administered. For these reasons, prophylactic antibiotics should not be prescribed to be given "on call to the OR," which can occur 2 or more hours prior to the initial incision, nor should concurrent therapeutic antibiotics be relied on to provide adequate protection. In both situations, the chance for improperly timed doses is high.

Despite the importance of appropriately timed prophylactic antibiotic therapy, few patients receive antibiotics at the optimal time in relation to surgery. Potential barriers include antibiotics ordered after the patient has arrived in the operating room, delayed antibiotic preparation or delivery, and use of antibiotics that require long infusion times. One study assessed the timing of prophylactic antibiotics in 100 patients and found that only 26% of patients received an antibiotic dose within 2 hours of the initial surgical incision.[33]

Although most studies comparing single versus multiple doses of prophylactic antibiotics have failed to show a benefit of multidose regimens, the duration of operations in these studies may not be as long as that frequently observed in clinical practice. Proponents of administering a second antibiotic dose during lengthy operations suggest that the risk for SSI is just as great at the end of surgery (during wound closing) as it is during the initial incision.[34] One study of patients undergoing clean-contaminated operations suggests that procedures longer than 3 hours require a second intraoperative dose of cefazolin or substitution of cefazolin with a longer-acting antimicrobial agent.[4] A second study of patients undergoing elective colorectal surgery suggests that low serum antimicrobial concentrations at the time of surgical closure is the strongest predictor of postoperative SSI.[35] Studies of patients undergoing cardiac surgery also have demonstrated a higher infection rate among patients with undetectable antibiotic serum concentrations at the conclusion of the procedure.[36]

One strategy to ensure appropriate redosing of prophylactic antibiotics during long operations is use of a visual or auditory reminder system. One hospital reported its experience with such a system, finding that an automated reminder improved compliance and reduced SSIs. However, even with the reminder system, intraoperative redosing was done in only 68% of eligible patients.[37] Another strategy currently being evaluated is the role of continuous infusions of cefazolin, which one pilot study has found to be a feasible way to ensure adequate serum concentrations of antibiotic during prolonged surgeries.[38] Further trials are required before such an intervention can be recommended.

Underlying disease states that may affect antibiotic metabolism and/or elimination should be considered when developing a prophylactic regimen. For example, patients with thermal burn and spinal cord injuries eliminate certain classes of antibiotics, primarily the aminoglycosides and β-lactams, at unusually high rates compared with controls.[39] Individuals undergoing cardiac bypass may have altered antibiotic disposition related to increased volume of distribution and reduced total body clearance and thus require special dosing consideration.[40]

ANTIMICROBIAL CHOICE

❺ The choice of prophylactic antibiotic depends on the type of surgical procedure, the most frequent pathogens seen with this procedure, safety and efficacy profiles of the antimicrobial agent, current literature evidence supporting its use, and cost. Although most SSIs involve the patient's normal flora, antimicrobial selection also must take into account the susceptibility patterns of nosocomial pathogens within each institution. Typically, gram-positive coverage should be included in the choice of surgical prophylaxis because organisms such as *S. aureus* and *S. epidermidis* are encountered commonly as skin flora. The decision to broaden antibiotic prophylaxis to agents with gram-negative and anaerobic spectra of activity depends on both the surgical site (e.g., upper respiratory tract, gastrointestinal tract, genitourinary tract) and whether the operation will transect a hollow viscous or mucous membrane that may contain resident flora.[3]

Although antimicrobial prophylaxis can be administered through a variety of routes (e.g., oral, topical, intramuscular), the parenteral route is favored because of the reliability by which adequate tissue concentrations may be acheived.[41] Cephalosporins are the most commonly prescribed agents for surgical prophylaxis because of their broad antimicrobial spectrum, favorable pharmacokinetic profile, low incidence of adverse side effects, and low cost. First-generation cephalosporins, such as cefazolin, are the preferred choice for surgical prophylaxis, particularly for clean surgical procedures.[3,4,7] In cases where broader gram-negative and anaerobic coverage is desired, antianaerobic cephalosporins, such as cefoxitin and cefotetan, are appropriate choices. Although third-generation cephalosporins (e.g., ceftriaxone) have been advocated for prophylaxis because of their increased gram-negative coverage and prolonged half-lives, their inferior gram-positive and anaerobic activity in addition to their high cost have discouraged the widespread use of these agents.[3,4,7]

Allergic reactions are the most common side effects associated with cephalosporin use. Reactions can range from minor skin manifestations at the site of infusion to rash, pruritus, and rarely anaphylaxis (<0.02%). The structural similarity between penicillins and cephalosporins (each contains a β-lactam ring) has led to considerable confusion about the cross-allergenicity between these two classes of drugs. Twenty percent of the general population is labeled "penicillin allergic," yet of these patients, only 10% to 20% have positive results of a penicillin skin test.[42] The rate of cross-reactivity is approximately 2%, but as only 20% of all "penicillin-allergic" patients truly are penicillin allergic, the true incidence of cross-reactivity likely is less than 1%. Routine penicillin skin testing is not cost effective.[42] In summary, the administration of cephalosporins is both safe and cost effective for many patients who are labeled "penicillin allergic," and they can be used by patients who have not experienced an immediate or type I penicillin allergy.

Vancomycin can be considered for prophylactic therapy in surgical procedures involving implantation of a prosthetic device in which the rate of MRSA is high.[23,43] If the risk of MRSA is low and a β-lactam hypersensitivity exists, clindamycin can be used for many procedures instead of cefazolin in order to limit vancomycin use. Infusion-related side effects, such as thrombophlebitis and hypotension, particularly with vancomycin, usually can be controlled by adequate dilution and slower administration rates.[44]

Pseudomembranous colitis secondary to cephalosporins is uncommon and generally easily treated with a short course of oral metronidazole. Although infrequent, bleeding abnormalities related to cephalosporin use have been reported.[45] The primary hematologic effect appears to be inhibition of vitamin K–dependent clotting factors that results in prolongation of the prothrombin time. The mechanism for this effect, most commonly seen with cefotetan, is related to the methylthiotetrazole side chain of the β-lactam molecule. Patients at greatest risk for this hypoprothrombinemic effect have received a prolonged course of these agents and have underlying risk factors for vitamin K deficiency, such as malnutrition.[46]

Because inappropriate prophylactic antibiotic use not only can induce antibiotic resistance but also can negatively affect an institution's antibiotic budget, initiatives to curtail inappropriate antibiotic use have become the focus of many drug use evaluation efforts. Potential sources of inappropriate antibiotic prophylaxis include the use of broad-spectrum antimicrobials when a narrow-spectrum agent is warranted, extending prophylaxis for durations beyond that recommended in published guidelines, and using expensive antibiotics when equivalent, less expensive agents are available. The most effective tools for ensuring appropriate prophylactic antibiotic prescribing are knowledge of the institutional postoperative infection rate for each type of surgical procedure and the bacterial epidemiology patterns for each surgical population. Individualized institutional guidelines that take into account best literature evidence, institution-based antibiotic susceptibility data, and surgeon preference are important tools for rationalizing antibiotic prophylaxis use.[47]

RECOMMENDATIONS FOR SPECIFIC TYPES OF SURGERY

Guidelines for surgical prophylaxis usually are structured according to the tissues affected during an operation. Although many different surgical procedures may be performed at any one anatomic site, this method of categorization still is optimal because the factors related to the success of a prophylactic regimen, such as the endogenous flora that are expected and the pharmacokinetics, pharmacodynamics, and spectrum of selected antimicrobials, generally are constant for a particular surgical site (see antimicrobial Choice above). The choice of antimicrobial prophylaxis is always best evaluated using the results of properly conducted clinical trials. In the absence of studies specific to the procedure in question, extrapolation from data on regimens for different procedures in the same anatomic site in question usually can be made. Subsequent modifications to each prophylactic regimen should be based on intraoperative findings or events.

❻ A comprehensive review of the surgical prophylaxis literature is beyond the scope of this chapter, but important factors are reviewed here for each type/site of surgery. Specific recommendations are summarized in Table 127–6. The reader is referred to published guidelines and review articles.[3,7,4,41,48]

GASTROINTESTINAL SURGERY

Gastrointestinal surgery can be categorized according to surgical site and infectious risk. Gastroduodenal surgery and hepatobiliary surgery generally are considered to be clean or clean-contaminated surgeries, with SSI rates generally less than 5%. Colorectal surgery, including appendectomies, is considered contaminated owing to the large quantities and polymicrobial nature of bacterial flora within the colon. SSI rates for these types of surgeries generally range from 15% to 30%. Emergent abdominal surgery involving bowel perforation or peritonitis is considered a dirty surgical procedure, associated with a greater than 30% risk of SSI, and should be treated with *therapeutic* rather than *prophylactic* antibiotics.[3]

Gastroduodenal Surgery

Insignificant numbers of bacteria usually are found in the stomach and duodenum because of their acidity. The rate of SSIs in gastroduodenal surgery generally is low, so procedures in this region can be classified as clean procedures. The risk for an SSI in this population increases with any condition that can lead to bacterial overgrowth, such as obstruction, hemorrhage, or malignancy, or increasing the pH of gastroduodenal secretions with concomitant acid suppression therapy. Antimicrobial prophylaxis is of clinical benefit only in this high-risk population. In most cases, a single dose of intravenous cefazolin will provide adequate prophylaxis.[48] For patients with a β-lactam allergy, oral ciprofloxacin is as efficacious as parenteral cefuroxime as prophylactic therapy for gastroduodenal surgery.[49] Antimicrobial prophylaxis is indicated in esophageal surgery only in the presence of obstruction. Postoperative *therapeutic* antibiotics may be indicated if perforation is detected during surgery, depending on whether an established infection is present.

Use of antibiotic prophylaxis for percutaneous endoscopic gastrostomy placement is controversial.[50] Although postoperative peristomal infection can occur in up to 30% of patients, clinical trials with cefazolin given 30 minutes preoperatively in this population are conflicting.[50] A pharmacoeconomic study that incorporated a meta-analysis of available studies to determine efficacy suggested that antibiotic prophylaxis was cost effective for patients undergoing percutaneous endoscopic gastrostomy placements.[51]

Hepatobiliary Surgery

Although bile normally is sterile and the SSI rate after biliary surgery is low, antibiotic prophylaxis is of benefit in this population. Bile contamination (bactobilia) can increase the frequency of SSIs and is present in many patients (e.g., those with acute cholecystitis, biliary obstruction, advanced age).[48] In general, however, the correlation between bactobilia in surgical specimens and the subsequent pathogens implicated in an SSI is poor. The most frequently encountered organisms are *E. coli, Klebsiella* spp., and Enterococci. *Pseudomonas* is an uncommon finding in the absence of cholangitis. Trials comparing first-, second-, and third-generation cephalosporins have not demonstrated benefit over single-dose cefazolin prophylaxis even in high-risk patients (e.g., age >60 years, previous biliary surgery, acute cholecystitis, jaundice, obesity, diabetes, common bile duct stones).[52] Ciprofloxacin and levofloxacin are effective alternatives for β-lactam–allergic patients undergoing open cholecystectomy.[53,54] In fact, orally administered levofloxacin appears to provide similar intraoperative gallbladder tissue concentrations.[54] For low-risk patients undergoing elective laparoscopic cholecystectomy, antibiotic prophylaxis is not of benefit and is not recommended.[55] The risk for SSIs in cirrhotic patients undergoing transjugular intrahepatic portosystemic shunt surgery may be reduced with a single prophylactic dose of ceftriaxone[56] but not with single doses of shorter-acting cephalosporins.[57]

Although surgeons may use *presumptive* antibiotic therapy for patients with acute cholecystitis or cholangitis and defer surgery until the patient is afebrile in an effort to decrease the risk of subsequent infections, this practice is controversial. Detection of an active infection during surgery (e.g., gangrenous gallbladder, suppurative cholangitis) is an indication for a course of postoperative *therapeutic* antibiotics. In either case, antibiotics with additional antianaerobic activity (e.g., cefoxitin or cefotetan) are indicated.[58]

Appendectomy

Suspected appendicitis is a frequent cause of abdominal surgery. Numerous antibiotic regimens, all with activity against gram-positive and gram-negative aerobes and anaerobic pathogens, are effective in reducing SSI incidence.[48] A cephalosporin with antianaerobic activity, such as cefoxitin or cefotetan, is recommended as first-line therapy; however, a comparative trial of cefoxitin and cefotetan suggests that cefotetan may be superior, possibly because of its longer duration of action.[59] In patients with β-lactam allergy, metronidazole in combination with gentamicin is an effective regimen. Broad-spectrum antibiotics covering nosocomial pathogens (e.g., *Pseudomonas*) do not further reduce SSI risk and instead may increase the cost of therapy and promote bacterial resistance.[60] Although single-dose therapy with cefotetan is adequate, prophylaxis with cefoxitin may require intraoperative dosing if the procedure extends beyond 3 hours. Established intraabdominal infections (e.g., gangrenous or perforated appendix) require an appropriate course of postoperative *therapeutic* antibiotics. Laparoscopic appendectomy produces lower postoperative infection rates that open appendectomy; however, antimicrobial prophylaxis was used for all patients in these studies; thus, the role for prophylaxis in this population remains poorly studied.[61]

Colorectal Surgery

In the absence of adequate prophylactic therapy, the risk for SSI after colorectal surgery is high because of the significant bacterial counts in fecal material present in the colon (frequently $>10^9$ per gram). Anaerobes and gram-negative aerobes predominate, but gram-positive aerobes also may play an important role. Reducing this bacterial load with a thorough bowel preparation regimen (4 L of polyethylene glycol solution or 90 mL of sodium phosphate solution administered orally the day before surgery) is controversial; however, 99% of surgeons in a survey routinely use mechanical preparation.[62] Risk factors for SSIs include age older than 60 years, hypoalbuminemia, poor preoperative bowel preparation, corticosteroid therapy, malignancy, and operations lasting longer than 3.5 hours.[7]

CLINICAL CONTROVERSY

A randomized trial of 380 patients undergoing elective colorectal surgery suggests that SSIs are not reduced by preoperative mechanical bowel preparation.[63] This finding was confirmed in a meta-analysis showing that mechanical bowel preparation does not reduce the risk of anastomotic leakage or other complications, including postoperative infection.[64] Despite this new evidence, mechanical bowel preparations continue to be a standard of practice prior to elective bowel surgery.

TABLE 127-6 Most Likely Pathogens and Specific Recommendations for Surgical Prophylaxis

Type of Operation	Likely Pathogens	Recommended Prophylaxis Regimen[a]	Comments	Grade of Recommendation[b]
Gastrointestinal surgery				
Gastroduodenal	Enteric gram-negative bacilli, gram-positive cocci, oral anaerobes	Cefazolin 1 g × 1 (see text for recommendations for percutaneous endoscopic gastrostomy)	High-risk patients only (obstruction, hemorrhage, malignancy, acid suppression therapy, morbid obesity)	IA
Cholecystectomy	Enteric gram-negative bacilli, anaerobes	Cefazolin 1 g × 1 for high-risk patients Laparoscopic: None	High-risk patients only (acute cholecystitis, common duct stones, previous biliary surgery, jaundice, age >60 y, obesity, diabetes mellitus)	IA
Transjugular intrahepatic portosystemic shunt (TIPS)	Enteric gram-negative bacilli, anaerobes	Ceftriaxone 1 g × 1	Longer-acting cephalosporins preferred	IA
Appendectomy	Enteric gram-negative bacilli, anaerobes	Cefoxitin or cefotetan 1 g × 1	Second intraoperative dose of cefoxitin may be required if procedure lasts longer than 3 h	IA
Colorectal	Enteric gram-negative bacilli, anaerobes	PO: Neomycin 1 g + erythromycin base 1 g at 1 PM, 2 PM, and 11 PM 1 day preoperatively plus mechanical bowel preparation IV: Cefoxitin or cefotetan 1 g × 1	Benefits of oral plus IV is controversial except for colostomy reversal and rectal resection	IA
Gastrointestinal Endoscopy	Variable depending on procedure but typically enteric gram-negative bacilli, gram-positive cocci, oral anaerobes	PO: Amoxicillin 2 g × 1 IV: Ampicillin 2 g × 1 or cefazolin 1 g × 1	Only recommended for high-risk patients undergoing high-risk procedures (see text)	IA
Urologic surgery				
Prostate resection, bladder resection, cystoscopy	*Escherichia coli*	Cefazolin 1 g × 1	Generally not recommended for patients with sterile preoperative urine cultures	IB
Gynecological surgery				
Cesarean section	Enteric gram-negative bacilli, anaerobes, group B streptococci, enterococci	Cefazolin 2 g × 1	Can be given before initial incision or after cord is clamped	IA
Hysterectomy	Enteric gram-negative bacilli, anaerobes, group B streptococci, enterococci	Vaginal: Cefazolin 1 g × 1 Abdominal: Cefotetan 1 g × 1 or Cefazolin 1 g × 1	Metronidazole 1 g IV × 1 is recommended alternative for penicillin allergy	IA
Head and neck surgery				
Maxillofacial surgery	*Staphylococcus aureus*, streptococci oral anaerobes	Cefazolin 2 g or clindamycin 600 mg	Repeat intraoperative dose for operations longer than 4 h	IA
Head and neck cancer resection	S. aureus, streptococci oral anaerobes	Clindamycin 600 mg at induction and every 8 h × 2 more doses	Add gentamicin for clean–contaminated procedures	IA
Cardiothoracic surgery				
Cardiac surgery	*S. aureus*, *Staphylococcus epidermidis*, *Corynebacterium*	Cefazolin 1 g every 8 h × 48 h	Patients >80 kg should receive 2 g of cefazolin instead; in areas with high prevalence of *S. aureus* resistance, vancomycin should be considered	IA
Thoracic surgery	*S. aureus*, *S. epidermidis*, *Corynebacterium*, enteric gram-negative bacilli	Cefuroxime 750 mg IV every 8 h × 48 h	First-generation cephalosporins are deemed inadequate and shorter durations of prophylaxis have not been adequately studied	IA
Vascular surgery				
Abdominal aorta and lower extremity vascular surgery	*S. aureus*, *S. epidermidis*, enteric gram-negative bacilli	Cefazolin 1 g at induction and every 8 h × 2 more doses	Although complications from infections may be infrequent, graft infections are associated with significant morbidity	IB
Orthopedic surgery				
Joint replacement	*S. aureus*, *S. epidermidis*	Cefazolin 1 g × 1 preoperatively, then every 8 h × 2 more doses	Vancomycin reserved for penicillin-allergic patients or where institutional prevalence of methicillin-resistant *Staphylococcus aureus* warrants use	IA
Hip fracture repair	*S. aureus*, *S. epidermidis*	Cefazolin 1 g × 1 preoperatively, then every 8 h for 48 hours	Compound fractures are treated as if infection is presumed	IA
Open/compound fractures	*S. aureus*, *S. epidermidis*, gram-negative bacilli, polymicrobial	Cefazolin 1 g × 1 preoperatively, then every 8 h for a course of presumed infection	Gram-negative coverage (i.e., gentamicin) often indicated for severe open fractures	IA
Neurosurgery				
Cerebrospinal fluid shunt procedures	*S. aureus*, *S. epidermidis*	Cefazolin 1 g every 8 h × 3 doses or ceftriaxone 2 g × 1	No agents have been shown to be better than cefazolin in randomized comparative trials.	IA
Craniotomy	*S. aureus*, *S. epidermidis*	Cefazolin 1 g × 1 or cefotaxime 1 g × 1	Trimethoprim–sulfamethoxazole (160/800mg) IV × 1 can be substituted for patients with penicillin allergy	IA
Spinal surgery	*S. aureus*, *S. epidermidis*	Cefazolin 1 g × 1	Limited number of clinical trials comparing different treatment regimens	IB

[a]One-time doses are optimally infused at induction of anesthesia except as noted. Repeat doses may be required for long procedures. See text for references.
[b]Strength of recommendations:
Category IA: Strongly recommended and supported by well-designed experimental, clinical, or epidemiologic studies.
Category IB: Strongly recommended and supported by some experimental, clinical, or epidemiologic studies and strong theoretical rationale.
Category II: Suggested and supported by suggestive clinical or epidemiologic studies or theoretical rationale.

Antimicrobial prophylaxis reduced mortality from 11.2% to 4.5% in a pooled analysis of trials comparing antimicrobial prophylaxis with no prophylaxis for colon surgery.[65] Effective antibiotic prophylaxis reduces even further the risk for an SSI. Several oral regimens designed to reduce bacterial counts in the colon have been studied.[48] The combination of 1 g neomycin and 1 g erythromycin base given orally 19, 18, and 9 hours preoperatively is the regimen most commonly used in the United States.[66] Neomycin is poorly absorbed but provides intraluminal concentrations that are high enough to effectively kill most gram-negative aerobes. Oral erythromycin is only partially absorbed but still produces concentrations in the colon that are sufficient to suppress common anaerobes. If surgery is postponed, the antibiotics must be readministered to maintain efficacy. Optimally, the bowel preparation regimen should be completed prior to starting the oral antibiotic regimen. This is of particular concern because most procedures now are performed electively on a "same-day surgery" basis. In this case, the bowel preparation regimen is self-administered by the patient at home on the day prior to hospital admission, and compliance cannot be monitored carefully.

Patients who cannot take oral medications should receive parenteral antibiotics. Cefoxitin or cefotetan is used most commonly, but other second-generation and some third-generation cephalosporins also are effective.[67] The role of metronidazole in combination with cephalosporin therapy is unclear. Only retrospective evidence suggests that the addition of metronidazole to a cephalosporin or extended-spectrum penicillin provides additional benefit.[68] Until this finding is confirmed in prospective studies, metronidazole should be reserved for combination therapy with cephalosporins with poor anaerobic coverage (e.g., cefazolin). At this time, the evidence recommending the addition of metronidazole to cephalosporins with anaerobic activity (e.g., cefotaxime, cefoxitin, and ceftriaxone) is insufficient. For β-lactam–allergic patients, perioperative doses of gentamicin and metronidazole have been used.[69] Whether the addition of preoperative parenteral antibiotics to the standard preoperative oral antibiotic regimen described earlier will decrease SSI rates lower than oral prophylaxis alone is controversial; however, combination therapy is superior to parenteral therapy alone.[70] Postoperative antibiotics generally are unnecessary in the absence of any untoward events or findings during surgery. Intravenous antibiotics are required for colostomy reversal and rectal resection because enterally administered antibiotics will not reach the distal segment that is to be reanastomosed or resected.[71]

Gastrointestinal Endoscopy

Despite the large number of endoscopic procedures performed each year, the rate of postprocedural infection is relatively low. The highest bacteremia rates have been reported in patients undergoing esophageal dilatation for stricture or sclerotherapy for management of esophageal varices. Although postprocedural bacteremia can occur in as many as 22% of patients, the bacteremia usually is transient (<30 minutes) and rarely results in clinically significant infection. Therefore, antimicrobial prophylaxis is routinely recommended only for high-risk patients (prosthetic heart valves, history of endocarditis, systemic–pulmonary shunt, synthetic vascular graft <1 year old, complex cyanotic congenital heart disease, obstructed bile duct, liver cirrhosis, immunocompromised patients) undergoing high-risk procedures (stricture dilation, variceal sclerotherapy, endoscopic retrograde cholangiopancreatography).[72] Single-dose preprocedural regimens similar to those for endocarditis prophylaxis are most common (amoxicillin for patients who can tolerate oral premedication or either ampicillin or cefazolin administered intravenously). A meta-analysis of antimicrobial prophylaxis for endoscopic placement of percutaneous feeding tubes also suggests that a single preoperative dose of antibiotics reduces the risk of postoperative infection compared to no antibiotic (6.4% vs 24%).[73] Consensus guidelines have adopted this recommendation and suggest a single dose of cefazolin within 30 minutes prior to the procedure.[72]

UROLOGIC SURGERY

Preoperative bacteruria is the most important risk factor for development of an SSI after urologic surgery. All patients should have a preoperative urinalysis and should receive *therapeutic* antibiotics if bacteruria is detected. Patients with sterile urine preoperatively are at low risk for developing an SSI, and the benefit of *prophylactic* antibiotics in this setting is controversial.[74] Antibiotic prophylaxis is warranted in high-risk patients (e.g., prolonged indwelling catheterization, positive urine cultures, and neutropenia) undergoing transurethral, perineal, or suprapubic resection of the prostate, resection of bladder tumors, or cystoscopy.[74] The exact incidence of SSIs in this population is obscured by the frequent use of postoperative urinary catheters and the subsequent risk of bacteriuria. *E. coli* is the most frequently encountered organism. Routine use of broad-spectrum antibiotics, such as third-generation cephalosporins and fluoroquinolones, does not decrease SSI rates more than cefazolin, so such regimens are not recommended. One comparative trial determined that a single dose of oral ciprofloxacin was as effective as intravenous cefazolin and suggests that this may be a cheaper and easier alternative for outpatient urologic surgery.[75] Regimens consisting of more a single dose do not improve outcome. Urologic procedures requiring an abdominal approach, such as a nephrectomy or cystectomy, require antibiotic prophylaxis similar to that used for a clean-contaminated abdominal procedure.[74]

OBSTETRIC AND GYNECOLOGIC SURGERIES

Cesarean Section

Cesarean section is the most frequently performed surgical procedure in the United States.[7] Prophylactic antibiotics are given to prevent endometritis, the most commonly occurring SSI. In the past, antibiotics were recommended for only high-risk patients, including those with premature membrane rupture or those not receiving prenatal care. Several large trials, as well as a meta-analysis of 81 trials, have shown benefit in administering prophylactic antibiotics to all women undergoing emergent or elective cesarean section regardless of their underlying risk factors.[76] Cefazolin remains the drug of choice despite the wide spectrum of potential pathogens, and a single 2-g dose appears to be superior to single or multiple 1-g doses.[77] Providing a broader spectrum of coverage with cefoxitin (for anaerobes) or piperacillin (for *Pseudomonas* or Enterococci) does not further reduce postoperative infection rates. For patients with a β-lactam allergy, preoperative metronidazole is an acceptable alternative.[76]

CLINICAL CONTROVERSY

During a cesarean section, unlike other surgical procedures, the most appropriate timing of antibiotic administration is controversial. Traditionally, antimicrobials were administered after the initial incision and when the umbilical cord was clamped in an attempt to minimize infant drug exposure, which theoretically could mask the signs of neonatal sepsis and select resistant organisms in infants who develop infections. A randomized controlled trial compared single-dose cefazolin administration at or before the initial incision to administration after cord clamp and found no significant difference in postpartum maternal or neonatal infection, suggesting that either strategy is appropriate.[78] However, there was a trend toward a reduction in the incidence of endometritis in patients randomized to preoperative antibiotics, and the study has been criticized as being underpowered to detect this difference.

Hysterectomy

The most important factor affecting the incidence of SSI after hysterectomy is the type of procedure performed. Vaginal hysterectomies are associated with a high rate of postoperative infection when performed without the benefit of prophylactic antibiotics because of the polymicrobial flora normally present at the operative site.[79] As with cesarean sections, cefazolin is the drug of choice for vaginal hysterectomies despite the wide spectrum of possible pathogens.[79] The American College of Obstetricians and Gynecologists (ACOG) recommends a single dose of either cefazolin or cefoxitin.[80] For patients with a β-lactam allergy, a single preoperative dose of either metronidazole or doxycycline also is effective.[80]

Prophylactic antibiotics are recommended for abdominal hysterectomy despite the lack of bacterial contamination from the vaginal flora. Both cefazolin and antianaerobic cephalosporins (e.g., cefoxitin and cefotetan) have been studied extensively. Single-dose cefotetan is superior to single-dose cefazolin,[81] and the investigators suggest that cefotetan should be the drug of choice for abdominal hysterectomies. However, other investigators suggest that either agent is appropriate, provided 24 hours of antimicrobial coverage is not exceeded.[7] The ACOG guidelines suggest that first-, second-, or third-generation cephalosporins can be used for prophylaxis.[80] Metronidazole also is effective and can be used if patients are allergic to β-lactam antibiotics.[79] Antibiotic prophylaxis may not be required in laparoscopic gynecologic surgery or tubal microsurgery.[82] Similar to other surgical procedures, perioperative events and findings may require use of *therapeutic* antibiotics after surgery.

HEAD AND NECK SURGERY

Use of prophylactic antibiotics during head and neck surgery depends on the procedure type. Clean procedures (per NRC definition), such as parotidectomy or simple tooth extraction, are associated with a low incidence of SSI. Head and neck procedures involving an incision through a mucosal layer are associated with a higher risk for SSI. The normal flora of the mouth is polymicrobial; both anaerobes and gram-positive aerobes predominate. Although typical doses of cefazolin usually are ineffective for anaerobic infections, a 2-g dose produces concentrations high enough to inhibit these organisms. A pharmacokinetic study suggested that a single dose of clindamycin is adequate for prophylaxis in maxillofacial surgery unless the procedure lasts longer than 4 hours, when a second dose should be administered intraoperatively.[83] For most head and neck cancer resection surgeries, including free-flap reconstruction, 24 hours of clindamycin is appropriate, and no additional benefit of extending therapy beyond 24 hours is seen. A combination of clindamycin and gentamicin to cover aerobic, anaerobic, and gram-negative bacteria in clean-contaminated oncologic surgery is recommended.[84] Topical therapy with clindamycin, amoxicillin–clavulanate, and ticarcillin–clavulanate has been described in small trials, but the exact role of topical antibiotics is not defined.[85] Antimicrobial prophylaxis is not indicated for endoscopic sinus surgery without nasal packing.[41]

CARDIOTHORACIC SURGERY

Although cardiac surgery generally is considered a clean procedure, antibiotic prophylaxis lowers SSI incidence.[48] The substantial morbidity related to an SSI in this population, coupled with the routine implementation of prosthetic devices, further justifies the routine use of prophylaxis.[86] Patients who develop SSIs after coronary artery bypass graft surgery have a mortality rate of 22% at 1 year compared with 0.6% for those who do not develop an SSI.[87] Risk factors for developing an SSI after cardiac surgery include obesity, renal insufficiency, connective tissue disease, reexploration for bleeding, and poorly timed administration of antibiotics.[86] Skin flora pathogens predominate; gram-negative organisms are rare.

Cefazolin has been studied extensively and is considered the drug of choice. Although several studies and a meta-analysis advocate the use of second-generation cephalosporins (e.g., cefuroxime) rather than cefazolin, various methodologic flaws in these studies have limited the extrapolation of these results to practice. Cefazolin was as effective as cefuroxime in a large randomized trial of 702 patients undergoing open heart surgery and thus remains the standard of care.[88] Both patient weight and timing of cefazolin administration relative to surgery must be considered when developing a dosing strategy. Patients weighing more than 80 kg should receive 2 g cefazolin rather than 1 g. Doses should be administered no earlier than 60 minutes before the first incision and no later than the beginning of induction.[84] Extending therapy beyond 48 hours does not further reduce SSI rates. Single-dose cefazolin therapy may be sufficient but is not recommended by the Society of Thoracic Surgeons at this time pending further study.[89]

Routine vancomycin administration may be justified in hospitals having a high incidence of MRSA or when sternal wounds are to be explored surgically for possible mediastinitis. However, a large comparative trial enrolling almost 900 patients in a single center with a high prevalence of MRSA infections found that both cefazolin and vancomycin had similar efficacy in preventing SSI in patients undergoing cardiac surgery that required sternotomy.[90] Mediastinitis constitutes a failure of a prior prophylactic regimen. Continued postoperative vancomycin should be guided by culture and sensitivity data.[42] Subsequent antibiotic therapy is guided by intraoperative findings.

Pulmonary resection is associated with significant SSI risk, and prophylactic antibiotics have an established role in preventing postoperative infectious morbidity. Pleuropulmonary infections are much more common than wound infections, and pathogenic organisms likely migrate from the oral cavity or pharynx.[91] First-generation cephalosporins are inadequate; 48 hours of cefuroxime is preferred. A regimen of ampicillin–sulbactam is superior to first-generation cephalosporins, but further studies are required before this agent can be recommended as first-line prophylactic therapy.[92]

VASCULAR SURGERY

Vascular surgery, like cardiac surgery, generally is considered a clean surgery by NRC criteria. Although vascular graft infections occur infrequently (3%–5%), the associated morbidity and mortality are extensive because treatment often requires surgical graft removal along with *therapeutic* antibiotic therapy.[93] Prophylactic antibiotics are of benefit, particularly for procedures involving the abdominal aorta and the lower extremities. Cefazolin is regarded as the drug of choice.[94] Twenty-four hours of prophylaxis with cefazolin is adequate; longer courses may lead to bacterial resistance.[95] For patients with β-lactam allergy, 24 hours of oral ciprofloxacin has been shown to be effective.[93]

ORTHOPEDIC SURGERY

Most orthopedic surgery is clean by definition; thus, prophylactic antibiotics generally are indicated only when prosthetic materials (e.g., pins, plates, and artificial joints) are implanted.[20] A late-occurring infectious complication in this surgical population can result in substantial morbidity and may lead to prosthesis failure and subsequent removal. Staphylococci are the most frequently encountered pathogens; gram-negative aerobes are infrequent. Use of cefazolin is supported by substantial literature evidence and therefore is the prophylactic agent of choice. Vancomycin, although effective, is not recommended for routine use unless a patient has a documented history of a serious allergy to β-lactams or the propensity for MRSA infections at a particular institution necessitates its use. The current recommended duration of prophylaxis for joint replacement and hip fracture surgery is 24 hours.[7] Antibiotic-impregnated cement and beads have been used to lower SSI rates, but conclusive data regarding their efficacy are lacking.[20]

Patients suffering open (compound) fractures are particularly susceptible to infection because bacterial contamination almost always has occurred already. Under these circumstances, use of antibiotics is *presumptive*. In this setting cefazolin often is combined with an aminoglycoside, but controlled trials are lacking.[96] A clinical trial comparing clindamycin and cloxacillin suggests that clindamycin is superior and may be appropriate as monotherapy for Gustilo type I and II open fractures but not for type III fractures, for which added gram-negative activity is recommended.[97] Duration of antibiotic therapy is highly variable and depends on surgical findings during debridement, results of intraoperative cultures, and clinical status. A prospective trial comparing short (<24 hours) and long (>24 hours) courses of antimicrobial prophylaxis for severe trauma suggests that longer courses of antibiotics do not offer additional benefit and may be associated with the development of resistant infections.[98] However, established joint infections and osteomyelitis require an extended course of *therapeutic* antibiotics.

NEUROSURGERY

Definitive recommendations on the role of antibiotic prophylaxis in neurosurgery cannot be made at this time.[99] Although the rates of SSI after these generally clean operations are low, the morbidity and mortality of SSI, should they occur, are high. Procedures involving cerebrospinal fluid (CSF) shunt placement should be considered separately because this procedure involves placement of a foreign body and is associated with higher infection rates. When choosing an antibiotic, considerations include not only the spectrum of activity but also the penetration of the agent into the site of action (CSF). A meta-analysis suggested that single doses of cefazolin or, where required, vancomycin appear to lower SSI risk after craniotomy.[100] The largest prospective randomized trial to date of 826 patients undergoing clean neurosurgical procedures suggested that a single dose of ceftizoxime was as effective as a combination regimen of single-dose vancomycin and gentamicin. The authors also reported that ceftizoxime was better tolerated and more consistently achieved adequate CSF levels to inhibit the most common organisms.[101] A study of 780 patients undergoing neurosurgical procedures that included shunt surgery reported that single doses of cefotaxime and trimethoprim–sulfamethoxazole were equally effective in preventing SSIs.[102] Most studies of procedures involving a shunt have been small in size and do not consistently show lower infection rates with antibiotic prophylaxis, although the results of a systematic review and meta-analysis suggest that a significant improvement in the incidence of shunt infection with 24 hours of systemic antibiotics (i.e., cefazolin) and use of antibiotic impregnated catheters independently.[103]

SSIs associated with spinal surgery are rare but devastating when they occur. Use of antimicrobial prophylaxis in this setting is warranted and recommended by a meta-analysis.[104] Large randomized controlled trials are lacking, but cefazolin is the antibiotic recommended most commonly. Cephalosporin penetration into the vertebral disc has been questioned. Some small studies suggest that the addition of gentamicin, which has better penetration, might be warranted; however, there is a paucity of clinical trials comparing these two regimens.[105]

MINIMALLY INVASIVE AND LAPAROSCOPIC SURGERY

Laparoscopic surgeries are being performed more frequently for a variety of different operations, including gynecologic, orthopedic, and biliary surgeries. This minimally invasive technique is associated with smaller wounds, fewer infectious complications, smaller inflammatory response, and therefore a better-preserved immune response to infection compared with the open surgical approach.[106] The role of antimicrobial prophylaxis in this setting depends on the type of surgery performed and preexisting risk factors for infection. Unfortunately, few large prospective, placebo-controlled trials have determined in which patients and surgeries antimicrobial prophylaxis is warranted.

In addition to the recommendations for previously mentioned laparoscopic procedures, there is a variety of levels of evidence for prophylaxis in other laparoscopic and endoscopic procedures. Patients undergoing endoscopic retrograde cholangiopancreatography do not need antimicrobial prophylaxis unless biliary obstruction is evident. In these situations, a single 1-g dose of cefazolin will suffice.[107] The role of antimicrobial prophylaxis for transurethral resection of the prostate is better established. A third-generation cephalosporin such as ceftriaxone (or cotrimoxazole for severely β-lactam–allergic patients) can be recommended as single-dose prophylaxis, especially for patients with nonsterile urine preoperatively or indwelling catheters.[107] Insertion of peritoneal dialysis catheters by laparoscopic technique is associated with significantly lower rates of postoperative infection. With SSI rates less than 5%, prophylactic antimicrobial therapy may not be warranted, but this has not been studied in a sufficiently large placebo-controlled trial. If the decision to provide antimicrobial prophylaxis is made, a single dose of cefazolin will suffice.[107]

NONPHARMACOLOGIC INTERVENTIONS

Strategies other than antimicrobial strategies and aseptic technique for reducing postoperative infections have been investigated in different types of surgeries. The most commonly cited and practiced interventions include intraoperative maintenance of normothermia, provision of supplemental oxygen in the perioperative period, and aggressive perioperative glucose control.

Core body temperature can fall by 1°C to 1.5°C intraoperatively in patients under general anesthesia. Intraoperative hypothermia has been associated with impaired immune function, decreased blood flow to the surgical site, decreased tissue oxygen tension, and an increased risk of SSI. Efforts to maintain intraoperative normothermia should be exercised and may include the use of warming blankets and intravenous fluid warmers to maintain core body temperature above 36°C (97°F). One prospective trial of 200 patients undergoing colorectal surgery found that maintenance of normothermia reduced postoperative infection rates along with other morbidity parameters, including length of stay.[108]

Low oxygen tension in the tissues that make up the surgical site increases the risk of bacterial colonization and subsequent SSI by decreasing the efficiency of neutrophil activity. Administration of high concentrations of oxygen (80% via ventilator or 12 L/min via a nonrebreather mask) reduced postoperative infection rates significantly in a multicenter randomized trial of 500 patients undergoing colorectal surgery.[109]

Diabetes and poor glucose control are well-known risk factors for SSI. The increased risk of infection is thought to be due to both macrovascular (vasculopathy and venoocclusive disease) and microvascular (subtle immunologic deficiencies, including neutrophil dysfunction and reduced complement and antibody activity) complications. Aggressive control of perioperative blood glucose level decreases the incidence of SSI in diabetics undergoing cardiac surgery and is being evaluated in other types of surgery and in nondiabetic patients.[110]

CLINICAL CONTROVERSY

Although interventions to maintain normothermia intraoperatively, provide supplemental oxygen in the perioperative period, and aggressively control perioperative glucose show a significant reduction in SSI, they cannot be generalized to all types of surgeries. However, given the simplicity and low cost of these interventions, many clinicians consider applying these measures outside of the studied population(s). At this time, pending further research, these interventions can be recommended for routine use only in the type of patient or surgery for which they were studied.

QUALITY ASSURANCE AND PHARMACOECONOMIC IMPLICATIONS

The recommendations and literature reviewed in this chapter indicate that SSIs are preventable with appropriately chosen and timed prophylactic therapy in combination with meticulous aseptic technique and a variety of nonantimicrobial methods. Despite this practice, infection is the most common complication seen postoperatively. For this reason, many organizations, including the Centers for Medicare and Medicaid Service (CMS), CDC, and Joint Commission on Accreditation of Healthcare Organizations (JCAHO), have mandated a formalized approach to improving patient safety and reducing SSIs. Quality assurance data collected from Medicare inpatients found that two of the three performance measures of the National Surgical Infection Project (SIP), implemented by CMS and the CDC in 2002, are not consistently being met.[111] Although 92.6% of patients were given a prophylactic antimicrobial regimen consistent with published guidelines, only 55.7% of these surgical patients have parenteral antimicrobial prophylaxis initiated within 1 hour prior to incision, and the prophylactic antimicrobial was discontinued within 24 hours after surgery end time in only 40.7% of patients.[111] Strategies have been investigated and shown to improve surgical antibiotic prophylaxis practices for these three outcomes as part of the SIP. These three performance outcomes have been adopted as core measures by JCAHO as publicly reported quality measure by the Hospital Quality Alliance. However, in light of a lack of clear guidance on what constitutes "high rates" of MRSA in published SIP guidelines, the national shortage of antibiotics recommended for patients undergoing general abdominal colorectal surgery (e.g., cefotetan, cefoxitin), and conflicting recommendations for prevention of endocarditis in patients undergoing surgery who have coexisting valvular heart disease, the CMS and JCAHO have temporarily suspended the public reporting of these SIP quality measures.[112] Standardized institutional guidelines can effectively ensure appropriate prophylactic antimicrobial therapy and ultimately reduce SSIs at individual institutions. Strategies for improving such programs are outlined in Table 127–7.[113]

TABLE 127-7 Strategies for Implementing an Institutional Program to Ensure Appropriate Use of Antimicrobial Prophylaxis in Surgery

1. Educate
Develop an educational program that enforces the importance and rationale of timely antimicrobial prophylaxis.
Make this educational program available to all healthcare practitioners involved in the patient's care.
2. Standardize the ordering process
Establish a protocol (e.g., a preprinted order sheet) that standardizes antibiotic choice according to current published evidence, formulary availability, institutional resistance patterns, and cost.
3. Standardize the delivery and administration process
Use system that ensures antibiotics are prepared and delivered to the holding area in a timely fashion.
Standardize the administration time to less than 1 hour preoperatively.
Designate responsibility and accountability for antibiotic administration.
Provide visible reminders to prescribe/administer prophylactic antibiotics (e.g., checklists).
Develop a system to remind surgeons/nurses to readminister antibiotics intraoperatively during long procedures.
4. Provide feedback
Follow up with regular reports of compliance and infection rates.

It is paramount to consider the cost implications of pharmacotherapy guidelines that affect a large number of patients. Although investigators have incorporated basic financial analysis into the results of antibiotic prophylaxis comparative trials,[42,47,50,87] robust pharmacoeconomic studies of various regimens of antimicrobial prophylaxis in surgery are lacking. Most of these studies are cost minimization studies because only drug acquisition costs are considered. Studies that incorporate all relevant drug and treatment costs in relation to pertinent patient outcomes, such as incidence of SSIs, hospital length of stay, and antibiotic-related adverse events, are needed.

EVALUATION OF THERAPEUTIC OUTCOMES

When evaluating the outcome of surgical antibiotic prophylaxis, it is important to differentiate any potential SSI from other postoperative infection or complication. Although fever and leukocytosis are common in the immediate postoperative period, they typically resolve with prompt ambulation, timely removal of invasive devices, prevention and/or resolution of atelectasis through optimal respiratory care, and effective analgesia. It is important to remember that the emergence of distal infections, such as pneumonia, does not constitute a failure of surgical prophylaxis. Prophylaxis should be as short as possible because prolonged prophylactic regimens may contribute to the selection of resistant organisms and may make any infection more difficult to treat.

Surgical site appearance is the most important determinant of the presence of an infection. Drainage of pus from the incision accompanied by redness, warmth, and pain or tenderness is highly suggestive of an SSI. By definition, any surgical site that requires incision and drainage by the surgeon is considered infected regardless of appearance. Failure to heal and wound dehiscence also are seen commonly with SSIs, although surgical technique and nutritional status may be important contributing factors.

The presentation of signs and symptoms consistent with an SSI in relation to previous surgery is an important consideration when evaluating therapeutic outcomes after surgical prophylaxis. Many SSIs will not be evident during acute hospitalization. In fact, SSIs may not become evident until up to 30 days later or, in the case of prosthesis implantation, up to 1 year later. Thus, the true incidence of SSI can be determined only by completing comprehensive postdischarge surveillance. All studies investigating the efficacy of surgical prophylaxis must include adequate postdischarge followup in order to be able to thoroughly assess the success of any prophylactic regimen.

ABBREVIATIONS

ACOG: American College of Obstetricians and Gynecologists

ASA: American Society of Anesthesiologists

CDC: Centers for Disease Control and Prevention

CSF: cerebrospinal fluid

JCAHO: Joint Commission on Accreditation of Healthcare Organizations

MIC: minimum inhibitory concentration

MRSA: methicillin-resistant *Staphylococcus aureus*

MSSA: methicillin-sensitive *Staphylococcus aureus*

NNIS: National Nosocomial Infections Surveillance System

NRC: National Research Council

SENIC: Study on the Efficacy of Nosocomial Infection Control

SSI: surgical site infection

VRE: vancomycin-resistant enterococci

REFERENCES

1. Mitka M. Preventing surgical infection is more important than ever. JAMA 2000;283:44–45.
2. de Lalla F. Antimicrobial chemotherapy in the control of surgical infectious complications. J Chemother 1999;11:440–445.
3. Mangram AJ, Horan TC, Pearson ML, et al. Guideline for prevention of surgical site infection, 1999. Centers for Disease Control and Prevention (CDC) Hospital Infection Control Practices Advisory Committee. Am J Infect Control 1999;27:97–132.
4. Hendrick TL, Anastacio MM, Sawyer RG. Prevention of surgical site infection. Expert Rev Anti Infect Ther 2006;4:223–33.
5. National Academy of Sciences, National Research Council. Postoperative wound infections: The influence of ultraviolet irradiation of the operating room and of various other factors. Ann Surg 1964;160:32–135.
6. Cruse PJE, Foord R. A five-year prospective study of 23,649 surgical wounds. Arch Surg 1973;107:206–210.
7. ASHP Commission on Therapeutics. ASHP therapeutic guidelines on antimicrobial prophylaxis in surgery. In: Deffenbaugh J, ed. Best Practices for Health System Pharmacy. Bethesda, MD: ASHP, 1999:349–396.
8. Furnary AP, Zerr KJ, Grunkemeier GL, Starr A. Continuous intravenous insulin infusion reduces the incidence of deep sternal wound infection in diabetic patients after cardiac surgical procedures. Ann Thorac Surg 1999;67:352–360.
9. Dionigi R, Rovera F, Dionigi G, et al. Risk factors in surgery. J Chemother 2001;13:6–11.
10. Perl TM, Cullen JJ, Wenzel RP, et al. Intranasal mupirocin to prevent postoperative Staphylococcus aureus infections. N Engl J Med 2002; 346:1871–7.
11. Haley RW, Culver DH, Morgan WM, et al. Identifying patients at high risk of surgical wound infection: A simple multivariate index of patient susceptibility and wound contamination. Am J Epidemiol 1985;127:206–215.
12. Wilson AP, Hodgson B, Liu M, et al. Reduction in wound infection rates by wound surveillance with postdischarge follow-up and feedback. Br J Surg 2006;93:630–8.
13. Gaynes RP, Culver DH, Horan TC, et al. Sugical site infection (SSI) rates in the United States, 1992–1998 : The national nosocomial infections surveillance system basic SSI risk index. CID 2001;33(Suppl 2):S69–77.
14. National Nosocomial Infections Surveillance (NNIS) System Report, data summary from January 1992 through June 2004 issued October 2004. Am J Infect Control 2004;32:470–85.
15. Owens WD, Felts JA, Spitznagel EL. ASA physical status classifications: A study of consistency of ratings. Anesthesiology 1978;49:239–243.
16. Elek SD, Conen PE. The virulence of Staphylococcus pyogenes for man: A study of the problems of wound infection. Br J Exp Pathol 1958;38:573–586.
17. Burke JF. Identification of the sources of staphylococci contaminating the surgical wound during operation. Ann Surg 1963;158:898–904.
18. Kaiser AB, Kernodle DS, Parker RA. Low-inoculum model of surgical wound infection. J Infect Dis 1992;166:393–399.
19. Esposito S. Immune system and surgical site infection. J Chemother 2001;13:12–16.
20. De Lalla F. Antibiotic prophylaxis in orthopedic prosthetic surgery. J Chemother 2001;13:48–53.
21. Halwani M, Solaymani-Dodaran M, Grundman H, et al. Cross transmission of nosocomial pathogens in an adult intensive care unit: Incidence and risk factors. J Hosp Infect 2006;63:39–46.
22. Murray BE. Vancomycin-resistant enterococcal infections. N Engl J Med 2000;342:710–721.
23. Hospital Infection Control Practices Advisory Committee. Recommendations for preventing the spread of vancomycin resistance. MMWR 1995;44:1–13.
24. Centers for Disease Control and Prevention. Interim guidelines for prevention and control of Staphylococcus aureus infection associated with reduced susceptibility to vancomycin. MMWR 1997;46:626–635.
25. Cosgrove SE, Qi Y, Kaye KS, et al. The impact of methicillin resistance in Staphylococcus aureus bacteremia on patient outcomes: Mortality, length of stay, and hospital charges. Infect Control Hosp Epidemiol 2005;26:166–74.
26. Manian FA, Meyer PL, Setzer J, et al. Surgical site infections associated with methicillin-resistant Staphylococcus aureus: Do postoperative factors play a role? Clin Infect Dis 2003;36:863–8.
27. Lowy FD, Waldhausen JA, Miller M, et al. Report of the National Heart, Lung and Blood Institute-National Institute of Allergy and Infectious Diseases working group on antimicrobial strategies and cardiothoracic surgery. Am Heart J 2004:147:575–81.
28. Munoz P, Burrillo A, Bouza E. Criteria used when initiating antifungal therapy against Candida spp. in the intensive care unit. Int J Antimicrob Agents 2000;15:83–90.
29. Lipsett PA. Surgical critical care: Fungal infections in surgical patients. Crit Care Med 2006;34:S25–24.
30. McKinnon PS. Goff DA, Kern JW, et al. Temporal assessment of Candida risk factors in the surgical intensive care unit. Arch Surg 2001;136:1401–8.
31. Classen DC, Evans RS, Pestotnik SL, et al. The timing of prophylactic administration of antibiotics and the risk of surgical wound infection. N Engl J Med 1992;326:281–286.
32. Garey KW, Dao T, Chen, et al. Timing of vancomycin prophylaxis for cardiac surgery patients and the risk for surgical site infections. J Antimicrob Chemother 2006;58:645–50.
33. Bratzler DW, Houck PM, Richards C, et al. Use of antimicrobial prophylaxis for major surgery: Baseline results from the National Surgical Infection Prevention Project. Arch Surg 2005;140:174–82.
34. Esposito S. Is single-dose antibiotic prophylaxis sufficient for any surgical procedure? J Chemother 1999;11:556–564.
35. Zelenitzky SA, Ariano RE, Harding GKM, et al. Antibiotic pharmacodynamics in surgical prophylaxis: an association between intraoperative antibiotic concentrations and efficacy. Antimicrob Agents Chemother 2002;46:3026–3030.
36. Goldman DA, Hopkins CC, Karchmer AW. Cephalothin prophylaxis in cardiac valve surgery: A prospective, double-blind comparison of two-day and six-day regimen. J Thorac Cardiovasc Surg 1977;73:470–479.
37. Zanetti G, Flanagan HL Jr, Cohn LH, et al. Improvement of intraoperative antibiotic prophylaxis in prolonged cardiac surgery by automated alerts in the operating room. Infect Control Hosp Epidemiol 2003; 24:7–9.
38. Waltrip T, Lewis R, Young V, et al. A pilot study to determine the feasibility of continuous cefazolin infusion. Surg Infect 2002;3:5–9.
39. Weinbren MJ. Pharmacokinetics of antibiotics in burn patients. J Antimicrob Chemother 1999;44:319–327.
40. Caffarelli AD, Holden JP, Baron EJ, et al. Plasma cefazolin during cardiovascular surgery: Effects of cardiopulmonary bypass and profound hypothermic circulatory arrest. J Thorac Cardiovasc Surg 2006;131:1338–43.
41. Weed HG. Antimicrobial prophylaxis in the surgical patient. Med Clin North Am 2003;27:59–75.
42. Salkind AR, Cuddy PG, Foxworth JW. The rational clinical examination: Is this patient allergic to penicillin? An evidence-based analysis of the likelihood of penicillin allergy. JAMA 2001;285:2498–2505.
43. Gemmel CG, Edwards DI, Fraise AP, et al. Guidelines for the prophylaxis and treatment of methicillin Staphylococcus aureus (MRSA) infections in the UK. J Antimicrob Chemother 2006;57:589–608.
44. Hadaway L, Chamallas SN. Vancomycin: New perspectives on an old drug. J Infus Nurs 2003;26:278–284.

45. Wong RS, Cheng G, Chang NP, et al. Use of cefoperazone still needs a caution for bleeding from induced vitamin K deficiency. Am J Hematol 2006;81:76.
46. Williams KJ, Bax RP, Brown H, Machin SJ. Antibiotic treatment and associated prolonged prothrombin time. J Clin Pathol 1991;44:738–741.
47. Frighetto L, Marra CA, Stiver HG, et al. Economic impact of standardized orders for antimicrobial prophylaxis program. Ann Pharmacother 2000;34:154–160.
48. Bratzler DW, Houck PM. Antimicrobial prophylaxis for surgery: An advisory statement from the National Surgical Infection Prevention Project. Clin Infect Dis 2004;38:1706–1715.
49. McArdle CS, Morran CG, Anderson JR, et al. Oral ciprofloxacin as prophylaxis in gastroduodenal surgery. J Hosp Infect 1995;30:211–216.
50. Sharma VK, Howden CW. Meta-analysis of randomized, controlled trials of antibiotic prophylaxis before percutaneous endoscopic gastrostomy. Am J Gastroenterol 2000;95:3133–3136.
51. Kulling D, Sonnenberg A, Fried M, Bauerfeind P. Cost analysis of antibiotic prophylaxis for PEG. Gastrointest Endosc 2000;51:152–156.
52. Jewesson PJ, Stiver G, Wai A, et al. Double-blind comparison of cefazolin and ceftizoxime for prophylaxis against infections following elective biliary tract surgery. Antimicrob Agents Chemother 1996;40:70–74.
53. Agrawal CS, Sehgal R, Singh RK, Gupta AK. Antibiotic prophylaxis in elective cholecystectomy: A randomized, double-blinded study comparing ciprofloxacin and cefuroxime. Ind J Physiol Pharmacol 1999; 43:501–504.
54. Swoboda S, Oberdorfer K, Klee F, et al. Tissue and serum concentrations of levofloxacin 500 mg administered intravenously or orally for antibiotic prophylaxis in biliary surgery. J Antimicrob Chemother 2003;51:459–462.
55. Koc M, Zulfikaroglu B, Kece C, et al. A prospective, randomized study of prophylactic antibiotics in elective laparoscopic cholecystectomy. Surg Endosc 2003;17:1716–1718.
56. Gulberg V, Deibert P, Ochs A, et al. Prevention of infectious complications after transjugular intrahepatic portosystemic shunt in cirrhotic patients with a single dose of ceftriaxone. Hepatogastroenterology 1999;46:1126–1130.
57. Deibert P, Schwartz S, Olschewski M, et al. Risk factors and prevention of early infection after implantation or revision of transjugular intrahepatic portosystemic shunts: Results of a randomized study. Dig Dis Sci 1998;43:1708–1713.
58. Sheen-Chen SM, Chen WJ, Eng HL, et al. Bacteriology and antimicrobial choice in hepatolithiasis. Am J Infect Control 2000;28:298–301.
59. Liberman MA, Greason KL, Frame S, Ragland JJ. Single-dose cefotetan or cefoxitin versus multiple-dose cefoxitin as prophylaxis in patients undergoing appendectomy for acute nonperforated appendicitis. J Am Coll Surg 1995;180:77–80.
60. Colliza S, Rossi S. Antibiotic prophylaxis and treatment of surgical abdominal sepsis. J Chemother 2001;13:193–201.
61. Chung RS, Rowland DY, Li P, Diaz J. A meta-analysis of randomized, controlled trials of laparoscopic versus conventional appendectomy. Am J Surg 1999;177:250–256.
62. Zmora O, Wexner SD, Hajjar L, et al. Trend in preparation for colorectal surgery: Survey of the members of the American Society of Colon and Rectal Surgeons. Am Surg 2003;69:150–154.
63. Zmora O, Mahajna A, Bar-Zakai B, et al. Colon and rectal surgery without mechanical bowel preparation: A randomized, prospective trial. Ann Surg 2003;237:363–367.
64. Guenaga KF, Matos D, Castro AA, et al. Mechanical bowel preparation for elective colorectal surgery. Cochrane Database Syst Rev 2005;1:CD001544.
65. Baum ML, Anish DS, Chalmers TC, et al. A survey of clinical trials of antibiotic prophylaxis in colon surgery: Evidence against further use of no-treatment controls. N Engl J Med 1981;305:795–799.
66. Solla JA, Rothenberger DA. Preoperative bowel preparation: A survey of colon and rectal surgeons. Dis Colon Rectum 1990;33:154–159.
67. Jewesson P, Chow A, Wai A, et al. A double-blind, randomized study of three antimicrobial regimens in the prevention of infections after colorectal surgery. Diagn Microbiol Infect Dis 1997;29:155–165.
68. Mittelkotter U. Antimicrobial prophylaxis for abdominal surgery: Is there a need for metronidazole? J Chemother 2001;13:27–34.
69. McDonald PJ, Karran SJ. A comparison of intravenous cefoxitin and a combination of gentamicin and metronidazole as prophylaxis in colorectal surgery. Dis Colon Rectum 1983;26:661–664.
70. Lewis RT. Oral versus systemic antibiotic prophylaxis in elective colon surgery: A randomized study and meta-analysis send a message from the 1990s. Can J Surg 2002;45:173–180.
71. Ghorra SG, Rzeczycki TP, Natarajan R, Pricolo VE. Colostomy closure: Impact of preoperative risk factors on morbidity. Am Surg 1999;65:266–269.
72. Hirota WK, Petersen K, Baron TH, et al. Guidelines for antibiotic prophylaxis for GI endoscopy. Gastrointest Endosc 2003;58:475–482.
73. Sharma VK, Howden CW. Meta-analysis of randomized, controlled trials of antibiotic prophylaxis before percutaneous endoscopic gastrostomy. Am J Gastroenterol 2001;96:1951–1952.
74. Olson ES, Cookson BD. Do antimicrobials have a role in preventing septicaemia following instrumentation of the urinary tract? J Hosp Infect 2000;45:85–97.
75. Christiano AP, Hollowell CM, Kim H, et al. Double-blind, randomized comparison of single-dose ciprofloxacin versus intravenous cefazolin in patients undergoing outpatient endourologic surgery. Urology 2000;55:182–185.
76. Smaill F, Hofmeyr GJ. Antibiotic prophylaxis for cesarean section. Cochrane Database Syst Rev 2002;2:CD000933.
77. Rouzi AA, Khalifa F, Ba'aqeel H, et al. The routine use of cefazolin in cesarean section. Int J Gynaecol Obstet 2000;69:107–112.
78. Thigpen BD, Hood WA, Chouhan S, et al. Timing of prophylactic antibiotic administration in the uninfected labouring gravida: A randomized clinical trial. Am J Obstet Gynecol, 2005;192:1864–8.
79. Guaschino S, De Santo D, De Seta F. New perspectives in antibiotic prophylaxis for obstetric and gynaecological surgery. J Hosp Infect 2002;50(Suppl A):S13–S16.
80. American College of Obstetricians and Gynecologists. Antibiotic prophylaxis for gynecologic procedures. Obstet Gynecol 2006;108:225–234.
81. Hemsell DL, Johnson ER, Hemsell PG, et al. Cefazolin is inferior to cefotetan as single dose prophylaxis for women undergoing elective total abdominal hysterectomy. Clin Infect Dis 1995;20:677–684.
82. Sturlese E, Retto G, Pulia A, et al. Benefits of antibiotic prophylaxis in laparoscopic gynaecological surgery. Clin Exp Obstet Gynecol 1999;26:217–218.
83. Meuller SC, Henkel KO, Neumann J, et al. Perioperative antibiotic prophylaxis in maxillofacial surgery: Penetration of clindamycin into various tissues. J Craniomaxillofac Surg 1999;27:172–176.
84. Simo R, French G. The use of prophylactic antibiotics in head and neck oncological surgery. Curr Opin Otolaryngol Head Neck Surg 2006;14:55–61.
85. Grandis JR, Vickers RM, Rihs JD, et al. Efficacy of topical amoxicillin plus clavulanate-ticarcillin plus clavulanate and clindamycin in contaminated head and neck surgery: Effect of antibiotic spectra and duration of therapy. J Infect Dis 1994;170:729–732.
86. Roy MC. Surgical-site infections after coronary artery bypass graft surgery: Discriminating site-specific risk factors to improve prevention efforts. Infect Control Hosp Epidemiol 1998;19:229–233.
87. Hollenbeak CS, Murphy DM, Koenig S, et al. The clinical and economic impact of deep chest surgical site infections following coronary artery bypass graft surgery. Chest 2000;118:397–402.
88. Curtis JJ, Boley TM, Walls JT, et al. Randomized, prospective comparison of first- and second-generation cephalosporins as infection prophylaxis for cardiac surgery. Am J Surg 1993;166:734–737.
89. Edwards FH, Egleman RM, Houck P, et al. The Society of Thoracic Surgeons Practice Guidelines Series: Antibiotic prophylaxis in cardiac surgery, part 1: duration. Ann Thorac Surg 2006;81:397–404.
90. Finkelstein R, Rabino G, Masiah T, et al. Vancomycin versus cefazolin prophylaxis for cardiac surgery in the setting of a high prevalence of methicillin-resistant staphylococcal infections. J Thorac Cardiovasc Surg 2002;123:326–332.
91. Sok M, Dragas AZ, Erzen J, et al. Sources of pathogens causing pleuropulmonary infections after lung cancer resection. Eur J Cardiothorac Surg 2002;22:23–27.
92. Boldt J, Piper S, Uphus D, et al. Preoperative microbiologic screening and antibiotic prophylaxis in pulmonary resection operations. Ann Thorac Surg 1999;68:208–211.
93. Pratesi C, Russo D, Dorigo W, et al. Antibiotic prophylaxis in clean surgery: Vascular surgery. J Chemother 2001;13:123–128.
94. Marroni M, Cao P, Fiorio M, et al. Prospective, randomized, double-blind trial comparing teicoplanin and cefazolin as antibiotic prophy-

laxis in prosthetic vascular surgery. Eur J Clin Microbiol Infect Dis 1999;18:175–178.
95. Terpstra S, Noorkhoek GT, Voesten HG, et al. Rapid emergence of resistant coagulase-negative staphylococci on the skin after antibiotic prophylaxis. J Hosp Infect 1999;43:195–202.
96. Gillespie WJ, Walenkamp G. Antibiotic prophylaxis for surgery for proximal femoral and other closed long bone fractures. Cochrane Database Syst Rev 2001;1:CD000244.
97. Vasenius J, Tulikoura I, Vainionpaa S, Rokkanen P. Clindamycin versus cloxacillin in the treatment of 240 open fractures: A randomized, prospective study. Ann Chir Gynaecol 1998;87:224–228.
98. Velmahos GC, Toutouzas KG, Sarkisyan G, et al. Severe trauma is not an excuse for prolonged antibiotic prophylaxis. Arch Surg 2002;137:537–541.
99. Hosein IK, Hill DW, Hatfield RH. Controversies in the prevention of neurosurgical infection. J Hosp Infect 1999;43:5–11.
100. Barker FG. Efficacy of prophylactic antibiotics for craniotomy: A meta-analysis. Neurosurgery 1994;35:484–492.
101. Pons VG, Denlinger SL, Guglielmo BJ, et al. Ceftizoxime versus vancomycin and gentamicin in neurosurgical prophylaxis: A randomized, prospective, blinded clinical trial. Neurosurgery 1993;33:416–422.
102. Whitby M, Johnson BC, Atkinson RL, et al. The comparative efficacy of intravenous cefotaxime and trimethoprim/sulfamethoxazole in preventing infection after neurosurgery: A prospective, randomized study. Brisbane Neurosurgical Infection Group. Br J Neurosurg 2000;14:13–18.
103. Ratilal B, Costa J, Sampaio C. Antibiotic prophylaxis for surgical introduction of intracranial ventricular shunts. Cochrane Database Syst Rev 2006;3:CD005365.
104. Barker FG. Efficacy of prophylactic antibiotic therapy in spinal surgery: A meta-analysis. Neurosurgery 2002;51:391–400.
105. Riley LH 3d. Prophylactic antibiotics for spine surgery: Description of a regimen and its rationale. J South Orthop Assoc 1998;7:212–217.
106. Balague Ponz C, Trias M. Laparoscopic surgery and surgical infection. J Chemother 2001;13:17–22.
107. Wilson APR. Antibiotic prophylaxis in endoscopic and minimally invasive surgery. J Chemother 2001;13:102–107.
108. Kurz A, Sessler DI, Lenhardt R. Perioperative normothermia to reduce the incidence of surgical-wound infection and shorten hospitalization. Study of Wound Infection and Temperature Group. N Engl J Med 1996;334:1209–1215.
109. Greif R, Akca O, Horn EP, et al. Supplemental perioperative oxygen to reduce the incidence of surgical-wound infection. Outcomes Research Group. N Engl J Med 2000;342:161–167.
110. Furnary AP, Zerr KJ, Grunkemeier GL, et al. Continuous intravenous insulin infusion reduces the incidence of deep sternal wound infection in diabetic patients after cardiac surgical procedures. Ann Thorac Surg 1999;67:352–360.
111. Braztler DW, Houck PM, Richards C, et al. Use of antimicrobial prophylaxis for major surgery: Baseline results from the National Surgical Infection Prevention Project. Arch Surg 2005;190:9–15.
112. Braztler DW, Hunt DR. The surgical infection prevention and surgical care improvement projects: National initiatives to improve outcomes for patients having surgery. Clin Infect Dis 2006;43:322–30.
113. Joint Commission on Accreditation of Healthcare Organizations. Surgical infection prevention core performance measures for national implementation. *http//www.jcaho.org/pms/core+measures/10asipmeaslistpop.pdf.*

CHAPTER 128

Vaccines, Toxoids, and Other Immunobiologics

MARY S. HAYNEY

KEY CONCEPTS

1. Live vaccines may confer lifelong immunity but cannot be administered to immunosuppressed patients.
2. Inactivated and subunit vaccines and toxoids often require multiple doses to provide protection from infection, and booster doses generally are needed after the primary series.
3. Children younger than 2 years are unable to mount a T-cell–independent immune response that is elicited by polysaccharide vaccines.
4. Severely immunocompromised individuals should not receive live vaccines, and their responses to inactivated, polysaccharide, toxoid, and recombinant vaccines may be poor.
5. The childhood and adolescent immunization schedules, which are updated frequently and published annually, can be used to develop an immunization plan for children.
6. Annual influenza immunization is recommended for individuals with many chronic medical conditions, all individuals older than 50 years, pregnant women, young children aged 6 to 59 months, healthcare workers, and household contacts of high-risk individuals.
7. Pneumococcal immunization is achieved with two different types of vaccines: the conjugate heptavalent vaccine used in infants and the pneumococcal polysaccharide vaccine used in the elderly and other individuals with high-risk medical conditions.
8. Immune globulin provides rapid postexposure protection from measles, hepatitis A, varicella, and other infections, but the protection wanes over time.
9. Immune globulin adverse effects often are secondary to infusion rate. Slowing the intravenous infusion rate ameliorates chills, nausea, and fever that may develop during administration.
10. $Rh_0(D)$ immune globulin prevents Rh-negative mothers from mounting an immune response that results in hemolytic disease of the newborn. Hemolytic disease of the newborn results when Rh-negative mothers are sensitized to the Rh(D) antigen on the red blood cells of their fetuses.

Learning objectives, review questions, and other resources can be found at **www.pharmacotherapyonline.com.**

Immunization is defined as rendering a person protected from an infectious agent. Immunity to an infectious agent can be acquired by exposure to the disease, by transfer of antibodies from mother to fetus, through administration of immune globulin, and from vaccination. Immunization is the process of introducing an antigen into the body to induce protection against the infectious agent without causing disease. An *antigen* is a substance that induces an immune response. An *antibody* produced by the humoral arm of the immune system usually is the response that is measured as evidence of successful vaccination. However, the cellular immune response, which is much more difficult to measure, is also an important aspect of vaccine response.

This chapter introduces three groups of agents: vaccines, toxoids, and immune sera (together known as *immunobiologics*). Agents with a limited scope of use, such as agents for bioterrorism or travel, are beyond the scope of this chapter.

PRODUCTS TO PRODUCE IMMUNIZATION

Vaccines and toxoids are separate and distinct products. However, both types of products induce active immunity—that is, immunity generated by a natural immunologic response to an antigen. Vaccines can be live attenuated or killed. Killed vaccines may consist of whole or split particles derived from the pathogen. Bacterial vaccines generally are killed whole bacteria or specific bacterial antigens or conjugates. Live-attenuated vaccines induce an immunologic response more consistent with that occurring with natural infection. ❶ Because the organisms in live-attenuated vaccines undergo limited replication in the vaccinated individual after administration, they may confer lifelong immunity with one dose (as does a primary natural infection). ❷ Multiple doses of killed vaccines usually are needed to induce long-lasting, effective immunity. Additional doses at varying time intervals (booster doses) often are required to maintain immunity. Booster doses of such vaccines elicit memory responses from the B cells that produce immunoglobulin G (IgG). The immune system already has developed an array of antibodies to the antigen. Upon restimulation with a booster dose, the B cells, which produce the most specific antibodies against the antigen, are activated. Restimulation allows the most active antibodies against the antigen to be selected and maintained in the "immunologic memory." Thus, the booster dose results in a rapid, intense antibody response that is long-lasting. Killed vaccines also can differ in immunity potential, depending on their composition. For example, polysaccharide vaccines tend to be poorly immunogenic in infants, whereas protein–polysaccharide conjugated vaccines of the same antigen tend to be highly immunogenic (e.g., pneumococcal polysaccharide vaccine vs pneumococcal conjugated vaccine). ❸ A T-cell–independent immune response is made to polysaccharide antigens that stimulate B cells directly.[1] There is no maturation or booster response with a T-cell–independent immune response, and children younger than 2 years cannot make this type of response. Protein–polysaccharide conjugate vaccines stimulate T cells and promote interactions between T cells and B cells when producing the protective immune responses consisting of immunologic memory and high-affinity IgG.

Toxoids are inactivated bacterial toxins that generally are combined with aluminum salts to enhance their antigenicity by prolonging antigen absorption and exposure. These adjuvants also increase local tissue irritation when injected. Toxoids stimulate the production of antibodies against the bacterial toxins rather than the infecting bacterial pathogens.

Immune sera are sterile solutions containing antibody derived from human (immunoglobulin) sources. Immunoglobulins are derived from donor pools of blood plasma and are processed using cold ethanol fractionation in order to inactivate known potential pathogens. These sera are indicated for induction of passive immunity (temporary immunity to infection as a result of administration of antibodies not produced by the host; see Other Immunobiologics below).

In addition to the active component in an immunobiologic, other active and inert ingredients are often present. Suspending agents, such as water, saline, or complex fluids containing proteins (e.g., albumin), are used as the vehicle for the immunobiologic agent. Preservatives, stabilizers, and antibiotics may be added to help maintain the integrity of the product. Immunized individuals may respond with allergic reactions not to the immunobiologic agent itself but to the other components of the pharmaceutical preparation. Different manufacturers of the same immunobiologic may have different active and inert ingredients or different quantities of these ingredients in their products.

Use of combination vaccines can decrease the number of injections required at a single visit. For this reason, combination vaccines can increase patient, parent, and healthcare provider compliance with the immunization schedule. Also, combination vaccines can decrease the cost of stocking and administering vaccines by protecting against multiple diseases with a single product. Licensed combination vaccines should be used whenever any of their components are indicated.[2]

Certain vaccines manufactured by various companies are considered interchangeable. Hepatitis A and hepatitis B vaccines are considered interchangeable. It is preferable to use diphtheria, tetanus toxoids, and acellular pertussis (DTaP) vaccine from the same manufacturer to complete the entire primary series. However, immunization should not be delayed if the particular type of vaccine administered for the initial doses cannot be ascertained easily. Finally, all licensed *Haemophilus influenzae* type b (Hib) conjugate vaccines are considered interchangeable for the primary series of three doses of vaccine.[3]

In general, vaccines and toxoids must be kept refrigerated because breaking the "cold chain" may result in loss of potency. Varicella vaccine, and zoster vaccines must be stored frozen. However, freezing most vaccines can result in loss of potency. Immune sera generally should be kept refrigerated and not frozen except for lyophilized human intravenous immunoglobulin (IVIG), which can be stored at room temperature. Careful attention to appropriate storage of all vaccines and immunobiologics is absolutely imperative. Directions for appropriate storage can be found in the package inserts.

FACTORS AFFECTING RESPONSE TO IMMUNIZATION

Various factors are known to affect response to vaccines and toxoids. Viability of the antigen is an important factor (live attenuated vs killed), as discussed previously. Total dose also is important because there seems to exist a threshold dose above which no further increase in antibody titer is seen. The interval between immunization doses, number of doses given, or both may change immune response to an agent. Among hepatitis B vaccine nonresponders, a significant proportion of individuals mount a vaccine response when given additional doses of vaccine.[2] In contrast, additional doses of influenza vaccine are minimally effective in immunocompetent elderly individuals, individuals with human immunodeficiency virus (HIV) infection, and patients with cancer.[3–5] Generally, intervals longer than those recommended between vaccine doses do not reduce immune response.[1]

The route and site of administration of the immunobiologic are important. This is best illustrated by the hepatitis B vaccine, which elicits a satisfactory antibody response when given in the deltoid muscle but not a consistent response when administered in the gluteal area.[6] Injections should be administered at a site with little likelihood of site damage. Immunobiologics containing adjuvants should be given into a muscle mass because they can cause irritation when given subcutaneously or intradermally.[1]

Host factors influence vaccine response. Immunodeficiency, increasing age, underlying disease, and genetic background have been associated with poor response rates.[7–10]

VACCINE ADMINISTRATION

Subcutaneous injections should be administered into the thigh of infants and in the upper arm area of older children and adults. A $^5/_8$-inch, 25-gauge needle should be used, taking care not to administer the dose intradermally or intramuscularly (IM). For IM injection, the anterolateral aspect of the upper thigh (infants and toddlers) or the deltoid muscle of the upper arm (children and adults) should be used. When giving an IM injection to an adult, at least a 1-inch needle should be used for persons weighing less than 90 kg and a 1.5-inch needle for persons weighing more than 90 kg to ensure injection in the muscle.[7] The buttock should not be used because of the potential for inadequate immunologic response and the potential risk of injury to the sciatic nerve. When the buttock must be used (as for large doses of immunoglobulin), only the upper outer quadrant should be used, with the needle inserted anteriorly.

The rotavirus vaccine is administered orally. The tube of vaccine should be squeezed inside the infant's mouth toward the inner cheek until the dosing tube is empty. If the infant regurgitates or spits out the vaccine, readministration is not recommended.[11]

LAIV is administered intranasally. A specially designed sprayer is inserted just inside the nostril, and the dose is sprayed by depressing the plunger of the sprayer. The clip is removed from the plunger so that the second half of the dose can be administered into the other nostril. The vaccinated individual should breathe normally. The dose does not need to be repeated if the individual sneezes during or shortly after administration.[12]

Questions often arise concerning the simultaneous administration of vaccines. In general, inactivated and live-attenuated vaccines can be administered simultaneously at separate sites. If two or more inactivated vaccines cannot be administered simultaneously, they can be administered without regard to spacing between doses. Inactivated and live vaccines can be administered simultaneously or, if they cannot be administered simultaneously, at any interval between doses, except for cholera (killed) and yellow fever (live) vaccines, which should be given at least 3 weeks apart. If live vaccines are not administered simultaneously, their administration should be separated by at least 4 weeks. Live viral vaccines may interfere with purified protein derivative response; thus, tuberculin testing should be postponed 4 to 6 weeks after administration of live-virus vaccine.[1]

Simultaneous administration of immunoglobulin and live-attenuated vaccines may inhibit host antibody response because of impairment of viral replication. A dose relationship exists between administration of immunoglobulin and inhibition of immune

TABLE 128-1 Suggested Intervals between Administration of Antibody-Containing Products for Different Indications and Measles-Containing Vaccine and Varicella Vaccine[a]

Product/Indication	Dose, Including Milligrams of Immunoglobulin G per Kilogram of Body Weight[a]	Recommended Interval before Measles or Varicella (months)
Respiratory syncytial virus IG[b]	15 mg/kg IM	None
Tetanus IG	250 units (10 mg IgG/kg) IM	3
Hepatitis A IG		
Contact prophylaxis	0.02 mL/kg (3.3 mg IgG/kg) IM	3
International travel	0.06 mL/kg (10 mg IgG/kg) IM	3
Hepatitis B IG	0.06 mL/kg (10 mg IgG/kg) IM	3
Rabies IG	20 international units/kg (22 mg IgG/kg) IM	4
Varicella IG	125 units/10 kg (20–40 mg IgG/kg) IM	5
Measles prophylaxis IG		
Standard (i.e., nonimmunocompromised) contact	0.25 mL/kg (40 mg IgG/kg) IM	5
Immunocompromised contact	0.50 mL/kg (80 mg IgG/kg) IM	6
Blood transfusion		
Red blood cells (RBCs), washed	10 mL/kg negligible IgG/kg	None
RBCs, adenine-saline added	10 mL/kg (10 mg IgG/kg) IV	3
Packed RBCs (hematocrit 65%)[c]	10 mL/kg (60 mg IgG/kg) IV	6
Whole blood (hematocrit 35%–50%)[c]	10 mL/kg (80–100 mg IgG/kg) IV	6
Plasma/platelet products	10 mL/kg (160 mg IgG/kg) IV	7
Cytomegalovirus intravenous immune globulin (IVIG)	150 mg/kg maximum	6
Respiratory syncytial virus prophylaxis IVIG	750 mg/kg	9
IVIG		
Replacement therapy for immune deficiency[d]	300–400 mg/kg IV[d]	8
Idiopathic (immune) thrombocytopenic purpura	400 mg/kg IV 1,000 mg/kg IV	8 10
Kawasaki's disease	2 g/kg IV	11

[a]This table is not intended for determining the correct indications and dosages for using antibody-containing products. Unvaccinated persons might not be fully protected against measles during the entire recommended interval, and additional doses of immune globulin or measles vaccine might be indicated after measles exposure. Concentrations of measles antibody in an immune globulin preparation can vary by manufacturer's lot. Rates of antibody clearance after receipt of an immune globulin preparation also might vary. Recommended intervals are extrapolated from an estimated half-life of 30 days for passively acquired antibody and an observed interference with the immune response to measles vaccine for 5 months after a dose of 80 mg IgG/kg. (Data from Mason W, Takahashi M, Schneider T. Persisting passively acquired measles antibody following gamma globulin therapy for Kawasaki's disease and response to live virus vaccination (abstract 311). Presented at the 32nd meeting of the Interscience Conference on Antimicrobial Agents and Chemotherapy, Los Angeles, California, October 1992.)

[b]Contains antibody only to respiratory syncytial virus.

[c]Assumes serum immunoglobulin G (IgG) concentration of 16 mg/mL.

[d]Measles and varicella vaccination is recommended for children with asymptomatic or mildly symptomatic human immunodeficiency virus (HIV) infection but is contraindicated for persons with severe immunosuppression from HIV or any other immunosuppressive disorder.

From MMWR 2006;55(2).

response to a vaccine (Table 128–1). Whole blood and other blood products containing antibodies may interfere with the response to the measles, mumps, and rubella (MMR) and varicella vaccines. For rubella-seronegative women who are immediately postpartum and have received a blood product in the last trimester or anti-Rh_o(D) immunoglobulin at the time of delivery, vaccination with MMR should be done immediately, with rubella antibody testing at least 3 months later to determine vaccine response. In any patient, if vaccination with MMR or varicella is followed by emergency immunoglobulin administration, the vaccine can be repeated or seroconversion to viral antigens can be confirmed after sufficient time has elapsed (see Table 128–1). Immunoglobulin does not interfere with the response to oral vaccines or yellow fever vaccine.[1]

Simultaneous administration of inactivated vaccines along with immunoglobulins is not contraindicated. However, different sites are recommended for killed vaccine and immunoglobulin administration. Increasing the dose or number of vaccines in this circumstance is not recommended.

IMMUNIZATION OF SPECIAL POPULATIONS

NEONATES, INFANTS, AND PREGNANT WOMEN

The age of the recipient is an important determining factor in vaccine and toxoid response. In the first few months of life, maternal antibodies acquired via transplacental transfer during the third trimester of gestation protect an infant. However, the maternal antibodies also inhibit the immune response to live vaccines because the circulating antibodies neutralize the vaccine before the infant has the opportunity to mount an immune response. For this reason, live vaccines are not administered until maternal antibodies have waned, generally by infant age 12 months.[1]

Premature infants should be vaccinated at the same chronologic age using the same schedule and precautions for full-term infants. The full recommended doses of vaccines should be used, regardless of age or birth weight. Hepatitis B vaccine should be administered to preterm, low birth weitht infants at one month of age. Breast-fed infants should be vaccinated according to standard pediatric schedules.

Most vaccines are pregnancy category C. As with most drugs, the vaccines are given this category assignment not because of a known risk to the fetus but because of lack of information. No birth defect has ever been attributed to vaccine exposure.[1] For example, no cases of congenital rubella syndrome from inadvertent administration of rubella vaccine to a pregnant woman have ever been reported. Despite this, vaccination of pregnant women generally is deferred until after delivery because of concern over potential risk to the fetus.

Universal influenza immunization is recommended for women who will be pregnant during influenza season. Tetanus-diphtheria (Td) vaccine is recommended for pregnant women who have not received a Td booster in the past 10 years. Although live vaccines generally are avoided because of the theoretical risk of transmission of the vaccine organism to the fetus, inactivated vaccines may be administered to pregnant women when the benefits outweigh the risks.[3] Hepatitis B, hepatitis A, meningococcal, inactivated polio, and pneumococcal polysaccharide vaccines should be administered to pregnant women who are at risk for contracting these infections.[13]

IMMUNOCOMPROMISED HOSTS

Vaccination in compromised hosts (e.g., those with chronic disease, such as diabetes or connective tissue disease, alcoholics, or those with cancer or HIV disease) must be individualized based on the disease state and its treatment. ❹ In general, severely immunocompromised individuals should not receive live vaccines. Administration of other vaccines may be indicated, but responses may be suboptimal.

Patients with chronic pulmonary, renal, hepatic, or metabolic disease who are not receiving immunosuppressants can receive both live-attenuated and killed vaccines and toxoids to induce active immunity. These patients often need higher doses of vaccines or more frequent dosing to induce immunity. Generally, immunization should be considered early in the course of the disease in an attempt to induce immunity at a point when the disease is less severe.

Patients with active malignant disease can receive killed vaccines or toxoids but should not be given live vaccines. The MMR vaccine is not contraindicated for close contacts, however. Live-virus vaccines can be administered to persons with leukemia who have not received chemotherapy for at least 3 months. Vaccines should be timed so that they do not coincide with the start of chemotherapy or radiation therapy. Annual influenza vaccine should be administered 2 weeks prior to chemotherapy or between cycles.[3] If vaccines cannot be given at least 2 weeks before the start of these therapies, immunization should be postponed until 3 months after the therapy has been completed. Passive immunization with immunoglobulin can be used in place of active immunization regardless of the history of immunization.

Glucocorticoids may cause suppressed responses to vaccines. For the purposes of immunization, the immunosuppressing dose of corticosteroids is prednisone 20 mg or more daily or 2 mg/kg daily, or an equivalent dose of another steroid, for at least 2 weeks. Patients receiving long-term alternate-day steroid therapy with short-acting agents, administration of maintenance physiologic doses of steroids (e.g., 5–10 mg/day of prednisone) via topical, aerosol, intraarticular, bursal, or tendon steroid injections require no special consideration for immunization. If patients have been receiving high-dose corticosteroids or have had a course lasting longer than 2 weeks, then at least 1 month should pass before immunization with live-virus vaccines.[1]

Patients with HIV infection require special consideration. Responses to live and killed antigens generally are suboptimal and decrease as the disease progresses because HIV produces defects in cell-mediated immunity and humoral immunity. For children up to age 16 years with HIV infection, immunization following the standard schedules is recommended for hepatitis B, DTaP (up to age 7 and Td for children older than 7 years), heptavalent pneumococcal conjugate vaccine (PCV7), Hib, inactivated polio vaccine (IPV), and annual influenza. Two doses of MMR vaccine should be administered at least 1 month apart as soon as possible after the first birthday. MMR and varicella virus should be administered only to children who have no or only moderate evidence of immunosuppression.[14] Two doses of varicella vaccine separated by 3 months are recommended only for children with no evidence of immunosuppression.[14] Children with HIV infection are at high risk for invasive pneumococcal disease, so children aged 24 to 59 months who did not receive the primary series as infants should receive two doses of PCV7 separated by at least 2 months. These children also should receive pneumococcal polysaccharide vaccine (PPV23). Other killed vaccines can be used without concern for increased risk.

TRANSPLANT PATIENTS

Solid-Organ Transplant Patients

Organ transplantation has become routine treatment of end-stage organ disease of many causes. Although the number of organ transplants performed is severely limited by the availability of donor organs, survival of transplant recipients is increasing. Solid-organ transplant patients remain on immunosuppressive regimens for the rest of their lives. These immunosuppressive regimens result in a higher risk of infection and decrease the protection conferred by immunization.[15]

Whenever possible, transplant patients should be immunized prior to transplantation. Live vaccines generally are not given after transplantation. Posttransplantation diphtheria, tetanus, pneumococcal, and influenza vaccine responses are unpredictable. Decreased immune response has been documented following hepatitis B vaccine.

Hematopoietic Stem Cell Transplant Patients

Reimmunization of patients with hematopoietic stem cell transplantation is necessary because antibody concentrations wane rapidly. Annual influenza immunization may begin as soon as 6 months after successful engraftment. Reimmunization with DTaP vaccine if the child is 7 years or younger, Hib, inactivated polio, hepatitis B, and pneumococcal polysaccharide vaccines should begin approximately 12 months after hematopoietic stem cell transplantation. MMR can be administered at 24 months. Varicella, meningococcal, and pneumococcal conjugate vaccines are not recommended. Immunization of household contacts and healthcare workers also is necessary.[1]

CONTRAINDICATIONS AND PRECAUTIONS

There are few contraindications to the use of vaccines except those outlined earlier. The contraindications include a history of anaphylactic reactions to the vaccine or a component of the vaccine or an unexplained encephalopathy occurring within 7 days of a dose of pertussis vaccine. Immunosuppression and pregnancy are temporary contraindications to live vaccines. An interval of time must elapse based on the dose of immunoglobulin before a live vaccine can be administered (see Table 128–1). Precautions for DTaP administration include hypotonic hyporesponsive episode, fever of 40.5°C (104.9°F) or greater, crying lasting more than 3 hours within 48 hours of a previous dose, and seizures with or without fever within 3 days after a dose.[3] Generally, mild to moderate local reactions, mild acute illnesses, concurrent antibiotic use, prematurity, family history of adverse events, diarrhea, and breast-feeding are not contraindications to immunization.

OBTAINING AN IMMUNIZATION HISTORY

An immunization history should be obtained from every patient, regardless of the reason for the healthcare visit. Ideally, any history provided by the patient from memory should be verified by reviewing the patient's personal written immunization record or a database that contains the complete immunization history. State-based immunization registries are being developed to improve immunization coverage by allowing healthcare providers access to records at any contact with the healthcare system. Registries are aimed primarily at facilitation of childhood immunization records.[16] If an official written record is not available, patient characteristics (e.g., military service, travel history, and occupation) may provide clues to the immunization history. Serologic testing for immunity against certain diseases can provide specific information but is used routinely for only a few selected diseases (e.g., measles, rubella, hepatitis A and B, and varicella) and selected circumstances (e.g., employment in a healthcare facility). If a written record does not exist, one should be generated at the time of initiation of immunization. Patients without a written record should be considered susceptible, and an immunization program started and completed unless a serious adverse reaction occurs. As a general rule, the risks associated with overimmunization are minimal relative to the risks associated with contracting vaccine-preventable diseases.[3]

VACCINE DELIVERY

Shortfalls in vaccine coverage targets exist in both adult and pediatric populations.[17] Among children, those of preschool age historically have been the most neglected. Entry into public school is contingent on receipt of certain required immunizations, resulting in vaccine coverage rates greater than 97% in children 6 years of age and older. However, the lack of a similar enforcement mechanism in younger patients has contributed to exceptionally low immunization rates (<50%), particularly in children younger than 2 years. From 1989 to 1991, the United States experienced a national measles epidemic largely caused by inadequately immunized preschool-aged children. Additionally, other segments of the population (i.e., adolescents and senior citizens) have been identified as needing better vaccine coverage.[17–19]

According to the Centers for Disease Control and Prevention (CDC), every healthcare visit, regardless of its purpose, should be viewed as an opportunity to review a patient's immunization status and to administer needed vaccines. Immunization is perhaps the most cost-effective medical practice available. Each visit should encompass assessment of individuals' vaccine needs, administration of indicated agents, and documentation of immunization histories. The outcome measurement of what percentage of patients in a particular practice site is completely immunized is extremely important because the benefits of optimal vaccine use extend beyond the individual patient to the public as a whole.

NATIONAL VACCINE INJURY COMPENSATION ACT

The National Child Vaccine Injury Act of 1986 was passed by the U.S. Congress in response to reports of vaccine side effects and liability concerns of vaccine manufacturers and healthcare providers. With vaccine safety being questioned and manufacturers ceasing the development and marketing of vaccines, the National Vaccine Injury Compensation Program was instituted to offer a no-fault alternative means to compensate victims for injury due to vaccination. The program offers liability protection to manufacturers and an efficient means of recovering damages for individuals potentially injured by vaccines. Compensation for vaccine-related injuries is outlined in the Vaccine Injury Table (available at *http://www.hrsa.gov/vaccinecompensation/*). The act also instituted mandatory record keeping by healthcare providers in the permanent medical record. Specifically, the manufacturer and lot number of the vaccine, date of administration, and name, address, and title of the person giving the vaccine must be recorded. Additionally, the act mandates that healthcare providers report to their local health department or to the Food and Drug Administration (FDA) any occurrence of adverse reactions.

Healthcare providers must report all events requiring medical attention within 30 days of vaccination to the Vaccine Adverse Event Reporting System (VAERS), which serves as a central depot for vaccine-related adverse effects. Only a temporal association between the adverse event and vaccine administration needs to be made. No adverse event rates can be determined because only the number of adverse events reported is known; the number of vaccines administered is not known. This database can be used to determine changes in the frequencies of adverse events, to evaluate risk factors for adverse events, and to find rare adverse events.[29] VAERS report forms can be obtained by calling 1-800-822-7967, or reports can be made online at *www.vaers.hhs.gov*.

USE OF VACCINES AND TOXOIDS

❺ Appendices 128–1 and 128–2 show the recommended schedules for routine immunization of children and adults. Many states require children to be fully immunized prior to entering elementary school; however, optimal protection is achieved by immunizing at the recommended ages, which requires special attention to children younger than 2 years. Adults and adolescents also require vaccination and often are unaware of this need. An early adolescent preventive health visit is recommended. This visit is an opportunity to catch up on missed immunizations and to administer meningococcal conjugate, DTaP, and human papillomavirus (HPV) vaccines. Adults should receive routine Td boosters and be immune to measles, mumps, rubella, and varicella by either immunization or history of infection. Older adults need an annual influenza vaccine after age 50 years, zoster vaccine after age 60 years, and pneumococcal polysaccharide vaccine after age 65 years. Certain individuals with conditions or lifestyles that put them at high risk for vaccine-preventable diseases also should be immunized as described in the following text and outlined in the immunization schedules in the appendices.

TOXOIDS

DIPHTHERIA TOXOID ADSORBED AND DIPHTHERIA ANTITOXIN

Diphtheria is an acute illness caused by the toxin released by a *Corynebacterium diphtheriae* infection. The toxin inhibits cellular protein synthesis, and membranes form on mucosal surfaces. Systemic toxemia can result in myocarditis, neuritis, and thrombocytopenia. Membrane formation can cause respiratory obstruction, and significant toxin absorption can lead to severe illness and death.

Diphtheria toxoid adsorbed is a sterile suspension of modified toxins of *C. diphtheriae* that induces immunity against the exotoxin of this organism. Two strengths of diphtheria toxoid are available in the United States: pediatric strength (D) and adult strength (d), which contains less antigen because of the higher rate of adverse effects seen when the pediatric strength is used in adult patients.[20] The widespread use of diphtheria toxoid essentially has eliminated diphtheria from the United States.

Primary immunization with diphtheria toxoid (D) is indicated for children older than 6 weeks. The usual dose is 0.5 mL IM at rotating sites. Generally, the toxoid is given in combination with tetanus toxoid and acellular pertussis vaccine (as DTaP or in combination with hepatitis B surface antigen and IPV) at age 2, 4, and 6 months. Additional doses are given at age 15 to 18 months and again at age 4 to 6 years.[21] Completing the primary diphtheria toxoid immunization series usually induces immunity of at least 10 years' duration in 90% of persons. Booster doses should be given every 10 years.

If primary immunization is given to an immunosuppressed patient, an additional dose of diphtheria toxoid should be administered 1 month after the return to normal immune status. Diphtheria toxoid can be administered to persons with mild febrile illnesses and with other live or killed vaccines.[20]

For unimmunized adults, a complete three-dose series of diphtheria toxoid should be administered, with the first two doses given at least 4 weeks apart and the third dose given 6 to 12 months after the second. The combined Td preparation is recommended for adults because it contains less diphtheria toxoid than the pediatric dose and is associated with fewer reactions to the diphtheria component. All adults should receive booster doses of Td every 10 years. Adverse effects of diphtheria toxoid include mild to moderate tenderness, erythema, and induration at the injection site. Systemic reactions occur very rarely.[20]

TETANUS TOXOID, TETANUS TOXOID ADSORBED, AND TETANUS IMMUNOGLOBULIN

Tetanus is a severe acute illness caused by the exotoxin of *Clostridium tetani*. Sustained muscle contractions are characteristic of tetanus. Tetanus toxin interferes with neurotransmitters that promote muscle relaxation, leading to continuous muscle spasms. Death can be due to the tetanus toxin itself or secondary to a

TABLE 128-2 Tetanus Prophylaxis

	Wound Type			
	Clean, Minor		*All Other*	
Vaccination history	Td[a]	TIG	Td[a]	TIG
Unknown or fewer than three doses	Yes	No	Yes	Yes
Three or more doses	No[a,b]	No	No[a,c]	No

TIG, tetanus immune globulin.
[a]A single dose of diptheria, tetanus toxoids, and acellular pertussis (DTaP) should be used for the next dose of tetanus-diphtheria (Td) toxoid
[b]Yes if more than 10 years since last dose.
[c]Yes if more than 5 years since last dose.

complication such as aspiration pneumonia, dysregulation of the autonomic nervous system, or pulmonary embolism.[22]

Tetanus toxoid and tetanus toxoid adsorbed (adsorbed onto aluminum hydroxide, phosphate, or potassium sulfate to increase antigenicity) are sterile suspensions of the toxoid derived from *C. tetani.* Both toxoids are used to promote active immunity against tetanus; however, tetanus toxoid adsorbed is the preferred agent because it elicits a greater immune response and is associated with fewer adverse reactions.

A series of three 0.5-mL doses of tetanus toxoid elicits protection in 90% of vaccinees. Primary vaccination provides protection for at least 10 years. Additional doses of tetanus toxoid (combined with diphtheria toxoid, i.e., Td) are recommended as part of wound management if a patient has not received a dose of tetanus toxoid within the preceding 5 years. For minor or clean wounds, no dose is given. Table 128–2 summarizes these recommendations. Tetanus immunoglobulin should be given to individuals who have received fewer than three doses of tetanus toxoid and have more serious wounds. It can be administered with tetanus toxoid, provided that separate syringes and separate injection sites are used.[22]

In children, primary immunization against tetanus usually is offered in conjunction with diphtheria and pertussis vaccination (using DTaP or a combination vaccine that includes hepatitis B and polio vaccines). A 0.5-mL dose is recommended at age 2, 4, 6, and 15 to 18 months, but the first dose can be administered as early as age 6 weeks.[21] In children 7 years and older and in adults who have not been immunized previously, a series of three 0.5-mL doses of Td is administered IM initially. The first two doses are given 1 to 2 months apart, and the third dose is recommended at 6 to 12 months after the second dose. Boosters are recommended every 10 years, and unless there is contraindication to diphtheria toxoid, Td should be used. Tetanus toxoid can be given simultaneously with other killed and live vaccines, and, if indicated, it can be given to immunosuppressed patients.

Adverse reactions to tetanus toxoid include mild to moderate local reactions at the injection site, such as warmth, erythema, and induration. Rarely, fever, malaise, aches and pains, or neurologic disorders have been reported. In general, major local reactions occur within 2 to 8 hours of administration to patients with high serum tetanus antitoxin levels. This type of reaction is indicative of high preexisting antibody concentrations, and additional doses of toxoid should not be given any sooner than 10 years. Local reactions do not limit the use of the toxoid for further dosing. Although safety during pregnancy has not been definitely established, tetanus toxoid has been administered to pregnant women for prevention of neonatal tetanus. Generally, waiting until the second trimester is suggested.

Tetanus immune globulin is a sterile, concentrated, nonpyrogenic solution of immunoglobulins prepared from hyperimmunized humans. It is used to provide passive immunity to tetanus after the occurrence of traumatic wounds in nonimmunized or suboptimally immunized persons (see Table 128–2). A dose of 250 to 500 units IM should be administered. When administered with tetanus toxoid, separate sites for administration should be used. Tetanus immune globulin also is used for treatment of tetanus. In this setting, a single dose of 3,000 to 6,000 units IM is administered.

Adverse effects of tetanus immune globulin include pain, tenderness, erythema, and muscle stiffness at the injection site, which may persist for several hours. Systemic reactions occur rarely. IV administration has been associated with severe adverse reactions and is not recommended.

VACCINES

HAEMOPHILUS INFLUENZAE TYPE B VACCINES

Before 1995, Hib was responsible for thousands of cases of serious illnesses (e.g., meningitis, epiglottitis, pneumonia, sepsis, and septic arthritis). The incidence of Hib disease has declined more than 99% since introduction of the conjugate vaccines based on the organism's capsular substance, polyribosylribitol phosphate (PRP).[23]

The Hib vaccines used are conjugate products consisting of either a polysaccharide or an oligosaccharide of PRP covalently linked to a protein carrier. The protein carrier is important because it provides for T-lymphocyte–dependent immunologic response, whereas earlier Hib vaccines that consisted of only unconjugated PRP elicited a response that was T-cell independent. T-cell involvement in the response provides for (a) a greater antibody response regardless of the age of the patient receiving the vaccine, (b) immunologic response at an earlier age (including infants), and (c) a booster effect on subsequent exposure to the Hib capsule, whether through revaccination or natural exposure. The protein carrier is not considered a vaccine and should not be substituted for immunization against tetanus, diphtheria, or *Neisseria meningitidis.*

Hib conjugate vaccines are stable at 2°C to 8°C (35.6°F–46.4°F) and should not be frozen. They are indicated for routine use in all infants and children younger than 5 years. Additionally, these three products differ in their immunogenicity and schedule of administration (Table 128–3). The primary series of Hib vaccination consists of a 0.5-mL IM dose at ages 2, 4, and 6 months if HbOC (HibTITER) or PRP-T (ActHIB) is used. If PRP-OMP is being used, the primary series consists of doses given at ages 2 and 4 months. The series should not be initiated in an infant younger than 6 weeks. Although use of one product for the entire primary series is desirable, adequate protection is achieved even when different products are used during the initial doses. Following the primary series, a booster dose is recommended at age 12 to 15 months. Any of the Hib conjugate vaccines are suitable for the booster dose regardless of which conjugate was used for the primary series of doses.[1,21]

Schedules are more complex for infants who do not begin Hib immunization at the recommended age or who have fallen behind in the immunization schedule. For infants 7 to 11 months of age who have not been vaccinated, three doses of HbOC, PRP-OMP, or PRP-T should be given: two doses spaced 4 weeks apart and then a booster dose at age 12 to 15 months (but at least 8 weeks since the second dose). For unvaccinated children ages 12 to 14 months, two

TABLE 128-3 *Haemophilus influenzae* Type b Conjugate Vaccine Products

Vaccine	Trade Name	Protein Carrier
HbOC	HibTITER (Wyeth Vaccines)	Mutant diphtheria toxin protein
PRP-T	ActHIB (Aventis Pasteur)	Tetanus toxoid
PRP-OMP	PedvaxHIB (Merck)	*Neisseria meningitides* serogroup B outer membrane protein

The polysaccharide is polyribosylribitol-phosphate (PRP).

doses should be given, with an interval of 2 months between doses. In a child older than 15 months, a single dose of any of the four conjugate vaccines is indicated.[21] The American Academy of Pediatrics has made recommendations for children with lapsed immunization. For infants 7 to 11 months who have received one or two doses of Hib vaccine, one dose of vaccine with a booster dose at least 8 weeks later at age 12 to 15 months should be given. For children 12 to 14 months who received two doses, a single dose is indicated. If the child received only one dose before age 12 months, two additional doses separated by 8 weeks should be given. A single dose of vaccine is needed for a child 15 to 59 months old who has received any incomplete schedule.[24]

Vaccines for Hib are recommended for routine use only for patients up to age 59 months; beyond this age, most individuals will have natural immunity to Hib infection. Patients with certain underlying conditions (e.g., HIV infection, IgG_2 subclass deficiency, sickle cell disease, splenectomy, and hematopoietic stem cell transplants and those receiving chemotherapy for malignancies) are at higher than normal risk for Hib infection, and use of at least one dose of vaccine in these patients should be considered, although efficacy data in most of these situations are lacking.[1,25]

Adverse reactions to the Hib vaccine are uncommon. Erythema and induration at the injection site occur in approximately 25% of children and resolve within 24 hours. Fever, diarrhea, and vomiting are reported occasionally. Fever greater than 38°C (100.4°F) is reported in 2.4% of children.

HEPATITIS VACCINES

Information on vaccination for viral hepatitis is given in Chapter 42.

HUMAN PAPILLOMAVIRUS VACCINE

HPV infections are the most common sexually transmitted infections, with the highest prevalence of infection in sexually active young adults.[26] Although more than 120 different HPV types have been identified, at least 40 different types of HPV infect the anogenital tract. These 40 different viruses are grouped into low-risk and high-risk types. Low-risk types can cause genital warts and mild abnormalities on Papanicolaou (Pap) tests. The low-risk types are relatively harmless and temporary, and they do not increase the risk of cervical cancer. As many as 18 types are considered high risk. They cause abnormal Pap test results and may lead to cancer of the cervix, vulva, vagina, anus, or penis. High-risk HPV infections are necessary but not sufficient for the development of cervical cancer and for the majority of other anogenital and oral squamous cell cancers.

Most HPV infections are asymptomatic, and diagnosis is not pursued. HPV infection may cause precancerous changes in the cervix, which can be diagnosed primarily with a Pap test.[27] Additionally, HPV DNA in women older than 30 years with mild Pap test abnormalities can be detected. Because HPV infection usually resolves without complications, routine screening to determine if a patient has been infected is not recommended.

The Advisory Committee on Immunization Practices (ACIP) recommended the quadrivalent HPV vaccine as a three-dose series for all females 11 to 12 year old. The vaccine is licensed for females aged 9 to 26 years. Females aged 13 to 26 years also may benefit from immunization, and its use in this population is recommended. The vaccine series of three doses administered at 0, 2, and 6 months should be completed before sexual debut, but those who are sexually active also can be immunized because the vaccine series may protect them from HPV types to which they have not been exposed. The quadrivalent vaccine contains recombinant virus-like particles of the HPV capsid proteins from types 6, 11, 16, and 18.[28] Types 6 and 11 are low-risk viruses associated with anogenital warts. Types 16 and 18 cause approximately 70% of cervical cancers. Both of these vaccines induce high antibody responses and protect against cervical cell dysplasia and cancer.[29] The vaccine is well tolerated, with injection-site reactions and systemic reactions (e.g., headache and fatigue) occurring as commonly in immunized individuals as in the group receiving placebo.

This effective vaccine is an important advance, but the need for a Pap test for cervical cancer screening remains. Although 4.5 years of protection following the vaccine series has been documented, the need for future booster doses is not yet known.[30] Also, the usefulness of the vaccine in protecting males from HPV infection and anogenital warts has not been fully evaluated.

INFLUENZA VIRUS VACCINE

Influenza is respiratory illness characterized by abrupt onset of fever, myalgia, headache, severe malaise, cough, sore throat, and rhinitis. The illness typically resolves in several days but can exacerbate a chronic medical condition or lead to secondary bacterial pneumonia. Influenza activity each winter results in increased numbers of physician visits, hospitalizations, and deaths.

The ACIP makes yearly recommendations on the use and composition of influenza virus vaccine. The recommendations are published annually in *Morbidity and Mortality Weekly Report*. The reader should refer to these annual guidelines as a supplemental update to this chapter.

Influenza is classified as type A or B, with influenza A further subtyped based on hemagglutinin (H) and neuraminidase (N) surface antigens. Influenza A causes significant disease in humans, and the virus is subject to mutation by a phenomenon known as *antigenic drift and shift*, resulting in the development of different influenza strains. Previous exposure to or vaccination against one strain does not confer protection against other strains. Influenza B, also a significant cause of human disease, is less likely to mutate. The antigenic composition of influenza vaccine is determined from year to year by the predominant circulating strains worldwide and generally changes on a yearly basis.

Influenza vaccines are available as inactivated trivalent split or subunit vaccine or as a live-attenuated vaccine administered intranasally. Although both types of influenza vaccine probably are equally effective in protection from infection, they are indicated for distinct populations and should not be considered interchangeable.[12]

The inactivated influenza vaccine preparations generally contain 45 mcg antigen in 15-mcg trivalent units per 0.5 mL and are administered by IM injection. Children 6 to 35 months old receive 0.25 mL of inactivated influenza vaccine. Two doses of vaccine administered at least 1 month apart are necessary for all children younger than 9 years who are receiving the vaccine for the first time.[12] Preservative-free vaccine is available in 0.25- and 0.5-mL doses for use in young children.

LAIV is derived from a master influenza vaccine strain that has been adapted to grow at 25°C (77°F) most efficiently. LAIV is administered by spraying into each nostril of the vaccine recipient. The vaccine virus undergoes limited replication in the upper respiratory tract, inducing a local and systemic response. LAIV is indicated for healthy individuals aged 2 to 49 years. It should not be used in individuals who are at high risk for complications from influenza infection. Two doses separated by at least 4 weeks are needed for children aged 5 to 8 years who are receiving the vaccine for the first season. LAIV is packaged in a prefilled sprayer that must be refrigerated until use.[31,32]

Response to influenza vaccine generally is measured in terms of antibody response and, more important, efficacy. The elderly and individuals with chronic diseases are less likely to develop antibody levels that are considered protective and may remain susceptible to influenza infection. However, vaccination confers protection from secondary complications and reduces the risk of hospitalization or pneumonia by 50% to 60% and death by 80%. Influenza vaccine is cost effective in nursing home populations, in the elderly who live in the community, in young children, and in healthy working adults.[33–35]

❻ Annual influenza vaccination is strongly recommended for individuals older than 6 months who have chronic medical conditions that place them at increased risk for the complications of influenza. Annual influenza vaccination should be given to (a) all individuals 50 years and older; (b) residents of nursing homes; (c) adults and children with chronic cardiovascular or pulmonary diseases, including asthma; (d) adults and children with chronic metabolic disease, renal dysfunction, hemoglobinopathies, or immunosuppression (including immunosuppression from medications or HIV); (e) children and teenagers receiving chronic aspirin therapy; and (f) pregnant women. Children younger than 2 years have a risk of hospitalization equivalent to of other individuals with high-risk conditions. Young children up to age 5 years are very likely to require medical attention for influenza infection, so immunization of children aged 6 to 59 months is recommended.[36] The inactivated influenza vaccine has not been studied in infants younger than 6 months. Immunization of their household contacts and out-of-home caregivers may decrease the risk of influenza infection in these young infants. In addition, the influenza vaccination should be recommended for the following groups that can transmit influenza to high-risk groups: (a) healthcare workers in inpatient and outpatient settings, (b) employees of residential care facilities for high-risk patients, and (c) household members (including children) of persons in high-risk groups. Finally, influenza vaccination should be offered to anyone wishing to avoid influenza infection.[12] The optimal time period in the United States for influenza vaccination administration is October and November. However, the vaccine can be administered to unvaccinated individuals in high-risk groups throughout the influenza season, which typically lasts until April. Administration of influenza vaccines is contraindicated in persons with known anaphylactic reaction to eggs or other components of the vaccine. Vaccination need not be delayed in individuals with minor illness with or without fever.

Adverse reactions to the vaccine include local tenderness and low-grade fever in 3% to 5% of vaccinees beginning 6 to 12 hours postimmunization and lasting 1 to 2 days. Treatment with salicylates or acetaminophen is recommended. A slight increase in the risk of Guillain-Barré syndrome may follow in the weeks after influenza vaccination. The risk is estimated to be one case of Guillain-Barré syndrome per million doses of influenza vaccine administered.[37] Runny nose is the most commonly reported adverse reaction in both adults and children after administration of LAIV. Adults complained of headache and sore throat more frequently after receiving LAIV than after placebo. Children experienced higher rates of fever, vomiting, abdominal pain, and myalgias with vaccine than placebo.[12]

MEASLES VACCINE

Measles (rubeola) is a highly contagious viral illness characterized by rash and high fever. Complications of measles infections include severe diarrhea, otitis media, pneumonia, and encephalitis. Measles results in one to two deaths per 1,000 cases, with a much higher death rate in developing countries. With widespread vaccination, measles is on the verge of elimination in the Americas.

The measles vaccine is a live-attenuated viral vaccine that produces a subclinical, noncommunicable infection. Approximately 95% of vaccine recipients seroconvert after a single dose, and most individuals are protected for life.[38] Most persons who do not respond to the initial dose of measles vaccine will seroconvert after receiving a second dose, and this forms the basis for the two-dose vaccine strategy that was implemented in the United States in 1989.

The measles vaccine is administered subcutaneously as a 0.5-mL dose in the arm (or in the thigh if the patient is younger than 15 months). The vaccine is administered routinely for primary immunization to persons 12 to 15 months of age, usually as the MMR vaccine. The measles vaccine is not administered earlier than 12 months (except in certain outbreak circumstances) because persisting maternal antibody that was acquired transplacentally late in gestation can neutralize the vaccine virus before the vaccinated person can mount an immune response. A second dose of MMR is recommended when children are 4 to 6 years old.[21] The second dose of vaccine results in seroconversion in 95% of individuals who were first-dose nonresponders.[39]

Measles-containing vaccine should not be given to pregnant women or immunosuppressed patients. The one exception is HIV-infected patients, who are at very high risk for severe complications if they develop measles.[31] Persons with HIV infection who have never had measles or have never been vaccinated against it should be given measles-containing vaccine unless there is evidence of severe immunosuppression. The second dose should be given 1 month later rather than waiting for entry to school.

Recent administration of immunoglobulin interferes with measles vaccine response, so the recommended interval between the immunoglobulin and vaccine is determined by the dose of immunoglobulin (see Table 128–1).[1] Live vaccines not administered during the same visit must be delayed for at least 30 days following measles or MMR vaccine. Live measles vaccine may suppress a positive tuberculin skin test for up to 6 weeks postadministration.[1] Persons with a history of anaphylactic reaction to egg protein were considered to be at high risk for serious reactions to measles vaccine, a product derived from chick embryo fibroblasts. However, the risk of measles vaccination to egg-allergic patients is exceedingly low. Therefore, individuals requiring the measles vaccine should receive it regardless of a history of egg allergy.[38] A history of serious neomycin hypersensitivity remains a contraindication to measles vaccine use because each 0.5-mL dose contains 25 mcg neomycin. Finally, mild febrile illness and upper respiratory tract infections are not contraindications to vaccination.[38]

Measles vaccination is indicated in all persons born after 1956 or in those who lack documentation of wild virus infection by either history or antibody titers. Persons who received killed measles vaccine alone, who were given live vaccine within 3 months of receiving killed vaccine, or who received a vaccine of unknown type between 1963 and 1967 should be revaccinated. Two doses of a measles-containing vaccine are required for college students and healthcare workers who were born in 1957 or later. If two doses are needed (the person has never been vaccinated), the doses should be given at least 1 month apart.[25]

The measles vaccine has an excellent safety record. The most common side effect following vaccination is fever, which occurs in 5% to 15% of vaccinees. Transient generalized rash may occur in approximately 5% of vaccine recipients. These reactions generally appear 5 to 12 days postvaccination and last 2 to 5 days. Other adverse effects, such as headache, cough, sore throat, eye pain, malaise, and transient thrombocytopenia, occur less frequently. Local reactions at the injection site are rare but may occur in subjects who have been vaccinated previously with killed vaccine. After extensive study, no association between MMR vaccination and the development of autism has been made.[40]

MENINGOCOCCAL POLYSACCHARIDE AND CONJUGATE VACCINES

N. meningitidis is a leading cause of meningitis and sepsis in children and young adults in the United States. The vast majority of cases are sporadic, although the frequency of outbreaks, most often involving serogroup C, is increasing.

A quadrivalent vaccine containing capsular polysaccharides for serotypes A, C, Y, and W-135 has been available since the early 1970s. A conjugate vaccine containing the same serotypes was licensed for use in individuals 2 to 55 years old. Although serogroup B causes approximately one third of all cases, it has not been incorporated into the vaccine because group B polysaccharide is not immunogenic. The meningococcal conjugate vaccine is recommended for all children 11 to 12 years old and others at high risk for invasive meningococcal infection, including high school students and college freshmen who live in dormitories. The meningococcal polysaccharide vaccine is indicated in high-risk populations, such as those exposed to the disease, those in the midst of uncontrolled outbreaks, travelers to areas with epidemic or hyperendemic meningococcal disease, and individuals who have terminal complement component deficiencies or asplenia. Meningococcal polysaccharide vaccine is used primarily for individuals younger than 11 years or older than 55 years for whom meningococcal immunization is indicated. The polysaccharide preparation can be used for the immunization of college students and adults between 20 and 55 years of age, but the conjugate vaccine is preferred.[41]

College freshmen, particularly those living in dormitories or residence halls, are at modestly increased risk for invasive meningococcal disease compared with the rest of the population in this age group.[42,43] The ACIP recommends that healthcare providers inform students and parents about the increased risk and that a safe, effective vaccine is available.[43] The meningococcal conjugate vaccine should be made easily available for college freshmen wishing to decrease their risk for meningococcal disease. Most states now have legislation requiring college and universities to provide students and their parents with information about meningococcal disease and the availability of a vaccine. A few states require meningococcal immunization of college students.

Meningococcal polysaccharide vaccine is administered subcutaneously as a single 0.5-mL dose. Vaccinees should be older than 2 years of age because of the difficulty younger patients have responding to polysaccharide antigens. However, younger children may produce sufficient antibody levels against serogroup A if given two doses 3 months apart. Antibody levels thought to be protective are attained within 10 to 14 days. Revaccination can be considered in 2 to 3 years in high-risk children younger than 4 years at initial vaccination because of rapid antibody decline. Older children and adults who remain at high risk should be revaccinated after 3 to 5 years. Meningococcal conjugate vaccine is administered by IM injection. Currently, only a single dose is recommended.

A possible association between the meningococcal conjugate vaccine and Guillain-Barré syndrome has been reported. Although confidence in the estimated rate of this rare illness is lacking, an adolescent who recently was immunized with meningococcal conjugate vaccine incurs an approximately 1:1,000,000 increased risk for developing Guillain-Barré syndrome.[44] Injection-site reactions are the most common adverse effects following administration of either the meningococcal conjugate or polysaccharide vaccine.[41]

MUMPS VACCINE

Mumps is a viral illness that classically causes bilateral parotitis 16 to 18 days after exposure. Fever, headache, malaise, myalgia, and anorexia may precede the parotitis. Serious complications are rare but more common in adults. The mumps vaccine is a lyophilized live-attenuated vaccine prepared from chick embryo cultures. Each 0.5-mL dose of the vaccine also contains 25 mcg neomycin. The vaccine is available alone or in combinations with measles and rubella vaccines. The mumps vaccine is used to produce active immunity while producing a subclinical, noncommunicable infection.

The vaccine usually is given in combination with measles and rubella vaccines (as MMR) and is administered as a 0.5-mL subcutaneous injection in the upper arm. Dosing recommendations coincide with those for measles vaccine, with the first dose administered at age 12 to 15 months and the second dose prior to the child's entry into elementary school. Two doses of mumps-containing vaccine are recommended for school-aged children, international travelers, college students, and healthcare workers born after 1956.[45] A single dose of vaccine is acceptable documentation of immunity to mumps for other adults considered at lower risk of mumps infection, including adults born after 1956 and those with an uncertain history of wild virus infection.

Mumps vaccine should not be given to pregnant women or immunosuppressed patients. Additionally, conception should be avoided for 28 days following vaccination.[1] Anaphylactic reactions to mumps-containing vaccines are very rare and generally not associated with hypersensitivity to eggs. Therefore, egg allergy is not a contraindication to vaccination. The effect of immunoglobulin preparations on mumps vaccine response is unknown, but the response to measles and rubella is compromised if the vaccine is administered after immunoglobulins. The recommended interval between the immunoglobulin and vaccine is determined by the dose of immunoglobulin (see Table 128–1).[1] The vaccine should not be given to individuals with anaphylactic reactions to neomycin.

Serious adverse reactions to the vaccine are reported rarely. Parotitis, rash, pruritus, and purpura occur rarely. Local reactions, including soreness, burning, and stinging, may occur at the injection site.

PERTUSSIS VACCINE

Pertussis is caused by a bacterial infection with *Bordetella pertussis.* The illness is characterized by paroxysms of coughing to expel thick mucus. Prior to the availability of a vaccine, pertussis was a common childhood infection and was a significant cause of childhood mortality. Pertussis is most contagious in the early stage of the disease, can infect people of all ages, but is most serious in infants and young children.[46]

Acellular pertussis vaccines contain selective components of the *B. pertussis* organism. All acellular vaccines contain pertussis toxin, and some contain one or more additional bacterial components (e.g., filamentous hemagglutinin, pertactin [a 69-kDa outer membrane protein], and fimbriae types 2 and 3). Acellular pertussis vaccine is recommended for all doses of the pertussis schedule at 2, 4, 6, and 15 to 18 months of age. A fifth dose of pertussis vaccine is given to children 4 to 6 years of age.[46] Pertussis vaccine is administered in combination with diphtheria and tetanus (DTaP). Administration of an acellular pertussis–containing vaccine is also recommended for adolescents once between ages 11 and 18 years. Also, adults up to age 64 years should receive a pertussis-containing vaccine with their next dose of Td toxoids.

Local administration site reactions are relatively common. Systemic reactions, such as moderate fever, occur in 3% to 5% of vaccinees. Very rarely, high fever, febrile seizures, persistent crying spells, and hypotonic hyporesponsive episodes occur following vaccination. Allergy to a vaccine component and encephalopathy without known cause within 7 days of a pertussis vaccine are contraindications to future doses of vaccine. Efficacy of the vaccine is estimated to be approximately 80%.[47]

PNEUMOCOCCAL VACCINES

S. pneumoniae is a common pathogen with a range of manifestations, including asymptomatic upper respiratory tract colonization, sinusitis, acute otitis media, pharyngitis, pneumonia, meningitis, and bacteremia. Rates of invasive infections are highest in children younger than 2 years (approximately 200 per 100,000 population). The incidence increases again to 61 per 100,000 population in the elderly. Between the two age extremes, the incidence of invasive disease is approximately 24 per 100,000 population. Invasive pneumococcal infections cause approximately 40,000 deaths annually. Most of the deaths occur in the elderly or in those with underlying medical conditions. Approximately half the deaths could be preventable by vaccine. Two pneumococcal vaccine preparations, PCV7 and 23-valent pneumococcal polysaccharide vaccine (PPV23) are available. The vaccines have different indications and are not interchangeable.

Pneumococcal Polysaccharide Vaccine

Pneumococcal polysaccharide vaccine (Pneumovax 23) is a mixture of highly purified capsular polysaccharides from 23 of the most prevalent or invasive types of *S. pneumoniae* seen in the United States. Serotypes included are 1, 2, 3, 4, 5, 6B, 7F, 8, 9N, 9V, 10A, 11A, 12F, 14, 15B, 17F, 18C, 19A, 19F, 20, 22F, 23F, and 33F. These 23 types represent 85% to 90% of all blood isolates and 85% of pneumococcal isolates from other generally sterile sites seen in the United States. The vaccine is administered IM or subcutaneously as a single 0.5-mL dose. Each 0.5-mL dose of vaccine contains 25 mcg of each polysaccharide type dissolved in isotonic saline solution (for a total of 575 mcg polysaccharide) and 0.25% phenol as preservative.[48]

7 PPV23 is recommended for the following immunocompetent persons[48]:

- Persons 65 years and older (if an individual received vaccine more than 5 years earlier and was younger than 65 years at the time of administration, revaccination should be given)
- Persons aged 2 to 64 years with a chronic illness
- Persons aged 2 to 64 years with functional or anatomic asplenia (when splenectomy is planned, PPV23 should be given at least 2 weeks before surgery; a single revaccination is recommended at 5 years in subjects older than 10 years and at 3 years in subjects younger than 10 years)
- Persons aged 2 to 64 years of age living in environments where the risk of invasive pneumococcal disease or its complications is increased (this does not include daycare center employees and children)
- Persons with cochlear implants

PPV23 is recommended for immunocompromised persons 2 years and older with (a) HIV infection, (b) leukemia, (c) lymphoma, (d) Hodgkin's disease, (e) multiple myeloma, (f) generalized malignancy, (g) chronic renal failure or nephrotic syndrome, (h) patients receiving immunosuppressive therapy including corticosteroids, and (i) organ and bone marrow transplant recipients. A single revaccination should be given if 5 years or more have passed since the first dose in subjects older than 10 years. In subjects 10 years of age and younger, revaccination should be given 3 years after the previous dose.

PPV23 induces type-specific antibodies (T-cell–independent mechanisms) with a twofold rise within 2 to 3 weeks in 80% of young healthy adults. No correlation of antibody levels and protection has been determined. Antibody levels to these strains remain elevated for at least 5 years. In certain individuals, these levels decline within 10 years. Children may be protected for only 3 to 5 years. Elderly individuals and patients with chronic disease may have lower antibody levels produced with the vaccine. Children younger than 2 years do not respond adequately to the vaccine.

A number of other groups, including immunocompromised patients (e.g., leukemia, lymphoma, and multiple myeloma), dialysis patients, and patients with acquired immune deficiency syndrome, have reduced antibody production with the vaccine. Asymptomatic HIV-infected patients respond sufficiently to the vaccine. Patients with Hodgkin's disease respond to the vaccine better before splenectomy, chemotherapy, or radiation therapy.

PPV23 vaccine efficacy has been debated in the literature. Although prelicensure trials in young, healthy gold miners in South Africa showed a reduction in nonbacteremic disease rates, randomized clinical trials performed in the postmarketing period on elderly persons with chronic disease did not confirm these findings.[48] A large study of elderly individuals demonstrated a decreased risk of pneumonia caused by *S. pneumoniae* in vaccinated individuals but showed no change in the risk of community-acquired pneumonia even though most community-acquired pneumonias are caused by *S. pneumoniae*.[49] For invasive disease, reduction rates of 56% to 81% with the vaccine have been shown. Adults hospitalized with community-acquired pneumonia are significantly less likely to die if they have been immunized. In addition, immunized patients were less likely to have respiratory failure and had hospitalization stays that were shorter by 2 days.[50] A meta-analysis of nine randomized controlled trials concluded that the vaccine was efficacious in reducing the frequency of bacteremic pneumococcal disease among adults in low-risk groups and that the vaccine was cost effective.[48]

Although the safety of PPV23 during the first trimester of pregnancy has not been evaluated, no adverse effects have been seen in newborns whose mothers received the vaccine during pregnancy.[48]

PPV23 safety is well documented. Local reactions occur frequently within the first 48 hours and generally are mild. Local erythema and induration (30%), local discomfort (40%), and local swelling (3%) are the side effects observed most commonly. Revaccination has been associated with self-limited injection-site reactions more commonly than after the first dose.[51] Severe systemic reactions occur rarely and consist of weakness, myalgia, headache, photophobia, chills, and fever. In patients with HIV infection, pneumococcal vaccine may cause a transient increase in viral replication, but the importance of this finding is unknown.

Pneumococcal Conjugate Polysaccharide Vaccine

Invasive pneumococcal disease occurs even more frequently in children younger than 2 years than in those older than 65 years. The infection ranges goes from nasopharyngeal carriage to bacteremia and meningitis. Because of the lack of immune responsiveness in children younger than 2 years when exposed to polysaccharide vaccines, a conjugate vaccine was developed to protect young children from certain strains of *S. pneumoniae*.

Currently, a heptavalent vaccine (Prevnar) is available for use in children. This vaccine contains the conjugated capsular polysaccharides of serotypes 4, 6B, 9V, 14, 18C, 19F, and 23F, which cause approximately 80% of pediatric pneumococcal bacteremias in the United States.[52] The vaccine elicits a primary T-cell–dependent antibody response with the first dose and an immunologic memory effect after four doses. In clinical use, the vaccine is associated with a dramatic decline in invasive disease not only in immunized young children but also in individuals in all age groups.[53] In addition, a decline in the rate of disease caused by penicillin-resistant isolates has been noted.[54]

7 PCV7 is administered as a 0.5-mL IM injection at 2, 4, and 6 months of age and between 12 and 15 months of age. PCV7 also should be used in older children aged 24 to 59 months who are at high risk. Children with sickle cell disease or splenic dysfunction, HIV infection, immunocompromising conditions, or chronic illnesses should be immunized. PPV23 can be used in conjunction with PCV7. PPV23 should be administered after age 2 years and at least 2 months after the last dose of PCV7.

The vaccine series generally is well tolerated. Injection-site reactions and fever are the most commonly reported adverse effects.[52] Widespread use of PCV7 in infants and young children has resulted in a decreased incidence of invasive pneumococcal disease in the entire population and a decreased incidence of infection with penicillin-resistant *S. pneumoniae*.[53]

POLIOVIRUS VACCINES

Poliomyelitis is a contagious viral infection that usually causes asymptomatic infection; however, in its serious form it causes acute flaccid paralysis. Poliovirus is spread via the fecal–oral route. The virus replicates in the upper respiratory tract, gastrointestinal tract, and local lymphatics. The vast majority of polio infections are subclinical and asymptomatic. Indigenous polio has been absent from the United States since 1979, and the last case in the Americas was reported in 1991. Global eradication efforts are entering the final stages, and the eradication of polio should be accomplished in the next few years.

An inactivated trivalent vaccine developed by Jonas Salk was licensed for use in 1955. In 1987, an enhanced-potency IPV was introduced and has replaced the original inactivated vaccine. A live-attenuated oral polio vaccine (OPV) was developed by Albert Sabin in 1962. OPV was the primary immunizing agent for poliovirus infection. Widespread OPV use is responsible for eradication of wild-type polio in most of the world. However, with no poliovirus circulation in the United States for years, IPV is the recommended vaccine for the primary series and booster dose for children. OPV will continue to be used in areas of the world that have circulating poliovirus. The CDC maintains a stockpile of OPV to be used only in case of an outbreak.[55]

The IPV series is administered routinely to children at ages 2, 4, and 6 to 18 months, and 4 to 6 years. Protective antibodies to all three serotypes develop in 90% to 100% of children after two doses of vaccine. After three doses, 99% to 100% develop protective immunity, and the fourth dose results in long-term immunity.[55]

Primary poliomyelitis immunization is recommended for all children up to age 18 years. Primary immunization of adults over age 18 years is not recommended routinely because a high level of immunity already exists in this age group and the risk of exposure in developed countries is exceedingly small. However, unimmunized adults who are at increased risk for exposure because of travel, residence, or occupation should receive IPV series. Incompletely immunized adults or children should complete the series of IPV regardless of the interval since initiation of primary immunization. Adults do not need a booster dose routinely unless they are at increased risk of exposure (travel), in which case a single dose of IPV can be given.[55]

Allergies to any component of IPV, including streptomycin, polymyxin B, and neomycin, are contraindications to vaccine use. No serious side effects are attributable to IPV. Pregnant women should be given IPV only if there is a clear need, such as women who will be traveling or living in an area with endemic or epidemic poliovirus. IPV is recommended for immunodeficient individuals and their household contacts. Although the response may be lower, some protection against infection may be conferred.

The routine use of OPV in the United States has been discontinued because OPV is rarely associated with vaccine-associated paralytic poliomyelitis in vaccinees (one in 6.2 million doses) or contacts (one in 7.6 million doses). Because individuals with primary immune deficiency are at increased risk for this adverse reaction, OPV is not recommended for persons who are immunodeficient or for normal individuals who reside in a household with an immunocompromised person. The use of OPV is reserved for polio outbreak control.[55]

RABIES VACCINE

Human diploid cell vaccine (HDCV), rabies vaccine adsorbed (RVA), and purified chick embryo cell (PCEC) rabies vaccine are killed vaccines used for preexposure and postexposure rabies virus prophylaxis. Transmission of rabies can occur via percutaneous, permucosal, or airborne exposure to the rabies virus. Circumstances favoring such transmission include animal bites and attacks and contamination of scratches, cuts, abrasions, and mucous membranes with saliva or other infectious material (brain tissue). Unprovoked attacks and daytime attacks by nocturnal animals are considered highly suspect. Common wild animal transmitters include skunks, coyotes, foxes, and raccoons. Almost 60% of human rabies deaths in the United States since 1980 were associated with bat contact. Canine rabies is very common in many foreign countries (most of Asia, Africa, and Latin America). Rodents, rabbits, and hares are infected rarely. A few cases of person-to-person transmission have been reported.[56,57]

Preexposure indications for using HDCV, RVA, or PCEC rabies vaccine include persons whose vocation or avocation place them at high risk for rabies exposure, such as veterinarians, animal handlers, laboratory workers in rabies research laboratories, and field personnel (trappers, hunters, cave explorers). Travelers who will be in a country or area of a country where there is a constant threat of rabies, whose stay is likely to extend beyond 1 month, and who may not have readily available medical services (e.g., Peace Corps workers and missionaries) should be considered for preexposure prophylaxis.[57] Rabies immunization of immunocompromised individuals should be postponed until the immunosuppression has resolved, or activities should be modified to minimize the potential exposure to rabies. If the vaccine is used in immunocompromised persons, antibody titers should be checked postimmunization. Pregnancy is not a contraindication if the risk of rabies is great. A rabies immunization series should be completed with the same product because no data exist on interchangeability of products. All three vaccine preparations can be administered for preexposure prophylaxis as a three-dose series of 1 mL IM on days 0 and 7 and once between days 21 and 28.

Individuals with ongoing risk of exposure—either continuous risk (e.g., research laboratory staff or those involved in rabies biologics production) or individuals with frequent exposures (e.g., those involved with rabies diagnosis, spelunkers, veterinarians, animal control workers, and wildlife workers in rabies-enzootic areas)—should undergo serologic testing every 6 months and 2 years, respectively, to monitor rabies antibody concentrations. A booster dose is recommended if the complete virus neutralization is <1:5 serum dilution by the rapid fluorescent focus inhibition test.

Preexposure prophylaxis does not eliminate the need for postexposure therapy. Persons previously immunized with HDCV, RVA, or PCEC rabies vaccine or those who previously received postexposure prophylaxis should receive two 1-mL IM doses of HDCV, RVA, or PCEC rabies vaccine on postexposure days 0 and 3. Rabies immunoglobulin should not be given to this group.

Postexposure prophylaxis should be given after percutaneous or permucosal exposure to saliva or other infectious material from a high-risk source. Each case must be considered individually. Consideration needs to be given to the geographic area, species of animal, circumstances of the incident, and type of exposure. Local or state health departments should be contacted for assistance. Thorough cleansing of the wound with soap and water followed by irrigation with a virucidal agent such as povidone–iodine solution is an extremely important part of the management of rabies-prone wounds. Individuals who have not been immunized previously should receive the recommended regimen of rabies immunoglobulin (see Rabies Immunoglobulin below) and five doses of HDCV, RVA, or PCEC rabies vaccine 1 mL IM on days 0, 3, 7, 14, and 28 after exposure.[57]

IM vaccine should be given in the deltoid muscle in adults and in the anterolateral thigh in children. The gluteal region should not be used.

Adverse reactions to HDCV, RVA, and PCEC rabies vaccine are less common and less serious with the currently available vaccines compared with previously used preparations. Injection-site reactions, including pain, erythema, swelling, and itching, are reported frequently. Another 5% to 40% of vaccinees may have headache, nausea, abdominal pain, muscle aches, dizziness, or a combination of these effects. Systemic allergic reactions ranging from hives to anaphylaxis occur in a very small number of subjects. Given the lack of alternative therapy and the fact that rabies infection is almost always fatal, persons exposed to rabies who do have adverse reactions should continue the vaccine series in a setting with medical support services. In persons receiving booster doses of HDCV, an immune complex–like disease has been seen 2 to 21 days later in as many as 6% of vaccinees.[57]

Rabies Immunoglobulin

Human rabies immunoglobulin is used in conjunction with rabies vaccine as part of postexposure rabies management for previously unvaccinated individuals. The product is derived from plasma obtained from donors who have been hyperimmunized with rabies vaccine and have high titers of circulating antibody.

In persons who previously have not been immunized against rabies, rabies immunoglobulin is given simultaneously with HDCV, RVA, or PCEC rabies vaccine to provide optimal coverage in the interval before immune response to the vaccine occurs. The efficacy of this regimen has been clearly demonstrated. In situations where a vaccine has been used alone, mortality rates of 50% to 60% have been observed. Mortality after the combination vaccine and rabies immunoglobulin regimens is exceedingly rare; however, deaths have been reported when the wound was not infiltrated with rabies immunoglobulin.[58]

Rabies immunoglobulin does not interfere with vaccine-induced antibody formation. Its use is not recommended beyond 8 days after initiation of the vaccine series nor in persons previously immunized to rabies.

Human rabies immunoglobulin is administered in a dose of 20 international units/kg (0.133 mL/kg). If anatomically feasible, the entire dose should be infiltrated around the wound(s). Any remaining volume should be administered IM at a site distant from the rabies vaccination site. This product should never be administered by the intravenous route. Because other antibodies in the rabies immunoglobulin may interfere with the response to live-virus vaccines (MMR and varicella), it is recommended that these immunizations be delayed for 3 months.[57]

Side effects are rare but may include local soreness at the wound or IM injection site and mild temperature elevations. Caution is advised when administering the product to persons with known systemic allergies to immunoglobulin or thimerosal. Pregnancy is not a contraindication to its use.

RUBELLA VACCINE

Rubella (German measles) is characterized by an erythematous rash, lymphadenopathy, arthralgia, and low-grade fever. As many as 20% to 50% of rubella infections are asymptomatic.[59] The most important consequence of rubella infection occurs during pregnancy, particularly during the first trimester. Congenital rubella syndrome is associated with auditory, ophthalmic, cardiac, and neurologic defects. Rubella infection during pregnancy also can result in miscarriage or stillbirth. The primary goal of rubella immunization is to prevent congenital rubella syndrome. Rubella is no longer endemic in the United States, but high immunization rates are necessary to prevent rubella outbreaks from imported cases.

Rubella vaccine contains lyophilized live-attenuated rubella virus grown in human diploid cell culture. The vaccine is available alone or in combination with measles vaccine, mumps vaccine, or both. Each 0.5-mL dose also contains 25 mcg neomycin and is administered subcutaneously.

Rubella vaccine induces antibodies that are protective against wild-virus infection. The duration of immunity has not been established. A second dose is recommended, however, at the same time measles vaccine is administered (as a second dose of MMR). The vaccine is indicated for children older than 1 year age. Although individuals born before 1957 are assumed to be immune to rubella, this assumption is not sufficient for women who could become pregnant. Therefore, all women of childbearing potential should have documentation of receiving at least one dose of a rubella-containing vaccine or laboratory evidence of immunity.[59] Recent administration of immunoglobulin interferes with rubella vaccine response for at least 3 months and depends on the dose of immunoglobulin that is administered.[1,38,59] Table 128–1 can be used as a guide for the recommended interval. The vaccine should not be given to immunosuppressed individuals, although MMR vaccine should be administered to young children with HIV infection without severe immunosuppression as soon as possible after their first birthday.[38] The vaccine should not be given to individuals who have experienced anaphylactic reactions to neomycin.[38]

Adverse effects of the rubella virus vaccine tend to increase with the age of the recipient. Symptoms are similar to wild-virus infection and include lymphadenopathy, rash, urticaria, fever, malaise, sore throat, headache, myalgias, and paresthesias of the extremities. These symptoms occur 7 to 12 days after vaccination and last 1 to 5 days. Joint symptoms occur more often in susceptible postpubertal females. Arthralgia occurs in 25% of vaccinees, and 10% have arthritis-like symptoms. These symptoms usually begin 1 to 3 weeks after vaccination and persist for 1 day to 3 weeks. A very small excess risk of chronic arthropathy exists.[60] The vaccine may cause suppression of tuberculin skin tests for up to 6 weeks after vaccination. The vaccine virus may be excreted in nose and throat secretions, but it is not contagious.

The rubella vaccine has never been associated with congenital rubella syndrome, but its use during pregnancy is contraindicated. However, routine pregnancy testing prior to vaccination is not recommended. Women should be counseled not to become pregnant for 4 weeks following vaccination.[61] Termination of pregnancy is not indicated in women who are accidentally given the vaccine or who become pregnant during the month after vaccination.

VARICELLA AND ZOSTER VACCINES

Varicella is a highly contagious disease caused by varicella-zoster virus. The clinical illness is characterized by the appearance of successive waves of pruritic vesicles that rapidly crust over. Malaise and fever are common and last for 2 to 3 days. The virus remains dormant in the dorsal ganglia and reactivates as herpes zoster, also known as *shingles.* Although the exact stimulus for reactivation is unknown, a decrease in varicella-specific cell-mediated immunity associated with age or immunosuppression appears to be necessary but not sufficient for reactivation.

Varicella Vaccine

Live-attenuated varicella vaccine contains the Oka/Merck strain of varicella virus, which was attenuated by propagation through several different cell culture lines. Varicella vaccine is a lyophilized product that must be kept frozen and protected from light. Once reconstituted, it must be administered subcutaneously within 30 minutes. Each 0.5-mL dose contains a minimum of 1,350 plaque-forming units of virus as well as 12.5 mg of hydrolyzed gelatin and trace amounts of neomycin, fetal bovine serum, and residual components from cell culture.[14]

The varicella vaccine is safe and immunogenic in healthy children and adults. In clinical studies, varicella vaccine has been 70% to more than 95% effective in preventing chickenpox. Vaccinated individuals who develop chickenpox typically experience milder disease, with low or no fever and fewer skin lesions, many of which do not vesiculate. Similarly, vaccinated individuals who develop breakthrough infections transmit the varicella virus to others at a lower rate.[14]

The duration of protection provided by varicella vaccine is unknown but is believed to be long. Potential self-boosting of vaccinated individuals as the latent vaccine virus reactivates in individuals with the lowest varicella antibody titer is one possibility for conferring lifelong immunity. Additionally, children who are immunized against varicella and then are exposed to wild virus experience an immunologic boost.[62] As varicella vaccine use becomes more widespread, the circulation of wild virus can be expected to diminish and the opportunity for immunologic boosting as a result of natural exposure also will decline. Whether additional doses will be needed under these circumstances or if reactivation of latent vaccine virus will be sufficient to confer long-term protection is not known. Long-term studies assessing the duration of protection and the advisability of additional doses are ongoing.

The varicella vaccine is recommended for all children at 12 to 18 months of age, with a second dose prior to entering school between ages 4 and 6 years. It is also recommended for patients older than this age if they have not already had chickenpox. Varicella vaccine can be used for postexposure prophylaxis. The vaccine is effective in the prevention or modification of varicella infection when given within 3 days and possibly 5 days of exposure.[63] Because the varicella vaccine is a live vaccine, it is contraindicated in pregnant women and in immunocompromised individuals. An exception is children with asymptomatic or mildly symptomatic HIV infection, who should receive two doses of varicella vaccine 3 months apart. Also, children with humoral immune deficiencies may be immunized. Varicella vaccination is contraindicated in individuals with a history of anaphylactic reaction to any component of the vaccine. Persons who have received blood, plasma, or immunoglobulin products in the recent past should not receive varicella vaccine because of concern that passively acquired antibody will interfere with response to the vaccine. The recommended time interval between antibody-containing products and varicella vaccine depends on the dose of immune globulin (see Table 128–1). Although no adverse events associated with salicylate use after vaccination have been reported, salicylates should be avoided for 6 weeks after vaccination because of the association of salicylate use and Reye syndrome following varicella infection.[14]

The varicella vaccine has an excellent safety record. Pain, local swelling, and erythema at the injection site occur in up to 32% of patients and fever in 10% to 15%. A varicella-like rash occurs in approximately 4% of vaccinees, accompanied by few, if any, systemic symptoms. The rash may be localized at the injection site or generalized. Lesions usually are few in number (2–10) and often papular rather than vesicular. Transmission of vaccine virus to susceptible close contacts has occurred but is rare and believed to occur only when the vaccinee develops a rash. Because the risk of vaccine virus transmission is very low and primary infection can be very severe, vaccination of household contacts of immunocompromised patients is recommended to prevent introduction of varicella into the household.[14]

Zoster Vaccine

After the primary infection with varicella-zoster virus manifested as chicken pox, the virus remains latent in the dorsal ganglia. Herpes zoster, more commonly known as *shingles*, occurs upon reactivation of varicella-zoster virus replication. Herpes zoster can occur at any age, but the incidence dramatically increases with increasing age. The rate of disease increases sharply beginning in the fifth decade. The disease rate in individuals aged 80 to 89 years is 1,010 per 100,000 persons per year.[64] Patients with HIV, cancer, or other conditions associated with immunosuppression are at increased risk for disease.[65] The development of the disease is associated with declining cellular immunity to varicella-zoster virus.[66]

The clinical presentation of herpes zoster usually is a vesicular eruption limited to one dermatome. The most common complication is postherpetic neuralgia, which is pain that persists after the skin lesions have healed. The duration and severity of the pain varies. Postherpetic neuralgia can persist for weeks to years. The risk of postherpetic neuralgia increases dramatically with age. Virtually no risk of developing postherpetic neuralgia with herpes zoster exists prior to age 50 years, but the risk increases to 50% to 75% after ages 60 and 75 years, respectively.[67] The pain can be so severe as to limit activities of daily living and quality of life.[68]

The zoster vaccine contains 19,000 units of Oka/Merck strain live varicella-zoster virus.[69] Although the same strain of vaccine virus is contained in the childhood varicella vaccines, the doses of vaccine virus are dramatically different, and the vaccines are *not* interchangeable.

A large, placebo-controlled, double-blinded clinical trial with approximately 19,000 participants older than 60 years in each group demonstrated the efficacy of the zoster vaccine. All 38,000 subjects were followed for the development of herpes zoster for a median of 3 years. The primary end point of the study was the burden of disease, which was defined as a composite measure considering incidence, severity, and duration of herpes zoster. The burden of disease was reduced by 61% in the vaccine group. The vaccine decreased the incidence of zoster by 51% and the development of postherpetic neuralgia by 67%.[70]

The zoster vaccine is recommended for immunocompetent individuals older than 60 years. This live vaccine should not be used in immunocompromised individuals, including those with HIV or malignancies. The vaccine should not be used in individuals who have an allergy to any component of the vaccine preparation, by pregnant women, or by patients with untreated active tuberculosis.[69] No evidence of transmission of the live vaccine virus exists, but transmission of the varicella vaccine virus has been documented. Postmarketing surveillance will be used to establish if the theoretical risk is a small clinical problem.

The duration of protection is unknown but in one clinical trial was shown to be at least 4 years.[70] Future doses may be required for continued protection. The live zoster vaccine is not indicated for treatment of herpes zoster or postherpetic neuralgia.

Varicella-Zoster Immunoglobulin

Varicella-zoster immunoglobulin is used after exposure to varicella for passive immunization of susceptible immunodeficient patients or other susceptible individuals at particularly high risk for complications of varicella infection. Varicella-zoster immunoglobulin is available only under an investigational new drug protocol.[71]

Postexposure prophylaxis with varicella-zoster immunoglobulin is indicated for the following susceptible individuals: (a) immunocompromised patients, (b) neonates whose mothers develop varicella within 5 days before or 2 days after delivery, (c) preterm infants (<28 weeks' gestation or weight <1,000 g) who are exposed to varicella while hospitalized, and (d) susceptible pregnant women.[71] If varicella is prevented, vaccination should be offered at a later date. Exposure to varicella is defined as direct indoor contact for more than 1 hour with an infectious person. A negative history of clinical disease is not a reliable indicator of varicella susceptibility. Most people with a negative clinical history will have detectable antibody on laboratory testing. Caution is warranted when interpreting a low positive result in an immunosuppressed patient who has received blood products or immunoglobulin because the circulating antibody may be acquired passively.

For maximum effectiveness, varicella-zoster immunoglobulin must be given as soon as possible and not more than 96 hours following exposure. Because this agent may only attenuate infection, patients who receive varicella-zoster immunoglobulin still may have a period of communicability, and varicella-zoster immunoglobulin may prolong the incubation period to 28 days. Antiviral therapy can be initiated if signs and symptoms of varicella infection become apparent.

Administration of varicella-zoster immunoglobulin is by the IM route at doses of 125 units per 10 kg of body weight up to 625 units (five vials) for patients weighing more than 40 kg. The dose for newborn infants is 125 units.

OTHER IMMUNOBIOLOGICS

IMMUNOGLOBULIN

Immunoglobulin is available as both an intramuscular (IMIG) and an intravenous (IVIG) preparation. The IMIG preparation, or the Cohn fraction II, is prepared from pooled plasma of several thousand donors by cold ethanol fractionation. It typically contains greater than 95% IgG and trace amounts of IgM, IgA, and other plasma proteins. Because Ig is harvested from a large donor pool, it contains a wide spectrum of IgG antibodies to the pathogens prevalent in the area from which the donors were obtained. In the fractionation process, high-molecular-weight IgG aggregates are formed, which can activate complement in the absence of antigen and precipitate anaphylactoid reactions. For this reason, IMIG is unsuitable for IV administration. IMIG typically contains 15% to 18% protein and not less than 90% IgG. A number of IVIG preparations are available commercially in the United States. Generally, these preparations contain greater than 90% IgG monomers and trace to small amounts of IgA. These products are available as lyophilized powders or solutions.

When administered either IV or IM, immunoglobulin distributes in approximately 5% of the body weight of the recipient. The plasma half-life of immunoglobulin ranges from 18 to 32 days. This range of half-life probably is attributable to the variation in the half-life of IgG subclasses. Peak serum concentrations occur immediately with IVIG but within 2 days with IMIG. After the initial period of equilibration, circulating IgG levels are superimposable between IV and IM equivalent dosages. No dosage adjustment is necessary in patients with renal insufficiency, hepatic insufficiency, or both, dialysis patients, or geriatric patients.

8 Immunoglobulin is indicated in a wide variety of circumstances to provide passive immunity to individuals.[72] The indications for IMIG differ from those for IVIG. IMIG is indicated for providing passive immunity in patients with hepatitis A infections, hepatitis B exposures (however, hepatitis B immunoglobulin is significantly more effective), measles, varicella, and primary immunodeficiency diseases. Although IMIG is indicated for treatment of primary immunodeficiency, IVIG is better tolerated and is more effective. IMIG is not indicated for prevention of rubella, mumps, or poliomyelitis. Table 128–4 lists the suggested dosages of IMIG for prevention or attenuation of various infectious diseases.

There are many approved indications, as well as off-label uses, for IVIG. The therapeutic dose of IVIG is set empirically at 2 g/kg,[72–74] often given as five daily doses of 400 mg/kg each. However, it may be preferable to divide the total dose into two daily doses of 1 g/kg if the patient can tolerate the volume of the infusion. Mechanisms of IVIG action for treatment of these conditions have been hypothesized.

- *Primary Immunodeficiency States.*[75] In primary immunodeficiency states, monthly doses of between 100 and 800 mg/kg are administered; the average dose is 200 to 400 mg/kg. The immunodeficiency states for which IVIG is indicated include both antibody deficiencies and combined immune deficiencies. Significant reactions can occur in patients with low intrinsic levels of IgA given IVIG with greater amounts of IgA. An IVIG product with very low amounts of IgA should be used for these patients. IVIG is indicated for some patients with HIV infection; however, the data supporting IVIG use are better for the pediatric population.[76] With the advent of new antiretroviral agents and combination therapies, the usefulness of IVIG may be even more limited.

TABLE 128-4 Indications and Dosage of Intramuscular Immune Globulin in Infectious Diseases

Primary immunodeficiency states	1.2 mL/kg IM, then 0.6 mL/kg every 2–4 weeks
Hepatitis A exposure	0.02 mL/kg IM within 2 weeks
Hepatitis A prophylaxis	0.02 mL/kg IM for exposure <3 months' duration
	0.06 mL/kg IM for exposure up to 5 months' duration
Hepatitis B exposure	0.06 mL/kg (hepatits B immunoglobulin preferred in known exposures)
Measles exposure	0.25 mL/kg (maximum dose 15 mL) as soon as possible
	0.5 mL/kg (maximum dose 15 mL) as soon as possible for immunocompromised individuals
Varicella exposure	0.6–1.2 mL/kg as soon as possible when varicella-zoster immunoglobulin not available

- *Idiopathic (Immune) Thrombocytopenic Purpura.* For treatment of hemorrhage associated with idiopathic (immune) thrombocytopenic purpura (ITP), doses of 1 g/kg daily for 2 to 3 days plus high-dose methylprednisolone are indicated. Rh_o(D) immunoglobulin can be used in Rh-positive individuals as an alternative to IVIG (see Rh_o(D) Immunoglobulin below). Adults tend to respond less well to IVIG than do children. IVIG is acceptable for treatment of both chronic and acute ITP, and IVIG has been used for ITP associated with pregnancy without adverse effects on the fetus. Corticosteroids remain the drugs of choice for adult ITP.[79] In thrombotic thrombocytopenia purpura, IVIG is reported to be effective in patients who do not respond to plasmapheresis. Other platelet disorders in which IVIG may be useful include neonatal immune thrombocytopenia, perinatal autoimmune thrombocytopenia, drug-induced thrombocytopenia, thrombocytopenia secondary to infection, and transfusion-refractory thrombocytopenia; however, the data supporting these uses are minimal.[72,74]
- *Chronic Lymphocytic Leukemia.* IVIG is used as a prophylactic measure in patients with chronic lymphocytic leukemia who have had a serious bacterial infection. Doses of 400 mg/kg every 3 to 4 weeks are used.
- *Kawasaki's Disease (Mucocutaneous Lymph Node Syndrome).* This disease, which generally occurs in children, carries the hallmark of development of coronary artery abnormalities. Generally, the American Academy of Pediatrics recommends that if the strict criteria for Kawasaki's disease are met, an IVIG dose of 400 mg/kg/day for 4 consecutive days be used or, preferably, 2 g/kg as a single dose. The dose should be administered within 10 days of disease onset. Aspirin therapy also should be initiated.[78]
- *Bone Marrow Transplant.* IVIG is approved for reducing graft-versus-host disease and infections in patients older than 20 years. Patients receive 500 mg/kg 7 and 2 days before transplantation and weekly up to 3 months after. At 100 days posttransplant, patients receive a monthly dose of IVIG for 1 year. Following this regimen, infection (e.g., cytomegalovirus [CMV], fungal, bacterial, and interstitial pneumonia) decreased from 51% to 34% in bone marrow transplant patients. IVIG is not indicated in patients younger than 20 years.

- *Varicella-Zoster.* Another approved indication for IVIG is for prophylaxis of varicella-zoster if varicella-zoster immunoglobulin is not available.

A number of other proposed uses of IVIG have been identified. It is important to note that these uses are off-label but may be generally accepted in the medical community for routine treatment.[72] Off-label uses include the following:

- *Neonatal Sepsis.* Neonatal sepsis can cause significant morbidity within 24 hours of birth. Group B *Streptococcus* and *Escherichia coli* are the primary infecting organisms, but other bacteria and fungi may be associated with sepsis. IVIG appears to be effective in neonates older than 34 weeks' gestational age or who weigh less than 1,500 g. Routine use is not recommended; however, IVIG may be useful in neonates with recurrent infections.
- *Guillain-Barré Syndrome.* IVIG is effective and is considered an alternative to plasmapheresis.[73]
- *Autoimmune Diseases.* IVIG may be effective in self-limited immunoregulatory diseases but less effective in chronic diseases such as systemic lupus erythematosus. Overall, little evidence indicates that IVIG is useful for management of autoimmune diseases, except for patients with severe active disease who have not responded to or tolerated other interventions.[79]
- *Intractable Epilepsy.* IVIG may be useful for patients with confirmed IgG deficiency. IVIG may be considered for certain syndromes, such as West's or Lennox-Gastaut's syndrome.[73]
- *Chronic Inflammatory Demyelinating Polyneuropathy.* Although steroids are the first-line therapy, IVIG may be used in patients who do not respond to or do not tolerate steroids.[73]
- *CMV Infection.* Use of CMV-IVIG is recommended instead of use of IVIG.

Adverse effects of immunoglobulin vary with the route of administration. Following IMIG, pain, tenderness, and muscle stiffness persisting for hours or days are common. Repeat courses may cause sensitization with resulting allergic reactions. ❾ With IVIG, adverse effects occur in fewer than 1% of immunocompetent patients and in fewer than 10% of other patients. Chills, fever, nausea, and vomiting often are related to the rate of the infusion. Infusion should be given at a rate of 0.01 to 0.02 mL/kg/min for 30 minutes. If no reactions occur, then the rate can be increased to 0.02–0.04 mL/kg/min. If reactions do occur, the infusion should be stopped for 30 minutes and restarted at a lower rate. Although recommendations for infusion rate vary slightly depending on the preparation, the guidelines presented can be followed for the various IV preparations.

Most adverse reactions are mild and transient. Arthralgia, myalgia, fever, pruritus, nausea, vomiting, chest tightness, palpitations, diaphoresis, dizziness, pallor, and respiratory distress have been reported. Rarely, aseptic meningitis has occurred from a few hours to 2 days after high-dose infusion. The syndrome resolves within days without sequelae. Acute renal failure has been reported, primarily in individuals with underlying renal dysfunction, diabetes, sepsis, volume depletion, or other nephrotoxic drugs or in patients older than 65 years. To minimize the risk, ensure adequate hydration prior to infusion and choose an IVIG product that does not contain high sucrose concentrations for individuals at high risk.[80]

Immunoglobulin products are derived from human blood. Precautions such as donor screening and fractionation procedures and solvent-detergent treatment during the manufacturing process render the IVIG products free of HIV and hepatitis B and C viruses. Although no manufacturing process can guarantee no viral contamination, the potential infection risk from immunoglobulin preparations is very small.[81]

RH_O(D) IMMUNOGLOBULIN

Second only to the ABO blood group system, Rhesus antigen D [Rh_o(D)] is an important antigen in human blood. The Rh_o(D) locus encodes this antigen, but this locus is absent in approximately 15% of the population. ❿ Individuals lacking the Rh_o(D) locus are Rh_o(D) negative and have the potential to mount an antibody response to erythrocytes with the Rh_o(D) present. Rh_o(D) incompatibility during pregnancy can lead to sensitization of the mother. The maternal antibodies developed following normal fetal leakage of erythrocytes to the mother can cause hemolytic disease of the newborn during subsequent pregnancies.

Rh_o(D) immunoglobulin is a sterile solution of immunoglobulins prepared from human sera with high titers of Rh_o(D) antibody. Rh_o(D) immunoglobulin suppresses the antibody response and formation of anti-Rh_o(D) in Rh_o(D)-negative women exposed to Rh_o(D)-positive blood. Administration of Rh_o(D) immunoglobulin prevents hemolytic disease of the newborn in subsequent pregnancies with a Rh_o(D)-positive fetus. When administered within 72 hours of delivery of a full-term infant, Rh_o(D) immunoglobulin reduces active antibody formation from 12% to 1% to 2%. The reduction in antibody formation is lower when Rh_o(D) immunoglobulin is given beyond 72 hours postpartum. Smaller doses of Rh_o(D) immunoglobulin are used after abortion, miscarriage, amniocentesis, or abdominal trauma. In addition, Rh_o(D) immunoglobulin is used in the case of a premenopausal woman who is Rh_o(D) negative and has inadvertently received Rh_o(D)-positive blood or blood products.

The dosage of Rh_o(D) immunoglobulin varies with the indication. A standard dose of 300 mcg is given within 72 hours of a term delivery. Occasionally, when the fetus is known to be Rh_o(D) positive, a 300-mcg dose is given at 28 weeks' gestation and within 72 hours after delivery. For postpregnancy termination occurring up to 13 weeks' gestation, one microdose (50 mcg) vial is given within 72 hours. For pregnancy termination after 13 weeks, one standard dose (300 mcg) is given within 72 hours. In other circumstances, such as in abdominal trauma, amniocentesis, or transfusion accidents, the dosage (number of standard dose vials) is based on the estimated packed red blood cell volume of fetal/maternal hemorrhage divided by 15. Rh_o(D) immunoglobulin is administered IM only.

When considering use of Rh_o(D) immunoglobulin use, the mother's Rh_o(D) antigen status must be known with certainty. Rh_o(D) immunoglobulin should not be given to individuals positive for this antigen or to those with anti-Rh_o(D) antibodies. Occasionally, a large fetal bleed of Rh_o(D)-positive blood may make crossmatching of the mother difficult. In these cases, Rh_o(D) immunoglobulin should be given only if previous tests have shown that the mother is Rh_o(D) negative with no anti-Rh_o(D) antibody.

Adverse reactions to Rh_o(D) immunoglobulin include injection-site tenderness and fever. Rh_o(D) does not interfere with response to rubella vaccine. Rubella-seronegative women should be immunized at hospital discharge even if they received Rh_o(D) immunoglobulin postpartum.

CYTOMEGALOVIRUS IMMUNOGLOBULIN

CMV causes a generally mild infection in immunocompetent individuals. However, immunocompromised individuals are at risk for serious complications, including pneumonia, retinitis, gastrointestinal manifestations, and hepatitis. CMV causes a latent infection that can be transmitted from a previously infected solid organ donor to a seronegative recipient. CMV-IVIG contains IgG antibodies obtained from healthy persons with high titers of antibodies to CMV.

Attenuation of primary CMV disease associated with solid-organ transplantation in seronegative recipients of seropositive organs is the indication for CMV-IVIG. It is dosed using a tapering schedule that varies depending on the type of transplant. CMV-IVIG is administered intravenously every 2 weeks, with the final dose administered 16 weeks posttransplantation. Use of CMV-IVIG has resulted in a significant decrease in CMV-related syndromes. Additional studies are needed to determine the efficacy of CMV-IVIG in bone marrow transplantation. CMV-IVIG has been effective in some studies but ineffective in others.

Adverse effects of CMV-IVIG are seen in fewer than 5% of recipients and include flushing, chills, muscle cramps, back pain, chest tightness, fever, nausea, vomiting, hypotension, and tachycardia. These adverse events may be related to the infusion rate and can be managed by temporarily discontinuing the infusion. The infusion can be restarted at a decreased rate. Anaphylaxis occurs rarely and should be considered if hypotension develops during the infusion. Because CMV-IVIG contains other antibodies, live-virus vaccines should be withheld until 3 months after CMV-IVIG administration.

VACCINE INFORMATION RESOURCES

The field of vaccinology is developing ever more rapidly, with numerous changes in recommendations for vaccine use made each year. Keeping up to date with the current recommendations can be a challenge. The childhood, adolescent, and adult immunization schedules are updated frequently and published annually. Recommendations for the use of influenza vaccine are issued annually. Healthcare providers involved in primary care and immunization delivery must keep themselves abreast of these changes in a systematic way. Reading electronic newsletters and browsing reliable websites are efficient methods for obtaining information (Table 128–5). Although several excellent, reliable, and timely websites exist, hundreds of sites with misleading and incorrect information also exist. Many of these sites are targeted at parents.

Vaccines are the only class of medications to which nearly every patient is exposed. Knowledge of these agents is critical to providing pharmaceutical care. Dramatic progress in public health has been made through the appropriate use of immunization. Additional improvements in quality of life and mortality can be made through continued increases in vaccination coverage with careful attention to this aspect of care by all healthcare providers.

TABLE 128-5 Web Resources for Vaccine Information

Recommended internet sites for vaccine information	
www.cdc.gov/vaccines	Centers for Disease Control and Prevention: Vaccines and Immunizations
www.cdc.gov/ncidod/diseases/hepatitis	Centers for Disease Control and Prevention's National Center for Infectious Diseases Viral Hepatitis
www.immunize.org	Immunization Action Coalition
www.vaccines.org	The Vaccine Page
www.nfid.org/	National Foundation for Infectious Diseases
www.cdc.gov/mmwr/	Morbidity and Mortality Weekly Report
www.hrsa.gov/vaccinecompensation	Vaccine Injury Compensation Program
www.vaers.hhs.gov	Vaccine Adverse Event Reporting System
www.iom.edu/	Institute of Medicine of the National Academies
www.immunizationinfo.org/	National Network for Immunization Information
Recommended electronic newsletters	
www.immunize.org/express	Immunization Action Coalition's newsletter
www.cdc.gov/mmwr/	Morbidity and Mortality Weekly Report

ABBREVIATIONS

ACIP: Advisory Committee on Immunization Practices
CDC: Centers for Disease Control and Prevention
CMV-IVIG: cytomegalovirus intravenous immunoglobulin
DTaP: diphtheria-tetanus-acellular pertussis
HDCV: human diploid cell vaccine
Hib: *Haemophilus influenzae* type b
IMIG: intramuscular immunoglobulin
IPV: inactivated polio vaccine
ITP: idiopathic (immune) thrombocytopenic purpura
IVIG: intravenous immunoglobulin
LAIV: live-attenuated influenza vaccine
MMR: measles-mumps-rubella
OPV: oral polio vaccine
PCEC: purified chick embryo cell
PCV: pneumococcal conjugate vaccine
PPV: pneumococcal polysaccharide vaccine
PRP: polyribosylribitol phosphate
RVA: rabies vaccine absorbed
Td: tetanus-diphtheria
VAERS: Vaccine Adverse Event Reporting System

REFERENCES

1. Centers for Disease Control and Prevention. General recommendations on immunization. Recommendations of the Advisory Committee on Immunization Practices (ACIP) and the American Academy of Family Physicians (AAFP). MMWR Morb Mortal Wkly Rep 2006;55:1–47.
2. Poland GA. Hepatitis B immunization in health care workers. Dealing with vaccine nonresponse. Am J Prev Med 1998;15:73–77.
3. Arrowood JR, Hayney MS. Immunization recommendations for adults with cancer. Ann Pharmacother 2002;36:1219–1229.
4. Miotti P, Nelson K, Dallabetta G, Farzadegan H, Margolick J, Clements M. The influence of HIV infection on antibody responses to a two-dose regimen of influenza vaccine. JAMA 1998;262:779–783.
5. Poland GA. Lessons from the influenza vaccine recall of 1996–1997. JAMA 1997;278:1022–1023.
6. Poland GA, Borrud A, Jacobson RM, et al. Determination of deltoid fat pad thickness. Implications for needle length in adult immunization. JAMA 1997;277:1709–1711.
7. Weber DJ, Rutala WA. Immunization of immunocompromised persons. Immunol Allergy Clin North Am 2003;23:605–634 v–vi.
8. Hayney MS. Pharmacogenomics and infectious diseases: Impact on drug response and applications to disease management. Am J Health Syst Pharm 2002;59:1626–1631.
9. Alimonos K, Nafziger AN, Murray J, Bertino JS Jr. Prediction of response to hepatitis B vaccine in health care workers: Whose titers of antibody to hepatitis B surface antigen should be determined after a three-dose series, and what are the implications in terms of cost-effectiveness? Clin Infect Dis 1998;26:566–571.
10. Dorrell L, Hassan I, Marshall S, Chakraverty P, Ong E. Clinical and serological responses to an inactivated influenza vaccine in adults with HIV infection, diabetes, obstructive airways disease, elderly adults and healthy volunteers. Int J STD AIDS 1997;8:776–779.
11. Centers for Disease Control and Prevention. Prevention of rotavirus gastroenteritis among infants and children. Recommendations of the Advisory Committee on Immunization Practices. MMWR Morb Mortal Wkly Rep 2006;55:1–13.
12. Centers for Disease Control and Prevention. Prevention and control of influenza. Recommendations of the Advisory Committee on Immunization Practices (ACIP). MMWR Morb Mortal Wkly Rep 2007;56(5):1–53.

13. Centers for Disease Control and Prevention. Guidelines for vaccinating pregnant women from the Recommendation of the Advisory Committee on Immunization Practices (ACIP): U.S. Department of Health & Human Services, 1998:1–11, updated May 2007.
14. Centers for Disease Control and Prevention. Prevention of varicella. Recommendations of the Advisory Committee on Immunization Practices (ACIP). MMWR. 2007;56(4):1–38.
15. Ballout A, Goffin E, Yombi JC, Vandercam B. Vaccinations for adult solid organ transplant recipient: Current recommendations. Transplant Proc 2005;37:2826–2827.
16. Centers for Disease Control and Prevention. Development of community- and state-based immunization registries. CDC response to a report from the National Vaccine Advisory Committee. MMWR Morb Mortal Wkly Rep 2001;50:1–17.
17. U.S. Department of Health and Human Services. Healthy People 2010: Understanding and Improving Health. Washington, DC: U.S. Government Printing Office, 2000:62.
18. Middleman AB, Rosenthal SL, Rickert VI, Neinstein L, Fishbein DB, D'Angelo L. Adolescent immunizations: A position paper of the society for adolescent medicine. J Adolesc Health 2006;38:321–326.
19. Centers for Disease Control and Prevention. Recommended childhood and adolescent immunization schedule—United States, January–June 2004. MMWR Morb Mortal Wkly Rep 2004;53:Q1–Q4.
20. Diphtheria. In: Atkinson W, Hanborsky J, Lynne M, Wolfe CS, eds. Epidemiology and Prevention of Vaccine-Preventable Diseases. Washington, DC: Public Health Foundation, 2006:57–68.
21. Centers for Disease Control and Prevention. Recommended childhood and adolescent immunization schedule—United States, 2007. MMWR Morb Mortal Wkly Rep 2007;55:Q1–Q4.
22. Tetanus. In: Atkinson W, Hanborsky J, Lynne M, Wolfe CS, eds. Epidemiology and Prevention of Vaccine-Preventable Diseases. Washington, DC: Public Health Foundation, 2006:69–78.
23. Centers for Disease Control and Prevention. Progress toward elimination of *Haemophilus influenzae* type b invasive disease among infants and children—United States, 1998–2000. MMWR Morb Mortal Wkly Rep 2002;51:234–237.
24. *Haemophilus influenza* type b. In: Atkinson W, Hanborsky J, Lynne M, Wolfe CS, eds. Epidemiology and Prevention of Vaccine-Preventable Diseases. Washington, DC: Public Health Foundation, 2006:111–123.
25. Centers for Disease Control and Prevention. Recommended adult immunization schedule—United States, October 2007-September 2008. MMWR Morb Mortal Wkly Rep 2007;56:Q1-Q4.
26. Trottier H, Franco EL. The epidemiology of genital human papillomavirus infection. Vaccine 2006;24:S4–S15.
27. Meningococcal disease. In: Atkinson W, Hanborsky J, Wolfe C, eds. Epidemiology and Prevention of Vaccine-Preventable Diseases. Washington, DC: Public Health Foundation, 2004:247–255.
28. Merck & Co. Inc. Gardasil® [Quadrivalent Human Papillomavirus (Types 6, 11, 16, 18) Recombinant Vaccine]. Package Insert, 2006.
29. Chen RT, DeStefano F, Pless R, Moobrey G, Kramarz P, Hibbs B. Challenges and controversies in immunization safety. Infect Dis Clin North Am. 2001;15(1):21–39.
30. Harper DM, Franco EL, Wheeler CM, et al. Sustained efficacy up to 4.5 years of a bivalent L1 virus-like particle vaccine against human papillomavirus types 16 and 18: Follow-up from a randomised control trial. Lancet 2006;367:1247–1255.
31. Belshe RB, Mendelman PM, Treanor J, et al. The efficacy of live attenuated, cold-adapted, trivalent, intranasal influenzavirus vaccine in children. N Engl J Med 1998;338:1405–1412.
32. Nichol KL, Mendelman PM, Mallon KP, et al. Effectiveness of live, attenuated intranasal influenza virus vaccine in healthy, working adults: A randomized controlled trial. JAMA 1999;282:137–144.
33. Nichol KL, Lind A, Margolis KL, et al. The effectiveness of vaccination against influenza in healthy, working adults. N Engl J Med 1995;333:889–893.
34. Salo H, Kilpi T, Sintonen H, Linna M, Peltola V, Heikkinen T. Cost-effectiveness of influenza vaccination of healthy children. Vaccine 2006;24:4934–4941.
35. Nichol KL, Nordin J, Mullooly J, Lask R, Fillbrandt K, Iwane M. Influenza vaccination and reduction in hospitalizations for cardiac disease and stroke among the elderly. N Engl J Med 2003;348:1322–1332.
36. Poehling KA, Edwards KM, Weinberg GA, et al. The underrecognized burden of influenza in young children. N Engl J Med 2006;355:31–40.
37. Lasky T, Terracciano GJ, Magder L, et al. The Guillain-Barré syndrome and the 1992–1993 and 1993–1994 influenza vaccines. N Engl J Med 1998;339:1797–1802.
38. Centers for Disease Control and Prevention. Measles, mumps, and rubella—Vaccine use and strategies for elimination of measles, rubella, and congenital rubella syndrome and control of mumps: Recommendations of the Advisory Committee on Immunization Practices (ACIP). MMWR Morb Mortal Wkly Rep 1998;47:1–57.
39. Poland GA, Jacobson RM, Thampy AM, et al. Measles reimmunization in children seronegative after initial immunization. JAMA 1997;277:1156–1158.
40. Institute of Medicine. Immunization Safety Review. Vaccines and Autism. Washington, DC: The National Academies Press, 2004:1–200.
41. Centers for Disease Control and Prevention. Prevention and Control of Meningococcal Disease. Recommendations of the Advisory Committee on Immunization Practices (ACIP). MMWR Morb Mortal Wkly Rep 2005;54:1–21.
42. Bruce MG, Rosenstein NE, Capparella JM, Shutt KA, Perkins BA, Collins M. Risk factors for meningococcal disease in college students. JAMA 2001;286:688–693.
43. Centers for Disease Control and Prevention. Prevention and control of meningococcal disease and Meningococcal disease and college students: Recommendations of the Advisory Committee on Immunization Practices (ACIP). MMWR Morb Mortal Wkly Rep 2000;49:1–20.
44. Centers for Disease Control and Prevention. Update: Guillain-Barré Syndrome Among Recipients of Menactra® Meningococcal Conjugate Vaccine —United States, June 2005–September 2006. MMWR Morb Mortal Wkly Rep 2006;55:1120–1124.
45. Centers for Disease Control and Prevention. Updated recommendations of the Advisory Committee on Immunization Practices (ACIP) for the control and elimination of mumps. MMWR Morb Mortal Wkly Rep 2006;55:629–630.
46. Centers for Disease Control and Prevention. Preventing tetanus, diphtheria, and pertussis among adolescents: Use of tetanus toxoid, reduced diphtheria toxoid and acellular pertussis vaccines. Recommendations of the Advisory Committee on Immunization Practices (ACIP). MMWR Morb Mortal Wkly Rep 2006;55:1–42.
47. Centers for Disease Control and Prevention. Pertussis vaccination: Use of acellular pertussis vaccines among infants and young children. Recommendations of the Advisory Committee on Immunization Practices (ACIP). MMWR Morb Mortal Wkly Rep 1997;46:1–25.
48. Centers for Disease Control and Prevention. Prevention of pneumococcal disease: Recommendations of the Advisory Committee on Immunization Practices (ACIP). MMWR Morb Mortal Wkly Rep 1997;46:1–24.
49. Jackson LA, Neuzil KM, Yu O, et al. Effectiveness of pneumococcal polysaccharide vaccine in older adults. N Engl J Med 2003;348:1747–1755.
50. Fisman DN, Abrutyn E, Spaude KA, Kim A, Kirchner C, Daley J. Prior pneumococcal vaccination is associated with reduced death, complications, and length of stay among hospitalized adults with community-acquired pneumonia. Clin Infect Dis 2006;42:1093–1101.
51. Jackson LA, Benson P, Sneller VP, et al. Safety of revaccination with pneumococcal polysaccharide vaccine. JAMA 1999;281:243–248.
52. Centers for Disease Control and Prevention. Preventing pneumococcal disease among infants and young children: Recommendations of the Advisory Committee on Immunization Practices (ACIP). MMWR Morb Mortal Wkly Rep 2000;49:1–35.
53. Centers for Disease Control and Prevention. Direct and indirect effects of routine vaccination of children with 7-valent pneumococcal conjugate vaccine on incidence of invasive pneumococcal disease—United States, 1998–2003. MMWR Morb Mortal Wkly Rep 2005;54:893–897.
54. Whitney CG, Farley MM, Hadler J, et al. Decline in invasive pneumococcal disease after the introduction of protein-polysaccharide conjugate vaccine. N Engl J Med 2003;348:1737–1746.
55. Centers for Disease Control and Prevention. Poliomyelitis prevention in the United States: Updated recommendations of the Advisory Committee on Immunization Practices (ACIP). MMWR Morb Mortal Wkly Rep 2000;49:1–22.
56. Centers for Disease Control and Prevention. Compendium of animal rabies prevention and control, 2005. MMWR Morb Mortal Wkly Rep 2005;55:1–8.

57. Centers for Disease Control and Prevention. Human rabies prevention—United States, 1999. Recommendations of the Advisory Committee on Immunization Practices (ACIP). MMWR Morb Mortal Wkly Rep 1999;48:1–21.
58. Wilde H, Sirikawin S, Sabcharoen A, et al. Failure of postexposure treatment of rabies in children. Clin Infect Dis 1996;22:228–232.
59. Centers for Disease Control and Prevention. Control and prevention of rubella: Evaluation and management of suspected outbreaks, rubella in pregnant women, and surveillance for congenital rubella syndrome. MMWR Morb Mortal Wkly Rep 2001;50:1–23.
60. Tingle AJ, Mitchell LA, Grace M, et al. Randomised double-blind placebo-controlled study on adverse effects of rubella immunisation in seronegative women. Lancet 1997;349:1277–1281.
61. Centers for Disease Control and Prevention. Revised ACIP recommendation for avoiding pregnancy after receiving a rubella-containing vaccine. MMWR Morb Mortal Wkly Rep 2001;50:1117.
62. Krause PR, Klinman DM. Varicella vaccination: Evidence for frequent reactivation of the vaccine strain in healthy children. Nat Med 2000;6:451–454.
63. Watson B, Seward J, Yang A, et al. Postexposure effectiveness of varicella vaccine. Pediatrics 2000;105:84–88.
64. Hope-Simpson RE. The nature of herpes zoster: A long-term study and a new hypothesis. Proc R Soc Lon B Biol Sci 1965;58:9–20.
65. Insinga RP, Itzler RF, Pellissier JM, Saddier P, Nikas AA. The Incidence of herpes zoster in a United States Administrative Database. J Gen Intern Med 2005;20:748–753.
66. Raeder CK, Hayney MS. Immunology of varicella immunization in the elderly. Ann Pharmacotherapy 2000;34:228–234.
67. Ragozzino MW, Melton LJd, Kurland LT, Chu CP, Perry HO. Population-based study of herpes zoster and its sequelae. Medicine 1982;61:310–316.
68. Johnson RW. Consequences and management of pain in herpes zoster. J Infect Dis 2002;186(Suppl 1):S83–S90.
69. Merck & Co. Inc. Zoster Vaccine Live (Oka/Merck) Zostavax®. Package Insert, 2006.
70. Oxman MN, Levin MJ, Johnson GR, et al. A vaccine to prevent herpes zoster and postherpetic neuralgia in older adults. N Engl J Med 2005;352:2271–2284.
71. Centers for Disease Control and Prevention. A new product (VariZIG^{TM}) for postexposure prophylaxis of varicella available under an investigational new drug application expanded access protocol. MMWR Morb Mortal Wkly Rep 2006;55:209–210.
72. Ratko TA, Burnett DA, Foulke GE, Matuszewski KA, Sacher RA. Recommendations for off-label use of intravenously administered immunoglobulin preparations. University Hospital Consortium Expert Panel for Off-Label Use of Polyvalent Intravenously Administered Immunoglobulin Preparations. JAMA 1995;273:1865–1870.
73. Dalakas MC. Intravenous immunoglobulin in autoimmune neuromuscular diseases. JAMA 2004;291:2367–2375.
74. Chen C, Danekas LH, Ratko TA, Vlasses PH, Matuszewski KA. A multicenter drug use surveillance of intravenous immunoglobulin utilization in US academic health centers. Ann Pharmacother 2000;34:295–299.
75. Durandy A, Wahn V, Petteway S, Gelfand EW. Immunoglobulin replacement therapy in primary antibody deficiency diseases—maximizing success. Int Arch Allergy Immunol 2005;136:217–229.
76. Centers for Disease Control and Prevention. Guidelines for preventing opportunistic infections among HIV-infected persons—2002. MMWR Morb Mortal Wkly Rep 2002;51:1–52.
77. Bromberg ME. Immune thrombocytopenic purpura: The changing therapeutic landscape. N Engl J Med 2006;355:1643–1645.
78. Freeman AF, Shulman ST. Kawasaki's disease: Summary of the American Heart Association guidelines. Am Fam Physician 2006;74:1141–1148.
79. Kieseier BC, Hartung HP. Therapeutic strategies in the Guillain-Barré syndrome. Semin Neurol 2003;23:159–168.
80. Centers for Disease Control and Prevention. Renal insufficiency and failure associated with immune globulin intravenous therapy—United States, 1985–1998. MMWR Morb Mortal Wkly Rep 1999;48:581–521.
81. Orbach H, Katz U, Sherer Y, Shoenfeld Y. Intravenous immunoglobulin: Adverse effects and safe administration. Clin Rev Allergy Immunol 2005;29:173–184.

Appendix 128-1

2007 Childhood and Adolescent Immunization Schedules

Recommended Immunization Schedule for Persons Aged 0–6 Years—UNITED STATES • 2007

Vaccine▼ Age▶	Birth	1 month	2 months	4 months	6 months	12 months	15 months	18 months	19–23 months	2–3 years	4–6 years
Hepatitis B[1]	HepB	HepB	HepB	*see footnote 1*	HepB	HepB	HepB	HepB	HepB Series	HepB Series	HepB Series
Rotavirus[2]			Rota	Rota	Rota						
Diphtheria, Tetanus, Pertussis[3]			DTaP	DTaP	DTaP		DTaP	DTaP			DTaP
Haemophilus influenzae type b[4]			Hib	Hib	*Hib[4]*	Hib	Hib	Hib	Hib	Hib	Hib
Pneumococcal[5]			PCV	PCV	PCV	PCV	PCV			PCV / PPV	PCV / PPV
Inactivated Poliovirus			IPV	IPV	IPV	IPV	IPV	IPV			IPV
Influenza[6]					Influenza (Yearly)	Influenza (Yearly)	Influenza (Yearly)	Influenza (Yearly)	Influenza (Yearly)	Influenza (Yearly)	Influenza (Yearly)
Measles, Mumps, Rubella[7]						MMR	MMR				MMR
Varicella[8]						Varicella	Varicella				Varicella
Hepatitis A[9]						HepA (2 doses)	HepA (2 doses)	HepA (2 doses)	HepA (2 doses)	HepA Series	HepA Series
Meningococcal[10]										MPSV4	MPSV4

Range of recommended ages

Catch-up immunization

Certain high-risk groups

This schedule indicates the recommended ages for routine administration of currently licensed childhood vaccines, as of December 1, 2006, for children aged 0–6 years. Additional information is available at http://www.cdc.gov/nip/recs/child-schedule.htm. Any dose not administered at the recommended age should be administered at any subsequent visit, when indicated and feasible. Additional vaccines may be licensed and recommended during the year. Licensed combination vaccines may be used whenever any components of the combination are indicated and other components of the vaccine are not contraindicated and if approved by the Food and Drug Administration for that dose of the series. Providers should consult the respective Advisory Committee on Immunization Practices statement for detailed recommendations. Clinically significant adverse events that follow immunization should be reported to the Vaccine Adverse Event Reporting System (VAERS). Guidance about how to obtain and complete a VAERS form is available at **http://www.vaers, hhs.gov** or by telephone, **800-822-7967**.

1. **Hepatitis B vaccine (HepB).** *(Minimum age: birth)*
   At birth:
   - Administer monovalent HepB to all newborns before hospital discharge.
   - If mother is hepatitis surface antigen (HBsAg)-positive, administer HepB and 0.5 mL of hepatitis B immune globulin (HBIG) within 12 hours of birth.
   - If mother's HBsAg status is unknown, administer HepB within 12 hours of birth. Determine the HBsAg status as soon as possible and if HBsAg-positive, administer HBIG (no later than age 1 week).
   - If mother is HBsAg-negative, the birth dose can only be delayed with physician's order and mother's negative HBsAg laboratory report documented in the infant's medical record.

   After the birth dose:
   - The HepB series should be completed with either monovalent HepB or a combination vaccine containing HepB. The second dose should be administered at age 1–2 months. The final dose should be administered at age ≥24 weeks. Infants born to HBsAg-positive mothers should be tested for HBsAg and antibody to HBsAg after completion of ≥3 doses of a licensed HepB series, at age 9–18 months (generally at the next well-child visit).

   4-month dose:
   - It is permissible to administer 4 doses of HepB when combination vaccines are administered after the birth dose. If monovalent HepB is used for doses after the birth dose, a dose at age 4 months is not needed.
2. **Rotavirus vaccine (Rota).** *(Minimum age: 6 weeks)*
   - Administer the first dose at age 6–12 weeks. Do not start the series later than age 12 weeks.
   - Administer the final dose in the series by age 32 weeks. Do not administer a dose later than age 32 weeks.
   - Data on safety and efficacy outside of these age ranges are insufficient.
3. **Diphtheria and tetanus toxoids and acellular pertussis vaccine (DTaP).** *(Minimum age: 6 weeks)*
   - The fourth dose of DTaP may be administered as early as age 12 months, provided 6 months have elapsed since the third dose.
   - Administer the final dose in the series at age 4–6 years.
4. ***Haemophilus influenzae*** **type b conjugate vaccine (Hib).** *(Minimum age: 6 weeks)*
   - If PRP-OMP (PedvaxHIB® or ComVax® [Merck]) is administered at ages 2 and 4 months, a dose at age 6 months is not required.
   - TriHiBit® (DTaP/Hib) combination products should not be used for primary immunization but can be used as boosters following any Hib vaccine in children aged ≥12 months.
5. **Pneumococcal vaccine.** *(Minimum age: 6 weeks for pneumococcal conjugate vaccine [PCV]; 2 years for pneumococcal polysaccharide vaccine [PPV])*
   - Administer PCV at ages 24–59 months in certain high-risk groups. Administer PPV to children aged ≥2 years in certain high-risk groups. See *MMWR* 2000;49(No. RR-9):1–35.
6. **Influenza vaccine.** *(Minimum age: 6 months for trivalent inactivated influenza vaccine [TIV]; 5 years for live, attenuated influenza vaccine [LAIV])*
   - All children aged 6–59 months and close contacts of all children aged 0–59 months are recommended to receive influenza vaccine.
   - Influenza vaccine is recommended annually for children aged ≥59 months with certain risk factors, health-care workers, and other persons (including household members) in close contact with persons in groups at high risk. See *MMWR* 2006;55(No. RR-10):1–41.
   - For healthy persons aged 5–49 years, LAIV may be used as an alternative to TIV.
   - Children receiving TIV should receive 0.25 mL if aged 6–35 months or 0.5 mL if aged ≥3 years.
   - Children aged <9 years who are receiving influenza vaccine for the first time should receive 2 doses (separated by ≥4 weeks for TIV and ≥6 weeks for LAIV).
7. **Measles, mumps, and rubella vaccine (MMR).** *(Minimum age: 12 months)*
   - Administer the second dose of MMR at age 4–6 years. MMR may be administered before age 4–6 years, provided ≥4 weeks have elapsed since the first dose and both doses are administered at age ≥12 months.
8. **Varicella vaccine.** *(Minimum age: 12 months)*
   - Administer the second dose of varicella vaccine at age 4–6 years. Varicella vaccine may be administered before age 4–6 years, provided that ≥3 months have elapsed since the first dose and both doses are administered at age ≥12 months. If second dose was administered ≥28 days following the first dose, the second dose does not need to be repeated.
9. **Hepatitis A vaccine (HepA).** *(Minimum age: 12 months)*
   - HepA is recommended for all children aged 1 year (i.e., aged 12–23 months). The 2 doses in the series should be administered at least 6 months apart.
   - Children not fully vaccinated by age 2 years can be vaccinated at subsequent visits.
   - HepA is recommended for certain other groups of children, including in areas where vaccination programs target older children. See *MMWR* 2006;55(No. RR-7):1–23.
10. **Meningococcal polysaccharide vaccine (MPSV4).** *(Minimum age: 2 years)*
    - Administer MPSV4 to children aged 2–10 years with terminal complement deficiencies or anatomic or functional asplenia and certain other highrisk groups. See *MMWR* 2005;54(No. RR-7):1–21.

Adapted from materials approved by the Advisory Committee on Immunization Practices (http://www.cdc.gov/nip/acip), the American Academy of Pediatrics (http://www.aap.org), and the American Academy of Family Physicians (http://www.aafp.org).

Recommended Immunization Schedule for Persons Aged 7–18 Years—UNITED STATES • 2007

Vaccine▼ Age▶	7–10 years	11–12 years	13–14 years	15 years	16–18 years
Tetanus, Diphtheria, Pertussis[1]	*see footnote 1*	Tdap	Tdap		
Human Papillomavirus[2]	*see footnote 2*	HPV (3 doses)	HPV Series		
Meningococcal[3]	MPSV4	MCV4		MCV4 MCV4	
Pneumococcal[4]	PPV				
Influenza[5]	Influenza (Yearly)				
Hepatitis A[6]	HepA Series				
Hepatitis B[7]	HepB Series				
Inactivated Poliovirus[8]	IPV Series				
Measles, Mumps, Rubella[9]	MMR Series				
Varicella[10]	Varicella Series				

Range of recommended ages

Catch-up immunization

Certain high-risk groups

This schedule indicates the recommended ages for routine administration of currently licensed childhood vaccines, as of December 1, 2006, for children aged 7–18 years. Additional information is available at **http://www.cdc.gov/nip/recs/child-schedule.htm**. Any dose not administered at the recommended age should be administered at any subsequent visit, when indicated and feasible. Additional vaccines may be licensed and recommended during the year. Licensed combination vaccines may be used whenever any components of the combination are indicated and other components of the vaccine are not contraindicated and if approved by the Food and Drug Administration for that dose of the series. Providers should consult the respective Advisory Committee on Immunization Practices statement for detailed recommendations. Clinically significant adverse events that follow immunization should be reported to the Vaccine Adverse Event Reporting System (VAERS). Guidance about how to obtain and complete a VAERS form is available at **http://www.vaers.hhs.gov** or by telephone, **800-822-7967**.

1. **Tetanus and diphtheria toxoids and acellular pertussis vaccine (Tdap).** *(Minimum age: 10 years for BOOSTRIX® and 11 years for ADACEL™)*
   - Administer at age 11–12 years for those who have completed the recommended childhood DTP/DTaP vaccination series and have not received a tetanus and diphtheria toxoids vaccine (Td) booster dose.
   - Adolescents aged 13–18 years who missed the 11–12 year Td/Tdap booster dose should also receive a single dose of Tdap if they have completed the recommended childhood DTP/DTaP vaccination series.
2. **Human papillomavirus vaccine (HPV).** *(Minimum age: 9 years)*
   - Administer the first dose of the HPV vaccine series to females at age 11–12 years.
   - Administer the second dose 2 months after the first dose and the third dose 6 months after the first dose.
   - Administer the HPV vaccine series to females at age 13–18 years if not previously vaccinated.
3. **Meningococcal vaccine.** *(Minimum age: 11 years for meningococcal conjugate vaccine [MCV4]; 2 years for meningococcal polysaccharide vaccine [MPSV4])*
   - Administer MCV4 at age 11–12 years and to previously unvaccinated adolescents at high school entry (at approximately age 15 years).
   - Administer MCV4 to previously unvaccinated college freshmen living in dormitories; MPSV4 is an acceptable alternative.
   - Vaccination against invasive meningococcal disease is recommended for children and adolescents aged ≥2 years with terminal complement deficiencies or anatomic or functional asplenia and certain other high-risk groups. See *MMWR* 2005;54(No. RR-7):1–21. Use MPSV4 for children aged 2–10 years and MCV4 or MPSV4 for older children.
4. **Pneumococcal polysaccharide vaccine (PPV).** *(Minimum age: 2 years)*
   - Administer for certain high-risk groups. See *MMWR* 1997;46(No. RR-8):1–24, and *MMWR* 2000;49(No. RR-9):1–35.
5. **Influenza vaccine.** *(Minimum age: 6 months for trivalent inactivated influenza vaccine [TIV]; 5 years for live, attenuated influenza vaccine [LAIV])*
   - Influenza vaccine is recommended annually for persons with certain risk factors, health-care workers, and other persons (including household members) in close contact with persons in groups at high risk. See *MMWR* 2006;55(No. RR-10):1–41.
   - For healthy persons aged 5–49 years, LAIV may be used as an alternative to TIV.
   - Children aged <9 years who are receiving influenza vaccine for the first time should receive 2 doses (separated by ≥4 weeks for TIV and ≥6 weeks for LAIV).
6. **Hepatitis A vaccine (HepA).** *(Minimum age: 12 months)*
   - The 2 doses in the series should be administered at least 6 months apart.
   - HepA is recommended for certain other groups of children, including in areas where vaccination programs target older children. See *MMWR* 2006;55 (No. RR-7):1–23.
7. **Hepatitis B vaccine (HepB).** *(Minimum age: birth)*
   - Administer the 3-dose series to those who were not previously vaccinated.
   - A 2-dose series of Recombivax HB® is licensed for children aged 11–15 years.
8. **Inactivated poliovirus vaccine (IPV).** *(Minimum age: 6 weeks)*
   - For children who received an all-IPV or all-oral poliovirus (OPV) series, a fourth dose is not necessary if the third dose was administered at age ≥4 years.
   - If both OPV and IPV were administered as part of a series, a total of 4 doses should be administered, regardless of the child's current age.
9. **Measles, mumps, and rubella vaccine (MMR).** *(Minimum age:12 months)*
   - If not previously vaccinated, administer 2 doses of MMR during any visit, with ≥4 weeks between the doses.
10. **Varicella vaccine.** *(Minimum age: 12 months)*
    - Administer 2 doses of varicella vaccine to persons without evidence of immunity.
    - Administer 2 doses of varicella vaccine to persons aged <13 years at least 3 months apart. Do not repeat the second dose, if administered ≥28 days after the first dose.
    - Administer 2 doses of varicella vaccine to persons aged ≥13 years at least 4 weeks apart.

Adapted from materials approved by the Advisory Committee on Immunization Practices (http://www.cdc.gov/nip/acip), the American Academy of Pediatrics (http://www.aap.org), and the American Academy of Family Physicians (http://www.aafp.org).

Catch-up Immunization Schedule — UNITED STATES • 2007

for Persons Aged 4 Months—18 Years Who Start Late or Who Are More Than 1 Month Behind

The table below provides catch-up schedules and minimum intervals between doses for children whose vaccinations have been delayed. A vaccine series does not need to be restarted, regardless of the time that has elapsed between doses. Use the section appropriate for the child's age.

Vaccine	Minimum Age for Dose 1	Minimum Interval Between Doses			
		Dose 1 to Dose 2	Dose 2 to Dose 3	Dose 3 to Dose 4	Dose 4 to Dose 5
CATCH-UP SCHEDULE FOR PERSONS AGED 4 MONTHS–6 YEARS					
Hepatitis B[1]	**Birth**	**4 weeks**	**8 weeks** (and 16 weeks after first dose)		
Rotavirus[2]	**6 wks**	**4 weeks**	**4 weeks**		
Diphtheria, Tetanus, Pertussis[3]	**6 wks**	**4 weeks**	**4 weeks**	**6 months**	**6 months[3]**
Haemophilus influenzae type b[4]	**6 wks**	**4 weeks** if first dose administered at age <12 months **8 weeks (as final dose)** if first dose administered at age 12–14 months **No further doses needed** if first dose administered at age ≥15 months	**4 weeks[4]** if current age <12 months **8 weeks (as final dose)[4]** if current age ≥12 months and second dose administered at age <15 months **No further doses needed** if previous dose administered at age ≥15 months	**8 weeks (as final dose)** This dose only necessary for children aged 12 months–5 years who received 3 doses before age 12 months	
Pneumococcal[5]	**6 wks**	**4 weeks** if first dose administered at age <12 months and current age <24 months **8 weeks (as final dose)** if first dose administered at age ≥12 months or current age 24–59 months **No further doses needed** for healthy children if first dose administered at age ≥24 months	**4 weeks** if current age <12 months **8 weeks (as final dose)** if current age ≥12 months **No further doses needed** for healthy children if previous dose administered at age ≥24 months	**8 weeks (as final dose)** This dose only necessary for children aged 12 months–5 years who received 3 doses before age 12 months	
Inactivated Poliovirus[6]	**6 wks**	**4 weeks**	**4 weeks**	**4 weeks[6]**	
Measles, Mumps, Rubella[7]	**12 mos**	**4 weeks**			
Varicella[8]	**12 mos**	**3 months**			
Hepatitis A[9]	**12 mos**	**6 months**			
CATCH-UP SCHEDULE FOR PERSONS AGED 7–18 YEARS					
Tetanus, Diphtheria/ Tetanus, Diphtheria, Pertussis[10]	**7 yrs[10]**	**4 weeks**	**8 weeks** if first dose administered at age <12 months **6 months** if first dose administered at age ≥12 months	**6 months** if first dose administered at age <12 months	
Human Papillomavirus[11]	**9 yrs**	**4 weeks**	**12 weeks**		
Hepatitis A[9]	**12 mos**	**6 months**			
Hepatitis B[1]	**Birth**	**4 weeks**	**8 weeks** (and 16 weeks after first dose)		
Inactivated Poliovirus[8]	**6 wks**	**4 weeks**	**4 weeks**	**4 weeks[6]**	
Measles, Mumps, Rubella[7]	**12 mos**	**4 weeks**			
Varicella[8]	**12 mos**	**4 weeks** if first dose administered at age ≥13 years **3 months** if first dose administered at age <13 years			

1. **Hepatitis B vaccine (HepB).** *(Minimum age: birth)*
   - Administer the 3-dose series to those who were not previously vaccinated.
   - A 2-dose series of Recombivax HB® is licensed for children aged 11–15 years.
2. **Rotavirus vaccine (Rota).** *(Minimum age: 6 weeks)*
   - Do not start the series later than age 12 weeks.
   - Administer the final dose in the series by age 32 weeks. Do not administer a dose later than age 32 weeks.
   - Data on safety and efficacy outside of these age ranges are insufficient.
3. **Diphtheria and tetanus toxoids and acellular pertussis vaccine (DTaP).** *(Minimum age: 6 weeks)*
   - The fifth dose is not necessary if the fourth dose was administered at age ≥4 years.
   - DTaP is not indicated for persons aged ≥7 years.
4. **Haemophilus influenzae type b conjugate vaccine (Hib).** *(Minimum age: 6 weeks)*
   - Vaccine is not generally recommended for children aged ≥5 years.
   - If current age <12 months and the first 2 doses were PRP-OMP (PedvaxHIB® or ComVax® [Merck]), the third (and final) dose should be administered at age 12–15 months and at least 8 weeks after the second dose.
   - If first dose was administered at age 7–11 months, administer 2 doses separated by 4 weeks plus a booster at age 12–15 months.
5. **Pneumococcal conjugate vaccine (PCV).** *(Minimum age: 6 weeks)*
   - Vaccine is not generally recommended for children aged ≥5 years.
6. **Inactivated poliovirus vaccine (IPV).** *(Minimum age: 6 weeks)*
   - For children who received an all-IPV or all-oral poliovirus (OPV) series, a fourth dose is not necessary if third dose was administered at age ≥4 years.
   - If both OPV and IPV were administered as part of a series, a total of 4 doses should be administered, regardless of the child's current age.
7. **Measles, mumps, and rubella vaccine (MMR).** *(Minimum age: 12 months)*
   - The second dose of MMR is recommended routinely at age 4–6 years but may be administered earlier if desired.
   - If not previously vaccinated, administer 2 doses of MMR during any visit with ≥4 weeks between the doses.
8. **Varicella vaccine.** *(Minimum age: 12 months)*
   - The second dose of varicella vaccine is recommended routinely at age 4–6 years but may be administered earlier if desired.
   - Do not repeat the second dose in persons aged <13 years if administered ≥28 days after the first dose.
9. **Hepatitis A vaccine (HepA).** *(Minimum age: 12 months)*
   - HepA is recommended for certain groups of children, including in areas where vaccination programs target older children. See *MMWR* 2006;55(No. RR-7):1–23.
10. **Tetanus and diphtheria toxoids vaccine (Td) and tetanus and diphtheria toxoids and acellular pertussis vaccine (Tdap).** *(Minimum ages: 7 years for Td, 10 years for BOOSTRIX®, and 11 years for ADACEL™)*
    - Tdap should be substituted for a single dose of Td in the primary catch-up series or as a booster if age appropriate; use Td for other doses.
    - A 5-year interval from the last Td dose is encouraged when Tdap is used as a booster dose. A booster (fourth) dose is needed if any of the previous doses were administered at age <12 months. Refer to ACIP recommendations for further information. See *MMWR* 2006;55(No. RR-3).
11. **Human papillomavirus vaccine (HPV).** *(Minimum age: 9 years)*
    - Administer the HPV vaccine series to females at age 13–18 years if not previously vaccinated.

Information about reporting reactions after immunization is available online at http://www.vaers.hhs.gov or by telephone via the 24-hour national toll-free information line 800-822-7967. Suspected cases of vaccine-preventable disease should be reported to the state or local health department. Additional information, including precautions and contraindications for immunization, is available from the National Center for Immunization and Respiratory Diseases at http://www.cdc.gov/nip/default.htm or telephone, 800-CDC-INFO (800-232-4636).

Appendix 128-2
2007 Adult Immunization Schedule

Recommended Adult Immunization Schedule

Note: These re-commendations must be read with the feetsnotes that fallow.

Figure 1. Recommended adult immunization schedule, by vaccine and age group
United States, October 2007–September 2008

<table>
<tr><th>Age group (yrs)▶
Vaccine▼</th><th>19–49 years</th><th>50–64 years</th><th>≥65 years</th></tr>
<tr><td rowspan="2">Tetanus, diphtheria, pertussis (Td/Tdap)[1*]</td><td colspan="3">1 dose Td booster every 10 yrs</td></tr>
<tr><td colspan="2">Substitute 1 dose of Tdap for Td</td><td></td></tr>
<tr><td>Human papillomavirus (HPV)[2*]</td><td>3 doses females (0, 2, 6 months)</td><td></td><td></td></tr>
<tr><td>Measles, mumps, rubella (MMR)[3*]</td><td>1 or 2 doses</td><td colspan="2">1 dose</td></tr>
<tr><td>Varicella[4*]</td><td colspan="3">2 doses (0, 4–8 wks)</td></tr>
<tr><td>Influenza[5*]</td><td>1 dose annually</td><td colspan="2">1 dose annually</td></tr>
<tr><td>Pneumococcal (polysaccharide)[6,7]</td><td colspan="2">1–2 doses</td><td>1 dose</td></tr>
<tr><td>Hepatitis A[8*]</td><td colspan="3">2 doses (0, 6–12 mos, or 0, 6–18 mos)</td></tr>
<tr><td>Hepatitis B[9*]</td><td colspan="3">3 doses (0, 1–2, 4–6 mos)</td></tr>
<tr><td>Meningococcal[10]</td><td colspan="3">1 or more doses</td></tr>
<tr><td>Zoster[11]</td><td></td><td colspan="2">1 dose</td></tr>
</table>

Figure 2. Vaccines that might be indicated for adults based on medical and other indications
United States, October 2007–September 2008

<table>
<tr><th rowspan="2">Indication ▶
Vaccine ▼</th><th rowspan="2">Pregnancy</th><th rowspan="2">Immuno-compromising conditions (excluding human immunodeficiency virus [HIV]), medications, radiation[13]</th><th colspan="2">HIV infection[1,12,13] CD4+ T lymphocyte count</th><th rowspan="2">Diabetes, heart disease, chronic pulmonary disease, chronic alcoholism</th><th rowspan="2">Asplenia[12] (Including elective splenectomy and terminal complement component deficiencies)</th><th rowspan="2">Chronic liver disease</th><th rowspan="2">Kidney failure, end-stage renal disease, receipt of hemodialysis</th><th rowspan="2">Health-care personnel</th></tr>
<tr><th><200 cells/μL</th><th>≥200 cells/μL</th></tr>
<tr><td rowspan="2">Tetanus, diphtheria, pertussis (Td/Tdap)[1*]</td><td colspan="9">1-dose Td booster every 10 yrs</td></tr>
<tr><td></td><td colspan="8">Substitute 1 dose of Tdap for Td</td></tr>
<tr><td>Human papillomavirus (HPV)[2*]</td><td></td><td colspan="8">3 doses for females through age 26 years (0, 2, 6 mos)</td></tr>
<tr><td>Measles, mumps, rubella (MMR)[3*]</td><td colspan="3">Contraindicated</td><td colspan="6">1 or 2 doses</td></tr>
<tr><td>Varicella[4*]</td><td colspan="3">Contraindicated</td><td colspan="6">2 doses (0, 4–8 wks)</td></tr>
<tr><td>Influenza[5*]</td><td colspan="8">1 dose TIV annually</td><td>1 dose TIV or LAIV annually</td></tr>
<tr><td>Pneumococcal (polysaccharide)[6,7]</td><td>1–2 doses</td><td colspan="7">1–2 doses</td><td>1–2 doses</td></tr>
<tr><td>Hepatitis A[8*]</td><td colspan="9">2 doses (0, 6–12 mos, or 0, 6–18 mos)</td></tr>
<tr><td>Hepatitis B[9*]</td><td colspan="9">3 doses (0, 1–2, 4–6 mos)</td></tr>
<tr><td>Meningococcal[10]</td><td colspan="9">1 or more doses</td></tr>
<tr><td>Zoster[11]</td><td colspan="3">Contraindicated</td><td></td><td colspan="5">1 dose</td></tr>
</table>

*Covered by the Vaccine Injury Compensation Program.

Legend	
Light bar	For all persons in this category who meet the age requirements and who lack evidence of immunity (e.g. lack documentation of vaccination or have as evidence of prior infection)
Dark bar	Recommended if some other risk factor is present (e.g., on the basis of medical, occupational, lifestyle, or other indications)

These schedules indicate the recommended age groups and medical indications for which administration of currently licensed vaccines is commonly indicated for adults ages 19 years and older, as of October 1, 2007. Licensed combination vaccines may be used whenever any components of the combination are indicated and when the vaccine's other components are not contraindicated. For detailed recommendations on all vaccines, including those used primarily for travelers or that are issued during the year, consult the manufacturers' package inserts and the complete statements from the Advisory Committee on Immunization Practices (www.cdc.gov/vaccines/pubs/acip-list.htm).

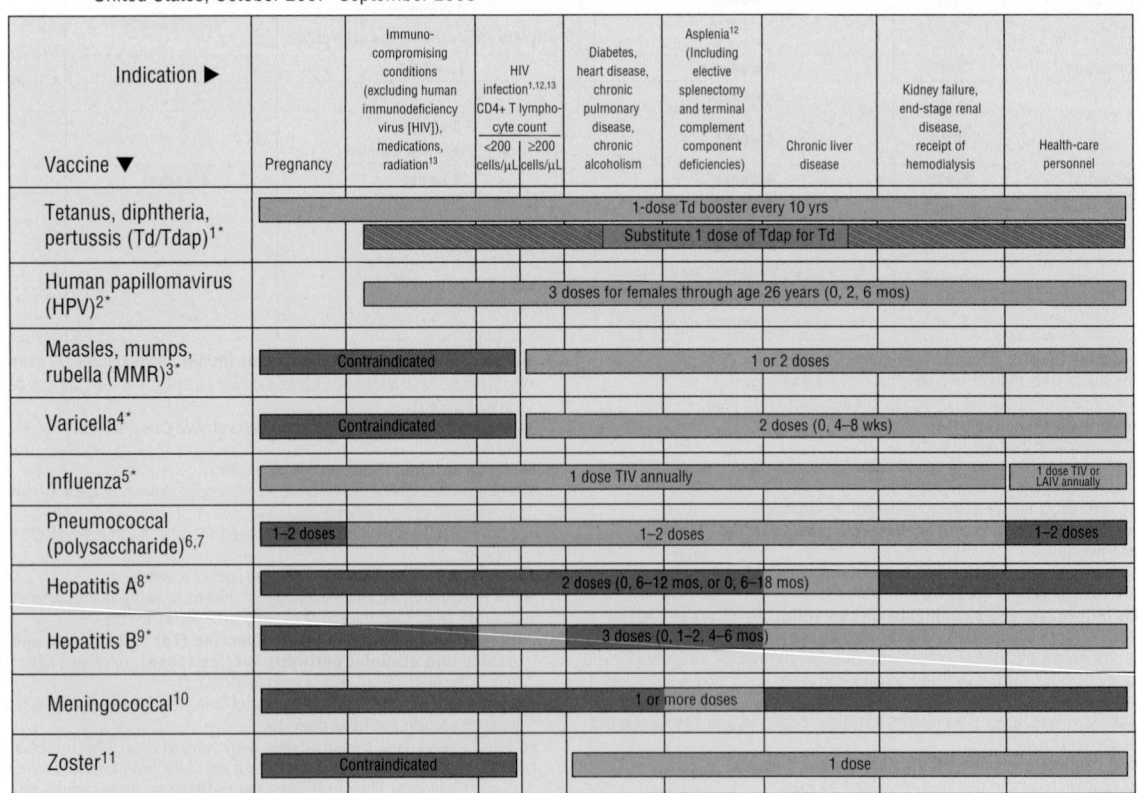

Footnotes

Recommended Adult Immunization Schedule • United States, October 2007 – September 2008

For complete statements by the Advisory Committee on Immunization Practices (ACIP), visit www.cdc.gov/vaccines/pubs/ACIP-list.htm.

1. Tetanus, diphtheria, and acellular pertussis (Td/Tdap) vaccination

Tdap should replace a single dose of Td for adults aged <65 years who have not previously received a dose of Tdap. Only one of two Tdap products (Adacel®[sanofi pasteur]) is licensed for use in adults.

Adults with uncertain histories of a complete primary vaccination series with tetanus and diphtheria toxoid–containing vaccines should begin or complete a primary vaccination series. A primary series for adults is 3 doses of tetanus and diphtheria toxoid–containing vaccines; administer the first 2 doses at least 4 weeks apart and the third dose 6–12 months after the second. However, Tdap can substitute for any one of the doses of Td in the 3-dose primary series. The booster dose of tetanus and diphtheria toxoid–containing vaccine should be administered to adults who have completed a primary series and if the last vaccination was received ≥10 years previously. Tdap or Td vaccine may be used, as indicated.

If the person is pregnant and received the last Td vaccination ≥10 years previously, administer Td during the second or third trimester; if the person received the last Td vaccination in <10 years, administer Tdap during the immediate postpartum period. A one-time administration of 1 dose of Tdap with an interval as short as 2 years from a previous Td vaccination is recommended for postpartum women, close contacts of infants aged <12 months, and all health-care workers with direct patient contact. In certain situations, Td can be deferred during pregnancy and Tdap substituted in the immediate postpartum period, or Tdap can be administered instead of Td to a pregnant woman after an informed discussion with the woman.

Consult the ACIP statement for recommendations for administering Td as prophylaxis in wound management.

2. Human papillomavirus (HPV) vaccination.

HPV vaccination is recommended for all females aged ≤26 years who have not completed the vaccine series. History of genital warts, abnormal Papanicolaou test, or positive HPV DNA test is not evidence of prior infection with all vaccine HPV types; HPV vaccination is still recommended for these persons.

Ideally, vaccine should be administered before potential exposure to HPV through sexual activity; however, females who are sexually active should still be vaccinated. Sexually active females who have not been infected with any of the HPV vaccine types receive the full benefit of the vaccination. Vaccination is less beneficial for females who have already been infected with one or more of the HPV vaccine types.

A complete series consists of 3 doses. The second dose should be administered 2 months after the first dose; the third dose should be administered 6 months after the first dose.

Although HPV vaccination is not specifically recommended for females with the medical indications described in Figure 2, "Vaccines that might be indicated for adults based on medical and other indications," it is not a live-virus vaccine and can be administered. However, immune response and vaccine efficacy might be less than in persons who do not have the medical indications described or who are immunocompetent.

3. Measles, mumps, rubella (MMR) vaccination.

Measles component: Adults born before 1957 can be considered immune to measles. Adults born during or after 1957 should receive ≥1 dose of MMR unless they have a medical contraindication, documentation of ≥1 dose, history of measles based on health-care provider diagnosis, or laboratory evidence of immunity.

A second dose of MMR is recommended for adults who 1) have been recently exposed to measles or are in an outbreak setting; 2) have been previously vaccinated with killed measles vaccine; 3) have been vaccinated with an unknown type of measles vaccine during 1963–1967; 4) are students in postsecondary educational institutions; 5) work in a health-care facility; or 6) plan to travel internationally.

Mumps component: Adults born before 1957 can generally be considered immune to mumps. Adults born during or after 1957 should receive 1 dose of MMR unless they have a medical contraindication, history of mumps based on health-care provider diagnosis, or laboratory evidence of immunity.

A second dose of MMR is recommended for adults who 1) are in an age group that is affected during a mumps outbreak; 2) are students in postsecondary educational institutions; 3) work in a health-care facility; or 4) plan to travel internationally. For unvaccinated health-care workers born before 1957 who do not have other evidence of mumps immunity, consider administering 1 dose on a routine basis and strongly consider administering a second dose during an outbreak.

Rubella component: Administer 1 dose of MMR vaccine to women whose rubella vaccination history is unreliable or who lack laboratory evidence of immunity. For women of childbearing age, regardless of birth year, routinely determine rubella immunity and counsel women regarding congenital rubella syndrome. Women who do not have evidence of immunity should receive MMR vaccine upon completion or termination of pregnancy and before discharge from the health-care facility.

4. Varicella vaccination.

All adults without evidence of immunity to varicella should receive 2 doses of single-antigen varicella vaccine unless they have a medical contraindication. Special consideration should be given to those who 1) have close contact with persons at high risk for severe disease (e.g., health-care personnel and family contacts of immunocompromised persons) or 2) are at high risk for exposure or transmission (e.g., teachers; child care employees; residents and staff members of institutional settings, including correctional institutions; college students; military personnel; adolescents and adults living in households with children; nonpregnant women of childbearing age; and international travelers).

Evidence of immunity to varicella in adults includes any of the following: 1) documentation of 2 doses of varicella vaccine at least 4 weeks apart; 2) U.S.-born before 1980 (although for health-care personnel and pregnant women birth before 1980 should not be considered evidence of immunity); 3) history of varicella based on diagnosis or verification of varicella by a health-care provider (for a patient reporting a history of or presenting with an atypical case, a mild case, or both, health-care providers should seek either an epidemiologic link with a typical varicella case or to a laboratory-confirmed case or evidence of laboratory confirmation, if it was performed at the time of acute disease); 4) history of herpes zoster based on health-care provider diagnosis; or 5) laboratory evidence of immunity or laboratory confirmation of disease.

Assess pregnant women for evidence of varicella immunity. Women who do not have evidence of immunity should receive the first dose of varicella vaccine upon completion or termination of pregnancy and before discharge from the health-care facility. The second dose should be administered 4–8 weeks after the first dose.

5. Influenza vaccination.

Medical indications: Chronic disorders of the cardiovascular or pulmonary systems, including asthma; chronic metabolic diseases, including diabetes mellitus, renal or hepatic dysfunction, hemoglobinopathies, or immunosuppression (including immunosuppression caused by medications or human immunodeficiency virus [HIV]); any condition that compromises respiratory function or the handling of respiratory secretions or that can increase the risk of aspiration (e.g., cognitive dysfunction, spinal cord injury, or seizure disorder or other neuromuscular disorder); and pregnancy during the influenza season. No data exist on the risk for severe or complicated influenza disease among persons with asplenia; however, influenza is a risk factor for secondary bacterial infections that can cause severe disease among persons with asplenia.

Occupational indications: Health-care personnel and employees of long-term care and assisted-living facilities.

Other indications: Residents of nursing homes and other long-term care and assisted-living facilities; persons likely to transmit influenza to persons at high risk (e.g., in-home household contacts and caregivers of children aged 0–59 months, or persons of all ages with high-risk conditions); and anyone who would like to be vaccinated. Healthy, nonpregnant adults aged ≤49 years without high-risk medical conditions who are not contacts of severely immunocompromised persons in special care units can receive either intranasally administered live, attenuated influenza vaccine (FluMist®) or inactivated vaccine. Other persons should receive the inactivated vaccine.

6. Pneumococcal polysaccharide vaccination.

Medical indications: Chronic pulmonary disease (excluding asthma); chronic cardiovascular diseases; diabetes mellitus; chronic liver diseases, including liver disease as a result of alcohol abuse (e.g., cirrhosis); chronic alcoholism, chronic renal failure or nephrotic syndrome; functional or anatomic asplenia (e.g., sickle cell disease or splenectomy [if elective splenectomy is planned, vaccinate at least 2 weeks before surgery]); immunosuppressive conditions; and cochlear implants and cerebrospinal fluid leaks. Vaccinate as close to HIV diagnosis as possible.

Other indications: Alaska Natives and certain American Indian populations and residents of nursing homes or other long-term care facilities.

7. Revaccination with pneumococcal polysaccharide vaccine.

One-time revaccination after 5 years for persons with chronic renal failure or nephrotic syndrome; functional or anatomic asplenia (e.g., sickle cell disease or splenectomy); or immunosuppressive conditions. For persons aged ≥65 years, one-time revaccination if they were vaccinated ≥5 years previously and were aged <65 years at the time of primary vaccination.

8. Hepatitis A vaccination.

Medical indications: Persons with chronic liver disease and persons who receive clotting factor concentrates.

Behavioral indications: Men who have sex with men and persons who use illegal drugs.

Occupational indications: Persons working with hepatitis A virus (HAV)–infected primates or with HAV in a research laboratory setting.

Other indications: Persons traveling to or working in countries that have high or intermediate endemicity of hepatitis A (a list of countries is available at wwwn.cdc.gov/travel/contentdiseases.aspx) and any person seeking protection from HAV infection.

Single-antigen vaccine formulations should be administered in a 2-dose schedule at either 0 and 6–12 months (Havrix®), or 0 and 6–18 months (Vaqta®). If the combined hepatitis A and hepatitis B vaccine (Twinrix®) is used, administer 3 doses at 0, 1, and 6 months.

9. Hepatitis B vaccination.

Medical indications: Persons with end-stage renal disease, including patients receiving hemodialysis; persons seeking evaluation or treatment for a sexually transmitted disease (STD); persons with HIV infection; and persons with chronic liver disease.

Occupational indications: Health-care personnel and public-safety workers who are exposed to blood or other potentially infectious body fluids.

Behavioral indications: Sexually active persons who are not in a long-term, mutually monogamous relationship (e.g., persons with more than 1 sex partner during the previous 6 months); current or recent injection-drug users; and men who have sex with men.

Other indications: Household contacts and sex partners of persons with chronic hepatitis B virus (HBV) infection; clients and staff members of institutions for persons with developmental disabilities; international travelers to countries with high or intermediate prevalence of chronic HBV infection (a list of countries is available at wwwn.cdc.gov/travel/contentdiseases.aspx); and any adult seeking protection from HBV infection.

Settings where hepatitis B vaccination is recommended for all adults: STD treatment facilities; HIV testing and treatment facilities; facilities providing drug-abuse treatment and prevention services; health-care settings targeting services to injection-drug users or men who have sex with men; correctional facilities; end-stage renal disease programs and facilities for chronic hemodialysis patients; and institutions and nonresidential daycare facilities for persons with developmental disabilities.

Special formulation indications: For adult patients receiving hemodialysis and other immunocompromised adults, 1 dose of 40 μg/mL (Recombivax HB®), or 2 doses of 20 μg/mL (Engerix-B®) administered simultaneously.

10. Meningococcal vaccination.

Medical indications: Adults with anatomic or functional asplenia, or terminal complement component deficiencies.

Other indications: First-year college students living in dormitories; microbiologists who are routinely exposed to isolates of *Neisseria meningitidis*; military recruits; and persons who travel to or live in countries in which meningococcal disease is hyperendemic or epidemic (e.g., the "meningitis belt" of sub-Saharan Africa during the dry season [December–June]), particularly if their contact with local populations will be prolonged. Vaccination is required by the government of Saudi Arabia for all travelers to Mecca during the annual Hajj.

Meningococcal conjugate vaccine is preferred for adults with any of the preceding indications who are aged ≤55 years, although meningococcal polysaccharide vaccine (MPSV4) is an acceptable alternative. Revaccination after 3–5 years might be indicated for adults previously vaccinated with MPSV4 who remain at increased risk for infection (e.g., persons residing in areas in which disease is epidemic)

11. Herpes zoster vaccination

A single dose of zoster vaccine is recommended for adults aged ≥60 years regardless of whether they report a prior episode of herpes zoster. Persons with chronic medical conditions may be vaccinated unless a contraindication or precaution exists for their condition.

12. Selected conditions for which *Haemophilus influenzae* type b (Hib) vaccine may be used

Hib conjugate vaccines are licensed for children aged 6 weeks–71 months. No efficacy data are available on which to base a recommendation concerning use of Hib vaccine for older children and adults with the chronic conditions associated with an increased risk for Hib disease. However, studies suggest good immunogenicity in patients who have sickle cell disease, leukemia, or HIV infection or who have had splenectomies; administering vaccine to these patients is not contraindicated.

13. Immunocompromising conditions.

Inactivated vaccines are generally acceptable (e.g., pneumococcal, meningococcal, and influenza [trivalent inactivated influenza vaccine]), and live vaccines generally are avoided in persons with immune deficiencies or immune suppressive conditions. Information on specific conditions is available at www.cdc.gov/vaccines/pubs/acip-list.htm.

CHAPTER 129 Human Immunodeficiency Virus Infection

PETER L. ANDERSON, THOMAS N. KAKUDA, AND
COURTNEY V. FLETCHER

KEY CONCEPTS

1. Infection with human immunodeficiency virus (HIV) occurs through three primary modes: sexual, parenteral, and perinatal. Sexual intercourse, primarily receptive anal and vaginal intercourse, is the most common method for transmission.

2. HIV infects cells expressing cluster of differentiation 4 (CD4) receptors, such as T-helper lymphocytes, monocytes, macrophages, dendritic cells, and brain microglia. Infection occurs via an interaction between glycoprotein 160 (gp160) on HIV with CD4 (primary interaction) and chemokine coreceptors (secondary interactions) present on the surfaces of these cells.

3. The hallmark of untreated HIV infection is profound CD4 T-lymphocyte depletion and severe immunosuppression that puts patients at significant risk for infectious diseases caused by opportunistic pathogens. Opportunistic infections in settings without access to antiretroviral drugs are the chief cause of morbidity and mortality associated with HIV infection.

4. General principles for the management of opportunistic infections include preventing or reversing immunosuppression with antiretroviral therapy, preventing exposure to pathogens, vaccination, prospective immunologic monitoring, primary chemoprophylaxis, treatment of acute episodes, secondary chemoprophylaxis, and discontinuation of such prophylaxes following antiretroviral therapy and subsequent immune recovery.

5. Complete eradication of HIV currently is not possible. Therefore, the goal of antiretroviral therapy is to achieve maximal and durable suppression of HIV replication, interpreted to be a sustained plasma viral load less than the lower limit of quantitation. Another equally important outcome is an increase in CD4 lymphocytes because this closely correlates with the risk for developing opportunistic infections.

6. Current recommendations for the initial treatment of HIV advocate a minimum of three active antiretroviral agents. The typical regimen consists of two nucleoside analogs with either a protease inhibitor (pharmacologically enhanced with low-dose ritonavir) or a nonnucleoside reverse transcriptase inhibitor.

7. Clinical use of antiretroviral agents is complicated by drug–drug interactions. Some interactions are beneficial and used purposely; others may be harmful, leading to dangerously elevated or inadequate drug concentrations. For these reasons, clinicians involved in the pharmacotherapy of HIV infection must exercise constant vigilance and maintain a current knowledge of drug interactions.

8. Inadequate suppression of viral replication allows HIV to select for antiretroviral-resistant HIV variants, the major factor limiting the ability of antiretroviral drugs to inhibit virus replication and delay disease progression.

9. Current recommendations for treating drug-resistant HIV include choosing at least two drugs to which the patient's virus is susceptible. Susceptibility can be assessed using either (virtual) genotypic or phenotypic resistance testing.

10. The longer life span conferred by antiretroviral treatment has given rise to new medical issues. First, a wide spectrum of metabolic abnormalities have become common, some of which are adverse effects from antiretroviral drugs. Second, hepatitis C virus coinfection has emerged as an important cause of morbidity and mortality. Medical management of these contemporary HIV complications is constantly evolving.

Learning objectives, review questions,
and other resources can be found at
www.pharmacotherapyonline.com.

Acquired immune deficiency syndrome (AIDS) was first recognized by the medical community as a distinct clinical entity in 1981. This syndrome was described initially in a cohort of young, previously healthy homosexual men with new-onset profound immunologic deficits, *Pneumocystis carinii* (now *Pneumocystis jiroveci*) pneumonia (PCP), and Kaposi sarcoma.[1] A retrovirus, human immunodeficiency virus type 1 (HIV-1), is the major cause of AIDS.[2] A second retrovirus, HIV-2, also is recognized to cause AIDS, although it is less virulent, transmissible, and prevalent than HIV-1. These retroviruses are transmitted primarily by sexual contact and by contact with contaminated blood or blood products. Several risk behaviors for the acquisition of HIV infection have been identified in the United States, most notably the practice of anorectal intercourse and the sharing of blood-contaminated needles by injection-drug users. In many developing countries, the majority of HIV transmission occurs via heterosexual intercourse and from childbearing women to their offspring. Initially, the medical management of HIV consisted of repeated treatments for opportunistic infections (OIs) and eventual palliative care. In the mid 1990s, a new era in the pharmacotherapy for HIV, known as *combination antiretroviral therapy* (ART), was born. ART consists of combinations of antiretroviral agents that potently and durably suppress HIV replication, delay the onset of AIDS, reverse HIV-associated immunologic deficits, and significantly prolong patient survival.[3,4] Unfortunately, therapeutic challenges remain in the ART era and include the need for continuous adherence to medication, drug–drug interactions, drug-resistant HIV, acute and long-term drug toxicities, and other complications associated with a prolonged life span. Global statistics on the prevalence, incidence, and treatment access for this disease remain grim. No strategies to date have been successful in curing HIV, and no vaccine is available. This chapter provides an overview of the pathophysiology and pharmacotherapy of HIV.

HUMAN IMMUNODEFICIENCY VIRUS

EPIDEMIOLOGY

The epidemiologic characteristics of HIV infection differ according to geographic region and depend upon the mode of transmission, governmental prevention efforts and resources, and cultural factors.[5]

Transmission

❶ Infection with HIV occurs through three primary modes: sexual, parenteral, and perinatal. Sexual intercourse, primarily receptive anal and vaginal intercourse, is the most common method for transmission. No sex act between individuals can be considered absolutely safe. HIV transmission can occur from artificial insemination with infected semen. The probability of HIV transmission from receptive anorectal intercourse is estimated at 0.1% to 3% per sexual act.[6] For receptive vaginal intercourse, the risk is approximately 0.1% to 0.2%. The risk from insertive sex acts is lower, approximately 0.01% to 0.4% for insertive anal intercourse and approximately 0.05% to 0.1% for insertive vaginal intercourse.[6,7] Oral intercourse can transmit HIV; again receptive intercourse carries higher risk.[6] Condom use reduces risk of transmission by approximately 20-fold.[6] Other factors that affect the probability of infection include vaginal bleeding during intercourse and the stage of HIV disease in the index partner. For example, there is a 2.5-fold relative risk of transmission for each $\log_{10}$ increase in virus load in the blood.[6] Individuals with genital ulcers or sexually transmitted diseases, such as syphilis, chancroid, herpes, gonorrhea, chlamydia, and trichomoniasis, are at greater risk for contracting HIV. HIV incidence and prevalence are lower in cultures that advocate male circumcision, which is estimated to reduce risk of HIV transmission by 60%. The mechanism of increased risk in uncircumcised males may be due to high lymphocyte concentrations and susceptibility to skin tears in foreskin apparatus.[8] Casual contact with patients with AIDS or with HIV infection is not a significant risk factor for HIV transmission.[9]

Prevention of sexual transmission has focused primarily on education that encourages abstinence (especially for adolescents), use of condoms, and reduction of high-risk behavior (anal intercourse and promiscuity).[5] Additional strategies include treating other sexually transmitted diseases. A combined approach has been advocated for successful prevention. Prevention strategies under investigation include interventional male circumcision, HIV vaccines, topical vaginal microbicides, and preexposure prophylaxis with antiretroviral agents.

Parenteral transmission of HIV broadly encompasses infections due to contaminated blood exposure from needle sticks, intravenous injection with used needles, receipt of blood products, and organ transplants. Use of contaminated needles or other injection-related paraphernalia by drug abusers has been the main cause of parenteral transmissions. The risk of HIV transmission from sharing needles is approximately 0.67% per episode.[10] Prevention strategies include stopping drug abuse, obtaining needles from credible sources (e.g., pharmacies), never reusing any paraphernalia, using sterile procedures in all injecting activities, and safely disposing of used paraphernalia. When sterile paraphernalia is not available, the equipment should be boiled or disinfected with bleach.[6]

Before widespread screening, HIV was readily transmitted in blood products. However, today blood and tissue products in the healthcare system are rigorously screened. The estimated risk for receiving tainted blood or blood products in the United States is approximately 1:2,000,000 and that for receiving a tainted tissue transplant is 1:55,000.[11,12] Healthcare workers have a small but definite occupational risk of contracting HIV through accidental injury. Most cases of occupationally acquired HIV have been the result of a percutaneous needle stick injury, which carries an estimated 0.3% risk of transmitting HIV. Mucocutaneous exposures (e.g., tainted blood splash in eyes, mouth, nose) carries a transmission risk of approximately 0.09%.[13] Significant risk factors for seroconversion with a needle stick include deep injury, injury with a device visibly contaminated with blood, and advanced HIV disease in the index patient. The risk of transmission from an HIV-infected healthcare worker to a patient is extremely remote.[9] Comprehensive medical guidelines have been developed to minimize the hazard of HIV exposure for healthcare workers and for persons exposed by rape or other means.[10,13]

Perinatal infection, or vertical transmission, is the most common cause of pediatric HIV infection.[14] Most infections occur during or near to the time of birth, although a fraction can occur in utero. The risk of mother-to-child transmission is approximately 25% in the absence of breast-feeding and antiretroviral therapy. Factors that increase the likelihood of vertical transmission include prolonged rupture of membranes, chorioamnionitis, genital infection during pregnancy, preterm delivery, vaginal delivery, birth weight less than 2,500 g, illicit drug use during pregnancy, and high maternal viral load. Breast-feeding also can transmit HIV. The estimated frequency of breast milk transmission in one study was 16.2%, with the majority of infections developing within the first 6 months.[15] Formula feeding prevents HIV infections but may not improve mortality from other causes early in life.[16] Whenever feasible, HIV-infected mothers are recommended not to breast-feed. A separate and comprehensive set of guidelines have been developed to minimize the hazard of mother-to-child HIV transmission.[14] These guidelines are discussed in the Treatment of Special Population section.

Persons with HIV infection are broadly categorized as those living with HIV and those with an AIDS diagnosis. An AIDS diagnosis is made when the cluster of differentiation 4 (CD4; T-helper cell) count drops below 200 cells/μL or after an AIDS indicator condition is diagnosed.[17] Further distinctions regarding the stage of HIV and AIDS are given in the Centers for Disease Control and Prevention (CDC) surveillance case definition (Table 129–1).[18] In the United States, new HIV/AIDS cases are reported by healthcare providers to a public health department.[17] The cumulative number of reported AIDS diagnoses at the end of December 2005 was 956,019; 550,394 (more than half) have already died.[19] The estimated prevalence of HIV infections including AIDS cases in the United States is just over one million individuals. Each year the CDC estimates that 40,000 new cases of HIV infection occur in the United States. Approximately 25% of persons with HIV are unaware of their infection. The epidemic in the United States initially was established in white men who have sex with men, and the prevalence of HIV in this population still is high. Overall cases in men outnumber women by approximately 6:1. New trends in transmission include more cases in women and African Americans and Hispanics, a proportion of whom are not well linked to appropriate prevention, care, and treatment services. Approximately half of new cases occurred in African Americans (who make up only 12% of the general population), about one third in whites, and less than one fourth in Hispanics. The main risk factor for transmission in women is heterosexual intercourse (80% of cases) and injection-drug use (20% of cases). For men the main risks are men who have sex with men (65%), heterosexual sex (15%), and injection-drug use (15%).

Worldwide, approximately 65 million people have been infected with HIV, and approximately 25 million of these persons have already died as of 2006. Today, approximately 39 million people are

TABLE 129-1 Centers for Disease Control and Prevention 1993 Revised Classification System for HIV Infection in Adults and AIDS Surveillance Case Definition

CD4⁺ T-Cell Categories (Absolute Number and Percentage)	(A) Asymptomatic, Acute (Primary) HIV or PGL	(B) Symptomatic, Not (A) or (C) Conditions	(C) AIDS Indicator Conditions
≥500/μL or ≥29%	A1	B1	C1
200–499/μL or 14%–28%	A2	B2	C2
<200/μL or <14%	A3	B3	C3

AIDS indicator conditions	
Candidiasis of bronchi, trachea, or lungs	Lymphoma, Burkitt
Candidiasis, esophageal	Lymphoma, immunoblastic
Cervical cancer, invasive	Lymphoma, primary, or brain
Coccidioidomycosis, disseminated or extrapulmonary	*Mycobacterium avium* complex or *Mycobacterium kansasii,* disseminated or extrapulmonary
Cryptococcosis, extrapulmonary	*Mycobacterium tuberculosis*, any site (pulmonary or extrapulmonary)
Cryptosporidiosis, chronic intestinal (duration >1 month)	*Mycobacterium*, other species or unidentified species, disseminated or extrapulmonary
Cytomegalovirus disease (other than liver, spleen, or nodes)	*Pneumocystis carinii* pneumonia
Cytomegalovirus retinitis (with loss of vision)	Pneumonia, recurrent
Encephalopathy, HIV-related	Progressive multifocal leukoencephalopathy
Herpes simplex: chronic ulcer(s) (duration >1 month); or bronchitis, pneumonitis, or esophagitis	*Salmonella* septicemia, recurrent Toxoplasmosis of brain
Histoplasmosis, disseminated or extrapulmonary	Wasting syndrome due to HIV
Isosporiasis, chronic intestinal (duration >1 month)	
Kaposi sarcoma	

AIDS, acquired immune deficiency syndrome; HIV, human immunodeficiency virus; PGL, persistent generalized lymphadenopathy.

living with HIV/AIDS, including 2.5 million children (younger than 15 years).[20] The new infection rate is approximately five million per year, including 700,000 children. The highest concentration of HIV/AIDS cases is in sub-Saharan Africa, where approximately 25 million people are infected. Some African countries have HIV prevalence rates of 33% or more (e.g., Swaziland); however, other African countries have declining prevalence rates (e.g., Kenya) due to successful prevention strategies. Heterosexual transmission is the most common mode of transmission in Sub-Saharan Africa and worldwide (85% of cases). Women in sub-Saharan Africa and developing countries are at disproportionately high risk for acquiring HIV because of higher transmission risk with receptive intercourse and cultural factors that foster HIV transmission, such as sex between younger women and older men.[5,20] Other important epidemiologic features of the HIV epidemic include growing prevalence in eastern Europe (e.g., Russian Federation), central Asia (e.g., Ukraine), eastern Asia (e.g., India), and China. Injection-drug use is fueling several of these epidemics.

ETIOLOGY

HIV is an enveloped single-stranded RNA virus and a member of the Lentivirinae (*lenti,* meaning "slow") subfamily of retroviruses. Lentiviruses are characterized by their indolent infectious cycle. There are two related but distinct types of HIV: HIV-1 and HIV-2. HIV-2, found mostly in western Africa, consists of seven phylogenetic lineages designated as subtypes (clades) A through G.[21] HIV-1 also can be categorized based on phylogeny. Three groups of HIV-1 currently are recognized: M (main or major), N (non-M, non-O), and O (outlier). The nine subtypes of HIV-1 group M are identified as A through D, F through H, and J and K. Mixtures of subtypes are referred to as *circulating recombinant forms.* Group M, subtype B, is primarily responsible for the epidemic in North America and western Europe.

The origin of HIV is of considerable interest. The accumulated evidence suggests that HIV in humans was the result of a cross-species transmission (zoonosis) from primates infected with simian immunodeficiency virus (SIV).[22] Phylogenetic and geographic relationships suggest that HIV-2 arose from SIV that infects sooty mangabeys. The origin of HIV-1 is less clear, but similarities exist between SIVcpz, a virus that infects chimpanzees (*Pan troglodytes troglodytes*), and HIV-1 groups M and N. Group O may have arisen from a SIV variant that infects wild gorillas.[23] Cultural practices, such as preparation and eating of bush meat or keeping animals as pets, may have allowed the virus to jump from primate to humans. The earliest known human infection with HIV has been traced to central Africa in 1959. Modern transportation, promiscuity, and drug abuse have caused the rapid spread of the virus within the United States and throughout the world.[5,22] This chapter focuses on HIV-1 group M, which is the predominant strain likely to be encountered in the western world.

DETECTION OF HIV AND SURROGATE MARKERS OF DISEASE PROGRESSION

The most common laboratory method for diagnosing HIV-1 infection is an enzyme-linked immunosorbent assay (ELISA), which detects antibodies against HIV-1. ELISA is both highly sensitive (>99%) and highly specific (>99%), but rare false-positive results can occur in multiparous women; recent recipients of hepatitis B, HIV, influenza, or rabies vaccine; patients with multiple blood transfusion, liver disease, and renal failure; or those undergoing chronic hemodialysis. False-negative results may occur and most commonly are attributed to new infection where antibody production is not yet adequate. The minimum time to develop antibodies is 3 to 4 weeks from initial exposure, with greater than 95% of individuals developing antibodies after 6 months. Convenient methods for obtaining an ELISA sample have been developed, including an oral collection device (OraSure), an over-the-counter home fingerstick blood collection test system (Home Access), a urine test (Calypte), and a rapid (20–40 minutes) turnaround test (OraQuick). The rapid test improves upon the number of persons who agree to be tested and who actually receive the results.[24]

Positive ELISA results are repeated in duplicate, and if one or both tests are reactive, a confirmatory test is performed for final diagnosis. Western blot is the most commonly used confirmatory test, although an indirect immunofluorescence assay is available. A reactive ELISA test and a positive confirmatory test indicate an established HIV infection. If the confirmatory test is indeterminate, the dilemma can be resolved by retesting the individual after 30 days or performing a viral load assay if the patient is at high risk or symptomatic.[25]

HIV testing is recommended when HIV infection is suspected because of symptoms and/or high-risk behavior. Additionally, the CDC now recommends routine HIV screening in all healthcare settings in persons 13 to 64 years, a new policy called "opt-out" testing.[26] The policy states that consent for medical care will imply consent for HIV testing; however, the person must be informed of the test and can opt out of taking it. The rationale for this strategy is to diagnose those who unknowingly carry HIV so as to improve their prognosis and reduce further transmission.

Once diagnosed, HIV disease is monitored primarily by two surrogate markers, viral load and CD4 cell count.[27] The viral load test quantifies the degree of viremia by measuring the number of copies of viral RNA (HIV RNA) in the plasma. Methods for determining HIV RNA include reverse-transcription polymerase chain reaction (RT-PCR), branched-chain DNA, transcription-mediated amplification, and nucleic acid sequence–based assay. RT-PCR and branched DNA are used more widely than the other techniques. Irrespective of the method used, viral load is reported as the number of viral RNA copies per milliliter of plasma. Each assay has its own lower limit of sensitivity to viral subtypes, and results can vary from one assay method to the other; therefore, it is recommended that the same assay method be used consistently within patients. Results also may vary by the type of blood collection tube used. Reductions in viral load often are reported in base 10 logarithm. For example, if a patient presents initially with a viral load of 100,000 copies/mL (10^5 copies/mL) and subsequently has a viral load of 10,000 copies/mL (10^4 copies/mL), the decrease in viral load is 1 $\log_{10}$. Given that HIV RNA varies within patients, a clinical response is generally considered when the decline in viral load is more than 0.5 $\log_{10}$.[27] Viral load assays have greater than 99% specificity and can be used to detect most strains of HIV. More important, viral load is a major prognostic factor for monitoring disease progression and the effects of treatment.

Because HIV attacks and leads to the destruction of cells bearing the CD4 receptor, the number of CD4 lymphocytes (T-helper cells) in the blood is a critical surrogate marker of disease progression. The normal adult CD4 lymphocyte count ranges from 500 to 1,600 cells/mm,[3] or 40% to 70% of all lymphocytes. CD4 counts in children are age dependent, with younger children having higher CD4 counts. The hallmark of HIV disease is depletion of CD4 cells and the associated development of OIs and malignancies.[28]

PATHOGENESIS

❷ Understanding the life cycle of HIV (Fig. 129–1) is necessary because the current strategies used for treatment of HIV target various points in this cycle.[29,30] Once HIV enters the human body, the outer glycoprotein (gp160) on its surface, which is composed of two subunits (gp120 and gp41) has affinity for CD4 receptors, proteins present on the surface of T-helper lymphocytes, monocytes, macrophages, dendritic cells, and brain microglia. The gp120 subunit is responsible for CD4 binding. Once initial binding occurs, the intimate association of HIV with the cell is enhanced by further binding to chemokine coreceptors. The two major chemokine receptors used by HIV are CCR5 and CXCR4. HIV isolates may contain a mixture of viruses that target one or the other of these coreceptors, and some viral strains may be dual-tropic (i.e., can use both coreceptors). The HIV strain that preferentially uses CCR5, R5 viruses, are macrophage-tropic and nonsyncytium-inducing (syncytium is cell clumping). The R5 virus typically is implicated in most cases of sexually transmitted HIV. The HIV strain that targets CXCR4, designated X4 virus, is T-cell–tropic and often is predominant in the

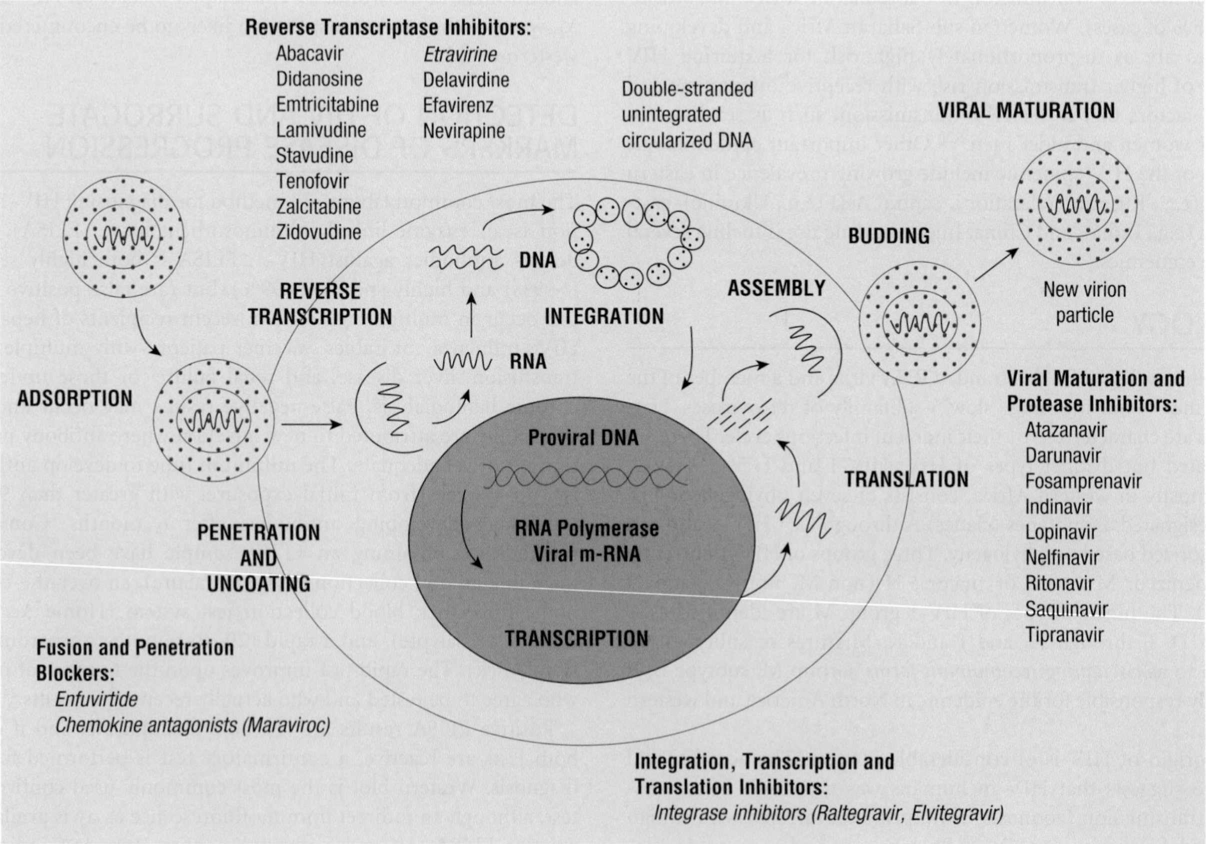

FIGURE 129-1. Life cycle of human immunodeficiency virus with potential targets where replication may be interrupted. *(Reprinted with permission, Courtney V. Fletcher, 2007.)*

later stage of disease. X4 virus is syncytium-inducing. CD4 and coreceptor attachment of HIV to the cell promotes membrane fusion, which is mediated by gp41, and finally internalization of the viral genetic material and enzymes necessary for replication.

After internalization, the viral protein shell surrounding the nucleic acid (capsid) is uncoated in preparation for replication.[29,30] The genetic material of HIV is positive-sense (5′ to 3′) single-stranded RNA; the virus must transcribe this RNA into DNA (transcription normally occurs from DNA to RNA; HIV works backward, hence the name *retrovirus*). To do so, HIV is equipped with the unique enzyme RNA-dependent DNA polymerase (reverse transcriptase). Reverse transcriptase first synthesizes a complementary strand of DNA using the viral RNA as a template. The RNA portion of this DNA–RNA hybrid is then partially removed by ribonuclease H (RNase H), allowing reverse transcriptase to complete the synthesis of a double-stranded DNA molecule. Unfortunately, the fidelity of reverse transcriptase is poor, and many mistakes are made during the process. These errors in the final DNA product contribute to the rapid mutation of the virus, which enables the virus to evade the immune response (which complicates vaccine development), and promotes drug resistance to evolve. Following reverse transcription, the final double-stranded DNA product migrates into the nucleus and is integrated into the host cell chromosome by integrase, another enzyme unique to HIV.

The integration of HIV into the host chromosome is troublesome. Most notably, HIV can establish a persistent, latent infection, particularly in long-lived cells of the immune system such as memory T lymphocytes.[31] The virus is effectively hidden in these cells, and this characteristic has greatly inhibited the ability to cure HIV infection. Second, random integration of HIV may cause cellular abnormalities and induce apoptosis.

After integration, HIV preferentially replicates in activated cells.[28–30] Activation by antigens, cytokines, or other factors stimulates the cell to produce nuclear factor kappa B (NF-κB), an enhancer-binding protein. NF-κB normally regulates the expression of T-lymphocyte genes involved in growth but also can inadvertently activate replication of HIV. HIV encodes six regulatory and accessory proteins: Tat, Nef, Rev, Vpu, Vif, and Vpr, which enhance replication and inhibit innate immunity. For example, the Tat protein is a potent amplifier of HIV gene expression; it binds to a specific RNA sequence of HIV that initiates and stabilizes transcription elongation. Vif is viral protein that binds human ABOBEC3, a cytosine deaminase that converts viral RNA cytosine to uracil and thereby provides innate cellular immunity.[32] Assembly of new virion particles occurs in a stepwise manner beginning with the coalescence of HIV proteins beneath the host cell lipid bilayer. The nucleocapsid subsequently is formed with viral single-stranded RNA and other components packaged inside. Once packaged, the virion then buds through the plasma membrane, acquiring the characteristics of the host lipid bilayer. After the virus buds, the maturation process begins. Within the virion, protease, another enzyme unique to HIV, begins cleaving a large precursor polypeptide (gag-pol) into functional proteins that are necessary to produce a complete virus. Without this enzyme, the virion is immature and unable to infect other cells.

HIV-1 exhibits a very high turnover rate, with an estimated 10 billion new viruses produced each day. More than 99% of these viruses are produced in newly infected activated cells.[28] Ultimately, most infected cells and some uninfected bystander cells will be destroyed from a number of mechanisms, including cell lysis by newly budding virions, cytotoxic T-lymphocyte–induced cell killing, syncytia formation, and apoptosis. Syncytia formation occurs when viral proteins expressed on the surface of the infected cell act as ligands for receptors expressed on uninfected cells. Uninfected cells clump onto the infected cell and fuse into a giant multinucleated cell. The syncytium-inducing X4 virus phenotype may develop later in disease and is associated with more rapid disease progression. Destruction of the CD4 cells leads to profoundly compromised immune function and consequently AIDS.

CLINICAL PRESENTATION

Clinical presentation of primary HIV infection varies, but most patients (40%–90%) have an acute retroviral syndrome or mononucleosis-like illness (Table 129–2).[33] Symptoms often last 2 weeks, and hospitalization may be required for 15% of patients. Primary infection is associated with a high viral load (>10^6 copies/mL) and a precipitous drop in CD4 cells. A reservoir of latently infected cells is established at this time.[28] Virus disseminates to and replicates in the lymph tissues (mucosa, lymph nodes, and gut-associated lymph tissue). After several weeks an immune response is mounted, the amount of HIV RNA in plasma falls substantially, and symptoms resolve gradually. However, this clinically latent period is not virologically latent because HIV replication is continuous (10 billion viruses per day) and immune system destruction is ongoing. A persistent decrease in CD4 cells is the most measurable aspect of this immune system deterioration. Plasma viral load, on the other hand, will appear to have stabilized at a particular level or "set point." The set point that is established correlates directly with the time to AIDS and morbidity. The Multicenter AIDS Cohort Study measured viral load in 181 HIV-positive men and followed them for as long as 11 years. Only 8% of patients with viral loads of less than 4,530 copies/mL progressed to AIDS within 5 years, whereas the 5-year progression rate for patients with initial viral loads greater than 36,270 copies/mL was 62%. The mortality rates within 5 years were 5% and 49%, respectively. Thus, a higher viral set point is associated with poorer prognosis.[34]

Most children born with HIV are asymptomatic. On physical examination, children often present with unexplained physical signs, such as lymphadenopathy, hepatomegaly, splenomegaly, failure to thrive, weight loss or unexplained low birth weight (in prenatally exposed infants), and fever of unknown origin. Laboratory findings include anemia, hypergammaglobulinemia (primarily immunoglobulin [Ig]A and IgM), altered mononuclear cell function, and altered T-cell subset ratios. Of note, the normal range for CD4 cell counts in young children is much different from the range in adults (Table 129–3).[35] Children have different susceptibility and/or exposures to OIs compared with adults. Bacterial infections, including *Streptococcus pneumoniae, Salmonella* spp., and *Mycobacterium tuberculosis,* may be more prevalent in children with AIDS than in adults with the disease. Kaposi sarcoma is rare in children. Children with HIV infection may develop lymphocytic interstitial pneumonitis without evidence of *P. jiroveci* or other pathogens on lung biopsy. Some children present with progressive, unexplained neurologic deterioration, including late-onset seizures, loss of developmental milestones, cessation of brain growth, and diffuse unexplained encephalopathy. A

TABLE 129-2 Clinical Presentation of Primary Human Immunodeficiency Virus Infection in Adults

Symptoms
Fever, sore throat, fatigue, weight loss, myalgia
40% to 80% of patients exhibit a morbilliform or maculopapular rash usually involving the trunk
Diarrhea, nausea, vomiting
Lymphadenopathy, night sweats
Aseptic meningitis (fever, headache, photophobia, stiff neck) may be present in 25% of presenting cases
Other
High viral load (may exceed 1,000,000 copies per milliliter)
Persistent decrease in CD4 lymphocytes

TABLE 129-3 Centers for Disease Control and Prevention 1994 Revised Classification System for Human Immunodeficieny Virus Infection in Children Younger Than 13 Years

Immunologic Categories	12 Month CD4 Cells/μL (%[a])	1–5 Years CD4 Cells/μL (%[a])	6–12 Years CD4 Cells/μL (%[a])	
1. No evidence of suppression	≥1,500 (≥25%)	≥1,000 (≥25%)	≥500 (≥25%)	
2. Evidence of moderate suppression	750–1,499 (15%–24%)	500–999 (15%–24%)	200–499 (15%–24%)	
3. Severe suppression	<750 (<15%)	<500 (<15%)	<200 (<15%)	
Immunologic Categories	**N: No Signs/Symptoms**	**A: Mild Signs/Symptoms**	**B: Moderate Signs/Symptoms**	**C: Severe Signs/Symptoms**
1. No evidence of suppression	N1	A1	B1	C1
2. Evidence of moderate suppression	N2	A2	B2	C2
3. Severe suppression	N3	A3	B3	C3

[a]Percentage of total lymphocytes.

presentation of recurrent or persistent bacterial, fungal, or viral infections, which may be chronic and initially subclinical or slowly progressive, has been observed. Included in this group are children with recurrent bacterial sepsis, meningitis, and chronic otitis media and children with chronic oral candidiasis and presumed disseminated histoplasmosis. The current CDC pediatric AIDS surveillance definition (see Table 129–3) excludes children with congenital or perinatally acquired cytomegalovirus or other identified causes of congenital immunodeficiency.[35] General management of the HIV-infected child involves principles similar to those used for the adult: antiretroviral therapy, treatment and prophylaxis of OIs, and supportive care.[36]

TREATMENT

DESIRED OUTCOME

5 The central goal of antiretroviral therapy is to decrease morbidity and mortality. The most important and effective way to achieve this goal is maximal suppression of HIV replication, which is interpreted as plasma HIV RNA less than the lower limit of quantitation (i.e., undetectable; usually <50 copies/mL).[27] Such a profound reduction in HIV RNA is associated with long-term response to therapy (i.e., durability).[37] Another equally important outcome is an increase in CD4 lymphocytes because this closely correlates with the risk for developing OIs.[27] Undetectable HIV RNA almost always corresponds with a rise in CD4 lymphocytes, although patients occasionally respond virologically or immunologically without the other.[27]

GENERAL APPROACH TO TREATMENT

Prior to 1996, HIV infection was treated with single or dual antiretroviral agents, which were generally not effective at controlling viremia.[3] Thus, the mainstay of treatment was pharmacologic management of OIs and palliative care. At that time, the prognosis for HIV infection was dire and most patients were disabled and eventually died. From 1995 to 1996, a new class of antiretrovirals, the protease inhibitors (PIs), was introduced, and a new paradigm in HIV treatment was born. Combinations of three active antiretroviral agents from two pharmacologic classes were shown to profoundly inhibit HIV replication, prevent and reverse immune deficiency, and substantially decrease morbidity and mortality—constituting the ART era.[3] At the same time, multiple other major medical advances were introduced, such as the discovery that HIV establishes a long-lived reservoir in chronically infected cells, and the viral load test. With this backdrop of dramatic changes, in 1997 the National Institutes of Health Office of AIDS Research convened a panel to define the scientific principles that might serve as a guide for the clinical use of antiretroviral agents.[38] The 11 principles presented here are an amalgamation of knowledge of the life cycle of HIV, the consequences of HIV replication, clinical trials of antiretroviral agents, and scientific opinion. These foundational principles are still relevant today.

1. Ongoing HIV replication leads to immune system damage and progression to AIDS. HIV infection is always harmful, and true long-term survival free of clinically significant immune dysfunction is unusual.
2. Plasma HIV RNA levels indicate the magnitude of HIV replication and its associated rate of CD4 cell destruction, whereas CD4 cell counts indicate the extent of HIV-induced immune damage already suffered. Regular periodic measurement of plasma HIV RNA levels and CD4 cell counts is necessary to determine the risk of disease progression in an HIV-infected individual and to determine when to initiate or modify antiretroviral treatment regimens.
3. Because rates of disease progression differ among individuals, treatment decisions should be individualized by level of risk indicated by plasma HIV RNA levels and CD4 cell counts.
4. Use of potent combination antiretroviral therapy to suppress HIV replication to below the levels of detection of sensitive plasma HIV RNA assays limits the potential for selection of antiretroviral-resistant HIV variants, the major factor limiting the ability of antiretroviral drugs to inhibit virus replication and delay disease progression. Therefore, maximum achievable suppression of HIV replication should be the goal of therapy.
5. The most effective means for accomplishing durable suppression of HIV replication is simultaneous initiation of combinations of effective anti-HIV drugs with which the patient has not been treated previously and that are not cross-resistant with antiretroviral agents with which the patient has been treated previously.
6. Each of the antiretroviral drugs used in combination therapy regimens always should be used according to optimal schedules and dosages.
7. The available effective antiretroviral drugs are limited in number and mechanism of action, and cross-resistance between specific drugs has been documented. Therefore, any change in antiretroviral therapy increases future therapeutic constraints.
8. Women should receive optimal antiretroviral therapy regardless of pregnancy status.
9. The same principles of antiretroviral therapy apply to both HIV-infected children and adults, although treatment of HIV-infected children involves unique pharmacologic, virologic, and immunologic considerations.
10. Persons with acute primary HIV infections should be treated with combination antiretroviral therapy to suppress virus

replication to levels below the limit of detection of sensitive plasma HIV RNA assays.

11. HIV-infected persons, even those with viral loads below detectable limits, should be considered infectious and should be counseled to avoid sexual and drug-use behaviors that are associated with transmission or acquisition of HIV and other infectious pathogens.

CLINICAL CONTROVERSY

Treatment of persons with acute primary HIV infection with combination antiretroviral therapy to suppress virus replication to levels below the limit of detection of sensitive plasma HIV RNA assays is controversial. Well-designed trials with clinical end points that define the long-term safety and efficacy of initiating combination antiretroviral therapy during acute HIV infection are lacking. Theoretical benefits are decreasing the severity of acute disease; perhaps lowering the initial viral load setpoint, which affects progression rates; preserving immune function; and reducing the risk for viral transmission. However, these potential benefits must be weighed against the issues imposed by early intervention of chronic therapy, which would be many years ahead of normal initiation of therapy (discussed below).

The extent to which these 11 principles will stand the test of time is unknown; new information on the pathogenesis and treatment of HIV accrues constantly.[27,39] Twenty-two distinct antiretroviral compounds are now approved by the Food and Drug Administration (FDA), and more are certain to come. Healthcare professionals involved in the care of HIV-infected persons must consult the most current literature on the principles and strategies for therapy. An excellent source for information on treatment guidelines, which is regularly updated, is available at *www.AIDSinfo.NIH.gov*. With these caveats, Table 129–4 presents the state of the art for treatment of HIV-infected individuals as of January 2007.[27] Treatment is recommended for all HIV-infected persons with a history of an AIDS-defining event, symptomatic disease, or a CD4 lymphocyte count below 200 cells/mm^3. Asymptomatic patients with CD4 counts between 201 and 350 cells/mm^3 should be offered therapy. In persons with CD4 counts above 350 cells/mm^3, therapy is generally not recommended, although some clinicians initiate treatment when the HIV RNA count is >100,000 copies/mL.

CLINICAL CONTROVERSY

The precise time to start therapy is controversial. Early in the ART era, the mantra was "hit early and hit hard," with hopes that the drugs would be well tolerated and the virus could be eradicated. When it became clear that treatment was long term and that the drugs had potential long-term side effects, the mantra changed to a drug-sparing paradigm where therapy was initiated as late as possible. The benefits of early therapy include preventing the known detriments of unchecked viral replication, including irreversible immune damage and increased likelihood of viral transmission. The potential risks of initiating combination antiretroviral therapy include the lifestyle demands of continuous therapy, drug toxicities, and development of antiretroviral drug resistance.

■ PHARMACOLOGIC THERAPY

Conceptually the four primary methods of therapeutic intervention against HIV are inhibition of viral replication, virucides to prevent HIV infection, vaccination to stimulate a more effective immune response, and restoration of the immune system with immunomodulators; the latter three approaches are mostly investigational. Several approaches for an HIV vaccine are in development, including whole killed virus, subunit and peptide vaccination, recombinant live vector, and naked DNA delivery. Although clinical studies of vaccines have been performed, at this time a viable vaccine is not within reach. Genetic variability in HIV and a nascent understanding of the role of the immune system in suppressing viral replication are significant barriers to the development of an effective HIV vaccine with long-lasting and protective immunity.[40] Immunomodulators, such as interleukin-2 (aldesleukin), provide mild benefits in terms of increased CD4 cells, however, interleukin-2 is also associated with significant toxicities.[41] Virucides for use vaginally or rectally to prevent sexual transmission of HIV are in early development.[5]

Antiretroviral Agents

Inhibiting viral replication with combinations of potent antiretroviral agents has been the most clinically successful strategy. Three primary groups of drugs are used today: entry inhibition, reverse transcriptase inhibitors, and PIs (Table 129–5).[27] Reverse transcriptase inhibitors consist of two classes: those that are chemical derivatives of purine- and pyrimidine-based nucleosides and nucleotides (nucleoside/nucleotide reverse transcriptase inhibitors [NtRTIs]) and those that are not (nonnucleoside reverse transcriptase inhibitors [NNRTIs]). NtRTIs include the thymidine analogs stavudine (d4T) and zidovudine (AZT or ZDV); the cytosine analogs emtricitabine (FTC), lamivudine (3TC), and zalcitabine (ddC); the guanosine analog abacavir sulfate (ABC); and the adenosine analogs inosine derivative didanosine (ddI) and tenofovir disoproxil fumarate (TDF or PMPA,) an adenosine-derived nucleotide analog (nucleotide is a nucleoside with one or more phosphates). Note that drug abbreviations are provided here and below for reference, but their use is discouraged because they may lead to prescribing or administration errors. As a class, the NtRTIs require phosphorylation to the 5′-triphosphate moiety to be active.[42] Intracellular phosphorylation occurs by cytoplasmic or mitochondrial kinases and phosphotransferases (not viral kinases). Following prodrug activation, the 5′-triphosphate moiety acts in two ways: (a) it competes with endogenous deoxynucleotides for the catalytic site of reverse transcriptase, and (b) it prematurely terminates DNA elongation owing to the modified 3′-hydroxyl group. Although nucleoside reverse transcriptase inhibitor (NRTI) triphosphates are specific for HIV reverse transcriptase, their adverse effects may be caused in part by inhibition of human DNA polymerases, particularly mitochondrial DNA polymerase γ.[42] Toxicities include peripheral neuropathy, pancreatitis, lipoatrophy (subcutaneous fat loss), myopathy, anemia, and rarely life-threatening lactic acidosis with fatty liver.[43] Use of stavudine and zalcitabine has declined in favor of more tolerable NtRTIs (e.g., lamivudine and tenofovir); in fact, zalcitabine is no longer manufactured.[27] With some exceptions, NtRTIs are mainly eliminated by the kidney. Resistance has been reported for all NtRTIs, including cross-resistance within the class as multiple and/or specific mutations accrue.[44]

NNRTIs are a chemically heterogeneous group of agents that bind noncompetitively to reverse transcriptase adjacent to the catalytic site. Unlike NRTIs, NNRTIs do not require intracellular activation, do not compete against endogenous deoxynucleotides, and do not have strong antiviral activity against HIV-2. Given the different site of binding to reverse transcriptase, NNRTIs can be used with NtRTIs effectively. Available NNRTIs include efavirenz (EFV), delavirdine (DLV), and nevirapine (NVP).[27] As a class, the NNRTIs are generally associated with rash and elevated liver function tests, including life-threatening cases rarely, particularly for nevirapine.[43] NNRTIs are mainly cleared by liver and/or gut-mediated metabolism (cytochrome P450 [CYP] 2B6 and 3A). The NNRTIs are unique in that a

TABLE 129-4 Treatment of Human Immunodeficiency Virus Infection: Antiretroviral Regimens Recommended in Antiretroviral-Naïve Persons

	Agents	Limitation
Nonnucleoside reverse transcriptase inhibitor (NNRTI) for combination with dual NRTIs (strength of recommendation in parentheses)		
Preferred	Efavirenz (AII)	Efavirenz is not recommended in pregnant women or in women without adequate contraception
Alternative	Nevirapine (BII)	Nevirapine should not be initiated in women with CD4⁺ T-cell count >250 cells/μL or in men with CD4⁺ T-cell count >400 cells/μL because of increased risk of symptomatic hepatic events in these patients
Protease inhibitor (PI)–based regimens		
Preferred	Atazanavir + ritonavir (AIII)	Drug interaction with proton pump inhibitors, unconjugated hyperbilirubinemia
	or	
	Fosamprenavir + ritonavir (twice daily) (AII)	Twice daily dosing, lipids
	or	
	Lopinavir/ritonavir (twice daily) (coformulated) (AII)	Twice-daily dosing, lipids
Alternatives	Atazanavir (BII)	See above (ritonavir recommended when given with tenofovir)
	o	
	Fosamprenavir (BII)	
	o	
	Fosamprenavir + ritonavir (once daily) (BII)	Fewer head-to-head data with once-daily fosamprenavir–ritonavir and lopinavir–ritonavir, as well as saquinavir (Invirase) + ritonavir
	or	
	Lopinavir/ritonavir (once daily) (coformulated) (BII)	
	or	
	Saquinavir (Invirase) + ritonavir (CII)	
Dual nucleoside (nucleotide) reverse transcriptase inhibitor (NtRTI) backbones		
Preferred	Lamivudine[a] *plus* zidovudine (coformulated) (AII)	Twice daily, nausea and anemia with zidovudine
	or	
	Tenofovir *plus* emtricitabine[a] (coformulated) (AII)	Potential tenofovir nephrotoxicity in susceptible patients
Alternative	Abacavir *plus* lamivudine[a] (coformulated) (BII)	Abacavir hypersensitivity in ~5% of patients
	o	
	Didanosine plus lamivudine[a] (BII)	Didanosine-associated pancreatitis and peripheral neuropathy
Triple nucleoside (nucleotide) reverse transcriptase inhibitor (NtRTI) regimens		
(Only as an alternative to NNRTI- or PI-based regimens when these cannot be used as preferred therapy)		
Alternative	Abacavir *plus* lamivudine *plus* zidovudine (CII)	See above

NRTI, nucleoside reverse transcriptase inhibitor.
Evidence-Based Rating Definition
Rating Strength of Recommendation:
A, Both strong evidence for efficacy and substantial clinical benefit support recommendation for use; should always be offered.
B, Moderate evidence for efficacy or strong evidence for efficacy but only limited clinical benefit, supports recommendation for use; should usually be offered.
C, Evidence for efficacy is insufficient to support a recommendation for or against use, or evidence for efficacy might not outweigh adverse consequences (e.g., drug toxicity, drug interactions) or cost of treatment under consideration; use is optional.
D, Moderate evidence for lack of efficacy or for adverse outcome supports recommendation against use; should usually not be offered.
E, Good evidence for lack of efficacy or for adverse outcome supports a recommendation against use; should never be offered.
Rating Quality of Evidence Supporting the Recommendation:
I, Evidence from at least one correctly randomized, controlled trial.
II, Evidence from at least one well-designed clinical trial without randomization and with laboratory results, from cohort or case-controlled analytic studies (preferably from more than one center), or from multiple time-series studies, or dramatic results from uncontrolled experiments.
III, Evidence from opinions of respected authorities based on clinical experience, descriptive studies, or reports of consulting committees.
[a]Lamivudine and emtricitabine are considered interchangeable.
From Department of Health and Human Services (DHHS) Panel on Antiretroviral Guidelines for Adults and Adolescents. Guidelines for the use of antiretroviral agents in HIV-infected adults and adolescents. October 10, 2006, http://AIDSinfo.NIH.gov.

single mutation is needed to confer high-level cross-resistance for the class, which has been termed a *low-genetic barrier* to resistance.[44]

The PIs include amprenavir (APV) and its prodrug fosamprenavir (FPV), atazanavir (ATV), darunavir (DRV), indinavir (IDV), lopinavir (LPV), nelfinavir (NFV), ritonavir (RTV), saquinavir (SQV), and tipranavir (TPV). PIs competitively inhibit the cleavage of the gag-pol polyprotein, which is a crucial step in the viral maturation process, thereby resulting in the production of immature, noninfectious virions. PIs are generally associated with gastrointestinal distress and metabolic changes, such as increased lipids, insulin insensitivity, and changes in body fat distribution.[43] PIs are cleared by liver and/or gut-mediated metabolism (mainly CYP3A). Resistance to the PIs generally requires the buildup of multiple mutations, termed a *high-genetic barrier*. Multiple mutations can lead to cross-resistance.[44]

Enfuvirtide (ENF, T-20, or pentafuside) is the only fusion inhibitor available at this time. Enfuvirtide is a synthetic 36-amino-acid peptide that binds gp41, which inhibits fusion of HIV with the target cell. Because of the peptide nature of enfuvirtide, oral delivery is impossible, and subcutaneous injection is the preferred route of administration.[45] Injection-site reactions are the most common adverse effect. Enfuvirtide is cleared via protein catabolism and amino acid recycling. Similar to NNRTIs, enfuvirtide appears to have a low genetic barrier to resistance.[46]

Many novel antiviral agents in the classes listed above and novel agents in new drug classes that exploit other steps in the HIV life cycle (see Fig. 129–1) are in development, with a focus on activity against drug-resistant virus.[47] For instance, chemokine receptor antagonists (CCR5 and CXCR4 inhibitors) that abort the viral entry step are being developed. Optimal use of these drugs may require a viral tropism test to determine whether CCR5 or CXCR4 is the predominant strain. Integrase inhibition is another important strategy in development, and promising new agents are under study. Drugs that block steps in the maturation or assembly of HIV other than protease cleavage are viable antiviral candidates. Several of these new antiretroviral compounds currently are available by expanded access. Multiple new antiretrovirals, including new drug classes, will reach the market in the next several years.

TABLE 129-5 Pharmacologic Characteristics of Antiretroviral Compounds

Drug	F (%)	$t_{1/2}$ (h)[a]	Adult Dose[b] (doses/day)	Plasma C_{max}/C_{min} (μM)	Distinguishing Adverse Effect
Nucleoside (Nucleotide) reverse transcriptase inhibitors (NtRTIs)					
Abacavir	83	1.5/20	300 mg (2)	5.2/0.03	Hypersensitivity
			or		
			600 mg (1)	7.4[c]	
Didanosine	42	1.4/24	200 mg (2)	2.8/0.03	Peripheral neuropathy, pancreatitis
			or		
			400 mg (1)	5.6[c]	
Emtricitabine	93	10/39	200 mg (1)	7.3/0.04	Pigmentation on soles and palms in non-whites
Lamivudine	86	5/22	150 mg (2)	6.3/1.6	Headache, pancreatitis (children)
			or		
			300 mg (1)	10.5/0.5	
Stavudine	86	1.4/7	40 mg (2)	2.4/0.04	Lipoatrophy, peripheral neuropathy
Tenofovir	40	17/60	300 mg (1)	1.04/0.4	Renal toxicity (proximal tubule)
Zalcitabine	85	2/3.5	0.75 mg (3)	0.05/0.001	Oral ulcers, peripheral neuropathy
Zidovudine	64	1.1/7	200 mg (3)	2/0.2	Anemia, neutropenia,myopathy
			or		
			300 mg (2)	3[c]	
Nonnucleoside reverse transcriptase inhibitors (NNRTIs)					
Delavirdine	85	5.8	400 mg (3)	35/14	Rash, elevated liver function tests
			or		
			600 mg (2)		
Efavirenz	43	48	600 mg (1)	12.9/5.6	Central nervous system disturbances and teratogenicity
Nevirapine	93	25	200 mg (2)[d]	22/14	Potentially serious rash and hepatotoxicity
Protease inhibitors (PIs)					
Amprenavir[e]	?	9	1400 mg (2)[e]	9.5/0.7	Rash
or			*or*		
Forsamprenavir[e]			1400 mg (1)[e,f]	14.3/2.9	
Atazanavir	68	7	400 mg (1)	3.3/0.23	Unconjugated hyperbilirubinemia
			or		
			300 mg (1)[f]	6.2/0.9	
Darunavir	82	15	600 mg (2)[f]	11.9/6.5	Hyperlipidemia, rash
Indinavir	60	1.5	800 mg (3)	13/0.25	Nephrolithiasis
			or		
			400–800 mg (2)[f]		
Lopinavir[g]	?	5.5	400 mg (2)	13.6/7.5	Hyperlipidemia
Nelfinavir	?	2.6	750 mg (3)	5.3/1.76	Diarrhea
			or		
			1250 mg (2)	7/1.2	
Ritonavir	60	3–5	600 mg (2)[d]	16/5	Gastrointestinal intolerance
			o		
			"Boosting doses"		
Saquinavir	4	3	1,000 mg (2)[f]	3.9/0.55	Mild nausea, bloating
Tipranavir	?	6	500 mg (2)[f]	77.6/35.6	Hepatoxocity, intracranial hemorrhage
Entry inhibitors					
Enfuvirtide	84	3.8	90 mg (2)	1.1/0.73	Injection-site reactions

C_{max}, maximum plasma concentration; C_{min}, minimum plasma concentration; F, bioavailability; $t_{1/2}$, elimination half-life.
[a]NtRTIs: Plasma NtRTI $t_{1/2}$/intracellular (peripheral blood mononuclear cells) NtRTI-triphosphate $t_{1/2}$; plasma $t_{1/2}$ only for other classes.
[b]Dose adjustment may be required for weight, renal or hepatic disease, and drug interactions.
[c]C_{min} concentration typically below the limit of quantification.
[d]Initial dose escalation recommended to minimize side effects.
[e]Fosamprenavir is a tablet phosphate prodrug of amprenavir. Amprenavir is available only as oral solution.
[f]Must be boosted with low doses of ritonavir (100–200 mg).
[g]Available as coformulation 4:1 lopinavir to ritonavir.
Data from Panel on Clinical Practices for the Treatment of HIV Infection,[27] Anderson et al.,[42] and product information for agents.

Interestingly, the antimalarials chloroquine and hydroxychloroquine exert anti–HIV-1 and anti–HIV-2 activity through interference with gp120 (HIV envelope glycoprotein) during assembly.[48] Foscarnet, an anticytomegalovirus pyrophosphate analog, exhibits modest anti-HIV activity via inhibition of HIV reverse transcriptase.[49]

Drug Interactions

❼ Medical use of antiretroviral agents is complicated by clinically significant drug–drug interactions that can occur with many of these agents.[27] Some interactions are beneficial and used purposely; others may be harmful, leading to dangerously elevated or inadequate drug concentrations. Clinicians involved in the pharmacotherapy of HIV must understand the mechanistic basis for these interactions and maintain a current knowledge of drug interactions for these reasons.

Many clinically significant antiretroviral-associated drug interactions involve CYP3A (3A4 and 3A5)-mediated metabolism and clearance. The PIs, except nelfinavir, and the NNRTI delavirdine are avidly metabolized by CYP3A. In general, efavirenz and nevirapine are inducers of CYP3A, whereas delavirdine and the PIs inhibit CYP3A. Ritonavir is a potent inhibitor of CYP3A-mediated metabolism and is now used almost exclusively at lower doses as a pharmacokinetic enhancer of other PIs.[50] Darunavir, lopinavir, saquinavir hard-gel formulation, and tipranavir must be taken with ritonavir to achieve optimal plasma concentrations. Atazanavir, fosamprenavir, and indinavir are also primarily used with ritonavir for the same reason. Nelfinavir is not effectively boosted by ritonavir given CYP2C19-mediated metabolism. Many potential concomitant drugs on the market are also metabolized by CYP3A and therefore susceptible to clinically relevant drug interactions with PIs and NNRTIs.[27] Agents with narrow therapeutic indices and/or that exhibit major changes in pharmacokinetics with CYP3A inhibition are most important in this regard. Examples include, but are not limited to, simvastatin, lovastatin, ergot derivatives, and some antiarrhythmics. The drug interaction potential of antimycobacterium agents, specifically the rifamycins, are particularly relevant given the high potential for such infections in HIV patients.[51] Rifampin, a potent inducer of CYP3A metabolism, is contraindicated with use of most PIs because PI concentrations are reduced substantially even with ritonavir enhancement. However, ritonavir enhancement generally allows coadministration of PIs and rifabutin. In such cases, the rifabutin dose will require adjustment given its CYP3A-mediated clearance.

The herbal product St. John's wort (*Hypericum perforatum*) is a potent inducer of metabolism and is contraindicated with PIs and NNRTIs. It must be stressed that the pharmacology of CYP3A interactions may be complicated by simultaneous induction/inhibition of drug transporter-mediated (e.g., P-glycoprotein) clearance and or other phase I or phase II enzymes. Thus, it is clear that clinicians who treat HIV must stay abreast of antiretroviral drug interaction data. The Department of Health and Human Services guidelines for antiretroviral use provide, and regularly update, excellent summaries of known clinically relevant drug interactions.[27]

NtRTIs are not metabolized by CYP3A, but other drug interaction considerations are important. Generally, NtRTIs of the same nucleobase should not be coadministered. For example, zidovudine and stavudine both are thymidine analogs and are phosphorylated by the same cellular enzymes. Antagonism occurs between these two drugs both in vitro and in vivo; thus, the two should never be given together.[52] Similarly, cytosine analogs should not be coadministered. The adenosine analogs didanosine and tenofovir exhibit a plasma drug interaction whereby didanosine concentrations are significantly increased. Furthermore, the two adenosine analogs are less effective together compared with other recommended NRTI regimens and there is concern for CD4 lymphotoxicity, a toxicity that appears unique to this combination.[53,54] Coadministration of didanosine and tenofovir is not recommended.

Landmarks in the Evolution of Antiretroviral Therapy

Antiretroviral therapy has undergone major changes over the past 20 years. Illustrating these changes is important for a thorough understanding of current treatment strategies. The fundamental landmarks in the use of antiretroviral agents are as follows:

- An early study demonstrated that zidovudine monotherapy confers a survival benefit in persons who have AIDS.[55] This study showed that a single drug provided moderate clinical benefit.
- Further investigation showed that combination regimens of two NtRTIs (e.g., zidovudine and didanosine or zalcitabine) are superior to zidovudine monotherapy in immunologic and virologic parameters, particularly in patients with no previous antiretroviral therapy, and confer a superior survival benefit [AIDS Clinical Trials Group (ACTG) 175].[56] This study established that monotherapy was inferior to dual therapy.
- Use of triple therapy with combinations of two NtRTIs with NNRTIs or PIs has been associated with a reduced incidence of OIs and improved survival.[4] A pivotal study established that dual therapy was inferior to triple therapy.[4]
- Evolution of triple-therapy regimens showed superior virologic efficacy of pharmacokinetically enhanced PIs and efavirenz versus single PIs and triple NtRTI regimens.[57,58] Two studies demonstrated that certain three-drug regimens provided better virologic efficacy than other three-drug regimens.[57,58]

❻ Taken together, the pivotal studies described established that HIV should not be treated with single or dual NtRTIs. Current recommendations for initial treatment of HIV infection advocate a minimum of three active antiretroviral agents: two NtRTIs and either a ritonavir-boosted PI or NNRTI. [27,39] The dual NtRTI backbone should include tenofovir plus emtricitabine (coformulated as Truvada) or zidovudine plus lamivudine (coformulated as Combivir). Abacavir plus lamivudine (coformulated as Epzicom) is an alternative. Recommended initial PIs include atazanavir–ritonavir, lopinavir–ritonavir, or fosamprenavir–ritonavir. Efavirenz is the recommended NNRTI except for women who plan to become pregnant or who not have adequate contraception, owing to potential teratogenicity. Atripla is a once-daily coformulation of efavirenz–tenofovir–emtricitabine. The antiretroviral regimens are listed in Table 129–4. Several factors contribute to whether the patient will mount a durable response to initial therapy, including adherence, pharmacologic effectiveness, and tolerability. Furthermore, variability in the potential for failure of the initial drugs to limit the effectiveness of subsequent drugs gives importance to the sequencing of regimens.

The simplest definition of adherence is the patient's ability to take medication as directed. Antiretroviral therapy is complex and long term, and the risk for virologic failure increases as adherence decreases. Patients with greater than 95% adherence on a PI regimen had better virologic and immunologic outcomes and a lower hospitalization rate than those with adherence levels even slightly below this threshold.[59] As clinicians, it is critical to establish a relationship of trust with the patient and to communicate to the patient the importance of proper medication taking. Education should be aimed at understanding the disease process, monitoring, and goals of therapy. An individual's "readiness" to take medications should be clearly established before any treatment is initiated.[27,39] Caregivers, friends, and/or family members should be included in this process because social and psychological support are among the most important factors that influence adherence in this patient population. A special adherence section is included in the latest guidelines for antiretroviral therapy.[60]

Several large, randomized, comparative (head-to-head) trials are providing insights into differences in efficacy among antiretroviral combinations. A double-blind, placebo-controlled trial of 637 antiretroviral-naive patients randomized to lopinavir–ritonavir 400/100 mg twice daily or nelfinavir 750 mg three times daily (both with 40 mg stavudine and 150 mg lamivudine twice daily). After 48 weeks, 75% of patients treated with lopinavir–ritonavir achieved viral loads less than 400 copies/mL versus 63% of nelfinavir-treated patients.[58] The mean increases in CD4 cell counts were similar for both agents: 195 cells/mm^3 with nelfinavir and 207 cells/mm^3 with lopinavir–ritonavir. Tolerability was similar between the two agents. This study demonstrated the virologic superiority of a ritonavir-enhanced PI-based regimen (specifically, lopinavir–ritonavir) compared with a single PI regimen. In another randomized, double-blinded, multicenter clinical trial, 1,147 antiretroviral naive patients were randomized to a triple NRTI regimen (abacavir–lamivudine–zidovudine) versus an NNRTI-based regimen (efavirenz–lamivudine–zidovudine) or a NNRTI plus triple NRTI regimen (efavirenz–abacavir–lamivudine–zidovudine).[57] The virologic response rate and safety between the two efavirenz-based arms after 3 years of followup were not significantly different. However, an interim analysis showed that the triple NRTI regimen was virologically inferior to the pooled efavirenz-based arms. After a median of 32 weeks of therapy, 21% of subjects randomized to triple NtRTIs experienced virologic failure (two successive HIV RNA >200 copies/mL after 16 weeks) versus only 11% of subjects randomized to either of the two efavirenz-based arms. This trial solidified the standing of efavirenz plus two NRTIs as a preferred initial therapy and indicated that the addition of another NRTI (abacavir) did not improve upon response.

A large randomized clinical trial (n = 878) demonstrated the noninferiority of twice-daily fosamprenavir–ritonavir compared with lopinavir–ritonavir, both with an NRTI backbone of once-daily abacavir–lamivudine over 48 weeks.[61] Another randomized clinical trial (n = 810) found that unboosted atazanavir was noninferior to efavirenz with a zidovudine–lamivudine backbone after 48 weeks.[62] Nevertheless, many clinicians and treatment guidelines recommend ritonavir-boosted atazanavir because it provides pharmacokinetic security in cases of potential drug interactions, such as between atazanavir and histamine$_2$-blockers or tenofovir.[27,39] Finally, an overview of 53 clinical trials of 14,264 patients provided additional support for the current recommendations for initial therapy. Regimens that included an NNRTI (mostly efavirenz) or ritonavir-boosted PI outperformed regimens with a single PI or triple NRTIs in terms of virologic response.[63]

An interesting observation from several ritonavir-boosted PI clinical trials is that PI resistance is unexpectedly rare in patients who experience virologic failure during their initial ritonavir-boosted PI regimen.[58,61] This is in contrast to virologic failure of regimens with single PIs. The mechanism for this phenomenon is not well understood.

Trials that compare dual NRTI backbones also offer insights into subtle differences in efficacy and safety. An open-labeled trial of 517 antiretroviral naïve patients randomized to tenofovir–emtricitabine versus zidovudine–lamivudine both with efavirenz demonstrated that significantly more patients in the tenofovir–emtricitabine arm achieved less than 400 copies/mL at 48 weeks (84%) compared with patients randomized to zidovudine–lamivudine (73%).[64] Part of this difference was attributed to more patients discontinuing zidovudine–lamivudine due to adverse events compared with tenofovir–emtricitabine. Nevertheless, many clinical trials and more than a decade of clinical experience support the overall safety and efficacy of zidovudine–lamivudine.[27] The dual NRTI backbone of stavudine–didanosine is associated with more frequent serious mitochondrial-associated adverse events, such as lipoatrophy, peripheral neuropathy, pancreatitis, and lactic acidemia with fatty liver compared with zidovudine–lamivudine.[65] Generally, stavudine, didanosine, and zalcitabine (termed the "d" drugs ddI, d4T, and ddC) are associated with high incidences of these toxicities and thus are not recommended as first-line therapy and particularly not in combination.[27]

Use of triple NRTIs is not advocated, except in unusual circumstances, such as to avoiding drug–drug interactions with concomitant rifamycins during HIV–tuberculosis coinfections. In such cases, zidovudine–lamivudine–abacavir is advocated, as this regimen has been studied most extensively. As mentioned earlier, abacavir–lamivudine–zidovudine was virologically inferior to efavirenz-based regimens; however, 61% of subjects randomized to triple NRTIs had less than 50 copies/mL at 48 weeks (compared with 83% of those randomized to an efavirenz-based arm).[57] Thus, abacavir–lamivudine–zidovudine provided considerable virologic potency, albeit less than efavirenz-based regimens in this study. Triple NRTI regimens of tenofovir–lamivudine and either abacavir or didanosine have exhibited unexpected and unacceptably poor virologic efficacy and rapid development of resistance in several clinical studies.[66,67] These latter regimens are not recommended.

The durability and sequencing of the regimen are important. Since the advent of ART, patients have been living longer with improved quality of life. As a consequence, patients will have to rely on their treatment for years to come, not months. Data on the long-term (>5 years) durability of ART are scarce. One randomized clinical trial tested sequencing various combinations of efavirenz and/or nelfinavir with zidovudine–lamivudine or stavudine–didanosine using a factorial design.[65] The primary end point was the time to virologic failure of the second three-drug regimen. The regimen of zidovudine–lamivudine–efavirenz was associated with the longest time to virologic failure of the second regimen and was deemed the best initial regimen in this study. Unfortunately, multitudes of sequencing combinations are possible, and few data support other sequencing strategies.

Resistance

❽ Regimen failure is commonly associated with antiretroviral resistance, and testing for such resistance is a useful clinical tool.[44] The two types of resistance tests are phenotype and genotype. A phenotype test determines the concentration of antiretroviral necessary to inhibit 50% replication of the patient's viral isolate (inhibitory concentration of 50% [IC_{50}]) in a recombinant in vitro viral assay. Results usually are expressed as a fold change in susceptibility (IC_{50}) compared with a wild-type laboratory strain virus. Although an increase in the fold change suggests reduced susceptibility to that antiretroviral agent, resistance is never absolute, and partial susceptibility may remain. Theoretically, drug levels may be increased to overcome reduced susceptibility; this strategy is currently under evaluation. Genotyping assesses genetic mutations and associated codon changes in gp41, reverse transcriptase, or protease in the patient's virus and compares it to the wild-type sequence. Mutations, when present, are listed by the wild-type amino acid followed by the position in the genetic sequence of the protein or enzyme and end with the mutation found in the patient. For example, a common mutation caused by lamivudine and emtricitabine is the M184V mutation: a substitution of valine (V) for methionine (M) at the 184 position of reverse transcriptase. New genetic mutations are discovered occasionally and interpretation of genotypes is complex, so the reader is encouraged to consult the most recent guidelines on HIV resistance testing.[44]

As with any medication, adverse effects occur with antiretroviral agents that may limit the patient's ability to tolerate medication. A detailed discussion on the specific presentation and management of these adverse effects is beyond the scope of this chapter but can be found elsewhere.[27,39,42,43]

TREATMENT

Treatment of Special Populations

■ PREGNANCY

Several considerations are relevant to the treatment of pregnant women, including the health of the mother, prevention of HIV transmission to the fetus, potential for teratogenicity, and dosing issues based on pharmacokinetic changes during pregnancy. Treatment recommendations have been made and should be consulted to address the specific requirements for HIV-infected pregnant women and the prevention of vertical transmission.[14] Generally, pregnant women should be treated as would nonpregnant women, with some exceptions. For example, efavirenz should not be used, particularly in the first trimester, because of potential teratogenicity. In terms of prevention of HIV transmission, ACTG protocol 076 is a landmark study that underpins current treatment recommendations for pregnancy.[68] This trial randomized 477 HIV-infected pregnant women (14–34 weeks' gestation) to either zidovudine or placebo. The zidovudine regimen consisted of antepartum zidovudine (100 mg five times daily) plus a continuous infusion of zidovudine during labor (2 mg/kg intravenously over 1 hour followed by 1 mg/kg/h), and zidovudine for the newborn (2 mg/kg orally every 6 hours for 6 weeks). The HIV transmission rate was 25.5% among those who received placebo but was 8.3% when the mothers and their babies received zidovudine.[68] Adverse reactions associated with zidovudine therapy in the study were minimal: hemoglobin concentrations were significantly lower at birth in infants whose mothers received zidovudine, but this difference disappeared by 12 weeks of age. Although zidovudine exposure in utero appears generally safe over the short term, longer followup studies assessing safety later in life are underway.[69] Zidovudine prophylaxis is generally recommended as part of treatment regimens for pregnant women. Currently, HIV transmission rates have been reduced to approximately 1% for women who are treated with ART and zidovudine prophylaxis.[14]

In resource-poor settings or when HIV infection is detected very close to delivery, an abbreviated course of zidovudine (i.e., given during labor or in the first 48 hours of the baby's life) also can reduce transmission substantially and may be easier for the patient to take. Alternatively, single-dose nevirapine given to the mother during labor and to the baby within 3 days of birth can reduce transmission of HIV; however, the risk of nevirapine resistance in the mother is considerable, occurring in more than 40% of cases.[70] The high risk likely is due to the low genetic barrier to resistance for the drug coupled with the long decay half-life and subsequent prolonged suboptimal concentrations. Resistance from single-dose nevirapine in mothers can be reduced from approximately 60% to 12% with the addition of zidovudine–lamivudine for 4 to 7 days.[71]

■ POSTEXPOSURE PROPHYLAXIS

Protection of healthcare workers from accidental exposure to HIV and in cases of rape or high-risk postcoital and postinjection drug-use episodes are important concerns. The CDC has issued guidelines governing treatment of occupational and other high risk HIV exposures.[10,13] The principles of the guidelines are to grade the exposure risk and treat as soon as possible after high-risk exposures. The makeup of the treatment depends upon the risk. Postexposure prophylaxis with a triple-drug regimen consisting of two NRTIs and a boosted-PI is recommended for percutaneous blood exposure involving significant risk (large-bore needle, visible blood from patients with advanced AIDS). Two NRTIs may be offered to the healthcare worker with lower risk of exposure, such as cases involving small blood exposures to the mucous membrane or broken skin. Treatment is not necessary if the source of exposure is urine or saliva. The optimal duration of treatment is unknown, but at least 4 weeks of therapy is advocated. Treatment ideally should be initiated within 1 to 2 hours of exposure, but treatment is recommended up to 72 hours postexposure. Expert consultation is needed when exposure to drug-resistant virus is suspected or confirmed, but this should not delay initiation of postexposure prophylaxis.

Preexposure prophylaxis is an investigational strategy for reducing HIV transmission.[72] The concept is to prevent HIV infection by treating persons at high risk for HIV exposure with antiretrovirals before they are actually exposed. An example involves chronic tenofovir therapy in at-risk sex workers, which is under study in areas with high HIV prevalence. At this time, this strategy cannot be recommended without safety and efficacy information.

EVALUATION OF THERAPEUTIC OUTCOMES

Two laboratory tests are used to evaluate response to antiretroviral therapy: the plasma HIV RNA and the CD4 count.[27,39] After therapy is initiated, patients are generally monitored at 3-month intervals, although an assessment at 2 to 8 weeks is warranted to document early response. The two main indications for a change in therapy are significant toxicity and treatment failure. Should a single agent be responsible for an intolerable side effect, that agent often can be singly changed out of the regimen, for example, the patient who experiences intolerable central nervous system disturbances during initiation of efavirenz can switch to lopinavir–ritonavir without changing the dual NRTI backbone. Caution must be exercised when drugs in the regimen have overlapping toxicities, which makes changing a single agent problematic. Serious and life-threatening toxicities warrant cessation of the whole regimen before deciding upon a subsequent therapy.

As a general guide, the following events indicate treatment failure and should prompt consideration for changing therapy:

1. Less than 1 $\log_{10}$ reduction in HIV RNA 1 to 4 weeks after initiation of therapy or a failure to achieve less than 400 copies/mL by 24 weeks or less than 50 copies/mL by 48 weeks.
2. After HIV RNA suppression, repeated detection of HIV-RNA.
3. Failure to achieve a rise in CD4 of 25 to 50 cells/mm^3 by 48 weeks.
4. Clinical disease progression, usually the development of a new OI.

THERAPEUTIC FAILURE

❾ Therapeutic failure in HIV therapy may be the result of nonadherence to medication, development of drug resistance, intolerance to one or more medications, adverse drug–drug or drug–food interactions, or pharmacokinetic–pharmacodynamic variability.[27] In cases of therapeutic failure, these potential causes should be investigated and addressed, if possible. Drug resistance testing is recommended while the patient is undergoing the failing regimen or within 4 weeks after stopping the regimen as long as the HIV RNA count is greater than 1,000 copies/mL, which is the threshold for resistance assays. Most clinicians use the genotype assay because it is less expensive and results typically are available sooner compared with the phenotype assay. Resistance results usually require expert interpretation. In general, patients who do not respond to their first regimen should be treated with at least one new class (e.g., if the patient was treated initially with a PI, consider an NNRTI-based regimen). Several recently approved drugs are active against highly resistant HIV. For example, the two newest PIs darunavir and tipranavir and the fusion inhibitor enfuvirtide are active against multidrug-resistant HIV. The guiding principles (numbers 5 and 7) recommend changing to a minimum of two new antiretroviral drugs to which the patient's virus is susceptible. Recent clinical trials with darunavir and tipranavir in highly treatment-experienced patients with multidrug-resistant HIV support these principles. A subanalysis of two randomized clinical trials of highly treatment-experienced patients comparing tipranavir–ritonavir to a comparator–PI–ritonavir (not including darunavir) showed that in patients who were enfuvirtide naïve, 59% of patients who received tipranavir–ritonavir and enfuvirtide (i.e., two new agents) experienced a protocol-defined virologic response at 48 weeks compared with only 22% who received comparator–PI–ritonavir with enfuvirtide (i.e., one new agent).[73] Similarly, a subanalysis of two randomized clinical trials of highly treatment-experienced patients comparing darunavir–ritonavir to comparator–PI–ritonavir showed that approximately 50% of subjects who received darunavir–ritonavir plus at least one other active agent (including enfuvirtide) achieved less than 50 copies/mL versus approximately 15% who did not have at least one other active agent in their regimen.[74] These data demonstrate the efficacy of these two new ritonavir-enhanced PIs for drug-resistant HIV and underscore the need for additional active agents in these regimens.

Other strategies for therapeutic failure, which are investigational at this time, include drug holidays, structured or strategic treatment interruptions, and structured intermittent therapy. The overall premise of these strategies is similar: stop all antiretrovirals and allow the patient time off medication—the drug-sparing paradigm. Reinitiation of therapy is intended to reestablish control of the disease, as wild-type virus is expected to predominate. However, a recent landmark clinical trial tested the hypothesis that episodic antiretroviral therapy guided by the CD4 count, the drug-sparing paradigm, would lower morbidity and mortality, including that associated with drug toxicity compared with continuous therapy.[75] The patients randomized to episodic therapy (drug-sparing) experienced significantly increased risk of opportunistic disease or death from any cause, including drug-related causes. Most morbidity and mortality were consequences of lowering the CD4 count and increasing the viral load, but increased drug-related toxicity also was observed. Thus, this episodic drug-sparing approach did not reduce the risk of adverse events that have been associated with antiretroviral therapy, and drug-sparing approaches are not advocated outside the research setting. Furthermore, it is important to consider the implications of stopping all drugs simultaneously for regimens with drugs having short half-lives (e.g., zidovudine) and drugs having long half-lives (e.g., efavirenz and nevirapine). The result may be functional monotherapy for the drug with a long half-life and the risk of resistance mutations, especially for drugs with low genetic barriers (e.g., NNRTIs).[76] At this time, the optimal time sequence for staggered component discontinuation has not been determined.

CLINICAL CONTROVERSY

There is a compelling theoretical rationale for therapeutic drug monitoring in the experienced patient, but this approach is currently controversial. Drug susceptibility is founded on the premise that increasing drug concentration corresponds with stronger inhibition of replication up to a maximal effectiveness. This principle holds for drug-resistant variants, except higher drug concentrations are needed for the same levels of inhibition. Therefore, drug concentration monitoring could guide dose adjustments needed to attain the higher target drug concentrations required for optimal viral inhibition. Currently, therapeutic drug monitoring is suggested as a consideration for patients with multidrug-resistant HIV as well as in other select clinical situations. However, limitations to therapeutic drug monitoring include the lack of established target concentrations, intrapatient pharmacokinetic variability, lack of randomized clinical trials proving benefit or cost effectiveness, and few analytical laboratories and experts available for interpretation. Most antiretrovirals are not suitably formulated for minor dose adjustments.

COMPLICATIONS OF HIV INFECTION AND AIDS

❸ In the pre-ART era, the major therapeutic focus was prevention and treatment of opportunistic infections associated with uncontrolled HIV replication and a steady decline in CD4 cells.[3] Uncontrolled HIV is an insidious disease; persons infected often present with OIs, a consequence of the weakened immune system rather than HIV per se. Most OIs are caused by organisms that are common in the environment and often represent the reactivation of quiescent, hidden infections common in the population. The probability of developing specific OIs is closely related to CD4 count thresholds (Fig. 129–2). These CD4 thresholds serve as a basis for initiating primary OI chemoprevention.[77]

❹ In the ART era, the main principle in the management of OIs is treating HIV infection to enable CD4 cell recovery and maintenance above safe levels.[78] Additional important principles regarding management of OIs are as follows:

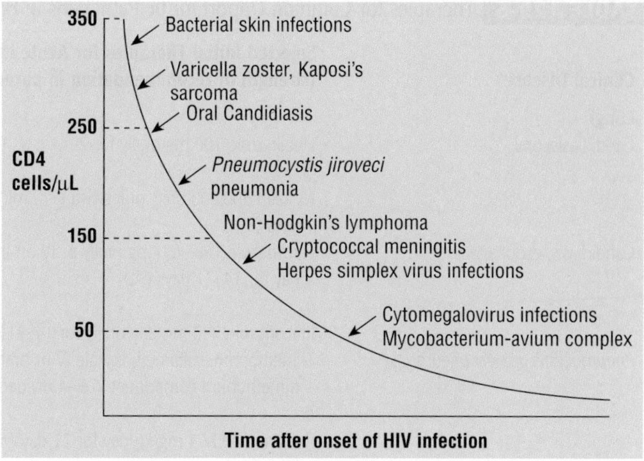

FIGURE 129-2. Natural history of opportunistic infections associated with human immunodeficiency virus infection. *(Reprinted with permission, © Courtney V. Fletcher, 2007.)*

1. Prevent exposure to opportunistic pathogens
2. Vaccinations to prevent first-episode disease (consult HIV-specific guidelines)
3. Primary chemoprophylaxis at certain CD4 thresholds to prevent first-episode disease
4. Treat emergent OI
5. Secondary chemoprophylaxis to prevent disease recurrence
6. Discontinuation of certain prophylaxes with sustained ART-associated immune recovery

Several considerations are required for the patient who presents with an OI and is simultaneously diagnosed with HIV and who thus needs both OI and ART treatment.[78] Immediate initiation of ART is indicated for OIs that respond to CD4 recovery, such as, cryptosporidiosis, progressive multifocal leukoencephalopathy, and Kaposi sarcoma. However, for other OIs such as tuberculosis, *Mycobacterium avium* complex (MAC), and PCP, several potential problems complicate the timing of when to initiate ART relative to OI therapy. First, the numerous possible drug–drug interactions and the complexity of adhering to concomitant regimens can be daunting. Second, potentially overlapping drug toxicities can hand-tie clinicians trying to stop specific drugs thought to be eliciting the toxicity event. Third, an immune reconstitution syndrome (IRIS) has been associated with initiation of ART in the presence of underlying OIs.[79] IRIS is characterized by fever and worsening of OI manifestations in the initial weeks after ART. An ART-associated rapid-onset immune reconstitution against the OI pathogen is thought to be the mechanism of IRIS. Thus, clinicians often will treat the OI first, await a response, then consider ART. However, clinicians must make such decisions on a case-by-case basis.

The three major OIs (PCP, MAC, and cytomegalovirus retinitis) all have decreased substantially in incidence with the advent of ART.[3] Furthermore, primary and secondary chemoprophylaxes for OIs have contributed to the same decreases. Nevertheless, opportunistic diseases continue to be complications of HIV disease and occur at low CD4 lymphocyte counts. For example, the risk of an OI was almost six fold higher in persons receiving ART with a baseline CD4 count less than 50 cells/μL compared with more than 200 cells/μL.[80]

The spectrum of OIs observed in HIV-infected individuals and recommended first-line regimens for treatment are given in Table 129–6. Recommended therapies for primary prophylaxis are given in Table 129–7.[77,78] An exhaustive review of all OIs associated with

TABLE 129-6 Therapies for Common Opportunistic Pathogens in HIV-Infected Individuals

Clinical Disease	Selected Initial Therapies for Acute Infection in Adults (strength of recommendation in parentheses)	Common Drug- or Dose-Limiting Adverse Reactions
Fungi		
Candidiasis, oral	Fluconazole 100 mg orally for 7–14 days (AI)	Elevated liver function tests, hepatotoxicity, nausea and vomiting
	or	
	Nystatin 500,000 units oral swish (~5 mL) four times daily for 7–14 days (BII)	Taste, patient acceptance
Candidiasis, esophageal	Fluconazole 100–400 mg orally or IV on the first day, then 100 mg/day for 14–21 days (AI)	Same as above
	o	
	Itraconazole 200 mg/day orally for 14–21 days (AI)	Elevated liver function tests, hepatotoxicity, nausea and vomiting
Pneumocystis jiroveci pneumonia	Trimethoprim–sulfamethoxazole IV or orally 15–20 mg/kg/day as trimethoprim component in 3–4 divided doses for 21 days[a] (AI)	Skin rash, fever, leucopenia Thrombocytopenia
	or	
	Pentamidine IV 4 mg/kg/day for 21 days[a] (AI)	Azotemia, hypoglycemia, hyperglycemia, arrhythmias
	Mild episodes	
	Atovaquone suspension 750 mg (5 mL) orally twice daily with meals for 21 days[a] (BI)	Rash, elevated liver enzymes, diarrhea
Cryptococcal meningitis	Amphotericin B 0.7 mg/kg/day IV for a minimum of 2 weeks *with* or *without* flucytosine 100 mg/kg/day orally in four divided doses (AI)	Nephrotoxicity, hypokalemia, anemia, fever, chills Bone marrow suppression
	followed by	Elevated liver enzymes
	Fluconazole 400 mg/day, orally for 8 weeks or until CSF cultures are negative (AI)[a]	Same as above
Histoplasmosis	Amphotericin B 0.7 mg/kg/day IV for 3 to 10 days (AI) *followed by* Itraconazole 200 mg twice daily, orally for 12 weeks (AII)[a]	Same as above
Coccidioidomycosis	Amphotericin B 0.5–1 mg/kg/day IV until clinical improvement (usually after 500–1,000 mg) (AII)[a]	Same as above
	or	
	Fluconazole 400–800 mg once daily (meningeal disease) (AII)[a]	Same as above
Protozoa		
Toxoplasmic encephalitis	Pyrimethamine 200 mg orally once, then 50–75 mg/day	Bone marrow suppression
	plus	
	Sulfadiazine 1–1.5 g orally four times daily	Allergy, rash, drug fever
	and	
	Leucovorin 10–20 mg orally daily for 6 weeks (AI)[a]	
Isosporiasis	Trimethoprim and sulfamethoxazole: 160 mg trimethoprim and 800 mg sulfamethoxazole orally or IV four times daily for 10 days (AII)[a]	Same as above
Bacteria		
Mycobacterium avium complex	Clarithromycin 500 mg orally twice daily, *plus* ethambutol 15 mg/kg/day orally (AI), *and*	Gastrointestinal intolerance, optic neuritis, peripheral neuritis
	For advanced disease, rifabutin 300 mg/day (dose may need adjustment with ART) (AI)[a]	Rash, gastrointestinal intolerance Neutropenia, discolored urine, uveitis
Salmonella enterocolitis or bacteremia	Ciprofloxacin 500–750 mg orally twice daily for 14 days (longer duration for bacteremia or advanced HIV) (AIII)	Gastrointestinal intolerance
Campylobacter enterocolitis	Ciprofloxacin 500 mg orally twice daily for 7 days (or 14 days with bacteremia) (BIII)	Same as above
Shigella enterocolitis	Ciprofloxacin 500 mg orally twice daily for 5 days (or 14 days for bacteremia) (AIII)	Same as above
Viruses		
Mucocutaneous herpes simplex	Acyclovir 5 mg/kg IV every 8 hours until lesions regress, then acyclovir 400 mg orally three times daily until complete healing (famciclovir or valacyclovir is alternative) (AII)	Gastrointestinal intolerance, crystalluria
Primary varicella-zoster	Acyclovir 30 mg/kg/day IV in 3 divided doses for 7–10 days, then switch to oral acyclovir 800 mg four times daily after defervescence (famciclovir or valacyclovir is alternative) (AIII)	Obstructive nephropathy, central nervous system symptomatology
Cytomegalovirus (retinitis)	Ganciclovir intraocular implant *plus* valganciclovir 900 mg once daily until immune recovery from ART (AI)[a]	Neutropenia, thrombocytopenia
Cytomegalovirus esophagitis or colitis	Ganciclovir 5 mg/kg IV every 12 hours or foscarnet 180 mg/kg/day in two or three divided doses IV for 21 to 28 days (BII)	Same as above Nephrotoxicity, hypohypercalcemia, hypophosphatemia, anemia

ART, antiretroviral therapy; CSF, cerebrospiral fluid; HIV, human immunodeficiency virus.

[a]Maintenance therapy is recommended.

See Table 129-4 for levels of evidence-based recommendations.

From reference 78.

TABLE 129-7 Therapies for Prophylaxis of First-Episode Opportunistic Diseases in Adults and Adolescents

Pathogen	Indication	First Choice (strength of recommendation in parentheses)
I. Standard of care		
Pneumocystis jiroveci	$CD4^+$ count <200/μL *or* oropharyngeal candidiasis	Trimethoprim–sulfamethoxazole, one double-strength tablet orally once daily (AI) or 1 single-strength tablet orally once daily (AI)
Mycobacterium tuberculosis		
Isoniazid-sensitive	TST reaction ≥5 mm *or* prior positive TST result without treatment *or* contact with case of active tuberculosis	Isoniazid 300 mg orally plus pyridoxine, 50 mg orally once daily for 9 months (AII) *or* Isoniazid 900 mg orally plus pyridoxine 100 mg orally twice weekly for 9 months (BII)
Isoniazid-resistant	Same as isoniazid-sensitive; high probability of exposure to isoniazid-resistant tuberculosis	Rifampin 600 mg orally once daily (AIII) or rifabutin 300 mg orally once daily (BIII) for 4 months
Toxoplasma gondii	Immunoglobulin G antibody to *Toxoplasma* and $CD4^+$ count <100/μL[3]	Trimethoprim–sulfamethoxazole one double-strength tablet orally once daily (AII)
Mycobacterium avium complex	$CD4^+$ count <50/μL[3]	Azithromycin 1,200 mg orally once weekly (AI) or clarithromycin 500 mg orally twice daily (AI)
Varicella zoster virus (VZV)	Significant exposure to chicken pox or shingles for patients who have no history of either condition or, if available, negative antibody to VZV	Varicella-zoster immune globulin, five vials (1.25 mL each) intramuscularly administered ideally within 48 hours of exposure but ≤96 hours (AIII)
II. Usually recommended		
Streptococcus pneumoniae	CD4 count ≥200 cells/μL[3]	23-valent polysaccharide vaccine, 0.5 mL intramuscularly (BII)
Hepatitis B virus	All susceptible (antihepatitis B core antigen negative) patients	Hepatitis B vaccine, three doses (BII)
Influenza virus	All patients (annually, before influenza season)	Inactivated trivalent influenza virus vaccine (annual): 0.5 mL intramuscularly (BII)
Hepatitis A virus	All susceptible (anti–hepatitis A virus–negative) patients at increased risk for hepatitis A infection (e.g., illegal drug users, men who have sex with men, hemophiliacs) or patients with chronic liver disease including chronic hepatitis B or C	Hepatitis A vaccine: two doses (BIII)
III. Indicated for use only in selected circumstances		
Bacteria	Neutropenia	Granulocyte colony-stimulating factor (G-CSF), 5–10 mcg/kg subcutaneously once daily for 2–4 weeks; or granulocyte-macrophage colony-stimulating factor (GM-CSF), 250 mcg/m^2 subcutaneously for 2–4 weeks (CII)
Cryptococcus neoformans	$CD4^+$ count <50/μL[3]	Fluconazole 100–200 mg orally once daily (CI)
Histoplasma capsulatum	$CD4^+$ count < 100/μL[3], endemic geographic area	Itraconazole capsule, 200 mg orally once daily (CI)
Cytomegalovirus	$CD4^+$ count <50/μL[3] and cytomegalovirus antibody positivity	Oral ganciclovir, 1 g orally three times daily (valganciclovir should be used in place of ganciclovir due to better bioavailability) (CI)

TST, tuberculin skin test.
See Table 129-4 for levels of evidence-based recommendations.
From Kaplan et al.[77]

HIV infection is beyond the scope of this chapter. The following discussion of PCP provides an overview of the epidemiology, diagnosis, clinical manifestations, and results of treatment and serves as an illustration for the principles discussed earlier. Readers desiring more specific information, either for the diseases or agents mentioned, can consult additional references.[77,78]

PNEUMOCYSTIS CARINII (PNEUMOCYSTIS JIROVECI) PNEUMONIA

PCP is the most common life-threatening OI in patients with AIDS. *P. jiroveci* was formerly named *P. carinii*; the name change was made to distinguish the organism that infects humans (*P. jiroveci*) from the strain that infects rodents (*P. carinii*). The acronym PCP is still used today. Early in the AIDS epidemic, approximately 60% of patients with AIDS had PCP as their AIDS-defining event, and 80% experienced PCP at some point during their lifetime.[78,81] The advent of ART and effective prophylaxis for PCP have substantially decreased the relative incidence of PCP. However, PCP still occurs in persons unaware of their HIV infection, and breakthrough PCP can occur in those with variable adherence to ART and/or prophylaxis.[78]

P. jiroveci is a fungus that has protozoan characteristics as well.[81] Exposure to *P. jiroveci* is widespread; two thirds of the population has developed serum antibodies by age 2 to 4 years. The organism appears to reside without consequence in humans unless the host becomes immunologically compromised. Disease associated with immunosuppression probably occurs from both new acquisition and reactivation. Ninety percent of PCP cases in AIDS patients occurred in those with CD4 counts less than 200 cells/mm^3. Other risk factors include oral thrush, recurrent bacterial pneumonia, unintentional weight loss, and high plasma HIV RNA. Past episodes of PCP increase risk for future episodes, which provides the basis for secondary chemoprophylaxis, as described below.[77,78]

The presentation of PCP in AIDS often is insidious.[77,78,81] Characteristic symptoms include fever and dyspnea. Clinical signs are tachypnea with or without rales or rhonchi and a nonproductive or mildly productive cough occurring over a period of weeks, although more fulminant presentations can occur. Chest radiographs may show florid or subtle infiltrates but occasionally are normal. Infiltrates usually are interstitial and bilateral, however. Arterial blood gases may show minimal hypoxia (PaO_2 80–95 mm Hg) but in more advanced disease may be markedly abnormal. The diagnosis of PCP usually is made by identification of the organism in induced sputum or in specimens obtained from bronchoalveolar lavage. Less commonly, transbronchial or open lung biopsy is used to locate the organism. Diagnostic PCR tests are in development.

Untreated PCP has a mortality rate of nearly 100%. Several potential treatments are available for PCP, but the treatment of choice is trimethoprim–sulfamethoxazole (or cotrimoxazole), which is associated with a response rate of 60% to 100%.[78] Parenteral pentamidine is equally efficacious but significantly more toxic. Trimethoprim–sulfamethoxazole is also the regimen of choice for primary and secondary prophylaxis of PCP in patients with and without HIV.[77]

When used for treatment of PCP, the dose of trimethoprim–sulfamethoxazole is 15 to 20 mg/kg/day (based on the trimethoprim component) as three to four divided doses.[78] Treatment duration typically is 21 days but also must be based on clinical response. Trimethoprim–sulfamethoxazole usually is initiated by the intravenous route, although oral therapy may suffice in mildly ill and reliable outpatients or for completion of a course of therapy after a response has been achieved with intravenous administration. Patients with moderate to severe PCP should be treated with corticosteroids as soon as possible after starting PCP therapy and certainly within 72 hours, in order to blunt the deterioration seen just after initiation of PCP therapy.[78,81] Furthermore, as mentioned above, if the patient presents with PCP as their HIV diagnosis, IRIS and other complications may arise with early initiation of ART. Some clinicians will complete the PCP therapy before initiating ART.

Adverse reactions to trimethoprim–sulfamethoxazole and pentamidine are common, occurring in 20% to 85% of patients in this setting.[78] The more common adverse reactions seen with trimethoprim–sulfamethoxazole are rash (including Stevens-Johnson syndrome), fever, leukopenia, elevated serum transaminase levels, and thrombocytopenia. The incidence of these adverse reactions is higher in HIV-infected individuals than in those not infected with HIV.[82] Mild rashes should be watched closely for progression to more severe reactions but are not an absolute contraindication to continuing therapy.[78] This highlights the potential problem of overlapping toxicities with antiretrovirals such as abacavir and nevirapine, which also are associated with rash and hypersensitivity, including life-threatening cases. For pentamidine, side effects include hypotension, tachycardia, nausea, vomiting, severe hypoglycemia or hyperglycemia, pancreatitis, irreversible diabetes mellitus, elevated serum transaminase levels, nephrotoxicity, leukopenia, and cardiac arrhythmias. Some of these reactions appear to be related to the infusion rate (e.g., hypotension and tachycardia) and can be minimized by infusing pentamidine over 1 hour or more.[81] The overall incidence of adverse reactions to pentamidine appears to be similar between individuals infected with HIV and those not infected. Dosage modification or pharmacokinetic monitoring can reduce the toxicity of both pentamidine and trimethoprim–sulfamethoxazole.[83] Dose reduction of pentamidine from 4 to 3 mg/kg/day appears to be successful in minimizing further rises in serum creatinine levels.[78,81] Maintenance of serum trimethoprim concentrations between 5 and 8 mcg/mL may help to prevent severe myelosuppression.[83] Early addition of adjunctive corticosteroid therapy to anti-PCP regimens decreases the risk of respiratory failure and improves survival in patients with AIDS and moderate to severe PCP (PaO_2 ≤70 mm Hg or alveolar-arterial gradient ≥35 mm Hg).[78] The adverse effects associated with corticosteroid therapy in these patients were minimal, primarily an increased incidence of herpetic lesions, although some concerns exist about the potential for reactivation of tuberculosis or cytomegalovirus or long-term effects on bones.[81,84]

Prevention of PCP is clearly a preferable treatment strategy. The relative risk of PCP in 1,665 HIV-infected participants who did not have AIDS was 4.9 in those with CD4 lymphocyte counts less than 200 cells/mm^3.[85] Primary prophylaxis is recommended for any HIV-infected person who has a CD4 lymphocyte count less than 200 cells/mm^3 (or CD4 percentage of total lymphocytes <14%) or a history of oropharyngeal candidiasis.[77] Secondary PCP prophylaxis is recommended for all HIV-infected individuals who have had a previous episode of PCP.

Trimethoprim–sulfamethoxazole is the preferred therapy for both primary and secondary prophylaxis of PCP in adults and adolescents.[77] Trimethoprim–sulfamethoxazole is the most effective and least expensive agent for prophylaxis. It also appears to confer cross-protection against toxoplasmosis and many bacterial infections. The recommended dose in adults and adolescents is one double-strength tablet daily, although other regimens, such as one double-strength tablet thrice weekly or one single-strength tablet daily and gradual dose escalation using liquid trimethoprim–sulfamethoxazole, have been used in an attempt to reduce the incidence of adverse reactions and improve compliance. Alternative prophylactic regimens are available if trimethoprim–sulfamethoxazole cannot be tolerated.

In the ART era, the profound reduction in HIV replication and restoration in CD4 cell count to levels rarely associated with the development of OIs provides a basis for the discontinuation of primary and secondary prophylaxis.[77] For PCP, primary prophylaxis should be discontinued in patients receiving and responding to ART who have a CD4 cell count greater than 200 cells/mm^3 sustained for at least 3 months. Primary prophylaxis should be reinstated if the CD4 count drops to less than 200 cells/mm^3. The same criteria apply for both discontinuation and reinitiation of secondary prophylaxis of PCP. However, continued secondary prophylaxis should be considered when the original PCP episode occurred at a CD4 count greater than 200 cells/mm^3.

In summary, comprehensive recommendations are available for management of PCP, which are contained within two thorough sets of guidelines for the overall management of OIs in the context of HIV infection including prevention and treatment.[77,78] Readers are advised that data continue to emerge on new OI therapies, the safety of stopping primary and secondary prophylaxis, as well as criteria for when to restart secondary prophylaxes. The most current guidelines always should be consulted. Similar OI guidelines have been developed that are specific to children.[86]

COMPLICATIONS IN THE ART ERA

⑩ Medical issues have emerged in the ART era as HIV patients live longer and are exposed to antiretrovirals for many years. A recent medical issue of concern is HIV-associated lipodystrophy.[84,87] Components of this syndrome include dyslipidemia (increased triglycerides and low-density lipoproteins [LDLs] and decreased high-density lipoproteins), abnormal glucose homeostasis (insulin resistance and impaired glucose tolerance), bone disorders (osteopenia and osteonecrosis), body fat abnormalities (lipoatrophy of the face and extremities and central lipoaccumulation), and lactic acidosis with hepatosteatosis. These metabolic abnormalities often occur in combination. The cause of these signs and symptoms and the reason for combinations of them are not known. Some abnormalities are associated with the HIV infection itself, such as hypertriglyceridemia, insulin resistance, and osteopenia. However, the same metabolic abnormalities are associated with antiretroviral therapy, and distinguishing the contribution of disease versus drug and ascertaining whether one abnormality precipitates the development of other abnormalities are difficult.[84,87] Various mechanistic hypotheses have been put forward, including effects from immune system dysregulation, NtRTI-induced mitochondrial toxicity, and PI interactions with various cellular processes, such as glucose uptake, adipocyte differentiation, and lipolysis.[88] Generally, NNRTIs (mostly efavirenz), PIs (except atazanavir), and the NtRTIs stavudine and zidovudine are linked with dyslipidemia.[27] PIs and some NtRTIs (e.g., stavudine) are associated with insulin resistance. Body fat changes are associated with PIs and NtRTIs (especially stavudine and, to a lesser extent, zidovudine). A cross-sectional study of 17,852 patients demonstrated that patients treated with either an NNRTI (mostly efavirenz) or PI had several-fold higher incidences of total cholesterol ≥240 mg/dL versus antiretroviral-naive patients. Triglycerides ≥200 mg/dL were significantly more common in all treatment groups (NtRTIs-only, NNRTI-based, and PI-based regimens versus antiretroviral-naive patients), whereas changes in body fat was more common by eight-fold or more in all treatment groups versus antiretroviral-naive patients.[89] Other studies have reported changes in body fat in up to 50% of ART-treated patients.[88]

These metabolic complications create several challenges and concerns. First, the metabolic abnormalities may increase the risk of adverse cardiovascular events, and some evidence gives credence to this concern. A large observational prospective cohort study of 23,468 HIV-infected patients applied the Framingham cardiovascular risk algorithm and compared the estimated cardiovascular event rate with the actual event rate.[90] The algorithm takes into account known risk factors, many of which are associated with ART, such as diabetes and dyslipidemia as well as sex, age, smoking, and blood pressure. The study showed that the estimated event rate paralleled the actual event rate, and both increased with years on ART. This finding suggests that increased cardiovascular risk can be explained by conventional risk factors, which are induced by ART. Therefore, the metabolic abnormalities precipitated by ART and HIV should be treated as cardiovascular disease risk factors and may warrant medical intervention.

A second concern and challenge is how to manage the changes in body fat distribution, which can be disfiguring and upsetting to patients.[84,87] Some strategies have led to a mild return of subcutaneous fat for those with severe peripheral lipoatrophy. Controlled trials of antiretroviral substitution have demonstrated that patients randomized to switch away from stavudine to either abacavir or tenofovir have had small gains in subcutaneous fat.[91] Small controlled studies have demonstrated small but inconsistent gains in subcutaneous fat with thiazolidinedione therapy.[92] Central fat accumulation is difficult to treat. Metformin reduces central fat accumulation, but lean body mass and subcutaneous fat may exhibit unwanted declines.[92] Lifestyle changes, such as reducing calorie intake and increasing aerobic exercise, may reduce central fat. Unfortunately, both lipoatrophy and fat accumulation eventually may lead to reconstructive surgery strategies in severe or refractory cases. Perhaps the best management of body fat changes is prevention through initiation of regimens less likely to cause such changes (see current recommendations for initial therapy).

Another challenge involves ART-associated hyperlipidemia. Antiretroviral substitution studies have shown lipid improvements after switching away from PIs to either NNRTIs or atazanavir, but direct pharmacologic intervention often is required.[92] Elevated LDL may respond to β-hydroxy-β-methylglutaryl-coenzyme A (HMG-CoA) reductase inhibitor (statin) therapy. However, serious concerns exist regarding drug–drug interactions between PIs and statins, including atorvastatin, lovastatin, rosuvastatin, and simvastatin.[27,92] The plasma area under the concentration time curve of these statins can be increased multiple-fold and may increase the risk for rhabdomyolysis. Generally, fluvastatin, pravastatin (except with darunavir–ritonavir), or low-dose atorvastatin is recommended for chemotherapy of ART-associated LDL elevations. HIV-specific guidelines have been developed for treating ART-associated dyslipidemia with recommendations lifestyle modifications, such as use of fibrates, niacin, and fish oil for isolated hypertriglyceridemia.[27] Current guidelines should always be consulted, as new information regarding the special concerns and challenges associated with HIV lipodystrophy continue to accrue.[92]

Another emergent ART-era issue is hepatitis C virus (HCV)–HIV coinfection. HIV–HCV coinfection is common because of the shared blood-borne route of transmission.[93,94] Approximately 30% of HIV-infected patients in the United States have HIV–HCV (approximately 300,000 individuals). Up to 72% of injection-drug users and 85% of hemophiliacs with HIV have HIV–HCV.

Multiple challenges and concerns complicate therapy for HIV–HCV-infected patients. First, HIV worsens the prognosis of HCV by reducing the chance of HCV clearance and accelerating HCV progression. After acute HCV infection, approximately 20% of patients without HIV will clear HCV compared with only 5% to 10% of those who also have HIV.[93,94] With chronic HCV infection, progression to fibrosis and cirrhosis is several-fold faster in HIV–HCV patients versus HCV-monoinfected patients. Whether HCV alters HIV disease is unclear, as the evidence to date is mixed. However, it is clear that end-stage liver disease from HCV has become an important cause of morbidity and death in HIV–HCV-infected patients.[93]

Randomized controlled trials have demonstrated lower response rates to standard-of-care HCV therapy (ribavirin and pegylated interferon-α) in HIV–HCV-infected patients compared with similar studies in HCV-monoinfected patients.[94,95] HIV–HCV patients in these studies had high levels of CD4 cells (average approximately 500 cells/mm^3) and either were taking ART or had stable HIV disease. Sustained virologic responses for HCV were only 27% to 44% overall (14%–29% for HCV genotype I), which compares poorly with response rates in HCV-monoinfected patients (>50% overall and >40% for HCV genotype I).[94,96,97] In HCV monoinfection, non-genotype I can be treated for 24 weeks, whereas HIV–HCV patients may need 48 weeks of treatment for the same genotypes. Generally, HIV-induced immunologic defects may complicate HCV disease and response, but the precise underlying mechanism(s) of this attenuated HCV response in HIV–HCV patients has not been elucidated.

Another challenge in HIV–HCV patients is liver toxicity to ART. Coinfected patients have several-fold higher risk of ART-associated transaminase elevations versus patients infected with HIV but not HCV.[93,94,97] Nevirapine and full-dose ritonavir appear to carry highest risk of transaminitis, whereas stavudine has been linked with steatosis. Ritonavir-boosted PIs generally do not carry the same elevated risk as full-dose ritonavir with the exception of tipranavir, which is associated with risk of clinical hepatitis and hepatic decompensation, especially in those with HCV or hepatitis B infections. Liver function must be monitored with extra vigilance if tipranavir is used in this population.[27] However, with the exception of the specific antiretrovirals noted above, the general threat of major liver toxicity is low, and this concern should not dissuade the use of ART in HIV–HCV-coinfected persons.[97]

Finally, two potentially dangerous drug–drug interactions exist between ART and HCV therapies. Didanosine should not be used with HCV therapy because of increased risk for pancreatitis and/or lactic acidosis.[97] The mechanism for this increase risk is not clear. Ribavirin inhibits inosine 5′-monophosphate dehydrogenase in vitro, which enables higher intracellular levels of dideoxyadenosine triphosphate (the active anabolite of didanosine) and potentially more mitochondrial toxicity.[94,98] However, interferon increases the risk of didanosine-associated pancreatitis.[99] The other potentially dangerous interaction is severe anemia when zidovudine is used with ribavirin and interferon.[94,97] This appears to be a pharmacodynamic interaction, as zidovudine and ribavirin both affect red blood cell integrity and/or output. At this time, zidovudine is not contraindicated with ribavirin and interferon, but close hematologic monitoring is needed, including potential adjunctive erythropoietin.[94,97]

As with the many other special circumstances and considerations that apply in the management of HIV-infected patients discussed in this chapter, specific guidelines have been established for managing HCV in HIV–HCV-coinfected patients, including recommendations for managing ART-associated liver toxicity.[97,100] The most current recommendations should always be consulted, as new knowledge and treatment strategies accrue continuously.

CONCLUSIONS

Irrefutable progress has been made in the management of HIV. Disease progression can be delayed, survival can be prolonged, and the risk of maternal-to-fetal HIV transmission can be reduced substantially. However, a cure and an effective vaccine remain out of reach. Twenty-two distinct antiretroviral agents are available now for clinical use, and additional compounds will follow. There continues to be significant deficits in our understanding of the virologic and immunologic processes associated with HIV infection and the clinical pharmacology of anti-HIV compounds. Particular issues include the ever-present need for simpler and more potent regimens, strategies for drug-resistant viral isolates, and better understanding of the inexorably progressive nature of HIV infection in some patients despite antiretroviral therapy. The medical management of OIs associated with HIV disease has changed dramatically since the recognition of AIDS early in the 1980s and changes continue today. The approach to PCP is illustrative. Chronologic landmarks in the evolution of PCP management include treatment of only established PCP disease to treatment in which primary and secondary prophylaxis based on CD4 lymphocyte count are standards of care, and finally to treatment where prophylaxis should be discontinued with sustained CD4 recovery on ART. Such evolution reflects progress in both understanding the risk factors for OIs and pharmacologic therapy. Collectively, three important general lessons have been learned from the treatment of HIV and associated OIs: need for prospective immunologic and virologic monitoring and early recognition of HIV infection, use of potent combinations of antiretroviral agents to maximally inhibit viral replication and restore immune function, and primary and secondary prophylaxis of OIs. Observance of these principles, coupled with carefully controlled investigations of novel agents and therapeutic strategies, will continue to offer definite benefit and improve the quality of life for HIV-infected individuals and yield an advantage over this pernicious virus that causes AIDS.

ACKNOWLEDGMENTS

Supported by Grants RO1 AI64029, RO3 AI68438, RO1 AI33835, UO1 AI41089, and UO1 AI38858 from the National Institute of Allergy and Infectious Disease.

ABBREVIATIONS

ACTG: AIDS Clinical Trials Group

AIDS: acquired immunodeficiency syndrome

ART: combination antiretroviral therapy

CD: cluster of differentiation

CDC: Centers for Disease Control and Prevention

CYP: cytochrome P450

ELISA: enzyme-linked immunosorbent assay

gp: glycoprotein

HCV: hepatitis C virus

HIV: human immunodeficiency virus

IC_{50}: concentration of antiretroviral agent necessary to inhibit 50% of viral replication

IRIS: immune reconstitution syndrome

LDL: low-density lipoprotein

MAC: *Mycobacterium avium* complex

NNRTI: nonnucleoside reverse transcriptase inhibitor

NtRTI: nucleoside/nucleotide reverse transcriptase inhibitor

OI: opportunistic infection

PCP: *Pneumocystis jiroveci (carinii)* pneumonia

PI: protease inhibitor

RT-PCR: reverse-transcription polymerase chain reaction

SIV: simian immunodeficiency virus

VZV: varicella-zoster virus

REFERENCES

1. Centers for Disease Control and Prevention. Kaposi's sarcoma and Pneumocystis pneumonia among homosexual men: New York and California. MMWR 1981;30:305–308.
2. Gallo R, Salahuddin S, Popovic M, et al. Frequent detection and isolation of cytopathic retroviruses (HTLV-III) from patients with AIDS and at risk for AIDS. Science 1984;224:500–503.
3. Walensky RP, Paltiel AD, Losina E, et al. The survival benefits of AIDS treatment in the United States. J Infect Dis 2006;194:11–19.
4. Palella FJ Jr, Delaney KM, Moorman AC, et al. Declining morbidity and mortality among patients with advanced human immunodeficiency virus infection. N Engl J Med 1998;338:853–860.
5. Simon V, Ho DD, Abdool Karim Q. HIV/AIDS epidemiology, pathogenesis, prevention, and treatment. Lancet 2006;368:489–504.
6. Incorporating HIV prevention into the medical care of persons living with HIV. Recommendations of Centers for Disease Control and Prevention, the Health Resources and Services Administration, the National Institutes of Health, and the HIV Medicine Association of the Infectious Diseases Society of America. MMWR Recomm Rep 2003;52(RR-12):1–24.
7. Comparison of female to male and male to female transmission of HIV in 563 stable couples. European Study Group on Heterosexual Transmission of HIV. BMJ 1992;304:809–813.
8. Auvert B, Taljaard D, Lagarde E, Sobngwi-Tambekou J, Sitta R, Puren A. Randomized, controlled intervention trial of male circumcision for reduction of HIV infection risk: The ANRS 1265 Trial. PLoS Med 2005;2:e298.
9. Centers for Disease Control and Prevention. HIV and Its Transmission. 1999, *http://www.cdc.gov/hiv/resources/factsheets/transmission.htm*.
10. Smith DK, Grohskopf LA, Black RJ, et al. Antiretroviral postexposure prophylaxis after sexual, injection-drug use, or other nonoccupational exposure to HIV in the United States: Recommendations from the U.S. Department of Health and Human Services. MMWR Recomm Rep 2005;54(RR-2):1–20.
11. Stramer SL, Glynn SA, Kleinman SH, et al. Busch MP. Detection of HIV-1 and HCV infections among antibody-negative blood donors by nucleic acid-amplification testing. N Engl J Med 2004;351:760–768.
12. Zou S, Dodd RY, Stramer SL, Strong DM. Probability of viremia with HBV, HCV, HIV, and HTLV among tissue donors in the United States. N Engl J Med 2004;351:751–759.
13. Panlilio AL, Cardo DM, Grohskopf LA, Heneine W, Ross CS. Updated U.S. Public Health Service guidelines for the management of occupational exposures to HIV and recommendations for postexposure prophylaxis. MMWR Recomm Rep 2005;54(RR-9):1–17.
14. Public Health Services Task Force. Recommendations for Use of Antiretroviral Drugs in Pregnant HIV-1-Infected Women for Maternal Health and Interventions to Reduce Perinatal HIV-1 Transmission in the United States: Living Document. October 12, 2006, *http://www.AIDSinfo.NIH.gov*.
15. Nduati R, John G, Mbori-Ngacha D, et al. Effect of breastfeeding and formula feeding on transmission of HIV-1. JAMA 2000;283:1167–1174.
16. Thior I, Lockman S, Smeaton LM, et al. Breastfeeding plus infant zidovudine prophylaxis for 6 months vs formula feeding plus infant zidovudine for 1 month to reduce mother-to-child HIV transmission in Botswana: A randomized trial: The Mashi Study. JAMA 2006;296:794–805.
17. Centers for Disease Control and Prevention. Guidelines for National HIV case surveillance, including monitoring for HIV infection and acquired immunodeficiency syndrome. MMWR 1999;48(RR-13):1–31.
18. Centers for Disease Control and Prevention. 1993 revised classification system for HIV infection and expanded surveillance case definitions for AIDS among adolescents and adults. MMWR 1992;41(RR-17):1–19.

19. Centers for Disease Control and Prevention. HIV/AIDS surveillance report, 2005. Vol. 17. U.S. Department of Health and Human Services, Centers for Disease Control and Prevention. *http://www.cdc.gov/hiv/topics/surveillance/resources/reports/*.
20. UNAIDS. 2006 Report on the Global AIDS Epidemic: A UNAIDS 10th Anniversary Special Edition. *http://www.unaids.org/en/*.
21. Robertson DL, Anderson JP, Bradac JA, et al. HIV-1 nomenclature proposal. Science 2000;288:55–56.
22. Hahn BH, Shaw GM, De Cock KM, Sharp PM. AIDS as a zoonosis: Scientific and public health implications. Science 2000;287:607–614.
23. Van Heuverswyn F, Li Y, Neel C, et al. Human immunodeficiency viruses: SIV infection in wild gorillas. Nature 2006;444:164.
24. San Antonio-Gaddy M, Richardson-Moore A, Burstein GR, Newman DR, Branson BM, Birkhead GS. Rapid HIV antibody testing in the New York State Anonymous HIV Counseling and Testing Program: Experience from the field. J Acquir Immune Defic Syndr 2006;43:446–450.
25. Mylonakis E, Paliou M, Lally M, Flanigan TP, Rich JD. Laboratory testing for infection with the human immunodeficiency virus: Established and novel approaches. Am J Med 2000;109:568–576.
26. Branson BM, Handsfield HH, Lampe MA, et al. Revised recommendations for HIV testing of adults, adolescents, and pregnant women in health-care settings. MMWR Recomm Rep 2006;55(RR-14):1–17.
27. Panel on Clinical Practices for the Treatment of HIV Infection. Guidelines for the Use of Antiretroviral Agents in HIV-Infected Adults and Adolescents. 2006, *http://www.AIDSinfo.NIH.gov*.
28. Douek DC, Picker LJ, Koup RA. T cell dynamics in HIV-1 infection. Annu Rev Immunol 2003;21:265–304.
29. Tang H, Kuhen KL, Wong-Staal F. Lentivirus replication and regulation. Annu Rev Genet 1999;33:133–170.
30. Frankel AD, Young JAT. HIV-1: Fifteen proteins and an RNA. Annu Rev Biochem 1998;67:1–25.
31. Pierson T, McArthur J, Siliciano RF. Reservoirs for HIV-1: Mechanisms for viral persistence in the presence of antiviral immune responses and antiretroviral therapy. Annu Rev Immunol 2000;18:665–708.
32. Cullen BR. Role and mechanism of action of the APOBEC3 family of antiretroviral resistance factors. J Virol 2006;80:1067–1076.
33. Kahn JO, Walker BD. Acute human immunodeficiency virus type 1 infection. N Engl J Med 1998;339:33–39.
34. Mellors JW, Rinaldo CR Jr, Gupta P, White RM, Todd JA, Kingsley LA. Prognosis in HIV-1 infection predicted by the quantity of virus in plasma. Science 1996;272:1167–1170.
35. Centers for Disease Control and Prevention. 1994 revised classification system for human immunodeficiency virus infection in children less than 13 years of age. MMWR 1994;43(RR-12):1–10.
36. The Working Group on Antiretroviral Therapy and Medical Management of HIV-Infected Children. Guidelines for the Use of Antiretroviral Agents in Pediatric HIV Infection. October 26, 2006, *http://www.AIDSinfo.NIH.gov*.
37. Raboud JM, Montaner JS, Conway B, et al. Suppression of plasma viral load below 20 copies/ml is required to achieve a long-term response to therapy. AIDS 1998;12:1619–1624.
38. Center for Disease Control and Prevention. Report of the NIH Panel to Define Principle of Therapy of HIV Infection. MMWR 1998;47(No. RR-5).
39. Hammer SM, Saag MS, Schechter M, et al. Treatment for adult HIV infection: 2006 recommendations of the International AIDS Society—USA panel. Top HIV Med 2006;14:827–843.
40. McMichael AJ. HIV vaccines. Annu Rev Immunol 2006;24:227–255.
41. Piscitelli SC, Bhat N, Pau A. A risk-benefit assessment of interleukin-2 as an adjunct to antiviral therapy in HIV infection. Drug Saf 2000;22:19–31.
42. Anderson PL, Kakuda TN, Lichtenstein KA. The cellular pharmacology of nucleoside- and nucleotide-analogue reverse-transcriptase inhibitors and its relationship to clinical toxicities. Clin Infect Dis 2004;38:743–753.
43. Carr A. Toxicity of antiretroviral therapy and implications for drug development. Nat Rev Drug Discov 2003;2:624–634.
44. Hirsch MS, Brun-Vezinet F, Clotet B, et al. Antiretroviral drug resistance testing in adults infected with Human Immunodeficiency Virus type 1:2003 Recommendations of an International AIDS Society–USA Panel. Clin Infect Dis 2003;37:113–128.
45. Fletcher CV. Enfuvirtide, a new drug for HIV infection. Lancet 2003; 361:1577–1578.
46. Gallant JE. Antiretroviral drug resistance and resistance testing. Top HIV Med 2005;13:138–142.
47. AIDSINFO Drug Database. *www.aidsinfo.nih.gov*.
48. Romanelli F, Smith KM, Hoven AD. Chloroquine and hydroxychloroquine as inhibitors of human immunodeficiency virus (HIV-1) activity. Curr Pharm Des 2004;10:2643–2648.
49. Acosta EP, Fletcher CV. Agents for treating human immunodeficiency virus infection. Am J Hosp Pharm 1994;51:2251–2267.
50. Flexner C. Dual protease inhibitor therapy in HIV-infected patients: Pharmacologic rationale and clinical benefits. Annu Rev Pharmacol Toxicol 2000;40:649–674.
51. Centers for Disease Control and Prevention. TB/HIV Drug Interactions: Updated Guidelines for the Use of Rifamycins for the Treatment of Tuberculosis Among HIV-Infected Patients Taking Protease Inhibitors or Nonnucleoside Reverse Transcriptase Inhibitors. 2004, *http://www.cdc.gov/nchstp/tb/tb_hiv_drugs/toc.htm*.
52. Havlir DV, Tierney C, Friedland GH, et al. In vivo antagonism with zidovudine plus stavudine combination therapy. J Infect Dis 2000;182:321–325.
53. Maitland D, Moyle G, Hand J, et al. Early virologic failure in HIV-1 infected subjects on didanosine/tenofovir/efavirenz: 12-week results from a randomized trial. AIDS 2005;19:1183–1188.
54. Negredo E, Molto J, Burger D, et al. Unexpected CD4 cell count decline in patients receiving didanosine and tenofovir-based regimens despite undetectable viral load. AIDS 2004;18:459–463.
55. Fischl MA, Richman DD, Grieco MH, et al. The efficacy of azidothymidine (AZT) in the treatment of patients with AIDS and AIDS-related complex. N Engl J Med 1987;317:185–191.
56. Hammer SM, Katzenstein DA, Hughes MD, et al. A trial comparing nucleoside monotherapy with combination therapy in HIV-infected adults with CD4 cell counts from 200 to 500 per cubic millimeter. N Engl J Med 1996;335:1081–1090.
57. Gulick RM, Ribaudo HJ, Shikuma CM, et al. Triple-nucleoside regimens versus efavirenz-containing regimens for the initial treatment of HIV-1 infection. N Engl J Med 2004;350:1850–1861.
58. Walmsley S, Bernstein B, King M, et al. Lopinavir-ritonavir versus nelfinavir for the initial treatment of HIV infection. N Eng J Med 2002;346:2039–2046.
59. Paterson DL, Swindells S, Mohr J, et al. Adherence to protease inhibitor therapy and outcomes in patients with HIV infection. Ann Intern Med 2000;133:21–30.
60. Panel on Clinical Practices for the Treatment of HIV Infection. Supplement: Guidelines for Promoting Treatment Adherence, Including Adapting Patient-, Clinician-, and Regimen-Based Approaches. 2004, *http://www.AIDSinfo.NIH.gov*.
61. Eron J Jr, Yeni P, Gathe J Jr, et al. The KLEAN study of fosamprenavir-ritonavir versus lopinavir-ritonavir, each in combination with abacavir-lamivudine, for initial treatment of HIV infection over 48 weeks: A randomised non-inferiority trial. Lancet 2006;368:476–482.
62. Squires K, Lazzarin A, Gatell JM, et al. Comparison of once-daily atazanavir with efavirenz, each in combination with fixed-dose zidovudine and lamivudine, as initial therapy for patients infected with HIV. J Acquir Immune Defic Syndr 2004;36:1011–1019.
63. Bartlett JA, Fath MJ, Demasi R, et al. An updated systematic overview of triple combination therapy in antiretroviral-naive HIV-infected adults. AIDS 2006;20:2051–2064.
64. Gallant JE, DeJesus E, Arribas JR, et al. Tenofovir DF, emtricitabine, and efavirenz vs. zidovudine, lamivudine, and efavirenz for HIV. N Engl J Med 2006;354:251–260.
65. Robbins GK, De Gruttola V, Shafer RW, et al. Comparison of sequential three-drug regimens as initial therapy for HIV-1 infection. N Engl J Med 2003;349:2293–2303.
66. Gallant JE, Rodriguez AE, Weinberg WG, et al. Early virologic nonresponse to tenofovir, abacavir, and lamivudine in HIV-infected antiretroviral-naive subjects. J Infect Dis 2005;192:1921–1930.
67. Jemsek J HP, Harper E. Poor virologic responses in early emergence of resistance in treatment naive, HIV-infected patients receiving a once daily triple nucleoside regimen of didanosine, lamivudine and tenofovir DF [abstract 51]. 11th Conference of Retroviruses and Opportunistic Infections; San Francisco, CA, February 8–11, 2004.
68. Connor EM, Sperling RS, Gelber R, et al. Reduction in maternal-infant transmission of human immunodeficiency virus type 1 with zidovudine treatment. N Engl J Med 1994;331:1173–1180.

69. Public Health Services Task Force. Supplement: Safety and Toxicity of Individual Antiretroviral Agents in Pregnancy. 2006, *http://www.AIDSinfo.NIH.gov*.
70. Guay LA, Musoke P, Fleming T, et al. Intrapartum and neonatal single-dose nevirapine compared with zidovudine for prevention of mother-to-child transmission of HIV-1 in Kampala, Uganda: HIV-NET 012 randomised trial. Lancet 1999;354:795–802.
71. McIntyre J, Martinson N, Gray G. Addition of short course Combivir to single dose Viramune for the prevention of mother to child transmission of HIV-1 can significantly decrease the subsequent development of maternal and paediatric NNRTI-resistant virus [abstract tufo0204]. 3rd International AIDS Society Conference on HIV Pathogenesis and Treatment, Rio de Janeiro, Brazil, July 24–27 2005.
72. Derdelinckx I, Wainberg MA, Lange JM, Hill A, Halima Y, Boucher CA. Criteria for drugs used in pre-exposure prophylaxis trials against HIV infection. PLoS Med 2006;3:e454.
73. Hicks CB, Cahn P, Cooper DA, et al. Durable efficacy of tipranavir-ritonavir in combination with an optimised background regimen of antiretroviral drugs for treatment-experienced HIV-1-infected patients at 48 weeks in the Randomized Evaluation of Strategic Intervention in multi-drug reSistant patients with Tipranavir (RESIST) studies: An analysis of combined data from two randomised open-label trials. Lancet 2006;368:466–475.
74. Bellos N, Falcon R, Hill A. Durability of viral load suppression with darunavir/ritonavir in treatment-experienced patients: POWER 1 and 2 combined week 48 analysis [abstract 958]. 44th Annual Meeting of the Infectious Diseases Society of America; Toronto, Canada, October 12–15 2006.
75. El-Sadr WM, Lundgren JD, Neaton JD, et al. Rappoport C. CD4+ count-guided interruption of antiretroviral treatment. N Engl J Med 2006;355:2283–2296.
76. Taylor S, Allen S, Fidler S, White D, et al. Stop Study: After discontinuation of efavirenz, plasma concentrations may persist for 2 weeks or longer [abstract 131]. 11th Conference on Retroviruses and Opportunistic Infections; San Francisco, CA, February 8–11, 2004.
77. Kaplan JE, Masur H, Holmes KK. Guidelines for preventing opportunistic infections among HIV-infected persons—2002. Recommendations of the U.S. Public Health Service and the Infectious Diseases Society of America. MMWR Recomm Rep 2002;51(RR-8):1–52.
78. Panel on Clinical Practices for the Treatment of HIV Infection. Treating Opportunistic Infections Among HIV-Infected Adults and Adolescents Recommendations from Center for Disease Control and Prevention, the National Institutes of Health, and the HIV Medicine Association/Infectious Diseases Society of America. December 17, 2004, *http://www.AIDSinfo.NIH.gov*.
79. Lipman M, Breen R. Immune reconstitution inflammatory syndrome in HIV. Curr Opin Infect Dis 2006;19:20–25.
80. Ledergerber B, Egger M, Erard V, Weber R, Hirschel B, Furrer H. AIDS-related opportunistic illnesses occurring after initiation of potent antiretroviral therapy. JAMA 2000;282:2220–2226.
81. Santamauro J, Stover D. *Pneumocystis carinii* pneumonia. Med Clin North Am 1997;81:299–318.
82. Wofsy C. Use of trimethoprim-sulfamethoxazole in the treatment of Pneumocystis carinii pneumonitis in patients with acquired immunodeficiency syndrome. Rev Infect Dis 1987;9(Suppl 2):S184–S194.
83. Wharton J, Coleman D, Wofsy C, et al. Trimethoprim-sulfamethoxazole or pentamidine for *Pneumocystis carinii* pneumonia in the acquired immunodeficiency syndrome. Ann Intern Med 1986;105:37–44.
84. Morse CG, Kovacs JA. Metabolic and skeletal complications of HIV infection: The price of success. JAMA 2006;296:844–854.
85. Phair J, Munoz A, Detels R, et al. The risk of *Pneumocystis carinii* pneumonia among men infected with human immunodeficiency virus type 1. N Engl J Med 1990;322:161–165.
86. Mofenson LM, Oleske J, Serchuck L, Van Dyke R, Wilfert C. Treating opportunistic infections among HIV-exposed and infected children: Recommendations from Center for Disease Control and Prevention, the National Institutes of Health, and the Infectious Diseases Society of America. MMWR Recomm Rep 2004;53(RR-14):1–92.
87. Koutkia P, Grinspoon S. HIV-associated lipodystrophy: Pathogenesis, prognosis, treatment, and controversies. Annu Rev Med 2004;55:303–317.
88. Grinspoon S, Carr A. Cardiovascular risk and body-fat abnormalities in HIV-infected adults. N Engl J Med 2005;352:48–62.
89. Friis-Moller N, Weber R, Reiss P, et al. Cardiovascular disease risk factors in HIV patients—association with antiretroviral therapy. Results from the DAD study. AIDS 2003;17:1179–1193.
90. Law MG, Friis-Moller N, El-Sadr WM, et al. The use of the Framingham equation to predict myocardial infarctions in HIV-infected patients: Comparison with observed events in the D.A:D Study. HIV Med 2006;7:218–230.
91. Moyle GJ, Sabin CA, Cartledge J, et al. A randomized comparative trial of tenofovir DF or abacavir as replacement for a thymidine analogue in persons with lipoatrophy. AIDS 2006;20:2043–2050.
92. Wohl DA, McComsey G, Tebas P, et al. Current concepts in the diagnosis and management of metabolic complications of HIV infection and its therapy. Clin Infect Dis 2006;43:645–653.
93. Andersson K, Chung RT. Hepatitis C Virus in the HIV-infected patient. Clin Liver Dis 2006;10:303–320 viii.
94. Hughes CA, Shafran SD. Treatment of hepatitis C in HIV-coinfected patients. Ann Pharmacother 2006;40:479–489.
95. Torriani FJ, Rodriguez-Torres M, Rockstroh JK, et al. Peginterferon Alfa-2a plus ribavirin for chronic hepatitis C virus infection in HIV-infected patients. N Engl J Med 2004;351:438–450.
96. Yee HS, Currie SL, Darling JM, Wright TL. Management and treatment of hepatitis C viral infection: Recommendations from the Department of Veterans Affairs Hepatitis C Resource Center program and the National Hepatitis C Program office. Am J Gastroenterol 2006;101:2360–2378.
97. Tien PC. Management and treatment of hepatitis C virus infection in HIV-infected adults: Recommendations from the Veterans Affairs Hepatitis C Resource Center Program and National Hepatitis C Program Office. Am J Gastroenterol 2005;100:2338–2354.
98. Balzarini J, Lee CK, Herdewijn P, De Clercq E. Mechanism of the potentiating effect of ribavirin on the activity of 2',3'-dideoxyinosine against human immunodeficiency virus. J Biol Chem 1991;266:21509–21514.
99. Kovacs JA, Bechtel C, Davey RT Jr, et al. Combination therapy with didanosine and interferon-alpha in human immunodeficiency virus-infected patients: Results of a phase I/II trial. J Infect Dis 1996;173:840–848.
100. Sulkowski MS, Thomas DL. Hepatitis C in the HIV-infected person. Ann Intern Med 2003;138:197–207.

SECTION 17
ONCOLOGIC DISORDERS

CHAPTER 130

Cancer Treatment and Chemotherapy

PATRICK J. MEDINA AND CHRIS FAUSEL

KEY CONCEPTS

1 Carcinogenesis is a multistep process that includes initiation, promotion, conversion, and progression. The growth of both normal and cancerous cells is genetically controlled by the balance or imbalance of oncogene, protooncogene, and tumor suppressor gene protein products. Multiple genetic mutations are required to convert normal cells to cancerous cells. Apoptosis and cellular senescence (aging) are normal mechanisms for cell death.

2 Because patients with clinically evident metastatic cancer can rarely be cured, early detection is critical. Screening programs are designed to detect cancers in asymptomatic people who are at risk of a specific type of cancer. Knowing the early warning signs of cancer is also important in early detection, when cancers are most likely to be localized.

3 Treatment for cancer should not begin until the presence of cancer is confirmed by a tissue (i.e., histologic) diagnosis. Clinical cancer staging provides prognostic information, and in conjunction with the patient's treatment goals, guides the selection of cancer treatment. The goals of cancer treatment include cure, prolongation of life, and relief of symptoms. Surgery and radiation therapy provide the best chance of cure for patients with localized cancers, but systemic treatment methods are required for disseminated cancers.

4 Adjuvant therapy is systemic therapy that is administered to treat any existing micrometastases remaining after surgical excision of localized disease. Because adjuvant therapy is given to patients with no remaining clinical evidence of cancer, the benefit of the treatment cannot be proven for an individual patient, but only for patient populations. Treatment decisions are based largely on an assessment of the presence of risk factors in an individual patient and the patient's estimated risk for cancer recurrence. The effectiveness of adjuvant therapies is measured by the relative and absolute reduction in the risk of recurrence.

5 Traditional chemotherapy agents target rapidly proliferating cells. Agents can be either "cell-cycle phase-specific," targeting one specific phase of the cell cycle, or "cell-cycle phase-nonspecific," targeting all proliferating cells regardless of their place in the cell cycle. Cell-cycle phase-specific agents are generally given more frequently or as continuous infusions, whereas cell-cycle phase-nonspecific agents are given as a single dose.

6 Monoclonal antibodies in cancer treatment recognize an antigen that is expressed preferentially on cancer cells or target growth factors responsible for cancer growth. These agents can vary in the amount of foreign component that can be used to predict tolerability of the agents. Monoclonal antibodies that target cellular antigens induce cell death by a variety of mechanisms that involve the host immune system. These agents can also be used to deliver drugs or radioisotopes to the antigen-expressing cells.

7 The HER (human epidermal growth factor receptor) contains four known receptor subtypes that regulate cell proliferation pathways through signal transduction. The HER family is dysregulated in many common tumors. Several agents have been developed to prevent signal transduction through this pathway. Monoclonal antibodies, which competitively bind to extracellular receptors, and small molecular inhibitors, which target intracellular signal transduction pathways, are commercially available for several malignancies.

8 Tumors must develop new blood vessels through the process of angiogenesis in order to grow. This process, regulated by proangiogenic and antiangiogenic factors, becomes dysregulated in several malignancies and can lead to tumor growth, invasion, and metastasis. New anticancer agents can target this process and decrease tumor growth.

9 Understanding the mechanism of chemotherapy drug toxicities can lead to more effective prevention and treatment of these toxicities. Prospective dose modification of some cancer drugs is essential in patients with impaired renal or hepatic function, to reduce the risk of severe toxicities. Identification of genetic variations that affect drug activation and metabolism may per-

Learning objectives, review questions, and other resources can be found at **www.pharmacotherapyonline.com.**

mit the development of individualized drug therapy regimens that optimize effectiveness and minimize toxicity.

10 Myelosuppression is the acute dose-limiting toxicity for most nonspecific cancer drugs. Anemia can cause fatigue in cancer patients, whereas risk of infection in patients is related to the depth and duration of neutropenia. Unexplained fever in neutropenic patients requires prompt initiation of empiric antibiotic therapy. Colony-stimulating factors are available to improve fatigue in patients with anemia and reduce the risk of febrile neutropenia. Evidence-based clinical guidelines should direct the use of costly supportive care resources such as hematopoietic growth factors.

Cancer is a group of more than 100 different diseases that are characterized by uncontrolled cellular growth, local tissue invasion, and distant metastases.[1] It is now the leading cause of mortality in Americans younger than age 85 years. About 1.4 million cases of cancer will be diagnosed in 2007, and cancer will claim an estimated 559,650 lives in the United States.[2] Figure 130–1 illustrates the estimated incidence of common cancers and cancer-related deaths. The four most common cancers are prostate, breast, lung, and colorectal cancer. The most common cause of cancer-related deaths in the United States is lung cancer, which accounts for about 160,000 deaths each year. These cancers are discussed in further detail in the chapters that follow.

The roles of healthcare professionals in the management of cancer patients can be very diverse. Thorough knowledge of antineoplastic drug pharmacology and pharmacokinetics is essential to prevent and to manage drug-induced toxicities. Supportive-care issues, such as nutritional support, pain management, infection, and nausea and vomiting, require application of clinical, pharmacologic, and economic principles. Provision of drug information to other healthcare professionals and to patients and their families is another critical role. Experienced healthcare professionals are able to fulfill these roles and to make valuable contributions to patient care in the oncology setting.

This chapter introduces the basic concepts of carcinogenesis, tumor growth, and cancer treatment, provides general information on the pharmacology and clinical use of the antineoplastic agents, and presents an overview of supportive care issues in the oncology patient.

Estimated New Cases

Males			Females		
Prostate	218,890	29%	Breast	178,480	26%
Lung & bronchus	114,760	15%	Lung & bronchus	98,620	15%
Colon & rectum	79,130	10%	Colon & rectum	74,630	11%
Urinary bladder	50,040	7%	Uterine corpus	39,080	6%
Non-Hodgkin lymphoma	34,200	4%	Non-Hodgkin lymphoma	28,990	4%
Melanoma of the skin	33,910	4%	Melanoma of the skin	26,030	4%
Kidney & renal pelvis	31,590	4%	Thyroid	25,480	4%
Leukemia	24,800	3%	Ovary	22,430	3%
Oral cavity & pharynx	24,180	3%	Kidney & renal pelvis	19,600	3%
Pancreas	18,830	2%	Leukemia	19,440	3%
All sites	**768,860**	**100%**	**All Sites**	**678,060**	**100%**

Males			Females		
Lung & bronchus	89,510	31%	Lung & bronchus	70,880	26%
Prostate	27,050	9%	Breast	40,460	15%
Colon & rectum	26,000	9%	Colon & rectum	26,180	10%
Pancreas	16,840	6%	Pancreas	16,530	6%
Leukemia	12,320	4%	Ovary	15,280	6%
Liver & Intrahepatic bile duct	11,280	4%	Leukemia	9,470	4%
Esophagus	10,900	4%	Non-Hodgkin lymphoma	9,060	3%
Urinary bladder	9,630	3%	Uterine corpus	7,400	3%
Non-Hodgkin lymphoma	9,600	3%	Brain & other nervous system	5,590	2%
Kidney & renal pelvis	8,090	3%	Liver & Intrahepatic bile duct	5,500	2%
All Sites	**289,550**	**100%**	**All Sites**	**270,100**	**100%**

FIGURE 130-1. Estimated 2007 cancer incidences *(top)* and deaths *(bottom)* in the United States for males and females. *(Reproduced with permission from Jemal et al.[2])*

ETIOLOGY OF CANCER

CARCINOGENESIS

❶ The mechanisms by which cancers occur are incompletely understood. A cancer, or neoplasm, is thought to develop from a cell in which the normal mechanisms for control of growth and proliferation are altered. Current evidence supports the concept of carcinogenesis as a multistage process that is genetically regulated.[3–6] The first step in this process is *initiation*, which requires exposure of normal cells to carcinogenic substances. These carcinogens produce genetic damage that, if not repaired, results in irreversible cellular mutations. This mutated cell has an altered response to its environment and a selective growth advantage, giving it the potential to develop into a clonal population of neoplastic cells. During the second phase, known as *promotion*, carcinogens or other factors alter the environment to favor growth of the mutated cell population over normal cells. The primary difference between initiation and promotion is that promotion is a reversible process. Because it is reversible, the promotion phase may be the target of future chemoprevention strategies, including changes in lifestyle and diet. At some point, however, the mutated cell becomes cancerous (*conversion* or *transformation*). Depending on the type of cancer, 5 to 20 years may elapse between the carcinogenic phases and the development of a clinically detectable cancer. The final stage of neoplastic growth, called *progression*, involves further genetic changes leading to increased cell proliferation. The critical elements of this phase include tumor invasion into local tissues and the development of metastases.

Substances that may act as carcinogens or initiators include chemical, physical, and biologic agents.[5] Exposure to chemicals may occur by virtue of occupational and environmental means, as well as lifestyle habits. The association of aniline dye exposure and bladder cancer is one such example. Benzene is known to cause leukemia. Some drugs and hormones used for therapeutic purposes are also classified as carcinogenic chemicals (Table 130–1). Physical agents that act as carcinogens include ionizing radiation and ultraviolet light. These types of radiation induce mutations by forming free radicals that damage DNA and other cellular components. Viruses are biologic agents that are associated with certain cancers. The Epstein-Barr virus is believed to be an important factor in the initiation of Burkitt's lymphoma. Likewise, infection with human papilloma virus is known to be a major cause of cervical cancer. All the previously mentioned carcinogens, as well as age, gender, diet, growth factors, and chronic irritation, are among the factors considered to be promoters of carcinogenesis.

TABLE 130-1 Selected Drugs and Hormones Known to Cause Cancer in Humans

Drug or Hormone	Type of Cancer Caused
Alkylating agents (e.g., chlorambucil, mechlorethamine, melphalan, nitrosoureas)	Leukemia
Anabolic steroids	Liver
Analgesics containing phenacetin	Renal, urinary bladder
Anthracyclines (e.g., doxorubicin)	Leukemia
Antiestrogens (tamoxifen)	Endometrium
Coal tars (topical)	Skin
Estrogens	
Nonsteroidal (diethylstilbestrol)	Vagina/cervix, endometrium, breast, testes
Steroidal (estrogen replacement therapy, oral contraceptives)	Endometrium, breast, liver
Epipodophyllotoxins (etoposide, teniposide)	Leukemia
Immunosuppressive drugs (cyclosporine, azathioprine)	Lymphoma, skin
Oxazaphosphorines (cyclophosphamide, ifosfamide)	Urinary bladder, leukemia

Adapted from Compagni and Christofori[4] and Cotran et al.[6]

GENETIC AND MOLECULAR BASIS OF CANCER

❶ In recent years there has been marked progress in our understanding of the genetic changes that lead to the development of cancer, largely because of improvements in research techniques and new information generated as part of the Human Genome Project.[3,5–7] Two major classes of genes are involved in carcinogenesis: oncogenes and tumor suppressor genes. Figure 130–2 illustrates the acquired capabilities of cancer cells that differ from normal cellular function.[8] Oncogenes develop from normal genes, called protooncogenes, and may have important roles in all phases of carcinogenesis. Protooncogenes are present in all cells and are essential regulators of normal cellular functions, including the cell cycle. Genetic alteration of the protooncogene through point mutation, chromosomal rearrangement, or gene amplification activates the oncogene. These genetic alterations may be caused by carcinogenic agents such as radiation, chemicals, or viruses (somatic mutations), or they may be inherited (germ-line mutations). Once activated, the oncogene produces either excessive amounts of the normal gene product or an abnormal gene product. The result is dysregulation of normal cell growth and proliferation, which imparts a distinct growth advantage to the cell and increases the probability of neoplastic transformation. An exam-

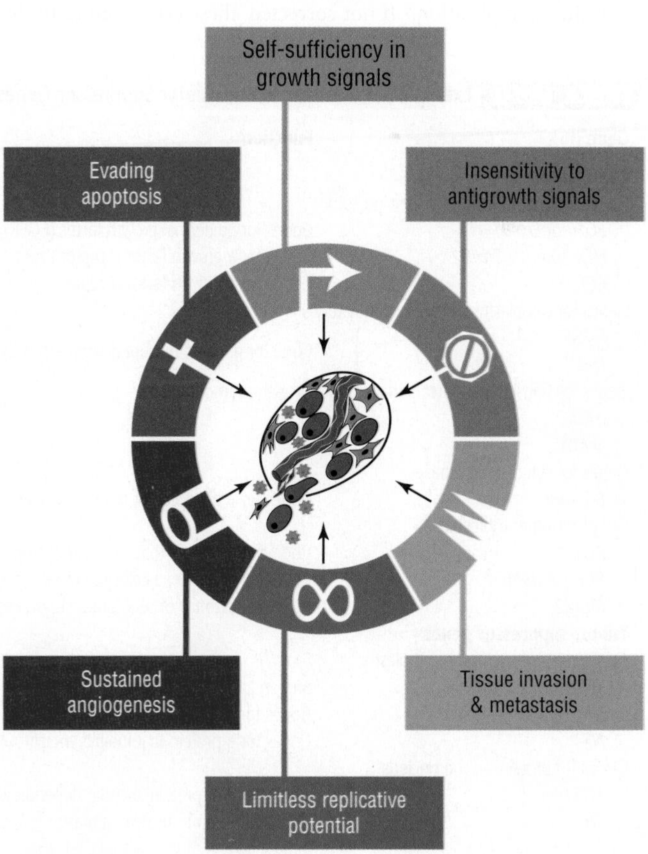

FIGURE 130-2. Functional capabilities acquired by cancer cells including angiogenesis, self-proliferation, insensitivity to antigrowth signals and limitless growth potential, metastasis; and antiapoptotic effects. It is thought that most, if not all cancer cells acquire these functions through a variety of mechanisms, including activation of oncogenes and mutations in tumor suppressor genes. *(This article was published in Cell, Vol. 100(1), Hanahan D, Weinberg RA, The Hallmarks of Cancer, Pages 57–70, Copyright Elsevier.)*

ple is the human epidermal growth factor receptor (HER) family of oncogenes. This family of receptor tyrosine kinases contains four members: ErbB-1, also known as epidermal growth factor receptor (EGFR), HER-2, HER-3, and HER-4. When activated, these receptors mediate cell proliferation and differentiation of cells through activation of intracellular tyrosine kinase receptors and downstream signaling pathways. As an oncogene, the gene product is overexpressed or amplified, resulting in excessive cellular proliferation, metastasis, angiogenesis, and cell survival in several cancers. Table 130–2 lists examples of oncogenes by their cellular function.[9]

In contrast, tumor suppressor genes regulate and inhibit inappropriate cellular growth and proliferation.[3,6,7] Gene loss or mutation results in loss of control over normal cell growth. Two common examples of tumor suppressor genes are the retinoblastoma and *p53* genes. Mutation of *p53* is one of the most common genetic changes associated with cancer, and is estimated to occur in half of all malignancies.[7] The normal gene product of *p53* is responsible for negative regulation of the cell cycle, allowing the cell cycle to halt for repairs, corrections, and responses to other external signals. Inactivation of *p53* removes this checkpoint, allowing mutations to occur. Mutation of *p53* is linked to a variety of malignancies, including brain tumors (astrocytoma); carcinomas of the breast, colon, lung, cervix, and anus; and osteosarcoma. Another important function of *p53* may be modulation of cytotoxic drug effects. Loss of *p53* is associated with antineoplastic drug resistance.

Another group of genes important in carcinogenesis are the DNA repair genes. The normal function of these genes is to repair DNA that is damaged by environmental factors, or errors in DNA that occur during replication.[6] If not corrected, these errors can result in mutations that activate oncogenes or inactivate tumor suppressor genes. As more mutations in the genome occur, the risk for malignant transformation increases. The DNA repair genes have been classified as tumor suppressor genes because a loss in their function results in increased risk for carcinogenesis. Deficiencies in DNA repair genes have been discovered in familial colon cancer (hereditary nonpolyposis colon cancer) and breast cancer syndromes.

❶ Oncogenes and tumor suppressor genes provide the stimulatory and inhibitory signals that ultimately regulate the cell cycle.[3,7] These signals converge on a molecular system in the nucleus known as the cell-cycle clock. The function of the clock in normal tissue is to integrate the signal input and to determine if the cell cycle should proceed. The clock is composed of a series of interacting proteins, the most important of which are cyclins and cyclin-dependent kinases. Cyclins (especially cyclin D_1) and cyclin-dependent kinases promote entry into the cell cycle and are overexpressed in several cancers, including breast cancer. Cyclin-dependent kinase inhibitors have been identified as important negative regulators of the cell cycle.

❶ When the normal regulatory mechanisms for cellular growth fail, backup defense systems may be activated. The secondary defenses include apoptosis (programmed cell death or suicide) and cellular senescence (aging). Apoptosis is a normal mechanism of cell death required for tissue homeostasis.[3,7,10] This process is regulated by oncogenes and tumor suppressor genes and is also a mechanism of cellular death after exposure to cytotoxic agents. Overexpression of oncogenes responsible for apoptosis may produce an "immortal" cell, which has increased potential for malignancy. The *bcl-2* oncogene is an example. The most common chromosomal abnormality found in lymphoid malignancies is the t(14;18) translocation. The

TABLE 130-2 Examples of Oncogenes and Tumor Suppressor Genes

Gene	Function	Associated Human Cancer
Oncogenes		
Genes for growth factors or their receptors		
EGFR or *Erb-B1*	Codes for epidermal growth factor (EGFR) receptor	Glioblastoma, breast, head and neck, and colon cancers
HER-2/neu or *Erb-B2*	Codes for a growth factor receptor	Breast, salivary gland, prostate, bladder, and ovarian cancers
RET	Codes for a growth factor receptor	Thyroid cancer
Genes for cytoplasmic relays in stimulatory signaling pathways		
K-RAS	Code for guanine nucleotide-proteins with GTPase activity	Lung, ovarian, colon, pancreatic binding cancers
N-RAS		Neuroblastoma, acute leukemia
Genes for transcription factors that activate growth-promoting genes		
c-MYC		Leukemia and breast, colon, gastric, and lung cancers
N-MYC		Neuroblastoma, small cell lung cancer, and glioblastoma
Genes for cytoplasmic kinases		
BCR-ABL	Codes for a nonreceptor tyrosine kinase	Chronic myelogenous leukemia
Genes for other molecules		
BCL-2	Codes for a protein that blocks apoptosis	Indolent B-cell lymphomas
BCL-1 or PRAD1	Codes for cyclin D_1, a cell-cycle clock stimulator	Breast, head, and neck cancers
MDM2	Protein antagonist of p53 tumor suppressor protein	Sarcomas
Tumor-suppressor genes		
Genes for proteins in the cytoplasm		
APC	Step in a signaling pathway	Colon and gastric cancer
NF-1	Codes for a protein that inhibits the stimulatory Ras protein	Neurofibroma, leukemia, and pheochromocytoma
NF-2	Codes for a protein that inhibits the stimulatory Ras protein	Meningioma, ependymoma, and schwannoma
Genes for proteins in the nucleus		
MTS1	Codes for p16 protein, a cyclin-dependent kinase inhibitor	Involved in a wide range of cancers
RB1	Codes for the pRB protein, a master brake of the cell cycle	Retinoblastoma, osteosarcoma, and bladder, small cell lung, prostate, and breast cancers
p53	Codes for the p53 protein, which can halt cell division and induce apoptosis	Involved in a wide range of cancers
Genes for protein whose cellular location is unclear		
BRCA1	DNA repair, transcriptional regulation	Breast and ovarian cancers
BRCA2	DNA repair	Breast cancer
VHL	Regulator of protein stability	Renal cell cancer
MSH2, MLH1, PMS1, PMS2, MSH6	DNA mismatch repair enzymes	Hereditary nonpolyposis colorectal cancer

Adapted from Calvo et al.,[3] Cotran et al.,[6] and Weinberg.[7]

bcl-2 protooncogene is normally located on chromosome 18. Translocation of this protooncogene to chromosome 14 in proximity to the immunoglobulin heavy chain gene leads to overexpression of *bcl-2*, which decreases apoptosis and confers a survival advantage to the cell. Studies show that *p53* is also a regulator of apoptosis. Loss of *p53* disrupts normal apoptotic pathways, imparting a survival advantage to the cell. Recent evidence also has revealed an important role for apoptosis as a mechanism of inherent resistance to chemotherapy.[10]

Cellular senescence is another important defense mechanism.[6,7] Laboratory studies demonstrate that once a cell population has undergone a preset number of doublings, growth stops and cells die. This is known as senescence, a process that is regulated by telomeres. Telomeres are the DNA segments or caps at the ends of chromosomes. They are responsible for protecting the end of the DNA from damage. With each replication, the length of the telomeres is shortened. After the telomeres are shortened to a critical length, senescence is triggered. In this way, telomeres tally and limit the number of cell doublings. In cancer cells, the function of telomeres is overcome by overexpression of an enzyme known as telomerase. Telomerase replaces the portion of the telomeres that is lost with each cell division, thereby avoiding senescence and permitting an infinite number of cell doublings. Telomerase is a target for antineoplastic drug development.

❶ As information regarding the role of oncogenes and tumor suppressor genes accumulated, it became evident that a single mutation is probably insufficient to initiate cancer.[4–7] Scientists postulate that combinations of mutations are required for carcinogenesis and that each mutation is inherited by the next generation of cells. Thus, several detectable genetic mutations may be present in an established tumor. Early mutations are found in both premalignant lesions and in established tumors, whereas later mutations are found only in the established tumor. This theory of sequential genetic mutations resulting in cancer has been demonstrated in colon cancer. In colon cancer, the initial genetic mutation is believed to be loss of the adenomatous polyposis coli gene, which results in formation of a small benign polyp. Oncogenic mutation of the *ras* gene is often the next step, leading to enlargement of the polyp. Loss of function of DNA mismatch repair enzymes may occur at many points in the progression of malignant transformation. Loss of the *p53* gene and another gene, believed to be the "deleted in colorectal cancer" gene, complete the transformation into a malignant lesion. Loss of *p53* is thought to be a late event in the development and progression of the malignancy.

Identification of genes and other proteins involved in carcinogenesis has several important clinical implications. They may be used in cancer screening to identify individuals at increased risk for cancer and are being used to design new anticancer agents and gene therapies, several of which have recently been approved for use. Specific genetic abnormalities are so commonly associated with some types of cancers that the presence of that abnormality aids in the diagnosis of that cancer. If the presence of these genes (i.e., gene expression profile) can reliably predict the clinical course of a cancer or response to certain cancer therapies, then genetic analysis may also become an important prognostic and treatment decision tool. An example of this is overexpression of HER-2 predicting response to trastuzumab.[9]

PATHOLOGY OF CANCER

TUMOR ORIGIN

Tumors may arise from any of four basic tissue types: epithelial tissue, connective tissue (i.e., muscle, bone, and cartilage), lymphoid tissue, and nerve tissue. Although some malignant cells are atypical of their cells of origin, the involved cells usually retain enough of their parent's traits to identify their origin. Benign tumors are named by adding the suffix *-oma* to the name of the cell type. Hence, adenomas are benign growths of glandular origin, or growths that exhibit a glandular pattern. Table 130–3 lists common tumor nomenclature by tissue type.[6]

TABLE 130-3 Tumor Classification by Tissue Type

Tissue of Origin	Benign	Malignant
Epithelial		
Surface epithelium	Papilloma	Carcinoma (squamous, epidermoid)
Glandular tissue	Adenoma	Adenocarcinoma
Connective tissue		
Fibrous tissue	Fibroma	Fibrosarcoma
Bone	Osteoma	Osteosarcoma
Smooth muscle	Leiomyoma	Leiomyosarcoma
Striated muscle	Rhabdomyoma	Rhabdomyosarcoma
Fat	Lipoma	Liposarcoma
Lymphoid tissue and hematopoietic cells		
Bone marrow elements		Leukemias
Lymphoid tissue		Hodgkin's and non-Hodgkin's lymphoma
Plasma cell		Multiple myeloma
Neural tissue		
Glial tissue	"Benign" gliomas	Glioblastoma multiforme, astrocytoma
Nerve sheath	Neurofibroma	Neurofibrosarcoma
Melanocytes	Pigmented nevus (mole)	Malignant melanoma
Mixed tumors		
Gonadal tissue	Teratoma	Teratocarcinoma

Adapted from Cotran et al.[6]

Some cancers are preceded by cellular changes that are abnormal, but not yet malignant. Correction of these early changes could potentially prevent the occurrence of a cancer. Precancerous lesions may be described as consisting of either hyperplastic or dysplastic cells. Hyperplasia is an increase in the number of cells in a particular tissue or organ, which results in an increased size of the organ. It should not be confused with hypertrophy, which is an increase in the size of the individual cells. Hyperplasia occurs in response to a stimulus and reverses when the stimulus is removed. Dysplasia is defined as an abnormal change in the size, shape, or organization of cells or tissues. Hyperplasia and dysplasia may precede the appearance of a cancer by several months or years.

Malignant cells are divided into those of epithelial origin or the other tissue types. Carcinomas are malignant growths arising from epithelial cells. Malignant growths of muscle or connective tissue are called sarcomas. An adenocarcinoma is a malignant tumor arising from glandular tissue. Another term used frequently in the description of malignancy is *carcinoma in situ*. In this instance, the cancer is limited to the epithelial cells of origin; it has not yet invaded the basement membrane. Carcinoma in situ is a preinvasive stage of malignancy, and most tumors have progressed well beyond this stage at diagnosis. Like all classification systems, there are exceptions to these rules. Malignancies of hematologic origin, such as leukemias and lymphomas, are classified separately. Leukemias and lymphomas are discussed in later chapters.

TUMOR CHARACTERISTICS

Tumors may be either benign or malignant. Benign tumors are noncancerous growths that are often encapsulated, localized, and indolent. Cells of benign tumors resemble the cells from which they developed. These masses seldom metastasize, and once removed they rarely recur. In contrast, malignant tumors invade and destroy the surrounding tissue. The cells of malignant tumors are genetically unstable, and loss of normal cell architecture results in cells that are atypical of their tissue or cell of origin. These cells lose the ability to perform their usual functions. This loss of structure and function is defined as anaplasia. In contrast to benign tumors, malignant tumors tend to metastasize, and consequently, recurrences are common after removal or destruction of the primary tumor.

INVASION AND METASTASIS

❷ Metastasis is the spread of neoplastic cells from the primary tumor site to distant sites.[5,11] Despite advances in diagnostic techniques and screening for cancer, many patients have detectable metastatic disease at diagnosis. Once clinically evident distant metastases are present, cancers are seldom curable. Newly diagnosed cancer patients may also have microscopic cancer metastases. Although clinically undetectable, these small clusters of diseased cells must be present, because many patients subsequently relapse at distant sites despite removal of the primary tumor. Some patients with micrometastatic disease may be cured with systemic chemotherapy.

The two primary pathways of metastasis are hematogenous and lymphatic. Other less-common modes of disease spread include dissemination via cerebrospinal fluid and transabdominal spread within the peritoneal cavity. Tumors are constantly shedding neoplastic cells into the systemic circulation or surrounding lymphatics. This process may begin early in the life of the tumor and often increases with time. The time course for metastasis depends largely on the biology of the tumor. Breast cancer, for example, tends to metastasize very early. Not all of the shed cancer cells, or "seeds," result in a metastatic lesion. The "seed" must first find the appropriate "soil," or an environment suitable for growth.[11] This process is illustrated in the diverse patterns of metastasis that are characteristic of individual types of cancer. An example is prostate cancer, which commonly metastasizes to bone, but rarely to the brain.

The process of invasion and metastasis involves several essential steps. After neoplastic transformation, the malignant cells and surrounding host tissue secrete substances that stimulate the formation of new blood vessels to provide oxygen and nutrients. This process is known as *angiogenesis* or *neovascularization*.[12] Tumor cells must then detach from the primary mass and invade surrounding blood and lymph vessels. The tumor cells or cell aggregates detach and embolize through these vessels, but most do not survive circulation. The disseminated cells must then attach to the vascular endothelium. The cells may proliferate within the lumen of the vessel, but most commonly extravasate into the surrounding tissue. The local microenvironment may provide growth factors that can serve as "fertilizer" to potentiate the proliferation of the metastasis. At every step of the way, the potential metastatic cell must fight the host immune system. Last, the metastasis must again initiate angiogenesis to ensure continued growth and proliferation. Because angiogenesis has been recognized as a critical element in primary tumor growth as well as metastasis, it has become a target for development of new anticancer agents, which will be described later in the chapter. Figure 130–3 summarizes the functions acquired by a cell to survive as well as mechanisms by which the cancer cell achieves this function.[8]

DIAGNOSIS AND STAGING

SCREENING

❷ Because cancers are most curable with surgery or radiation before they have metastasized, early detection and treatment have

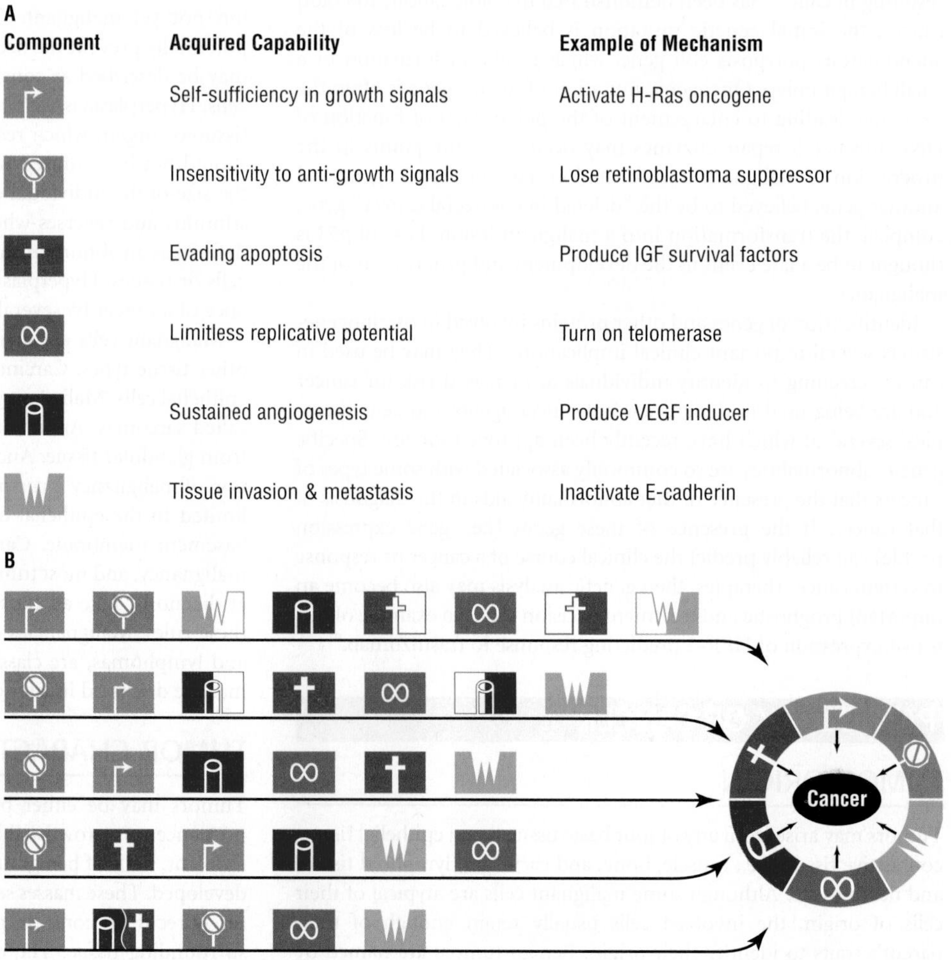
A
Component
Acquired Capability
Example of Mechanism
Self-sufficiency in growth signals
Activate H-Ras oncogene
Insensitivity to anti-growth signals
Lose retinoblastoma suppressor
Evading apoptosis
Produce IGF survival factors
Limitless replicative potential
Turn on telomerase
Sustained angiogenesis
Produce VEGF inducer
Tissue invasion & metastasis
Inactivate E-cadherin
B
Cancer

FIGURE 130-3. The mechanisms of tumorigenesis exhibited by most cancers. (IGF, insulin-like growth factor; VEGF, vascular endothelial growth factor.) *(This article was published in Cell, Vol. 100(1), Hanahan D, Weinberg RA, The Hallmarks of Cancer, Pages 57–70, Copyright Elsevier.)*

TABLE 130-4 Screening Guidelines for Early Detection of Cancer in Asymptomatic People

Disease	Test or Procedure	Sex	Age (y)	Frequency
Breast cancer	Breast self-examination	F	20 and over	Monthly[a]
	Clinical breast examination	F	20–39	Every 3 years
			40 and over	Every year
	Mammography	F	40 and over	Every year[b]
Colorectal cancer	One of the following examination schedules should be followed:			
	Fecal occult blood test (FOBT) or fecal immunochemical test (FIT)	M and F	50 and over	Every year
	Flexible sigmoidoscopy	M and F	50 and over	Every 5 years
	Annual FOBT or FIT and flexible sigmoidoscopy[c]	M and F	50 and over	Every 5 years
	Colonoscopy	M and F	50 and over	Every 10 years
	Double contrast barium enema	M and F	50 and over	Every 5 years
Prostate cancer	Digital rectal exam and prostate-specific antigen (PSA) blood test	M	50 and over	Every year[d]
Cervical cancer	Pap test or liquid-based test	F	3 years after beginning vaginal intercourse	Every year[e]
				Every 2 years
Endometrial cancer	Information on risks and symptoms	F	Menopause	Once[f]
Cancer-related check-up	Health counseling and physical examination[g]	M and F	20–40	Every 3 years
			40 and over	Every year

[a]Beginning in their early 20s, women should be told about the benefits and limitations of breast self-examination (BSE). The importance of prompt reporting of any new breast symptoms to a healthcare professional should be emphasized. It is acceptable for women to choose not to do BSE or to do BSE irregularly.

[b]Women at increased risk (e.g., family history, genetic tendency, or past breast cancer) should talk with their physician about benefits and limitations of starting earlier, having additional tests, or more frequent examinations.

[c]Flexible sigmoidoscopy together with FOBT or FIT is preferable to either test alone, although annual FOBT/FIT alone and flexible sigmoidoscopy every 5 years without FOBT/FIT has some benefit. People at moderate-to-high risk for colorectal cancer should discuss a different testing schedule with their physician.

[d]Digital rectal examination and PSA testing should be offered annually to men with a life expectancy of at least 10 years. Men at high risk (e.g., African American men and men with a strong family history) should begin testing at age 45 years.

[e]At or after age 30 years, women with three consecutive normal tests may be screened at less-frequent intervals (every 2–3 years). Alternatively, human papollomavirus DNA testing and conventional or liquid-based testing could be performed every 3 years. Women at high risk (e.g., human immunodeficiency virus infection or weak immune system) may be screened more frequently. Women older than age 70 years may stop screening if they had three normal tests in the last 10 years.

[f]Women with or at risk for hereditary nonpolyposis colon cancer should begin annual endometrial biopsy starting at age 35 years.

[g]To include examination for cancers of the mouth, thyroid, testicles, skin, lymph nodes, and ovaries, as well as health counseling about tobacco, sun exposure, diet and nutrition, risk factors, sexual practices, and environmental and occupational exposures.

From Smith et al.[13]

obvious potential benefits. In addition, small tumors are more responsive to chemotherapy, as discussed previously. Early diagnosis is difficult for many cancers because they do not produce clinical signs or symptoms until they have become large or have metastasized. Cancer screening programs are designed to detect signs of cancer in people who have not yet developed symptoms from cancer. Lack of effective screening methods for some cancers and inaccessibility of some anatomic sites further complicate the process. Education of the public on the early warning signs of common cancers is extremely important for facilitating early detection. For some cancers, effective screening procedures do exist. The Papanicolaou (Pap) smear test, for example, is an effective tool to detect cervical cancer in its early stages. Self-examination of the breasts in women and of the testicles in men may lead to early diagnosis of cancers in these organs. The American Cancer Society has published guidelines for routine screening examinations (Table 130–4).[13]

DIAGNOSIS

The presenting signs and symptoms of cancer vary widely and depend on the type of cancer. The presentation in adults may include any of cancer's seven warning signs (Table 130–5), as well as pain or loss of appetite.[14] The warning signs of cancer in children are different, and reflect the types of tumors more common in this patient population (Table 130–6).[14] Even with increased public awareness, the fear of a cancer diagnosis can deter patients from seeking medical attention. The definitive diagnosis of cancer relies on the procurement of a sample of the tissue or cells suspected of malignancy and pathologic assessment of this sample. This sample can be obtained by numerous methods, including biopsy, exfoliative cytology, or fine-needle aspiration. A tissue diagnosis is essential, because many benign conditions can masquerade as cancer. Definitive treatment should not begin without a pathologic diagnosis.

STAGING AND WORKUP

❸ In addition to tissue diagnosis, tumors should be staged to determine the extent of disease before any definitive treatment is initiated. The process is dictated by knowledge of the biology of the tumor and by the signs and symptoms elicited in the history and physical examination. Staging provides information on prognosis and guides treatment selection. After treatment is implemented, the staging workup is usually repeated to evaluate the effectiveness of the treatment. Uniform staging criteria are imperative in clinical research

TABLE 130-5 Cancer's Seven Warning Signs

Change in bowel or bladder habits
A sore that does not heal
Unusual bleeding or discharge
Thickening or lump in breast or elsewhere
Indigestion or difficulty in swallowing
Obvious change in wart or mole
Nagging cough or hoarseness
If YOU have a warning signal, see your doctor!

American Cancer Society Study Communicating Cancer Information Through Mass Distribution Leaflets—an American Cancer Society Study. CA Cancer J Clin 1967;17:291–293.

TABLE 130-6 Cancer's Warning Signs in Children

Continued, unexplained weight loss
Headaches with vomiting in the morning
Increased swelling or persistent pain in bones or joints
Lump or mass in abdomen, neck, or elsewhere
Development of a whitish appearance in the pupil of the eye
Recurrent fevers not caused by infections
Excessive bruising or bleeding
Noticeable paleness or prolonged tiredness

Data from http://www.cancer.org/docroot/CRI/content/CRI_2_2_3x_Can_Childhood_Cancers_Be_Detected_Early.asp?sitearea=CRI

aimed at evaluating cancer treatment regimens. Staging has been valuable in learning more about the biology of various tumor types. A staging workup may involve radiographs, computed tomography scans, magnetic resonance imaging, positron emission tomography scans, ultrasonograms, bone-marrow biopsies, bone scans, lumbar puncture, and a variety of laboratory tests, including appropriate tumor markers. Some cancers produce antigens or other substances that are characteristic of that particular cancer. These so-called tumor markers are often nonspecific and may be elevated in many different cancer types, or in patients with nonmalignant diseases. As a result, tumor markers are generally more useful for monitoring response and detecting recurrence than as diagnostic tools. Examples are the measure of human chorionic gonadotropin and alpha-fetoprotein in patients with testicular cancer, or prostate-specific antigen in prostate cancer.[6]

The most commonly applied staging system for solid tumors is the TNM classification, where T = tumor, N = node, and M = metastases. A numerical value is assigned to each letter to indicate the size or extent of disease. The designated rating for tumor describes the size of the primary mass and ranges from T_1 to T_4. Carcinoma in situ is designated T_{is}. Nodes are described in terms of the extent and quality of nodal involvement (N_0 to N_3). Metastases are generally scored depending on their presence or absence (M_0 or M_1). To simplify the staging process, most cancers are classified according to the extent of disease by a numerical system involving stages I through IV. Stage I usually indicates localized tumor, stages II and III represent local and regional extension of disease, and stage IV denotes the presence of distant metastases. The assigned TNM rating translates into a particular stage classification. For example, $T_3N_1M_0$ describes a moderate- to large-sized primary mass, with regional lymph node involvement and no distant metastases, and for most cancers is stage III. The criteria for classifying disease extent are quite specific for each different type of cancer.[15] For some tumors, alternative alphabetical systems (stage A, B, C, or D) are used in clinical practice.

TREATMENT

Modalities of Cancer Treatment

Four primary modalities are employed in the approach to cancer treatment: surgery, radiation, chemotherapy, and biologic therapy. The oldest of these is surgery, which plays a major role in the diagnosis and treatment of cancer. Surgery remains the treatment of choice for most solid tumors diagnosed in the early stages. Radiation therapy was first used for cancer treatment in the late 1800s and remains a mainstay in the management of cancer. Although very effective for treating many types of cancer, surgery and radiation are local treatments. These modalities are likely to produce a cure in patients with truly localized disease. But because most patients with cancer have metastatic disease at diagnosis, localized therapies often fail to completely eliminate the cancer. In addition, systemic diseases such as leukemia cannot be treated with a localized modality. Chemotherapy (including hormonal therapy) accesses the systemic circulation and can theoretically treat the primary tumor and any metastatic disease. Biologic therapies are currently considered in the broader sense of immunotherapy or "targeted therapies." Immunotherapy, the earliest important form of biologic therapy, usually involves stimulating the host's immune system to fight the cancer. The agents used in immunotherapy are usually naturally occurring cytokines, which have been produced with recombinant DNA technology. Examples of agents used in immunotherapy include interferons and interleukins (ILs). Targeted therapies include monoclonal antibodies, tyrosine kinase inhibitors, proteosome inhibitors, and others.

❹ Many cancers appear to be eliminated by surgery or radiation. However, the high incidence of later recurrence implies that the primary tumor began to metastasize before it was removed. These early metastases are too small to detect with currently available diagnostic tests and are known as micrometastases. Adjuvant therapy is defined as the use of systemic agents to eradicate micrometastatic disease following localized modalities such as surgery or radiation or both. The goal of systemic therapy given in this setting is to reduce subsequent recurrence rates and prolong long-term survival. Thus, adjuvant therapy is given to patients with potentially curable malignancies who have no clinically detectable disease after surgery or radiation. Because adjuvant therapy is given at a time that the cancer is undetectable (i.e., no measurable disease), its effectiveness cannot be measured by response rates; instead, it is evaluated by recurrence rates and survival. The value of adjuvant therapy is best established in colorectal and breast cancers. Drug therapy may also be given in the neoadjuvant or preoperative setting. The goals in this instance are to make other treatment modalities more effective by reducing tumor burden and to destroy micrometastases. For example, in head and neck cancer, neoadjuvant chemotherapy is employed in an attempt to shrink large tumors and to make them more amenable to later surgical resection, and possibly spare critical organs, such as the larynx.

The management of most types of cancer involves the use of combined modalities. Early stage breast cancer is a good example of the use of a combined-modality approach. The primary tumor is removed surgically, and radiation therapy is delivered to the remaining breast (after lumpectomy) or to the axilla (if there is marked lymph node involvement). Adjuvant therapy (chemotherapy, targeted therapy, and/or hormonal therapy) is then administered to eradicate any micrometastatic disease.

TREATMENT

Principles of Drug Therapy

■ PURPOSES OF CHEMOTHERAPY

The era of modern cancer chemotherapy was born in 1941, when Goodman and Gilman first administered nitrogen mustard to patients with lymphoma.[16] Since then, numerous antineoplastic agents have been developed, and a variety of chemotherapy regimens have been investigated in every type of cancer. Table 130–7 lists tumors and their responsiveness to chemotherapy.[6,17] Cancer chemotherapy may be indicated as a primary, palliative, adjuvant, or neoadjuvant treatment modality. Treatment with cytotoxic drugs is the primary curative modality for a few diseases, including leukemias, lymphomas, choriocarcinomas, and testicular cancer. Most solid tumors are not curable with chemotherapy alone, either because of the biology of the tumor or because of advanced disease at presentation. Chemotherapy in this setting is often initiated for palliative purposes. It is often possible to decrease tumor size or to retard growth enough to reduce untoward symptoms caused by the tumor. Adjuvant and neoadjuvant chemotherapy are defined in the previous section.

MOLECULAR AND CELLULAR BASIS FOR DRUG THERAPY

PRINCIPLES OF TUMOR GROWTH

The study of tumor growth forms the foundation for many of the basic principles of modern cancer chemotherapy. The growth of most tumors is illustrated by the gompertzian tumor growth curve (Fig. 130–4).[6,17,18] Gompertz was an insurance actuary who described the relationship between age and expected death. This mathematical

TABLE 130-7 The Role of Chemotherapy in the Treatment of Cancer

Chemotherapy used alone with curative intent	
Acute lymphocytic leukemia	Acute myelogenous leukemia
Burkitt's lymphoma	Diffuse large cell lymphoma
Hodgkin's lymphoma	Testicular cancer
Choriocarcinoma (gestational trophoblastic neoplasm)	
Chemotherapy used as adjuvant therapy with curative intent	
Breast cancer	Colorectal cancer
Ewing's sarcoma	Osteosarcoma
Wilms tumor	Ovarian cancer
Chemotherapy used as neoadjuvant therapy	
Anal carcinoma[a]	Bladder cancer
Breast cancer (locally advanced)[a]	Cervical cancer
Esophageal cancer	Head and neck cancers[a]
Osteosarcoma[a]	Rectal cancer
Soft tissue sarcoma[a]	
Chemotherapy used to palliate symptoms in advanced disease	
Bladder cancer[a]	Brain tumors
Breast cancer[a]	Carcinoid tumors
Cervical cancer	Chronic lymphocytic leukemia
Chronic myelogenous leukemia[a]	Colorectal cancer[a]
Endometrial cancer	Esophageal cancer
Gastric cancer	Head and neck cancers
Hairy cell leukemia[a]	Kaposi's sarcoma
Indolent lymphomas	Metastatic melanoma
Multiple myeloma[a]	Mycosis fungoides
Neuroblastoma[a]	Non–small cell lung cancer
Osteosarcoma	Ovarian cancer[a]
Pancreatic cancer	Prostate cancer
Small cell lung cancer[a]	Soft-tissue sarcoma
Chemotherapy has little or no effect on palliation	
Hepatocellular cancer	Renal cell carcinoma
Thyroid cancer	

[a]Significant increase in survival is achieved.
Adapted from Cotran et al.[6] and Buick.[17]

model also approximates tumor cell proliferation. In the early stages, tumor growth is exponential, which means that the tumor takes a constant amount of time to double its size. During this early phase, a large portion of the tumor cells is actively dividing. This population of cells is called the *growth fraction*. The doubling time, or time required for the tumor to double in size, is very short. Because most anticancer drugs have greater effect on rapidly dividing cells, tumors are most sensitive to the effects of chemotherapy when the tumor is small and the growth fraction is high. However, as the tumor grows, the doubling time is slowed.[17,18] The growth fraction is decreased, probably owing to the tumor outgrowing its blood and nutrient supply or the inability of blood and nutrients to diffuse throughout the tumor mass. Wide variability exists in measured doubling times for different cancers. The doubling time of most solid tumors is about 2 to 3 months. However, some tumors have doubling times of only days (e.g., aggressive lymphomas) and others have even longer doubling times (e.g., some salivary gland tumors).[6]

Figure 130–4 also illustrates the impact of tumor burden. It takes about 10^9 cancer cells (1-g mass, 1 cm in diameter) for a tumor to be clinically detectable by palpation or radiography. Such a tumor has undergone about 30 doublings in cell number. It only takes 10 additional doublings for this 1-g mass to reach 1 kg in size. A tumor possessing 10^{12} cancer cells (1-kg mass) is considered lethal. Thus a tumor is clinically undetectable for most of its life span. Tumor burden also impacts response to chemotherapy. The cell kill hypothesis states that a certain percentage of cancer cells (not a certain number of cells) will be killed with each course of chemotherapy. For example, if a tumor consists of 1,000 cancer cells and the chemotherapy regimen kills 90% of the cells, then 10% or 100 cancer cells remain. The second chemotherapy course kills another 90% of cells, and again only 10% or 10 cells remain. According to this hypothesis, the tumor burden will never reach zero. Tumors consisting of less than 10^4 cells are believed to be small enough for elimination by host factors, including immunologic mechanisms, and these factors must be in place for a cure to be possible. The limitations of this theory are that it assumes all cancers are equally responsive and that drug resistance and metastases do not occur.[1,6,17,18]

TUMOR PROLIFERATION

Both cancer cells and normal cells reproduce in a series of steps known as the cell cycle. Figure 130–5 depicts the cell cycle and the phases of activity for commonly used antineoplastic agents.[17,18] The first phase

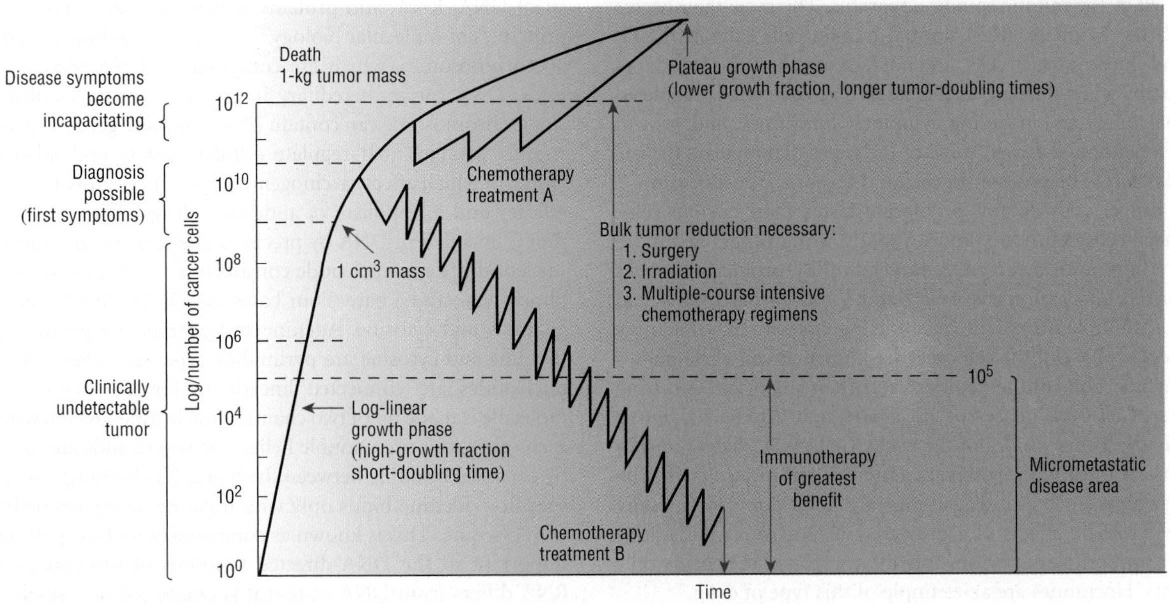

FIGURE 130-4. Gompertzian kinetics tumor-growth curve: relationship to symptoms, diagnosis, and various treatment regimens. *(Reproduced with permission from Buick.[17])*

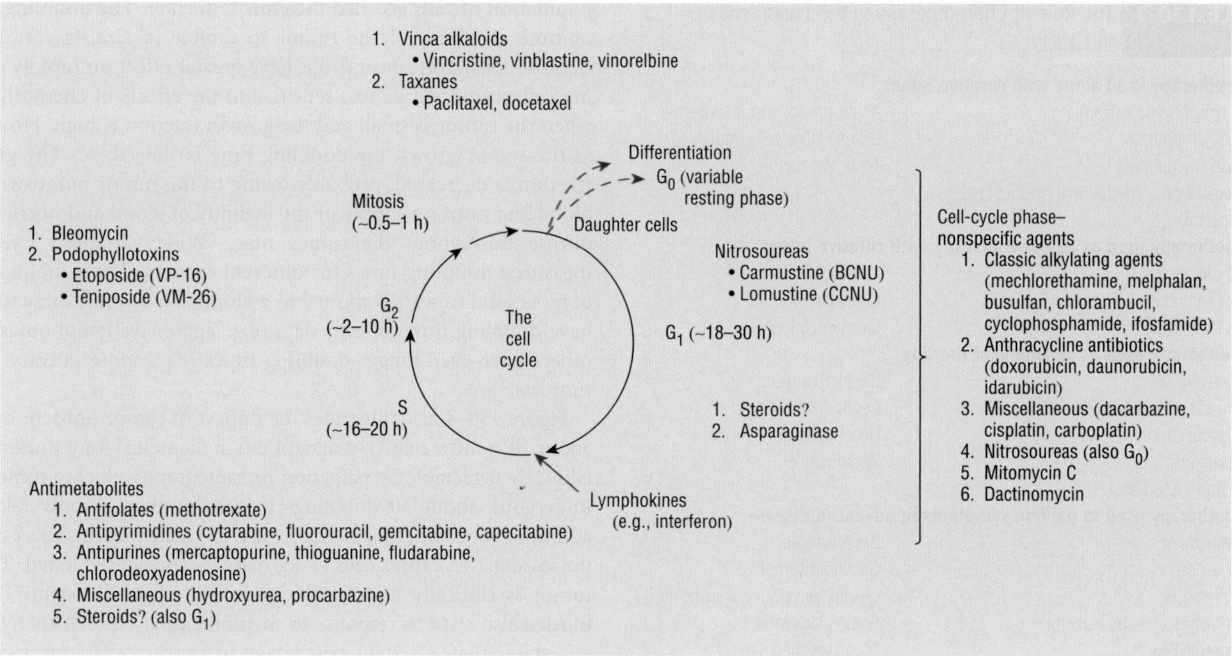

FIGURE 130-5. Cell-cycle activity for anticancer drugs. Cell-cycle phase-specific agents appear to be most active during a particular phase, but may also be active in another phase. Cell-cycle phase-nonspecific agents may have greater activity in one phase than another, but not to the degree of cell-cycle (phase)-specific agents. In many cases, it is likely that drug cytotoxicity involves multiple intracellular sites of action and may not be linked to specific cell-cycle events.

is mitosis (M). Mitosis lasts for about 30 to 60 minutes and during this phase, cell division occurs. After mitosis, the cell might enter a dormant phase (G_0), or might proceed to the first gap phase (G_1). G_0 is the largest variable in the cell cycle, and during this resting phase, the cell is not actively committed to cell division. Some stimulus causes the cell to enter the first gap phase (G_1). During G_1, the cell prepares for DNA synthesis by manufacturing necessary enzymes. DNA synthesis (S) occurs next, and this phase lasts 10 to 20 hours. The percentage of cells in the S phase can be measured by flow cytometry and is an indicator of the rate of tumor-cell proliferation. Tumors with a high percentage of S-phase cells are aggressively growing. The synthesis phase is followed by a second gap or premitotic phase (G_2), lasting 2 to 10 hours. During this second gap, the cell prepares for mitosis by producing ribonucleic acid (RNA) and specialized proteins, as well as the mitotic spindle apparatus. The cycle then begins again with the M phase. Most normal human cells exist in the G_0 phase, and most cancer cells are not sensitive to the effects of chemotherapy when they are in this stage. The cell cycle is regulated by external mitogens, including cytokines, hormones, and growth factors. As mentioned earlier, some of the genes that regulate the cell cycle are known to be protooncogenes and tumor suppressor genes.

❺ All cancer cells do not proliferate faster than normal cells; some cancer cells reproduce more rapidly while others are more indolent. Many anticancer drugs target rapidly proliferating cells (both normal and cancerous cells), and these agents may act at selective or multiple sites of the cell cycle. Agents with major activity in a particular phase of the cell cycle are known as cell-cycle phase-specific agents. The antimetabolites exert their major effect during the S phase. Cell-cycle phase-specific agents may also be active to a lesser extent in other phases of the cycle. Cell-cycle phase-nonspecific agents are those with significant activity in multiple phases. The alkylating agents, such as nitrogen mustard, are examples. In many cases, the cytotoxic effects of a drug may result from interactions with other intracellular activities and are not related to specific cell-cycle events. Hormones are an example of this type of drug.

Knowledge of cell-cycle specificity has been applied to the scheduling of chemotherapy administration. By definition, cell-cycle phase-specific agents exert their major activity when cells are in a particular phase of the cell cycle. At any given time, the heterogeneous cell populations within a tumor are at various phases in the cell cycle. By giving phase-specific agents as a continuous infusion or in multiple repeated fractions, clinicians can theoretically target more cells as they progress into the drug-sensitive phase. Thus cell-cycle phase-specific agents are also termed *schedule dependent.* In contrast, cell-cycle phase-nonspecific drugs are active in many phases, and consequently are not schedule dependent. The activity of this group of drugs depends on the dose, and these drugs are termed *dose dependent.*

MOLECULAR BIOLOGY

Because many antineoplastic agents interfere with the cellular synthesis of DNA, RNA, and proteins, it is important to review the basic principles of molecular biology.[3,19] Each normal human cell contains 46 chromosomes, which are composed of DNA (deoxyribonucleic acid). DNA carries hereditary information in units called genes. A single chromosome can contain 20,000 or more genes. Genes code for specific proteins that regulate cellular activity and inherited traits (some of which affect carcinogenesis and cancer growth, as well as the efficacy and metabolism of anticancer drugs). The genetic information is encoded in DNA by precise sequencing of subunits known as nucleotides. Each nucleotide consists of a sugar (deoxyribose), phosphoric acid, and a base. Four bases exist in DNA: adenine, thymine, guanine, and cytosine. Adenine and guanine are purine-type bases; thymine and cytosine are pyrimidine-type bases (Fig. 130–6). These nucleotides are connected linearly to form a chain. Each DNA molecule is made up of two chains of nucleotides, which wind around each other to form a double helix. The two strands are held together by chemical bonding between the bases. The bonding process is very specific—adenine binds only with thymine, and guanine binds only with cytosine. This is known as complementary base pairing. RNA is important in the DNA-directed synthesis of proteins or enzymes. RNA differs from DNA in that it is composed of a single strand of nucleotides, the sugar is ribose, and the base uracil is substituted for thymine. There are three known types of RNA: messenger RNA (mRNA), transfer RNA (tRNA), and ribosomal RNA (rRNA).

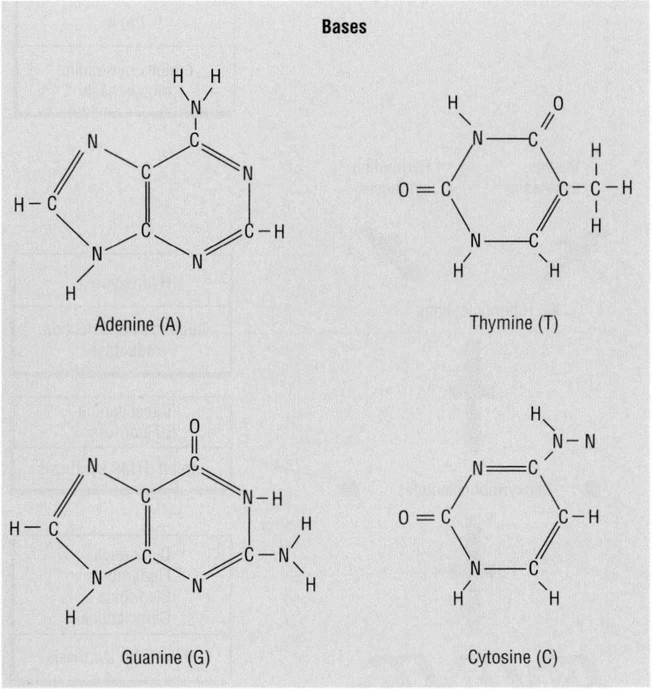

FIGURE 130-6. Structures of DNA constituents.

DNA SYNTHESIS

During the DNA synthesis phase, which takes place in the cell nucleus, the DNA unwinds and exposes its nucleotides. When DNA unwinds for replication or protein synthesis, only the portion of the molecule containing the needed nucleotides needs to be exposed. Rather than unwinding the entire strand, topoisomerase I and II enzymes cleave the DNA strands to facilitate unwinding of the section that is needed. The enzyme DNA polymerase matches free complementary nucleotides from the environment to the exposed nucleotides of the DNA. The newly created strands rewind, resulting in two complete double helices. The topoisomerase enzymes are also responsible for resealing the cleaved DNA strands.

PROTEIN SYNTHESIS

The synthesis of proteins is a more complex process. Proteins consist of chains of amino acids in very specific sequences. As in DNA synthesis, the double helix must unwind. However, in protein synthesis, only the portion of the DNA molecule that codes for the desired protein is exposed. The enzyme RNA polymerase matches free complementary RNA nucleotides to the exposed DNA nucleotides, and the resultant chain of nucleotides is called mRNA. This process is called transcription. The mRNA travels to ribosomes in the cytoplasm, where protein synthesis occurs. Each three nucleotides of the mRNA chain compose a codon, whose sequence is specific for a particular amino acid. The codon is recognized by tRNA, which then carries the amino acid to the ribosome, where it is added to the growing peptide chain. This process is known as translation. The completed protein is then ready for its intended use as an enzyme or as a structural component.

CLINICAL PHARMACOLOGY OF CHEMOTHERAPY AND ENDOCRINE AGENTS

Agents used in cancer chemotherapy are commonly categorized by their mechanism of action or by their origin. The alkylating agents exert their effects on DNA and protein synthesis by binding to DNA and preventing the unwinding of the DNA molecule. The antimetabolites resemble naturally occurring nuclear structural components ("metabolites"), such as the nucleotide bases, or inhibit enzymes involved in the synthesis of DNA and proteins. Antitumor antibiotics derive their name from their source; they are fermentation products of *Streptomyces* species. Figure 130–7 shows the sites of action of common categories of antineoplastic agents. The following section addresses these and other classes of agents used in the treatment of cancer. The clinical uses, mechanisms, side effects, and practical patient management suggestions for commonly used agents in each class are detailed. Table 130–8 summarizes dose modifications of individual agents.

ANTIMETABOLITES

Fluorinated Pyrimidines

Fluorouracil Originally synthesized in the late 1950s, fluorouracil (5-FU) is a fluorinated analog of the naturally occurring pyrimidine uracil. It is a prodrug and must be metabolized to the nucleotide form, fluorodeoxyuridine monophosphate, to be active. In the presence of folates, fluorodeoxyuridine monophosphate binds tightly to and interferes with the function of thymidylate synthase. This enzyme is required for synthesis of thymidine, one of the four essential building blocks of DNA. Another metabolite of 5-FU, the triphosphate nucleotide, is incorporated into RNA as a false base, and interferes with its function. Interference with both thymidine formation and RNA function is important in producing the cytotoxic effects of 5-FU. Although 5-FU nucleotides can also be incorporated directly into DNA and affect its stability, the contribution to cell damage remains unclear. The method of administration influences the mechanism of action, with thymidylate synthesis inhibition playing a greater role in continuous-infusion regimens, and incorporation into RNA being more important for intermittent bolus schedules.[20]

Several pharmacologic strategies have been attempted to increase the cytotoxicity of 5-FU against tumor cells and to decrease its toxicity to normal cells. The most successful of these attempts at biochemical modulation is combinations of fluorouracil and the reduced folate leucovorin. Folates increase the stability of the fluorodeoxyuridine monophosphate–thymidylate synthase complex, thereby increasing the cytotoxicity and clinical usefulness of the drug.[20]

Oral Fluoropyrimidines Capecitabine is an orally active pyrimidine analog of uracil and is a prodrug of 5-FU. Because capecitabine is enzymatically converted to 5-FU, it shares the same mechanisms of action. It generates higher levels of 5-FU selectively within some tumors compared with healthy tissues. Because chronic twice-daily oral dosing of capecitabine produces sustained 5-FU levels similar to continuous intravenous infusions of 5-FU, the toxicity pattern is similar to that of 5-FU infusions.[20,21] Several other oral fluoropyrimidine products are under investigation.

Cytidine Analogs

Cytarabine Cytarabine (ara-C) is an arabinose analog of cytosine. Cytarabine was originally isolated from sponges, but is now produced synthetically. Ara-C is phosphorylated to its active triphosphate form (ara-CTP) within tumor cells. Ara-CTP inhibits DNA polymerase, an enzyme responsible for strand elongation. It is also incorporated directly into DNA, where it inhibits the replication of DNA and acts as a chain terminator to prevent DNA elongation. Activation of ara-C is opposed by deaminase enzymes, particularly cytidine deaminase, which degrades ara-C to an inactive form, ara-U.[20,22,23]

Cytidine deaminase levels are very low in the CNS. Cytotoxic concentrations are maintained in the CNS for several hours after intrathecal administration of traditional cytarabine formulations,

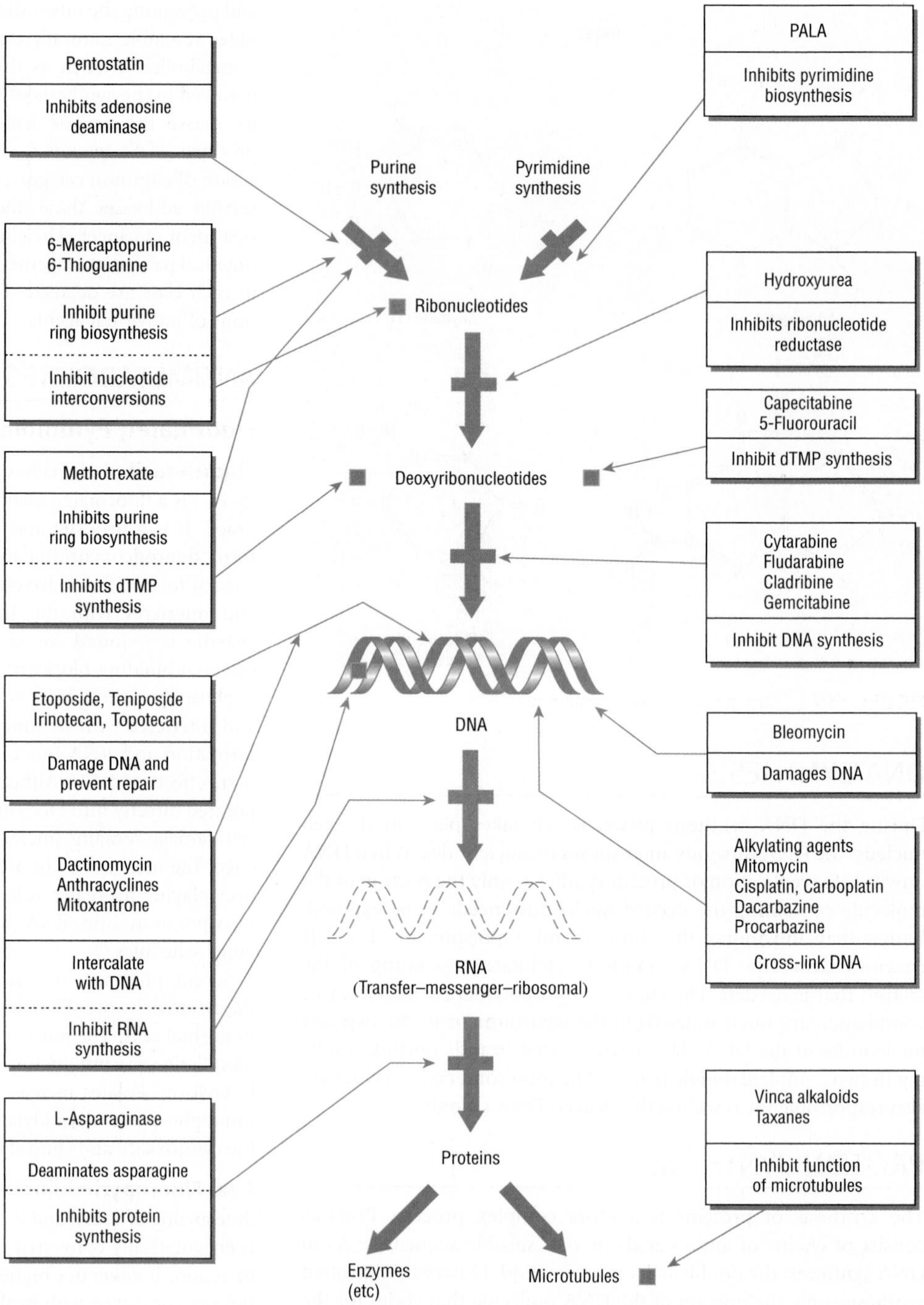

FIGURE 130-7. Mechanisms of action of commonly used antineoplastic agents. (dTMP, deoxythymidylic acid; PALA, *N*-phosphonacetyl-L-aspartate.) *(From Chabner BA, Ryan DP, Paz-Ares L, Garcia-Carbonero R, Calabresi P. Antineoplastic agents. In: Hardman JG, Limbird LE, Gilman AG, eds. Goodman & Gilman's The Pharmacologic Basis of Therapeutics, 10th ed. New York: McGraw-Hill, 2001: 1381.)*

and for more than 2 weeks following administration of depot formulated cytarabine intrathecally.

The toxicity of cytarabine is dose dependent. The most characteristic toxicity of high-dose ara-C (>1 g/m^2 per dose) regimens is a cerebellar syndrome of dysarthria, nystagmus, and ataxia. Risk of CNS toxicity is strongly correlated with advanced age and renal dysfunction. Renal insufficiency permits accumulation of high levels of ara-CTP, which is believed to be neurotoxic. Hepatic dysfunction, high cumulative doses, and bolus dosing may also increase the risks of neurotoxicity.[20,22,23]

Gemcitabine Gemcitabine is a fluorine-substituted deoxycytidine analog related structurally to cytarabine. Its activation and mechanism of action are similar to those of cytarabine. Gemcitabine is incorporated into DNA, where it inhibits DNA polymerase activity. It also inhibits ribonucleotide reductase, which is the enzyme required to convert ribonucleotides into the deoxyribonucleotide forms required for both DNA synthesis and repair. Compared with cytarabine, gemcitabine achieves intracellular concentrations about 20 times higher than does ara-C, secondary to increased penetration of cell membranes, and greater affinity for the activating enzyme deoxycytidine kinase. Gemcitabine that is incorporated into DNA has a prolonged intracellular half-life. Its stereo configuration causes another normal base pair to be added next to the fraudulent gemcitabine base pair in the DNA strand. This "masked chain termination" protects the gemcitabine from excision and elimination.[20,22,24]

Azacytidine and Decitabine Azacytidine was approved in 2004 and decitabine in 2006 for the treatment of patients with myelodysplastic syndrome, a disorder of hematopoietic cell maturation that can progress to acute myeloid leukemia. Both of these agents are nucleoside analogs, and they are believed to exert their pharmacodynamic effects by direct incorporation into DNA and inhibition of DNA methyltransferase which cause hypomethylation of DNA. Cellular differentiation and apoptosis are believed to result from this effect. The cytotoxicity of these agents may also be attributed to

TABLE 130-8 Empiric Dose Modifications in Patients with Renal and Hepatic Disease[a]

Agent	Organ Dysfunction	Suggested Dose Modification
Methotrexate, cisplatin	Renal impairment	In proportion to lowered creatinine clearance (normal = 60 mL/min per m^2) Cl_{cr} <10 mL/min, contraindicated
Carboplatin	Renal impairment	See Table 130-9 for dosing guideline
Cyclophosphamide	Renal failure	Cl_{cr} <25 mL/min; reduce dose by 50%
Bleomycin	Renal failure	Cl_{cr} <25 mL/min; reduce dose by 50% to 75%
Capecitabine	Renal impairment	Cl_{cr} 30–50 mL/min; reduce dose by 25% Cl_{cr} <30 mL/min, contraindicated
Cytarabine (high dose: >1 g/m^2)	Renal impairment	For creatinine 1.5–1.9 mg/dL, reduce dose by 50% For creatinine >2.0 mg/dL, reduce dose by 95%
Topotecan	Renal impairment	Cl_{cr} 20–39 mL/min; reduce dose by 25%
Cladribine, fludarabine	Renal impairment	In proportion to lowered creatinine clearance
Hydroxyurea, doxorubicin, daunorubicin, vincristine, vinblastine	Hepatic dysfunction	For bilirubin >1.5 mg/dL, reduce dose by 50%; for bilirubin >3.0 mg/dL, reduce dose by 75%
Vinorelbine	Hepatic dysfunction	For bilirubin >2.0 mg/dL, reduce dose by 50% For bilirubin >3.0 mg/dL, reduce dose by 75%
Gemcitabine	Hepatic dysfunction	For bilirubin >1.6 mg/dL, reduce dose by 20%
Idarubicin, mitoxantrone	Hepatic dysfunction	Consider dose reductions; no published guidelines available
Docetaxel	Hepatic dysfunction	Contraindicated in patient with bilirubin >1.5 × ULN or transaminases >1.5 × ULN or alkaline phosphatase >2.5 × ULN
Irinotecan	Hepatic dysfunction	Contraindicated in patients with bilirubin >2 mg/dL, or transaminases >3 × ULN (without liver metastases), >5 × ULN (with liver metastases)
Paclitaxel	Hepatic dysfunction	Reduce dose by ≥50% for moderate to severe increases in bilirubin or transaminases

Cl_{cr}, creatinine clearance; ULN, upper limit of normal laboratory values.
[a]Only approximate guidelines can be given. See text for explanations and limitations.
Adapted from Chabner[1] and package inserts.

the formation of covalent adducts between DNA methyltransferase and active drug being incorporated into DNA, particularly in cells actively dividing. Hypomethylation of DNA also appears to normalize the function of genes that control cell differentiation and proliferation, promoting normal cell maturation.[25,26]

These agents have demonstrated efficacy in slowing the progression of myelodysplastic syndrome to acute myelogenous leukemia (AML), reducing transfusion requirements and allowing for the improvement of normal hematopoiesis over time. The primary toxicity is myelosuppression, particularly during early phases of treatment as the malignant clone driving myelodysplastic syndrome is cleared from the bone marrow and normal hematopoiesis is slowly restored. Mild gastrointestinal toxicity and infectious complications are also reported with these agents.

Purines and Purine Antimetabolites

6-Mercaptopurine and 6-Thioguanine Some of the oldest and newest anticancer agents are synthetic analogs of the naturally occurring purines guanine and adenine. 6-Mercaptopurine (6-MP) was the first purine analog to be used in cancer chemotherapy. 6-Thioguanine is the two-amino analog of 6-MP. Both drugs are rapidly converted to ribonucleotides that inhibit purine biosynthesis. They also undergo purine interconversion reactions needed to supply purine precursors for synthesis of nucleic acids. Clinical cross-resistance is generally observed.[20]

6-MP depends on xanthine oxidase for an initial oxidation step. Its metabolism is markedly decreased by concomitant administration of the xanthine oxidase inhibitor allopurinol, and serious toxicity may result. Oral 6-MP doses must be reduced when allopurinol is administered together with 6-MP.[20]

Fludarabine Monophosphate Fludarabine monophosphate is an analog of the purine adenine. Like cytarabine, fludarabine interferes with DNA polymerase, causing chain termination. Unlike ara-C, fludarabine is also incorporated into RNA, resulting in inhibited transcription. The usual dose-limiting toxicity is myelosuppression. Fludarabine is also immunosuppressive, with associated opportunistic infections resulting from fludarabine's effect on T cells and a subsequent decrease in CD4 counts; prophylactic antibiotics and antiviral medications are recommended and should continue until CD4 counts normalize.[20,27]

Cladribine and Pentostatin Cladribine and pentostatin are purine nucleoside analogs with slightly different mechanisms of action. Cladribine is resistant to inactivation by adenosine deaminase and triphosphorylated to an active form that is incorporated into DNA, resulting in inhibition of DNA synthesis and early chain termination. Cladribine's antitumor activity is unusual for an antimetabolite in that it affects both actively dividing and resting cancer cells. Pentostatin is a potent inhibitor of adenosine deaminase. Adenosine deaminase is an enzyme critical in purine base metabolism and is found in high concentrations in lymphatic tissue. Like fludarabine, these agents possess immunosuppressive effects that place patients at risk for serious opportunistic infections.[20,22]

Antifolates

Folate vitamins are essential cofactors in DNA synthesis. They carry one-carbon groups in transfer reactions that are required for purine and thymidylic acid synthesis, and, in turn, for formation of DNA and for cell division. Natural folates circulating in the blood have a single glutamic acid group, but within cells they are converted to polyglutamates, which are more efficient cofactors and which are preferentially retained inside the cells.[28]

Dietary folates must be chemically reduced to their tetrahydro forms, with four hydrogens on the pteridine ring, to be active. The enzyme responsible for this reduction is dihydrofolate reductase (DHFR), a key enzyme whose actions are inhibited by methotrexate and other antifolates. The result of this inhibition is depletion of intracellular pools of reduced folates (tetrahydrofolates) essential for thymidylate and purine synthesis. Lack of either thymidine or purines prevents synthesis of DNA. The DHFR-mediated effects of antifolate drugs on normal and probably also on cancerous cells may be neutralized by supplying reduced folates exogenously. The reduced folate used clinically for "rescue" is leucovorin (folinic acid), which bypasses the metabolic block induced by DHFR inhibitors.[28]

Methotrexate The folic acid analog methotrexate (MTX) is the best understood of all drugs in the broad category of antimetabolites. It has been in clinical use for more than 50 years. Like physiologic folates, MTX is transported intracellularly by an active transport system. In high doses, passive diffusion may overcome tumor cell resistance caused by saturated active transport systems. Resistance to the antifolates can also be caused by amplification of DHFR. Other potential causes of resistance are slow rates of thymidylate synthesis, decreased affinity of DHFR for MTX, and lack of polyglutamation within tumor cells. Polyglutamated forms of folates are better retained within cells. Malignant cells may achieve greater MTX polyglutamate levels than normal cells, which may, in part, explain the selective effects of MTX on malignant versus normal cells.[28]

Accurate and readily available assays for serum MTX levels have made therapeutic drug monitoring of MTX a valuable clinical tool. The threshold for cytotoxic effects of MTX is approximately 5×10^{-8} M. Toxicity and efficacy relates not only to peak concentrations, but more importantly, to time that concentrations remain above this threshold level. For MTX doses requiring leucovorin rescue (generally doses greater than 1,000 mg/m^2), leucovorin must be administered until levels fall below 5×10^{-8} M. Therapeutic drug monitoring is also an effective means of increasing the likelihood of therapeutic success, by individualizing doses based on target levels.[28]

Pemetrexed Pemetrexed is a multitargeted antifolate that inhibits at least three biosynthetic pathways in thymidine and purine synthesis. In addition to inhibition of DHFR, it also inhibits thymidine synthase and glycinamide ribonucleotide formyltransferase, decreasing the risk of development of drug resistance. Severe hematologic toxicity and deaths associated with neutropenic sepsis have been reported in clinical trials with pemetrexed. Elevated baseline cystathionine or homocysteine concentrations correlated with this unexpected toxicity. Routine supplementation of folic acid and vitamin B_{12} lowers levels of these substances and lowers the risk of mortality related to neutropenic sepsis. The FDA labeled use of pemetrexed requires administration of folic acid and vitamin B_{12} throughout the duration of treatment with the drug.[28]

MICROTUBULE-TARGETING DRUGS

Vinca Alkaloids

Vincristine, vinblastine, and vinorelbine are natural alkaloids derived from the periwinkle (vinca) plant. They act as mitotic inhibitors, or "spindle poisons." Although the alkaloids are very similar structurally, they have different activities and patterns of toxicity. Vinorelbine and vinblastine are associated with dose-limiting myelosuppression, whereas vincristine causes mild myelosuppressive effects but is more neurotoxic.

Vinca alkaloids bind to tubulin, the structural protein that polymerizes to form microtubules. These are the hollow tubes that make up the mitotic spindle and that are also important in nerve conduction and neurotransmission. Vinca alkaloids disrupt the normal balance between polymerization and depolymerization of microtubules, inhibiting assembly of microtubules and disrupting microtubule dynamics. This interferes with formation of the mitotic spindle and causes cells to accumulate in mitosis. They also disturb a variety of microtubule-related processes in cells, and induce apoptosis. Resistance to the vinca alkaloids develops primarily from P-glycoprotein–mediated multidrug resistance, which decreases drug accumulation and retention within tumor cells.[29]

Taxanes

Paclitaxel and docetaxel are taxane plant alkaloids with antimitotic activity. Paclitaxel was isolated from the bark of the Pacific yew tree, *Taxus brevifolia*, but is now produced semisynthetically from the needles of the European yew, *Taxus baccata*. Docetaxel is a semisynthetic taxoid extracted from 10-deacetyl baccatin III, a noncytotoxic precursor found in the renewable needle biomass of yew plants.[29]

Paclitaxel and docetaxel both act by binding to tubulin, but unlike the vincas do not interfere with tubulin assembly. Instead, the taxanes promote microtubule assembly and therefore interfere with microtubule disassembly. They induce tubulin polymerization, resulting in formation of inappropriately stable, nonfunctional microtubules. The stability of the microtubules damages cells, because the dynamics of microtubule-dependent structures required for mitosis and other cellular functions are disrupted. Taxanes also have some nonmitotic actions that can promote cancer cell death, such as inhibition of angiogenesis. Resistance to the antitumor effects of the taxanes is attributable to alterations in tubulin or tubulin binding sites, or to P-glycoprotein–mediated multidrug resistance. Although paclitaxel and docetaxel have very similar mechanisms of action, cross-resistance between the two agents is incomplete.[29] Myelosuppression is common with both agents but other adverse effects can differ. Increased fluid retention is seen with docetaxel, whereas increased neurotoxicity and hypersensitivity reactions are seen with paclitaxel.[30]

To circumvent the hypersensitivity reactions with paclitaxel, and perhaps increase the efficacy, paclitaxel was recently formulated to be bound to albumin (nab-paclitaxel). This new dosage form is devoid of the Cremophor excipient that is believed to mediate the hypersensitivity reactions and exacerbate myelosuppression with the conventional formulation. This formulation appears to be selectively activated by tumor cells to the active paclitaxel compound.[31] In comparative clinical trials, this novel compound has shown comparable activity to original formulations of paclitaxel with a lower incidence of hypersensitivity reactions. Peripheral neuropathies remain a common adverse effect with this formulation.

Estramustine

Estramustine is an unusual drug because it structurally combines the alkylating agent *nor*-nitrogen mustard with the hormone estradiol. It was designed with the intent that the estradiol portion of the molecule would facilitate uptake of the alkylating agent into hormone-sensitive prostate cancer cells. Despite the inclusion of an alkylator, estramustine does not function in vivo as an alkylating agent. Estrogens are released after its administration and are responsible for most of the toxicity of estramustine, but are not believed to contribute to its cytotoxic effect. In the mid-1980s, estramustine was redefined as an antimicrotubule agent. It binds covalently to microtubule-associated proteins that are part of the structural support for microtubules. The binding causes the separation of microtubule-associated proteins from the microtubules, inhibiting microtubule assembly and eventually causing their disassembly.[32]

TOPOISOMERASE INHIBITORS

Topoisomerases are essential enzymes involved in maintaining DNA topologic structure during replication and transcription. DNA topoisomerase enzymes relieve torsional strain during DNA unwinding by producing strand breaks. They cleave DNA strands and form intermediates with the strands, producing a gap through which DNA strands can pass, then reseal the strand breaks. Topoisomerase I produces single-strand breaks; topoisomerase II produces double-strand breaks.[33] Several important anticancer agents target topoisomerase enzymes: camptothecins, anthracyclines, and the epipodophyllotoxins.

Camptothecin Derivatives

Camptothecin, a plant alkaloid derived from *Camptotheca acuminata*, is a potent inhibitor of DNA topoisomerase I. Clinical trials failed to show expected antitumor activity, and the drug produced severe, unpredictable toxicity. The camptothecin analogs irinotecan and topotecan were synthesized to reduce toxicity and improve therapeutic effects. Both topotecan and irinotecan, through its active metabolite SN-38, inhibit the activity of the topoisomerase I enzymes. Topoisomerase I enzymes stabilize DNA single-strand breaks and inhibit strand resealing.[33–35]

Etoposide and Teniposide

Etoposide and teniposide are semisynthetic podophyllotoxin derivatives. Podophyllin is extracted from the mayapple or mandrake plant. Like the vinca alkaloids, podophyllin itself binds to tubulin and interferes with microtubule formation. Unlike the parent compound, however, etoposide and teniposide damage tumor cells by causing strand breakage through inhibiting topoisomerase II.[33] Resistance may be caused by differences in topoisomerase II levels, by increased cell ability to repair strand breaks, or by increased levels of P-glycoproteins. Etoposide and teniposide are usually clinically cross-resistant. They are cell-cycle phase-specific and arrest cells in the S or early G_2 phase. As a result, activity is much greater when they are administered in divided doses over several days, rather than in large single doses.

Anthracene Derivatives

The most widely used and best understood anthracene derivative is doxorubicin, also commonly known by its earliest trade name, Adriamycin or "Adria." Other members of the anthracene group include daunorubicin (daunomycin), idarubicin, epirubicin, and mitoxantrone. All of these agents, except mitoxantrone, are anthracyclines and share a common, four-membered anthracene ring complex with an attached aglycone or sugar portion. The ring complex is a chromophore and accounts for the intense colors of these compounds. Doxorubicin differs from its parent compound daunorubicin by the addition of a hydroxyl group on the attached sugar, and it is sometimes referred to as hydroxydaunorubicin. A hydroxyl group on epirubicin is in the *epi* conformation compared with doxorubicin (epidoxorubicin), and idarubicin is demethoxydaunorubicin. Mitoxantrone is an anthracenedione rather than an anthracycline, and has no sugar group attached to the three-membered anthracene ring complex.[33,36]

Doxorubicin, Daunorubicin, Idarubicin, and Epirubicin

Anthracyclines have been classified as antitumor antibiotics, but it is more accurate to refer to them as intercalating topoisomerase inhibitors. Intercalating agents are compounds that insert or stack between base pairs of DNA. Although it is well established that the planar groups of the anthracene ring complex do intercalate with DNA, causing structural changes that interfere with DNA and RNA synthesis, this is not their primary mechanism of cytotoxicity. The anthracyclines are primarily topoisomerase II inhibitors, producing double-strand DNA breaks.[33,36]

The anthracyclines also undergo electron reductions to reactive compounds that can damage DNA and cell membranes. Free radicals formed from reduction of the anthracyclines first donate electrons to oxygen to make superoxide, which can react with itself to make hydrogen peroxide. Cleavage of hydrogen peroxide produces the highly reactive and destructive hydroxyl radical. This last step requires iron, and the anthracyclines are potent iron binders. Iron–anthracycline complexes can bind to DNA and react rapidly with hydrogen peroxide to produce the hydroxyl radicals that actually cleave DNA. Human cells have natural defenses against oxygen radical damage, in the form of enzymes that can convert the radicals to less reactive compounds, or that can repair DNA damage. Differences in distribution of these defensive enzymes may account for the cardiotoxicity of the anthracyclines. For example, cardiac muscle has low levels of defensive enzymes and high levels of enzymes that activate anthracyclines. Oxygen free-radical formation is firmly established as a cause of cardiac damage and extravasation injury, but is not a major mechanism of tumor-cell killing. Resistance to the anthracyclines is usually secondary to P-glycoprotein–dependent multidrug resistance, causing the anthracyclines to be actively pumped out of tumor cells. Altered topoisomerase II activity may also be clinically important.[33,36]

Mitoxantrone The anthracenedione mitoxantrone was synthesized in an attempt to develop agents with comparable antitumor activity to doxorubicin, but with an improved safety profile. Like the anthracyclines, mitoxantrone is an intercalating topoisomerase II inhibitor, but its potential for free-radical formation is much less than that of the anthracyclines. This decreased tendency for free-radical formation may explain the reduced risks of cardiac toxicity and ulceration after extravasation.[33,36]

ALKYLATING AGENTS

The alkylating agents are among the oldest and most useful of antineoplastic drugs. Their clinical use evolved from the observation of bone marrow suppression and lymph node shrinkage in soldiers exposed to sulfur mustard gas warfare during World War I. In an effort to develop similar agents that might be useful in treating cancerous overgrowths of lymphoid tissues, less-reactive derivatives were synthesized. Their effectiveness as anticancer agents was confirmed by clinical trials in the middle 1940s.

All of the alkylating agents work through the covalent bonding of highly reactive alkyl groups or substituted alkyl groups with nucleophilic groups of proteins and nucleic acids. Some alkylating agents react directly with biologic molecules; others form an intermediate compound that reacts with the targets. The most common binding site for alkylating agents is the seven-nitrogen group of guanine. These covalent interactions result in cross-linking between two DNA strands or between two bases in the same strand of DNA. Reactions between DNA and RNA and between drug and proteins may also occur, but the main insult that results in cell death is inhibition of DNA replication, because the interlinked strands do not separate as required. Because the alkylating agents can damage DNA during any phase of the cell cycle, they are not cell-cycle phase specific. However, their greatest effect is seen in rapidly dividing cells.

As a class, alkylators are cytotoxic, mutagenic, teratogenic, carcinogenic, and myelosuppressive. Resistance to these agents can occur from increased DNA repair capabilities, from decreased entry into or accelerated exit from cells, from increased inactivation of the agents inside cells, or from lack of cellular mechanisms to result in cell death following DNA damage. They react with water and are inactivated by hydrolysis, making spontaneous degradation an important component of their elimination.[37]

Cyclophosphamide and Ifosfamide

Cyclophosphamide and ifosfamide are nitrogen mustard derivatives, and are widely used alkylating agents. They are closely related in structure, clinical use, and toxicity. Neither agent is active in its parent form and must be activated by mixed hepatic oxidase enzymes including the cytochrome P450 (CYP) 2B6 and CYP3A4/5 isoenzymes. The active metabolite of cyclophosphamide is phosphoramide mustard. Another metabolite, 4-hydroxycyclophosphamide is cytotoxic, but is not an alkylating agent. Ifosfamide is hepatically activated to ifosfamide mustard. Acrolein, a metabolite of both cyclophosphamide and ifosfamide, has little antitumor activity, but is responsible for the hemorrhagic cystitis of these agents.[37]

Nitrosoureas

The nitrosoureas are alkylating agents characterized by lipophilicity and ability to cross the blood–brain barrier. Carmustine or bischloroethylnitrosourea (BCNU) and lomustine (CCNU) are commercially available. BCNU is available as an intravenous preparation and as a drug-impregnated biodegradable wafer (Gliadel) for direct application to residual tumor tissue following surgical resection of brain tumors. The nitrosoureas decompose to reactive alkylating metabolites and to isocyanate compounds that have several effects on reproducing cells.[37]

Nonclassic Alkylating Agents

Several other cytotoxic agents appear to act as alkylators, although their structures do not include the classic alkylating groups. They are capable of binding covalently to cellular components and include procarbazine, dacarbazine, temozolomide, the heavy metal compounds, and some antitumor antibiotics.[37]

Dacarbazine and Temozolomide Dacarbazine (DTIC) and temozolomide are nonclassic alkylating agents. Both compounds undergo demethylation to the same active intermediate (monomethyl triazeno-imidazole-carboxamide [MTIC]) that interrupts DNA replication by causing methylation of guanine. Unlike dacarbazine, temozolomide does not require the liver for activation, and is chemically degraded to MTIC at physiologic pH. Both drugs inhibit DNA, RNA, and protein synthesis.[37,38]

Important pharmacokinetic differences exist between the two drugs. Dacarbazine is poorly absorbed, and must be administered by intravenous infusion. Temozolomide is rapidly absorbed after oral administration, and is nearly 100% bioavailable when given on a completely empty stomach. Dacarbazine penetrates the CNS poorly, but temozolomide readily crosses the blood–brain barrier, achieving therapeutically active concentrations in cerebrospinal fluid and brain tumor tissues.[37,38]

HEAVY METAL COMPOUNDS

Cisplatin, Carboplatin, and Oxaliplatin

The platinum derivatives—cisplatin, carboplatin, and oxaliplatin—are anticancer agents with remarkable usefulness in cancer treatment. Recognition of cisplatin's cytotoxic activity was the result of a serendipitous observation that bacterial growth in culture was altered when an electric current was delivered to the media through platinum electrodes. The growth change was noted to be similar to that produced by alkylating agents and radiation. It was found that a platinum–chloride complex, now known as cisplatin, generated by the current was responsible for the changes. Carboplatin is a structural analog of cisplatin in which the chloride groups of the parent compound are replaced by a carboxycyclobutane moiety. It shares a similar spectrum of clinical activity with cisplatin, and cross-resistance is common. Oxaliplatin is an organoplatinum compound in which the platinum is complexed with an oxalate ligand as the leaving group and to diaminocyclohexane. Its spectrum of activity differs substantially from the other platinum compounds, and includes notable activity against colorectal cancers.[37,39]

The cytotoxicity of the platinum derivatives depends on platinum binding to DNA and the formation of intrastrand cross-links or adducts between neighboring guanines. These intrastrand links cause a major bending of the DNA. They may cause cellular damage by distorting the normal DNA conformation and preventing bases that are normally paired from lining up with each other. Interstrand cross-links also occur.[37,39]

The cytotoxic form of cisplatin is the aquated species, in which hydroxyl groups or water molecules replace the two chloride groups. This reaction occurs readily in low concentrations of chloride, such as the concentrations present within cells, and produces a positively charged compound that can react with DNA. The aquated species is responsible for both the efficacy and toxicity of cisplatin. Carboplatin also undergoes aquation, but at a slower rate. Oxaliplatin becomes active when the oxalate ligand is displaced in physiologic solutions.[37,39]

TABLE 130-9 Dosing Formulas for Chemotherapy Agents[a]

DuBois and DuBois
BSA (m^2) = $Wt\ (kg)^{0.425} \times Ht\ (cm)^{0.725} \times 0.007184$
Mosteller
BSA (m^2) = $\sqrt{(Ht\ (cm) \times Wt\ (kg)/3600)}$
Calvert (for carboplatin)
Dose (mg)[a] = $AUC^b \times (Cl_{cr}{}^c + 25)$

AUC, area-under-the-curve; BSA, body surface area; Cl_{cr}, creatinine clearance; Ht, height; Wt, weight.
[a]Note that the dose is in total milligrams to be administered, not mg/m².
[b]AUC needs to be stated in the dosing protocol.
[c]Cockcroft and Gault equation used.
Data from Haskell CM. Principles of cancer chemotherapy. In: Haskell CM, ed. Cancer Treatment. 5th ed. Philadelphia: WB Saunders. 2001;62–86.

Resistance to the therapeutic effects of platinum compounds may occur through several mechanisms. The ability to repair platinum-induced DNA damage may be increased, or the agents may be inactivated by increased levels of intracellular glutathione, metallothioneins, or other thiol-containing proteins. Altered uptake into cells may also affect sensitivity to platinum compounds.[37,39]

Cisplatin is a highly toxic antineoplastic agent that can cause serious nephrotoxicity, ototoxicity, peripheral neuropathy, emesis, and anemia. The significant efficacy of cisplatin against many tumor types makes it a valuable agent despite these toxicities, most of which can be prevented or managed with aggressive supportive care measures.[37] In contrast, carboplatin administration is limited by hematologic toxicity. Patients with compromised renal function require dose reductions to limit myelosuppressive toxicity.[37,39] The most widely used dosage schema, the Calvert formula (Table 130–9), uses a target area-under-the-curve and renal function parameters to estimate the carboplatin dose. Carboplatin's potential to cause renal damage, peripheral neuropathy, ototoxicity, and nausea and vomiting is much less than that of comparable cisplatin doses.[37] Oxaliplatin is not nephrotoxic or ototoxic, is moderately emetogenic, but produces peripheral neuropathies and unique cold-induced neuropathies.[40] All of the platinum derivatives have potential to cause hypersensitivity reactions, including anaphylaxis.

ENDOCRINE THERAPIES

Perhaps the earliest successful approach to target the growth processes of cancerous cells was the use of endocrine therapies. Endocrine manipulation is an option for management of cancers from tissues whose growth is under gonadal hormonal control, especially breast, prostate, and endometrial cancers. These cancers may regress if the "feeding" hormone is eliminated or antagonized. Major organ system toxicity is uncommon from hormonal treatment, making it the least toxic of systemic anticancer therapies. Increasingly specific agents such as the selective estrogen receptor modulators and aromatase inhibitors have increased the utility of hormonal therapies in the treatment of cancer.[41–46] These agents are discussed in detail in Chapters 131 and 134.

Corticosteroid hormones are also useful anticancer agents because of their lymphotoxic effects. Their primary use is in management of hematologic malignancies, especially lymphomas, lymphocytic leukemias, and multiple myeloma. In addition to their cytotoxic effects, corticosteroids have many other applications in supportive care of cancer patients. Corticosteroids have diverse toxicities in chronic or high-dose use, but are generally well tolerated in the short-term therapies usually used in cancer patient care.[47]

MISCELLANEOUS AGENTS

Bleomycin

Bleomycin or "bleo" is an antitumor antibiotic. It is a mixture of peptides from fungal *Streptomyces* species, and its strength is expressed in units of drug activity. One unit is roughly equal to 1 mg of polypeptide protein. The predominant peptide is bleomycin A2, which makes up approximately 70% of the commercial product. Bleomycin's cytotoxicity is secondary to DNA strand breakage, or scission, which it produces via free-radical formation. Cytotoxicity depends on binding of an bleomycin–iron complex to DNA. The bleomycin–iron complex then reduces molecular oxygen to free oxygen radicals that cause primarily single-strand breaks in DNA. Bleomycin has greatest effect on cells in the G_2 phase of the cell cycle and in mitosis.[48]

Bleomycin is inactivated within cells by the enzyme aminohydrolase. This enzyme is widely distributed, but is present in only low concentrations in the skin and the lungs, explaining the predominant toxicities of bleomycin to those sites. The presence of hydrolase enzymes in tumor cells is the primary mechanism of resistance to bleomycin. Cells can also become resistant by repairing the DNA breaks produced by bleomycin.[48]

Hydroxyurea

Hydroxyurea is a unique drug that inhibits ribonucleotide reductase. Cells accumulate in the S phase because DNA synthesis is inhibited, and only abnormally short DNA strands are produced.[20] This drug is often used to cause a rapid decline in a patient's white blood cells prior to initiating more potent chemotherapy agents.

L-Asparaginase

L-Asparaginase is unique among cytotoxic drugs in its unusual mechanism of action, patterns of toxicity, and source. It is an enzyme produced by *Escherichia coli* and other bacteria. L-Asparagine is a nonessential amino acid that can be synthesized by most mammalian cells, except for those of certain lymphoid human malignancies, which lack or have very low levels of the synthetase enzyme required for L-asparagine formation. L-Asparagine is degraded by the enzyme L-asparaginase, which depletes existing supplies and inhibits protein synthesis. Increased L-asparagine synthetase activity within tumor cells causes resistance to L-asparaginase treatment.[49]

Arsenic Trioxide

Arsenic is an organic element and a well-known poison that is an effective treatment for acute promyelocytic leukemia.[50] As an antineoplastic, arsenic trioxide acts as a differentiating agent, inducing the growth progression of cancerous cells into mature, more normal cells. It also induces programmed cell death or apoptosis.

Mitomycin C

Mitomycin C is a natural product that is sometimes classified as an antitumor antibiotic.[37,51] It has similarities to nitrogen mustard compounds and may function as an alkylating agent, although its toxicity pattern differs from conventional alkylating agents.

CLINICAL PHARMACOLOGY OF TARGETED AND BIOLOGIC AGENTS

Most anticancer drugs lack selectivity for tumor cells and are lethal to both tumor and normal cells. Although a few, such as methotrexate, capecitabine, L-asparaginase, and the immune therapies demonstrate some degree of selectivity for malignant cells, the selectivity is incomplete, and dose-limiting damage to normal cells also occurs. Exploiting targets and pathways critical for the survival and growth of cancer cells allows for the rational development of targeted and molecular therapies. Several anticancer agents that target malignant cells or the biochemical processes that control cancerous cell growth are available to treat both solid and hematologic malignancies. These agents are designed to improve outcomes while minimizing adverse effects.

MONOCLONAL ANTIBODIES

❻ The monoclonal antibodies have become established agents in the treatment of cancer. Monoclonal antibodies (MoABs) consist of immunoglobulin sequences that are known to recognize a specific antigen or protein on the surface of cells. There are five classes of immunoglobulins (IgA, IgD, IgE, IgG, and IgM), with IgG the most commonly used therapeutically. The fundamental structure of all antibodies is identical and consists of two heavy and two light chains joined to form a molecule that resembles the letter Y. The variable region (Fab fragment) of antibodies differs greatly and is composed of three complementary determining regions. The Fab portion is composed of heavy (V_H) and light chains (V_L) which are responsible for binding to antigens. The constant region (Fc fragment) determines the effector function of the antibody.[52]

Two main classes of MoABs are used in the treatment of cancer, the most common of which are unconjugated or naked MoABs. The other class is immunoconjugates, which are MoABs conjugated to a toxin (immunotoxin), chemotherapy agent, or radioactive particle (radioimmunoconjugate). MoABs may also be divided into agents that target cell surface antigens and induce cell death and those that target growth factor receptors or ligands.[52] Standardized nomenclature exists for naming MoABs and can provide information to the clinician.[53] The suffix -mab is used for all MoABs and fragments and is always preceded by the identification of the animal source of the product. The letters "o," "u," "xi," and "zu" before the -mab suffix indicate a murine, human, chimeric, and humanized source, respectively. The general disease state the MoAB is treating precedes the source and is identified using a code. Currently, most approved MoABs used in cancer have the code syllabus -tu(m) which designates it for use against miscellaneous tumors. If the product is conjugated to another chemical, such as a toxin, or is radiolabeled, a separate word is added for this designation. In addition, the name of the isotope, element symbol, and isotope number should precede the name of the MoAB. For example, iodine I-131-tositumomab is a murine MoAB designated for use in cancer that is conjugated to the radioisotope iodine 131.

❻ The first MoABs used in humans were murine, but most of the MoABs used today are chimeric, humanized, or fully human. These agents differ in the amount of foreign component. Hypersensitivity and infusion-related reactions, with or without the development of human antimouse antibodies (HAMAs), are generally greatest with murine antibodies and least with humanized antibodies.[52,54] Human antibodies would not be expected to cause HAMA reactions. However, clinicians should be careful when administering any MoAB as rare HAMA-like reactions have occurred to chimeric and humanized MoABs. The severity of these reactions can range from mild (e.g., fever, chills, nausea, and rash) to severe, life-threatening anaphylaxis with cardiopulmonary collapse. Many patients also experience chest or back pain during the infusion. Patients with circulating tumor cells in the bloodstream are at highest risk for more severe reactions. For these reasons, patients must be monitored closely during drug infusion. The reactions tend to be more severe with the initial infusion, and subside with subsequent treatment. Most agents require premedication with antihistamines and acetaminophen. Recommended infusion rates are usually lower for the initial dose, with incremental increases as tolerated by the patient. For patients experiencing signs or symptoms of infusion-related reactions, the infusion should be interrupted and prompt treatment with antihistamines, corticosteroids, and other supportive measures should be initiated. Pulmonary toxicity may occur as part of the infusion-related reaction or may occur as a distinct entity.[52,54,55]

HAMA reactions can also increase the clearance of the MoAB from the body by targeting the murine portion of the antibody as foreign. This will decrease the half-life of the MoAB and may decrease the ability of the MoAB to bind to its target antigen and potentially decrease its efficacy over time.

Additionally, the toxicities of the MoABs will be determined by the selectivity of the target antigen. Antibodies against antigens found on normal and tumor cells will have increased toxicity compared to tumor-specific antigens found only on tumor tissues. The specific location of the target antigen will also dictate the specific toxicity of the MoAB. For example, gemtuzumab targets CD33+ antigen, which is found on tumor and early myeloid cells. As a result, prolonged myelosuppression is an anticipated adverse effect of gemtuzumab.[56]

❻ There are several mechanisms by which MoABs may induce death of cancer cells. Unconjugated MoABs that target antigens on the cell surface of cancer cells may directly mediate cell killing through complement activation (complement-dependent cytotoxicity [CDC]), antibody-dependent cellular toxicity (ADCC), or signaling the cascade of events that lead to tumor cell apoptosis.[52,54,57] CDC results when the Fc portion of the MoAB activates the complement system leading to tumor cell lysis. In ADCC, effector cells which contain Fc receptors bind to the Fc portion of the MoAB and either lyses or phagocytosizes the antibody-containing cell. Natural killer cells, monocytes, and macrophages are all capable of mediating ADCC. Finally, antibody binding may result in the transmission of signals that induce apoptosis, or programmed cell death in the targeted cell.

❻ In addition to the mechanisms of cell death above, immunoconjugates deliver a chemotherapy drug or radioactive particle to the site of disease. Once bound to target antigens, the chemotherapy drug conjugated to the MoAB is internalized by the target cell and kills tumor cells through traditional mechanisms of action.[58] MoABs conjugated to radiation deliver radiation targeted to the site of tumor involvement, resulting in cell death. In addition to killing the target cell, radioimmunoconjugates are capable of killing antigen-negative tumors through radiation crossfire sometimes termed the "innocent bystander" effect. Both types of immunoconjugates are able to deliver therapy to specific sites of disease while limiting systemic exposure to the chemotherapy agent or radiation.

Finally, MoABs have been developed that target the underlying mechanism of cell growth and proliferation. These agents are discussed later in the chapter but have similar structure, nomenclature, and potential adverse effects as agents that target antigens present on malignant cells.

CELL SURFACE GLYCOPROTEIN MONOCLONAL ANTIBODIES

Gemtuzumab Ozogamicin

Gemtuzumab ozogamicin consists of a recombinant humanized anti-CD33 MoAB conjugated to the calicheamicin derivative *N*-acetyl-gamma calicheamicin, a cytotoxic antitumor antibiotic, by the linker ozogamicin.[54] The myeloid cell-surface antigen CD33 is expressed on the surface of leukemic blasts in more than 80% of patients with AML.[56] CD33 is also expressed on normal and leukemic myeloid colony-forming cells, including leukemic precursors. The binding of the Fab fragment of gemtuzumab ozogamicin to the CD33 antigen results in the formation of a complex that is internalized into CD33+ cells. Upon internalization, the calicheamicin derivative is cleaved from the antibody and released inside the cell. The released calicheamicin derivative binds to DNA in the minor groove resulting in DNA double-strand breaks and cell death.[54,59]

Gemtuzumab ozogamicin is indicated in elderly patients with CD33+ AML and who have failed at least one chemotherapy regimen. The recommended dose of gemtuzumab ozogamicin is 9 mg/m^2 administered as a 2-hour intravenous infusion.[56] Patients should receive diphenhydramine 50 mg and acetaminophen 650 to 1,000 mg 1 hour before gemtuzumab to prevent infusion-related reactions. These symptoms usually occurred at the end of the 2-hour infusion and are temporary. Patient vital signs should be monitored during the infusion and for 4 hours following therapy for these reactions. Fewer infusion-related events are observed after the second dose of gemtuzumab ozogamicin and patients may not need prolonged monitoring. The recommended treatment course with gemtuzumab ozogamicin is a total of 2 doses with 14 days between the doses with recovery from hematologic toxicities not a requirement for administration of the second dose.

Myelosuppression is the most severe toxicity associated with gemtuzumab ozogamicin.[60] Virtually all patients will have platelet nadirs of less than 25,000 cells/mm^3, with the time to platelet recovery (>25,000 cells/mm^3) ranging from 35 to 75 days. Greater than 90% of patients will have severe neutropenia (absolute neutrophil count [ANC] <1,000 cells/mm^3), with the median time to neutrophil recovery (ANC >500 cells/mm^3) about 40 days. Finally, 50% of patients experience anemia (hemoglobin <8 g/dL).

Tumor lysis syndrome including secondary renal failure secondary has been reported in association with the use of gemtuzumab ozogamicin. Leukoreduction with hydroxyurea or leukapheresis to reduce the white blood cell (WBC) count to ≤30,000 cells/mm^3 prior to administration of gemtuzumab ozogamicin and appropriate preventive measures such as hydration and allopurinol may be considered to decrease the likelihood of tumor lysis syndrome.

Hepatotoxicity, including severe venoocclusive disease, has also been reported in association with the use of gemtuzumab ozogamicin.[59,60] Risk factors include receiving gemtuzumab before or after stem cell transplantation, underlying hepatic disease or abnormal liver function, and patients receiving gemtuzumab ozogamicin in combination with chemotherapy. Patients should be monitored for rapid weight gain, right upper quadrant pain, hepatomegaly, ascites, and elevations in bilirubin and/or liver enzymes to identify and treat venoocclusive disease if it develops.

Rituximab

Rituximab was the first MoAB approved as an anticancer agent by the FDA (November 1997). Rituximab is a chimeric MoAB directed against the CD20 antigen found on the surface of normal and malignant B cells.[61] The exact function of CD20 is unknown but it appears to regulate an early step in the activation, differentiation, and growth of B cells. The Fab domain of Rituximab binds to the CD20 antigen on B lymphocytes and the Fc domain recruits immune effector functions to mediate B-cell lysis.[61] Although the exact mechanism of action is unknown, possible explanations for its antitumor effect include CDC- and ADCC-mediated killing of malignant B cells along with a direct apoptotic effect.[61]

Rituximab was initially FDA-approved for the treatment of patients with relapsed or refractory, low-grade or follicular, CD20+, B-cell non-Hodgkin lymphomas (NHLs). It recently received FDA approval for first-line therapy of both aggressive and indolent NHLs in combination with chemotherapy. Other therapeutic roles for rituximab therapy include other malignancies with CD20-

antigen expression (e.g., chronic lymphocytic leukemia) alone and in combination with standard chemotherapy.[61,62] Rituximab is also FDA approved for the treatment of refractory rheumatoid arthritis and has an evolving role in a variety of immune-mediated diseases such as Waldenström's macroglobulinemia, aplastic anemia, and others.

Following the first infusion of rituximab there is a rapid and sustained depletion of circulating and tissue B cells. This may account for the shorter half-life and increased adverse effects seen with the initial doses of rituximab. With subsequent infusions of rituximab, there is a corresponding increase in half-life, clearance, and maximum serum concentrations, which has been correlated to both a decrease in adverse effects and an increase in response rates with subsequent rituximab infusions.[61,62]

Most of rituximab's adverse events occur during the first infusion and are components of an infusion-related complex related to the amount of circulating B cells. After the first infusion, the incidence and the severity of these reactions decrease dramatically.[61,62] The most common events in the infusion-related complex are transient fever, chills, nausea, asthenia, and headache. Prior to the rituximab infusion, patients should receive diphenhydramine and acetaminophen as premedications. Rituximab should be administered by slow IV infusion only, with close monitoring of patients during the infusion. The first rituximab infusion is started at 50 mg/h and can be escalated as tolerated in 50 mg/h increments every 30 minutes to a maximum rate of 400 mg/h.[62] If the patient experiences infusion reactions consisting of fever and chills or rigors, the infusion should be temporarily slowed or interrupted and continued at one-half the previous rate upon improvement of patient symptoms. The rate of subsequent infusions may be increased (initiate at 100 mg/h, increase by 100 mg/h increments at 30-minute intervals to a maximum of 400 mg/h) if the patient tolerated the first infusion well.[62] Although rituximab targets B cells, which are responsible for humoral immunity, infection and severe hematologic events with rituximab are infrequent with neutropenia, anemia, and thrombocytopenia occurring in less than 1% of patients.[61]

Ibritumomab Tiuxetan

Ibritumomab tiuxetan is an immunoconjugate that consists of the murine anti-CD20 MoAB ibritumomab and tiuxetan, a linker-chelator, that allows the attachment of indium-111 (used for imaging and dosimetry) and yttrium-90 (active radiotherapy).[63] As described earlier, the CD20 antigen is found on normal and circulating B cells.

The ibritumomab therapeutic regimen consists of two steps.[59] In each step rituximab is given to decrease the number of circulating B cells before the radioimmunoconjugate is administered. Step one is the dosimetry (the calculations required for determining the radiation dose to be delivered) and imaging step performed to ensure appropriate distribution of the radiolabeled compound for safety and efficacy reasons. The initial dose of rituximab is followed by In-111 ibritumomab tiuxetan, used for imaging. Next, Y-90–ibritumomab is administered to patients after a second dose of rituximab if adequate distribution of In-111 was demonstrated. Y-90–ibritumomab is the therapeutic radiation isotope and selectively delivers radiation to B cells that express the CD20 antigen.

The radiation induced cytotoxicity delivered by Y-90–ibritumomab not only affects the tumor cells it binds to but also other cells that are within the pathlength of the radioisotope's emissions (innocent bystander effect).[58,59,63] Consequently, Y-90–ibritumomab can induce cell death in CD-20–positive and –negative tumors and eradicate a large number of tumor cells. Additionally, ibritumomab induces ADCC, CDC, and apoptosis in target cells.[58,59,63]

Ibritumomab tiuxetan is indicated for the treatment of relapsed or refractory low-grade, follicular, or transformed B-cell NHL, including rituximab-refractory NHL. Because ibritumomab is derived from murine sources, only one course of therapy is recommended to prevent the development of HAMA reactions.

Adverse reactions associated with the ibritumomab tiuxetan treatment regimen include severe infusion-related reactions, including life-threatening anaphylaxis.[58,59,63] These severe reactions typically occur during the first rituximab infusion. Signs and symptoms in these patients may include hypotension, angioedema, hypoxia, or bronchospasm, and require the interruption of rituximab, In-111 ibritumomab tiuxetan, or Y-90–ibritumomab tiuxetan administration. The premedications and infusion titration schedule for rituximab described earlier should be followed, including the availability of emergency supplies for the treatment of anaphylactic reactions.

Unlike rituximab, myelosuppression is common with ibritumomab as a consequence of the radioisotope component of the antibody.[58,63] Ibritumomab tiuxetan results in prolonged thrombocytopenia and neutropenia in patients with platelet counts greater than 150,000 cells/mm^3 prior to treatment and increases in patients with mild thrombocytopenia at baseline (platelet count 100,000 to 149,000 cells/mm^3).[63] Consequently, the Y-90–ibritumomab tiuxetan dose should be reduced in these patients. It is not recommended to give ibritumomab tiuxetan to patients with platelet counts less than 100,000 cells/mm^3 or with more than 25% bone marrow involvement. The median durations of thrombocytopenia and neutropenia were 24 and 22 days, respectively and monitoring and management of cytopenias, along with their complications (e.g., febrile neutropenia, bleeding) is necessary for up to 3 months after the completion of treatment.[59,63]

Tositumomab

Tositumomab is another murine CD20 monoclonal antibody radioimmunoconjugate, similar to ibritumomab. One important difference is that tositumomab is combined with the radioisotope iodine I-131 which has therapeutic and safety implications. The tositumomab therapeutic regimen also consists of two steps.[58] The first uses naked tositumomab (without the I-131) to decrease the number of circulating B cells prior to the administration of the radioimmunoconjugate. Because the I-131 isotope can be used for imaging and dosimetry, both steps in the administration of tositumomab use this radioisotope (in different doses). If imaging and dosimetry studies with the lower I-131 dose indicate adequate distribution of the radioimmunoconjugate, the second step consisting of a larger dose of I-131 tositumomab is administered 7 to 14 days after the first. The mechanisms of cell death are similar to ibritumomab as is the indication for use in patients with refractory NHL.

Most adverse effects are similar to ibritumomab with infusion-related reactions requiring appropriate premedications along with prolonged myelosuppression, primarily neutropenia and thrombocytopenia. Complete blood counts should be obtained weekly for 10 to 12 weeks to assess recovery of normal blood counts. One unique adverse effect to ibritumomab relates to the use of I-131 as the radioisotope. To prevent iodine uptake by the thyroid gland, and subsequent delivery of ionizing radiation to the thyroid gland, thyroid protective agents such as saturated solution of potassium iodide (4 drops three times per day) should be initiated at least 24 hours prior to the start of the tositumomab regimen and continued for 14 days after the therapeutic dose.[58,64]

Alemtuzumab

Alemtuzumab is a recombinant humanized MoAB that is directed against CD52. CD52 is expressed on the surface of B and T lymphocytes, natural killer cells, monocytes, and macrophages.[65] Alemtuzumab's therapeutic effect comes from binding to the CD52 antigen present on leukemic lymphocytes in chronic lymphocytic leukemia and inducing cell lysis and death.[65]

Alemtuzumab is indicated for the treatment of B-cell chronic lymphocytic leukemia in patients who have been treated with alkylating agents and who have failed fludarabine therapy. Because of alemtuzumab's ability to deplete B and T lymphocytes, alemtuzumab is also being investigated as part of conditioning regimens for stem cell transplants, treatment of autoimmune hematologic disorder, indolent lymphomas, and treatment of graft-versus-host disease.[59,65]

Alemtuzumab is administered by intravenous infusion. The initial dose is 3 mg administered over 2 hours daily until tolerated (≤ grade 2 infusion-related reactions), at which time daily doses are increased to 10 mg and continued until infusion reactions are tolerated. A maintenance dosage of 30 mg three times a week is then initiated. Maintenance therapy is continued for up to 12 weeks.

Alemtuzumab is associated with severe infusion-related reactions, hematologic toxicity, and opportunistic infections that are severe enough to warrant a black-box warning in the package insert.[65] Infusion reactions include severe rigors, and fever in most patients along with mild to moderate nausea, vomiting, and rash. As with other MoABs, these reactions are most common during the first week of therapy and decline with continued administration. More severe infusion-related reactions such as hypotension, shortness of breath, and bronchospasm are possible with alemtuzumab administration and require appropriate precautions. Pretreatment with diphenhydramine and acetaminophen before the first dose and at each dose escalation is recommended.

Hematologic toxicity consisting of severe prolonged neutropenia (ANC <1,000 cells/mm^3) and thrombocytopenia (platelets <50,000 cells/mm^3) occur in most patients. Clinicians should monitor blood counts prior to alemtuzumab administration to determine if the dose needs to be delayed or reduced.[59,65]

Because CD52 is expressed on lymphocytes, alemtuzumab can induce profound lymphopenia including a decrease in CD4 and CD8 counts. This decrease is usually seen through the first 4 weeks of therapy, with a gradual increase through week 12.[65] However, in some cases the CD4 and CD8 counts did not return to baseline after more than a year after treatment with alemtuzumab. Patients should receive prophylaxis for *Pneumocystis jirovecii* pneumonia (trimethoprim-sulfamethoxazole DS given twice a day, three times a week) and herpes virus (acyclovir) which should be continued for up to 6 months after alemtuzumab therapy or until CD4 counts reach 200 cells/mm^3 to prevent complications.

AGENTS THAT TARGET GROWTH FACTOR RECEPTORS AND LIGANDS

Recent advances in molecular biology have identified a number of pathways and potential targets related to cancer cell growth and survival. Targeting the HER pathway is currently used to treat a variety of solid tumor malignancies. MoABs have been developed to target the extracellular receptors of the HER family. In addition, small molecular inhibitors that target intracellular signal transduction pathways are available to clinicians for several malignancies. Additional agents target the vascular endothelial growth factor (VEGF) ligand or receptor and other downstream signaling targets.

❼ As mentioned previously, the HER family of receptors contains four known members, which upon binding to growth factor ligands result in intracellular phosphorylation of transcription factors and cell proliferation (Fig. 130–8).[9,66,67] HER-1 (more commonly called EGFR) and HER-2 are known to be overexpressed in several cancers, including breast, lung, and colon cancers. Activation of these receptors leads to uncontrolled cellular growth and proliferation, tumor metastasis, and the prevention of apoptosis in malignant cells.[66] The roles of HER-3 and HER-4 in cancer growth and proliferation are still under investigation. All members of this family contain a transmembrane glycoprotein extracellular ligand binding site, a transmembrane domain, and a cytosolic tyrosine kinase tail. Members of the HER family are inactive by themselves, and must form a dimer (a molecule composed of two subunits), either with a member of the same family (homodimer), or with a member of a different subtype of the HER family (heterodimer).[67] Dimerization of the receptor leads to tyrosine kinase phosphorylation and subsequent activation of downstream pathways required to activate signal transduction and cell growth.

Based on these identified cellular targets, several agents have been developed to prevent signal transduction through this pathway. MoABs which competitively bind to extracellular receptors of the HER family and prevent ligand binding and subsequent dimerization of receptors are available to clinicians. In addition, small molecules that target intracellular tyrosine kinase receptors are approved for use in a variety of tumors. These agents allow growth factor receptors to dimerize but prevent the phosphorylation of tyrosine kinase domains. The net effect of both strategies is to prevent downstream activation of the signal transduction resulting in a decrease in cell proliferation (Fig. 130–9).

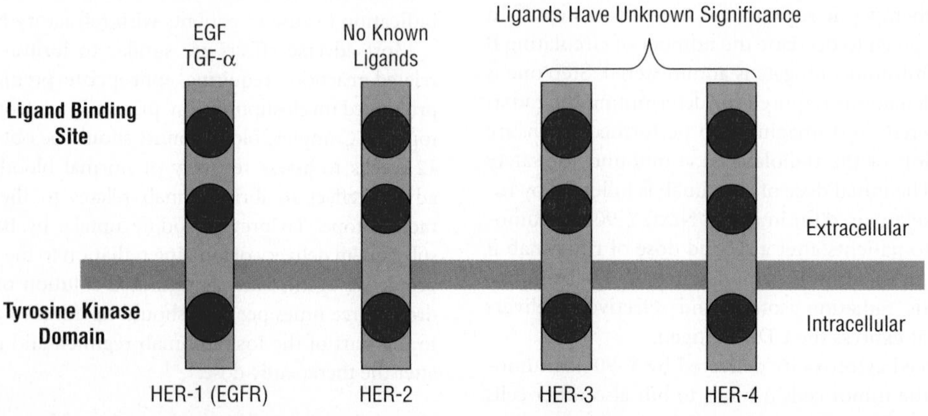

FIGURE 130-8. The HER family of growth factor receptors. All members of the human epidermal growth factor receptor (HER) contain a transmembrane glycoprotein, an extracellular ligand binding site, and a hydrophobic intracellular portion with a tyrosine kinase domain. HER-1 (or more commonly called EGFR [epidermal growth factor receptor]) has several known ligands (commonly implicated in cancer are EGF [epidermal growth factor] and TGF-α [transforming growth factor-α]); HER-2 has no known ligands; while the significance of ligands for HER-3 and HER-4 are unknown at this time. Once the molecule binds to another member of the HER family the tyrosine kinase domain is phosphorylated and genes regulating proliferation, antiapoptosis, and cell transformation are turned on.

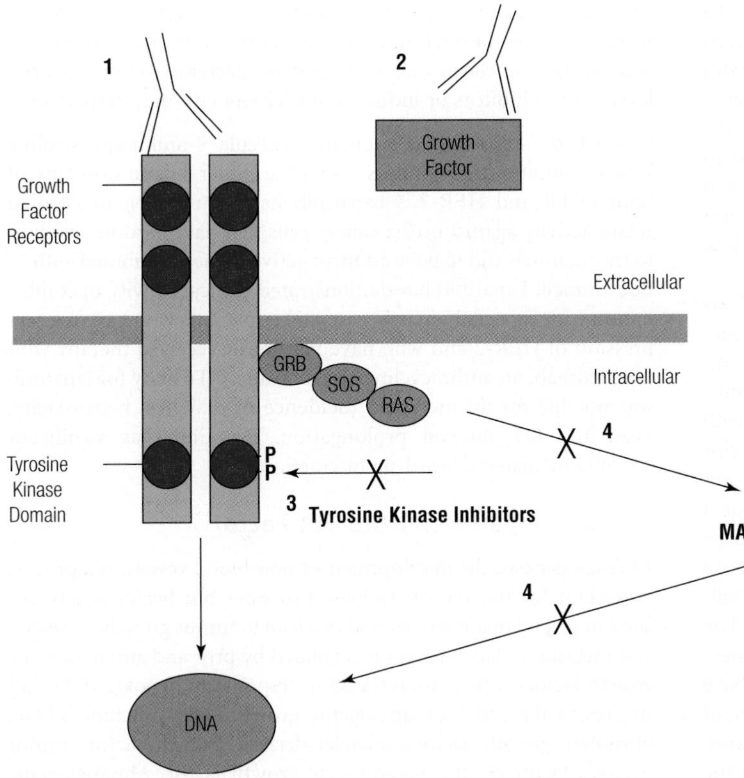

FIGURE 130-9. Strategies against growth factor receptors include (1) MoABs against the growth factor receptor; (2) MoABs against the growth factor itself; (3) molecules that target intracellular tyrosine kinases and prevent phosphorylation of tyrosine residues and subsequent activation of downstream signals; and (4) targeting downstream signals such as the MAP (mitogen activation protein) kinase pathway. All of these targets have the same goal of decreasing cell proliferation and increasing cell death of tumor cells.

Human Epidermal Growth Factor Receptor Family

Cetuximab Cetuximab is a recombinant chimeric MoAB that binds specifically to the extracellular domain of EGFR.[54,68,69] Cetuximab is composed of the Fv regions of a murine anti-EGFR antibody with human IgG_1 heavy and kappa light chain constant regions. Cetuximab binds specifically to the EGFR on both normal and tumor cells and competitively inhibits the binding of epidermal growth factor and other ligands, such as transforming growth factor-α.[69] Binding of cetuximab to the EGFR blocks dimerization of the receptors and downstream phosphorylation and activation of receptor-associated kinases. This results in inhibition of cell growth, induction of apoptosis, and inhibition of VEGF production. Patients with EGFR-expressing metastatic colorectal cancer who fail, or could not tolerate, irinotecan-based chemotherapy are candidates for cetuximab. The clinical controversy surrounding the requirement that colon tumors be EGFR positive is discussed in Chap. 133. The recommended dose of cetuximab, in combination with irinotecan or as monotherapy, is 400 mg/m^2 as an initial loading dose administered as a 120-minute IV infusion. The recommended weekly maintenance dose is 250 mg/m^2 infused over 60 minutes.[69,70] Cetuximab is also approved for use in head and neck cancer either by itself or in combination with radiation.[71]

The most serious adverse events associated with cetuximab are infusion-related reactions and development of an acne-like rash.[69,70] Severe, potentially fatal, infusion reactions include the rapid onset of airway obstruction and hypotension. In studies in advanced colorectal cancer, severe infusion reactions were observed in patients receiving cetuximab plus irinotecan and patients receiving cetuximab monotherapy.[70] Premedication with diphenhydramine is recommended to minimize the occurrence of infusion reactions and appropriate medical resources for the treatment of severe infusion reactions should be available during cetuximab infusions.

Skin reactions occur in most patients receiving cetuximab and can be severe. This reaction is similar between all EGFR inhibitors regardless of the site of action (extracellular or intracellular) and appears to be related to the function of EGFR in skin follicles.[72] Skin reactions appear most commonly on the face, upper chest, and back, but can extend to the extremities. These reactions are characterized by multiple follicular or pustular appearing lesions that generally appear within the first 2 weeks of therapy. Although the reactions usually resolve following cessation of treatment, resolution can be slow, continuing beyond 28 days in nearly one-half of cases. In patients who develop severe rash, dose modifications may be necessary. Interestingly, a trend for improved responses with increasing severity of skin reactions has been reported and requires further followup to assess the clinical importance of these reactions.[70,72] Other common adverse events with cetuximab include fatigue, GI complaints (nausea, vomiting, diarrhea, and constipation), and abdominal pain.[69,70]

Trastuzumab Trastuzumab is a recombinant humanized MoAB that selectively binds to HER-2.[62,73] The antibody is an IgG_1 kappa antibody that contains human framework regions and murine complementarily determining regions that binds to HER-2. HER-2 is overexpressed in about one-third of patients with breast cancer and to varying degrees in a variety of other malignancies (e.g., ovarian, lung, prostate).[9,62] Trastuzumab inhibits cell-cycle progression by decreasing cells entering the S phase of the cell cycle, leading to downregulation of HER-2 receptors on tumor cells and decreased cell proliferation.[73] Trastuzumab also leads to ADCC and CDC, along with directly inducing apoptosis in cells overexpressing the HER-2 protein.[73] In addition, synergy between trastuzumab and traditional chemotherapeutic agents has been demonstrated, resulting in trastuzumab often being used in combination with traditional chemotherapy agents.

Trastuzumab is approved in the treatment of metastatic breast cancer as a single agent or in combination with paclitaxel. Trastuzumab has also demonstrated a benefit in the adjuvant treatment of HER-2 positive breast cancer and is given for 1 year in combination with chemotherapy.[74] The combination of trastuzumab with other chemotherapy agents including vinorelbine, carboplatin, and others has shown synergistic effects and is under clinical investigation.[62] The addition of trastuzumab to anthracycline therapy is not recommended because of concerns of additive cardiotoxicity of the regimen.

Trastuzumab can be administered as a loading dose of 4 mg/kg given intravenously over 90 minutes, followed by weekly infusions of 2 mg/kg over 30 minutes as a single-agent or in combination with chemotherapy.[73] Trastuzumab has been administered every 3 weeks in combination with various chemotherapy agents to simplify the chemotherapy regimen; response rates and safety appear similar to those seen in the approved weekly trastuzumab regimen. When administered every 3 weeks with chemotherapy, the most common dose of trastuzumab is 8 mg/kg administered as a loading dose followed by 6 mg/kg given intravenously over 90 minutes.[75]

The most serious adverse reactions caused by trastuzumab include cardiomyopathy, infusion-related reactions, hypersensitivity reactions (including anaphylaxis), and increased myelosuppression. An evaluation of cardiac function should be performed prior to administration and extreme caution should be exercised in patients with preexisting cardiac dysfunction and in those who have received prior anthracyclines. In patients who develop a clinically significant decrease in left ventricular function (ejection fraction <50% or a greater than 10% decrease), discontinuation of therapy should be considered. Approximately 40% of patients treated will experience a symptom complex consisting of mild-to-moderate fever and/or chills during the administration of the first cycle of trastuzumab.[73] The symptoms generally resolve with treatment with acetaminophen, diphenhydramine, and meperidine. Rare anaphylactic reactions have been reported and appropriate medical resources for the treatment of these reactions should be available during trastuzumab infusions. Similar to most MoABs, the symptoms are most common with the initial infusions of trastuzumab and occur infrequently thereafter.

Myelosuppression is infrequent following the administration of trastuzumab as a single agent, but the incidence of neutropenia and febrile neutropenia is higher when trastuzumab is given with myelosuppressive chemotherapy as compared to giving the chemotherapy alone.[73]

Erlotinib and Gefitinib These agents are both orally active, selective EGFR-tyrosine kinase inhibitors that block signal transduction pathways involved in proliferation, survival, and metastases of cancer cells.[76,77] These agents inhibit EGFR activity by competing with adenosine triphosphate for its binding site on the EGFR tyrosine kinase cytosolic domain, which blocks the tyrosine kinase cascade of downstream signaling, and ultimately interferes with the proliferation and growth of cancer cells.

Gefitinib was originally approved based on response data for the treatment of inoperable non–small cell lung cancer (NSCLC).[76] However, subsequent data failed to demonstrate a survival benefit for patients taken gefitinib and the drug is only approved in the United States as monotherapy for the continued treatment of patients with inoperable NSCLC after failure of both platinum-based and docetaxel chemotherapies who have previously benefited from gefitinib and will not be discussed further.

Erlotinib has demonstrated both a survival advantage and a clinical benefit in clinical trials and is indicated for the treatment of patients with locally advanced or metastatic NSCLC as a second-line agent.[77] Erlotinib is also approved for use in pancreatic cancer in combination with gemcitabine. Reasons for the difference in clinical activity between gefitinib and erlotinib are unclear but may be the result of differences in drug levels achieved or the mutational status of the EGFR receptor.[78] Erlotinib has also demonstrated activity in a variety of other tumors such as head and neck and brain tumors. The recommended dose of erlotinib is 150 mg a day taken 1 hour before or 2 hours after a meal for NSCLC and 100 mg a day for pancreatic cancer.

Rash and diarrhea are the most common adverse events reported with erlotinib. Some studies suggest that the development of a rash may be predictive of a response to therapy and correlates with clinical benefit.[72] The rash that develops is similar to cetuximab and is treated similarly. Interstitial lung disease is a rare adverse effect reported in patients taken erlotinib. Drug interactions include increased international normalized ratio levels for patients on concomitant warfarin and increased or decreased erlotinib drug levels with inhibitors or inducers of CYP3A4 enzymes, respectively.

Lapatinib Lapatinib is a small molecule 4-anilinoquinazoline kinase inhibitor that inhibits the intracellular kinase domains of both EGFR and HER-2.[79] Lapatinib has been shown in vitro to retain activity against breast cancer cells that have become resistant to trastuzumab and to have additive activity when combined with 5-fluorouracil. Lapatinib has demonstrated clinical activity in combination with capecitabine in breast cancer patients who have overexpression of HER-2 and who have previously received therapy with trastuzumab, an anthracycline and a taxane.[79] Toxicity for lapatinib was notable for an increased incidence of diarrhea, hepatoxicity, rash, and QT interval prolongation. Lapatinib has significant CYP450 mediated drug–drug interactions.

Vascular Endothelial Growth Factor

❽ Angiogenesis, the development of new blood vessels, is a process important for normal physiologic processes but becomes unregulated in several malignancies and can lead to tumor growth, invasion, and metastasis. This process is regulated by pro- and antiangiogenic growth factors, which are released in response to hypoxia and other stresses to the cell.[80] Proangiogenic growth factors include VEGF, fibroblast growth factors, platelet-derived growth factor, tumor necrosis factor-α, and keratinocyte growth factor. Antiangiogenic growth factors include interleukin-12, the interferons, platelet factor-4, and tissue inhibitors of metalloproteinase.[80]

The best studied of the proangiogenic factors is VEGF, whose elevated levels have been associated with a poor prognosis and an increased risk of metastases in a variety of malignancies, including acute myeloid leukemia, breast cancer, hepatocellular carcinoma, NSCLC, ovarian cancer, and colon cancer.[80] Similar to other growth factors, VEGF binds to specific receptors located on the extracellular domain of growth factor receptors. There are three known receptors of VEGF: VEGFR-1, -2, and -3.[80] The VEGFR-1 and VEGFR-2 receptors are expressed primarily in endothelial cells and in some tumor cells, and mediate the biologic effects of VEGF. Each of the receptors induces a different signal transduction pathway. These pathways eventually result in the generation of proteases that are necessary for the breakdown of the extracellular matrix, the first step of angiogenesis. Interference with their ability to develop new blood vessels by means of antiangiogenic drugs can limit or prevent tumor growth.[80]

Drugs can interfere with angiogenesis in many different ways. Examples are targeting vascular growth factors, or the production and control of the endothelial cells that make up the vessel linings. Most antiangiogenic drugs are cytostatic rather than truly cytotoxic, as they prevent new vessel growth and thus cause growth delay of the tumors. Some vascular targeting agents, however, can destroy existing blood vessels and may have cytotoxic properties.[80]

Bevacizumab Bevacizumab is a recombinant humanized MoAB directed against circulating VEGF.[80] It is a chimeric antibody with an amino acid sequence that is 93% human IgG and 7% murine antibody. Bevacizumab binds to all biologically active circulating isoforms of VEGF and prevents the activation and promotion of angiogenesis.[80]

Bevacizumab is approved, in combination with 5-fluorouracil-based chemotherapy, for the initial treatment of colorectal cancer.[81] It was also recently FDA-approved for first-line treatment, in combination with carboplatin and paclitaxel, of patients with unresectable, locally advanced, recurrent or metastatic nonsquamous NSCLC. Bevacizumab is being studied in a number of other solid tumors including breast, renal cell, ovarian, pancreatic, head and neck, and cervical cancers.

The recommended dose of bevacizumab in colon cancer is 5 mg/kg given every 14 days as an intravenous infusion; the dose in other tumors depends on the schedule of chemotherapy being administered with bevacizumab.[81,82] The initial bevacizumab dose should be delivered over 90 minutes as an intravenous infusion following chemotherapy; subsequent infusions may be administered over 30 minutes if the first is well tolerated.

The three most frequent adverse effects associated with bevacizumab are hypertension, bleeding episodes, and thrombotic events.[81,82] Hypertension associated with bevacizumab is more common in patients with a previous history of hypertension and responds to oral antihypertensive medications. The most common type of bleeding associated with bevacizumab is transient nosebleeds. However, fatal CNS and gastrointestinal hemorrhages have been reported with bevacizumab administration. The manufacturer has issued a black box warning regarding the risk of gastrointestinal perforation, wound dehiscence, and fatal hemoptysis.[82] Bevacizumab is not recommended for use within 28 days of major surgery and patients should be instructed to report abdominal pain (an initial sign of GI hemorrhage) to their healthcare provider immediately. Paradoxically, bevacizumab also has been found to cause thrombotic events, including deep vein thrombosis, pulmonary embolism, and myocardial infarction, especially in elderly patients with a history of cardiac events. Another rare adverse effect associated with bevacizumab is proteinuria and patients should be monitored for the development or worsening of proteinuria by checking urine dipsticks for protein. Patients with a 2+ or greater urine dipstick reading should undergo further assessment to determine if bevacizumab is safe to administer.

Sunitinib and Sorafenib Most targeted agents approved to date have been developed against a single target associated with either the tumor or its growth and survival. Two similar agents, sunitinib and sorafenib, were recently FDA approved. They inhibit multiple tyrosine kinases, with the goal of enhanced antitumor activity. These agents are inhibitors of VEGFR-2 and platelet-derived growth factor receptor, which are involved in angiogenesis; c-KIT involved in gastrointestinal stromal tumors; and FLT3 involved in leukemia. In addition, sorafenib inhibits several isoforms of the serine/threonine kinase Raf, which is part of the mitogen-activated protein kinase signaling pathway involved in cell proliferation.[83]

Gastrointestinal adverse effects such as diarrhea are common with both agents, as is rash, fatigue, and hypertension. Unique adverse events include congestive heart failure with sunitinib and hand–foot syndrome with sorafenib.

Both of these agents are approved for use in advanced renal cell cancers and sunitinib is also approved for gastrointestinal stromal tumors after imatinib failures. Ongoing trials are evaluating both of these agents in a multitude of tumors.

Miscellaneous Targeted Agents

Imatinib and Dasatinib Imatinib mesylate is a selective inhibitor of the tyrosine kinase activity of BCR-ABL fusion gene, the product of the Philadelphia chromosome.[84] The Philadelphia chromosome is the hallmark finding of chronic myeloid leukemia (CML) and is a translocation of genetic material between chromosome 9 and 22. Imatinib mesylate binds to the kinase binding site of the BCR-ABL gene, competitively blocking access to adenosine triphosphate. This prevents tyrosine-kinase phosphorylation of the gene and downstream activation of cellular proliferation.[84] Imatinib mesylate also causes apoptosis or arrest of growth in hematopoietic cells expressing BCR-ABL. An additional effect of imatinib mesylate is its ability in blocking the tyrosine kinase activity of c-KIT (stem-cell factor receptor) and platelet-derived growth factor receptor.[54,84]

Imatinib mesylate is a standard treatment option for newly diagnosed Philadelphia chromosome-positive (Ph+) CML and for c-KIT (CD117)-positive gastrointestinal stromal tumors. A major advance seen with imatinib mesylate therapy is its ability to eliminate the Philadelphia chromosome in patients receiving therapy resulting in cytogenetic responses (elimination of the genetic defect), thus achieving the goal of all targeted therapies; the attack and elimination of the underlying cancer biology.

Adverse effects to imatinib mesylate are usually mild to moderate in severity. Severe fluid retention (pleural effusion, pericardial effusion, and ascites) occurs in less than 10% of patients taking imatinib mesylate. Patients should be monitored regularly for early signs and symptoms of fluid retention (leg swelling, shoes no longer fitting, and shortness of breath) and instructed to call their healthcare clinicians when symptoms first develop. Additional adverse effects for imatinib mesylate include mild or moderate superficial edema, elevation of liver enzymes, nausea, muscle cramps, headache, and rash.[85] Rash may require early intervention as rare cases of Stevens-Johnson's syndrome have been reported with imatinib mesylate and may require permanent discontinuation of therapy.[85]

Imatinib mesylate is metabolized by and is an inhibitor of the CYP3A4 enzyme system and caution should be exercised when substrates, inducers, or inhibitors of CYP3A4 are used concomitantly with imatinib mesylate.[85] Additionally, imatinib mesylate is an inhibitor of the CYP2D6 and levels of CYP2D6 substrates can increase.

Dasatinib is a next-generation tyrosine kinase inhibitor that shares the same binding site on the BCR-ABL tyrosine kinase adenosine triphosphate-binding domain with imatinib. In contrast, dasatinib maintains clinical activity in CML and Philadelphia chromosome-positive acute lymphocytic leukemia patients with mutations in the BCR-ABL binding site that confer imatinib resistance. It recently received FDA-approval for the treatment of patients with CML resistant to imatinib or other therapies. Dasatinib also inhibits a family of tyrosine kinases called SRC kinases that are believed to mediate cellular differentiation, proliferation, and survival; SRC kinases have been implicated in modulating multiple oncogenic signal transduction pathways.[84]

Dasatinib has a toxicity profile similar to that of imatinib with myelosuppression, nausea and vomiting, headache, and fluid retention being commonly reported. Dasatinib has also been reported to cause hypocalcemia and pleural effusions. Similar to other tyrosine kinase inhibitors, dasatinib has extensive drug–drug interactions with agents metabolized by the CYP3A4 isoenzyme.

Bortezomib The proteasome is an enzyme complex that is responsible for degrading proteins that control the cell cycle. Some of the proteins degraded by proteosomes regulate critical functions for cancer growth, such as regulation of the cell cycle, transcription factors, apoptosis, angiogenesis, and cell adhesion.[86,87] One proteosome inhibitor, bortezomib, is commercially available. Bortezomib has very specific affinity for the catalytic portion of the proteosome. It can induce apoptosis in cancer cells indirectly. Bortezomib is a specific inhibitor of the 26S proteasome; one consequence of 26S proteasome inhibition is the accumulation of IκB, an inhibitor of the major transcription factor NF-κB. NF-κB induces transcription of genes that block cell death pathways and promote cell proliferation. Its activity depends on its release from its inhibitory partner protein, IκB, in the cytoplasm and move to the nucleus. When IκB fails to degrade, through the actions of bortezomib, NF-κB remains in the cytoplasm, preventing it from transcribing the genes that promote cancer growth. Bortezomib is approved for the treatment of patients with multiple myeloma and mantle cell lymphoma.[86,87]

The most commonly reported adverse events are asthenia (fatigue, malaise, and weakness), nausea, and diarrhea occurring in over half of patients. Additional adverse effects include decreased appetite, GI complaints (nausea and constipation), myelosuppression (thrombocytopenia, anemia, and neutropenia), peripheral neuropathies, and fever.[86] Most of these adverse effects are mild to moderate and managed with supportive care measures. Of these common adverse effects, severe adverse effects were limited to thrombocytopenia, neutropenia, asthenia, and peripheral neuropathies.

Temsirolimus Mammalian target of rapamycin (mTOR) is a component of intracellular signaling pathways involved in the growth and proliferation of cells. mTOR receives input from upstream signaling pathways, including growth factors and hormones. Once activated, mTOR stimulates protein synthesis by phosphorylating translation regulators. mTOR also contributes to protein degradation and angiogenesis.[88]

Temsirolimus binds to FKBP-12 and the protein–drug complex inhibits the activity of mTOR by blocking its kinase activity.[88,89] mTOR inhibition suppresses the production of proteins that regulate progression through the cell cycle and angiogenesis. mTOR inhibition also results in reduced levels of cell growth factors involved in angiogenesis such as VEGF. Temsirolimus is approved for metastatic renal cell carcinoma, in which angiogenesis is a prominent clinical feature.

The most common adverse reactions with temsirolimus are rash, fatigue, mucositis, nausea, edema, and loss of appetite. The most common laboratory abnormalities are increases in serum creatinine and liver function tests, thrombocytopenia, and neutropenia. Additionally, hyperglycemia and hyperlipidemia that require monitoring of glucose and lipid profiles should be expected.[88,89] Rare, but potentially serious adverse effects include interstitial lung disease, immunosuppression (and infection), and renal failure. Temsirolimus is metabolized by the CYP3A4 isozyme, and possible drug interactions requiring dosage adjustments may be necessary.

Thalidomide and Lenalidomide Thalidomide, the infamous drug that caused severe limb deformities (phocomelia or "seal limbs") when used by pregnant women as a nonprescription sedative in the 1960s, is approved for treatment of leprosy and has orphan drug status for multiple myeloma. It also has documented clinical activity in several other types of cancer. Thalidomide is a glutamic acid derivative, and is broadly classed as an immunomodulatory agent. Lenalidomide, is a novel 4-amino-glutarimide analog of thalidomide with similar therapeutic activity, but a different adverse effect profile.[90] These agents have many potential mechanisms of action, with the main hypothesis thought to be through angiogenesis inhibition, an action also linked to its teratogenic effects. Other possible mechanisms include direct inhibition of cancer cells, free radical oxidative damage to DNA, interfering with adhesion of cancer cells, inhibiting tumor necrosis factor- production, or altering secretion of cytokines that affect the growth of cancer cells.[90]

The most common adverse events for thalidomide include somnolence, constipation, dizziness, orthostatic hypotension, rash, and peripheral neuropathies. Neutropenia is extremely rare. In contrast, lenalidomide is associated with much less somnolence and neuropathies compared to thalidomide.[90] Neutropenia, thrombocytopenia, and thrombotic issues are most prevalent with lenalidomide use. Because thalidomide is teratogenic, great care must be taken to prevent their use during pregnancy and several members of the healthcare team are required by the FDA to assist in this goal. All pharmacies and prescribers must be enrolled in the System for Thalidomide Education and Prescribing Safety (S.T.E.P.S.) program to dispense thalidomide and lenalidomide is only available under a special restricted distribution program called RevAssist.

BIOLOGIC AND IMMUNE THERAPIES

Retinoids

Vitamin A and its metabolites, collectively referred to as the retinoids, play important roles in numerous biologic processes, including normal cellular differentiation. Because cancerous growth is characterized by abnormal cellular differentiation, retinoids may play important therapeutic roles in the treatment and perhaps in the prevention of cancers. Tretinoin (all-*trans*-retinoic acid) is a naturally occurring derivative of vitamin A (retinol). Other retinoids indicated for treatment of cancers include alitretinoin (9-*cis*-retinoic acid), available in gel form for topical management of Kaposi sarcoma lesions, and bexarotene (Targretin) gel or capsules for treatment of cutaneous T-cell lymphoma.[91]

Retinoids are classed as morphogens, small molecules released from one type of cell that can affect the growth and differentiation of neighboring cells. Their normal roles in the human body are to induce differentiation of some cells, stop the differentiation of others, and both suppress and induce apoptosis in different cell types. Their diverse actions come from the diversity of their receptors. The two classes of retinoid receptors are retinoid X receptors (RXRs) and retinoic acid receptors (RARs), each with α, β, and γ subclasses. RXRs are versatile; they bind to RARs and to other nuclear receptors such as thyroid hormone receptors. Once activated, the receptors act as transcription factors that, in turn, regulate the expression of genes that control cellular growth and differentiation.[91]

Tretinoin binds primarily to the RAR-α receptors. Alitretinoin is considered a panagonist, which means that it binds to all known retinoid receptors, producing diverse regulatory effects. Bexarotene is synthetic and is classed as a rexinoid. It is the first RXR-selective retinoid agonist. The exact mechanism of action of alitretinoin and bexarotene as anticancer agents is unknown.[91]

Immune Therapies

An intact immune system is believed to play an important role in the control of cancer growth, as evidenced by the high incidence of cancers in immunosuppressed patients such as solid-organ transplant recipients or those with human immunodeficiency virus infections. There are also rare but well documented spontaneous remissions of immunologically-linked cancers, particularly melanoma and renal cell carcinoma. Immune therapies attempt to harness the immune system to treat cancer.[92,93]

Interferons The interferons (IFNs) are a family of proteins produced by nucleated cells and by recombinant DNA technology, with antiviral, antiproliferative, and immunoregulatory activities. They are classified as α, β, or γ interferons based on antigenic, biologic, and pharmacologic properties. Many subtypes of IFN-α are known. IFN-α_{2a} and IFN-α_{2b}, approved for anticancer indications, are very similar single-species recombinant products.

The mechanisms of IFN-α's antitumor action are complex. IFN increases the activity of cytotoxic cells within the immune system, but they also have direct antiproliferative effects. IFNs prolong the cell cycle, which results in cytostasis, an increase in cell size, and apoptosis. They can inhibit new blood vessel formation in tumors and can increase the expression of antigens on tumor cell surfaces, making the cancerous cells more easily recognized by immune effector cells. They also inhibit or block certain oncogenes that can direct the unregulated cell growth that is characteristic of cancerous cells. Alterations in gene expression may change the levels of receptors for other cytokines, or the concentration of regulatory proteins on immune cells, or may activate enzymes that alter cellular growth and function.[92]

Interleukin-2 (Aldesleukin) Interleukin-2 (aldesleukin; IL-2) is a lymphokine produced by recombinant DNA technology that promotes B- and T-cell proliferation and differentiation and initiates a cytokine cascade with multiple interacting immunologic effects. The IL-2 receptor is expressed in increased amounts on activated T cells and mediates most of the effects of IL-2. Antitumor effects depend on proliferation of cytotoxic immune cells that can recognize and destroy tumor cells without damaging normal cells. Some of these cytotoxic cells are natural killer cells, lymphokine-activated killer (LAK) cells, and tumor-infiltrating lymphocytes (TILs).[93]

The toxicity of IL-2 is related to dose, route, and duration of therapy, but IL-2 is toxic therapy that requires vigorous supportive care. The most common dose-limiting toxicities are hypotension, fluid retention, and renal dysfunction. IL-2 decreases peripheral vascular resistance, producing peripheral vasodilation, tachycardia, and hypotension. A characteristic vascular- or capillary-leak syndrome produces fluid retention, which, in turn, can cause respiratory compromise. These toxicities require administration of vasopressors in most patients, judicious use of fluid support and diuretics, and supplemental oxygen. Patients with underlying cardiovascular or renal abnormalities are more susceptible to these adverse effects, making careful patient selection important.[93] Most patients treated with IL-2 in full doses experience thrombocytopenia, anemia, eosinophilia, reversible cholestasis, and skin erythema with burning and pruritus, and some have neuropsychiatric changes, hypothyroidism, and bacterial infections.[93] In general, the toxicities from IL-2 therapy reverse quickly once therapy is stopped, and can be managed or prevented by careful prospective monitoring and pharmacologic supportive care.

Denileukin Diftitox Denileukin diftitox (Ontak) is a recombinant fusion protein that combines the active sections of both IL-2 and diphtheria toxin. Unconjugated diphtheria toxin is much too toxic to administer to humans. As the "payload" of the fusion protein, however, its cytotoxic effects are directed toward cells that express the high-affinity form of the IL-2 receptor, such as cancer cells of some patients with cutaneous T-cell lymphoma. Once denileukin diftitox interacts with the IL-2 receptors, the toxin inhibits protein synthesis in the cancer cells and causes cell death.[94]

Although denileukin diftitox is directed therapy, its targeting of cells that express high-affinity IL-2 receptors is not specific because these receptors are expressed on cells other than cancer cells. Denileukin diftitox produces acute hypersensitivity reactions, flu-like symptoms, sometimes with prominent diarrhea, and vascular-leak syndrome. It differs from the vascular-leak syndrome produced by high-dose IL-2 in that it occurs in fewer patients, is delayed in onset, is usually self-limited, and does not consistently recur on retreatment.[93,94] Patients with an albumin less than 3 g/dL are at increased risk for vascular-leak syndrome and use in these patients is not recommended.

RESPONSE CRITERIA

The response to chemotherapy and other treatment modalities may be described as a cure, complete response, partial response, stable disease, or progression.[95] These terms are used routinely in oncology to define the response to chemotherapy and other treatment modalities. A cure implies that the patient is entirely free of disease and has the same life expectancy as a cancer-free individual. Because of our inability to detect small numbers of tumor cells, we can never be absolutely certain that an individual patient is cured. Cancers that are curable with treatment are characterized by a stable plateau in the survival curve where the risk of relapse is very low. For most of these curable cancers, the survival curve has plateaued by about 5 years. Therefore, patients with one of these curable cancers who are alive 5 years from the time of diagnosis without disease recurrence are often considered "cured" of their cancer. However, patients with some malignancies, such as breast cancer and melanoma, for example, are still at significant risk for relapse after 5 years.

In an attempt to simply and unify response definitions in both clinical practice and published reports, the World Health Organization response criteria was updated in 2000 and are now termed the RECIST (Response Evaluation Criteria in Solid Tumors) criteria.[95] *Complete response* (CR) means complete disappearance of all cancer without evidence of new disease for at least 1 month after treatment. The terms *cure* and *CR* are not synonymous. Although an individual must have a CR to be cured, many individuals who achieve a CR will eventually relapse. A *partial response* is defined as a 30% or greater decrease in the tumor size or other objective disease markers, and no evidence of any new disease for at least 1 month. Overall objective response rates for a given treatment are calculated by adding the CR and partial response rates. *Progressive disease* is defined as a 20% increase in the tumor size or the development of any new lesions while receiving treatment. A patient whose tumor size neither grows nor shrinks by the above criteria is termed to have *stable disease*. Some patients may experience subjective improvement in the symptoms caused by their cancer without a defined response. Although clinically important, this does not indicate an objective response. The term *clinical benefit response* was recently developed to document these subjective responses; it refers to patients who have clinical benefit as measured by decreases in pain or analgesic consumption, or improved quality of life or performance status.

These response definitions are applicable to solid tumors, but diseases such as leukemias and multiple myeloma are not characterized by discrete, measurable masses. Responses in these diseases are measured by elimination of abnormal cells (e.g., return to normal hematology parameters and normal bone marrow in leukemia), return of tumor markers to normal levels (e.g., normal serum protein electrophoresis in multiple myeloma), or improved function of affected organs (e.g., improved renal function after obstructive uropathy). Cytogenetic markers and molecular techniques have an increasingly important role in determining whether all cancer has been truly eliminated. For example, in chronic myelogenous leukemia, the Philadelphia chromosome can be detected by polymerase chain reaction techniques, even when no leukemia is evident in the bone marrow or bloodstream. Patients without evidence of the Philadelphia chromosome are classified as a *complete cytogenetic response*. Measuring cytogenetic responses is increasingly common in patients with known cytogenetic abnormalities and absence of complete cytogenetic responses may predict disease relapse.

Finally, different survival end points may be used to assess treatment response. Overall survival is considered as the gold standard but increasing emphasis is being placed on other survival end points that consider quality of life. These end points include disease-free survival and progression-free survival, which measure the time the patient "survives" free of disease (i.e., cancer) or progression, respectively.

FACTORS AFFECTING RESPONSE TO CHEMOTHERAPY

These include tumor burden, tumor-cell heterogeneity, drug resistance, dose intensity, and patient-specific factors. The significance of tumor burden was discussed earlier in the Prinicples of Tumor Growth section. Tumors consist of a heterogeneous population of cell types. Because of the genetic instability of cancer cells as compared to normal cells, mutations commonly occur during cell division. Large tumors have undergone many cell divisions and express multiple cell mutations resulting in genetically varied cell populations.[6,17] In 1979, Goldie and Coldman proposed that these cytogenetic changes were not completely random and were highly associated with the development of the ability of tumors to develop drug resistance.[1,6,17] The probability of developing resistant cell populations increases as tumor size increases. It is believed that a small percentage of resistant cancer cells may survive initial chemotherapy. Resistant populations later proliferate and eventually become the dominant cell types, which may explain the common pattern of an initial response to chemotherapy, followed by progressive tumor regrowth despite continuing the same treatment regimen.

Drug resistance may be either an acquired or inherited property of a neoplastic cell. Mechanisms of drug resistance include decreased activation of prodrugs, decreased uptake of drugs secondary to alterations in drug transport systems, changes in target enzymes, alterations in the ability to repair drug-induced damage, increased drug inactivation, and decreased apoptosis.[6,10,17] One focus of research in this area is pleiotropic drug resistance or multidrug resistance.[17,96] When some cancer cells are exposed to increasing concentrations of a specific antineoplastic agent in vitro, they become resistant to that agent. Surprisingly, these same cells also become resistant to other structurally unrelated antineoplastic agents and are therefore considered multidrug resistant. Cytotoxic agents derived from natural products, such as the anthracyclines, actinomycin D, mitomycin C, the vinca alkaloids, the epipodophyllotoxins, and the taxanes, produce multidrug resistance. The resistant cancer cells possess a membrane-associated protein known as P170 or P-glycoprotein, which appears to enhance the export of toxins, such as chemotherapy agents, out of the cell (Fig. 130–10). The gene that encodes for P-glycoprotein is known as the *mdr-1* gene. Expression of this gene is amplified in cells that are resistant to the natural products listed previously. P-glycoprotein is also found in high concentrations in tumors that are traditionally resistant to chemotherapy (e.g., renal cell cancer and NSCLC) and thus may also be an important mechanism of intrinsic or inherited drug resistance. Several drugs have been investigated as possible inhibitors of this efflux pump, such as the calcium channel blockers, quinidine, cyclosporine, and the phenothiazines. Another efflux pump, known as the multidrug resistance-associated protein (MRP), was also recently identified. Other potential mechanisms of drug resistance include inactivation of chemotherapy agents by glutathione metabolism, upregulation of target enzymes such as topoisomerases or dihydrofolate reductase, and decreased apoptosis after exposure to chemotherapy. The last mechanism can be mediated by *bcl-2* oncogene overexpression or loss of the *p53* gene, as discussed in the oncogene section. The interplay between apoptosis and drug resistance is an area of intense research.

The relationship between dose and response has been extensively explored in cancer chemotherapy.[1] Dose is believed to be a critical factor in determining response for many types of cancers. *Dose intensity* is defined as the dose delivered to the patient over a specified period of time. The three main variables that determine delivered dose intensity are the dose per course, the interval between doses, and the total cumulative dose. *Dose density* refers to shortening of the usual interval between doses (e.g., every 2 weeks instead of every 3 weeks) and is designed to maximize the drugs' effects on tumor growth kinetics. This strategy has been most extensively studied in breast cancer, with positive results in adjuvant therapy of patients with high-risk node-positive disease. The delivery of optimal dose intensity is often compromised by the toxicities of the oncologic drugs. Treatment cycles are commonly delayed because of inadequate recovery from drug toxicity, especially myelosuppression. Subsequent doses of chemotherapy are often reduced to prevent or reduce the severity of these toxicities. The impact of this issue on patient outcome has been proven in studies showing reduced rates of response and survival in individuals receiving less-than-optimal chemotherapy doses.[1] Understanding the pathophysiology of drug-induced toxicities has led to the development of more effective agents for prevention and management of these toxicities. The development of drug- and toxicity-specific chemoprotective agents has facilitated application of dose-intensity principles.[1] The colony-stimulating factors avert neutropenia and permit delivery of dose-intensive or dose-dense regimens that are myelosuppressive. The issue of dose intensity is particularly important in the setting of high-dose chemotherapy with autologous hematopoietic stem cell support. Although lethal myelosuppression is avoided by administering hematopoietic stem cells, other severe end-organ toxicities emerge as antineoplastic drug doses are increased.

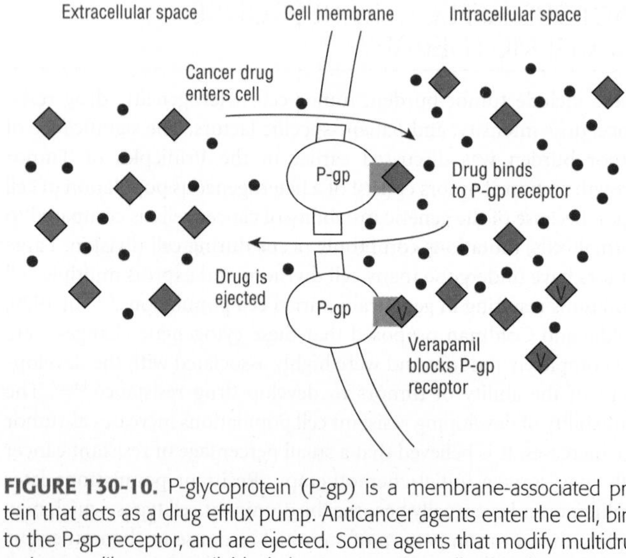

FIGURE 130-10. P-glycoprotein (P-gp) is a membrane-associated protein that acts as a drug efflux pump. Anticancer agents enter the cell, bind to the P-gp receptor, and are ejected. Some agents that modify multidrug resistance, like verapamil, block the P-gp receptor, allowing the anticancer agent to remain in the cell.

Patient-specific factors create unpredictable variability in response to chemotherapy. The biology of cancer is strongly affected by host characteristics and genetics. The pathway of genetic mutations that resulted in malignancy can also affect response to therapy. For example, breast cancers that overexpress the HER-2 oncogene are often sensitive to anthracycline-based regimens.[73] Likewise, patients with EGFR mutations that result in enhanced tyrosine kinase activity are more likely to respond to the tyrosine kinase inhibitor gefitinib.[78] Interindividual variations in drug absorption, disposition, elimination, or metabolism may lead to sub- or supratherapeutic levels of antineoplastic agents and their metabolites. As a result, both drug efficacy and drug toxicity can be affected. Until recently, healthcare professionals in oncology have modified dose based on variations in body size, blood counts, and renal and hepatic function. Prospective dose modifications based on these parameters are still very important to optimize the effectiveness of therapy and minimize toxicity. But more specific tools are becoming available, as we learn how to identify and apply differences in people's genetic makeup to their cancer drug therapy. *Pharmacogenomics* is the study of the role of inheritance in individual variation in drug response.[97] In oncology, several clinically relevant genetic polymorphisms, or variations, have been identified that can affect drug pharmacokinetics and pharmacodynamics. Examples include polymorphisms in genes responsible for the activity of the enzymes dihydropyrimidine dehydrogenase (responsible for 5-fluorouracil metabolism), thiopurine *S*-methyltransferase (responsible for thiopurine metabolism), and uridine diphosphate-glucuronosyltransferase 1A1 (responsible for irinotecan metabolism).[97] Patients with deficiencies in these enzymes can experience significant, and possibly life-threatening, toxicity. Screening for these genetic abnormalities will permit individualization of regimens to avoid toxicity and maximize antitumor effects. Monitoring of antineoplastic drug concentrations may also improve the therapeutic index. Pharmacokinetic and pharmacodynamic modeling is associated with improved responses and decreased toxicity in children with acute lymphoblastic leukemia.

The presence of other disease states (i.e., comorbidities) may also affect response to treatment by limiting treatment options. The overall functional status of a patient may be assessed using performance status scales, such as the Karnofsky and Eastern Cooperative Oncology Group scales (Table 130–10).[98] These scales can be used to predict patient tolerance of chemotherapy and to assess the

TABLE 130-10 Performance Status Scales

Description: Karnofsky Scale	Karnofsky Scale (%)	Zubrod Scale (ECOG)	Description: ECOG Scale
No complaints; no evidence of disease	100	0	Fully active, able to carry on all predisease activity
Able to carry on normal activity; minor signs or symptoms of disease	90		
Normal activity with effort, some signs or symptoms of disease	80	1	Restricted in strenuous activity, but ambulatory and able to carry out work of a light or sedentary nature
Cares for self; unable to carry on normal activity or to do active work	70		
Requires occasional assistance but is able to care for most personal needs	60	2	Out of bed more than 50% of time; ambulatory and capable of self-care, but unable to carry out any work activities
Requires considerable assistance and frequent medical care	50		
Disabled; requires special care and assistance	40	3	In bed more than 50% of time; capable of only limited self-care
Severely disabled; hospitalization indicated, although death not imminent	30		
Very sick; hospitalization necessary; requires active supportive treatment	20	4	Bedridden; cannot carry out any self-care; completely disabled
Moribund; fatal processes progressing rapidly	10		
Dead	0		

ECOG, Eastern Cooperative Oncology Group.
Adapted from reference 98.

effects of chemotherapy on the patient's level of activity and quality of life. For many cancers, performance status at diagnosis is the most important prognostic indicator.

Today's oncology clinician has a wealth of information to consider when designing a treatment approach for an individual patient. Patient-specific factors (e.g., performance status, comorbidities, renal and hepatic function, and pharmacogenomics), tumor-specific factors (e.g., pathology, stage, and molecular profile), and treatment goals (e.g., palliation and cure) are all considered when determining the best treatment option. Treatment cost can also be an important consideration.

COMBINATION CHEMOTHERAPY

Although single-agent therapy is sometimes employed, the more common approach to chemotherapy involves administration of multiple agents to overcome factors for decreased patient response noted previously.[1,16,98] Initially, this approach was based on the Goldie-Coldman hypothesis, which addresses the issue of tumor cell heterogeneity and the inevitable development of drug resistance. Combination chemotherapy is given to target as many types of cells in the tumor as possible. Selection of agents for combination chemotherapy regimens involves consideration of drug-specific factors such as mechanism of action, antitumor activity, and toxicity profile. Drugs that possess minimally overlapping mechanisms of action and toxicities are combined, when possible. Myelosuppressive combinations are sometimes alternated with nonmyelosuppressive combinations to allow bone marrow recovery, while gaining additive antitumor effects. The selected agents should each have significant activity against the tumor that is to be treated. If a synergistic reaction is known to exist for two agents, they may be combined in various treatment regimens.

With the availability of new targeted therapies, one area of research is to determine the optimal ways to combine these agents, both with traditional chemotherapy agents and other targeted agents. In theory, these agents make ideal combination agents because they target the underlying cancer biology while usually avoiding typical chemotherapy adverse effects. Clinicians must be careful in combining these agents based on clinical data that demonstrate additive or synergistic benefit. Combinations of chemotherapy and targeted agents have proven successful in breast and colon cancer but have failed to demonstrate an advantage in NSCLC. It is now known that tyrosine kinase inhibitors may be antagonistic with chemotherapy in lung cancer patients who have tumor cells that predominately express wild-type EGFR, whereas patients with tumor cells identified to have somatic mutations in EGFR may experience synergy and benefit from the combination.[99] Therefore predictive markers are needed to identify which patients may benefit from combinations of chemotherapy and targeted agents and how best to give them.

ADMINISTRATION OF CHEMOTHERAPY

DOSING AND ADMINISTRATION

Healthcare practitioners should monitor several clinical and laboratory values prior to the administration of chemotherapy. In general, a WBC count ≥3,000/mm^3 or an ANC of ≥1,500/mm^3 and a platelet count of ≥100,000/mm^3 are usually required prior to administering chemotherapy. In addition, a chemistry panel is drawn to assess renal and hepatic function, especially for agents eliminated via those routes. Table 130–8 lists agents that require dosing adjustments and require specific laboratory tests prior to administration; failure to do so may result in overdosing and excessive toxicity from the agent.

Once it is determined that it is safe to administer, chemotherapy is generally dosed based on body surface area (BSA).[100] BSA is commonly used as an estimate of cardiac output and subsequent distribution to the liver and kidneys, the primary determinants of drug elimination. The most common methods used to determine BSA are the Mosteller and DuBois formulas, which are listed in Table 130–9.

CLINICAL CONTROVERSY

The use of actual versus ideal body weight for calculating BSA is a source of debate in oncology. Although actual body weight is most often used, some clinicians prefer to use an adjusted body weight in obese patients. Clinicians need to clearly state the weight used in the BSA calculation. New methods of dosing using individual patient- and tumor-specific-factors are an area of active research.

When determining the dose to be administered, healthcare practitioners should use with caution extreme values in BSA (values greater than 2 m^2) and assess patient clinical factors. New dosing methods are being developed to improve the accuracy of chemotherapy dosing and prevent both over- and underdosing. Carboplatin is now commonly dosed based on the patient's estimated glomerular filtration rate. This method, listed in Table 130–9, is known as the Calvert formula and has been demonstrated to achieve adequate levels of carboplatin without excessive toxicity.[101] Chemotherapy may also be dosed based on weight or drug levels and clinicians should be proficient in these calculations prior to dosing and administering any chemotherapy. Additional methods using pharmacogenomic testing are being studied to individualize chemotherapy doses.

SAFETY AND HANDLING ISSUES

The cytotoxic drugs used to treat cancer are carcinogenic, mutagenic, and teratogenic. Consequently, these drugs should be handled with care to avoid inadvertent exposure of healthcare professionals.[102] All pharmacies should have written procedures for handling these drugs safely, and all personnel should be oriented to these procedures. The United States Pharmacopeia (USP) chapter 797 regulates the preparation of extemporaneously compounded sterile preparations and should be used by centers that prepare chemotherapy.[102]

The most common avenue of exposure is via inhalation of aerosolized drug. Individuals preparing chemotherapy should work in a class II biologic safety cabinet and wear gowns and powder-free disposable latex gloves. The gowns should be made of lint-free, low-permeability fabric with a solid front, long sleeves, and tight-fitting elastic cuffs. Negative-pressure techniques should be employed in drug preparation to minimize aerosolization. Healthcare workers administering these agents should take similar precautions to avoid exposure. Kits for cleaning up chemotherapy spills should be located in all areas of the institution in which chemotherapy is handled. Cytotoxic waste should be disposed of properly, and patients should be informed of proper methods of disposing of potentially contaminated body excreta and cytotoxic waste.

GENERAL SUPPORTIVE CARE ISSUES

9 The treatment of cancer with most antineoplastic drugs is complicated by the risk of multiple serious toxicities, many of which are life-threatening. Drug-specific toxicities, such as doxorubicin-induced cardiotoxicity and bleomycin-related pulmonary toxicity, were summarized earlier. Several adverse effects are common to many antineoplastic agents. These include nausea and vomiting, myelosuppression, mucositis, alopecia, infertility, and carcinogenesis. With the addition of targeted therapies, new toxicities such as rash have become issues for healthcare practitioners to address. Nutritional support and pain management are also important supportive care issues, although malnutrition and pain are not usually direct results of drug toxicity. The management of chemotherapy-induced nausea and vomiting and the basic principles of nutritional support and pain management are discussed in detail in other chapters.

Because many antineoplastic drugs affect DNA synthesis, all rapidly proliferating cells are more sensitive to the toxic effects of chemotherapy. Normal tissues such as the bone marrow, intestinal mucosa, and hair follicles are such tissue sites where drug effects are manifested.

MYELOSUPPRESSION

10 Although not seen with all antineoplastic agents, myelosuppression is the most common dose-limiting side effect of cytotoxic agents. Bone marrow suppression does not usually occur immediately after chemotherapy administration. Blood components that have already been produced must be consumed before the effect is evident. WBCs, especially neutrophil precursors, are most significantly affected because of their rapid proliferation and short life span (6 to 12 hours). Platelets (5- to 10-day life span) are also affected, but to a much less degree than neutrophils. Erythrocytes, with a 120-day life span, are affected the least. Usual nadirs, or lowest blood cell counts, occur at 10 to 14 days following chemotherapy administration, with recovery by 3 to 4 weeks. There are some exceptions to this general rule. The nitrosoureas, mitomycin C, gemtuzumab, and radiolabeled antibodies exhibit a delayed pattern of nadir (4 to 6 weeks) and recovery (6 to 8 weeks). Planned courses of chemotherapy may have to be delayed while waiting for the granulocyte count to return to normal. Patients with leukemia or receiving a stem cell transplant may have a more rapid nadir of about 5 to 7 days. A guide for suggested blood counts for a patient to safely receive myelosuppressive chemotherapy is listed in the previous section on chemotherapy administration.

Myelotoxicity is a desired therapeutic effect in leukemia patients during induction chemotherapy. However, myelosuppression, particularly with fever, is an undesirable side effect during chemotherapy for other malignancies. If significant myelosuppression has occurred with prior courses of chemotherapy, the doses of the offending agent(s) in subsequent courses may be reduced. The magnitude of dose reduction is dictated by the degree of myelosuppression incurred and the incidence and severity of infection or bleeding. Empiric dosage reductions may be made for the first chemotherapy treatment if the patient has a low baseline WBC or platelet count, has diminished bone marrow reserve, has impaired drug-elimination capabilities, or is to receive a combination of several drugs that cause myelosuppression. Patients who have received multiple prior courses of other myelotoxic chemotherapy regimens or extensive radiation therapy, especially to the pelvis, may have a decreased bone marrow reserve. They are more sensitive to the myelosuppressive effects of chemotherapy, and normal doses may produce profound marrow toxicity. The pharmacokinetic profile of a myelosuppressive agent is also important in determining the appropriate dose. For example, the anthracyclines produce bone marrow suppression as an acute dose-limiting toxicity, and these agents depend on biliary excretion as their primary route of elimination. A patient with biliary obstruction may have compromised elimination of anthracyclines and is at increased risk for severe bone marrow suppression if the dose is not appropriately adjusted (see Table 130–8).

However, in some tumors (e.g., breast cancer or lymphoma) dosage reduction may compromise antitumor response, leading to worse patient outcomes.[1] In patients who are responding well to treatment, some degree of myelosuppression is accepted by most healthcare practitioners if it is not compromising the patient's quality-of-life and the tumor is responding to therapy. In these patients, empiric use of hematopoietic growth factors provides an alternative to dose reduction.

Anemia

10 Although usually not life-threatening, anemia is the most common hematologic complication of cancer chemotherapy.[103] The incidence of anemia depends on several factors, including the type and duration of therapy and the type and stage of the underlying malignancy. For example, carboplatin is more commonly associated with anemia than many other chemotherapeutic agents. Multiple conditions are known to cause anemia in cancer patients, including chronic gastrointestinal blood loss, nutrient deficiency (e.g., iron and folate), chemotherapy and radiation therapy, bone marrow invasion by the tumor, hemolysis, renal dysfunction, and anemia of chronic disease. Of all the signs and symptoms of anemia, fatigue is most common in cancer patients.[103] In fact, fatigue is the most commonly reported symptom overall in patients undergoing chemotherapy. The presence of fatigue is correlated with the severity of anemia; treatment of anemia results in improvement in fatigue and quality-of-life. Anemia is only one of many possible causes of fatigue in patients with cancer. Other common causes of fatigue include insomnia, depression, unrelieved pain, and the underlying malignancy.

Previously, the only option for the treatment of chemotherapy-related anemia was red blood cell transfusions. This intervention is still the mainstay of acute management, but the availability of the recombinant human erythropoietic products—epoetin alfa and darbepoetin alfa—has provided another therapeutic option.[103] Several studies have documented the efficacy of these agents in the anemia associated with chemotherapy. Both epoetin alfa and darbepoetin alfa increase hemoglobin and hematocrit, decrease transfusion requirements, and improve quality-of-life. One difference between the products is that darbepoetin has a threefold longer half-life, which allows for less-frequent administration of darbepoetin in the clinical setting.[104]

Clinical practice guidelines to guide the appropriate use of erythropoietic agents have been developed.[103] The first step is to evaluate the underlying cause of the anemia and initiate specific therapy as indicated. For example, patients with iron-deficiency anemia should receive iron supplementation. Patients with chronic bleeding or hemolysis should not receive erythropoietic therapy, as this does not target the underlying cause of their anemia. Epoetin alfa and darbepoetin alfa should be considered for chemotherapy- or cancer-related anemia only after otherwise treated causes of anemia have been ruled out. The 2007 National Comprehensive Cancer Network guidelines suggest starting symptomatic patients when their hemoglobin is less than 11 g/dL with a target hemoglobin of 11 to 12 g/dL to achieve maximum benefit.[103] Several early indicators of response have been proposed, including an increase in hemoglobin of 1 g/dL above baseline, a decline in ferritin, or an increase in the absolute reticulocyte count after 2 to 4 weeks of therapy. These surrogate end points can be used to identify nonresponders early, so that therapy may be modified or discontinued, as indicated. Serum erythropoietin levels have minimal utility in predicting response or monitoring therapy and are often not measured in clinical practice.

Patients are most commonly started on either epoetin alfa 40,000 units once each week or darbepoetin alfa at a dose of 200 mcg every other week or 500 mcg every 3 weeks. Other dosing strategies are effective but generally less convenient for patients. After 4 to 6 weeks, the hemoglobin should be reassessed. In patients who do not achieve at least a 1 g/dL rise in hemoglobin, the 2007 National Comprehensive Cancer Network guidelines recommend to increase the epoetin alfa dose to 60,000 units once a week and the darbepoetin alfa dose to 300 mcg every other week.[103] Iron stores should be checked to rule out iron deficiency as a cause of treatment failure. Supplemental oral or intravenous iron may be administered to increase the response to erythropoietic therapy. Treatment should be discontinued in patients who do not respond after 4 to 6 weeks at the higher dose. Adverse effects related to erythropoietic products are rare and generally mild and include pain at injection site, rash, flu-like symptoms, and hypertension. However, serious adverse effects such as thrombotic events and pure red cell aplasia are possible. These events have generally occurred when the target hemoglobin of 12 g/dL is exceeded or the hemoglobin rises too quickly. The 2007 National Comprehensive Cancer Network guidelines recommend that if hemoglobin increases by more than 1 g/dL in a 2-week period, the dose of either product should be reduced by 25%. If hemoglobin levels exceed 12 g/dL while on therapy, healthcare practitioners should hold therapy and reinitiate therapy at a 25% dose reduction if the patients hemoglobin falls below 12 g/dL.[103]

Neutropenia

⑩ When the ANC falls below 500/mm^3, infection risk increases.[105] The ANC may be calculated by multiplying the percentage of neutrophils (segmented plus banded neutrophils) by the total WBC count. The risk of infection is also directly proportional to the duration of neutropenia. Other risk factors for infection include alteration in the integrity of physical defense barriers and the functional integrity of WBCs. The patient's underlying cancer and treatment with cytotoxic drugs and radiation can affect neutrophil function. The diagnosis of infection in the neutropenic patient is complicated by the lack of WBCs. Usual signs and symptoms of infection, such as pus, abscesses, and infiltrates on chest radiography, are often absent as a result of the lack of WBCs. Clinicians must rely on fever as an indication of infection in these patients. Definitive culture results may take days, and a septic neutropenic cancer patient can die within hours if not treated. Therefore the basic approach to the management of the febrile neutropenic cancer patient is prompt initiation of empiric antibiotics. The antibiotics are chosen based on reliable coverage of the most likely organisms, antibiotic sensitivities at the institution, the patient's signs and symptoms (if present), side-effect profiles, and cost.[105] The most common source of infection in these patients is self-infection with body flora, which includes both gram-positive and gram-negative bacteria. Specific treatment of infections in immunocompromised hosts is discussed in another chapter.

Numerous methods have been explored to prevent infections in cancer patients. Colony-stimulating factors (CSFs) are commonly employed for this purpose.[105] These hormones are naturally occurring proteins that are essential for the normal growth and maturation of blood cell components (Fig. 130–11). The CSFs have the ability to enhance the production and also the function of their target cells. Two agents, G-CSF (granulocyte colony-stimulating factor) and GM-CSF (granulocyte-macrophage colony-stimulating factor) are commercially available in the United States. G-CSF (filgrastim) specifically stimulates the production of neutrophilic granulocytes. GM-CSF (sargramostim) promotes the proliferation of granulocytes (neutrophils and eosinophils) and monocytes/macrophages.[106] Although GM-CSF stimulates megakaryocytes, no consistent effect on platelet production has been observed in clinical trials. Both agents initially enhance demargination and mobilization of mature cells from the marrow and then provide constant stimulation of stem cell progenitors. CSFs are produced by recombinant DNA technology, and several host cells are used to produce CSFs, including bacteria (*E. coli*), yeast, and mammalian cells (Chinese hamster ovary cells). Products derived from yeast or mammalian sources are glycosylated to varying degrees, as are naturally occurring CSFs, while those derived from *E. coli* are nonglycosylated.[106] This difference does not result in any clinically significant effects on neutrophil production. Pegfilgrastim is a long-acting CSF, created by addition of a polyethylene glycol molecule to G-CSF.[107] Clinical trials have demonstrated that a single dose of pegfilgrastim provides equivalent effects to 10 to 11 days of daily G-CSF, with similar side-effect profiles.

The CSFs reduce the incidence, magnitude, and duration of neutropenia when used as preventive therapy following a variety of myelosuppressive chemotherapy regimens.[105,108] These effects have been accompanied by a modest decrease in febrile days, infections, and days on antibiotics. In some studies, use of CSFs also resulted in a decrease in the incidence of mucositis. Growth factors have also permitted the administration of subsequent chemotherapy courses on schedule, resulting in enhanced dose intensity. However, the increased dose intensity provided by the CSFs has not consistently translated into improved tumor response or survival. Because of lack of impact on response rates and survival, decisions regarding appropriate use of growth factors should be based on weighing proven clinical benefits against economic considerations. The American Society of Clinical Oncology has developed evidence-based clinical practice guidelines to promote appropriate use of the CSFs.[108]

Growth factors may be used in either primary or secondary prophylaxis of neutropenia. Primary prophylaxis refers to the use of CSFs to prevent neutropenia with the first cycle of chemotherapy. Recently, the American Society of Clinical Oncology stated that this strategy is clinically and economically appropriate for patients who are receiving a chemotherapy regimen with a 20% or higher risk of

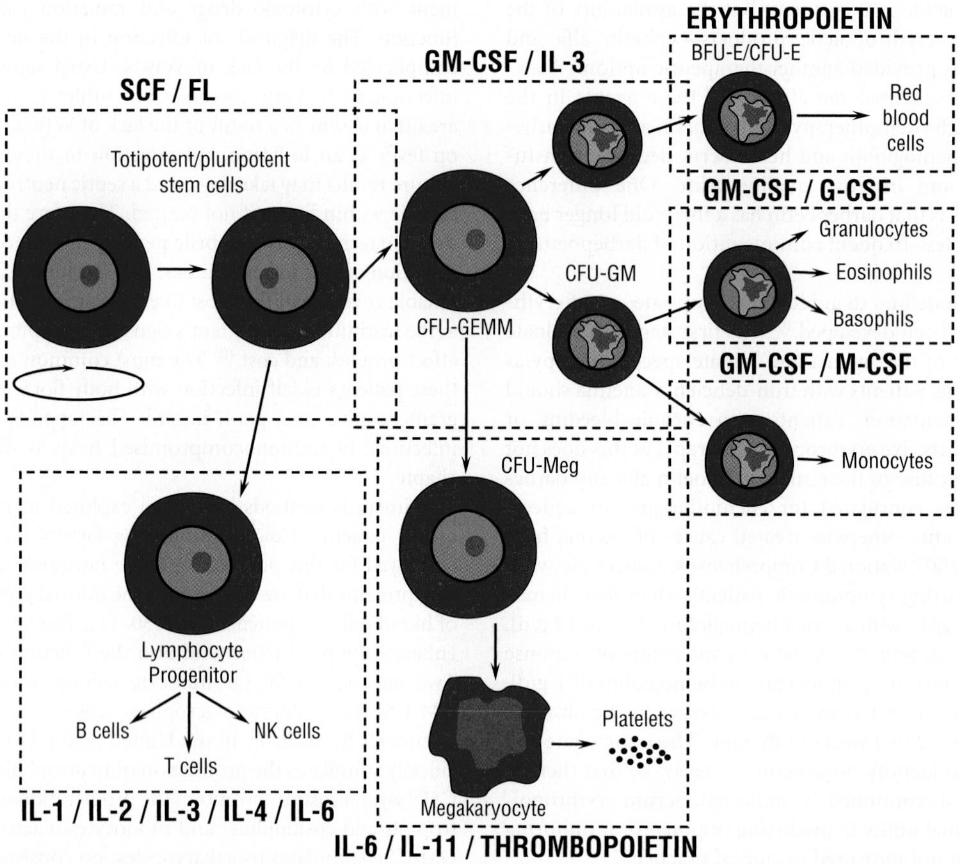

FIGURE 130-11. Sites of action of hematopoietic growth factors in the differentiation and maturation of marrow cell lines. A self-sustaining pool of marrow stem cells differentiates under the influence of specific hematopoietic growth factors to form a variety of hematopoietic and lymphopoietic cells. Stem cell factor (SCF), FTL-3 ligand (FL), interleukin-3 (IL-3), and granulocyte/macrophage colony-stimulating factor (GM-CSF), together with cell–cell interactions in the marrow, stimulate stem cells to form a series of burst-forming units (BFU) and colony-forming units (CFU): CFU-GEMM, CFU-GM, CFU-Meg, BFU-E, and CFU-E (GEMM, granulocyte, erythrocyte, monocyte, and megakaryocytes; GM, granulocyte and macrophage; Meg, megakaryocyte; E, erythrocyte). After considerable proliferation, further differentiation is stimulated by synergistic interactions with growth factors for each of the major cell lines—granulocyte colony-stimulating factor (G-CSF), monocyte/macrophage-stimulating factor (M-CSF), thrombopoietin, and erythropoietin. Each of these factors also influences the proliferation, maturation, and, in some cases, the function of the derivative cell line. *(Adapted from Hillman RS. Hematopoietic agents: Growth factors, minerals and vitamins. In: Hardman JG, Limbird LE, Gilman AG, eds. Goodman & Gilman's The Pharmacologic Basis of Therapeutics, 10th ed. New York: McGraw-Hill, 2001:1489.)*

febrile neutropenia.[108] Secondary prophylaxis refers to the use of growth factors to prevent recurrent neutropenia in patients who had experienced neutropenia with the prior cycle of chemotherapy. It is recommended that secondary prophylaxis be reserved for patients with chemosensitive cancers where dose reduction may affect disease-free or overall survival.[108]

Pegfilgrastim, G-CSF, and GM-CSF are used clinically to prevent febrile neutropenia after administration of standard doses of chemotherapy although only pegfilgrastim and G-CSF are FDA-approved for this indication. One exception is in acute myelogenous leukemia, in which both G-CSF and GM-CSF have been demonstrated to reduce the duration of neutropenia, often accompanied by modest decreases in hospitalization and infectious complications, after induction chemotherapy. Benefits have been most clearly documented in patients older than age 55 years. Similar data are available for G-CSF in the treatment of patients with acute lymphoblastic leukemia. These beneficial effects, however, have not resulted in improved response rates or overall survival.[108]

The role of CSFs in the treatment of established neutropenia is less-well defined. Most studies suggest no or only minimal clinical benefit from use of CSFs in treating neutropenia; therefore, CSFs should not be routinely employed in patients with established neutropenia, regardless of the presence of fever. However, certain high-risk patients with fever and neutropenia may benefit from CSFs: neutropenia >10 days, ANC <100/mm^3, age >65 years, infectious complications (pneumonia, sepsis, or invasive fungal infections), and patients who are hospitalized at the time of the development of neutropenic fever.[105,108]

Both G-CSF and GM-CSF have also proven effective in acceleration of hematopoietic engraftment and in treatment of graft failure following hematopoietic stem cell transplantation. Other uses for the CSFs include peripheral blood stem cell mobilization, neutropenia in patients with acquired immune deficiency syndrome, myelodysplastic syndromes, congenital neutropenia, and aplastic anemia. Growth factors should not be used in patients receiving concomitant chemotherapy and radiotherapy, especially if the radiation involves the mediastinum. These patients appear to experience more significant thrombocytopenia when administered CSFs.

At currently recommended doses, the CSFs are well tolerated. Side effects are more commonly seen with GM-CSF and may be related to the drug's ability to enhance binding of neutrophils to endothelial cells or to activation of monocytes/macrophages, which may stimulate the release of cytokines such as IL-1 and tumor necrosis factor.[106] The most common toxicity of the CSFs is bone pain (20% to 25% of patients), which can be treated with acetaminophen. Other side effects of G-CSF include an increase in lactate dehydrogenase, alkaline phosphatase, and uric acid levels. Additional toxicities of GM-CSF include constitutional symptoms, such as low-grade fever, myalgia, arthralgia, lethargy, and mild headache. GM-CSF may also produce an elevation in liver transaminases. At higher doses of GM-CSF, pleural and pericardial effusions, capillary-leak syndrome, and thrombus formation may occur. A first-dose reaction described after GM-CSF administration has been reported more commonly with the *E. coli*-derived product (molgramostim), which is not commercially available in the United States. This reaction is more common after intravenous infusion and consists of dyspnea, facial flushing, hypotension, hypoxia, and tachycardia. Both G-CSF and GM-CSF may produce mild erythema at subcutaneous injection sites, as well as a generalized maculopapular rash with either subcutaneous or intravenous administration. Pegfilgrastim adverse effects are similar to G-CSF and are treated the same.[106]

The dosing and administration of CSFs approved for prophylaxis of chemotherapy-induced neutropenia after standard dose chemotherapy is as follows: G-CSF 5 mcg/kg until the ANC reaches 10,000/mm^3 (or clinically safe) or pegfilgrastim 6 mg as a single dose. Both agents should be started between 24 and 72 hours after chemotherapy; G-CSF can be stopped the day before chemotherapy whereas pegfilgrastim needs to be stopped within 14 days of the next dose because of its long half-life. The dose for other uses varies, for instance in the setting of peripheral blood stem cell mobilization doses of 10 mcg/kg per day are usually used. The recommended dose of GM-CSF is 250 mcg/m^2 per day. Pharmacokinetic data favor subcutaneous injection as the most effective route. However, in patients in whom subcutaneous injections are not feasible (e.g., anasarca), G-CSF and GM-CSF may be given intravenously. Pegfilgrastim should not be given intravenously. Because of the high cost associated with CSF use, alternative dosing regimens have been explored. These regimens attempt to decrease the total amount of CSF used by either delaying the start of CSFs (e.g., to day 3 after chemotherapy), decreasing the dose (e.g., to 3 mcg/kg per day of G-CSF), or decreasing the duration of CSF therapy. Standardized doses of 300 mcg or 480 mcg of G-CSF and 500 mcg of GM-CSF, based on product vial sizes, are often used to minimize waste. Specifically, the posttreatment target ANC of 10,000/mm^3 recommended by product information is often reduced in clinical practice to 5,000/mm^3 or lower. For patients receiving pegfilgrastim, it is important that additional CSFs not be administered for the 10 days following administration, as additional benefit is not realized.[107]

Thrombocytopenia

Chemotherapy-induced thrombocytopenia puts the patient at risk for significant bleeding. To date, platelet transfusions remain the mainstay of management. At most centers, platelet transfusions are reserved for patients with a platelet count of <10,000 cells/mm^3 unless they are actively bleeding, must undergo a surgical procedure, or have documented infections or fever in which the threshold is higher. For patients with nonmyeloid malignancies who experienced significant thrombocytopenia with a prior cycle of chemotherapy, oprelvekin (IL-11) may be considered as secondary prophylaxis.[109] When used after chemotherapy regimens associated with a high risk of thrombocytopenia, oprelvekin decreased the need for platelet transfusions, as well as the numbers of platelets required for transfusion. Unfortunately, oprelvekin is associated with some significant adverse effects, mostly related to fluid retention (e.g., edema, dilutional anemia, dyspnea, and pleural effusions). Cardiac toxicity, especially tachycardia, and atrial fibrillation and flutter also have been observed. Prophylactic oprelvekin also is significantly more expensive than platelet transfusions.[110] Considering the modest clinical benefit, the adverse effects, and the high cost, oprelvekin use should be reserved for patients who are at high risk for severe thrombocytopenia from chemotherapy where dose reduction is known to compromise disease response. Other CSFs, such as interleukins-1, -3, and -6, have also been studied, but significant impact on platelet counts with an acceptable adverse effect profile has not been demonstrated.[109] The discovery and development of thrombopoietin, a megakaryocyte-stimulating factor, may represent the most significant factor in the future of thrombocytopenia treatment.

MUCOSITIS

The gastrointestinal mucosa is composed of epithelial cells with a high mitotic index and rapid turnover rate, making it a common site of chemotherapy-induced toxicity.[111] The subsequent inflammation, or mucositis, can lead to painful ulcerations, local infection, and inability to eat, drink, or swallow. Disruption of the GI mucosal barrier may also provide an avenue for systemic microbial invasion. The time course for development and resolution of mucositis often parallels that of neutropenia. Agents most commonly associated with mucositis include 5-FU, doxorubicin, and methotrexate. Currently, the most effective means of preventing mucositis is through good oral hygiene. Patients who are at high risk for this toxicity (those with poor dentition, high-dose chemotherapy, or radiation therapy involving the oropharynx) should be evaluated by a dentist prior to chemotherapy and should be instructed to rinse their mouths frequently with baking soda and salt water or plain saline rinses during and between courses of chemotherapy. Clinical practice guidelines for the prevention and treatment of cancer therapy-induced mucositis were recently published.[111] The benefit of chlorhexidine rinses over saline rinses is unclear. In patients undergoing radiation therapy to the head and neck region, chlorhexidine rinses have detrimental effects on the oral mucosa. For patients receiving 5-FU treatment, the use of ice (oral cryotherapy) may decrease the risk for mucositis by decreasing drug delivery to the oral mucosa. A better understanding of the pathophysiology of mucositis has resulted in identification of promising new agents to better prevent mucositis. The keratinocyte growth factor palifermin is approved for use in patients receiving high-dose chemoradiotherapy prior to hematopoietic stem cell transplantation. Palifermin is given intravenously at a dose of 60 mcg/kg per day for 3 consecutive days immediately before the initiation of conditioning therapy and then again for 3 days after hematopoietic stem cell transplantation.[112] The effect of palifermin on solid-tumor growth is unknown and its use in nonhematologic cancers is not recommended.

After mucositis has developed, treatment is mainly supportive, including use of topical or systemic analgesics and oral hygiene (including the rinses described).[111] Viscous lidocaine, diphenhydramine liquid, and dyclonine are topical anesthetics commonly employed. Severe cases of mucositis may lead to dehydration and require intravenous hydration and pain medications including patient-controlled analgesia pumps. Local infections caused by *Candida* species and reactivation of herpes simplex viruses are common in these patients. Suspicious lesions should be cultured, and appropriate antifungal and/or antiviral treatment should then be instituted. Antifungal therapy may be delivered topically for mild infections (thrush) with clotrimazole troches or nystatin oral suspension. For more severe oral or esophageal fungal infections, systemic treatment with oral fluconazole or intravenous antifungals is indicated.

Mucosal damage can occur at any point along the entire length of the GI tract. In the lower portion of the GI tract, this damage is usually manifested as diarrhea (mild to life-threatening in nature) and abdominal pain. Support with intravenous fluids and electrolyte supplementation should be initiated promptly in severe cases. After infectious causes have been ruled out, diarrhea can safely be treated with antispasmodics such as Lomotil or loperamide. The somatostatin analog octreotide has also been used successfully to treat severe cases of chemotherapy-induced diarrhea; guidelines exist to assist practitioners in treating this toxicity.[111,113]

CUTANEOUS REACTIONS

Cutaneous reactions to chemotherapy are generally reversible and self-limiting upon chemotherapy dose reductions or delays. Common reactions include localized rash, photosensitivity, skin hyperpigmentation, nail changes, and hand–foot syndrome, but can be associated with severe hypersensitivity reactions. Common agents known to cause rash in patients include cytarabine, 5-FU, and bleomycin.

In targeted therapies, particularly those that target the EGFR receptor, rash is often the most common adverse effect associated with therapy and requires prompt recognition by healthcare professionals to prevent drug discontinuation. Some studies suggest that the rash may be a surrogate marker of response to these agents, perhaps indicating a genetic predisposition to response with EGFR targeted agents. Rash occurs in up to two-thirds of patients on EGFR inhibitors, most commonly in the first month on treatment with the typical site of presentation being the face and upper torso. Although no clear guidelines exist for the treatment of this rash, patients should be supported based on their presentation.[72] Anecdotal reports indicate that emollients help if patients complain of dry skin, topical and systemic antibiotics may help if the rash becomes infected, and steroids may help prevent itching and inflammation.[72]

ALOPECIA

Although not a life-threatening side effect of chemotherapy, the toxicity that many patients find most distressing is alopecia. Alopecia from chemotherapy is usually temporary, and the degree of hair loss varies widely.[114] Loss of hair is not limited to the scalp; any area of the body may be affected. Patients receiving a taxane as part of their chemotherapy regimen are especially prone to total-body alopecia. Hair loss usually begins 1 to 2 weeks after chemotherapy, and regrowth may begin before the chemotherapy courses are completed. Cryotherapy (local application of ice) and scalp tourniquets have both been investigated as methods of preventing alopecia. Both techniques produce vasoconstriction, resulting in decreased exposure of hair follicles to the chemotherapy agents. These techniques are not uniformly effective and are contraindicated in patients with cancers that may metastasize to the scalp, such as leukemia and lymphoma.

EXTRAVASATION

Vesicants are antineoplastic agents that may cause severe tissue damage if they escape from the vasculature.[115] These agents include the anthracyclines, actinomycin D, the vinca alkaloids, mitomycin C, nitrogen mustard, and the taxanes. The anthracyclines are the most notorious agents, and the most extensively investigated. The tissue damage may result in prolonged pain, tissue sloughing, infection, and loss of mobility. Prompt initiation of the appropriate interventions is important to minimize morbidity. Unfortunately, most information on extravasation management is anecdotal; few controlled clinical studies have been conducted to determine optimal intervention strategies. Consequently, prevention is the focus of extravasation management. The most important method of prevention is good administration technique, but extravasations may occur despite good administration technique.[115] The vein selected for administration should be on the distal portion of the arm. The large veins of the forearm are desirable because if a drug does extravasate, there is adequate soft-tissue coverage to protect crucial structures like nerves and tendons, and joint function is not put at risk. Peripherally administered vesicants should be given slowly via intravenous injection (IV push) through the side arm of a running IV. The person administering the vesicant should verify needle stability and adequate blood return after each 1 to 2 mL of drug is injected. Vesicants should not be administered by intravenous infusion unless the patient has a central venous catheter. For extravasation of vesicants, one of the most important interventions is the application of ice packs to the affected area. One exception to this rule is the vinca alkaloids, which are better managed with application of heat. Only a few antidotes to vesicant agents are employed clinically. Sodium thiosulfate is used to neutralize nitrogen mustard extravasations, and hyaluronidase (if available) can improve the outcome after extravasation of vinca alkaloids, etoposide, and taxanes. Topical application of dimethyl sulfoxide may be an effective method for managing anthracycline and mitomycin C extravasations.[115]

INFERTILITY

Advances in the treatment of some cancers, such as Hodgkin disease and testicular cancer, have produced long-term survivors and the opportunity to examine the late consequences of chemotherapy administration. Infertility and secondary cancers have emerged as important late effects. The gonadal toxicities of chemotherapy have not received much attention in the past because they are not life-threatening. High rates of fertility deficits and sexual dysfunction have been noted for both men and women.[116] In men, antitumor drugs produce severe oligospermia or azoospermia as well as infertility. Serum testosterone levels are only rarely altered. The recovery of spermatogenesis after completion of chemotherapy is unpredictable. Men receiving combination chemotherapy appear to sustain more long-lasting adverse effects on fertility than do men receiving single-agent therapy. Age, total dose, duration of therapy, and type of drug are other important variables. In women, toxic effects on the ovaries result clinically in amenorrhea, vaginal epithelial atrophy, and menopausal symptoms. These effects are related to dose and age. Younger patients are more resistant to the effects on the ovaries. As with men, the recovery of fertility is unpredictable, but women younger then 25 years of age appear to have the best outcomes. The effects of the alkylating agents on fertility have been extensively studied. This group of drugs exerts profound and consistently detrimental effects on reproductive function.[116] Less is known about commonly used agents such as doxorubicin, taxanes, and platinum compounds. The risk of infertility should be discussed with all patients prior to receiving chemotherapy and they should be informed about options for fertility preservation.

SECONDARY MALIGNANCIES

Secondary cancers induced by chemotherapy and radiation are a serious long-term complication.[117] Although many types of solid tumors have been reported as chemotherapy-induced malignancies, AML or myelodysplastic syndromes are the most common secondary cancers. AML or myelodysplastic syndrome has been reported following successful treatment of Hodgkin lymphoma, acute leukemias, NHL, multiple myeloma, breast cancer, and advanced ovarian cancer. For curable cancers, the relatively small risk for occurrence of secondary malignancies is far outweighed by the benefits of survival in large numbers of patients. However, for cancers such as ovarian cancer, the risk of leukemia is not offset by improved survival in patients treated with chemotherapy. The issue of secondary malignancies is of particular concern in patients receiving adjuvant chemotherapy. As with the late complication of infertility, the antineoplastic agents primarily associated with secondary cancers are the alkylating agents. Etoposide, teniposide, radionucleotides, and the anthracyclines also are linked to secondary leukemias. Solid tumors as secondary malignancies occur more commonly after treatment with radiation than with chemotherapy.

ABBREVIATIONS

ADCC: antibody dependent cellular cytotoxicity
AML: acute myelogenous leukemia
ANC: absolute neutrophil count
ara-C: cytarabine
ara-CTP: active triphosphate form of cytarabine
BCNU: carmustine
BSA: body surface area
CCNU: lomustine
CDC: complement dependent cytotoxicity
CML: chronic myeloid leukemia
CR: complete response
CSF: colony-stimulating factor
DHFR: dihydrofolate reductase
DNA: deoxyribonucleic acid
EGFR: epidermal growth factor receptor
5-FU: fluorouracil
G_0: dormant phase of the cell cycle
G_1: first gap phase of the cell cycle
G_2: second gap or premitotic phase of the cell cycle
G-CSF: granulocyte colony-stimulating factor
GM-CSF: granulocyte-macrophage colony-stimulating factor
HAMA: human antimouse antibodies
HER: human epidermal growth factor receptor
IL: interleukin
IFN: interferon
6-MP: 6-mercaptopurine
M: mitosis
MoAB: monoclonal antibody
mRNA: messenger RNA
MTIC: monomethyl triazeno imidazole carboxamide
mTOR : mammalian target of rapamycin
MTX: methotrexate
NF-κB: nuclear factor-κB
NHL: non-Hodgkin lymphoma
NSCLC: non–small cell lung cancer
RAR: retinoic acid receptor
RNA: ribonucleic acid
rRNA: ribosomal RNA
RXR: retinoid X receptor
S: DNA synthesis phase of the cell cycle
tRNA: transfer RNA
VEGF: vascular endothelial growth factor
WBC: white blood cell

REFERENCES

1. Chabner BA. Clinical strategies for cancer treatment: The role of drugs. In: Chabner BA, Longo DL, eds. Cancer Chemotherapy and Biotherapy: Principles and Practice, 4th ed. Philadelphia: Lippincott Williams & Wilkins, 2006:1–14.
2. Jemal A, Siegel R, Ward E, et al. Cancer statistics, 2007. CA Cancer J Clin 2007;57:43–66.
3. Calvo KR, Petricoin EF, Liotta LA. Genomics and proteomics. In: DeVita VT, Hellman S, Rosenberg SA, eds. Cancer: Principles and Practice of Oncology, 7th ed. Philadelphia: Lippincott Williams & Wilkins, 2005:51–72.
4. Compagni A, Christofori G. Recent advances in research on multistage tumorigenesis. Br J Cancer 2000;83:1–5.
5. Weston A, Harris CC. Chemical carcinogenesis. In: Kufe DW, Pollock RE, Weichselbaum RR, eds. Cancer Medicine, 6th ed. Hamilton, Ont: BC Decker, 2003:267–278.
6. Cotran RS, Kumar V, Collins T. Neoplasia. In: Cotran RS, Kumar V, Collins T, eds. Robbins' Pathologic Basis of Disease. Philadelphia: WB Saunders, 1999:260–328.
7. Weinberg RA. How cancer arises. Sci Am 1996;275:62–71.
8. Hanahan D, Weinberg RA. The hallmarks of cancer. Cell 2000;100(1):57–70.
9. Gross ME, Shazer RL, Agus DB. Targeting the HER-kinase axis in cancer. Semin Oncol 2004;31(Suppl 3):9–20.
10. Johnstone RW, Ruefli AA, Lowe SW. Apoptosis: A link between cancer genetics and chemotherapy. Cell 2002;108:153–164.
11. Stetler-Stevenson WG. Invasion and Metastases. In: DeVita VT, Hellman S, Rosenberg SA, eds. Cancer: Principles and Practice of Oncology, 7th ed. Philadelphia: Lippincott Williams & Wilkins, 2005:113–127.
12. Folkman J, Kalluri R. Tumor angiogenesis. In: Kufe DW, Pollock RE, Weichselbaum RR, eds. Cancer Medicine, 6th ed. Hamilton, Ont: BC Decker, 2003:161–194.
13. Smith RA, Cokkinides V, Eyre HJ. American Cancer Society guidelines for the early detection of cancer, 2006. CA Cancer J Clin 2006;56:11–25.
14. American Cancer Society. Warning Signs of Cancer. Atlanta, GA: American Cancer Society, 2007.
15. Fleming ID, et al., eds. AJCC Cancer Staging Manual, 6th ed. New York: Springer-Verlag, 2002:209–217.
16. Calabresi P, Chabner BA. Chemotherapy of neoplastic disease. In: Hardman JG, Limbird LE, Molinoff PB, eds. Goodman & Gilman's The Pharmacologic Basis of Therapeutics, 10th ed. New York: McGraw-Hill, 2001:1381–1388.
17. Buick RN. Cellular basis of chemotherapy. In: Dorr RT, Von Hoff DD, eds. Cancer Chemotherapy Handbook, 2nd ed. New York: Elsevier, 1994:3–14.
18. Dang C, Gilweski TA, Sarbone A, Norton L. Chemotherapy: Cytokinetics. In: Kufe DW, Pollock RE, Weichselbaum RR, eds. Cancer Medicine, 6th ed. Hamilton, Ont: BC Decker, 2003:645–668.
19. Ross J. Structure and function of the gene. In: Abeloff MD, Armitage JO, Lichter AS, Niederhuber JE, eds. Clinical Oncology, 2nd ed. Philadelphia: Churchill Livingstone, 2000:3–9.
20. Pizzorno G, Diasio RB, Cheng Y-C. Pyrimidines and purine antimetabolites. In: Kufe DW, Pollock RE, Weichselbaum RR, eds. Cancer Medicine, 6th ed. Hamilton, Ont: BC Decker, 2003:739–757.
21. Wagstaff AJ, Ibbotson T, Goa KL. Capecitabine: A review of its pharmacology and therapeutic efficacy in the management of advanced breast cancer. Drugs 2003;63:217–236.
22. Johnson SA. Clinical pharmacokinetics of nucleoside analogues: Focus on haematological malignancies. Clin Pharmacokinet 2000;39:5–26.
23. Smith GA, Damon LE, Rugo HS, et al. High-dose cytarabine dose modification reduces the incidence of neurotoxicity in patients with renal insufficiency. J Clin Oncol 1997;15:833–839.
24. Venook AP, Egorin MJ, Rosner GL, et al. Phase I and pharmacokinetic trial of gemcitabine in patients with hepatic or renal dysfunction: Cancer and Leukemia Group B 9565. J Clin Oncol 2000;18:2780–2787.
25. Silverman LR, Demakos EP, Peterson BL, et al. Randomized controlled trial of azacitidine in patients with the myelodysplastic syndrome: A study of the cancer and leukemia group B [see comment]. J Clin Oncol 2002;20:2429–2440.
26. McKeage K, Croom KF. Decitabine: In myelodysplastic syndromes [see comment]. Drugs 2006;66:951–958.
27. Plosker GL, Figgitt DP. Oral fludarabine [see comment]. Drugs 2003;63:2317–2323.
28. Kamen BA, Cole PD, Bertino JR. Folate antagonists. In: Kufe DW, Pollock RE, Weichselbaum RR, eds. Cancer Medicine, 6th ed. Hamilton, Ont: BC Decker, 2003:727–738.

29. Rowinsky E. Microtubule-targeting natural products. In: Kufe DW, Pollock RE, Weichselbaum RR, eds. Cancer Medicine, 6th ed. Hamilton, Ont: BC Decker, 2003:791–810.
30. Krieger JA, Stanford BL, Ballard EE, Rabinowitz I. Implementation and results of a test dose program with taxanes. Cancer J 2002;8:337–341.
31. Gradishar WJ, Tjulandin S, Davidson N, et al. Phase III trial of nanoparticle albumin-bound paclitaxel compared with polyethylated castor oil-based paclitaxel in women with breast cancer. J Clin Oncol 2005;23:7794–7803.
32. Kitamura T, Nishimatsu H, Hamamoto T, et al. EMP combination chemotherapy and low-dose monotherapy in advanced prostate cancer. Expert Rev Anticancer Ther 2002;2:59–71.
33. Rubin EH, Hait WN. Anthracylines and DNA intercalators/epipodophyllotoxins/camptothecins/DNA topoisomerases. In: Kufe DW, Pollock RE, Weichselbaum RR, eds. Cancer Medicine, 6th ed. Hamilton, Ont: BC Decker, 2003:781–790.
34. Ulukan H, Swaan PW. Camptothecins: A review of their chemotherapeutic potential. Drugs 2002;62:2039–2057.
35. Raymond E, Boige V, Faivre S, et al. Dosage adjustment and pharmacokinetic profile of irinotecan in cancer patients with hepatic dysfunction. J Clin Oncol 2002;20:4303–4312.
36. Danesi R, Fogli S, Gennari A, et al. Pharmacokinetic-pharmacodynamic relationships of the anthracycline anticancer drugs. Clin Pharmacokinet 2002;41:431–444.
37. Colvin M. Alkylating agents and platinum antitumor compounds. In: Kufe DW, Pollock RE, Weichselbaum RR, eds. Cancer Medicine, 6th ed. Hamilton, Ont: BC Decker, 2003:759–779.
38. Stupp R, Gander M, Leyvraz S, Newlands E. Current and future developments in the use of temozolomide for the treatment of brain tumours. Lancet Oncol 2001;2:552–560.
39. Guminski AD, Harnett PR, deFazio A. Scientists and clinicians test their metal—Back to the future with platinum compounds. Lancet Oncol 2002;3:312–318.
40. Grothey A, Goldberg RM. A review of oxaliplatin and its clinical use in colorectal cancer. Expert Opin Pharmacother 2004;5:2159–2170.
41. Jordan VC. Estrogens and antiestrogens. In: Kufe DW, Pollock RE, Weichselbaum RR, eds. Cancer Medicine, 6th ed. Hamilton, Ont: BC Decker, 2003:939–946.
42. Osborne CK, Zhao H, Fuqua SA. Selective estrogen receptor modulators: Structure, function, and clinical use. J Clin Oncol 2000;18: 3172–3186.
43. Schally AV, Comaru-Schally AM. Hypothalamic and other peptide hormones. In: Kufe DW, Pollock RE, Weichselbaum RR, eds. Cancer Medicine, 6th ed. Hamilton, Ont: DC Becker, 2003:911–926.
44. Buzdar AU, Harvey HA. Aromatase inhibitors. In: Kufe DW, Pollock RE, Weichselbaum RR, eds. Cancer Medicine, 6th ed. Hamilton, Ont: DC Becker, 2003:947–959.
45. Denmeade SR, Isaacs JT. Androgen deprivation strategies in the treatment of advanced prostate cancer. In: Kufe DW, Pollock RE, Weichselbaum RR, eds. Cancer Medicine, 6th ed. Hamilton, Ont: DC Becker, 2003:967–979.
46. McCarty KSJ, Nichols M, McCarty DSS. Progestins. In: Kufe DW, Pollock RE, Weichselbaum RR, eds. Cancer Medicine, 6th ed. Hamilton, Ont: DC Becker, 2003:961–966.
47. McKay LI, Cidlowski JA. Corticosteroids. In: Kufe DW, Pollock RE, Weichselbaum RR, eds. Cancer Medicine, 6th ed. Hamilton, Ont: DC Becker, 2003:927–938.
48. Lazo JS. Bleomycin. Cancer Chemother Biol Response Modif 1999;18:39–45.
49. Kurtzberg J, Yousem D, Beauchamp N Jr. Asparaginase. In: Kufe DW, Pollock RE, Weichselbaum RR, eds. Cancer Medicine, 6th ed. Hamilton, Ont: DC Becker, 2003:823–830.
50. Soignet SL, Frankel SR, Douer D, et al. United States multicenter study of arsenic trioxide in relapsed acute promyelocytic leukemia. J Clin Oncol 2001;19:3852–3860.
51. Bradner WT. Mitomycin C. A clinical update. Cancer Treat Rev 2001;27:35–50.
52. Scheinberg DA, Mulford DA, Jurcic JG, et al. Antibody therapies of cancer. In: Chabner BA, Longo DL, eds. Cancer Chemotherapy and Biotherapy: Principles and Practice, 4th ed. Philadelphia: Lippincott Williams & Wilkins, 2006:666–698.
53. American Medical Association. Monoclonal antibodies. 2006 February 14, 2006 [cited 2006 September 30,2006]. 2006, *http://www.ama-assn.org/ama/pub/category/13280.html.*
54. Rotea W Jr, Saad ED. Targeted drugs in oncology: New names, new mechanisms, new paradigm. Am J Health Syst Pharm 2003;60:1233–1243; quiz 1244–1245.
55. Harris M. Monoclonal antibodies as therapeutic agents for cancer. Lancet Oncol 2004;5:292–302.
56. Giles F, Estey E, O'Brien S. Gemtuzumab ozogamicin in the treatment of acute myeloid leukemia. Cancer 2003;98:2095–2104.
57. Villamor N, Montserrat E, Colomer D. Mechanism of action and resistance to monoclonal antibody therapy. Semin Oncol 2003;30:424–433.
58. Cheson BD. Radioimmunotherapy of non-Hodgkin lymphomas. Blood 2003;101:391–398.
59. Cersosimo RJ. Monoclonal antibodies in the treatment of cancer, Part 2. Am J Health Syst Pharm 2003;60:1631–1641; quiz 1642–1643.
60. Mylotarg (Gemtuzumab). Product information. Philadelphia: Wyeth Pharmaceuticals, 2006.
61. Plosker GL, Figgitt DP. Rituximab: A review of its use in non-Hodgkin's lymphoma and chronic lymphocytic leukaemia. Drugs 2003;63:803–843.
62. Cersosimo RJ. Monoclonal antibodies in the treatment of cancer, Part 1. Am J Health Syst Pharm 2003;60:1531–1548.
63. Hernandez MC, Knox SJ. Radiobiology of radioimmunotherapy with 90Y ibritumomab tiuxetan (Zevalin). Semin Oncol 2003;30(Suppl 17):6–10.
64. Kaminski MS, Zelenetz AD, Press OW, et al. Pivotal study of iodine I 131 tositumomab for chemotherapy-refractory low-grade or transformed low-grade B-cell non-Hodgkin's lymphomas [see comment]. J Clin Oncol 2001;19:3918–3928.
65. Frampton JE, Wagstaff AJ. Alemtuzumab. Drugs 2003;63:1229–1243; discussion 1245–1246.
66. Syed S, Rowinsky E. The new generation of targeted therapies for breast cancer. Oncology (Williston Park) 2003;17:1339–1351; discussion 52.
67. Rowinsky EK. Signal events: Cell signal transduction and its inhibition in cancer. Oncologist 2003;2006;8(Suppl 3):5–17.
68. Finley RS. Overview of targeted therapies for cancer. Am J Health Syst Pharm 2003;60(Suppl 9):S4–S10.
69. Reynolds NA, Wagstaff AJ. Cetuximab: In the treatment of metastatic colorectal cancer. Drugs 2004;64:109–118; discussion 119–121.
70. Cunningham D, Humblet Y, Siena S, et al. Cetuximab monotherapy and cetuximab plus irinotecan in irinotecan-refractory metastatic colorectal cancer [see comment]. N Engl J Med 2004;351:337–345.
71. Bonner JA, Harari PM, Giralt J, et al. Radiotherapy plus cetuximab for squamous-cell carcinoma of the head and neck [see comment]. N Engl J Med 2006;354:567–578.
72. Perez-Soler R, Saltz L. Cutaneous adverse effects with HER1/EGFR-targeted agents: Is there a silver lining? J Clin Oncol 2005;23:5235–5246.
73. Treish I, Schwartz R, Lindley C. Pharmacology and therapeutic use of trastuzumab in breast cancer. Am J Health Syst Pharm 2000;57:2063–2076; quiz 2077–2079.
74. Romond EH, Perez EA, Bryant J, et al. Trastuzumab plus adjuvant chemotherapy for operable HER2-positive breast cancer. N Engl J Med 2005;353:1673–1684.
75. Leyland-Jones B, Gelmon K, Ayoub JP, et al. Pharmacokinetics, safety, and efficacy of trastuzumab administered every three weeks in combination with paclitaxel [see comment]. J Clin Oncol 2003;21:3965–3971.
76. Cersosimo RJ. Gefitinib: A new antineoplastic for advanced non-small-cell lung cancer[see comment]. Am J Health Syst Pharm 2004;61:889–898.
77. Tang PA, Tsao M-S, Moore MJ. A review of erlotinib and its clinical use. Expert Opin Pharmacother 2006;7:177–193.
78. Janne PA, Johnson BE. Effect of epidermal growth factor receptor tyrosine kinase domain mutations on the outcome of patients with non-small cell lung cancer treated with epidermal growth factor receptor tyrosine kinase inhibitors. Clin Cancer Res 2006;12(Pt 2):4416s–4420s.
79. Geyer CE, Forster J, Lindquist D, et al. Lapatinib plus capecitabine for HER2-positive advanced breast cancer. N Engl J Med 2006;355:2733–2743.
80. Zondor SD, Medina PJ. Bevacizumab: An angiogenesis inhibitor with efficacy in colorectal and other malignancies. Ann Pharmacother 2004;38:1258–1264.

81. Hurwitz H, Fehrenbacher L, Novotny W, et al. Bevacizumab plus irinotecan, fluorouracil, and leucovorin for metastatic colorectal cancer [see comment]. N Engl J Med 2004;350:2335–2342.
82. Avastin (Bevacizumab). Product information. San Francisco, CA: Genentech, 2006.
83. Eto M, Naito S. Molecular targeting therapy for renal cell carcinoma. Int J Clin Oncol 2006;11:209–213.
84. Deininger M, Buchdunger E, Druker BJ. The development of imatinib as a therapeutic agent for chronic myeloid leukemia. Blood 2005;105:2640–2653.
85. Gleevec (Imatinib Mesylate). Product information. East Hanover, NJ: Novartis Pharmaceutical Corporation, January 2004.
86. Richardson PG, Barlogie B, Berenson J, et al. A phase 2 study of bortezomib in relapsed, refractory myeloma [see comment]. N Engl J Med 2003;348:2609–2617.
87. Mitchell BS. The proteasome—An emerging therapeutic target in cancer [comment]. N Engl J Med 2003;348:2597–2598.
88. Pantuck AJ, Thomas G, Belldegrun AS, Figlin RA. Mammalian target of rapamycin inhibitors in renal cell carcinoma: Current status and future applications. Semin Oncol 2006;33:607–613.
89. Hudes G, Carducci M, Tomczak P, et al. Temsirolimus, interferon alfa, or both for advanced renal-cell carcinoma. N Engl J Med 2007;356:2271–2281.
90. Rajkumar SV, Kyle RA. Multiple myeloma: Diagnosis and treatment. Mayo Clin Proc 2005;80:1371–1382.
91. Sporn MB, Lippman SM. Chemoprevention of cancer. In: Kufe DW, Pollock RE, Weichselbaum RR, eds. Cancer Medicine, 6th ed. Hamilton, Ont: DC Becker, 2003:414–422.
92. Borden EC. Interferons. In: Kufe DW, Pollock RE, Weichselbaum RR, eds. Cancer Medicine, 6th ed. Hamilton, Ont: DC Becker, 2003:831–841.
93. Ekmekcioglu S, Grimm EA. Cytokines: Biology and applications in cancer medicine. In: Kufe DW, Pollock RE, Weichselbaum RR, eds. Cancer Medicine, 6th ed. Hamilton, Ont: DC Becker, 2003:843–851.
94. Foss F. Clinical experience with denileukin diftitox (ONTAK). Semin Oncol 2006;33(Suppl 3):S11–S16.
95. Therasse P, Arbuck SG, Eisenhauer EA, et al. New guidelines to evaluate the response to treatment in solid tumors. J Natl Cancer Inst 2000;92:205–216.
96. Kellen JA. The reversal of multidrug resistance: An update. J Exp Ther Oncol 2003;3:5–13.
97. Lee W, Lockhart AC, Kim RB, Rothenberg ML. Cancer Pharmacogenomics: Powerful tools in cancer chemotherapy and drug development. Oncologist 2005;10:104–111.
98. Haskell CM. Principles of cancer chemotherapy. In: Haskell CM, ed. Cancer Treatment, 5th ed. Philadelphia: WB Saunders, 2001:62–86.
99. Johnson DH. Targeted therapies in combination with chemotherapy in non–small cell lung cancer. Clin Cancer Res 2006;12(Pt 2):4451s–4457s.
100. Vu TT. Standardization of body surface area calculations. J Oncol Pharm Pract 2002;8:49–54.
101. Calvert AH, Newell DR, Gumbrell LA, et al. Carboplatin dosage: Prospective evaluation of a simple formula based on renal function. J Clin Oncol 1989;7:1748–1756.
102. American Society of Hospital Pharmacists. ASHP guidelines on handling hazardous drugs. Am J Health Syst Pharm 2006;63:1172–1193.
103. The NCCN Cancer- and Treatment-Related Anemia Clinical Practice Guidelines in Oncology (Version 3.2007). 2007 National Comprehensive Cancer Network, Inc. 2007, *http://www.nccn.org*.
104. Siddiqui MAA, Keating GM. Darbepoetin alfa: A review of its use in the treatment of anaemia in patients with cancer receiving chemotherapy. Drugs 2006;66:997–1012.
105. Hughes WT, Armstrong D, Bodey GP, et al. 2002 Guidelines for the use of antimicrobial agents in neutropenic patients with cancer [see comment]. Clin Infect Dis 2002;34:730–751.
106. Nemunaitis J. A comparative review of colony-stimulating factors. Drugs 1997;54:709–729.
107. Wolf T, Densmore JJ. Pegfilgrastim use during chemotherapy: Current and future applications. Curr Hematol Rep 2004;3:419–423.
108. Smith TJ, Khatcheressian J, Lyman GH, et al. 2006 Update of recommendations for the use of white blood cell growth factors: An evidence-based clinical practice guideline. J Clin Oncol 2006;24:3187–3205.
109. Demetri GD. Pharmacologic treatment options in patients with thrombocytopenia. Semin Hematol 2000;37(Suppl 4):11–18.
110. Cantor SB, Elting LS, Hudson DV Jr, Rubenstein EB. Pharmacoeconomic analysis of oprelvekin (recombinant human interleukin-11) for secondary prophylaxis of thrombocytopenia in solid tumor patients receiving chemotherapy. Cancer 2003;97:3099–3106.
111. Rubenstein EB, Peterson DE, Schubert M, et al. Clinical practice guidelines for the prevention and treatment of cancer therapy-induced oral and gastrointestinal mucositis. Cancer 2004;100(Suppl):2026–2046.
112. Spielberger R, Stiff P, Bensinger W, et al. Palifermin for oral mucositis after intensive therapy for hematologic cancers. N Engl J Med 2004;351:2590–2598.
113. Benson AB, III, Ajani JA, Catalano RB, et al. Recommended guidelines for the treatment of cancer treatment-induced diarrhea. J Clin Oncol 2004;22:2918–2926.
114. Berger AM, Karakunnell J. Hair loss. In: DeVita V, Hellman S, Rosenberg SA, eds. Cancer Principles and Practice of Oncology, 7th ed. Philadelphia: Lippincott Williams & Wilkins, 2005:2556–2559.
115. Albanell J, Baselga J. Systemic therapy emergencies. Semin Oncol 2000;27:347–361.
116. Lee SJ, Schover LR, Partridge AH, et al. American Society of Clinical Oncology recommendations on fertility preservation in cancer patients. J Clin Oncol 2006;24:2917–2931.
117. Van Leeuwen FE, Travis LB. Second cancers. In: DeVita VT, Hellman S, Rosenberg SA, eds. Cancer Principles and Practice of Oncology, 7th ed. Philadelphia: Lippincott Williams & Wilkins, 2005:2575–2601.

CHAPTER 131 Breast Cancer

LAURA BOEHNKE MICHAUD, JANET L. ESPIRITO, AND FRANCISCO J. ESTEVA

KEY CONCEPTS

1. Breast cancer is usually diagnosed in early stages, when it is a highly curable malignancy.
2. Local therapy of early-stage breast cancer consists of modified radical mastectomy or lumpectomy plus external beam radiation therapy. The surgical approach to the ipsilateral axilla may consist of a full level I/II axillary lymph node dissection or a lymph node mapping procedure with sentinel lymph node biopsy.
3. Adjuvant endocrine therapy reduces the rates of relapse and death in patients with hormone receptor-positive early breast cancer tumors. Adjuvant chemotherapy reduces the rates of relapse and death in all patients with early stage breast cancer.
4. The choice of chemotherapy regimen, dose, schedule and duration of therapy, and the choice of endocrine therapy are controversial and rapidly changing as results from ongoing randomized clinical trials are reported.
5. Neoadjuvant chemotherapy is appropriate for patients with locally advanced or inflammatory breast cancer, followed by local therapy and further adjuvant systemic therapy.
6. Initial therapy of metastatic breast cancer in women with hormone receptor-positive tumors should consist of hormonal therapy.
7. Women with metastatic breast cancer who have hormone receptor-positive tumors and respond to an initial hormonal manipulation will usually respond to a second hormonal manipulation.
8. Approximately 40% of women with metastatic breast cancer will respond to chemotherapy regimens; anthracycline- and taxane-containing regimens are the most active.
9. The goal of adjuvant chemotherapy is curative, whereas the goal of chemotherapy in the metastatic setting is palliative.
10. Although controversial, annual screening mammography in women younger than 50 years of age is clearly beneficial and many national and international studies demonstrate a 20% to 40% reduction in breast cancer mortality from annual or biannual screening mammography in women ages 50 to 70 years.

Breast cancer is the most common site of cancer and is second only to lung cancer as a cause of cancer death in American women. It is estimated that 178,480 new cases of breast cancer will be diagnosed and that 40,460 women will die of breast cancer in 2007.[1] In addition to invasive breast cancers, it is estimated that 62,030 cases of noninvasive, or in situ, cancer will be diagnosed among women in the United States in 2007.

Learning objectives, review questions, and other resources can be found at **www.pharmacotherapyonline.com.**

Female breast cancer incidence rates vary considerably across racial and ethnic groups. The average annual age-adjusted incidence rate from 2000 to 2003 was 134 cases per 100,000 among white females, 118 cases among African Americans, 89 cases in Hispanics, 89 cases among Asian-Americans/Pacific Islanders, and 74 cases in American Indians/Alaska Natives.[2] Reasons for the higher incidence rates in whites than in other racial and ethnic groups may include differences in reproductive and lifestyle factors, and access to and use of screening.[3]

Female breast cancer incidence rates have increased for all women combined since 1980, although the rate of increase slowed in the 1990s, and has leveled off since 2001. Factors that may explain the increase in incidence include increased use of screening mammography and use of postmenopausal hormone-replacement therapy (HRT).[1] The incidence of ductal carcinoma in situ (DCIS) also increased rapidly between the early and late 1980s, and continues to increase. The increase in DCIS is largely attributed to increased use of screening mammography, because most cases of DCIS manifest solely as clustered microcalcifications seen on mammography.[3]

(1) For all racial and ethnic groups, most breast cancers are diagnosed at an early stage, when tumors are small and localized. However, a higher proportion of disease is diagnosed at more advanced stages in African American and other minority women than in white women. The death rate is also higher among African American women than white women despite the lower incidence. From 2000 to 2003, the breast cancer death rate was highest in African Americans (34.3 cases per 100,000 women), followed by whites (25.3), Hispanics (16.2), American Indians/Alaska Natives (13.4), and Asian-Americans/Pacific Islanders (12.6).[2] The disparity between white and African American women can be explained by differences in timely diagnosis through mammography screening and limited access to prompt treatment.[3] Despite these differences, overall mortality rates from breast cancer in the United States have declined since 1990. These declines have been attributed to increased use of screening and effectiveness of adjuvant treatment.[4,5] Figure 131–1 shows the temporal trends in incidence and mortality by race.

The median age for the diagnosis of breast cancer is between the ages of 60 and 65 years.[2] Although lung cancer is the leading cause of cancer deaths for women regardless of age, breast cancer is the leading cause of cancer deaths for females between the ages of 20 and 59 years.[1]

EPIDEMIOLOGY AND ETIOLOGY

The two variables most strongly associated with the occurrence of breast cancer are gender and age. Although one commonly thinks of

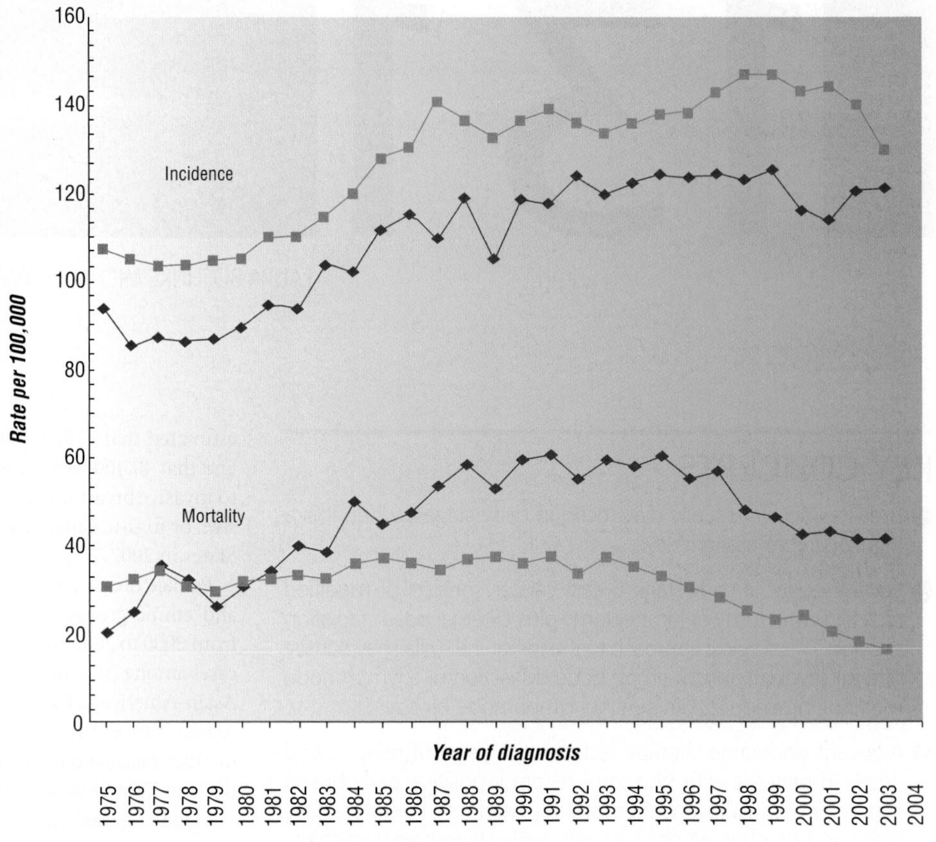

FIGURE 131-1. Breast cancer incidence and mortality rates by race, 1975–2003. *(From reference 2.)*

breast cancer as a disease confined to women, about 2,030 cases of male breast cancer will be diagnosed in the United States in 2007.[1] Male gender had been considered a poor prognostic factor in some investigations, but it is now believed that higher mortality rates in men are attributable to more advanced disease at the time of diagnosis. When stage and other known prognostic factors are controlled for, the clinical outcome for men with breast cancer is comparable to women.[6] Likewise, treatment of male breast cancer is similar to treatment of breast cancer in females.

The incidence of breast cancer increases with advancing age. A frequently quoted breast cancer statistic is that 1 in 8 women will develop breast cancer during their lifetime. It should be emphasized that this is a cumulative lifetime risk of developing the disease from birth to death. The 1-in-8-women figure is often misinterpreted by women who assume that it translates into 1 in 8 women being diagnosed with breast cancer each year. A more useful method of presenting the risk data is based on age intervals.[7] Table 131–1 shows that the risk of a woman developing breast cancer before the age of 40 years is about 1 in 233, and more than half the risk occurs after age 60 years.

An understanding of the relationship between age and the incidence of breast cancer is particularly relevant when one discusses "risk factors" or factors other than age that increase a woman's probability of developing breast cancer. The relative risk (RR) of developing breast cancer for an individual woman in a defined risk group is usually multiplied by the probability of a woman developing breast cancer during her lifetime, and this figure is taken as the cumulative lifetime risk of that individual developing breast cancer. However, the risk of developing breast cancer depends on age. Therefore a more meaningful way to counsel patients regarding their risk of developing breast cancer based on the presence of a known risk factor incorporates an age-specific incidence rate, not cumulative lifetime risk. For example, if a 40-year-old woman with a strong family history of breast cancer has a RR ratio of 2.0, her risk of developing breast cancer by the age of 50 is only 2.9% (2 × 1.44) not 25.34% (2 × 12.67) (see Table 131–1). It is also important to note that recognized risk factors are not additive in a simple mathematical sense. Finally, it should be emphasized that most women with breast cancer have no identifiable major risk factor, indicating that the search for the etiology of this disease is largely incomplete.

A number of calculators are available to estimate a patient's risk of developing breast cancer. The National Cancer Institute has an online version of the Breast Cancer Risk Assessment Tool (*www.cancer.gov/bcrisktool/Default.aspx*). This tool is based on a statistical model known as the Gail Model, derived from data from the Breast Cancer Detection and Demonstration Project, a mammography screening project conducted in the 1970s. The Breast Cancer Risk Assessment Tool was designed for healthcare professionals to project a woman's

TABLE 131-1 Risk of Developing Breast Cancer in SEER Areas, Women, All Races 2001–2003

Age Interval (years)	Probability (%) of Developing Invasive Breast Cancer during the Interval
30–40	0.43 or 1 in 233
40–50	1.44 or 1 in 69
50–60	2.63 or 1 in 38
60–70	3.65 or 1 in 27
From birth to death	12.67 or 1 in 8

SEER, Surveillance Epidemiology and End Results.
From Ries LAG, Harkins D, Krapcho M, eds. SEER Cancer Statistics Review: 1975–2003. Bethesda, MD. http://seer.cancer.gov/csr/1975–2003/

individualized risk for invasive breast cancer over a 5-year period and over her lifetime. This model has been shown to provide accurate estimates in white women, but it has not been validated for other racial and ethnic groups, and other subgroups including those with genetic risk factors. Other risk assessment models also exist, each taking into account different risk factors. These empiric models may not be as useful for women with a history suggestive of hereditary breast cancer. Thus, no one model is appropriate for every patient.

ENDOCRINE FACTORS

A number of endocrine factors have been linked to the incidence of breast cancer.[8,9] Many of these relate to the total duration of menstrual life. Early menarche, generally defined as menstruation beginning before age 12 years, increases the cumulative lifetime risk of breast cancer development. Similarly, most studies demonstrate an increased risk in women with a late age of natural menopause (age 55 years or later). Conversely, bilateral oophorectomy prior to age 40 years reduces the relative risk of developing breast cancer.

Nulliparity and a late age at first birth (≥30 years) are reported to increase the lifetime risk of developing breast cancer. It is suggested that the period between the onset of menses and the age of first pregnancy provides a "window of initiation" for the development of breast cancer. This is a time when an unbalanced hormonal environment reacts with the abundant and highly responsive breast tissue. Investigators postulate that international differences in age of menarche, age at menopause, and childbearing may account for a substantial part of the international differences in the incidence of breast cancer.

Many studies have evaluated the relationship between exogenous hormones and development of breast cancer. Postmenopausal estrogen replacement therapy has been the subject of several epidemiologic studies and meta-analyses, with conflicting results. The NCI-sponsored Women's Health Initiative (WHI) is a set of clinical trials designed to investigate the risks and benefits of treatment strategies that could affect women's health issues, such as breast cancer. The WHI trials of hormone therapy were two large parallel, randomized, double-blind, placebo-controlled trials that evaluated estrogen plus progestin in combination or estrogen alone in postmenopausal women. The estrogen plus progestin trial randomized more than 16,000 postmenopausal women to take conjugated equine estrogen combined with medroxyprogesterone or a placebo.[10] This study reported an increased risk of breast cancer (38 vs. 30 cases per 10,000 person years [RR = 1.26, 95% Confidence Interval (CI) 1.00–1.59]) in women taking combined estrogen/progestin for an average of 5.2 years were compared to those receiving placebo. In the estrogen alone trial, over 10,000 women who had a hysterectomy and therefore did not require progestin therapy due to a decreased risk of endometrial carcinoma, were randomized to estrogen alone or placebo.[11] The risk of breast cancer was not increased in women who received estrogen alone as compared to placebo. Differences in dosages, formulations, and routes of administration of various hormonal preparations available make interpretation of these studies complex. However, most of the current evidence does show a causal relationship between HRT and breast cancer.[12] Unresolved issues remain as to whether lower doses or short-term use for menopausal symptoms can be safe and effective. Longer duration of use of HRT and concurrent use of progestins appear to contribute to breast cancer risk.

The use of postmenopausal HRT in women with a history of breast cancer is generally contraindicated. Because of the association of estrogen and risk of breast cancer, many clinicians believe that patients with a strong family history or other risk factors for breast cancer should not receive postmenopausal HRT. Women who are considering HRT should carefully consider the risks versus benefits (see Chap. 85 for a detailed discussion of hormone replacement therapy).

Epidemiologic studies of oral contraceptives do not show a consistent relationship between use of birth control pills and breast cancer risk. Results are conflicting and assessment of the studies should consider the particular oral contraceptive products involved, daily and cumulative doses of the hormones administered, and the latency for development of breast cancer. Newer formulations of oral contraceptives contain lower hormone concentrations, with different routes of administration (e.g. patch, injections, etc.). Reassuring data that oral contraceptives do not increase breast cancer risk later in life have recently been published.[13,14] Although it is not entirely possible to rule out a promotional effect of oral contraceptives on breast cancer development in young patients, most experts believe that the safety and benefits of low-dose oral contraceptives currently outweigh the potential risks. Oral contraceptives are known to reduce the risk of ovarian and endometrial cancers.

GENETIC FACTORS

Both personal and family histories influence a woman's risk of developing breast cancer. A past medical history of breast cancer is associated with an increased risk of contralateral breast cancer. Cancer of the uterus and ovary is also associated with an increased risk for the development of breast cancer. Breast cancer is also observed as part of cancer family syndromes in association with other tumors.

Many women have "lumpy breasts" and have a clinical diagnosis of fibrocystic breast disease or benign breast disease. Fibrocystic disease encompasses a heterogeneous group of processes with various degrees of breast cancer risks, and therefore is not clinically meaningful for counseling patients regarding individual risk of breast cancer. Benign breast conditions are classified as nonproliferative, proliferative without atypia, or atypical hyperplasia. Nonproliferative lesions do not increase the risk of breast cancer. Proliferative lesions without atypia include fibroadenomas, and are associated with a mildly elevated breast cancer risk of about 1.5 to 2.0 times the general population. Atypical hyperplasias are classified as either ductal or lobular units, and these lesions may increase a woman's risk for breast cancer to about 3.5 to 5.0 times the general population.

Dense breast tissue reduces the sensitivity of mammography for detecting breast cancer, and is also associated with an increased risk of breast cancer. Genetic factors may play a role in this finding because mammographic breast density has been shown to have high heritability and is also strongly associated with a positive family history of breast cancer. Many variables including age, weight, menopausal status, HRT, and parity can influence mammographic breast density. The risk of breast cancer in women with dense breasts (defined by mammography) has been estimated to be between 2 and 6 times that of women of the same age with little density.[15]

It has been recognized for some time that a family history of breast cancer is associated with a woman's own risk for developing the disease. The percentage of all breast cancers in the population that can be attributed to family history is approximately 10%. Empirical estimates of the risks associated with particular patterns of family history of breast cancer indicate the following[16]:

1. Having any first-degree relative with breast cancer increases a woman's risk of breast cancer about 1.5- to 3-fold. Risk increases with increasing numbers of affected first-degree relatives.
2. The risk is affected by both a woman's own age and the age of the relative when diagnosed. A higher RR is seen when a woman and her relative at diagnosis are younger than 50 years.

3. The risk associated with having any second-degree relative with breast cancer is complex, and depends on other family history patterns. However, the risk is generally lower than that of first-degree relatives.
4. Affected family members on both the maternal and the paternal sides are important to consider in evaluation of risk.

Although women with a family history of breast cancer are at increased risk for the disease, the diagnosis of breast cancer is still uncommon in young women, even with a positive family history. Although family history is an important risk factor to consider, other risk factors should also be considered as most women who develop breast cancer do not have a family history. Nonetheless, increasing knowledge about the genetics of the disease continues to add to our knowledge.

In the early 1990s, pedigree analysis of 23 high-risk families for breast and ovarian cancer provided evidence for a rare autosomal dominant allele.[17] Further studies identified an abnormal gene on the long arm of chromosome 17 (17q21) in a large percentage of these hereditary breast and ovarian cancer patients. Isolation of the *BRCA1* gene was initially reported in 1994. A second breast cancer gene, called *BRCA2*, has been mapped to chromosome 13. These genes function as tumor suppressor genes, maintaining genomic integrity and DNA repair. Germ-line mutations in either *BRCA1 or BRCA2* are associated with an increased risk for breast and ovarian cancer. Compared to an average woman's 13% lifetime risk of developing breast cancer, the probability of developing breast or ovarian cancer by the age of 70 years in women with a *BRCA1* or *BRCA2* mutation is estimated to be 35% to 84% for breast cancer and 10% to 50% for ovarian cancer.[18,19] The risk of ovarian cancer is considered higher among carriers of *BRCA1* mutations than for carriers of *BRCA2* mutations.

The probability of being a *BRCA* gene-mutation carrier is related to ethnicity and family history. Particular family history patterns are associated with an increased risk, including the number of affected and unaffected family members who had breast and/or ovarian cancer, including first- and second-degree relatives; younger age (<50 years) at which breast cancer is diagnosed; the presence of bilateral breast cancer; and a history of breast cancer in a male relative. Both maternal and paternal family histories are relevant. Specific gene mutations can also be seen more often among certain ethnic groups. Jewish people of Eastern European decent (Ashkenazi Jews) have an unusually high (2.5%) carrier rate of germ-line mutations in *BRCA1* and *BRCA2* as compared to the rest of the U.S. population. Three particular *BRCA* founder mutations are most often identified in women of Jewish ancestry.[17]

Since the discovery of *BRCA1* and *BRCA2*, genetic testing for mutations in these genes has become available. The question of who should receive screening for *BRCA* gene mutations is unresolved. It is estimated that clinically significant *BRCA* mutations occur at a frequency of about 1 in 500 persons in the general, non-Jewish U.S. population.[19] Risk tools to predict for the presence of a clinically significant *BRCA* mutation exist. Because many of these tools were developed from data in previously tested women with existing cancer, their applicability and effectiveness for screening in the general population are unknown. Several organizations have published recommendations on genetic susceptibility testing for individuals who meet the criteria for increased risk.[18,20,21] Testing is generally recommended only when there is personal or family history suggestive of hereditary cancer, when the test can be adequately interpreted, and when results will assist with diagnosis and management. Genetic counseling is recommended to assist individuals in making informed decisions.

The management of women who test positive for a known deleterious mutation in *BRCA1* or *BRCA2* is controversial. Options include prophylactic mastectomy and/or oophorectomy, chemoprevention, and/or intensive screening.[18,19,22,23] Bilateral total mastectomy and/or oophorectomy reduce the risk of breast cancer occurrence, but both breast and ovarian cancers have been reported in patients who have had prophylactic removal of these organs. The benefit of tamoxifen or raloxifene for chemoprevention in *BRCA* mutation carriers is not clear.[22] Although tamoxifen reduces the risk of estrogen receptor-positive breast cancers, breast cancers associated with *BRCA1* mutations tend to be estrogen receptor negative.[24] Similar data regarding this subset of patients are not yet available with raloxifene. In patients with *BRCA* mutations, annual screening mammography has poor sensitivity and may miss aggressive cancers. Descriptive studies suggest an increased risk for interval cancers (occurring between mammograms) in this population of women. Magnetic resonance imaging (MRI) has demonstrated higher sensitivity than mammography in *BRCA* mutation carriers. Annual breast MRI screening is now recommended by the American Cancer Society as an adjunct to mammography for known *BRCA* mutation carriers, for untested individuals who have a first-degree relative with a *BRCA* mutation, or for women with a 20% or greater lifetime risk of breast cancer based on models that largely depend on family history.[25] Thus, for women who do not opt for surgical prophylaxis, intensive surveillance with annual mammogram and breast MRI screening, along with clinical breast examinations every 6 months is an option.[21,23]

The clinical significance of other unclassified variant gene mutations is unknown. Testing negative for a *BRCA* gene mutation does not necessarily rule out a hereditary form of breast cancer. In cases where there is significant personal or family history, a negative test may be considered an uninformative negative, as it may be a result of mutations undetected by currently available screening techniques, or a result of mutations in other, unidentified genes. Other genes that have been identified as being associated with hereditary breast cancer include TP53, CHK2, PTEN, and ATM.[17]

ENVIRONMENTAL AND LIFESTYLE FACTORS

Breast cancer incidence rates vary considerably between countries, which suggests that environmental and lifestyle factors play an important role in the etiology. Compelling evidence is derived from studies of Asian women who migrated to the United States. Although the incidence of breast cancer in Asian women is quite low, the incidence of breast cancer in Asian women who were born in the United States, or who migrated from Asia to the United States, gradually increases to equal that of the white population in the same geographic area.[9]

Diet is an obvious environmental factor, and possible relationships between fat intake and steroid hormone metabolism have led to an emphasis on dietary fat as a possible etiologic agent for breast cancer. Epidemiologic data show a positive correlation between higher dietary fat intake and breast cancer risk. The correlation is stronger in postmenopausal than in premenopausal women. A low-fat diet is linked to low blood estrogen levels and lower breast cancer risk. Studies in laboratory animals provide further evidence of a relationship between dietary fat intake and breast cancer. Despite these compelling indirect data, case control and cohort studies report mixed results. In a meta-analysis of 31 case-control and 14 cohort studies on dietary fat and breast cancer, Boyd et al. reported a small but significant RR of 1.13 (95% CI 1.03 to 1.25) when comparing highest and lowest fat intake categories.[26]

Additional investigated dietary factors include food-derived heterocyclic amines, which are known carcinogens found commonly in cooked meat. Experimental and epidemiologic data suggest an association between breast cancer and the Western diet, which typically includes a large amount of cooked meats and fat. In the meta-analysis by Boyd et al., saturated fat and meat intake were also associated with a small, but significant increased risk in breast cancer.[26] Other studies have found no significant association between breast cancer and the Western diet. Effects may depend on menopausal status, as studies of premenopausal women suggest a possible increased risk.[27]

Many studies have also examined the association between breast cancer and intake of dietary fiber and micronutrients, including β-carotene, and vitamins A, C, and E. The relationship between vitamins and breast cancer is unclear. Studies of breast cancer risk in relation to fruit and vegetable intake suggest some protective effect, as they are food sources of micronutrients and fiber. A meta-analysis of 21 case-control and 5 cohort studies reported a significant reduction in breast cancer risk with higher vegetable consumption, with no significant difference seen with fruit intake.[28] Additional reviews of prospective, cohort studies reported no significant associations with either vegetable or fruit intake and breast cancer risk.[29] Thus, results of studies investigating the effects of fruit, vegetable, fiber, and meat consumption on breast cancer incidence are inconclusive.

One dietary factor that deserves mention is the possible effect of phytoestrogens on breast cancer risk. Phytoestrogens are natural plant estrogens found in soybean products, seeds, berries, and nuts. Interest in the study of these compounds has largely been based on observational studies showing lower rates of breast cancer in Asian countries, where soy consumption is high.[30] Because these compounds exhibit weak estrogenic properties, some experts believe that they may function as relative antiestrogens by displacing natural estradiol. However, studies have also reported a potential stimulatory effect on breast tissue. Nonetheless, the effect of phytoestrogens on breast cancer is very controversial, and further research is needed.

The hypothesis that low dietary fat intake reduces breast cancer risk was tested in the Women's Health Initiative Randomized Controlled Dietary Modification Trial.[31] This study is the first large-scale, prospective, controlled trial to study the relationship between diet and breast cancer. It randomized more than 48,000 postmenopausal women to a dietary intervention that consisted of reducing total fat intake to 20% of energy, consuming at least five servings of fruits and vegetables daily and six servings of grains daily, versus a comparison group without any dietary interventions. Risk factors for breast cancer were evenly balanced between groups. Over an 8-year mean followup period, 3.35% of women in the intervention group developed invasive breast cancer versus 3.66% of women in the comparison group (annualized incidence rate 0.42% vs. 0.45%, hazard ratio 0.91; 95% CI 0.83 to 1.01). Although the difference was not statistically significant, a trend toward a decreased incidence over time was seen, suggesting the need for longer followup. Limitations from this study include the inability to separate out the effects on breast cancer attributed to dietary fat reduction as compared to that attributed to increased fruit, vegetable, and grain intake. Because the Women's Health Initiative trial only evaluated women who adopted dietary changes after menopause, it is unknown what the effects would be in younger women or girls who make these dietary interventions sooner in life. Although there is still much to be learned about the effects of diet on the risk of developing breast cancer, a low-fat diet may reduce the risk of recurrence and improve relapse-free survival in women with early stage, resected breast cancer.[32]

Both body weight and height are associated with developing breast cancer. High body mass index and obesity are related to breast cancer risk in a complex way that differs by age and menopausal status. Most studies of premenopausal women show either no relationship with body weight, or slightly declining breast cancer risks with increasing body weight. One plausible biologic mechanism to explain this observation is reduced ovarian activity in obese women. Most studies in postmenopausal women, however, show increasing breast cancer risks with increasing body weight. In addition to obesity, the distribution of body fat also may play an independent role in the development of breast cancer. Upper body (central or abdominal) adiposity increases the risk of breast cancer independent of overall obesity. This association may be related to the excess levels of free-circulating estrogen resulting from the conversion of androstenedione to estradiol in peripheral adipose tissue.[33] Although height is not a modifiable risk factor, weight and body composition are modifiable and should be studied further.

Many studies report an inverse association between physical activity and breast cancer risk.[34] A review of 19 cohort and 29 case-control studies suggests that the association is stronger for postmenopausal breast cancer than for premenopausal breast cancer. Exercise may provide modest protection against breast cancer, but the relationship is complex. Possible explanations include the effects of physical activity on menstrual characteristics (in premenopausal women), body size, weight, and serum hormone levels. Thus estrogen-related pathways or other metabolic hormones such as insulin or insulin-like growth factors may play a role. Exercise in women following a diagnosis of breast cancer may also increase the likelihood of overall survival.[35]

Many epidemiologic studies have evaluated the relationship between alcohol and breast cancer. Alcohol is the only dietary factor that has shown consistent results in clinical trials. Studies indicate both a modest positive association between alcohol and breast cancer and a dose–response relationship.[36,37] The risk increases with consumption of alcohol in general, regardless of the beverage type or woman's menopausal status. Potential biologic mechanisms for this association include increased levels of estrogen or other reproductive steroid hormones; increased production of insulin-like growth factors by the liver; and altered hepatic metabolism of carcinogens. Although a causal relationship between alcohol consumption and breast cancer has not been proven in a prospective trial, the weight of the evidence suggests that a relationship, direct or indirect, may exist. As alcohol consumption is a modifiable risk factor, use in moderation is a sensible approach.

Radiation is associated with an increased risk of breast cancer, particularly with exposure at a young age (<20 years), which again suggests that a "window of initiation" for breast cancer occurs at a relatively early age. Much of the knowledge about radiation-related breast cancer comes from epidemiologic studies of patients exposed to diagnostic or therapeutic radiation, and of survivors of the Japanese atomic bomb.[38] Women treated with chest irradiation for childhood and adolescent Hodgkin's lymphoma, as well as survivors of other childhood cancers (where radiation is used as a mainstay of therapy) are among the populations at greater risk for secondary breast cancers. The risk increases linearly with radiation dose. Exposure to diagnostic x-rays including annual screening mammography does not impart a sufficient dose of radiation for clinical concern in the general population. The risk of breast cancer after radiation exposure in those with genetic risk factors is unclear and is an ongoing area of research.

In conclusion, numerous studies have been performed to investigate potential causative factors in the etiology of breast cancer. Several endocrine, genetic, environmental, and lifestyle factors are associated with the development of breast cancer to varying degrees. Some factors are modifiable, whereas others are not. Additionally, the impact of individual risk factors may vary depending on other confounding variables such as age, family history, estrogen use, and menopausal status. Although epidemiologic studies provide a large body of the current evidence, each has its limitations and results are varied. Meta-analyses can summarize the numerous study results, but heterogeneity of studies can be a limitation. Additional prospective, randomized controlled trials will add to our knowledge of factors that affect the risk of developing breast cancer.

CLINICAL PRESENTATION

General

- The patient may not have any symptoms, as breast cancer may be detected in asymptomatic patients though routine screening mammography.

Local Signs and Symptoms

- A painless, palpable lump is most common.
- Less common: pain; nipple discharge, retraction or dimpling; skin edema, redness or warmth.
- Palpable local-regional lymph nodes may also be present.

Signs and Symptoms of Systemic Metastases

- Depends on the site of metastases, but may include bone pain, difficulty breathing, abdominal pain or enlargement, jaundice, mental status changes.

Laboratory Tests

- Tumor markers such as cancer antigen (CA 27.29) or carcinoembryonic antigen (CEA) may be elevated.
- Alkaline phosphatase or liver function tests may be elevated in metastatic disease.

Other Diagnostic Tests

- Mammogram (with or without ultrasound, breast MRI, or both).
- Biopsy for pathology review and determination of tumor estrogen/progesterone receptor (ER/PR) status and *HER2* status.
- Systemic staging tests may include: chest x-ray, chest CT, bone scan, abdominal CT or ultrasound or MRI.

CLINICAL PRESENTATION

A painless lump is the initial sign of breast cancer in most women. The typical malignant mass is solitary, unilateral, solid, hard, irregular, and nonmobile. In small numbers of cases, stabbing or aching pain is the first symptom. Less commonly, nipple discharge, retraction, or dimpling may herald the onset of the disease. In more advanced cases, prominent skin edema, redness, warmth, and induration of the underlying tissue may be observed.

The breast is a complex organ composed of skin, subcutaneous tissue, fatty tissue, and branching ductal and glandular structures (Fig. 131–2). Various diseases that affect these structures can produce a palpable mass. In addition, the physiologic changes associated with the menstrual cycle can cause breast abnormalities. Common causes of breast masses in young women are fibroadenoma, fibrocystic disease, carcinoma, and fat necrosis.

Many women will detect some breast abnormality themselves, underscoring the importance of breast self-examination. But in the United States, it is increasingly common for breast cancer to be detected during routine screening mammography in asymptomatic women. It is widely accepted that the smaller the mass, the higher the likelihood of cure. Thus as the number of breast cancer cases found by screening mammography increases, overall survival of breast cancer patients has improved, albeit this decreasing mortality is also related to improved systemic therapy.

Breast cancer that is confined to a localized breast lesion is often referred to as *early, primary, localized,* or *curable.* Breast cancer that has spread to local-regional lymph nodes is still considered early stage (Fig. 131–3). Unfortunately, breast cancer cells often spread by contiguity, lymph channels, and through the blood to distant sites. This often occurs early in breast cancer growth, and deposits of tumor cells form in distant sites that cannot be detected with current diagnostic methods and equipment (micrometastases). When breast cancer cells can be detected clinically or radiologically in sites distant from the breast, the disease is referred to as *advanced* or *metastatic* breast cancer. Tissues most commonly involved with metastases are lymph nodes (other than local–regional lymph nodes), skin, bone, liver, lungs, and brain. Symptoms of bone pain, difficulty breathing, abdominal enlargement, jaundice, and mental status changes may herald the clinical presentation of metastatic breast cancer. A small percentage of women have signs and symptoms of distant metastases when they first seek treatment. In virtually all of them, a breast mass has been present for several months to years. In addition, about one-half of all patients who initially are treated for localized disease will eventually develop signs and symptoms of metastatic breast cancer.

DIAGNOSIS

Initial workup for a woman presenting with a lesion or symptoms suggestive of breast cancer should include a careful history, physical examination of the breast, three-dimensional mammography, and possibly other breast imaging techniques such as ultrasonography. Most breast cancers can be visualized on a mammogram as a mass, a cluster of calcifications, or a combination. Specific mammographic features associated with the highest risk of malignancy include masses with spiculated margins and/or irregular shape, and calcifications with a linear and/or segmental distribution.[39] Factors that affect the ability of mammography to detect cancer include breast density (the fat-to-glandular tissue ratio of the breast) which may be affected by age, menopausal status, and HRT. Ultrasonography, MRI, and digital mammography are alternate imaging methods that are being investigated for women with dense breasts. The technical quality of the examination and the expertise of the radiologist are also important factors.

The Breast Imaging Reporting and Data System (BI-RADS) was developed by the American College of Radiology to standardize mammographic reporting.[40,41] Table 131–2 presents BI-RADS classifications and management recommendations. There are seven assessment categories with four possible recommendations: (a) additional imaging evaluation, (b) routine interval screening, (c) short-term followup, and (d) biopsy. The probability of a biopsy positive for malignancy increases from <2% for BI-RADS category 3 mammograms to 20% to 30% for category 4 mammograms, to >95% for category 5 mammograms.

Breast biopsy is indicated for a mammographic abnormality that suggests malignancy or for a palpable mass on physical examination. Three techniques are available: fine-needle aspiration, core-needle biopsy, and excisional biopsy.[42] Excisional biopsy, which completely removes the abnormal tissue, is performed with either a local or general anesthetic, and is usually done as an outpatient operative procedure. Needle biopsies are performed percutaneously, and include both core-needle biopsy (which removes a core of tissue) and fine-needle aspiration (which removes cells from the suspicious site). These are generally office procedures that are associated with minimal discomfort and anxiety, few complications, no disfigurement, and decreased costs when compared to surgical excisional biopsy. The accuracy of fine-needle aspiration is good in experienced hands, but its limitations include false negatives, specimens with insufficient material for diagnosis, and the inability to distinguish invasive from in situ cancer. Core-needle biopsy is the preferred biopsy method for mammographically detected, nonpalpable abnormalities. Core-needle biopsy offers a more definitive histologic diagnosis, avoids inadequate samples, and can distinguish invasive from in situ breast cancer. Following confirmation of malignancy via core-needle biopsy, subsequent surgical procedures are performed to assure complete removal of the abnormal tissue.

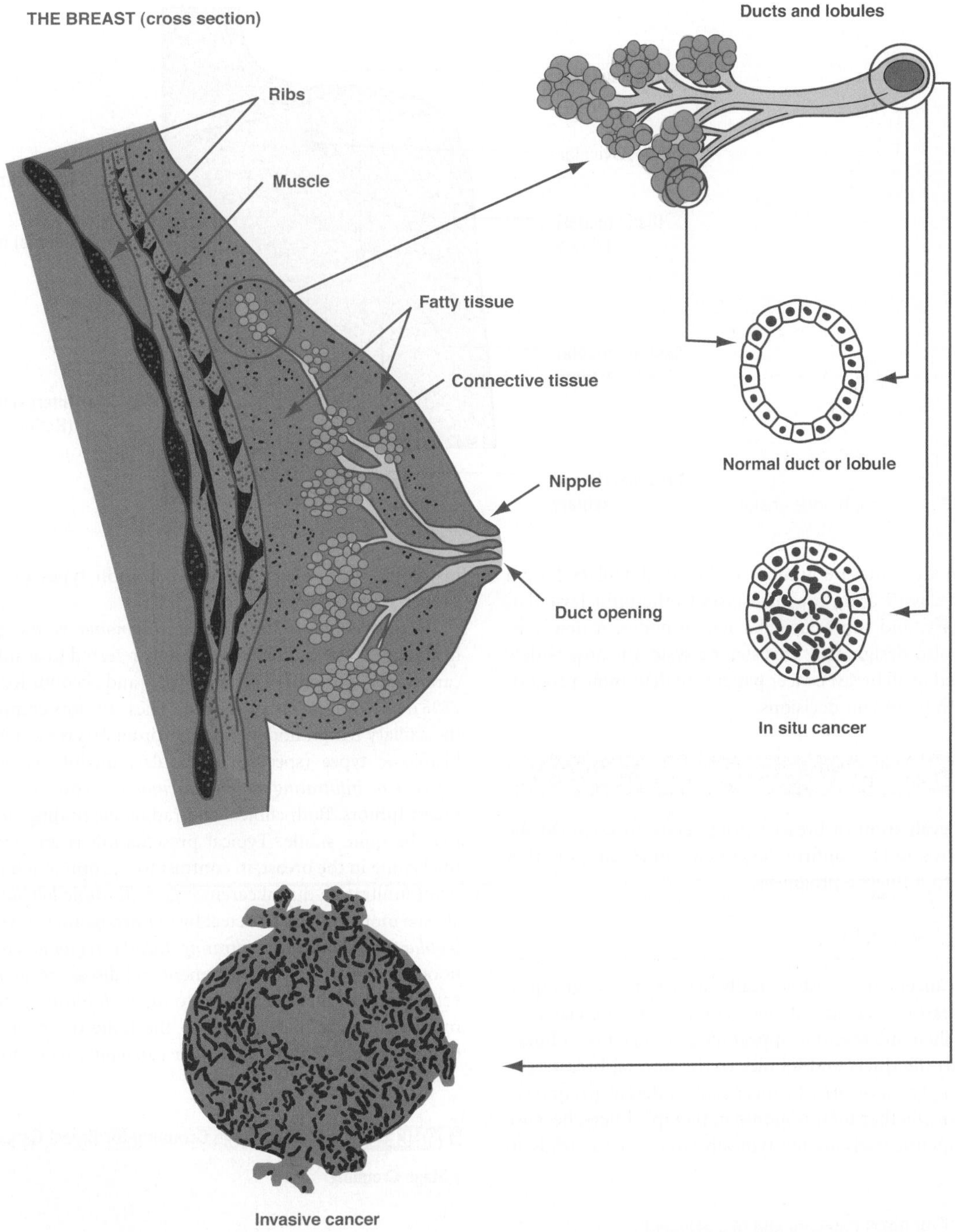

FIGURE 131-2. Breast anatomy.

STAGING AND PROGNOSIS

Few malignant diseases illustrate the importance of the relationship of stage (anatomic extent of disease) at the time of diagnosis and overall survival more clearly than breast cancer. Stage is defined on the basis of the primary tumor extent and size (T_{1-4}), presence and extent of lymph node involvement (N_{1-3}), and presence or absence of distant metastases (M_{0-1}) (Table 131–3 and Fig. 131–4). Although many possible combinations of T and N are possible within a given stage, simplistically, stage 0 represents carcinoma in situ (T_{is}) or disease that has not invaded the basement membrane of the breast tissue. Stage I represents a small primary invasive tumor without lymph node involvement, and stage II disease usually involves regional lymph nodes. Stages I and II are often referred to as *early breast cancer.* It is in these early stages that the disease is highly curable. Stage III, also referred to as *locally advanced disease,* usually represents a large tumor with extensive nodal involvement in which either node or tumor is fixed to the chest wall. Stage IV disease is characterized by the presence of metastases to organs distant from the primary tumor and is often referred to as *advanced or metastatic disease* as described earlier. Most breast cancer today presents in early stages where the prognosis is favorable (Table 131–4).

The American Joint Committee for Cancer published new staging criteria for breast cancer that were officially implemented in January 2003.[43] Tumor staging systems are periodically updated to incorporate new diagnostic and therapeutic advances that affect risk of disease recurrence and survival. Major changes included in the 2003 staging system from the 1988 version included size-based discrimination between micrometastases and isolated tumor cells, classifica-

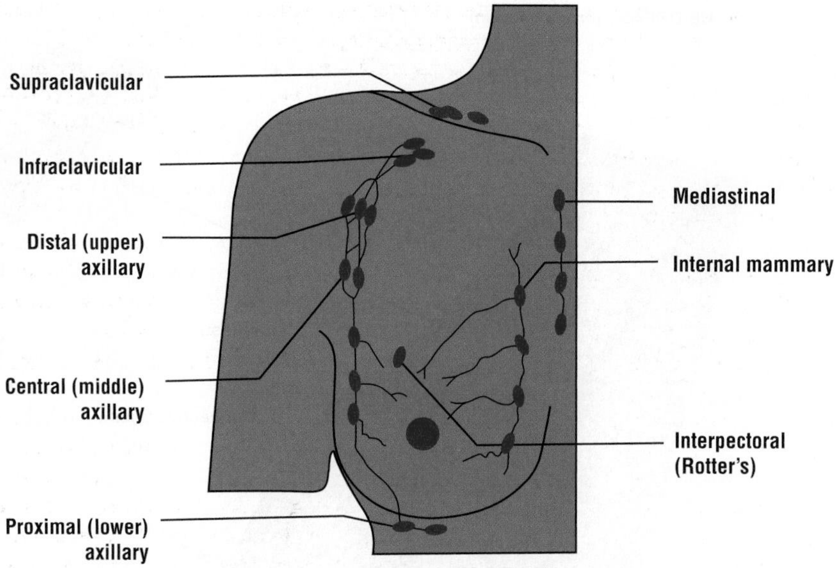

FIGURE 131-3. Lymph node anatomy.

tion of lymph node status by number of involved axillary lymph nodes, and new classification for metastases to the infraclavicular, internal mammary, and supraclavicular lymph nodes. A new substage, IIIC, was also designated. This staging system is now widely accepted and used in all breast cancer patients to determine prognosis and assist with treatment decisions.

PATHOLOGY

The pathologic evaluation of breast lesions serves to establish the histologic diagnosis and to confirm the presence or absence of other factors believed to influence prognosis.

INVASIVE CARCINOMA

Invasive breast cancers are a histologically heterogeneous group of lesions. Most breast cancers are adenocarcinomas and are classified on the basis of their microscopic appearance as ductal or lobular, corresponding to the ducts and lobules of the normal breast. The various histologic types of breast cancer have different prognoses, but it is unknown whether their response to therapy differs, because patients in therapeutic trials are not typically stratified according to histologic type. The five most common types of invasive breast cancer are briefly described.[44]

Invasive or *infiltrating ductal carcinoma* is the most common histology. These tumors are generally referred to as infiltrating ductal carcinoma "not otherwise specified," and account for approximately 75% of all invasive breast cancers. These tumors commonly spread to the axillary lymph nodes and their prognosis is poorer than for other histologic types (specifically tubular, medullary, and mucinous). *Invasive or infiltrating lobular carcinoma* accounts for 5% to 10% of breast tumors. Both clinical and radiologic findings for these tumors may be quite subtle. Typical presentation is an area of ill-defined thickening in the breast, in contrast to a prominent lump characteristic of infiltrating ductal carcinoma. *Infiltrating lobular carcinoma* can also be more difficult to detect by mammography. Overall, *infiltrating lobular carcinoma* and *infiltrating ductal carcinoma* have similar likelihoods of axillary node involvement and disease recurrence and death, yet the sites of metastases tend to differ. *Infiltrating ductal carcinoma* more frequently metastasizes to the bone or to the liver, lung, or brain, whereas *infiltrating lobular carcinoma* tends to metastasize to

TABLE 131-2 BI-RADS Category and Management Recommendations for Mammograms

BI-RADS Category	Assessment	Recommendations
0	Assessment incomplete	Need additional imaging evaluation and/or prior mammograms for comparison
1	Negative	Continue routine screening
2	Benign finding(s)	Continue routine screening
3	Probably benign finding	Initial short-term followup mammogram at 6 months, followed by additional examinations until longer-term stability demonstrated (2 or more years)
4	Suspicious abnormality	Biopsy should be considered
5	Highly suggestive of malignancy	Appropriate action should be taken; biopsy and treatment as indicated
6	Known biopsy-proven malignancy	Appropriate action should be taken; Assure that definitive treatment is completed

BI-RADS, Breast Imaging Reporting and Data Systems.
From ACR Breast Imaging Reporting and Data System, Breast Imaging Atlas. Reston, VA:. American College of Radiology, 2003.

TABLE 131-3 TNM Stage Grouping for Breast Cancer

Stage Grouping			
0	T_{is}	N_0	M_0
I	T_1^a	N_0	M_0
IIA	T_0	N_1	M_0
	T_1^a	N_1	M_0
	T_2	N_0	M_0
IIB	T_2	N_1	M_0
	T_3	N_0	M_0
IIIA	T_0	N_2	M_0
	T_1^a	N_2	M_0
	T_2	N_2	M_0
	T_3	N_1	M_0
	T_3	N_2	M_0
IIIB	T_4	N_0	M_0
	T_4	N_1	M_0
	T_4	N_2	M_0
IIIC	Any T	N_3	M_0
IV	Any T	Any N	M_1

TNM, tumor, node, metastasis.
[a] T_1 includes T_1mic.
Singletary SE, et al. Revision of the American Joint Committee on Cancer Staging System for Breast Cancer. J Clin Oncol 2002;20:3631. Reprinted with permission from the American Society of Clinical Oncology.

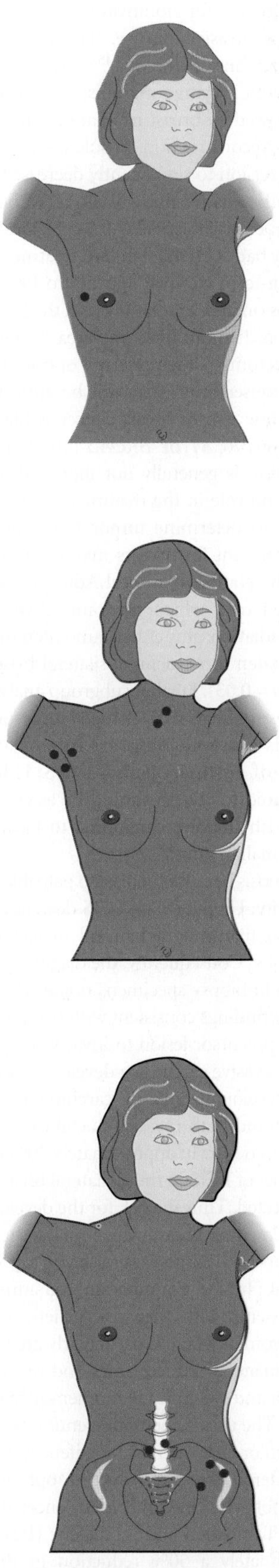

T_x Primary tumor cannot be assessed
T_0 No evidence of tumor
T_{is} Carcinoma in situ
T_1 ≤2 cm
- T_1 mic ≤0.1 cm
- T_{1a} > 0.1–0.5 cm
- T_{1b} > 0.5–1 cm
- T_{1c} > 1–2 cm

T_2 >2–5 cm
T_3 >5 cm
T_4 Any size; with direct extension to chest wall or skin
T_{4a} Extension to chest wall (not including pectoralis muscle)
T_{4b} Edema (including peau d'orange) or ulceration of skin or satellite skin nodules
T_{4c} Both $T_{4a}$and T_{4b}
T_{4d} Inflammatory carcinoma

Clinical Nodes (N)
N_X Regional lymph nodes cannot be assessed (e.g., previously removed)
N_0 No regional lymph node metastasis
N_1 Metastasis in movable ipsilateral axillary lymph node(s)
N_2 Metastases in ipsilateral axillary lymph nodes fixed or matted, or in clinically apparent ipsilateral internal mammary nodes in the absence of clinically evident axillary lymph node metastasis
- N_{2a} Metastasis in ipsilateral axillary lymph nodes fixed to one another (matted) or to other structures
- N_{2b} Metastasis only in clinically apparent ipsilateral internal mammary nodes and in the absence of clinicall evident axillary lymph node metastasis

N_3 Metastasis in ipsilateral infraclavicular lymph node(s), or in clinically apparent ipsilateral internal mammary lymph node(s) and in the presence of clinically evident axillary lymph node metastasis; or metastasis in ipsilateral supraclavicular lymph node(s) with or without axillary or internal mammary lymph node involvement
- N_{3a} Metastasis in ipsilateral infraclavicular lymph node(s) and axillary lymph node(s)
- N_{3b} Metastasis in ipsilateral internal mammary lymph node(s) and axillary lymph node(s)
- N_{3c} Metastasis in ipsilateral supraclavicular lymph node(s)

Pathologic Nodes (pN)†
pN0 No regional lymph node metastasis histologically
pN1mi Micrometastasis (>0.2 mm, none >2.0 mm)
pN1 Metastasis in one to three axillary lymph nodes and/or internal mammary nodes with microscopic disease detected by sentinel lymph node dissection but not clinically apparent
pN2 Metastasis in four to nine axillary lymph nodes, or in clinically apparent internal mammary lymph nodes in the absence of axillary lymph node metastasis
pN3 Metastasis in 10 or more axillary lymph nodes, or in infraclavicular lymph nodes, or in clinically apparent ipsilateral internal mammary lymph nodes in the presence of one or more positive axillary lymph nodes; or in more than three axillary lymph nodes with clinically negative microscopic metastasis in internal mammary lymph nodes; or in ipsilateral supraclavicular lymph nodes

†Based on axillary lymph node dissection with or without sentinel lymph node dissection

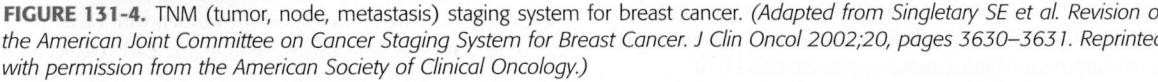

Metastasis (M)
M_X Distant metastasis cannot be assessed
M_0 No distant metastases
M_1 Distant metastasis

FIGURE 131-4. TNM (tumor, node, metastasis) staging system for breast cancer. *(Adapted from Singletary SE et al. Revision of the American Joint Committee on Cancer Staging System for Breast Cancer. J Clin Oncol 2002;20, pages 3630–3631. Reprinted with permission from the American Society of Clinical Oncology.)*

the leptomeninges, peritoneal surfaces, retroperitoneum, gastrointestinal tract, reproductive organs, and other unusual sites.

The three most common special types of invasive cancer are *medullary, mucinous, and tubular.* Prognosis may be more favorable with these unusual histologies. *Medullary carcinoma* accounts for less than 7% of all breast carcinomas, *mucinous (or colloid) carcinoma* constitutes approximately 3%, *and tubular carcinoma* accounts for approximately 2% of all breast cancers. Histologies rarely reported

TABLE 131-4 Estimated Stage at Diagnosis and 5-Year Relative Survival Rates

Stage at Diagnosis	Percentage of Cases	5-Year Survival[d]
Localized[a]	61%	98%
Regional[b]	31%	83%
Distant[c]	6%	26%
Unknown	2%	–

[a]Confined to primary site. Includes stages I and II.
[b]Regional spread to lymph nodes or directly beyond primary site. Includes stages II and III.
[c]Distant metastasis. Stage IV.
[d]With conventional local and systemic therapy.
From Ries LAG, Harkins D, Krapcho M, eds. SEER Cancer Statistics Review: 1975–2003. Bethesda, MD. http://seer.cancer.gov/csr/1975–2003/

include adenocystic carcinoma, carcinosarcomas, metaplastic, cribriform, and papillary carcinoma.

Special situations seen clinically and histologically include Paget's disease of the breast, phyllodes tumors, and inflammatory breast cancer. Paget's disease of the breast occurs in 1% to 4% of all patients with breast cancer, and is characterized by neoplastic cells in the nipple areolar complex. The patient presents clinically with eczematous changes in the nipple with itching, burning, oozing, bleeding, or some combination of these. In most cases, the nipple changes are associated with an underlying carcinoma in the breast that is usually palpable.

Phyllodes tumors of the breast (also known as cystosarcoma phyllodes) are rare tumors with subtypes that range from benign to malignant. These tumors often enlarge rapidly, are painless, and can appear radiographically as fibroadenomas.[45]

Inflammatory breast cancer is characterized clinically by prominent skin edema, redness and warmth, and induration of the underlying tissue. Biopsies of the involved skin reveal cancer cells in the dermal lymphatics. Inflammatory breast cancer typically has a very rapid onset and is often mistaken for an infectious cellulitis or mastitis. Although it may look somewhat similar to a neglected mass, its presentation with rapid onset and progression of local symptoms distinguishes it from other cases of locally advanced breast cancer. Prognosis of patients with inflammatory breast cancer is poor, even if the disease is apparently localized.[46]

NONINVASIVE CARCINOMA

As with invasive carcinoma, the noninvasive lesions may be divided broadly into ductal and lobular categories. Evidence supports that the development of malignancy is a multistep process and that invasive breast cancer has a preinvasive phase. During the carcinoma in situ phase, normal epithelial cells undergo genetic alterations that result in malignant transformation. Transformed epithelial cells proliferate and pile up within lobules or ducts, but lack the required genetic alterations that enable the cells to penetrate the basement membrane. Therefore carcinoma in situ is diagnosed when malignant transformation of cells has occurred, but the basement membrane is intact.

The widespread use of screening mammography and subsequent biopsy and greater recognition of noninvasive breast carcinoma by pathologists has resulted in a significant increase in the diagnosis of in situ breast cancer during the past decade. The natural history of these disorders is not well described, and thus the debate continues regarding carcinoma in situ: Is carcinoma in situ preinvasive cancer or simply a marker of unstable epithelium that represents an increased risk for the development of subsequent aggressive cancer?[47,48]

DCIS is more frequently diagnosed than lobular carcinoma in situ (LCIS). Most cases of DCIS today are found by biopsies performed for clustered microcalcifications seen on screening mammography. Five distinct histologic patterns of DCIS have been identified: comedo, cribriform, micropapillary, papillary, and solid.

The ultimate goal of treatment for noninvasive carcinomas is to prevent the development of invasive disease. Treatment of DCIS depends on its location, size, and pathology.[45] Treatment options include: (1) local excision with negative margins; (2) local excision (with negative margins) followed by breast irradiation; and (3) traditional total mastectomy with reconstruction. Whole breast irradiation is recommended following excision to significantly decrease the risk of local recurrence. Excision with negative margins alone, without radiation may be considered in patients with small (<0.5 cm), localized, and low-grade DCIS. Mastectomy had been the standard treatment of DCIS for several decades, but long-term survival appears to be equivalent with mastectomy versus excision and irradiation, and the latter option allows for breast conservation. If more than one area of the breast is involved with DCIS, a mastectomy is the preferred option. It has also been suggested that breast conservation may not be appropriate for younger women whose lifetime risk of breast cancer is high given a diagnosis of DCIS, including *BRCA1* or *BRCA2* mutation carriers. Axillary lymph node dissection is generally not indicated. Currently cytotoxic chemotherapy has no role in the treatment of patients with pure DCIS. It is important to determine tumor hormone receptor status because tamoxifen treatment for 5 years may be considered in some women with DCIS. The National Surgical Adjuvant Breast and Bowel Project (NSABP) B-24 trial, which randomized women with DCIS to lumpectomy with radiation plus either tamoxifen or placebo, showed a benefit with tamoxifen in reducing ipsilateral breast cancer recurrence (44% reduction, $p = 0.03$). Further subgroup analysis of this trial suggests a benefit for those patients with estrogen receptor-positive DCIS. Ongoing clinical trials are evaluating the role of aromatase inhibitors in the treatment of postmenopausal DCIS. Followup of women who have been treated for DCIS should be as comprehensive as that of a woman with invasive carcinoma to facilitate early detection of any subsequent malignancy.[48]

LCIS is a microscopic diagnosis because there is no palpable mass and no specific clinical abnormality. Unlike DCIS, LCIS does not generally demonstrate calcifications on mammography, and in fact is usually undetectable by mammography. Consequently, the diagnosis of LCIS is usually an incidental finding in biopsy specimens obtained because of symptoms or mammography findings consistent with benign lesions. It is unclear whether LCIS is a precursor lesion to invasive carcinoma or serves as a marker of risk for invasive carcinoma developing somewhere in the breast. The risk for developing invasive carcinoma is approximately 0.5% to 1% per year, and both invasive ductal carcinoma and invasive lobular carcinoma can occur. In approximately 30% to 50% of patients, there are multiple foci of LCIS in the ipsilateral breast, and the contralateral breast is also affected. Thus the risk for the development of breast cancer is equally high in either breast, which makes the management of LCIS very controversial.[47] Some experts favor a program of observation, with semiannual physical examination and annual mammography.[45] In selected patients with high-risk genetic mutations, strong family history, or in women who are particularly anxious about the development of cancer, bilateral mastectomies and reconstruction may be considered. Radiation and systemic chemotherapy have no role in the management of LCIS. The use of chemoprevention with tamoxifen in premenopausal women or tamoxifen or raloxifene in postmenopausal women can be considered as a risk reduction option. Patients with LCIS were included in both the NSABP Breast Cancer Prevention Trial (P1) and the Study of Tamoxifen and Raloxifene (P2) trials.[49,50] Both trials showed approximately a 50% reduction in the risk of developing invasive breast cancer for women with LCIS receiving either tamoxifen or raloxifene (see Prevention and Early Detection below).

PROGNOSTIC FACTORS

The natural history of breast cancer varies between patients, with some having an extremely aggressive disease that progresses rapidly, whereas others follow a more indolent course. The ability to predict prognosis is extremely important in designing treatment recommendations to maximize quantity and quality of life. A number of pathologic prognostic and predictive factors have been identified. Prognostic factors are characteristics or measurements available at diagnosis or time of surgery, that in the absence of adjuvant therapy are associated with recurrence rate, death rate, or other clinical outcomes. Predictive factors are measurements available at diagnosis that are associated with response to a specific therapy. Prognostic and predictive factors fall into three categories: patient characteristics that are independent of the disease such as age; disease characteristics such as tumor size or histologic type; and biomarkers that are measurable parameters in tissues, cells, or fluids, such as hormone receptor status.[51,52]

Age at diagnosis and ethnicity are patient characteristics that may affect prognosis. Some younger patients, particularly those younger than 35 years of age, have more aggressive forms of disease and a worse prognosis. African American women also have decreased survival compared to white women. The cause of this racial disparity is more than likely multifactorial, relating to access to care, higher stages at diagnosis, and more aggressive biologic features.

Disease characteristics that have been shown to provide important prognostic information include lymph node status, tumor size, histologic subtype, nuclear or histologic grade, lymphatic and vascular invasion, and proliferation indices.

Tumor size and the presence and number of involved lymph nodes are established primary factors in assessing the risk for breast cancer recurrence and subsequent metastatic disease. Table 131–5 shows 5-year survival rates according to size of the primary tumor and axillary node involvement. The major factor that influences the likelihood of recurrence is the presence of positive lymph nodes. However, regardless of lymph node status, the size of the primary tumor remains an independent prognostic factor for disease recurrence.

The number of affected lymph nodes is directly related to disease recurrence. The revised staging system for breast cancer recognizes the absolute number of positive nodes as a prognostic factor: N_1 represents 1 to 3 positive nodes, N_2 represents 4 to 9 positive nodes, and N_3 represents 10 or more positive nodes in its pathologic staging system.[43]

Certain histologic subtypes and clinical presentation of breast cancer have prognostic importance. As mentioned earlier, because women with pure *tubular* or *mucinous* tumors have more favorable outcomes than *invasive ductal carcinomas*, treatment recommendations may differ.[45] Inflammatory breast cancer, although a clinical designation and not a distinct histologic subtype, is associated with a poor prognosis.

Nuclear grade and tumor (histologic) differentiation are known independent prognostic indicators. Several histologic grading systems have been developed, most of which grade tumors with a score from 1 to 3: grade 1 (well differentiated); grade 2 (moderately differentiated); grade 3 (poorly differentiated). Higher-grade tumors are associated with higher rates of distant metastasis and poorer survival. This factor aids in making treatment decisions, particularly for patients with small tumors and negative lymph nodes.

TABLE 131-5 Five-Year Survival Rates (%) According to Tumor Size and Axillary Lymph Node Status (in percent)

	Tumor Size		
Lymph Node Status	***<2 cm***	***2–5 cm***	***>5 cm***
Negative	96	89	82
1–3 positive	87	80	73
≥4 positive	66	59	46

Data from Schnitt SJ, Guidi AJ. Pathology of invasive breast cancer. In: Harris JR, Lippman ME, Morrow M, Osborne CK, eds. Diseases of the Breast, 3rd edition. Philadelphia: Lippincott Williams & Wilkins, 2004:567.

Lymphatic and vascular invasion, defined as evidence of tumor emboli in lymphatic or vascular spaces, has emerged in recent years as having prognostic significance for the risk of recurrence. This factor helps identify node-negative patients who are at increased risk for lymph node involvement and metastases.

The rate of tumor cell proliferation also has prognostic significance in breast cancer recurrence. Rate of cell proliferation can be evaluated with various techniques, including mitotic index, which counts the number of mitotic bodies; thymidine-labeling index or S-phase fraction with DNA flow cytometry, which determines the percentage of tumor cells actively dividing; or through the use of monoclonal antibodies to antigens present on proliferating cells, such as Ki-67. These proliferation indices are additional factors that may be useful in decision making, and may also be predictive markers for responsiveness to chemotherapy, although this is still controversial.

Hormone receptors are not strong prognostic markers, but are used clinically to predict response to hormone therapy. Hormone receptors are nuclear transcription factors that, upon ligand binding, activate a variety of signal transduction pathways that result in cell growth and proliferation. The hormone receptors clinically useful in discussions of breast cancer include the estrogen receptor (ER) and the progesterone receptor (PR). Determination of both ER and PR status is an established procedure that is important in the management of breast cancer. Immunohistochemistry is used to determine the level (i.e., quantity) of hormone receptors, which is important for predictive ability. Although the ER has received the most attention, the presence of the PR protein is important for the functional effects of the ER protein to occur. Hormone receptors are most valuable in predicting response to hormone therapy. Approximately 60% to 70% of patients with ER-positive and PR-positive tumors will respond to hormonal manipulation. Patients with ER-negative and PR-negative tumors rarely respond to hormonal manipulation. The response rate in patients with ER-positive and PR-negative or ER-negative and PR-positive tumors is somewhere in between, but significant benefit may still be gained with hormonal therapy in these patients.

Approximately 50% to 70% of patients with primary or metastatic breast cancer have hormone receptor (HR)-positive tumors. HR positivity, more common in postmenopausal women, is associated with a superior response to hormone therapy and a longer disease-free survival.

The *HER2/neu (HER2)* gene is located on chromosome 17q21 and encodes a 185-kilodaton transmembrane tyrosine kinase growth factor receptor. The *HER2* protein is normally expressed at low levels in the epithelial cells of normal breast tissue. *HER2* is a member of the erbB (or HER) growth factor receptor family and its overexpression is associated with transmission of growth signals that control aspects of normal cell growth and division. *HER2* overexpression occurs in approximately 20% to 30% of breast cancers, and is associated with increased tumor aggressiveness, increased rates of recurrence, and increased mortality. In some studies, *HER2* gene amplification and protein overexpression, measured by fluorescence in situ hybridization (FISH) and immunohistochemistry (IHC), respectively, correlates with factors associated with a poor prognosis. Clearly, a *HER2*-positive status predicts response to trastuzumab therapy, which is a monoclonal antibody directed against the *HER2* receptor. A final controversy surrounds the testing method employed to determine *HER2* status. Although there are many methods, *HER2* gene amplification measured by FISH (reported as either positive, equivocal, or negative) and overexpression of the *HER2* protein product measured by IHC (reported as 0, 1+, 2+, or 3+) are the most commonly used methods. *HER2* status should be determined for all invasive breast cancers, and guidelines for testing are available.[53] Positive for HER2 is either IHC 3+ or FISH positive. Available data do not demonstrate the superiority of one test over the other. For equivocal results of IHC 2+ or FISH, confirmatory testing with the alternate test is recommended. While *HER2* gene amplification or protein overexpression has traditionally been considered a poor prognostic factor, the outcomes of patients with *HER2*-positive breast cancer may be changing with the advent of targeted therapies such as trastuzumab being used in the treatment of early stage disease.

Although there is a growing understanding of the prognostic significance of individual factors, it is not clear how each contributes to the overall prognosis for an individual patient. Computer-aided models, including Adjuvant! (*www.adjuvantonline.com*) are available that combine patient- and tumor-related variables to estimate overall prognosis for individual patients with early stage breast cancer and aid in decisions regarding adjuvant systemic therapy.[54] Such programs have limitations, and should be used by healthcare professionals and not directly by patients because of the importance of accurate data entry, selection of different treatment options, and understanding of results (see Systemic Adjuvant Therapy below).

Genetic profiling is also being used to provide prognostic and predictive information on clinical outcomes of breast cancer. The Oncotype DX assay uses a reverse-transcription polymerase chain reaction assay of 21 genes to predict the likelihood of distant recurrence in lymph node-negative and ER-positive breast cancer patients treated with tamoxifen.[55] A recurrence score is calculated to categorize patients into low-, intermediate-, or high-risk groups. MammaPrint is another molecular prognostic test that uses DNA microarray analysis to measure the activity of a set of 70 genes to determine the likelihood of breast cancer recurrence in women with stage I or II breast cancer, tumor size 5 cm or less, and no lymph node involvement. To predict the risk of breast cancer metastasis, an algorithm is used to issue a score that indicates whether the patient is at low or high risk.[56] These tools provide additional prognostic information to aid in decision making regarding treatment for these subgroups of patients with otherwise favorable prognostic features. Genetic profiling is also being studied for predicting responsiveness or resistance to treatment, and has immense potential for improving prognostic and predictive accuracy.

Novel molecular markers that have shown prognostic and predictive significance include urokinase-type plasminogen activator and its inhibitor, plasminogen activator inhibitor type 1, cyclin E, and presence of tumor cells in bone marrow and/or circulating blood. Completion of prospective validation studies will provide further information as to whether these tests are suitable for use in making treatment decisions in individual patients.

In summary, lymph node status and tumor size are two significant prognostic factors that assist clinicians in estimating prognosis and making treatment recommendations for most breast cancer patients (see also Systemic Adjuvant Therapy below). Although the risk of recurrence is clearly high in patients with large primary tumors or lymph node-positive disease, many patients with small primary tumors and lymph node-negative disease will still develop metastases, yet our ability to accurately identify these individual patients is limited. Evaluation of additional prognostic factors can help identify which patients will have a good outcome with local therapy alone, as well as those patients with aggressive features who would benefit from more aggressive, multimodality treatment.

TREATMENT

■ EARLY BREAST CANCER (STAGE I AND II)

Local-Regional Therapy

❷ Most patients presenting with breast cancer today have either an in situ tumor, a small invasive tumor with negative lymph nodes (stage I), or a small invasive tumor with axillary lymph node involvement (stage II) cancer. Surgery alone can cure most, if not all, patients with in situ cancers, 70% to 80% of patients with stage I, and about half of all patients with stage II cancers. The choice of surgical procedures has changed drastically over the past 50 years. This is partly a result of changes in our understanding of the biology of breast cancer, and is partly a result of a series of well-conducted clinical trials performed over this time period.

The Halstedian theory and concept of tumor growth, formulated at the end of the 19th century, held that breast cancer was a local–regional disease that spread to involve larger contiguous areas of the breast, chest wall, and adjacent lymph nodes. This hypothesis gave rise to the Halsted radical mastectomy, a surgical approach based on the rationale that cure of early disease could best be achieved with expansive, meticulously performed surgical procedures. *Radical mastectomy* involves removal of the breast and both major and minor pectoralis muscles. The axillary nodes on the same side (ipsilateral) as the breast lesion are also removed. Substantial morbidity is associated with this procedure. Muscle resection decreases strength and range of motion, and removal of axillary lymph nodes can produce edema of the arm and resected breast area. This procedure was often followed by external beam radiation therapy to the involved area.

During the 1960s, it was recognized that breast cancer is often microscopically disseminated at the time of initial diagnosis. This evolutionary concept that breast cancer is not only a local, but also a systemic disease, resulted in major changes in local and systemic therapy. The modified radical mastectomy, also termed *total mastectomy with axillary lymph node dissection,* became the standard surgical approach in the 1970s and was not as precisely defined or standardized as the radical mastectomy. The pectoralis minor muscle may be excised, divided, or left intact, and more importantly, there may be variation in the extent of axillary lymph node dissection, ranging from sampling to full dissection (including levels I and II ipsilateral axillary lymph nodes). Despite the lack of standardization, the modified radical mastectomy procedure is associated with significantly less morbidity and long-term complications compared to its radical counterpart.

Results of several large trials have since repudiated the Halsted theory and supported the alternative systemic hypothesis. Over the years these trials have investigated reducing the amount of surgery required to maintain acceptable cosmetic results and rates of local and distant recurrence and mortality. Breast-conserving therapy (BCT) includes removal of part of the breast, surgical evaluation of the axillary lymph node basin, and radiation therapy to the breast. The amount of breast tissue removed as a part of BCT varies from just removing the cancerous "lump" (a lumpectomy) with a small margin of adjacent normal-appearing tissue, to removing the "lump" with a wider excision of adjacent normal-appearing tissue (a wide local excision), to removing the entire quadrant of the breast that includes the cancerous "lump" (a quadrantectomy). All of these techniques are referred to as a *segmental or partial mastectomy.* In 1990, the National Institutes of Health Consensus Development Conference reviewed six trials comparing modified radical mastectomy with BCT.[57] Those patients who underwent BCT had removal of only part of the breast, and an axillary lymph node dissection followed by radiation therapy to the whole breast. From this analysis, the National Institutes of Health conference concluded that "BCT is an appropriate method of primary therapy for the majority of women with stage I and stage II breast cancer and is preferable because it provides survival equivalent to total mastectomy and axillary dissection while preserving the breast."[57] The median followup for these trials was 6.5 years at the time the National Institutes of Health conference was convened and this recommendation was made.

In a meta-analysis of updated information from these same six trials, now with a median followup of 14.7 years, the authors conclude that there remains no difference in overall survival between mastectomy and BCT.[58] However, with longer followup it does appear that local recurrence rates are significantly higher with BCT (pooled data odds ratio 1.56; 95% CI 1.29 to 1.89; p <0.001). This observation was also demonstrated in previous meta-analyses, including one by Morris et al. reported in 1997[59] and the Early Breast Cancer Trialists' Collaborative Group (EBCTCG) overview completed in 2000.[60] Although local–regional recurrences are concerning, it is not clear what impact they have on overall survival. In the Jatoi meta-analysis, no impact on overall survival was seen with more than 4,000 patients included in the analysis.[58] But in the EBCTCG meta-analysis, which included 25,000 women, increased locoregional recurrences were associated with increased breast cancer mortality.[60] Collectively, these data indicate that any negative impact on survival, if present, is probably very small, and competing causes of death from adverse effects related to cancer therapy and comorbid diseases must be considered to determine the overall risks associated with BCT for an individual patient. These risks should be weighed against the potential benefits of any local therapy. Also, most patients with early stage breast cancer receive systemic adjuvant therapy (to be discussed later; see Systemic Adjuvant Therapy below), which further reduces the risk of recurrence and death from breast cancer, possibly negating any potential increase in recurrence attributed to BCT. Because the studies included in all of these meta-analyses are quite heterogeneous and of varying quality, it is difficult to draw sound conclusions. Other clinical trials have investigated methods to better identify patients at high risk for recurrence to better define who might be appropriate candidates for BCT compared with mastectomy. Some clinical trials appear to indicate that young age (<35 years) is predictive for ipsilateral breast recurrences, but these trials also indicate a similar survival with BCT compared with mastectomy in this same population.[61,62] Women with a family history of breast cancer or an identified mutation in *BRCA1* or *BRCA2* are more likely to exist in this younger population, which may confound the independent contribution of age and treatment on clinical outcome.[63] This may be a result of the high risk of another cancer developing in the remaining breast tissue rather than a recurrence of the previously diagnosed cancer. However, despite the lack of sound clinical evidence to support the recommendation, the National Comprehensive Cancer Network (NCCN) has recommended that women who are 35 years of age or younger, or who are premenopausal and a carrier of a known *BRCA1* or *BRCA2* mutation, undergo mastectomy and consider additional risk reduction strategies (e.g., bilateral mastectomies).[45] Most experts agree that BCT is an appropriate option for local therapy of early stage breast cancer. BCT is appropriate for most women, but full disclosure of the risks and benefits should be made and thoroughly discussed, and the patient's clinical situation and preferences should be carefully considered prior to undergoing any such procedure.

Most patients diagnosed today with breast cancer can be treated with BCT. Several factors should be considered in selecting patients for BCT. Multiple sites of cancer within the breast and the inability to attain negative pathologic margins on the excised breast specimen are predictive for an increased risk of recurrence with BCT and are indications for mastectomy. Some preexisting collagen vascular diseases (e.g., scleroderma and systemic lupus erythematosus) are relative contraindications for the use of BCT because of an increased risk of radiation-related adverse effects. Although local recurrence following BCT has not been consistently associated with increased mortality, it is distressing to the patient and requires surgical removal of the breast. In addition, reconstructive therapy is often not feasible in a breast that has previously received irradiation. Another major consideration in selecting patients for BCT is the expected cosmetic result. Although tumor size is not an important consideration for breast cancer recurrence if negative margins can be achieved, the relationship of the size of the tumor to the total breast volume is an important cosmetic consideration. If the volume of the tissue removed encompasses a significant portion of the breast, better results may be obtained with mastectomy and reconstruction. Additionally, for some patients, preservation of a limited amount of breast tissue may not justify the inconvenience of radiation therapy. Another approach to therapy for these patients is primary (neoadjuvant) systemic therapy to potentially shrink the tumor and minimize surgery (see section on Locally Advanced Breast Cancer for further details). Aside from the probability of local recurrence and the ability to achieve a satisfactory cosmetic result, consideration must be given to the availability of an external beam radiation facility and the patient's willingness to comply with the prescribed course of radiotherapy. In most instances, external beam radiation therapy used in conjunction with breast-conserving procedures involves 4 to 6 weeks of radiation therapy directed to the entire breast tissue (a total of 5,000 cGy administered in daily 200-cGy doses) to eradicate residual disease. Complications associated with radiation therapy to the breast are minor and include reddening and erythema of the breast tissue and subsequent shrinkage of total breast mass beyond that predicted on the basis of breast tissue removal.

Although the current standard of care is to include local radiation therapy to the whole breast as a required component of BCT, current clinical trials are investigating the use of partial breast irradiation or no radiation after segmental mastectomy for certain patient populations with a very low risk of recurrence. The underlying goal of local therapy is to minimize complications while maximizing outcomes that are relevant to the patient (e.g., cosmetic results, local and distant recurrence rates, mortality).

Postmastectomy radiation therapy to the chest wall may also be required in certain situations where tumors are large or the number of positive axillary lymph nodes is high (see section on Locally Advanced Breast Cancer). However, these criteria are also widely debated and are the subject of several meta-analyses. Despite the controversy, it is clear that some women may benefit from local radiation therapy even after removal of the entire breast (i.e., total mastectomy). The NCCN Guidelines state that women with the following criteria should undergo postmastectomy radiation therapy: (a) positive surgical margins, (b) a tumor larger than 5 cm in greatest dimension, or (c) four or more positive axillary lymph nodes.[45] Patients with close margins (<1 mm of normal adjacent tissue) or one to three positive ipsilateral axillary lymph nodes should consider postmastectomy chest wall radiation therapy, but the benefits are controversial. Patients with surgical margins of at least 1 mm, tumor size of 5 cm or less and negative axillary lymph nodes do not require postmastectomy chest wall radiation therapy. The optimal sequence of radiation therapy and chemotherapy is somewhat controversial. Concurrent administration of chemotherapy and radiation therapy is usually avoided because of an increase in local adverse effects. Most clinicians administer systemic chemotherapy immediately following surgery given the hypothetical presence of systemic micrometastases that cannot be eradicated by local radiation therapy. Radiation therapy is then administered after chemotherapy, leaving hormone therapy (which is given for many years) for the end (see section on Adjuvant Biologic Therapy for discussion of sequencing trastuzumab).

The role of axillary lymph node dissection is being reevaluated as more women are being diagnosed with early stage breast cancer. Axillary lymph node dissection with histopathologic study of the full axillary specimen, including level I and II lymph nodes, was the gold standard for detecting axillary nodal involvement and determining the number of lymph nodes containing tumor. The number of positive axillary lymph nodes remains the most powerful predictor of breast cancer recurrence and survival, but other benefits may include a therapeutic effect of removing the lymph nodes and obtaining information to guide treatment selection. However, axillary dissection is associated with significant morbidity, with an acute complication rate as high as 20% to 30% and rates of chronic lymphedema as high as 20% to 30%.[64,65] Recent studies indicate that approximately 60% of patients with early stage breast cancer present with lymph node-negative disease, which indicates that many women would derive no therapeutic benefit, but would be exposed to the complications from the procedure.

For these reasons, a procedure involving lymphatic mapping and sentinel lymph node biopsy is increasingly accepted at many centers across the United States and guidelines regarding recommendations for this procedure are now available.[66–68] The sentinel lymph node(s) is the first lymph node(s) that receives lymph drainage from the primary tumor. Injection of a vital blue dye, a radiocolloid, or both around the primary breast tumor identifies the sentinel lymph node(s) in most patients, and the status of this lymph node(s) may predict the status of the remaining nodes in the nodal basin. While only one randomized clinical trial has compared this technique to the standard axillary dissection, the procedure has become the standard of care for certain groups of patients.

Many uncontrolled studies support the use of sentinel lymph node biopsy. Despite differences in the mapping technique, the experience of the surgeon, or the patient populations studied, recent studies show that the technique identified the sentinel lymph node(s) in more than 90% of patients.[68] In studies that incorporated completed axillary dissections for comparison, the sentinel procedure accurately predicted the status of the remaining axillary nodes in more than 90% of patients. Considerable controversy exists over the use of this procedure in women with large tumors (>5 cm) or locally advanced disease, palpable axillary lymph nodes, a multifocal or multicentric breast tumor, prior neoadjuvant (preoperative) chemotherapy, or prior surgery involving the breast and/or axilla. Patients who are pregnant or lactating are generally not considered candidates for this procedure.

Another factor that should be considered is the experience and mastery of the procedure by the surgical team. It has been shown that an individual surgeon must perform at least 20 procedures to attain competency and the American Society of Breast Surgeons has incorporated this caveat into its *2005 Consensus Statement on Guidelines for Performing Sentinel Lymph Node Dissection for Breast Cancer.*[69] The false-negative rate with this procedure appears to inversely correlate with the rate of identification of the sentinel lymph node and may also be an early indicator of accuracy within an institution.[68]

The long-term outcome of patients who are undergoing this procedure alone (without axillary dissection) is unknown. Ongoing clinical trials will hopefully answer these questions, but this is a very controversial subject with much debate amongst even the most highly regarded breast surgeons. Despite the absence of long-term data, total mastectomy with sentinel lymph node biopsy (without axillary lymph node dissection) may be a reasonable alternative for women who wish to avoid the inconvenience of radiation therapy and preserve their option for breast reconstruction in the future. The decision of whether to use the sentinel lymph node procedure or a full axillary dissection is very complex and the reader is referred to excellent reviews and guidelines for further information.[66–69]

Simple or *total mastectomy* involves removal of the entire breast without dissection of the underlying muscle or axillary nodes. The major disadvantage of this procedure is that axillary nodal status is not determined, and therefore important prognostic information may be lost. This procedure is used in patients with carcinoma in situ, in whom there is a 1% incidence of axillary node involvement, or in cases of in-breast recurrences following breast-conservation therapy.

The early trials investigating less-extensive surgical approaches to breast cancer are widely credited with the finding that BCT is an appropriate primary therapy for most women with stages I and II disease, and is preferable because it arguably provides survival rates equivalent to those of modified radical mastectomy. But these trials provided valuable information regarding the natural history of the disease and identified pathologic prognostic factors associated with early cancer spread. The preponderance of information available regarding selection of women most likely to benefit from systemic adjuvant therapy was derived from pathologic evaluation of tissues archived from these early trials. It is hoped that further investigation into less-extensive local therapy (now focused on the surgical approach to the axilla and radiation therapy) will continue to provide valuable information for the future.

Systemic Adjuvant Therapy

❸ *Systemic adjuvant therapy* is defined as the administration of systemic therapy following definitive local therapy (surgery, radiation, or a combination of these) when there is no evidence of metastatic disease, but a high likelihood of disease recurrence. The concept of breast cancer being a systemic disease and the rationale of adjuvant chemotherapy was based on a series of laboratory and clinical investigations conducted during the 1960s and 1970s that were directed primarily toward achieving a better understanding of tumor metastases. Table 131–6 illustrates the laboratory findings, clinical abnormalities, and biologic hypotheses that lead to recognition of breast cancer as a systemic disease and documented the value of adjuvant chemotherapy. The earliest adjuvant trials in breast cancer consisted of perioperative administration of alkylating agents with the intent of eradicating micrometastases that were disseminated at the time of surgical excision of the tumor. Many collaborative research groups have conducted stepwise series of studies designed to identify appropriate candidates for systemic adjuvant therapy, and the optimal regimens and duration of therapy. Several hundred randomized clinical trials evaluating various systemic adjuvant modalities have been reported. Most published results confirm that chemotherapy, hormonal therapy, or both, result in improved disease-free survival (DFS) and/or overall survival (OS) for all treated patients, or more commonly for patients in specific prognostic subgroups (e.g., nodal involvement, menopausal status, hormonal receptor status, or *HER2* status). The huge amounts of data generated by these trials have resulted in a great deal of controversy, with different conclusions being reached by various experts.

Interpretation of results of systemic adjuvant therapy is difficult because of differences in the patient populations studied, the varia-

TABLE 131-6 Laboratory Findings, Clinical Observations, and Biologic Hypothesis of Breast Cancer as a Systemic Disease and the Value of Adjuvant Chemotherapy

- By the time cancer becomes clinically detectable, it is advanced (about 30 doublings) and has had ample opportunity to establish distant micrometastases.
- There is no orderly pattern of tumor cell dissemination, and the bloodstream is of considerable importance in tumor spread.
- Operable breast cancer is often a systemic disease and variations in local–regional therapy have not substantially affected survival. Only by control of distant disease can there be an improvement in the outcome of breast cancer patients.
- Likelihood of disease recurrence is related to size of tumor mass and axillary node involvement at diagnosis.
- Recurrence of breast cancer following local–regional therapy is most commonly at sites distant from the breast.
- Tumor growth fraction is inversely related to tumor population site. Therefore, optimal kinetic conditions to achieve cure with chemotherapy exist in the setting of micrometastatic disease.
- Efficacy of chemotherapy is dose dependent and optimal doses of combination chemotherapy can be more safely and effectively administered in the adjuvant setting as opposed to the setting of advanced disease.

TABLE 131-7 Fifteen-Year Results of the Overview Analysis

	Tamoxifen vs. None[a]		Polychemotherapy vs. None	
	Reduction in Annual Odds		Reduction in Annual Odds	
Age (years)	*Recurrence (%)*	*Death (%)*	*Recurrence (%)*	*Death (%)*
All patients	39 ± 3	32 ± 4	23 ±2	17 ± 2
<40	44 ± 10	39 ±12	40 ± 6	29 ± 7
40–49	29 ± 7	24 ± 9	36 ± 4	30 ± 5
50–59	34 ± 5	24 ± 7	23 ± 3	15 ± 4
60–69	45 ± 5	35 ±6	13 ±3	9 ± 4
≥70	51 ± 12	37 ± 15	12 ± 11	13 ±12

[a]Estrogen-receptor positive or unknown disease with about 5 years of tamoxifen versus no adjuvant therapy.

Adapted from reference 5.

tion in natural history of breast cancer, the absence of information regarding pathologic prognostic factors in many studies, and differences in treatment approach and methods of analysis. It is important to remember that because the goal of systemic adjuvant therapy is cure, patients in these studies must be followed for long periods of time before results can be determined. In addition, because most patients with early breast cancer (50% to 90%) in the various trials are cured with local–regional therapy alone, large numbers of patients are required to show a statistically significant difference that can be attributed to systemic adjuvant therapy. For these reasons, several groups around the world have conducted meta-analyses of similar breast cancer trials in hopes of gaining more insight regarding adjuvant systemic therapy than a single study can provide. One such effort, organized by the EBCTCG, is based on a worldwide collaboration involving multiple randomized trials and is continually updated with results from new clinical trials.[5] The EBCTCG overview analyses are updated every 5 years and have been published in 1988, 1992, 1998, and 2005. The most recent update, published in 2005 as a result of analyses that took place in 2000, reflects the 10-year and 15-year effects on breast cancer recurrence and survival, respectively. Many important questions regarding the optimal way to administer adjuvant chemotherapy and hormonal therapy, and the magnitude of benefit as measured by DFS or OS to clinically relevant subsets of patients, have been answered by these overview analyses. Simply stated, the results of these analyses support the use of adjuvant hormonal therapy in all patients with positive HR status, regardless of age, menopausal status, involvement of axillary lymph nodes, or tumor size. The results of these overview analyses also support the use of adjuvant chemotherapy in most women with lymph node metastases or with primary breast cancers larger than 1 cm in diameter (both node-negative and node-positive).[5] It is important to note that data from clinical trials incorporating the taxanes, modern aromatase inhibitors, or trastuzumab into adjuvant chemotherapy regimens were not included in these analyses, as trials with these agents were not started by 1995, the cut-off for data inclusion.[5] Results from these more recent clinical trials are discussed later (see sections on Adjuvant Chemotherapy, Adjuvant Biologic Therapy, Adjuvant Endocrine Therapy).

It is important to understand the relative and absolute magnitude of benefit associated with adjuvant systemic therapy in breast cancer. Table 131–7 shows the proportional reduction in the annual odds of recurrence and death by age for adjuvant polychemotherapy and adjuvant tamoxifen given for 5 years in women with tumors that are positive for hormone receptors based on the results of these overview analyses. Throughout these reports, the results are presented as they are in Table 131–7, as proportional benefits that compare the effects of two groups, in this case, chemotherapy or hormonal therapy versus no chemotherapy or hormonal therapy. A proportional reduction of 25% might equivalently be described as

TABLE 131-8 Absolute Reduction in Mortality at 10 Years per 100 Patients Treated

Estimated 10-year Death Rate with No Therapy	Hypothetical Proportional Reduction in Mortality as a Result of Treatment				
	50%	*40%*	*30%*	*20%*	*10%*
50% (5-cm tumor, one positive node)	25	20	15	10	5
30% (4-cm tumor, negative nodes)	15	12	9	6	3
10% (1.5-cm tumor, negative nodes)	5	4	3	2	1

an odds ratio, RR, or hazard ratio of 0.75; a RR or odds reduction of 25%; or a 25% reduction in the risk of death or death rate. For a given proportional reduction in death rate, the absolute improvement in 15-year survival will depend on the baseline risk of death with no treatment, which varies based on prognostic factors that include patient characteristics, disease characteristics and biomarkers identified earlier in this chapter. Table 131–8 shows the number of deaths avoided per 100 patients treated in several hypothetical subsets of patients with different estimated 15-year survivals without adjuvant therapy, as a function of different estimates of treatment benefit shown as the proportional reductions in mortality if they did receive adjuvant therapy. About 15 of every 100 patients benefited at 15 years from adjuvant therapy when a 30% proportional reduction in mortality is observed in the highest-risk subgroups (50% death rate with no adjuvant therapy). In contrast, the same 30% proportional reduction in mortality translated into a benefit for only 3 of 100 patients in the lowest-risk subset (10% death rate with no adjuvant therapy). Thus the absolute benefit of adjuvant therapy depends on both the proportional reduction in mortality and the risk of disease recurrence, with the greatest benefit observed in the highest-risk treatment groups. Table 131–9 uses data from the overview analyses to show the absolute benefits of adjuvant chemotherapy in terms of age and nodal status. In the highest-risk group, node-positive women younger than 50 years of age, only 42.8% were alive at 10 years with no polychemotherapy as compared to 54.2% with polychemotherapy, which translates into an absolute survival benefit of 11.4%. However, in the node-negative group, patients younger than 50 years old where survival with no polychemotherapy was highest (i.e., 76.3%), the addition of polychemotherapy produced an absolute benefit of only 4.8%. It

TABLE 131-9 Absolute Benefits of Adjuvant Chemotherapy by Age and Nodal Status

	With Polychemotherapy (%)	With No Polychemotherapy (%)	Absolute Benefit (%)
Disease-free survival			
Age <50 years			
Node-negative	72.6	62.3	10.3
Node-positive	47.4	34.1	13.3
Age 50–69 years			
Node-negative	74.9	70.0	4.9
Node-positive	47.0	42.8	4.2
Overall survival			
Age <50 years			
Node-negative	81.1	76.3	4.8
Node-positive	54.2	42.8	11.4
Age 50–69 years			
Node-negative	79.3	76.0	3.3
Node-positive	52.9	50.2	2.7

Adapted from reference 5.

should be pointed out that all of these differences in survival are highly statistically significant and form the basis for national and international guidelines that recommend offering cytotoxic chemotherapy to most women with early stage breast cancer.[45,70,71] However, the absolute benefit in node-positive women 50 to 69 years old is quite small (2.7%), and depending on other disease characteristics and comorbid conditions, patients may elect not to pursue treatment. Although a 2% absolute reduction in death attributable to polychemotherapy may appear small, at least two investigators report that most patients with breast cancer would accept severe toxicity from treatment to achieve as little as a 1% to 5% absolute improvement in survival.[72,73]

Several international and national groups have developed guidelines for treatment of early stage breast cancer based on specific patient and disease characteristics and the results of the overview analyses. In January 2005, an international group of researchers met in St. Gallen, Switzerland, for the Ninth International Expert Consensus Conference on the Primary Therapy of Early Breast Cancer.[70] At the conclusion of the conference, a consensus panel of experts reviewed and modified its previous guidelines and recommendations for selection of adjuvant systemic therapies in specific patient populations outside of the framework of clinical trials. Table 131–10 shows these recommendations based on risk of relapse, predicted response, results of treatment from randomized clinical trials, and patient preferences concerning risks and benefits of effective therapy. Patient populations are categorized into groups based on risk of relapse. The panel defined risk categories for patients with operable breast cancer as follows: (a) low-risk includes node-negative patients with tumors ≤2 cm, and all of the following: histologic or nuclear grade 1, no peritumoral vascular invasion, *HER2*-negative status, and age ≥35 years; (b) intermediate-risk includes node-negative patients with at least one of the following: pathologic tumor size >2 cm, histologic or nuclear grade 2 or 3, peritumoral vascular invasion, *HER2*-positive status, or age <35 years; (c) intermediate-risk also includes node positive (1 to 3 involved nodes) if *HER2* negative; (d) high-risk includes node positive (1 to 3 involved nodes) if *HER2* positive or node positive (≥4 involved nodes). Patients are further classified into endocrine responsive (HR positive), endocrine response uncertain (HR unknown or uncertain), or endocrine nonresponsive (HR negative), based on the presence or absence of hormone receptors.

The NCCN has also developed practice guidelines for the treatment of breast cancer. These guidelines, which are updated annually, reflect the increasing trend toward the use of chemotherapy in postmenopausal (age >50 years) patients, in addition to its established use in premenopausal (age <50 years) patients, hormonal therapy in all HR-positive women regardless of age or menopausal status, and the combination of both chemotherapy and hormonal therapy.[45] These guidelines differ from the St. Gallen expert consensus guidelines in the recommendation of chemotherapy for women with node-negative tumors 1 to 2 cm or 0.6 to 1 cm in size. If the characteristics of these tumors are unfavorable (angiolymphatic invasion, high nuclear or histologic grade, *HER2* overexpression, or HR-negative), then chemotherapy is recommended with or without hormonal therapy, depending on HR status.

Intensive research efforts are directed toward identifying those characteristics of the primary tumor (e.g., pathologic or molecular prognostic factors) that may predict for a higher or lower likelihood of distant metastases and death in node-negative patients. Although many prognostic factors are being investigated, no single factor or combination of factors sufficiently identifies those at risk of metastases or is sufficiently standardized to be reproducibly applicable to all patients. Currently, two commercially available genetic tests are being prospectively validated as decision-support tools for adjuvant chemotherapy. Oncotype DX is one of these tests which screens for expression of 21 genes using reverse-transcription polymerase chain

TABLE 131-10 St. Gallen Consensus Recommendations for Adjuvant Treatment of Early-Stage Breast Cancer

Patient Group	Low Risk[a]	Intermediate Risk[a]	High Risk[a]
Premenopausal			
HR positive[b]	• Tam or none[c] • or LHRH[c]	• Tam[e] ± OAS ± Chemo, or • Chemo → Tam[e] (± OAS), or • Tam alone, or • OA/OS	• Chemo → Tam[e] or • Chemo → Tam[e] + OAS, or • Chemo ± (OAS + AI)
HR unknown/uncertain[b]	• Tam or none[c] • or LHRH[c]	• Chemo → Tam[e] (± OAS), or • Tam[e] ±OAS (± Chemo), or • Chemo → (OAS + AI) • OAS	• Chemo → Tam[e], or • Chemo → Tam[e] + OAS, or • Chemo → (OAS + AI)
HR negative[b]	• Not applicable	• Chemo	• Chemo
Postmenopausal			
HR positive[b]	• Tam or AI or none[c]	• Tam, or • AI, or • Chemo → Tam[e], or • Chemo → AI • Switch to AI after Tam; exemestane or anastrozole after 2–3 years, and letrozole after 5 years.	• Chemo → Tam[e], or • Chemo → AI • Switch to AI after Tam; exemestane or anastrozole after 2–3 years, and letrozole after 5 years.
HR unknown/uncertain[b]	• Tam or AI or none[c]	• Chemo → AI, or • Chemo → Tam[e] • Switch to AI after Tam; exemestane or anastrozole after 2–3 years, and letrozole after 5 years.	• Chemo → AI, or • Chemo → Tam[e] • Switch to AI after Tam; exemestane or anastrozole after 2–3 years, and letrozole after 5 years.
HR negative[b]	• Not applicable	• Chemo	• Chemo

AI, aromatase inhibitor (anastrozole, exemestane, letrozole); Chemo, chemotherapy (see text for specific regimen information); LHRH, leuteinizing hormone releasing hormone (goserelin is most extensively studied); OAS, ovarian ablation or suppression; Tam, tamoxifen.

Parentheses indicate research questions that are currently being addressed in ongoing clinical trials.

[a]See text for definition of risk categories.

[b]See text for definitions of hormone receptor status and responsiveness to endocrine therapies.

[c]Indicates alternative treatment option in cases of medical contraindications or patient/physician preferences.

[d]Some experts recommend that all patients with node-positive disease should be treated as high risk patients and that AC and CMF should be eliminated from the list of acceptable regimens.

[e]Tamoxifen should not be given concurrently with chemotherapy; sequential administration is preferred.

Data from reference 70.

reaction and results in a recurrence score that can be used to determine the risk of recurrence and/or death from breast cancer in women with ER-positive, node-negative, invasive breast cancer.[55] The tumor tissue used for this test is paraffin-embedded tumor from archived samples. This tool is somewhat controversial given that it has only been validated in patients receiving adjuvant tamoxifen therapy and inconsistent results have been reported from some validation trials. Ongoing clinical trials hope to further elucidate the role of Oncotype DX in the future management of breast cancer. A second test, MammaPrint, was recently approved to estimate prognosis in breast cancer patients with early-stage disease, regardless of HR status. MammaPrint screens the tumor for 77 genes using microarray technology. The assay requires fresh-frozen tissue and reports the predicted rates of recurrence as high or low. This information has been shown to accurately predict for recurrence in a subset of patients not receiving systemic adjuvant therapy.[56] The MINDACT (Microarray In Node-negative Disease may Avoid ChemoTherapy) trial, ongoing in Europe, will compare the predictive capabilities of MammaPrint against the standard prognostic factors to assess which patients with node-negative, ER-positive breast cancer will benefit from adjuvant chemotherapy. We await further information to guide the use of these novel pharmacogenomic tools.

A clinical tool that is gaining favor is an Internet-based tool called Adjuvant! (*www.adjuvantonline.com*), which helps clinicians and patients make informed decisions regarding adjuvant therapy for breast, colon, and lung cancers. The tool allows healthcare professionals to estimate the risks of negative outcomes (e.g., cancer recurrence and/or death), and the potential benefits of therapy (e.g., reduction of risks of recurrence and/or death). This is a validated, evidence-based tool which incorporates multiple prognostic and predictive factors into a mathematical model in which each factor is weighted based on established evidence from clinical trials and is placed in the background of the Surveillance, Epidemiology, and End Results (SEER) database for patients living in the United States.[74] By entering the patient's age, comorbidities, ER status, tumor grade, tumor size, and nodal status, the clinician can use the tool to estimate the breast cancer mortality and/or recurrence risk at 10 years and determine the impact of chemotherapy, hormone therapy or both on these risks. The results are then projected in a graphic format which is easy to understand and explain to patients. Some of the limitations of Adjuvant! include the limited information regarding outcome in patients with tumors that are smaller than 1 cm and no axillary lymph node involvement; it does not incorporate the *HER2* status of the primary tumor; and it does not consider potential adverse effects of therapy. For a more in-depth discussion of the issues and controversies regarding adjuvant therapy of breast cancer, the reader is referred to two excellent reviews.[75,76]

The use of preoperative systemic therapy is gaining favor in both early stage and locally advanced breast cancers. This approach to therapy, referred to as *neoadjuvant* or *primary systemic therapy*, usually consists of chemotherapy, but in special circumstances may also include hormonal therapy (e.g., in inoperable patients with significant comorbidities). Advantages of preoperative systemic therapy include (a) a decrease in the size of the tumor to minimize surgery; (b) determining the response to chemotherapy/hormone therapy in vivo (an important prognostic indicator); and (c) other theoretical advantages (e.g., delivery of chemotherapy through an intact vascular system). In a pivotal study conducted by the NSABP (Trial B18), preoperative chemotherapy was compared to traditional chemotherapy given after surgery (same chemotherapy and same number of cycles).[77,78] Although no difference was found in DFS or OS, rates of BCT were higher in the group receiving preoperative chemotherapy (67.8% vs. 59.8%).[78] This study also identified a small subset of patients (13%) who had a pathologic complete response (no tumor left at surgery) after chemotherapy. These patients went on to have a significantly longer DFS as compared with patients who did not achieve a pathologic complete response (p <0.0001).[78] While this approach to therapy is generally reserved for patients with inoperable tumors (locally advanced), early-stage breast cancer patients who meet the criteria for BCT except for size of the tumor may be considered for preoperative systemic therapy in order to decrease the size of the tumor, allowing for less radical surgery and better cosmetic results.

❹ Adjuvant Chemotherapy Cytotoxic drugs that have been used alone and in combination as adjuvant therapy in breast cancer include doxorubicin, epirubicin, cyclophosphamide, methotrexate, fluorouracil, paclitaxel, docetaxel, melphalan, prednisone, vinorelbine, and vincristine. Table 131–11 lists some of the most common combination chemotherapy regimens employed in the adjuvant and metastatic settings.

The basic principle of adjuvant therapy for any cancer type is that the regimen with the highest response rate in advanced disease should be the optimal regimen for use in the adjuvant setting. However, results from individual clinical trials investigating specific regimens in the adjuvant setting are required to identify the benefits and risks in a specific patient population. Early administration of effective combination chemotherapy at a time when the tumor burden is low should increase the likelihood of cure and minimize the emergence of drug-resistant tumor cell clones. Historically, combination chemotherapy regimens (polychemotherapy) have been more effective than single-agent chemotherapy. Because anthracyclines (doxorubicin and epirubicin) historically have been considered as the most active class of chemotherapy agents in the treatment of metastatic breast cancer, many experts assume that anthracycline-containing regimens are associated with a higher cure rate than non–anthracycline-containing regimens when used in the adjuvant setting. The overview analysis of polychemotherapy (discussed previously) investigated this question, analyzing results from 17 trials that directly compared an anthracycline-containing regimen with a cyclophosphamide, methotrexate, fluorouracil (CMF)-type regimen and demonstrated a significant advantage for the anthracycline regimens.[5] In that meta-analysis, anthracycline-containing regimens were modestly superior in reducing recurrence and death as compared to regimens without anthracyclines. An 11% ± 3% reduction in annual odds of recurrence and a 15% ± 3% reduction in annual odds of death were reported in the 2005 update, which translated into an absolute difference in OS of 3% at 5 years and 4% at 10 years.[5]

The taxanes (paclitaxel and docetaxel) are a newer class of agents that rival the anthracyclines in their activity in metastatic breast cancer, becoming (arguably) the most active class of chemotherapy for this disease. Because these agents are relatively new, adjuvant studies including them have not yet been incorporated into the published EBCTCG overview analyses. An updated overview analysis with inclusion of these results is expected to be published in 2009. However, results from several individual clinical trials with substantial followup provide meaningful information. In a pooled analysis of 15,500 patients from 9 trials, the addition of a taxane resulted in significant increases in DFS and OS (RR 0.86, 95% CI 0.81 to 0.90, p <0.00001; RR 0.84, 95% CI 0.79 to 0.89, p <0.0001, respectively).[79] These trials included both sequential and concurrent taxane therapy (paclitaxel or docetaxel) in conjunction with other drugs that are routinely given in the adjuvant setting (anthracyclines, cyclophosphamide, fluorouracil, and/or methotrexate). Regardless of administration (e.g., weekly, every 3 weeks, prolonged or short infusions) or type of taxane, DFS and OS were consistently and significantly improved. Most of these trials enrolled node-positive patients only, but some also included high-risk node-negative patients. Although the definition of this group of patients differed between studies, the improvement in DFS and OS was consistent across all subgroups analyzed.

TABLE 131-11 Common Chemotherapy Regimens for Breast Cancer

Adjuvant Chemotherapy Regimens	
AC[a] Doxorubicin 60 mg/m^2 IV, day 1 Cyclophosphamide 600 mg/m^2 IV, day 1 Repeat cycles every 21 days for 4 cycles	**AC → Paclitaxel[b]** Doxorubicin 60 mg/m^2 IV, day 1 Cyclophosphamide 600 mg/m^2 IV, day 1 Repeat cycles every 21 days for 4 cycles Followed by: Paclitaxel 175 mg/m^2 IV over 3 hours Repeat cycles every 21 days for 4 cycles
FAC[c] Fluorouracil 500 mg/m^2 IV, days 1 and 4 Doxorubicin 50 mg/m^2 IV continuous infusion over 72 hours[w] Cyclophosphamide 500 mg/m^2 IV, day 1 Repeat cycles every 21–28 days for 6 cycles	**TAC[d]** Docetaxel 75 mg/m^2 IV, day 1 Doxorubicin 50 mg/m^2 IV bolus, day 1 Cyclophosphamide 500 mg/m^2 IV, day 1 (Doxorubicin should be given first) Repeat cycles every 21 days for 6 cycles (must be given with growth factor support)
CAF[e] Cyclophosphamide 600 mg/m^2 IV, day 1 Doxorubicin 60 mg/m^2 IV bolus, day 1 Fluorouracil 600 mg/m^2 IV, day 1 Repeat cycles every 21–28 days for 6 cycles	**Paclitaxel → FAC[f]** Paclitaxel 80 mg/m^2 per week IV over 1 hour every week for 12 weeks Followed by: Fluorouracil 500 mg/m^2 IV, days 1 and 4 Doxorubicin 50 mg/m^2 IV continuous infusion over 72 hours[w] Cyclophosphamide 500 mg/m^2 IV, day 1 Repeat cycles every 21–28 days for 4 cycles[f]
FEC[g] Fluorouracil 500 mg/m^2 IV, day 1 Epirubicin 100 mg/m^2 IV bolus, day 1 Cyclophosphamide 500 mg/m^2 IV, day 1 Repeat cycle every 21 days for 6 cycles	**CMF[h,i]** Cyclophosphamide 100 mg/m^2 per day orally, days 1–14 Methotrexate 40 mg/m^2 IV, days 1 and 8 Fluorouracil 600 mg/m^2 IV, days 1 and 8 Repeat cycles every 28 days for 6 cycles ***or*** Cyclophosphamide 600 mg/m^2 IV, day 1 Methotrexate 40 mg/m^2 IV, day 1 Fluorouracil 600 mg/m^2 IV, days 1 and 8 Repeat cycles every 21 days for 6 cycles
CEF[j] Cyclophosphamide 75 mg/m^2 per day orally on days 1–14 Epirubicin 60 mg/m^2 IV, days 1 and 8 Fluorouracil 600 mg/m^2 IV, days 1 and 8 Repeat cycles every 21 days for 6 cycles (requires prophylactic antibiotics or growth factor support)	**Dose-Dense AC → Paclitaxel[k]** Doxorubicin 60 mg/m^2 IV bolus, day 1 Cyclophosphamide 600 mg/m^2 IV, day 1 Repeat cycles every 14 days for 4 cycles (must be given with growth factor support) Followed by: Paclitaxel 175 mg/m^2 IV over 3 hours Repeat cycles every 14 days for 4 cycles (must be given with growth factor support)[w]
Metastatic Single-Agent Chemotherapy	
Paclitaxel[l,m] Paclitaxel 175 mg/m^2 IV over 3 hours Repeat cycles every 21 days ***or*** Paclitaxel 80 mg/m^2 per week IV over 1 hour Repeat dose every 7 days	**Vinorelbine[n]** Vinorelbine 30 mg/m^2 IV, days 1 and 8 Repeat cycles every 21 days ***or*** Vinorelbine 25–30 mg/m^2 per week IV Repeat cycles every 7 days (adjust dose based on absolute neutrophil count; see product information)
Docetaxel[o,p] Docetaxel 60–100 mg/m^2 IV over 1 hour Repeat cycles every 21 days ***or*** Docetaxel 30–35 mg/m^2 per week IV over 30 minutes Repeat dose every 7 days	**Gemcitabine[q]** Gemcitabine 600–1,000 mg/m^2 per week IV, days 1, 8, and 15 Repeat cycles every 28 days (may need to hold day 15 dose based on blood counts)[q]
Capecitabine[r] Capecitabine 2,000–2,500 mg/m^2 per day orally, divided twice daily for 14 days Repeat cycles every 21 days	**Liposomal doxorubicin[s]** Liposomal doxorubicin 30–50 mg/m^2 IV over 90 minutes Repeat cycles every 28 days

(continued)

TABLE 131-11 Common Chemotherapy Regimens for Breast Cancer (continued)

Metastatic Combination Chemotherapy Regimens	
Docetaxel + capecitabine[t]	**Paclitaxel + Gemcitabine**[u]
Docetaxel 75 mg/m² IV over 1 hour, day 1	Paclitaxel 175 mg/m² IV over 3 hours, day 1
Capecitabine 2,000–2,500 mg/m² per day orally divided twice daily for 14 days	Gemcitabine 1250 mg/m² IV days 1 and 8
Repeat cycles every 21 days	Repeat cycles every 21 days

AC, Adriamycin (doxorubicin), Cytoxan (cyclophosphamide); CAF, Cytoxan (cyclophosphamide), Adriamycin (doxorubicin), 5-fluorouracil; CEF, cyclophosphamide, epirubicin, 5-fluorouracil; CMF, cyclophosphamide, methotrexate, 5-flourouracil; FAC, 5-fluorouracil, Adriamycin (doxorubicin), cyclophosphamide; FEC, 5-fluorouracil, epirubicin, cyclophosphamide; TAC, Taxol (paclitaxel), Adriamycin (doxorubicin) cyclophosphamide

[a]From Fisher B, Brown AM, Dimitrov NV, et al. J Clin Oncol 1990;8:1483.
[b]From Henderson CI, Berry DA, Demetri GD, et al. J Clin Oncol 2003;21:976.
[c]From Buzdar AU, Hortobagyi GN, Singletary SE, et al. In: Salmon S, ed. Adjuvant Therapy of Cancer, VIII. Philadelphia: Lippincott-Raven, 1997:93–100.
[d]From Martin M, Dienkowski T, Mackey J, et al. NEJM 2005;352:2302.
[e]From Wood WC, et al. N Engl J Med 1994;330:1253.
[f]From reference 84
[g]French Adjuvant Study Group. J Clin Oncol 2001;19:602.
[h]From Bonadonna G, Brusamolino E, Valagussa P, et al. N Engl J Med 1976;294:405.
[i]From Fisher B, Redmond C, Dimitrov NV, et al. N Engl J Med 1989;32:473.
[j]From Levine MN, Bramwell VH, Pritchard KI, et al. J Clin Oncol 1998;16:2651.
[k]From reference 873
[l]From Taxol (paclitaxel) product information. Princeton, NJ: Bristol-Myers Squibb, March 2003.
[m]From Perez EA, Vogelci, Irwin DH, et al. Clin Oncol 2001;19:4216.
[n]From Zelek L, Bartheir S, Riofrio M, et al. Cancer 2001;92:2267.
[o]From Taxotere (docetaxel) product information. Bridgewater, NJ: Sanofi-aventis, November 2007.
[p]From Hainsworth JD, Burris HA 3rd, Erlaud JB, et al. J Clin Oncol 1998;16:2164.
[q]From Carmichael J, Possinger K, Philip P, et al. J Clin Oncol 1995;13:2731.
[r]From reference 132
[s]From reference133
[t]From reference 135.
[u]From reference 136
[v]FAC may also be given with bolus doxorubicin administration, and the fluorouracil dose is then given on days 1 and 8.
[w]Another way to give these agents in a dose-dense manner is A → P → C as sequential single agents, in the same doses indicated above, every 14 days for 4 cycles each with growth factor support (see reference 83 for details).

CLINICAL CONTROVERSY

Although incorporation of taxanes into many different adjuvant chemotherapy regimens, both sequentially and concurrently, has led to a shift in therapy for node-positive breast cancer patients, the use of taxane-containing regimens in node-negative patients remains controversial. The use of an anthracycline-containing regimen is established for both node-negative and node-positive breast cancer patients.

There is no apparent biologic reason why node-negative disease should respond differently to the taxanes than node-positive disease. However, the absolute benefits for this population may not be large enough to warrant a change from the standard of care. Further followup from these trials will continue to address this issue. Specific data regarding toxicities related to the addition of a taxane in the adjuvant setting are still largely debated. In the pooled analysis, the authors were unable to ascertain the adverse events from the published information and therefore did not analyze this aspect of the trials.[79] But the addition of a taxane may predispose patients to some transient peripheral neuropathy, myelosuppression, and alopecia. The long-term adverse events related to these regimens are yet to be determined. Also, the cost-effectiveness of adding a taxane to an adjuvant regimen is still largely debated given the paucity of reliable information addressing this issue.

No validated predictive factors exist for response to chemotherapy, but some studies suggest that *HER2* status and ER negativity may be useful predictors of response. Retrospective studies suggest that the benefit of anthracycline-containing regimens over CMF-like regimens is limited to those tumors that overexpress *HER2*. However, this is based on retrospective data and should be viewed with caution. The use of trastuzumab, a monoclonal antibody directed against the *HER2* receptor, in the adjuvant setting with chemotherapy is now considered standard of care for the treatment of patients with *HER2*-positive tumors (see Adjuvant Biologic Therapy below). ER status has also been evaluated as a predictor of response. Several clinical trials have attempted to correlate ER-negative status with response to adjuvant chemotherapy, but the results of these studies are inconsistent and decisions concerning chemotherapy should not be based on ER status at this time. Several investigators have attempted to predict response to specific chemotherapy regimens (e.g., taxane-containing regimens) with microarray technology, which uses DNA from the tumor to test for thousands of genetic mutations. Although these types of genetic tests need to be validated in prospective clinical trials, they may serve in the future to help determine what chemotherapy regimen a patient should receive to gain the most benefit.

Although the optimal duration of adjuvant chemotherapy administration is unknown, it appears to be on the order of 12 to 24 weeks and depends on the regimen being used. Chemotherapy is usually initiated within 3 weeks of surgical removal of the primary tumor. "Dose intensity" and "dose density" appear to be critical factors in achieving optimal outcomes in adjuvant breast cancer therapy. *Dose intensity* is defined as the amount of drug administered per unit of time and is typically reported in milligrams per square meter of body surface area per week (mg/m² per week). Increasing dose, decreasing time, or both can increase dose intensity. *Dose density* is one way of achieving dose intensity, but not by increasing the amount of drug given, as occurs with dose escalation, but instead by decreasing the time between treatment cycles. The importance of dose intensity first received wide attention in 1981, when the Milan group reported in a retrospective analysis of their original CMF adjuvant study that only those patients who received at least 85% of their planned CMF dose benefited significantly from adjuvant therapy, while those receiving less than 65% of the planned dose had the same DFS and OS as the group of control patients treated by surgery alone.[80] These observations led to prospective clinical trials of standard anthracycline-containing regimens with higher doses of cyclophosphamide or doxorubicin. A study by the Cancer and Leukemia Group B (CALGB) randomized 1,572 women to three treatment groups given different doses and schedules of cyclophosphamide, doxorubicin, and 5-fluorouracil.[81] The high-dose arm had twice the dose intensity and twice the drug dose as the low-dose arm (basically representing what we now consider "standard dose" cyclophosphamide, doxorubicin, 5-fluorouracil). The moderate-dose arm had two-thirds the dose intensity as the high-dose arm, but the same total drug dose. At a median followup of 9 years, DFS and OS for patients on the moderate- and high-dose arms were superior to those for the patients in the low-dose arm, but no difference in DFS or OS was observed between the moderate- and the high-dose arms. In a more recent study conducted by the CALGB, the doxorubicin dose was escalated (60 mg/m^2, 75 mg/m^2, or 90 mg/m^2) in combination with cyclophosphamide at a fixed dose of 600 mg/m^2.[82] No benefits were seen with the higher dose levels in this trial. Thus dose reductions for standard treatment regimens should be avoided, unless necessitated by severe toxicity. But increasing doses beyond those contained in standard treatment regimens does not appear to be beneficial and may be harmful.

Several studies investigating the impact of *dose density* have now been reported. Interest in this approach to adjuvant therapy was stimulated when the CALGB reported results from their trial 9741 which tested not only dose density, but also the question of using sequential versus combination chemotherapy regimens. Using a 2 × 2 factorial design, investigators randomized node-positive breast cancer patients after surgery to compare sequential versus concurrent chemotherapy, and standard dose versus dose density.[83] The arms of the study were (group 1) sequential doxorubicin (A) for four cycles, followed by paclitaxel (P) for four cycles, followed by cyclophosphamide (C) for four cycles, with all cycles given every 3 weeks; (group 2) sequential A for four cycles, followed by P for four cycles, followed by C for four cycles, with all cycles given every 2 weeks with filgrastim; (group 3) concurrent AC for four cycles, followed by P for four cycles, with all cycles given every 3 weeks; and (group 4) concurrent AC for four cycles, followed by P for four cycles, with all cycles given every 2 weeks with filgrastim. After a median followup of 36 months, the patients receiving every-2-week chemotherapy had a significantly prolonged DFS (at 3 years: 85% vs. 81%; RR 0.74, $p = 0.01$) and OS (92% vs. 90%; RR 0.69, $p = 0.013$) as compared with every 3-week chemotherapy.[83] The use of sequential versus concurrent chemotherapy did not show a benefit for one over the other in terms of DFS or OS, but sequential therapy did appear to be less toxic. Patients in the concurrent every-2-week group (group 4) had significantly more regimen-related toxicity, including a very high rate of red blood cell transfusions for anemia (13% of cycles).[83] Red blood cell transfusions are rarely required with most other standard adjuvant chemotherapy regimens used for breast cancer. Previous data with paclitaxel given weekly versus every 3 weeks indicates that this drug is more effective when given weekly in the neoadjuvant setting.[84] Thus some speculate that the different paclitaxel schedule is the primary reason for the success with this approach to therapy.

Other investigators have tested similar dose-dense regimens with different outcomes. The GONO-MIG (Gruppo Oncologico Nord Ovest—Mammella Intergruppo) trial compared six cycles of 5-fluorouracil, epirubicin, and cyclophosphamide administered every 3 weeks with the same regimen administered every 2 weeks with filgrastim support.[85] The event-free survival and OS were not significantly different between the two arms (hazard ratio 0.88, 95% CI 0.71 to 1.08; hazard ratio 0.87, 95% CI 0.67 to 1.13, respectively). However, the study was relatively small (n = 1,214) and inadequately powered because of a lower-than-expected overall event rate. A noticeable difference between this study and the CALGB trial 9741 was the absence of a taxane, which may explain why dose-density was successful in the CALGB 9741 trial. Another trial, the North American Breast Cancer Intergroup Trial E1199, randomized patients in a 2 × 2 factorial design to receive doxorubicin and cyclophosphamide for 4 cycles every 3 weeks followed by either weekly or three-weekly paclitaxel or docetaxel.[86] While this study does not directly address the question of dose density because of the lower doses given in the weekly arms, it has been suggested that the pharmacologic advantage of a taxane given more frequently may be the essential factor driving the beneficial outcomes seen with "dose density" in the CALGB trial. Although no differences in DFS or OS were observed between the weekly or three-weekly schedule or the different taxanes, a subgroup analysis indicated that the weekly paclitaxel arm appeared to fare the best in terms of DFS (P3 vs. P1; hazard ratio 1.20; $p = 0.06$), but this advantage was not statistically significant.[86] Although other trials have attempted to investigate dose-dense regimens, they also have other variables that were altered that could potentially impact the outcomes. Consequently, they do not directly address the question and their results may be influenced by factors other than dose density. A detailed discussion of these nuances is beyond the scope of this chapter and the reader is referred to excellent references on this topic for further information.[87,88] Nonetheless, despite a relatively short followup, unclear overall benefit compared to conventional regimens, and potentially more toxicity, the dose-dense regimens may be considered as options for adjuvant therapy for node-positive breast cancer. Thorough discussion regarding the risks and benefits each individual patient may face is imperative given the uncertainty surrounding these regimens.

A major focus of clinical investigations in the past was the use of high-dose chemotherapy regimens as adjuvant therapy. Because bone marrow suppression is the dose-limiting toxicity for most chemotherapeutic agents, high-dose chemotherapy regimens followed by colony-stimulating factors or reinfusion of autologous hematopoietic stem cells were developed. Trials to define the effectiveness of high-dose regimens were justified given the positive response rates seen in the metastatic breast cancer setting and the very poor prognosis associated with disease that involves 4 to 9, and particularly 10 or more, axillary lymph nodes. Several cooperative groups have conducted trials of high-dose chemotherapy versus conventional adjuvant therapy. None of the trials showed a significant difference in DFS or OS. Based on the available evidence, this approach to therapy is currently not recommended outside the context of a clinical trial.

The short-term toxic effects of chemotherapy used in the adjuvant setting are generally well tolerated. Although a number of investigators have demonstrated a reduction in quality-of-life, most patients are able to maintain a reasonable level of function and emotional and social well being during treatment.[89,90] Supportive therapy of the patient receiving systemic adjuvant chemotherapy has improved over the past decades. Increased attention to the impact of symptoms on quality-of-life may account for some of this improvement. In addition, more effective antiemetics have become available to assist in managing chemotherapy-induced nausea and vomiting, and colony-stimulating factors are often helpful in preventing febrile neutropenia, particularly in elderly patients or patients receiving high-dose and dose-dense chemotherapy regimens. Despite the use of newer antiemetics for prevention of nausea and vomiting, many women still have difficulty with this side effect and delayed nausea and vomiting remains problematic in some patients. Aprepitant, a novel neurokinin-1 antagonist, may be considered in addition to serotonin receptor antagonists and dexamethasone to improve outcomes for some patients, but clinicians should be aware of the potential for clinically significant drug–drug interactions between aprepitant and other drugs, including chemotherapy. The use of growth factors to support some adjuvant chemotherapy regimens may be required (with dose-dense regimens), but should also be used with caution. Granulocyte colony-stimulating factor and erythropoietin have potential effects on cancer cells and the cellular environment that may negatively impact the antitumor effects of chemotherapy or enhance adverse effects related to the chemotherapy.[88] Although these effects are very controversial, the addition of growth factors to a regimen should be undertaken only after all risks and benefits are thoroughly considered.

Many other side effects are common with the chemotherapy regimens employed for treatment of early stage breast cancer and patients should be appropriately counseled regarding the likelihood of alopecia, weight gain, and fatigue. Patients who are menstruating will often experience a cessation of menses that may not return; cessation of menses may be accompanied by signs and symptoms of menopause. Deep vein thrombosis has been reported in women receiving combination chemotherapy regimens.[91] Leukemia and other hematologic disorders have long been associated with the alkylating agents (e.g., cyclophosphamide) and the topoisomerase II inhibitors (e.g., doxorubicin and epirubicin). Several studies have estimated a 0% to 1.5% cumulative incidence of leukemia and/or myelodysplasia after adjuvant chemotherapy with median followup of 3 to 11 years.[92] To date, the dose-dense regimens have not been associated with an excess rate of leukemias, but the followup on these trials is relatively short.

Cardiomyopathy induced by doxorubicin occurs in less than 1% of women whose total dose of doxorubicin is less than 320 mg/m^2.[293] This risk may be further decreased by use of continuous infusion doxorubicin. It should be noted that epirubicin in the adjuvant setting is usually given at a dose of 100 to 120 mg/m^2.[94] At this dose, epirubicin has an equal chance of causing cardiomyopathy as standard doxorubicin doses when both agents are given as bolus or short infusions. Taxanes are often associated with hypersensitivity reactions, peripheral neuropathy and/or myalgias and arthralgias for a few days following the infusion.

It is important to note that the magnitude of survival benefit for adjuvant chemotherapy in stages I and II breast cancer is modest, with an absolute reduction in mortality of only 5% at 10 years for patients with negative axillary lymph nodes and 10% for patients with positive axillary lymph nodes. In addition, it is currently not possible to accurately predict who will attain this survival benefit. However, studies have reported that most breast cancer patients would accept severe toxicity from treatment to achieve as little as a 1% to 5% improvement in survival.[72,73] Thus in the absence of the ability to predict who will benefit, it is likely that most patients with stage I and stage II breast cancer would choose adjuvant chemotherapy. The optimal chemotherapy regimen for use in the adjuvant setting has yet to be identified and the choice depends on many patient and tumor characteristics.

Adjuvant Biologic Therapy As biologic agents continue to demonstrate significant activity against metastatic breast cancer, they are subsequently tested in the adjuvant setting. Trastuzumab is a monoclonal antibody targeted against the *HER2* receptor protein. It has demonstrated significant survival benefits when administered with chemotherapy in women with metastatic, *HER2*-positive breast cancer. Several recently published or presented studies support the use of trastuzumab in combination with adjuvant chemotherapy for patients with early-stage, *HER2*-positive breast cancer (Table 131–12).[95–98] Results from these trials report up to a 50% reduction in the risk of recurrence with the addition of trastuzumab to an adjuvant chemotherapy regimen. While similar benefits are seen in the published trials to date, the chemotherapy regimens, sequence of administration and duration of trastuzumab differ (Table 131–12).

Most of the regimens investigated include an anthracycline and a taxane given concurrently with trastuzumab or sequentially prior to trastuzumab. From the available evidence, it appears that administration of a taxane with trastuzumab may be more effective than trastuzumab administered after chemotherapy. However, sequential administration of trastuzumab still offers significant benefit over regimens without trastuzumab. The adjuvant use of trastuzumab without any anthracycline has been reported in one trial (Breast Cancer International Research Group 006) and from preliminary analyses appears to provide similar benefit with diminished adverse effects as compared with traditional anthracycline-containing adjuvant trastuzumab regimens. The duration of trastuzumab therapy ranges from 9 to 52 weeks in the published studies. The optimal duration of therapy is unknown. In the United States, trastuzumab was approved for adjuvant therapy of early-stage, *HER2*-positive breast cancer when given in combination with doxorubicin and cyclophosphamide followed by paclitaxel and the trastuzumab was

TABLE 131-12 Adjuvant Trastuzumab Trials

Trial	N9831/B-31[95] (n = 3,779)		HERA[96] (n = 1,694)		FinHer[97] (n = 232)		BCIRG 006[98] (n = 3,222)		
Design	AC × 4 → P[a] × 12 wks	AC × 4 → PH[a] × 12 wks → H[a] × 40 wks	Chemo → obs	Chemo → H[b] × 1 year	T/V[c] × 9 wks → FEC[c] × 3	TH/VH[c] × 9 wks → FEC[c] × 3	AC × 4 → T[d] × 4	AC × 4 → TH[d] × 4	TCH[d] × 6
Median F/U	2 years		1 year		3 years		3 years		
DFS HR (95% CI)	0.48 (0.39–0.59)[e]		0.54 (0.43–0.67)[e]		0.42 (0.21–0.83)[e]		Control vs. AC→TH 0.61 (0.48–0.76)[e] Control vs. TCH 0.67 (0.54–0.83)[e]		
OS HR (95% CI)	0.67 (0.48–0.93)[e]		0.76 (0.47–1.23)		0.41 (0.16–1.08)		Control vs. AC→TH 0.59 (0.42–0.85)[e] Control vs. TCH 0.66 (0.47–0.93)[e]		
AE/Comments	CHF 0.8% vs. 4.1%; rare cases of interstitial pneumonitis-trastuzumab (9 patients)		Symptomatic CHF 0.06% vs 1.73% (p <0.0001); decrease LVEF 2.21% vs. 7.08% (p <0.001).		No significant increase in toxicity with trastuzumab		CHF: AC → T (4 patients); AC→TH (20 patients); TCH (4 patients)[e]		

AC, doxorubicin plus cyclophosphamide; AE, adverse events; BCIRG, Breast Cancer International Research Group; Chemo, chemotherapy; CHF, congestive heart failure; CI, confidence intervals; DFS, disease-free survival; FEC, fluorouracil, epirubicin, cyclophosphamide; FinHer, Finland Herceptin study; F/U, followup; H, trastuzumab; HERA, Herceptin Adjuvant Trial; HR, hazard ratios; N9831/B-31, North Central Cancer Treatment Group and NSABP trials (see text); LVEF, left ventricular ejection fraction; OS, overall survival; P, paclitaxel; T, docetaxel; TCH, docetaxel, carboplatin, trastuzumab; V, vinorelbine; wks, weeks.

[a]Paclitaxel given either every 3 weeks for 4 cycles or weekly for 12 weeks; trastuzumab given weekly × 12 weeks, then either weekly or every 3 weeks for a total of 52 weeks of therapy.

[b]Trastuzumab given every 3 weeks for 1 year; third arm of the trial administered trastuzumab for 2 years (results not reported).

[c]Patients randomized to docetaxel every 3 weeks × 3 or vinorelbine weekly × 8 weeks (last week of vinorelbine omitted prior to FEC); FEC given with epirubicin at 60 mg/m^2 every 3 weeks × 3 cycles.

[d]Docetaxel (T) administered at 100 mg/m^2 every 3 weeks × 4 cycles; in TH arm trastuzumab administered weekly × 52 weeks (after chemotherapy trastuzumab may have been administered every 3 weeks); TCH administered docetaxel at 75 mg/m^2 with carboplatin at an area-under-the-curve of 6 and weekly trastuzumab (after chemotherapy trastuzumab may have been administered every 3 weeks).

[e]p <0.01.

initiated with the taxane and continued for 1 year (total duration of trastuzumab is 52 weeks). This approval was based largely on the results of the NSABP/NCCTG (North Central Cancer Treatment Group) combined analysis published in the *New England Journal of Medicine*. This has become the standard duration of therapy in the United States and many other countries, at least until other data become available to further guide this practice. The HERA (Herceptin Adjuvant) trial was the only study design to incorporate the question of duration of therapy. Published results from that trial reported on the 1-year arm of the trial versus observation. Patients on the 2-year trastuzumab arm are still blinded and continue to be followed; results from this pending analysis will help to determine the optimal duration of trastuzumab in this setting. Shorter durations of trastuzumab therapy have been reported (FinHER [Finland Herceptin] trial) but are not directly compared with the standard duration. Therefore, conclusions regarding the comparative efficacy of trastuzumab regimens that are shorter than 1 year are difficult to ascertain through indirect comparisons.

The incidence of adverse cardiac effects associated with the addition of trastuzumab appears to increase when an anthracycline is included in the regimen prior to administration of trastuzumab. In the NSABP/NCCTG analysis, the cumulative incidence of New York Heart Association class III or IV congestive heart failure or death from cardiac causes was significantly higher in the trastuzumab arm (4.1% vs. 0.8%).[95] However, the higher risk of cardiac complications may be acceptable given the significant reductions in breast cancer recurrence and death rates. Sequential administration of trastuzumab after chemotherapy (as in the HERA trial) appears to produce a lower incidence of cardiac toxicity (severe congestive heart failure = 1.73% with trastuzumab). However, the definition of cardiac events in each trial was different. Rare cases of interstitial pneumonitis were reported in the trastuzumab arm (nine patients) in the combined NSABP/NCCTG trial only. The causality of these events is unclear, but may be related to trastuzumab. Chemotherapy-related adverse effects are slightly more frequent with the addition of trastuzumab, including neutropenia, infection and diarrhea, but these toxicities are easily managed and do not preclude the use of trastuzumab in patients with early stage breast cancer.

All of these adjuvant trials continued trastuzumab administration during adjuvant radiation therapy and hormonal therapy. Therefore, issues related to combining these treatment modalities also exist. The optimal trastuzumab-containing regimen has yet to be determined, but all factors related to efficacy and safety should be considered and discussed with the patient.

CLINICAL CONTROVERSY

Trastuzumab clearly has improved the outcome for women with early-stage, *HER2*-positive breast cancer. However, the optimal trastuzumab-containing regimen remains unknown. Questions remain regarding optimal concurrent chemotherapy; optimal dose, schedule, and duration of trastuzumab therapy; and use of other concurrent therapeutic modalities. Many ongoing clinical trials hope to answer these questions. Also, while the addition of trastuzumab has improved DFS and OS, it is not effective for all women and issues regarding trastuzumab resistance are becoming more complex.

Many questions remain regarding the optimal use of trastuzumab in the adjuvant therapy of early stage breast cancer. Some of the studies included patients with high-risk, node-negative disease. While this group of patients also benefited from therapy with trastuzumab, the FDA has not approved the use of trastuzumab in the United States in this group of women.[99] FDA approval is limited to node-positive patients based on the results of the NCCTG and NSABP trials. In these trials less than 10% of patients included were node negative. In addition, the pharmacoeconomics of this addition to therapy has yet to be fully elucidated. In the United States, only one study has analyzed the cost-effectiveness of this approach. Hillner et al. estimated an incremental cost of about $50,000 per life-year gained based on data from the NCCTG/NSABP and HERA trials combined.[100] This figure is well below what has typically been considered acceptable for other therapeutic advances in the United States (e.g., dialysis, adjuvant chemotherapy for early-stage breast cancer), but borders on unacceptable for other countries with nationalized healthcare. While this type of discussion is far beyond the scope of this chapter, the reader is referred to the following reviews for further discussion regarding this topic.[101,102] Nonetheless, trastuzumab is a very effective but costly addition to adjuvant therapy, with apparent risks that should be discussed in detail with all patients with *HER2*-positive breast cancer prior to undergoing therapy. A similar approach has been used in the neoadjuvant treatment of *HER2*-positive breast cancer as well (see section on Locally Advanced Breast Cancer).

Adjuvant Endocrine Therapy ❹ Hormonal therapies that have been studied in the treatment of primary or early stage breast cancer include tamoxifen, toremifene oophorectomy, ovarian irradiation, luteinizing hormone-releasing hormone (LHRH) agonists and aromatase inhibitors. Choice of agent(s) depends on menopausal status and is based on a multitude of clinical trials completed in this setting that establish different roles for different therapies.

Tamoxifen was traditionally the gold standard adjuvant hormonal therapy and has been used in the adjuvant setting for three decades. Tamoxifen is antiestrogenic in breast cancer cells, but it appears to have estrogenic properties in other tissues and organs.[103,104] More recent studies show that tamoxifen and other similar drugs have many estrogenic and antiestrogenic effects that depend on the tissue and the gene in question, and they are more appropriately called selective estrogen receptor modulators (SERMs). Women receiving adjuvant tamoxifen therapy have reduced risk of recurrence and mortality as compared to women not receiving adjuvant tamoxifen therapy.[5] This observation, coupled with evidence of tamoxifen's tolerability including beneficial estrogenic effects on the lipid profile and bone density, led to tamoxifen being the hormonal agent of choice for both pre- and postmenopausal women. Premenopausal patients may derive equivalent benefit from ovarian ablation via surgery or administration of LHRH agonists when compared with tamoxifen.[5] In the United States, tamoxifen is generally considered the adjuvant hormonal therapy of choice for premenopausal women. However, many ongoing clinical trials are investigating the use of the LHRH agonists or oophorectomy instead of or in addition to tamoxifen in this group of women.

The optimal dose of tamoxifen is unclear. The EBCTCG overview showed that more is not necessarily better for response rates.[5] Lower doses of tamoxifen may be effective, but no clinical trials have addressed this question. Therefore the current recommended dose for tamoxifen in the adjuvant, metastatic, and preventive settings is 20 mg/day. Because tamoxifen has a long biologic half-life, it can be administered as a single daily dose. Adjuvant tamoxifen therapy is generally initiated shortly after surgery or as soon as pathology results are known and the decision to administer tamoxifen as adjuvant therapy is made.

When adjuvant tamoxifen is given with chemotherapy, it should be given after chemotherapy is completed. This recommendation is based on laboratory and clinical evidence from a phase III trial suggesting tamoxifen administered concurrently with chemotherapy may antagonize the beneficial effect of chemotherapy.[105] In the phase III clinical trial, after a median followup of 8.5 years, sequential tamoxifen resulted in an estimated DFS advantage of 18% (hazard ratio 1.18) as compared to concurrent use of tamoxifen with chemotherapy.[105] Some clinicians also advocate the initiation of tamoxifen following completion of radiation therapy, but this subject is very controversial and few trials have addressed the issue of concurrent versus sequential hormone therapy and radiation therapy.

The optimal duration of tamoxifen therapy in the adjuvant setting is currently 5 years. Studies of prolonged administration (e.g., 10 years) have failed to demonstrate any advantage and in fact may be associated with a slightly worse survival.[106]

The most reliable information regarding the side effects of tamoxifen comes from the NSABP Breast Cancer Prevention Trial (P1).[49] This trial randomized 13,388 women 35 years of age or older who were at increased risk for breast cancer to placebo (n = 6,707) or to 20 mg/day of tamoxifen (n = 6,681) for 5 years. Although the primary finding of this study is that tamoxifen reduces the risk of invasive breast cancer by 49%, this study also provides an excellent opportunity to determine the risk of side effects associated with tamoxifen. Information was prospectively collected with regard to the occurrence of hot flashes, vaginal discharge, irregular menses, fluid retention, nausea, skin changes, diarrhea, and weight gain or loss. The self-administered depression scale and a global quality of life and a sexual function scale were administered at each followup visit. The only symptomatic differences noted between the placebo and tamoxifen group were related to hot flashes and vaginal discharge, both of which occurred more often in the tamoxifen group. No important differences between the two groups were observed in the various self-reporting instruments. Tamoxifen did not increase the risk of ischemic heart disease, but reduced the risk of hip radius and spine fractures. Of note, the rates of stroke, pulmonary embolism, and deep vein thrombosis were elevated in the tamoxifen group (stroke, RR 1.59; pulmonary embolism, RR 3.01; and deep vein thrombosis, RR 1.60), particularly in women age 50 years or older. The rate of endometrial cancer was increased in the tamoxifen group (RR 2.53), and this increased risk occurred predominantly in women age 50 years or older. The increased risk of endometrial carcinoma is similar in magnitude to that associated with postmenopausal estrogen replacement therapy and is likely a consequence of an estrogenic effect of tamoxifen on the endometrium. Some experts argue that this risk is acceptable because the endometrial cancer induced by tamoxifen is low-stage, low-grade, and easily treated with surgery or other means and does not pose a life-threatening risk to women. Tamoxifen was also associated with an increased risk of uterine sarcomas (a more aggressive form of endometrial cancer), but this risk appears to be lower than the more common endometrial cancers identified in the NSABP P-1 study.[107] Routine endometrial biopsy is not currently recommended for women receiving tamoxifen therapy. However, women receiving tamoxifen therapy should be counseled to have regular gynecologic examinations and immediately report unusual vaginal bleeding to their primary clinicians for further evaluation.

Toremifene is another marketed antiestrogen whose primary advantage is a lower estrogenic-to-antiestrogenic ratio as compared to tamoxifen (based on laboratory data).[108] Toremifene (60 mg orally daily) has been found to have efficacy similar to that of tamoxifen in metastatic disease and a generally similar side-effect profile.[109] Toremifene is currently indicated as an alternative to tamoxifen in patients with metastatic breast cancer, but studies are ongoing to evaluate its safety and efficacy in the adjuvant setting. Preliminary results from these trials indicate similar efficacy and safety, with possibly inferior bone protection with toremifene.[110,111] However, further followup is required to determine the long-term effects of toremifene in the adjuvant setting.

In premenopausal women, the use of LHRH-agonists or other means of ovarian ablation provides benefit in the adjuvant setting. In the EBCTCG overview analysis published in 2005, the overall benefit of ovarian ablation or suppression was significant compared with no treatment, but smaller than previously reported in 1996 (reduction in annual odds of recurrence = 25% ± 12% in women <40 years old and 29% ± 6% in women 40 to 49 years old).[5] Many of the ongoing trials with the LHRH agonists were not yet included in this analysis and most of the clinical trials analyzed included patients with HR-positive, -negative, and -unknown status. In a subsequent systematic review of 11 randomized trials, similar benefit was observed with goserelin as compared with CMF chemotherapy in hormone-sensitive premenopausal breast cancer patients.[112] It is not clear whether the benefit of chemotherapy in this population is a result of the actual effects of chemotherapy or a result of the endocrine effects of chemotherapy-induced menopause. Consequently, some studies have investigated the benefits of adding ovarian ablation or suppression to chemotherapy, either with or without tamoxifen. Results from these studies clearly indicate a benefit from ceasing menses, regardless of whether this is caused by chemotherapy or ovarian ablation or suppression.[112] It is not clear whether the addition of an LHRH agonist to tamoxifen is advantageous in women with HR-positive tumors who continue to menstruate after chemotherapy. Multiple ongoing trials are attempting to answer this question; these trials include an LHRH agonist alone, with tamoxifen or with an aromatase inhibitor.

In postmenopausal women, aromatase inhibitors are gradually replacing tamoxifen in the adjuvant setting. Three different approaches to therapy have been undertaken with these new agents: (a) direct comparison with tamoxifen for adjuvant hormonal therapy, (b) sequential use after 5 years of adjuvant tamoxifen therapy, and (c) sequential use after 2 to 3 years of adjuvant tamoxifen. Anastrozole and letrozole have been directly compared with tamoxifen as initial therapy in postmenopausal women with HR-positive, early stage breast cancer (ATAC [Arimidex, Tamoxifen, Alone or in Combination] trial and BIG [Breast International Group] 1–98 Trial).[113,114] These comparisons show an advantage with the aromatase inhibitors over tamoxifen in terms of DFS. The other approach to adjuvant hormonal therapy with the aromatase inhibitors is sequential use of newer agents after the optimal 5 years of tamoxifen or only 2 to 3 years of tamoxifen. In a highly publicized study reported in the *New England Journal of Medicine*, 5 additional years of letrozole was compared with placebo in postmenopausal breast cancer patients who had completed 5 years of tamoxifen therapy.[115] After a median followup of 2.4 years, letrozole was associated with superior estimated 4-year DFS as compared with placebo (93% vs. 87%; $p < 0.001$). Because of this difference, patients were unblinded and allowed to crossover to the active arm of therapy. Although that decision will limit the ability of the trial to show any differences in OS, further followup will continue to evaluate safety and DFS in those patients randomized to letrozole from the beginning of the trial. In a pooled analysis of trials investigating a switch to an aromatase inhibitor, patients who had completed 2 to 3 years of adjuvant tamoxifen therapy were randomized to continue tamoxifen or crossover to anastrozole or exemestane for the remainder of 5 years.[116] These trials all show longer DFS in patients who switched to an aromatase inhibitor as compared to those who continued with tamoxifen alone.

Although the followup from these trials is also relatively short, most national and international guidelines currently recommend incorporation of an aromatase inhibitor into the adjuvant hormonal therapy regimen for all postmenopausal, hormone-sensitive breast cancers.[45] The current NCCN guidelines for breast cancer management state that any of the following are acceptable endocrine therapy regimens for these women: (a) anastrozole or letrozole for 5 years; (b) tamoxifen for 2 to 3 years followed by anastrozole or exemestane for a total of 5 years of endocrine therapy; or (c) tamoxifen for 5 years followed by letrozole for another 5 years (total of 10 years of endocrine therapy).[45] The optimal hormonal therapy regimen in the adjuvant setting has yet to be determined. In the BIG 1–98 trial mentioned earlier with letrozole compared with tamoxifen, two separate arms are also investigating the value of switching from tamoxifen to an aromatase inhibitor or vice versa. Results from this trial are eagerly awaited and will help to more clearly define a treatment strategy for women facing this clinical dilemma.

Aromatase inhibitors are generally well tolerated. Adverse effects include hot flashes, myalgia/arthralgia, vaginal dryness/atrophy, and mild headaches and diarrhea. Although concerns surrounding loss of bone density and an increased risk of osteoporosis are evident in these adjuvant trials, the overall impact on quality-of-life and long-term survival has yet to be determined. Bisphosphonates are coadministered with the aromatase inhibitors in many patients in the metastatic setting and may also be beneficial in the adjuvant setting. Other adverse events that are worrisome include questionable effects on the cardiovascular system (e.g., hypercholesterolemia), cognitive functioning and joint health. Longer followup from these trials will continue to provide valuable information to guide treatment decisions and side effect management.

CLINICAL CONTROVERSY

The optimal use of antiaromatase agents in the adjuvant setting for postmenopausal women with HR-positive tumors is controversial. Multiple studies have been published with results indicating a benefit to regimens that include an aromatase inhibitor as initial therapy or after tamoxifen. However, many questions remain as to the optimal drug, dose, sequence, and duration of therapy for these agents.

In summary, tamoxifen has been used in the adjuvant setting for nearly 30 years and has a very-well-defined safety and efficacy profile in this setting. Although it is difficult to define the role of new therapies given the lengthy history of tamoxifen, the role of tamoxifen in the adjuvant setting is changing with the incorporation of newer agents either concurrently (e.g., LHRH agonists) or sequentially (e.g., aromatase inhibitors).

■ LOCALLY ADVANCED BREAST CANCER (STAGE III)

❺ *Locally advanced breast cancer* generally refers to breast carcinomas with significant primary tumor and nodal disease, but in which distant metastases cannot be documented. A wide variety of clinical scenarios can be seen within this group of patients, including neglected tumors that have spread locally, to inflammatory breast cancers that are a unique clinical entity. Inflammatory breast cancer is associated with similar clinical findings as compared to other neglected, locally advanced breast tumors (e.g., erythema representing skin involvement). The distinction between the two diagnoses lies in the rapidity of onset of symptoms. Many locally advanced breast cancers are diagnosed in patients who have had symptoms for months to years and have neglected to seek medical attention. Although these women have a poor prognosis because of the delay in diagnosis, they are not classified as inflammatory breast cancer. The hallmark of inflammatory breast cancers is the rapid onset of symptoms within weeks to months, including erythema of the skin with or without a detectable underlying breast mass. These patients are often inappropriately treated for cellulitis with antibiotics for several weeks to months. Because of the aggressive nature of this disease, a delay in diagnosis can be fatal for some of these women.

The natural history of locally advanced breast cancer showed that even when local-regional control was accomplished, systemic relapse and death from breast cancer eventually occurred in most patients.[117] That observation led to interest in the use of neoadjuvant or primary chemotherapy in locally advanced breast cancer, which renders inoperable tumors resectable, and can increase rates of BCT. Other potential benefits related to early initiation of systemic therapy include delivery of drugs through an intact vasculature, in vivo assessment of response to therapy, and the opportunity to study the biologic effects of the systemic treatment. However, this approach to therapy also results in a loss of standard, well-validated pathologic prognostic markers, such as initial tumor size (measured by pathologic examination) and the number of axillary lymph nodes involved. Also, as discussed earlier, OS with adjuvant as compared with neoadjuvant chemotherapy is similar. However, in light of other benefits gained with neoadjuvant therapy, these two factors may not be enough to continue to drive the practice of primary surgery. The topic of adjuvant versus neoadjuvant systemic therapy is fraught with controversy, but the many advantages of neoadjuvant, primary systemic therapy are continuing to drive an increase in the number of operable patients offered this treatment modality.[118] For patients with inoperable breast cancer, including inflammatory breast cancer, the initial approach to therapy should be chemotherapy with the goal of achieving resectability. The NCCN guidelines addressing the management of locally advanced disease recommend primary chemotherapy with either an anthracycline- or taxane-containing regimen.[45]

After neoadjuvant chemotherapy, most tumors respond with more than a 50% decrease in tumor size; approximately 70% of patients experience a reduction in their stage of disease. The chemotherapy regimens used in this setting are similar to those used in the adjuvant setting, but the regimens usually include an anthracycline, incorporate a taxane in some manner, and may have higher dose-density or dose-intensity. For patients with *HER2*-positive tumors, the incorporation of trastuzumab with chemotherapy is appropriate.[119] For more detailed information regarding the specific regimen-related information, the reader is referred to a recently published review.[120] Neoadjuvant endocrine therapy may be an option for patients who have unresectable HR-positive tumors who are unable to receive chemotherapy (e.g., multiple comorbid conditions).[121]

Local therapy usually follows chemotherapy, and the extent of surgery is determined by response to chemotherapy, the wishes of the patient, and the cosmetic results likely to be achieved. However, many patients may be able to have BCT if an acceptable response to chemotherapy is achieved. Adjuvant radiation therapy should be administered to all locally advanced breast cancer patients to minimize local recurrences, regardless of the type of surgery used for that individual patient (e.g., mastectomy or segmental mastectomy). Inoperable tumors that are unresponsive to systemic chemotherapy may require radiation therapy for local management and may not be eligible for surgical resection after radiation. These patients are not commonly seen, but have a very poor prognosis. For most patients in this category, cure is still the primary goal of therapy and can be achieved in a large number of patients when all treatment modalities are employed.

■ METASTATIC BREAST CANCER (STAGE IV)

❻ The goal of therapy with early and locally advanced breast cancer is to cure the disease. After it has advanced beyond local–regional disease, breast cancer is currently incurable. The goals of treatment of metastatic breast cancer are to improve symptoms and quality of life and extend survival. Thus it is important to choose therapy with good activity while minimizing toxicities. Treatment of metastatic breast cancer with cytotoxic, biologic, or endocrine therapy often results in regression of disease and improvements in quality-of-life. In patients who respond to therapy, duration of survival is also increased. The choice of therapy for metastatic disease is based on the site of disease involvement and presence or absence of certain characteristics. The most important factor predicting response to endocrine therapy is the presence of estrogen and progesterone receptors in the primary tumor tissue. Fifty percent to 60% of patients with ER-positive tumors and 75% to 80% of patients with ER- and PR-positive tumors will respond to hormonal therapy, whereas those with ER- and PR-negative tumors have a less than 10% response rate. Thus the most important factor determining choice of endocrine versus cytotoxic chemotherapy is the presence of hormone receptors in the primary breast tumor. Site of disease is also important because endocrine therapy is more likely to be effective in patients with bone and soft-tissue metastases. Patients with asymptomatic visceral involvement (e.g., liver or lung) may be candidates for hormonal therapy, depending on the clinical circumstance (hormones usually work more slowly than chemotherapy). Patients with symptomatic visceral and/or central nervous system involvement generally have more rapidly growing cancers that require chemotherapy. Endocrine therapy is the treatment of choice for patients with HR-positive tumors who exhibit the first sign of metastatic disease in soft tissue, bone, or pleura, because of the equal probability of response to hormonal therapy as compared to chemotherapy, and the lower toxicity profile of endocrine therapy.

❼ Patients who respond to initial endocrine therapy often respond to a second (or even third) hormonal manipulation. But the response rate is lower and duration of response is shorter with second (and third) hormonal manipulations. Patients are sequentially treated with endocrine therapy until their tumors cease to respond, at which time cytotoxic chemotherapy can be given. Concurrent administration of different hormonal therapies or chemotherapy plus hormones is not used in the setting of metastatic breast cancer because of lack of increased efficacy and evidence of increased toxicity. Women with HR-negative tumors, with rapidly progressive or symptomatic lung, liver, or bone marrow involvement, and those with progressive disease while on initial endocrine therapy are usually treated initially with cytotoxic chemotherapy. Patients with tumors that have *HER2* protein overexpression or gene amplification should be considered for treatment with trastuzumab alone or with chemotherapy.

Endocrine Therapy

❻ The pharmacologic goal of endocrine therapy for breast cancer is to either decrease circulating levels of estrogen or prevent the effects of estrogen at the breast cancer cell (targeted therapy) by blocking the hormone receptors or downregulating the presence of those receptors. Achievement of the first goal depends on the menopausal status of the patient, but achievement of the second goal is independent of menopausal status. Many endocrine therapies are available to target either goal of therapy, and combinations of drugs with different mechanisms of action can also be given. Unfortunately, combinations have not demonstrated any efficacy benefits over single-agent hormone therapy, but have increased toxicity. Therefore combinations of endocrine agents for breast cancer are not recommended outside the context of a clinical trial. Sequential use of these agents is now becoming popular in the adjuvant setting and may play a role in the metastatic setting when a patient is progressing on one agent after an initial response. These patients are often treated with a series of endocrine agents, usually over several years, before chemotherapy is considered.

Until recently, there was little evidence that the response or survival benefit from one endocrine therapy was clearly superior to that achieved with other therapies. Randomized controlled trials showed that antiestrogens, progestins, aminoglutethimide, estrogens, and androgens; and surgical procedures including oophorectomy, adrenalectomy, and hypophysectomy were equivalent in patients with metastatic breast cancer. Consequently, the choice of a particular endocrine therapy was based primarily on toxicity and patient preference (Table 131–13). Based on these criteria, tamoxifen is the preferred initial agent when metastases are present, except when the patient is receiving adjuvant tamoxifen at the same time or within 1 year of occurrence of metastatic disease. In these cases, other agents are generally employed.

Over the past decade, results of clinical trials of third-generation aromatase inhibitors have changed the treatment of metastatic breast cancer, as well as of early-stage breast cancer (as was noted previously). In postmenopausal and castrated women, the main source of estrogen is derived from the peripheral conversion of androstenedione, produced by the adrenal gland, into estrone and estradiol. This conversion requires the enzyme aromatase. Aromatase also catalyzes the conversion of androgens to estrogens in the ovary in premenopausal women and in extraglandular tissue, including the breast and breast cancer cells, in postmenopausal women. Therefore aromatase inhibitors effectively reduce the levels of circulating estrogens and estrogens in the target organ. Aminoglutethimide was the prototype aromatase inhibitor, but was a nonspecific, weak enzyme inhibitor associated with many toxicities. Several analogs and derivatives of aminoglutethimide, as well as novel compounds, have been tested over the years to try and improve on the therapeutic ratio of this agent. Third-generation aromatase inhibitors now available include anastrozole, letrozole, and exemestane. These agents have far greater

TABLE 131-13 Endocrine Therapies Used for Metastatic Breast Cancer

Class	Drug	Dose	Side Effects
Aromatase inhibitors			
Nonsteroidal	Anastrozole	1 mg orally daily	Hot flashes, arthralgias, myalgias, headaches, diarrhea, mild nausea
	Letrozole	2.5 mg orally daily	
Steroidal	Exemestane	25 mg orally daily	
Antiestrogens			
SERMs	Tamoxifen	20 mg orally daily	Hot flashes, vaginal discharge, mild nausea, thromboembolism, endometrial cancer
	Toremifene	60 mg orally daily	
SERDs	Fulvestrant	250 mg IM every 28 days	Hot flashes, injection site reactions, possibly thromboembolism.
LHRH analogs	Goserelin	3.6 mg SC every 28 days	Hot flashes, amenorrhea, menopausal symptoms, injection site reactions (extended formulations are not recommended for the treatment of breast cancer)
	Leuprolide	3.75 mg IM every 28 days	
	Triptorelin	3.75 mg IM every 28 days	
Progestins	Megestrol acetate	40 mg orally four times a day	Weight gain, hot flashes, vaginal bleeding, edema, thromboembolism
	Medroxyprogesterone	400–1000 mg IM every week	
Androgens	Fluoxymesterone	10 mg orally twice a day	Deepening voice, alopecia, hirsutism, facial/truncal acne, fluid retention, menstrual irregularities, cholestatic jaundice
Estrogens	Diethylstilbestrol	5 mg orally three times a day	Nausea/vomiting, fluid retention, anorexia, thromboembolism, hepatic dysfunction
	Ethinyl estradiol	1 mg orally three times a day	
	Conjugated estrogens	2.5 mg orally three times a day	

LHRH, luteinizing hormone-releasing hormone; SC, subcutaneous; SERD, selective estrogen receptor downregulator SERM, selective estrogen receptor modulator.

selectivity and higher potency for the aromatase enzyme than aminoglutethimide. A major advantage of these newer compounds is their reduced toxicity profile, which consists mainly of mild nausea, hot flashes, arthralgias/myalgias, and mild fatigue. Anastrozole and letrozole are nonsteroidal compounds that exhibit reversible, competitive inhibition of aromatase. These are triazole compounds and have no intrinsic hormonal activity. Exemestane is a steroidal compound which binds irreversibly to aromatase, forming a covalent bond. While this mechanism may have theoretical advantages to the reversible binding seen with the nonsteroidal agents, there is no clinical evidence that this drug is superior to other agents in this class. Exemestane does possess some androgenic properties at doses that are much higher than those used clinically.

These third-generation aromatase inhibitors have been compared with megestrol acetate as second-line therapy in postmenopausal women with positive or unknown HR status who have progressed while on tamoxifen therapy. Although response rates with these agents have not been significantly better, time to progression and OS are significantly better with at least two of the three aromatase inhibitors (anastrozole and exemestane).[122] Rates of clinical benefit (objective response + stabilization of disease for 24 weeks) are also improved with the aromatase inhibitors. Clinical benefit, a category of response used in metastatic breast cancer clinical trials, is another clinically relevant end point because it is associated with similar OS compared with patients who have objective responses.[123] Tolerability is also improved with the aromatase inhibitors compared with megestrol acetate. Toxicity patterns showed more nausea, vomiting, and hot flashes with the aromatase inhibitor and more weight gain, fluid retention, and thromboembolism with megestrol acetate. All three agents are approved for second-line therapy of advanced breast cancer in postmenopausal women, and have largely replaced megestrol acetate for second-line therapy.

Both anastrozole and letrozole are also approved for first-line therapy of advanced breast cancer in postmenopausal women. Large randomized trials have compared these agents to tamoxifen and found similar response rates and a longer median time to progression for patients receiving the selective aromatase inhibitor.[122] A consistent finding in these trials was a lower incidence of thromboembolic events and vaginal bleeding in patients who received selective aromatase inhibitors. Based on these results, many experts have concluded that the new aromatase inhibitors are superior to tamoxifen as first-line therapy for advanced breast cancer in postmenopausal women. Although not FDA-approved for this indication, exemestane has been compared with tamoxifen as front-line therapy for hormone-sensitive metastatic breast cancer. In that small randomized phase II trial, exemestane demonstrated an advantage over tamoxifen in terms of response rates and time to progression.[122] Use of a steroidal aromatase inhibitor (exemestane) after a patient progresses on a nonsteroidal inhibitor (anastrozole or letrozole) may provide some benefit and is a common practice based on limited data. The opposite sequence also has shown some benefit; thus patients may receive two aromatase inhibitors (first-line and second-line, sequentially), especially those patients who progress while on adjuvant tamoxifen therapy.

The aromatase inhibitors should only be used in postmenopausal women. Pre- or perimenopausal women, whose ovaries are functioning, are inappropriate candidates for these therapies, at least based on the available evidence. Use of the aromatase inhibitors in addition to ovarian ablation (e.g., oophorectomy or LHRH agonists) is under investigation. Interestingly, the use of aromatase inhibitors in men with advanced breast cancer should be avoided because these agents increase circulating levels of testosterone, which may negate the therapeutic effects of the drug.[124] The use of an aromatase inhibitor combined with an LHRH agonist (which will decrease testosterone production) has been suggested, but until further clinical trials are completed the efficacy and safety of this treatment approach is unknown.

Antiestrogens bind to estrogen receptors, which inhibit receptor-mediated gene transcription and therefore block the effect of estrogen on the end target. This class of agents is now subdivided into two pharmacologic categories, SERMs and pure antiestrogens. SERMs include tamoxifen and toremifene and demonstrate tissue-specific activity, both estrogenic and antiestrogenic, as described previously. The agonistic activity is thought to be responsible for many of the adverse reactions seen with these agents, including the increased risk of endometrial cancer, and has led to the development of pure estrogen receptor antagonists that lack estrogen agonist activity. Pure antiestrogens are a new class of agents and are also referred to as selective estrogen receptor downregulators (SERDs). These molecules bind to the ER, inhibit estrogen binding, and degrade the drug-ER complex, thus decreasing the amount of ER on the tumor cell surface. Fulvestrant is currently the only pure antiestrogen commercially available in the United States.

Tamoxifen is generally considered to be the antiestrogen of choice in premenopausal women with metastatic breast cancer who have HR-positive tumors. Tamoxifen is usually administered in 20-mg once-daily doses. A tamoxifen dose of 20 mg/day reaches a steady-state concentration after about 4 months of therapy. The half-life of tamoxifen during chronic dosing is 7 days. Serum tamoxifen concentrations can be detected 6 weeks after discontinuation of therapy. Thus the maximum beneficial effects of tamoxifen are not observed for at least 2 months following initiation of therapy, and it is unlikely that symptoms of metastatic disease will return, even if patients miss several doses. The toxicities of tamoxifen are described in the Adjuvant Endocrine Therapy section above. The only additional toxicity that may be observed in the setting of metastatic breast cancer (specifically bone metastases) is a tumor flare and/or hypercalcemia, which occurs in approximately 5% of patients following the initiation of any SERM therapy and is not an indication to discontinue SERM therapy. It is generally accepted that this reaction is associated with response to endocrine therapy, but patients who do not experience such a reaction may still respond. This reaction is seen less frequently with the concurrent use of bisphosphonates as a result of their inhibition of osteoclasts, subsequently preventing the release of calcium from the bone.

Toremifene is another commercially available SERM for the treatment of breast cancer. It exhibits similar efficacy and tolerability compared with tamoxifen in the metastatic setting and is given at a dose of 60 mg daily. The same issues apply to toremifene as were discussed with tamoxifen. Cross-resistance to toremifene has been demonstrated in patients with tamoxifen-refractory disease.[125] Thus at the current time, toremifene appears to be an alternative to tamoxifen in postmenopausal patients with positive or unknown HR status with metastatic breast cancer. Raloxifene, another SERM, received approval in December 1997 for prevention of osteoporosis in postmenopausal women. Available data with raloxifene as a treatment for breast cancer show very low response rates and no clinical benefit. Consequently, use of this agent for breast cancer treatment should be discouraged. Investigation into the use of raloxifene for prevention of breast cancer in high-risk women has recently been reported (see Prevention and Early Detection).

Fulvestrant is approved for the second-line therapy of postmenopausal metastatic breast cancer patients with HR-positive tumors. It is given as an intramuscular injection every 28 days and is marketed as a single injection of 5 mL or two injections of 2.5 mL each. Studies have compared this agent to anastrozole in the treatment of postmenopausal women with metastatic breast cancer. Biologically, fulvestrant should produce similar outcomes in premenopausal women, but no data exist to confirm the safety or efficacy in premenopausal women. In the comparative trials with fulvestrant and anastrozole, similar efficacy and safety were demonstrated with both agents when given after patients progressed on tamoxifen therapy.[126] When compared directly with tamoxifen, time-to-progression was slightly shorter in the fulvestrant arm but the difference did not reach statistical significance.[126] That trial failed to confirm statistical noninferiority, which indicates that the trial could not show that fulvestrant was equivalent to tamoxifen. Adverse events related to fulvestrant include injection-site reactions, hot flashes, asthenia, and headaches. The dose of fulvestrant is 250 mg given intramuscularly every 28 days. This agent is covered by Medicare and is a good option for patients who are unable to take an oral medication. Ongoing clinical trials addressing comparative efficacy with exemestane and other dosing strategies will hopefully further define the role of this agent.

Another goal of hormonal therapy in premenopausal women is to reduce estrogen production with surgery, irradiation, or medication. No difference in the overall response rate has been found in two randomized trials of tamoxifen and oophorectomy in premenopausal women. However, the secondary response rate to oophorectomy after tamoxifen treatment was somewhat higher than the response to tamoxifen after primary oophorectomy (33% vs. 11%).[127] Based on this finding, some experts suggest that tamoxifen does not completely antagonize available estrogen, particularly in premenopausal women. Ovarian ablation (surgically or chemically) is still commonly used in some parts of the United States and is considered by many specialists to be the endocrine therapy of choice in premenopausal women. The mortality rate with surgical oophorectomy is low, usually less than 3% in appropriately selected patients. Irradiation of the ovaries was a means of castration many years ago, but was associated with multiple complications and is no longer performed for these purposes. Chemical castration with LHRH analogs is increasingly used instead of oophorectomy in premenopausal women.

Medical castration with LHRH analogs is used in premenopausal metastatic breast cancer patients and induces remission in about one-third of unselected cases. The mechanism of action of LHRH analogs in breast cancer is downregulation of LHRH receptors in the pituitary. Decreased levels of luteinizing hormone subsequently lead to a decrease in estrogen to castrated levels. Thus the effect of LHRH analogs on circulating estrogen levels in premenopausal breast cancer simulates oophorectomy. The three agents available in the United States are leuprolide, goserelin, and triptorelin, but only goserelin is approved for the treatment of metastatic breast cancer. These agents are administered as an injection every 4 weeks (all products have extended formulations, lasting 3 months to 1 year, but they are not recommended for the treatment of breast cancer) and are associated with minimal side effects including amenorrhea, hot flashes, and occasional nausea (see Table 131–13). LHRH agonists may also produce a flare response because of an initial surge in leuteinizing hormone and estrogen production for the first 2 to 4 weeks. This flare response is similar to that seen with tamoxifen and patients should be monitored for increasing pain and/or hypercalcemia during the initiation period. A meta-analysis was conducted of several trials that combined tamoxifen and LHRH agonists versus LHRH agonists alone in premenopausal patients with metastatic breast cancer.[128] With a median followup of 6.8 years, there was a significant survival benefit and progression-free survival benefit in favor of the combined treatment. The overall response rate was significantly higher with combined endocrine treatment. However, this analysis did not compare tamoxifen alone to the combination of an LHRH agonist with tamoxifen. Therefore if an LHRH agonist is used as first-line therapy for metastatic breast cancer, it should be used in combination with tamoxifen. But if tamoxifen is used as first-line therapy for metastatic breast cancer, the addition of a LHRH agonist is controversial because of the lack of clinical data to support it.

Progestins such as megestrol acetate and medroxyprogesterone acetate have been compared with tamoxifen in randomized trials and have been found to yield equal response rates. Medroxyprogesterone acetate is more frequently used in Europe, while megestrol acetate is more frequently used in the United States. Based on efficacy and tolerability, these agents are generally reserved as third-line therapy after patients have failed an aromatase inhibitor and an antiestrogen (tamoxifen, toremifene, or fulvestrant). The most common dose used for megestrol acetate is 160 mg/day. The most common side effect is weight gain, occurring in 20% to 50% of patients. Patients experiencing weight gain may also have fluid retention, but fluid retention is not totally responsible for the weight gain. In cachectic cancer patients, the weight gain may be desirable, but this is not uniformly true of all patients with metastatic breast cancer. Other side effects associated with progestins include vaginal bleeding in 5% to 10% of patients either while taking the progestational agent or when it is discontinued, and less than a 10% incidence of hot flashes. Thromboembolic complications are also associated with these agents.

High-dose estrogens and androgens are rarely used today because of their side effect profile and the availability of better tolerated alternatives (e.g., aromatase inhibitors). About one-third of patients placed on high-dose estrogens will discontinue them because of side effects, the most important of which are thromboembolic events, vomiting, and fluid retention. Less-common side effects include areolar hyperpigmentation, breast tenderness and engorgement, vaginal discharge, incontinence, hot flashes, and phlebitis. All the effective androgens cause masculinizing effects, including hirsutism and acne, in more than 50% of patients. The mechanism by which these agents exert a therapeutic effect in breast cancer is unknown. Approximately 20% response rates were reported in clinical trials conducted in the 1960s and 1970s in unselected groups of breast cancer patients.

Cytotoxic Therapy

❽ Cytotoxic chemotherapy is eventually required in most patients with metastatic breast cancer. Patients with HR-negative tumors require chemotherapy as initial therapy of metastases. Patients with hormone-sensitive tumors who initially respond to hormonal manipulations eventually cease to respond and go on to require chemotherapy. Combination chemotherapy results in an objective response in approximately 60% of patients previously unexposed to chemotherapy. Most patients have partial responses, and complete disappearance of disease occurs in fewer than 10% of patients treated. The median duration of response is 5 to 12 months, but some patients will have an excellent response to an initial course of chemotherapy and may live 5 to 10 years or longer without evidence of disease. Median survival of patients after treatment with commonly used drug combinations for metastatic breast cancer ranges between 14 and 33 months. The median time to response ranges from 2 to 3 months in most studies, but this period depends on the site of measurable disease and can range from 3 weeks (skin and lymph node metastases) to 18 weeks (bone metastases). Once a chemotherapy regimen has been initiated, it is usually continued until there is unequivocal evidence of progressive disease.

Factors associated with an increased likelihood of response include a good performance status, a limited number (one to two) of disease sites (or involved organ systems), and a prolonged previous response to chemotherapy or hormonal therapy (i.e., long disease-free interval). Patients who have progressive disease during chemotherapy have a lower likelihood of response to a different type of chemotherapy. However, this is not necessarily true for patients who are given chemotherapy after some interval during which they have received no chemotherapy. Patients may actually be retreated with a regimen they received earlier if some time has passed since receiving the similar drugs (e.g., several years), but this is rarely done because of large number of agents now available to treat breast cancer. Patients who do not respond to endocrine therapy are as likely to respond to chemotherapy as patients who are treated with chemotherapy as their initial treatment modality. Age, menopausal status, and receptor status do not appear to be associated with response to chemotherapy.

A number of chemotherapeutic agents have demonstrated activity in the treatment of breast cancer, including doxorubicin, epirubicin, paclitaxel (conventional and protein-bound), docetaxel, capecitabine, fluorouracil, cyclophosphamide, methotrexate, vinblastine, vinorelbine, gemcitabine, mitoxantrone, mitomycin-C, thiotepa, and melphalan. The most active classes of chemotherapy in metastatic breast cancer are the anthracyclines and the taxanes, producing response rates as high as 50% to 60% in patients who have not received prior chemotherapy for metastatic disease.[129] Paclitaxel was FDA-approved in 1994 for single-agent treatment of metastatic breast cancer for patients who had relapsed following therapy with a doxorubicin-containing regimen. Weekly administration of paclitaxel results in higher response rates and less toxicity as compared with every-3-week administration.[84] The most useful weekly dose in the metastatic setting appears to be 80 mg/m^2 per week with no breaks in therapy. With this approach, the toxicity profile of paclitaxel changes with less myelosuppression and delayed onset of peripheral neuropathy, but slightly more fluid retention and skin and nail changes. Although the incidence of hypersensitivity reactions is also slightly less at these lower doses, requiring fewer premedications, it remains at approximately 3%, even with all available preventive measures.

Docetaxel has also demonstrated high single-agent activity against metastatic breast cancer. It received FDA-approval in 1995 for treatment of metastatic breast cancer for patients with relapse following therapy with doxorubicin-containing regimens. Impressive overall response rates of 54% to 68% were reported in four studies of docetaxel 100 mg/m^2 as first-line chemotherapy. As compared with paclitaxel (175 mg/m^2 over 3 hours every 3 weeks), docetaxel (100 mg/m^2 every 3 weeks) was associated with longer time-to-progression (hazard ratio 1.64; p <0.0001) and OS (hazard ratio 1.41, p = 0.03).[130] Myelosuppression is the major dose-limiting toxicity of docetaxel. Nonhematologic toxicities include fatigue, mucosal toxicity, mild-to-moderate nausea and vomiting, diarrhea, and neurosensory complaints. Results from the comparative randomized trial mentioned above show that although docetaxel is associated with less neuropathy, myalgia, and hypersensitivity than paclitaxel given every 3 weeks, febrile neutropenia, fluid retention, and skin reactions appear to occur more frequently with docetaxel.[130]

A new formulation of paclitaxel has now been approved by the FDA. This protein-bound paclitaxel (Abraxane) is covalently bound to albumin, then microemulsified into nanoparticles to improve solubility of the chemotherapeutic agent. In a randomized trial of protein-bound paclitaxel versus conventional paclitaxel (each given every 3 weeks), the protein-bound paclitaxel was associated with improved response rates and time-to-progression in patients with taxane-naive metastatic breast cancer.[131] Myelosuppression was more pronounced in the conventional paclitaxel arm, whereas peripheral neuropathy was more frequently observed in the protein-bound paclitaxel arm. Weekly administration of the protein-bound paclitaxel also has been reported to be efficacious and safe. Final results from comparative studies with docetaxel or weekly conventional paclitaxel have yet to be reported. Many ongoing clinical trials will help to further elucidate the role of protein-bound paclitaxel in the clinical management of both metastatic and early breast cancer.

After patients have been treated with an anthracycline and a taxane, single-agent capecitabine, vinorelbine or gemcitabine have resulted in response rates of 20% to 25%.[132] Decisions regarding which agent to choose are based on patient characteristics, expected toxicities and previous exposure to chemotherapy. An increasing number of patients diagnosed with metastatic breast cancer have been exposed to adjuvant chemotherapy consisting of an anthracycline and a taxane. If metastases are found within 6 to 12 months of completing treatment with these agents, many clinicians will choose treatment from a different chemotherapy class. If it has been longer since their adjuvant therapy, then retreating with the same agents may be considered. However, given the cardiotoxicity associated with the anthracyclines, the use of these agents in the metastatic setting has been generally avoided until the availability of the liposomal anthracyclines. Pegylated liposomal doxorubicin is associated with less cardiotoxicity and similar efficacy compared to conventional doxorubicin and is a viable option for women who recur more than 1 year after their adjuvant anthracycline regimen.[133]

Since the anthracyclines, taxanes and capecitabine are all approved for metastatic breast cancer and have very specific indications for their use. Patients who initially respond to these classic agents progress later, are usually in fairly good health and have few effective options at this juncture in the course of their disease. One class of drugs that show promise in this resistant population is the epothilones. Epothilones are natural compounds first identified from soil-derived *Sorangium cellulosum* myxobacterium. They are classified as microtubule stabilizing agents (MSAs). The mechanism of action of the epothilones is similar to but distinct from the taxanes, binding to beta-microtubulin in a unique manner but ultimately leading to microtubule stabilization and cell death in similar manner compared to the taxanes. These natural compounds are very lipophilic and unstable in solution, leading to development of semisynthetic analogues. One of these analogues, BMS 247550 or ixabepilone, has shown significant activity in metastatic breast cancer patients who have received a taxane, anthracycline and capecitabine and was recently approved by the FDA. Single agent datra with ixabepilone demonstrated a 22% to 57% objective response rate in patients who were heavily to minimally pretreated, respectively.[134] In combination with capecitabine, ixabepilone was found to increase response rates (35% vs 14%, p <0.0001) and time-to-progression (5.8 months vs 4.2 months, p = 0.0003) compared to capecitabine alone in metastatic breast cancer patients who had received a prior taxane and ananthracycline.[134] Adverse effects associated with ixabepilone include myelosuppression, peripheral neuropathy, myalgias/arthralgias, alopecia, mild nausea and skin/nail changes.[134] Other epothilones are currently in clinical trials and could lead to significant advances on many other cancers as well.

Combination chemotherapy regimens are associated with higher response rates than are single-agent therapies in the treatment of metastatic breast cancer, but the higher response rates have not usually translated into significant differences in time-to-progression and OS. The use of sequential single-agent chemotherapies versus the combination regimens is widely debated for metastatic breast cancer.

CLINICAL CONTROVERSY

The benefits of combination chemotherapy regimens for metastatic breast cancer over sequential single agents have not been clearly defined. A few trials have compared combination regimens to single-agent chemotherapy, with higher response rates seen with the combination. However, these trials failed to include an arm with the same agents given sequentially. Thus it is not clear whether sequential single agents or combination regimens are optimal in this setting.

One trial investigating the combination of doxorubicin with paclitaxel versus each single agent with crossover to the other agent upon progression set out to help answer the question of which approach is more effective.[135] While response rates were higher with the combination regimen, time-to-progression and OS were similar between all arms of the study. This was probably because most patients who progressed on their first single agent went on to receive the second-line single agent, thereby negating any potential survival benefits seen with improved response rates. In another study comparing single-agent docetaxel to the combination of docetaxel with capecitabine, the combination arm produced higher response rates, time to progression, and OS than did the single agent.[136] However, because only 15% of patients in the docetaxel-alone arm received capecitabine after progression, this study does not answer the question of whether combination therapy is better than sequential single-agent therapy. Other studies also have demonstrated similar results, but none of them adequately answer the question of whether sequential administration of single-agent chemotherapy or concurrent combination chemotherapy is optimal.

Combination regimens are associated with greater toxicity. In the palliative metastatic setting, the least toxic approach is preferred when efficacy is considered equal. In clinical practice, patients who require a rapid response to chemotherapy (e.g., those with symptomatic bulky metastases) often receive combination therapy despite the added toxicity. This decision is complex and should be made on an individual patient basis.

Biologic or Targeted Therapy

Therapies that focus on molecular targets through novel mechanisms are often referred to as biologic therapy. These agents, while using the biologic knowledge gained from decades of research, are designed to specifically target cancer cells while generally sparing normal tissues. For breast cancer, several agents that focus on a myriad of targets that are differentially expressed in breast cancer cells and play a critical role in their proliferation and survival are available in this class.

The first agent to show promise with this approach to therapy was trastuzumab (Herceptin). Trastuzumab is a humanized monoclonal antibody that binds with a specific epitope of the *HER2* protein. Mechanisms of action of trastuzumab include disruption of HER receptor dimerization, disruption of downstream signaling pathways (e.g., PI3K/Akt), G_1 arrest and reduced proliferation, induction of apoptosis, suppression of angiogenesis, induction of immune-mediated responses (e.g., antibody-dependent cellular cytotoxicity), inhibition of *HER2* extracellular domain proteolysis and inhibition of DNA repair. These biologic effects lead to inhibition of cellular growth, decreased malignant potential, and possibly reversal of resistance to certain chemotherapies and endocrine therapy. Single-agent treatment with trastuzumab has a response rate of 15% to 20% and a clinical benefit rate of nearly 40% of patients with *HER2*-overexpressing cancers.[137] Moreover, the results of a large randomized trial demonstrated that trastuzumab has at least additive, and perhaps synergistic, activity with other chemotherapeutic agents.[138] In this pivotal trial comparing chemotherapy in combination with trastuzumab versus chemotherapy alone, the addition of trastuzumab increased response rates, time-to-progression, and OS when compared to chemotherapy alone. Patients who were anthracycline naive were treated with an anthracycline (mostly doxorubicin, some epirubicin) plus cyclophosphamide, and patients who had received an adjuvant anthracycline regimen were treated with paclitaxel. During this trial, patients who received the anthracycline-trastuzumab combination had a very high incidence of cardiotoxicity (27%), leading to discontinuation of this arm of the study and a black box warning regarding this contraindication in the product information for trastuzumab. Many investigators are attempting to circumvent this toxicity while giving these two classes of agents together (e.g., liposomal doxorubicin, continuous-infusion doxorubicin, lower-dose epirubicin). However, until further information regarding the safety of these approaches becomes available, this combination should not be given outside the context of a clinical trial.

Many other chemotherapy agents have successfully been administered with trastuzumab. Only one other phase III trial has been published comparing chemotherapy alone versus chemotherapy plus trastuzumab. Marty et al. compared docetaxel alone versus docetaxel with trastuzumab in patients with previously untreated *HER2*-positive metastatic breast cancer.[139] That trial demonstrated significant advantages to the combination over chemotherapy alone in terms of response rates, time-to-progression, and OS.

Other chemotherapy agents that have been evaluated in several phase II trials in combination with trastuzumab include vinorelbine, gemcitabine, capecitabine, and the platinum agents (cisplatin and carboplatin). In phase II trials, vinorelbine in combination with trastuzumab has shown very high response rates, even in heavily pretreated patients.[140] In a postmarketing surveillance study presented at the San Antonio (TX) Breast Cancer Symposium in December 2006, cohorts treated with taxane-trastuzumab and vinorelbine-trastuzumab combinations had similar progression-free survival.[141] The two combinations are being compared in a head-to-head phase III clinical trial to determine which regimen is superior as front-line therapy for metastatic breast cancer. In another phase III trial, the triplet combination of paclitaxel, carboplatin, and trastuzumab was compared with paclitaxel and trastuzumab as dual therapy.[142] This study demonstrated superior response rates and time-to-progression with the triplet regimen versus the doublet regimen. A similar trial designed to confirm this data using docetaxel instead of paclitaxel failed to demonstrate any advantage with the addition of carboplatin to a taxane-trastuzumab regimen.[143] These conflicting results indicate that the benefit of adding a platinum compound to these regimens remains questionable. Toxicities with the addition of carboplatin are significantly greater in terms of myelosuppression and nausea, which should be considered when making treatment decisions in the setting of metastatic breast cancer where quality-of-life is paramount.

Trastuzumab is generally well tolerated. The most common adverse effects are infusion-related, primarily fever and chills, and occur in approximately 40% of patients during the initial infusion. Other infusion-related reactions include nausea, vomiting, pain at tumor sites, rigors, headaches, dizziness, dyspnea, hypotension, rash, and asthenia, which are much less common.[101] These reactions are generally mild-to-moderate and last about 1 to 2 hours after the infusion is started and usually do not recur with subsequent infusions. Acetaminophen and diphenhydramine may be given and/or the infusion rate reduced to help alleviate the symptoms related to these reactions. If infusion-related symptoms occur, subsequent doses should be infused over 90 minutes. Infusion over 30 minutes is appropriate if symptoms subside. A rare, but more severe reaction consisting of severe hypersensitivity and/or pulmonary reactions has been reported. It is important to educate patients regarding the pulmonary reactions, as these may occur up to 24 hours after the infusion and can be fatal if not promptly treated. Trastuzumab may increase the incidence of infection, diarrhea, and/or other adverse events when given with chemotherapy, but most of these increases are not clinically significant for the individual patient.

The most serious adverse effect of trastuzumab is cardiotoxicity. As mentioned earlier, the incidence of heart failure is approximately 5% with single-agent trastuzumab and the risk is unacceptably high when trastuzumab is given with an anthracycline. Fortunately, the heart failure seen with trastuzumab is somewhat reversible with pharmacologic management and some patients have continued therapy with trastuzumab after their left ventricular ejection fraction has returned to normal. Although there are no guidelines for cardiac monitoring with this agent, close monitoring for clinical signs and symptoms of heart failure is recommended in order to intervene with appropriate cardiac treatments.

Trastuzumab is administered as an initial loading dose of 4 mg/kg, followed by a 2-mg/kg dose administered weekly. A phase II study has demonstrated successful administration of trastuzumab on a 3-week schedule with a 8-mg/kg loading dose followed 3 weeks later with a 6-mg/kg maintenance dose given every 3 weeks.[144] Every-3-weeks administration is more convenient than weekly administration, but comparative data with this dose and schedule versus the standard dose and schedule are not available at this time. When patients progress on therapy with trastuzumab, many clinicians will continue the trastuzumab and change the chemotherapy regimen despite the lack of evidence to support this practice. Attempts to answer this question in a clinical trial have failed because of poor patient accrual and patients' unwillingness to be randomized to stop trastuzumab therapy. This practce is changing with the availability of lapatinib, which is effective in trastuzumab-resistant disease (see below).

It should be noted that only 20% to 30% of patients with metastatic breast cancer overexpress *HER2,* and commercially available IHC tests that are reported as 2+ for *HER2* are often negative by the more sensitive and specific FISH technique. To date, there is no benefit associated with the administration of trastuzumab to patients with *HER2*-negative tumors (IHC score of 0 to 1+, or FISH-negative), and a very questionable benefit associated with administration of trastuzumab to women with tumors that are 2+ for *HER2* by IHC staining alone. The patients who benefit most from trastuzumab therapy include those whose tumors express *HER2* protein at the 3+ level or who clearly demonstrate gene amplification by FISH testing. Further analyses investigating what other predictive markers for response to trastuzumab may be clinically useful are currently ongoing.

Lapatinib is a tyrosine kinase inhibitor that dually targets *HER2* and the epidermal growth factor receptor (*EGFR* or *HER1*). This small molecule works intracellularly to actively shut down the signaling pathway from these two receptors and thus inhibit cell growth and division. Lapatinib is an oral agent with modest activity against breast cancer as a single agent. However, in combination with capecitabine in women with *HER2*-positive metastatic breast cancer who were previously treated with an anthracycline, a taxane, and trastuzumab, it improves response rates (22% vs. 14%; $p = 0.09$) and time to progression (8.4 vs. 4.4 months; hazard ratio 0.49; 95% CI 0.34 to 0.71, $p < 0.001$) as compared to capecitabine alone.[145] Based on this evidence, the FDA recently approved lapatinib in this setting. Adverse events associated with the addition of lapatinib are primarily rash and diarrhea. Because of concerns regarding the role of HER2 in normal cardiac functioning, lapatinib may also increase the risk for cardiac dysfunction. However, in a review of more than 2,800 patients who received lapatinib in phase I to III trials, cardiotoxicity occurred in only 1.3% of patients.[146] Although these data are reassuring, it does not rule out the possibility of expanded toxicity when this agent is used in patients not included in the clinical trials such as those with underlying cardiac risks. Lapatinib is currently being investigated in numerous clinical trials, the results of these trials will further elucidate the role of this agent in the management of both early and late stages of the disease.

Targeting tumor blood vessels is another strategy to fight breast cancer. One of the most important growth factors that regulate the development of new blood vessels (angiogenesis) is vascular endothelial growth factor. Bevacizumab is a monoclonal antibody targeted against vascular endothelial growth factor and is FDA-approved for use with irinotecan-containing chemotherapy regimens for the management of metastatic colorectal cancer. Bevacizumab has also been tested in clinical trials with capecitabine and paclitaxel in metastatic breast cancer patients. In the first clinical trial reported in breast cancer patients, bevacizumab was given every 3 weeks in combination with capecitabine in women who had failed both anthracycline- and taxane-containing regimens.[147] While response rates were significantly higher in the bevacizumab arm of this trial, time-to-progression and OS remained the same as with capecitabine alone. In a subsequent trial, newly diagnosed metastatic breast cancer patients were randomized to receive weekly paclitaxel with or without bevacizumab (given every other week).[148] That trial demonstrated significantly better response rates and time to progression with the addition of bevacizumab. These two trials differed in their patient populations, choice of chemotherapy and bevacizumab dose and schedule. Based on these conflicting results, the role of bevacizumab is not clearly defined for the management of metastatic breast cancer. Nonetheless, the NCCN has incorporated the bevacizumab/paclitaxel regimen into their guidelines as one option for the management of metastatic breast cancer.[45]

Many other biologic or targeted agents are being investigated and may end up changing the overall management of breast cancer for both early and metastatic disease.

Radiation Therapy

Radiation is an important modality in the treatment of symptomatic metastatic disease. The most common indication for treatment with radiation therapy is painful bone metastases or other localized sites of disease refractory to systemic therapy. Radiation therapy provides significant pain relief to approximately 90% of patients who are treated for painful bone metastases. Radiation is also an important modality in the palliative treatment of metastatic brain lesions and spinal cord lesions, which respond poorly to systemic therapy, as well as eye or orbit lesions and other sites where significant accumulation of tumor cells occurs. Skin and/or lymph node metastases confined to the chest wall area may also be treated with radiation therapy for palliation (e.g., open wounds or painful lesions).

PREVENTION AND EARLY DETECTION

Current efforts at breast cancer prevention are directed toward the identification and removal of risk factors. Unfortunately, a number of risk factors associated with development of breast cancer, such as family history of breast cancer or personal history of breast or other gynecologic malignancies, cannot be modified. Isolation and cloning of breast cancer susceptibility genes now allows screening of women with histories suggestive of "breast cancer families" and identification of appropriate candidates for prophylactic bilateral mastectomy. This surgery is considered for women who are at very high risk for the development of breast cancer, particularly if the women's breasts are difficult to evaluate by both physical examination and mammography and if they have persistent disabling fears that they will be diagnosed with the disease.

In the past 10 years, there has been increasing interest in chemoprevention of breast cancer. Two important classes of agents being studied for breast cancer chemoprevention are the retinoids and SERMs. Retinoids (all vitamin A and its isomer derivatives and synthetic analogs) are biologic regulators of orderly epithelial cell development, and are therefore potentially ideal agents for controlling abnormal epithelial proliferation that occurs in carcinogenesis. Because only preclinical data are available to suggest a benefit with these types of therapies, clinical trials are needed to further investigate the role of the retinoids in prevention of breast cancer.

The drugs currently receiving the most attention as chemopreventive agents for breast cancer are the SERMs, tamoxifen and raloxifene. As previously described, tamoxifen is useful as an adjunct after treatment of primary breast cancer. In randomized trials of tamoxifen as an adjuvant treatment for breast cancer, women who received tamoxifen were also found to have a reduced incidence of contralateral primary breast carcinomas.[5] In a large, randomized, placebo-controlled study, the NSABP demonstrated significant reductions in risk of invasive and noninvasive breast cancers with 5 years of tamoxifen therapy (20 mg/day) in women at high risk for developing the disease.[49] Although this study is controversial, other studies from around the world also have been reported that investigated the role of tamoxifen in chemoprevention. A meta-analysis of these trials indicates a consistent benefit with tamoxifen in reducing the incidence of ER-positive breast cancers (48% reduction; 95% CI 36% to 58%; p <0.0001).[149] Tamoxifen has been repeatedly shown to be a relatively safe drug with an acceptable toxicity profile when used to treat patients with breast cancer. However, its estrogenic effects on the uterus and the coagulation system increase the risk of serious adverse effects that may be critical for patients taking this agent in the chemoprevention setting. Toxicities associated with tamoxifen were previously described in the Adjuvant Endocrine Therapy section above. Any decision to use tamoxifen for chemoprevention should be made after a thorough discussion of the woman's risk of breast cancer, the potential benefits of tamoxifen, and the potential serious adverse events associated with tamoxifen.

A similar trial now has been reported that compared tamoxifen to raloxifene in a similar population of high-risk women. The Study of Tamoxifen and Raloxifene (STAR or P2) was published in 2006 and demonstrated a similar rate of invasive breast cancers with the two drugs.[150] However, the rates of noninvasive breast cancer were numerically higher in the raloxifene arm of the trial, although this difference did not reach statistical significance. It is not clear what long-term outcome will be related to this difference, but further followup will be required to draw any sound conclusions. Rates of endometrial cancer and deep venous thromboses were more frequent in the tamoxifen arm, but overall quality of life was similar between the two agents.[150] Based on these results, the FDA approved raloxifene for breast cancer risk reduction in women at high risk of the disease. A similar reduction in the incidence of contralateral primary breast cancers was demonstrated with anastrozole in the adjuvant ATAC study (discussed previously), leading to the premise that aromatase inhibitors may also play a role in chemoprevention of breast cancer.[113] No data are yet available investigating the aromatase inhibitors in the setting of prevention, but clinical trials are underway.

⑩ The rationale for early detection of breast cancer is based on the relationship between stage of breast cancer at diagnosis and the probability for cure. If all breast cancer cases could be detected at a very early stage of the disease (i.e., small primary tumor and negative lymph nodes), then more patients could be cured of their disease. Screening guidelines for early detection of breast cancer in women at average risk have been developed by several organizations, including the American Cancer Society, the United States Preventive Services Task Force, and the National Cancer Institute.[151–153] The American Cancer Society guidelines are most commonly cited.

The American Cancer Society currently recommends that all women older than age 20 years be informed of the benefits and limitations of breast self-examinations (BSEs).[151] Several studies have investigated the benefits of BSE. These trials were primarily conducted prior to the routine use of mammographic screening and demonstrated an inferential benefit in diagnosis of earlier stages of breast cancer. One trial, the Shanghai trial, appeared to indicate no benefit, but there was a higher rate of biopsies in women who were taught BSE than in women who were not taught BSE.[154] The investigators from this trial caution that this was a study of BSE instruction and not BSE performance. Compliance and competency with the BSE were neither guaranteed nor evaluated in this trial. Because of the lack of direct evidence to support or refute a benefit with BSE, the American Cancer Society has taken the position that it is not recommended, but women of all ages should be instructed and encouraged to be aware of their breasts in order to recognize any changes and promptly report these to a health professional.[151]

Recommendations for breast examination by a healthcare professional (clinical breast examination) vary among the three available screening guidelines. The rate of breast cancer detection using clinical breast examination (CBE) alone is low, with even lower rates in younger women and women with higher body weight.[151] Randomized clinical trials have reported inconsistent results and often evaluated CBE in conjunction with mammograms. The American Cancer Society recommends CBE in conjunction with mammography for women ages 40 years and older.[151] For younger patients, it is recommended as part of a periodic health examination every 3 years, but this recommendation is based on weak evidence.

The most controversial screening recommendation for breast cancer is related to annual mammography. Most, if not all, guidelines recommend annual mammography for women 50 years of age and older. Nearly 75% of all breast cancers occur in women 50 years of age or older, and it has been conclusively demonstrated that regular use of screening mammography can reduce mortality from breast cancer by 20% to 40% in this age group. Controversy regarding the use of screening mammography is largely confined to women younger than 50 years of age. After many years of debate, most available guidelines recommend mammograms in this age group of women every 1 to 2 years.[151–153] Although the absolute mortality benefits of screening a younger population are clearly smaller, screening mammography reduces mortality in women ages 40 to 49. There are also many other debates within this controversial area and the reader is referred to these references for further details.[151–153] Other radiologic methods of breast imaging are also being investigated (e.g., ultrasonography and MRI). Recommendations for women with a high risk of breast cancer are not fully established. However, the American Cancer Society recently updated their recommendations to include breast screening MRI as an adjunct to mammography for the following groups of women: (1) known *brca* mutation carriers; (2) untested inidividuals with a first degree relative with a *brca* mutation; (3) women with a 20% or greater lifetime risk of breast cancer based on models that largely depend on family history.[25]

It should also be noted that there are risks associated with any screening procedure and they should be discussed with each patient so they are able to make an informed decision regarding these procedures. The risks involved with screening mammograms include false-negative results, false-positive results, overdiagnosis (true positives that will not become clinically significant), and radiation risk. The rate of false-negative results with the current technology is approximately 20%, which explains why CBE is an important adjunct to screening for many women. Although the specificity of mammography is quite high (90%), most abnormal examinations are false positives, leading to additional biopsies and psychological distress. The issue of overdiagnosis refers primarily to the growth in detection of DCIS from screening mammography. The biologic significance of these tumors is unknown because only some of them would become invasive if left in place. So the question remains: Are we treating women who do not require treatment? Experts in the field continue to debate this issue. Radiation exposure also has been discussed in the context of screening mammography, but the small doses of radiation exposure with mammograms (2 to 4 mGy per standard two-view examination) appears to be overshadowed by other benefits in terms of reduction in mortality as a consequence of early cancer detection.[153]

Significant advances in the safety and efficacy of screening mammography have occurred during the past two decades. These advances have enabled superior visualization of breast and breast tissue with a lower dose of radiation being delivered. Despite these advances, approximately 10% of all palpable masses are not detected by mammography. This is most commonly observed in premenopausal women, and may be directly related to the increased density of breast tissue in this estrogen-rich environment.

Although the safety and efficacy of screening mammography in terms of image quality and dosimetry are very acceptable, the American College of Radiology has recognized for some years the need for greater quality control in mammography. The Mammography Quality Standards of 1992 assures that all mammographic facilities achieve a common high standard of quality assurance. Responsibility for operation of the act has been given to the FDA and all facilities that offer mammography must be FDA-certified to remain open. Passage of this landmark legislation, as well as provision of appropriate levels of funding to conduct this program, represents an important contribution to the health of women. Similar quality assurance measures will need to be implemented for breast MRI's, given the recommendations to utilize this imagining method for early detection high-risk women. All women should be aware that breast MRIs are not currently regulated and should choose to have these tests performed at a reputable facility to insure quality.

EVALUATION OF THERAPEUTIC OUTCOMES

❾ The desired therapeutic outcome of adjuvant therapy of breast cancer differs significantly from that of metastatic disease. Adjuvant therapy—chemotherapy, biologic therapy, and hormonal therapy—is administered with curative intent. The rationale for adjuvant therapy is that breast cancer, even when diagnosed in early stages when clinical evidence of distant spread is not apparent, is a systemic disease that spreads early to distant sites. Adjuvant therapy is intended to eradicate micrometastases and thus cure the patient of breast cancer. Therefore, the overall goal of adjuvant therapy is to cure the disease, which is something that cannot be fully evaluated for years following initial diagnosis and treatment. In addition, because disease cannot be detected at the time adjuvant therapy is started, assessment of disease response is not possible. Instead, a predetermined number of cycles of adjuvant therapy and/or years of biologic or hormonal therapy are administered. Adjuvant chemotherapy is often associated with significant toxicity. Maintaining dose intensity has been demonstrated to be important in the cure of disease, and therefore optimizing supportive care measures such as antiemetics and growth factors is highly recommended. The concept of dose density, using growth factors to maintain blood counts while decreasing the interval between chemotherapy administrations, is very controversial in the management of early-stage breast cancer. Multiple studies investigating this approach to adjuvant chemotherapy have been conducted with conflicting results and many more trials continue to be analyzed in hopes of determining the long-term outcomes related to this approach to therapy. The goals of therapy with neoadjuvant chemotherapy are slightly different. These goals focus on earlier end points of tumor response so as to minimize surgery, determine prognosis, and potentially conserve the breast tissue for a better cosmetic result. The other outcomes discussed with adjuvant therapy also apply to this scenario, in terms of improving survival and decreasing recurrences as compared to no systemic therapy.

Palliation is the therapeutic outcome in treatment of metastatic breast cancer. In general, the least-toxic therapies are used initially, with increasingly aggressive therapies applied in a sequential fashion and in a manner that does not significantly compromise the quality of the patient's life. Tumor response to a particular treatment regimen may be measured by clinical chemistry such as liver enzyme elevation in a patient with hepatic metastases, or imaging techniques such as bone scans or chest radiographs. However, assessment of the patient's clinical status and symptom control is often adequate to evaluate response to the therapy administered. In the patient with metastatic breast cancer, it is common to initiate hormonal therapy or chemotherapy and continue administration until signs and symptoms of disease progression or new signs and symptoms present. Optimizing quality-of-life is the therapeutic end point in the treatment of patients with metastatic breast cancer. A number of valid and reliable tools are available for objective assessment of quality-of-life in patients with breast cancer.

CONCLUSIONS

Breast cancer is the most commonly occurring cancer in women in the United States, and is second only to lung cancer as the most common cancer cause of death. The etiology of breast cancer is unknown, but a number of factors that increase a woman's chances of developing the disease have been identified. These risk factors suggest a complex interplay between hormones, genetic factors, environment, and lifestyle. The identification of the *BRCA1* and *BRCA2* genes, tumor suppressor genes important in the development of inherited and perhaps sporadic breast and ovarian cancer, has been instrumental in identifying patients who are at high risk, as well as improving our basic understanding of the causes of breast and ovarian cancer.

Most breast cancers are diagnosed in early stages before the disease has disseminated to sites distant from the breast. Treatment of early-stage breast cancer consists of local management, as well as systemic adjuvant therapy with chemotherapy, biologic and hormonal therapy, or a combination of these. BCT, which consists of complete removal of the tumor (lumpectomy), combined with breast irradiation and axillary lymph node staging, is currently the preferred method of treatment for most patients with localized breast cancer. Patients who are not candidates for breast conservation or who do not choose this local therapy will generally receive the modified radical mastectomy.

It is apparent from clinical and laboratory experiments and observation that spread of breast cancer via the bloodstream occurs early in the course of the disease, which can result in patients relapsing with systemic metastatic disease following local curative therapy. The likelihood of later development of metastatic disease is related to the size of the primary tumor, presence of lymph node involvement and number of nodes affected, and a number of additional pathologic prognostic factors, which include proliferative capacity, nuclear grade, hormone receptor status, and presence or absence of oncogenes and other protein products. Systemic adjuvant therapy is commonly administered to patients with localized breast cancer following surgical procedures to diminish the risk of or delay disease recurrence. The NCCN and other groups have developed guidelines for adjuvant systemic therapy for early stage breast cancer based on expert consensus and evidence, and these treatment recommendations continue to evolve as new data become available.

Advanced breast cancer includes locally advanced breast cancer (stage III) and metastatic breast cancer (stage IV). Treatment of stage III breast cancer generally consists of a combination of surgery, radiation, and chemotherapy administered in an aggressive approach. Although response rates and survival have improved, there is still much progress to be made in stage III breast cancer. Metastatic breast cancer is usually incurable with available therapies, and patients should be encouraged to participate in clinical trials of novel agents or therapeutic approaches. It is interesting to note that some long-term responses have been observed in a subset of patients with metastatic disease who have a complete or near complete response to conventional chemotherapy. Unfortunately, this represents a small number of the total population of patients with metastatic breast cancer. Metastatic breast cancer is treated with endocrine therapy, chemotherapy or biologic therapy. Patients who are HR-positive will generally receive initial endocrine therapy followed by chemotherapy when endocrine therapy fails. Patients who are HR-negative or who have symptomatic disease involving the liver, lung, or central nervous system will generally receive chemotherapy as first-line therapy of metastatic disease. Chemotherapy will result in an objective response in approximately 50% to 60% of patients previously unexposed to chemotherapy. Most patients have partial responses, and complete disappearance of disease occurs in fewer than 10% of patients treated. Median duration of response is 5 to 12 months; although some patients will have an excellent response to an initial course of chemotherapy and may live 5 to 10 years without evidence of disease. In general, median survival of patients after treatment with commonly used drug regimens for metastatic breast cancer ranges from 14 to 33 months. The response rate to second- and third-line chemotherapy varies from 20% to 40%, depending on the previous chemotherapy regimens the patient has received. Development of novel targeted agents (e.g., trastuzumab) has also changed the outlook for patients whose tumors overexpress *HER2*. Through continued research, other biologic or targeted agents may also improve outcomes for breast cancer patients.

Current efforts at breast cancer prevention are directed toward the identification and removal of risk factors and chemoprevention with drug therapy. Two classes of agents, the retinoids and SERMs, are being evaluated for their ability to prevent breast cancer. Tamoxifen and raloxifene have demonstrated efficacy in decreasing rates of invasive breast cancer in women who are at high risk of developing the disease. Early detection of breast cancer remains important for decreasing breast cancer mortality. The rationale for early detection of breast cancer is based on the clear relationship between stage of breast cancer at diagnosis and the probability of a cure. The American Cancer Society and other groups have developed screening guidelines for early detection of breast cancer. Although these guidelines differ slightly, the overall benefits of screening mammography are apparent in their recommendations. Incorporation of newer screening methods (e.g., MRI) into these guidelines has occurred and will continue to evolve as new data become available.

Intensive research efforts are ongoing in all aspects of breast cancer etiology, detection, prevention, and treatment. Thanks to the thousands of patients who volunteered for these clinical trials, a substantial reduction in mortality has been seen in select patient subsets. It is hoped that the information obtained in the next decade will result in the knowledge required to significantly reduce mortality from breast cancer for all women. Only through these continued efforts and participation of patient volunteers will advances be made in the management of this disease.

ABBREVIATIONS

BCT: breast-conserving therapy

BSE: breast self-examination

CALGB: Cancer and Leukemia Group B

CBE: clinical breast examination

CMF: cyclophosphamide, methotrexate, fluorouracil (regimen)

DCIS: ductal carcinoma in situ

DFS: disease-free survival

ER: estrogen receptor

FISH: fluorescence in situ hybridization

HR: hormone receptor

IHC: immunohistochemistry

LCIS: lobular carcinoma in situ

LHRH: luteinizing hormone-releasing hormone

NCCN: National Comprehensive Cancer Network

NSABP: National Surgical Adjuvant Breast and Bowel Project

OS: overall survival

PR: progesterone receptor

RR: relative risk

SERD: selective estrogen receptor downregulator

SERM: selective estrogen receptor modulators

REFERENCES

1. Jemal A, Siegel R, Ward E, et al. Cancer statistics 2007. CA Cancer J Clin 2007;1990;57:43–66.
2. Ries LAG, Harkins D, Krapcho M, et al., (eds). SEER Cancer Statistics Review, National Cancer Institute. 1975–2003 [cited 2006 10/2/2006]. 2003, *http://seer.cancer.gov/csr/1975_2003/*.
3. Ghafoor A, Jemal A, Ward E, et al. Trends in breast cancer by race and ethnicity. CA Cancer J Clin 2003;53:342–355.
4. Berry DA, Cronin KA, Plevritis SK, et al. Effect of screening and adjuvant therapy on mortality from breast cancer. N Engl J Med 2005;353:1784–1792.
5. Effects of chemotherapy and hormonal therapy for early breast cancer on recurrence and 15-year survival: An overview of the randomised trials. Lancet 2005;365:1687–1717.
6. Giordano SH, Buzdar AU, Hortobagyi GN, Breast cancer in men. Ann Intern Med 2002;137:678–687.
7. Fay MP, Pfeiffer R, Cronin KA, et al. Age-conditional probabilities of developing cancer. Stat Med 2003;22:1837–1848.
8. Clemons M, Goss P. Estrogen and the risk of breast cancer. N Engl J Med 2001;344:276–285.
9. Velie EM, Nechuta S, Osuch JR. Lifetime reproductive and anthropometric risk factors for breast cancer in postmenopausal women. Breast Dis 2005;24:17–35.
10. Rossouw JE, Anderson GL, Prentice RL, et al. Risks and benefits of estrogen plus progestin in healthy postmenopausal women: Principal results From the Women's Health Initiative randomized controlled trial. JAMA 2002;288:321–333.
11. Anderson GL, Limacher M, Assaf AR, et al. Effects of conjugated equine estrogen in postmenopausal women with hysterectomy: The Women's Health Initiative randomized controlled trial. JAMA 2004;291:1701–1712.
12. Colditz GA. Estrogen, estrogen plus progestin therapy, and risk of breast cancer. Clin Cancer Res 2005;11(Pt 2):909s–917s.
13. Marchbanks PA, McDonald JA, Wilson HG, et al. Oral contraceptives and the risk of breast cancer. N Engl J Med 2002;346:2025–2032.
14. Vessey M, Painter R. Oral contraceptive use and cancer. Findings in a large cohort study, 1968–2004. Br J Cancer 2006;95:385–389.
15. McCormack VA, dos Santos Silva I. Breast density and parenchymal patterns as markers of breast cancer risk: A meta-analysis. Cancer Epidemiol Biomarkers Prev 2006;15:1159–1169.
16. Collaborative Group on Hormonal Factors in Breast Cancer. Familial breast cancer: Collaborative reanalysis of individual data from 52 epidemiological studies including 58,209 women with breast cancer and 101,986 women without the disease. Lancet 2001;358:1389–1399.
17. Narod SA, Foulkes WD. BRCA1 and BRCA2: 1994 and beyond. Rev Cancer 2004;4:665–676.
18. U.S. Preventive Services Task Force. Genetic risk assessment and BRCA mutation testing for breast and ovarian cancer susceptibility: Recommendation statement. Ann Intern Med 2005;143:355–361.
19. Nelson HD, Huffman LH, Fu R, et al. Genetic risk assessment and BRCA mutation testing for breast and ovarian cancer susceptibility: Systematic evidence review for the US Preventive Services Task Force. Ann Intern Med 2005;143:362–379.

20. ASCO Working Group on Genetic Testing for Cancer Susceptibility. American Society of Clinical Oncology policy statement update: Genetic testing for cancer susceptibility. J Clin Oncol 2003;21:2397–2406.
21. NCCN Clinical Practice Guidelines in Oncology: Genetic/Familial High-Risk Assessment: Breast and Ovarian v.1.2006. NCCN Clinical Practice Guidelines in Oncology 2006. 2006, *http://www.nccn.org/professionals/physician_gls/PDF/genetics_screening.pdf.*
22. Calderon-Margalit R, Paltiel O. Prevention of breast cancer in women who carry BRCA1 or BRCA2 mutations: A critical review of the literature. Int J Cancer 2004;112:357–364.
23. Smith RA, Saslow D, Sawyer KA, et al. American Cancer Society guidelines for breast cancer screening: Update 2003. CA Cancer J Clin 2003;53:141–169.
24. King MC, Wieand S, Hale K, et al. Tamoxifen and breast cancer incidence among women with inherited mutations in BRCA1 and BRCA2: National Surgical Adjuvant Breast and Bowel Project (NSABP-P1) Breast Cancer Prevention Trial. JAMA 2001;286:2251–2256.
25. Saslow D, Boetes C, Burke W, et al. American cancer society guidelines for breast screening with MRI as an adjunct to mammography. CA Cancer J Clin 2007;57:75–89.
26. Boyd NF, Stone J, Vogt KN, et al. Dietary fat and breast cancer risk revisited: A meta-analysis of the published literature. Br J Cancer 2003;89:1672–1685.
27. Cho E, Chen WY, Hunter DJ, et al. Red meat intake and risk of breast cancer among premenopausal women. Arch Intern Med 2006; 166:2253–2259.
28. Gandini S, Merzenich H, Robertson C, et al. Meta-analysis of studies on breast cancer risk and diet: The role of fruit and vegetable consumption and the intake of associated micronutrients. Eur J Cancer 2000;36:636–646.
29. van Gils CH, Peeters PH, Bueno-de-Mesquita HB, et al. Consumption of vegetables and fruits and risk of breast cancer. JAMA 2005;293:183–193.
30. Trock BJ, Hilakivi-Clarke L, Clarke R. Meta-analysis of soy intake and breast cancer risk. J Natl Cancer Inst 2006;98:459–471.
31. Prentice RL, Caan B, Chlebowski RT, et al. Low-fat dietary pattern and risk of invasive breast cancer: The Women's Health Initiative Randomized Controlled Dietary Modification Trial. JAMA 2006;295:629–642.
32. Chlebowski RT, Blackburn GL, Thomson CA, et al. Dietary fat reduction and breast cancer outcome: Interim efficacy results from the Women's Intervention Nutrition Study. J Natl Cancer Inst 2006;98:1767–1776.
33. Connolly BS, Barnett C, Vogt KN, et al. A meta-analysis of published literature on waist-to-hip ratio and risk of breast cancer. Nutr Cancer 2002;44:127–138.
34. Monninkhof EM, Elias SG, Vlems FA, et al. Physical activity and breast cancer: A systematic review. Epidemiology 2007;18:137–157.
35. Holmes MD, Chen WY, Feskanich D, et al. Physical activity and survival after breast cancer diagnosis. JAMA 2005;293:2479–2486.
36. Key J, Hodgson S, Omar RZ, et al. Meta-analysis of studies of alcohol and breast cancer with consideration of the methodological issues. Cancer Causes Control 2006;17:759–770.
37. Hamajima N, Hirose K, Tajima K, et al. Alcohol, tobacco and breast cancer—collaborative reanalysis of individual data from 53 epidemiological studies, including 58,515 women with breast cancer and 95,067 women without the disease. Br J Cancer 2002;87:1234–1245.
38. Ronckers CM, Erdmann CA, Land CE. Radiation and breast cancer: A review of current evidence. Breast Cancer Res 2005;7:21–32.
39. Helvie MA. Imaging analysis: Mammography, In: Harris JR, Lippman ME, Morrow M, et al., eds. Diseases of the Breast, 3rd ed. Philadelphia, Lippincott Williams & Wilkins, 2004:131–148.
40. Eberl MM, Fox CH, Edge SB, et al. BI-RADS classification for management of abnormal mammograms. J Am Board Fam Med 2006;19:161–164.
41. NCCN Clinical Practice Guidelines in Oncology: Breast Cancer Screening and Diagnosis Guidelines v.1.2007. NCCN Clinical Practice Guidelines in Oncology 2007. 2007, *http://www.nccn.org/professionals/physician_gls/PDF/breast-screening.pdf.*
42. Brenin DR. Management of the palpable breast mass. In: Harris JR, Lippmann ME, Morrow M, et al., eds. Diseases of the Breast, 3rd ed. Philadelphia, Lippincott Williams & Wilkins, 2004:33–46.
43. Singletary SE, Allred C, Ashley P, et al. Revision of the American Joint Committee on Cancer staging system for breast cancer. J Clin Oncol 2002;20:3628–3636.
44. Schnitt SJ, Guidi AJ. Pathology of invasive breast cancer. In: Harris JR, Lippman ME, Morrow M, et al., eds. Diseases of the Breast, 3rd ed. Philadelphia, Lippincott Williams & Wilkins, 2004:541–584.
45. NCCN Clinical Practice Guidelines in Oncology: Breast Cancer v.1.2007. NCCN Clinical Practice Guidelines in Oncology. 2007, *http://www.nccn.org/professionals/physician_gls/PDF/breast.pdf.*
46. Merajver SD, Sabel MS. Inflammatory breast cancer. In: Harris JR, Lippman ME, Marrow M, et al., eds. Diseases of the Breast, 3rd ed. Philadelphia, Lippincott Williams & Wilkins, 2004:971–982.
47. Newman LA. Lobular carcinoma in situ: Clinical management. In: Harris JR, Lippman ME, Morrow M, et al., eds. Diseases of the Breast, 3rd ed. Philadelphia, Lippincott Williams & Wilkins, 2004;497–506.
48. Morrow M, Harris JR. Ductal carcinoma in situ and microinvasive carcinoma. In: Harris JR, Lippman ME, Morrow M, et al., eds. Diseases of the Breast, 3rd ed. Philadelphia, Lippincott Williams & Wilkins, 2004;521–540.
49. Fisher B, Costantino JP, Wickerham DL, et al. Tamoxifen for prevention of breast cancer: Report of the National Surgical Adjuvant Breast and Bowel Project P-1 Study. J Natl Cancer Inst 1998;90:1371–1388.
50. Vogel VG, Costantino JP, Wickerham DL, et al. Effects of tamoxifen vs raloxifene on the risk of developing invasive breast cancer and other disease outcomes: The NSABP Study of Tamoxifen and Raloxifene (STAR) P-2 trial. JAMA 2006;295:2727–2741.
51. Cianfrocca M, Goldstein LJ. Prognostic and predictive factors in early-stage breast cancer. Oncologist 2004;9:606–616.
52. Kapoor A, Vogel VG. Prognostic factors for breast cancer and their use in the clinical setting. Expert Rev Anticancer Ther 2005;5:269–281.
53. Wolff AC, Hammond ME, Schwartz JN, et al. American Society of Clinical Oncology/College of American Pathologists guideline recommendations for human epidermal growth factor receptor 2 testing in breast cancer. J Clin Oncol 2007;25:118–145.
54. Ravdin PM, Siminoff LA, Davis GJ, et al. Computer program to assist in making decisions about adjuvant therapy for women with early breast cancer. J Clin Oncol 2001;19:980–991.
55. Paik S, Shak S, Tang G, et al. A multigene assay to predict recurrence of tamoxifen-treated, node-negative breast cancer. N Engl J Med 2004;351:2817–2826.
56. Buyse M, Loi S, van't Veer L, et al. Validation and clinical utility of a 70-gene prognostic signature for women with node-negative breast cancer. J Natl Cancer Inst 2006;98:1183–1192.
57. NIH Consensus Development Conference on the Treatment of Early-Stage Breast Cancer. Bethesda, MD, June 18–21. J Natl Cancer Inst Monogr 1992:1–187.
58. Jatoi I, Proschan MA, Randomized trials of breast-conserving therapy versus mastectomy for primary breast cancer: A pooled analysis of updated results. Am J Clin Oncol 2005;28:289–294.
59. Morris AD, Morris RD, Wilson JF, et al. Breast-conserving therapy vs mastectomy in early-stage breast cancer: A meta-analysis of 10-year survival. Cancer J Sci Am 1997;3:6–12.
60. Clarke M, Collins R, Darby S, et al. Effects of radiotherapy and of differences in the extent of surgery for early breast cancer on local recurrence and 15-year survival: An overview of the randomised trials. Lancet 2005;366:2087–2106.
61. Komoike Y, Akiyama F, Iino Y, et al. Ipsilateral breast tumor recurrence (IBTR) after breast-conserving treatment for early breast cancer: Risk factors and impact on distant metastases. Cancer 2006;106:35–41.
62. Zhou P, Gautam S, Recht A. Factors affecting outcome for young women with early stage invasive breast cancer treated with breast-conserving therapy. Breast Cancer Res Treat 2007;10151–57.
63. Golshan M, Miron A, Nixon AJ, et al. The prevalence of germline BRCA1 and BRCA2 mutations in young women with breast cancer undergoing breast-conservation therapy. Am J Surg 2006;192:58–62.
64. Ivens D, Hoe AL, Podd TJ, et al. Assessment of morbidity from complete axillary dissection. Br J Cancer 1992;66:136–138.
65. Keramopoulos A, Tsionou C, Minaretzis D, et al. Arm morbidity following treatment of breast cancer with total axillary dissection: A multivariated approach. Oncology 1993;50:445–449.
66. Lyman GH, Giuliano AE, Somerfield MR, et al. American Society of Clinical Oncology guideline recommendations for sentinel lymph node biopsy in early-stage breast cancer. J Clin Oncol 2005;23:7703–7720.
67. Ferrari A, Rovera F, Dionigi P, et al. Sentinel lymph node biopsy as the new standard of care in the surgical treatment for breast cancer. Expert Rev Anticancer Ther 2006;6:1503–1515.

68. Kim T, Giuliano AE, Lyman GH. Lymphatic mapping and sentinel lymph node biopsy in early-stage breast carcinoma: A metaanalysis. Cancer 2006;106:4–16.
69. Consensus Statement on Guidelines for Performing Sentinel Lymph Node Dissection in Breast Cancer October 19, 2003. 2005, *http://www.breastsurgeons.org/slnd.shtml.*
70. Goldhirsch A, Glick JH, Gelber RD, et al. Meeting highlights: International expert consensus on the primary therapy of early breast cancer 2005. Ann Oncol 2005;16:1569–1583.
71. Pestalozzi BC, Luporsi-Gely E, Jost LM, et al. ESMO Minimum Clinical Recommendations for diagnosis, adjuvant treatment and follow-up of primary breast cancer. Ann Oncol 2005;16(Suppl 1):i7–i9.
72. Ravdin PM, Siminoff IA, Harvey JA. Survey of breast cancer patients concerning their knowledge and expectations of adjuvant therapy. J Clin Oncol 1998;16:515–521.
73. Lindley C, Vasa S, Sawyer WT, et al. Quality of life and preferences for treatment following systemic adjuvant therapy for early-stage breast cancer. J Clin Oncol 1998;16:1380–1387.
74. Olivotto IA, Bajdik CD, Ravdin PM, et al. Population-based validation of the prognostic model ADJUVANT! for early breast cancer. J Clin Oncol 2005;23:2716–2725.
75. Cianfrocca M, Gradishar WJ. Controversies in the therapy of early stage breast cancer. Oncologist 2005;10:766–779.
76. Piccart MJ, de Valeriola D, Dal Lago L, et al. Adjuvant chemotherapy in 2005: Standards and beyond. Breast 2005;14:439–445.
77. Fisher B, Brown A, Mamounas E, et al. Effect of preoperative chemotherapy on local-regional disease in women with operable breast cancer: Findings from National Surgical Adjuvant Breast and Bowel Project B-18. J Clin Oncol 1997;15:2483–2493.
78. Fisher B, Bryant J, Wolmark N, et al. Effect of preoperative chemotherapy on the outcome of women with operable breast cancer. J Clin Oncol 1998;16:2672–2685.
79. Bria E, Nistico C, Cuppone F, et al. Benefit of taxanes as adjuvant chemotherapy for early breast cancer: Pooled analysis of 15,500 patients. Cancer 2006;106:2337–2344.
80. Bonadonna G, Valagussa P, Moliterni A, et al. Adjuvant cyclophosphamide, methotrexate, and fluorouracil in node-positive breast cancer: The results of 20 years of follow-up. N Engl J Med 1995;332:901–906.
81. Wood WC, Budman DR, Korzun AH, et al. Dose and dose intensity of adjuvant chemotherapy for stage II, node-positive breast carcinoma. N Engl J Med 1994;330:1253–1259.
82. Henderson IC, Berry DA, Demetri GD, et al. Improved outcomes from adding sequential Paclitaxel but not from escalating Doxorubicin dose in an adjuvant chemotherapy regimen for patients with node-positive primary breast cancer. J Clin Oncol 2003;21:976–983.
83. Citron ML, Berry DA, Cirrincione C, et al. Randomized trial of dose-dense versus conventionally scheduled and sequential versus concurrent combination chemotherapy as postoperative adjuvant treatment of node-positive primary breast cancer: First report of Intergroup Trial C9741/Cancer and Leukemia Group B Trial 9741. J Clin Oncol 2003;21:1431–1439.
84. Green MC, Buzdar AU, Smith T, et al. Weekly paclitaxel improves pathologic complete remission in operable breast cancer when compared with paclitaxel once every 3 weeks. J Clin Oncol 2005;23:5983–5992.
85. Venturini M, Del Mestro L, Aitini E, et al. Dose-dense adjuvant chemotherapy in early breast cancer patients: Results from a randomized trial. J Natl Cancer Inst 2005;97:1724–1733.
86. Sparano JA, Wang M, Martino S, et al. Phase III study of doxorubicin-cyclophosphamide followed by paclitaxel or docetaxel given every 3 weeks or weekly in patients with axillary node-positive or high-risk node negative breast cancer: Results of North American Breast Cancer Intergroup Trial E1199. In San Antonio Breast Cancer Symposium, December 2005. San Antonio, Texas; 2005.
87. Kummel S, Rezai M, Kimmig R, et al. Dose-dense chemotherapy for primary breast cancer. Curr Opin Obstet Gynecol 2007;19:75–81.
88. Orzano JA, Swain SM. Concepts and clinical trials of dose-dense chemotherapy for breast cancer. Clin Breast Cancer 2005;6:402–411.
89. Moore HC. Impact on quality of life of adjuvant therapy for breast cancer. Curr Oncol Rep 2007;9:42–46.
90. Groenvold M, Fayers PM, Petersen MA, et al. Breast cancer patients on adjuvant chemotherapy report a wide range of problems not identified by healthcare staff. Breast Cancer Res Treat 2007;103:185–195.
91. Levine MN, Gent M, Hirsh J, et al. The thrombogenic effect of anticancer drug therapy in women with stage II breast cancer. N Engl J Med 1988;318:404–407.
92. Matesich SM, Shapiro CL. Second cancers after breast cancer treatment. Semin Oncol 2003;30:740–748.
93. Henderson IC, Sloss LJ, Jaffe N, et al. Serial studies of cardiac function in patients receiving Adriamycin. Cancer Treat Rep 1978;62:923–929.
94. Ellence (epirubicin) product information. 2005, *http://www.pfizer.com/pfizer/download/uspi_ellence.pdf.*
95. Romond EH, Perez EA, Bryant J, et al. Trastuzumab plus adjuvant chemotherapy for operable HER2-positive breast cancer. N Engl J Med 2005;353:1673–1684.
96. Piccart-Gebhart MJ, Procter M, Leyland-Jones B, et al. Trastuzumab after adjuvant chemotherapy in HER2-positive breast cancer. N Engl J Med 2005;353:1659–1672.
97. Joensuu H, Kellokumpu-Lehtinen PL, Bono P, et al. Adjuvant docetaxel or vinorelbine with or without trastuzumab for breast cancer. N Engl J Med 2006;354:809–820.
98. Slamon D, Eiermann W, Robert N, et al. Phase III trial comparing AC-T with AC-TH and with TCH in the adjuvant treatment of HER2 positive early breast cancer patients: Second interim efficacy analysis. In San Antonio Breast Cancer Symposium, December 14, 2006. San Antonio, Texas, 2006.
99. Herceptin (trastuzumab) product information. 2006, *http://www.gene.com/gene/products/information/oncology/herceptin/insert.jsp.*
100. Hillner B. Clinical and cost-effectiveness implications of the adjuvant trastuzumab in HER2+ breast cancer trials. San Antonio Breast Cancer Symposium, December 10, 2005. San Antonio, Texas, 2005.
101. Plosker GL, Keam SJ. Trastuzumab: A review of its use in the management of HER2-positive metastatic and early-stage breast cancer. Drugs 2006;66:449–475.
102. Norum J. The cost-effectiveness issue of adjuvant trastuzumab in early breast cancer. Expert Opin Pharmacother 2006;7:1617–1625.
103. Love RR, Wiebe DA, Newcomb PA, et al. Effects of tamoxifen on cardiovascular risk factors in postmenopausal women. Ann Intern Med 1991;115:860–864.
104. Love RR, Mazess RB, Barden HS, et al. Effects of tamoxifen on bone mineral density in postmenopausal women with breast cancer. N Engl J Med 1992;326:852–856.
105. Albain KS, Green SJ, Ravdin PM, et al. Adjuvant chemohormonal therapy for primary breast cancer should be sequential instead of concurrent: Initial results from intergroup trial 0100 (SWOG-8814). In Proceedings of the American Society of Clinical Oncology Annual Meeting, 2002:A143.
106. Fisher B, Dignam J, Bryant J, et al. Five versus more than five years of tamoxifen for lymph node-negative breast cancer: Updated findings from the National Surgical Adjuvant Breast and Bowel Project B-14 randomized trial. J Natl Cancer Inst 2001;93:684–690.
107. Nolvadex (tamoxifen) product information. 2003. *http://www.fda.gov/medwatch/SAFETY/2003/03Jan_labels/Nolvadex_01-03.PDF.*
108. Fareston (toremifene) product information. 2004. *http://www.fareston.com/pdfs/Prescribing_Info.pdf.*
109. Hayes DF, Van Zyl JA, Hacking A, et al. Randomized comparison of tamoxifen and two separate doses of toremifene in postmenopausal patients with metastatic breast cancer. J Clin Oncol 1995;13:2556–2566.
110. Pagani O, Gelber S, Price K, et al. Toremifene and tamoxifen are equally effective for early-stage breast cancer: First results of International Breast Cancer Study Group Trials 12–93 and 14–93. Ann Oncol 2004;15:1749–1759.
111. Holli K. Tamoxifen versus toremifene in the adjuvant treatment of breast cancer. Eur J Cancer 2002;38(Suppl 6):S37–S38.
112. Sharma R, Beith J, Hamilton A. Systematic review of LHRH agonists for the adjuvant treatment of early breast cancer. Breast 2005;14:181–191.
113. Howell A, Cuzick J, Baum M, et al. Results of the ATAC (Arimidex, Tamoxifen, Alone or in Combination) trial after completion of 5 years' adjuvant treatment for breast cancer. Lancet 2005;365:60–62.
114. Coates AS, Keshaviah A, Thurlimann B, et al. Five years of letrozole compared with tamoxifen as initial adjuvant therapy for postmenopausal women with endocrine-responsive early breast cancer: Update of study BIG 1–98. J Clin Oncol 2007;25:486–492.

115. Goss PE, Ingle JN, Martino S, et al. A randomized trial of letrozole in postmenopausal women after five years of tamoxifen therapy for early-stage breast cancer. N Engl J Med 2003;349:1793–1802.
116. Bria E, Ciccarese M, Giannarelli D, et al. Early switch with aromatase inhibitors as adjuvant hormonal therapy for postmenopausal breast cancer: Pooled-analysis of 8794 patients. Cancer Treat Rev 2006;32:325–332.
117. Giordano SH. Update on locally advanced breast cancer. Oncologist 2003;8:521–530.
118. Kaufmann M, Hortobagyi GN, Goldhirsch A, et al. Recommendations from an international expert panel on the use of neoadjuvant (primary) systemic treatment of operable breast cancer: An update. J Clin Oncol 2006;24:1940–1949.
119. Buzdar AU, Ibrahim NK, Francis D, et al. Significantly higher pathologic complete remission rate after neoadjuvant therapy with trastuzumab, paclitaxel, and epirubicin chemotherapy: Results of a randomized trial in human epidermal growth factor receptor 2-positive operable breast cancer. J Clin Oncol 2005;23:3676–3685.
120. Hanrahan EO, Hennessy BT, Valero V. Neoadjuvant systemic therapy for breast cancer: An overview and review of recent clinical trials. Expert Opin Pharmacother 2005;6:1477–1491.
121. Macaskill EJ, Renshaw L, Dixon JM. Neoadjuvant use of hormonal therapy in elderly patients with early or locally advanced hormone receptor-positive breast cancer. Oncologist 2006;11:1081–1088.
122. Altundag K, Ibrahim NK. Aromatase inhibitors in breast cancer: An overview. Oncologist 2006;11:553–562.
123. Robertson J LD. Static disease of long duration (greater than 24 weeks) is an important remission criterion in breast cancer patients treated with the aromatase inhibitor "Arimidex" (anastrozole). Breast Cancer Res Treat 1997;46:214.
124. Mauras N, O'Brien KO, Klein KO, et al. Estrogen suppression in males: Metabolic effects. J Clin Endocrinol Metab 2000;85:2370–2377.
125. Stenbygaard LE, Herrstedt J, Thomsen JF, et al. Toremifene and tamoxifen in advanced breast cancer—a double-blind cross-over trial. Breast Cancer Res Treat 1993;25:57–63.
126. Howell A. Pure oestrogen antagonists for the treatment of advanced breast cancer. Endocr Relat Cancer 2006;13:689–706.
127. Ingle JN, Krook JE, Green SJ, et al. Randomized trial of bilateral oophorectomy versus tamoxifen in premenopausal women with metastatic breast cancer. J Clin Oncol 1986;4:178–185.
128. Klijn JG, Blamey RW, Boccardo F, et al. Combined tamoxifen and luteinizing hormone-releasing hormone (LHRH) agonist versus LHRH agonist alone in premenopausal advanced breast cancer: A meta-analysis of four randomized trials. J Clin Oncol 2001;19:343–353.
129. Michaud LB, Valero V, Hortobagyi G. Risks and benefits of taxanes in breast and ovarian cancer. Drug Saf 2000;23:401–428.
130. Jones SE, Erban J, Overmoyer B, et al. Randomized phase III study of docetaxel compared with paclitaxel in metastatic breast cancer. J Clin Oncol 2005;23:5542–5551.
131. Gradishar WJ, Tjulandin S, Davidson N, et al. Phase III trial of nanoparticle albumin-bound paclitaxel compared with polyethylated castor oil-based paclitaxel in women with breast cancer. J Clin Oncol 2005;23:7794–7803.
132. Gralow JR. Optimizing the treatment of metastatic breast cancer. Breast Cancer Res Treat 2005;89(Suppl 1):S9–S15.
133. O'Brien ME, Wigler N, Inbar M, et al. Reduced cardiotoxicity and comparable efficacy in a phase III trial of pegylated liposomal doxorubicin HCl (CAELYX/Doxil) versus conventional doxorubicin for first-line treatment of metastatic breast cancer. Ann Oncol 2004;15:440–449.
134. Fornier MN. Ixabepilone, first in a new class of antineoplastic agents: the natural epothilones and their analogues. Clin Breast Cancer 2007;7(10):757–763.
135. Sledge GW, Neuberg D, Bernardo P, et al. Phase III trial of doxorubicin, paclitaxel, and the combination of doxorubicin and paclitaxel as front-line chemotherapy for metastatic breast cancer: An intergroup trial (E1193). J Clin Oncol 2003;21:588–592.
136. O'Shaughnessy J, Miles D, Vukelja S, et al. Superior survival with capecitabine plus docetaxel combination therapy in anthracycline-pretreated patients with advanced breast cancer: Phase III trial results. J Clin Oncol 2002;20:2812–2823.
137. Cobleigh MA, Vogel CL, Tripathy D, et al. Multinational study of the efficacy and safety of humanized anti-HER2 monoclonal antibody in women who have HER2-overexpressing metastatic breast cancer that has progressed after chemotherapy for metastatic disease. J Clin Oncol 1999;17:2639–2648.
138. Slamon DJ, Leyland-Jones B, Shak S, et al. Use of chemotherapy plus a monoclonal antibody against HER2 for metastatic breast cancer that overexpresses HER2. N Engl J Med 2001;344:783–792.
139. Marty M, Cognetti F, Maraninchi D, et al. Randomized phase II trial of the efficacy and safety of trastuzumab combined with docetaxel in patients with human epidermal growth factor receptor 2-positive metastatic breast cancer administered as first-line treatment: The M77001 study group. J Clin Oncol 2005;23:4265–4274.
140. Burstein HJ, Harris LN, Marcom PK, et al. Trastuzumab and vinorelbine as first-line therapy for HER2-overexpressing metastatic breast cancer: Multicenter phase II trial with clinical outcomes, analysis of serum tumor markers as predictive factors, and cardiac surveillance algorithm. J Clin Oncol 2003;21:2889–2895.
141. Kaufman PA, Mayer M, Paik S, et al. registHER: Trastuzumab-based taxane or vinorelbine treatment selection in patients with HER2-positive metastatic breast cancer: Patient characteristics and preliminary outcomes (Meeting Abstract). In San Antonio Breast Cancer Symposium, December 15, 2006. San Antonio, TX; 2006:A2066.
142. Robert N, Leyland-Jones B, Asmar L, et al. Randomized phase III study of trastuzumab, paclitaxel, and carboplatin compared with trastuzumab and paclitaxel in women with HER-2–overexpressing metastatic breast cancer. J Clin Oncol 2006;24:2786–2792
143. Forbes JF, Kennedy J, Pienkowski T, et al. BCIRG 007: Randomized phase III trial of trastuzumab plus docetaxel with or without carboplatin first line in HER2 positive metastatic breast cancer (MBC) (Meeting Abstract). J Clin Oncol, 2006 ASCO Annual Meeting Proceeding Part I. Vol 24, No. 18S (June 20 Supplement), 2006: LBA516.
144. Leyland-Jones B, Gelmon K, Ayoub JP, et al. Pharmacokinetics, safety, and efficacy of trastuzumab administered every three weeks in combination with paclitaxel. J Clin Oncol 2003;21:3965–3971.
145. Geyer CE, Forster J, Lindquist D, et al. Lapatinib plus capecitabine for HER2-positive advanced breast cancer. N Engl J Med 2006;355:2733–2743.
146. Perez EA, Byrne AJ, Hammond IW, et al. Results of an analysis of cardiac function in 2,812 patients treated with lapatinib (Meeting Abstract). J Clin Oncol, 2006 ASCO Annual Meeting Proceedings Part I. Vol 24, No. 18S (June 20 Supplement), 2006:583.
147. Miller KD, Chap LI, Holmes FA, et al. Randomized phase III trial of capecitabine compared with bevacizumab plus capecitabine in patients with previously treated metastatic breast cancer. J Clin Oncol 2005;23:792–799.
148. Miller KD, Wang M, Gralow J, et al. A randomized phase III trial of paclitaxel versus paclitaxel plus bevacizumab as first-line therapy for locally recurrent or metastatic breast cancer: A trial coordinated by the Eastern Cooperative Oncology Group (E2100). In San Antonio Breast Cancer Symposium, December 8, 2005. San Antonio, TX; 2005:A3.
149. Cuzick J, Powles T, Veronesi U, et al. Overview of the main outcomes in breast-cancer prevention trials. Lancet 2003;361:296–300.
150. Land SR, Wickerham DL, Costantino JP, et al. Patient-reported symptoms and quality of life during treatment with tamoxifen or raloxifene for breast cancer prevention: The NSABP Study of Tamoxifen and Raloxifene (STAR) P-2 trial. JAMA 2006;295:2742–2751.
151. Smith RA, Cokkinides V, Eyre HJ. American Cancer Society guidelines for the early detection of cancer, 2006. CA Cancer J Clin 2006;56:11–25; quiz 49–50.
152. US Preventive Services Task Force. Breast Cancer Screening. 2002, *http://www.ahrq.gov/clinic/uspstf/uspsbrca.htm.*
153. National Cancer Institute. Breast Cancer Screening Recommendations. 2006, *http://www.cancer.gov/cancertopics/pdq/screening/breast/healthprofessional.*
154. Thomas DB, Gao DL, Self SG, et al. Randomized trial of breast self-examination in Shanghai: Methodology and preliminary results. J Natl Cancer Inst 1997;89:355–365.

CHAPTER 132 Lung Cancer

JEANNINE S. MCCUNE AND DEBORAH A. FRIEZE

KEY CONCEPTS

1. Lung cancer is the leading cause of cancer deaths in both men and women in the United States. The overall 5-year survival rate for all types of lung cancer is approximately 15%.

2. Cigarette smoking is responsible for most lung cancers. Smoking cessation should be encouraged, particularly in those receiving curative treatment (i.e., stages I to IIIA non–small cell lung cancer and limited-stage small cell lung cancer).

3. Non–small cell lung cancer (NSCLC) is diagnosed in most (80%) lung cancer patients. NSCLC typically has a slower growth rate and doubling time than small cell lung cancer (SCLC).

4. No screening test is recommended to identify lung cancer patients at earlier stages, when the cure rates are much higher than that at more advanced stages. Thus, many lung cancers go undetected until they are advanced because individuals who have a long history of cigarette smoking are unlikely to notice the early symptoms of cough or dyspnea. It is often symptoms associated with large tumors or metastatic disease that prompt medical attention.

5. Surgery is potentially curative in patients with early stage NSCLC, but its role is more limited in those with SCLC. Radiotherapy is used for patients with either disease, particularly in those with symptomatic metastases. Chemotherapy has been used in patients with SCLC for more than 25 years. The role of chemotherapy in NSCLC has traditionally been more controversial. However, cytotoxic chemotherapy is now the standard of care for those with unresectable stage III and stage IV NSCLC and a good performance status (i.e., able to perform functions of daily living). Results from recently published trials show that adjuvant chemotherapy increases overall survival in patients with earlier stages of NSCLC.

6. The most appropriate treatment for NSCLC is determined by the size and location of the tumor, extent of lymph node spread, presence or absence of metastatic sites, and the performance status of the patient. Surgery and adjuvant chemotherapy are the treatments of choice for early stage NSCLC (stage I or II); some patients may benefit from postoperative radiation.

7. In patients with locally advanced NSCLC (stage III), chemotherapy with or without radiation followed by surgery improves survival over radiation followed by surgery. Doublet chemotherapy including cisplatin or carboplatin and another active drug (i.e., vinorelbine, paclitaxel, docetaxel, or gemcitabine) is recommended for patients with unresectable stage III or stage IV disease. The addition of bevacizumab to doublet chemotherapy improves 1-year survival in selected patients with advanced NSCLC.

8. Docetaxel, pemetrexed, and erlotinib are appropriate treatment options for unresectable stage III or IV NSCLC patients with a good performance status who have relapsed after initial (i.e., first-line) cytotoxic chemotherapy.

9. Because SCLC has the propensity to disseminate early on in the disease, surgery is not usually indicated. SCLC is radiosensitive, and radiotherapy is used in combination with chemotherapy in patients with limited stage SCLC. Prophylactic cranial irradiation is used in selected patients to reduce the risk of central nervous system (CNS) metastases. Combination chemotherapy prolongs median survival in SCLC patients. The most widely used chemotherapy regimens for SCLC include cisplatin or carboplatin plus etoposide. Despite very high response rates to chemotherapy, most patients with SCLC eventually have disease progression and die from their disease.

Learning objectives, review questions, and other resources can be found at **www.pharmacotherapyonline.com.**

Lung cancer is a major cause of morbidity and mortality. It has reached epidemic proportions in many industrialized countries and is the most frequently fatal malignancy in the world. The American Cancer Society estimates nearly 213,380 new cases of lung cancer will be diagnosed in the United States in 2007.[1] Despite major advances in the understanding and management of lung cancer, the overall 5-year survival rate for all types of lung cancer remains a dismal 15%.[2] In the United States, lung cancer is estimated to account for approximately 15% of all newly diagnosed cancers in adults.[1] (1) It remains the leading cause of cancer death in both adult men and women, with about 160,390 deaths expected in 2007.[1] The incidence and death rate caused by lung cancer are declining in men, but the incidence recently plateaued and mortality continues to increase in women.[1] Since 1987, lung cancer has surpassed breast cancer as the primary cause of cancer death in American women.[1] In comparison to whites, the incidence of lung cancer is greater in African Americans and the mortality rate is greater in African American men but lower in African American women.[1]

The incidence of lung cancer increases with age, with the peak age of diagnosis being between 55 and 65 years. Among patients 40 years of age and older, the likelihood that a solitary pulmonary nodule seen on chest radiography is a carcinoma is high and this probability increases proportionately with age. Patients with lung cancer may undergo surgery, chemotherapy, radiation, or multimodality therapy, depending on the histologic type of the tumor, its size and location, and the presence of metastases at diagnosis. Two leading oncology groups representing leading clinicians in the

United States have published clinical practice guidelines for the treatment of lung cancer. The National Comprehensive Cancer Network (NCCN) has developed consensus-based guidelines that provide recommendations regarding the screening, staging, and treatment of both small cell lung cancer (SCLC) and non–small cell lung cancer (NSCLC).[3,4] The American Society of Clinical Oncology first published evidence-based guidelines regarding the staging and treatment of NSCLC in 1997, which were subsequently updated in 2003.[5] In addition, the Agency for Healthcare Research and Quality has published an evidence report regarding the management of SCLC.[6] The American College of Chest Physicians (ACCP) also recently published evidence-based clinical practice guidelines.[95]

ETIOLOGY

Lung carcinomas arise from normal bronchial epithelial cells that have acquired multiple genetic lesions and are capable of expressing a variety of phenotypes.[7] Recently, significant advances have been made in understanding the molecular genetic changes involved in lung cancer pathogenesis.[7] A large variety of molecular lesions result in abrogation of key cellular regulatory and growth control pathways.[7] Activation of protooncogenes, inhibition or mutation of tumor suppressor genes, and production of autocrine (self-stimulatory) growth factors contribute to cellular proliferation and malignant transformation.[7] Many of the autocrine loops, and protooncogene and tumor suppressor gene changes are common to both SCLC and NSCLC, but certain mutations are found more frequently in each subtype of lung cancer. These unique tumor characteristics may offer more targeted interventions to prevent or treat lung cancer. For example, of the autocrine loops, SCLC frequently overexpresses KIT, whereas NSCLC frequently overexpresses epidermal growth factor receptor (EGFR). This is notable as EGFR inhibitors, such as erlotinib, are used clinically to treat NSCLC (see Human Epidermal Growth Factor Receptor Inhibitors) and offer a potential method of lung cancer chemoprevention.[7,8] Properly designed clinical trials are necessary, however, as demonstrated by the lack of efficacy of imatinib in the treatment of SCLC. Although imatinib inhibits KIT kinase in several SCLC lines, no responses occurred in patients with SCLC overexpressing c-KIT.[9]

❷ Smoking is a major cause of lung cancer, with approximately 80% of lung cancer deaths in the United States directly attributed to tobacco abuse.[7,10] Tobacco smoke contains many substances, including tumor promoters, carcinogens and cocarcinogens. Many of these carcinogens cause lung tumors in laboratory animals or humans and are likely to be involved in induction of lung cancer.[7] Most cases of NSCLC and SCLC are caused by cigarette smoking, although cigars and pipes are also carcinogenic.[10–12] Smoking cessation is associated with a gradual decrease in the risk, but more than 5 years is necessary before an appreciable decline in risk occurs.[10,12] Although smoking cessation substantially reduces the risk of lung cancer, the risk never reaches that of a nonsmoker and almost 50% of all lung cancers in the United States are diagnosed in former smokers.[10] Because of the public health implications, the United States has several mainly state-led tobacco control efforts including antismoking campaigns, increased tobacco taxes, and smoke-free areas in many public areas.[10] State tobacco control efforts inversely correlate with lung cancer death rates.[10] Continued efforts are needed as the prevalence of cigarette smoking has plateaued at 23% since the mid-1990s and there is a trend of greater proportion of adolescents, particularly girls, starting to smoke cigarettes.[11] The association between environmental tobacco smoke (ETS, also referred to as passive smoking) and lung cancer risk in nonsmokers is not as clear.[10] Nonsmokers exposed to ETS excrete tobacco-specific carcinogens in the urine at 1% to 5% the amount detected in smokers, which are consistent with the relative risks of lung cancer in ETS-exposed nonsmokers and to active smokers.[10] In nonsmokers, ETS contributes to 25% of all lung cancers and the risk of lung cancer is proportional to the level of ETS exposure.[10]

Although most cases of lung cancer are attributable to cigarette smoking, less than 20% of smokers develop lung cancer which suggests that other risk factors are relevant. An increased risk of lung cancer has been associated with exposure to other environmental respiratory carcinogens (e.g., asbestos, benzene).[10] Genetic risk factors are also important, with an increased risk of lung cancer observed in those with first-degree relatives diagnosed with the disease.[10] Lung cancer risk is associated with polymorphisms affecting the expression and/or function of enzymes regulating metabolism of tobacco carcinogens, DNA repair or inflammation.[10] Patients with a history of tuberculosis, pulmonary fibrosis, chronic bronchitis and emphysema, chronic obstructive airway disease and in adults with asthma are at an increased risk for lung cancer.[12] Gathering data to better identify which patients are at highest risk of developing lung cancer will be key for new lung cancer screening trials and in chemoprevention trials.

HISTOLOGIC CLASSIFICATION

Before treatment begins, it is critical that an experienced lung cancer pathologist reviews the pathologic material because of the vastly different treatment regimens for NSCLC and SCLC. ❸ NSCLC is diagnosed in most (80%) lung cancer patients. NSCLC typically has a slower growth rate and doubling time than SCLC. On microscopic examination, SCLC can be confused with NSCLC.[3,13] Immunohistochemistry and electron microscopy are invaluable techniques for diagnosis and subclassification, but most lung tumors can be classified by light microscopic criteria. The World Health Organization Classification of Lung Cancer is widely accepted (Table 132–1). In the most recent update of this classification, adenocarcinoma was further subclassified, the definition of bronchioalveolar carcinoma was restricted to noninvasive tumors and large cell neuroendocrine carcinoma was recognized as a histologically high-grade non–small cell carcinoma.[14]

Four major cell types of carcinomas (squamous cell, adenocarcinoma, large cell, and small cell) account for more than 90% of all lung tumors. Because squamous cell, adenocarcinoma, and large cell carcinomas have a similar overall prognosis and treatment strategy, they are frequently grouped together and referred to as NSCLC. Until recently, NSCLCs were treated similarly until the recent data showing an increased frequency of bleeding in squamous cell lung cancer patients receiving bevacizumab.[15,16] Although once the most common type of NSCLC, squamous cell (or epidermoid) carcinoma now accounts for less than 30% of all lung cancers, and is distinguished histologically by evidence of squamous differentiation. This tumor historically arose centrally but its presentation in the peripheral lung is increasing.[14] Squamous cell carcinomas (along with SCLC) have a much higher incidence among smokers and among males and appear to have a strong dose–response relationship to tobacco exposure.[10,11] Although they can grow rapidly, most squamous cell carcinomas tend to be slow growing and confined to the lungs (especially early in the disease course). Such tumors may eventually metastasize to the hilar and mediastinal lymph nodes, liver, adrenal glands, kidneys, bone, and gastrointestinal tract.

Adenocarcinoma accounts for about one-half of lung cancers and is increasing in frequency.[14] Mixed histologies predominate, including acinar, papillary, and bronchioloalveolar carcinoma (nonmucinous and mucinous); variants include well-differentiated fetal adenocarcinoma, mucinous (colloid) adenocarcinoma, mucinous cystadenocarcinoma, signet ring adenocarcinoma, and clear cell adenocarcinoma.[14] Although the diagnostic criteria for bronchioloalveolar carcinoma varied widely in the past, the current World Health Organization/International Association for the Study of

TABLE 132-1 The World Health Organization/International Association for the Study of Lung Cancer Histologic Classification of Non–Small Cell Lung Carcinomas

1. Squamous cell carcinoma
   - Papillary
   - Clear cell
   - Small cell
   - Basaloid
2. Adenocarcinoma
   - Acinar
   - Papillary
   - Bronchioloalveolar carcinoma
     - Nonmucinous
     - Mucinous
     - Mixed mucinous and nonmucinous or indeterminate cell type
   - Solid adenocarcinoma with mucin
   - Adenocarcinoma with mixed subtypes
   - Variants
     - Well-differentiated fetal adenocarcinoma
     - Mucinous (colloid) adenocarcinoma
     - Mucinous cystadenocarcinoma
     - Signet ring adenocarcinoma
     - Clear cell adenocarcinoma
3. Large cell carcinoma
   - Variants
     - Large cell neuroendocrine carcinoma
     - Combined large cell neuroendocrine carcinoma
     - Basaloid carcinoma
     - Lymphoepithelioma-like carcinoma
     - Clear cell carcinoma
     - Large cell carcinoma with rhabdoid phenotype
4. Adenosquamous carcinoma
5. Carcinomas with pleomorphic, sarcomatoid, or sarcomatous elements
   - Carcinomas with spindle and/or giant cells
   - Spindle cell carcinoma
   - Giant cell carcinoma
   - Carcinosarcoma
   - Pulmonary blastoma
6. Carcinoid tumor
   - Typical carcinoid
   - Atypical carcinoid
7. Carcinomas of salivary gland type
   - Mucoepidermoid carcinoma
   - Adenoid cystic carcinoma
   - Others
8. Unclassified carcinoma

Adapted from reference 13 which is based on reference 14.

Lung Cancer definition is much more restrictive because it is limited only to noninvasive tumors.[14] If stromal, vascular, or pleural invasion is identified in an adenocarcinoma that has an extensive bronchioloalveolar carcinoma component, the tumor would be classified as an adenocarcinoma of mixed subtype with predominant bronchioloalveolar pattern and either a focal acinar, solid, or papillary pattern, depending on which pattern is seen in the invasive component. The presentation and natural history of adenocarcinomas are quite variable. These tumors can present as a single nodule, multifocal nodules, or rapidly progressing, bilateral, diffuse processes. They are likely to metastasize at an early stage (often before the diagnosis of the primary tumor) and spread widely to distant sites including the contralateral lung, liver, bone, adrenal glands, kidneys, and central nervous system. As a result, adenocarcinoma has a worse prognosis than squamous cell carcinoma.

Large cell carcinomas are undifferentiated epithelial tumors, which are often a diagnosis of exclusion.[14] These tumors tend to be large and bulky tumors arising in the periphery of the lung, have a propensity to metastasize in a pattern quite similar to adenocarcinomas, and are associated with a similar poor prognosis.

Small cell carcinomas account for approximately 15% of all lung tumors.[4] Nearly all SCLCs are immunoreactive for keratin, epithelial membrane antigen, thyroid transcription factor 1 and many stain positively for markers of neuroendocrine differentiation.[4] They are distinguished by a proliferation of neoplastic cells with round to oval nuclei. These tumors occur in both the major bronchi and in the periphery of the lung.[14] SCLC is a very aggressive and rapidly growing tumor with approximately 60% to 70% of patients initially presenting with disseminated disease outside of the hemithorax.[11] These tumors commonly express neuroendocrine differentiation, which may account for some of the paraneoplastic syndromes frequently associated with this disease. SCLC secretes gastrin-releasing peptide that acts as an autocrine growth factor. Secretion of other peptide hormones, cytogenetic abnormalities, and amplification and increased expression of oncogenes are also common. This disease has a propensity to metastasize to the lymph nodes, opposite lung, liver, adrenal glands and other endocrine organs, bone, bone marrow, and central nervous system.

Lung tumors frequently exhibit more than one histologic cell type, and it is now evident that all types of lung cancer share a common pluripotent stem cell. Studies of lung cancer cells have also shown that cell lines may spontaneously change phenotype, which may explain the mixed histology. Occasionally, patients can also have multiple lung nodules arising in different lobes or the contralateral lung. This is referred to as *synchronous tumors,* and the nodules may be of similar or different cell types. This usually worsens the patient's overall prognosis.

CLINICAL PRESENTATION

❹ At the time of diagnosis, 16% of lung cancers are localized, 37% have regional spread, and 39% have distant metastases.[1] Location and extent of the tumor determine the presenting signs and symptoms. A lesion in the central portion of the bronchial tree is more likely to cause symptoms at an earlier stage as compared to a lesion in the periphery of the lung, which may remain asymptomatic until the lesion is large or has spread to other areas. The most common initial signs and symptoms include cough, dyspnea, chest pain, sputum production, and hemoptysis. Unfortunately, many patients with lung cancer also have chronic pulmonary and/or cardiovascular diseases (usually related to smoking), and such symptoms may go unnoticed or be attributed to the concomitant disease. Many patients also exhibit systemic symptoms of malignancy such as anorexia, weight loss, and fatigue.[10,11] Disseminated disease can cause extrapulmonary signs and symptoms such as neurologic deficits resulting from CNS metastases, bone pain or pathologic fractures secondary to bone metastases, or liver dysfunction resulting from tumor involvement in the liver.

CLINICAL PRESENTATION OF LUNG CANCER

Local Signs and Symptoms Associated with Primary Tumor or Regional Spread within the Thorax

- Cough
- Hemoptysis
- Dyspnea
- Rust-streaked or purulent sputum
- Chest, shoulder, or arm pain
- Wheeze and stridor
- Superior vena cava obstruction
- Pleural effusion or pneumonitis
- Dysphagia (secondary to esophageal compression)

- Hoarseness (secondary to laryngeal nerve paralysis)
- Horner's syndrome
- Phrenic nerve paralysis
- Pericardial effusion/tamponade
- Tracheal obstruction

Extrapulmonary Signs and Symptoms Associated with Metastatic Involvement

- Bone pain and/or pathologic fractures
- Liver dysfunction
- Neurologic deficits
- Spinal cord compression

Paraneoplastic Syndromes

- Weight loss
- Cushing's syndrome
- Hypercalcemia (most commonly in squamous cell lung cancer)
- Syndrome of inappropriate secretion of antidiuretic hormone (most commonly in SCLC)
- Pulmonary hypertrophic osteoarthropathy
- Clubbing
- Anemia
- Eaton-Lambert's myasthenic syndrome
- Hypercoagulable state

Paraneoplastic syndromes are signs and symptoms that occur at sites away from the primary tumor or its metastases and are not associated with direct tumor involvement. They may be caused by the production of biologically active substances (e.g., peptide hormones) or antibodies, or by other undefined mechanisms. Paraneoplastic syndromes occur more frequently with lung cancer than with any other tumor. These syndromes may be the first signs of a tumor and may prompt the search for an underlying malignancy.

SCREENING AND PREVENTION

Because lung cancer is usually diagnosed at later stages, early detection as a result of screening may offer the best opportunity to decrease lung cancer mortality. During the 1970s, three trials were initiated to evaluate lung cancer screening: two that compared chest radiography alone to chest radiography and sputum cytology and a third trial that compared annual to quarterly screening with a chest radiography and sputum cytology. None of these trials showed a reduction in lung cancer mortality.[2] Several methodologic deficiencies in the trial designs have been recognized, including the exclusion of women, tobacco use not high enough to insure a population at sufficiently high risk for lung cancer, and inadequate power.[2] An annual chest radiograph was a standard component of healthcare at that time, so a truly nonscreened control group would have been difficult to achieve.[2]

Although there is no accepted screening for lung cancer, ongoing research is evaluating novel methods for lung cancer screening, such as polymerase chain reaction-based assays of sputum cytology samples, and low-dose computed tomography (CT) scans.[2,17] In 1993, the Early Lung Cancer Action Project initiated a clinical trial to evaluate early lung cancer diagnosis with annual spiral CT screening in 31,567 participants who were at risk for lung cancer because of a history of cigarette smoking, occupational exposure, or ETS.[18] Screening led to a lung cancer diagnosis in 484 participants, most (85%) of whom had stage I lung cancer and an estimated 10-year survival rate of 88%.[18] However, a separate study suggested that annual CT screening did not decrease lung cancer mortality.[19] Randomized controlled trials evaluating the role of CT scanning are ongoing.[19,20] Currently, asymptomatic individuals should not be screened outside a clinical screening trial.[19,21,96]

Diet was associated with lung cancer risk in several epidemiologic studies.[12] Increased intake of fresh fruit and vegetables lower risk in both men and women regardless of their smoking status.[12] The specific chemopreventive nutrients have yet to be identified, with provitamin A carotenoids, particularly β-carotene, being the most studied.[12] The effects of β-carotene on lung cancer risk were evaluated in three large-scale, randomized, chemoprevention trials, specifically ATBC (α-tocopherol β-carotene), CARET (Carotene and Retinol Efficacy Trial), and the Physicians' Health Study.[12] The ATBC trial was a primary prevention trial in 29,000 male smokers 50 to 69 years old who received either placebo, α-tocopherol (vitamin E) 50 international units daily, β-carotene 20 mg daily, or both supplements for 5 to 8 years.[22] Supplementation with α-tocopherol had no effect on lung cancer incidence or mortality, whereas β-carotene administration resulted in a *higher* incidence of lung cancer and *increased* mortality.[22] The CARET trial was a primary prevention trial in 18,000 high-risk men and women (i.e., current and recent smokers and men who were asbestos-exposed workers) who received either placebo or the combination of β-carotene 30 mg daily and retinyl palmitate 25,000 international units daily for 5 to 8 years.[12] Those receiving β-carotene and retinyl palmitate had an *increased* lung cancer and all-cause mortality, with the excess risk of lung cancer mainly being within women.[23] The Physicians' Health Study evaluated the effects of aspirin, β-carotene (50 mg every other day) in 22,000 healthy males, of which 11% were current smokers and another 39% were former smokers.[12] After an average followup of 12.5 years, β-carotene did not affect lung cancer incidence.[12] Thus, β-carotene appears to be harmful only in high-risk heavy smokers or those with previous asbestos exposure and therefore these individuals should avoid β-carotene supplementation. Several hypotheses are being evaluated to explain the contradictory findings of the epidemiologic studies with these three chemoprevention trials.[12] The chemopreventative effects of selenium, the EGFR inhibitor gefitinib, the cyclooxygenase-2 inhibitor celecoxib, and the farnesyl transferase inhibitor lonafarnib are being evaluated.[8]

DIAGNOSIS

A patient suspected to have lung cancer should undergo a multidisciplinary (including surgeons, radiologists, and medical oncologists) diagnostic evaluation. All patients must also have a thorough history and physical examination with emphasis on detecting signs and symptoms of the primary tumor, regional spread of the tumor, distant metastases, and paraneoplastic syndromes. The patient's performance status should be assessed to determine whether or not a patient may be able to withstand aggressive surgery or chemotherapy. Weight loss, performance status and smoking history are key findings that will direct treatment. Baseline pulmonary function tests should also be obtained.

Chest radiographs, endobronchial ultrasound, CT scans, and positron emission tomography (PET) scans are among the most valuable diagnostic tests.[95] Chest radiography is the primary method of lung cancer detection, and may also be used to measure tumor size, establish gross lymph node enlargement, and detect other tumor-related findings, such as pleural effusion, lobar collapse, and metastatic bone involvement of ribs, spine, and shoulders. In addition, CT may be helpful in the evaluation of parenchymal lung abnormalities, detection of masses only suspected on the chest radiograph, and assessment of mediastinal and hilar lymph nodes. PET scans are reported to be more accurate than CT scans in distinguishing malignant from benign lesions, detecting mediastinal lymph node metastases, and identifying metastatic spread.[24] Most recently, the use of integrated CT-PET technology has been reported to improve the diagnostic accuracy in the staging of NSCLC over either CT or PET technology alone.[24,25]

Pathologic examination of sputum cytology and/or tumor biopsy by bronchoscopy, mediastinoscopy, percutaneous needle biopsy, or open-lung biopsy may be necessary to establish the diagnosis of lung cancer.[95] Mediastinal lymph node sampling via mediastinoscopy or dissection at the time of surgery is important to confirm the presence or absence of lymph node involvement. If mediastinal lymph nodes are found to be involved at the time of surgery, a complete lymph node dissection should be done. Once the diagnosis is established, imaging of additional anatomic locations (e.g., brain) are obtained based on signs and symptoms of the patient and the anticipated treatment plan.

STAGING

The extent (or stage) of the tumor involvement is important because it is used to select therapy, estimate the probability of cure and survival, and facilitate comparison of the individual patient to large-scale clinical trials.

NON–SMALL CELL LUNG CANCER

The World Health Organization has established a TNM staging classification for NSCLC based on the primary tumor size and extent (T), regional lymph node involvement (N), and presence or absence of distant metastases (M) (Table 132–2).[14] For comparison of various therapeutic modalities, a simpler stage grouping system is also used in which stage I refers to tumors confined to the lung without lymphatic spread; stage II refers to large tumors with ipsilateral peribronchial or hilar lymph node involvement; stage III includes other lymph node and regional involvement; and stage IV includes any tumor with distant metastases.[14]

The primary tumor is assessed with chest radiographs and fiberoptic bronchoscopy, whereas lymphatic spread is usually assessed by mediastinoscopy, gallium-67 citrate scanning, and CT and/or PET scans.[10] If the history and physical examination or other routine clinical studies (e.g., complete blood cell count and liver function tests) suggest the possibility of metastatic disease, then additional scans (e.g., bone, brain, or liver) or biopsies (e.g., bone marrow or liver) may be necessary for staging, particularly if the patient is considering aggressive treatment.[10]

SMALL CELL LUNG CANCER

A two-stage classification established by the Veterans Administration Lung Cancer Study Group is widely used in the United States to stage SCLC.[11] Limited stage is classified as disease confined to one hemithorax and to the regional lymph nodes. All other disease is classified as extensive. Approximately 60% to 70% of patients initially present with extensive stage disease. The initial pretreatment evaluation of a SCLC patient should include a medical history, a clinical examination including neurologic examination, laboratory tests (i.e., complete blood cell count with differential, serum electrolytes, liver function tests, calcium, lactate dehydrogenase, blood urea nitrogen, and serum creatinine), and chest radiography.[4,26] Additional testing is guided by suspicious signs or symptoms detected during the physical examination along with common sites of SCLC metastases. Small cell lung cancer cells are detected in an extensive number of sites (e.g., liver 69%; adrenals 65%; bone and bone marrow 54%; pancreas 51%; brain 28% to 50%) during autopsy of patients diagnosed with SCLC.[26] In those with presumed limited-stage SCLC, a CT scan of the chest and abdomen, bone scan, and CT scan or magnetic resonance imaging of the brain are needed.[4,26] A bone marrow biopsy may be obtained if no extrathoracic disease is detected.[4,26]

TABLE 132-2 Tumor (T), Node (N), Metastasis (M) Staging for Non–Small Cell Lung Carcinoma

Primary tumor (T)	
T_x	Positive malignant cells but primary tumor cannot be assessed
T0	No evidence of primary tumor
TIS	Carcinoma in situ
T_1	Tumor ≤3 cm in greatest dimension, surrounded by lung or visceral pleura without bronchoscopic evidence of invasion more proximal than lobar bronchus (i.e., not in the main bronchus)
T_2	Tumor with any of the following features: >3 cm in greatest dimension; involvement of main bronchus, 2 cm or more distal to the carina; invasion of visceral pleura; or associated atelectasis or obstructive pneumonitis extending to hilar region but not including entire lung
T_3	Tumor of any size that direct invades any of the following: chest wall (including superior sulcus tumors), diaphragm, mediastinal pleura, parietal pericardium; or tumor in main bronchus less than 2 cm distal to the carina; or associated atelectasis or obstructive pneumonitis of the entire lung
T_4	Tumor of any size that invades the mediastinum, heart, great vessels, trachea, esophagus, vertebral body, or carina; or separate tumors in same lung; or tumor with a malignant pleural effusion
Regional lymph nodes (N)	
Nx	Regional lymph nodes cannot be assessed
N_0	No regional lymph node involvement
N_1	Metastasis in ipsilateral peribronchial and/or ipsilateral hilar lymph node(s), including direct extension
N_2	Metastasis in ipsilateral mediastinal and/or subcarinal lymph node(s)
N_3	Metastasis in contralateral mediastinal, contralateral hilar, ipsilateral or contralateral scalene, or supraclavicular lymph node(s)
Distant metastasis (M)	
M_x	Distant metastases cannot be assessed
M_0	No distant metastases
M_1	Distant metastases, including separate tumor nodule(s) in a different lobe (ipsilateral or contralateral)

	Stage Groupings			5-Year Survival (%)
Stage IA	T_1	N_0	M_0	67
Stage IB	T_2	N_0	M_0	57
Stage IIA	T_1	N_1	M_0	55
Stage IIB	T_2	N_1	M_0	39
	T_3	N_0	M_0	
Stage IIIA	T_1–T_3	N_2	M_0	23
	T_3	N_1	M_0	
Stage IIIB	Any T	N_3	M_0	3
	T_4	Any N	M_0	7
Stage IV	Any T	Any N	M_1	1

Data from AJCC Cancer Staging Manual, 6th edition, 2002 published by Springer-Verlag, New York. www.cancerstaging.net.

TREATMENT

Non–Small Cell Lung Cancer

❺ If left untreated, most patients with NSCLC will die within 1 year of diagnosis. Surgery, radiation therapy, and systemic therapy with cytotoxic chemotherapy or targeted therapies are all used in the management of NSCLC patients. The application of these various treatment modalities are determined by the stage of NSCLC and the patient's comorbidities and performance status. It is critical that the intent of treatment—whether curative or palliative—is clearly understood prior to starting treatment, as it will influence the aggressiveness of therapy. Favorable prognostic factors for survival include early stage disease, performance status ≤2 based on the Eastern Cooperative Group (ECOG) scale, no more than 5% unintentional weight loss, and female gender.[3] Table 132–3 lists commonly used chemotherapy regimens for NSCLC and SCLC treatment.

Stages I and II Non–Small Cell Lung Cancer

❺ ❻ Surgical resection (pneumonectomy or lobectomy) is first-line treatment for patients with stages I and II ($T_{1-2}N_0$ and $T_{1-2}N_1$) NSCLC with the exception of T_3N_0, for which the treatment is discussed with stage III disease. Overall, about 60% to 70% of patients with stage I and 40% to 50% of patients with stage II disease who undergo complete surgical resection survive 5 years without disease recurrence.[25] The most important prognostic factors for patients undergoing surgical resection are the size of the tumor, the presence or absence of lymph node involvement, and residual tumor in the surgical margins.[3]

Removal of the involved lobe of the lung (e.g., lobectomy) is the recommended surgical procedure for stage I tumors, but some studies show that pneumonectomy may reduce the rate of local recurrences for patients with larger-size stage IB tumors.[27] Pneumonectomy, or removal of the entire lung (versus lobectomy), is the recommended surgical procedure for stage II disease with lymph node involvement ($T_{1-3}N_1$). Despite complete resection, many patients with stage II disease develop recurrent disease and die within 2 years.[10]

Clinical trials of adjuvant radiotherapy in early stage NSCLC have yielded conflicting results.[25,28,29] The postoperative radiotherapy meta-analysis in 2,128 patients showed a 21% *increase* in the relative risk of death for those receiving radiotherapy with the most deleterious effects in patients with N_0 or N_1 disease.[29] Consequently, adjuvant radiotherapy is recommended only in those patients with detectable NSCLC cells at the edge of the resected lung tissue (termed *positive margins*) when a second resection is not possible. By eliminating the residual disease and reducing the risk of local disease recurrence, radiotherapy in this setting is curative.

The role of adjuvant cytotoxic chemotherapy in early stage NSCLC has been subject to much debate. Early clinical trials, including the Adjuvant Lung Cancer Project Italy (ALPI) and Big Lung Trial (BLT), failed to demonstrate a survival benefit to adjuvant chemotherapy.[30,31] However, recently published trials report that adjuvant cytotoxic chemotherapy is beneficial in early stage NSCLC (i.e., stages I to IIIA). The International Adjuvant Lung Cancer Trial (IALT) Collaborative Group reported a 17% relative improvement in disease-free survival and a 4.1% absolute increase in overall survival for patients receiving cisplatin-based adjuvant therapy versus those receiving no adjuvant therapy.[32] This trial included 1,867 patients with stages I, II, and III NSCLC who received cisplatin in combination with etoposide, vinblastine, vinorelbine, or vindesine, as chosen by the treating oncologist. Radiation therapy was administered after chemotherapy based on the preference of the treating physician. Additional trials have been conducted to clarify the role of adjuvant chemotherapy for the treatment of early stage NSCLC including the Cancer and Leukemia Group B (CALGB), Adjuvant Navelbine International Trialist Association (ANITA), and the National Cancer Institute of Canada (NCIC) JBR.10. Both the ANITA and JBR.10 trials report a statistically significant improvement in 5-year overall survival (Table 132–4). The absolute benefit in 5-year overall survival of adjuvant chemotherapy was 4.1% in the IALT trial, 8.6% in the ANITA trial, and 15% in the JBR.10 trial,[33] all of which exceed the 3.2% absolute benefit in 5-year overall survival with adjuvant chemotherapy for early stage breast cancer.[32] The role of adjuvant chemotherapy in patients with stage IB NSCLC is not clear. Adjuvant chemotherapy failed to improve survival in the stage IB subgroup of the ANITA and JBR.10 trials. The

TABLE 132-3 Common Chemotherapy Regimens Used to Treat Lung Cancer

Non-small cell lung carcinoma[3]	
Cisplatin/paclitaxel (CP)	Cisplatin 75 mg/m² IV day 1 Paclitaxel 175 mg/m² over 24 hours IV day 1 repeat cycle every 21 days[42] *or* Cisplatin 80 mg/m² IV day 1 Paclitaxel 175 mg/m² IV over 3 hours day 1 repeat cycle every 21 days[87]
Gemcitabine/cisplatin (GC)	Gemcitabine 1,000 mg/m² IV days 1, 8, 15 Cisplatin 100 mg/m² IV day 1 repeat cycle every 28 days[42]
Gemcitabine/cisplatin (GCq21)	Gemcitabine 1,200 mg/m² days 1 and 8 Cisplatin 80 mg/m² IV day 1 repeat cycle every 21 days[88] *or* Gemcitabine 1,250 mg/m² days 1 and 8 Cisplatin 80 mg/m² IV day 1 repeat cycle every 21 days[87]
Docetaxel/cisplatin (DC)	Docetaxel 75 mg/m² IV day 1 Cisplatin 75 mg/m² IV day 1 repeat cycle every 21 days[42]
Paclitaxel/carboplatin (PCb)	Paclitaxel 225 mg/m² over 3 hours IV day 1 Carboplatin AUC 6 mcg*h/mL IV day 1 repeat cycle every 21 days[42,43] *or* Paclitaxel 175 mg/m² IV over 3 hours day 1 Carboplatin AUC 6 mcg*h/mL IV day 1 repeat cycle every 21 days for 6 cycles[89]
Vinorelbine/cisplatin (VC)	Vinorelbine 25 mg/m² IV weekly Cisplatin 100 mg/m² IV day 1 repeat cycle every 28 days[43] *or* Vinorelbine 30 mg/m² IV days 1 and 8 Cisplatin 80 mg/m² IV day 1 repeat cycle every 21 days[88]
Etoposide/cisplatin (EP)	Etoposide 100 mg/m² IV days 1, 2, and 3 Cisplatin 100 mg/m² IV day 1 repeat cycle every 28 days[32]
Vinorelbine/gemcitabine (VG)	Vinorelbine 25 mg/m² IV days 1 and 8 Gemcitabine 1,000 mg/m² days 1 and 8 Repeat cycle every 21 days[88,90]
Paclitaxel/gemcitabine (PG)	Paclitaxel 175 mg/m² IV over 3 hours day 1 Gemcitabine 1,250 mg/m² days 1 and 8 repeat cycle every 21 days[87]
Gemcitabine/docetaxel (GD)	Gemcitabine 1,000 mg/m² IV days 1 and 8 Docetaxel 100 mg/m² IV day 8 repeat cycle every 21 days[91]
Paclitaxel/vinorelbine (PV)	Paclitaxel 135 mg/m² IV day 1 Vinorelbine 25 mg/m² IV day 1 repeat cycle every 14 days for 9 cycles[89]
Small cell lung carcinoma[4]	
Etoposide/cisplatin (EP)	Cisplatin 80 mg/m² IV day 1 Etoposide 100 mg/m² IV days 1, 2, and 3 repeat cycle every 3 weeks[83,92] *or* Cisplatin 60 mg/m² IV day 1 Etoposide 120 mg/m² IV days 1, 2, and 3 repeat cycle every 3 weeks[84]
Cisplatin/irinotecan (IP)	Cisplatin 60 mg/m² IV day 1 Irinotecan 60 mg/m² IV days 1, 8, and 15 repeat cycle every 4 weeks[83,92] *or* Cisplatin 30 mg/m² IV day 1 Irinotecan 65 mg/m² IV days 1 and 8 repeat cycle every 3 weeks[84]

TABLE 132-4 Adjuvant Chemotherapy for Early Stage Lung Cancer

Trial	Stage	N	Treatment Arms	Number of Cycles	Postoperative Radiotherapy	5-Year Survival	P Value
BLT[30,31]	I–IV	381	Observation		Per individual institutional policy	60% (2-year)	0.90
			Cisplatin plus vindesine; mitomycin/ifosfamide; mitomycin/vinblastine; or vinorelbine	3		74% (2-year)	
IALT[32]	I–III	1867	Observation		Per individual institutional policy	40.4%	0.03
			Cisplatin-based doublet (etoposide, vindesine, vinorelbine, vinblastine)			44.5%	
ALPI[30,31]	I–IIIA	1209	Observation		Per individual institutional policy	No difference seen in overall survival	0.585
			Cisplatin, mitomycin, and vindesine	3			
ANITA[35,93]	I–IIIA	840	Observation		Per individual institutional policy	43%	0.017
			Vinorelbine/cisplatin	4		51%	
JBR.10[33]	IB–II	482	Observation		None	54%	0.002
			Vinorelbine/cisplatin	4		69%	
CALGB 9633[94]	IB	344	Observation		None	57%	0.32
			Paclitaxel/carboplatin	4		60%	

ALPI, Adjuvant Lung Cancer Project Italy; ANITA, Adjuvant Novelbine International Trialist Association; BLT, Big Lung Trial; CALGB, Cancer and Leukemia Group B; IALT, International Adjuvant Lung Cancer Trial; JBR.10, National Cancer Institute of Canada JBR10.10.

CALGB trial was designed to evaluate the role of adjuvant chemotherapy in stage IB NSCLC patients. Preliminary results of that trial show a significant improvement in 3-year survival (79% vs. 70%, $p = 0.045$), but no difference in 5-year overall survivial. Several hypotheses have been offered to explain the difference in results amongst the trials: Both the ALPI and BLT trials used older, less active chemotherapy regimens (e.g. mitomycin-vindesine-cisplatin), while the BLT was underpowered and had a short duration of followup. Other differences include cisplatin dosing, number of dropouts, and number of patients receiving radiotherapy. Although the answer is unclear, in light of several trials reporting a survival benefit with adjuvant chemotherapy, a paradigm shift for patients with stage IB, II, or IIIA NSCLC has occurred.[3,34] The benefit of adjuvant therapy in patients with stage I disease is not as clear and requires further research. Thus, cisplatin-based systemic chemotherapy without radiation therapy following surgical resection is recommended for patients with stage II NSCLC.[3,95]

CLINICAL CONTROVERSY

The benefit of adjuvant cytotoxic chemotherapy for patients with stage I NSCLC is unclear. Adjuvant cytotoxic chemotherapy improves overall survival in patients with later stages (i.e., stage II to IIIA) NSCLC. However, there are limited numbers of patients with stage IA enrolled in these trials and the data does not suggest a survival benefit. Additional clinical trials of the role of adjuvant cytotoxic chemotherapy is needed in patients with stage IA NSCLC.

Patients with stages I and II NSCLC who refuse surgery or who are considered poor surgical candidates because of concomitant illness or minimal pulmonary reserve, are treated with radiotherapy alone (i.e., without chemotherapy or surgery).[3] Radiotherapy is also used when the tumor is unresectable because of fixation to a major blood vessel, the trachea, or the esophagus. Of those patients, the 2- and 5-year survival rates appear to be highest for patients whose tumors would otherwise be considered resectable. Patients who have recurrent disease following surgical resection are usually managed similarly to those who present with stage IV disease (see Unresectable Stage IIIB and Stage IV Non–Small Cell Lung Cancer).

Stages IIB and III Non–Small Cell Lung Cancer

❼ The prognosis for patients with either stage IIIA or IIIB NSCLC is poor, with 5-year survival rates ranging from 10% to 40%, depending on tumor size, tumor location, and lymph node involvement.[10] Optimal management of patients with locally advanced NSCLC stage IIB (T_3N_0), IIIA ($T_{1-3}N_2$, T_3N_1), and potentially resectable IIIB (T_4N_{0-1}) tumors is controversial. Improvements in diagnostic imaging of NSCLC has led to more accurate staging of NSCLC patients and many patients who were classified as stage III NSCLC in earlier studies would most likely be diagnosed with stage IV disease today. Evaluation of the results from earlier clinical trials must consider this stage shift. Presently, there is wide variability in this group of patients and also their treatment. All three treatment modalities—surgery, radiation, and chemotherapy—are used for most stage III patients, although the timing of their application varies based on the physical location and size of the primary tumor and nodal status.

As with early stage NSCLC, surgery followed by postoperative radiotherapy and/or cisplatin-based chemotherapy is an acceptable treatment plan, although the role of both radiation and chemotherapy is not as well defined.[3] The use of postoperative radiotherapy varied in the adjuvant chemotherapy trials (see Table 132–4), providing little guidance for its use. As mentioned above, the 1998 meta-analysis of postoperative radiotherapy showed a detrimental effect in stages I/II disease, yet despite an improvement in locoregional control, neither a positive or negative effect on survival was seen in stage III disease.[29] One major criticism of the 1998 postoperative radiotherapy meta-analysis is the radiation techniques used in those trials are antiquated, leading to more toxicity and potentially more treatment-related deaths. Given the improvement in modern radiation delivery, postoperative radiotherapy remains a reasonable treatment plan to improve locoregional disease.[3] Radiotherapy given without chemotherapy, however, does not impact overall survival rates because many of these patients develop systemic (distant) metastases.[28] Thus, adjuvant chemotherapy is used to prevent distant recurrence. Patients with stage IIIA disease were included in many of the adjuvant chemotherapy trials (ANITA 39%, BLT 26%, and IALT 39%).[31,32,35] Both the IALT and ANITA trials demonstrated a significant survival improvement with adjuvant chemotherapy in stage IIIA patients. Based on these data, adjuvant chemotherapy is likely to provide a 5% to 10% improvement in survival.[36] Because other studies have failed to show the same advantage and given the inconsistent use of postoperative radiotherapy in these trials, more data are needed to clearly define optimal adjuvant therapy.

In patients with surgically resectable (N_{0-1} or limited N_2 disease), locally advanced stages IIB, IIIA, and a rare subset of IIIB disease, neoadjuvant chemotherapy with or without concurrent radiotherapy, followed by surgery, improves local and regional control and overall survival when compared to preoperative radiation followed by surgery.[3,4,28] The possible advantages of neoadjuvant therapy include earlier treatment of systemic disease, tumor regression that increases the likelihood of a complete surgical resection, improved patient compliance, and the ability to pathologically assess the response to chemotherapy, which may help guide future treatment.[36] Neoadjuvant cisplatin-based doublet combinations are generally recommended.[10] Superior sulcus tumors (T_{3-4}, N_{0-1}) are treated with radiotherapy and concurrent chemotherapy followed by surgery, if resectable.[3] If the tumor is not resectable, NCCN guidelines recommend treatment with definitive concurrent chemoradiation.[3]

Given the vast heterogeneity and the multiple treatment modalities available, patients with N_2 disease require evaluation for the possibility of distant metastasis in order to determine the timing and role of surgery. If distant metastasis are not present and patient has $T_{1-2}N_2$ disease, neoadjuvant chemotherapy with or without radiation is recommended.[3] If N_2 disease is not identified until surgery, adjuvant chemotherapy with or without concurrent radiotherapy is used to reduce the risk of systemic and local disease recurrence. Large phase III trials continue to evaluate various combinations of neoadjuvant therapy versus initial surgery followed by adjuvant therapy. Both neoadjuvant and adjuvant therapies use cisplatin-based doublets with or without radiotherapy. Accurate disease staging, consistent eligibility criteria, and multidisciplinary communication are essential to the success of these trials in elucidating the role of future neoadjuvant therapy in locally advanced NSCLC, as well as the ideal adjuvant therapy. Patients who recur following localized treatment for stage III NSCLC are managed similarly to those with newly diagnosed stage IV NSCLC.

Unresectable Stage IIIB and Stage IV Non–Small Cell Lung Cancer

❼ About two-thirds of NSCLC patients present with advanced (i.e., unresectable stage IIIB and IV) disease at the time of diagnosis. Most of these advanced tumors are not surgically resectable as a result of disseminated (multiple sites) metastatic disease or metastatic sites that are not amenable to surgery. Patients with single metastatic sites may undergo surgical resection of both the primary tumor in the lung and the metastatic site.[3]

Chemotherapy is the first-line therapy for most patients with advanced NSCLC. The intent of chemotherapy is to palliate symptoms, improve quality of life, and increase the duration of survival. Improved response rates, a modest increase in survival, and decreased toxicity profiles observed with many of the newer chemotherapy agents and combination regimens have led experts to agree that most patients with stage IV disease should receive at least one chemotherapy regimen.[3–5]

In the setting of advanced NSCLC, the potential benefits—both in terms of overall survival and quality of life—of cytotoxic chemotherapy were not clearly established until the 1990s. The Non–Small Cell Lung Cancer Collaborative Group reported the pivotal results of a large meta-analysis encompassing more than 25 years and 52 clinical trials of chemotherapy in the management of NSCLC.[37] The results of this meta-analysis and other evidence suggest that chemotherapy, when combined with either surgery and/or radiotherapy, improves median survival for patients with advanced stage NSCLC by 2 to 4 months and increases the 1-year survival rate by 10% to 20%.[25,37] Several studies have compared chemotherapy to the best supportive care and have shown consistently better outcomes for chemotherapy.[10,37]

Both the NCCN and American Society of Clinical Oncology guidelines recommend first-line chemotherapy consisting of a doublet with a platinum (i.e., cisplatin or carboplatin) and a newer agent (i.e., gemcitabine, paclitaxel, docetaxel and vinorelbine) (see Table 132–3). Older non–platinum-containing regimens and regimens containing alkylating agents generally produced inferior outcomes.[25]

The results of first-line chemotherapy in patients with advanced NSCLC depend on the patient's current performance status and comorbidities.[10] An initial favorable performance status (ECOG performance status of 0 to 2) appears to be the most consistent predictor of a better response and improved survival after chemotherapy. All patients with good performance status without significant comorbidities, including elderly patients, should receive first-line doublet chemotherapy. Single-agent chemotherapy should be considered in those patients with an ECOG performance status 2 (PS-2) or significant comorbidities. Patients with poor ECOG performance status (≥PS-3) do not respond well to chemotherapy.[10] Patients with an unfavorable prognosis (poor performance status or significant concomitant diseases) should receive best supportive care and palliative radiation when necessary.[3,4,25]

First-line platinum-based doublet chemotherapy is usually administered for a total number of four to six cycles in those patients whose NSCLC is stable or responding to chemotherapy.[3–5] The optimal number of cycles remains controversial. Response rates and quality of life were not improved with the administration of six, as compared to three, cycles of mitomycin, cisplatin and vinblastine.[38] For those receiving paclitaxel-carboplatin (PCb), administration of chemotherapy until disease progression had no clinically significant benefit in survival, response rate, or quality of life, but increased toxicity as compared to administration of four cycles.[39]

Second-line chemotherapy is usually offered to those patients with an ECOG performance status of 0 to 2 who experience disease progression to or after first-line chemotherapy. Third-line therapy can be offered if disease progression continues in a patient with adequate performance status. Best supportive care is recommended by the NCCN guidelines for those patients with disease progression and an ECOG performance status worse than 2.[3]

Single-Agent Chemotherapy Single-agent chemotherapy is an alternative in elderly patients or those with an ECOG performance status of 2.[3] First-line, single-agent chemotherapy has objective response rates of 5% to 25% with no significant effect on overall survival.[10] Complete responses are rare and those that do occur are of brief duration (i.e., 2 to 4 months).[10] Among the most active cytotoxic chemotherapy agents in NSCLC are cisplatin, carboplatin, docetaxel, paclitaxel, etoposide, gemcitabine, ifosfamide, irinotecan, topotecan, mitomycin, vinblastine, vinorelbine, and pemetrexed. The EGFR inhibitor, erlotinib, is also active as a single agent, as discussed later in Human Epidermal Growth Factor Receptor Inhibitors.

Combination Chemotherapy Response rates for combination chemotherapy regimens are generally higher than for single-agent therapy, but improvement in overall survival rates has not been consistently observed.[40] Combination chemotherapy regimens that have consistently reported response rates exceeding 30% have used various combinations of cisplatin, carboplatin, gemcitabine, ifosfamide, or mitomycin, and vinblastine, vindesine, or vinorelbine (Tables 132–3 and 132–5). Some studies show that cisplatin dose may have an impact on tumor response, and the most widely recommended first-line regimens now include a platinum—either cisplatin or carboplatin—with a newer cytotoxic chemotherapy agent.

Until the mid-1990s, first-line chemotherapy with etoposide and cisplatin (EP) was regarded as the most active regimen in the treatment of advanced NSCLC.[10] Subsequently, numerous randomized controlled clinical trials demonstrated that a platinum-based doublet with a newer cytotoxic chemotherapy agent had superior response rates or median survival rates. Each of these newer chemotherapeutic agents had single-agent activity of greater than 20% in NSCLC and include plant alkaloids (i.e., vinorelbine), taxanes (i.e.,

TABLE 132-5 First-Line Combination Regimens in Stage IIIB or IV Non–Small Cell Lung Cancer

Reference	Number Evaluable/ Performance Status	Regimen	Overall Response Rate (%)	Median Survival Duration	Median 1-Year Survival (%)	Time to Disease Progression
Schiller et al. (ECOG 1594)[42]	1,155	CP	21%	7.8 mo	31%	3.4 mo
	1,083 PS-0–1, 63 PS-2	GC	22%	8.1 mo	36%	4.2 mo[a]
		DC	17%	7.4 mo	31%	3.7 mo
		PCb	17%	8.1 mo	34%	3.1 mo
Kelly et al. (SWOG)[43]	408	PCb	PR 27%	8 mo	36%	NR
	All PS-0–1	VC	PR 27%	8 mo	33%	NR
		EP	22%	7.2 mo	NR	7.2 mo
Gridelli et al.[88]	503	VG	25%	8 mo	31%	4.3 mo
	PS-0–2	GCq21	30%	9.5 mo	38%	5.8 mo
		VCq21				
Smit et al. (EORTC)[87]	458	CP	32%	8.1 mo	36%	4.2 mo
	PS-0–2	GCq21	37%	8.9 mo	33%	5.1 mo
		PG	28%	6.7 mo	27%	3.5 mo[b]
Georgeoulias et al.[91]	389	GD	30%	9 mo	34%	4 mo
	PS-0–2	VC	39%	9.7 mo	41%	5 mo
Stathopoulos et al.[89]	360	PV	43%	10 mo	38%	6 mo
	PS-0–2	PCb	46%	11 mo	43%	7 mo

CP, cisplatin and paclitaxel; DC, docetaxel and cisplatin; ECOG, Eastern Cooperative Oncology Group; EORTC, European Organziation for Research and Treatment of Cancer; EP, etoposide and cisplatin; GC, gemicitabine and cisplatin; GCq21, gemcitabine and cisplatin repeated every 21 days; GD, gemcitabine and docetaxel; NR, not reported; PCb, paclitaxel and carboplatin; PG, paclitaxel and gemcitabine; PR, partial response; PS, performance status; PV, paclitaxel and vinorelbine; SWOG, Southwest Oncology Group; VC, vinorelbine and cisplatin; VG, vinorelbine and gemcitabine.

[a]Statistically significant difference.

[b]Statistically significant difference between CP and PG, but not CP and GCq21.

From National Comprehensive Cancer Network.[3]

paclitaxel and docetaxel), antimetabolites (i.e., gemcitabine), antifolates (i.e., pemetrexed), and topoisomerase I inhibitors (i.e., topotecan and irinotecan).[41] Results from many published trials combining these new chemotherapy agents with platinum-based regimens suggest improved 1-year survival rates in advanced NSCLC of 30% to 40% versus 15% to 25% with the older cisplatin-based combination regimens.[42–44] Table 132–5 lists the results of selected phase III trials of chemotherapy in patients with advanced NSCLC.

Similar survival and response rates have been reported with platinum-based doublet chemotherapy regimens that include one of these newer cytotoxic chemotherapy agents.[42] The efficacy and toxicity of the control arm—cisplatin and paclitaxel (CP)—were compared to that of three platinum-containing regimens (i.e., cisplatin and either gemcitabine [GC] or docetaxel [DC]) versus PCb in a large, randomized, controlled clinical trial conducted by ECOG. The trial enrolled 1,155 patients with poor-prognosis stage IIIB (pleural or pericardial effusion refractory to radiotherapy) or stage IV NSCLC. Patients were stratified by performance status and baseline weight loss. Patients with performance status 0 to 2 were initially eligible for the trial, but an interim analysis revealed that patients with a performance status of 2 experienced increased toxicity with the cisplatin-containing regimens, and the study was subsequently limited to patients with performance status 0 or 1. There were no significant differences between the control arm of CP and the other three regimens in response rate, median survival, or 1-year survival (see Table 132–5) The GC regimen resulted in a modest 1-month advantage in time-to-disease progression (P = 0.002) and had the lowest incidence of severe neutropenia and febrile neutropenia. However, the GC regimen had a higher incidence of severe thrombocytopenia and moderate-to-severe renal dysfunction. Moderate nausea was a problem for all of the cisplatin-containing regimens and was the greatest in the GC regimen with the higher dosage of cisplatin (100 mg/m^2 vs. 75 mg/m^2). The PCb regimen was the best-tolerated regimen, but it also had the lowest response rate and time to disease progression. Overall, the results of the four regimens were similar in this trial, and no clear advantage was observed for one regimen over another.[42] This trial helped to move research in advanced NSCLC toward targeted therapies, as it documented that the best available cytotoxic chemotherapy led to a plateau in survival rates.

In the palliative setting of treating advanced NSCLC, several trials have evaluated if less-toxic carboplatin has similar efficacy to cisplatin. In a large phase III trial, Rosell et al. randomized patients to receive paclitaxel 200 mg/m^2 (3-hour infusion) with either cisplatin 80 mg/m^2 (CP) or carboplatin AUC (area-under-the-curve) 6 mcg*h/mL (PCb). While the response rates were not significantly different (28% for CP vs. 25% for PCb), median survival was significantly longer in the CP arm as compared with the PCb arm (9.8 vs. 8.2 months, $P = 0.019$). Patients treated with CP had more gastrointestinal and renal toxicities, while those treated with PCb had more hematologic toxicities. Overall quality of life was similar between the arms.[45] In a meta-analysis of eight randomized trials of a cisplatin-based versus a carboplatin-based regimen (N = 2,948), cisplatin-based regimens were associated with a higher objective response rate (odds ratio = 1.36, $P < 0.001$) and an improved overall survival that was not statistically significant. Subset analysis of five trials comparing cisplatin plus a newer agent versus carboplatin and a newer agent resulted in an 11% improvement in survival (P = 0.039) with the cisplatin-containing regimens.[46] Based on the above trials, many clinicians prefer cisplatin over carboplatin in combination with a newer agent in patients with a good performance status.

Nonplatinum doublets (e.g., gemcitabine-paclitaxel) have also been evaluated in the setting of first-line therapy of advanced NSCLC. The results of a meta-analysis comparing platinum-based regimens with either the same regimen without the platinum or with the platinum replaced by another agent demonstrated the importance of the platinum in the chemotherapy regimen.[47] Thirty-seven trials with a total of 7,633 patients were included in the meta-analysis. The overall 1-year survival was 34% and 29% in the platinum-containing regimens and nonplatinum regimens, respectively. A significant improvement in 1-year survival was noted when comparing platinum-based regimens to single-agent nonplatinum regimens (35% vs. 25%, P = 0.001) or nonplatinum combination regimens (37% vs. 31%, P = 0.0057). However, no significant difference was demonstrated when single-agent regimens were excluded and platinum-based combination regimens were compared to nonplatinum combination regimens (36% vs. 35%, P = 0.17).[47] Although platinum-based combination regimens remain the standard of care, further information is needed to elucidate the role of non–platinum-containing combination regimens. Table 132–3 lists examples of such combinations.

Addition of a third drug to platinum-based doublets has not consistently demonstrated benefit and in some cases has been associated with increased toxicity.[48] One trial to date has demonstrated a survival benefit with a three-drug combination. In that phase III trial, 324 patients were randomized to paclitaxel-carboplatin-gemcitabine (PCG) or PCb.[49] The response rates were 46% and 20% (P <0.0001), median overall survival 10.8 months and 8.3 months (P = 0.032), and 1-year overall survival rates were 45% and 34% (P = 0.032) for PCG and PCb arms, respectively. Grades 3 and 4 hematologic toxicities were significantly higher in the PCG arm, resulting in significantly more platelet (6% vs. 0%, P = 0.004) and red cell transfusions (21.5% vs. 8.4%, P = 0.002). In contrast, a number of novel agents, including tirapazamine and a matrix metalloproteinase inhibitor, have been added to PCb with no improvement in survival and a substantial increase in toxicity.[50,51] Vascular endothelial growth factor (VEGF) inhibitors, as discussed below, in combination with doublet chemotherapy, may offer benefit to some patient populations.

Historically, ECOG PS-2 patients were excluded from NSCLC trials because of excessive toxicity with minimal benefit from combination cytotoxic therapy. With better supportive care therapies, 63 patients were enrolled in ECOG 1594, but accrual of PS-2 patients was halted early in the trial because of a perceived increase in toxicity.[42] To clarify the role of platinum-based doublet chemotherapy, a phase II trial was conducted in advanced-stage PS-2 NSCLC patients in which patients were randomized to dose attenuated PCb or GC.[52] Overall response rate and disease control rates were 23% versus 14% and 55% versus 53% in the PCb and GC arms, respectively. Patients in the PCb arm experienced more neutropenia and sensory neuropathy, whereas the GC arm had more thrombocytopenia, nausea/vomiting, fatigue, and elevation in serum creatinine. Consequently, PS-2 patients may be considered for combination cytotoxic therapy.

In summary, cisplatin-based doublets improve survival and quality of life as compared to best supportive care or single-agent chemotherapy in patients with advanced NSCLC. The optimal combination regimen has not yet been identified. The role of non–platinum-based combination regimens and triple-combination regimens remains to be defined.

Second-Line Chemotherapy ❽ Docetaxel, pemetrexed, and erlotinib are options for second-line therapy in patients with a good performance status who progress during or after first-line chemotherapy. Docetaxel was the first agent to receive FDA approval for the treatment of advanced NSCLC after failure of a platinum-based chemotherapy regimen. The initial docetaxel dose of 100 mg/m^2 (D 100) IV over 1 hour every 21 days was decreased to 75 mg/m^2 (D 75) after an interim analysis showed a greater risk of severe neutropenia with the higher dose. Docetaxel, at the D 75 dose, was superior to best supportive care in terms of time-to-disease progression (10.6 weeks vs. 6.7 weeks; P = 0.001), median survival (7.5 months vs. 4.6 months; P = 0.047), and 1-year survival (37% vs. 11%; P = 0.003).[53] D75 and D100 had a statistically significant improvement in 1-year survival when compared to a control regimen of vinorelbine or ifosfamide (32%, 21%, and 19%, respectively).[54]

Subsequently, pemetrexed (Alimta) was FDA approved for second-line treatment of advanced NSCLC based on results of a phase III trial. In that trial, 571 patients were randomized to receive either pemetrexed 500 mg/m^2 with folate and cyanocobalamin supplementation or D 75. There was no significant difference seen in overall response rate, stable disease, or median survival for the pemetrexed and docetaxel arms. Docetaxel had significantly more hematologic toxicities as compared to pemetrexed, leading to more hospitalizations and use of growth factors and erythropoiesis stimulating agents. Patients receiving docetaxel had a significantly higher rate of alopecia, while patients receiving pemetrexed had a significantly higher elevation in alanine aminotransferase.[55]

CLINICAL CONTROVERSY

There is no consensus regarding the optimal second-line treatment of patients with NSCLC. Pemetrexed and docetaxel have similar response and survival rates. These two cytotoxic chemotherapy agents have differing toxicity profiles which may help choose treatment for an individual patient.

Although not FDA approved for NSCLC, oral topotecan has demonstrated efficacy similar to docetaxel as a second-line agent. The toxicity profiles of the two agents are different in that topotecan is associated with more anemia, thrombocytopenia, nausea, vomiting and diarrhea, while docetaxel is associated with more neutropenia, alopecia, pyrexia, cough and neuropathy.[56]

Human Epidermal Growth Factor Receptor Inhibitors The human epidermal growth factor receptor (HER) family consists of four receptors that are amplified to a varying degree in several different solid tumors. HER-2/*neu* is the second receptor within the family and is overexpressed in 20% to 30% of breast cancers. Given the success seen with the use of trastuzumab (Herceptin) in breast cancer and the presence of HER-2/*neu* overexpression in NSCLC, a phase II trial was conducted to evaluate the tolerability and efficacy of trastuzumab in combination with PCb. The addition of trastuzumab did not alter the toxicity profile of PCb alone and response rates were similar to historical data of chemotherapy alone. Several early phase trials were conducted with trastuzumab, but more mature and prospective data are needed.[57]

The EGFR (also known as HER1) was the first tyrosine kinase receptor within the HER family to be discovered. Signals initiated by cell surface membrane EGFRs are vital in the proliferation and survival of cancer cells. Recognition that many NSCLCs overexpress the EGFR has led to the evaluation of several EGFR inhibitors in the management of NSCLC.[58,59] These agents include small molecules that block the intracellular tyrosine kinase portion of the EGFR (i.e., gefitinib, erlotinib) and anti-EGFR monoclonal antibodies (i.e., cetuximab and panitumumab).

Gefitinib (Iressa) was the first EGFR inhibitor to be approved by the FDA, with its indication as a single agent for patients with advanced NSCLC whose disease progressed despite both platinum-based doublet and docetaxel regimens. Early clinical trials in heavily pretreated patients showed that gefitinib was well tolerated and resulted in antitumor responses in 12% to 18% of patients.[60,61] However, the Iressa Survival Evaluation in Lung Cancer (ISEL), a postmarketing trial required by the FDA, failed to demonstrate a survival advantage for those receiving gefitinib as compared with best supportive care.[62] Thus, the FDA restricted the use of gefitinib to patients who continue to benefit from the medication or who are enrolled in a clinical trial.

A second EGFR inhibitor, erlotinib (Tarceva), was approved by the FDA in November 2004 as a single agent for patients with locally advanced or metastatic NSCLC after failure of at least one prior chemotherapy regimen. Its approval was based on an international, multicenter, randomized, double-blind phase III trial (BR.21) in 731 patients with locally advanced or metastatic NSCLC who had failed at least one prior chemotherapy regimen.[63] Patients were randomized to receive either erlotinib 150 mg or placebo orally once daily. Patients in the erlotinib group had a significantly higher objective response rate (9% vs. 1%, P <0.001) and longer median progression-free and overall survival (9.9 weeks vs. 7.9 weeks, P <0.001 and 6.7 months vs. 4.7 months [hazard ratio = 0.73], P <0.001, respectively) than those in the placebo group. Patients in the erlotinib group also had significantly improved symptom control, specifically time to deterioration of cough, dyspnea, and pain.

Because of their benefit in the second- or third-line setting, the potential benefit of adding erlotinib or gefitinib to doublet platinum-based chemotherapy was studied.[64,65] Two large, randomized phase III studies failed to demonstrate improved response rates or survival when gefitinib was added to chemotherapy as compared to chemotherapy alone.[64,65] The TRIBUTE study randomly assigned 1,079 patients with advanced stage, previously untreated NSCLC to PCb with or without erlotinib 150 mg daily. The addition of erlotinib did not improve response rate, time to progression, or overall survival. A subset analysis of never smokers showed an significant improvement in survival with erlotinib of 22.5 months as compared to 10.1 months in the placebo arm (hazard ratio = 0.49, 95% CI 0.28 to 0.85). No survival difference was observed in the chemotherapy-alone arm for those who never smoked compared to smokers.[66] Similar results were seen when erlotinib was added to GC in the Tarceva Lung Cancer Investigation Trial (TALENT) trial.[59]

Several factors correlate with response to EGFR inhibitors. Analyses of the gefitinib trials showed that responses were more common in women, patients who had never smoked, and in patients with bronchoalveolar carcinomas or adenocarcinomas with bronchoalveolar features. Interestingly, the intensity of immunohistochemical staining of the tumor for EGFR did not correlate with the likelihood of a response.[59] Tumors with heterozygous mutations within the tyrosine kinase portion of the EGFR are more likely to respond to gefitinib.[67] These mutations appear to activate growth factor signaling as a result of enhanced stabilization between the tyrosine kinase and adenosine triphosphate or its competitive inhibitor, gefitinib. Prospective evaluation of this molecular marker may assist clinicians in selecting patients who are most likely to respond to this targeted therapy. One small prospective study in Japan examined 75 patients for an EGFR mutation, specifically a somatic mutation in exons 18 to 23. EGFR mutations were identified in 25 patients (33%), most of whom were female (P <0.01) and either never smoked or were light smokers (P <0.01). Of the 16 patients who were enrolled in the study, partial responses were observed in 12 patients (75%) and stable disease in two patients (12.5%).[68] Two additional small studies demonstrated similar results.[69] Similar to the gefitinib data, multivariate analysis of BR.21 identified never smoking, Asian origin, and adenocarcinoma as independent predictors of survival to erlotinib therapy.[63]

Subsequent work on predictors of response to erlotinib suggested that those with tumors overexpressing EGFR had an improvement in overall survival for those treated with erlotinib compared to placebo.[59,70] EGFR mutations are also associated with an improvement in clinical response to erlotinib, but no increase in survival. Almost 200 EGFR mutations have been identified in NSCLC throughout exons 18 through 21, with the majority resulting from deletions that lead to the elimination of four amino acids (LREA) encoded by exon 19 and a point mutation in exon 21 (L858R).[69] Mutations are most commonly seen in NSCLC tumors from women, never smokers, adenocarcinoma, and patients of East Asian decent.[59]

Cetuximab is an immunoglobulin G_1 monoclonal antibody that binds to the extracellular portion of the EGFR.[58] Cetuximab may be advantageous to the tyrosine kinase inhibitors of EGFR because it also may exhibit antibody dependent cellular cytotoxicity and down-regulation of the receptor by internalization. Early trials demonstrated that cetuximab is safe and well tolerated when added to paclitaxel-carboplatin (CPC) as well as gemcitabine-carboplatin (CGC).[58,71] The CPC regimen was studied in 31 chemotherapy-naive NSCLC patients, while 35 chemotherapy-naive patients received the CGC regimen. Complete or partial response was shown in 26% and 29% and a 1-year survival rate was 40% and 46% in the CPC and GCG regimens, respectively. Both studies included patients with immunohistochemical evidence of EGFR expression (≥1+) and demonstrated a response rate similar to historical controls of chemotherapy alone. Randomized studies are ongoing to further elucidate the addition of cetuximab to chemotherapy in NSCLC patients.

Vascular Endothelial Growth Factor Inhibitors The VEGF is important for the development of vasculogenesis and angiogenesis required for tumor cell growth and metastasis, thus making it a key therapeutic target. Bevacizumab (Avastin) is the recombinant, humanized monoclonal antibody that neutralizes VEGF. Preclinical trials demonstrate synergy when bevacizumab is combined with cytotoxic therapy in a number of malignancies without untoward adverse effects. A phase II trial randomized 99 chemotherapy-naive patients with advanced or recurrent NSCLC to bevacizumab 7.5 mg/kg or 15 mg/kg plus PCb or PCb alone.[72] Patients with CNS metastasis, non-healing wounds, significant cardiovascular disease, significant peripheral vascular disease, active secondary malignancy, pregnancy, or major surgery within 4 weeks of starting therapy, and those requiring anticoagulation were excluded from the trial because of concern over excessive toxicity to the angiogenesis inhibitor. An independent review faculty evaluated the data and found a response rate of 40%, 22%, and 31%, and a median survival of 17.7 months, 11.6 months, and 14.9 months for the high-dose bevacizumab arm, the low-dose bevacizumab arm, and the control arm, respectively. Nineteen patients in the control arm crossed over to bevacizumab monotherapy upon disease progression. Five patients had disease stabilization and 12-month survival was 47% following crossover. Adverse effects of chemotherapy were not significantly different with the addition of bevacizumab. Leucopenia, diarrhea, fever, headache, rash, and chills were slightly more common in the bevacizumab-containing arms. In addition, several patients in the bevacizumab arms developed hypertension, proteinuria, and bleeding. Bleeding events included minor mucocutaneous hemorrhage (most commonly grade 1 or 2 epistaxis) and major hemoptysis. Four patients died as a result of hemoptysis or hematemesis, two others experienced life-threatening bleeding complications. All six patients had centrally located tumors, five had cavitation or necrosis of tumors, and four of the patients had squamous cell carcinoma. A prospective, randomized trial evaluating the addition of bevacizumab 15 mg/kg to PCb was conducted by ECOG.[52] As a result of bleeding complications seen in the phase II trial, patients with squamous cell carcinoma or brain metastasis were excluded. The addition of bevacizumab led to an improvement of progression-free survival from 4.5 months to 6.2 months (P <0.001), median survival from 10.3 months to 12.3 months (P = 0.003), and 1-year survival from 44% to 51%. There were significantly more bleeding events in the bevacizumab-containing arm (4.4% vs. 0.7%, P <0.001). Seventeen treatment-related deaths occurred during the study: 2 in the PCb group and 15 in the PCb-bevacizumab group. Other adverse events seen more frequently in the PCb-bevacizumab group include hypertension, neutropenia, febrile neutropenia, thrombocytopenia, hyponatremia, rash, and headache (P <0.05). NCCN guidelines recommend the addition of bevacizumab to chemotherapy for patients with advanced NSCLC of non–squamous cell histology, no history of hemoptysis, no CNS metastasis, and not receiving therapeutic anticoagulation.[3]

Radiation Therapy ❺ Palliative radiotherapy with chemotherapy may be helpful in selected patients to control local and systemic disease and to reduce disease-related symptoms. Brain metastases are also commonly treated with radiotherapy; in the case of a solitary brain lesion, surgical resection may be used in conjunction with whole-brain radiation.

Adverse effects of radiotherapy frequently result in severe esophagitis, pneumonitis, skin desquamation, myelopathies, cardiac abnormalities, and pulmonary toxicity in the surrounding normal tissues. Improved radiotherapy delivery techniques, such as multiple daily radiation fractions (hyperfractionated accelerated radiation therapy) and three-dimensional treatment planning, allow delivery of greater dosage fractions specifically to the tumor site while decreasing the toxicity to surrounding normal tissues, as compared to standard radiotherapy. A phase III trial randomized patients with unresectable NSCLC to receive two cycles of PCb followed by either once-daily radiation 64 Gy delivered in 32 2-Gy fractions or hyperfractionated accelerated radiation therapy delivered three times a day for 15 days with a total dose of 57.6 Gy.[73] Of the 141 patients, the median survival for hyperfractionated accelerated radiation therapy arm was 20.3 months compared to 14.9 months in the daily radiation arm (P = 0.28). Only 42% of the target accrual was met as a consequence of low patient accrual, difficulty in delivering hyperfractionated accelerated radiation therapy, mucosal toxicity, and data from other trials demonstrating the benefit of concurrent over the sequential radiotherapy.

Concurrent radiotherapy plus chemotherapy with radiosensitizing agents, such as cisplatin, paclitaxel, and gemcitabine, improve survival but further complicate the risks for severe toxicity, especially esophagitis.[74] Several trials have evaluated the use of sequential and concurrent chemoradiation, but the results of only one trial have been published. In that trial, Faruse et al. randomized 320 patients to chemotherapy (cisplatin, vindesine, and mitomycin) and radiation (56 Gy delivered in 28 fractions) beginning on either day 2 of chemotherapy or following the completion of chemotherapy. After a median followup of 5 years, median survival was significantly improved with concurrent chemoradiation when compared to sequential chemotherapy followed by radiotherapy (16.5 vs. 13.3 months, $P = 0.04$).[75] Myelosuppression was increased in the concurrent arm as opposed to the sequential arm, while nonhematologic toxicities were similar between the two groups. Numerous randomized combined modality trials continue to evaluate the optimal delivery method, schedule, and dosages for radiotherapy in concert with cisplatin and the newer chemotherapy agents.

EVALUATION OF THERAPEUTIC OUTCOMES IN NSCLC PATIENTS

Patients who have undergone surgical resection with or without chemotherapy, radiation, or both, a physical examination and chest radiography are recommended every 3 to 4 months for the first 2 years, then every 6 months for 3 years, and then annually. In addition, a low-dose spiral chest CT scan is recommended annually to monitor for evidence of locoregional recurrence. Suspicious symptoms or physical findings (e.g., bone pain, visual abnormalities or headache, or elevated liver function tests) should prompt an evaluation to rule out distant metastases.[3]

Tumor response to chemotherapy is generally evaluated at the end of the second or third cycle and at the end of every second cycle thereafter. Patients with stable disease, with objective response, or with measurable decrease in tumor size (complete or partial response) should continue until four to six cycles have been administered.[38,39] Following initial therapy for NSCLC, patients must be monitored for evidence of disease recurrence.

TREATMENT

Small Cell Lung Cancer

5 9 Combination chemotherapy regimens significantly increase the median survival in SCLC patients. With treatment, median survival rates for patients with limited and extensive disease are 14 to 20 months and 9 to 11 months, respectively.[4] Prognostic factors used to determine the appropriate therapy for SCLC patients include the stage of disease (i.e., limited vs. extensive disease) and performance status (e.g., an ECOG performance status of 0, or ability to carry out all normal activity without restriction). Patients with a better performance status at the time of initial diagnosis also have an improved prognosis.[11] Additional prognostic factors that have been identified as adverse prognostic factors in some studies include male gender, older age, the total number of metastatic sites, development of Cushing's syndrome as a paraneoplastic manifestation, and abnormal lactate dehydrogenase.[11]

■ SURGERY AND RADIATION THERAPY

The role of surgery in SCLC has been evaluated in various clinical trials of heterogenous populations who also received outdated chemotherapy regimens.[6] Thus, the Agency for Healthcare Research and Quality Evidence Report stated that no conclusion can be drawn regarding the role of surgery in SCLC.[6] In clinical practice, only the rare patient with small, isolated lesions undergoes surgery.[4,11]

5 9 Because SCLC is considered to be a very radiosensitive tumor, radiotherapy is used in combination with chemotherapy to treat limited-disease SCLC or used alone for management of symptomatic metastases. Radiotherapy decreases local recurrences in patients with limited-disease SCLC with modest improvements in survival.[11,76] The optimal dose and scheduling of thoracic radiotherapy plus chemotherapy have not been fully defined.[6] Although survival is increased by twice-daily radiotherapy concurrent with chemotherapy, it is rarely used because of the inconvenience and the high incidence of severe esophagitis.[76] Sequential therapy, in which radiotherapy begins after completion of chemotherapy administration, is inferior to concurrent chemoradiotherapy with the frequently used EP regimen.[77] It is not clear whether to initiate thoracic radiotherapy with earlier cycles (i.e., cycle 1) compared to later cycles (i.e., cycle 6) of cisplatin-based chemotherapy.[6,76] NCCN guidelines recommend the use of concurrent chemoradiotherapy over sequential therapy started with chemotherapy cycle 1 or 2 in limited-disease SCLC patients.[4]

For SCLC patients, radiotherapy is also used to prevent and treat brain metastases. Brain metastases are found in less than 10% of SCLC patients at the time of diagnosis.[11] Brain metastases are clinically debilitating and are frequently the sole site of relapse in those diagnosed with limited-stage SCLC.[11] It is estimated that brain metastases will present in 50% to 80% of limited-stage patients who survive 2 years and do not receive radiation therapy to the central nervous system. The role of prophylactic cranial irradiation (PCI) is based on the theory that eradication of microscopic or subclinical brain metastases would prevent or delay the onset of brain metastases. However, PCI has been associated with neurologic and intellectual impairment although the effects of potential contributing factors such as chemotherapy, possible paraneoplastic syndromes, and the effects of chronic cigarette and alcohol abuse have not been well understood.[6,11] The Prophylactic Cranial Irradiation Overview Collaborative Group conducted a meta-analysis of seven trials that enrolled patients after 1985. The analysis included data from 987 patients with SCLC in complete remission after initial therapy, and compared overall survival with the addition of PCI to an observation group. The pooled relative risk of death in the patients receiving PCI compared to the observation group was 0.84, which corresponded to a modest 5.4% absolute increase in overall survival at 3 years (15.3% alive in the observation group vs. 20.7% alive in the PCI group; $P = 0.01$).[78] In addition, PCI increased disease-free survival and decreased the incidence of brain metastases with a trend toward greater benefit with earlier delivery of PCI. Based on this analysis, in patients without significant cognitive impairment or cerebral atrophy, PCI is recommended in those with limited stage in complete response, and should be considered in those with extensive stage in complete response.[4] PCI is not recommended in patients with multiple comorbidities, poor performance status or impaired mental function.[4] Doses ranging from 25 Gy in 10 fractions to 36 Gy in 18 fractions are recommended.[4]

For patients with symptomatic brain metastases, therapeutic dosages of cranial irradiation usually control the CNS disease. Dexamethasone (to decrease intracranial pressure) and anticonvulsants are routinely administered to patients with brain metastases for symptomatic control and seizure prevention, respectively. Combination chemotherapy should also be administered, with administration occurring after whole-brain irradiation in those patients with symptomatic brain metastases.[4,11]

■ CHEMOTHERAPY

A number of cytotoxic agents have demonstrated significant single-agent activity in chemotherapy-naive patients with limited- and extensive-disease SCLC, but the activity in recurrent or refractory SCLC is modest. Cisplatin, carboplatin, etoposide, irinotecan, and topotecan are among the more commonly used chemotherapy agents in first-line treatment of SCLC patients. Single-agent chemotherapy is inferior to doublet chemotherapy.[25]

❾ In the United States, the most frequently used regimens in newly diagnosed patients are: PE (or EP): cisplatin (P) + etoposide (E); EC (CE): etoposide (E) + carboplatin (C); and IP: irinotecan (I) + cisplatin (P).[4,25] Overall response rates (70% to 90% vs. 60% to 70%) and survival durations (14 to 20 months vs. 9 to 11 months) are generally superior for patients with limited stage versus those with extensive stage disease.[4] According to the NCCN guidelines, chemotherapy with concurrent radiation is recommended for patients with limited-disease SCLC and good performance status (a category 1 recommendation, which indicates uniform consensus based on high-level evidence).[4] The same recommendation was made for patients with limited-disease SCLC with poor performance status, although the grade of evidence was lower (category 2A, which indicates uniform consensus based on lower-level evidence including clinical experience).[4] The 2-year disease-free survival rate for patients with limited stage at diagnosis is approximately 40%.[4] In comparison, very few patients with extensive stage at diagnosis are alive at 2 years without disease.[4] Because the duration of response is usually brief (less than 1 year) for patients achieving a complete response, drug-resistant cells are often responsible for treatment failure.

A relative plateau in overall survival rates in SCLC has occurred over the past two decades. In hopes of improving outcomes in these patients, multiple approaches have been studied in clinical trials, including (a) use of alternating chemotherapy; (b) dose-intense or dose-dense chemotherapy; (c) triplet chemotherapy; and (d) maintenance therapy. The Goldie-Coldman theory predicts that cycling of two active, non–cross-resistant chemotherapy regimens may overcome this problem.[79] However, disease-free and overall survival did not improve with alternating or sequential chemotherapy regimens in SCLC patients.[4,11] Experimental animal and human tumor data suggest that the amount of drug administered over a unit of time (i.e., mg/m^2 per week) may be critical to the degree of tumor cell kill. The importance of dose-intensity has been evaluated in many types of human cancer, particularly those like SCLC, which are initially responsive to chemotherapy, but are not usually curable with conventional therapies. Many clinical trials evaluated the role of dose-intensity, and the results of these trials showed a small, clinically insignificant improvement in median survival in extensive-disease SCLC patients.[4] Similarly, survival was not improved by increasing dose intensity via shortening the interval between cycles (i.e., dose density).[4] The incidence and severity of toxicities such as granulocytopenia, febrile neutropenia, mucositis, and weight loss are significantly higher in patients who receive dose-intensive treatment regimens. Currently, dose-intensive chemotherapy regimens should not be considered as standard oncology practice and should be reserved for clinical trials in patients with limited-disease SCLC and for the evaluation of newer agents. The addition of other active chemotherapy agents to doublet chemotherapy have provided minimal improvement in survival.[4] The addition of paclitaxel to EP resulted in minimal improvements in overall survival, with increased myelosuppression and grades 3 and 4 neurotoxicity, diarrhea, and asthenia.[80] Maintenance chemotherapy after induction appears to offer minimal benefit.[4] Maintenance with the targeted therapy marimastat, a matrix metalloproteinase inhibitor, did not improve progression-free or overall survival, but diminished quality of life in limited- and extensive-disease SCLC.[81]

Novel doublet regimens are currently being investigated. In patients with extensive-stage SCLC, the combination of oral topotecan with IV cisplatin resulted in similar response rates and overall survival rates and shorter time to progression than EP.[82] Overall toxicities were similar and patients treated with the EP regimen had slightly better, but of uncertain clinical significance, resolution of symptoms related to lung cancer. The most promising advance in chemotherapy for SCLC patients has been doublet chemotherapy regimens that include irinotecan. The Japanese Clinical Oncology Group compared IP (irinotecan 60 mg/m^2 IV on days 1, 8, and 15 combined with cisplatin 60 mg/m^2 IV day 1 given every 28 days for four cycles) versus EP (etoposide and cisplatin given every 21 days for four cycles) in 154 patients with extensive-disease stage SCLC.[83] Study enrollment was halted after the interim analysis results showed a statistically significant difference in median survival (12.8 vs. 9.4 months, respectively) and 1-year survival in the IP arm (19.5% vs. 5.2%). IP was well tolerated, with significantly less moderate-to-severe neutropenia (66% vs. 92%) and thrombocytopenia (5% vs. 18%) versus the EP arm. As expected, moderate-to-severe diarrhea was reported in 16% of patients receiving IP. Confirmatory trials were initiated because of the relatively small number of patients in the Japanese Clinical Oncology Group trial, potential pharmacogenomic differences between Japanese and white patients, and the use of cisplatin and irinotecan doses that differed from those commonly given in the United States.[84] The results of one of the two confirmatory studies have been reported, and showed that treatment with IP did not improve survival.[84] In that study, IP (irinotecan 65 mg/m^2 IV on days 1 and 8 combined with cisplatin 30 mg/m^2 IV day 1 given every 21 days for four cycles) was compared with EP (etoposide and cisplatin given every 21 days for four cycles) in 323 patients with extensive-disease stage SCLC.[84] Median survival was 9.3 months versus 10.2 months with IP versus EP, respectively, and 2-year overall survival was 7.9% and 8.0%, respectively. The dose intensities of cisplatin and irinotecan were similar between the two trials, and it has been hypothesized that differences in polymorphisms in uridine diphosphate-glucuronosyltransferase, which metabolizes irinotecan, or molecular differences in lung cancer may explain the differences in study results between Asian and United States populations.[84] Consequently, the optimal first-line chemotherapy regimen in newly diagnosed SCLC patients is unclear until further data are available.

CLINICAL CONTROVERSY

Patients with newly diagnosed extensive-disease SCLC should receive cisplatin with either etoposide (EP) or irinotecan (IP). Initial data suggested IP had a survival benefit over EP, which has been the standard of care for more than 15 years. However, data from a confirmatory trial suggested similar survival between EP and IP. Consequently, either regimen is used in patients with newly diagnosed extensive-disease SCLC.

Second-Line Chemotherapy

SCLC patients who relapse or progress after first-line chemotherapy have a median survival of 4 to 5 months.[4,6] Unfortunately, when disease recurs, it is usually less sensitive to chemotherapy. The agent of choice for second-line chemotherapy is often based on the length of time between completion of the induction chemotherapy regimen and relapse.[4] The likelihood of response is associated with the time from first-line therapy to relapse. If this interval is less than 3 months, the patient has refractory SCLC and is unlikely to respond to second-line therapy. NCCN guidelines include ifosfamide, paclitaxel, docetaxel, and gemcitabine as options for those with refractory SCLC and a good performance status (i.e., performance status 0 to 2).[4] If greater than 3 months have elapsed since first-line chemotherapy and disease relapse, the expected response rate to chemotherapy is 25%. In these patients, NCCN guidelines include topotecan, irinotecan, CAV (cyclophosphamide, doxorubicin, and vincristine), gemcitabine, paclitaxel, docetaxel, and vinorelbine as treatment options. The original chemotherapy regimen is used for those who have a long duration of disease control (i.e., >6 months between induction chemotherapy and relapse).[4]

EVALUATION OF THERAPEUTIC OUTCOMES IN SCLC PATIENTS

The effectiveness of first-line therapy is evaluated after two to three cycles of treatment. At this point, therapy is continued for patients with a complete or partial response or stable disease, and discontinued or changed to a non–cross-resistant regimen in patients demonstrating evidence of progressive disease. The induction chemotherapy regimen is administered for four to six cycles if the SCLC disease is responsive. In those with a complete response, PCI is offered as discussed above. After recovery from first-line therapy, followup visits should occur every 3 months for years 1, 2, and 3, then every 4 to 6 months for years 4 and 5, then annually for patients with either a partial or complete response.[4]

COMPLICATIONS AND SUPPORTIVE CARE

Patients with lung cancer frequently have numerous concurrent medical problems. Such problems may be related to invasion of the primary tumor and its metastases, paraneoplastic syndromes (see Clinical Presentation above), chemotherapy and radiotherapy toxicity, or concomitant disease states (e.g., cardiac disease, renal dysfunction, chronic obstructive pulmonary disease, asthma, or diabetes). Depression is also common and sometimes persistent in patients with SCLC and NSCLC and should be treated. Identification, diagnosis, and treatment of the patient as a whole may improve the patient's overall quality of life and tolerance to cancer treatments.

The chemotherapy regimens used in the management of lung cancer are intensive and are associated with a wide variety of toxic effects. Nausea and vomiting may be severe. Cisplatin-containing regimens require the use of aggressive acute and delayed antiemetic regimens containing a serotonin antagonist, dexamethasone and aprepitant.[85] Patients experiencing protracted nausea and vomiting may require intravenous hydration and nutritional support. Myelosuppression is often the dose-limiting toxicity associated with chemotherapy. Granulocytopenia places patients at a high risk for serious infections. Other toxic effects associated with these chemotherapy regimens include mucositis, anemia, nephrotoxicity, peripheral neuropathies, and ototoxicity.

Approximately 30% to 65% of advanced-stage NSCLC patients will develop bone metastases, which may lead to significant bone pain, pathologic fractures, spinal cord compression, and hypercalcemia.[86] Zoledronic acid, an intravenously administered bisphosphonate, has been shown to reduce skeletal-related events in patients with bone metastases at a dose of 4 mg over 15 minutes infused every 3 weeks. Although the data does not show a significant reduction in skeletal-related events, time to first event is significantly increased (230 vs. 163 days for placebo, $P = 0.023$) thereby making zoledronic acid a viable therapy for patients with bone metastasis.

Patients receiving radiation therapy may experience complications including severe esophagitis, fatigue, radiation pneumonitis, and cardiac toxicity. These toxicities are usually more common and severe when radiation is combined with chemotherapy. The patient's baseline performance status and the degree of pulmonary dysfunction (e.g., chronic obstructive pulmonary disease from years of tobacco use) must be considered in the decision of radiation dosage and fractionation.

It is readily apparent that many lung cancer patients receive complex pharmacologic regimens that may include chemotherapeutic agents, antiemetics, antibiotics, analgesics, anticoagulants, bronchodilators, corticosteroids, anticonvulsants, and cardiovascular agents. Such regimens necessitate intensive therapeutic monitoring in order to avoid drug-related and radiotherapy-related toxic effects and to optimize therapeutic outcome for individual patients.

ABBREVIATIONS

AUC: area-under-the-curve

CT: computed tomography

ECOG: Eastern Cooperative Oncology Group

EGFR: epidermal growth factor receptor

NCCN: National Comprehensive Cancer Network

NSCLC: non-small cell lung cancer

PCI: prophylactic cranial irradiation

PET: positron emission tomography

SCLC: small cell lung cancer

VEGF: vascular endothelial growth factor

REFERENCES

1. Jemal A, Siegel R, Ward E, Murray T, Xu J, Thun MJ. Cancer statistics, 2007. CA Cancer J Clin 2007;57:43–66.
2. Miller YE, Petty TL, Lam S. The early detection of lung cancer using bronchoscopy and cytologic analysis. In: Pass HI, Carbone DP, Johnson DH, Minna JD, Turrisi AT, eds. Lung Cancer: Principles and Practice, 3rd ed. Philadelphia: Lippincott, Williams & Wilkins, 2005:189–199.
3. National Comprehensive Cancer Network. NCCN Clinical Practice Guidelines in Oncology—Non–Small Cell Lung Cancer. 2007, *http://www.nccn.org/professionals/physician_gls/default.asp*.
4. National Comprehensive Cancer Network. NCCN Clinical Practice Guidelines in Oncology—Small Cell Lung Cancer. 2007, *http://www.nccn.org/professionals/physician_gls/default.asp*.
5. Pfister DG, Johnson DH, Azzoli CG, et al. American Society of Clinical Oncology treatment of unresectable non–small-cell lung cancer guideline: Update 2003. J Clin Oncol 2004;22:330–353.
6. Seidenfeld J, Samson DJ, Bonnell C, Ziegler KM, Aronson N. Management of small cell lung cancer. In: Agency for Healthcare Research and Quality. 2006, *http://www.ahrq.gov/clinic/tp/lungcantp.htm*.
7. Sekido Y, Fong WM, Minna JD. Molecular biology of lung cancer. In: DeVita VT Jr, Hellman S, Rosenberg SA, eds. Cancer: Principles & Practice of Oncology, 7th ed. Philadelphia: Lippincott Williams & Wilkins, 2005:745–752.
8. Kim ES, Lippman SM, Hong WK. Chemoprevention of lung cancer. In: Pass HI, Carbone DP, Johnson DH, Minna JD, Turrisi AT, eds. Lung Cancer: Principles and Practice, 3rd ed. Philadelphia: Lippincott, Williams & Wilkins, 2005:220–228.

9. Dy GK, Miller AA, Mandrekar SJ, et al. A phase II trial of imatinib (ST1571) in patients with c-kit expressing relapsed small-cell lung cancer: A CALGB and NCCTG study. Ann Oncol 2005;16:1811–1816.
10. Schrump DS, Altorki NK, Henschke CL, Carter D, Turrisi AT, Guthrerez ME. Non–small cell lung cancer. In: DeVita VT Jr, Hellman S, Rosenberg SA, eds. Cancer: Principles & Practice of Oncology, 7th ed. Philadelphia: Lippincott Williams & Wilkins, 2005:753–809.
11. Murren JR, Turrisi AT, Pass HJ. Small Cell Lung Cancer. In: DeVita VT Jr, Hellman S, Rosenberg SA, eds. Cancer: Principles & Practice of Oncology, 7th ed. Philadelphia: Lippincott Williams & Wilkins, 2005:810–825.
12. Schottenfeld D, Searle JG. The etiology and epidemiology of lung cancer. In: Pass HI, Carbone DP, Johnson DH, Minna JD, Turrisi AT, eds. Lung Cancer: Principles and Practice, 3rd ed. Philadelphia: Lippincott, Williams & Wilkins, 2005:3–24.
13. NCI. Non-Small Cell Lung Cancer (PDQ): Treatment Health Professional Version. In: Last Modified: 05/17/2006, *http://www.cancer.gov/cancertopics/pdq/treatment/non-small-cell-lung/healthprofessional*.
14. Travis WD, Colby TV, Corrin B, Shimosato Y, Brambilla E. Pathology Panels of the World Health Organization and the International Association for the Study of Lung Cancer, 3rd ed. Berlin: Springer Verlag, 1999.
15. Ramalingam SS, Dahlberg SE, Langer CJ, et al. Outcomes for elderly, advanced-stage non small-cell lung cancer patients treated with bevacizumab in combination with carboplatin and paclitaxel: analysis of Eastern Cooperative Oncology Group Trial 4599. J Clin Oncol 2008:26:60–65.
16. Sandler A, Gray R, Perry MC, et al. Paclitaxel-carboplatin alone or with bevacizumab for non–small-cell lung cancer. N Engl J Med 2006; 355:2542–2550.
17. Henschke CI, Yankelvitz DF, Wisnivesky JP, Smith JP, Libby D, Pasmantier M. CT screening for lung cancer: The diagnostic-prognostic or dual-gnostic approach. In: Pass HI, Carbone DP, Johnson DH, Minna JD, Turrisi AT, eds. Lung Cancer: Principles and Practice, 3rd ed. Philadelphia: Lippincott, Williams & Wilkins, 2005:210–219.
18. Henschke CI, Yankelevitz DF, Libby DM, Pasmantier MW, Smith JP, Miettinen OS. Survival of patients with stage I lung cancer detected on CT screening. N Engl J Med 2006;355:1763–1771.
19. Bach PB, Jett JR, Pastorino U, Tockman MS, Swensen SJ, Begg CB. Computed tomography screening and lung cancer outcomes. JAMA 2007;297:953–961.
20. Unger M. A pause, progress, and reassessment in lung cancer screening. N Engl J Med 2006;355:1822–1824.
21. Black WC, Baron JA. CT screening for lung cancer: Spiraling into confusion? JAMA 2007;297:995–997.
22. Virtamo J, Pietinen P, Huttunen JK, et al. Incidence of cancer and mortality following alpha-tocopherol and beta-carotene supplementation: A postintervention follow-up. JAMA 2003;290:476–485.
23. Goodman GE, Thornquist MD, Balmes J, et al. The Beta-Carotene and Retinol Efficacy Trial: Incidence of lung cancer and cardiovascular disease mortality during 6-year follow-up after stopping beta-carotene and retinol supplements. J Natl Cancer Inst 2004;96:1743–1750.
24. Lardinois D, Weder W, Hany TF, et al. Staging of non-small-cell lung cancer with integrated positron-emission tomography and computed tomography. N Engl J Med 2003;348:2500–2507.
25. Spira A, Ettinger DS. Multidisciplinary management of lung cancer. N Engl J Med 2004;350:379–392.
26. Argiris S, Murren JR. Staging and prognostic factors in small cell lung cancer. In: Pass HI, Carbone DP, Johnson DH, Minna JD, Turrisi AT, eds. Lung Cancer: Principles and Practice, 3rd ed. Philadelphia: Lippincott, Williams & Wilkins, 2005:387–399.
27. Deslauriers J, Gregoire J. Surgical therapy of early non-small cell lung cancer. Chest 2000;117(Suppl 1):104S–109S.
28. Effects of postoperative mediastinal radiation on completely resected stage II and stage III epidermoid cancer of the lung. The Lung Cancer Study Group. N Engl J Med 1986;315:1377–1381.
29. Postoperative radiotherapy in non-small-cell lung cancer: Systematic review and meta-analysis of individual patient data from nine randomised controlled trials. PORT Meta-analysis Trialists Group. Lancet 1998;352:257–263.
30. Scagliotti GV. The ALPI Trial: The Italian/European experience with adjuvant chemotherapy in resectable non-small lung cancer. Clin Cancer Res 2005;11(Pt 2):5011s–5016s.
31. Waller D, Peake MD, Stephens RJ, et al. Chemotherapy for patients with non-small cell lung cancer: The surgical setting of the Big Lung Trial. Eur J Cardiothorac Surg 2004;26:173–182.
32. Arriagada R, Bergman B, Dunant A, Le Chevalier T, Pignon JP, Vansteenkiste J. Cisplatin-based adjuvant chemotherapy in patients with completely resected non-small-cell lung cancer. N Engl J Med 2004;350:351–360.
33. Winton T, Livingston R, Johnson D, et al. Vinorelbine plus cisplatin vs. observation in resected non-small-cell lung cancer. N Engl J Med 2005;352:2589–2597.
34. Visbal AL, Leighl NB, Feld R, Shepherd FA. Adjuvant chemotherapy for early-stage non-small cell lung cancer. Chest 2005;128:2933–2943.
35. Douillard JY, Rosell R, De Lena M, et al. Adjuvant vinorelbine plus cisplatin versus observation in patients with completely resected stage IB-IIIA non-small-cell lung cancer (Adjuvant Navelbine International Trialist Association [ANITA]): A randomised controlled trial. Lancet Oncol 2006;7:719–727.
36. Kelsey CR, Werner-Wasik M, Marks LB. Stage III lung cancer: Two or three modalities? The continued role of thoracic radiotherapy. Oncology 2006;20:10.
37. Chemotherapy in non-small cell lung cancer: A meta-analysis using updated data on individual patients from 52 randomised clinical trials. Non-small Cell Lung Cancer Collaborative Group. BMJ 1995;311:899–909.
38. Smith IE, O'Brien ME, Talbot DC, et al. Duration of chemotherapy in advanced non-small-cell lung cancer: A randomized trial of three versus six courses of mitomycin, vinblastine, and cisplatin. J Clin Oncol 2001;19:1336–1343.
39. Socinski MA, Schell MJ, Peterman A, et al. Phase III trial comparing a defined duration of therapy versus continuous therapy followed by second-line therapy in advanced-stage IIIB/IV non-small-cell lung cancer. J Clin Oncol 2002;20:1335–1343.
40. Lilenbaum RC, Herndon JE 2nd, List MA, et al. Single-agent versus combination chemotherapy in advanced non-small-cell lung cancer: The cancer and leukemia group B (study 9730). J Clin Oncol 2005;23:190–196.
41. Bonomi P, Kim K, Fairclough D, et al. Comparison of survival and quality of life in advanced non-small-cell lung cancer patients treated with two dose levels of paclitaxel combined with cisplatin versus etoposide with cisplatin: Results of an Eastern Cooperative Oncology Group trial. J Clin Oncol 2000;18:623–631.
42. Schiller JH, Harrington D, Belani CP, et al. Comparison of four chemotherapy regimens for advanced non-small-cell lung cancer. N Engl J Med 2002;346:92–98.
43. Kelly K, Crowley J, Bunn PA, Jr, et al. Randomized phase III trial of paclitaxel plus carboplatin versus vinorelbine plus cisplatin in the treatment of patients with advanced non—small-cell lung cancer: A Southwest Oncology Group trial. J Clin Oncol 2001;19:3210–3218.
44. Kosmidis P, Mylonakis N, Nicolaides C, et al. Paclitaxel plus carboplatin versus gemcitabine plus paclitaxel in advanced non-small-cell lung cancer: A phase III randomized trial. J Clin Oncol 2002;20:3578–3585.
45. Rosell R, Gatzemeier U, Betticher DC, et al. Phase III randomised trial comparing paclitaxel/carboplatin with paclitaxel/cisplatin in patients with advanced non-small-cell lung cancer: A cooperative multinational trial. Ann Oncol 2002;13:1539–1549.
46. Hotta K, Matsuo K, Ueoka H, Kiura K, Tabata M, Tanimoto M. Meta-analysis of randomized clinical trials comparing Cisplatin to Carboplatin in patients with advanced non-small-cell lung cancer. J Clin Oncol 2004;22:3852–3859.
47. D'Addario G, Pintilie M, Leighl NB, Feld R, Cerny T, Shepherd FA. Platinum-based versus non-platinum-based chemotherapy in advanced non-small-cell lung cancer: A meta-analysis of the published literature. J Clin Oncol 2005;23:2926–2936.
48. Delbaldo C, Michiels S, Syz N, Soria JC, Le Chevalier T, Pignon JP. Benefits of adding a drug to a single-agent or a 2-agent chemotherapy regimen in advanced non-small-cell lung cancer: A meta-analysis. JAMA 2004;292:470–484.
49. Paccagnella A, Oniga F, Bearz A, et al. Adding gemcitabine to paclitaxel/carboplatin combination increases survival in advanced non-small-cell lung cancer: Results of a phase II-III study. J Clin Oncol 2006;24:681–687.

50. Williamson SK, Crowley JJ, Lara PN, Jr, et al. Phase III trial of paclitaxel plus carboplatin with or without tirapazamine in advanced non-small-cell lung cancer: Southwest Oncology Group Trial S0003. J Clin Oncol 2005;23:9097–9104.
51. Leighl NB, Paz-Ares L, Douillard JY, et al. Randomized phase III study of matrix metalloproteinase inhibitor BMS-275291 in combination with paclitaxel and carboplatin in advanced non-small-cell lung cancer: National Cancer Institute of Canada-Clinical Trials Group Study BR 18. J Clin Oncol 2005;23:2831–2839.
52. Langer C, Li S, Schiller J, Tester W, Rapoport BL, Johnson DH. Randomized phase II trial of paclitaxel plus carboplatin or gemcitabine plus cisplatin in Eastern Cooperative Oncology Group performance status 2 non-small-cell lung cancer patients: ECOG 1599. J Clin Oncol 2007;25:418–423.
53. Shepherd FA, Dancey J, Ramlau R, et al. Prospective randomized trial of docetaxel versus best supportive care in patients with non-small-cell lung cancer previously treated with platinum-based chemotherapy. J Clin Oncol 2000;18:2095–2103.
54. Fossella FV, DeVore R, Kerr RN, et al. Randomized phase III trial of docetaxel versus vinorelbine or ifosfamide in patients with advanced non-small-cell lung cancer previously treated with platinum-containing chemotherapy regimens. The TAX 320 Non-Small Cell Lung Cancer Study Group. J Clin Oncol 2000;18:2354–2362.
55. Hanna N, Shepherd FA, Fossella FV, et al. Randomized phase III trial of pemetrexed versus docetaxel in patients with non-small-cell lung cancer previously treated with chemotherapy. J Clin Oncol 2004;22: 1589–1597.
56. Ramlau R, Gervais R, Krzakowski M, et al. Phase III study comparing oral topotecan to intravenous docetaxel in patients with pretreated advanced non-small-cell lung cancer. J Clin Oncol 2006;24:2800–2807.
57. Langer CJ, Stephenson P, Thor A, Vangel M, Johnson DH. Trastuzumab in the treatment of advanced non-small-cell lung cancer: Is there a role? Focus on Eastern Cooperative Oncology Group study 2598. J Clin Oncol 2004;22:1180–1187.
58. Robert F, Blumenschein G, Herbst RS, et al. Phase I/IIa study of cetuximab with gemcitabine plus carboplatin in patients with chemotherapy-naive advanced non-small-cell lung cancer. J Clin Oncol 2005;23:9089–9096.
59. Pao W, Miller VA. Epidermal growth factor receptor mutations, small-molecule kinase inhibitors, and non-small-cell lung cancer: Current knowledge and future directions. J Clin Oncol 2005;23:2556–2568.
60. Fukuoka M, Yano S, Giaccone G, et al. Multi-institutional randomized phase II trial of gefitinib for previously treated patients with advanced non-small-cell lung cancer (The IDEAL 1 Trial) [corrected]. J Clin Oncol 2003;21:2237–2246.
61. Kris MG, Natale RB, Herbst RS, et al. Efficacy of gefitinib, an inhibitor of the epidermal growth factor receptor tyrosine kinase, in symptomatic patients with non-small cell lung cancer: A randomized trial. JAMA 2003;290:2149–2158.
62. Thatcher N, Chang A, Parikh P, et al. Gefitinib plus best supportive care in previously treated patients with refractory advanced non-small-cell lung cancer: Results from a randomised, placebo-controlled, multicentre study (Iressa Survival Evaluation in Lung Cancer). Lancet 2005;366:1527–1537.
63. Shepherd FA, Rodrigues Pereira J, Ciuleanu T, et al. Erlotinib in previously treated non-small-cell lung cancer. N Engl J Med 2005; 353:123–132.
64. Giaccone G, Herbst RS, Manegold C, et al. Gefitinib in combination with gemcitabine and cisplatin in advanced non-small-cell lung cancer: A phase III trial—INTACT 1. J Clin Oncol 2004;22:777–784.
65. Herbst RS, Giaccone G, Schiller JH, et al. Gefitinib in combination with paclitaxel and carboplatin in advanced non-small-cell lung cancer: A phase III trial—INTACT 2. J Clin Oncol 2004;22:785–794.
66. Herbst RS, Prager D, Hermann R, et al. TRIBUTE. A phase III trial of erlotinib hydrochloride (OSI-774) combined with carboplatin and paclitaxel chemotherapy in advanced non-small-cell lung cancer. J Clin Oncol 2005;23:5892–5899.
67. Lynch TJ, Bell DW, Sordella R, et al. Activating mutations in the epidermal growth factor receptor underlying responsiveness of non-small-cell lung cancer to gefitinib. N Engl J Med 2004;350:2129–2139.
68. Inoue A, Suzuki T, Fukuhara T, et al. Prospective phase II study of gefitinib for chemotherapy-naive patients with advanced non-small-cell lung cancer with epidermal growth factor receptor gene mutations. J Clin Oncol 2006;24:3340–3346.
69. Sequist LV, Bell DW, Lynch TJ, Haber DA. Molecular predictors of response to epidermal growth factor receptor antagonists in non-small-cell lung cancer. J Clin Oncol 2007;25:587–595.
70. Tsao MS, Sakurada A, Cutz JC, et al. Erlotinib in lung cancer—Molecular and clinical predictors of outcome. N Engl J Med 2005;353:133–144.
71. Thienelt CD, Bunn PA Jr, Hanna N, et al. Multicenter phase I/II study of cetuximab with paclitaxel and carboplatin in untreated patients with stage IV non-small-cell lung cancer. J Clin Oncol 2005;23:8786–8793.
72. Johnson DH, Fehrenbacher L, Novotny WF, et al. Randomized phase II trial comparing bevacizumab plus carboplatin and paclitaxel with carboplatin and paclitaxel alone in previously untreated locally advanced or metastatic non-small-cell lung cancer. J Clin Oncol 2004;22:2184–2191.
73. Belani CP, Wang W, Johnson DH, et al. Phase III study of the Eastern Cooperative Oncology Group (ECOG 2597): Induction chemotherapy followed by either standard thoracic radiotherapy or hyperfractionated accelerated radiotherapy for patients with unresectable stage IIIA and B non-small-cell lung cancer. J Clin Oncol 2005;23:3760–3767.
74. Johnson DH. Locally advanced, unresectable non-small cell lung cancer: New treatment strategies. Chest 2000;117(Suppl 1):123S–126S.
75. Furuse K, Fukuoka M, Kawahara M, et al. Phase III study of concurrent versus sequential thoracic radiotherapy in combination with mitomycin, vindesine, and cisplatin in unresectable stage III non-small-cell lung cancer. J Clin Oncol 1999;17:2692–2699.
76. Perry MC. Thoracic radiation therapy in limited stage small-cell lung cancer: Timing is everything...Isn't it? J Clin Oncol 2006;24:3815–3816.
77. Takada M, Fukuoka M, Kawahara M, et al. Phase III study of concurrent versus sequential thoracic radiotherapy in combination with cisplatin and etoposide for limited-stage small-cell lung cancer: Results of the Japan Clinical Oncology Group Study 9104. J Clin Oncol 2002;20:3054–3060.
78. Auperin A, Arriagada R, Pignon JP, et al. Prophylactic cranial irradiation for patients with small-cell lung cancer in complete remission. Prophylactic Cranial Irradiation Overview Collaborative Group. N Engl J Med 1999;341:476–484.
79. Goldie JH, Coldman AJ, Gudauskas GA. Rationale for the use of alternating non-cross-resistant chemotherapy. Cancer Treat Rep 1982;66:439–449.
80. Mavroudis D, Papadakis E, Veslemes M, et al. A multicenter randomized clinical trial comparing paclitaxel-cisplatin-etoposide versus cisplatin-etoposide as first-line treatment in patients with small-cell lung cancer. Ann Oncol 2001;12:463–470.
81. Shepherd FA, Giaccone G, Seymour L, et al. Prospective, randomized, double-blind, placebo-controlled trial of marimastat after response to first-line chemotherapy in patients with small-cell lung cancer: A Trial of the National Cancer Institute of Canada-Clinical Trials Group and the European Organization for Research and Treatment of Cancer. J Clin Oncol 2002;20:4434–4439.
82. Eckardt JR, von Pawel J, Papai Z, et al. Open-label, multicenter, randomized, phase III study comparing oral topotecan/cisplatin versus etoposide/cisplatin as treatment for chemotherapy-naive patients with extensive-disease small-cell lung cancer. J Clin Oncol 2006;24:2044–2051.
83. Noda K, Nishiwaki Y, Kawahara M, et al. Irinotecan plus cisplatin compared with etoposide plus cisplatin for extensive small-cell lung cancer. N Engl J Med 2002;346:85–91.
84. Hanna N, Bunn PA Jr, Langer C, et al. Randomized phase III trial comparing irinotecan/cisplatin with etoposide/cisplatin in patients with previously untreated extensive-stage disease small-cell lung cancer. J Clin Oncol 2006;24:2038–2043.
85. NCCN Clinical Practice Guidelines: Antiemesis, 2007. 2007, *http://www.nccn.org/professionals/physician_gls/default.asp.*
86. Rosen LS, Gordon D, Tchekmedyian S, et al. Zoledronic acid versus placebo in the treatment of skeletal metastases in patients with lung cancer and other solid tumors: A phase III, double-blind, randomized trial—the Zoledronic Acid Lung Cancer and Other Solid Tumors Study Group. J Clin Oncol 2003;21:3150–3157.

87. Smit EF, van Meerbeeck JP, Lianes P, et al. Three-arm randomized study of two cisplatin-based regimens and paclitaxel plus gemcitabine in advanced non-small-cell lung cancer: A phase III trial of the European Organization for Research and Treatment of Cancer Lung Cancer Group—EORTC 08975. J Clin Oncol 2003;21:3909–3917.
88. Gridelli C, Gallo C, Shepherd FA, et al. Gemcitabine plus vinorelbine compared with cisplatin plus vinorelbine or cisplatin plus gemcitabine for advanced non-small-cell lung cancer: A phase III trial of the Italian GEMVIN Investigators and the National Cancer Institute of Canada Clinical Trials Group. J Clin Oncol 2003;21:3025–3034.
89. Stathopoulos GP, Veslemes M, Georgatou N, et al. Front-line paclitaxel-vinorelbine versus paclitaxel-carboplatin in patients with advanced non-small-cell lung cancer: A randomized phase III trial. Ann Oncol 2004;15:1048–1055.
90. Lilenbaum RC, Chen CS, Chidiac T, et al. Phase II randomized trial of vinorelbine and gemcitabine versus carboplatin and paclitaxel in advanced non-small-cell lung cancer. Ann Oncol 2005;16:97–101.
91. Georgoulias V, Ardavanis A, Tsiafaki X, et al. Vinorelbine plus cisplatin versus docetaxel plus gemcitabine in advanced non-small-cell lung cancer: A phase III randomized trial. J Clin Oncol 2005;23:2937–2945.
92. Lara PN Jr, Gandara DR, Natale RB. Randomized phase III trial of cisplatin/irinotecan versus cisplatin/etoposide in patients with extensive-stage small-cell lung cancer. Clin Lung Cancer 2006; 7:353–356.
93. Douillard J, Rosell R, De Lena M, et al. Adjuvant vinorelbine plus cisplatin versus observation in patients with completely resected stage IB-IIIA non-small-cell lung cancer (Adjuvant Navelbine International Trialist Association [ANITA]): A randomized controlled trial. Lancet Oncol 2006;7:719–727.
94. Pignon JP, Tribodet H, Scagliotti GV, et al. Lung Adjuvant Cisplatin Evaluation (LACE): A pooled analysis of five randomized clinical trials including 4,584 patients. 2005 ASCO Annual Meeting Proceedings Part I [abstract #7008]. J Clin Oncol 2005;23(16 Suppl):366s.
95. Alberts WM. American College of Chest Physicians. Diagnosis and management of lung cancer executive summary: ACCP evidence-based clinical practice guidelines (2nd Edition). Chest 2007; 132(Suppl):1S–19S
96. Bach PB, Silverstri GA, Hanger M, et al. American College of Chest Physicians. Screening for lung cancer: ACCP evidence-based clinical practice guidelines (2nd Edition). Chest 2007;132(Suppl):69S–77S.

CHAPTER 133

Colorectal Cancer

PATRICK J. MEDINA, WEIJING SUN, AND LISA E. DAVIS

KEY CONCEPTS

1. Maintaining a diet with high-fiber and low fat intake has not been proven to reduce colorectal cancer risk, but is beneficial for reducing risk of other chronic diseases.

2. Regular use of aspirin and other nonsteroidal antiinflammatory drugs, estrogen replacement therapy, and calcium and vitamin D supplementation may reduce risk of colorectal cancer in certain selected populations, but they are not currently recommended for cancer prevention.

3. Effective colorectal cancer screening programs incorporate regular examination of the entire colon starting at age 50 years for average-risk individuals. Colorectal adenomas can progress to cancer and should be removed.

4. The histologic stage of colorectal cancer upon diagnosis—determined by depth of bowel invasion, lymph node involvement, and presence of metastases—is still the most important prognostic factor for disease recurrence and survival.

5. The treatment goal for stages I, II, and III colon cancer is cure; surgery should be offered to all eligible patients for this purpose. Six months of fluoropyrimidine-based adjuvant chemotherapy significantly reduces the risk of cancer recurrence and overall mortality as compared to observation alone in patients with stage III disease.

6. Adjuvant therapy consisting of fluoropyrimidine-based chemosensitized radiation therapy should be offered to patients with stage II or III cancer of the rectum. Adjuvant fluoropyrimidine-based chemotherapy plus radiation decreases risk of local and distant disease recurrence as compared to observation alone.

7. Chemotherapy is palliative for metastatic disease. Fluoropyrimidine-based chemotherapy regimens, administered in a variety of schedules, provide a modest improvement in survival and can be highly beneficial in reducing patient symptoms.

8. Bevacizumab plus chemotherapy as initial therapy for metastatic disease is considered standard of care and provides a survival benefit compared to combination chemotherapy alone. A fluoropyrimidine with oxaliplatin or irinotecan improves survival compared to fluoropyrimidine monotherapy, and should be offered to patients who are candidates for aggressive treatment. The ability for patients to receive all active cytotoxic agents (e.g., fluoropyrimidine, oxaliplatin, irinotecan) during the course of their disease improves their overall survival.

9. Capecitabine is an acceptable alternative to intravenous fluorouracil in both adjuvant therapy and in the setting of metastatic disease, as it provides similar efficacy and its oral dosing may offer greater patient convenience.

10. Individuals whose disease progresses during or is refractory to irinotecan may benefit from cetuximab, either alone or combined with continuing irinotecan. Positive tumor epidermal growth factor receptor (EGFR) immunohistochemistry test results do not appear to predict tumor response to anti-EGFR monoclonal antibodies.

Learning objectives, review questions, and other resources can be found at **www.pharmacotherapyonline.com.**

Colorectal cancer involves the colon, rectum, and the anal canal. It is one of the three most common cancers occurring in adult men and women in the United States, and accounts for about 1 in 9 cancer diagnoses. In 2007, an estimated 153,760 new cases will be diagnosed, of which 112,340 will involve the colon and 41,420 the rectum.[1] An additional 4,650 new cases of cancer involve the anus, anal canal, or anorectum.[1]

For both adult men and women, colorectal cancer is the third leading cause of cancer-related deaths in the United States. An estimated 52,180 deaths will occur during 2007.[1]

Mortality and incidence rates associated with colorectal cancer in the United States have decreased over the past decades. These contrast with an increasing rate of incidence in countries where overall risk was relatively low (e.g., Japan and parts of Asia) and a stabilizing rate of incidence in high-risk countries in Northern and Western Europe.[2] Colorectal cancer mortality rates are comparable between the United States, Western Europe, and Japan.[2]

Multiple factors are associated with the development of colorectal cancer, including acquired and inherited genetic susceptibility, environmental elements, and lifestyle choices. Overall, approximately 39% of affected individuals undergo a surgical procedure alone intended for cure. An additional 36% of individuals can potentially be cured by undergoing surgery followed by adjuvant radiation therapy (XRT), chemotherapy, or both. Curability is influenced primarily by extent of tumor invasion into adjacent tissues or organs, involvement of lymph nodes, and presence of metastatic disease. Five-year survival rates are close to 91% and 88% for persons with early stages of colon and rectal cancer, respectively.[3] After the tumor has spread regionally to adjacent lymph nodes or tissues, 5-year survival rates drop to 69% for colon cancer and to 63% for cancer of the rectum; 5-year survival for individuals with metastatic disease is approximately 10%.

Treatment modalities for colorectal cancer include surgery, XRT, chemotherapy, and other targeted molecular therapies (e.g., angiogenesis inhibitors, epidermal growth factor receptor inhibitors). Surgery is the important and definitive procedure associated with cure; XRT can improve curability following surgical resection in rectal cancer and may reduce symptoms and complications associated with advanced disease. Chemotherapy is used in adjuvant treatment regimens as well as in treatment for advanced stages of disease. Much progress has been made in the treatment of advanced disease, in the ability to identify candidates for potentially curative surgical procedures, and the availability of active drug regimens that can improve patients' survival.

EPIDEMIOLOGY

Colorectal cancer is the third most common malignancy worldwide, accounting for an estimated 1,023,256 new cases annually.[4] The variation in colorectal cancer occurrence worldwide is at least 25-fold.[2] The highest incidence rates occur in the most highly developed areas such as Australia, New Zealand, North America, Japan, and Western and Northern Europe. The lowest incidence rates are seen in less-developed areas such as Africa, South Central Asia, and Central America. The influence of environmental factors on colorectal cancer risk has become evident through studies of migrants, where the incidence of colorectal cancer increases rapidly within first-generation immigrants who migrate from low- to high-risk areas.[2] However, colorectal cancers are known to develop more frequently in certain families and genetic predisposition to this disease is also well-recognized.

The incidence of colon cancer is greatest among males, who have an age-adjusted incidence rate of 40.0 per 100,000, as compared to females for whom the rate is 31.5 per 100,000.[3] Cancer of the rectum occurs less frequently; the incidence rate is 16.7 and 10.3 per 100,000 for males and females, respectively. Differences in colorectal cancer incidence exist among ethnic groups in American men and women. Although cancer of the colon and rectum is the third most frequent malignancy among white, African American, Asian American/Pacific Islander, and American Indian/Alaska Native males, it ranks second among Hispanic/Latino males. In women, cancer of the colon and rectum is the second most frequent malignancy in African American, Asian American/Pacific Islander, and American Indian/Alaska Native females, but third most common cancer in white and Hispanic/Latino females.[1] Cultural and genetic factors, as well as disparities in access to healthcare services, may influence risk among population groups.[1]

The overall incidence of colon and rectal cancers in the United States continues to decline, with an annual percent decrease of 1.5% from 1995–2004.[3] In almost every ethnic group, the decline in cancer incidence accelerated from 1998 to 2004. An increase in screening and polyp removal may contribute to a part of this trend. Figure 133–1 displays trends for incidence and mortality rates among white and African-American males and females in the United States.

The median age at diagnosis is 71 years, with fewer than 10% of patients diagnosed younger than age 54 years.[3] An individual's risk increases with increasing age, and 75% of cases develop in adults older than 65 years of age. The stage of disease at presentation is similar among different ethnic groups, although the tendency to present with later-stage disease is slightly higher for African Americans than in whites.

Cancer of the colon and rectum accounts for approximately 10% of all cancer deaths in the United States. It is estimated that 52,180 individuals will die of colorectal cancer in the United States in 2007, which represents a continued decline in overall combined mortality for both colon and rectal cancer observed during the last 20 years. For women, the decline in colorectal cancer mortality rates has been evident since 1950, whereas death rates among men did not start to decline until the late 1970s.[3] Overall mortality rates are also higher among African American males and females, and the rates of decline are lower as compared to those among white, American Indian/Alaska Native, Asian/Pacific Islander, and Hispanic males and females.[3] Factors contributing to the overall decline in colorectal cancer mortality likely include decreasing incidence rates, screening programs with early polyp removal, and more effective and better-tolerated treatments. Differences among different world geographic regions, as well as in population groups in the United States, may also reflect variations in underlying tumor biology, stage at diagnosis, and availability of effective treatments.[4]

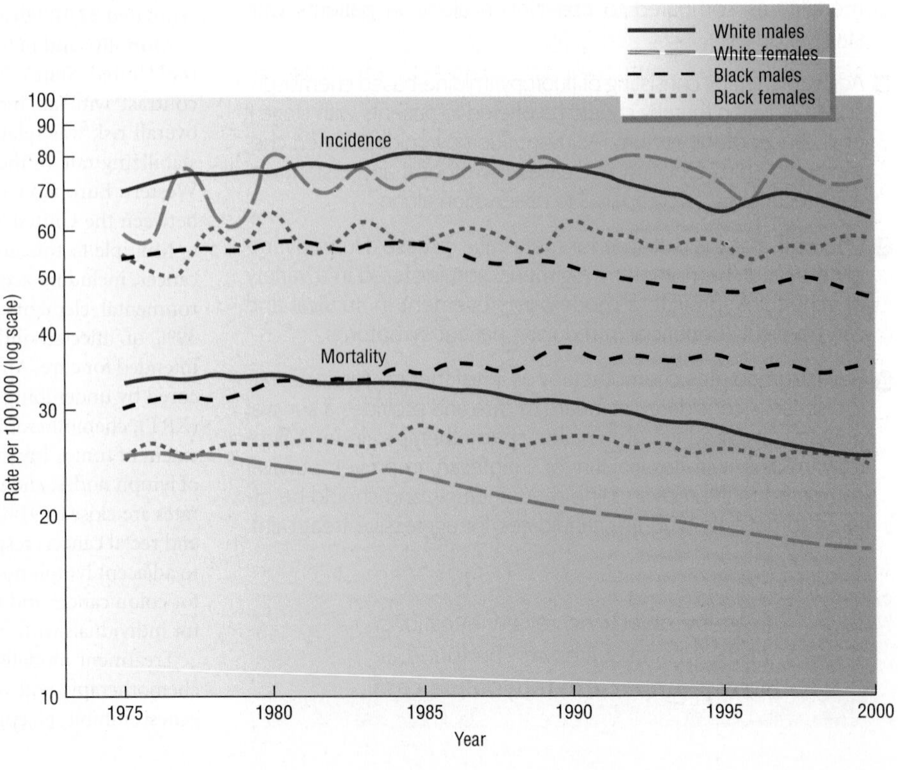

FIGURE 133-1. Surveillance, Epidemiology, and End Results (SEER) incidence and mortality rates for invasive colon and rectum cancer, 1975 to 2004, age-adjusted and age-specific. Rates are per 100,000 and age-adjusted to the 2000 U.S. standard population. *(From reference 3.)*

ETIOLOGY AND RISK FACTORS

Numerous studies suggest that the development of colorectal cancer is related to dietary or environmental factors that affect the bowel, lifestyle choices, and certain comorbid conditions, in addition to physical and genetic susceptibilities.

DIETARY INTAKE AND NUTRIENTS

❶ Epidemiologic studies of worldwide incidence of colorectal cancer suggest that economic development and dietary habits strongly influence its development. Although findings based on epidemiologic data are subject to potential biases, as well as inconsistencies in how dietary factors are categorized and measured, numerous studies have attempted to ascertain the true contribution of dietary habits as independent risk factors for colon cancer development.

Fiber

❶ Dietary fiber is composed of remnants of plant cells that are not processed by normal human digestive enzymes.[5] Fibers are frequently classified as either water soluble (pectins, gums, agar, and mucilages) or insoluble (celluloses, hemicellulose, and lignins). The insoluble fibers are most likely to protect against cancer.[5] Foods that are high in fiber include vegetables, fruit, grains, and cereals. Dietary fiber is postulated to reduce colonic mucosal cell exposure to carcinogens through the dilution or reduced absorption of carcinogens in the bowel, reduced fecal pH, reduced bowel transit time, alterations in bile acid metabolism, or increased production of short-chain fatty acids.[5–7] Fiber degradation products may further serve to reduce activity of tumor promoting substances. A protective effect from a diet high in fruits and vegetables is biologically plausible because certain constituents (e.g., micronutrients, protease inhibitors, organosulfides, isothiocyanates) may reduce oxidative damage to DNA and lipids, induce drug-metabolizing enzymes, or enhance DNA repair processes.[8]

Results of observational studies have not shown a consistent association between dietary fiber, fruit, vegetable, and whole grains intake and risk of colorectal adenomas or carcinoma. Two large studies reported an inverse relationship between fiber intake and colorectal cancer, with a 25% to 27% reduction in the risk of colorectal cancer among participants in the highest quintile of dietary fiber intake as compared to those in the lowest quintile.[7] These findings were confirmed in a pooled analysis of 13 prospective cohort studies in age-adjusted analysis, but after other dietary risk factors were accounted for, high dietary fiber intake did not reduce colorectal cancer risk.[7] In the National Institutes of Health–American Association of Retired Persons (NIH-AARP) Diet and Health Study, the risk of colorectal cancer for the highest quintile of vegetable intake was reduced for men but not for women.[8] Fruit intake was not related to colorectal cancer risk in men or women. In contrast, frequent fruit consumption was associated with a lower risk of colorectal adenomas in men and women who participated in the Health Professionals Follow-Up Study and from the Nurses' Health Study.[6] Whether these dietary factors might influence the development of colorectal cancer at certain aspects of adenoma development, recurrence, or progression to malignancy is unknown.[6]

Thus, the evidence that increased dietary fiber—and possibly fruit or vegetable—consumption reduces colorectal cancer risk is suggestive, but not conclusive, and the amount, type, and duration of fiber intake may determine who benefits.

Fat

❶ Epidemiologic studies suggest that a relationship exists between dietary fat intake and colorectal cancer risk, although this has not been consistently seen.[6] This may have resulted from the use of dietary evaluations that focused on the quantity, origin, or type (saturated, monounsaturated, and polyunsaturated) of fat rather than on specific fatty acids ingested. The association between red meat consumption and colorectal cancer is strongest, which may be related to the heterocyclic amines and polycyclic aromatic hydrocarbons formed during cooking or the presence of specific fatty acids in red meat such as arachidonic acid. Processed meat products containing certain preservatives may increase exogenous exposure to carcinogenic *N*-nitroso compounds. Also, individuals who consume diets that are rich in meats not only eat less fiber, but also eat less fish.[9] Animal and in vitro studies suggest that n-3 long-chain polyunsaturated fatty acids, which are present in fish oils and cold-water fish, may play a protective role in colorectal carcinogenesis.[9] In a prospective study of 478,040 men and women, colorectal cancer risk was associated with high consumption of red and processed meat (hazard ratio [HR] 1.35, 95% confidence interval (CI) 0.96 to 1.88 for >160 g/day vs. <20 g/day) but inversely associated with fish intake (HR 0.69, 95% CI 0.45 to 0.88, >80 g/day vs. <10 g/day).[9]

The role of dietary fat in cancer development may be a result of its effect on fecal bile acid concentrations. The release of bile acids is stimulated following ingestion of dietary fat. These acids are then converted by colonic flora to secondary bile acids, which are associated with bowel mucosal irritation and cell proliferation responses and may promote tumor growth.[10]

Although data suggest that red and processed meat and saturated fat intake are associated with an increased risk of colorectal cancer, the exact nature and magnitude of this risk has not been determined.

Calcium and Vitamin D

❷ An inverse association between dietary calcium and vitamin D intake and colorectal cancer risk has been reported in several observational studies that have led to randomized trials.[11] Calcium may exert antiproliferative effects by binding to bile and fatty acids in the small intestine, thereby reducing colonic epithelial cell exposure to mutagens.[11] In addition, calcium induces differentiating, proapoptotic, and direct growth-restraining activities on both normal and tumor cells in the gastrointestinal tract.[11] Vitamin D has antiproliferative and differentiation and apoptosis-inducing effects on cells of the large intestine. Most of its actions are mediated through a high-affinity receptor, VDR, and the expression of this receptor is altered during different phases of colon cancer development.[11] Thus, cellular responsiveness to vitamin D is unlikely limited to dietary intake alone. Vitamin D and calcium appear to interact synergistically to protect against adenoma recurrence and colorectal cancer.[12]

Folate and Other Micronutrients

An inverse relationship between folate and colorectal cancer risk has been demonstrated in experimental animal and human studies, but the underlying basis for this is complex. Folate is a key constituent of dark-green vegetables, citrus fruits, and dried beans, and the contribution of these dietary components is considered beneficial. Decreased dietary folate intake alters cellular DNA methylation patterns and impairs DNA biosynthesis.[11] Because DNA methylation status plays an influential role on nuclear transcription inhibition, inappropriate hypo- or hypermethylation can result in oncogene activation or inactivation of tumor suppressor genes.[11] These effects as mechanisms of oncogenic transformation and tumor progression have been described in colon cancer. Data suggest that an adequate dietary folate intake may be enough to lower the risk of colon cancer, and exceeding normal intake may not be beneficial. Folate supplementation may also have a promoting effect on established colorectal cancer.[13] Deficiencies in other dietary micronutrients may increase colorectal cancer risk, including selenium, vitamin C, vitamin E, and carotenoids, but, as with folate, there is no convincing evidence that routine dietary supplementation is beneficial.[10,13]

Coffee, Tea, and Caffeine Consumption

The association between coffee, tea, and caffeine consumption and colorectal cancer risk remains controversial, despite some findings from several small case-control and cohort studies.[14,15] Coffee and tea contain several constituents that have anticarcinogenic properties in vitro and in animal studies, but evidence in humans is limited. In a meta-analysis of 25 studies that addressed black and green tea consumption and colorectal cancer risk, there was inadequate evidence that either type of tea is protective against colorectal cancer.[15] Data from the Nurses' Health Study and the Health Professionals' Follow-Up Study were used to determine relationships between caffeinated or decaffeinated coffee and tea and cancer risk.[14] Although caffeinated coffee, caffeinated tea, and total caffeine consumption were not associated with colon or rectal cancer risk, individuals who regularly consumed decaffeinated coffee had a 52% lower risk (95% CI 19% to 71%) of rectal cancer. This observation has yet to be confirmed by other studies.

LIFESTYLE FACTORS

Nonsteroidal Antiinflammatory Drug and Aspirin Use

❷ Several lifestyle factors are known to affect colorectal cancer risk (Table 133–1). Observational studies have demonstrated that regular (at least two doses per week) nonsteroidal antiinflammatory drug (NSAID) and aspirin use is associated with a reduced risk of colorectal cancer. In an average-risk individual, regular aspirin use is associated with a 13% to 28% reduction in the risk of colorectal adenoma, and the pooled relative risk reduction in colorectal cancer from cohort studies is approximately 22%.[16] The reduction in risk appears greater for individuals with a history of adenoma. The dose of aspirin may be important, as low-dose aspirin was not beneficial in reducing colorectal cancer incidence in either the Physician's Health Study or the Women's Health Study.[17]

TABLE 133-1 Lifestyle Factors Associated with Colorectal Cancer Risk

Factor	Comments
Alcohol intake	Colorectal cancer risk increased by 50% with heavy (greater than 10-14 drinks/week) alcohol use; risk increases by 15% for an increase of 100 g/week (5–7 drinks/week)
Aspirin and non-aspirin NSAID use	Regular aspirin use associated with 22% reduction in colorectal cancer risk; regular NSAID use reduces colorectal cancer risk by 30%–40%
Calcium and vitamin D intake	Vitamin D 400 international units and calcium intake of 1,000 mg/day (adults <50 years) or 1,200 mg/day (adults >50 years) may be sufficient to reduce colorectal cancer risk
Type 2 diabetes mellitus	Associated with 30% increase in risk of colorectal cancer
Obesity and physical inactivity	Elevated BMI, waist circumference, waist-to-hip ratio, and physical inactivity associated with increased risk
Postmenopausal hormone use	Exogenous hormone intake decreases risk of colon and rectal cancer by about 20%
Tobacco use	Use of tobacco products contributes to approximately 12% of colorectal cancer deaths annually
Western diet	High fat, red, and processed meat consumption, low fish intake, and low fiber (fruit, vegetables, whole grains) intake linked to increased risk

BMI, body mass index; NSAID, nonsteroidal antiinflammatory drug.

Benefit has also been seen with NSAID and cyclooxygenase-2 inhibitor (COX-2) users. NSAID use is associated with protection against adenomas and colorectal cancer, with a 30% to 40% reduction in the risk of colorectal cancer.[17] Although COX-2 inhibitors reduce the incidence of colorectal adenoma recurrence, there is no evidence to show that they reduce colorectal cancer risk or mortality.[17]

The protective effects of these agents appear to be related to their inhibition of COX-2 and free radical formation. COX-2 overexpression is seen in precancerous and cancerous lesions in the colon and is associated with decreased colon cancer cell apoptosis and increased production of angiogenesis-promoting factors.[18] Up to 40% of colorectal adenomas and 90% of sporadic colon carcinomas have elevated levels of COX-2.[18,19] COX-2 appears to play a role in polyp formation and COX-2 inhibition suppresses polyp growth. In contrast, cyclooxygenase-1 (COX-1) levels remain normal in both normal and malignant tissue, although COX-1 inhibition may also be important.[20] Inhibition of COX by NSAIDs, aspirin, and cyclooxygenase inhibitors restores apoptosis and decreases expression of proangiogenic factors.

Exogenous Hormone Use

❷ Exogenous postmenopausal hormone use, particularly postmenopausal estrogen-replacement therapy, is associated with a significant reduction in colorectal cancer risk in most studies.[21–23] A meta-analysis of postmenopausal hormone replacement therapy showed a 19% to 20% reduction in risk of colorectal cancer in women who received hormone-replacement therapy as compared to women who never used hormone-replacement therapy.[23] The risk is reduced in postmenopausal women receiving both estrogen only and combined estrogen and progestin therapy, and persists for about 10 years after therapy is discontinued. Risk reduction appears greatest among women who are currently receiving hormone-replacement therapy. The Women's Health Initiative showed that the incidence of colorectal cancer was reduced by 39% with combined estrogen/progestin use, although colorectal cancers were diagnosed at a more advanced stage in women who took hormones than in women who received placebo.[24]

Several mechanisms for a protective effect of estrogens on the bowel have been identified.[21,24] Declining estrogen levels associated with aging are associated with estrogen receptor hypermethylation, resulting in reduced expression of the estrogen receptor gene and dysregulated colonic mucosal cell growth. In addition, estrogen may interact with bile acids, or alter levels of insulin and insulin-like growth factor-1, an important mitogen that influences cell-cycle progression in certain cells.

Obesity and Physical Inactivity

Physical inactivity and elevated body mass index (BMI), independent of level of physical activity, are associated with an elevated risk of colon adenoma, colon cancer, and rectal cancer.[10] Individuals with a total higher level of activity throughout life have the lowest risk. Hypotheses for these relationships include the observation that physical activity stimulates bowel peristalsis, resulting in decreased bowel transit time, and the possibility that exercise-induced alterations in body glucose, insulin levels, and perhaps other hormones may reduce tumor cell growth.[21]

In most studies, BMI was associated with increased risk of colorectal cancer in men, but the relationship is weaker and less consistent for women, possibly because of interactions with age or hormone-replacement therapy. Differences in body composition and distribution of fat weight among men and women could contribute to this discrepancy.[25] In the European Prospective Investigation into Cancer and Nutrition, body weight and BMI were associated with a greater risk of colon cancer in men (relative risk [RR] 1.55, 95% CI 1.12 to 2.15) for men in the highest versus the lowest quintile of BMI.[25] Although measures of fat distribution, such as waist circumference and waist-to-hip ratio, were associated with risk of colon cancer in men and women, these relationships were not observed among postmenopausal women who took hormone replacement therapy. In a cohort of men and women from the NIH-AARP Diet and Health Study, increased risk of colon, but not rectal cancer was associated with BMI in men and women.[26] Hormone-replacement therapy in women or physical activity in men did not modify this association. However, the association between BMI and colon cancer risk was observed in younger (ages 50 to 66 years) but not in older women (ages 67 to 71 years). Thus, the relationship between obesity and colorectal cancer among women may diminish with age. Premenopausal obese women appear to be at the greatest risk as compared to postmenopausal obese women.

Several mechanisms that link body size to colorectal cancer risk have been proposed, including insulin resistance, chronic inflammation, and alterations in growth factors or steroid hormones.[27] Type 2 diabetes mellitus, independent of body mass size and physical activity level, is associated with increased colorectal cancer risk, although previous findings have been heterogeneous with regard to sex and cancer subsite.[28] In a meta-analysis of 15 studies, diabetes was associated with a 30% increase in risk of colorectal cancer and increased risk of colorectal cancer mortality (RR 1.26, 95% CI 1.05 to 1.50).[28] Features associated with type 2 diabetes, such as hyperinsulinemia, factors related to insulin resistance, increased bowel transit time, and elevated levels of fecal bile acids, may serve to promote colorectal carcinogenesis.[28]

The hypothesis that metabolic syndrome might be associated with colorectal cancer risk was tested in a population-based cohort of 14,109 men and women.[29] An association between metabolic syndrome and colorectal cancer was stronger for men compared to women. The physiologic features of metabolic syndrome may serve to promote cancer development and warrant further study.

Alcohol and Tobacco Use

Alcohol consumption increases the risk of colorectal cancer, but stronger associations have been observed for men than for women, possibly because alcohol consumption is generally greater in men than in women.[30] In a meta-analysis of 16 prospective studies, the risk of colorectal cancer was approximately 50% greater for individuals who consumed the highest amount of alcohol per week (>200 g) as compared to individuals with the lowest intake (<100 g/week). A dose–response relationship was also observed, with a 15% increase in colorectal cancer risk for an increase of 100 g of alcohol (which corresponds to 5 to 7 drinks) consumed per week.

Smoking tobacco products, including cigarettes, cigars, and pipes, may contribute to as much as 12% of all colorectal cancer deaths.[31] Risk for hyperplastic polyps, adenomas, or concurrent hyperplastic and adenomatous polyps with current tobacco use, estimated by the odds ratio, was 4.4, 1.8, and 6.2, respectively, in participants of the Prostate, Lung, Colorectal, and Ovarian Trial who underwent flexible sigmoidoscopy.[32] Increased cancer risk was also observed in ex-smokers, although the effects were weaker.

CLINICAL RISK FACTORS

Chronic Inflammatory Diseases

Chronic ulcerative colitis, particularly when it involves the entire large intestine, predisposes individuals to colorectal cancer at a rate that is 5- to 10-fold greater than average.[33] The risk is even greater for young individuals and increases for all affected individuals with increasing extent of bowel involvement and disease duration. The cumulative risk of colorectal cancer is low early in life, but increases from 2% at 10 years after diagnosis to 8% and 18% at 20 and 30 years, respectively.[33] Although a precise causative link has not been established, chronic underlying inflammation may be a significant predisposing factor. The progressive dysplastic changes that bowel mucosa undergo are similar to those observed in adenomatous polyps. Similarly, patients with Crohn's disease are also at increased risk, and the risk is believed to be about that of patients with ulcerative colitis.[33] As compared to sporadic colon cancer or cancer associated with ulcerative colitis, colon cancer in patients with Crohn's disease tends to arise in the proximal colon.[33] This is most likely related to the area of bowel affected by the chronic inflammatory process in individuals with Crohn's disease. Overall, persons diagnosed with either disease constitute approximately 1% to 2% of all new cases of colorectal cancer each year.

GENETIC SUSCEPTIBILITY

Hereditary

Three specific patterns of colon cancer occurrence are generally observed: sporadic, inherited, and familial.[34,35] Although most cases of colon cancer are sporadic in nature, as many as 10% of cases are thought to be hereditary. The two most common forms of hereditary colon cancer are familial adenomatous polyposis (FAP) and hereditary nonpolyposis colorectal cancer (HNPCC). Each of these results from a specific germ line mutation.[34] FAP is a rare autosomal dominant trait caused by inactivating mutations of the adenomatous polyposis coli (*APC*) gene and accounts for 0.2% to 1% of all colorectal cancers. The disease is manifested by hundreds to thousands of tiny sessile adenomatous polyps that carpet the colon and rectum, typically arising during adolescence.[36] The polyps continue to proliferate throughout the colon, with eventual transformation to malignancy. The risk of developing colorectal cancer for individuals with untreated FAP is virtually 100%; most will develop colorectal cancer between the fourth and fifth decades of life.[35] Several variants of FAP exist and are associated with different extracolonic manifestations.[36,37]

HNPCC, also referred to as Lynch syndrome, is an autosomal dominant inherited syndrome that accounts for up to 5% of colon cancer cases.[37] Multiple generations within a family are affected and colorectal cancer develops early in life, with a mean age at time of diagnosis of about 45 years of age.[35] Germ line mutations in one of the DNA mismatch-repair (MMR) genes, most commonly *MLH1*, *MSH2*, or *MSH6*, are responsible for HNPCC.[35,37–39] In contrast to FAP, adenomatous polyps are not a primary manifestation of the HNPCC. Polyps that do form tend to be located primarily in the right-sided, or proximal colon. Because the clinical presentation of HNPCC is difficult to distinguish from "sporadic" forms of colorectal cancer, the diagnosis of HNPCC can be confirmed by the presence of germ line mutations in a family of genes responsible for DNA MMR. Criteria for diagnosis of HNPCC have been established, and it is important to identify carriers of these MMR mutations so that they can be counseled and followed appropriately.[39] Carriers of a germ line mutation have an estimated 70% risk of developing colorectal cancer by the age of 70 years.[39] In addition, these individuals have a moderately increased risk of developing cancers in other organs.

Familial colon cancer represents the least-understood pattern of colorectal cancer. Approximately 20% of patients who develop colorectal cancer will have a family history of colorectal cancer.[35] In these families, the frequency of colorectal cancer is too high to be considered sporadic, but the pattern is not consistent with an inherited syndrome. First-degree relatives of patients diagnosed with colorectal cancer have an increased risk of the disease that is at least two to four times that of persons in the general population without a family history.[36]

Enzyme Polymorphisms

Increasing evidence suggests that genetic polymorphisms in drug-metabolizing enzymes, such as *N*-acetyltransferases (NAT1 and NAT2), cytochrome P450 (CYP) isoenzymes, glutathione-*S*-transferase (GST) enzymes, methylenetetrahydrofolate reductase (MTHFR), and hemochromatosis gene mutations may confer genetic susceptibility to colorectal cancer.[21] Individuals with certain variations in NAT1, NAT2, CYP1A2, CYP1A1, and CYP2E1 enzyme genotypes may be particularly susceptible to carcinogenic effects of a high dietary intake of meat, tobacco smoke, or other environmental factors.[40,41] The *MTHFR* C677T genotype may influence the association of colorectal cancer risk through interactions with dietary folate, alcohol, or vitamin B_{12} intake. Mutations in the hemochromatosis gene are associated with increased colon cancer risk with increasing age and total iron intake.

SUMMARY OF RISK FACTORS

In summary, multiple factors are associated with colorectal cancer risk. Lifestyle factors related to economic development, such as obesity, physical inactivity, chronic hyperinsulinemia, and alcohol and tobacco use, increase risk of colorectal cancer. Observational studies report associations between high dietary intake of processed and red meats and fat, and a diet low in fiber, folate, fruit and vegetables with increased risk of colorectal cancer. Regular aspirin and NSAID use and postmenopausal hormone replacement therapy decrease risk, but recommendations have not been made because of unresolved issues regarding risk-to-benefit considerations. Inherited genetic susceptibilities and clinical risk factors, such as inflammatory bowel disease, are well known risks for colon cancer.

PATHOPHYSIOLOGY

ANATOMY AND BOWEL FUNCTION

The large intestine consists of the cecum; ascending, transverse, descending, and sigmoid colon; and the rectum (Fig. 133–2). In adults, it extends about 1.5 m and has a diameter ranging from 8 cm in the cecum to 2 cm in the sigmoid colon. The function of the large intestine is to receive 500 to 2,000 mL of ileal contents per day. Absorption of fluid and solutes occurs in the right colon or the segments proximal to the middle of the transverse colon, with movement and storage of fecal material in the left colon and distal segments of the colon. Mucus secretion from goblet cells into the intestinal lumen lubricates the mucosal surface and facilitates movement of the dehydrated feces. It also serves to protect the luminal wall from bacteria and colonic irritants such as bile acids.

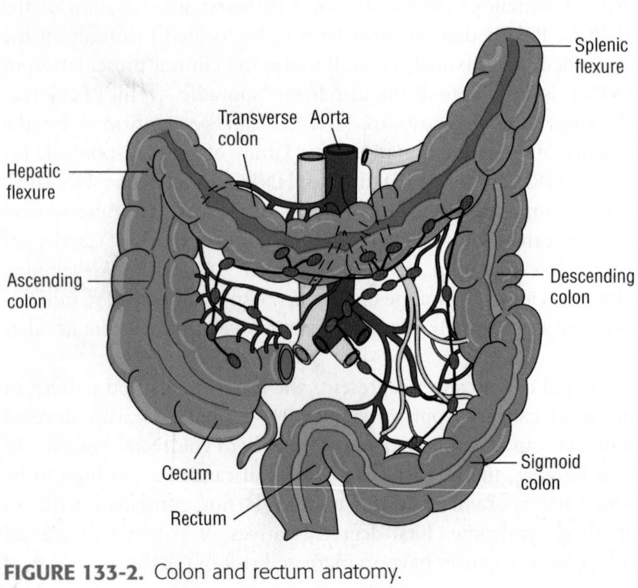

FIGURE 133-2. Colon and rectum anatomy.

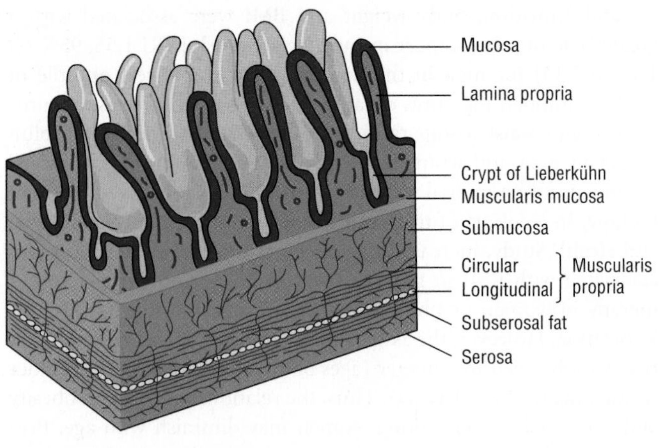

FIGURE 133-3. Cross-section of bowel wall.

Four major tissue layers, from the lumen outward, form the large intestine: the mucosa, submucosa, muscularis externa, and serosa (Fig. 133–3). Embedded in the submucosa and muscularis externa is a rich lymphatic capillary system. Lymphatic channels do not extend into the mucosa. The muscularis externa consists of circular smooth muscle and three outer longitudinal smooth muscle bands. Contraction of these muscle groups moves colonic material toward the anal canal. The outermost layer of the colon, the serosa, secretes a fluid that allows the colon to slide easily over nearby structures within the peritoneum. The serosa covers only the anterior and lateral aspects of the upper third of the rectum. The lower third lies completely extraperitoneal and is surrounded by fibrofatty tissue as well as adjacent organs and structures.

The surface epithelium of the colonic mucosa undergoes continual renewal, and complete replacement of epithelial cells occurs every 4 to 8 days. Cell replication normally takes place within the lower third of crypts, the tubular glands located within the intestinal mucosa. The cells then mature and differentiate to either goblet or absorptive cells as they migrate toward the bowel lumen. The total number of epithelial cells remains relatively constant as the number of cells migrating from the crypts is balanced by the rate of exfoliation of cells from the mucosal surface. This two-phase process is critical to the malignant transformation of the epithelial cells. The number of dysplastic and hyperplastic aberrant crypt foci increases with increasing age; as the mass of abnormal cells accumulates at the top of the crypt and starts to protrude into the stream of fecal matter, their contact with fecal mutagens can lead to further cell mutations and eventual adenoma formation.[21]

COLORECTAL TUMORIGENESIS

The development of a colorectal neoplasm is a multistep process of several genetic and phenotypic alterations of normal bowel epithelium structure and function, leading to unregulated cell growth, proliferation, and tumor development. Because most colorectal cancers develop sporadically, with no inherited or familial disposition, efforts have been directed toward identifying these alterations and learning whether detection of such changes may lead to improved cancer detection and/or treatment outcomes.

Colorectal tumorigenesis involves multiple genetic events, including gene mutations, epigenetic silencing of gene transcription through promotor hypermethylation, loss of heterozygosity, and

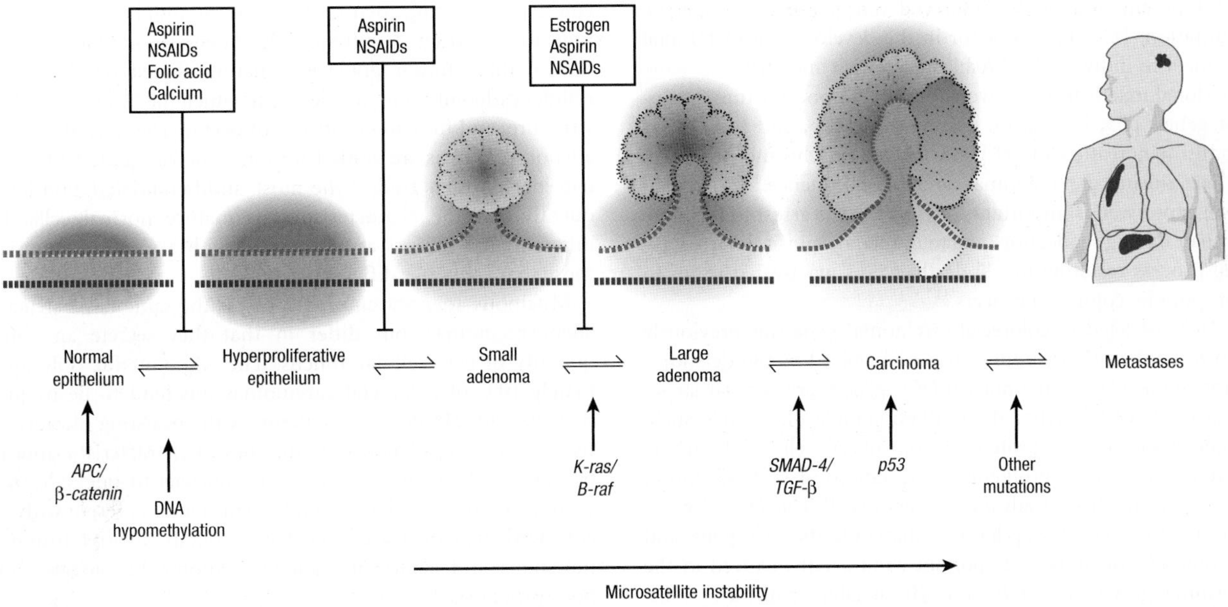

FIGURE 133-4. Genetic changes associated with the adenoma–carcinoma sequence in colorectal cancer. The accumulation of genetic changes in the pathogenesis of colorectal cancer includes DNA hypomethylation across the genome, mutation in the adenomatous polyposis coli (*APC*) gene or abnormalities in *β*-catenin; mutational activation of cyclooxygenase-2 (COX-2); *k-Ras* or *B-raf* oncogene activation; tumor suppressor gene deletions in chromosome 18q (SMAD-4 mutations) and disruption of transforming growth factor-*β* receptor type II signaling; and defects in *p53* function. Shown also are points of possible chemopreventive activity by various agents. (NSAIDs, nonsteroidal antiinflammatory drugs.) *(From references 42, 43, and 50.)*

gene amplification. A genetic model has been proposed for colorectal tumorigenesis that describes a process of transformation from adenoma to carcinoma. However, at least three separate additional molecular pathways to developing colorectal cancer have been identified.[21] These include a pathway for HNPCC, an ulcerative colitis–dysplasia carcinoma sequence, and a pathway involving hypermethylation. Some of the molecular processes are common to more than one pathway.

Figure 133–4 is an overview of the adenoma–carcinoma model. The adenoma–carcinoma sequence of tumor development reflects an accumulation of mutations within colonic epithelium which confer a selective growth advantage to the affected cells. Key elements of this process include hyperproliferation of epithelial cells to form a small benign neoplasm or adenoma in conjunction with cellular gene mutations.[42] These mutations occur early and frequently in sporadic cases of both adenomas and colorectal cancer. Somatic mutations must occur in at least four or five genes to produce the malignant transformation.[34]

Genetic changes include activation of oncogenes, inactivation of tumor suppressor genes, and defects in DNA MMR genes. Table 133–2 lists specific genetic mutations that cause colorectal cancer. Activating mutations of *ras* protooncogenes, primarily involving the K-*ras* and N-*ras* genes, occur frequently in colorectal cancer. The *ras* family of genes is responsible for encoding proteins involved in transmission of extracellular growth signals to the nucleus. Activation of *ras* leads to a constitutive activity of the protein, resulting in continuous stimulus of cell proliferation and other activities that promote carcinogenesis.

Deletion or inactivation of tumor suppressor genes may facilitate transformation of normal cells to cancerous cells. One of the earliest genetic changes in colorectal tumorigenesis involves the mutation or loss of the *APC* gene, a tumor suppressor gene localized on the long arm of chromosome 5q21. The *APC* gene encodes for a protein that binds to *α*- and *β*-catenin, which belong to a family of proteins associated with intracellular adhesion.[42] *β*-Catenin, an essential component of the Wnt signaling pathway, binds to the cytoplasmic domain of E-cadherin, an important molecule responsible for cell–cell adhesion. These activities, among others, are believed to be involved in regulation of cell shape and cell-to-cell communication, and may affect cell-cycle regulation or apoptosis. Alterations in *β*-catenin may also lead to abnormal epithelial proliferation and differentiation of cells. Inactivation of the *APC* gene is the single gene defect responsible for FAP, and is frequently an early event in

TABLE 133-2 Genetic Mutations Associated with Colorectal Cancer

Type of Mutation	Disease	Genes
Germ line	Familial adenomatous polyposis (FAP)	*APC*
	MYH-associated polyposis (MAP)	*MYH*
	Hereditary nonpolyposis colorectal cancer (HNPCC)	DNA mismatch-repair genes:
		MSH2
		MLH1
		PMS1
		PMS2
		MSH6
		MSH3
		IGF1
Somatic	Sporadic colorectal cancer	Oncogenes:
		ras
		B-raf
		myc
		src
		Tumor suppressor genes:
		p53
		SMAD-4
		APC
Low-penetrance susceptibility alleles	CRC in Ashkenazi Jewish population	*APC*I1307K*
		BLM
	Familial CRC	*TGF-βRI*
		HRAS1-VNTR
		MTHFR

APC, adenomatous polyposis coli; CRC, colorectal cancer; HRAS1-VNTR, Harvey ras-1 variable number tandem repeat; IGF1, insulin-like growth factor-1; MTHFR, methylenetetrahydrofolate reductase; TGF-*β*RI, transforming growth factor-*β* receptor type I.
From references 34 , 36, and 137.

the development of sporadic colorectal cancer cases.[34] A specific *APC* mutation, I1307K, is a factor in the development of familial colon cancer in individuals of Ashkenazi Jewish ancestry.[36]

Mutational inactivation of two additional important tumor suppressor genes, *p53*, located on chromosome 17p, and the *DPC-4* (deleted in pancreatic cancer) gene, located on chromosome 18q, occur later during the adenoma–carcinoma sequence.[43,42] Normal *p53* gene expression is important for G_1 cell-cycle arrest to facilitate DNA repair during replication, and to induce apoptosis, an irreversible cell process resulting in cell death. *p53* is inactivated in up to 75% of sporadic colorectal cancers.[34]

The *DCC* (deleted in colorectal carcinoma) gene was previously thought to be the tumor suppressor gene involved in 18q deletions. The protein encoded by the normal *DCC* gene shares similar structural features to certain types of cell adhesion molecules, and as such, may interact with various proteins to control cell–cell or cell–matrix interactions and cellular proliferation. Mutations of *DCC* are found in approximately 50% of advanced adenomas.[34] The *DPC-4* gene, also referred to as *SMAD-4*, is located adjacent to the *DCC* gene, and has become identified as an important component involved in the transforming growth factor-β (TGF-β) signaling pathway.[43] This signaling pathway involves SMAD proteins and TGF-β receptors type I (TGF-βRI) and type II (TGF-βRII). In normal epithelium, TGF-β has an antiproliferative role and induces growth arrest and apoptosis. Alterations in *SMAD* or TGF-β receptors lead to a loss of the normal growth inhibitory response to TGF-β. The frequency of *SMAD-4* mutations in colorectal cancer is reported to be from 6% to 30%.[43]

A distinct group of genetic traits has also been identified for individuals with HNPCC, but they also occur in sporadic cases of colorectal cancer. Replication errors occur frequently and represent widespread alterations in the length of a series of repeated nucleotides, or microsatellites, within tumor DNA. Mutations of those genes that appear to recognize and regulate DNA mismatch-repair errors, or MMR genes, contribute to microsatellite instability and colorectal tumorigenesis.[42] Failure to repair DNA mismatches results in microsatellite instability, which accelerates further gene mutations, leading to oncogene activation or tumor suppressor gene inactivation. Tumor progression may then be facilitated through a link between DNA repair defects and mutations of critical growth regulatory genes. Inactivation of TGF-βRII has been demonstrated in cells with replication errors.[36]

Several additional genes and protein receptors are probably important in colorectal tumorigenesis, although their roles have not been completely determined. COX-2, which is induced in colorectal cancer cells, influences apoptosis and other cellular functions. The peroxisome proliferator-activated receptor (PPAR) gene, a nuclear receptor that serves as a transcription factor, may interact with the COX pathway and affect tumorigenesis.[34] The PPARδ isoform is upregulated in colorectal cancer, and its activation promotes tumor growth. COX-derived prostaglandins indirectly activate PPARδ, which further enhances adenoma growth. The protooncogene c-*erb*-B is activated in a high percentage of human tumors, including colorectal cancer, and encodes for expression of epidermal growth factor receptor (EGFR), a transmembrane glycoprotein involved in signaling pathways that affect cell growth, differentiation, proliferation, and angiogenesis. EGFR, which is overexpressed in a high proportion (72% to 82%) of colorectal cancers, is associated with increased cell proliferation and metastasis.[44] These mechanisms are potentially important because of the availability of pharmacologic agents that can influence these processes and affect cell growth.

HISTOLOGY

Adenocarcinomas account for more than 90% of tumors of the large intestine.[45] Other histologic types such as mucinous adenocarcinoma, signet-ring adenocarcinoma, carcinoid simplex, and carcinoid tumors occur less frequently. Adenocarcinomas are assigned one of three tumor grade designations based on the degree of cellular differentiation, the degree to which the tumor resembles the structure, and function of its cell of origin. The most differentiated adenocarcinomas are grade I tumors, whereas grade III tumors are considered "high grade," the most undifferentiated, and have frequently lost the characteristics of mature normal cells. Poorly differentiated tumors are associated with a worse prognosis than those that are better differentiated.[45]

Mucinous adenocarcinomas possess the same basic structure as adenocarcinomas, but differ in that they secrete an abundant quantity of extracellular mucus. They account for only approximately 10% of colorectal carcinomas but tend to be frequent in patients with HNPCC and patients with coexisting ulcerative colitis.[45] Signet-ring adenocarcinomas have a characteristic appearance because of the displacement of the nucleus to one side by large vacuoles of intracellular mucin. Patients tend to present with a more advanced stage of disease and have a highly invasive tumor. Both mucinous and signet-ring adenocarcinoma histologies confer a poor prognosis.[46]

PREVENTION AND SCREENING

Cancer prevention efforts can be considered as either primary or secondary. Primary prevention strategies aim to prevent the development of colorectal cancer in a population at risk. Secondary prevention approaches are undertaken to prevent malignancy in a population that has already manifested an initial disease process. The basis for primary prevention depends on identification of risk factors followed by eradication or alteration of their effects on carcinogenesis. Primary prevention also includes lifestyle and diet modification. Several primary preventive measures have undergone or are currently undergoing study; Table 133–3 lists some strategies.

TABLE 133-3 Prevention Strategies for Colorectal Cancer

Prevention Strategy	Proposed Mechanism of Protective Effect
High-fiber diet supplementation[a]	Decreases fecal bile acids; decreases bowel transit time; direct binding to fecal mutagens; dilution of fecal material
Dietary fat reduction[a]	Decreases fecal bile acids; reduces consumption of heterocyclic amines and other carcinogens that are produced through meat preparation and processing techniques
Nonsteroidal anti-inflammatory agents[b,c]	Inhibit COX-2; induce apoptosis via 15-LOX-1
Selenium	Antioxidant effects
Calcium	Direct binding to bile and fatty acids; inhibits epithelial cell proliferation
Estrogens[c]	Decrease synthesis of secondary bile acids; decrease production of IGF-1; direct antiproliferative effects on colorectal epithelium.
Ursodeoxycholic acid	Modulates bile acid composition; inhibits cell proliferation
Eflornithine	Inhibits cellular proliferation through alterations in polyamine metabolism
Curcumin	Induces glutathione *S*-transferase (GST) enzymes; inhibits COX-2 expression

COX-2, cyclooxygenase-2; 15-LOX-1, 15-lipoxygenase-1; IGF-1, insulin-like growth factor 1.
[a]To date, findings from randomized trials have failed to demonstrate a protective effect of low-fat high-fiber fruit and vegetable dietary intake in reducing risk of recurrence of colorectal adenomas or colorectal cancer.
[b]Includes COX-2 inhibitors.
[c]Risk of use may outweigh benefit.
Data from Hawk ET, Levin B. Colorectal Cancer Prevention. J Clin Oncol 2005;23:378–391.

DIET

❶ Although early studies suggest that a substantial increase in daily dietary fiber and/or decrease in dietary fat intake might significantly reduce colorectal cancer risk, results from recent randomized trials are inconsistent. The role of a diet high in fiber, or the use of fiber supplementation, as a prevention strategy requires further investigation.

CHEMOPREVENTION

❷ The most widely studied agents for the chemoprevention of colorectal cancer are aspirin, nonaspirin NSAIDs, and COX-2 inhibitors, but their use as chemopreventive agents in the general population has not been established. Nonaspirin NSAIDs and COX-2 inhibitors reduced the incidence of colorectal adenomas in cohort and case-control studies (RR 0.64 and 0.54, respectively) and COX-2 inhibitors were also effective in controlled trials (RR 0.72, CI 0.68 to 0.77).[17] However, the United States Preventive Services Task Force has concluded that potential harms associated with their use outweigh the benefits of aspirin and NSAIDs for prevention of colorectal cancer in the general population.[47]

In randomized studies of individuals with FAP, sulindac and celecoxib reduced the size and number of adenomatous polyps, but they are not viewed as alternatives to surgery. Sulindac can induce regression of existing adenomas, but in a randomized study of newly diagnosed patients with FAP it did not prevent new adenoma formation.[48] In 1999, the FDA approved the use of celecoxib to reduce the number of adenomatous colorectal polyps in FAP, as an adjunct to usual care. This approval was based primarily on results from a trial of 77 patients with FAP who received celecoxib, 400 mg orally twice daily, or placebo, for 6 months. Celecoxib administration significantly reduced the mean polyp number (28% vs. 4.5%) and polyp burden (30.7% vs. 4.9%) as compared to placebo.[19] Recently, celecoxib was shown to decrease sporadic adenoma formation by more than 30% as compared to placebo, but the risk of cardiovascular events was increased in the treatment group and its use in the general population cannot be recommended at this time.[49] In addition, its benefits are likely to be transient, because patients receiving sulindac experienced an increase in size and number of polyps within 3 months after the sulindac was discontinued.[50]

The use of aspirin as both a primary and secondary chemopreventive agent remains controversial. Regular use of aspirin reduced the incidence of colorectal cancer in cohort studies by 22%, and reduced the incidence of adenomas in randomized controlled trials, case-control studies, and cohort studies.[16] The benefits appear greatest with high-dose rather than low-dose (325- vs. 81-mg) aspirin and with administration for periods longer than 10 years, but the risk of bleeding complications is also greater.[16] In addition, aspirin use appears to reduce the risk of colorectal cancers that overexpress COX-2 but not those with absent or weak COX-2 expression.[51]

Randomized trials of calcium and folate supplementation as chemoprevention have also been conducted and findings do not support their use at this time. In the placebo-controlled Calcium Poly Prevention Study, patients with a previous colorectal adenoma who received calcium carbonate supplementation for 5 years experienced a moderate reduction (adjusted RR 0.63, CI 0.46 to 0.87) in risk of recurrent colorectal adenomas.[52] In another randomized trial, protection was limited to individuals with higher serum vitamin D levels. These findings are in contrast with results from a large, randomized trial of calcium plus vitamin D supplementation for 7 years in 36,282 women from the Women's Health Initiative, which did not demonstrate any difference in the incidence of invasive colorectal cancer between treatment or placebo.[53] Because of the long latency period associated with cancer development, the 7-year duration of this trial may have been too short. However, there is no evidence that calcium intake greater than that recommended to reduce osteoporosis is protective against colorectal cancer. Although calcium intake appears to be inversely related to colon cancer, its role as a chemopreventive agent is still under investigation.

Additional intervention trials of various micronutrients, including selenium and folic acid, and other chemopreventive agents have been completed or are ongoing.[50] A randomized, placebo-controlled trial of folate 1 mg daily for up to 6 years as primary prevention of colorectal adenomas did not show a reduction in adenoma risk.[54] Furthermore, folate supplementation appeared to be associated with an increased risk of adenomas, and this observation requires further exploration. As such, folate supplementation to reduce colorectal cancer risk is not recommended at this time. Because of their different mechanisms of action and sites of influence on the process of colorectal carcinogenesis, certain populations of individuals may benefit most from selected agents.

SURGICAL RESECTION

Surgical resection remains an option to prevent colon cancer in individuals at extremely high risk for its development. Despite the potential for NSAIDs to reduce adenoma development and to induce adenoma regression in individuals with FAP, their effects are incomplete and their use cannot replace surgical resection as an important means of cancer prevention for these high-risk individuals. Individuals with FAP who are found to have polyposis on lower endoscopy screening examinations should undergo total proctocolectomy and ileal pouch–anal anastomosis or subtotal colectomy with an ileorectal anastomosis.[55] Because of the high incidence of metachronous cancers (45%) in patients with HNPCC, prophylactic subtotal colectomy with an ileorectal anastomosis is recommended for those individuals.[55] Colonoscopic polypectomy, removal of polyps detected during screening colonoscopy, is considered the standard of care for all individuals to prevent the progression of premalignant adenomatous polyps to adenocarcinomas.

SCREENING

❸ Based on the recognized incidence of colorectal cancer, identification of high-risk individuals, and the high rate of curability associated with localized lesions, screening recommendations for early detection of colorectal cancer have been established.[56,57] This section reviews available screening techniques for colon cancer.

Fecal Occult Blood Testing

❸ The use of fecal occult blood tests (FOBTs) annually or biannually, results in an increased number of asymptomatic individuals diagnosed with early stages of disease. Results from four randomized, controlled trials with a combined enrollment of over 320,000 patients show that repeated FOBTs reduce the risk of colorectal cancer mortality by 16% (RR 0.84, CI 0.78 to 0.90).[58] Two main methods are available to detect occult blood in the feces: guaiac dye or derivative, and immunochemical methods. The Hemoccult II is the most commonly used FOBT in the United States. This is a guaiac-based test that detects pseudoperoxidase activity in hemoglobin when hemoglobin comes in contact with a guaiac-impregnated paper. When a solution containing hydrogen peroxide is poured over the paper, a blue color appears if the test is positive. The testing process is complex and requires specific patient counseling to avoid inaccurate results (Table 133–4).

The Hemoccult Sensa, another guaiac-based test, is preferred by some organizations because it may have increased sensitivity and specificity as compared to the Hemoccult II. Clinical guidelines

TABLE 133-4 Patient Counseling Points Prior to Hemoccult II Testing

To Avoid False Positives	To Avoid False Negatives
1. Dietary restrictions • Avoid rare red meat and vegetables with peroxidase activity (turnips, broccoli, cauliflower, and radishes) for 3 days prior to testing 2. Medical restrictions • Avoid iron products, rectal administration of medications and digital rectal examinations for 3 days prior to testing • Avoid nonsteroidal antiinflammatory drugs for up to 7 days prior to testing	• Avoid vitamin C for 3 days prior to testing • Avoid testing dehydrated samples (rehydrating of samples is not recommended)
Procedure for Hemoccult II testing	
Patient applies two separate samples of three different stools to six test card windows	

have been developed for performing and interpreting results of FOBT.[56] The limitations associated with fecal occult blood screening remain an issue of active concern. Many early stage tumors do not bleed, and therefore the false-negative rates are approximately 70% for cancer and 90% for polyps. In addition, the test results may not be valid because the test is often poorly performed in both the home and physician office settings.[57] However, these concerns are addressed through continued serial screening with FOBT. In addition, approximately 1% to 5% of randomly selected individuals will have a positive test result and approximately 2% to 17% of those individuals will be found to have colorectal cancer.[56,59] False-positive results can prove to be very expensive and inconvenient for a patient because of the followup tests required to confirm a positive result. Nevertheless, studies evaluating the effects of FOBT as a screening modality have established that their annual use reduces colorectal cancer mortality by up to 33%.[56]

Newer tests, such as immunochemical assays, were developed to reduce the rate of false-positive results associated with the guaiac-based tests. Fecal immunochemical tests (FIT) (InSure and others) use antibodies to detect the globin protein portion of human hemoglobin. These FITs have the advantage of improved specificity and sensitivity.[60] A potential increase in patient compliance is expected because these tests do not react with dietary factors or medications. To date, these FITs have not found widespread use in the United States because of commercial and technical reasons, although they, along with guaiac-based tests, are recommended in some screening protocols.

Flexible Sigmoidoscopy

❸ Sigmoidoscopy can examine the lower 35% to 60% of the bowel, depending on the instrument, and thus increases the detection rate by about two- to threefold.[56] A 60-cm flexible sigmoidoscope can be used to reach the splenic flexure so as to detect 50% to 60% of cancers, but it requires more operator training, is associated with increased risk, and is not tolerated as well as the 35-cm instrument. The combination of sigmoidoscopy plus FOBT appears to improve sensitivity for lesions that will be missed by sigmoidoscopy alone, but the true benefit of this approach to general practice has not been established.[56] Whether this will improve patient outcomes requires further study.

Total Colonic Examination

❸ Total colonic examination can be accomplished with colonoscopy or double-contrast barium enema. A colonoscope facilitates examination of the whole bowel to the cecum in most patients, and allows for simultaneous removal of premalignant lesions. Although it allows for greater visualization of the colon, colonoscopy involves greater risk and inconvenience to patients. However, it is the preferred screening method based on its superior ability to detect lesions in the proximal colon as compared to sigmoidoscopy.[56,59] This may become increasingly important, as the proportion of tumors occurring in the proximal or right (cecum, ascending, and transverse colon) side of the colon has increased over the past 30 years, with fewer occurring in the rectum and distal or left (descending and sigmoid colon) side. It remains somewhat controversial whether this observation reflects a change in the biology of the disease or the nature of screening techniques. Most lesions, however, still occur in the distal colon.

A double-contrast barium enema produces an image of the entire colon in most examinations, and the retained barium outlines small polyps and mucosal lesions. This approach is the least-expensive method of examining the entire colon, but is considered inferior to colonoscopy for detecting polyps and colorectal cancer.[57] In addition, a supplemental colonoscopy is required if suspicious lesions are identified. Because of these limitations, the combination of double-contrast barium enema with flexible sigmoidoscopy is used to increase the sensitivity for detecting a colorectal malignancy versus double-contrast barium enema alone, and is generally reserved for use when a colonoscopy is not feasible.

Novel Screening Strategies

Molecular screening strategies analyze stool samples for presence of potential markers of malignancy in cells that are shed from premalignant polyps or adenocarcinomas in the bowel.[60] These include abnormalities or mutations in DNA, RNA expression patterns that are characteristic of malignancy, and the presence of proteins or other molecular cellular components. Of these, DNA testing has undergone the most testing. In a large-scale comparison of fecal DNA analysis to FOBT in asymptomatic individuals at average-risk, neither test was able to identify most of the neoplastic lesions found with colonoscopy, but fecal DNA analysis detected a greater proportion of lesions than did FOBT without compromising specificity.[61] Additional work is ongoing to identify the role of novel molecular markers in colorectal cancer detection, but none to date have shown improvement over FIT. Genetic testing is an important cancer-screening approach for family members of individuals diagnosed with FAP or HNPCC, and is appropriate for selected individuals, but should only be offered in conjunction with genetic counseling.

Computed tomography (CT) colonography (virtual colonoscopy) is an imaging procedure that creates two- or three-dimensional images of the colon by combining multiple helical CT scans. Initial tests are promising, although patients still require bowel cleansing and colonoscopy to remove detected lesions.[60]

Screening Summary

Table 133–5 outlines the current American Cancer Society guidelines for screening and surveillance for early detection of colorectal polyps and cancer. Men and women who are 50 years of age and are at average risk (their only risk factor is age >50 years) should be screened with annual FOBT or FIT with examination of the colon every 5 to 10 years, depending on the type of test used.[57] Although several methods for examining the colon are available, there is no evidence that one test should be chosen over another.[59] However, colonoscopy is the preferred modality of the American Society for Gastrointestinal Endoscopy.[56] More rigorous (usually starting at an earlier age) screening recommendations are recommended for moderate- to high-risk individuals.

DIAGNOSIS

SIGNS AND SYMPTOMS

The signs and symptoms associated with colorectal cancer can be extremely varied, subtle, and nonspecific. Patients with early stage

TABLE 133-5 American Cancer Society Guidelines for Screening and Surveillance for Early Detection of Colorectal Polyps and Cancer

Risk Category	Recommendation[a]	Age to Begin (Years)	Interval
Average risk	FOBT or FIT	50	Annually
	or		
	Flexible sigmoidoscopy	50	Every 5 years
	or		
	FOBT (or FIT) plus flexible sigmoidoscopy[b]	50	Annual FOBT (or FIT) with flexible sigmoidoscopy every 5 years
	or		
	DCBE	50	Every 5 years
	or		
	Colonoscopy	50	Every 10 years
Increased risk			
People with one or two, small (<1 cm) tubular adenomas with low-grade dysplasia	Colonoscopy[c]	5–10 years after initial polypectomy	If examination is normal, screening as for average risk person
People with large (≥1 cm) or multiple (3 to 10) adenomatous polyps, or adenomas with high-grade dysplasia or villous features	Colonoscopy[c]	Within 3 years after initial polypectomy	If normal, repeat in 3 years; if still normal or shows only one or two adenomas, then repeat every 5 years
Patients with more than 10 adenomas at a single examination	Colonoscopy	Within 3 years after initial polypectomy	If normal, repeat in 3 years; consider possibility of familial syndrome
Personal history of curative-intent resection of colorectal cancer	Colonoscopy[c]	Within 1 year after resection	If normal, repeat in 3 years; if still normal, repeat every 5 years
Colorectal cancer or adenomatous polyps in first-degree relative younger than age 60 years or in two or more first-degree relatives at any ages	Colonoscopy[c]	Age 40 or 10 years before the youngest case in family, whichever is earlier	Every 5–10 years
High risk			
Family history of familial adenomatous polyposis (FAP)	Early surveillance with endoscopy, and counseling to consider genetic testing	Puberty	If genetic test positive, colectomy is indicated
Family history of hereditary nonpolyposis colon cancer (HNPCC)	Colonoscopy and counseling to consider genetic testing	Age 21	If genetic test positive, or if the patient has not had genetic testing, every 1–2 years until age 40, then annually
Inflammatory bowel disease; chronic ulcerative colitis; Crohn's disease	Colonoscopy biopsies for dysplasia	8 years after the start of pancolitis or 12–15 years after the start of left-sided colitis	Every 1–2 years

DCBE, double-contrast barium enema; FOBT, fecal occult blood testing; FIT, fecal immunochemical testing.
[a]Digital rectal examination should be done at the time of each sigmoidoscopy, colonoscopy, or DCBE.
[b]FOBT together with flexible sigmoidoscopy is preferred over FOBT or flexible sigmoidoscopy alone.
[c]If colonoscopy is not available or feasible, DCBE alone or together with flexible sigmoidoscopy are acceptable alternatives.
From references 57 and 139–141.

colorectal cancer are often asymptomatic and lesions are usually found as a result of screening studies. Any change in bowel habits (e.g., constipation, diarrhea, or alteration in size or shape of stool), vague abdominal discomfort, abdominal pain, or distension may all be warning signs of a malignant process. Obstructive symptoms and changes in bowel habits frequently develop with tumors located in the transverse and descending colon. Bleeding may be acute or chronic and most commonly appears as bright red blood mixed with stool. Iron-deficiency anemia, presenting as weakness and occasionally as high-output congestive heart failure, frequently develops as a result of chronic occult blood loss.

PRESENTATION OF COLORECTAL CANCER

General

- Patient symptoms are usually nonspecific and can vary drastically among patients.

Symptoms

- Change in bowel habits (generally an increase in frequency) or rectal bleeding.
- Constipation, depending on the location of the tumor.
- Nausea, vomiting, and abdominal discomfort.
- Fatigue may be present if anemia is severe.

Signs

- Blood in the stool is the most common sign.
- Hepatomegaly and jaundice in advanced disease.
- Leg edema as a consequence of lymph node involvement, thrombophlebitis, fistula formation, weight loss, and pain in the lower back or radiating down the legs are indicative of widespread disease.

Laboratory Tests

- Positive guaiac stool test and anemia (iron deficiency) from blood loss.
- Elevated carcinoembryonic antigen (most patients).
- Elevated liver enzymes may be present with metastatic disease.

Approximately 20% of patients with colorectal cancer present with metastatic disease.[3] Metastatic spread occurs as a result of direct tumor invasion of adjacent tissues or by lymphatic or hematogenous spread. The venous drainage of the colon and rectum influences the pattern of metastases most commonly seen. The most common site of metastasis is the liver, often the only site of metastatic disease in 40% of patients, followed by the lungs and then bones, specifically the sacrum, coccyx, pelvis, and lumbar vertebrae. Liver metastases are present in 5% to 10% of patients at presentation.

WORKUP

When a patient is suspected of having colorectal carcinoma, a careful history and physical examination should be performed. The patient history should include a past medical history and family

TABLE 133-6 Recommended Pretreatment Evaluation for Patients with Potentially Curable Colorectal Cancer

- Personal medical history and family history of colorectal polyps, cancer, or other malignancies
- Physical examination, including evaluation for lymphadenopathy, hepatomegaly, and ascites; women should have appropriate evaluations to rule out breast, ovarian, or endometrial cancers
- Complete blood count, liver chemistries, and serum carcinoembryonic antigen
- Total colonic evaluation with colonoscopy or flexible sigmoidoscopy with double-contrast barium enema
- Chest radiography
- Chest/abdominal/pelvic computed tomography scan
- Additional studies as indicated

Data from Skibber JM, Minsky BD, Hoff PM. Cancer of the colon. In: DeVita VT, Hellman S, Rosenberg SA (ed). Cancer: Principles and Practice of Oncology, 6/e. Philadelphia, Lippincott, Williams & Wilkins, 2001.

history, especially noting the presence of inflammatory bowel disease, colorectal cancer, polyps, and cancers of the breast, ovary, and endometrium. A complete physical examination includes careful abdominal examination for the presence of masses or ascites, a rectal examination, and an assessment for possible hepatomegaly and lymphadenopathy. A breast and pelvic examination is recommended in all women, especially in women with a history of breast, ovarian, or endometrial cancer. Table 133–6 summarizes the recommended tests for pretreatment evaluation of patients with potentially curable colorectal cancer.

An unexplained anemia in an older patient requires surveillance of the entire large bowel, especially the right colon. Red blood cell indices (e.g., hemoglobin, hematocrit, mean corpuscular volume, and reticulocyte count) and a workup of iron status (e.g., serum ferritin, serum iron, and total iron-binding capacity) may be useful to confirm acute or chronic blood loss and/or iron-deficiency anemia. An evaluation of the entire large bowel is undertaken with either colonoscopy or sigmoidoscopy and a double-contrast barium enema. A barium enema may be preferred in situations in which a partially obstructing lesion prohibits passage of the endoscope, but it should be avoided if complete obstruction or perforation of the bowel is suspected. A characteristic finding indicative of colon cancer seen on barium enema is an apple core-shaped lesion with tumor involving the circumference of the bowel. When possible, the endoscope is used to collect tissue for a histologic evaluation and provide a preliminary diagnosis following the procedure.

Baseline laboratory tests should be obtained and include a complete blood cell count, platelet count, prothrombin time, activated partial thromboplastin time, and liver and renal function tests. Abnormal liver function tests may suggest liver involvement with tumor. However, patients with metastatic disease to the liver may have normal liver function tests, and abnormal liver function tests are not always indicative of metastatic disease.

Additional laboratory tests may include a baseline carcinoembryonic antigen (CEA) level if it is likely to augment staging and treatment plans.[62] CEA belongs to a group of cell-surface glycoproteins termed *oncofetal proteins*, which are expressed during embryonic development and reexpressed on the cell surfaces of many carcinomas, particularly those of the gastrointestinal tract. CEA concentrations can be measured in the blood and can therefore potentially serve as a marker for colorectal cancer. But not all colorectal cancers produce CEA, and elevated concentrations are more frequent in patients with metastatic disease. It is important to recognize, however, that several concomitant disease states are associated with an elevated CEA: liver diseases, gastritis, peptic ulcer disease, diverticulitis, chronic obstructive pulmonary disease, chronic or acute inflammatory conditions, and diabetes.[62] Most commercially available assays list a value of less than 5 ng/mL as the upper limit of normal. Although CEA measurement is too insensitive and nonspecific to be used as a screening test for early stage colorectal cancer, it is the marker of choice for monitoring colorectal cancer response to treatment, particularly if the pretreatment concentration is elevated.[62] The CEA test also has preoperative prognostic implications because it has been shown to correlate with the size and degree of differentiation of the carcinoma. Elevated preoperative CEA levels correlate with a poor survival and may predict likelihood of recurrence, regardless of tumor stage at diagnosis. However, it should not be used to determine whether a patient should receive adjuvant therapy. After a potentially curative resection, CEA levels should return to normal within 4 to 6 weeks. Persistently elevated CEA levels may indicate residual disease, while elevations after normalization may indicate relapsed disease.

Radiographic imaging studies evaluate the extent of disease involvement. Although a chest radiograph is recommended to rule out the presence of metastatic spread to the lungs, a CT scan of the chest is preferred. A CT scan of the abdomen and pelvis is often performed to evaluate hepatic and retroperitoneal involvement and occult abdominal and pelvic disease, and to determine the depth of tumor penetration into the bowel wall and/or invasion to adjacent organs. Detection of lymph node involvement with either study is limited by the difficulty of distinguishing inflammatory or reactive lymph nodes from those infiltrated with tumor. Because CT scans may not adequately detect peritoneal seeding, small distant lymph node metastasis, or liver metastasis in colon cancer, an occasional patient may need to undergo a laparotomy, spiral CT, magnetic resonance imaging, or glucose analog [^{18}F]-fluorodeoxyglucose-positron emission tomography (PET) scan in order to confirm metastatic disease. PET imaging can provide functional information to discriminate between benign and malignant disease by detecting tumor-related metabolic alterations in affected tissues. PET scans are commonly used for the detection of recurrent colorectal cancer in patients with rising CEA levels and inconclusive findings on standard imaging studies. It is often combined with or followed by a CT scan because anatomical localization of a lesion using PET alone can be difficult.

Endoscopic ultrasound is a technique that is becoming more widely available for the evaluation of patients with rectal cancer. It is useful for detecting the depth of tumor penetration, and like pelvic CT scans, is fair to good in determining lymph node involvement. Cystoscopy or IV pyelography studies are rarely indicated except for very large rectal tumors found on examination, if the patient exhibits symptoms, or if a CT scan suggests bladder involvement. Intraluminal and hepatic magnetic resonance imaging studies may also provide useful information.

Radioimmunoscintigraphy uses tumor-directed antibodies labeled with γ-producing radionuclides such as ^{99m}technetium or ^{111}indium to detect malignant cells.[63] Several tumor-associated proteins have been identified within or on the surface membrane of colorectal malignant cells to which monoclonal antibodies have been targeted. Of these, TAG-72 and CEA are commonly used. Radiolabeled monoclonal antibodies directed against these antigens are used in clinical studies for both external immunoscintigraphy as well as intraoperative localization of tumor. OncoScint, an ^{111}indium-labeled B72.3 monoclonal antibody targeted to the TAG-72 cell-surface antigen, is an FDA-approved diagnostic imaging agent available for determining the location and extent of extrahepatic disease in patients with colorectal cancer. CEA-Scan is a ^{99m}Tc-labeled fragment of the anti-CEA antibody for the assessment of recurrent colorectal carcinoma. The use of these tests is generally reserved for those patients who have completed standard diagnostic imaging tests, but may still require additional information regarding the extent of disease. They may also play an important role in identifying metastatic or recurrent disease in individuals with rising CEA levels and negative standard radiographic studies.

TABLE 133-7 TNM Staging Definitions for Colorectal Cancer

Criteria	Classification	Definition
Primary tumor (T)	T_X	Primary tumor cannot be assessed
	T_0	No evidence of primary tumor
	T_{is}	Carcinoma in situ: intraepithelial or invasion of the lamina propria[a]
	T_1	Tumor invades submucosa
	T_2	Tumor invades muscularis propria
	T_3	Tumor invades through the muscularis propria into the subserosa, or into the nonperitonealized pericolic or perirectal tissues
	T_4	Tumor directly invades other organs or structures and/or perforates the visceral peritoneum[b,c]
Regional lymph nodes (N)	N_X	Regional nodes cannot be assessed
	N_0	No regional lymph node metastasis
	N_1	Metastasis in one to three regional lymph nodes
	N_2	Metastasis in four or more regional lymph nodes
Distant metastasis (M)	M_X	Distant metastasis cannot be assessed
	M_0	No distant metastasis
	M_1	Distant metastasis

[a] T_{is} includes cancer cells confined within the glandular basement membrane (intraepithelial) or lamina propria (intramucosal) with no extension through the muscularis mucosae into the submucosa.
[b] Direct invasion in T_2 includes invasion of other segments of the colorectum by way of the serosa; for example, invasion of the sigmoid colon by a carcinoma of the cecum.
[c] Tumor that is adherent to other organs or structures macroscopically is classified T_2. However, if no tumor is present in the adhesion microscopically, the classification should be pT_3. The V and L substaging should be used to identify the presence or absence of vascular or lymphatic invasion.
From reference 142. Used with the permission of the American Joint Committee on Cancer (AJCC), from AJCC Cancer Staging Manual. With kind permission of Springer Science and Business Media.

STAGING

❹ The purpose of the staging examinations is to determine the extent of disease, which allows the oncologist to develop treatment options and estimate overall prognosis. Traditionally, the Dukes classification, originally published in 1932, was used in the staging of colorectal cancers.[45] Since its original publication, it has undergone several modifications; a modified Astler-Coller version is now used more commonly. In an effort to standardize the staging system for colorectal cancer, the American Joint Committee on Cancer and the International Union Against Cancer jointly recommend the TNM classification system. This classification takes three aspects of cancer growth: T (tumor size), N (lymph node involvement), and M (presence or absence of metastases) into account. The TNM classification also allows for various subdivisions within each of the three categories, which is then used for determining the disease stage. Table 133–7 summarizes the staging definitions using the TNM system. Table 133–8 shows the stage assignment based on TNM classifications and corresponding 5-year survival by stage. Figure 133–5 shows the relationship between the modified Astler-Coller and American Joint Committee on Cancer/International Union Against Cancer staging systems.

PROGNOSIS

❹ The stage of colorectal cancer upon diagnosis is the most important independent prognostic factor for survival and disease recurrence. Table 133–9 compares the stage of disease on presentation and relative survival rates for individuals with colon and rectum cancer.

TABLE 133-8 Colon Cancer Stage by TNM Classification and Associated 5-Year Survival

Stage	T	N	M	Dukes[a]	MAC[a]	Survival (%)
0	T_{is}	N_0	M_0	–	–	
I	T_1	N_0	M_0	A	A	93.2
	T_2	N_0	M_0	A	B_1	
IIA	T_3	N_0	M_0	B	B_2	84.7
IIB	T_4	N_0	M_0	B	B_3	72.2
IIIA	T_1–T_2	N_1	M_0	C	C_1	83.4
IIIB	T_3–T_4	N_1	M_0	C	C_2/C_3	64.1
IIIC	Any T	N_2	M_0	C	$C_1/C_2/C_3$	44.3
IV	Any T	Any N	M_1	–	D	8.1

[a] Dukes B is a composite of better ($T_3 N_0 M_0$) and worse ($T_4 N_0 M_0$) prognostic groups, as is Dukes C (any T N_1 M_0 and any T N_2 M_0). MAC is the modified Astler-Coller classification.
From references 46, 142, and 143.

Clinical factors present at time of diagnosis that are associated with a poor prognosis and decreased survival include bowel obstruction or perforation, rectal bleeding, high preoperative CEA level, distant metastases, and location of the primary tumor in the rectum or rectosigmoid area.[45] Along with resection of the primary tumor, a minimum of 12 lymph nodes must be examined to accurately determine regional lymph node involvement and predict lymph node-negative disease.[46] The pathologic assessment also includes determination of TNM stage, tumor type and histologic grade, presence of vascular invasion, and whether the resected margins are free of tumor. Consideration of these factors plays an important role in determining optimal strategies for treatment and appropriate followup.

Additional stage-independent pathologic variables that have negative prognostic or predictive value with regard to adjuvant therapy include: presence of lymphatic or perineural invasion; mucinous or signet-ring histology; high tumor proliferation indices; tumor aneuploidy; absence of host immune response to the tumor; and presence of certain molecular markers (18q/*DCC* mutation or loss of heterozygosity, microsatellite stability [MSS], *ras* mutations, elevated thymidylate synthase [TS] expression, and *p53* mutation or loss).[45,46,64] Of these, the highest level of evidence supports the consideration of lymphatic invasion as a prognostic factor. The next level of evidence, which is supporting but requires additional validation, is for 18q/*DCC* mutation or loss of heterozygosity and MSS.

Colorectal cancers with allelic loss of heterozygosity on chromosome 18q or absent DCC protein are associated with a worse prognosis within stage II disease, and may predict response to adjuvant chemotherapy, but data are insufficient to warrant its use at this time.[62] MSS can be determined through DNA sequencing or by immunohistochemistry staining for protein products of the *MSH2* or *MLH1* genes. Colorectal cancers that demonstrate high frequency MSS appear to be associated with a more favorable outcome and may respond better to fluorouracil.[65] Although findings from several

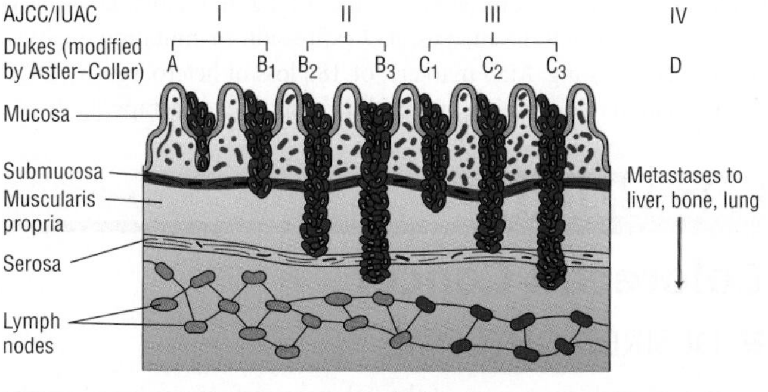

FIGURE 133-5. Staging systems for colorectal cancer. (AJCC, American Joint Committee for Cancer; IUAC, International Union Against Cancer.)

TABLE 133-9 Colon and Rectal Cancer Disease Stage and Survival Rates (SEER Data, 1996–2003)

Tumor Stage at Diagnosis	Stage Distribution (%)[a]		5-Year Relative Survival (%)	
	Colon	*Rectum*	*Colon*	*Rectum*
Localized	37	45	90.8	87.8
Regional	37	34	69.4	63.4
Distant	21	15	10.8	8.5
All stages	–	–	63.5	65.0

SEER, Surveillance, Epidemiology, and End Results.
[a]Approximately 4% and 6% of cancers of the colon and rectum, respectively, were unstaged.
From reference 3.

studies suggest that MSS status may predict efficacy of adjuvant fluoropyrimidine therapy, this finding must be confirmed in a prospective study before its use can be recommended.[62] Trials that account for MSS are ongoing.

Tumors that overexpress mutant *p53* demonstrate a high degree of resistance to radiation, fluorouracil, and certain other chemotherapeutic agents and are associated with a less-favorable prognosis. However, because of heterogeneous and conflicting results of reported studies, often attributable to methodologies that do not address the functional status of both *p53* alleles, *p53* status does not appear useful as a guide for treatment decisions.[62]

Tumors that overexpress TS, an enzyme that converts deoxyuridine monophosphate to deoxythymidine monophosphate, an essential step for DNA synthesis, are less sensitive to fluorouracil chemotherapy. Patients whose colon cancers have higher levels of TS appear to have a significantly worse overall 5-year survival than patients whose cancers have a low level of TS.[45] The importance of elevated TS and type of therapeutic interventions is unclear. No large cooperative group trial has identified a subgroup of patients who failed to benefit from fluorouracil plus leucovorin therapy based on tumor TS levels. Consideration of tumor TS expression in several adjuvant therapy trials is ongoing.

Tumors that have a high rate of proliferation are generally associated with a poor prognosis. Ki-67 is expressed in cells actively engaged in the cell cycle and has also been used as a measure of colon cancer proliferation. Interestingly, for unknown reasons, high levels of Ki-67 were associated with an increase in overall survival in patients with early stage colon cancer. EGFR testing of colorectal tumor cells with immunohistochemistry has been a standard component of pathologic analysis, but the value of EGFR positive staining in predicting response to anti-EGFR treatment is still unclear. Whereas EGFR overexpression may be linked to more advanced disease or predict risk of metastasis, its relationship to overall survival is controversial.[44] Whether other methods to assess EGFR status prove useful remains to be determined.

Evaluation of these factors may provide important clues as to which patients will benefit most from more aggressive therapy, individuals who may not in the future require systemic chemotherapy, and new therapeutic targets for the treatment of colorectal cancer, but further study is required. The current American Society of Clinical Oncology (ASCO) guidelines do not recommend the use of DNA ploidy, DNA flow cytometric proliferation analysis, *p53* expression or mutation analysis, *ras* oncogene testing, MSS markers, or 18q loss of heterozygosity/DCC determination to determine prognosis or response to therapy.[62]

TREATMENT

Colorectal Cancer

■ DESIRED OUTCOME

Treatment goals for cancer of the colon or rectum are based on the stage of disease at presentation. Stages I, II, and III disease are considered potentially curable, and are managed with the intent of eradicating micrometastases that may be present. Based on the numbers and site(s) of metastases, approximately 20% to 30% of patients with metastatic colorectal cancer may be cured, if their metastases are considered resectable. Most patients with stage IV disease are not curable, and treatments for metastatic disease are considered palliative to reduce symptoms, avoid disease-related complications, and prolong survival.

■ GENERAL APPROACH TO TREATMENT

Although advanced age is not an absolute contraindication for relatively aggressive therapies, the age of the patient, concomitant disease states, lifestyle factors, and the patient's preferences must be considered in the treatment planning process. Special or emergent conditions, such as bowel perforation, spinal cord compression, and severe pain, anemia, or other symptomatic problems, need to be addressed acutely, after which time a more long-term disease-specific plan can be developed. The treatment approaches for colorectal cancer reflect two primary treatment goals: curative therapy for localized disease and palliative therapy for metastatic cancer.

For patients for whom treatment intent is curative, surgical resection of the primary tumor is the most important component of therapy. Depending on the extent of disease and whether the tumor originated in the colon or rectum, further adjuvant chemotherapy or chemotherapy plus XRT may be appropriate. For selected patients with resectable metastases, surgical resection may be an option. However, for most patients with metastases, systemic chemotherapy is the mainstay of treatment; XRT may also be useful for disease palliation of localized symptoms or when chemotherapy is no longer effective. Patients with metastatic disease who are asymptomatic may benefit from initiation of therapy and treatment should not be withheld until they develop symptoms.

■ OPERABLE DISEASE

Surgery

❺ Individuals with operable—stages I, II, and III—colorectal cancer should undergo complete surgical resection of the primary tumor mass with regional lymphadenectomy as a curative approach for their disease.[45] The surgical approach for colon cancer generally involves complete resection of the tumor with an appropriate margin of tumor-free bowel and a regional lymphadenectomy. A total colectomy is rarely needed in colon cancer, but may be indicated for selected patients with FAP or chronic ulcerative colitis.

Surgery for rectal cancer depends on the region of tumor involvement. A low anterior resection is the procedure of choice in patients with lesions in the middle to upper rectum.[66] Patients with lesions in the lower portion of the rectum may require an abdominoperineal resection if either the amount of unaffected bowel is insufficient for a resection far enough away from the tumor, or too close to areas that cannot permit an anastomosis. Excision of the mesorectum, the surrounding tissue that contains perirectal fat and draining lymph nodes, has also been advocated. Newer surgical techniques have been developed in an attempt to retain function of the rectal sphincter and still achieve complete tumor resection. Individuals who are not candidates for sphincter-sparing resections or have extensive local spread of tumor will require an abdominoperineal resection. This involves removal of the distal sigmoid, rectosigmoid, rectum, and anus with the establishment of a permanent sigmoid colostomy. Less than one-third of patients will require a permanent colostomy for rectal cancer.[66] Other complications that occur frequently with surgery for rectal cancer include urinary retention, incontinence, impotence, and locoregional recurrence.

Overall, surgery for colorectal cancer is associated with a morbidity and mortality rate of 8% to 15% and 1% to 2%, respectively, depending on the type and extent of procedure.[45,66] Common complications associated with colorectal surgery include infection, anastomotic leakage, obstruction, adhesion formation, and malabsorption syndromes. Laparoscopic colectomy has become an accepted procedure for colon cancer and there are limited data for patients with rectal cancer.[67] This technique appears to produce similar oncologic results to conventional surgery, with the benefits of a smaller surgical incision, shorter hospital stay, and reduced pain.

Adjuvant Therapy for Colon Cancer

❺ Adjuvant therapy in colorectal cancer is administered to selected individuals after complete tumor resection in an attempt to eliminate residual micrometastatic disease, thereby decreasing tumor recurrence and improving survival rates. Because more than 90% of patients with stage I colon or rectal cancer are cured by surgical resection alone, adjuvant therapy is not indicated.[45] The role of adjuvant chemotherapy for stage II colon cancer is less clear because the results of studies in patients with stage II disease are conflicting. Adjuvant chemotherapy for patients with stage II disease has not been shown to be superior to surgery alone with the exception of high-risk patients who are ill defined. The ASCO guideline does not recommend routine use of adjuvant chemotherapy in patients with stage II disease unless it is administered in conjunction with a clinical trial.[68] Stage II patients who are at higher risk for relapse include those with inadequate lymph node sampling, perforation of the bowel at presentation, poorly differentiated tumors, and T_4 lesions. Adequate examination of the lymph nodes for tumor involvement is most important for appropriate staging of the patient with colorectal cancer. Various tumor molecular genetic factors (e.g., chromosome 18q deletion, tumor ploidy, mutations of protooncogenes or tumor suppressor genes, tumor TS expression, and MSS) are also being studied in an effort to identify subsets of patients with stage II disease who have an increased risk of relapse. Despite the lack of a consensus regarding the use of adjuvant chemotherapy for individuals with high-risk stage II colon cancer, many practitioners offer this therapy to selected patients. Optimal dosing, administration schedule, and duration of therapy have yet to be determined, but most practitioners use the same treatment approach as for patients with stage III colon cancer.

Adjuvant chemotherapy is standard therapy for patients with stage III colon cancer. The presence of lymph node involvement with tumor places patients with stage III colon cancer at high risk for recurrence, and the risk of death within 5 years of surgical resection alone is as high as 70%, depending on the number of lymph nodes involved.[45] In this population of patients, adjuvant chemotherapy significantly decreases risk of cancer recurrence and death and is standard of care.

Adjuvant XRT plus chemotherapy is considered standard treatment for patients with stage II/III rectal cancer.[66] Tumors arising in the rectum are technically more difficult to resect with wide circumferential margins, and lead to local recurrences more frequently than that seen with colon cancers. Therefore, XRT is an important aspect of adjuvant therapy for rectal cancer to reduce risk of local tumor recurrence.

Adjuvant Radiation Therapy Adjuvant XRT has no definite role in colon cancer because most recurrences are extrapelvic and occur in the abdomen.[45] Although local recurrence and debilitating pelvic pain are uncommon, a subset of patients with T_3 or T_4 tumors located in the cecum and in hepatic and splenic flexures, are at increased risk of local recurrence and may benefit from postoperative XRT and chemotherapy. Early trials with whole-abdominal XRT were limited by considerable toxicity.[66] However, results from studies combining abdominal XRT plus fluorouracil are promising. To date, postoperative local XRT may reduce the risk of local recurrence and improve survival compared to adjuvant chemotherapy alone, but should only be considered for select patients with colon cancer.[45]

In patients undergoing surgery for rectal cancer, XRT is used to reduce risk of local tumor recurrence. Radiation therapy is given prior to or following surgery and can be delivered with a variety of dosing regimens, administration schedules, and techniques.[66] Preoperative XRT may be used to reduce the initial size of the tumor to such an extent that the tumor can be reclassified to a lower stage, or "downstaged," and therefore rendered more resectable. This might lead to improved patient survival or result in the need for a less-extensive surgical procedure. Preoperative XRT is also administered to reduce the amount of tumor seeding that can occur during surgery, but this approach is more likely to affect a greater area than is necessary.[66] Postoperative administration of XRT may more adequately treat a defined area, but is associated with more toxicity because of a greater amount of bowel being present in the treatment field.

Adverse effects associated with XRT in colorectal cancer can be acute or chronic. Acute effects primarily include hematologic depression, dysuria, diarrhea, abdominal cramping, and proctitis. Chronic symptoms that sometimes persist for months following discontinuation of XRT include persistent diarrhea, proctitis or enteritis, small bowel obstruction, perineal tenderness, and impaired wound healing.

Adjuvant Chemotherapy ❺ For more than 40 years, fluorouracil has been the most widely used chemotherapeutic agent for the adjuvant treatment of colorectal cancer, both as a single agent and in combination with other agents. Newer agents such as oxaliplatin and capecitabine have been incorporated into combination chemotherapy regimens for the adjuvant treatment of colon cancer. Investigational chemotherapy agents, biologic therapies that target the underlying tumor biology, and new administration methods are also being developed. Current adjuvant trials focus on combination chemotherapy regimens with newer targeted agents added.

Based on their activity for metastatic colon cancer, fluorouracil and floxuridine were investigated as single-agent chemotherapy agents for use after surgery. In 1988, a meta-analysis was published that evaluated phase III trials that compared adjuvant fluorouracil to surgery alone.[69] A small, statistically insignificant improvement in survival was noted with fluorouracil-based regimens. Since then, most trials focused on improving the efficacy of fluorouracil in the adjuvant colon cancer.

Historical Perspective. In 1990, the National Institutes of Health Consensus Development Conference recommended that the use of fluorouracil and levamisole be considered standard therapy for patients with surgically treated stage III colon cancer. Levamisole is a synthetic, oral anthelmintic drug with immunomodulatory properties and minimal, generally reversible toxicities. Levamisole was administered in 3-day cycles with fluorouracil for a period of 1 year.

❻ Concurrently it was discovered that the pharmacology of fluorouracil provides several opportunities to increase its antitumor activity. The addition of leucovorin increases the binding affinity of the active fluorouracil metabolite to TS, thus enhancing its cytotoxic activity. The combination of fluorouracil plus leucovorin has undergone extensive study in the adjuvant setting, based on the observation that fluorouracil plus leucovorin substantially improves response rates as compared to fluorouracil alone for metastatic disease. Several large randomized trials have evaluated the efficacy of fluorouracil plus leucovorin as adjuvant therapy for patients with stage II or III colon cancer. The International Multicentre Pooled Analysis of Colon Cancer Trials analyzed pooled data from three ongoing trials comparing surgery alone to adjuvant fluorouracil (370 to 400 mg/m^2 per day) plus high-dose leucovorin (200 mg/m^2 per day) given daily for 5 consecutive days, repeated every 28 days for 6 cycles (6 months).[70] The recurrence and death rates were reduced by 35% and 22%,

TABLE 133-10 Chemotherapy Regimens for the Adjuvant Treatment of Colorectal Cancer

Regimen	Agents	Comment
FOLFOX4[120]	Oxaliplatin 85 mg/m² IV day 1 Folinic acid 200 mg/m² per day IV over 2 hours days 1 and 2 Fluorouracil 400 mg/m² IV bolus, after folinic acid then 600 mg/m² CIV over 22 hours days 1 and 2 • Repeat every 14 days	Improved DFS as compared to infusional fluorouracil-leucovorin–based regimens.
FLOX[144]	Oxaliplatin 85 mg/m² IV administered on weeks 1, 3, and 5 Fluorouracil 500 mg/m² IV bolus weekly × 6 Folinic acid 500 mg/m² IV weekly × 6 • Each cycle lasts 8 weeks and is repeated for 3 cycles	Improved DFS as compared to bolus fluorouracil-leucovorin–based regimens.
Capecitabine	Capecitabine 1,250 mg/m² po twice daily on days 1 through 14 every 21 days	Equivalent DFS as compared to the Mayo Clinic regimen with improved tolerability.
Fluorouracil-based regimens		
Roswell Park regimen[145]	Fluorouracil 600 mg/m² per day IV, day 1 Folinic acid 500 mg/m² per day IV over 2 hours • Repeat weekly for 6 of 8 weeks	
Mayo Clinic regimen[146]	Fluorouracil 425 mg/m² per day IV, days 1–5 Folinic acid 20 mg/m² per day IV, days 1–5 • Repeat every 4 to 5 weeks	
de Gramont regimen[97]	Fluorouracil 400 mg/m² per day IV bolus, followed by 600 mg/m² CIV over 22 hours, days 1 and 2 for 2 consecutive days Folinic acid 200 mg/m² per day IV over 2 hours days 1 and 2 • Repeat every 2 weeks	Improved safety as compared to the Mayo Clinic regimen.

CIV, continuous intravenous infusion; DFS, disease-free survival.

respectively. These studies were initiated when a surgery-alone control group was appropriate for stage III colon cancer, before the results were available from the fluorouracil plus levamisole adjuvant trial.

In the United States, the Roswell Park regimen and the Mayo Clinic regimen were most commonly used, while in Europe, treatments such as the de Gramont regimen favor a continuous intravenous schedule of fluorouracil (Table 133–10). The weekly fluorouracil plus high-dose leucovorin (Roswell Park) and the daily fluorouracil plus low-dose leucovorin (Mayo Clinic) regimens were compared in a four-arm U.S. Intergroup trial (INT-0089) that randomized patients with high-risk stage II and stage III colon cancer to either regimen, fluorouracil plus levamisole, or a combination of fluorouracil, leucovorin, and levamisole.[71] The standard fluorouracil plus levamisole regimen was administered over 12 months and the leucovorin-containing regimens were given for 6 cycles over a time period of 6 to 8 months. Overall survival (OS) was the primary end point with disease-free survival (DFS) as a secondary end point. The high-dose leucovorin regimen was not superior to the low-dose leucovorin regimen, and the three-drug combination was not superior to fluorouracil plus leucovorin alone. In addition, 6 months of adjuvant therapy with fluorouracil plus leucovorin was as effective as 12 months of fluorouracil plus levamisole. Other large trials have consistently shown 6 months of fluorouracil plus leucovorin to be at least equivalent to 12-month regimens containing levamisole.[72,73] Thus, a 6-month regimen of fluorouracil plus leucovorin was defined as the standard duration of chemotherapy for patients with stage III colon cancer. Levamisole is no longer included in chemotherapy regimens for colon cancer.

The schedule of fluorouracil and leucovorin administration varies in the different regimens. Clinical studies comparing the efficacy of bolus and continuous infusion schedules generally favor continuous infusion of fluorouracil, which is probably related to its short plasma half-life and S-phase specificity for optimal TS inhibition. Continuous IV infusions also permit increased fluorouracil dose intensity, which may account for the higher response rates observed with prolonged infusions of fluorouracil. In most of the commonly used combination regimens, fluorouracil is administered by both IV bolus injection and continuous IV infusion.

Clinically significant differences in toxicity also differ based on the dose, route, and schedule of fluorouracil administration. Leukopenia is the primary dose-limiting toxicity of IV bolus fluorouracil, although diarrhea, stomatitis, and nausea and vomiting can also occur.[74] The incidence and severity of stomatitis can be significantly reduced with the use of oral cryotherapy. In this approach, the patient is required to chew and hold ice chips in the mouth during the period between 5 minutes prior to and 30 minutes following the bolus injection of fluorouracil. The protective effects of this procedure is probably related to the local vasoconstriction caused by the ice chips, which temporarily reduces blood flow to the oral mucosa, thereby reducing drug exposure to the oral mucosa.

Although continuous IV infusion fluorouracil is generally well tolerated, dose-limiting toxicities can be substantial. A distinct toxicity, palmar–plantar erythrodysesthesia ("hand–foot syndrome"), and stomatitis occur most frequently with this route of administration.[74] Hand–foot syndrome occurs in 24% to 40% of patients receiving extended continuous IV infusions and is characterized by painful swelling and erythroderma of the soles of the feet, palms of the hands, and distal fingers. The skin toxicity is fully reversible upon interruption of therapy or dose reduction and is not life-threatening, but it can be significant and acutely disabling. The incidence of stomatitis, diarrhea, and hematologic toxicity is not substantial at standard doses, but increases with increasing fluorouracil doses. No significant difference is noted in the incidence of mucositis, diarrhea, nausea and vomiting, or alopecia between continuous and bolus IV fluorouracil administration.[74]

An additional determinant of fluorouracil toxicity, regardless of the method of administration, is related to its catabolism and pharmacogenomic factors. Dihydropyrimidine dehydrogenase (DPD) is the main enzyme responsible for the catabolism of fluorouracil to inactive metabolites. A rare pharmacogenetic disorder characterized by complete or near-complete deficiency of this enzyme has been identified in cancer patients. Patients with this enzyme deficiency develop severe toxicity, including death, after fluorouracil administration. Molecular studies have identified a relationship between allelic variants in the *DPYD* gene (the gene that encodes DPD) and a deficiency in DPD activity.[75] Approximately 3% of patients may be genotypically heterozygous for a mutant DPYD allele, although differences between sex and races are unknown at this time.

In summary, fluorouracil and leucovorin can be administered in a variety of treatment schedules, but none has proven superior with regard to overall patient survival. Table 133–10 lists examples of some of these regimens.

Despite the activity of fluorouracil-based adjuvant chemotherapy, the results obtained thus far indicate need for continued improvement. New chemotherapy agents and chemotherapy regimens are constantly being investigated in an attempt to improve on the response and safety of fluorouracil plus leucovorin in the adjuvant setting. Most attempts to improve the adjuvant therapy for colon cancer add a third active chemotherapy agent to a fluoropyrimidine-based regimen.

Fluorouracil Plus Oxaliplatin. The role of oxaliplatin in adjuvant chemotherapy was evaluated based on its activity in metastatic disease. In the Multicenter International Study of Oxaliplatin/5-Fluorouracil/Leucovorin in the Adjuvant Treatment of Colon Cancer (MOSAIC) trial, 2,246 patients with stage II or III colon cancer were randomized to receive fluorouracil plus leucovorin or FOLFOX4 (fluorouracil/leucovorin plus oxaliplatin) postoperatively.[76] The addition of oxaliplatin resulted in a 23% risk reduction in disease recurrence and increased 3-year overall DFS (78.2% vs. 72.9%) as compared to fluorouracil plus leucovorin alone. With a median followup of 56 months, the addition of oxaliplatin resulted in an absolute 4-year OS difference of 2.1%, which was not statistically significant. The addition of oxaliplatin was associated with increased paresthesia, neutropenia, and GI toxicity (nausea, vomiting, diarrhea) that were manageable with supportive care. Further supporting the role of oxaliplatin in the adjuvant setting are the results of the recently reported National Surgical Adjuvant Breast and Bowel Project C-07 trial, which compared the Roswell Park regimen of bolus fluorouracil/leucovorin with or without oxaliplatin. Three-year DFS was improved by 4.9% (HR = 0.79, P = 0.004) with oxaliplatin added to the fluorouracil backbone. As expected, neurotoxicity was increased with oxaliplatin.[77]

Although a significant difference in OS has not yet been observed, consistent improvement in 3-year DFS, a recently accepted end point of adjuvant colon cancer trials, with oxaliplatin led to the approval of oxaliplatin in the adjuvant setting. The 2007 National Comprehensive Cancer Network (NCCN) guidelines recommend oxaliplatin-based regimens as an option for patients with stage III colon cancer who can tolerate combination therapy, and most practitioners incorporate oxaliplatin into adjuvant treatment regimens.

Further modifications of the FOLFOX4 regimen may also improve tolerability. Capecitabine, an oral prodrug of fluorouracil, and other oral pyrimidines are also being evaluated in adjuvant studies as a replacement for fluorouracil in an attempt to improve the safety and ease of administration of the chemotherapy regimens.

Capecitabine. In addition to being investigated as a replacement for fluorouracil in combination regimens, capecitabine is FDA approved as a single agent in the adjuvant setting. The Xeloda in Adjuvant Colon Cancer Therapy (X-ACT) trial compared capecitabine to the Mayo Clinic regimen of bolus fluorouracil/leucovorin in the adjuvant treatment of 1,987 patients with stage III colon cancer.[78] Both regimens were given for 6 months. This trial was designed to show noninferiority of capecitabine to bolus fluorouracil. DFS between the groups was found to be equivalent. Secondary end points of relapse-free survival (HR 0.86; 95% CI 0.74 to 0.99; $P = 0.04$) and safety were improved with capecitabine. In particular, the incidence of diarrhea, stomatitis and neutropenia was decreased with capecitabine, but the incidence of hand–foot syndrome was increased with capecitabine.

Investigational Approaches. Despite its proven benefit in the metastatic setting, irinotecan has not shown a benefit in the adjuvant setting and should not be used outside of clinical trials at this time. Three trials have evaluated the addition of irinotecan to bolus or continuous infusion fluorouracil/leucovorin and all have failed to demonstrate a DFS benefit. Cancer and Leukemia Group B 89803 compared the irinotecan plus fluorouracil/leucovorin (IFL) regimen to bolus fluorouracil/leucovorin; not only was there no DFS benefit but the IFL regimen was associated with significant toxicity.[79] The Third Pan-European Trial in Adjuvant Colon Cancer (PETACC-3) and ACCORD studies, which used infusional regimens similar to folinic acid, fluorouracil and irinotecan (FOLFIRI), also found no difference in DFS as compared with infusional fluorouracil/leucovorin.[80,81]

With the success of cetuximab and bevacizumab in the metastatic setting, most current adjuvant trials are evaluating monoclonal antibodies in combination with the previously mentioned regimens. FOLFOX ± bevacizumab or cetuximab are part of large phase III trials currently enrolling in cooperative groups to assess the benefit in this setting. Patients should be encouraged to enroll in these important trials.

Approach to Selecting an Adjuvant Regimen. Selecting a specific regimen from those listed in Table 133–10 requires an assessment of several patient specific factors, including the performance status of the patient, comorbid conditions that may exist, and patient preferences for treatment based on lifestyle factors important to the patient. If a clinical trial is not an option, most patients with good performance status will receive oxaliplatin in combination with fluorouracil/leucovorin. Capecitabine may be the preferred option for patients with preexisting neuropathies, such as diabetic patients, or those patients wishing not to receive IV chemotherapy for any other reason. Fluorouracil/leucovorin has limited use at this time but is an acceptable option for patients who cannot receive oxaliplatin and are unable to tolerate or take oral capecitabine. For example, patients who develop severe hand–foot syndrome may tolerate bolus fluorouracil/leucovorin as this toxicity is minimal with this administration method.

Adjuvant Therapy for Rectal Cancer

6 Rectal cancer involves those tumors found below the peritoneal reflection in the most distal 15 cm of the large bowel, and as such is distinct from colon cancer in that it has a propensity for both local and distant recurrence. The higher incidence of local failure and overall poorer prognosis associated with rectal cancer is a result of anatomic limitations in excising adequate radial margins around the rectal tumor. Although an abdominoperineal resection of the tumor and adjacent tissues results in a high probability of local control and long-term survival, the sequelae, including need for a permanent colostomy and high incidence of sexual and genitourinary dysfunction, has led to investigation of approaches that use multimodal therapies that preserve the integrity of the anal sphincter.[82] In addition, adjuvant therapy after surgical resection is an important aspect of treatment of the primary tumor. The effectiveness of postoperative XRT and fluorouracil-based chemotherapy for stage II or III rectal cancer is well established. Although T_1 tumors with a favorable histology may be treated successfully with local excision alone, adjuvant XRT plus chemotherapy should be offered for larger lesions. Similar to adjuvant therapy for colon cancer, fluorouracil provides the basis for chemotherapy regimens for rectal cancer. The XRT decreases the rate of local pelvic recurrences, whereas the fluorouracil decreases the risk of distant tumor recurrence and enhances the effectiveness of the XRT. The optimal delivery schedule for these two therapies is the subject of ongoing investigation, but many trials have demonstrated improved local control and survival for patients who receive a combination of postoperative XRT and chemotherapy as compared to surgery alone. In 1990, based on results from the Gastrointestinal Tumor Study Group and the Mayo Clinic–North Central Cancer Treatment Group studies, the National Cancer Institute Consensus Conference recommended that standard postoperative adjuvant treatment for patients with stage II or III rectal tumors should consist of six cycles of fluorouracil-based chemotherapy with concurrent pelvic XRT.[83] The Gastrointestinal Tumor Study Group trial was designed to evaluate adjuvant postoperative treatment for patients with stage II or III rectal cancer and demonstrated that combined chemotherapy and radiation therapy improved recurrence rate and survival compared

to chemotherapy or radiotherapy alone.[84] The Mayo Clinic–North Central Cancer Treatment Group trial compared postoperative XRT alone, postoperative XRT with concurrent fluorouracil plus semustine chemotherapy, and pre- and postirradiation chemotherapy in a similar population of 204 patients with rectal cancer.[85] This was the first randomized trial in which one cycle of combination chemotherapy was given before and after XRT in addition to the administration of fluorouracil during XRT. The use of combined chemotherapy and XRT significantly affected local recurrence, relapse-free survival, and OS as compared to XRT alone. These studies established fluorouracil plus XRT as the foundation for adjuvant therapy in stages II and III rectal cancer.

Additional trials have sought to determine optimal combinations of concurrent radiation and fluorouracil. Many treatment centers now administer continuous-infusion fluorouracil throughout the 5- or 6-week schedule of postoperative XRT for rectal cancer. Several schedules for combining fluorouracil with postoperative XRT provide similar relapse-free survival and OS but differ with regard to toxicity profile and catheter requirements for drug administration.[86] The integration of capecitabine as an alternative to fluorouracil and the incorporation of other agents available in the treatment of colorectal cancer into adjuvant therapy for rectal cancer is under investigation.

Preoperative (Neoadjuvant) Therapy ❻ Interest in preoperative or neoadjuvant therapy has increased based on advances in imaging techniques to more accurately stage rectal tumors preoperatively and the success of combined XRT plus fluoropyrimidine-based chemotherapy administered in the postoperative setting. Preoperative XRT, by shrinking and thereby downstaging the tumor prior to surgical resection, improves sphincter preservation, but the primary concern with this approach is potential overtreatment with XRT in some patients.

Neoadjuvant chemoradiotherapy may further enhance tumor shrinkage and improve the rate of tumor resectability with rectal sphincter preservation. The European Organization for Research and Treatment of Cancer 22921 trial evaluated the addition of fluorouracil plus leucovorin to preoperative XRT and showed an improvement in tumor shrinkage with lower lymph node involvement. However, long-term local control and survival outcomes need to be assessed.[87] The 2007 NCCN guidelines for rectal cancer indicate that postoperative infusional fluorouracil-based chemotherapy plus XRT is the preferred treatment for resectable T_3N_0 or any T_2N_{1-2} lesions (category 1 recommendation).[88] Neoadjuvant fluorouracil or capecitabine chemoradiation followed by abdominoperineal resection or low anterior resection should be considered for locally unresectable tumors. Postoperative therapy, either as chemotherapy alone or combined chemoradiotherapy should be administered to all patients who received preoperative chemotherapy for rectal cancer.[88]

■ METASTATIC DISEASE

Initial Therapy

❼ Several advances have been made in developing efficacious treatment options for metastatic colorectal cancer. Whereas surgery and XRT are usually used to manage isolated sites of tumor, chemotherapy is most useful for patients with disseminated disease and is the primary treatment modality for unresectable metastatic colorectal cancer.

Surgery Complete surgical resection of discrete hepatic, pulmonary, abdominal, or brain metastases in patients with colorectal cancer, if possible, may offer selected patients an opportunity to experience extended DFS. Patients who have from one to three small nodules isolated to the liver, lungs, or abdomen have the most favorable outcomes. Up to 25% of patients will present with hepatic metastases at time of diagnosis, and 60% of patients with colorectal cancer will develop hepatic metastases sometime during the course of their disease. Approximately 35% of patients who undergo resection of hepatic-limited metastases can be cured.[89] These results are drastically better than those in patients with unresectable metastatic colorectal cancer, in whom 5-year survival is uncommon. Patients with no significant general medical risk factors, fewer than four hepatic lesions, CEA levels less than 200 ng/mL, small tumor size, lack of extrahepatic tumor, and adequate surgical margins have the best opportunity for an improved long-term outcome. The primary site of tumor should also be completely resected. Ablative therapies that involve destroying the tumor through freezing and thawing (cryoablation), heat (radiofrequency), or alcohol injection may be useful for patients who have very small hepatic lesions and are unable to undergo liver resection surgery, but are less successful than surgical interventions. Outcomes associated with resection of isolated pulmonary, abdominal, and brain metastases have been less studied, but this approach is potentially curative and should be considered for patients with resectable disease who are appropriate surgical candidates.

Because about two-thirds of patients who undergo resection of hepatic metastases will have disease recurrence, postsurgery therapies (e.g., adjuvant systemic and hepatic arterial infusion chemotherapy) have been studied in an attempt to improve long-term outcomes. A randomized trial that compared 6 months of hepatic floxuridine and dexamethasone plus IV fluorouracil with leucovorin to IV fluorouracil with leucovorin alone following resection of hepatic metastases in 156 patients showed improved 2-year DFS (86% vs. 72%) and hepatic recurrence-free survival at 2 years (90% vs. 60%) with the combined therapy.[90] Many practitioners offer adjuvant chemotherapy to selected patients following potentially curative hepatic resection, but further studies, especially those involving more active agents, are needed to determine an optimal treatment regimen.[91]

Radiation Symptom control is the primary goal of XRT for patients with advanced or metastatic colorectal cancer.

Chemotherapy ❼ Accepted initial chemotherapy regimens for metastatic colorectal cancer consist of oxaliplatin plus fluorouracil and leucovorin, irinotecan plus fluorouracil and leucovorin, bevacizumab plus a fluorouracil-based regimen, capecitabine alone, or fluorouracil plus leucovorin alone (Table 133–11). The site(s) of tumor involvement and history of prior chemotherapy help to define an appropriate management strategy. In general, treatment options are similar for metastatic cancer of the colon and rectum.

Currently, most metastatic colorectal cancers are incurable and treatment goals are to reduce patient symptoms, improve quality-of-life, and extend survival. Two recent meta-analyses have estimated the magnitude of benefit and harm associated with palliative chemotherapy for metastatic colorectal cancer. In a pooled analysis of randomized trials comparing chemotherapy to observation or supportive care alone, a total of nine trials that included 614 patients were evaluated.[92] All trials used fluorouracil-based chemotherapy, but three trials in which hepatic arterial or portal vein administration was used were also included. Several trials allowed delayed or discretionary use of chemotherapy in patients assigned to observation or supportive care alone; 12% to 57% of control patients received at least one course of chemotherapy. Despite these discrepancies, chemotherapy was associated with a significant reduction in mortality at 1 (RR 0.69) but not 2 years (RR 0.93). The second meta-analysis analyzed individual patient data and summary statistics from 13 randomized trials that included 1,365 patients.[93] Eligible trials compared palliative chemotherapy given via any route of administration to supportive care alone or treatments not involving chemotherapy. Trials that allowed chemotherapy use in control patients were not excluded. In the analysis of seven trials in which individual patient data were available, palliative chemotherapy was

TABLE 133-11 Chemotherapeutic Regimens for Metastatic Colorectal Cancer

	Regimen	Major Dose-Limiting Toxicities/Comments
Initial therapy		
Oxaliplatin plus fluorouracil plus leucovorin		
Oxaliplatin plus bimonthly infusional fluorouracil; FOLFOX4[97]	Oxaliplatin 85 mg/m² IV day 1 plus bolus fluorouracil 400 mg/m² IV plus leucovorin 200 mg/m² IV followed by fluorouracil 600 mg/m² IV in 22-hour infusion on days 1 and 2, every 2 weeks	Sensory neuropathy, neutropenia
mFOLFOX6	Oxaliplatin 85 mg/m² IV day 1 plus leucovorin 400 mg/m² IV on day 1 followed by fluorouracil 400 mg/m² IV bolus on day 1, then 1200 mg/m²/day × 2 days (total 2,400 mg/m² over 46–48 hours) continuous infusion, repeat every 2 week	Sensory neuropathy, neutropenia; easier administration as compared to FOLFOX4
Irinotecan plus fluorouracil plus leucovorin		
Irinotecan plus infusional fluorouracil; FOLFIRI[104]	Irinotecan 180 mg/m² IV plus leucovorin 400 mg/m² IV plus bolus fluorouracil 400 mg/m² IV, followed by fluorouracil 2,400 mg/m² continuous IV infusion over 46 hours on day 1, repeated every 2 weeks	Nausea, diarrhea, mucositis, neutropenia
Biweekly irinotecan plus infusional fluorouracil[99]	Irinotecan 180 mg/m² IV day 1 plus leucovorin 400 mg/m² then fluorouracil 400 mg/m² IV, followed by fluorouracil 600 mg/m² continuous IV infusion over 22 hours, days 1 and 2, repeated every 2 weeks	Neutropenia, diarrhea
Irinotecan plus bolus fluorouracil; IFL; Saltz regimen[100]	Irinotecan 125 mg/m² IV plus fluorouracil 500 mg/m² IV plus leucovorin 20 mg/m² IV weekly for 4 of 6 weeks	Diarrhea (increased as compared to FOLFIRI), neutropenia
Bevacizumab		
Bevacizumab plus fluorouracil-based regimens	Bevacizumab 5 mg/kg IV every 2 weeks plus fluorouracil and leucovorin (given in any schedule below) or IFL or FOLFOX or FOLFIRI	Hypertension, thrombosis, proteinuria from bevacizumab added to toxicities of regimen chosen
Capecitabine		
Capecitabine monotherapy[106]	See Table 133–10[a]	Diarrhea, hand–foot syndrome
CapOx	Oxaliplatin 130 mg/m² day 1 plus capecitabine 850 mg/m² twice a day for 14 days, repeat every 3 weeks	Diarrhea, hand–foot syndrome, neuropathies
Fluorouracil plus leucovorin only		
Weekly, high-dose leucovorin; Roswell Park regimen[146]	See Table 133–10[a]	Diarrhea, mucositis
Consecutive day, low-dose leucovorin; Mayo Clinic regimen[146]	See Table 133–10[a]	Mucositis, neutropenia
Bolus plus infusional fluorouracil; (LV5FU2)[97]; de Gramont regimen	See Table 133–10[a]	Neutropenia, mucositis
Salvage therapy[b]		
Irinotecan		
Weekly irinotecan[100]	Irinotecan 125 mg/m² IV every week for 4 of 6 weeks	Neutropenia, diarrhea
Every 3-weeks irinotecan[116]	Irinotecan 350 mg/m² IV every 3 weeks	Neutropenia, diarrhea (less-than-weekly irinotecan)
Oxaliplatin plus fluorouracil plus leucovorin		
Oxaliplatin plus bimonthly infusional fluorouracil; FOLFOX4[147]	Same as FOLFOX4 above	Sensory neuropathy, neutropenia
Cetuximab		
Cetuximab plus irinotecan[c,122]	Continue irinotecan as previously dosed, plus cetuximab 400 mg/m² IV loading dose, then cetuximab 250 mg/m² IV weekly thereafter	Asthenia, diarrhea, nausea, acneiform rash, vomiting
Cetuximab[d,122]	Cetuximab 400 mg/m² IV loading dose, then cetuximab 250 mg/m² IV weekly thereafter	Papulopustular, follicular rash, asthenia, constipation, diarrhea
Fluorouracil		
Protracted continuous infusion[117]	Fluorouracil 250–300 mg/m² per day continuous IV infusion until disease progression	Mucositis, hand–foot syndrome
Investigational		
CapOx[148]	Same as CapOx above.	Diarrhea, sensory neuropathy
CapIri[148]	Capecitabine 1,000 mg/m² orally twice daily days 1–14 plus irinotecan 100 mg/m² IV days 1 and 8; repeat every 3 weeks	Diarrhea, neutropenia

[a]Doses and schedules the same as those in the adjuvant setting.
[b]See Fig. 133–6 for comments on salvage regimens.
[c]If irinotecan-refractory disease.
[d]If patient cannot tolerate irinotecan.

shown to reduce the risk of death by 35%, which translates to a prolongation of median survival by 3.7 months. The investigators were unable to determine the effect of treatment on toxicities or quality-of-life because of inadequate data. However, the results of both analyses suggest that palliative chemotherapy is beneficial and improves survival in metastatic colorectal cancer. Because many patients assigned to control arms eventually received chemotherapy, the magnitude of survival benefit associated with chemotherapy could be underestimated.

Fluorouracil continues to be incorporated into current first-line chemotherapy regimens used for metastatic colorectal cancer. When administered in bolus injection treatment schedules, fluorouracil is given most frequently with leucovorin. The addition of irinotecan to fluorouracil plus leucovorin significantly improves response rates, progression-free survival (PFS), and median survival. Oxaliplatin in combination with fluorouracil and leucovorin has shown improvements in median survival when compared to the combination of irinotecan plus fluorouracil and leucovorin in the initial treatment of metastatic colon cancer. The addition of bevacizumab to fluorouracil-based regimens improves efficacy compared to chemotherapy alone. Either of these three- or four-drug combinations may be considered as first-line therapy for metastatic colorectal cancer. Ongoing trials are evaluating the sequencing of these regimens and comparing the efficacy of combinations of fluorouracil plus leucovorin, to investigational treatments with capecitabine, oral fluoropyrimidines and newer agents, such as cetuximab. Table 133–12 summarizes comparative outcome data from potentially useful chemotherapeutic treatments for metastatic colorectal cancer.

7 ***Fluorouracil-Based Regimens.*** Fluorouracil has been administered as a single agent by IV bolus injection but response rates are only 10% to 20%.[94] As such, IV bolus fluorouracil as a single agent is considered ineffective for metastatic colorectal cancer. A variety of continuous IV infusion fluorouracil regimens have been developed to increase the duration of drug exposure during the S-phase of the cell cycle and increase cytotoxicity. Despite differences in dose intensity among the different regimens, no clear survival advantages or trends are observed for any particular regimen. However, in comparison to IV bolus fluorouracil, response rates with continuous infusion fluorouracil are about doubled. In a meta-analysis of six randomized trials evaluating 1,219 patients with advanced colorectal cancer that compared continuous infusion and bolus IV fluorouracil, a significantly higher tumor response rate (22% vs. 14%) and OS benefit (overall HR 0.88) were observed in patients

TABLE 133-12 Comparative Outcomes from Selected Trials in Metastatic Colorectal Cancer

Trial	Number	Outcome Measures	Results
First-line			
Goldberg et al.[103]	795	Primary: TTP; secondary: OS, RR, time to treatment discontinuation	Median TTP: IFL vs. FOLFOX 6.9 vs. 8.7 months ($P = 0.0014$). Median survival 15.0 months with IFL vs. 19.5 months with FOLFOX ($P = 0.001$). Response rate with FOLFOX (45%) higher compared to IFL (31%; $P = 0.002$) and IROX (35%, $P = 0.03$). TTP and OS with IROX (6.5 and 17.4 months) no different from FOLFOX.
de Gramont et al.[147]	420	Primary: PFS; secondary: RR, OS, tolerability, QOL	Median PFS: 9.0 vs. 6.2 months ($P = 0.0003$); RR: 50.7 vs. 22.3% ($P = 0.0001$), oxaliplatin plus LV5FU2 vs. LF5FU2 alone; no difference in OS (16.2 vs. 14.7 months) or QOL between oxaliplatin plus LV5FU2 vs. LV5FU2 alone
Saltz et al.[100]	683	Primary: PFS; secondary: RR, OS	Median PFS longer with IFL (7.0 months) vs. FU/LV (4.3 months; $P = 0.004$); PFS similar with irinotecan alone (4.2 months) compared to FU/LV; RR higher with IFL vs. FU/LV (50 vs. 28%; $P < 0.001$); median survival longer with IFL (14.8 months) vs. 12.6 months with FU/LV ($P = 0.04$), which was similar to irinotecan (12.0 months)
Douillard et al.[99]	387	Primary: RR; secondary: TTP, response duration, TTF, OS, QOL	Significantly higher RR with infusional IFL vs. infusional FU/LV alone (35 vs 22%; $P < 0.005$) by ITT; TTP longer with IFL (6.7 vs. 4.4 months; $P < 0.001$) and OS longer with IFL vs. infusional FU/LV alone (17.4 vs. 14.1 months; $P = 0.031$)
Tournigand et al.[104]	226	Test the best sequence of FOLFIRI vs. FOLFOX6; primary: second PFS; secondary: PFS, OS, RR, safety	Median survival 21.5 months with FOLFIRI then FOLFOX6 vs. 20.6 months with FOLFOX6 then FOLFIRI; median PFS also no different (14.2 vs. 10.9 months), or RR or median PFS with first treatment: FOLFOX6 54% and 8.0 months, vs. 56% and 8.5 months with FOLFIRI
Hurwitz et al.[107]	925	Primary: OS; secondary: PFS, RR, response duration, QOL	Bevacizumab plus IFL increased median survival (20.3 months) vs. IFL alone (15.6 months; $P = 0.00003$), PFS (10.6 vs. 6.24 months; $P < 0.00001$), RR (45% vs. 35%; $P = 0.0029$), and duration of response (10.4 vs. 7.1 months; $P = 0.0014$)
Twelves[106]	1,207	Primary: RR; secondary: TTP, OS, response duration	Tumor response to capecitabine greater than with FU/LV (25.7 vs. 16.7%; $P < 0.0002$), but no difference in median TTP (4.6 vs. 4.7 months) or median survival (392 vs. 391 days)
Hochster[108]	360	Primary: toxicity; secondary RR, TTP, OS	Grade 3/4 toxicity not increased with bevacizumab. TTP, RR, and OS all greater when bevacizumab added to CAPOX, FOLFOX or bolus fluorouracil/leucovorin. Median survival with bevacizumab containing regimens was 24.4 months vs. 18.4 months without bevacizumab (not a randomized trial)
Second-line			
Rougier et al.[117]	267	Primary: OS; secondary: PFS, RR, symptom-free survival, adverse effects, QOL	Irinotecan improved median PFS (4.2 vs. 2.9 months; $P = 0.030$) compared to infusion fluorouracil and 1-year survival (45% vs. 35%; $P = 0.035$) but not median OS (10.8 vs. 8.5 months). Median pain-free survival was similar ($P = 0.06$; 10.3 vs. 8.5 months) between irinotecan and fluorouracil, as was QOL
Cunningham et al.[116]	279	Primary: OS; secondary; performance status, body weight, tumor-related symptoms, QOL	Compared to best supportive care, OS was improved with irinotecan (13.8% 1-year survival vs. 36.2%; $P = 0.0001$); survival without deterioration in performance status, weight loss greater than 5%, and pain-free survival were also improved with irinotecan
Cunningham et al.[122]	329	Primary: RR; secondary: TTP, OS	Addition of cetuximab to continuing irinotecan associated with 22.9% response rate compared to 10.9% with cetuximab alone ($P = 0.0074$); median survival with cetuximab plus irinotecan similar to cetuximab alone (8.6 vs. 6.9 months; $P = 0.48$), but TTP was longer with cetuximab plus irinotecan (4.1 vs. 1.5 months; hazard ratio 0.54; 95% CI, 0.42–0.71)
Giantonio et al.[120]	829	Primary: OS; secondary: PFS, RR, toxicity	Addition of bevacizumab to FOLFOX4 in patients previously treated with irinotecan and a fluoropyrimidine improved median OS (12.2 vs. 10.8 months; $P = 0.001$), PFS (7.3 vs. 4.7 months; $P < 0.0001$), and overall RR (22.7% vs. 8.6%, $P < 0.0001$) compared to FOLFOX4 alone
Van Cutsem et al.[149]	463	Primary: PFS; secondary: objective RR, OS, safety	Panitumumab plus BSC prolonged PFS compared to BSC alone, with a median PFS of 8 weeks with panitumumab (hazard ratio 0.54; 95% CI, 0.44–0.66)

BSC, best supportive care; FU5LV2, bolus plus infusional fluorouracil and leucovorin; FU/LV, fluorouracil plus leucovorin; IFL, irinotecan plus fluorouracil plus leucovorin; IROX, irinotecan plus oxaliplatin; ITT, intention to treat; OS, overall survival; PFS, progression-free survival; QOL, quality-of-life; RR, response rate; TTF, time-to-treatment failure; TTP, time-to-tumor progression.

receiving fluorouracil by continuous IV infusion.[95] However, these effects are generally considered as marginal. Increased acceptance and added clinical benefit with continuous infusion fluorouracil has been demonstrated when fluorouracil is administered with other agents and is becoming more commonplace in clinical practice.

Numerous studies have evaluated various doses and administration schedules of fluorouracil plus leucovorin in an attempt to improve treatment response rates and survival in metastatic colorectal cancer. Response rates of 14% to 58% have been observed with a variety of doses of fluorouracil in combination with leucovorin at doses ranging from 20 to 500 mg/m^2.[45] The administration sequence and timing of leucovorin may be important factors in the efficacy of biochemical modulation with leucovorin. Leucovorin administration prior to fluorouracil is the most effective approach to enable intracellular-reduced folates to accumulate prior to fluorouracil administration. Despite significantly higher response rates and improved PFS achieved with leucovorin-modulated fluorouracil regimens, their effect on OS is modest.

The Mayo Clinic regimen was the reference regimen in metastatic colon cancer for many years, but the limitations of this regimen are becoming more apparent. A collaborative trial compared the Mayo Clinic regimen to the Roswell Park regimen in 372 patients with metastatic disease.[96] No differences in tumor response (35% vs. 31%), median survival (9.3 months vs. 10.7 months), or palliative responses were observed. The Mayo Clinic regimen was associated with significantly more leukopenia and stomatitis, whereas the Roswell Park regimen caused more diarrhea and required more hospitalizations to manage toxicity.

The Mayo Clinic regimen has also been compared to bimonthly and weekly regimens of infusional fluorouracil. Higher response rates of 24% to 54% have been noted in bimonthly regimens of fluorouracil administered first as an IV bolus infusion followed by a 22-hour continuous infusion in combination with high-dose leucovorin administered over 2 hours.[110] Although the bimonthly combined IV bolus and continuous infusion fluorouracil schedule (de Gramont regimen) did not improve median survival as compared to the Mayo Clinic schedule, it was associated with a lower incidence of severe granulocytopenia, diarrhea, and mucositis.[97] High response rates (39% to 58%) have also been observed in previously untreated and treated patients receiving weekly fluorouracil as a continuous 24-hour infusion in combination with high-dose leucovorin given over 2 to 24 hours. In a recent trial of untreated metastatic colorectal cancer, 497 patients were randomly assigned to receive the Mayo Clinic regimen of fluorouracil/leucovorin or fluorouracil 2,600 mg/m^2 as a 24-hour continuous infusion alone or in combination with high-dose leucovorin weekly.[98] Although median survival rates were not different between groups, PFS was prolonged when weekly fluorouracil was administered with high-dose leucovorin. Similar to other toxicity results, leukopenia and mucositis were more frequent in patients receiving bolus fluorouracil plus leucovorin (Mayo Clinic regimen), whereas patients receiving continuous infusion fluorouracil plus leucovorin experienced more diarrhea and hand–foot syndrome.

In summary, the Mayo Clinic regimen of fluorouracil plus low-dose leucovorin remains an acceptable regimen, but a weekly schedule of leucovorin plus fluorouracil (either bolus or continuous infusion) may be more convenient for the patient in terms of fewer scheduled clinic appointments, less interference with work schedules, and ease of dose adjustments based on toxicity. Bimonthly infusions of fluorouracil given over 2 days produce higher response rates when compared to daily regimens and are gaining in acceptability. However, the incorporation of newer agents into treatment regimens rather than continual adjustments of fluorouracil and leucovorin doses and administration schedules have led to the greatest advances in drug therapy for metastatic colorectal cancer.

❼ ***Fluorouracil and Leucovorin Plus Irinotecan.*** Based on irinotecan's activity against untreated and fluorouracil-resistant colorectal cancer, several investigations have been completed to determine whether the addition of irinotecan to fluorouracil plus leucovorin as initial therapy for metastatic disease could further improve survival. In a randomized trial of 387 previously untreated patients with advanced colorectal cancer, irinotecan plus fluorouracil and leucovorin was compared to fluorouracil plus leucovorin with regard to tumor response, survival, and quality-of-life (see Table 133–12).[99] Patients randomized to fluorouracil plus leucovorin could receive weekly fluorouracil (2,600 mg/m^2) as a 24-hour IV infusion plus leucovorin (500 mg/m^2), or the de Gramont regimen of IV bolus and infusional fluorouracil. For the three-drug treatment, a weekly regimen of irinotecan (80 mg/m^2) with a 24-hour infusion of fluorouracil (2,300 mg/m^2) plus leucovorin 500 mg/m^2, or an every 2-week regimen consisting of irinotecan (180 mg/m^2) on day 1 with IV bolus fluorouracil (400 mg/m^2) followed by a 22-hour IV infusion (600 mg/m^2) plus leucovorin (200 mg/m^2 given on days 1 and 2) can be used. Tumor response, median time-to-disease progression, and OS were all greater in the irinotecan group. Diarrhea and neutropenia were the most common toxicities and were worse in the irinotecan-containing groups. Diarrhea was the most common reason for dose reduction or treatment discontinuation with the weekly regimens, and led to hospital admission for 32% of patients receiving irinotecan as compared to 12% of patients who received only fluorouracil plus leucovorin. Neutropenia was the most common cause of dose reductions with the every-2-week regimens. Results from questionnaires indicated that quality-of-life consistently declined later in the irinotecan group.

A second randomized trial compared the addition of irinotecan (125 mg/m^2) to weekly fluorouracil plus leucovorin (fluorouracil 500 mg/m^2 IV bolus plus leucovorin 20 mg/m^2 IV bolus, each given weekly for 4 weeks, repeated every 6 weeks) to the Mayo Clinic regimen and to irinotecan alone (125 mg/m^2 IV weekly for 4 weeks, repeated every 6 weeks) as first-line therapy in 683 patients with metastatic colorectal cancer.[100] The combination of irinotecan, fluorouracil, and leucovorin resulted in significantly increased tumor response rates and improved PFS and OS as compared to fluorouracil plus leucovorin and irinotecan alone, respectively. The combined incidence of grade 3 or 4 diarrhea was 22.7% with the three-drug combination, as compared to 13.2% with fluorouracil plus leucovorin and 31% with irinotecan alone. However, the incidence of grade 3 diarrhea was almost threefold greater with triple-drug therapy as compared to the two-drug regimen. Midcycle dose reductions caused by neutropenia, which were more common with the three-drug treatment, could potentially have lowered subsequent risk of grade 4 diarrhea. Mucositis was more frequent in the fluorouracil plus leucovorin group. Quality-of-life analyses did not indicate that the addition of irinotecan to fluorouracil plus leucovorin compromised quality-of-life.

The most common adverse effects of irinotecan in these regimens are diarrhea, neutropenia, nausea and vomiting, asthenia, abdominal pain, and alopecia; diarrhea and neutropenia are dose limiting.[99,100] Two distinct patterns of diarrhea have been described. Early-onset diarrhea occurs during or within 2 to 6 hours after irinotecan administration and is characterized by lacrimation, diaphoresis, abdominal cramping, flushing, and/or diarrhea. These cholinergic symptoms, thought to be caused by inhibition of acetylcholinesterase, respond to atropine 0.25 to 1 mg given intravenously or subcutaneously. Approximately 10% of patients experience the acute symptoms during or shortly following the irinotecan. More commonly, late-onset diarrhea occurs 1 to 12 days after irinotecan administration, and may last for 3 to 5 days. Late-onset diarrhea may require hospitalization or discontinuation of therapy, and fatalities have been reported. The incidence of late-onset diarrhea was as high as 39% in some studies, but is now much lower with aggressive antidiarrheal intervention.[45] Aggressive intervention with high-dose loperamide therapy should consist of 4 mg taken at the first sign of soft or watery stools, followed by 2 mg orally every 2 hours until symptom-free for 12 hours; this regimen can be modified to 4 mg every 4 hours taken during the night.

The severity of delayed diarrhea has been correlated with the systemic exposure (i.e., area under the concentration-versus-time curve) of irinotecan and SN-38 (irinotecan's active metabolite) and with genetic polymorphisms in the enzyme uridine diphosphate-glucuronosyltransferase (UGT1A1), which is responsible for the glucuronidation of SN-38 to inactive metabolites. Reduced or deficient levels of the UGT1A1 enzyme are observed in Gilbert syndrome, a familial hyperbilirubinemia disorder, and correlate with irinotecan-induced diarrhea and neutropenia.[101] A test for deficiency in this enzyme was recently approved and clinicians can consider obtaining these results for individual patients prior to initiating irinotecan-based therapy to see if a dose-reduction is warranted.

Based on these studies, the addition of irinotecan to fluorouracil plus leucovorin (FOLFIRI or IFL) increases survival when compared to fluorouracil plus leucovorin in the first-line treatment of metastatic colorectal cancer. These data support the current consensus that the three-drug treatment regimen be considered a first-line option for metastatic colorectal cancer. Accordingly, irinotecan received FDA approval in 2000 as first-line therapy for metastatic colorectal cancer in combination with fluorouracil and leucovorin. FOLFIRI is preferred for most patients because it has fewer toxicities than IFL.

8 ***Fluorouracil and Leucovorin Plus Oxaliplatin.*** Oxaliplatin, a 1,2-diaminocyclohexane platinum carrier ligand with a mechanism of action similar to cisplatin, in combination with infusional fluorouracil plus leucovorin, is FDA-approved for use in first-line and salvage regimens for metastatic colorectal cancer (see Table 133–11). Oxaliplatin differs from cisplatin in that the DNA damage induced by oxaliplatin may not be as easily recognized by the DNA MMR complex.[102] Thus oxaliplatin-induced DNA damage may play a particularly important role in colorectal cancers that are associated with defects in MMR genes, which are common in HNPCC. Oxaliplatin's incorporation into fluorouracil-based regimens as first-line therapy for metastatic colorectal cancer is associated with higher response rates, improved PFS, and variable effects on OS. A comparison of the de Gramont regimen, with or without oxaliplatin 85 mg/m^2 as a 2-hour infusion on day 1 (FOLFOX4 regimen), was designed to evaluate PFS as a primary end point in 420 previously untreated patients with metastatic disease.[93] Tumor response (50.7% vs. 22.3%) and PFS (median: 9 months vs. 6.2 months) were improved with oxaliplatin compared to fluorouracil plus leucovorin alone; the difference in OS did not reach statistical significance (median: 16.2 months vs. 14.7 months). Although the three-drug regimen was associated with higher frequencies of grade 3 and 4 toxicities, primarily neutropenia, diarrhea, and neurosensory toxicity, they did not significantly impair quality-of-life.

Intergroup Trial N9741, a comparison of oxaliplatin plus fluorouracil and leucovorin (FOLFOX4) to weekly irinotecan plus IV bolus fluorouracil and leucovorin (IFL), and a combination of irinotecan plus oxaliplatin (IROX) in 795 patients with previously untreated metastatic colorectal cancer showed superior efficacy with FOLFOX4.[103] The IROX arm showed no advantage over either of the other two arms. Significant improvements in response rates, PFS, and median survival were seen with FOLFOX4 as compared to IFL (see Table 133–12).[103] The study design allowed patients who failed either regimen to crossover to irinotecan or oxaliplatin, depending on their initial treatment assignment. Sixty percent of patients who failed FOLFOX4 received salvage irinotecan, whereas 24% of IFL failures received salvage oxaliplatin. The impact that this crossover had on survival is unknown, but may have resulted in improved survival for the FOLFOX4 arm. In addition, the method of fluorouracil administration, and its impact on study results, has been called into question. Patients on the IFL arm received weekly IV bolus fluorouracil, while patients on the FOLFOX4 arm were administered fluorouracil as IV bolus followed by continuous infusion IV, which is known to increase response rates. Consequently, it is not possible to evaluate the true contributions of oxaliplatin and irinotecan combined with fluorouracil plus leucovorin in this study. The deletion of fluorouracil (or any fluorinated pyrimidine) from a first-line regimen may be undesirable.

In a phase III cooperative group study, a simplified combined bolus and infusional fluorouracil regimen with irinotecan (FOLFIRI) was compared to oxaliplatin combined with the same fluorouracil plus leucovorin schedule (FOLFOX6) in previously untreated patients with advanced colorectal cancer to determine whether the sequence of administration of both regimens differed with regard to efficacy and toxicities.[104] Patients were randomized to receive initial treatment with FOLFIRI or FOLFOX6, and at disease progression the patients then received the alternate regimen. Both sequences resulted in similar response rates, PFS, and median survival, but the grade 3 or 4 toxicity profiles were different. Neurotoxicity, neutropenia, and thrombocytopenia were more common with FOLFOX6, while febrile neutropenia, nausea/vomiting, mucositis, and fatigue were significantly more frequent with FOLFIRI.

Oxaliplatin has minimal renal toxicity, myelosuppression, and nausea and vomiting when compared to other platinum-based drugs. Oxaliplatin is associated with both acute and persistent neuropathies.[105] The acute neuropathies occur with 1 to 2 days of dosing and resolve within 2 weeks. The neuropathies usually occur peripherally, but may also occur in the jaw and tongue. A rare acute syndrome of pharyngolaryngeal dysesthesia (1% to 2% of patients) is characterized by subjective sensations of difficulty in swallowing and shortness of breath. Overall, acute neuropathies occur in approximately 90% of patients, and are precipitated or exacerbated by exposure to cold temperatures or cold objects. Thus patients should be instructed to avoid cold drinks and use of ice, and to cover skin before exposure to cold or cold objects. Several prophylactic and treatment strategies have been studied with varying degrees of success. Carbamazepine, gabapentin, amifostine, and calcium and magnesium infusions have been used to both prevent and treat oxaliplatin-induced neuropathies. Persistent neuropathy is typically a cumulative adverse effect, occurring after 8 to 10 cycles, and is seen mostly in patients who are responding to therapy.[103] The neuropathy is characterized by paresthesia, dysesthesia, and hypoesthesia, but may also include deficits in proprioception that can interfere with daily activities (e.g., writing, buttoning, swallowing, and difficulty walking as a result of impaired proprioception), and occur in half of patients receiving oxaliplatin with infusional fluorouracil plus leucovorin, but usually resolve with dosage reductions or cessation of oxaliplatin therapy.[105]

CLINICAL CONTROVERSY

The results of N9741 have been debated between clinicians since their presentation. Whether an irinotecan-containing regimen (IFL or FOLFIRI) or FOLFOX4 should be the first regimen used in metastatic colon cancer is an unanswered question. Sequencing trials suggest that it does not matter and most patients should receive both irinotecan- and oxaliplatin-containing regimens at some point during treatment for their disease.

9 ***Capecitabine.*** Capecitabine (Xeloda) is an oral, tumor-activated and tumor-selective fluoropyrimidine carbamate. Capecitabine is converted to fluorouracil through a three-step activation process, the final step being activation by thymidine phosphorylase, which is present in greatest concentrations at the tumor site. These activation steps lead to about a 3-fold increase in tumor and 1.4-fold increase in hepatic fluorouracil levels. Capecitabine was compared to fluorouracil plus leucovorin as first-line therapy for metastatic colorectal cancer in two randomized phase III trials. In a pooled analysis of 1,207 patients randomized to capecitabine (1,250 mg/m^2 orally twice daily for 14 days, repeated every 3 weeks) or the Mayo Clinic regimen, tumor response to capecitabine was superior to that of fluorouracil plus leucovorin (25.7% vs. 16.7%).[106] Time-to-tumor-progression and median survival, however, were no different. Hand–foot syndrome was more common with capecitabine, whereas grade 3 or 4 neutropenia and stomatitis were more common with fluorouracil plus leucovorin. The convenience of oral administration and different toxicity profile make capecitabine a useful alternative to IV fluorouracil regimens in the setting of metastatic disease. However, because the IV treatment arm in these comparative studies could be considered more toxic than the weekly IV fluorouracil plus leucovorin treatment schedule, it is premature to conclude that capecitabine is as efficacious as and less toxic than all parenteral fluorouracil-based regimens. Infusional fluorouracil is generally considered to be superior to bolus administration, and oral capecitabine may mimic this method of fluorouracil administration. These data, along with capecitabine's ease of administration, and data that irinotecan and oxaliplatin appear to have a greater effect when combined with infusional fluorouracil has led to capecitabine being evaluated as a replacement for infusional fluorouracil.

Both irinotecan and oxaliplatin have been combined with capecitabine and preliminary data suggest these combinations will be safe and effective in the initial treatment of metastatic colorectal cancer. The current FDA-approved indication for capecitabine in metastatic colon cancer is when therapy with a fluoropyrimidine alone is desired. Replacement of fluorouracil-leucovorin with capecitabine in other regimens is not currently approved, although longer follow-up of completed trials may show that capecitabine is a suitable replacement for infusional fluorouracil in combination with either irinotecan or oxaliplatin.

8 ***Biologic Therapy.*** Bevacizumab (Avastin) is a recombinant, humanized monoclonal antibody that inhibits vascular endothelial growth factor. Bevacizumab, in combination with intravenous fluorouracil-based chemotherapy, was FDA approved in 2004 for initial treatment of patients with metastatic colorectal cancer. This represents the third available combination regimen for first-line treatment. Results from two randomized trials show increased benefit as compared to chemotherapy alone.

A phase III trial of bevacizumab in combination with IFL as first-line therapy in patients with metastatic colorectal cancer has also been completed. Patients were randomized to receive IFL plus placebo or IFL plus bevacizumab 5 mg/kg every 2 weeks.[107] The addition of bevacizumab to IFL therapy resulted in an increase in response rate (34.7% vs. 44.9%) and median (15.6 vs. 20.3 months) and PFS (6.24 vs. 10.6 months) as compared to IFL alone. The frequency of typical adverse effects associated with IFL chemotherapy was not increased with the addition of bevacizumab. Grade 3 hypertension was significantly increased in the bevacizumab group. The incidence of other safety concerns with bevacizumab, such as bleeding, thromboembolism, and proteinuria, were not increased in the bevacizumab group as compared to placebo. The hypertension is easily managed with oral antihypertensive agents. The risk of gastrointestinal perforation was increased by the addition of bevacizumab to IFL, and patients complaining of abdominal pain associated with vomiting or constipation should be considered for this rare, but potentially fatal complication. Bevacizumab is also associated with a twofold increased risk of arterial thrombotic events, with patients who are older than age 65 years or who have a prior history of arterial thrombotic events at greatest risk. Nevertheless, because these individuals derive the same survival benefits with bevacizumab as other patients, they may be appropriate candidates to receive bevacizumab.

The use of bevacizumab with FOLFOX4 in the initial treatment of metastatic colon cancer was recently reported. In this trial, the first cohort of patients were randomized to three oxaliplatin-based regimens (TREE-1 [arm 1: oxaliplatin plus infusional 5-FU; arm 2: oxaliplatin plus bolus 5-FU; arm 3: oxaliplatin plus oral capecitabine]) while the second cohort of patients (TREE-2) received the same regimens plus bevacizumab as their first-line treatment for metastatic colon cancer. The addition of bevacizumab was associated with increased overall response rate and longer time to progression and median survival, although these differences were not significant as a consequence of the small sample size. Overall median survival with the addition of bevacizumab was 18.4 months in the TREE-1 cohort and 24.4 months in the TREE-2 cohort.[108] In a separate phase III trial, the addition of bevacizumab to oxaliplatin-based chemotherapy (XELOX or FOLFOX) significantly improved PFS.[109] Studies to compare the addition of bevacizumab to FOLFOX4 versus irinotecan-based combinations of bevacizumab are ongoing.

Investigational Approaches

Targeted Agents. Preliminary results with cetuximab in the first-line metastatic setting combined with either FOLFOX or FOLFIRI suggest that the combination improves response rates to either chemotherapy regimen without adding substantial toxicity.[110] Similar results have been reported with panitumumab,[111] but for reasons that are not well-understood, the addition of panitumumab to bevacizumab plus irinotecan- or oxaliplatin-containing chemotherapy *reduced* PFS in the Panitumumab Advanced Colorectal Cancer Evaluation Study (PACCE) trial. Whether two monoclonal antibodies can be safely and effectively combined with standard chemotherapy in the first-line treatment of metastatic colorectal cancer remains to be determined.

Hepatic Artery Infusion. Although hepatic chemotherapy infusion for metastatic colorectal cancer remains an area of investigation, it has not been shown to be superior to systemic chemotherapy. The rationale for hepatic artery infusion (HAI) is based on the principle that normal liver hepatocytes and early micrometastases obtain their primary blood supply from the portal vein. In contrast, tumors in the liver are thought to receive most of their blood supply via the hepatic artery.[91] Consequently, drug administration via the hepatic artery should result in delivery of high drug concentrations to the tumor cells with a much lower exposure to normal liver tissue.

Because the liver is a common site of colorectal cancer metastasis, and the only site of metastatic involvement in up to one-third of patients, hepatic-directed therapies continue to be explored. Historically, floxuridine and fluorouracil have undergone the most study for hepatic artery infusion, but other active agents such as irinotecan and oxaliplatin have also been studied. Trials involving HAI have been conducted in patients with unresectable liver metastases and as adjuvant therapy following curative resection of isolated metastases.

Regional HAI can be accomplished using a hepatic arterial port, a totally implantable pump, or a percutaneously placed catheter into the hepatic artery that is connected to an external pump. Early trials of HAI revealed objective response rates ranging from 30% to 88%, many of which were observed in previously treated patients, and increased survival rates as compared to historic controls. Because supportive care alone is no longer considered standard of care for metastatic disease, when HAI was compared to systemic chemotherapy, most comparisons did not yield a survival benefit.[91] Furthermore, most studies allowed patients in the systemic therapy treatment groups to crossover to HAI upon tumor progression; therefore the impact of these treatments on survival is difficult to interpret. Most recently, HAI was compared to systemic fluorouracil plus leucovorin in patients with hepatic-only metastasis.[112] HAI was associated with significantly longer OS (median: 24.4 vs. 20 months, $P = 0.0034$) and time-to-hepatic-progression (median: 9.8 vs. 7.3 months, $P = 0.034$) as compared to systemic chemotherapy. As expected, time-to-extrahepatic-progression was longer (14.8 vs. 7.7 months, $P = 0.029$) with systemic chemotherapy. This study has been criticized for the systemic chemotherapy treatment arm, which is considered less-than-optimal therapy by current standards.

Given the significant improvements with systemic chemotherapy for metastatic disease achieved with systemic chemotherapy over the past several years, attention has been directed to HAI with nonfluoropyrimidines, including irinotecan, oxaliplatin, and biologic agents. Early studies show promising results, but it is not clear whether this approach offers any advantage compared to systemic therapy.

Because of toxicities associated with HAI, most patients require some transient interruption of therapy, a decrease in dosage, or discontinuation of therapy. Furthermore, extrahepatic disease progression with HAI therapy alone remains a clinical problem. Although increased response rates and a trend toward improved survival have been reported, the costs and toxicities with this approach are significant. Therefore, for the minority of patients who present with unresectable disease to the liver only, HAI may represent a reasonable therapeutic option, but it is not considered standard therapy at this time.

Approach to Selecting an Initial Metastatic Regimen Practitioners can select first-line treatment for metastatic colorectal cancer from among four treatments: oxaliplatin plus fluorouracil plus leucovorin (FOLFOX); irinotecan plus fluorouracil plus leucovorin (FOLFIRI or IFL); bevacizumab plus fluorouracil-based chemotherapy; and capecitabine-based therapy. The most important factor in patient survival is not the initial regimen but whether or not patients receive all three active chemotherapy drugs (fluorouracil, irinotecan, and oxaliplatin) at some point in their treatment course.[113] Based on the comparable results of FOLFIRI versus FOLFOX6, combined with the inferiority of IFL to FOLFOX4, either of these regimens is considered the reference standard in metastatic colorectal cancer. The IFL regimen is rarely used in clinical practice. Similar to the adjuvant setting, patient-specific factors may lead practitioners to choose between FOLFOX and FOLFIRI. Preexisting neuropathies may lead to FOLFIRI being chosen initially, whereas increased bilirubin or known UGT1A1 deficiency (known risk factors for delayed diarrhea) may lead to FOLFOX as the initial choice. The 2007 NCCN guidelines recommend the addition of bevacizumab to any initial fluorouracil-based regimen unless contraindicated.[114]

Capecitabine may be an appropriate substitute for intravenous fluorouracil in these combination regimens; the 2007 NCCN guidelines list CapOx plus bevacizumab as an acceptable initial regimen based on preliminary data demonstrating equivalence to oxaliplatin plus continuous infusion 5-FU.[115] Fluorouracil plus leucovorin alone or capecitabine monotherapy is also appropriate first-line treatment for those individuals who cannot tolerate three-drug combination regimens.

Second-Line Therapy

Systemic chemotherapy represents the mainstay of therapy for patients whose disease progresses following initial treatment for metastatic disease. Figure 133–6 depicts an algorithm for treatment of refractory metastatic disease. Treatment options are based on the type of and response to prior treatments, the site and extent of disease, and patient factors and treatment preferences.

Systemic Chemotherapy On disease progression following standard initial therapy, appropriate treatment options may include oxaliplatin plus fluorouracil and leucovorin with or without bevacizumab, irinotecan plus cetuximab, cetuximab, irinotecan, continuous-infusion fluorouracil, capecitabine plus oxaliplatin, capecitabine, intrahepatic therapy for selected patients, supportive care, or participation in a clinical trial. The choice of specific agents depends primarily on the type of prior therapy received. Because most patients will have received a combination of a pyrimidine with either irinotecan or oxaliplatin, second-line therapy with the alternate regimen should be considered. Patient survival can exceed 2 years.

Irinotecan. Two important trials have delineated an appropriate standard of care for patients who experience disease progression with fluorouracil therapy for metastatic colorectal cancer.[116,117] The results of these trials demonstrate a survival benefit associated with irinotecan, which was FDA approved in 1996 as second-line therapy for recurrent or progressive disease following fluorouracil. In phase II studies of previously treated patients with metastatic colorectal cancer, objective response rates of 13% to 27% have been observed.[116,117]

In a phase III trial of 189 patients with metastatic colorectal cancer that had progressed within 6 months of treatment with fluorouracil, irinotecan was compared to supportive care alone with regard to survival, quality-of-life, and other clinical variables.[116] Irinotecan was administered as 350 mg/m^2 IV every 3 weeks; the dose was reduced to 300 mg/m^2 for individuals who were 70 years of age or older, had a World Health Organization performance status of 2, or who had clinical risk factors for developing excessive treatment-related toxicity. Supportive care could include any symptomatic therapy with the exception of irinotecan or any other topoisomerase I inhibitor. With the exception of more patients with poor performance status in the supportive care group, baseline patient characteristics were similar between groups. Median survival was 9.2 months with irinotecan, as compared to 6.5 months with supportive care alone. One-year survival was significantly greater with irinotecan (36.2% vs. 13.8%) and was not associated with significantly worse quality-of-life scores except for diarrhea. Clinical variables such as cognitive functioning, pain, dyspnea, and appetite loss were in favor of irinotecan therapy. The most common grade 3 or 4 side effects with irinotecan included leukopenia and neutropenia (22%), diarrhea (22%), nausea (14%), and vomiting (14%). Seventy-two percent of patients receiving irinotecan required hospital admission for adverse events, as compared to 63% of supportive care patients. Thus irinotecan was associated with an improved survival and quality-of-life as compared to supportive care alone that appeared to balance treatment-related toxicities.

A comparison of irinotecan to continuous-infusion fluorouracil in a similar population of 267 patients allocated patients to irinotecan, 300 to 350 mg/m^2 IV every 3 weeks, or one of three continuous-infusion fluorouracil regimens: leucovorin 200 mg/m^2 IV over 2 hours followed by IV bolus fluorouracil (400 mg/m^2) and 22-hour continuous-infusion fluorouracil (600 mg/m^2), given the first 2 days of every 2-week period; fluorouracil 250 to 300 mg/m^2 as prolonged continuous IV infusion until disease progression; or fluorouracil 2,600 to 3,000 mg/m^2 per day IV over 24 hours, with or without leucovorin (20 to 500 mg/m^2 IV), given weekly for 6 weeks, with a 2-week rest period between cycles.[117] Median followup after 15 months revealed a longer 1-year survival (45% vs. 32%) and median survival (10.8 months vs. 8.5 months) with irinotecan, as compared to fluorouracil. Sixty-nine percent of patients receiving irinotecan experienced at least one grade 3 or 4 toxicity, as compared to 54% of patients receiving fluorouracil. The most common toxicities with irinotecan were diarrhea, neutropenia, pain, vomiting, and asthenia, while pain, asthenia, diarrhea, and dermatologic toxicities were most common with fluorouracil. There was no difference in hospitalization requirement for adverse effects between treatments.

Based on these results, irinotecan should be considered standard second-line therapy for patients who have failed prior treatment with fluorouracil-based regimens. Initial administration of irinote-

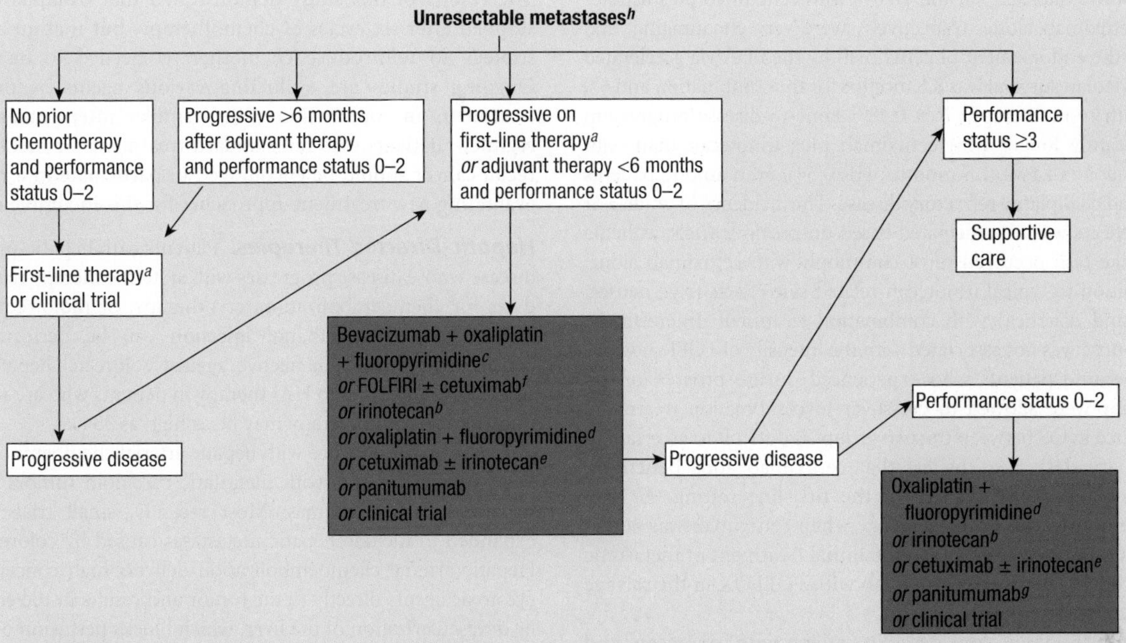

[a] Bevacizumab + oxaliplatin + fluoropyrimidine (e.g., infusional 5-FU/LV (FOLFOX) *or* capecitabine (CapeOx)); *or* bevacizumab + irinotecan + infusional 5-FU/LV (FOLFIRI); *or* bevacizumab + 5FU/LV; *or* capecitabine ± bevacizumab; *or* 5-FU/LV ± bevacizumab.

[b] If no prior irinotecan.

[c] If first-line regimen did not contain bevacizumab or oxaliplatin.

[d] If no prior oxaliplatin.

[e] If irinotecan-refractory or intolerant and no prior cetuximab.

[f] If first-line regimen did not contain irinotecan.

[g] If no prior cetuximab or panitumumab.

[h] Initial unresectable metastases may be converted to resectable disease in selected patients who exhibit a good tumor response to systemic chemotherapy. Those patients may be candidates for surgical tumor resection followed by adjuvant chemotherapy.

FIGURE 133-6. Algorithm for treatment of unresectable or refractory metastatic colorectal cancer.

can at the lower dose should be considered for patients who have received significant prior pelvic or abdominal irradiation. Protracted continuous-infusion fluorouracil could be considered for those individuals with disease that no longer responds to bolus IV fluorouracil plus leucovorin or irinotecan.

Oxaliplatin. For patients who received primary treatment with irinotecan and fluorouracil, oxaliplatin plus fluorouracil and leucovorin should be considered. Despite the low activity of single-agent oxaliplatin against fluorouracil-refractory disease, when oxaliplatin has been administered in a bimonthly regimen with high-dose leucovorin and continuous fluorouracil infusion, a 20.6% response rate with a median survival in excess of 10 months has been reported.[118] The combination of oxaliplatin plus fluorouracil and leucovorin is also effective as salvage therapy after initial treatment with irinotecan plus fluorouracil and leucovorin, with a response rate of approximately 20%.[119] Although irinotecan can be used effectively as a single agent in colorectal cancer, it should be noted that oxaliplatin does not have substantial activity alone, and should only be given in combination with a fluoropyrimidine.

In patients who did not receive bevacizumab in their initial treatment, FOLFOX plus bevacizumab is recommended based on phase III data. Results from Eastern Cooperative Group 3200 demonstrated that bevacizumab, in combination with FOLFOX4, improved survival in patients with previously treated advanced colorectal cancer.[120] It should be noted that patients were excluded if they received prior oxaliplatin or bevacizumab and the dose of bevacizumab was 10 mg/kg instead of 5 mg/kg. Median survival was improved from 10.7 to 12.5 months ($P = 0.0018$). There are no substantial data to support the use of bevacizumab after progression on first-line bevacizumab.

⑩ ***Biologic Therapy.*** Cetuximab (IMC-C225, Erbitux) is a chimeric monoclonal antibody directed against an EGFR that received FDA approval in 2004. Cetuximab may be administered in combination with irinotecan, but can be used as a single agent in patients who cannot tolerate irinotecan-based chemotherapy.

In a phase II study, patients with EGFR-expressing metastatic colorectal cancer who had failed an irinotecan-based regimen received open-label cetuximab, 400 mg/m^2 IV as a loading dose, followed by weekly infusions of 250 mg/m^2 IV until disease progression.[121] Of 57 patients treated, 5 achieved a partial response, with a minor response or stable disease developing in 21 additional patients. The median survival was 6.4 months. The most common grade 3 or 4 adverse events were papulopustular, follicular skin rash (18% grade 3) and adverse effects characterized as asthenia, lethargy, malaise, or fatigue (9% grade 3).

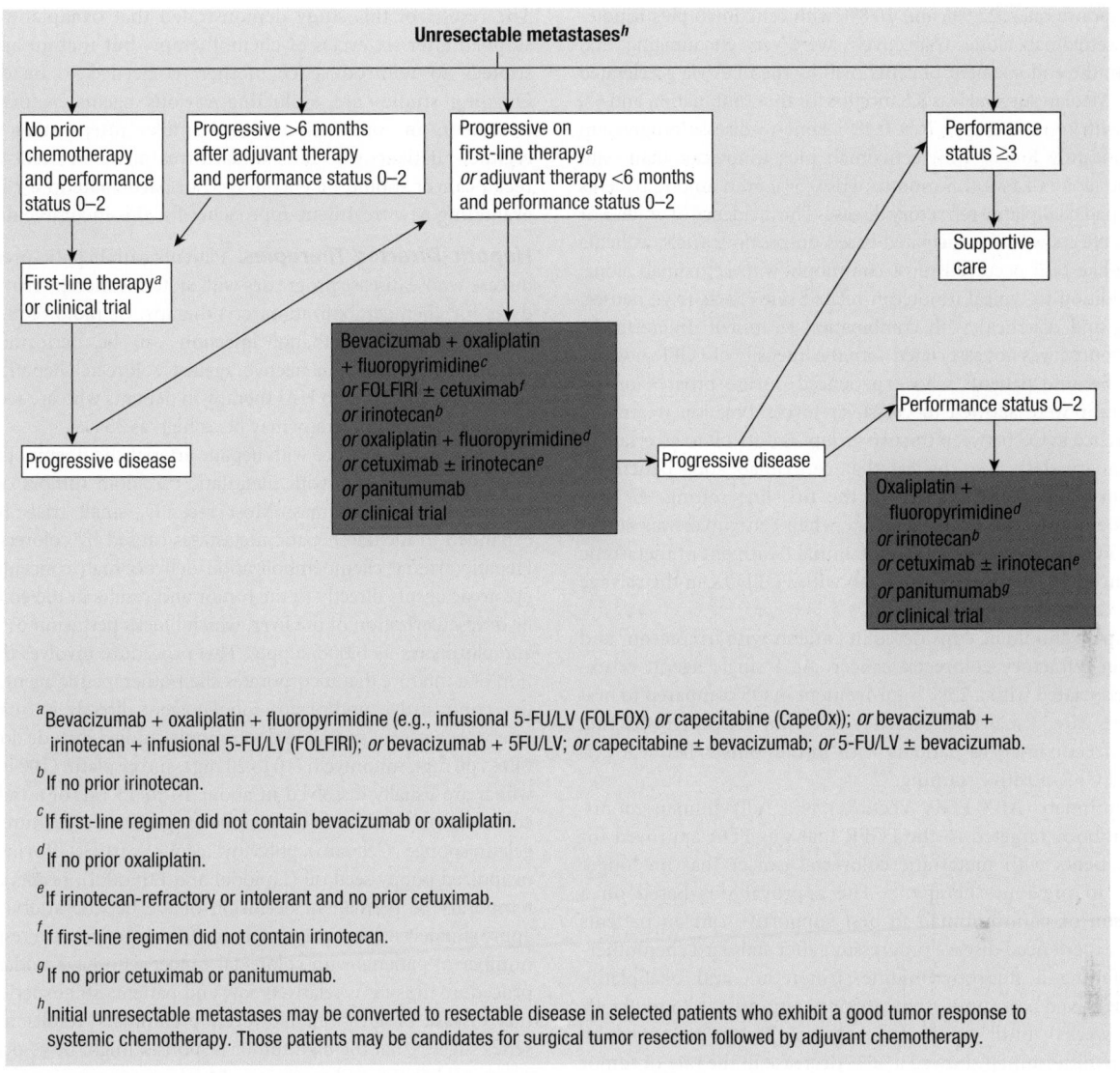

The combination of cetuximab plus irinotecan was also compared to cetuximab as a single agent in patients with EGFR-positive colorectal cancer that had progressed on irinotecan. Three hundred and twenty-nine patients were randomized in a 2:1 ratio to receive cetuximab plus continuation of the irinotecan or cetuximab alone.[122] The objective tumor response rates, 22.9% and 10.8% with cetuximab plus irinotecan and cetuximab alone, respectively, were very encouraging, and resulted in the endorsement of cetuximab by the FDA via accelerated approval. Median survival was 8.6 months for the combination and 6.9 months with monotherapy ($P = 0.48$). Time-to-disease-progression was significantly longer with cetuximab plus irinotecan than with cetuximab alone (4.1 vs. 1.5 months; HR 0.54), even among patients who also had oxaliplatin-refractory disease. The incidence of grade 3 or 4 adverse effects was as anticipated based on previous trials; asthenia and acne-like rash occurred most commonly with cetuximab alone, and in addition to typical irinotecan-related side effects (e.g., nausea, vomiting, and diarrhea) with combination treatment. Interestingly, tumor response was not associated with the intensity of EGFR-positive staining. Because patients who experienced disease progression on monotherapy were allowed to crossover to combination treatment, any difference in OS between the two groups is difficult to ascertain.

Preliminary data also suggest that cetuximab adds benefit to oxaliplatin-based regimens and in the first-line setting. A 2006 abstract demonstrated similar efficacy when cetuximab was added to either FOLFOX or FOLFIRI in the initial treatment of metastatic colon cancer.[110] The use of cetuximab with FOLFOX in the salvage setting is currently unknown.

Cetuximab should be considered in patients with irinotecan- and oxaliplatin-refractory colorectal cancer. As a single agent, cetuximab is associated with a 23% improvement in OS compared to best supportive care.[150] Current evidence does not support restricting the use of cetuximab to patients with immunohistochemical evidence of EGFR-positive staining.[114]

Panitumumab (ABX-EGF, Vectibix) is a fully human monoclonal antibody targeted to the EGFR that was FDA approved for use in patients with metastatic colorectal cancer that no longer responds to previous therapy.[123] The approval was based on a comparison of panitumumab to best supportive care in patients who had experienced disease progression after standard chemotherapy, including a fluoropyrimidine, irinotecan, and oxaliplatin. Patients received best supportive care or panitumumab (6 mg/kg IV every 2 weeks) until tumor progression. Those patients who received panitumumab showed a 46% decrease in the rate of tumor progression compared to those who only received best supportive care (HR 0.54, 95% CI 0.44 to 0.66). As expected, dermatologic toxicities were observed in patients receiving panitumumab, as well as fatigue, abdominal pain, nausea, and diarrhea. Only one hypersensitivity reaction was reported. As with cetuximab, EGFR-positivity with immunohistochemistry should not be used to determine appropriate candidates for panitumumab. Additional studies with investigational monoclonal antibodies are ongoing.

CLINICAL CONTROVERSY

Currently, cetuximab and panitumumab are only approved by the FDA for patients with documented EGFR-positive tumors. Mounting clinical evidence suggests that patients with EGFR-negative tumors may derive the same benefit,[124] but insurance coverage for patients with EGFR-negative tumors may be difficult to obtain.

Miscellaneous Salvage Chemotherapy. Similar to initial treatment of metastatic colon cancer, capecitabine is being investigated as a replacement for infusional fluorouracil in salvage regimens in combination with irinotecan or oxaliplatin.

One interesting subject of debate is whether treatment could be suspended once disease stabilization occurs and restarted upon disease progression. In the OPTIMOX study, patients were randomized to receive continuous FOLFOX4 until disease progression, or a simplified regimen, FOLFOX7, with intermittent oxaliplatin.[125] The results of this study demonstrated that oxaliplatin could be stopped after six cycles of chemotherapy, but that an appropriate strategy to reintroduce chemotherapy needed to be developed. Ongoing studies are evaluating various agents as maintenance treatments in conjunction with a similar intermittent treatment regimen. Patients who fail standard treatment for metastatic colorectal cancer should be encouraged to participate in a clinical trial evaluating new treatment approaches for this incurable disease.

Hepatic-Directed Therapies. Patients with hepatic-predominant disease whose disease progresses with systemic therapy may be candidates for chemoembolization, cryotherapy, or radiofrequency ablation. Percutaneous ethanol injection can be performed but is considered relatively ineffective against colorectal hepatic metastases.[126] Response rates to HAI therapy in patients who are refractory to fluorouracil-based therapy may be as high as 33%.

The largest experience with hepatic arterial chemoembolization has been seen in patients with metastatic carcinoid tumors or primary hepatocellular carcinomas. Most recently, small trials have been expanded to include hepatic metastases caused by colorectal cancer. Hepatic arterial chemoembolization delivers high concentrations of cytotoxic agents directly to the tumor and results in the embolization or devascularization of the liver, which blocks perfusion of the tumor and eliminates its blood supply. This procedure involves the instillation of a mixture that incorporates chemotherapeutic agents, radioactive contrast dye, and/or an embolic agent directly into the hepatic artery. Agents and doses most commonly studied include doxorubicin (40 to 60 mg), mitomycin (10 to 20 mg), and cisplatin (100 to 150 mg), which are usually dissolved in about 10 to 15 mL of a radiographic contrast dye.[127] Addition of an embolic agent to the mixture, such as a gelatin sponge (Gelfoam), polyvinyl alcohol particles, bovine collagen, or iodized poppy seed oil (Lipiodol and Ethiodol), results in either a temporary or permanent occlusion of the hepatic artery. Although approximately 80% of patients in one trial experienced a response, the number of patients with colorectal cancer who have undergone this procedure thus far is relatively low and patients still experience eventual disease progression. However, preliminary results from small series suggest that the high tumor responses might be associated with a survival benefit, and randomized trials comparing systemic therapy to hepatic chemoembolization for unresectable disease are ongoing.

Cryosurgery involves placement of a cryoprobe into the tumor, either percutaneously or intraoperatively, and then lowering the probe temperature to 100°C (148°F).[126] This is repeated in cycles, resulting in formation of an ice ball that causes tumor destruction. Cryosurgery may be used alone or in conjunction with other localized procedures, such as radiofrequency ablation, which is becoming increasingly used for colorectal liver metastases. The technique involves placement of a chilled perfusion electrode needle into the tumor with subsequent application of alternating electrical current through the electrode, resulting in thermal coagulative necrosis of the tumor.[126] Laser interstitial thermal therapy represents an alternate method for causing tumor coagulative necrosis using a laser. Radiofrequency ablation is also being evaluated in conjunction with HAI, in an effort to reduce local recurrence of metastatic tumors. Procedure-related complications can include bleeding, coagulopathy, liver abscess, biliary stricture, and pleural effusion.[126] Although these approaches represent potential treatment strategies for patients with unresectable, yet limited hepatic metastases, additional experience is needed to determine long-term outcomes. Furthermore, extrahepatic sites of disease continue to be a problem even for those individuals in whom the liver tumors can be eradicated.

New Strategies and Agents in Development

At present, fluorouracil plus leucovorin, bevacizumab, capecitabine, irinotecan, oxaliplatin, and cetuximab are the most frequently used chemotherapeutic agents for cancer of the colon and rectum. New chemotherapy agents have been studied in an attempt to further improve antitumor efficacy and reduce treatment toxicities. Oral fluorinated pyrimidines and TS inhibitors, such as fluorouracil prodrugs and inhibitors of fluorouracil catabolism, can prolong in vivo fluorouracil exposure and enhance antitumor effects without the use of continuous IV infusions. But traditional chemotherapy agents, which target rapidly dividing cells, kill both malignant and nonmalignant cells, and new cancer therapies are needed to improve therapeutic outcomes. In particular, targeted therapies aimed at the underlying cancer pathology are increasingly being developed and used in colorectal cancer treatment. A variety of agents targeted toward augmenting the host immune system response have undergone, or are currently undergoing, study for colorectal cancer, including monoclonal antibodies and tumor vaccines. Another potential strategy is regulating tumor growth through the inhibition of various cell signal-transduction pathways. Agents that can alter microenvironmental factors that support angiogenesis and tumor metastases may also be of benefit.

In addition, observations that various tumor characteristics (e.g., TS expression), patient drug-metabolizing enzymes (e.g., DPD and plasma uracil-to-dihydrouracil ratio), and molecular markers (e.g., chromosome 18q allelic loss, microsatellite instability, and *p53* mutation or loss) may predict prognosis and response to certain therapies and provide the rationale for pharmacogenomic strategies to select first-line therapies for individual patients.[128–130] Although patients who are deficient in DPD experience severe and potentially life-threatening toxicities with conventional doses of fluorouracil, determination of DPD activity is relatively time-consuming and the techniques are not amenable to routine clinical practice. As an alternative, plasma ratio determinations of uracil and dihydrouracil, which are more easily obtainable, can identify individuals with DPD deficiency and who are at risk of developing significant toxicities. Of factors predictive for tumor sensitivity to fluorouracil, TS expression has been most studied. Results from in vitro studies demonstrate that pretreatment intratumoral TS levels are inversely correlated to tumor response to fluorouracil. Whether increased tumor TS expression reflects a biologically more aggressive tumor or is directly related to fluorouracil resistance is unknown. Studies are underway to use this and other information to identify rational therapeutic approaches for select patients.

PHARMACOECONOMIC CONSIDERATIONS

The estimated expenditures for colorectal cancer in the United States alone are between $5.3 and $6.5 billion per year.[131] The total lifetime cost for managing a patient with cancer of the colon based on North American data is close to $100,000.[131] Costs for patients with rectal cancer are approximately 15% higher because of the added expense of XRT. The highest of costs of treatment are incurred during the initial and terminal phases of care. Thus, a long-term approach is needed to accurately estimate the cost of treating patients diagnosed with colorectal cancer. In addition, long-term cancer-related excess costs were calculated with the Surveillance, Epidemiology, and End Results (SEER)-Medicare–linked database as $33,700 and $36,500 for colon and rectal cancer, respectively.[131] The impact of changes in clinical practice on treatment costs, such as increased use of adjuvant therapy, changes in duration of hospital stay and outpatient delivery of health services, and incorporation of costly agents into standard treatment regimens, must also be continually considered.

The cost of the drugs alone (based on 95% of Average Wholesale Price (AWP) in 2004) were estimated for a 70-kg, 170-cm tall patient with colorectal cancer for a typical treatment period of 8 weeks.[131] The cost of biweekly infusional fluorouracil plus leucovorin (LV5FU2) is only about $263, but the incorporation of irinotecan (FOLFIRI) or oxaliplatin (FOLFOX) increases drug costs to $9,381 and $11,889, respectively. Total drug costs are about $21,000 with the addition of bevacizumab; an 8-week treatment course of standard cetuximab-containing regimens costs about $31,000. Thus, while the availability of these newer cytotoxic and biologic agents has extended median survival of patients with metastatic colorectal cancer, the economic impact of drug therapy alone on the healthcare system is of increasing importance.

The cost-effectiveness of therapeutic regimens in various treatment settings has also been evaluated. The addition of irinotecan to fluorouracil and leucovorin as first-line therapy for metastatic disease was supported in the United Kingdom based on an incremental cost-effectiveness ratio of £14,794 per life-year gained.[132] A comparison of the costs and effects of FOLFOX compared to IFL, based on the perspective of a United States payer, showed total costs of $94,693 for FOLFOX and $66,231 for IFL, with a gain in survival of 4.4 months with FOLFOX at an incremental cost-effectiveness ratio of $80,410 per life-year gained.[132] The associated $11,890 per quality-adjusted life-year gained is considered an acceptable oncology intervention within the United States healthcare system.

In adjuvant treatment, a cost-effectiveness analysis of FOLFOX4 compared to LV5FU2 from a Medicare perspective showed an incremental cost-effectiveness ratio with FOLFOX4 of $20,603 per life-year gained and $22,804 per quality-adjusted life-year gained.[133] At a threshold of $50,000 per quality-adjusted life-year, FOLFOX4 would be viewed as cost-effective adjuvant therapy for stage III colon cancer. Substitution of intravenous fluorouracil with oral capecitabine may have positive economic effects, but data are limited.[132] Reduced costs for capecitabine with regard to drug administration and drug-related adverse effects offset its higher acquisition cost as compared to fluorouracil plus leucovorin in adjuvant therapy for stage III colon cancer, but a cost-effectiveness analysis was not reported.[134]

The cost-effectiveness of combination chemotherapy with cetuximab, bevacizumab, or panitumumab in the United States has not been established. A report by the National Institute for Health and Clinical Excellence (NICE) suggests that neither first-line bevacizumab nor second-line or subsequent treatment cetuximab would be considered cost-effective.[132]

Colorectal cancer screening is regarded as cost-effective, but only approximately 35% of the population age 50 years and older undergoes regular screening.[135] The cost-effectiveness of standard methods varies. Base-case estimates, adjusted to year 2000 dollars, were $6,300 to $19,700 per life-year saved, $13,600 to $36,300 per life-year saved, and $7,300 to $22,000 per life-year saved for FOBT, sigmoidoscopy, and colonoscopy, respectively.[135] When adjusted average cost-effectiveness ratios were calculated and compared among FOBT, colonoscopy, and sigmoidoscopy, colonoscopy was the most cost-effective screening strategy when performed every 10 years. Based on an average estimated adherence rate with FOBT or sigmoidoscopy of approximately 50%, the ability to offer patients a choice of screening alternatives has been proposed in an attempt to increase acceptance of screening.[135] A base-rate estimate of the cost-effectiveness of offering a choice of cancer screening options to individuals age 50 years and older is $11,900 per life-year gained.[135] Because most accepted screening strategies have cost-effectiveness ratios that are well below the accepted benchmark of $50,000 per life-year saved, this strategy is considered cost-effective. As many as 12,000 deaths each year might be prevented if all individuals who were candidates for colorectal screening participated in a regular program.[135]

EVALUATION OF THERAPEUTIC OUTCOMES

The goal of monitoring is to evaluate whether the patient is receiving any benefit from the management of the disease or to detect recurrence. Similarly, followup examinations help to determine whether preventive interventions or screening studies effectively reduce an individual's risk for developing colorectal cancer or presenting with an advanced stage of disease. During treatment for active disease, patients should undergo monitoring for measurable tumor response, progression, or new metastases; these tests may include chest CT scans or radiographs, abdominal or pelvic CT scans or radiographs, depending on the site of disease being evaluated for response, and CEA measurements every 3 months if the CEA is or was previously elevated. In addition, a complete blood cell count should be obtained prior to each course of chemotherapy administration to ensure that hematologic indices are adequate. Baseline liver function tests and an assessment of renal function should be evaluated prior to and periodically during therapy. These tests and other selected serum chemistries should also be evaluated with the development of any new symptoms or significant change in disease status. Patients should be evaluated during every treatment visit for the presence of anticipated side effects, which generally include loose stools or diarrhea, nausea or vomiting, mouth sores, fatigue, and fever, as well as other side effects such as neuropathy and skin rash that are typically associated with oxaliplatin and cetuximab, respectively. Patients receiving bevacizumab should be evaluated for hypertension and proteinuria.

Symptoms of recurrence such as pain syndromes, changes in bowel habits, rectal or vaginal bleeding, pelvic masses, anorexia, and weight loss develop in less than 50% of patients. A greater percentage of recurrences are detected in asymptomatic patients because of increased serum CEA levels that lead to further examination. Although the value of CEA monitoring for asymptomatic disease recurrence is questioned by some because of the related expense and emotional stress associated with false-positive elevations, CEA monitoring plays an important role in postoperative followup studies for most individuals. A PET scan can be considered to identify localized sites of metastatic disease when a rising CEA level suggests metastatic disease but CT scans and other imaging studies are negative.

Patients who undergo curative surgical resection, with or without adjuvant therapy, require close followup based on the premise that early detection and treatment of recurrence could still render them cured. In addition, early treatment for asymptomatic metastatic colorectal cancer appears superior to delayed therapy. Specific practice guidelines for postoperative surveillance examinations were developed by ASCO (Table 133–13). These guidelines also recommend against routinely monitoring liver function tests, complete blood cell count, FOBT, annual chest radiographs in asymptomatic patients.[136]

Recent advances in the treatment for cancer of the colon and rectum now offer the potential to improve patient survival but for many patients, improved DFS and PFS represent equally important therapeutic outcomes. Although treatment approaches for metastatic colorectal cancer have been historically assessed by their ability to produce a measurable objective tumor response, which is generally believed necessary for any treatment to improve survival, the effects of therapies on survival are clinically more meaningful than their

TABLE 133-13 Major Features of the American Society of Clinical Oncology Postoperative Surveillance Practice Guidelines for Colon and Rectal Cancer

- History and physical examination every 3 to 6 months for the first 3 years, every 6 months during years 4 and 5, and subsequently at the discretion of the physician
- Annual computed tomographic scan of the chest and abdomen for 3 years after primary therapy for patients who are at higher risk of recurrence and who could be candidates for curative-intent surgery
- Colonoscopy at 3 years after operative treatment, and, if results are normal, every 5 years thereafter

Data from Desch EC, Benson AB, III, Somerfield MR, et al. Colorectal Cancer Surveillance: 2005 Update of an American Society of Clinical Oncology Practice Guideline. J Clin Oncol 2005;23:8512–8519.

ability to induce a tumor response. However, with the availability of multiple active treatments for metastatic disease, and the likelihood that patients will receive more than one during the course of their treatment, improvements in OS with new therapies will be increasingly difficult to determine.

In the absence of the ability of a specific treatment to demonstrate improved survival, important outcome measures should include the effects of the treatment on patient symptoms, daily activities and performance status, and other quality-of-life indicators, as well as progression-free survival and time to treatment failure. Because most metastatic colorectal cancers are incurable, a specific decision regarding an individual patient's care ultimately will be required. This decision should be based on a careful assessment of the balance between risks associated with treatment (or lack thereof) and benefits of treatment. Effort should also be made to ensure that the costs of screening, diagnostic tests, treatments, and procedures for colorectal cancer are consistent with their value in improving patient outcomes.

ABBREVIATIONS

APC: adenomatous polyposis coli (gene)

ASCO: American Society of Clinical Oncology

BMI: body mass index

CAPOX: capecitabine, oxaliplatin

CEA: carcinoembryonic antigen

COX: cyclooxygenase

CT: computed tomography

CYP: cytochrome P450 isoenzyme

DFS: disease-free survival

DPD: dihydropyrimidine dehydrogenase

EGFR: epidermal growth factor receptor

FAP: familial adenomatous polyposis

FIT: fecal immunochemical test

FOBT: fecal occult blood test

FOLFIRI: fluorouracil, leucovorin, irinotecan

FOLFOX: fluorouracil, leucovorin, oxaliplatin

5-FU: fluorouracil

HAI: hepatic artery infusion

HNPCC: hereditary nonpolyposis colorectal cancer

HR: hazard ratio

IFL: irinotecan plus fluorouracil plus leucovorin

MMR: mismatch-repair (gene)

MTHFR: methylenetetrahydrofolate reductase

NCCN: National Comprehensive Cancer Network

NSAID: nonsteroidal antiinflammatory drug

OS: overall survival

PET: positron emission tomography

PFS: progression-free survival

RR: relative risk

TGF-β: transforming growth factor-β

TS: thymidylate synthase

UGT1A1: uridine diphosphate-glucuronosyltransferase

XELOX: capecitabine, oxaliplatin

XRT: radiation therapy

REFERENCES

1. Jemal A, Siegel R, Ward EEA. Cancer statistics, 2007. CA Cancer J Clin 2007;57:43–66.
2. Parkin D, Bray F, Ferlay J, et al. Global cancer statistics, 2002. CA Cancer J Clin 2005;55:74–108.
3. Ries L, Melbert D, Krapcho M, et al., eds. SEER Cancer Statistics Review, 1975–2004. National Cancer Institute. Bethesda, MD, http://seer.cancer.gov/csr/1975–2004, Accessed November 1, 2007.
4. Kamangar F, Dores G, Anderson W. Patterns of cancer incidence, mortality, and prevalence across five continents: Defining priorities to reduce cancer disparities in different geographic regions of the world. J Clin Oncol 2006;24:2137–2150.
5. Asano T, McLeod R. Dietary fibre for the prevention of colorectal adenomas and carcinomas. Cochrane Database Syst Rev, 2002. Issue 1. Art. No.: CD003430. DOI: 10:1002/14651858. CD003430.
6. Michels K, Giovannucci E, Chan A, et al. Fruit and vegetable consumption and colorectal adenomas in the Nurses' Health Study. Cancer Res 2006;66:3942–3953.
7. Park Y, Hunter D, Spiegelman D, et al. Dietary fiber intake and risk of colorectal cancer. A pooled analysis of prospective cohort studies. JAMA 2005;294:2849–2857.
8. Park Y, Subar A, Kipnis V, et al. Fruit and vegetable intakes and risk of colorectal cancer in the NIH-AARP Diet and Health Study. Am J Epidemiol 2007.
9. Norat T, Bingham S, Ferrari P, et al. Meat, fish, and colorectal cancer risk: The European Prospective Investigation into Cancer and Nutrition. J Natl Cancer Inst 2005;97:906–916.
10. Giovannucci E. Modifiable risk factors for colon cancer. Gastroenterol Clin North Am 2002;31:925–943.
11. Lamprecht SA, Lipkin M. Chemoprevention of colon cancer by calcium, vitamin D and folate: Molecular mechanisms. Nat Rev Cancer 2003;3:601–614.
12. Hartman T, Albert P, Snyder K, et al. The association of calcium and vitamin D with risk of colorectal adenomas. J Nutr 2005;135:252–259.
13. Kim Y-I. Folate and colorectal cancer: An evidence-based critical review. Mol Nutr Food Res 2007;51:267–292.
14. Michels KB, Willett WC, Fuchs CS, Giovannucci E. Coffee, tea, and caffeine consumption and incidence of colon and rectal cancer. J Natl Cancer Inst 2005;97:282–292.
15. Sun C-L, Yuan J-M, Koh W-P, Yu MC. Green tea, black tea and colorectal cancer risk: A meta-analysis of epidemiologic studies. Carcinogenesis 2006;27:1301–1309.
16. Dube C, Rostom A, Lewin G, et al. The use of aspirin for primary prevention of colorectal cancer: A systematic review prepared for the U.S. Preventive Services Task Force. Ann Intern Med 2007;146:365–375.
17. Rostom A, Dube C, Lewin G, et al. Nonsteroidal anti-inflammatory drugs and cyclooxygenase-2 inhibitors for primary prevention of colorectal cancer: A systematic review prepared for the U.S. Preventive Services Task Force. Ann Intern Med 2007;146:376–389.
18. Thun MJ, Henley SJ, Patrono C. Nonsteroidal anti-inflammatory drugs as anticancer agents: mechanistic, pharmacologic, and clinical issues. J Natl Cancer Inst 2002;94:252–266.
19. Steinbach G, Lynch PM, Phillips RKS, et al. The effect of celecoxib, a cyclooxygenase-2 inhibitor, in familial adenomatous polyposis. N Engl J Med 2000;342:1946–1952.
20. Flossmann E, Rothwell PM. Effect of aspirin on long-term risk of colorectal cancer: Consistent evidence from randomised and observational studies. Lancet 2007;369:1603–1613.
21. Potter JD. Colorectal cancer: Molecules and populations. J Natl Cancer Inst 1999;91:916–932.
22. Chan JA, Meyerhardt JA, Chan AT, Giovannucci EL, Colditz GA, Fuchs CS. Hormone replacement therapy and survival after colorectal cancer diagnosis. J Clin Oncol 2006;24:5680–5686.
23. Grodstein F, Newcomb PA, Stampfer MJ. Postmenopausal hormone therapy and the risk of colorectal cancer: A review and meta-analysis. Am J Med 1999;106:574–582.
24. Chlebowski RT, Wactawski-Wende J, Ritenbaugh C, et al. Estrogen plus progestin and colorectal cancer in postmenopausal women. N Engl J Med 2004;350:991–1004.
25. Pischon T, Lahmann PH, Boeing H, et al. Body size and risk of colon and rectal cancer in the European Prospective Investigation Into Cancer and Nutrition (EPIC). J Natl Cancer Inst 2006;98:920–931.
26. Adams KF, Leitzmann MF, Albanes D, et al. Body mass and colorectal cancer risk in the NIH–AARP Cohort. Am J Epidemiol 2007;166:36–45.
27. Gunter MJ, Leitzmann MF. Obesity and colorectal cancer: Epidemiology, mechanisms and candidate genes. J Nutr Biochem 2006;17:145–156.
28. Larsson SC, Orsini N, Wolk A. Diabetes mellitus and risk of colorectal cancer: A meta-analysis. J Natl Cancer Inst 2005;97:1679–1687.
29. Ahmed RL, Schmitz KH, Anderson KE, et al. The metabolic syndrome and risk of incident colorectal cancer. Cancer 2006;107:28–36.
30. Moskal A, Norat T, Ferrari P, et al. Alcohol intake and colorectal cancer risk: A dose-response meta-analysis of published cohort studies. Int J Cancer 2007;120:664–671.
31. Chao A, Thun MJ, Jacobs EJ, Henley SJ, Rodriguez C, Calle EE. Cigarette smoking and colorectal cancer mortality in the Cancer Prevention Study II. J Natl Cancer Inst 2000;92:1888–1896.
32. Ji B-T, Weissfeld JL, Chow W-H, et al. Tobacco smoking and colorectal hyperplastic and adenomatous polyps. Cancer Epidemiol Biomarkers Prev 2006;15:897–901.
33. Collins P, Mpofu C, Watson A, Rhodes J. for detecting colon cancer and/or dysplasia in patients with inflammatory bowel disease. Cochrane Database Syst Rev 2006;(2):CD000279.
34. Calvert PM, Frucht H. The genetics of colorectal cancer. Ann Intern Med 2002;137:603–612.
35. Lynch HT, de la Chapelle A. Hereditary colorectal cancer. N Engl J Med 2003;348:919–932.
36. Chapelle ADL. Genetic predisposition to colorectal cancer. Nat Rev Cancer 2004;4:769–780.
37. Vasen HFA, Moslein G, Alonso A, et al. Guidelines for the clinical management of Lynch syndrome (hereditary non-polyposis cancer). J Med Genet 2007;44:353–362.
38. Lagerstedt Robinson K, Liu T, Vandrovcova J, et al. Lynch syndrome (hereditary nonpolyposis colorectal cancer) diagnostics. J Natl Cancer Inst 2007;99:291–299.
39. Lindor NM, Petersen GM, Hadley DW, et al. Recommendations for the care of individuals with an inherited predisposition to lynch syndrome: A systematic review. JAMA 2006;296:1507–1517.
40. Reszka E, Wasowicz W, Gromadzinska J. Genetic polymorphism of xenobiotic metabolising enzymes, diet and cancer susceptibility. Br J Nutr 2006;96:609–619.
41. Goode EL, Potter JD, Bamlet WR, Rider DN, Bigler J. Inherited variation in carcinogen-metabolizing enzymes and risk of colorectal polyps. Carcinogenesis 2007;28:328–341.
42. Robbins DH, Itzkowitz SH. The molecular and genetic basis of colon cancer. Med Clin North Am 2002;86:1467–1495.
43. Arends JW. Molecular interactions in the Vogelstein model of colorectal carcinoma. J Pathol 2000;190:412–416.
44. Italiano A. Targeting the epidermal growth factor receptor in colorectal cancer: Advances and controversies. Oncology 2006;70:161–167.
45. Skibber J, Minsky B, Hoff P. Cancer of the colon. In: DeVita V, Hellman S, Rosenberg S, eds. Cancer: Principles and Practice of Oncology, 6th ed. Philadelphia: Lippincott Williams & Wilkins, 2001:1216–1270.
46. Compton CC. Colorectal carcinoma: Diagnostic, prognostic, and molecular features. Mod Pathol 2003;16:376–388.
47. U.S. Preventive Services Task Force. Routine aspirin or nonsteroidal anti-inflammatory drugs for the primary prevention of colorectal cancer: U.S. Preventive Services Task Force Recommendation Statement. Ann Intern Med 2007;146:361–364.
48. Giardiello FM, Yang VW, Hylind LM, et al. Primary chemoprevention of familial adenomatous polyposis with sulindac. N Engl J Med 2002;346:1054–1059.
49. Bertagnolli MM, Eagle CJ, Zauber AG, et al. Celecoxib for the prevention of sporadic colorectal adenomas. N Engl J Med 2006;355:873–884.
50. Janne PA, Mayer RJ. Chemoprevention of colorectal cancer. N Engl J Med 2000;342:1960–1968.
51. Chan AT, Ogino S, Fuchs CS. Aspirin and the risk of colorectal cancer in relation to the expression of COX-2. N Engl J Med 2007;356:2131–2142.
52. Grau MV, Baron JA, Sandler RS, et al. Prolonged effect of calcium supplementation on risk of colorectal adenomas in a randomized trial. J Natl Cancer Inst 2007;99:129–136.

53. Wactawski-Wende J, Kotchen JM, Anderson GL, et al. Calcium plus vitamin D supplementation and the risk of colorectal cancer. N Engl J Med 2006;354:684–696.
54. Cole BF, Baron JA, Sandler RS, et al. Folic acid for the prevention of colorectal adenomas: A randomized clinical trial. JAMA 2007;297:2351–2359.
55. Kwak E, Chung D. Hereditary colorectal cancer syndromes: An overview. Clin Colorectal Cancer 2007;6:340–344.
56. Davila R, Rajan E, Baron T, et al. ASGE guideline: Colorectal cancer screening and surveillance. Gastrointest Endosc 2006;63:546–557.
57. Smith RA, Cokkinides V, Eyre HJ. Cancer Screening in the United States, 2007: A review of current guidelines, practices, and prospects. CA Cancer J Clin 2007;57:90–104.
58. Hewitson P, Glasziou P, Irwig L, et al. Screening for colorectal cancer using the faecal occult blood test, Hemoccult. Cochrane Database Syst Rev 2007. Issue 1. Art. No.: CD001216. DOI: 10.1002/14651858. CD001216.pub 2.
59. Walsh JME, Terdiman JP. Colorectal cancer screening: Scientific review. JAMA 2003;289:1288–1296.
60. Levin B, Brooks D, Smith RA, Stone A. Emerging technologies in screening for colorectal cancer: CT colonography, immunochemical fecal occult blood tests, and stool screening using molecular markers. CA Cancer J Clin 2003;53:44–55.
61. Imperiale TF, Ransohoff DF, Itzkowitz SH, Turnbull BA, Ross ME, the Colorectal Cancer Study G. Fecal DNA versus fecal occult blood for colorectal-cancer screening in an average-risk population. N Engl J Med 2004;351:2704–2714.
62. Locker GY, Hamilton S, Harris J, et al. ASCO 2006 update of recommendations for the use of tumor markers in gastrointestinal cancer. J Clin Oncol 2006;24:5313–5327.
63. Saunders TH, Mendes Ribeiro HK, Gleeson FV. New techniques for imaging colorectal cancer: The use of MRI, PET and radioimmunoscintigraphy for primary staging and follow-up. Br Med Bull 2002;64:81–99.
64. Pages F, Berger A, Camus M, et al. Effector memory T cells, early metastasis, and survival in colorectal cancer. N Engl J Med 2005;353:2654–2666.
65. Ribic CM, Sargent DJ, Moore MJ, et al. Tumor microsatellite-instability status as a predictor of benefit from fluorouracil-based adjuvant chemotherapy for colon cancer. N Engl J Med 2003;349:247–257.
66. Skibber J, Hoff P, Minsky B. Cancer of the rectum. In: DeVita V, Hellman S, Rosenberg S, eds. Cancer: Principles and Practice of Oncology, 6th ed. Philadelphia: Lippincott Williams & Wilkins, 2001:1271–1318.
67. Kahnamoui K, Cadeddu M, Farrokhyar F, Anvari M. Laparoscopic surgery for colon cancer: A systematic review. Can J Surg 2007;50:48–57.
68. Benson AB, III, Schrag D, Somerfield MR, et al. American Society of Clinical Oncology recommendations on adjuvant chemotherapy for stage II colon cancer. J Clin Oncol 2004;22:3408–3419.
69. Buyse M, Zeleniuch-Jacquotte A, Chalmers T. Adjuvant therapy of colorectal cancer. Why we still don't know. JAMA 1988;259:3571–3578.
70. Efficacy of adjuvant fluorouracil and folinic acid in colon cancer. International Pooled Analysis of Colon Cancer Trials (IMPACT) Investigators. Efficacy of adjuvant fluorouracil and folinic acid in colon cancer. Lancet 1995;345:939–944.
71. Haller DG, Catalano PJ, Macdonald JS, et al. Phase III study of fluorouracil, leucovorin, and levamisole in high-risk stage II and III colon cancer: Final report of Intergroup 0089. J Clin Oncol 2005;23:8671–8678.
72. Wolmark N, Rockette H, Mamounas E, et al. Clinical trial to assess the relative efficacy of fluorouracil and leucovorin, fluorouracil and levamisole, and fluorouracil, leucovorin, and levamisole in patients with Dukes' B and C carcinoma of the colon: Results from National Surgical Adjuvant Breast and Bowel Project C-04. J Clin Oncol 1999;17:3553–3559.
73. O'Connell MJ, Laurie JA, Kahn M, et al. Prospectively randomized trial of postoperative adjuvant chemotherapy in patients with high-risk colon cancer. J Clin Oncol 1998;16:295–300.
74. Meta-Analysis Group in Cancer. Toxicity of fluorouracil in patients with advanced colorectal cancer: Effect of administration schedule and prognostic factors. J Clin Oncol 1998;16:3537–3541.
75. van Kuilenburg ABP, Haasjes J, Richel DJ, et al. Clinical implications of dihydropyrimidine dehydrogenase (DPD) deficiency in patients with severe 5-fluorouracil-associated toxicity: Identification of new mutations in the DPD gene. Clin Cancer Res 2000;6:4705–4712.
76. Andre T, Boni C, Mounedji-Boudiaf L, et al. Oxaliplatin, fluorouracil, and leucovorin as adjuvant treatment for colon cancer. N Engl J Med 2004;350:2343–2351.
77. Land SR, Kopec J, Cecchini R, et al. Neurotoxicity from oxaliplatin combined with weekly bolus fluorouracil and leucovorin as surgical adjuvant chemotherapy for stage II and III colon cancer: NSABP C-07. J Clin Oncol 2007;25: 2205–2211.
78. Twelves C, Wong A, Nowacki MP, et al. Capecitabine as adjuvant treatment for Stage III colon cancer. N Engl J Med 2005;352:2696–2704.
79. Saltz LB, Niedzwiecki D, Hollis D, et al. Irinotecan fluorouracil plus leucovorin is not superior to fluorouracil plus leucovorin alone as adjuvant treatment for stage III colon cancer: results of CALGB 89803. J Clin Oncol 2007;25:3456–3461.
80. Cutsem EV, Labianca R, Hossfeld D, et al. Randomized phase III trial comparing infused irinotecan / 5-fluorouracil (5-FU)/folinic acid (IF) versus 5-FU/FA (F) in stage III colon cancer patients (pts). (PETACC 3). In: 2005 ASCO Annual Meeting Proceedings. J Clin Oncol 2005;23(Suppl 16):8.
81. Ychou M, Raoul J, Douillard J, et al. A phase III randomized trial of LV5FU2+CPT-11 vs. LV5FU2 alone in adjuvant high risk colon cancer (FNCLCC Accord02/FFCD9802). In: 2005 ASCO Annual Meeting Proceedings. J Clin Oncol 2005;23(Suppl 16):3502.
82. Baxter NN, Garcia-Aguilar J. Organ preservation for rectal cancer. J Clin Oncol 2007;25:1014–1020.
83. NIH consensus conference. Adjuvant therapy for patients with colon and rectal cancer. JAMA 1990;264:1444–1450.
84. Prolongation of the disease-free interval in surgically treated rectal carcinoma. Gastrointestinal Tumor Study Group. N Engl J Med 1985;312:1465–1472.
85. Krook JE, Moertel CG, Gunderson LL, et al. Effective surgical adjuvant therapy for high-risk rectal carcinoma. N Engl J Med 1991;324:709–715.
86. Smalley SR, Benedetti JK, Williamson SK, et al. Phase III trial of fluorouracil-based chemotherapy regimens plus radiotherapy in postoperative adjuvant rectal cancer: GI INT 0144. J Clin Oncol 2006;24:3542–3547.
87. Bosset J-F, Collette L, Calais G, et al. Chemotherapy with preoperative radiotherapy in rectal cancer. N Eng J Med 2006;355:1114–1123.
88. The NCCN Rectal Cancer Clinical Practice Guidelines in Oncology (Version 1.2007). Copyright 2007 National Comprehensive Cancer Network, Inc. 2007, *http://www.nccn.org*. To view the most recent and complete version of the guideline, go online to *www.nccn.org*.
89. Gill S, Blackstock AW, Goldberg RM. Colorectal cancer. Mayo Clin Proc 2007;82:114–129.
90. Kemeny N, Huang Y, Cohen AM, et al. Hepatic arterial infusion of chemotherapy after resection of hepatic metastases from colorectal cancer. N Engl J Med 1999;341:2039–2048.
91. Cohen AD, Kemeny NE. An update on hepatic arterial infusion chemotherapy for colorectal cancer. Oncologist 2003;8:553–566.
92. Jonker D, Maroun J, Kocha W. Survival benefit of chemotherapy in metastatic colorectal cancer: A meta-analysis of randomized controlled trials. Br J Cancer 2000;82:1789–1794.
93. Colorectal Cancer Collaborative G. Palliative chemotherapy for advanced colorectal cancer: Systematic review and meta-analysis. BMJ 2000;321:531–535.
94. Sobrero AF, Aschele C, Bertino JR. Fluorouracil in colorectal cancer—A tale of two drugs: Implications for biochemical modulation. J Clin Oncol 1997;15:368–381.
95. Efficacy of intravenous continuous infusion of fluorouracil compared with bolus administration in advanced colorectal cancer. Meta-Analysis Group in Cancer. J Clin Oncol 1998;16:301–308.
96. Buroker TR, O'Connell MJ, Wieand HS, et al. Randomized comparison of two schedules of fluorouracil and leucovorin in the treatment of advanced colorectal cancer. J Clin Oncol 1994;12:14–20.
97. de Gramont A, Bosset JF, Milan C, et al. Randomized trial comparing monthly low-dose leucovorin and fluorouracil bolus with bimonthly high-dose leucovorin and fluorouracil bolus plus continuous infusion for advanced colorectal cancer: A French intergroup study. J Clin Oncol 1997;15:808–815.
98. Kohne CH, Wils J, Lorenz M, et al. Randomized phase III study of high-dose fluorouracil given as a weekly 24-hour infusion with or without leucovorin versus bolus fluorouracil plus leucovorin in advanced colorectal cancer: European Organization of Research and Treatment of

Cancer Gastrointestinal Group Study 40952. J Clin Oncol 2003;21:3721–3728.

99. Douillard J, Cunningham D, Roth A, et al. Irinotecan combined with fluorouracil compared with fluorouracil alone as first-line treatment for metastatic colorectal cancer: A multicentre randomised trial. Lancet 2000;355:1041–1047.
100. Saltz LB, Cox JV, Blanke C, et al. Irinotecan plus fluorouracil and leucovorin for metastatic colorectal cancer. N Engl J Med 2000;343:905–914.
101. O'Dwyer PJ, Catalano RB. Uridine diphosphate glucuronosyltransferase (UGT) 1A1 and irinotecan: Practical pharmacogenomics arrives in cancer therapy. J Clin Oncol 2006;24:4534–4538.
102. Raymond E, Faivre S, Chaney S, Woynarowski J, Cvitkovic E. Cellular and molecular pharmacology of oxaliplatin. Mol Cancer Ther 2002;1:227–235.
103. Goldberg RM, Sargent DJ, Morton RF, et al. A randomized controlled trial of fluorouracil plus leucovorin, irinotecan, and oxaliplatin combinations in patients with previously untreated metastatic colorectal cancer. J Clin Oncol 2004;22:23–30.
104. Tournigand C, Andre T, Achille E, et al. FOLFIRI Followed by FOLFOX6 or the reverse sequence in advanced colorectal cancer: A randomized GERCOR Study. J Clin Oncol 2004;22:229–237.
105. Grothey A. Oxaliplatin-safety profile: Neurotoxicity. Semin Oncol 2003;30:5–13.
106. Twelves C. Capecitabine as first-line treatment in colorectal cancer. Eur J Cancer 2002;38:15–20.
107. Hurwitz H, Fehrenbacher L, Novotny W, et al. Bevacizumab plus irinotecan, fluorouracil, and leucovorin for metastatic colorectal cancer. N Engl J Med 2004;350:2335–2342.
108. Hochster HS, Hart LL, Ramanathan RK, Hainsworth JD, Hedrick EE, Childs BH. Safety and efficacy of oxaliplatin/fluoropyrimidine regimens with or without bevacizumab as first-line treatment of metastatic colorectal cancer (mCRC): Final analysis of the TREE-Study. In: 2006 ASCO Annual Meeting Proceedings. J Clin Oncol 2006;24(Suppl 18):3510.
109. Saltz L, Clark S, Diaz-Rubio E, et al. Bevacizumab (Bev) in combination with XELOX or FOLFOX4: Updated efficacy results from XELOX-1/ NO16966 a randomized phase III trial in first-line metastatic colorectal cancer. In: 2007 ASCO Annual Meeting Proceedings. J Clin Oncol 2007;25(Suppl 18):4028.
110. Venook A, Niedzwiecki D, Hollis D, et al. Phase III study of irinotecan/ 5FU/LV (FOLFIRI) or oxaliplatin/5FU/LV (FOLFOX) ± cetuximab for patients (pts) with untreated metastatic adenocarcinoma of the colon or rectum (MCRC): CALGB 80203 preliminary results. In: 2006 ASCO Annual Meeting Proceedings. J Clin Oncol 2006;24(Suppl 18):3509.
111. Hecht J, Posey J, Tchekmedyian S, et al. Panitumumab in combination with 5-fluorouracil, leucovorin, and irinotecan (IFL) or FOLFIRI for first-line treatment of metastatic colorectal cancer (mCRC). In: 2006 ASCO Gastrointestinal Cancers Symposium, 2006, Abstract 237.
112. Kemeny NE, Niedzwiecki D, Hollis DR, et al. Hepatic arterial infusion versus systemic therapy for hepatic metastases from colorectal cancer: A randomized trial of efficacy, quality of life, and molecular markers (CALGB 9481). J Clin Oncol 2006;24:1395–1403.
113. Grothey A, Sargent D. Overall survival of patients with advanced colorectal cancer correlates with availability of fluorouracil, irinotecan, and oxaliplatin regardless of whether doublet or single-agent therapy is used first line. J Clin Oncol 2005;23:9441–9442.
114. The NCCN Colon Cancer Clinical Practice Guidelines in Oncology (Version 2.2007). Copyright 2007 National Comprehensive Cancer Network, Inc. 2007, *http://www.nccn.org*. To view the most recent and complete version of the guideline, go online to *www.nccn.org*.
115. Díaz-Rubio E, Tabernero J, Gómez-España A, et al. Phase III trial of capecitabine and oxaliplatin (XELOX) vs. continuous infusion 5-fluorouracil plus oxaliplatin (FUFOX) as first-line therapy in metastatic colorectal cancer: Final report of the Spanish TTD group trial. J Clin Oncol 2007;25:4224–4230.
116. Cunningham D, Pyrhönen S, James R, et al. Randomised trial of irinotecan plus supportive care versus supportive care alone after fluorouracil failure for patients with metastatic colorectal cancer. Lancet 1998;352:1413–1418.
117. Rougier P, Van Cutsem E, Bajetta E, et al. Randomised trial of irinotecan versus fluorouracil by continuous infusion after fluorouracil failure in patients with metastatic colorectal cancer. Lancet 1998;352:1407–1412.
118. Andre T, Bensmaine MA, Louvet C, et al. Multicenter phase II study of bimonthly high-dose leucovorin, fluorouracil infusion, and oxaliplatin for metastatic colorectal cancer resistant to the same leucovorin and fluorouracil regimen. J Clin Oncol 1999;17:3560–3568.
119. Kouroussis C, Souglakos J, Mavroudis D, et al. Oxaliplatin with high-dose leucovorin and infusional 5-fluorouracil in irinotecan-pretreated patients with advanced colorectal cancer (ACC). Am J Clin Oncol 2002;25:627–631.
120. Giantonio BJ, Catalano PJ, Meropol NJ, et al. Bevacizumab in combination with oxaliplatin, fluorouracil, and leucovorin (FOLFOX4) for previously treated metastatic colorectal cancer: Results from the Eastern Cooperative Oncology Group Study E3200. J Clin Oncol 2007;25:1539–1544.
121. Saltz LB, Meropol NJ, Loehrer PJ Sr, Needle MN, Kopit J, Mayer RJ. Phase II trial of cetuximab in patients with refractory colorectal cancer that expresses the epidermal growth factor receptor. J Clin Oncol 2004;22:1201–1208.
122. Cunningham D, Humblet Y, Siena S, et al. Cetuximab monotherapy and cetuximab plus irinotecan in irinotecan-refractory metastatic colorectal cancer. N Engl J Med 2004;351:337–345.
123. Saadeh CE, Lee HS. Panitumumab: A fully human monoclonal antibody with activity in metastatic colorectal cancer. Ann Pharmacother 2007;41:606–613.
124. Chung KY, Shia J, Kemeny NE, et al. Cetuximab shows activity in colorectal cancer patients with tumors that do not express the epidermal growth factor receptor by immunohistochemistry. J Clin Oncol 2005;23:1803–1810.
125. Tournigand C, Cervantes A, Figer A, et al. OPTIMOX1: A randomized study of FOLFOX4 or FOLFOX7 with oxaliplatin in a stop-and-go fashion in advanced colorectal cancer—A GERCOR study. J Clin Oncol 2006;24:394–400.
126. Dick EA, Taylor-Robinson SD, Thomas HC, Gedroyc WMW. Ablative therapy for liver tumours. Gut 2002;50:733–739.
127. Fraker D, M S. Regional therapy of hepatic metastases. Hematol Oncol Clin North Am 2002;16:947–967.
128. Marsh S. Pharmacogenetics of colorectal cancer. Expert Opin Pharmacother 2005;6:2607–2616.
129. Ruzzo A, Graziano F, Loupakis F, et al. Pharmacogenetic profiling in patients with advanced colorectal cancer treated with first-line FOLFOX-4 chemotherapy. J Clin Oncol 2007;25:1247–1254.
130. Del Rio M, Molina F, Bascoul-Mollevi C, et al. Gene expression signature in advanced colorectal cancer patients select drugs and response for the use of leucovorin, fluorouracil, and irinotecan. J Clin Oncol 2007;25:773–780.
131. Jansman FGA, Postma M, Brouwers JRBJ. Cost considerations in the treatment of colorectal cancer. Pharmacoeconomics 2007;25:537–562.
132. Krol M, Koopman M, Uyl-de Groot C, Punt CJA. A systematic review of economic analyses of pharmaceutical therapies for advanced colorectal cancer. Expert Opin Pharmacother 2007;8:1313–1328.
133. Aballea S, Chancellor JVM, Raikou M, et al. Cost-effectiveness analysis of oxaliplatin compared with 5-fluouracil/leucovorin in adjuvant treatment of stage III colon cancer in the US. Cancer 2007;109:1082–1089.
134. Twelves C. Xeloda in Adjuvant Colon Cancer Therapy (X-ACT) trial: Overview of efficacy, safety, and cost-effectiveness. Clin Colorectal Cancer 2006;6:278–287.
135. Maciosek MV, Solberg LI, Coffield AB, Edwards NM, Goodman MJ. Colorectal cancer screening: Health impact and cost effectiveness. Am J Prev Med 2006;31:80–89.
136. Desch CE, Benson AB, III, Somerfield MR, et al. Colorectal cancer surveillance: 2005 update of an American Society of Clinical Oncology practice guideline. J Clin Oncol 2005;23:8512–8519.
137. Houlston RS, Tomlinson IPM. Polymorphisms and colorectal tumor risk. Gastroenterology 2001;121:282–301.
138. Hawk ET, Levin B. Colorectal cancer prevention. J Clin Oncol 2005;23:378–391.
139. Smith RA, Cokkinides V, Eyre HJ. American Cancer Society Guidelines for the early detection of cancer, 2003. CA Cancer J Clin 2003;53:27–43.
140. Rex DK, Kahi CJ, Levin B, et al. Guidelines for colonoscopy surveillance after cancer resection: A Consensus update by the American Cancer Society and US Multi-Society Task Force on Colorectal Cancer. CA Cancer J Clin 2006;56:160–167.

141. Winawer SJ, Zauber AG, Fletcher RH, et al. Guidelines for Colonoscopy Surveillance after Polypectomy: A Consensus Update by the US Multi-Society Task Force on Colorectal Cancer and the American Cancer Society. CA Cancer J Clin 2006;56:143–159.
142. Colon and rectum. In: Greene Page DL, Fleming ID, et al., eds.: American Joint Committee on Cancer. AJCC Cancer Staging Manual, 6th ed. New York, NY: Springer, 2002, pp 113–124.
143. O'Connell JB, Maggard MA, Ko CY. Colon cancer survival rates with the new American Joint Committee on Cancer sixth edition staging. J Natl Cancer Inst 2004;96:1420–1425.
144. Kuebler JP, Wieand HS, O'Connell MJ, et al. Oxaliplatin combined with weekly bolus fluorouracil and leucovorin as surgical adjuvant chemotherapy for stage II and III colon cancer: Results from NSABP C-07. J Clin Oncol 2007;25:2198–2204.
145. Wolmark N, Rockette H, Fisher B, et al. The benefit of leucovorin-modulated fluorouracil as postoperative adjuvant therapy for primary colon cancer: Results from National Surgical Adjuvant Breast and Bowel Project protocol C-03. J Clin Oncol 1993;11:1 879–1887.
146. O'Connell MJ, Mailliard JA, Kahn MJ, et al. Controlled trial of fluorouracil and low-dose leucovorin given for 6 months as postoperative adjuvant therapy for colon cancer. J Clin Oncol 1997;15:246–250.
147. de Gramont A, Figer A, Seymour M, et al. Leucovorin and fluorouracil with or without oxaliplatin as first-line treatment in advanced colorectal cancer. J Clin Oncol 2000;18:2938–2947.
148. Grothey A, Jordan K, Kellner O, et al. Capecitabine/irinotecan (CapIri) and capecitabine/oxaliplatin (CapOx) are active second-line protocols in patients with advanced colorectal cancer (ACRC) after failure of first-line combination therapy: Results of a randomized phase II study. J Clin Oncol 2004;22(14S)(Suppl):3534.
149. Van Cutsem E, Peeters M, Siena S, et al. Open-label phase III trial of panitumumab plus best supportive care compared with best supportive care alone in patients with chemotherapy-refractory metastatic colorectal cancer. J Clin Oncol 2007;25:1658–1664.
150. Jonker DJ, O'Callaghan CJ, Karapetis CS, et al. Cetuximab for the treatment of colorectal cancer. N Engl J Med 2007; 357:2040-2048.

CHAPTER 134 Prostate Cancer

JILL M. KOLESAR

KEY CONCEPTS

1. Prostate cancer is the most frequent cancer in American men. African American ancestry, family history, and increased age are the primary risk factors for prostate cancer.
2. Prostate-specific antigen is a useful marker for detecting prostate cancer at early stages, predicting outcome for localized disease, defining disease-free status, and monitoring response to androgen-deprivation therapy or chemotherapy for advanced-stage disease.
3. The prognosis for prostate cancer patients depends on the histologic grade, the tumor size, and disease stage. More than 85% of patients with stage A_1 disease but less than 1% of those with stage D_2 disease can be cured.
4. Androgen ablation therapy, with orchiectomy, a luteinizing hormone-releasing hormone (LHRH) agonist alone or a LHRH agonist plus an antiandrogen (combined hormonal blockade), can be used to provide palliation for patients with advanced (stage D_2) prostate cancer. The effects of androgen deprivation are most pronounced in patients with minimal disease at diagnosis.
5. Antiandrogen withdrawal, for patients with progressive disease while receiving combined hormonal blockade with an LHRH agonist plus an antiandrogen, can provide additional symptomatic relief. Mutations in the androgen receptor can cause antiandrogen compounds to act like receptor agonists.
6. Androgen ablation with a LHRH agonist plus an antiandrogen should be used prior to radiation therapy for patients with locally advanced prostate cancer to improve outcomes over radiation therapy alone.
7. Chemotherapy with docetaxel and prednisone improves survival in patients with hormone-refractory prostate cancer. Patients with hormone-refractory prostate cancer should be considered for entry into clinical trials investigating new therapies for prostate cancer.

Prostate cancer is the most commonly diagnosed cancer in American men.[1] Most men with prostate cancer have an indolent course and treatment options for early disease include expectant management, surgery, and radiation. With expectant management, patients are monitored for disease progression or development of symptoms. Localized prostate cancer can be cured by surgery or radiation therapy, but advanced prostate cancer is not yet curable. Treatment for advanced prostate cancer can provide significant disease palliation for many patients for several years after diagnosis. The endocrine dependence of this tumor is well documented, and hormonal manipulation to decrease circulating androgens remains the basis for the treatment of advanced disease.

EPIDEMIOLOGY

1 In the United States, it is estimated that 218,890 new cases of prostatic carcinoma will be diagnosed and more than 27,050 men will die from this disease in 2007.[1] Between 2000 and 2004 the median age at prostate cancer diagnosis was 68 years and the median age at death caused by prostate cancer was 80 years.[2] Both prostate cancer incidence and mortality vary with ethnicity. The incidence for all races in the United States is 168 cases diagnosed per 100,000 men. Blacks are at higher than average risk of prostate cancer with an incidence of 256 per 100,000, whereas individuals of Asian and Native American descent are at lower risk with 97 cases per 100,000 and 62 per 100,000, respectively. Whites and Hispanics are at intermediate risk with 161 and 142 cases per 100,000 men, respectively. The number of deaths caused by prostate cancer for all races in the United State is 28 deaths per 100,000 men. Blacks are at the highest risk of prostate cancer death, with a cancer death rate of 62 per 100,000 men, as compared to individuals of Native American descent (22 per 100,000), whites (26 per 100,000), Hispanics (21 per 100,000), and individuals of Asian descent (11 per 100,000 men). Although prostate cancer incidence increased during the late 1980s and early 1990s because of widespread prostate-specific antigen (PSA) screening, deaths from prostate cancer have been continuously declining since 1995.[1]

ETIOLOGY

Table 134–1 summarizes the possible factors associated with prostate cancer.[3,4] The only widely accepted risk factors for prostate cancer are age, race-ethnicity, and family history of prostate cancer.[3,4] The disease is rare in persons younger than 40 years, but the incidence sharply increases with each subsequent decade, most likely because the individual has had a lifetime exposure to testosterone, a known growth signal for the prostate.[4]

RACE AND ETHNICITY

The incidence of prostate cancer varies across geographic regions. Scandinavian countries and the United States report the highest incidence of prostate cancer, whereas the disease is relatively rare in Japan and other Asian countries.[5] African American men have the

TABLE 134-1 Risk Factors Associated with Prostate Cancer

Factor	Possible relationship
Probable risk factors	
Age	More than 70% of cases are diagnosed in men older than 65 years
Race	African Americans have higher incidence and death rate
Genetic	Familial prostate cancer inherited in an autosomal dominant manner
	Polymorphisms in the CAG repeat in the androgen receptor (AR) gene, CYP17, SRDA2, MSR1, a deletion of the GSTT1 gene
Possible risk factors	
Environmental	Clinical carcinoma incidence varies worldwide
	Latent carcinoma similar between regions. Nationalized males adopt intermediate incidence rates between that of the United States and their native country
Occupational	Increased risk associated with cadmium exposure
Diet	Increased risk associated with high-meat and high-fat diets
	Decreased intake of 1,25-dihydroxyvitamin D, vitamin E, lycopene, and β-carotene increases risk
Hormonal	Does not occur in eunuchs
	Low incidence in cirrhotic patients. Up to 80% are hormonally dependent. African Americans have 15% increased testosterone
	Japanese have decreased 5 α-reductase activities
	Polymorphic expression of the androgen receptor

Compiled from references 2, 4, 5, 6.

highest rate of prostate cancer in the world, and prostate cancer mortality in African Americans is more than twice that seen in white populations in the United States.[2] Hormonal, dietary, and genetic differences, and differences in access to healthcare may contribute to the altered susceptibility to prostate cancer in these populations.[3,4] Testosterone, commonly implicated in the pathogenesis of prostate cancer, is 15% higher in African American men as compared with white males. Activity of 5α-reductase, the enzyme that converts testosterone to its more active form, dihydrotestosterone (DHT), in the prostate, is decreased in Japanese men as compared with African Americans and whites.[3,4] In addition, genetic variations in the androgen receptor exist. Activation of the androgen receptor is inversely correlated with CAG repeat length. Shorter CAG repeat sequences have been found in African Americans. Therefore the combination of increased testosterone and increased androgen receptor activation may account for the increased risk of prostate cancer for African American men.[3,4] The Asian diet generally is considered to be low in fat and high in fiber with a high concentration of phytoestrogens, potentially explaining their decreased risk.[5,6]

FAMILY HISTORY

A familial clustering of prostate cancer is observed and a recent comprehensive linkage analysis of 54 pedigrees identified a region at chromosome 22q12.3 comprised of 11 possible genes likely to be associated with hereditary prostate cancer.[7]

An alternative explanation for the familial clustering may be polymorphisms in genes important for prostate cancer function and development.[6] Candidate polymorphisms include a polymorphism in the androgen receptor, which has two different nucleotide repeat variants, the CAG and the GCC. The CAG repeat varies in repeat number from 11 to 31 repeats in healthy individuals, and the number of repeats is inversely proportional to the activity of the androgen receptor. Some studies show that shorter CAG repeats are associated with increased prostate cancer risk. Another candidate polymorphism is SRD5A2, which is the gene that codes for 5α-reductase, the enzyme that converts testosterone to the more active DHT. A variant in SRD5A2, the Ala49Thr, increases the activity and may increase prostate cancer risk.[6]

A large study performed in the CAPS (Cancer Prostate in Sweden) population, including more than 1,200 subjects with prostate cancer, evaluated a number of polymorphisms previously reported to be associated with prostate cancer risk. Six polymorphisms located in five different genes were significantly associated with risk of prostate cancer, three polymorphisms were in the androgen biosynthesis and response pathway including the CAG repeat in the androgen receptor (AR) gene ($p = 0.03$), one SNP in the CYP17 gene ($p = 0.04$), two SNPs in the SRD5A2 gene ($p = 0.02$ and 0.02, respectively), a deletion of the GSTT1 gene ($p = 0.006$), and one SNP in the MSR1 gene, IVS5–59C > A ($p = 0.009$).[8]

DIET

A number of epidemiologic studies support an association between high fat intake and risk of prostate cancer. A strong correlation between national per capita fat consumption and prostate cancer mortality has been reported, and prospective case-control studies suggest that a high-fat diet is associated with a two-fold higher risk of prostate cancer.[9]

Other dietary factors implicated in prostate cancer include retinol, carotenoids, lycopene, and vitamin D consumption.[6] Retinol, or vitamin A, intake, especially in men older than age 70 years, is associated with an increased risk of prostate cancer, whereas intake of its precursor, β-carotene, has a protective or neutral effect. Lycopene, obtained primarily from tomatoes, decreases the risk of prostate cancer in small cohort studies. The antioxidant vitamin E also may decrease the risk of prostate cancer. Men who developed prostate cancer in one cohort study had lower levels of 1,25$(OH)_2$-vitamin D than did matched controls, although a prospective study did not confirm this finding. Dietary intervention may be promising in prostate cancer prevention.

OTHER FACTORS

Benign prostatic hyperplasia (BPH) is a common problem of elderly men, affecting more than 40% of men older than age 70 years. BPH results in the urinary symptoms of hesitancy and frequency. Since prostate cancer affects a similar age group and often has similar presenting symptoms, the presence of BPH often complicates the diagnosis of prostate cancer, although it does not appear to increase the risk of developing prostate cancer.[3,10]

Smoking has not been associated with an increased risk of prostate cancer, but smokers with prostate cancer have an increased mortality resulting from the disease when compared with nonsmokers with prostate cancer (relative risk 1.5 to 2), suggesting that although smokers are not more likely to develop prostate cancer, they are at increased risk of death as a consequence of other smoking-related illnesses.[3] In a prospective cohort study, alcohol consumption was not associated with the development of prostate cancer.

CHEMOPREVENTION

Currently, the most promising agent for the prevention of prostate cancer is finasteride, a 5α-reductase inhibitor used for benign prostatic hypertrophy.[10] When compared to placebo, the point prevalence of prostate cancer was reduced for those on finasteride by 25% (95% confidence interval [CI] 18.6 to 30.6%, hazard ratio = 0.75). However, patients in the finasteride group who developed prostate cancer had more high-grade (Gleason grade 7 to 10) tumors than those in the placebo group. Overall, finasteride did reduce the risk of prostate cancer, but the prostate cancers that were diagnosed in the finasteride group were more aggressive. Consequently, the use of finasteride to prevent prostate cancer is controversial.[11] Because of its established role in the treatment of BPH, the 20% to 30% of men older than age 50 years with BPH may derive the additional benefit of prostate cancer prevention and should be offered treatment with finasteride. In the 70% to 80% of men without BPH, the benefits, side effects (primarily impotence), and risks of finasteride should be discussed prior to initiating therapy.

Other agents, including selenium, a naturally occurring trace element that is essential in the human diet, vitamin E, vitamin D, lycopene, green tea, nonsteroidal antiinflammatory agents, isoflavones, and statins are being investigated for prevention of prostate cancer. Although the results of these studies are promising, none are currently recommended for routine use outside of a clinical trial.[12]

SCREENING

Early detection of potentially curable prostate cancers is the goal of prostate cancer screening. For cancer screening to be beneficial, it must reliably detect cancer at an early stage, when intervention would decrease mortality. Whether prostate cancer screening fits these criteria has generated considerable controversy.[13]

The common approach to prostate cancer screening, as recommended by the American Cancer Society, is to offer a baseline PSA and digital rectal examination (DRE) beginning at age 50 years to all men of normal risk with a 10-year or greater life expectancy.[14] Men at high risk (African American men and men with a strong family of one or more first-degree relatives), should begin testing at age 45 years. Men at even higher risk, secondary to multiple first-degree relatives affected at an early age, could begin testing at age 40 years. Routine screening of all men is not recommended. Providers should describe the potential benefits and known risks of screening, diagnosis, and treatment, listen to the patient's concerns, and then decide with the patient on an individual's screening method.

The recommendation to *consider*, rather than perform, prostate cancer screening is based on the still unproven benefits of prostate cancer screening. A recent Cochrane review identified only two completed randomized clinical trials comparing prostate cancer screening to no intervention.[15] A meta-analysis of the data from these studies indicated that men randomized to screening had prostate cancer detected more often, but did not have a reduction in prostate cancer specific mortality (relative risk 1.01, 95% CI 0.80 to 1.29). Neither study assessed the effect of prostate cancer screening on quality of life, all-cause mortality, or cost-effectiveness. Because PSA measurements can identify small, subclinical prostate cancers, where no intervention may be required, detecting prostate cancer in those not needing therapy not only increases the cost of care through unnecessary screening and workups, but also increases the toxicity of therapy, by subjecting some patients to unnecessary therapy.[16] The ongoing Prostate, Lung, Colon, and Ovarian (PLCO) screening trial is designed to determine if prostate cancer screening is effective in reducing prostate cancer mortality and the results of that trial will help resolve this controversy.[17]

The DRE has been recommended since the early 1900s for the detection of prostate cancer. The primary advantage of DRE is its specificity, reported at greater than 85%, for prostate cancer. Other advantages of DRE include low cost, safety, and ease of performance. However, DRE is relatively insensitive and is subject to interobserver variability. DRE as a single screening method has poor compliance and had little effect on preventing metastatic prostate cancer in one large case-control study.[18]

❷ PSA is a glycoprotein produced and secreted by the epithelial cells of the prostate gland. The physiologic function of PSA is to liquefy ejaculate and it is primarily confined to the seminal plasma, although it is also measurable in the plasma.[19] PSA exists as a complex with the proteases α_1-antichymotrypsin, α_1-antitrypsin and α_2-macroglobulin. Several different assays, measuring free (i.e., unbound) PSA and complexed PSA (PSA bound to α_1-antichymotrypsin) are available.

Total PSA measurements are used widely for prostate cancer screening in the United States.[19] The normal range for total PSA is ≤4 ng/mL and this cut-off is primarily based on a prospective study by Gann et al., which demonstrated that a single PSA level >4 ng/mL had a sensitivity of 73%, with a specificity of 91% in detecting prostate cancer within 4 years.[20] The complexed PSA test may also be used for PSA testing (upper level of normal range is 3.4 ng/mL).[21]

PSA may be decreased by approximately 50% after 6 to 12 months of treatment with finasteride, dutasteride and androgen receptor blockers.[22] When assessing a PSA value in men on these medications, the clinician should double the actual value. Because both ejaculation and DRE can influence PSA levels, the PSA level should be drawn prior to the DRE and patients should be advised to abstain from ejaculation for 48 hours prior to PSA measurement. Additionally, PSA is influenced by acute urinary retention, acute prostatitis, and prostatic ischemia or infarction, as well as BPH, a nearly universal condition in men who are at risk for prostate cancer. PSA elevations between 4 and 10 ng/mL cannot distinguish between BPH and prostate cancer, which limits the usefulness of PSA alone for the early detection of prostate cancer. The free PSA test is used in men with a total PSA ranging between 4 and 10 ng/mL; those with a free PSA percentage of <15% are more likely to have prostate cancer and should have a biopsy, whereas those in this range with a free PSA >25% are most likely have BPH and may not require a biopsy. Individuals with a free PSA between 15% and 25% may have a biopsy or be watched further, depending on other clinical characteristics, such as age.[23]

PSA velocity, or the rate of change in PSA levels over time, may be another predictor of prostate cancer risk.[24] In a recent report, men with an initial PSA of <4 ng/mL but with a PSA velocity >0.35 ng/mL per year had a higher relative risk of prostate cancer death as compared to men with a PSA velocity of ≤0.35 ng/mL per year (relative risk 4.7, 95% CI 1.3 to 16.5; $p = 0.02$).[25] Based on these results, some experts recommend further workup for individuals with a PSA less than 4 ng/mL, if their PSA velocity is >0.35 ng/mL per year.

PATHOPHYSIOLOGY

The prostate gland is a solid, rounded, heart-shaped organ positioned between the neck of the bladder and the urogenital diaphragm (Fig. 134–1). Normal growth and differentiation of the prostate depends on the presence of androgens, specifically DHT.[26,27] The testes and the adrenal glands are the major sources of circulating androgens. Hormonal regulation of androgen synthesis is mediated through a series of biochemical interactions between the hypothalamus, pituitary, adrenal glands, and testes (Fig. 134–2). Luteinizing hormone-releasing hormone (LHRH) released from the hypothalamus stimulates the release of luteinizing hormone (LH) and follicle-stimulating hormone (FSH) from the anterior pituitary gland. LH complexes with receptors on the Leydig cell testicular membrane and stimulates the production of testosterone and small amounts of estrogen. FSH acts on the Sertoli cells within the testes to promote the maturation of LH receptors and to produce an androgen-binding protein. Circulating testosterone and estradiol influence the synthesis of LHRH, LH, and FSH by a negative feedback loop operating at the hypothalamic and pituitary level.[27–29] Prolactin, growth hormone, and estradiol appear to be important accessory regulators for prostatic tissue permeability, receptor binding, and testosterone synthesis.

Testosterone, the major androgenic hormone, accounts for 95% of the androgen concentration. Although the primary source of testosterone is the testes, 3% to 5% of the testosterone concentra-

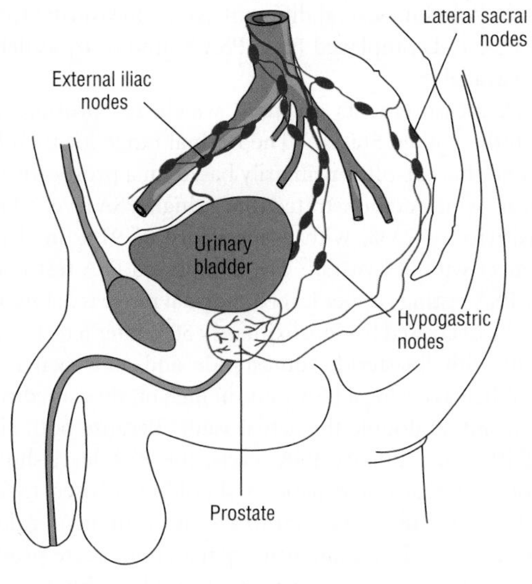

FIGURE 134-1. The prostate gland.

TABLE 134-2 Hormonal Manipulations in Prostate Cancer	
Androgen source ablation	Antiandrogens
Orchiectomy	Flutamide
Adrenalectomy	Bicalutamide
Hypophysectomy	Nilutamide
LHRH or LH inhibition	Cyproterone acetate[b]
Estrogens	Progesterones
LHRH agonists	5α-Reductase inhibition
Progesterones[a]	Finasteride[b]
Cyproterone acetate[b]	
Androgen synthesis inhibition	
Aminoglutethimide	
Ketoconazole	
Progesterones[a]	

LH, luteinizing hormone; LHRH, luteinizing hormone-releasing hormone.
[a]Minor mechanisms of action.
[b]Investigational compounds or uses.

tion is derived from direct adrenal cortical secretion of testosterone or C19 steroids such as androstenedione.[26,27,30]

Hormonal manipulations to ablate or reduce circulating androgens can occur through several mechanisms (Table 134–2).[26,27] The organs responsible for androgen production can be removed surgically (orchiectomy, hypophysectomy, or adrenalectomy). Hormonal pathways that modulate prostatic growth can be interrupted at several steps (see Fig. 134–2). Interference with LHRH or LH can reduce testosterone secretion by the testes (estrogens, LHRH agonists, progestogens, and cyproterone acetate). Estrogen administration reduces androgens by directly inhibiting LH release, by acting directly on the prostate cell, or by decreasing free androgens by increasing steroid-binding globulin levels.[26,27,30]

Isolation of the naturally occurring hypothalamic decapeptide hormone LHRH has provided another group of effective agents for advanced prostate cancer treatment.[28] The physiologic response to LHRH depends on both the dose and the mode of administration. Intermittent pulsed LHRH administration, which mimics the endogenous release pattern, causes sustained release of both LH and FSH, whereas high-dose or continuous intravenous administration of LHRH inhibits gonadotropin release caused by receptor downregulation.[27] Structural modification of the naturally occurring LHRH and innovative delivery have produced a series of LHRH agonists that cause a similar downregulation of pituitary receptors and a decrease in testosterone production.[29]

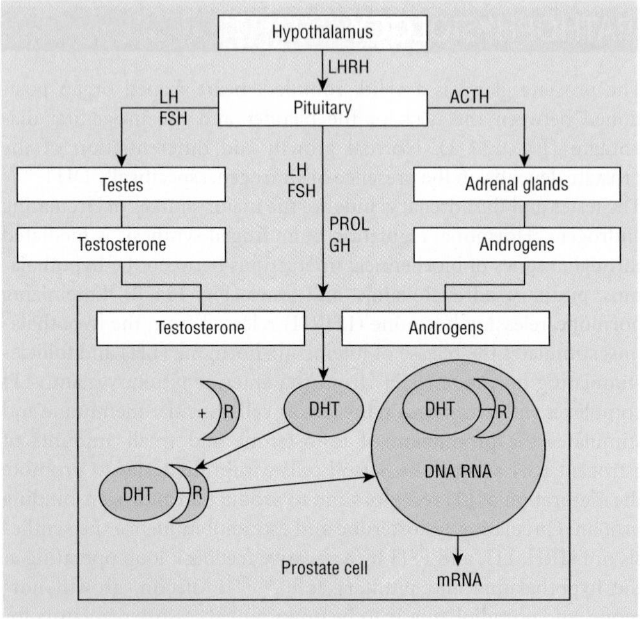

FIGURE 134-2. Hormonal regulation of the prostate gland. (A, androgen; ACTH, adrenocorticotropic hormone; DHT, dihydrotestosterone; FSH, follicle-stimulating hormone; GH, growth hormone; LH, luteinizing hormone; LHRH, luteinizing hormone-releasing hormone; mRNA, messenger ribonucleic acid; PROL, prolactin; R, receptor; T, testosterone.)

Androgen synthesis can be inhibited in the testes or in the adrenal gland. Aminoglutethimide inhibits the desmolase-enzyme complex in the adrenal gland, thereby preventing the conversion of cholesterol to pregnenolone. Pregnenolone is the precursor substrate for all adrenal-derived steroids, including androgens, glucocorticoids, and mineralocorticoids.[29] Ketoconazole, an imidazole antifungal agent, causes a dose-related reversible reduction in serum cortisol and testosterone concentration by inhibiting both adrenal and testicular steroidogenesis.[29,30] As a secondary mechanism to its antiandrogen action, megestrol acetate inhibits the synthesis of androgens. This inhibition appears to occur at the adrenal level, but circulating levels of testosterone also are reduced, which suggests that inhibition at the testicular level also may occur.[29,30]

Antiandrogens inhibit the formation of the DHT-receptor complex and thereby interfere with androgen-mediated action at the cellular level.[30] Megestrol acetate, a progestational agent, also is available and has antiandrogen actions.[30] Finally, the conversion of testosterone to DHT may be inhibited by 5α-reductase inhibitors.[10]

PATHOLOGY

The normal prostate is composed of acinar secretory cells arranged in a radial shape and surrounded by a foundation of supporting tissue. The size, shape, or presence of acini is almost always altered in the gland that has been invaded by prostatic carcinoma. Adenocarcinoma, the major pathologic cell type, accounts for more than 95% of prostate cancer cases.[22,31] Rare tumor types include small cell neuroendocrine cancers, sarcomas, and transitional cell carcinomas.

Prostate cancer can be graded systematically according to the histologic appearance of the malignant cell and then grouped into well, moderately, or poorly differentiated grades.[31,32] Gland architecture is examined and then rated on a scale of 1 (well differentiated) to 5 (poorly differentiated). Two different specimens are examined, and the score for each specimen is added. Groupings for total Gleason score are 2 to 4 for well-differentiated, 5 or 6 for moderately differentiated, and 7 to 10 for poorly differentiated tumors. Poorly differentiated tumors grow rapidly (poor prognosis), whereas well-differentiated tumors grow slowly (better prognosis).

Metastatic spread can occur by local extension, lymphatic drainage, or hematogenous dissemination.[26,32] Lymph node metastases are more common in patients with large, undifferentiated tumors that invade the seminal vesicles. The pelvic and abdominal lymph node groups are the most common sites of lymph node involvement (see Fig. 134–1). Skeletal metastases from hematogenous spread are the most common sites of distant spread. The bone lesions are usually osteoblastic or a combination of osteoblastic and osteolytic. The most common site of bone involvement is the lumbar spine. Other sites of bone involvement include the proximal femurs, pelvis, thoracic spine, ribs, sternum, skull, and humerus. The lung, liver, brain, and adrenal glands are the most common sites of visceral involvement, although these organs are usually not involved initially. Approximately 25% to 35% of patients will have evidence of lymphangitic or nodular pulmonary infiltrates at autopsy. The prostate is a rare site for metastatic involvement from other solid tumors.

CLINICAL PRESENTATION

Localized Disease

- Asymptomatic

Locally Invasive Disease

- Ureteral dysfunction, frequency, hesitancy, and dribbling
- Impotence

Advanced Disease

- Back pain
- Cord compression
- Lower-extremity edema
- Pathologic fractures
- Anemia
- Weight loss

The information obtained from the diagnostic tests is used to stage the patient. There are two commonly recognized staging classification systems (Table 134–3). The formal international classification system (tumor, node, metastases [TNM]), adopted by the International Union Against Cancer in 1974, was updated in 1992 in an effort to provide congruence with the classical American Urologic System staging system for prostate cancer.[33] The American Urologic System classification is the most commonly used staging system in the United States (Table 134–3). Patients are assigned to stages A through D and corresponding subcategories based on size of the tumor (T), local or regional extension, presence of involved lymph node groups (N), and presence of metastases (M).[33] Based on men diagnosed with prostate cancer at Walter Reed Army Medical Center from 1988 to 1998, which included more than 2,042 prostate cancer diagnoses, localized prostate cancer (stage T_1 and T_2) was diagnosed more frequently (89% vs. 68%), and advanced disease (stages T_3, T_4, and D) was diagnosed less frequently (11% vs. 32%) when comparing the 1998 to the 1988 incidence rates.

❸ The most important prognostic factor appears to be the histologic grade, because the degree of differentiation ultimately determines the stage of disease. Poorly differentiated tumors are highly associated with both regional lymph node involvement and distant metastases.[31]

During 1992 to 1999, 5-year overall survival rates were estimated at 98% for whites and 93% for African Americans.[1] During this same period, the survival rates for localized or regional disease (100%), and distant disease (33%) in white males were about the same as the survival rates for localized or regional disease (100%), and distant disease (26%) in African American males.[1] A 6.3% decline in age-adjusted mortality was documented for the period 1991 to 1995.[34] Ten-year cancer-specific survival is approximately 95% for stage A_1,

TABLE 134-3 Staging and Classification Systems for Prostate Cancer

AUS[a] Stage (A–D)	AJC-UICC[b] Classification (TNM)
A (Occult, nonpalpable)	$T_xN_xM_x$ (Cannot be assessed)
A_1: Focal	$T_0N_0M_0$ (Nonpalpable)
A_2: Diffuse	T_0: Focal or diffuse
B (Confined to prostate)	$T_1N_0M_0$, $T_2N_0M_0$
B_1: Single nodule in one lobe, less than 1.5 cm	T_1 (Clinically inapparent tumor not palpable or visible by imaging)
	T_{1a}: Tumor incidental histologic finding in 5% or less of tissue resected
	T_{1b}: Tumor incidental histologic finding in 5% or more of tissue resected
	T_{1c}: Tumor identified by needle biopsy (e.g., because of elevated prostate-specific antigen)
B_2: Diffuse involvement of whole gland, greater than 1.5 cm	T_2: (Tumor confined within the prostate[c])
	T_{2a}: Tumor involves half of a lobe or less
	T_{2b}: Tumor involves more than half a lobe, but not both lobes
	T_{2c}: Tumor involves both lobes
C (Localized to periprostatic area)	$T_3N_0M_0$, $T_4N_0M_0$
C_1: No seminal vesicle involvement, less than 70 g	T_3: (Tumor extends through the prostatic capsule[d])
	T_{3a}: Unilateral extracapsular extension
	T_{3b}: Bilateral extracapsular extension
	T_{3c}: Tumor invades the seminal vesicle(s)
C_2: Seminal vesicle involvement, greater than 70 g	T_4: (Tumor is fixed or invades adjacent structures other than the seminal vesicles)
	T_{4a}: Tumor invades any of bladder neck, external sphincter, or rectum
	T_{4b}: Tumor invades levator muscles and/or is fixed to the pelvic wall
D (Metastatic disease)	Any T, N_{1-4}, M_0, or N_{0-4}, M_1
D_1: Pelvic lymph nodes or ureteral obstruction	N_1: Metastasis in a single lymph node, 2 cm or less in greatest dimension
D_2: Bone, distant lymph node, organ, or soft tissue metastases	N_2: Metastasis in single lymph node more than 2 cm but not more than 5 cm in greatest dimension; or multiple lymph node metastases, none more than 5 cm in greatest dimension
	N_3: Metastasis in lymph node more than 5 cm in greatest dimension
	M_{1a}: Nonregional lymph node(s)
	M_{1b}: Bone(s)
	M_{1c}: Other site(s)

[a]American Urologic System.

[b]American Joint Committee–International Union Against Cancer.

[c]Tumor found in one or both lobes by needle biopsy, but not palpable or visible by imaging, is classified as T_{1c}.

[d]Invasion into the prostatic apex or into (but not beyond) the prostatic capsule is not classified as T_3 but as T_2.

80% for stages A_2 to B_2, 60% for stage C, 40% for stage D_1, and 10% for stage D_2.[35] More than 85% of patients with stage A_1 can be cured, whereas fewer than 1% of patients with stage D_2 will be cured.

TREATMENT

Prostate Cancer

■ DESIRED OUTCOME

The desired outcome in early stage prostate cancer is to minimize morbidity and mortality caused by prostate cancer while minimizing toxicity associated with prostate cancer treatments.[36] Unfortunately, the most appropriate therapy of early stage prostate cancer is unknown. Early stage disease may be treated with surgery, radiation, or watchful waiting. Although surgery and radiation are potentially curative, they are associated with significant morbidity and mortality. Because the overall goal is to minimize morbidity and mortality associated with the disease, watchful waiting is appropriate in selected individuals. Advanced prostate cancer (stage D) is not currently curable, and treatment should focus on providing symptom relief and maintaining quality of life.[37]

NONPHARMACOLOGIC THERAPY

Expectant Management

Expectant management, also known as observation or watchful waiting, involves monitoring the course of disease and initiating treatment if the cancer progresses or the patient becomes symptomatic. A PSA and DRE are performed every 6 months, with a repeat biopsy at any sign of disease progression. The advantages of expectant management are avoiding the adverse effects associated with definitive therapies such as radiation and radical prostatectomy, and minimizing the risk of unnecessary therapies. The major disadvantage of expectant management is the risk that the cancer progresses and requires a more intensive therapy.[36]

Orchiectomy

Bilateral orchiectomy, or removal of the testes, rapidly reduces circulating androgens to castrate levels (<50 ng/dL).[22] However, many patients are not surgical candidates because of their advanced age, and other patients find this procedure psychologically unacceptable.[22] Orchiectomy is the preferred initial treatment in patients with impending spinal cord compression or ureteral obstruction.

Radiation

The two commonly used methods for radiation therapy are external beam radiotherapy and brachytherapy.[36] In external beam radiotherapy, either 3D conformal radiation or intensity-modulated radiotherapy should be used to deliver doses of 70 to 75 Gy in 35 to 41 fractions in patients with low-grade prostate cancer and 75 to 80 Gy for those with intermediate- or high-grade prostate cancer. Brachytherapy involves the permanent implantation of radioactive beads of 145 Gy ^{125}Iodine or 124 Gy of ^{103}Palladium and is generally reserved for individuals with low-risk cancers.

Radical Prostatectomy

Complications from radical prostatectomy include blood loss, stricture formation, incontinence, lymphocele, fistula formation, anesthetic risk, and impotence. Nerve-sparing radical prostatectomy can be performed in many patients; 50% to 80% regain sexual potency within the first year. Acute complications from radiation therapy include cystitis, proctitis, hematuria, urinary retention, penoscrotal edema, and impotence (30% incidence).[22] Chronic complications include proctitis, diarrhea, cystitis, enteritis, impotence, urethral stricture, and incontinence.[22] Because radiation and prostatectomy have significant and immediate mortality when compared with observation alone, many patients may elect to postpone therapy until symptoms develop.

PHARMACOLOGIC THERAPY

Drug Treatments of First Choice

Luteinizing Hormone-Releasing Hormone Agonists LHRH agonists are a reversible method of androgen ablation and are as effective as orchiectomy in treating prostate cancer.[40] Currently available LHRH agonists include leuprolide, leuprolide depot, leuprolide implant, triptorelin depot, triptorelin implant, and goserelin acetate implant.[27] Leuprolide acetate is administered once daily, whereas leuprolide depot and goserelin acetate implant can be administered either once monthly, once every 12 weeks, or once every 16 weeks (leuprolide depot, every 4 months). The leuprolide depot formulation contains leuprolide acetate in coated pellets. The dose is administered intramuscularly, and the coating dissolves at different rates to allow sustained leuprolide levels throughout the dosing interval. Goserelin acetate implant contains goserelin acetate dispersed in a plastic matrix of D,L-lactic and glycolic acid copolymer and is administered subcutaneously. Hydrolysis of the copolymer material provides continuous release of goserelin over the dosing period. A recently approved leuprolide implant is a miniosmotic pump that delivers 120 mcg of leuprolide daily for 12 months. After 12 months the implant is removed, and a different implant can be placed. Triptorelin LA is administered as an intramuscular injection of 11.25 mg every 84 days. Triptorelin depot is administered as an intramuscular injection of 3.75 mg once every month.

Several randomized trials have demonstrated that leuprolide, goserelin and triptorelin are effective agents when used alone in patients with advanced prostate cancer.[27] Response rates of around 80% have been reported, with a lower incidence of adverse effects compared with estrogens.[27] No head-to-head trials have directly compared the currently available LHRH agonists or the dosage formulations, but a meta-analysis reported no difference in efficacy or toxicity between leuprolide and goserelin.[41] Triptorelin is a more recent addition, but is generally considered equally effective.[42] Consequently, the choice between the three agents is usually made based on cost and patient and physician preference for a dosing schedule.

The most common adverse effects reported with LHRH agonist therapy include a disease flareup during the first week of therapy, hot flashes, erectile impotence, decreased libido, and injection-site reactions.[27] The disease flareup is thought to be caused by initial induction of LH and FSH by the LHRH agonist, and manifests clinically as either increased bone pain or increased urinary symptoms.[27] This flare reaction usually resolves after 2 weeks and has a similar onset and duration pattern for the depot LHRH products.[43,44]

LHRH agonist monotherapy can be used as initial therapy, with similar response rates to orchiectomy and estrogen administration expected.[44] LHRH therapy is associated with a lower incidence of cardiovascular-related adverse effects as compared with estrogen administration. Patients should be counseled to expect worsening symptoms during the first week of therapy, and caution should be exercised when initiating LHRH agonist therapy in patients with widely metastatic disease involving the spinal cord or having the potential for ureteral obstruction because irreversible complications may occur.

Antiandrogens Three antiandrogens—bicalutamide,[45,46] nilutamide,[47] and flutamide[48]—are currently available (Table 134–4). Antiandrogens have been used as monotherapy in previously untreated patients, but a recent meta-analysis determined that patients who received monotherapy with antiandrogens have a shorter survival than patients treated with LHRH agonist therapy (hazard ratio 1.13, 95% CI 0.915 to 1.386) or orchiectomy.[44] Therefore, for advanced prostate cancer, until androgen monotherapy demonstrates at least equivalent survival outcome to LHRH therapy, antiandrogens are indicated only in combination with androgen-ablation therapy; flutamide and bicalutamide are indicated in combination with an LHRH agonist, and nilutamide is indicated in combination with orchiectomy.[29]

Table 134–4 lists the most common antiandrogen-related adverse effects. In the only randomized comparison of bicalutamide plus an LHRH agonist versus flutamide plus an LHRH agonist, diarrhea was more common in flutamide-treated patients. Antiandrogens can reduce the symptoms from the flare phenomenon associated with LHRH agonist therapy.

TABLE 134-4 Antiandrogens

Antiandrogen	Usual Dose	Adverse Effects
Flutamide	750 mg/day	Gynecomastia Hot flushes Gastrointestinal disturbances (diarrhea) Liver function test abnormalities Breast tenderness Methemoglobinemia
Bicalutamide	50 mg/day	Gynecomastia Hot flushes Gastrointestinal disturbances (diarrhea) Liver function test abnormalities Breast tenderness
Nilutamide	300 mg/day for first month then 150 mg/day	Gynecomastia Hot flushes Gastrointestinal disturbances (nausea or constipation) Liver function test abnormalities Breast tenderness Visual disturbances (impaired dark adaptation) Alcohol intolerance Interstitial pneumonitis

Combined Hormonal Blockade Although up to 80% of patients with advanced prostate cancer will respond to initial hormonal manipulation, nearly all patients will progress within 2 to 4 years after initiating therapy.[22] Two mechanisms have been proposed to explain this tumor resistance. The tumor could be heterogeneously composed of cells that are hormone dependent and hormone independent, or the tumor could be stimulated by extratesticular androgens that are converted intracellularly to DHT. The rationale for combination hormonal therapy is to interfere with multiple hormonal pathways to completely eliminate androgen action. In clinical trials, combination hormonal therapy, sometimes also referred to as *maximal androgen deprivation* or total androgen blockade, has been used. The combination of LHRH agonists or orchiectomy with antiandrogens is the most extensively studied combined androgen-deprivation approach.

Many studies have compared combined androgen blockade (CAB) with conventional medical or surgical castration.[48–50] In studies with LHRH agonists, the results have varied, with no consistent benefit demonstrated for CAB. A recently completed NCI intergroup trial involving 1,387 evaluable stage D_2 prostate cancer patients failed to show any significant survival benefits for the combination of orchiectomy plus flutamide over orchiectomy alone.[51] Like other studies of CAB, overall survival was longest in patients with minimal disease. Diarrhea, elevated liver function tests, and anemia were more common in those patients who received flutamide.

The most recent meta-analysis of 27 randomized trials in 8,275 patients (4,803 treated with flutamide, 1,683 treated with nilutamide, and 1,784 treated with cyproterone) comparing maximal androgen blockade with conventional medical or surgical castration showed a small survival benefit at 5 years for those treated with flutamide or nilutamide (27.6%) compared to those with castration alone (24.7%; $p = 0.0005$).[50]

In one of the few combination androgen-deprivation studies comparing two different antiandrogens (bicalutamide vs. flutamide), the time-to-treatment-failure (the main study end point), time-to-progression (as defined by appearance of new or worsening bone or extraskeletal lesions), and time-to-death were equivalent, suggesting that the two treatments are equally effective.[52]

Although some experts now consider CAB to be the initial hormonal therapy of choice for newly diagnosed patients, the clinician is left to weigh the costs of combined therapy against potential benefits in light of conflicting results in the randomized trials[29] and the modest benefit seen in the meta-analysis.[50] For those trials that did show an advantage for CAB, whether these effects are specific to the testosterone-deprivation method (orchiectomy vs. leuprolide vs. goserelin), the antiandrogen, the duration of therapy, or patient selection is not clear. Until further carefully designed studies that use survival, time-to-progression, quality of life, patient preference, and cost as end points are conducted, it is appropriate to use either LHRH agonist monotherapy or CAB as initial therapy for metastatic prostate cancer. CAB may be most beneficial for improving survival in patients with minimal disease and for preventing tumor flare, particularly in those with advanced metastatic disease. All other patients may be started on LHRH monotherapy, and an antiandrogen may be added after several months if androgen ablation is incomplete.

CLINICAL CONTROVERSY

The use of combined androgen blockade is controversial. Meta-analysis shows a small survival advantage when comparing CAB to orchiectomy or LHRH agonist alone. However, this modest benefit is achieved at significant financial cost and with additional toxicities.

There is still considerable debate concerning when to start hormonal-deprivation therapy in patients with advanced prostate cancer.[36] The original recommendation to start therapy when symptoms appeared was based on the Veterans Administration Cooperative Urologic Research Group (VACURG) trials, in which no overall survival difference was demonstrated in patients who either started diethylstilbestrol initially or crossed over to active treatment when symptoms appeared.[52] Because LHRH agonists and antiandrogens are considered suitable alternatives with less cardiovascular toxicity, it is no longer clear whether delaying therapy is justified. Reanalysis of the original VACURG data[53] and recent combined androgen-deprivation trials[54,55] demonstrate a survival advantage for young, good-performance-status, minimal-disease patients treated initially with hormonal therapy, which supports early intervention before symptoms appear.[53] The issue of when best to start hormonal therapy is the subject of several ongoing clinical trials.[53]

CLINICAL CONTROVERSY

Older data with diethylstilbestrol showed that initiation of hormonal therapy at symptom onset yielded equivalent survival to starting hormonal therapy at initial diagnosis. With equivalent survival, decreased costs, and decreased toxicity from diethylstilbestrol, the standard of practice was to delay initiation of hormonal therapy until symptoms developed. The favorable toxicity profile of LHRH agonists led to the re-evaluation of the starting time for therapy; current research shows that younger men with a good performance status may benefit from initiation of hormonal therapy at diagnosis, rather than waiting for symptoms to develop.

Alternative Drug Treatments

The selection of secondary or salvage therapies for patients who progress after their initial therapy depends on what was used for initial management.[36] For patients initially diagnosed with localized prostate cancer, radiotherapy can be used in the case of failed radical prostatectomy. Alternatively, androgen ablation can be used in patients who progress after either radiation therapy or radical prostatectomy.

Secondary Hormonal Manipulations Secondary hormonal manipulations, such as the addition of an antiandrogen to a patient who incompletely suppresses testosterone secretion with an LHRH agonist, or withdrawal of antiandrogens in a patient receiving combination therapy, or use of agents that inhibit androgen synthesis, can be attempted in patients initially treated with one hormonal modality. Supportive care, chemotherapy, or local radiotherapy can be used in patients who have failed all forms of androgen-ablation manipulations because these patients are considered to have androgen-independent disease.

For patients who initially received an LHRH agonist alone, castration testosterone levels should be documented. Patients with inadequate testosterone suppression (plasma testosterone remains >20 ng/dL) can be treated by adding an antiandrogen or performing an orchiectomy. If castration testosterone levels have been achieved, the patient is considered to have androgen-independent disease, and palliative androgen-independent salvage therapy can be used.

❹ If the patient initially received combined androgen blockade with an LHRH agonist and an antiandrogen, then androgen withdrawal is the first salvage manipulation.[36] Objective and subjective responses have been noted following the discontinuation of flutamide,[53] bicalutamide,[54] or nilutamide[55] in patients receiving these agents as part of combined androgen ablation with an LHRH agonist. Mutations in the androgen receptor allow antiandrogens such as flutamide, bicalutamide, and nilutamide (or their metabolites) to become agonists and activate the androgen receptor.[56] Patient responses to androgen withdrawal manifest as significant PSA reductions and improved clinical symptoms. Androgen withdrawal responses lasting 3 to 14 months have been noted in up to 35% of patients, and response seems to be most closely related to longer androgen exposure times.[52] Incomplete cross-resistance has been noted in some patients who received bicalutamide after they had progressed while receiving flutamide.[45] The addition of an agent that blocks adrenal androgen synthesis, such as aminoglutethimide, at the time that androgens are withdrawn may produce a better response than androgen withdrawal alone.[56] Because of the potential for response immediately after antiandrogen withdrawal, a sufficient observation and assessment period (usually 4 to 6 weeks) is usually required before a patient can be enrolled on a clinical trial evaluating a new agent or therapy for advanced prostate cancer.

Androgen synthesis inhibitors, such as aminoglutethimide or ketoconazole, can provide symptomatic relief for a short time in approximately 50% of patients with progressive disease despite previous androgen-ablation therapy.[29] Adverse effects during aminoglutethimide therapy occur in approximately 50% of patients.[29] Central nervous system effects that include lethargy, ataxia, and dizziness are the major adverse reactions. A generalized morbilliform, pruritic rash has been reported in up to 30% of patients treated. The rash is usually self-limiting and resolves within 5 to 8 days with continued therapy. Adverse effects from ketoconazole include gastrointestinal intolerance, transient rises in liver and renal function tests, and hypoadrenalism.

Supportive Care After all hormonal manipulations are exhausted, the patient is considered to have androgen-independent disease. At this point, either chemotherapy or palliative supportive therapy is appropriate.[36] Most patients with advanced prostate cancer have metastatic disease to the bone, which results in pain and skeletal events, such as fractures. Palliation can be achieved by pain management, using radioisotopes such as strontium-89[57] or samarium-153 lexidronam[58] for bone-related pain, analgesics, corticosteroids, bisphosphonates,[59] or local radiotherapy.[36]

Bisphosphonates have been evaluated in patients with prostate cancer since the 1980s.[60] A recent Cochrane review that included 1,955 patients from 10 clinical trials evaluated pain response as the primary outcome measure with secondary outcomes including analgesic consumption, skeletal events, prostate cancer death, disease progression, radiologic response, PSA response, adverse events, performance status, and quality of life, and comparisons between different routes, doses, and types of bisphosphonates. A variety of bisphosphonates have been studied, including clodronate (seven studies), zoledronic acid (one study), pamidronate (one study) and etidronate (one study). In all studies, participants received concurrent hormonal therapy, chemotherapy, or radiation therapy. In the meta-analysis, bisphosphonates did not decrease pain or analgesic consumption, improve disease response, prolong survival, or improve quality of life. However, bisphosphonates are effective overall in decreasing skeletal-related events (odds ratio 0.79, 95% CI 0.62 to 1.00; $P = 0.05$), and toxicity, with the exception of nausea, which was greater in patients receiving bisphosphonates, was similar to placebo.[60]

Zoledronic acid is currently indicated for use in prostate cancer patients with bone metastases after failing one hormonal therapy, based on a study demonstrating that patients receiving zoledronic acid had significantly less skeletal morbidity than those on the placebo arm both by the proportions analysis (33% vs. 44%, respectively; $P = 0.021$) and time-to-first-skeletal-related event analysis ($P = 0.011$) in patients with bone metastases.[61] Zoledronic acid should be avoided in individuals with a serum creatinine >3 mg/dL. Although not approved for this indication, pamidronate is also widely used. The usual dose of pamidronate is 90 mg every month and the usual dose of zoledronic acid is 4 mg every 3 to 4 weeks. Both drugs can cause renal failure, and the risk of renal failure depends on the dose and duration of infusion. To minimize the risk of renal failure, zoledronic acid should be administered as a 4-mg dose over 15 minutes. A trial of pamidronate or zoledronic acid can be initiated in prostate cancer patients with bone pain; if no benefit is observed, the drug may be discontinued.[59]

Bisphosphonates such as pamidronate and zoledronic acid may prevent skeletal morbidity, such as pathologic fractures and spinal cord compression, in men with hormone-refractory metastatic prostate cancer with clinically significant bone loss, as measured by serial bone mineral density testing.[62] To determine if bisphosphonates can slow metastatic disease progression, the PR05 trial evaluated 311 patients with newly diagnosed bony metastatic disease who received standard hormone therapy and were randomly assigned to receive 3 years of sodium clodronate or placebo.[63] The clodronate group did not demonstrate decreased analgesic consumption or improved bone progression free survival or overall survival when compared to the control group, but were less likely to have a worsened World Health Organization performance status (hazard ratio 0.71, 95% CI 0.56 to 0.92; $P = 0.008$).

In a similar trial, the PR04 study randomized 508 men who were within 3 years of initial prostate cancer diagnosis with no evidence of metastases to clodronate or placebo to determine if early intervention with bisphosphonates could prevent development of metastases. The clodronate group received no benefit in bone metastases free survival or overall survival as compared to the placebo group with an increased risk of adverse events.[64]

Chemotherapy ❺ Historically, hormone refractory prostate cancer has been considered resistant to chemotherapy, with response rates of less than 9% for all regimens evaluated.[65] In 1996, the combination of mitoxantrone with prednisone was reported to induce a palliative response in 29% of patients with symptomatic disease, compared to 12% receiving prednisone alone, while improving quality of life, and was approved by the FDA despite having no impact on overall survival.[66]

More recently, the combination of docetaxel 75 mg/m^2 every 3 weeks and prednisone 5 mg twice a day has been shown to prolong survival in hormone-refractory metastatic prostate cancer (Table 134–5).[67] The most common adverse events reported with this regimen are nausea, alopecia, and bone marrow suppression. In addition, fluid retention and peripheral neuropathy, known effects of docetaxel, are observed. The combination of estramustine (280 mg three times a day, days 1 to 5) and docetaxel (60 mg/m^2 on day

TABLE 134-5 First-Line Chemotherapy Regimens for Metastatic Hormone-Independent Prostate Cancer

Regimen	Usual Dose	Adverse Effects	Dose Adjustments
Docetaxel	75 mg/m² every 3 weeks	Fluid retention, alopecia, mucositis, myelosuppression, hypersensitivity	Hepatic Do not administer if AST/ALT greater than 1.5 times the upper limit of normal and alkaline phosphatase greater than 2.5 upper limit of normal Hematologic Assure complete blood count recovered
Estramustine	280 mg three times daily on days 1–5	Edema, gynecomastia, leucopenia, increased risk of thromboembolic events	Hematologic Assure complete blood count recovered

ALT, alanine aminotransferase; AST, aspartate aminotransferase.

2, every 3 weeks) also improves survival in hormone-refractory metastatic prostate cancer.[68] Estramustine causes a decrease in testosterone and a corresponding increase in estrogen, which results in an increase in thromboembolic events, gynecomastia, and decreased libido. Both docetaxel (in combination with prednisone) and estramustine are FDA-approved for the treatement of metastatic prostate cancer.

Estramustine is an oral capsule and should be refrigerated. Calcium inhibits the absorption of estramustine. Although both the docetaxel-prednisone and the docetaxel-estramustine regimens are effective in hormone-refractory prostate cancer, most clinicians, supported by a recent Cochrane review,[65] prefer the docetaxel-prednisone regimen because of the cardiovascular adverse effects associated with estramustine. In addition, androgen ablation is usually continued when chemotherapy is initiated.[36]

GENERAL APPROACH TO TREATMENT

The initial treatment for prostate cancer depends primarily on the disease stage, the Gleason score, the presence of symptoms, and the life expectancy of the patient.[36] Prostate cancer is usually initially diagnosed by PSA and DRE and confirmed by a biopsy, where the Gleason score is assigned. Asymptomatic patients with a low risk of recurrence, those with a T_1 or T_{2a}, Gleason score of 2 through 6, and a PSA <10 ng/mL can be managed by expectant management, radiation, or radical prostatectomy.[36] As patients with asymptomatic early stage disease generally have an excellent 10-year survival, immediate morbidities of treatment must be balanced with the likelihood of dying from prostate cancer. In general, more aggressive treatments of early stage prostate cancer are reserved for younger men, although patient preference is a major consideration in all treatment decisions.

Estimation of life expectancy is an important component for both prostate cancer screening and treatment. Life expectancy may be estimated from social security tables (*www.ssa.gov/OACT/STATS/table4c6.html*), which reports the life expectancy of the population by age. After determining an approximate life expectancy based on age, the clinician can adjust for individual health status by adding 50% for individuals in the top 25% for overall health, decreasing it by 50% for those in the bottom 25% for overall health and making no adjustment for those in the middle quartiles.[36] In a patient with an estimated normal life expectancy of <10 years, expectant management or radiation therapy may be offered. In those with an estimated normal life expectancy of ≥10 years, either expectant management, radiation (external beam or brachytherapy), or radical prostatectomy with a pelvic lymph node dissection may be offered. Radical prostatectomy and radiation therapy generally are considered therapeutically equivalent for localized prostate cancer, although neither has been proven to be better than observation alone.[36–38] Complications from radical prostatectomy include blood loss, stricture formation, incontinence, lymphocele, fistula formation, anesthetic risk, and impotence. Nerve-sparing radical prostatectomy can be performed in many patients—50% to 80% regain sexual potency within the first year. Acute complications from radiation therapy include cystitis, proctitis, hematuria, urinary retention, penoscrotal edema, and impotence (30% incidence).[16] Chronic complications include proctitis, diarrhea, cystitis, enteritis, impotence, urethral stricture, and incontinence.[31] Because radiation and prostatectomy have significant and immediate mortality when compared with expectant management alone, many patients may elect to postpone therapy until symptoms develop.

Individuals with T_{2b} or T_{2c} disease, a Gleason score of 7, or a PSA ranging from 10 to 20 ng/mL are considered at intermediate risk for prostate cancer recurrence.[36] Individuals with <10-year expected survival may be offered expectant management, radiation therapy, or radical prostatectomy with or without a pelvic lymph node dissection, and those with a ≥10-year life expectancy may be offered either radical prostatectomy with or without a pelvic lymph node dissection or radiation therapy.

Patients who are at high risk of recurrence (T_3 disease, a Gleason score ranging from 8 to 10, or a PSA value >20 ng/mL) should be treated with androgen ablation for 2 to 3 years combined with radiation therapy.[26] Select individuals with a low tumor volume may receive a radical prostatectomy with or without a pelvic lymph node dissection.

❻ Patients with T_{3b} and T_4 disease have a very high risk of recurrence and are not candidates for radical prostatectomy because of extensive local spread of disease.[36] Androgen ablation should be instituted at diagnosis rather than waiting for symptomatic disease or progression to occur. In a clinical trial enrolling 500 men with locally advanced prostate cancer who were randomized to either immediate initiation of androgen ablation with either orchiectomy or androgen ablation, or deferred hormonal therapy, individuals with immediate therapy had a median actuarial cause-specific survival duration of 7.5 years for immediate treatment compared to 5.8 years for deferred treatment.[39]

❼ Estrogens were once widely used, but the most widely used estrogen, diethylstilbestrol, was withdrawn from the United States market in 1997 because of increased cardiovascular risk. Secondary hormonal manipulations, cytotoxic chemotherapy, or supportive care is used for the patient who progresses after initial therapy.[29]

PHARMACOECONOMIC CONSIDERATIONS

The main economic concerns for prostate cancer focus on prostate cancer screening for asymptomatic men, initial therapy of clinically localized disease, surgical versus medical castration, and the use of combined hormonal blockade as treatment for advanced disease.

Prostate cancer screening remains highly controversial because the survival benefits and the associated costs are not well defined.[69] Krahn et al.[70] determined that annual screening of all eligible men would cost 45 million Canadian dollars, or 0.15% of total healthcare expenditures. Available cost-utility studies estimate that the cost per crude or quality-adjusted life-year gained from prostate cancer screening ranges from $3,000 to $729,000.[69–72] As the cost-effectiveness of prostate cancer screening cannot be determined until the benefits are documented, it is important to incorporate economic analysis into the large, ongoing, screening studies.

Treatment options for clinically localized prostate cancer include radiation therapy, surgery, or watchful waiting. There is currently no evidence to suggest which therapy is the most clinically effective, and treatment choice is often made by patient or physician preference. However, there are large economic differences in the therapies, with the cost of a radical prostatectomy $12,000 more expensive than watchful waiting, and radiation therapy $15,000 more expensive than watchful waiting.[73]

Surgical castration (by removal of the testes) and medical castration with LHRH agonists yield similar clinical results, although the majority of patients prefer medical castration. In two economic analyses, the primary cost of the surgical castration was hospital length of stay and medical castration drug costs. Both analyses found that in patients surviving 18 to 24 months, a surgical castration was more cost-effective.[74]

Table 134–6 lists the costs for the initial hormonal therapies for stage D_2 prostate cancer. Using a societal perspective and data from the original leuprolide plus flutamide versus leuprolide alone trial to calculate the incremental cost per life-year gained, Hillner et al.[71] concluded that CAB has an incremental cost-effectiveness of $25,300 per life-year gained, which is within current accepted benchmarks. The cost dropped to $13,700 per life-year gained in patients with minimal disease.

In a followup study, this same group used physician focus group estimates to generate quality-of-life factors and incorporated these factors into an economic model.[73] The incremental cost per quality-adjusted life-year gained seemed reasonable when data from the original CAB were used: $25,000 for patients with minimal disease and $18,000 for patients with severe disease. However, these incremental costs increased dramatically to $53,700 for patients with minimal disease and to $41,000 for patients with severe disease when the same model was applied to survival data from a meta-analysis.

Because there is considerable debate about the value of using CAB for advanced prostate cancer, continued economic assessments of this therapy are crucial to help policymakers and clinicians decide on the most appropriate therapy. It also is increasingly important to incorporate economic analyses into chemotherapy trials, particularly those that include clinical benefit response as a main end point.

TABLE 134-6 Comparative Costs of Hormonal Therapy for Advanced Prostate Cancer

Drug	Dose	Annual Cost (Based on AWP)
Leuprolide depot	7.5 mg/month	$709.20/month for annual cost of $8,510
Leuprolide depot	22.5 mg/12 weeks	$2,127.59/12 weeks for annual cost of $8,510
Leuprolide depot	30 mg/16 weeks	$2,836.79/16 weeks for annual cost of $8,510
Goserelin implant	3.6 mg every 28 days	$469.99/month for annual cost of $5,640
Goserelin implant	10.8 mg/12 weeks	$1,409.98/12 weeks for annual cost of $5,640
Triptorelin depot	3.75mg q 28 days	$582.00/month for annual cost of $6,984
Triptorelin LA depot	11.25 mg q 84 days	$1,746.00/84 days for annual cost of $6,984
Flutamide	750 mg/day	$376.60/month for annual cost of $4,519
Bicalutamide	50 mg/day	$484.44/month for annual cost of $5,813
Nilutamide	300 mg/day for first month then 150 mg/day	$728.80 for first month, then $364.40/month for annual cost of $4,373.80 for chronic therapy
Combined Androgen Blockade		**Cost Per 3 Months of Therapy (Based on AWP)**
Leuprolide depot 22.5 mg/12 weeks		
+ flutamide	750 mg/day	$3,257
+ bicalutamide	50 mg/day	$3,581
+ nilutamide	150 mg/day	$3,221
Goserelin depot 10.8 mg/12 weeks		
+ flutamide	750 mg/day	$2,540
+ bicalutamide	50 mg/day	$2,863
+ nilutamide	150 mg/day	$2,503
Triptorelin LA depot 11.25 mg every 84 days		
+ flutamide	750 mg/day	$2,876
+ bicalutamide	50 mg/day	$3,199
+ nilutamide	150 mg/day	$2,839

AWP, average wholesale price; LA, long acting.
Compiled from Thomson PDR, Red Book, Montvale, NJ, 2006.

EVALUATION OF THERAPEUTIC OUTCOMES

Monitoring of prostate cancer depends on the stage of the cancer.[36] When definitive, curative therapy is attempted, objective parameters to assess tumor response include assessment of the primary tumor size, evaluation of involved lymph nodes, and the response of tumor markers such as PSA to treatment. Following definitive therapy, the PSA level is checked every 6 months for the first 5 years, then annually. Local recurrence in the absence of a rising PSA may occur, so the DRE is also performed. In the metastatic setting, clinical benefit responses can be documented by evaluating performance status changes, weight changes, quality of life, and analgesic requirements, in addition to the PSA or DRE at 3-month intervals.

ABBREVIATIONS

BPH: benign prostatic hyperplasia

CAB: combined androgen blockade

DHT: dihydrotestosterone

DRE: digital rectal examination

FSH: follicle-stimulating hormone

LH: luteinizing hormone

LHRH: luteinizing hormone–releasing hormone

PSA: prostate-specific antigen

VACURG: Veterans Administration Cooperative Urologic Research Group

REFERENCES

1. Jemal A, Siegel J, Ward E, et al. Cancer statistics, 2007. CA Cancer J Clin 2007;57:43–66.
2. Ries LAG, Melbert D, Krapcho M, et al. (eds). SEER Cancer Statistics Review, 1975–2004. Bethesda, MD: National Cancer Institute. 2007, *http://seer.cancer.gov/csr/1975_2004/*, based on November 2006 SEER data submission, posted to the SEER website, 2007.
3. Hsieh K, Albertsen PC. Populations at high risk for prostate cancer. Urol Clin North Am 2003;30:669–676.
4. Odedina FT, Ogunbiyi JO, Ukoli FA. Roots of prostate cancer in African-American men. J Natl Med Assoc 2006;98:539–543.
5. Denis L, Morton MD, Griffiths K. Diet and its preventative role in prostate cancer. Eur Urol 1999;35:377–387.
6. Crawford ED. Epidemiology of prostate cancer. Urology 2003;62(6 Suppl 1):3–12.
7. Camp NJ, Cannon-Albright LA, Farnham JM, et al. Compelling evidence for a prostate cancer gene at 22q12.3 by the International

Consortium for Prostate Cancer Genetics. Hum Mol Genet 2007; 16:1271–1278.

8. Lindstrom S, Zheng SL, Wiklund F, et al. Systematic replication study of reported genetic associations in prostate cancer: Strong support for genetic variation in the androgen pathway. Prostate 2006;66:1729–1743.
9. Bostwick DG, Burke HB, Djakiew D, et al. Human prostate cancer risk factors. Cancer 2004;101(10 Suppl):2371–2490.
10. Thompson IM, Goodman PJ, Tangen CM, et al. The influence of finasteride on the development of prostate cancer. N Engl J Med 2003;349:215–224.
11. Marberger M, Adolfsson J, Borkowski A, et al. The clinical implications of the prostate cancer prevention trial. BJU Int 2003;92:667–671.
12. Neill MG, Fleshner ME. An update on chemoprevention strategies in prostate cancer for 2006. Curr Opin Urol 2006;16:132–137.
13. Schmid HP, Prikler L, Semjonow A. Problems with prostate-specific antigen screening: A critical review. Recent Results Cancer Res 2003;163:226–231.
14. Smith RA, Cokkinides V, Eyre HJ. American Cancer Society guidelines for the early detection of cancer, 2006. CA Cancer J Clin 2006;56:11–25.
15. Ilic D, O'Connor D, Green S, Wilt T. Screening for prostate cancer. Cochrane Database Syst Rev 2006;3:CD004720.
16. Ross KS, Carter HB, Pearson JD, Guess HA. Comparative efficacy of prostate specific antigen screening strategies for prostate cancer detection. JAMA 2000;284:1399–1405.
17. Andriole GL, Levin DL, Crawford ED, et al. Prostate cancer screening in the Prostate, Lung, Colorectal and Ovarian (PLCO) Cancer Screening Trial: Findings from the initial screening round of a randomized trial. J Natl Cancer Inst 2005;97:433–438.
18. Galic J, Karner I, Cenan L, et al. Role of screening in detection of clinically localized prostate cancer. Coll Antropol 2003;27(Suppl 1):49–54.
19. Wilson SS, Crawford ED. Screening for prostate cancer: Current recommendations. Urol Clin North Am 2004;31:219–226.
20. Gann PH, Hennekens CH, Stampfer MJ. A prospective evaluation of plasma prostate-specific antigen for detection of prostatic cancer. JAMA 1995;273:289–294.
21. Okihara K, Cheli CD, Partin AW, et al. Comparative analysis of complexed prostatic specific antigen, free prostate specific antigen, and their ratio in detecting prostate cancer. J Urol 2002:167:2017–2024.
22. Khauli RB. Prostate cancer: Diagnostic and therapeutic strategies with emphasis on the role of PSA. J Med Liban 2005;53:95–102.
23. Catalona WJ, Partin AW, Slawin KM, et al. Use of the percentage of free prostate-specific antigen to enhance differentiation of prostate cancer from benign prostatic disease: A prospective multicenter clinical trial. JAMA 1998;279:1542–1547.
24. Thompson IM, Pauler DK, Goodman PJ, et al. Prevalence of prostate cancer among men with a prostate-specific antigen level less than or equal to 4.0 ng per milliliter. N Engl J Med 2004;350:2239–2246.
25. Carter HB, Ferrucci L, Kettermann A, et al. Detection of life-threatening prostate cancer with prostate-specific antigen velocity during a window of curability. J Natl Cancer Inst 2006;98:1521–1527.
26. Culig Z. Role of the androgen receptor axis in prostate cancer. Urology 2003;62(5 Suppl 1):21–26.
27. Marks LS. Luteinizing hormone-releasing hormone agonists in the treatment of men with prostate cancer: Timing, alternatives, and the 1-year implant. Urology 2003;62(6 Suppl 1):36–42.
28. Huggins C, Hodges CV. Studies on prostatic cancer: 1. The effect of castration, of estrogen, and of androgen injection on serum phosphatases in metastatic carcinoma of the prostate. Cancer Res 1941;1:293–297.
29. Oh WK. Secondary hormonal therapies in the treatment of prostate cancer. Urology 2002;60(3 Suppl 1):87–92.
30. Anderson J. The role of antiandrogen monotherapy in the treatment of prostate cancer. BJU Int 2003;91:455–461.
31. Iczkowski KA. Current prostate biopsy interpretation: Criteria for cancer, atypical small acinar proliferation, high-grade prostatic intraepithelial neoplasia, and use of immunostains. Arch Pathol Lab Med 2006;130:835–843.
32. De Marzo AM. Meeker AK, Zha S, et al. Human prostate cancer precursors and pathobiology. Urology 2003;62(5 Suppl 1):55–62.
33. Montie JE. Staging of prostate cancer: Current TNM classification and future prospects for prognostic factors. Cancer 1995;75(Suppl):1814–1818.
34. Hoeksema M, Law C. Cancer mortality rates fall: A turning point for the nation. J Natl Cancer Inst 1996;88:1706–1707.
35. Leach FS, Koh MS, Chan Y, et al. Prostate specific antigen as a clinical biomarker for prostate cancer: What's the take home message? Cancer Biol Ther 2005;4(4):371–375.
36. Scardino PT, D'Amico A, Eastham JA, et al. National Comprehensive Cancer Network. National Comprehensive Cancer Network guidelines for the management of prostate cancer. Prostate Cancer v 1.2007. 2007, *http://www.nccn.org*.
37. Schroder FH, de Vries SH, Bangma CH. Watchful waiting in prostate cancer: Review and policy proposals. BJU Int 2003;92:851–859.
38. Scher HI. Prostate carcinoma: Defining therapeutic objectives and improving overall outcomes. Cancer 2003;97(3 Suppl):758–771.
39. Medical Research Council Prostate Cancer Working Party Investigators Group. Immediate versus deferred treatment for advanced prostate cancer: Initial results of the Medical Research Council Trial. Br J Urol 1997;79:235–246.
40. Prostate Cancer Trialist's Collaborative Group. Maximum androgen blockade in advanced prostate cancer: An overview of the randomised trials. Lancet 2000;355:1491–1498.
41. Alloul K, Sauriol L, Lafortune L. Meta-analysis and economic evaluation of LHRH agonists' depot formulations in advanced prostatic carcinoma. Can J Urol 1998;5:585–594.
42. Heyns CF, Simonin MP, Grosgurin P, Schall R, Porchet HC. For the South African Triptorelin Study Comparative efficacy of triptorelin pamoate and leuprolide acetate in men with advanced prostate cancer. BJU Int 2003;92:226–231.
43. Hedlund PO, Henriksson P. Parenteral estrogen versus total androgen blockade in the treatment of advanced prostate carcinoma: Effects of overall survival and cardiovascular mortality. Urology 2000;55:328–333.
44. Seidenfield J, Samson DJ, Hasselblad V, et al. Single therapy androgen suppression in men with advanced prostate cancer: A systematic review and meta analysis. Ann Intern Med 2000;132:566–577.
45. Scher H, Leibertz C, Kelly W, et al. Bicalutamide for advanced prostate cancer: The natural history versus treated history of disease. J Clin Oncol 1997;15:2928–2938.
46. Bales G, Chodak G. A controlled trial of bicalutamide versus castration in patients with advanced prostate cancer. Urology 1996;47:38–43.
47. Decensi A, Bocardo F, Guarneri D, et al. Monotherapy with nilutamide, a pure nonsteroidal antiandrogen, in untreated patients with metastatic carcinoma of the prostate. J Urol 1991;146:377–381.
48. Labrie F, Dupont A, Cusan L, et al. Combination therapy with flutamide and medical (LHRH agonist) or surgical castration in advanced prostate cancer: 7-year clinical experience. J Steroid Biochem Mol Biol 1990;37:943–950.
49. Tyrell CJ, Altwein Je, Klippel F, et al. Comparison of an LHRH analogue with combined androgen blockade in advanced prostate cancer. Eur Urol 2000;37:205–211.
50. Moul JW, Fowler JE Jr. Evolution of therapeutic approaches with luteinizing hormone-releasing hormone agonists in 2003. Urology 2003;62(6 Suppl 1):20–28.
51. Eisenberger MA, Blumenstein BA, Crawford ED, et al. Bilateral orchiectomy with or without flutamide for metastatic prostate cancer. N Engl J Med 1998;339:1036–1042.
52. The Veterans Administration Cooperative Urological Research Group. Carcinoma of the prostate: Treatment comparisons. J Urol 1967;98:516–522.
53. Scher HI, Kelly WK. Flutamide withdrawal syndrome: Its impact on clinical trials in hormone refractory prostate cancer. J Clin Oncol 1993;11:1566–1572.
54. Small E, Srinivas S. The androgen withdrawal syndrome: Experience in a large cohort of unselected patients with advanced prostate cancer. Cancer 1995;76:1428–1434.
55. Huan SD, Gerridzen RG, Yau JC, Stewart DJ. Antiandrogen withdrawal syndrome with nilutamide. Urology 1997;49:632–634.
56. Sartor O, Cooper M, Weinberger M, et al. Surprising activity of flutamide withdrawal, when combined with aminoglutethimide, in treatment of hormone-refractory prostate cancer. J Natl Cancer Inst 1994;86:222–227.
57. Crawford ED, Kozlowski JM, Debruyne FM, et al. The use of strontium 89 for palliation of pain from bone metastases associated with hormone-refractory prostate cancer. Urology 1994;44:481–485.

58. Resche I, Chatal JF, Pecking A, et al. A dose-controlled study of 153Sm-ethylenediaminetetramethylenephosphonate (EDTMP) in the treatment of patients with painful bone metastases. Eur J Cancer 1997;33:1583–1591.
59. Posadas EM, Dahut WL, Gulley J. The emerging role of bisphosphonates in prostate cancer. Am J Ther 2004;11:60–73.
60. Yuen KK, Shelley M, Sze WM, Wilt T, Mason MD. Bisphosphonates for advanced prostate cancer. Cochrane Database Syst Rev 2006;(4), CD 006250.
61. Ibrahim A, Scher N, Williams G, et al. Approval summary for zoledronic acid for treatment of multiple myeloma and cancer bone metastases. Clin Cancer Res 2003;9:2394–2399.
62. Saad F, Higano CS, Sartor O, et al. The role of bisphosphonates in the treatment of prostate cancer: Recommendations from an expert panel. Clin Genitourin Cancer 2006;4:257–262.
63. Dearnaley DP, Sydes MR, Mason MD, et al. A double-blind, placebo-controlled, randomized trial of oral sodium clodronate for metastatic prostate cancer (MRC PR05 Trial). J Natl Cancer Inst 2003;95:1300–1311.
64. Mason MD, Sydes MR, Glaholm J, et al. Oral sodium clodronate for nonmetastatic prostate cancer—Results of a randomized double-blind placebo-controlled trial: Medical Research Council PR04 (ISRCTN61384873). J Natl Cancer Inst 2007;99:765–776.
65. Shelley M, Harrison C, Coles B, Staffurth J, Wilt TJ, Mason MD. Chemotherapy for hormone-refractory prostate cancer. Cochrane Database Syst Rev 2006;(4):CD005247.
66. Tannock IF, Osoba D, Stockler MR, et al. Chemotherapy with mitoxantrone plus prednisone or prednisone alone for symptomatic hormone-resistant prostate cancer: A Canadian randomized trial with palliative end points. J Clin Oncol 1996;14:1756–1764.
67. Tannock IF, de Wit R, Berry WR, et al. Docetaxel plus prednisone or mitoxantrone plus prednisone for advanced prostate cancer. N Engl J Med 2004;351:1502–1512.
68. Petrylak DP, Tangen CM, Hussain MH, et al. Docetaxel and estramustine compared with mitoxantrone and prednisone for advanced refractory prostate cancer. N Engl J Med 2004;351:1513–1520.
69. Benoit RM, Naslund MJ. The economics of prostate cancer screening. Oncology (Williston Park) 1997;11:1533–1543.
70. Krahn MD, Coombs AB, Levy IG. Current and projected annual direct costs of screening asymptomatic men for prostate cancer using prostate specific antigen. CMAJ 1999;160:49–57.
71. Hillner BE, McLeod DG, Crawford ED, Bennett CL. Estimating the cost-effectiveness of total androgen blockade with flutamide in M1 prostate cancer. Urology 1995;45:633–640.
72. Bennett CL, Matchar D, McCrory D, et al. Cost-effective models for flutamide for prostate carcinoma patients: Are they helpful to policy makers? Cancer 1996;77:1854–1861.
73. Turini M, Redaelli A, Gramegna P, Radice D. Quality of life and economic considerations in the management of prostate cancer. Pharmacoeconomics 2003;21:527–541.
74. Hummel S, Paisley S, Morgan A, et al. Clinical and cost-effectiveness of new and emerging technologies for early localised prostate cancer: A systematic review. Health Technol Assess 2003;7:iii, ix–x, 1–157.

CHAPTER 135 Lymphomas

VAL R. ADAMS AND GARY C. YEE

KEY CONCEPTS

1. Patients with Hodgkin's lymphoma present with a painless, rubbery lymph node, which most commonly resides in the neck (cervical or supraclavicular nodes).

2. Patients with early-stage Hodgkin's lymphoma should be treated with combination chemotherapy with or without involved-field radiation and in special circumstances radiation alone.

3. Combination chemotherapy with doxorubicin (Adriamycin), bleomycin, vinblastine, and dacarbazine (ABVD) is the primary treatment for patients with advanced-stage Hodgkin's lymphoma. Patients with advanced unfavorable disease may be treated with more aggressive regimens that have greater activity, but are associated with a higher risk of secondary malignancies.

4. Some patients with Hodgkin's lymphoma will be refractory to initial therapy or will have a recurrence following a complete remission. Response to salvage therapy depends on the extent and site of recurrence, previous therapy, and duration of initial remission. High-dose chemotherapy and autologous hematopoietic stem cell transplantation should be considered in patients with refractory or relapsed disease.

5. The current classification system for non-Hodgkin's lymphoma is the World Health Organization classification system, which is based on the principle that non-Hodgkin's lymphomas can be classified into specific disease entities, defined by a combination of morphology, immunophenotype, genetic features, and clinical features.

6. As compared with Hodgkin's lymphoma, the clinical presentation of non-Hodgkin's lymphoma is more variable because of disease heterogeneity and more frequent extranodal involvement.

7. The Ann Arbor staging system correlates poorly with prognosis in non-Hodgkin's lymphoma because the disease does not spread through contiguous lymph nodes and often involves extranodal sites.

8. Several prognostic models have been developed to estimate prognosis in patients with non-Hodgkin's lymphoma. The International Prognostic Index (IPI) score is a well-established model for patients with aggressive non-Hodgkin's lymphoma. The Follicular Lymphoma International Prognostic Index (FLIPI) is a similar model used for patients with follicular and other indolent lymphomas.

9. The clinical behavior and degree of aggressiveness can be used to categorize non-Hodgkin's lymphoma into indolent and aggressive lymphomas. Patients with an indolent lymphoma usually have a relatively long survival, with or without aggressive chemotherapy. Although these lymphomas respond to a wide range of therapeutic approaches, few if any of these patients are cured of their disease. In contrast, aggressive lymphomas are rapidly growing tumors and patients have a short survival if appropriate therapy is not initiated. Most patients with aggressive lymphomas respond to intensive chemotherapy and many are cured of their disease.

10. Patients with localized follicular lymphoma can be cured with radiation therapy alone. Advanced follicular lymphoma is not curable, and there are many treatment options, including watchful waiting, extended-field radiation therapy, single-agent alkylating agents, anthracycline-containing combination chemotherapy, purine analogs, interferon-α, anti-CD20 monoclonal antibodies, and high-dose chemotherapy with hematopoietic stem cell rescue.

11. Patients with localized aggressive lymphomas can be cured with several cycles of R-CHOP (rituximab, cyclophosphamide, hydroxydaunorubicin, Oncovin, prednisone) chemotherapy and involved-field irradiation. Patients with bulky stage II, stage III, or stage IV aggressive lymphomas can be cured of their disease with R-CHOP chemotherapy.

12. Conventional-dose salvage therapy can induce responses in patients with aggressive lymphomas who relapse, but long-term survival and cure is uncommon. Some patients with aggressive lymphoma who relapse and respond to salvage therapy can be cured with high-dose chemotherapy and autologous hematopoietic stem cell transplantation.

Learning objectives, review questions,
and other resources can be found at
www.pharmacotherapyonline.com.

Lymphomas are a heterogeneous group of malignancies that arise from malignant transformation of immune cells that reside predominantly in lymphoid tissues. They most commonly present as a solid tumor, but can sometimes present as circulating tumor cells in peripheral blood. The differing histology of lymphoma cells has led to classification of Hodgkin's lymphoma (Reed-Sternberg cells) or non-Hodgkin's lymphoma (B- or T-cell lymphocyte markers). Non-Hodgkin's lymphomas (NHLs) are further classified into distinct clinical entities, which are defined by a combination of morphology, immunophenotype, genetic features, and clinical features. Chemotherapy is the mainstay of treatment in patients with lymphoma, especially those with widespread disease. Overall cure rates are high for many subtypes of lymphomas, even when patients present with advanced disease.

HODGKIN'S LYMPHOMA

Thomas Hodgkin's first described the mysterious disease of the lymph system that bears his name in 1932. Hodgkin's disease is a form of lymphoma, the cause of which is still unknown, and is fatal in more than 90% of patients untreated for 2 to 3 years. The prognosis with treatment is generally good, but is not well predicted by stage alone. The International Prognostic Index (IPI) was created to better predict an individual's risk of recurrence, which influences treatment decisions. Patients with Hodgkin's lymphoma can be categorized into four prognostic groups: early favorable disease, early unfavorable disease, advanced favorable disease, and advanced unfavorable disease. These groups are defined by patient age, gender, tumor size and spread (stage), presence or absence of systemic symptoms, and laboratory test results. When appropriate therapy is given, more than 75% of all newly diagnosed Hodgkin's lymphoma patients will be cured. This extraordinary success has not been without cost. The treatment programs are intense, technically demanding, and associated with considerable acute toxicity and long-term complications. The long-term effects, particularly secondary malignancies, account for a higher cumulative mortality than Hodgkin's lymphoma 15 to 20 years after treatment. Long-term toxicities with standard chemotherapy regimens have been more fully documented in recent years and are shaping future therapies.[1–4]

EPIDEMIOLOGY AND ETIOLOGY

It is estimated that 8,190 new cases of Hodgkin's lymphoma will be diagnosed in the United States in 2007, which represents less than 1% of all known cancers. It is expected that there will be 1,070 deaths associated with Hodgkin's lymphoma during this same time.[5] This disease occurs slightly more frequently in males than in females. Once thought to be only a disease of the young, it is now recognized that Hodgkin's lymphoma exhibits a bimodal distribution in industrialized countries. The first peak occurs between the ages of 15 and 44 years (highest from 20 to 29 years of age) and again in those older than 55 years.[1] The 5-year overall survival for all stages according to the Surveillance, Epidemiology, and End Results (SEER) database is approximately 85%.[6] Death rates as a consequence of recurrent Hodgkin's lymphoma are less than those from other causes 15 years after treatment.[7,8]

The etiology of Hodgkin's lymphoma is unknown and remains elusive for several reasons. Tissue taken from a Hodgkin's lymphoma mass reveals that only 1% to 2% of the cells are Reed-Sternberg cells (malignant), which has made it difficult to study.[1] The only risk factors that have consistently been associated with the disease include viral exposure and immune function. Infection has been considered a potential cause of Hodgkin's lymphoma since the disease was first described. Studies suggest an increased risk of Hodgkin's lymphoma in patients who have been infected with the Epstein-Barr virus (EBV). Reed-Sternberg cells (large, bilobate, multinuclear cells), the malignant cells in Hodgkin's lymphoma, are linked to EBV, particularly in patients older than age 50 years.[1,9] The increased risk associated with EBV infection appears to dissipate over about 20 years.[10] Immunosuppressed individuals are also at an increased risk of developing Hodgkin's lymphoma. This includes patients with congenital immunosuppression, solid-organ transplantation recipients, and human immunodeficiency virus (HIV)-infected patients. Although the risk of developing Hodgkin's lymphoma is about sevenfold greater in patients with HIV, the risk is not nearly as great as for non-Hodgkin's lymphoma and does not appear to be correlated with CD4 count.[11]

Genetic factors also predispose people to Hodgkin's lymphoma. The risk of Hodgkin's lymphoma is increased in people with ataxia telangiectasia. The strongest evidence suggesting that genes are important in the etiology of Hodgkin's lymphoma comes from identical twin studies, which show that the unaffected identical twin has about a 100-fold increase in risk. Other environmental risk factors are linked with Hodgkin's lymphoma, but only appear to play a minor role.[1,9]

PATHOPHYSIOLOGY

Hodgkin's lymphoma is a clonal malignant lymphoid disease of transformed lymphocytes. The malignant cell in Hodgkin's lymphoma is known as "Reed-Sternberg" after Drs. Carl Sternberg and Dorothy Reed, who are credited with the first definitive microscopic description of Hodgkin's lymphoma in 1898 and 1902, respectively.[1] The origin of the Reed-Sternberg cell has eluded scientists because of the inability to isolate and analyze these cells to the necessary depth. A typical Hodgkin's lymphoma mass occurs in a lymph node and contains normal reactive and inflammatory cells, fibrosis, and a relatively small percentage (1% to 2%) of Reed-Sternberg cells. In recent years, new laboratory techniques have led to significant progress in identifying the origin of the Reed-Sternberg cell. Single-cell polymerase chain reaction and DNA microarray analysis indicate that nearly all classic Hodgkin's lymphoma cases and all nodular lymphocyte-predominant Hodgkin's lymphomas have immunoglobulin gene rearrangements, which indicates a germinal center or postgerminal center B-cell origin (Table 135–1).[1,9] Interestingly, nearly all Reed-Sternberg cells fail to express B-cell specific cell surface proteins.

During malignant transformation, B-cell transcriptional processes are disrupted, which prevent B-cell surface marker expression and production of immunoglobulin messenger ribonucleic acid. The normal cellular consequence of failure to express immunoglobulin is apoptosis, but because of alterations in the normal apoptotic pathways, cell survival and proliferation are favored. Reed-Sternberg cells overexpress nuclear factor-κB, which is associated with cell proliferation and antiapoptotic signals. Infections with viral and bacterial pathogens upregulate nuclear factor-κB and consequently are hypothesized to be involved with the etiology of Hodgkin's lymphoma.[1,9] This hypothesis is supported by the finding of EBV in many Hodgkin's lymphoma tumors, but it is important to note that not all tumors are associated with EBV.[1,12] As molecular techniques continue to improve, our understanding of the pathophysiology of Hodgkin's lymphoma will also improve.

The histopathologic classification of Hodgkin's lymphoma has undergone numerous changes over the last three decades. The current classification system used today is the World Health Organization (WHO) modification of the Revised European-American Classification of Lymphoid Neoplasms (Table 135–2).[13] This classification divides Hodgkin's lymphoma into two major groups: classical Hodgkin's

TABLE 135-1 B-Cell Development and the Corresponding Neoplasm Derived at Each Stage

		B Cells	Corresponding Neoplasm
Foreign antigen independent	Bone marrow	Stem cell	
		Pro-B cell	
		Pre-B cell	B-LBL/ALL
↓	↓	Immature B cell	
Foreign antigen dependent	Peripheral lymphoid tissue	Mature naive B cell	B-CLL, MCL
		Germinal center	BL, FL, LPHL, DLBCL, cHL
↓		Memory B cell	MZL, B-CLL
Terminal differentiation		Plasma cell	Plasmacytoma/myeloma

ALL, acute lymphocytic leukemia; BL, Burkitt's lymphoma; B-CLL, B-cell chronic lymphocytic leukemia; B-LBL, B-cell lymphoblastic lymphoma; cHL, classic Hodgkin's lymphoma; DLBCL, diffuse large B-cell lymphoma; FL, follicular lymphoma; LPHL, lymphocyte-predominant Hodgkin's lymphoma; MCL, mantle cell lymphoma; MZL, marginal zone B-cell lymphoma.
Adapted from Harris et al.[48]

TABLE 135-2 WHO Classification of Lymphoid Malignancies

B Cell	T Cell	Hodgkin's Lymphoma
Precursor B-cell neoplasm	Precursor T-cell neoplasm	Nodular lymphocyte-predominant Hodgkin's lymphoma
Precursor B-lymphoblastic leukemia/lymphoma (precursor B-cell acute lymphoblastic leukemia)	**Precursor T-lymphoblastic lymphoma/leukemia (precursor T-cell acute lymphoblastic leukemia)**	Classic Hodgkin's lymphoma
Mature (peripheral) B-cell neoplasms	Mature (peripheral) T-cell neoplasms	Nodular sclerosis Hodgkin's lymphoma
B-cell chronic lymphocytic leukemia/small lymphocytic lymphoma	T-cell prolymphocytic leukemia	Lymphocyte-rich classic Hodgkin's lymphoma
B-cell prolymphocytic leukemia	T-cell granular lymphocytic leukemia	Mixed-cellularity Hodgkin's lymphoma
Lymphoplasmacytic lymphoma	Aggressive NK cell leukemia	Lymphocyte-depletion Hodgkin's lymphoma
Splenic marginal zone B-cell lymphoma (± villous lymphocytes)	Adult T-cell lymphoma/leukemia (HTLV-I +)	
Hairy cell leukemia	Extranodal NK/T-cell	
Plasma cell myeloma/plasmacytoma	Enteropathy-type T-cell lymphoma	
Extranodal marginal zone B-cell lymphoma of MALT type	Hepatosplenic $\gamma\delta$ T-cell lymphoma	
Mantle cell lymphoma	Subcutaneous panniculitis-like T-cell lymphoma	
Follicular lymphoma	**Mycosis fungoides/Sézary syndrome**	
Nodal marginal zone B-cell lymphoma (± monocytoid B cells)	Anaplastic large cell lymphoma primary cutaneous type	
Diffuse large B-cell lymphoma	**Peripheral T-cell lymphoma, not otherwise specified (NOS)**	
Burkitt's lymphoma/Burkitt's cell leukemia	**Angioimmunoblastic T-cell lymphoma**	
	Anaplastic large cell lymphoma, primary systemic type	

Bold type represents those malignancies that occur in at least 1% of patients.
HTLV, human T-cell lymphotropic virus; MALT, mucosa-associated lymphoid tissue; NK, natural killer; WHO, World Health Organization.
Adapted from Harris et al.[48]

lymphoma and nodular lymphocyte-predominant Hodgkin's disease, which constitute approximately 95% and 5% of cases, respectively. Classical Hodgkin's lymphoma is further divided into four subtypes: nodular sclerosis, mixed cellularity, lymphocyte-depletion, and lymphocyte-rich. The subtypes in these classification systems are based on characteristics of the Reed-Sternberg cell, the surrounding cells, and connective tissue. Nodular sclerosis has features that make it distinct from the other three subtypes, which represent a continuum of background cellularity, with lymphocyte-predominance being the most cellular and lymphocyte-depletion being the least cellular. Nodular lymphocyte-predominant Hodgkin's lymphoma is separated because of its distinct immunophenotype: $CD15^-$, $CD20^+$, $CD30^-$, and $CD45^+$ (the opposite of classical Hodgkin's disease).[1] With the introduction of extensive staging, sophisticated megavolt radiotherapy, and effective combination chemotherapy, the prognostic value of these subtypes is becoming less clear. The true value of understanding these subtypes is likely tied to the pathogenesis of the disease and potential prevention in the future.

CLINICAL PRESENTATION

❶ Approximately 70% of patients with Hodgkin's lymphoma present with a painless, rubbery lymph node and commonly have mediastinal nodal involvement. Hodgkin's lymphoma is occasionally diagnosed in asymptomatic patients who have a mediastinal mass found with chest radiography or other imaging procedure. Asymptomatic adenopathy of the inguinal and axillary regions may be present at diagnosis but is less common, whereas involvement of Waldeyer ring and the epitrochlear nodes rarely occurs (Fig. 135–1).[14] Approximately 25% of patients with Hodgkin's lymphoma present with constitutional symptoms (B symptoms) and pruritus is commonly noted but its presence does not appear to have significant prognostic value.[1]

DIAGNOSIS, STAGING, AND PROGNOSTIC FACTORS

Diagnostic and staging procedures are based on recommendations made at the Ann Arbor and Cotswolds conferences and new scientific advances, as described in the National Comprehensive Cancer Network (NCCN) guidelines.[15] The diagnosis and pathologic classification of Hodgkin's lymphoma can only be made by review of a biopsy (preferably an excisional biopsy) of the enlarged node by an expert hematopathologist. In addition to a careful physical examination and routine laboratory tests, chest radiography and computed tomography (CT) scans of the chest, abdomen, and pelvis are routinely performed. Positron emission tomography (PET) scanning is more sensitive and specific than CT scanning, but its impact on survival and role staging is unclear.[1,16] Bone marrow biopsy is recommended in patients with more advanced-stage disease.

Staging can be based on clinical or pathologic findings. Clinical stage is based on all noninvasive procedures (history, physical examination, laboratory tests, and radiologic findings), whereas pathologic stage is based on the biopsy findings of strategic sites (muscle, bone, skin, spleen, and abdominal nodes) with an invasive procedure such as a laparoscopy or laparotomy. Those patients with extranodal disease (muscle, skin, bone, or Waldeyer ring) contiguous to involved nodes are classified with the subscript "E" in the Cotswolds staging system.[15] As a result of improved imaging techniques, pathologic workup and staging that can be associated with toxicity is rarely performed.

The Ann Arbor staging classification, which was developed at the 1970 Ann Arbor conference, has proven to be a good workable scheme. At the Cotswolds meeting in 1989, the Ann Arbor classification was modified to account for new diagnostic techniques (e.g., CT and magnetic resonance imaging), and the understanding that prognosis is associated with the bulk of the disease and the number of involved nodal sites (Table 135–3).[1,17] After careful staging, about one-half of patients have localized disease (stages I, II, and II_E) and the remainder have advanced disease (stage III or IV). Approximately 10% to 15% present with metastatic disease (stage IV). It is important to note that Hodgkin's lymphoma appears to follow a predictable pattern of nodal spread that is not seen with the NHLs.[1,15,17]

Patient prognosis is predominately driven by age and stage. Patients who are older than ages 65 to 70 years are about one-half as likely to be cured as younger patients. The difference in cure rates may be related to the high rate of comorbid diseases and decreased organ function, which impairs the patient's ability to tolerate intensive chemotherapy. Stage is the other dominant factor in predicting survival; patients with limited-stage disease (stages I to II) have a 90% to 95% cure rate, whereas those with advanced disease (stages III to IV) have only a 65% to 70% cure rate.[1,15,17]

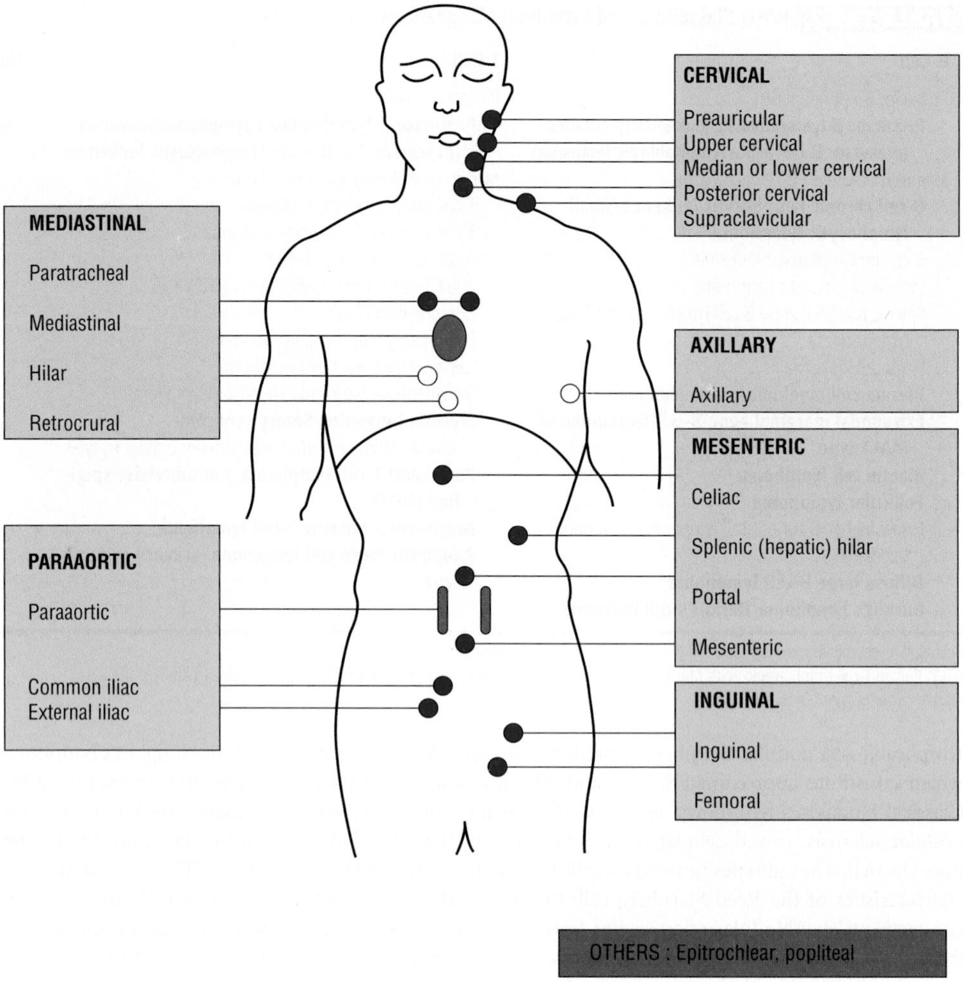

FIGURE 135-1. Areas of lymph nodes used in the staging of Hodgkin's and non-Hodgkin's lymphoma. Each rectangle corresponds to a nodal area. *(This research was originally published and modified from Blood. Solal-Celigny P, Roy P, Colombat P, et al. Follicular lymphoma international prognostic index. Blood 2004;104:1258–1265. Copyright © American Society of Hometology.)*

TABLE 135-3 The Cotswolds Staging Classification of Hodgkin's Lymphoma

Stage I	Involvement of a single lymph node region or structure (I) or of a single extralymphatic organ or site (I_E)
Stage II	Involvement of two or more lymph node regions on the same side of the diaphragm (II) or localized involvement of an extralymphatic organ or site and of one or more lymph node regions on the same side of the diaphragm (II_E). The number of nodal regions involved should be indicated by a subscript (e.g., II_2)
Stage III	Involvement of lymph node regions on both sides of the diaphragm (III), which may also be accompanied by localized involvement of an extralymphatic organ or site (III_E) or by involvement of the spleen (IIIS) or both ($IIIS_E$). III1: with or without splenic, hilar, celiac, or portal node involvement. III2: with paraaortic, iliac, or mesenteric node involvement
Stage IV	Diffuse or disseminated involvement of one or more extralymphatic organs or tissues with or without associated lymph node enlargement
	A–No symptoms
	B–Fever, night sweats, weight loss (>10%)
	X–Bulky disease
	>One-third the width of the mediastinum
	>10 cm maximal dimension of nodal mass
	E–Involvement of extralymphatic tissue on one side of the diaphragm by limited direct extension from an adjacent, involved lymph node region
	S–Involvement of the spleen
	CS–Clinical stage
	PS–Pathologic stage

Data from Staging and selection of treatment modality in patients with Hodgkin's disease. In: Up to Date Online 15.1.2007. (Accessed March 12, 2007)

Additional risk factors have been identified that improve the prognostic accuracy and impact therapeutic choices. An international collaborative effort identified seven adverse prognostic factors with similar impact on survival (each factor reduced survival by 7% to 8% per year), which can be combined to generate an International Prognostic Score that is used to predict progression-free and overall survival (Table 135–4).[18]

TABLE 135-4 The International Prognostic Factors Project Score for Advanced Hodgkin's Lymphoma

Risk Factors
Serum albumin (<4 g/dL)
Hemoglobin (<10.5 g/dL)
Male gender
Stage IV disease
Age (≥45 years)
White blood cell (WBC) count (≥15,000/mm^3)
Lymphocytopenia (<600/mm^3 or <8% of WBC count)

Number of Factors	Freedom from Progression[a]	Overall Survival[a]
0	84 ± 4	89 ± 2
1	77 ± 3	90 ± 2
2	67 ± 2	81 ± 2
3	60 ± 3	78 ± 3
4	51 ± 4	61 ± 4
≥5	42 ± 5	56 ± 5

[a]Percentage of patients at 5 years.
Data from Hasenclever D, Diehl V. A prognostic score for advanced Hodgkin's disease. International Prognostic Factors Project on Advanced Hodgkin's Diease. N Engl J Med 1998;339:1506–1514.

TREATMENT

Hodgkin's Lymphoma

The current goal in the treatment of Hodgkin's lymphoma is to maximize curability while minimizing short- and long-term treatment-related complications. According to the SEER database, the 5-year age-adjusted relative survival is greater than 80%.[6] The development of effective therapies for all stages of Hodgkin's lymphoma remains one of the most remarkable achievements in modern cancer care.

Although multiple treatment modalities are used to treat Hodgkin's lymphoma, surgery has a limited therapeutic role regardless of stage. It is, however, important for diagnosis (excisional biopsy), and on some occasions, such as placement of a central line.[1]

Combination chemotherapy is the primary treatment modality for most Hodgkin's lymphoma patients. In general, patients with early-stage Hodgkin's lymphoma are treated with combination chemotherapy (and radiation), whereas patients with advanced-stage disease are treated with combination chemotherapy with or without radiation therapy. For patients with refractory or recurrent disease, salvage therapy consists of multiagent chemotherapy with or without high-dose chemotherapy and autologous hematopoietic stem cell transplantation (HSCT), which can be curative.[1]

Radiation is often an integral part of the treatment plan. Selected patients with early-stage disease (usually nodular lymphocyte-predominant histology) can receive radiation as the only treatment modality, whereas most patients will receive chemotherapy and radiation. Although radiation is a local therapy, many patients with advanced disease will also receive radiation therapy to residual or bulky disease sites after chemotherapy. The major concern with radiation therapy is its long-term effects, such as cardiovascular disease and secondary malignancies, which commonly occur in the lung, breast, gastrointestinal tract, and connective tissue.[1,3,19] To avoid these toxicities, several studies have been completed and others are ongoing to maximize efficacy while minimizing the extent of radiation (radiation field) and the dose of radiation.[20] Radiation to a single field that contains Hodgkin's lymphoma is called *involved-field radiation*; radiation to the involved field and a second uninvolved area is termed *extended-field radiation* or *subtotal nodal irradiation*; and radiation of all areas is called *total nodal irradiation*.[21] When given with chemotherapy (the most common scenario), typically only involved-field radiation is used to avoid the increased toxicity associated with extended-field radiation. The following sections review treatment of early-stage favorable disease, early-stage unfavorable disease, advanced-stage favorable disease, advanced-stage unfavorable disease, and salvage therapy.

■ TREATMENT OF EARLY-STAGE FAVORABLE DISEASE

Patients with early-stage favorable disease have stage IA or IIA disease and no adverse risk factors (extranodal disease, bulky disease, three or more sites of nodal involvement, or an erythrocyte sedimentation rate of ≥50). Until recently, extended-field radiation was considered to be the treatment of choice for stages IA and IIA disease. This treatment produces disease-free survival rates ranging from 65% to 85% and overall survival rates ranging from 75% to 93%.[1,22,23]

In an effort to avoid the long-term effects of extended-field radiation and improve treatment results, several studies have evaluated a combined modality approach that involves the use of short-duration chemotherapy and involved-field radiation. Based on favorable results of these studies, most clinicians no longer treat patients with early-stage favorable disease with radiation alone.[1,15,22,23]

❷ Clinical trials comparing radiation alone to radiation plus chemotherapy show lower relapse rates in patients treated with combined modality therapy (radiation and chemotherapy), but no change in overall survival.[1,23,24] Current studies focus on questions such as the optimal number of chemotherapy cycles and the volume of radiation that must be used to obtain optimal patient outcomes. Results of recent studies suggest that as few as two to four cycles of chemotherapy are adequate. Different combination chemotherapy regimens have been used in these studies, and no one regimen is clearly superior to another.[20,22–24]

The current NCCN guidelines recommend that patients with early-stage favorable disease be treated with two cycles of the Stanford V regimen (doxorubicin, vinblastine, mechlorethamine, etoposide, vincristine, bleomycin, and prednisone) or four cycles of the ABVD (doxorubicin [Adriamycin], bleomycin, vinblastine, and dacarbazine) regimen, followed by consolidative involved-field radiation.[15] With this approach, 5-year progression-free and overall survival rates of >90% can be achieved.

In selected patients, those with nodular lymphocyte-predominant Hodgkin's lymphoma, who choose to omit chemotherapy, or who cannot tolerate chemotherapy, radiation therapy alone is an option and does not appear to adversely affect survival.[1,15,22,23] The disadvantage of radiation therapy alone as compared to combination chemotherapy and radiation is the higher relapse rate. The lack of difference in survival rates is a result of the fact that patients who relapse after radiation alone (20% to 25%) can be successfully salvaged with chemotherapy. If the decision is made to use radiation alone, extended-field radiation appears to be superior to involved-field radiation, based on a meta-analysis conducted by Specht et al.[25] Results of that analysis showed that more extensive radiation reduces the risk of treatment failure at 10 years (31% vs. 43%), although it does not improve 10-year overall survival (77% vs. 77.1%).

■ TREATMENT OF EARLY-STAGE UNFAVORABLE DISEASE

Patients with early-stage disease who have certain features associated with a poor prognosis (B symptoms, extranodal disease, bulky disease, three or more sights of nodal involvement, or an erythrocyte sedimentation rate >50) are defined as having unfavorable disease. Current guidelines recommend combined modality therapy (combination chemotherapy and involved-field radiation) to reduce the relapse rate and avoid the toxicity associated with extended-field radiation.[1,15,22,23]

❷ Although randomized trials show that combined modality therapy reduces the relapse rate in patients with early-stage unfavorable disease, questions concerning the appropriate radiation volume, most effective chemotherapy regimen, and number of chemotherapy cycles remain.[23] A number of studies have compared extended-field radiation to involved-field radiation. In the largest trial (German Hodgkin Study Group [GHSG] HD8 n = 1,204),[26] patients with early-stage unfavorable Hodgkin's lymphoma treated with chemotherapy and involved-field radiation had similar outcomes in terms of freedom from treatment failure and overall survival as those treated with the same chemotherapy regimen and extended-field radiation. Because toxicity was greater with extended-field radiation, the accepted standard is chemotherapy and involved-field radiation.

Several ongoing trials compare different chemotherapy regimens or number of chemotherapy cycles.[1,20,23] Mechlorethamine, vincristine, procarbazine, and prednisone (MOPP) was one of the first highly effective regimens introduced to treat Hodgkin's lymphoma. MOPP or MOPP-like regimens then were given alternately or hybridized with a combination of ABVD. In advanced disease, ABVD was found to be less toxic than alternating MOPP/ABVD, and both were found to be superior to MOPP alone. Consequently,

ABVD has become the standard regimen used to treat patients with early-stage unfavorable disease. It has established effectiveness in patients with advanced-stage disease and a favorable toxicity (both acute and chronic) profile.[1]

Despite the excellent results from treatment with ABVD and radiation, approximately 5% of patients will not respond to initial treatment and another 15% of patients will relapse following an initial response. Several ongoing studies are evaluating more aggressive regimens or more cycles of therapy. Two large European trials are evaluating ABVD versus a more intense combination of bleomycin, etoposide, doxorubicin, cyclophosphamide, vincristine, procarbazine, and prednisone (BEACOPP), 4 versus 6 cycles of chemotherapy, and 20 versus 30 Gy involved-field radiation.[1,20,23] Preliminary analysis at 40 and 64 months indicates no difference in treatment failure or overall survival between groups. The current NCCN guideline lists the Stanford V regimen as an acceptable option, which also uses more drugs than the ABVD regimen.[15] However, none of these more aggressive regimens has proven to be more effective than ABVD and each is associated with more toxicity.[27] Therefore, ABVD and involved-field radiation remain the standard at this time.

In summary, most patients with early stage disease will be treated with two to four cycles of ABVD chemotherapy and involved-field radiation. The number of cycles administered is based on favorable versus unfavorable disease. When radiation is completely omitted, six cycles of ABVD are recommended.[15] Although this approach results in excellent outcomes, studies are ongoing to maximize efficacy while minimizing acute and long-term toxicity.

■ TREATMENT OF ADVANCED-STAGE DISEASE

Advanced-stage disease consists of stages III and IV disease. In some studies, stage IIB with a large mediastinal mass or extranodal disease is also considered advanced-stage disease (see Table 135–3). By definition, stages III and IV patients have tumor on both sides of the diaphragm, which almost always precludes the use of radiation alone as a therapeutic modality. Intensive combination chemotherapy is the mainstay of treatment, although some patients will benefit from radiation following chemotherapy. The prognosis of advanced-stage disease is excellent with 5-year overall survival rates ranging from less than 56% to 90%. Prognostic factors have been identified and standardized to provide a more accurate individual prognosis (see Table 135–4).[1,18] Historically, all patients with advanced disease have been treated the same and studies have typically enrolled all advanced-stage patients regardless of prognosis.

Combination Chemotherapy

One of the initial combination chemotherapy regimens introduced in the early 1960s that was shown to produce cures in advanced Hodgkin's lymphoma was the MOPP regimen (Table 135–5).[28] MOPP chemotherapy was a mainstay of treatment for patients with stages III and IV advanced Hodgkin's lymphoma. It produced complete remissions in 84% of patients and has a 10-year cure rate of 54%.[29]

Ever since MOPP therapy was introduced and the efficacy confirmed, researchers tried to modify the regimen in an attempt to improve efficacy and decrease toxicity.[28] Some MOPP variations including MVPP (vinblastine substituted for vincristine), CVPP (cyclophosphamide substituted for mechlorethamine), and ChlVPP (chlorambucil substituted for mechlorethamine, and vinblastine substituted for vincristine) were attractive alternatives to MOPP because they offered equal efficacy and differing or less severe toxicities.

❸ The development of ABVD by Bonnadonna et al. at the Milan Cancer Institute about a decade later represents the next important step in the evolution of therapy for Hodgkin's lymphoma (see Table 135–5). ABVD was initially shown to be effective in MOPP failures and was later compared directly to MOPP in advanced disease, where it produced an 82% complete response rate, as compared with a 67% complete response rate with MOPP. Improved failure-free survival was demonstrated with ABVD, but no significant differences in 5-year overall survival were noted.[30] Because ABVD was less toxic and provided similar or better outcomes than MOPP, it replaced MOPP as the standard regimen for advanced-stage Hodgkin's lymphoma.

In the early 1980s, the Goldie-Coldman hypothesis proposed that chemotherapy resistance was related to spontaneous mutation rates and the development of resistant clones. To test that hypothesis, researchers designed several clinical trials to evaluate the efficacy of alternating non–cross-resistant drug combinations in patients with Hodgkin's lymphoma.[31]

The initial approach investigators took was to alternate or combine the MOPP and ABVD regimens. When MOPP and ABVD (or ABV) are combined in a monthly cycle, it is referred to as a hybrid regimen. Besides a potential benefit in efficacy, another potential benefit of alternating or hybrid regimens is decreased risk of long-term toxicities. In the alternating MOPP/ABVD regimen, the cumulative doses of procarbazine and mechlorethamine are reduced by 50% and the cumulative doxorubicin dose is reduced by 50%. In the hybrid regimen the cumulative doxorubicin dose is reduced by 33% and the cumulative bleomycin dose is reduced by 50%.

Several clinical trials have been performed to evaluate the efficacy of alternating or hybrid MOPP/ABVD regimens. The results of these trials show that alternating and hybrid regimens are superior to MOPP but not to ABVD.[1,23,30] Another approach was to administer sequential cycles of MOPP and ABVD (MOPP → ABVD). Results of an intergroup trial showed sequential MOPP and ABVD to be inferior to the MOPP/ABV hybrid regimen in terms of response and survival.[32] In another randomized comparison of the MOPP/ABV hybrid regimen and ABVD, the complete remission rate, failure-free survival, and overall survival were similar between the two regimens.[33] However, that trial was closed prematurely because of an increased number of treatment-related deaths and secondary malignancies in the patients who received the MOPP/ABV hybrid regimen.

More aggressive regimens such as Stanford V and BEACOPP have been evaluated as alternatives to MOPP or ABVD. The Stanford V regimen generated significant interest because of the results of phase II trials.[23] However, a randomized controlled trial that compared the Stanford V, ABVD, and a MOPP/ABV hybrid-like regimen (MOPPEBVCAD) found the Stanford V to be inferior in terms of failure-free survival.[27] Developed by the GHSG, BEACOPP uses similar drugs as in the COPP/ABVD regimen (a combination of bleomycin, etoposide, doxorubicin, cyclophosphamide, vincristine, procarbazine, and prednisone), but rearranges the drugs in a shorter 3-week cycle. Several different versions of BEACOPP have been developed: standard-dose BEACOPP (BEACOPP baseline), higher-dose BEACOPP (BEACOPP-escalated), and dose-dense BEACOPP (BEACOPP-14).[20] Granulocyte colony-stimulating factor support is required for the BEACOPP-escalated and BEACOPP-14 regimens. A recent trial randomized 1,201 patients to COPP/ABVD (alternating), BEACOPP, or an increased-dose BEACOPP.[34] Most patients had advanced favorable disease and after chemotherapy, all patients received radiation to sites of bulky or residual disease. Freedom from treatment failure at 5 years was 69%, 76%, and 87% for COPP/ABVD, standard-dose BEACOPP, and increased-dose BEACOPP, respectively ($P < 0.001$ for comparison of increased-dose BEACOPP with the COPP/ABVD group and with the BEACOPP group). Five-year overall survival was 83%, 88%, and 91%, for COPP/ABVD, standard-dose BEA-

TABLE 135-5 Combination Chemotherapy Regimens for Hodgkin's Lymphoma

Drug	Dosage (mg/m²)	Route	Days
MOPP			
Mechlorethamine	6	IV	1, 8
Vincristine	1.4	IV	1, 8
Procarbazine	100	Oral	1–14
Prednisone	40	Oral	1–14
Repeat every 21 days			
ABVD			
Adriamycin (doxorubicin)	25	IV	1, 15
Bleomycin	10	IV	1, 15
Vinblastine	6	IV	1, 15
Dacarbazine	375	IV	1, 15
Repeat every 28 days			
MOPP/ABVD			
Alternating months of MOPP and ABVD			
MOPP/ABV hybrid			
Mechlorethamine	6	IV	1
Vincristine	1.4	IV	1
Procarbazine	100	Oral	1–7
Prednisone	40	Oral	1–14
Doxorubicin	35	IV	8
Bleomycin	10	IV	8
Vinblastine	6	IV	8
Repeat every 28 days			
Stanford V			
Doxorubicin	25	IV	Weeks 1, 3, 5, 7, 9, 11
Vinblastine	6	IV	Weeks 1, 3, 5, 7, 9, 11
Mechlorethamine	6	IV	Weeks 1, 5, 9
Etoposide	60	IV	Weeks 3, 7, 11
Vincristine	1.4[a]	IV	Weeks 2, 4, 6, 8, 10, 12
Bleomycin	5	IV	Weeks 2, 4, 6, 8
Prednisone	40	Oral	Every other day for 12 weeks; begin tapering at week 10
One course (12 weeks)			
BEACOPP (baseline)			
Bleomycin	10	IV	8
Etoposide	100	IV	1–3
Adriamycin (doxorubicin)	25	IV	1
Cyclophosphamide	650	IV	1
Oncovin (vincristine)	1.4[a]	IV	8
Procarbazine	100	Oral	1–7
Prednisone	40	Oral	1–14
Repeat every 21 days			
BEACOPP (escalated)			
Bleomycin	10	IV	8
Etoposide	200	IV	1–3
Adriamycin (doxorubicin)	35	IV	1
Cyclophosphamide	1250	IV	1
Oncovin (vincristine)	1.4[a]	IV	8
Procarbazine	100	Oral	1–7
Prednisone	40	Oral	1–14
Granulocyte colony-stimulating factor		Subcutaneously	8+
Repeat every 21 days			

[a]Vincristine dose capped at 2 mg.

COPP, and increased-dose BEACOPP, respectively ($P = 0.002$ for comparison of COPP/ABVD vs. increased-dose BEACOPP). Although most of these patients had favorable disease, patients with unfavorable disease showed an improvement in 5-year freedom from treatment failure (59%, 74%, and 82%, respectively) and overall survival (67%, 81%, and 82%, respectively), in COPP/ABVD, standard-dose BEACOPP, and increased-dose BEACOPP. Increased-dose BEACOPP appears to be the best regimen from this study, but it was also more toxic. Despite filgrastim support, 90% of patients in the increased-dose BEACOPP group had grade IV leukopenia, as compared to 19% in patients in the COPP/ABVD arm and 37% in the standard-dose BEACOPP arm. The higher rate of acute toxicity did not translate into a difference in acute treatment-related fatalities (<2% for all three regimens). The improvements in efficacy have been tempered because of a 2.5% leukemia rate at 5 years, which is higher than the 0.4% in the COPP-ABVD arm. These and other long-term complications are a major concern for patients with a good prognosis, and these more aggressive regimens have not been widely adopted.[22,23] Longer follow-up of this trial is required to determine whether the survival gain with increased-dose BEACOPP is maintained and outweighs the increased risk of long-term toxicities such as secondary malignancies.[23] Because long-term follow-up will take years, some experts recommend that these more intensive regimens be considered in patients with high-risk disease. Recently, the NCCN guidelines[15] and National Cancer Institute treatment Physician Data Query (PDQ)[35] suggest that patients with advanced-stage disease should be divided into favorable and unfavorable disease.

Risk-Adapted Therapy

Advanced-stage favorable disease patients are described based on stage and the presence of 3 or less poor prognostic factors from the international prognostic index (Table 135–4). This group of patients has about a 60% likelihood of being free from treatment failure at 5 years with traditional combination chemotherapy.[35] Patients with unfavorable disease are described based on stage and the presence of 4 or more poor prognostic factors from the international prognostic index (Table 135–4).[18] This group of patients has less than a 50% likelihood of being free from treatment failure at 5 years with traditional combination chemotherapy.[35] Because of the high treatment failure rate, the therapeutic focus for this group of patients is efficacy rather than long-term toxicity. Until recently, all advanced-stage patients were grouped together. But the current NCCN guidelines[15] and National Cancer Institute PDQ treatment statement[35] suggest that escalated-dose BEACOPP be considered for patients with unfavorable disease because of the increase in efficacy. The guidelines recommend that advanced-stage favorable disease patients be treated with ABVD because of less-acute toxicity, no sterility, and a low risk of secondary acute myeloid leukemia/myelodysplastic syndrome.[15,35]

Radiation

The role of low-dose consolidative radiation when added to chemotherapy for the treatment of advanced-stage Hodgkin's lymphoma is controversial.[23] The rationale for its use is based on the radiosensitivity of Hodgkin's lymphoma, a 20% to 40% relapse rate, and the tendency of Hodgkin's lymphoma to relapse at sites of initial involvement.[36] Many clinical trials were conducted to evaluate the benefit of additional radiation in patients who have a complete response to combination chemotherapy. The results of these studies were inconsistent, and a meta-analysis of 14 randomized trials showed a modest improvement in disease control at 10 years, but no difference in overall survival.[37] In one study, patients with advanced disease were randomized to receive either involved-field radiation after MOPP/ABV hybrid chemotherapy or no further therapy. Eight-year event-free survival has been reported for patients achieving a complete response randomized to receive radiation or no radiation and a group of partial responders who received radiation (73% vs. 77% and 76%, respectively). These results suggest that radiation provides no benefit for patients who achieve a complete remission with chemotherapy; radiation was also associated with a higher risk of secondary cancers (12.9% vs. 5.6% in the radiation and no radiation arms, respectively). It does, however, show a significant role for consolidative radiation in patients who have a partial response after chemotherapy.[38]

Summary

In summary, the standard treatment of advanced-stage favorable Hodgkin's lymphoma is six to eight cycles of ABVD chemotherapy. BEACOPP should be considered for patients with unfavorable disease. Although not yet prospectively tested, this risk-adapted approach should result in approximately 70% to >90% of patients achieving a complete remission and approximately 60% to 80% of patients being cured of their disease. No further treatment is needed for patients attaining a complete remission. Patients achieving a partial remission should receive consolidative radiation to residual sites of disease.

CLINICAL CONTROVERSY

Some clinicians believe that increased-dose BEACOPP is superior to ABVD in the treatment of patients with advanced-stage Hodgkin's lymphoma. Increased-dose BEACOPP has been shown to be superior to COPP/ABVD, which is similar to MOPP/ABVD. Other experts believe that ABVD is still the treatment of choice because increased-dose BEACOPP has not been tested directly against it. They also express concern over the long-term toxicity with increased-dose BEACOPP. This controversy will be answered with currently ongoing randomized studies and longer followup of the increased-dose BEACOPP trial.

TREATMENT OF REFRACTORY OR RELAPSED DISEASE

❹ The goal of salvage therapy is cure regardless of the site(s) of recurrence or primary therapy. With the increasing use of chemotherapy with or without radiation, regardless of disease extent, the rate of primary refractory disease is decreasing. Patients who do not achieve a complete remission with the initial regimen are considered to have primary refractory disease. These patients have a poor prognosis when treated with salvage chemotherapy, and therefore are candidates for high-dose chemotherapy and autologous HSCT.[1,22,23,39]

Patients who relapse after an initial complete response can be treated with the same regimen, a different potentially non–cross-resistant regimen, radiation, or high-dose chemotherapy and autologous HSCT (often preceded by conventional-dose chemotherapy). The response to salvage therapy depends on the extent and site of recurrence, previous therapy, and duration of initial remission. Patients who relapse after radiation therapy alone have a good chance of being cured with combination chemotherapy, although fewer patients are being treated with radiation alone. Other patient groups who have a favorable prognosis following salvage therapy include patients who experience a local recurrence in a nonirradiated location and those who relapse more than 1 year after completion of their initial chemotherapy. Patients who experience late relapses can be cured with retreatment with the same chemotherapy regimen, treatment with a different, potentially non–cross-resistant regimen, or high-dose chemotherapy and autologous HSCT. The National Cancer Institute has reported on its long-term followup of MOPP-retreated patients. Patients with long initial remissions had a 45% disease-free survival rate at 10 years.[40]

Patients who have an early relapse (less than 1 year after treatment) generally respond poorly to standard-dose salvage chemotherapy, with cure occurring in less than 20% of patients. High-dose chemotherapy and autologous HSCT is more effective, but also produces a higher risk of treatment-related mortality. The choice of salvage treatment should therefore consider the patient's tolerance for a particular set of chemotherapeutic agents and treatment approach (standard-dose chemotherapy vs. high-dose chemotherapy and autologous HSCT).[23]

High-dose therapy should be considered in patients who relapse within 12 months of initial remission and in those who are refractory to first-line chemotherapy.[23] Although no one preparative regimen has been shown to be superior to another, most regimens do not include total-body irradiation because of its potential pulmonary toxicity. Most patients are already at higher risk for pulmonary toxicity because of previous exposure to one or more of the following: bleomycin, thoracic radiation, and nitrosoureas. High-dose chemotherapy with autologous HSCT produces long-term progression-free survival rates in patients with refractory and relapsed disease.[23] A recent study on the efficacy of HSCT for relapsed or recurrent Hodgkin's lymphoma reported 5- and 10-year overall survival rates of 53% and 47%, respectively. They also identified three factors that predicted progression-free survival: chemoresistant disease, residual disease at transplant, and B symptoms at pretransplant relapse. Patients with zero or one risk factor had a 5-year progression-free survival of 67%, those with two risk factors had a 37% progression-free survival, and those with all three risk factors only had a 9% progression-free survival rate.[39] Chapter 142 provides more details about high-dose chemotherapy and HSCT.

LONG-TERM COMPLICATIONS

A variety of acute and chronic toxicities may occur as a result of treatment for Hodgkin's lymphoma. Long-term complications of radiation therapy, chemotherapy, and combined modality therapy have become more evident as the curability and long-term survival of Hodgkin's lymphoma patients has improved.[19,23] Gonadal dysfunction, secondary malignancies, and cardiac disease have become important considerations in the treatment of this malignancy. Almost all men and up to 50% of premenopausal women treated with six cycles of regimens containing alkylating agents become sterile. This appears to be a dose-related phenomenon. For men, even a single dose of nitrogen mustard or chlorambucil can cause sterility, so if fertility is a major concern, ABVD may be the best alternative.[41]

Now that 10-, 15-, and 20-year survival data are available, evaluation of secondary malignancies can be made. Recent reports show that after treatment for Hodgkin's lymphoma, the relative risk for secondary cancers is increased by about threefold. The risk of developing leukemia carries the highest increase in risk and is seen with radiotherapy, chemotherapy, and chemoradiotherapy. Radiotherapy alone increases the risk modestly, while multimodality therapy increases the risk the most (relative risk = 31.6). The incidence of solid tumors, most commonly gastrointestinal tumors, lung cancer, and breast cancer is also increased. The risk of gastrointestinal tumors is increased the greatest (relative risk = 3.3) by chemoradiotherapy, the risk of lung cancer was also increased with all treatment modalities, with the highest being from chemoradiotherapy (relative risk = 4.3), while the breast cancer risk is increased only after radiotherapy (relative risk = 2.5). The increase in relative risk varies with age and type of treatment. The risks are the highest for patients who are younger than age 25 years at the time of treatment.[42] The relative risk also varies with specific therapies; for example patients who receive MOPP or increased-dose BEACOPP therapy appear to have a higher risk of secondary acute leukemia as compared with ABVD.[23]

Although chemoradiotherapy is associated with a higher risk of secondary malignancies, a meta-analysis of 37 randomized trials showed that its use as first-line therapy in patients with early-stage Hodgkin's lymphoma may actually be associated with a *lower* risk of secondary malignancies as compared with radiotherapy alone (odds ratio = 0.78) by reducing relapse and need for salvage therapy.[43] However, first-line chemoradiotherapy was associated with a higher risk of secondary malignancies as compared with chemotherapy alone (odds ratio = 1.38) in patients with Hodgkin's lymphoma, most of whom had advanced-stage disease.

NON-HODGKIN'S LYMPHOMA

The NHLs are a heterogeneous group of lymphoproliferative disorders that affect individuals from early childhood to late adulthood. Advances in molecular biology techniques and our understanding of the human immune system have led to major progress in understanding the pathogenesis and treatment of the lymphomas. NHLs are classified into distinct clinical entities that are defined by a combination of morphology, immunophenotype, genetic features, and clinical features. These differences influence the natural history, and approach and response to treatment. The use of extensive combination chemotherapeutic regimens shows dramatic improvement in survival and cure in patients with a disease that once was considered incurable. The 5-year survival rate for patients with NHL has increased from 48% to 64% over the past 25 years, and the mortality rate actually *declined* from 1997 to 2004.[5,6] Further improvement in survival is anticipated with the continued expansion of our therapeutic armamentarium, including high-dose chemotherapy and biologic therapy.

EPIDEMIOLOGY AND ETIOLOGY

NHL is the fifth most common cause of newly diagnosed cancer in the United States and accounts for approximately 4% of all cancers. An estimated 63,190 new cases will be diagnosed in 2007, and it is estimated that 18,660 people will die from NHL during this same period.[5] Although the average age of patients at the time of diagnosis is about 67 years, NHL can occur at any age. The incidence rate generally increases with age, and is higher in men than in women and in whites than in blacks.[6] The age-adjusted incidence rate of NHL increased by more than 80% in the United States since the early 1970s, from about 11 cases per 100,000 in 1975 to nearly 20 cases per 100,000 in 2003 and 2004.[6] The incidence of NHL increased by 3% to 4% from 1975 to 1991, but appears to have stabilized since reaching its peak in 1994. The increase in the incidence of NHL over the past three decades is second only to melanoma and has been referred to as an epidemic of NHL. Although the increased incidence has been particularly noted among the elderly and patients with acquired immune deficiency syndrome (AIDS), much of this increase cannot be explained by known risk factors.

The etiology of NHL is unknown, although several genetic diseases, environmental agents, and infectious agents are associated with the development of NHL.[44–46] An increased incidence of NHL is seen in many congenital and acquired immunodeficiency states, supporting the role of immune dysregulation in the etiology of NHL. Patients with congenital immunodeficiency disorders such as Wiskott-Aldrich syndrome, ataxia, and telangiectasia; acquired immunodeficiency disorders such as AIDS, acquired hypogammaglobulinemia, and graft-versus-host disease; and those receiving chronic pharmacologic immunosuppression in the setting of solid-organ transplantation are predisposed to the development of NHL. Autoimmune diseases (Hashimoto thyroiditis, Sjögren's syndrome) cause chronic inflammation in the mucosa-associated lymphoid tissue (MALT), which predisposes patients to subsequent lymphoid malignancies. Other autoimmune diseases, such as systemic lupus erythematosus and rheumatoid arthritis, are also associated with the development of NHL, but the use of immunosuppressive agents in these diseases makes the pathologic cause less clear.

Certain infections are associated with the development of lymphoma.[44–46] EBV was discovered in cell lines from tumors of patients with African (endemic) Burkitt's lymphoma, and EBV DNA is associated with nearly all cases of endemic Burkitt's lymphoma. However, EBV is associated with sporadic Burkitt's lymphoma in only approximately 20% to 30% of cases. EBV is also associated with posttransplant lymphoproliferative disorders and some lymphomas in patients with AIDS or congenital immunodeficiencies. The human T-cell lymphotropic virus type 1 was the first human retrovirus associated with a malignancy. Infection with human T-cell lymphotropic virus type 1, especially in early childhood, is strongly associated with an aggressive form of T-cell lymphoma, known as adult T-cell leukemia/lymphoma. Human T-cell lymphotropic virus type 1 is endemic in southern Japan, Africa, and the Caribbean. In endemic areas, more than 50% of all NHL cases are adult T-cell leukemia/lymphoma. A third virus associated with NHL is human herpes virus 8. This virus was originally isolated from Kaposi's sarcoma lesions in AIDS patients. Finally, gastric infection with

Helicobacter pylori, a gram-negative bacteria that leads to chronic gastritis, is associated with gastric MALT lymphomas.

A number of physical agents are also associated with the development of NHL.[44–46] Exposure to herbicides, particularly phenoxyl herbicides, is associated with the development of NHL. These observations may explain why certain occupations, such as farmers, forestry workers, and agricultural workers, are associated with a higher risk of NHL. Exposure to lawn-care pesticides is also increasing in the general population. A higher risk of NHL is also associated with exposure to other chemical solvents and dyes, exposure to radiation from nuclear explosions, and high intake of meats and dietary fats. Smoking or alcohol consumption is not strongly associated with an increased risk of NHL.

MOLECULAR ABNORMALITIES

Chromosomal translocations have become a hallmark of many lymphoid malignancies.[47,48] The presence of these specific translocations can be helpful in the diagnosis and classification of lymphoid malignancies. The mechanisms leading to the translocations are unknown, but they usually involve the antigen receptor loci. In contrast to most myeloid and some lymphoid leukemias, NHLs usually place a structurally intact cellular protooncogene under the regulatory influence of highly expressed immunoglobulin or T-cell receptor genes, leading to effects on cell growth, cellular differentiation, or apoptosis. The most common chromosomal translocations involve t(8;14), t(14;18), and t(11;14); each translocation involves the immunoglobulin heavy-chain gene locus on chromosome 14 at 14q32. The translocation t(8;14) that involves c-*MYC*, a well-characterized oncogene clearly associated with malignancy, is implicated in nearly all cases of Burkitt's lymphoma. The translocation t(14;18) that involves *BCL*-2, one of several putative B-cell lymphoma-associated oncogenes, is found in approximately 90% of follicular B-cell lymphomas. The translocation t(11;14) that involves *BCL*-1, is found in most patients with mantle cell lymphoma. Another putative B-cell lymphoma-associated oncogene, *BCL*-6, is found in about a third of diffuse large B-cell lymphomas.

Although mutations in the *p53* tumor suppressor gene have been recognized in many human neoplasms, such mutations have not been consistently found in patients with lymphoma, which suggests that it may occur late in malignant evolution.

Detection of oncogenes, such as *BCL*-2 in follicular lymphomas, can be used clinically to monitor for minimal residual disease. In patients with follicular lymphoma who received monoclonal antibody-purged autologous bone marrow transplantation, those whose bone marrow was negative by polymerase chain reaction for the *BCL*-2 rearrangement after purging had significantly longer freedom from recurrence than those whose bone marrow remained polymerase chain reaction-positive.[49]

Because of their role in the pathogenesis of lymphoma, oncogenes are attractive molecular targets for the development of new and novel therapies.[50]

PATHOLOGY AND CLASSIFICATION

NHLs are neoplasms derived from the monoclonal proliferation of malignant B or T lymphocytes and their precursors. Approximately 85% of NHLs in the United States are of B-cell origin. Proliferation of malignant cells results in the replacement of the normal cells and architecture of lymph nodes or bone marrow with a relatively uniform population of lymphoid cells. The classification of NHLs has evolved over the last five decades, as advances in immunology and genetics have allowed scientists to recognize a number of previously unrecognized subtypes of NHLs (Table 135–6).[46,51] The current classification schemes characterize the NHLs according to the cell of origin (B cell vs. T cell), clinical features, and morphologic features. Additional immunohistochemical markers, cytogenetic features, and genotypic characteristics may also be of help to further classify NHL into subtypes.

TABLE 135-6 Evolution in the Classification of Non-Hodgkin's Lymphomas

Time	Classification System	Basis for Classification
1950s–1960s	Rappaport	Morphology
1970s–1980s	Luke-Collins	Morphology and immunophenotype
1970s–1980s	Kiel	Morphology and immunophenotype
1980s–1990s	International Working Formulation	Morphology and clinical behavior
1990s	REAL	Disease entities
2001	WHO	Disease entities

REAL, Revised European-American Classification of Lymphoid Neoplasms developed by the International Lymphoma Study Group; WHO, World Health Organization.

Morphology

The macroscopic and microscopic appearance of the involved tissue remains one of the most important factors in the diagnosis and classification of NHLs. In the 1950s, Rappaport et al. proposed a morphologic classification of malignant lymphomas based on two features: (a) that the malignant cell would disrupt the nodal architecture in a *nodular* or *diffuse* manner, and (b) that lymphomas of histiocytic origin existed. The Rappaport classification gained rapid acceptance in the United States because of its precision, simplicity, and prognostic significance. Application of the system divided NHLs into those with large (i.e., incorrectly called "histiocytes") or small cells, with or without a nodular (i.e., follicular) growth pattern.

Immunology

In the 1970s, it became apparent that NHLs were tumors of the immune system and were derived from B or T lymphocytes. The availability of techniques using antibodies to antigens on the surface of lymphoid cells (i.e., immunophenotype) and cytochemical assays led to the following conclusions: (a) most NHLs were of B-cell origin; (b) all follicular or nodular lymphomas were of follicle center cell origin; and (c) most lymphomas previously classified as reticulum cell sarcoma, clasmatocytic lymphoma, or histiocytic lymphoma had the immunologic characteristics of transformed lymphocytes. Using this new information, expert pathologists independently developed new classification schemes for NHL in the 1970s and 1980s.[46,51] The Kiel classification was based primarily on the work of Lennert and became widely used in Europe. In North America, the Lukes and Collins classification scheme was used briefly, but was soon superseded by the Working Formulation. Like the Rappaport classification, divisions within the Working Formulation were based largely on cell size (large ["histiocytic"] vs. small [lymphocytic]), cell shape (round vs. not round), and growth pattern (follicular [nodular] vs. diffuse). Both the Kiel and Working Formulation classification schemes also considered the histologic grade of the tumor, but only the Working Formulation considered actual survival curves of patients with the various subtypes of NHL. "Low-grade" indicated longer median survival (i.e., indolent) whereas "intermediate-grade" and "high-grade" indicated shorter median survival (i.e., aggressive). In the 1980s and early 1990s, the Working Formulation became the most widely used classification scheme in North America, whereas the Kiel classification was widely used in Europe.[51] It was based on the premise that NHL was a single disease with a range of histologic grade and clinical aggressiveness.

New Disease Entities

In the 1980s and early 1990s, rapid advances in immunology and genetics allowed scientists to recognize a number of previously unrecognized subtypes of NHLs. Cytogenetic and molecular genetic analyses identified the presence of many chromosomal translocations, oncogenes, and their gene products in patients with NHL (see Molecular Abnormalities section). In addition, diseases that would have been lumped together as "low-grade" or "intermediate/high grade" in the Working Formulation showed marked differences in survival, which prompted scientists to reevaluate lymphoma classification schemes.

Information from these studies allowed scientists to further classify B-cell lymphomas as malignant expansions of cells from either the germinal center, mantle zone, or marginal zone of normal lymph nodes (see Table 135–1).[48,52] Germinal centers are complex structures that form in spleen and lymph nodes in response to antigenic challenge. In addition to B cells, germinal centers contain antigen-presenting cells and helper T cells that cooperate in mediating the B-cell changes that result in a more potent secondary immune response. Malignant transformation often occurs or is initiated in germinal center B cells. Follicular, Burkitt's, and most large cell lymphomas are believed to be tumors of germinal center B cells. Three histologically distinct microenvironments have been described within the germinal center: a mantle zone surrounding interior dark, and light zones. The mantle zone contains small resting B cells that have not been exposed to antigen ("naive"). Tumors of cells from the mantle zone are usually clinically indolent and histologically low grade. Antigen-triggered activation of the densely packed B cells of the dark zone causes cells to proliferate and subjects genomic DNA to somatic hypermutation. Surviving clones from within the dark zone then enter the light zone where proliferation slows and affinity selection occurs. During affinity selection, only cells with surface immunoglobulin receptors with high affinity for the antigen survive. Antigen-specific B cells generated in the germinal center reaction leave the follicle and reappear in the outer mantle zone, to form a marginal zone. Marginal zones are particularly prominent in mesenteric lymph nodes, Peyer patches, and the spleen. These postgerminal center B cells include memory B cells of the marginal zone and plasma cells. Marginal cell B-cell lymphomas tend to be indolent and may be either extranodal or nodal; extranodal marginal cell B-cell lymphomas are also referred to as MALT lymphomas.

T-cell lymphomas can be classified on the basis of antigen expression as either precursor (thymic) or mature (peripheral) in origin. These classifications clinically translate to precursor lymphoblastic lymphomas or to a heterogeneous group of peripheral T-cell lymphomas. Tumors of natural killer or natural killer-like T cells are uncommon.

The International Lymphoma Study Group, an informal group of 19 hematopathologists from the United States, Europe, and Asia, adopted a new approach to lymphoma classification in 1993. Because it represented a revision of current or prior European and American lymphoma classifications, it was called the Revised European-American Classification of Lymphoid Neoplasms (REAL). The REAL classification system is based on the principle that a classification is a list of "real" disease entities, which are defined by a combination of morphology, immunophenotype, genetic features, and clinical features.[51,53] The relative importance of each of these criteria for both definition and diagnosis differs among different diseases. Morphology is always important, and some diseases are primarily defined by morphology alone (e.g., follicular lymphoma), although immunophenotype can be helpful in difficult cases. Some diseases have a specific immunophenotype (e.g., mantle cell lymphoma, small lymphocytic lymphoma) that is virtually diagnostic of that disease. A specific genetic abnormality is important in some lymphomas—t(11;14) in mantle cell lymphoma, t(8;14) in Burkitt's lymphoma, and t(14;18) in follicular lymphoma—whereas other lymphomas lack specific genetic abnormalities (e.g., MALT lymphoma, diffuse large B-cell lymphoma). Finally, other lymphomas consider clinical features (e.g., extranodal vs. nodal presentation in marginal zone lymphoma and peripheral T-cell lymphoma). A recent retrospective study of the REAL classification confirmed the clinical relevance of this approach.[54]

Since 1995, members of the European and American Hematopathology societies have worked to develop a new WHO classification of hematologic malignancies. The final classification was published in 2001.[13] The WHO classification uses an updated version of the REAL classification and expands the principles of the REAL classification to the classification of myeloid and histiocytic malignancies.

❺ The WHO classification categorizes lymphoid malignancies into three major categories: B-cell lymphomas, T-cell (and putative natural killer cell) lymphomas, and Hodgkin's lymphoma (see Table 135–2).[51,53] Within the B-cell and T-cell neoplasm category there are two major categories: "precursor" neoplasms, which correspond to the earliest stages of differentiation (lymphoblastic), and "peripheral" neoplasms, which correspond to the more differentiated B- and T-cell stages. The WHO classification uses the term *grade* to refer to histologic parameters such as cell and nuclear size, density of chromatin, and proliferation fraction, and the term *aggressiveness* to denote clinical behavior of a tumor. This classification scheme includes both lymphomas and lymphoid leukemias because there is no distinction between the solid and circulating forms of these diseases. The WHO classification includes several previously unrecognized types of lymphomas, including mantle cell lymphoma, monocytoid B-cell lymphoma, extranodal lymphoma of MALT, splenic marginal zone lymphoma, primary mediastinal large B-cell lymphoma, and a variety of T-cell lymphomas. New entities not specifically recognized in the Working Formulation account for approximately 20% to 25% of the cases.

The WHO classification has broad clinical implications. The WHO Clinical Advisory Committee has agreed that clinical groupings of lymphoid neoplasms into prognostic categories are neither necessary nor desirable because such arbitrary groupings are of no practical value and may be misleading.[55] Treatment of a specific patient should be determined not by the broad prognostic group into which the patient's neoplasm falls but by the specific type of neoplasm, with the addition of grade *within* the tumor type (if applicable), and clinical prognostic factors.

CLINICAL PRESENTATION

❻ Patients with NHL present with a wide variety of symptoms, depending on the site of involvement and whether tumor involvement is nodal or extranodal.[56] Sites of involvement and dissemination of the malignant cells can sometimes be predicted based on the cell of origin and the tendency of tumors to frequently disseminate to areas where the normal counterparts of the lymphoma cells are located. For example, B-cell lymphomas involve areas of the lymphoid system normally populated by B-lymphocytes, such as lymph nodes, spleen, and bone marrow. T-cell lymphomas commonly disseminate to various extranodal sites, such as the skin and lungs.

PRESENTATION OF NON-HODGKIN'S LYMPHOMA

General

- Patients with NHL present with a wide variety of symptoms, depending on the site of involvement and whether tumor involvement is nodal or extranodal

Symptoms

- Approximately 40% of patients present with fever, night sweats, and weight loss (i.e., B symptoms)
- Fatigue, malaise, and pruritus

Signs

- More than two-thirds of patients present with peripheral lymphadenopathy

Laboratory Tests

- A complete blood count, tests of renal and liver function, and serum electrolytes should be obtained
- Serum β_2-microglobulin and lactate dehydrogenase levels may be useful as prognostic factors and for monitoring response to therapy

Other Diagnostic Tests

- Varies depending on sites of involvement

Most patients present with peripheral lymphadenopathy. The lymphadenopathy may be either localized or generalized, and the involved nodes are often painless, rubbery, and discrete, and usually located in the cervical and supraclavicular regions as in Hodgkin's lymphoma (see Fig. 135–1). Rapid and progressive lymphadenopathy is more characteristic of aggressive lymphomas. Waxing and waning of lymph nodes, including their complete disappearance and reappearance, is more characteristic of indolent lymphomas. Massive lymphadenopathy can sometimes lead to organ dysfunction. For example, patients with NHL may present with acute renal failure from retroperitoneal adenopathy causing ureteral obstruction or from metabolic abnormalities such as hyperuricemia with uric acid nephropathy.

Approximately 40% of patients with NHL present with fever (temperature >38°C [100.4°F]), weight loss (unexplained weight loss of 10% of body weight over the past 6 months), or night sweats (drenching night sweats). If one of more of these symptoms is present, the patient is noted to have B symptoms, and a B is added to the stage of disease (discussed in Diagnosis, Staging, and Prognostic Factors section in Hodgkin's Lymphoma). B symptoms are more commonly observed in patients with aggressive NHLs.

Patients with Hodgkin's lymphoma rarely present with extranodal (i.e., extralymphatic) disease, but 10% to 35% of patients with NHL have primary extranodal disease at the time of diagnosis.[56] The frequency of extranodal presentation varies dramatically among different subtypes. The most common extranodal sites are the gastrointestinal tract followed by the skin. The liver or spleen may be enlarged in patients with generalized adenopathy. Patients with mesenteric or gastrointestinal involvement may present with signs and symptoms of nausea, vomiting, obstruction, abdominal pain, a palpable abdominal mass, or gastrointestinal bleeding. Patients with bone marrow involvement may have symptoms related to anemia, neutropenia, or thrombocytopenia. Other sites of extranodal disease include the testes and bone. The incidence of solitary brain lymphoma is increasing, especially in patients with AIDS.

DIAGNOSIS, STAGING, AND PROGNOSTIC FACTORS

As with Hodgkin's lymphoma, the diagnosis of NHL must be established by pathologic review of tissue obtained by biopsy.[56] The preferred procedure is an excisional biopsy, where the entire involved lymph node is removed for review by an experienced hematopathologist. This procedure should be done carefully to prevent distortional artifact of the architecture, which could lead to an inaccurate diagnosis. Needle biopsy of the node can sometimes provide adequate tissue for pathologic diagnosis, if an excisional biopsy cannot be performed. When adenopathy is not present, diagnosis may be established by biopsy of cutaneous lesions, bone marrow biopsy and aspiration in patients with unexplained myelosuppression, liver biopsy in patients with hepatomegaly or elevated liver function transaminases, or biopsy of involved extranodal organs, such as bone, Waldeyer ring, lung, and testis.

After the diagnosis is established, further workup is required to determine the extent of involvement.[46,56,57] Clinical staging always begins with a thorough history and physical examination. Patients should be questioned about the presence or absence and extent of fever, night sweats, and weight loss. A detailed history of lymphadenopathy should also be obtained, including when and where the lymph nodes were first noted, and their rate of growth. A complete physical examination is performed to assess the extent of disease involvement, with special attention given to all nodal areas (see Fig. 135–1). All patients should have a complete blood count, serum chemistries including liver and renal profiles, a chest radiograph, and bone marrow aspiration and biopsy. The likelihood of bone marrow involvement varies among the different histologic types of lymphoma (Table 135–7). Lumbar puncture to evaluate the cerebrospinal fluid is recommended in patients who have histologic types of lymphoma that often spread to the CNS.

Imaging studies are usually important in the staging workup.[56,57] CT scanning can identify both nodal and extranodal sites of disease, and has largely replaced lymphangiography for the evaluation of retroperitoneal lymphadenopathy. The abdominal and pelvic CT

TABLE 135-7 Clinical Characterstics of Patients with Common Types of Non-Hodgkin's Lymphomas

Disease	Median Age (Years)	Frequency in Children	% Male	Stage I/II vs. III/IV (%)	B Symptoms (%)	Bone Marrow Involvement (%)	Gastrointestinal Tract Involvement (%)	% Surviving 5 years
B-cell chronic lymphocytic leukemia/small lymphocytic lymphoma	65	Rare	53	9 vs. 91	33	72	3	51
Mantle cell lymphoma	63	Rare	74	20 vs. 80	28	64	9	27
Extranodal marginal zone B-cell lymphoma of MALT type	60	Rare	48	67 vs. 33	19	14	50	74
Follicular lymphoma	59	Rare	42	33 vs. 67	28	42	4	72
Diffuse large B-cell lymphoma	64	≈25% of childhood NHL	55	54 vs. 46	33	16	18	46
Burkitt's lymphoma	31	≈30% of childhood NHL	89	62 vs. 38	22	33	11	45
Precursor T-cell lymphoblastic lymphoma	28	≈40% of childhood NHL	64	11 vs. 89	21	50	4	26
Anaplastic large T-/null cell lymphoma	34	Common	69	51 vs. 49	53	13	9	77
Peripheral T-cell non-Hodgkin's lymphoma	61	≈5% of childhood NHL	55	20 vs. 80	50	36	15	25

MALT, mucosa-associated lymphoid tissue; NHL, non-Hodgkin's lymphoma

From Kasper DL, Braunwald E, Fauci AS, et al. eds. Harrison's Principles of Internal Medicine. 16th ed. New York: McGraw-Hill,2005:648.

scan can identify mesenteric and retrocrural node involvement. CT scans can also detect tumor involvement of organs, including the kidneys, ovary, spleen, and liver. PET is strongly recommended in patients with potentially curable aggressive NHLs, but it is expensive and not available at all centers.[58] Magnetic resonance imaging is of limited usefulness in the staging of NHL. Gallium scans are sometimes used as part of the staging work up. Other tests, such as liver–spleen scan, bone scan, upper gastrointestinal series, and intravenous pyelogram, are sometimes useful in patients with organ symptomatology or serum chemistry abnormalities.

Although staging laparotomy was widely used in the late 1960s and 1970s as part of the staging workup in patients with lymphoma, it is rarely used today because of technical improvements in imaging studies and the morbidity and potential mortality associated with the procedure.

The Ann Arbor staging classification developed for the clinical staging of Hodgkin's lymphoma is also used to stage patients with NHL (see Table 135–3). After completion of the staging workup, most patients will be found to have advanced disease (stages III and IV). The frequency of localized disease at the time of diagnosis varies depending on the histologic type of lymphoma (see Table 135–7). Stage is a more important prognostic factor in Hodgkin's lymphoma than in NHL.

❼ The Ann Arbor system emphasizes the distribution of nodal disease sites because Hodgkin's lymphoma usually spreads through contiguous lymph nodes and does not involve extranodal sites. But NHL is a disease with tremendous heterogeneity that does not spread through contiguous lymph nodes and that often involves extranodal sites. As a result of these clinical differences between Hodgkin's lymphoma and NHL, Ann Arbor stage correlates poorly with prognosis.

❽ This lack of accuracy with the Ann Arbor staging system in NHL has led to several international projects to develop prognostic models for the most common types of NHLs—diffuse large B-cell lymphomas and follicular lymphomas. The International Non-Hodgkin's Lymphoma Prognostic Factors Project was based on more than 2,000 patients with diffuse aggressive lymphomas treated with an anthracycline-containing combination chemotherapy regimen in the United States, Europe, and Canada.[59] The Project identified five risk factors that correlated with low response to chemotherapy and poor survival: (a) age >60 years, (b) reduced performance status ≥2, (c) abnormal serum lactate dehydrogenase (LDH) levels, (d) two or more extranodal sites of disease, and (e) advanced tumor stage (Ann Arbor stages III or IV; Table 135–8). In patients ≤60 years old, three risk factors correlated with low response to chemotherapy and poor survival: (a) reduced performance status, (b) abnormal serum LDH levels, and (c) Ann Arbor stage. It is unclear whether the effect of serum LDH level is related to a tumor or a host event. LDH likely measures cellular catabolism (the enzyme is released from injured cells), or the product of tumor burden and proliferation. Because each of the factors has about the same impact (e.g., relative risk) on prognosis, the number of adverse risk factors is summed to provide the IPI. Patients could, therefore, have a score of 0 to 5. Table 135–8 shows the correlation between four risk groups based on the IPI score and complete response rate and 5-year survival. For patients ≤60 years old, a simplified IPI score can be developed based on Ann Arbor stage, serum LDH, and performance status.

As prognosis improves as a result of more effective therapy, it is important to reevaluate prognostic factors. The IPI was based on patients treated from 1982 to 1987 with anthracycline-based combination chemotherapy; none of the patients received rituximab. In a reexamination of the IPI in a cohort of patients treated with rituximab-containing chemotherapy, Sehn et al. found that the IPI remained predictive but it only identified two, rather than four, risk groups.[60] When the number of risk factors is redistributed, three risk groups are identified that correlate with prognosis. This revised IPI score may more accurately predict prognosis in patients treated with rituximab-containing combination chemotherapy, but needs to be validated in a larger group of patients.

TABLE 135-8 Risk Factors and Survival According to the International Non-Hodgkin's Lymphoma Prognostic Factors Project

All Patients	Patients ≤60 Years of Age
Age >60 years of age	LDH > normal
LDH > normal	Performance status ≥2
Performance status ≥2	Ann Arbor stage III or IV
Ann Arbor stage III or IV	
Extranodal involvement ≥2 sites	

Risk Group	Number of Risk Factors	Complete Response Rate (%)	5-Year Survival Rate (%)
Patients of all ages (% of patients)			
Low (35)	0, 1	87	73
Low intermediate (27)	2	67	51
High intermediate (22)	3	55	43
High (16)	4, 5	44	26
Patients ≤60 years of age (% of patients)			
Low (22)	0	92	83
Low intermediate (32)	1	78	69
High intermediate (32)	2	57	46
High (14)	3	46	32

LDH, lactic dehydrogenase.

Data from The International Non-Hodgkin's Lymphoma Prognostic Factors Project. A predictive model for aggressive non-Hodgkin's lymphoma. N Engl J Med 1993;329:987–994. Copyright © 1993 Massachusetts Medical Society.

Although the IPI is often used to predict prognosis in patients with other NHL subtypes, the IPI has several shortcomings when applied to patients with indolent lymphomas. Because only patients with diffuse aggressive lymphomas were used to develop the IPI system, some important prognostic factors may have been missed. Furthermore, the IPI system has limited discriminating power in follicular lymphoma because only approximately 10% of patients are categorized as high-risk in the IPI system. To address these concerns, an international cooperative study was designed to develop a prognostic model similar to the IPI in patients with follicular lymphoma. The results of that study, which was based on more than 4,000 patients with follicular lymphoma diagnosed between 1985 and 1992, was recently published.[61] Five factors were identified that correlated with poor survival: (a) age >60 years, (b) advanced tumor stage (Ann Arbor stage III or IV), (c) low hemoglobin level (<12 g/dL), (d) five or more nodal sites of disease (see Fig. 135–1), and (e) an abnormal serum LDH level. Analogous to the IPI, the number of adverse risk factors is summed to provide the Follicular Lymphoma International Prognostic Index (FLIPI). Three prognostic groups were identified: low-risk (0 to 1 factors), intermediate-risk (2 factors), and high-risk (≥3 factors). The new system appeared to have higher discriminating power among groups as compared with the IPI system. Table 135–9 shows the correlation between the FLIPI score and overall survival.

Although IPI and FLIPI are clinically useful tools to estimate prognosis, the factors used to calculate these scores probably represent clinical surrogates for the biologic heterogeneity among NHLs and many researchers are interested in determining the prognostic importance of certain phenotypic and molecular characteristics of NHLs. For example, markers of apoptosis, cell-cycle regulation, cell lineage, and cell proliferation are being evaluated as potentially clinically useful prognostic factors.[62] Gene expression profiling with microarrays may also correlate with survival. Using gene expression profiling, investigators identified at least two molecularly distinct

TABLE 135-9 Risk Factors and Survival According to the Follicular Lymphoma International Prognostic Index

All patients
Age >60 years of age
Ann Arbor stage III or IV
Number of nodal sites ≥5
Abnormal lactate dehydrogenase level
Hemoglobin <12 g/dL

Risk Group (% of Patients)	Number of Risk Factors	5-Year Overall Survival (%)	10-Year Overall Survival (%)
Low (36)	0–1	91	71
Intermediate (37)	2	78	51
High (27)	≥	53	36

Adapted from reference 61.

forms of diffuse aggressive lymphomas based on gene expression patterns indicative of different stages of B-cell differentiation: germinal center B-cell and activated peripheral blood B-cell.[63] Patients with the germinal center B-cell profile had significantly better overall survival independent of IPI score after treatment with CHOP (cyclophosphamide, hydroxydaunorubicin, Oncovin, prednisone) or CHOP-like chemotherapy. The investigators used 17 genes to construct a model that correlated with overall survival after chemotherapy. In another study of diffuse aggressive lymphomas, investigators were able to develop a predictive model based on only six genes.[64] Two molecularly distinct profiles of follicular lymphoma also have been identified; the first included genes encoding for T-cell markers and genes highly expressed in macrophages, and the second included genes that are preferentially expressed in macrophages, dendritic cells, or both.[65] Patients with the first molecular signature had a more favorable outcome than those with the second signature. These results suggest that molecular classification of tumors on the basis of gene expression may allow identification of clinically significant subtypes of cancer.

TREATMENT

Non-Hodgkin's Lymphoma

■ GENERAL TREATMENT PRINCIPLES

The primary goals in the treatment of NHL are to relieve symptoms, cure the patient of their disease whenever possible, and minimize the risk of serious toxicities. The treatment strategy depends on many factors, including patient's age, concomitant disease, disease type, stage of disease, site of disease, and patient preference.

❾ Historically, both the clinical behavior and degree of aggressiveness are often used to describe NHLs. Indolent lymphomas, which make up approximately 25% to 40% of all NHLs, are characterized by their slow-growth behavior. Patients with an indolent lymphoma usually have a relatively long survival (measured in years), with or without aggressive chemotherapy. Although these lymphomas respond to a wide range of therapeutic approaches, there is no convincing evidence of a survival plateau, which indicates that patients are rarely cured of their disease. In contrast, aggressive lymphomas, which make up approximately 60% to 75% of all NHLs, are characterized by rapid growth rate and short survival (measured in weeks to months), if appropriate therapy is not initiated. Despite their more aggressive nature, many patients with aggressive lymphomas who respond to chemotherapy can experience prolonged disease-free survival and some are cured of their disease. Therefore, the terminology for the NHLs represents a paradox, where "indolent" is bad and "aggressive" is good in terms of the likelihood for cure.

Therapeutic approaches to NHL include radiation therapy, chemotherapy, and biologic agents.[46] The role of radiation therapy in the treatment of NHL differs from its role in the treatment of Hodgkin's lymphoma. Although the disease responds to radiation therapy, only a small percentage of patients with NHL present with truly localized disease that can be treated with local or regional radiation therapy. Radiation therapy is used more commonly in advanced disease, primarily as a palliative measure to control local bulky disease.

Effective chemotherapy for NHL ranges from single-agent therapy in indolent lymphomas to aggressive, complex chemotherapy regimens in aggressive lymphomas. The most active agents used in the treatment of NHL include the alkylating agents (e.g., cyclophosphamide, chlorambucil), bleomycin, doxorubicin, purine analogs, etoposide, methotrexate, vincristine, and corticosteroids (e.g., prednisone, dexamethasone). The most aggressive chemotherapy approaches are dose-dense chemotherapy or high-dose chemotherapy followed by autologous or allogeneic HSCT.

B-cell lymphomas have served as a model for immunotherapy with monoclonal antibodies for more than 20 years, beginning with the successful use of custom-made monoclonal antibodies targeted against the idiotype present on the patient's cancer cells.[66] These encouraging results lead to the development of monoclonal antibodies against a more "generic" target, a molecule on the surface of B cells that would be present on tumor cells.[66] One potential target, the CD20 molecule, is present only on cells in the B-lymphocyte lineage. It is expressed on the surface of both normal and malignant B cells, but not on other normal tissues. Rituximab (Rituxan) is a chimeric monoclonal antibody directed at the CD20 molecule.[66] Since rituximab was approved in November 1997 to treat relapsed or refractory indolent or follicular $CD20^+$ lymphomas, it has become one of the most widely used therapies for NHL. More recently, two radiolabeled monoclonal antibodies (i.e., radioimmunoconjugates) targeted against the CD20 antigen were approved. With the availability of monoclonal antibodies and radioimmunoconjugates for the therapy of lymphoma, nearly all patients with NHL will receive one or more biologic agents during the course of their disease.

Objective response to therapy for NHL should be defined according to the International Workshop to Standardize Response Criteria for Non-Hodgkin's Lymphoma, which was recently updated to incorporate the results of newer tests to monitor response such as PET, immunohistochemistry, and flow cytometry.[58] The revised guidelines describe criteria for response (e.g., complete response, partial response, and stable disease) and survival (e.g., overall, disease-free, event-free, progression-free).

Appropriate therapy for NHL depends on the patient's age, histologic type, stage of disease, site of disease, and presence of adverse prognostic factors (as measured by IPI or FLIPI score), and patient preferences. In general, treatment of lymphoma can be divided into limited disease and advanced disease. Limited disease includes those patients with localized disease (Ann Arbor stages I and II). Advanced disease is defined as all Ann Arbor stage III or IV patients, and also frequently includes Ann Arbor stage II patients with poor prognostic features (see Tables 135–8 and 135–9).[59,61]

The following section discusses the clinical characteristics and therapy of the most common disease entities.

■ INDOLENT LYMPHOMAS

Follicular Lymphomas

The combined group of follicular lymphomas makes up the second most common histologic type of NHL in the United States, comprising approximately 20% of all NHLs worldwide and up to 70% of indolent lymphomas reported in American and European clinical trials.[54,67] These lymphomas are classified as *follicular small cleaved cell, follicular mixed cell, and follicular large cell lymphoma* in the

Working Formulation.[51] The WHO classification includes criteria for grading follicular lymphoma based on the number of centroblasts per high-power field: grade 1 (0 to 5 centroblasts/high-power field), grade 2 (6 to 15 centroblasts/high-power field), and grade 3 (>15 centroblasts/high-power field).[13] The clinical behavior and treatment outcome of grades 1 and 2 follicular lymphoma are similar, and they are usually treated as indolent lymphomas. In contrast, grade 3 follicular lymphoma is synonymous with what is often referred to as follicular large cell lymphoma and is usually treated as an aggressive lymphoma.

Follicular lymphomas tend to occur in older adults, with a slight female predominance (see Table 135–7). Most patients have advanced disease at diagnosis, but approximately 25% to 33% of patients have localized disease (clinical stage I or II) at diagnosis.[54] Extranodal disease, bulky disease, and B symptoms are uncommon features at diagnosis. Most patients with follicular lymphoma have the chromosomal translocation t(14;18) at the time of diagnosis.

The clinical course is generally indolent, with median survivals of 8 to 10 years. But the natural history of follicular lymphoma can be unpredictable. Spontaneous regression of objective disease has been noted in as many as 20% to 30% of patients.[68] There is also a high conversion rate of follicular lymphoma to a more aggressive histology over time that steadily increases after diagnosis and reaches 40% to 70% at 8 to 10 years.[46,68] At autopsy, 95% of patients with follicular lymphoma have some evidence of diffuse large B-cell lymphoma. Patients with transformed indolent lymphoma should be treated in the same way as an aggressive lymphoma.

Most patients have dramatic responses to initial therapy, and their disease course is characterized by multiple relapses, with responses to salvage therapy becoming progressively shorter after every relapse, eventually leading to death from disease-related causes.[68] This pattern of constant relapses over time without evidence of a survival plateau and the failure of randomized controlled trials to show a survival benefit with aggressive chemotherapy led to the conclusion that therapy does not prolong overall survival and patients are not cured of their disease. However, several recently published studies suggest that the use of biologic agents, particularly rituximab, has changed the natural history of the follicular lymphoma. In a study of patients enrolled in Southwest Oncology Group (SWOG) trials over a period of more than 20 years, patients treated with CHOP and a monoclonal antibody had a significantly longer 4-year overall survival than those treated with CHOP alone (91% vs. 69%).[69] Similar results were reported in patients treated over a 30-year period at the M.D. Anderson Cancer Center.[70] That study also showed an apparent plateau in the failure-free survival curve.

Certain subsets of patients with follicular lymphoma have a much better or worse prognosis.[62] Some studies suggest that the natural history of follicular large cell lymphoma (i.e., grade 3 follicular lymphoma) is similar to that of other aggressive lymphomas and that treatment with intensive combination chemotherapy regimens may result in long-term disease-free survival, including a possible plateau in the survival curve.[67,71] The recent development of the FLIPI prognostic model should help clinicians to identify patients in different prognostic groups based on disease characteristics at the time of diagnosis.[61] Patients who are predicted to have a poor prognosis (i.e., high-risk) could then be offered aggressive or experimental therapy, whereas those who are predicted to have a good prognosis (i.e., low-risk) would be treated with standard therapy, avoiding unnecessary toxicity.

Treatment of Localized Disease (Stages I and II) Radiation therapy is the standard treatment for early stage follicular lymphoma. Involved-field, extended-field, and total nodal irradiation have been used. Carefully staged patients with either stage I or contiguous stage II disease treated with radiation therapy alone can achieve disease-free survival rates of 40% to 50% and overall survival rates of 60% to 70% at 10 years.[67,72] Late relapses are uncommon; only 10% of patients who reached 10 years without relapse subsequently experienced a recurrence.

Chemotherapy is not usually given in most patients with localized follicular lymphoma, but it may be helpful in some patients with high-risk stage II disease (e.g., multiple sites of involvement or bulky disease).[73]

⑩ Approximately 40% to 60% of patients with clinical stage I or II follicular lymphoma are cured of their disease with radiation therapy alone.[67,72] Most centers use radiation at a dose of 30 to 40 Gy to either involved (i.e., local) or regional fields, which would consist of irradiation to the involved nodal region plus one additional uninvolved region on each side of the involved nodes. Extended-field irradiation is not usually used because of the absence of a survival benefit and possible increased risk of secondary malignancies. In addition, previous use of extended-field irradiation compromises the ability of that patient to receive subsequent chemotherapy. The current NCCN guidelines state that locoregional radiation therapy, chemotherapy followed by radiation therapy, or extended-field radiation therapy are appropriate options for patients with early-stage follicular lymphoma.[57]

Treatment of Advanced Disease (Stages III and IV) ⑩ The management of stages III and IV indolent lymphomas remains controversial because until recently, no therapeutic approaches had been shown to prolong overall survival despite the high complete remission rates to initial therapy. However, the results of recently published studies suggest that the initial use of biologic therapy such as rituximab is associated with longer overall survival.[69,70] More than 80% of patients with stage III or IV follicular lymphoma are alive at 5 years, and the median survival ranges between 7 and 10 years.

Therapeutic options for these patients are diverse and include watchful waiting, radiation therapy, single-agent chemotherapy, combination chemotherapy, biologic therapy, radioimmunotherapy, and combined-modality therapy.[46,67,72,74] Although complete remission can be achieved in 50% to 80% of patients with various treatments, the median time to relapse is usually only 18 to 36 months. Approximately 20% of patients who have a complete response remain in remission for longer than 10 years. After relapse, patients are retreated and, again, high remission rates can be achieved. Unfortunately, response rates and duration of response both decrease with each retreatment.

Two different initial treatment approaches exist and are described as conservative or aggressive. Patients treated with the conservative approach receive no initial therapy followed by single-agent chemotherapy, rituximab, or radiation therapy when treatment is needed. Candidates for the conservative approach are usually older, asymptomatic, and have minimal tumor burden. Patients with symptoms, extensive extranodal involvement, bulky disease, or impaired end-organ function at the time of diagnosis are not candidates for conservative treatment. With the aggressive approach, patients usually receive combination chemotherapy, with or without rituximab, or radioimmunotherapy early in the disease course. Both conservative and aggressive approaches are listed as possible options in the current NCCN guidelines, but the guidelines recommend that initial therapy should include rituximab unless contraindicated.[57] Patients who respond to induction therapy may receive maintenance therapy with single-agent rituximab.

At the time of relapse, many treatment options are available,[57,67,75] and the following factors must be considered: age, symptomatic status of the patient, tumor burden, rate of regrowth (based on previous assessment of active disease sites), presence or absence of characteristics suggesting transformation or biologic progression, prior therapy, degree and duration of response to prior therapy, availability of clinical trials, and patient preferences.

No Initial Therapy. Because there are no convincing data that standard treatment approaches have improved survival, some clinicians have adopted a "watch-and-wait" approach for asymptomatic patients where therapy is delayed until the patient experiences systemic symptoms or disease progression such as rapidly progressive or bulky adenopathy, anemia, thrombocytopenia, or disease in threatening sites such as the orbit or spinal cord.[74,76] The median time until treatment was required is 3 to 5 years, and approximately 20% of patients do not require therapy for up to 10 years. The 10-year survival is 73%, which is not significantly different from patients who received therapy at the time of diagnosis. In a randomized study of asymptomatic patients with indolent lymphomas (mostly follicular), patients who underwent watchful waiting had similar cause-specific and overall survival as compared with those who received immediate chlorambucil.[77] With a median length of followup of 16 years, approximately 17% of patients who were randomized to the watchful waiting group died of other causes without receiving chemotherapy and an additional 9% are alive and have not yet had chemotherapy. As described above, patients with follicular lymphoma who are followed without therapy sometimes have spontaneous regressions that can be complete while the disease in other patients can convert to a more aggressive histology. If the watchful waiting approach is chosen, the patient should be evaluated at least every 2 months for the first year and quarterly thereafter, so that intervention can occur before serious problems occur.

Radiation. Follicular lymphoma is sensitive to radiation therapy, and total lymphoid irradiation or whole-body irradiation has been used to treat patients with advanced follicular lymphoma. Although the results with total lymphoid irradiation have been excellent in selected patients with limited-stage III follicular lymphoma,[67] extensive radiation therapy is rarely used for patients with advanced follicular lymphoma requiring systemic therapy because of concerns regarding prolonged myelosuppression and difficulties in administering future treatments. Total lymphoid irradiation has been given in combination with chemotherapy, but studies fail to show a survival advantage for combined modality treatment.[67] As a result, new high-dose chemotherapy regimens usually do not include the use of total lymphoid irradiation.

Chemotherapy. Oral alkylating agents, given either alone or combined with prednisone, have been the mainstay of treatment for follicular lymphoma. More intensive chemotherapy has not been shown to improve patient outcome. In a randomized trial of oral chlorambucil (0.1 to 0.2 mg/kg/day), oral cyclophosphamide (1.5 to 2.5 mg/kg/day), or CVP (cyclophosphamide, vincristine, and prednisone) in patients with indolent lymphoma, no significant difference in overall survival or freedom-from-relapse between the three groups was observed.[68] In a more recently published randomized trial of single-agent cyclophosphamide (100 $mg/m^2/day$) versus CHOP-B (cyclophosphamide, doxorubicin, vincristine, prednisone, and bleomycin), no significant difference in overall time to failure or overall survival was observed at 10 years.[78] The dosage of single-agent chlorambucil or cyclophosphamide is usually adjusted to maintain a platelet count above 100,000 $cells/mm^3$ and a white blood cell count above 3,000 $cells/mm^3$. Although single-agent alkylating agents have a high initial complete remission rate, the time required to achieve a complete response is slow (median time is 9 to 12 months). Complete responses occur more rapidly with combination chemotherapy, particularly with doxorubicin-containing regimens. Many clinicians will therefore give CHOP or CHOP-like chemotherapy when a rapid response is necessary. The development of the CHOP regimen is described in more detail in Aggressive Lymphomas below. Table 135–10 shows the CHOP regimen that is widely used in the treatment of NHL. In those who achieve a complete response, the duration of response is relatively short (about 2.5 years). There is no benefit of maintenance therapy with chemotherapy. After the "best" response is achieved, many experts will discontinue therapy and observe.

TABLE 135-10 CHOP Regimen

Drug	Dose (mg/m^2)	Route	Treatment Days
Cyclophosphamide	750	IV	1
Doxorubicin	50	IV	1
Vincristine	1.4	IV	1
Prednisone	100	Oral	1–5
One cycle is 21 days			

Another name for doxorubicin is hydroxydaunorubicin.

Both single-agent alkylating agents and CVP are well tolerated by most patients. The advantages of oral chlorambucil are no hair loss, little or no nausea, and minimal myelosuppression. Because of its mild side effect profile, oral chlorambucil is usually recommended for older patients who are minimally symptomatic or who have other comorbidities. There are some concerns with the risk of secondary acute leukemia in patients receiving continuous exposure to alkylating agents.

Purine Analogs. Several studies report encouraging results with two adenosine analogus, fludarabine phosphate and cladribine (2-chlorodeoxyadenosine), in previously untreated and relapsed advanced follicular lymphoma.[79] The mechanism of action for both drugs is not well understood, but both agents accumulate in lymphocytes and are resistant to adenosine deaminase. In patients with relapsed or refractory indolent lymphoma, single-agent fludarabine has an overall response rate of almost 50% and a complete response rate of 10% to 15%. Response rates are higher in previously untreated patients, with overall and complete response rates of 70% and almost 40%, respectively. The median time to progression is less than 6 months for relapsed disease and more than 12 months for previously untreated patients. Although the response rates to 2-chlorodeoxyadenosine in previously untreated patients is similar to those with fludarabine, the duration of response appears to be shorter with 2-chlorodeoxyadenosine.

Combination regimens that include one of these purine analogs are also being investigated.[79] Fludarabine and mitoxantrone (FN) and fludarabine, mitoxantrone, and dexamethasone (FND), given with or without rituximab, are examples of fludarabine-containing regimens that show encouraging results in patients with indolent lymphoma.

Purine analogs usually do not cause nausea and vomiting or hair loss, but they are associated with cumulative and prolonged myelosuppression and profound immunosuppression, which increases the risk of opportunistic infections, such as fungal infections, *Pneumocystis jiroveci* pneumonia, and viral infections. Because the use of fludarabine-based regimens may impair stem cell mobilization and collection, some experts avoid fludarabine-based regimens for patients who are potential candidates for autologous HSCT.

Interferon Alfa. Single-agent interferon-α (IFN-α) is active in the treatment of follicular lymphoma, but is not curative.[80] Several randomized controlled trials have evaluated the potential benefit of adding IFN-α to combination chemotherapy. Based on the results of one of these trials, IFN-α_{2b} (Intron A) was granted FDA approval as initial treatment for patients with clinically aggressive follicular lymphoma and a large tumor burden, in combination with an anthracycline-containing regimen. Its approval was based on the Groupe d'Etude des Lymphomes Folliculaires (GELF) trial, which compared CHVP (cyclophosphamide, doxorubicin, teniposide, and prednisone) to CHVP and IFN-α_{2b}.[81] CHVP was given monthly for six cycles, then every 2 months for six more cycles, whereas IFN-α_{2b} was given at a dose of 5 million units three times a week for 18 months. Patients who received concurrent IFN-α_{2b} had a significantly higher response rate (85% vs. 69%), which translated into significant differences in median progression-free survival (2.9 years vs. 1.5 years) and overall survival (not reached vs. 5.6 years).

At least 10 randomized controlled trials in the United States and Europe have evaluated the role of IFN-α either during induction, as maintenance therapy, or in both settings. The results of these trials have been inconsistent.[82] In a meta-analysis of more than 1,500 newly diagnosed patients from the various randomized trials, the efficacy of IFN-α depended on the intensity of the initial chemotherapy regimen and the IFN-α dose.[83] The major conclusion of the meta-analysis was that IFN-α was probably beneficial in patients receiving relatively intensive initial chemotherapy (anthracycline- or anthracene-containing regimen) and at a dose of ≥5 million units (≥36 × 10^6 units per month).

In the most recent randomized controlled trial, 571 patients with stage III or IV indolent NHL (mostly follicular) were studied as part of a SWOG trial. Patients who responded to intensive chemotherapy that consisted of six to eight cycles of prednisone, methotrexate, doxorubicin, cyclophosphamide, and etoposide/mechlorethamine, vincristine, procarbazine, and prednisone (ProMACE-MOPP) or chemotherapy plus irradiation therapy were randomized to receive either consolidation IFN-α_{2b} (2 million units/m^2 given subcutaneously three times weekly) for 2 years or observation.[84] With a median follow-up of more than 6 years, no difference in progression-free or overall survival was observed.

The reasons for the divergent results cannot be easily explained.[82] Based on these negative results, the significant cost and toxicities associated with this agent and the recent availability of other treatment options, most clinicians no longer use IFN-α in patients with indolent lymphomas.

Rituximab. The approval of rituximab is arguably the most important recent development in the treatment of NHL. Its initial approval in 1997 was based on an open-label multicenter study that enrolled 166 patients with relapsed or recurrent indolent lymphoma.[85] Rituximab, given intravenously at a dose of 375 mg/m^2 weekly for 4 weeks, resulted in an overall response of 48% (complete response: 6%, partial response: 42%). Median time to progression for responders was 13.2 months and median duration of response was 11.6 months. Other studies of single-agent rituximab in patients with relapsed or refractory indolent NHL have reported overall response rates of 40% to 60% and complete response rates of 5% to 10%.[86]

Based on the activity of rituximab in relapsed or refractory patients, it is increasingly being used as first-line therapy, either alone or in combination with chemotherapy.[86,87] When given as a single-agent to patients with previously untreated indolent NHL, the overall response rate is 60% to 70% and the complete response rate is 20% to 30%. It is interesting to note that many of these patients remain in molecular remission (i.e., polymerase chain reaction–negative) at 12 months.

The rationale for the use of rituximab in combination with conventional agents is based on clinical activity of both agents/regimens, non–cross-resistant mechanisms of action, nonoverlapping toxicities, and synergistic antitumor activity in vitro. Many clinical trials have evaluated the use of rituximab in combination with other chemotherapy agents.[86,87] In a phase II trial of six courses of rituximab and CHOP chemotherapy (R-CHOP), the overall and complete response rate in 40 patients with previously untreated or relapsed indolent lymphoma was 95% and 55%, respectively.[88] More than 70% of patients were progression-free after 4 years of followup. In an updated analysis, median time-to-progression was reached at 82 months.[89] Based on these encouraging results, several randomized controlled trials have evaluated rituximab in combination with various chemotherapy regimens in first-line therapy for follicular or other indolent lymphomas.[72,87] In the R-CHOP versus CHOP trial, patients who were randomized to receive R-CHOP as initial therapy had significantly higher overall response rates (96% vs. 90%), reduced risk for treatment failure (relative risk = 0.4), and longer time-to-treatment-failure and overall survival.[90] In another randomized trial of R-CHOP versus CHOP in relapsed or resistant follicular lymphoma, patients treated with R-CHOP had higher overall and complete response rates (85% vs. 72% and 30% vs. 16%, respectively) and lower risk of treatment failure (hazard ratio = 0.65), but no significant difference in overall survival was observed.[91] Similar results were reported when rituximab was added to other combination regimens.[72,87] In a meta-analysis of all randomized controlled trials, patients with indolent lymphoma treated with rituximab and chemotherapy had a significantly higher overall response rate and reduced risk of treatment failure (hazard ratio [HR] = 0.62) and death (HR = 0.65).[92] In 2006, rituximab was FDA-approved for first-line therapy for follicular lymphoma in combination with CVP chemotherapy.

Rituximab and CHOP chemotherapy can be combined in many different ways.[93] In the R-CHOP regimen developed by Czuczman et al., two doses of rituximab are given before the start of CHOP therapy; two more doses are given in the middle of the six cycles of CHOP; and two additional doses are given at the end of CHOP therapy.[88] However, in most NHL protocols and in clinical practice, rituximab is given on day 1 of CHOP chemotherapy.[93] In some protocols, rituximab is given on the day before chemotherapy (i.e., day 0) or rituximab is given on day 1 and the other drugs are given on day 3.

In patients who respond to rituximab, either alone or combined with chemotherapy, maintenance therapy with single-agent rituximab is often given to prolong the duration of remission. In a phase II study, patients with indolent lymphoma who responded to first-line single-agent rituximab received maintenance rituximab, given at a dose of 375 mg/m^2 weekly for 4 weeks every 6 months, in an attempt to improve the initial therapeutic response and prolong duration of remission.[94] With continued maintenance therapy, the final response rate increased to 73%, with 37% complete responses. Median progression-free survival was 34 months. Based on these encouraging results, several randomized controlled trials were initiated in previously untreated or chemotherapy-treated patients with indolent lymphoma.[74,87] Patients in these trials received induction therapy with either single-agent rituximab or combination chemotherapy with or without rituximab. Several different maintenance rituximab schedules have been used: 375 mg/m^2 weekly for 4 weeks every 6 months for 2 years or 375 mg/m^2 every 2 to 3 months for 1 to 2 years.[87,93] Administration every 2 to 3 months is supported by the observation that therapeutic rituximab levels are maintained for about 3 months.[93] The results of these trials show that maintenance single-agent rituximab significantly prolongs progression-free and overall survival as compared with observation or rituximab retreatment at the time of disease progression.[87] In 2006, rituximab was FDA-approved as maintenance therapy for patients with stable disease or who achieve a partial or complete response following induction chemotherapy.

Most of the adverse effects of rituximab are infusion-related, particularly after the first infusion, and consist of fever, chills, respiratory symptoms, fatigue, headache, pruritus, and angioedema.[87] Premedication with oral acetaminophen 650 mg and diphenhydramine 50 mg is usually given 30 minutes before rituximab infusion.

Radioimmunotherapy. The recent approval of the anti-CD20 radioimmunoconjugates—^{131}I-tositumomab (Bexxar) and ^{90}Y-ibritumomab tiuxetan (Zevalin)—has provided clinicians with a novel treatment option for patients with indolent NHLs.[72,95,96] Both ^{131}I-tositumomab and ^{90}Y-ibritumomab tiuxetan are mouse antibodies linked to a radioisotope, either iodine-131 (^{131}I) or yttrium-90 (^{90}Y). Indolent lymphomas are known to be responsive to radiation therapy (i.e., radiosensitive), and the rationale of radioimmunotherapy is that the antibody will act as a "guided missile" to deliver its payload (i.e., radiation) to its target (i.e., lymphoma cells that express the CD20 antigen). The specificity of the monoclonal antibody allows delivery of the radiation selectively to the tumor (and adjacent normal tissues).

Radioimmunoconjugates have some advantages and disadvantages over unlabeled ("naked") monoclonal antibodies such as rituximab. Tumor cell kill following rituximab depends on binding of the antibody to the tumor cell and the host immune system. Therefore, tumor cells that do not express the target antigen are not accessible to the antibody, or those that are resistant to immune-mediated attacks may escape treatment. Radioimmunoconjugates, because of their ability to deliver radiation over a distance from a source, can not only kill tumor cells that are in contact with the antibody, but also adjacent tumor cells which may not have been in contact with the antibody or may not express the target antigen. This effect is sometimes referred to as the relevant bystander or "crossfire" effect. However, one disadvantage of radioimmunotherapy is that it can also damage adjacent normal tissues, such as bone marrow cells.

Both ^{131}I-tositumomab and ^{90}Y-ibritumomab tiuxetan have shown activity in relapsed and refractory patients with indolent or transformed lymphomas.[72,95,96] In patients who respond to radioimmunotherapy, the duration of remission can be more than several years. Based on these encouraging results, some clinicians consider radioimmunotherapy earlier in the disease course, including patients with previously untreated disease. In a phase II study, patients with previously untreated follicular lymphoma were treated with six cycles of CHOP chemotherapy followed 4 to 8 weeks later by ^{131}I-tositumomab.[97] The overall response rate to the entire treatment regimen was 91%, including 69% complete remissions, and the 5-year progression-free survival is estimated to be 67%. Similar results were reported in a phase II trial of ^{131}I-tositumomab given without induction CHOP chemotherapy in previously untreated patients with advanced-stage follicular lymphoma.[98] A current multicenter cooperative group study (SWOG S0016) randomizes previously untreated patients with advanced indolent lymphomas to either CHOP or rituximab (given concurrently, based on the Czuczman regimen[88]) or CHOP and ^{131}I-tositumomab (given sequentially).

Radioimmunotherapy is generally well-tolerated. The major acute toxicities with both radioimmunoconjugates are infusion-related reactions and myelosuppression. ^{131}I-tositumomab can also cause thyroid dysfunction. The primary concern with radioimmunotherapy is the development of treatment-related myelodysplastic syndrome or acute myelogenous leukemia.[99]

The decision to use radioimmunotherapy must be made carefully because of the complexity, risks, and costs of the treatment regimen. Because of safety concerns related to delivery of radiation to bone marrow, candidates for radioimmunotherapy usually have limited bone marrow involvement and adequate absolute neutrophil and platelet counts. Although medical oncologists usually select patients for therapy, the radioimmunotherapy regimen must be administered at a radiation oncology or nuclear medicine facility.

Hematopoietic Stem Cell Transplantation. High-dose chemotherapy, followed by autologous or allogeneic HSCT, is another option for patients with relapsed follicular lymphoma.[72,75,100] In patients who are transplanted at the time of initial treatment failure, 5-year event-free survival is approximately 40% to 50%. Although the rate of recurrence is lower after allogeneic HSCT as compared with autologous HSCT, that benefit is offset by increased treatment-related mortality after allogeneic HSCT.[100] The presence of a survival plateau after allogeneic HSCT suggests that some patients may be cured of their disease. In a recently published randomized trial, patients with relapsed follicular lymphoma who received autologous HSCT had significantly longer progression-free and overall survival than those who received additional courses of combination chemotherapy.[101]

Based on these encouraging results, some studies have evaluated autologous HSCT as consolidation therapy after CHOP or CHOP-like chemotherapy in patients with poor-risk follicular lymphoma.[72] Preliminary results of several randomized controlled trials show that autologous HSCT does not consistently prolong progression-free or overall survival. None of the induction regimens in these trials included rituximab, which further complicates interpretation of these results. Based on these results, autologous HSCT cannot be recommended as first-line consolidation therapy.

Rituximab is being evaluated in the setting of autologous HSCT.[86,102] It is given pretransplant as an in vivo purging agent prior to stem cell collection. In other studies, rituximab is given as posttransplant consolidation.

High-dose myeloablative transplants are usually reserved for younger patients without serious comorbidities, but nonmyeloablative allogeneic transplants may be an option for older patients who would not otherwise be eligible for autologous or allogeneic HSCT.

Investigational Therapies. As discussed above, the idiotype present on the patient's tumor cells serves as a potential target for immunotherapy. This idiotype can be used to manufacture a patient-specific vaccine.[103] Vaccines would potentially produce both humoral and cellular immune responses, and would also be longer acting than passive immunotherapy. Several vaccines are being evaluated in clinical trials.[66]

Other Indolent Lymphomas

Marginal zone B-cell lymphomas, MALT (extranodal) and nodal types, are two of the new forms of NHL not previously recognized in the Working Formulation.[104] Extranodal and nodal types of marginal zone B-cell lymphomas represent approximately 7.6% and 1.8%, respectively, of new cases of NHLs.[54] Clinically, MALT lymphomas tend to be indolent. Most patients present with localized disease involving extranodal sites, which involves glandular epithelial tissues of various sites, such as the stomach, lungs, parotid gland, thyroid, and orbit. The stomach is the most frequent site and gastric MALT lymphomas are frequently associated with chronic gastritis and *H. pylori* infection. Because MALT lymphomas tend to remain localized for long periods, local treatment (surgery or local/regional radiation therapy) is effective and offers the opportunity for cure. Patients with gastric MALT lymphomas who are positive for *H. pylori* should be treated for their infection (e.g., antibiotics). Patients with disseminated MALT lymphoma should be treated with the same type of chemotherapy used in patients with follicular lymphoma.

■ AGGRESSIVE LYMPHOMAS

Diffuse Large B-Cell Lymphoma

Diffuse large B-cell lymphomas (DLBCLs) are the most common lymphoma in the International NHL Classification Project, accounting for approximately 30% of all NHLs.[54] Most DLBCLs are classified as *diffuse large cell cleaved, noncleaved,* or *immunoblastic* or *diffuse mixed cell* in the Working Formulation.[51] DLBCLs are characterized by the presence of large cells, which are similar in size to or larger than tissue macrophages and usually more than twice the size of normal lymphocytes. The median age at the time of diagnosis is in the seventh decade, but DLBCL can affect individuals of all ages, from children to the elderly. Patients often present with a rapidly enlarging symptomatic mass, with B symptoms in approximately 30% to 40% of the cases.[56,105] Approximately 30% to 40% of patients with DLBCL present with extranodal disease; common sites include the head and neck, gastrointestinal tract, skin, bone, testis, and CNS. DLBCL is the most common type of diffuse aggressive lymphomas, which share in common an aggressive clinical behavior that leads to death within weeks to months if the tumor is not treated. Diffuse aggressive lymphomas are also sensitive to many chemotherapeutic agents, and some patients treated with chemotherapy can be cured of their disease.

Several factors have been shown to correlate with response to chemotherapy and survival in patients with aggressive lymphoma.[62] Because the IPI was originally developed based on patients with aggressive lymphoma, IPI score correlates with prognosis (see Table 135–8).[59] As described above, the revised IPI score may more accurately predict prognosis in patients receiving rituximab-containing combination chemotherapy.[60]

Therapy of DLBCL is based on the Ann Arbor stage, IPI (or revised IPI) score, and other prognostic factors.[46,105,106] About one-half of patients present with localized (stage I or II) disease. However, many patients present with large bulky masses (i.e., larger than 10 cm), and patients with bulky stage II disease are treated with the same approach as that used with those with advanced disease (stage III or IV).

Treatment of Localized Disease (Stages I and II) Before 1980, radiation therapy was the primary treatment for patients with localized DLBCL. Five-year disease-free survival with radiation therapy alone was approximately 50% and 20% in patients with stage I and stage II disease, respectively.[105,107] Randomized trials in the 1980s showed that radiation therapy followed by chemotherapy resulted in significantly longer disease-free and overall survival as compared with radiation therapy alone. Other studies reported excellent results with a short course of chemotherapy (three cycles) followed by involved-field radiotherapy or six to eight cycles of CHOP chemotherapy, with or without consolidation radiotherapy. With either of these approaches, 5-year progression-free survival was >90% for patients with stage I disease and approximately 70% for patients with stage II disease.[105,107]

⓫ Because it was not clear which approach was more effective, the SWOG performed a randomized trial that compared three cycles of CHOP and involved-field radiotherapy or eight cycles of CHOP in patients with stage I and nonbulky stage II aggressive lymphoma.[108] Patients treated with three cycles of CHOP plus radiotherapy had significantly better 5-year progression-free (77% vs. 64%) and overall (82% vs. 72%) survival than did patients treated with CHOP alone. The incidence of life-threatening toxicity was higher in patients who received CHOP alone. But with longer followup, more patients who received abbreviated chemotherapy experienced late relapses and the differences in progression-free or overall survival were no longer significant between the two arms. Further subgroup analysis of that trial identified several prognostic factors that led to the development of the stage-modified IPI score.[107] Four adverse risk factors comprise the score: nonbulky stage II disease (bulky stage II disease is considered advanced disease), age >60 years, elevated LDH levels, or performance status ≥2.

The stage-modified IPI score is often used to identify patients with localized aggressive NHL who may have a poor prognosis. Based on the results of this trial, the current standard for therapy of most patients with localized nonbulky aggressive lymphoma without any adverse risk factors is three to four cycles of R-CHOP followed by locoregional radiation therapy (30 to 40 Gy).[57,105] Five-year median survival in this favorable group of patients exceeds 90%.[107]

Five-year median survival is reduced to approximately 70% in patients with at least one adverse risk factor in the stage-modified IPI score.[107] Patients in this high-risk subgroup may benefit from more aggressive chemotherapy (six to eight cycles of R-CHOP) followed by locoregional radiation therapy.[57]

Treatment of Advanced Disease (Bulky Stage II, Stages III and IV) It has been known since the late 1970s that intensive combination chemotherapy can cure some patients with disseminated DLBCL.[46,105] Initial studies with COP (same as CVP) produced a plateau on the survival curve of just 10%, with a median survival of less than 1 year. Based on the activity of single-agent doxorubicin, McKelvey et al. developed the CHOP regimen (see Table 135–10).[109] A few years later, a SWOG study showed that CHOP was more active than COP, and CHOP chemotherapy rapidly became the treatment of choice for patients with aggressive lymphomas.[110] Studies in larger numbers of patients showed that approximately 50% of patients had a complete remission to CHOP chemotherapy, and 50% to 75% of the patients who had a complete response (about one-third of all patients) experienced long-term disease-free survival and cure of their disease.

In an effort to improve these results, many investigators used several general approaches to develop second- and third-generation regimens in the 1980s and early 1990s.[46,105] Results of phase II trials suggested that these second- and third-generation regimens were more active than CHOP, with slightly higher complete response rates and improved disease-free survival rates. However, they were also more difficult to administer, more toxic, and more expensive. Based on these results, many oncologists adopted one of these second- or third-generation combination regimens as their standard regimen for patients with advanced aggressive lymphomas.

Many randomized studies have compared different combination regimens in patients with aggressive lymphoma.[46,105] Although the results of these studies show that no one regimen is clearly superior to another, they show the superiority of anthracycline-containing regimens over those that do not contain an anthracycline. In the largest and most widely quoted study, the SWOG initiated a randomized trial in 1986 that compared CHOP to three of the most commonly used third-generation regimens in nearly 900 patients with bulky stage II, stage III, or stage IV aggressive NHL. At the time of the initial publication (median followup: 35 months), no differences in disease-free and overall survival were observed between the four groups.[111] Furthermore, no significant differences in disease-free or overall survival were observed in any subgroup of patients. But the risk of treatment-related mortality was higher in patients receiving one of the third-generation regimens. Extended followup of that trial shows that approximately 35% of patients who participated in that trial are probably cured of their disease, regardless of the initial combination chemotherapy regimen.[107] Interestingly, the overall survival is approximately 10% higher than the disease-free survival, which probably reflects the effectiveness of salvage high-dose chemotherapy with autologous HSCT (see Treatment of Refractory or Relapsed Disease section below).

Based on the lack of survival benefit with the newer combination chemotherapy regimens, the less complicated and less expensive CHOP regimen was considered as the treatment of choice for most patients with DLBCL and other aggressive NHLs for many years. Even with CHOP chemotherapy, however, less than 50% of patients with DLBCL were cured of their disease and most patients who relapse after an initial response do so in the first 2 years. New treatment approaches were clearly needed.

Several studies attempted to improve treatment results by increasing chemotherapy dose (i.e., dose-intensity), shortening the interval between chemotherapy cycles (i.e., dose-density), or both. Because of the increased risk of severe neutropenia, these approaches require growth factor support. Although results of these studies have not consistently shown improved survival, encouraging results from several recently published studies suggest that these approaches be evaluated in future randomized trials.[112,113]

Based on the encouraging results of R-CHOP in indolent lymphomas, several studies evaluated this combination in aggressive lymphomas.[87,106,107] The first randomized controlled trial that established the efficacy of R-CHOP in advanced-stage DLBCL showed that R-CHOP significantly increased complete response rates and overall survival in elderly (≥60 years old) patients as compared with CHOP alone (discussed in Treatment of Elderly Patients with Advanced Disease section later).[114] Although the results of that study established R-CHOP as standard therapy in older patients, the role of R-CHOP in the treatment of younger patients was not clear. That issue was recently addressed in the MabThera International Trial, which enrolled younger (18 to 60 years old) patients with good-prognosis DLBCL.[115] Patients randomized to receive rituximab plus CHOP-like chemotherapy had significantly higher complete response rates (86% vs. 68%) and longer 3-year event-free and overall survival (79% vs. 59% [HR = 0.44] and 93% vs. 84% [HR = 0.40], respectively). Furthermore, in a population-based study conducted in British Columbia, institution of a policy recommending R-CHOP for all patients with newly diagnosed advanced-stage DLBCL resulted in significant improvements in progression-free and overall survival.[116] Based on these trial results, rituximab received FDA approval for first-line treatment in combination with CHOP or CHOP-like chemotherapy and R-CHOP is recommended for most patients with advanced-stage DLBCL in the current NCCN Guideline.

Treatment outcomes for high-risk patients according to the IPI (or revised IPI) score are unsatisfactory. High-risk groups generally include all patients older than 60 years and those with an IPI score of ≥3 (or an age-adjusted IPI score of ≥2). Because progression-free survival is only approximately 50% in these high-risk patients treated with R-CHOP,[60,117] other more aggressive treatments, preferably as part of a clinical trial, should be considered in these patients. Examples of more aggressive approaches include dose-intense or dose-dense chemotherapy with growth factor support, usually combined with rituximab, or high-dose chemotherapy with autologous HSCT.[105–107,118]

One approach is to give high-dose chemotherapy with autologous HSCT as intensive consolidation in high-risk patients with DLBCL who achieve a remission with standard chemotherapy.[119] Several randomized controlled trials have been conducted in patients with aggressive NHLs, and the results of these trials have been critically reviewed by two independent panels of experts.[120,121] Based on a review of the available evidence, it was concluded that high-dose chemotherapy with autologous HSCT is effective in high-risk (based on IPI score) patients who have a complete remission to conventional therapy (first complete remission in high-risk patients) and in untreated high-risk patients (high-dose sequential therapy in untreated high-risk patients).[121] There was inadequate evidence to make a treatment recommendation for the other possible clinical situations, such as in patients who do not respond to standard induction therapy (primary refractory disease) or in patients who have a partial remission to standard induction therapy (first partial remission after full-course induction therapy). A recently published meta-analysis of all randomized controlled trials of autologous HSCT as intensive consolidation in aggressive NHL concluded that there was no evidence that autologous HSCT improved outcomes in good-risk patients.[122] The evidence for high-risk patients was inconclusive.

CLINICAL CONTROVERSY

Because of high relapse rate in patients who have a complete response to R-CHOP, some experts believe that high-dose chemotherapy with autologous HSCT should be considered as consolidation therapy in high-risk patients with aggressive NHLs who have a complete remission to R-CHOP chemotherapy. Other experts, however, believe that the evidence supporting high-dose chemotherapy with autologous HSCT in this setting is inconclusive and that autologous HSCT should be reserved for patients who relapse.

⓫ In summary, all patients with bulky stage II, stage III, or stage IV disease should be treated with R-CHOP or rituximab and CHOP-like chemotherapy until a complete response is achieved (usually four cycles).[57] Clinicians are encouraged to adopt the revised response criteria proposed by the International Working Group.[58] In patients who have a positive pretreatment PET scan, PET scanning can be useful in response assessment. A rapid response to chemotherapy (i.e., a complete response achieved in the first three treatment cycles) is associated with a more durable remission compared with patients requiring longer treatment cycles. Two or more cycles of chemotherapy should be given following attainment of a complete response (total of six to eight cycles). The use of long-term maintenance therapy following a complete response has not been shown to improve survival. Treatment outcomes for high-risk patients according to the IPI (or revised IPI) score are unsatisfactory and alternative treatment approaches, preferably as part of a clinical trial, should be considered in these patients.[57] High-dose chemotherapy with autologous HSCT should be considered in high-risk patients who respond to standard chemotherapy and are candidates for autologous HSCT.

Treatment of Elderly Patients with Advanced Disease More than one-half of patients with NHL are older than 60 years of age at diagnosis, and about one-third are older than age 70 years. The International Non-Hodgkin's Lymphoma Prognostic Factors Project showed that patients older than 60 years of age had a significantly lower complete response rate and overall survival.[59] The reasons for the poorer outcome in elderly patients are not clear. Older patients do not tolerate intensive chemotherapy as well as younger patients, and some studies report that older patients have a higher risk of treatment-related mortality. As a result, many clinicians treat elderly patients with reduced dose or less-aggressive chemotherapy regimens. In general, these less-intensive regimens have used anthracyclines with less cardiotoxicity than doxorubicin, have substituted mitoxantrone for doxorubicin, or have used short-duration weekly therapy.[105]

Over the past few years, several nonrandomized and randomized trials have evaluated different treatment approaches in older patients with aggressive NHL.[105] The results of these studies suggest that carefully selected elderly patients with good performance status and without significant comorbidities can tolerate aggressive anthracycline-containing regimens as well as younger patients. These patients should be treated initially with full-dose R-CHOP or similar regimens; dosages can be reduced later if severe toxicity occurs. Hematopoietic growth factors may allow elderly patients to maintain dose intensity.

The combination of rituximab and CHOP (R-CHOP) has replaced CHOP as standard treatment for elderly patients with aggressive lymphoma, based on the results of the Groupe d'Etude des Lymphomes de l'Adulte (GELA) study.[114] In that study of 399 elderly patients with DLBCL, patients who were randomized to receive R-CHOP had a significantly higher complete response rate (76% vs. 63%) and longer event-free and overall survival as compared with those who received CHOP. In an updated analysis of that trial, significant differences in 5-year event-free survival (47% vs. 29%) and overall survival (58% vs. 45%) were observed between the two treatment groups.[117] In another randomized controlled trial conducted primarily in the United States (Eastern Cooperative Group 4494), elderly (≥60 years old) patients who received rituximab, either as induction or maintenance with CHOP chemotherapy, had significantly longer failure-free survival as compared to those not given rituximab during their treatment course.[123] Maintenance therapy with single-agent rituximab did not provide any additional benefit in patients who received R-CHOP as induction therapy. It is important to note that rituximab is given differently in the two studies. In the GELA study, rituximab is given on day 1 (the same day that cyclophosphamide, doxorubicin, and vincristine are administered) with each cycle of CHOP chemotherapy.[114] In the Eastern Cooperative

Group 4494 study, R-CHOP was modeled after the regimen developed by Czuczman et al:[88] two doses of rituximab are given before cycle 1, and one dose is given before cycles 3, 5, and 7 (if administered).[123] In most NHL protocols and in clinical practice, rituximab is given on day 1 of CHOP chemotherapy.[93]

Treatment of Refractory or Relapsed Disease Although many patients with aggressive NHL experience long-term survival and cure with intensive chemotherapy, approximately 20% to 30% of patients fail to achieve a complete remission and, of those patients who do achieve a complete remission, approximately 20% to 30% subsequently relapse. Therefore, approximately 30% to 40% of all patients with aggressive NHL will require salvage therapy at some point during their disease course. Response to salvage therapy depends on the initial responsiveness of the tumor to chemotherapy. Patients who achieve an initial complete remission and then relapse generally have a better response to salvage therapy than those who are primarily or partially resistant to chemotherapy.

Many conventional-dose salvage chemotherapy regimens have been used in patients with relapsed or refractory NHL. Many patients who respond to salvage therapy (i.e., chemosensitive relapse) will then receive high-dose chemotherapy with autologous HSCT. In an effort to avoid cross-resistance, most salvage regimens incorporate drugs not used in the initial therapy. Some of the more commonly used salvage regimens include DHAP (dexamethasone, cytarabine, cisplatin), ESHAP (etoposide, methylprednisolone, cytarabine, cisplatin), and MINE (mesna, ifosfamide, mitoxantrone, etoposide), and no one regimen appears to be clearly superior to any other regimen.[105,124] Rituximab is sometimes added to these salvage regimens. With these salvage regimens, approximately 25% to 35% of patients achieve a complete response, with a median duration of remission of 1 to 2 years. Only approximately 5% to 10% of patients will have long-term disease-free survival.

ICE (ifosfamide, carboplatin, and etoposide) chemotherapy is a newer regimen that has been used in patients with refractory disease. Some clinicians believe that ICE is better tolerated than older cisplatin-based regimens, particularly in older patients. The combination of ICE and rituximab (RICE) is currently being evaluated as a salvage regimen, and early results are encouraging.[125] Rituximab is given before the first dose of ICE and then weekly during the regimen.

⓬ To improve the cure rate, many studies have evaluated high-dose chemotherapy with autologous HSCT as intensive consolidation therapy in patients who respond to salvage therapy.[119–121] In the PARMA study, 215 patients with relapsed aggressive NHL who had a response to DHAP salvage therapy were randomized to receive either high-dose chemotherapy or continued DHAP therapy.[126] Patients who received high-dose chemotherapy had significantly longer 5-year disease-free survival (46% vs. 12%) and overall survival (53% vs. 32%) than did those treated with conventional salvage therapy. Further analysis of that study showed that patients who relapsed within 12 months of their initial diagnosis were less likely to benefit from high-dose chemotherapy than were patients who relapsed after 12 months. Based on a review of the available evidence, including the PARMA study, it was concluded that high-dose chemotherapy with autologous HSCT is effective in patients who relapse for the first time and who have responded to salvage therapy (first chemotherapy-sensitive relapse).[120,121] Unfortunately, there was inadequate evidence to make a treatment recommendation for patients who relapse and have not responded to salvage therapy (chemotherapy-resistant relapse). Based on these studies, high-dose chemotherapy with autologous HSCT is considered to be the treatment of choice in younger patients with chemotherapy-sensitive relapse.[57,105] High-dose chemotherapy with autologous HSCT is not recommended in patients with untested or chemotherapy-refractory relapse.

Rituximab is being evaluated in the setting of autologous HSCT.[86,102,119] It is given pretransplant as an in vivo purging agent prior to stem cell collection. In one study of patients with aggressive lymphoma, two courses of rituximab (starting at day 42 and 6 months after transplantation) were given as posttransplant consolidation.[102]

Other Aggressive Lymphomas

Mantle cell lymphoma (MCL) is one of the new disease entities that was previously unrecognized by other classification systems.[107,127,128] This histologic type was found in 6% of cases in the International Lymphoma Classification Project.[54] The chromosomal translocation t(11;14) occurs in most cases of MCL. MCL usually occurs in older adults, particularly in men, and most patients have advanced disease at the time of diagnosis (see Table 135–7). Extranodal involvement is found in approximately 90% of cases. The course of the disease is moderately aggressive; the median overall survival is about 3 years, with no evidence of a survival plateau.

Patients with disseminated MCL are usually treated with the same intensive combination chemotherapy regimens that are used in diffuse aggressive lymphomas. One widely used combination regimen is HyperCVAD (cyclophosphamide, vincristine, doxorubicin, dexamethasone) alternating with methotrexate and cytarabine. Overall response rates to these regimens is approximately 80%, with about one-half of patients achieving a complete response.[107,127,128] Median progression-free and overall survival was 20 and 36 months, respectively. Because MCL usually expresses CD20, rituximab, either alone or combined with CHOP, has been used with some success in patients with newly diagnosed and relapsed MCL.[87,107,127,128] In a meta-analysis of randomized controlled trials, the addition of rituximab to combination chemotherapy was associated with improved overall survival (HR = 0.60).[92] Despite the high response rates, MCL is not considered curable with standard chemotherapy. Consequently, younger patients who have an initial response to chemotherapy often undergo autologous or allogeneic HSCT as consolidation therapy.[127,128] The NCCN Guideline recommends that patients with advanced-stage MCL be treated initially with rituximab and combination chemotherapy, followed by autologous or allogeneic HSCT as first-line consolidation therapy.[57] Unfortunately, most patients with MCL eventually relapse and are treated with salvage therapy or enrolled in trials of investigational agents, some of which are aimed at molecular targets.[50,107] Bortezomib (Velcade) received FDA approval in 2006 for treatment of relapsed or refractory MCL based on the results of a phase II study that showed a 33% response rate.[129]

Primary mediastinal large B-cell lymphoma is a distinct clinicopathologic entity, accounting for approximately 7% of all DLBCLs and 2.4% of all NHLs in the International NHL Classification Project.[54] This type of lymphoma tends to occur in younger patients (median age at presentation is 30 years old) and has a female predominance (see Table 135–7).[130] Patients present with a locally invasive mediastinal mass originating in the thymus, with frequent airway compromise and superior vena cava syndrome. Although the disease course is similar to that of other aggressive lymphomas, the biologic features of primary mediastinal large B-cell lymphoma clearly differentiate it from other types of DLBCL.[130] Patients with primary mediastinal large B-cell lymphoma should be treated similar to other patients with localized DLBCL.

NON-HODGKIN'S LYMPHOMA IN ACQUIRED IMMUNE DEFICIENCY SYNDROME

The risk of NHL for patients with AIDS is increased more than 100-fold as compared to the general population.[131,132] AIDS-related lymphoma arises as a consequence of long-term stimulation and proliferation of B lymphocytes from HIV and the reactivation of prior EBV infection as a consequence of HIV-induced immunosuppression. AIDS-related lymphoma usually occurs late in the course of HIV infection and is the cause of death in approximately 15% of HIV-infected individuals. Although HIV infects T cells, more than 95% of AIDS-related lymphomas are B-cell neoplasms. Most cases of AIDS-related lymphomas are classified as Burkitt's or DLBCL.

The clinical presentation is similar to that observed in other immunocompromised states. Most patients with AIDS-related lymphoma present with B symptoms and have advanced-stage (III or IV) disease at the time of diagnosis.[131] Involvement of extranodal sites is common. The clinical course of AIDS-related lymphoma is usually aggressive and has improved with the availability of highly active antiretroviral therapy (HAART). Improved survival has been observed, primarily in patients with DLBCL. Patients with AIDS-related lymphoma treated with intensive therapy have a median survival that is similar to the survival of patients with HIV-negative NHLs.[132] In the post-HAART era, many of the prognostic factors have also changed and only lymphoma-related factors such as the IPI remain as independent predictors of prognosis.

The treatment of patients with AIDS-associated lymphomas is difficult because the immunocompromised state of these patients increases their risk of significant toxicity as a consequence of myelosuppressive therapy. Except for primary CNS lymphoma, AIDS-related lymphoma is never considered truly localized and systemic chemotherapy is indicated. For patients with adequate immune function and without a history of an opportunistic infection, chemotherapy regimens similar to that used for aggressive lymphomas may be used.[46,131,132] However, many patients with AIDS-related lymphoma were previously treated with less-intensive regimens because of the increased risk of treatment-related toxicity. In the post-HAART era, however, most clinicians believe that standard doses of chemotherapy can be safely administered to patients who achieve a virologic response to HAART.

The results of treatment with standard chemotherapy regimens have been disappointing, particularly in patients with Burkitt's lymphoma. In patients with DLBCL, the complete response rate with combination chemotherapy is approximately 40% to 50%, with 5-year overall survival rates of approximately 20% to 30%. Newer approaches, such as the dose-adjusted EPOCH (etoposide, prednisone, vincristine, cyclophosphamide, and doxorubicin) regimen developed at the National Cancer Institute and rituximab-containing combination chemotherapy, appear promising.[132]

The optimal timing for HAART is not clear in patients with AIDS-related lymphoma.[132] If HAART is given concurrently with chemotherapy, patients should be monitored closely for possible pharmacokinetic interactions between HAART and chemotherapy. Some experts suggest that HAART should be withheld until the completion of chemotherapy to allow administration of full chemotherapy doses and to avoid the risk of pharmacokinetic interactions. Prophylactic antibiotics should be continued during chemotherapy and intrathecal chemotherapy should be administered to prevent CNS relapses.

EVALUATION OF THERAPEUTIC OUTCOMES

Hodgkin's and non-Hodgkin's lymphomas tend to respond well to radiation, chemotherapy, and biologic therapy. The goal of therapy for patients with Hodgkin's and aggressive non-Hodgkin's lymphoma is long-term survival and cure. The therapeutic goal in patients with indolent NHLs is less clear because of the indolent nature of the disease and the lack of convincing evidence showing that therapy prolongs survival. Therapeutic responses should be evaluated based on physical examination, radiologic evidence, PET scanning, and other positive findings at baseline.[58] Patients with Hodgkin's and aggressive non-Hodgkin's lymphomas are usually evaluated for response at the end of four cycles of therapy or at the end of treatment if fewer than four cycles of therapy are planned. If patients are treated with chemotherapy alone, two additional cycles of chemotherapy are given after the patient has achieved a complete remission. The rapidity of response to therapy in patients with indolent NHL depends on the choice of therapy. Responses occur slowly with therapy with oral alkylating agents, but occur much more rapidly with aggressive therapies such as combination chemotherapy with or without rituximab. If radiation alone is used, then a therapeutic evaluation should occur at the end of treatment.

CONCLUSIONS

Several decades ago, lymphomas were considered a fatal disease. Today, most patients with Hodgkin's lymphoma and many patients with aggressive NHLs can be cured with radiation therapy, chemotherapy, or a combination of radiation and chemotherapy. Our ability to achieve long-term survival and cure in these patients is the result of many factors, including development of accurate and reproducible classification systems; a more uniform approach to the staging of lymphoma; and advances in treatment strategies, especially the use of intensive combination chemotherapy. The routine use of hematopoietic growth factors allows oncologists to maintain dose intensity, which may be important for the treatment of aggressive lymphomas. The use of high-dose chemotherapy with autologous HSCT as intensive consolidation therapy for selected patients with aggressive NHLs who respond to initial induction therapy or as salvage therapy after relapse for patients with Hodgkin's lymphoma or aggressive NHLs has also contributed to increased cure rates.

New treatment approaches are needed, particularly for indolent NHLs. One of the most exciting therapies is biologic therapy with anti-CD20 monoclonal antibodies. The recent approval of radiolabeled anti-CD20 antibodies (i.e., radioimmunoconjugates) provides another therapeutic option for these patients. There is some evidence that these new therapies have changed the natural history of the disease. It is important to better understand how to use these new agents, either alone or combined with standard chemotherapy. Although about one-third of patients with aggressive lymphomas can be cured of their disease, most patients will relapse and eventually die of their disease. More effective induction chemotherapy regimens are needed for newly diagnosed patients, and more active salvage therapy is needed for patients with relapsed aggressive NHLs.

The goal for the future is to develop treatment modalities to achieve cure in a larger number of patients. But the acute and chronic toxicities associated with treatment must also be considered, particularly in elderly patients and those with significant comorbidities. Consideration of long-term toxicities is of particular concern to patients with Hodgkin's lymphoma because of the high cure rate.

Finally, a better understanding of the pathogenesis of NHL through continued research in molecular biology and immunology will hopefully lead to the development of specific therapies aimed at molecular targets. In addition, gene expression profiling may also allow researchers to identify new clinically important subtypes of NHL and to identify subgroups of patients who do respond poorly to standard therapy.

REFERENCES

1. Connors JM. Hodgkin's lymphoma. In: Abeloff MD, Armitage JO, Niederhuber JE, Kastan MB, McKenna WG, eds. Clinical Oncology. Philadelphia: Elsevier Churchill Livingstone, 2004: 3rd edition, pp 2985–3014.
2. Mauch PM, Weiss L, Armitage JO. Hodgkin's disease. In: Kufe D, Pollock R, Weichselbaum R, et al., eds. Cancer Medicine. Lewiston: BC Decker, 2003: 6th edition, pp 2163–2188.

3. Gustavsson A, Osterman B, Cavallin-Stahl E. A systematic overview of radiation therapy effects in Hodgkin's lymphoma. Acta Oncol 2003;42:589–604.
4. Josting A, Heidecke C, Dieh V. Overview of the Sixth International Symposium on Hodgkin's disease—recent advances in basic and clinical trials. Eur J Haematol Suppl 2005;75:1–5.
5. Jemal A, Siegel R, Ward E, Murray T, Xu J, Thun MJ. Cancer statistics, 2007. CA Cancer J Clin 2007;57:43–66.
6. Ries LAG, Melbert D, Krapcho M, Mariotto A, et al. (eds). SEER Cancer Statistics Review, 1975–2004, National Cancer Institute. Bethesda, MD, *http://seer.cancer.gov/csr/1975_2004/*, based on November 2006 SEER data submission, posted to the SEER web site, 2007.
7. Aleman BM, van den Belt-Dusebout AW, Klokman WJ, Van't Veer MB, Bartelink H, van Leeuwen FE. Long-term cause-specific mortality of patients treated for Hodgkin's disease. J Clin Oncol 2003;21:3431–3439.
8. Mauch P, Ng A, Aleman B, et al. Report from the Rockefeller Foundation Sponsored International Workshop on reducing mortality and improving quality of life in long-term survivors of Hodgkin's disease: July 9–16, 2003, Bellagio, Italy. Eur J Haematol Suppl 2005;75:68–76.
9. Papadaki T, Stamatopoulos K. Hodgkin disease immunopathogenesis: Long-standing questions, recent answers, further directions. Trends Immunol 2003;24:508–511.
10. Hjalgrim H, Askling J, Sorensen P, et al. Risk of Hodgkin's disease and other cancers after infectious mononucleosis. J Natl Cancer Inst 2000;92:1522–1528.
11. Goedert JJ, Cote TR, Virgo P, et al. Spectrum of AIDS-associated malignant disorders. Lancet 1998;351:1833–1839.
12. Keegan THM, Glaser SL, Clarke CA, et al. Epstein-Barr virus as a marker of survival after Hodgkin's lymphoma: A population-based study. J Clin Oncol 2005;23:7604–7613.
13. Jaffe ES, Harris NL, Stein H, Vardiman JW. World Health Organization Classification of Tumours: Pathology and Genetics of Tumours of the Haematopoietic and Lymphoid tissues. Lyon: IARC Press, 2001.
14. Mauch PM. Clinical presentation and patterns of disease distribution in Hodgkin's lymphoma in adults. In: UpToDate, Rose BD (ed), UpToDate, Walthem, MA, 2007.
15. NCCN Clinical Practice Guidelines in Oncology. Hodgkin Disease/Lymphoma, (version 1.2007) *http://www.nccn.org*.
16. Hutchings M, Eigtved AI, Specht L. FDG-PET in the clinical management of Hodgkin lymphoma. Crit Rev Oncol Hematol 2004;52:19–32.
17. Mauch PM, Canellos GP. Staging and selection of treatment modality in patients with Hodgkin's disease. In: UpToDate, Rose BD (ed), UpToDate, Walthem, MA, 2007.
18. Hasenclever D, Diehl V. A prognostic score for advanced Hodgkin's disease. International Prognostic Factors Project on Advanced Hodgkin's Disease. N Engl J Med 1998;339:1506–1514.
19. Brusamolino E, Baio A, Orlandi E, et al. Long-term events in adult patients with clinical stage ia-iia nonbulky Hodgkin's lymphoma treated with four cycles of doxorubicin, bleomycin, vinblastine, and dacarbazine and adjuvant radiotherapy: A single-institution 15-year follow-up. Clin Cancer Res 2006;12:6487–6493.
20. Klimm B, Diehl V, Pfistner B, Engert A. Current treatment strategies of the German Hodgkin Study Group (GHSG). Eur J Haematol Suppl 2005;75:125–134.
21. Lee CK. Evolving role of radiation therapy for hematologic malignancies. Hematol Oncol Clin North Am 2006;20:471–503.
22. Ansell SM, Armitage JO. Management of Hodgkin lymphoma. Mayo Clin Proc 2006;81:419–426.
23. Connors JM. State-of-the-art therapeutics: Hodgkin's lymphoma. J Clin Oncol 2005;23:6400–6408.
24. Press OW, LeBlanc M, Lichter AS, et al. Phase III randomized intergroup trial of subtotal lymphoid irradiation versus doxorubicin, vinblastine, and subtotal lymphoid irradiation for stage IA to IIA Hodgkin's disease. J Clin Oncol 2001;19:4238–4244.
25. Specht L, Gray RG, Clarke MJ, Peto R. Influence of more extensive radiotherapy and adjuvant chemotherapy on long-term outcome of early-stage Hodgkin's disease: A meta-analysis of 23 randomized trials involving 3,888 patients. International Hodgkin's Disease Collaborative Group. J Clin Oncol 1998;16:830–843.
26. Engert A, Schiller P, Josting A, et al. Involved-field radiotherapy is equally effective and less toxic compared with extended-field radiotherapy after four cycles of chemotherapy in patients with early-stage unfavorable Hodgkin's lymphoma: Results of the HD8 trial of the German Hodgkin's Lymphoma Study Group. J Clin Oncol 2003;21:3601–3608.
27. Gobbi PG, Levis A, Chisesi T, et al. ABVD versus modified Stanford V versus MOPPEBVCAD with optional and limited radiotherapy in intermediate- and advanced-stage Hodgkin's lymphoma: Final results of a multicenter randomized trial by the Intergruppo Italiano Linfomi. J Clin Oncol 2005;23:9198–9207.
28. Diehl V, Stein H, Hummel M, Zollinger R, Connors JM. Hodgkin's Lymphoma: Biology and treatment strategies for primary, refractory, and relapsed disease. Hematology 2003;2003:225–247.
29. Longo DL, Young RC, Wesley M, et al. Twenty years of MOPP therapy for Hodgkin's disease. J Clin Oncol 1986;4:1295–1306.
30. Canellos GP, Anderson JR, Propert KJ, et al. Chemotherapy of advanced Hodgkin's disease with MOPP, ABVD, or MOPP alternating with ABVD. N Engl J Med 1992;327:1478–1484.
31. Goldie JH, Coldman AJ, Gudauskas GA. Rationale for the use of alternating non-cross-resistant chemotherapy. Cancer Treat Rep 1982;66:439–449.
32. Glick JH, Young ML, Harrington D, et al. MOPP/ABV hybrid chemotherapy for advanced Hodgkin's disease significantly improves failure-free and overall survival: The 8-year results of the intergroup trial. J Clin Oncol 1998;16:19–26.
33. Duggan DB, Petroni GR, Johnson JL, et al. Randomized comparison of ABVD and MOPP/ABV hybrid for the treatment of advanced Hodgkin's disease: Report of an intergroup trial. J Clin Oncol 2003;21:607–614.
34. Diehl V, Franklin J, Pfreundschuh M, et al. Standard and increased-dose BEACOPP chemotherapy compared with COPP-ABVD for advanced Hodgkin's disease. N Engl J Med 2003;348:2386–2395.
35. National Cancer Institute. Adult Hodgkin's Lymphoma (PDQ): Treatment. 2007, *http://www.cancer.gov/cancertopics/pdq/treatment/adulthodgkins/healthprofessional*.
36. Prosnitz LR. Consolidation radiotherapy in the treatment of advanced Hodgkin's disease: Is it dead? Int J Radiat Oncol Biol Phys 2003;56:605–608.
37. Loeffler M, Brosteanu O, Hasenclever D, et al. Meta-analysis of chemotherapy versus combined modality treatment trials in Hodgkin's disease. International Database on Hodgkin's Disease Overview Study Group. J Clin Oncol 1998;16:818–829.
38. Aleman BMP, Raemaekers JMM, Tomisic R, et al. Involved-field radiotherapy for patients in partial remission after chemotherapy for advanced Hodgkin's lymphoma. Int J Radiat Oncol Biol Phys 2007;67:19–30.
39. Majhail NS, Weisdorf DJ, Defor TE, et al. Long-term results of autologous stem cell transplantation for primary refractory or relapsed Hodgkin's lymphoma. Biol Blood Marrow Transplant 2006;12:1065–1072.
40. Longo DL, Duffey PL, Young RC, et al. Conventional-dose salvage combination chemotherapy in patients relapsing with Hodgkin's disease after combination chemotherapy: The low probability for cure. J Clin Oncol 1992;10:210–218.
41. Kulkarni SS, Sastry PS, Saikia TK, Parikh PM, Gopal R, Advani SH. Gonadal function following ABVD therapy for Hodgkin's disease. Am J Clin Oncol 1997;20:354–357.
42. Swerdlow AJ, Barber JA, Hudson GV, et al. Risk of second malignancy after Hodgkin's disease in a collaborative British cohort: The relation to age at treatment. J Clin Oncol 2000;18:498.
43. Franklin J, Pluetschow A, Paus M, et al. Second malignancy risk associated with treatment of Hodgkin's lymphoma: Meta-analysis of the randomised trials. Ann Oncol 2006;17:1749–1760.
44. Hartge P, Wang SS. Overview of the etiology and epidemiology of lymphoma. In: Mauch PM, Armitage JO, Coiffier B, Dalla-Favera R, Harris NL, eds. Non-Hodgkin's Lymphoma. Philadelphia: Lippincott Williams & Wilkins, 2004:711–727.
45. Vose JM, Chiu BC-H, Cheson BD, Dancey J, Wright J. Update on epidemiology and therapeutics for non-Hodgkin's lymphoma. Hematology (Am Soc Hematol Educ Program) 2002:241–262. Available online at *http://asheducationbook.org*.
46. Lister TA, Coiffier B, Armitage JO. Non-Hodgkin's lymphoma. In: Abeloff MD, Armitage JO, Kastan MB, Niederhuber JE, McKenna WG, eds. Clinical Oncology, 3rd ed. New York: Churchill Livingstone, 2004, pp 3015–3076.
47. Macintyre E, Willerford D, Morris SW. Non-Hodgkin's lymphoma: Molecular features of B cell lymphoma. Hematology (Am Soc Hematol

Educ Program) 2000:180–204. Available online at *http://asheducationbook.org*.
48. Harris NL, Stein H, Coupland SE, et al. New approaches to lymphoma diagnosis. Hematology (Am Soc Hematol Educ Program) 2001:194–220. Available online at *http://asheducationbook.org*.
49. Freeman AS, Neuberg D, Mauch P, et al. Long-term follow-up of autologous bone marrow transplantation in patients with relapsed follicular lymphoma. Blood 1999;94:3325–3333.
50. Hachem A, Gartenhaus RB. Oncogenes as molecular targets in lymphoma. Blood 2005;106:1911–1923.
51. Trumper LH, Brittinger G, Diehl V, Harris NL. Non-Hodgkin's lymphoma: A history of classification and clinical observations. In: Mauch PM, Armitage JO, Coiffier B, Dalla-Favera R, Harris NL, eds. Non-Hodgkin's Lymphomas. Philadelphia: Lippincott Williams & Wilkins, 2004:3–19.
52. Kuppers R, Klein U, Hansmann M-L, Rajewsky K. Cellular origins of human B-cell lymphomas. N Engl J Med 1999;341:1520–1529.
53. Harris NL. Revised European-American and World Health Organization classifications of non-Hodgkin's lymphoma. In: Mauch PM, Armitage JO, Coiffier B, Dalla-Favera R, Harris NL, eds. Non-Hodgkin's Lymphoma. Philadelphia: Lippincott Williams & Wilkins, 2004:45–58.
54. The Non-Hodgkin's Lymphoma Classification Project. A clinical evaluation of the International Lymphoma Study Group classification of non-Hodgkin's lymphoma. Blood 1997;89:3909–3918.
55. Harris NL, Jaffe ES, Diebold J, et al. World Health Organization Classification of neoplastic diseases of the hematopoietic and lymphoid tissues: Report of the Clinical Advisory Committee meeting. Airlie House, Virginia, November 1997. J Clin Oncol 1999;17:3835–3849.
56. Freedman AS, Friedberg JW. Approach to the diagnosis of non-Hodgkin's lymphoma. In: UpToDate, Rose BD (ed), UpToDate Waltham, MA, 2007.
57. NCCN Clinical Practice Guidelines in Oncology. Non-Hodgkin's Lymphoma (version 3.2007). *http://www.nccn.org*.
58. Cheson BD, Pfistner B, Juweid ME, et al. Revised response criteria for malignant lymphoma. J Clin Oncol 2007;25:579–586.
59. The International Non-Hodgkin's Lymphoma Prognostic Factors Project. A predictive model for aggressive non-Hodgkin's lymphoma. N Engl J Med 1993;329:987–994.
60. Sehn LH, Berry B, Chhanabhai M, et al. The revised International Prognostic Index (R-IPI) is a better predictor of outcome than the standard IPI for patients with diffuse large B-cell lymphoma treated with R-CHOP. Blood 2007;109:1857–1861.
61. Solal-Celigny P, Roy P, Colombat P, et al. Follicular lymphoma international prognostic index. Blood 2004;104:1258–1265.
62. Sehn LH. Optimal use of prognostic factors in non-Hodgkin's lymphoma. Hematology (Am Soc Hematol Educ Program) 2006:295–302. Available online at *http://asheducationbook.org*.
63. Rosenwald A, Wright G, Chan WC, et al. The use of molecular profiling to predict survival after chemotherapy for diffuse large-B-cell lymphoma. N Engl J Med 2002;346:1937–1947.
64. Lossos IS, Czerwinski DK, Alizadeh AA, et al. Prediction of survival in diffuse large-B-cell lymphoma based on the expression of six genes. N Engl J Med 2004;350:1828–1837.
65. Dave SS, Wright G, Tan B, et al. Prediction of survival in follicular lymphoma based on molecular features of tumor-infiltrating immune cells. N Engl J Med 2004;351:2159–2169.
66. Maloney DG. Immunotherapy for non-Hodgkin's lymphoma: Monoclonal antibodies and vaccines. J Clin Oncol 2005;23:6421–6428.
67. Freedman AS, Friedberg JW, Mauch PM, Dalla-Favera R, Harris NL. Follicular lymphoma. In: Mauch PM, Armitage JO, Coiffier B, Dalla-Favera R, Harris NL, eds. Non-Hodgkin's Lymphoma. Philadelphia: Lippincott Williams & Wilkins, 2004:367–388.
68. Horning SJ. Natural history of and therapy for the indolent non-Hodgkin's lymphomas. Semin Oncol 1993;20(Suppl 5):75–88.
69. Fisher RI, LeBlanc M, Press OW, Maloney DG, Unger JM, Miller TP. New treatment options have changed the survival of patients with follicular lymphoma. J Clin Oncol 2005;23:8477–8452.
70. Liu Q, Fayad L, Cabanillas F, et al. Improvement of overall and failure-free survival in stage IV follicular lymphoma: 25 years of treatment experience at The University of Texas M.D. Anderson Cancer Center. J Clin Oncol 2006;24:1582–1589.
71. Ganti AK, Weisenburger DD, Smith LM, et al. Patients with grade 3 follicular lymphoma have prolonged relapse-free survival following anthracycline-based chemotherapy: The Nebraska Lymphoma Study Group Experience. Ann Oncol 2006;17:920–927.
72. Hiddemann W, Buske C, Dreyling M, Weigert O, Lenz G, Unterhalt M. Current management of follicular lymphomas. Br J Haematol 2006;136:191–202.
73. Seymour JF, Pro B, Fuller LM, et al. Long-term follow-up of a prospective study of combined modality therapy for stage I-II indolent non-Hodgkin's lymphoma. J Clin Oncol 2003;21:2115–2122.
74. Gribben JG. How I treat indolent lymphoma. Blood 2007;109:4617–4626.
75. Cabanillas F, Horning S, Kaminski M, Champlin R. Managing indolent lymphomas in relapse: Working our way through a plethora of options. Hematology (Am Soc Hematol Educ Program) 2000:166–179. Available online at *http://asheducationbook.org*.
76. McLaughlin P. Progress and promise in the treatment of indolent lymphomas. Oncologist 2002;7:217–225.
77. Ardeshna KM, Smith P, Norton A, et al. Long-term effect of a watch and wait policy versus immediate systemic treatment for asymptomatic advanced-stage non-Hodgkin's lymphoma: A randomised controlled trial. Lancet 2003;362:516–522.
78. Peterson BA, Petroni GR, Frizzera G, et al. Prolonged single-agent versus combination chemotherapy in indolent follicular lymphomas: A study of the Cancer and Leukemia Group B. J Clin Oncol 2003;21:5–15.
79. Di Bella N, Ravandi F. Purine analogue combinations for indolent lymphomas. Semin Hematol 2006;43(Suppl 2):S11–S21.
80. van Besien K, Schouten H. Follicular lymphoma: A historical overview. Leuk Lymphoma 2007;48:232–243.
81. Solal-Celigny P, Lepage E, Brousse N, et al. Doxorubicin-containing regimen with or without interferon alfa-2b for advanced follicular lymphoma: Final analysis of survival and toxicity in the Groupe d'Etude des Lymphomes Folliculaires 86 Trial. J Clin Oncol 1998;16:2332–2338.
82. Cheson BD. The curious case of the baffling biological. J Clin Oncol 2000;18:2007–2009.
83. Rohatiner AZS, Gregory WM, Peterson B, et al. Meta-analysis to evaluate the role of interferon in follicular lymphoma. J Clin Oncol 2005;34:2215–2223.
84. Fisher RI, Dana BW, LeBlanc M, et al. Interferon alfa consolidation after intensive chemotherapy does not prolong the progression-free survival of patients with low-grade non-Hodgkin's lymphoma: Results of the Southwest Oncology Group Randomized Phase III Study 8809. J Clin Oncol 2000;18:2010–2016.
85. McLaughlin P, Grillo-Lopez AJ, Link BK, et al. Rituximab chimeric anti-CD20 monoclonal antibody therapy for relapsed indolent lymphoma: Half of patients respond to a four-dose treatment program. J Clin Oncol 1998;16:2825–2833.
86. Cohen Y, Solal-Celigny P, Polliack A. Rituximab therapy for follicular lymphoma: A comprehensive review of its efficacy as primary treatment, treatment for relapsed disease, re-treatment and maintenance. Haematologica 2003;88:811–823.
87. Cvetkovic RS, Perry CM. Rituximab: A review of its use in non-Hodgkin's lymphoma and chronic lymphocytic leukemia. Drugs 2006;66:791–820.
88. Czuczman MS, Grillo-Lopez AJ, White CA, et al. Treatment of patients with low-grade B-cell lymphoma with the combination of chimeric anti-CD20 monoclonal antibody and CHOP chemotherapy. J Clin Oncol 1999;17:268–276.
89. Czuczman MS, Weaver R, Alkuzweny B, Berlfein J, Grillo-Lopez AJ. Prolonged clinical and molecular remission in patients with low-grade or follicular non-Hodgkin's lymphoma treated with rituximab plus CHOP chemotherapy: 9-year follow-up. J Clin Oncol 2004;22:4711–4716.
90. Hiddemann W, Kneba M, Dreyling M, et al. Frontline therapy with rituximab added to the combination of cyclophosphamide, doxorubicin, vincristine, and prednisone (CHOP) significantly improves the outcome for patients with advanced-stage follicular lymphoma compared with therapy with CHOP alone: Results of a prospective randomized study of the German Low-Grade Lymphoma Study Group. Blood 2005;106:3725–3732.
91. van Oers MHJ, Klasa R, Marcus RE, et al. Rituximab maintenance improves clinical outcome of relapsed/resistant follicular non-Hodgkin's lymphoma in patients both with and without rituximab during induction: Results of a prospective randomized phase 3 intergroup trial. Blood 2006;108:3295–3301.

92. Schulz H, Bohlius JF, Trelle S, et al. Immunochemotherapy with rituximab and overall survival in patients with indolent or mantle cell lymphoma: A systematic review and meta-analysis. J Natl Cancer Inst 2007;99:706–714.
93. Ghielmini M. Multimodality therapies and optimal schedule of antibodies: Rituximab in lymphoma as an example. Hematology (Am Soc Hematol Educ Program) 2005:321–328. Available online at *http://asheducationbook.org*.
94. Hainsworth JD, Litchy S, Burris HA, et al. Rituximab as first-line and maintenance therapy for patients with indolent non-Hodgkin's lymphoma. J Clin Oncol 2002;20:4261–4267.
95. Cheson BD. Radioimmunotherapy of non-Hodgkin lymphomas. Blood 2003;101:391–398.
96. Emmanouilldes C. Radioimmunotherapy for non-Hodgkin's lymphoma. Semin Oncol 2003;30:531–544.
97. Press OW, Unger JM, Braziel RM, et al. Phase II trial of CHOP chemotherapy followed by tositumomab/iodine I-131 tositumomab for previously untreated follicular non-Hodgkin lymphoma: Five-year follow-up of Southwest Oncology Group Protocol S9911. J Clin Oncol 2006;24:4143–4149.
98. Kaminski MS, Tuck M, Estes J, et al. ^{131}I-tositumomab therapy as initial treatment for follicular lymphoma. N Engl J Med 2005;352:441–449.
99. Armitage JO, Carbone PP, Connors JM, Levine AM, Bennett JM, Kroll S. Treatment-related myelodysplasia and acute leukemia in non-Hodgkin's lymphoma patients. J Clin Oncol 2003;21:897–906.
100. van Besien K, Loberiza FR, Bajorunaite R, et al. Comparison of autologous and allogeneic hematopoietic stem cell transplantation for follicular lymphoma. Blood 2003;102:3521–3529.
101. Schouten HC, Qian W, Kvaloy S, et al. High-dose therapy improves progression-free survival and survival in relapsed follicular non-Hodgkin's lymphoma: Results from the randomized European CUP trial. J Clin Oncol 2003;21:3918–3927.
102. Horwitz SM, Negrin RS, Blume KG, et al. Rituximab as adjuvant to high-dose therapy and autologous hematopoietic cell transplantation for aggressive non-Hodgkin lymphoma. Blood 2004;103:777–783.
103. Levy R. Karnofsky lecture: Immunotherapy of lymphoma. J Clin Oncol 1999;17(Suppl):7–13.
104. Cavalli F, Isaacson PG, Gascoyne RD, Zucca E. MALT lymphomas. Hematology (Am Soc Hematol Educ Program) 2001:241–258. Available online at *http://asheducationbook.org*.
105. Armitage JO, Mauch PM, Harris NL, Dalla-Favera R, Bierman PJ. Diffuse large B-cell lymphoma. In: Mauch PM, Armitage JO, Coiffier B, Dalla-Favera R, Harris NL, eds. Non-Hodgkin's Lymphoma. Philadelphia: Lippincott Williams & Wilkins, 2004:427–453.
106. Coiffier B. Standard treatment of advanced-stage diffuse large B-cell lymphoma. Semin Hematol 2006;43:213–220.
107. Fisher RI, Miller TP, O'Connor OA. Diffuse aggressive lymphoma. Hematology (Am Soc Hematol Educ Program) 2004:221–236. Available online at *http://asheducationbook.org*.
108. Miller TP, Dahlberg S, Cassady JR, et al. Chemotherapy alone compared with chemotherapy plus radiotherapy for localized intermediate- and high-grade non-Hodgkin's lymphoma. N Engl J Med 1998;339:21–26.
109. McKelvey EM, Gottleib JA, Wilson HE, et al. Hydroxyldaunomycin (Adriamycin) combination chemotherapy in malignant lymphoma. Cancer 1976;38:1484–1493.
110. Jones SE, Grozea PN, Metz EN, et al. Superiority of Adriamycin containing combination chemotherapy in the treatment of diffuse lymphoma: A Southwest Oncology Group study. Cancer 1979;43:417–425.
111. Fisher RI, Gaynor ER, Dahlberg S, et al. Comparison of a standard regimen (CHOP) with three intensive chemotherapy regimens for advanced non-Hodgkin's lymphoma. N Engl J Med 1993;328:1002–1006.
112. Blayney DW, LeBlanc ML, Grogan T, et al. Dose-intense chemotherapy every 2 weeks with dose-intense cyclophosphamide, doxorubicin, vincristine, and prednisone may improve survival in intermediate- and high-grade lymphoma: A phase II study of the Southwest Oncology Group (SWOG 9349). J Clin Oncol 2003;21:2466–2473.
113. Coiffier B. Increasing chemotherapy intensity in aggressive lymphoma: A renewal? J Clin Oncol 2003;21:2457–2459.
114. Coiffier B, Lepage E, Briere J, et al. CHOP chemotherapy plus rituximab compared with CHOP alone in elderly patients with diffuse large-B-cell lymphoma. N Engl J Med 2002;346:235–242.
115. Pfreundschuh M, Trümper L, Österborg A, et al. CHOP-like chemotherapy plus rituximab versus CHOP-like chemotherapy alone in young patients with good-prognosis diffuse large-B-cell lymphoma: A randomised controlled trial by the MabThera International Trial (MInT) Group. Lancet Oncol 2006;7:379–391.
116. Sehn LH, Donaldson J, Chhanabhai M, et al. Introduction of combined CHOP plus rituximab therapy dramatically improved outcome of diffuse large B-cell lymphoma in British Columbia. J Clin Oncol 2005;22:5027–5033.
117. Feugier P, Van Hoof A, Sebban C, et al. Long-term results of the R-CHOP study in the treatment of elderly patients with diffuse large B-cell lymphoma: A study by the Groupe d'Etude des Lymphomes de l'Adulte. J Clin Oncol 2005;23:4117–4126.
118. Held G, Schubert J, Reiser M, et al. Dose-intensified treatment of advanced-stage diffuse large B-cell lymphomas. Semin Hematol 2006;43:221–229.
119. Nademanee A, Forman SJ. Role of hematopoietic stem cell transplantation for advanced-stage diffuse large B-cell lymphoma. Semin Hematol 2006;43:240–250.
120. Shipp MA, Abeloff MD, Antman KH, et al. International consensus conference on high-dose therapy with hematopoietic stem cell transplantation in aggressive non-Hodgkin's lymphomas: Report of the jury. J Clin Oncol 1999;17:423–429.
121. Haln T, Wolff SN, Czuczman M, et al. The role of cytotoxic therapy with hematopoietic stem cell transplantation in the therapy of diffuse large cell B-cell non-Hodgkin's lymphoma: An evidence-based review. Biol Blood Marrow Transplant 2001;7:308–331.
122. Greb A, Bohlius J, Trelle S, et al. High-dose chemotherapy with autologous stem cell support in first-line treatment of aggressive non-Hodgkin lymphoma: Results of a comprehensive meta-analysis. Cancer Treat Rev 2007:338–346.
123. Habermann TM, Weller EA, Morrison VA, et al. Rituximab-CHOP versus CHOP alone or with maintenance rituximab in older patients with diffuse large B-cell lymphoma. J Clin Oncol 2006;24:3121–3127.
124. Seyfarth B, Josting A, Dreyling M, Schmitz N. Relapse in common lymphoma subtypes: Salvage treatment options for follicular lymphoma, diffuse large cell lymphoma and Hodgkin disease. Br J Haematol 2006;133:3–18.
125. Kewalramani T, Zelenetz AD, Nimer SD, et al. Rituximab and ICE as second-line therapy before autologous stem cell transplantation for relapsed or primary refractory diffuse large B-cell lymphoma. Blood 2004;103:3684–3688.
126. Philip T, Guglielmi C, Hagenbeek A, et al. Autologous bone marrow transplantation as compared with salvage chemotherapy in relapses of chemotherapy-sensitive non-Hodgkin's lymphoma. N Engl J Med 1995;333:1540–1545.
127. Hiddemann W, Lenz G, Weisenburger DD, Dreyling MH. Mantle cell lymphoma. In: Mauch PM, Armitage JO, Coiffier B, Dalla-Favera R, Harris NL, eds. Non-Hodgkin's Lymphoma. Philadelphia: Lippincott Williams & Wilkins, 2004:461–476.
128. Witzig TE. Current treatment approaches for mantle-cell lymphoma. J Clin Oncol 2005;23:6409–6414.
129. Fisher RI, Bernstein SH, Kahl BS, et al. Multicenter phase II study of bortezomib in patients with relapsed or refractory mantle cell lymphoma. J Clin Oncol 2006;24:4867–4874.
130. van Besien K, Kelta M, Bahaguna P. Primary mediastinal B-cell lymphoma: A review of pathology and management. J Clin Oncol 2001;19:1855–1864.
131. Levine AM, Said JW. Management of acquired immunodeficiency syndrome-related lymphoma. In: Mauch PM, Armitage JO, Coiffier B, Dalla-Favera R, Harris NL, eds. Non-Hodgkin's Lymphoma. Philadelphia: Lippincott Williams & Wilkins, 2004:613–627.
132. Mounier N, Spina M, Gisselbrecht C. Modern management of non-Hodgkin's lymphoma in HIV-infected patients. Br J Haematol 2007;136:685–698.

CHAPTER 136

Ovarian Cancer

JUDITH A. SMITH AND JUDITH K. WOLF

KEY CONCEPTS

1. Ovarian cancer is denoted "the Silent Killer" because of the nonspecific signs and symptoms that contribute to the delay in diagnosis. The few patients who present with disease still confined to the ovary will have a 5-year survival rate greater than 90%, but most patients present with advanced disease and have a 5-year survival rate of 10% to 30%.

2. Ovarian cancer is a sporadic disease with less than 10% of cases of ovarian cancer attributed to heredity. However, a history of two or more first-degree relatives with ovarian cancer increases a woman's risk of developing ovarian cancer by more than 50%.

3. CA-125 is a nonspecific inflammatory antigen used as a tumor marker for diagnosis and monitoring epithelial ovarian carcinoma. If CA-125 is elevated at the time of diagnosis, changes in CA-125 titers correlate with disease response and progression.

4. Ovarian cancer is staged surgically according to the International Federation of Gynecology and Obstetrics (FIGO) staging algorithm. Tumor debulking and total abdominal hysterectomy-bilateral oophorectomy surgery are the primary surgical interventions for ovarian cancer. After the completion of the staging and primary surgical treatment, the current standard of care is six cycles of a taxane-platinum–containing chemotherapy regimen.

5. Although most patients will achieve a complete response to initial treatment, more than 50% will have recurrence within the first 2 years. If recurrence occurs less than 6 months after completion of chemotherapy, the tumor is considered to be platinum-resistant. The antitumor activity of second-line chemotherapy regimens is similar and the choice of treatment for recurrent platinum-resistant ovarian cancer depends on residual toxicities, physician preference, and patient convenience. Participation in a clinical trial is also a reasonable option for these patients.

Ovarian cancer is a gynecologic cancer that usually arises from disruption or mutations in the epithelium of the ovary.[1] It is associated with the highest mortality among the gynecologic cancers, primarily because most patients present with advanced disease. ❶ Ovarian cancer is denoted "the Silent Killer" because of the nonspecific signs and symptoms that often lead to a delay in diagnosis. The few patients who present with disease still confined to the ovary will have a 5-year survival rate greater than 90%, but most patients present with advanced disease and have a 5-year survival rate of 10% to 30%. Primary treatment includes tumor-debulking surgery followed by six cycles of a taxane-platinum chemotherapy regimen. Although 70% of patients achieve an initial complete response to chemotherapy, more than 50% of these patients will have recurrence within the first 2 years from diagnosis.[2] Ovarian cancers often metastasize via the lymphatic and blood systems to the liver and/or lungs. Common complications of advanced and progressive ovarian cancer include ascites and small bowel obstruction.

Learning objectives, review questions, and other resources can be found at **www.pharmacotherapyonline.com.**

ETIOLOGY AND EPIDEMIOLOGY

It is estimated that 22,430 new cases of ovarian cancer will be diagnosed and 15,280 women will die of the disease in 2007.[3] Ovarian cancer is associated with the highest mortality rate among the gynecologic cancers and is the fifth leading cause of cancer-related deaths in woman. The mortality rate associated with ovarian cancer has not changed significantly over the past three decades. The high mortality rate is related to the insidious onset of nonspecific symptoms and the lack of adequate screening tools, which allows the disease to go undiagnosed until it has progressed beyond the pelvic cavity.

As with many other cancers, the risk of ovarian cancer increases with increasing age. A woman's risk increases from 15.7 to 54 per 100,000 as her age advances from 40 to 79 years, and the median age at diagnosis is 59.[3] Most cases of ovarian cancer present during the peri- and postmenopausal phase of women's reproductive life span.[4]

❷ Hereditary accounts for less than 10% of all ovarian cancer cases. Family history is an important risk factor in the development of ovarian cancer. If one family member has a diagnosis of ovarian cancer, the associated lifetime risk is 9%, but this risk increases to greater than 50% if there are two or more first-degree relatives (e.g., her mother and sister) with a diagnosis of ovarian cancer or multiple cases of ovarian and breast cancer within the same family.[1,2]

BRCA1 and *BRCA2* are the tumor suppressor genes thought to be involved in one or more pathways of DNA damage recognition and repair. The *BRCA1* gene is located on chromosome 17q12–21 and the *BRCA2* gene is located on chromosome 13q12–13. Both *BRCA1* and *BRCA2* mutations are associated with ovarian cancer. However, *BRCA1* is more prevalent, being associated with 90% of inherited and 10% of sporadic cases of ovarian cancer.[5] Patients with *BRCA1*-associated ovarian cancer are usually considerably younger than patients with *BRCA2* mutations, with a mean age of 54 years.[6] Patients usually present with advanced stage at diagnosis, and the *BRCA1*-linked ovarian cancers are more aggressive tumors that typically are serous histology, moderate to high grade. As *BRCA1* and *BRCA2* are thought to be involved in DNA damage or repair, their inactivation/mutations may be associated with an increased resistance of ovarian cancer cells to cytotoxic agents with mechanisms of action involving induction DNA damage.

Hereditary breast and ovarian cancer syndrome is one of the two different forms of hereditary ovarian cancer and is associated with germ-line mutations in *BRCA1* and *BRCA2*.[5,7] The hereditary nonpolyposis colorectal cancer or Lynch's syndrome is a familial syndrome with germ-line mutations causing defects in enzymes involved in DNA mismatch repair, which is associated with up to 12% of hereditary ovarian cancer cases.[5]

Hormone exposure, specifically estrogen, and reproductive history also are associated with the risk of developing ovarian cancer. Conditions that increase the total number of ovulations in women's reproductive history, such as nulliparity, early menarche, or late menopause, are associated with an increasing risk for epithelial ovarian cancers.[8,9] Conversely, those conditions that limit ovulations are associated with a protective effect. Each time ovulation occurs, the ovarian epithelium is broken, followed by cellular repair. According to the *incessant ovulation hypothesis*, the risk of mutations and, ultimately, cancer increases each time the ovarian epithelium undergoes cell repair.

Finally, ovarian cancer is associated with certain dietary and environmental factors. A diet that is high in galactose, animal fat, and meat may increase the risk of ovarian cancer, whereas a vegetable-rich diet may decrease the risk of ovarian cancer.[7,10] Although controversial, exogenous factors such as asbestos and talcum powder use in the perineal area also are associated with an increased risk of ovarian cancer.[7,10]

PATHOLOGY AND CLASSIFICATION

Ovarian carcinomas can be separated into three major entities: epithelial carcinomas, germ cell tumors, and stromal carcinomas. Most ovarian tumors (85% to 90%) are derived from the epithelial surface of the ovary.[11] The classification of common epithelial tumors has been developed by the World Health Organization and the International Federation of Gynecology and Obstetrics.[12] The nomenclature considers cell type, location of the tumor, and the degree of the malignancy, which ranges from benign tumors to tumors of low malignancy to invasive carcinomas. Epithelial tumors classified as low malignancy ("borderline malignancy") are characterized by epithelial papillae with atypical cell clusters, cellular stratification, nuclear atypia, and increased mitotic activity, and have a much better prognosis than those classified as invasive carcinomas. Malignant tumors are characterized by an infiltrative destructive growth pattern with malignant cells growing in a disorganized manner and dissection into stromal planes.

Invasive epithelial adenocarcinomas are characterized by histologic subtype and grade, which measures the degree of cellular differentiation. Although the histologic type of the tumor is not a significant prognostic factor, with the exception of clear cell, the histopathologic grade is an important prognostic factor. Undifferentiated tumors are associated with a poorer prognosis than those lesions that are considered to be well or moderately differentiated. A universal grading system for ovarian cancer was established that combines mitotic score, nuclear atypia score, and architectural score based on the histologic pattern.[13]

The histologic subtypes of adenocarcinomas include papillary serous, mucinous, endometrioid, clear cell, mixed epithelial, transition-cell, and undifferentiated.[2,4,13] Papillary serous adenocarcinoma is the most common type of epithelial ovarian cancer and accounts for approximately 46% of cases. The peak age of diagnosis ranges from 45 to 65 years with 63 years as the median age of diagnosis.[14] Serous carcinomas typically display complex papillary and solid patterns and qualify as high-grade carcinomas. Endometrioid carcinomas are seen in women 40 to 50 years of age and comprise approximately 8% of ovarian carcinomas, of which approximately 6% are surface epithelial neoplasms.[14] Endometrioid tumors are usually diagnosed as stage I disease and have a better prognosis than tumors with serous histology. Mucinous carcinomas occur in women between 40 and 70 years of age and account for approximately 36% of all ovarian cancers. The overall prognosis for mucinous carcinoma is better than for serous carcinoma because most patients present with stage I disease. Clear cell carcinoma comprises approximately 3% of ovarian carcinomas in women, with a mean age of 57 years. Although clear cell carcinoma is the least-common ovarian neoplasm, it is most commonly associated with paraneoplastic-related hypercalcemia.[14]

Germ cell tumors of the ovary, including malignant teratoma and dysgerminomas, are rare, comprising approximately 2% to 3% of all ovarian cancers in Western countries with an increased incidence in black and Asian women.[15,16] These tumors are highly curable and affect primarily young women. In contrast to epithelial tumors, approximately 60% to 70% of germ cell tumors are stage I at diagnosis, which is related to earlier detection and response to symptoms in this younger patient population.[16] Serum markers (human β-chorionic gonadotropin and alpha-fetoprotein) are helpful to confirm the diagnosis and monitor response to treatment.

Finally, ovarian sex cord-stromal tumors account for 7% of all ovarian cancers and tend to be diagnosed at stage I.[12] Sex cord-stromal tumors are associated with hormonal effects, such as precocious puberty, amenorrhea, and postmenopausal bleeding. Because these tumors are rare, the optimal treatment of ovarian sex cord-stromal tumors is not clear. The current recommended standard of care is surgery followed by treatment with a platinum-based chemotherapy regimen.

Ovarian cancer is usually confined to the abdominal cavity, but spread can occur to the lung, liver, and, less commonly, to the bone or brain. Disease is spread by direct extension, peritoneal seeding, lymphatic dissemination, or by blood-borne metastasis. Lymphatic seeding is the most common pathway and frequently causes ascites.

SCREENING AND PREVENTION

SCREENING

Ovarian cancer is an uncommon disease with no known preinvasive component, which has made it difficult to screen patients to detect early disease. In addition, the risk factors for developing ovarian cancer are not well understood, which also makes it difficult to identify a high-risk group of individuals. At the present time, there are no effective screening tools for early detection of ovarian cancer.

Pelvic examinations are noninvasive and well accepted, and can detect large tumors with a sensitivity of 67% for detecting all tumors.[15] However, because pelvic examinations cannot detect minimal or microscopic disease, they do not usually detect ovarian cancer until it is in advanced stage. As a result of these limitations, routine pelvic examinations are not an effective screening tool and do not decrease overall mortality.[15]

Transvaginal ultrasound (TVUS) creates an image of the ovary by releasing sonic sound waves and can be used to evaluate the size and shape and to detect the presence of cystic or solid masses or abdominal fluid. TVUS can also evaluate blood flow within ovarian mass. Normal ovarian size cutoff parameters range from 1.25 cm^2 for women 55 to 59 years of age to 1.0 cm^2 for women older than age 65 to 69 years.[17,18] TVUS is sensitive in identifying ovarian lesions and abnormalities, but its use as a routine screening test is limited by a lack of specificity and an inability to detect peritoneal cancer or cancer in normal size ovaries.[19,20]

Serum cancer antigen-125 (CA-125) is a nonspecific inflammatory antigen that can be elevated in numerous conditions associated with inflammation in the abdominal cavity. CA-125 has been extensively studied as a potential tumor marker for ovarian cancer based on the observation that CA-125 levels in a woman without ovarian cancer tend to stay the same or decrease over time, whereas levels associated with malignancy tend to gradually increase over time.[19] However, CA-125 is a nonspecific test that can be elevated in number of benign conditions, including other gynecologic conditions, such as endometriosis, and many nongynecologic conditions, such as diverticulitis and peptic ulcer disease. CA-125 levels are an unreliable predictor of the presence or absence of disease. Because of these limitations, CA-125 levels are not recommended as a routine screening test for detection of ovarian cancer. Numerous other serologic markers such as carcinoembryonic antigen and lipid-associated sialic acid have been evaluated but cannot be recommended for routine screening for ovarian cancer.

The United States Preventive Services Task Force found fair evidence to support screening with CA-125 or TVUS and concluded that earlier detection would likely have a small effect, at best, on mortality from ovarian cancer.[21] Unfortunately, because of the low prevalence of ovarian cancer and the invasive nature of diagnostic testing after a positive screening test, the United States Preventive Services Task Force also found fair evidence that screening could likely lead to important harms. The United States Preventive Services Task Force concluded that the potential harms outweigh the potential benefits and recommended against any form of routine screening with CA-125 or TVUS for ovarian cancer.

In high-risk women, as defined by family history, most clinicians use a multimodality approach for ovarian cancer screening that includes an annual TVUS in combination with CA-125 blood test every 6 months. Changes in CA-125 are monitored over time and changes such as a persistent elevation or consistent increases in CA-125 levels in conjunction with TVUS abnormalities are evaluated further.

PREVENTION

As with most cancers, it is difficult to make recommendations for prevention for the general population because ovarian cancer is a sporadic disease with no established risk factors. Noninvasive measures, such as chemoprevention, have demonstrated some benefit in decreasing the risk of developing ovarian cancer. Ovulation itself is considered a potential insult to the ovarian epithelium, increasing its susceptibility to damage and, ultimately, to cancer. Interventions or reproductive conditions associated with decreasing the number of ovulations, including multiparity, may have a protective effect for the prevention of ovarian cancer. However, the more invasive prevention interventions, such as prophylactic surgery and genetic screening, should be reserved for those women identified to be at high risk for developing ovarian cancer.

Chemoprevention

Although a number of agents have been investigated as chemoprevention of ovarian cancer, including oral contraceptives, aspirin, nonsteroidal antiinflammatory agents, and retinoids, none of these agents is currently accepted as standard treatment for the prevention of ovarian cancer. Oral contraceptives inhibit ovulation, which reduces the opportunity for potential for damage to the ovarian epithelium. Oral contraceptives decrease the relative risk to less than 0.4 in women who used oral contraceptives for longer than 10 years.[22,23] Because oral contraceptive use is associated with an increased risk of breast cancer, women with a family history of breast cancer are not candidates for this use of oral contraceptives as chemoprevention of ovarian cancer.[22,23]

Nonsteroidal antiinflammatory drugs, aspirin, and acetaminophen also have been suggested for use in the chemoprevention of different cancers, especially hereditary nonpolyposis colon cancer.[24] Although the results of observational studies show that the use of nonsteroidal antiinflammatory drugs, aspirin, and acetaminophen reduces the risk of ovarian cancer, these findings have not been confirmed in prospective clinical studies. The proposed mechanism of these agents is the antiinflammatory effect on normal ovulation and inhibition of ovulation.[24,25]

Prophylactic Surgery

Prophylactic surgical interventions for the prevention of ovarian cancer are reserved for patients with a significant family history and/or with known genetic mutations such as *BRCA1* and should be postponed until after childbearing is completed. The goal is to remove healthy, at-risk organs before any carcinogenic activity is initiated, ultimately reducing the risk of developing cancer. These surgeries include prophylactic oophorectomy or bilateral salpingo-oophorectomy and tubal ligation. These procedures will cause surgical menopause which can be associated with severe hot flashes, vaginal dryness, sexual dysfunction and increased risk for development of osteoporosis and heart disease in these women. Because of the potential impact on quality of life and increased health risks, prophylactic surgery is not recommended as a general prevention intervention for the general population.

Although prophylactic surgical interventions are associated with significant reduction in risk of developing ovarian cancer, patients who choose to have a prophylactic oophorectomy/bilateral salpingo-oophorectomy completed need to be informed that complete protection is not guaranteed.[15,23,26] Although a 67% risk reduction has been shown, a potential 2% to 5% risk of primary peritoneal cancer remains.[27,28] Primary peritoneal cancers have identical histology of ovarian tumors with diffuse involvement of peritoneal surfaces. Often primary peritoneal cancers can result from "seeding" during the prophylactic surgery. It is recommended for peritoneal washings to be completed during the prophylactic surgery to check for presence of peritoneal surfaces. If positive, then prophylactic surgery would change to staging and treatment surgery to determine extent of disease and remove any other possible lesions.

Tubal ligation is another procedure that can potentially reduce the risk for developing ovarian cancer. In a case-control study, Narod et al. reported that tubal ligation in *BRCA*-positive women was associated with a 63% reduction in risk of developing ovarian cancer.[29] However, it is not recommended as a sole procedure in prophylaxis. The mechanism for its protective effect is not clear but it has been proposed that tubal ligation may limit exposure of the ovary to environmental carcinogens.

GENETIC SCREENING

Genetic screening should be considered for those women with a significant family history of ovarian cancer. Patients should be evaluated for the presence of genes such as *BRCA1*, *BRCA2*, or other genes such as those associated with hereditary nonpolyposis colorectal cancer or the hereditary breast ovarian cancer (hereditary breast and ovarian cancer syndrome) syndrome.[29–32] Prior to genetic screening, appropriate patient/family counseling and genetic counseling should be available to help women prepare and deal with the health and psychosocial implications of the genetic screening results.

CLINICAL PRESENTATION

Patients with early ovarian cancer are often asymptomatic and the ovarian mass is often detected incidentally during their annual pelvic examinations. Patients with ovarian cancer often present with nonspecific, vague symptoms.[2,4,33] These symptoms can easily be confused with symptoms of common benign gastrointestinal disorders. Patients will often not seek medical attention until these symptoms become unrelenting and bothersome, which allows the disease to progress. Patients with advanced disease may report symptoms such as pain, abdominal distension, and ascites.[2,33]

Several groups have partnered together to educate women about early signs and symptoms of ovarian cancer. Goff et al. recently developed a symptom index total, based on a comparison of symptoms experienced in patients with ovarian cancer and a matched control group.[34] Symptoms that were correlated with ovarian cancer were persistent or recurrent bloating, pelvic or abdominal pain, difficulty eating or feeling full quickly, and urinary symptoms (either urgency or frequency). The Gynecologic Cancer Foundation, Society of Gynecologic Oncologists, and American Cancer Society recommend that women who have any of those problems nearly every day for more than 2 or 3 weeks should see a gynecologist, especially if the symptoms are new and quite different from her usual state of health.

CLINICAL PRESENTATION OF OVARIAN CANCER

General

- Ovarian cancer is sometimes referred to as "the Silent Killer" because of the vague nonspecific signs and symptoms that contribute to the delay in diagnosis.

Symptoms

- The patient may complain of abdominal discomfort, nausea, dyspepsia, flatulence, bloating, fullness, early satiety, urinary frequency, change in bowel function (diarrhea or constipation), weight change, and digestive disturbances.
- Several oncology groups have partnered to educate women about the following early symptoms: bloating, pelvic or abdominal pain, difficulty eating or feeling full quickly, and feeling a frequent or urgent need to urinate.

Signs

- Abdominal or pelvic mass may be palpable.
- Lymphadenopathy may be present.
- Vaginal bleeding may be irregular.
- Patient may have signs of ascites (abdominal distension, shifting, and dullness to percussion—may present like a "pregnant abdomen").

Laboratory Tests

- CA-125 may be elevated (normal level is less than 35 units/mL).
- Abnormalities in liver function tests may suggest hepatic involvement.
- Abnormalities in renal function tests may suggest compression of the renal system by the tumor.

DIAGNOSIS

The diagnostic workup for suspected ovarian cancer includes a careful physical examination including a Papanicolaou (Pap) smear, pelvic and a rectovaginal examination.[7] The presence of a pelvic mass that is unilateral or bilateral, solid, irregular, fixed, or nodular is highly suggestive of ovarian cancer. Unfortunately, by the time pelvic mass can be palpitated on physical exam, the disease is already advanced beyond pelvic cavity. A detailed family history should be taken, especially noting the number and pattern of first degree relatives with malignancies.

A complete blood count, chemistry profile (including liver and renal function tests), and CA-125, carcinoembryonic antigen, and CA19 levels should be performed. ❸ Although CA-125 is a nonspecific antigen, it is the best current tumor marker for epithelial ovarian carcinoma. A normal CA-125 value is less then 35 units/mL. If CA-125 is elevated at the time of diagnosis, changes in CA-125 titers correlate with tumor burden. Rising CA-125 titers are often associated with disease progression, but CA-125 can be elevated in various other conditions such as different phases of the menstrual cycle, diverticulitis, endometriosis, as well as other non-gynecologic cancers. When patient presents with an abdominal mass, it is important to rule out other cancers in the abdominal cavity. Carcinoembryonic antigen and CA19–9 are markers for other gastrointestinal cancers and may be helpful in the differential diagnosis.

Other diagnostic tests should include a transvaginal or abdominal ultrasonography, chest radiography, computed tomography, magnetic resonance imaging, or positron emission tomography scan. An upper GI series, intravenous pyelogram, cystoscopy, proctoscopy, or barium enema is sometimes indicated to confirm diagnosis and extent of disease.

TREATMENT

Ovarian Cancer

■ GENERAL APPROACH TO TREATMENT

❺ A multimodality approach that includes comprehensive surgery and chemotherapy is used for the initial treatment of ovarian cancer with curative intent. Although most patients will initially achieve a complete response, more than 50% will recur within the first 2 years.[2,35] A clinical complete response to treatment is defined as no evidence of disease by physical examination or diagnostic tests and a normal CA-125 titer.

Chemotherapy regimens for ovarian cancer have evolved over the past four decades. Treatment regimens began with single-agent melphalan followed by single-agent cyclophosphamide. Shortly after cisplatin was introduced into clinical practice, it was added to cyclophosphamide and this combination was the "standard of care" for over a decade until the introduction of paclitaxel in the 1980s. Paclitaxel soon replaced cyclophosphamide and paclitaxel plus cisplatin became the standard of care. Carboplatin was then substituted for cisplatin because of its improved toxicity profile and paclitaxel plus carboplatin was adopted. During this same period, many researchers have conducted numerous clinical trials of intraperitoneal (IP) chemotherapy. These advances in chemotherapy for the treatment of ovarian cancer have not translated into major changes in overall 5-year survival, which remains less then 20%.

Certain subgroups of patients have a better or worse response to chemotherapy. The histologic subtype of the tumor is a prognostic factor; clear cell histology is more likely to be poorly differentiated, faster growing, and have intrinsic drug resistance.[2,37] However the extent of residual disease, size larger than 1 cm, and tumor grade are better predictors of response to chemotherapy and overall survival.[2]

In general, younger patients have a better performance status and tolerate chemotherapy better than elderly patients. For unknown reasons, white women tend to have a worse prognosis and response to therapy as compared to other ethnic backgrounds.[2,6,7]

In patients with recurrent ovarian cancer, the goals of treatment are to relieve symptoms such as pain or discomfort from ascites, slow disease progression, and prevent serious complications such as small bowel obstructions.

■ SURGERY

Surgery is the primary treatment intervention for ovarian cancer.[37–41] Surgery may be curative for selected patients with limited stage IA disease.

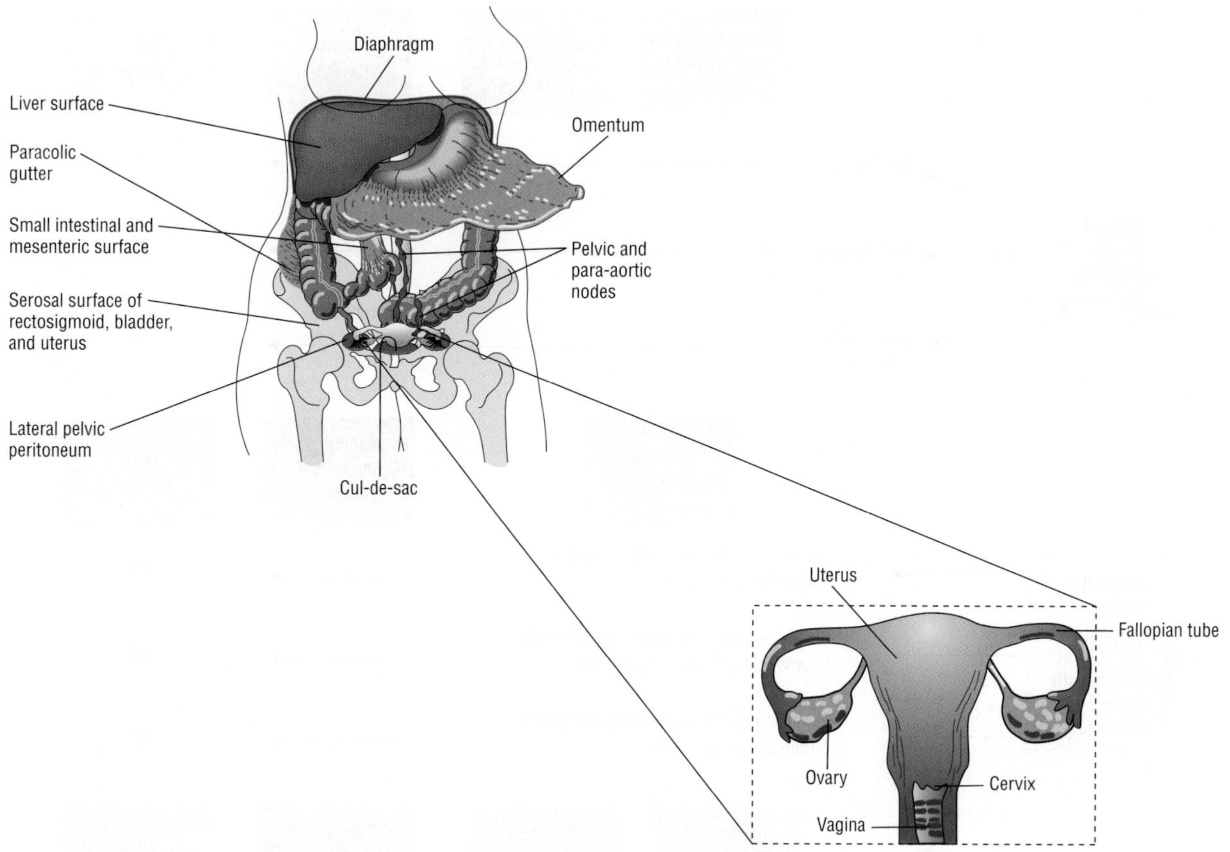

FIGURE 136-1. Staging laparotomy for ovarian cancer with diagram of female reproductive tract (uterus, fallopian tubes, ovaries, vagina). Dash line box outlines what is removed during the total abdominal hysterectomy with bilateral salpingo-oophorectomy.

Primary surgical treatment includes a total abdominal hysterectomy with bilateral salpingo-oophorectomy, omentectomy, and lymph node dissection (Fig. 136–1).[37,41] The primary objective of the surgery is to optimally debulk the tumor to less than 1 cm of residual disease.[42] Long-term followup studies confirm that residual disease smaller than 1 cm correlates with higher complete response rates to chemotherapy and longer overall survival as compared to patients with bulky residual disease (larger than 1 cm).[40,41]

A comprehensive exploratory laparotomy is vital for the accurate confirmation of diagnosis and staging of ovarian cancer.[37–39] ❹ Unlike other cancers that are typically diagnosed by biopsy and/or laboratory results and clinically staged by results from imaging tests, gynecologic cancers, such as ovarian cancer, are surgically diagnosed and then staged according to the International Federation of Gynecology and Obstetrics (FIGO) staging algorithm (Fig. 136–2). The FIGO staging system requires a fairly extensive surgery by an experienced gynecologic oncologist. The skill of the surgeon has a significant impact on prognosis, with definitive benefit of a trained gynecologic oncologist performing surgery as compared to a gynecologist or general surgeon.[43] The reasons for this approach include (a) pelvic tumors cannot be readily biopsied without risk of "tumor seeding," which can increase the risk of recurrence, and (b) surgical staging takes into account the presence of microscopic disease in samples obtained by pelvic washing and lymph node dissection and read by a pathologist during the surgical procedure. It is recommended that the initial surgical staging and tumor-debulking surgery be completed by a trained gynecologic oncology surgeon when ovarian cancer is suspected to prevent understaging and to optimize overall outcome.[44]

Secondary cytoreduction or interval debulking is when surgery is performed after completion of some or all chemotherapy to remove residual disease. Some protocols include additional cycles of chemotherapy after the surgical procedure. The importance of cytoreduction before, during or after chemotherapy is still controversial but it has been recommended to facilitate response to chemotherapy and improve overall survival. Randomized trials of secondary surgical cytoreduction have reported conflicting results. In an older randomized trial, van der Burg et al. performed interval debulking surgery on 140 stage IIB to stage IV suboptimally debulked (less than 1 cm of residual disease) ovarian cancer patients after receiving three cycles of cisplatin plus cyclophosphamide.[45] Patients then received an additional three cycles of these same drugs after surgery. Patients randomized to the nonsurgical treatment arm received six cycles of chemotherapy. Interval debulking surgery significantly prolonged overall and progression-free survival and reduced the risk of death by 33%. However, in a recently published study of 550 women with stage III or IV disease treated with primary cytoreductive surgery and three cycles of paclitaxel and cisplatin, patients randomized to receive secondary cytoreductive surgery followed by three more cycles of chemotherapy had similar progression-free survival and overall survival as compared with those randomized to receive three more cycles of chemotherapy alone.[46]

The overall effect of interval debulking is influenced by several factors including initial response to chemotherapy, the amount of residual disease before and after second-look surgery, and the presence of microscopic residual disease. The results of recent trials suggest that secondary surgical cytoreduction does not prolong survival in patients who are treated with maximal primary cytoreductive surgery followed by appropriate postoperative chemotherapy.

"Second-look surgery" is an elective surgical procedure performed in patients who achieve a clinical complete response after primary chemotherapy to determine if any visible or microscopic disease is present in the peritoneal cavity. The benefit of "second-look laparotomy" to evaluate residual disease after completing chemotherapy remains controversial because it has been difficult to establish any impact on overall survival. It has questionable benefit

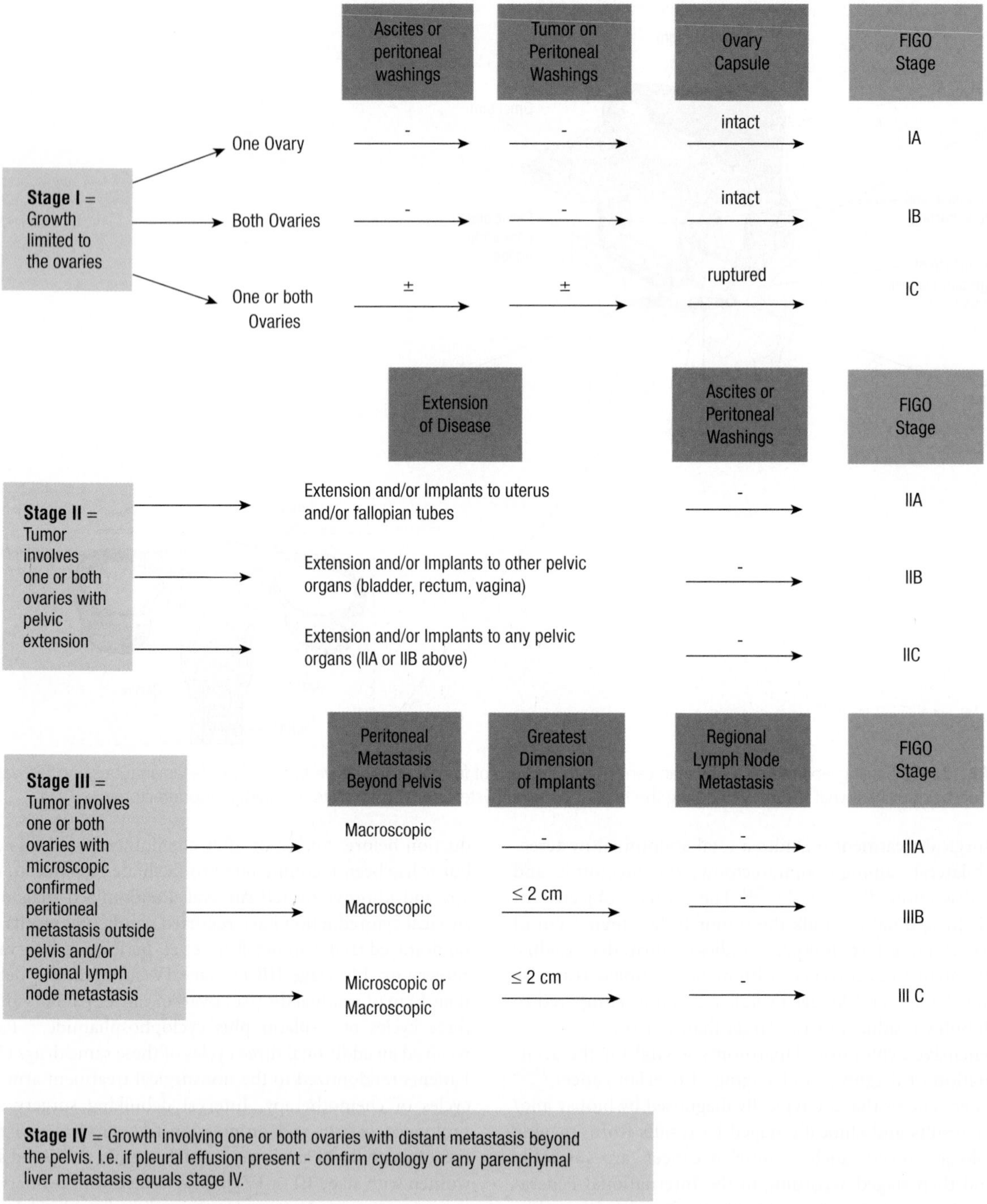

FIGURE 136-2. International Federation of Gynecology and Obstetrics (FIGO) staging algorithm.

because approximately 50% of those with a negative second look still relapsed.[3] If visible or microscopic disease is detected during second look, then the clinician may decide to give additional chemotherapy. But if no visible or microscopic disease is detected during second look, the clinician may decide to observe and monitor the patient. Use of laparoscopic surgical techniques is controversial for initial surgery but is sometimes considered in debulking of recurrent or advanced disease when the intent is palliative rather than curative.[40] In patients with recurrent disease, the goal of debulking surgery is to relieve symptoms associated with complications such as small bowel obstructions and help improve the patient's quality of life.

■ RADIATION

Radiation has a limited role in the management of ovarian cancer. Use of radiation for treatment of early stage disease has had no benefit or impact on overall survival.[47] Radiation therapy is most beneficial for palliation of symptoms in patients with recurrent pelvic disease, often associated with small bowel obstructions. The two forms of radiation therapy used in ovarian cancer are external beam whole-abdominal irradiation and intraperitoneal isotopes such as ^{32}P. Alleviation of symptoms with external beam whole-abdominal irradiation is associated with a significant improvement in the patient's quality of life. The recommended dose ranges from 35 to 45 Gy, depending on the treatment history and ability to tolerate radiation treatments.

■ CHEMOTHERAPY

First-Line Treatment

Systemic chemotherapy with a taxane-platinum regimen following optimal surgical debulking is the standard of care for treatment of

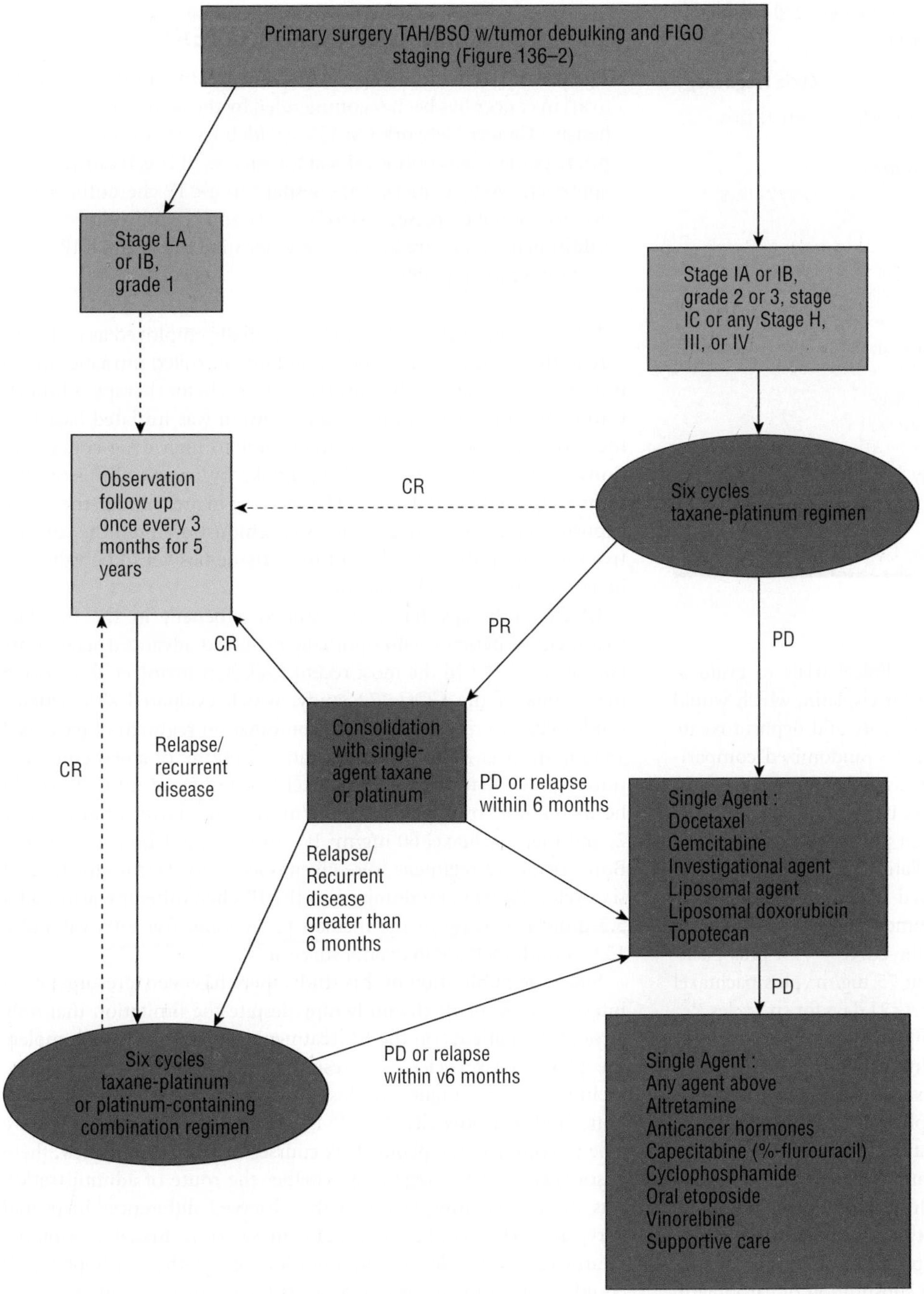

FIGURE 136-3. Management of newly diagnosed, refractory and progressive epithelial ovarian cancer. All recommendations are category 2A unless otherwise indicated. (BSO, bilateral salpingo-oophorectomy; CR, complete response; PD, progression of disease; PR, partial response; TAH, total abdominal hysterectomy; USO, unilateral salpingo-oophorectomy.)

epithelial ovarian cancer (Fig. 136–3). Table 136–1 summarizes the chemotherapeutic regimens used as the initial treatment of newly diagnosed epithelial ovarian cancer. More than 60 randomized, controlled clinical trials have evaluated combination chemotherapy regimens for the treatment of advanced ovarian cancer and a meta-analysis of these trials confirmed the efficacy of platinum/taxane regimens over other regimens.[48,49]

Historically, single-agent alkylating agents such as melphalan, and later cyclophosphamide, were used for the treatment of advanced ovarian cancer until the introduction of cisplatin in the 1970s. Combination chemotherapy regimens containing cisplatin and cyclophosphamide achieved higher response rates and overall survival than regimens without cisplatin in patients with advanced ovarian cancer.[50] Based on the results of these trials, the combination of cisplatin plus cyclophosphamide remained the standard of care for the treatment of ovarian cancer until the early 1990s.

The next major advance in the therapy of advanced ovarian cancer occurred with the introduction of paclitaxel into chemotherapy regimens. McGuire et al. reported the results of Gynecologic Oncology Group (GOG)-111 study that found the combination of paclitaxel 135 mg/m^2 over 24 hours and cisplatin 75 mg/m^2 achieved higher response rates and longer survival than did cyclophosphamide 750 mg/m^2 and cisplatin 75 mg/m^2 in patients with newly diagnosed, suboptimally debulked, stages III and IV ovarian cancer.[51] Survival improved significantly in the paclitaxel arm, with an increase in median progression-free survival (18 months vs. 13 months) and overall survival (38 months vs. 24 months). Neutropenia, alopecia, and peripheral neuropathy were more severe in the paclitaxel/cisplatin group. Similar results were reported in a large European-Canadian Intergroup Phase III randomized trial study (OV10) that also confirmed superior response rates with the paclitaxel 135 mg/m^2 over 24 hours with cisplatin 75 mg/m^2 regimen as compared to cyclophosphamide 750 mg/m^2 with cisplatin 75 mg/m^2 regimen.[52] Based on the results of these studies, paclitaxel plus cisplatin was widely adopted and became the accepted standard of care.

TABLE 136-1 Chemotherapeutic Regimens for the Initial Treatment of Epithelial Ovarian Cancer

Drug(s)	Dose(s)	Cycle Frequency
Paclitaxel + carboplatin	175 mg/m² IV (3-hour infusion) day 1 Dosed to AUC 5–7.5 IV day 1	Every 21 days
Paclitaxel + cisplatin (IV)	135 mg/m² IV (24-hour infusion) day 1 75 mg/m² IV day 1	Every 21 days
Paclitaxel + cisplatin (IP)	Day 1: paclitaxel 135 mg/m² IV infused over 24 hours + Day 2: cisplatin 100 mg/m² IP infused over 1 hour + Day 8: paclitaxel 60 mg/m² IP infused over 1 hour. Regimen is given once every 21 days × six cycles.	Every 21 days
Cisplatin + cyclophosphamide	50–100 mg/m² IV day 1 500–1,000 mg/m² IV day 1	Every 21–28 days
Docetaxel + carboplatin	75 mg/m² IV day 1 Dosed to AUC 5 IV day 1	Every 21 days

AUC, area-under-the-curve; IP, intraperitoneal.

The availability of carboplatin lead to clinical trials to evaluate whether carboplatin could be substituted for cisplatin, which would spare patients from the significant neurotoxicity and nephrotoxicity associated with cisplatin. Several prospective randomized comparisons of carboplatin plus paclitaxel versus cisplatin plus paclitaxel in patients with advanced ovarian cancer have been conducted.[53–56] The results of these trials show that carboplatin plus paclitaxel is equally efficacious and better tolerated than cisplatin and paclitaxel. In the GOG-158 study, 840 previously untreated patients with optimally resected stage III disease (no residual tumor nodule >1 cm) were randomized to carboplatin (area-under-the-curve = 7.5) plus paclitaxel 175 mg/m² over 3 hours, or cisplatin 75 mg/m² plus paclitaxel 135 mg/m² over 24 hours administered every 21 days for six cycles.[53,55] The results of that trial showed no difference in progression-free survival between the two treatment arms with a median time to progression of 19.4 months in the paclitaxel plus cisplatin arm versus 20.7 months in the paclitaxel plus carboplatin arm. As expected, the incidence of leukopenia, fever, gastrointestinal toxicity, and metabolic toxicity was higher in patients in the cisplatin arm, whereas patients in the carboplatin arm experienced more thrombocytopenia and pain. Although the incidence of neurotoxicity was similar in the two treatment arms, it was more severe in the paclitaxel plus cisplatin arm. The results of this study showed that the substitution of carboplatin for cisplatin in the regimen does not compromise efficacy and improves tolerability. These findings were confirmed in two other large randomized controlled studies.[55,56] Based on these results, paclitaxel plus carboplatin became the accepted standard of care.

Other clinical trials have evaluated the use of docetaxel as a substitute for paclitaxel. In the Scottish Randomized Trial in Ovarian Cancer trial, Vasey et al. compared carboplatin (area-under-the-curve = 5) combined with either docetaxel (75 mg/m² over 1 hour) or paclitaxel (175 mg/m² over 3 hours) administered every 21 days for six cycles as first-line chemotherapy for stages IC to IV epithelial ovarian cancer.[57] The results of this study showed that the substitution of docetaxel for paclitaxel does not compromise efficacy and improves tolerability, particularly neurotoxicity. These findings have not yet been confirmed in another randomized control trial. Based on the results of this study, the combination of docetaxel plus carboplatin is considered a reasonable treatment option for patients with advanced ovarian cancer. Six cycles of paclitaxel plus carboplatin following tumor debulking surgery remains the current standard of care for treatment of advanced ovarian cancer.

CLINICAL CONTROVERSY

The use of IP chemotherapy as first-line treatment of advanced ovarian cancer has been recommended by the National Comprehensive Cancer Network (NCCN) guidelines. However, appropriate patient selection is critical for success of this treatment approach. Many clinicians are hesitant to use IP chemotherapy because of the increased risk of toxicity and complications. Additional studies are ongoing to determine the optimal IP chemotherapy regimen.

Intraperitoneal chemotherapy was initially employed as palliative care in the management of ascites and uncontrolled intraabdominal tumors. In the late 1970s, intraperitoneal chemotherapy administration at a primary treatment intervention was initiated based on the rationale that exposure of the tumor to high drug concentrations would increase tumor drug uptake by passive diffusion and ultimately cancer cell death.[58] The increase in area-under-the-curve exposure in the peritoneal cavity was demonstrated but the correlative increase in drug uptake in tumor tissue has yet to be validated in any preclinical or clinical study.

IP chemotherapy has demonstrated a benefit in the first-line treatment of patients with optimally debulked advanced stage ovarian cancer.[49,59–62] In the most recent trial, Armstrong et al. reported the results of the GOG-172 study, which evaluated 415 patients randomized to receive either the combination regimen of paclitaxel 135 mg/m² over 24 hours and cisplatin 75 mg/m² or a new combination regimen that included paclitaxel 135 mg/m² IV infused over 24 hours followed by cisplatin 100 mg/m² IP infused over 1 hour on day 2, and then paclitaxel 60 mg/m² IP infused over 1 hour on day 8.[57] Both treatment regimens were given once every 21 days for total of six cycles. Patients randomized to the IP chemotherapy arm had a 5.5-month increase in the median progression-free survival and a 15.9-month increase in overall survival.[59]

Since the publication of this study, there has been a resurgence of interest in use of IP chemotherapy despite the limitation that only 42% of the patients on the IP treatment arm were able to complete the planned six cycles as a result of significantly more toxicity, including pain, fatigue, myelosuppression, gastrointestinal, metabolic, and neurotoxicity.[59,60,63,64] Because only 42% of patients were able to complete the planned six courses of IP chemotherapy, there is some controversy regarding whether the route of administration was the contributing factor in the observed differences in overall survival.[59] The significant increase in systemic toxicity, primarily neurotoxicity, has led to the question of whether carboplatin IP could be substituted for cisplatin. Although these platinum agents have demonstrated equal efficacy when administered IV to ovarian cancer patients, based on the concept that drug passively diffuses into the tumor, the difference in molecular size of cisplatin versus carboplatin makes it difficult to extrapolate IP activity of cisplatin to carboplatin.

The NCCN 2007 guidelines recommend that IP chemotherapy be considered and offered to patients as appropriate first-line treatment of optimally debulked, ≥1 cm residual disease, ovarian cancer.[65] The National Cancer Institute also released a position statement in January 2006 supporting the role of IP chemotherapy as first-line treatment for advanced ovarian cancer.[66] Because of the significant toxicities associated with IP therapy, only carefully selected patients should receive IP therapy. Ideal candidates for IP therapy are younger patients with good performance status, minimal comorbidities, adequate renal and liver function, and optimally debulked disease without significant bowel resection.[59,64]

In patients who are poor surgical candidates because of comorbidities or bulky tumors, neoadjuvant chemotherapy can be given prior to any surgical interventions.[67] In patients with bulky disease, the goal of neoadjuvant chemotherapy is to reduce tumor burden to make surgery more feasible and optimal tumor debulking more likely. The typical regimen used in neoadjuvant chemotherapy is three cycles of a taxane combined with a platinum agent followed by surgery. After surgery, patients usually receive another three to six cycles, depending on their response to chemotherapy. In patients who are poor candidates for surgery because of comorbidities, the primary intent of neoadjuvant chemotherapy is to relieve symptoms and slow disease progression. In this setting, palliative chemotherapy alone has not been curative for patients with advanced ovarian cancer.[67] If tolerated, these patients will receive the standard taxane-platinum chemotherapy regimen once every 3 to 4 weeks. Another option for palliative neoadjuvant chemotherapy, especially in elderly patients, is single-agent carboplatin once every 4 weeks.

Consolidation Therapy

If patients do not achieve a clinical complete response after completion of six cycles of taxane-platinum regimen, then consolidation chemotherapy should be considered in an attempt to achieve a complete response (see Fig. 136–3). If the patient has a partial response to first-line chemotherapy, as measured by a greater than 50% decline in CA-125 (as compared with the presurgery level) or tumor regression, the cancer is still considered taxane-platinum sensitive. The typical regimens for consolidation chemotherapy are the taxane-platinum regimen or single-agent therapy with either a taxane or platinum agent.[68] If the patient had a poor response to taxane and/or platinum agents, then alternative second-line agents can be considered.[65] Additional cycles of chemotherapy are given until complete response is achieved. Another alternative in the setting of no or minimal measurable disease after completion of primary chemotherapy is to just observe the patient and provide supportive care as indicated until disease progresses then reinitiate chemotherapy at that time.[65]

Because the initial clinical complete response observed in first-line treatment has not been durable, optimization of first-line therapy is under investigation. Numerous options have been evaluated, including the use of additional cycles or maintenance chemotherapy and dose intensity.

CLINICAL CONTROVERSY

GOG-178 evaluated 3 versus 12 cycles of paclitaxel maintenance chemotherapy after completion of first-line chemotherapy. This study was closed early after the interim analysis reported a significant improvement in progression-free survival. Because most patients who were randomized to receive 3 cycles of maintenance therapy crossed over to the 12-cycle arm after the interim analysis, the impact on overall survival is unknown. The benefit of maintenance chemotherapy after achieving a complete response has led to much debate among gynecologic oncology clinicians.

Maintenance Chemotherapy Maintenance chemotherapy is similar to consolidation chemotherapy except it is given to those patients who have achieved a clinically complete response. The goal of maintenance chemotherapy is to eradicate any residual microscopic disease that may be present to extend progression-free and, ultimately, overall survival.

Maintenance chemotherapy has gained popularity after the publication of the results of the collaborative Southwest Oncology Group and GOG 178 study that compared single-agent paclitaxel 175 mg/m^2 over 3 hours once every 21 days for 3 additional cycles versus an additional 12 cycles.[69,70] Eligible patients had to have been in complete clinical remission after at least five to six cycles of a taxane-platinum regimen. This study was closed after the interim analysis by the Southwest Oncology Group Safety Monitoring Committee because patients receiving the additional 12 cycles had 7-month longer progression-free survival than those receiving 3 cycles of single-agent paclitaxel (28 vs. 21 months). After the results were reported, many patients randomized to the three-cycle arm chose to receive nine additional cycles of paclitaxel, which reduced the ability of the trial to show a difference in overall survival.[71] Because this study was closed early and did not demonstrate an overall survival benefit, another randomized, controlled trial through the GOG was initiated to confirm the improvement in progression-free survival and to attempt to determine the impact on overall survival. Until these confirmatory trials are completed, the role of maintenance chemotherapy is controversial in the management of advanced ovarian cancer patients. Maintenance chemotherapy is listed as an option in the 2007 NCCN guidelines (2B recommendation).[65]

High-Dose Chemotherapy with Hematopoietic Stem Cell Rescue High-dose chemotherapy with autologous or allogeneic hematopoietic stem cell transplantation (HSCT) is an option for selected patients with chemosensitive disease, few comorbidities, and good performance status. Although high response rates have been reported in patients with recurrent ovarian cancer treated with autologous HSCT, the duration of response is usually short and few patients have experienced long-term progression-free survival.[72,73] Allogeneic HSCT has been also been evaluated in recurrent ovarian cancer to induce an immune response against the tumor ("graft-versus-tumor" effect).

Based on the activity of autologous HSCT in recurrent ovarian cancer, Goncalves et al. evaluated the modality for first-line treatment of patients with optimally debulked ovarian cancer. In this multicenter phase II study, 34 patients received two cycles of high-dose cyclophosphamide-epirubicin once every 21 days followed by two cycles of high-dose carboplatin (days 42 and 98).[74] Each dose of high-dose carboplatin was followed by hematopoietic stem cell infusion. The results of this study failed to show an improvement in the rate of pathologic complete response with upfront autologous HSCT as compared to standard taxane-platinum chemotherapy. Additional studies are ongoing to determine the role of autologous or allogeneic HSCT in the treatment of advanced ovarian cancer.

Treatment of Recurrent Disease

5 Although most patients will achieve a complete response to initial treatment, most patients will eventually have recurrence of their disease. When a patient relapses, the prognostic factors are similar to the factors after initial surgery except that the disease-free interval—defined as the length of time that has lapsed since the completion of chemotherapy—should be considered to determine if the tumor is likely to be drug resistant. If recurrence occurs less than 6 months after completion of chemotherapy, or if the patient progresses during platinum-based chemotherapy, the tumor is defined as platinum-resistant. Patients with platinum-sensitive disease generally have a better prognosis than platinum-resistant patients.

Because the chemotherapy agents used for second-line treatment of recurrent or refractory platinum-resistant disease have similar response rates that average less than 30%, the selection of the agent depends on the toxicity profile of the agent, physician preference, patient performance status, residual toxicities, and patient convenience (see Fig. 136–3). Participation in a clinical trial of an investigational agent is also a reasonable option for these patients. If the patient has a clinical complete response to first-line chemotherapy and the recurrence occurs more than 6 months after chemotherapy is completed, the tumor is considered platinum-sensitive. Table 136–2 summarizes some of the chemotherapeutic regimens used in the treatment of recurrent or refractory ovarian cancer.

TABLE 136-2 Chemotherapeutic Regimens for Recurrent or Refractory Ovarian Cancer

Drug(s)	Dose(s)	Cycle Frequency
Docetaxel	75 mg/m² IV day 1	Every 21 days
Pegylated-liposomal doxorubicin	40 mg/m² IV day 1	Every 28 days
Gemcitabine	800–1,000 mg/m² IV days 1, 8, and 15	Every 28 days
Paclitaxel	60–80 mg/m² IV (1-h infusion) day 1	Every week
Paclitaxel	135–175 mg/m² IV day 1	Every 21 days
Carboplatin	AUC 5 IV day 1	Every 21–28 days
Cisplatin	75 mg/m² IV day 1	Every 21–28 days
Topotecan	1.3–1.5 mg/m² IV once daily for 5 days	Every 21 days
Topotecan	4 mg/m² IV once a week × 3 weeks, then 1 week off	Every 21 days
Etoposide	50 mg/m² orally once daily days 1–10 repeat every 21 days	Every 28 days
Capecitabine	1,800–2,000 mg/m² in divided doses twice a daily for 2 weeks on, 1 week off	Every 21 days
Altretamine	260 mg/m² orally (total daily dose divided in four doses) for 14–21 days	Every 28 days
Tamoxifen	20 mg orally twice a day	Continuous
Letrozole	2.5 mg orally once daily	Continuous

AUC, area-under-the-curve.

CLINICAL CONTROVERSY

In patients with recurrent ovarian cancer that is platinum-sensitive, some clinicians recommend retreatment with a chemotherapy regimen that includes a platinum agent. Other clinicians suggest that the platinum-free interval for these patients should be extended and recommend that recurrent disease first be treated with a nonplatinum regimen (i.e., pegylated-liposomal doxorubicin), reserving the platinum agent until the next relapse.

Platinum-Sensitive Disease Retreatment with a platinum-containing regimen should be considered in patients with platinum-sensitive disease. The International Collaborative Ovarian Neoplasm 4 and Arbeitsgemeinschaft Gynaekologische randomized 802 patients with recurrent platinum-sensitive ovarian cancer to either single-agent platinum, a non–taxane-platinum combination, or a taxane-platinum combination.[75] Patients treated with the paclitaxel plus platinum regimen had significantly longer progression-free (29 vs. 24 months) and overall survival (hazard ratio = 0.82 [95% CI 0.69 to 0.97]) as compared to the other two treatment arms.[75] Although the combination taxane-platinum was clearly superior in this European study, it is difficult to extrapolate these results to patients treated in the United States because of differences in first-line treatment. At the time that International Collaborative Ovarian Neoplasm 4 was conducted, the standard of care in Europe for first-line treatment was single-agent carboplatin, so most patients enrolled on this study had no prior exposure to a taxane agent. However, the standard of care in the United States has been combination taxane-platinum since the early 1990s. Confirmatory data is needed to evaluate if combination regimens would also be more beneficial in these patients for treatment of recurrent ovarian cancer.

The 2007 NCCN guidelines recommend the combination of carboplatin with either gemcitabine or paclitaxel for treatment of platinum-sensitive recurrent ovarian cancer.[65] Carboplatin alone or any of the second-line agents is recommended for patients with platinum-sensitive disease who are unable to tolerate additional combination chemotherapy regimens because of residual toxicity or poor performance status.[65,76]

Platinum-Resistant Disease Unfortunately many patients develop recurrent drug-resistant disease after initial platinum-based therapy and cytoreductive surgery.[77,78] Patients who progress on a platinum agent or have no response are considered "platinum-refractory," whereas those patients who have recurrence within 6 months of completing a platinum-containing regimen are considered "platinum-resistant."[79] The 2007 NCCN guidelines list many possible treatment options for recurrent platinum-resistant/-refractory ovarian carcinoma.[65] The optimal chemotherapeutic agent or regimen in the treatment of platinum-resistant disease is currently unclear. Ideally, the agent should be active in ovarian cancer and non–cross-resistant with taxanes or platinum agents. Unfortunately, the response rate is low for all of the agents in platinum-refractory/-resistant ovarian cancer. Patients should usually be evaluated for response after treatment with at least three cycles of the chemotherapy agent or regimen. Because partial responses are rare, stable disease is considered a treatment success. If no response is observed, then an alternative chemotherapy regimen may be selected.

Topotecan, an analog of the plant alkaloid 20(S)-camptothecin, is active in patients with metastatic ovarian cancer and is non–cross-resistant with platinum-based chemotherapy.[80] Preclinical studies suggest that protracted schedules of administration with low doses achieve the greatest antitumor response.[81] Topotecan has demonstrated activity in phase II trials as second-line and salvage therapy in patients who have relapsed after, or progressed during, platinum-based therapy.[80,81,83] A randomized phase III trial compared topotecan and paclitaxel in patients with advanced ovarian cancer who had failed one platinum-based regimen.[82] Patients were randomized to receive topotecan 1.5 mg/m² per day as a 30-minute infusion for 5 days repeated every 21 days or paclitaxel 175 mg/m² as a 3-hour infusion every 21 days. The overall response rate was 20.5% and 13.2% for the topotecan- and paclitaxel-treated groups, respectively. The median time to progression for topotecan-treated patients (32 weeks) was not significantly different than for paclitaxel-treated patients (20 weeks). Median survival was 61 weeks in the topotecan-treated group and 43 weeks in the paclitaxel-treated group. Topotecan was well tolerated with minimal nonhematologic toxicities.[80,82,83]

Pegylated liposomal doxorubicin is one of the primary agents used for second-line therapy of recurrent ovarian cancer.[84–86] The drug tends to be better tolerated than topotecan, which is important for heavily pretreated patients with advanced disease. A large, randomized phase III study compared pegylated liposomal doxorubicin 50 mg/m² every 4 weeks to topotecan 1.5 mg/m² per day for 5 days repeated every 21 days in patients who failed first-line platinum therapy.[86] A total of 474 patients were randomized, 239 to pegylated liposomal doxorubicin and 235 to topotecan. The overall confirmed response rates for the pegylated liposomal doxorubicin and topotecan groups were 20% and 17%, respectively. Overall survival tended to favor pegylated liposomal doxorubicin, with a median of 108 weeks versus 71.1 weeks for topotecan. Differences in toxicity were observed between the arms, with more hematologic toxicity occurring in the topotecan arm and more palmar-plantar erythrodysesthesia (PPE) in the pegylated liposomal doxorubicin arm. However, the incidence of PPE has decreased in current clinical practice because the standard dose of pegylated liposomal doxorubicin used currently, 40 mg/m², is less than the dose that was used in the initial clinical trials and approved by the FDA.[87,88]

Gemcitabine, a novel pyrimidine antimetabolite, is also a widely used agent used in the treatment of recurrent platinum-resistant ovarian cancer. Although the overall response rate is only approximately 13% to 22% with single-agent gemcitabine in patients with platinum-refractory recurrent ovarian cancer, an additional 16% to 50% of patients have stable disease for a median of 7 months.[89,90] The main toxicities include myelosuppression, fatigue, myalgia, and skin rash. Because of its non–cross-resistant activity and in vivo synergy with platinum agents, gemcitabine is being evaluated in doublet regimens in patients with refractory disease and with carboplatin/taxane regimens in previously untreated patients.[90] The combination of gemcitabine with taxanes have demonstrated response rates from 36% to 90%, which if confirmed, is extremely encouraging.[90]

Other agents that have shown an overall response rate of 10% to 25% in patients with recurrent ovarian cancer include altretamine, etoposide, capecitabine, tamoxifen, letrozole, vinorelbine, and oxaliplatin.[91] Response rates tend to be higher in the platinum-sensitive subgroups. Most of these agents are available in oral formulations, which allows for outpatient administration in the palliative care setting.

Although there are no guidelines for the selection of agents for the treatment of recurrent platinum-resistant ovarian cancer, the three most commonly used agents in clinical practice include pegylated liposomal doxorubicin, gemcitabine, and topotecan. These agents have demonstrated efficacy when used as a single agent and in combination with other agents. A phase II GOG study is ongoing to help define the optimal chemotherapy combination for treatment of recurrent or refractory platinum-resistant ovarian cancer.

Additional research continues to identify new agents and new targets for the treatment of ovarian cancer. Because platinum agents and taxanes have been identified as the most active classes of agents for treatment of ovarian cancer, drug development has focused on new platinum derivatives, taxanes and taxane analogs, and agents that exert cytotoxic activity by interacting with DNA directly. Specifically, new cytotoxic agents such as Yondelis, TLK-286, pemetrexed, and epothilones; monoclonal antibodies such as bevacizumab and cetuximab; and small molecule tyrosine inhibitors such as erlotinib, gefitinib, and lapatinib, are being evaluated in patients with ovarian cancer.[92–94]

PHARMACOECONOMIC CONSIDERATIONS

Healthcare at the end of life is associated with higher costs than at any other time, and, unfortunately, most patients with ovarian cancer will eventually die from the disease.[95] In the past, cost-to-benefit analyses have demonstrated palliative care, despite the limited benefit, is cost-effective based on patients' expectations and "willingness to pay."[96,97] Economic analyses of new chemotherapy agents usually measure cost-effectiveness, where effectiveness is measured as changes in survival (i.e. overall survival, progression-free survival) or quality-adjusted life-years.[98]

The paclitaxel plus platinum regimen is the current accepted standard of care for first-line treatment of advanced ovarian cancer. When paclitaxel was initially evaluated as first-line treatment, several economic analyses showed that the cost-effectiveness ratio of paclitaxel and cisplatin was within the range of other accepted medical interventions and supported its adoption as first-line treatment of advanced ovarian cancer.[98,99] In another cost-benefit study, Dranitsaris et al. reported that patients were willing to pay a mean of $64 which was marginally lower than the incremental cost of $87 to receive docetaxel rather than paclitaxel to reduce their risk of toxicity, primarily neuropathy.[100]

In the setting of recurrent ovarian cancer, Smith et al. performed a retrospective cost minimization analysis of pegylated liposomal doxorubicin versus topotecan.[101] The results of that analysis showed that pegylated liposomal doxorubicin was the preferred second-line agent, based on lower costs because of reduced toxicities as compared to topotecan.[101]

EVALUATION OF THERAPEUTIC OUTCOMES

Patients receiving a taxane or platinum chemotherapy regimen should be monitored for signs of hypersensitivity or infusion-related reactions. Patients treated with paclitaxel often experience infusion-related reactions which have been attributed to the Cremophor diluent. Premedications including an H_1-blocker, H_2-blocker, and steroid should be administered prior to each chemotherapy administration to prevent hypersensitivity reactions. If a patient has a reaction, paclitaxel desensitization can be attempted with 24 hours of premedications (H_1-blocker, H_2-blocker, and steroids) followed by paclitaxel given as a titrated infusion (1:1000 → 1:100 →1:10 → full dose) over 8 hours. With repeated exposure (i.e., seven cycles or more) to carboplatin, patients can develop a delayed hypersensitivity reaction. A similar protocol can be used for carboplatin desensitization.

Ovarian cancer patients receive multiple courses of chemotherapy that can have varying effects on kidney and liver function. Appropriate laboratory tests should be ordered to assess organ function so that chemotherapy doses can be adjusted as indicated. Patients on platinum-containing regimens often can experience electrolyte wasting, so patients should be monitored for electrolytes intravenous or oral replacement is indicated. The use of myeloid growth factors should be considered to prevent treatment delays and/or dose reductions. Prevention of nausea and vomiting, both acute and delayed, is critical for patients receiving emetogenic chemotherapy regimens such as paclitaxel-carboplatin.

During initial taxane-platinum chemotherapy, a CA-125 level should be obtained with each cycle and monitored for at least a 50% reduction in CA-125 after completion of four cycles, which is related to an improved prognosis. Patients who achieve a complete response after completion of first-line treatment should have followup once every 3 months, including CA-125, physical examination, pelvic examination, and appropriate diagnostic scans (i.e., computed tomography, magnetic resonance imaging, or positron emission tomography), which should be evaluated for presence of disease. In addition to routine followup examinations, clinicians should monitor for resolution of any residual chemotherapy-related side effects, including neuropathies, nephrotoxicity, ototoxicity, myelosuppression, and nausea/vomiting.

In the progressive disease or recurrent setting, CA-125 levels can still be used to monitor for response and should be checked with each cycle, although no change in therapy is recommended until after completion of at least three cycles of the second-line chemotherapy. In addition to laboratory monitoring, appropriate diagnostic scans (i.e., computed tomography, magnetic resonance imaging, or positron emission tomography) should be done once every three cycles. Again, patients need to be monitored with each cycle of chemotherapy to evaluate for new or persistent of toxicities such as neuropathies, fluid retention, PPE, myelosuppression, and nausea/vomiting.

Eventually most ovarian cancer patients will progress through all chemotherapy regimens and investigational treatment options, after which the best supportive care measures should be provided to maintain patient comfort and quality of life. Develop a plan for treatment of common complications of advanced/progressive ovarian cancer, including thrombosis, ascites, uncontrollable pain, and small bowel obstruction. The primary goal at the end of life for patients with progressive ovarian cancer is to provide any measures necessary to maintain patient comfort and quality of life.

CONCLUSIONS

Ovarian cancer remains one of the major challenges in gynecologic oncology. Key issues for improving outcome are patient education and awareness of the signs and symptoms of ovarian cancer. Earlier diagnosis is associated with a significant improvement in prognosis and overall survival. Although some milestones have been reached in extending progression-free and overall survival over the past few decades, there are still many unresolved issues. More data is needed to determine the optimal agents to be used for IP chemotherapy and the usefulness of maintenance chemotherapy and their impact on overall survival. Research needs to identify and develop new approaches to the prevention of recurrence and new options for the treatment of advanced primary as well as recurrent and refractory ovarian cancer, such as agents to modulate or overcome drug resistance, new molecular targets and optimize chemotherapy regimens.

ABBREVIATIONS

BRCA1: breast cancer activator gene 1

BRCA2: breast cancer activator gene 2

CA-125: CA antigen 125

CA-19: cancer antigen 19

FIGO: International Federation of Gynecology and Obstetrics

GOG: Gynecologic Oncology Group

NCCN: National Comprehensive Cancer Network

PPE: palmar-plantar erythrodysesthesia

REFERENCES

1. Shepherd JE. Current strategies for prevention, detection, and treatment of ovarian cancer. J Am Pharm Assoc 2000;40:392–401.
2. Cannistra SA. Cancer of the ovary. N Engl J Med 2004;351:2519–2529.
3. Jemal A, Siegel R, Ward E, Murray T, Xu J, Smigal C, Thun MJ. Cancer statistics, 2007 CA Cancer J Clin 2007;57:43–66.
4. Colomob N, VanGorp T, Parma G, et al. Ovarian cancer. Crit Rev Oncol Hematol 2006;60:159–179.
5. Lux MP, Fashing PA, Beckmann MW. Hereditary breast and ovarian cancer: Review and future perspectives. J Mol Med 2006;84: 16–28.
6. Boyd J, Sonoda Y, Federici MG, et al. Clinicopathologic features of BRCA-linked and sporadic ovarian cancer. JAMA 2000;283:2260–2265.
7. Runnebaum IB, Stickeler E. Epidemiological and molecular aspects of ovarian cancer risk. J Cancer Res Clin Oncol 2001;127:73–79.
8. Martin VR. Ovarian cancer. Semin Oncol Nurs 2002;18:174–183.
9. Pecorelli S, Odicino F, Maisonneuve P, et al. Carcinoma of the ovary. Annual report on the results of treatment in gynaecological cancer. J Epidemiol Biostat 1998;3:75–102.
10. Edmondson RJ, Monaghan JM. The epidemiology of ovarian cancer. Int J Gynecol Cancer 2001;11:423–429.
11. Holschneider CH, Berek JS. Ovarian cancer: Epidemiology, biology, and prognostic factors. Semin Surg Oncol 2000;19:3–10.
12. Ozols RF, Schwartz PE, Eifel PJ. Ovarian cancer, fallopian tube carcinoma, and peritoneal carcinoma. In: Devita VT, Hellman S, Rosenberg SA, eds. Cancer: Principles and Practice of Oncology, 6th ed. Philadelphia: Lippincott Williams & Wilkins, 2001:1597–1632.
13. Silverberg SG, Histopathologic grading of ovarian carcinoma: A review and proposal. Int J Gynecol Pathol 2000;19:7–15.
14. Seidman JD, Kuman RJ. Pathology of ovarian carcinoma. Hematol Oncol Clin North Am 2003;17:909–925.
15. Cherry C, Vacchiano SA. Ovarian cancer screening and prevention. Semin Oncol Nurs 2002;18:167–173.
16. Patterson DM, Rustin GJS. Controversies in the management of germ cell tumours of the ovary. Curr Opin Oncol 2006;18:500–506.
17. Sherman ME, Lacey JV, Buys SS, et al. Ovarian volume: Determinants and associations with cancer among postmenopausal women. Cancer Epidemiol Biomarkers Prev 2006;15:1550–1554.
18. Pavlik EJ, DePriest PD, Gallion HH, et al. Ovarian volume related to age. Gynecol Oncol 2000;77:410–412.
19. Edwards BK, Brown ML, Wingo PA, et al. Annual report to the nation on the status of cancer 1975–2002 featuring population-based trends in cancer treatment. J Natl Cancer Inst 2005;97:1407–1427.
20. Munkarah A, Chatterjee M, Tainsky MA. Update on ovarian cancer screening. Curr Opin Obstet Gynecol 2007;19:22–26.
21. U.S. Preventive Services Task Force. Screening for ovarian cancer: Recommendation statement. Ann Fam Med 2004;2:260–262.
22. Parazzini F, Chatenoud L, Chiantera V, Benzi G, Surace M, La Vecchia C. Population attributable risk for ovarian cancer. Eur J Cancer 2000;36:520–524.
23. Barnes MN, Grizzle WE, Grubbs CJ, Partridge EE. Paradigms for primary prevention of ovarian carcinoma. CA Cancer J Clin 2002;52:216–225.
24. Cramer DW, Harlow BL, Titus-Ernstoff L, et al. Over-the-counter analgesics and risk of ovarian cancer. Lancet 1998;351:104–107.
25. Tavani A, Gallus S, La Vecchia C, Cont E, Montella M, Franceschi S. Aspirin and ovarian cancer: An Italian case-control study. Ann Oncol 2000;11:1171–1173.
26. Domchek SM, Rebbeck TR. Prophylactic oophorectomy in women at increased cancer risk. Curr Opin Obstet Gynecol 2007;19:27–30.
27. Meeuwissen PAM, Seynaeve C, Brekelmans CTM, Meijers-Heijboer HJ, Klijn JGM, Burger CW. Outcome of surveillance and prophylactic salpingo-oophorectomy in asymptomatic women at high risk for ovarian cancer. Gynecol Oncol 2005;97:476–482.
28. Piver MS, Jishi MF, Tsukada Y, et al. Primary peritoneal carcinoma after prophylactic oophorectomy in women with a family history of ovarian cancer. A report of the Gilda Radner Familial Ovarian Cancer Registry. Cancer 1993;71:2751–2755.
29. Narod SA, Sun P, Ghadirian P, et al. Tubal ligation and risk of ovarian cancer in carriers of BRCA1 and BRCA2 mutations: A case control study. Lancet 2001;357:1467–1470.
30. Lux MP, Fashing PA, Beckmann MW. Hereditary breast and ovarian cancer: Review and future perspectives. J Mol Med 2006;84(1):16–28.
31. Coukos, G. Gene therapy for ovarian cancer. Oncology 2001;15:1197–1208.
32. Tait DL, Obermiller PS, Hatmaker AR. Relin-Frazier S, Holt JT. Ovarian cancer BRCA1 gene therapy: Phase I and II trial differences in immune response and vector stability. Clin Cancer Res 1999;5:1708–1714.
33. Goff BA, Mandel LS, Melancon CH, Muntz HG. Frequency of symptoms of ovarian cancer in women presenting to primary care clinics. JAMA 2004;291:2705–2712.
34. Goff BA, Mandel LS, Drescher CW, et al. Development of an ovarian cancer symptom index. Cancer 2007;109:221–227.
35. Salzberg M, Thurlimann B, Bonnefois H, et al. Current concepts of treatment strategies in advanced or recurrent ovarian cancer. Oncology 2005;68:293–298.
36. Pectasides D, Pectaside E, Psyrri A, Economopoulos T. Treatment issues in clear cell carcinoma of the ovary: A different entity? Oncologist 2006;11:1089–1094.
37. Stratton JF, Tidy JA, Paterson MEL. The surgical management of ovarian cancer. Cancer Treat Rev 2001:27;111–118.
38. Dauplat J, Le Bouedec G, Pomel C, Scherer C. Cytoreductive surgery for advanced stages of ovarian cancer. Semin Surg Oncol 2000;19:42–48.
39. Stratton JF, Tidy JA, Paterson MEL. The surgical management of ovarian cancer. Cancer Treat Rev 2001:27;111–118.
40. Bristow RE, Tomacruz RS, Armstrong DK, Trimble EL, Montz FJ. Survival Effect of maximal cytoreductive surgery for advanced ovarian carcinoma during platinum era: A meta analysis. J Clin Oncol 2002;20: 1248–1259.
41. Hoffman MS, Griffin D, Tebes S, et al. Sites of bowel resected to achieve optimal ovarian cancer cytoreduction: Implications regarding surgical management. Am J Obstet Gynecol 2005;193:582–588.
42. Bhoola S, Hoskins WJ. Diagnosis and management of epithelial ovarian cancer. Obstet Gynecol 2006;107:1399–1410.
43. Mayer AR, Chambers SK, Graves E, et al. Ovarian cancer staging: Does it require a gynecologic oncologist? Gynecol Oncol 1992;47: 223–227.
44. Nguyen HN, Averette HE, Hoskins W, et al. National survey of ovarian carcinoma. Part V. The impact of physician's specialty on patients' survival. Cancer 1993;72:3663–3670.
45. van der Burg ME, van Lent M, Buyse M, et al. The effect of debulking surgery after induction chemotherapy on the prognosis in advanced epithelial ovarian cancer. Gynecological Cancer Cooperative Group of the European Organization for Research and Treatment of Cancer [see comments]. N Engl J Med 1995;332:629–634.
46. Rose PG, Nerenstone S, Brady MF, et al. Secondary surgical cytoreduction for advanced ovarian carcinoma. N Engl J Med 2004;351:2489–2497.
47. Berek JS, Trope C, Vergote I. Surgery during chemotherapy and at relapse of ovarian cancer. Ann Oncol 1999;10(Suppl 1):3–7.

48. Marsden DE, Friedlander M, Hacker NF. Current management of epithelial ovarian carcinoma: A review. Semin Surg Oncol 2000;19:11–19.
49. Kyrgiou M, Salanti G, Pavlidis N, Paraskevaidis E, Ioannidis JPA. Survival benefits with diverse chemotherapy regimens for ovarian cancer: Meta-analysis or multiple treatments. J Natl Cancer Inst 2006;98:1655–1663.
50. Ozols R. Systemic therapy for ovarian cancer: Current status and new treatments. Semin Oncol 2006;33(Suppl 6):S3–S11.
51. McGuire WP, Hoskins WJ, Brady MF, et al. Cyclophosphamide and cisplatin compared with paclitaxel and cisplatin in patients with stage III and stage IV ovarian cancer. N Engl J Med 1996;334:1–6.
52. Piccart MJ, Bertelsen K, Stuart G, et al. Long-term follow-up confirms a survival advantage of the paclitaxel-cisplatin regimen over the cyclophosphamide-cisplatin combination in advanced ovarian cancer. Int J Gynecol Cancer 2003;13(Suppl 2):144–148.
53. Bookman MA, Greer BE, Ozols RF. Optimal therapy of advanced ovarian cancer: Carboplatin and paclitaxel vs. cisplatin and paclitaxel (GOG 158) and an update on GOG0 182-ICON5. Int J Gynecol Cancer 2003;136:735–740.
54. Ozols RF, Bundy BN, Green BE, et al. Phase III trial of carboplatin and paclitaxel compared with cisplatin and paclitaxel in patients with optimally resected stage III ovarian cancer: A Gynecologic Oncology Group Study. J Clin Oncol 2003;21:3194–3200.
55. du Bois A, Luck HJ, Meier W, et al. A randomized clinical trial of cisplatin/paclitaxel versus carboplatin/paclitaxel as first-line treatment of ovarian cancer. J Natl Cancer Inst 2003;3;95:1320–1329.
56. Neijt JP, Engelholm SA, Tuxen MK, et al. Exploratory phase III study of paclitaxel and cisplatin versus paclitaxel and carboplatin in advanced ovarian cancer. J Clin Oncol 2000;18:3084–3092.
57. Vasey PA, Jayson GC, Gordon A, et al. Phase III randomized trial of docetaxel-carboplatin versus paclitaxel-carboplatin as first-line chemotherapy for ovarian carcinoma. J Natl Cancer Inst 2004;1796: 1682–1691.
58. Fujiwara K, Armstrong D, Morgan M, Markman M. Principles and practice of intraperitoneal chemotherapy for ovarian cancer. Int J Gynecol Cancer 2007;17:1–20.
59. Armstrong DK, Bundy B, Wenzel L, et al. Intraperitoneal cisplatin and paclitaxel in ovarian cancer. N Engl J Med 2006;354:34–43.
60. Jaaback K, Johnson N. Intraperitoneal chemotherapy for the initial management of primary epithelial ovarian cancer. Cochrane Database Syst Rev 2006;3:1–28.
61. Markman M, Bundy BN, Alberts DS, et al. Phase III trial of standard-dose intravenous cisplatin in small-volume stage III ovarian carcinoma: An intergroup study of the gynecologic oncology group, southwestern oncology group, and eastern cooperative oncology group. J Clin Oncol 2001;19:1001–1007.
62. Alberts DS, Liu PY, Hannigan EV, et al. Intraperitoneal cisplatin plus intravenous cyclophosphamide versus intravenous cisplatin plus intravenous cyclophosphamide for stage III ovarian cancer. N Engl J Med 1996;335:1950–1955.
63. Walker JL, Armstrong DK, Huang HQ, et al. Intraperitoneal catheter outcomes in a phase III trial of intravenous versus intraperitoneal chemotherapy in optimal stage III ovarian and primary peritoneal cancer: A Gynecologic Oncology Group Study. Gynecol Oncol 2006;100:27–32.
64. Markman M, Walker JL. Intraperitoneal chemotherapy of ovarian cancer: A review, with a focus on practical aspects of treatment. J Clin Oncol 2006;24:988–994.
65. National Comprehensive Cancer Network (NCCN) Practice Guidelines in Oncology—Ovarian Cancer, V1.2007. 2007, *http://www.nccn.org.*
66. NCI Clinical Announcement. Intraperitoneal Chemotherapy for Ovarian Cancer. Released on January 5, 2006. 2006, *http://ctep.cancer.gov/highlights/clin_annc_010506.pdf.*
67. Salzberg M, Thurlimann B, Bonnefois H, et al. Current concepts of treatment strategies in advanced or recurrent ovarian cancer. Oncology 2005;68:293–298.
68. Gadducci A, Cosio S, Conte PF, Genazzani AR. Consolidation and maintenance treatments for patients with advanced epithelial ovarian cancer in complete response after first-line chemotherapy: A review of the literature. Crit Rev Oncol Hematol 2005;55:153–166.
69. Markman M, Liu PY, Wilczynski, et al. Phase III randomized trial of 12 versus 3 months of maintenance paclitaxel in patients with advanced ovarian cancer who attained a clinically-defined complete response to platinum/paclitaxel-based chemotherapy: A Southwest Oncology Group and Gynecology Oncology Group trial. J Clin Oncol 2003;21:2460–2465.
70. Gadducci A, Cosio S, Conte PF, Genazzani AR. Consolidation and maintenance treatments for patients with advanced epithelial ovarian cancer in complete response after first-line chemotherapy: A review of the literature. Crit Rev Oncol Hematol 2005;55:153–166.
71. Markman M. Unresolved issues in the chemotherapeutic management of gynecologic malignancies. Semin Oncol 2006;33(Suppl 6): S33–S38.
72. Mulder PO, Willemse PH, Aalders JG, et al. High-dose chemotherapy with autologous bone marrow transplantation in patients with refractory ovarian cancer. Eur J Cancer Clin Oncol 1989;25:645–649.
73. Stiff PJ, Veum-Stone J, Lazarus HM, et al. High-dose chemotherapy and autologous stem cell transplantation for ovarian cancer: An autologous blood and marrow transplant registry report. Ann Intern Med 2000;133:504–515.
74. Goncalves A, Delva R, Fabbro M, et al. Post-operative sequential high-dose chemotherapy with haematopoietic stem cell support as front-line treatment in advanced ovarian cancer: A multicenter study. Bone Marrow Transplant 2006;37:651–659.
75. ICON and AGO Collaborators. Paclitaxel plus platinum-based chemotherapy versus conventional platinum-based chemotherapy in women with relapsed ovarian cancer: The ICON4/AGO-OVAR-2.2 trial. Lancet 2003;361:2099–2106.
76. Gronlund B, Hogdall C, Hansen HH, Engelholm SA. Performance status rather than age is the key prognostic factor in second-line treatment of elderly patients with epithelial ovarian carcinoma. Cancer 2002;94:1961–1967.
77. Ozols RF. Recurrent ovarian cancer: Evidence-based treatment. J Clin Oncol 2002;20:1151–1163.
78. Markman M, Bookman MA. Second-line treatment for ovarian cancer. Oncologist 200;5;26–35.
79. Herzog TJ, Pothuri B. Ovarian cancer: A focus on management of recurrent disease. Nat Clin Pract Oncol 2006;3:604–611.
80. Swisher EM, Mutch DG, Rader JS, et al. Topotecan in platinum- and paclitaxel-resistant ovarian cancer. Gynecol Oncol 1997;66:480–486.
81. Markman M. Topotecan: An important new drug in the management of ovarian cancer. Semin Oncol 1997;24:S5–S11.
82. ten Bokkel Huinink W, Gore M, Carmichael J, et al. Topotecan versus paclitaxel for the treatment of recurrent epithelial ovarian cancer. J Clin Oncol 1997;15:2183–2193.
83. Creemers GJ, Bolis G, Gore M, et al. Topotecan, an active drug in the second-line treatment of epithelial ovarian cancer: Results of a large European phase II study [see comments]. J Clin Oncol 1996;14:3056–3061.
84. Muggia FM, Hainsworth JD, Jeffers S, et al. Phase II study of liposomal doxorubicin in refractory ovarian cancer: Antitumor activity and toxicity modification by liposomal encapsulation. J Clin Oncol 1997;15:987–993.
85. Gordon AN, Cranai CO, Rose PG, et al. Phase II study of liposomal doxorubicin in platinum- and paclitaxel refractory epithelial ovarian cancer. J Clin Oncol 2000;18:3093–3100.
86. Gordon AN, Fleagle JT, Guthrie D, et al. Recurrent epithelial ovarian carcinoma: A randomized phase III trial of pegylated liposomal doxorubicin versus topotecan. J Clin Oncol 2001;19:3312–3322.
87. Wilailk S, Linasmita V. A study of pegylated liposomal doxorubicin in platinum-refractory epithelial ovarian cancer. Oncology 2004;67:183–186.
88. Drake RD, Lin WM, King M, Farrar D, Miller DS, Coleman RL. Oral dexamethasone attenuates Doxil-induced palmer-plantar erythrodysesthesias in patients with recurrent gynecologic malignancies. Gynecol Oncol 2004;94:320–324.
89. Lund B, Hansen P, Theilade K, et al. Phase II study of gemcitabine (2x, 2x-dilfuorodeoxycytidine in previously treated ovarian cancer patients. J Natl Cancer Inst 1994;6:1530–1533.
90. Poveda A. Gemcitabine in patients with ovarian cancer. Cancer Treat Rev 2005;31(Suppl 4):S29-S37.

91. Cannistra SA, Bast RC, Berek JS, et al. Progress in the management of gynecologic cancer: Consensus summary statement. J Clin Oncol 2003;21(Suppl):129S–132S.
92. Ozols RF, Systemic therapy for ovarian cancer: Current status and new treatments. Semin Oncol 2006;33(Suppl 6):S3–S11.
93. Kurzeder C, Sauer G, Deissler H. Molecular targets of ovarian carcinomas with acquired resistance to platinum/taxane chemotherapy. Curr Cancer Drug Targets 2006;6:207–227.
94. Cannistra SA, Bast RC, Berek JS, et al. Progress in the management of gynecologic cancer: Consensus summary statement. J Clin Oncol 2003;21(Suppl):129s–132s.
95. Higginson IJ, Edmonds P. Services, costs and appropriate outcomes in end of life care. Ann Oncol 1999;10:135–136.
96. Patnaik A, Doyle C, Oza AM. Palliative therapy in advanced ovarian cancer: Balancing patient expectations, quality of life and cost. Anticancer Drugs 1998;9:869–878.
97. Ferguson JS, Summerhayes M, Masters S, Schey S, Smith IE. New treatments for advanced cancer: An approach to prioritization. Br J Cancer 2000;83:1268–1273.
98. Cowens A, Boucher S, Roche, et al. Is paclitaxel and cisplatin a cost effective first line therapy for advanced ovarian carcinoma. Cancer 1996;77:2086–2091.
99. Young M, Plosker GL. Paclitaxel: A pharmacoeconomic review of its use in the treatment of ovarian cancer. Pharmacoeconomics 2001; 19:1227–1259.
100. Dranitsaris G, Elia-Pacitti J, Cottrell W. Measuring treatment preferences and willingness to pay for docetaxel in advanced ovarian cancer. Pharmacoeconomics 2004;22:375–387.
101. Smith DH, Adam JR, Johnston SRD, Gordan A, Drummond MF, Bennett CL. A comparative economic analysis of pegylated liposomal doxorubicin versus topotecan in ovarian cancer in the USA and the UK. Ann Oncol 2002;13:1590–1597.

CHAPTER 137 Acute Leukemias

HELEN L. LEATHER AND BETSY BICKERT POON

KEY CONCEPTS

1. Acute leukemias are the most common malignancies in children and the leading cause of cancer-related death in patients younger than age 35 years.
2. The World Health Organization recently developed a new classification system for myeloid neoplasms, but the French-American-British (FAB) classification remains the most widely used.
3. To establish a definitive diagnosis of acute leukemia, the following diagnostic components are required: bone marrow biopsy and aspirate (with >20% blasts), cytogenetics, and immunophenotyping.
4. Several risk factors correlate with prognosis for acute lymphoblastic leukemia (ALL). Poor prognostic factors include high white blood cell count at presentation, very young or very old age at diagnosis, delayed remission induction and presence of certain cytogenetic abnormalities (e.g., Philadelphia [Ph^+] chromosome).
5. For children with ALL, remission induction therapy includes vincristine, a corticosteroid, and asparaginase, with or without an anthracycline. For adults with ALL, vincristine, prednisone, and an anthracycline are given, and asparaginase is sometimes added.
6. All patients with ALL require prophylactic therapy to prevent CNS disease because of the high risk of central nervous system relapse. The choice for therapy includes a combination of the following: cranial irradiation, intrathecal chemotherapy, or high-dose systemic chemotherapy with drugs that cross the blood–brain barrier.
7. Long-term maintenance therapy for 2 to 3 years is essential to eradicate residual leukemia cells and prolong the duration of remission. Maintenance therapy consists of oral methotrexate and mercaptopurine, with or without monthly pulses of vincristine and a corticosteroid.
8. Disease-free survival is lower in adults with ALL and has been attributed to greater drug resistance, poor side-effect tolerance with subsequent nonadherence, and possibly less-effective therapy. This population is also more likely to have Ph^+ ALL, which is associated with a worse outcome.
9. Colony-stimulating factors can be safely and effectively used with myelosuppressive chemotherapy for acute leukemias. The benefits can include reduced incidence of serious infections, reduced hospital stays, and fewer treatment delays, but do not include prolonged disease-free survival or overall survival.
10. There are several poor prognostic factors for adult acute myeloid leukemia (AML): older age, organ impairment, certain FAB subtypes, presence of extramedullary disease, and presence of certain cytogenetic and molecular abnormalities.
11. Therapy of AML usually includes induction therapy with an anthracycline and cytarabine. Postremission therapy is required in all patients and can include either consolidation chemotherapy with or without maintenance therapy, or hematopoietic stem cell transplantation.
12. It is estimated that up to 10^8 to 10^9 malignant cells remain following attainment of a complete remission. Postremission therapy with either chemotherapy or hematopoietic stem cell transplantation is essential in AML.
13. Treatment of acute promyelocytic leukemia consists of induction therapy, followed by consolidation and maintenance therapy. Induction includes tretinoin and an anthracycline; consolidation therapy consists of two to three cycles of anthracycline-based therapy; maintenance consists of pulse doses of tretinoin, mercaptopurine, and methotrexate for 2 years.

Learning objectives, review questions, and other resources can be found at **www.pharmacotherapyonline.com.**

The leukemias are heterogeneous hematologic malignancies characterized by unregulated proliferation of the blood-forming cells in the bone marrow. These immature proliferating leukemia cells (blasts) physically "crowd out" or inhibit normal cellular maturation in bone marrow, resulting in anemia, neutropenia, and thrombocytopenia. Leukemic blasts may also infiltrate a variety of tissues such as lymph nodes, skin, liver, spleen, kidney, testes, and the central nervous system.

The term *leukemia* was coined by Virchow to describe the "white blood" of some patients that he saw under the microscope in 1845.[1] Historically, leukemia has been classified as acute or chronic based on differences in cell of origin and cell line maturation, clinical presentation, rapidity of progression of the untreated disease, and response to therapy. Four major leukemias are recognized: acute lymphoblastic (or lymphocytic) leukemia (ALL), acute myeloid leukemia (AML), chronic lymphocytic leukemia, and chronic myeloid leukemia. Undifferentiated immature cells that proliferate autonomously characterize acute leukemias. Chronic leukemias also proliferate autonomously, but the cells are more differentiated and mature.[1] Untreated, the acute leukemias are rapidly progressive, resulting in death within 2 to 3 months.

EPIDEMIOLOGY

1 It is estimated that 18,610 new cases of acute leukemias—13,410 cases of AML and 5,200 cases of ALL—will be diagnosed in the

United States in 2007, accounting for 1.3% of the total cancer incidence.[2] The incidence has been relatively stable for two decades. An estimated 10,410 deaths per year, representing approximately 2% of all cancer deaths, are caused by acute leukemias. The acute leukemias are the leading cause of cancer-related deaths in persons younger than age 35 years, but an uncommon cause of cancer-related death after age 35 years.[1,2] Among adults, acute and chronic leukemias occur at equal rates. More than 90% of the cases of acute and chronic leukemia occur in adults. AML accounts for most cases of acute leukemia in adults, and occurs with increasing frequency in elderly patients. There are about 4 cases of AML and 1.4 cases of ALL per 100,000 individuals.[3] The median age at diagnosis of patients with AML is about 65 years, whereas the median age for ALL patients is about 10 years.[1–3] The incidence of AML rises with age from 1.8 per 100,000 in individuals younger than age 65 years to 17.9 per 100,000 in those 65 years or older.[3,4] Acute leukemia is slightly more common in males than in females. In the United States, acute leukemia is more common among whites than among African Americans, American Indians, and Hispanic ethnicities.[1,3]

Despite the low incidence rate, the acute leukemias are the most common malignancy in persons younger than 15 years of age, accounting for approximately 30% of all childhood malignancies.[3] In the United States, 9,850 persons younger than 15 years of age are diagnosed with cancer each year; approximately 2,500 of them have ALL.[4] AML accounts for approximately 20% of all childhood leukemias, and the chronic leukemias account for less than 5%.[3] Childhood ALL is 30% more common in males than in females, peaks at 2 to 5 years of age, and is twice as likely to affect white children as African American children.[3,5] The incidence of childhood AML is highest in the Hispanic population and occurs throughout childhood without any peak age period. Acute leukemia during the first year of life (infant leukemia) is twice as likely to be ALL as AML.[3]

Chemotherapy has dramatically improved the outlook of patients with acute leukemia. More than 85% of children and young adults with acute leukemia achieve an initial complete remission (CR) of their disease. Overall, 65% to 85% of adults achieve an initial CR.[1,4] For persons younger than 20 years of age, the 5-year survival rate is 83% for ALL and 50% for AML.[3] The prognosis of adult acute leukemia is generally worse than that of childhood leukemia, with only 30% to 40% of patients becoming long-term survivors.[1,4]

ETIOLOGY

The exact cause of the acute leukemias is unknown. A multifactorial process involving genetics, environmental and socioeconomic factors, toxins, immunologic status, and viral exposures is likely. Table 137–1 summarizes the major factors that have been linked to acute leukemias. Infectious and genetic factors have the strongest associations to date.[1,6–8] In pediatric ALL, a number of environmental factors are inconsistently linked to the diseases: exposure to ionizing radiation, toxic chemicals, herbicides and pesticides; maternal use of contraceptives, diethylstilbestrol, or cigarettes; parental exposure to drugs (amphetamines, diet pills, and mind-altering medications), diagnostic radiographs, alcohol consumption, or chemicals before and during pregnancy; and chemical contamination of groundwater.[6,8] Ionizing radiation and benzene exposure are the only environmental risk factors strongly associated with ALL or AML.[8] A few studies have reported a possible link between electromagnetic fields of high-voltage power lines and the development of leukemia, but larger studies could not confirm this association. In most patients who develop leukemia, a causative agent cannot be identified.

Childhood AML is associated with Hispanic ethnicity, prior exposure to alkylating agents or epidophyllotoxins, and in utero exposure to ionizing radiation.[1,8] Maternal alcohol consumption, parental and child pesticide exposure, and parental benzene exposure are also associated with childhood AML.

TABLE 137-1 Risk Factors for Acute Leukemia

Drugs	**Chemical**
Alkylating agents	Benzene
Epidophyllotoxins	**Pesticides**
Genetic conditions	**Pyrethroid-based shampoo**
Ataxia telangiectasia	**Radiation**
Bloom's syndrome	Ionizing radiation
Diamond-Blackfan's anemia	**Virus**
Down's syndrome	Epstein-Barr virus
Familial monosomy 7	Human T-lymphocyte virus (HTLV-1 and HTLV-2)
Fanconi's anemia	**Social habits**
Klinefelter's syndrome	Cigarette smoking
Kostmann's syndrome	Maternal marijuana use
Langerhans cell histiocytosis	Maternal ethanol use
Neurofibromatosis type 1	
Schwachman's syndrome	
Severe combined immunodeficiency syndrome	
Wiskott-Aldrich's syndrome	

PATHOPHYSIOLOGY

A basic understanding of normal hematopoiesis is needed before one can understand the pathogenesis of leukemia. Chapter 103 has a detailed discussion of hematopoiesis. Normal hematopoiesis consists of multiple well-orchestrated steps of cellular development. A pool of pluripotent stem cells undergoes differentiation, proliferation, and maturation, to form the mature blood cells seen in the peripheral circulation. These pluripotent stem cells initially differentiate to form two distinct stem cell pools. The myeloid stem cell gives rise to six types of blood cells (erythrocytes, platelets, monocytes, basophils, neutrophils, and eosinophils), while the lymphoid stem cell differentiates to form circulating B and T lymphocytes. Leukemia may develop at any stage and within any cell line.

Two features are common to both AML and ALL: first, both arise from a single leukemic cell that expands and acquires additional mutations, culminating in a monoclonal population of leukemia cells. Second, there is a failure to maintain a relative balance between proliferation and differentiation, so that the cells do not differentiate past a particular stage of hematopoiesis. Cells (lymphoblasts or myeloblasts) then proliferate uncontrollably. Proliferation, differentiation, and apoptosis are under genetic control, and leukemia can occur when the balance between these processes is altered. New antileukemia drug therapies are being developed that are specifically targeted to the biologic processes involved in proliferation and differentiation.

AML probably arises from a defect in the pluripotent stem cell or a more committed myeloid precursor, resulting in partial differentiation and proliferation of immature precursors of the myeloid blood-forming cells. In older patients, trilineage leukemic involvement is common, suggesting that the cell of origin is probably a stem or very early progenitor cell. In younger patients, a more differentiated progenitor becomes malignant, allowing maturation of some granulocytic and erythroid populations. These two forms of AML exhibit different patterns of resistance to chemotherapy, with resistance more evident in the older adults with AML. ALL is a disease characterized by proliferation of immature lymphoblasts. In this type of acute leukemia, the defect is probably at the level of the lymphopoietic stem cell or a very early lymphoid precursor.[1]

Leukemic cells have growth and/or survival advantages over normal cells, leading to a "crowding out" phenomenon in the bone marrow. This growth advantage is not caused by more rapid prolif-

TABLE 137-2 Morphologic (FAB) Classification of Acute Myeloid Leukemia

	Subtype	Adults (%)	Frequency of FAB Subtype[a] Children <2 years (%)	Children >2 years (%)
M0	Acute myeloblastic leukemia, without maturation	5	Low	Low
M1	Acute myeloblastic leukemia with minimal maturation	15	17	25
M2	Acute myeloblastic with maturation	25		27
M3	Acute promyelocytic leukemia	10		5
M4	Acute myelomonocytic leukemia	25	30	26
M5a	Acute monoblastic leukemia, poorly differentiated	5	52	16
M5b	Acute monoblastic leukemia, well differentiated	5		
M6	Acute erythroleukemia	5		2
M7	Acute megakaryoblastic leukemia	10		5–7

FAB, French-American-British.
[a]Percentages should be compared vertically, not horizontally.

eration as compared with normal cells. Some studies suggest that it is caused by factors produced by leukemic cells that either inhibit normal cellular proliferation and differentiation, or reduce apoptosis as compared with normal blood cells.

The types of genetic alterations that lead to leukemia have only recently become evident. The genetic defects may include (a) activation of a normally suppressed gene (protooncogene) to create an oncogene that produces a protein product that signals increased proliferation; (b) loss of signals for the blood cell to differentiate; (c) loss of tumor suppressor genes that control normal proliferation; and (d) loss of signals for apoptosis. Most normal cells are programmed to die eventually through apoptosis, but the appropriate programmed signal is often interrupted in cancer cells, leading to continued survival, replication, and drug resistance. Signal transduction, RNA transcription, cell-cycle control factors, cell differentiation, and programmed cell death may all be affected.

LEUKEMIA CLASSIFICATION

❷ The French-American-British (FAB) classification system identifies eight different subtypes of AML based on granulocytic differentiation and maturation (Table 137–2), and this system is used to determine prognosis and choice of therapy. However, it does not consider clinical characteristics, clonal cytogenetic abnormalities, immunophenotyping, or response to therapy. The World Health Organization and the Society of Hematopathology have proposed a new classification system for myeloid neoplasms (Table 137–3).[9] This new classification system incorporates not only morphologic findings, but also genetic, immunophenotypic, biologic, and clinical features. It has long been known that certain cytogenetic abnormalities have prognostic significance, but did not always correlate well with the FAB classification system.[10] In addition, this new classification attempts to formally incorporate the relationship between AML and myelodysplastic syndrome (MDS). A limitation of the World Health Organization classification is that it does not account for some of the myeloid disorders of childhood. There are recommendations to expand the myelodysplastic/myeloproliferative disorders to include additional subclasses such as juvenile myelomonocytic leukemia and patients with Down syndrome.[11]

Lymphoid leukemias are not addressed in the current World Health Organization classification system. Markers on the cell surface or membrane of the lymphoblast can be used to classify ALL. ALL may also be described by cytogenetic abnormalities. Chromosome alterations include numerical (hyperdiploidy and hypodiploidy), and structural abnormalities due to exchanges of genetic information within (inversion) or between (translocation) chromosomes.[12] ALL is also subclassified based on cell type into mature B-cell, precursor B-cell, and T-cell disease. Eighty percent of childhood ALL derives from precursor B cells and approximately 15% from T cells. The remainder is either mixed lineage or from mature B cells.

ACUTE LYMPHOBLASTIC LEUKEMIA

CLINICAL PRESENTATION

❸ Common signs and symptoms at presentation result from malignant cells replacing and suppressing normal hematopoietic progenitor cells and infiltration into extramedullary spaces. In addition to clinical presentation, laboratory and pathology evaluations are required for a definitive diagnosis of leukemia. An abnormal complete blood count is usually the diagnostic test that initiates a leukemia diagnostic workup. The most important test is a bone marrow biopsy and aspirate, which is submitted to hematopathology for numerous evaluations. A lumbar puncture is performed to determine if there are blasts in the central nervous system (CNS). A

TABLE 137-3 World Health Organization Classification of Acute Myeloid Leukemia

Acute myeloid leukemia (AML) with recurrent genetic abnormalities
AML with t(8;21)(q22;q22), (AML1/ETO)
AML with abnormal bone marrow eosinophils and inv(16)(p13;q22) or t(16;16)(p13;q22), (CBFβ/MYH11)
Acute promyelocytic leukemia with t(15;17)(q22;q12), (PML/RARα) and variants
AML with 11q23 (MLL) abnormalities
Acute myeloid leukemia with multilineage dysplasia
Following MDS or MDS/MPD disorder
Without antecedent MDS or MDS/MPD, but with dysplasia in at least 50% of cells or two or more lineages
Acute myeloid leukemia and MDS, therapy-related
Alkylating agent/radiation-related type
Topoisomerase II inhibitor-related type (some may be lymphoid)
Others
Acute myeloid leukemia, not otherwise categorized, classify as
Acute myeloid leukemia, minimally differentiated
Acute myeloid leukemia without maturation
Acute myeloid leukemia with maturation
Acute myelomonocytic leukemia
Acute monoblastic/acute monocytic leukemia
Acute erythroid leukemia (erythroid/myeloid and pure erythroleukemia)
Acute megakaryocytic leukemia
Acute basophilic leukemia
Acute panmyelosis with myelofibrosis
Myeloid sarcoma

MDS, myelodysplastic syndrome; MLL, mixed lineage leukemia; MPD, myeloproliferative disease; PML, promyelocytic leukemia; RAR, retinoic acid receptor-α.
From Vardiman et al.[9]

chest radiograph is performed to screen for a mediastinal mass (most common in T-cell disease).

Leukemia is suspected if the bone marrow contains greater than 5% blasts. Cytochemical stains are helpful to determine if the acute leukemia is of myeloid or lymphoid lineage. Immunophenotyping analyzes specific antigens, known as clusters of differentiation, often abbreviated "CD," present on the surface of hematopoietic cells. Although no leukemia-specific antigens have been identified, the pattern of cell-surface antigen expression reliably distinguishes between lymphoid and myeloid leukemia.[1] Cytogenetic analysis of the marrow to determine the presence of nonrandom numerical and structural chromosomal abnormalities in leukemic cells is also helpful for diagnosis, establishing prognosis, and evaluating response to therapy.[1,5,6,12] Chromosome translocations can result in abnormal expression and/or function of cellular oncogenes. Unique translocations can identify specific subtypes of acute leukemia. Recently, technically difficult cytogenetic analysis has been supplemented with fluorescent in situ hybridization, which allows for quick, sensitive analysis of samples that might be inadequate for karyotyping. Fluorescent in situ hybridization is a process in which specific genes in an intact cell are visualized with fluorescent-labeled probes. Molecular tests may be used to identify products of specific translocations.

CLINICAL PRESENTATION[1,5,6]

General

- Recent history of vague symptoms such as tiredness, lack of exercise tolerance, and "feeling unwell," but in no obvious distress.

Symptoms

- Patient's commonly report fever, pallor, weight loss, malaise, fatigue, palpitations, and bone pain. Other possible symptoms include epistaxis, palpitations, dyspnea on exertion, seizures, headache, or diplopia.

Signs

- Temperature is often elevated and may be caused by disease or infection; ecchymoses or petechiae; painless testicular enlargement; splenomegaly, hepatomegaly, and/or lymphadenopathy; and, rarely, small, blue-green collections of leukemia cells under the skin (chloromas).

Laboratory Tests

- Complete blood count with differential. Anemia (43% <7 g/dL) is normochromic and normocytic (without a compensatory increase in reticulocytes). Thrombocytopenia (severe, <20,000 cells/mm^3) is present in 28% of cases. Leukopenia/leukocytosis: 17% of patients will present with a white blood cell (WBC) count ≥50,000 cells/mm^3 and 53% with a WBC <10,000 cells/mm^3.
- Uric acid may be elevated because of rapid cellular turnover and is more common in patients presenting with elevated WBC count.
- Electrolytes: potassium and phosphate may be elevated with a compensatory decrease in calcium.

Other Diagnostic Tests

- Bone marrow aspirate and biopsy: send for morphologic examination, cytochemical staining, immunophenotyping, and cytogenetic (chromosome) analysis. All patients should have a screening lumbar puncture performed to assess CNS involvement.

RISK CLASSIFICATION

❹ Many clinical and laboratory features at diagnosis are associated with response to treatment, as measured by the CR rate, duration of remission, and long-term survival. Identification of these risk factors allows the clinician to better understand the disease and to tailor treatment according to risk of disease recurrence (i.e., risk-adapted therapy). For example, if a patient has many clinical and laboratory features that are associated with a good response to chemotherapy ("standard-risk"), then the clinician may choose to give less-intensive therapy to reduce the risk of long-term side effects. Conversely, if a patient is unlikely to respond well to standard therapy ("high-risk" or "very-high-risk"), then the clinician may choose to give more-intensive chemotherapy.

The National Cancer Institute developed an ALL risk stratification to create a standard for comparison in children.[13] Remission induction therapy is initially selected based on this classification, which divides children into standard- or high-risk categories based on age, WBC count, and karyotype (Fig. 137–1). Recently, more sophisticated biologic studies have allowed more refined risk stratification.[14] For example, it incorporates treatment response through the measurement of subclinical minimal residual disease by either flow cytometry or polymerase chain reaction.

The strongest prognostic factor for outcome for ALL is response to therapy. Traditionally this was measured morphologically in bone marrow specimens. More recently molecular measurement of minimal residual disease has enabled detection of leukemic cells not visible on morphologic examination.[15] This technique allows detection of 1 leukemia cell in 10,000 normal cells, which is about 100-fold more sensitive than morphologic examination. If minimal residual disease is detected at the end of induction therapy, the clinician may decide to give more-intensive therapy to decrease the risk of relapse.

The Children's Oncology Group has proposed a risk- and response-based classification of childhood ALL (see Fig. 137–1).[14] That classification system uses the National Cancer Institute risk assignment to initially categorize patients into standard- or high-risk groups. Patients with T-cell ALL are automatically categorized as very-high-risk, regardless of age, WBC count, or other factors. Following remission induction therapy, risk is reclassified based on the rapidity and completeness of response to therapy, the presence or absence of cytogenetic abnormalities, testicular involvement, or CNS involvement (see Fig. 137–1). Children may have their therapy augmented if the bone marrow has more than 5% blasts on day 15 of therapy. Children will have therapy reduced if they have either triple trisomies (chromosomes 4, 10, and 17) or TEL-AML1 (translocation ETS leukemia-acute myeloid leukemia-1) fusions and have less than 5% blasts by day 8 or 15 or 29 of induction in conjunction with less than 0.1% minimal residual disease on day 29. Children who have the Philadelphia chromosome [Ph$^+$ disease, t(9;22)], hypodiploidy, T-cell disease, induction failures, mixed lineage leukemia (MLL), or a slow response to induction therapy are considered very high-risk.

Other prognostic factors have been identified but are not the basis for therapy changes. Females have a better prognosis than males. Race is controversial, with older studies indicating worse outcomes for minorities. Hepatosplenomegaly and mediastinal mass are both associated with worse outcomes.

TREATMENT

Acute Lymphoblastic Leukemia

■ TREATMENT GOALS

The short-term goal of treatment for acute leukemia is to rapidly achieve a complete clinical and hematologic remission. CR is defined as the disappearance of all physical and bone marrow

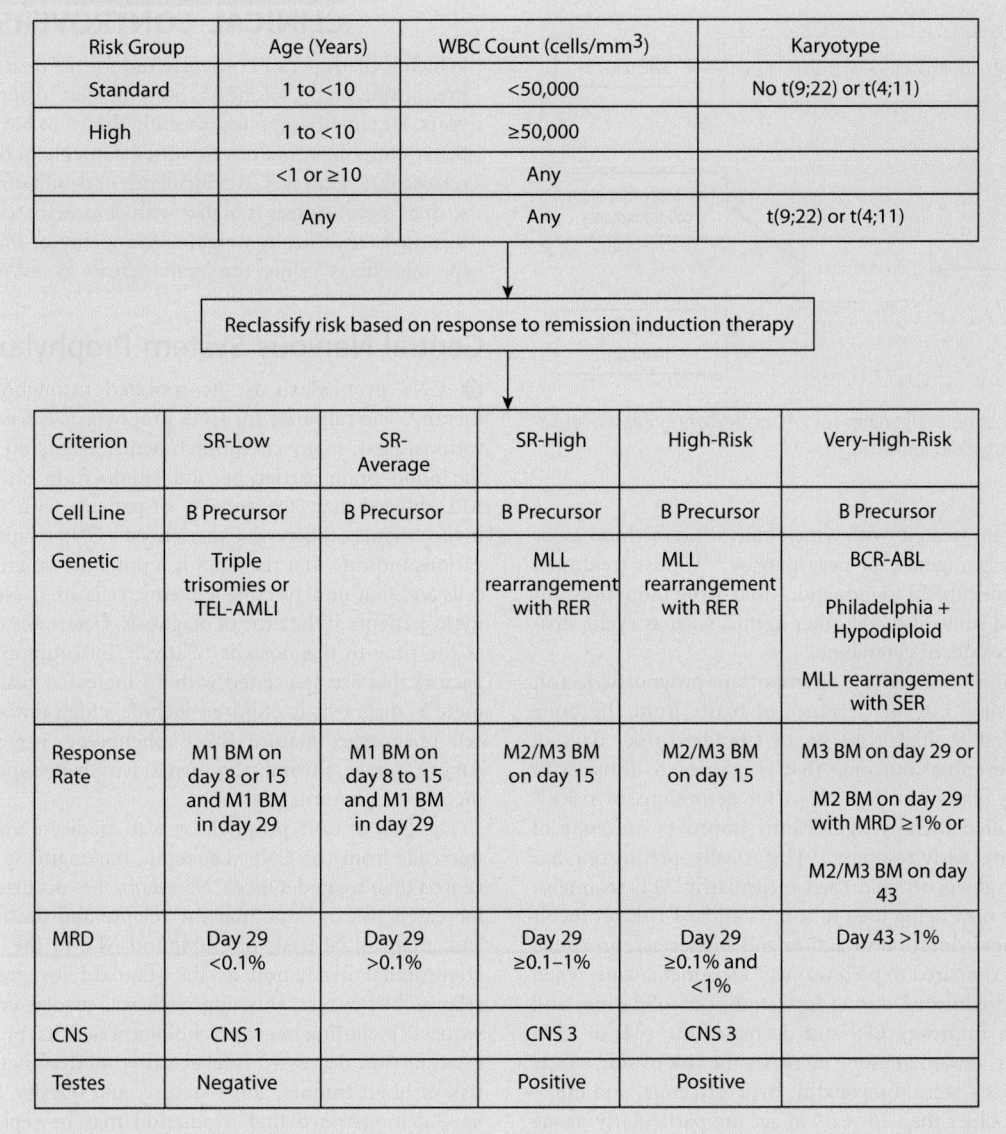

Risk Group	Age (Years)	WBC Count (cells/mm^3)	Karyotype
Standard	1 to <10	<50,000	No t(9;22) or t(4;11)
High	1 to <10	≥50,000	
	<1 or ≥10	Any	
	Any	Any	t(9;22) or t(4;11)

Reclassify risk based on response to remission induction therapy

Criterion	SR-Low	SR-Average	SR-High	High-Risk	Very-High-Risk
Cell Line	B Precursor	B Precursor	B Precursor	B Precursor	B Precursor
Genetic	Triple trisomies or TEL-AMLI		MLL rearrangement with RER	MLL rearrangement with RER	BCR-ABL Philadelphia + Hypodiploid MLL rearrangement with SER
Response Rate	M1 BM on day 8 or 15 and M1 BM in day 29	M1 BM on day 8 to 15 and M1 BM in day 29	M2/M3 BM on day 15	M2/M3 BM on day 15	M3 BM on day 29 or M2 BM on day 29 with MRD ≥1% or M2/M3 BM on day 43
MRD	Day 29 <0.1%	Day 29 >0.1%	Day 29 ≥0.1–1%	Day 29 ≥0.1% and <1%	Day 43 >1%
CNS	CNS 1		CNS 3	CNS 3	
Testes	Negative		Positive	Positive	

FIGURE 137-1. Risk- and response-based classification of childhood ALL. *Note:* Patients with T-cell ALL are automatically categorized as very-high-risk regardless of other factors. (BM, bone marrow; CNS 1, no lymphoblasts; CNS 3, lymphoblasts with ≥5 WBC/mm^3 or clinical signs of CNS disease; M1, <5% blasts, M2, 5–25% blasts, M3, >25% blasts; MLL, mixed lineage leukemia; MRD, minimal residual disease; RER, rapid early response; SER, slow early response; SR, standard risk; TEL-AML1, translocation ETS leukemia-acute myeloid leukemia-1; WBC, white blood cell.)

evidence (normal cellularity with <5% blasts) of leukemia, with restoration of normal hematopoiesis (neutrophils ≥1,500 cells/mm^3 and platelets >100,000 cells/mm^3). After a CR is achieved, the goal is to maintain the patient in continuous CR. In general, a child is considered to be "cured" after being in continuous CR for 5 to 10 years.

Successful treatment of ALL was first developed in children. Current regimens induce CR in 98% of children with ALL.[12] Children who do not achieve a CR by the end of induction have an overall event-free survival (EFS) of 16%.[5] Cure rates in children have risen from less than 5% with treatments used in the 1960s to approximately 90% by 2005.[12] The reason for this improvement lies largely in improved scheduling of existing drugs, as relatively few new drugs have come to the market since the 1960s.

Although treatment results with adult ALL are worse than those with childhood ALL, recent use of aggressive chemotherapy in adult ALL has increased the CR rate to 60% to 85%. Long-term disease-free survival (DFS) in this population, however, remains low (between 30% and 40%) because of the higher proportion of adults presenting with poor-risk disease. CR rates and DFS vary according to a number of poor prognostic factors and certain types of ALL are associated with a very poor outcome.

Therapy for childhood ALL is divided into five phases: (a) remission induction; (b) consolidation therapy; (c) interim maintenance; (d) delayed intensification; and (e) maintenance therapy (Fig. 137–2). CNS prophylaxis is a mandatory component of ALL treatment regimens and is administered longitudinally during all phases of treatment.

■ TREATMENT PHASES

Remission Induction

❺ The goal of remission induction is to rapidly induce a complete clinical and hematologic remission, where hematologic remission is defined as reducing the leukemia cell burden below morphologic detection following recovery of normal blood counts. The CR rate

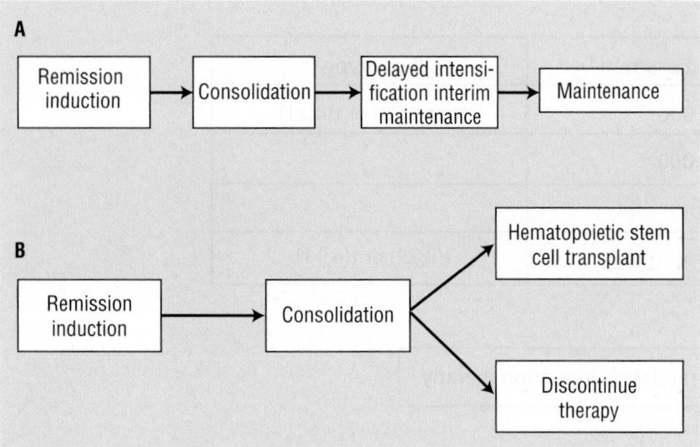

FIGURE 137-2. Treatment algorithm for *(A)* acute lymphoblastic leukemia and *(B)* acute myeloid leukemia.

is 98% in children treated with vincristine, dexamethasone or prednisone, and asparaginase or pegaspargase.[1,12] Most treatment protocols add daunorubicin to induction (four-drug induction) for high-risk ALL, and some also add other agents, such as cyclophosphamide, methotrexate, or cytarabine.

The rate of clearance of blasts is an important prognostic factor. Children with a slow rate of clearance of blasts from the bone marrow in the first 8 (high-risk) or 15 (standard-risk) days of therapy have an eventual outcome that is inferior to those with rapid clearance of blasts (see Fig. 137–1 for definitions of risk).[16] Additional intensified therapy significantly improves outcome of children with a slow early response.[16] Historically, prednisone has been the primary glucocorticoid used in pediatric ALL regimens. Dexamethasone is now being used in some standard-risk protocols because of its longer duration of action and higher cerebrospinal fluid penetration compared to prednisone.[12] Dexamethasone, when used in place of prednisone during induction, consolidation, and maintenance, also improves EFS and decreases the risk of CNS relapse.[17] However, dexamethasone increases the risk of side effects such as osteonecrosis, steroid myopathy, hyperglycemia, and infections.[17,18] Patients older than 10 years of age are particularly prone to osteonecrosis and receive dexamethasone intermittently (7 days on, 7 days off) to minimize these effects. Because patients with Down syndrome have increased infections and mortality with dexamethasone, prednisone is substituted in these patients.

Asparaginase is available in three forms. Asparaginase and pegaspargase are isolated from *Escherichia* coli while crisantaspase (investigational agent available if allergic to the other products) is isolated from *Erwinia chrysanthemi*. Pegaspargase is pegylated *E. coli* asparaginase; pegylation prolongs its duration of activity and allows it to be given less frequently. Pegaspargase is preferred over asparaginase because of fewer intramuscular injections, decreased antibody formation, and superior response rates. Asparaginase products are the chemotherapeutic agents most likely to cause hypersensitivity reactions (10% to 40%). The reaction is delayed with pegaspargase and usually occurs 6 to 12 hours following a dose. The hypersensitivity reaction to pegaspargase may also be prolonged and frequently requires hospitalization for 5 to 7 days.

Ph^+ ALL is associated with a poor long-term outcome and is treated as very-high-risk disease. This includes a four-drug induction and a matched related-donor allogeneic hematopoietic stem cell transplant (HSCT) if available. The availability of imatinib mesylate, a signal transduction inhibitor that inhibits BCR-ABL kinase, has stimulated much research to try and improve responses in the 10% to 20% of children who are Ph^+ and refractory to a four-drug induction.[19] Imatinib is currently incorporated into childhood treatment trials for Ph^+ ALL in Europe and the United States.

CLINICAL CONTROVERSY

Which is the superior corticosteroid for the treatment of ALL? Prednisone/prednisolone has been the steroid of choice for many years. Dexamethasone was recently shown to have better CNS penetration than prednisone with a consequent decrease in CNS relapse rate. However, the incidence of debilitating side effects such as osteonecrosis is higher with dexamethasone. Many investigators have difficulty weighing the quality-of-life decrease from the side effects against the small increase in survival.

Central Nervous System Prophylaxis

❻ CNS prophylaxis is incorporated throughout all phases of therapy. The rationale for CNS prophylaxis is based on two observations. First, many chemotherapeutic agents do not readily cross the blood–brain barrier. Second, results from early clinical trials of ALL showed that 50% to 85% of patients with ALL and no CNS involvement at diagnosis experienced a CNS relapse.[5,6] These observations indicate that the CNS is a potential sanctuary for leukemic cells and that undetectable leukemic cells are present in the CNS in many patients at the time of diagnosis. Detectable CNS involvement at the time of diagnosis is relatively uncommon (<5%) in ALL.[5] Factors that are associated with an increased risk of CNS involvement at diagnosis in children include a high initial WBC count, T-cell phenotype, mature B-cell phenotype, age ≤1 year, African American race, thrombocytopenia, lymphadenopathy, and hepatomegaly or splenomegaly.[5,12]

The goal of CNS prophylaxis is to eradicate undetectable leukemic cells from the CNS. Leukemic meningitis is more easily prevented than treated. Once CNS relapse has occurred, patients are at increased risk of bone marrow relapse and death from refractory leukemia. Initial trials of childhood ALL in the 1960s established craniospinal irradiation as the standard for prevention of CNS relapse.[12] However, this approach was associated with long-term sequelae including neuropsychological deficits, precocious puberty, osteoporosis, decreased intellect, thyroid dysfunction, an increased risk of brain tumors, short stature, and obesity. Subsequent trials have demonstrated that irradiation may be replaced by frequent administration of intrathecal chemotherapy in most children with ALL.[12] Only patients with very-high-risk disease still receive prophylactic cranial radiation in the United States as a consequence of the long-term sequelae.

The selection of a CNS prophylaxis regimen must consider efficacy, toxicity, and risk of CNS disease. Intrathecal chemotherapy, cranial irradiation, and high-dose intravenous methotrexate or cytarabine can be used to treat or prevent CNS disease. Current treatment approaches have reduced isolated CNS relapses to less than 5% among children.[5,20] Risk factors for CNS relapse include male sex, hepatomegaly, CNS2 disease (the presence of leukemic blasts in a cerebrospinal fluid sample that contains <5 WBC/mm^3), age younger than 2 years or older than 6 years, and a bloody diagnostic lumbar puncture.[5,20] Intrathecal therapy consists of methotrexate and cytarabine, given either alone or in combination. When given together, hydrocortisone is commonly added (triple intrathecal therapy) to decrease the incidence of arachnoiditis. For standard-risk ALL, triple intrathecal therapy reduces CNS relapse rates by 2.5% in comparison to intrathecal methotrexate, but has no effect on overall survival.[20] The doses of intrathecal chemotherapy used in pediatric ALL patients must be individualized based on age because of differences in the volume of cerebrospinal fluid at various ages. Liposomal cytarabine induces CNS remission in 57% of relapsed patients, but is associated with a high incidence of arachnoiditis and other CNS-related side effects.[21] Currently its use is limited to refractory or relapsed CNS disease.

Consolidation Therapy

Consolidation therapy in ALL is started after a CR has been achieved, and refers to continued intensive chemotherapy in an attempt to eradicate clinically undetectable disease in order to secure (consolidate) the remission. Regimens usually incorporate either non–cross-resistant drugs that are different from the induction regimen, or more dose-intensive use of the same drugs.

Randomized trials show that consolidation therapy clearly improves patient outcome in children, but its benefit in adults is less clear.[1,12] The relative benefit of individual components of treatment regimens is difficult to demonstrate because of the overall complexity of therapy in ALL. Standard consolidation lasts 4 weeks and usually consists of vincristine, mercaptopurine, and intrathecal methotrexate. Children with testicular disease usually receive radiation during this phase of therapy if a complete clinical response in the testes is not achieved by the end of induction. In children, the intensity of consolidation therapy is based on the child's risk classification and rate of cytoreduction during induction. Patients who respond slowly to induction therapy are at higher risk of relapse if they are not treated on more aggressive regimens. Consolidation may be intensified for slow early responders or high-risk patients to include cyclophosphamide, low-dose cytarabine, and pegaspargase. Children with Ph^+ ALL or infants with t(4;11) mixed lineage leukemia (MLL), or children who only achieve a partial remission may receive a HSCT in first remission if a suitable donor is available.[1] Imatinib has been incorporated into consolidation for children with Ph^+ disease.

Delayed Intensification/Interim Maintenance

One or two delayed intensification phases separated by low-intensity interim maintenance cycles have been added to maintain remission and to decrease cumulative toxicity. Delayed intensification usually consists of dexamethasone, vincristine, doxorubicin, pegaspargase, cyclophosphamide, thioguanine or mercaptopurine, low-dose cytarabine, and intrathecal methotrexate. Interim maintenance usually consists of dexamethasone, vincristine, weekly methotrexate, mercaptopurine, and intrathecal methotrexate. The addition of these delayed intensified cycles improved results with a 6-year 76% EFS for a single delayed intensification and 83% for two cycles in intermediate-risk patients.[22] A single delayed intensification improved 7-year EFS by 6% in low-risk patients.[23] Current studies are testing similar regimens in standard-risk patients. The antimetabolite-based regimens may have a reduced risk of late toxicities, but the more intensive regimens appear to result in better survival for some patients, especially those with higher-risk disease.

Maintenance Therapy

❼ Maintenance therapy allows long-term drug exposure to slowly dividing cells, allows the immune system time to eradicate leukemia cells, and promotes apoptosis (programmed cell death). The goal of maintenance therapy is to further eradicate residual leukemic cells and prolong remission duration. Although maintenance therapy is clearly beneficial in childhood ALL, the possible benefit in adults has only recently been demonstrated.

Maintenance therapy usually consists of daily mercaptopurine and weekly methotrexate for 12-week courses, at doses that produce relatively little myelosuppression, with monthly "pulses" of vincristine and a steroid for 5 days per month. In an effort to determine the long-term outcome of the duration and intensity of maintenance therapy, the Childhood ALL Collaborative Group published findings from a large meta-analysis involving 12,000 randomized children from 42 trials initiated prior to 1987.[24] That analysis revealed that longer maintenance, pulses of vincristine and prednisone, and the inclusion of one or two intensive reinduction courses significantly reduced the total number of deaths or relapse. However, only intensive reinduction improved survival.

Based on the results of studies that show a trend toward an increase in late relapse (excluding isolated testicular relapse) among male children treated for 2 years versus 3 years, some centers treat female children for 2 years while males receive maintenance to complete a total of 3 years of therapy. Interpatient variability in the pharmacokinetics of oral methotrexate and mercaptopurine may also be an important determinant of the effectiveness and toxicity of maintenance therapy. Patients who take their oral methotrexate and mercaptopurine on an evening versus a morning schedule appear to have a superior outcome. Mercaptopurine cannot be given with milk or milk products because of the presence of xanthine oxidase. To account for the interpatient variability, most clinicians will titrate the dose of either agent to maintain an absolute neutrophil count of 750 to 1,500 cells/mm^3. Some protocols circumvent bioavailability and poor adherence issues by administering methotrexate intravenously or intramuscularly. The importance of these pharmacokinetic issues in adults is less-well defined.

Genetic polymorphisms may affect drug metabolism, receptor expression, drug transportation, drug disposition, and pharmacologic response. These alterations may contribute to acute and chronic toxicity from ALL therapy as well as differences in treatment outcome. The most studied polymorphism involves thiopurine metabolism. Thiopurines are inactivated by *S*-methylation by cellular thiopurine *S*-methyltransferase (TPMT). Approximately 10% of the population has intermediate TPMT activity as a result of heterozygous polymorphisms in the gene encoding for TPMT, and 1 in 300 has extremely low activity as a result of homozygous presence of this TPMT polymorphism.[25] Deficiency of TPMT activity results in excessive myelosuppression from mercaptopurine and thioguanine. Patients with low activity (homozygous mutant TPMT genotype) may require 85% to 90% dose reductions.[25] Prospective evaluation of TPMT status was complicated in the past, as many ALL patients receive transfusions prior to definitive diagnosis. TPMT status can now be determined directly by DNA-based testing, which may become a standard of care in the near future.

■ T-CELL DISEASE

Patients with T-cell leukemia have an inferior response rate to standard-risk therapy and are automatically categorized as very-high-risk (see Fig. 137–1). Patients with T-cell leukemia have an increased incidence of CNS disease and benefit from systemic therapy that penetrates the CNS such as high-dose methotrexate.[18] Patients with T-cell disease have lower methotrexate polyglutamate accumulation and seem to benefit from these higher doses.

Nelarabine is a prodrug of ara-G that preferentially accumulates in T-lymphoblasts as ara-GTP. Children and young adults in first bone marrow relapse had a 55% complete or partial response in the phase II trial.[26] Nelarabine is currently incorporated into a high-risk backbone for initial therapy of childhood T-cell ALL.

■ ACUTE LYMPHOBLASTIC LEUKEMIA IN INFANTS

ALL and AML in infants younger than 1 year of age accounts for less than 5% of the reported acute leukemias in childhood, but they are associated with poor outcomes. EFS in infant ALL is 20% to 40%.[27] Sixty percent to 70% of infants with acute leukemia have a translocation that involves the MLL gene located at 11q23.[27] In infant ALL, the t(4;11) is most common and has been associated with an extremely poor outcome in the past, with only 10% to 20% EFS.[27] Other poor prognostic factors in infant ALL include age less than 6 months, a high WBC count, hepatosplenomegaly, and CNS disease. These factors are also closely associated with MLL translocations.

Patients with infant ALL may have greater drug resistance to asparaginase and prednisone, but increased sensitivity to cytarabine.[27] Although intensive regimens such as high-dose methotrexate and high-dose cytarabine have improved survival rates, unacceptably high mortality rates have also been observed with some regimens. Lack of pharmacokinetic data for chemotherapy in infants has contributed to toxicity from inappropriate dosing of doxorubicin and vincristine. To reduce neuropsychological complications, most protocols avoid cranial irradiation. The use of allogeneic HSCT for infants with ALL remains controversial due to a lack of donors, concerns over the long-term toxicity of total body irradiation, and excessive mortality in some series.

■ ACUTE LYMPHOBLASTIC LEUKEMIA IN ADULTS

❽ Because most adults are considered high-risk, adults usually receive more-intensive remission induction regimens. Complete remission is achieved in 70% to 90% of adults with a four-drug regimen containing daunorubicin or doxorubicin, vincristine, L-asparaginase, and prednisone.[1,6] DFS is considerably lower and is achieved in 30% to 40% of patients. The value of adding more drugs to the basic three- or four-drug induction regimen is unclear. Equally unclear is the value of higher doses of standard combinations of drugs for remission induction. Some studies suggest that high-dose methotrexate and cytarabine alternating with fractionated cyclophosphamide plus vincristine, doxorubicin, and dexamethasone (hyperCVAD) may improve response and survival in adults with ALL.[28] Poorer outcomes in adults have been attributed to greater drug resistance, poor side-effect tolerance with subsequent nonadherence, and possibly less-effective therapy.

A considerable number of ALL cases occur in patients older than age 60 years, and treatment of this group of patients is an even greater challenge. The response to therapy and durability of response seem less than in younger adults or children. Treatment-related mortality rates during remission induction therapy are also higher in this population. Older patients are more likely to be Ph^+ positive, with the Ph^+ present in more than 50% patients age 55 years and older. Older patients are less likely to have T-cell ALL.[6] Based on data demonstrating improved and sustained responses in Ph^+ chronic myeloid leukemia with the tyrosine kinase inhibitor imatinib, several groups have evaluated the addition of imatinib to conventional chemotherapy in Ph^+ ALL patients.[29–32] Although no randomized trials have compared imatinib and conventional chemotherapy versus conventional chemotherapy alone, several single-center uncontrolled trials have reported improved overall survival (OS) with the addition of imatinib.[29,30] This approach also appears to be tolerated in the elderly.[31] Two other tyrosine kinase inhibitors, dasatinib and nilotinib, have also been evaluated in imatinib-resistant Ph^+ leukemias. Responses are achieved, although are short-lived, with relapses occurring within 6 months.[33,34] A primary concern with the tyrosine kinase inhibitors is the emergence of resistance, specifically T315I mutations.

■ TREATMENT OF RELAPSED ACUTE LYMPHOBLASTIC LEUKEMIA

The most common site for relapse is the bone marrow, although isolated relapses can occur in the CNS or testicles. Because marrow relapse usually follows isolated CNS or testicular relapses, patients with isolated extramedullary relapses are treated with localized radiation (cranial or testicular) and aggressive systemic chemotherapy similar to that given to patients with a marrow relapse.[5,35]

Patients who have completed treatment and who have stayed in remission for longer periods are more likely to be reinduced into remission again. Patients with more favorable risk factors initially, and those who received less intensive initial treatments, are more likely to respond well to reinduction/salvage regimens. Although 80% to 90% of children can achieve a second remission with anthracycline, corticosteroid, vincristine, and asparaginase/pegaspargase, the 3-year OS following bone marrow (28%), CNS (60%), and testicular relapse (60%) is not optimal.[35] Survival is only 8% for children achieving a third remission after a second bone marrow relapse.[35] Clofarabine, a purine antimetabolite, achieves a 12.5% complete response rate, but the duration of response is less than 6 months.

Allogeneic HSCT (alloHSCT) is the treatment of choice for early bone marrow relapse (first CR [CR1] less than 36 months).[35] Children who relapse more than 36 months after completion of initial therapy have reasonable outcomes with chemotherapy alone.[12,35] For patients with initial remissions less than 36 months, alloHSCT performed while in second CR (CR2) is associated with a 8-year DFS of 41%, versus 23% with chemotherapy.[36] Patients who undergo alloHSCT are less likely to relapse, but are more likely to experience treatment-related morbidity and mortality if total-body irradiation is included in the conditioning regimen.[37]

Historically high-risk adult patients with a human leukocyte antigen (HLA)-matched sibling have been offered alloHSCT, but recent data suggest that there is no benefit to alloHSCT in this population (with the exception of Ph^+ ALL). High treatment-related mortality in this group may offset any benefit from a lower relapse rate.[38] Most elderly patients are not candidates for standard alloHSCT but are candidates for nonmyeloablative alloHSCT. Whether this approach will reduce treatment-related mortality and result in more favorable outcomes is currently unknown. The National Marrow Donor Program and the American Society for Blood and Marrow Transplantation have developed guidelines for transplant consultation based on current clinical practice and evidence-based medicine. The following groups of ALL patients are at risk for progression and should be referred for transplant evaluation: high-risk ALL, including patients with high-risk cytogenetics (i.e., Ph^+), high WBC count (>30,000 to 50,000 cells/mm^3) at diagnosis, CNS or testicular leukemia, no CR within 4 weeks of initial treatment, remission induction failures, and those patients in CR2 and beyond.[39,40]

■ ROLE OF COLONY-STIMULATING FACTORS IN ACUTE LYMPHOBLASTIC LEUKEMIA

❾ The use of granulocyte colony-stimulating factor colony-stimulating factor in children and adults administered during, after, or between courses has been shown to shorten the duration of neutropenia by 2 to 10 days.[41,42] Standard-risk ALL therapy in children is not myelosuppressive and does not warrant the use of colony-stimulating factors. In the adult ALL population, one trial has demonstrated an improved CR rate, but this has not been confirmed in other large randomized studies.[42] No trial has shown improved EFS or OS in either the pediatric or adult populations. Several studies reported a decrease in the incidence of febrile neutropenia, duration of hospitalization, and duration of antibiotic use, although the effects on these end points are inconsistent among trials.[42]

The current American Society of Clinical Oncology guidelines recommend the initiation of colony-stimulating factors after completion of the first few days of chemotherapy of either the initial induction or first remission course to shorten the duration of neutropenia by at least a week.[42]

■ LATE EFFECTS OF ACUTE LYMPHOBLASTIC LEUKEMIA

Certain late effects associated with cranial or craniospinal irradiation and/or corticosteroids were discussed earlier. The Childhood Cancer Survivor Study tracks the health status of adults treated for childhood cancer between 1970 and 1986 and has yielded invaluable information on how to monitor adult survivors.[43] Leukemia survivors have a relative risk of 2.2 for developing a chronic health condition as compared with healthy siblings, and a relative risk of 4.1 for severe or disabling chronic conditions. Former ALL regimens that incorporated intensive use of topoisomerase II inhibitors (etoposide and teniposide) are associated with unacceptably high risks of development of secondary leukemia.[12] High cumulative doses of anthracyclines used in high-risk or relapsed patients can cause cardiomyopathy. Cranial irradiation has also been found to cause learning deficits, especially in patients younger than 5 years of age at the time of treatment. Patients who received cranial radiation as children also have higher unemployment rates and lower marital rates among females two decades after diagnosis.[44] The Children's Oncology Group has recently developed long-term followup guidelines for survivors of childhood, adolescent, and young adult cancers (*www.survivorshipguidelines.org*).

ACUTE MYELOID LEUKEMIA

CLINICAL PRESENTATION

❸ Common signs and symptoms at presentation are described below. In addition to clinical presentation, laboratory and pathology evaluations are required for a definitive diagnosis of leukemia. The most important test is a bone marrow aspirate and biopsy, which is submitted to hematopathology for testing and evaluation. Cytochemical stains are helpful to determine if the acute leukemia is of myeloid or lymphoid lineage. Immunophenotyping is necessary and was described in the ALL clinical presentation above. Cytogenetic analysis of the marrow to determine the presence of nonrandom numerical and structural chromosomal abnormalities in leukemic cells is also helpful for diagnosis, establishing prognosis, and evaluating response to therapy.[10] Chromosome translocations can result in abnormal expression and/or function of cellular oncogenes. Unique translocations can identify specific subtypes of acute leukemia. For example, acute promyelocytic leukemia (APL) is characterized by a specific translocation between chromosomes 15 and 17: t(15;17). Recently, technically difficult cytogenetic analysis has been supplemented with fluorescent in situ hybridization that allows for quick, sensitive analysis of samples that might be inadequate for karyotyping. Molecular tests may be used to identify products of specific translocations, such as promyelocytic leukemia (PML) retinoic acid receptor-α (RARα) in APL and AML1-ETO and CBFβ/MYH 11 in other subtypes of AML. The results of some of these molecular tests correlate with prognosis and are discussed in Risk Classification below.

CLINICAL PRESENTATION[1,4]

General

- Recent history of vague symptoms such as tiredness, lack of exercise tolerance, chest pain, and "feeling unwell" but in no obvious distress.

Symptoms

- The patient may report weight loss, malaise, fatigue, and palpitations and dyspnea on exertion. They may also present with fever, chills, and rigors suggestive of infection; bruising (excessive vaginal bleeding, epistaxis, ecchymoses, and petechiae); gum hypertrophy (AML M4 and AML M5 subtypes); bone pain; seizures; headache; and diplopia.

Signs

- Temperature may be elevated because of low neutrophil count; petechiae.

Laboratory Tests

- Complete blood cell count (with differential). Anemia is usually present and is normochromic and normocytic (without a compensatory increase in reticulocytes). Thrombocytopenia (severe, <50,000 cells/mm^3) is present in approximately 50% of cases. Leukopenia/leukocytosis: approximately 20% of patients will present with an elevated WBC count, 20% with a low WBC count, and the rest with normal counts. Even patients with elevated counts can be considered functionally neutropenic.
- Uric acid may be elevated as a result of rapid cellular turnover (more common in patients presenting with elevated WBC counts).
- Electrolytes: potassium and phosphate are usually elevated.
- Coagulation: elevated prothrombin time, partial thromboplastin time, D-dimers; hypofibrinogenemia.

Other Diagnostic Tests

- Bone marrow biopsy and aspirate: send for morphologic examination, cytochemical staining, immunophenotyping, and cytogenetic (chromosome) analysis. At diagnosis the marrow is typically hypercellular, with normal erythropoiesis being replaced by leukemic blasts. To be diagnosed with AML, there needs to be more than 20% blasts. Molecular testing for FMS-like tyrosine kinase 3 (FLT3) mutations is warranted.
- For patients presenting with CNS signs, a diagnostic lumbar puncture should be performed. This is typically performed once there is clearance of blasts from the peripheral blood. CNS involvement is common with AML M4 and M5 subtypes.

RISK CLASSIFICATION

❿ Many clinical and laboratory features at diagnosis are associated with response to treatment, as measured by the CR rate, duration of remission, and long-term survival. Identification of these risk factors may allow the clinician to better understand the disease and to tailor treatment according to risk of disease recurrence. For example, if a patient has many clinical and laboratory features that are associated with a good response to chemotherapy ("good-risk"), then the clinician may choose to give less-intensive therapy to reduce the risk of long-term toxic effects. Conversely, if a patient is unlikely to respond well to therapy ("high-risk"), then the clinician may choose to give more intensive chemotherapy that might include HSCT.

Several prognostic factors have been identified for adults with AML. The most important patient factor is age, with younger patients more likely to achieve a CR than older patients (older than age 60 years).[1,4,7] The lower CR rate in older patients results from an increased frequency of fatal infection and bleeding complications and resistance to conventional chemotherapy. The duration of remission is also shorter in older patients as compared to younger patients. Other patient-specific prognostic factors include concurrent infection and any major organ impairment.[4] FAB morphologic subtype may be important, with some subtypes associated with a worse outcome. Patients with extramedullary disease, CNS involvement, or underlying MDS have a worse prognosis. Certain cytogenetic abnormalities are also known to worsen the response rate and survival of patients with AML (Table 137–4).[1,4,10] In addition, patients who develop a "secondary" leukemia after treatment of another malignancy usually have a very poor response to antileukemic chemotherapy.

Prognostic factors associated with pediatric AML have been reported but few have been shown to consistently predict treatment outcome. Historically, poor prognostic factors include an initial WBC count greater than 100,000 cells/mm^3, FAB subtype M1 without Auer

TABLE 137-4 Risk Category According to Cytogenetic Abnormalities Present

	Risk Category		
Disease	***Good-Risk***	***Intermediate-Risk***	***High-Risk***
AML	t(8;21)(q22;q22); inv(16); t(15;17); t(9;11) trisomy 21	Normal karyotype; trisomy 8; 11q23; del(7q); del(9q); trisomy 22	Complex karyoptype; –5; –7; del(5q); inv(3p)
Probability of relapse	≤25%	50%	>70%
4-Year survival	≥70%	40–50%	≤20%
ALL	Hyperdiploidy; t(10;14); or 6q		t(9;22); t(8;14); t(4;11); t(1;9)

ALL, acute lymphoblastic leukemia; AML, acute myeloid leukemia.
Data from Hasle et al.[11] *and Thomas et al.*[29]

rods, certain chromosomal abnormalities (see Table 137–4), age younger than 5 years, and having AML secondary to prior chemotherapy or radiation therapy. A recent report from the Children's Cancer Group identified both poor and favorable prognostic factors. Poor prognostic factors at diagnosis included male gender, platelet count ≤20,000 cells/mm^3, hepatomegaly, MDS, FAB subtype M5, greater than 15% bone marrow blasts at day 14 of induction therapy, and trisomy 8.[45] Abnormal chromosome 16 was associated with a higher rate of CR.[45]

More recently, several genetic molecular abnormalities have been identified in adults with AML that have prognostic significance. Abnormalities that are associated with a poor outcome include FLT3 abnormalities; MLL; brain and acute leukemia gene, cytoplasmic (BAALC) and Wilms tumor gene (WT-1).[46] Nucleophosmin mutations, member1 (NPM1) (in the absence of FLT3 abnormalities) are associated with an improved relapse-free survival and OS.[46] The future of AML treatment may lie in a prognostically prioritized molecular classification. There are proposed algorithms for patient management based on the presence or absence of these abnormalities but they are not currently incorporated into standard practice.[46]

TREATMENT

Acute Myeloid Leukemia

■ TREATMENT GOALS

⓫ The short-term goal of treatment for AML is to rapidly achieve a complete clinical and hematologic remission. In the absence of a CR, a rapid and fatal outcome is inevitable. CR is defined as the disappearance of all clinical and bone marrow evidence (normal cellularity >20% with <5% blasts) of leukemia, with restoration of normal hematopoiesis (neutrophils ≥1,000 cells/mm^3 and platelets >100,000 cells/mm^3).[47] Partial remission is a significant response to treatment (a decrease of at least 50% of blasts), but evidence of residual disease in the bone marrow remains (5% to 25% blasts) and is considered a treatment failure requiring additional therapy. The definition of response for adult AML was reevaluated in 2003, and changes in the definition of response were proposed to include not only CR, but also morphologic CR (patient independent of transfusion), CR with incomplete count recovery, cytogenetic CR (patient with normal cytogenetics in which cytogenetics were previously abnormal), and molecular CR (molecular studies negative).[47]

After a CR is achieved, the goal is to maintain the patient in continuous CR. As discussed later, the occurrence of leukemic relapse in the bone marrow significantly reduces the likelihood of curing the disease. Most patients who will die from acute leukemia die within the first 6 years; the survival curve (percentage alive versus time) beyond the sixth year after therapy does not continue to decline as rapidly ("survival plateau"), and at this time patients can be considered "cured."[1]

With recent advances in chemotherapy and supportive care, 65% to 85% of all patients with AML achieve a CR, and 20% to 40% become long-term survivors.[1,4] Overall, the median duration of remission is 1 to 2 years. In patients older than 60 years of age, the percentage of patients achieving a CR is lower (39% to 64%), and the median duration of remission is shorter than 1 year.[48] In contrast to ALL, effective therapies used in AML cause severe and often prolonged myelosuppression, with the exception of tretinoin. As a result, patients with AML, particularly patients older than 60 years of age, are at greater risk for treatment-related fatal infectious and bleeding complications.

The 5-year survival in children with AML has increased from 17% in 1976 to 50% in 2000.[3] Children with Down syndrome and AML receive less-intense therapy and have an EFS of 68% to 100%.[49] Treatment of AML, unlike that of ALL, usually only consists of induction and intensive postremission therapy (see Fig. 137–2). CNS prophylaxis is not routinely given in adult AML, but is generally administered to pediatric patients.

■ TREATMENT PHASES

Remission Induction

⓫ As with ALL, the goal of remission induction for AML is to rapidly induce a CR with associated restoration of normal hematopoiesis. Compared to ALL, however, fewer patients with AML achieve CR. Because the CR rate in AML is related to the intensity of the remission induction regimen, the drugs used in AML are given at doses that uniformly cause severe marrow hypoplasia (except tretinoin). One reason for the lower CR rate in AML as compared to ALL is the inability to give optimal doses of chemotherapy because of marrow toxicity. With continued improvement of supportive care for patients undergoing chemotherapy, more intensive treatment regimens are being given in an effort to reduce the high rate of leukemic relapse and increase the proportion of long-term survivors. Most patients achieve a CR after one or two courses of chemotherapy. Patients who require additional chemotherapy to achieve a CR have been reported to have a poor prognosis, even if remission is ultimately achieved.[1]

The most active single agents in AML are the anthracycline antibiotics (daunorubicin, doxorubicin, and idarubicin), anthracenediones (mitoxantrone), and the antimetabolite cytarabine. The most common regimen ("7+3") combines daunorubicin administered as a short infusion of 45 to 60 mg/m^2 per day on days 1 to 3, along with cytarabine administered as a continuous 24-hour infusion of 100 mg/m^2 per day on days 1 to 7.[4,50,51] The CR rate with the 7+3 regimen is 65% to 75% in patients ages 18 to 60 years. The remission rate decreases to 40% to 50% in patients older than 60 years of age.

Several trials have attempted to improve upon conventional 7+3 therapy, but have shown no improvement by (a) increasing cytarabine to 10 days, (b) shortening cytarabine to 5 days, (c) substituting doxorubicin for daunorubicin, (d) adding thioguanine, or (e) increasing cytarabine dosage to 200 mg/m^2 per day (given by continuous infusion).[4] Other clinical trials have evaluated idarubicin or mitoxantrone as alternatives to daunorubicin in combination with standard continuous infusion cytarabine. Trials in younger patients reported improved CR rates with these newer anthracyclines/anthracenediones and one trial demonstrated prolonged survival. Among older adults the CR rate and OS does not appear to be different among the different anthracyclines/anthracenediones.[50,51] In a review of long-term followup results from randomized trials evaluating idarubicin versus daunorubicin, only one trial maintained a significant difference favoring idarubicin. The effect of anthracycline choice on the CR rates in the elderly was studied by the Eastern Cooperative Oncology Group (ECOG).[52] Elderly AML patients were randomized to standard doses of cytarabine combined with either daunorubicin (45 mg/m^2 for 3 days), idarubicin (12 mg/m^2 for 3 days), or mitoxantrone (12 mg/m^2 for 3 days). No difference in DFS, OS, or toxicity was seen between the three induction regimens.[52]

CLINICAL CONTROVERSY

Is there a superior anthracycline to use as part of the induction regimen for AML? Some clinicians believe that idarubicin is superior in attaining a complete remission following one cycle of induction compared to alternative anthracyclines or anthracenediones. Randomized trials in the elderly show similar remission rates with all anthracyclines and anthracenediones. Whether there is a difference in younger patient's remains to be seen.

Thus the anthracycline of choice for the standard 7+3 regimen remains controversial, with many centers adopting idarubicin into the induction regimen in younger AML patients, and the choice in the elderly is based on individual clinician preference and institutional acquisition costs.

Other strategies that have been evaluated include adding another agent such as etoposide to the induction regimen.[4,50,51] A comparison of the standard 7+3 regimen with or without etoposide on days 1 to 7 ("7+3+7") in newly diagnosed AML patients ages 15 to 70 years demonstrated no difference in CR rates or OS. A subset analysis of patients younger than 55 years of age demonstrated a doubling of the duration of remission and OS in the etoposide-containing arm. The 7+3+7 regimen was more toxic in patients older than 55 years of age. These results have been confirmed in other studies, but as yet are to be adopted in the United States as part of standard therapy. Based on experimental tumor models that showed a steep dose–response curve for cytarabine, higher doses of cytarabine have also been evaluated as a means to enhance the outcome of remission induction therapy. Several groups, including the Southwest Oncology Group and the Australian Leukemia Study Group, have evaluated the impact of adding high-dose cytarabine to induction therapy. This strategy does not improve the CR rate or OS, but does improve DFS. A retrospective study conducted by the European Group for Blood and Marrow Transplantation demonstrated that the cytarabine dose administered during induction and/or consolidation did not influence the outcome in patients who ultimately went on to receive allogeneic or autologous HSCT.[53] These data suggest that high doses of cytarabine during induction may not be needed in patients scheduled to receive a HSCT as postremission therapy. In summary, the role of high-dose cytarabine during induction remains controversial. If used during induction, high-dose cytarabine is more appropriate in younger patients than in elderly patients because of poor tolerance by elderly patients.

The National Comprehensive Cancer Network (NCCN) has published guidelines for the treatment of AML.[54] The classic 7+3 regimen may be inadequate in adults younger than 60 years of age because the duration of remission is less than that reported in some studies that employed high-dose cytarabine in induction.[54] The NCCN guideline recommends that adults younger than 60 years of age without an antecedent hematologic disorder (i.e., no preexisting hematologic malignancy such as MDS) be treated with either the 7+3 regimen or more aggressive chemotherapy including high-dose cytarabine with an anthracycline or anthracenedione. In patients 60 years of age and older with good performance status, the conventional 7+3 regimen should be used or the patient should be enrolled in available clinical trials. The approach in patients with an antecedent hematologic disorder differs, and younger patients (<60 years) should be offered available clinical trials or proceed to alloHSCT (provided a suitable donor is available). Older patients (≥60 years) with an antecedent hematologic disorder or those with significant comorbidities unrelated to leukemia should be offered a clinical trial or best supportive care because of the dismal outcomes associated with conventional chemotherapy. All adult patients who present with CNS symptoms, and all AML M4 and AML M5 patients who are not symptomatic, should have a diagnostic lumbar puncture, and if it is positive, should be treated for disease. Methotrexate 12 to 15 mg, with or without cytarabine, should be administered intrathecally twice a week until clearance of leukemic blasts from the cerebrospinal fluid, and then monthly for about 6 months.

Intensive Postremission Therapy

⓬ Although most adults with AML achieve a CR, the duration of remission is short (4 to 8 months) if no further treatment is given. Relapse is presumably a consequence of the presence of residual, but clinically undetectable, leukemic cells after remission induction therapy. The goal of intensive postremission therapy is to eradicate these residual leukemic cells and to prevent the emergence of drug-resistant disease. The need for postremission therapy is based on postmortem analysis and cell kinetic data suggesting that nearly 10^9 residual leukemic cells remain after effective remission induction therapy. Strategies evaluated as postremission therapy include (a) low-dose, prolonged maintenance therapy, (b) short-course intensive chemotherapy-alone regimens, and (c) high-dose chemotherapy with or without radiation therapy followed by alloHSCT or autologous HSCT (autoHSCT).

Chemotherapy In the treatment of AML, postremission therapy is often referred to as consolidation therapy. Results of randomized trials in adults clearly show that postremission therapy following remission induction therapy prolongs survival versus no therapy, although the exact duration of postremission therapy is controversial.[4,50,51]

The intensity of postremission therapy is important.[55] In a large Cancer and Leukemia Group B (CALGB) trial, all patients received standard 7+3 induction, and once a CR was achieved, were randomized to receive one of three cytarabine-based consolidation regimens: 100 mg/m^2 per day or 400 mg/m^2 per day as a continuous 24-hour infusion, or 3,000 mg/m^2 every 12 hours on days 1, 3, and 5.[56] For adults younger than age 60 years, the probability of remaining in CR after 4 years was significantly higher in patients who received high-dose cytarabine (25% vs. 29% vs. 44%, respectively).[56] Elderly patients had lower response rates in all arms and did not benefit from the administration of higher doses of cytarabine, probably because they were unable to tolerate the high-dose regimen. Dose-limiting neurotoxicity in the high-dose arm was greater in elderly patients.[56]

It is not clear whether the same agents (cytarabine and an anthracycline) given for remission induction should be used for postremission therapy in higher doses, or whether different agents should be given. If leukemic relapse is caused by a resistant cell line, then the use of different agents that are non–cross-resistant with drugs used in induction might be beneficial.

High-dose cytarabine appears to be a key part of postremission therapy, particularly if not used in induction therapy. However, many questions remain, such as the optimal dose (g/m^2), number of doses per cycle, and number of cycles of high-dose cytarabine. Among patients with core-binding factor AML, defined as the presence of either t(8;21) or inv(16), it is clear that multiple cycles are beneficial, generally three to four cycles.[57,58] The NCCN guideline recommends four cycles of high-dose cytarabine for adults younger than 60 years of age and with good cytogenetics or, alternatively, one cycle of high-dose cytarabine followed by autoHSCT.[54] Patients with intermediate-risk cytogenetics should receive 4 cycles of high-dose cytarabine or undergo either an autoHSCT or an allogeneic (sibling) HSCT.[54] If a patient is 60 years of age or older, standard-dose cytarabine with or without anthracycline for one to two cycles, a reduced-dose high-dose cytarabine regimen (1 to 1.5 g/m^2 per day for four to six doses) for one to two cycles, or enrollment in a clinical trial is recommended. Patients with high-risk cytogenetics, underlying MDS, or secondary AML should either be enrolled in a clinical trial or be referred for either a matched sibling or alternative donor alloHSCT.[54]

CLINICAL CONTROVERSY

Intensive postremission therapy is clearly necessary to prevent relapse and those regimens containing high-dose cytarabine appear to be a key part of postremission therapy. However, the optimal dose of high-dose cytarabine, the number of doses per cycle, and the number of cycles to give remain unknown.

Allogeneic Hematopoietic Stem Cell Transplantation

AlloHSCT represents the most aggressive approach to postremission therapy in the management of AML. Much controversy surrounds this treatment approach, specifically the appropriateness, timing, treatment design, and donor selection.

The antileukemic activity of alloHSCT is based on the administration of pretransplant high-dose chemotherapy (or chemoradiotherapy) and the development of a posttransplant immune-based antileukemic response. The immune-based response, referred to as a graft-versus-leukemia (GVL) effect, often accompanies the graft-versus-host disease (GVHD) reaction. The immune-based benefit of alloHSCT has been demonstrated through the observation of consistently lower relapse rates with alloHSCT as compared to autologous or syngeneic HSCT. This potential benefit of alloHSCT can be offset by the risk of posttransplant complications such as GVHD, venoocclusive disease, graft failure, and infections.

AlloHSCT was first evaluated as a treatment modality for AML in refractory patients, but because of initial success in small numbers of patients, it has also been evaluated as intensive postremission therapy in AML patients in first or subsequent remission. Nonrandomized trials of HLA-identical sibling alloHSCT performed in AML patients in CR1 reported 5-year survival rates of 45% to 60% with relapse rates of 10% to 20%.[4,50,51] Transplant-related mortality following HLA-matched sibling alloHSCT is 15% to 25% in most series. As clinicians have gained more experience in this intensive form of therapy and been provided with more effective immunosuppressive and antibiotic regimens, transplant-related mortality rates have decreased and survival rates have increased. Bone marrow registry data indicate that long-term survival rates in AML patients who receive a matched sibling alloHSCT while in first remission have increased from approximately 45% in the early 1980s to approximately 60% in the mid-1990s.[1]

Table 137–5 presents the results of randomized comparisons of alloHSCT to autoHSCT or intensive consolidation chemotherapy alone.[4,51] AlloHSCT from an HLA-matched sibling donor for AML patients in CR1 results in long-term DFS in 43% to 55% of patients. Although the results vary, some of the studies show longer DFS and lower relapse rates with alloHSCT in AML in CR1 as compared to chemotherapy-alone postremission regimens.

AlloHSCT is still generally restricted to patients younger than 60 years of age, which limits the number of patients eligible for treatment of a disease that primarily affects older adults. One new approach, termed nonmyeloablative stem cell transplant (NST), uses less-toxic nonmyeloablative preparative regimens and is now being evaluated in AML patients, particularly in older patients and those with comorbid illnesses that would limit their eligibility for conventional alloHSCT. NST is designed to provide enough immunosuppression in the preparative regimen to allow for engraftment of donor cells, and depends heavily on the development of a GVL effect as a means to treat and prevent relapse of AML. Initial results of NST in AML indicate that the procedure is well tolerated in a wide age range of patients, and that it is associated with low rates of regimen-related toxicity.[59,60] Evaluations in larger numbers of patients are necessary to determine the comparative impact of NST on GVHD, DFS, and OS. Because only 30% of patients have an HLA-matched sibling donor, alloHSCT is further restricted as a treatment alternative for AML patients.[61] Matched unrelated donor transplantation with a phenotypically HLA-matched donor identified from bone marrow registries is also a treatment option in young adults and pediatric AML patients. This approach is associated with long-term DFS rates of 30% to 40%, which are slightly lower than in AML patients undergoing HLA-matched sibling alloHSCT because of a higher risk of treatment-related mortality with the procedure.[4,51,62]

The decision to transplant a patient depends a great deal on which biological risk group the patient belongs. Among patients with favorable risk AML, alloHSCT does not result in better outcomes as compared to high-dose cytarabine-based therapy. All patients with high-risk AML, including those with an antecedent hematologic disorder, treatment-related MDS, or induction failure, should undergo evaluation for HSCT. Similarly patients in CR1 with high-risk cytogenetics and patients in CR2 and beyond should undergo evaluation for alloHSCT.[39]

Autologous Hematopoietic Stem Cell Transplantation

Compared to alloHSCT, autoHSCT has the advantage of a lower risk of posttransplant complications because of lack of immunosup-

TABLE 137-5 Comparative Trials of Allogeneic HSCT (AlloHSCT) or Autologous HSCT (AutoHSCT) or Chemotherapy (Chemo) Alone as Postremission Therapy for AML in First Complete Remission

	Disease-Free Survival at 4 Years (%)			Overall Survival at 4 Years (%)		
	AlloHSCT	*AutoHSCT*	*Chemo*	*AlloHSCT*	*AutoHSCT*	*Chemo*
Zittoun et al. (EORTC-GIMEMA)	55%[a]	48%[b]	30%	59%	56%	46%
Harousseau et al. (GOELAM)	44%	44%	40%	53%	50%	54%
Cassileth et al. (Intergroup)	43%	35%	35%	46%	43%	52%[c]
Burnett et al. (UK MRC)	47%	50%	40%–58%	53%	52%	46%–52%

AML, acute myeloid leukemia; HSCT, hematopoietic stem cell transplantation.
[a] $p < 0.01$ (vs chemo)
[b] $p = 0.05$ (vs chemo)
[c] $p = 0.05$ (vs autoHSCT), $p = 0.04$ (vs alloHSCT)
Data from references 4 and 51.

pression and GVHD, and more broad applicability because of a lack of donor limitations and fewer age restrictions. Although the preparative regimen still provides antileukemic activity, autoHSCT is associated with a higher risk of relapse because of a lack of a GVL effect and potential tumor contamination with autologous stem cells. DFS following autoHSCT for AML in CR1 ranges from 40% to 60%, with treatment-related mortality of 5% to 15% and relapse rates of 30% to 50%.[63] Long-term response rates decrease proportionally as autoHSCT is employed in second or subsequent CR.

Controversies in autoHSCT include the optimal timing of therapy, the amount of consolidation therapy needed prior to HSCT, the dose of stem cells needed, and the impact of posttransplant therapy.[63] Table 137–5 compares autoHSCT versus other postremission therapies.

Comparisons of Postremission Therapy Options Several randomized trials in AML patients in CR1 have compared outcomes following alloHSCT, autoHSCT, and/or intensive consolidation chemotherapy (see Table 137–5).[51] In most trials, eligible patients based on age and donor availability received an alloHSCT and the remaining patients were randomized between autoHSCT and chemotherapy alone. The European Organization for Research and Treatment of Cancer-GIMEMA (Gruppo Italiano Malattie Ematologiche Maligne dell'Adulto) trial observed a DFS advantage and reduced relapse risk for alloHSCT or autoHSCT as compared to chemotherapy alone, but no differences in OS.[4,51] Survival rates were comparable because of a higher relapse rate in the chemotherapy group as compared to a higher treatment-related mortality rate in the alloHSCT group. This is the only trial that has demonstrated superior 4-year DFS with transplantation versus chemotherapy. Interestingly, the response rates in the conventional chemotherapy arm in this trial were lower than those reported in other studies, which may account for the survival benefit in the transplant group. Several other trials have shown no difference in DFS or OS between autoHSCT, alloHSCT, and conventional chemotherapy. In aggregate, these trials show that either autoHSCT or alloHSCT can reduce the risk of relapse, although this has not translated into a survival benefit. One trial design issue that might explain this lack of survival benefit was the low percentage of patients who progressed to transplantation when randomized, thus diluting the effect of transplantation. The effect of stem cell source on DFS and OS is controversial. Several comparative trials of bone marrow versus peripheral blood have been completed in patients with hematologic malignancies, and a meta-analysis of nine randomized trials demonstrated a lower relapse rate for those patients receiving peripheral blood stem cells.[64]

Most transplant centers base their decision to transplant on cytogenetic risk category.[4] Patients with high-risk cytogenetics do poorly with conventional chemotherapy or autoHSCT (DFS <15%), making alloHSCT the treatment of choice in this population. Patients with good-risk cytogenetics should not proceed to transplant in CR1, as neither auto- nor alloHSCT is superior to conventional chemotherapy. The optimal treatment of choice in patients with intermediate-risk cytogenetics is not clear and is based on clinician preference. Many centers consider a relapse probability of 40% to 50% sufficiently high so as to warrant the risk of transplantation-related mortality. The decision to proceed with HSCT in this group may rest on the results of molecular testing. As discussed in Risk Classification above, several genetic molecular abnormalities have been identified in adults with AML that have prognostic significance. Abnormalities that are associated with a poor outcome include FLT3 abnormalities; myeloid/lymphoid or MLL abnormalities; BAALC; and WT-1.

According to the NCCN guidelines, the decision to proceed to HSCT depends on cytogenetics.[54] If the patient has a good-risk cytogenetic profile and is younger than age 60 years, then high-dose cytarabine for four cycles or one cycle of high-dose cytarabine-based therapy followed by autoHSCT is preferred over alloHSCT. If the patient has a high-risk cytogenetic profile and is younger than 60 years of age, then alloHSCT transplantation should be considered early after remission induction. Patients with intermediate-risk cytogenetics should be entered into a clinical trial, but if a clinical trial is not available, either a matched sibling alloHSCT or an autoHSCT should be considered. AutoHSCT can be used if a hematologic and cytogenetic remission is achieved. For patients 60 years and older, the NCCN guidelines do not favor HSCT and recommend either enrollment into a clinical trial, or consideration of conventional dose cytarabine with or without an anthracycline or intermediate dose cytarabine. Clinicians increasingly consider autoHSCT as a treatment option, and for selected patients older than 60 years of age, NST is being used more frequently.[59,60] For the AML patient who relapses early after induction therapy, if a sibling or matched related donor is available, then alloHSCT is the primary reinduction therapy because conventional chemotherapy offers little benefit. If the relapse occurs late, then HSCT can be used as postremission consolidation after conventional induction therapy.[54]

■ CHILDHOOD ACUTE MYELOID LEUKEMIA

The most effective remission induction regimens for children include an anthracycline plus cytarabine, and either thioguanine or etoposide, yielding a remission rate of 75% to 85%.[65] Intensified therapy regimens, which include more antileukemic agents or compress the time in which the agents are delivered, improve survival rates. In compressed or intensified treatment regimens, the second course of therapy is given 6 days after the first, without waiting for marrow recovery to occur. Although intensive therapy is associated with an increased mortality rate as compared with standard chemotherapy in children with AML, the long-term EFS is significantly better in the intensive-therapy group (49% vs. 35%).[65,66] The Children's Oncology Group is assessing the benefit of adding gemtuzumab to current therapy.

Following induction therapy, patients should be evaluated for a response. A proportion of children will not achieve a CR, and will require additional chemotherapy called *reinduction*. Typically a bone marrow biopsy is performed 7 to 10 days after the completion of chemotherapy (or day 14 from the start of chemotherapy) to document disease eradication. If there is persistent disease, a second course of therapy is administered. The second course may be identical to the initial induction regimen, or include high-dose cytarabine and asparaginase, or mitoxantrone and cytarabine. If the marrow is aplastic, a repeat marrow biopsy should be performed upon hematologic recovery to document a CR.

An evidence-based review of the role of HSCT in the treatment of pediatric AML concluded that HSCT was indicated in the following settings: (a) CR1: alloHSCT is superior to autoHSCT and chemotherapy; (b) CR2: alloHSCT is preferable to chemotherapy and autoHSCT.[67] Children with no suitable stem cell donor should receive consolidation chemotherapy, with which survival results are similar to those seen with autoHSCT.[68]

Infant AML is usually myelomonoblastic or monoblastic in morphology. Poor prognostic factors include t(1;22), high WBC count, and CNS disease. Neonates with Down syndrome may develop transient myeloproliferative disease that usually spontaneously resolves without treatment within a few months. Infants with AML receive the same therapy as children of other ages, with the dosing per kilogram and not per body surface area.

■ ACUTE MYELOID LEUKEMIA IN THE ELDERLY

As the median age at diagnosis is in the range of 65 to 70 years, AML is a disease of the elderly. Unfortunately, long-term DFS is lower in older patients, ranging from 5% to 15%, as compared to 40% in younger patients.[48] In patients older than age 55 years, a review of ECOG studies reported the median duration of survival to be 6 to 9 months, as compared to 11 months in patients younger than age 55 years. The actual response and survival rates may be even lower, as many elderly patients with AML are not included in clinical trials because of a lack of eligibility and poor performance status.[4,48]

Elderly patients with AML have a poor outcome as a result of the frequent presence of unfavorable prognostic factors, including high-risk cytogenetic features, preceding myelodysplasia, and a higher incidence of inherent drug resistance.[4] Greater than 70% of de novo AML patients older than age 55 years will express the multidrug resistance phenotype associated with chemotherapy resistance, including resistance to the leukemia-active anthracyclines and etoposide.[48] Older patients with AML may also have poor outcome because of the inability to withstand aggressive therapy as a result of poor organ function, poor performance status, or existing comorbidities. Although older patients with AML may be able to tolerate aggressive remission induction therapy, they often cannot tolerate intensive postremission therapy, which increases their likelihood of leukemic relapse.

The potential therapeutic strategies in elderly AML patients include (a) no chemotherapy (i.e., best supportive care or palliative care therapy), (b) attenuated chemotherapy, (c) investigational therapy, or (d) standard-dose chemotherapy.[4] The palliative approach is most appropriate in patients with slowly progressive leukemia ("smoldering leukemia"). The difficulty lies in the ability to reliably identify these patients at diagnosis. Although initially accepted in older patients, palliative care approaches in older patients with AML with moderate-to-good performance status and organ function are now considered inappropriate. An ECOG-CALGB study randomized patients to either conventional chemotherapy or to observation in which patients could receive modest doses of chemotherapy for symptom palliation. Survival was twice as long in the chemotherapy group. The quality-of-life of each group was similar, with patients in each group spending approximately 50% of the study time in the hospital.[69]

These results show that chemotherapy prolongs survival without significantly decreasing the quality-of-life for elderly patients. Thus chemotherapy is a viable treatment option for elderly patients, although the best chemotherapy regimen and overall treatment approach are controversial. One approach is to attenuate the dose of chemotherapy, preferably with oral agents where possible, or lower doses of intravenous agents. Agents used in this strategy include oral etoposide, low-dose subcutaneous cytarabine, and other oral agents such as thioguanine and idarubicin (oral idarubicin is not currently commercially available in the United States). The United Kingdom AML Study Group recently published a comparative trial of low-dose subcutaneous cytarabine twice daily versus hydroxyurea. Low-dose cytarabine produced a greater number of complete remissions compared to placebo, and prolonged 1-year survival.[70]

Another approach is to use the same remission induction regimens that would be used in younger adults. With this approach, the complete remission rate in older AML patients ranges from 41% to 62%, as compared with 65% to 73% in adults younger than 60 years of age, and are very short-lived (5 to 10 months). Treatment-related mortality ranges from 15% to 20%. More elderly patients than younger patients will require two courses of remission induction therapy to achieve a complete remission. In an effort to improve response rates, some trials have attempted to determine the optimal anthracycline and the appropriate dose. Unlike younger patients, comparative data in elderly patients do not suggest any efficacy or toxicity advantages of idarubicin or mitoxantrone over daunorubicin for AML induction therapy.[71] Mitoxantrone in combination with etoposide results in worse survival compared to daunorubicin and cytarabine.[72] Early uncontrolled trials reported high morbidity and mortality rates during remission induction in elderly AML patients who received aggressive doses of daunorubicin (>45 mg/m^2 per day for 3 days), but more recent trials suggest that older AML patients can safely tolerate higher doses of daunorubicin (60 to 90 mg/m^2 per day), which may be a result of improvements in supportive care.[69,73] Older patients with AML also do not experience added benefit when etoposide is incorporated into an anthracycline and cytarabine-containing regimen, or when etoposide is substituted for cytarabine in induction.[74,75]

Postremission strategies in elderly AML patients are less-well defined.[4] Although high-dose cytarabine is a standard component of postremission therapy in younger patients, it has not been shown to be beneficial in elderly AML patients. In the elderly, attenuated-dose cytarabine during remission induction decreases remission and survival rates while decreasing treatment-related mortality rates, which raises the concern that attenuated-dose cytarabine during postremission therapy may cause similar outcomes. In the CALGB trial that compared postremission cytarabine doses, higher doses of cytarabine (3,000 mg/m^2) was not as effective in patients older than age 60 years as it was in younger patients.[56] Serious toxicities, particularly neurotoxicity, were more frequent in elderly patients, and these toxicities limited the ability to deliver the planned four courses of therapy. A recent ECOG review concluded that lower doses of cytarabine (1,500 mg/m^2 for 6 to 12 doses) in older AML patients are well tolerated, with a treatment-related mortality rate of only 2% and median survival at 2 years of 30%.[73] Based on these data, some clinicians suggest that attenuated high-dose regimens (such as 1,500 mg/m^2) may be sufficient for elderly AML patients. The appropriate number of cycles of postremission consolidation therapy is unknown and currently under investigation in a randomized ECOG trial. An alternative approach to intensive postconsolidation therapy is the administration of multiple courses of chemotherapy in the ambulatory setting. The Acute Leukemia French Association recently demonstrated improved overall survival among patients receiving six monthly courses of outpatient chemotherapy (daunorubicin or idarubicin day 1; low-dose subcutaneous cytarabine for 5 days) compared to intensive consolidation (daunorubicin or idarubicin days 1 to 4; cytarabine continuous infusion).[76]

Although maintenance therapy is considered inferior to intensive consolidation chemotherapy in younger patients, its role in older patients with AML is still undefined. Some studies suggest that maintenance therapy following consolidation prolongs DFS but not OS as compared to no maintenance therapy.[77] Because older patients may not be able to tolerate more aggressive postremission strategies such as HSCT, maintenance therapy may play an important role in improving outcomes.

More novel immunomodulatory approaches to postremission therapy have been evaluated in elderly patients with AML. Results with interleukin-2 as a means to enhance the antileukemic activity of immune cells are promising. A recently completed randomized trial of interleukin-2/histamine hydrochloride versus control as postconsolidation immunotherapy resulted in increased DFS.[78] The CALGB is currently conducting a randomized trial in the elderly comparing 90 days of postremission low-dose, subcutaneous interleukin-2 versus observation. FLT3 ligand is another immunomodulatory cytokine that enhances recovery and activity of hematopoietic and dendritic cells and is currently under investigation as postremission therapy in elderly AML patients.

Several FLT3 inhibitors are in clinical development, including ABT-869, lestaurtinib (CEP-701), and midostaurin (PKC 412). Inhibition of farnesyl transferase is another treatment target. Tipifarnib has been the most extensively evaluated, demonstrating CR rates of 14%.[79] Other approaches include antiangiogenic therapies (e.g., lenalidomide, semaxanib [SU5416], axitinib [AG013736], bevacizumab, arsenic trioxide), proteasome inhibition and antiapoptotic therapies (e.g., bortezomib, oblimersen), epigenetic therapies (e.g., azacitidine, decitabine), and novel alkylating agents such as cloretazine.[80] Response rates with these new approaches in the elderly range from 0% to 59%. Whether they can modify the course of disease resulting in prolonged survival is unclear. Gemtuzumab ozogamicin is an immunoconjugate that consists of a monoclonal antibody linked to calicheamicin, a potent antineoplastic agent. Based on its activity in relapsed and refractory AML, it is being evaluated in combination with chemotherapy in untreated patients. It is unknown whether these improved CR rates will translate into longer DFS and OS.

NST is another therapeutic option in elderly patients with AML and MDS. Two small studies suggest this is a feasible option, with actuarial OS and EFS rates of 44% to 69% and 37% to 56%, respectively.[59,60] The advantage of this approach is less toxicity as a result of less-intensive chemotherapy, with the immune system providing the major antileukemic effect via GVHD/GVL mechanisms (see Chap. 142).

■ TREATMENT OF RELAPSED OR REFRACTORY ACUTE MYELOID LEUKEMIA

The most common cause of treatment failure in AML patients receiving chemotherapy alone or undergoing HSCT is relapse. In addition, many patients, particularly elderly patients, have refractory disease as defined by the inability to achieve a CR after two courses of induction therapy. In most cases, the preferred method of treatment for relapsed or refractory disease is HSCT. Prolonged DFS is observed in 30% to 40% of patients receiving allo- or autoHSCT in first relapse or CR2. Unfortunately, only a small percentage of relapsed or refractory adult patients will be eligible for HSCT, particularly alloHSCT, because of age and donor restrictions. The role of NST is also being evaluated in this setting.

The timing of HSCT to treat relapse is controversial. Some studies suggest that outcomes of HLA-matched, related alloHSCT are similar regardless of whether the transplant is performed at the time of early first relapse or in CR2. The difficulty with this approach is identifying a patient in "early relapse," as often the patient will present in a florid relapse. While performing the alloHSCT in first relapse eliminates the need for and toxicity of salvage chemotherapy, the feasibility of this approach is limited by the lead time required to activate a donor search. An International Bone Marrow Transplant Registry study demonstrated that alloHSCT was superior to chemotherapy for treatment of relapse occurring 1 to 2 years following induction.[81] Prolonged leukemia-free survival occurred in at least twofold more alloHSCT recipients as compared to patients receiving chemotherapy. In the treatment of refractory disease, alloHSCT is superior to autoHSCT in adults younger than age 55 years.

Patients who relapse following alloHSCT have a poor outcome, with a median survival of about 3 to 4 months.[1,82] In this setting, treatment options depend on performance status, clinical condition, and the time since alloHSCT. Patients relapsing less than 100 days following alloHSCT are unlikely to respond to current therapies, and salvage attempts are often associated with a high treatment-related mortality. For selected patients relapsing more than 1 year after alloHSCT, a second alloHSCT may be an alternative, but the likelihood of prolonged survival is generally less than 10% with a second transplant.[1] Other strategies being investigated for the treatment of relapse after alloHSCT include immune manipulation to stimulate a GVL effect through donor lymphocyte infusions, and premature discontinuation of calcineurin inhibitors and other immunosuppressants.

AutoHSCT is an option at the time of first relapse if cells have been previously collected and stored during first remission. If such cells were not collected, then it is necessary to achieve a second CR in order to proceed to autoHSCT. Prolonged DFS of 30% and 20% are reported when autoHSCT is performed in CR2 and CR3, respectively. The advantages of autoHSCT are the lack of donor limitations and fewer age-based restrictions; the disadvantage is the need to achieve a CR, which requires exposure to more cytotoxic chemotherapy. If patients relapse following autoHSCT, alloHSCT from a related or unrelated donor is preferred in selected younger patients. NST or other investigational therapies can be considered for older patients who relapse after autoHSCT.

If patients with relapsed or refractory disease are not candidates for HSCT, until recently the primary mode of treatment was salvage chemotherapy. The ability to achieve a second CR with salvage chemotherapy is related to the duration of the first remission. Approximately 50% to 60% of patients who relapse longer than 2 years after induction therapy will achieve a second CR, often with the same induction regimen.[4,51] If the patient relapses 1 to 2 years after induction therapy, the second CR rate decreases to 40%, and only 10% to 20% of patients who relapse within 6 to 12 months following induction are able to achieve a second CR with alternate salvage chemotherapy regimens. Long-term survival at 3 years ranges from zero in patients who relapse early to 20% to 25% in those who experience a prolonged duration of initial remission. Based on these data, a risk-adapted approach should be taken when considering treatment options.

The most commonly used salvage regimens include high-dose cytarabine given at doses of 2,000 to 3,000 mg/m^2 every 12 hours for 8 to 12 doses. High-dose cytarabine schedules that use once-daily doses or alternate-day doses have also been used in an attempt to minimize toxicity.[1,51] Cytarabine has been administered alone or in combination with various agents, including etoposide, fludarabine, topotecan, clofarabine, and an anthracycline, as treatment of relapsed or refractory AML. Response rates to such salvage regimens range from 30% to 50%, but are often short-lived. Patients who received high-dose cytarabine during remission induction may be less likely to benefit from such a regimen for treatment of relapse, and thus require alternate salvage strategies. Patients with remission duration of longer than 1 year appear to benefit most from high-dose cytarabine regimens.[4,51]

Approximately 70% of relapsed or refractory AML express the multidrug resistance phenotype, which confers a high degree of chemotherapy resistance because of its encoding and overexpression of P-glycoprotein. P-glycoprotein is a membrane protein capable of removing certain antineoplastics from the intracellular to extracellular space. Antagonists of P-glycoprotein, such as cyclosporine, the cyclosporine analog valspodar (formerly PSC 833), and zosuquidar, have been investigated as a strategy to overcome resistance in these patients.[83–85] In addition to inhibiting P-glycoprotein, cyclosporine may also affect the disposition of agents such as anthracyclines, and thus increase the exposure to cytotoxic agents. Valspodar is 10-fold more effective in inhibiting P-glycoprotein than cyclosporine and lacks cyclosporine's renal toxicity. Unfortunately, randomized trials in previously untreated or relapsed/refractory patients have shown no advantages and more regimen-related deaths in patients older than age 60 years receiving the multidrug resistance modulator.[83,84] Similarly zosuquidar did not result in improvements in OS, although more patients with a poor performance score were randomized to the intervention group and may in part be the reason for the adverse outcome.[85]

Monoclonal antibodies have the potential to deliver targeted therapy to the malignant cell. Gemtuzumab ozogamicin is an anti-CD33 antibody complexed to the antitumor antibiotic calicheamicin. Because CD33 is expressed in 90% of leukemic blasts, this anti-CD33–directed product provides targeted cell kill to leukemic cells. Patients with AML in first untreated relapse treated with gemtuzumab (9 mg/m^2 for two doses separated by 14 days) attained a CR in 16% of patients, with an additional 13% of patients having normalization of blood counts with the exception of persistent platelet counts <100,000 cells/mm^3.[86] Toxicity can be problematic with gemtuzumab. Common adverse effects include infusion-related reactions (fever and chills), prolonged neutropenia and thrombocytopenia, and transient elevations in hepatic enzymes. A more serious adverse event associated with gemtuzumab therapy is venoocclusive disease. It was initially thought that this only occurred in patients receiving gemtuzumab following HSCT, but has now been described in several patients who never underwent HSCT. Patients treated with gemtuzumab should have their weight and liver function tests, particularly bilirubin, monitored. Because gemtuzumab lacks specific dose-limiting organ toxicities, it has also been investigated in combination with other chemotherapy agents.[87] The United Kingdom Medical Research Council AML15 trial evaluated the benefit of adding gemtuzumab to remission induction chemotherapy (i.e., cytarabine-daunorubicin-etoposide or daunorubicin-cytarabine or fludarabine-cytarabine-filgrastim-idarubicin). Although the CR rates were similar, the combination of gemtuzumab plus conventional chemotherapy was associated with an improved DFS.[87] Gemtuzumab therapy in pediatric patients has been limited by the high risk of venoocclusive disease of the liver when given prior to HSCT. Other antibodies are under investigation in salvage regimens and high-dose preparative regimens for AML.

Several classes of new agents are being investigated as alternate treatment approaches for relapsed or refractory AML, including the ubiquitin-proteasome pathway inhibitors (bortezomib), new novel nucleoside analogs (troxacitabine), hypomethylating agents (decitabine and 5-azacitidine), histone deacetylase inhibitors (phenylbutyrate, vorinostat), and angiogenesis modulators (bevacizumab and thalidomide).[88] Arsenic trioxide, which is effective in the treatment of APL, is being investigated for the treatment of AML via its modulation of apoptotic and chromatin remodeling pathways. Imatinib mesylate, the tyrosine kinase inhibitor used in the treatment of chronic myeloid leukemia, also inhibits AML cell lines and is currently undergoing clinical trials in AML.[89]

In children with AML, the duration of CR1 predicts response to salvage chemotherapy. The BFM (Berlin-Frankfurt-Munster) group reported that patients who relapse within 1.5 years of initial diagnosis have a 5-year survival of 10%, versus 40% for those who relapse later than 1.5 years after initial diagnosis.[90] In children with relapsed or refractory AML, a regimen of mitoxantrone 12 mg/m^2 per day for 4 days starting on the third day of treatment and cytarabine 1,000 mg/m^2 per dose every 12 hours for eight doses can achieve a second CR rate of 76% with only a 3% mortality rate.[91] However, the 2-year OS rate was only 24%. Patients were eligible to receive intensification with high-dose cytarabine and etoposide at the investigator's discretion, and this arm was closed as a consequence of a toxic death rate of 10%. Currently, most pediatric patients in CR2 receive alloHSCT if a suitable donor is available.

■ LATE EFFECTS OF THERAPY FOR ACUTE MYELOID LEUKEMIA

Because of the intense therapy received by children with AML, they are at risk for a variety of long-term sequelae. A recent study reported that more than 50% of survivors have growth abnormalities.[92] Other findings include neurocognitive deficits, transfusion-associated hepatitis, endocrine disorders, cataracts, and cardiomyopathy (median cumulative anthracycline dose 335 mg/m^2). The 20-year cumulative risk for a second malignancy is estimated to be 1.8%.

TREATMENT

Acute Promyelocytic Leukemia

⓭ APL is a subclass of AML (FAB M3) that accounts for approximately 10% of all cases, and is the most curable of the AML subtypes. Most patients are diagnosed between the ages of 15 and 60 years. Five-year DFS rates of 70% to 80% are reported with APL.[93] APL is clinically unique from the other subclasses because of the common occurrence of severe coagulopathy (characterized by disseminated intravascular coagulation) at diagnosis and during remission induction therapy. In APL, differentiation and maturation arrest are caused by alterations in the RAR because of the translocation of chromosomes 15 and 17. The discovery of t(15;17) now provides a cytogenetic marker of the disease and is predictive of response to differentiation therapy with tretinoin (commonly referred to as all-*trans* retinoic acid). This translocation leads to a fusion protein of the PML gene on chromosome 15 and the RARα on chromosome 17.

Prior to the availability of tretinoin, treatment of APL consisted of the same combination chemotherapy regimens used in the treatment of other subclasses of AML. Such standard regimens produced CR rates of 50% to 60%, but were associated with a high treatment-related mortality rate caused by hemorrhagic complications. The introduction of molecularly targeted therapy with tretinoin allows for high CR rates with a significant reduction in life-threatening bleeding complications.

■ TREATMENT PHASES

Remission Induction

Tretinoin, an oral vitamin A analog, is usually given orally in a dose of 45 mg/m^2 per day, as a single dose or divided into two doses, given after a meal. Tretinoin-based regimens achieve CR rates as high as 95% in APL patients within 1 to 3 months. Because tretinoin does not cross the blood–brain barrier, leukemic meningitis should be treated with conventional intrathecal chemotherapy.

Although devoid of myelosuppressive effects, tretinoin therapy is associated with headache, skin and mucous membrane reactions, bone pain, nausea, and the retinoic acid syndrome. When tretinoin is started, rapid onset of differentiation of promyelocytes occurs, which can lead to leukocytosis and retinoic acid syndrome. The retinoic acid syndrome (fever, respiratory distress, interstitial pulmonary infiltrates, pleural effusions, and weight gain) is now referred to as the APL differentiation syndrome or APL hyperleukocytosis syndrome, because it is associated with other treatment modalities in the management of APL. Among tretinoin-treated patients, this syndrome is fatal in 5% to 29% of cases. A combination of chemotherapy with tretinoin induction decreases the risk of APL differentiation syndrome, and rapid initiation of dexamethasone 10 mg (0.2 mg/kg per dose in children) twice daily for 3 days upon development of symptoms decreases associated mortality.[93]

A number of clinical trials have evaluated treatment regimens for APL since the discovery of tretinoin.[93] These trials demonstrated that tretinoin induction therapy, followed by consolidation chemotherapy, produced similar CR rates but decreased relapse and increased EFS and OS as compared to chemotherapy alone for remission induction and consolidation. However, a significant proportion of patients receiving tretinoin in that study relapsed by 4 years, and 25% of patients experienced the APL differentiation syndrome. In an effort to extend the duration of remission and decrease tretinoin-associated toxicity, other trials have evaluated the sequential and concurrent administration of tretinoin with chemotherapy during remission induction therapy. The United Kingdom Medical Research Council trial compared concurrent administration of tretinoin with chemotherapy to sequential tretinoin during induction (given 5 days before anthracycline-based remission induction chemotherapy) with the hope of reducing coagulopathy-related complications. Concurrent administration was superior in terms of CR rates, early death, and EFS and OS at 3 years. The French study demonstrated similar CR rates with concurrent or sequential tretinoin and standard induction chemotherapy, but noted a better DFS and EFS at 2 years in the concurrent administration group (suggesting a synergistic or additive effect for the combination).[93] Based on these data, the current recommendations for induction therapy for newly diagnosed APL patients include tretinoin 45 mg/m^2 per day until a CR is achieved, in combination with an anthracycline (either daunorubicin 50 to 60 mg/m^2 per dose for 3 days, or idarubicin 12 mg/m^2 per dose every other day for four doses).[93] Similar CR rates are observed with daunorubicin or idarubicin. APL cells appear to be more sensitive to anthracyclines, perhaps as a consequence of decreased P-glycoprotein expression.

It is important to note that chemotherapy regimens used in combination with tretinoin differ from standard AML regimens, primarily as a result of the lack of a cytarabine backbone. Several studies have evaluated the role of cytarabine in remission induction regimens for APL. In earlier trials, the addition of cytarabine did not improve the CR rate.[93] Children should also be treated with tretinoin and an anthracycline, with results similar to those achieved in adults.

Arsenic trioxide is a compound with demonstrated efficacy in relapsed APL. It has been evaluated as part of remission induction therapy in several small studies. The concept of a "chemotherapy-free" regimen in this disease is attractive. Administration of arsenic trioxide with or without tretinoin (± chemotherapy) results in high initial CR rates and molecular response rates.[94–96] Larger studies are needed before this can be adopted as a standard of care.

Intensive Postremission Therapy

Consolidation chemotherapy should be administered to patients with APL because of the high relapse rate. Consolidation therapy usually consists of an anthracycline-based regimen in combination with tretinoin. The role of high-dose cytarabine in consolidation is still controversial. Although one European trial has demonstrated increased relapse risk if cytarabine is not incorporated,[93] these results have not been confirmed by other groups. Current recommendations reserve high-dose cytarabine regimens for patients who remain polymerase chain reaction-positive after consolidation with an anthracycline-containing regimen.[93]

Arsenic trioxide has also been evaluated in consolidation therapy. The CALGB recently released the results of a randomized trial that compared standard chemotherapy plus tretinoin followed by arsenic trioxide to standard chemotherapy plus tretinoin followed by standard postremission therapy. The addition of arsenic trioxide resulted in longer EFS and OS.[97]

Maintenance Therapy

Unlike other subtypes of AML, maintenance therapy is an important component of therapy for APL. Before the advent of tretinoin, nonrandomized trials suggested a benefit of continuous low-dose methotrexate and mercaptopurine in prevention of relapse of APL. Larger prospective randomized trials have demonstrated decreased relapse rates in patients who received maintenance therapy (either tretinoin or combination chemotherapy), and some trials have demonstrated increased EFS and OS.[93] In a study that compared maintenance with tretinoin, chemotherapy, or tretinoin plus chemotherapy versus observation, observation was associated with the highest relapse rate and tretinoin plus chemotherapy with the lowest relapse rate.[93] Current recommendations for maintenance therapy in adult APL patients include tretinoin 45 mg/m^2 per day for 15 days every 3 months, in addition to mercaptopurine 100 mg/m^2 orally daily and methotrexate 10 mg/m^2 per week, for 2 years in all patients.[93] The NCCN guidelines similarly recommend tretinoin maintenance therapy with or without 6-mercaptopurine and methotrexate.[54]

TREATMENT OF RELAPSED ACUTE PROMYELOCYTIC LEUKEMIA

Relapsed APL can also be effectively treated with tretinoin therapy. Patients relapsing after tretinoin-based therapy can achieve a second CR with tretinoin-based reinduction. For patients resistant to induction or reinduction with tretinoin-based regimens, alternative strategies include arsenic trioxide, and allo- or autoHSCT. Outcomes with autoHSCT depend on the disease status of the patient at the time of transplant. AutoHSCT in CR2 (versus CR1) is associated with a lower OS, leukemia-free survival, and increased treatment-related mortality. Based on the sensitive nature of patients to chemotherapy, autoHSCT in CR1 is currently not warranted, but offers an excellent option for polymerase chain reaction PML/RARα-negative patients in CR2. AlloHSCT should not be offered to patients in CR1, as the mortality associated with alloHSCT outweighs the risks of conventional chemotherapy. However, it is an appropriate choice in CR2 as consolidation after reinduction with either arsenic trioxide or tretinoin.[98]

Arsenic trioxide has induced clinical remissions in relapsed APL through its induction of apoptosis and differentiation.[99,100] The recommended dose is 0.15 mg/kg per day IV until bone marrow remission, not to exceed 60 doses, followed by consolidation beginning 3 to 6 weeks after completion of induction at the same dose for a total of 25 doses over a period up to 5 weeks. Arsenic trioxide therapy is associated with two specific toxicities. First, it can cause the APL hyperleukocytosis syndrome, similar to that seen with tretinoin. Management is similar: corticosteroids at first signs of pulmonary distress or a rapidly rising WBC count. The second toxicity is a prolongation of the QT_c interval. Consequently, it is important to obtain a baseline 12-lead electrocardiogram prior to starting therapy with arsenic trioxide, and correct any electrolyte abnormalities, including potassium, calcium, and magnesium. Other medications known to prolong the QT_c interval should be avoided, if possible, during arsenic trioxide therapy. The QT_c interval should not exceed 500 milliseconds at baseline, and if it increases to >500 milliseconds during therapy, the patient should be reevaluated. Do not reintroduce the arsenic trioxide until the QT_c is <460 milliseconds. Following induction of a second CR with arsenic trioxide in relapsed patients, postremission therapy with combination arsenic trioxide and chemotherapy can result in molecular remissions and improved DFS, as compared to chemotherapy or arsenic trioxide alone following remission.[100] Additional investigations are underway to evaluate the role of arsenic trioxide in multidrug postremission regimens.

PATIENT MONITORING

In comparison to non-APL AML, molecular and cytogenetic testing at the end of remission induction therapy in APL has no prognostic value. Clinicians should not make decisions based on the presence or absence of any genetic abnormalities at this time. Because terminal differentiation of blasts in APL requires more than 40 days, results of a bone marrow biopsy obtained at the end of remission induction can be misleading because insufficient time has elapsed to determine response. Molecular and cytogenetic response assessment should occur after the completion of consolidation treatment.

Detection of residual PML/RARα transcripts in the bone marrow at the end of consolidation therapy is strongly associated with subsequent hematologic relapse. Achievement of PML/RARα-negative status is associated with a higher probability of cure. The use of this molecular technique allows the clinician to assess response to therapy and also detect relapse earlier, which might prevent the development of overt disease recurrence and is associated with improved outcome compared with delaying treatment until overt morphologic relapse.[93] Most experts recommend that APL patients should be routinely evaluated for continuous remission status. Suggested followup includes polymerase chain reaction for PML/RARα every 3 to 6 months for 2 years, and then every 6 months for 2 years.[93]

■ ROLE OF COLONY-STIMULATING FACTORS IN ACUTE MYELOID LEUKEMIA

9 Colony-stimulating factors have been evaluated in AML patients to enhance chemotherapy cytotoxicity, shorten the duration of neutropenia, and reduce the incidence and severity of infection following induction and consolidation chemotherapy. Most studies show limited benefit with the use of colony-stimulating factors as "priming" agents administered during remission induction therapy in an effort to recruit leukemia cells into the cycle to enhance susceptibility to cell-cycle–specific chemotherapy agents, leading to increased cell kill. A recent trial demonstrated similar response rates, but those patients in CR following remission induction chemotherapy had a higher DFS if they received filgastrim.[101] No effect on OS was observed. Subgroup analysis demonstrated improved OS and DFS for patients with standard-risk AML receiving filgrastim. Results from the French Association (ALFA)-9000 trial were recently published. In that trial, the addition of sargramostim to induction and consolidation courses resulted in higher CR rates and EFS, but no effect on OS was observed.[102] Use of colony-stimulating factors concurrently during chemotherapy administration is discouraged outside the setting of a clinical trial and is not recommended for this use in the American Society of Clinical Oncology guidelines.[42]

CLINICAL CONTROVERSY

Colony-stimulating factors were investigated a decade ago as "priming agents" to recruit cells into the cycle, so theoretically there was a greater leukemia cell kill. Although most studies showed no difference in the CR rate, recent data suggest this approach may improve DFS in certain subgroups of patients.

Both filgrastim and sargramostim are FDA approved to prevent neutropenic complications in adult AML patients receiving intensive chemotherapy. The original package inserts listed myeloid malignancies as a contraindication to the use of filgrastim or sargramostim. Myeloid blast cells have receptors for granulocyte colony-stimulating factor and granulocyte-macrophage colony-stimulating factor, and there was initial concern that the use of these factors would stimulate regrowth of the myeloid leukemia. Although subsequent studies have addressed these concerns, many pediatric clinicians do not initiate filgrastim until an initial remission is achieved.

A number of randomized trials, primarily in elderly patients, consistently demonstrate that filgrastim or sargramostim reduces the duration of neutropenia following AML induction chemotherapy.[42] While neutropenia can be reduced from 2 to 12 days depending on the trial, results vary in terms of improvements in infectious morbidity and mortality, resource use, and disease response rates. The American Society of Clinical Oncology Guidelines for the Use of White Blood Cell Growth Factors considers the use of colony-stimulating factors after initial induction therapy reasonable, with the understanding that the effects on length of hospitalization and incidence of severe infection are modest.[42] Patients older than age 55 years appear to derive the greatest benefit, and use is appropriate in this population where more rapid marrow recovery might decrease the duration of hospitalization.[42] Following consolidation therapy, patients receiving colony-stimulating factors have a more profound shortening of the duration of severe neutropenia resulting in a reduction in infection rates and an associated reduction in the use of antibiotic therapy.[42] Use of growth factors after consolidation do not affect CR duration or OS. Further pharmacoeconomic data are required in this setting, but the body of evidence supports their use following consolidation therapy in adults. Other controversial issues surrounding colony-stimulating factor use in AML include which colony-stimulating factor to use, what dose, which day to start after chemotherapy, how long to continue, and should the marrow be examined for leukemia prior to starting a colony-stimulating factor. All growth factors have been evaluated in patients with AML, including sargramostim, filgrastim, and pegfilgrastim. Although pegfilgrastim is not FDA approved for this indication, preliminary results show that it can be used in this setting.[103,104] The use of colony-stimulating factors can also interfere with the interpretation of the day 14 bone marrow examination. Growth factors should be discontinued at least 7 days prior to a bone marrow aspirate and biopsy to avoid interfering with the interpretation of the results (i.e., may see immature myeloid forms that would suggest residual disease).

SUPPORTIVE CARE

The most common and significant toxic effect of antileukemic agents is marrow suppression. With the exception of corticosteroids, tretinoin, asparaginase/pegaspargase, and vincristine, antineoplastic agents used to treat acute leukemia cause myelosuppression. During AML remission induction and postremission therapy, daily monitoring of the complete blood count and the absolute neutrophil count is necessary to determine when red cell and platelet transfusions are needed and when neutropenia is achieved. Less-frequent monitoring may be sufficient during ALL induction. Marrow hypoplasia from the myelosuppressive regimens usually reaches its lowest point (nadir) after 1 to 2 weeks of therapy and lasts for another 1 to 2 weeks. During this period of hypoplasia, infectious and bleeding complications are major causes of death in leukemic patients. As typical signs and symptoms of infection may be absent in the neutropenic host, frequent monitoring of vital signs (especially fever) and daily physical examination are important.[105] Infection control strategies often include routine hand washing; dietary restrictions; reverse isolation and laminar-air flow rooms; fungal, *Pneumocystis*, and bacterial prophylaxis; and the empiric use of broad-spectrum antibiotics when fever occurs (see Chap. 126).[105] In contrast to the practice at many institutions, the NCCN guidelines do not recommend prophylactic antimicrobials or gut decontamination during induction or consolidation, and leave the choice to the discretion of the treating facility based on local infection patterns and concerns.[54] Several groups have analyzed the literature surrounding the use of prophylactic antibacterials. In general, prophylactic antibacterials should be reserved for patients who are expected to have prolonged (more than 7 days) and profound (absolute neutrophil count <100 cells/mm^3) neutropenia. Based on these criteria, prophylaxis following induction chemotherapy is warranted and postconsolidation therapy is warranted on a case-by-case basis.

In children, prophylactic antibiotics have not proven useful and have resulted in increased resistance. Pediatric ALL patients on standard induction regimens, which generally are minimally myelosuppressive, often have recovered blood counts earlier and do not require very aggressive measures. However, they do require close monitoring of vital signs and blood counts until their counts recover. Pediatric AML patients are usually admitted for at least 1 month during induction and again for consolidation. Regardless of therapy, children with AML have a 10% to 20% induction mortality rate caused by infection and bleeding complications.[106] The incidence of viridans streptococci has increased with the intensity of therapy and is most associated with high-dose cytarabine. These infections can lead to meningitis or delayed acute respiratory distress syndrome.

Pneumocystis jiroveci prophylaxis (usually trimethoprim-sulfamethoxazole) is begun in all adults and children with ALL by the end of induction and continues until 6 months after therapy is discontinued.

Acute leukemia patients, particularly those patients with an initial elevated WBC count, are at risk for tumor lysis syndrome. Preventive measures include allopurinol or rasburicase, and adequate hydration (with or without sodium bicarbonate) prior to and during chemotherapy to prevent the development of urate nephropathy from rapid destruction of WBCs. In adults, 300 mg of allopurinol once daily, started 1 to 2 days prior to chemotherapy, is usually adequate. Children should receive 10 mg/kg per day of allopurinol in three divided doses. Rasburicase, a recombinant urate-oxidase enzyme produced by genetic modification of *Saccharomyces cerevisiae,* catalyzes the enzymatic oxidation of uric acid into the inactive soluble metabolite, allantoin. In children, rasburicase 0.15 to 0.2 mg/kg per day more rapidly reduces uric acid levels in patients with aggressive malignancies compared to allopurinol, and reduces the need for dialysis.[107–109] Rasburicase has been evaluated in adults, and some studies in adults show that fixed dosing produces equivalent outcomes to a mg/kg dosing strategy.[110] Because of its cost, this product is usually limited to patients with ALL who have a high WBC count or bulky extramedullary disease, aggressive lymphoma, or patients with AML with a high presenting WBC. Most institutions also include an elevated uric acid as part of the criteria for use. Because of the rapid onset of action and long duration of action of rasburicase, many institutions also limit its use to a single dose and allow repeat doses when the criteria for use are met again. Rasburicase is contraindicated in patients with glucose-6-phosphate dehydrogenase deficiency.

Tumor lysis syndrome may lead not only to hyperuricemia, but also to hyperkalemia, hyperphosphatemia, and hypocalcemia. Hematologic support consists primarily of platelet and packed red blood cell transfusions. Platelet transfusions are often given for peripheral counts below 5,000 to 10,000 cells/mm^3 or clinical signs of bleeding. Transfusions of packed red cells may also be indicated for a hematocrit less than 25%, profound fatigue, shortness of breath, tachycardia, or chest pain. APL can release procoagulants that can cause disseminated intravascular coagulation, necessitating close monitoring and replacement of coagulation factors with cryoprecipitate. Because of the gastrointestinal toxic effects of chemotherapy, parenteral nutrition may be required. Patients are frequently receiving infusions of antibiotics, fluids, hyperalimentation, and blood products simultaneously. To provide the total support needed for these patients, a multiple-lumen central venous access device such as a Hickman catheter can be placed at the start of therapy.

EVALUATION OF THERAPEUTIC OUTCOMES

Appropriate development of a pharmaceutical care plan for the acute leukemia patient begins with establishing the diagnosis and prognosis for the patient. Long-term therapeutic goals for the patient may include long-term DFS, although palliative care is a possibility in some patients. The desired short-term outcome is the establishment of remission. The return of hematologic values to normal and a repeat bone marrow biopsy that demonstrates no evidence of disease serve as documentation that remission has been achieved. Monitoring guidelines for induction or consolidation are similar (Table 137–6). After the appropriate postremission therapy has been completed, the patient may return monthly for 1 year, and then every 3 months, to check hematologic values. If no evidence of disease exists after 5 years from the diagnosis and the patient has been in continuous CR, the patient is considered cured.

Intense monitoring of fevers, hematologic and chemistry laboratory values, microbiology reports, and the patient's physical condition are necessary to identify infection, risk of bleeding, and tumor lysis syndrome early. A coagulation screening panel will identify patients with ongoing disseminated intravascular coagulation, a particular risk with APL.

During therapy, the pharmacist can be an important provider of patient education. Patients should receive information regarding acute and chronic toxicities of the chemotherapy being administered, as well as possible treatments for those toxicities. The pharmacist can also be an important resource for information regarding antibiotics, antiemetics, nutritional support, colony-stimulating factors, and other supportive care issues.

Pharmacists need to be involved in checking drug doses and any dose modifications for organ dysfunction or prior toxicity. Pharmacists are often in the best position to recognize the potential for medication errors and drug interaction and to help avoid them. Similarly, pharmacists are often able to identify the possibility that patient problems are secondary to drug treatments.

Numerous late sequelae from leukemia therapy have been recognized and should be included in the monitoring plan after therapy is completed. Chapter 142 discusses the long-term consequences of HSCT.

TABLE 137-6 Acute Myeloid Leukemia Assessment and Monitoring

Baseline Workup	Monitoring during Therapy	Postremission Monitoring
History and physical examination	Daily physical examination	Routine physical examination at clinic visit
CBC with differential, platelets	CBC with differential, platelets	CBC with differential, platelets
Serum chemistries (creatinine, bilirubin, AST, ALT to assess organ function)	Serum chemistries (including uric acid, K^+, Ca^{+2}, PO_4, S_{cr} during tumor lysis syndrome risk period[a])	Bone marrow biopsy and aspirate at set intervals to evaluate ongoing remission and if peripheral blood counts are abnormal or if they fail to recover within 5 weeks of treatment
Coagulation (PT, PTT, D-dimers, fibrinogen)	Coagulation (PT, PTT, D-dimers, fibrinogen [if APL])	PML/RARα monitoring [if APL]
Bone marrow biopsy and aspirate with cytogenetics	Bone marrow biopsy and aspirate 7–10 days after end of chemotherapy. Repeat bone marrow biopsy and aspirate upon hematologic recovery to document complete response (with cytogenetics if initially abnormal)	
Immunophenotyping and cytochemistry	Temperature curve (initiate antibiotics when febrile)	
Human leukocyte antigen (HLA) typing	Lumbar puncture (with intrathecal chemotherapy) if initial lumbar puncture was positive for leukemia)	
Cardiac workup (MUGA or echocardiogram; ECG)		
Intravascular access		
Lumbar puncture (if symptomatic or AML M4 or M5)		
Chest radiography		
Height and weight		
Molecular testing for genetic aberrations (FLT3, NPM1)		

ALT, alanine aminotransferase; APL, acute promyelocytic leukemia; AST, aspartate aminotransferase; CBC, complete blood cell count; ECG, electrocardiogram; FLT3, FMS-related tyrosine kinase 3; MUGA, multiple-gated acquisition (blood pool scan); NMP1, nucleophosmin; PML/RARα, promyelocytic-leukemia retinoic acid receptor-α; PT, prothrombin time; PTT, partial thromboplastin time; S_{cr}, serum creatinine.
[a]Risk for tumor lysis syndrome during induction therapy only.

ABBREVIATIONS

autoHSCT: autologous hematopoietic stem cell transplantation
BAALC: brain and acute leukemia gene, cytoplasmic
CALGB: Cancer and Leukemia Group B
CR: complete remission
CR1: first complete remission
CR2: second complete remission
CR3: third complete remission
DFS: disease-free survival
ECOG: Eastern Cooperative Oncology Group
EFS: event-free survival
FAB: French–American–British classification system
GVHD: graft-versus-host disease
GVL: graft-versus-leukemia (effect)
HLA: human leukocyte antigen
HSCT: hematopoietic stem cell transplantation
MDS: myelodysplastic syndrome
MLL: mixed lineage leukemia
NCCN: National Comprehensive Cancer Network
NPM1: nucleophosmin mutations, member 1
NST: nonmyeloablative stem cell transplant
OS: overall survival
Ph^+: Philadelphia chromosome
PML: promyelocytic leukemia (gene)
RAR: retinoic acid receptor-α
TPMT: thiopurine methyltransferase
WBC: white blood cell

REFERENCES

1. Scheinberg DA, Maslak P, Weiss M. Acute leukemias. In: DeVita VT, Hellman S, Rosenberg SA, eds. Cancer: Principles and Practice of Oncology, 7th ed. Philadelphia: Lippincott Williams & Wilkins, 2005:2088–2120.
2. Jemal A, Siegel R, Ward E, et al. Cancer statistics, 2007. CA Cancer J Clin 2007;57:43–66.
3. Ries LAG, Eisner MP, Kosary CL, et al. SEER Cancer Statistics Review, 1975–2003. Bethesda, MD: National Cancer Institute. 2006, *http://seer.cancer.gov/csr/1975_2003/*.
4. Estey E, Dohner H. Acute myeloid leukaemia. Lancet 2006;368:1894–1907.
5. Margolin JF, Steuber CP, Poplack DG. Acute lymphoblastic leukemia. In: Pizzo PA, Poplack DG, eds. Principles and Practices of Pediatric Oncology, 5th ed. Philadelphia: Lippincott Williams & Wilkins, 2006:538–590.
6. Faderl S, Jeha S, Kantarjian HM. The biology and therapy of adult acute lymphoblastic leukemia. Cancer 2003;98:1337–1354.
7. Deschler B, Lubbert M. Acute myeloid leukemia: Epidemiology and etiology. Cancer 2006;107:2099–2107.
8. Belson M, Kingsley B, Holmes A. Risk factors for acute leukemia in children: A review. Environ Health Perspect 2007;115:138–145.
9. Vardiman JW, Harris NL, Brunning RD. The World Health Organization (WHO) classification of the myeloid neoplasms. Blood 2002;100:2292–2302.
10. Byrd JC, Mrozek K, Dodge RK, et al. Pretreatment cytogenetic abnormalities are predictive of induction success, cumulative incidence of relapse, and overall survival in adult patients with de novo acute myeloid leukemia: Results from Cancer and Leukemia Group B (CALGB 8461). Blood 2002;100:4325–4336.
11. Hasle H, Niemeyer CM, Chessells JM, et al. A pediatric approach to the WHO classification of myelodysplastic and myeloproliferative disease. Leukemia 2003;17:277–282.
12. Pui CH, Evans WE. Treatment of acute lymphoblastic leukemia. N Engl J Med 2006;354:166–178.
13. Smith M, Arthur D, Camitta B, et al. Uniform approach to risk classification and treatment assignment for children with acute lymphoblastic leukemia. J Clin Oncol 1996;14:18–24.
14. Schultz KR, Pullen J, Sather HN, et al. Risk- and response-based classification of childhood B-precursor acute lymphoblastic leukemia: A combined analysis of prognostic markers from the Pediatric Oncology Group (POG) and Children's Cancer Group (CCG). Blood 2007;109:926–935.
15. Mandrell BN and Pritchard M. Understanding the clinical implications of minimal residual disease in childhood leukemia. J Pediatr Oncol Nurs 2006;23:38–44.
16. Nachman J, Sather HN, Gaynon PS, et al. Augmented Berlin-Frankfurt-Munster therapy abrogates the adverse prognostic significance of slow early response to induction chemotherapy for children and adolescents with acute lymphoblastic leukemia and unfavorable presenting features: A report from the Children's Cancer Group. J Clin Oncol 1997;15:2222–2230.
17. Mitchell CD, Richards SM, Kinsey SE, et al. Benefit of dexamethasone compared with prednisolone for childhood acute lymphoblastic leukemia: Results of the UK Medical Research Council ALL 97 randomized trial. Br J Haematol 2005;129:734–745.
18. Ravindranath Y. Recent advances in pediatric acute lymphoblastic and myeloid leukemia. Curr Opin Oncol 2003;15:23–35.
19. Jones LK and Saha V. Philadelphia positive acute lymphoblastic leukemia of childhood. Br J Haematol 2005;130:489–500.
20. Maltoub Y, Lindemulder S, Gaynon PS, et al. Intrathecal triple therapy decreases central nervous system relapse but fails to improve event-free survival when compared with intrathecal methotrexate: Results of the Children's Cancer Group (CCG) 1952 study for standard-risk acute lymphoblastic leukemia, reported by the Children's Oncology Group. Blood 2006;108:1165–1173.
21. Bomgaars L, Geyer JR, Franklin J, et al. Phase I trial of intrathecal liposomal cytarabine in children with neoplastic meningitis. J Clin Oncol 2004;22:3916–3921.
22. Lange BJ, Bostrom BC, Cherlow JM, et al. Double-delayed intensification improves EFS for children with intermediate-risk acute lymphoblastic leukemia: A report from the Children's Cancer Group. Blood 2002;99:825–833.
23. Hutchinson RJ, Gaynon PS, Sather H, et al. Intensification of therapy for children with lower-risk acute lymphoblastic leukemia: Long-term follow-up of patients treated on Children's Cancer Group trial 1881. J Clin Oncol 2003;21:1790–1797.
24. Richards S, Gray R, Peto R, et al. Duration and intensity of maintenance chemotherapy in acute leukemia: Overview of 42 trials involving 12,000 randomised children. Childhood ALL Collaborative Group. Lancet 1996;347:1783–1788.
25. Wall AM, Rubnitz JE. Pharmacogenomic effects on therapy for acute lymphoblastic leukemia in children. Pharmacogenomics J 2003;3:128–135.
26. Berg SL, Blaney SM, Devidas M, et al. Phase II study of nelarabine (Compound 506U78) in children and young adults with refractory T-cell malignancies: A report from the Children's Oncology Group. J Clin Oncol 2005;23:3376–3382.
27. Biondi A, Cimino G, Pieters R, et al. Biological and therapeutic aspects of infant leukemia. Blood 2000;96:24–33.
28. Kantarjian HM, O'Brien S, Smith TL, et al. Results of treatment with hyper-CVAD, a dose-intensive regimen, in adult acute lymphocytic leukemia. J Clin Oncol 2000;18:547–561.
29. Thomas DA, Faderl S, Cortes J, et al. Treatment of Philadelphia chromosome-positive acute lymphocytic leukemia with hyper-CVAD and imatinib mesylate. Blood 2004;103:4396–4407.
30. Yanada M, Takeuchi J, Sugiura I, et al. High complete remission rate and promising outcome by combination of imatinib and chemotherapy for newly diagnosed BCR-ABL-positive acute lymphoblastic leukemia: A phase II study by the Japan Adult Leukemia Study Group. J Clin Oncol 2006;24:460–466.
31. Delannoy A, Delabesse E, Lheritier V, et al. Imatinib and methylprednisolone alternated with chemotherapy improve the outcome of elderly

patients with Philadelphia-positive acute lymphoblastic leukemia: Results of the GRAALL AFR09 study. Leukemia 2006;20:1526–1532.

32. Wassmann B, Pfeifer H, Goekbuget N, et al. Alternating versus concurrent schedules of imatinib and chemotherapy as front-line therapy for Philadelphia-positive acute lymphoblastic leukemia (Ph+ ALL). Blood 2006;108:1469–1477.
33. Talpaz M, Shah NP, Kantarjian H, et al. Dasatinib in imatinib-resistant Philadelphia chromosome-positive leukemias. N Engl J Med 2006; 354:2531–2541.
34. Kantarjian H, Giles F, Wunderle L, et al. Nilotinib in imatinib-resistant CML and Philadelphia chromosome-positive ALL. N Engl J Med 2006;354:2542–2551.
35. Gaynon PS. Childhood acute lymphoblastic leukaemia and relapse. Br J Haematol 2005;131:579–587.
36. Eapen M, Raetz E, Zhang M-J, et al. Outcome after HLA-matched sibling transplantation or chemotherapy in children with B-precursor acute lymphoblastic leukemia in second remission: A collaborative study of the Children's Oncology Group and the Center for International Blood and Marrow Transplant Research. Blood 2006;107:4961–4967.
37. Hahn T, Wall D, Camitta B, et al. The role of cytotoxic therapy with hematopoietic stem cell transplantation in the therapy of acute lymphoblastic leukemia in children: An evidence-based review. Biol Blood Marrow Transplant 2005;11:823–861.
38. Goldstone AH, Richards SM, Lazarus HM, et al. In adults with standard-risk acute lymphoblastic leukemia (ALL) the greatest benefit is achieved from matched sibling allogeneic transplant in first complete remission (CR) and an autologous transplant is less effective than conventional consolidation/maintenance chemotherapy in ALL patients: Final results of the international ALL trial (MRC UKALL XII/ECOG E2993). Blood 2008;111:1827–1833.
39. National Marrow Donor Program website. *http://www.nmdp.org.*
40. Hahn T, Wall D, Camitta B, et al. The role of cytotoxic therapy with hematopoietic stem cell transplantation in the therapy of acute lymphoblastic leukemia in adults: An evidence-based review. Biol Blood Marrow Transplant 2006;12:1–30.
41. Wittman B, Horan J, Lyman GH. Prophylactic colony stimulating factors in children receiving myelosuppressive chemotherapy: A meta-analysis of randomized controlled trials. Cancer Treat Rev 2006;32:289–303.
42. Smith TJ Khatcheressian J, Lyman GH, et al. 2006 Update of recommendations for the use of white blood cell growth factors: And evidence based clinical practice guideline. J Clin Oncol 2006;24:3187–3205.
43. Oeffinger KC, Mertens AC, Sklar CA, et al. Chronic health conditions in adult survivors of childhood cancer. N Engl J Med 2006;355:1572–1582.
44. Pui CH, Cheng C, Leung W, et al. Extended follow-up of long-term survivors of childhood acute lymphoblastic leukemia. N Engl J Med 2003;349:640–649.
45. Wells RJ, Arthur D, Srivastava A, et al. Prognostic variables in newly diagnosed children and adolescents with acute myeloid leukemia: Children's Cancer Group Study 213. Leukemia 2002;16:601–607.
46. Mrozek K, Marcucci G, Paschka P, Whitman SP, Bloodfield CD. Clinical relevance of mutations and gene-expression changes in adult acute myeloid leukemia with normal cytogenetics: Are we ready for a prognostically prioritized molecular classification? Blood 2007;109:431–448.
47. Cheson B, Bennett JM, Kopecky KJ, et al. Revised recommendations of the International Working Group for diagnosis, standardization or response criteria, treatment outcomes, and reporting standards for therapeutic trials in acute myeloid leukemia. J Clin Oncol 2003;21:4642–4649.
48. Buchner T, Berdel WE, Wormann B, et al. Treatment of older patients with acute myeloid leukemia. Crit Rev Oncol Hematol 2005;56:247–259.
49. Langmuir PB, Aplenc R, Lange BJ. Acute myeloid leukaemia in children. Best Pract Res Clin Haematol 2001;14:77–93.
50. Kolitz JE. Current therapeutic strategies for acute myeloid leukemia. Br J Haematol 2006;134:555–572.
51. Milligan DW, Grimwade D, Cullis JO, et al. Guidelines on the management of acute myeloid leukaemia in adults. Br J Haematol 2006;135:450–474.
52. Rowe JM, Neuberg D, Friedenberg W, et al. A phase 3 study of three induction regimens and of priming with GM-CSF in older adults with acute myeloid leukemia: A trial by the Eastern Cooperative Oncology Group. Blood 2004;103:479–485.
53. Cahn JY, Labopin M, Sierra J, et al. No impact of high-dose cytarabine on the outcome of patients transplanted for acute myeloblastic leukaemia in first remission. Acute Leukaemia Working Party of the European Group for Blood and Marrow Transplant (EBMT). Br J Haematol 2000;110:308–314.
54. National Comprehensive Cancer Network Clinical Practice Guidelines in Oncology. Acute Myeloid Leukemia. Version 2.2007. 2007, *http://www.nccn.com/physician_gls/f_guidelines.html.*
55. Kern W, Estey EH. High-dose cytosine arabinoside in the treatment of acute myeloid leukemia. Review of three randomized trials. Cancer 2006;107:116–124.
56. Mayer RJ, Davis RB, Schiffer CA, et al. Intensive postremission chemotherapy in adults with acute myeloid leukemia. Cancer and Leukemia Group B. N Engl J Med 1994;331:896–903.
57. Byrd JC, Dodge RK, Carroll A, et al. Patients with t(8;21)(q22;q22) and acute myeloid leukemia have superior failure-free and overall survival when repetitive cycles of high-dose cytarabine are administered. J Clin Oncol 1999;17:3767–3775.
58. Byrd JC, Ruppert AS, Mrozek K, et al. Repetitive cycles of high-dose cytarabine benefit patients with acute myeloid leukemia and inv(16)(p13q22) or t(16;16)(p13;q22): Results from CALGB 8461. J Clin Oncol 2004;22:1087–1094.
59. Alyea EP, Kim HT, Ho V, et al. Comparative outcome of nonmyeloablative and myeloablative allogeneic hematopoietic cell transplantation for patients older than 50 years of age. Blood 2005;105:1810–1814.
60. Aoudjhane M, Labopin M, Gorin NC, et al. Comparative outcome of reduced intensity and myeloablative conditioning regimen in HLA identical sibling allogeneic haematopoietic stem cell transplantation for patients older than 50 years of age with acute myeloblastic leukaemia: A retrospective survey from the Acute Leukemia Working Party (ALWP) of the European group for Blood and Marrow Transplantation (EBMT). Leukemia 2005;19:2304–2312.
61. Estey E, de Lima M, Tibes R, et al. Prospective feasibility analysis of reduced-intensity conditioning (RIC) regimens for hematopoietic stem cell transplantation (HSCT) in elderly patients with acute myeloid leukemia (AML) and high-risk myelodysplastic syndrome (MDS). Blood 2007;109:1395–1400.
62. Bertz H, Potthoff K, Finke J. Allogeneic stem-cell transplantation from related and unrelated donors in older patients with myeloid leukemia. J Clin Oncol 2003;21:1480–1484.
63. Breems DA, Lowenberg B. Autologous stem cell transplantation in the treatment of adults with acute myeloid leukemia. Br J Haematol 2005;130:825–833.
64. Stem Cell Trialists' Collaborative Group. Allogeneic peripheral blood stem-cell compared with bone marrow transplantation in the management of hematologic malignancies: An individual patient data meta-analysis of nine randomized trials. J Clin Oncol 2005;23:5074–5087.
65. Gregory J, Arcecci R. Acute myeloid leukemia in children: A review of risk factors and recent trials. Cancer Invest 2002;20:1027–1037.
66. Woods WG. Curing childhood acute myeloid leukemia at the half-way point: Promises to keep and miles to go before we sleep. Pediatr Blood Cancer 2006;46:565–569.
67. Oliansky DM, Rizzo JD, Aplan PD, et al. The role of cytotoxic therapy with hematopoietic stem cell transplantation in the therapy of acute myeloid leukemia in children: An evidence-based review. Biol Blood Marrow Transplant 2007;13:1–25.
68. Woods WG, Neudorf S, Gold S, et al. A comparison of allogeneic bone marrow transplantation, autologous bone marrow transplantation, and aggressive chemotherapy in children with acute myeloid leukemia in remission. Blood 2001;97:56–62.
69. Löwenberg B, Zittoun R, Kerkhofs H, et al. On the value of intensive remission-induction chemotherapy in elderly patients of 65+ years with acute myeloid leukemia: A randomized phase III study of the European Organization for Research and Treatment of Cancer Leukemia Group. J Clin Oncol 1989;7:1268–1274.
70. Burnett A, Milligan D, Prentice A, et al. , on behalf of the National Cancer Research Institute Haematological Oncology Study Group Acute Leukemia Working Party. A comparison of low-dose cytarabine and hydroxyurea with or without all-trans-retinoic acid for acute myeloid leukemia and high-risk myelodysplastic syndrome in patients not considered fit for intensive treatment. Cancer 2007;109:1114–1124.
71. AML Collaborative Group. A systematic collaborative review of randomized trials comparing idarubicin with daunorubicin (or other

anthracyclines) as induction therapy for acute myeloid leukemia. Br J Haematol 1998;103:100–109.
72. Anderson JE, Kopecky KJ, Willman CL, et al. Outcome after induction chemotherapy for older patients with acute myeloid leukemia is not improved with mitoxantrone and etoposide compared to cytarabine and daunorubicin: A Southwest Oncology Group study. Blood 2002;100:3869–3876.
73. Rowe JM, Andersen JW, Mazza JJ, et al. Randomized placebo-controlled phase III study of granulocyte-macrophage colony stimulating factor in adult patients (>55–70 years) with acute myelogenous leukemia: A study of the Eastern Cooperative Oncology Group (E1490). Blood 1995;86:457–462.
74. Bishop JF, Lowenthal RM, Joshua D, et al. Etoposide in acute nonlymphocytic leukemia. Australian Leukemia Study Group. Blood 1990;75:27–32.
75. Anderson JE, Kopecky KJ, Willman CL, et al. Outcome after induction chemotherapy for older patients with acute myeloid leukemia is not improved with mitoxantrone and etoposide compared to cytarabine and daunorubicin: A Southwest Oncology Group study. Blood 2002;100:3869–3876.
76. Gardin C, Turlure P, Fagot T, et al. Postremission treatment of elderly patients with acute myeloid leukemia in first complete remission after intensive induction chemotherapy: Results of the multicenter randomized Acute Leukemia French Association (ALFA) 9803 trial. Blood 2007;109:5129–5135.
77. Buchner T, Berdel WE, Schoch C, et al. Double induction containing either one course of high-dose cytarabine plus mitoxantrone and postremission therapy by either autologous stem cell transplantation or by prolonged maintenance for acute myeloid leukemia. J Clin Oncol 2006;24:2480–2489.
78. Brune M, Castaigne S, Catalano J, et al. Improved leukemia-free survival after postconsolidation immunotherapy with histamine dihydrochloride and interleukemi-2 in acute myeloid leukemia: Results of a randomized phase 3 trial. Blood 2006;108 :88–96.
79. Lancet JE, Gojo I, Grotlib J, et al. A phase 2 study of the farnesyltransferase inhibitor tipifarnib in poor-risk and elderly patients with previously untreated acute myelogenous leukemia. Blood 2007;109:1387–1394.
80. Giles F, Rizzieri D, Karp J, et al. Cloretazine (VNP40101M), a novel sulfonylhydrazine alkylating agent, in patients age 60 years or older with previously untreated acute myeloid leukemia. J Clin Oncol 2007;25:25–31.
81. Gale RP, Horowitz MM, Rees JKH, et al. Chemotherapy versus transplants for acute myelogenous leukemia in second remission. Leukemia 1996;10:13–19.
82. Michallet M, Thomas X, Vernant JP, et al. Long-term outcome after allogeneic hematopoietic stem cell transplantation for advanced stage acute myeloblastic leukemia: A retrospective study of 379 patients reported to the Societe Francaise de Greffe de Moelle (SFGM). Bone Marrow Transplant 2000;26:1157–1163.
83. Greenberg PL, Lee SJ, Advani R, et al. Mitoxantrone, etoposide, and cytarabine with or without valspodar in patients with relapsed or refractory acute myeloid leukemia and high-risk myelodysplastic syndrome: A phase III trial (E2995). [Erratum in: J Clin Oncol 2004;22:2747.] J Clin Oncol 2004;22:1078–1086.
84. Baer MR, George SL, Dodge RK. Phase 3 study of the multidrug resistance modulator PSC-833 in previously untreated patients 60 years of age and older with acute myeloid leukemia: Cancer and Leukemia Group B Study 9720. Blood 2002;100:1224–1232.
85. Cripe LD, Li X, Litzow M, et al. A randomized placebo-controlled, double-blind trial of the MDR modulator, Zosuquidar, during conventional induction and post-remission therapy for patients >60 years of age with newly diagnosed acute myeloid leukemia (AML) or high-risk myelodysplastic syndrome (MR-MDS): ECOG 3999 [abstract]. Blood 2006;108:423.
86. Larson RA, Sievers EL, Stadtmauer EA, et al. Final report of the efficacy and safety of gemtuzumab ozogamicin (Mylotarg) in patients with CD33-positive acute myeloid leukemia in first recurrence. Cancer 2005;104:1442–1452.
87. Burnett AL, Kell WJ, Goldstone AH, et al. The addition of gemtuzumab ozogamicin to induction chemotherapy for AML improves disease free survival without extra toxicity: Preliminary analysis of 1115 patients in the MRC AML15 trial [abstract]. Blood 2006;108:13.
88. Tallman MS. New agents for the treatment of acute myeloid leukemia. Best Pract Res Clin Haematol 2006;19:311–320.
89. Heidel F, Cortes J, Rucker FG, et al. Results of a multicenter phase II trial for older patients with c-kit positive acute myeloid leukemia (AML) and high-risk myelodysplastic syndrome (HR-MDS) using low-dose Ara-C and imatinib. Cancer 2007;109:907–914.
90. Stahnke K, Boos J, Bender-Gotze C, et al. Duration of first remission predicts remission rates and long-term survival in children with relapsed acute myelogenous leukemia. Leukemia 1998;12:1534–1538.
91. Wells RJ, Adams MT, Alonzo TA, et al. Mitoxantrone and cytarabine induction, high-dose cytarabine, and etoposide intensification for pediatric patients with relapsed or refractory acute myeloid leukemia: Children's Cancer Group Study 2951. J Clin Oncol 2003;21:2940–2947.
92. Leung W, Hudson MM, Strickland DK, et al. Late effects of treatment in survivors of childhood acute myeloid leukemia. J Clin Oncol 2000;18:3273–3279.
93. Sanz MA. Treatment of acute promyelocytic leukemia. Hematology Am Soc Hematol Educ Program 2006:147–155.
94. Estey E, Garcia-Manero G, Ferrajoli A, et al. Use of all-trans retinoic acid plus arsenic trioxide as an alternative to chemotherapy in untreated acute promyelocytic leukemia. Blood 2006;107:3469–3473.
95. Shen ZX, Shi ZZ, Fang J, et al. All-trans retinoic acid/As_2O_3 combination yields a high quality remission and survival in newly diagnosed acute promyelocytic leukemia. Proc Natl Acad Sci U S A 2004;101:5328–5335.
96. Ghavamzadeh A, Alimoghaddam K, Ghaffari SH, et al. Treatment of acute promyelocytic leukemia with arsenic trioxide without ATRA and/or chemotherapy. Ann Oncol 2006;17:131–134.
97. Powell BL, Moser B, Stock W, et al. Effect of consolidation with arsenic trioxide on event-free survival and overall survival among patients with newly diagnosed acute promyelocytic leukemia: North American Intergroup Protocol C9710 [abstract]. J Clin Oncol 2007 ASCO Annual Meeting Proceedings (Part 1);25:2.
98. Nabhan C, Mehta J, Tallman M. The role of bone marrow transplantation in acute promyelocytic leukemia. Bone Marrow Transplant 2001;28:219–226.
99. Soignet S, Maslak P, Wang Z, et al. Complete remission after treatment of acute promyelocytic leukemia with arsenic trioxide. N Engl J Med 1998;339:1341–1348.
100. Soignet S, Frankel S, Douer D, et al. United States multicenter study of arsenic trioxide in relapsed acute promyelocytic leukemia. J Clin Oncol 2001;19:3852–3860.
101. Lowenberg B, van Putten W, Theobald M, et al. Effect of priming with granulocyte colony-stimulating factor on the outcome of chemotherapy for acute myeloid leukemia. N Engl J Med 2003;349:743–752.
102. Thomas X, Raffoux E, de Botton S, et al. Effect of priming with granulocyte-macrophage colony-stimulating factor in younger adults with newly diagnosed acute myeloid leukemia: A trial by the Acute Leukemia French Association (ALFA) Group. Leukemia 2007;21:453–461.
103. Schlenk RF, Dohner K, Groner S, et al. Impact of Pegfilgrastim on Hematological Reconstitution and Incidence of Neutropenic Fever after Consolidation Therapy with High-Dose Cytarabine in Acute Myeloid Leukemia: Comparative Analysis between AMLSG 07–04 and the German AML Intergroup Trial [abstract]. Blood 2006;108:2020.
104. Thomas X, Chelghoum Y, Thiebaut A, et al. Intensive timed sequential chemotherapy followed by a single pegfilgrastim (Neulasta) administration in patients with high-risk acute myeloid leukemia (AML): Preliminary results of the EMA-2000/Neu Trial [abstract]. Blood 2006;108:4558.
105. Hughes WT, Armstrong D, Bodey GP, et al. 2002 guidelines for the use of antimicrobial agents in neutropenic patients with cancer. Clin Infect Dis 2002;34:730–751.
106. Langmuir PB, Aplenc R, Lange BJ. Acute myeloid leukaemia in children. Best Pract Res Clin Haematol 2001;14:77–93.
107. Pui CH, Jeha S, Irwin D, Camitta B, et al. Recombinant urate oxidase (rasburicase) in the prevention and treatment of malignancy-associated hyperuricemia in pediatric and adult patients: Results of a compassionate-use trial. Leukemia 2001;15:1505–1509.
108. Pui CH, Mahmoud HH, Wiley JM, et al. Recombinant urate oxidase for the prophylaxis or treatment of hyperuricemia in patients with leukemia or lymphoma. J Clin Oncol 2001;19:697–704.
109. Bosly A, Sonet A, Pinkerton CR, et al. Rasburicase (recombinant urate oxidase) for the management of hyperuricemia in patients with cancer: Report of an international compassionate use study. Cancer 2003;98:1048–1054.
110. Trifilio S, Gordon L, Singhal S, et al. Reduced-dose rasburicase (recombinant xanthine oxidase) in adult cancer patients with hyperuricemia. Bone Marrow Transplant 2006;37:997–1001.

CHAPTER 138 Chronic Leukemias

AMY M. PICK, MARCEL DEVETTEN, AND TIMOTHY R. MCGUIRE

KEY CONCEPTS

1. Chronic myelogenous leukemia (CML) is characterized by the presence of the Philadelphia chromosome (Ph), a translocation between chromosomes 9 and 22. The resulting abnormal fusion protein, p210 *BCR-ABL*, phosphorylates tyrosine kinase residues and is constitutively active, resulting in uncontrolled cell proliferation.
2. Three phases of CML have been identified: chronic phase, accelerated phase, and blast crisis. At the time of diagnosis, most patients have chronic phase CML.
3. Imatinib is a tyrosine kinase inhibitor and is the most commonly used therapy in the treatment of chronic phase CML. Most patients on imatinib achieve a complete cytogenetic response within 9 to 12 months of initiation.
4. Interferon alfa (IFN-α) plays a minor role in the current treatment of CML and is reserved for patients who fail tyrosine kinase inhibitors and are ineligible for transplant.
5. Allogeneic hematopoietic stem cell transplantation is the only curative treatment for CML and is most often used when patients have suboptimal responses to imatinib therapy.
6. The management of CLL is highly variable and includes observation in asymptomatic older patients, the use of well-tolerated single agent chemotherapy in symptomatic older patients, and more aggressive therapy in younger patients.
7. Alemtuzumab may be used in patients who fail fludarabine and alkylator-based therapy. Its role in combination therapy is currently under investigation.
8. The combination of fludarabine, cyclophosphamide, and rituximab in CLL achieves higher response rates than single-agent chemotherapy.
9. Allogeneic hematopoietic stem cell transplantation in patients with CLL appears to achieve long-term disease-free survival in some patients, but late relapses occur and its role remains controversial.

Chronic leukemia includes chronic myelogenous leukemia (CML), chronic lymphocytic leukemia (CLL), hairy cell leukemia, and prolymphocytic leukemia. Chronic leukemia differs from acute leukemia in that its clinical course is indolent. Most patients with chronic leukemia survive for several years after their initial diagnosis, even without treatment. Conversely, most patients with acute leukemia die of their disease within weeks to months if not treated. This chapter focuses on the two most common types of chronic leukemia, CML and CLL.

Learning objectives, review questions, and other resources can be found at **www.pharmacotherapyonline.com.**

CHRONIC MYELOGENOUS LEUKEMIA

CML is a myeloproliferative disease that results from a malignant transformation of an early hematopoietic progenitor cell. This leads to abnormal proliferation and accumulation of progenitor and mature myeloid cells in the bone marrow and peripheral blood.[1] The clinical course of CML has three phases: chronic phase, accelerated phase, and blast crisis. The disease begins in the chronic phase in which signs and symptoms can be controlled with chemotherapy. CML then progresses to a transition phase, known as accelerated phase, in which blast counts in the bone marrow and peripheral blood increase despite ongoing therapy. Finally, there is blast crisis, a terminal phase that is similar to acute leukemia that can lead to rapid clinical deterioration and death.

EPIDEMIOLOGY AND ETIOLOGY

It is estimated that 4,570 new cases of CML will be diagnosed in the United States in 2007, representing 15% of all leukemias.[2] CML patients have a median age at diagnosis of 67 years.[3] This age, collected from the Surveillance, Epidemiology, and End Results database, is higher than the median age of 45 to 55 years reported from most institutional studies.[1]

For most newly diagnosed cases of CML, the etiology is unclear. Ionizing radiation and heavy occupational exposure to benzene are known risk factors. The increased risk of CML from radiation exposure was evident in atomic bomb survivors and in patients who received radiation therapy for ankylosing spondylitis.[1] CML is not associated with any known oncogenic viruses.

PATHOPHYSIOLOGY

CML was first described in 1845, but extensive research into the genetic and molecular characteristics of the disease began with the discovery of the Philadelphia chromosome (Ph) in 1960 by Nowell and Hungerford. Research in the 1980s identified the molecular changes that occur as a result of the Ph when an oncogenic protein was identified and implicated in the pathophysiology of CML.[4–6]

Ph is the first karyotypic abnormality specifically implicated in the pathogenesis of cancer, and its discovery has resulted in extensive research into the molecular biology of CML.[1] This chromosomal abnormality is characteristic of CML and is present in approximately 95% of patients with a presumptive diagnosis of the disease. It can also occur in

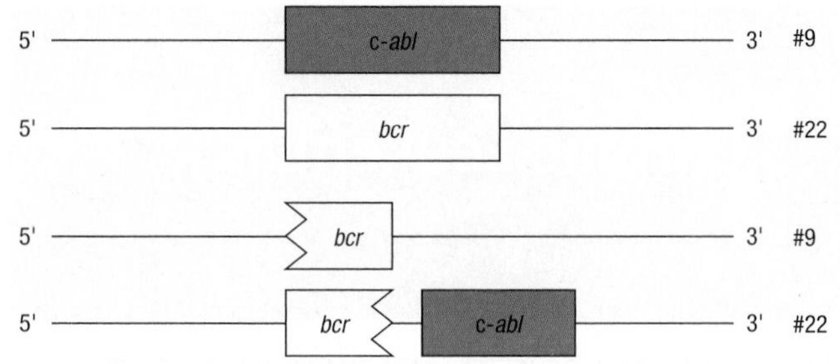

FIGURE 138-1. Diagram of the chromosomal translocation that results in the Philadelphia chromosome. (*Fishleder AK. Oncogenes and cancer: Clinical applications. Cleve Clin J Med 1990;57:721–726. Reprinted with permission. Copyright ©1990. Cleveland Clinic. All rights reserved.)*

as many as 20% of adults and 5% of children with acute lymphoblastic leukemia, and in rare cases of acute myelogenous leukemia.[1,7]

❶ Ph, identified as a shortened long arm of chromosome 22, is found in granulocyte and erythrocyte progenitors, macrophages, megakaryocytes, and, occasionally, lymphocytes.[1] The Ph is the consequence of breaks in chromosomes 9 and 22, resulting in a transposition that relocates the 3 end of *abl*, the Abelson protooncogene, from its normal site on chromosome 9 at band 34 to the 5 end of the breakpoint cluster region *(bcr)* on chromosome 22 at band 11.[1,7] This reciprocal translocation is symbolized as t(9;22)(q34;q11) and results in the formation of the hybrid *bcr-abl* fusion gene (Fig. 138–1). Through this chromosomal translocation, the *abl* protooncogene is able to escape the normal genetic controls on its expression and is activated into a functional oncogene, directing the transcription of an 8.5-kilobase messenger ribonucleic acid (mRNA) molecule. The translated 210-kilodalton protein, known as p210*BCR-ABL*, is unique and has higher tyrosine phosphokinase activity than the 145-kilodalton protein translated by the mRNA of the normal *abl* gene. The enzymatic activities of normal tyrosine kinases are under tight control and become activated only with physiologic activating signals. But p210*BCR-ABL* is constitutively (i.e., constantly) active, and this unregulated activity results in cell proliferation, inhibition of programmed cell death, and accumulation of the malignant clone.[4,6] Although p210*BCR-ABL* is the most common tyrosine kinase found in CML, variations in the breakpoints in the *abl* gene encode different size proteins. For example, a smaller protein, p190*BCR-ABL*, is involved in two-thirds of adults with Ph-positive acute lymphoblastic leukemia, although rarely found in CML patients.[1,7,8]

Because CML begins with the malignant transformation of a single cell, it is considered a clonal disease. This alteration gives the transformed progenitor cell an inheritable growth advantage, leading to the proliferation of a neoplastic, monoclonal population of pluripotent stem cells.[1,4] The Ph can be found in both myeloid and lymphoid cells, which suggests that the transformed cell of CML is a pluripotent stem cell. Granulocytosis, usually present in CML, results from the increased growth rate of the transformed clone and disruption of normal hematopoietic cell maturation. Disrupted maturation leads to additional divisions by CML progenitor cells before reaching a nonproliferative stage; the resulting number of circulating granulocytes may be many times higher than normal. Later in the clinical course of CML, cytopenias may occur in association with fibrotic changes in the bone marrow.[1,4]

The *bcr-abl* fusion gene encodes for a mutant tyrosine kinase that is involved in both the increased proliferation of the CML clone and the reduction in FAS-mediated apoptosis.[1,4] Characterization of the adenosine triphosphate binding site on the tyrosine kinase has led to the development of tyrosine kinase inhibitors. The first of these inhibitors, imatinib mesylate (Gleevec), was approved by the FDA in 2001 for patients in chronic phase who had failed interferon-α (IFN-α) or who were in accelerated phase or blast crisis. It received additional FDA approval in 2002 for first-line treatment in newly diagnosed CML. More potent inhibitors with a higher binding affinity and selectivity for *abl* kinase have been developed, including dasatinib (Sprycel) and nilotinib (Tasigna), and are likely to be used in imatinib-resistant CML.[9–12] The clinical results associated with the newer generation tyrosine kinase inhibitors are discussed in more detail in Treatment below.

CLINICAL PRESENTATION

CLINICAL PRESENTATION OF CML[1]

General

- 90% of patients are diagnosed in chronic phase
- 50% are asymptomatic in chronic phase and often diagnosed following abnormal complete blood count[1]

Signs and Symptoms

- Fatigue
- Left upper quadrant pain
- Abdominal pain or distension
- Weight loss
- Night sweats

Physical Examination

- Splenomegaly
- Hepatomegaly

Laboratory Tests

- Peripheral blood
  - Leukocytosis
  - Thrombocytosis
  - Basophilia
  - Low or undetectable leukocyte alkaline phosphatase
  - Elevated uric acid and lactate dehydrogenase
- Molecular testing
  - Presence of *bcr-abl* by reverse-transcription polymerase chain reaction
- Bone marrow
  - Hypercellular
  - Fully mature myeloid cells
  - Increased megakaryocytes
  - <10% blasts in chronic phase
- Cytogenetics
  - Presence of the Ph chromosome
  - Additional abnormalities

CLINICAL COURSE

❷ Three clinical phases of CML have been identified: chronic phase, accelerated phase, and blast crisis. Nearly all patients are in chronic phase at the time of diagnosis.[13] In chronic phase CML, nontransplant therapies suppress the CML clone and normalize the white blood cell (WBC) count. As the disease progresses, other mutations develop and treatment becomes less effective. Clinical evidence of disease progression, the accelerated phase of CML, begins to emerge as the patient's WBC count becomes increasingly difficult to control with therapy. Physical symptoms of acceleration include a resurgence of splenic enlargement, unexplained fever, and persistent bone pain. The rate of progression of CML is variable. In about one-third of patients, blast crisis occurs without

TABLE 138-1 Newly Proposed System for Defining Phase of Chronic Myelogenous Leukemia

Chronic Phase	Accelerated Phase	Blast Crisis
• <10% blasts in peripheral blood or bone marrow	• 10–29% blasts in peripheral blood or bone marrow • Platelets <100,000 cells/mm^3 or >1,000,000 cells/mm^3 Additional findings • Cytogenetic evolution • Progressive Splenomegaly	• >30% blasts in peripheral blood or bone marrow • Large clusters of blasts on bone marrow biopsy • Presence of extramedullary infiltrates Additional findings • Fever • Malaise • Splenomegaly

Data from Cortes JE, Talpaz M, O'Brien S, et al. Staging of chronic myeloid leukemia in the imatinib era. Cancer 2006;106:1306–1315.

an apparent accelerated phase.[14,15] Blast crisis is the final stage of CML and is marked by the presence of rapidly proliferating blast cells that have lost the ability to differentiate into mature cells.[1,16] The proliferative advantage of blast cells over normal hematopoietic cells is much greater than that of chronic phase leukemic cells. A poor response to treatment is seen, which is not exclusively a result of drug resistance but also from the high proliferative rate of the blastic clone.[17] The increased proliferative rate in blast crisis CML is the consequence of a number of factors in addition to *bcr-abl*, such as the activation of the RAC- and RAS-signaling pathways and loss of tumor suppressors such as p53.[1,14] In blast crisis, about two-thirds of patients experience myeloid leukemia and the other third transform to a lymphoid leukemia.

Although the three phases of CML are well recognized, the criteria used to define them varies greatly. Clinical trials of imatinib have used different classification criteria for the various phases, with all staging criteria developed prior to the development of imatinib. In 2001, the World Health Organization proposed a new classification system that included new criteria for accelerated phase and blast crisis.[18] In a comparison of the World Health Organization criteria with that used in imatinib trials, approximately 10% of patients had to be reclassified to a different phase.[19] Based on that analysis, a new classification system was proposed to distinguish the phases of CML (Table 138–1).

PROGNOSIS

The overall survival of the patient depends on the phase of CML at the time of diagnosis. Most patients with CML are diagnosed in chronic phase and can be maintained on imatinib for many years. The duration of accelerated phase is shorter than chronic phase and typically lasts a few months before progression to blast crisis. The median survival for patients in blast crisis is 7 to 10 months, with most treatment options providing modest or no survival advantage.[4,20]

There are currently no biomarkers available to predict disease progression for CML. Important poor prognostic factors include older age, splenomegaly, high platelet count, and a high percentage of circulating blasts at diagnosis. These features have been used to categorize patients into three risk groups: low, intermediate, and high. This scoring system, known as the Sokal score, was developed in the 1970s and is able to predict disease progression based on specified risk factors.[1] Although the scoring system was developed prior to the use of imatinib, the Sokal score predicted the likelihood of success with imatinib (Treatment).

TREATMENT

Chronic Myelogenous Leukemia

The ultimate goal in the treatment of CML is eradication of the Ph clone. Most, if not all, patients will initially be placed on imatinib therapy following a diagnosis of CML. More than 85% of patients will achieve a complete cytogenetic response on imatinib and will remain on imatinib until disease progression.[13,21,22] A small percentage of patients will choose allogeneic hematopoietic stem cell transplantation (HSCT), which is the only treatment shown to permanently eliminate the Ph-positive malignant clone. Table 138–2 shows the effect of various treatment modalities on survival in chronic-phase CML.

Three types of treatment responses have been described: hematologic, cytogenetic, and molecular (see Fig. 138–2). *Hematologic* response is defined as the normalization of peripheral blood counts and is the earliest type of response. *Cytogenetic* responses are based on the percentage of cells positive for Ph in the bone marrow, with *complete* cytogenetic remission defined as the elimination of Ph and *major* cytogenetic response defined as fewer than 35% Ph-positive cells. Patients who have a major or complete cytogenetic response have an improved survival compared to those who fail to achieve a cytogenetic response.[1,23]

Because most patients on imatinib achieve a complete cytogenetic response, more sensitive tests to monitor disease status are increasingly used. *Molecular* responses are determined by quantitative reverse-transcriptase polymerase chain reaction (RT-PCR), which is several logs more sensitive than methods used to measure cytogenetic remissions. A complete molecular response is the absence of *bcr-abl* transcripts by RT-PCR. Caution must be used as RT-PCR assays have various sensitivities and may show a complete molecular remission even when low levels of *bcr-abl* transcripts are present.[23] Quantitative RT-PCR should be performed on every patient prior to initiating therapy and throughout therapy to monitor residual disease. Because there is good correlation between bone marrow and peripheral blood *bcr-abl* mRNA levels, peripheral blood can often be used for this analysis.[13,23,24] Figure 138–2 illustrates the residual disease that remains after various types of responses and the response rates obtained with the common therapies for CML.

■ CONVENTIONAL CHEMOTHERAPY

Conventional cytotoxic chemotherapy can be used in chronic-phase CML to reduce high circulating WBCs, but has only modest effects on median survival.[1] Historically, the two agents used to normalize WBCs are busulfan (Myleran) and hydroxyurea (Hydrea). Busulfan is rarely used because randomized trials show that hydroxyurea treatment provides a significant survival advantage over busulfan.[25]

Hydroxyurea rapidly lowers high circulating WBCs in chronic-phase CML. Hydroxyurea inhibits the enzyme ribonucleotide reduc-

TABLE 138-2 Effect of Therapy on Survival in Patients with Early Chronic-Phase Chronic Myelogenous Leukemia

Therapy	5-Year Survival (%)	Median Survival (Months)
Busulfan[25]	30–40	40–50
Hydroxyurea[25]	40–50	50–60
IFN-α[1]	50–70	60–80
IFN-α + ara-C[1]	60–80	NR
Allogeneic transplantation		
Matched sibling[1,55]	60–80	NR
Matched unrelated[1,7]	40–70	NR
Imatinib[21]	89	NR

NR, not yet reached.

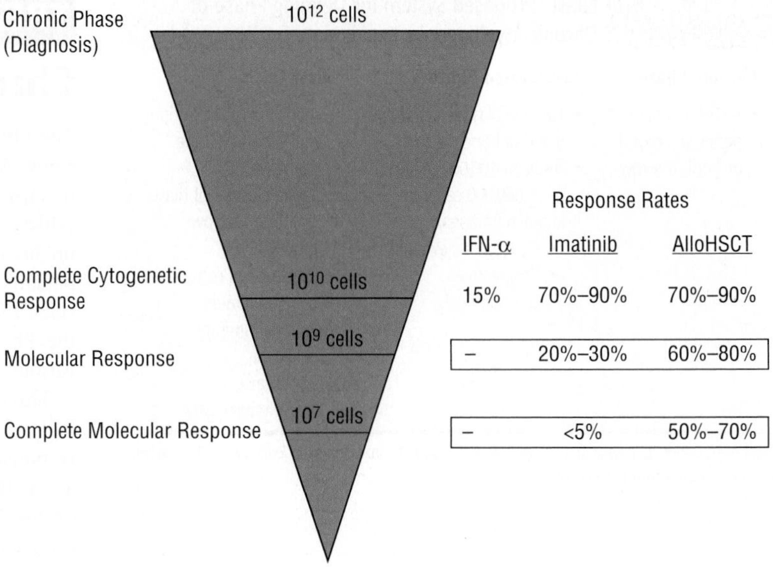

FIGURE 138-2. Type and frequency of response associated with common CML therapies. (AlloHSCT, allogeneic hematopoietic stem cell transplantation; IFN, interferon.) *(Adapted from Lowenberg B. Minimal residual disease in chronic myeloid leukemia. N Engl J Med 2003;349(15): 1399–1401. Copyright © 2003 Massachusetts Medical Society. All rights reserved.)*

tase, which inhibits DNA synthesis, eliminates cells in the S phase of the cell cycle, and synchronizes cells in the G_1 or pre-DNA synthesis phase.[1] The drug is usually administered daily and can be initiated at 40 to 50 mg/kg/day in divided doses until the WBC count falls below 10,000 cells/mm^3. At this point, the dose can be decreased to a maintenance level of 20 mg/kg/day but is usually discontinued as imatinib alone can maintain WBC count. Imatinib is often the sole agent used if rapid reduction in WBCs is not required. Unlike hydroxyurea, imatinib suppresses the malignant clone in the bone marrow and has a direct impact on long-term disease-free survival.[25–27]

■ IMATINIB MESYLATE (GLEEVEC)

The development of imatinib has revolutionized the treatment of CML. The pivotal discovery in imatinib's development was the characterization of the adenosine triphosphate binding site on the *bcr-abl* tyrosine kinase. From the numerous tyrosine kinase inhibitors developed in the 1990s, STI571 (STI stands for signal transduction inhibitor), better known as imatinib, emerged as the drug with the best oral bioavailability and selectivity for the *bcr-abl* tyrosine kinase.[28,29] In 2001, imatinib mesylate (Gleevec) received FDA approval for patients in chronic phase who had failed IFN-α and in accelerated phase or blast crisis. In 2002, it received FDA approval for first-line treatment in newly diagnosed CML.

Imatinib inhibits several tyrosine kinases including *bcr-abl*, KIT, and platelet-derived growth factor receptor. It is the inhibition of the *bcr-abl* tyrosine kinase that leads to differentiation and apoptosis of the CML clone. Imatinib competitively binds to the adenosine triphosphate-binding site on *bcr-abl*, which inhibits the phosphorylation of proteins involved with CML clone proliferation.[27,30] Table 138–3 summarizes the clinical results of imatinib in CML patients in chronic phase, accelerated phase, and blast crisis. Early phase I and phase II studies of imatinib, designed to determine maximum tolerated dose and safety, showed higher-than-expected response rates in all CML patient populations.[27,31] The impressive activity in these early trials led to FDA approval of imatinib, prior to the completion of a large phase III trial, for patients with previously treated CML. Subsequent trials examined imatinib in newly diagnosed CML patients. Today, imatinib is the treatment of choice for nearly all patients with chronic-phase CML.[10,12,22,32]

Chronic Phase

A large phase III randomized trial, known as the International Randomized Study of Interferon vs. STI571 (IRIS) study compared 400 mg imatinib to IFN-α plus low-dose subcutaneous cytarabine. After a median followup of 19 months, patients who received imatinib had a significantly higher rate of complete hematologic remissions, as well as of complete and major cytogenetic remissions. Additionally, a significantly lower percentage of patients had progressed to blast crisis or were intolerant to therapy.[33] The study was designed so that patients could crossover to the other arm for lack of activity or intolerance. After 60 months of followup, only 3% of patients who were originally randomized to receive IFN-α remained on their initial regimen.[21] Because of this nearly complete crossover to the imatinib arm, it is not possible to determine the relative survival benefit of imatinib when compared to IFN-α.

The 5-year followup data from the IRIS trial was recently published.[21] The estimated 5-year overall survival of the 553 patients who were originally randomized to receive imatinib was 89%. Eighty-seven percent of patients achieved a complete cytogenetic response while on imatinib. There were differences in the rate of complete cytogenetic responses among risk groups when the Sokal scoring system was used. The complete cytogenetic response rates were 89%, 82%, and 69% in low-risk, intermediate-risk, and high-risk patients, respectively, The risk of disease progression while on imatinib has remained fairly constant and quite low, ranging between 1.5% and 2.8% during the first 3 years to less than 1% in years 4 and 5. The risk of disease progression was associated with the Sokal score; the rates of progression were 3%, 8%, and 17% in low-risk, intermediate-risk, and high-risk patients, respectively. However, the Sokal score was not associated with disease progression in patients who had a complete cytogenetic response. Indicators for disease progression include a lack of a major cytogenetic response at 12 months and lack of complete cytogenetic response at 18 months.[21]

TABLE 138-3 Cytogenetic Response Associated with Imatinib in Chronic Myelogenous Leukemia

Disease Status	Daily Dose	MCR	CCR	Median Followup
CML-CP				
Newly Diagnosed[21]	400 mg	92%	87%	60 months
	800 mg	96%	90%	30 months
CML-AP[38]	600 mg	49%	43%	12 months
	400 mg	16%	11%	
CML-BC[20,39]	400–800 mg	16%	7.4%	–

CCR, complete cytogenetic response; CML, chronic myelogenous leukemia; CML-AP, accelerated phase; CML-BC, blast crisis; CML-CP, chronic phase; MCR, major cytogenetic response.

❸ Imatinib effectively reduces WBC count in chronic-phase CML. Declines in the WBC count are usually observed after 1 to 2 weeks and complete hematologic responses are achieved in the first 6 weeks. More time is required to achieve a cytogenetic response, with many patients requiring 9 to 12 months to obtain a complete cytogenetic response.[13,22] Although most patients on imatinib achieve a complete cytogenetic response, very few patients achieve a complete molecular remission. In a study by Hughes et al., less than 5% of patients on imatinib have undetectable levels of *bcr-abl* when analyzed by RT-PCR.[34] Recent studies suggest that the level of residual disease is predictive of progression-free survival. A decline in *bcr-abl* mRNA by 2 logs within 3 months after achieving a complete cytogenetic response is reported to be a predictor of longer progression-free survival.[35] Consequently, careful monitoring of *bcr-abl* levels by RT-PCR is required to help clinicians determine modifications in therapy. The 2008 National Comprehensive Cancer Network (NCCN) guidelines suggest that *bcr-abl* levels should be measured at baseline and then every 3 months to assess response.[22] If patients fail to achieve a decline in *bcr-abl* transcripts, other interventions should be considered, such as increasing the imatinib dose, dasatinib, nilotinib, or clinical trial. The lack of a complete and permanent molecular remission is the primary reason why imatinib is not considered a cure in CML.

The imatinib dose depends on the phase of CML. The NCCN guidelines and the European Leukemia Network recommend imatinib as the preferred treatment for most patients in chronic phase.[22,32] Most, if not all, newly diagnosed patients in chronic phase will be started on imatinib 400 mg daily and nearly 90% of these patients will achieve a complete cytogenetic response (see Table 138–3). Because most patients fail to achieve a complete molecular response with 400 mg daily, studies are evaluating the role of higher doses of imatinib. Historical data suggests that higher cytogenetic responses can be seen with 800 mg daily versus 400 mg daily in newly diagnosed chronic-phase CML.[36] This dosing issue remains unsettled. The 2008 NCCN guidelines suggests that newly diagnosed patients with poor prognostic factors or high-risk Sokal scores may consider starting on higher doses of imatinib.[22] The European Leukemia Network does not recommend starting on higher doses of imatinib for any patient until prospective randomized studies confirm there is a response or survival benefit over imatinib 400 mg.[32]

Accelerated Phase/Blast Crisis

The response rate of imatinib is lower in accelerated phase or blast crisis as compared with chronic phase. In a phase II study, the complete hematologic and cytogenetic response rates for imatinib in accelerated phase were reported to be 82% and 43%, respectively, and patients treated with imatinib had a significantly improved survival when compared to historical controls.[37,38] In blast crisis, 24% of patients treated with imatinib have a hematologic response and 16% a major cytogenetic response.[39] Unlike the long duration of response seen with imatinib in chronic phase, the duration in accelerated phase and blast crisis is much shorter. In the studies mentioned above, the estimated median duration of response for patients receiving imatinib in accelerated phase was 13.4 months.[38] In blast crisis, the estimated median duration of response with imatinib was 10 months.[39] Although clinical responses are seen, many patients cannot tolerate the side effects of higher doses of imatinib required for response in patients not in chronic phase.[26,40] Several ongoing clinical trials are investigating the use of imatinib in combination with other therapies.[32,40]

The maximum dose tolerated of imatinib in phase I trials was 1,000 mg, but doses as high as 1,200 mg are being evaluated in resistant patients.[26,40] Studies have examined these higher doses in this population. Higher response rates have been reported with 600 mg of imatinib compared to 400 mg in advanced disease.[27,37] Because of the lack of prospective data, the dosing for advanced phases is not specifically addressed by the NCCN guidelines or the European Leukemia Network.[22,32] Typically, higher doses of 600 to 800 mg daily are used in patients with accelerated phase or blast crisis CML.[11,13,20,22,37]

Imatinib Resistance

Some patients will experience disease progression despite imatinib therapy. Imatinib resistance is categorized based on the time to onset of nonresponsive disease. Intrinsic or primary resistance occurs when patients fail to achieve a hematologic response to therapeutic doses of imatinib (lack of efficacy). Acquired or secondary resistance occurs when there is a loss of efficacy over time.[17,40] Mutations in *bcr-abl* are the most common mechanism of resistance, occurring in 42% to 90% of cases and are typically found in advanced disease.[32,40] The most common mutations are *bcr-abl* domain point mutations that impair imatinib binding. It is estimated that 89% of patients with *bcr-abl* mutations will relapse in chronic phase.[40,41] Approximately 10% of imatinib resistance is associated with overproduction of *bcr-abl*.[1] The overproduction of *bcr-abl* is caused by genomic amplification of additional *bcr-abl* transcripts.[42] In the case of *bcr-abl* over-expression, dose escalation may be the best approach. Higher doses of imatinib may be the optimal approach for avoiding imatinib resistance.[40,41] Therefore, clinical trials are evaluating the role of imatinib 800 mg in unresponsive or advanced disease CML.[1,17] The use of more potent *bcr-abl* tyrosine kinase inhibitors such as dasatinib or nilotinib may effectively overcome imatinib resistance.[11,40]

Imatinib Monitoring

Imatinib therapy should be frequently monitored to assess response or disease progression. Recommendations for monitoring include baseline molecular and cytogenetic assessment. A complete hematologic response is expected within 3 months of starting imatinib in chronic phase patients. If patients appear to be responding to treatment, then *bcr-abl* transcripts should be evaluated by RT-PCR every 3 months and bone marrow cytogenetics performed every 6 to 12 months.[16,22–24] Most patients will achieve a cytogenetic response and will remain on imatinib therapy. Treatment options for patients who have disease progression include imatinib dose escalation, dasatinib, nilotinib, allogeneic HSCT, and a clinical trial.[22,32]

Side Effects and Drug Interactions

Imatinib is associated with hematologic and nonhematologic side effects. Myelosuppression is one of the most common side effects. Moderate-to-severe (grade 3 or 4) myelosuppression occurs in approximately 5% to 10% of patients with chronic-phase CML and in 50% to 60% of patients in accelerated phase or blast crisis.[1,14,27] The myelosuppression usually occurs during the first 2 to 4 weeks of therapy and is more common in patients with advanced disease (i.e., high blastic involvement of the bone marrow) and those with low hemoglobins.[43] Because hematopoiesis in patients with CML depends on the Ph-positive progenitors, some degree of myelosuppression should be expected when the clone is suppressed. However, a recent study reported that imatinib also suppresses normal hematopoiesis, which suggests that myelosuppression associated with imatinib is probably related to effects on the Ph clone and normal progenitors.[26,44] During imatinib therapy, patients should have blood work drawn every 1 to 2 weeks to monitor for severe myelosuppression. Appropriate initial management of myelosuppression is to interrupt imatinib treatment, not dose reduce, as dose reductions below 300 mg daily do not fully inhibit *bcr-abl* and may lead to the emergence of imatinib resistance.[1,14,22,27]

Imatinib is also associated with nonhematologic toxicities.[10,22,26,27] Dose-related nausea and vomiting is the most common side effect and can be managed by taking the drug with a meal. Higher doses of imatinib should be split in half and taken twice daily to reduce GI side effects. Diarrhea is another common side effect that is dose-related and can be controlled with antidiarrheal medications. Dose-related edema and fluid retention often manifests as periorbital edema. Rarely, fluid retention can be severe, leading to pulmonary and cerebral edema. Risk factors for edema include female gender, age older than 65 years and a history of heart and kidney disease. Approximately 20% to 40% of patients complain of musculoskeletal symptoms, which tend to occur during the first month of therapy and decline in severity over time. Calcium and magnesium supplements may provide symptomatic relief. Drug rash can frequently occur but is usually mild and can be managed with antihistamines or topical steroids. Severe rash, while uncommon, has been reported as an important cause for discontinuation of therapy. Hepatotoxicity can occur with imatinib, and the drug should be withheld if liver function tests exceed five times normal. After the tests normalize, imatinib can be restarted at a reduced dose of not less than 300 mg per day. The drug is then escalated upward to the prior dose if the liver function tests do not rise during 6 to 12 weeks of treatment at the reduced dose.[26] One death as a consequence of liver failure has been reported in a patient receiving large doses of acetaminophen and imatinib. It is recommended that patients on imatinib limit their use of acetaminophen to 1,300 mg daily.[22] Clinicians should evaluate the patient's medication history for all drugs that may contribute to hepatotoxicity.

Imatinib is metabolized by CYP3A4 and inducers of this enzyme may decrease imatinib concentrations. For example, a patient in the original phase I trial of imatinib who was also on phenytoin had a suboptimal response and was found to have a 75% reduction in plasma imatinib concentrations as compared to patients not on phenytoin. The clinical significance of this interaction was confirmed by rapid disease response when phenytoin therapy was withdrawn.[31] Imatinib may increase the concentrations of other drugs metabolized by CYP3A4. For example, imatinib has been reported to increase blood levels of cyclosporine and simvastatin. Other agents that should be closely monitored include aprepitant, dexamethasone, St. John's wort, and warfarin.[22]

OTHER TYROSINE KINASE INHIBITORS

Dasatinib (Sprycel) and nilotinib (Tasigna) are two recently approved tyrosine kinase inhibitors used to overcome resistance in CML. Dasatinib is an oral *bcr-abl* tyrosine kinase inhibitor that was FDA approved in 2006 for the treatment of imatinib-resistant CML. Dasatinib is an oral tyrosine kinase inhibitor of five critical oncogenic enzymes, including *bcr-abl*. Unlike imatinib, dasatinib binds to both the active and inactive forms of *bcr-abl* kinase and can overcome most *bcr-abl* mutations responsible for imatinib resistance. Preclinical data show that dasatinib is 300 times more potent than imatinib and has been active in all imatinib-resistant clones studied to date except for the T315I mutant.[11,41] The drug received accelerated approval based on hematologic and cytogenetic responses seen in imatinib-resistant or imatinib-intolerant patients.[45] In a phase II study of 186 patients with imatinib-resistant or -intolerant chronic phase CML, 90% and 52% of patients achieved a complete hematologic response and major cytogenetic response, respectively.[46] Responses were also observed in patients with more advanced disease.[45] In another phase II trial, patients with imatinib-resistant chronic phase CML were randomized to receive either dasatinib or high-dose (800 mg) imatinib.[47] Dasatinib-treated patients had a significantly higher major and complete cytogenetic response rate than those treated with high-dose imatinib (52% vs. 33%). The complete cytogenetic response rate was also significantly higher with dasatinib (40% vs. 16%). The dose used in those trials was 70 mg twice daily. A phase III dose-optimization study showed that dasatinib 100 mg once daily was equivalent to dasatinib 70 mg twice daily in patients with chronic-phase CML.[45] Patients with more advanced disease should be treated with dasatinib at a dose of 70 mg twice daily.

Nilotinib is an oral tyrosine kinase inhibitor of the inactive form of *bcr-abl* that was FDA approved in 2007 for the treatment of imatinib-resistant CML. Nilotinib is 10 to 30 times more potent in inhibiting *bcr-abl* than imatinib as a result of a modification of the methylpiperazinyl group of imatinib.[11,41] In clinical trials, nilotinib inhibited 32 of the 33 imatinib-resistant *bcr-abl* mutations. Like imatinib and dasatinib, nilotinib does not inhibit the kinase activity of the T315I *bcr-abl* mutation. The drug received accelerated approval based on hematologic and cytogenetic responses in imatinib-resistant and imatinib-intolerant patients.[48] In a phase II trial of 280 patients with imatinib-resistant or -intolerant chronic phase CML, 48% of patients achieved a major cytogenetic response.[49] Responses were also observed in patients with accelerated phase CML.[50] The nilotinib dose used in these trials was 400 mg twice daily; the drug should not be given with food. The dosing in clinical trials has been 400 to 600 mg twice daily for imatinib-resistant CML.

The side-effect profile of other tyrosine kinase inhibitors is similar to imatinib. Reversible myelosuppression is the most common side effect seen with dasatinib and nilotinib, and sometimes requires temporary interruption of therapy. Other side effects for dasatinib include nausea, vomiting, diarrhea, edema, and pleural effusions.[11,45-47] Edema or pleural effusions has not been reported in early clinical trials with nilotinib, but elevations in indirect bilirubin has been noted in 10% to 15% of patients.[11,48-50] Future studies and longer followup time will be needed to examine additional side effects of these two drugs.

Like imatinib, dasatinib and nilotinib are metabolized by CYP3A4. Clinicians need to be aware of possible drug interactions with inducers and inhibitors of the CYP3A4 pathway.[22] Dasatinib and nilotinib may prolong the QT interval. Until further data is available, patients should avoid concomitant therapy with other drugs that are known to prolong the QT interval, such as antiarrhythmics, macrolide antibiotics, and phenothiazines. In vitro data also suggest that long-term suppression of gastric acid decreases dasatinib absorption. Patients should refrain from taking concomitant H_2-blockers or proton pump inhibitors while on dasatinib until further studies can determine the clinical relevance.[45] The bioavailability of nilotinib is increased when given with a meal.[48]

The precise role of dasatinib and nilotinib in the treatment of CML needs to be fully elucidated. The 2008 NCCN guidelines recommend that dasatinib or nilotinib be considered when patients do not achieve a complete hematologic response in 3 months or no cytogenetic response in 6 months. If patients continue to have a partial response or have disease progression while on imatinib, then a change in therapy to dasatinib or nilotinib should be considered.[22]

The results from the early studies of dasatinib and nilotinib are quite promising for those who have imatinib-resistant CML. The development of the new generation tyrosine kinase inhibitors may further improve the prognosis of CML. Ongoing studies are investigating their use as frontline therapy and in combination with other therapies.

INTERFERON ALFA

Prior to the introduction of imatinib, IFN-α was the preferred agent in the treatment of CML. Today it is reserved for patients who fail tyrosine kinase inhibitor therapies and are not candidates for HSCT.

The interferons are a family of glycoproteins involved in many of the functional aspects of the hematopoietic system. Two recombinant forms of IFN-α are currently marketed: IFN-α_{2a} (Roferon

A) and IFN-α_{2b} (Intron A). In addition, two polyethylene glycol-conjugated products were developed in an attempt to improve the toxicity profile and decrease the frequency of injections of IFN-α (PEG-IFN-α_{2b} and PEG-IFN-α_{2a}). Although PEG-IFN-α_{2b} is not more effective and has a similar toxicity profile to the nonpegylated drug in CML patients,[51] PEG-IFN-α_{2b} can be administered weekly as compared with daily administration for the nonpegylated formulation.[52]

❹ The past enthusiasm for the use of IFN-α in the treatment of chronic-phase CML was based on reports that 20% to 50% of patients achieve a major cytogenetic response, which led to prolonged survival.[7] In the 10% to 15% of patients achieving a complete cytogenetic response, the median survival was more than 10 years.[22,32] The unimpressive results of IFN-α in the IRIS trial in comparison to imatinib has limited the agent's use in CML. Only 14% of patients treated with IFN-α achieved a complete cytogenetic response, as compared to 76% of patients treated with imatinib.[21] Although imatinib has generally replaced IFN-α as initial treatment of chronic-phase CML, some patients continue to receive IFN-α. These patients include those who had achieved a cytogenetic response to IFN-α and continue to receive the drug as maintenance therapy. With the introduction of new *bcr-abl* tyrosine kinase inhibitors to treat patients who fail imatinib, the usage of IFN-α will probably continue to decline.

IFN-α use is also limited by its toxicity profile.[53] IFN-α use is associated with both short-term constitutional toxicities and potentially dose-limiting long-term toxicities. In the IRIS trial, 26% of patients discontinued IFN-α as a result of intolerable side effects.[21] The most predictable early toxicity is a flu-like syndrome characterized by fever, chills, myalgia, headache, and anorexia. These dose-dependent effects may be a result of IFN-α–induced leukocytosis and release of inflammatory cytokines. This acute flu-like syndrome can be ameliorated by starting IFN-α dosing at 50% of the final dose during the first week, giving the drug at bedtime, and coadministering acetaminophen or indomethacin with each IFN-α dose.[53] Reduction of initial WBC counts to about 10,000 cells/mm^3 with hydroxyurea may also reduce these symptoms. Despite these methods of ameliorating toxicity, the flu-like syndrome is an important source of morbidity, occasionally requiring termination of therapy. Cardiovascular toxicities (tachycardia, hypotension) are seen in approximately 15% of patients in the first few weeks. Long-term adverse effects include weight loss, alopecia, neurologic effects (paresthesia, cognitive impairment, depression), and immune-mediated complications (hemolysis, thrombocytopenia, nephrotic syndrome, systemic lupus erythematosus, hypothyroidism), which can be dose limiting in approximately 5% to 20% of patients.[1,53]

The role of IFN-α in the treatment of CML is quite limited with the introduction of tyrosine kinase inhibitors. According to the 2008 NCCN guidelines and European Leukemia Network, patients who are unable to tolerate other therapies may consider IFN-α.[22,32] However, despite its limited use, IFN-α is a disease-modifying agent and ongoing clinical trials are investigating the use of imatinib and IFN-α in combination for the treatment of CML.[32,54]

■ HEMATOPOIETIC STEM CELL TRANSPLANTATION

❺ Allogeneic HSCT remains the only therapy proven to cure patients with CML, with many patients alive and disease-free decades after transplant. Patients undergoing allogeneic HSCT from a human leukocyte antigen (HLA)-matched sibling donor have 5-year survival rates ranging from 60% to 80% and long-term survival of approximately 50%.[1,32,55,56] In most long-term survivors, the *bcr-abl* translocation is absent in all diagnostic tests including RT-PCR. Prognostic risk factors associated with survival outcomes include age, phase of disease and disease duration. Increasing age is associated with poorer prognosis, with higher transplant-related mortality in patients older than age 50 years. Patients with early disease who receive transplantations have better outcomes than those in accelerated phase or blast crisis. The time from diagnosis to transplantation also affects outcomes. Patients who undergo matched-sibling allogeneic HSCT within the first year of diagnosis have a better 5-year survival rate than those who undergo transplantation more than 1 year after their diagnosis (70% to 80% vs. 50% to 60%).[1,32,55,56]

Unfortunately, fewer than 30% of patients eligible for allogeneic HSCT will have an HLA-matched sibling donor, and alternative donors must be considered. The most common alternative donor is an HLA-matched unrelated individual. Results from several studies show that using matched unrelated donors, 40% to 70% of patients are alive at 5 years posttransplant, which is only slightly lower than the results reported for matched-sibling transplantations.[7,55,56]

The remarkable activity of imatinib has resulted in fewer transplant for CML and has stimulated debate as to which, if any, subgroup should be treated with allogeneic HSCT as primary therapy. The difficulty is identifying those patients who will have suboptimal responses and might benefit from early transplantation. A recent study by the German CML Study Group reported that survival with drug therapy (IFN-α or imatinib) is superior to early allogeneic HSCT for low-risk patients, but no difference in survival was observed in high-risk patients.[57] The results from this study suggest allogeneic HSCT should be reserved for high-risk patients. The use of imatinib prior to transplantation is also controversial. Although imatinib is probably not curative for most patients, nearly all patients with newly diagnosed chronic-phase CML are started on imatinib therapy at the time of their diagnosis. Recent studies show that imatinib use prior to transplantation does not negatively affect survival.[58,59] These studies suggest that patients must be monitored carefully for early signs of imatinib nonresponse or relapse.

The European Leukemia Network expert recommendations lists allogeneic HSCT as one of two strategies (the other being imatinib) used in high-risk patients with low transplant-related mortality. It is also considered an option when patients fail imatinib or other therapies.[32] The 2008 NCCN guidelines no longer list allogeneic HSCT as a potential front-line option for patients.[22] All patients should be informed that imatinib probably is not curative and disease progression can occur at any time, sometimes without warning. Patients who should consider allogeneic HSCT are newly diagnosed CML patients who are young enough to tolerate the procedure and who have a HLA-matched related or unrelated donor; patients who do not achieve a hematologic remission within 3 months of therapy; patients who do not achieve a cytogenetic response after 6 to 12 months; and patients who are in accelerated phase or blast crisis CML. With the median age of onset for CML being in the sixth decade of life and the high risk of mortality in patients older than 50 years of age, more than half of CML patients will be excluded from allogeneic HSCT based on age alone. Even when all the criteria are met (matched donor and younger age), 100-day mortality after allogeneic HSCT is between 10% and 20% in established transplant centers. This risk of early mortality associated with allogeneic HSCT may be too high in the imatinib era where most patients have complete cytogenetic responses without significant toxicity. The clinical decision is further complicated by the observation that there is a recognized window when transplantation is optimally performed. Better outcomes are observed when a patient undergoes transplantation within the first 2 years of diagnosis.[22,32] Consequently, delaying transplantation might negatively impact survival outcomes. Ongoing studies need to investigate whether this concern is valid in the imatinib era.

CLINICAL CONTROVERSY

Although the controversy of whether to use imatinib or allogeneic HSCT as initial therapy is relevant to fewer than 30% of newly diagnosed CML patients, it continues to be controversial. Because early versus late transplantation is associated with better outcomes, one reasonable approach is to evaluate hematologic remission at 3 months in patients receiving imatinib. If patients do not have a complete hematologic remission and are eligible for transplantation, it should be considered. Cytogenetic responses should be evaluated every 3 months and those who obtain a complete cytogenetic remission on imatinib within 9 to 12 months of diagnosis should remain on imatinib. Delaying the transplantation might compromise the success of the allogeneic HSCT or lead to disease progression, in which transplantation outcomes are poorer.

Treatment options in patients who relapse after transplantation include inducing a graft-versus-leukemia (GVL) effect, imatinib, or IFN-α. The infusion of donor lymphocytes as a form of adoptive immunotherapy can induce a GVL effect. In relapsed CML, donor lymphocytes induce durable responses and these responses strongly correlate with the development of graft-versus-host disease (GVHD).[60,61] Tumor burden also predicts the likelihood of response to donor lymphocyte infusion in relapsed CML. A study by Raiola stratified the response rate of donor lymphocyte infusion according to relapse type. The response rate to donor lymphocytes was 100% in patients with molecular relapse, 90% in patients with cytogenetic relapse, 75% with relapsed chronic phase, and 35% in patients with relapsed accelerated phase or blast crisis.[62] The dose, timing, and method of administration of donor lymphocytes may also impact effectiveness. In one study, there was a significantly lower incidence of GVHD with escalating doses of donor lymphocyte infusion (fractionated dosing) rather than single-dose donor lymphocytes while maintaining a similar 70% to 90% complete cytogenetic remission rate.[63] This study suggests that the administration of donor lymphocytes in fractionated doses rather than a single large dose after the patient recovers from tissue damage may induce a GVL effect while minimizing GVHD. The optimal method of administering donor lymphocytes remains unclear, but these data suggest it may be possible to partially separate the GVL effect from GVHD.

Imatinib has been used in patients who have residual disease after allogeneic HSCT. Most patients respond to imatinib with complete molecular response of 70% without development of acute GVHD, which is often associated with donor lymphocyte infusions.[64] Although more work needs to be done on imatinib salvage after allogeneic HSCT, this high response rate is promising.

It is too early to define the role of nonmyeloablative transplants in CML but early results suggest equivalent efficacy to myeloablative transplants. Although early mortality is low following nonmyeloablative transplantation, transplant-related mortality is approximately 25% at 2 years.[65,66]

EVALUATION OF THERAPEUTIC OUTCOMES

Because nearly all patients with newly diagnosed chronic-phase CML will receive imatinib therapy, the goal of disease monitoring in CML is to identify patients who have optimally responded to an initial course of imatinib. A suboptimal response to imatinib is defined as no complete hematologic response at 3 months or lack of a complete cytogenetic response at 9 to 12 months. Recently published guidelines suggest that monitoring of *bcr-abl* transcripts is currently the best available test to monitor disease response.[23,24] These guidelines suggest that *bcr-abl* levels should be measured at baseline and then every 3 months to assess response.[22,32] The increase in *bcr-abl* levels may allow practitioners to identify patients who have progressive disease and may need a change in therapy. Imatinib dose escalation, dasatinib, nilotinib, or allogeneic HSCT should be considered in patients who do not respond or fail to maintain a molecular response.[22,32]

CHRONIC LYMPHOCYTIC LEUKEMIA

CLL is a lymphoproliferative disorder characterized by accumulation of functionally incompetent clonal B lymphocytes.[67] CLL is the most common form of leukemia in the United States, but is rare in other countries, such as Japan and China. It is estimated that about 15,340 new cases of CLL will be diagnosed in the United States in 2007.[2] Occasional family clusters have been recognized, and first-degree relatives of patients with CLL are at three times the risk of developing a lymphoid malignancy as compared to the general population. CLL is a disease of the elderly, with a median age of onset between 65 and 75 years, although 20% to 30% of CLL occurs in patients who are younger than 55 years of age.[3] Etiologic factors have not been identified in CLL, and there is no data supporting either radiation or viral oncogenesis.[1]

CLINICAL PRESENTATION OF CHRONIC LYMPHOCYTIC LEUKEMIA

Constitutional Symptoms

- Fever, fatigue, weight loss

Physical Examination

- Lymphadenopathy (87%)
- Splenomegaly (54%)
- Hepatomegaly (14%)

Laboratory Tests

- Peripheral blood
  - Lymphocytosis
  - Coombs-positive autoimmune hemolytic anemia
  - Hyper- or hypogammaglobulinemia
  - Monoclonal gammopathy
  - Anemia
  - Thrombocytopenia
- Bone marrow
  - Hypercellular
  - Increased mature lymphocytes
  - Increased megakaryocytes
- Molecular markers
  - Cytogenetics (17p-)
  - ZAP-70 mutations

STAGING AND PROGNOSIS

Survival times for patients with CLL are widely variable, with some patients dying within 2 years and others living two decades from the time of diagnosis. Two systems are used to estimate prognosis: the Rai and the Binet staging systems. Prognosis depends on stage and tumor burden at diagnosis. The Rai staging system has been combined into a risk classification scheme: low risk (stage 0), intermediate risk (stages I and II), and high risk (stages III and IV) with median survivals of greater than 10 years, 7 years, and 2 to 4 years, respectively.[1,68] The other common staging system is the Binet system, which is more commonly used in Europe.

Despite the prognostic importance of staging, the disease course varies within each stage so that one patient may have an indolent course with long survival time, while another patient may have more aggressive disease and a relatively short survival time. Because staging systems, such as the Rai system, incompletely predict for individual patients who progress rapidly within each stage, additional parameters are being developed to accurately identify patients who have poorer prognosis. Some of the more promising biologic markers include CD38 expression, ZAP-70 expression, and cytogenetic changes such as deletion of the short arm of chromosome 17 (17p-) corresponding to p53 silencing. CD38 is a cell-surface marker that is associated with early progression, significantly shorter overall survival and a poor response to fludarabine.[67–70] ZAP-70 is an intracellular protein with tyrosine kinase activity. Once considered as simply a surrogate marker for the unmutated variable region of the immunoglobulin heavy chain gene (IgVH), ZAP-70 appears to predict for rapid CLL disease progression and independently correlates with prognosis. Patients who have elevated ZAP-70 expression by flow cytometry have poorer prognosis.[68,71,72] These newer biomarkers, like ZAP-70 and CD38 expression, may help identify high-risk patients. The cytogenetic abnormality, 17p-, may be the most consistent of the prognostic markers identifying poor-risk patients who respond poorly to fludarabine-based therapy.

CLINICAL CONTROVERSY

Certain molecular and cellular markers have been identified that may predict CLL disease progression. ZAP-70 expression, CD38 expression, IgVH mutations, and 17p- are associated with a more aggressive form of CLL, although current treatment guidelines do not indicate when and how to initiate treatment based on these biologic markers. Controversy surrounds whether or not treatment should be based on these biologic markers alone. 17p- is the most consistent poor prognostic marker and results in a loss of the tumor suppressor gene, p53. One approach may be to treat young patients with these adverse prognostic markers with more aggressive combination therapy or consider allogeneic transplantation. For older patients, it may be reasonable to consider initiating less-intensive therapy, or if the patient is asymptomatic, waiting until symptoms arise. Although there is limited data supporting this approach, the hope is that early treatment may achieve complete remission and improve overall survival in those with aggressive disease.

TREATMENT

Chronic Lymphocytic Leukemia

Because CLL is considered to be an incurable disease, the primary goals of treatment are to improve quality and duration of life. ❻ The management of patients with CLL is highly variable, with some patients receiving therapy immediately and delaying therapy in others. The decision to begin treatment is based on several factors, including age of the patient, symptoms, aggressiveness of the tumor, and high-risk molecular features. Treatment is often instituted after signs and symptoms of progressive disease, autoimmune complications, symptomatic splenomegaly, bulky lymph nodes, severe lymphocytosis (greater than 100,000 to 200,000 cells/mm^3), and increased infectious complications.[67,73,74]

Most stage 0 patients do not require treatment and can be managed with observation. In patients with stage I or II disease, treatment is controversial. A consistent survival benefit from early therapy has not been reported in asymptomatic patients.[74,75] Cytotoxic chemotherapy in early stage CLL is usually reserved for patients who have disease characteristics consistent with a more aggressive course, such as short lymphocyte doubling times and presence of biologic markers such as ZAP-70 or high-risk cytogenetics. In stages III and IV disease, treatment is required, with the goal of achieving a partial or complete remission. Survival is improved in those patients who achieve a complete remission and is longest in those who become minimal residual disease negative. Table 138–4 reviews the current drug therapies used in newly diagnosed and previously treated CLL.[73,74,76,77]

TABLE 138-4 Treatment for Newly Diagnosed and Previously Treated Chronic Lymphocytic Leukemia

Treatment	Overall Response	Complete Response
Chlorambucil		
Untreated	37%	4%
Fludarabine alone		
Untreated	60–80%	20–30%
Previously treated	13–59%	3–37%
Fludarabine + cyclophosphamide		
Untreated	80–90%	25–40%
Previously treated	60–70%	10–15%
Rituximab alone		
Untreated	50–60%	10–20%
Previously treated	80–90%	20–40%
Fludarabine + rituximab		
Untreated	80–100%	30–50%
Previously treated	80–90%	20–40%
Fludarabine + cyclophosphamide + rituximab		
Untreated	95%	70%
Previously treated	73%	25%
Alemtuzumab alone		
Untreated	80–90%	20–30%
Previously treated	30–50%	0–20%
Alemtuzumab + fludarabine		
Previously treated	83%	17–30%

Adapted from Abbott,[67] Wienda,[73] Robak and Kaznicki,[76] and Gribben.[80]

CYTOTOXIC CHEMOTHERAPY

Orally administered alkylating agents such as chlorambucil and cyclophosphamide can be used as primary treatment for CLL. The timing of therapy is controversial. Results from a meta-analysis involving 2,048 patients from six randomized controlled studies evaluated low-dose alkylating agents in CLL. The analysis showed that delayed treatment in asymptomatic patients did not adversely effect 10-year survival. More importantly, if only deaths caused by CLL were considered, significantly longer survival was observed when treatment was deferred.[75] Chlorambucil continues to be widely used in elderly, symptomatic patients as initial treatment for CLL, but its use is based on a small number of studies with no demonstrable survival advantage.[1,67] Commonly used dosing schedules for chlorambucil are intermittent pulse dosing of 15 to 40 mg/m^2 orally every 28 days or daily doses of 4 to 8 mg/m^2 per day.[76] The dose of chlorambucil is often titrated to minimize myelosuppression. The addition of prednisone to chlorambucil is likely to increase infectious risk with no advantage in the treatment of CLL, but prednisone may have value in patients with autoimmune blood dyscrasias.[1]

Cyclophosphamide produces a similar response rate as chlorambucil (overall response rate: 40% to 60%; complete response: 4%) and can be used in patients who cannot tolerate chlorambucil or in whom response is not optimal.[1] Some patients who don't respond to chlorambucil do respond to single-agent cyclophosphamide. Cyclophosphamide is typically given orally at a daily dose of 1 to 3 mg/kg. Oral cyclophosphamide is less-commonly used compared to chlorambucil because of the risk of hemorrhagic cystitis and bladder cancer with prolonged treatment.

Fludarabine-based therapy is a common initial treatment in CLL. It is particularly useful in younger patients and in those patients who can tolerate immunosuppressive chemotherapy. Fludarabine, along with the other purine analogs, 2-chlorodeoxyadenosine (cladribine) and 2-deoxycoformycin (pentostatin), is highly active in CLL, with fludarabine being the most widely studied purine analog in the treatment of CLL.[73,74,77,78] Most patients receive fludarabine 20 mg/m^2 intravenously daily for 5 days when used as single-agent chemotherapy. Cladribine and pentostatin have similar activity, although head-to-head trials comparing these three nucleosides have not been conducted.[67,73,76,77,79]

Fludarabine was initially studied in CLL patients who were refractory to chlorambucil. Several trials reported overall response rates to fludarabine in previously treated patients ranging from 13% to 59% and complete response rates of 3% to 37%.[80,81] The most durable responses occurred in patients with lower-stage disease.[81] Based on these encouraging results in patients with refractory disease, fludarabine was studied in chemotherapy-naive patients. Three large phase II trials conducted in symptomatic, untreated CLL patients confirmed the efficacy of fludarabine. In these trials, fludarabine produced higher overall response rates and complete remissions than did alkylating-based therapies. In one of the randomized studies that compared fludarabine to chlorambucil in chemotherapy-naive patients, fludarabine-treated patients had a higher complete remission rate as compared with chlorambucil (20% vs. 5%).[82] However, the higher complete remission rate did not translate into a significant difference in overall survival, and patients treated with fludarabine had a higher rate of severe neutropenia and infection. The study allowed chlorambucil failures to cross over to the fludarabine arm, which may have reduced the ability to show a survival advantage in patients treated with fludarabine. Based off the following studies, there have been concerns about the higher incidence of opportunistic infections seen with fludarabine. A recent review of younger patients enrolled in a large phase III trial showed 33% of patients receiving fludarabine or fludarabine-based therapy had infectious complications.[83] An increase in *Pneumocystis* infections was not observed, but a 6% increase in herpes and varicella zoster infection was documented. Dose reductions occurred frequently during the infectious episode.[83] Based on the increased risk of infectious complications, some practitioners recommend antiviral and antibacterial prophylaxis to prevent these infections.[84,85]

■ BIOLOGIC THERAPY

Monoclonal antibodies, such as rituximab and alemtuzumab, are increasingly being used in the treatment of CLL. Rituximab is a chimeric monoclonal antibody that targets the CD20 antigen expressed on B lymphocytes. Rituximab was originally studied in patients with non-Hodgkin's lymphoma. The results from early trials of rituximab in CLL showed limited efficacy, with a 10% to 15% partial response rate.[86] This finding was attributed to the lower CD20 expression on the surface of the CLL cells as compared to non-Hodgkin's lymphoma and a more rapid clearance of rituximab in CLL, possibly through shedding of CD20.[73,87] When rituximab was used as the sole therapy in CLL, higher doses than those used in indolent non-Hodgkin's lymphoma had to be given to overcome these biologic features. Subsequent studies with higher rituximab doses (up to 2,250 mg/m^2) have reported increased overall response rates to 40% to 75% in previously treated patients.[73,87,88]

❼ Alemtuzumab is a monoclonal antibody that targets the CD52 antigen found on B and T lymphocytes. It was FDA approved in 2001 for the treatment of patients with CLL who had been treated with alkylating agents and had failed fludarabine therapy. Alemtuzumab has generally been used in CLL patients who are refractory to other available therapies, although data as first-line therapy are accumulating.[73,89,90] Alemtuzumab is often titrated to a maintenance dose of 30 mg intravenously given three times a week for 12 weeks. As a single agent, alemtuzumab has produced response rates from 33% to 53% in patients with refractory disease, but the complete response rates have been low.[73,78,90] Results from a randomized phase III trial comparing alemtuzumab to chlorambucil in chemotherapy-naive patients with symptomatic CLL showed higher complete response rates with alemtuzumab than with chlorambucil, 24% vs. 2%, respectively.[91] These differences in response rate translated into a significant difference in progression-free survival (hazard ratio 0.58, 95% confidence interval 0.43-0.77). Based on these results, alemtuzumab received FDA approval in 2007 as first-line treatment for CLL. Alemtuzumab may also have a role in clearing minimal residual disease after patients have been treated with chemotherapy. O'Brien et al. reported that 38% of patients with residual disease after fludarabine could achieve a molecular remission following alemtuzumab therapy and some of these remissions appeared to be durable.[92] Currently it is not known whether eliminating residual disease improves overall survival outcomes in CLL. Investigations are ongoing with the expectation that undetectable residual disease will correlate with improved remission duration and survival.[73] The activity of alemtuzumab in CLL is encouraging, but the drug is also associated with serious, potentially life-threatening toxicities, including pancytopenia, infusion reactions, and opportunistic infections. Because of alemtuzumab's profound immunosuppression, the 2008 NCCN guidelines recommend antibacterial and antiviral prophylaxis to prevent *Cytomegalovirus* reactivation and *Pneumocystis* infections.[85] Prophylaxis with trimethoprim-sulfamethoxazole and famciclovir or valacyclovir is recommended with the use of alemtuzumab.[1,86]

Infusion-related reactions are one of the most frequently reported toxicities with alemtuzumab. The reactions experienced with intravenous administration include fever, rigors, and hypotension. Although alemtuzumab is FDA approved for intravenous administration, the use of subcutaneous alemtuzumab has been explored to reduce the frequency of these reactions.[73,90,93] In a study by Lundin et al., 41 patients received 30 mg of subcutaneous alemtuzumab three times a week for 12 weeks. The response rate was 87%. The responses occurred after 18 weeks of therapy, which is longer than intravenous therapy. The major adverse event was grades 1 and 2 skin reactions, which was seen in 90% of patients, but fever, rigors, and hypotension were rare.[94] Approximately 10% of patients had reactivation of *Cytomegalovirus* and required ganciclovir treatment. It appears that antiviral and antibacterial prophylaxis is warranted with subcutaneous alemtuzumab.[90,94]

The exact role of rituximab or alemtuzumab in CLL is still being investigated. The 2008 NCCN guidelines recommend that rituximab be used in combination with other agents for first-line treatment of CLL in those patients who can tolerate aggressive chemotherapy. The guidelines do not recommend single-agent rituximab.[85] Alemtuzumab is primarily used as second-line therapy for CLL after failing combination-based therapy. The 2008 NCCN guidelines recommend that alemtuzumab be used as first-line therapy in high-risk patients with the 17 p- mutation. Clinicians must assess the risk-to-benefit ratio with alemtuzumab for reactivation of *Cytomegalovirus* can be deleterious.[85] Appropriate infection prophylaxis must be given.

■ COMBINATION THERAPY

The high single-agent activity of fludarabine has led to fludarabine-based combination regimens in patients with CLL. The most widely studied combination is fludarabine with cyclophosphamide, which produces complete response rates between 25% and 40% in treatment-naive patients as compared to 20% to 30% for single-agent fludarabine.[73,78,86] Although improved response rates and progression-free survival have been reported with fludarabine and cyclophosphamide combinations compared with fludarabine alone, no benefit in overall survival has yet been observed.[73,78]

Combination fludarabine and rituximab has promising activity. In vitro studies suggest that rituximab is synergistic with fludarabine and cyclophosphamide and has led investigators to evaluate this combination in clinical trials.[73,86] ❽ Results from an uncontrolled trial of fludarabine, cyclophosphamide, and rituximab reported a complete remission rate of 70% in previously untreated CLL patients. This is the highest complete remission rate reported for any treatment of CLL.[86] This same combination was impressive in previously treated patients, with a complete remission rate of 25%.[95]

Combinations with alemtuzumab have also been studied. The combination of fludarabine and alemtuzumab achieved an overall response rate of 83% in heavily pretreated patients.[96] Combinations of alemtuzumab and rituximab produced a response rate of 53% in a group of CLL patients. The response rates were higher (63%) in patients who had not received prior antibody therapy.[97] The investigators did note that more than half the patients experienced an infection suggesting severe treatment-related immunosuppression. The treatment of CLL increasingly involves fludarabine combined with monoclonal antibody therapy. Patient selection is critical given the high risk of serious infection. Most younger patients will be candidates for fludarabine-monoclonal antibody based combination therapy. Symptomatic elderly patients with aggressive disease who can tolerate immunosuppressive therapy may also be candidates for this regimen.[74]

HEMATOPOIETIC STEM CELL TRANSPLANTATION

There is limited experience with the use of HSCT in CLL. Early mortality with autologous and allogeneic HSCT is approximately 10% and 40%, respectively.[67,80,98] ❾ Patients treated with allogeneic HSCT achieve higher rates of molecular remission and appear to have a longer duration of disease-free survival, but at the expense of high treatment-related mortality.[98] Contrary to the high mortality reported in most studies, a randomized phase II study of high-risk CLL patients comparing allogeneic and autologous HSCT reported 100-day mortality of 4% in both arms. After 6 years of followup, no difference in overall survival (58% autologous and 55% allogeneic) was observed.[99] This low early mortality must be interpreted carefully, given that only 25 carefully selected patients received allogeneic HSCT as compared to 137 who received autologous transplantation. Also, T-cell depletion was performed on the allogeneic grafts, which may reduce early mortality at the cost of increased relapse as a consequence of reduced GVL effect.[99]

Although this modality of treatment may hold some promise of cure, the advanced age of most CLL patients and the associated high treatment-related mortality limits the use of allogeneic HSCT in CLL. HSCT is an option for younger patients with aggressive disease. Older patients who are not candidates for full-intensity allogeneic HSCT may be candidates for nonmyeloablative allogeneic HSCT.[80]

EVALUATION OF THERAPEUTIC OUTCOMES

CLL is considered an incurable indolent disease and the goal of therapy is to increase the duration and quality of life. Careful risk-to-benefit analysis should be applied in older patients with indolent disease. A reasonable strategy in asymptomatic patients is observation (i.e., no therapy). Therapy should be considered in patients with symptomatic disease. Younger patients with aggressive disease should receive a fludarabine-based therapy, possibly in combination with rituximab and cyclophosphamide.[85]

TREATMENT SUMMARY OF CHRONIC LEUKEMIA

The treatments used for CML and CLL are vastly different with tyrosine kinase inhibitors used in CML and biologics playing an increasingly important role in CLL. For the vast majority of patients with chronic-phase CML, imatinib is used as initial therapy. In patients who do not achieve an adequate response, dose escalation of imatinib, allogeneic HSCT, other tyrosine kinase inhibitors, or clinical studies should be considered. Allogeneic HSCT still remains the only curative therapy for CML. IFN-α is no longer a first-line option for CML based on its inferior activity as compared with imatinib and is reserved to those who can not tolerate tyrosine kinase inhibitors.

The goal in the treatment of CLL is to optimize quality of life rather than to use aggressive, toxic therapy. Observation is appropriate in asymptomatic patients with low-risk disease characteristics. Treatment should be reserved for patients with symptomatic or high-risk disease. In the older patient, the use of chlorambucil may still be preferred over fludarabine because of the lower infectious risk and ease of administration. In the younger patient, fludarabine-based combination therapy is often given with the goal of obtaining complete remissions. The combination of fludarabine, cyclophosphamide, and rituximab has reported the highest response rates in CLL. Alemtuzumab is most frequently used in previously treated patients, but is being studied as part of initial therapy in patients with high risk disease. The use of alemtuzumab is limited by its severe immunosuppressive profile.

ABBREVIATIONS

CLL: chronic lymphocytic leukemia

CML: chronic myelogenous leukemia

GVHD: graft-versus-host disease

GVL: graft-versus-leukemia (effect)

HLA: human leukocyte antigen

HSCT: hematopoietic stem cell transplantation

IgVH: immunoglobulin heavy chain gene

IFN-α: interferon alfa

IFN-α_{2a}: interferon alfa$_{2a}$

IFN-α_{2b}: interferon alfa$_{2b}$

IRIS: International Randomized study of Interferon vs. STI571 trial

NCCN: National Comprehensive Cancer Network

Ph: Philadelphia chromosome

RT-PCR: reverse transcriptase-polymerase chain reaction

WBC: white blood cell

ZAP-70: zeta-associated protein-70

REFERENCES

1. Druker BJ, Lee SJ, O'Brien S, Keating MJ. Chronic leukemias. In: Devita VT, Hellman S, Rosenberg SA, eds. Cancer: Principles and Practice of Oncology, 7th ed. Philadelphia: Lippincott Williams & Wilkins, 2005:2121–2143.
2. Jemal A, Siegel R, Ward E, et al. Cancer statistics, 2007. CA Cancer J Clin 2007;57:43–66.
3. Ries LAG, Harkins D, Krapcho M, et al., eds. SEER Cancer Statistics Review, 1975–2003. Bethesda, MD: National Cancer Institute. 2006, *http://seer.cancer.gov/csr/1975_2003/*, based on November 2005 SEER data submission.

4. Clarkson B, Strife A, Wisniewski D, et al. Chronic myelogenous leukemia as a paradigm of early cancer and possible curative strategies. Leukemia 2003;17:1211–1262.
5. Nowell PC. Progress with chronic myelogenous leukemia: A personal perspective over four decades. Annu Rev Med 2002;53:1–13.
6. Goldman JM, Melo JV. Chronic myeloid leukemia—Advances in biology and new approaches to treatment. N Engl J Med 2003;349:1451–1464.
7. Quintas-Cardama A, Cortes JE. Chronic myelogenous leukemia: Diagnosis and treatment. Mayo Clin Proc 2006;81:973–988.
8. Sawyers CL. Chronic myeloid leukemia. N Engl J Med 1999;340:1330–1340.
9. Savona M, Talpaz M. Chronic myeloid leukemia: Changing the treatment paradigms. Oncology (Williston Park) 2006;20:707–711.
10. Schiffer CA. BCR-ABL tyrosine kinase inhibitors for chronic myelogenous leukemia. N Engl Med 2007;357:258–265.
11. Jabbour E, Cortes J, O'Brien S, et al. New targeted therapies for chronic myelogenous leukemia: Opportunities to overcome imatinib resistance. Semin Hematol 2007;44(Suppl 1):S25–S31.
12. Goldman JM. How I treat chronic myeloid leukemia in the imatinib era. Blood 2007;110:2828–2837.
13. Deininger MW. Management of early stage disease. Hematology (Am Soc Hematol Educ Program) 2005;174–182.
14. Alvarez RH, Kantarjian H and Cortes JE. The biology of chronic myelogenous leukemia: Implications for imatinib therapy. Semin Hematol 2007;44(Suppl 1):S4–S14.
15. Jabbour E, Kantarjian H, O'Brien S, et al. Sudden blastic transformation in patients with chronic myelogenous leukemia treated with imatinib mesylate. Blood 2006;107:480–482.
16. Ilaria RL Jr. Pathobiology of lymphoid and myeloid blast crisis and management issues. Hematology (Am Soc Hematol Educ Program) 2005;188–194.
17. Shah NP. Loss of response to imatinib: Mechanisms and management. Hematology (Am Soc Hematol Educ Program) 2005;183–187.
18. Vardiman JW, Harris NL, Brunning RD. The World Health Organization (WHO) classification of myeloid neoplasms. Blood 2002;100:2292–2302.
19. Cortes JE, Talpaz M, O'Brien S, et al. Staging of chronic myeloid leukemia in the imatinib era. Cancer 2006;106:1306–1315.
20. Sawyers CL, Hochhaus A, Feldman E, et al. Imatinib induces hematologic and cytogenetic responses in patients with chronic myelogenous leukemia in myeloid blast crisis: Results of a phase II study. Blood 2002;99:3530–3539.
21. Druker BJ, Guilhot F, O'Brien S, et al. Five-year follow-up of patients receiving imatinib for chronic myelogenous leukemia. N Engl J Med 2006;355:2408–2417.
22. The NCCN Chronic Myelogenous Leukemia Clinical Practice Guideline (Version 3. 2008). Available at: http://www.nccn.org. Accessed Jan 20, 2008.
23. Hughes T, Deininger M, Hochhaus A, et al. Monitoring CML patients responding to treatment with tyrosine kinase inhibitors: Review and recommendations for harmonizing current methodology for detecting *BCR-ABL* transcripts and kinase domain mutations and for expressing results. Blood 2006;108:28–37.
24. Hughes T. ABL kinase inhibitor therapy for CML. Baseline assessments and response monitoring. Hematology (Am Soc Hematol Educ Program) 2006;211–218.
25. Hehlmann R, Heimpel H, Hasford J, et al. Randomized comparison of busulfan and hydroxyurea in chronic myelogenous leukemia: Prolongation of survival by hydroxyurea. The German CML Study Group. Blood 1993;82:398–407.
26. Deininger MW, O'Brien SG, Ford JM, Druker BJ. Practical management of patients with chronic myeloid leukemia receiving imatinib. J Clin Oncol 2003;21:1637–1647.
27. Moen MD, McKeage K, Plosker LG, Siddiqui MAA. Imatinib: A review of its use in chronic myeloid leukemia. Drugs 2007;67:299–320.
28. Deininger MWN, Druker BJ. Specific targeted therapy at chronic myelogenous leukemia with imatinib. Pharmacol Rev 2003;55:401–423.
29. Deininger M, Buchdunger E, Druker BJ. The development of imatinib as a therapeutic agent for chronic myeloid leukemia. Blood 2005;105:2640–2653.
30. Kurzrock R, Kantarjian HM, Druker BJ, Talpaz M. Philadelphia chromosome-positive leukemias: From basic mechanisms to molecular therapeutics. Ann Intern Med 2003;138:819–830.
31. Druker BJ, Talpaz M, Resta DJ, et al. Efficacy and safety of a specific inhibitor of the *BCR-ABL* tyrosine kinase in chronic myeloid leukemia. N Engl J Med 2001;344:1031–1037.
32. Baccarani M, Saglio G, Goldman J, et al. Evolving concepts in the management of chronic myeloid leukemia: Recommendations from an expert panel on behalf of the European Leukemia Network. Blood 2006;108:1809–1820.
33. O'Brien SG, Guilhot F, Larson RA, et al. Imatinib compared with interferon and low-dose cytarabine for newly diagnosed chronic-phase chronic myeloid leukemia. N Engl J Med 2003;348:994–1004.
34. Hughes TP, Kaeda J, Branford S, et al. Frequency of major molecular responses to imatinib or interferon alfa plus cytarabine in newly diagnosed chronic myeloid leukemia. N Engl J Med 2003;349:1423–1432.
35. Press RD, Love Z, Tronnes AA, et al. *BCR-ABL* mRNA levels at and after the time of a complete cytogenetic response (CCR) predict the duration of CCR in imatinib mesylate-treated patients with CML. Blood 2006;107:4250–4256.
36. Kantarjian H, Talpaz M, O'Brien S, et al. High-dose imatinib mesylate therapy in newly diagnosed Philadelphia chromosome-positive chronic phase chronic myeloid leukemia. Blood 2004;103:2873–2878.
37. Talpaz M, Silver RT, Druker BJ, et al. Imatinib induces durable hematologic and cytogenetic responses in patients with accelerated phase chronic myeloid leukemia: Results of a phase 2 study. Blood 2002;99:1928–1937.
38. Kantarjian H, Talpaz M, O'Brien S, et al. Survival benefit with imatinib mesylate therapy in patients with accelerated phase chronic myelogenous leukemia comparison with historic experience. Cancer 2005;103:2099–2108.
39. Druker BJ, Sawyers CL, Kantarjian H, et al. Activity of a specific inhibitor of the *BCR-ABL* tyrosine kinase in the blast crisis of chronic myeloid leukemia and acute lymphoblastic leukemia with the Philadelphia chromosome. N Engl J Med 2001;344:1038–1042.
40. Hochhaus A, Erben P, Ernst T, Mueller MC. Resistance to targeted therapy in chronic myelogenous leukemia. Semin Hematol 2007;44(Suppl 1):S15–S24.
41. Kantarjian HM, Talpaz M, Giles F, O'Brien S, Cortes J. New insights into the pathophysiology of chronic myeloid leukemia and imatinib resistance. Ann Intern Med 2006;145:913–923.
42. Gadzicki D, Von Neuhoff N, Steinemann D, et al. BCR-ABL gene amplification and overexpression in a patient with chronic myeloid leukemia treated with imatinib. Cancer Genet Cytogenet 2005;159:164–167.
43. Quintas-Cardama A, Kantarjian H, O'Brien S, et al. Granulocyte colony-stimulating factor may overcome imatinib induced neutropenia in patients with chronic phase chronic myelogenous leukemia. Cancer 2004;100:2592–2597.
44. Agis H, Jaeger E, Doninger C, et al. In vivo effects of imatinib mesylate on human hematopoietic progenitor cells. Eur J Clin Invest 2006;36:402–408.
45. SPRYCEL (dasatinib) tablets. Product information. Bristol-Myers Squibb, Princeton, NJ. November 2007.
46. Hochhaus A, Kantarjian HM, Baccarani M, et al. Dasatinib induces notable hematologic and cytogenetic responses in chronic-phase chronic myeloid leukemia after failure of imatinib therapy. Blood 2007;109:2303–2309.
47. Kantarjian H, Pasquini R, Hamerschlak N, et al. Dasatinib or high-dose imatinib for chronic-phase chronic myeloid leukemia after failure of first-line imatinib: A randomized phase 2 trial. Blood 2007;109:5143–5150.
48. TASIGNA (nilotinib) tablets. Product information. Novartis, East Hanover, NJ, October 2007.
49. Kantarjian HM, Giles F, Gattermann N, et al. Nilotinib (formerly AMN107), a highly selective BCR-ABL tyrosine kinase inhibitor, is effective in patients with Philadelphia chromosome-positive chronic myelogenous leukemia in chronic phase following imatinib resistance and intolerance. Blood 2007;110:3540–3546.
50. Le Coutre P, Ottmann OG, Giles F, et al. Nilotinib (formerly AMN107), a highly selective BCR-ABL tyrosine kinase inhibitor, is active in patients with imatinib-resistant or -intolerant accelerated phase chronic myelogenous leukemia. Blood 2008;111:1834–1839.
51. Michallet M, Maloisel F, Delain M, et al. Pegylated recombinant interferon alpha-2b vs recombinant interferon alpha-2b for the initial treatment of chronic-phase chronic myelogenous leukemia: A phase III study. Leukemia 2004;18:309–315.

52. Bukowski RM, Tendler C, Cutler C, et al. Treating cancer with PEG Intron. Cancer 2002;95:389–396.
53. Jonasch E, Haluska FG. Interferon in oncological practice: Review of interferon biology, clinical applications and toxicities. Oncologist 2001;6:34–55.
54. Baccarani M, Martinelli G, Rosti G, et al. Imatinib and pegylated human recombinant interferon-a2b in early chronic-phase chronic myeloid leukemia. Blood 2004;104:4245–4251.
55. Gratwohl A, Brand R, Apperley J, et al. Allogeneic hematopoietic stem cell transplantation for chronic myeloid leukemia in Europe 2006: Transplant activity, long-term data and current results. An analysis by the Chronic Leukemia Working Party of the European Group for Blood and Marrow Transplantation (EBMT). Haematologica 2006;91:513–521.
56. van Rhee F, Szydlo RM, Hermans J, et al. Long-term results after allogenic bone marrow transplantation for chronic myelogenous leukemia in chronic phase: A report from the Chronic Leukemia Working Party of the European Group for Blood and Marrow Transplantation. Bone Marrow Transplant 1997;20:553–560.
57. Hehlmann R, Berger U, Pfirrmann M, et al. Drug treatment is superior to allografting as first-line therapy in chronic myeloid leukemia. Blood 2007;109:4686–4692.
58. Deininger M, Schleuning M, Greinix H, et al. The effect of prior exposure to imatinib on transplant-related mortality. Haematologica 2006;91:452–459.
59. Oehler VG, Gooley T, Snyder DS, et al. The effects of imatinib treatment with allogeneic transplant for chronic myelogenous leukemia. Blood 2007;109:1782–1789.
60. Porter D, Levine JE. Graft-versus host disease and graft-versus leukemia after donor leukocyte infusion. Semin Hematol 2006;43:53–61.
61. Apperley JF. Managing the patient with chronic myeloid leukemia through and after allogeneic stem cell transplantation. Hematology (Am Soc Hematol Educ Program) 2006;226–232.
62. Raiola AM, Van Lint MT, Valbonesi M, et al. Factors predicting response and graft-versus-host disease after donor lymphocyte infusions: A study on 593 infusions. Bone Marrow Transplant 2003;31:687–693.
63. Dazzi F, Szydlo RM, Craddock C, et al. Comparison of single-dose and escalating-dose regimens of donor lymphocyte infusion for relapse after allografting for chronic myeloid leukemia. Blood 2000;95:67–71.
64. Hess G, Bunjes D, Siegert W, et al. Sustained complete molecular remissions after treatment with imatinib mesylate in patients with failure after allogeneic stem cell transplantation for chronic myelogenous leukemia: Results of a prospective phase II open label multicenter study. J Clin Oncol 2005;23:7583–7593..
65. Scott BL, Sandmaier BM. Reduced intensity allogeneic transplant: Outcomes with myeloid malignancies. Hematology (Am Soc Hematol Educ Program) 2006;381–389.
66. Or R, Shapira MY, Resnick I, et al. Nonmyeloablative allogeneic stem cell transplantation for treatment of chronic myelogenous leukemia in first chronic phase. Blood 2003;101:441–445.
67. Abbott BL. Chronic lymphocytic leukemia: Recent advances in diagnosis and treatment. Oncologist 2006;11:21–30.
68. Montserrat E. New prognostic markers in CLL. Hematology (Am Soc Hematol Educ Program) 2006;279–84.
69. Matria Z. CD38 as a prognostic marker in CLL. Hematology 2005;10:39–46.
70. Deaglio S, Vaisitti T, Aydin S, Ferrero E, Malavasi F. In-tandem insight from basic science combined with clinical research: CD38 as both marker and key component of the pathogenetic network underlying chronic lymphocytic leukemia. Blood 2006;108:1135–1144.
71. Rassenti LZ, Huynh L, Toy TL, et al. ZAP-70 compared with immunoglobulin heavy-chain gene mutation status as a predictor of disease progression in chronic lymphocytic leukemia. N Engl J Med 2004;351:893–901..
72. Orchard J, Ibbotson R, Best G, Parker A, Oscier D. ZAP-70 in B cell malignancies. Leuk Lymphoma 2005;46:1689–1698.
73. Wierda WG. Current and investigation therapies for patients with CLL. Hematology (Am Soc Hematol Educ Program) 2006;285–94.
74. Shanafelt TD, Byrd JC, Call TG, Zent CS, Kay NE. Narrative review: Initial management of newly diagnosed, early-stage chronic lymphocytic leukemia. Ann Intern Med 2006;145:435–447.
75. Chemotherapeutic options in chronic lymphocytic leukemia: A meta-analysis of the randomized trials. CLL Trialists' Collaborative Group. J Natl Cancer Inst 1999;91:861–868.
76. Robak T, Kaznicki N. Alkylating agents and nucleoside analogues in the treatment of B cell chronic lymphocytic leukemia. Leukemia 2002;16:1015–1027.
77. Lamanna N, Weiss MA. Purine analogue-based chemotherapy regimens for second-line therapy in patients with chronic lymphocytic leukemia. Semin Hematol 2006;43:S44-S49.
78. Hallek M. Chronic lymphocytic leukemia (CLL): First-line treatment. Hematology (Am Soc Hematol Educ Program) 2005;285–91.
79. Robak T, Blonski JZ, Kasznicki M, et al. Cladribine with or without prednisone in the treatment of previously treated and untreated B-cell chronic lymphocytic leukaemia—Updated results of the multicentre study of 378 patients. Br J Haematol 2000;108:357–368.
80. Gribben JG. Salvage therapy for CLL and the role of stem cell transplantation. Hematology (Am Soc Hematol Educ Program) 2005;292–298.
81. Sorensen JM, Vena DA, Fallavollita A, et al. Treatment of refractory chronic lymphocytic leukemia with fludarabine phosphate via the group C protocol mechanism of the National Cancer Institute: Five-year follow-up report. J Clin Oncol 1997;15:458–465.
82. Rai KR, Peterson BL, Appelbaum FR, et al. Fludarabine compared with chlorambucil as primary therapy for chronic lymphocytic leukemia. N Engl J Med 2000;343:1750–1757.
83. Eichhorst BF, Busch R, Schweighofer C, et al. Due to the low infection rates no routine anti-infective prophylaxis is required in younger patients with chronic lymphocytic leukemia during fludarabine-based first line therapy. Br J Haematol 2007;136:63–72.
84. Keating MJ, O'Brien S, Kontoyiannis D, et al. Results of first salvage therapy for patients refractory to a fludarabine regimen in chronic lymphocytic leukemia. Leuk Lymphoma 2002;43:1755–1762.
85. The NCCN non-Hodgkin's Lymphoma Clinical Practice Guideline (Version 3. 2007). Available at: http://www.nccn.org. Accessed Jan 20, 2008.
86. Keating MJ, O'Brien S, Albitar M, et al. Early results of a chemoimmunotherapy regimen of fludarabine, cyclophosphamide, and rituximab as initial therapy for chronic lymphocytic leukemia. J Clin Oncol 2005;23:4079–4088.
87. Keating M, O'Brien S, Albitar M. Emerging information on the use of rituximab in chronic lymphocytic leukemia. Semin Oncol 2002;29(Suppl 2):70–74.
88. Hillmen P. Advancing therapy for chronic lymphocytic leukemia—The role of rituximab. Semin Oncol 2004;31(Suppl 2):22–26.
89. Ravandi F, O'Brien S. Alemtuzumab in CLL and other lymphoid neoplasms. Cancer Invest 2006;24:718–725.
90. Rai KR. Novel therapeutic strategies with alemtuzumab for chronic lymphocytic leukemia. Semin Oncol 2006;33(Suppl 5):S15–S22.
91. Hillmen P, Skotnicki AB, Robak T, et al. Alemtuzumab compared with chlorambucil as first-line therapy for chronic lymphocytic leukemia. J Clin Oncol 2007;35:5616-5623
92. O'Brien SM, Kantarjian HM, Thomas DA, et al. Alemtuzumab as treatment for residual disease after chemotherapy in patients with chronic lymphocytic leukemia. Cancer 2003;98:2657–2663.
93. Osterborg A, Karlsson C, Lundin J, Kimby E, Mellstedt H. Strategies in the management of alemtuzumab-related side effects. Semin Oncol 2006;33(Suppl 5):S29–S35.
94. Lundin J, Kimby E, Bjorkholm M, et al. Phase II trial of subcutaneous anti-CD52 monoclonal antibody alemtuzumab (Campath-1H) as first-line treatment for patients with B-cell chronic lymphocytic leukemia (B-CLL). Blood 2002;100:768–773.
95. Wierda W, O'Brien S, Wen S, et al. Chemoimmunotherapy with fludarabine, cyclophosphamide, and rituximab for relapsed and refractory chronic lymphocytic leukemia. J Clin Oncol 2005;23:4070–4078.
96. Elter T, Borchmann P, Schulz H, et al. Fludarabine in combination with alemtuzumab is effective and feasible in patients with relapsed or refractory B-cell chronic lymphocytic leukemia: Results of a phase II trial. J Clin Oncol 2005;23:7024–7031.
97. Faderl S, Thomas DA, O'Brien S, et al. Experience with alemtuzumab plus rituximab in patients with relapsed and refractory lymphoid malignancies. Blood 2003;101:3413–3415.
98. Dreger P, Montserrat E. Autologous and allogeneic stem cell transplantation for chronic lymphocytic leukemia. Leukemia 2002;16:985–992.
99. Gribben JG, Zahrieh D, Stephans K, et al. Autologous and allogeneic stem cell transplantation for poor risk chronic lymphocytic leukemia. Blood 2005;106:4389–4396.

CHAPTER 139 Multiple Myeloma

TIMOTHY R. MCGUIRE

KEY CONCEPTS

1. Multiple myeloma (MM) is a cancer that develops in plasma cells leading to excessive production of a monoclonal immunoglobulin (M protein).

2. Most patients have skeletal involvement at the time of diagnosis with associated bone pain and fractures. Anemia, hypercalcemia, and renal failure may also be present. A bone marrow biopsy with 10% or more plasma cells and a M-protein spike on plasma or urine electrophoresis confirm the diagnosis.

3. Most patients will require treatment after diagnosis but treatment can be deferred in patients with smoldering (asymptomatic) or stage I MM. Treatment of patients with symptomatic or stage II or III disease produces benefits in various measures of survival and quality of life.

4. Thalidomide plus dexamethasone is a commonly used induction regimen. It produces higher complete remission rates as compared to melphalan plus prednisone but at the cost of greater grade III and IV toxicity which can include venous thromboembolism (VTE) and neuropathy.

5. Bortezomib is an FDA-approved treatment for relapsed MM and is being studied as initial therapy combined with dexamethasone or chemotherapy. Bortezomib may have superior activity in chromosome 13 deletion patients.

6. Lenalidomide is a more potent, and perhaps less toxic, thalidomide analog that is being studied as initial therapy combined with dexamethasone or chemotherapy.

7. Autologous hematopoietic stem cell transplantation (autoHSCT) is used after induction in patients with reasonably good performance status to maximize complete remissions and prolong survival.

8. The use of myeloablative allogeneic hematopoietic stem cell transplantation (alloHSCT) produces high early mortality but the use of nonmyeloablative alloHSCT may offer a chance for long-term disease-free survival.

9. Bisphosphonates are used to treat bone disease associated with MM, which results in decreased pain and skeletal-related events and improvement in quality of life.

10. Salvage therapy for patients with relapsed or refractory MM can include any of the prior listed therapies, depending on performance status of the patient and prior treatments used for induction.

Learning objectives, review questions, and other resources can be found at **www.pharmacotherapyonline.com.**

Multiple myeloma (MM) is a relatively common hematologic malignancy that develops in plasma cells or immunoglobulin-producing B lymphocytes.[1,2] The plasma cells produce excessive monoclonal immunoglobulins that can be measured in the plasma or urine. Because of the various bone-mobilizing cytokines secreted from the MM clone and bone marrow stromal cells, patients often have skeletal involvement at diagnosis. The lytic bone lesions result from the double insult of pathologic activation of osteoclasts (bone mobilizing cells) and inhibition of osteoblasts (bone-forming cells). MM is initially sensitive to chemotherapy but drug resistance often develops rapidly, primarily because of upregulation of multidrug resistant proteins such as P-glycoprotein and regulators of apoptosis such as *bcl-2*. Although therapy is not curative, several new agents have been developed that have improved the duration and quality of life of MM patients.

Disease progression is influenced by cytokines that are able to stimulate plasma cell growth and angiogenesis. Several of these cytokines, including interleukin-6 (IL-6), basic fibroblast growth factor (bFGF), tumor necrosis factor-α (TNF-α), and vascular endothelial growth factor (VEGF), have become targets for new therapies such as thalidomide, its congener lenalidomide, and bortezomib.

EPIDEMIOLOGY AND ETIOLOGY

In the United States, it is estimated that 19,900 cases of MM will be diagnosed in 2007, with 10,790 deaths. It is a disease that affects older adults with a median age at diagnosis of 70 years. MM occurs more frequently in males and African Americans.[1–3]

No cause can be identified in most patients. Exposure to high doses of radiation increases the risk of developing MM.[1,2] Although not proven, there may be a hereditary component to MM, given the reports of familial associations. The relationship between viral infection and risk of MM is controversial. Human herpes virus-8 is often reported to be a likely candidate virus for development of MM.[1] However, a recent study was unable to isolate human herpes virus-8 from patients with MM and it is unlikely that human herpes virus-8 is an etiologic agent in this disease.[4] Patients with human immunodeficiency virus-1 infections have 4.5 times the risk of developing MM, which suggests a role for human immunodeficiency virus-1 as a viral cofactor. Human immunodeficiency virus-1–positive patients develop MM at an earlier age and with disease that has aggressive characteristics leading to poorer outcomes.[5]

PATHOPHYSIOLOGY

MM presents a very complex picture of multistep malignant transformation. A precursor condition called monoclonal gammopathy of undetermined significance (MGUS) is associated with monoclonal immunoglobulin in the blood (≤3 g/dL) without clinical manifestations of the complications of MM.[6,7] The conversion rate of MGUS to MM is approximately 1% per year. The molecular changes associated with the conversion of MGUS to MM are not clear, but genome-wide studies have identified several candidate genes for disease progression.[8] Smoldering MM is asymptomatic disease with low tumor burden and an indolent course.[1,9] In patients with smoldering MM, the risk of progression is approximately 10% per year for the first 5 years after diagnosis, approximately 3% per year for the next 5 years, and approximately 1% per year for the next 10 years.[9]

In early MM, the balance between apoptotic and antiapoptotic genes is disrupted with overexpression of antiapoptotic genes.[10] As the disease progresses, a greater number of gene products that confer resistance, such as mutated p53, are overexpressed.[11] Molecules such as IL-6 and the transcriptional regulator nuclear factor kappa B (NF-κB) also stimulate clonal growth and promote resistance to therapy.[12] Given their imprecise but important role in initiation and progression of MM, IL-6 and NF-κB are targets for both old and new therapies.

❶ MM is characterized by the accumulation of malignant plasma cells in the bone marrow and the production of a monoclonal immunoglobulin (M protein). These proteins, secreted by the malignant clone, are frequently referred to as paraproteins.[1] Both MM and normal plasma cells are produced from differentiated B cells after antigen stimulation. Normal plasma cells will die within days to weeks after differentiation whereas MM plasma cells are immortalized.[1,2] MM cells are seldom seen in large quantities in the peripheral blood because of their interaction with bone marrow stromal cells. This interaction between MM cells and bone marrow stroma is mediated by adhesion molecules within an abnormal bone marrow microenvironment and is required for growth and disease progression.[13] Figure 139–1 describes several of the factors involved in disease pathogenesis and progression and potential molecular drug targets.

The major target for the newer therapies is NF-κB. The effects of NF-κB are pleiotropic and integral to MM progression. NF-κB activation is high in MM and results in an abnormally high production of MM growth factors such as IL-6 and adhesion molecules in the bone marrow. Thalidomide is a potent inhibitor of TNF-α, which is a cytokine with important NF-κB-inducing activity. Thalidomide also has direct NF-κB-inhibiting activity by conserving inhibitor of NF-κB (IκB), the cytosolic inhibitor of NF-κB. Lenalidomide has similar mechanisms of action as thalidomide but is significantly more potent. Thalidomide and lenalidomide also activate important antimyeloma immune responses. Bortezomib is the most specific of the NF-κB inhibitors. Through its inhibition of the protease complex, the proteasome, bortezomib prevents IκB degradation and termination of NF-κB signal. Understanding the targets of these newer agents has led to a better understanding of the pathophysiology of MM.

CLINICAL PRESENTATION

❷ Most MM patients present with complaints of bone pain and fatigue at diagnosis. Approximately 10% to 20% of patients are asymptomatic at the time of diagnosis, most of whom will have either smoldering or stage I disease.[14] Most patients show evidence of end-organ damage at the time of diagnosis. Initial laboratory evaluation often reveals hypercalcemia, renal insufficiency, anemia, and abnormalities in various disease markers, such as albumin and

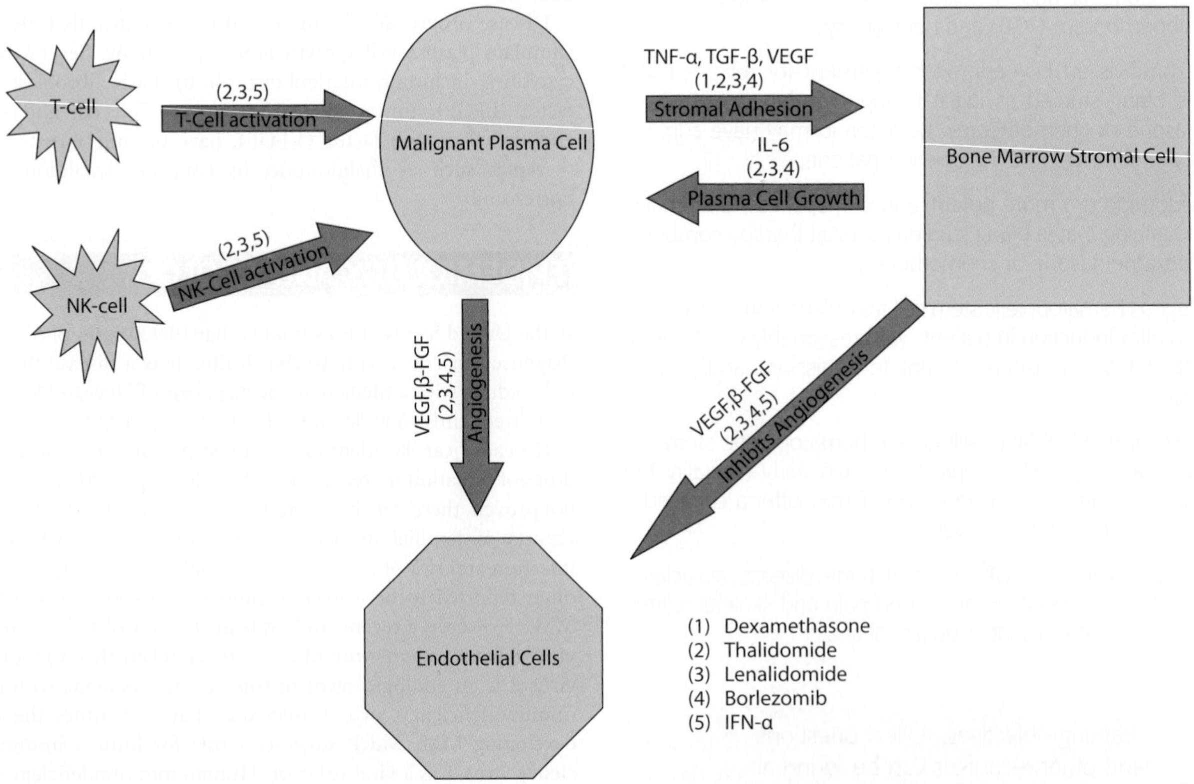

FIGURE 139-1. Sites of action of selected drugs used in the treatment of multiple myeloma. (bFGF, basic fibroblast growth factor; IFN-α, interferon alfa; IL, interleukin; NK, natural killer; TNF-α, tumor necrosis factor; TGF–β, transforming growth factor; VEGF, vascular endothelial growth factor.)

β_2-microglobulin. Skeletal evaluation shows gross abnormalities in most patients. Bone scans show abnormalities that often include lytic lesions, osteoporosis, and fractures. This group of findings (hypercalcemia, renal insufficiency, anemia, and bone lesions) is often referred to as CRAB.[6] A bone marrow biopsy with 10% or more plasma cells and an M-protein spike on plasma or urine electrophoresis confirms the diagnosis.[15] Immunofixation after electrophoresis identifies the M-protein isotype being secreted. In approximately 20% of patients, no M protein can be detected in the plasma but is found in the urine, requiring that urine be examined as part of a complete diagnostic workup. Approximately 60% of patients will have intact monoclonal immunoglobulin G, 20% will have monoclonal immunoglobulin A, and the remaining 20% will secrete only monoclonal light chains. Antibodies are composed of two light chains where antigen binds and two heavy chains. Light-chain immunoglobulin alone can be secreted by the MM clone. Free monoclonal light chains in the urine are called Bence Jones proteins because they were first described by Dr. Henry Bence Jones and are primarily responsible for MM-associated renal failure.[1,15]

CLINICAL PRESENTATION OF MULTIPLE MYELOMA

General Criteria

- 80% of patients present with symptomatic disease

Signs and Symptoms

- Bone pain (fractures, lytic lesions)
- Fatigue (anemia)
- Infection (reduced polyclonal response)
- Neurologic symptoms (nerve compression)
- Polyuria (hypercalcemia)
- Nausea and vomiting (hypercalcemia)

Laboratory Parameters

- Elevated paraproteins
  - Plasma electrophoresis
  - Urine electrophoresis
  - Immunofixation
- Elevated serum creatinine
- Hypercalcemia
- Low hemoglobin
- Low albumin
- Elevated β_2-microglobulin
- Elevated C-reactive protein

Bone Marrow

- ≥10% plasma cells

Cytogenetics

- Chromosome 13 deletion
- Translocation (4;14)
- Del (17p)

The skeleton is involved at the time of diagnosis in most patients with MM.[16] Bone scans show abnormalities that often include lytic lesions, osteoporosis, or fractures. The effects of MM on the skeleton result from abnormal production of cytokines including IL-1, IL-6, TNF-α, and the receptor for activation of NF-κB ligand (RANK-L). Bone disease is the net effect of the activation of osteoclasts and inhibition of osteoblastogenesis.[17]

In addition to bone disease, patients are frequently anemic from infiltration of the bone marrow with the MM clone and poor erythropoietin response. Those patients with low erythropoietin levels benefit most from erythropoietic therapy. Patients can have clinically important hypercalcemia, which results from calcium mobilization from the bone. Renal failure can occur as a result of high protein load from the monoclonal protein secretion as well as dehydration.

TABLE 139-1 The International Staging System (ISS) for Multiple Myeloma

Stage	Characteristics	Median Survival (Months)
I	Serum β_2-microglobulin <3.5 mcg/mL Serum albumin ≥3.5 g/dL	62
II	Not stage I or stage III	44
III	Serum β_2-microglobulin ≥5.5 mcg/mL	29

From Greipp PR, Miguel JS, Durie BG, et al. International staging system for multiple myeloma. J Clin Oncol 2005;23:3412–3420. Reprinted with premission from the American Society of Clinical Oncology.

STAGING AND PROGNOSTIC FACTORS

Some patients with MM are asymptomatic and have no evidence of end-organ damage at the time of diagnosis. These patients are categorized as having smoldering (or asymptomatic) MM.[1,9] Most patients will have evidence of end-organ damage (hypercalcemia [>10.5 g/dL], renal impairment [>2.0 mg/dL], anemia [<10 g/dL or >2 g/dL below normal], or bone disease) at the time of diagnosis and are categorized as having active (symptomatic) disease. Patients with asymptomatic disease have an indolent course, with a median survival of about 5 years.[9]

A new International Staging System (ISS) uses serum β_2-microglobulin and albumin concentrations to stage patients.[18] These two routine laboratory tests are powerful prognostic discriminators. Using the ISS, researchers have shown that older age negatively affects survival. ISS predicts survival in patients treated with either conventional treatment or autologous hematopoietic stem cell transplantation (autoHSCT). An older staging system, Durie-Salmon, uses hemoglobin, serum calcium, bone involvement, and M protein to categorize patients in one of three stages. Table 139–1 describes the ISS and median survival for each of the three ISS stages.

Several negative prognostic factors have been proposed for MM, including chromosome 13 deletion and other cytogenetic abnormalities, elevated β_2-microglobulin, elevated C-reactive protein, high plasma cell labeling index, low albumin, and high bone marrow microvessel density.[1] Some of these prognostic factors are incorporated into the ISS. These prognostic factors generally represent the underlying pathologic changes associated with MM including genetic damage (chromosome 13 deletion), proinflammatory changes (C-reactive protein), tumor load (β_2-microglobulin) and dysregulated cellular growth (labeling index and marrow microvessel density).

TREATMENT

Multiple Myeloma

OVERVIEW OF INITIAL THERAPY

3 MM is not a curable disease. The role of therapy is to prolong progression-free and overall survival and improve quality of life. Patients with more active (symptomatic) or advanced disease (stages II and III) require therapy.[1,14,19] In patients with smoldering (asymptomatic) or stage I disease, watchful waiting is the general practice despite a systematic review that suggests early treatment with chemotherapy slows disease progression and may decrease vertebral compression.[20] These benefits are offset by the absence of convincing

TABLE 139-2 Drug Therapy in Newly Diagnosed Multiple Myeloma

Induction Regimen	Level of Evidence
Regimens in Non-AutoHSCT Candidates	***Category***
Melphalan + prednisone (MP)	2A
Melphalan + prednisone + thalidomide (MPT)	1
Melphalan + prednisone + bortezomib (MPV)	2B
Regimens Regardless of AutoHSCT Eligibility	
Vincristine + doxorubicin + dexamethasone	2A
Dexamethasone	2A
Thalidomide + dexamethasone	2A
Liposomal doxorubicin + vincristine + dexamethasone (DVD)	2A
Lenalidomide + dexamethasone	2B
Bortezomib + dexamethasone	2B
Bortezomib + doxorubicin + dexamethasone	2B
Bortezomib + thalidomide + dexamethasone	2B

Category 1: Uniform NCCN consensus based on high level evidence.
Category 2A: Uniform NCCN consensus based on lower evidence, including clinical experience.
Category 2B: Nonuniform NCCN consensus but no major disagreement.
Data from NCCN Guidelines NCCN. Clinical Practice Guidelines in Oncology. Multiple Myeloma. Version 2007. http://www.NCCN.org.

evidence that early treatment improves overall survival and important toxicities associated with therapy. The National Comprehensive Cancer Network (NCCN) Guidelines support watchful waiting for smoldering or stage I MM.[14]

Initial management of symptomatic MM depends on high-risk features of the disease (cytogenetics), patient age, performance status, and whether autoHSCT is planned. Although current treatments are not curative, median survival has increased significantly from about 7 months to 24 to 36 months primarily as a result of improved treatment of symptomatic MM and supportive care.[1] There is no standard initial or induction therapy for the treatment of symptomatic MM. Table 139–2 lists commonly used regimens, which are categorized based on whether or not the patient is an autoHSCT candidate. The age restriction for autoHSCT has changed because of low transplant-related mortality, but autoHSCT is generally reserved for patients ≤65 years of age.

The choice of induction therapy in autoHSCT candidates include VAD (vincristine, doxorubicin, and dexamethasone) or VAD-like chemotherapy, dexamethasone combined with thalidomide, lenalidomide, or bortezomib, and high-dose dexamethasone alone. Melphalan is usually avoided in patients who are eligible for autoHSCT because of its adverse effect on stem cell mobilization. When autoHSCT is not an option, melphalan plus prednisone is an acceptable choice for induction therapy but many clinicians add thalidomide to melphalan and prednisone (MPT) based on the results of randomized controlled trials that show significantly higher response rates and longer progression-free survival with MPT. MPT is listed as a preferred first-line therapy in the NCCN Guidelines and a recently published Mayo Clinic Consensus Statement (Table 139–3).[14,19] Maintenance therapy is not recommended outside of the context of a clinical trial.

CLINICAL CONTROVERSY

For patients who are autoHSCT candidates, induction therapy has usually involved the administration of 4 months of VAD. High-dose dexamethasone alone is also an option, given that most of the activity of VAD resides with dexamethasone. Newer agents, such as thalidomide, bortezomib, or lenalidomide, combined with dexamethasone show promising activity and are increasingly being used as induction therapy. However, thalidomide or lenalidomide combined with high-dose dexamethasone have increased toxicity as compared to high-dose dexamethasone alone. The elevated risk of venous thromboembolism requires prophylaxis, which makes these regimens less convenient. The Mayo Clinic Consensus Statement lists the combination of lenalidomide plus low-dose dexamethasone as a preferred induction regimen in autoHSCT candidates because of its high activity and lower incidence of venous thromboembolism.[19] Bortezomib is generally well tolerated but is associated with significant rates of neuropathy and requires intravenous administration. There are no convincing data to show that the higher response rates associated with these newer regimens lead to improved outcomes in patients undergoing autoHSCT. Therefore, none of the available induction regimens can be considered standard of care, and VAD and high-dose dexamethasone induction remain acceptable options.

TABLE 139-3 Evidence-Based Treatment Recommendations for Newly Diagnosed Multiple Myeloma

Recommendation	Strength of Recommendation and Level of Evidence[a]
Melphalan, prednisone, and thalidomide (MPT) should be used as initial therapy for standard-risk patients ineligible for autoHSCT	A I–II
MPT (as an alternative, consider a bortezomib-containing regimen to maximal response) should be used as initial therapy for high-risk patients ineligible for autoHSCT	D III (for MPT) D III–IV (for considering bortezomib-based regimen)
Lenalidomide and low-dose dexamethasone should be used as induction therapy for standard- and high-risk patients eligible for autoHSCT	B II–III
Early autoHSCT, followed by a second HSCT (if the patient does not achieve a very good partial response or better with the first HSCT) should be used as consolidation therapy for standard-risk patients eligible for HSCT	B I

autoHSCT, autologous hematopoietic stem cell transplantation.
[a]Strength of recommendations: A, evidence of type I or consistent findings from multiple studies of types II, III, or IV; B, evidence of types II, III, or IV, and findings are generally consistent; C, evidence of types II, III, or IV, but findings are inconsistent; D, little or no systematic empirical evidence. Quality of evidence: I, evidence from meta-analysis of multiple, well-designed, controlled studies, randomized trials with low false-positive and low false-negative errors (high power); II, evidence from at least one well-designed experimental study, randomized trials with high false-positive and/or negative errors (low power); III, evidence from well-designed, quasiexperimental studies, such as nonrandomized, controlled single-group, prepost, cohort, time, or matched case-control studies; IV, evidence from case reports and clinical examples.
Data from Dispenzieri A, Rajkumar SV, Gertz MA, et al. Treatment of newly diagnosed multiple myeloma based on Mayo Stratification of Myeloma and Risk-adapted Therapy (mSmart): Concensus statement. Mayo Clin Proc 2007:82:323–341.

Clinical response to therapy is generally defined by a reduction in paraprotein in blood and urine.[1] Clinical complete response is defined as elimination of plasma paraprotein, as measured by electrophoresis and immunofixation, and plasma cells (≤5%) in the bone marrow. Complete responses are uncommon in MM and lesser responses, including minor response, partial response, and very good partial response, are more commonly attained. These lesser responses can be important because they may correlate with improved survival. Table 139–4 describes the most common types of responses that are used clinically.[14]

DRUGS USED IN THE MANAGEMENT OF MULTIPLE MYELOMA

Conventional Chemotherapy

Two of the common conventional chemotherapy regimens used to treat MM are melphalan plus prednisone (MP) and VAD (Table 139–5).[21] The use of conventional-dose melphalan has an adverse effect on stem cell mobilization and subsequent autoHSCT. Mel-

TABLE 139-4 Definition of Clinical Response in Multiple Myeloma

Type of Response	Definition[a]
Minor response (MR)	• 25%–49% decrease in serum M protein • Reduction in 24-hour urine light chain by 50–89%
Partial response (PR)	• ≥50% decrease in serum M protein • Reduction in 24-hour urine light chain by ≥90%
Very good partial remission (vgPR)	• Serum and urine M protein detected on immunofixation but not electrophoresis
Complete remission (CR)	• Negative immunofixation on serum and urine • No soft-tissue plasmacytomas • <5% plasma cells in the bone marrow

[a]Maintained for a minimum of 6 weeks.

phalan may also lead to the development of myelodysplastic syndrome.[22] Despite these adverse effects, MP remains an acceptable initial therapy for older patients who are not eligible for autoHSCT.[14]

The use of VAD (or VAD-like) chemotherapy as initial treatment became more common because of these concerns with melphalan. However, the slightly higher response rates with VAD and similar combination chemotherapy did not translate into improved survival as compared to melphalan.[23]

Dexamethasone accounts for most of the antimyeloma activity of VAD (see Table 139–5), which led to the use of dexamethasone alone as upfront therapy. However, a recent study reported that melphalan plus prednisone produced similar response rates and survival as compared to dexamethasone. The higher rate of infection and CNS toxicity in patients treated with dexamethasone led these investigators to conclude that high-dose dexamethasone be used with caution as upfront therapy, particularly in older patients who are not eligible for autoHSCT and who would usually receive MP.[24] Increasingly, patients who are autoHSCT candidates receive dexamethasone and thalidomide to maximize initial response rates. In addition, newer therapies, such as bortezomib and lenalidomide, continue to be investigated as upfront therapy.[14,19,25]

Thalidomide (Thalomid)

Thalidomide was first used clinically in Europe in the late 1950s as a sedative and antiemetic but its use was largely abandoned when

TABLE 139-5 Initial Therapies for Multiple Myeloma

	Type of Response		
Regimen	***OR (%)***	***CR (%)***	***CR + near CR (%)***
Melphalan + prednisone[25,35]	40–50	1–2	5–10
Dexamethasone[24,34]	40–50	1	
Thalidomide[32]	34–40		
Thalidomide + dexamethasone[30,33,34]	50–70	5	
Melphalan, prednisone, and thalidomide[30,35,36]	70–80	15–30	20–40
VAD and related chemotherapy[56,59]	50–60		
Doxorubicin combinations + thalidomide[30,37]	70–90	10–30	40-50
Single autoHSCT[55,58,59]	80–90	10–40	40–50
Tandem autoHSCT[64,65,66]	80–90	20–40	30–50
AutoHSCT followed by RI-alloHSCT[72,73]	80–90	50–60	60
Bortezomib[48]	40–50	3	12
Bortezomib + dexamethasone[48,49]	80–90	5–20	20–30
Bortezomib + chemotherapy[25]	89	32	43
Lenalidomide + dexamethasone[30]	90	6	38
Lenalidomide + chemotherapy[25]	85	17	41

alloHSCT, allogeneic hematopoietic stem cell transplantation; autoHSCT, autologous hematopoietic stem cell transplantation; CR, complete response; OR, overall response (at least PR); RI, reduced intensity; VAD, vincristine, doxorubicin, and dexamethasone.

teratogenicity was reported. Its immunomodulatory effects became evident with its use in Hansen's disease (or leprosy), and it continues to be used for this rare indication. These clinical benefits are thought to be related to the anti-TNF activity of thalidomide. Because of the role of inflammatory cytokines in the pathophysiology of MM, thalidomide was first studied in refractory MM in 1999. The realization that thalidomide had activity against myeloma rejuvenated it as an important therapeutic agent.[26]

Thalidomide has multiple immune effects including inhibition of inflammatory mediators, antiangiogenic activity, and T-cell modulating activity.[27] Thalidomide destabilizes TNF-α messenger RNA leading to increased destruction of the transcripts and reduction in TNF-α production. One potential explanation for thalidomide's anti-myeloma activity is inhibition of TNF-mediated NF-κB activation, which results in increased apoptosis of the MM clone. Thalidomide also has TNF-independent effects; it protects the cytosolic IκB and prevents signal transduction to the nucleus, resulting in a decline in MM growth factors.[26,27]

Myeloma bone marrow has a high rate of neovascularization, which makes it susceptible to antiangiogenic therapy. Bone marrow microvessel density has been identified as an independent prognostic factor in MM.[28] One explanation for the angiogenesis that occurs in MM is the paracrine release of TNF-α by the myeloma clone and bone marrow stromal cells, which leads to the release of angiogenic factors, including VEGF, IL-8, bFGF, and IL-1, through NF-κB induction. Thalidomide treatment can reduce bone marrow microvessel density, which may contribute to its antimyeloma activity.

The role of TNF-α inhibition is supported by a small study that showed that TNF-α polymorphisms predicted for thalidomide response in patients with MM.[29] High producers of TNF-α had significantly higher response rates and improved survival with thalidomide therapy as compared to patients without the hypersecretory phenotype. These results may be explained by inhibition of TNF-α as a required growth factor in patients with the TNF-α hypersecretory phenotype. The authors commented that larger studies are required to confirm and explain these results. Figure 139–1 shows that thalidomide inhibits proliferation and angiogenesis, stimulates T lymphocytes, and modifies the cytokine-secreting ability of bone marrow stromal cells.

Single-agent thalidomide has been extensively evaluated in refractory MM where it produces overall response rates (includes minor responses) in the 30% to 40% range with rare complete remissions.[30] Although minor and partial responses are the most common types of responses, these end points result in improvement in survival.[31]

❹ With the activity of thalidomide in refractory MM established, subsequent studies evaluated its activity in newly diagnosed patients and in combination with other therapies, including dexamethasone and chemotherapy. Partial response rates with single-agent thalidomide in untreated patients are approximately 30% to 40%, and response rates increase to 60% to 70% when minor responses are included.[32] When dexamethasone is added to thalidomide in untreated patients, response rates increase to approximately 90% if minor responses are included.[33] The higher response rate with thalidomide plus dexamethasone makes this an attractive combination for initial therapy. However, the higher rate of thromboembolism with this combination (15% to 20%) is a concern.[34] In addition, the complete remission rate remains low (<5%).

The addition of thalidomide to chemotherapy also increases response rates (see Table 139–5). Two randomized controlled trials in newly diagnosed MM showed that the addition of thalidomide to MP results in an increased response rate.[35,36] In the first randomized trial, the overall response rate with MPT was 76% with a complete and near-complete response rate of greater than 15%.[35] The higher response rates with MPT translated into superior 2-year event-free (54% vs. 27%; $P = 0.0006$) and a trend in improved 3-year survival

(80% vs. 64%; $P = 0.19$).[35] The second randomized trial was stopped early because MPT showed clear improvements over the other treatment arms. Results of that trial also showed significantly improved median progression-free (27.5 vs. 17.8 months) and overall survival (51.6 vs. 33.2 months) with MPT.[36] Based on these impressive results, some have recommended that MPT be the new standard induction therapy in older patients ineligible for autoHSCT (see Table 139–3).[19,25] The increased response rate of MPT is at the expense of higher rates of grades III and IV toxicity (48% vs. 25%), particularly venous thromboembolism (VTE), peripheral neuropathy, and infection.[35]

The combination of thalidomide, dexamethasone, and pegylated liposomal doxorubicin produces a high overall response rate of 98% and a complete remission rate of 34%. The major grades III and IV toxicities were VTE (14%) and infection (22%). Toxicity was acceptable, even in patients older than 65 years of age.[37] Although the activity of doxorubicin plus thalidomide compares favorably with other combinations (see Table 139–5), one disadvantage of this regimen is that pegylated liposomal doxorubicin requires intravenous administration. The high response rate of thalidomide plus pegylated liposomal doxorubicin combinations needs to be confirmed in a randomized trial that compares it with an accepted standard.

Thalidomide dose correlates with response and toxicity. In one large trial of single-agent thalidomide, a higher response rate was observed when more than 42 g of thalidomide was administered over a 3-month period, which is equivalent to a daily dose of about 450 mg.[31] As expected, the higher dose was associated with higher rates of thalidomide-related toxicity. When thalidomide is combined with chemotherapy, thalidomide doses of 100 mg/day are associated with high complete remission rates.[35,37] Neuropathy, one of the important dose limiting toxicities, may correlate with cumulative thalidomide doses. Thalidomide-induced neuropathy is usually, but not always, reversible and is associated with demyelinating changes in peripheral neurons. Approximately 10% to 20% of patients are unable to tolerate thalidomide and neuropathy is often the toxicity associated with discontinuation of therapy.[31,38] Unfortunately, no effective methods have been identified to prevent or treat thalidomide-induced neuropathy.

Other common toxicities associated with thalidomide include constipation, sedation, and rash. While these toxicities can be problematic, they rarely require discontinuation of thalidomide treatment. Stimulant laxatives can be used to prevent severe constipation. Constipation and rash appear to be dose-related while sedation occurs at all dose levels. The severity of constipation and sedation declines over time in many patients.[30,38]

The rate of VTE with single-agent thalidomide is relatively low (1% to 3%) and may not exceed the baseline incidence for MM patients. VTE prophylaxis is not recommended in patients receiving single-agent thalidomide.[19] When thalidomide is combined with dexamethasone, MP, or doxorubicin, the risk of thrombosis is elevated. The underlying mechanism for thrombosis in these patients is unknown but rates in several studies of combination therapy were as high as 10% to 30%.[36,39,40] VTE prophylaxis is recommended and preventive strategies include therapeutic doses of warfarin or low-molecular-weight heparin.[19] Warfarin is associated with bleeding complications and should be reserved for patients with a history of VTE. Aspirin (81 mg or 325 mg) may be beneficial in preventing thrombosis, but large, well-controlled studies are required. Aspirin should be reserved for those patients at high risk of bleeding on warfarin or low-molecular-weight heparin.[34,41]

Bortezomib (Velcade)

❺ Bortezomib is a proteasome inhibitor approved for use in refractory MM. The proteasome is a protease complex responsible for degrading cytosolic proteins that are conjugated to ubiquitin. Ubiquitin is a 8.5-kilodalton polypeptide that tags various proteins for destruction.[42] By reversibly binding to the chymotrypsin site in the catalytic core of the 26S proteasome, bortezomib inhibits the degradation of these targeted proteins.

In MM, NF-κB activity is increased, resulting in increased transcription of inflammatory cytokines such as IL-6 and TNF-α, which are involved in the pathogenesis and progression of MM. In the cytosol, NF-κB is bound to and inhibited by IκB. The proteasome degrades IκB. When the proteasome is inhibited with bortezomib, cytosolic concentrations of IκB remain high and NF-κB is retained in the cytosol as an inactive complex. The resulting inhibition of NF-κB signal leads to a reduction in cytokine production and growth inhibition of the MM clone. Other proteins involved in cell-cycle regulation and apoptotic signaling that may be affected by bortezomib include p53, JNK proteins, and capase-3.[42]

In phase I studies in patients with refractory hematologic malignancies, bortezomib was administered twice weekly for 2 consecutive weeks followed by a week of rest. The responses observed in those studies included a complete response in 1 of 8 patients who completed the first course of therapy and minor responses in two patients. These responses were impressive for a phase I trial and confirmed the promising activity in preclinical studies.[43]

Patients with refractory MM were enrolled into a phase II trial and received 1.3 mg/m^2 of bortezomib twice weekly for 2 weeks followed by a week of rest. Patients received up to eight cycles. The overall response rate was 35% (includes minor responses) with 7 (3.6%) patients achieving a complete response.[44] In a second phase II study, the overall response rate increased to 50% (includes minor responses) when bortezomib was combined with dexamethasone. Based on the phase I and II studies, bortezomib was approved in May 2003 under the FDA's accelerated approval process for relapsed or refractory MM in patients who had failed at least two prior therapies.[45]

Subsequently, a large phase III study (Assessment of Proteasome Inhibition for Extending Remissions [APEX] trial) demonstrated that bortezomib had superior activity as compared to high-dose dexamethasone in relapsed MM.[46] Bortezomib-treated patients had higher complete and partial response rates (38% vs. 18%), longer median time to progression (6.2 vs. 3.5 months), and improved 1-year overall survival (80% vs. 66%) as compared to patients receiving dexamethasone. The differences in each of these end points were statistically significant. The results from this study led to expanded FDA approval in 2005 to include patients who had relapsed after one therapy.

Combination therapy with bortezomib has shown promising results in relapsed MM in a number of small phases I and II studies. It had been observed that patients who had suboptimal response to bortezomib responded after the addition of dexamethasone. Subsequent studies reported improved results with the combination of bortezomib and corticosteroids with the complete and near complete response rate ranging between 5% and 15%.[47] The combination of bortezomib with either doxorubicin or melphalan is being evaluated, with early results suggesting similar or higher overall response rates than when it is combined with dexamethasone.[47]

There are limited data on bortezomib in newly diagnosed patients (see Table 139–5). Bortezomib alone produces about a 40% response rate (complete remission plus partial response) with approximately 3% of patients obtaining a complete remission. When combined with dexamethasone, the overall response rate increases to approximately 90% (complete remission plus partial response) with complete remissions of 5% to 20%.[48,49] In a phase II study of bortezomib combined with MP in newly diagnosed elderly MM patients, the overall response rates of 89% and complete remission rates of 32% are among the highest reported with induction therapies.[50] Based on these results, the Mayo Clinic Consensus Statement recommends that a bortezomib-containing regimen be considered as initial therapy for high-risk patients who are not eligible for hematopoietic stem cell transplantation (see Table 139–3).[19]

Bortezomib is a relatively well-tolerated drug. The most common toxicities include mild-to-moderate fatigue and gastrointestinal toxicities. Neuropathy occurs less frequently but is the most common cause for discontinuation of therapy. In the APEX trial, the rate of neuropathy was 36% in the bortezomib group versus 9% in the dexamethasone group.[46] Eight percent of patients with refractory or relapsed MM required discontinuation of therapy because of severe neuropathy. Newly diagnosed patients tolerate bortezomib better than patients with relapsed or refractory MM, with only 1% to 2% discontinuing therapy. Other important toxicities included thrombocytopenia, fever, neutropenia, and infection. An increased incidence of shingles was reported in bortezomib-treated patients, and the NCCN Guidelines recommend that herpes zoster prophylaxis be considered.[14] VTE prophylaxis is not required with bortezomib-containing regimens.

Lenalidomide (Revlimid)

❻ Lenalidomide is a thalidomide analog that shares a similar mechanism of action with thalidomide, but is significantly more potent than thalidomide. Because of differences in the toxicity profile, the use of lenalidomide is likely to increase. In a phase II study, patients with relapsed, refractory MM were randomized to two doses of lenalidomide (15 vs. 30 mg). Overall response rates were 24% in this group of heavily pretreated patients who were generally resistant to thalidomide.[51] The 30-mg dose was well tolerated and had better complete response rates as compared to the 15 mg dose (0 vs 6%).

The addition of lenalidomide to high-dose dexamethasone has been shown to increase response rate and prolong survival in patients with relapsed MM. In 2006, lenalidomide received FDA approval based on the results of two recently published randomized controlled trials.[52,53] One trial was conducted in North America while the other trial was conducted outside of North America. In both trials, patients were randomized to receive a combination of either lenalidomide (25 mg per day on days 1 to 21 of a 28-day cycle) or an identical placebo and high-dose dexamethasone. In the North American trial, patients in the lenalidomide and dexamethasone group had overall (complete, near-complete, or partial) and complete response rates of 61% and 14%, as compared to 20% and 0.6% in the dexamethasone alone group ($p < 0.001$).[53] These improved response rates translated into longer median overall survival in the lenalidomide and dexamethasone group (29.6 vs. 20.5 months). Similar results were reported in the trial conducted outside of the United States.[52]

Lenalidomide has been studied as upfront therapy in newly diagnosed MM (see Table 139–5). Preliminary results of phase I and phase II studies of lenalidomide plus dexamethasone report an overall response rate of 90% and a complete response rate of 18%.[30] These rates are higher than those reported with thalidomide plus dexamethasone. Lenalidomide causes less neurotoxicity and constipation but more myelosuppression than thalidomide.[51–53] When used as part of combination therapy, the risk of VTE with lenalidomide is similar to that observed with thalidomide and VTE prophylaxis is recommended. Preliminary results from a phase III trial in newly diagnosed MM reported that patients randomized to lenalidomide plus high-dose dexamethasone had an 25% incidence of VTE as compared to a 9% rate in those randomized to the lenalidomide plus low-dose dexamethasone arm.[54] That trial also reported superior 18 month survival in the lenalidomide plus low-dose dexamethasone group (91% vs. 80%) and this regimen could become the new standard induction regimen for patients undergoing autoHSCT. Based on these results, the Mayo Clinic Consensus Statement lists lenalidomide plus low-dose dexamethasone as the preferred induction regimen in patients undergoing autoHSCT because of its low toxicity profile and its activity in relapsed patients (see Table 139–3).[19] The low risk of VTE in the lenalidomide plus low-dose dexamethasone arm may allow for VTE prophylaxis with aspirin alone.[19]

Summary of Newer Therapy Combinations as Initial Therapy

Increasingly, chemotherapy is being added to thalidomide, lenalidomide, or bortezomib as upfront therapy. Melphalan and prednisone can be the backbone to which these newer drugs are added if the patient is not a candidate for autoHSCT. As previously discussed, MPT produces high response rates and bortezomib added to melphalan plus prednisone produces similar results.[25,35,36] Based on the results of phase III trials demonstrating superiority of MPT over MP, many experts believe that MPT is the preferred induction regimen in patients who are ineligible for autoHSCT, at least until results of randomized controlled trials with lenalidomide or bortezomib are available (see Table 139–3).[14,19] The addition of bortezomib to melphalan and prednisone may be particularly useful in MM patients with high-risk cytogenetics (chromosome 13 deletion, t(4;14), and 17p-).

If autoHSCT is planned after induction therapy, melphalan plus prednisone should be avoided, and thalidomide, bortezomib, or lenalidomide can be added to dexamethasone or VAD-like chemotherapy. The NCCN Guidelines lists several induction therapies (see Table 139–2). Because there is no standard induction regimen, clinicians can select from a wide range of possible induction regimens (see Table 139–5). Although some experts recommend lenalidomide and low-dose dexamethasone in patients who are autoHSCT candidates (see Table 139–3), thalidomide plus dexamethasone remains a reasonable choice until more data are available. Patients with chromosome 13 or 17p deletion may benefit most from bortezomib-containing induction regimens because of its activity in these high-risk patients.[19] Because patients with high-risk cytogenetics may have poorer outcomes after autoHSCT, bortezomib-containing regimens should be considered in this group of patients, regardless of their eligibility for autoHSCT (see Table 139–3).[19]

Several ongoing phase III trials should determine the comparative efficacy of the various induction regimens. Thalidomide plus MP is being compared to lenalidomide plus MP in a United States Intergroup trial, while bortezomib plus MP is being compared to MP in the VISTA (Velcade as Initial Standard Therapy in multiple myeloma: Assessment with melphalan and prednisone) trial. The results of these trials are eagerly awaited for treatment of elderly MM patients.

■ AUTOLOGOUS HEMATOPOIETIC STEM CELL TRANSPLANTATION

Although MM is a chemosensitive tumor with significant response rates after treatment with conventional chemotherapy, complete remission rates are low and the duration of response is short. In an attempt to improve outcomes with chemotherapy, high-dose chemotherapy regimens that require stem cell support have been used after initial induction therapy. The intent of the induction therapy prior to transplant is to reduce tumor load but it remains controversial whether or not the quality of response (partial vs. complete) associated with induction is predictive of outcomes when followed by transplantation.

Several well-designed, randomized, controlled trials have evaluated the role of high-dose chemotherapy followed by autoHSCT. Previously untreated patients were usually randomized to induction therapy alone versus the same induction therapy followed by high-dose chemotherapy and autoHSCT. The results generally showed that autoHSCT improved progression-free survival with a more variable effect on overall survival.[55–57] No survival plateau has been observed in the group treated with autoHSCT, which suggests that few, if any, patients are cured of their disease. Despite these variable effects on overall survival, MM has become the leading indication for autoHSCT worldwide.

7 A systematic review of autoHSCT in newly diagnosed MM was published in 2007.[57] The review pooled results from 9 studies comprising 2,411 patients randomized to either autoHSCT or standard therapy. The combined hazard ratio for overall survival with autoHSCT was 0.92 (95% confidence interval 0.74 to 1.13) and for progression-free survival was 0.75 (95% confidence interval 0.59 to 0.96). These results indicate that high-dose therapy with autoHSCT significantly improves progression-free survival but does not significantly improve overall survival. This benefit in progression-free survival was at the expense of greater transplant-related mortality. Patients who received autoHSCT had a threefold higher risk of treatment-related death as compared to conventional dose chemotherapy. The authors concluded that for every 26 patients who received a transplant, there would be one excess death from autoHSCT as compared to conventional chemotherapy.

Two of the randomized trials comparing autoHSCT to standard therapy in newly diagnosed MM included in the systematic review were recently updated. Barlogie et al. reported that progression-free and overall survival were equivalent between high-dose and conventional-dose groups.[58] This is different than the conclusions of the systematic review, which reported a significant improvement in progression-free survival. That study has been criticized for using total-body irradiation plus melphalan rather than the more commonly used high-dose melphalan alone. However, several other studies that used total-body irradiation in addition to melphalan have reported variable results, which suggest that the differences in the preparative regimen do not explain these negative results. In the second study, Fermand et al. showed a benefit in event-free survival but no benefit in overall survival. These results were consistent with the systematic review. This study used standard high-dose melphalan and compared it to conventional therapy in previously untreated patients.[59]

Although the use of autoHSCT as upfront therapy has become standard of care in patients younger than age 65 years, it is associated with higher treatment-related mortality and there is no convincing evidence that it prolongs overall survival. The widespread adoption of autoHSCT as standard therapy is related to the significant improvement in progression-free survival. But as conventional therapy continues to improve, response rates and progression-free survival are likely to approach those seen with autoHSCT without the elevated risk of transplant-related mortality.

Most patients are treated with autoHSCT as initial therapy after a short course of induction chemotherapy. However, a smaller number of patients receive autoHSCT as salvage therapy after patients have failed conventional treatments. A study in the early 1990s compared autoHSCT with chemotherapy in previously treated MM patients.[60] The results of that study showed that high-dose therapy was no better then VAD alone. However, more recent studies report benefit from autoHSCT in both primary treatment failures and relapsed MM.[61,62] The NCCN Guidelines list autoHSCT as one of the acceptable options in the salvage setting. Responses to autoHSCT in the salvage setting can occur even in patients who have relapsed after prior successful autoHSCT.[14]

The optimal timing of autoHSCT (early vs. late) in MM was investigated in a randomized controlled trial. Patients were randomized to early (N = 91) or late transplantation (N = 94) and no significant difference in 5-year overall survival was observed between the groups.[63] Event-free survival, however, was significantly longer in the early transplantation group (39 months vs. 13 months). In an analysis that factors in the time without symptoms, treatment, or treatment toxicity (TWisTT), patients receiving early transplantation had a longer time in a state associated with good quality of life (27.8 vs. 22.3 months). The results of this study support early autoHSCT because of its effects on event-free survival and quality of life.

A specialized form of autoHSCT is tandem transplantation, which involves the use of two separate autoHSCT procedures separated by a rest period of several months. In a heterogeneous group of 1,000 newly diagnosed and previously treated patients receiving autoHSCT for MM, 70% were able to receive a second autoHSCT. The complete remission rate was 44% with a 5-year event-free survival of 25% and 5-year overall survival of 40%.[64] Transplant-related mortality was low but was higher in patients receiving both transplants (2.7% vs. 4.8%). Approximately 10% to 15% of patients who did not achieve a complete remission with the first transplantation, attained it with the second transplantation.[64,65] Because of this increased risk of mortality with tandem transplantation, it would be helpful to identify those patients who would benefit most. The French group reported that patients who did not achieve at least a very good partial response after the first transplantation benefited most from the second transplant.[66] That study reported an estimated 7-year overall survival of 21% in the single-transplantation arm and a 42% survival in the double-transplantation arm.

Because nearly all patients treated with either single or tandem transplantations will eventually relapse, maintenance therapy after autoHSCT has been studied. Maintenance therapy after autoHSCT may be the ideal situation as maintenance is likely to be most effective in patients with minimal residual disease. Variable results and high toxicities have been reported with IFN-α and dexamethasone and neither drug can be recommended outside of a clinical trial.[67] Thalidomide has also been studied as maintenance after autoHSCT. In the largest study to date, 593 patients were randomized to receive either no maintenance, pamidronate alone, or the combination of thalidomide plus pamidronate. Patients randomized to the thalidomide group had significantly longer event-free and overall survival as compared with those who received no thalidomide.[68] The median duration of thalidomide maintenance was 15 months and the average dose was 200 mg per day. Nearly 40% of patients had to discontinue thalidomide as a consequence of toxicity. In a subgroup analysis, patients with deletion of chromosome 13 did not benefit and other maintenance therapies need to be found for this high-risk group. Maintenance trials are ongoing with bortezomib and lenalidomide, which may be more effective in these high-risk MM patients. Bortezomib and lenalidomide may also be better tolerated than thalidomide. The NCCN Guidelines indicate that there is no consensus on the use of dexamethasone and IFN-α maintenance. Thalidomide, lenalidomide, or bortezomib should be used as maintenance therapy in the context of a clinical trial.[14,19]

The primary conclusion that can be drawn from the current data on autoHSCT in MM is that it should be used in younger patients with good performance status as part of initial therapy.[14,19] Prior to transplant, all patients should receive induction therapy to reduce tumor burden. Because of higher transplant-related mortality, a second autoHSCT or allogeneic hematopoietic stem cell transplantation (alloHSCT) should only be considered in patients who do not achieve a very good partial response or better with the first autoHSCT (see Table 139–3).

■ ALLOGENEIC HEMATOPOIETIC STEM CELL TRANSPLANTATION

AlloHSCT uses a stem cell source other than the patient themselves and is therefore a transplant across immunologic barriers. The major posttransplant complications associated with transplanting across these barriers, are graft failure and acute and chronic graft-versus-host disease. Acute or chronic graft-versus-host disease may be associated with a graft-versus-myeloma effect. The graft-versus-myeloma effect, which is mediated by antitumor effector cells from the graft-versus-host disease reaction, reduces relapse risk and may offer the patient the best chance for long-term disease-free survival.[69] Unlike autoHSCT, which is simply a method of increasing the dose-intensity of chemotherapy, alloHSCT is an immune therapy. This is supported by the success of nonmyeloablative alloHSCT in some leukemias, where reduced-intensity preparation provides sufficient immunosuppression for the graft to survive and mediate a graft-versus-tumor effect.[70]

❽ Despite data reporting lower relapse rates in MM patients, myeloablative alloHSCT produces high transplant-related mortality (20% to 50%), leading to overall survival rates similar to autoHSCT.[62] The reasons for the high transplant-related mortality in alloHSCT are not entirely clear. One possible explanation is that MM patients come to transplantation heavily pretreated, at an older age, and with greater existing organ damage as compared to other cancers. However, a study was closed prematurely in MM patients younger than 55 years of age with minimal pretreatment because of unacceptably high transplant-related mortality (approximately 50%).[65]

With the high transplant-related mortality associated with myeloablative alloHSCT, the use of nonmyeloablative alloHSCT is an attractive option to reduce early posttransplant mortality. Several conclusions can be made based on the available data on the use of nonmyeloablative alloHSCT in MM patients. First, the transplant-related mortality associated with nonmyeloablative alloHSCT is lower than that reported with myeloablative alloHSCT.[65,71] Second, the cytoreductive activity of the reduced-intensity preparation may be insufficient for the graft-versus-myeloma effect to have its full impact.[65] Most immune therapies, including the graft-versus-myeloma reaction, are most effective when patients have minimal residual disease and nonmyeloablative alloHSCT may have insufficient antitumor activity to achieve important tumor reduction. The need for cytoreduction may be accomplished by autoHSCT preceding the reduced-intensity alloHSCT procedure. Two recent trials of this novel approach produced conflicting results when comparing tandem autoHSCT to single autoHSCT followed by reduced-intensity alloHSCT. In a trial by Garban et al., neither event-free nor overall survival differed between tandem autoHSCT and single autoHSCT followed by reduced-intensity alloHSCT.[72] However, a more recent trial reported significantly improved event-free and overall survival when autoHSCT was combined with reduced-intensity alloHSCT.[73] These conflicting results may relate to the inclusion of particularly high-risk patients and the use of more aggressive immunosuppression in the negative trial. In both trials, transplant-related mortality was not higher in the combined autoHSCT and reduced-intensity alloHSCT arm.[72,73] Until more data is available, combining autoHSCT with reduced intensity alloHSCT cannot be recommended outside of a clinical trial.[65]

■ SUPPORTIVE CARE

Bisphosphonates

Along with the anti-MM therapy described thus far in this chapter, supportive care measures are aggressively used to stabilize skeletal abnormalities. Bisphosphonates have been used for more than a decade in the management of MM. Once a well-accepted standard of care, the optimal use of bisphosphonates has become more controversial as a result of osteonecrosis of the jaw (ONJ), a rare, but serious adverse effect of bisphosphonate use in MM.

❾ Bisphosphonates have a major role in the treatment of bone-related complications associated with MM. Bone resorption is a manifestation of the disease process and is mediated in part by inflammatory molecules including IL-6, IL-1, and TNF-α.[1] Bone disease is not seen in MGUS but occurs in approximately 80% of MM patients at diagnosis.[74] Although the classic cytokine mediators of bone loss are important, a newer view involves excessive production of RANK-L, which activates NF-κB through its receptor (RANK).[75] As previously stated, NF-κB is a transcriptional regulator that increases the production of various inflammatory molecules. Normally, RANK-L mediated activation is in equilibrium with osteoprotegerin, which inhibits NF-κB by serving as a decoy receptor for RANK-L.[75,76] In the bone marrow of MM patients, excess RANK-L is produced particularly from stromal cells, which, when coupled with a decline in osteoprotegerin from both stromal cells and osteoblasts, leads to osteoclast activation and bone destruction. Macrophage inflammatory protein α_1, macrophage colony-stimulating factor, and VEGF may also play important roles in MM bone disease by stimulating the production and activation of osteoclasts.[77] Macrophage inflammatory protein α_1 is also an important chemotactic factor released by MM cells; it attracts osteoclast precursors, enabling myeloma cells to influence the maturation and activation of osteoclasts, which suggests that antimyeloma drugs can have a beneficial effect on MM bone disease.[77,78] Although MM bone disease may involve many cell types and many soluble and cell-bound molecules, it is useful to simplify its pathophysiology and consider it to be an imbalance between RANK-L and osteoprotegerin.

Activation of osteoclasts leads to a net loss of bone mass and to many of the common clinical features of MM, including fractures, hypercalcemia, and bone pain. The bone resorption is influenced by the MM cells in proximity to the osteolytic lesions and is associated with recruitment of osteoclasts.[78,79] The disruptive effect on skeletal integrity can lead to direct mortality, but more commonly has a major impact on morbidity and quality of life.[1]

Bisphosphonates are analogs of endogenous pyrophosphate but are more resistant to hydrolysis than pyrophosphate. Like endogenous pyrophosphate, the bisphosphonates bind to crystalline calcium in the bone and is then phagocytized by osteoclasts.[80] The best described effect of the bisphosphonates is the inhibition of osteoclast activity, which likely occurs by direct osteoclast cytotoxicity.[81] In addition to osteoclast inhibition, bisphosphonates may also promote apoptosis in MM cells. This effect may result from the inhibition of the mevalonic acid pathway, which produces several molecules required for growth of the MM clone.[82] The inhibition of mevalonic acid pathway is similar to the activity of the statins which have been shown to induce apoptosis in osteoclasts and MM cells. In addition, other potential antimyeloma effects of bisphosphonates may include modifying the cytokine microenvironment, inhibiting the adhesion of MM cells to bone marrow matrix cells, and inhibiting angiogenesis.[80] Although it is possible that bisphosphonates have an antimyeloma effect, there is little direct clinical evidence to support this activity.

The use of bisphosphonates in MM is based on the results from two large, randomized, controlled trials. In a pamidronate study, the drug was compared to placebo in a group of MM patients undergoing their first or second course of chemotherapy.[83] Several clinical end points were found to be positively impacted by pamidronate therapy. The investigators reported that patients in the pamidronate group had a lower risk of skeletal-related events, lower pain scores, and improved quality of life. Importantly, a survival advantage was observed in the pamidronate-treated patients who had already received one or more courses of antimyeloma chemotherapy. This finding of improved survival in subgroup analysis is part of the circumstantial evidence to propose an antimyeloma effect for the bisphosphonates.

Guidelines for the use of zoledronic acid in MM are based largely on a randomized study in MM and breast cancer. In patients with bone metastases, zoledronic acid was compared to pamidronate with the intent of demonstrating clinical equipoise.[84] The study did show equivalence between pamidronate and zoledronic acid. The lack of a placebo arm because of ethical concerns of restricting an effective therapy complicates interpretation of this study. Despite this limitation, pamidronate and zoledronic acid appear to have equivalent clinical benefit in stabilizing the skeleton.

Other randomized, controlled trials have been conducted, and the results of these trials were pooled in a systematic review.[85] Eleven randomized trials were included, which accounted for 1,113 MM patients receiving bisphosphonate therapy along with 1,070 MM patients in a control arm who received no bisphosphonate therapy. The risk of vertebral fractures was significantly lower in the bisphosphonate-treated patients as compared to controls (odds ratio = 0.59; 95% CI 0.45 to 0.78). Pain scores were also reduced (odds ratio = 0.59; 95% CI 0.46 to 0.76). Given that the aggregate data in the systematic review agreed with the large controlled studies described above, the effect on vertebral fractures and pain are well-supported benefits of bisphosphonate therapy.

Clinical practice guidelines for the use of bisphosphonates in MM were recently updated by an expert panel under the auspices of the American Society of Clinical Oncology Health Services Research Committee.[16] The evidence-based guidelines recommend that symptomatic MM patients be placed on bisphosphonate therapy at the time of diagnosis to reduce pain and skeletal-related events, and to improve quality of life. No firm recommendation was made on the duration of bisphosphonate therapy and which of the two agents should be used. However, the expert panel recommended a duration of bisphosphonate use of 2 years in those patients with responsive or stable disease. Reinstituting bisphosphonate therapy at relapse or progression is at the discretion of the clinician.[16]

CLINICAL CONTROVERSY

Although bisphosphonates are indicated in MM patients with bone disease, controversies surrounding the selection of agent and duration of therapy remain. Because of recent reports of ONJ in MM patients, a more cautious approach on bisphosphonate use is being considered. ONJ is associated with patients undergoing dental procedures, those receiving the more potent bisphosphonates, and those receiving longer than 2 years of bisphosphonate therapy. Clinical practice guidelines developed by Mayo Clinic recommend that all dental procedures be performed prior to the administration of bisphosphonates, that therapy be given for no more than 2 years, and that pamidronate rather than zoledronic acid be used in newly diagnosed patients.[86] Given the benefit of bisphosphonates on skeletal-related events, limiting therapy to 2 years remains controversial. The preference of pamidronate over zoledronic acid is also controversial given that ONJ also has been reported with pamidronate and the higher risk of ONJ with zoledronic acid is based on observational studies and not head-to-head randomized comparisons.

Although a good case can be made for the use of bisphosphonates early after the diagnosis of MM, many controversies remain, including whether an antimyeloma effect exists, how long patients should remain on this expensive therapy, and, most importantly, the risk of ONJ. The recent association between bisphosphonates and ONJ suggests a more cautious approach with bisphosphonate therapy.

ONJ is characterized by an area of exposed necrotic bone and often affects the mandible and the maxilla, but can also affect the soft palate. The development of ONJ may be related to dental disease and tooth extraction, and appears to be more common with zoledronic acid than with pamidronate. The relationship with zoledronic acid is sufficiently strong to lead the Mayo Clinic to recommend that pamidronate be used in newly diagnosed MM patients.[86] The incidence of ONJ is unknown but may be as high as 10% in MM patients receiving zoledronic acid for extended periods of time. Because the risk of ONJ during the first 2 years of pamidronate appears to be very low, the Mayo Clinic Guidelines recommend monthly infusions of pamidronate for 2 years after diagnosis.

Pamidronate and zoledronic acid are usually well tolerated. Flu-like symptoms can occur following the administration of bisphosphonates. Acute renal dysfunction can occur with both agents and is related to both infusion time and dose. For zoledronic acid, the risk of acute renal dysfunction is higher with the 8-mg dose (vs. 4 mg) and when the duration of infusion is 5 minutes (vs. 15 minutes). Similarly pamidronate should be dosed at 90 mg and infused over at least 2 hours. Patients with moderate renal dysfunction (creatinine clearance: 30 to 60 mL/min) should have the dose of zoledronic acid adjusted downward by 25% (3 mg). This recommendation was included in the zoledronic acid package insert and is based on a greater renal toxicity in patients with preexisting renal dysfunction.[16] Randomized studies suggest that renal effects are similar between pamidronate and zoledronic acid, and for this reason patients on bisphosphonate therapy should have serum creatinine measured at baseline and then periodically thereafter.[16,87]

SALVAGE THERAPY

⑩ The same drugs used to treat MM initially can also be used as salvage therapy in MM patients who have relapsed. Salvage therapy is used at relapse, regardless of whether the patient had received a previous transplant. Patients who relapse 6 months after initial induction therapy can have that induction therapy repeated. Bortezomib is an effective salvage therapy. When bortezomib was compared to high-dose dexamethasone, response rates were 38% versus 18%, respectively.[46] The activity of bortezomib in patients with high-risk cytogenetics is particularly useful because these high-risk patients are more likely to relapse and require salvage therapy. Lenalidomide plus dexamethasone is also approved for treating patients in the salvage setting, based on the results of two phase III trials.[52,53] Thalidomide can also be used at relapse with overall response rates that are somewhat lower than bortezomib and lenalidomide.[31] Thalidomide, bortezomib, and lenalidomide can be combined with chemotherapy in the salvage setting to improve responses.

The combination of bortezomib and pegylated liposomal doxorubicin is another active regimen in relapsed or refractory MM. In a recently published phase III trial, patients randomized to the bortezomib and pegylated liposomal doxorubicin arm had significantly longer median time-to-progression (9.3 vs. 6.5 months, hazard ratio = 0.55; 95% Cl 0.43 to 0.71) and 15-month survival (76% vs. 65%) as compared with patients randomized to receive bortezomib alone.[88] It is interesting to note that the overall (complete and partial) response rate was only slightly higher in the bortezomib and pegylated liposomal doxorubicin group (44% vs. 41%). Based on the results of this study, the combination of bortezomib and pegylated liposomal doxorubicin received FDA approval in 2007 for patients with previously treated MM and is listed as a category I recommendation in the NCCN Guidelines.[14] As expected, patients who received the combination experienced more adverse effects.

Cycling therapies may be important in maximizing response rates. Patients who relapse after a specific induction therapy probably should not receive that same regimen as salvage therapy. The NCCN Guidelines offer many options for salvage, including thalidomide, lenalidomide, or bortezomib with or without dexamethasone or chemotherapy. In addition, autoHSCT or nonmyeloablative alloHSCT may have a role as salvage therapy in some patients.[14]

EVALUATION OF THERAPEUTIC OUTCOMES

Because MM is currently not a curable disease, the goals of therapy are to prolong survival and to improve quality of life. Patients with asymptomatic MM are usually followed and not treated. Asymptomatic patients are assessed every 3 to 6 months for disease progression, which would then require therapy. Assessment involves measurement of M protein in blood and urine and laboratory tests that include complete blood count, serum creatinine, and calcium. Patients are treated as the disease produces symptoms. Disease response is defined by a decline in M protein. After completion of the initial course of therapy and response is obtained, patients should be monitored every 3 months. Bone surveys are performed yearly or as required because of changes in symptoms. Various other tests are performed on an as-needed basis to evaluate disease status, including bone marrow biopsy, magnetic resonance imaging, and positron emission tomography, or computed tomography scan.

CONCLUSIONS

MM remains an incurable disease despite significant therapeutic advances. Thalidomide plus dexamethasone or lenalidomide plus dexamethasone are reasonable upfront regimens for those that require treatment and are candidates for autoHSCT. Chemotherapy is a reasonable alternative to these regimens in autoHSCT-ineligible patients, with melphalan and prednisone with or without thalidomide the most likely regimen. Younger patients with good performance status should receive autoHSCT after a short course of induction. The use of maintenance therapy after autoHSCT should be considered as part of a clinical trial. Nonmyeloablative alloHSCT may produce long-term disease-free survival but may require that the patient achieve a minimal residual disease state prior to the transplant procedure. When patients progress after initial therapy, salvage therapy may include regimens that contain thalidomide, lenalidomide, or bortezomib; autoHSCT and alloHSCT may be used in patients who are able to tolerate transplantation. Although there now are multiple therapies that can be used and there has been improvement in survival times and quality of life, MM remains a fatal disease that requires continued treatment advances.

ABBREVIATIONS

AlloHSCT: allogeneic hematopoietic stem cell transplantation

AutoHSCT: autologous hematopoietic stem cell transplantation

bFGF: basic fibroblast growth factor

IL: interleukin

IκB: inhibitor of NF-κB

ISS: International Staging System

MGUS: monoclonal gammopathy of undetermined significance

MM: multiple myeloma

MP: melphalan plus prednisone

MPT: melphalan, prednisone, plus thalidomide

NF-κB: nuclear factor kappa-B

ONJ: osteonecrosis of the jaw

RANK-L: receptor for activation of NF-κB ligand

TNF-α: tumor necrosis factor-α

VAD: vincristine, doxorubicin, dexamethasone

VEGF: vascular endothelial growth factor

REFERENCES

1. Munshi NC, Tricot G, Barlogie B. Plasma cell neoplasms. In: Devita VT, Hellman S, Rosenberg SA, eds. Cancer Principles and Practice of Oncology, 7th ed. Philadelphia: Lippincott Williams & Wilkins, 2005:2465–2499.
2. Barlogie B, Shaughnessy J, Epstein J, et al. Plasma cell myeloma. In: Lichtan MA, Beutler E, Kipps TJ, et al. Hematology, 7th Ed. New York: McGraw-Hill, 2006:1501–1533.
3. Jemal A, Siegel R, Ward E, et al. Cancer statistics, 2007. CA Cancer J Clin 2007;57:43–66.
4. Brander C, Raje N, O'Connor PG, et al. Absence of biologically important Kaposi sarcoma associated herpesvirus gene products and virus-specific cellular responses in multiple myeloma. Blood 2002;100:698–700.
5. Cheung MC, Pantanowitz L, Dezube BJ. AIDS-related malignancies: Emerging challenges in the era of highly active anti-retroviral therapy. Oncologist 2005;10:412–426.
6. Kyle RA, Rajkumar S. Multiple Myeloma. N Engl J Med 2004;351:1860–1873.
7. Kyle RA, Therneau TM, Rajkumar SV, et al. Prevalence of monoclonal gammopathy of undetermined significance. N Engl J Med 2006;354:1362–1369.
8. Walker BA, Leone PE, Jenner MW, et al. Integration of global SNP-based mapping and expression arrays reveals key regions, mechanisms, and genes important to the pathogenesis of multiple myeloma. Blood 2006;108:1733–1743.
9. Kyle RA, Remstein ED, Thereau TM, et al. Clinical course and prognosis of smoldering (asymptomatic) multiple myeloma. N Engl J Med 2007;356:2582–2590.
10. Spets H, Stromberg T, Georgii-Hemming P, et al. Expression of the bcl-2 family of pro- and anti-apoptotic genes in multiple myeloma and normal plasma cells. Eur J Haematol 2002;69:76–89.
11. Liebisch P, Dohner H. Cytogenetics and molecular cytogenetics in multiple myeloma. Eur J Cancer 2006;42:1520–1529.
12. Tosi P, Gamberi B, Giuliani N. Biology and treatment of multiple myeloma. Biol Blood Marrow Transplant 2006;12:81–86.
13. Pagnucco G, Cardinale G, Gervasi F. Targeting multiple myeloma cells and their bone marrow microenvironment. Ann N Y Acad Sci 2004;1028:390–399.
14. The NCCN Multiple Myeloma. Clinical Practice Guidelines in Oncology. (Version 1.2008, Available at *http://www.NCCN.org*.
15. San Miguel JF, Gutierrez NC, Mateo G, Orfao A. Conventional diagnostics in multiple myeloma. Eur J Cancer 2006;42:1510–1519.
16. Kyle RA, Yee GC, Somerfield MR, et al. American Society of Clinical Oncology 2007 Clinical Practice Guideline update on the role of bisphosphonates in multiple myeloma J Clin Oncol 2007;25:2462–2472.
17. Yeh HS, Berenson JR. Myeloma bone disease and treatment options. Eur J Cancer 2006;42:1554–1563.
18. Greipp PR, Miguel JS, Durie BG, et al. International staging system for multiple myeloma. J Clin Oncol 2005;23:3412–3420.
19. Dispenzieri A, Rajkumar SV, Gertz MA, et al. Treatment of newly diagnosed multiple myeloma based on Mayo Stratification of Myeloma and Risk-adapted therapy (mSmart): Consensus statement. Mayo Clin Proc 2007;82:323–341.
20. He Y, Wheatley K, Clark O, et al. Early versus deferred treatment for early stage multiple myeloma. Cochrane Database of Systemic Reviews 2003, Issue 1. Art. No.: CD004023. DOI: 10.1002/14651858.CD004023.
21. Kyle RA, Rajkumar V. Treatment of multiple myeloma: An emphasis on new developments. Ann Med 2006;38:111–115.
22. Ishii Y, Hsiao HH, Sashida G, et al. Derivative (1;7)(q10;p10) in multiple myeloma. A sign of therapy-related hidden myelodysplastic syndrome. Cancer Genet Cytogenet 2006;167:131–137.
23. Kumar A, Loughran T, Alsina M, et al. Management of multiple myeloma: A systematic review and critical appraisal of published studies. Lancet Oncol 2003;4:293–304.
24. Facon T, Mary JY, Pegourie B, et al. Dexamethasone-based regimens versus melphalan prednisone for elderly multiple myeloma patients ineligible for high dose therapy. Blood 2006;107:1292–1298.
25. Orlowski RZ. Initial therapy of multiple myeloma patients who are not candidates for stem cell transplantation. Hematology (Am Soc Hematol Educ Program) 2006:338–347.
26. Gordan JN, Goggin PM. Thalidomide and its derivative emerging from the wilderness. Postgrad Med J 2003;79:127–132.
27. Hwang JJ, Ghobrial IM, Anderson KC. New frontiers in the treatment of multiple myeloma. ScientificWorldJournal 2006;6:1475–1503.
28. Rajkumar SV, Leong T, Roche PC, et al. Prognostic value of bone marrow angiogenesis in multiple myeloma. Clin Cancer Res 2000;6:3111–3116.
29. Neben K, Mytilineos J, Moehler TM, et al. Polymorphisms of the TNF-α gene promoter predict for outcome after thalidomide therapy in relapsed and refractory multiple myeloma. Blood 2002;100:2263–2265.

30. Kumar S, Rajkumar SV. Thalidomide and lenalidomide in the treatment of multiple myeloma. Eur J Cancer 2006;42:1612–1622.
31. Barlogie B, Desikan R, Eddlemon P, et al. Extended survival in advanced and refractory multiple myeloma after single-agent thalidomide: Identification of prognostic factors in a phase 2 study of 169 patients. Blood 2001;98:492–494.
32. Rajkumar SV, Gertz MA, Lacy MQ, et al. Thalidomide as initial therapy for early stage myeloma. Leukemia 2003;17:775–779.
33. Rajkumar SV, Hayman S, Gertz MA, et al. Combination therapy with thalidomide plus dexamethasone for newly diagnosed myeloma. J Clin Oncol 2002;20:4319–4323.
34. Rajkumar SV, Blood E, Vesole D, et al. Phase III clinical trial of thalidomide plus dexamethasone compared with dexamethasone alone in newly diagnosed multiple myeloma: A clinical trial coordinated by Eastern Cooperative Oncology Group. J Clin Oncol 2006;24:431–436.
35. Palumbo A, Bringhen S, Caravita T, et al. Oral melphalan with prednisone chemotherapy plus thalidomide compared with melphalan and prednisone alone in elderly patients with multiple myeloma: Randomized controlled trial. Lancet 2006;367:825–831.
36. Facon T, Mary JY, Hulin C, et al. Melphalan and prednisone plus thalidomide versus melphalan and prednisone alone or reduced-intensity autologous stem cell transplantation in elderly patients with multiple myeloma (IFM 99-06): a randomised trial. Lancet 2007;370:1209–1218.
37. Offidani M, Corvatta L, Piersantelli M, et al. Thalidomide, dexamethasone, and pegylated liposomal doxorubicin for patients older than 65 years with newly diagnosed multiple myeloma. Blood 2006;108:2159–2164.
38. Ghobrial IM, Rajkumar SV. Management of thalidomide toxicity. J Support Oncol 2003;1:194–205.
39. Bennett CL, Angelotta C, Yarnold PR, et al. Thalidomide and lenalidomide associated thromboembolism among patients with cancer. JAMA 2006;296:2558–2560.
40. Zangari M, Siegel E, Barlogie B, et al. Thrombogenic activity of doxorubicin in myeloma patients receiving thalidomide: Implications for therapy. Blood 2002;100:1168–1171.
41. Rajkumar SV. Thalidomide therapy and deep venous thrombosis in multiple myeloma. Mayo Clin Proc 2005;80:1549–1551.
42. Joazeirs C, Anderson KC, Hunter T. Proteasome inhibitor drugs on the rise. Cancer Res 2006;66:7840–7842.
43. Orlowski RZ, Stinchcombe TE, Mitchell BS, et al. Phase 1 trial of the proteasome inhibitor PS341 in patients with refractory hematologic malignancies. J Clin Oncol 2002;20:4420–4427.
44. Richardson P, Barlogie B, Berenson J, et al. A Phase II study of bortezomib in relapsed, refractory myeloma. N Engl J Med 2003;348:2609–2617.
45. Jagannath S, Barlogie B, Berenson J, et al. A phase 2 study of two doses of bortezomib in relapsed or refractory myeloma. Br J Haematol 2004;127:165–172.
46. Richardson PG, Sonneveld P, Schuster MW, et al. Bortezomib or high dose dexamethasone in relapsed multiple myeloma. N Engl J Med 2005;352:2487–2498.
47. Richardson PG, Mitsiades C, Ghobrial I, Anderson K. Beyond single agent bortezomib: Combination regimens in relapsed multiple myeloma. Curr Opin Oncol 2006;18:598–608.
48. Jagannath S, Durie BG, Wolf J, et al. Bortezomib therapy alone and in combination with dexamethasone for previously untreated symptomatic multiple myeloma. Br J Haematol 2005;129:776–783.
49. Harousseau JL, Attal M, Leleu X, et al. Bortezomib plus dexamethasone as induction treatment prior to autologous stem cell transplant in patients with newly diagnosed multiple myeloma: Results of an IFM Phase II study. Haematologica 2006;91:1498–1505.
50. Mateos MV, Hernandez JM, Hernandez MT, et al. Bortezomib plus melphalan and prednisone in elderly untreated patients with multiple myeloma: Results of a multivariate Phase I/II study. Blood 2006;108:2165–2172.
51. Richardson PG, Blood E, Mitsiades CS, et al. A randomized phase 2 study of lenalidomide therapy for patients with relapsed or relapsed and refractory multiple myeloma. Blood 2006;108:3458–3464.
52. Dimopoulous M, Spencer A, Attal M, et al. Lenalidomide plus dexamethasone for relapsed or refractory multiple myeloma. N Engl J Med 2007;357:2123–2132.
53. Weber DM, Chen C, Niesvizky R, et al. Lenalidomide plus dexamethasone for relapsed multiple myeloma in North America. N EngL J Med 2007;357:2133–2142.
54. Rajkumar SV, Jacobus S, Callander N, et al. A randomized trial of lenalidomide plus high-dose dexamethasone versus lenalidomide plus low-dose dexamethasone in newly diagnosed multiple myeloma (E4A03): A trial coordinated by the Eastern Cooperative Oncology Group. Blood 2007;110:31A (abstract #74).
55. Child JA, Morgan GJ, Davies FE, et al. High-dose chemotherapy with hematopoietic stem cell rescue for multiple myeloma. N Engl J Med 2003;348:1875–1883.
56. Attal M, Harousseau JL, Stoppa AM, et al. A prospective, randomized trial of autologous bone marrow transplantation and chemotherapy in multiple myeloma. N Engl J Med 1996;335:91–97.
57. Koreth J, Cutler CS, Djulbegovic B, et al. High-dose therapy with single autologous transplantation versus chemotherapy for newly diagnosed multiple myeloma: A systematic review and meta-analysis of randomized controlled trials. Biol Blood Marrow Transplant 2007;12:183–196.
58. Barlogie B, Kyle RA, Anderson KC, et al. Standard chemotherapy compared with high dose chemotherapy for multiple myeloma: Final results of phase III US Intergroup Trial S9321. J Clin Oncol 2006;24:929–936.
59. Fermand JP, Katsahian S, Divine M, et al. High dose therapy and autologous blood stem cell transplantation compared with conventional treatment in multiple myeloma patients aged 55 to 65 years: Long-term results of a randomized control trial from the Group Myeloma-Autograffe. J Clin Oncol 2005;23:9227–9233.
60. Alexanian R, Dimopoulos M, Smith T, et al. Limited value of myeloablative therapy for late multiple myeloma. Blood 1994:83: 512–516.
61. Kumar S, Lacy MQ, Dispenzieri A, et al. High-dose therapy and autologous stem cell transplantation for multiple myeloma poorly responsive to initial therapy. Bone Marrow Transplant 2004;34:161–167.
62. Pant S, Copeland EA. Hematopoietic stem cell transplantation in multiple myeloma. Biol Blood Marrow Transplant 2007;13:877–885.
63. Fermand JP, Ravaud P, Chevaer S, et al. High dose therapy and autologous peripheral blood stem cell transplantation in multiple myeloma: Up-front or rescue treatment? Results of a multicenter sequential randomized clinical trial. Blood 1998;92:3131–3136.
64. Desikan R, Barlogie B, Sawyer J, et al. Results of high-dose therapy for 1000 patients with multiple myeloma: Durable complete remission and superior survival in the absence of chromosome 13 abnormalities. Blood 2000;95:4008–4010.
65. Vesole DH, Simic A, Lazarus HM. Controversy in multiple myeloma transplants: Tandem autotransplants and mini-allografts. Bone Marrow Transplant 2001;28:725–735.
66. Attal M, Harousseau JL, Facon T, et al. Single versus double autologous stem cell transplantation for multiple myeloma. N Engl J Med 2003;349:2495–2502.
67. Mihelic R, Kaufman JL, Lonial S. Maintenance therapy in multiple myeloma. Leukemia 2007;1–8.
68. Attal M, Harousseau JL, Leyvraz S, et al. Maintenance therapy with thalidomide improves survival in patients with multiple myeloma. Blood 2006;108:3289–3294.
69. Laterveer L, Verdonck LF, Peeters T, et al. Graft-versus-myeloma may overcome the unfavorable effect of deletion of chromosome 13 in multiple myeloma. Blood 2003;101:1201–1202.
70. Champlin R, Khouri I, Anderlini P, et al. Nonmyeloablative preparative regimens for allogeneic hematopoietic transplantation. Oncology 2003;17:94–100.
71. Lee C, Badros A, Barlogie B, et al. Prognostic factors in allogeneic transplantation for patients with high-risk multiple myeloma after reduced intensity conditioning. Exp Hematol 2003;31:73–80.
72. Garban F, Attal M, Michallet M, et al. Prospective comparison of autologous stem cell transplantation followed by dose reduced allograft with tandem autologous stem cell transplant in high risk de novo multiple myeloma. Blood 2006;107:3474–3480.
73. Bruno B, Rotta M, Patriarcia F, et al. A comparison of allografting with autografting for newly diagnosed myeloma. N Engl J Med 2007; 356:1110–1120.
74. Hernandez JM, Suquia B, Queizan TA, et al. Bone remodeling markers are useful in the management of monoclonal gammopathies. Hematol J 2004;5:480–488.
75. Sezer O, Heider U, Zavrski, et al. RANK ligand and osteoprotegerin in myeloma bone disease. Blood 2003;101:2094–2098.

76. Hjertner O, Standal M, Borset A, et al. Identification of new targets for therapy of osteolytic bone disease in multiple myeloma. Curr Drug Targets 2005;6:701–711.
77. Terpos E, Dimopoulos MA. Myeloma bone disease: Pathophysiology and management. Ann Oncol 2005;16:1223–1231.
78. Giuliani N, Rizzoli V, Roodman GD. Multiple myeloma bone disease: Pathophysiology of osteoblast inhibition. Blood 2006;108:3992–3996.
79. Epstein J. New insights into myeloma lytic bone disease. Blood 2003;102:5.
80. Russell RG. Bisphosphonates: From bench to bedside. Ann N Y Acad Sci 2006;1068:367–401.
81. Papapoulos SE. Bisphosphonate actions: Physical chemistry revisited. Bone 2006;38:613–616.
82. Baulch-Brown C, Molloy TJ, Yeh SL, et al. Inhibitor of the mevalonate pathway as potential therapeutic agents in multiple myeloma. Leuk Res 2007;31:341–352.
83. Berenson JR, Lichtenstein A, Porter L, et al. Long-term pamidronate treatment of advanced multiple myeloma patients reduces skeletal events. Myeloma Aredia Study Group. J Clin Oncol 1998;16:593–602.
84. Rosen LS, Gordon D, Antonio BS, et al. Zoledronic acid versus pamidronate in the treatment of skeletal metastases in patients with breast cancer or osteolytic lesions of multiple myeloma: A phase III, double blind, comparative trial. Cancer J 2001;7:377–387.
85. Djulbegovic B, Wheatley K, Ross J, et al. Bisphosphonates in multiple myeloma. Cochrane Database Systematic Reviews 2002, Issue 4. Art No.: CD003188. DOI: 10.1002/14651858.CD003188.
86. Lacy MQ, Dispenzieri A, Gertz MA, et al. Mayo clinic consensus statement for the use of bisphosphonates in multiple myeloma. Mayo Clin Proc 2006;81:1047–1053.
87. Guarueri V, Donati S, Nicolini M, et al. Renal safety and efficacy of intravenous bisphosphonates in patients with skeletal metastases treated for up to ten years. Oncologist 2005;10:842–848.
88. Orlowski RZ, Nagler A, Sonnveld P, et al. Randomized phase III study of pegylated liposomal doxorubicin plus bortezomib compared with bortezomib alone in relapsed or refractory multiple myeloma: Combination therapy improves time to progression. J Clin Oncol 2007; 25:3892–3901.

CHAPTER 140 Myelodysplastic Syndromes

JULIANNA A. BURZYNSKI AND TREVOR MCKIBBIN

KEY CONCEPTS

1. Myelodysplastic syndromes (MDSs) are primarily a disease of the elderly, with a median age at diagnosis between 60 and 75 years.
2. MDS are associated with environmental, occupational, and therapeutic exposures to chemicals or radiation.
3. The manifestations of MDS are due to a combination of immune dysregulation and genomic instability, which creates a dysplastic, clonal population of cells in a milieu unable to support normal hematopoiesis.
4. Most patients with MDS present with fatigue and lethargy or symptoms related to tissue hypoxia due to anemia.
5. The prognosis of patients with MDS is variable. Overall survival ranges from a few months to several years and can be estimated with the International Prognostic Scoring System (IPSS) or World Health Organization Classification-based Scoring System (WPSS).
6. Palliation of symptoms and improvement in quality of life are the goals of therapy for most patients.
7. Patients with MDS with low or intermediate-1 IPSS risk, serum erythropoietin level less than 500 IU/L, and low requirement for red blood cell (RBC) transfusions are most likely to respond to erythropoietin.
8. Allogeneic hematopoietic stem cell transplantation (HSCT) offers potentially curative therapy to patients with MDS who have a donor and are healthy enough for the procedure.
9. Hypomethylating agents are appropriate for patients with transfusion-dependent or symptomatic MDS who are not candidates for allogeneic HSCT.
10. Antithymocyte globulin is an appropriate treatment option for patients with low or intermediate-1 IPSS risk MDS who express human leukocyte antigen DR15 with symptomatic anemia that is unlikely to respond to erythropoietic agents.
11. Lenalidomide is recommended as a treatment option for patients with symptomatic anemia and low-risk MDS expressing a 5q deletion.

WWW The complete chapter, learning objectives, and other resources can be found at **www.pharmacotherapyonline.com.**

Myelodysplastic syndromes (MDS) encompass a spectrum of clonal myeloid disorders characterized by ineffective hematopoiesis that results in anemia, thrombocytopenia, leukopenia, or a combination of peripheral cytopenias.[1,2] MDS are frequently associated with clonal chromosomal abnormalities, qualitative disorders of blood cells, and a variable propensity for progression to acute myeloid leukemia (AML). The clinical course of patients with MDS varies along a continuum from a rapid progression to AML to years of slowly progressive bone marrow failure.[3,4]

Our understanding of MDS and the available treatment options have advanced in recent years. In 1999, the World Health Organization (WHO) developed a classification system in an attempt to make the categories of MDS more homogenous with respect to natural history of the disease.[2] The International Prognostic Scoring System (IPSS) for MDS was developed to better enable clinicians to categorize patients according to risk for progression to AML and predict median survival from the time of diagnosis.[3] Until 2004, supportive care was the most common therapy for most patients because no medications for treatment of MDS were approved by the Food and Drug Administration (FDA). Three medications (azacitidine, decitabine, and lenalidomide) currently are approved by the FDA for treatment of MDS, and several more are being investigated. The change in classification of MDS, improvement in risk stratification, and development of new treatment options represent steps forward in our understanding and management of MDS.

EPIDEMIOLOGY

❶ MDS are primarily a disease of the elderly, with a median age at diagnosis between 60 and 75 years.[5] Males predominate, with an estimated male-to-female ratio of approximately 1.7:1.[6] Overall, an estimated 3 to 12 cases of MDS are diagnosed per 100,000 persons per year. The incidence of MDS increases with age; in patients older than 70 years, an estimated 15 to 50 new cases per 100,000 persons occur per year.[5] Approximately 10,300 new cases are diagnosed in the United States each year, making MDS roughly as common as chronic lymphocytic leukemia.[6] Many experts predict that the prevalence of MDS is likely to increase as the population of the United States ages and clinicians become more aware of MDS.

CHAPTER 141 Skin Cancer

ROWENA N. SCHWARTZ AND LINDSAY J. CORPORON

KEY CONCEPTS

1. Cutaneous melanoma is an increasingly common malignancy, but it is a cancer that can be cured if detected early. Public education about screening and early detection is one strategy for controlling the increase in incidence and the mortality associated with cutaneous melanoma.
2. Surgical resection can cure patients with early-stage melanoma.
3. The toxicities associated with interferon-α_{2b} therapy are significant and require patient education, close patient monitoring, and appropriate dose modification based on toxicity.
4. Patients with locally advanced disease should be evaluated for adjuvant therapy; recommended options include interferon-α_{2b} or participation in a clinical trial.
5. High-dose aldesleukin (interleukin-2) is an option for some individuals with metastatic melanoma. The toxicities associated with this regimen are significant and warrant close patient selection. Individuals receiving high-dose aldesleukin require close monitoring and management by an experienced healthcare team. A small subset of patients experiences a durable response with this therapy, although the question of risk versus benefit should be assessed on an individualized basis.
6. Metastatic melanoma remains a clinical challenge. At this time, there is not a single standard treatment approach for individuals with metastatic disease. Dacarbazine and temozolomide are considered the most active chemotherapy and can be used as single agents. Combination chemotherapy has not been shown to be superior to single-agent therapy with dacarbazine.
7. As the biology of melanoma has been further delineated, a growing number of potential targets for drug therapy have been identified. Recent work has focused on drugs that target specific pathways of melanoma development and progression.
8. Nonmelanoma skin cancers, including basal cell carcinoma and squamous cell carcinoma, are the most common forms of skin cancer. The most effective treatment is surgery.

The incidence of skin cancer has steadily increased in recent years. Although nonmelanoma skin cancers (NMSCs) are the most common malignancies of the skin, cutaneous melanoma accounts for most skin cancer-related deaths. As the incidence of skin cancer increases and the mortality rates associated with melanoma rise, it is essential to consider issues of care beyond that of disease treatment. Skin cancer prevention and screening have a major impact on public health and on the success of treatment for those individuals diagnosed with both NMSC and melanoma. Skin cancers tend to occur more frequently in older individuals (e.g., median age at diagnosis for melanoma is 45–55 years). As the population continues to age, there is need to find effective strategies to prevent, detect, and treat individuals with these cancers.

Learning objectives, review questions, and other resources can be found at **www.pharmacotherapyonline.com.**

MELANOMA

The incidence and mortality rates of cutaneous melanoma have increased during the past several decades and continue to increase dramatically.[1] In men, the incidence of melanoma is increasing more rapidly than any other malignancy. In women, lung cancer is the only malignancy that has a higher increase in its incidence rate. In the year 2007, it is estimated that approximately 59,940 new cases of melanoma will be diagnosed in the United States. Unfortunately, this estimate is not accurate because many superficial and in situ melanomas are managed in facilities that do not routinely report their cases to cancer registries.[2] In the last decade of the 20th century, the rate of increase of melanoma in select subgroups of the United States population (e.g., women) has declined although the incidence overall has continued to increase. It has been suggested that the increase in cutaneous melanoma over time is due to a cohort effect. It appears that individuals born before 1950 show increased risk, whereas those born after 1950 show a stable or declining rate.[3] More simply stated, the rate of increase in the incidence of melanoma may be declining in younger patients, but the incidence and mortality in older individuals have increased, particularly in men over age 65 years.[4] Childhood and adolescent melanoma is rare, but in young adults between the ages of 15 and 19 years melanoma accounts for approximately 7% of all cancers.[5]

Of all the skin cancers, melanoma has the highest mortality. It is estimated that in 2007 approximately 8,110 individuals will die of melanoma.[2] Melanoma is second only to adult leukemia in terms of the loss of years of potential life for cancers. The incidence and mortality of melanoma vary worldwide. The overall mortality rate from melanoma appears to have stabilized and possibly declined in recent years in Australia, the United States, and Europe.[1] The stabilization of mortality rates appears to be related to efforts at both primary and secondary prevention of melanoma in addition to advances in the management of melanoma patients, such as adjuvant treatment. Importantly, this change in mortality rate overall has not been seen throughout the population. Mortality rates have increased 157% in older men (7.5 to 19.3 per 100,000) in the United States.[4]

TABLE 141-1 Risk Factors for Melanoma

Host risk factors
Adulthood (age >15 years)
History of cutaneous melanoma
Dysplastic nevi
Cutaneous melanoma in first-degree relative
Immunodeficiency/immunosuppression
High density of common nevi and atypical nevi
High degree of freckling
Sunburns easily/tans rarely
Blonde or red hair
Blue, green, or gray eyes
Socioeconomic status (higher > lower)
White (vs. black) race
External risk factors
Intense intermittent sun exposures
History of sunburn
More than four painful sunburns before age 15 years
Outdoor leisure

ETIOLOGY AND EPIDEMIOLOGY

The etiology of melanoma, like most other malignancies, is not fully understood. A number of host factors and environmental factors have been identified (Table 141–1), and it is likely that these factors alone or in combination increase the occurrence of cutaneous melanomas.

A number of genes have been implicated in melanoma development and progression, and molecular profiling studies have identified several distinct molecular subclasses of melanoma.[6] Familial atypical multiple mole syndrome or hereditary dysplastic nevus syndrome is a hereditary disease characterized by a predisposition to develop dysplastic nevi and cutaneous melanoma. Only approximately 8% to 10% of cases of melanoma are thought to be associated with a family history or hereditary dysplastic nevus syndrome. Older case-control studies of patients with familial atypical multiple mole syndrome suggest a risk for melanoma of 400- to 1,000-fold higher than that seen in the general population. The mode of inheritance is somewhat controversial and is believed to be polygenic.

Genetic studies of this heritable trait in families led to the identification of CDKN2A as the familial melanoma gene, located at chromosome 9p21. CDKN2A encodes two distinct proteins: inhibitor of cyclin-dependent kinase 4 (INK4A; also known as $p16^{INK4a}$) and ARF. INK4A inhibits the G_1 cyclin-dependent kinases that phosphorylate and inactivate the retinoblastoma protein, allowing the cell to go into the S phase. ARF (also known as $p14^{ARF}$ in humans) inhibits p53 degradation; therefore, loss of ARF inactivates p53.

The genomic complexity of the 9p21 locus has raised questions of the importance of neighboring genes, such as CDKN2B.[7] Growing evidence implicates hyperactive receptor tyrosine kinase signaling in the development and progression of melanoma. One of the major signaling mediators of receptor tyrosine kinase is the mitogen-activated protein kinase pathway resulting in activation of RAS and BRAF. Activating BRAF mutations are the most common somatic genetic event in human melanoma, occurring in 25% to 70% of melanoma patients. BRAF does not appear to be an inherited disposition gene, but the high prevalence of BRAF mutations in cutaneous melanoma appear to be an epidemiologic link between ultraviolet (UV) radiation and melanoma. BRAF mutations are common in melanomas arising from skin with intermittent sun exposure but is not as commonly seen in melanomas in chronically sun-exposed areas.[8]

Individuals with germ-line inactivation of the retinoblastoma gene are predisposed to melanoma.[6] Individuals with a history of bilateral retinoblastoma have a 4- to 80-fold higher lifetime risk of melanoma. Of interest, these melanomas do not occur at the site of radiation for treatment of retinoblastoma.

Sunlight is one of the most important environmental factors in the pathogenesis of melanoma, and the incidence of melanoma has been associated with latitude and the intensity of solar exposure among susceptible populations. Radiation in the ultraviolet B (UVB) range (280–320 nm) is historically considered to be the critical factor linking sunlight and melanoma, although prolonged exposure to ultraviolet A (UVA) radiation (320–400 nm) also may be important. Use of older UVB-blocking sunscreens may not be as protective as once thought because they allow more sustained sun exposure without any clinical symptoms of burn (e.g., erythema or pain), ultimately resulting in intense irradiation of the skin by UVA light.[9]

Individual physical characteristics can determine responses to UV radiation. White persons with fair-colored hair (red and blond), light-colored eyes (blue and green), and high degrees of freckling and those who have a tendency to burn and rarely tan with exposure to sunlight appear especially at risk.[1,10] Epidemiologic research has not been able to show a relationship between cumulative exposure to sunlight and occurrence of cutaneous melanoma, although cumulative exposure does appear to play a role in NMSC. Studies have demonstrated a lower risk for development of melanoma in outdoor workers compared to indoor workers.[9] Intermittent overexposure to sunlight, blistering sunburns, and the time of life of exposure to the sun now are believed to be the more critical factors for development of cutaneous melanoma. Individuals who have a history of severe sunburns appear to have a higher risk for development of melanoma than do individuals who have had chronic sun exposure without a history of burning. The risk with sunlight and UV radiation seems to be greatest during childhood and adolescence. Intensive exposure to sunlight during infancy and early adolescence is more hazardous than exposure during adult life.

One of the most important risk factors for melanoma is the number of melanocytic nevi (pigmented lesions) on the body. A second risk factor is the presence of atypical melanocytic nevi.[1] Small congenital melanocytic nevi are present in up to 1% of newborns.[5] Acquired melanocytic nevi often appear after infancy and often are located in sun-exposed areas. The risk of melanoma may be related to the number of melanocyte nevi acquired during childhood.[5]

Immunocompromised patients are at an increased risk for development of cutaneous melanoma.[5,10] Immunodeficiency includes individuals with ataxia telangiectasia, chronic lymphocytic leukemia, Hodgkin's lymphoma, and immunosuppression following organ transplant. Acquired immunodeficiency syndrome has been shown to increase the risk of developing cutaneous melanoma, and the disease often is more aggressive.[11] Personal history of nonmelanoma or melanoma skin cancers is a risk factor for subsequent melanoma.

A rare but important risk for melanoma is maternal–fetal transfer of melanoma. Although melanoma is not the most common cancer in pregnancy, it is the cancer most likely to metastasize to the placenta and the fetus.[12] Maternal–fetal transmission of melanoma results in approximately 25% mortality risk to babies born to mothers with placental involvement. Neonates delivered with concomitant placental involvement but without clinical evidence of disease still are considered to be at increased risk for development of disease.

PATHOGENESIS

Melanomas most often arise within epidermal melanocytes of the skin, although they also can arise from noncutaneous melanocytes. Human melanocytes are dendritic pigmented cells that arise from the neural crest tissue during early fetal development and migrate over a predictable route to a variety of sites within the body, including the skin, uveal tract, meninges, and ectodermal mucosa. In adults, most melanocytes are located at the epidermal–dermal junction of the skin and the choroid of the eye, but they can be found in other tissues such as the meninges and the alimentary and respiratory tract. Primary melanoma can arise in any area of the body with melanocytes. The skin is the most frequent site of melanoma; cutaneous melanoma constitutes 90% of all melanoma. Primary melanoma can arise in the eye (ocular melanoma)[13] and less frequently in the meninges, respiratory tract, colon, and gallbladder.[14]

Normal melanocytes arise from melanoblasts and undergo a series of differentiation events before reaching a final end-cell differentiation state. Normal melanocytes can be arrested in their differentiation process at any given state of maturation without loss of their proliferation capacity. Melanocytes adhere to the basement membrane of the epidermis and, despite a resting state, maintain a lifelong proliferation potential. The existence of melanoma stem cells has been suggested from work with cells from melanoma lines.[6]

Melanocytes synthesize melanin to protect various tissues, such as the skin, from UV radiation (UVR)–induced damage and reach the keratinocytes in the upper layers of the epidermis via dendrites. Tyrosinase is an essential enzyme within melanosomes that synthesizes melanin.

Skin melanocytes transform from preexisting nevocellular nevi in the development of melanoma. A series of distinct steps are involved in the development and progression of melanoma from melanocytes. The pathologic components of the progression in human melanoma involve a series of morphologic stages: (a) acquired or congenital melanocytic nevus, (b) melanocytic nevus with architectural atypia, (c) histologically dysplastic nevus with cytologic atypia and architectural atypia, (d) primary melanoma in the radial growth phase in which limited growth and radial expansion of the nevi may occur without metastatic competence (nontumorigenic melanoma), (e) primary melanoma in the vertical growth phase with or without in-transit metastases in which there appears to be uncontrolled proliferation and increased angiogenesis, (f) regional lymph node metastatic melanoma (lymphatic), and (g) distant metastatic melanoma (hematogenous).[15] Primary melanoma is characterized by radial growth and limited vertical thickness (<0.75 mm). Primary melanoma demonstrates little tendency to metastasize. Melanoma has a potential for metastasis formation with the onset of a vertical growth phase. Therefore, the thickness of a primary melanoma is an important prognostic factor and is used in the staging classification of cutaneous melanoma. Of note, melanomas can skip steps in this development pathway.

Normal melanocytes require growth factors for proliferation, but melanoma cells can proliferate without growth factors.[16] Melanoma cells secrete a variety of growth autocrine and paracrine factors that may facilitate proliferation. Additionally, with disease progression, melanoma cells increase production of certain growth factors and cytokines. The phosphatidylinositol 3-kinase (PI3K)–AKT pathway often is overactive in melanoma. Integrins and growth factors promote growth and survival of melanoma through these pathways.

Basic fibroblast growth factors (bFGFs) are thought to be important mediators of growth stimulation and cell survival and act as motility factors for melanoma cells. In addition, bFGFs upregulate serine proteinases and metalloproteinases. Melanoma cells are strong producers of chemoattractive proteins such as interleukin-8. Vascular endothelial growth factor can be triggered in the vertical growth phase.[17] Most of these changes occur between the radial growth phase and vertical growth phase of primary melanoma, and metastatic cells often show the highest cytokine production.

Understanding the biology of melanoma has provided potential targets for drug therapy.[18,19] For example, the role of bFGF in the pathogenesis of melanoma has led to investigation of antisense oligonucleotides to block bFGF. Other pathways, such as mitogen-activated protein kinase pathway has been targeted by RAF and MEK inhibitors and the PI3K/AKT pathway by TOR inhibitors. As pathways are identified and as agents that inhibit these pathways enter clinical trials and practice, there is growing excitement about the opportunities to impact treatment of melanoma in new and effective ways.

Immune factors appear to be involved in the progression of melanoma more often than in most other solid tumors.[10,16] Spontaneous cancer regressions are rare but are a well-documented phenomenon seen in melanoma. Focal regression in primary melanoma has been reported. Tumor regression appears to be associated with host immunity.

A number of different tumor antigens have been identified in the cellular membrane and cytoplasm of melanoma cells and are referred to as melanoma-associated antigens. Ganglioside antigens have been of particular interest in the development of immunotherapy for melanoma. A large number of monoclonal antibodies to melanoma-associated antigens have been developed and are being evaluated in clinical trials for diagnosis of and therapy for melanoma.

The humoral and cellular responses of individuals with melanoma who express melanoma-associated antigen have been described and provide the rationale for immunotherapy in the management of metastatic melanoma.[10] Melanoma-directed antibodies have been isolated in the sera of patients with melanoma. The presence of antimelanoma antibodies in the sera of patients correlates with the clinical status of the patients, and the antibodies gradually disappear from the serum as the disease progresses. This phenomenon may be explained by the possible formation of anti-idiotype antibodies directed against the antimelanoma antibodies, an increase in the circulation of soluble tumor antigens that saturate all antibody combining sites, increased levels of immunosuppression, or absorption of antibodies on the tumor mass.

Interest has focused on the role of cell-mediated immune response in melanoma. Specific cell-mediated responses may play a role in tumor regression, but the role of specific cells, such as cytotoxic T lymphocytes (CTLs), is not fully understood. Tumor-infiltrating lymphocytes (TILs) have been shown in vivo and in vitro to possess antitumor reactivity. TILs contain a large number of mature tumor-specific lymphocytes and have been a target for manipulation in immunotherapeutic approaches for melanoma.[10] Two recently identified targets are cytotoxic T lymphocyte antigen 4 (CTLA-4) and toll-like receptor 9 (TLR9). CTLA-4 is a glycoprotein expressed on the surface of activated T cells that appears to have an inhibitory effect on T cells. Blocking the effect of CTLA-4 could be an effective strategy for increasing the T-cell antitumor response.[20]

HISTOLOGIC SUBTYPES OF MELANOMA

Dysplastic nevi are believed to be a link between benign nevi and melanoma. Dysplastic nevi are defined by a number of architectural and cytologic criteria.[21] Dysplastic nevi may appear as flat macules with asymmetry, border irregularity, color variation, and usually a diameter greater than 5 mm. Compared to melanoma lesions, dysplastic nevi appear less evolved.

Cutaneous melanomas are categorized by growth patterns. Four major histologic subtypes or growth patterns of primary cutaneous melanoma have been identified: superficial spreading melanoma, nodular melanoma, lentigo maligna melanoma, and acral lentiginous melanoma. Desmoplastic melanoma is a less common subtype but is more commonly seen in older individuals. Desmoplastic melanoma is of concern because the clinical presentation is similar to that seen in NMSC. If a biopsy of the lesion is not obtained, the disease may be mismanaged. Clinical outcomes of the four major melanoma subtypes are similar, if the comparison controls for depth of penetration or tumor thickness. Any of the four subtypes can present as an amelanotic variant. Amelanotic melanomas appear to be devoid of clinically apparent pigmentation. Uveal melanoma is considered a separate disease from cutaneous melanoma.

The ability to predict the metastatic potential of melanomas would be a valuable prognostic tool. An attempt to predict the likelihood for metastasis is based on radial and vertical growth phases. Radial growth phase describes the early stage of melanoma when the tumor is thin and primarily intraepidermal in location.[22] By definition, malignant melanoma in situ is a form of radial growth phase melanoma. Vertical growth phase is the stage of melanoma with clear metastatic potential.

Superficial spreading melanoma is the most common morphologic type of cutaneous melanoma, accounting for approximately 70% of all melanomas.[10,22] The lesions usually arise from a preexisting nevus, known as a *precursor lesion*, and evolve slowly over 1 to 5 years. At some point, superficial spreading melanoma may progress to a more rapid growth phase. Early in lesion development, the superficial spreading melanoma is flat, but the surface becomes irregular and asymmetrical as the lesion progresses. The lesion enlarges when it enters into a rapid growth phase, and the edges appear notched or lacy. The lesions can be blue, black, or pink. Areas within the lesion may be hypopigmented. These patches of color variation, specifically the hypopigmented areas, are thought to be associated with tumor regression within the lesion or pigment inconsistency. The clinical differential diagnosis of superficial spreading melanoma includes both benign and malignant skin disease. This subtype is sometimes confused with seborrheic keratoses or pigmented basal cell carcinoma (BCC). Superficial spreading melanoma may occur at any anatomic site on the body, but they are more commonly seen on the back in men and on the legs in women. This subtype of melanoma is more common in women. The mean age of diagnosis of superficial spreading melanoma is 50 years, which is earlier than that seen for other subtypes. Superficial spreading melanoma usually occurs after puberty.

Lentigo maligna melanoma represents a small percentage of melanomas. It is unique from other histologic subtypes because it does not have the same propensity to metastasize.[10,22] Lentigo maligna melanoma arises on chronically sun-exposed sites in older individuals and presents as a freckle-like lesion. Lentigo maligna melanomas are generally large (>3 cm), flat, and tan-colored lesions with shades of brown and black. The lesions gradually grow and develop darker, with asymmetric flecks in areas. Lentigo maligna melanoma is uncommon before age 50 years and may have been present for more than 5 years. Like some forms of NMSC, lentigo maligna melanoma is linked to cumulative sun exposure. Only approximately 5% to 8% of lentigo maligna melanoma evolve into invasive melanoma, which is characterized by nodular development within the flat precursor lesion. Lentigo maligna melanoma can be difficult to distinguish from solar lentigo, which typically is a smaller and evenly pigmented flat-appearing lesion.

Nodular melanoma is the second most common growth pattern of melanoma, occurring in 15% to 30% of patients. Nodular melanoma is a pure vertical growth phase disease. In nodular melanoma, a small expansive nodule in the papillary dermis invades the reticular dermis and subcutis. The radial growth phase is absent at all times. Nodular melanomas are more aggressive and develop more rapidly than superficial spreading melanoma. Nodular melanomas are dark blue–black and often uniform in color with a shiny surface, although a small percentage of nodular melanomas are amelanotic and have a fleshy appearance. Nodular melanomas are raised and often symmetric. Nodular subtype of melanoma accounts for most thick lesions at the time of diagnosis.[23] They can occur at any age (median age 53 years) and are most common on the trunk, head, and neck. Nodular melanomas are more common in men. Of note, nodular melanomas can resemble a traumatized nevi.

Acral lentiginous melanoma presents as three distinct clinical subtypes: melanoma on the palms of the hands or soles of the feet, subungual melanoma, and mucosal melanoma.[10,22] Most acral lentiginous melanomas are located on the soles of the feet and look like a large tan or brown stain. The lesions often have irregular convoluted borders. The initial macular component of palmar/plantar melanomas can be masked by the thickened stratum corneum at these sites. Many of these lesions look verrucous in appearance, making them difficult to distinguish from warts by the untrained eye. Suspicious lesions on the palms or soles of the feet should be evaluated. Acral lentiginous melanoma includes subungual melanoma, which arises in the nail matrix or nail bed. The most common presentation is a brown or black line in the great toe or the thumbnail. Mucosal melanoma is rare but can occur on any mucosal surface. Mucosal melanoma occurs most commonly in the oropharyngeal mucosa, followed by the anal/rectal mucosa, genital mucosa, and urinary mucosa. Unfortunately, mucosal melanoma often does not become clinically apparent until the mass is large or the lesion bleeds. Acral lentiginous melanoma occurs in less than 10% of white people with melanoma but is the most common type of melanoma reported in individuals with a dark complexion (e.g., African Americans, Asians, and Hispanics).

Unusual subtypes of primary melanoma include desmoplastic/neurotropic melanoma, mucosal melanoma, malignant blue nevus, melanoma arising in giant congenital nevus, and clear cell sarcoma. These subtypes account for less than 5% of primary melanomas.[10]

Uveal melanoma is the most common primary intraocular malignancy seen in adults but is an uncommon tumor.[24] Unlike cutaneous melanoma, the frequency and mortality of uveal melanoma have remained steady. This melanoma arises from the pigmented epithelium of the choroid. Iris melanoma is a subset of uveal melanoma and tends to have a more benign course. The risk of metastasis varies with the histologic type and size of the tumor as well as the location in the eye. Metastases occur most frequently in the liver but have been documented in a variety of tissues.

CLINICAL PRESENTATION

The initial clinical presentation of melanoma often is a cutaneous lesion (see Chap. 99). The lesion can be located anywhere on the body but is most commonly discovered on the lower extremities in women and on the back and trunk in men. The cardinal clinical feature of a cutaneous melanoma is a pigmented skin lesion that changes over a period of time. The clinical features used to describe or evaluate a questionable lesion are highlighted by the mnemonic "ABCDE." Unlike benign pigmented lesions, the shape of a melanoma lesion is often (A) *asymmetric*. Benign lesions tend to have regular margins, whereas melanoma lesions often have irregular (B) *borders*. The (C) *color* of melanoma lesions is often variegated, ranging in color from tan to blue-black, and at times the lesion is intermingled with colors of red, purple, and white. The size or (D) *diameter* of a melanoma lesion is frequently 6 mm or greater when identified, whereas benign lesions usually are smaller. Early melanoma lesions may be diagnosed at a smaller size, and size of a lesion should not be used as "the trigger" to have a suspicious lesion evaluated. Another warning sign of a potential melanoma is the *evolution* (E) in preexisting nevi. Changes such as a sudden or continuous enlargement of a lesion, an elevation of a lesion, or any change in the skin surrounding a nevus, including redness or swelling, are important clinical signs. Uncommonly, the sensation of the lesion may become itchy or tender and painful. Friability of the lesion resulting in bleeding or oozing is a danger sign. Perhaps the most important warning sign of danger is the evolution in any characteristic of a lesion.

The clinical appearance of a melanoma depends on the histologic subtype and the stage of development of the lesion. It usually is possible to distinguish three variants of cutaneous melanoma: flat melanoma, nodular melanoma, and flat melanoma with a nodular area. Flat melanoma usually corresponds to the histologic classification of superficial spreading melanoma.

The diagnosis of melanoma is complicated by a number of pigmented moles (melanocytic nevi) and nonmelanocytic lesions that resemble melanoma. An average of 10 to 40 ordinary nevi can be found on the skin of white adults. These lesions usually are absent at birth, increase in number through adult life,[5] and then gradually decline in number. They appear as tiny pinpoint macules and usually are uniform in color but increase in size to a maximum of 4 to 6 mm. Nonmelanocytic pigmented lesions, such as seborrheic keratoses, pigmented BCC, and vascular lesions, also can appear similar to a melanoma lesion.

❶ Improved survival rates for melanoma have been attributed to the identification and treatment of disease at an early stage, when the disease is limited and has not yet metastasized. It follows that one strategy to improve survival rates would be to increase efforts to identify early-stage melanoma. The cost effectiveness of massive screening for all adults by a physician has never been demonstrated. A number of agencies, such as the American Academy of Dermatology and the American Cancer Society, have sponsored free annual screenings. Routine examination of the skin by physicians is recommended for individuals at high risk. The entire cutaneous surface, including the scalp, should be examined.

It has been estimated that approximately 50% of the initial melanoma lesions found are discovered by self-examination. Therefore, one of the most direct strategies to improve early detection would be a method to increase effective skin self-examination (SSE) by the individual, the individual's partner, and/or a caregiver. Identification of early melanoma allows the opportunity to treat the lesions when they are thin and curable. Persons who perform SSE present for care at an earlier stage in the disease process and have 50% less advanced melanoma and lower mortality from the disease.[25] Healthcare individuals who routinely work with the public, such as community pharmacists, have an opportunity to increase public awareness concerning the benefits and appropriate methods for SSE. Educational pamphlets describing SSE (Table 141–2) for the public are widely available through the American Cancer Society, American Academy of Dermatology, and Skin Cancer Foundation. If a newly discovered pigmented lesion is identified or if a preexisting pigmented lesion changes, the individual should be evaluated by a physician immediately. As with adults, a change in the appearance of a pigmented lesion in a child is the most common clinical presentation in pediatric and adolescent populations. In children, any change in a mole, such as bleeding or change in color or size, should be evaluated.[5]

SSE is of special interest in the elderly. As the population of older adults (65 years and older) increases, it is expected that the mortality from melanoma also will increase. Barriers to successful SSE in the elderly, such as failing eyesight, lack of partners, and poor memory, impact the older adult in detecting new or changing lesions. These barriers, coupled with the higher incidence of melanoma in males, present a challenge and an opportunity for the healthcare professional to target education on this growing segment of our population.

A biopsy of the lesion is critical to establish diagnosis of melanoma. Subsequent pathologic interpretation of the biopsy will help provide information on prognosis and treatment options. An excisional biopsy with a margin of normal-appearing skin is recommended for a suspicious lesion and should include a portion of underlying subcutaneous fat for microstaging. Although a biopsy is recommended for large lesions where an excisional biopsy is impractical, an incisional biopsy can be performed but should include a core of full-thickness skin and subcutaneous tissue. When excisional biopsies are not appropriate, as with the face or palmar surface of the hands, a full-thickness incisional or punch biopsy is preferred over a shave biopsy.

Evaluation of any individual with a suspected melanoma includes a complete history and total body skin examination. The focus of the patient history is identifying potential risk factors. Risk-related questions include an assessment of family history of melanoma, personal history of skin cancer and/or nevus excisions, sun exposure, and phototype. Total dermatologic examination is necessary to determine melanoma risk factors (e.g., mole pattern, mole type, or freckling) and for staging. For patients with melanomas 1 mm or more in thickness, a baseline chest x-ray film and liver chemistries are generally recommended even though these tests are relatively insensitive at detecting clinically occult distant disease. The appropriate workup of individuals with early-stage disease is controversial.[10] Lactate dehydrogenase should be measured because elevated serum lactate dehydrogenase level is an independent predictor of decreased survival in published studies, even after accounting for site and number of metastases.[26] Any clinical indication of regional lymph node involvement should be confirmed with fine-needle aspiration or on biopsy of the enlarged lymph node. Additionally, any other signs or symptoms suggestive of metastatic disease should be completely evaluated.

STAGING AND PROGNOSTIC FACTORS

The size of a primary melanoma lesion is associated with the likelihood of metastases. The prognostic factor originally used to determine survival was based on the cross-sectional profile of the primary tumor. The cross-sectional profile could be evaluated if the deepest invasive tumor cells lay above or below the sweat glands. This assessment was further clarified by Clark,[27] who described the relationship of depth of invasion of the cancer cells to the standard anatomic landmarks of the skin (Table 141–3). Clark's classification is a practical approach for patients with more superficial tumors, because tumors classified as Clark levels I through III seldom metastasize. The classification system has been criticized because of problems associated with practical measurements. Melanoma lesions that occur in the presence of lymphoid infiltration, fibrosis, or even the cells of preexisting nevi are difficult to assess with classic reference landmarks.

Breslow[28] replaced Clark's classification of reference landmarks with the use of thickness of the primary melanoma lesion. Tumor thickness is quantified to the nearest tenth of a millimeter using an ocular micrometer, measuring from the top of the granular layer of the overlying epidermis to the deepest contiguous invasive melanoma cell. The correlation between tumor thickness and probability of tumor metastases is strong but does not include aspects such as tumor satellites, defined rather arbitrarily as skin involvement within 2 cm of the primary lesion, and vascular invasion. It was once thought that

TABLE 141-2 Self-Examination of Suspicious Moles

1. Examine your body front and back in the mirror, and then right and left sides with arms raised.
2. Bend the elbows and look carefully at the forearms and upper arms and palms.
3. Look at the backs of the legs and feet. Look specifically in the spaces between toes and at the soles of the feet.
4. Examine the back of the neck and scalp with the help of a hand-held mirror; part hair (or use a blow dryer) to lift hair and give yourself a closer look.
5. Check the back and buttocks with a hand-held mirror.

Derived from publications of the American Academy of Dermatology.

TABLE 141-3 Clark's Classification

Clark Level	Anatomic Landmark
N	Epidermis
I	Dermal-epidermal junction
II	Papillary dermis
III	Interface between papillary dermis and reticular dermis
IV	Reticular dermis and subcutaneous fat

the presence of satellite nodule(s) had the same impact on prognosis as a high-risk primary lesion (tumor thickness >4 mm). It is now thought that patients with satellitosis have a worse prognosis than patients with thick primary lesions, and prognosis is more similar to that of patients with nodal metastases. A number of prognostic factors, in addition to tumor thickness and level of invasion, are associated with the risk for developing metastatic disease.[29]

The American Joint Committee on Cancer (AJCC) developed a staging system for melanoma that divides patients with localized melanoma into four stages according to microstaging criteria of Breslow and Clark.[30] In addition to consideration of the primary lesion, the AJCC staging system includes aspects of the tumor satellite, extent of lymph node involvement, and presence of metastatic disease.[30] Analysis of several large databases worldwide identified areas in which the AJCC staging system, which was published in 1997, did not reflect the natural history of melanoma. Issues such as the appropriate cutoff values for primary tumor thickness, ulceration of the melanoma, and satellite lesions of the primary tumor should be considered when making decisions about therapy.[29] The cutoff values initially proposed by Breslow for primary tumor thickness were initially used in the AJCC staging system, but it appears that cutoff depths of 1, 2, and 4 mm of thickness may better predict overall survival. Melanoma ulceration is associated with increased mitotic rate within a primary melanoma. The presence of ulceration of the primary lesion has been correlated with poorer survival for patients with very thin or thick lesions, but ulceration of the melanoma was not included in the 1997 AJCC staging system.

A revised staging system for cutaneous melanoma was developed by the AJCC and has been used for several years.[31] It is important to carefully examine older clinical trials to determine which staging system was used to determine patient inclusion and exclusion criteria, as results may differ based on these patient criteria. Revisions of the new melanoma staging system include (a) melanoma thickness and ulceration for all tumors (except T1 tumors); (b) number of metastatic lymph nodes versus gross dimensions and delineation of clinically occult versus clinically apparent nodal metastases; (c) site of distant metastases and presence of elevated serum lactate dehydrogenase for metastatic disease; (d) upstaging of all patients with stage I, II, and III disease when a primary melanoma is ulcerated; and (e) new convention for separating clinical and pathologic staging to include information obtained from intraoperative lymphatic mapping and sentinel node biopsy. Clinical staging includes microstaging of the primary melanoma and clinical and radiologic evaluation. It is used after complete excision of the primary melanoma with clinical assessment for regional and distant metastasis. Pathologic staging includes microstaging of the primary melanoma and pathologic information about the regional nodes after partial or complete lymphadenectomy. At this time, it appears that patients with very limited disease (stage 0) do not require pathologic evaluation of lymph nodes (Tables 141–4 and 141–5). As with other solid tumors, the presence of regional lymph node involvement is a powerful predictor of tumor burden and patient outcome. In the past, the primary method for determining nodal status was surgical resection and analysis of the lymph nodes via a regional lymph node dissection. The extent of lymph node dissection was determined by the anatomy of the area of the lesion. In recent years, preoperative lymphoscintigraphy and intraoperative sentinel node mapping have become more widely used methods for identifying the first or sentinel lymph node in the direct pathway of lymph drainage from the primary cutaneous melanoma. Sentinel lymph node biopsy (SLNB) is a minimally invasive procedure that is used to determine if a patient is a candidate for a complete lymph node dissection. The rationale for lymphatic mapping and subsequent sentinel node biopsy is based on the observation that regions of the skin have patterns of lymphatic drainage to specific lymph nodes in the regional lymphatic basin. The sentinel lymph node is believed to be the first node in the lymphatic basin into which the primary melanoma drains. Unlike other solid tumors, melanoma appears to progress in an orderly nodal distribution. Evaluation of sentinel nodes has been used for detection of micrometastases in breast cancer and in melanoma. SLNB allows for more thorough examination of a single sentinel node than is possible when examining multiple lymph nodes with a lymph node dissection and may be most useful for melanomas located in ambiguous drainage sites such as the head and neck areas. SLNB is associated with low false-negative rates and low complication rates.[32] Detection of clinically undetectable disease in a lymph node basin that is not directly adjacent to the primary lesion may allow for upstaging of patients who initially are believed to have node-negative disease.

There is great interest in further developing methods to improve the detection of occult micrometastases in biopsied lymph nodes

TABLE 141-4 Melanoma TNM Classification

T Classification	Thickness	Ulcerative Status
TX	Primary tumor cannot be addressed (e.g., shave biopsy)	
T0	No evidence of primary tumor	
Tis	Melanoma in situ	
T1	≤1 mm	A: No ulceration and level II/III B: With ulceration or level IV/V
T2	1.01–2 mm	A: No ulceration B: With ulceration
T3	2.01–4 mm	A: No ulceration B: With ulceration
T4	>4 mm	A: No ulceration B: With ulceration
N Classification	**No. of Metastatic Nodes**	**Nodal Metastatic Mass**
NX	Regional lymph nodes cannot be assessed	
N0	No regional lymph nodes	
N1	1 node	A: Micrometastasis B: Macrometastasis
N2	2–3 nodes	A: Micrometastasis B: Macrometastasis C: In-transit metastases/ satellite(s) without metastatic nodes
N3	≥4 metastatic lymph nodes, matted nodes, ulcerated melanoma, metastatic lymph nodes, or intransit metastatic or satellite lesions	
M Classification	**Site**	**Serum Lactate Dehydrogenase**
MX	Distant metastases cannot be assessed	
M0	No distant metastasis	
M1a	Distant skin, subcutaneous tissue, or nodal metastatic disease	Normal
M1b	Lung metastases	Normal
M1c	All other visceral metastases or distant metastasis at any site associated with elevated serum lactic dehydrogenase	Normal
	Any distant metastasis	Elevated

Micrometastases are diagnosed after sentinel or elective lymphadenectomy.
Macrometastases are defined as clinically detectable lymph node metastases confirmed by therapeutic lymphadenectomy or when any lymph node metastasis exhibits extracapsular extension.
Data from Barch CM, Buzaid AC, Soong SJ, et al. Final version of the American Joint Committee on cancer staging system for cutaneous melanoma. J Clin Oncol 2001;19:3635–3648.

TABLE 141-5 American Joint Committee on Cancer Tumor (T), Node (N), Metastasis (M) Stage Grouping for Cutaneous Melanoma

Pathologic Stage	T	N	M	Clinical Stage	T	N	M
0	Tis	N0	M0	0	Tis	N0	M0
IA	T1a	N0	M0	IA	T1a	N0	M0
IB	T1b	N0	M0	IB	T1b	N0	M0
	T2a	N0	M0		T2a	N0	M0
IIA	T2b	N0	M0	IIA	T2b	N0	M0
	T3a	N0	M0		T3a	N0	M0
IIB	T3b	N0	M0	IIB	T3b	N0	M0
	T4a	N0	M0		T4a	N0	M0
IIC	T4b	N0	M0	IIC	T4b	N0	M0
IIIA	T1–4a	N1a	M0	IIIA	Any T1–4a	N1b	M0
IIIB	T1–4a	N1b	M0	IIIB	Any T1–4a	N2b	M0
	T1–4a	N2a	M0				
IIIC	Any T	N2b, N2c	M0	IIIC	Any T	N2c	M0
	Any T	N3	M0		Any T	N3	M0
IV	Any T	Any N	M1	IV	Any T	Any N	M1

with more sensitive reverse-transcription polymerase chain reaction assays to detect the presence of tyrosinase messenger RNA. Early results of this technique for detection of occult melanoma cells in the blood of patients with small clinical lesions have not been as successful as hoped, but strategies that combine several methods are being evaluated.[1,33] Polymerase chain reaction–based detection of melanoma cells in sentinel lymph nodes of patients with melanoma also is being evaluated as a prognostic tool.[34]

The stage of melanoma at the time of diagnosis is one of the primary indicators of natural history of the disease. Other factors such as tumor growth phase, mitotic rate, density of TILs infiltrating the tumor tissue, anatomic site of the primary tumor, gender, and age, also have been reported to have an impact on survival (Table 141–6). In addition, a number of additional prognostic factors have been identified in patients with advanced disease. The number of metastatic sites, disease involvement of the gastrointestinal tract, liver, pleura, or lung, Eastern Cooperative Oncology Group (ECOG) performance status ≥1, male gender, and patients with prior immunotherapy have been associated with poor prognosis.

TREATMENT

Melanoma

Treatment of cutaneous melanoma depends on the stage of disease. Local disease is managed, and often cured, with surgical ablation. Regional disease is treated with surgical resection of the primary lesion and, depending on the risk of recurrence, possibly adjuvant therapy. Use of adjuvant therapy after surgical resection and the role of interferon-α as adjuvant therapy remain controversial. Treatment of disseminated melanoma remains a challenge. Although numerous clinical trials have evaluated single-agent and combination chemotherapy, immunotherapy, targeted therapy, and biochemotherapy regimens, there is not a single standard approach for management of the individual with metastatic melanoma.[1,10,35,36]

TABLE 141-6 Prognostic Factors for Cutaneous Melanoma

Tumor-related factors
Tumor thickness
Level of tumor invasion
Anatomic site of primary tumor (increased survival in tumors of extremities vs. axial, neck, head, and trunk tumors)
Mitotic rate (correlated with decreased survival)
Angiogenesis
Occurrence of microsatellites
Area of tumor regression
Presence of tumor-infiltrating lymphocytes (correlated with increased survival)
Patient-related factors
Age (decreased survival in patients >60 years old)
Gender (survival: female > male)

SURGERY

❷ Patients who present with a suspicious pigmented lesion should undergo a full-thickness excisional biopsy, if possible. Sites at which excisional biopsy is inappropriate include the face, palm of the hand, sole of the foot, distal digit, and subungual lesions. A full-thickness incisional or punch biopsy is preferred in these cases to provide microstaging and ultimately to determine therapy.

Localized cutaneous melanoma often can be cured with surgical excision. The extent of the excision margin is important in preventing local recurrence and ultimate survival. For melanoma in situ, excision of the visible lesion or biopsy site with a 0.5- to 1-cm border of clinically normal skin and a layer of subcutaneous tissue with confirmation of histologically negative peripheral margins is recommended. The recommended clinical margin for invasive melanoma depends on the tumor thickness. Excision with a 1-cm margin of clinically normal skin and underlying subcutaneous tissue is recommended for invasive melanomas ≤1 mm thick.[35,37] This recommendation is a significant reduction from the previous practice of a large 5-cm margin. The appropriate margin of excision for melanomas between 1 and 2 mm in thickness is controversial. A study suggests the risk of locoregional recurrence is higher when melanomas that are at least 2 mm thick are excised with a 1-cm margin rather than a 2-cm margin.[38] Current National Comprehensive Cancer Network (NCCN) guidelines recommend a 1- to 2-cm margin for melanoma with tumor thickness of 1.01 to 2 mm.[35] Lesions that are 2 to 4 mm thick should be excised with a 2-cm margin. Primary tumors more than 4 mm thick require at least a 2-cm margin, but whether a larger margin is beneficial is not clear.[39] Surgical management of lentigo maligna melanoma is problematic, as subclinical extension of atypical junctional melanocytic hyperplasia may extend beyond the visible margins. Complete excision of these lesions is important.

When isolated regional lymph nodes are detected via physical examination in the absence of distant disease, therapeutic lymphadenectomy is recommended. The extent of therapeutic lymph node dissection often is modified according to the anatomic area of the lymphadenopathy. The role of lymphadenectomy is not as established when the regional lymph nodes do not appear to be involved under clinical examination. Although a subgroup of patients with early-stage melanoma will have microscopic metastatic disease in nonpalpable lymph nodes, prophylactic regional lymph node dissection does not prolong survival or decrease time to relapse in randomized clinical trials.[10,36] Selective regional lymphadenectomy performed after scintigraphic and dye lymphographic identification of the affected sentinel draining lymph node(s) is becoming increasingly available and common. If the sentinel node is found to have micrometastatic melanoma, regional dissection of the involved nodal basin is performed. Lymphatic mapping with sentinel node biopsy, if available, should be considered in patients with melanomas that are more than 1 mm thick. If the lesion is 0.75 to 1 mm in thickness with ulceration or is Clark level IV or V, lymphatic mapping with sentinel node biopsy may be considered based on patient characteristics such as ulceration of the tumor.[36] Of note, the likelihood of detecting metastatic disease in the sentinel lymph node depends on tumor thickness. The likelihood of detecting metastatic disease is approximately 1% in tumors that are less than 0.8 mm but increases to more than 30% in tumors 4 mm thick.[35]

One of the most important aspects of surgical management of cutaneous melanoma is the role of patient follow-up.[1,35] Postsurgical follow-up of patients who have had a melanoma excised is essential to monitor for undetected metastatic disease and the development of a second primary cutaneous melanoma or nonmelanoma primary malignancy. Scheduled screening in addition to routine surgical follow-up are required for any patient with a melanoma; the recommended frequency and duration depend on the stage of melanoma. The optimal duration of follow-up remains controversial. Most patients who are going to have recurrent disease will do so in the first 5 years after treatment, but late recurrences more than 10 years after surgery have been observed. The increased lifetime risk of developing a second primary melanoma supports lifetime dermatologic surveillance for all patients.

Curative surgery usually is limited to patients with early-stage disease. A patient with stage III melanoma usually has lymph node involvement, but in-transit metastases also may occur. In-transit metastasis is the clinical manifestation of tumor that develops in lymphatics between the primary melanoma and the regional lymph node basin.[10] In-transit metastases are more than 2 cm from the original lesion. In-transit metastases are more common in individuals with thick ulcerated lesion. Surgery is used for management of in-transit lesions, and the goal is complete resection. Unfortunately, subsequent recurrence in the same extremity often occurs after initial resection of in-transit metastases. When in-transit metastases occur in extremities, local therapy with isolated limb perfusion or isolated limb infusion has been used.[10]

The role of surgery beyond that of cure is less clear, although surgery may offer palliation for patients with isolated metastases.[40] Resection of isolated lesions in the brain and lungs may be appropriate in certain cases and should be evaluated based on individual patient criteria. Surgery can be an option in situations where the lesion is accessible and where the lesion may cause problems if not removed. Surgery can extend survival in select patients with metastatic disease. Patients whose metastases can be completely resected may experience improved quality of life, improved overall survival, and occasionally long-term disease control.[40]

Brain metastases is a frequent complication of advanced melanoma. Approximately 20% to 50% of patients with stage IV disease will develop clinically apparent central nervous system involvement. Surgical resection, with or without radiation, has been used in select individuals. More recently, high control rates of brain metastases have been achieved with focal radiation therapy such as linear accelerator-based stereotactic radiosurgery or gamma-knife technologies.[41,42] Melanoma in the gastrointestinal tract can lead to bowel obstruction, and appropriate resection or bypass may allow the patient significant relief of symptoms. Despite the lack of controlled clinical trials, the impact on palliative surgery should be evaluated in the context of a patient's comfort and quality of life. Surgery may be an appropriate option if the perceived outcome is to provide patient comfort. On the other hand, surgery may constitute a significant physical challenge or financial burden to a patient with a limited life expectancy. The clinical scenarios involving surgical resection should be fully evaluated in terms of overall quality of life.

The risk of relapse and death after resection of a local or regional cutaneous melanoma is the primary determinant for use of adjuvant therapy after primary resection. Adjuvant trials have focused on patients at intermediate or high risk for recurrence.

■ IMMUNOTHERAPY

Melanoma is considered one of the most immunogenic solid tumors, and it appears to interact with and respond to the immune system of the host in which it arises. Spontaneous regressions of melanoma suggest the importance of the immune system in disease modulation. Lymphoid infiltration into the primary melanoma also suggests that immunomodulation may impact the biology of melanoma. Early work showed that nonspecific immunomodulators, such as levamisole and bacillus Calmette-Guérin, for treatment of melanoma were associated with some regression of the tumor, although many of these responses were limited and short-lived. Because melanoma is one of the cancers most resistant to traditional treatment modalities such as radiation and chemotherapy, immunotherapy offers an avenue of treatment. Although the complete response rate seen in patients with melanoma treated with biotherapy is relatively low, the durability of responses in individuals who respond can be significant. Remaining unanswered questions are what is the best approach to biotherapy in a patient with melanoma and can biotherapy be combined with other available and emerging antineoplastic therapy.

Interferon

One of the oldest, and most controversial, immunotherapy approaches to treatment of melanoma is the use of interferons.[1] The *interferons* are a group of proteins with diverse immunomodulatory and antiangiogenic properties. A number of studies have evaluated various doses and schedules of recombinant interferon for treatment of metastatic melanoma. Response rates in metastatic melanoma range from 10% to 30%, and overall response rates are approximately 15% for interferon-α. Unfortunately, the optimal dose, treatment schedule, and treatment combination/regimens have not been established for management of metastatic melanoma.[10]

In clinical trials of interferon therapy for patients with metastatic melanoma, response rates were highest in patients with minimal disease. Responses were seen at all sites of disease but were most frequent in subcutaneous, lymph node, and pulmonary metastases. The success of interferon in patients with minimal disease encouraged investigators to evaluate the role of adjuvant interferon after curative surgical resection in patients who were at high risk for recurrent disease (bulky disease or regional lymph node involvement). Early trials of short-term or low-dose regimens of interferon-α did not demonstrate a survival benefit in the adjuvant setting. In an attempt to optimize response in the adjuvant setting, maximum tolerated doses of interferon-α were administered for 1 month, followed by prolonged therapy of interferon-α at more tolerable doses for 48 weeks. The rationale for the intensive induction phase was to provide peak interferon levels sufficient to inhibit tumor growth and avoid the development of anti-interferon antibodies. A large, multicenter cooperative group trial (E1684) of adjuvant interferon-α_{2b} versus observation was designed for 287 patients with high-risk (stage IIB and III disease based on the 1997 AJCC staging criteria) melanoma following curative surgical resection.[43] Interferon-α_{2b} was given intravenously as an induction therapy at maximum tolerated doses of 20 million international units/m^2 per dose 5 days per week for 4 weeks in an

TABLE 141-7 Results of Eastern Cooperative Oncology Group Trials of Adjuvant High-Dose Interferon-α_{2b} Therapy in Melanoma Patients at High Risk for Recurrence

Trial	Regimen	5-Year Relapse-Free Survival	5-Year Overall Survival	Reference
E1684	High-dose IFN[a]	37%	46%	Kirkwood et al.[43]
	Observation	26%	37%	
E1690	High-dose IFN[b]	44%	52%	Kirkwood et al.[45]
	Low-dose IFN	40%	53%	
	Observation	35%	55%	

[a]High-dose interferon (IFN) 20 million international units/m²/day IV for 1 month and 10 million international units/m² three times per week subcutaneously (SC) for 48 weeks.
[b]High-dose IFN 20 million international units/m²/day 5 days per week IV for 4 weeks and 10 million international units/m² three times per week subcutaneously (SC) for 48 weeks.

outpatient setting; treatment was continued for 48 weeks with subcutaneous interferon-α_{2b} 10 million international units/m² per dose three times per week at home. This therapy now is often referred to as *high-dose interferon* (HDI). With a median follow-up of 6.9 years, patients treated with HDI had significantly longer relapse-free and overall survival compared to patients who were observed following surgical resection (1.72 vs 0.98 years and 3.8 vs 2.8 years, respectively).[43] Table 141–7 shows 5-year relapse-free and overall survival results. With longer follow-up (median 12.6 years), however, the difference in overall survival was no longer significant.[44] Further analysis of the hazard function showed that the greatest reduction in melanoma recurrence occurred during the first few months of treatment. Subgroup analysis of this study indicated that patients with large primary tumors and node-negative disease (T4N0M0) did not receive the same benefit from therapy, but the small number of patients in this group made it difficult to draw definite conclusions about the role of interferon for adjuvant therapy in this subgroup.

HDI treatment is associated with multiple toxicities, including flu-like syndrome. Other toxicities include depression, nausea, weight loss, fatigue, myelosuppression, elevations in liver function tests, and renal insufficiency. Toxicities of interferon therapy in the adjuvant HDI trials were common and severe, and most patients required dose reductions and/or delays at some point during treatment. Dose modifications were required for dose-limiting constitutional symptoms, myelosuppression, and hepatic toxicities, but 74% of patients were able to complete the year of therapy in an outpatient setting.

One of the strategies for reducing the toxicities associated with interferon was to modify the dose and duration. A subsequent ECOG trial (E1690) of low-dose interferon (LDI; three million units per dose given subcutaneously three times weekly) for 24 months compared to the HDI regimen described above versus observation did not demonstrate an overall survival advantage of HDI versus observation.[45] At median followup of 52 months, the 5-year estimated relapse-free survival rates for HDI, LDI, and observation were 44%, 40%, and 35%, respectively. Relapse-free survival was significantly longer in the HDI group, prolonging the median time to relapse by 10 months compared to observation and LDI. With longer follow-up, however, the difference in relapse-free survival was no longer significant.[44] A significant overall survival benefit was not seen for HDI or LDI compared to observation, although the investigators speculated that this analysis of survival was affected by the number of patients in the observation arm who received interferon therapy after disease progression.[45]

Use of interferon in the adjuvant setting remains controversial. Although the HDI regimen is used in the United States, the LDI strategy remains standard in many European countries.[1] In a pooled analysis of 713 patients who participated in two randomized controlled trials (E1684 and E1690), HDI was associated with a significant reduction in relapse-free survival compared with observation (P <0.006).[44] No benefit in overall survival was observed in the pooled analysis. The results of nine randomized clinical trials of adjuvant HDI or LDI versus observation in melanoma were included in a systematic review. The systematic review observed a trend toward reduction of risk of recurrence of melanoma and of death among the interferon-treated patients in nearly all studies.[46] Adjuvant interferon-α has been evaluated in a number of clinical trials in patients with intermediate- to very-high-risk melanoma after surgical resection. A systematic review evaluated nine randomized controlled trials of high- and low-dose regimens.[46] Due to differences in dose, frequency, and duration of interferon-α treatments in the various trials, the review was not able to compare LDI versus HDI. Furthermore, the wide variability in number of patients enrolled, end points, patient selection, quality, type of therapy, duration of treatment, and follow-up precluded statistical analysis of the pooled results. Although the differences in overall survival were not always statistically significant, HDI remains the only adjuvant treatment shown to prolong survival in prospective randomized trials. Interferon-α_{2b} is approved by the Food and Drug Administration (FDA) for treatment of patients with primary melanomas larger than 4 mm (stage IIB and IIC) and in patients with melanoma involving regional lymph nodes who are disease-free following lymph node dissection (stage III).

Although interferon is widely used in the adjuvant setting, there are concerns over the considerable treatment toxicities and the lack of consistent overall survival advantage of a toxic and expensive regimen. In addition, whether the results from the HDI trials should be extrapolated to patients with local recurrences, satellite lesions, or in-transit metastases is not clear. Remaining questions include the following: (a) Are the toxicities associated with HDI treatment worth the potential benefits for patients? (b) What are the mechanism(s) and best approaches to managing interferon toxicity? (c) Is the regimen/schedule of interferon used in the initial positive trial (HDI) necessary to achieve the benefits seen in this study? Aggressive toxicity evaluation and individualized management are essential to help preserve quality of life in individuals receiving interferon therapy.

❸ A mechanism for optimizing the care of patients receiving interferon is to effectively prevent and manage treatment-related toxicities. A common syndrome seen with interferon-α therapy is a diverse group of side effects referred to as *constitutional symptoms,* which can include acute symptoms such as fever, chills, myalgia, and fatigue, and can encompass some of the more chronic toxicities such as fatigue, anorexia, and depression.[47] Acetaminophen can be used to prevent or minimize acute dose-related symptoms such as fever, myalgia, and chills. Opiates such as meperidine are often required when patients experience severe chills or rigors, most commonly during the initial month of the HDI induction phase. Nonsteroidal antiinflammatory drugs (NSAIDs) have been used to manage interferon-related myalgia but may have overlapping side effects with interferon, such as a decrease in renal blood flow and nausea. NSAIDs, like acetaminophen, may mask fevers that occur in patients who experience neutropenia while undergoing therapy. Fatigue is one of the most frequently observed dose-limiting toxicities seen with interferon therapy.[47] The mechanisms of interferon-induced fatigue are not fully understood and may be multifactorial in individual patients. Interferon-induced fatigue appears to be dose related and may worsen with continued therapy. Pharmacologic (e.g., amantadine) and nonpharmacologic interventions (e.g., exercise, psychosocial techniques, distraction, energy management, and dietary modifications) for treatment cancer-related fatigue and now interferon-related fatigue are being evaluated.[47,48] Anorexia was reported in approximately 70% of patients receiving adjuvant interferon therapy for melanoma and is thought to be mediated through direct effects on hypothalamic neurons, modification of normal hypothalamic neurotransmitters/neuropeptides, or effects from stimulation of other cytokines.[47,49] Depression is common and should be fully evaluated and treated based on patient-related symptoms.[47] Contributing factors such as interferon-induced hypothyroidism and/or concomitant interferon symptoms (e.g., nausea and fatigue) should be evaluated concurrently with depression symptoms to optimize treatment decisions. Taste alterations may contribute to anorexia. Investigational strategies for ameliorating interferon-induced anorexia include nutritional intervention, use of appetite stimulants such as megestrol acetate, and patient education. Glucocorticoids should not be used for appetite stimulation or as part of an antiemetic therapy because they may adversely impact the immunomodulatory effects of interferon. Other toxicities such as hematologic or hepatic toxicities require monitoring and appropriate dose modification.

Because of the associated toxicity and adverse effects seen with interferon-α therapy, there has been worldwide concern about the usefulness of this intensive adjuvant therapy for melanoma despite the possible benefits in relapse-free and overall survival.[50] A subsequent report from the cooperative group study demonstrated a quality-of-life benefit with interferon therapy based on the quality-of-life-adjusted survival analysis.[51] This analysis calculates the quality-of-life-adjusted years gained as a result of interferon-α treatment or the clinical benefit of time without toxicities and without disease.

❹ The role of interferon as adjuvant therapy is not clear at this time. If adjuvant interferon is given, what product (e.g. pegylated interferon), dose, and duration of therapy should be used are not clear. The issues of patient side effects and cost must be carefully weighed against the potential disease-free survival benefit. Because HDI is the only therapy to demonstrate benefit in large comparative trials, it should be considered for patients with high-risk disease. The 2008 NCCN Guidelines for melanoma list interferon-α as one of several options for select patients with high-risk disease.[35] Other options include observation and probably, most importantly, clinical trials. Individuals should be prescreened for potential problems associated with therapy; relative contraindications to HDI therapy include autoimmune diseases, immunosuppression, decompensated liver disease, severe neuropsychiatric diseases, and life-threatening infection.[47] Efforts continue to better define the optimal treatment regimen for HDI versus other strategies in well-designed clinical trials.

CLINICAL CONTROVERSY

The role of interferon-α as adjuvant therapy for high-risk patients after surgical resection of melanoma is controversial. Assessment of patient risk factors, availability of clinical trials, and cost of therapy should be evaluated prior to initiation of therapy.

The role of interferon in advanced disease is even less clear, especially for patients who have recurred after treatment with adjuvant interferon therapy. Interferon-α has been used as a single agent in patients with metastatic disease who have not received adjuvant therapy and in combination with chemotherapy and/or other biotherapy for metastatic melanoma. The challenges of combination therapy are that many of the toxicities seen with interferon can be exacerbated by concomitant chemotherapy (e.g., nausea, vomiting, and neutropenia).

Interleukin-2

Interleukin-2 (IL-2) is a glycoprotein produced by activated lymphocytes.[52] IL-2 was first identified as a T-cell growth factor, but now IL-2 clearly is a growth factor for a variety of cells including lymphocytes, T cells, and natural killer (NK) cells. IL-2 also may be immunosuppressive. The role of each of these effects of IL-2 on disease control in melanoma is not clear.

The precise mechanism of cytotoxicity of IL-2 is unknown. High concentrations of IL-2 have not been shown to have a direct antitumor effect on cancer cells in vitro. In vitro and in vivo, IL-2 stimulates the production and release of many secondary monocyte-derived and T-cell–derived cytokines, including IL-4, IL-5, IL-6, IL-8, tumor necrosis factor-α, granulocyte-macrophage colony-stimulating factor, and interferon-γ, which may have direct or indirect antitumor activity. In addition, IL-2 stimulates the cytotoxic activities of NK cells, monocytes, lymphokine-activated killer (LAK) cells, and CTLs. IL-2 also appears to activate endothelial cells, which results in increased expression of adhesion molecules.[52]

❺ Based on preclinical studies that demonstrated a dose–response relationship between recombinant IL-2 (aldesleukin) and tumor response, initial clinical trials of aldesleukin in patients with melanoma used relatively high doses of the drug as a single agent or in combination with LAK cells. The response rates seen in these trials ranged from 15% to 25%, and 2% to 5% of patients achieved complete responses, some of which were durable. Responses were seen at a number of metastatic sites, such as lung, liver, bone, lymph nodes, and subcutaneous tissue. Based on reevaluation of early clinical trials,[53] aldesleukin received FDA approval for treatment of metastatic melanoma. Overall, objective response rates were approximately 16%, but in some cases responses were durable and were observed in patients with large tumor burdens. The high doses of aldesleukin used in the initial clinical trials and recommended in the labeling of the drug are associated with serious toxicities and may limit the practicality of therapy for individual patients and broad application in certain healthcare systems. The high-dose aldesleukin regimen used for treatment of metastatic melanoma is 600,000 international units/kg per dose every 8 hours for 14 doses maximum in a 5-day period given for two cycles, with a 10- to 14-day rest period between cycles. At these doses, cytokine-induced capillary leak syndrome is a common problem and often is accompanied by significant hypotension, visceral edema, dyspnea, tachycardia, and arrhythmias. Increased permeability of capillary walls allows for a fluid shift from the intravascular space into tissue. As the patient becomes intravascularly dehydrated, hypotension may occur, resulting in reflex tachycardia and arrhythmias. In addition, the decrease in blood volume may result in decreased renal blood flow and urine output, manifesting as an increase in blood urea nitrogen, serum creatinine, edema, weight gain, and a decrease in urine output (input greater than output). Visceral edema can result in pulmonary congestion, pleural effusions, and edema. The management of patients receiving high-dose aldesleukin requires careful monitoring and a staff trained in aspects of critical care such as hypotension management. Although patients initially receiving high-dose aldesleukin are treated in an intensive care unit, most patients can be managed on a designated oncology unit if the staff is familiar with the toxicities and management strategies of the toxicities. Additional side effects seen with aldesleukin include constitutional symptoms, pruritus, eosinophilia, bone marrow suppression including thrombocytopenia, increased liver function tests, and nausea.[54]

CLINICAL CONTROVERSY

Although aldesleukin has been associated with long-term durable responses in a small subset of patients with metastatic melanoma, the toxicity profile, intensity of therapy, and cost have limited its acceptance in the United States. Patients should be evaluated for treatment prior to initiation of therapy.

In an attempt to reduce treatment-related toxicities, a number of studies have evaluated continuous-infusion aldesleukin and lower doses of aldesleukin, given either alone or combined with chemotherapy and interferon therapy. Although initial reports were encouraging, survival has not been significantly affected. At this time, direct head-to-head comparisons of various dosing schedules and regimens are needed to determine the optimum approach to aldesleukin therapy in metastatic melanoma. Coadministration of LAK cells with aldesleukin does not appear to significantly improve clinical response.[55] Although some studies have suggested improved response with coadministration of TILs with recombinant IL-2, the therapy is technically difficult and costly, and the overall clinical benefit has not been clearly demonstrated.[56]

One of the greatest treatment challenges in treatment of metastatic melanoma is determining the role of aldesleukin therapy for each patient. Based on reports of long-term responses (>10 years) experienced by some patients, the risk certainly is worth the benefit for those individuals. Unfortunately, at this time it is difficult to determine which individuals will respond to aldesleukin therapy, as no biologic or immunologic parameters have been found to correlate with response. The decision to treat an individual with high-dose aldesleukin should be based on an analysis of an individual patient's risk versus potential benefit. Patients with inadequate pulmonary function, cardiac function, renal insufficiency, active infection, or poor performance status are poor candidates for this therapy. Aldesleukin can be safely administered with a properly trained healthcare team and is one of only two approved therapies for treatment of metastatic melanoma.

Vaccines

The rationale for vaccination as a therapeutic modality is based on the observation that antigens expressed on the surface of tumor cells differ from normal cells and the hope that vaccines might induce effective tumor-specific immune responses with fewer toxicities than conventional chemotherapy or other immunotherapies. Greater knowledge about tumor antigens and the mechanism of antigen presentation and immune response to antigens has led to the development of several vaccination strategies for treatment of early and advanced melanoma.

A variety of melanoma vaccines based on whole tumor cells, peptides, proteins, and tumor lysates have been evaluated for treatment of patients with metastatic disease and for intermediate- and high-risk patients after surgical resection of disease.[57–60] Although tumor responses with some of these approaches have been observed in phase I and II trials, none of the vaccine responses have been confirmed in phase III trials.[59] These early trials have focused on safety, feasibility, and immunogenicity of the vaccine. Vaccines are a promising but still experimental approach in the treatment of melanoma.

Vaccination is a form of active specific immunotherapy directed against a particular cellular target or specific membrane antigen. The ideal tumor vaccine would generate an active, systemic, long-lived immune response in the cancer-bearing host against tumors; protect against primary development or subsequent relapse of cancer; or induce regression of established cancer. Obstacles in the development of a vaccine include identifying appropriate antigens to target and generating immune responses against tumor antigens to which the immune system has been already exposed.

Whole-cell tumor vaccines can be derived from cell lines that are already established (allogeneic vaccines) or from the patient's own tumor cells (autologous). Whole-cell vaccines are challenging to produce for several reasons: a new vaccine must be prepared for each patient, patients must have sufficient tumor available to provide adequate material, and considerable delay may exist between time of tumor removal and vaccine administration.[57] In addition there are technical challenges to producing the vaccine in the laboratory.[58] Currently no autologous tumor cell vaccine has been successfully studied in a phase III randomized clinical trial. An example of a whole-cell tumor vaccine that is being studied is Canvaxin. Canvaxin (CancerVax, Carlsbad, CA) is an allogeneic whole-cell vaccine that uses bacillus Calmette-Guérin as a immune adjuvant. Small trials have shown improvements in survival compared with historical controls, and some objective clinical responses have been seen in patients with metastatic melanoma. Two large randomized trials have compared Canvaxin to observation, one in patients with metastatic melanoma and one in stage III melanoma. The results of these trials have not yet been published, but have been reported to show no significant differences between the vaccine and observation.[59]

Antigen vaccines use individual antigens to stimulate immune responses, as compared with whole-cell vaccines, which contain many thousands of antigens.[60] These antigens usually are proteins or pieces of proteins called *peptides*. Antigen vaccines may be specific for a certain type of cancer, but they are not made for a specific patient. Vaccines against GM2 ganglioside, a glycolipid expressed on most melanomas, are examples of vaccines targeted against an antigen. Two randomized controlled trials with anti-GM2 vaccines have failed to show any benefit with the vaccine.[59]

Peptide antigen vaccines match the patient's haplotype with the spectrum of immunity that he or she expresses. T cells recognize antigens as peptide epitopes on the surface of major histocompatibility complex (MHC) molecules. Antigenic peptides can be mixed with an immunologic adjuvant and administered with the goal of loading empty MHC molecules in vivo. To date the most commonly used peptides have shown activity only in patients who express human leukocyte antigen (HLA)-A2. However, because not all patients express this HLA antigen, many patients would not be eligible for this vaccine.[57] Additional peptide antigens that are compatible in other haplotypes have been identified, and eventually this disadvantage may be overcome. Peptide vaccination can generate quantifiable and functional tumor-reactive T cells, but clinical responses are rare and do not consistently correlate with CTL response.

Because protein antigen vaccines have a slightly broader spectrum of antigen diversity, all patients with melanoma potentially could be eligible for vaccination with this particular type of vaccine. Proteins intrinsically produced by the cell are presented only to $CD8^+$ T cells, whereas proteins taken up by antigen-presenting cells are presented only to $CD4^+$ T cells. Under certain conditions, antigen-presenting cells can present protein-derived antigens to both $CD4^+$ and $CD8^+$ in a process known as *cross-presentation*.[57]

Tumor lysates can be generated from tumor cells by mechanical disruption or enzymatic digestion.[57] Tumor cells that shed antigens in culture can be purified and used as an antigen source for vaccines. Production of a vaccine from these sources raises concern because standardization of production and verification of purity and biological activity are more difficult.

Vaccines in combination with other biologic therapies are being evaluated. In a randomized trial of 604 patients with resected stage III cutaneous melanoma, LDI combined with an allogeneic melanoma lysate vaccine (2 years) was compared with HDI alone (1 year).[63] Median overall survival was not significantly different between the two treatment arms ($P = 0.56$). Five-year relapse-free and overall survival were similar in the two treatment arms. The incidence of serious treatment-related adverse events was similar in the two arms, but more severe neuropsychiatric toxicity was observed in patients receiving HDI. Although the results of this trial suggest that the vaccine has some activity in melanoma, the study was not powered sufficiently to show either equivalency or small differences in efficacy. HLA typing was optional based on whether the centers were able to perform the typing. With ongoing research, hopefully standards can be made and additional trials performed with this vaccine specifically in patients with certain HLA types.

Occasional clinical responses have been observed in clinical trials of melanoma vaccines, which demonstrate the potential of this form of treatment. Many clinical trials with vaccine therapy in melanoma patients are ongoing. The results of completed clinical trials have not yet shown definitive evidence of improved survival. Further research is needed to improve vaccine responses and to determine how to apply treatment to melanoma patients.

Other Approaches

Dendritic cells are potent antigen-presenting cells that initiate antigen-specific immune responses. Dendritic cells express high levels of MHC class I and class II molecules, which are essential in antigen presentation. Activation of T cells and recruitment of non–antigen-specific effectors, such as NK cells and macrophages, result in a broad immune response. One strategy that uses dendritic cells for inducing antitumor immune responses is peptide-pulsed dendritic cells. Antimelanoma CTLs can be generated from healthy donors and patients with melanoma with dendritic cells pulsed with melanoma-derived peptides. A number of clinical trials are evaluating dendritic cell–based immunotherapy.[58,59]

Monoclonal antibodies have been used for diagnosis and treatment of melanoma. Monoclonal antibodies can be used to target biologic pathways (e.g., bevacizumab to target angiogenesis) that are associated with tumor progression and as a delivery system for antineoplastic drugs. Monoclonal antibodies have been conjugated to cytotoxic agents, radioisotopes, and toxins such as ricin A.[10,20] More recently, monoclonal antibodies have been developed to target processes that are involved in the host immune response to melanoma. Cytotoxic T-lymphocyte antigen-4 (CTLA4) is a transmembrane protein that suppresses the induction of immune responses against tumor antigens.[61,62] CTLA4 blockade may represent a novel approach to enhance the immune response against melanoma antigens. Ipilimumab (MDX-010) and tremelimumab (CP-675206; formerly known as ticilimumab) are two monoclonal antibodies against CTLA4 that are in clinical development. Preliminary results of clinical trials show promising activity in malignant melanoma. MDX-010 is a fully human immunoglobulin G_1 monoclonal antibody in clinical trials that targets CTLA-4, which results in increased antitumor activity mediated by T cells.[20]

Gene therapy of human melanoma is in its infancy but suggests several exciting approaches to management of metastatic melanoma. Several strategies for gene therapy are under investigation for treatment of melanoma. One approach to gene therapy for melanoma is modification of melanoma cells with insertion of one or more cytokine genes and then administration of these altered allogeneic or autologous cells as a vaccine. Cytokine gene transduction has been accomplished with a number of cytokines, including aldesleukin (IL-2), tumor necrosis factor-α, IL-4, and interferon. It is hoped that insertion of cytokine genes into melanoma cells will significantly increase the cells' immunogenicity.

Genes can be transferred in vitro into TILs associated with melanoma in an attempt to potentiate the cytotoxicity of these cells. Rosenberg et al. were the first to attempt to transduce the gene coding for resistance to neomycin into human TILs.[56] This approach has since been used to transfer the tumor necrosis factor gene into TILs.

Thalidomide and thalidomide analogs are being evaluated for management of melanoma. Thalidomide, given either as a single agent or in combination with chemotherapy or cytokines, is being evaluated in a variety of studies. Thalidomide analogs also are being evaluated in an attempt to avoid toxicities associated with the parent compound. The thalidomide analogs are grouped into two classes: selective cytokine inhibitory drugs and immunomodulatory derivatives. Both classes appear to have antiangiogenic and antiinflammatory properties, but the selective cytokine inhibitory drugs are phosphodiesterase inhibitors. Immunomodulatory derivatives also have effects on T-cell stimulation and inhibition of tumor necrosis factor-α. Several of these agents are being evaluated in clinical trials of metastatic melanoma.[64]

CHEMOTHERAPY

A number of antineoplastic agents have demonstrated in vitro activity against melanoma, but only a few drugs have consistently shown a response rate greater than 10% in individuals with metastatic melanoma. Most clinical trials that evaluate new agents in melanoma measure activity in terms of response rates, which often include partial response rates in addition to complete response. It is important to understand that these response rates do not always correlate with survival and do not evaluate benefit to the patient. Response rates also do not represent the toxicities and the complications of therapy. Complete responses can be durable in a small number of patients.

❻ *Dacarbazine*, a cytotoxic drug thought to exert its antitumor effect through alkylation, currently is the most effective single agent for treatment of melanoma. Dacarbazine remains the only FDA-approved chemotherapeutic agent for treatment of metastatic melanoma in the United States.[64,65] Prospective controlled clinical trials have observed response rates of 10% to 25%, with an average duration of response of 5 to 7 months. Complete responses are uncommon, with less than 5% of patients treated with single-agent dacarbazine sustaining long-term complete responses. There does not appear to be a survival benefit for dacarbazine relative to other treatments or supportive care. Patients with skin, subcutaneous tissue, and lymph node involvement respond most frequently, whereas patients with metastatic disease to the liver, bone, and central nervous system often are unresponsive. The optimum dose schedule of dacarbazine has never been determined; therefore, single-dose regimens are often preferred for patient convenience. Common side effects of dacarbazine therapy include moderate myelosuppression, severe nausea and vomiting, and a flu-like syndrome after large doses. Nausea and vomiting can be prevented and managed with available antiemetics and is not a major complication. At this time, dacarbazine has no defined role in the adjuvant setting.

Temozolomide is one of a series of imidazole tetrazine derivatives that was developed as a potential alternative to dacarbazine.[64] Temozolomide is an oral prodrug of the active metabolite of dacarbazine. Dacarbazine requires hepatic transformation to its active intermediate, whereas at physiologic pH, temozolomide chemically degrades to the cytotoxic monomethyltriazenoimidazole carboxamide (MTIC). Temozolomide is administered orally and appears to be less emetogenic than dacarbazine, although nausea can be a challenging chronic toxicity. Temozolomide appears to cross into the central nervous system and so initially was thought to have benefit for patients with central nervous system metastases. In chemotherapy-naive individuals with metastatic melanoma, temozolomide showed efficacy at least equivalent to that of dacarbazine in terms of objective response rates, time to progression, and overall and disease-free survival. There was suggestion that temozolomide may have been associated with improvement in some aspects of quality of life in this phase III trial, although overall disease control was similar to dacarbazine.[66]

A potential advantage of temozolomide is the convenience of the oral dosing form, which allows a potentially more effective dosing schedule (e.g., multiple doses per day or a multiple-day administration). It is believed that prolonged administration may help to overcome some of the chemotherapy drug-resistance mechanisms of intermittent dosing temozolomide or dacarbazine. The active metabolite of dacarbazine and temozolomide, MTIC, methylates guanine residues in DNA at the O^6 position. Resistance to agents that produce O^6 methylation is partly due to increased levels of O^6-alylguanine-DNA alkyltransferase. Temozolomide administration results in decreased activity of alkyltransferase for at least 24 hours. Daily administration of temozolomide may be a strategy to increase the cytotoxicity of the drug.[67] Clinical evaluations of prolonged administration of temozolomide are ongoing, often in combination with other agents such as interferon.[68,69]

The *nitrosoureas* are active against melanoma. Nitrosoureas, such as carmustine and lomustine, have antitumor activity similar to that of dacarbazine, with reported response rates between 10% and 20%. Sites of responses are similar to those seen with dacarbazine. It was initially hoped that use of the lipophilic nitrosoureas would provide added benefit against a malignancy that can metastasize to the brain. Unfortunately, despite the ability of these agents to cross the blood–brain barrier, the commercially available nitrosoureas have not been shown to have increased activity against melanoma in the central nervous system. Fotemustine, a nitrosourea available in Australia and some European countries, appears to cross the blood–brain barrier more rapidly than do other nitrosoureas. Response rates of 30% have been reported in previously untreated patients, with response rates of 25% of patients who had cerebral metastases. Fotemustine is considered standard therapy in some countries.[70] The most common toxicity of the nitrosoureas is delayed myelosuppression, particularly thrombocytopenia. Leukopenia and thrombocytopenia may be seen as long as 3 to 5 weeks after drug administration and may limit the inclusion of these agents to multidrug regimens.

Cisplatin and related compounds have been evaluated in the management of metastatic melanoma. The effectiveness of platinum compounds as single agents is limited, with reported response rates of 10% to 15% with a short median duration. The activity of cisplatin in melanoma may be dose dependent, and higher response rates have been seen with higher doses of cisplatin in single-institution studies.[71] The toxicities of cisplatin can be problematic, especially in higher doses, and include acute and delayed nausea and vomiting, renal toxicity, and neurotoxicity. Other platinum analogs, such as carboplatin and oxaliplatin, are being evaluated for treatment of melanoma.

Taxanes have demonstrated encouraging results in initial trials of metastatic melanoma. Response rates of 15% to 17% have been seen in initial phase II trials with paclitaxel and docetaxel. Abraxane, the albumin-bound nanoparticle formulation of paclitaxel, has shown encouraging results in a very small phase II trials and is being evaluated in a randomized phase III trial.[72] At this time, these agents are not routinely used as single-agent therapy for melanoma but are being incorporated into multidrug strategies undergoing evaluation for use against metastatic melanoma.

In an attempt to improve the limited responses seen with single-agent chemotherapy, a variety of combination chemotherapy regimens (Table 141–8) have been evaluated in both small and large clinical trials. Response rates as high as 30% to 50% were reported in single-institution phase II trials of patients with metastatic melanoma. The combination of dacarbazine with other chemotherapy, most commonly cisplatin, increased the response rates reported with dacarbazine alone, but the survival benefit has been minimal. Responses often were limited to metastases in soft tissue, lymph nodes, and the lung, the sites most likely to respond to single-agent dacarbazine therapy. The concern with combination chemotherapy is increased toxicity, and any reports of increased response rates should be weighed against the effect of toxicities on overall quality of life. The initial reports with the cisplatin, vinblastine, and dacarbazine (CVD) regimen were exciting, with reported response rates greater than 50%, 4% complete response rate, median response duration 9 months, and acceptable toxicities.[73] Comparisons of this regimen to dacarbazine alone have been conflicting. Subsequent reports showed no difference in response rates or survival.

The Dartmouth regimen is a combination that includes carmustine, dacarbazine, cisplatin, and tamoxifen. Initial reports from uncontrolled phase II trials of this combination have demonstrated high response rates of 20% to 50%, but few patients achieve long-term survival. The benefit of tamoxifen to this regimen has been controversial, but a controlled clinical trial from the National Cancer Institute of Canada demonstrated no benefit in response or survival from tamoxifen in this combination.[74] Careful analysis of the initial studies demonstrates that the criteria used to measure response were not consistent with standards used in large multicenter studies. Phase III trials have shown no benefit of the Dartmouth regimen compared to single-agent dacarbazine.[75,76] Response rates were 15%, and median survival was approximately 7 months in both studies. Of concern, toxicities were higher with the combination study and included bone marrow suppression, nausea, vomiting, and fatigue.

TABLE 141-8 Combination Chemotherapy Regimens for Metastatic Melanoma

Dartmouth regimen (CDBT): Repeated every 3–4 weeks
Cisplatin 25 mg/m^2 IV daily × 3 (days 1, 2, and 3)
Dacarbazine 220 mg/m^2 IV daily × 3 (days 1, 2, and 3)
Carmustine 150 mg/m^2 IV daily × 1 (day 1)
Tamoxifen 10 mg orally twice a day
CVD
Cisplatin 20 mg/m^2 IV daily × 4 (days 2, 3, 4, 5)
Vinblastine 1.6 mg/m^2 IV daily × 5 (days 1, 2, 3, 4, 5)
Dacarbazine 800 mg/m^2 IV daily × 1 (day 1)

TARGETED THERAPY

❼ The role of protein kinases in the regulation and proliferation signals in cancer cells is becoming a key focus for anticancer agents. The role of protein kinase inhibitors has emerged as standard therapy for malignancies such as renal cell carcinoma, chronic myelogenous leukemia, and gastrointestinal stromal tumors. As the biology of melanoma continues to unfold, there has been an increasing excitement about the development of targeted therapies against targets important for the development and progression of melanoma.[20,77] There now is greater interest in identifying potential targets in melanoma and determining the applicability in specific patients and/or patient subsets.

Mutations of BRAF have been described in melanoma cell lines, and it appears that approximately 50% to 70% of melanomas exhibit BRAF alteration.[18,78] Sorafenib, a biaryl urea originally synthesized as a BRAF and CRAF inhibitor, is being evaluated in melanoma. Sorafenib inhibits both wild-type and mutant BRAF, in addition to other tyrosine kinases involved in angiogenesis and tumor progression. Preclinical studies demonstrated activity against human melanoma tumor xenografts in preclinical trials, modest activity as a single agent in phase II clinical trials in refractory metastatic melanoma, and promising results in combination trials with chemotherapy.[64,78,79] Early results from phase II studies look promising for the combination of sorafenib and other anticancer agents. Based on these early promising results from phase II trials, a number of phase II trials are evaluating the efficacy of sorafenib with carboplatin and paclitaxel. It will be important to evaluate the efficacy of the addition of sorafenib to the "untested" combination of carboplatin and paclitaxel for treatment of metastatic melanoma.

Another agent of interest is imatinib mesylate, an oral agent that inhibits c-Kit and PDGFR. Expression of c-Kit has been observed in nearly 50% of early stage melanomas, but it appears that *c-Kit* expression is progressively reduced as the cells transform to a more highly metastatic phenotype.[80] PDGFR is also highly expressed on melanoma cells. Imatinib has been shown to suppress melanoma cell growth in preclinical studies. In a phase II study, high-dose imatinib was shown to be inactive in metastatic melanoma.[81]

ENDOCRINE THERAPY

The role of endocrine therapy in the management of melanoma has been debated over the last decade.[10] Initial reports that described high-affinity cytoplasmic estrogen receptors in patients with metastatic melanoma caused some experts to speculate about the possibility that antiestrogens or other hormonal manipulation may be beneficial in modulating the biology of melanoma. Additionally, estrogens have been shown to suppress T-lymphocyte activity and to suppress or stimulate the activities of B lymphocytes, macrophages, and NK cells, supporting a hypothesis that estrogens influence the immunologic mechanisms that appear to be important in melanoma.

In a randomized trial, tamoxifen was shown to have a response and survival benefit when combined with dacarbazine in patients with metastatic melanoma; this benefit was most pronounced in women.[82] Well-designed prospective randomized studies demonstrate that tamoxifen does not significantly enhance the antitumor effect of dacarbazine alone or the combination of dacarbazine with cisplatin and carmustine.[10,83] As discussed previously, subsequent trials have not been able to confirm the initial reported benefit of the antiestrogen when combined with chemotherapy, and tamoxifen is no longer routinely included in chemotherapy regimens.[64]

■ BIOCHEMOTHERAPY

Low overall response rates and toxicity have limited the routine use of chemotherapy alone or immunotherapy alone in the management of metastatic disease. Over the past decade, the strategy of a combination of chemotherapy and cytokines, aldesleukin, and/or interferon, often termed *biochemotherapy*, has been a major focus of investigation in the management of metastatic melanoma and more recently in the adjuvant setting. The primary rationale is to combine two therapies with some biologic activity to increase overall activity and perhaps response rates. Additionally, some preclinical trials suggest potential synergistic interactions between cytokines and some chemotherapy agents. As with other treatment strategies in melanoma, the results from initial trials suggested a higher response rate with biochemotherapy than the rates seen with either chemotherapy or biotherapy alone. Although several studies have suggested an increase in response rate with the addition of interferon-α to chemotherapy, results of most studies have shown that the addition of interferon-α does not increase the antitumor effect of dacarbazine but does increase toxicity and cost. Similarly, the combination of aldesleukin to chemotherapy has not been consistently shown to increase response or survival. The most encouraging results have been seen with combination chemotherapy and combination biotherapy, but the results of phase III studies have not demonstrated a clear advantage of biochemotherapy compared to chemotherapy alone. A recently published meta-analysis of 18 randomized trials of chemotherapy versus biochemotherapy showed that biochemotherapy was associated with a significantly higher response rate in treatment of metastatic melanoma.[84] However, these differences in response rates did not translate into a significant difference in overall survival. Toxicities can be severe and are consistent with the individual agents in the regimen.

One of the problems with most studies of biochemotherapy is the relatively short duration of response. Recurrence rates among patients who respond to therapy are as high as 50% within 18 to 24 months. Strategies such as subcutaneous low-dose aldesleukin are being investigated in an effort to prolong overall survival and time to progression in patients who do respond to treatment. Initial response rates, durable complete remission, and activity in patients in whom HDI therapy was not successful has stimulated interest in evaluating biochemotherapy in the adjuvant setting for high-risk patients with node-positive disease as compared to HDI.

A more recent strategy for biochemotherapy is substitution of newer agents into the combination. For example, a small phase II trial of patients with metastatic melanoma evaluated the substitution of temozolomide for dacarbazine.[86,87]

■ LIMB PERFUSION AND LIMB INFUSION

Isolated limb perfusion is a surgical procedure of regional intravascular delivery of chemotherapy and/or biotherapy into an extremity with cutaneous melanoma.[88,89] Isolated limb perfusion is a method for escalating the dose of chemotherapeutic drugs to a specific region of the body while limiting the systemic toxicities of the agent. Most perfusions can be performed with drug exposures of less than 2%. The most significant side effect of isolated limb perfusion is regional toxicity; all of the skin, subcutaneous tissue, and tissue of the extremity receives the same dose and is subjected to the same perfusion conditions as the tumor located within the extremity. After regional perfusions, objective response rates greater than 50% in treated limbs have been reported, with overall response rates possibly as high as 80%. The role of hyperthermia (39°C–40°C [102°F–104°F]) with regional isolated perfusion is not clearly defined. Although most clinical trials have used melphalan, whether the combination of melphalan with other agents may improve results is not known.[90] Agents that have been combined with melphalan include actinomycin D, nitrogen mustard, thiotepa, and cisplatin. Work with biologic response modifiers, such as tumor necrosis factor-α, have been encouraging.[91] A simplified form of isolated limb perfusion, called isolated limb infusion), is a low-flow isolated limb perfusion performed under hypoxic conditions via small-caliber arterial and venous catheters. It has been proposed that the hypoxia that develops during isolated limb infusion may be beneficial with certain cytotoxic agents such as melphalan.

■ TREATMENT BY STAGE

Treatment of cutaneous melanoma is determined by many factors, including disease-related and patient-related issues. Most available reviews[36,64] and guidelines[35] provide treatment recommendations based on stage of disease. Most patients present with localized disease.[35] Treatment of localized disease is surgical excision, with the extent of excision based on the tumor size. Wide excision is recommended for in situ melanoma and wide excision with SLNB for stage IA, IB, and II disease. Long-term survival of individuals with early-stage disease and thin tumors (<1 mm) is good, but survival is negatively impacted as tumor thickness increases.

The role of adjuvant therapy in the management of individuals with high risk for recurrence remains controversial. One controversy is determination of which patients are appropriate candidates for treatment after resection of the primary tumor. Although adjuvant therapy has been considered historically in patients with locally advanced disease (stages II and III), it is increasingly being considered after surgical resection of an isolated distant metastases.

Another controversy with adjuvant therapy is the choice of therapy. HDI has the most evidence supporting its use and is FDA approved for this indication. The challenges with this therapy have been discussed, and the therapy has limited worldwide acceptance. The most appropriate option is a clinical trial, if available. New therapies and combinations must be evaluated to help answer the questions that remain about adjuvant therapy in melanoma. Clinical trials of chemotherapy, immunotherapy, vaccines, and emerging therapies are ongoing and often are available through academic health centers and within the community through oncologist office-based practices.

Another treatment challenge is the management of patients with advanced disease. The 2008 NCCN guidelines list a variety of systemic therapies for advanced or metastatic melanoma, including dacarbazine, temozolomide, high-dose aldesleukin, and combination therapies of biochemotherapy that include dacarbazine or temozolomide.[35] Of note, the preferred treatment is participation in a clinical trial. Best supportive care is also an option in some individuals. Data suggest that surgical treatment of metastatic melanoma should be considered in select individuals based on the extent and location of disease.

An important consideration for treatment of melanoma is the presentation of the disease. As discussed, treatment of melanoma isolated to the limb may be most appropriately treated with regional therapy. Treatment options for metastatic uveal melanoma include strategies for managing hepatic metastasis, such as chemoembolization to the liver and intrahepatic chemotherapy. [92]

Prevention and Detection

The results of early treatment emphasize the role of early detection and prevention. The American Academy of Dermatology recommends monthly self-examination of skin to serve as a mechanism for recognizing moles or marks on the skin that may be melanoma. Patients with a strong family history should have a clinical examination and, in some cases, screening photography to document the size, shape, and location of moles.

There are three different strategies for chemoprevention for melanoma. Primary chemoprevention is used to prevent occurrences of melanoma in healthy individuals. Secondary chemoprevention is used to prevent premalignant melanoma precursors from becoming melanoma. Tertiary chemoprevention is used to prevent melanoma recurrence in individuals who were treated for melanoma and have no evidence of disease. A variety of agents have been studied in human and in vitro models, with varying results and no clear choice for any of these agents (Table 141–9).[93] The mainstay of melanoma prevention remains strategies to protect individuals from harmful effects of the sun.

UV light exposure plays a complex role in melanoma development. Childhood sunburns and intermittent sun exposure correlate positively with melanoma risk. Education and reeducation about the importance of sun protection have the potential to help decrease the rising incidence of this disease. More recently, the method of sun protection has become an area of controversy.

Historically, patients have been counseled that the risk of skin cancer can be limited by the use of sunscreens with a sun protection factor (SPF) of 15 or greater. Although some studies have found a decreased risk of melanoma in sunscreens users, others have demonstrated no association and even increased melanoma risk with sunscreen use. Methodologic difficulties may explain the discrepancy in study results. Factors that include variables in sun exposure, sunscreen use, and sun sensitivity are very difficult to control in these trials. In addition, all sunscreens are not the same. Sunscreens traditionally have been designed to prevent erythema by blocking UVB, leaving users relatively unprotected from wavelengths such as UVA. Use of sunscreens, especially those with higher SPFs, may lead to the ability of individuals to increase their time in the sun without clinical indication of sunburn. Another concern is that irregular use of sunscreens increases the risk of intermittent UV exposure.

It is important to counsel patients about the appropriate use of sunscreens to optimize benefits from these products. One study noted that most consumers typically apply less sunscreen than is needed to establish the SPF number on the bottle; the actual SPF received is 20% to 50% that of number.[94,95] Sunscreens should be applied 15 to 30 minutes before going into the sun and should be reapplied every 2 hours, after swimming, and after perspiring heavily. Sun protection must be used regularly and not limited to times of recreation or anticipated "prolonged" exposure. Times of season changes, when the potential for sun exposure can be perceived as erratic, are possible times for the "first-of-the-season sunburn."

TABLE 141-9 Sunscreens

Physical Blockers (Reflectants)	Chemical Absorbers
Zinc oxide	Ultraviolet B absorbers
Talc	Salicylates
Titanium dioxide	Cinnamates
Red petrolatum	Camphor derivatives
	Aminobenzoates
	Ultraviolet A absorbers
	Benzopehnone-6
	Dibenzoylmethanes

The other question concerning sunscreen lotions is product selections. Older sunscreen lotions are more efficient in protecting against shorter UV wavelengths that lead to sunburns than in protecting against the longer wavelengths in the UVA range that may lead to skin damage and skin cancers such as melanoma. UVA radiation, unlike UVB, is consistent. Newer forms of sunscreens combine protection for UVA and UVB. Unfortunately, no currently approved system rates products for UVA protective capabilities. SPF is a measure of protection from UVB radiation only. The impact of the use of high-potency sunscreens on the incidence of melanoma is not clear at this time, because the lag time for melanoma is approximately two decades and high-potency sunscreens have only been popular for approximately 10 years.

One strategy for sun protection is use of protective clothing to minimize damage to the skin for individuals who spend time in the sun. The slogan "Slip! Slop! Slap!" (slip on a shirt, slop on the sunscreen, and slap on a hat), initially developed for public health campaigns in Australia, provides a more comprehensive approach to sun protection. Clothing designed to protect an individual from sun exposure but allows physical activities such as water sports and hiking are widely available. The clothes are designed for skin protection, but it is important to realize that not all clothing provides sufficient protection from UV radiation. Clothes with tight weaves provide greater protection. Hats are important (slap on a hat!), especially hats with a brim to protect ears, neck, and nose. Other strategies, such as sun avoidance, especially during peak hours of sun intensity (10 AM to 4 PM), and staying in the shade when outdoors, are important education concepts for individuals who are in the sun for prolonged periods and/or who are at high risk for burning.[96] Skiers and winter sports enthusiasts should be cautioned about exposure to UV radiation, as the reflection off snow and high altitude contribute to increased UV exposure.

EVALUATION OF THERAPEUTIC OUTCOMES

The outcome of patients treated with melanoma depends on the stage of disease at presentation. The prognosis of patients with thin tumors (<1 mm in thickness) and localized disease is good, with long-term survival in more than 90% of patients. The risk of regional nodal involvement increases with increasing tumor thickness, so survival rates decrease in patients with nodal involvement. Long-term survival in patients with distant metastases is even lower. Therefore, early diagnosis and appropriate treatment of early disease are essential. Patients with suspicious pigmented lesions should be evaluated and the lesion excised whenever possible. Treatment is determined by patient factors and stage of disease.

There is no clear recommendation regarding appropriate follow-up of patients with melanoma. Clinical practice guidelines published by the NCCN provide some guidance for follow-up of patients with melanoma.[35] Intensive surveillance has the benefit of early detection of recurrent disease, which may lead to better options of surgical resection. Emphasis on evaluation of locoregional areas is important. For patients with in situ melanoma, periodic skin examinations for life are recommended, although frequency is determined based on patient risk factors. Local recurrence is associated with aggressive tumor biology and frequently is a manifestation of an aggressive primary tumor. If a local recurrence occurs after inadequate primary disease, the patient should undergo a workup based on the lesion thickness of the original melanoma. Patients with nodal recurrence should be evaluated for lymph node metastases. Patients with systemic recurrence should be evaluated and treated in a fashion similar to patients presenting with systemic disease.

NONMELANOMA SKIN CANCER

8 Nonmelanoma skin cancers (NMSCs), which are malignant growths of the external surface or epithelia layer of the skin, are the most common form of cancer in the United States and the most common form of skin cancer. The incidence of NMSC is increasing each year, although the absolute incidence is not known because NMSCs often are excluded from cancer registry statistics. More than one million cases of basal cell and squamous cell skin cancers are expected to be diagnosed in 2007. The incidence rate has been increasing worldwide at a rate of 3% to 8% per year since 1964, with greater increases near the equator.[2,97] There is a wide geographic variation in the incidence of NMSC, believed to be due to the differences in climate and the skin type of local populations. As with melanoma, the incidence is increasing in older persons, but of concern is the increase of NMSC in younger individuals.[98] BCC accounts for approximately 80% of NMSCs. Squamous cell carcinoma (SCC) is the second most common form of skin cancer, with more than 200,000 new cases estimated to occur each year in the United States.

NMSCs have a good prognosis when detected and treated early. Although these skin cancers have low mortality, they may produce significant morbidity and healthcare cost.[99]

BCC, like SCC, develops within the epidermis. BCC derives from the basal layer of keratinocytes, which is the deepest cell layer of the epidermis. SCC arises from the more superficial layers of keratinocytes. Keratinocyte damage secondary to exposure to UV radiation is thought to be a primary cause of NMSC, and the risk for skin cancer is highest in susceptible individuals. Damage to keratinocytes results in actinic keratosis (AK), solar lentigo, and dermatoheliosis (photoaging). AKs are sun-induced premalignant skin lesions and can develop into SCC. Some argue that AK should be considered a very-early-stage SCC. Approximately 5% to 20% of AK will transform into SCC within 10 to 25 years, with no means available for determining which AK lesions will transform.

BASAL CELL CANCER

BCC is the most common form of skin cancer. The true incidence is unknown because a diagnosis may not be possible in individuals with multiple primaries or in those with no determined histology. Age-standardized yearly rates in the United States have been estimated at 407 cases of BCC per 100,000 white men and 212 cases per 100,000 white women.[100] As with melanoma, rates are highest in elderly men.

The genetics of BCC are not fully understood. Certain genetic syndromes predispose individuals to NMSC, specifically those that affect the impact of sunlight on the individual (e.g., albinism). In the majority of BCCs, there is a mutation in the tumor suppressor PTCH gene system found on chromosome 9q.

A major risk factor for BCC is exposure to UV radiation; pattern and amount of exposure to UV radiation appears to be important. Intense intermittent exposure to the sun is associated with a higher risk for BCC versus continuous exposure. As with melanoma, physical characteristics such as light skin color, light eyes (green or blue), and blond or red hair have been identified as independent risk factors. Additionally, immunosuppression increases the risk for BCC. For example, renal transplant recipients have a 10 times higher risk for BCC than do individuals who did not undergo renal transplantation.[101] The incidence of subsequent cases of BCC is increased by a factor of 10 for individuals after an initial BCC compared to the general population.

The hallmark of BCC is a waxy, translucent, or pearly appearance (see Chap. 99). Often the lesions have central ulcerations and a raised pale border. Telangiectasias are common and lead to lesion friability, poor healing, and bleeding. Pigmented BCCs are not common and may be confused with melanoma. BCCs most often arise in areas of the body exposed to sun; the most common presentation is a lesion on the head or neck area, followed by the trunk, arms, and legs. These cancers can be found in other areas of the body. There are a variety of histologic subtypes of BCC, and lesions can often be a mixed histology.[102] The most common form of BCC is nodular BCC, which presents as a pearly papule or nodule with overlying telangiectasia. Superficial BCC may present as a scaly erythematous patch. Melanin may be present in either form of BCC lesions, so the lesion may present with a dark blue or black coloring. Amelanotic or minimally pigmented melanomas can appear similar to BCC.

BCCs do not tend to metastasize but can be very locally destructive. Although BCCs often are considered a skin cancer that remains localized, left untreated these cancers can spread. Risk factors for extensive spread include diameter greater than 2 cm, location on the central part of the face or ears, long-standing duration, incomplete excision, aggressive histologic pattern of growth, and perivascular involvement.[103] Some histologic subtypes of BCC are associated with aggressive behavior; micronodular, infiltrative, sclerosing, and morpheaform patterns are more likely to recur than nodular and superficial BCCs.

Treatment

The goal of primary treatment of BCC is cure . Because BCCs do not tend to metastasize, the goals of treatment are local control and preservation of the function and cosmetic appearance of the area. Treatment of BCC often is surgical. Individuals who have low-risk disease in whom surgery or radiation is not an option may benefit from local topical therapies, such as topical 5-fluorouracil. Few randomized trials have compared different treatments. When evaluating new treatments, the clinician should critically evaluate issues such as duration of followup and impact of treatment on the primary lesion versus recurrent disease.

BCCs are most commonly treated with surgery. Surgical approaches include curettage and electrodesiccation, cryosurgery, excision, and Mohs micrographic surgery. Factors that determine the most appropriate surgical approach include the individual's age and overall health, histologic subtype, lesion location and size, and whether the lesion is a primary or recurrent tumor.

Curettage and electrodesiccation are methods commonly used for management of BCCs that are small in diameter. The tumor is scraped with a curette and the area is treated with electrosurgery to control bleeding and eradicate cancer cells that may remain. Often multiple treatments are used to completely remove the tumor. Scarring is a risk with this procedure. Curettage and electrodesiccation are used for low-risk tumors but should not be used in hair-bearing regions or if fat is reached during the procedures. Five-year cure rates are greater than 90% with curettage and electrodesiccation and cryosurgery when used for individuals with low-risk lesions.

Excisional treatments include Mohs surgery and excision with postoperative margin assessment. Postoperative margin assessment is an option if the lesion can be excised with 4-mm clinical margins and repair to the area. If the margins are positive, then resection is expanded or radiation is recommended. Primary lesions of any size on the neck, trunk, arms, or leg have a very high 5-year cure rate with surgical excision (>99%), whereas excision of lesions on the head is less effective with increasing tumor size.[101] Mohs micrographic surgery with intraoperative frozen section assessment is a specialized surgical procedure recommended for all high-risk tumors or tumors with positive margins during excision. If any part of the specimen shows infiltration of the margin, serial excisions can be done to the area affected. Mohs micrographic surgery is used for individuals with large (>2 cm) tumors, high-risk histologic subtypes, recurrent BCC, and at locations that are cosmetically sensitive (e.g., face). The availability of surgical margin assessment during the procedure allows for margin control of affected margins and tissue conservation of nonaffected margins. The disadvantage of Mohs micrographic surgery is that specialization and/or training are required to perform the procedure. Complications of Mohs micrographic surgery are mainly postoperative and associated with the procedures, especially bleeding. Scarring and cosmetic effects depend on the extent and location of surgery and postsurgical management. Mohs micrographic surgery has the lowest 5-year recurrence rate compared to other surgical procedures. Recurrent BCC is often treated with Mohs micrographic surgery. Cryosurgery is a cytodestructive technique that involves the use of liquid nitrogen spray or probe to induce cell necrosis by exposing tissue to low temperatures.

Nonsurgical approaches of BCC include radiotherapy, local (e.g., topical or local drug injection) therapy, and photodynamic therapy. Radiation therapy is used for management of BCC, often for individuals who are not good surgical candidates (i.e., because of lesion location). Radiation is not recommended for younger individuals, based on the potential for carcinogenesis and long-term cosmetic effect. Radiation is contraindicated for patients with genetic conditions that predispose to skin cancer.

Topical 5-fluorouracil, an antimetabolite antineoplastic agent used intravenously for a variety of cancers, has been used topically in solutions and cream formulations for treatment of BCC when conventional methods are not practical. 5-Fluorouracil monotherapy is often associated with low clearance rates; the actual rate depends on many patient and drug therapy (e.g., concentration) factors. Topical 5-fluorouracil has been used in combination with surgical strategies such as curettage and electrodesiccation, but the benefit of this strategy is not clear. Some challenges with topical 5-fluorouracil are the side effects of local reactions, including pain and burning, pruritus, inflammation, tenderness, and scarring at the site of application. Special instructions for safe handling of the product should be provided for the patient and any caregivers.

Imiquimod is a topical immune response modifier used for treatment of small (<2 cm in diameter) superficial lesions on the trunk, neck, legs, and arms of some patients with a normal immune system. Imiquimod activity is mediated through activation of macrophages and other cells by binding of cell surface receptors (TLR7), which induces proinflammatory cytokines such as interferon-γ and tumor necrosis factor-α. Imiquimod 5% cream may induce Fas receptor–mediated apoptosis in BCC.[104] Imiquimod currently is approved for treatment of external genital and perianal warts and AK on the face and scalp. The optimal regimen for treatment of superficial BCC is imiquimod administered daily for 5 days per week for 6 weeks.[105] Higher dosing regimens have been used but are limited by cutaneous reactions. Longer treatment regimens have not yet shown benefit. The treatment regimens used for nodular BCC often include daily treatment (i.e., 7 days per week) for a longer duration. Side effects usually are mild to moderate skin reactions, including erythema, crusting, flaking, and erosion.

Topical photodynamic therapy involves the use of light to activate a photosensitizer, resulting in the formation of a cytotoxic reactive oxygen species that is selectively destructive to tumor.[106] Photodynamic therapy with methyl 5-aminolevulinate as a photosensitizer has been shown be effective for superficial BCC but has been shown to be associated with high rates of recurrence.

As with melanoma, the issues with NMSC, such as BCC, extend beyond treatment. Cancer prevention and early detection are important concerns. Early detection efforts extend beyond identification of initial BCCs, with additional focus on identification of any recurrence or secondary primary. Identification and aggressive followup of groups at high risk for recurrence, individuals with truncal BCC, or those presenting with tumor clusters may impact on the overall success of any treatment program.[107]

SQUAMOUS CELL CANCER

SCC is a type of nonmelanoma skin cancer that shows malignant characteristics, including anaplasia, rapid growth, local invasion, and metastatic potential. This type of NMSC is a tumor of the epidermis that grows by expansion and infiltration of the surrounding skin and structures. SCCs, unlike most BCCs, may metastasize via lymphatic or hematogenous spread.

SCC is the second most common form of skin cancer, with more than 200,000 new cases estimated to occur each year in the United States. Risk factors for developing SCC include fair complexion, poor tanning ability, and predisposition to sunburn. UV light is an important risk factor for SCC. A study found that UV exposure correlates with the risk of SCC and the aggressiveness of the SCC.[108] SCC appears to be the skin cancer most associated with chronic exposure to sun. In dark-skinned ethnic groups, SCC is the most common cutaneous malignancy and arises most often on sites of preexisting inflammatory sites, burn injuries, scars, prior sites of radiation therapy, or trauma.[109] Similar to other skin cancers, the risk of SCC is higher in individuals on immunosuppressive medications after organ transplantation.[110] Another high-risk group includes patients treated with psoralens and UVA light for psoriasis.[111]

SCC appears as a slightly raised, red, hyperkeratotic macule or papule on sun-exposed sites but may occur anywhere (see Chap. 99). SCCs arising from AK are scaly but tend to be thicker. The lesions may appear like a patch, plaque, nodule, or scaling. Unlike BCC, the edges tend to be fleshy in appearance. SCC most commonly occurs on the face, ear, neck, lip, and back of the hands.

Appropriate biopsy should be performed on any lesion suspected of being SCC, considering the potential for invasive disease. A shave biopsy is sufficient and will not lead to spread of the cancer. A grading system has been devised to classify SCC with respect to percentage of differentiated cells: grade 1 tumors have greater than 75% well-differentiated cells, grade 2 tumors have 50% to 75% well-differentiated cells, grade 3 tumors have 25% to 50% well-differentiated cells, and grade 4 tumors have less than 25% well-differentiated cells. The prognosis of patients with SCC worsens as the percentage of well-differentiated cells decreases.[112]

The type of treatment should be selected based on lesion size, anatomic location, depth of invasion, degree of cellular differentiation, and history of treatment. The three general approaches to treatment of SCC are destruction by curettage and electrodesiccation or cryosurgery; removal by traditional excisional surgery or Mohs surgery, and radiation. Invasive SCC can be a potentially lethal neoplasm that warrants close followup. Most cases of SCC are treated by successful complete excision, although patients have a lifelong risk of developing second primary skin cancers, which require repeated surgical resections and reconstructive procedures.[113]

Although rarely fatal, SCC has tremendous social and economic burden due to high medical costs. Advanced cases have been shown to result in diminished quality of life, functional impairment, and other serious consequences.[114] SCCs are more likely than BCCs to metastasize and lead to mortality. Risk factors that can predict aggressive disease behavior and poor clinical outcome are lesion size at least 4 cm, histologic evidence of perineural and deep invasions into underlying tissues, and inadequate initial treatment of patients with nodal involvement.[115] Long-term prognosis for metastatic disease is extremely poor. Ten-year survival rates are less than 20% for patients with regional lymph node involvement and less than 10% for patients with distant metastases.[116]

Basosquamous carcinomas, which are lesions with microscopic features of both BCC and SCC, should be excised completely because of the aggressive nature of this cancer.

CHEMOPREVENTION OF NONMELANOMA SKIN CANCER

Chemoprevention is the oral or topical use of a dietary or pharmacologic agent to inhibit or reverse the development of cancer. The first step in the development of many skin cancers is exposure to UV radiation. One step in chemoprevention is the protection of individuals against exposure, or "unsafe" exposure to UV radiation. Other strategies target the many steps between exposure to the UV radiation and development of cancer. The retinoids have been shown to be chemopreventive in patients with xeroderma pigmentosum, renal transplant recipients, and individuals with risk associated with premalignant lesions (>10 AKs). In addition, oral retinoids (acitretin and isotretinoin) has been shown to reduce the development of precancers and skin cancers in high-risk patients, specifically individuals with a history of SCC and BCC.[117] Side effects of retinoids depend on dose and range from mucocutaneous reactions to elevations in cholesterol, triglycerides, and liver function tests. Chronic use of retinoids causes skeletal changes associated with demineralization and calcification of ligaments and vertebral disks. These agents are associated with toxicities, and their therapeutic effects are limited to the time the individual is taking the drug. When the medication is stopped, the benefit is diminished. Approaches to optimizing safety and effectiveness of theses agents have been published.[118]

Potential agents for chemoprevention of NMSC include a variety of substances, including many over-the-counter topical or oral preparations. Vitamin E, β-carotene, and selenium once were thought to prevent skin cancer but now are not considered effective.[117]

ABBREVIATIONS

AJCC: American Joint Committee on Cancer
ARF: alternative reading frame
bFGF: basic fibroblast growth factor
BCC: basal cell carcinoma
CTL: cytotoxic T lymphocyte
CTLA-4: cytotoxic T lymphocyte antigen 4
ECOG: Eastern Cooperative Oncology Group
HDI: high-dose interferon
HLA: human leukocyte antigen
IL-2: interleukin-2
INK4A: inhibitor of cyclin-dependent kinase 4
LAK: lymphokine-activated killer
LDI: low-dose interferon
NMSC: nonmelanoma skin cancer
NSAID: nonsteroidal antiinflammatory drug
SCC: squamous cell cancer
SLNB: sentinel lymph node biopsy
SPF: sun protection factor
TIL: tumor-infiltrating lymphocyte
TLR9: toll-like receptor 9
UVA: ultraviolet A
UVB: ultraviolet B

REFERENCES

1. Garbe C, Eigentler TK. Diagnosis and treatment of cutaneous melanoma: State of the art 2006. Melanoma Res 2007;17:117–127.
2. Jemal A, Siegel R, Ward E, et al. Cancer statistics, 2007. CA Cancer J Clin 2006;57:1:43–66.
3. Berwick M, Weinstock MA. Epidemiology current trends. In: Balch CM, Houghton AN, Sober AJ, Soong S, eds. Cutaneous Melanoma. St. Louis: Quality Medical Publishing, 2003:15–23.
4. Swetter SM, Geller AC, Kirkwood JM. Melanoma in the older person. Oncology 2004;1187–1196.
5. Pappo AS. Melanoma in children and adolescents. Eur J Cancer 2003;39:2651–2661.
6. Chin L, Garraway LA, Fisher DE. Malignant melanoma: Genetics and therapeutics in the genomic era. Genes Dev 2006;20:2149–2182.
7. Meltzer PS. Genetic diversity in melanoma. N Engl J Med 2005;353:2104–2107.
8. Maldonado JL, Fridlyand J, Patel H, et al. Determinant of BRAF mutations in primary melanomas. J Natl Cancer Inst 2003;95:1878–1890.
9. Gallagher RP, Elwood JM, Yang P. Is chronic sunlight exposure important in accounting for increases in melanoma incidence? Int J Cancer 1989;44:813–815.
10. Balch CM, Atkins MB, Sober AJ. Cutaneous melanoma. In: DeVita VT, Hellman S, Rosenberg SA, eds. Cancer: Principles and Practice of Oncology, 7th ed. Philadelphia: Lippincott Williams & Wilkins, 2005:1754–1825.
11. Wilkins K, Turner R, Dolev JC, et al. Cutaneous malignancy and human immunodeficiency virus disease. J Am Acad Dermatol 2006;54:189–206.
12. Alexander A, Samlowski WE, Grossman D, et al. Metastatic melanoma in pregnancy: Risk of transplacental metastases in the infant. J Clin Oncol 2003;21:2179–2186.
13. Damato B. Treatment of primary intraocular melanoma. Expert Rev Anticancer Ther 2006;6:493–506.
14. Mori D, Satoh T, Nakafusa Y, et al. Primary colonic malignant melanoma. Pathol Int 2006;56:744–748.
15. Dore JF, Carrel S. Biology of melanoma differentiation and progression. In: Lejeune FJ, Chaudhuri PK, Das Gupta K, eds. Malignant Melanoma: Medical and Surgical Management. New York: McGraw-Hill, 1994:9–26.
16. Bogenrieder T, Elder DE, Herlyn M. Molecular and cellular biology. In: Balch CM, Houghton AN, Sober AJ, Soong S, eds. Cutaneous Melanoma. St. Louis: Quality Medical Publishing, 2003:15–23.
17. Mahabeleshwar GH, Byzova TV. Angiogenesis in melanoma. Semin Oncol 2007;34:555–565.
18. Gray-Schopfer V, Wellbrock C, Marais R. Melanoma biology and new targeted therapy. Nature 2007;445:851–857.
19. Lejeune FJ, Rimoldi D, Speiser D. New approaches in metastatic melanoma: Biological and molecular targeted therapies. Expert Rev Anticancer Ther 2007;7:701–713.
20. Queirolo P, Acquati M. Targeted therapies in melanoma. Cancer Treat Rev 2006;32:524–531.
21. Clemente C, Cochran AJ, Elder DE, et al. Histopathologic diagnosis of dysplastic nevi: Concordance among pathologist convened by the World Health Organization Melanoma Programme. Hum Pathol 1991;22:313–319.
22. Liu V, Mihm MC. Pathology of malignant melanoma. Surg Clin North Am 2003;83:31–60.
23. Chamberlain AJ, Fritschi L, Giles GG, et al. Nodular type and older age are the most significant associations of thick melanoma in Victoria, Australia. Arch Dermatol 2002;138:609–614.
24. Avery RB, Mehta MP, Auchter RM, Albert DM. Intraocular melanoma. In: DeVita VT, Hellman S, Rosenberg SA, eds. Cancer: Principles and Practice of Oncology, 7th ed. Philadelphia: Lippincott Williams & Wilkins, 2005:1809–1825.
25. Berwick M, Begg CM, Fine JA, Roush CG, Barnhill RL. Screening for cutaneous melanoma by skin self-examination. J Natl Cancer Inst 1996;88:17–23.
26. Balch CM, Soong SJ, Buzaid AC, et al. The new melanoma staging system and factors predicting melanoma survival. Clin Oncol Update 2002;5:3.1–19.
27. Clark WH Jr. A classification of malignant melanoma in man correlated with histogenesis and biologic behavior. In: Montagna W, Hu F,

eds. Advances in Biology of the Skin. The Pigmentary System. London: Pergamon, 1967:621–645.

28. Breslow A. Thickness, cross-sectional areas and depth of invasion in the prognosis of cutaneous melanoma. Ann Surg 1970;172:1902–1908.
29. Balch CM, Soong SJ, Gershenwald JE, et al. Prognostic factors analysis of 17,600 melanoma patients: Validation of the American Joint Committee on Cancer melanoma staging system. J Clin Oncol 2001;19:3622–3634.
30. Flemming ID, Cooper JS, Henson DE, et al, eds. AJCC Cancer Staging Manual, 5th ed. Philadelphia: Lippincott-Raven, 1997:163–167.
31 Balch CM, Buzaid AC, Soong SJ, et al. Final version of the American Joint Committee on cancer staging system for cutaneous melanoma. J Clin Oncol 2001;19:3635–3648.
32. Morton DL, Thompson JF, Cochran AJ, et al. Sentinel-node biopsy or nodal observation in melanoma. N Engl J Med 2006;355:1307–1317.
33. Hoon DS, Wang Y, Dale PS, et al. Detection of occult melanoma cells in blood with a multiple-marker polymerase chain reaction assay. J Clin Oncol 1995;13:2109–2116.
34. Mocellin S, Hoon DSB, et al. Sentinel lymph node molecular ultrastaging in patients with melanoma: A systematic review and meta-analysis of prognosis. J Clin Oncol 2007;25:1588–1595.
35. NCCN Melanoma Clinical Practice Guidelines in Oncology (Version 1.2008). Available at *http://www.nccn.org*. Accessed Jan 21, 2008.
36. Tsao H, Atkins MB, Sober AJ. Management of cutaneous melanoma. N Engl J Med 2004;351:998–1012.
37. Balch CM, Urist MM, Karakousis CP, et al. Efficiency of 2-cm surgical margins for intermediate-thickness melanomas (1–4 mm): Results of a multi-institutional randomized surgical trial. Ann Surg 1993;218:262–269.
38. Meirion Thomas K, Newton-Bishop J, A'Hern R, Coombes G, et al. Excision margins in high-risk malignant melanoma. N Engl J Med 2004;350:757–766.
39. Mos ME, Balch CM, Cascinelli N, Edwards MJ. Excision of primary melanoma. In: Balch CM, Houghton AN, Sober AJ, Soong S, eds. Cutaneous Melanoma. St. Louis: Quality Medical Publishing, 2003:209–230.
40. Young SE, Martinez ST, Essner R. The role of surgery in treatment of stage IV melanoma. J Surg Oncol 2006;94:344–351.
41. Ulm AJ, Friedman WA, Bova FJ, et al. Linear accelerator radiosurgery in the treatment of brain metastases. Neurosurgery 2004;55:1076–1085.
42. Kondziolka D, Martin JJ, Flickinger JC, et al. Long-term survivors after gamma knife radiosurgery for brain metastases. Cancer 2005;104:2784–2791.
43. Kirkwood JM, Straderman MH, Ernstoff MS, et al. Interferon alfa-2b adjuvant therapy of high-risk resected cutaneous melanoma: The Eastern Cooperative Oncology Group Trial EST 1684. J Clin Oncol 1996;14:7–17.
44. Kirkwood JM, Manola J, Ibrahim J, Sondak V, Ernstoff MS, Rao U. A pooled analysis of Eastern Cooperative Oncology Group and Intergroup trials of adjuvant high-dose interferon for melanoma. Clin Cancer Res 2004;10:1670–1677.
45. Kirkwood JM, Ibrahim JG, Sondak VK, et al. High- and low-dose interferon alfa-2b in high risk melanoma: First analysis of intergroup trial E1690/S9111/C9190. J Clin Oncol 2000;18:2444–2458.
46. Lens MB, Dawes M. Interferon alfa therapy for malignant melanoma: A systematic review of randomized controlled trials. J Clin Oncol 2002;20:1818–1825.
47. Kirkwood JM, Bender C, Agarwala S, et al. Mechanisms and management of toxicities associated with high-dose interferon alfa-2b therapy. J Clin Oncol 2002;20:3703–3718.
48. Dalakas MC, Mock V, Hawkins MJ. Fatigue: Definitions, mechanisms, and paradigms for study. Semin Oncol 1998;25(Suppl 1):48–53.
49. Plata-Salaman CR. Cytokines and anorexia: A brief overview. Semin Oncol 1998;25(Suppl 1):64–72.
50. Moschos SJ, Kirkwood JM. Present status and future prospects for adjuvant therapy of melanoma: Time to build upon the foundation of high-dose interferon alfa-2b. J Clin Oncol 2004;22:11–14.
51. Cole BF, Gelber RD, Kirkwood JM, et al. A quality-of-life-adjusted survival analysis of interferon alfa-2b adjuvant treatment for high-risk resected cutaneous melanoma: An Eastern Cooperative Oncology Group Study (E1684). J Clin Oncol 1996;14:2666–2673.
52. Bukowski RM, Tannenbaum CS, Finke JH. Clinical pharmacokinetics of interleukin 1 interleukin 2 interleukin 4 tumor necrosis factor, interleukin 12 and macrophage colony-stimulating factor. In: Chabner B, Longo DL, eds. Cancer Chemotherapy & Biotherapy: Principles and Practice, 3rd ed. Lippincott Williams & Wilkins, 2001:779–828.
53. Atkins MB, Lotze MT, Dutcher JP, et al. High-dose recombinant interleukin-2 therapy for patients with metastatic melanoma: Analysis of 270 patients between 1985 and 1993. J Clin Oncol 1999;17:2105–2116.
54. Schwartz RN, Stover L, Dutcher J. Managing toxicities of high-dose interleukin-2. Oncology 2002;16(Suppl 13):11–20.
55. Law TM, Motzer RJ, et al. Phase III randomized trial of interleukin-2 with or without lymphokine-activated killer cells in the treatment of patient with advanced renal cell carcinoma. Cancer 1995;76:824–832.
56. Rosenberg SA, Yannelli JR, et al. Treatment of patients with metastatic melanoma with autologous tumor-infiltrating lymphocytes and interleukin 2. J Natl Cancer Inst 1994;86:1159–1166.
57. Faries MB, Morton DL. Therapeutic vaccines for melanoma. Biodrugs, 2005;19:247–260.
58. Terando AM, Faries MB, Morton DL. Vaccine therapy for melanoma: Current status and future directions. Vaccine 2007;25(Suppl 2):B4–16.
59. Chapman PB. Melanoma vaccines. Semin Oncol 2007;34:516–523.
60. Mirev BR. Melanoma vaccines. Semin Oncol 2002;29:479–493.
61. Cranmer LD, Hamid O, Urba WJ. Targeting cytotoxic T-lymphocyte antigen-4 (CTLA-4): A novel strategy for the treatment of melanoma and other malignancies. Cancer 2007;110:2614–2627.
62. O'Day SJ, Hamid O, Urba WJ. Targeting cytotoxic T-lymphocyte antigen-4 (CTLA-4): A novel strategy for the treatment of melanoma and other malignancies. Cancer 2007;110:2614–2627.
63. Mitchell MS, Abrams J, Thompson JA, et al. Randomized trial of allogeneic melanoma lysate vaccine with low-dose interferon alfa-2b compared with high-dose interferon alfa-2b for resected stage III cutaneous melanoma. J Clin Oncol 2007;25:2078–2085.
64. Gogas HJ, Kirkwood JM, Sondak VK. Chemotherapy for metastatic melanoma. Time for a change? Cancer 2007;109:455–464.
65. Serrone L, Zeuli M, Sega FM, Cognetti F. Dacarbazine-based chemotherapy for metastatic melanoma: Thirty-year experience overview. J Exp Clin Cancer Res 2000;19:21–34.
66. Middleton M, Grob J, Aaronson N, et al. Randomized Phase III study of temozolomide versus dacarbazine in the treatment of patients with advanced metastatic malignant melanoma. J Clin Oncol 2000;18:158–166.
67. Lee SM, Thatcher N, Margison GP. O–alkylguanine-DNA alkyltransferase depletion and regeneration in human peripheral lymphocytes following dacarbazine and fotemustine. Cancer Res 1991;51:619–623.
68. Hwu WJ, Panageas KS, Menell JH, et al. Phase II study of temozolomide plus pegylated interferon–α-2b for metastatic melanoma. Cancer 2006;106:2445–2451.
69. Garcia M, Garcia del Muro X, Tres A, et al. Phase II multicentre study of temozolomide in combination with interferon alpha-2b in metastatic malignant melanoma. Melanoma Res 2006;16:365–370.
70. Jacquillat C, Khayat D, Banzet P, et al. Final report of the French multicenter phase II study of the nitrosourea fotemustine in 153 evaluable patients with disseminated malignant melanoma including patients with cerebral metastases. Cancer 1990;66:1873–1878.
71. Glover D, Ibrahim J, Kirkwood J, et al. Phase II randomized trial of cisplatin and WR-2721 versus cisplatin alone for metastatic melanoma: An Eastern Cooperative Oncology Group study (E1686). Melanoma Res 2003;13:619–626.
72. Hersch E, O'Day S, Gonzales R, et al. Phase II trial of ABI-007 (Abraxane) in previously treated and chemotherapy naïve patients with metastatic melanoma [abstract]. Melanoma Res 2006;16:S78.
73. Legha SS, Ring S, Papadopoulos N, et al. A prospective evaluation of a triple-drug regimen containing cisplatin, vinblastine and DTIC (CVD) for metastatic melanoma. Cancer 1989;64:2024–2029.
74. Rusthoven JJ, Quirt IC, Iscoe NA, et al. Randomized, double-blind, placebo-controlled trial comparing the response rates of carmustine, dacarbazine, and cisplatin with and without tamoxifen in patients with metastatic melanoma. National Cancer Institute of Canada clinical trials group. J Clin Oncol 1996;14:2083–2090.
75. Chapman PB, Einhorm L, Meyeres ML, et al. Phase III multicenter randomized trial of the Dartmouth regimen versus dacarbazine in patients with metastatic melanoma. J Clin Oncol 1999;17:2745–2751.
76. Middleton MR, Lorigan P, Owen J, et al. A randomized phase III study comparing dacarbazine, BCNU, cisplatin and tamoxifen with dacarbazine and interferon in advanced melanoma. Br J Cancer 2000;82:1158–1162.

77. Becker JC, Kirkwood JM, Agarwala SS, et al. Molecularly targeted therapy for melanoma. Cancer 2006;107:2317–2327.
78. Haluska F, Pemberton T, Ibrahim N, Kalinsky K. The RTK/RAS/BRAF/PI3K pathways in melanoma: Biology, small molecule inhibitors, and potential applications. Semin Oncol 2007;34:546–554.
79. Takimoto CH, Awada A. Safety and anti-tumor activity of sorafenib (Nexavar) in combination with other anti-cancer agents: A review of clinical trials. Cancer Chemother Pharmacol 2008;61:535–548.
80. Janku F, Novotny J, Julisova JI, et al. KIT receptor is expressed in more than 50% of early-stage malignant melanoma: A retrospctive study of 261 patients. Melanoma Res 2005;15:251–256.
81. Wyman K, Atkins MB, Prieto V, et al. Multicenter phase II trial of high-dose imatinib mesylate in metastatic melanoma. Cancer 2006;106:2005–2011.
82. McClay EF, McClay ME. Tamoxifen: Is it useful in the treatment of patients with metastatic melanoma. J Clin Oncol 1994:12:617–626.
83. Agarwala SS. A phase III randomized trial of dacarbazine and carboplatin with and without tamoxifen in the treatment of patients with metastatic melanoma. Cancer 1999;85:1979–1984.
84. Ives NJ, Stowe RL, Lorigan P, Whearley K. Chemotherapy compared with biochemotherapy for the treatment of metastatic melanoma. A meta-analysis of 18 trials involving 2,621 patients. J Clin Oncol 2007;25:5426–5434.
85. Shah GD, Chapman PB. Adjuvant therapy of melanoma. Cancer J 2007;13:217–222.
86. Gonazalez Cao M, Malvehy J, Marti R, et al. Biochemotherapy with temozolomide, cisplatin, vinblastine, subcutaneous interleukin-2 and interferon-α in patients with metastatic melanoma. Melanoma Res 2006;16:59–64.
87. Majer M, Jensen RL, Shrieve DS, et al. Biochemotherapy of metastatic melanoma in patients with recently diagnosed brain metastases. Cancer 2007;110:1329–1337.
88. Rossi CR, Foletto M, Pilati P, Mocellin S, Lise M. Isolated limb perfusion in locally advanced cutaneous melanoma. Semin Oncol 2002;29:400–409.
89. Kroon BBR. Regional isolation perfusion in melanoma of the limbs: Accomplishments, unsolved problems, future. Eur J Surg Oncol 1998;14:101–110.
90. Sanki A, Kam PCA, Thompson JF. Long-term results of hyperthermic isolated limb perfusion for melanoma. Ann Surg 2007;245:591–596.
91. Lejeune FJ, Eggermont AMM. Hyperthermic isolated limb perfusion with tumor necrosis factor is a useful therapy for advanced melanoma of the limbs. J Clin Oncol 2007;25:1449–1450.
92. Feldman ED, Finkpank JF, Alexander HR. Regional treatment options for patients with ocular melanoma metastatic to the liver. Ann Surg Oncol 2004;11:290–297.
93. Francis SO, Mahlberg MJ, Johnson KR, et al. Melanoma chemoprevention. J Am Acad Dermatol 2006;55:849–861.
94. Westerdahl J, Olsson H, Masback A, et al. Is the use of sunscreens a risk factor for malignant melanoma? Melanoma Res 1995;5:59–65.
95. Stokes R, Diffey B. How well are sunscreen users protected? Photodermatol Photoimmunol Photomec 1997;13:186–188.
96. Marks R, Hill D. Prevention of skin cancer. In: Sober AJ, Haluska FG, eds. American Cancer Society Atlas of Clinical Oncology Skin Cancer. Ontario, Canada: BC Decker, 2001:325–339.
97. Bivens MM, Bhosle M, Balkrishnan R, et al. Nonmelamona skin cancer: Is the incident really increasing among patients younger than 40? A reexamination using 25 years of US outpatient data. Derm Surg 2006;32:1473–1479.
98. Christenson LJ, Borrowman TA, Vachon CM, et al. Incidence of basal cell and squamous cell carcinomas in a population younger than 40 years. JAMA 2005;294:681–690.
99. Joseph AK, Mark TL, Mueller C. The period prevalence and costs of treating nonmelanoma skin cancers in patients over 65 years of age covered by Medicare. Dermatol Surg 2001;27:955- 959.
100. Miller DL, Weinstock MA. Nonmelanoma skin cancer in the United States: Incidence. J Am Acad Dermatol 1994;30:774–778.
101. Rubin AI, Chen EH, Ratner D. Basal-cell carcinoma. N Engl J Med 2005;353:2262–2269.
102. Sexton M, Jones DB, Maloney ME. Histologic pattern analysis of basal cell carcinoma: Study of a series of 1039 consecutive neoplasms. J Am Acad Dermatol 1990;23:1118–1126.
103. Walling HW, Fosko SW, Geraminejad PA, et al. Aggressive basal cell carcinoma: Presentation, pathogenesis, and management. Cancer Metastasis Rev 2004;23:389–401.
104. Berman B, Sullican T, De Araujo T, et al. Expression of Fas-receptor on basal cell carcinoma after treatment with imiquimod 5% cream or vehicle. Br J Dermatol 2003;149(Suppl 66):59–61.
105. Ceilley RI, Del Rosso JQ. Current modalities and new advances in the treatment of basal cell carcinoma. Int J Dermatol 2006;45:489–498.
106. Braathen LR, Szeimies RM, Basset-Sequin N, et al. Guidelines on the use of photodynamic therapy for nonmelanoma skin cancers: An international consensus. J Am Acad Dermatol 2007;56:125–143.
107. Madan V, Hoban P, Stange RC, et al. Genetics and risk factors for basal cell carcinoma. Br J Dematol 2006(Suppl 1);154:5–7.
108. Ramos J, Villa J, Ruiz A, et al. UV Dose determines key characteristics of nonmelanoma skin cancer. Cancer Epidemiol Biomarkers Prev 2004;13:2006–2011.
109. Gloster HM, Neal K. Skin cancer and skin of color. J Am Acad Dermatol 2006;55:741–760.
110. Leienring W, Friedman DL, Flowers MED, et al. Nonmelanoma skin and mucosal cancers after hematopoietic stem cell transplantation. J Clin Oncol 2006;24:1119–1126.
111. Stern RS, Lunder EJ. Risk of squamous cell carcinoma and methoxsalen (psoralen) and UV-A radiations (PUVA). A meta-analysis. Arch Dermatol 1998;134:1582–1585.
112. Rowe DE, Carroll RJ, Day CL Jr. Prognostic factors for local recurrence, metastasis, and survival rates in squamous cell carcinoma of the skin, ear, and lip. Implications for treatment modality selection. J Am Acad Dermatol 1992;26:976–990.
113. Glass AG, Hoover RN. The emerging epidemic of melanoma and squamous cell skin cancer. JAMA 1989;262:2097–2100.
114. Chen JG, Fleishcer AB Jr, Smith ED, et al. Cost of nonmelanoma skin cancer treatment in the United States. Dermatol Surg 2001;27:1035–1038.
115. Clayman GL, Lee JJ, Holsinger C, et al. Mortality risk from squamous cell skin cancer. J Clin Oncol 2005;23:759–765.
116. Dinehart SM, Pollack SV. Metastases from squamous cell carcinoma of the skin and lip: An analysis of twenty-seven cases. J Am Acad Dermatol 1989;21:241–248.
117. Wright TI, Spencer JM, Flowers FP. Chemoprevention of nonmelanoma skin cancer. J Am Acad Dermatol 2006;54:933–946.
118. Otley CC, Stasko T, Tope WD, et al. Chemoprevention of nonmelanoma skin cancer with systemic retinoids: Practical dosing and management of adverse effects. Dermatol Surg 2006;32:562–568.

CHAPTER 142

Hematopoietic Stem Cell Transplantation

JANELLE B. PERKINS AND GARY C. YEE

KEY CONCEPTS

1. Hematopoietic stem cell transplantation (HSCT) is a process that involves intravenous infusion of hematopoietic stem cells from a donor into a recipient, after the administration of chemotherapy with or without radiation. The rationale is to increase tumor cell kill by increasing the dose of chemotherapy. Immune-mediated effects contribute to the tumor cell kill observed after allogeneic HSCT.

2. Hematopoietic stem cells used for transplantation can come from the recipient (autologous) or from a related or unrelated donor (allogeneic). If the related donor is a twin, the transplant is referred to as a syngeneic transplant.

3. Human leukocyte antigen (HLA) mismatching of allogeneic donor/recipient pairs at either a class I or class II locus correlates with the risk of graft failure, graft-versus-host disease (GVHD), and survival. The ideal donor is matched at HLA-A, HLA-B, HLA-C, HLA-DRB1, and HLA-DQB1.

4. Hematopoietic stem cells are found in the bone marrow, peripheral blood, and umbilical cord blood. Because of their rarity and their similarity to other cells, hematopoietic stem cells are difficult to isolate and measure. These stem cells express the CD34 antigen, and quantification of the number of $CD34^+$ cells has become a clinically useful measure of the number of hematopoietic stem cells.

5. Because of clinical and economic advantages, peripheral blood has replaced bone marrow as the source of hematopoietic stem cells in the autologous and adult allogeneic HSCT setting. Bone marrow continues to be the primary graft source in children undergoing allogeneic HSCT.

6. The purpose of the preparative (or conditioning) regimen in traditional myeloablative transplants is two-fold: (a) maximal tumor cell kill and (b) immunosuppression of the recipient to reduce the risk of graft rejection (allogeneic HSCT only).

7. Reduced-intensity conditioning regimens (including those that are nonmyeloablative) have been developed in order to reduce early posttranslant morbidity and mortality while maximizing the graft-versus-tumor (GVT) effect of the allogeneic graft. The advantage of this approach is that patients who otherwise would not be eligible for allogeneic HSCT now can be offered a potentially curative therapy.

8. Posttransplant immunotherapy is based on the GVT effect caused by certain subsets of T cells responsible for eradication of malignant cells. Posttransplant immunotherapy includes the use of donor lymphocyte infusions, immunomodulatory cytokines, monoclonal antibodies, or antitumor vaccines.

9. Transplant-related mortality associated with allogeneic HSCT ranges from 10% to 80%, depending mostly on age, donor, and disease status. Major causes of death include infection, organ toxicity, and GVHD. The most common cause of death after autologous HSCT is disease relapse. Transplant-related mortality usually is less than 5%, depending on the conditioning regimen, age, and disease status.

10. Treatment of acute GVHD often is unsuccessful, and the resulting complications can be fatal. Patients undergoing allogeneic HSCT are given prophylactic immunosuppressive therapy, which inhibits T-cell activation and/or proliferation. The most commonly used GVHD prophylaxis regimen is cyclosporine or tacrolimus and methotrexate.

11. Initial treatment of both acute and chronic GVHD consists of prednisone, either alone or combined with cyclosporine or tacrolimus. Treatment of patients with steroid-refractory GVHD is problematic.

Learning objectives, review questions, and other resources can be found at **www.pharmacotherapyonline.com.**

(1) Hematopoietic stem cell transplantation (HSCT) is a process that involves intravenous infusion of hematopoietic stem cells from a compatible donor into a recipient, usually after administration of high-dose chemotherapy. Hematopoietic stem cells can be derived from the bone marrow, peripheral blood, or umbilical cord blood. The rationale for HSCT for treatment of malignant disease is based on studies showing that most anticancer drugs have a steep dose–response relationship and that bone marrow suppression limits the chemotherapy dosage that can be safely administered. Although standard-dose chemotherapy can prolong survival in many cancer patients, most patients are not cured of their disease (Fig. 142–1). Infusion of hematopoietic stem cells allows administration of very high doses of chemotherapy (as much as 10-fold higher). If tumor cells that are resistant to standard doses are sensitive to higher doses of chemotherapy, then tumor cell kill will be greatly increased, and the likelihood of cure would be higher with HSCT. However, the chemotherapy dose cannot be escalated indefinitely because of the risk for death caused by nonhematopoietic toxicity. The success and increasing use of reduced-intensity regimens (including those used in nonmyeloablative transplants [NMT]) show that immune-mediated effects contribute to the tumor cell kill observed after allogeneic HSCT.

High-dose chemotherapy followed by HSCT has become an important modality for treatment of a variety of malignant and nonmalig-

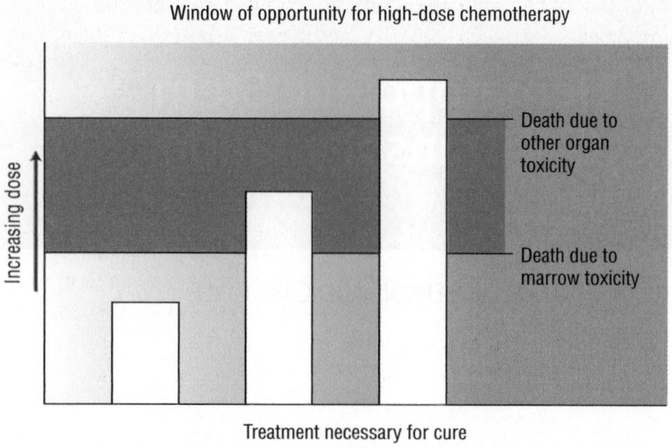

FIGURE 142-1. Patients represented by the middle column are the best candidates for hematopoietic stem cell transplantation because the technique allows for administration of chemotherapy or radiation in doses that otherwise would be intolerable because of severe myelosuppression.

nant diseases. It is estimated that 50–60,000 transplants are performed worldwide each year, primarily for malignant diseases.[1] Approximately 40% of these transplants are performed in North America. The number of transplants has declined in the last decade because of declining use of autologous transplants for breast cancer and increasing use of tyrosine kinase inhibitors for treatment of chronic myelogenous leukemia. However, this decline is being offset in part by an increase in the number of patients receiving umbilical cord blood (UCB) transplants and patients older than 55 years being transplanted after reduced-intensity conditioning regimens.

Historically, the most common type of donor was a genetically nonidentical individual, such as a histocompatible sibling (referred to as allogeneic HSCT [alloHSCT]). However, the number of autologous transplants in which the patient serves as his or her own donor has increased dramatically, and the number of autologous transplants (autoHSCT) performed (approximately 35,000) currently exceeds the number of alloHSCTs (approximately 20,000) performed each year.[1] This chapter focuses on the application of HSCT for treatment of malignant disease, but it is important to note that many nonmalignant diseases—including aplastic anemia, thalassemia, sickle cell anemia, immunodeficiency disorders, and other genetic disorders—are potentially curable with alloHSCT. Transplantation is also being investigated as a treatment modality for patients with life-threatening autoimmune diseases, such as rheumatoid arthritis, systemic and multiple sclerosis, and systemic lupus erythematosus.

This chapter summarizes the procedures involved in HSCT, current issues in the field of HSCT, and application of HSCT in the treatment of malignant diseases. More detailed information on HSCT can be found in published reviews and books.[2–5] Information on HSCT also can be found on several websites (Center for International Blood and Marrow Transplant Research [CIBMTR; *www.cibmtr.org*] and National Marrow Donor Program [*www.marrow.org*]).

DONORS AND HISTOCOMPATIBILITY TESTING

❷ Different types of donors are used in HSCT. In *autologous* transplants, patients receive their own hematopoietic stem cells, which were collected and stored before intensive cytotoxic therapy. In *syngeneic* transplants, an identical twin serves as the donor. In *allogeneic* transplants, the donor is genetically not identical to the recipient but shares some common tissue antigens. Immunologic compatibility is evaluated by studies of cell surface antigens (human leukocyte antigens [HLAs]) encoded by genes of the major histocompatibility complex (MHC), which is located on the sixth chromosome.[6] The genes of the HLA system are clustered in three distinct regions designated as class I, class II, and class III. Class I and class II antigens function as major transplantation antigens; products of class III genes have other important roles in the immune system. The major class I loci in humans are referred to as HLA-A, HLA-B, and HLA-C. The one major class II locus is HLA-D. Class II genes encode for the α and β polypeptide chains of the class II molecules. The designation of class II genes consists of three letters: the first (D) indicates the class, the second (M, O, P, Q, or R) the family, and the third (A or B) the chain (α and β, respectively). Class I and class II antigens differ in their tissue distribution, structure, and function. Class I antigens are expressed on virtually all nucleated cells and serve as the primary targets for cytotoxic T lymphocytes. Class II antigens normally are expressed only on macrophages, B lymphocytes, and activated T lymphocytes, and they serve as the primary targets for helper T lymphocytes.

HLA genes are closely linked to one another within the MHC and generally are inherited together. The series of HLA alleles occurring on a single chromosome is termed a *haplotype*. The combination of two parental haplotypes inherited by an individual determines an individual's *genotype*. For a given HLA locus, an individual generally has two different corresponding antigens expressed in their genotype (e.g., HLA-A2 and HLA-A3; HLA-B44 and HLA-B7; HLA-DR4 and HLA-DR2).

Historically, the most important HLA loci in allogeneic HSCT were HLA-A, HLA-B, and HLA-D (or HLA-DR [D-Related]). Typing for HLA-A and HLA-B traditionally was performed by serologic typing with standard microcytotoxicity assays having panels of antisera containing HLA molecules.[7] HLA types determined by this method were reported as the locus (A or B), followed by a number that designated the cell surface HLA antigen (e.g., HLA-A2). Typing for the HLA-D was performed with cellular typing methods, such as the mixed lymphocyte reaction (MLR) or mixed lymphocyte culture (MLC). A "positive" MLR or MLC indicated incompatibility somewhere in the HLA-D region. Individuals who had a low degree of reactivity in the MLR or MLC (expressed as a low percent relative response), and who met other selection criteria, could serve as donors.

Serologic methods of HLA typing have been replaced by DNA-based techniques that use polymerase chain reaction (PCR) amplification of specific HLA genes from genomic DNA. DNA typing methods are categorized by the level of discrimination they provide in defining the sequence of an HLA gene. *Low-resolution* methods provide limited sequence information about a particular HLA gene and allow identification only to the antigen level, much like older serologic methods. Results of low-resolution typing are given in the form HLA-A*02, where the asterisk denotes DNA-based typing and the corresponding serologic equivalent of the antigen is labeled as a two-digit number. Low-resolution typing typically is used to identify sibling donors. However, neither serologic nor low-resolution techniques can distinguish the extremely polymorphic nature of many of the HLA antigens. For example, more than 2,800 alleles have been defined, approximately 1,900 HLA class I alleles and approximately 900 HLA class II alleles (*www.ebi.ac.uk/imgt/hla/stats.html*). Each of these alleles may correspond to a unique HLA molecule. Different alleles can be distinguished only by *high-resolution* typing techniques. Results of high-resolution techniques are reported as the corresponding HLA antigen, followed by an asterisk and a four-digit number identifying the allele. For example, the HLA-A*02 antigen may be encoded by alleles HLA-A*0201, A*0202, A*0203, etc. (up to A*0249). In some cases, the four-digit allele name includes several alleles. For example, HLA-B*4006 includes B*40060101 and B*40060102. Methods that define the HLA type A beyond the serologic level but short of the allele level are termed *intermediate-*

resolution. For example, this method might identify the presence of either HLA-A*0201 or A*0205 but may not be able to discriminate one allele from the other.

❸ HLA mismatching at either the class I and II locus correlates with the risk of graft failure, graft-versus-host disease (GVHD), and survival.[7] HLA *antigen* mismatches, particularly when they involve both class I and II antigens, are generally more important risk factors than *allele* mismatches. In an analysis of 1,874 patients who received matched unrelated donor transplants under the auspices of the National Marrow Donor Program (NMDP), low-resolution mismatches at HLA-A, HLA-B, HLA-C, and HLA-DRB1 each were similarly associated with increased risk of GVHD and mortality.[8] High-resolution mismatches, particularly at HLA-A and HLA-DRB1, also were associated with increased mortality. In addition, among patients who received transplants from "6 antigen-matched" (HLA-A, HLA-B, and HLA-DRB1 matched) donors, the number of allele mismatches correlated with the risk of grades III to IV acute GVHD and survival. The observation concerning the prognostic value of HLA-C was particularly important, since until that time the locus was omitted from most matching algorithms. HLA-C typing now is included in standard typing protocols.

The most common donor for alloHSCT is an HLA-identical sibling. The odds that any one full sibling will match a patient are 1:4. Only approximately 30% of Americans have an HLA-identical sibling. In an effort to offer alloHSCT to patients who lack an HLA-identical sibling donor, alternative donors are being used. Rarely, a parent is HLA identical with his or her child. A relative can be a zero- (rare), one-, two-, or three-loci antigen mismatch (assuming testing for HLA-A, HLA-B, and HLA-DR antigens). Although some patients who receive transplants from mismatched related donors experience long-term survival, their risks of graft failure and acute GVHD are higher than for recipients of matched-sibling transplants.[9] It is estimated that only another 10% of patients will have a closely HLA-matched related donor.

The most common type of alternative donor is an individual unrelated to the recipient who is fully or closely HLA-matched. To facilitate identification of these donors, the NMDP (*www.marrow.org*) was started in 1986 with initial funding from a U.S. Navy contract. To date, the NMDP has registered more than seven million donors in the United States, and the NMDP has facilitated more than 30,000 matched unrelated donor transplants. Patients searching the NMDP Registry have access to an additional four million donors through agreements with international cooperative registries. Approximately one third of the alloHSCTs performed worldwide are from unrelated donors.[1] The NMDP currently requires that the recipient be typed by high-resolution methodology at HLA-A, HLA-B, HLA-C, and HLA-DRB1. The NMDP also suggests typing other DR and DQ alleles when developing a search strategy. Although it is the transplant center's responsibility to select the donor, the NMDP *recommends* that selected donor and recipient be matched at HLA-A, HLA-B, HLA-C, and HLA-DRB1 by high-resolution typing, when possible. To permit an NMDP donor as a source for transplant, the NMDP *requires* a low-resolution match for at least five of six HLA antigens at HLA-A, HLA-B, and HLA-DR for marrow or peripheral blood transplants and four of six for UCB transplants. The following guidelines should be used for unrelated donor selection: (a) assume that HLA-A, HLA-B, HLA-C, and HLA-DRB1 are equally important; (b) avoid antigen mismatches, if possible; (c) accept one allele mismatch over one antigen mismatch; and (d) minimize the number of allele mismatches.[10]

The likelihood of any one unrelated individual being an antigen-level match ranges from 1:100 to 1:1,000,000, depending on the prevalence of the patient's HLA type and ethnic background. With the current size of the NMDP registry, the matching likelihood is higher than 80% for white people. Because most minorities are not as well represented as whites in the program, the likelihood of finding a donor for patients from certain ethnic groups is lower. Agreements between NMDP and international registries may improve the likelihood of finding donors for patients who are not white. Another limitation is the time needed to search for a potential donor. Some donor searches take up to 3 to 4 months, and many patients with acute leukemia may relapse while waiting for completion of the search. Cost is a concern, with the cost for donor search and marrow procurement ranging from $25,000 to $50,000. The clinical results of alloHSCT with unrelated donors are encouraging. With improved HLA typing techniques and better supportive care, most reported outcomes are no longer significantly different than with related sibling donors.[7,11,12]

COLLECTION OF HEMATOPOIETIC STEM CELLS

Hematopoietic stem cells serve as "mother" cells for all blood cells, including erythrocytes, leukocytes, and platelets (see Chap. 103).[13] Stem cells have varying degrees of "stemness." True *pluripotent* stem cells are capable of replicating indefinitely and can give rise to stem and progenitor cells of *all* tissues. *Multipotent* stem cells, such as hematopoietic stem cells, have the capacity for self-renewal and can differentiate into more than one cell type in a particular tissue lineage. Because of their capacity for self-renewal, hematopoietic stem cells are capable of repopulating the recipient's marrow.

❹ Hematopoietic stem cells are rare cells, composing less than 0.01% of all bone marrow cells. Isolation and quantitative measurement of stem cells is extremely difficult because of their rarity and their similar appearance to other cells. For these reasons, surrogate markers are used to measure the number of stem cells. Determination of the number of cells expressing the CD34 antigen ($CD34^+$ cells), as determined by flow cytometry, has become the standard method of measuring hematopoietic stem cell content.[14] CD34 is an antigen expressed on hematopoietic stem cells and other early progenitor cells.

Hematopoietic stem cells are found in the bone marrow, peripheral blood, and UCB. Hematopoietic stem cells from the bone marrow are obtained by multiple aspirations from the anterior and posterior iliac crests while the donor is under general anesthesia. The procedure takes approximately 1 hour and yields 200 to 1,500 mL, depending on the size of the donor. The marrow is transferred into tissue culture medium containing preservative-free heparin. The pooled marrow is passed through a series of stainless steel screens to break up aggregated particles, resulting in an essentially single-cell suspension. In alloHSCT, the marrow stem cells are given to the recipient 12 to 24 hours after harvest. In autoHSCT, the marrow is frozen and stored until needed. After intravenous infusion, the marrow stem cells enter the systemic circulation and find their way to the bone marrow cavity, where they reseed and grow in the bone marrow microenvironment. Although the donor experiences local soreness for a few days, the procedure usually is well tolerated, with no delayed complications resulting from the marrow aspiration. The major risk of serving as a marrow donor is the risk of undergoing general anesthesia.

Hematopoietic stem cells in peripheral blood (peripheral blood progenitor cells or peripheral blood stem cells [PBSCs]) are found in the mononuclear fraction of white blood cells (lymphocytes and monocytes) and are collected by a procedure called *leukapheresis* (or *apheresis*). In this outpatient procedure, approximately 9 to 14 L of blood is processed over several hours during each daily leukapheresis session. Most of the blood cells are returned to the donor, and each leukapheresis yields approximately 200 mL of cells.

The number of hematopoietic stem cells that circulate in peripheral blood normally is too low for this approach to be technically

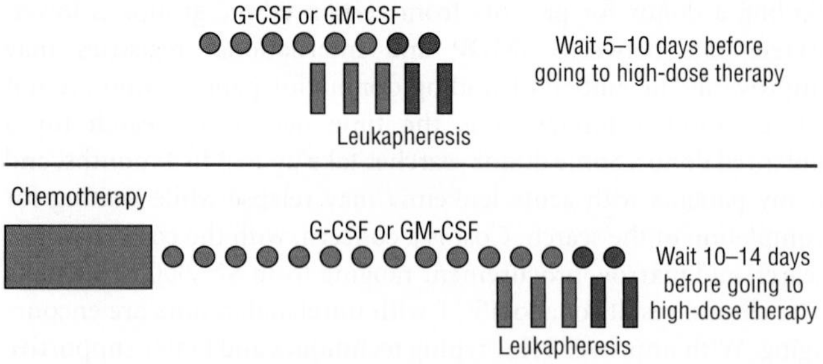

FIGURE 142-2. Schema for collection of peripheral blood progenitor cells after hematopoietic growth factor administration (top) or after chemotherapy and hematopoietic growth factor administration (bottom). Symbols with gray shading represent procedures performed only if adequate numbers of CD34+ cells have not been collected. (G-CSF, granulocyte colony-stimulating factor; GM-CSF, granulocyte-macrophage colony-stimulating factor.)

feasible. Without mobilization techniques, at least six leukaphereses usually are required to collect a sufficient number of PBSCs. Several methods have been used clinically to "mobilize" hematopoietic stem cells from the bone marrow into peripheral blood.[14–17] The first method is administration of chemotherapy, which can briefly increase the number of PBSCs as much as 100-fold. The second and most common method is administration of a recombinant hematopoietic growth factor such as granulocyte colony-stimulating factor (G-CSF; filgrastim) or granulocyte-macrophage colony-stimulating factor (GM-CSF; sargramostim). Each agent has its own potential advantages and disadvantages.[18] Both agents are approved by the Food and Drug Administration for this indication, but G-CSF is the most commonly used growth factor. Commonly used dosages are 5 to 16 mcg/kg/day for G-CSF and 250 mcg/m^2/day for GM-CSF. The combination of chemotherapy followed by a hematopoietic growth factor increases the number of PBSCs to a greater extent than either method alone. This approach is more expensive and is associated with more adverse effects than a growth factor alone, but the number of leukaphereses is reduced, and the additional chemotherapy may further reduce the tumor burden before transplant. With current mobilization techniques, most HSCT centers collect sufficient PBSCs with three or fewer leukaphereses. Figure 142–2 shows representative schemas for mobilization and collection of PBSCs.

Several studies show that the number of CD34$^+$ cells infused correlates significantly with the rate of neutrophil and platelet recovery after high-dose chemotherapy.[14–16] Rapid neutrophil recovery usually is observed in patients who receive at least 2×10^6 CD34$^+$ cells/kg (body weight of recipient). More rapid platelet recovery is observed when at least 5×10^6 CD34$^+$ cells/kg are transplanted compared to lower cell doses. As a result, most transplant centers use 2×10^6 CD34$^+$ cells/kg as a minimum number to collect for autologous transplant, with an optimal target of 5×10^6 CD34$^+$ cells/kg. Some studies suggest clinical and economic benefits are associated with infusion of higher CD34$^+$ cell doses.[19,20] Although the difference in the *median* number of days to neutrophil or platelet recovery usually is no more than 1 to 2 days in patients who receive more than 5×10^6 CD34$^+$ cells/kg compared to those who receive less than 5×10^6 CD34$^+$ cells/kg, fewer patients who receive more than 5×10^6 CD34$^+$ cells/kg have delayed engraftment. This small effect may be important, because patients with delayed engraftment consume a disproportionate share of healthcare resources, such as additional transfusions, hospital days, and drugs (e.g., antibiotics and growth factors).

The optimal regimen for mobilizing PBSCs is not clear.[15–17] Results of some randomized studies show that G-CSF alone provides higher yields of CD34$^+$ cells than GM-CSF alone.[17,18] Higher doses of G-CSF or twice-daily administration of G-CSF also may mobilize more CD34$^+$ cells. Many cytokines and other novel agents, given either alone or in combination with G-CSF, are being evaluated for use in mobilization regimens.[16–18,21]

In some otherwise-eligible transplant candidates, an optimal number of CD34$^+$ cells will not be obtained with standard mobilization methods. Risk factors associated with poor mobilization include the amount (greater than six cycles) and type of prior chemotherapy (alkylating agents) and prior radiation therapy.[15–17] Older age and some diagnoses also are associated with poor mobilization. Several strategies for overcoming the obstacle of poor mobilization have been evaluated, including remobilization with the same or higher doses of the same hematopoietic growth factor, a combination of hematopoietic growth factors, or a combination of chemotherapy and a hematopoietic growth factor. Bone marrow harvest is an option but often is of limited value.

❺ Use of peripheral blood instead of bone marrow as a source of hematopoietic stem cells offers several clinical and economic advantages. The most clinically important advantage is that patients who receive mobilized PBSCs experience more rapid hematopoietic engraftment. Although engraftment of all lineages is more rapid when PBSCs are used, the most significant effect is observed with platelet recovery. Patients who receive mobilized PBSCs experience platelet recovery as much as 2 to 3 weeks earlier and require fewer platelet transfusions than those who receive bone marrow stem cells. As a result, patients usually are discharged earlier from the hospital, so the overall cost of autoHSCT is reduced with the use of PBSCs. Another advantage is that the donor does not experience the discomfort associated with marrow aspirations and is not exposed to the risk associated with general anesthesia. PBSCs may be less likely to be contaminated with malignant cells compared with marrow stem cells. Finally, because PBSCs are collected from the mononuclear cell fraction, a fraction that also contains immunocompetent cells (e.g., natural killer [NK] cells and T lymphocytes), some investigators believe that infusion of PBSCs represents a form of "adoptive immunotherapy." In this model, NK cells and lymphocytes targeted against tumor cells help to kill residual tumor cells. As a result of these clinical and economic advantages, peripheral blood has replaced bone marrow as the source of stem cells in the autologous setting.

Peripheral blood is increasingly being used as a source of hematopoietic stem cells in alloHSCT.[22,23] Approximately 75% of alloHSCTs performed in adults currently come from PBSCs harvested from normal donors, despite early concerns that the increased numbers of T lymphocytes found in peripheral blood could increase the risk of GVHD.[1] Concerns also were raised over the safety and ethics of administering G-CSF to normal individuals volunteering as donors. G-CSF is generally well tolerated. Short-term effects are similar to those seen in cancer patients (e.g., bone pain, headache, fever, arthralgias, malaise). Although there are concerns about increased risk of acute leukemia in healthy subjects given G-CSF, no higher risk has been observed.[24]

Randomized controlled trials and large registry studies show that patients who received allogeneic PBSC transplants from HLA-identical siblings experienced more rapid hematopoietic recovery and required fewer transfusions compared to patients receiving bone marrow.[22,23,25] The difference in the rate of engraftment may be related to the three-fold higher numbers of CD34$^+$ cells infused in recipients of PBSC transplants. Although most of these studies did not report an increased risk of acute GVHD or transplant-related mortality in patients receiving allogeneic PBSC transplants, a higher incidence of chronic GVHD has been observed. In a meta-analysis of nine randomized trials, the risk of chronic GVHD was nearly two-fold higher for patients who received allogeneic PBSC transplants compared to those who received bone marrow transplantation (BMT).[26] Some studies have reported a correlation between CD34$^+$ cell dose and the risk of chronic GVHD, which suggests that the higher CD34$^+$ cell dose explains, in part, the increased risk of chronic GVHD.[27] Use of PBSCs from unrelated donors is being investigated.[23] Approximately 25% of the matched unrelated transplants coordinated by the NMDP use PBSCs.

In addition to bone marrow and peripheral blood, hematopoietic stem cells are found in UCB. UCB is an attractive source for several reasons.[28,29] Because the stem cells are collected from placental blood, there is no risk to the mother or the baby and a very low risk of transmissible infectious diseases, such as cytomegalovirus and Epstein-Barr virus. The cells are available immediately because the donor does not have to be located and the material harvested. UCB initially was obtained from siblings, but now recipients of transplants from unrelated donors account for almost all patients who receive UCB transplants. More than 8,000 unrelated UCB transplants have been performed worldwide.

Results of uncontrolled studies show that recipients of UCB transplantation have a lower risk of GVHD but a higher risk of graft failure compared with recipients of BMT.[28] Recipients of UCB transplantation usually receive a $CD34^+$ cell dose more than 1 log lower than that given to recipients of BMT, and this difference in $CD34^+$ cell dose may explain the delayed engraftment in recipients of UCB transplantation. The number of infused total nucleated and $CD34^+$ cells correlates with outcomes following UCB transplantation. Although no randomized comparisons have been performed, a recently published analysis of data from the CIBMTR and the New York Blood Center showed similar survival in children with acute leukemia who underwent either unrelated UCB transplantation or BMT.[30]

A major limitation of UCB transplants is the small volume of blood collected, usually 60 to 150 mL. Although the relatively low numbers of hematopoietic cells may be adequate for hematopoietic engraftment in children and small adults, it may not be adequate for larger recipients. Efforts to expand the number of hematopoietic stem cells include culturing them ex vivo with combinations of hematopoietic growth factors or "pooling" several units of UCB for one recipient. Preliminary results with unrelated UCB transplants in adult recipients are encouraging,[28,29] but more experience is needed with adult recipients before this procedure can be recommended for that population.

APPROACHES TO ERADICATE MALIGNANT CELLS

MYELOABLATIVE CONDITIONING REGIMENS

❻ Nearly all patients who receive HSCT must be prepared (or "conditioned") before infusion of hematopoietic stem cells.[31] In patients with malignant disease, the goal of the preparative or conditioning regimen is to kill as many malignant cells as possible. Myeloablative conditioning regimens usually include commonly used anticancer drugs given at very high doses, doses that would be associated with severe and life-threatening bone marrow suppression if hematopoietic stem cells were not infused. In patients undergoing alloHSCT, another purpose of the conditioning regimen is to suppress the immune system of the recipient so that the graft is not rejected.

In some conditioning regimens, the only drug given is cyclophosphamide, a drug with both immunosuppressive and cytotoxic effects. Because of the inadequate antitumor activity of cyclophosphamide in some types of cancers, other drugs are often added. Examples of drugs that are included in preparative regimens are cytarabine (ara-C), busulfan, thiotepa, etoposide (VP-16), carboplatin, cisplatin, carmustine (BCNU), melphalan, and ifosfamide.[31]

Total-body irradiation (TBI) is sometimes used in pretransplant conditioning regimens, particularly in patients with leukemia.[32] In patients with malignant disease, the rationale is to eradicate malignant cells located in areas inaccessible to the systemic circulation and thus to the cytotoxic agents. TBI also has significant immunosuppressive activity. Historically, the standard TBI regimen involved administration of a midline tissue dose of approximately 1,000 cGy (1 cGy = 1 rad), which is more than twice the lethal dose of radiation for a normal person. Many centers currently give fractionated (split over several days, once or twice a day) rather than single-dose TBI to patients with malignant disease. The rationale for this approach is an improved therapeutic ratio, that is, destruction of more leukemic cells and marrow stem cells while sparing other normal tissues. The acute toxicities of TBI consist of fever, nausea, vomiting, diarrhea, mucositis, and tender swelling of the parotid gland. Long-term complications of TBI-containing regimens include cataract formation, growth retardation, carcinogenesis, permanent reproductive sterility, and secondary malignancies.

Leukemia

Most patients with leukemia undergoing alloHSCT receive either cyclophosphamide and TBI (CyTBI) or busulfan and cyclophosphamide (BuCy). When given with TBI, cyclophosphamide usually is given first as two doses of 60 mg/kg/day, followed by TBI. TBI can be given as a single dose or fractionated over several days. One variation of the regimen is administration of hyperfractionated TBI first, followed by cyclophosphamide. In that regimen, which is used primarily in patients with acute lymphoblastic leukemia (ALL), 11 TBI doses of 120 cGy are given; doses are given three times per day on days –7 to –5 (*Note:* Day 0 is designated as the day of transplant) and twice per day on the last day (day –4). After TBI, two doses of cyclophosphamide are given intravenously once per day at a dosage of 60 mg/kg on days –3 and –2.

Because of the many acute and chronic toxicities of TBI, the need for specialized equipment, and the lack of convincing evidence showing superiority over non–TBI-containing regimens, most protocols no longer include TBI in the conditioning regimen. One widely used conditioning regimen that does not include TBI is busulfan and cyclophosphamide (BuCy). In the original regimen (BuCy4), busulfan was given orally at a dosage of 1 mg/kg every 6 hours (4 mg/kg/day) for 16 doses on days –9 to –6, followed by four doses of cyclophosphamide given intravenously once daily at a dosage of 50 mg/kg on days –5 to –2. In one widely used modification of the regimen (BuCy2), the total cyclophosphamide dosage is reduced from 200 (50×4) to 120 (60×2) mg/kg. Plasma busulfan concentrations are monitored at some centers because some studies suggest that systemic exposure correlates with outcome,[33] and use of a targeted busulfan and cyclophosphamide preparative regimen may improve patient outcome.[34] A commercially available intravenous form of busulfan (Busulfex) reduces some of the interpatient variability in systemic exposure.[35] Use of intravenous busulfan may reduce the risk of sinusoidal obstruction syndrome. The dose of intravenous busulfan approved for pretransplant conditioning regimens is 0.8 mg/kg every 6 hours for 4 days. Once-a-day dosing regimens that may facilitate outpatient administration of intravenous busulfan have been developed.

CLINICAL CONTROVERSY

Based on studies showing that busulfan concentrations correlate with outcomes, some centers routinely monitor busulfan concentrations in patients undergoing alloHSCT. However, the busulfan assay is not available at most centers because it is technically difficult and the number of patients receiving BuCy is small. Therefore, therapeutic drug monitoring of busulfan usually is inconvenient and expensive because samples must be sent to another center. Some centers have switched to intravenous busulfan to reduce the interpatient variability in pharmacokinetics and avoid the need for monitoring busulfan concentration.

Several prospective randomized studies have compared CyTBI to BuCy in patients with acute or chronic myelogenous leukemia undergoing alloHSCT.[36–38] The results of these studies show that BuCy has similar or greater antileukemic activity than CyTBI in patients with chronic myelogenous leukemia (CML). However, some studies suggest that the CyTBI regimen in patients with acute myelogenous leukemia (AML) was associated with slightly better disease-free survival rates than BuCy. However, none of the patients in these studies who were randomized to BuCy received busulfan doses adjusted on the basis of plasma concentrations. In children with ALL, a retrospective study showed higher survival among children who received CyTBI as a preparative regimen.[39] Long-term toxicities between the two regimens appear to be comparable.

Other drugs have been evaluated in addition to or instead of cyclophosphamide in the preparative regimen.[31,38] Examples include cytarabine or etoposide in combination with TBI. No convincing data indicate that any of these regimens is superior to CyTBI or BuCy. The same preparative regimens usually are given to patients undergoing autoHSCT for leukemia.

Lymphoma

Based on experience in patients with leukemia, CyTBI was the initial regimen used for many patients with Hodgkin's and non-Hodgkin's lymphoma, particularly in alloHSCT. Most preparative regimens used in autoHSCT for lymphoma include an alkylating agent (either cyclophosphamide or melphalan), carmustine, and etoposide.[31,40] TBI usually is not included in the conditioning regimen because many patients with lymphoma have received prior radiotherapy. One widely used regimen in autoHSCT is the CBV regimen, which consists of cyclophosphamide, carmustine (BCNU), and etoposide (VP-16). In that original regimen, cyclophosphamide was given at a dosage of 1.5 g/m^2 on days –6 to –3, carmustine at a dosage of 300 mg/m^2 on day –6, and etoposide at a dosage of 100 mg/m^2 every 12 hours for six doses on days –6 to –4. Some centers have modified the original CBV regimen by changing the dosage of some of the drugs or adding or substituting other drugs, including cytosine arabinoside, etoposide, melphalan, lomustine, and thioguanine. Other widely used nitrosourea-based regimens are BEAC (BCNU, etoposide, ara-C, and cyclophosphamide) and BEAM (BCNU, etoposide, ara-C, and melphalan). No single preparative regimen is clearly superior to other regimens for treatment of lymphoma.

Although TBI usually is not included in the conditioning regimen, some form of radiation therapy is often given, depending on the type, location, and extent of disease. Instead of TBI, some patients receive localized radiation in high doses to areas of residual or bulky disease. Many patients with Hodgkin's lymphoma have received thoracic radiation as primary therapy for their disease, so TBI usually is avoided in these patients. Conversely, most patients with indolent non-Hodgkin's lymphoma receive TBI as part of their preparative regimen because of the known sensitivity of these tumors to low doses of radiation.[41]

One disadvantage of TBI is that it delivers as much radiation to normal organs as it does to tumor cells. The availability of anti-CD20–radiolabeled monoclonal antibodies offers the potential to deliver more radiation to tumor cells and less to normal organs. In these trials, ^{131}I-tositumomab was given, either alone or combined with high-dose cyclophosphamide and etoposide, with autoHSCT in patients with non-Hodgkin's lymphoma.[42,43] With this approach, very high radiation doses could be delivered to sites of disease. Preliminary results with this approach are encouraging.[44]

Solid Tumors

Most conditioning regimens in autoHSCT include at least one alkylating agent because of their steep dose–response curve. Many regimens include more than one alkylating agent, based on preclinical studies showing that resistance to a specific alkylating agent does not impart cross-resistance to other alkylating agents. Other anticancer drugs that modulate the activity of alkylating agents in a synergistic manner, such as etoposide, are attractive drugs for inclusion in high-dose preparative regimens. The dose of nonalkylating agents with antitumor activity has been increased in patients with solid tumors based on tumor-specific activity. Examples include mitoxantrone, paclitaxel, and topotecan. Whether these regimens offer any clinical advantages to those that include only alkylating agents is not clear.

REDUCED-INTENSITY CONDITIONING REGIMENS

❼ The primary goal of myeloablative conditioning regimens is to eradicate malignant cells by administering very high doses of anticancer drugs. It was later discovered that donor T cells contributed to the tumor cell kill observed after alloHSCT, an effect referred to as the *graft-versus-tumor* (GVT) *effect*. Evidence for the GVT effect is based on retrospective studies showing that patients who developed GVHD had a lower risk of leukemic relapse than those who did not develop GVHD.[45] However, the overall survival rate was not different because of the increased nonrelapse mortality associated with GVHD. Other anecdotal evidence supporting a T-cell–mediated GVT effect was the increased risk of relapse found with T-cell–depleted transplants compared to unmodified transplants and the difference in relapse rates between recipients of syngeneic and HLA-identical sibling transplants.

Attempts to deliver higher doses of chemotherapy or TBI generally did not improve survival but increased regimen-related toxicities. In the early 1990s, researchers began to evaluate reduced-intensity conditioning (RIC) regimens as a method to take advantage of the GVT effect. The rationale for RIC is based on the assumption that most of the tumor cell kill associated with alloHSCT is the result of the GVT effect and not the result of the myeloablative doses of chemotherapy or radiation (Fig. 142–3).[46–49] If this assumption is correct, the major role of the conditioning regimen is to suppress the host immune system, thus allowing engraftment of donor hematopoietic stem cells and donor T-cell cytotoxicity. Approximately 30% of allogeneic transplants are performed with RIC regimens.[1]

RIC often is used synonymously with "nonmyeloablative," and NMTs refer to transplants performed with these conditioning regimens. A *nonmyeloablative regimen* is defined based on the following characteristics: (a) no eradication of host hematopoiesis and reversible myelosuppression (usually less than 28 days) without stem cell support, (b) presence of mixed chimerism upon engraftment, and (c) low rates of nonhematologic toxicity.[48] Based on these criteria, not all RIC regimens should be considered nonmyeloablative. A major advantage of this approach is that potentially curative transplants are being offered to patients who typically would not be considered for alloHSCT because of their unacceptably high risk of transplant-related complications (e.g., increased age or moderately compromised organ function). More than 60% of patients receiving RIC regimens are older than 50 years compared to less than 20% of those receiving myeloablative regimens.[1] In addition, because of the lower rate of toxicity, alloHSCT with RIC can be offered to patients who have relapsed after traditional myeloablative autologous or allogeneic transplants.

A number of RIC regimens that vary in their cytotoxic (and thus myelosuppressive) and immunosuppressive activity have been developed.[46–49] Most regimens include fludarabine (125–240 mg/m^2) because of its potent immunosuppressive activity, combined with either low-dose TBI (at doses up to 8 Gy) or an alkylating agent, such as cyclophosphamide (2–3.6 g/m^2 or 120–200 mg/kg), busulfan (up to 10 mg/kg), or melphalan (up to 180 mg/m^2). Antithymocyte globulin or alemtuzumab is sometimes given for additional immuno-

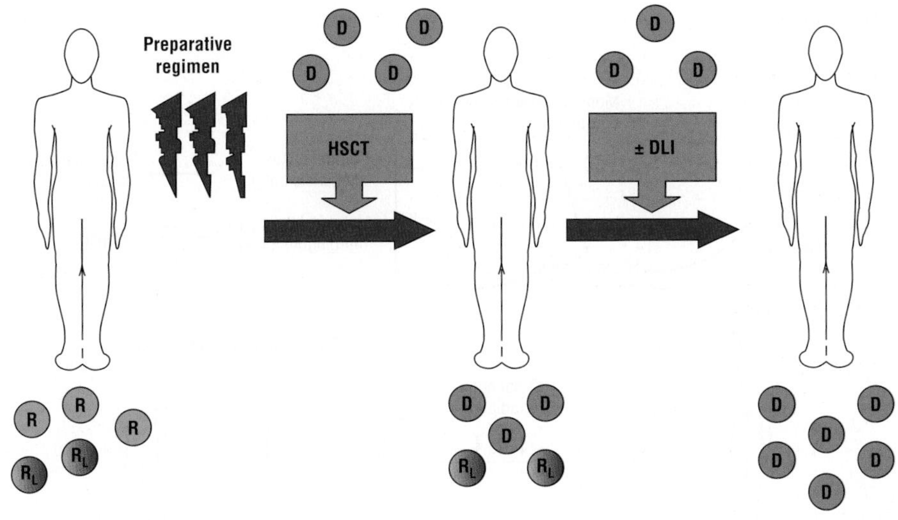

FIGURE 142-3. Schema for nonmyeloablative transplantation for hematologic malignancy. Recipients (R) receive a nonmyeloablative conditioning regimen and an allogeneic hematopoietic stem cell transplant (HSCT). Initially, mixed chimerism is present with the coexistence of donor (D) cells and recipient-derived normal and leukemia/lymphoma (R_L) cells. Donor-derived T cells mediate a graft-versus-host hematopoietic effect that eradicates residual recipient-derived normal and malignant hematopoietic cells. Donor lymphocyte infusions (DLI) can be administered to enhance graft-versus-tumor effects. *(Adapted from Champlin R, Khouri I, Anderlini P, et al. Nonmyeloablative preparative regimens for allogeneic hematopoietic transplantation: Biology and current indications. Oncology 2003;17:94–100.)*

suppression, and other purine analogs (e.g., pentostatin or cladribine) are sometimes used instead of fludarabine.

Because some RIC regimens are not completely myeloablative, host hematopoiesis can persist and lead to mixed chimerism (blood cells from both donor and recipient are present; see Fig. 142–3).[50] Several studies have reported significant correlations between donor T-cell chimerism levels and the risk of graft rejection, GVHD, and relapse. For example, a low percentage of donor T and NK cells present on day 14 has been associated with graft rejection, whereas high T-cell donor chimerism on day 28 has been associated with acute GVHD.[46] Achievement of full donor chimerism was associated with better progression-free survival. These data suggest that monitoring donor chimerism posttransplant may allow early interventions to prevent graft rejection or relapse.

Several clinical studies have reported the results of RIC regimens from HLA-matched related or unrelated donors.[46–49] In the largest series, 253 patients received HLA-matched-related NMT at one of several transplant centers that are part of an international consortium of transplant centers led by the Fred Hutchinson Cancer Research Center.[51,52] All patients had a hematologic malignancy. The source of hematopoietic stem cells was G-CSF–mobilized PBSCs. Median age was 54 years; the oldest patient was 73 years. Median followup was 13 months. The first 58 patients were conditioned with TBI alone (2 Gy); 17% of these patients experienced nonfatal graft rejection. Fludarabine was added to the conditioning regimen in the remaining patients, and the incidence of graft rejection decreased to less than 5%. A combination of cyclosporine and mycophenolate mofetil was given as GVHD prophylaxis. Most patients did not require platelet transfusions, and only approximately two thirds of patients required RBC transfusions. Most of the transplants were performed entirely in the ambulatory care setting. Typical side effects, such as mucositis, diarrhea, and organ toxicities, were absent. Although the risk of infection in the first 100 days appeared to be lower than that seen with myeloablative alloHSCT, the risk of late viral and fungal infections persisted.[53,54] GVHD, although delayed compared to historical controls, still was a significant problem.[55] Transplant-related mortality was only 5% at day 100. Compared with matched controls, patients who received NMT had significantly lower transplant-related mortality at day 100 and at 1 year.[56]

Under a similar protocol, the same consortium of transplant centers treated 89 patients with HLA-matched unrelated NMT.[57] Durable engraftment was observed in 85% of patients who received G-CSF–mobilized PBSCs but only in 56% of marrow recipients. Transplant-related mortality was 11% at day 100. Patients who received PBSCs had improved progression-free and overall survival compared with marrow recipients.

Progression-free survival varies depending on the specific RIC regimen, disease type and status at the time of transplant, donor type, and patient age and comorbidities. Patients with indolent lymphoid malignancies had the lowest relapse rate after NMT, whereas those with advanced myeloid and lymphoid malignancies had the highest relapse rate.[58] Patients transplanted while in remission had lower relapse rates than those who were not in remission at the time of transplant. Direct comparison of the results of NMT versus myeloablative transplants is difficult because patients undergoing NMT tend to be older and have more comorbidities. In two retrospective comparisons of RIC regimens versus standard myeloablative transplants in patients with AML who were older than 50 years, nonrelapse mortality was lower in the RIC-treated patients, but leukemia-free survival was equivalent due to the higher relapse rate seen in the RIC groups.[59,60] Studies evaluating "disease-targeted" therapy (radiolabeled monoclonal antibody, imatinib, or rituximab) combined with NMT to improve outcomes in specific malignancies are ongoing.[46]

CLINICAL CONTROVERSY

Although RIC regimens reduce transplant-related mortality, whether this approach results in improved survival compared with myeloablative regimens is not clear. Also unclear is whether this approach improves survival compared with conventional chemotherapy. Direct comparison of the results of NMT versus myeloablative transplants is difficult because patients undergoing NMT tend to be older and have more comorbidities. Randomized controlled trials addressing these questions are ongoing, and the results of these studies should better define the role of RIC regimens and NMT.

Antitumor responses have been observed with RIC regimens in patients with renal cell carcinoma, melanoma, breast cancer, and other solid tumors.[46,61] In order to improve on the efficacy seen in this setting, some investigators are evaluating novel approaches that enhance allogeneic immune responses against tumor-associated antigens (if available), such as posttransplant vaccination.

In summary, transplants with RIC regimens from HLA-matched related or unrelated donors are a promising treatment modality for patients who are not candidates for myeloablative alloHSCT because of their age, comorbidities, or poor organ function. Myelosuppression is mild, and most patients do not develop severe neutropenia or thrombocytopenia. Because of the reduced intensity of the conditioning regimen, early transplant-related mortality is

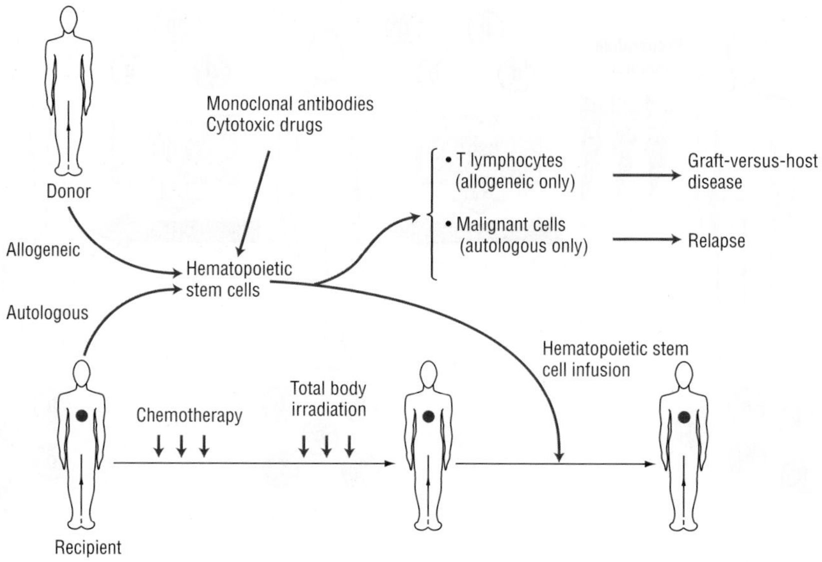

FIGURE 142-4. Use of ex vivo marrow purging to remove or destroy T cells (allogeneic only) or residual malignant cells (autologous only).

less than that seen with myeloablative alloHSCT. GVHD and infections, although occurring later after transplant, continue to be a significant cause of morbidity and mortality. Antitumor responses have been observed in hematologic malignancies and solid tumors.

PURGING THE STEM CELL PRODUCT

One disadvantage of autoHSCT is that the stem cell product (graft) may be contaminated with malignant cells. Infusion of these malignant cells may contribute to tumor relapse. Many approaches have been developed to eliminate ("purge") the marrow of these tumor cells.[62] The most common approach is addition of substances, such as chemicals or monoclonal antibodies, to the stem cell product while it is outside of the body (ex vivo; Fig. 142–4). Because the substances are removed before the stem cells are infused, nonhematopoietic tissues are not exposed to the substances and therefore are not damaged. However, these substances can remove or damage hematopoietic stem cells, which are essential for complete and rapid engraftment, and purging has been associated with delayed marrow recovery. Ex vivo marrow purging also is performed in alloHSCT in an attempt to eliminate T lymphocytes believed to be responsible for acute GVHD (Fig. 142–4). Results with this approach are discussed in the section on Graft-versus-Host Disease.

One approach is the addition of one or more monoclonal antibodies that are directed against specific antigens present on the tumor cells but are absent on nearly all other cells.[43,63] Although this approach is theoretically attractive, it is limited because not all cells from patients with the same type of cancer express a specific antigen. Furthermore, for some types of cancers, identifying antigens distinct from those present on normal hematopoietic stem cells is difficult. To date, this strategy has been used most commonly in patients with lymphoid malignancies, either ALL or non-Hodgkin's lymphoma.

Another method of ex vivo purging involves adding chemicals or drugs to kill the tumor cells.[64] The advantage of this technique is that it can be used for a broader range of tumor types. However, chemical purging is not completely selective for tumor cells, so the precise amount of chemical or drug that kills sufficient numbers of tumor cells while sparing the largest number of hematopoietic stem cells must be added. The chemical most commonly used for purging is 4-hydroperoxycyclophosphamide (4-HC, or perfosfamide), a congener of cyclophosphamide. 4-HC is a stable compound that enters cells and is rapidly reduced to 4-hydroxycyclophosphamide, which serves as the precursor to the reactive phosphoramide mustard. The level of aldehyde dehydrogenase, the enzyme that inactivates 4-hydroxycyclophosphamide, appears to be highest in early hematopoietic progenitors and decreases as these cells differentiate. This observation may explain why 4-HC appears to have an acceptable therapeutic index. Other analogs of cyclophosphamide (e.g., mafosfamide) also are being investigated as chemical purging agents.

Although ex vivo purging has been extensively studied, convincing evidence that it improves transplant outcomes is lacking. The techniques can be cumbersome and add cost to the transplant procedure, so their use should be restricted to clinical trials.

Rituximab has been used pretransplant for in vivo purging of the stem cell graft prior to autoHSCT in patients with non-Hodgkin's lymphoma.[41,43] When used for in vivo purging, rituximab usually is given before each leukapheresis. Although use of rituximab was effective in reducing the number of tumor cells in the stem cell graft, whether this approach improves disease-free survival after autoHSCT is not clear.

POSTTRANSPLANT IMMUNOTHERAPY

❽ The rationale for posttransplant immunotherapy is based on observations that certain subsets of T cells are responsible for eradication of malignant cells. This is referred to as the *graft-versus-leukemia* or *graft-versus-tumor* (GVT) effect.

Donor Lymphocyte Infusions

Perhaps the most commonly used form of posttransplant immunotherapy is donor lymphocyte infusions (DLI) for treatment of disease relapse after alloHSCT.[65,66] Lymphocytes are collected from the same donor who provided hematopoietic stem cells. Most experiences with DLI have been cases of patients with CML. More than 80% of patients who are in cytogenetic or molecular relapse respond to DLI. The response rate of patients in more advanced phases is approximately 15% to 30%. Although the time to response is delayed (median 3–4 months), patients often have a durable molecular remission to DLI.

Response rates to DLI of patients with other myeloid malignancies, such as AML and myelodysplasia, are generally lower (25%–30%) than the rates of patients with CML.[65–67] This may be related to the rapid proliferation of acute leukemia within the often prolonged time to response after DLI or to the lack of suitable target antigens on non-CML cells for recognition by donor cytotoxic T cells. Patients with relapsed AML post-HSCT are more likely to achieve a complete response to DLI if they had a longer remission period after transplant and had some GVHD after the DLI.[65,68]

Administration of induction chemotherapy prior to DLI administration may improve the antitumor activity of DLI in patients with AML, but this method has not been tested in a randomized study. DLI has been shown to have limited benefit in patients with relapsed ALL after transplant.

DLI appears to be effective in patients with multiple myeloma who relapse after alloHSCT, with reported response rates of 40% to 50%.[65–67] Unfortunately, these responses tend to be transient and associated with the occurrence of GVHD. Anecdotal evidence suggests a graft-versus-lymphoma effect in patients with indolent non-Hodgkin's lymphoma and chronic lymphocytic leukemia (a disease entity closely related to indolent non-Hodgkin's lymphoma).

DLI is sometimes given posttransplant for treatment of residual or progressive disease in patients with mixed chimerism after NMT. Preliminary results show that DLI in this setting is effective and is associated with acceptable toxicity (mostly GVHD) in patients with early signs of disease persistence or progression.[66,69] Prophylactic DLI to eradicate residual disease and reduce the risk of relapse is being investigated.

The most serious complications of DLI are pancytopenia and GVHD. The cytopenias generally are transient and can be treated with hematopoietic growth factors. A small percentage of patients may have a more prolonged course of aplasia with associated risk of infection, bleeding, and anemia. These patients may benefit from another infusion of donor stem cells. Acute GVHD (grade II or greater) occurs in 40% to 60% patients receiving DLI. Although the severity of GVHD has been correlated with the GVT effect, complete responses have been seen in the absence of GVHD, suggesting that the effects can be separated. DLI is associated with 10% to 15% nonrelapse mortality at 1 year.

Because of the potential of DLI to cure some patients with certain hematologic malignancies, investigators are evaluating strategies to separate the GVT effect from the GVH effect, which would make DLI more tolerable. Other investigators are developing methods that would expand the efficacy of DLI to other malignancies. Some of these strategies include T-cell depletion from the stem cells, followed by delayed T-cell add-back transplant for patients with evidence of residual disease approximately 3 months posttransplant; selective depletion of $CD8^+$ cells from the DLI; in vivo or in vitro T-cell activation with interleukin (IL)-2; and infusion of T cells that are selected to recognize tumor-specific antigens.[65,67]

Immunomodulatory Cytokines

Another approach to inducing a GVT effect in patients who relapse after HSCT is posttransplant administration of a cytokine with immunomodulatory activity, such as IL-2.[45,70,71] Some benefit in terms of effects on NK cells and other important antitumor immune responses has been observed with the use of IL-2. Toxicities have been tolerable in most patients but can be serious and life-threatening. Studies that will define the role of these cytokines in prolonging relapse-free survival after HSCT are necessary.

Monoclonal Antibodies

Rituximab is being evaluated as adjuvant therapy in patients with non-Hodgkin's lymphoma treated with autoHSCT.[43,72] The timing and number of doses of rituximab therapy vary. The Stanford program reported promising results with two 4-week courses starting at day 42 and 6 months posttransplant.[72] Neutropenia was observed in approximately 50% of the patients treated.

TRANSPLANT-RELATED COMPLICATIONS

9 Although many patients with cancer who are treated with high-dose chemotherapy and autoHSCT or alloHSCT experience long-term survival and cure of their disease, this modality is associated with many serious and potentially life-threatening complications. In the early 1970s, early posttransplant mortality was extremely high, and most HSCT patients did not survive beyond 100 days. During those early years of alloHSCT, death usually was related to infection, GVHD, interstitial pneumonia, and leukemic relapse. Today, largely because of the availability of improved broad-spectrum antibiotics, immunosuppressive drugs, antiviral drugs, and hematopoietic growth factors, transplant-related mortality after alloHSCT with HLA-matched sibling donors has been reduced to less than 30% at most centers. Mortality is even lower with the use of RIC regimens. Causes of death usually are related to transplant-related organ toxicity, GVHD, or immunosuppression. Until recently, alloHSCT usually was restricted to patients younger than 50 years with an HLA-identical sibling donor. With advances in the prevention and treatment of transplant-related complications and the availability of RIC regimens, alloHSCT now is being offered to many patients older than 50 years. The risk of transplant-related mortality after high-dose chemotherapy with autoHSCT is less than 5% at many centers, depending on patient population and conditioning regimen. Mortality is lower with autologous transplants because of the lack of GVHD and associated complications of immunosuppression. Transplant-related mortality in autoHSCT usually is caused by conditioning regimen organ toxicity or infection.

Table 142–1 lists the dose-limiting nonhematologic toxicities for several drugs that are commonly included in conditioning regimens. These toxicities may be uncommon or rare with administration of conventional doses of specific drugs. When these agents are given in high doses, the toxicities seen with conventional doses (e.g., mucositis, enteritis, nausea, vomiting, hematuria) can be more frequent and/or severe. Several unusual and severe manifestations of regimen-related toxicities are discussed in this section.

SINUSOIDAL OBSTRUCTION SYNDROME

Sinusoidal obstruction syndrome (SOS), formerly known as hepatic venoocclusive disease, occurs as a result of chemotherapy-induced dilation of hepatic sinusoids, necrosis of perivenular hepatocytes, and collagenization of the hepatic sinusoids and venules. These histologic changes can lead to portal hypertension and hepatic failure.[73] Clinical signs of SOS include fluid retention (resulting in sudden weight gain

TABLE 142-1 Dose-Limiting Nonhematologic Toxicities for Selected Chemotherapeutic Agents Included in Myeloablative Conditioning Regimens in Hematopoietic Stem Cell Transplantation

Drug	Conventional Dose[a] (mg/m²)	HSCT Dose (mg/m²)	Dose-Limiting Toxicity
Busulfan (oral)	2	450	Hepatic
Carboplatin	400	2,000	Hepatic, renal
Carmustine	200	1,200	Pulmonary, hepatic
Cisplatin	100	200	Renal, peripheral neuropathy
Cyclophosphamide	1,000	7,500	Cardiomyopathy
Etoposide	300–600	2,400	Mucositis
Ifosfamide	5,000	18,000	Renal
Melphalan	40	225	Mucositis
Thiotepa	20–50	1125	Mucositis, central nervous system

HSCT, hematopoietic stem cell transplantation.

[a]Doses are approximate and are for drugs used as single agents. When combinations are used, doses may need to be decreased.

Modified from Eder JP, Elias A, Shea TC, et al. A phase I–II study of cyclophosphamide, thiotepa, and carboplatin with autologous bone marrow transplantation in solid tumor patients. J Clin Oncol 1990;8:1242.

and ascites), hepatomegaly (sometimes painful), and hyperbilirubinemia/jaundice. SOS usually occurs within the first 3 weeks after transplant. The incidence of SOS ranges from 5% to 20% in most published series. Severe SOS is fatal in 50% to 75% of patients who develop the condition. Factors that reportedly increase the risk of SOS include use of TBI-containing conditioning regimens (dose-dependent), individual variability in cyclophosphamide metabolism, and elevated liver function tests pretransplant. Pretransplant exposure to gemtuzumab ozogamicin (Mylotarg) has been implicated in the development of SOS in patients undergoing alloHSCT.[74] Use of some drugs in the conditioning regimen, such as busulfan, cyclophosphamide, or carmustine, may increase the risk of SOS.

The pharmacokinetics of busulfan or cyclophosphamide may correlate with the risk of SOS. Because busulfan concentrations have been correlated with the risk of SOS, many HSCT centers adjust busulfan doses based on plasma concentrations.[33] Use of IV busulfan reduces the interpatient variation in systemic exposure associated with the oral formulation and has been associated with a reduced risk of SOS.[35] Exposure to the O-carboxyethyl-phosphoramide mustard metabolite of cyclophosphamide has been reported to correlate with the risk of SOS and nonrelapse mortality.[75] In addition, when busulfan and cyclophosphamide are given in combination, the order in which they are given may contribute to the risk of SOS. Presumably because of the effect of busulfan on cyclophosphamide pharmacokinetics (increased exposure to active and/or toxic metabolites), liver toxicity appears to be worse when busulfan is given first, as traditionally given in the BuCy regimen.[76]

Some studies suggest that prostaglandin E_1, unfractionated and low-molecular-weight heparin, or ursodiol may be partially effective in preventing SOS.[77] In a systematic review of three randomized trials comparing prophylactic ursodiol versus no treatment, Tay et al.[78] found a reduced risk of SOS (relative risk 0.34, 95% confidence interval 0.17–0.66) with prophylactic ursodiol. These studies were conducted in patients undergoing myeloablative transplants. Transplant-related mortality was reduced (relative risk 0.58, 95% confidence interval 0.35–0.95). Other outcomes, such as relapse and overall survival, were not affected. Prophylactic defibrotide may also be effective.[79]

Treatment is generally supportive. Recombinant tissue plasminogen activator has been given to patients with severe SOS because of the possible role of the coagulation cascade in the pathogenesis of SOS. Responses have been reported, but patients also experienced a higher risk of bleeding.[77] Defibrotide may also be beneficial.[80]

PULMONARY COMPLICATIONS

Pulmonary complications following HSCT can be categorized as infectious and noninfectious (infectious complications are discussed in Chap. 126). Noninfectious complications are categorized as early (first 100 days posttransplant) and late (>100 days posttransplant). Patients who receive high-dose BCNU are also at risk for pulmonary fibrosis as a result of direct pulmonary tissue damage caused by this agent. Early complications include diffuse alveolar hemorrhage, engraftment syndrome, and idiopathic interstitial pneumonitis.[81] Diffuse alveolar hemorrhage is characterized by dyspnea, hypoxia, dry cough, and fever. Chest x-ray film usually shows diffuse infiltrates in an alveolar pattern. Diffuse alveolar hemorrhage is diagnosed by examination of bronchoalveolar lavage fluid, which reveals progressively bloodier fluid with each instilled aliquot, and negative findings on microbiologic analysis. Although the condition can be life-threatening or fatal, prompt treatment with high doses of corticosteroids is sometimes beneficial.

Fever, erythrodermatous skin rash, and noncardiogenic pulmonary edema can occur during neutrophil recovery after HSCT. Because these clinical manifestations usually occur immediately before or at the time of neutrophil engraftment, this clinical entity has been referred to as *engraftment syndrome*.[82] The incidence of engraftment syndrome is not known because of the lack of uniform diagnostic criteria, although some series report that approximately 10% of patients who receive autoHSCT develop the syndrome. Engraftment syndrome can progress to life-threatening respiratory failure with or without multiple organ failure. Corticosteroids are effective in some patients.

Idiopathic interstitial pneumonitis (also called idiopathic pneumonia syndrome) is defined as widespread alveolar injury in the absence of active lower respiratory tract infection following HSCT. Patients with idiopathic interstitial pneumonitis are clinically indistinguishable from patients with interstitial pneumonitis related to infection. Idiopathic interstitial pneumonitis is postulated to have a multifactorial etiology, including toxic effects of myeloablative conditioning, immunologic cell-mediated injury, inflammatory cytokine-induced lung damage, and occult pulmonary infections. The risk is similar in recipients of autoHSCT or alloHSCT but appears to be higher in patients who are conditioned with a TBI-containing regimen or who have acute GVHD. Mortality as high as 70% has been reported, and treatment consists of supportive care only. The incidence of idiopathic interstitial pneumonitis may be lower after RIC compared to conventional regimens.[83]

Late pulmonary complications cover a wide spectrum of disorders and include both obstructive and restrictive lung diseases. Included in these disorders are bronchiolitis obliterans with or without organizing pneumonia, diffuse alveolar damage, and lymphocytic interstitial pneumonia.[81,84,85] Therapy consists of steroids, which are approximately 50% effective. Patients with mild-to-moderate airflow impairment appear to have the best response. Mortality from these disorders is approximately 40%.

GRAFT FAILURE

Initial engraftment after high-dose chemotherapy conditioning regimens usually occurs in the first 2 to 4 weeks posttransplant. Engraftment is evidenced by rising peripheral blood counts and the presence of hematopoietic precursor cells in the marrow. In alloHSCT, the presence of donor cells (i.e., chimerism) is confirmed by fluorescent in situ hybridization of sex chromosomes and PCR-based analysis of polymorphic DNA sequences.[50] Full chimerism is defined as greater than 95% of T cells of donor origin. In most patients, engraftment is sustained with complete recovery of hematopoiesis.

Graft failure can occur after autologous, syngeneic, and allogeneic HSCT. It can be the result of an immunologic reaction between donor and host, heavy pretreatment with chemotherapy and/or radiation therapy, infusion of insufficient numbers of hematopoietic stem cells, viral infection, recurrence of primary hematologic malignancy, drug reaction (e.g., to ganciclovir), or development of a secondary myelodysplasia. Two syndromes have been observed. Early graft failure occurs when the rate of hematopoietic recovery is delayed (primary graft failure or delayed engraftment), whereas late graft failure is characterized by a decline in peripheral blood counts after initial engraftment (secondary graft failure). With widespread use of PBSCs and posttransplant growth factors, primary graft failure is rare after autologous and HLA-matched related alloHSCT. Graft failure that occurs after alloHSCT, characterized by regrowth of immunocompetent host cells and a simultaneous loss of donor cells, is referred to as *graft rejection*. Graft rejection occurs rarely after HLA-matched related alloHSCT. An increased risk of graft rejection has been observed in recipients of hematopoietic stem cells from HLA-mismatched related or unrelated donors, recipients of T-cell–depleted marrow, and patients with severe aplastic anemia.[7,9,86]

The long-term prognosis of patients with graft failure is poor. Despite supportive care, death may result from infection or bleeding. In some patients with an allogeneic donor, a second infusion of stem cells can be attempted. The most effective therapy for graft failure is G-CSF or GM-CSF.

Hematopoietic growth factors usually are given posttransplant to patients who receive autoHSCT, although some clinicians believe that posttransplant G-CSF or GM-CSF is unnecessary because of the already rapid engraftment seen after mobilized PBSC transplants.[87,88] The usual dosage of GM-CSF is 250 mcg/m^2/day. Many different dosages and schedules of G-CSF have been used after autoHSCT. Originally, G-CSF was given at a dose of 5 to 10 mcg/kg/day beginning on the day of or the day after infusion of stem cells and continued until neutrophil recovery to greater than an arbitrary number of neutrophils (500–1,000 cells/mm^3). In one study of three different G-CSF dosages (5, 10, and 16 mcg/kg/day), no significant difference in the rate of hematopoietic recovery between the different dosages was observed.[89] In another study, delayed initiation of G-CSF at a dosage of 5 mcg/kg/day until day 5 posttransplant did not impair hematopoietic recovery after autoHSCT.[90] Pegfilgrastim in the transplant setting is being studied.

Hematopoietic growth factors accelerate the rate of hematopoietic recovery in patients undergoing alloHSCT. However, laboratory studies show that growth factors can modify T-cell and dendritic cell function, and one retrospective study of patients with acute leukemia reported that G-CSF use after allogeneic BMT was associated with significantly increased risk of acute GVHD and death.[91] No detrimental effects of G-CSF were noted in patients receiving allogeneic PBSC transplants. In a meta-analysis of 34 randomized controlled trials, no increased risk of acute GVHD or treatment-related mortality was observed when G-CSF or GM-CSF was used after alloHSCT.[92] In another retrospective analysis of 2,719 patients from the CIBMTR, no association between G-CSF use and acute or chronic GVHD, transplant-related mortality, or survival was observed in recipients of HLA-identical sibling bone marrow, recipients of HLA-identical sibling peripheral blood, and recipients of HLA-matched unrelated donor bone marrow.[93] As a result of these concerns, use of growth factors after alloHSCT is not considered standard of care.[88]

None of the commercially available hematopoietic growth factors has a significant effect on platelet recovery. Results of studies with investigational platelet growth factors, such as thrombopoietin and IL-11, given posttransplant have been disappointing.[87] Platelet transfusions remain the standard of care in patients with thrombocytopenia below a given threshold (e.g., 10,000 cells/mm^3) or in patients with significant bleeding.

Anemia may be problematic in the posttransplant setting, especially in patients receiving alloHSCT. The etiology is unclear and most likely is multifactorial. Erythropoietin administration may be useful in reducing the need for red blood cell transfusions and may be given in regimens similar to those given for malignancy-associated anemia.[87]

GRAFT-VERSUS-HOST DISEASE

GVHD is caused by immunocompetent donor T cells reacting against recipient/host antigens presented by antigen-presenting cells. In that setting, donor T cells recognize histocompatibility antigens of the host as genetically foreign, become activated, proliferate, and attack recipient tissue, thereby producing the clinical syndrome of GVHD.[94]

Two different clinical GVHD syndromes (acute and chronic) are recognized, depending on the time of onset and clinical presentation.[95–97] *Acute* GVHD usually presents prior to day 100 posttransplant (*classic* acute GVHD), but it can be *persistent, recurrent,* or *late-onset* with clinical manifestations occurring after day 100. Acute GVHD observed after day 100 usually is the result of immunosuppression withdrawal for relapsed or persistent malignancy or administration of DLI, or occurs in the setting of NMT. *Chronic* GVHD usually occurs after day 100, either with or without characteristics of acute GVHD. Chronic GVHD without characteristics of acute GVHD (*classic* chronic GVHD) occurs after resolution of acute GVHD (quiescent or interrupted) or de novo (no prior acute GVHD). An "overlap syndrome" may occur in which features of both acute and chronic GHVD are present simultaneously, usually when chronic GVHD develops prior to resolution of acute GVHD (progressive onset). Acute GVHD usually is limited to the gastrointestinal tract, skin, and liver, whereas signs and symptoms of chronic GVHD resemble an autoimmune disorder and can affect many organ systems.

A "hyperacute" form of GVHD may occur in patients with multiple HLA mismatches and in patients who receive T-cell–replete transplants without adequate GVHD prophylaxis, especially in myeloablative regimens.[98,99] Descriptions of hyperacute GVHD vary but usually include fever, generalized erythroderma, desquamation, and edema. More severe forms with accompanying organ failure have been seen in haploidentical donors. Hyperacute GVHD typically occurs approximately 1 week after transplant before engraftment of neutrophils. The response rate to first-line therapy appears to be lower in patients with hyperacute GVHD compared to patients who develop GVHD later posttransplant, but no difference in survival has been observed.[99]

Acute Graft-Versus-Host Disease

The pathophysiology of acute GVHD has been described as a three-step process.[94] In step 1, the high-dose conditioning regimen damages host tissues. Damage to the intestinal mucosa leads to release of lipopolysaccharides into the systemic circulation, which stimulates secretion of inflammatory cytokines such as IL-1 and tumor necrosis factor-α (TNF-α). These cytokines upregulate MHC gene products and host antigen-presenting cells such as dendritic cells, which play a critical role in this immune response. In step 2, donor T cells are activated, and secretion of other cytokines (IL-2 and interferon-γ) by activated T cells results in recruitment of macrophages and alteration of target cells in the gastrointestinal tract and skin so that they are more susceptible to damage. In step 3, multiple cytotoxic effector cells (T cells and macrophages) are generated and contribute to target tissue injury by secreting more inflammatory cytokines that cause target cell apoptosis. The term *cytokine storm* is sometimes used to describe the critical role of inflammatory cytokines in this process.

Based on this three-step model, three general approaches can be used to prevent GVHD in humans.[94] The first is to reduce host tissue damage with the use of RIC regimens. The second and most widely used approach is to modulate donor T cells by reducing T-cell numbers (T-cell depletion), activation (most immunosuppressive agents), or proliferation (antiproliferative agents). The third approach is to block inflammatory stimulation and effectors (e.g. TNF-α inhibitors, IL-1 receptor antagonist).

The principal target organs in acute GVHD are the skin, liver, and gastrointestinal tract.[95,98] Acute GVHD is classified into four grades, depending on the number of organs involved and the degree of involvement of each organ (Table 142–2). Grade I disease involves only the skin. Grades II through IV involve the skin and either the liver, gastrointestinal tract, or both. The initial sign of acute skin GVHD usually is a generalized maculopapular rash that initially involves the face, ears, palms, soles, and upper trunk. The skin rash can spread to the rest of the body and, if untreated or refractory to treatment, will progress to bullae formation and desquamation, much like a burn injury. Gastrointestinal GVHD is manifested as diarrhea but may progress to abdominal pain/cramping and ileus. GVHD of the upper intestinal tract has been described presenting as nausea, vomiting, anorexia, and dyspepsia. The diagnosis of gastrointestinal GVHD should be made by biopsy of the intestinal tract (stomach, duodenum, or rectum). Hepatic GVHD usually is asymptomatic, consisting of hyperbilirubinemia and elevated alkaline phosphatase

TABLE 142-2 Consensus Grading of Acute Graft-Versus-Host Disease

	Organ/Extent of Involvement		
	Skin	***Liver***	***Intestinal Tract***
Stage			
1	Rash on <25% of skin[a]	Bilirubin 2–3 mg/dL[b]	Diarrhea >500 mL/day[c] or persistent nausea[d]
2	Rash on 25–50% of skin	Bilirubin 3–6 mg/dL	Diarrhea >1,000 mL/day
3	Rash on >50% of skin	Bilirubin 6–15 mg/dL	Diarrhea >1,500 mL/day
4	Generalized erythroderma with bulla formation	Bilirubin >15 mg/dL	Severe abdominal pain with or without ileus
Grade			
0	None	None	None
I	Stage 1–2	None	None
II	Stage 3	or Stage 1	or Stage 1
III	–	Stage 2–3	or Stage 2–4
IV[e]	Stage 4	or Stage 4	–

[a]Use the "rule of nines" to determine body surface area involvement.
[b]Range given as total bilirubin. Downgrade one stage if an additional cause of elevated bilirubin has been documented.
[c]Volume of diarrhea applies to adults. For pediatric patients, the volume of diarrhea should be based on body surface area.
[d]Persistent nausea with histologic evidence of graft-versus-host disease in the stomach or duodenum.
[e]Grade IV may include lesser organ involvement but with extreme decrease in performance status.
This article was published in Semin Hematol, Vol. 43, Deeg HJ, Artin JH. The clinical spectrum of acute graft-verus-host disease, pages 24–31. Copyright Elsevier 2006.

levels; increases in serum aminotransferases occur less consistently. The diagnosis can be made by biopsy, although many patients cannot provide biopsy samples because of the inherent risk of hemorrhage.

The overall incidence of moderate to severe (grades II–IV) acute GVHD ranges from 10% to more than 80%.[95] Mortality directly attributable to acute GVHD or its treatment occurs in 10% to 20% of patients. The incidence of GVHD is related to the degree of histocompatibility, number of T cells in the graft, donor and recipient age, intensity of the conditioning regimen, source of hematopoietic cells (bone marrow vs peripheral blood), and prophylactic regimen. Acute GVHD can occur in patients receiving DLI for treatment of relapsed disease following HSCT.[66,69] The risk of acute GVHD is lower in recipients of UCB transplants.[28] The most severe acute GVHD is observed in alloHSCT with non–HLA-identical donors. In these settings, the incidence of grades II to IV acute GVHD exceeds 50% despite aggressive GVHD prophylaxis.

Multiorgan acute GVHD and the drugs given to prevent or treat the disease are associated with delayed immunologic recovery and increased susceptibility to infections. Infection is often the primary cause of death in patients with GVHD. Patients with GVHD treated with an immunosuppressive regimen should receive prophylactic antiviral, antibacterial, and antifungal therapy and be monitored routinely for the occurrence of these infections.

⑩ Because treatment of established acute GVHD often is unsatisfactory, aggressive preventive measures usually are taken. The most common strategy used to prevent acute GVHD is blocking the activation of T cells by administration of immunosuppressive agents.[94,95,100] Several immunosuppressive agents have been used, including methotrexate, cyclosporine, tacrolimus, mycophenolate mofetil, antithymocyte globulin, corticosteroids, and monoclonal antibodies directed at T cells. The pharmacology of these drugs is reviewed elsewhere.[101] Most GVHD prophylaxis regimens combine two or more immunosuppressive agents that affect different stages of T-cell activation. Another strategy is removing or depleting most T cells from donor bone marrow ex vivo prior to transplant by physical separation (i.e., lectin agglutination) or by treatment with monoclonal antibodies directed at T cells (see Fig. 142–4).[86]

In alloHSCT with HLA-matched donors, the combination of cyclosporine or tacrolimus and either methotrexate or corticosteroids reduces the incidence of grades II to IV acute GVHD to 25% to 40%. Intravenous cyclosporine or tacrolimus usually is started a few days before or on day 0. Cyclosporine is given at an initial dosage of 3–5 mg/kg/day and tacrolimus at 0.02–0.03 mg/kg/day. Dosages are adjusted based on trough concentrations. Patients are converted to oral formulations when they can be tolerated. Cyclosporine and tacrolimus typically are given at full doses until days 50 to 100, gradually tapered in the absence of GVHD, and discontinued by day 180. Methotrexate is given intravenously on days 1, 3, 6, and 11 posttransplant. The methotrexate dosage is 10 mg/m^2, except for the first dose given on day 1 (15 mg/m^2). Alternatively, some centers use 5 mg/m^2 (same schedule). The day 11 dose is sometimes omitted because of the drug's myelosuppressive effects, severe mucositis, or development of conditions that may prolong methotrexate systemic exposure (e.g., renal failure or third spacing). When corticosteroids are used, methylprednisolone or prednisone usually is started during the first 2 weeks posttransplant, given at full dosages for several weeks, and gradually tapered in the absence of GVHD. Although the efficacy of methotrexate-based regimens and corticosteroid-based regimens appears to be similar, use of methotrexate may increase the risk of delayed engraftment and is associated with significant mucositis, and corticosteroid administration is associated with a higher incidence of infections. Three-drug regimens composed of cyclosporine, methotrexate, and corticosteroids have been studied but have not been shown to be more efficacious in HLA-matched transplants.[95,100]

Two large multicenter randomized trials compared cyclosporine and methotrexate with tacrolimus and methotrexate. One study was performed in patients undergoing HLA-identical sibling alloHSCT,[102] whereas the other study was performed in patients undergoing matched unrelated alloHSCT.[103] Both studies found the tacrolimus combination to be significantly superior to the cyclosporine combination in preventing grades II to IV acute GVHD. The incidence of renal impairment was higher in patients receiving tacrolimus, and more tacrolimus-treated patients in the HLA-identical sibling alloHSCT trial required hemodialysis. The incidence of hypertension was significantly higher in cyclosporine-treated patients in the HLA-matched sibling alloHSCT trial. No difference in the overall or relapse-free survival rate was reported in the two trials. However, in the subgroup of patients with advanced disease in the HLA-identical sibling alloHSCT trial, cyclosporine-treated patients had significantly better overall and disease-free survival rates at 2 years compared to patients who received tacrolimus. The authors explained that lowering the target blood levels to less than 20 ng/mL might reduce the renal toxicity of tacrolimus. Based on the results of these two studies, many transplant centers use tacrolimus and methotrexate as first-line acute GVHD prophylaxis.

Because of the gastrointestinal and hematologic toxicities of methotrexate, a GVHD prophylaxis regimen that uses sirolimus in place of methotrexate in combination with tacrolimus has been developed by investigators at the Dana-Farber Cancer Institute. In an uncontrolled study of 53 patients receiving myeloablative alloHSCT, the combination of sirolimus and tacrolimus was associated with rapid engraftment and low incidences of grades II to IV acute GVHD and treatment-related mortality.[104] Randomized trials comparing this regimen to standard methotrexate-containing regimens are needed.

Acute GVHD prophylaxis regimens used in NMT usually are similar to those used in myeloablative alloHSCT. However, some centers have developed novel prophylactic regimens specifically for patients undergoing NMT. An example of such a regimen is cyclosporine and mycophenolate mofetil,[51,52] which was developed based on preclinical studies.[105]

The role of ex vivo T-cell depletion from donor grafts is controversial (see Fig. 142–4).[86] Although use of T-cell–depleted marrow can reduce the incidence and severity of acute GVHD, it is associated with an increased risk of graft failure, delayed immune reconstitution, leukemic relapse, cytomegalovirus reactivation, and Epstein-Barr virus–related lymphoproliferative disorders. As a result, this approach does not improve the survival rate in recipients of HLA-identical sibling donor marrow. These observations suggest that important cell populations are being eliminated in the depletion process. Various approaches that selectively remove the T cells responsible for GVHD while leaving those cells that mediate engraftment, antileukemic effect, and suppression of Epstein-Barr virus–transformed lymphocytes are being investigated.[100] Another approach is infusion of the T cells originally depleted from the graft later in the posttransplant period to prevent leukemic relapse.[106] Because of the higher risk of GVHD in alloHSCT with HLA-mismatched donors, T-cell depletion is sometimes included as part of the GVHD prophylaxis regimen in that setting.

With alternative donors, the risk of moderate-to-severe (grades II–IV) acute GVHD is 50% or higher with conventional two-drug prophylaxis. Several approaches are used to reduce the risk of acute GVHD in this high-risk group of patients: three-drug GVHD prophylaxis, pretransplant administration of antithymocyte globulin, or ex vivo T-cell depletion of donor bone marrow (see Fig. 142–4). Encouraging results have been reported with the addition of novel immunosuppressive agents, such as sirolimus, to two-drug prophylaxis regimens.[107] The addition of antilymphocyte/antithymocyte globulin to the pretransplant conditioning regimen reduced the risk of acute and chronic GVHD but increased the risk of serious infections.[108] Uncontrolled studies suggest that ex vivo T-cell depletion significantly reduces the risk of early graft failure and acute GVHD, with apparent preservation of the graft-versus-leukemia effect.[86]

If a patient develops grades II to IV GVHD, prophylactic agents are continued and high-dose corticosteroids in the form of intravenous methylprednisolone are given.[109] The usual dosage is 1 to 2 mg/kg/day, given in two divided doses. The initial dosage is as high as 10 mg/kg/day in some protocols, although there is no convincing evidence that higher dosages are more effective. Approximately 25% to 40% of patients with established acute GVHD respond to high-dose corticosteroids. If the patient responds, the corticosteroid dose is tapered gradually over several weeks, depending on response. In patients who experience a flare in GVHD during the taper phase, therapy consists of increasing the steroid dose and then tapering more slowly. Oral beclomethasone dipropionate, a topically active corticosteroid, has been shown to reduce the frequency of gastrointestinal GVHD relapses when continued after prednisone taper.[110] Administration of beclomethasone has been associated with a better survival at 200 days and 1 year after transplant. GVHD-associated mortality is strongly correlated to response to initial treatment and ranges from approximately 25% in patients who had a complete response to approximately 80% in patients who had no response or progressive disease.

Several randomized trials have evaluated other agents combined with methylprednisolone as initial therapy for acute GVHD.[95,109] In particular, the addition of anti–T-cell antibodies, such as antithymocyte globulin or monoclonal antibodies (e.g., daclizumab), has not been shown to improve patient outcome.[109,111] Similarly, the combination of methylprednisolone and the anti–TNF-α monoclonal antibody infliximab has not been shown to increase response rate compared to methylprednisolone alone.

If the manifestations of acute GVHD in any organ worsen over 3 days of treatment or if the skin does not improve by 5 days, the patient likely will not respond and secondary therapy should be considered.[109] Most clinicians continue administration of steroids and add another agent, such as antithymocyte globulin, denileukin diftitox, a monoclonal antibody, or another immunosuppressive agent (e.g., mycophenolate mofetil, sirolimus, or pentostatin).[95,109] One approach that has shown benefit as steroid-sparing therapy is extracorporeal photopheresis. During this procedure, the patient's blood is exposed extracorporeally to 8-methoxypsoralen followed by ultraviolet A radiation, and then returned to the patient. This process is thought to result in suppression of T-cell reactivity and induction of regulatory T cells. Clinical results have been positive, especially in patients with skin GVHD.[109] In addition, a variety of humanized monoclonal antibodies or fusion proteins, such as denileukin diftitox (Ontak), daclizumab (Zenapax), infliximab (Remicade), and etanercept (Enbrel), are being evaluated for treatment of steroid-refractory acute GVHD.[109]

CLINICAL CONTROVERSY

Optimal treatment of steroid-refractory GVHD is unclear. Comparative trials are needed to determine a standard approach to this difficult condition.

Chronic Graft-Versus-Host Disease

Chronic GVHD is the major determinant of late transplant-related morbidity and mortality.[95,112,113] The pathophysiology of chronic GVHD is poorly understood but is generally thought to be a result of pathogenic donor T cells that proliferate unchecked by normal mechanisms. These T cells are responsible for tissue damage through direct cytolytic attack, stimulation of inflammatory cytokines, or B-cell activation and antibody production. Chronic GVHD is often considered an autoimmune disease because of its similarity to other autoimmune disorders.

The incidence of chronic GVHD in patients who survive more than 150 days ranges from 20% to 70%.[95] The risk of chronic GVHD increases with increasing donor and recipient age and is higher in patients who receive transplants from HLA-nonidentical donors and in patients who receive PBSC transplants (especially with higher CD34 cell doses). Chronic GVHD can occur in patients receiving DLI posttransplant.[66] A meta-analysis reported that the risk of chronic GVHD is increased by nearly two-fold in patients who receive allogeneic PBSC transplants compared with BMT.[26] The risk of chronic GVHD is lower after UCB transplantation.[28,114] The incidence of chronic GVHD is rising because of increasing use of alternative donors, use of PBSCs as the graft source, use of DLI for treatment of recurrence, and older recipient age. Previous acute GVHD increases the risk of chronic GVHD, but approximately 20% to 30% of patients who develop chronic GVHD after HLA-matched alloHSCT have no history of acute GVHD ("de novo"). Unlike acute GVHD, prophylactic immunosuppression does not appear to reduce the incidence or severity of chronic GVHD.

Chronic GVHD resembles autoimmune diseases and can affect any organ or tissue of the body.[95–97,115] The most common sites involved are the skin, mouth, liver, and eye. The National Institutes of Health Consensus Development Project developed standardized criteria for the diagnosis of chronic GVHD and proposed a new clinical scoring system for the evaluation of patients with chronic GVHD.[96] The Working Group recommends that the diagnosis of chronic GVHD be made with the presence of at least one *diagnostic* clinical sign of chronic GVHD (e.g., poikiloderma or esophageal web) or a *distinctive* manifestation (e.g. keratoconjunctivitis sicca) confirmed by biopsy or other test (e.g., Schirmer test). In addition, a consensus scoring system was developed to measure the severity of involvement of individual organs.

The most widely used staging system for chronic GVHD prior to the National Institutes of Health Consensus Development Project was the limited/extensive classification proposed by the Seattle HSCT program.[95,112] In that system, chronic GVHD is classified as limited or extensive, depending on pathologic findings and the extent of systemic involvement. *Limited* chronic GVHD indicates localized skin involvement, mild hepatic dysfunction, or both. Most patients have *extensive* disease, with involvement of the skin, liver, eyes, mouth, esophagus, or other organs. Many patients with extensive chronic GVHD will die of infections or become disabled.

Several investigators have proposed improved staging systems based on large numbers of patients.[96,116] The National Institutes of Health Consensus Working Group recommends a global staging system that categorizes chronic GVHD into mild, moderate, and severe.[96] *Mild* chronic GVHD involves only one or two organs or sites (except the lung) with no clinically significant functional impairment (maximum score of 1 in all affected organs or sites). *Moderate* chronic GVHD involves at least one organ or site with clinically significant but no major disability (maximum score of 2 in any affected organ or site), or three or more organs or sites with no clinically significant functional impairment (maximum score of 1 in all affected organs or sites), or lung score of 1. *Severe* chronic GVHD indicates major disability caused by chronic GVHD (score of 3 in any organ or site) or lung score of 2 or greater.

The long-term survival rate is worse in certain subgroups of patients, such as patients with extensive skin involvement, thrombocytopenia, progressive onset of chronic GVHD (development of chronic GVHD prior to the resolution of acute GVHD), and those who do not respond to immunosuppressive therapy.[95]

⓫ If no functional impairment is present, patients with mild skin-only disease can be treated with a variety of topical preparations, such as clobetasol, tacrolimus, and pimecrolimus.[117] Initial treatment of patients with more severe or systemic involvement of chronic GVHD consists of prednisone 1 mg/kg/day.[95,97,112] To reduce the amount of corticosteroid exposure, many clinicians use either alternate-day prednisone or add cyclosporine. However, a randomized trial showed no differences in response or survival between prednisone alone or in combination with cyclosporine in standard-risk patients (platelet counts >100,000 cells/mm^3).[68] Treatment is continued until signs and symptoms of the disease have resolved and then are tapered gradually, usually over a period of several months to years. Approximately 50% of patients will require long-term immunosuppression to control chronic GVHD.

In addition to topical therapy for skin manifestations, other treatments can be applied to lessen the symptoms of chronic GVHD.[117] Patients should be educated on the use of sunscreens (and/or avoidance of sun exposure) to reduce skin injury and exacerbation of GVHD skin lesions. Nonsclerotic skin lesions without erosions or ulcerations may respond well to topical steroids and emollients. Patients should be advised to maintain good oral hygiene with routine dental care. Saliva substitutes can be given for dry mouth symptoms, and topical corticosteroid gels can be used for localized and symptomatic oral lesions. Artificial tears or, if necessary for more severe symptoms, cyclosporine or steroid eye drops are useful for patients with chronic GVHD manifesting as dry eyes or conjunctivitis. Physical therapy is recommended to reduce functional loss as a result of steroid myopathy, joint contractures, and deconditioning.

Patients who do not respond to initial therapy have a very poor prognosis. Noncomparative trials have investigated several therapies with varying degrees of success, including thalidomide, ultraviolet A irradiation after oral treatment with β-methoxypsoralen, extracorporeal photophoresis, tacrolimus, sirolimus, pentostatin, mycophenolate mofetil, hydroxychloroquine, rituximab, and others.[95,97,112,113] In a trial of 21 patients with steroid-refractory chronic GVHD, the clinical response rate to rituximab was 70%.[118] Some of these agents are being tested in phase III randomized trials of patients with newly diagnosed chronic GVHD.

Infection is the primary cause of death in patients with chronic GVHD, and antimicrobial prophylaxis is an important component of the care of patients being treated for chronic GVHD. Patients should receive oral trimethoprim–sulfamethoxazole, penicillin, an antifungal azole agent, and acyclovir to prevent infections commonly seen in immunocompromised patients.[95,97,115,117,119] Routine monitoring for cytomegalovirus reactivation should be performed. Some HSCT centers also administer intravenous immunoglobulin to patients with low serum immunoglobulin G levels.

INFECTION

Patients undergoing high-dose chemotherapy with autoHSCT or alloHSCT are severely immunocompromised and therefore are at high risk for bacterial, fungal, and viral infection. Management of these infections is discussed in detail in Chapter 126. Comprehensive guidelines for monitoring, prophylaxis, and treatment of infections in HSCT recipients are available at *www.cdc.gov/mmwr/preview/mmwrhtml/rr4910a1.htm* and *www.nccn.org*.

LATE COMPLICATIONS

With the success of HSCT, the number of long-term survivors has grown. Many survivors experience delayed complications of transplantation, especially those receiving alloHSCT, and primary care physicians will care for these patients.[120] Major late complications include restrictive and obstructive pulmonary disease; bone and joint disease (including avascular necrosis); cataract formation; endocrine dysfunction, including sterility and thyroid dysfunction; impaired growth and development; infections; cardiovascular disease; cirrhosis as a result of chronic hepatitis C infection; and secondary malignancies.[121,122] Physical recovery tends to occur earlier than psychological or work recovery.[123] Full recovery usually takes several years, and approximately two-thirds of patients do not have major limitations by 5 years.

ABBREVIATIONS

4-HC: 4-hydroperoxycyclosphosphamide

ALL: acute lymphoblastic leukemia

AlloHSCT: allogenic HSCT

AML: acute myelogenous leukemia

AutoHSCT: autologous HSCT

BMT: bone marrow transplant

BuCy: busulfan and cyclophosphamide

CIBMTR: Center for International Blood and Marrow Transplant Research

CML: chronic myelogenous leukemia

DLI: donor lymphocyte infusion

G-CSF: granulocyte colony-stimulating factor

GM-CSF: granulocyte-macrophage colony-stimulating factor

GVHD: graft-versus-host disease

GVT: graft-versus-tumor (effect)

HLA: human leukocyte antigen

HSCT: hematopoietic stem cell transplantation

MHC: major histocompatibility complex

MLC or MLR: mixed lymphocyte culture or reaction

NK: natural killer (cells)

NMDP: National Marrow Donor Program

NMT: nonmyeloablative transplantation

PBSC: peripheral blood stem cell

RIC: reduced-intensity conditioning

SOS: sinusoidal obstruction syndrome

TBI: total-body irradiation

TNF-α: tumor necrosis factor-α

UCB: umbilical cord blood

REFERENCES

1. Pasquini MC, Wang Z, Schneider L. Current use and outcome of hematopoietic stem cell transplantation: Part I - CIBMTR Summary Slides, 2007. CIBMTR Newsletter 2007;13:5-9. Available at: *http://www.cibmtr.org/PUBLICATIONS/Newsletter/DOCS/2007Dec.pdf*. Accessed on January 10, 2008.
2. Armitage JO, Antman KH. High-dose cancer therapy: Pharmacology, hematopoietins, stem cells, 4th ed. Philadelphia: Lippincott Williams & Wilkins, 2000.
3. Blume KG, Forman SJ, Appelbaum FR. Thomas' Hematopoietic Cell Transplantation, 3rd ed. Malden, MA: Blackwell Sciences, 2004.
4. Appelbaum FR. The current status of hematopoietic cell transplantation. Annu Rev Med 2003;54:491–512.
5. Copelan EA. Hematopoietic stem-cell transplantation. N Engl J Med 2006;354:1813–1826.
6. Klein J, Sato A. The HLA system. N Engl J Med 2000;343:702–709.
7. Petersdorf EW. Hematopoietic cell transplantation from unrelated donors. In: Blume KG, Forman SJ, Appelbaum FR, eds. Thomas' Hematopoietic Cell Transplantation, 3rd ed. Malden, MA: Blackwell Science, 2004:1132–1149.
8. Flomenberg N, Baxter-Lowe LA, Confer D, et al. Impact of HLA class I and class II high resolution matching on outcomes of unrelated donor bone marrow transplantation: HLA-C mismatching is associated with a strong adverse effect on transplant outcome. Blood 2004;104:1923–1930.
9. Anasetti C, Velardi A. Hematopoietic cell transplantation from HLA partially matched related donors. In: Blume KG, Forman SJ, Appelbaum FR, eds. Thomas' Hematopoietic Cell Transplantation, 3rd ed. Malden, MA: Blackwell Science, 2004:1116–1131.
10. Hurley CK, Lowe LB, Logan B, et al. National Marrow Donor Program HLA-matching guidelines for unrelated marrow transplants. Biol Blood Marrow Transplant 2003;9:610–615.
11. Yakoub-Agha I, Mesnil F, Kuentz M, et al. Allogeneic marrow stem-cell transplantation from human leukocyte antigen-identical siblings versus human leukocyte antigen-allelic-matched unrelated donors (10/10) in patients with standard-risk hematologic malignancy: A prospective study from the French Society of Bone Marrow Transplantation and Cell Therapy. J Clin Oncol 2006;24:5695–5702.
12. Moore J, Nivison-Smith I, Goh K, et al. Equivalent survival for sibling and unrelated donor allogeneic stem cell transplantation for acute myelogenous leukemia. Biol Blood Marrow Transplant 2007;13:601–607.
13. Manz MG, Akashi K, Weissman IL. Biology of hematopoietic stem and progenitor cells. In: Blume KG, Forman SJ, Appelbaum FR, eds. Thomas' Hematopoietic Cell Transplantation, 3rd ed. Malden, MA: Blackwell Science, 2004:69–95.
14. Siena S, Schiavo R, Pedrazzoli P, Carlo-Stella C. Therapeutic relevance of $CD34^+$ cell dose in blood cell transplantation for cancer therapy. J Clin Oncol 2000;18:1360–1377.
15. Kessinger A, Sharp JG. The whys and hows of hematopoietic progenitor and stem cell mobilization. Bone Marrow Transplant 2003;31:319–329.
16. Fruehauf S, Seggewiss R. It's moving day: Factors affecting peripheral blood stem cell mobilization and strategies for improvement. Br J Haematol 2003;122:360–375.
17. Ng-Cashin J, Shea T. Mobilization of autologous peripheral blood hematopoietic cells for support of high-dose cancer therapy. In: Blume KG, Forman SJ, Appelbaum FR, eds. Thomas' Hematopoietic Cell Transplantation, 3rd ed. Malden, MA: Blackwell Science, 2004:576–587.
18. Cashen AF, Lazarus HM, Devine SM. Mobilizing stem cells from normal donors: Is it possible to improve upon G-CSF? Bone Marrow Transplant 2007;39:577–588.
19. Glaspy JA. Economic considerations in the use of peripheral blood progenitor cells to support high-dose chemotherapy. Bone Marrow Transplant 1999;23(Suppl 2):S21–S27.
20. Schulman KA, Birch R, Zhen B, Pania N, Weaver CH. Effect of $CD34^+$ cell dose on resource utilization in patients after high-dose chemotherapy with peripheral blood stem cell support. J Clin Oncol 1999;17:1227–1233.
21. Flomenberg N, Devine SM, DiPersio JE, et al. The use of AMD3100 plus G-CSF for autologous hematopoietic progenitor cell mobilization is superior to G-CSF alone. Blood 2005;106:1867–1874.
22. Couban S, Barnett M. The source of cells for allografting. Biol Blood Marrow Transplant 2003;2003:669–673.
23. Schmitz N. Peripheral blood hematopoietic cells for allogeneic transplantation. In: Blume KG, Forman SJ, Appelbaum FR, eds. Thomas' Hematopoietic Cell Transplantation, 3rd ed. Malden, MA: Blackwell Science, 2004:588–598.
24. Tigue CC, McKoy JM, Evens AM, Trifilio SM, Tallman MS, Bennett CL. Granulocyte-colony stimulating factor administration to healthy individuals and persons with chronic neutropenia or cancer: An overview of safety considerations from the Research on Adverse Drug Effects and Reports project. Bone Marrow Transplant 2007;40:185–192.
25. Schmitz N, Eapen M, Horowitz M, et al. Long-term outcome of patients given transplants of mobilized blood or bone marrow: A report from the International Bone Marrow Transplant Registry and the European Group for Blood and Marrow Transplantation. Blood 2006;108:4288–4290.
26. Group SCTsC. Allogeneic peripheral blood stem-cell compared with bone marrow transplantation in the management of hematologic malignancies: An individual patient data meta-analysis of nine randomized trials. J Clin Oncol 2005;23:5074–5087.
27. Heimfeld S. HLA-identical stem cell transplantation: Is there an optimal CD34 cell dose? Bone Marrow Transplant 2003;31:839–845.
28. Brunstein CG, Setubal DC, Wagner JE. Expanding the role of umbilical cord blood transplantation. Br J Haematol 2007;137:20–35.
29. Schoemans H, Theunissen K, Maertens J, Boogaerts M, Verfaillie C, Wagner J. Adult umbilical cord blood transplantation: A comprehensive review. Bone Marrow Transplant 2006;38:83–93.
30. Eapen M, Rubinstein P, Zhang MJ, et al. Outcomes of transplantation of unrelated donor umbilical cord blood and bone marrow in children with acute leukaemia: A comparison study. Lancet 2007;369:1947–1954.
31. Bensinger WI, Spielberger R. Preparative regimens and modification of regimen-related toxicities. In: Blume KG, Forman SJ, Appelbaum FR, eds. Thomas' Hematopoietic Cell Transplantation, 3rd ed. Malden, MA: Blackwell Science, 2004:158–177.
32. Shank B, Hoppe RT. Radiotherapeutic principles of hematopoietic cell transplantation. In: Blume KG, Forman SJ, Appelbaum FR, eds. Thomas' Hematopoietic Cell Transplantation, 3rd ed. Malden, MA: Blackwell Science, 2004:178–197.
33. McCune JS, Gibbs JP, Slattery JT. Plasma concentration monitoring of busulfan: Does it improve outcome? Clin Pharmacokinet 2000;39:155–165.
34. Radich JP, Gooley T, Bensinger W, et al. HLA-matched related hematopoietic cell transplantation for chronic-phase CML using a targeted busulfan and cyclophosphamide preparative regimen. Blood 2003;102:31–35.
35. Kashyap A, Wingard J, Cagnoni P, et al. Intravenous versus oral busulfan as part of a busulfan/cyclophosphamide preparative regimen for allogeneic hematopoietic stem cell transplantation: Decreased incidence of hepatic venoocclusive disease (HVOD), HVOD-related mortality, and overall 100-day mortality. Biol Blood Marrow Transplant 2002;8:493–500.
36. Socie G, Clift RA, Blaise D, et al. Busulfan plus cyclophosphamide compared with total-body irradiation plus cyclophosphamide before marrow transplantation for myeloid leukemia: Long-term follow-up of 4 randomized studies. Blood 2001;98:3569–3574.
37. Ferry C, Socie G. Busulfan-cyclophosphamide versus total body irradiation-cyclophosphamide as preparative regimen before allogeneic hematopoietic stem cell transplantation for acute myeloid leukemia: What have we learned? Exp Hematol 2003;31:1182–1186.
38. Gupta V, Lazarus HM, Keating A. Myeloablative conditioning regimens for AML allografts: 30 years later. Bone Marrow Transplant 2003;32:969–978.
39. Davies SM, Ramsay NKC, Klein J, et al. Comparison of preparative regimens in transplants for children with acute lymphoblastic leukemia. J Clin Oncol 2000;18:340–347.

40. Mounier N, Gisselbrecht C. Conditioning regimens before transplantation in patients with aggressive non-Hodgkin's lymphoma. Ann Oncol 1998;9(Suppl 1):S15–S21.
41. Hunault-Berger M, Ifrah N, Solal-Celigny. Intensive therapies in follicular non-Hodgkin's lymphomas. Blood 2002;2002:1141–1151.
42. Press OW. Radioimmunotherapy for non-Hodgkin's lymphomas: A historical perspective. Semin Oncol 2003;30(Suppl 4):10–21.
43. Malek SN, Flinn IW. Incorporating monoclonal antibodies in blood and marrow transplantation. Semin Oncol 2003;30:520–530.
44. Gopal AK, Gooley TA, Maloney DG, et al. High-dose radioimmunotherapy versus conventional high-dose therapy and autologous hematopoietic stem cell transplantation for relapsed follicular non-Hodgkin's lymphoma: A multivariate cohort analysis. Blood 2003;102:2351–2357.
45. Fefer A. Graft-versus-tumor responses. In: Blume KG, Forman SJ, Appelbaum FR, eds. Thomas' Hematopoietic Cell Transplantation, 3rd ed. Malden, MA: Blackwell Science, 2004:369–379.
46. Sandmaier BM, Mackinnon S, Childs RW. Reduced intensity conditioning for allogeneic hematopoietic cell transplantation: Current perspectives. Biol Blood Marrow Transplant 2007;13:87–97.
47. Slavin S, Morecki S, Weiss L, Shapira MY, Resnick I, Reuven O. Nonmyeloablative stem cell transplantation: Reduced-intensity conditioning for cancer immunotherapy—From bench to patient bedside. Semin Oncol 2004;31:4–21.
48. Giralt S. Reduced-intensity conditioning regimens for hematologic malignancies: What have we learned over the last 10 years? Hematology (Am Soc Hematol Educ Program) 2005:384–389.
49. Barrett AJ, Savani BN. Stem cell transplantation with reduced-intensity conditioning regimens: A review of ten years experience with new transplant concepts and new therapeutic agents. Leukemia 2006;20:1661–1672.
50. Baron F, Sandmaier BM. Chimerism and outcomes after allogeneic hematopoietic cell transplantation following nonmyeloablative conditioning. Leukemia 2006;20:1690–1700.
51. Mielcarek M, Storb R. Non-myeloablative hematopoietic cell transplantation as immunotherapy for hematologic malignancies. Cancer Treat Rev 2003;29:283–290.
52. Sandmaier BM, Storb R. Nonmyeloablative therapy and hematopoietic cell transplantation for hematologic disorders. In: Blume KG, Forman SJ, Appelbaum FR, eds. Thomas' Hematopoietic Cell Transplantation, 3rd ed. Malden, MA: Blackwell Science, 2004:1165–1176.
53. Junghanss C, Marr KA, Carter RA, et al. Incidence and outcome of bacterial and fungal infections following nonmyeloablative compared with myeloablative allogeneic hematopoietic stem cell transplantation: A matched control study. Biol Blood Marrow Transplant 2002;8:512–520.
54. Junghanss C, Boeckh M, Carter RA, et al. Incidence and outcome of cytomegalovirus infections following nonmyeloablative compared with myeloablative allogeneic stem cell transplantation: A matched control study. Blood 2002;99:1978–1985.
55. Mielcarek M, Martin PJ, Leisenring W, et al. Graft-versus host disease after nonmyeloablative versus conventional hematopoietic stem cell transplantation. Blood 2003;102:756–762.
56. Diaconescu R, Flowers CR, Storer B, et al. Morbidity and mortality with nonmyeloablative compared to myeloablative conditioning before hematopoietic cell transplantation from HLA matched related donors. Blood 2004;104:1550–1558.
57. Maris MB, Niederwieser D, Sandmaier BM, et al. HLA-Matched unrelated donor hematopoietic cell transplantation after nonmyeloablative conditioning for patients with hematologic malignancies. Blood 2003;102:2021–2030.
58. Kahl C, Storer BE, Sandmaier BM, et al. Relapse risk in patients with malignant disease given allogeneic hematopoietic cell transplantation after nonmyeloablative conditioning. Blood 2007:110:2744–2748.
59. Alyea EP, Kim HT, Ho V. Comparative outcomes of nonmyeloablative and myeloablative allogeneic hematopoietic cell transplantation for patients older than 50 years of age. Blood 2005;105:1810–1814.
60. Aoudjhane M, Labopin M, Gorin N-C, et al. Comparative outcome of reduced intensity and myeloablative conditioning regimen in HLA identical sibling allogeneic haematopoietic stem cell transplantation for patients older than 50 years of age with acute myeloblastic leukaemia: A retrospective survey from the Acute Leukemia Working Party (ALWP) of the European group for Blood and Marrow Transplantation (EBMT). Leukemia 2005;19:2304–2312.
61. Bregni M, Ueno NT, Childs R. The second international meeting on allogeneic transplantation in solid tumors. Bone Marrow Transplant 2006;38:527–537.
62. Roman-Unfer S, Cook B, Nieto Y, Shpall E. Negative and positive stem cell selection. In: Armitage JO, Antman KH, eds. High-Dose Cancer Therapy, 3rd ed. Philadelphia: Lippincott Williams & Wilkins, 2000: 331–353.
63. Gribben JG. Antibody-mediated purging. In: Blume KG, Forman SJ, Appelbaum FR, eds. Thomas' Hematopoietic Cell Transplantation, 3rd ed. Malden, MA: Blackwell Science, 2004:244–253.
64. Colvin OM. Pharmacologic purging of bone marrow. In: Blume KG, Forman SJ, Appelbaum FR, eds. Thomas' Hematopoietic Cell Transplantation, 3rd ed. Malden, MA: Blackwell Science, 2004:254–257.
65. Kolb HJ, Schmid C, Barrett AJ, Schendel DJ. Graft-versus-leukemia reactions in allogeneic chimeras. Blood 2004;103:767–776.
66. Porter DL, Levine JE. Graft-versus-host disease and graft-versus-leukemia after donor leukocyte infusion. Semin Hematol 2006;45:53–61.
67. Collins RH. Management of relapse after allogeneic transplantation. In: Blume KG, Forman SJ, Appelbaum FR, eds. Thomas' Hematopoietic Cell Transplantation, 3rd ed. Malden, MA: Blackwell Science, 2004:1150–1163.
68. Levine JE, Braun T, Penza SL, et al. Prospective trial of chemotherapy and donor leukocyte infusions for relapse of advanced myeloid malignancies after allogeneic stem cell transplantation. J Clin Oncol 2002;20:405–412.
69. Bethge A, Hegenbart U, Stuart MJ, et al. Adoptive immunotherapy with donor lymphocyte infusions after allogeneic hematopoietic cell transplantation following nonmyeloablative conditioning. Blood 2004;103:790–795.
70. Stein AS, O'Donnell MR, Slovak ML, et al. Interleukin-2 after autologous stem cell transplantation for adult patients with acute myeloid leukemia in first complete remission. J Clin Oncol 2003; 21:615–623.
71. Negrin RS. Prevention and therapy of relapse following autologous hematopoietic cell transplantation. In: Blume KG, Forman SJ, Appelbaum FR, eds. Thomas' Hematopoietic Cell Transplantation, 3rd ed. Malden, MA: Blackwell Science, 2004:1394–1405.
72. Horwitz SM, Negrin RS, Blume KG, et al. Rituximab as adjuvant to high-dose therapy and autologous hematopoietic cell transplantation for aggressive non-Hodgkin's lymphoma. Blood 2004;103:777–783.
73. McDonald GB. Management of hepatic disease following haematopoietic cell transplant. Aliment Pharmacol Ther 2006;24:441–452.
74. Wadleigh M, Richardson PG, Zahrieh D, et al. Prior gemtuzumab ozogamicin exposure significantly increases the risk of veno-occlusive disease in patients who undergo myeloablative allogeneic stem cell transplantation. Blood 2003;102:1578–1582.
75. McDonald GB, Slattery JT, Bouvier ME, et al. Cyclophosphamide metabolism, liver toxicity, and mortality following hematopoietic stem cell transplantation. Blood 2003;101:2043–2048.
76. McCune JS, Batchelder A, Deeg HJ, et al. Cyclophosphamide following targeted oral busulfan as conditioning for hematopoietic cell transplantation: Pharmacokinetics, liver toxicity, and mortality. Biol Blood Marrow Transplant 2007;13:853–862.
77. Kumar S, DeLeve LD, Kamath PS, Tefferi A. Hepatic veno-occlusive disease (sinusoidal obstruction syndrome) after hematopoietic stem cell transplantation. Mayo Clin Proc 2003;78:589–598.
78. Tay J, Timmouth A, Fergusson D, Huebsch L, Allan DS. Systematic review of controlled clinical trials on the use of ursodeoxycholic acid for the prevention of hepatic venoocclusive disease in hematopoietic stem cell transplant. Biol Blood Marrow Transplant 2007;13:206–217.
79. Chalandon Y, Roosnek E, Mermillod B, et al. Prevention of veno-occlusive disease with defibrotide after allogeneic stem cell transplantation. Biol Blood Marrow Transplant 2004;10:347–354.
80. Richardson PG, Murakami C, Jin Z, et al. Multi-institutional use of defibrotide in 88 patients after stem cell transplantation with severe veno-occlusive disease and multisystem organ failure: Response without significant toxicity in a high-risk population and factors predictive of outcome. Blood 2002;100:4337–4343.
81. Horak DA. Pulmonary complications after hematopoietic cell transplantation. In: Blume KG, Forman SJ, Appelbaum FR, eds. Thomas' Hematopoietic Cell Transplantation, 3rd ed. Malden, MA: Blackwell Science, 2004:873–882.

82. Spitzer TR. Engraftment syndrome following hematopoietic stem cell transplantation. Bone Marrow Transplant 2001;27:893–898.
83. Fukuda T, Hackman RC, Guthrie KA, et al. Risks and outcomes of idiopathic pneumonia syndrome after nonmyeloablative compared to conventional conditioning regimens for allogeneic hematopoietic stem cell transplantation. Blood 2003;102:2777–2785.
84. Palmas A, Tefferi A, Meyers JL, et al. Late-onset noninfectious pulmonary complications after allogeneic bone marrow transplantation. Br J Haematol 1998;100:680–687.
85. Dudek AZ, Mahaseth H, DeFor TE, Weisdorf DJ. Bronchiolitis obliterans in chronic graft-versus-host disease: Analysis of risk factors and treatment outcomes. Biol Blood Marrow Transplant 2003;9:657–666.
86. Soiffer RJ. T-cell depletion to prevent graft-versus-host disease. In: Blume KG, Forman SJ, Appelbaum FR, eds. Thomas' Hematopoietic Cell Transplantation, 3rd ed. Malden, MA: Blackwell Science, 2004:221–233.
87. Finke J, Mertelsmann R. Recombinant growth factors after hematopoietic cell transplantation. In: Blume KG, Forman SJ, Appelbaum FR, eds. Thomas' Hematopoietic Cell Transplantation, 3rd ed. Malden, MA: Blackwell Science, 2004:613–623.
88. Smith TJ, Khatcheressian J, Lyman GH, et al. 2006 update of recommendations for the use of white blood cell growth factors: An evidence-based clinical practice guidelines. J Clin Oncol 2006;24:3187–3205.
89. Bolwell B, Goomastic M, Dannley R, et al. G-CSF post-autologous progenitor cell transplantation: A randomized study of 5, 10 and 16 mcg/kg/day. Bone Marrow Transplant 1997;19:215–219.
90. Bolwell B, Pohlman B, Andresen S, et al. Delayed G-CSF after autologous progenitor cell transplantation: Prospective randomized trial. Bone Marrow Transplant 1998;21:369–373.
91. Ringden O, Labopin M, Gorin N-C, et al. Treatment with granulocyte colony-stimulating factor after allogeneic bone marrow transplantation for acute leukemia increases the risk of graft-versus-host disease and death: A study from the Acute Leukemia Working Party of the European Group for Blood and Marrow Transplantation. J Clin Oncol 2004;22:416–423.
92. Dekker A, Bulley S, Beyene J, et al. Meta-analysis of randomized controlled trials of prophylactic granulocyte colony-stimulating factor and granulocyte-macrophage colony-stimulating factor after autologous and allogeneic stem cell transplantation. J Clin Oncol 2006;24:5207–5215.
93. Khoury HJ, Loberiza FR, Ringden O, et al. Impact of posttransplantation G-CSF on outcomes of allogeneic hematopoietic stem cell transplantation. Blood 2006;107:1712–1716.
94. Ferrara JLM, Reddy P. Pathophysiology of graft-versus host disease. Semin Hematol 2006;43:3–10.
95. Sullivan KM. Graft-versus-host disease. In: Blume KG, Forman SJ, Appelbaum FR, eds. Thomas' Hematopoietic Cell Transplantation, 3rd ed. Malden, MA: Blackwell Science, 2004:635–664.
96. Filipovich AH, Weisdorf DJ, Pavletic S, et al. National Institutes of Health Consensus Development Project on Criteria for Clinical Trials in Chronic Graft-versus-Host Disease: I. Diagnosis and Staging Working Group Report. Biol Blood Marrow Transplant 2005;11:945–955.
97. Gilman AL, Serody J. Diagnosis and treatment of chronic graft-versus-host disease. Semin Hematol 2006;43:70–80.
98. Deeg HJ, Antin JH. The clinical spectrum of acute graft-versus-host disease. Semin Hematol 2006;43:24–31.
99. Saliba RM, deLima M, Giralt S, et al. Hyper-acute GVHD. Risk factors, outcomes, and clinical applications. Blood 2007;109:2751–2758.
100. Chao NJ, Chen BJ. Prophylaxis and treatment of acute graft-versus-host disease. Semin Hematol 2006;43:32–41.
101. Chao NJ. Pharmacology and the use of immunosuppressive agents after hematopoietic cell transplantation. In: Blume KG, Forman SJ, Appelbaum FR, eds. Thomas' Hematopoietic Cell Transplantation, 3rd ed. Malden, MA: Blackwell Science, 2004:209–220.
102. Ratanatharathorn V, Nash RA, Przepiorka D, et al. Phase III study comparing methotrexate wand tacrolimus (Prograf, FK506) with methotrexate and cyclosporine for graft-versus-host disease prophylaxis after HLA-identical sibling bone marrow transplantation. Blood 1998;92:2303–2314.
103. Nash RA, Antin JH, Karanes C, et al. Phase 3 study comparing methotrexate and tacrolimus with methotrexate and cyclosporine for prophylaxis of acute graft-versus-host disease after marrow transplantation from unrelated donors. Blood 2000;96:2062–2068.
104. Cutler C, Li S, Ho VT, et al. Extended follow-up of methotrexate-free immunosuppression using sirolimus and tacrolimus in related and unrelated donor peripheral blood stem cell transplantation. Blood 2007;109:3108–3114.
105. Yu C, Seidel K, Nash RA, et al. Synergism between mycophenolate mofetil and cyclosporine in preventing graft-versus-host disease among lethally irradiated dogs given DLA-identical unrelated marrow grafts. Blood 1998;91:2581–2587.
106. Elmaagacli AH, Peceny R, Steckel N, et al. Outcome of transplantation of highly purified peripheral blood $CD34^+$ cells with T-cell add-back compared with unmanipulated bone marrow or peripheral blood stem cells from HLA-identical sibling donors in patients with first chronic phase chronic myeloid leukemia. Blood 2003;101:446–453.
107. Antin JH, Kim HT, Cutler C, et al. Sirolimus, tacrolimus, and low-dose methotrexate for graft-versus-host disease prophylaxis in mismatched related donor or unrelated donor transplantation. Blood 2003;102:1601–1605.
108. Bacigalupo A. Antilymphocyte/thymocyte globulin for graft-versus-host disease prophylaxis: Efficacy and side effects. Bone Marrow Transplant 2006;35:225–231.
109. Deeg HJ. How I treat refractory acute GVHD. Blood 2007;109:4119–4126.
110. Hockenbery DM, Cruickshank S, Rodell TC, et al. A randomized, placebo-controlled trial of oral beclomethasone dipropionate as a prednisone-sparing therapy for gastrointestinal graft-versus-host disease. Blood 2007;109:4557–4563.
111. Lee SJ, Zahrieh D, Agura E, et al. Effect of up front daclizumab when combined with steroids for the treatment of acute graft versus host disease: Results of a randomized trial. Blood 2004;104:1559–1564.
112. Vogelsang GB. Chronic graft-versus-host disease. Br J Haematol 2004;125:435–454.
113. Lee SJ. New approaches for preventing and treating chronic graft-versus-host disease. Blood 2005;105:4200–4206.
114. Grewal SS, Barker JN, Davies SM, Wagner JE. Unrelated donor hematopoietic cell transplantation: Marrow or umbilical cord blood? Blood 2003;101:4233–4244.
115. Lee SJ, Vogelsang G, Flowers MED. Chronic graft-versus-host disease. Biol Blood Marrow Transplant 2003;9:215–233.
116. Akpek G, Lee SJ, Flowers ME, et al. Performance of a new clinical grading system for chronic graft-versus-host disease: A multicenter study. Blood 2003;102:802–809.
117. Couriel D, Carpenter PA, Cutler C, et al. Ancillary Therapy and Supportive Care of Chronic Graft-versus-Host Disease: National Institutes of Health Consensus Development Project on Criteria for Clinical Trials in Chronic Graft-versus Host Disease: V. Ancillary Therapy and Supportive Care Working Group Report. Biol Blood Marrow Transplant 2006;12:375–396.
118. Cutler C, Miklos D, Kim HT, et al. Rituximab for steroid-refractory chronic graft-versus-host disease. Blood 2006;108:756–762.
119. Bhushan V, Collins RH. Chronic graft-vs-host disease. JAMA 2003;290:2599–2603.
120. Antin JH. Long-term care after hematopoietic-cell transplantation in adults. N Engl J Med 2002;347:36–42.
121. Socie G, Salooja N, Cohen A, et al. Nonmalignant late effects after allogeneic stem cell transplantation. Blood 2003;101:3373–3385.
122. Flowers MED, Deeg HJ. Delayed complications after hematopoietic cell transplantation. In: Blume KG, Forman SJ, Appelbaum FR, eds. Thomas' Hematopoietic Cell Transplantation, 3rd ed. Malden, MA: Blackwell Science, 2004:944–961.
123. Syrjala KL, Langer SL, Abrams JR, et al. Recovery and long-term function after hematopoietic cell transplantation for leukemia and lymphoma. JAMA 2004;291:2335–2343.

SECTION 18
NUTRITION DISORDERS

CHAPTER 143

Assessment of Nutrition Status and Nutrition Requirements

KATHERINE HAMMOND CHESSMAN AND VANESSA J. KUMPF

KEY CONCEPTS

1. Classification of nutrition status is often desired as a means to identify those who are nutritionally at risk or malnourished.
2. Nutrition screening programs should identify those at risk for poor nutrition-related outcomes as a consequence of either over- or undernutrition.
3. Nutrition assessment is the first step in formulating a patient-specific nutrition care plan for a patient who is found to be nutritionally at risk or malnourished.
4. A nutrition-focused medical, surgical, and dietary history and a nutrition-focused physical examination are key components of nutrition assessment and will reveal risk factors for and the likelihood of malnutrition and nutrient deficiencies.
5. Appropriate anthropometric measurements are essential in a complete nutrition assessment and should be evaluated based on published standards.
6. Biochemical (laboratory) tests are also essential for nutrition assessment but must be interpreted in the context of the physical findings, medical and surgical history, and clinical status of the patient, as well as specific test limitations.
7. Nutrient deficiencies involving micronutrients (e.g., vitamins or trace elements) or macronutrients (e.g., fat, protein, or carbohydrate) are possible, and a comprehensive nutrition assessment will identify the presence of these.
8. When determining patient-specific nutrition requirements, goals should be established based on the patient's clinical condition and the need for maintenance or repletion in adults, as well as for continued growth and development in children.
9. Drug-nutrient interactions can affect a patient's nutrition status as well as the response to and adverse effects seen with drug therapy, and must be considered when evaluating a patient's nutrition care plan.
10. An initial nutrition assessment and determination of nutrition requirements only defines an empirical starting point for a nutrition care plan. Close monitoring is required so that timely adjustments to the nutrition care plan can be made based on patient-specific responses to ensure appropriate nutrition-related outcomes.

Learning objectives, review questions, and other resources can be found at **www.pharmacotherapyonline.com.**

Nutrition care is a vital component of quality patient care. This chapter reviews the tools most commonly used for nutrition screening and accurate, relevant, and cost-effective nutrition assessment. Determination of patient-specific macro- and micronutrient requirements and potential drug-nutrient interactions are also discussed.

CLASSIFICATION OF NUTRITION DISEASE

❶ Undernutrition usually results from starvation (inadequate nutrient intake), impaired absorption of nutrients or altered metabolism (inappropriate use of ingested nutrients).[1] An alteration in nutrient metabolism exists when the cell has altered substrate demands or use, such as cachexia associated with inflammatory or neoplastic conditions. In such situations, enhancing nutritional intake may not be sufficient to meet the increased demand.[1] Regardless of the cause, undernutrition results in changes in subcellular, cellular, and/or organ function that expose the individual to increased risks of morbidity and mortality (see Chap. 144). In general, deficiency states can be categorized as those involving protein and calories or single nutrients such as individual vitamins or trace elements. Protein-calorie malnutrition can be classified as marasmus, kwashiorkor, or mixed marasmus/kwashiorkor.

Marasmus is a chronic condition resulting from prolonged inadequate intake or use of protein and calories. Somatic protein (skeletal muscle) and adipose tissue (subcutaneous fat) wasting occurs, but visceral protein production (e.g., albumin and transferrin) is usually preserved. Weight loss typically exceeds 10% of usual body weight (UBW; typical weight). When severe, cell-mediated immunity, measured by delayed cutaneous hypersensitivity (DCH), and muscle function are impaired. Patients with wasting diseases such as cancer commonly have marasmus and a prototypical starved, wasted appearance.

Kwashiorkor develops when there is adequate calorie but inadequate protein intake. These patients generally appear well nourished but are extremely catabolic, usually secondary to trauma, infection, or burns. There is depletion of visceral (and to some degree somatic) protein stores with relative adipose tissue preservation, and hypoalbuminemia and edema are commonly seen. In the setting of severe metabolic stress and protein deprivation, kwashiorkor may develop rapidly and may result in impaired immune function.

Mixed marasmus/kwashiorkor is a form of severe protein-calorie malnutrition that develops in chronically ill, starved patients during periods of hypermetabolic stress. There is reduced visceral protein synthesis superimposed on wasting of somatic protein and energy (adipose tissue) stores. Immunocompetence is lowered, increasing the incidence of infection, and wound healing is compromised.

Obesity (overnutrition) is a major healthcare concern in the United States. Recently, 66% of American adults were estimated to be overweight (defined as a body mass index [BMI] of 25 kg/m^2 or greater), while 32% of American adults were noted to be obese (BMI of 30 kg/m^2 or greater).[2] Additionally, approximately 15% of children and adolescents (ages 6 to 19 years) are obese (BMI at or above the 95th percentile for age[3] on the gender-appropriate BMI-for-age growth chart published by the Centers for Disease Control National Center for Health Statistics [NCHS]).[4] Many more children are considered to be at-risk for obesity (BMI at or above the 85th percentile for age). Nutrition assessment allows identification of obese individuals or those at risk of becoming obese. The consequences of obesity are numerous and include type 2 diabetes mellitus, cardiovascular disease, and stroke (see Chap. 148).

NUTRITION SCREENING

❷ Because it is neither practical nor warranted to conduct a comprehensive nutrition assessment on every patient, nutrition screening provides a systematic way to identify individuals who are overweight, obese, malnourished, or at risk for malnutrition,[5] and to predict the probability of their outcome as a result of nutrition factors.[6] Risk factors for undernutrition include any disease state, complicating condition, treatment, or socioeconomic condition that may result in a decreased nutrient intake, altered metabolism, and/or malabsorption. Risk factors for obesity include family history of obesity, certain medical diagnoses, poor dietary habits, lack of exercise, and some drug therapies. Nutrition screening is typically a rapid and simple process that can be done in the home by the patient or home healthcare professional, in long-term care facilities, in ambulatory care clinics, or in a hospital. Various rating and classification systems have been proposed to assess nutrition risk and guide subsequent interventions.[5–8] Checklists are used in many clinical settings to quantify a person's food and alcohol consumption habits; ability to buy, prepare, and eat food; weight history; diagnoses; or medical/surgical procedures. Depending on the specific criteria evaluated, the presence of three to four risk factors may increase a person's risk for malnutrition. Pediatric screening programs most often evaluate growth parameters against the NCHS growth charts and medical conditions known to increase nutrition risk. Hospital screening programs must also identify patients receiving specialized nutrition support (enteral or parenteral nutrition) prior to admission.

Nutrition screening using simple tools in the community or outpatient setting, especially in young children and the elderly, can identify potential nutrition issues early before they become significant problems.[4–8] The Joint Commission, formerly called the Joint Commission on Accreditation of Healthcare Organizations, includes nutrition screening and assessment in their performance standards for institutions.[9] For inpatients, a nutrition screening process that uses institution-specified criteria should be conducted within 24 to 72 hours of admission. Patients initially determined to be "not at risk" should be reevaluated every 7 to 14 days to detect deterioration in nutrition status secondary to changes in food intake or clinical condition. By identifying at-risk individuals, nutrition screening can be a cost-effective way to help decrease complications and length of hospital stay. In any setting, patients determined to be "at nutrition risk" should receive a subsequent comprehensive assessment that includes formulation of a nutrition care plan.

ASSESSMENT OF NUTRITION STATUS

❸ A comprehensive nutrition assessment is the first step in formulating a patient-specific nutrition care plan. Nutrition assessment has four major goals: (a) identification of the presence of factors associated with an increased risk of developing malnutrition, including disorders resulting from macro- or micronutrient deficiencies (undernutrition), obesity (overnutrition), or impaired metabolism; (b) determination of risk of malnutrition-associated complications; (c) establishment of estimated nutrition needs; and (d) establishment of baseline parameters against which to measure nutrition therapy outcomes.

A comprehensive nutrition assessment should include a nutrition-focused medical, surgical and dietary history, a nutrition-focused physical examination including anthropometrics and laboratory measurements. Nutrition assessment provides a basis for determining the patient's nutrition requirements and the optimal type and timing of nutrition intervention.

CLINICAL EVALUATION

❹ Clinical evaluation of nutrition status correlates well with objective evaluations (e.g., laboratory and anthropometric measurements). The medical, surgical, and dietary history components of the clinical evaluation provide information regarding those factors that predispose to malnutrition (e.g., prematurity, chronic diseases, gastrointestinal [GI] malfunction, and alcohol abuse) and overnutrition (e.g., poor dietary habits, limited exercise, chronic diseases, and family history). The clinician should direct the interview to elicit any history of weight gain or loss, anorexia, vomiting, diarrhea, and decreased or unusual food intake (Table 143–1).

The nutrition-focused health history and physical examination takes a systems approach to assess lean body mass (LBM) and findings of vitamin, trace element, or essential fatty acid deficiencies or excesses. The assessment should include documentation of the presence and degree of muscle wasting, edema, loss of subcutaneous fat, dermatitis, glossitis, cheilosis, and/or jaundice (Table 143–2).[5,8]

Since the 1980s, the subjective global assessment, a simple, reproducible, cost-effective approach to nutrition assessment, has been used by many practitioners. Five aspects of the medical and dietary history make up the subjective global assessment: weight changes in the previous 6 months, dietary intake changes, GI symptoms, functional capacity of the GI tract, and the presence of disease states. Weight loss of less than 5% of UBW is considered a "small" loss, 5% to 10% loss is a "potentially significant loss," and more than a 10% loss is a "definitely significant loss." Dietary intake should be characterized as either normal or abnormal, and the length of time and degree of abnormal intake should be noted. The presence of GI symptoms (e.g., anorexia, nausea, vomiting, or diarrhea) on a daily basis for longer than 2 weeks is significant. Functional capacity assesses the patient's energy level and whether the patient is active or bedridden. Finally, disease states present are assessed as to their impact on metabolic demands (i.e., no stress, low, moderate, or high stress). Four physical examination findings are rated as normal, mild, moderate, or severe: loss of subcutaneous fat (triceps and chest), muscle wasting (quadriceps and deltoids), edema (ankle and sacral), and ascites. The clinician then ranks the patient's nutrition

TABLE 143-1 Pertinent Data from Nutrition-Focused Medical, Surgical, and Dietary History

Nutrition intake and dietary habits
Anorexia
Unusual or absent taste
Dietary intake and special diets, including enteral or parenteral nutrition
Supplemental vitamin, mineral, or herbal intake
Food allergies or intolerance
Underlying pathology with nutritional effects
Chronic infections or inflammatory states
Neoplastic diseases
Endocrine disorders
Chronic illness including pulmonary disease, cirrhosis, and kidney failure
Hypermetabolic states such as trauma, burns, and sepsis
Digestive or absorptive disease, nausea, vomiting, diarrhea, constipation
Hyperlipidemia
End-organ effects
Weight changes
Skin or hair changes
Exercise intolerance, fatigue
Gastrointestinal tract symptoms: diarrhea, vomiting, constipation
Gastrointestinal surgery
Bariatric surgery
Small bowel and/or colon resection
Gastrectomy
Miscellaneous
Catabolic medications or therapies: corticosteroids, immunosuppressive agents, radiation, or chemotherapy
Other medications: diuretics, laxatives, or anabolic steroids
Genetic background: body habitus of parents, siblings, and family
Alcohol or drug abuse

status as adequately nourished, moderately malnourished, or severely malnourished.[8,10] Other nutrition assessment tools have been developed and evaluated in various populations.[8,11]

ANTHROPOMETRIC MEASUREMENTS

❺ Anthropometric measurements, gross measurements of body cell mass, are used to evaluate LBM and fat stores. The most common measurements are weight, stature (height or length, depending on age), head circumference (for children younger than 3 years of age), and measurements of limb size, such as skinfold thickness, midarm muscle circumference, wrist circumference, and waist circumference. Bioelectrical impedance analysis (BIA) is also an anthropometric assessment tool. These parameters are used to compare an individual with normative standards for a population and as repeated measurements in an individual to monitor response to a nutrition care plan. In adults, nutrition-related changes in anthropometric measurements occur slowly; several weeks or more are usually required before detectable changes are noted. In infants and young children, however, changes may occur more quickly. Acute changes in anthropometric measurements, specifically weight and skinfold thickness, usually reflect changes in hydration status, which must be considered when interpreting these parameters, particularly in hospitalized patients.

WEIGHT, STATURE, AND HEAD CIRCUMFERENCE

Body weight is a nonspecific measure of body cell mass, representing skeletal mass, body fat, and the energy-using component referred to as LBM. Change in weight over time, particularly in the absence of edema, ascites, and voluntary losses, is an important indicator of altered LBM. Interpretation of actual body weight (ABW) should take into consideration ideal weight-for-height, also referred to as ideal body weight (IBW), UBW, fluid status, and age (Table 143–3).[8] The UBW is intended to describe an individual's typical weight and is generally more useful when assessing weight loss or gain than comparing the current weight to an IBW or desirable weight. Dehydration will result in decreased ABW but not a loss in LBM. Once the patient is rehydrated, rechecking the weight is important to establish the baseline weight to use for nutrition evaluation. The presence of edema or ascites increases total body

TABLE 143-2 Physical Findings Suggestive of Malnutrition

General appearance
Edema (especially ankle and sacral)
Cachexia or obesity
Ascites
Signs and symptoms of dehydration: poor skin turgor, sunken eyes, orthostasis, or dry mucous membranes
Muscle wasting or loss of subcutaneous fat
Skin and mucous membranes
Thin, shiny, dry or scaly skin
Decubitus ulcers
Ecchymoses or perifollicular petechiae
Poor healing of surgical or traumatic wounds
Pallor or redness of gums or fissures at mouth edge
Glossitis, stomatitis, or cheilosis
Musculoskeletal
Retarded growth
Bone pain or tenderness or epiphyseal swelling
Muscle mass less than expected for habitus, genetic history, and level of exercise
Neurologic
Ataxia, positive Romberg test, or decreased vibratory or position sense
Nystagmus
Convulsions or paralysis
Encephalopathy
Failure to meet age-appropriate developmental milestones
Hepatic
Jaundice
Hepatomegaly

TABLE 143-3 Evaluation of Body Weight

Actual body weight (ABW) compared to ideal body weight (IBW)	
ABW <69% IBW	Severe malnutrition
ABW 70–79% IBW	Moderate malnutrition
ABW 80–89% IBW	Mild malnutrition
ABW 90–120% IBW	Normal
ABW >120% IBW	Overweight
ABW ≥150% IBW	Obese
ABW ≥200% IBW	Morbidly obese
Actual body weight (ABW) compared to usual body weight (UBW)	
ABW 85–95% UBW	Mild malnutrition
ABW 75–84% UBW	Moderate malnutrition
ABW <75% UBW	Severe malnutrition
Body mass index (BMI) (kg/m^2) or (lb/in^2)	**Interpretation**
Adults	
<16	Severe malnutrition
16–16.9	Moderate malnutrition
17–18.5	Mild malnutrition
19–25	Healthy (19–34 years of age)
21–27	Healthy (older than 35 years of age)
25–30	Overweight (19–34 years of age)
27.5–29.9	Overweight (older than 35 years of age)
30–40	Moderate obesity
>40	Severe or morbid obesity
Children	
BMI-for-age <5th percentile	Underweight
BMI-for-age 5th–85th percentile	Healthy
BMI-for-age >85th percentile	At risk for overweight
BMI-for-age ≥95th percentile	Overweight

water (TBW), thus increasing ABW. Weights of patients with severe edema and ascites should not be used for nutrition assessment without taking the extra water weight into consideration. Subtle changes in fluid status that may affect ABW can be detected by monitoring the patient's daily fluid intake and output.

The IBW provides one population reference standard against which the ABW can be compared to detect both over- and undernutrition states. The IBW for a given height is the weight that correlates with maximum longevity. Numerous reference tables have been generated based on various population statistics. In clinical practice, mathematical equations based on gender and height are used commonly to estimate IBW. IBW is calculated as 50 kg + [2.3 × (inches over 5 feet)] for adult men, and for adult women as 45.5 kg + [2.3 × (inches over 5 feet)]. For obese adults, an adjusted IBW may be used for nutrition-related calculations: adjusted IBW = [(ABW–IBW) × 0.25] + IBW. The IBW of children can be calculated as [(height in cm)^2 × 1.65]/1,000. Alternatively, IBW-for-height in children can be determined by identifying the weight corresponding to the same growth percentile as the child's measured stature (length or height) on the appropriate NCHS growth chart.[4]

Change in weight over time can be calculated as the percentage of UBW, where percent change = (ABW/UBW) × 100 (see Table 143–3).[8] Use of the UBW as a reference point provides a more accurate reflection of clinically and nutritionally significant weight changes. Determining a patient's UBW, however, depends on patient or family recall, which may be inaccurate. The use of UBW avoids the problems of normative tables, and it documents comparative changes in body weight. The change in weight also should be interpreted relative to time. In adults, unintentional weight loss of more than 10% in less than 6 months correlates with a poor clinical outcome.

Stature is determined by genetics and nutrition intake. If it is not possible to obtain a standing height, other methods to estimate height may be used. The measurement of demispan, the distance from the sternal notch to the web between the middle and ring fingers measured along a horizontally outstretched arm with the wrist in neutral rotation and zero extension or flexion, can be obtained in the seated position. Demispan may more accurately assess height in the elderly, especially those with kyphosis and/or vertebral collapse. Once the demispan is measured, height can be estimated using the following equations: women: height (cm) = 1.35 × demispan (cm) + 60.1; men, height (cm) = 1.4 × demispan (cm) + 57.8. Knee height may also be used to estimate height and is especially helpful in patients with limb contractures, such as patients with cerebral palsy.[12,13] The knee height is measured from just under the heel to the anterior surface of the thigh just proximal to the patella. Using the average of two measurements rounded to the nearest 0.1 cm, height is estimated using the following equations: women: height (cm) = 84.88 (0.24 × age [years]) + (1.83 × knee height [cm]); men, height (cm) = 64.19 (0.04 × age [years]) + (2.02 × knee height [cm]).[13]

The best indicator of adequate nutrition in a child is appropriate rate of growth. At each medical encounter, weight, stature, and head circumference should be plotted on the appropriate NCHS gender- and age-based growth curve. These charts were developed in 1977 from a large population of healthy, primarily white children and recently revised to better reflect the ethnic mix of the United States' population. Special growth charts are available for assessment of short- and long-term growth of premature infants[14,15] and children with Down's syndrome.[16] For premature infants with corrected postnatal age of 40 weeks or more, the NCHS growth charts can be used; however, weight-for-age and length-for-age should be plotted according to corrected postnatal age until 2 years and 3.5 years of age, respectively.

Recommended intervals between measurements are weight, 7 days; length, 4 weeks; height, 8 weeks; and head circumference, 7 days in infants and 4 weeks in children up to 3 years of age. Growth velocity can be used to assess growth at intervals too close to plot accurately on a growth chart (Table 143–4).[4] In newborns, average weight gain is 10 to 20 g/kg per day (24 to 35 g/day in term infants and 10 to 25 g/day in preterm infants). Weight gain declines considerably after 2 to 3 months of age.[4] Head growth (measured by head circumference), which is usually 0.5 cm/week during the first year of life, can be compromised during periods of critical illness or malnutrition. Sustained head growth during these periods, especially at a rate above expected, suggests hydrocephalus.

TABLE 143-4 Expected Growth Velocities in Term Infants and Children

Age	Weight (g/day)	Height (cm/month)
0–3 months	24–35	2.8–3.4
4–6 months	15–21	1.7–2.4
7–12 months	10–13	1.3–1.6
1–3 years	5–9	0.6–1
4–6 years	5–6	0.5–0.6
7–10 years	7–11	0.4–0.5

Example of growth assessment:

Age: 2 months; weight: 3.9 kg; weight at 1 month of age, 3.1 kg; days since last wt: 30

Growth velocity = [(3.9 kg–3.1 kg) × 1,000 g/kg]/30 days = 26.7 g/day

Interpretation: normal growth

Growth failure or failure-to-thrive is defined as weight-for-age or weight-for-height (or length) below the 5th percentile or a falloff of two or more major percentiles (major percentiles are defined as 95th, 90th, 75th, 50th, 25th, 10th, and 5th). Weight-for-height evaluation is age-independent and helps differentiate the stunted child (chronic malnutrition) from the wasted child (acute malnutrition). Short stature, which is associated with many chronic diseases, is a manifestation of chronic undernutrition. Short stature in the absence of malnutrition suggests an endocrinopathy such as growth hormone deficiency but may also be a normal variant.

BODY MASS INDEX

BMI, which is most commonly defined as body weight in kilograms divided by the square of the height in meters (kg/m^2), is another index of weight-for-height. Using pounds and inches, BMI (lbs/in^2) can also be estimated as (weight [pounds]/height [inches^2]) × 703. BMI is more highly correlated with body fat than any other indicator using height and weight. It can be used to categorize both obesity and undernutrition in adults and children. Various tables listing BMI stratified by height and weight are available for quick reference. According to the World Health Organization and others, a person with a BMI greater than 25 kg/m^2 is overweight and one with a BMI of 30 kg/m^2 or higher is obese. BMI has also been used to assess undernutrition with a BMI less than 18.5 kg/m^2 indicating undernutrition (see Table 143–3).[8,17–19]

In general, a healthy weight is one associated with a reduction in disease risk. A BMI greater than 25 kg/m^2 is considered a risk factor for premature death and disability as consequences of being overweight and of obesity (see Chap. 148). These health risks increase as the BMI increases. Although BMI correlates strongly with total body fat, individual variation, especially in very muscular persons, may lead to erroneous classification of either obesity or malnutrition when BMI alone is used to assess nutrition status. BMI should be interpreted based on individual characteristics including gender, frame size, and age.[18] A major advantage of the revised NCHS growth charts for children 2 years of age and older is the addition of age- and gender-specific BMI charts. Use of these charts helps to heighten parental and healthcare provider awareness of children whose BMI and family history put them at risk for adult obesity and its associated risks.[4]

CLINICAL CONTROVERSY

Clinicians disagree whether an individual's nutrition status is best evaluated using IBW, ABW, adjusted IBW, or BMI. Frame size and muscle mass, as well as gender and height, can influence both IBW and BMI, leading to misclassification of nutrition status. Use of adjusted IBW in obese individuals may lead to under- or overestimation of needs.

SKINFOLD THICKNESS AND MIDARM MUSCLE CIRCUMFERENCE

Skinfold thickness measurement provides an estimate of subcutaneous fat, whereas midarm muscle circumference estimates skeletal muscle mass. Although simple and noninvasive, these anthropometric measurements are not used commonly in clinical practice but can be used for both population analysis and individual long-term monitoring. Triceps skinfold thickness is the most commonly used skinfold measurement, although reference standards also exist for subscapular and iliac sites. More than 50% of the body's fat is subcutaneous, and changes in subcutaneous fat usually reflect changes in total body fat. Careful technique in the use of pressure-regulated calipers is essential for reproducibility and reliability in measuring triceps skinfold thickness. Midarm muscle circumference is a calculated value based on the measurement of the midarm circumference and triceps skinfold thickness.

Individual anthropometric measurements should be interpreted cautiously because standards do not account for individual variations in bone size, muscle mass, hydration status, or skin compressibility; reference standards do not account for obesity, ethnicity, illness, and increased age; and technique is critical (interobserver error can be as high as 30%). Furthermore, these parameters are slow to change in adults, often requiring weeks before significant alterations from baseline can be detected.

WAIST CIRCUMFERENCE

Waist circumference is used to assess abdominal fat content. Excess abdominal fat that is disproportionate to total body fat is an independent predictor of risk for obesity-related complications. Waist circumference is determined by measuring the distance around the smallest area below the rib cage and the top of the iliac crest. Interpretation varies with age. Men are considered at risk if the waist circumference is greater than 40 inches; women are at risk if the waist circumference is greater than 35 inches. These standards do not apply if the patient is less than 5 feet tall or has a BMI of 35 kg/m^2 or greater.[19]

WAIST-TO-HIP RATIO

The waist-to-hip ratio is also associated with undesirable health consequences. For most people, extra weight around the waist confers more of a health risk than extra weight around the hips and thighs. The waist-to-hip ratio is determined by dividing the waist circumference by the hip circumference (maximal posterior extension of the buttocks). For both men and women, a waist-to-hip ratio of 1 or greater is considered a risk factor for adverse health consequences. A ratio of less than 1 in men or 0.8 or less in women is considered "not-at-risk."[19]

BIOELECTRICAL IMPEDANCE

BIA is a simple, noninvasive, and relatively inexpensive technique used to measure LBM.[20,21] The technology is based on the fact that lean tissue has a higher electrical conductivity (less resistance) than fat, which is a poor current conductor because of its greater fluid and electrolyte content. By applying a very small electric current to appendages (wrist and ankle or both feet), impedance (resistance) to flow can be measured. Assessment of LBM, TBW, and water's distribution into compartments can be determined with BIA. Increased TBW decreases impedance; therefore, it is important to evaluate fluid status along with BIA measurements. Other potential limitations of BIA include variability with electrolyte imbalance, interference by large fat masses (obesity), and the lack of reference standards that reflect variations in individual body size and clinical condition. Although BIA equations have high validity when used in the population in which they were developed (mostly young, healthy adults), BIA calculations are subject to considerable errors if applied to other populations. BIA is not superior to BMI as a predictor of overall adiposity in the general population and is therefore currently used primarily as a research tool.[21]

BIOCHEMICAL ASSESSMENT OF LEAN BODY MASS

❻ LBM includes skeletal muscle, somatic protein, and functional proteins such as the circulating and visceral proteins. Biochemically, LBM can be assessed by measuring the serum visceral proteins, albumin (ALB), transferrin (TFN), and prealbumin (thyroxine-binding prealbumin or transthyretin). Retinol-binding protein, fibronectin (an opsonic protein), and somatomedin-C (insulin-like growth factor-1), proteins with a very short half-life (less than 12 to 24 hours), have also been evaluated as indicators of nutrition status. However, the clinical availability of these alternative tests is limited, and their relevance to nutrition status and patient outcome is debatable. Creatinine-height index has historically been used to assess LBM but is seldom used today because of the lack of evidence to support its usefulness in assessing muscle mass.[8,22]

Visceral Proteins

Measurement of serum concentrations of the transport proteins synthesized by hepatocytes can be used to assess the visceral protein compartment. It is assumed that a low serum protein concentration in states of undernutrition reflects the hepatic protein synthetic mass, and therefore indirectly reflects the functional protein mass of other organs such as heart, lung, kidney, and intestines. The visceral proteins with the greatest relevance for nutrition assessment are serum ALB, TFN, and prealbumin. Many factors other than nutrition may affect the serum concentration of these proteins, including age, abnormal kidney (nephrotic syndrome) or GI tract (protein-losing enteropathy) losses, hydration status (dehydration results in hemoconcentration, overhydration in hemodilution), hepatic function (because this is the primary synthesis site), and metabolic stress (sepsis, trauma, surgery, and/or infection). Visceral protein concentrations must be interpreted relative to the individual's overall clinical condition (Table 143–5).[5,8,22,23]

Albumin remains one of the most widely used biochemical markers of malnutrition and has long been used in population studies. It is, however, a relatively insensitive index of early protein malnutrition because there is a large amount normally found in the body (4 to 5 g/kg of body weight), it is highly distributed in the extravascular compartment (60%), and it has a long half-life (18 to 20 days). However, chronic protein deficiency in the setting of adequate nonprotein calorie intake leads to marked hypoalbuminemia because of a net ALB loss from the intravascular and extravascular compartments. Serum ALB concentrations also are affected by moderate-to-severe calorie deficiency; hepatic, kidney, and GI disease; and infection, trauma, stress, and burns. In many cases, interpretation of serum ALB concentrations relative to nutrition status is difficult; however, a positive correlation between decreased

TABLE 143-5 Visceral Proteins Used for Assessment of Lean Body Mass

Serum Protein	Half-Life (Days)	Function	Factors Resulting in Increased Values	Factors Resulting in Decreased Values
Albumin	18–20	Maintains plasma oncotic pressure; transports small molecules	Dehydration, anabolic steroids, insulin, infection	Overhydration, edema, kidney dysfunction, nephrotic syndrome, poor dietary intake, impaired digestion, burns, congestive heart failure, cirrhosis, thyroid/adrenal/pituitary hormones, trauma, sepsis
Transferrin (TFN)	8–9	Binds Fe in plasma; transports Fe to bone	Fe deficiency, pregnancy, hypoxia, chronic blood loss, estrogens	Chronic infection, cirrhosis, burns, enteropathies, nephrotic syndrome, cortisone, testosterone
Prealbumin (transthyretin)	2–3	Binds T_3 and to a lesser extent T_4; carrier for retinol-binding protein	Kidney dysfunction	Cirrhosis, hepatitis, stress, surgery, inflammation, hyperthyroidism, cystic fibrosis, kidney dysfunction, zinc deficiency

Fe, iron; T_3, triiodothyronine; T_4, thyroxine.

serum ALB concentrations and poor clinical outcome has been demonstrated in most of the above mentioned settings. Additionally, serum ALB concentrations of 2.5 g/dL or less can be expected to exacerbate ascites and peripheral, pulmonary, and GI mucosal edema as a result of decreased colloid oncotic pressure.

TFN is a glycoprotein that binds and transports ferric iron to the liver and reticuloendothelial system for storage. As a surrogate marker of nutrition status, TFN will decrease in response to protein depletion before serum ALB concentrations decrease because it has a shorter biologic half-life (8 days), and there is less of it in the body (less than 100 mg/kg of body weight). Serum TFN concentrations may be determined by direct measurement or can be estimated indirectly from measurement of total iron-binding capacity, where TFN = (total iron-binding capacity × 0.8) − 43. Critical illness, hydration status, and iron stores affect the serum TFN concentration. In iron deficiency, hepatic TFN synthesis is increased, resulting in increased serum TFN concentrations unrelated to protein status.

Prealbumin is the transport protein for thyroxine and a carrier for retinol-binding protein. The body's content of prealbumin is low (10 mg/kg of body weight), and it has a very short biologic half-life (2 to 3 days). Prealbumin may be reduced in as few as 3 days after calorie and protein intake is significantly decreased, or when hypercatabolism or severe metabolic stress (trauma or burns) is present. Because of its short half-life, it is most useful in monitoring the short-term, acute effects of nutrition support or deficits. As with ALB and TFN, serum prealbumin concentrations are depressed in those with liver disease as a consequence of decreased hepatic synthesis. Increased serum prealbumin concentrations have been noted in patients with kidney disease as a result of impaired excretion.

Serum visceral proteins are of greatest value in assessing uncomplicated semistarvation and recovery. During severe acute stress (trauma, burns, or sepsis), these proteins are relatively poor markers of nutrition status because their synthesis is downregulated as the liver increases the production of acute-phase reactants such as C-reactive protein, α_1-acid glycoprotein, and α_1-antitrypsin.

IMMUNE FUNCTION TESTS

The frequency of impaired immunocompetence and an increased incidence of infection in malnourished patients suggests that certain immune function tests can be used as nutrition status markers. Nutrition affects immune status either directly, affecting primarily the lymphoid system, or indirectly by affecting cellular metabolism or organ systems that are involved with immune system regulation. Immune function tests used in nutrition assessment are the total lymphocyte count and DCH reactions. Both tests are simple, readily available, and inexpensive. Total lymphocyte count reflects the number of circulating T and B lymphocytes. Tissues that generate T cells are very sensitive to malnutrition and undergo involution resulting in decreased T-cell production and eventually lymphocytopenia. Total lymphocyte count is calculated from a complete blood count with differential: total lymphocyte count = (% lymphocytes × total number of white blood cells). Values of less than 1,500 cells/mm^3 and 900 cells/mm^3 are associated with moderate and severe nutrition depletion, respectively.[24]

DCH is commonly assessed using antigens to which the patient was previously sensitized. The recall antigens used most frequently in nutrition assessment are mumps, *Candida albicans,* streptokinase-streptodornase, *Trichophyton,* coccidioidin, and purified protein derivative. Anergy is associated with severe malnutrition, and immune response may be restored with nutrition repletion. Other more sophisticated immune function tests have been used to evaluate nutrition status in research settings, including lymphocyte surface antigens (CD4 and CD8 counts, CD4:CD8 ratio), T-lymphocyte responsiveness, and serum interleukin concentrations. Nonnutrition factors that affect total lymphocyte count include infection (e.g., human immunodeficiency virus/acquired immunodeficiency syndrome, pertussis, viruses, and tuberculosis), immunosuppressive drugs (e.g., corticosteroids, cyclosporine, chemotherapy, and antilymphocyte globulin), leukemia, and lymphoma. DCH can be affected by a number of factors, including fever, viral illness, recent live virus vaccination, critical illness, irradiation, immunosuppressive drugs, diabetes mellitus, human immunodeficiency virus/acquired immunodeficiency syndrome, cancer, and surgery. This lack of specificity currently limits the usefulness of these tests as nutrition status markers. Nutrients such as arginine, omega-3 fatty acids, and nucleic acids given in pharmacologic doses have been shown to improve immune function. Monitoring the efficacy of a nutrition care plan that includes these potentially immunomodulating nutrients may need to include immune function assessment with these or other immune function indicators.[25,26]

SPECIFIC NUTRIENT DEFICIENCIES

7 A comprehensive nutrition assessment must include an evaluation of possible trace element, vitamin, and essential fatty acid deficiencies. Because of their key role in metabolic processes (as coenzymes and cofactors), a deficiency of any of these nutrients may result in altered metabolism and cell dysfunction and may interfere with metabolic processes necessary for nutritional repletion. The evaluation of single nutrient deficiency states includes an accurate history to identify symptoms and risk factors that may indicate deficiency or predispose the patient to developing a deficiency state. A nutrition-focused physical examination for signs of deficiencies and biochemical assessment to confirm a suspected diagnosis also should be done. Ideally, biochemical assessment would be based on the nutrient's function (e.g., metalloenzyme activity) rather than simply measuring the nutrient's serum concentration. Unfortunately, few practical methods to assess micronutrient function are available, and most assays measure serum concentrations of the individual nutrient.

TABLE 143-6 Assessment of Trace Element Status

Trace Element	Signs of Deficiency	Signs of Toxicity	Factors Associated with Altered Plasma Concentrations
Chromium	Glucose intolerance, peripheral neuropathy, increased free fatty acid concentrations, low RQ, weight loss, increased LDL-C, glucosuria, impaired protein utilization	Industrial exposure: skin/nasal septum lesions, allergic dermatitis, increased incidence of lung cancer	Decreased: long-term inadequate intake Increased: kidney failure
Copper	Neutropenia, leukopenia, hypochromic anemia, osteoporosis, hair/skin depigmentation, dermatitis, anorexia, diarrhea, mental deterioration, hypercholesterolemia	Wilson's disease: liver cirrhosis, diarrhea, vomiting, metallic taste	Decreased: high iron or vitamin C intake, corticosteroid use Increased: infection, rheumatoid arthritis, pregnancy, oral contraceptives, decreased biliary excretion
Iodine	Hypothyroid goiter, neuromuscular impairment, deaf-mutism, increased embryonic and postnatal mortality, cognitive impairment, impaired fertility, cretinism (severe cases)	Thyrotoxicosis: nodular goiter, weight loss, tachycardia, muscle weakness, warm skin	Decreased: long-term inadequate intake
Iron	Microcytic, hypochromic anemia (weakness, pallor, fatigue), glossitis, headache, dysphagia, nail changes, gastric atrophy, paresthesia, decreased cognitive function	Liver cirrhosis, cardiomyopathy, pancreatic damage, skin pigmentation	Increased: blood transfusion Decreased: blood loss
Manganese	Nausea, vomiting, dermatitis, hair color changes, hypocholesterolemia, growth retardation, defective carbohydrate and protein metabolism	Parkinsonian-like symptoms, hyperirritability, hallucinations, libido disturbances, ataxia	Increased: decreased biliary excretion, high iron or vitamin C intake
Molybdenum	Tachycardia, tachypnea, altered mental status, visual changes, headache, nausea, vomiting	Gout-like syndrome, increased urinary copper	Decreased: low birth weight, excessive GI losses
Selenium	Muscle weakness/pain, cardiomyopathy	Nausea, vomiting, hair/nail loss, tooth decay, skin lesions, irritability, fatigue, peripheral neuropathy	Decreased: malignancy, liver failure, pregnancy Increased: reticuloendothelial neoplasia
Zinc	Dermatitis, hypogeusia, alopecia, diarrhea, apathy, depression, growth retardation, impaired wound healing, immunosuppression, acrodermatitis enteropathica	Acute: gastric distress, nausea, dizziness, death with large intravenous doses Chronic: immunosuppression, decreased HDL-C, copper deficiency	Decreased: infection, burns, stress, hypoalbuminemia, corticosteroids, pregnancy, inflammation Increased: tissue injury, hemolysis, contaminated collection tube

HDL-C, high-density-lipoprotein cholesterol; LDL-C, low-density-lipoprotein cholesterol; RQ, respiratory quotient.

TRACE ELEMENTS

Clinical syndromes are associated with deficiency states of the essential trace elements zinc, copper, manganese, selenium, chromium, iodine, fluoride, molybdenum, and iron in children and adults. Each element is involved in a variety of biologic functions and is necessary for normal metabolism, serving as a coenzyme and/or playing a role in hormonal metabolism or erythropoiesis. Other essential trace elements for which deficiency states have not been recognized include tin, nickel, vanadium, cobalt, gallium, aluminum, arsenic, boron, bromine, cadmium, germanium, and silicon. Toxicities can occur with excess intake of some trace elements. With the current public interest in alternative and complementary medicine, clinicians must ask patients about their use of nutrition supplements and assess for signs and symptoms of toxicities (overdose) as well as deficiencies (Table 143–6).

Zinc is a component of many enzymes and proteins and is involved in the regulation of gene expression. Zinc deficiency is characterized by several signs and symptoms, including a moist eczematous dermatitis that is most apparent in the nasolabial folds and around orifices (see Table 143–6).[27,28] Zinc deficiency occurs most frequently with abnormal GI losses, such as in Crohn's disease, malabsorptive states (e.g., short-bowel syndrome), and extensive ostomy or fistula losses, or from prolonged inadequate intake, such as with zinc-free or inadequately zinc-supplemented parenteral nutrition. Zinc deficiency can be documented by the presence of low plasma zinc concentrations. However, plasma zinc concentrations decrease in acute stress states such as trauma, surgery, burns, or sepsis and generally remain depressed until stress resolves. Also, because zinc is a normal contaminant of most blood collection tubes, special zinc-free collection tubes must be used for plasma assays. Hair zinc analysis by atomic absorption spectroscopy or neutron activation analysis may be a good indicator of zinc status in children,[29] and lymphocyte 5'-nucleotidase activity and leukocyte zinc content are better indicators of zinc status in adults, but these assays are not widely available.

Copper is a component of enzymes involved in iron metabolism. The signs and symptoms of copper deficiency include anemia, skeletal demineralization, and hypercholesterolemia (see Table 143–6).[27,28] In severe cases, such as in Menkes syndrome, copper deficiency is further manifested as hypothermia, hair and skin depigmentation, progressive mental deterioration, and growth retardation. Factors predisposing to copper deficiency include malabsorption states, protein-losing enteropathy, nephrotic syndrome, and copper-free parenteral nutrition.[30,31] The chronic ingestion of too much copper or inadequate elimination can result in liver cirrhosis (e.g., Wilson disease). Copper deficiency is assessed most frequently using plasma copper or ceruloplasmin concentrations. As with zinc, serum copper concentrations may not accurately reflect total body copper status because serum concentrations may be altered by a variety of conditions and may remain normal even when hepatic stores are deficient (see Table 143–6). Copper function also may be assessed by measuring activity of the cuproenzymes—erythrocyte superoxide dismutase or cytochrome-C oxidase—in platelets or leukocytes. Enzyme activity is decreased significantly in copper deficiency. However, measurement of enzyme activity is method and technique sensitive and not routinely available.

Chromium is an important cofactor, along with insulin, in the maintenance of normal blood glucose concentrations. Chromium deficiency is characterized by glucose intolerance and impaired protein utilization. Patients with chromium deficiency also may have increased free fatty acid concentrations and a low respiratory quotient (RQ) (see Table 143–6). Chromium deficiency has only been identified in patients receiving long-term parenteral nutrition with inadequate chromium intake.[27,28,32,33] Plasma chromium concentrations do not accurately reflect total body chromium status, presumably because the biologically active form of chromium is an organic substance known as the glucose tolerance factor. Chromium toxicity is not a common clinical concern and has been reported only with contaminated drinking water or industrial exposure. Chromium picolinate supplementation as an adjunct for weight loss has not been proven effective. Manganese is important in the function of many enzymes, including arginase (amino acid metabolism), pyruvate carboxylase (carbohydrate metabolism), and superoxide dismutase (cholesterol metabolism; antioxidant), and in bone formation. Manganese deficiency has only been reported in association with the ingestion of chemically defined manganese-deficient oral diets.[27,28] Table 143–6 lists common symptoms associated with manganese deficiency. Manganese toxicity is more concerning and has been described in several patients receiving long-term parenteral nutrition supplemented with a standard trace element preparation.[34–38] Manganese appears to accumulate in brain tissue, especially in the setting of chronic cholestasis and short-bowel syndrome. Clinical toxicity is evidenced primarily by extrapyramidal symptoms mimicking Parkinson's disease. Serum manganese concentrations do not correlate well with the clinical presentation, but magnetic resonance imaging of the basal ganglia may show hyperintensity areas, especially in the globus pallidus. In most reported cases, discontinuation of manganese in the parenteral nutrition solution resulted in resolution of neurologic symptoms in 6 months with partial or total normalization of the magnetic resonance image after 1 to 2 years. Other methods of evaluating manganese status include measuring the manganese content of mononuclear blood cells[37] and the activity of manganese superoxide dismutase, a mitochondrial antioxidant enzyme.[37] These methods are good indicators of manganese status but are not widely available.

Selenium, as selenocysteine, is incorporated into several enzymes: glutathione peroxidase (antioxidant), iodothyronine deiodinase (thyroid hormone regulation), and selenoprotein P (vitamin C metabolism). Prematurity, acute illness, chronic GI losses, and long-term selenium-free parenteral nutrition are associated with low serum selenium concentrations and decreased glutathione peroxidase activity.[27,28,39–43] The clinical significance of reduced serum selenium concentrations is unclear. Selenium deficiency has been described in patients receiving long-term selenium-free parenteral nutrition. Muscle pain and weakness are the most frequently observed signs and symptoms (see Table 143–6), but severe biochemical deficiency is not always accompanied by these symptoms. Fatal cardiomyopathy has been reported in several cases.

Selenium toxicity or selenosis generally only occurs in those with long-term exposure to foods grown in selenium-rich soil (e.g., Great Plains area of the United States) and may occur when intake exceeds 400 mcg per day for prolonged periods. Selenium status may be assessed by measuring plasma selenium concentrations, which will reflect recent selenium intake. Decreased concentrations may indicate selenium deficiency, but reductions also have been observed in patients with malignancies, liver failure, and pregnancy. Assays that measure the activity of the selenium-containing enzyme glutathione peroxidase in erythrocytes or the plasma concentration of selenoprotein P may be more sensitive indicators of selenium status because they reflect chronic ingestion, but neither is widely available.

Molybdenum is a cofactor for enzymes involved in catabolism of sulfur amino acids, purines, and pyrimidines (i.e., xanthine, aldehyde, and sulfite oxidases). Molybdenum deficiency is rare. One case of molybdenum deficiency has been reported in a patient receiving long-term parenteral nutrition who presented with symptoms that included tachycardia, tachypnea, headache, night blindness, nausea, vomiting, central scotomas, lethargy, disorientation, and ultimately coma (see Table 143–6). Symptoms were reversed when molybdenum was added to the parenteral nutrition solution.[44] Factors predisposing to molybdenum deficiency appear to be low birth weight, excessive loss via the GI tract, such as with short-bowel syndrome, and long-term inadequate intake, such as with molybdenum-free parenteral nutrition. Biochemical abnormalities expected in molybdenum deficiency include very low serum and urine uric acid concentrations (low xanthine oxidase activity) and low urine inorganic sulfate concentrations (low sulfate oxidase activity).[45]

Deficiency of iodine, a component of thyroid hormones, may result in goiter formation (see Chap. 78). However, not everyone with an iodine-deficient diet will develop a goiter. Thyroxine (T_4) and triiodothyronine (T_3) can be used to assess iodine status (see Table 143–6). Intravenous iodine supplements typically are not necessary except during long-term parenteral nutrition with minimal enteral intake. Iodine needs generally are met by cutaneous absorption of iodine from germicides (e.g., povidone-iodine) used in catheter care or consumption of iodized salt.[46,47] Use of povidone-iodine as a topical antiseptic has decreased with the increased use of chlorhexidine for catheter care, thus the need for iodine supplementation must be individualized. Iodine excess is rarely a clinical concern when thyroid function is normal.

Iron is an important component of hemoglobin, myoglobin, and cytochrome enzymes; it is important in oxygen transport, muscle iron storage, and cellular energy production. Patients with iron-deficiency anemia generally present with fatigue, weakness, and pallor, but they may have other symptoms (see Chap. 104). Inadequate iron intake, malabsorption, and blood loss are the principal causes of iron-deficiency anemia. Iron toxicity (overload) with possible organ damage can occur when chronic iron intake exceeds requirements such as in patients receiving frequent blood transfusions. Iron deficiency or overload is confirmed by assessment of body iron stores, as reflected indirectly by measurement of hemoglobin, serum iron, total iron-binding capacity, and serum ferritin, or directly by marrow staining and liver biopsy. Although the direct methods are the most accurate, they are invasive, and indirect measurements are used more commonly. Because indirect parameters may be altered by chronic illness independent of iron stores, concomitant illness must be considered in their interpretation.

VITAMINS

Vitamins act as both catalysts (cofactors) and substrates in essential metabolic reactions in the body. A comprehensive nutrition-focused history and physical examination is the most valuable means of assessing patients for vitamin deficiency or toxicity (Table 143–7). A thorough review of all the complex interrelationships of vitamins and their effects on nutrition and metabolism, however, is beyond the scope of this chapter.[48] Although it is uncommon to see a single-vitamin deficiency as multiple vitamin deficiencies are most often associated with generalized malnutrition, single-vitamin deficiencies may occasionally be noted. Thiamine deficiency may result in lactic acidosis and encephalopathy,[49] whereas pernicious anemia caused by vitamin B_{12} (cyanocobalamin) deficiency has been reported with increasing frequency, especially in the elderly, as a consequence of decreased gastric acidity. Recently, the incidence of vitamin D deficiency was reported to be increased, especially in children[50] and the elderly.[51,52] Laboratory assessment may be useful to confirm the clinical suspicion of a deficiency state. The first indication of a deficiency is usually a fall in circulating serum concentrations of the vitamin or its coenzyme. Subsequently, there is a decrease in urinary excretion of the vitamin, which, in turn, is followed by diminished tissue concentrations of the vitamin. The most common measurements of vitamin status are assays of circulating amounts in plasma or serum. Assays of biochemical or metabolic function of the vitamin are more likely to reflect body stores than are serum concentrations. Most of these functional assays use erythrocyte or leukocyte extracts to determine apoenzyme activity, which is dependent on the vitamin coenzyme (Table 143–7). Vitamin toxicity can occur, especially with

TABLE 143-7 Assessment of Vitamin Status

Vitamin	Signs of Deficiency	Laboratory Assay	Comments
Water-soluble vitamins			
Thiamine (B_1)	Early: anorexia, fatigue, depression, impaired memory/concentration	Whole blood or erythrocyte transketolase activity	Increased need with hemodialysis, peritoneal dialysis, alcoholism, malabsorption, hypermetabolism
	Late: paresthesia, nystagmus, lactic acidosis, congestive heart failure, Wernicke-Korsakoff's syndrome, peripheral neuritis, beriberi	Blood thiamin	
Riboflavin (B_2)	Mucositis, dermatitis, cheilosis, photophobia, corneal vascularization, lacrimation, decreased vision, impaired wound healing, normocytic anemia	Urinary riboflavin	
Pantothenic acid	Fatigue, malaise, headache, insomnia, vomiting, abdominal cramps	Serum pantothenic acid	
Niacin	Pellagra: dermatitis, dementia, glossitis, diarrhea, memory loss, headaches	Urinary niacin metabolites	Flushing and GI distress can be seen with supplements; increased need with hemo- and peritoneal dialysis, malabsorption
Pyridoxine (B_6)	Dermatitis, glossitis, distal limb numbness/paresthesia, convulsions, sideroblastic anemia	Serum pyridoxal 5'-phosphate Plasma B_6	Sensory neuropathy with high supplement intake
Folic acid	Megaloblastic anemia, diarrhea, glossitis, cheilosis, angular stomatitis, fatigue, difficulty concentrating, irritability, headache, palpitations, shortness of breath, heart failure, tachycardia, postural hypotension, lactic acidosis, neural tube defects	Serum folate Serum homocysteine	Decreased with increased cellular/tissue turnover (pregnancy, malignancy, hemolytic anemia); masks neurologic complications of vitamin B_{12} deficiency; decreases risks of neural tube defects
Cyanocobalamin (B_{12})	Pernicious anemia, glossitis, spinal cord degeneration, peripheral neuropathy	Serum B_{12} Serum methylmalonic acid	Decreased absorption in the elderly, distal ileal resection, loss of gastric intrinsic factor
Biotin	Dermatitis, depression, lassitude, somnolence	Urinary biotin	
Ascorbic acid (C)	Enlargement/keratosis of hair follicles, impaired wound healing, anemia, lethargy, depression, bleeding, ecchymosis	Plasma ascorbic acid	GI disturbances, kidney stones, excess iron absorption with excess intake; smokers need 35 mg/day more than nonsmokers
Fat-soluble vitamins			
Retinol (A)	Dermatitis, night blindness, xerophthalmia, Bitot spots,[a] pruritus, follicular hyperkeratosis, excessive deposition of periosteal bone, hair changes, poor growth Irreversible: punctuate keratopathy, keratomalacia, corneal perforation	Serum vitamin A	Teratogenic effects, liver toxicity with excessive intake; alcohol intake, liver disease, hyperlipidemia, and severe protein malnutrition increase susceptibility to adverse effects of high intake; β-carotene supplements recommended only for those at risk of deficiency (fat malabsorption)
D	Rickets, osteomalacia, muscle weakness, poor growth, hypocalcemia	Plasma 25-hydroxy vitamin D	Elevated intake causes hypercalcemia; decreased in uremia, elderly (especially in winter), fat malabsorption
α-tocopherol (E)	Hemolysis	Serum vitamin E	Excess intake: hemorrhagic toxicity; increased risk of bleeding with anticoagulants
K	Bleeding (ecchymosis, petechiae, hematomas)	Prothrombin time	Anticoagulant therapy can be affected by supplements or diet

[a]Bitot spots are spots located superficially in the conjunctiva, which are oval, triangular, or irregular in shape.

the fat-soluble vitamins (A, D, E, and K), which are stored in the body. Excessive dietary intake of vitamin A (hypervitaminosis A) is linked to an increased risk of hip fractures in both men and women.[53–55] With the exception of cyanocobalamin, which is stored in the liver, water-soluble vitamins are not stored in the body; consequently, the risk of toxicity is considered minimal unless ingested in very high individual doses. Recent evidence, however, suggests that even water-soluble vitamins may be associated with adverse events when taken chronically in high doses. Although administration of folic acid is definitively associated with a reduction in neural tube defects, its ability to improve some cardiac outcomes (a result of its effect on homocysteine concentrations) is less-well established.[56,57] The administration of folic acid, vitamin B_6 (pyridoxine), and vitamin B_{12} after coronary artery stenting is associated with an increase in the risk of in-stent restenosis.[58] With the current use of nutrition supplements by Americans, the clinician should be alert for the signs of hypervitaminosis (Table 143–7).

ESSENTIAL FATTY ACIDS

The body can synthesize all fatty acids except α-linoleic acid (an omega-6 fatty acid) and linolenic acid (an omega-3 fatty acid). Consequently, intake of approximately 2% to 4% of total calories as these fatty acids is essential to prevent deficiency. Symptoms of essential fatty acid deficiency include dermatitis (dry, cracked, scaly skin), alopecia, impaired wound healing, growth failure, thrombocytopenia, and anemia. Essential fatty acid deficiency is rare in adults and children but can occur with prolonged use of lipid-free parenteral nutrition, with severe fat malabsorption, with very-low-fat enteral feeding formulations or diets, and with severe malnutrition, especially in stressed patients.[59,60] In critically ill adults and older children with increased metabolic demands, biochemical evidence of essential fatty acid deficiency can occur within 1 week of starting lipid-free parenteral nutrition.[59,60] Because newborns, especially those born prematurely, have limited fat stores, they may develop essential fatty acid deficiency more rapidly than adults. Biochemical essential fatty acid deficiency has been noted within 72 hours after birth in preterm infants receiving fat-free intravenous solutions.[61]

Linoleic acid normally is converted to arachidonic acid (a tetraene fatty acid). If linoleic acid is unavailable, oleic acid will be substituted, which results in production of eicosatrienoic acid (a triene fatty acid) as the metabolic end product, enabling an essential fatty acid deficiency to be detected on the basis of decreased tetraene production and increased triene production. Normally, the ratio of trienes to tetraenes is less than 0.4; when this ratio becomes greater than 0.4, the diagnosis of essential fatty acid deficiency is established. However, because analysis of plasma fatty acids is expensive and not widely available, diagnosis is generally made on clinical findings.

CARNITINE

Carnitine is a quaternary amine required for transport of long-chain fatty acids into the mitochondria for β-oxidation and energy production. Carnitine also binds acyl residues and helps in their elimination (detoxification), thereby decreasing the number conjugated with coenzyme A and increasing the ratio of free to acetylated coenzyme A. Carnitine is available from a wide variety of dietary sources (especially meats) and can be synthesized by the liver and kidneys from lysine and methionine. Hepatic synthesis is decreased in premature infants, and low plasma carnitine concentrations and/or overt carnitine deficiency have been documented in premature infants receiving parenteral nutrition or carnitine-free diets, as well as in those with inborn errors of metabolism.[62–64] Other predisposing factors for carnitine deficiency include chronic kidney or liver disease, vitamin C deficiency, chronic use of valproic acid and zidovudine, and a vegetarian diet.

The clinical presentation of carnitine deficiency includes generalized skeletal muscle weakness, fatty liver, and fasting hypoglycemia. Carnitine status can be assessed by measurement of plasma, urine, or red blood cell total and free carnitine concentrations. Plasma and urine carnitine concentrations are most helpful in primary carnitine deficiency (an inborn error of metabolism). Plasma concentrations constitute less than 1% of the total body carnitine.[63] Acylcarnitine concentrations are more helpful in secondary causes of carnitine deficiency. When only total and free concentrations are available, the free is subtracted from the total to give the acylcarnitine concentration.

MUSCLE FUNCTION TESTS

A relatively new approach in nutrition assessment is evaluation of muscle function as an end-organ response. Hand-grip strength (forearm muscle dynamometry), respiratory muscle strength, and muscle response to electrical stimulation have been used. Measuring hand-grip strength is a relatively simple, noninvasive, and inexpensive (most hand-grip dynamometers cost less than $400) procedure that correlates with patient outcome.[65–67] Ulnar nerve stimulation causes measurable muscle contraction and is currently used in the intensive care unit to monitor the adequacy of neuromuscular blockade. In the setting of malnutrition, increased fatigue and a slowed muscle relaxation rate have been noted; these indices return to normal after refeeding. Both these parameters have the advantage of being indicators of tissue function rather than composition. Their usefulness in clinical practice is currently hampered by a lack of appropriate reference standards and limited data confirming their sensitivity and specificity for nutrition assessment.

OTHER NUTRITION ASSESSMENT TOOLS

Various methods to determine body composition have been used in the research setting. These methods generally are complex, require expensive technology, and at present are limited to research centers. One of the most promising for routine clinical practice is dual-energy x-ray absorptiometry (DXA). DXA is best known for its use in measuring bone density for the evaluation of osteoporosis, but DXA can be used to quantify the mineral, fat, and LBM compartments of the body.[68–71] DXA is available in most hospitals and many clinics. Equipment for central DXA scans requires a fair amount of space and is expensive; that is, $40,000 to $160,000 depending on complexity of the scanner. Portable (or peripheral) DXA devices that use ultrasound and infrared interactance can be used to measure bone density in peripheral bones such as the wrist, fingers, or heel, and have also been used to assess subcutaneous fat. These portable DXA scanners are much less expensive ($10,000 to $20,000 or less) and are amenable for use in community screenings in malls, health fairs, and pharmacies. Further research is needed to determine if DXA will be useful clinically in nutrition assessment.

Magnetic resonance imaging and computed tomography can measure subcutaneous, intraabdominal, and regional fat distribution. Neutron activation is a means of measuring body nitrogen, calcium, sodium, chloride, and phosphorus. These measurements can then be used to calculate total body fat, bone, and protein. Isotope dilution methods determine TBW and underwater weighing determines density. In addition, these methods can be used to estimate LBM and body fat. LBM also can be estimated using total body electrical conductivity and by measuring the naturally occurring isotope ^{40}K. These techniques are used primarily in research and seldom in clinical practice.

ASSESSMENT OF NUTRIENT REQUIREMENTS

❽ Nutrition requirements depend on an individual's clinical condition and the need for continued maintenance of adequate nutrition, or whether starvation or ongoing metabolic stress dictates a need for repletion. For obese patients, usual nutrition requirements may be altered because of the need for weight loss. In children, there is the added consideration of sustaining or reestablishing normal growth and development. Organ function (e.g., intestine, kidney, liver, and pancreas) may affect nutrient utilization.

Nutrient requirements vary with age, gender, size, disease state, clinical condition, nutrition status, and physical activity level. An estimate of nutrient requirements must be made using guidelines interpreted in the context of these patient-specific factors. The recommended dietary allowances (RDAs) initially were intended as guidelines for preventing nutrition deficiencies in a healthy population of individuals, but they have often been used inappropriately to evaluate the diets of individuals. In the early 1990s, the Food and Nutrition Board began the task of revising the RDAs and created a new family of nutrition reference values, the dietary reference intakes (DRIs) which include seven nutrient groups.[72]

The four categories of the new DRIs are estimated average requirements, RDAs, adequate intakes, and tolerable upper intake levels. Estimated average requirements can be used for planning nutrient intakes for groups, as they are defined as the amount of the nutrient that meets the needs of 50% of persons in a given group. The RDA is designated as nutrient intake that meets the needs of almost all persons in the designated group. The RDA is approximately two standard deviations above the estimated average requirement for nutrients for which the requirement is well defined, and 1.2 times the estimated average requirement for nutrients for which there is more variability. To evaluate an individual's daily intake, the RDA is the most appropriate comparator. Adequate intakes are defined as the average intake of a designated group that appears to sustain a particular nutrition state, growth, or other functional indication of health. This category is reserved for nutrients for which no estimated average requirement or RDA has been determined. Finally the tolerable upper intake level is the maximum nutrient intake that is unlikely to pose adverse affects in almost all persons in a designated group. DRIs have been established for six of the seven established nutrient groups: (a) calcium, phosphorus, magnesium, vitamin D, and fluoride; (b) folate and other B vitamins; (c) antioxidants (e.g., selenium and vitamins C and E); (d) trace elements; (e) macronutrients (e.g., protein, fat, carbohydrates, and fiber); and (f) electrolytes and water.[72] Recommendations for group seven, which includes other food components (e.g., phytoestrogens), are still in development.

ENERGY REQUIREMENTS

The DRIs for macronutrients recommend that adults consume 45% to 65% of their total calories as carbohydrates, 20% to 35% as fat, and 10% to 35% as protein.[73] The recommendations for children are similar: carbohydrate, 45% to 65%; fat, 30% to 40%; and, protein, 10% to 30%. Infants, especially premature infants, need a higher proportion of fat (approximately 40% to 50% of total calories) in their diets to ensure normal neurologic development. An RDA for total carbohydrates of 130 g/day for adults and children is included in the most recent DRIs.[72–74]

CLINICAL CONTROVERSY

Clinicians continue to debate whether an individual's energy requirements should be expressed as total or nonprotein calories. Proponents of nonprotein calories argue that sufficient energy must be provided from nonprotein sources (dextrose and fat) to spare protein from conversion to energy to be used for wound healing and LBM maintenance. Supporters of total calories state that the nonprotein calorie approach overestimates energy needs because 15% of daily energy expenditure is derived from protein breakdown. Even with adequate energy intake, protein metabolism is not necessarily prioritized for anabolism, especially during stress. Additionally, standard equations for estimating energy needs were derived using total energy-expenditure measurements. Regardless of the method chosen, the practitioner should consistently document which method was used.

Estimating Energy Expenditure

There are numerous published methods for determining an individual's total energy or calorie (kcal) requirement. The most commonly used methods to determine energy requirements use population estimates of calories per kilogram of body weight (kcal/kg), equations that estimate an individual's energy expenditure, or indirect calorimetry. The simplest method to assess energy requirements is to use population estimates of calories required per kilogram of body weight. This method assumes standard values for the energy requirements associated with various disease states or clinical conditions, as well as the additional requirements for repletion of a malnourished individual. It does not take into consideration age- or gender-related differences in energy needs. Daily adult requirements determined by this method, using ABW or adjusted IBW in kilograms, are accepted to be:

Healthy, normal nutrition status: 20 to 25 kcal/kg per day

Malnourished or metabolically stressed: 25 to 30 kcal/kg per day

Major burn injury (>50% total body surface area): 30 to 40 kcal/kg per day

Table 143–8 shows suggested calorie intakes for maintenance and normal growth of healthy infants and children.[72,73] For children, these maintenance energy requirements are approximately 150% of basal metabolic rate, with the additional calories needed to support activity and growth. Caloric requirements increase with fever, sepsis, major surgery, trauma, burns, and long-term growth failure, and in the presence of chronic conditions such as bronchopulmonary dysplasia, congenital heart disease, and cystic fibrosis. Energy needs may decrease with obesity and neurologic disability (e.g., cerebral palsy). Clinical judgment and close monitoring are essential to ensure that the desired nutrition therapy outcomes are attained.

Various equations are used to estimate energy needs of adults and children (see Table 143–9).[60,73,75] The Harris-Benedict equations are a popular means for assessing energy requirements in adults. They have the advantage of taking into consideration the patient's age, height, weight, gender, and clinical condition. These equations were derived from oxygen (O_2) consumption measurements made on normally nourished individuals who were in a fasting and resting state. Although these equations are commonly referred to as the "BEE (basal energy expenditure) equations," they actually estimate resting energy expenditure (REE), the amount of energy expended at rest by a fasting, awake individual in a temperature-controlled environment performing only basal functions such as breathing, circulation, and metabolic processes. Table 143–9 shows the Harris-Benedict equations.

Because these equations approximate REE, their results must be modified by a factor that is most representative of the individual's clinical condition. For example, an individual who is confined to bed

TABLE 143-8 Dietary Reference Intakes for Energy and Protein in Healthy Children

Age (Reference Age/Weight)	Estimated Energy Requirement (kcal/day) Boy	Girl	Protein RDA (g/kg/day)[a]
0–6 months (3 months/6 kg)	570	520	1.52[b]
7–12 months (9 months/9 kg)	743	676	1.5
1–2 years (24 months/12 kg)	1,046	992	
1–3 years (24 months/12 kg)			1.1
3–8 years (6 years/20 kg)	1,742	1,642	
4–8 years (6 years/20 kg)			0.95
9–13 years (11 years/M: 36 kg; W: 37 kg)	2,279	2,071	0.95
14–18 years (16 years/M: 61 kg; W: 54 kg)	3,152	2,368	0.85

M, men; RDA, recommended dietary allowance; W, women.
[a]Protein requirements in metabolically stressed children increase by 50% or more.
[b]Adequate intake (AI).
Adapted from Food and Nutrition Board.[72,73]

TABLE 143-9 Equations to Estimate Energy Expenditure in Adults and Children[a]

Adults

Harris-Benedict (kcal/day)

Men: BEE = 66 + [(13.7W(kg)] + [5H(cm)] – (6.8A)

Women: BEE = 655 + [(9.6W(kg)] + [1.8H(cm)] – (4.7A)

DRI equations (kcal/day)

Men: EER = 662 – 9.53A + (PA × 15.91W) + 539.6H(m)

Women: EER = 354 – 6.91A + (PA × 9.36W) + 726H(m)

PA = 1 if sedentary; 1.12 if low active; 1.27 if active; and 1.45 if very active.

Children

FAO/WHO/UNU (kcal/day)

0–3 years of age

Boys: BMR = 60.9W – 54

Girls: BMR = 61W – 51

4–10 years of age

Boys: BMR = 22.7W + 495

Girls: BMR = 22.5W + 499

11–18 years of age

Boys: BMR = 17.5W + 651

Girls: BMR = 12.2W + 746

DRI equations (kcal/day)

Birth through 2 years of age

EER = (89W – 100) + GF

GF = 175 kcal if 0–3 months; 56 kcal if 4–6 months; 22 kcal if 7–12 months; 20 kcal if 13–35 months

3–18 years of age

Boys: EER = 88.5 – (61.9A) + PA [26.7W + 903H(m)] + GF

Girls: EER = 135.3 – (30.8A) + PA [10W + 934H(m)] + GF

GF = 20 kcal if 3–8 years; 25 kcal if 9–18 years.

PA = 1 if sedentary; 1.13–1.16 if low activity; 1.26–1.31 if normal activity; and 1.42–1.56 if very active

A, age in years; BEE, basal energy expenditure; BMR, basal metabolic rate; DRI, Dietary Reference Intakes; EER, estimated energy requirement; FAO/WHO/UNU, Food and Agriculture Organization/World Health Organization/United Nations University; GF, growth factor, H, height in centimeters (cm) or meters (m), as indicated; PA, physical activity factor; W, weight in kilograms.
[a]No real consensus exists as to which formula is best in all situations. Many clinicians use both to calculate a range of acceptable intakes.

TABLE 143-10 Stress Factors for Use in Children and Adults

Condition	Factor
No stress	
Confined to bed	1.2
Out of bed: normal activity	1.3
Catch-up growth	1.5
Mild stress	
Postoperative recovery: uncomplicated surgery	1
Trauma: mild (e.g., long-bone fracture)	1.2
Moderate stress	
Sepsis (moderate)	1.3
Trauma: central nervous system (sedated)	1.3
Trauma: moderate to severe	Children: 1.5 Adults: 1.3
Severe stress	
Sepsis (severe)	Children: 1.6 Adults: 1.3
Trauma: central nervous system (severe)	Children: Up to 2.0 Adults: up to 1.3
Burns (proportionate to burned area)	Up to 2.0

may require a calorie intake that is only 20% to 30% above the REE, whereas a person who is suffering from a severe burn injury may require 150% to 200% of the calculated REE. Some clinicians multiply the calculated REE by both a stress factor and an activity factor. Because in validation studies in healthy subjects these equations have been shown to overestimate REE by 6% to 15%, the calculated REE should be multiplied by either a stress factor or an activity factor to avoid further overestimation of the individual's energy needs.[72] It should also be noted that ABW (up to a BMI of 57 kg/m^2 in men and 40 kg/m^2 in women), not IBW or adjusted IBW, was used to generate the original data with these equations.[72] The metabolic response to stress in children appears to be similar to that seen in critically ill adults, and the "stress factors" used in adults and shown in Table 143–10 can be used in children once the REE has been determined using one of the equations shown in Table 143–9.[76,77] Controversy exists over the accuracy and reliability of predicting energy expenditure based on these equations because clinical judgments of stress level or activity level will vary between clinicians.[69,77]

Measuring Energy Expenditure

The most accurate method to determine energy expenditure is to measure it using indirect calorimetry, also referred to as metabolic gas monitoring. Indirect calorimetry methodology is based on the fact that when substrates (carbohydrates, fat, and protein) are oxidized, O_2 is consumed and carbon dioxide (CO_2) is produced in varying amounts depending on the substrate being oxidized. Indirect calorimetry is a noninvasive procedure where oxygen consumption (VO_2, mL/min) and carbon dioxide production (VCO_2, mL/min) are measured, and the measured resting energy expenditure (MREE; kcal/day) is calculated using the abbreviated Weir equation as ($MREE = 3.9VO_2 + 1.1VCO_2) \times 1.44$.[77–80]

MREE represents the total energy expended by the patient during the time period over which the measurements were taken. It is often extrapolated to a 24-hour period to approximate daily energy requirements. MREE reflects alterations in energy requirements as a result of disease or clinical condition, but does not include energy required for nutritional repletion of a malnourished individual or growth in a child. The energy intake required for these functions is accounted for by multiplying MREE by a metabolic or activity factor: mechanically ventilated, critically ill, 1; critically ill, no mechanical ventilation, 1 to 1.1; adult acute noncritically ill, 1.1 to 1.4 depending on activity; adult needing repletion or a child, 1.3 to 1.5; adult outpatient, 1.1 to 2 depending on activity; and adult depletion (weight loss), less than 1.[79]

The data obtained from indirect calorimetry also can be used to determine an RQ which reflects substrate oxidation, characterizes substrate use, and is calculated as VCO_2/VO_2. RQ values for nutrient substrates are fat, 0.7; carbohydrate, 1; protein, 0.8; and mixed substrate (fat, carbohydrate, and protein), 0.85. An RQ value of greater than 1 represents either lipogenesis or hyperventilation; an RQ value of less than 0.7 may indicate a ketogenic diet, fat gluconeogenesis, or ethanol oxidation. Values outside the 0.67 to 1.3 range should raise doubts as to the test's validity. Clinically, the RQ is used to determine if a patient is being overfed, which is indicated by an RQ value greater than 1.

CLINICAL CONTROVERSY

Clinicians do not agree on the best method for estimating energy requirements for a specific individual. Numerous equations and "stress" factors have been published, but none has been shown to be superior in all situations. These equations are probably adequate, however, for determining most individuals' needs. Measuring energy expenditure with indirect calorimetry is potentially more accurate, especially for the stressed, hospitalized, and ventilated patient, but it is neither appropriate nor available for all patients. Regardless of the method chosen, careful monitoring of the response to nutrition intervention is imperative.

There are limitations to the use of indirect calorimetry.[60,78,79] Not all institutions have metabolic carts available or personnel trained to use them. Calibration errors are common, and indirect calorimetry overestimates REE for patients with hyperventilation, metabolic acidosis, overfeeding, and air leaks anywhere in the system. Underestimates of REE are likely with hypoventilation, metabolic alkalosis, underfeeding, and gluconeogenesis. Mechanically ventilated patients are technically easier to study because the indirect calorimeter circuit can be integrated into the ventilator circuit. The patient must be at complete rest for 1 hour, must not receive bolus feedings either by feeding tube or orally for 4 hours, should have no changes in substrate delivery for 12 hours, must be on a fraction of inspired O_2 of less than 0.6, and the positive end-expiratory pressure must be less than 5 cm H_2O to ensure a steady-state reading. Unfortunately, many of the patients in whom indirect calorimetry would be most useful will not meet these requirements.

PROTEIN

Daily protein requirements are based on age, nutrition status, disease state, and clinical condition. Table 143–8 lists the RDA for protein for children; for individuals older than 18 years of age, the RDA is 0.8 g/kg per day, which is less than most people typically consume.[72,73] In adults older than 60 years of age, protein needs are increased to 1 g/kg per day to help reduce loss of LBM that occurs with aging, and up to 1.5 to 2 g/kg per day may be needed in states of metabolic stress, such as infection, trauma, and surgery, to prevent loss of LBM.[73,81] Protein requirements are also higher in pregnant and lactating women (1.1 g/kg per day).[72,73]

Protein metabolism depends on both kidney and liver function; and protein requirements are altered with kidney or liver dysfunction (see Chap. 147). Critical illness (e.g., sepsis, burns, or trauma) results in a hypercatabolic state in which there is increased protein synthesis and degradation. Consequently, protein requirements are increased to 1.5 to 2 g/kg per day. In burned patients, protein requirements may be as high as 2.5 to 3 g/kg per day or 20% to 25% of total calories in children. Liver failure typically results in the need for protein restriction (0.5 g/kg per day) except if a hypercatabolic state is also present, in which case the requirement may be increased to 1.5 g/kg per day. Protein needs in kidney failure are variable and affected by the various kidney replacement therapies available. The application of these guidelines requires both clinical judgment and frequent monitoring of kidney and liver function, serum chemistries, clinical condition, and nutrition outcomes (see Chap. 147).

Nitrogen is found only in protein and at a relatively constant ratio of 1 g nitrogen per 6.25 g protein. This ratio may vary somewhat for enteral and parenteral feeding formulations, depending on the biologic value of the protein source. Adequacy of protein intake can be assessed clinically by measuring urinary nitrogen excretion and comparing it with nitrogen intake—a nitrogen balance study. Nitrogen balance indirectly reflects an individual's protein use or protein catabolic rate, which increases with hypercatabolism. As the stress level increases, a concomitant increase in protein catabolism results in an increase in urinary nitrogen excretion. Usually the amount of urea nitrogen is measured in a 24-hour urine urea collection. In healthy individuals, the quantity of urine urea nitrogen accounts for 80% to 90% of the total urine nitrogen excreted. Nitrogen output (g/day) can be approximated as 24-hour urine urea nitrogen + 4, where 4 is a factor representing usual skin, fecal, and respiratory nitrogen losses.[82] Alternatively, if available, total urine nitrogen can be measured and may be more accurate. If total urine nitrogen is used, then the best estimate of nitrogen output is total urine nitrogen × 1.05.[82] In patients with kidney failure, in which case neither urine urea nitrogen nor total urine nitrogen represents nitrogen generation, protein turnover can be approximated with equations based on urea kinetics that estimate the rate of urea production.[22]

FAT

The daily adequate intake for men and women for α-linolenic acid is 1.6 and 1.1 g, respectively; for linoleic acid, it is 14 to 17 g/day for men and 11 to 12 g/day for women. Overall, fat should represent no more than 10% to 35% of total calories, with the recommendation that saturated fatty acids, *trans* fatty acids, and dietary cholesterol intake be kept as low as possible while consuming a nutritionally adequate diet.[72,73] As mentioned previously, fat intake in children younger than 2 years of age is critical for proper central nervous system growth and development; generally, no fat restriction (e.g., skim milk) should be imposed until after the age of 2 years.

FIBER

Maintenance of normal bowel habits, lower blood pressure, and lower cholesterol serum concentrations is attributed to dietary fiber intake. Some evidence also suggests that fiber has a role in the prevention of colon cancer and promotion of weight control through its effect on satiety. Men and women 50 years of age and younger should ingest 38 g/day and 25 g/day, respectively, of total fiber. For men and women older than 50 years of age, the recommended intakes are 30 g/day and 21 g/day, respectively.[72,73,81] For children younger than 16 years of age, the "age + 5" rule is often used. The recommended daily intake of fiber is calculated by adding 5 g to the child's age in years. For example, a 6-year-old child should ingest 11 g/day of dietary fiber.[72,73,83,84]

FLUID

The daily fluid requirement for an adult depends on many factors but is generally 30 to 35 mL/kg. It also can be estimated as 1 mL/kcal ingested or as 1,500 mL/m^2 per 24 hours. Fluid requirements per kilogram are higher for children and even higher for preterm infants because of their higher percentage of TBW and basal energy needs. Additionally, premature neonates have increased fluid requirements because of greater insensible losses and the kidney's inefficiency in concentrating urine. The Holliday-Segar method is a commonly employed, quick, and simple method for estimating minimum daily fluid needs of children that also can be applied to adults. Children who weigh less than 10 kg should receive at least 100 mL/kg per day. An additional 50 mL/kg per day should be provided for each kilogram of body weight between 11 kg and 20 kg, and 20 mL/kg per day for each kilogram above 20 kg. Thus daily fluid needs for a child weighing 8 kg would be at least 800 mL/day, whereas at least 1,350 mL/day would be needed for a 17-kg child.

TABLE 143-11 Factors That Alter Fluid Requirements

Increased Requirements	Decreased Requirements
Fever	Fluid overload
Radiant warmers	Cardiac failure
Diuretics	Decreased urinary output
Vomiting	Heat shields
Nasogastric suction	Relatively high humidity
Ostomy/fistula drainage	Humidified air via endotracheal tube
Diarrhea	Kidney failure
Glycosuria	Hypoalbuminemia with starvation
Phototherapy	Syndrome of inappropriate secretion of antidiuretic hormone (SIADH)
Increased ambient temperatures	
Hyperventilation	
Prematurity	
Excessive sweating	
Increased metabolism (e.g., hyperthyroidism)	
Diabetes insipidus	

Table 143–11 lists factors that alter fluid needs for both adults and children. All sources of fluid intake should be assessed (e.g., fluid vehicles for intravenous medications and intravenous or feeding tube flushes) when determining fluid requirements. Monitoring of urine output and specific gravity as well as serum electrolytes and weight changes can be used to assess fluid status. A urine output of at least 1 mL/kg per hour (in children) and approximately 50 mL per hour (in adults) is considered adequate to ensure tissue perfusion. Urine output should be higher if large fluid volumes or high renal solute loads (e.g., parenteral nutrition or concentrated enteral feeding formulations) are being administered. Urine specific gravity depends on the kidney's concentrating and diluting capabilities. Concomitant diuretic therapy as a result of increased solute excretion limits the usefulness of urine specific gravity as an index of fluid status.

MICRONUTRIENTS

Requirements for micronutrients (e.g., electrolytes, trace elements, and vitamins) vary with age, gender, and the route by which the nutrient is ingested (Table 143–12).[5,72,85] The variability between oral and parenteral requirements is a result of bioavailability considerations. Micronutrients poorly absorbed via the GI tract usually are required in greater doses enterally than parenterally. However, many water-soluble micronutrients are excreted more rapidly via the kidneys when administered intravenously. In these situations, the intravenous dose is greater than the oral dose. Other factors that affect micronutrient requirements include GI losses through diarrhea, vomiting, or high-output fistula; wound healing; and hypermetabolism/catabolism. Cutaneous micronutrient losses (e.g., zinc, copper, and selenium) also may be significant after major burn injury. Sodium, potassium, magnesium, and phosphorus are particularly dependent on kidney function, and in the setting of kidney failure, intake will likely need to be restricted. Calcium needs, on the other hand, may be increased in these patients. Patients who are severely malnourished will have increased electrolyte requirements during early refeeding owing to preexisting deficiencies and/or rapid intracellular uptake with anabolism. Failure to provide adequate electrolytes during refeeding has resulted in death from the refeeding syndrome.[86]

TABLE 143-12 Recommended Daily Electrolytes, Trace Elements, and Vitamins[a]

	Adult (≥19 years of age)		Pediatric	
Nutrient	***Enteral***	***Parenteral***	***Enteral***	***Parenteral***
Electrolytes and minerals				
Acetate[b]	–	–	–	–
Calcium	1,000–1,200 mg	0–15 mEq	0–12 months: 210–270 mg 1–3 years: 500 mg 4–8 years: 800 mg 9–18 years: 1,300 mg	Premature: 2–4 mEq/kg Other: 1–2.5 mEq/kg
Chloride[b]	–	–	–	2–6 mEq/kg
Magnesium	M: 400–420 mg W: 310–320 mg	10–20 mEq	0–6 months: 30 mg 7–12 months: 75 mg 1–3 years: 80 mg 4–8 years: 130 mg 9–18 years: 240–410 mg	0.25–1 mEq/kg
Phosphorus	700 mg	20–45 mmol	0–6 months: 100 mg 7–12 months: 275 mg 1–8 years: 460–500 mg 9–18 years: 1,250 mg	Premature: 1–2 mmol/kg Others: 0.5–1 mmol/kg
Potassium[c,d]	4,700 mg	60–100 mEq (1–2 mEq/kg)	0–6 months: 400 mg 7–12 months: 700 mg 1–8 years: 3,000–3,800 mg 9–18 years: 4,500–4,700 mg	2–5 mEq/kg
Sodium[c,d]	1,200–1,500 mg	60–100 mEq (1–2 mEq/kg)	0–6 months: 120 mg 7–12 months: 370 mg 1–8 years: 1,000–1,200 mg 9–18 years: 1,500 mg	2–6 mEq/kg
Trace elements				
Chromium[e] (mcg)	20–35	10–15	0–6 months: 0.2 7–12 months: 5.5 1–8 years: 11–15 9–18 years: 21–35	0.14–0.2 mcg/kg (max 5 mcg)
Copper[f] (mcg)	900	0.3–1.5	0–12 months: 200–220 1–8 years: 340–440 9–18 years: 700–890	20 mcg/kg (max 300 mcg)
Fluoride	3–4 mg	–	0–6 months: 0.01 mg 7–12 months: 0.5 mg 1–8 years: 0.7–1 mg 9–18 years: 2–3 mg	–
Iodine[g] (mcg)	150	70–140 (not well defined)	0–12 months: 110–130 1–8 years: 90 9–18 years: 120–150	1 mcg/kg
Iron (mg)	M: 8 W (≤50 years): 18 W (>50 years): 8	Varies	0–6 months: 0.27 7 months–8 years: 7–11 M (9–18 years): 8–11 F (9–13): 8 F (14–18): 15	Varies
Manganese[f] (mg)	1.8–2.3	0.15–1	0–6 months: 0.003 7–12 months: 0.6 1–8 years: 1.2–1.5 9–18 years: 1.6–2.2	1 mcg/kg (maximum 50 mcg)
Molybdenum (mcg)	45	100–200	0–12 months: 2–3 1–8 years: 17–22 9–18 years: 34–43	0.25 mcg/kg (maximum 5 mcg)
Selenium (mcg)	55	20–60	0–12 months: 15–20 1–8 years: 20–30 9–18 years: 40–55	1.5–3 mcg/kg (maximum 30 mcg)
Zinc[h] (mg)	8–11	2.5–5	0–12 months: 2–3 1–8 years: 3–5 9–18 years: 8–11	Premature: 300–400 mcg/kg Other: 50–250 mcg/kg
Vitamins				
Ascorbic acid (mg) (Vitamin C)	75–90	100	0–12 months: 40–50 1–8 years: 15–25 9–18 years: 45–75	80
Biotin (mcg)	30	60	0–12 months: 5–6 1–8 years: 8–12 9–18 years: 20–25	20

(continued)

TABLE 143-12 Recommended Daily Electrolytes, Trace Elements, and Vitamins[a] (continued)

	Adult (≥19 years of age)		Pediatric	
Nutrient	***Enteral***	***Parenteral***	***Enteral***	***Parenteral***
Choline (mg)	425–550	Not established	0–12 months: 125–150 1–8 years: 200–250 9–18 years: 375–550	Not established
Cobalamin (mcg) (Vitamin B_{12})	2.4	5	0–12 months: 0.4–0.5 1–8 years: 0.9–1.2 9–18 years: 1.8–2.4	1
Folic acid (mcg)	400	400	0–12 months: 65–80 1–8 years: 150–200 9–18 years: 300–400	140
Niacin (mg NE)	14–16	40	0–12 months: 2–4 1–8 years: 6–8 9–18 years: 12–16	17
Pantothenic acid (mg)	5	15	0–12 months: 1.7–1.8 1–8 years: 2–3 9–18 years: 4–5	5
Pyridoxine (mg) (Vitamin B_6)	1.3–1.7	4	0–12 months: 0.1–0.3 1–8 years: 0.5–0.6 9–18 years: 1–1.3	1
Riboflavin (mg)	1.1–1.3	3.6	0–12 months: 0.3–0.4 1–8 years: 0.5–0.6 9–18 years: 0.9–1.3	1.4
Thiamin (mg)	1.1–1.2	3	0–12 months: 0.2–0.3 1–8 years: 0.5–0.6 9–18 years: 0.9–1.2	1.2
Vitamin A (mcg RE) (Retinol)	700–900	600–1,000 (3,300–5,500 international units)	0–12 months: 400–500 1–8 years: 300–400 9–18 years: 600–900	700 (2300 international units)
Vitamin D (mcg)	≤50 years: 5 (200 IU) 51–70 years: 10 (400 international units) >70 years: 15 (600 international units)	5 (200 international units)	All ages: 5 (200 international units)	5–10 (200–400 international units)
Vitamin E (mg TE) (α-tocopherol)	15 (15 international units)	10 (10 international units)	0–12 months: 4–5 (4–5 international units) 1–8 years: 6–7 9–18 years: 11–15	7 (7 international units)
Vitamin K (mcg)	90–120	0.7–2.5 mg	0–12 months: 2–2.5 1–8 years: 30–55 9–18 years: 60–75	200

M, men; NE, niacin equivalents; RE, retinol equivalents; TE, tocopherol equivalent; W, women.
[a]Data from references 5, 49, and 55. Data represent either the recommended dietary allowance or the adequate intake for each nutrient where established.
[b]Not established; as needed to maintain acid–base balance.
[c]Newborns and low-birth-weight or very-low-birth-weight infants or with concomitant disease (e.g., necrotizing enterocolitis) may have higher requirements. Intake in nonhealthy children must be individualized.
[d]No recommended dietary allowance or adequate intake has been established.
[e]An additional 20 mcg of chromium per day is recommended in patients with significant intestinal losses.
[f]May accumulate in cholestasis.
[g]Long-term parenteral nutrition only if no topicals containing iodide or iodized table salt are used.
[h]An additional 12.2 mg zinc/L of small bowel fluid lost and 17.1 mg zinc/kg of stool or ileostomy output is recommended; add an additional 2 mg zinc per day for acute catabolic stress.

DRUG–NUTRIENT INTERACTIONS

❾ Drug-induced nutrient deficiency, poor therapeutic response, enhanced drug toxicity, and failure to achieve desired nutrition outcomes can occur if either nutrition support or drug therapy is stopped as a consequence of adverse effects.[87–91] Patient outcomes may be enhanced when an effective screening method to identify significant drug–nutrient interactions is coupled with a patient-counseling program. An important part of the screening process is to recognize risk factors that influence drug–nutrient interactions. The potential for drug–nutrient interactions is greatest in pediatric and elderly individuals, those with poor nutrition status (obesity and marasmus), those receiving multiple drug therapies, and those receiving tube feedings.

Mineral and electrolyte serum concentrations may change because of drug therapy. For example, with diuretics, urine sodium, potassium, and magnesium wasting may occur, causing a reduction in their respective serum concentrations (see Chaps. 52 to 54). Serum electrolyte concentrations also may increase as a direct result of the drug's mechanism (e.g., potassium-sparing diuretics) or because of the drug's salt form. Corticosteroids and cyclosporine are known to cause hyperglycemia, whereas other drugs are prescribed to pharmacologically lower blood glucose concentrations, for example, insulin and oral hypoglycemics (see Chap. 77).

Vitamin status also may be affected by drugs (Table 143–13). For example, sulfasalazine therapy causes a decrease in folic acid, isoniazid therapy causes pyridoxine deficiency, and furosemide therapy may result in decreased thiamin concentrations. Drug therapy outcomes also may be affected by vitamin intake. The ingestion of high doses of folic acid may decrease methotrexate's therapeutic effect, whereas changes in an individual's usual vitamin K or vitamin E intake may cause variability in warfarin's anticoagulation effects.

Drug-delivery vehicles also may contain nutrients. Most intravenous therapies (maintenance intravenous fluids, drugs, and electro-

TABLE 143-13 Drug Effects on Vitamin Status

Drug	Effect
Antacids	Thiamin deficiency
Antibiotics	Vitamin K deficiency
Anticonvulsants	Vitamin D and folic acid malabsorption
Antineoplastics	Folic acid antagonism and malabsorption
Antipsychotics	Decreased riboflavin
Cathartics	Increased requirements for vitamins D, C, and B_6
Cholestyramine	Vitamins A, D, E, and K, β-carotene malabsorption
Colestipol	Vitamins A, D, E, and K, β-carotene malabsorption
Corticosteroids	Decreased vitamins A, D, and C
Diuretics (loop)	Thiamin deficiency
Histamine$_2$ antagonists	Vitamin B_{12} deficiency
Isoniazid	Vitamin B_6 deficiency
Mineral oil	Vitamins A, D, E, and K malabsorption
Orlistat	Vitamins A, D, E, and K malabsorption
Pentamidine	Folic acid deficiency
Proton pump inhibitors	Vitamin B_{12} deficiency

lyte replacements) are delivered using either dextrose (e.g., dextrose 5% in water) or sodium (e.g., 0.9% normal saline) in the admixture. Lipid emulsion (10%) is used as the vehicle for the anesthetic agent propofol and may contribute a large amount of fat calories when continuous propofol infusions are used. In these instances, nutrition-support regimens must be adjusted to accommodate the calories and other nutrients delivered through these therapies.

PRACTICAL GUIDELINES FOR NUTRITION ASSESSMENT

⑩ The value of any given marker used for nutrition assessment is only as great as its ability to accurately identify the patient with malnutrition and to correlate with malnutrition-associated complications. Most of the currently available markers of nutrition status were first used in epidemiologic studies to define large populations suffering from malnutrition caused by famine. The response of the various nutrition status markers to nutrition therapy and the correlation between improvement in these markers and decreased morbidity and mortality further support their validity. However, when applied to an individual, most of these markers lack specificity and sensitivity, which makes the development of a clinically useful, cost-effective approach to individual patient nutrition assessment challenging.

The importance of the nutrition-focused history and physical examination in both nutrition screening and nutrition assessment cannot be overemphasized. The least amount of objective data that can further substantiate the clinical impression and provide a baseline for subsequent monitoring are those markers that show the best correlation with outcome: weight and serum albumin concentration. The cost-effectiveness of the addition of further biochemical parameters is yet to be determined. The assessment of other anthropometric measures is most useful in the setting of anticipated long-term nutrition support in which these measurements will serve as a longitudinal marker of an individual's response to the nutrition care plan.

Initially, nutrition requirements are determined on the basis of assumptions made about the patient's clinical condition and the nutrition needs associated with repletion or growth, if needed. Once a nutrition intervention has been initiated, periodic reassessment of nutrition status is critical to determine the accuracy of the initial estimate of nutrition requirements. Also, nutrition requirements are dynamic in the setting of acute or critical illness—as the patient's clinical status changes, so will protein and energy requirements, further emphasizing the need for continued reassessment.

Better markers of nutrition status and methods for determining patient-specific nutrition requirements are needed to allow further refinement of estimates of an individual's nutrition needs. Functional tests and simple, noninvasive tests for body composition analysis hold promise for the future. However, until better methods of assessment become available clinically and are demonstrated to be cost-effective, the currently available battery of tests will continue to be the mainstay of nutrition assessment.

Information in this chapter can be used to establish empiric goals for a nutrition care plan. However, as with other forms of therapy, continuous monitoring and reassessment are required to determine if these goals are appropriate for an individual patient.

ABBREVIATIONS

ABW: actual body weight

ALB: albumin

BIA: bioelectrical impedance analysis

BMI: body mass index

DCH: delayed cutaneous hypersensitivity

DRI: dietary reference intake

DXA: dual-energy x-ray absorptiometry

IBW: ideal body weight

LBM: lean body mass

MREE: measured resting energy expenditure

NCHS: National Center for Health Statistics

RDA: recommended dietary allowance

REE: resting energy expenditure

RQ: respiratory quotient

TBW: total body water

TFN: transferrin

UBW: usual body weight

V_{CO_2}: carbon dioxide production

V_{O_2}: oxygen consumption

REFERENCES

1. Kotler DP. Cachexia. Ann Intern Med 2000;133:622–634.
2. Ogden CL, Carroll MD, Curtin LR, et al. Prevalence of overweight and obesity in the United States, 1999–2004. JAMA 2006;295:1459–1555.
3. Ogden CL, Flegal KM, Carroll MD, Johnson CL. Prevalence and trends in overweight among US children and adolescents, 1999–2000. JAMA 2002;288:1728–1732.
4. Centers for Disease Control and Prevention, National Center for Health Statistics. CDC growth charts: United States, 2000. *http://www.cdc.gov/growthcharts/*.
5. ASPEN Board of Directors and the Clinical Guidelines Task Force. Guidelines for the use of parenteral and enteral nutrition in adult and pediatric patients. JPEN J Parenter Enteral Nutr 2002;26 (suppl 1):1SA-138SA.
6. Kondrup J, Allison SP, Elia M, et al. ESPEN guidelines for nutrition screening 2002. Clin Nutr 2003;22:415–421.
7. Kovacevich DS, Boney AR, Braunschweig CL, et al. Nutrition risk classification: A reproducible and valid tool for nurses. Nutr Clin Pract 1997;12:20–25.
8. Russell MK, Mueller C. Nutrition screening and assessment. In: Gottschlich MM, ed. The A.S.P.E.N. Nutrition Support Core Curriculum: A Case-Based Approach—The Adult Patient. Silver Spring, MD: America Society for Parenteral and Enteral Nutrition, 2007:163–186.
9. Joint Commission on Accreditation of Healthcare Organizations. Comprehensive Accreditation Manual for Hospitals: The Official Handbook, 2006. Oakbrook Terrace, IL: Joint Commission Resources, 2006.

10. Barbosa-Silva MCG, Barros AJD. Indications and limitations of the use of subjective global assessment in clinical practice: An update. Curr Opin Clin Nutr Metab Care 2006;9:263–269.
11. Hudgens J, Langkamp-Henken B. The mini nutritional assessment as an assessment tool in elders in long-term care. Nutr Clin Pract 2004;19:463–470.
12. Bell KL, Davies PS. Prediction of height from knee height in children with cerebral palsy and non-disabled children. Ann Hum Biol 2006; 33:493–499.
13. Chumlea WC, Guo SS, Steinbaugh ML. Prediction of stature from knee height for black and white adults and children with application to mobility-impaired or handicapped persons. J Am Diet Assoc 1994;94:1385–1388.
14. Guo SS, Roche AF, Chumlea WC, et al. Growth in weight, recumbent length, and head circumference for preterm low-birthweight infants during the first three years of life using gestation-adjusted ages. Early Hum Dev 1997;47:305–325.
15. Ehrenkranz RA, Younes N, Lemons JA, et al. Longitudinal growth of hospitalized very low birth weight infants. Pediatrics 1999;104:280–289.
16. Cronk C, Crocker AC, Pueschel SM, et al. Growth charts for children with Down syndrome: 1 month to 18 years of age. Pediatrics 1988;81:102–110.
17. World Health Organization. Obesity: Preventing and managing the global epidemic. WHO Technical Report Series, no. 894. Geneva: WHO, 1998.
18. Cook Z, Kirk S, Lawrenson S, Sandford S. Use of BMI in the assessment of undernutrition in older subjects: Reflecting on practice. Proc Nutr Soc 2005;64:313–317.
19. Dickey RA, Baluska DG, Bray GW, et al. AACE/ACE Position Statement on the Prevention, Diagnosis, and Treatment of Obesity, 1998 revision. *http://www.aace.com/clin/guidelines/obesityguide.pdf*.
20. Buchholz AC, Bartok C, Schoeller DA. The validity of bioelectrical impedance models in clinical populations. Nutr Clin Pract 2004;19:433–446.
21. Willett K, Jiang R, Lenart E, et al. Comparison of bioelectrical impedance and BMI in predicting obesity-related medical conditions. Obesity (Silver Spring) 2006;14:480–490.
22. Russell MK, McAdams MP. Laboratory monitoring of nutritional status. In: Matarese LE, Gottschlich MM. Contemporary Nutrition Support Practice: A Clinical Guide. Philadelphia: WB Saunders, 1998:47–63.
23. Erstad BL, Campbell DJ, Rollins CJ, Rappaport WD. Albumin and prealbumin concentrations in patients receiving postoperative parenteral nutrition. Pharmacotherapy 1994;14:458–462.
24. Chandra RK, Sarchielli P. Nutritional status and immune response. Clin Lab Med 1993;13:455–461.
25. Grimble RF. Immunonutrition. Curr Opin Gastroenterol 2006;21:216–222.
26. Kudsk KA. Immunonutrition in surgery and critical care. Annu Rev Nutr 2006;26:463–479.
27. Boosalis, MG. Micronutrients. In: Gottschlich MM, ed. The Science and Practice of Nutrition Support: A Case-Based Core Curriculum, America Society for Parenteral and Enteral Nutrition. Dubuque, IA: Kendall/Hunt, 2001:85–106.
28. Shenkin A. Micronutrients. In: Rombeau JL, Rolandelli RH, eds. Clinical Nutrition: Enteral and Tube Feeding, 3rd ed. Philadelphia: WB Saunders, 1997:96–111.
29. Weber CW, Nelson GW, Vasquez-de-Vaquera M, et al. Trace elements in the hair of healthy and malnourished children. J Trop Pediatr 1990;36:230–234.
30. Tamura H, Hirose S, Watanabe O, et al. Anemia and neutropenia due to copper deficiency in enteral nutrition. JPEN J Parenter Enteral Nutr 1994;18:185–189.
31. Hurwitz M, Garcia MG, Poole RL, Kerner JA. Copper deficiency during parenteral nutrition: A report of four pediatric cases. Nutr Clin Pract 2004;19:305–308.
32. Stoeker BJ. Chromium. In: Ziegler EE, Filer LJ, eds. Present Knowledge in Nutrition, 7th ed. Washington, DC: ILSI Press, 1996:344–352.
33. Verhage AH, Cheong WK, Jeejeebhoy KN. Neurologic symptoms due to possible chromium deficiency in long-term parenteral nutrition that closely mimic metronidazole-induced syndromes. JPEN J Parenter Enteral Nutr 1996;20:123–127.
34. Dickerson RN. Manganese intoxication and parenteral nutrition. Nutrition 2001;17:689–693.
35. Iinuma Y, Kubota M, Uchiyama M, et al. Whole-blood manganese levels and brain manganese accumulation in children receiving long-term home parenteral nutrition. Pediatr Surg Int 2003;19:268–272.
36. Keen CL, Zidenbery-Cherr S, Lonnerdal B. Nutritional and toxicological aspects of manganese intake: An overview. In: Mertz W, Abernathy CO, Olin SS, eds. Risk Assessment of Essential Elements. Washington, DC: ILSI Press, 1994:221–235.
37. Siepler JK, Nishikawa RA, Diamantidis T, et al. Asymptomatic hypermagnesemia in long-term home parenteral nutrition patients. Nutr Clin Pract 2003;18:370–373.
38. Bertinet DB, Tinivella M, Balzola FA, et al. Brain manganese deposition and blood levels in patients undergoing home parenteral nutrition. JPEN J Parenter Enteral Nutr 2000;24:223–227.
39. Abrams CK, Siram SM, Galsim C, et al. Selenium deficiency in long-term total parenteral nutrition. Nutr Clin Pract 1992;7:175–178.
40. Lockitch G, Jacobson B, Quigley G, et al. Selenium deficiency in low birth weight neonates: An unrecognized problem. J Pediatr 1989;114:865–870.
41. Rannem T, Ladefoged K, Hylander E, et al. The effect of selenium supplementation on skeletal and cardiac muscle in selenium-depleted patients. JPEN J Parenter Enteral Nutr 1995;19:351–355.
42. Levander OA, Burk PF. Selenium. In: Ziegler EE, Filer LJ, eds. Present Knowledge in Nutrition, 7th ed. Washington, DC: ILSI Press, 1996:320–328.
43. Geoghegan M, McAuley D, Eaton S, Powell-Tuck J. Selenium in critical illness. Curr Opin Crit Care 2006;12:136–141.
44. Friel JK, MacDonald AC, Mercer CN, et al. Molybdenum requirements in low-birth-weight infants receiving parenteral and enteral nutrition. JPEN J Parenter Enteral Nutr 1999;23:155–159.
45. Sardesai VM. Molybdenum: An essential trace element. Nutr Clin Pract 1993;8:277–281.
46. Nichoalds GE. Iodine. In: Baumgartner TG, ed. Clinical Guide to Parenteral Micronutrition, 3d ed. Deerfield, IL: Fujisawa USA, 1997:361–374.
47. Moukarzel AA, Buchman AL, Salas JS, et al. Iodine supplementation in children receiving long-term parenteral nutrition. J Pediatr 1992;121:252–254.
48. Clark SF. Vitamins and trace elements. In: Gottschlich MM, ed. The A.S.P.E.N. Nutrition Support Core Curriculum: A Case-Based Approach—The Adult Patient. Silver Spring, MD: America Society for Parenteral and Enteral Nutrition, 2007:129–162.
49. Centers for Disease Control and Prevention. Lactic acidosis traced to thiamin deficiency related to nationwide shortage of multivitamins for total parenteral nutrition—United States, 1997. JAMA 1997;278:109–111.
50. Gartner LM, Greer FR, Section on Breastfeeding and Committee on Nutrition, American Academy of Pediatrics. Prevention of rickets and vitamin D deficiency: New guidelines for vitamin D intake. Pediatrics 2003;111:908–910.
51. Lyman D. Undiagnosed vitamin D deficiency in the hospitalized patient. Am Fam Physician 2005;71:299–304.
52. Liu BA, Gordon M, Labranche JM, et al. Seasonal prevalence of vitamin D deficiency institutionalized older adults. J Am Geriatr Soc 1997;45:598–603.
53. Melhus H, Michaëlsson K, Kindmark A, et al. Excessive dietary intake of vitamin A is associated with reduced bone mineral density and increased risk for hip fracture. Ann Intern Med 1998;129:770–778.
54. Peskanich D, Singh V, Willett WC, Colditz GA. Vitamin A intake and hip fractures among postmenopausal women. JAMA 2002;287:47–54.
55. Michaëlsson K, Lithell H, Vessby B, Melhus H. Serum retinol levels and the risk of fracture. N Engl J Med 2003;348:287–294.
56. Willett WC, Stampfer MJ. What vitamins should I be taking, doctor? N Engl J Med 2001;345:1819–1824.
57. The Heart Outcomes Prevention Evaluation (HOPE) 2 Investigators. Homocysteine lowering with folic acid and B vitamins in vascular disease. N Engl J Med 2006;354:1567–1577.
58. Lange H, Suryapranata H, De Luca G, et al. Folate therapy and in-stent restenosis after coronary stenting. N Engl J Med 2004;350:2673–2681.
59. Adolph M, Hailer S, Echart J. Serum phospholipid fatty acids in severely injured patients on total parenteral nutrition with medium chain/long chain triglyceride emulsions. Ann Nutr Metab 1995;39:251–260.
60. Wooley JA, Frankenfield D. Energy. In: Gottschlich MM, ed. The A.S.P.E.N. Nutrition Support Core Curriculum: A Case-Based Approach—The Adult Patient. Silver Spring, MD: America Society for Parenteral and Enteral Nutrition, 2007:19–32.
61. Foote KD, MacKinnon MJ, Innis SM. Effect of early introduction of formula versus fat-free parenteral nutrition on essential fatty acid status of preterm infants. Am J Clin Nutr 1991;54:93–97.

62. Tibboel D, Delemarre FMC, Przyrembel H, et al. Carnitine deficiency in surgical neonates receiving total parenteral nutrition. J Pediatr Surg 1990;25:418–421.
63. Borum PR. Carnitine. In: Baumgartner TG, ed. Clinical Guide to Parenteral Micronutrition, 3rd ed. Deerfield, IL: Fujisawa USA, 1997:629–641.
64. Scaglia F. Carnitine deficiencies. EMedicine.com, Inc. July 26, 2006, *http://www.emedicine.com/ped/topic321.htm*.
65. Cerra FB, Benitez MR, Blackburn GL, et al. Applied nutrition in ICU patients: A consensus statement of the American College of Chest Physicians. Chest 1997;111:769–778.
66. Kalfarentzos F, Spiliotis J, Velimezis G, et al. Comparison of forearm muscle dynamometry with nutritional prognostic index, as a preoperative indicator in cancer patients. JPEN J Parenter Enteral Nutr 1989;13:34–36.
67. Kerr A, Syddall HE, Cooper C, et al. Does admission grip strength predict length of stay in hospitalized older patients? Age Ageing 2006;35:82–84.
68. Genton L, Hans D, Kyle UG, Pichard C. Dual-energy x-ray absorptiometry and body composition: Difference between devices and comparison with reference models. Nutrition 2002;18:66–70.
69. King S, Wilson J, Kotsimbos T, Bailey M, Nyulasi I. Body composition assessment in adults with cystic fibrosis: Comparison of dual-energy x-ray absorptiometry with skinfolds and bioelectrical impedance analysis. Nutrition 2005;21:1087–1094.
70. Liu LF, Roberts R, Moyer-Mileur L, Samson-Fang L. Determination of body composition in children with cerebral palsy: Bioelectrical impedance analysis and anthropometry vs dual-energy x-ray absorptiometry. J Am Diet Assoc 2005;105:794–797.
71. Steiner MC, Barton RL, Singh SJ, Morgan MDL. Bedside methods versus dual energy x-ray absorptiometry for body composition measurement in COPD. Eur Respir J 2002;19:626–631.
72. Food and Nutrition Board, Institute of Medicine, National Academy of Sciences. Dietary Reference Intakes (DRIs): Recommended Intakes for Individuals, 2004. *http://www.iom.edu/Object.File/Master/21/372/0.pdf*.
73. Food and Nutrition Board, Institute of Medicine, National Academy of Sciences. Dietary Reference Intakes for Energy, Carbohydrate, Fiber, Fat, Fatty Acids, Cholesterol, Protein, and Amino Acids, 2005. *http://www.nap.edu/books/0309085373/html/R2.html*.
74. Skipper A, Tupesis N. Is there a role for nonprotein calories in developing and evaluating the nutrient prescription? Nutr Clin Pract 2005;20:321–324.
75. World Health Organization. Energy and Protein Requirements. WHO Technical Report Series No. 724. Geneva: World Health Organization, 1985.
76. Dimand RJ. Parenteral nutrition in the critically ill infant and child. In: Baker RD, Baker SS, Davis AM, eds. Pediatric Parenteral Nutrition. New York: Chapman & Hall, 1997:273–300.
77. Malone AM. Methods of assessing energy expenditure in the intensive care unit. Nutr Clin Pract 2002;17:21–28.
78. Moreira de Rocha EE, Alves VGF, da Fonseca RBV. Indirect calorimetry: Methodology, instruments and clinical application. Curr Opin Clin Nutr Metab Care 2006;9:247–256.
79. Holdy KE. Monitoring energy metabolism with indirect calorimetry: Instruments, interpretation, and clinical application. Nutr Clin Pract 2004;19:447–454.
80. Rubenbauer JR, Johannsen DL, Baier SM, Litchfield R, Flakoll PJ. The use of a handheld calorimetry unit to estimate energy expenditure during different physiological conditions. JPEN J Parenter Enteral Nutr 2006;30:246–250.
81. McGee M, Binkley J, Jensen GL. Geriatric nutrition. In: Gottschlich MM, ed. The Science and Practice of Nutrition Support: A Case-Based Core Curriculum, America Society for Parenteral and Enteral Nutrition. Dubuque, IA: Kendall/Hunt, 2001:373–389.
82. Velasco N, Long CL, Otto DA, et al. Comparison of three methods for the estimation of total nitrogen losses in hospitalized patients. JPEN J Parenter Enteral Nutr 1990;14:517–522.
83. Marlett JA, McBurney MI, Slavin JL, American Dietetic Association. Position of the American Dietetic Association: Health implications of dietary fiber. J Am Diet Assoc 2002;102:993–1000.
84. Dwyer JT. Dietary fiber for children: How much? Pediatr 1995;96:1019–1022.
85. Greene HL, Hambidge KM, Schanler R, Tsang RC. Guidelines for the use of vitamins, trace elements, calcium, magnesium, and phosphorus in infants and children receiving total parenteral nutrition: Report of the Subcommittee on Pediatric Parenteral Nutrient Requirements from the Committee on Clinical Practice Issues of the American Society for Clinical Nutrition. Am J Clin Nutr 1988;48:1324–1342.
86. Kraft MD, Btaiche IF, Sacks GS. Review of the refeeding syndrome. Nutr Clin Pract 2005;20:625–633.
87. Jefferson JW. Drug and diet interactions: Avoiding therapeutic paralysis. J Clin Psychiatry 1998;59:31–39.
88. Saito M, Hirata-Koizumi M, Matsumoto M, et al. Undesirable effects of citrus juice on the pharmacokinetics of drugs: Focus on recent studies. Drug Saf 2005;28:677–694.
89. Santos CA, Boullata JI. An approach to evaluating drug-nutrient interactions. Pharmacotherapy 2005;25:1789–1800.
90. Singh BN. Effects of food on clinical pharmacokinetics. Clin Pharmacokinet 1999;37:213–255.
91. McCabe BJ. Prevention of food–drug interactions with special emphasis on older adults. Curr Opin Clin Nutr Metab Care 2004;7:21–26.

CHAPTER 144 Prevalence and Significance of Malnutrition

GORDON SACKS AND CATHERINE M. CRILL

KEY CONCEPTS

1. Weight loss is a hallmark sign of malnutrition in the cancer patient and correlates with decreased survival for some cancer types.
2. Nutritional problems in human immunodeficiency virus/acquired immunodeficiency syndrome (HIV/AIDS) patients have shifted from complications of severe wasting to metabolic changes associated with subcutaneous fat atrophy, visceral fat accumulation, hypertriglyceridemia, and insulin resistance.
3. Immune function, growth, and survival can be improved in HIV-positive children with aggressive nutritional and antiviral therapy.
4. Enteral nutrition (EN) decreases septic complications when compared with parenteral nutrition (PN) in severely injured trauma patients.
5. EN promotes remission in the majority of patients with acute Crohn's disease.
6. Adults with less than 60 cm remaining of small bowel after massive surgery will require PN for months to years.
7. EN supplemented with immune-enhancing nutrients lowers metabolic and infectious complications in adult surgical patients.
8. Maintaining adequate nutrition status contributes to improved outcomes in patients with cystic fibrosis (CF).
9. Optimizing nutritional status of pediatric solid organ transplant patients pre- and posttransplantation can improve outcomes and reduce morbidity.
10. Malnutrition is associated with increased use of healthcare resources and nutritional interventions can contribute to cost savings by reducing length of hospital stay and morbidity associated with malnutrition.

The term malnutrition has been used to characterize a broad range of altered nutritional states. Overnutrition is the term used to describe excess nutrient intake, whereas undernutrition is used to describe insufficient intake or substrate use. Both of these nutritional states can contribute to the poor outcome of many disease states. Unless specifically stated otherwise, in this chapter malnutrition is considered to be synonymous with undernutrition (refer to Chap. 148 for a discussion on overnutrition/obesity). In children, malnutrition is defined by a variety of criteria. Stages (e.g., Waterlow stages) were developed to define the severity of protein-energy malnutrition. Anthropometric evaluations, using established age-based growth curves, can also be used to define acute and chronic malnutrition using either Z scores or height and weight percentiles. In general, malnutrition in children is defined as growth that is below the fifth percentile for age or less than 90% to 95% of the median value for age. In this chapter, the prevalence of malnutrition is characterized and the significant impact of abnormalities in nutrition assessment parameters on the morbidity and mortality of adult and pediatric patients with selected disease states is presented. Interventional strategies for the prevention and management of malnutrition are characterized and the economic consequences of malnutrition are also presented.

Learning objectives, review questions, and other resources can be found at **www.pharmacotherapyonline.com.**

PREVALENCE

Although malnutrition occurs throughout the world, it is most prevalent in underdeveloped countries, where food supply, ignorance, poverty, overcrowding, and poor sanitation are contributing factors. The most susceptible individuals in developed and underdeveloped countries are infants (especially premature infants), pregnant or lactating women, and the elderly. The predominant factors that contribute to malnutrition in developed countries include poor maternal nutrition before and during pregnancy, misconceptions about the use of certain foods, fad diets, maternal illiteracy, household poverty, and alcohol or drug abuse. The relationship between malnutrition and breast-feeding is time-dependent. The benefit of breast-feeding during the first 6 months of life in reducing mortality and improving growth is well known and advocated by the American Academy of Pediatrics. Prolonged breast-feeding (beyond 6 months to 1 year), however, has been associated with an increased risk of malnutrition. This association may be a result of the lower use of complementary foods in economically and educationally disadvantaged households, rather than breast-feeding per se.[1]

Malnutrition in adults is associated most commonly with exacerbations of chronic disease or an onset of an acute illness and thus is quite prevalent in the hospital setting. Recognition of the scope of the problem coincides with the systematic application of nutrition assessment techniques to hospitalized individuals in the last three decades. The heightened awareness of nutritional disease and better in-hospital nutrition management since the mid-1970s has contributed to a decline in its prevalence.[2] The prevalence of previously unrecognized malnutrition in hospitalized adult patients from varying socioeconomic backgrounds is still high and ranges from 40% to 55% in a variety of institutions.[3] Worldwide, approximately 200 million children are moderately to severely underweight, while 70 million are severely malnourished.[4] The overwhelming majority of these children live in South Asia or sub-Saharan Africa.[5] More than one-half of global childhood deaths of children younger than 5 years of age is attributable—directly or indirectly—to malnutrition.[6,7] Chronic malnutrition in children younger than 2 years of age is an independent predictor of poor cognitive development lasting up to 11 years of age.[8] Severe malnutrition is both a medical and social disorder and successful management requires attention to both of these factors. The first of the United Nations' Millennium Development Goals, drafted in 2002, was to halve the number of people suffering from hunger.[6] Fortunately, the global trend indicates a modest but consistent decline in malnutrition-associated mortality in children younger than 5 years of age.[9]

Because children have both limited body stores and high metabolic demands, they are at particular risk for developing malnutrition, especially during illness. Although the majority of undernourished children are from underdeveloped countries, malnutrition is also prevalent in the United States and other industrial countries. In 1974, a publicly funded health and nutrition program known as the Pediatric Nutrition Surveillance System was established to generate data on the prevalence of malnutrition in low-income U.S. children (<5 years of age). Several advances were observed during the period of 1995 through 2004, most notably a decrease in high birth weight and anemia and an increase in the percentage of infants ever breastfed and those breastfed for at least 6 months.[10] Prevalence of short stature (height for age) and low birth weight remained stable. The prevalence of underweight status of 4.7%, which is lower than the expected value of 5%, suggests that the prevalence of acute malnutrition in this population is low. The prevalence of overweight children, however, increased from 11% in 1995 to 14.8% in 2004. The focus on malnutrition has now been shifted to the prevention and treatment of childhood obesity, which has reached epidemic proportions (see Chap. 148).

Children with chronic disease and those in periods of rapid growth have the highest prevalence of malnutrition. Hendricks et al. characterized the change in prevalence of protein-energy malnutrition in hospitalized children over a 15-year period.[11] Overall prevalence was high, but significant reductions were detected in acute malnutrition (weight for height <90% of median) from 33.6% to 24.5%, and chronic malnutrition (weight for height <95% of median) from 46.8% in 1976 to 27.3% in the 1990s.

PHYSIOLOGIC RESPONSE TO STARVATION

During the first few days of starvation, hepatic glycogen stores are used for energy and skeletal muscle proteolysis provides amino acids as a source for new glucose production (i.e., gluconeogenesis) creating fuel substrates for glucose-dependent tissues, such as the brain, renal medulla, and red blood cells. When glycogen stores are depleted, skeletal muscle is scavenged for amino acids and fatty acids are mobilized from adipose tissue. With prolonged starvation (i.e., >5 days), metabolic pathways shift to derive energy from ketone production (i.e., β-hydroxybutyrate and acetoacetate) as a result of free fatty acid oxidation while sparing protein mobilization from skeletal muscle. Protein conservation is evidenced clinically by a reduction in urinary urea nitrogen from a normal value of 12 g/day to 3 to 5 g/day by 5 to 6 weeks.[12] Inadequate nutrient intake is accompanied by reductions in basal metabolic rate and the synthetic capacity of the liver. Endocrine adaptive functions occur in response to severe energy and protein deficiencies, including a decline in insulin secretion and increases in glucagon and epinephrine concentrations.

The outcome of prolonged malnutrition is an inappropriate reduction in lean body mass resulting in alterations in the function of essentially every organ. The clinical significance of the effect will depend on the specific anatomic structure or system and on the degree of malnutrition. For example, with mild malnutrition, loss of skeletal muscle mass may be apparent as weakness or a decreased level of physical activity. However, alterations in cardiac function, circulatory failure and decreased cardiac output which usually are only seen in advanced malnutrition and can result in impaired renal plasma flow and glomerular filtration rates. Major defects in T-lymphocyte function and the complement system result from atrophy of the thymus gland. Ultimately, the malnourished patient becomes more susceptible to infections (Table 144–1). Until recently, the effect of early malnutrition (fetal and neonatal) on organ and cellular function was only recognized in terms of short-term growth and development outcomes. Now it is known that "fetal programming" or "metabolic imprinting" is linked to adult health. Specifically, maternal body composition and dietary balance during pregnancy can influence the risk of adult-onset cardiac disease, type 2 diabetes, and obesity.[9,13,14]

Malnourished patients have an increased likelihood of developing wound infections and the wound healing rates have also been noted to be slower in those with poor nutritional status.[1] Protein is essential for the integrity of the structural components of skin (i.e., collagen) and severe protein deficiency can result in edema secondary to the reduction in circulating proteins, such as albumin.[15] Deficiency of arginine, vitamin C, vitamin A, or zinc also may contribute to decreased wound healing (Table 144–2). Supplemental vitamin A promotes wound healing in animal models in the presence of deficiency, and arginine has improved markers of wound healing (i.e., protein and hydroxyproline in the wound bed) in elderly healthy human volunteers.[16] However, supplementation of these nutrients is

TABLE 144-1 Immune Response Mechanisms in Malnutrition

Parameter	Observation in Malnutrition
Cell-mediated immune response	
Delayed cutaneous hypersensitivity	Decreased
Lymphocyte transformation	Decreased
Polymorphonuclear leukocyte response	
Phagocytosis	Normal or decreased
Metabolism	Decreased
Bactericidal capacity	Decreased
Chemotaxis	Decreased
Total lymphocyte count	Decreased
T cells	
CD4	Decreased
CD8	Decreased
Helper to suppressor ratio	Decreased
Humoral response	
Complement activity (CH50)	Decreased
Secretory immunoglobulin A	Decreased
Serum complement	Decreased or normal
Serum immunoglobulins	Normal
Serum opsonization	Normal

TABLE 144-2 Nutritional Disorders and Wound Healing

Nutritional Disorder	Effect on Wound Healing
Arginine deficiency	Altered collagen formation
Copper deficiency	Impaired lysyl oxidase activity
Protein-energy malnutrition	Decreased wound strength because of reduced hydroxyproline content of wound; decreased rate of wound healing; increased incidence of wound infection
Vitamin C deficiency	Decreased fibroblast maturation with failure of collagen synthesis; decreased angiogenesis
Vitamin A deficiency	Decreased collagen accumulation; formation of abnormal collagen
Zinc deficiency	Impaired DNA and protein synthesis; impaired mitosis and cell proliferation

only recommended in the presence of documented deficiencies as supplementation in nondeficient individuals may actually be harmful. For example, excess vitamin E antagonizes the promotion of wound healing by vitamin A, and excess zinc will displace copper and interfere with lysyl oxidase (the enzyme necessary for collagen cross-link formation). Finally, ingestion of excessive amounts of vitamin A may cause liver damage, hemorrhage, and even coma.[15]

DISEASE-SPECIFIC CONSEQUENCES

Malnutrition seldom exists as an isolated disease state; rather, it is usually found in patients with other preexisting illnesses. Often the primary disease or complications of the disease predispose an individual to the development of malnutrition. The primary factors that enhance the likelihood of developing malnutrition include decreased dietary intake (e.g., as a consequence of nausea, vomiting, or anorexia), malabsorption (e.g., as a result of short-bowel syndrome, severe diarrhea, or high-output fistula), and altered metabolism (hypermetabolic and catabolic states caused by sepsis, trauma, cancer, or AIDS). Malnutrition is also associated with the failure of major organs such as the kidney, liver, heart, and lungs (see Chap. 147).

CANCER

❶ Patients with cancer have many factors that contribute to their increased likelihood of developing malnutrition (Table 144–3). The frequency is highest (>80%) in patients with gastric and pancreatic tumors, and lowest in patients with hematologic malignancies.[17] Unintentional weight loss, a sign of malnutrition, occurs in 30% to 80% of adult cancer patients. A significant relationship between weight loss and reduced survival has been demonstrated for some (lung, prostate, and colon cancer), but not all tumor types.[17] The degree of reduction in median survival is statistically significant for many cancers and ranges from 49% to 79%.

Current clinical practice guidelines state that routine use of enteral and parenteral nutrition (i.e., specialized nutrition support [SNS]) is not indicated in well-nourished or mildly malnourished patients undergoing surgical interventions, chemotherapy, or radiation therapy for neoplastic disease. Use of parenteral nutrition (PN) in this population may actually result in more complications and a poor response to cancer treatment.[18] Specialized nutrition support is indicated in malnourished cancer patients who have a life expectancy of at least 3 to 6 months and who have been unable to ingest and/or absorb adequate nutrients for longer than 7 days.[19] In addition, PN may be of benefit in a select group of patients with inoperable malignant bowel obstruction (i.e., ovarian cancer) who lack significant involvement of vital organs, have a good performance status, and are expected to survive longer than 6 months.[20]

TABLE 144-3 Risk Factors for Malnutrition in Cancer Patients

Risk Factor	Nutrition Consequence
Primary disease	
Tumor type	Weight loss, anorexia, altered taste, altered metabolism
Complicating conditions	
Malabsorption	Impaired absorption of all or selected nutrients, diarrhea
Bowel obstruction	Nausea and vomiting, inability to ingest nutrients orally or by enteral nutrition
Infection	Increased energy expenditure and protein requirements, altered metabolism, anorexia, malabsorption
Psychological response	Anorexia, food aversion
Treatments	
Chemotherapy	Taste and appetite alterations, nausea and vomiting, mucositis, esophagitis, diarrhea, constipation
Surgery	
Radical resection of oropharyngeal region	Problems with chewing and swallowing
Esophageal reconstruction	Gastric stasis and hypochlorhydria secondary to vagotomy; diarrhea and steatorrhea
Gastrectomy	Dumping syndrome, malabsorption, lack of intrinsic factor, hypoglycemia
Intestinal resection	Malabsorption, renal oxalate stones, metabolic acidosis, diarrhea
Pancreatectomy	Malabsorption, diabetes mellitus
Radiation	
Head and neck	Stomatitis, dysgeusia, xerostomia
Abdomen and pelvis	Bowel obstruction, fistulae, radiation enteritis (diarrhea, protein-losing enteropathy, malabsorption)

Malnutrition in children with cancer is common, and the prevalence is greater in those with Ewing sarcoma and neuroblastoma, than in those with leukemias and lymphomas.[21,22] While undernutrition has historically been an independent prognostic factor in the long-term outcome of children with certain cancers, not all researchers agree and it remains an area of continued research.[23–25] Although advancements in cancer treatment strategies have greatly improved outcomes for children, many of the complications of treatment protocols, including surgery, combination chemotherapy, and radiation therapy, are associated with an increased prevalence of malnutrition.[19,26] Theoretically, early recognition and aggressive management of malnutrition may minimize the nutritional consequences, improve tumor response, reduce side effects of therapy, and improve survival. Indeed cancer patients treated with bone marrow transplantation have shown improved tumor response and clinical outcome with PN compared with those who were not receiving PN.[27] Of note, survivors of childhood acute lymphoblastic leukemia, particularly those who received cranial irradiation therapy, are at increased risk for obesity later in life.[28]

Improved nutrition status enhances survival and improves treatment tolerance in many but not all children.[26,29] Malnutrition as a consequence of simple starvation, characterized by normal metabolism but inadequate nutrient intake or malabsorption, appears to be more responsive to nutrition intervention[30] than malnutrition as a result of cancer cachexia, which is characterized by altered nutrient use despite adequate supply.[31,32]

CLINICAL CONTROVERSY

The goal of enteral nutrition (EN) and PN support in patients with cancer is to prevent or reverse protein-calorie malnutrition and cancer cachexia. In terminally ill children and adults, the use of EN and PN is controversial. Some clinicians believe their use is warranted in these patients only if an improved quality of life can be attained.

AIDS

❷ Generalized wasting and malnutrition were common characteristics of HIV/AIDS during the early years of this epidemic. In many patients, weight loss and wasting were often the earliest symptoms, along with opportunistic infection. Malnutrition was often progressive and contributed to death in some patients.[19,33] Poor nutrition status as indicated by weight loss and decreased serum prealbumin concentrations has been shown to be a predictor of mortality in adult AIDS patients.[34,35] Furthermore, simultaneous micronutrient deficiencies such as vitamin A, vitamin B_{12}, zinc, and selenium are significantly associated with HIV-related mortality, independent of CD4 counts and changes in CD4 over time. When the individual effect of these micronutrient deficiencies is further delineated, selenium deficiency was found to be the only independent predictor of HIV-related prognosis.[35] Recently, nutritional problems have shifted from the characteristic lethal wasting associated with opportunistic infections to a syndrome of subcutaneous fat atrophy (lipoatrophy), fat accumulation (lipohypertrophy) in the abdomen or over the back of the neck ("buffalo hump"), hypertriglyceridemia, and insulin resistance.[36] The etiology is unclear but appears to be associated with both protease inhibitor and nucleoside analog therapy, particularly when these drugs are combined.[37] The implications of these metabolic and body compositional changes on outcome and development of comorbidities (i.e., atherosclerosis) are unclear at this time.

❸ Most HIV-positive children will experience nutritional deficits and growth abnormalities.[38] Infants with perinatal-acquired HIV have normal birth weights, but show signs of growth delay as early as 4 months.[39] Failure to thrive is reported in up to 33% of HIV-infected children.[40] Impaired linear growth also appears to correlate with periods of rapid viral replication and lower CD4 T-lymphocyte counts during the first 18 months of life.[41,42] There is a direct relationship between these growth abnormalities and morbidity and mortality.[38] Prior to the use of highly active antiretroviral therapy, EN rehabilitation increased CD4 count and body weight in children with AIDS.[44] Fortunately, immune function, growth velocity, and survival can be improved markedly if aggressive nutritional therapy and antiviral therapy are initiated.[38]

The response to nutrition intervention in adults with AIDS is variable. Supplemental dietary intake of selected micronutrients is associated with a reduction in mortality in HIV-1 seropositive homosexual/bisexual men. High intakes of B-group vitamins (B_1, B_6, and niacin) and β-carotene are associated with improved survival, whereas an increased intake of zinc is associated with worse survival.[45] Cyanocobalamin (vitamin B_{12}) deficiency is common among HIV patients and is associated with neurologic changes, peripheral neuropathy, and decreased performance in problem-solving skills. Whether the deficiency is a result of malabsorption or protease inhibitor therapy, yearly determinations of serum cyanocobalamin are recommended and cyanocobalamin parenteral therapy should be initiated for those with serum concentrations <350 pg/mL.[46] In the presence of persistent weight loss, nutritional counseling with oral supplements may improve caloric intake and lean body mass.[47] If weight loss persists despite aggressive dietary oral intake, EN via a feeding tube can be attempted. Lean body mass repletion in AIDS patients with weight loss and inadequate food intake has been reported when EN was the sole source of nutrient intake.[47] Kotler et al. compared the effects of PN and an oral semielemental diet on body weight, body composition, survival, quality of life, and medical costs in AIDS outpatients with malabsorption syndromes.[48] At the end of 3 months, the PN group gained more weight and significantly more fat, but body cell mass measurements and survival did not differ between the groups. However, the group receiving an oral diet scored significantly better on the quality-of-life physical-functioning subscale. The most dramatic differences were in medical costs, with a fourfold cost increase in patients receiving PN versus oral diet therapy.[49]

With earlier diagnosis and initiation of treatment for HIV-positive status prior to the full development of AIDS, the prevalence of malnutrition may ultimately decline. New treatment modalities for AIDS are also being developed that may affect the prevalence of malnutrition and the response to nutrition intervention in this patient population. For example, 12 weeks of recombinant human growth hormone treatment was evaluated in 178 HIV-infected patients with unintentional weight loss of ≥10%. In this trial, growth hormone administration resulted in a mean increase of 3 kg of lean body mass with a decrease of about 1.7 kg of body fat. These changes in body composition were accompanied by an improvement in functional performance, reflected by treadmill work output.[50] However, concerns regarding the development of hyperglycemia and diabetes associated with long-term use of growth hormone have tempered its use. Other agents, including thalidomide,[51] testosterone,[52] nandrolone decanoate,[53] and oxandrolone,[54] also show promise in reversing cachexia associated with AIDS.

CRITICAL ILLNESS, TRAUMA, AND BURN INJURY

Trauma, burn injury, and sepsis are all catalysts for the release of mediators that initiate and regulate the hypermetabolic response. The metabolic consequences of this response include altered carbohydrate metabolism, increased protein synthesis and degradation, and increased lipid oxidation, which ultimately result in net loss of protein and lean body mass.[55] In a previously well-nourished individual, critical illness can result in the onset of kwashiorkor-like malnutrition within 5 to 7 days, whereas in a previously malnourished individual, critical illness can precipitate severe mixed marasmus-kwashiorkor within 3 to 5 days. In a prospective study of 129 adult patients admitted to the intensive care unit, 43% were malnourished.[49] Malnourished patients had an increased length of stay in the intensive care unit (a mean of 27 vs. 19 days) and a statistically significantly increased incidence of complications (55% vs. 40%) compared with well-nourished patients with a similar severity of illness.

❹ The goal of nutrition support in critically ill patients is to prevent the development of or worsening of malnutrition as positive patient outcomes such as better tissue repair and organ function may be improved when SNS is initiated for these patients.[55] EN initiated within 24 to 48 hours of injury may attenuate the hypermetabolic response.[57] EN also results in fewer septic complications than does PN.[58] Three meta-analyses suggest that critically ill patients derive the greatest benefit when enterally fed an immune-enhanced formula that contains pharmacologic doses of immune-modulating nutrients such as arginine, glutamine, nucleic acids, and omega-3 fatty acids.[59–61] Supplementation of micronutrients, such as zinc and selenium, early in the recovery phase of burn and traumatic injuries also improves outcomes. Clinical benefits are most likely linked to enhancement of antioxidant defense mechanisms and immunity.[62]

During critical illness in the pediatric population, the catabolic response limits the capacity for somatic growth.[19,63,64] To avoid overfeeding during acute illness, the American Society for Parenteral and Enteral Nutrition (ASPEN) recommends that requirements for growth (i.e., caloric provision above measured or predicted energy requirements) not be included in daily caloric provision.[19]

INFLAMMATORY BOWEL DISEASE

Malnutrition has been reported in 20% to 85% of patients with inflammatory bowel disease: malabsorption, increased gastrointestinal losses, and poor oral intake are the predominant causes of malnutrition. The risks are not the same with all diseases in this category as evidenced by the findings that the nutrition consequences in patients with ulcerative colitis tend to be less severe than those with Crohn's disease.[65] Decreased food intake may be a result of pain, anorexia, or altered taste; malabsorption may be caused by mucosal abnormalities, bacterial overgrowth, or diminished absorptive surface area after surgical resection of diseased bowel; and hypermetabolism may be a consequence of fever and infection. Various nutrient abnormalities, such as anemia, metabolic bone disease, and vitamin and trace mineral deficiencies, have been observed in inflammatory bowel disease patients.[65] Growth failure, characterized by retarded skeletal maturation and delayed development of secondary sex characteristics, occurs in as many as 35% of children with Crohn's disease and up to 10% of children with ulcerative colitis.[66,67]

❺ Specialized nutrition support, including both EN and PN, has been used in the past as supportive and primary treatment modalities. Use of supportive SNS has been directed at reversing nutritional deficiencies associated with Crohn's disease. Enteral nutrition as a primary therapy has been investigated in limited clinical trials and via meta-analyses of available data. The results have consistently shown that conventional corticosteroids are more effective than exclusive use of a liquid diet, either orally or enterally, in the treatment of active Crohn's disease.[68] The response rate to standard EN was, however, greater than the 18% to 42% placebo-response rate observed in many controlled clinical trials. Although the reasons for the therapeutic effects of EN are not well understood, it seems unlikely that the mechanism is merely the consequence of nutrition repletion. Proposed hypotheses include alteration in intestinal microbial flora, elimination of dietary antigen uptake, and reduction of intestinal synthesis of inflammatory mediators.[68] A unique oral nutrient supplement combining omega-3 fatty acids and fructooligosaccharides when given to patients with mild to moderate ulcerative colitis for 6 months has been shown to be associated with a significant decrease in the dose of prednisone required to control clinical symptoms as compared with a placebo group.[69] As a result some clinicians now believe that dietary manipulation may not only interrupt the inflammatory process but also serve as a useful adjunct in the management of patients with active inflammatory bowel disease.

In addition, EN therapy has been shown to improve linear growth and mucosal healing in pediatric patients with Crohn's disease and to induce response rates of 50% to 60% in those with active Crohn's disease.[19,68] Although SNS may be used to maintain weight and nutrition status in patients with ulcerative colitis, it has not been shown to induce or maintain remission.

CHRONIC INTESTINAL PSEUDOOBSTRUCTION

The patient with pseudoobstruction, a hypomotility or dysmotility disorder of the gastrointestinal tract that is thought to be a neuromuscular disorder of the smooth muscle and/or its innervation, often presents with symptoms indistinguishable from those associated with a bowel obstruction. Prolonged dysmotility can result in malnutrition, as well as growth failure, in children.[70] Primary factors contributing to a risk of malnutrition are anorexia, nausea, vomiting, and obstruction, which may recur over years. Approximately 15% to 30% of patients with pseudoobstruction require SNS with either PN or EN.[70]

SHORT-BOWEL SYNDROME

Short-bowel syndrome is the result of the surgical resection or disease-associated functional loss of a large portion of the intestinal tract. The degree of nutrition impairment depends on the amount and location of excised bowel. Malabsorption is present to some extent immediately following surgery and may be permanent. Bowel adaptation will occur over time (up to 1 to 2 years), but may not result in restoration of the full absorptive capacity of the intestine.[19,71] Intestinal adaptation occurs more frequently in children than in adults.[72] Two institutions reported longitudinal experience with intestinal adaptation in infants and children with short-bowel syndrome.[73,74] Premature infants may have the best adaptive response to short-bowel syndrome due to rapid intestinal growth during late gestation, when the jejunum, ileum, and colon more than double in length.[75] For this reason, the use of a percentage of expected small-bowel length, rather than absolute remnant length, for assessing the ability for adaptation and successful wean from PN might be more appropriate in infants with short-bowel syndrome.[73]

❻ Adults who have 600 to 700 cm of ileum remaining after surgical resection (i.e., 100 to 200 cm of ileum resected) require vitamin B_{12}, calcium, and magnesium supplementation. Massive resection of the small bowel, leaving less than 60 cm in adults and less than 10 cm in children, results in severe malabsorption of all nutrients and these patients require total or supplemental PN for months or years postoperatively.[72,76,77] Removal of the colon with the retention of <50 cm of jejunum and ileum may require that patients remain on PN for life.[76] One long-term study of 124 adults with nonmalignant short-bowel syndrome maintained on PN demonstrated that the presence of terminal ileum in continuity with the colon enhanced the probability of weaning from PN and survival.[78] In the absence of SNS, malnutrition is inevitable and can be life-threatening. For those children with intestinal failure resulting from extensive bowel loss or life-threatening complications from prolonged PN, innovative surgical procedures including bowel lengthening, serial transverse enteroplasty, and transplantation (small bowel with or without a liver) can improve the gut's adaptive process and reduce the need for PN.[72,79–81]

SURGICAL PATIENTS

❼ Malnourished patients tend to have a greater risk of postoperative morbidity and mortality than do well-nourished patients. Several nutrition assessment parameters predict morbidity and mortality in surgical patients. In a classic study by Mullen et al., the value of 16 nutritional and immunologic variables was examined and serum concentrations of albumin and transferrin, as well as delayed cutaneous hypersensitivity reactions, were found to be the most reliable predictors of outcome.[82] These factors have been confirmed by several authors to correlate with morbidity and mortality.[83,84] A retrospective study by Kudsk et al.[85] extended these findings by showing that operative site, in addition to the preoperative albumin concentration, was an independent risk factor in predicting clinical outcome: patients who underwent a colectomy and gastrectomy tolerated greater degrees of hypoalbuminemia than did those patients who underwent esophagectomy or pancreatectomy. The subjective global assessment, developed by Detsky et al., is a clinical method that can aid in the recognition of undernutrition by evaluating a patient's nutritional status based on features of the medical history and physical examination.[86] In prospective studies, subjective global assessment was very successful in predicting complications in surgical patients. The use of preoperative PN in patients with malnutrition, particularly when associated with a low serum albumin concentration, reduced the incidence of major postoperative complications in several patient populations.[87] Parenteral nutrition administered solely after surgery is actually associated with an increased incidence of complications in approximately 10% of patients. However, perioperative SNS delivered prior to and following major abdominal or thoracic surgical procedures is beneficial in malnourished patients.[88] In a multiinstitutional Veterans Administration Cooperative Study, 395 malnourished patients were randomly assigned to receive PN administered 1 to 2 weeks before surgery and up to 3 days afterward or no perioperative PN (control group). Differences in mortality at 30 and 90 days were not statistically significant, and there was no significant reduction in complication rate. The incidence of noninfectious complications was higher in those with the greatest degree of malnutrition. In the PN group, the highest incidence of infectious complications was in the borderline or mildly malnourished patients, but severely malnourished PN patients had significantly less noninfectious complications than controls (5% vs. 49%, $P = 0.03$). The investigators concluded that perioperative PN did not result in an improved postoperative course except in patients who were severely malnourished preoperatively. In patients who were mildly to moderately malnourished, the incidence of infectious complications associated with the use of PN outweighed the benefits. As with critically ill patients, EN with immune-enhanced formulas appears to promote the best nutrition and clinical outcome with fewer metabolic and infectious complications for surgical patients.[89]

CYSTIC FIBROSIS

8 The predominant clinical findings of cystic fibrosis (CF) are related to altered pulmonary function and pancreatic exocrine function. Historically, growth retardation and failure to thrive have been classic features of CF. Over the past decade, the nutritional status of children with CF has improved, largely as a result of nutritional interventions aimed at improving pulmonary function and clinical outcome. However, the most recent Patient Registry data from 2004 reported that 15% of children with CF were still below the 5th percentile in height for age and another 15% below the 5th percentile in weight for age.[90]

A longitudinal study confirmed that nutrition and lung function are codependent variables in CF.[91] Other factors that contribute to nutrition disorders associated with CF include an increased energy expenditure, malabsorption, anorexia, gastroesophageal reflux, pharmacotherapy, CF-related diabetes, ineffective pancreatic enzyme supplementation, and inadequate pulmonary toilet.[92] Increased energy requirements in CF patients are the result of the increased amount of work required to breathe and an elevated resting energy expenditure during pulmonary exacerbations. Children with mild to moderate lung disease may be spared from this rise in resting energy expenditure during an acute exacerbation.[93] It is also theorized that the genetic defect that causes CF affects metabolism causing an increase in energy requirements. The physical pounding on the back of the patient while in a partially inverted position (i.e., pulmonary toilet) is designed to loosen the thickened bronchial secretions that impair breathing. It may be performed numerous times throughout the day and may result in an increase in energy expenditure. It also interferes with the feeding schedule, which needs to be designed to ensure that the stomach is empty or nearly empty before the pulmonary toilet process begins, to prevent pulmonary aspiration of stomach contents.

As life expectancy of patients with CF increases, the recognition of CF-associated diseases has also increased. Cystic fibrosis-related diabetes mellitus is now a well-recognized problem and further complicates the nutritional management of these individuals.[94] Altered pancreatic function is common and more than 90% of CF patients need pancreatic enzyme supplementation. Insufficiency of pancreatic enzyme secretion into the intestine reduces the absorption of fat and fat-soluble vitamins. Consequently, more than two-thirds of CF centers in North America use a hydrolyzed (semielemental) enteral formula with low fat content for CF infants. However, the nutrition benefits of this expensive hydrolyzed formula over a conventional cow's milk formula have been challenged.[95,96] Nutritional management typically focuses on the use of oral pancreatic enzymes (e.g., Viokase and Pancrease), supplemental fat-soluble vitamins, and a high-protein, high-calorie diet.[92] If nutrition status cannot be maintained with these measures, supplemental EN or PN may be indicated.

SOLID-ORGAN FAILURE

9 Malnutrition with growth impairment is a well-recognized complication of renal, hepatic, and cardiac failure in children that is associated with an increased risk of morbidity and mortality. Mechanisms responsible for malnutrition include reduced energy intake, increased resting energy rates, and increased total energy expenditure.[97–99] Early clinical onset of organ failure can have profound effects on growth and development, especially in children with end-stage liver disease. Among children diagnosed with hereditary renal disorders, 50% had marked growth retardation (mean age at observation: 10 years).[99] Prevalence of malnutrition in hospitalized children with cardiac disease varies with age and type of cardiac lesion. Seventy-nine percent of infants with heart disease had evidence of acute malnutrition, compared with less than 30% in all other age groups. The prevalence of chronic malnutrition was common in all age groups. An inverse relationship to age was observed with 82%, 84%, 61%, 58%, and 38% of infants, toddlers, preschool children, school-age children, and adolescents, respectively, being malnourished.[100] Children with complex cardiac disease or left-to-right intracardiac shunts had the highest prevalence of both acute and chronic malnutrition (38% to 80%). Catch-up growth in children with chronic renal failure, complex congenital heart lesions, and advanced cirrhosis can be attained with aggressive feeding regimens, including EN.[101] Optimizing nutritional status during the pre- and posttransplantation phase can improve outcomes and reduce morbidity.[102,103] After liver transplantation, catch-up growth can occur, but final height often remains 0.5 to 1 standard deviation below normal.[104]

FAILURE TO THRIVE

Pediatricians have traditionally used the term failure to thrive to characterize children who do not achieve normative weight and height milestones. Geriatricians recently transposed this term to describe elderly patients who fail to maintain their functional status, as reflected by weight loss, declines in physical and cognitive function, and the general appearance of hopelessness.[105] Estimates of undernutrition as high as 65% in residents of long-term care facilities have been noted, compared with a rate of 5% to 15% in community-dwelling persons older than 65 years of age. Factors contributing to this anorexia and weight loss include underlying medical conditions, such as cardiac failure and gastritis, which are associated with decreased oral intake. A variety of medications may interfere with taste and sense of smell, resulting in a lack of appetite. Distortion of a taste sensation has been reported with angiotensin-converting enzyme inhibitors and calcium channel blockers. β-Blockers and the quinolones alter sense of smell in the elderly.[106] Management strategies may include sugarless chewing gum, lozenges, or substituting a different medication in the same therapeutic class. Nutritional intervention is reserved for individuals who are unable to reverse their unintentional weight loss and have a body mass index less than 18 kg/m^2. Commercially available oral supplements successfully improve caloric intake and promote weight gain in undernourished homebound elders. Enteral nutrition administered through a feeding tube should only be considered for older individuals who are unable to orally consume adequate nutrients. Parenteral nutrition is appropriate for older persons with intestinal failure who are undernourished but who have a reasonable expectation of recovery from the underlying problem (e.g., Crohn's disease, bowel obstruction, severe pancreatitis). Enteral or parenteral nutrition used solely for the purpose of postponing death is strongly discouraged. Specialized nutrition support is justified in older individuals with a reasonable duration and quality of life.

Infants and children not meeting expected growth parameters are typically given the diagnosis of failure to thrive. A recent study evaluated the definitions of failure to thrive in the medical literature and found that, consistent with a 1985 Consensus recommendation, the definition of failure to thrive in all of the evaluated sources was based on anthropometrics alone; however, many dissimilarities existed as to which anthropometric parameters were used.[107] Failure to thrive has been suggested to be either organic (medical), nonorganic (psychosocial), or mixed in etiology.[107] There are numerous medical and psychosocial causes of failure to thrive (Table 144–4). ASPEN recommends that the term pediatric undernutrition be used in place of failure to thrive and that the degree of undernutrition be assessed as either moderate or severe.[19] Evaluation should include a thorough patient history, including nutrition, social, and family history, and physical examination to rule out medical causes. To optimize nutrition and improve growth velocity, patients with failure

TABLE 144-4 Causes of Pediatric Undernutrition

Medical	Psychosocial
Prematurity	Family stress
Gastroesophageal reflux disease	Poverty
Feeding difficulty	External demands
Colic	Parental Issues
Orofacial abnormality	Maternal physical and emotional deprivation
Chronic diarrhea	Maternal depression
Excessive juice intake	Beliefs on feeding/nutrition practices
Food allergy	Education level
Gastroenteritis	Mental capacity
Parasitic infection	Emotional disturbance
Malabsorption syndromes	History of drug/alcohol abuse
Gluten sensitivity (celiac disease)	History of childhood abuse/neglect
Lactase deficiency	Child neglect
Milk-protein allergy	Child abuse
Pancreatic enzyme deficiency	
Protein-losing enteropathy	
Delayed introduction of complementary foods	
Cystic fibrosis	
Biliary disease	
Inflammatory bowel disease	
End-organ disease (cardiac, renal, hepatic, pulmonary)	
Endocrine disorder	
Immunodeficiency	
Human immunodeficiency virus/acquired immune deficiency syndrome	
Immunoglobulin deficiency	
Severe combine immunodeficiency	
Inborn errors of metabolism	
Congenital syndromes	
Lead poisoning	
Malignancy	
Anorexia/bulimia	

to thrive should be closely monitored on a designated nutrition plan, with routine assessment of anthropometrics using growth curves.[19]

NEONATES

Regardless of the disease process, pediatric patients, particularly neonates and infants, are at greater risk for nutrition disorders and develop the most severe consequences more frequently. Pharmacologic and technologic advances in neonatal medicine have improved the survival of premature, extremely low birth weight infants (<1,000 g). These premature neonates are at increased risk for malnutrition as well as developing disease states such as necrotizing enterocolitis and bronchopulmonary dysplasia (BPD) that may further complicate nutrition status.

Premature neonates have decreased protein and fat stores and have an increased protein catabolic rate, which may be further increased by sepsis and critical illness. Early administration (i.e., within the first 24 hours) of amino acids has been found to result in positive nitrogen balance, as well as a decreased incidence of hyperglycemia.[109–111] Because hyperglycemia is also associated with increased morbidity and mortality during the neonatal period, attempts to prevent and/or treat hyperglycemia should be taken.[112–114]

Although the successful achievement of catch-up growth has been related to improved neurodevelopmental outcomes,[115,116] recent data suggest that rapid early weight gain may be associated with cardiovascular disease later in life (abnormal lipid profile, insulin and leptin resistance, increased blood pressure).[117] Barker's hypothesis of "fetal origins of adult disease" suggests that adaptations the infant makes when malnourished or stressed (i.e., toward energy conservation) may result in central obesity, diabetes, and cardiovascular disease later in life.[118]

Bronchopulmonary Dysplasia

BPD or chronic lung disease is a clinical, pathologic, and radiographic disease of the newborn resulting from prolonged exposure to positive-pressure ventilation and elevated oxygen concentrations. Risk factors for developing BPD include the degree of prematurity, nutrition, and immunologic status. Characteristics of BPD include pulmonary edema and tissue destruction with subsequent repair, fibrosis, and inflammation. Growth failure and altered body composition are common in infants with BPD when compared with their peers without BPD.[119] The persistence of this altered body composition can last into the first years of life. Estimates of growth failure after hospital discharge range between 30% and 67%.[120] The origin of growth failure is multifactorial and is associated with elevations in both resting and total energy expenditure, use of corticosteroids, intrauterine growth retardation, and feeding problems.[121,122] Given that pulmonary edema is common, fluid restriction is often necessary. This restriction further impedes provision of adequate calories and may contribute to poor growth.[121] Optimal oxygen therapy during the first year of life in infants with BPD can result in growth patterns similar to those seen in infants without BPD.[123] Growth failure during the first 2 years of life, early childhood, and beyond has been reported, but it appears that prematurity and sociodemographic factors rather than BPD per se are most predictive of future growth.[124,125] Catch-up growth can be attained faster when infants are fed higher intakes of protein, calcium, phosphorus, and zinc.[126] Because vitamin A deficiency is associated with BPD, supplementation is given for the prevention of BPD and sepsis in preterm infants.[127,128] Benefits of vitamin A supplementation (i.e., a trend toward reduction in ventilatory support) must be weighed against the risks of repeated intramuscular injections and the potential for vitamin A toxicity (i.e., posthemorrhagic hydrocephalus or liver disease). The concern over these risks has prevented its widespread use at this time.

THERAPEUTIC OPTIONS TO MINIMIZE THE SIGNIFICANCE OF MALNUTRITION

The increased awareness of the prevalence and significance of untreated protein-calorie malnutrition has provided a strong incentive for a more rigorous evaluation of abnormalities of nutrition status and prompt initiation of SNS for malnourished patients. If nutrition assessment (see Chap. 143) reveals no malnutrition, then the patient or the patient's caregiver should be counseled on appropriate maintenance goals for nutrition intake.

If mild to moderate malnutrition is present, an anabolic feeding regimen should be initiated using oral supplements. If anorexia is a major contributing factor, EN may be indicated. Intact nutrients can be administered enterally when normal bowel function is present, but a specially designed formula that has a modified fat content, is lactose-free, contains fiber, and/or is calorie or protein enriched may be indicated if intestinal function is compromised (see Chap. 146). If malabsorption is a major contributing factor, EN using a disease-specific formula, or, alternatively, supplemental PN, may be indicated. In the presence of severe malnutrition, an anabolic feeding regimen should be initiated either enterally or parenterally depending on intestinal function and malabsorption.[19] Data from international studies show the median mortality rate secondary to severe malnutrition in children younger than 5 years of age is 25% and has not changed for the last five decades.[129] The findings in some institutions of a mortality rate of less than 5% suggests that treatment strategy and practices employed are critical to optimize patient outcomes. The World Health Organization has published guidelines for the management of severe malnutrition in children.[129] Table 144–5 summarizes the management principles endorsed in these guidelines.

TABLE 144-5 Management Principles for Severe Pediatric Malnutrition

1. Recognize the physiologic effects of reductive adaptation. Every organ system has adapted to starvation and cannot tolerate aggressive reintroduction of nutrition.
2. Treat or prevent hypoglycemia, hypothermia, and dehydration (days 1 to 3). Initiate small, frequent feedings (every 2 to 3 hours) and provide only enough calories to meet basic metabolic demands.
3. Avoid a high-protein diet (days 1 to 3) secondary to liver incompetence.
4. Correct electrolyte imbalance (day 1 through week 6).
5. Assume the child has an infection and empirically treat with antibiotics (days 1 to 7).
6. Avoid cardiac failure secondary to aggressive rehydration. Parenteral rehydration should be avoided at all costs and only used if the child is in shock. Avoid diuretics during the first 1 to 5 days even if edema is evident.
7. Advance enteral feeding to recover lost weight and provide for "catch-up growth" (day 7 through week 26).
8. Correct micronutrient deficiencies with vitamins and minerals (without iron on days 1 to 7 and with iron on day 7 through week 6).
9. Correct emotional and social disorders.

When bowel obstruction or short-bowel syndrome is present, PN is indicated. Equivocal data exist whether EN is absolutely contraindicated in hypoperfusion of the gut. The most recent recommendations advocate holding EN when patients have sustained hypotension (<70 mm Hg), a need for increasing doses of pressor agents to maintain the mean arterial pressure ≥70 mm Hg, increasing ventilatory support requirements, or worsening signs of GI intolerance to the enteral nutrition (i.e., sudden abdominal distension, abrupt increases in nasogastric output, and sudden abdominal pain).[130] The anticipated duration of the need for parenteral support will dictate whether one uses the peripheral or central venous route of administration (see Chap. 145). Routine reevaluation of the response to nutrition therapy and attainment of nutrition goals should be incorporated into the overall patient care plan.

PHARMACOECONOMIC CONSIDERATIONS

⑩ Malnourished patients have increased complications during their hospital course, among them an increased length of stay, thereby incurring increased healthcare costs.[3,131] Although the evidence is strong that malnutrition is associated with increased healthcare costs, it has been more difficult to establish the cost-to-benefit or cost savings of nutrition intervention. Tucker and Miguel confirmed the association between poor nutritional status and prolonged length of hospital stay, and also determined that when nutrition intervention occurred (oral, enteral, or parenteral nutrition), the average length of stay was decreased by 2.1 days.[131]

Trauma patients are at an unusually high risk for developing malnutrition because of the hypermetabolic and hypercatabolic state associated with underlying injury. Although several clinical trials have compared the efficacy of EN versus PN, little data are available regarding the cost-effectiveness of these two routes of administration. Trice et al.[132] assessed the economic impact of the delivery of EN versus PN to trauma patients. Their evaluation of the data from nine prospective, randomized clinical trials revealed that postoperative PN was associated with an almost fourfold increased risk of infectious complications and 15-fold greater risk of catheter sepsis compared with EN. Estimated total costs were 4- to 12.5-fold greater in patients receiving PN than in those receiving EN. Thus the decision to prescribe PN over EN should be evaluated carefully.

Economic savings also have been achieved when SNS teams are involved with the provision of EN.[133] A benefit of $4.20 was realized for every $1 invested in nutrition support team management. Furthermore, management by the nutrition support team resulted in reductions in mortality rate, length of hospital stay, readmission rates, and complications, compared with management by a nonteam group. Thus intervention by specially trained healthcare practitioners, including pharmacists, can lower costs associated with nutrition intervention without compromising the quality of patient care.

CONCLUSIONS

Although the cost-to-benefit analysis of nutrition intervention is weak, the issue that seems clear is that malnutrition is associated with significant morbidity and mortality in numerous disease states and clinical settings. Furthermore, it is likely that improved patient outcomes can be achieved by a systematic approach to identify the presence of risk factors for malnutrition, quantitate the degree of malnutrition, and initiate nutrition management.[19] The clinician's responsibilities in the management of nutrition disease include the following: identifying patients at risk for malnutrition; identifying candidates for nutrition intervention; designing patient-specific nutrition-support regimens; evaluating and managing drug–nutrient interactions; and, finally, initiating a monitoring plan to evaluate all clinical and laboratory data so as to optimize the safety and efficacy of the specialized nutrition support regimen.

ABBREVIATIONS

AIDS: acquired immunodeficiency syndrome

BPD: bronchopulmonary dysplasia

CF: cystic fibrosis

EN: enteral nutrition

HIV: human immunodeficiency virus

PN: parenteral nutrition

PNI: prognostic nutritional index

REFERENCES

1. Fawzi WW, Herrera MG, Nestel P, et al. A longitudinal study of prolonged breastfeeding in relation to child undernutrition. Int J Epidemiol 1998;27:255–260.
2. Coats KG, Morgan SL, Bartolucci AA, Weinsier RL. Hospital-associated malnutrition: A re-evaluation 12 years later. J Am Diet Assoc 1993;93:27–33.
3. Gallagher-Allred DR, Voss AC, Finn SC, et al. Malnutrition and clinical outcomes: The case for medical nutrition therapy. J Am Diet Assoc 1996;96:361–366.
4. Iyengar GV, Nair PP. Global outlook on nutrition and the environment: Meeting challenges of the next millennium. Sci Total Environ 2000;249:331–346.
5. UNICEF. Progress for Children. A Report Card on Nutrition. New York: UNICEF, 2006;4:1–34.
6. UNICEF. The State of the World's Children 2006. New York: UNICEF, 2006.
7. UN Millennium Project 2005. Halving Hunger: It Can Be Done. Summary Version of the Report of the Task Force on Hunger. New York: The Earth Institute at Columbia University, 2005.
8. Mendez MA, Adair LS. Severity and timing of stunting in the first two years of life affect performance on cognitive tests in late childhood. J Nutr 1999;129:1555–1562.
9. Caballero B. Global patterns of child health: The role of nutrition. Ann Nutr Metab 2002;46(Suppl 1):3–7.
10. Polhamus B, Thompson D, Dalenius K, et al. Pediatric Nutrition Surveillance 2004 Report. Atlanta, GA: U.S. Department of Health and Human Services, Centers for Disease Control and Prevention, 2006.
11. Hendricks KM, Duggan C, Gallagher L, et al. Malnutrition in hospitalized pediatric patients. Arch Pediatr Adolesc Med 1995;149:1118–1122.
12. Cahill GF. Fuel metabolism in starvation. Annu Rev Nutr 2006;26:1–22.

13. Sawaya Al, Martins P, Hoffman D, Roberts SB. The link between childhood undernutrition and risk of chronic diseases in adulthood: A case study of Brazil. Nutr Rev 2003;61(5 Pt 1):168–175.
14. Godfrey KM, Barker DJ. Fetal programming and adult health. Public Health Nutr 2001;4:611–624.
15. Scholl D, Langkamp-Henken B. Nutrient recommendations for wound healing. J Intraven Nurs 2001;24:124–132.
16. Kirk SJ, Hurson M, Regan MC, et al. Arginine stimulates wound healing and immune function in elderly human beings. Surgery 1993;114:155–160.
17. Dewys WD, Begg C, Lavin PT, et al. Prognostic effect of weight loss prior to chemotherapy in cancer patients. Am J Med 1980;69:491–497.
18. Koretz RL, Lipman TO, Klein S. AGA technical review on parenteral nutrition. Gastroenterology 2001;121:970–1001.
19. ASPEN Board of Directors and the Clinical Guidelines Task Force. Guidelines for the use of parenteral and enteral nutrition in adult and pediatric patients. JPEN J Parenter Enteral Nutr 2002;26(Suppl):1SA–138SA.
20. Moynihan T, Kelly DG, Fisch MJ. To feed or not to feed: Is that the right question? J Clin Oncol 2005;23:6256–6259.
21. Van Eys J. Malnutrition in children with cancer. Cancer 1979;43:2030–2035.
22. Sala A, Pencharz P, Barr RD. Children, cancer, and nutrition—A dynamic triangle in review. Cancer 2004;100:677–687.
23. Barr RD, Gibson B. Nutritional status and cancer in childhood. J Pediatr Hematol Oncol 2000;22:491–494.
24. Pedrosa F, Bonilla M, Liu A, et al. Effect of malnutrition at the time of diagnosis on the survival of children treated for cancer in El Salvador and Northern Brazil. J Pediatr Hematol Oncol 2000;22:502–505.
25. Lobato-Mendizabal E, Lopez-Martinez B, Ruiz-Arguelles GJ. A critical review of the prognostic value of the nutritional status at diagnosis in the outcome of therapy of children with acute lymphoblastic leukemia. Rev Invest Clin 2003;55:31–35.
26. Mauer AM, Burgess JB, Donaldson SS, et al. Special nutritional needs of children with malignancies: A review. JPEN J Parenter Enteral Nutr 1990;14:315–324.
27. Weisdorf SA, Lysne J, Wind D, et al. Positive effect of prophylactic total parenteral nutrition on long-term outcome of bone marrow transplantation. Transplantation 1987;43:833–838.
28. Mayer EI, Reuter M, Dopfer RE, Ranke MB. Energy expenditure, energy intake and prevalence of obesity after therapy for acute lymphoblastic leukemia during childhood. Horm Res 2000;53:193–199.
29. Holcomb GW, Ziegler MM. Nutrition and cancer in children. Surg Annu 1990:22:129–142.
30. Klein S, Simes J, Blackburn G. TPN and cancer clinical trials. Cancer 1986;58:1378–1386.
31. Brennan MF. Uncomplicated starvation versus cancer cachexia. Cancer Res 1977;37:2359–2364.
32. Kern KA, Norton JA. Cancer cachexia. JPEN J Parenter Enteral Nutr 1988;12:286–298.
33. Kotler D, Tierney A, Wang J, et al. Magnitude of body-cell-mass depletion and the timing of death from wasting in AIDS. Am J Clin Nutr 1989;50:444–447.
34. Guenter P, Muurahainen N, Simons G, et al. Relationships among nutritional status, disease progression, and survival in HIV infection. J Acquir Immune Defic Syndr 1993;6:1130–1138.
35. Baum MK, Shor-Posner G. Micronutrient status in relationship to mortality in HIV-1 disease. Nutr Rev 1998;56(1 Pt 2):S135–S139.
36. Kotler DP, Rosenbaum K, Wang J, et al. Studies of body composition and fat distribution in HIV-infected and control subjects. J Acquir Immune Defic Syndr Hum Retrovirol 1999;20:228–237.
37. Lichtenstein KA, Ward DJ, Moorman AC, et al. Clinical assessment of HIV-associated lipodystrophy in an ambulatory population. AIDS 2001;15:1389–1398.
38. Miller TL. Nutritional aspects of HIV-infected children receiving highly active antiretroviral therapy. AIDS 2003;17:S130–S140.
39. McKinney RE, Robertson JWR. Effect of human immunodeficiency virus infection on the growth of young children. J Pediatr 1993;123:579–582.
40. Winter H. Gastrointestinal tract function and malnutrition in HIV-infected children. J Nutr 1996;126:2620S–2622S.
41. Pollack H, Glasberg H, Lee E, et al. Impaired early growth of infants perinatally infected with human immunodeficiency virus: Correlation with viral load. J Pediatr 1997;130:915–922.
42. Miller TL, Easley KA, Zhang W, et al. Maternal and infant factors associated with failure to thrive in children with vertically transmitted human immunodeficiency virus-1 infection: The prospective, P2C2 human immunodeficiency virus multicenter study. Pediatrics 2001;108:1287–1296.
43. Brettler DB, Forsberg A, Bolivar E, et al. Growth failure as a prognostic indicator for progression to acquired immunodeficiency syndrome in children with hemophilia. J Pediatr 1990;117:584–588.
44. Guarino A, Spagnuolo MI, Giacomet V, et al. Effects of nutritional rehabilitation on intestinal function and on CD4 cell number in children with HIV. J Pediatr Gastroenterol Nutr 2002;34:366–371.
45. Tang AM, Graham NMH, Saah AJ. Effects of micronutrient intake on survival in human immunodeficiency virus type 1 infection. Am J Epidemiol 1996;143:1244–1256.
46. Coyne-Meyers K, Trombley LE. A review of nutrition in human immunodeficiency virus infection in the era of highly active antiretroviral therapy. Nutr Clin Pract 2004;19:340–355.
47. Berneis K, Battegay M, Bassetti S, et al. Nutritional supplements combined with dietary counseling diminish whole body protein catabolism in HIV-infected patients. Eur J Clin Invest 2000;30:87–94.
48. Kotler DP, Tierney AR, Ferraro R, et al. Enteral alimentation and repletion of body cell mass in malnourished patients with acquired immunodeficiency syndrome. Am J Clin Nutr 1991;53:149–154.
49. Kotler DP, Fogleman L, Tierney AR. Comparison of total parenteral nutrition and an oral, semielemental diet on body composition, physical function, and nutrition-related costs in patients with malabsorption due to acquired immunodeficiency syndrome. JPEN J Parenter Enteral Nutr 1998;22:120–126.
50. Schambelan M, Mulligan K, Grunfeld C, et al. Recombinant human growth hormone in patients with HIV-associated wasting: A randomized, placebo-controlled trial. Ann Intern Med 1996;125:873–882.
51. Kaplan G, Thomas S, Fierer DS. Thalidomide for the treatment of AIDS-associated wasting. AIDS Res Hum Retroviruses 2000;16:1345–1355.
52. Grinspoon S, Corcoran C, Anderson E. Sustained anabolic effects of long-term androgen administration in men with AIDS-wasting. Clin Infect Dis 1999;28:634–636.
53. Miller K, Corcoran C, Armstrong C. Transdermal testosterone administration in women with acquired immunodeficiency syndrome wasting: A pilot study. J Clin Endocrinol Metab 1998;83:2717–2725.
54. Earthman CP, Reid PM, Harper IT, et al. Body cell mass repletion and improved quality of life in HIV-infected individuals receiving oxandrolone. JPEN J Parenter Enteral Nutr 2002;26:357–365.
55. Frankenfield D. Energy expenditure and protein requirements after traumatic injury. Nutr Clin Pract 2006;21:430–437.
56. Giner M, Laviano A, Meguid MM, Gleason JR. In 1995 a correlation between malnutrition and poor outcome in critically ill patients still exists. Nutrition 1996;12:23–29.
57. Todd SR, Kozar RA, Moore FA. Nutrition support in adult trauma patients. Nutr Clin Pract 2006;21:421–429.
58. Kudsk KA, Croce MA, Fabian TC, et al. Enteral versus parenteral feeding: Effects on septic morbidity after blunt and penetrating abdominal trauma. Ann Surg 1992;215:503–513.
59. Heys SD, Walker LG, Smith I, et al. Enteral nutritional supplementation with key nutrients in patients with critical illness and cancer: A meta-analysis of randomized controlled clinical trials. Ann Surg 1999;229:467–477.
60. Beale RJ, Bryg DJ, Bihari DJ. Immunonutrition in the critically ill: A systematic review of clinical outcome. Crit Care Med 1999;27:2799–2805.
61. Heyland DK, Novak F, Drover J, et al. Should immunonutrition become routine in critically ill patients? A systematic review of the evidence. JAMA 2001;286:944–953.
62. Berger MM. Antioxidant micronutrients in major trauma and burns: Evidence and practice. Nutr Clin Pract 2006;21:438–449.
63. Letton RW, Chwals WJ, Jamie A, Charles B. Early postoperative alterations in infant energy use increase the risk of overfeeding. J Pediatr Surg 1995;30:988–992.
64. White MS, Shepherd RW, McEniery JA. Energy expenditure in 100 ventilated, critically ill children: Improving the accuracy of predictive equations. Crit Care Med 2000;28:2307–2312.
65. Gassul MA, Cabre E. Nutrition in inflammatory bowel disease. Curr Opin Clin Nutr Metab Care 2001;4:561–569.
66. Kleinman RE, Bladassano RN, Caplan A, et al. Nutrition support for pediatric patients with inflammatory bowel disease: A clinical report of

the North American Society for Pediatric Gastroenterology, Hepatology and Nutrition. J Pediatr Gastroenterol Nutr 2004;39:15–27.
67. Kim SC, Ferry GD. Inflammatory bowel diseases in pediatric and adolescent patients: Clinical, therapeutic, and psychosocial considerations. Gastroenterology 2004;126:1550–1560.
68. Griffiths AM. Enteral nutrition in the management of Crohn's disease. JPEN J Parenter Enteral Nutr 2005;29:S108–S117.
69. Seidner DL, Lashner BA, Brzezinski A, et al. An oral supplement with fish oil, soluble fiber, and antioxidants for corticosteroid sparing in ulcerative colitis: A randomized, controlled clinical trial. Clin Gastroenterol Hepatol 2005;3:358–369.
70. Vargas JH, Sachs P, Ament ME. Chronic intestinal pseudo-obstruction syndrome in pediatrics: Results of a national survey by members of the North American Society for Pediatric Gastroenterology and Nutrition. J Pediatr Gastroenterol Nutr 1988;7:323–332.
71. American Gastroenterological Association Clinical Practice Committee. AGA technical review on short bowel syndrome and intestinal transplantation. Gastroenterology 2003;124:1111–1134.
72. Thompson JS, Langnas AN, Pinch LW, et al. Surgical approach to short-bowel syndrome: Experience in a population of 160 patients. Ann Surg 1995;222:600–607.
73. Spencer AU, Neaga A, West B, et al. Pediatric short bowel syndrome. Redefining predictors of success. Ann Surg 2005;242:403–412.
74. Quiros-Tejeira RE, Ament ME, Reyen L, et al. Long-term parenteral nutritional support and intestinal adaptation in children with short bowel syndrome: A 25-year experience. J Pediatr 2004;145:157–163.
75. Touloukian RJ, Walker Smith GJ. Normal intestinal length in preterm infants. J Pediatr Surg 1983;18:720–723.
76. Wilmore DW, Robinson MK. Short bowel syndrome. World J Surg 2000;24:1486–1492.
77. Jeejeebhoy KN. Short bowel syndrome: A nutritional and medical approach. CMAJ 2003;16:1297–1302.
78. Messing B, Crenn P, Beau P, et al. Long-term survival and parenteral nutrition dependence in adult patients with the short bowel syndrome. Gastroenterology 1999;117:1043–1050.
79. Figueroa-Colon R, Harris PR, Birdsong E, et al. Impact of intestinal lengthening on the nutritional outcome for children with short bowel syndrome. J Pediatr Surg 1996;31:912–916.
80. Duggan C, Piper H, Javid PJ, et al. Growth and nutritional status in infants with short-bowel syndrome after the serial transverse enteroplasty procedure. Clin Gastroenterol Hepatol 2006;4:1237–1241.
81. Venick RS, Farmer DG, Saikali D, et al. Nutritional outcomes following pediatric intestinal transplantation. Transplant Proc 2006;38:1718–1719.
82. Mullen JL, Gertner MH, Buzby GP, et al. Implications of malnutrition in the surgical patient. Arch Surg 1979;114:121–125.
83. Rudman D, Feller AB, Nagraj HS, et al. Relation of serum albumin concentration to death rate in nursing home men. JPEN J Parenter Enteral Nutr 1987;11:360–363.
84. Buzby GP, Mullen JL, Mathews DC, et al. Prognostic nutritional index in gastrointestinal surgery. Am J Surg 1980;139:160–166.
85. Kudsk KA, Tolley EA, DeWitt RC, et al. Preoperative albumin and surgical site identify surgical risk for major postoperative complications. JPEN J Parenter Enteral Nutr 2003;27:1–9.
86. Detsky AS, Baker JP, O'Rourke K, et al. Predicting nutrition-associated complications for residents undergoing gastrointestinal surgery. JPEN J Parenter Enteral Nutr 1987;11:440–446.
87. Klein S, Kinney J, Jeejeebhoy K, et al. Nutrition support in clinical practice: Review of published data and recommendations for future research directions. JPEN J Parenter Enteral Nutr 1997;21:133–156.
88. The Veterans Affairs Total Parenteral Nutrition Cooperative Study Group. Perioperative total parenteral nutrition. N Engl J Med 1991;325:525–532.
89. Sacks GS, Genton L, Kudsk KA. Controversy of immunonutrition for surgical, critical-illness patients. Curr Opin Crit Care 2003;9:300–305.
90. Lai HJ. Classification of nutritional status in cystic fibrosis. Curr Opin Pulm Med 2006;12:422–427.
91. Steinkamp G, Wiedemann B. Relationship between nutritional status and lung function in cystic fibrosis: Cross sectional and longitudinal analyses from the German CF quality assurance (CFQA) project. Thorax 2002;57:596–601.
92. Borowitz D, Baker RD, Stallings V. Consensus report on nutrition for pediatric patients with cystic fibrosis. J Pediatr Gastroenterol Nutr 2002;35:246–259.
93. Stallings VA, Fung EB, Hofley PM, Scanlin TF. Acute pulmonary exacerbation is not associated with increased energy expenditure in children with cystic fibrosis. J Pediatr 1998;132:493–499.
94. Wilson DC, Kalnins D, Stewart C, et al. Challenges in the dietary treatment of cystic fibrosis related diabetes mellitus. Clin Nutr 2000;19:87–93.
95. Erskine JM, Lingard CD, Sontage MK, Accurso FJ. Enteral nutrition for patients with cystic fibrosis: Comparison of a semi-elemental and non-elemental formula. J Pediatr 1998;132:265–269.
96. Ellis L, Kalnins D, Corey M, et al. Do infants with cystic fibrosis need a protein hydrolysate formula? A prospective, randomized, comparative study. J Pediatr 1998;132:270–276.
97. Haffner D, Weinfurth A, Manz F, et al. Long-term outcome of paediatric patients with hereditary tubular disorders. Nephron 1999;83:250–260.
98. Greer R, Lehnert M, Lewindon P, et al. Body composition and components of energy expenditure in children with end-stage liver disease. J Pediatr Gastroenterol Nutr 2003;36:358–363.
99. Leitch CA. Growth, nutrition and energy expenditure in pediatric heart failure. Prog Pediatr Cardiol 2000;11:195–202.
100. Cameron JW, Rosenthal A, Olson AD. Malnutrition in hospitalized children with congenital heart disease. Arch Pediatr Adolesc Med 1995;149:1098–1102.
101. Claris-Appiani A, Ardissino GL, Dacco V, et al. Catch-up growth in children with chronic renal failure treated with long-term enteral nutrition. JPEN J Parenter Enteral Nutr 1995;19:175–178.
102. Varan B, Tokel K, Yilmaz G. Malnutrition and growth failure in cyanotic and acyanotic congenital heart disease with and without pulmonary hypertension. Arch Dis Child 1999;81:49–52.
103. McDiarmid SV. Risk factors and outcomes after pediatric liver transplantation. Liver Transpl Surg 1996;2:44–45.
104. Sokal EM, Cleghorn G, Goulet O, et al. Liver and intestinal transplantation in children: Working group report of the first world congress of pediatric gastroenterology, hepatology and nutrition. J Pediatr Gastroenterol Nutr 2002;25:S159–S172.
105. Sarkisian CA, Lachs MS. "Failure to thrive" in older adults. Ann Intern Med 1996;124:1072–1078.
106. Sacks GS. Nutritional considerations in the elderly. JPSW 2004;8–11.
107. Olsen EM. Failure to thrive: Still a problem. Clin Pediatr (Phila) 2006;45:1–6.
108. Bauchner H. Failure to thrive. In: Behrman RE, Kliegman RM, Jenson HB, eds. Nelson Textbook of Pediatrics, 17th ed. Philadelphia: WB Saunders, 2004;133–134.
109. Poindexter BB. Early amino acid administration for premature neonates. J Pediatr 2005;147:420–421.
110. Te Braake FWJ, van den Akker CHP, Wattimena DJL, et al. Amino acid administration to premature infants following birth. J Pediatr 2005;147:457–461.
111. Thureen PJ, Melara D, Fennessey PV, Hay WW Jr. Effect of low versus high intravenous amino acid intake on very low birth weight infants in the early neonatal period. Pediatr Res 2003;53:24–32.
112. Regan FA, Cutfield WS, Jefferies C, et al. The impact of early nutrition in premature infants on later childhood insulin sensitivity and growth. Pediatrics 2006;118:1943–1949.
113. Hays SP, O'Brian Smith E, Sunehag AL. Hyperglycemia is a risk factor for early death and morbidity in extremely low birth-weight infants. Pediatrics 2006;118:1811–1818.
114. Alaedeen DI, Walsch MC, Chwals WJ. Total parenteral nutrition-associated hyperglycemia correlated with prolonged mechanical ventilation and hospital stay in septic infants. J Pediatr Surg 2006;41:239–244.
115. Hack M, Merkatz IR, Gordon D, et al. The prognostic significance of postnatal growth in very low birth weight infants. Am J Obstet Gynecol 1982;143:693–699.
116. Latal-Hajnal B, Von Sibenthal K, Kovari H, et al. Postnatal growth in VLBW infants: Significant association with neurodevelopmental outcome. J Pediatr 2003;143:163–170.
117. Singhal A, Lucas L. Early origins of cardiovascular disease: Is there a unifying hypothesis? Lancet 2004;363:1642–1645.
118. Godfrey KM, Barker DJ. Fetal nutrition and adult disease. Am J Clin Nutr 2000;71:1344S–1352S.
119. Huysman WA, de Ridder M, de Bruin NC, et al. Growth and body composition in preterm infants with bronchopulmonary dysplasia. Arch Dis Child Fetal Neonatal Ed 2003;88:F46–F51.

120. Johnson DB, Cheney C, Monsen ER. Nutrition and feeding in infants with bronchopulmonary dysplasia after initial hospital discharge: Risk factors for growth failure. J Am Diet Assoc 1998;98:649–656.
121. Atkinson SA. Special nutritional needs of infants for prevention of and recovery from bronchopulmonary dysplasia. J Nutr 2001;131:942S–946S.
122. Abrams SA. Chronic pulmonary insufficiency in children and its effects on growth and development. J Nutr 2001;131:938S–941S.
123. Chye JK, Gray PH. Rehospitalization and growth of infants with bronchopulmonary dysplasia: A matched control study. J Paediatr Child Health 1995;31:105–111.
124. Robertson CMT, Etches PC, Goldson E, Kyle JM. Eight-year school performance, neurodevelopmental, and growth outcome of neonates with bronchopulmonary dysplasia: A comparative study. Pediatrics 1992;89:365–372.
125. Vrienich LA, Bozynski MEA, Shyr Y, et al. The effect of bronchopulmonary dysplasia on growth at school age. Pediatrics 1995;95:855–859.
126. Brunton JA, Saigal S, Atkinson SA. Growth and body composition in infants with bronchopulmonary dysplasia up to 3 months corrected age: A randomized trial of high-energy nutrient-enriched formula fed after hospital discharge. J Pediatr 1998;133:340–345.
127. Atkinson SA, Abrams SA. Symposium: Pediatric pulmonary insufficiency: Nutritional strategies for prevention and treatment-special nutritional needs of infants for prevention of and recovery from bronchopulmonary dysplasia. J Nutr 2001;131:9335–9345.
128. Darlow BA, Graham PJ. Vitamin A supplementation for preventing morbidity and mortality in very low birthweight infants. Cochrane Database Syst Rev 2001;ICD00501.
129. Ashworth A, Khanum S, Jackson A, Schofield C. Guidelines for the Inpatient Treatment of Severely Malnourished Children. World Health Organization, Geneva, Switzerland, 2003.
130. McClave SA, Chang W-K. Feeding the hypotensive patient: Does enteral feeding precipitate or protect against ischemic bowel. Nutr Clin Pract 2003;18:279–284.
131. Tucker HN, Miguel SG. Cost containment through nutrition intervention. Nutr Rev 1996;54:111–121.
132. Trice S, Melnik G, Page CP. Complications and costs of early postoperative parenteral versus enteral nutrition in trauma patients. Nutr Clin Pract 1997;12:114–119.
133. Hassell JT, Games AD, Shaffer B, Harkins LE. Nutrition support team management of enterally fed patients in a community hospital is cost-beneficial. J Am Diet Assoc 1994;94:993–998.

CHAPTER 145 Parenteral Nutrition

TODD W. MATTOX AND PAMELA D. REITER

KEY CONCEPTS

1. Four steps to developing a successful nutrition plan include definition of nutrition goals, determination of nutrition requirements, determination of appropriate route of nutrient delivery, and subsequent monitoring of the nutrition regimen to evaluate suitability of the regimen as a patient's clinical condition changes and to minimize or treat complications early.
2. The appropriate route of nutrition support depends on the functional condition of the patient's gastrointestinal (GI) tract, risk of aspiration, expected duration of nutrition therapy, and clinical condition.
3. Identifying the patient who is most likely to benefit from parenteral nutrition (PN) therapy includes consideration of the patient's age, nutrition status, expected duration of GI dysfunction, and potential risks of initiating therapy.
4. PN formulations include intravenous sources of protein, dextrose, fat, water, electrolytes, vitamins, trace elements, and other additives.
5. PN solutions may be appropriately formulated for administration by peripheral or central venous access.
6. PN solutions may be infused continuously or intermittently.
7. Biochemical and clinical measurements considered necessary for effective monitoring of patients receiving PN include serum chemistries, vital signs, weight, total daily fluid intake and losses, and nutritional intake.
8. Non–catheter-related complications of PN therapy are minimized with application of age-appropriate nutrient dosing guidelines, frequent monitoring, and rational adjustments to the PN regimen when metabolic abnormalities occur.
9. Expenses associated with PN therapy may be minimized by using PN in appropriate patients, appropriate use of laboratory measurements associated with PN therapy, maximizing efficient purchasing practices for PN solutions and compounding supplies, streamlining compounding procedures, and minimizing PN waste.

Maintenance of adequate nutrition status during illness has been recognized for more than 50 years as an integral part of the medical treatment plan for patients who are unable to use normal physiologic means of nourishment. Successful techniques for providing intravenous (IV) nutrition support were introduced to clinical practice in adults and subsequently, infants in the late 1960s.[1] Use of central venous access was investigated to reduce risk of metabolic complications associated with fluid overload and electrolyte imbalances. The use of larger vessels permitted infusion of concentrated formulas, which decreased the fluid volume required and avoided the phlebitis that commonly occurred when hypertonic infusions were given peripherally.

Learning objectives, review questions, and other resources can be found at **www.pharmacotherapyonline.com.**

Further clinical experience and research fostered development of protocols that promoted better patient care and resulted in a decline in complications associated with parenteral nutrition (PN) therapy.[2] The scope of practice for nutrition support clinicians has broadened as a result of increasing knowledge regarding the metabolic consequences associated with acute injury and chronic disease states. The pharmacist's role in providing safe and effective nutrition-support care requires knowledge of the principles of patient selection, initial therapy design, preparation and dispensing of the nutritional formulations, and outcome monitoring. Other responsibilities of the nutrition support pharmacist may include development of policy and procedures, as well as quality improvement activities for patient care and operational processes associated with providing parenteral and enteral nutrition.[3–6] However, the role of other healthcare professionals may be similar because of the evolving interdisciplinary approach to nutritional support.[5–10] This chapter reviews indications for PN, components of PN formulations, routes of IV administration, practical aspects of regimen design, solution admixture, outcome monitoring, and management of complications for both adult and pediatric (neonates, infants, and children) patients.

DESIRED OUTCOMES

1 The primary objective of nutrition support therapy is to promote positive clinical outcomes of an illness and improve a patient's quality of life. Four fundamental steps are key to providing optimal care for patients who require nutrition support. They are definition of nutrition goals, determination of nutrient requirements for achievement of the nutrition goals, delivery of the required nutrients, and subsequent assessment of the nutrition regimen.[5–7]

A patient's nutrition goals can be established after a thorough nutritional assessment (see Chap. 143). Nutrient requirements and an appropriate route for delivery of the required nutrients can then be determined (see Chaps. 144 and 146). Nutrition support goals include correction of the patient's caloric and nitrogen imbalances, and any fluid or electrolyte abnormalities, or known vitamin or trace element abnormalities. An additional goal is to lessen the metabolic response to injury by minimizing oxidant stress and favorably modulating immune response. These interventions should not cause or worsen other metabolic complications.

Specific caloric goals include (a) adequate energy intake to promote normal growth and development in neonates, infants, and children, (b) energy equilibrium and preservation of fat calorie stores in well-nourished adults, and (c) positive energy balance in malnourished patients with depleted endogenous fat stores. Obese patients with excess endogenous fat stores (greater than 120% of ideal body weight) may require less caloric support than nonobese patients with the same clinical condition.[11] Specific nitrogen goals are positive nitrogen balance or nitrogen equilibrium and improvement in the serum concentration of visceral protein markers such as transferrin or prealbumin.

❷ The gastrointestinal (GI) tract is the optimal route for providing nutrients unless obstruction, severe pancreatitis, or other GI complications are present (see Chap. 143).[12] Other considerations that may impact determination of an appropriate route for delivery of nutrition support include expected duration of nutrition therapy and risk of aspiration. Patients who have nonfunctional GI tracts or are otherwise not candidates for enteral nutrition may benefit from PN. Nutrition support provide by the IV route is also commonly referred to as total parenteral nutrition or hyperalimentation. Routine monitoring is necessary to ensure that the nutrition regimen is suitable for a given patient as the patient's clinical condition changes and to minimize or treat complications early.

INDICATIONS FOR PARENTERAL NUTRITION SUPPORT

The association between malnutrition and development of complications and mortality is well documented in adult and pediatric patients.[13,14] Although improvement in nutrition status as defined by various clinical nutrition markers has been reported in patients who received PN, the impact on clinical outcome is difficult to demonstrate in many adult populations. Several investigations have reported a positive effect of PN on complications and mortality, whereas others have failed to demonstrate any difference.[13,15] Early studies have been criticized for defects in study design, such as small sample sizes, inappropriate randomization, and inconsistent baseline nutrition status among the study group, which hindered demonstration of the effectiveness of PN therapy. The impact of PN on clinical outcome has been more successfully demonstrated in critically ill infants and children, particularly those with acquired or congenital GI tract anomalies.[17] Consensus guidelines for PN use in adults (Table 145–1) and pediatric (Table 145–2) patients are based on clinical experience and investigations in specific patient populations.[15,17,18] Unfortunately, conflicting data have resulted in a lack of consistency in published guidelines from different sources, which complicates identification of the patient who is most likely to benefit from PN. However, these published reports may serve as resources for development of institution-specific standards.

❸ The decision to initiate PN is based on the assessment that the patient cannot meet his or her nutritional requirements through the GI tract. This assessment must include an evaluation of the patient's nutrition status, clinical status, age, and potential risks of initiating therapy, such as infection and other metabolic abnormalities. The appropriate length of time to wait prior to starting PN therapy is not well defined.[12]

CLINICAL CONTROVERSY

The most appropriate time to initiate PN in adults differs between various consensus reports because few data specifically address this issue. Some recommend initiating PN in patients who are not candidates for enteral nutrition as early as after 7 days of inadequate oral intake, whereas others recommend waiting up to 14 days in previously well-nourished or moderately malnourished patients.

TABLE 145-1 Indications for Adult Parenteral Nutrition

1. Inability to absorb nutrients via the GI tract because of one or more of the following:
   a. Massive small bowel resection: usually patients with less than 100 cm of small bowel distal to the ligament of Treitz without a colon, or less than 50 cm of small bowel with an intact colon
   b. Intractable vomiting when adequate EN is not expected for 7–14 days.
   c. Severe diarrhea
   d. Bowel obstruction
   e. GI fistulae: PN is indicated in patients with prolonged inadequate nutritional intake longer than 5–7 days who are not candidates for EN
2. Cancer: antineoplastic therapy, radiation therapy, or HSCT
   a. PN may be used in moderately to severely malnourished patients receiving active anticancer treatment who are not candidates for EN
   b. PN is not routinely indicated for well-nourished or mildly malnourished patients undergoing surgery, chemotherapy, or radiation therapy
   c. PN is unlikely to benefit patients with advanced cancer whose malignancy is unresponsive to treatment. However, use may be appropriate for carefully selected patients who have failed trials of less-invasive medical therapies and have good performance status, an estimated life expectancy of longer than 40–60 days, and strong social and financial support
3. Pancreatitis: PN may be used in patients with severe pancreatitis with prolonged inadequate nutritional intake longer than 5–7 days who are not candidates for EN. PN should be used when EN exacerbates abdominal pain, ascites, or fistula output
4. Critical Care
   a. PN should be used in those patients in whom EN is contraindicated or is unlikely to provide adequate nutritional requirements within 5–10 days
   b. Organ failure (liver, renal, or respiratory): PN should be used in patients with moderate to severe catabolism when EN is contraindicated
   c. Burns: PN should be used in those patients in whom EN is contraindicated or is unlikely to provide adequate nutritional requirements within 4–5 days
5. Perioperative PN
   a. Preoperative: for 7–14 days for patients with moderate to severe malnutrition who are undergoing major GI surgery, if the operation can be safely postponed
   b. Postoperative: PN should be used in patients in whom EN is contraindicated or is unlikely to provide adequate nutritional requirements within 7–10 days
6. Hyperemesis gravidarum: when EN is not tolerated
7. Eating disorders: PN should be considered for patients with anorexia nervosa and severe malnutrition who are unable or unwilling to ingest adequate nutrition

EN, enteral nutrition; GI, gastrointestinal; HSCT, hematopoietic stem cell transplantation; PN, parenteral nutrition; SBS, short-bowel syndrome.
From references 12 and 17.

Adult PN therapy is not an emergent intervention and should not be initiated until the patient is hemodynamically stable.[12] In general, adults who are not candidates for enteral nutrition should be considered candidates for PN after 7 to 14 days of suboptimal nutritional intake.[12] Guidelines for use in infants and children are primarily influenced by age. The most appropriate time to initiate therapy in infants and children varies with age and nutritional status. Early PN

TABLE 145-2 Indications for Pediatric Parenteral Nutrition

1. When enteral nutrition is unlikely to provide adequate nutritional requirements
   a. Premature infant within 24–48 hours
   b. Other pediatric patients within 5–7 days
2. When the GI tract is not functional or cannot be assessed
   a. Massive small bowel resection resulting in short-bowel syndrome
   b. Neonatal necrotizing enterocolitis
   c. Severe inflammatory bowel disease
   d. Intractable diarrhea and/or vomiting
   e. Graft-versus-host disease
   f. Postchemotherapy
3. Infants and children requiring extracorporeal membrane oxygenation
4. Organ failure (liver, renal, pulmonary, pancreas) when enteral nutrition is contraindicated and child is catabolic

From references 16 and 18.

within the first 24 hours of life has been recommended for infants with a birth weight less than 1,500 grams.[19–21] Protein loss in extremely low-birth-weight infants can be twofold higher than in term infants, and frequently results in a negative nitrogen balance that cannot be corrected by glucose as a sole nutrient. Early aggressive PN in neonates can enhance protein accretion and somatic growth.[22] However, many clinicians hesitate to initiate early PN because of concern of adverse effects associated with protein intolerance. Withholding PN for 2 to 3 days after birth, coupled with a slow advancement of substrate, only appears to contribute to the acute semistarvation and growth failure seen in many neonates.[21,23] PN should be initiated within 5 to 7 days in other pediatric patients who are unable to meet their nutrient requirements with enteral nutrition.[16,20] Earlier intervention should be considered in term infants (within 2 to 3 days), critically ill children (within 3 to 5 days), and children with preexisting malnutrition. Guidelines for older children are similar to those in adults.

COMPONENTS OF PARENTERAL NUTRITION

❹ PN formulations include intravenous sources of protein, dextrose, fat, water, electrolytes, vitamins, trace elements, and other additives. PN solutions should provide the optimal combination of macro- and micronutrients to provide a patient's specific nutritional requirements. Macronutrients include water, protein, dextrose, and intravenous fat emulsion (IVFE) (Table 145–3). Micronutrients include vitamins, trace elements, and electrolytes. Both macronutrients and micronutrients are necessary for maintenance of normal metabolism. In general, macronutrients are used for energy (dextrose and fat) and as structural substrates (protein and fat). Micronutrients are required to support a variety of metabolic activities necessary for cellular homeostasis such as enzymatic reactions, fluid balance, and regulation of electrophysiologic processes. These components usually require individualized adjustments as the patient's clinical condition affects changes in metabolic stress, organ function, fluid and electrolyte balance, and acid–base status.

TABLE 145-3 Macronutrient Components of PN Solutions

Nutritional Substrate	Intravenous Source	Description
Fluid	Sterile water for injection USP	
Nitrogen	Crystalline amino acids	
	Standard solutions	Contain a balanced profile of essential, semiessential, and nonessential L-amino acids
	Disease-specific solutions	
	Hepatic encephalopathy	Amino acid profile includes higher BCAA concentrations and lower AAA and methionine concentrations
	Renal failure	Amino acid profile includes higher EAA and histidine concentrations
	Metabolic stress/trauma	Amino acid profile provides standard essential, semiessential, and nonessential amino acids with higher BCAA concentrations
	Pediatrics	Amino acid profile includes standard essential, semiessential, and nonessential amino acids with lower methionine, phenylalanine, and glycine concentrations; these solutions also contain taurine, glutamate, and aspartate
Energy		
Carbohydrate	Dextrose	
	Glycerol	Used in ProcalAmine (B. Braun Medical, Inc.)
Fat	Intravenous fat emulsion	
	LCT emulsions	Oil source is soybean or soybean and safflower combination

AAA, aromatic amino acids (includes phenylalanine and tyrosine); BCAA, branched-chain amino acids (leucine, isoleucine, and valine); EAA, essential amino acids (leucine, isoleucine, valine, phenylalanine, tryptophan, methionine, threonine, and lysine); LCT, long-chain triglycerides; PN, parenteral nutrition.

AMINO ACIDS

Protein in PN solutions is provided in the form of crystalline amino acids (CAAs), which are used primarily for protein synthesis. When oxidized for energy, 1 g of protein yields 4 calories. However, including the caloric contribution from protein when calculating calories provided by the PN regimen is controversial.[24]

CLINICAL CONTROVERSY

Although sufficient energy substrate should be provided to support amino acid use for protein synthesis, amino acid oxidation for energy has been demonstrated in critically ill patients and is thought to occur because of altered metabolism associated with severe metabolic stress. Hence some practice settings may express calories provided by PN as total calories (protein, carbohydrate, fat calories), whereas others may use nonprotein calories (carbohydrate and fat).

Commercially available CAA solutions may be categorized as standard amino acid solutions or modified amino acid solutions. Standard CAA solutions are designed for use in patients with "normal" organ function and nutritional requirements (see Table 145–3). Although standard CAA solutions differ in the proportion of specific amino acids, they contain a balanced profile of essential, semiessential, and nonessential L-amino acids. Despite these differences, similar effects on markers of protein use have been reported.[25] The protein concentration, total nitrogen, and electrolyte content is also different between products. Because the nitrogen concentration of dietary protein is approximately 16%, 6.25 (100 g protein/16 g nitrogen) is commonly accepted as the conversion figure for calculating the nitrogen amount provided by CAA protein. Differences in nitrogen content per gram of amino acids among CAA products may affect calculation of nitrogen amounts infused when determining nitrogen balance.[25,26] The clinical significance of these differences in determining nitrogen balance for routine clinical use is unknown.[26]

Electrolyte composition of standard CAA solutions varies from small, obligatory amounts, to the provision of maintenance requirements of most electrolytes for an adult. Electrolytes provided by CAA solutions must be considered when determining a patient's individual requirements. CAA are available in several different concentrations, which facilitates compounding of patient-specific PN regimens. Highly concentrated products (15% to 20%) are attractive for use in critically ill patients who typically require fluid restriction but have large protein needs. Modified amino acid solutions are designed for use in patients who have altered protein requirements, such as those with hepatic encephalopathy, renal failure, and metabolic stress or trauma, as well as neonates and pediatric patients (see Table 145–3) These solutions tend to be more expensive than standard CAA solutions. The rationale for and clinical efficacy of modified amino acids in disease-specific PN regimens is controversial (see Chap. 147).

Several commercially available CAA solutions are designed to provide conditionally essential amino acids, which are considered nonessential during health because they are produced from other amino acids. However, under certain physiologic conditions, such as prematurity or sepsis, these amino acids cannot be synthesized in sufficient quantities.[25] CAA solutions specifically designed for use in neonates and pediatric patients contain increased amounts of taurine, aspartic acid, and glutamic acid. Other conditionally essential amino acids, such as cysteine, carnitine, and glutamine, are not available in commercial CAA solutions in pharmacologic amounts because they are relatively unstable or poorly soluble.[25]

Consequently, PN solutions may need to be modified by clinicians to provide the desired amount of supplemental conditionally essential amino acids. Cysteine is a conditionally essential amino acid in preterm and term infants that may be added to PN solutions at the time of compounding. Cysteine supplementation also enhances calcium and phosphate solubility in PN solutions by decreasing the solution's pH.[27] Carnitine is a quaternary amine required for free fatty acid transport into the mitochondria for β-oxidation and energy production. Newborns are at risk for carnitine deficiency because of their immature synthetic and conservation mechanisms. Decreased plasma carnitine concentrations are associated with impaired lipid metabolism in patients receiving IVFE.[28] Supplemental carnitine may be added to the PN solution at the time of compounding. Carnitine use in neonatal PN regimens is generally reserved for patients receiving sole PN support for more than 2 weeks because the effect of short-term carnitine supplementation on clinical outcomes such as weight gain and lipid use is not clear.[28]

Glutamine is the most abundant free amino acid in the body and is an important intermediate for many metabolic processes. Glutamine is reported to have an important role in maintaining intestinal integrity, immune function, and protein synthesis during conditions of metabolic stress.[25,29] Investigations in humans and animals have reported positive effects on nutritional markers such as nitrogen balance, whereas others have reported significant improvement in other outcome markers, such as decreased length of hospitalization, incidence of infections, and GI toxicities associated with chemotherapy or radiation.[30] However, the best adult candidate for response to glutamine therapy has not been clearly identified.[30] The clinical usefulness of glutamine in neonates is less clear.[31] Plasma glutamine concentrations increase with supplementation, but no beneficial effect on sepsis, enteral feeding tolerance, necrotizing enterocolitis, growth or mortality has been reported.[29–33] The clinical use of glutamine is further complicated because there is no commercially available IV glutamine formulation. Currently available CAA solutions do not contain glutamine because of poor solubility and instability. Use of IV glutamine requires special manufacturing techniques not readily available in many institutional pharmacies.[34] Additional controlled trials are warranted to characterize the risks and costs associated with extemporaneous compounding before routine IV glutamine use can be recommended.[30,34] Dipeptide amino acids are a potential parenteral source for conditionally essential amino acids that may provide a solution to the instability and solubility limitations. Dipeptides are synthesized by combining two amino acids with a peptide bond. The resulting protein is more soluble and stable than the individual amino acids.[25] Intravenous dipeptide formulations would be advantageous clinically because they incorporate higher concentrations of some specific amino acids, as well as some low-solubility, low-stability amino acids that are omitted or present in small quantities in current CAA solutions. In addition, dipeptide use would allow formulation of CAA solutions with a higher nitrogen content. Further studies are needed to assess long-term safety and optimal combinations of amino acids in different disease states.

DEXTROSE

The primary energy source in PN solutions is carbohydrate, usually in the form of dextrose monohydrate, which is available in concentrations ranging from 5% to 70%. When oxidized, each gram of hydrated dextrose provides 3.4 kcal. The appropriate IV dextrose dose depends on the patient's age, estimated caloric requirements, and clinical condition. For example, minimum dextrose requirements in neonates is estimated to be approximately 6 to 10 mg/kg/min.[35] However, IV dextrose infusion rates should not exceed 12 to 14 mg/kg per minute in infants and 4 to 7 mg/kg per minute in adults.[35–37] The recommended dextrose dose for routine clinical care rarely exceeds 5 mg/kg per minute in older critically ill children (1 to 11 years old) and adults.[38,39] Maintaining an age-appropriate dextrose infusion rate is necessary to minimize risk of adverse effects. If the dextrose infusion rate exceeds the glucose oxidation rate, metabolically expensive pathways, such as glycogen repletion and lipid synthesis, are favored, resulting in increased energy expenditure, increased oxygen consumption, and increased carbon dioxide production. Excessive dextrose infusion rates also may contribute to the development of hyperglycemia, excess carbon dioxide production, and increased biochemical markers for liver function associated with fatty infiltration of the liver.[38–40]

Non–insulin-dependent carbohydrate sources have been investigated as an alternative to dextrose to improve glycemic control in patients with impaired insulin secretion or activity who require PN. Glycerol, a sugar alcohol that provides 4.3 kcal/g, is the only dextrose alternative commercially available for clinical use. It is available as an isotonic, 3% solution in combination with 3% amino acids and supplemental electrolytes (ProcalAmine, B. Braun Medical, Irvine, CA). Although the solution may be peripherally infused, a major disadvantage of this formula is the dilute amino acid and carbohydrate concentrations. Most adult patients require up to 3 to 4 L/day of ProcalAmine solution together with IVFE as a caloric source to provide minimum energy requirements.[41] Intravenous glycerol use in catabolic adults is safe and effective, but similar data are not available for infants and children.[42]

INTRAVENOUS FAT EMULSION

IVFE is used as a concentrated source of calories and essential fatty acids. Commercially available IVFE products differ in triglyceride source (soybean oil or a combination of soybean oil and safflower oil), fatty acid content, and commercially available concentrations (10%, 20%, and 30%). These products also contain egg phospholipids as an emulsifying agent and glycerol to make the emulsion isotonic. Although the caloric contribution of fat is 9 kcal/g, the caloric content of IVFE is 1.1 kcal/mL for 10% emulsion, 2 kcal/mL for 20% emulsion, and 3 kcal/mL for 30% emulsion because of the caloric contribution of the egg phospholipid and glycerol.[43] The triglyceride source of IVFEs differ in fatty acid composition. Emulsions containing soybean oil are made of approximately 50% to 55% linoleic acid and 4% to 9% linolenic acid, whereas IVFEs that contain safflower oil are made of approximately 66% linoleic acid and 4% linolenic acid.[43] Linolenic acid, an omega-3 fatty acid, and linoleic acid, an omega-6 fatty acid, are both polyunsaturated long-chain triglycerides (LCTs).[44] IVFE products also differ in phospholipid and triglyceride concentrations. Higher-concentrated IVFEs (20% and 30%) have a lower phospholipid-to-triglyceride ratio compared with 10% IVFE.[45] Because higher amounts of circulating phospholipids are associated with impaired triglyceride clearance in neonates and infants, 20% IVFE is the preferred product for this population.[34,40,45,46]

Both IVFE types are effective for treatment or prevention of essential fatty acid deficiency (EFAD). EFAD is the result of a biochemical deficiency of linoleic acid and arachidonic acid, which are considered essential in humans.[47] Since linolenic acid may be essential, all commercially available IVFEs contain soybean oil as a predominant linolenic acid source. These fatty acids are important for a variety of functions such as cellular integrity, platelet function, postnatal brain development, and wound healing.[47] Normally, linoleic acid is converted to the tetraene arachidonic acid. When linoleic acid is not present in sufficient amounts, oleic acid is converted to the triene 5,8,11-eicosatrienoic acid, a fatty acid of lesser physiologic integrity, and EFAD occurs. EFAD may be prevented by providing 2% to 5% of total calories as linoleic acid and 0.25% to 0.5% of total calories as linolenic acid.[34] This may be achieved in most adult patients by giving approximately 100 g IVFE weekly.[34,48] Neonates and infants require a minimum of 0.5 to 1 g/kg daily.[40]

Plasma IVFE clearance is directly related to gestational age of infants and appears to be influenced by the infusion rate and the patient's clinical status.[45,46] The risk of developing hypertriglyceridemia decreases with longer infusion times.[34,40,45] Rapid IVFE infusions are reported to contribute to decreased oxygenation in neonates.[40] Adverse pulmonary effects are thought to be caused by polyunsaturated fatty acid (PUFA)-driven prostaglandin production, which results in altered vascular tone. However, the association between IVFE and pulmonary dysfunction is not clear.[40] In addition, data in animals and humans also suggest that rapid infusion of long-chain fatty acid formulations may have a negative impact on immunocompetence by saturating the reticuloendothelial system.[44,46]

CLINICAL CONTROVERSY

Initiation of IVFE earlier than 4 to 7 days of life in infants with a birth weight less than 800 g remains controversial because of the potential increased risk of chronic lung disease and death. Some clinicians advocate initiating IVFE at 1 to 1.5 g/kg/day within the first week of life and advancing the dose after the second week of life.

As a caloric source, IVFE use may facilitate provision of adequate calories and minimize complications of nutrition therapy such as hyperglycemia, hepatotoxicity, or increased carbon dioxide production.[44] Although the frequency of acute adverse effects is reported to be less than 1% with current formulations, patients receiving their first IVFE dose should be monitored for dyspnea, chest tightness, palpitations, and chills. Headache, nausea, and fever also have been reported and might be associated with a rapid infusion rate. In general, IVFE use is contraindicated in patients with an impaired ability to clear fat emulsion, such as patients with pathologic hyperlipidemia and hypertriglyceridemia associated with pancreatitis.[46] Finally, patients with a reported egg allergy should be evaluated carefully for the nature and severity of the reaction before deciding to initiate a fat-based PN regimen.

Commercially available 10% and 20% IVFE products may be administered either by the central or peripheral route. They may be added directly to the PN solution as a total nutrient admixture (TNA) or 3-in-1 system (lipids, protein, glucose, and additives), or they may be piggybacked with the CAA-dextrose solution.[34,43,44] The more concentrated 30% IVFE is only approved for use in the preparation of TNA and is not intended for direct IV administration.

The negative effects of LCTs on immune function have stimulated a search for new lipid sources.[44] Medium-chain triglycerides (MCTs) may offer several advantages, especially for critically ill patients. MCTs are hydrolyzed and cleared more rapidly than LCTs, and they do not accumulate in the liver. In addition, MCTs do not require carnitine for entrance into mitochondria for oxidation. However, MCTs are not a source of essential fatty acids. Subsequent studies of IV MCT-LCT mixtures in a number of patients demonstrate safety and efficacy comparable with standard LCT emulsions.[44,47,49] Several MCT-LCT products are available in Europe, although no IV MCT formulations are currently available commercially in the United States. Other IV lipid formulations currently being investigated contain omega-3 PUFAs.[44] Current IVFEs contain omega-6 PUFAs as linoleic acid and omega-3 PUFAs as linolenic acid. Omega-3 PUFAs are metabolized to cytokine mediators, which may be less inflammatory and immunosuppressive than those derived from omega-6 PUFAs. The effect of IVFE administration on immune function, as well as patient morbidity and mortality, is not clear.[40,50,51] However, investigations of enteral solutions with a higher concentration of omega-3 PUFAs have reported decreased infections and improvement in in vitro immunologic indices in critically ill patients.[47,52] Although IVFE products remain the most common source of parenteral fat, a number of drugs have been introduced that contain lipid as either a vehicle for delivery or as a portion of the drug molecular formulation. Propofol, an IV anesthetic, is delivered in a soybean oil-in-water emulsion that is essentially the same as Intralipid 10%. This agent is used commonly for continuous sedation of ventilated patients and should be considered a potentially significant source of calories that may require adjustment of a patient's nutrition regimen.[53] The antifungal amphotericin B is available in several lipid-containing combinations such as liposomal and lipid complex formulations. The caloric contribution from these products when used in standard doses generally is small and is not relevant clinically.

VITAMINS

Maintenance guidelines for daily parenteral vitamin supplements have been established by the Nutrition Advisory Group of the American Medical Association (NAG-AMA) for adults, children, and infants.[54] The NAG-AMA identified 13 essential vitamins that include 4 fat-soluble vitamins and 9 water-soluble vitamins. These guidelines are based on the recommended daily allowances, which are designed to meet requirements of healthy people. Vitamin requirements for preterm infants and patients with metabolic stress or specific organ failures are controversial.[40,55–57] Revised NAG-AMA recommendations for parenteral vitamin requirements in infants and children primarily reflect changes for preterm infants requiring PN.[57]

Adult parenteral multiple-vitamin products formulated to comply with the NAG-AMA guidelines are available commercially, while there are two commercially available parenteral vitamin products for use in pediatric patients. MVI-Pediatric (Mayne Pharma, Paramus, NJ) and Infuvite Pediatric (Baxter Healthcare Corporation, Deerfield, IL) are formulated to meet the revised NAG-AMA guidelines for infants weighing less than 1 kg to children up to 11 years old. However, there are no commercially available IV multivitamin products designed to specifically meet the unique requirements of premature infants, including higher vitamin A and lower doses of vitamins B_1, B_2, B_6, and B_{12} compared to recommendations for term infants and older children.

In the past, parenteral multiple-vitamin formulations for adults contained only 12 essential vitamins. Vitamin K was not included to minimize the risk of a drug–nutrient interaction in patients receiving anticoagulants, which antagonize vitamin K-dependent coagulation factors. However, in 2000, the U.S. Food and Drug Administration (FDA) mandated reformulation of adult parenteral multiple-vitamin products to include 150 mcg of vitamin K in addition to higher doses of vitamins B_1, B_6, and C.[58] The NAG-AMA recommendation for vitamin K in adults is 2 to 4 mg weekly. Other practitioners recommend larger doses of 0.5 to 1 mg/day or 5 to 10 mg weekly.[34] An investigation of patients receiving long-term IVFE-containing PN with vitamin K-free parenteral multivitamins at home suggests that supplemental vitamin K may not be necessary to maintain normal prothrombin times and plasma vitamin K concentrations.[59] Vegetable oils such as soybean and safflower oils used in IVFEs are a natural source of phylloquinone (vitamin K_1). However, the vitamin K concentration depends on the type and concentration of vegetable oil in the IVFE.[58–60] Mean concentrations of 13.2 and 26.5 mcg/100 mL were reported for 10% and 20% Liposyn II (Abbott Laboratories, Abbott Park, IL), which contains both soybean and safflower oil.[60]

Mean concentrations of 30.9 and 67.5 mcg/100 mL were reported for 10% and 20% Intralipid (Baxter Healthcare Corporation, Deerfield, IL), which contains only soybean oil. The bioavailability of vitamin K_1 from IVFEs is unknown. Although hospitalized patients who received no additional vitamin K supplementation during short-term PN that included a low vitamin K-containing IVFE experienced minimal effects on international normalized ratio, supplemental vitamin K may be given intramuscularly or subcutaneously or added to the PN solution if needed.[58,61] Current recommendations suggest supplemental vitamin K is unnecessary when a vitamin K-containing multiple-vitamin product is used.[34] A parenteral multiple-vitamin formulation containing no vitamin K is commercially available for use in patients receiving home parenteral nutrition and warfarin anticoagulation. (MVI-12, multi-vitamin infusion without vitamin K, Mayne Pharma, Paramus, NJ.)

Vitamin requirements may be altered in malnutrition and other specific disease states or with certain drug therapies. Individual and combination products are available to provide additional or tailored supplementation, which may be necessary to prevent development of vitamin toxicities or deficiencies caused by altered metabolism or drug therapy.

TRACE ELEMENTS

Many trace elements are an important part of metalloenzymes and also function as cofactors in a variety of regulatory metabolic pathways.[55,57] Although 17 trace elements have demonstrated biologic importance, clear deficiency syndromes in humans have been described only for iron, iodine, cobalt (as vitamin B_{12}), zinc, and copper.[57,62,63] The NAG-AMA recognized zinc, copper, and chromium as being essential for IV supplementation in patients receiving PN.[64] Although a clear deficiency syndrome for manganese has not been reported in humans, the NAG-AMA considered manganese essential based on case reports of patients receiving PN with metabolic complications that corrected after manganese supplementation.[64] Reports of syndromes associated with selenium and molybdenum deficiency suggest that they also may be essential.[57,62] Recommendations for trace elements in pediatric patients receiving PN have been revised as well.[57]

Intravenous trace elements are available as single-mineral solutions and as multiple-mineral combinations with or without electrolytes. Most products provide the daily requirements for the trace minerals considered essential by the NAG-AMA (zinc, copper, chromium, and manganese), whereas some also include iodide, molybdenum, or selenium. Combination products are available for pediatric patients that provide manganese, copper, chromium, zinc, and selenium.

Requirements for trace elements also change depending on the clinical condition of the patient. For example, higher doses of supplemental zinc likely are necessary in patients with high-output ostomies or diarrhea because the GI tract is the predominant excretion route for zinc. Manganese and copper are excreted through the biliary tract, whereas chromium, molybdenum, and selenium are excreted renally. Hence these trace elements should be restricted or withheld from PN solutions in patients with cholestatic liver disease and renal failure, respectively.

ELECTROLYTES

Electrolytes such as sodium, potassium, calcium, magnesium, phosphorus, chloride, and acetate are necessary PN components for the maintenance of numerous cellular functions. Electrolytes may be given to maintain normal serum concentrations or to correct deficits. Patients who have "normal" organ function and relatively normal serum concentrations of any electrolyte should receive normal maintenance electrolyte doses when PN is initiated and daily thereafter. Specific electrolyte requirements vary according to the patient's age, disease state, organ function (see Chap. 147), previous and current drug therapy, nutrition status, and extrarenal losses. Electrolytes are available commercially as single- and multiple-nutrient solutions. Multiple-electrolyte solutions are useful in stable patients with normal organ function who are receiving PN. Concentrated multiple-electrolyte solutions designed for addition to PN solutions generally contain only sodium, potassium, calcium, and magnesium. Phosphorus must be added as a separate additive. Further information regarding metabolism and requirements of vitamins, trace elements, and electrolytes is given elsewhere.[34,65]

DESIGNING A PARENTERAL NUTRITION REGIMEN

5 Several factors, including the patient's venous access, fluid status, and macronutrient and micronutrient requirements, are important considerations when designing the PN regimen. A patient's venous access and fluid status determines how concentrated the PN solution may be compounded and hence have an impact on the nutrient amount that may be provided. PN solutions may be administered by central or peripheral venous access. The patient's clinical condition determines which route is most appropriate (Fig. 145–1).

PN solutions may be provided as a 2-in-1 formulation that contains dextrose, CAA, and other necessary micronutrients, or as a TNA that contains dextrose, CAA, and IVFE, as well as other necessary micronutrients. Use of TNA solutions offers several potential advantages, including reduced inventory (infusion pumps, tubing, and other related supplies), decreased time for compounding and administration, a potential decrease in manipulations of the infusion line (which should correspond with a decreased risk of catheter contamination), and ease of delivery and storage for patients receiving home PN.[66] Potential disadvantages include increased risk of infections and stability and compatibility concerns. For example, the stability of TNA solutions is less predictable than that of 2-in-1 solutions, which makes their use less desirable in specific patient populations such as neonates and infants.[34]

ROUTES OF PARENTERAL NUTRITION ADMINISTRATION

Peripheral Route

Peripheral parenteral nutrition (PPN) is an option for mild to moderately stressed patients in whom central access is unavailable or undesirable and function of their GI tract is expected to return within 10 to 14 days.[67] Potential PPN candidates should not be fluid restricted or require large nutrient amounts. Lower concentrations of amino acid (3% to 5% final concentration), dextrose (5% to 10% final concentration), and micronutrients compared to central parenteral nutrition (CPN) are necessary for peripheral administration. Because PPN solutions are relatively dilute, larger volumes are usually necessary to provide nutrient requirements. Additionally, many patients who receive PPN likely will require the use of IVFE to increase caloric support to levels more consistent with CPN regimens. The primary advantages of PPN include a lower risk of infectious, metabolic, and technical complications.[67] However, several other factors may complicate PPN use in many patient populations. Patients who have received multiple courses of chemotherapy, malnourished patients, premature infants, elderly patients, and others with an illness of long duration who have already been subjected to multiple venous accesses for fluid and medication administration are likely to have limited peripheral venous access. PPN use is also

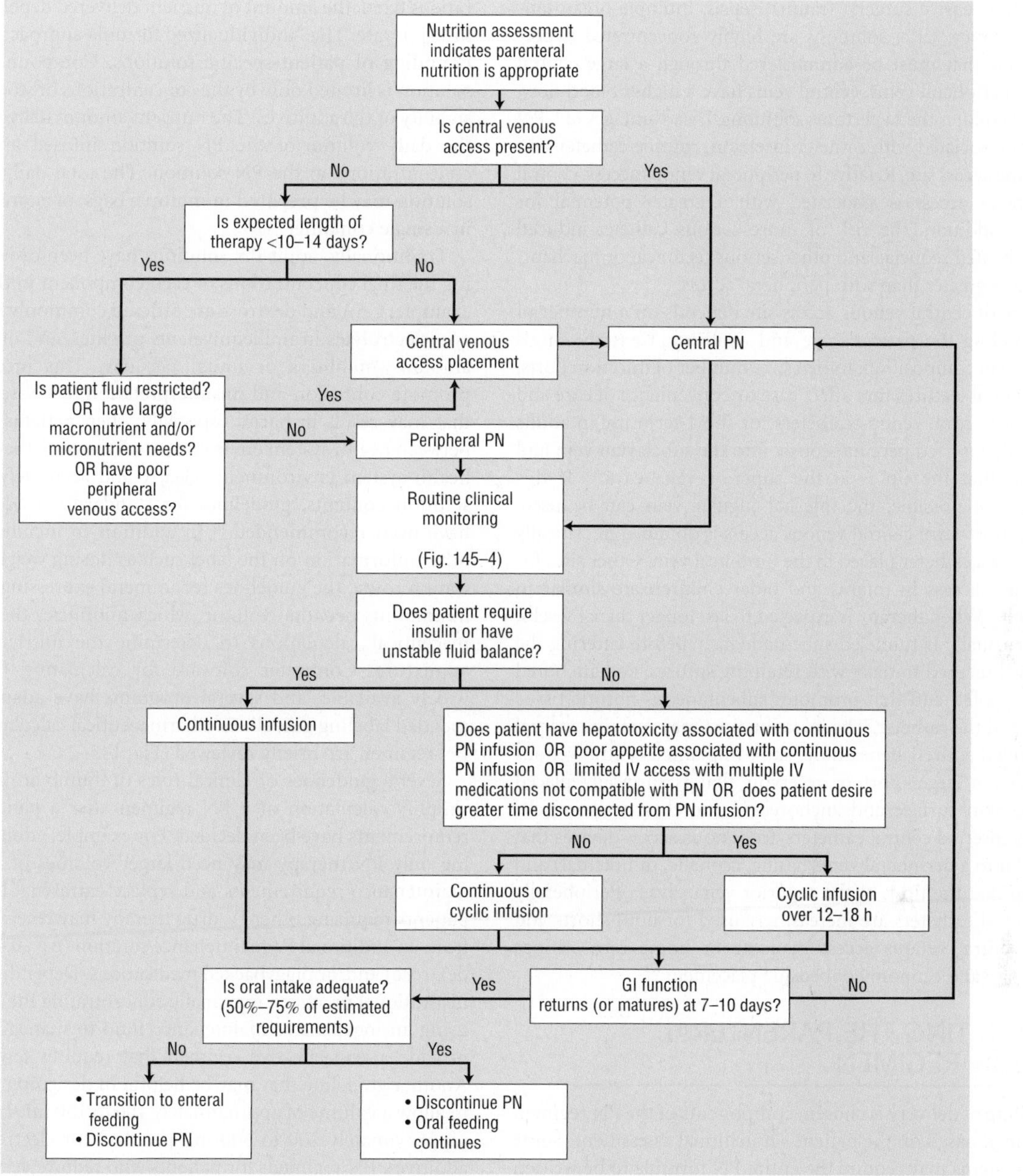

FIGURE 145-1. The route of parenteral nutrition (PN) and the infusion type depend on the patient's clinical status and the expected length of therapy.

limited by relatively poor peripheral vein tolerance to hypertonic solutions. Thrombophlebitis is a commonly reported complication in patients receiving PPN. Although the risk of developing phlebitis is greater with solution osmolarities greater than 600 to 900 mOsm/L, peripherally administered TNA with much higher osmolarities have been associated with low infusion-site complications in some centers.[67] Efforts to minimize development of phlebitis and/or infiltration sequelae in patients receiving PPN include addition of IVFE to the regimen as a possible venous lumen protectant, subtherapeutic heparin doses (0.5 to 1 unit/mL) to prevent thrombus formation, and/or small doses of hydrocortisone (5 mg/L) to minimize access site inflammation.[67] Midline catheter use may offer some advantage with reducing the risk of thrombophlebitis.[68] Although these catheters are not central venous access devices, they are longer and infuse into larger venous vessels which may dilute the PN solution to a more tolerable osmolarity. The osmolarity of a PN solution may be estimated by using the guidelines for osmolarities of selected PN components in Table 145–4.

Central Route

CPN is the preferred choice for PN delivery and is used predominantly for patients who require PN for periods of greater than 7–14 days during hospitalization or indefinitely at home.[68] These patients may have large nutrient requirements, poor peripheral venous access, and/or fluctuating fluid requirements, such as metabolically stressed

TABLE 145-4 Osmolarities of Selected Parenteral Nutrients

Nutrient	Osmolarity
Amino acid	100 mOsm/%
Dextrose	50 mOsm/%
Lipid emulsion	1.7 mOsm/%
Sodium (acetate, chloride, phosphate)	2 mOsm/mEq
Potassium (acetate, chloride, phosphate)	2 mOsm/mEq
Magnesium sulfate	1 mOsm/mEq
Calcium gluconate	1.4 mOsm/mEq

patients with extensive surgery, trauma, sepsis, multiple-organ failure, or malignancy. CPN solutions are highly concentrated hypertonic solutions that must be administered through a large central vein. Unlike peripheral veins, central veins have a higher blood flow, which quickly dilutes the hypertonic solutions. Disadvantages of CPN include risks associated with catheter insertion, routine catheter use, and care of the access site. Relative to peripheral venous access, central venous catheter access is associated with a greater potential for infection. In addition, the risk of more serious catheter-induced trauma and related sequelae and other serious technical or mechanical problems is greater than with peripheral access.

The choice of central venous access site depends on a number of factors, including the patient's age and anatomy. Central venous catheters vary in composition, lumen size, number of injection ports, and other special features that affect ease or convenience of care and maintenance. Central venous catheters for short-term use in adults are commonly inserted percutaneously into the subclavian vein and advanced so that the tip is at the superior vena cava.[68] If this approach is not possible, the internal jugular vein can be used. Frequently, short-term central venous access is obtained in critically ill neonates via a catheter placed in the umbilical vein. Other sites for central venous access in infants and older children are similar to those in adults. When therapy is expected to last longer than 4 weeks, the catheter usually is tunneled subcutaneously before entering the central vessel, secured initially with retaining sutures, and anchored in place with a felt cuff that promotes subcutaneous fibrotic tissue growth around the catheter. The injection port may remain external or be concealed entirely beneath the skin. Implanted central venous catheters have a larger port or reservoir that is surgically placed beneath the skin surface and anchored in the chest wall muscle. Peripherally inserted central catheters are venous access devices that are inserted into a peripheral vein (basilic, cephalic, or brachial) and advanced so that the tip is at the superior vena cava.[68] Peripherally inserted central catheters are increasingly used for both short- and long-term central venous access in acute or home care settings because of ease and economy of bedside placement.[69]

CONSTRUCTING THE PARENTERAL NUTRITION REGIMEN

Once the route of delivery is chosen, components of the PN regimen are determined based on the patient's nutritional assessment. Some healthcare systems may require the entire PN formula to be written in individual components and additives without the use of a standard order form. More commonly, the ordering process has been simplified by the use of order forms designed specifically for PN. These standardized order forms promote education of practitioners by providing brief guidelines for initiating PN and foster cost-efficient nutrition support by minimizing errors in ordering, compounding, and administration.[70,71] Standardized order forms also may include options for ordering certain related procedures, laboratory tests, protocols for patient management, or consultations with other medical services related to the patient's nutrition support. Standardized forms and protocols should be reviewed and updated periodically to reflect changes in the practices and patient population of a practice setting and also advances in technology that may affect provision of nutrition support.

Adult Parenteral Nutrition Solutions

In general, there are two methods for ordering adult PN. The "standard formula approach" offers a variety of base formulations with a fixed nonprotein calorie–to-nitrogen ratio. This method usually includes different formulas designed for mild to moderately stressed patients, renal failure patients, fluid-restricted patients, and liver failure patients. Because the nonprotein calorie-to-nitrogen ratio is fixed, the amount of nutrient delivered depends solely on the infusion rate. The "individualized formula approach" permits compounding of patient-specific solutions. Compounding of the PN solution is limited only by the concentrations of stock solutions and stability of the additives. The nutrient amount delivered depends on the daily volume of the PN solution infused and the nutrient concentrations in the PN solution. The total daily amount of PN solution may be prepared in multiple bags, or more cost-effectively in a single container.[34]

Traditionally, adult PN solutions have been ordered by expressing the final concentrations of each component in the solution. For example, CAA and dextrose are ordered commonly in final percentage, electrolytes in milliequivalents per liter, and other additives in amount (milliliters or units) per day. This inconsistency may promote confusion and misinterpretation of PN solution contents that may result in harm, especially when patients are transferred between health system environments. To ensure that PN labels in all health system environments clearly and accurately reflect the PN solution contents, guidelines for standardized adult PN labeling have been recommended.[34] In addition to including a variety of other information on the label such as dosing weight and administration route, the guidelines recommend expressing PN ingredients in amounts per total volume, which minimizes the need for pharmaceutical calculations to determine the nutrient value of the admixture. Computer software for calculating PN solutions is widely available, and several programs have adapted the recommended labeling guidelines. Pharmaceutical calculations of a 2-in-1 PN regimen are briefly reviewed (Fig. 145–2).

Several guidelines or clinical rules of thumb are available to help simplify calculation of a PN regimen after a patient's nutritional requirements have been decided. For example, adult patients receiving only PN therapy may need larger volumes of fluid to provide maintenance requirements and replace extrarenal losses. However, patients requiring other IV drug therapy may receive adequate fluid from an additional IV maintenance solution (e.g., 0.45% NaCl in 5% dextrose) and/or piggybacked medications. Depending on individual institutional practices, maximally concentrating the PN solution and using an inexpensive maintenance fluid to manage hydration may provide a cost-effective regimen that requires fewer adjustments. Another guideline that may be helpful in designing a PN regimen is to allow a volume of approximately 100 to 150 mL/L of base solution (approximately 200 to 300 mL per day) for electrolytes and other additives. PN regimens for patients who require very small amounts of additives, such as patients with renal failure, may be further concentrated.

Pediatric Parenteral Nutrition Solutions

Pediatric PN solutions are typically ordered using an individualized approach because clinical practice guidelines often recommend nutrient intakes based on the patient's weight. To simplify pediatric PN ordering many institutions use a pediatric-specific PN order form that expresses daily nutrient amount based on weight. For example, protein and fat are ordered as grams per kilogram per day, dextrose as milligrams per kilogram per minute, and electrolytes as milliequivalents per kilogram per day. However, some institutions may order macronutrients by expressing the final concentration of each component in the solution. Current safe practice guidelines suggest that the pediatric PN label identify components as an "amount per day" with a secondary expression of components as "amount per kilogram per day."[34] Auxiliary labels may be needed when the format between PN ordering and PN labeling is different. Calculations for determining a pediatric PN solution are reviewed to illustrate fundamental concepts for ordering pediatric PN solutions (Fig. 145–3). Additional features of the pediatric PN label include the dosing weight, administration date and time, expiration date, infu-

Calculation of an Adult Parenteral Nutrition Regimen

Patient case: A patient's daily nutritional requirements have been estimated to be 100 g protein and 2,000 total kcal. The patient has a central venous access and reports no history of hyperlipidemia or egg allergy. The patient is not fluid restricted. The PN solution will be compounded as an individualized regimen using a single-bag, 24-hour infusion of a 2-in-1 solution with intravenous fat emulsion (IVFE) piggybacked into the PN infusion line. Determine the total PN volume and administration rate by calculating the macronutrient stock solution volumes required to provide the desired daily nutrients. The stock solutions used to compound this regimen are 10% crystalline amino acids (CAA), 70% dextrose, and 20% IVFE.

1. Determine the daily IVFE calories and volume
   - 2,000 kcal/day × 30%–40% of total calories as fat = 600–800 kcal/day
     Choose IVFE 20% 250 mL/day × 2 kcal/mL = 500 kcal/day
2. Determine the 70% dextrose stock solution volume
   - Determine dextrose calories
     Dextrose calories = TOTAL – IVFE – Protein
     2,000 kcal – 500 kcal IVFE – (4 kcal/g × 100 g CAA) = 1,100 kcal
   - Calculate required dextrose (grams)
     1,100 kcal ÷ 3.4 kcal/g dextrose = 324 g dextrose
   - Determine 70% dextrose volume
     70 g/100 mL = 324 g/X mL 70% dextrose; X = 463 mL 70% dextrose
3. Calculate the 10% CAA stock solution volume
   - 10 g/100 mL = 100 g/X mL 10% CAA; X = 1,000 mL 10% CAA
4. Determine the 2-in-1 PN volume and administration rate
   - Calculate CAA/dextrose volume
     463 mL 70% dextrose + 1,000 mL 10% CAA = 1,463 mL CAA–dextrose
   - Add 100–200 mL for additives
     Total 2-in-1 volume = approximately 1,600–1,700 mL/day
   - Calculate the administration rate
     1,600–1,700 mL/day ÷ 24 hours = 67–71 mL/hour; round to 65–70 mL/hour
5. Choose final 2-in-1 PN regimen and determine provided nutrient amounts:
   - Final 2-in-1 regimen
     100 g CAA/324 gm dextrose in 1,680 mL/day to infuse at 70 mL/hour
     + 20% IVFE 250 mL to infuse at 2 mL/hour
   - Calculate macronutrient calories

20% IVFE calories:	250 mL × 2 kcal/mL =	500 kcal
Dextrose calories:	324 g × 3.4 kcal/g =	1,102 kcal
Protein calories:	100 g × 4 kcal/g =	400 kcal
Total kcal:		2,002 kcal
Nonprotein kcal:		1,602 kcal

FIGURE 145-2. Calculation of an adult parenteral nutrition (PN) regimen.

sion rate, and duration of infusion. Because infants and children generally receive daily maintenance fluid from the PN regimen, supplemental IV solutions are rarely needed. Pediatric PN may be provided as a 2-in-1 or TNA formulation. However, the TNA system is not recommended for use when compounding neonatal PN because of IVFE instability with higher calcium and phosphorus concentrations.[34] The labeling guidelines for IVFE in children are similar to those in adults.

ADMINISTRATION TECHNIQUES

PN solutions should be administered with an infusion pump. The IV administration line for CAA-dextrose solutions should include a 0.22-micron inline filter to remove particulate matter, air, and any microorganisms that may be present in the solution. IVFEs administered separately from the CAA-dextrose solution must be piggybacked into the PN line at a site beyond the inline filter because the average size of IVFE particles is approximately 0.5 microns.[34] Routine use of inline filters (greater than 0.22 microns) with TNA solutions is controversial.[68,72] However, the FDA recommends use of a 1.2-micron filter, which may be effective in preventing catheter occlusion caused by precipitates or lipid aggregates.[34] This filter size is also reported to remove *Candida albicans.*

INITIATING AND ADVANCING THE PARENTERAL NUTRITION INFUSION

ADULT PARENTERAL NUTRITION

The patient's nutrition status, current clinical status, history of glucose tolerance, and dextrose concentration in the formula will dictate

Calculation of a Pediatric Parenteral Nutrition Regimen

Patient Case: A 28-week gestational age infant's (weight 1.3 kg) estimated nutritional requirements are 3.5 g/kg/day protein, 3.5 g/kg/day intravenous fat emulsion (IVFE) and 120 nonprotein kcal/kg/day. The infant has central venous access and reports no history of hyperlipidemia or egg allergy. The PN solution will be compounded as an individualized regimen using a single-bag, 24-hour infusion of a 2-in-1 solution with IVFE piggybacked into the PN infusion line. Determine if the desired daily crystalline amino acids (CAA) and dextrose can be provided in the determined daily volume using 10% CAA, and 70% dextrose stock solutions. The IV fat source will be 20% IVFE.

1. Determine the 2-in-1 PN volume and administration rate
   - PN volume is based on maintenance fluid requirements
     150 mL/kg × 1.3 kg = 195 mL/day
   - PN Infusion rate
     195 mL ÷ 24 hours = 8.1mL/hour
2. Determine the daily protein amount and the corresponding 10% CAA volume
   - Calculate daily protein amount
     3.5 g/kg/day × 1.3 kg = 4.55 g/day
   - Calculate the 10% CAA stock solution volume
     10 g/100 mL = 4.55 g/X mL 10% CAA   X = 45.5 mL 10% CAA
3. Determine the daily dextrose amount and the corresponding 70% dextrose volume
   - Calculate daily dextrose amount to provde approximately 14 mg/kg/day
     (14 mg x 1.3 kg × 1,440 minutes/day) ÷ 1,000 mg/g = 26.2 g
   - Calculate the 70% CAA stock solution volume
     70 g/100 mL = 26.2 g/X mL 70% CAA   X = 37.4 mL 70% dextrose
   - Calculate the dextrose (final) concentration in the volume determined in step 1.
     26.2 g/195 mL = X g/100 mL   X = 13.4% dextrose
4. Determine the daily IVFE amount, volume, and administration rate
   - Calculate daily IVFE amount
     3.5 g/kg × 1.3 kg = 4.6 g/day
   - Calculate 20% IVFE volume
     20 g/100 mL = 4.6 g/X   X = 23 mL/day of 20% IVFE
   - Calculate the IVFE administration rate
     23 mL 20% IVFE ÷ 24 hours = 0.95 mL/hour
5. Determine final 2-in-1 PN regimen and provided nutrient amounts
   - Final PN regimen
     3.5 g/kg/d CAA/ 13.5% dextrose to infuse at 8.1 mL/hour
     + 20% IVFE 3.5 g/kg/day to infuse at 0.95 mL/hour
   - Calculate macronutrient calories

20% IVFE calories:	23 mL × 2 kcal/mL =	46 kcal
Dextrose calories:	26.2 g × 3.4 kcal/g =	89 kcal
Protein calories:	4.55 g × 4 kcal/g =	18 kcal
Total kcal:		153 kcal
Nonprotein kcal:		135 kcal

FIGURE 145-3. Calculation of a pediatric parenteral nutrition (PN) regimen.

the infusion rate at which the adult PN solution should be initiated. Stable patients with normal organ function and stable baseline serum glucose concentrations have demonstrated minimal effect on serum glucose concentrations when abruptly initiating or discontinuing PN therapy.[73–75] However, another approach is to begin the PN infusion and increase the rate gradually over 12 to 24 hours to the desired rate. The infusion rate is likewise reduced in a stepwise fashion, such as decreasing the rate by 50% for 1 hour prior to discontinuation, when the PN therapy ends.[74] This approach should prevent development of hyperglycemia and rebound hypoglycemia, respectively. Tapered initiation and cessation has been recommended for patients receiving intermittent subcutaneous regular insulin, patients with severe renal or hepatic disease, patients with other disease states that may increase the risk for development of hypoglycemia, such as severe diabetes or pancreatic malignancy, and patients who are receiving concurrent drug therapy that may predispose to development of hypoglycemia or mask the cardiovascular symptoms of hypoglycemia (β-blockers).[73]

Although the IVFE dose should not exceed 2.5 g/kg per day or 60% of total daily calories, lower doses of 1 g/kg per day not to exceed 30% of calories have been recommended to minimize negative effects associated with long-chain fatty acids.[34] Manufacturer's information recommends IVFE infusion over 4 to 8 hours for adults. However, infusion over 12 to 24 hours appears to be the best clinical strategy to promote IVFE clearance and minimize risk of negative effects on pulmonary and immune function.[45,46]

The manufacturer's guidelines recommend initiating IVFE in adults with a test dose of 0.5 to 1 mL/min for the first 15 to 30 minutes because of the potential for an immediate hypersensitivity reaction. In most patients, this is probably not necessary because of the relatively low incidence and benign nature of acute adverse reactions. In addition, infusion over 12 to 24 hours eliminates the need for a test dose because the infusion rate is within the range of the test dose rates recommended by the manufacturer. Appropriate electrolytes should be provided to patients with normal organ function based on standard nutrient ranges.[34] Adjustments may be necessary depending on the patient's clinical condition. Adults and children older than 11 years of age should receive daily amounts of trace elements and an adult vitamin formulation.

PEDIATRIC PARENTERAL NUTRITION

Pediatric PN solutions are typically initiated with a volume calculated to provide the patient's daily maintenance fluid requirements on the first day of therapy. Individual substrates are then advanced daily as tolerated with the goal PN regimen generally being achieved by day 3 of therapy. PN should be initiated with the goal protein dose. The initial dextrose dose for older infants and children is based on previous glucose tolerance. Although practices may vary, one approach is to start with (final concentration) 10% dextrose and advance the concentration in 5% increments daily as tolerated to a goal not to exceed 5 to 7 mg/kg per minute. Initial dextrose doses for premature infants should approximate fetal nutrient delivery rates of 5 to 6 mg/kg per minute. Frequently this mathematically translates into a final concentration range of 5% to 10% dextrose. The dextrose concentration for the neonatal PN should be advanced daily by 1% to 2.5% or by 2 to 4 mg/kg/min increments to a goal that does not exceed 12 to 14 mg/kg/min. IVFE is usually initiated at 0.5 g/kg per day in neonates and 0.5 to 1 g/kg per day in older children, and increased daily by 0.5 to 1 g/kg per day to a maximum of 3 to 4 g/kg per day. Incremental increases of IVFE dose allows daily serum triglyceride evaluation and early detection of those with impaired fat clearance. The IVFE dose should not exceed 60% of total daily calories for neonates and 30% of total calories for children. The best clinical strategy for minimizing the risk of adverse effects associated with rapid IVFE administration, and promoting IVFE clearance is to infuse IVFE over 20 to 24 hours or at a rate of 0.15 g/kg per hour.[45,46] This slow infusion also eliminates the need for a test dose because the infusion rate is less than the test-dose rate recommended by the manufacturer.

CLINICAL CONTROVERSY

Clinical investigations of PN in critically ill neonates report clinical benefits and low risk of adverse effects when PN is initiated within the first 24 hours of life. However, some clinicians continue to withhold PN therapy for 2 to 3 days after birth because of concerns for protein intolerance manifested by hyperammonemia, azotemia, and metabolic acidosis.

Intravenous electrolytes, vitamins, and trace elements should be initiated on the first day of therapy and continued as a daily component of the PN solution.[34] Children younger than age 11 years should receive a vitamin product formulated for pediatric patients. Two multivitamin dosing schemas have been suggested for infants and children.[34] One method recommends 2 mL/kg per day for infants weighing less than 2.5 kg and 5 mL per day for infants and children weighing more than 2.5 kg. The other suggests 30% of a vial (1.5 mL/day) for infants weighing less than 1 kg, 65% of a vial (3.25 mL/day) for infants weighing 1 to 3 kg, and 100% of the vial (5 mL/day) for children weighing more than 3 kg (up to 11 years of age). Adult IV vitamin formulations should not be used in infants because of potential neurotoxicity from accumulation of polysorbate and propylene glycol preservatives. Pediatric trace element formulations are dosed based on the child's weight. The usual recommended intake is 0.3 mL/kg for children weighing less than 3 kg and 0.2 mL/kg (maximum 5 mL/day) for children weighing more than 3 kg. Children weighing more than 25 kg should receive an adult trace element formulation. Pediatric patients receiving PN commonly transition from PN support to enteral nutrition by gradually, over a period of days to weeks, decreasing the PN infusion rate while increasing the enteral intake. The PN infusion rate should be reduced for 1 to 2 hours prior to stopping the infusion for neonates and infants because of their immature counterregulatory mechanisms which contribute to an increased risk for developing rebound hypoglycemia.[16] Blood glucose concentrations should be checked within 15 to 60 minutes after the PN infusion ends.

CONTINUOUS VERSUS CYCLIC INFUSIONS

❻ Continuous infusions are attractive for use in patients with unstable fluid balance or glucose control (see Fig. 145–1). The intermittent or cyclic infusion of PN over a period of time less than 24 hours, usually for 12 to 18 hours each day, is useful in hospitalized patients with limited venous access in whom administration of multiple other medications requires interruption of the PN infusion.[74] Cyclic PN also may prevent or treat hepatotoxicities associated with continuous PN therapy. In addition, this delivery mode allows patients receiving PN at home the ability to resume a relatively normal lifestyle.[74] Various protocols have been reported that suggest incremental increases to the maximum infusion rate for a desired period of time followed by a gradual taper to discontinue the solution.[16,73,74] However, metabolically stable adults and older children (older than age 2 years) receiving fat-based PN regimens are likely candidates for abrupt initiation and discontinuation of their intermittent PN regimen.[16,73,74] Cyclic PN is not optimal for all patients and should be used with caution in those with severe glucose intolerance or diabetes, or unstable fluid balance.

EVALUATION OF THERAPEUTIC OUTCOMES

❼ Thorough and consistent monitoring of patients who are receiving PN is necessary to ensure that the desired nutritional outcomes are achieved and to prevent the occurrence of adverse effects or complications. Routine evaluation should include the assessment of the patient's clinical condition with a focus on nutritional and metabolic effects of the PN regimen. Serial documentation of a patient's response to a particular regimen is a helpful guide for determining appropriate adjustments in fluid, electrolyte, and nutrient therapies.

Several biochemical and clinical measurements are necessary for effective monitoring of patients receiving PN. Serum concentrations of electrolytes, hematologic indices, and biochemical markers for renal function, liver function, and nutrition status should be measured prior to PN initiation and periodically thereafter depending on the patient's age, nutrition status, and clinical condition. The frequency of blood laboratory measurements in neonates and infants tends to be more conservative as a result of their smaller circulating blood volumes and, in some cases, lack of central vascular access. Other important clinical measurements include vital signs, weight, total fluid intake and losses, and nutritional intakes. Weekly height/

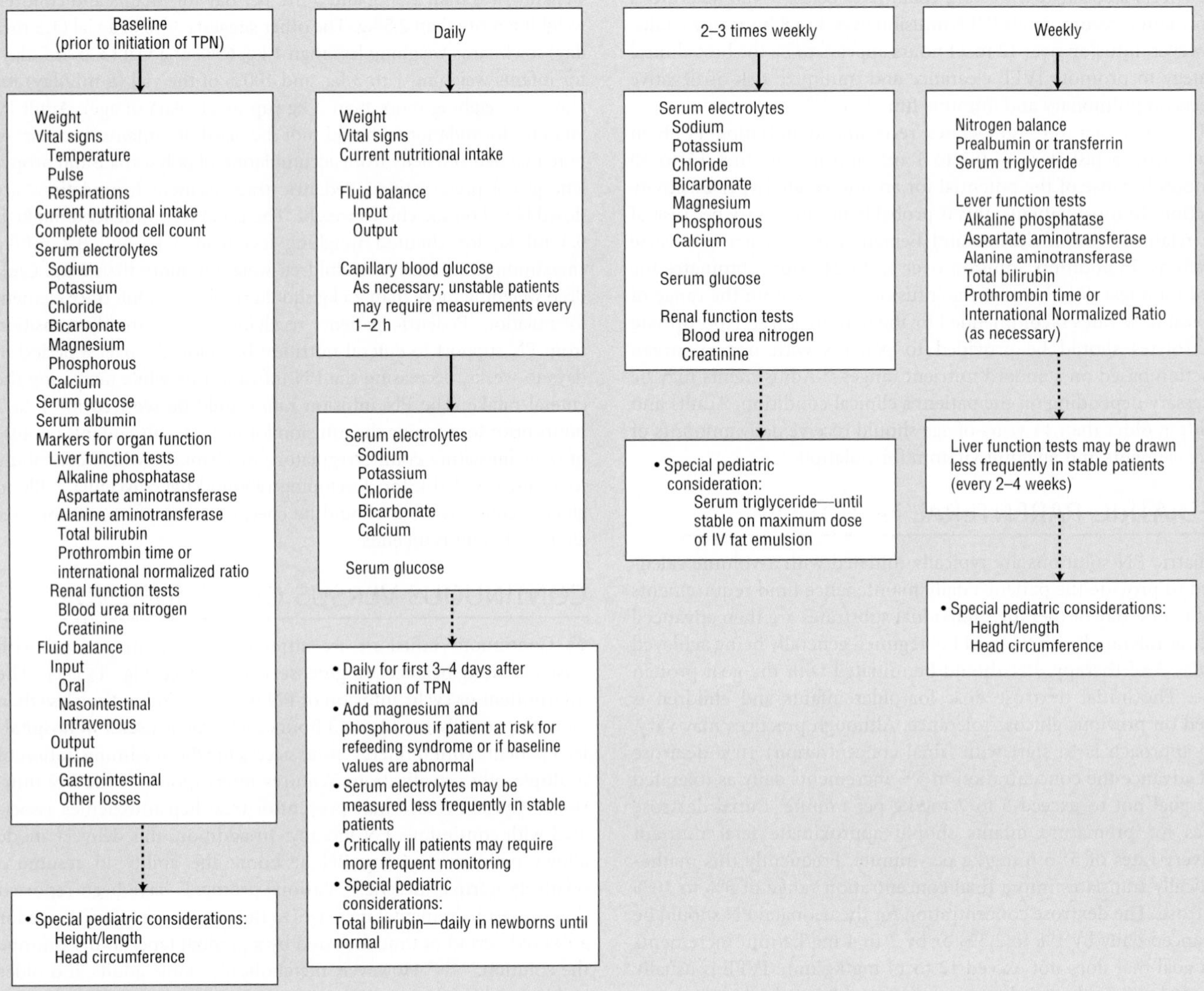

FIGURE 145-4. Monitoring strategy for patients receiving parenteral nutrition (PN).

length and head circumference measurements are helpful for monitoring nutritional changes in neonates. Monitoring parameters considered important for patients receiving PN and the suggested frequency of measurement for each are outlined in Fig. 145–4. Appropriate assessment and evaluation of patient data can identify potential complications that may be avoided or treated early. Monitoring protocols should be developed and tailored for the patient population, medical practices, and resources of individual practice settings.

COMPOUNDING, STORAGE, AND INFECTION CONTROL

The United States Pharmacopeia Chapter 797 details the procedures and requirements for compounding sterile preparations including PN formulations.[76] These standards apply to all healthcare settings in which sterile preparations are compounded and is used by boards of pharmacy, the FDA, and accreditation organizations such as the Joint Commission. Compounded sterile preparations are defined by risk level (high, medium, low) based on the probability of microbial, chemical, or physical contamination. PN solutions are classified as a medium-risk compounded sterile preparation. In general, PN solutions should be prepared using aseptic technique under a properly maintained laminar flow hood.[68,76] The hood should be situated such that the contaminant potential of normal work traffic and air currents is minimized. Personnel must be trained adequately and must practice strict aseptic technique. Supervision by a pharmacist experienced in compounding IV solutions and knowledgeable about stability, compatibility, and storage of PN solutions is also necessary. Quality assurance procedures should be developed to maintain safe and accurate admixture preparation. The potential risk of sepsis associated with PN solution contamination can be decreased greatly when pharmacy-based admixture programs follow specific guidelines developed to ensure proper compounding of PN solutions.[76]

In general, the type of solution being prepared dictates the methods of compounding, storage, and infusion. Currently, the two most commonly used types of PN solutions are 2-in-1 solutions with or without IVFE piggybacked into the PN line, and TNAs. Methods for compounding PN solutions vary based on a healthcare system's patient population and medical practices and the number of PN solutions that need to be prepared. PN base solutions may be prepared by using gravity-driven transfer of CAA stock solutions to partially filled bags of concentrated dextrose stock solutions.[34,77] Other practice settings may use commercially prepared CAA-dextrose products that are separated within a single bag and then mixed prior to use.[34] Advances in compounding technology have facilitated use of automated compounders for preparing PN solutions. Automated compounders are computer-based systems that perform the calculations necessary to determine volumes of nutrient stock solutions for PN formulations. In addition, most automated compounder systems include software that communicates the determined calculations directly to a transfer pump device that delivers fluid from the source container to the final container by either a volumetric or gravimetric fluid pumping system.[77] Advantages associated with automated compounders include reduced personnel time and compounding materials and improved compounding accuracy. Disadvantages include the potential for equipment failure and power outages.

Assurance of solution sterility during compounding, storage, and administration is necessary to reduce the risk of infection and related complications. Several studies demonstrated that because of their acidic pH and hypertonicity, CAA-dextrose PN solutions are poor media for bacterial growth.[78] However, growth of *Pseudomonas aeruginosa, Escherichia coli,* and fungi such as *C. albicans* has been reported in CAA-dextrose solutions.[78] In general, TNA solutions appear to support growth of bacteria less than IVFEs, but more than CAA-dextrose solutions. However, investigations of TNAs hung for up to 24 hours demonstrate that the risk of contamination was no greater than that reported with CAA-dextrose solutions.[44,68]

Because IVFEs also support growth of gram-positive and gram-negative bacteria as well as fungi, the Centers for Disease Control and Prevention recommend that IVFE infusions not exceed 12 hours, unless volume considerations require more time, in which case IVFE infusions should be completed within 24 hours.[68] However, these recommendations conflict with FDA-approved guidelines for handling procedures for the IVFE-containing anesthetic agent propofol, which restrict infusion time to 12 hours after the bottle has been spiked and require infusion tubing change every 12 hours.[79] Other clinical investigations of IVFE solutions infused for up to 24 hours in patients receiving PN demonstrated no correlation between risk of infection and length of hang time, so some institutions allow expiration times of up to 24 hours.[80] The Centers for Disease Control and Prevention guidelines recommend use of administration sets for 2-in-1 PN for up to 72 hours, but those used for TNA solutions and IVFE should be changed every 24 hours.

Frequently neonates require considerably smaller volumes of IVFE than are commercially available. For some patients, the volumes may be as low as 2 mL/day. To facilitate safe and accurate infusion of these small volumes, some institutions aseptically transfer IVFE into plastic syringes for syringe pump infusion. Use of transferred IVFE preparations has been associated with increased risk of bacteremia because of increased contamination risk during compounding or infusion line manipulation.[81] There are no consistent recommendations for acceptable infusion time of compounded IVFE preparations for non-TNA use. The Centers for Disease Control and Prevention recommendations do not address use of IVFE preparations transferred from the original container.[68] However, FDA-approved guidelines for propofol handling procedures restrict infusion times for doses provided in syringes to 6 hours.[79] Recent data reports a contamination risk of less than 0.1% during aseptic compounding of IVFE in syringes.[82] However, contamination risk during IVFE infusion when tubing is changed at 24-hour intervals is higher, but similar to or less than the contamination rate reported with the use of IVFE in the manufacturer's original container.[81,82] In view of the lack of consensus for acceptable infusion times for these preparations, and the clinical rationale for longer IVFE infusion times in pediatric patients who are receiving PN therapy, many institutions allow infusion times between 12 and 24 hours.[68,82]

STABILITY AND COMPATIBILITY

Comprehensive current information regarding compatibility and stability of PN solutions can be found in several reference sources such as *Trissel's Handbook on Injectable Drugs*, which is published every 2 years with supplements during alternating years, and the *King Guide to Parenteral Admixtures*, which is updated quarterly.[83,84] In many cases, the exact answer to a compatibility question may not be readily available, and a review of the primary literature may be necessary. When information is not available, clinical judgment and experience must be used carefully to resolve the situation.

CAA-dextrose solutions generally are stable for 1 to 2 months if refrigerated at 4°C (39.2°F) and protected from light.[27] However, TNA formulations are complex mixtures that are inherently unstable. Several factors affect stability of TNA solutions, including pH, electrolyte charges, temperature, and time after compounding.[27] The United States Pharmacopeia 797 standards recommend storage times of not more than 30 hours at controlled room temperature (15°C [59°F] to 30°C [86°F]) and not more than 9 days at refrigerated temperatures (2°C [35.6°F] to 4°C [39.2°F]) for all medium-risk compounded sterile preparations, including PN solutions.[85]

Because of differences in pH among various CAA products and differences in phospholipid content among IVFE products, specific manufacturers should be consulted for compatibility and stability information prior to routine mixing of components. One approach to compounding TNA formulations manually is to first combine CAA, dextrose, and sterile water (if necessary). Add electrolytes, vitamins, and trace elements and then visually inspect the solution for precipitate or other particulates. Finally, add IVFE and visually inspect the solution to ensure a uniform emulsion exists.[27,86,87] However, mixing components in this specific order and time sequence may not be possible with the use of automated compounders. The compounder's manufacturer should be consulted for the optimal mixing sequence to ensure safe compounding of TNA solutions.

The precipitation of calcium and phosphorus is a common interaction that is potentially life-threatening.[27,34] Factors that enhance the risk of precipitate formation include high concentrations of calcium and phosphorus salts, use of the chloride salt of calcium, decreased amino acid and dextrose concentrations, increased solution temperature, increased solution pH, use of an improper sequence when mixing calcium and phosphorus salts, and the presence of other additives including IVFEs.[27,34] Electrolyte stability in TNA solutions is difficult to assess because of poor visualization of a precipitate should one occur. PN solutions for neonates and infants tend to have larger calcium and phosphorus amounts, as well as other divalent cations, that limit the use of TNA formulations. Because of the relatively limited amount of published stability information, the use of a 2-in-1 formulation with separate administration of IVFEs is recommended for neonates and infants.[34] In general, alternative methods of delivering electrolytes or other medications should be pursued in any clinical situation in which compatibility information involving a TNA solution is lacking. Because the addition of bicarbonate to acidic PN solutions may result in the formation of carbon dioxide gas and insoluble calcium and magnesium carbonates, sodium bicarbonate use in PN solutions is not recommended.[34] Use of a bicarbonate precursor salt such as acetate usually is preferred.

Vitamins may be affected adversely by changes in solution pH, presence of other additives, storage time, solution temperature, and exposure to light.[27] Because of variable stabilities of individual vitamins, IV vitamin solutions should be added to the PN solution as near to the time of administration as is clinically feasible, and should not be in the PN solution longer than 24 hours.

Increased peroxide concentrations have been reported in IVFE and dextrose-amino acid solutions after addition of IV multivitamins and/or exposure to air or light.[88] Peroxide formation in dextrose-amino acid solutions depends on the concentration of IV multivitamins, CAA, and dextrose, and the presence of IVFEs.[88] Multiple in vitro experiments have reported negative effects of peroxides and associated metabolites on organ and immune function.[88,89] Peroxides are associated with neonatal hypoxic–ischemic encephalopathy, intraventricular hemorrhage, periventricular leukomalacia, chronic lung disease, retinopathy of prematurity, and necrotizing enterocolitis.[89] Neonates and infants are at increased risk for harmful effects of peroxides because they receive a higher daily peroxide load from PN solutions and they have lower endogenous antioxidant levels compared to adults.[88] Protecting PN and IVFE solutions from light is recommended to minimize peroxide formation and reduce the risk of negative metabolic effects from peroxide infusion.[20,88,89]

Many patients receiving PN at home or in a hospital also receive other IV medications. The compatibility of these medications and other intravenous IV solutions is an important concern in delivering safe and effective drug and nutritional therapy. Intravenous medications are infused most often as a separate admixture piggybacked in the PN line. However, some medications may be added directly to the PN solution and administered at the same rate as the PN infusion. Because of the potential for ineffective drug therapy or other complications associated with physiochemical incompatibility and stability of the PN solution, specific criteria should be considered before medications are added directly to the PN solution.[90] The dosage regimen should be stable for each 24-hour period and should have pharmacokinetic properties appropriate for continuous infusion. There should be documented chemical and physical compatibility of the medication with PN mixture components and other medications that may be piggybacked concomitantly into the PN line. Finally, the PN regimen should be infused continuously over 24 hours. Advantages of using PN admixtures as drug vehicles include consolidation of dosage units, improved pharmacotherapy for certain drugs, conservation of fluid in volume-restricted patients, fewer venous catheter violations, and decreased compounding and administration times.[90] However, a major disadvantage to the use of PN solutions as drug-delivery vehicles is the lack of compatibility and stability data for the PN solutions that are used commonly in clinical practice. Medications frequently added to PN solutions include regular insulin and histamine$_2$ antagonists.[83,84,90]

COMPLICATIONS OF PARENTERAL NUTRITION

MECHANICAL OR TECHNICAL COMPLICATIONS

Mechanical or technical complications include malfunctions in the system used for IV delivery of the solution, such as infusion pump failure, problems with administration sets or tubing, and problems with the catheter. Catheter-related complications are potentially life-threatening. Pneumothorax, catheter misdirection or migration into the wrong vein or improperly positioned within the cardiac chambers, arterial puncture, bleeding, and hematoma formation may occur during surgical placement of the catheter. Many of these complications, in addition to venous thrombosis and air embolism, also can occur after insertion. Catheters occasionally occlude or break during use. If these problems cannot be rectified easily, the catheter may need to be surgically replaced.

INFECTIOUS COMPLICATIONS

Infectious complications can be a major hazard in patients receiving CPN. Often these patients are predisposed to infection as a result of compromised immunity and/or concomitant infection. Frequent use of broad-spectrum antibiotic therapy and malnutrition are also predisposing factors for development of infection. Infection rarely develops secondary to solution contamination.[68,91] However, strict adherence to specific protocols for preparation of PN solutions should minimize this occurrence.[76,78] A more common source of systemic infection is catheter-related infection. Catheter-related bloodstream infection is defined as the presence of bacterial or fungal growth from the catheter tip and peripheral blood cultures. Catheter infection or a colonized catheter is defined as microbial growth from the catheter tip or from a blood culture drawn from the catheter with no growth of the same organism in the peripheral blood culture.[68] Patients with catheter-related infections may exhibit typical signs of sepsis syndrome such as fever, chills, mental status changes, hypotension, or glucose intolerance. These infections occur when the catheter becomes colonized by direct microbial invasion of the skin at the insertion site or at the infusion site of the catheter. For example, colonization may occur after multiple manipulations of the line used for PN administration, which can occur when the PN line is used to administer other medications. Other examples include failure of in-line bacterial filters, poor placement technique, and poor care of the insertion site.[68]

When no other source of infection is apparent in symptomatic patients, the catheter should be evaluated as the potential source. Blood cultures are usually drawn from a peripheral site and from the central catheter. Appropriate antimicrobial therapy is initiated. The fate of the central catheter depends on the patient's severity of illness, the suspected or identified pathogen and the type of catheter involved. The catheter may be removed and replaced in the same site; the catheter may be removed and replaced at a different anatomic location or it may not be replaced.[91]

METABOLIC AND NUTRITIONAL COMPLICATIONS

Metabolic and nutritional complications associated with PN therapy are numerous, and if left untreated, are potentially fatal. Unfortunately, the etiologies of metabolic abnormalities associated with PN are frequently multifactorial. Metabolic abnormalities related to substrate intolerance, fluid and electrolyte disorders, and acid–base disorders are summarized in multiple reviews (Table 145–5).[34,40,47,48,65,74,92–104]

PN-associated hepatic dysfunction, as evidenced by elevations in serum liver function measurements such as total bilirubin, aspartate aminotransferase, alanine aminotransferase, and alkaline phosphatase, is well documented.[93–95] No single etiology has been identified, although several risk factors have been reported. Risk factors for children include degree of prematurity, sepsis, hypoxia, lack of enteral nutrition, small bowel bacterial overgrowth, GI conditions requiring surgical intervention, duration of PN therapy, and long-term administration of excessive calories.[40,94,95] PN-associated hepatic dysfunction in infants is characterized clinically by a serum direct bilirubin concentration greater than 2 mg/dL.[95] Taurine deficiency has been

TABLE 145-5 Metabolic Abnormalities Associated with PN Macronutrients

Abnormality	Possible Etiologies
Hyperglycemia	Metabolic stress, infection, corticosteroids, pancreatitis, diabetes mellitus, peritoneal dialysis, excessive dextrose administration
Hypoglycemia	Abrupt dextrose withdrawal, excessive insulin
Excess carbon dioxide production	Excess dextrose administration
Hypertriglyceridemia	Metabolic stress, familial hyperlipidemia, pancreatitis, excess IVFE dose; rapid IVFE infusion rate
Abnormal liver function tests (elevated ALT, AST, Alk Phos, Bili)	Metabolic stress, infection, excess carbohydrate intake, excess caloric intake, EFAD; long-term PN therapy

ALT, alanine aminotransferase (SGPT); AST, aspartate aminotransferase (SGOT); Alk Phos, alkaline phosphatase; Bili, bilirubin; EFAD, essential fatty acid deficiency; EN, enteral nutrition; IVFE, intravenous fat emulsion; PN, parenteral nutrition.

proposed as an etiology of cholestasis in preterm infants and neonates.[95] Taurine is a conditionally essential amino acid that is not present in standard CAA solutions but which is important in neonatal and infant bile metabolism. However, the effectiveness of PN regimens with CAA solutions containing supplemental taurine is unclear.[94,95] Risk factors for PN-associated hepatic dysfunction in adults include preexisting liver diseases, sepsis, preexisting malnutrition, extensive bowel resection, duration of PN therapy, lack of enteral intake, nutrient deficiencies such as choline deficiency, and long-term administration of excessive calories.[93,94] PN-associated hepatic dysfunction in adults typically presents as steatosis and steatohepatitis on biopsy.[93,94] Clinically, PN-associated hepatic dysfunction is characterized by mild elevations in serum liver enzymes, usually less than three times the upper limit of normal, with peak enzyme levels usually occurring between 1 and 4 weeks after initiating PN.[93,94] In many cases, the liver abnormalities improve or resolve with manipulation of substrate intake or discontinuation of PN therapy. However, in severe cases, liver dysfunction may progress to overt failure and death.[94] Intestinal transplant with or without liver transplantation has become a treatment option for those PN-dependent patients who have failed available therapies for reversing progression of severe PN-associated liver dysfunction.[94]

Hypertriglyceridemia, defined as serum triglyceride concentrations of 400 to 500 mg/dL in adults and 150 to 200 mg/dL in preterm infants, neonates, and older pediatric patients, may occur in patients receiving IVFE-based PN. Risk factors include preexisting liver or pancreatic dysfunction, sepsis, multiple-organ failure, degree of prematurity, IVFE infusion rate, and dose.[37,45,46]

IVFE-associated hypertriglyceridemia generally is thought to be caused by defective lipid clearance.[45] Premature infants and neonates have relatively slower lipid clearance than do adults because of immature metabolic pathways, including decreased lipoprotein lipase activity.[37,45,46] Reducing the IVFE infusion rate or dose or withholding IVFE therapy should be considered when patients present with hypertriglyceridemia or lipemic serum.[45,46] Use of low-dose heparin to stimulate lipoprotein lipase activity has been suggested as a potential therapeutic intervention to treat IVFE-associated hypertriglyceridemia.[16,45] The role of carnitine for treatment of IVFE-associated hypertriglyceridemia is not clear.[16,45,46]

Severe and rapid declines in serum phosphate, potassium and magnesium concentrations, fluid retention, and other micronutrient deficiencies are common features of the refeeding syndrome.[96,97] Individuals at risk for refeeding syndrome include those who are severely malnourished with significant weight loss who receive aggressive nutritional supplementation. Other examples of patients receiving PN therapy who may be at risk for developing refeeding syndrome abnormalities include those who are unfed for 7 to 10 days with evidence of stress or nutritional depletion, those with chronic diseases causing undernutrition such as cancer, cardiac cachexia, chronic obstructive pulmonary disease or cirrhosis, and those with previous morbid obesity and massive weight loss.[97] The mechanism of the electrolyte abnormalities appears to be related to acute provision of macronutrient substrates that promote anabolism in an environment of depleted total body stores of phosphorus, potassium, and magnesium. Recommendations for initiating PN in adults at risk for refeeding syndrome include providing 25% to 50% of the calculated nonprotein caloric requirements initially. The dextrose dose should be initiated at approximately 100 to 200 g/day. Calories should be advanced over 3 to 4 days to the desired goal. Because the metabolic abnormalities described with refeeding syndrome appear to be related primarily to acute provision of large dextrose amounts, the goal protein dose may be provided with the initial PN infusion.[96] Pediatric PN regimens are usually advanced over several days as a general practice for all pediatric patients. However, additional recommendations for minimizing the risk of refeeding syndrome in pediatric patients includes provision of additional phosphorus and potassium above standard nutrient requirements at the time PN is initiated.[40]

Other nutritional complications of PN therapy may develop over a prolonged course of therapy (weeks to months) as a result of inappropriate intake of a particular nutrient. Certain conditions, such as metabolic stress in a previously malnourished patient, may elicit symptoms of deficiency much earlier if a nutrient is not appropriately provided. For example, lactic acidosis and other life-threatening complications associated with severe thiamine deficiency have been reported in patients who received PN solutions without multivitamin supplementation.[98] At least maintenance doses of vitamins, trace elements, and essential fatty acids should be provided to all patients with normal age-related organ function receiving PN.

Patients receiving PN regimens without IVFEs for extended periods (weeks to months) are at risk for development of EFAD. Clinical signs of EFAD include hair loss, desquamative dermatitis, thrombocytopenia, and malabsorption and diarrhea resulting from changes in intestinal mucosa.[34,47,48] EFAD also may be diagnosed by evaluating plasma fatty acid profiles. A triene-to-tetraene ratio more than 0.4 is biochemical evidence for EFAD. Although the time in which EFAD may develop is dependent on the patient's nutrition status, disease state, and age, these manifestations may occur 2 to 4 weeks after initiation of fat-free PN in adults and within 72 hours in premature infants.[37,47]

Metabolic bone disease is a complication usually reported in adults and children receiving long-term home PN.[93,99] This disorder in adults is characterized by osteomalacia with or without osteoporosis that may present without associated clinical, radiologic, or biochemical abnormalities. The diagnosis may not be made in premature infants until after the development of bone fractures or overt rickets. The etiology is poorly understood and likely multifactorial. Treatment options include pharmacologic intervention, calcium and vitamin D supplementation, and exercise. Others have recommended removal of vitamin D from the PN in patients with low serum parathyroid hormone and 1,25-hydroxyvitamin D concentrations.[99]

Clinical symptoms of trace element deficiencies, although rare, have been reported in patients receiving PN. More commonly, decreased serum trace element concentrations have been reported in a variety of patient populations. However, the clinical significance of decreased concentrations of many trace elements is not known because serum concentrations often do not correlate with total body stores.[62,63] Clinical signs and symptoms of trace element deficiencies are reviewed elsewhere.[62,63]

Occasionally, patients may develop nutrient-induced toxicities, most commonly as a result of the accumulation of fat-soluble vitamins or trace elements as a result of either excessive intake or decreased excretion. Certain disease states (e.g., severe renal or hepatic failure) may necessitate reduction in vitamin and trace element intake.

Many trace elements are present in PN components as contaminants.[54,100,101] The content varies among components and manufacturers. Some investigations of patients with normal organ function who were receiving PN have reported concern with elevated serum concentrations of particular trace elements such as chromium and manganese.[67,100,101] Aluminum is a common contaminant of many sterile IV solutions, including those used for compounding PN. Calcium and phosphorus solutions are among those components with higher levels of aluminum contamination.[102,103] Aluminum accumulation may occur during long-term PN therapy, especially in patients with renal insufficiency, and is associated with abnormal neurologic and hematologic function and metabolic bone disease in adults and premature infants.[99,102,103] Preterm infants are at higher risk of aluminum toxicities because they receive larger doses (micrograms per kilogram) from PN solutions than adults.[99,102,103] Preterm infants are also more likely to retain aluminum because of immature renal function. Although the maximum safe level of IV aluminum intake is unknown, the FDA has defined parenteral doses of 4 to 5 mcg/kg per day as amounts associated with central nervous system and bone toxicity in patients with impaired renal function, including premature neonates.[103,104] Even lesser amounts may result in tissue accumulation but no documented toxicity.

Recent data suggest that the aluminum content of sterile solutions used for compounding PN has declined as a result of awareness of toxicity and improvements in industrial PN component preparation.[103] However, in 2004 the FDA implemented a restriction of aluminum content in large-volume PN stock solutions (CAA, dextrose, sterile water for injection, IVFE) to a maximum of 25 mcg/L and a requirement for manufacturers to indicate the maximum aluminum concentration at expiration for both large and small volume parenteral products used for PN.[103,104]

HOME PARENTERAL NUTRITION

Advances in technology for the delivery of IV solutions have allowed medically stable patients who require extended PN therapy to be maintained indefinitely on IV nutrition. An increasing concern for cost containment of healthcare services has fostered use of sophisticated infusion devices to provide PN at home. Numerous programs are now available outside the traditional healthcare setting to support patients with various long-term or permanent medical conditions. Standards have been developed to promote safe and effective care.[6] Home PN services may be coordinated and administered through a hospital, or by a commercially operated corporation.

Many factors are considered in selecting candidates for home PN therapy. Significant benefit must be expected from placing a patient into the program. Additionally, the patient and the patient's caregiver must be willing to complete training successfully and assume numerous other responsibilities that are important for managing a new daily routine in the home. Other logistics such as funding, procurement of solutions and supplies, and clinical management and followup must be evaluated, resolved, and implemented for each patient in order to achieve the desired outcomes.[6]

Patients with Crohn's disease, ischemic bowel disease, severe GI motility disorders, extensive intestinal obstruction, and congenital bowel dysfunction have been maintained successfully with home PN.[105]

Patients commonly receive premixed PN solutions from the hospital or a commercial vendor. Intravenous vitamins or other additives may be added daily by the patient or caregiver, depending on the arrangement with the PN provider. The solution generally is administered through the night by infusion pump over 10 to 12 hours.[74] A cycled regimen allows the patient time away from the pump during daylight hours and provides many patients with the freedom to have a reasonably normal daily routine. Clinical management and followup are performed periodically according to the needs of the patient and the protocol of the care provider. A coordinated effort among several healthcare professionals, including physicians, pharmacists, nurses, social workers, and the patient and the patient's caregiver, as well as the suppliers, is paramount to providing safe and effective management. Home PN affords some patients the potential for an ambulatory lifestyle while maintaining an IV feeding regimen that was previously only available in the hospital setting. For others, home PN may contribute to a better quality of life in the comfort of their home.[105]

PHARMACOECONOMIC CONSIDERATIONS

9 Because numerous variables have an impact on the provision of PN support and the response to therapy, determining the true cost of PN is difficult.[105–108] In general, PN is an expensive intervention, and cost varies depending on the underlying indication for treatment and whether PN is provided at home or in an acute care setting.[105–108] Expenses associated with PN therapy may be categorized as direct and indirect costs.[107,108] Direct costs may be further categorized as fixed or variable costs. Fixed costs do not depend on the volume of patients receiving therapy. For example, an automatic compounder and the tubing sets required to transfer volumes of stock solutions to the administration bag would be considered fixed costs in many practice settings. These costs per patient tend to be highest in low-volume environments. Variable costs such as PN administration bags depend directly on the number of patients receiving PN. Other direct costs include ancillary services required by patients receiving PN and costs related to the management of nutritionally associated complications.

Benefits and other clinical effects of PN (i.e., length of stay and frequency of complications) in specific patient populations have been evaluated.[15–18] Few investigations have reported an economic assessment of the therapy. However, economic data from many of these reports would not necessarily reflect current costs. Indeed, the direct cost of PN solution components generally has declined over the past decade. Attempting to measure the cost or cost savings associated with reported benefits of PN therapy and other clinical effects based on results of controlled clinical trials is difficult.[106,107] Clinical outcomes measurements and hence economic outcomes are influenced by multiple factors, including experimental design, sample size, and specific health system practices. Several investigations used for determining costs and benefits of PN therapy have been criticized for such biases.[108]

Although the results of economic analyses of PN remain controversial, similarities among several reports provide a basis for methods of limiting the costs of PN therapy. These similarities include the following:

1. Use PN only for the most appropriate patients as described by institution-specific criteria based on current consensus statements.[110] The costs and complications associated with enteral nutrition are demonstrated to be less than those associated with PN.[111]
2. Reassess the need for routine laboratory measurements used for monitoring PN therapy. In general, the level of laboratory monitoring should decrease as a patient's clinical condition stabilizes.
3. Minimize the direct cost of PN by using efficient purchasing practices for PN solutions and compounding supplies through contract purchasing, streamlined compounding procedures, standardized administration times, and 24-hour hang times to reduce waste, single-bag PN solutions, and optimized monitoring plans.

CONCLUSIONS

Appropriate patient selection, assessment, and monitoring are key to successful PN therapy and the prevention of unnecessary complications. Because pharmacists are actively involved in the provision of PN at many levels, including direct patient care, education, and research, nutrition support is recognized as a pharmacy practice specialty.[112] In addition, as the interdisciplinary approach to specialized nutrition support has evolved, standards of practice have been defined for pharmacists, as well as for other healthcare professionals who provide nutrition support care.[4,8–10] Standardized order forms and monitoring protocols are useful tools to ensure appropriate administration and monitoring of PN therapy. The future of PN therapy and the role of the nutrition-support clinician will be affected primarily by new insights from clinical research and economic challenges in the healthcare environment.

ABBREVIATIONS

CAA: crystalline amino acid
CPN: central parenteral nutrition
EFAD: essential fatty acid deficiency
FDA: Food and Drug Administration
GI: gastrointestinal
IVFE: intravenous fat emulsion
IV: intravenous
LCT: long-chain triglyceride
MCT: medium-chain triglyceride
NAG-AMA: Nutrition Advisory Group of the American Medical Association
PN: parenteral nutrition
PPN: peripheral parenteral nutrition
PUFA: polyunsaturated fatty acid
TNA: total nutrient admixture

REFERENCES

1. Dudrick SJ. Early developments and clinical applications of total parenteral nutrition. JPEN J Parenter Enteral Nutr 2003;27:291–299.
2. Schneider PJ. Nutrition support teams: An evidence-based practice. Nutr Clin Pract 2006;21:62–67.
3. Holcombe BJ, Thorne DB, Strausburg KM, et al. Pharmacy practice insights: Analysis of the practice of nutrition support pharmacy specialists. Pharmacotherapy 1995;15:806–813.
4. American Society for Parenteral and Enteral Nutrition. Standards of practice for nutrition support pharmacists. Nutr Clin Pract 1999;14:275–281.
5 American Society for Parenteral and Enteral Nutrition Board of Directors and Task Force on Standards for Specialized Nutrition Support for Hospitalized Adult Patients. Standards for Specialized Nutrition Support: Adult Hospitalized Patients. Nutr Clin Pract 2002;17:384–391.
6. American Society for Parenteral and Enteral Nutrition Board of Directors and the Standards for Specialized Nutrition Support Task Force. Standards for specialized nutrition support: home care patients. Nutr Clin Pract 2005;20:579–590.
7. American Society for Parenteral and Enteral Nutrition Board of Directors and Task Force on Standards for Specialized Nutrition Support for Hospitalized Pediatric Patients. Standards for specialized nutrition support: hospitalized pediatric patients Nutr Clin Pract 2005;20:103–116.
8. ASPEN Board of Directors. Standards of practice for nutrition support dietitians. Nutr Clin Pract 2000;15:53–59.
9. ASPEN Board of Directors. Standards of practice for nutrition support nurses. Nutr Clin Pract 2001;16:56–62.
10. ASPEN and the Task Force on Standards for Nutrition Support Physicians. Standards of practice for nutrition support physicians. Nutr Clin Pract 2003;18:270–275.
11. Dickerson RN. Hypocaloric feeding of obese patients in the intensive care unit. Curr Opin Clin Nutr Metab Care 2005;8:189–196.
12. ASPEN Board of Directors and the Clinical Guidelines Taskforce. Administration of specialized nutrition support. JPEN J Parenter Enteral Nutr 2002;26:18SA–21SA.
13. ASPEN Board of Directors and the Clinical Guidelines Taskforce. Nutrition assessment—Adults. JPEN J Parenter Enteral Nutr 2002;26:9SA–12SA.
14. ASPEN Board of Directors and the Clinical Guidelines Taskforce. Nutrition Assessment-pediatrics. JPEN J Parenter Enteral Nutr 2002;26:13SA–18SA.
15. Koretz RL, Lipman TO, Klein S. AGA technical review on parenteral nutrition. Gastroenterology 2001;121:970–1001.
16. ASPEN Board of Directors and the Clinical Guidelines Taskforce. Administration of specialized nutrition support—Issues unique to pediatrics. JPEN J Parenter Enteral Nutr 2002;26:97SA–110SA.
17. ASPEN Board of Directors and the Clinical Guidelines Taskforce. Specific guidelines for disease—Adults. JPEN J Parenter Enteral Nutr 2002;26:61SA–96SA
18. ASPEN Board of Directors and the Clinical Guidelines Taskforce. Specific guidelines for disease—Pediatrics. JPEN J Parenter Enteral Nutr 2002;26:111SA–138SA
19. Ibrahim HM, Jeroudi MA, Baier RJ, et al. Aggressive early total parental nutrition in low-birth-weight infants. J Perinatol 2004;24:482–486.
20. Koletzko B, Goulet O, Hunt J, et al. Guidelines on paediatric parenteral nutrition of the European Society of Paediatric Gastroenterology, Hepatology and Nutrition (ESPGHAN) and the European Society for Clinical Nutrition and Metabolism (ESPEN), supported by the European Society of Paediatric Research (ESPR). J Pediatr Gastroenterol Nutr 2005;41 Suppl 2:S1–87.
21. Thureen PJ, Hay WW. Early aggressive nutrition in preterm infants. Semin Neonatol 2001;6:403–415.
22. Poindexter BB, Langer JC, Dusick AM, Ehrenkranz RA; National Institute of Child Health and Human Development Neonatal Research Network. Early provision of parenteral amino acids in extremely low birth weight infants: Relation to growth and neurodevelopmental outcome. J Pediatr 2006;148:300–305.
23. Clark RH, Wagner CL, Merritt RJ, et al. Nutrition in the neonatal intensive care unit: How do we reduce the incidence of extrauterine growth restriction? J Perinatol 2003;23:337–344.
24. Miles JM, Klein JA. Should protein be included in caloric calculations for a TPN prescription? Point-counterpoint. Nutr Clin Pract 1996;11:204–206.
25. Furst P, Stehle P. Are intravenous amino acid solutions unbalanced? New Horizons 1994;2:215–223.
26. Dickerson RN. Using nitrogen balance in clinical practice. Hosp Pharm 2005; 40:1081–1085.
27. Trissel LA. Amino acid injection In: Trissel LA. Handbook on Injectable Drugs, 14th ed. Bethesda, MD: American Society for Hospital Pharmacists, 2007:50–97.
28. Cairns PA, Stalker DJ. Carnitine supplementation of parenterally fed neonates. Cochrane Database Syst Rev 2000;(4):CD000950.
29. Des Robert C, Le Bacquer O, Piloquet H, et al. Acute effects of intravenous glutamine supplementation on protein metabolism in very low birth weight infants: a stable isotope study. Pediatr Res 2002;51:87–93.
30. Buchman AL. Glutamine: Commercially essential or conditionally essential? A critical appraisal of the human data. Am J Clin Nutr 2001;74:25–32.
31. Tubman TR, Thompson SW. Glutamine supplementation for preventing morbidity in preterm infants. Cochrane Database Syst Rev 2000;2:CD001457.
32. Poindexter BB, Ehrenkranz RA, Stoll BJ, et al. Parenteral glutamine supplementation does not reduce the risk of mortality or late-onset sepsis in extremely low birth weight infants. Pediatrics 2004;113:1209–1215.
33. Ball PA, Hardy G. Glutamine in pediatrics: Where next? Nutrition 2002;18:451–454.
34. Taskforce for the Revision. Safe Practices for Parenteral Nutrition. JPEN J Parenter Enteral Nutr 2004;28:539–570.
35. Hay WW. Early postnatal nutritional requirements of the very preterm infant based on a presentation at the NICHD-AAP workshop on research in neonatology. J Perinatol 2006,S13–18.
36. Rosemarin DK, Wardlaw GM, Mirtallo JM. Hyperglycemia associated with high, continuous infusion rates of total parenteral nutrition dextrose. Nutr Clin Pract 1996;11:151–156.
37. Thureen PJ, Hay WW Jr. Intravenous nutrition and postnatal growth of the micropremie. Clin Perinatol 2000;27:197–219.
38. Sheridan RL, Yu YM, Prelack K, et al. Maximal parenteral glucose oxidation in hypermetabolic young children: A stable isotope study. JPEN J Parenter Enteral Nutr 1998;22:212–216.
39. Btaiche IF, Khalidi N. Metabolic complications of parenteral nutrition in adults, part 1. Am J Health Syst Pharm 2004;61:1938–1949.
40. Shulman RJ, Phillips S. Parenteral nutrition in infants and children. J Pediatr Gastroenterol Nutr 2003;36:587–607.
41. Waxman K, Day AT, Stellin GP, et al. Safety and efficacy of glycerol and amino acids in combination with lipid emulsion for peripheral parenteral nutrition support. JPEN J Parenter Enteral Nutr 1992;16:374–378.

42. ProcalAmine. Product information. Irvine, CA: B. Braun Medical, 2003.
43. Intravenous fat emulsions. In: Wickersham RM, Novak KK, managing eds. Drug Facts and Comparisons. St. Louis: Wolters Kluwer Health, 2006:120–121
44. Driscoll DF, Adolph M, Bistrian BR. Lipid emulsions in parenteral nutrition. In: Rombeau JL, Rolandelli RH, eds. Clinical Nutrition: Parenteral Nutrition, 3rd ed. Philadelphia: WB Saunders, 2001:35–59.
45. Kerner JA Jr, Poole RL. The use of IV fat in neonates. Nutr Clin Pract 2006;21:374–380.
46. Sacks GS, Mouser JF. Is IV lipid emulsion safe in patients with hypertriglyceridemia? Nutr Clin Pract 1997;12:120–123.
47. Bistrian BR. Clinical aspects of essential fatty acid metabolism: Johnathon Rhoads Lecture. JPEN J Parenter Enteral Nutr 2003;27–168–175.
48. Dickerson RN. Essential fatty acid deficiency: An "old" disorder that should not be forgotten. Hosp Pharm 1998;33:1435–1440.
49. Lai HS, Chen WJ. Effects of medium-chain and long-chain triacylglycerols in pediatric surgical patients. Nutrition 2000;16:401–406.
50. Waitzberg DL, Lotierzo PH, Logullo AF, et al. Parenteral lipid emulsions and phagocytic systems. Br J Nutr 2002;87:S49–S57.
51. McCowen KC, Friel C, Sternberg J, et al. Hypocaloric total parenteral nutrition: Effectiveness in prevention of hyperglycemia and infectious complications. A randomized clinical trial. Crit Care Med 2000; 28:3606–3611.
52. Heyland DK, Novak F, Drover JW, et al: Should immunonutrition become routine in critically ill patients? A systematic review of the evidence. JAMA 2001:286:944–953.
53. Roth MS, Martin AB, Katz JA. Nutritional implications of prolonged propofol use. Am J Health Syst Pharm 1997;54:694–695.
54. American Medical Association Department of Foods and Nutrition. Multivitamin preparations for parenteral use: A statement by the nutritional advisory group. JPEN J Parenter Enteral Nutr 1979;3:258–262.
55. Demling RH, DeBiasse MA. Micronutrients in critical illness. Crit Care Clin 1995;11:651–673.
56. Greer FR. Vitamin metabolism and requirements in the micropremie. Clin Perinatol 2000;27:95–118.
57. Green HL, Hambidge KM, Schanler R, Tsang RC. Guidelines for the use of vitamins, trace elements, calcium, magnesium, and phosphorus in infants and children receiving total parenteral nutrition: Report of the Subcommittee on Pediatric Parenteral Nutrient Requirements from the Committee on Clinical Practice Issues of the American Society for Clinical Nutrition. Am J Clin Nutr 1988;48:1324–1342.
58. Helphingstine CJ, Bistrian BR. New food and drug administration requirements for inclusion of vitamin K in adult parenteral multivitamins. JPEN J Parenter Enteral Nutr 2003;27:220–224.
59. Chambrier C, Lellerq M, Saudin F, et al. Is vitamin K_1 supplementation necessary in long-term parenteral nutrition? JPEN J Parenter Enteral Nutr 1998;22:87–90.
60. Lennon C, Davidson KW, Sandowski JA, Mason JB. The vitamin K content of intravenous lipid emulsion. JPEN J Parenter Enteral Nutr 1993;17:142–144.
61. Duerksen DR, Papineau N. Is routine vitamin K supplementation required in hospitalized patients receiving parenteral nutrition? Nutr Clin Pract 2000;15:81–83.
62. Misra S, Kirby DF. Micronutrient and trace element monitoring in adult nutrition support. Nutr Clin Pract 2000;15:120–126.
63. Aggett PJ. Trace elements of the micropremie. Clin Perinatol 2000;27:119–129.
64. American Medical Association. Guidelines for essential trace element preparations for parenteral use: A statement by the Nutrition Advisory Group. JPEN J Parenter Enteral Nutr 1979;3:263–267.
65. Kraft MD, Btaiche IF, Sacks GS, Kudsk KA. Treatment of electrolyte disorders in adult patients in the intensive care unit Am J Health Syst Pharm 2005;62:1663–1682.
66. Campos ACL, Paluzzi M, Meguid MM. Clinical use of total nutrient admixtures. Nutrition 1990;6:347–356.
67. Culebras JM, Garcia-de-Lorenzo A, Zarazaga A, Jorquera F. Peripheral parenteral nutrition. In Rombeau JL, Rolandelli RH, eds. Clinical Nutrition: Parenteral Nutrition, 3rd ed. Philadelphia: WB Saunders, 2001:580–587.
68. O'Grady NP, Alexander M, Dellinger EP, et al. Guidelines for the prevention of intravascular catheter-related infections. MMWR Morb Mortal Wkly Rep 2002;51(RR10):1–26.
69. ASPEN Board of Directors and The Clinical Guidelines Taskforce. Access for administration of nutrition support. JPEN J Parenter Enteral Nutr 2002;26:33SA–41SA.
70. Cerulli J, Malone M. Can changes to a total parenteral nutrition order form improve prescribing? Nutr Clin Pract 2000;15:143–151.
71. Peverini RL, Beach DS, Wan KW, Vyhmeister NR. Graphical user interface for a neonatal parenteral nutrition decision support system. Proc AMIA Symp 2000:650–654.
72. Mirtallo JM. The complexity of mixing calcium and phosphate. Am J Hosp Pharm 1994;51:1535–1536.
73. Dickerson RN. How fast can I taper a TPN in a hospitalized patient? Hosp Pharm 1985;20:620–621.
74. Speerhas R, Wang J, Seidner D, Steiger E. Maintaining normal blood glucose concentrations with total parenteral nutrition: Is it necessary to taper total parenteral nutrition? Nutr Clin Pract 2003;18:414–416.
75. Krzyda EA, Andris DA, Whipple JK, et al. Glucose response to abrupt initiation and discontinuation of total parenteral nutrition. JPEN J Parenter Enteral Nutr 1993;17:64–67.
76. USP General Information Chapter. Pharmaceutical Compounding: Sterile Preparations (797). USP 27/NF 22. Rockville, MD: United States Pharmacopeia Convention, 2003.
77. American Society for Health-System Pharmacists. ASHP guidelines on the safe use of automated compounding devices for the preparation of parenteral nutrition admixtures. Am J Health Syst Pharm 2000;57:1343–1348.
78. Thompson B, Robinson LA. Infection control of parenteral nutrition solutions. Nutr Clin Pract 1991;6:49–54.
79. Propofol injectable emulsion 1%. Product information. Bedford, OH: Bedford Laboratories, 2005.
80. Ebbert ML, Farraj M, Hwang LT. The incidence and clinical significance of intravenous fat emulsion contamination during infusion. JPEN J Parenter Enteral Nutr 1987;11:42–45.
81. Sacks GS, Driscoll DF. Does lipid hang time make a difference? Time is of the essence. Nutr Clin Pract 2002;17:284–290.
82. Reiter PD, Robles J, Dowell EB. Effect of 24-hour intravenous tubing set change on the sterility of repackaged fat emulsion in neonates. Ann Pharmacother 2004;38:1603–1607.
83. Trissel LA. Handbook on Injectable Drugs, 14th ed. Bethesda, MD: American Society for Hospital Pharmacists, 2007.
84. King JC, Catania PN, ed. King Guide to Parenteral Admixtures, 36th ed. Napa, CA: King Guide Publications, 2007.
85. Proposed revisions to general chapter 797 pharmaceutical compounding-sterile preparations. Pharmacopeial Forum (PF) 2006:32; May-June.
86. Intralipid 20%. Product information. Deerfield, IL: Baxter Healthcare Corporation, 2000.
87. Trissel LA, Gilbert DL, Martinez JF, et al. Compatibility of medications with 3-in-1 parenteral nutrition admixtures. JPEN J Parenter Enteral Nutr 1999:67–74.
88. Laborie S, Lavoie JC, Pineault M, Chessex P. Contribution of multivitamins, air and light in the generation of peroxides in adult and neonatal parenteral nutrition solutions. Ann Pharmacother 2000;34:440–445.
89. Baird LL. Protecting TPN and lipid infusions from light: reducing hydroperoxides in NICU patients. Neonatal Netw 2001;20(2):17–22.
90. Driscoll DF, Baptista RJ, Mitrano FP, et al. Parenteral nutrient admixtures as drug vehicles: Theory and practice in the critical care setting. DICP 1991;25:276–283.
91. Mermel LA, Farr BM, Sherertz RJ, et al. Guidelines for the management of intravascular catheter-related infections. Clin Infect Dis 2001;32:1249–1272.
92. McMahon MM. Management of parenteral nutrition in acutely ill patients with hyperglycemia. Nutr Clin Pract 2004;19:120–128.
93. Btaiche IF, Khalidi N. Metabolic complications of parenteral nutrition in adults, part 2. Am J Health Syst Pharm 2004;61:2050–2057.
94. Buchman AL, Iyore K, Fryer J. Parenteral nutrition-associated liver disease and the role for isolated intestine and intestine/liver transplantation. Hepatology 2006;43:9–19.
95. Btaiche IF, Khalidi N. Parenteral nutrition-associated liver complications in children. Pharmacotherapy 2002;22:188–211.
96. Brooks MJ, Melnik G. The refeeding syndrome: An approach to understanding its complications and preventing its occurrence. Pharmacotherapy 1995;15:713–726.
97. Kraft MD, Btaiche IF, Sacks F. Review of the refeeding syndrome. Nutr Clin Pract 2005;20:625–633.

98. Centers for Disease Control. Lactic acidosis traced to thiamine deficiency related to nationwide shortage of multivitamins for total parenteral nutrition—United States, 1997. MMWR Morb Mortal Wkly Rep 1997;46:523–528.
99. Buchman AL, Moukarzel A. Metabolic bone disease associated with total parenteral nutrition. Clin Nutr 2000;19:217–231.
100. Mouser JF, Hak EB, Helms RA, et al. Chromium and zinc concentrations in pediatric patients receiving long-term parenteral nutrition. Am J Health Sys Pharm 1999;56:1950–1956.
101. Dickerson RN. Manganese intoxication and parenteral nutrition. Nutrition 2001;17:689–693.
102. Davis A, Spillane R, Zublena L. Aluminum: A problem trace metal in nutrition support. Nutr Clin Pract 1999;14:227–231.
103. Gura KM, Puder M. Recent developments in aluminum contamination of products used in parenteral nutrition. Curr Opin Clin Nutr Metab Care 2006;9:239–246.
104. Food and Drug Administration. Aluminum in large and small volume parenterals used in total parenteral nutrition. Fed Regist 2000;65:4103–4111.
105. Howard L. Home parenteral nutrition: Survival, cost, and quality of life. Gastroenterology 2006;130:S52–S59.
106. Lipman TO. The cost of TPN: Is the price right? JPEN J Parenter Enteral Nutr 1993;17:199–200.
107. Eisenberg JM, Glick HA, Buzby GP, et al. Does perioperative total parenteral nutrition reduce medical care costs? JPEN J Parenter Enteral Nutr 1993;17:201–209.
108. Twomey PL, Patching SC. Cost effectiveness of nutritional support. JPEN J Parenter Enteral Nutr 1985;9:3–10.
109. Eisenberg JM, Glick H, Hillman AL, et al. Measuring the economic impact of perioperative total parenteral nutrition: Principles and design. Am J Clin Nutr 1988;47:382–391.
110. Trujillo EB, Young LS, Chertow GM, et al. Metabolic and monetary costs of avoidable parenteral nutrition use. JPEN J Parenter Enteral Nutr 1999;23:109–113.
111. Zaloga GP. Parenteral nutrition in adult inpatients with functioning gastrointestinal tracts: Assessment of outcomes. Lancet 2006;367:1101–1111.
112. Holcomb BJ, Thorn DB, Strausburg KM, et al. Analysis of the practice of nutrition support pharmacy specialists. Pharmacotherapy 1995:15:806–813.

CHAPTER 146 Enteral Nutrition

VANESSA J. KUMPF AND KATHERINE HAMMOND CHESSMAN

KEY CONCEPTS

1. The gastrointestinal (GI) tract defends the host from toxins and antigens by both immunologic and nonimmunologic mechanisms, collectively referred to as the gut barrier function. Whenever possible, enteral nutrition (EN) is preferred over parenteral nutrition (PN) because it is as effective, may reduce metabolic and infectious complications, and is less expensive.

2. Candidates for EN are those who cannot or will not eat, those who exhibit a sufficiently functioning GI tract to allow adequate nutrient absorption, and in whom enteral access can be safely obtained.

3. The most common route for both short-term and long-term EN access is directly into the stomach. The method of delivery may be either continuously via an infusion pump, intermittently via a pump or gravity drip, or by bolus administration.

4. Patients unable to tolerate feeding directly into the stomach because of impaired gastric motility and for those at high risk of aspiration, feeding tube tip placement into the duodenum or jejunum may be indicated. When feeding into the small bowel, the continuous method of delivery via an infusion pump is required in order to enhance tolerance.

5. Selection of the enteral feeding formulation depends on nutritional requirements, the patient's primary disease state and related complications, and nutrient digestibility and absorption. A standard polymeric formulation will meet the needs of the majority of adult patients and children older than 10 years of age.

6. Measurement of gastric residual volumes can be used to monitor GI tolerance in patients receiving gastric feeding. Although not always reliable, excessive residual volumes may be associated with nausea, abdominal distension, and increased risk for aspiration.

7. Management of diarrhea in patients receiving EN should focus on identification and correction of the most likely cause(s). Tube feeding-related causes include too rapid delivery or advancement of formula, intolerance to the formula composition, and occasionally formula contamination.

8. Prior to administering medications through a feeding tube, the feeding tube tip location should be verified (stomach or small bowel) and the most suitable dosage form selected. Medications that should not be crushed and administered through a tube include enteric-coated or sustained-release capsules or tablets and sublingual or buccal tablets.

9. The coadministration of medications with EN can result in alterations in bioavailability and/or changes in the desired pharmacologic effects of several medications, including phenytoin, warfarin, selected antibiotics, antacids, and omeprazole.

Learning objectives, review questions, and other resources can be found at **www.pharmacotherapyonline.com.**

Enteral nutrition (EN) is defined as the delivery of nutrients by tube or by mouth into the GI tract. This chapter focuses on nutrient delivery through a feeding tube rather than the oral ingestion of food. The terms EN and tube feeding are thus used interchangeably in this context. The goal of EN is to provide calories, macronutrients, and micronutrients to those patients who are unable to achieve these requirements from an oral diet. Over the past 20 to 30 years, EN has replaced parenteral nutrition (PN) as the preferred method of specialized nutrition support in many patients who are at risk of malnutrition. Improvements in enteral access techniques and feeding formulations, and the recognition of methods to prevent and manage complications have resulted in an increased use of EN across all healthcare settings.

In this chapter, the principles and practices related to the successful use of EN support are described. Digestive and absorptive physiology is reviewed and the beneficial effects of EN are presented. The indications for EN, and descriptions of various enteral access and administration methods are also summarized. Characteristics of commercially available enteral feeding formulations are presented, as well as initiation and monitoring guidelines to prevent and manage complications. Clinical therapeutic controversies are highlighted and discussed. In addition, issues of drug compatibility, drug–nutrient interactions, and drug administration via enteral feeding tubes are discussed. Finally, the effectiveness and pharmacoeconomics of EN in enhancing nutrition and disease outcome goals are reviewed.

GASTROINTESTINAL TRACT PHYSIOLOGY

DIGESTION AND ABSORPTION

Digestion and absorption are GI processes that generate the body's usable fuels.[1–3] Digestion consists of the stepwise conversion of a complex chemical and physical nutrient into a molecular form which is absorbable by the intestinal mucosa. Absorption from the GI tract is a multistep process that includes the transfer of a nutrient across the intestinal cell membrane. The nutrient ultimately reaches the systemic circulation through the portal venous or splanchnic lymphatic systems, provided the GI or biliary tract does not excrete

TABLE 146-1 Gastrointestinal Enzymes and Hormones

Enzyme/Hormone	Site of Secretion	Main Actions
Amylase	Salivary glands, pancreas	Converts carbohydrates, starch, and glycogen to simple disaccharides
Cholecystokinin (CCK)	Duodenum, jejunum	Stimulates pancreatic enzyme secretion and gallbladder contraction
Chymotrypsinogen	Pancreas	Breaks down proteins into proteases and peptides
Enteroglucagon	Duodenum, small intestine	Inhibits pancreatic enzyme secretion and bowel motility
Gastric inhibitory peptide (GIP)	Small intestine	Decreases gastric motility and stimulates insulin secretion
Gastrin	Stomach, duodenum	Stimulates gastric acid secretion and mucosal growth
Glucagon	Pancreas	Stimulates hepatic glycogenolysis and inhibits motility
Lipase	Pancreas	Hydrolyzes short-chain and medium-chain triglycerides, involved in fat absorption
Pancreatic polypeptide	Pancreas	Inhibits gallbladder contraction and pancreatic and biliary secretion
Pepsinogen	Stomach	Converts large proteins into polypeptides
Secretin	Small intestine	Stimulates hepatic and pancreatic water and bicarbonate release
Trypsinogen	Pancreas	Breaks down proteins into proteases and peptides
Vasoactive inhibitory peptide (VIP)	Small intestine, pancreas	Vasodilator; stimulates water and bicarbonate secretion, release of insulin and glucagon, and production of small intestinal juice

it. Ingested nutrients are primarily large polymers that cannot be absorbed by the intestinal cell membrane unless they are transformed into an absorbable molecular form. In addition, a coordinated interplay of GI motility and neurohormonal secretion is required to facilitate adequate digestion and absorption.

Nutrient digestion involves the complex coordination of multiple mechanical, enzymatic, and physicochemical processes.[1–3] Mechanical dissolution of food occurs by chewing, mixing, and grinding of the stomach contents. Food stimulates the secretion of numerous neurohormones and enzymes from the salivary glands, stomach, liver and biliary system, pancreas, and intestines (Table 146–1). As food passes along the gut lumen, these neurohormones modulate GI motility and the secretions from subsequent organs of the digestive system. Nutrient digestion occurs within the gut lumen and is a specific function of the intestinal cell membrane, which is comprised of finger-like projections called villi. Each individual villus is made up of epithelial cells called enterocytes. The enterocyte surface contains special luminal projections called microvilli, which provide an increased surface area that is referred to as the brush-border membrane.

Figure 146–1 illustrates the digestion and absorption of carbohydrate, fat, and protein within the small intestine. Carbohydrates are presented to the small intestine as either a digestible or nondigestible form. Polysaccharides (starches) and oligosaccharides (sucrose and lactose) undergo enzymatic digestion within the small intestine to produce simple sugars. The simple sugars are absorbed via active and passive transport mechanisms and are eventually released into the portal vein. Polysaccharides such as cellulose complexes and other fiber components pass undigested to the colon, where they are digested by bacteria and enzymes to short-chain fatty acids.[4] Absorption of short-chain fatty acids by the colon stimulates sodium and water reabsorption, serves as an energy source, and provides nourishment to the colonic mucosa cells.

Fat is presented to the small intestine as long-chain triglycerides.[5] Its digestion requires pancreatic enzyme release and formation of mixed bile salt micelles, which then facilitate absorption across the intestinal enterocyte. Within the enterocyte, triglycerides are reesterified and packaged into chylomicrons for release into the lymphatic system. Medium-chain triglycerides (MCTs) can be absorbed intact by the mucosal membrane and are acted on by intracellular lipase within the enterocyte to release free fatty acids that pass directly into the portal vein.

Protein is presented to the small intestine primarily as large polypeptides and to a small extent as free amino acids because of the denaturation of protein within the stomach. Luminal polypeptide digestion generates oligopeptides, which are further hydrolyzed to dipeptides and tripeptides. Absorption of peptides occurs via a peptide transport system, while free amino acids are carried via specific amino acid transport systems. The carriers for the peptides are very efficient, whereas absorption of free amino acids appears to be more

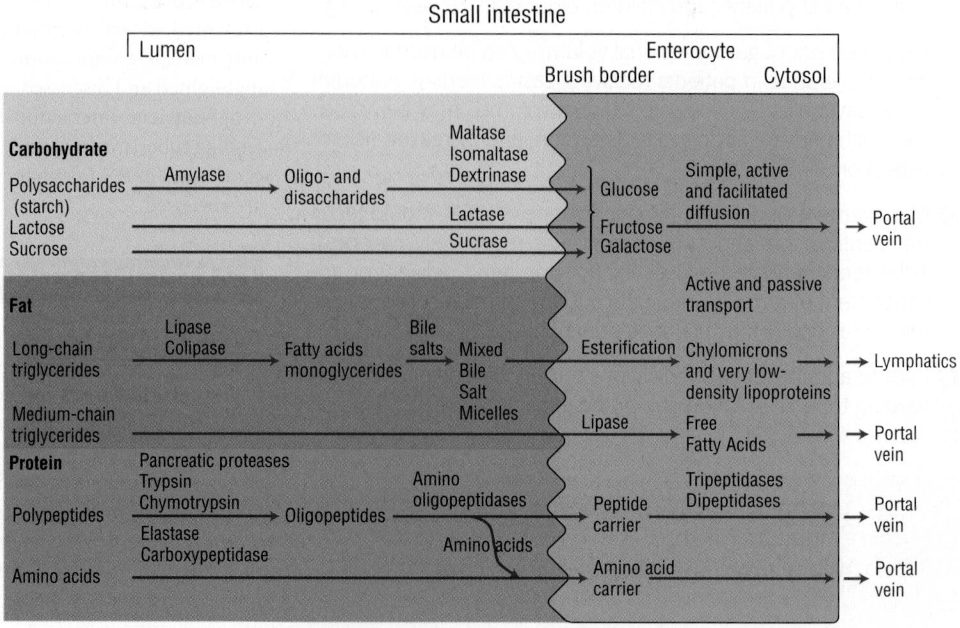

FIGURE 146-1. Schematic of carbohydrate, fat, and protein digestion.

limited and less efficient.[3] Understanding the mechanisms of digestive and absorptive physiology can greatly enhance the rational use of EN during conditions of normal or altered GI anatomy and/or function. Several circumstances may alter the efficacy of nutrient digestion and absorption. For example, the functional immaturity of the neonatal gut may lead to clinical problems associated with inadequate digestion and absorption of EN. These factors, as they relate to successful EN practice, are discussed in detail throughout this chapter.

GUT HOST DEFENSE MECHANISMS

❶ Besides digesting and absorbing nutrients to maintain nutritional health, the GI tract is actively involved in defending the host from toxins and antigens by means of nonimmunologic and immunologic mechanisms.[6] These gut host defense mechanisms are also collectively referred to as the gut barrier function. The gut barrier acts to prevent the spread of intraluminal bacteria and endotoxin to systemic organs and tissues. Hydrochloric acid secreted by the stomach kills the majority of the bacteria ingested with food. Under normal circumstances, a mucus gel layer coats the intestinal epithelium and thereby alters the adherence of bacteria to the cells of the GI tract and provides a favorable environment for anaerobic bacteria. Anaerobic bacteria, which normally colonize the mucus layer, aid in preventing tissue colonization by potential pathogens. Small-bowel peristalsis further prevents bacterial stasis and overgrowth. The gut barrier function is also maintained by the intestinal immune system, known as the gut-associated lymphoid tissue. This gut-associated lymphoid tissue regulates the local immune response to antigens within the GI tract. Specific immunoglobulins are secreted to kill remaining organisms and neutralize any toxins they produce. The hepatic Kupffer cells help to maintain gut barrier function by clearing the portal blood of gut-derived bacteria and endotoxins. The integrity of gut barrier function may be affected by numerous pathogenic insults such as physiologic stress and ischemia, and a variety of drugs, including chemotherapeutic agents. The nutritional aspects that influence the maintenance of the gut barrier are addressed in the Benefits of Enteral Nutrition and Enteral Feeding Formulation Selection sections of this chapter.

INDICATIONS FOR ENTERAL NUTRITION

❷ The decision to initiate EN is based on a variety of factors. Suitable candidates are those who cannot or will not eat a sufficient amount to meet nutritional requirements, those who exhibit a sufficient functioning GI tract to allow the absorption of nutrients, and those in whom a method of enteral access can be safely obtained.[7–9] Enteral nutrition may be indicated in a variety of conditions or disease states (Table 146–2). For example, patients who have neurologic disorders, such as a cerebrovascular accident, and have difficulty swallowing often require EN. Patients unable to eat because of conditions such as facial or jaw injuries, lesions of the oral cavity or esophagus, esophageal stricture, or head and neck cancer may also be candidates for EN delivered distal to the affected site. Extreme prematurity necessitates tube feeding because the suck–swallow mechanism has not yet developed sufficiently to allow safe oral intake.

Critically ill patients who are endotracheally intubated for mechanical ventilation represent a large percentage of patients requiring EN. Many of these patients may have reduced gastric motility and emptying caused by sepsis, GI surgery, anesthetic agents, opioid analgesics, and underlying pathology such as diabetic gastroparesis. However, successful EN can often be achieved by bypassing the stomach and placing the tip of the feeding tube beyond the pylorus into the duodenum, or preferably into the jejunum.

The use of EN during acute pancreatitis has increased. Concerns that feeding may exacerbate the disease process by stimulating exocrine pancreatic secretion historically led to the widespread use of PN and bowel rest in these patients. However, EN has been associated with a significant reduction in infectious complications compared to PN in patients with acute pancreatitis.[10] The degree of pancreatic stimulation depends on the location of the tip of the feeding tube and the composition of the feeding formulation.[11] The more distally the feeding is delivered, the less pancreatic stimulation occurs. When patients with pancreatitis require specialized nutrition support, EN should be attempted prior to initiating PN.[7]

The only absolute contraindications for EN are mechanical obstruction[8] and necrotizing enterocolitis.[12] However, conditions such as severe diarrhea, protracted vomiting, enteric fistulae, severe GI hemorrhage, and intestinal dysmotility may result in significant challenges to the successful use of EN.

TABLE 146-2 Potential Indications for Enteral Nutrition

Neoplastic disease	**Gastrointestinal disease**
Chemotherapy	Inflammatory bowel disease
Radiation therapy	Short bowel syndrome
Upper gastrointestinal tumors	Esophageal motility disorder
Cancer cachexia	Pancreatitis
Organ failure	Fistulas
Hepatic	Gastroesophageal reflux disease
Renal	Esophageal or intestinal atresia
Cardiac cachexia	**Neurologic impairment**
Pulmonary	Comatose state
Bronchopulmonary dysplasia	Cerebrovascular accident
Congenital heart disease	Demyelinating disease
Hypermetabolic states	Severe depression
Closed head injury	Failure to thrive
Burns	Cerebral palsy
Trauma	**Other indications**
Postoperative major surgery	Acquired immune deficiency syndrome
Sepsis	Anorexia nervosa
	Complications during pregnancy
	Geriatric patients with multiple chronic diseases
	Organ transplantation
	Inborn errors of metabolism
	Cystic fibrosis
	Extreme prematurity

BENEFITS OF ENTERAL NUTRITION

The importance of maintaining nutrient delivery through the GI tract in patients without a contraindication to its use is well supported. The beneficial effects of EN, specifically in the critically ill patient, is further enhanced if EN is initiated within 24 to 48 hours of admission to an intensive care unit.

ENTERAL VERSUS PARENTERAL NUTRITION

Clinical studies comparing EN to PN in the critically ill demonstrate a decrease in infectious complications and thereby improved outcomes with the use of EN.[13–15] The mechanism for the apparent beneficial effects is not clear although animal evidence suggests that EN prevents bacterial translocation across the gut. Without intraluminal fuels, it has been proposed that the integrity and function of the GI tract may deteriorate, and under stress, allow for the translocation of microbes or endotoxins.[16–18] It is further proposed that endotoxin release can activate inflammatory pathways and thereby contribute to the development of multisystem organ failure. Provision of enteral nutrients appears to help maintain intestinal mucosal structure and function, which may prevent translocation of gut bacteria to the portal or lymphatic circulation. Thus enteral nutrition appears to play a role in maintaining gut mucosal growth and development to preserve gut barrier function.

Critical reviews of available randomized controlled trials comparing EN to PN in the critically ill adult patient with an intact GI tract suggest a significant reduction in infectious complications associated with EN.[7,13,15] Decreased infectious complications have been documented in patients with abdominal trauma, burns, or severe head injury given EN compared to PN. EN is thus preferred over PN for the feeding of critically ill patients requiring specialized nutrition support.[7,15]

Enteral nutrition is more physiologic than PN in terms of nutrient utilization and therefore is generally associated with fewer metabolic complications, such as glucose intolerance and elevated insulin requirements to maintain normoglycemia.[19] It has been proposed that better blood glucose control occurs during enteral administration because the insulin released is absorbed with the glucose via the portal vein and is then metabolized by the liver. An additional physiologic benefit of enteral feeding is that it stimulates bile flow through the biliary tract and hence reduces the risk of developing cholestasis, gallbladder sludge, and gallstones, conditions which have been associated with long-term PN and bowel rest.[20] Also, EN avoids the potential infectious and technical complications associated with the placement and use of a central venous access device required for PN. Finally, EN is less costly than PN when all factors are considered.

EARLY VERSUS DELAYED INITIATION

The optimal timing of initiation of EN is a controversial issue. It has been suggested that initiating EN early in the course of illness may attenuate the stress response and improve feeding tolerance. Clinical studies demonstrating a decrease in infectious complications with the use of EN compared to PN in the critically ill patient initiated feeding within 24 to 48 hours of hospital admission.[13,15,21] The benefits of decreased infectious complications are not apparent when the initiation of EN is delayed. A review of available studies comparing early versus delayed EN in critically ill patients showed a trend toward a reduction in infectious complications with early EN.[15] In addition, a trend toward reduction in mortality associated with early EN has also been noted.[15,22]

In critically ill patients who are hemodynamically unstable, early EN may result in gut ischemia because of poor gut blood flow and increased oxygen demand. Consequently, it is recommended that initiation of EN be delayed until the patient is fluid resuscitated and has an adequate perfusion pressure. Once this goal is achieved, often within 6 hours of hospitalization, the initiation of EN at a low infusion rate is considered appropriate, along with clinical monitoring to assure GI tolerance.[23,24] Therefore, early EN (within 24 to 48 hours after hospital admission) is recommended in critically ill patients.[15] Early initiation of EN is not warranted for the mild to moderately stressed patient who is otherwise well nourished. It is reasonable to delay the initiation of EN in these patients until oral intake is inadequate for 7 to 14 days.[7]

ENTERAL ACCESS

Recent advances in enteral access techniques have contributed to the expanded use of EN for conditions in which PN had previously been used. In particular, improved methods of achieving jejunal access for feeding have allowed for the use of EN during the early postoperative and postinjury period when gastric motility is typically delayed. As outlined in Table 146–3, various factors influence the selection of enteral access site and device, including anticipated duration of use (short-term or long-term) and whether to feed into the stomach or small bowel. Figure 146–2 illustrates the predominant enteral access options.

SHORT-TERM ACCESS

❸ Short-term enteral access is generally easier to initiate, less invasive, and less costly than the establishment of long-term access.[25] The most frequently used routes for short-term enteral access are established by inserting a tube through the nose and passing the tip into the stomach (nasogastric [NG]), duodenum (nasoduodenal), or jejunum (nasojejunal). In general, these tubes are used in the hospitalized patient when the anticipated tube feeding duration is less than 4 to 6 weeks. The orogastric route is generally reserved for patients in whom the nasopharyngeal area is inaccessible or in young infants who are obligate nasal breathers. Because these routes do not require surgical intervention, they are the least invasive. The feeding tube is frequently held in place only by a piece of tape on the nose or face, and therefore can be inadvertently pulled out relatively easily.

TABLE 146-3 Options and Considerations in the Selection of Enteral Access

Access	Indications	Tube Placement Options	Advantages	Disadvantages
Nasogastric or orogastric	Short-term Intact gag reflex Normal gastric emptying	Manually at bedside	Ease of placement Allows for all methods of administration Inexpensive Multiple commercially available tubes and sizes	Potential tube displacement Potential increased aspiration risk
Nasoduodenal or nasojejunal	Short-term Impaired gastric motility or emptying High risk of GER or aspiration	Manually at bedside Fluoroscopically Endoscopically	Potential reduced aspiration risk Allows for early postinjury or postoperative feeding Multiple commercially available tubes and sizes	Manual transpyloric passage requires greater skill Potential tube displacement or clogging Bolus or intermittent feeding not tolerated
Gastrostomy	Long-term Normal gastric emptying	Surgically Endoscopically Radiologically Laparoscopically	Allows for all methods of administration Large-bore tubes less likely to clog Multiple commercially available tubes and sizes Low-profile buttons available	Attendant risks associated with each type of procedure Potential increased aspiration risk Requires stoma site care
Jejunostomy	Long-term Impaired gastric motility or gastric emptying High risk of GER or aspiration	Surgically Endoscopically Radiologically Laparoscopically	Allows for early postinjury or postoperative feeding Potential reduced aspiration risk Multiple commercially available tubes and sizes	Attendant risks associated with each type of procedure Bolus or intermittent feeding not tolerated Requires stoma site care

GER, gastroesophageal reflux.

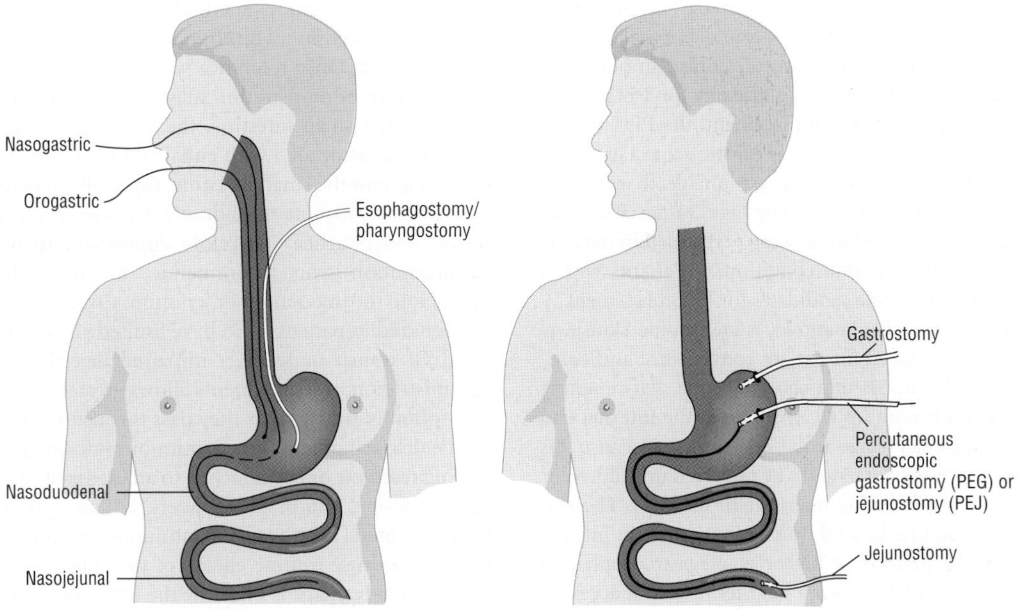

FIGURE 146-2. Access sites for tube feeding.

Nasogastric tubes vary in diameter size and stiffness. The large-bore (≥14 French [F]) rigid NG tubes are used primarily to decompress the stomach but can also be used for feeding. There is a low incidence of clogging with these tubes, and they provide a reliable way to measure gastric residual volumes. The major disadvantage associated with the use of these tubes is patient discomfort. Small-bore nasal tubes designed solely for feeding are available in varying lengths (16 to 60 inches) and diameter sizes (4F to 12F) to accommodate both pediatric (including neonates) and adult patients. The tip of the tube can be placed into the stomach, duodenum, or jejunum. These tubes consist of a lightweight, pliable silicone or polyurethane material that is more comfortable for the patient. A disadvantage of the small-bore tubes is that they may become easily occluded, often as a result of improper medication administration or tube flushing technique. Another disadvantage to the use of these tubes is that they do not allow a reliable way to monitor gastric residual volumes, as they will collapse when aspiration of gastric contents is attempted. Therefore, when the monitoring of gastric residual volumes is important, such as in a critically ill patient, a large-bore NG tube is preferred.

❹ In general, the stomach is the least expensive and the least labor-intensive access site to use for enteral feeding; however, feeding into the stomach is not as well tolerated. Patients with impaired gastric motility may be predisposed to aspiration and pneumonia when feedings are delivered into the stomach. Many critically ill, injured, and postoperative patients exhibit delayed gastric emptying, limiting their ability to tolerate gastric feeding. In addition, patients with diabetic gastroparesis or patients with severe gastroesophageal reflux disease or intractable vomiting are at a higher risk for aspiration of gastric contents resulting in pneumonia. In these patients, placing the tip of the tube into the duodenum or jejunum (also referred to as transpyloric placement) may be required to enable successful enteral feeding. However, studies have yet to prove definitively that transpyloric tube feedings actually do decrease the risk of aspiration and pneumonia. One meta-analysis of studies comparing gastric to transpyloric feeding in critically ill patients demonstrated no difference in the incidence of pneumonia,[26] whereas another critical review of the same patient population suggested that small-bowel feedings were associated with a reduction in gastroesophageal regurgitation and a lower rate of ventilator-associated pneumonia.[27] Thus, the true difference in aspiration and pneumonia risk between gastric and small-bowel feeding remains unclear. However, the transpyloric route may be beneficial in patients who do not tolerate gastric feeding. Its use may enable the successful use of EN in patients who would have otherwise failed and required PN.

Nasoenteric feeding tubes can be inserted at the patient's bedside by trained medical personnel. However, greater skill is required to advance the tip of the feeding tube beyond the pylorus. Several techniques have been described in the literature to help facilitate bedside placement. Prokinetic agents, such as metoclopramide and erythromycin, when given prior to insertion increase GI motility and facilitate spontaneous passage of the tube from the stomach into the small intestine.[28,29] Variable success rates have been reported with these techniques and are largely dependent on clinician experience. Alternatively, a variety of endoscopic and fluoroscopic techniques have been described to insert transpyloric tubes.[25] Radiographic confirmation of appropriate tip placement for feeding tubes inserted by bedside techniques should be obtained prior to use.[7]

LONG-TERM ACCESS

Feeding tubes used for short-term enteral access are usually not optimal for long-term use because of patient discomfort, long-term complications, and mechanical failures that develop over time. Long-term access should generally be considered when EN is anticipated for longer than 4 to 6 weeks. Many techniques can be used to establish long-term enteral access, including laparotomy, laparoscopy, endoscopy, and fluoroscopy. The ability to perform the various techniques will be somewhat dependent on the expertise and facilities available within each institution. Long-term enteral access options include gastrostomy, jejunostomy, esophagostomy, and pharyngostomy.

A gastrostomy is the most common type of long-term enteral access. It eliminates the nasal irritation and discomfort associated with nasoenteric feeding tubes and inadvertent removal is uncommon. In addition, because feeding gastrostomies use large-bore tubes, clogging is less of a problem. Multiple techniques for insertion of a gastrostomy tube have been described, including surgical laparotomy, endoscopy, radiography, and laparoscopy. The most common technique is the percutaneous endoscopic gastrostomy (PEG). It is minimally invasive and can be performed safely and cost-effectively in an endoscopy suite or at the bedside using conscious sedation and local anesthesia. Small children, however, will usually require general anesthesia for the procedure. Numerous kits are available for PEG placement in both children and adults and vary in size (12F to 28F; 1- to 4.5-cm shaft lengths), material used, internal and external bolsters, and insertion techniques. There are, however, ethical implications regarding determination of appropriate candidates for PEG placement.[30–32] Because of its relative ease of placement, the PEG tube is often placed inappropriately based on unrealistic expectations of what EN can accomplish in patients who are unable to eat. PEG placement is associated with an unexpectedly high 30-day mortality rate, which suggests that the procedure is being performed in patients who have multiple coexisting morbid conditions.[30] Patients with a poor prognosis are not appropriate candidates for PEG placement.

Once the gastrostomy tract has matured, a low-profile skin-level gastrostomy device may be placed for patient convenience and comfort. The "gastric button" consists of a short, silicone, self-retaining conduit with either a mushroom tip or a balloon at the internal end and a one-way valve and small flange at the skin surface. Because this averts the external tube presence, it tends to be preferred in children or ambulatory adults who are receiving intermittent feedings. The exit site of all gastrostomies requires general stoma care to prevent inflammation and infection. In patients at high risk of gastroesophageal reflux disease and aspiration who require long-term enteral access, a jejunostomy may be the most appropriate option.[33] Jejunostomies may also be indicated in patients unable to tolerate gastric feeding as a result of impaired gastric motility or delayed gastric emptying. These tubes can be inserted surgically, endoscopically, radiologically, or laparoscopically. The most appropriate technique depends on the expertise and facilities available. A surgical jejunostomy may be preferred if the patient requires a laparotomy or laparoscopy for other reasons. Endoscopic placement of a jejunostomy can be done by various methods. Typically, a small-bore jejunal extension tube (6F, 8F, or 10F) is inserted through a PEG and advanced through the pylorus into the duodenum or jejunum. This procedure has been referred to as percutaneous endoscopic jejunostomy, but this is misleading. The percutaneous endoscopic jejunostomy designation implies a direct opening from the skin into the jejunum. The more appropriate name is percutaneous endoscopic gastrojejunostomy or PEG with a jejunal extension tube. Also described in the literature are laparoscopically and radiologically placed jejunostomies.[33] Because jejunostomies use smaller-bore tubes, occlusion occurs more commonly than with gastrostomy tubes.

Pharyngostomies and esophagostomies are invasive because the tube is located in the neck and passes through the skin into the pharynx or esophagus, respectively. Historically, they have been used in patients with head and neck malignancies, and in patients with impaired swallowing caused by neuromuscular disorders. However, better long-term enteral access techniques have replaced the need for the pharyngostomy and esophagotomy routes. They are rarely performed today because of the high complication rate and extreme difficulty associated with their care.[30]

ADMINISTRATION METHODS

Enteral nutrition may be administered by continuous, cyclic (i.e., a continuous rate over a portion of the day), or bolus methods and may be accomplished by syringe, gravity, or infusion pump-controlled techniques. The method of delivery depends on the location of the tip of the feeding tube, the clinical condition and intestinal function of the patient, the environment in which the patient resides, and the patient's tolerance to the tube feeding.

CONTINUOUS

In the hospitalized patient, the continuous administration of EN is most commonly used for initiation, and is generally the preferred method in critically ill patients.[34,35] When initiating feeding into the stomach, the continuous method of delivery is less likely to result in abdominal distension, vomiting, and diarrhea than the intermittent bolus method. Once tolerance is established, a conversion to intermittent bolus administration may be warranted. When EN is delivered into the small intestine, the continuous method is preferred because it is associated with enhanced tolerance. The rapid delivery of feeding into the small intestine, especially hyperosmotic formulations, may contribute to abdominal distension, cramps, hyperperistalsis, and diarrhea. Therefore conversion to intermittent bolus administration is not recommended for those who have an access placed into the duodenum or jejunum. Continuous feeding may also be preferred in patients who have limited absorptive capacity due to rapid GI transit or severely impaired digestion. Slow continuous administration in such patients allows greater time for digestion and absorption of nutrients as they pass through the intestine.

The delivery system for a continuous infusion generally includes a feeding reservoir or bag attached to an extension set that is connected to an infusion pump. The delivery system is then attached to the patient's enteral access tube. Continuous infusion may increase nursing time because routine checks of the enteral infusion are needed, but this disadvantage is offset by the improved tolerance. For adults, EN infusion rates generally range from 50 to 125 mL/h, although higher infusion rates have been used without complications. In children, EN infusion rates of 1 to 2 mL/kg per hour can be started with advancements every 4 to 8 hours until the goal rate needed to meet caloric needs is achieved with good GI tolerance. The primary disadvantage to this method of administration is the cost and inconvenience associated with the pump and administration sets. In the home care setting, battery-operated ambulatory enteral pumps are available to allow the patient greater mobility.

CYCLIC

A patient who is not eating well during the day because of complaints of fullness and lack of appetite may benefit from a trial of cyclic EN wherein the enteral feeding is held during the day and infused only at night. In addition, the infusion of EN only at night will free the patient from the pump during the day and allow for greater mobility. This increased mobility may be particularly useful for the home patient or patient requiring rehabilitation. Because a pump controls the rate of infusion, this method of administration may be used in patients with either gastric or small bowel access.

BOLUS

The bolus administration of EN is most commonly used for patients in long-term care settings who have a gastrostomy. This administration technique involves the delivery of the enteral feeding formulation, usually over 5 to 10 minutes. Essentially the only equipment needed is a syringe to instill the feeding solution into the tube. Depending on the patient's nutritional requirements, an instillation volume of 240 to 500 mL is generally used and repeated four to six times per day. From a convenience standpoint, it is generally preferable to adjust the bolus volume in increments of the feeding formulation can size (usually 240 mL). The volume given in children is usually 20 to 25 mL/kg per feeding until their caloric requirements or adult volumes are reached. Although many patients tolerate this approach, the bolus technique may result in cramping, nausea, vomiting, aspiration, and diarrhea, especially in those who have duodenal or jejunal access. Its use should be avoided in patients with delayed gastric emptying and in patients who are at high risk of aspiration.

INTERMITTENT

If a patient is experiencing intolerance to bolus administration over 5 to 10 minutes, it may be helpful to administer the prescribed volume over a longer time period, generally 20 to 60 minutes. For this method, the desired volume of feeding formulation is emptied into a reservoir bag or container and infused by an infusion pump or gravity drip using a roller clamp. The bolus method of administration is more consistent physiologically with normal eating patterns than the continuous method. One study in infants demonstrated that normal gallbladder emptying did not occur with continuous infusion feedings, but was present in those infants receiving bolus feedings.[36] Thus those patients who need long-term EN and PN, especially children, may benefit when this approach is used because it minimizes the development of cholestatic liver disease.

ENTERAL FEEDING FORMULATION SELECTION

Historically, enteral formulas were created to provide essential nutrients. Over the years, enhancements have been made to meet specific patient needs and improve tolerance. For example, enteral formulas have been modified in nutrient composition by changing the content of the amino acids (such as glutamine and arginine), changing the omega-3 polyunsaturated fatty acid content, and adding ribonucleic acid to enhance immune function and improve disease outcome. These specific nutrients have been called nutraceuticals or pharmaconutrients because of the intent to use them to modify the disease process and improve clinical outcome. Currently, enteral feeding formulations are categorized by the U.S. Food and Drug Administration (FDA) as medical foods. They are considered components of supportive care and are simply regulated to ensure sanitary manufacture. Unfortunately, they are not subject to rules governing health claims, and the issue of the promotion of medical foods for therapeutic intent is currently not regulated by the FDA.[37,38]

The macronutrient content of enteral formulas (namely, protein, carbohydrate, and fat) varies in nutrient complexity (Table 146–4). Nutrient complexity refers to the amount of hydrolysis and digestion a substrate source requires prior to intestinal absorption. Polymeric or intact substrates are of similar molecular form as the food we eat. Enteral formulas that contain partially hydrolyzed or elemental substrates are characterized as elemental, or defined-formula diets. The caloric contribution of each of the macronutrients is as follows: carbohydrates, 4 kcal/g; protein, 4 kcal/g; and fat, 9 kcal/g. Micronutrients, including electrolytes, vitamins, trace elements, and water, do not contribute to caloric content.

TABLE 146-4 Enteral Formula Nutrient Complexity

Nutrient	Polymeric or Intact	Partially Hydrolyzed or Elemental
Carbohydrate	Starches	Oligosaccharides
	Fruit, vegetable, cereal solids	Maltodextrins
	Glucose polymers	Disaccharides
	Corn syrup solids	Maltose, sucrose, lactose
	Polysaccharides	Monosaccharides
		Glucose
		Galactose
Fat	Long-chain triglycerides	Medium-chain triglycerides
	Polyunsaturated fatty acids	Coconut oil
	Corn oil	Palm kernel oil
	Safflower oil	Free fatty acids
	Soybean oil	Linoleic
	Butterfat	
	Menhaden oil	
	Fish oils	
Protein	Whole	Oligopeptides
	Egg, milk, wheat, whey	Dipeptides
	Isolates	Tripeptides
	Caseinate salts	L-Amino acids
	Lactalbumin	

PROTEIN COMPOSITION

The essential amino acid content of the protein source determines the quality of the protein, and most commercially available enteral feeding formulations contain proteins of high quality. The molecular form of the protein source in enteral formulas will determine the amount of digestion that is required for absorption within the small bowel. Polymeric or intact protein sources require digestion to smaller peptides and free amino acids before they are absorbed from the GI tract. Therefore enteral formulation protein sources such as meat, milk, eggs, and caseinates require digestion by hydrochloric acid, specific protein enzymes, and pancreatic enzymes. Enteral formulations may also contain protein sources that are partially hydrolyzed as peptides or L-amino acids. As the molecular form of protein is reduced in size, the osmotic load within the enteral formula is increased. Many commercially available enteral feeding formulations contain combinations of intact and partially hydrolyzed protein sources.

CONDITIONALLY ESSENTIAL AMINO ACIDS

Glutamine and arginine are generally considered nonessential amino acids. However, during periods of high physiologic stress, patients may become deficient; consequently, these amino acids are characterized as conditionally essential. Because they are usually present in low amounts in most enteral feeding formulations, those formulations targeted for the critically ill may be supplemented with glutamine and/or arginine.

Glutamine serves as a key fuel for rapidly dividing cells, including enterocytes, endothelial cells, lymphocytes, and fibroblasts. The primary site of glutamine production is skeletal muscle. During critical illness, the catabolism of skeletal muscle provides an increased supply of glutamine, but this may not be enough to meet the high rate of glutamine use by cells of the immune system and other cells involved in recovery and repair. Glutamine depletion may result, particularly during prolonged periods of metabolic stress. However, it is unclear whether glutamine supplementation in enteral formulations plays a role in preserving normal intestinal morphology and function or preserving immune function.[39,40] Further research and investigation are required to determine the potential benefits and harm associated with glutamine-enriched enteral feeding formulations.

Arginine has been added to selected enteral formulations in concentrations that range from 4.5 to 14 g/L. However, the supplementation of arginine remains controversial, especially in patients with sepsis.[13,15,41,42] Many of the physiologic effects of arginine are mediated by its conversion to nitric oxide, which, in turn, modulates immune function, inflammation, and response to sepsis. Some of the effects may be potentially harmful in the patient with sepsis, especially when higher arginine intakes are used. Unfortunately, human studies evaluating arginine alone are limited. There is currently no consensus on whether arginine-supplemented enteral formulations should be used in septic patients.[13,15,41,42]

CARBOHYDRATE COMPOSITION

The carbohydrate component of enteral feeding formulations usually provides the major source of calories. Polymeric or intact enteral formulations contain starches and numerous types of glucose polymers, which require digestion to monosaccharide moieties prior to intestinal absorption (see Fig. 146–1). As the hydrolysis of carbohydrate increases within an enteral formulation, the osmolality of the formulation increases. Elemental carbohydrates such as glucose and galactose contribute significantly to the osmolality of enteral formulations, which is associated with feeding intolerance. Consequently, polymeric entities, rather than elemental sugars, are preferred in enteral formulas. Glucose polymers provide a useful carbohydrate source that is tolerated by most individuals (see Table 146–4). The polymers are large chains that provide minimal osmotic load, yet are absorbed easily in the intestine. The one shortcoming of glucose polymers and oligosaccharides is that they are not as sweet as simple glucose and thus may decrease the palatability of orally consumed products. Finally, almost all commercially available enteral feeding formulations used in adults and older children are lactose-free because some ethnic populations are lactase deficient and disaccharidase production within the gut lumen is reduced during illness or bowel rest. Infant formulas are available with or without lactose.

FAT AND FATTY ACID COMPOSITION

Fat is an important constituent in the diet because it provides a concentrated calorie source and serves as a carrier for fat-soluble vitamins. Sufficient linoleic acid is required to prevent essential fatty acid deficiency and should approximate 1% to 3% of total daily calories. The most common sources of fat in enteral feeding formulations are vegetable oils (soy or corn) rich in polyunsaturated fatty acids. The concentration of fat varies between less than 2% to 45% of total calories. High fat content of the diet is associated with delayed gastric emptying. Enteral feeding formulations can also contain fat in the form of MCTs, derived from palm kernel or coconut oils. Because MCTs do not contain linoleic acid, most enteral formulations that contain MCTs will also contain a source of long-chain triglycerides to provide essential fatty acids. Potential advantages of MCTs compared to long-chain triglycerides are that they are more water soluble, undergo rapid hydrolysis, require little to no pancreatic lipase or bile salt for absorption, and do not require carnitine for transport into the mitochondria where they are converted to energy. They also do not require chylomicron formation for small-bowel enterocyte absorption.

The source of long-chain fat within some enteral formulations has been modified from omega-6 to omega-3 fatty acids in an effort to modulate the inflammatory response to metabolic stress.[43] The omega-6 fatty acids serve as precursors to certain cytokines that are potent inflammatory mediators and also decrease cell-mediated immune response. The omega-6 fatty acids are high in linoleic acid and are derived from vegetable oil, whereas the omega-3 fatty acids, derived from cold water fish oils, are high in linolenic acid. It has been proposed that if the dietary proportion of omega-3 fatty acids is increased and omega-6 fatty acids is decreased, less inflammation and immunosuppression may occur during metabolic stress.

Docosahexaenoic acid (DHA) and arachidonic acid (ARA) are two fatty acids abundant in human milk, but until recently, were not contained in commercial infant formulas. Although the role of ARA supplementation is unclear, DHA is known to be important in both brain and eye development. In some studies, DHA and ARA supplementation provided benefits to a child's visual function and/or cognitive and behavioral development.[44–47] Other studies showed no difference with DHA and ARA supplementation.[48] The FDA has classified the plant-based fatty acid blends of DHA and ARA (DHASCO and ARASCO; Martek Biosciences Corporation, Columbia, MD) as generally recognized as safe in infant formulas, and most infant formulas are now routinely supplemented with these fatty acids.

FIBER CONTENT

Fiber, in the form of soy polysaccharides, has been added to several enteral feeding formulations intended for use in both children and adults in amounts ranging from 5.9 g/L to 24 g/L of dietary fiber. Infant formulas do not contain fiber, with the exception of one formula intended for use in infants with diarrhea (Similac Isomil DF, Abbott Nutrition, Columbus, OH). Fiber supplementation is common in clinical practice, primarily because fiber-free enteral formulations are implicated as a contributing factor to both diarrhea and constipation. Ingested fiber undergoes bacterial degradation within the colon to produce short-chain fatty acids. Potential benefits of fiber are the trophic effects on the colonic mucosa as well as promotion of sodium and water absorption within the colon.[4] It may help regulate bowel function in both normal individuals and in those with altered colonic motility. In addition, the resulting short-chain fatty acids are an excellent energy source. Although beneficial effects of fiber supplementation have not been clearly proven in clinical studies, there is experimental evidence that fiber may play an integral role in normal human nutrition and risk is generally minimal.[49,50] Fiber supplementation may be beneficial when long-term EN is required or in patients who experience diarrhea or constipation while receiving a fiber-free enteral formulation. In intensive care units, however, drugs and metabolic stress seem to be more powerful determinants of bowel function than the presence or absence of fiber.

OSMOLALITY AND RENAL SOLUTE LOAD

The osmolality and the renal solute load can affect tolerance to enteral feeding formulations. The osmolality of a given enteral formulation is a function of the size and quantity of ionic and molecular particles, primarily related to the protein, carbohydrate, electrolyte, and mineral content within a given volume. The unit of measure of osmolality is milliosmoles per kilogram (mOsm/kg). Iso-osmolar is considered to be approximately 300 mOsm/kg. Enteral formulations with greater amounts of partially hydrolyzed or elemental substrates have a higher osmolality than formulations containing polymeric or intact substrate forms. Therefore formulations that contain sucrose or glucose, dipeptides and tripeptides, and amino acids are generally hyperosmolar. Increased caloric density also increases the osmolality of an enteral formulation. In general, the osmolality of commercially available enteral feeding formulations ranges from 300 to 900 mOsm/kg. The American Academy of Pediatrics recommends that enteral formulations for use in infants have an osmolality of approximately 450 mOsm/kg or less. An extensive tabulation of the osmolality of formulas and medications commonly used in neonatal intensive care units was published over a decade ago and an update is long overdue.[51]

Symptoms of gastric retention, diarrhea, abdominal distension, nausea, and vomiting have been attributed to enteral formulations having high osmolality based on the assumption that a higher osmolality will draw water into the gut lumen. However, clinical evidence to support the relationship between osmolality and GI tolerance is lacking.[51] The practice of diluting hyperosmolar formulations has not been shown to enhance tolerance and should be discouraged unless dilution is done to increase fluid intake.[35] Factors such as concurrent antibiotic therapy, method of enteral feeding administration, and the formulation's composition are likely to play a greater role in GI tolerance than the osmolality.

The renal solute load is determined by the protein, sodium, potassium, and chloride content of the enteral formulation. Formulations that contain a greater solute load increase the obligatory water loss via the kidney. It is estimated that 40 to 60 mL of water is the minimal amount necessary to excrete 1 g of nitrogen.[56] Those receiving high-protein enteral formulations unable to ingest more water, such as a geriatric patient or a patient with altered mental status, may be at risk for significant dehydration.

TABLE 146-5 Adult Enteral Feeding Formulation Classification System

Category	Features	Indications
Standard polymeric	Isotonic 1–1.2 kcal/mL NPC:N 125:1 to 150:1 May contain fiber	Designed to meet the needs of the majority of patients. Patients with functional GI tract. Not suitable for oral use.
High protein	NPC:N <125:1 May contain fiber	Patients with protein requirements >1.5 g/kg/day, such as trauma, burns, pressure sores, or wounds. Patients receiving propofol.
High caloric density	1.5–2 kcal/mL Lower electrolyte content per calorie Hypertonic	Patients requiring fluid and/or electrolyte restriction, such as renal insufficiency.
Elemental	High proportion of free amino acids Low in fat	Patients who require low fat. Use has generally been replaced by peptide-based formulations.
Peptide-based	Contains dipeptides and tripeptides Contains MCTs	Indications/benefits not clearly established. Trial may be warranted in patients who do not tolerate intact protein due to malabsorption.
Disease-specific		
Renal	Caloric dense Protein content varies Low electrolyte content	Alternative to high caloric density formulations, but generally more expensive.
Hepatic	Increased branched-chain and decreased aromatic amino acids	Patients with hepatic encephalopathy.
Pulmonary	High fat, low carbohydrate	Patients with compromised pulmonary function.
Diabetic	High fat, low carbohydrate	Alternative to standard, fiber-containing formulation in patients with uncontrolled hyperglycemia.
Immunomodulating	Supplemented with glutamine, arginine, nucleotides, and/or omega-3 fatty acids	Indications not clearly established. Select nutrients may be beneficial or harmful in subgroups of critically ill patients.
Oral supplement	Sweetened for taste Hypertonic	Patients who require supplementation to an oral diet.

MCT, medium-chain triglyceride; NPC:N, nonprotein calorie-to-nitrogen ratio.

CLASSIFICATION OF ENTERAL FEEDING FORMULATIONS

❺ Although the majority of patients' needs can probably be met using three or four different formulations, certain disease states or clinical conditions may warrant the use of a specialty feeding formulation. Development of an effective formulary system should avoid the duplication of enteral feeding formulations and use only those specialty formulations with an established role. Categorizing enteral feeding formulations according to therapeutic class is necessary in developing a formulary system for adults (Table 146–5) and children (Table 146–6).

STANDARD POLYMERIC

A large number of commercially available enteral feeding formulations fall within the category of a standard polymeric formulation. These formulations are approximately isotonic (300 mOsm/L), provide about 1 kcal/mL, and are composed of intact nutrients in a well-proportioned mix of carbohydrate, fat, and protein. They are provided with or without dietary fiber. The nutrient requirements of the majority of adult patients and children older than 10 years of age receiving EN can generally be met using feeding formulations in this category. The nonprotein calorie-to-nitrogen ratio of these products is approximately 125:1 to 150:1. This ratio is a useful parameter for assessing protein density in relation to calories provided. Certain feeding formulations in this category may be promoted as high nitrogen, but fall within standard protein amounts. To maintain their isotonicity, products within this category are not sweetened, making them not very palatable and generally only suited for tube feeding and not oral supplementation; however, flavored products are available.

HIGH PROTEIN

Enteral feeding formulations with a nonprotein calorie-to-nitrogen ratio less than 125:1 can be categorized as high protein. The lower the ratio, the higher the protein density in relation to calories provided. In patients with high protein requirements, it is generally unacceptable to use a feeding formulation with standard protein amounts because the volume necessary to meet protein requirements will often result in excessive calorie intake. Patients who may be candidates for a high-protein feeding formulation are those with trauma, burns, pressure sores, surgical wounds, high fistula output, and other critically ill patients. In general, adult patients with estimated protein requirements exceeding 1.5 g/kg per day may benefit from a high-protein formulation. High-protein formulations may also be beneficial in mechanically ventilated patients who are receiving propofol for sedation. The vehicle for propofol is a soybean fat emulation that contains 1.1 kcal/mL. At therapeutic dosages, the use of propofol can significantly contribute to caloric intake and a high protein formulation may be beneficial in allowing for the provision of protein requirements while minimizing the risk of overfeeding.

HIGH CALORIC DENSITY

High caloric density formulations are concentrated to provide less fluid and electrolyte intake in comparison to a standard polymeric formulation. They provide approximately 2 kcal/mL and will achieve similar calorie and protein intake to a standard polymeric formulation, using half the volume. High caloric density formulations are often necessary for patients who require fluid and/or electrolyte restriction, such as those with renal insufficiency or congestive heart failure. Although specialty enteral formulations targeted for acute and chronic renal failure are also available, many patients with renal failure can be managed using a product in this category (see Chap. 147).

TABLE 146-6 Pediatric Enteral Feeding Formulation Classification System

Formula Type	Features	Indications
Infants		
Cow's milk-based	Isotonic Standard energy density for feeding: 20–24 kcal/oz, but also available in concentrate (40 kcal/oz) and powder forms Standard formulation contains lactose, but also available as lactose-free Most contain ARA and DHA	Normal, healthy infant
Soy protein-based	Hypotonic Standard energy density for feeding: 20 kcal/oz, but also available in concentrate (40 kcal/oz) and powder forms Lactose-free Most contain added soy fiber	Lactase deficiency or intolerance, galactosemia
Prematurity	Isotonic Standard energy density for feeding: 24 kcal/oz, but also available in 20 kcal/oz form Provide increased protein, mineral, electrolytes, and vitamins compared to term infant formulations	Preterm infants weighing less than 2–3 kg
Transition	Hypotonic Standard energy density for feeding: 22 kcal/oz Provide higher calcium and phosphorus content compared to term infant formulations	Preterm infants weighing less than 3 kg ready for discharge
Semielemental	Typically hypertonic Standard energy density for feeding: 20 kcal/oz Hydrolyzed protein and free amino acids May contain ARA and DHA Lactose-free Typically contain MCTs ranging from 5%–86% of fat content	Malabsorption, cow's milk protein allergy, chylothorax, cystic fibrosis, biliary atresia, short-bowel syndrome
Special diets	Low electrolyte/mineral content	Renal disease
Children ages 1–10 years		
Standard	Isotonic Standard energy density for feeding: 30 kcal/oz (1 kcal/mL) Intact protein; 30–38 g/L May contain added fiber	Functioning GI tract requiring tube feedings
Elemental	Typically hypertonic Standard energy density for feeding: 20–30 kcal/oz Hydrolyzed protein and free amino acids Lactose-free MCTs range from 25%–60% of fat content	Malabsorption, cow's milk protein allergy, chylothorax, cystic fibrosis, biliary atresia

ARA, arachidonic acid; DHA, docosahexaenoic acid; MCT, medium-chain triglycerides.

ELEMENTAL/PEPTIDE BASED

Formulations in this category contain protein and/or fat components that are hydrolyzed into smaller, predigested forms. Traditionally, enteral formulations in this category were referred to as elemental and contained a high proportion of protein in the form of free amino acids and a low amount of fat. Although still commercially available, many of these formulations have been replaced in clinical practice with formulations containing a portion of the protein in the form of dipeptides and tripeptides and less free amino acids. These formulations are referred to as peptide based. The alteration in protein composition was made in an effort to optimize protein absorption in patients with impaired digestive or absorptive capacity. Results from human and animal intestinal perfusion studies indicate that the partially hydrolyzed sources of protein provide an absorptive advantage over formulas that contain free amino acids.[53] Peptide-based formulations are generally higher in fat than the older, elemental formulations, and use MCTs in varying proportions as the fat source.

Indications for use of peptide-based formulations are not clearly established. Unfortunately, there are few controlled data on the nutritional efficacy of the peptide-based or free amino acid formulations. The routine use of peptide-based or free amino acid formulations is generally not recommended. Patients who do not tolerate standard, intact nutrient formulations as a result of malabsorption might be candidates for a trial of a peptide-based formulation. In addition, elemental or peptide-based products that have higher percentages of MCTs and small amounts of long-chain triglycerides may be beneficial for patients with severe pancreatic insufficiency such as chronic pancreatitis and cystic fibrosis, severe abnormalities of the intestinal mucosa such as untreated celiac disease, biliary tract disease such as biliary atresia or severe cholestasis, or chylothorax.

DISEASE SPECIFIC

Newer enteral feeding formulations have been designed to meet specific nutrient requirements and manage metabolic abnormalities associated with specific disease states. Conditions for which specialized enteral feeding formulations exist include renal and hepatic failure, pulmonary disease including acute respiratory distress syndrome, diabetes mellitus, wound healing, and metabolic stress. Chapter 147 discusses specific nutrient concerns during organ failure. Unfortunately, scientific and clinical research supporting the efficacy of specialized enteral feeding formulations is minimal.

Specialized enteral formulations designed to modulate the inflammatory response in patients with severe metabolic stress have been referred to as immune-enhancing formulations or immunonutrition. These specialized formulations are supplemented with nutrients such as glutamine, arginine, branched-chain amino acids, nucleotides, and omega-3 polyunsaturated fatty acids, as a result of their potential role in regulating immune function; guidelines for their use in critically ill patients have been published.[15,54–58] In some surgical and critically ill patients, the use of immune-enhancing formulations were associated with a reduced infection rate and length of hospital stay. However, the results of these trials are conflicting and controversial. Positive results have been demonstrated in patients undergoing elective GI surgery, major cancer surgery of the head and neck, and patients with severe trauma. However, immune-enhancing formulations are associated with increased mortality in patients with preexisting severe sepsis. There may be subgroups of critically ill patients who do not benefit and are actually harmed by immune-enhancing formulations. More study is warranted to determine the benefit-to-risk ratio associated with the use of these formulations and to identify which, if any, of the supplemented immune-enhancing nutrients are contributing to improved clinical outcome.

CLINICAL CONTROVERSY

The role of immune-enhancing enteral formulations in critically ill patients is controversial. Although some clinicians recommend their use in subgroups of critically ill patients, others await more evidence to support safety. When immune-enhancing enteral formulations are used, the optimal duration of therapy is unclear, although some studies suggest a minimum duration of 5 days.

In patients with acute respiratory distress syndrome, improved outcomes from using a low carbohydrate formulation supplemented with specific fatty acids (eicosapentaenoic acid and γ-linolenic acid) and antioxidants have been documented.[59] When compared with a high fat formulation, the specialized diet was associated with fewer days of ventilatory support, fewer intensive care unit days, and fewer new organ failures. Consequently, it is recommended that this specialized formulation be considered for patients with acute respiratory distress syndrome.[15,56,58]

There are no disease-specific enteral products currently marketed for use in infants or children from 1 to 10 years of age. The use of modular supplements is often necessary in children with special nutrition needs (see Modular Products below).

ORAL SUPPLEMENTS

In general, oral supplements are not intended for tube feeding, but to enhance an oral diet. They are sweetened to improve taste and therefore are hypertonic (about 450 to 700 mOsm/kg). Osmolality is generally not a problem in the patient with a functioning GI tract. However, in the tube-fed patient, a sweetened product is unnecessary and may contribute to GI intolerance, particularly diarrhea. Powder supplements that are mixed with milk should be avoided in lactose-intolerant patients. In addition to liquid supplements, puddings, gelatins, bars, and milkshake-like supplements are available.

MODULAR PRODUCTS

A module is a powder or liquid form of nutrients (i.e., protein, carbohydrate, or fat) that is used to supplement a commercially available enteral formulation. Addition of a modular product may be necessary, especially in children, to achieve a nutrient mix not supplied by a single commercially available product.[60] Alternatively, formulations available in powder or concentrate can be mixed with less water than needed for the standard dilution to deliver more nutrients in less volume. Infant formulas generally are concentrated beyond their standard concentration in this way. The mixing process required for modular components increases the potential for bacterial contamination and incorrect preparation. Contamination is a particular concern with the use of blenders and reconstitution of powders.[61,62] Human milk fortifiers are available for supplementation of human milk so that it meets the needs of a premature infant. Human milk fortifiers add additional calories, protein, and minerals and have been shown to improve nutritional outcomes in human milk-fed premature infants.[63–65]

REHYDRATION

Oral rehydration formulations are useful in maintaining hydration or treating dehydration in adult and pediatric patients with high GI output. Such formulations are available commercially in powder or liquid form or can be extemporaneously compounded.[66] They can be administered orally or given via a feeding tube. The glucose content of oral rehydration solutions is important because it stimulates active transport systems, which, in turn, stimulates passive sodium and water uptake simultaneously with the glucose. Therefore oral or enteral administration of rehydration solutions may decrease fecal water loss and generate a positive electrolyte balance.

FORMULARY AND DELIVERY SYSTEM CONSIDERATIONS

The selection of product should be based on the patient's nutritional requirements. In general, no more than one product is necessary per category of enteral feeding formulation and it may be possible to omit certain categories based on the specific patient population within a given institution. Additional selection criteria include container size and type, liquid or powder form, shelf life, ease of use, and cost.

The majority of enteral products are available as ready-to-use, prepackaged liquids, a few are available in the powdered state and require reconstitution prior to use. Advantages of ready-to-use liquid formulations are convenience and lower susceptibility to microbiologic contamination. One disadvantage is that more storage space is required. The ease or convenience of a ready-to-use liquid is especially important for self-care patients, the disabled, and those who have difficulty reading or following printed instructions. Ready-to-use liquid enteral formulations are generally available in rigid containers, cans, or closed, ready-to-hang bags. Bolus administration of EN is usually achieved using formulas available in cans. However, when formula from a can is used for continuous or cyclic administration, it must first be poured into a bag or bottle to allow for infusion via a pump. This "open system" differs from the closed, ready-to-hang containers from the standpoint of microbial contamination risk. The use of a powder formula is also considered an open system of delivery.

Contaminated enteral feeding formulations are a potential source of infectious complications.[61,62,67,68] The GI tract may serve as a portal of entry for bacteria into the systemic circulation, especially in patients who are receiving multiple antibiotics, have undergone a surgical procedure, or have GI tract stasis from a variety of causes. The contamination of enteral feeding formulations is associated with a lack of attention to proper handling techniques, inability to disinfect preparation equipment, and nonsterile or contaminated tube feeding additives. Unlike liquid formulations, powdered products are not guaranteed to be sterile by the manufacturer because of the inability to properly sterilize the powder without destruction of some of its components. Contamination of one infant formula with *Enterobacter sakazakii* at the manufacturing site was implicated in the death of an infant in a neonatal intensive care unit, prompting FDA warnings regarding the use of powdered formulations in premature neonates and other immunocompromised infants. Because powder formulations require reconstitution, often in a blender that is difficult to sterilize, they are also more susceptible to contamination at the time of preparation. Stringent handling procedures are recommended during all aspects of enteral feeding preparation and delivery to minimize contamination risk. The closed-system containers supply a ready-to-hang, prefilled, sterile supply of formula in volumes of 1 to 1.5 L. Numerous, but not all, enteral formulations intended for use in adults are available in the closed-administration system. The closed-administration system also offers the advantage of not requiring refrigeration and allowing hang times beyond 24 to 36 hours, whereas the conventional open-delivery system necessitates hang times of generally 4 to 8 hours.

INITIATION AND ADVANCEMENT PROTOCOL

Guidelines for the initiation and advancement of enteral feeding formulations vary greatly and scientific support for any of the guidelines is weak or nonexistent. The typical recommendation for continuous administration of EN for adults is to start at 20 to 50 mL/h and advance by 10 to 25 mL/h every 4 to 8 hours until the desired goal is achieved. For intermittent administration, the typical recommendation is to start at 120 mL every 4 hours and advance by 30 to 60 mL every 8 to 12 hours.[35] In children, the recommendation for continuous administration is initiation of 1 to 2 mL/kg per hour or 20 to 25 mL/kg per bolus with advancement by 2 mL/kg per hour every 4 to 12 hours. In premature infants, feedings are initiated at lower rates usually 10 to 20 mL/kg per day. Schedules for progression of tube feeding from initial to target rates are important and may influence tolerance. If the protocol is too conservative, it may take an excessively long period of time to reach nutrient goals. As previously discussed, the practice of diluting enteral feeding formulations is not routinely recommended unless necessary to increase fluid intake.[35] The development of an EN protocol within an institution that outlines initiation and advancement criteria may be a useful strategy to optimize achievement of nutrient goals.[15] Such a protocol should allow nursing to advance the rate (i.e., 25 mL/h every 4 hours until goal rate achieved) based on GI tolerance. Clinical signs of intolerance include abdominal distension, abdominal cramping, high gastric residual volumes, aspiration, and diarrhea.

COMPLICATIONS AND MONITORING

The majority of complications associated with EN are metabolic, GI, and mechanical. The early detection and management of potential complications is necessary to allow for the successful use of EN. In addition, measures to avoid complications should be incorporated into the management of all patients receiving EN and require close monitoring (Table 146–7).

METABOLIC COMPLICATIONS

Metabolic complications associated with EN are similar to those associated with PN, but the incidence tends to be lower. EN is frequently administered at lower rates than PN, resulting in less risk of metabolic complications associated with overfeeding. In addition, EN is associated with the achievement of lower blood glucose concentrations than PN.[69] Complications related to hydration and electrolyte imbalance and altered glucose control are observed more frequently in critically ill patients, especially those with underlying organ dysfunction. The micronutrient and water content within enteral feeding formulations are in fixed amounts intended to meet recommended dietary allowances for the average patient. Consequently, the frequency of clinical and laboratory assessment to monitor hydration, electrolyte, organ function, and glucose control adequately for a patient who is critically ill is greater than for a stable patient residing in a rehabilitation unit or at home. Patients receiving long-term EN at home may only require laboratory monitoring every 2 to 3 months, depending on their clinical status. In addition to macronutrient content, it is important to evaluate the actual content of water and micronutrients provided by the enteral formulations, especially in critically ill patients at high risk for metabolic complications. Supplemental fluid and electrolytes may be required in some patients. Conversely, for patients who have fluid retention or increased serum electrolytes, the enteral formulation may need to be changed to one that is more concentrated or provides less of a particular nutrient.

TABLE 146-7 Suggested Monitoring for Patients on Enteral Nutrition (EN)

Parameter	During Initiation of EN Therapy	During Stable EN Therapy
Vital signs	Every 4–6 hours	As needed with suspected change (i.e., fever)
Clinical assessment		
Weight	Daily	Weekly
Length/height (children)	Weekly–monthly	Monthly
Head circumference (<3 y of age)	Weekly–monthly	Monthly
Total intake/output	Daily	As needed with suspected change in intake/output
Tube feeding intake	Daily	Daily
Enterostomy tube site assessment	Daily	Daily
GI tolerance		
Stool frequency/volume	Daily	Daily
Abdomen assessment	Daily	Daily
Nausea or vomiting	Daily	Daily
Gastric residual volumes	Every 4–8 hours (varies)	As needed when delayed gastric emptying suspected
Tube placement	Prior to starting, then ongoing	Ongoing
Laboratory		
Electrolytes, blood urea nitrogen/serum creatinine, glucose	Daily	Every 1–3 months
Calcium, magnesium, phosphorus	3–7 times/week	Every 1–3 months
Liver function tests	Weekly	Every 1–3 months
Trace elements, vitamins	If deficiency/toxicity suspected	If deficiency/toxitiy suspected

GASTROINTESTINAL COMPLICATIONS

❻ The GI complications associated with tube feeding include nausea, vomiting, abdominal distension, cramping, aspiration, diarrhea, and constipation. A gastric residual volume refers to the volume of contents in the stomach and is measured by using a syringe and aspirating from a large-bore NG or gastrostomy tube. For patients receiving tube feeding into the stomach, gastric residual volumes are widely used as an indicator of tolerance. It is believed, although not well documented, that patients with high gastric residual volumes are at higher risk of vomiting and/or aspiration. The frequency of measuring gastric residual volumes generally varies between 4 and 8 hours, and most institutions follow a protocol that directs nursing to the frequency of monitoring and when to hold tube feeding.[70]

CLINICAL CONTROVERSY

Clinicians argue about what constitutes an excessive gastric residual volume. In adults, the definition of a high residual volume ranges from greater than 200 mL to greater than 500 mL. In children, residual volumes greater than twice the bolus volume or twice the hourly infusion rate for continuous gastric feedings are considered excessive.

If high gastric residuals occur, the response is often to withhold the next scheduled tube feeding. However, frequent interruptions in the delivery of EN can adversely impact the attainment of nutrient goals. Because gastric residual volumes are unreliable, symptoms such as abdominal distension, fullness, bloating, and discomfort should also be assessed and they are generally more reliable indicators of EN intolerance. A trend in elevated gastric residual volumes is generally more important than an isolated high measurement. If symptoms are present and residual volumes are elevated, a decrease in tube feeding rate may be warranted. In general, abruptly stopping tube feeding should be reserved for patients with overt regurgitation or aspiration.[71] Gastric residual volumes should generally be returned to the patient unless they are excessive (greater than 500 mL in adults).[34,71] It may be beneficial to initiate a prokinetic agent such as metoclopramide to increase gastric emptying rate and decrease residual volume, thereby enhancing tolerance.[34,72,73] If high gastric residual volumes persist, a transpyloric feeding tube may be considered for feeding into the small bowel. Other interventions may include a trial of a proton pump inhibitor or histamine$_2$-receptor antagonist to decrease the volume of gastric secretions, and minimizing the use of narcotics, sedatives, or other agents that may delay gastric emptying.[34,35]

Aspiration pneumonia is considered the most serious complication associated with tube feeding and is potentially life-threatening. Although aspiration is a fairly common event for critically ill patients receiving tube feeding, progression to aspiration pneumonia is difficult to predict. Risk factors for aspiration include a previous aspiration episode, decreased level of consciousness, neuromuscular disease, structural airway or GI tract abnormalities, endotracheal intubation, vomiting, persistently high gastric residual volumes, and prolonged presence in the supine position.[34] Identification of these risk factors, along with close monitoring of gastric residual volumes, is recommended for the management of critically ill patients receiving tube feeding. Traditionally, blue food coloring had been added to enteral formulations in an attempt to detect aspiration. However, because of its low sensitivity for detection and association with several serious adverse events, including death, the addition of blue food dye to enteral formulations should no longer be used.[34,74] An alternative to blue dye is to test the tracheobronchial secretions for glucose (the glucose oxidase strip method). This method assumes that the glucose concentration of these secretions is normally less than 5 mg/dL and that higher concentrations are consistent with aspiration of a feeding formulation. Unfortunately, false positives can occur using this technique as a result of blood in the specimen or when formulas containing low glucose concentrations (i.e., <200 mg/dL) are used.[75]

Strategies to decrease aspiration risk include keeping the patient's head of the bed elevated to a 30° to 45° angle during feeding and for 30 to 60 minutes after intermittent boluses in addition to those mentioned above. This positioning makes it more difficult for the EN formulation to migrate up the esophagus against gravity. Changing from bolus or intermittent to continuous administration may also reduce the risk. Aspiration may also occur with improper feeding tube placement or displacement. Therefore regular assessment of tube position is recommended.[34]

The reported incidence of diarrhea in patients receiving EN ranges from 20% to 70% because of the lack of a standard definition and the number of contributing factors.[35,76,77] When monitoring for diarrhea, stool frequency, consistency, and volume should be evaluated and previous bowel habits should be considered. One commonly accepted definition of diarrhea is more than three to five liquid stools per day or more than 250 to 500 mL/day (10 mL/kg per day in children) stool output for at least 2 consecutive days.[76] A single loose stool does not constitute diarrhea or require intervention.

❼ Diarrhea in patients receiving tube feeding may be caused by a number of factors and management should be directed at identifying and correcting the most likely cause(s). Tube feeding-related factors that may contribute to diarrhea include too rapid delivery or advancement of formula, intolerance to the formula composition, administering large volumes of feeding into the small bowel, and formula contamination. Measures to prevent or manage the development of diarrhea related directly to the tube feeding should address these potential causes.[77] If diarrhea occurs when using a fiber-free formulation, consider switching to a fiber-containing formulation. If using a high-fat formulation, it may be beneficial to switch to a formulation lower in fat or having a proportion of the fat supplied as MCTs. If protein malabsorption is suspected, switching from an intact protein to a peptide-based source may be beneficial. Avoid lactose-containing enteral formulations, although the majority of products designed for tube feeding are lactose-free. Finally, assess the risk of bacterial contamination of the formula and take steps to minimize any potential risk factors. Once infectious etiologies have been excluded, pharmacologic intervention may be required to control severe diarrhea, including the use of opiates, diphenoxylate, and loperamide.

A common cause of diarrhea that is unrelated to the tube feeding is drug therapy, particularly the use of broad-spectrum antibiotics. Another drug-related cause is the sorbitol contained in many liquid medication formulations. Sorbitol is used as a sweetening agent to enhance palatability, but acts as an osmotic laxative. In addition, many drugs available in a liquid form are hyperosmolar, which may also contribute to diarrhea. Because many patients receiving tube feeding also receive medications in a liquid form, all medications should be evaluated for their potential contribution. Infectious causes of diarrhea, such as antibiotic-induced bacterial overgrowth by *Clostridium difficile* or other intestinal flora, need to be considered when diarrhea develops. Diarrhea also may occur as a result of malabsorption, secondary to the underlying disease state or condition.

MECHANICAL COMPLICATIONS

Mechanical complications of EN are those associated with the feeding tube, including tube occlusion or malposition, and nasopulmonary intubation. Feeding tube occlusion is usually a result of the improper administration of medications and/or flushing technique. Kinking of the tube also may cause occlusion. The tube should be flushed with at least 30 mL of water before and after administering any medication. The recommended volume used in children is generally less than 30 mL and depends on the size of the tube. The frequency of flushing should be at least every 8 hours during continuous feeding and before and after each intermittent feeding. If tube occlusion occurs, an attempt to irrigate the tube with warm water should be made. Other fluids such as colas and cranberry juice have been used to irrigate occluded tubes but have not been shown to be any better than warm water. Some success in reestablishing patency also has been shown with the use of pancreatic enzymes mixed in sodium bicarbonate.[78] In addition, declogging devices that are specifically designed to unclog feeding tubes are available. They have been designed to either mechanically break through or remove the occlusion or provide an applicator and syringe prefilled with pancreatic enzymes and various powders targeted to restore patency.

Inadvertent tube removal or displacement has been reported to occur in more than 50% of patients receiving enteral tube feeding.[79] An agitated or confused patient may pull at the feeding tube and cause its removal or malposition. Measures to decrease agitation and confusion should be attempted. Various manipulations done to the patient throughout the day may also cause malposition. Securing the tube with tape may be helpful, as well as marking the tube with permanent ink at the exit site to assess for change in position.

When a feeding tube is inserted nasally or orally, there is a risk that the tube may inadvertently enter the tracheobronchial tree. The risk may be higher in patients who have an impaired cough or gag reflex and when a stylet is used for tube insertion. Proper positioning of the tube should always be confirmed by radiography prior to feeding initiation to avoid inadvertent administration of enteral formula into the lung.

OTHER COMPLICATIONS

A unique complication of tube feedings in children, especially in the first year of life, is the development of feeding disorders as a consequence of oral hypersensitivity, poor oral/motor skills, and food aversion. In these children, transitioning from tube to oral nutrition is often difficult and protracted. The involvement of an occupational or speech therapist, behavioral psychologist, or other trained individual, as well as perseverance by the family, often is necessary to improve oral intake. Avoidance of a strict nothing by mouth (NPO) status, if possible, and oral stimulation programs for those children who must remain NPO are recommended to avoid this complication.[80]

DRUG DELIVERY VIA FEEDING TUBE

Using enteral feeding tubes to deliver drugs is a common practice and offers an alternative for patients unable to take drugs by the oral route. However, in addition to complications of tube occlusion, effects on drug bioavailability and other potential interactions need to be considered when using this route. Medications have been given as a concomitant bolus administration via the feeding tube or admixed with the enteral feeding formulation.

CONCOMITANT DRUG ADMINISTRATION

8 Concomitant administration of medications with enteral feedings requires awareness of certain limitations. Medications delivered directly into the stomach allow for the normal process of drug dissolution. Medications delivered into the small bowel may result in alterations of drug dissolution because the stomach is bypassed. In addition, therapeutic effect designed to occur within the stomach, such as with antacids and sucralfate, may be influenced by feeding tube route. Because many drugs are best absorbed in the fasted state, they should be administered on an empty stomach as much as possible. Patients receiving bolus gastric feedings may receive medications appropriately spaced between the feedings, but patients receiving continuous feeding will require interruption for drug administration.

Selecting the proper medication dosage form for coadministration with the tube feeding is another important consideration. Medications in sublingual form, sustained-released capsules or tablets, and enteric-coated tablets should not be crushed and therefore should not be administered via enteral feeding tubes. An extensive list of oral dosage forms that should not be crushed is available in the literature.[81,82] Solid dosage forms that are appropriate to crush should be prepared as a very fine powder and mixed with 15 to 30 mL of water or other appropriate solvent before administering through the tube. In addition, the content of many capsules may be opened and administered in the same manner. Pellets contained inside microencapsulated dosage forms should generally not be crushed. It may be acceptable to administer intact pellets through the feeding tube, provided that the pellets are small enough and drug absorption is not compromised.[83–85] To avoid the need to crush a solid dosage form and mix with water, liquid dosage preparations have been used for administration through the feeding tube. However, the risk of GI intolerance should be considered because of the hyperosmolality of the liquid formulation and possible sorbitol content.[83,84] Although the use of a liquid dosage preparation may be more convenient than a solid dosage form, it may not be the best choice if GI intolerance is an issue.

As previously mentioned, adherence to proper flushing technique is necessary to prevent occlusion when administering medication through a feeding tube. At least 30 mL of water in adults and usually 10 to 15 mL in children should be given before and after medication administration to clear the drug through the tube and help get the drug into the stomach. If more than one medication is scheduled for a given time, each should be administered separately and the tube should be flushed with at least 5 mL water between them.[82,83,85]

ADMIXTURE OF DRUGS WITH ENTERAL FEEDING

Mixing liquid medications with certain enteral feeding formulations is associated with several types of physical incompatibilities, including granulation, gel formation, separation, and precipitation.[82,83] Not only can these physical incompatibilities inhibit drug absorption, gel formation potentially may clog small-bore enteral feeding tubes. Physical incompatibility with medications is more common in formulations that contain intact protein than in those with hydrolyzed protein. Also, medication and enteral formula incompatibilities are more common with the use of acidic pharmaceutical syrups. The most prudent recommendation is to avoid the routine admixture whenever possible, especially for nonaqueous preparations and syrups. In the clinical setting, exceptions do exist, such as adding electrolyte injections of potassium or sodium to enteral formulas to assist in maintaining or repleting electrolytes.

DRUG–NUTRIENT INTERACTIONS

9 The most significant drug and nutrient interactions that can occur during continuous enteral feeding are those in which the bioavailability of the drug is reduced and the desired pharmacologic effect is not achieved (Table 146–8). Unfortunately, limited clinical studies are available to document the extent of this problem with enteral feeding. Most of the observations are anecdotal case reports involving few patients. One of the most studied interactions has been the interaction between phenytoin and enteral feeding that results in decreased phenytoin bioavailability. The interaction was first reported in 1982,[86] yet the precise mechanism for the interaction remains unclear. Phenytoin serum concentrations may decrease by as much as 50% to 75% when phenytoin is given concomitantly with EN, possibly as a result of the binding of phenytoin to calcium caseinates or protein hydrolysates in the enteral formulation. Patients typically require higher than normal phenytoin doses while receiving EN.[83,84,87] The patient's clinical response and phenytoin serum concentrations should be monitored closely if phenytoin is given enterally during continuous enteral feeding and after its discontinuation.

TABLE 146-8 Medications with Special Considerations for Enteral Feeding Tube Administration

Drug	Interaction	Comments
Phenytoin	Reduced bioavailability in the presence of enteral nutrition Possible binding of phenytoin to calcium caseinates or protein hydrolysates in enteral feeding	A suggestion to minimize interaction is to hold tube feeding 1–2 hours before and after phenytoin, but this has no proven benefit Adjust tube feeding rate to account for time held for phenytoin administration Monitor phenytoin serum concentrations and clinical response closely Consider switching to IV phenytoin route if unable to reach therapeutic serum concentration
Fluoroquinolones Tetracycline	Potential for reduced bioavailability because of complexation of drug with divalent and trivalent cations found in enteral feeding	Consider holding tube feeding before and after administration Avoid jejunal administration of ciprofloxacin Monitor clinical response
Warfarin	Decreased absorption of warfarin because of enteral feeding; therapeutic effect antagonized by vitamin K in enteral formulations	Adjust warfarin dose based on international normalized ratio Anticipate need to increase warfarin dose when enteral feedings are started and decrease dose when enteral feedings are stopped
Omeprazole Lansoprazole	Administration via feeding tube complicated by acid-labile medication within delayed-release, base-labile granules	Granules become sticky when moistened with water and may occlude small-bore tubes Suggested that granules be mixed with acidic liquid when given via a gastric feeding tube An oral liquid suspension can be extemporaneously prepared for administration via a feeding tube[a]

[a]*From references 89 and 90.*

CLINICAL CONTROVERSY

A number of methods to minimize the interaction between phenytoin and continuous enteral feeding have been suggested, but no consensus exists. Some clinicians choose to hold the feeding for 1 to 2 hours before and after phenytoin administration to minimize the interaction. But because this has not been proven effective and may result in suboptimal nutrition, others choose not to interrupt the feeding. Regardless of the method used, serum concentration monitoring is imperative.

Decreased bioavailability of certain antibiotics, particularly quinolones, has been documented when coadministered with enteral feeding.[83–85,88] Although the practice of holding tube feeding for 30 minutes before and 30 minutes after quinolone administration has been recommended, it has not been shown to ultimately improve drug absorption. There is evidence to suggest that ciprofloxacin absorption is significantly decreased when given via a jejunostomy tube, so this practice should be avoided.[88] Warfarin resistance has been documented during enteral feeding, possibly as a consequence of decreased absorption or the antagonist effects of vitamin K. Prior to 1980, it was thought that the content of vitamin K (up to 1,330 mcg/1,000 kcal of enteral feeding formula) was contributing to the pharmacologic interaction with warfarin. Subsequently, the vitamin K content within formulas intended for use in adults was reformulated to less than 200 mcg/1,000 kcal. However, warfarin resistance continues to be reported and a warfarin dosage increase may be required in patients receiving EN.[83,84] The patient's international normalized ratio should be closely monitored in patients receiving both warfarin and enteral feedings. Conversely, when EN is discontinued, a reduction in warfarin dose may be required.

NUTRITION OUTCOME GOALS

Nutrition outcome goals of EN are to promote an adequate nutritional state in adults and promote growth and development of infants and children. Assessing the outcome of EN includes monitoring objective measures of body composition, protein and energy balance, and subjective outcome for physiologic muscle function and wound healing. Besides an improvement in nutrition outcome, another goal of EN is to reduce disease-related morbidity and mortality. Measures of disease-related morbidity include length of hospital stay, infectious complications, and the patient's sense of well-being. Such clinical outcome goals are extremely difficult to document with the use of EN, in part because other factors such as age, underlying comorbidities, extent of injury, immunocompetence, and end-organ complications also affect disease outcome. However, no disease process improves significantly with prolonged starvation. Ultimately, the successful use of EN can avoid the need for PN in patients unable to meet nutrient requirements with an oral diet.

PHARMACOECONOMIC CONSIDERATIONS

EN has consistently been shown to be less expensive than PN. The pharmacoeconomic comparison between EN and PN should include an evaluation of therapeutic outcome relative to the cumulative cost associated with providing the therapy. Therapy costs should include costs related to placement and maintenance of enteral or parenteral access; costs of nutrients and related supplies; the time spent by professional staff in ordering, compounding, delivering, administering, and managing therapy; costs of laboratory monitoring; and costs of managing complications that result from therapy. However, it is very difficult to capture all of these costs and separate cost from charge-based estimates. None of the existing pharmacoeconomic analyses incorporate all costs related to EN and PN therapy, but selected cost comparisons derived from clinical research trials in institutional settings have been published.[91–93] The cost of EN has been reported to be approximately 25% to 50% that of PN. Incorporating the cost of managing complications related to therapy greatly increases the overall cost of PN compared with EN.[93] In situations in which improved outcome has not been demonstrated with PN, EN appears preferable on a cost basis.[7]

ABBREVIATIONS

ARA: arachidonic acid

DHA: docosahexaenoic acid

EN: enteral nutrition

FDA: Food and Drug Administration

MCT: medium-chain triglyceride

NG: nasogastric

NPO: nothing by mouth

PEG: percutaneous endoscopic gastrostomy

PN: parenteral nutrition

ACKNOWLEDGMENTS

We gratefully acknowledge Doug Janson, PharmD, BCNSP, for his contribution to the 5th edition of this chapter.

REFERENCES

1. Caspary WF. Physiology and pathophysiology of intestinal absorption. Am J Clin Nutr 1992;55:299S–308S.
2. DeLegge MH, Ridley C. Nutrient digestion, absorption, and excretion. In: Gottschlich MM, ed. The Science and Practice of Nutrition Support: A Case-Based Core Curriculum. Dubuque, IA: Kendall/Hunt, 2001:1–16.
3. Farrell JJ. Digestion and absorption of nutrients and vitamins. In: Feldman M, Tschumy WO, Friedman LS, Sleisenger MH, eds. Sleisenger & Fordtran's Gastrointestinal and Liver Disease: Pathophysiology/Diagnosis/Management, 7th ed. Philadelphia: WB Saunders, 2002:1715–1745.
4. Rombeau JL, Kripke SA. Metabolic and intestinal effects of short-chain fatty acids. JPEN J Parenter Enteral Nutr 1990;96;14(Suppl):181S–185S.
5. Frakenfield D. Energy and macrosubstrate requirements. In: Gottschlich MM, ed. The Science and Practice of Nutrition Support: A Case-Based Curriculum. Dubuque, IA: Kendall/Hunt, 2001:31–52.
6. Jabbar A, Chang WK, Dryden GW, McClave S. Gut immunology and the differential response to feeding and starvation. Nutr Clin Pract 2003;18:461–482.
7. A.S.P.E.N. Board of Directors and The Clinical Guidelines Task Force. Guidelines for the use of parenteral and enteral nutrition in adult and pediatric patients. JPEN J Parenter Enteral Nutr 2002;26(1 Suppl):1SA–138SA.
8. Kirby DF, DeLegge MH, Fleming CR. American Gastroenterological Association technical review on tube feeding for enteral nutrition. Gastroenterology 1995;108:1282–1301.
9. Stroud M, Duncan H, Nightingale J. Guidelines for enteral feeding in adult hospital patients. Gut 2003;52(Suppl VII):vii1–vii12.
10. McClave SA, Chang WK, Dhaliwal R, Heyland DK. Nutrition support in acute pancreatitis: A systematic review of the literature. JPEN J Parenter Enteral Nutr 2006;30:143–156.
11. Abou-Assi S, O'Keefe SJ. Nutrition support during acute pancreatitis. Nutrition 2002;18:938–943.
12. Lee JS, Polin RA. Treatment and prevention of necrotizing enterocolitis. Semin Neonatal 2003;8:449–459.
13. Dhaliwal R, Heyland DK. Nutrition and infection in the intensive care unit: What does the evidence show? Curr Opin Crit Care 2005;11:461–467.

14. Huckleberry Y. Nutrition support and the surgical patient. Am J Health Syst Pharm 2004;61:671–684.
15. Heyland DK, Dhaliwal R, Drover JW, et al. Canadian clinical practice guidelines for nutrition support in mechanically ventilated, critically ill adult patients. JPEN J Parenter Enteral Nutr 2003;27:355–373.
16. Lipman TO. Bacterial translocation and enteral nutrition in humans: An outsider looks in. JPEN J Parenter Enteral Nutr 1995;19:156–165.
17. Wernerman J, Hammarqvist F. Bacterial translocation: Effects of artificial feeding. Curr Opin Clin Nutr Metab Care 2002;5:163–166.
18. Alpers DH. Enteral feeding and gut atrophy. Curr Opin Clin Nutr Metab Care 2002;5:679–683.
19. van den Berghe G, Wouters PJ, Bouillon R, et al. Outcome benefit of intensive insulin therapy in the critically ill: Insulin dose versus glycemic control. Crit Care Med 2003;31:359–366.
20. Kumpf VJ. Parenteral nutrition-associated liver disease in adult and pediatric patients. Nutr Clin Pract 2006;21:279–290.
21. Artinian V, Krayem H, DiGiovine B. Effects of early enteral feeding on the outcome of critically ill mechanically ventilated medical patients. Chest 2006;129:960–967.
22. Marik PE, Zaloga GP. Early enteral nutrition in acutely ill patients: A systemic review. Crit Care Med 2001;29:2264–2270.
23. McClave SA, Wei-Kuo Chang. Feeding the hypotensive patient: Does enteral feeding precipitate or protect against ischemic bowel? Nutr Clin Pract 2003;18:279–284.
24. Zaloga GP, Roberts PR, Marik P. Feeding the hemodynamically unstable patient: A critical evaluation of the evidence. Nutr Clin Pract 2003;18:285–293.
25. Vanek VW. Ins and outs of enteral access. Part 1: Short-term enteral access. Nutr Clin Pract 2002;17:275–283.
26. Marik PE, Zaloga GP. Gastric versus post-pyloric feeding: A systematic review. Crit Care 2003;7:46–51.
27. Heyland DK, Drover JW, Dkaliwal R, Greenwood J. Optimizing the benefits and minimizing the risks of enteral nutrition in the critically ill: Role of small bowel feeding. JPEN J Parenter Enteral Nutr 2002;26(6 Suppl):S51–S55.
28. Heiselman DE, Hofer, T, Vidovich RR. Enteral feeding tube placement success with intravenous metoclopramide administration in ICU patients. Chest 1995;107:1686–1688.
29. Kalliafas S, Choban PS, Ziegler D, et al. Erythromycin facilitates postpyloric placement of nasoduodenal feeding tubes in intensive care unit patients: Randomized, double-blinded, placebo-controlled trial. JPEN J Parenter Enteral Nutr 1996;20:385–388.
30. Vanek VW. Ins and outs of enteral access. Part 2: Long-term access-esophagostomy and gastrostomy. Nutr Clin Pract 2003;18:50–74.
31. Angus F, Burakoff R. The percutaneous endoscopic gastrostomy tube. Medical and ethical issues in placement. Am J Gastroenterol 2003;98:272–277.
32. Gauderer MW. Percutaneous endoscopic gastrostomy and the evolution of contemporary long-term enteral access. Clin Nutr 2002;21:103–110.
33. Vanek VW. Ins and outs of enteral access. Part 3: Long-term access-jejunostomy. Nutr Clin Pract 2003;18:201–220.
34. McClave SA, DeMeo MT, DeLegge MH, et al. North American Summit on Aspiration in the Critically Ill Patient: Consensus statement. JPEN J Parenter Enteral Nutr 2002;26(6 Suppl):S80–S85.
35. Parrish CR. Enteral feeding: The art and the science. Nutr Clin Pract 2003;18:76–85.
36. Jawaheer G, Shaw NJ, Pierro A. Continuous enteral feeding impairs gallbladder emptying in infants. J Pediatr 2001;138:822–825.
37. Mueller C, Nestle M. Regulation of medical foods: Toward a rational policy. Nutr Clin Pract 1995;10:8–15.
38. Heymsfield SB. Enteral solutions: Is there a solution? Nutr Clin Pract 1995;10:4–7.
39. Buchman AL. Glutamine: Commercially essential or conditionally essential? A critical appraisal of the human data. Am J Clin Nutr 2001;74:25–32.
40. Wilmore DW. The effect of glutamine supplementation in patients following elective surgery and accidental injury. J Nutr 2001;131:2543S–2549S.
41 Heyland DK, Samis A. Does immunonutrition in patients with sepsis do more harm than good? Int Care Med 2003;29:669–671.
42. Zaloga GP, Siddiqui R, Terry C, Marik P. Arginine: Mediator or modulator of sepsis? Nutr Clin Pract 2004;19:201–215.
43. Barton RG. Immune-enhancing enteral formulas: Are they beneficial in critically ill patients? Nutr Clin Pract 1997;12:51–62.
44. O'Connor DL, Hall R, Adamkin D, et al. Growth and development in preterm infants fed long-chain polyunsaturated fatty acids: A prospective, randomized controlled trial. Pediatrics 2001;108:359–371.
45. Birch EE, Hoffman DR, Castañeda YS, et al. A randomized controlled trial of long-chain polyunsaturated fatty acid supplementation of formula in term infants after weaning at 6 weeks of age. Am J Clin Nutr 2002;75:570–580.
46. Lucas A, Stafford M, Morley R, et al. Efficacy and safety of long-chain polyunsaturated fatty acid supplementation of infant-formula milk: A randomised trial. Lancet 1999;354:1948–1954.
47. Innis SM, Adamkin DH, Hall RT, et al. Docosahexaenoic acid and arachidonic acid enhance growth with no adverse effects in preterm infants fed formula. J Pediatr 2002;140:547–554.
48. Heird WC. The role of polyunsaturated fatty acids in term and preterm infants and breastfeeding mothers. Pediatr Clin North Am 2001;48:173–188.
49. Scheppach WM, Bartram HP. Experimental evidence for and clinical implications of fiber and artificial enteral nutrition. Nutrition 1993;9:399–405.
50. Roy CC, Kien L, Bouthillier L, Levy E. Short-chain fatty acids: Ready for prime time? Nutr Clin Pract 2006;21:351–366.
51. Jew R, Owen D, Kaufman D, et al. Osmolality of commonly used medications and formulas in the neonatal intensive care unit. Nutr Clin Pract 1997;12:158–163.
52. MacBurney MM, Russell C, Young LS. Formulas. In: Rombeau JL, Caldwell MD, eds. Clinical Nutrition: Enteral and Tube Feeding, 2nd ed. Philadelphia: WB Saunders, 1990:149–173..
53. Silk DBA, Grimble GK. Relevance of physiology of nutrient absorption to formulation of enteral diets. Nutrition 1992;8:1–12.
54. Montejo JC, Zarazaga A, Lopez-Martinez J, et al. Immunonutrition in the intensive care unit. A systematic review and consensus statement. Clin Nutr 2003;22:221–233.
55 Beale RJ, Bryg DJ, Bihari DJ. Immunonutrition in the critically ill: A systematic review of clinical outcome. Crit Care Med 1999;27:2799–2805.
56. Kreymann KG, Berger MM, Deutz NEP, et al. ESPEN guidelines on enteral nutrition: Intensive care. Clin Nutr 2006;25:210–223.
57. Heyland DK, Novak F, Drover JW, et al. Should immunonutrition become routine in critically ill patients? A systematic review of the evidence. JAMA 2001;286:944–953.
58. Russell MK, Charney P. Is there a role for specialized enteral nutrition in the intensive care unit? Nutr Clin Pract 2002;17:156–168.
59. Gadek JE, DeMichele SJ, Karlstad MD, et al. Effect of enteral feeding with eicosapentaenoic acid, gamma-linolenic acid, and antioxidants in patients with acute respiratory distress syndrome. Crit Care Med 1999;27:1409–1420.
60. Davis A, Baker S. The use of modular nutrients in pediatrics. JPEN J Parenter Enteral Nutr 1996;20:228–236.
61. Navajas MF-C, Chacon DJ, Solvas JRG, et al. Bacterial contamination of enteral feeds as a possible risk of nosocomial infection. J Hosp Infect 1992;21:111–120.
62. Oliviera MH, Bonelli R, Aidoo KE, Batista CR. Microbiological quality of reconstituted enteral formulations used in hospitals. Nutrition 2000;16:729–733.
63. Atkinson SA. Human milk feeding of the micropremie. Clin Perinatol 2000;27:235–247.
64. Porcelli P, Schanler R, Greer F, et al. Growth in human milk-fed very low birth weight infants receiving a new human milk fortifier. Ann Nutr Metab 2000;44:2–10.
65. Sankaran K, Papageorgiou A, Ninan A, Sankaran R. A randomized, controlled evaluation of two commercially available human breast milk fortifiers in health preterm neonates. J Am Diet Assoc 1996;96:1145–1149.
66. Corkins MR, Scolapio J. Diarrhea. In: Merritt R, ed. The A.S.P.E.N. Nutrition Support Practice Manual, 2nd ed. Silver Spring, MD: A.S.P.E.N., 2005:203–210.
67. Mehall JR, Kite CA, Saltzman DA, et al. Prospective study of the incidence and complications of bacterial contamination of enteral feeding in neonates. J Pediatr Surg 2002;37:1177–1182.
68. Thurn J, Crossley K, Gerdts A, et al. Enteral hyperalimentation as a source of nosocomial infection. J Hosp Infect 1990;15:203–217.

69. Zaloga GP. Parenteral nutrition in adult inpatients with functioning gastrointestinal tracts: Assessment of outcomes. Lancet 2006;367:1101–1111.
70. Williams TA, Leslie GD. A review of the nursing care of enteral feeding tubes in critically ill adults: Part I. Intensive Crit Care Nurs 2004;20:330–343.
71. McClave SA, Snider HL. Clinical use of gastric residual volumes as a monitor for patients on enteral tube feeding. JPEN J Parenter Enteral Nutr 2002;26(6 Suppl):S43–S50.
72. MacLaren R. Intolerance to intragastric enteral nutrition in critically ill patients: Complications and management. Pharmacotherapy 2000;20:1486–1498.
73. Booth CM, Heyland DK, Paterson WG. Gastrointestinal promotility drugs in the critical care setting: A systematic review of the evidence. Crit Care Med 2002;30:1429–1435.
74. Maloney JP, Ryan TA, Brasel KJ, et al. Food dye use in enteral feedings: A review and a call for a moratorium. Nutr Clin Pract 2002;17:168–181.
75. Maloney JP, Ryan TA. Detection of aspiration in enterally fed patients: A requiem for bedside monitors of aspiration. JPEN J Parenter Enteral Nutr 2002;26(6 Suppl):S34–S42.
76. Bliss DZ, Guenter PA, Settle RG. Defining and reporting diarrhea in tube-fed patients—What a mess! Am J Clin Nutr 1992;55:753–759.
77. Eisenberg PG. Causes of diarrhea in tube-fed patients: A comprehensive approach to diagnosis and management. Nutr Clin Pract 1993;8:119–123.
78. Frankel EH, Enow NB, Jackson KC, et al. Methods of restoring patency to occluded feeding tubes. Nutr Clin Pract 1998;13:129–131.
79. Cabre E, Gassull MA. Complications of enteral feeding. Nutrition 1993;9:1–9.
80. Bayzyk S. Factors associated with transition to oral feedings in infants fed by nasogastric tubes. Am J Occup Ther 1990;44:1070–1078.
81. Mitchell JF. Oral dosage forms that should not be crushed: July 2007 Chart. In: Hospital Pharmacy. St. Louis: Wolters Kluwer Health, 2007.
82. Engle KK, Hannawa TE. Techniques for administering oral medications to critical care patients receiving continuous enteral nutrition. Am J Health Syst Pharm 1999;56:1441–1444.
83. Beckwith MC, Feddema SS, Barton RG, Graves C. A guide to drug therapy in patients with enteral feeding tubes: Dosage form selection and administration methods. Hosp Pharm 2004;39:225–237.
84. Dickerson RN. Medication administration considerations for patients receiving enteral tube feedings. Hosp Pharm 2004;39:84–89.
85. Magnuson BL, Clifford TM, Hoskins LA, Bernard AC. Enteral nutrition and drug administration, interactions, and complications. Nutr Clin Pract 2005;20:618–624.
86. Bauer LA. Interference of oral phenytoin absorption by continuous nasogastric feedings. Neurology 1982;32:570–572.
87. Gilbert S, Hatton J, Magnuson B. How to minimize interaction between phenytoin and enteral feedings: Two approaches. Nutr Clin Pract 1996;11:28–31.
88. Nyffeler MS. Ciprofloxacin use in the enterally fed patient. Nutr Clin Pract 1999;14:73–77.
89. Quercia RA, Fan C, Liu X, et al. Stability of omeprazole in an extemporaneously prepared oral liquid. Am J Health Syst Pharm 1997;54:1833–1836.
90. Dunn A, White M, Reddy P, et al. Delivery of omeprazole and lansoprazole granules through a nasogastric tube in vitro. Am J Health Syst Pharm 1999;56:2327–2330.
91. Senkel M, Mumme A, Eickhoff U, et al. Early postoperative enteral immunonutrition: Clinical outcome and cost-comparison analyses in surgical patients. Crit Care Med 1997;25:1489–1496.
92. McClave SA, Greene LM, Snider HL, et al. Comparison of the safety of early enteral vs parenteral nutrition in mild acute pancreatitis. JPEN J Parenter Enteral Nutr 1996;21:14–20.
93. Trice S, Melnik G, Page CP. Complications and costs of early postoperative parenteral versus enteral nutrition in trauma patients. Nutr Clin Pract 1997;12:114–119.

CHAPTER 147 Nutritional Considerations in Major Organ Failure

BRIAN M. HODGES AND MARK DELEGGE

KEY CONCEPTS

1. Carbohydrate calories absorbed and protein lost via renal replacement therapy must be accounted for when designing a parenteral or enteral nutrition regimen for patients with renal failure.
2. Administration of renally excreted or regulated electrolytes, such potassium, magnesium, and phosphorus, should be limited in patients with renal failure unless refeeding syndrome is present or continuous renal replacement therapies are used.
3. Hyperglycemia is common in cirrhosis. Patients with fulminant hepatitis are, however, instead prone to hypoglycemia.
4. Folic acid and thiamine supplementation is important in patients with liver disease for the prevention of anemia and Wernicke's encephalopathy, respectively.
5. In short-bowel syndrome, parenteral nutrition should be used to meet nutritional needs in the immediate postoperative period after intestinal resection.
6. Increased fluid and electrolyte replacement is often necessary in short-bowel syndrome patients to replace gastrointestinal losses. Patients may need increased calcium, magnesium, zinc, and other trace elements because of decreased absorption and/or excessive gastrointestinal losses.
7. Patients with ileal resection commonly develop vitamin B_{12} deficiency, necessitating therapy with parenteral cyanocobalamin.
8. As small-bowel adaptation occurs, some short-bowel syndrome patients receiving parenteral nutrition can be transitioned successfully to enteral nutrition. Early initiation of enteral intake affects adaptation because intraluminal nutrients are a stimulus for this process.
9. Care should be taken to avoid overfeeding of patients with respiratory failure, as excessive carbon dioxide production may limit the patients' ability to have mechanical ventilation discontinued.
10. Excessive fluid administration should be avoided in patients with pulmonary disease because it may worsen already compromised pulmonary function.

Learning objectives, review questions, and other resources can be found at **www.pharmacotherapyonline.com.**

Because organ failure may alter absorption, use, and excretion of nutrients, administration of standard nutrients to patients with organ dysfunction may be inappropriate. Individualization of a nutritional regimen for these patients often requires a planned, disease-specific approach. Different laboratory testing or more frequent monitoring of traditional markers may be necessary to ensure that the desired therapeutic goals are achieved. For example, it is impossible to collect a 24-hour urine specimen to measure urea nitrogen and nitrogen balance in an anuric patient. In this situation, an alternative method of calculating urea nitrogen appearance is required.

Patients with acute organ failure requiring nutrition support often are hospitalized in intensive care units (ICUs). With advances in treating chronic organ failure, increasing numbers of older, chronically ill patients will require nutritional support on a long-term basis. It therefore will become increasingly common for nutrition support to be provided in community and ambulatory settings. Regardless of the setting, the clinician needs a firm pathophysiologic foundation on which to build a pharmaceutical care plan to ensure appropriate outcomes for patients requiring nutritional support.

This chapter discusses the nutritional needs of patients with renal, hepatic, gastrointestinal, and pulmonary failure. The predominant approaches to ensure delivery of safe and efficacious nutrients to patients with these disorders are critically reviewed.

RENAL FAILURE

Major differences exist between the metabolic, fluid, and electrolyte management of patients with acute renal failure (ARF) versus those with stable chronic kidney disease (CKD) and those with an ARF episode that complicates preexisting CKD. For example, positive nitrogen balance is more difficult to achieve in patients with ARF because of the increased rate of protein catabolism. Additionally, patients with ARF are more likely to develop hyperglycemia during nutritional support and frequently are dialyzed by modalities that are not used commonly for the patient with end-stage kidney disease. Because of these differences, the nutritional management of patients with ARF is discussed separately.

ACUTE RENAL FAILURE

Epidemiology

ARF, as defined in Chap. 45, is a decrease in glomerular filtration rate occurring over hours to weeks that is associated with an increase in the serum concentrations of waste products, such as urea and creatinine. ARF has been observed in as many as 5% of hospitalized patients, and in up to 50% of patients receiving care in an ICU.[1] The mortality rate of ARF patients who require renal replacement therapy ranges from 40% to as high as 70%. A recent study in Austria demonstrated that despite the recent advancements made in renal replacement therapies and ICU care, the mortality rate of patients was still 62.8%.[2] Severe malnutrition has been documented in 42% of patients with ARF and is an independent predictor of in-hospital mortality and increased morbidity from sepsis, shock, dysrhythmias, and acute respiratory failure.[3] Because malnutrition is an important apparently independent contributor to mortality in patients with ARF, nutrition support remains a cornerstone in the treatment of these patients, despite a lack of evidence demonstrating improvement in patient survival.[1,4]

Pathophysiology

Energy Requirements ARF does not itself change patient energy requirements. Energy requirements in ARF are greatly influenced by comorbid critical illness and the types of renal replacement therapies used.[4,5] Energy requirements in this patient population ideally should be measured by indirect calorimetry (see Chap. 143) because energy expenditures of patients with ARF are highly variable. Energy expenditure is close to normal in patients with uncomplicated ARF, but resting energy expenditure (REE) increases of up to 30% have been reported in the presence of sepsis and ARF.[6] Typically, ARF patients without underlying hypermetabolic conditions should receive 20 to 30 kcal/kg per day. Those with underlying hypermetabolic conditions, such as thermal injury or head injury, usually need even greater caloric intake, up to 35 kcal/kg per day, unless indirect calorimetry indicates otherwise.[7] Patients with stage 4 or 5 chronic kidney disease and acute metabolic illness or injury should receive similar energy provisions.[5] Increasing energy provision beyond this to 40 kcal/kg/day is not associated with better nutritional outcomes and has been associated with more frequent metabolic complications.[8]

Carbohydrate Hyperglycemia and peripheral insulin resistance are common in ARF. These patients usually have a superimposed illness that exacerbates glucose intolerance. The etiology of glucose intolerance in ARF is thought to be a result of increased levels of glucagon, growth hormone, and catecholamines—all known antagonists of insulin. Other proposed mechanisms include an elevated glucagon-to-insulin ratio secondary to impaired degradation of these hormones and elevated secretion of inflammatory cytokines.

Fat Intolerance to intravenous lipid emulsion (IVLE), evidenced by increased serum triglyceride concentrations, is common in ARF. Hypertriglyceridemia is thought to be caused by decreased catabolism of triglycerides and increased triglyceride synthesis from free fatty acids.[1] Hepatic triglyceride lipase and peripheral lipoprotein lipase activity may be reduced significantly in ARF patients.[6] Insulin resistance and metabolic acidosis may contribute to this process by inhibiting lipoprotein lipase.[9] Triglyceride concentrations therefore should be measured before administering IVLE to patients with ARF.

Protein ARF is associated with marked protein catabolism and urea accumulation. Most patients with ARF have a primary stressful illness that results in ureagenesis, and thus protein breakdown is accelerated. Protein catabolism in ARF may be stimulated as the result of insulin resistance, metabolic acidosis, circulating proteases and inflammatory mediators, and the effects of uremic toxins.[1] The mechanism may be direct, via modulation of protein synthesis, or indirect, by inhibiting the action of anabolic hormones. Unlike healthy patients or those with CKD, protein catabolism in the presence of ARF is not significantly attenuated by the administration of exogenous nutrition support.[4]

Significant amounts of protein and amino acids are also removed by dialysis. Amino acid losses of 5.2 g per conventional hemodialysis (HD) treatment, 7.3 g per high-flux HD session, and up to 13 to 16 g/day during continuous renal replacement therapy (CRRT) have been reported.[10] In one study, CRRT removed urea nitrogen to the same degree as functionally normal kidneys.[11] The clearance of histidine and tryptophan are enhanced, whereas the clearance of phenylalanine and valine are reduced in nondialyzed patients with ARF.[12] In patients undergoing CRRT, glutamine represents roughly one-third of all amino acid dialysate losses. Serum glutamine concentrations decrease significantly early during CRRT, but may return to baseline subsequently, suggesting altered glutamine metabolism early in the course of CRRT.[13]

Fluid, Electrolyte, and Acid–Base Disorders The volume status of patients with ARF depends primarily on residual urine output and the type of dialysis received, if any. The patient with oliguric ARF will have impaired excretion of sodium and water. In nonoliguric ARF, considerable sodium may be lost in the urine, necessitating replacement to maintain sodium balance. This also applies to the patient who is losing considerable gastric fluids. Patients on CRRT will lose sodium via hemofiltration or dialysis and should be given sodium as part of their CRRT replacement fluid regimen. To maintain sodium balance, most replacement fluids contain between 140 and 154 mEq sodium/L. The rate of administration of these fluids varies based on the type of CRRT, the rate of ultrafiltration, and the patient's clinical condition.[14]

Hyperkalemia is observed frequently in ARF secondary to protein catabolism and intracellular potassium release, as discussed in Chap. 54. Hyperkalemia also results from the impaired secretion and excretion of potassium by the kidney and the endogenous release secondary to tissue breakdown. If this is severe, emergent dialysis may be indicated. Patients on CRRT, however, usually require potassium replacement to avoid hypokalemia as a consequence of the significant dialytic potassium losses.

Because phosphorus is excreted renally, hyperphosphatemia is common in ARF. Like potassium, large amounts of phosphorus are released into the circulation secondary to tissue breakdown during ARF. Control of hyperphosphatemia is important because as the calcium-phosphorus product (serum calcium in milligrams per deciliter multiplied by serum phosphorus in milligrams per deciliter) exceeds 55, the risk of developing metastatic calcification increases (see Chap. 53). Conversely, with initiation of dialysis, particularly CRRT, patients must be monitored for dialysis-induced hypophosphatemia. Hypophosphatemia may also be observed in patients with acute or chronic renal failure who continue to receive oral phosphate binders despite decreased oral phosphorus intake.

The net removal of calcium during the continuous dialysis modalities depends on the calcium concentration of the dialysate fluid. Severe hypocalcemia has been reported when regional citrate anticoagulation has been used for CRRT in ARF and hepatic failure patients.[14]

Hypermagnesemia is less common than other electrolyte abnormalities, but can occur in ARF secondary to impaired excretion and endogenous release from tissue breakdown. Both magnesium and calcium losses via CRRT have been quantified recently: average daily losses were 24 mmol and 70 mmol of magnesium and calcium, respectively.[11]

Patients with ARF usually have metabolic acidosis because of impaired excretion of organic acids. If potassium and sodium are needed in the parenteral nutrition (PN) regimen, they should be added as acetate salts, which are converted to bicarbonate in the liver. This increase in bicarbonate partially compensates their metabolic acidosis. Intermittent and continuous dialytic therapies also may help improve the metabolic acidosis accompanying ARF by increasing the removal of these endogenously generated acids, as well as by increasing serum bicarbonate levels as the result of diffusion from the dialysate into the blood. Correction of acidosis was greatest when lactate buffers (lactate > bicarbonate > acetate) were used in one study employing continuous venovenous hemofiltration.[15]

Trace Elements The requirements for trace elements during nutritional support of ARF patients are not well established because trace element accumulation or losses during ARF have not been characterized. Additionally, many of the trace element alterations in ARF may represent an "acute-phase reaction."[7] Zinc and chromium are excreted by the kidney and theoretically can accumulate because of reduced excretion and increased intake secondary to impurities in dialysate or intravenous fluids. In ARF patients undergoing CRRT, zinc intake via nutrition support exceeds patient losses.[11] Selenium concentrations are reduced in ARF patients and may result in a decrease in thyroxine concentrations.[16,17] Because manganese and copper are excreted in bile and zinc and copper are removed by peritoneal dialysis (PD) and HD, most ARF patients receiving PN should receive trace element supplementation; in addition, some recommend that additional selenium supplementation may be necessary.[4,17] Doses of 50 to 70 mcg/day may be necessary to maintain selenium balance.[7]

Vitamins Little information is available concerning alterations in vitamin requirements in ARF, and the known changes require monitoring but not routine changes to patient treatment.[18] Losses of vitamins via dialysis also must be considered. Traditional HD clears several water-soluble vitamins such as folic acid, vitamins C and B_{12}, and pyridoxine, but not the highly protein-bound vitamins A and D.[19] Significant reductions in the plasma concentrations of water soluble vitamins have also been observed in patients receiving CRRT.[13,17] Currently, it seems prudent to administer vitamins at least daily in doses recommended by the Nutrition Advisory Group of the American Medical Association for patients receiving PN (see Chap. 145).[7] Administration of ascorbic acid should be restricted to 50 to 100 mg/day to offset losses caused by renal replacement therapies, but to avoid secondary oxalosis which may worsen renal function.[5,20] If the enteral route is used for nutritional support, vitamin administration should at least meet the recommended daily allowances.

TREATMENT

Acute Renal Failure

DESIRED OUTCOME

The maintenance of lean muscle mass and prevention of disorders of macro- and micronutrient excess or deficiency are the primary goals in the nutritional management of the patient with ARF. Although it has yet to be proven that nutrition support is associated with a reduction in mortality of patients with ARF, the secondary goals of nutrition therapy are to optimize immunocompetence and promote wound healing. Additionally, the attenuation of the inflammatory state, metabolic derangements, and alterations of the patient's antioxidant capacity should also be considered in the design of specialized nutrition support for patients with ARF.[4]

GENERALIZED APPROACH TO TREATMENT

Enteral nutrition (EN) is the preferred route of nutrient delivery in patients with ARF. [4,5] The products used frequently during EN are the calorically dense, electrolyte-free or electrolyte-reduced formulas.[21] These formulas are useful in patients with fluid overload, hyperkalemia, hypermagnesemia, and hyperphosphatemia. EN is well tolerated by many patients with ARF,[22] and is associated with improved maintenance of gastrointestinal tract function and survival in nonrandomized studies of patients with ARF.[2,23] It is recommended that EN be used, even if PN must be used as a supplement to meet the patient's nutritional needs. Unfortunately, because of the high incidence of gastrointestinal complications, many patients may not tolerate EN and thus require PN support.[2]

PHARMACOLOGIC THERAPIES

Drug Treatments of First Choice

Patients with ARF and comorbid hypermetabolism typically require 25 to 35 kcal/kg per day.[24] Increasing energy provision beyond this does not improve nutritional outcomes and is associated with increasing metabolic complications and a greater net fluid imbalance.[8] A relatively conservative initial estimate of patient energy needs is appropriate since the result of slightly underfeeding the patient are far less serious than those associated with overfeeding.[4,25]

❶ In the absence of dialysis, the nutritional formula should be concentrated in a small volume and contain minimal sodium (Table 147–1). In the oliguric patient who is receiving renal replacement therapy, these restrictions may be less rigorous, but the formula generally will need to be concentrated.[5] When using these high-dextrose-concentration formulas, careful monitoring of glucose homeostasis (every 6 hours) is important because the maintenance of euglycemia has been associated with improved clinical outcomes of critically ill adults.[25] Additionally, CRRT, which is increasingly popular in the treatment of ARF (see Chap. 45), contributes significant calories to a nutritional regimen. This is a direct result of the absorption of glucose from the dialysate or ultrafiltrate replacement fluids: net uptakes of up to 355 g/day have been reported.[13] Total glucose intake should range from 3 to 7 g/kg/day.[5]

TABLE 147-1 Empiric Parenteral Nutrition Formulas for Patients with Organ Failure

	Acute Renal Failure	Chronic Renal Failure	Hepatic Failure	Short Bowel	Pulmonary Failure
Dextrose (%)[a]	40	30	25	20	20
Crystalline amino acids (%)[a]	Variable	4	5[b]	5	5
Lipids (%)[a]	1	2	2	2	3
NaCl (mEq/L)	0	0	0	80[c]	10
Na acetate (mEq/L)	0	30	0	0	0
Na phosphate (mEq/L)	0[d]	7.5	15	7.5	30
K acetate (mEq/L)	0[d]	0	50	60	20
K chloride (mEq/L)	0	10	0	0	20
Ca gluconate (mEq/L)	5[d]	5	5	10	5
Magnesium sulfate (mEq/L)	0[d]	6	16	10	5
Multivitamins (mL/day)	10	10	10	10	10
Zinc (mg/day)	3	3–6	8	10	3
Copper (mg/day)	1.2	1.2	<1.2	1.2	1.2
Manganese (mcg/day)	300	300	<300	≤300	300
Chromium (mcg/day)	12	12	<12	20	12
Selenium (mcg/day)	–	40	40	60	40

[a]Final concentrations after admixture.
[b]Hepatamine 4% when criteria for use are met.
[c]Does not include 0.45% sodium chloride injection or lipid.
[d]The continuous renal replacement therapies frequently require variable additions of electrolytes.

ARF is not a contraindication to IVLE use, despite the changes in lipid metabolism. When the serum triglyceride concentration is less than 300 mg/dL, IVLE is recommended to prevent essential fatty acid deficiency and to provide a balanced caloric intake. Typically, doses of less than 1 g fat/kg per day will not significantly worsen triglyceride concentrations.[7] Current recommendations call for patients to receive between 0.8 and 1.2 g/kg/day, but no more than 1.5 g/kg/day.[5]

Although individual patient assessment for presence of hypercatabolism and dialytic losses is necessary, it is not uncommon for patients to require 2.5 g/kg per day of protein or more to achieve a positive nitrogen balance.[26] Protein restriction, to reduce the urea nitrogen appearance rate from exogenous protein intake, should not be used unless the ARF is thought to be temporary (e.g., expected to resolve in 7 to 10 days) and hypercatabolism is not present.[5,7,24] Once dialysis therapy is instituted, protein intake should be liberalized to 1 to 1.5 g/kg per day for noncatabolic patients and at least 1.5 g/kg per day for hypercatabolic patients.[24] Patients undergoing CRRT with hypermetabolism may need to receive 1.5 to 1.8 g/kg/day[24] or more (up to 2.5 g/kg/day) to achieve positive nitrogen balance.[23] The safety and efficacy of this aggressive strategy remains to be confirmed before it can be routinely recommended.[5,27]

CLINICAL CONTROVERSY

There is debate as to the most appropriate protein provision for patients with ARF who are receiving CRRT. Although initial data has shown an association between higher protein intake (up to 2.5 g/kg/day) and improved survival, many express concern about the effectiveness and safety of this practice.

❷ Several electrolytes (i.e., phosphorus, magnesium, and potassium) warrant special attention in patients with ARF.[5] During early ARF, PN solutions should not contain potassium unless the patient is hypokalemic or undergoing CRRT. After several days, the serum potassium concentrations tend to decrease, often necessitating cautious addition of potassium to the PN solution. If the enteral route is used, formulas with minimal potassium may be needed. Serum potassium concentrations may decrease more rapidly in patients receiving CRRT. Potassium losses during CRRT are proportional to the potassium gradient between blood and dialysate. Therefore cautious additions of potassium may be considered early in the course of ARF for those patients treated with CRRT. Serum magnesium concentrations do not decrease as quickly as potassium concentrations in patients receiving electrolyte-free nutrition regimens. As serum concentrations decrease toward normal and/or renal function returns, magnesium should be added to the PN solution in small amounts (4 to 6 mEq/L).

Phosphorus can be omitted from the nutritional formula of patients receiving PN until the phosphorus level approaches normal (<5 mg/dL). It is prudent to monitor phosphorus concentrations daily and to add phosphorus in small doses once the serum concentration is below 4 mg/dL. Failure to do so can lead to severe hypophosphatemia (see Chap. 53) despite continued renal failure, especially in the patient who is treated with CRRT. Patients with persistently high serum phosphorus concentrations who have a functional gastrointestinal tract can be prescribed phosphate-binding therapy (see Chap. 47) and enteral feedings low in phosphorus to minimize the absorption of exogenous phosphorus.

Alternative Drug Treatments

Standard mixed amino acids rather than essential amino acid solutions should be used.[5,24] Improved survival and return of renal function were observed decades ago when essential amino acids plus glucose were compared with glucose alone in patients with ARF. This led to the marketing of parenteral amino acids containing predominantly or solely essential amino acids. These products were formulated on the hypothesis that significant nitrogen reuse (urea recycling) occurs during ARF to synthesize nonessential amino acids. Subsequently, several prospective, double-blind studies have indicated no significant reduction in mortality when the essential amino acid formulations were used.[1,5,24]

■ PHARMACOECONOMIC CONSIDERATIONS

While analyses of total costs of ARF care have been published,[28] no specific research has yet been published assessing the cost-effectiveness of nutrition support in patients with ARF. Some authors, however, extrapolate the results of critical care nutrition studies[29] indicating that EN results in significant cost savings compared to PN to strengthen their recommendation that EN should be preferred over PN.[1,4,22]

■ EVALUATION OF THERAPEUTIC OUTCOMES

Although the clinical and quality-of-life (QOL) outcomes for patients with ARF have been reported, data specifically analyzing the effects of nutrition support are limited.[28] To date, there is no clear consensus regarding the degree of benefit, if any, of nutrition support on the outcome parameters of renal recovery or mortality. Data suggest that malnourished ARF patients experience significantly higher mortality rates (odds ratio of in-hospital mortality of 7.21) than ARF patients without malnutrition.[3] In one retrospective analysis EN was associated with a survival benefit, even when controlling for severity of illness.[2] No prospective studies to date show a survival benefit from aggressive nutritional support in patients with ARF. When nutrition support is used, the evaluation tools used in monitoring ARF patients are similar to those used for other patients receiving PN and EN (see Chaps. 145 and 146).

CHRONIC KIDNEY DISEASE

CKD is defined by either structural or functional damage to the kidneys that is present for at least 3 months (see Chap. 46). Malnutrition secondary to reduced oral nutrient intake frequently is evident when the glomerular filtration rate drops below 20 to 25 mL/min. Stage 5 CKD has been associated with inflammatory and metabolic changes that increase the likelihood of malnutrition and increased nutrient losses have been documented in those receiving hemodialysis and peritoneal dialysis. Because of its chronicity, malnutrition in these patients is treated most frequently in the ambulatory setting with oral nutritional supplements and EN.

Epidemiology

Protein-energy malnutrition is very common in patients with CKD and is a significant predictor of morbidity and mortality. Significant malnutrition has been noted in 28% to 48% of predialysis patients, in 9% to 72% of patients undergoing HD, and in up to 45% of patients commencing PD.[30,31] In one of the larger studies to date (n = 1,397), mean dietary calorie and protein intake in those 50 years of age and older was 22 kcal/kg per day and 0.9 g/kg per day, respectively.[32] Both these values are lower than published recommendations for patients with CKD.[33] Protein-energy malnutrition and wasting at initiation of dialysis is a significant predictor of morbidity and mortality in most studies of patients with stage 5 CKD.[30] However, there appears to be a gender difference in nutritional status in stage 5 CKD patients: women tend to have a higher prevalence of malnutrition[31] and poorer nutritional outcomes, yet a lower mortality rate.[34]

Pathophysiology

Carbohydrate In general, stage 5 CKD patients are not as nutritionally stressed as patients with ARF; however, more than one-half of stage 5 CKD patients have insulin resistance and hyperglycemia. This is attributed to the increased glucagon-to-insulin ratio, resulting in protein breakdown and gluconeogenesis. In patients with normal peritoneal transport on peritoneal dialysis, roughly 60% of glucose in the dialysate is absorbed. One method of estimating the quantity of glucose absorbed is as follows: glucose absorbed (g/day) $= 0.89x$ (g/day) $- 43$, where x is the total amount of dialysate glucose instilled daily. This dialysate glucose absorption can worsen existing hyperglycemia and contribute significantly to the patient's energy intake, making kwashiorkor-type malnutrition common. Although glucose control is not problematic unless the patient is diabetic, infected, or subjected to operative stress, insulin can be added to chronic ambulatory peritoneal dialysis bags to control hyperglycemia (see Chap. 48).

Fat Hypertriglyceridemia is common in stage 5 CKD patients. This is mainly a result of decreased catabolism of triglycerides secondary to decreased hepatic lipoprotein lipase activity.[35] Most stage 5 CKD patients receiving HD also receive heparin, which activates lipoprotein lipase and converts triglycerides to free fatty acids and glycerol. Carnitine, an amino acid necessary for the transport of long-chain fatty acids across mitochondria where oxidation results in energy production, is removed by HD and PD, and therefore serum carnitine concentrations typically are reduced in stage 5 CKD.[36]

Current guidelines do not advocate carnitine administration for the treatment of hypertriglyceridemia.[37] Studies of carnitine for this indication have varied widely in duration and have used both oral and intravenous administration in varying doses (1 mg/kg to 2 g/day intravenously, 10 mg/kg per day to 3 g/day orally).

Leptin, which is produced and secreted by fat cells, regulates satiety and energy balance (see Chap. 148). Leptin concentrations often are elevated in stage 5 CKD patients, particularly those undergoing PD probably as the result of decreased renal degradation of leptin and increased production as the result of chronic inflammation. Hyperleptinemia in CKD is associated with decreased protein intake and weight loss. Further study is required to better define the relationship between leptin concentrations and nutrition status in patients with CKD.[38,39]

Protein Secondary analysis of the Modification of Diet in Renal Disease Study indicated that in nondiabetics, a reduction of dietary protein intake may slow the rate of renal disease progression and ultimately delay the onset of dialysis (see Chap. 46).[40] The recent National Kidney Foundation Kidney Disease Outcomes Quality Initiative (NKF K/DOQI) guidelines for nutrition in patients with CKD recommend a diet providing 0.6 g/kg of protein per day for those with a glomerular filtration rate of less than 25 mL/min.[37] Although the safety of low-protein diets has been questioned, it has been suggested that for carefully selected and monitored patients, protein intakes of as low as 0.3 g/kg per day supplemented with essential amino acids can be used safely.[5,24]

Stage 5 CKD patients receiving PD require special attention as a consequence of protein losses across the peritoneal membrane. Peritoneal protein losses typically range from 5 to 15 g/day in PD patients.[37] PD protein losses, however, do not predict risk for malnutrition (as measured by serum albumin concentration) in all patients.[37] The American Society for Parenteral and Enteral Nutrition (ASPEN) and K/DOQI guidelines suggest that dietary protein intake of at least 1.2 to 1.3 g/kg per day (at least 50% of high biologic value) is needed to consistently achieve neutral or positive nitrogen balance in nonacutely ill peritoneal dialysis patients and clinically stable HD patients.[37] Dialysate protein losses also must be considered for the stage 5 CKD patient undergoing HD. The amount of protein lost via HD depends on the dialysis membrane used and whether the dialyzer is being reused. Typical losses are 10 to 12 g per dialysis session, but this may be increased by up to 50% with dialyzer reuse.[37]

Fluid and Electrolytes Hyponatremia, often due to overhydration, is common in CKD patients (see Chap. 52). Regular dialysis is the principal means for control of body water and serum sodium concentration in the stage 5 CKD patient. Patients with CKD who develop hyperkalemia generally have ingested excessive potassium relative to the potassium-removing capacity of the failing kidney (and dialysis, in the case of stage 5 CKD patients). The undernourished CKD patient receiving PN, however, may require considerable potassium as new body cell mass is synthesized.

Patients with CKD often are treated for hyperphosphatemia with phosphorus-restricted diets and phosphate binding agents (see Chaps. 46 and 47). When these patients receive aggressive nutritional support, the combination of refeeding (cellular uptake of phosphorus for synthesis of body cell mass) and vigorous phosphate-binding therapy can result in hypophosphatemia.

Metabolic acidosis, a common complication of stage 5 CKD, is associated with increased protein degradation and decreased synthesis of albumin.[37] Correction of acidosis in stage 5 CKD patients may be associated with increases in serum albumin, body weight, and midarm muscle circumference, and fewer hospitalizations.[41] Stabilization of serum bicarbonate concentrations (>22 mEq/L) via alteration of the dialysate bicarbonate concentration or administration of oral bicarbonate salts is a prudent nutritional intervention in these patients (see Chaps. 47 and 55).

Trace Elements There are considerable data regarding trace element requirements in patients with stage 5 CKD.[19] Decreased zinc concentrations have been linked to taste disturbances and sexual dysfunction. Zinc supplementation, however, does not universally reverse these anomalies. Although serum concentrations of this trace element are decreased, total body stores of zinc in stage 5 CKD often are increased. This suggests a redistribution of zinc or increased need to maintain normal enzymatic function in stage 5 CKD patients.

Serum chromium concentrations are elevated in chronic HD and peritoneal dialysis patients, perhaps because the needles used during HD and the peritoneal and hemodialysate fluids are sources of chromium. Both HD and peritoneal dialysis patients have decreased selenium concentrations that can be increased with oral selenium supplements of 135 to 140 mcg/day in HD patients.[42] It appears that for patients undergoing HD, significant selenium losses occur during dialysis.[19]

Vitamins Vitamin status is better defined in CKD patients than those with ARF. CKD patients are prone to develop water-soluble vitamin deficiencies because of decreased dietary intake secondary to anorexia and restriction of many foods because of their protein, potassium, or phosphorus content. Additionally, in the stage 5 CKD patient, HD losses of ascorbic acid, folic acid, and pyridoxine are common. Plasma ascorbic acid concentrations are usually normal in PD patients. This decrease was recently associated with increased cardiovascular morbidity and mortality.[43] The highly protein-bound vitamins (A, D, and B_{12}) are not removed significantly by HD.[19] Vitamin D deficiency is correlated with decreased serum albumin concentrations, and supplementation of vitamin D has increased serum albumin concentrations significantly in deficient patients.[44] Vitamin A concentrations often are elevated in CKD and can lead to hypervitaminosis A and its cirrhosis-like syndrome. Conversely, vitamin E supplementation may have a distinct benefit to patients with stage 5 CKD. Increased oxidative stress in Stage 5 CKD patients may contribute to the accelerated atherosclerosis. Vitamin E in doses of 800 international units per day decreases low-density lipoprotein oxidation in patients with stage 5 CKD, especially in patients under-

TABLE 147-3 Routine Nutritional Monitoring in Patients with End-Stage Renal Disease

Parameter	Frequency
Predialysis serum albumin	Monthly
Percentage of usual postdialysis or postdrain body weight	Monthly
Subjective global assessment	Every 6 months
Protein equivalent of total nitrogen appearance (PNA)[a]	Monthly for HD, every 3–4 months for PD
Dietary interview and/or diary	Every 6 months
Predialysis prealbumin	As needed
Anthropometry	As needed
Dual-energy x-ray absorptiometry	As needed

BUN, blood urea nitrogen; PD, peritoneal dialysis; HD, hemodialysis.

[a]Beginning of week PNA = Co/[36.3 + (5.48) (spKt/V) + (53.5/spKt/V)] = 0.168, where Co is predialysis BUN and spKt/V, the single-pool index of hemodialysis adequacy = Ln(R – 0.08 × t) + [4 – (3.5 × R)] × UF/W (R is postdialysis:predialysis BUN ratio, t is dialysis session in hours, UF is ultrafiltration in liters, and W is postdialysis weight in kilograms). (See Chap. 48.)

Reprinted from AM J Kidney Sis, Vol. 35 (6 Suppl 2), K/DOQI, National Kidney Foundation, Clinical practice guidelines for nutrition in chronic renal failure, pages S1–S140, with permission from the National Kidney Foundation.

result of a significant decrease in erythropoietin requirements in the very-low-protein group.[51]

■ EVALUATION OF THERAPEUTIC OUTCOMES

The short- and long-term monitoring plan for the stage 5 CKD patient receiving PN or EN needs to be carefully tailored. Special attention should be paid to maintenance of fluid and electrolyte homeostasis. This can be achieved via frequent (daily) monitoring of serum electrolyte concentrations (e.g., sodium, potassium, phosphorus, magnesium, and calcium) and fluid balance. Serum glucose concentrations should be followed frequently (four times daily) in those who develop persistent hyperglycemia.

Because protein-energy malnutrition is a significant predictor of morbidity and mortality in stage 5 CKD patients, monitoring to ensure the effectiveness of the long-term nutritional plan becomes critical. Increased serum albumin concentrations are correlated with increased survival and thus monitoring of serum albumin concentrations is recommended for all HD and PD patients (Table 147–3).

HEPATIC FAILURE

The liver is the primary organ involved in the digestion, metabolism, and storage of nutrients. When functional capacity is depressed, profound nutrient intolerance (hyper- or hypoglycemia, hypertriglyceridemia, and hepatic encephalopathy) may result. Other sequelae that accompany the failing liver are fluid and electrolyte imbalances, vitamin deficiencies, and malnutrition. It is estimated that 65% to 90% of patients with advanced liver disease and almost 100% of patients awaiting liver transplantation have some degree of malnutrition, which increases morbidity and mortality. Nutritional support is an important component of the overall care of the patient with liver disease that may decrease complications and extend survival.[52]

EPIDEMIOLOGY

It is estimated that 30% of cirrhotic patients have protein-energy malnutrition, 40% have protein malnutrition, and 10% have energy malnutrition.[53] Changes in body composition such as decreases in body cell mass may be seen in early phases of the disease, and become more severe as cirrhosis progresses. In general, there is no significant difference in the incidence of malnutrition between those with cirrhosis caused by alcoholism and those with postviral cirrhosis. One study, however, found that abstinent patients with alcoholic cirrhosis had lower average measures of nutritional adequacy than those with cirrhosis caused by chronic hepatitis C.[54]

PATHOPHYSIOLOGY

Energy

A decrease in spontaneous oral intake is quite common in patients with cirrhosis and appears to be multifactorial in nature. Potential causes of decreased oral intake include altered taste, early satiety as a result of ascites and/or hyperleptinemia, impaired motility and bacterial overgrowth in the small intestine, malabsorption as a consequence of gastrointestinal dysfunction and treatment with neomycin or lactulose, nausea, and chronic encephalopathy.[24,52]

Resting energy requirements in stable cirrhotics can appear to be normal, but approximately one-third are hypometabolic and one-third are hypermetabolic when energy expenditure is corrected for alterations in lean body mass.[52] The Harris-Benedict equation for estimating caloric needs usually underestimates their needs by 15% to 20%.[55] The marked variability in energy expenditure underscores the need for patient-specific regimen design and monitoring, and may suggest the need for indirect calorimetry testing.[52] An initial energy provision of 35 to 40 kcal/kg per day is recommended by ESPEN for patients with alcoholic steatohepatitis and liver cirrhosis.[56]

Carbohydrate

❸ In healthy adults, approximately 60% of absorbed glucose is taken up by the liver and used for glycogen synthesis, triglyceride synthesis, and glycolysis. In general, glycogen synthesis and glycolysis are enhanced by insulin, whereas gluconeogenesis and glycogen breakdown are controlled by glucagon. Hyperglycemia is common in cirrhosis as a result of peripheral insulin resistance, which is mediated by a decreased binding to insulin receptors and defective postreceptor signal handling in peripheral tissues. Plasma concentrations of insulin are elevated with or without a glucose stimulus. This makes administration of large doses of glucose problematic because administration of insulin to control hyperglycemia may not improve its utilization substantially.

Patients with fulminant hepatitis are prone to hypoglycemia because hepatic glucose production is depressed secondary to decreased glycogen stores, diminished gluconeogenesis, and impaired degradation of insulin. A continuous intravenous infusion of 5% dextrose usually prevents hypoglycemia in acute hepatitis, but concentrations greater than 10% dextrose may be needed in more severe cases.

Fat

The liver is responsible for synthesis of cholesterol, high-density lipoproteins, and very-low-density lipoproteins. The enzymes lipoprotein lipase and lecithin-cholesterol acyltransferase are synthesized in the liver. Increased serum triglyceride and free fatty acid concentrations are thus encountered in patients with hepatic failure, primarily as a result of the increased lipolysis. The significant insulin resistance that can be seen in cirrhosis causes a shift to lipids as a primary fuel source.[52] Whereas only 35% of total calories are derived from fat in normal patients after an overnight fast, this can increase to 75% in patients with cirrhosis.[55] Incorporation of late-evening snacks in patients with liver cirrhosis may correct abnormal substrate metabolism, increase carbohydrate metabolism, and decrease fat oxidation rates.[57,58]

Patients with severe liver failure may be at increased risk for essential fatty acid deficiency; the ratio of nonessential to essential fatty acids was found to be increased in patients with acute and chronic liver failure. Poor oral intake of fat and dietary fat malabsorption in patients with cirrhosis both contribute to essential fatty acid deficiency.[59] The concentrations of linoleic acid can be increased with administration of an average of 33 g/day of IVLE supplementation.[60] Despite concerns of impaired clearance of long-chain triglycerides in IVLE as a consequence of impaired synthesis of apoprotein CII in cirrhotic patents, IVLE solutions have been given safely to patients with fulminant hepatic failure.[61]

Diarrhea and steatorrhea are common in patients with hepatic cholestasis because of intestinal malabsorption (partly as a result of mucosal edema from hypoalbuminemia), inadequate bile acid delivery to the duodenum, and pancreatic dysfunction with decreased secretion of lipase.[55] Because the micelle formation is impeded, the long-chain fatty acids pass through the colon, resulting in a foul-smelling, soapy diarrhea.

Protein

Nitrogen requirements for the patient with liver failure are similar to those of normal subjects, but intolerance to protein may limit the achievement of this goal. Thus some have advocated restriction of dietary protein intake. Recent research indicates, however, that protein restriction is not beneficial for patients with cirrhosis even in the midst of episodic hepatic encephalopathy.[62]

> **CLINICAL CONTROVERSY**
>
> The need for protein restriction in patients with hepatic encephalopathy has been questioned. While it has been a standard practice in the past, newer data has revealed that reducing protein intake to <1.2 g/kg/day in medically optimized patients with episodic encephalopathy may be unwarranted.

Because the liver metabolizes the aromatic amino acids (i.e., phenylalanine, tyrosine, and tryptophan), methionine, and glutamine, the plasma concentrations of these amino acids are elevated in cirrhotic patients. Plasma concentrations of the branched-chain amino acids (i.e., valine, leucine, and isoleucine) often are depressed because these amino acids are metabolized by skeletal muscle. This altered plasma aminogram most likely contributes to the development of hepatic encephalopathy.

Fluid and Electrolytes

Patients with severe cirrhosis often have ascites and peripheral edema. The excess of total body sodium in the presence of an even greater excess of total body water results in hyponatremia. Salt and fluid restrictions are required to avoid exacerbating this overhydrated state (see Chap. 52).

Hypokalemia is common in patients with liver failure who have normal renal function. Poor nutritional intake and vomiting may initiate this disorder. Severe vomiting may also lead to volume contraction metabolic alkalosis, with increased renal excretion of potassium (see Chap. 55). Secondary hyperaldosteronism, a common finding in liver failure patients with intravascular volume depletion, also increases renal excretion of potassium. Loop diuretic therapy causes increased renal excretion of potassium, whereas diarrhea from lactulose therapy increases fecal excretion of potassium. All these conditions can lead to profound hypokalemia. Therefore, potassium requirements in liver failure patients receiving specialized nutritional support may be substantially larger than those in otherwise healthy adults.

Poor nutritional intake secondary to alcohol abuse and increased excretion of magnesium secondary to diuretic therapy contribute to hypomagnesemia. Even in cirrhotic patients with normal serum magnesium concentrations, muscle magnesium is depleted and independently associated with hepatic encephalopathy.[63] During nutrition support, requirements for phosphorus are also substantially elevated because synthesis of body cell mass occurs, placing this population at risk for developing hypophosphatemia during refeeding.

Trace Elements

Many patients with liver failure have a malabsorption syndrome and chronic diarrhea. Chronic diarrhea causes zinc deficiency. Cytokines, such as tumor necrosis factor, interleukin-1, and interleukin-6, may stimulate metallothionein, an intestinal zinc-binding protein, thereby further inhibiting zinc absorption. Thus patients with chronic diarrhea should be suspected of having zinc deficiency; measurement of serum concentrations, however, are rarely used to confirm such deficiencies. Patients receiving a protein-restricted diet may be at additional risk because substantial amounts of zinc are found in red meat.

Because copper and manganese are excreted in the bile, it has been recommended that these two trace elements not be administered or be administered in reduced doses to patients with serious cholestasis. Direct measurements of manganese in the globus pallidus of cirrhotic patients who died in hepatic coma were two- to sevenfold higher than expected. These findings suggest that reduced quantities of manganese should be provided in the nutritional formulation to avoid exacerbating encephalopathy in the patient with chronic liver disease. There are no prospective evaluations, however, demonstrating benefits of low copper or manganese diets.

An association between alcoholism and low serum selenium concentrations has been reported. Because selenium is important in maintaining the enzyme glutathione peroxidase, a deficiency of this trace element has been implicated as a cause of hepatic injury in the alcoholic patient. However, because human serum contains at least three fractions of selenium, the use of serum selenium concentrations as a marker for selenium deficiency is controversial. At this time, maintaining a daily selenium intake of 40 mcg is the most appropriate approach in patients with chronic liver disease.

Vitamins

❹ Folic acid deficiency may lead to megaloblastic anemia, whereas thiamine deficiency may result in Wernicke's encephalopathy after rehydration with intravenous glucose. Depletion of hepatic stores of vitamin A, pyridoxine, folic acid, riboflavin, pantothenic acid, vitamin B_{12}, and thiamine have been reported in patients with hepatic failure. Poor intake and malabsorption are the principal causes of vitamin deficiencies in patients with chronic liver disease.

Because vitamin D is metabolized to 25-hydroxyvitamin D in the liver, low concentrations of this vitamin are seen in patients with biliary cirrhosis. Impaired absorption of dietary vitamin D as a consequence of decreased bile production may also contribute to these low serum concentrations and the resultant osteoporosis. The most appropriate approach at this time is to provide the daily recommended intake of these vitamins and consider additional supplementation when a deficiency is documented.

TREATMENT

Hepatic Failure

■ DESIRED OUTCOMES

The primary objective of nutrition support in patients with cirrhosis is the provision of the recommended amounts of energy and protein. Adequate nutrition support may slow disease progression, prevent morbidity, enhance the structure and function of the gastrointestinal tract, and decrease mortality.[52,56]

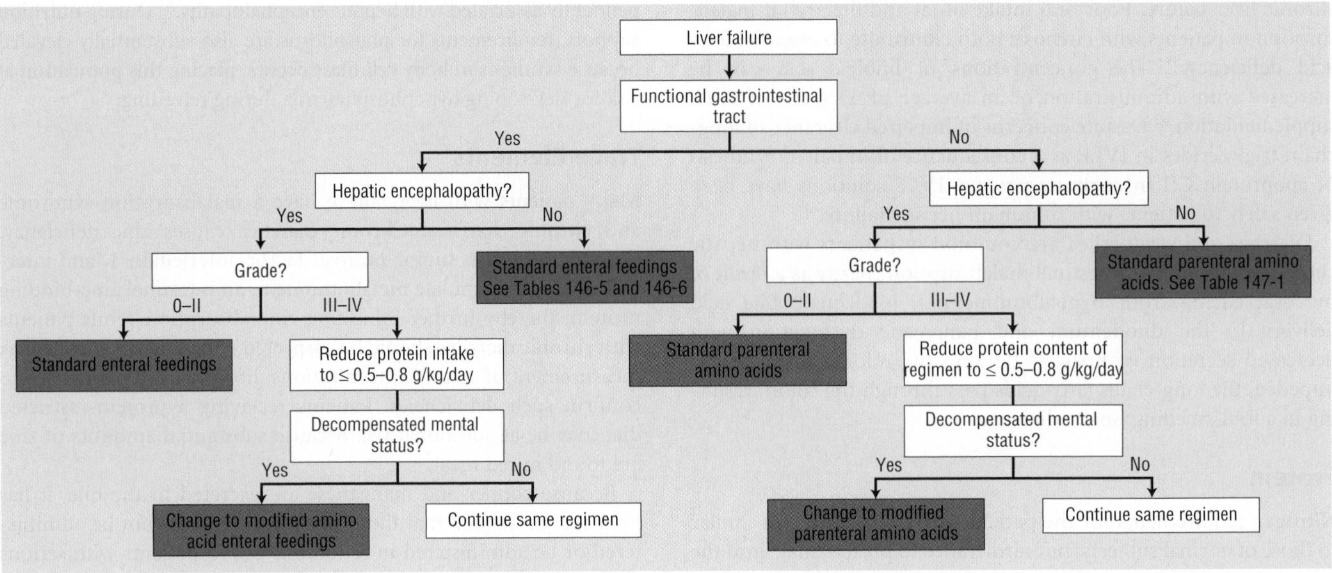

FIGURE 147-2. An algorithmic approach to nutritional support for the patient with hepatic failure.

■ GENERAL APPROACH TO TREATMENT

Enteral nutrition is preferred in patients with cirrhosis when the gastrointestinal tract is functional and accessible (Fig. 147–2). The recommendations in this figure are based on guidelines from ASPEN and ESPEN.[24,56] The indications for PN in the patient with liver failure are similar to those for general hospitalized patients. Because EN can contribute to hyperammonemia in cirrhotic patients with transjugular intrahepatic portosystemic shunts,[64] the use of PN in such patients might be preferable. In most cases, PN in the patient with liver failure can be accomplished via the administration of standard mixed amino acids (Fig. 147–2).

■ NONPHARMACOLOGIC THERAPIES

Dietary counseling makes patients aware of the risks that malnutrition poses for the progression of their disease and can provide strategies for patients to attain goal intakes, while being mindful of dietary restrictions. Many patients will have a higher likelihood of maintaining normal substrate utilization if they eat four or five small meals a day and a snack at bedtime. At least one study has found that intensive counseling is equivalent to providing oral nutritional supplements in increasing patient intake.[52] Cirrhotic patients may also derive up to a 26% increase in energy intake and a significant increase in lean body mass by receiving a transjugular intrahepatic portosystemic shunt.[65]

There is considerable interest in the use of vegetable-protein diets in the chronic management of patients with cirrhosis and hepatic encephalopathy. Enthusiasm for this therapy is based on the reduced amounts of aromatic amino acids and methionine in vegetable protein and a decrease in nitrogen absorption as the result of a decreased gastrointestinal transit time and an increase in fecal nitrogen excretion by colonic bacterial flora. However, compliance is more difficult to achieve with vegetable-based than animal-based protein diets. ASPEN recommends that a diet with vegetable-based protein be considered for those patients who do not tolerate at least 1 g/kg/day of protein from their normal diet.[24]

■ PHARMACOLOGIC THERAPIES

Drug Treatments of First Choice

In patients with liver disease who are unable to meet their nutritional needs despite dietary counseling, ESPEN guidelines recommend that EN be initiated with a goal of providing 35 to 40 kcal/kg/day and protein intake of 1.2 to 1.5 g/kg/day.[56] Indirect calorimetry quantification may be preferred to empiric estimates of caloric requirements in this setting. Excessive calorie provision actually may promote liver dysfunction and increased production of carbon dioxide with an associated increased work of breathing. Standard whole-protein formulas are recommended, but more concentrated formulations are appropriate to avoid excessive fluid overload in patients with ascites.[56]

When dextrose-based PN is started in those who cannot tolerate EN, additional thiamine may be needed to prevent Wernicke's encephalopathy. Standard mixed amino acids are appropriate for most patients. IVLE should be used in patients with liver failure only to prevent essential fatty acid deficiency when initial serum triglyceride concentrations exceed 300 mg/dL. If serum triglyceride concentrations are low or normal, IVLE may be used as a calorie source. Monitoring serum triglyceride concentration and free fatty acid oxidation (not available in all facilities) to ensure that lipid is both cleared and oxidized appropriately has been suggested. Oral medium-chain triglycerides have been used occasionally with success because they do not require pancreatic enzymes or micelle formation before absorption. However, these products do not provide essential fatty acids.

The electrolytes that warrant the most careful monitoring in liver disease include sodium, potassium, phosphorus, and magnesium. During fluid and salt restriction, patients (especially those receiving concurrent lactulose therapy for encephalopathy) should be observed for symptoms of volume depletion (e.g., increased pulse rate, decreased blood pressure, or dry mucous membranes). Magnesium concentrations as high as 24 mEq/L in the PN solution, which is two to three times the standard daily dose, may be required to maintain concentrations in the normal range.

Trace elements that warrant individual attention include zinc, copper, and manganese. For patients receiving PN, withholding copper from the solution until a copper serum concentration in the normal range is documented or the cholestasis resolves may be appropriate. Patients who have chronic cholestasis may require copper in reduced doses (e.g., 0.6 mg/day); however, they should have serum copper concentrations checked regularly (once per month in the acute care setting and every 6 months in the ambulatory setting). Manganese restriction also may be required in these patients. Table 147–4 lists the nutritional requirements of patients with liver failure secondary to cirrhosis and Table 147–1 presents an empiric PN formula for the patient with hepatic failure.[55,61]

TABLE 147-4 Nutrition Recommendations for Patients with Liver Disease

Patient Type	Calorie Energy (kcal/kg/day)	Protein (g/kg/day)	Comments
Compensated cirrhosis	25–35	1–1.2	Use a bedtime snack and frequent small meals
Decompensated cirrhosis[a]	25–35	0.5–1.5 for mild; 0.5 for severe	Use branched-chain amino acids for refractory cases of encephalopathy unresponsive to protein restriction
Decompenstated cirrhosis[a] with malnutrition	35–40	1.5	May have to temporarily decrease protein for encephalopathy worsening

[a]Decompensated cirrhosis: cirrhosis accompanied by significant ascites or encephalopathy.
Adapted from references 53 and 57.

Alternative Drug Treatments

The major controversy in nutritional support of the patient with liver failure has centered on the use of protein products. Modified amino acid solutions for PN (e.g., HepatAmine) are marketed for patients with liver failure and hepatic encephalopathy. They are enriched with branched-chain amino acids and have reduced amounts of aromatic amino acids and methionine. These products are formulated on the basis of the false neurotransmitter hypothesis, which postulates that hepatic encephalopathy may be a result of increased aromatic amino acid concentrations in the central nervous system.

NutriHep, a supplement for patients with hepatic encephalopathy, meets vitamin and mineral requirements, contains a high percentage of medium-chain triglycerides, and is supplemented with carnitine. Clinical trials using this and other branched-chain amino acid products have yielded promising outcomes, including decreases in morbidity and mortality. These results, however, have not been consistent. Enteral products with branched-chain amino acids also result in significant nonadherence because of poor taste.[52] This, coupled with the increased cost of these products, has led ASPEN and ESPEN to recommend reserving these products for patients with severe encephalopathy who decompensate on standard protein formulations despite continued lactulose-neomycin therapy.[24,56]

■ PHARMACOECONOMIC CONSIDERATIONS

Nutritional supplementation in patients with alcoholic cirrhosis reduces the frequency of hospitalizations.[66] Intuitively, this should be a cost-saving intervention, but without formal analysis the degree of benefit cannot be proven or quantified.

■ EVALUATION OF THERAPEUTIC OUTCOMES

Weight, albumin concentration, and prealbumin concentration are commonly used markers of nutrition status that may not be as reliable in patients with hepatic failure. Ascites, edema, and impaired hepatic protein synthesis make nutritional evaluation difficult in this patient population. Indeed, many of the commonly used markers of nutritional status correlate poorly with body cell mass in those with end-stage liver disease. Subjective global assessment, prognostic nutritional index, bioelectrical impedance, midarm muscle circumference, and handgrip strength have been tested as predictors of body cell mass.[52] Handgrip strength best correlates with malnutrition and is a better predictor of major complications in patients with cirrhosis.[67]

SHORT-BOWEL SYNDROME

Short-bowel syndrome (SBS) is generally a consequence of significant surgical resection of the small bowel that results in the malabsorption of nutrients and fluids. Morbidity and mortality caused by gastrointestinal failure in SBS patients has been improved with the provision of PN and EN. The goal of nutritional support with EN and PN is to maintain nutritional status, prevent or correct nutritional deficiencies, and enhance quality of life.[68]

EPIDEMIOLOGY

There are at least 10,000 patients who have SBS in the United States.[69] The most common etiologies in adults are surgical resections because of Crohn's disease, mesenteric vascular disease, and cancer. In infants, necrotizing enterocolitis, midgut volvulus, and intestinal atresia are the most common etiologies for resection leading to SBS.[69] SBS occurs more commonly in women than in men, most likely as a consequence of women having less small intestine length at baseline. This condition also may be functional as opposed to anatomic and occur in individuals who have not had resections, but who have a decreased small bowel absorptive capacity as a result of etiologies such as radiation enteritis or severe inflammatory bowel disease.[68] Symptoms of SBS generally include diarrhea, dehydration, electrolyte disturbances, and progressive malnutrition.[69]

PATHOPHYSIOLOGY

The average length of the small intestine, where the majority of nutrients are absorbed, in adults is 400 to 600 cm. The American Gastroenterological Association considers a patient to have SBS when the patient has 200 cm or less of functional small intestine.[70] Losing this absorptive capacity leads to deficiencies in multiple nutrients, requiring the initiation of interventional nutrition.

❺ PN must be used at least immediately following resection of the small intestine while the gastrointestinal tract is healing and adapting. Enteral nutrition may be used later during the transition to oral feedings, as the gastrointestinal tract is able to adapt with time, by increasing absorptive capacity, in approximately 50% of patients with SBS.[69] The length and type of nutritional support a patient may require is based on such factors as the length of remaining small intestine and the presence or absence of a functional colon. Adult patients have the highest likelihood of transitioning off of PN if the residual jejunum-ileum length is greater than 100 cm for individuals without a colon, or greater than 60 cm if a portion of the colon is in continuity with the remaining small intestine.[71] Factors that are predictive of a poor outcome include older age, disease in the residual bowel, and removal of the ileocecal valve, the physiologic sphincter that controls the rate of passage of intestinal contents from small to large bowel and prevents small bowel bacterial overgrowth.[72]

Intestinal Adaptation

The adaptation process of the residual small intestine to compensate for the loss of the resected area begins 24 to 48 hours after bowel resection and may continue to occur for 1 to 2 years.[73] Several factors act as stimuli for adaptation including enteral nutrients, pancreatic-biliary secretions, and intestinal hormones.[24] The ability of the remaining intestine to adjust after resection is also influenced by the area of bowel loss. The jejunum is the primary site for absorption of most nutrients, but if it is removed the ileum usually can accommodate and take on the structural characteristics and functional roles. Even with this compensation, patients with less than 50 to 60 cm of jejunum typically need indefinite PN. With ileal resection, the jejunum has a decreased capacity to adapt and perform the functions of the ileum.[73]

Energy Requirements

Caloric intake and energy needs of SBS patients are variable. Individuals who have lost more than 50% of their small intestine typically require 25 to 30 kcal per kg of ideal body weight, and when receiving enteral feedings, may need to ingest twice that number of calories to compensate for malabsorption.[70,74] This process is referred to as *adaptive hyperphagia*.[75] The average recommendation for patients with SBS who are receiving PN is also 25 to 30 kcal/kg of ideal body weight per day.[70]

Carbohydrate

Carbohydrate malabsorption plays a major role in diarrhea associated with SBS. Unabsorbed carbohydrates, especially simple carbohydrates, represent a substantial osmotic load in patients with SBS and are associated with an increased output. In patients with an intact colon, however, soluble fiber and complex carbohydrates are broken down by colonic bacteria to short-chain fatty acids, hydrogen, and methane. This fermentation causes flatulence; however, the colon is able to use the short-chain fatty acids as a source of energy. Thus, complex carbohydrates may provide a significant caloric source for patients with a massive resection and a preserved colon.[71]

Fat

Fat malabsorption also is common in SBS. The pathophysiology of this problem is complex and related to alterations in pancreatic enzyme secretion and bile salt absorption. The ileum is the major site of the latter process, and with its removal, bile salt malabsorption is common. Eventually, the total bile salt pool may be depleted, resulting in increased fat malabsorption and steatorrhea.[69] There has been much debate regarding the restriction of oral fats, which may decrease steatorrhea, number of stools, and stool weight in some patients. Fats have the highest number of kilocalories per gram, make the diet more palatable, and patients with SBS without a colon should not be restricted in the amount of fats they take in. For small-bowel patients with a healthy colon a diet higher in complex carbohydrates and lower in fat may result in lower stool volume and electrolyte loss, so this type diet may be more beneficial.[71] Medium-chain triglycerides have also been suggested for patients with SBS and an intact colon, as MCTs are better absorbed than long-chain triglycerides. MCTs may be especially useful in decreasing steatorrhea in patients with bile acid or pancreatic insufficiency. Care must be taken, however, because medium-chain triglycerides do not contain essential fatty acids.[69,71]

Protein

Protein is typically well tolerated as a caloric source in SBS patients. The optimal form for the delivery of protein to patients with SBS is the subject of much study and debate.[71] In the past, EN was often initiated with elemental formulas that contain free amino acids as the protein source because the efficiency of protein uptake was perceived to be better. However, total protein absorption is faster and more complete with dipeptide and tripeptide formulations. Absorption of free amino acids by the enteral route is a saturable process, whereas the absorption of small peptides is not. These more complex protein sources also may stimulate intestinal adaptation.[73] The American Gastroenterological Association now recommends that standard enteral formulas be used preferentially in SBS.[70]

Fluid, Electrolyte, and Acid–Base Disorders

❻ After substantial resections of the small bowel, the postoperative course is complicated by fluid and electrolyte imbalances that typically last 1 to 3 months.[73] Patients may have high-volume gastric fluid loss from nasogastric tubes and small intestine fluid loss from ostomies. Sodium content usually is elevated in these secretions, with concentrations reaching 80 to 100 mEq/L.[69] Acute gastric hypersecretion may occur after massive resection and contribute significantly to these deficits.[73] Secretory diarrhea (see Chap. 38) also results in fluid and electrolyte losses that may be difficult to quantify.

Patients with end jejunostomies or proximal ileostomies (surgically created openings into the jejunum and ileum, respectively, that divert the intestinal contents externally through a stoma) can have recurrent dehydration and electrolyte deficiencies. A high jejunostomy can produce fluid output of 3 to 4 L/day, with sodium loss of 90 mEq/L. To overcome the net secretion of sodium and water into the jejunum, the sodium content of fluids ingested by the patient needs to be approximately 90 mEq/L. In patients who have small intestine in continuity with the colon, the malabsorbed bile and fatty acids stimulate sodium and water excretion into the large bowel, but in general, these patients are at less risk for sodium and water depletion.[69]

Patients with a jejunostomy and individuals with long-term sodium depletion, magnesium deficiency, or excessive loss from diarrhea are at risk for hypokalemia.[68] Metabolic alkalosis, which may occur when a patient becomes dehydrated, accelerates the renal excretion of potassium, as all hydrogen ions are conserved in an attempt to correct the acid–base disorder. As bicarbonate ions are excreted renally, potassium is taken with them to maintain osmotic balance.

The unusually large amount of unabsorbed fatty acids within the remaining small intestine and colon of the patient with SBS will cause increased binding to calcium, resulting in a deficiency. This also may result in hyperoxaluria because dietary oxalate usually complexes with the intraluminal calcium and is excreted in the stool. As a result of decreased calcium available for binding, more oxalate is absorbed and available for renal excretion and thereby the risk of calcium oxalate renal stone formation is increased.[71] Vitamin D deficiency results in insufficient calcium absorption; thus SBS patients requiring long-term PN are at risk for metabolic bone disease. Magnesium deficiency is common in SBS patients with large ostomy or diarrheal losses. This deficiency should be corrected aggressively because of the correlation between low magnesium and potassium concentrations with the development of calcium oxalate stones. Serum concentrations are commonly monitored, but urinary magnesium concentrations may decrease earlier with deficiency, and may be a better estimate of total body stores than serum levels. Oral supplementation may be difficult because it can contribute to increased diarrhea or ostomy output. However, repletion is necessary to prevent complications and to effectively correct potassium deficits.[68]

SBS patients can lose substantial amounts of chloride (60 to 140 mEq/L) in addition to sodium from ostomy output. These individuals have a high risk of developing hypochloremic metabolic alkalosis. Patients who have SBS complicated by a pancreatic fistula and severe diarrhea lose considerable potassium and bicarbonate and may develop metabolic acidosis. Patients with severe diarrhea who have an intact colon will conserve sodium and chloride, resulting in considerable loss of potassium and bicarbonate and the development of metabolic acidosis. Quantifying fluid losses with particular attention to the sources of loss will aid in the acid–base management of these patients (see Chap. 55).

Lactic acidosis can occur in patients with SBS who have an intact colon and may result in symptoms of ataxia and delirium.[73] D-Lactic acid is produced by the fermentation of malabsorbed carbohydrates by colonic bacteria, and increased concentrations are associated with small bowel bacterial overgrowth. The diagnosis of D-lactic acidosis should be considered in patients with a functional colon who have an unexplained metabolic acidosis and an elevated anion gap.[73]

Trace Elements

Patients with SBS are particularly prone to zinc deficiency as a result of excessive losses from stool, ostomy outputs, and fistula drainage.

Although serum zinc concentrations are not always reflective of body zinc status, a low serum zinc concentration requires an adjustment in the replacement amount.[69] Significant bowel resection, GI losses, and impaired intestinal absorption also contribute to imbalances of other trace elements, such as copper, selenium, and manganese. Because trace element deficiencies are common, the need for supplementation of these micronutrients is essential for SBS patients, including those receiving PN, EN, or an adequate diet.[73]

Vitamins

❼ Patients with ileal resection commonly develop vitamin B_{12} deficiency, necessitating therapy with parenteral or intranasal cyanocobalamin. Most other water-soluble vitamins are absorbed in the proximal jejunum, and deficits of these vitamins are less common. There are reports, however, of SBS patients with symptomatic thiamine, folate, and biotin deficiencies.[69] Small bowel bacterial overgrowth can contribute to diminished vitamin B_{12} because bacteria may metabolize the nutrient within the intestine, decreasing its availability for absorption. SBS patients with fat malabsorption can acquire deficiencies in vitamins A, D, E, and K.[69]

TREATMENT

Short-Bowel Syndrome

DESIRED OUTCOMES

The desired outcomes of the nutritional management of patients with SBS are to provide effective energy, protein, micronutrients, and fluids in amounts adequate to maintain patient health and normal growth, avoid complications of SBS or the nutrition support regimen, and to optimize quality-of-life.[68] Finally, one wants to maximize the use of the gastrointestinal tract for nutrient provision to maintain gastrointestinal tract function.

GENERAL APPROACH TO TREATMENT

After intestinal resection, the clinical course and nutritional management of SBS patients may be described in three stages, or phases (Fig. 147–3). This algorithm is based on recommendations from the American Gastroenterological Association and a recent consensus conference on the management of patients with SBS.[70,72] The first stage, or acute phase, occurs during the initial postoperative period. This phase lasts at least 1 week, and may continue from 3 weeks to 3 months. It is complicated by major fluid and electrolyte losses (up to 5 L/day). The parenteral route should be used to supply nutritional needs.

❽ The second stage lasts from a few months to longer than a year, and institution of enteral or oral intake early during this stage is important because intraluminal nutrients are essential stimuli for intestinal adaptation. The amount of enteral/oral nutrition can be advanced as the patient tolerates; concomitantly, the duration and or rate of PN may be decreased. In the third and final stage, adaptation is maximized and many patients can be maintained with full enteral or oral nutrition. However, PN may not be required on a daily basis. If a PN regimen is to be reduced or discontinued, it should be done slowly; initially 1 to 2 nights of PN may be eliminated each week. Eventually, some patients may be able to tolerate administration on an every-other-night or every-third-night basis.[72,73] During the different phases of management, PN is administered through a peripherally inserted central catheter or surgically placed indwelling central venous catheter (see Chap. 145).

NONPHARMACOLOGIC THERAPY

Initially surgical management focuses on preventing GI resections and then preserving as much gastrointestinal tract as possible. Intestinal

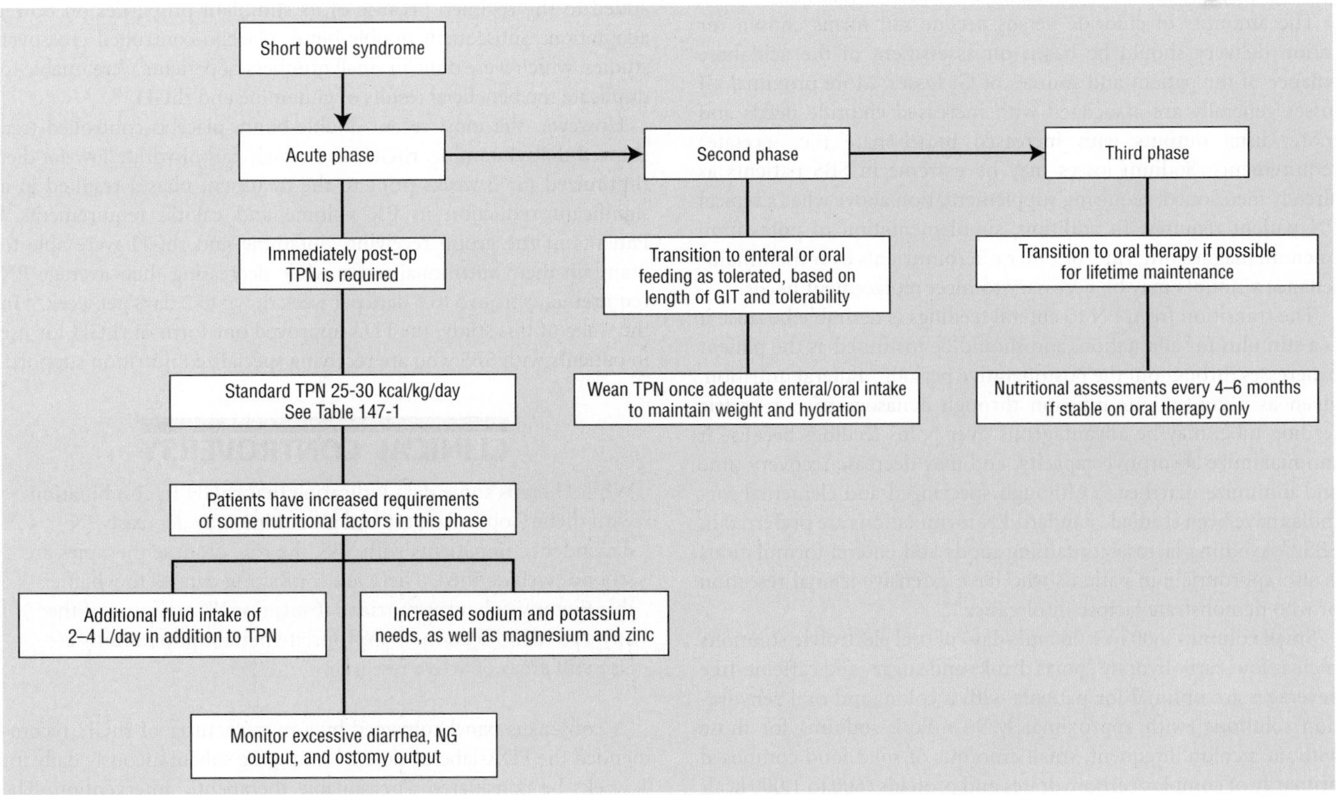

FIGURE 147-3. An algorithmic approach to nutritional support for the patient with short-bowel syndrome. (GIT, gastrointestinal tract; NG, nasogastric; TPN, total parenteral nutrition.)

transplantation is a surgical treatment option for patients with SBS, and approximately 1,200 such procedures have been performed.[68] With refinement of patient selection and surgical techniques, the 1-year survival rate after small-bowel transplantation is similar to that of those receiving home PN. Five-year survival, however, is still poorer than that reported in patients receiving home PN.[76] After transplantation, the majority of survivors are able to completely discontinue PN.[68] Consideration for small-bowel transplantation is currently reserved for those patients with SBS who fail therapy with PN because of recurrent line sepsis, loss of vascular access, PN-induced liver failure, or frequent severe dehydration.[70] As patient selection and immunosuppressive regimens continue to evolve, the indications for surgical treatment of SBS will likely expand.

■ PHARMACOLOGIC THERAPY

Drug Treatments of First Choice

The early phase of SBS is associated with large day-to-day variations in fluid and electrolyte losses. Strict output records should be assessed, as well as all intake, including intravenous medications. Initially, it is recommended to start a standard PN solution that meets the patient's maintenance metabolic, fluid, and electrolyte needs, and a separate intravenous replacement solution is typically necessary to keep the patient euvolemic based on actual fluid losses. Insensible losses should be estimated between 300 and 800 mL/day above measured output, and daily urine output should be kept at least 0.5 mL/kg/h. As fluid and electrolyte losses stabilize over time, it becomes possible to incorporate these replacement requirements into the PN solution. The American Gastroenterological Association recommends that the PN solution typically be composed of standard crystalline amino acids, glucose, and intravenous lipids. Energy provision of 25 to 30 kcal/kg ideal body weight per day is recommended, and may be administered as 1.0 to 1.5 g/kg of protein per day, approximately 20% to 30% of calories from intravenous lipids, and the remainder of calories from carbohydrates.[70] Table 147–1 gives an example of a PN formula for the patient with SBS.

The amounts of chloride versus acetate salt forms chosen for cation delivery should be based on assessment of the acid–base balance of the patient and sources of GI losses. More proximal GI losses generally are associated with increased chloride needs and more distal outputs with increased bicarbonate (i.e., acetate) requirements. Sodium losses may be extreme in SBS patients as already mentioned, requiring supplementation above what a typical PN patient requires. In addition, supplementation of potassium, calcium, magnesium, zinc, or other micronutrients over their maintenance amounts may be necessary to meet replacement needs.[73]

The transition from PN to enteral feedings is desirable because it is a stimulus for adaptation, and should be instituted as the patient progresses throughout the postoperative period.[69] Enteral nutrition, given as a continuous infusion through a nasogastric or gastric feeding tube, may be advantageous over bolus feedings because it can maximize absorptive capacity, and may decrease recovery time and minimize diarrhea.[73] Although specialized and elemental formulas have been studied, standard EN formulations are preferred in SBS.[70] Avoiding lactose-containing foods and enteral formulations is also appropriate in patients who have extensive jejunal resection or who demonstrate lactose intolerance.[69]

Small volumes (600 to 1,000 mL/day) of oral electrolyte solutions such as low-carbohydrate sports drinks and sugar- and caffeine-free beverages are optimal for patients with a colon, and oral rehydration solutions (with approximately 90 mEq/L sodium) for those without a colon. Frequent, small amounts of solid food composed primarily of complex carbohydrates and proteins (600 to 1,000 kcal/day) have been recommended, with avoidance of concentrated sweets and dairy products.[71] When a patient is able to maintain hydration and weight via EN and/or eating, PN may be tapered.[72] Many factors must be considered once a patient begins to transition off interventional nutrition when determining the content of a long-term oral diet for an SBS patient. Factors such as the site and length of remaining intestine, tolerance, and patient acceptance must be considered. Fat generally is not restricted in patients without a colon. However, patients with a colon may experience more diarrhea with a high-fat diet and may benefit from oral intake that has more calories from carbohydrates and less fat content.[71] The oral diet for patients with remaining functional colon also must account for oxalate content, and patients should avoid foods with high amounts of oxalate (e.g., spinach, parsley, rhubarb, cocoa, and tea) to decrease formation of calcium oxalate renal stones.[71] Finally, oral diets in SBS patients often need to be supplemented to maintain electrolyte, mineral, vitamin, and trace element balance.

The delivery of medications to patients with SBS may present many challenges, not the least of which is the questionable absorption of oral therapies. Oral products that contain sorbitol or mannitol should be avoided to minimize medication-related diarrhea. Loperamide and octreotide may be used to control diarrhea (see Chap. 38), and proton pump inhibitors and H_2-receptor antagonists are frequently required to reduce gastric hypersecretion (see Chap. 35). Because of erratic absorption, the dose of oral or enteral medications may need to be greater than recommended for patients with an intact gastrointestinal tract.

Alternative Drug Treatments

The use of specialized nutrients and growth factors to enhance small-bowel adaptation is a focus of intensive research. The amino acid glutamine is a fuel for intestinal cells, and may be necessary for maintaining intestinal structure in normal and physiologically stressed states. Initial uncontrolled research findings suggested that those who received glutamine in combination with rhGH and a high-carbohydrate/low-fat diet, may have a reduced PN dependence and increased nutrient absorption.[77] Recombinant growth hormone was added to the regimen because of its stimulant properties on bowel adaptation. Subsequent double-blind, placebo-controlled crossover studies, which were done in small numbers of patients were unable to duplicate the beneficial results of glutamine and rhGH.[78]

However, the most recent double-blind, placebo-controlled trial showed that glutamine, rhGH, and a high-carbohydrate/low-fat diet (optimized for 2 weeks prior to the treatment phase) resulted in a significant reduction in PN volume and caloric requirements.[74] Patients in the group receiving glutamine and rhGH were able to maintain their nutritional status while decreasing their average PN requirements from 5 to 6 days per week down to 2 days per week.[74] In the wake of this study, the FDA approved one form of rhGH for use in patients with SBS who are receiving specialized nutrition support.

CLINICAL CONTROVERSY

While there is some data indicating that rhGH in combination with dietary optimization and glutamine may decrease PN dependence in patients with SBS, the role of these therapies are still not well defined. There are conflicting data as to whether this therapy enhances nutrient absorption. The timing of therapy and identification of appropriate patient populations are also still areas of active research.

A consensus panel convened by a manufacturer of rhGH recommended the FDA-labeled dose of 0.1 mg/kg subcutaneously daily for 4 weeks be considered a reasonable therapeutic intervention. The panel suggested that appropriate patients are PN-dependent patients who are nutritionally stable and on an optimized diet and medication regimen, and that treatment be given 6 to 24 months after bowel resection.[78] This treatment, however, is not recommended by the American Gastroenterological Association.[70] Other experts question the benefit of rhGH and suggested that before incorporating it into SBS treatment, it should be studied during the adaptive phase of SBS.[69] The safety of prolonged use of rhGH is also unknown.

■ PHARMACOECONOMIC CONSIDERATIONS

Nutritional management of SBS is quite costly, especially in patients who require home PN. One year of home PN therapy is estimated to cost approximately $100,000.[76] This figure does not include home nursing, equipment, and the costs of intermittent hospitalizations. Significant savings may be realized in patients who are able to transition from PN, but this is unlikely to occur in patients who are still PN dependent after 2 years. No analyses have yet been published that describe the economic consequences of the potential PN-reducing effect of rhGH.[78] It has been reported that intestinal transplantation is a cost-effective intervention relative to the cost of home parenteral nutrition in patients who survive for 2 years postoperatively.[79]

■ EVALUATION OF THERAPEUTIC OUTCOMES

Therapeutic monitoring of SBS patients who are receiving PN for metabolic complications should follow the guidelines outlined in Chap. 145. This patient population differs in that serum electrolytes should be obtained daily until the patient has stabilized postoperatively. Special consideration should also be given to the fluid status of SBS patients, especially in the period immediately following surgery, when fluid losses are extreme. Monitoring of stool output is such a large factor that it must be taken into consideration for all SBS patients. Because many patients with SBS remain on PN for extended periods of time, clinicians must be careful to monitor for elevations in liver enzymes, and cycling PN for 12 to 14 hours daily should be considered in those patients to minimize these complications. Obtaining a serum fatty acid profile may be judicious in those patients on long-term PN without oral intake to ensure they do not have essential fatty acid deficiency.[80]

The most comprehensive and thorough analysis of the clinical outcomes of patients receiving home PN or EN comes from Medicare and the North American Home Parenteral and Enteral Patient Registry.[81] It was estimated that 40,000 and 152,000 patients in the United States were receiving home PN and EN support, respectively. Patients with GI failure, which included those with Crohn's disease, ischemic bowel disease, motility disorders, and congenital bowel defects, had relatively good clinical outcomes, especially when compared with the groups with cancer or acquired immune deficiency syndrome. The patients with GI failure had an 87% annual survival rate and a 50% to 75% likelihood of complete rehabilitation. Sepsis, metabolic disorders, and mechanical problems with catheters resulted in one to two hospitalizations per year for all patients.[81]

■ QUALITY-OF-LIFE ISSUES

Initially those patients on extended PN therapy have a significant gain in QOL when transitioning from the hospital to their home setting. This is often followed by the reality of restrictions in daily living, dehydration and malnutrition despite PN, and complications such as sepsis and liver dysfunction. Patients with SBS on home PN have reported that their QOL is significantly reduced in comparison to those with anatomic or functional SBS not on home PN.[78] There are currently no data assessing the effect of treatment with growth factors such as rhGH on QOL, although one might expect to see an improvement. Valid comparisons of home PN and intestinal transplantation are not available, as a consequence of the limited indications for transplantation.[79] Preparing patients and their caregivers for the possible stresses associated with this therapy (e.g., financial challenges, fatigue, depression, complications, and social or emotional problems) through education and referral to support groups, such as the Oley Foundation, may help to increase QOL.[82]

PULMONARY FAILURE

Nutrition support is an important aspect of preventing and treating both acute and chronic pulmonary failure. Malnourished patients are at increased risk of acute respiratory distress syndrome (ARDS), and malnutrition in patients with chronic obstructive pulmonary disease (COPD) is well documented. There is also a correlation between the outcomes of patients with alterations in nutritional status and concurrent pulmonary diseases.[83] Loss of lean muscle mass is detrimental because the depletion of diaphragm and intercostal muscles make the effort of breathing harder, and progression of weight loss leads to muscle fatigue and respiratory failure. The ventilatory drive, as well as compensation to hypoxia, is depressed in COPD patients who are malnourished, and nutritional support plays a key role in optimizing respiratory muscle function in patients with pulmonary disease.[84]

EPIDEMIOLOGY

More than 10% of the U.S. population older than 45 years of age suffers from COPD, resulting in significant cost to the healthcare system.[84] Weight loss and protein-calorie malnutrition may occur in up to one-half of those patients suffering from COPD, and weight loss often coincides with disease progression.[24,84] In those patients suffering from acute respiratory failure, nutritional abnormalities have been reported in up to 70%.[83] Engelen et al. studied body composition in patients with COPD, specifically emphysema and chronic bronchitis. They found a higher incidence of lean mass depletion in patients with emphysema than in those with chronic bronchitis. Body weight and body mass index were also lower in the group with emphysema.[85] In a further evaluation of these patients, the same investigators reported that skeletal muscle weakness was associated with wasting of extremity fat-free mass that was independent of COPD subtype.[86] Malnutrition is associated with an increased mortality rate in COPD patients with decreasing body mass index.[87]

PATHOPHYSIOLOGY

Energy Requirements

❾ Patients with COPD have highly variable REE, and commonly used predictive measures may underestimate their energy needs.[88] Those who are losing weight tend to have significantly higher REE adjusted for fat-free mass compared with weight-stable patients. Total daily energy expenditure also was found to be elevated in clinically stable COPD patients with both normal and increased REE. The cause of elevated total daily energy expenditure despite a normal REE is still unknown, although the oxygen cost of breathing, acute or chronic systemic inflammation, and medications may contribute.[83] Although the optimal approach to energy needs in COPD has not been identified, it is evident that there is no advantage to providing $1.7 \times$ REE compared to $1.3 \times$ REE.[89] Hypermetabolism likely contributes to the decreased body weight and fat-free mass, although it has been shown that in this patient population intake may be suboptimal. During meals hypoxic patients tend to experience decreases in oxygen saturation and increased dyspnea. Gastric filling may also be impaired because of diaphragmatic expansion and a false feeling of fullness.[83] These problems, combined with increased daily requirements, may result in the negative energy balance seen in many COPD patients. Several specialized equations have been developed to estimate energy requirements in this patient population, and indirect calorimetry may be used, but clinical benefit is questionable. Patients with acute respiratory failure also may have alterations in energy expenditure, but the situation is similar in that predictive formulas for energy needs exist, and indirect calorimetry may be used. Providing excess calories to the acutely ill patient in respiratory failure should be avoided because this may increase carbon dioxide production and the associated work of breathing.[24,84]

Carbohydrate

Malnutrition in patients with pulmonary disease has been consistently identified in the literature, and nutrition support should be considered as part of the overall treatment plan. However, increasing nutritional intake can be complicated because it may elevate the respiratory quotient, which may lead to a corresponding increase in work of breathing and resulting hypercapnia. The respiratory quotient is the ratio of the amount of CO_2 produced divided by the amount of O_2 consumed. When a subject is overfed, the amount of CO_2 produced markedly exceeds the amount of O_2 consumed, which can result in increased ventilatory demand.[90] Ventilatory drive may be improved in some patients with moderate infusions of carbohydrates; however, administration of glucose formulas at a rate greater than 5 mg/kg per minute has been shown to increase production of CO_2, and is associated with the inability to wean from mechanical ventilation.[84]

Fat

Fats have the lowest respiratory quotient, but administration of intravenous fat emulsions to mechanically ventilated patients has the potential to adversely affect pulmonary gas exchange in some clinical conditions.[91]

CLINICAL CONTROVERSY

There are conflicting data on the safety of administration of lipid emulsions to patients with ARDS. Discrepancies in trial data may be due to the use of differing lipid infusion rates and duration, as well as pre-existing lung function.

The administration of lipid emulsions to patients with ARDS may possibly decrease oxygenation. A recent trial assessing both long-chain triglyceride and combination long-chain triglyceride/medium-chain triglyceride administration showed that there was no deleterious effect on oxygenation. Discrepancies in trial data may be a result of differing lipid infusion rates and duration, and preexisting lung status.[92] Rapid administration of intravenous lipids should be avoided; a rate of 3 mg/kg per minute increases pulmonary vascular resistance in patients with ARDS.[92] A review of nutritional intervention in ambulatory COPD patients revealed that diets high in fat placed a lower demand on the respiratory system in comparison to diets with a higher carbohydrate content. In addition to an improvement in forced expiratory volume, the number of breaths needed per minute decreased within 3 weeks in COPD patients who switched to a high-fat/low-carbohydrate diet.[90] Although these effects are important, the most critical element in managing patients with pulmonary compromise is to avoid overfeeding.[24]

Protein

Undernourished patients demonstrate a blunted response to hypercapnia that improves after as little as 1 week of adequate nutritional support. This response is thought to result from protein administration, as evidenced by decreased partial CO_2 pressure, increased minute ventilation, and improved breathing patterns after the start of PN. Protein administration also may influence ventilatory demand by increasing ventilatory response to hypoxia and hypercapnia. This stimulation may be altered by the amino acid composition of the protein source, with increased amounts of branched-chain amino acids having a greater effect compared with standard amino acids. Although this protein effect is potentially beneficial in some patients, excessive protein administration could theoretically lead to increased work of breathing and fatigue.[84]

Fluid, Electrolyte, and Acid–Base Disorders

⑩ In patients with ARDS or pulmonary edema, excessive fluid intake should be avoided, and fluid accumulation is associated with a poor outcome. Patients in the ICU often receive substantial fluid loads from medication administration, and when possible it is important to limit intake by concentrating these sources.[24,84]

Alteration of micronutrient requirements in respiratory failure is commonly focused on phosphorus replacement. Phosphorus has an essential role in the synthesis of adenosine triphosphate and 2,3-diphosphoglycerate (2,3-DPG). Inadequate stores of adenosine triphosphate can lead to respiratory muscle weakness, and normal contractility of the diaphragm muscles is dependent on phosphate.[84] Finally, a significant percentage of critically ill patients experience hypophosphatemia from refeeding. Most patients with moderate to severe hypophosphatemia and respiratory failure should be treated with intravenous sodium or potassium phosphate (see Chap. 53). Correction of hypophosphatemia in ICU patients receiving nutritional support with a graduated weight-based dosing scheme of phosphorus replacement has been reported.[93]

Ventilator-dependent patients and those with stable COPD often have respiratory acidosis. A balanced mixture of chloride and acetate salts often is appropriate in these patients. The acid–base status of the ICU patient with pulmonary compromise should be monitored daily, whereas every 2 to 3 days may be adequate for the stable hospitalized COPD patient.

Vitamins and Trace Elements

Patients with pulmonary disease usually do not have significant alterations in vitamin and trace element requirements, and they can receive standard doses of these micronutrients. There are some data that support the additional supplementation of antioxidants vitamin C, vitamin E, and β-carotene because of a correlation with moderately improved pulmonary function. COPD patients may have an increased burden of oxidants from cigarette smoke or release of oxygen free radicals from inflammatory leukocytes in the lungs, and deficiencies of antioxidants may contribute to oxidant/antioxidant imbalances in these individuals.[94]

TREATMENT

Pulmonary Failure

■ DESIRED OUTCOMES

In patients with pulmonary failure, nutritional support should be given to meet energy and protein requirements and to limit wasting of respiratory muscles. In stable COPD patients, this may be done in addition to exercise rehabilitation programs to optimize weight and fat-free body mass. To date, nutrition support has not been shown to affect long-term survival in these patients.[95]

■ GENERAL APPROACH TO TREATMENT

When oral feedings are inadequate, ASPEN recommends that the enteral route be used in those who have a functional gut and can meet their needs through this route.[24] In acute respiratory failure, PN is often recommended when the GI tract is not usable, or as a supplement to EN if sufficient energy intake is otherwise not possible.[24,84]

Most general EN formulas contain an equal balance of nonprotein energy between carbohydrate and fat. Elemental or chemically defined products are the exception because they are intended to be high-carbohydrate, low-fat formulas to enhance absorption and digestion. In pulmonary patients administration of a high-carbohydrate formula may result in a significant increase in minute ventilation, heat production, and CO_2 production when compared with a high-fat formula. Because most general formulas contain balanced nonprotein calories, moderate doses of these products may be appropriate in most patients with pulmonary disease.[87] Patients who are fluid restricted should be given a higher energy formulation so as to maintain an appropriate fluid balance.[24]

■ NONPHARMACOLOGIC THERAPY

Patient education and nutritional counseling are essential to maximizing the health of patients with COPD. Education about appropriate energy and caloric intake and the proper use of oral nutritional supplements may enhance patient adherence to these practices. Ambulatory COPD patients may also benefit from a pulmonary rehabilitation program that integrates, diet, supplements, and exercise.[87]

■ PHARMACOLOGIC THERAPY

Drug Treatment of First Choice

Moderate doses of carbohydrate, fat, and protein given enterally are appropriate in most conditions. Total calorie provision 30% above basal energy expenditure does not have any untoward effects on pulmonary status. However, patients who are overfed, i.e. those who are receiving twice the basal energy expenditure, often produce excessive CO_2. Critically ill patients with respiratory failure can be fed 25 to 30 kcal/kg/day as they recover.[24,96] In patients with borderline ventilatory status the nutritional regimen should be monitored closely to prevent excessive CO_2 production, and increasing the proportion of nonprotein calories as fat relative to the amount of carbohydrates may be beneficial.[84] In general, patients with ARDS who need PN may receive nonprotein calories administered within the following ranges: 60% to 70% carbohydrate and 30% to 40% lipid. A reasonable protein dose is 1 to 1.5 g/kg per day for the patient with stable COPD. Patients who are mechanically ventilated with superimposed illness may require higher doses of protein (1.5 to 2.5 g/kg per day). Figure 147–4 illustrates an approach to the patient with acute respiratory failure requiring PN or EN support based on recommendations from ASPEN and ESPEN.[24,96] Table 147–1 includes an empirical PN formula for the patient with respiratory failure.

Alternative Drug Therapies

Enteral formulas (e.g., Pulmocare, NutriVent, and Respalor) marketed for use specifically in patients with pulmonary disease are commercially available. These products contain a higher percentage of nonprotein calories as fat (>50%). Several studies evaluated the use of these high-fat/low-carbohydrate products in patients with COPD and acute respiratory failure, and generally the outcomes were favorable.[90] These specialized pulmonary EN products are calorically dense (1.5 kcal/mL), which may be helpful for patients with severe ARDS or pulmonary edema, as well as others who may require fluid restriction. There are no data, however, indicating that these formulas result in improved clinical outcomes in patients with pulmonary failure. Nonspecialty formulations, and high concentration formulations for those requiring fluid restriction, are still preferred for routine use.[24,87]

An additional concentrated formula (Oxepa) has been marketed specifically for critically ill patients on mechanical ventilation, and studied in patients with acute lung injury and ARDS. The macronutrient composition of Oxepa is similar to that of the other specialized pulmonary enteral formulas, with 55% of the nonprotein caloric content being from fat. However, the lipid blend in the formula was altered with the goal being to decrease the production of proinflammatory cytokines by including eicosapentaenoic acid from fish oil and

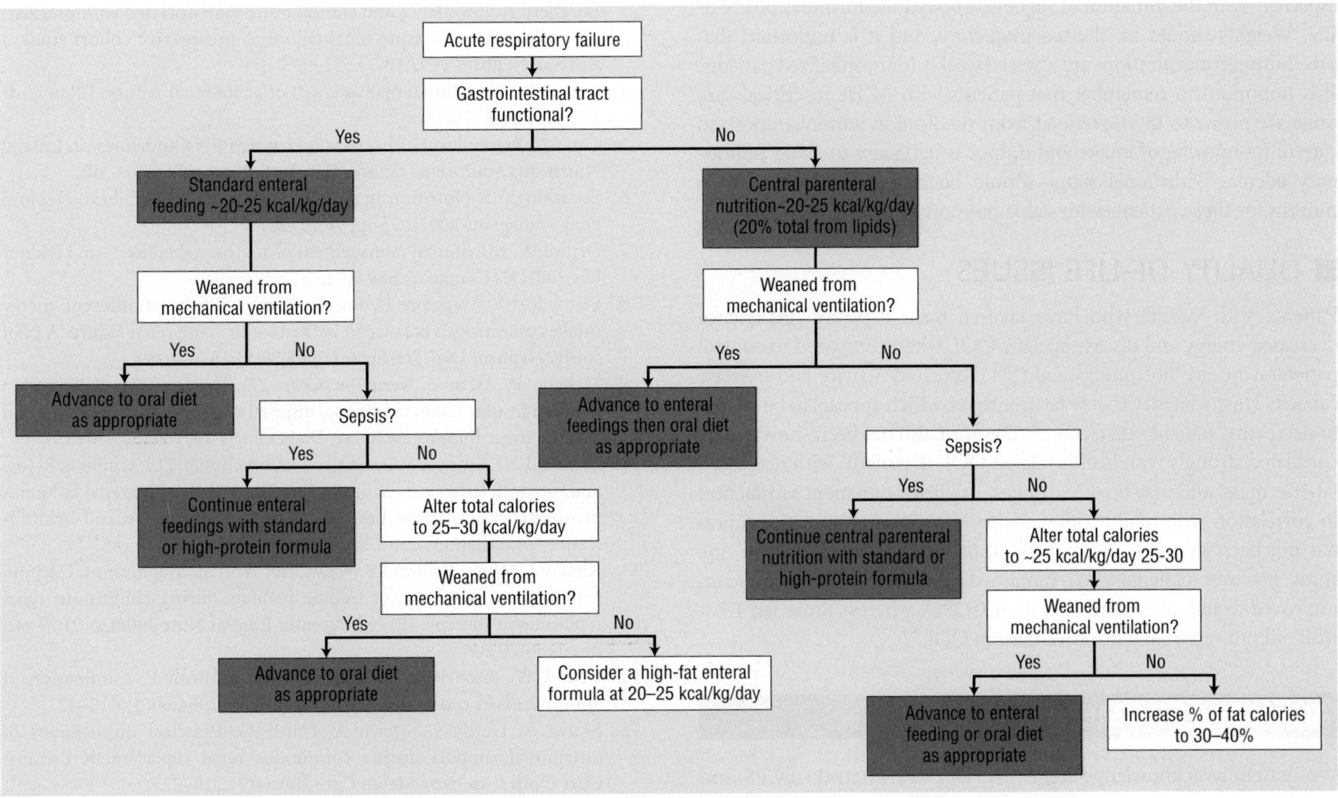

FIGURE 147-4. An algorithmic approach to nutritional support for the patient with acute respiratory failure.

γ-linolenic acid from borage oil. Nutrients with antioxidant properties (i.e., vitamin C, vitamin E, and β-carotene) also are supplemented in the product.[97,98] This formulation is associated with improved respiratory mechanics, decreased ventilatory dependence, and an attenuation of the inflammatory state in acute lung injury/ARDS. Although ASPEN and ESPEN recommend the use of this product, it has not yet been shown to improve survival in critically ill patients.[24,96]

rhGH is known to induce general muscle growth, lipolysis, and protein anabolism. When used as adjunctive therapy to EN support, COPD patients have shown improvements in lean body mass, maximal inspiratory pressure, and exercise capacity. The benefit of rhGH is debatable, with trials having differing results, but body mass and fat-free mass typically increase in patients after use of this product. The benefit in pulmonary patients as shown by improvements in respiratory muscle function and pulmonary function testing is questionable. The effects of anabolic steroids also have been evaluated for use in COPD as an adjunct to nutritional intervention. Patients on anabolic steroids tend to have larger increases in fat-free mass and more favorable distributions in weight gain in comparison to interventional nutrition alone.[99] More studies are needed to characterize the benefits of rhGH, as well as anabolic steroids, and to determine the risk to benefit ratio.

PHARMACOECONOMIC CONSIDERATIONS

There is no data available that establishes the pharmacoeconomic value of nutrition support in patients with respiratory failure.

EVALUATION OF THERAPEUTIC OUTCOMES

Because pulmonary patients are at extreme risk of malnutrition, monitoring the progression of the patient on interventional nutrition is extremely important. Therapeutic monitoring of pulmonary patients on PN for metabolic complications should follow the guidelines presented in Chap. 145. Patients on EN should be monitored as described in Chap. 146. Pulmonary status must be assessed for any changes, especially with the initiation of higher carbohydrate formulas of PN or EN. Weights should be charted frequently, and it is important that prealbumin concentrations are assessed weekly for hospitalized patients. It is important to remember that patients with ARDS in critical care units are prone to fluid overload from medication administration, so careful monitoring of intake and output is necessary to avoid pulmonary edema. Nutritional status should be monitored every 4 to 6 months for those patients with stable pulmonary disease and COPD.

QUALITY-OF-LIFE ISSUES

Patients with COPD who have fat-free mass depletion experience decreased energy and disease-specific QOL when compared to control patients who are not underweight.[100] Decreased activity and exercise capacity is associated with low fat-free mass, which appears to be related to decreasing patient satisfaction.[83] Dyspnea also has been shown to be correlated strongly with health-related QOL in patients with decreased fat-free mass, and may be the strongest predictor of patient satisfaction in correlation with malnutrition. Nutrition support supplementation has not been shown to definitively improve QOL in COPD. In one study, however, patients who maintained a diet of 1.3 × REE showed an improved feeling of control over their COPD, whereas those fed 1.7 × REE did not report any improvement in QOL.[89]

ACKNOWLEDGMENTS

We gratefully acknowledge Renee M. DeHart, PharmD BCPS and Sunshine Yocom, PharmD, for their contributions to the 6th edition of this chapter.

ABBREVIATIONS

ARDS: acute respiratory distress syndrome
ASPEN: American Society for Parenteral and Enteral Nutrition
ARF: acute renal failure
CKD: chronic kidney disease
COPD: chronic obstructive pulmonary disease
CRRT: continuous renal replacement therapy
EN: enteral nutrition
ESPEN: European Society for Parenteral and Enteral Nutrition
HD: hemodialysis
ICU: intensive care unit
IDPN: intradialytic parenteral nutrition
IVLE: intravenous lipid emulsion
NKF K/DOQI: National Kidney Foundation Kidney Disease Outcomes Quality Initiative
PD: peritoneal dialysis
PN: parenteral nutrition
QOL: quality-of-life
REE: resting energy expenditure
rhGH: recombinant human growth hormone
SBS: short-bowel syndrome

REFERENCES

1. Strejc JM, Strejc JM. Considerations in the nutritional management of patients with acute renal failure. Hemodial Int 2005;9(2):135–142.
2. Metnitz PG, Krenn CG, Steltzer H, et al. Effect of acute renal failure requiring renal replacement therapy on outcome in critically ill patients. Crit Care Med 2002;30(9):2051–2058.
3. Fiaccadori E, Lombardi M, Leonardi S, Rotelli CF, Tortorella G, Borghetti A. Prevalence and clinical outcome associated with preexisting malnutrition in acute renal failure: A prospective cohort study. J Am Soc Nephrol 1999;10(3):581–593.
4. Druml W. Nutritional management of acute renal failure. J Ren Nutr 2005;15(1):63–70.
5. Cano N, Fiaccadori E, Tesinsky P, et al. ESPEN Guidelines on Enteral Nutrition: Adult renal failure. Clin Nutr 2006;25(2):295–310.
6. Bozfakioglu S. Nutrition in patients with acute renal failure. Nephrol Dial Transplant 2001;16 Suppl 6:21–22.
7. Druml W. Nutritional management of acute renal failure. Am J Kidney Dis 2001;37(1 Suppl 2):S89–S94.
8. Fiaccadori E, Maggiore U, Rotelli C, et al. Effects of different energy intakes on nitrogen balance in patients with acute renal failure: A pilot study. Nephrol Dial Transplant 2005;20(9):1976–1980.
9. Maheux P, Azhar S, Kern PA, Chen YD, Reuven GM. Relationship between insulin-mediated glucose disposal and regulation of plasma and adipose tissue lipoprotein lipase. Diabetologia 1997;40(7):850–858.
10. Maxvold NJ, Smoyer WE, Custer JR, Bunchman TE. Amino acid loss and nitrogen balance in critically ill children with acute renal failure: A prospective comparison between classic hemofiltration and hemofiltration with dialysis. Crit Care Med 2000;28(4):1161–1165.
11. Klein CJ, Moser-Veillon PB, Schweitzer A, et al. Magnesium, calcium, zinc, and nitrogen loss in trauma patients during continuous renal replacement therapy. JPEN J Parenter Enteral Nutr 2002;26(2):77–92; discussion 93.
12. Druml W, Fischer M, Liebisch B, Lenz K, Roth E. Elimination of amino acids in renal failure. Am J Clin Nutr 1994;60(3):418–423.
13. Marin A, Hardy G, Marin A, Hardy G. Practical implications of nutritional support during continuous renal replacement therapy. Curr Opin Clin Nutr Metab Care 2001;4(3):219–225.
14. Mehta RL, Mehta RL. Acid-base and electrolyte management in continuous renal replacement therapy. Blood Purif 2002;20(3):262–268.

15. Heering P, Ivens K, Thumer O, et al. The use of different buffers during continuous hemofiltration in critically ill patients with acute renal failure. Intensive Care Med 1999;25(11):1244–1251.
16. Metnitz GH, Fischer M, Bartens C, Steltzer H, Lang T, Druml W. Impact of acute renal failure on antioxidant status in multiple organ failure. Acta Anaesthesiol Scand 2000;44(3):236–240.
17. Berger MM, Shenkin A, Revelly JP, et al. Copper, selenium, zinc, and thiamine balances during continuous venovenous hemodiafiltration in critically ill patients. Am J Clin Nutr 2004;80(2):410–416.
18. Druml W, Schwarzenhofer M, Apsner R, Horl WH. Fat-soluble vitamins in patients with acute renal failure. Miner Electrolyte Metab 1998;24(4):220–226.
19. Kalantar-Zadeh K, Kopple JD. Trace elements and vitamins in maintenance dialysis patients. Adv Ren Replace Ther 2003;10(3):170–182.
20. Bellomo R, Ronco C. How to feed patients with renal dysfunction. Curr Opin Crit Care 2000;6(4):239–246.
21. Wickersham R, ed. Drug Facts & Comparisons. St. Louis: Wolters Kluwer Health, 2006:81–88.
22. Fiaccadori E, Maggiore U, Giacosa R, et al. Enteral nutrition in patients with acute renal failure. Kidney Int 2004;65(3):999–1008.
23. Scheinkestel CD, Kar L, Marshall K, et al. Prospective randomized trial to assess caloric and protein needs of critically Ill, anuric, ventilated patients requiring continuous renal replacement therapy. Nutrition 2003;19(11–12):909–916.
24. ASPEN Board of Directors. Guidelines for the use of parenteral and enteral nutrition in adult and pediatric patients. JPEN J Parenter Enteral Nutr 2002;26(1 Suppl):1SA–138SA.
25. Van den Berghe G, Wouters PJ, Bouillon R, et al. Outcome benefit of intensive insulin therapy in the critically ill: Insulin dose versus glycemic control. Crit Care Med 2003;31(2):359–366.
26. Bellomo R, Tan HK, Bhonagiri S, et al. High protein intake during continuous hemodiafiltration: Impact on amino acids and nitrogen balance. Int J Artif Organs 2002;25(4):261–268.
27. Stein MY, Stein TP. High-protein feedings and the critically ill renal patient. Nutrition 2003;19(11–12):1030–1031.
28. Korkeila M, Ruokonen E, Takala J. Costs of care, long-term prognosis and quality of life in patients requiring renal replacement therapy during intensive care. Intensive Care Med 2000;26(12):1824–1831.
29. Gramlich L, Kichian K, Pinilla J, Rodych NJ, Dhaliwal R, Heyland DK. Does enteral nutrition compared to parenteral nutrition result in better outcomes in critically ill adult patients? A systematic review of the literature. Nutrition 2004;20(10):843–848.
30. Stratton RJ, Bircher G, Fouque D, et al. Multinutrient oral supplements and tube feeding in maintenance dialysis: A systematic review and meta-analysis. Am J Kidney Dis 2005;46(3):387–405.
31. Chung SH, Lindholm B, Lee HB. Influence of initial nutritional status on continuous ambulatory peritoneal dialysis patient survival. Perit Dial Int 2000;20(1):19–26.
32. Burrowes JD, Cockram DB, Dwyer JT, et al. Cross-sectional relationship between dietary protein and energy intake, nutritional status, functional status, and comorbidity in older versus younger hemodialysis patients. J Ren Nutr 2002;12(2):87–95.
33. Wiggins KL, Harvey KS. A review of guidelines for nutrition care of renal patients. J Ren Nutr 2002;12(3):190–196.
34. Sehgal AR. Outcomes of renal replacement therapy among blacks and women. Am J Kidney Dis 2000;35(4 Suppl 1):S148–52.
35. Vaziri ND, Moradi H. Mechanisms of dyslipidemia of chronic renal failure. Hemodial Int 2006;10(1):1–7.
36. Evans AM, Faull R, Fornasini G, et al. Pharmacokinetics of L-carnitine in patients with end-stage renal disease undergoing long-term hemodialysis. Clin Pharmacol Ther 2000;68(3):238–249.
37. American Kidney Foundation. Clinical practice guidelines for nutrition in chronic renal failure. K/DOQI, National Kidney Foundation. Am J Kidney Dis 2000;35(6 Suppl 2):S1–S140.
38. Mehrotra R, Kopple JD. Nutritional management of maintenance dialysis patients: Why aren't we doing better? Annu Rev Nutr 2001;21:343–379.
39. Mak RH, Cheung W, Cone RD, Marks DL. Leptin and inflammation-associated cachexia in chronic kidney disease. Kidney Int 2006;69(5):794–797.
40. Levey AS, Adler S, Caggiula AW, et al. Effects of dietary protein restriction on the progression of advanced renal disease in the Modification of Diet in Renal Disease Study. Am J Kidney Dis 1996;27(5):652–663.
41. Mehrotra R, Kopple JD. Protein and energy nutrition among adult patients treated with chronic peritoneal dialysis. Adv Ren Replace Ther 2003;10(3):194–212.
42. Temple KA, Smith AM, Cockram DB. Selenate-supplemented nutritional formula increases plasma selenium in hemodialysis patients. J Ren Nutr 2000;10(1):16–23.
43. Deicher R, Ziai F, Bieglmayer C, et al. Low total vitamin C plasma level is a risk factor for cardiovascular morbidity and mortality in hemodialysis patients. J Am Soc Nephrol 2005;16(6):1811–1818.
44. Yonemura K, Fujimoto T, Fujigaki Y, Hishida A. Vitamin D deficiency is implicated in reduced serum albumin concentrations in patients with end-stage renal disease. Am J Kidney Dis 2000;36(2):337–344.
45. Islam KN, O'Byrne D, Devaraj S, Palmer B, Grundy SM, Jialal I. Alpha-tocopherol supplementation decreases the oxidative susceptibility of LDL in renal failure patients on dialysis therapy. Atherosclerosis 2000;150(1):217–224.
46. Wrone EM, Hornberger JM, Zehnder JL, McCann LM, Coplon NS, Fortmann SP. Randomized trial of folic acid for prevention of cardiovascular events in end-stage renal disease. J Am Soc Nephrol 2004;15(2):420–426.
47. Serna-Thome MG, Padilla-Rosciano AE, Suchil-Bernal L. Practical aspects of intradialytic nutritional support. Curr Opin Clin Nutr Metab Care 2002;5(3):293–296.
48. How PP, Lau AH. Malnutrition in patients undergoing hemodialysis: Is intradialytic parenteral nutrition the answer? Pharmacotherapy 2004;24(12):1748–1758.
49. Li FK, Chan LY, Woo JC, et al. A 3-year, prospective, randomized, controlled study on amino acid dialysate in patients on CAPD. Am J Kidney Dis 2003;42(1):173–183.
50. Iglesias P, Diez JJ, Fernandez-Reyes MJ, et al. Recombinant human growth hormone therapy in malnourished dialysis patients: A randomized controlled study. Am J Kidney Dis 1998;32(3):454–463.
51. Di Iorio BR, Bellizzi V, Minutolo R, De Nicola L, Iodice C, Conte G. Supplemented very low-protein diet in advanced CRF. Is it money saving? Kidney Int 2004;65(2):742.
52. Henkel AS, Buchman AL. Nutritional support in patients with chronic liver disease. Nat Clin Pract Gastroenterol Hepatol 2006;3(4):202–209.
53. Moriwaki H, Tajika M, Miwa Y, et al. Nutritional pharmacotherapy of chronic liver disease: From support of liver failure to prevention of liver cancer. J Gastroenterol 2000;35 Suppl 12:13–17.
54. Caly WR, Strauss E, Carrilho FJ, Laudanna AA. Different degrees of malnutrition and immunological alterations according to the aetiology of cirrhosis: A prospective and sequential study. Nutr J 2003;2:10.
55. Dudrick SJ, Kavic SM. Hepatobiliary nutrition: History and future. J Hepatobiliary Pancreat Surg 2002;9(4):459–468.
56. Plauth M, Cabre E, Riggio O, et al. ESPEN Guidelines on Enteral Nutrition: Liver disease. Clin Nutr 2006;25(2):285–294.
57. Okamoto M, Sakaida I, Tsuchiya M, Suzuki C, Okita K. Effect of a late evening snack on the blood glucose level and energy metabolism in patients with liver cirrhosis. Hepatol Res 2003;27(1):45–50.
58. Miwa Y, Shiraki M, Kato M, et al. Improvement of fuel metabolism by nocturnal energy supplementation in patients with liver cirrhosis. Hepatol Res 2000;18(3):184–189.
59. Clemmesen JO, Hoy CE, Jeppesen PB, Ott P. Plasma phospholipid fatty acid pattern in severe liver disease. J Hepatol 2000;32(3):481–487.
60. Duerksen DR, Nehra V, Palombo JD, Ahmad A, Bistrian BR. Essential fatty acid deficiencies in patients with chronic liver disease are not reversed by short-term intravenous lipid supplementation. Dig Dis Sci 1999;44(7):1342–1348.
61. Matos C, Porayko MK, Francisco-Ziller N, DiCecco S. Nutrition and chronic liver disease. J Clin Gastroenterol 2002;35(5):391–397.
62. Cordoba J, Lopez-Hellin J, Planas M, et al. Normal protein diet for episodic hepatic encephalopathy: Results of a randomized study. J Hepatol 2004;41(1):38–43.
63. Chacko RT, Chacko A. Serum and muscle magnesium in Indians with cirrhosis of liver. Indian J Med Res 1997;106:469–474.
64. Plauth M, Roske AE, Romaniuk P, Roth E, Ziebig R, Lochs H. Post-feeding hyperammonaemia in patients with transjugular intrahepatic portosystemic shunt and liver cirrhosis: Role of small intestinal ammonia release and route of nutrient administration. Gut 2000;46(6):849–855.

65. Plauth M, Schutz T, Buckendahl DP, et al. Weight gain after transjugular intrahepatic portosystemic shunt is associated with improvement in body composition in malnourished patients with cirrhosis and hypermetabolism. J Hepatol 2004;40(2):228–233.
66. Hirsch S, Bunout D, de la Maza P, et al. Controlled trial on nutrition supplementation in outpatients with symptomatic alcoholic cirrhosis. JPEN J Parenter Enteral Nutr 1993;17(2):119–124.
67. Alvares-da-Silva MR, Reverbel da Silveira T. Comparison between handgrip strength, subjective global assessment, and prognostic nutritional index in assessing malnutrition and predicting clinical outcome in cirrhotic outpatients. Nutrition 2005;21(2):113–117.
68. Nightingale J, Woodward JM, on behalf of the Small Bowel and Nutrition Committee of the British Society of Gastroenterology. Guidelines for management of patients with a short bowel. Gut 2006;55(Suppl 4):iv1–12.
69. Buchman AL, Buchman AL. Etiology and initial management of short bowel syndrome. Gastroenterology 2006;130(2 Suppl 1):S5–S15.
70. American Gastroenterological Association. American Gastroenterological Association medical position statement: Short bowel syndrome and intestinal transplantation. Gastroenterology 2003;124(4):1105–1110.
71. Matarese LE, Steiger E. Dietary and medical management of short bowel syndrome in adult patients. J Clin Gastroenterol 2006;40(5 Suppl 2):S85–S93.
72. DiBaise JK, Matarese LE, Messing B, Steiger E. Strategies for parenteral nutrition weaning in adult patients with short bowel syndrome. J Clin Gastroenterol 2006;40(5 Suppl 2):S94–S98.
73. Sundaram A, Koutkia P, Apovian CM. Nutritional management of short bowel syndrome in adults. J Clin Gastroenterol 2002;34(3):207–220.
74. Byrne TA, Wilmore DW, Iyer K, et al. Growth hormone, glutamine, and an optimal diet reduces parenteral nutrition in patients with short bowel syndrome: A prospective, randomized, placebo-controlled, double-blind clinical trial. Ann Surg 2005;242(5):655–661.
75. Crenn P, Morin MC, Joly F, Penven S, Thuillier F, Messing B. Net digestive absorption and adaptive hyperphagia in adult short bowel patients. Gut 2004;53(9):1279–1286.
76. Sudan D. Cost and quality of life after intestinal transplantation. Gastroenterology 2006;130(2 Suppl 1):S158–S162.
77. Byrne TA, Persinger RL, Young LS, Ziegler TR, Wilmore DW. A new treatment for patients with short-bowel syndrome. Growth hormone, glutamine, and a modified diet. Ann Surg 1995;222(3):243–254; discussion 54–55.
78. Steiger E, DiBaise JK, Messing B, Matarese LE, Blethen S. Indications and recommendations for the use of recombinant human growth hormone in adult short bowel syndrome patients dependent on parenteral nutrition. J Clin Gastroenterol 2006;40(5 Suppl 2):S99–S106.
79. Abu-Elmagd KM. Intestinal transplantation for short bowel syndrome and gastrointestinal failure: Current consensus, rewarding outcomes, and practical guidelines. Gastroenterology 2006;130(2 Suppl 1):S132–S137.
80. Lord LM, Schaffner R, DeCross AJ, Sax HC. Management of the patient with short bowel syndrome. AACN Clin Issues 2000;11(4):604–618.
81. Howard L, Ament M, Fleming CR, Shike M, Steiger E. Current use and clinical outcome of home parenteral and enteral nutrition therapies in the United States. Gastroenterology 1995;109(2):355–365.
82. Albany: The Oley Foundation. 2006, *http://www.oley.org/*.
83. Schols AM, Wouters EF. Nutritional abnormalities and supplementation in chronic obstructive pulmonary disease. Clin Chest Med 2000;21(4):753–762.
84. Berry JK, Baum CL. Malnutrition in chronic obstructive pulmonary disease: Adding insult to injury. AACN Clin Issues 2001;12(2):210–219.
85. Engelen MP, Schols AM, Lamers RJ, Wouters EF. Different patterns of chronic tissue wasting among patients with chronic obstructive pulmonary disease. Clin Nutr 1999;18(5):275–280.
86. Engelen MP, Schols AM, Does JD, Wouters EF. Skeletal muscle weakness is associated with wasting of extremity fat-free mass but not with airflow obstruction in patients with chronic obstructive pulmonary disease. Am J Clin Nutr 2000;71(3):733–738.
87. Anker SD, John M, Pedersen PU, et al. ESPEN Guidelines on Enteral Nutrition: Cardiology and pulmonology. Clin Nutr 2006;25(2):311–318.
88. Slinde F, Ellegard L, Gronberg AM, Larsson S, Rossander-Hulthen L. Total energy expenditure in underweight patients with severe chronic obstructive pulmonary disease living at home. Clin Nutr 2003;22(2):159–165.
89. Planas M, Alvarez J, Garcia-Peris PA, et al. Nutritional support and quality of life in stable chronic obstructive pulmonary disease (COPD) patients. Clin Nutr 2005;24(3):433–441.
90. Cai B, Zhu Y, Ma Y, et al. Effect of supplementing a high-fat, low-carbohydrate enteral formula in COPD patients. Nutrition 2003;19(3):229–232.
91. Hasselmann M, Reimund JM. Lipids in the nutritional support of the critically ill patients. Curr Opin Crit Care 2004;10(6):449–455.
92. Faucher M, Bregeon F, Gainnier M, Thirion X, Auffray JP, Papazian L. Cardiopulmonary effects of lipid emulsions in patients with ARDS. Chest 2003;124(1):285–291.
93. Clark CL, Sacks GS, Dickerson RN, Kudsk KA, Brown RO. Treatment of hypophosphatemia in patients receiving specialized nutrition support using a graduated dosing scheme: Results from a prospective clinical trial. Crit Care Med 1995;23(9):1504–1511.
94. MacNee W. Oxidants/antioxidants and COPD. Chest 2000;117(5 Suppl 1):303S–317S.
95. Ferreira IM, Brooks D, Lacasse Y, et al. Nutritional supplementation for stable chronic obstructive pulmonary disease. Cochrane Database Syst Rev 2005(2):CD000998.
96. Kreymann KG, Berger MM, Deutz NE, et al. ESPEN guidelines on enteral nutrition: Intensive care. Clin Nutr 2006;25(2):210–223.
97. Gadek JE, DeMichele SJ, Karlstad MD, et al. Effect of enteral feeding with eicosapentaenoic acid, gamma-linolenic acid, and antioxidants in patients with acute respiratory distress syndrome. Enteral Nutrition in ARDS Study Group. Crit Care Med 1999;27(8):1409–1420.
98. Singer P, Theilla M, Fisher H, Gibstein L, Grozovski E, Cohen J. Benefit of an enteral diet enriched with eicosapentaenoic acid and gamma-linolenic acid in ventilated patients with acute lung injury. Crit Care Med 2006;34(4):1033–1038.
99. Schols AM. Nutrition in chronic obstructive pulmonary disease. Curr Opin Pulm Med 2000;6(2):110–115.
100. Katsura H, Yamada K, Kida K, Katsura H, Yamada K, Kida K. Both generic and disease specific health-related quality of life are deteriorated in patients with underweight COPD. Respir Med 2005;99(5):624–630.

CHAPTER 148 Obesity

JOHN V. ST. PETER AND CHARLES J. BILLINGTON

KEY CONCEPTS

1. Two clinical measures of excess body fat, regardless of sex, are the body mass index (BMI) and the waist circumference (WC). BMI and WC provide a better assessment of total body fat than weight alone and are independent predictors of obesity-related disease risk.
2. Excessive central adiposity increases risk for development of type 2 diabetes, hypertension, and dyslipidemia.
3. Weight loss of as little as 5% of total body weight can significantly improve blood pressure, lipid levels, and glucose tolerance in overweight and obese patients.
4. It is appropriate to consider medication therapy if 6 months of diet, exercise, and behavioral modification fail to stimulate weight loss.
5. A sufficient degree of obesity (BMI = 30 kg/m^2 and/or WC = 40 inches for males or 35 inches for females, or BMI of 27 to 30 kg/m^2 with concurrent risk factors) should be present before pharmacotherapy-facilitated weight loss is considered.
6. There is a high probability of weight regain when obesity pharmacotherapy is discontinued.
7. The FDA does not regulate labeling of herbal and food supplement diet agents, and content is not guaranteed.

It is now estimated that more than 95 million adults are overweight or obese in the United States.[1] Additionally, the number of adolescents who are overweight or obese has been increasing at an alarming rate during the last 30 years.[1,2] The presence of obesity and overweight is associated with a significantly increased risk for the development of many diseases (Table 148–1), poorer outcomes of comorbid disease states, and increased healthcare costs. Observational epidemiologic studies show that overall mortality parallels body weight increases above an optimal level.[3,4] This evidence is strongest for adults between the ages of 30 and 44 years. In older age groups, excess body weight increases the risk of death, but the degree of impact diminishes with age.[5] Annually, up to 35% of Americans have actively resolved to lose weight, spending between $30 and $50 billion on such attempts.[6] As of 2003, it is estimated that overweight and obesity account for 5% to 7% of total medical expenditures in the United States and the sum of direct and indirect costs is approaching $150 billion annually.[6] The recent report of the Surgeon General and the inclusion of several aggressive Healthy People 2010 goals have helped to stimulate national initiatives to reverse the rising rate of obesity through implementation of prevention strategies, consensus guidelines, and best practices.[7–10] This chapter reviews the epidemiology, pathophysiology, and therapeutic approaches for the management of obesity. Although nonpharmacologic treatment modalities are discussed, the pharmacotherapy of obesity is highlighted, and the role of pharmacotherapy relative to the other therapeutic options is critically reviewed.[11–14]

Learning objectives, review questions, and other resources can be found at **www.pharmacotherapyonline.com.**

EPIDEMIOLOGY

Obesity is increasing in prevalence in the United States. The National Health and Nutrition Examination Survey (NHANES) II data (1976–1980) estimated a prevalence of overweight persons in the United States at 25.4% of adults, representing 34 million individuals. During NHANES III (1988–1991), the prevalence had increased to 33.3%, representing 55 million American adults,[6,15] making the prevention of obesity a public health priority.[8] This is further emphasized by the continued pursuit of safe and effective long-term therapy for obesity. Individuals who were "fat" as children tend to remain overweight as adults.[1,16] In contrast to body weight, adult body mass index (BMI) was not well predicted from childhood weight. The fattest children had the highest risks of adult obesity. However, most obese adults had not been fat at earlier ages: Only 17% and 18% of obese 33-year-old men and women, respectively, had been fat at age 7 years. In contrast, early adulthood may be an important time for intervention to prevent future obesity; obesity increased in prevalence from 2% to 11% in men and from 3% to 12% in women during the 10-year period between ages 23 and 33 years.[16] The prevalence of overweight varies between races within the United States.[6,17–19] Mexican American women and black women had the highest prevalence, 48.1% and 49.1%, respectively. The prevalence of obesity also increases with age, reaching a maximum by the sixth decade in women and the seventh decade for men. Beyond this age, the prevalence progressively falls for both genders. Socioeconomic status also affects the prevalence of obesity in those between the ages of 25 and 54 years. The prevalence of overweight in nonpregnant women for each respective decade of life—25 to 34 years, 35 to 44 years, and 45 to 54 years—is 30.8%, 49.1%, and 54.1% of women with incomes below the poverty line versus 18.4%, 23.7%, and 30.3% of those above the poverty line.[16] Educational achievement, which is linked to socioeconomic status, is also correlated with the fraction of people who are overweight; prevalence of overweight is greatest in those with less than a high school education versus those with some college education.

TABLE 148-1 Conditions More Prevalent in Obese Populations

Cardiovascular	**Musculoskeletal**
Hypertension	Degenerative joint disease
Left ventricular hypertrophy	**Skin**
Congestive heart failure	Acanthosis nigricans
Coronary artery disease	Stretch marks
Stroke	Hirsutism
Pulmonary	Skin tags
Obstructive airway disease	**Gastrointestinal**
Sleep apnea	Cholelithiasis
Pulmonary hypertension	Esophageal reflux
Metabolic	Hiatus hernia
Hypercholesterolemia	**Psychological**
Hypertriglyceridemia	Eating disorders
Low serum high-density lipoprotein	Depression
Diabetes mellitus and glucose intolerance	Affective disorders
Hyperinsulinemia	Social stigma
Polycystic ovary syndrome	**Neoplasm**
Increased serum urate	Breast cancer
	Colon cancer

ETIOLOGY

The etiology of obesity in the vast majority of individuals can rarely be established. Obesity is a complex trait, and as such the etiology is multifactorial in origin, with genetic, environmental, and physiologic factors contributing to various degrees in different individuals. However, studies in twins confirm the presence of genetic contributions,[20] while the rapid increase in obesity prevalence in the last 30 years indicates a strong environmental contribution. In a small minority of individuals, diagnosis of an underlying medical condition contributing to the weight excess can be made. Even then, the diagnosed condition may or may not be treatable. One of the current areas of investigation is the extent that genetic traits influence the risk of developing obesity, as well as how these genetic traits interact with environmental factors to cause obesity.[21]

GENETIC PREDISPOSITION

Family studies show a clear correlation of body weight between parents and children. The correlation between siblings is even higher. In monozygotic twins, BMI is almost always identical, and there is a strong correlation in the accumulation of visceral fat. These twin studies demonstrate the strong role of genetics in determining both obesity and distribution of body fat. The incidence of obesity in adopted individuals relative to their adopted parents provides insight into the role of genetics versus family environment. A clear correlation between the BMI of adult adoptees and their biologic parents exists, but not between an adoptee and the adoptee's adoptive parent. These observations further support the notion that genes are primarily responsible for determining adult body weight. The relative impact of genetic versus environmental factors varies between persons. In some individuals, genetic factors are the primary determinants of obesity, whereas in others, the obesity may be caused primarily by environmental factors. The actual variance in body fat between individuals determined by genes is unknown. Estimates for this variance range from 20% to a high of almost 80%. A number of single-gene mutations producing obesity have been identified, but so far such mutations are rare and account for an extremely small number of the total cases of obesity.[22] The total number and identity of contributing genes is still being determined, as is the means by which the many potential "obesity" genes interact with each other, and with the environment, to produce the obesity phenotype. Clearly, without positive calorie balance, obesity cannot occur. The environment, now largely created by humans, interacts with underlying genetic traits for obesity, with the modern urban American environment apparently being an ideal one for obesity expression.

Syndromes in which obesity is a major component are extremely rare. Prader-Willi, Simpson-Goabi-Behmel, Cohen, Bardet-Biedl, Carpenter, Börjeson, and Wilson-Turner syndromes are all associated with obesity. Of these, Prader-Willi syndrome is the most common, with a frequency of 1 in 20,000 live births. Other phenotypic features include changes in stature, mental retardation, and developmental abnormalities (e.g., hypogonadism). Because the incidence of these syndromes is rare, even collectively they contribute very little to the incidence of obesity. The clinician evaluating a patient for obesity needs to be aware of their existence, and the physical examination of obese patients always should include an assessment for secondary causes of obesity, including genetic syndromes.

ENVIRONMENTAL FACTORS

Economic development is associated with lifestyle changes.[2] Many of these societal changes may contribute to the observed rise in the prevalence of obesity throughout the world. Those that are most probably related to obesity include reduced physical activity or work (sedentary lifestyle), abundant and readily available food supply, increased fat intake, increased consumption of refined simple sugars, increased consumption of pre-prepared and processed foods, and decreased ingestion of vegetables and fruits. These changes in our environment likely contribute to a state of positive energy balance in many individuals (Fig. 148–1).[23] Observations from public health studies support this concept. For example, the prevalence of obesity in Copenhagen remained stable during the period between 1925 and 1942 at approximately 0.1%. However, since the end of World War II, there has been a steady increase in the prevalence of obesity.[23] These observational data suggest an environmental role for the development of obesity.

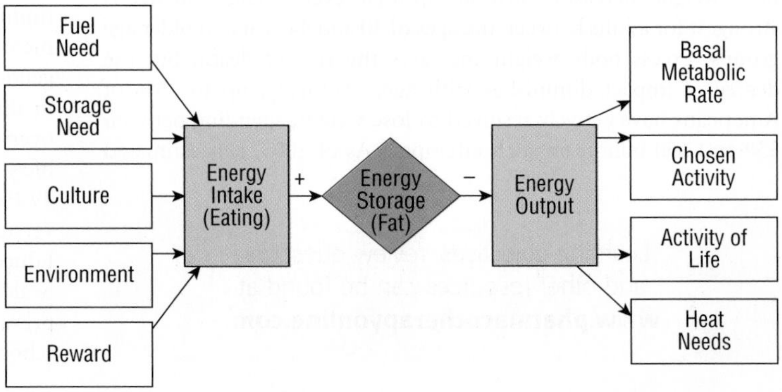

FIGURE 148-1. Net energy stores are determined by various inputs and outputs. Simply stated, obesity occurs when imbalance occurs between energy intake and expenditure.

NUTRITION

The appropriate diet that leads to long-term weight loss in ambulatory self-sufficient individuals is unknown. Weight regain is common, primarily because people return to their prediet food-intake patterns. It is clear that caloric intake in excess of habitual energy expenditure is a prerequisite to weight gain and obesity, but not all individuals with high caloric intake gain weight. The primary consideration is total calorie intake but macronutrient composition of the diet (i.e., percentage of calories as carbohydrates, protein, or fat) that is most favorable for maintaining healthy weight is still debatable. Of the three macronutrients, dietary fat has received the most attention. Both animals and humans prefer and often will seek out foods high in fat. High-fat foods have a desirable texture and sensory characteristics in the mouth. Although fat is itself tasteless, fats enhance the flavor of other foods. Clearly, one way that fatty foods promote weight gain is by increased energy intake because fat is more energy dense than other macronutrients. Furthermore, fats are stored with greater efficiency than protein or carbohydrates. Nutritional management of obesity as discussed in this chapter is based on reducing calorie intake. Because the Western diet is high in fat, and because fat contains more than twice the calories per gram of carbohydrate and protein, in most diets the total fat content is reduced by necessity.[24]

APPETITE

Appetite is a complex behavioral phenotype that results from processing of many inputs and values within a distributed brain network involving principally the hypothalamus, limbic system, brainstem, hippocampus, and elements of the cortex. Within this neural network, many neurotransmitters and neuropeptides have been identified that can stimulate or depress the brain's appetite network and thereby impact total caloric intake.

Biogenic Amines

The first receptor systems found to either stimulate or decrease food intake in animals and humans were the biogenic amines, and these neurotransmitters remain the basis for the most robust pharmacologic interventions for obesity. Serotonin, also known as 5-hydroxytryptamine (5-HT), and cells known to respond to 5-HT are found throughout the central nervous system and the periphery. At least seven distinct subfamilies of 5-HT receptors have been cloned to date, with each of these seven exhibiting one or more subtypes. Currently, two major noradrenergic receptor subtypes are recognized (α and β), each with multiple subtypes. Histamine and dopamine also demonstrate multiple receptor subtypes, but their role in regulation of human eating behaviors and food intake is less-well documented. Direct stimulation of 5-HT_{1A} and noradrenergic α_2-receptors will increase food intake, whereas the opposite occurs with 5-HT_{2C} and noradrenergic α_1- or β_2-receptor activation. In animal models, stimulating histamine receptor subtypes 1 or 3 and dopamine receptor subtypes 1 or 2 results in lowering of food intake. Table 148–2 summarizes the major effects of direct receptor stimulation, inhibition, or changes in synaptic cleft amine concentrations on food intake.

Neuropeptides

The hypothalamus is a crucial site within the brain's appetite network, and many neuropeptides, which influence appetite, have their main effects within the hypothalamus. Attention in the last several years has focused on the neural projection between parts of the hypothalamus, the arcuate nucleus sending signals to the paraventricular nucleus. The key peptides in this projection are currently thought to be neuropeptide Y and α-melanocyte–stimulating hormone, which engages melanocortin receptors in the paraventricular nucleus.[25] Neuropeptide Y is the most potent known stimulator of eating when it is active in arcuate to paraventricular projection,[26,27] while action at the melanocortin receptor is one of the crucial inhibitors of eating.[25] Melanocortin action to suppress eating is thought to be especially important in humans because melanocortin pathway genes are among those found to influence body weight.[22]

TABLE 148-2 Effects of Various Neurotransmitters, Receptors, and Peptides on Food Intake

Brain Site	Increased Eating	Decreased Eating
Arcuate Nucleus of Hypothalamus (ARC)	Ghrelin	Leptin Glucagon Like Peptide-1 (GLP-1) Peptide YY (PYY)
Paraventricular Nucleus of Hypothalamus (PVN)	Neuropeptide Y (NPY) Agouti Related Protein (AgRP) Opioids (especially mu) Galanin	Melanocyte Stimulating Hormone (MSH, Melanocortin) Corticotropin Releasing Hormone (CRH) Cholecystokinin (CCK)
Lateral Hypothalamus (LH)	Orexin Melanocyte Concentration Hormone (MCH)	
Hypothalamus	Norepinephrine α_2 Serotonin 5-HT_{1A}	Norepinephrine α_1 and β_2 Serotonin 5-HT_{1B} and 5-HT_{2C} Histamine H_1 and H_3
Nucleus Accumbens	Dopamine	
Amygdala	Opioids (especially mu)	
Brainstem (Hindbrain)	Neuropeptide Y (NPY) Agouti Related Protein (AgRP) Opioids (especially mu)	Leptin Melanocyte Stimulating Hormone (MSH, Melanocortin) Cholecystokinin (CCK)
Vagus Nerve	Ghrelin	Leptin Cholecystokinin (CCK) Glucagon Like Peptide-1 (GLP-1) Peptide YY (PYY)
Various or Undetermined	Cannabinoid CB_1	Dopamine D_1 and D_2

The lateral hypothalamus has been historically known as the hunger center within the brain, and peptides that potentially convey the hunger message have been identified in the lateral hypothalamus.[25] The most prominent of these lateral hypothalamic peptides, orexin, increases food intake stimuli within the lateral hypothalamus and from lateral to paraventricular hypothalamus.[27] Another peptidergic stimulator of eating that principally originates in the lateral hypothalamus is melanocyte-concentrating hormone. Neurons in the lateral hypothalamus use orexin and melanocyte-concentrating hormone to communicate with other neurons throughout the brain, affecting a number of functions beyond appetite.

Hunger and satiety, in the sense that these relate to the energy state of the body, are functions thought to be sited especially in the hypothalamus. Long-term energy state and body fat content are particularly important in the sensing and integrative functions of the hypothalamus. However, humans eat in response to a broader set of stimuli and values than energy need and fat mass. Reward, pleasure, learning, and memory are among the other important values processed within the brain that contribute to the decision to eat.

Many of the hedonic aspects of eating are handled within the broad category of brain sites referred to as the limbic system, and a different set of neurotransmitters and neuropeptides are thought to be important in the function of this system. Dopamine in the nucleus accumbens is the best known of these hedonic and eating-related neural peptides. It has also been implicated in the neural pathways underlying other behaviors, such as the use of drugs of abuse.[25] In the amygdala, other emotional aspects of eating are processed, and in part are influenced by endogenous opiates which mainly initiate their effect by altering mu opioid receptor-based signaling.[28] Also thought to be involved in the hedonics of eating are the endocannabinoids, although the brain site most important for this function is not yet clearly defined.[29]

Peripheral Appetite Related Signals to the Brain

Since the 1950s, it has been conjectured that body fat content must be sensed in some way at the level of the hypothalamus.[30] The protein product of the mouse obese gene (*ob*) called *leptin* (after *leptos*, the Greek word for "thin"), appears to be the signaling mechanism between fat and hypothalamic feeding centers.[30] The *ob/ob* genetically obese mouse does not produce leptin, and this animal's marked obesity and hyperphagia subsides with leptin supplementation. The human leptin homologue has been cloned, and unlike the leptin-deficient *ob/ob* mouse, obese human serum leptin levels increase as fat cell mass increases. In fact there is a direct relationship between serum leptin concentrations and various markers of obesity such as percentage of body fat, BMI, and serum insulin concentrations. Figure 148–2 shows the peripheral link that leptin appears to provide in signaling the central nervous system about the status of fat cell mass. Unlike endocrine feedback systems, leptin blood levels in humans mainly matter when they are low, and higher serum levels of leptin and even supplementary leptin do not have much affect on the brain appetite network function. Thus, it is not surprising that recent studies of leptin supplementation in humans have not significantly decreased obesity.[31] However, there is increasing evidence of the complicated nature of leptin effects both within and outside the central nervous system.[30,32,33]

Other peripheral signals important to the brain's processing of appetite include those from the gastrointestinal tract.[34] Several gut hormones are of current interest, notably those released by the intestine in response to passage of digesting food such as glucagon-related peptide-1, oxyntomodulin, and peptide YY. Each of these hormonal signals suppress eating in animals and humans. Glucagon-related peptide-1 also has other effects, most importantly as an incretin, which facilitates release of insulin by pancreatic β-cells in response to meal-related glucose. Interestingly, there is also a gut hormone, ghrelin, which is released from the distal stomach and duodenum when they are empty, and stimulates appetite.

An understanding of the relationships between the brain, its many neurotransmitters and neuropeptides, environmental stimulation of brain activities, and other hormones, such as insulin and glucocorticoids, is still evolving.[25,27] Exogenous manipulation of neural signals and associated peripheral hormones may provide future pharmacotherapeutic approaches to obesity management.[27]

ACTIVITY

It is generally accepted that increased physical activity is important in the management of obesity.[6,35] Similarly, a sedentary lifestyle predisposes to weight gain and obesity. Studies tend to show that obesity is associated with lower levels of physical activity, but it is unclear whether lower activity in the obese is a cause or consequence of the excess weight. It is clear that excess weight increases the physical cost of activity, and may offset, to some degree, the lower levels of activity with respect to energy balance. It is also clear that the obese can be physically active and there is evidence that increased fitness can protect the obese from some of the harm associated with their excess weight. Physical activity includes voluntary work, recreational activity, and spontaneous physical activity including involuntary movements. Some authors suggest that obese individuals have reduced levels of spontaneous physical activity leading to lower daily energy expenditure. However, results from studies designed to measure total daily energy expenditure remain controversial. A recent literature review found only a modest beneficial effect of exercise in preventing weight gain, with or without previous weight reduction.[36]

WEIGHT GAIN SECONDARY TO MEDICAL CONDITIONS

Occasionally patients present with obesity secondary to an identifiable acquired medical condition. Weight gain is often associated with hypothyroidism, although the majority of patients presenting with hypothyroidism are not overweight (see Chap. 78). Some of these patients lose weight within weeks of thyroxin-replacement therapy. However, many patients will not achieve a normal or ideal body

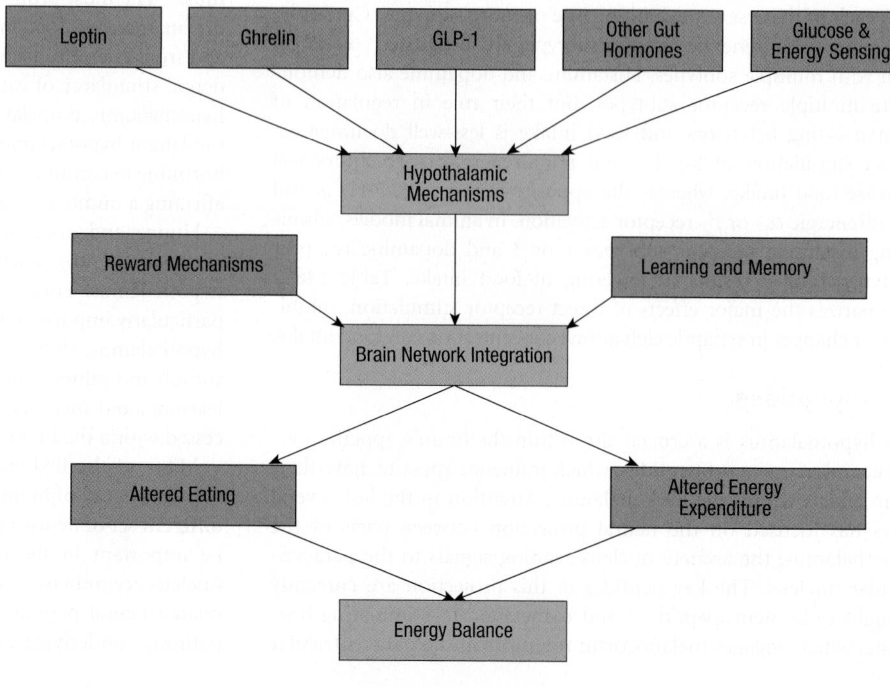

FIGURE 148-2. Intrinsic hypothalamic hunger and satiety mechanisms are modified by input from fat tissue via leptin; from gut via ghrelin, GLP-1 and other hormones; and by direct sensing of prevailing glucose and other energy signals. The hypothalamus generates signals that are integrated within brain networks, which are also receiving signals and food hedonics, learning and memory, and other motivations. The brain network affects change in energy balance by modifying food intake and energy expenditure.

weight despite adequate thyroid hormone replacement. Indeed, it is not uncommon for patients to request higher than physiologic replacement doses of thyroxin to artificially suppress their weight. It is important to remember that excess thyroid therapy can be associated with complications, including osteoporosis and cardiac disorders. Cushing's syndrome, another cause of obesity, is seen most commonly in patients receiving exogenous glucocorticoid therapy. These agents often are prescribed for a chronic condition such as chronic obstructive pulmonary disease, organ transplantation, and arthritis. Idiopathic Cushing's disease caused by excess endogenous steroid secretion is, in contrast, very rare. In both iatrogenic and idiopathic Cushing's disease, the weight gain is partly a result of fluid retention, as well as of increased adiposity. The adiposity associated with glucocorticoid excess has a particular body distribution in that it is central with relative loss of body muscle mass and thinning of the skin, leading to the characteristic purple skin striae and a buffalo hump behind the neck.

An increasing number of medications are associated with weight gain.[37] Most prominent among these are several of the treatments for diabetes, notably insulin, sulfonylureas, and thiazolidinediones. Some of the weight gain associated with diabetic treatments is thought to be caused by appetite-stimulated transient hypoglycemia, but it is likely that other mechanisms are also involved. More recently, weight gain was associated with a number of psychiatric medicines used for treatment of psychosis, mood disorders, and depression, and with several anticonvulsants. The most prominent weight gain problems have been seen with atypical antipsychotics, but it now seems clear that older antipsychotic agents are also sometimes implicated in weight gain. The pharmacologic mechanism responsible for the weight gain in patients who are receiving atypical and other antipsychotics, as well as most anticonvulsants has not been determined, but does not appear to be related to dopamine blockade. Interestingly, one anticonvulsant, topiramate, can cause weight loss, sometimes substantial weight loss.[38]

Occasionally patients can present with lesions of the hypothalamus that lead to hyperphagia and obesity. This disorder is rare and should not be confused with behavioral disorders of eating that are associated with psychopathology. These include binge eating disorders, which may respond to psychotherapy, and in some cases, to pharmacotherapy (see Chap. 66). Obesity is itself associated with a higher prevalence of affective disorders, which if untreated may impair the success of any weight-loss program. The clinician managing obesity must be aware of the presence of psychosocial disorders, both as a cause and as an effect of obesity. Counseling strategies need to be incorporated into the management of selected obese individuals.[12] Furthermore, medications used to manage affective disorders, such as the selective serotonin reuptake inhibitors, have not been studied extensively with regard to combination use with appetite suppressant agents.

PATHOPHYSIOLOGY

ENERGY BALANCE

The net balance of energy ingested relative to energy expended by an individual over time determines the degree of obesity. Figure 148–1 represents the interplay between energy intake and expenditure. Energy stores will increase if there is imbalance between intake and expenditure. An individual's metabolic rate is the single largest determinant of energy expenditure. It is important to determine metabolic rate under standardized conditions, giving rise to terms such as resting energy expenditure (REE) and basal metabolic rate (BMR). REE is defined as the energy expended by a person at rest under conditions of thermal neutrality. BMR is defined as the REE measured soon after awakening in the morning, at least 12 hours after the last meal. Metabolic rate increases after eating, based on the size and composition of the meal. It reaches a maximum approximately 1 hour after the meal is consumed and is essentially back to basal levels 4 hours after the meal. This increase in metabolic rate is known as the *thermogenic effect of food*. The REE may include the residual thermic effect of a previous meal and may be lower than BMR during quiet sleep. In practice, BMR and REE differ by less than 10%, and the terms frequently are used interchangeably. Physical activity is the other major portion of total energy expenditure, and is the most variable component. Even "sedentary" people expend some additional energy each day through their physical activity, but that amount is quite small relative to marathoners.

PERIPHERAL STORAGE AND THERMOGENESIS

Adipose tissue generally is divided into two major types, white and brown. The primary function of white adipose tissue is lipid manufacture, storage, and release. Lipid storage occurs in response to insulin with lipid release occurring during periods of calorie restriction, when insulin levels are suppressed. Brown-type tissue is notable for its ability to dissipate energy via a process of uncoupled mitochondrial respiration.[39] Currently, the exact roles of each of these tissue subtypes are better defined in animal models than in humans. Adipose tissue is highly innervated by the sympathetic nervous system, and adrenergic stimulation is known to activate lipolysis in fat cells as well as increase energy expenditure in adipose tissue and skeletal muscle. These properties provide a potential pharmacologic avenue for altering energy balance and changing weight status. A major focus of research in obesity pharmacotherapy has centered on the activity of adrenergic receptors and their effect on adipose tissue with respect to energy storage and expenditure or thermogenesis.[40] All three subtypes of β-adrenergic receptors (β_1, β_2, and β_3) appear to be active in fat cell function. The β_3-receptor appears to be less responsive than β_1 and β_2 with respect to activation via norepinephrine. This has led to the development of specific β_3-adrenoceptor agonists. However, apparent differences in selectivity and responsiveness between animal and human β_3-receptors have complicated the drug development process. In vivo studies in humans suggest that the β_3-receptor may be largely responsible for adipose tissue adrenergic-mediated increases in thermogenesis.[41] Genetic polymorphisms have been identified in both the β_2- and β_3-receptor systems that are associated with obesity or excess weight gain.[42] Thus genetic susceptibility for excess weight status may in part be related to adrenergic dysfunction. The development of effective pharmacotherapies involving these receptor systems may be delayed pending definitive identification of receptor subtype contributions.

CLINICAL PRESENTATION

❶ A consistent and reproducible description of weight status is essential in the diagnosis and management of obesity. Evidence-based guidelines issued by many groups, notably the World Health Organization and the National Institutes of Health, have established a stratification of weight excess based on associated medical risk.[43] The first increment of excess weight is termed *overweight*, with the term *obesity* reserved for the higher levels of weight excess. For use in the clinic, these levels of excess weight are defined on the basis of BMI, a measure of total body weight relative to height. Those with a BMI of 18.5 to 25 are considered to have "normal" weight; overweight, obese, and severely obese are reserved for those with a BMI of 25 to 30, 30 to 40, and over 40, respectively. Using metric units, BMI (kg/m^2) is defined as weight in kilograms divided by height in meters squared (kg/m^2). Using pounds and inches, BMI (lbs/in^2) is estimated as: weight [pounds]/height [inches^2] × 703. Because the BMI may overestimate the degree of excess body fat in some clinical situations (e.g., edematous states, extreme muscularity, muscle wasting, short-stature), the final decision is often based on clinical judgment.

BMI is an acceptable measure of obesity and is the practical method of defining obesity in the clinic and epidemiologic studies; however, it does not always correspond to excess fat. Ideally, obesity refers to a state of excess body fat as determined by measures of skinfold thickness, body density using underwater body weight, bioelectric impedance and conductivity, dual-energy x-ray absorptiometry, computed tomography, or magnetic resonance imaging. These measurement techniques that determine body fat directly are currently too expensive and time-consuming to be used in population studies or for application in the clinical setting.

Furthermore, all fat is not equal in its danger to health. Central obesity reflects high levels of intraabdominal or visceral fat, and this pattern of obesity is associated with an increased propensity for the development of hypertension, dyslipidemia, type 2 diabetes, and cardiovascular disease (sometimes referred to as the "metabolic syndrome"). Intraabdominal fat is best estimated by imaging techniques such as computed tomography and magnetic resonance imaging. The other broadly defined type of fat is subcutaneous fat, which may be heterogeneous in its metabolic effects. Superficial subcutaneous fat has a weak association with metabolic markers of insulin production, release, and resistance, whereas deep subcutaneous fat demonstrates a strong relationship with insulin resistance.[39] Thus, in addition to the absolute excess fat mass, the distribution of this fat regionally in the body has an important effect on the mortality of obese individuals.

Waist circumference (WC) is the most practical method of characterizing central or visceral adiposity. Clinically, WC is the narrowest circumference measured in the area between the last rib and the top of the iliac crest.[24] The current definition for high-risk WC is greater than 40 inches in males and greater than 35 inches in females.[24] Notably, epidemiologic studies demonstrate that WC adds little in terms of risk prediction once a patient's BMI reaches 35 kg/m^2. Thus, routine collection of WC should be implemented in those with BMIs between 25 and 35 kg/m^2. Although BMI and WC are related, each measure independently predicts disease risk. Both measurements should be taken at initial assessment and during routine followup of therapy for obesity.

The importance and clinical applicability of these measurements continue to evolve as there are probably racial and ethnic differences in the relationship between BMI, WC, and risk for development of disease and enhanced comorbidity.[17–19,44] Table 148–3 outlines the current classification of overweight and obesity using BMI and WC. The table identifies risk for development of type 2 diabetes, hypertension, or cardiovascular disease at various stages of BMI or WC. Note that increased WC confers increased risk even in normal-weight individuals.

TABLE 148-3 Classification of Overweight and Obesity by Body Mass Index (BMI), Waist Circumference, and Associated Disease Risk

			Disease Risk[a] (Relative to Normal Weight and Waist Circumference)	
	BMI (kg/m2)	Obesity Class	*Men ≤40 in* *Women ≤35 in*	*>40 in* *>35 in*
Underweight	<18.5		–	–
Normal[b]	18.5–24.9		–	–
Overweight	25.0–29.9		Increased	High
Obesity	30.0–34.9	I	High	Very high
	35.0–39.9	II	Very high	Very high
Extreme obesity	≥40	III	Extremely high	Extremely high

[a]Disease risk for type 2 diabetes, hypertension, and cardiovascular disease.
[b]Increased waist circumference can also be a marker for increased risk even in persons of normal weight.
Adapted from Preventing and Managing the Global Epidemic of Obesity. Report of the World Health Organization Consultation on Obesity. Geneva: World Health Organization, 1997. Reprinted with permission from NLH-NHLBI, http://www.nhlbi.nih.gov/guidelines/obesity/ob_home.htm.

COMORBIDITIES

❷ Obesity is associated with serious health risks and increased mortality. Several disease states and/or conditions are more prevalent in obese patients (see Table 148–1). Increased body fat, increased total body weight, and a central distribution of body fat are all associated with an increased incidence of mortality, primarily as a result of cardiovascular disease. Hypertension, hyperlipidemia, insulin resistance, and glucose intolerance are all known cardiac risk factors that tend to cluster in obese individuals. Therefore, the obese individual is exposed to multiple risk factors. Some of the earliest studies from Framingham have confirmed the relationship between obesity and increased risk of stroke and coronary heart disease in both men and women.[45] Increased mortality is seen even with modest excess body weight. Blood pressure frequently is elevated in obese individuals and may in part explain the increased incidence of stroke and cardiovascular disease observed with obesity. Hypertension in lean individuals is associated with concentric cardiac hypertrophy as a consequence of an increased afterload, which increases the risk of cardiac ischemia. In contrast with obesity, eccentric dilation is observed, leading to an increased volume load. This dilated cardiomyopathy is associated with a reduction in ventricular ejection fraction and a high-output cardiac state. The combination of obesity and hypertension is associated with thickening of the ventricular wall, ischemia, and increased heart volume. This leads more rapidly to heart failure an association that has been recognized for more than two decades.[46,47] Alterations in pulmonary function are common in patients with obesity. Sleep apnea is a significant and costly condition in terms of morbidity and mortality that is associated with obesity.[46,47] This disorder is more common in men. The exact mechanism by which obesity leads to sleep apnea is unknown, but weight loss often results in significant and sometimes dramatic improvements in sleep apnea.

Diabetes mellitus and impaired glucose tolerance are associated with insulin resistance and obesity. The cellular mechanism by which obesity causes insulin resistance is unknown. Proposed mechanisms include downregulation of insulin receptors, abnormal postreceptor signals, circulating antagonists to insulin such as fatty acids or cytokines, and impaired gene transcription in insulin-responsive cells. Regardless of the mechanism of the insulin resistance, as insulin response becomes impaired, the pancreatic β-cells respond by increasing insulin production and release, resulting in a state of relative hyperinsulinemia. Although hyperinsulinemia is known to be associated with an increased risk of cardiovascular disease, it is not known whether the increased insulin levels contribute directly to cardiac disease or if they are just a marker for the underlying defect of insulin resistance and glucose intolerance. Insulin resistance, in turn, also frequently leads to impaired lipid metabolism (increased cholesterol, increased triglycerides, and low circulating high-density lipoprotein) and hypertension. As with cardiovascular disease, fat distribution is an important factor in determining the risk of developing type 2 diabetes. Central obesity increases the risk of diabetes. Intentional weight loss reduces mortality substantially in obese individuals with diabetes.[48]

Osteoarthritis in weight-bearing joints, such as the knees, may be related directly to the mechanical effects of excess body weight and the resulting forces exerted on these joint surfaces. The increase of osteoarthritis in non–weight-bearing joints, however, suggests that obesity may lead to altered cartilage, collagen, and even bone metabolism. Osteoarthritis and its symptoms, such as pain, are a significant barrier to physical activity and a key impediment to sustained weight loss.

Obesity affects the human reproductive system in a number of ways. Obesity is associated with earlier menarche in girls and hyperandrogenism, hirsutism, and anovulatory menstrual cycles in women. In some women this disorder manifests as overt polycystic ovary syndrome.[49] Insulin resistance is common in these women. Weight loss, and more recently, therapy with insulin-sensitizing drugs such as the thiazolidinediones and biguanides, have been shown to restore normal ovulation in some women.[49] These observations suggest that insulin resistance plays a part in the causation of polycystic ovary syndrome-associated with obesity.

TREATMENT

Obesity

DESIRED OUTCOME

❸ Weight management is commonly considered successful when a predefined amount of weight has been lost such that a final goal is achieved. However, desired outcomes are fully dependent on the clinical situation. Success may also include end points of decreasing the rate of weight gain or maintaining a weight-neutral status. A significant number of web-based resources for supporting both patient and practitioner weight management activities are available.[8,10,24,50–52]

GENERAL APPROACH TO TREATMENT

The success of obesity therapy has been measured most often as weight loss over study periods of up to 12 months. Successful obesity treatment plans have incorporated diet, exercise, behavior modification (with or without pharmacologic therapy), and/or surgical intervention. Specific weight goals should be established that are consistent with medical needs and patient personal desire. For most obese patients, a weight loss goal of 5% to 10% to no more than 30% of initial weight is reasonable. An average rate of weight loss after the first month of therapy is around 1 lb per week. Patients should not be allowed to attain weight less than their estimated ideal weight.

Patients seeking help for obesity do so for many reasons, including improvement in their quality of life, a reduction in associated morbidity, and to prolong their life. Yet numerous individuals seek therapy for obesity primarily for cosmetic purposes and often have unreasonable goals and expectations. Aggressive marketing of weight-loss programs, therapies, and diets—parallel to the fashion industry's standards of desirable body profiles—has led many individuals to set impossible goals and expectations. In some cases, these persons will go to extreme measures to achieve weight loss. Consequently, clinicians must be careful to fully discuss risks of therapies and to clearly define achievable benefits and magnitude of weight loss. Criteria for weight loss vary from the most aggressive goal of trying to achieve an "ideal weight" to the more reasonable goals of modest (e.g., loss of 5% of body weight) but sustained weight loss. In practice, the goal has to be set based on many factors, including initial body weight, patient motivation and desire, presence of comorbid conditions, and age. For example, in patients with diabetes, even modest weight loss can improve glucose control and reduce mortality significantly,[48,49] yet in individuals with osteoarthritis, significantly more weight reduction may be required to improve symptoms. Indeed, dietary modification and exercise have been shown to ameliorate hyperglycemia, hyperlipidemia, and hypertension with weight loss of less than 5% of initial body weight. These data emphasize the importance of defining end points and measures of success in any weight-loss plan.

Weight-loss interventions must be founded on lifestyle changes such as a modification in eating practices, complemented by drug therapy if indicated, and in some cases surgery (Fig. 148–3). Prior to recommending any therapy, the clinician must evaluate the patient for the presence of secondary causes of obesity. If a secondary cause is suspected, then a more complete diagnostic workup and appropriate therapy are paramount. The next step in the patient evaluation is to determine the presence and severity of other medical conditions either directly associated with obesity (e.g., diabetes) or that have an impact on therapeutic decision making (e.g., history of liver disease or cardiac arrhythmia). Appropriate laboratory tests to exclude and/or quantify the degree of specific conditions such as diabetes, liver dysfunction, and nephropathy should be done as indicated by the history and physical examination. Based on the outcome of this medical evaluation, the patient then should be counseled on treatment options, benefits, and risks. The ultimate goals of treatment must be defined clearly. These goals may be absolute weight loss if obesity is present without other comorbid conditions. If improvement in blood glucose, blood cholesterol, and hypertension are primary goals, then these must be defined appropriately, and may include setting target levels for low-density-lipoprotein cholesterol, glycosylated hemoglobin, or blood pressure. For these patients, weight loss goals may be as little as 5% of starting weight. In contrast, if obesity is causing physical problems such as impaired mobility, osteoarthritis, or sleep apnea, then a weight loss goal of 10% to 20% of starting weight may be a more appropriate target. All too often patients expect to lose weight overnight, only to be disappointed. Thus it is important to set a time course for the plan. A reasonable rate of weight loss is typically about 0.5 kg per week.

NONPHARMACOLOGIC THERAPY

Behavioral Modification

❹ Behavior modification is common to almost all weight-loss interventions. The primary aim is to help patients choose lifestyles that are conducive to safe and sustained weight loss. Behavioral therapy is based on principles of human learning and thus attempts to substitute learned undesirable habits with desirable behaviors using a combination of stimulus control and reinforcement. Most such programs use self-monitoring of diet and exercise both to increase patient awareness of behavior, and as a tool for the clinician to determine patient compliance as well as patient motivation.[53,54] Behavior is reinforced by techniques including behavioral contracting, social support, relapse prevention, and in some cases booster treatments. Behavioral contracts are written agreements jointly developed by the patient and clinician. Components of these agreements include goals of therapy, methods to achieve these goals, and rewards for achieving these goals successfully. Social support requires the active participation of a close friend or relative who is involved in monitoring compliance and reinforcing behavior. Relapse prevention is geared to identifying high-risk situations for relapse such as social events, and training the individual to avoid these circumstances. Eventually, the patient is trained to deal with these situations actively, such as refusing high-fat foods assertively rather than avoiding such social events.

Diet

Numerous diet or nutrition plans exist to aid in weight loss.[54,55] The lay press is replete with many diet routines that fall into and out of favor.

CLINICAL CONTROVERSY

Because of the popularity of diets such as Atkin's New Diet Revolution (high fat, low carbohydrate, high protein) and The New Pritikin Program (low fat, high carbohydrate, medium protein), there is extensive discussion in the lay media and academic circles regarding the risks, benefits, and outcomes related to diets that preferentially employ macronutrient extremes (i.e., high protein vs. high carbohydrate vs. low fat). Ultimately, overall energy balance will determine the rate and extent of weight change.

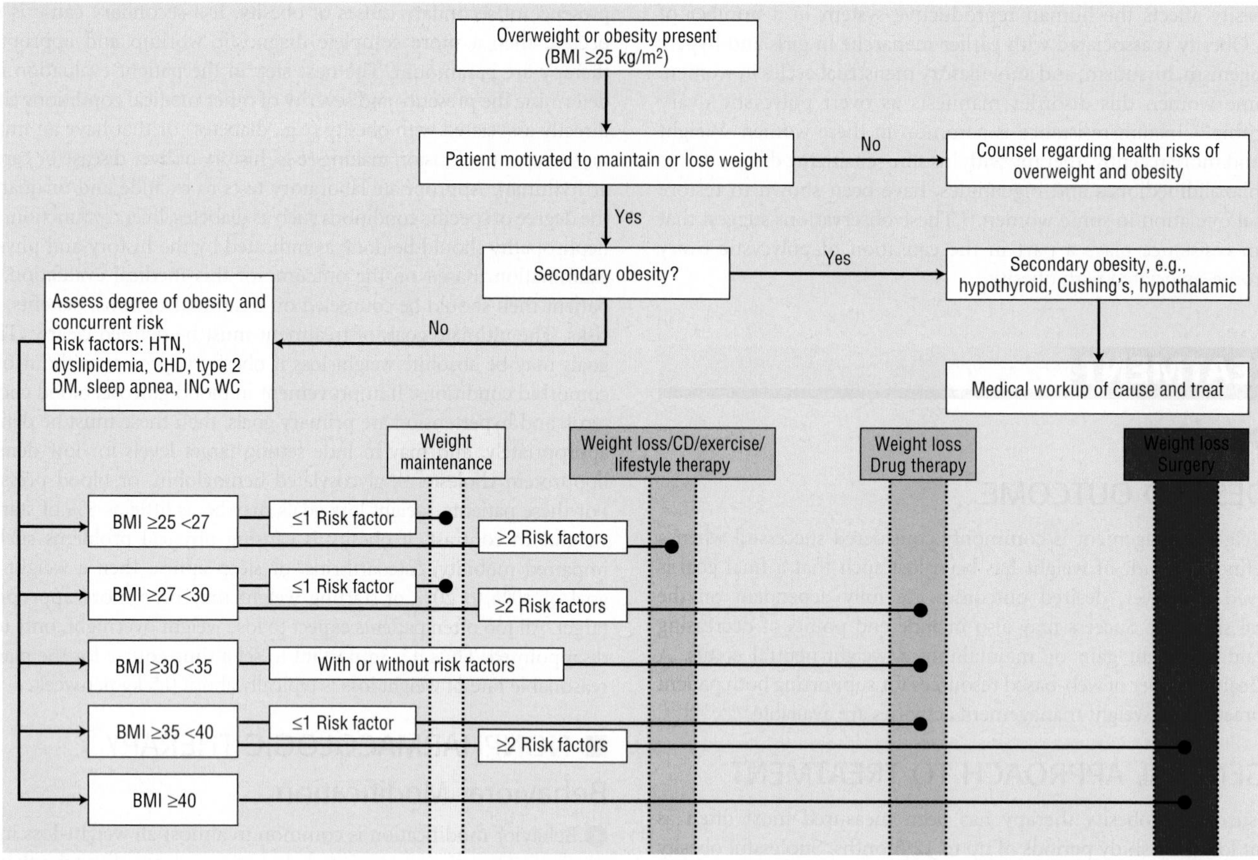

FIGURE 148-3. Pharmacotherapy treatment algorithm. A select population of individuals, based on BMI and WC together with concurrent risk factors, may benefit from medication therapy as an adjunct to a program of weight loss that includes diet, exercise, and behavioral modification. (WC, waist circumference; INC WC, >40 inches for males and >35 inches for females; BMI, body mass index; CHD, coronary heart disease; DM, diabetes mellitus; HTN, hypertension; LCD, low-calorie diet.)

Few, if any, of the popular "fad" diets have been objectively studied in a randomized, controlled fashion, with sufficient power to clearly determine their acute and chronic effects. Current data suggests that low carbohydrate diets achieve better weight loss than low protein diets for the first 6 months of treatment, but that the diets are equal in their effects at 1 year. Additionally, the relative efficiency of these diets for weight loss and chronic weight maintenance remain ill defined. However, recent efforts to better understand the acute and chronic effects of these extremes in macronutrient intake are being reported.[56,57] Whichever diet program is selected, it is clear that energy consumption must be less than energy expenditure to achieve weight loss (see Fig. 148–1). The challenge has been to develop a diet plan that leads to consistent adherence by the patient and therefore sustained weight loss and/or maintenance. Two broad categories of diet have been used in clinical practice: low calorie and very low calorie. The low-calorie diet or Step 1 Diet, is recommended as part of the recent National Heart, Lung, and Blood Institute's Obesity Education Initiative. This low-calorie diet recommends from 1,000 to 1,200 kcal/day for women and 1,200 to 1,600 kcal/day for men, based on estimated needs and weight maintenance or reduction goals. Very-low-calorie diets generally contain less than 800 kcal/day. These highly restrictive diets often result in early weight loss, but have been disappointing in the long-term, in part because it is difficult for individuals to maintain compliance. Additionally, very-low-calorie diets require intensive medical monitoring, and are possibly less effective, for long-term weight reduction than low-calorie diets. Other investigators have proposed total or modified fasts. The obvious problem with total fasts is that both fat and lean body mass are lost. In addition, because of diuresis, significant mineral losses occur. Because of the problem with total fasting, alternate regimens called protein-supplemented modified fasts, became popular. With a protein-supplemented modified fast, the protein is given in the form of either formula or natural foods such as fish or lean meat. The consensus is that it is dangerous to allow these diets to be continued for longer than 16 weeks at a time. Patients may lose 1.5 to 2.3 kg per week on these diets. When these types of severe calorie-restricted diets are employed individuals will need vitamin and mineral supplementation.[24,51]

A more reasonable goal for individuals is weight reduction of about 0.5 to 1 kg per week achieved by a negative calorie balance of approximately 500 to 1,000 kcal/day. This translates into a diet of approximately 20 kcal/kg of desirable body weight for most adults. The dietary regimen should be well balanced in fat, carbohydrates, and proteins, as well as in micronutrients. Generally 0.8 g of protein per kilogram of desirable body weight is recommended, with at most 30% of calories from fat.

Surgery

Surgery remains the most effective intervention for the treatment of obesity. However, because of its related morbidity and mortality, this intervention is reserved for those with BMI greater than 40 kg/m^2 or 35 kg/m^2 and significant comorbidity.[58–60] Surgical procedures mainly reduce stomach volume, complemented in some cases by a reduction of the absorptive surface of the alimentary tract, and often are associated with some degree of malabsorption. Currently, the three major types of procedures are stapled gastroplasty, adjustable gastric banding, and conventional Roux-en-Y gastric bypass.[61]

CLINICAL CONTROVERSY

The superiority of conventional Roux-en-Y bypass versus adjustable gastric banding in terms of efficacy, morbidity, and mortality is actively debated. However, given the nature of bariatric surgery and available alternatives, the probability that randomized controlled trials will be completed to answer these questions is low.

Gastroplasty and adjustable gastric banding are designed to reduce the volume of the stomach and thus restrict the rate of nutrient intake. Conventional bypass combines a restrictive approach with a degree of malabsorption induced by excluding 90% to 95% of the stomach, the entire duodenum, and a portion of the proximal jejunum. Conventional Roux-en-Y bypass yields greater and more long-lasting weight loss than the other two methods. Ultimately, reductions in total body weight of approximately 35% can be achieved. Less optimal weight loss, late weight gain, the need for surgical revision in 15% to 20% for outlet stenosis or severe reflux, and long-term failure rates of up to 80% have dampened interest in gastroplasty.[61] Similarly, gastric banding is plagued by frequent reoperation for stenosis and erosion or both of the band. Improvements in the peri- and postoperative care of gastric surgery patients has reduced morbidity and mortality with conventional bypass to approximately 10% and 1%, respectively.[61] Some of the most common early complications of conventional gastric bypass are deep venous thrombosis, anastomotic leaks, and wound infections. Approximately one-third of patients develop significant vitamin B_{12} and iron deficiency, with a large proportion demonstrating microcytic anemia. Dumping syndrome, characterized by colic, nausea, diarrhea, and bloating, does occur in a small number of patients and can complicate provision of drug therapy in some cases. Classically, Roux-en-Y gastric bypass was only performed as an open surgical procedure. However, recent developments in surgical technique have allowed this procedure to be performed via laparoscope.[60] Long-term results comparing the outcomes of open versus laparoscopic methods are not yet available. After experiencing weight loss, many gastric surgery patients are able to discontinue pharmacotherapy for glucose lowering, dyslipidemia, and hypertension. Frequently however, hypertension medications must be restarted at various time periods postsurgery, in spite of the fact that weight regain has not or has only minimally occurred. The reasons and mechanisms for this are unclear, but reiterate the need for intensive followup by all clinical specialties involved in the care of these patients.

Selection of the appropriate patients for surgery and subsequently identifying the most appropriate procedure for each patient is critical. The input of an experienced surgeon working with a multidisciplinary team is invaluable.

CLINICAL CONTROVERSY

The debate regarding the appropriateness of obesity pharmacotherapy remains heated, fueled by the recognized national need to treat a growing epidemic. Controversy about the standards by which to judge long-term outcomes studies, and the medical and litigious fallout from the failed use of fen-phen (fenfluramine-phentermine) and dexfenfluramine (Redux) have fueled the debate.

PHARMACOLOGIC THERAPY

5 The debate regarding the appropriateness of obesity pharmacotherapy remains heated, fueled by the recognized national need to treat a growing epidemic and the medical and litigious fallout from the failed use of fen-phen (fenfluramine-phentermine) and dexfenfluramine (Redux).[62,63] Strategies for the pharmacologic management of obesity have been focused on modulating central and/or peripheral sites that regulate human energy balance. Figure 148–4 depicts sites of action of these therapies within the energy intake, storage, and expenditure cycle. Table 148–4 lists the status of the most common classes of agents currently in use. Since the 1970s, numerous studies of the effects of central appetite suppressant agents on weight status have been completed.[64] The National Task

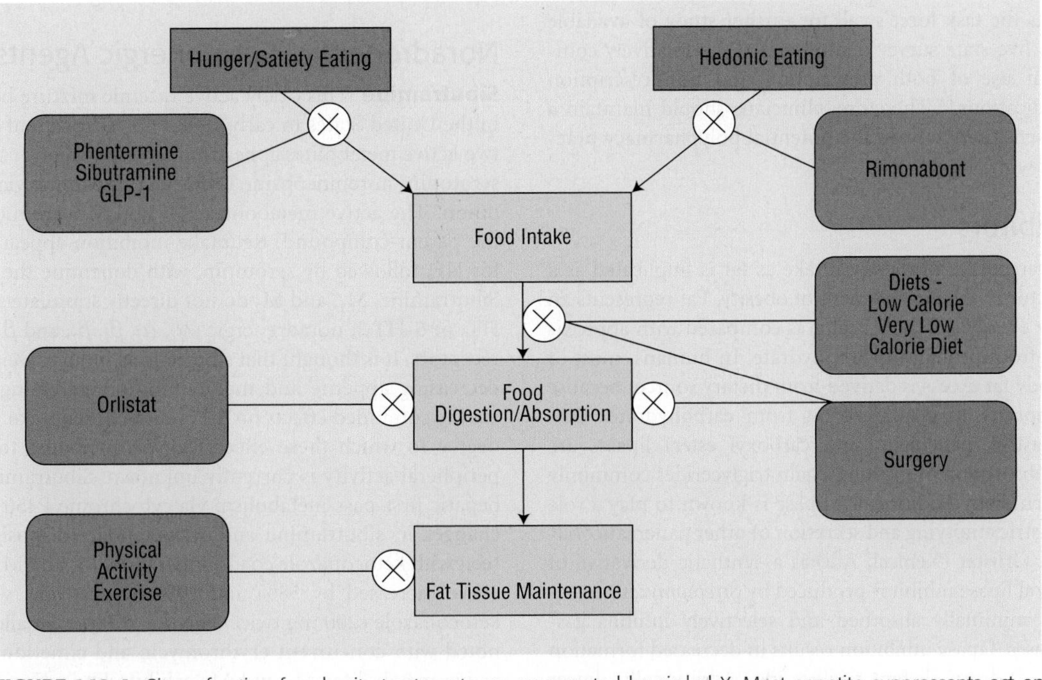

FIGURE 148-4. Sites of action for obesity treatments are represented by circled X. Most appetite suppressants act on hunger and satiety mechanisms, but the endocannabinoid antagomist rimonabont is an example of intervention that appears to affect hedonic properties of eating. Traditional diets act by limiting food intake, as does bariatric surgery. Orlistat interferes with fat absoprtion in the gut, while gastric bypass surgery interferes with absorption more generally.

TABLE 148-4 Pharmacotherapeutic Agents for Weight Loss

Class	Availability	Status	Daily Dosages (mg)
Gastrointestinal lipase inhibitor			
Orlistat (Xenical)	Rx	Long-term use	360
Noradrenergic/serotonergic agent			
Sibutramine (Meridia)	Rx	Long-term use	5–15
Noradrenergic agents			
Phendimetrazine (Prelu-2, Bontril, Plegine, X-Trazine)	Rx	Short-term use	70–105
Phentermine (Fastin, Oby-trim, Adipex-P, Ionamin)	Rx	Short-term use	15–37.5
Diethylpropion (Tenuate, Tenuate Dospan)	Rx	Short-term use	75
Cannabinoid receptor agent			
Rimonabant (Acomplia[a])	Rx	Approval pending in the United States	20

[a]Trade name in European markets.

Force on the Prevention and Treatment of Obesity concluded that short-term anorexic agent use was difficult to justify because of the predictable weight regain that occurs on discontinuation of pharmacotherapy.[65] However, long-term pharmacotherapy may have a place in the treatment of obesity for patients who have no obvious contraindications to available drug therapy.[24,66] Additionally, the American Association of Clinical Endocrinologists and the American College of Endocrinology have developed a guideline for multidisciplinary obesity team approach to the management of therapy.[67] More recently, the U.S. Preventive Services Task Force published an exhaustive summary of evidence related to screening and interventions for adult obesity that incorporates a graded assessment of obesity pharmacotherapy randomized controlled trials.[54] The discovery of cardiac valve disease in relation to serotonergic appetite suppressant use and its resulting multibillion dollar class action litigation affirms the task force's call for further study of available therapies.[62,63] A five-state survey demonstrated the relatively common concurrent use of both prescription and nonprescription weight loss medications.[68] Therefore, clinicians should maintain a high degree of sensitivity toward the potential polypharmacy practices of patients with obesity.

Lipase Inhibitors

Orlistat The percentage of dietary intake as fat is implicated as a contributing factor in the development of obesity. Fat represents an extremely dense energy source; 9 kcal/g as compared with approximately 4 kcal/g from protein or carbohydrate. In humans, most of accumulated body fat excess is derived from dietary sources because of a limited capacity to synthesize fat from carbohydrate. Gastrointestinal (gastric, pancreatic, and carboxyl ester) lipases are essential in the absorption of the long-chain triglycerides commonly found in Western diets. Additionally, lipase is known to play a role in facilitating gastric emptying and secretion of other pancreaticobiliary substances. Orlistat (Xenical, Alli) is a synthetic derivative of lipstatin, a natural lipase inhibitor produced by *Streptomyces toxytricini*. Orlistat is minimally absorbed and selectively inhibits gastrointestinal lipases. Lipase inhibition results in decreased formation of free fatty acids from dietary triglyceride. Additionally, lower luminal free fatty acid concentrations result in malabsorption of cholesterol. Orlistat induces weight loss by a persistent lowering of dietary fat absorption. Clinical studies employing orlistat as an adjunct to diet therapy demonstrate dose-dependent reductions in fat absorption. Up to 30% reduction in fat absorption occurred with daily doses of 360 mg.[11,14,69] No additional decreases in fat absorption occur with doses above 400 mg/day. The drug must be taken with foods that contain fat in order to exert its effect.

At least one gastrointestinal complaint (soft stools, abdominal pain/colic, flatulence, fecal urgency, or incontinence) is reported initially in up to 80% of individuals using orlistat. These complaints are most common in the first 1 to 2 months of therapy, are mild to moderate in severity, and tend to improve with continued orlistat use. Limiting dietary fat prior to initiation of orlistat therapy may be beneficial in decreasing initial gastrointestinal complaints. Orlistat-induced malabsorption of fat-soluble vitamins has been documented.[11,14,69] Therefore, vitamin supplementation should be considered during therapy with this agent. Orlistat does not appear to change the pharmacokinetic or dynamic profiles of numerous other agents including oral contraceptives, digoxin, glyburide, phenytoin, pravastatin, warfarin, nifedipine, captopril, atenolol, furosemide, and ethanol. A notable exception is cyclosporine, wherein case reports suggest significant decreases in cyclosporine serum concentrations with concurrent orlistat use.[69]

Overall, results from clinical trials demonstrate that orlistat effectively increases the amount of weight lost and decreases the amount of weight regained during medically supervised weight-loss programs.[11,14] Significant improvements in lipid profile, glucose control, and other markers of metabolism are seen in spite of the relatively small 2- to 4-kg differences in weight lost when using orlistat in addition to diet. In patients with impaired glucose tolerance, weight loss using orlistat significantly decreased the rate of conversion to type 2 diabetes. Additionally, improved glycemic control can be attained in patients with type 2 diabetes by inducing or increasing weight loss with orlistat in addition to diet management. In some cases, dosages or the number of agents required for glucose lowering may be deceased.[69] Orlistat is the first agent for the chronic treatment of obesity with an indication for use in adolescents aged 12 to 16 years. Finally, orlistat was recently approved in the United States for over-the-counter use without a prescription (trade name Alli, GlaxoSmithKline, Moon Township, PA) when ingested at a reduced daily dose of 180 mg.

Noradrenergic–Serotonergic Agents

Sibutramine This orally active racemic mixture became available in the United States in early 1998.[11,14,70] The parent compound and two active metabolites appear to increase synaptic concentrations of serotonin, norepinephrine (NE), and dopamine via reuptake inhibition. The active metabolites (M_1 and M_2) are more potent than the parent-compound. Reuptake inhibition appears to be greatest for NE, followed by serotonin, with dopamine the least inhibited. Sibutramine, M_1, and M_2 do not directly stimulate serotonergic (5-HT_1 or 5-HT_2), noradrenergic (α_1, α_2, β_1, β_2, and β_3), or dopamine receptors. It is thought that sibutramine induces weight loss by both decreasing appetite and maintaining or increasing thermogenesis via the combined effects on 5-HT and NE reuptake. In humans, the degree to which these effects can be attributed to central versus peripheral activity is currently unknown. Sibutramine is subject to hepatic first-pass metabolism via cytochrome P450 3A4. Moderate changes in sibutramine and/or metabolite disposition have been seen with ketoconazole coadministration. M_1 and M_2 area under the curve increased by 58% and 20%, respectively, with concurrent ketoconazole (200 mg twice daily for 7 days). Smaller changes were noted with concurrent erythromycin and cimetidine therapy. The active metabolites M_1 and M_2 exhibit elimination half-lives of 14 and 16 hours, respectively. Further metabolism of the active metabolites results in conjugates that are eliminated renally. The pharmacokinetics of sibutramine allow for once-daily oral dosing.

6 Sibutramine has been studied in clinical trials in doses from 1 to 30 mg daily and it demonstrates a relatively clear dose–response relationship. Weight loss from daily doses of 1 mg is, on average, no different than from placebo. The recommended starting dose is 10 mg daily, with a recommended dose range of 5 to 15 mg daily. Dry mouth, anorexia, insomnia, constipation, appetite increase, dizziness, and nausea were noted two- to threefold more frequently in sibutramine-treated subjects than in placebo-treated subjects. Statistically significant increases in both systolic and diastolic blood pressure, in the range of 2 mm mercury, and pulse rate have been noted with sibutramine use.[70] Baseline blood pressure should be established prior to beginning therapy, and close monitoring is required when using this agent. Sibutramine product labeling indicates that it should not be used in patients with a history of coronary artery disease, stroke, congestive heart failure, or arrhythmias. Like other centrally acting appetite suppressants, sibutramine should not be used in patients receiving monoamine oxidase (MAO) inhibitor therapies. Sibutramine is listed as a schedule IV prescription substance despite being noted as having no street value by recreational substance users. Primary pulmonary hypertension has not been reported with sibutramine use. Echocardiographic assessments of a small cohort of patients from clinical trials with approximately 6 months of exposure do not demonstrate the cardiac valve problems seen with the fenfluramine derivatives. Based on 12-month clinical trials, weight loss with sibutramine therapy appears to be most significant during the first 6 months of therapy. Twenty-nine percent of placebo-treated patients in these trials attained a 5% reduction in total body weight after 12 months whereas 56% and 65% of patients receiving 10 or 15 mg of sibutramine, respectively, achieved at least a 5% reduction in total body weight. A 10% reduction in body weight was achieved by 8% of placebo-treated patients, whereas 30% and 39% of those taking sibutramine 10 and 15 mg/day, respectively, acheived this level of weight reduction. As with other centrally active appetite suppressants, weight regain occurs with cessation of therapy.

Endocannabinoid System Agents

Rimonabant. During the last 20 years, arachidonic acid derivatives known as endocannabinoids were identified as endogenous substances that activate cannabinoid receptors.[71,72] A complex regulatory relationship exists between the endocannabinoid system, energy regulatory hormones, and neuropeptides.[71] The endocannabinoid system appears to be overactive in states of overweight and obesity. Additionally, the endocannabinoid system appears to be involved in the propagation of addictive behaviors related to ingestion of substances such as nicotine, cocaine, heroin, alcohol, and amphetamines.

Two distinct cannabinoid receptors are known and have been cloned, CB_1 and CB_2. The existence of a third, CB_3, is hypothesized.[72] These G-protein-coupled receptors have wide and differing tissue distribution. CB_1 receptors are found in high concentrations in brain and peripheral organs including; liver, gastrointestinal tract, adipocytes, skeletal and cardiac muscle.[71] Central and peripheral CB_1 receptors are involved in many aspects of energy balance; regulation of food intake, glucose and lipid metabolism and body composition. CB_2 receptors are mainly expressed within immune system tissues and are not currently recognized as affecting energy balance.

Rimonabant (SR141716A) first described in 1994 as an inhibitor of brain CB_1 receptors is now recognized as having potent central and peripheral effects on feeding, nutrient metabolism, and body composition.[14,72] An extensive series of randomized, double-blind, placebo-controlled clinical trials have been undertaken to assess rimonabant safety and efficacy for the treatment of obesity with and without comorbid diabetes and dyslipidemia. It is also being studied as an adjunct therapy for smoking cessation.

For weight-loss studies, rimonabant doses of 5 mg or 20 mg daily have been employed. Significant weight loss at 1 year over that with placebo occurs with both doses, approximately 2 kg with the 5-mg dose and 6 kg with the 20-mg dose. Notably, almost 60% of those receiving 20 mg of rimonabant sustained weight loss of greater than or equal to 5% of total body weight. Fewer patients, approximately 30%, achieved this goal at the 5-mg dose versus approximately 19% in placebo-treated arms. Significantly, about one-third of patients receiving 20 mg rimonabant sustained and maintained weight loss of greater than or equal to 10% of total body weight.

Statistically and clinically significant improvements in lipid profile have been noted with rimonabant exposure with increases in high-density lipoprotein and decreases in triglyceride concentrations. As with weight loss, the greatest effects are noted at rimonabant doses of 20 mg daily. In patients with comorbid type 2 diabetes, marked improvements in glycemic control were seen, with more than 40% of those receiving rimonabant 20 mg daily attaining hemoglobin A_{1c} levels of less than 6.5%. Weight loss produced by rimonabant can improve many of the significant comorbidities of obesity including effects on glycemia and lipids. Although these effects are expected with any form of weight loss, there is some evidence for additional mechanisms affecting these comorbidities with the endocannabinoid blockade.[72]

The FDA's Endocrinologic and Metabolic Drugs Advisory Committee in June 2007 agreed unanimously that rimonabant did not demonstrate a favorable enough risk-to-benefit profile to enable it to be approved for weight management in individuals with a BMI of ≥ 30 kg/m^2 or in individuals with a BMI of ≥ 27 kg/m^2 when accompanied by at least one comorbid condition.[73] The committee's concerns centered on what many concluded was a "clear" signal of increased risk of neurologic side effects—seizures, depression, anxiety, aggressiveness, and suicidal thoughts among patients randomized to rimonabant. Consequently, Sanofi-Aventis will have to gather more detailed safety information about rimonabant over the long-term, in larger patient numbers, before it can request further consideration for approval for marketing in the United States.

Noradrenergic Agents

Phentermine Phentermine is structurally similar to amphetamine, but it has less-severe CNS stimulation and a lower abuse potential. Its mechanism of action is related to enhanced NE and dopamine neurotransmission. Phentermine is available in both immediate-release and sustained-release formulations. However, the value of sustained-release formulations are questionable based on the reported phentermine plasma half-life of 12 to 24 hours.[74] Phentermine is an effective adjunct to diet, exercise, and behavior modification for producing weight loss in excess of that seen with placebo.[75] Intermittent phentermine therapy appears to elicit comparable weight loss when compared with continuous use. However, most individuals experience weight regains during therapy and generally always after discontinuing use.[74] A single dose of 30 mg once daily in the morning provides effective appetite suppression throughout the day. Divided doses of 8 mg immediately prior to meals, however, are common. Doses above 30 mg daily do not improve effectiveness.[75] Evening or nighttime dosing should be avoided because of insomnia. Significant increases in blood pressure, palpitations, and arrhythmias can occur with phentermine administration. Use is not advisable in hypertensive patients and those with unstable cardiovascular function. The potential for hypertensive crisis with coadministration of phentermine and MAO inhibitors is noted in product labeling because of the documented cases of this syndrome seen with coadministration of amphetamine or noradrenergic derivatives and MAO inhibitors.[76] Similar warnings have been noted regarding concomitant use of tricyclic antidepressants, but this is less-well documented. With MAO inhibitors, a minimum washout time of 14 days prior to use of any adrenergic agent is suggested to avoid excessive adrenergic stimulation syndromes. Phentermine use is contraindicated in patients who are abusers of substances such as cocaine, phencyclidine, and methamphetamine, again because of the potential for excessive adrenergic stimulation syndromes and abuse potential. Mydriasis from adrenergic stimulation can worsen glaucoma, and patients diagnosed with glaucoma should not receive phentermine. Diabetic patients may experience altered insulin or oral hypoglycemic dosage requirements soon after beginning therapy and prior to any substantial weight loss.

Phentermine currently remains on the market as a short-term pharmacotherapy for obesity despite recognition of cardiac valvulopathy in a high percentage of patients who used phentermine in combination with fenfluramine derivatives. Phentermine remains one of the most widely prescribed weight management medications in spite of product labeling that indicates short-term, monotherapy use only.[77] This usage pattern persists in spite of the current federal recommendations that promote only long-term drug intervention when obesity pharmacotherapy is appropriate.[51]

Mazindol Chemically distinct from amphetamines and phentermine, mazindol's tricyclic structure resulted in amphetamine-like appetite suppression.[11] Despite demonstrated efficacy as a short-term therapy for weight reduction, mazindol is no longer available in the United States.

Diethylpropion Diethylpropion stimulates norepinephrine release from presynaptic storage granules. Increased adrenergic neurotransmitter concentrations activate hypothalamic centers, which result in decreased appetite and food intake. This drug undergoes extensive first-pass hepatic metabolism. Active metabolites are eliminated renally and account for approximately 70% of the administered dose. The elimination half-life of these metabolites is approximately 8 hours.[75] Less than 10% of the parent compound is recovered in urine. No specific dosing recommendations exist for use in patients with renal or hepatic insufficiency. Diethylpropion can be taken in divided daily doses, generally 25 mg three times daily before meals. An extended-release formulation is also employed by some clinicians, usually as 75 mg taken once daily in the morning or midmorning. Both dosing regimens are effective in achieving short-term weight loss in excess of placebo.[11] Complaints of insomnia increase if late afternoon dosing is used. Diethylpropion causes less CNS stimulation than mazindol and generally causes less insomnia than phentermine. Patients with severe hypertension or significant cardiovascular disease should not receive diethylpropion. Diabetic patients may experience decreased insulin or oral hypoglycemic dosage requirements soon after beginning therapy and prior to any substantial weight loss. More frequent blood glucose self-monitoring and medical follow-up are warranted when treating diabetic patients with diethylpropion.

Amphetamines Appetite suppressant effects of the amphetamines were well recognized in the 1930s. Amphetamines activate central noradrenergic receptor systems as well as dopaminergic pathways at higher doses, by stimulating neurotransmitter release. Increases in blood pressure and mild bronchodilation are attributed to peripheral α- and β-receptor activation. The powerful stimulant and addictive potential of the amphetamines relative to other available agents has resulted in their general avoidance for the treatment of obesity.

Serotonergic Agents

Serotonin is an important neurotransmitter involved in many human physiologic systems. Sleep–wake cycles, sensitivity to pain, blood pressure, mood, and eating behaviors have links to serotonin activity. Increasing central serotonin levels decreases the amount of food consumed and prolongs the time between food intake. Some serotonergic agents increase central serotonin concentrations via stimulating release of presynaptic stores and/or inhibition of reuptake into storage granules. Additionally, either the parent compound or metabolites of these agents also may stimulate postsynaptic 5-HT receptors directly. Peripheral serotonin effects that have an impact on appetite, such as slowing gastric motility, also have been described. A major distinction between serotonergic and noradrenergic anorexiants is that serotonergic agents lack the central stimulant effects and thus the abuse potential seen with the noradrenergic compounds.[11,14] Conversely, decreased wakefulness, altered sleep patterns, and changes in affect can be seen.

Antidepressants: Selective Serotonin Reuptake Inhibitors It is interesting to note that some of the serotonergic appetite-suppressing agents were first studied as antidepressants and then noted subsequently to have effects on weight. As a class, the serotonin reuptake inhibitors generally are weight neutral as opposed to other commonly used compounds such as the tricyclic antidepressants (see Chap. 71). Patients receiving fluoxetine (60 mg/day) demonstrate initial weight loss of up to 2 to 4 kg on average, but weight regain occurs despite continued medication use such that no difference is noted between fluoxetine and placebo over periods of up to 1 year.[14] A direct relationship exists between amount of weight lost and the sum of fluoxetine and norfluoxetine plasma concentrations. Higher plasma concentrations are associated with greater weight loss. The antidepressant serotonin reuptake inhibitors are not approved by the FDA as weight management agents and are not recommended currently for routine treatment of obesity. Some practitioners have prescribed these agents for the treatment of obesity "off label" either alone or in combination with phentermine. The safety and efficacy of phentermine-serotonin reuptake inhibitor combinations is unclear. A case report of adverse experiences (e.g., impaired mentation, tremor, hyperreflexia, and gastrointestinal symptoms) with unintentional concurrent use of phentermine and fluoxetine reinforces the need for caution by prescribers of unlabeled combination therapy.[78] Serious adverse effects such as primary pulmonary hypertension and cardiac valve abnormalities in excess of background prevalence have not been reported in relation to selective serotonin reuptake inhibitor use for obesity therapy.

Not Recommended but of Historical Interest

Phenylpropanolamine Although commonly classified as a noradrenergic anorexic, phenylpropanolamine (PPA) is atypical with regard to its mechanism and site of action. PPA racemates, D- and L-norephedrine, have chemical structures quite similar to amphetamine.[11,14] PPA has been used for many years as a constituent of nonprescription appetite suppressants and various cough and cold preparations. However, because of persistent case reports of hemorrhagic stroke related to PPA exposure, the U.S. Food and Drug Administration and pharmaceutical manufacturers partnered to complete a case-control study known as the Hemorrhagic Stroke Project during the 1990s. In October 2000, the Nonprescription Drugs Advisory Committee discussed the Hemorrhagic Stroke Project report and concluded that PPA was not safe for continued use. Based on the accepted background prevalence of stroke and the odds ratios defined by the Hemorrhagic Stroke Project report, Kernan et al. estimate that 1 woman may experience PPA-related stroke for every 107,000 to 3,268,000 women exposed to PPA appetite suppressants.[79] Despite the very low risk of hemorrhagic stroke, the FDA believes that a favorable risk-to-benefit ratio no longer exists for any PPA-containing products. As such, PPA-containing products have either been reformulated without PPA or removed from the market in the United States. However, because of the voluntary nature of the request for reformulation or removal from the market, the FDA recommends that all consumers review product labels to ensure the absence of PPA from weight loss and cough or cold preparations.[80]

Ephedrine Ephedrine appears to suppress appetite and increase energy expenditure via release of presynaptic norepinephrine and direct stimulation of thermogenic β-adrenergic receptors.[14] The efficiency of ephedrine stimulation is somewhat blunted by physiologic feedback systems involving adenosine and various prostaglandins. This notion has stimulated research to characterize the effect of ephedrine in the presence of adenosine and prostaglandin antagonists such as caffeine and aspirin.[14] Ephedrine in combination with caffeine has enhanced appetite suppression and thermogenesis as compared with placebo and other anorectics over time periods of up to 6 months. Oral doses of 20 mg ephedrine and 200 mg caffeine up to three times daily have been studied. The spectrum of side effects with ephedrine and ephedrine-caffeine combinations is similar to that seen with other noradrenergic agents. Side effects are more notable at higher doses and most commonly include tremor, agitation, nervousness, increased sweating, and insomnia; palpitations and tachycardia have also been reported. Patients with diabetes, hypertension, or cardiovascular disease (including arrhythmic conditions) should not self-medicate with ephedrine-containing products without evaluation by a qualified physician. Ephedrine is available both with and without a prescription; neither form is labeled by the FDA for use as an obesity therapy.

■ COMPLEMENTARY AND ALTERNATIVE THERAPIES

❼ Many individuals choose to undertake weight-loss regimens that incorporate the ingestion of herbal, natural, or food supplement products without medical monitoring. It is important to remember that the FDA does not regulate the manufacture and labeling of these products. Some herbal and food supplement diet agents contain pharmacologically active substances that should be used with caution or avoided in obese patients with conditions such as diabetes, hypertension, and significant cardiovascular disease. Another problem with many of these marketed products is the lack of consistency in labeling versus actual product content. Table 148–5 lists some of the common constituents found in many of these products.

Chromium

The inclusion of chromium as an effective agent for weight loss is unclear. The hexavalent form of this trace element is thought to be carcinogenic, whereas the trivalent form found in human food sources is essentially nontoxic.[81] Chromium is considered an essential nutrient and experimentally in animals is an insulin cofactor active in carbohydrate, protein, and lipid metabolism.[81] In humans, insulin resistance has been reported in a few cases of apparent severe chromium deficiency during long-term total parenteral nutrition (see Chap. 145). Currently, there is no reliable means of assessing total body chromium status, making diagnosis of deficiency difficult. The tryptophan metabolite, picolinic acid, forms a complex with trivalent chromium, which improves bioavailability. Food sources with highly available chromium include brewer's yeast, calf liver, American cheese, and wheat germ.[81] A double-blind, placebo-controlled study of chromium picolinate as a supplement to aerobic exercise in the treatment of obesity failed to demonstrate any effectiveness.[82]

TABLE 148-5 Herbal/Natural Products and Food Supplements Used for Weight Loss[a]

Herbal/Natural/Food Supplements	Active Moiety	Proposed Mechanism
Chromium picolinate	Chromium	Unclear
St. John's wort	Hypericin	Serotonergic/monoamine oxidase inhibition
Hoodia	P57	Unclear
White willow bark	Salicylate	Inhibit norepinephrine breakdown
Calcium pyruvate	Pyruvate	Unclear
Guarana extract	Caffeine	Noradrenergic
Various tea extracts	Caffeine	Noradrenergic
Garcinia gambogia extract (citrin)	Hydroxycitric acid	Unclear
Chitosan	Cationic polysaccharide	Block fat absorption

[a]Safety and efficacy not documented.

Ephedra Alkaloids

Based on the known effects of ephedrine, dietary supplements claiming weight management effects have employed plant sources of ephedra alkaloids. Various parts of the Ephedraceae, ma huang, *Sida cordifolia*, and *Pinellia ternata* plants are known to produce ephedra alkaloids, including L-ephedrine, D-pseudoephedrine, L-norephedrine, D-norpseudoephedrine, L-*N*-methylephedrine, and D-*N*-methylpseudoephedrine.[83] Common names routinely included in dietary supplement labeling for these alkaloid sources include joint fir, popotillo, country mallow, sea grape, and yellow horse. From 1994 through July 1997, the FDA received more than 800 reports of serious adverse events, including seizures, stroke, and death, coincident with ephedrine alkaloid-containing dietary supplement use. An in-depth review of 140 reports of adverse events related to ephedrine alkaloid-containing dietary supplements demonstrated that approximately half the reports involved cardiovascular symptoms.[84] As of 2004, the FDA has determined that all sources of ephedra alkaloids must be excluded from dietary supplements because they present an unreasonable high health risk.[85]

St. John's Wort

A perennial flowering plant (*Hypericum perforatum*), St. John's wort has been employed as a medicinal herb for thousands of years. Its use in weight loss and herbal supplements probably is based on the proposed effects of its constituent naphthodianthrones (hypericin and pseudohypericin). These are thought to be inhibitors of MAO and would be expected to increase synaptic concentrations of monoamines such as serotonin and NE. Consistent with these assumptions, *Hypericum* extracts appear to be more effective than placebo in the treatment of depression.[86] However, in vitro studies have not been able to substantiate direct MAO inhibition at physiologic hypericin concentrations, and recognized antidepressant effects may be due to other constituents.[87] The risks of concurrent use of *Hypericum* derivatives and other adrenergic and serotonergic compounds have not been characterized. Currently, St. John's wort has not been studied with respect to its role in obesity management and cannot be recommended for routine use in self-management of obesity.

Pyruvate

Pyruvate is a commonly listed ingredient in many herbal weight management preparations. Multiple salt forms are used, including sodium, magnesium, potassium, and calcium. Other names include α-ketopropionic acid, 2-oxypropanoic acid, and acetylformic acid. Pyruvate is a three-carbon intermediate formed during normal glucose metabolism and/or during glycolysis. It is advertised in the lay press for its ability to "increase metabolism" and thus promote weight loss. Objective data documenting these effects are lacking.[88,89] Although most pyruvate nutritional weight management supplements contain less than 2 g per dose, large exposures (more than 20 g) are known to cause noticeable gastrointestinal side effects, including bloating and diarrhea.

Hoodia

Hoodia is a desert cactus of the Apocynaceae plant family. Natives indigenous to the Kalahari Desert are purported to consume the stems and roots of this plant for their appetite suppressant effects. Other names appearing on product labels include Kalahari cactus, Hoodia cactus or extract, Hoodia gordonii cactus, and Kalahari diet. Hoodia extract, sometimes also referred to as P57, is rumored to elicit weight loss; however, no peer-reviewed reports of effectiveness are currently available.

White Willow Bark

White willow bark is a source of salicylate, a prostaglandin inhibitor. Prostaglandin inhibition may enhance adrenergic stimulation via inhibition of NE breakdown.

Guarana Extract and Various Tea Extracts

Guarana and tea are sources of caffeine that have inherent adrenergic properties and increase the effects of stimulant substances such as ephedrine or ephedra alkaloids.

Chitosan

Chitosan is a cationic polysaccharide, specifically a partially *N*-deacetylated form of chitin. This nonhydrolyzable fiber exhibits properties similar to those of cellulose. In vitro and preclinical data indicate that chitosan may be effective in blocking absorption of fat from the gut. It has been suggested that orally administered chitosan may be an effective weight-reduction agent by blocking calories ingested as fat. Chitosan is a major constituent in several heavily advertised weight-management food supplements and nonprescription preparations. However, a small number of properly randomized and blinded or open-label investigations currently demonstrate that orally administered chitosan is not an effective inhibitor of fat absorption in humans.[88] While further research may be warranted with respect to the appropriate dose in humans needed to impair fat absorption, current claims of chitosan effectiveness in humans are unsubstantiated.

■ PHARMACOECONOMIC CONSIDERATIONS

There are few data regarding economic consequences of treating obesity. One study evaluated the savings in prescription costs following a 12-week weight reduction program in 40 type 2 diabetic patients. Patients lost an average of 33.7 lb over the study period. A cost analysis was completed on 32 of 40 patients who were taking antihypertensive and/or antidiabetic medications using the out-of-pocket costs for these medications at the beginning of the study and after 1 year. The patients sustained a mean weight loss of 19.8 lb over the next year. The average cost of these prescriptions at the beginning as compared to the 1-year followup was $63.30 versus $32.50 per month. The estimated annual average saving in prescription costs per patient was $443. A more objective assessment of costs related to orlistat use has been published based on data obtained from three peer-reviewed publications. In this report from the United Kingdom, the cost utility of orlistat was estimated at £46,000 (approximately $75,000) per quality-adjusted life-year gained. Sensitivity analysis from this report demonstrated marked variability in this estimate of £14,000 to £132,000 (approximately $23,000 to $215,200). The authors raised questions about the potential long-term value of pharmacotherapy for obesity.[90]

Finally, Martin et al. compared the costs associated with medical and surgical treatment of obesity.[91] Medical therapy groups received diet therapy only (no medications), and cost included weekly clinic visits for behavioral modification. A successful outcome was defined as loss of at least one-third of excess body weight above ideal body weight. They monitored all patients for 2 years and some for as long as 7 years so that long-term weight control could be addressed. As expected, the costs of surgery were much higher than medical therapy over the first 2 years ($24,000 vs. $3,000). However, when costs were extrapolated out to 6 years, the cost per pound lost for medical therapy exceeded surgical therapy (about $313 vs. $261 per pound lost). It is clear from the preceding data that weight loss can be expensive for the consumer. Prospectively designed cost-benefit or cost-effectiveness analyses are needed to determine if costs of weight loss therapy or surgery are balanced by lower costs of hospitalizations for other medical problems associated with obesity or the additional life years gained. Quality-of-life measures also need to be taken into consideration when evaluating these types of data.

Third-party payor and insurance reimbursement for provision of obesity treatment services continues to be inconsistent. However, these issues are under active discussion and specific information regarding reimbursement for obesity treatment from multiple different perspectives including the Centers for Medicaid and Medicare Services and the IRS are freely available via the Web.[92–94]

■ EVALUATION OF THERAPEUTIC OUTCOMES

Monitoring the Care Plan

Outcome Measures Assessment of patient progress should be documented in a healthcare setting once or twice monthly for 1 to 2 months and then monthly thereafter.[24,67] Each encounter should document weight, WC, BMI, blood pressure, medical history, and patient assessment of obesity medication tolerability.[24,67] Chronic use of obesity medications should be consistent with the approved product labeling. Medication therapy should be discontinued after 3 to 4 months if the patient has failed to demonstrate weight loss or maintenance of prior weight. A recent American Association of Clinical Endocrinologists/American College of Endocrinology statement on obesity provides a patient evaluation checklist, a validated survey of general well-being, and sample informed consent that could be used in screening and followup of patients receiving obesity pharmacotherapy as part of a weight loss program.[67] Additionally, numerous tools for both patient and practitioner are readily available through the Department of Human Services, NIH-NHLIB Obesity Education Initiative, and several other agencies.[10] The Short Form 36 (SF-36) also has been used as a quality-of-life evaluation tool for obese patients undergoing programmatic weight loss. Quarterly assessments of well-being and quality of life using validated assessment tools can be helpful in objectively quantifying the effectiveness of therapy, as well as potential drug-induced side effects (e.g., depression).[67]

Diabetic patients receiving weight loss medication require more intense medical monitoring and self-monitoring of blood glucose. Some centrally acting weight-loss agents, such as the serotonergic agents, have direct effects that immediately improve glucose tolerance, even prior to significant weight loss. Insulin therapy therefore may need to be adjusted with the start of obesity medication therapy. Peripherally active agents, such as orlistat, have also been shown to decrease oral hypoglycemic agent requirements in type 2 diabetic patients.[69] However, this effect was noted later in therapy and correlated more directly with weight loss. Some diabetic patients may require daily telephone contact with a healthcare provider to assist in adjusting their hypoglycemic therapy. Weekly patient visits to a healthcare setting may be necessary for 1 to 2 months until the effects of diet, exercise, and weight loss medication become more predictable. As frequent as quarterly assessment of hemoglobin A_{1c} may be appropriate in type 2 diabetics who lose weight to aid in adjustment of hypoglycemic therapy. Lipid profiles can normalize or improve with weight loss. Lipid status should be assessed semiannually or annually in patients with hyperlipidemia to determine need for continued hyperlipidemia therapies. Weight loss also can result in normalization of blood pressure in hypertensive obese patients.

Assessment of appropriateness of antihypertensive therapy should occur with each followup visit.

An expert committee of the National Heart, Lung, and Blood Institute of the National Institutes of Health has completed an extensive summary of clinical guidelines for the assessment and treatment of obesity.[51] This report provides guidance with evidence-based, graded assessment and treatment recommendations from an extensive meta-analysis of the available obesity literature. The evaluation and management of a patient with obesity requires careful clinical, biochemical, and if necessary, psychological evaluation. The evaluation must include an assessment of current medical conditions and medications the patient uses. Clearly, a multidisciplinary team including, but not limited to, a physician, nutritionist, psychologist, and pharmacist best achieves this. The algorithm in Figure 148–3 shows an approach to determining appropriate types of treatment for the overweight individual. The decision to treat any overweight/obese patient depends on the degree and distribution of obesity present, the motivation of the patient to lose weight, and the potential benefits and risks of weight loss. The initial step in this process should be to verify the presence of clinically significant excess body weight. In the clinical setting, this is done most often by measuring height, weight, and WC of the individual and calculating BMI. If the BMI is greater than 25 kg/m^2 and/or WC is greater than 40 inches for males or 35 inches for females, it is likely that the patient will benefit from weight maintenance or loss. The next step is to assess whether the patient actually is motivated to lose weight. No matter what the treatment options are, they all require significant effort on the part of the patient to change lifestyle and comply with the management plan. If it is clear that the patient is not yet ready to meet these expectations, then early counseling will reduce the chance of frustration for the patient, clinician, and in some cases other family members. This does not exclude the possibility of educating the patient about potential risks of obesity and the benefits of weight loss. This type of basic information in certain cases can lead to a significant change in motivation and desire to lose weight and improved compliance.

Pharmacotherapy may be appropriate for some overweight individuals (e.g., those with a BMI of 30 kg/m^2 or more without weight-related, immediate life-threatening medical conditions). It also should be considered for those with BMI of 27 kg/m^2 or more or an increased WC who have two or more risk factors. From the healthcare providers' perspective, drug therapy for obesity always should be considered as a supplement to an integrated program of diet, exercise, and behavior modification (including group support). A complete medical and medication history is essential in determining appropriate obesity drug therapy. Consideration must be given to alcohol, nicotine, caffeine, and herbal or food supplement use as well as prescription and nonprescription drugs.

CONCLUSIONS

The prevalence of obesity has increased dramatically in the last 30 years. Obesity is determined by a combination of genetic and environmental factors. Epidemiologic studies provide evidence for a causative role of environmental factors in the development of obesity in those individuals who are genetically susceptible. Furthermore, there are clear differences in racial susceptibility to obesity and its complications such as diabetes. The precise role of genetic and environmental factors in the development is unknown. It is clear, though, that obesity is a lifelong condition. Currently, orlistat and sibutramine are available in the United States and are indicated for the long-term treatment of overweight and obesity. However, clinicians should keep in mind that long-term results over periods of 3 or more years regarding these therapies will require further research. Weight regain challenges many individuals regardless of the therapeutic modalities used, especially when treatment is stopped. Nevertheless, in recent years, increasingly effective treatments have been developed, and there has been recognition that long term therapy, including long-term drug therapy, should be the standard in treatment of this chronic disease. These pharmaceutical agents have augmented the role of lifestyle changes and diet and therefore serve a useful role as adjunct therapies for obesity.

Every patient seeking help for the management of obesity should be evaluated for secondary causes of obesity. Although a secondary cause is rare, it is important to identify and manage. Treatment of obesity needs to be individualized. It is important to consider factors such as patient desires, age, degree and duration of obesity, and the presence or absence of medical conditions both directly related to obesity and those which may have an impact on the therapeutic decisions. Whatever combinations of therapeutic modalities are used, it is clear that management is a lifelong process requiring patient support and careful monitoring for safety and efficacy.

ABBREVIATIONS

5-HT: 5-hydroxytryptamine (serotonin)

BMI: body mass index

BMR: basal metabolic rate

MAO: monoamine oxidase

NHANES: National Health and Nutrition Examination Survey

PPA: phenylpropanolamine

REE: resting energy expenditure

WC: waist circumference

REFERENCES

1. Hedley AA, Ogden CL, Johnson CL, Carroll MD, Curtin LR, Flegal KM. Prevalence of overweight and obesity among US children, adolescents, and adults, 1999–2002. JAMA 2004;291(23):2847–2850.
2. Crespo CJ, Smit E, Troiano RP, Bartlett SJ, Macera CA, Andersen RE. Television watching, energy intake, and obesity in US children: Results from the third National Health and Nutrition Examination Survey, 1988–1994. Arch Pediatr Adolesc Med 2001;155(3):360–365.
3. Hu FB, Willett WC, Li T, Stampfer MJ, Colditz GA, Manson JE. Adiposity as compared with physical activity in predicting mortality among women. N Engl J Med 2004;351(26):2694–2703.
4. Lissner L, Odell PM, D'Agostino RB, et al. Variability of body weight and health outcomes in the Framingham population. N Engl J Med 1991;324(26):1839–1844.
5. Stevens J, Cai J, Pamuk ER, Williamson DF, Thun MJ, Wood JL. The effect of age on the association between body-mass index and mortality. N Engl J Med 1998;338(1):1–7.
6. Finkelstein EA, Ruhm CJ, Kosa KM, Finkelstein EA, Ruhm CJ, Kosa KM. Economic causes and consequences of obesity. Annu Rev Public Health 2005;26:239–257.
7. Office of the Surgeon General. Overweight and obesity. 2003, *http://www.surgeongeneral.gov/topics/obesity/*.
8. U.S. Department of Health and Human Services. Healthy People 2010; Chapter 19 Nutrition and Overweight. *http://www.healthypeoplegov/Document/HTML/Volume2/19Nutritionhtm#_edn162.*
9. U.S. Preventive Services Task Force. Screening for obesity in adults: Recommendations and rationale. Ann Intern Med 2003;139(11):930–932.
10. U.S. Department of Health and Human Services, NIH-NHLBI. Obesity Education Initiative. 2003, *http://www.nhlbi.nih.gov/about/oei/index.htm.*
11. Li Z, Maglione M, Tu W, et al. Meta-analysis: Pharmacologic treatment of obesity. Ann Intern Med 2005;142(7):532–546.
12. Wadden TA, Berkowitz RI, Womble LG, et al. Randomized trial of lifestyle modification and pharmacotherapy for obesity. N Engl J Med 2005;353(20):2111–2120.
13. Lakka TA, Bouchard C, Lakka TA, Bouchard C. Physical activity, obesity and cardiovascular diseases. Handb Exp Pharmacol 2005;(170):137–163.

14. Ioannides-Demos LL, Proietto J, McNeil JJ, Ioannides-Demos LL, Proietto J, McNeil JJ. Pharmacotherapy for obesity. Drugs 2005;65(10):1391–1418.
15. Kuczmarski RJ, Carroll MD, Flegal KM, Troiano RP. Varying body mass index cutoff points to describe overweight prevalence among U.S. adults: NHANES III (1988 to 1994). Obes Res 1997;5(6):542–548.
16. Power C, Lake JK, Cole TJ. Body mass index and height from childhood to adulthood in the 1958 British born cohort. Am J Clin Nutr 1997;66(5):1094–1101.
17. Fernandez JR, Allison DB. Understanding racial differences in obesity and metabolic syndrome traits. Nutr Rev 2003;61(9):316–319.
18. Fernandez JR, Heo M, Heymsfield SB, et al. Is percentage body fat differentially related to body mass index in Hispanic Americans, African Americans, and European Americans? Am J Clin Nutr 2003;77(1):71–75.
19. Park YW, Allison DB, Heymsfield SB, Gallagher D. Larger amounts of visceral adipose tissue in Asian Americans. Obes Res 2001;9(7):381–387.
20. Hainer V, Stunkard A, Kunesova M, Parizkova J, Stich V, Allison DB. A twin study of weight loss and metabolic efficiency. Int J Obes Relat Metab Disord 2001;25(4):533–537.
21. Comuzzie AG. The emerging pattern of the genetic contribution to human obesity. Best Pract Res Clin Endocrinol Metab 2002;16(4):611–621.
22. Rankinen T, Zuberi A, Chagnon YC, et al. The human obesity gene map: The 2005 update. Obesity (Silver Spring) 2006;14(4):529–644.
23. Hill JO, Peters JC. Environmental contributions to the obesity epidemic. Science 1998;280(5368):1371–1374.
24. U.S. Department of Health and Human Services, NIH-NHLBI. Clinical Guidelines on the Identification, Evaluation, and Treatment of Overweight and Obesity in Adults; Practical Guide. 2003, *http://www.nhlbi.nih.gov/guidelines/obesity/ob_home.htm*.
25. Berthoud HR. Multiple neural systems controlling food intake and body weight. Neurosci Biobehav Rev 2002;26(4):393–428.
26. Magni P. Hormonal control of the neuropeptide Y system. Curr Protein Pept Sci 2003;4(1):45–57.
27. Halford JC, Cooper GD, Dovey TM. The pharmacology of human appetite expression. Curr Drug Targets 2004;5(3):221–240.
28. Glass MJ, Billington CJ, Levine AS. Naltrexone administered to central nucleus of amygdala or PVN. Neural dissociation of diet and energy. Am J Physiol Regul Integr Comp Physiol 2000;279(1):R86–R92.
29. Kirkham TC. Endocannabinoids in the regulation of appetite and body weight. Behav Pharmacol 2005;16(5–6):297–313.
30. Harvey J, Ashford ML. Leptin in the CNS. much more than a satiety signal. Neuropharmacology 2003;44(7):845–854.
31. Proietto J, Thorburn AW. The therapeutic potential of leptin. Expert Opin Investig Drugs 2003;12(3):373–378.
32. Zabeau L, Lavens D, Peelman F, Eyckerman S, Vandekerckhove J, Tavernier J. The ins and outs of leptin receptor activation. FEBS Lett 2003;546(1):45–50.
33. Juge-Aubry CE, Meier CA. Immunomodulatory actions of leptin. Mol Cell Endocrinol 2002;194(1–2):1–7.
34. Small CJ, Bloom SR. Gut hormones and the control of appetite. Trends Endocrinol Metab 2004;15(6):259–263.
35. Slentz CA, Duscha BD, Johnson JL, et al. Effects of the amount of exercise on body weight, body composition, and measures of central obesity: STRRIDE—A randomized controlled study. Arch Intern Med 2004;164(1):31–39.
36. Fogelholm M, Kukkonen-Harjula K. Does physical activity prevent weight gain: A systematic review. Obes Rev 2000;1:95–111.
37. Malone M, Malone M. Medications associated with weight gain. Ann Pharmacother 2005;39(12):2046–2055.
38. Astrup A, Caterson I, Zelissen P, et al. Topiramate: Long-term maintenance of weight loss induced by a low-calorie diet in obese subjects. Obes Res 2004;12(10):1658–1669.
39. Avram AS, Avram MM, James WD, Avram AS, Avram MM, James WD. Subcutaneous fat in normal and diseased states: 2. Anatomy and physiology of white and brown adipose tissue. J Am Acad Dermatol 2005;53(4):671–683.
40. de Souza CJ, Burkey BF. Beta 3-adrenoceptor agonists as anti-diabetic and anti-obesity drugs in humans. Curr Pharm Des 2001;7(14):1433–1449.
41. Collins S, Surwit RS. The beta-adrenergic receptors and the control of adipose tissue metabolism and thermogenesis. Recent Prog Horm Res 2001;56:309–328.
42. Arner P, Hoffstedt J. Adrenoceptor genes in human obesity. J Intern Med 1999;245(6):667–672.
43. Anonymous. Clinical guidelines on the identification, evaluation, and treatment of overweight and obesity in adults—The evidence report. National Institutes of Health. Obes Res 1998;2006;6(Suppl 2):51S–209S.
44. Fernandez JR, Shriver MD, Beasley TM, et al. Association of African genetic admixture with resting metabolic rate and obesity among women. Obes Res 2003;11(7):904–911.
45. Hubert HB, Feinleib M, McNamara PM, Castelli WP. Obesity as an independent risk factor for cardiovascular disease: A 26-year follow-up of participants in the Framingham Heart Study. Circulation 1983;67(5):968–977.
46. Poirier P, Giles TD, Bray GA, et al. Obesity and cardiovascular disease: Pathophysiology, evaluation, and effect of weight loss: An update of the 1997 American Heart Association Scientific Statement on Obesity and Heart Disease from the Obesity Committee of the Council on Nutrition, Physical Activity, and Metabolism. Circulation 2006;113(6):898–918.
47. Poirier P, Giles TD, Bray GA, et al. Obesity and cardiovascular disease: Pathophysiology, evaluation, and effect of weight loss. Arterioscler Thromb Vasc Biol 2006;26(5):968–976.
48. Williamson DF, Thompson TJ, Thun M, Flanders D, Pamuk E, Byers T. Intentional weight loss and mortality among overweight individuals with diabetes. Diabetes Care 2000;23(10):1499–1504.
49. Diamanti-Kandarakis E, Zapanti E. Insulin sensitizers and antiandrogens in the treatment of polycystic ovary syndrome. Ann NY Acad Sci 2000;900:203–212.
50. U.S. Department of Health and Human Services, NIH-NHLBI. Aim for a healthy weight; Information for Patients and Health Professionals. *http://www.nhlbi.nih.gov/health/public/heart/obesity/lose_wt/index.htm*.
51. U.S. Department of Health and Human Services, NIH-NHLBI. Clinical Guidelines on the Identification, Evaluation, and Treatment of Overweight and Obesity in Adults; Full Report. 2003, *http://www.nhlbi.nih.gov/guidelines/obesity/ob_home.htm*.
52. American Heart Association. Physical Activity and Healthy Eating Program for Women. *http://www.s2mw.com/choosetomove/index.html*.
53. Williamson DA, Perrin LA. Behavioral therapy for obesity. Endocrinol Metab Clin North Am 1996;25(4):943–954.
54. McTigue KM, Harris R, Hemphill B, et al. Screening and interventions for obesity in adults: Summary of the evidence for the U.S. Preventive Services Task Force. Ann Intern Med 2003;139(11):933–949.
55. National Institute of Diabetes and Digestive and Kidney Diseases (NIDDK) Health Information. Weight Loss and Control. 2003, *http://www.niddk.nih.gov/health/nutrit/nutrit.htm*.
56. Hays NP, Starling RD, Liu X, et al. Effects of an ad libitum low-fat, high-carbohydrate diet on body weight, body composition, and fat distribution in older men and women: A randomized controlled trial. Arch Intern Med 2004;164(2):210–217.
57. Daousi C, Dunn AJ, Foy PM, MacFarlane IA, Pinkney JH. Endocrine and neuroanatomic features associated with weight gain and obesity in adult patients with hypothalamic damage. Am J Med 2005;118(1):45–50.
58. Waitman JA, Aronne LJ. Obesity surgery: Pros and cons. J Endocrinol Invest 2002;25(10):925–928.
59. O'Brien PE, Dixon JB. Laparoscopic adjustable gastric banding in the treatment of morbid obesity. Arch Surg 2003;138(4):376–382.
60. Cottam DR, Mattar SG, Schauer PR. Laparoscopic era of operations for morbid obesity. Arch Surg 2003;138(4):367–375.
61. Brolin RE. Bariatric surgery and long-term control of morbid obesity. JAMA 2002;288(22):2793–2796.
62. Khan MA, Herzog CA, St.Peter JV, et al. The prevalence of cardiac valvular insufficiency assessed by transthoracic echocardiography in obese patients treated with appetite-suppressant drugs. N Engl J Med 1998;339(11):713–718.
63. AHP Diet Drug Settlement. 2006, *http://www.settlementdietdrugs.com/*.
64. Greenway FL, Caruso MK, Greenway FL, Caruso MK. Safety of obesity drugs. Exp Opin Drug Saf 2005;4(6):1083–1095.
65. National Task Force on the Prevention and Treatment of Obesity. Long-term pharmacotherapy in the management of obesity. JAMA 1996;276(23):1907–1915.
66. Yanovski SZ. Pharmacotherapy for obesity—Promise and uncertainty. N Engl J Med 2005;353(20):2187–2189.
67. Bray GA. AACE/ACE Obesity statement. Endocr Pract 1997;3(3):163–208.

68. Blanck HM, Khan LK, Serdula MK. Use of nonprescription weight loss products: Results from a multistate survey. JAMA 2001;286(8):930–935.
69. Leung WY, Neil TG, Chan JC, Tomlinson B. Weight management and current options in pharmacotherapy: Orlistat and sibutramine. Clin Ther 2003;25(1):58–80.
70. Arterburn DE.Crane PK.Veenstra DL. The efficacy and safety of sibutramine for weight loss: A systematic review. Arch Intern Med 2004;164(9):994–1003.
71. Matias I, Bisogno T, Di M, V, Matias I, Bisogno T, Di Marzo V. Endogenous cannabinoids in the brain and peripheral tissues: Regulation of their levels and control of food intake. Int J Obes 2006;2007;30(Suppl 1):S7–S12.
72. Gelfand EV, Cannon CP. Rimonabant: A cannabinoid receptor type 1 blocker for management of multiple cardiometabolic risk factors. J Am Coll Cardiol 2006;47(10):1919–1926.
73. Diet Drug Acomplia/Zimulti Dealt Blow as FDA Panel Says Keep It Off U.S. Market. *http://www.acompliareport.com/News/news-061807.htm*.
74. Bray GA, Greenway FL. Current and potential drugs for treatment of obesity. Endocr Rev 1999;20(6):805–875.
75. Silverstone T. Appetite suppressants. A review. Drugs 1992;43(6):820–836.
76. Dawson JK, Earnshaw SM, Graham CS. Dangerous monoamine oxidase inhibitor interactions are still occurring in the 1990s. J Accid Emerg Med 1995;12(1):49–51.
77. Stafford RS, Radley DC. National trends in antiobesity medication use. Arch Intern Med 2003;163(9):1046–1050.
78. Bostwick JM, Brown TM. A toxic reaction from combining fluoxetine and phentermine. J Clin Psychopharmacol 1996;16(2):189–190.
79. Kernan WN, Viscoli CM, Brass LM, et al. Phenylpropanolamine and the risk of hemorrhagic stroke. N Engl J Med 2000;343(25):1826–1832.
80. Food and Drug Administration. Phenylpropanolamine (PPA) information page. 2006, *http://www.fda.gov/cder/drug/infopage/ppa/default.htm*.
81. National Research Council. Trace Elements. Recommended Dietary Allowances, 10th ed. Washington, DC: National Academy Press, 1998: 195–246.
82. Trent LK, Thieding-Cancel D. Effects of chromium picolinate on body composition. J Sports Med Phys Fitness 1995;35(4):273–280.
83. Betz JM, Gay ML, Mossoba MM, Adams S, Portz BS. Chiral gas chromatographic determination of ephedrine-type alkaloids in dietary supplements containing Ma Huang. J AOAC Int 1997;80(2):303–315.
84. Haller CA, Benowitz NL. Adverse cardiovascular and central nervous system events associated with dietary supplements containing ephedra alkaloids. N Engl J Med 2000;343(25):1833–1838.
85. Department of Health and Human Services, Food and Drug Administration. Final rule declaring dietary supplements containing ephedrine alkaloids as adulterated because they represent an unreasonable risk. Fed Regist 2004;69(28):6788–6854.
86. Linde K, Ramirez G, Mulrow CD, Pauls A, Weidenhammer W, Melchart D. St John's wort for depression—An overview and meta-analysis of randomised clinical trials. BMJ 1996;313(7052):253–258.
87. Cott JM. In vitro receptor binding and enzyme inhibition by *Hypericum perforatum* extract. Pharmacopsychiatry 1997;30(Suppl 2):108–112.
88. Pittler MH, Ernst E, Pittler MH, Ernst E. Dietary supplements for body-weight reduction: A systematic review. Am J Clin Nutr 2004;79(4):529–536.
89. Koh-Banerjee PK, Ferreira MP, Greenwood M, et al. Effects of calcium pyruvate supplementation during training on body composition, exercise capacity, and metabolic responses to exercise. Nutrition 2005;21(3):312–319.
90. Foxcroft DR, Milne R. Orlistat for the treatment of obesity: Rapid review and cost-effectiveness model. Obes Rev 2000;1:121–126.
91. Martin LF, Tan TL, Horn JR, et al. Comparison of the costs associated with medical and surgical treatment of obesity. Surgery 1995;118(4):599–606.
92. Porter S. Dealing with obesity: Reimbursement remains an obstacle. American Academy of Family Physicians. FP Report: December 2000;6(12). *http://www.aafp.org/fpr/2001200/10.html*.
93. Centers for Medicare & Medicaid Services. Obesity as an Illness (#CAG-00108N). Medicare Coverage Policy, National Coverage Determinations: Tracking Sheet and Coverage Issues Manual, sections 35–26,35–33. *http://www.cms.hhs.gov/mcd/viewtrackingsheet.asp?id=57*.
94. Internal Revenue Service. Publication 502: Medical and Dental Expenses for Use in Preparing 2005 Returns. 2005, *www.irs.gov*.

GLOSSARY

2,3-Bisphosphoglycerate: An intermediate in the Rapoport-Luebering shunt, formed between 1,3-bisphosphoglycerate and 3-phospho-glycerate; an important regulator of the affinity of hemoglobin for oxygen.

5-α-reductase: Enzyme responsible for conversion of testosterone to its active metabolite dihydrotesterone. Two types of this enzyme exist. Type 2 is predominant in prostate cells.

α-Amino-3-hydroxy-5-methylisoxazole-4-propionate: See *AMPA.*

α-Hydroxy acids: Exfoliating products such as lactic, glycolic, malic, mandelic, and tartaric acid used in cosmetics.

β-Hydroxy acid: Salicylic acid.

γ-Aminobutyric acid (GABA): The major inhibitory neurotransmitter in the central nervous system.

γ-Aminobutyric acid ($GABA_A$) receptors: Postsynaptic ionotropic receptors that bind to GABA and result in Cl^- influx and neuronal hyperpolarization. GABA is the main inhibitory neurotransmitter in the brain, and $GABA_A$ receptors mediate fast CNS inhibitory neurotransmission.

Abscess: A purulent collection of fluid separated from surrounding tissue by a wall comprised of inflammatory cells and adjacent organs. It usually contains necrotic debris, bacteria, and inflammatory cells.

Abstinence: Refraining from the indulgence in something, as sexual intercourse or substances, by one's own choice. The absence of genital contact that could permit a pregnancy (i.e., penile penetration into the vagina).

Acanthosis: Increased thickness of the prickle cell layer of the skin.

Acetabular: Relating to the acetabulum, the hollow, cuplike portion of the pelvis into which the head of the thigh bone (femur) fits.

Achalasia: Problem that occurs when a ring of muscle fibers, such as a sphincter of the esophagus, fail to relax.

Acne: Inflammatory eruption of the sebaceous gland.

Acnegenicity: Product effect that causes irritation of follicles resulting in papules and pustules.

Acquired resistance: See *Secondary resistance.*

Acromegaly: A pathologic condition characterized by excessive production of growth hormone.

Activities of daily living: Dressing, bathing, getting around inside the home, feeding, toileting, and grooming. See also *Instrumental activities of daily living.*

Acute coronary syndrome (ACS): Ischemic chest discomfort at rest most often accompanied by ST-segment elevation, ST-segment depression, or T-wave inversion on the 12-lead electrocardiogram and caused by plaque rupture and partial or complete occlusion of the coronary artery by thrombus. Acute coronary syndromes include infarction and unstable angina. Former terms used to describe types of ACS include *Q-wave myocardial infarction, non–Q-wave myocardial infarction,* and *unstable angina.*

Acute pain: Can be a useful physiologic process warning individuals of disease states and potentially harmful situations. Severe, unremitting, undertreated, acute pain, when it outlives its biologic usefulness, can produce many deleterious effects (e.g., psychological problems). It usually subsides when the healing process decreases the pain-producing stimuli.

Acute pancreatitis: Acute inflammation of the pancreas that can be mild with minimal or no organ dysfunction or severe with organ failure and local complications.

Acute stress disorder: A disorder characterized by anxiety, dissociative, and other symptoms that occurs within 1 month after exposure to an extreme traumatic stressor.

Acute tubular necrosis: Acute renal failure as the result of renal tubular epithelial cell damage, which can be caused by either direct toxic or ischemic effects of drugs.

Adaptive functioning: Individual effectiveness coping with everyday stressors compared to a peer with similar background, and socioeconomic and psychosocial opportunities.

Adaptive inflammation: Inflammatory pain that promotes the shifting from prevention of tissue damage to promotion of healing.

Addiction: A primary, chronic, neurobiologic disease, with genetic, psychosocial, and environmental factors influencing its development and manifestations. It is characterized by behaviors that include one or more of the following five Cs: *c*hronicity, impaired *c*ontrol over drug use, *c*ompulsive use, *c*ontinued use despite harm, and *c*raving.

Adjuvant analgesics: Agents that are useful in the treatment of pain but are usually not classified as analgesics.

Administrative burden: The demands placed on those who administer an instrument.

Adolescents: Pediatric patients who are 12 to 16 years of age.

Adoptive immunotherapy: Administration of immune cells for the purpose of cancer treatment.

Adrenergic: Neuronal or neurologic activity caused by neurotransmitters such as epinephrine, norepinephrine, and dopamine.

Adrenocorticotropic hormone (ACTH): A polypeptide hormone secreted by the anterior pituitary that controls secretion of cortisol from the adrenal glands.

Adverse drug events: Injuries resulting from administration of a drug or other circumstances surrounding use of the drug but not necessarily caused by the drug itself. See also *Adverse drug reaction.*

Adverse drug reaction: Any noxious, unintended, and undesired effect of a drug that occurs at doses used in humans for prophylaxis, diagnosis, or therapy.

Affect: Pattern of behaviors that a clinician can observe that expresses a person's current state of emotion.

Afterload: The pressure or the *load* the heart must generate to eject blood into the systemic circulation. Although approximated by the systemic vascular resistance, it is a complex measure that includes blood viscosity, aortic impedance, and ventricular wall thickness. Along with preload, it is an important determinant of cardiac output.

Aganglionosis: The state of being without ganglia.

Agnosia: Cardinal symptom of Alzheimer's disease; inability to recognize or identify a familiar object in the absence of impaired sensory function.

Agoraphobia: Anxiety about, or avoidance of, places or situations from which escape might be difficult (or embarrassing) or in which help might not be available in the event of having a panic attack or panic-like symptoms.

Akathisia: The sensation of inner restlessness resulting in the need to make movements such as pacing or moving the legs. Akathisia has subjective and objective components.

Albumin: The major protein in plasma, with a molecular weight of 65 kDa.

Albuminuria: A condition where a large amount of albumin (>300 mg/day) is present in the urine, often indicating glomerular damage in the kidney.

Alcohol ablation: Alcohol ablation of the septum is a nonsurgical procedure to improve outflow tract obstruction. It is a percutaneous catheter-based method to decrease septal thickness by therapeutic myocardial infarction.

Alcoholism: A chronic, progressive, and potentially fatal biogenic and psychosocial disease characterized by tolerance and physical dependence and manifested by a total loss of control, as well as diverse personality changes and social consequences.

Algorithm (treatment algorithm): Identifies and specifies sequences for treatment alternatives, with specific options and tactics for care. Based on scientific data and on expert consensus in areas where there is little scientific data, algorithms are divided into stages so that the simplest, most efficacious, and best-tolerated treatments available are tried first. If results are not optimal, treatment advances to the next stage. Unless a patient's illness fails to improve sufficiently with early stage treatments, he or she is spared treatments that are more complex, that might be less well tolerated, or that have more potential for drug interactions or serious side effects. Algorithms recommend key decision points in treatment decision making.

Allergic interstitial nephritis: Inflammation of the interstitial region of the kidney often associated with acute onset of renal insufficiency.

Allergic salute: Constant upward rubbing of the nose as a result of allergies.

Allergic shiners: Dark circles under the eyes as a result of nasal congestion leading to venous pooling.

Allodynia: Painful response to normally non-noxious stimuli.

Allogeneic transplantation: Transfer of cells between different individuals.

Allograft: An organ or tissue transplant from one human to another.

Alloimmunization: Rapid consumption of transfused platelets through an immune-mediated reaction.

Alternate forms: All modes of administration other than the mode for which the instrument was originally developed.

Amenorrhea: Lack of menstruation or the abnormal ending of the female menstrual cycle.

American Urological Association (AUA) Symptom Index: A validated questionnaire of seven questions that can be used by patients to assess the bothersomeness of their voiding symptoms. The total score range is 0 to 35. Higher scores are consistent with severely bothersome symptoms.

Amnesia: A pathologic impairment of memory.

AMPA/kainate receptors: Two of three types of ionotropic postsynaptic glutamate receptors. These receptors are similar and are often considered together. On binding glutamate, these receptors permit the influx of sodium ions (Na^+) and results in brain excitation. These are one of the two primary receptors for excitatory neurotransmission in the brain.

Amygdala: A small almond-shaped temporal lobe structure that plays a role in emotions and fear control.

Anaphylactoid: Anaphylaxis-like reactions that do not involve immunoglobulin E (IgE)-mediated mechanisms.

Anaphylaxis: Acute, life-threatening allergic reaction involving multiple organ systems.

Anastomosis: The surgical connection of two tubular structures, such as blood vessels, in a transplanted organ.

Andropause: Refers to a number of symptoms associated with decreased testosterone production by the testes in aging men. The symptoms include decreased libido, increased body fat, depressed mood, and osteoporosis. The symptoms of andropause generally worsen as the patient ages. Andropause in men parallels menopause in women.

Anemia of chronic disease: Mild to moderate anemia not associated with blood loss or hemolysis. Usually with normal cell size. Can be seen with chronic inflammation (e.g., rheumatoid arthritis, chronic infection) or malignancy.

Anemia of chronic kidney disease: A decrease in red blood cell production caused by a deficiency in the hormone erythropoietin normally produced by progenitor cells of the kidney. As kidney function declines, less erythropoietin is available to stimulate red blood cell production (erythropoiesis) in the bone marrow. Contributing factors include iron deficiency and a shortened, red-blood-cell life span.

Aneuploid: Deviation by a whole number in the total number of chromosomes in a cell compared to normal (46 in humans).

Angioedema: An allergic reaction characterized by edema of a tissue such as the lips, eyes, mouth, joints, or other structures because of leak of fluid from blood vessels.

Anhedonia: A lack of pleasure or interest in usual activities.

Anisocytosis: Considerable variation in the size of cells that are normally uniform, especially with reference to red blood cells.

Ankylosis: Bony fusion resulting from chronic joint inflammation.

Anomia: Cardinal symptom of Alzheimer's disease; inability to name objects or to recognize names.

Anorexia nervosa: A psychiatric disorder in which patients present with a fear of being obese. These patients often express a dislike or lack of interest in food; it is most common in young females and can disrupt normal menstrual cycles. It is associated with poor medication treatment response and can result in fatal medical complications.

Antenatal: Time between conception and birth; same as prenatal.

Anterograde amnesia: Inability to remember events or actions that occur after taking a sedative hypnotic medication.

Antibiogram: A summary of antimicrobial susceptibilities.

Anticipatory anxiety: The fear of having an anxiety attack, which is often a trigger by itself; "fear of fear."

Anticoagulant: Any substance that inhibits, suppresses, or delays the formation of blood clots. These substances occur naturally and regulate the clotting cascade. Several anticoagulants have been identified in a variety of animal tissues and have been commercially developed for medicinal use.

Antigenic drift: The creation of antigenic variants by point mutations in the surface antigens, hemagglutinin and/or neuraminidase, of a particular subtype of influenza.

Antigenic shift: Occurs when an influenza virus acquires a new hemagglutinin and/or neuraminidase.

Antimicrobial cycling: A predetermined change in an antimicrobial recommendation for empiric therapy of a specific infection at a predetermined time.

Antimycotic: Inhibiting fungal growth.

Antithrombotic: A pharmacologic agent that prevents thrombus/clot formation. This category includes both antiplatelet agents and anticoagulants.

Anuria: Production of less than 50 mL of urine/day.

Anxiety: A state of apprehension, uncertainty, and fear resulting from the anticipation of a realistic or fantasized threatening event or situation that often impairs physical and psychological functioning.

Aortic stenosis: Aortic stenosis is the obstruction of blood flow across the aortic valve. This disorder has several etiologies: congenital unicuspid or bicuspid valve, rheumatic fever, and degenerative calcific changes of the valve.

Aphasia: Cardinal symptom of Alzheimer's disease; inability to generate or comprehend spoken language.

Aphthous ulcer: A small superficial area of ulceration within the gastrointestinal mucosa, typically found in the oral cavity.

Apical pulse: Point at the apex (bottom portion) of the heart impacts the chest wall.

Apoptosis: Programmed cell death.

Appendageal: Referring to hair, sweat glands, and nails.

Apraxia: Cardinal symptom of Alzheimer's disease; inability to carry out a motor task in the absence of impaired motor function.

Arteriovenous (AV) fistula: In hemodialysis, a vascular access surgically created by connection of an artery directly to a vein, usually in the forearm.

Arteriovenous (AV) graft: In hemodialysis, a vascular access surgically created using a synthetic tube to connect an artery to a vein.

Arteriovenous malformations: A tangle of blood vessels, both arterial and venous, that can rupture and cause hemorrhage in the brain.

Arthrodesis: The surgical immobilization of a joint (i.e., joint fusion).

Arthropathy: Disease of the joints.

Ascites: Accumulation of serous fluid in the peritoneal cavity.

Asherman's syndrome: A cause for menstrual flow obstruction; often resulting from infection or surgery affecting the endometrium.

Asperger's disorder: A type of pervasive developmental disorder characterized by severe and sustained impairment in social interaction, restricted and repetitive patterns of behavioral/interested activities—similar to autism but without clinically significant delays in language and cognitive development or age-appropriate self-help skills.

Aspiration pneumonitis: The inflammation of lung tissue caused by the aspiration of fluids and gastric contents that often leads to dyspnea, pulmonary edema, secondary infections, and adult respiratory distress syndrome. Hydrocarbon pneumonitis is caused by the pulmonary aspiration of hydrocarbons such as kerosene and gasoline.

Assertive community treatment: A treatment program for the care of individuals with schizophrenia in which teams provide comprehensive wraparound services for the patient, including going to the home to provide support for daily living skills, housing, and supported employment. Team members are available 24 hours daily if needed to meet the patient's comprehensive care needs.

Asystole: The presence of a flat line on the electrocardiogram monitor.

Ataxia: Loss of the ability to coordinate muscular movement.

Atelectasis: Pulmonary parenchymal collapse caused by alveolar or bronchial obstruction.

Atopic dermatitis: Skin inflammation that causes itching, scales, and erythema.

Atopy: An allergic syndrome characterized by asthma, hay fever, and urticaria or eczema.

Atrial fibrillation: Rapid beating of the atria that results in variable ventricular rates.

Atropinism: Symptoms of poisoning by atropine or belladonna.

Aura: Sensory or somatosensory alteration without loss of consciousness.

Augmentation: Addition of a medication not usually used as monotherapy for a disorder to a core medication for a disorder in an attempt to enhance the patient's clinical response.

Auscultation: Listening to the heart or other organs with a stethoscope.

Autism/Autistic disorder: A type of pervasive developmental disorder with a neurobiologic etiology, characterized by impaired reciprocal social interaction, impaired communication skills, and a limited range of activities and interests; frequently associated with mental retardation; sometimes referred to as early infantile autism, childhood autism, or Kanner autism.

Autologous transplantation: Readministration of the same person's cells that were previously collected.

Autosomal: Pertaining to a chromosome.

Axonal transaction: Destroying or severing the axon so that electrical impulses are impeded along the nerve sheath or across the nerve synapse. Axonal damage is not reversible and leads to long-term disability and the formation of black holes.

Azotemia: Term referring to elevated levels of urea in the serum or blood.

Azotorrhea: An excessive loss of protein in the feces.

Bacteremia: Presence of viable bacteria (fungi) in the bloodstream.

Bacterial prostatitis: An inflammation of the prostate gland and surrounding tissue as a result of infection.

Bacteriuria: The presence of bacteria in the urine.

Barrett esophagus: Inflammatory changes in the esophagus resulting in replacement of epithelial lining by columnar-type cells that can lead to stricture or adenocarcinoma.

Basal ganglia and striatum: Parts of the brain regulating movements.

Behavioral phenotype: The actions or reactions of a person to internal or external environmental influences.

Benign prostatic hyperplasia: Nonmalignant enlargement of the prostate gland in elderly men.

Bilateral salpingo-oophorectomy: Surgical excision (removal) of both ovaries.

Biliverdin: A green bile pigment formed from the oxidation of heme.

Binge eating: Excessive intake of calorie-laden food over a short period of time.

Bioavailability: The fraction of drug absorbed into the systemic circulation after extravascular administration.

Biochemical markers: Intracellular macromolecules released into the peripheral circulation from necrotic myocytes as a result of myocardial cell death (infarction). These laboratory tests are used in the diagnosis of myocardial infarction. Examples include troponin I, troponin T, creatinine kinase myocardial band (MB), and myoglobin.

Biofilm: A population or community of microorganisms adhering to a surface by a secreted coating. This coating also reduces microorganism vulnerability to antibiotics.

Biopsy: A procedure in which a tiny piece of a body part, such as the kidney or bladder, is removed for examination under a microscope.

Bioterrorism agents: Organisms or toxins that can cause disease and death in humans, animals, or plants for the purpose of eliciting terror.

Bipolar I disorder: Characterized by one or more manic or mixed episodes, and is usually accompanied by major depressive episodes.

Bipolar II disorder: Characterized by one or more major depressive episodes and accompanied by at least one hypomanic episode.

Bleeding diathesis: A condition in which there is an unusual susceptibility or predisposition to bleeding.

Blood urea nitrogen (BUN): A waste product in the blood that comes from the breakdown of food protein. The kidneys filter blood to remove urea and thus maintain homeostasis. As kidney function decreases, the BUN level increases.

Blood–brain barrier: The relative lack of permeability of large molecules (and those molecules lacking lipid solubility) into the central nervous system because of the nonfenestrated capillary beds of the cerebral vasculature.

Borborygmi: Rumbling or gurgling noises produced by movement of gas, fluid, or both in the alimentary canal and audible at a distance.

Brachytherapy: A procedure in which radioactive material sealed in needles, seeds, wires, or catheters is placed directly into or near a tumor. Also called internal radiation, implant radiation, or interstitial radiation therapy.

Bradykinesia: Delay or slowness in initiating and performing purposeful, voluntary movement as seen in Parkinsonism.

Breakthrough bleeding: The unpredictable and irregular bleeding associated with hormone therapy.

Bronchiectasis: Dilation of a bronchus or bronchi, usually related to excessive secretions.

Bronchioles: A subdivision of bronchi; smaller in diameter and without cartilage.

Bronchiolitis: Inflammation of the bronchioles.

Bronchoalveolar lavage: Instilling and then removing a lavage fluid to reveal the secretory and/or cellular contents from deep in the lung.

Bronchorrhea: Excessive bronchial secretions that can impair pulmonary ventilation.

Bruit: An abnormal and often harsh sound heard over a blood vessel, usually an artery, on examination with a stethoscope caused by turbulent blood flow.

B-type natriuretic peptide: B-type natriuretic peptide is a 32-amino-acid polypeptide secreted by the ventricles in response to excessive myocyte stretching. Elevated levels are typically seen in patients with left ventricular dysfunction and can correlate with both the heart failure severity and the prognosis.

Bulimia nervosa: A psychiatric disorder manifested by episodes of consuming a large caloric load over a short period of time (binge eating), with subsequent self-induced vomiting, use of cathartics or diuretics, fasting, or excessive exercise to prevent weight gain.

BUN (blood urea nitrogen): A waste product in the blood that comes from the breakdown of food protein. The kidneys filter blood to remove urea. As kidney function decreases, the BUN level increases.

Bursitis: Inflammation of the bursa, a fluid-filled soft tissue structure that usually results in pain and swelling.

Caffeinism: A clinical syndrome produced by acute or chronic overuse of caffeine characterized by anxiety, psychomotor alterations, sleep disturbances, mood changes, and psychophysiologic complaints.

Calcimimetic: A class of agents that stimulate calcium-sensing receptors on the parathyroid gland and *mimic* the effects of extracellular calcium. They suppress parathyroid hormone (PTH) release and increase the sensitivity of the receptor to extracellular calcium.

Calcium-sensing receptor: The calcium receptor on the chief cells of the parathyroid gland, activation of which leads to suppression of PTH release.

Candidiasis: Fungal infection involving *Candida* species.

Carcinoid: A carcinoid is a slow-growing tumor usually located in the gastrointestinal system and sometimes in the lungs or other sites. Carcinoids can spread to the liver and can secrete serotonin or prostaglandins.

Cardiac index: Cardiac output standardized for body surface area. Mathematically, cardiac index = cardiac output/body surface area.

Cardiac output: The volume of blood pumped by the heart per unit of time. Cardiac output is the product of heart rate and stroke volume.

Cardioembolic stroke: An ischemic stroke thought to be caused by an embolism arising from the heart. Cardioembolic stroke can be assumed in patients with significant cardiovascular disease including atrial fibrillation, dilated cardiomyopathy, prosthetic valves, recent myocardial infarction (MI), and patent foramen ovale.

Cardiopulmonary arrest: The abrupt cessation of spontaneous and effective ventilation and circulation following a cardiac or respiratory event.

Cardiopulmonary bypass: The use of extracorporeal devices to pump blood and oxygenate the blood while the heart or lungs are not functional. Extracorporeal membrane oxygenation (ECMO) is a form of long-term cardiopulmonary bypass that is typically used for days to weeks.

Cardiopulmonary resuscitation: The provision of artificial ventilation and circulation until it is possible to provide advanced cardiac life support and reestablish spontaneous circulation.

Carotid Doppler: A technique that provides information about the presence and severity of atherosclerosis of the carotid artery using noninvasive sound wave technology.

Carotid endarterectomy: Removal of the atherosclerotic plaque from the inside of a stenotic carotid artery by a surgical technique. The vessel is surgically opened and sewn and/or patched after removal of the plaque.

Case-control study: An observational study of persons with the disease of interest (cases) and a suitable control group of persons without the disease to establish the extent of association between exposure(s) of interest and disease.

Cataplexy: Sudden loss of muscle control with retention of clear consciousness that follows a strong emotional stimulus (as elation, surprise, or anger) and is a characteristic symptom of narcolepsy.

Cellulitis: An acute, infectious process that initially affects the epidermis and dermis and can subsequently spread within the superficial fascia.

Centrilobular: Affecting the central portion of the lobe.

Cerebral autoregulation: The process by which cerebral blood flow is maintained in a tight range over a wide range of peripheral blood pressures. It is accomplished by reactive dilation and constriction of cerebral arteries.

Cerebral blood flow (CBF): The volume of blood perfusing a given brain mass as a function of time.

Cerebral blood volume (CBV): The total volume of blood within the cerebral vasculature at a given point in time.

Cerebral microdialysis: A sampling method that allows continuous acquisition of a small volume of cerebral extracellular fluid specimens using a microdialysis probe inserted into the brain.

Cerebral oxygen consumption ($CMRO_2$): The cerebral metabolic rate for oxygen consumption calculated as the mean hemispheric CBF and the arteriovenous oxygen content difference ($AVDO_2$).

Cerebral oxygen delivery (CDO_2): The product of CBF and arterial oxygen content.

Cerebral perfusion pressure: A critical monitoring parameter in traumatic brain injury patients defined as the difference between the mean arterial pressure and the intracranial pressure.

Cerebrospinal fluid: The clear, colorless fluid that bathes and cushions the brain and spinal cord.

Cervical cap: A thimble-shaped latex rubber device that is held on the cervix by suction, thus acting as a barrier to reduce the risk of pregnancy.

Cervical effacement: During the first stage of labor, as the cervix is opening, it is also thinning. The thinning of the cervix is termed *effacement*.

Cervical ripening: Prior to inducing labor, the cervix must be favorable, approximately 2 cm dilated and 80% thinned out. If this is not the case, an agent must be used to induce histochemical changes to make the cervix more favorable.

Cervical stenosis: A cause for menstrual flow obstruction; often caused by surgical interventions for cervical dysplasia.

Cervicitis: Inflammation of the cervix.

Chancre: A sore or ulcer, the dermal lesion of primary syphilis.

Chancroid: A venereal dermal lesion caused by agents other than syphilis.

Children: Pediatric patients who are 1 to 11 years of age.

Cholestatic hepatitis: Rare form of hepatitis marked by stopped or suppressed flow of bile; characterized by pruritus, dark urine, light-colored stools, elevated alkaline phosphatase, and conjugated bilirubin.

Cholinesterase inhibitors: Class of medication that inhibits enzymatic activity of acetylcholinesterase, butyrylcholinesterase, or both to prevent the degradation of acetylcholine.

Chronic condition: An illness or impairment that cannot be cured.

Chronic kidney disease (CKD): Slow and progressive loss of kidney function that takes several years, often resulting in permanent kidney failure requiring dialysis or transplantation.

Chronic pain/persistent pain: Pain persisting for months to years.

Chronic pancreatitis: Chronic inflammation of the pancreas caused by the many sequelae of long-standing pancreatic injury leading to irreversible pancreatic damage.

Chvostek's sign: A facial twitch produced by tapping on the cheek over the branches of the facial nerve.

Circumstantial speech: Speech pattern whereby the expressed ideas are characterized by unnecessary detail. The speaker ultimately makes their point, but in a very roundabout manner.

Clearance: The volume of blood per unit time (e.g., L/h, mL/min) completely cleared of a drug.

Clinical inertia: A clinical situation in which no therapeutic move was made to treat a medical condition in a patient who is not considered adequately treated, or at his or her treatment goal.

Clinical outcomes: Medical events that occur as a result of the condition or its treatment.

Clinical pharmacokinetics: Discipline that describes the absorption, distribution, metabolism, and elimination of drugs in patients.

Clinical proteinuria: Total protein in the urine in amounts greater than 300 mg/day.

Clinical resistance: Refers to failure of an antifungal agent in the treatment of a fungal infection that arises from factors other than microbial resistance, such as failure of the antifungal agent to reach the site of infection, or inability of a patient's immune system to eradicate a fungus whose growth is retarded by an antifungal agent.

Clinically isolated syndrome: The first attack of multiple sclerosis characterized by a neurologic syndrome such as optic neuritis and generally seen with silent or asymptomatic white matter lesions (seen on magnetic resonance imaging) suggestive of demyelination. Individuals that experience a clinically isolated syndrome are at high risk of developing definite multiple sclerosis.

Clotting cascade: A series of enzymatic reactions by clotting factors leading to the formation of a blood clot. The clotting cascade is initiated by several thrombogenic substances. Each reaction in the cascade is triggered by the preceding one, and the effect is amplified by positive feedback loops.

Clotting factor: Plasma proteins found in the blood that are essential to the formation of blood clots. Clotting factors circulate in inactive forms but are activated by their predecessor in the clotting cascade or a thrombogenic substance. Each clotting factor is designated by a Roman numeral (e.g., factor VII) and by the letter "a" when activated (e.g., factor VIIa).

Cluster headache: A primary headache disorder characterized by attacks of severe unilateral headache pain that occurs in series of weeks or months (cluster periods) separated by remission periods usually lasting months or years.

Cluster period: The time during which cluster-headache attacks occur regularly and at least once every other day.

Codon: A sequence of three consecutive nucleotides that specify an amino acid or amino acid chain termination.

Coelomic metaplasia: Transformation of normal cells into endometrial cells.

Cognitive behavioral therapy: A form of psychotherapy designed to replace distorted or inappropriate ways of thinking with healthy, more realistic thoughts to alter maladaptive moods and behavior. It is instructional in approach and is based on the theory that thoughts (not external influences such as people, situations, and events) cause feelings and behaviors. Patients learn to identify the thinking that causes the negative feelings and behaviors and then learn how to replace that thinking with thoughts that lead to more desirable feelings and behaviors.

Cogwheeling: A ratchet-like movement in the joints, characteristic of Parkinson disease.

Cohort study: Assembly of a group of persons without a disease(s) of interest at the onset of the study, determination of the exposure status of each person, and observation of the cohort over time to determine the development of disease in exposed and nonexposed persons.

Colectomy: Surgical removal of the colon.

Colonization resistance: Preservation of anaerobic flora by selective gut decontamination to prevent colonization by potentially pathogenic gram-negative organisms.

Colony-stimulating factors: Proteins that regulate the proliferation, maturation, and differentiation of stem cells to red blood cells, white blood cells, and platelets.

Coma: A state of unconsciousness whereby a patient is not opening his or her eyes, not obeying commands, and not uttering understandable words.

Comedo, comedones (pl.): Plug of sebum and keratinous material in a hair follicle; blackhead.

Comedogenicity: Product effect that causes follicular plugging resulting in comedones.

Comedolytic: Prevents shed keratinocytes from aggregating in follicle and clogging pores.

Comorbidity: A concomitant but unrelated pathologic or disease process.

Complex partial seizure: A seizure beginning in one hemisphere of the brain. It is manifested by automatisms, periods of memory loss, or aberrations of behavior.

Compulsion: Repetitive ritualistic behavior such as ordering or hand washing or a mental act such as repeating words silently with the intent of preventing or reducing distress or some dreaded event or situation.

Conceptual model: The rationale for and description of the concepts that a measurement instrument is intended to assess and the interrelationships of those concepts.

Condom: A sheath, usually made of thin rubber, used to cover the penis during sexual intercourse to prevent conception or infection.

Confounding: A situation in which the effects of two processes are not separated. The distortion of the apparent effect of an exposure on risk brought about by the association of other factors that can influence the outcome.

Constrictive pericarditis: Constrictive pericarditis is a disorder caused by inflammation of the pericardium with subsequent thickening, scarring, and contracture of the pericardium. The pericardium cannot stretch during contraction, thereby preventing chamber filling.

Construct validity: The strength of the relationship between measures purporting to measure or reflect the same underlying theoretical construct.

Content validity: Refers to how adequately the questions/items capture the relevant aspects of the domain or concept being measured.

Continuation therapy: The second phase in drug therapy during which the goal is to eliminate any remaining symptoms and prevent a relapse.

Continuous-combined estrogen-progestogen therapy: Daily administration of both estrogen and a progestogen.

Continuous long-cycle estrogen-progestogen therapy: Estrogen is given daily and a progestogen is given six times a year (every other month for 12 to 14 days).

Convection: The movement of solutes, or metabolic waste products, by bulk flow in association with fluid removal. Convective clearance is not dependent on concentration gradients, and the magnitude of its contribution to total clearance is directly related to the ultrafiltration (fluid removal) rate.

Convulsion: Specific seizure type where the seizure is manifested by involuntary muscle contractions.

Cor pulmonale: Right-sided heart failure caused by lung disease.

Corneocytes: Flattened, dead, keratin-filled epidermal cells.

Coronary artery bypass graft surgery (CABGS): Thoracic surgery where parts of a saphenous vein from a leg or internal mammary artery from the arm are placed as conduits to restore blood flow between the aorta and one or more coronary arteries to *bypass* the coronary artery stenosis (occlusion).

Corpus cavernosum: Two chambers on the dorsal side of the penis. Chambers composed of sinusoidal tissue, which can fill with arterial blood to produce an erection.

Corpus luteum: The small yellow endocrine structure that develops within a ruptured ovarian follicle and secretes progesterone and estrogen.

Corpus spongiosum: One chamber on the ventral side of the penis. Chamber is composed of sinusoidal tissue, which can fill with arterial blood to produce an erection. The urethra passes through the corpus spongiosum.

Cortical necrosis: Acute renal failure secondary to ischemic necrosis of the renal cortex usually caused by significantly diminished renal arterial perfusion.

Corticotropin-releasing hormone (CRH): A trophic hormone released by the hypothalamus that stimulates release of adrenocorticotropic hormone (ACTH).

Cost-effectiveness ratio: The outcome of cost-effective analysis. The numerator of the ratio summarizes the costs and financial savings associated with the therapy, including the costs of the therapy itself, side effects, medical costs, and savings from avoided illness and disability. The denominator of the cost-effectiveness ratio reflects the health effect of the intervention. The year of life saved is probably the most commonly used measure of the health effect.

Cranial nerve palsy: Paralysis of one or more of the 12 cranial (brain) nerves.

Craniectomy (for stroke): Removal of part of the skull overlying an area of injury to relieve the pressure of cerebral edema.

C-reactive protein: An endogenous marker released by the body in response to inflammation.

Creatine kinase, creatine kinase MB: Creatine kinase (CK) enzymes are found in many isoforms, with varying concentrations depending on the type of tissue. Creatine kinase is a general term used to describe the nonspecific total release of all types of CK, including that found in skeletal muscle (MM), brain (BB), and heart (MB). Creatine kinase MB is released into the blood from necrotic myocytes in response to infarction and is a useful laboratory test for diagnosing myocardial infarction. If the total CK is elevated, then the relative index (RI), or fraction of the total that is composed of CK-MB, is calculated as follows:

$$RI = (CK\text{-}MB/CK\ total) \times 100$$

A RI greater than 2 is typically diagnostic of infarction.

Creatinine (serum): A protein metabolic by-product obtained from the diet or generated from muscles of the body. Creatinine is removed from blood by the kidneys; as kidney disease progresses, the level of creatinine in the blood increases.

Creatinine clearance: A test that measures how efficiently the kidneys filter creatinine and other waste products from the blood. Low creatinine clearance (<60 mL/min) usually indicates the presence of kidney damage.

Crepitus: A crinkly, crackling, or grating feeling or sound in the joints, skin, or lungs.

Cronbach α-coefficient: Commonly used statistical measure to quantify internal consistency reliability for multi-item scales or tests.

Crossmatch: A test to determine if a recipient has antibodies against donor antigens. A positive crossmatch indicates that the recipient has antibodies against the donor, and the two are incompatible. A negative crossmatch means the recipient does not have antibodies against the donor, and the two are considered compatible.

Crust: Dried exudate, secretion, or hemorrhage; scab.

Crypt abscess: Neutrophilic infiltration of the intestinal glands (crypts of Lieberkühn); a characteristic finding in patients with ulcerative colitis.

Culture negative endocarditis: Describes a patient in whom a clinical diagnosis of infective endocarditis is likely, but blood cultures do not yield a pathogen.

Cutaneous: Pertaining to the skin.

Cutis: Skin.

Cyanopsia: A condition when a patient sees a blue halo around objects, or objects appear to be blue-colored.

Cyanosis: Bluish tint to the skin or mucous membranes because of lack of oxygen.

Cyclic estrogen-progestogen therapy: Estrogen is taken continuously, with a progestogen added cyclically the last 10 to 14 days during each 28-day cycle.

Cyst: Sac or closed cavity containing fluid, semifluid, or solid material.

Cystitis: Inflammation of the bladder, usually caused by infection.

Cytokines: Protein molecules that are released by one cell (e.g., T-lymphocytes) that can have an influence on other cells. These proteins are important in numerous cell functions, such as regulating the immune response and cell-to-cell communication.

Dactylitis: Erythema and swollen hands, feet, fingers, and toes. Also known as *hand-and-foot syndrome.*

Deep vein thrombosis: A disorder of thrombus formation causing obstruction of a deep vein in the leg, pelvis, or abdomen.

Defibrillation: The therapeutic use of electric current in an attempt to completely depolarize the myocardium and provide an opportunity for the natural pacemaker centers of the heart to resume normal activity.

Delayed cerebral ischemia: A worsening in neurologic function in a subarachnoid hemorrhage patient, occurring several days after the initial bleed, not due to another cause.

Delusion: Fixed, false beliefs that are not based in reality or consistent with the patient's religion or culture. Delusions can be classified as paranoid, somatic, or grandiose in nature. Delusions are often unshakable in spite of evidence to the contrary.

Dementia: A chronic progressive neurodegenerative syndrome characterized by a decline in memory and at least one other cognitive function.

Demyelination: Destruction of myelin in the spinal cord and brain leading to the formation of plaques that impair communication between neurons. Demyelination is classically found in the central nervous system of patients with multiple sclerosis and may be reversible.

Depersonalization: A change in an individual's self-awareness, during anxiety disorder, such that one feels detached from his or her own experiences, with the self, body, and mind seeming alien or distant. Persistent or recurrent experiences as if one is an outside observer of one's mental processes or body (e.g., feeling like one is in a dream).

Derealization: A feeling of estrangement or detachment from one's environment.

Dermatitis: Inflammation of the skin.

Dermatophyte: Fungal infection of the skin.

Dermis: The inner layer of skin between the epidermis and hypodermis.

Desensitization: Administration of increasing doses of drug to achieve patient tolerance and avoidance of hypersensitivity reactions.

Detoxification programs: A medically supervised treatment program for alcohol or drug addiction designed to purge the body of intoxicating or addictive substances. Such a program is used as a first step in overcoming physiologic or psychologic addiction.

Detumescence: Process by which an erect penis becomes flaccid.

Diagnostic overshadowing: Underestimating the significance of the emotional disturbances because of the presence of significant cognitive deficits.

Dialysate: The cleansing solution used in dialysis to remove excess fluids and waste products from the blood.

Dialysis: The process of removing toxic substances and fluid across a semipermeable membrane to maintain fluid, electrolyte, and acid–base balance.

Diaphragm: (1) A flexible ring covered with rubber or other plastic material, fitted over the cervix of the uterus to prevent pregnancy. (2) Muscular membrane separating the abdominal and thoracic cavities, used for respiration.

Diastolic blood pressure: The arterial blood pressure that occurs after cardiac contraction when the cardiac chambers are filling.

Diastolic heart failure: A condition caused by increased resistance to the filling of one or both ventricles; this leads to symptoms of congestion from the inappropriate upward shift of the diastolic pressure-volume relation.

Diffusion-weighted imaging: A type of magnetic resonance imaging (MRI) that can sensitively detect changes in water movement in tissue. It is particularly sensitive to the early changes seen during brain ischemia.

Digital clubbing: Rounded and swollen tip of finger usually associated with long-term pulmonary disease.

Dihydrotestosterone: The active androgen metabolite, which is formed inside various cells. In the case of benign prostatic hyperplasia (BPH), dihydrotestosterone is formed inside prostate cells by the action of 5-α-reductase, which converts testosterone to dihydrotestosterone. Dihydrotestosterone stimulates the glandular portion of the prostate to undergo hyperplasia.

Disinhibition: A physiologic effect that occurs during psychoactive substance use characterized by a loss of normal, executive functioning and normal behavior. An increase in behaviors with the propensity to harm the individual is common.

Dissociative amnesia: Inability to remember some important aspect of an event.

Diverticulitis: Inflammation of a diverticulum, especially of the small pockets in the wall of the colon that fill with stagnant fecal material and become inflamed; rarely, they can cause obstruction, perforation, or bleeding.

Dopamine: A monoamine neurotransmitter formed in the brain by the decarboxylation of dopa and essential to the normal functioning of the central nervous system.

Doppler imaging: With Doppler imaging, a probe generates sound waves typically at 2.5 MHz. When encountering an object, sound waves are scattered or reflected back toward the probe from the object's interface with adjacent structures; this is repeated in many times per second to build up a moving real-time image of the heart.

Drug abuse: A maladaptive pattern of substance use indicated by repeated adverse consequences related to the repeated use of the substance. Examples include failure to fulfill important obligations at work, school, or home; repeated use in situations in which it is physically dangerous, such as driving under the influence; legal problems; and social or interpersonal problems such as arguments and fights.

Drug addiction: A chronic disorder characterized by the compulsive use of a substance resulting in physical, psychologic, or social harm to the user and continued use despite that harm.

Dual diagnosis: A developmentally disabled person comorbid with a psychiatric disorder.

Dysentery: Diarrhea characterized by blood, mucus, and leukocytes in the stool with tenesmus and fever.

Dyskinesia: Choreiform abnormal involuntary movements involving usually the face, neck, trunk, and extremities.

Dysmenorrhea: Crampy pelvic pain occurring with or just prior to menses. *Primary* dysmenorrhea implies pain in the setting of normal pelvic anatomy, whereas *secondary* dysmenorrhea is secondary to underlying pelvic pathology.

Dyspareunia: Painful sexual intercourse.

Dyspepsia: Literally means "bad digestion," but refers to persistent or recurrent pain or discomfort centered in the upper abdomen. Symptoms can include epigastric pain, bloating, abdominal distention, postprandial fullness, early satiety, and nausea.

Dysphagia: Difficulty swallowing.

Dysphoria or dysphoric: A feeling of discomfort or an unpleasant mood, such as sadness, anxiety, or irritability.

Dyspnea: Dyspnea is referred to as shortness of breath or difficulty or distress in breathing.

Dystonia: Sustained muscular spasm or abnormal postures.

Early empirical therapy: The administration of systemic antifungal agents at the onset of fever and neutropenia.

Economic outcomes: The direct, indirect, and intangible costs compared with the consequences of a medical intervention.

Edema: Accumulation of fluid in tissues.

Effective renal plasma flow (ERPF): The flow of plasma through the kidneys; often measured by *p*-aminohippurate (PAH) clearance and expressed in volume per unit of time (mL/min). The ERPF is less than the true renal plasma flow (RPF) because plasma flow through renal connective and adipose tissue is not measured and the extraction of PAH, although high (>0.9), is not complete.

Ejaculatory dysfunction: This is a type of sexual dysfunction that can present as premature ejaculation (before orgasm has occurred), anejaculation (failure of emission), or retrograde ejaculation (when ejaculate moves backward into the bladder as opposed to forward and out of the body during orgasm). In some cases, ejaculatory dysfunction can decrease sexual enjoyment in the patient.

Ejection fraction: The ejection fraction is the percentage of blood ejected from the left ventricle with each heart beat.

Elation: An exaggerated feeling of well-being, euphoria, or elation.

Electroconvulsive therapy: A treatment for severe mental illness in which a precisely calculated electric stimulus is administered in a controlled medical setting to produce a generalized seizure.

Electroencephalograph (EEG): Used to evaluate brain electrical activity.

Electroencephalography: A test that measures electrical brain wave activity through the use of multiple scalp electrodes.

Electromyography: Test of muscle function because of either primary muscle disease or secondary to nerve injury.

Embolism: The sudden blockage of a vessel caused by a blood clot or foreign material that has been brought to the site by the flow of blood.

Embolization: The process by which a blood clot or foreign material dislodges from its site of origin, flows in the blood, and blocks a distant vessel.

Emergency contraception: Any method of contraception that acts after intercourse to prevent pregnancy.

Emesis: See *Vomiting.*

Empirical therapy: With systemic antifungal agents is administered to granulocytopenic patients with persistent or recurrent fever despite the administration of appropriate antimicrobial therapy.

Enanthem: Eruption on a mucous membrane (as the inside of the mouth) occurring as a symptom of a disease

Encephalitis: Inflammation of the brain tissue.

Encephalopathy: An altered brain state that can occur with altered brain structure. Many etiologies are associated with encephalopathy (toxins, cancer, metabolic disorders, CNS infections, increased cranial pressure, radiation, alcohol, psychotropic drugs, trauma, inadequate nutrition, decreased brain oxygen, and CNS injury). Consciousness is impaired with patients having a decreased/altered mental state and diffuse slowing of the EEG. Encephalopathy is often associated with seizures, loss of cognitive/memory, and personality changes, and can be associated with myoclonus and other neurologic impairments.

Endobronchitis: Inflammation of the epithelial lining of the bronchi.

Endocarditis: An infection of the endocardial surface of the heart, which can include one or more heart valves, the mural endocardium, or a septal defect.

Endometriosis: Presence of endometrial tissue outside the uterus.

Enkephalins: Pentapeptide endorphins, found in many parts of the brain, that bind to specific receptor sites, some of which can be pain-related opiate receptors.

Enteric fever: Intestinal inflammation and ulceration with high fever and abdominal complaints caused by infection.

Enterocolitis: Inflammation of the small intestine and colon.

Enterotoxin: A cholera-like disease that produces secretory diarrhea.

Enuresis: Urinary incontinence, especially at night.

Enzymuria: Presence of enzymes in the urine.

Epidermis: The outer layer of skin.

Epilepsy: Two or more unprovoked seizures; symptoms of disturbed electrical activity in the brain.

Epilepsy syndrome: The combination of seizure type with other components of the patient history such as age of onset, intellectual development, findings on neurologic examination, and results of neuroimaging.

Episodic: Recurring and remitting in a regular or irregular pattern.

Epistaxis: Nose bleed.

Epithelial cells: Cells that make up epithelium.

Epithelial tissue of the prostate: Also known as glandular tissue. This portion of the prostate is responsible for producing prostatic secretions, and this comprises only approximately 25% of the total volume of the enlarged prostate gland in patients with benign prostatic hyperplasia. Epithelial tissue is androgen dependent.

Epithelium: Layer of avascular cells covering body surfaces.

Erectile dysfunction: Also known as *impotence.* This is a failure of the penis to become rigid enough to allow for vaginal penetration of the sexual partner.

Erysipelas: Infection of the more superficial layers of the skin and cutaneous lymphatics.

Erythema: Redness.

Erythema multiforme: Symmetrical patches of raised, red skin.

Erythema nodosum: Raised, red, tender nodules on the skin that vary in size from 1 cm.

Erythroderma: Generalized redness of the skin.

Erythropoiesis: The production of erythrocytes (red blood cells) within the bone marrow.

Erythropoietic agents: Agents developed with recombinant DNA technology that have the same biologic activity as endogenous erythropoietin to stimulate red blood cell production. Available agents in the United States include epoetin alfa and darbepoetin alfa.

Erythropoietin: A hormone made by the kidneys that is required for red blood cell formation in the bone marrow. Lack of this hormone leads to anemia.

Eschar: Black, painless skin ulcer characteristic of cutaneous anthrax.

Esophageal: Involving the esophagus.

Esophageal stricture: A narrowing of the esophageal lumen because of acid reflux into the lower esophagus.

Esophagitis: Inflammation of the esophagus.

Essential or primary hypertension: Persistently elevated blood pressure that results from unknown pathophysiological etiology.

Estrogen therapy: Unopposed estrogen regimens administered to postmenopausal women following hysterectomy.

Euphoria: A mood state characterized by an exaggerated, superficial sense of well-being, characterized extreme happiness, sometimes more than is reasonable in a particular situation.

Euthymia or euthymic: A mood in a *normal* range without depression or mood elevation.

Evidence-based medicine (EBM): Evidence-based medicine emphasizes the consideration of results from clinical research as the basis for clinical decision making. Under this practice approach, unless individual patient-specific factors dictate otherwise, treatment should generally be guided by those approaches that have the best research evidence for efficacy, tolerability, and patient acceptance.

Evoked potentials: EEG-based technique involving measurement of brain-wave activity in response to stimuli, usually visual or auditory.

Exanthema: An eruption on the skin occurring as a symptom of a disease.

External beam radiotherapy: Treatment by radiation emitted from a source located at a distance from the body; also called beam therapy and external beam therapy.

Extrapyramidal: Regarding involuntary motor movement.

Extrapyramidal system: Neurotransmitter tracts in the midbrain with dopamine as the primary ascending neurotransmitter, with cell bodies in the substantial nigra and axons terminating in the basal ganglia (e.g., caudate nucleus, putamen). The extrapyramidal system is largely involved in the control of fine motor movements, and with some degree of emotional expression as well.

Fasciculations: The localized contractions of muscle groups, often visible through the skin, because of excessive neuronal discharge.

Fear: A direct, focused response to a specific event or object of which an individual is consciously aware.

Felty syndrome: Rheumatoid arthritis associated with splenomegaly and neutropenia.

Fibrin: An insoluble protein that is one of the principle ingredients of a blood clot. Fibrin strands bind to one another to form a fibrin mesh. The fibrin mesh often traps platelets and other blood cells.

Fibrosis: Formation of fibrous tissue as a reparative or reactive process.

First-generation (typical or traditional) antipsychotic: An antipsychotic medication with a mechanism of action thought to be primarily caused by the blockade of dopamine-2 (D_2) receptors. D_2-blockade is associated with hyperprolactinemia and extrapyramidal side effects.

Fistula: A communicating tubelike passage from one organ to another, or from an organ to an external surface; often seen in severe cases of Crohn's disease.

Flight of ideas: An accelerated flow of speech with thoughts that change rapidly from one topic to another.

Focal seizures: Partial seizures.

Follicle-stimulating hormone (FSH): A polypeptide hormone secreted by the anterior pituitary gland that promotes ovarian follicle development and stimulates estradiol and progesterone.

Fragile X syndrome: A genetic disorder commonly associated with mental retardation in which the tip of the long arms of the X chromosome separates from the rest of the genetic material; most males and 30% of females with fragile X syndrome have mental retardation; males develop enlarged testicles, enlarged ears, and a prominent jaw.

Freezing: Intermittent immobility lasting a few seconds, particularly in walking, seen in Parkinsonism.

Fulminant hepatitis: Acute hepatic failure; rare complication of viral hepatitis, it can also result from hepatotoxins, or drug sensitivity and causes massive necrosis of the liver; marked by a high fatality rate.

Functional analysis: Evaluation performed by a psychologist qualified in applied behavioral analysis to determine if a behavior is caused by some environmental factor.

Functional pain: Pain because of abnormal operation of the nervous system.

Functional psychiatric disorder: A mental disorder that is primarily defined by a constellation of symptoms and behaviors and for which the pathophysiologic etiology is still largely unknown.

Fungemia: The presence of fungi in the blood.

Gastroesophageal reflux disease (GERD): Symptomatic clinical condition or histologic alteration that results from episodes of gastroesophageal reflux.

Gene: Series of codons that specify a particular protein.

Generalized anxiety disorder (GAD): Excessive anxiety and worry occurring more days than not for a period of at least 6 months.

Generalized convulsive status epilepticus (GCSE): Most common and dangerous type of status epilepticus (SE). It consists of bilateral (both brain hemispheres) electrical seizure activity that manifests as tonic and/or clonic motor activity. The convulsions and/or brain discharges can be symmetrical or asymmetrical (i.e., parts of body and brain mirroring or not mirroring each other in activity). Consciousness is not maintained during the seizure episodes. The duration is sufficient enough in length to meet the definition of SE.

Generalized seizures: Seizures occurring in both hemispheres of the brain. They can be primary or secondarily generalized.

Generic/general measures: Instruments designed to be applicable across a wide variety of conditions/diseases, medical interventions, and populations.

Genotype: Genetic makeup of an organism or group of organisms with respect to a single trait or traits. Can also refer to parent-to-offspring gene transmission.

Genu valgum: A deformity marked by lateral angulation of the leg in relation to the thigh.

Genu varum: A deformity marked by medial angulation of the leg in relation to the thigh; an outward bowing of the legs.

Gestation: Time from fertilization of egg until birth.

Gigantism: Excess secretion of growth hormone prior to epiphyseal closure in children.

Glasgow coma scale: The most widely used system to grade the arousal and functional capacity of the cerebral cortex consisting of eye opening, motor responses, and verbal responses.

Glaucoma: Any of a group of ocular disorders that lead to an optic neuropathy characterized by changes in the optic nerve head (optic disk) that is associated with loss of visual sensitivity and field. Open angle and closed angle are the two major types of glaucoma.

Glomerular filtration rate (GFR): The primary index of overall kidney function; the volume of plasma that is filtered by the glomerulus per unit of time; often reported in mL/min or mL/min/1.73 m^2.

Glomerulonephritis: Glomerular lesions characterized by inflammation of the capillary loops in the glomerulus caused by immunologic, vascular, and other idiopathic diseases (may be diffuse or membranoproliferative).

Glomerulosclerosis: Fibrosis of the glomeruli.

Glomerulus: A coiled capillary bed in the kidney that is responsible for filtering water and small molecular weight substances from the blood.

Gonadotropin: A sex hormone that promotes gonadal growth and functioning in both males and females.

Gonadotropin-releasing hormone (GnRH): A trophic hormone released by the hypothalamus that stimulates release of follicle-stimulating hormone (FSH) and luteinizing hormone (LH).

Gout: A disease spectrum that includes hyperuricemia, recurrent attacks of acute arthritis associated with monosodium urate crystals in leukocytes found in synovial fluid, deposits of monosodium urate crystals in tissues (tophi), interstitial renal disease, and uric acid nephrolithiasis.

gp120: The glycoprotein structure on the surface of human immunodeficiency virus (HIV) that binds to CD4 on human cells.

Grandiosity: An inflated self-appraisal of one's status, power, or identity.

Granuloma inguinale: Granuloma lesions affecting the genital area.

Growth hormone (GH): A polypeptide hormone secreted by the anterior pituitary gland that stimulates insulinlike growth factor-1 (IGF-1) production and promotes growth of all body cells.

Growth hormone-releasing hormone (GHRH): A trophic hormone released by the hypothalamus that stimulates release of growth hormone.

Guillain-Barré's syndrome: A disorder characterized by progressive symmetrical paralysis and loss of reflexes, usually beginning in the legs. The paralysis typically involves more than one limb, is progressive, and usually proceeds from the end of an extremity toward the torso. Areflexia or hyporeflexia can occur in the limbs. It typically occurs after recovery from a viral infection.

Gumma: A granulomatous lesion found in organs or tissues as a result of syphilis.

Gynecomastia: Gynecomastia is the abnormal development of large breasts in men.

Half-life: The time required for serum concentrations to decrease by one-half after absorption and distribution are complete.

Hallucination: A sensory perception (e.g., auditory, gustatory, olfactory, somatic, tactile, visual) that occurs without external stimulation of the relevant sensory organ.

Haplotype: A set of polymorphisms that are inherited together.

Haptocorrin: A group of carrier proteins that bind with vitamin B_{12} in the blood and aid in its transport.

Haptoglobin: A group of α_2-globulins in human serum, so called because of their ability to combine with hemoglobin, preventing loss in the urine; levels are decreased in hemolytic disorders and increased in inflammatory conditions or with tissue damage.

Hay fever: See *Rhinitis.*

Health outcomes: The consequences or ends results of a disease and/or its treatment.

Health profiles: Generic instruments that provide an array of scores representing individual dimensions or domains of health-related quality of life (HRQOL) or health status.

Health-related quality of life (HRQOL): A person's perception of how health impacts his or her physical, social, and psychologic functioning and well-being.

Health state preference: The perceived relative desirability of a health state measured on a scale where 1.0 equals full health, and 0.0 equals dead.

Heart failure: A clinical syndrome that can result from any disorder that impairs the ability of the heart to fill with or eject blood. Although heart failure can be caused by numerous cardiac disorders, the primary clinical signs and symptoms of dyspnea, fatigue, and volume overload are similar regardless of the initial cause.

Heinz bodies: Intracellular inclusions usually attached to the red cell membrane composed of denatured hemoglobin.

Hemagglutinin: The major antigenic determinant of the influenza virus; a surface antigen that allows the influenza virus to enter host cells by attaching to sialic acid receptors.

Hematemesis: Vomiting up blood that can be bright red or similar to coffee grounds in appearance.

Hematochezia: Passage of visible bright red bloody stools.

Hematopoiesis: The formation and maturation of blood cells and their derivatives.

Hematopoietic growth factors: See *Colony-stimulating factors.*

Hematuria: Presence of red blood cells in the urine.

Hemochromatosis: Hemochromatosis is a disorder that interferes with iron metabolism, which results in excess iron deposition throughout the body.

Hemodialysis: A dialysis procedure during which blood is pumped outside the body through a dialyzer that acts like an artificial kidney; the dialyzer removes extra fluids and wastes from the blood and returns the clean blood to the body.

Hemolytic uremic syndrome: A condition characterized by the breakup of red blood cells (hemolysis) and kidney failure. Platelets clump together within the kidney's small blood vessels resulting in ischemia leading to kidney failure.

Hemosiderin: A golden yellow or yellow-brown insoluble protein produced by phagocytic digestion of hematin; found in most tissues, especially in the liver, spleen, and bone marrow, in the form of granules much larger than ferritin molecules (of which they are believed to be aggregates) but with a higher content, as much as 37%, of iron.

Hepatosplenic candidiasis: Clinical presentation often manifested only as fever while a patient remains neutropenic (<1,000 white blood cells/mm^3). When the white blood cell (WBC) count increases to >1000 cells/mm^3, imaging studies can detect the presence of abscess or microabscesses in the liver and spleen, often found with acute suppurative and granulomatous reactions. Infection can persist for months and ultimately cause the patient's death despite aggressive systemic therapy with antifungal agents. Also known as *chronic systemic candidiasis.*

Heterozygous: Presence of different (alleles) genes at one location.

Hippocampal sclerosis: A condition in which there are histopathologic changes in the hippocampus that have been associated with patients with a history of prolonged SE. There is an association with hippocampal sclerosis and temporal lobe epilepsy.

Hippocampus: A sea horse–shaped structure located within the brain that is an important part of the limbic system. The hippocampus is involved in some aspects of memory, in the control of the autonomic functions, and in emotional expression.

Hirsutism: Heavy, abnormal growth of hair on the face or body; excess body hair appearing on the lower abdomen, around the nipples, around the chin and upper lip, between the breasts, and on the lower back.

HLA (human leukocyte antigen): See *Human leukocyte antigen.*

Hollenhorst plaque: Cholesterol emboli that usually dislodges from the carotid arteries, or calcific fragments from a stenosed aortic valve that can be visualized on a retinal exam.

Homocysteine: A homolog of cysteine, produced by the demethylation of methionine, and an intermediate in the biosynthesis of l-cysteine from l-methionine through l-cystathionine. Elevated levels of homocysteine have been associated with certain forms of heart disease.

Homozygous: Presence of identical genes (alleles) at one location.

Hormone therapy: Either estrogen-only therapy or combined estrogen and progestogen therapy.

Hot flashes/flushes: A sensation of warmth, frequently accompanied by skin flushing and perspiration.

Human leukocyte antigen (HLA): The *self antigens* are the histocompatibility antigens found on human leukocytes and tissues that enable the body to differentiate *self* from *foreign* cells. The HLA antigens are used in histocompatibility testing to determine the suitability of an organ for transplant.

Humanistic outcomes: Patient-reported outcomes such as patient satisfaction and health-related quality of life.

Hydrocephalus: An uncharacteristic increase in the amount of cerebrospinal fluid within the skull, causing dangerous expansion of the cerebral ventricles.

Hyperalgesia: Exaggerated painful response to normally noxious stimuli.

Hyperarousal: A state of elevated or increased alertness, awareness, or wakefulness.

Hypercapnia: Elevation of carbon dioxide gas in the blood.

Hypercoagulable state: A disorder or state of excessive or frequent thrombus formation; also known as *thrombophilia.*

Hypereosinophilic syndrome: Hypereosinophilic syndrome is a group of leukoproliferative disorders characterized by an overproduction of eosinophils resulting in organ damage.

Hyperkalemia: Serum potassium concentration above 5.5 mEq/L.

Hypermagnesemia: Serum magnesium concentration above 1.8 mEq/L or 2.3 mg/dL.

Hyperpigmentation: Excess pigment in skin causing an area of darker color than surrounding skin.

Hyperprolactinemia: A state of persistent serum prolactin elevation characterized by prolactin concentrations greater than 20 mcg/L observed on multiple occasions.

Hyperresponsiveness: In the airways, the characteristic of an exaggerated response to stimuli.

Hypertensive crises: Clinical situations where blood pressure values are very elevated, typically greater than 180/120 mm Hg; they are categorized as either a hypertensive emergency or hypertensive urgency depending on the clinical presentation.

Hypertensive emergency: A clinical situation in which a patient has extremely high blood pressure values, typically greater than 180/120 mm Hg that is also accompanied by the presence of acute and/or progressing target-organ damage. Immediate but gradual reduction in blood pressure using intravenous antihypertensive agents is needed to prevent acute morbidity and/or mortality.

Hypertensive urgency: A clinical situation in which a patient has extremely high blood pressure values, typically greater than 180/120 mm Hg that is not accompanied by acute or progressing target-organ injury. These situations require oral antihypertensive therapy to reduce blood pressure to stage 1 values over a period of several hours to several days.

Hypertrophic cardiomyopathy: Hypertrophic cardiomyopathy is a genetic disorder characterized by disproportionate hypertrophy of the left ventricle, and occasionally of the right ventricle.

Hypervigilance: An enhanced state of sensory sensitivity accompanied by an exaggerated intensity of behaviors whose purpose it is to detect threats.

Hypnagogic hallucinations: Dreamlike experiences on the threshold of sleep that intrude into wakefulness.

Hypnopompic hallucinations: Dreamlike experiences on the threshold of awakening that intrude into wakefulness.

Hypochlorhydria: Presence of an abnormally small amount of hydrochloric acid in the stomach.

Hypokalemia: Serum potassium concentration below 3.5 mEq/L.

Hypomagnesemia: Serum magnesium concentration below 1.4 mEq/L or 1.7 mg/dL.

Hypomania: An abnormally and persistently elevated, expansive, or irritable mood that lasts at least 4 days but does not cause marked impairment in functioning.

Hypomimia: Decreased facial expression often associated with decreased blink rate.

Hypophonia: Decreased volume of speech.

Hypothalamus: A small region at the base of the brain that controls the release of hormones from the anterior and posterior regions of the pituitary gland and regulates limbic functions, fluid balance, body temperature, cardiovascular function, respiratory function, and diurnal rhythms.

Hysterectomy: Surgical removal of the uterus.

Hysteresis: A situation in which concentration-effect curves do not always follow the same pattern when serum concentrations increase as they do when serum concentrations decrease. Can result from tolerance to a drug (clockwise hysteresis) or accumulation of active metabolites (counterclockwise hysteresis).

Iatrogenesis or iatrogenic disease: A disease produced as a consequence of medical or surgical treatment.

Ictal: The period during a seizure.

Icteric: Relating to or marked by jaundice.

Idiopathic: Unknown etiology.

Ileitis: Inflammation of the ileus.

Illusions: Visual perceptions that are misinterpreted but have a real sensory stimulus.

Immunocompromised host: A patient with defects in host defenses that predisposes him or her to infection (risk factors can include neutropenia, immune system defects from disease or immunosuppressive drug therapy, compromise of natural host defenses, environmental contamination, and changes in normal flora of the host).

Immunoglobulin: Structurally related glycoproteins that function as antibodies and are divided into classes on the basis of structure/biologic activity.

Impaction: An immovable packing; a lodgment of something in a strait or passage of the body; as, impaction of the fetal head in the strait of the pelvis; impaction of food or feces in the intestines of man or beast.

Impending status epilepticus (SE): Any seizure that does not stop automatically within 5 minutes has been termed *impending SE.* This is a fairly new term that was created to recognize the importance of early treatment of SE. Pharmacologic and nonpharmacologic treatment of SE should be initiated for those seizures that do not spontaneously terminate within 5 minutes.

Impetigo: A superficial skin infection that is seen most commonly in children.

Implantable cardioverter-defibrillator (ICD): The ICD is a surgically implanted electronic device that monitors, detects, and treats potentially life-threatening ventricular tachycardia with rate-responsive ventricular pacing.

Inanition: Severe weakness and wasting as occurs from lack of food, defect in assimilation, or neoplastic disease.

Incubation period: The time between exposure of a biologic (i.e., pathogen), chemical, or radiologic substance and when symptoms first start to appear (also known as latency).

Induction: Administration of a highly intense level of immunosuppression in the perioperative period or use of antibody therapy to provide enough immunosuppression to delay administration of nephrotoxic calcineurin inhibitors.

Infant mortality: Deaths occurring in those younger than the age of 1 year per 1,000 live births.

Infants: Pediatric patients who are 1 month to 1 year of age.

Infection: Inflammatory response to invasion of normally sterile host tissue by the microorganisms.

Information bias: A flaw in measuring exposure or outcome data that results in systematic differences in the quality of information gathered for study and comparison groups. See also *Selection bias.*

Instrumental activities of daily living: Housekeeping chores, shopping, going outside, medication management. See also *Activities of daily living.*

Insulin-like growth factor-1: An anabolic peptide that acts as a direct stimulator of cell proliferation and growth in all body cells.

Integumentary system: Skin, subcutaneous tissue, and skin appendages.

Interleukin: A type of cytokine, usually influencing a white blood cell.

Intermittent-combined estrogen-progestogen therapy: A regimen that combines a daily estrogen with a progestogen administered intermittently in cycles of 3 days on and 3 days off (which is then repeated without interruption).

International normalized ratio (INR): A measure of coagulation calculated from the patient's prothrombin time (PT) measurement compared to the laboratory's mean normal control measurement and takes into account the sensitivity of the thromboplastin used to perform the test.

Interpersonal psychotherapy: A psychologic intervention that focuses on interpersonal relationships and psychosocial functioning.

Interpretability: The degree to which one can assign qualitative meaning to an instrument's quantitative scores.

Intertriginous areas: Body fold areas (e.g., between buttocks, beneath breasts, between toes, under arms).

Intoxication: The development of a substance-specific syndrome after recent ingestion and presence in the body of a substance; associated with maladaptive behavior during the waking state caused by the effect of the substance on the central nervous system.

Intracavernosal injection: Injection into the corpus spongiosum.

Intracranial hypertension: Excessive pressure (greater than 20 mm Hg) within the nondistensible intracranial cavity (i.e., skull) that can develop following traumatic brain injury.

Intracranial pressure: The pressure of the cerebral spinal fluid that is essentially the same as the pressure within the brain tissue (i.e., intraparenchymal pressure).

Intraperitoneal (IP): Situated within or administered by entering the peritoneum.

Intrauterine device: A device inserted in the uterus to prevent pregnancy, either through spermicidal action (copper device) or thickening cervical mucus to inhibit sperm penetration and migration (progesterone device).

Intrinsic resistance: See *Primary resistance.*

Intussusception: Invagination of one portion of the intestine into an adjacent part of the intestines.

Inulin: A fructose polysaccharide that is filtered by the glomerulus; its clearance is often used as an index of GFR.

Iothalamate: A nonradiolabeled or radiolabeled iodinated contrast agent that is filtered by the glomerulus; its clearance is often used as an index of GFR.

Irritable: Easily annoyed and provoked to anger.

Irritative voiding symptoms: Urinary urgency and frequency. This results from detrusor muscle decompensation that results from long-standing bladder outlet obstruction.

Isolated systolic hypertension: Patients with diastolic blood pressure values that are less than or equal to 90 mm Hg and systolic blood pressure values that are greater than or equal to 140 mm Hg.

Janeway lesion: These lesions appear as flat, painless, red to bluish-red spots on the palms and soles of patients with acute bacterial endocarditis.

Jarisch-Herxheimer reaction: An increase in symptoms of spirochetal disease caused by the initiation of treatment.

J-curve phenomenon (in hypertension): A theoretical situation where lowering blood pressure provides a reduced risk of cardiovascular events, but when blood pressure is lowered too much, can paradoxically increase the risk of cardiovascular events.

Jugular venous oxygen saturation (Sjv_{O_2}): Oxygen hemoglobin saturation of blood in the jugular bulb, which is a key element in estimating CMR_{O_2}.

K complexes: Electronegative waves followed by electropositive waves seen on the EEG during sleep.

Karyotyping: Chromosomal analysis.

Keratinization: Keratin formation.

Keratinized: Skin that has developed thicker areas of keratin in the stratum corneum.

Keratinocyte: Cell of the epidermis that produces keratin.

Keratoconjunctivitis sicca: Dry, itchy eyes that result from atrophy of the lacrimal ducts, which can be seen in inflammatory arthritis.

Keratolytic: Agent that solubilizes intracellular cement of keratin cells in the stratum corneum.

Ketogenic diet: A special antiseizure diet that is high in fat and low in carbohydrates and protein.

Kleptomania: An impulse control disorder characterized by frequent and repeated theft.

Kt/V: A measurement of how much urea is being removed from the blood during dialysis. The measurement takes into account the efficiency of the dialyzer (clearance, K), the treatment time (t), and the volume of distribution of urea (V).

Kussmaul sign: Kussmaul sign is a rise in jugular venous pressure on inspiration. Kussmaul sign is seen in conditions in which there is right ventricular filling.

Lactation: Production and secretion of breast milk.

Lanugo: Fine body hair normally found on a fetus. The hair develops in patients with anorexia nervosa when they are very underweight and malnourished.

Laparoscopic: Abdominal exploration or surgery employing a type of endoscope called laparoscope.

Laparotomy: Surgical opening of the abdominal cavity.

Laryngospasm: The spasmodic closure of the larynx because of a variety of causes such as allergic reactions, response to irritants, and pharmacologic actions.

Lavage: Washing out.

Laxative: A medication or agent used to produce a bowel movement.

Left ventricular ejection fraction: Also known simply as the ejection fraction, it is the fraction or percentage of the end diastolic blood volume ejected by the left ventricle during systole. It is a measurement of cardiac systolic function with a normal ejection being >60%. It can be determined noninvasively by an echocardiogram.

Left ventricular end diastolic volume: Left ventricular end diastolic volume refers to the volume of blood found in the left ventricular at the end of heart relaxation or diastole.

Left ventricular hypertrophy: Enlargement of the left ventricle, which is seen in heart failure and can give rise to arrhythmias.

Leptospirosis: A bacterial disease that affects humans and animals caused by the genus Leptospira.

Lewy bodies: Pink-staining spheres found inside neuronal cells of the substantia nigra and other brain regions, considered to be a histopathologic marker for Parkinson's disease.

Lichenification: Thickening of epidermis because of irritation.

Linear pharmacokinetics: The situation when changes in long-term daily doses of drugs result in proportional changes in steady state serum drug concentrations. Most drugs follow this pattern.

Linkage disequilibrium: Two or more polymorphisms that are inherited together more frequently than would be expected based on chance.

Lipid peroxidation: A pathophysiologic process involving the iron-catalyzed attack of lipid membranes by reactive oxygen species.

Liposomes: Spherical amphiphilic vesicles capable of sustained release of water-soluble substances.

Locus ceruleus: A small area in the brainstem containing norepinephrine neurons that is considered to be a key brain center for anxiety and fear.

Lower urinary tract symptoms: This term collectively refers to obstructive and irritative urinary voiding symptoms of benign prostatic hypertrophy (BPH).

Lumbar puncture: The procedure used to withdraw cerebrospinal fluid through a needle inserted in the lumbar region of the spinal column.

Luteinizing hormone (LH): A polypeptide hormone secreted by the anterior pituitary gland that stimulates ovulation and maintains the corpus luteum.

Luteolysis: Death of the corpus luteum.

Lymphangitis: An inflammation involving the subcutaneous lymphatic channels.

Lymphocytosis: Increased blood concentration of lymphocytes ($>4 \times 10^9$ cells/mm^3) commonly observed in mononucleosis, pertussis, measles, chickenpox, or lymphoid malignancies.

Lymphogranuloma venereum: Inflammation of the lymph nodes caused by *Chlamydia trachomatis* resulting in destruction and scarring of tissue.

Macule: Flat, nonpalpable, variable-colored lesion.

Maculopapular: Skin eruption containing both macules and papules.

Magnetic resonance angiography (MRA): A noninvasive method to evaluate the patency of blood vessels using magnetic resonance imaging.

Magnetic resonance imaging (MRI): An imaging technique based on the magnetic properties of the hydrogen atom. It provides an accurate, computer-processed image that can be more sensitive than computed tomography.

Major depression: A psychiatric disorder in which the patient can present with symptoms of depressed mood, a lack of interest in usual activities or inability to experience pleasure, changes in sleep and eating habits, guilt, reduced energy, thoughts of self-harm, and a sense of helplessness or hopelessness.

Major histocompatibility complex (MHC): A set of genes responsible for most of the proteins on the surface of cells in the body that are responsible for recognition of *self.*

Mania: An abnormally and persistently elevated, expansive, or irritable mood that lasts at least 1 week and causes marked impairment in functioning.

Mass effect: Distortion or displacement of the brain anatomy because of an implied or apparent mass (such as stroke or tumor).

Mastalgia or mastodynia: Pain in the breast.

Mean arterial pressure: The mean arterial pressure is the product of the cardiac output and systemic vascular resistance. Because the cardiac output is pulsatile, rather than continuous, and as two-thirds of the normal cardiac cycle is spent in diastole, the mean arterial pressure is not the arithmetic mean of the systolic and diastolic blood pressures. Mean arterial pressure = diastolic blood pressure + one-third (systolic blood pressure–diastolic blood pressure).

Measurement model: An instrument's scale and subscale structure and the procedures followed to create scale and subscale scores.

Meconium ileus: Intestinal obstruction caused by meconium.

Megakaryocytes: Precursors of platelets.

Melanin: Dark pigment that is part of determining skin color.

Melena: Dark-colored stools resulting from upper gastrointestinal bleed.

Membrane stripping: When the cervix is dilated, a practitioner can use a hand to separate the amniotic membranes from the uterus. This technique has been shown to reduce the need for labor induction.

Menarche: The time of the first menstrual period or flow.

Meningitis: Inflammation, usually infectious, of the meninges, a covering of the brain.

Menopause: The permanent cessation of menses following the loss of ovarian follicular activity.

Menorrhagia: Menstrual blood loss of greater than 80 mL per cycle; a more practical definition is heavy menstrual flow associated with problems of containment of flow, unpredictably heavy flow days, or other associated symptoms.

Menses: Periodic bloody discharge from the uterus.

Mental status examination: An objective patient evaluation conducted through a direct patient interview and used to make a diagnosis, assess the course of illness, or determine treatment response.

Mesolimbic pathway: A dopaminergic pathway in the brain that connects the ventral tegmental area in the midbrain to the nucleus accumbens in the striatum and is involved in motivation and reward.

Metabolic syndrome: A constellation of metabolic and cardiovascular changes consisting of at least three of the following: obesity, low high-density lipoprotein (HDL), elevated triglycerides, hypertension, and elevated fasting blood glucose.

Metastasis: Movement or spread of disease from one organ or part to a new location not directly connected.

Methemoglobin: A form of hemoglobin that occurs when its iron is oxidized to the +3 state, which decreases oxygen binding.

Methionine: The 1-isomer is a nutritionally essential amino acid and the most important natural source of *active methyl* groups in the body, hence usually involved in methylations in vivo.

Michaelis–Menten kinetics: The situation where changes in steady state serum drug concentrations of drugs are disproportional to changes in long-term daily doses because of alterations in drug metabolism.

Microalbuminuria: A condition in which a small amount of albumin (30–300 mg/day) is present in the urine; often indicates an early stage of chronic kidney disease (CKD).

Microcephalic: Abnormally small head.

Microcomedo: Microscopic lesion formed from the combination of sloughed, clumping keratinocytes reacting with sebum and fatty acids from the sebaceous gland.

Micrographia: Handwriting that is small, trails off in size, or very slow.

Midsystolic: Middle of systole.

Migraine aura: Early symptom of an attack of migraine with aura, which is the manifestation of focal cerebral dysfunction. The aura typically precedes the headache.

Mild cognitive impairment: A syndrome characterized by cognitive impairment that is not of sufficient severity to warrant a diagnosis of dementia.

Milia: Small, white cysts containing keratin.

Mixed states: Rapidly alternating mood states (mania and major depressive episodes) that last at least 1 week, and cause marked impairment in functioning.

Molds: Fungal organisms that grow as multicellular branching, thread-like filaments (hyphae) that are either *septate* (divided by transverse walls) or *coenocytic* (multinucleate without cross walls). On agar media, molds grow outward from the point of inoculation by extension of the tips of filaments, and then branch repeatedly, interweaving to form fuzzy, matted growths called *mycelium.* Germ tubes are the beginning of *hyphae*, which arise as perpendicular extensions from the yeast cell, with no constriction at their point of origin.

Molybdenum (Mo): A bioelement found in a number of proteins.

Monoamine neurotransmitters: Neurotransmitters that contain one amino group and are derived from amino acids such as tyrosine and tryptophan. Includes, among others, the catecholamines (dopamine and norepinephrine) and an indoleamine (serotonin).

Mood: A more pervasive and sustained emotional state that colors a person's perception of the world.

Morbilliform: Maculopapular lesions that become confluent on the face and body.

Mucolytic: The ability to break down mucus.

Mucositis: Inflammation of the mucosa.

Multiattribute health status classification systems: Preference-based HRQOL instruments for which health-state preferences have been derived from population studies. The instruments assess respondents' health status, and then population preferences are applied to produce the index score.

Multiparity: Condition of having given birth to multiple children.

Multiple-organ dysfunction syndrome (MODS): Presence of altered organ function requiring intervention to maintain homeostasis.

Multiple sclerosis (MS): A demyelinating disease, caused by inflammation, leading to neurologic deficits and often, disability.

Mutism: A state in which a person either has the inability or refuses to speak or vocalize sounds.

Mycotic: A fungal infection.

Myectomy: A surgical removal of the overgrown septal muscle to decrease the outflow tract obstruction.

Myocarditis: Inflammation of the cardiac muscle.

Myoclonic seizures: Brief shock-like muscular contractions of the face, trunk, and extremities. They usually begin in adolescence and are referred to as *juvenile myoclonic epilepsy* (JME).

Myoclonus: A sudden twitching of muscles or parts of muscles, without any rhythm or pattern.

Myositis: Inflammation of the muscle, characterized by pain, tenderness, and sometimes spasm in the affected area.

National Kidney Foundation (NKF): A major voluntary health organization that seeks to prevent kidney and urinary tract diseases, improve the health and well-being of individuals and families affected by these diseases, and increase the availability of all organs for transplantation.

Nausea: An unpleasant sensation associated with an awareness of the urge to vomit.

Necrosis: Local death of cells or tissue.

Necrotizing fasciitis: A rare, but very severe infection of the subcutaneous tissue that can be caused by aerobic and/or anaerobic bacteria and results in progressive destruction of the superficial fascia and subcutaneous fat.

Negative symptoms: Those symptoms of schizophrenia that are largely associated with a deficit in psychosocial functioning, emotional expression, and interpersonal interactions. Examples include blunted affect, alogia, decreased interest and involvement in social and occupational activities, and decreased grooming and hygiene.

Neonatal: Within the first 4 weeks (28 days) of life.

Neonates: Newborns who are 1 day to 1 month of age.

Nephritis: Inflammation of the kidney.

Nephrolithiasis: Presence of one or more stones in the renal pelvis, collecting system, or ureters.

Nephron: The working unit of the kidney that is comprised of a glomerulus and tubule. Each kidney is made up of approximately 1 million nephrons, which collectively remove drugs, toxins, and fluid from the blood.

Nephropathy: Refers to a pathologic alteration of the kidney.

Nephrotic range proteinuria: Proteinuria >3 g/day associated with glomerular disease and nephrotic syndrome.

Nephrotoxicity: Toxic insult to the kidney.

Nerve conduction studies: Measurement of the speed of electrical conduction through a nerve.

Neuraminidase: The second major antigenic determinant of the influenza virus; a surface antigen that allows the release of new viral particles from host cells by catalyzing the cleavage of linkages to sialic acid.

Neuritic plaques: Hallmark pathologic marker of Alzheimer's disease comprised of β-amyloid protein and masses of broken neurites.

Neurofibrillary tangles: Hallmark pathologic marker of Alzheimer's disease derived from abnormal phosphorylation of τ-protein filaments.

Neuropathic pain: Pain caused by nervous system damage.

Neutropenia: An abnormally reduced number of neutrophils circulating in peripheral blood; although exact definitions of neutropenia often vary, an absolute neutrophil count of <1000 cells/mm^3 indicates a reduction sufficient to predispose patients to infection.

New York Heart Association classification: The New York Heart Association classification provides a simple way of classifying the extent of heart failure. It places patients in one of four categories based on how much they are limited during physical activity.

***N*-methyl-D-aspartate antagonists:** Class of medications that decreases the activity of synaptic glutamate, thus decreasing the likelihood of cell death.

***N*-methyl-D-aspartate (NMDA) receptor:** An ionotropic subtype glutamate receptor that coexists with the α-amino-3-hydroxy-5-methylisoxazole-4-propionic acid (AMPA) receptor involved in excitatory neurotransmission; it is responsible for the slow opening and closing phase of the depolarization of the postsynaptic membrane involving sodium and calcium entry; a cellular receptor complex involved in the intracellular passage of calcium into CNS cells on stimulation by amines such as glutamate and aspartate; one of three types of ionotropic post-synaptic glutamate receptors. On binding glutamate, these receptors permit the influx of calcium ions (Ca^{+2}) and result in brain excitation. These are one of the two primary receptors for excitatory neurotransmission in the brain.

Nociceptive pain: Pain caused by physiologic processes that involve stimulation, transmission, perception, modulation, and adaptive inflammation.

Nocturia: Frequent nighttime urination (>2 micturitions per night).

Nodule: Elevated, palpable, solid, round or oval lesion more than 0.5 cm in diameter.

Nonarteritic, anterior, ischemic optic neuropathy: A disorder caused by an acute decrease of blood flow to the optic nerve, which results in sudden vision loss. If persistent, it can lead to permanent vision loss.

Nonconvulsive status epilepticus (NCSE): Believed to be less common and to have a better prognosis than GCSE. The most common two types are absence status epilepticus and complex partial status epilepticus. Both are associated with an impairment in consciousness. For the more common of the two, absence status, the patient appears in a twilight state to lethargy. For complex partial status epilepticus partial return to consciousness can occur, and it may or may not be associated with motor activity or automatisms. The duration is sufficient enough in length to meet the definition of SE.

Nonoliguria: Production of >450 mL urine/day.

Nonpolyposis: Absence of polyps.

Nonulcer dyspepsia: Ulcer-like dyspepsia that has been investigated, but endoscopic findings yield no evidence of mucosal injury (ulcer).

Norepinephrine (NE): A hormone secreted by the adrenal medulla and also released at synapses.

Nosocomial infection: An infection acquired in a healthcare facility.

NSAID: Nonsteroidal antiinflammatory drug.

***N*-terminal proBNP:** The biologically inactive fragment of B-type natriuretic peptide (BNP). Compared to BNP, *N*-terminal proBNP circulates at higher plasma concentrations and has a longer half-life.

Nulliparity: Condition of not having given birth to a child.

Oblique lie: The fetus is at an angle to the cervix. The head is not the presenting part, and often the patient will need to be delivered by cesarean section.

Obsession: Recurrent and persistent thoughts, images, or impulses experienced as intrusive and distressing.

Obsessive–compulsive disorder (OCD): An anxiety disorder characterized by obsessions and/or compulsions that are time-consuming and interfere significantly with normal routine, social or occupational functioning, or relationships.

Obstructive voiding symptoms: Decreased force of the urinary stream, hesitancy, incomplete bladder emptying, urinary dribbling. This results from bladder outlet obstruction as could be caused by benign prostatic hyperplasia.

Odynophagia: Painful swallowing.

Oligoanovulation: The condition of having few to no ovulatory menstrual cycles.

Oligomenorrhea: Reduced frequency of menses with a time interval between periods greater than 40 days but less than 6 months.

Oliguria: Diminished volume of urine output (volume <400 to 500 mL/day).

Omentumectomy: Excision of the double fold of peritoneum attached to the stomach and connecting it with abdominal viscera (omentum).

Onychomycosis: Fungal infection of the nail apparatus.

Open prostatectomy: In this surgical procedure, an enlarged prostate is removed in its entirety. Access to the prostate can be achieved by cutting through the bladder and reaching down to the prostate, or by cutting through the perineum (between the legs).

Ophthalmia neonatorum: Inflammation of the conjunctiva resulting from acquisition of gonococcal infection at birth.

Opioid addiction: A behavioral pattern manifesting as loss of control over opioid use, compulsive use, and continued use despite harm.

Opioid dependence: State that occurs subsequent to extended exposure to an opioid and manifests as withdrawal symptoms after abrupt dose reduction, discontinuation, or after the administration of an opioid antagonist.

Opioid tolerance: Decreased effectiveness of opioid over time because of opioid exposure.

Opportunistic infection (OI): Infection with microorganism that occurs because of altered physiologic state of the patient.

Orchiectomy: The surgical removal of the testicles.

Organic erectile dysfunction: Term used to refer to erectile dysfunction that is caused by vascular, neurologic, and/or hormonal causes.

Orthopnea: Difficulty breathing after lying down.

Orthostatic hypotension: A significant drop in blood pressure, defined as a systolic blood pressure decrease of greater than 20 mm Hg or a diastolic blood pressure decrease of greater than 10 mm Hg, that occurs when changing from a supine to a standing position.

Osler nodes: Osler nodes are red, raised tender nodules usually 5 mm in diameter on the pulps of toes or fingers. Seen in patients with endocarditis, they are thought to be caused by the deposition of immune complexes.

Osteogenesis imperfecta: Genetic disorder characterized by low trabecular and cortical bone density.

Osteomalacia: Abnormal bone mineralization, referred to as rickets in children.

Osteopenia: Low bone density, dual-energy x-ray absorptiometry (DXA) T-score of –1 to –2.5

Osteophyte: A bony outgrowth or protuberance.

Osteoporosis: Very low bone density, DXA T-score less than –2.5, with or without a low trauma fracture. National Osteoporosis Foundation definition: "A chronic, progressive disease characterized by low bone mass, microarchitectural deterioration and decreased bone strength, bone fragility and a consequent increase in fracture risk."

Osteotomy: The surgical cutting of a bone.

Otitis media: Inflammation of the middle ear.

Ovulation: Periodic ripening and rupture of mature follicle and the discharge of ovum from the cortex of the ovary.

Oxytocin: A polypeptide hormone secreted by the posterior pituitary gland that stimulates uterine contraction.

Paget's disease: Disorder of bone remodeling in discrete sections of bone.

PAH: *p*-aminohippurate, a small molecule that is completely secreted from the tubules into urine, so that blood leaving the kidney is virtually free of PAH; a marker that is often used to measure renal plasma flow (RPF).

Pain: An unpleasant sensory and emotional experience associated with actual or potential tissue damage or described in terms of such damage.

Palpation: Touching the skin to feel the outline of an organ.

Pan- or holosystolic: Throughout the end time of systole.

Pancolitis: Inflammation that involves the majority of the colon in patients with inflammatory bowel disease.

Pancreatitis: An acute or chronic inflammation of the pancreas with variable involvement of local tissues and remote organs.

Panel reactive antibody (PRA): The percentage of cells from a panel of donors with which a potential recipient's bloodstream reacts. The more antibodies in the recipient's bloodstream, the higher the PRA. The higher the PRA, the higher the risk for a positive crossmatch.

Panhypopituitarism: A condition of complete or partial loss of anterior and posterior pituitary function resulting in a complex disorder characterized by multiple pituitary-hormone deficiencies.

Panic attack: A discrete period in which there is the sudden onset of intense apprehension, fearfulness, or terror, often associated with feelings of impending doom.

Panic disorder: The presence of recurrent, unexpected panic attacks followed by at least 1 month of persistent concern about having another panic attack, worry about the possible implications or consequences of the panic attacks, or a significant behavioral change related to the attacks.

Panlobular: Affecting the entire lobe.

Papillary: Upper layer of the dermis.

Papilledema: Swelling around the optic nerve, usually caused by pressure on the nerve by a tumor or stroke.

Papule: Solid, elevated, lesion more than 0.5 cm in diameter.

Papulosquamous: Raised plaque or papule with scaling.

***p*-Aminohippurate (PAH):** A small molecule that is completely secreted from the tubules into urine, so that blood leaving the kidney is virtually free of PAH; a marker that is often used to measure renal plasma flow (RPF).

Paranoia: Ideation involving suspiciousness or the belief that one is being harassed, persecuted, or unfairly treated.

Parenchyma: Specific cells or tissue of an organ.

Paresthesia: An abnormal sensation, such as of burning, pricking, tickling, or tingling.

Parkinsonism: A constellation of symptoms with atypical features such that a diagnosis of idiopathic Parkinson disease cannot be made.

Parous: Having borne one or more children.

Paroxysmal nocturnal dyspnea: Onset of difficulty breathing after lying down for several hours.

Partial agonist: A drug with high binding affinity to a receptor and that elicits a weaker response than the endogenous neurotransmitter. At least theoretically, this causes an agonist effect in states of decreased endogenous neurotransmitter tone and an antagonist effect in the endogenous state of heightened neurotransmitter activity.

Partial seizure: A seizure that begins in one hemisphere of the brain. It can be simple, complex, or secondarily generalized.

Patch: Large macule (more than 2 cm in diameter).

Patient-reported outcomes: The consequences of the disease and/or its treatment as perceived and reported by the patient.

Pelvic inflammatory disease (PID): Infection of the lining of the uterus, the fallopian tubes, or the ovaries.

Penumbra (ischemic): The area of brain tissue around the core of the infarct that has decreased function but remains viable. It is proposed that reperfusion of this tissue will allow survival of the affected neurons and other brain cells.

Peptic ulcer: Cellular distribution of the gastrointestinal mucosa, submucosa, and muscular layer. Chronic peptic ulcers usually occur as a *single hole* and are found most often in the stomach and duodenum.

Percussion: Tapping on a structure to elicit a sound.

Percussion and postural drainage: Tapping on the thorax to physically loosen pulmonary secretions and posturing the body to facilitate expectoration.

Percutaneous coronary intervention (PCI): A minimally invasive procedure whereby access to the coronary arteries is obtained through the femoral artery up the aorta to the coronary os. Contrast media is used to visualize the coronary artery stenosis using a coronary angiogram. A guidewire is used to cross the stenosis and small balloon is inflated and/or stent is deployed to break up atherosclerotic plaque and restore coronary artery blood flow. The stent is left in place to prevent restenosis of the coronary artery.

Pericarditis: Inflammation of the pericardium, which is the fibroserous sac enclosing the heart.

Perimenopause: The period immediately prior to the menopause and the first year after menopause. Reflects the transition to menopause (with irregular menstrual cycles) and includes the 3 to 5 years before and 1 year after the cessation of menstrual flow.

Perinatal: Time shortly before and after birth.

Perioral dermatitis: Rash around the mouth. In patients with anorexia nervosa or bulimia nervosa, the rash is secondary to repeated vomiting that creates skin irritation from exposure to the gastric contents.

Peripheral arterial disease (PAD): Atherosclerotic occlusive disease of the extremities, usually diagnosed by symptoms (claudication) or assessment of the blood flow to an extremity.

Peripheral blood progenitor cells: Immature blood cells, which are capable of producing white blood cells, platelets, and red blood cells.

Peritoneal dialysis (PD): A dialysis procedure performed in the peritoneal cavity in which the peritoneum acts as the semipermeable membrane.

Peritonitis: The acute, inflammatory response of the peritoneal lining to microorganisms, chemicals, irradiation, or foreign body injury.

Perseveration: Persistent repetition of the same verbal or motor response despite differing stimuli.

Pervasive developmental disorder: A group of disorders characterized by severe and pervasive impairments in the development of socialization and communication skills, as well as behavioral repertoire, with a typical diagnosis younger than age 3 years; includes autistic disorder, Rett syndrome, pervasive development disorder not otherwise specified, childhood disintegrative disorder, and Asperger disorder.

Petechiae: Pinpoint, flat, round, red spots under the skin caused by intradermal hemorrhage.

Peyronie's disease: Disease of the penis associated with fibrous tissue scarring along the inside of the penile shaft resulting in significant and abnormal curvature of the erect penis. Associated with penile pain; deformity makes sexual intercourse difficult or impossible.

P-glycoprotein: An adenosine triphosphatase (ATPase)-dependent membrane transporter efflux pump coded for by the multidrug-resistance gene 1 (MDR1 or ABCB1 or PGY1) found in the human blood-brain barrier and intestine as well as other tissues; lipophilic molecules are good substrates for the ABCB1 efflux transport system at the blood–brain barrier.

Pharmacodynamics: The study of the relationship between the concentration of a drug and the response obtained in a patient.

Pharmacoepidemiology: The study of the use of and the effects of drugs in large numbers of people with the purpose of supporting safe and effective drug therapies. This type of observational research is useful when more rigorous, experimental designs are not feasible.

Pharmacogenetics: Genetic basis for interindividual differences in drug response.

Pharmacovigilance: The science and activities relating to the detection, assessment, understanding, and prevention of adverse effects or any other drug-related problems.

Pharyngitis: An acute infection of the oropharynx or nasopharynx.

Phase I reactions: Metabolic changes by the body that generally make the drug molecule more polar and water soluble so that it is prone to elimination by the kidney, such as oxidation, hydrolysis, and reduction.

Phase II reactions: Metabolic changes by the body that generally make the drug molecule more prone to elimination by the kidney, such as conjugation to form glucuronides, acetates, or sulfates.

Phenotypes: How a gene is expressed (e.g., eye color, height, drug metabolism capacity). The expression of genetic alleles (genotype) as an observable physical or biochemical trait.

Phobia: A persistent, abnormal, and irrational fear of a specific thing or situation that compels one to avoid it, despite the awareness and reassurance that it is not dangerous.

Phonophobia: Hypersensitivity to sound, usually causing avoidance.

Photic stimulation: Stimulation of the visual cortex through visual stimulation with bright and alternating light.

Photoallergy: Photosensitivity disorder of skin (light and photoallergic agent).

Photophobia: Hypersensitivity to light, usually causing avoidance.

Phototoxicity: Photosensitivity disorder of skin (light and phototoxic agent).

Physical dependence: A state of adaptation that is manifested by a drug class–specific withdrawal syndrome that can be produced by abrupt cessation, rapid dose reduction, decreasing blood level of the drug, and/or administration of an antagonist.

Pilonidal: Hair-containing cyst.

Pilosebaceous: Sebaceous gland and adjacent hair follicle.

Placenta previa: The placenta is located over the cervical opening. In this situation, the mother and baby can hemorrhage because the placenta will separate from the uterus before the baby is born. Women who have a placenta previa must be delivered by cesarean section.

Plaque: Raised, flat lesion (more than 2 cm in diameter).

Pneumonitis: Inflammation of lung tissue.

Poikilocytosis: The presence of irregularly shaped red blood cells in the peripheral blood.

Poikilothermia: Inability to maintain normal body temperature.

Polyarteritis nodosa: A systemic necrotizing vasculitis of small and medium-sized arteries.

Polycythemia: An increase in the number of red cells present in the blood.

Polymorphisms: Interindividual variations in the genetic code at the level of one nucleotide.

Porphyria: A group of disorders involving heme biosynthesis, characterized by excessive excretion of porphyrins or their precursors; can be inherited or can be acquired, as from the effects of certain chemical agents.

Porphyrins: Pigments widely distributed throughout nature (e.g., heme, bile pigments, cytochromes) consisting of four pyrroles joined in a ring (porphin) structure.

Positive symptoms: Those symptoms of schizophrenia, largely based on perceptual and thought disturbances, that are typically associated with psychosis. Examples are suspiciousness, paranoia, delusions, hallucinations, and disorganized thought processes.

Positron emission tomography (PET): Specialized nuclear scanning technique that allows the measurement of regional blood flow and glucose metabolism. With radiolabeled ligands, also allows for the measurement of the binding of drugs to receptors.

Posterior fossa: The cavity in the back part of the skull that contains the cerebellum, brainstem, and cranial nerves 5–12.

Postexposure prophylaxis: Dispensing or administering a medication (including a vaccine) to start immediately after exposure to a disease or organism, to prevent the disease from developing or spreading.

Postictal: The recovery period after a seizure, when a patient can be lethargic or confused. Duration can be variable.

Posttraumatic seizures: Seizure event(s) that can occur following a traumatic brain injury within the first 7 days postinjury (early) or beyond 7 days postinjury (late).

Postrenal acute renal failure (ARF): Acute renal failure with an anatomical cause that is in the urinary tract.

Posttraumatic stress disorder: An anxiety disorder in which exposure to an exceptional mental or physical stressor is followed by persistent reexperiencing of the event, avoidance of reminders of the event, and arousal symptoms.

Postvoid residual urine volume: Urine left in the bladder after the patient has been asked to completely empty urine out of the bladder. Normally the postvoid residual urine volume should be zero. A high postvoid residual urine volume is associated with recurrent urinary tract infection.

PRA (panel reactive antibody): The percentage of cells from a panel of donors with which a potential recipient's bloodstream reacts. The more antibodies in the recipient's bloodstream, the higher the PRA. The higher the PRA, the higher the risk for a positive crossmatch.

Preexposure vaccination: Administration of a protective vaccine to the public, military troops, or high-risk individuals prior to the potential exposure to an infectious disease.

Preference-based measures: Measures that provide an overall HRQOL index score based on a scale anchored by 1.0 (full health) and 0.0 (dead).

Prefrontal cortex: Part of the brain that integrates thought, emotion, and motivation.

Preload: Along with afterload, it is an important determinant of cardiac output. It is the degree of stretch of the myocardial fibers (sarcomeres) at the end of diastole. As the sarcomeres are stretched, the force of contraction increases. Preload is approximated by the left ventricular end diastolic volume or pressure.

Premature infants: Those born before 37 weeks of gestational age.

Premature ovarian failure: Amenorrhea, sex-steroid deficiency, and infertility in women younger than 40 years of age.

Premenstrual dysphoric disorder (PMDD): Severe psychiatric mood disorder with marked affective symptoms causing significant interference in work or relationships temporally associated with the luteal phase and not caused by an underlying psychiatric disturbance; a severe form of premenstrual syndrome and is listed in the appendix of the *Diagnostic and Statistical Manual of Mental Disorders, Fourth Edition Revised.* The diagnostic criteria require prospective documentation of symptoms, a specific constellation of symptoms, and functional impairment.

Premenstrual molimina: Includes premenstrual symptoms such as breast tenderness, pelvic heaviness or bloating, and food cravings that are not distressing and do not interfere with daily functioning.

Premenstrual syndrome (PMS): A constellation of symptoms including mild mood disturbance and physical symptoms that occur prior to the menses and resolve with initiation of menses.

Premonitory migraine symptoms: Symptoms preceding and forewarning of a migraine attack by 2 to 48 hours, occurring before the aura in migraine with aura and before the onset of pain in migraine without aura.

Prerenal ARF: Acute renal failure caused by a reduction of renal blood flow. Often associated with volume depletion or poor cardiac function.

Presbycusis: Progressive bilateral loss of hearing that occurs in the aged.

Pressured speech: More and faster speech that is difficult or impossible to interrupt.

Preterm: Before 37 weeks of gestation.

Priapism: Painful prolonged erection.

Primary amenorrhea: Absence of menses by age 16 years in the presence of normal secondary sexual development or absence of menses by age 14 years in the absence of normal secondary sexual development.

Primary hypogonadism: Failure of the testes to produce an adequate supply of testosterone to meet physiologic needs.

Primary lesion: Basic skin lesion that appears at the beginning of skin disorder.

Primary resistance: Refers to resistance recorded prior to drug exposure in vitro or in vivo, as determined by in-vitro susceptibility testing using standardized methodology.

Proctitis: Inflammation confined to the rectum in patients with inflammatory bowel disease.

Prodrome: Early symptom indicating that disease or further symptoms are imminent.

Progestogen: A term referring to progesterone and the synthetic progestational compounds (sometimes referred to as *progestins*).

Prolactin: A polypeptide hormone secreted by the anterior pituitary gland that stimulates lactation.

Proprioception: A sense or perception, usually at a subconscious level, of the movements and position of the body and especially its limbs, independent of vision; this sense is gained primarily from input from sensory nerve terminals in muscles and tendons and the fibrous capsule of joints combined with input from the vestibular apparatus.

Prostate-specific antigen (PSA): A clinical laboratory test; PSA is a tumor marker that is used to screen for, monitor response to treatment of, and determine degree of spread of prostate cancer. Normally, PSA blood levels should be low as PSA is passed out of the body in the ejaculate.

Prostatectomy: Removal of all or part of the prostate gland. There are two main types: (1) transurethral resection of the prostate (TURP)—removes part of the tissue surrounding the urethra that can be blocking the flow of urine; and (2) radical prostatectomy, which removes all of the prostate and the seminal vesicles.

Protease: An enzyme in HIV that cleaves large precursor polypeptides into functional proteins that are necessary to produce a complete virus.

Proteinuria: A condition in which the urine contains large amounts of protein (>150 mg/day); often a sign of glomerular or tubular damage in the kidney.

Proteolytic: The ability to break down protein.

Prothrombin: A clotting factor that is converted to thrombin; also known as factor II.

Prothrombin time (PT): A measure of coagulation representing the amount of time required to form a blood clot after the addition of thromboplastin to the blood sample; also known as Quick's test.

Pruritus: Itching.

Pseudoaddiction: A behavior pattern reflective of seeking relief of pain and resembling that of addictive behavior.

Pseudoallergic: Adverse reactions that appear like allergic reactions but do not have an immunologic mechanism.

Pseudocyst: Collection of pancreatic juice and tissue debris enclosed by a wall of fibrous or granulation tissue.

Pseudohypertension: A falsely elevated blood pressure measurement that is usually because of rigid, calcified brachial arteries; this can be seen in patients who are ≥65 years, have long-standing diabetes, or have chronic kidney disease.

Pseudomembranous colitis: Inflammation of the colon caused by the toxin of *Clostridium difficile* and resulting in bloody diarrhea.

Pseudopolyps: An area of hypertrophied gastrointestinal mucosa that resembles a polyp and contains nonmalignant cells.

Pseudoxanthoma elasticum: Pseudoxanthoma elasticum is a chronic degenerative disease of connection tissues of the skin, eyes, and cardiovascular system resulting from fragmentation and calcification of elastic fibers.

Psychoeducation: Education geared toward patients becoming more informed about their mental illness and treatment. Additional goals include self-monitoring, efforts to improve treatment adherence, interactions between patient and clinicians, and empowerment.

Psychogenic erectile dysfunction: Erectile dysfunction because of failure of central nervous system to perceive or process sexually stimulating information.

Psychometrics: The measurement of psychologic constructs, such as quality of life.

Psychomotor: Movement or muscular activity related to mental processes.

Psychomotor retardation: A slowing or limitation of motor functioning or muscular movements.

Psychosocial functioning: A person's level of functioning on a daily basis that encompasses all the domains of life experience (e.g., interpersonal relationships, work, school, recreation).

Psychosocial rehabilitation programs: Care programs oriented toward improving patient's daily adaptive functioning. Includes such interventions as basic living skills, social skills training, basic education, work programs, and supported housing.

Psychosocial stressor: Any significant life event or change that can be associated with the onset, occurrence, or exacerbation of a mental disorder.

Psychotherapy: A general term used to describe a form of treatment based on talking with a therapist. Psychotherapy aims to relieve distress by discussing and expressing feelings, to help the patient to change attitudes, behavior, and habits and to develop better ways of coping.

Pulmonary artery occlusion pressure: It is usually determined by a balloon-tipped Swan-Ganz catheter that is advanced into a distal branch of the pulmonary artery. Inflation of the balloon at the catheter tip occludes the pulmonary artery and allows measurement of the left atrial pressure that reflects the left ventricular diastolic pressure. Therefore, it is a measure of the left ventricular preload.

Pulmonary aspiration: The inhalation of fluids and gastric contents into the lungs that can cause aspiration pneumonitis.

Pulmonary embolism: A disorder of thrombus formation causing obstruction of a pulmonary artery or one of its branches and results in pulmonary infarction.

Pulsating: Throbbing or beating with a rhythm.

Pulseless electrical activity (PEA): The absence of a detectable pulse and the presence of some type of electrical activity other than ventricular fibrillation (VF) or paroxysmal ventricular tachycardia.

Purgatives: An agent used for purging the bowels.

Purpura: Discoloration of skin because of a hemorrhagic spot more than 0.5 cm in diameter.

Pustule: Small, raised lesion containing pus or exudates.

Pyelonephritis: An infection involving the kidneys and representing upper tract infection.

Pyoderma: Purulent skin disease.

Pyoderma gangrenosum: Skin ulceration with necrotic edges.

Pyuria: Presence of pus or white blood cells in the urine.

Quality-adjusted life-years (QALY): A health outcome summary measure in which quantity of life is adjusted for its quality. A year in full health is equivalent to 1.0 QALY. A year in a health state considered worse than full health, such as 0.5, would equal 0.5 QALY, which is equivalent to living half a year in full health.

Radionuclide ventriculography: Radionuclide ventriculography, also known as contrast ventriculography, provides imaging of a ventricle of the heart after the injection of a radioactive contrast medium. The technique is less invasive than cardiac catheterization and is used to assess ventricular function.

Rales: The clicking, rattling, or crackling noises heard on auscultation of the lungs during inhalation.

Rating scales: Tools used to objectively describe, assess, and measure subjective findings common in psychiatric illnesses. Rating scales are also used to diagnose specific psychiatric conditions.

Rational polytherapy: The concurrent use of two or more drugs for patients not responding to monotherapy. The combination of drugs is based on a consideration of mechanism of action, clinical pharmacokinetics, adverse reactions, and drug interactions.

Rebound insomnia: Sleep that is worsened compared to patients' baseline sleep for a few days after discontinuation of a sedative hypnotic medication.

Rebound vasodilation or congestion: See *Rhinitis medicamentosa.*

Refractory status epilepticus: SE is considered refractory when adequate doses of a benzodiazepine, hydantoin, or barbiturate have failed to terminate the seizures. That is, a patient must have failed two first-line therapies to be considered refractory.

Rejection: The response of the immune system, usually involving T- or B-lymphocytes, to the recognition of foreign antigens in transplanted tissue, which destroys the cells in the transplanted organ and ultimately leads to organ failure, if not treated successfully.

Relapse: New or old multiple sclerosis symptoms lasting 24 hours or longer often associated with demyelination or inflammation in the brain or spinal cord. Relapses are also referred to as an attack, exacerbation, or flare-up of multiple sclerosis.

Relapsing-remitting multiple sclerosis: The most common form of multiple sclerosis at the time of diagnosis. It is characterized by attacks usually with full or partial recovery and no disease progression between attacks.

Relative risk reduction: The amount of risk reduced when compared to a control. When one sees a 5% event rate in the control group and a 4% event rate in the treatment group, the relative risk reduction is 20%. The absolute risk reduction is 1%.

Reliability: The extent to which measures give consistent or accurate results.

Remote symptomatic: When the cause of the SE is from a previous neurologic injury or anatomic malformation, e.g., a patient with a prior stroke, head trauma, or brain tumor.

Renal osteodystrophy (ROD): The condition resulting from sustained metabolic changes that occur with chronic kidney disease including secondary hyperparathyroidism, hyperphosphatemia, hypocalcemia, and vitamin D deficiency. The skeletal complications associated with ROD include osteitis fibrosa cystica (high bone turnover disease), osteomalacia (low bone turnover disease), adynamic bone disease, and mixed bone disorders.

Renal replacement therapy: Any form of dialysis or hemofiltration used to support patients without adequate kidney function. Goals of renal replacement therapy are to remove excess fluid; remove waste products and toxins; and control electrolyte concentrations.

Renal: General term referring to the kidneys.

Renin-angiotensin aldosterone system: A complex endogenous humorally mediated system that is involved with most of the regulatory components involved with arterial blood pressure.

Renovascular: Pertaining to blood vessels located within the kidney, such as the afferent and efferent arterioles, and renal arteries.

Respiratory disturbance index: A summary measure that quantifies the number of apneas, hypopneas, and respiratory effort-related arousals per hour of sleep.

Respondent burden: The time, energy, and other demands placed on those to whom the instrument is administered.

Responsiveness: The ability or power of a measure to detect clinically important change when it occurs.

Resting tremor: Tremor that occurs or exacerbates when the affected body part is at rest; it decreases or disappears with active motions.

Restrictive cardiomyopathy: Restrictive cardiomyopathy is characterized by nondilated ventricles with impaired ventricular filling. Hypertrophy is typically absent, although the infiltrative and storage diseases can cause a left ventricular wall thickness elevation.

Retching: Contractions of the diaphragm, thoracic, and abdominal muscles without expulsion of gastric contents.

Retinitis: Inflammation of the retina, often caused by infection with cytomegalovirus.

Retrograde pyelography: A procedure where radiocontrast dye is injected into the ureter to produce detailed radiographs of the ureter and kidneys.

Rett's syndrome: A type of pervasive developmental disorder typically associated with severe to profound mental retardation, seen in females only, with the development of significant multiple progressively worsening deficits following a period of normal development (microcephaly, loss of purposeful hand motor skills, and acquisition of stereotyped hand movements, diminished social interests, and appearance of poorly coordinated gait or trunk movements).

Reverse transcriptase: The enzyme in HIV that synthesizes a complementary strand of DNA.

Reye's syndrome: Acute encephalopathy characterized by fever, vomiting, fatty infiltration of the liver, disorientation, and coma, occurring mainly in children and usually following a viral infection, such as chicken pox or influenza.

Rhabdomyolysis: The breakdown of muscle tissue and release of myoglobin and intracellular electrolytes into the circulation because of a variety of causes such as crush injuries, drug-induced immobilization, and status epilepticus. It often leads to acute renal failure.

Rheumatoid arthritis: A systemic, symmetric autoimmune disease with swelling, pain, and inflammation of joints as a key finding.

Rhinitis: Inflammation of the nasal mucous membrane. Can be seasonal (*hay fever*) or perennial (increasingly called *intermittent* or *persistent*).

Rhinitis medicamentosa: Nasal congestion associated with tolerance to and resulting overuse of topical decongestants. Also known as *rebound vasodilation* or *rebound congestion.*

Rickets: See *Osteomalacia.*

Rigidity: Increased resistance detectable with the passive movement of a limb.

Roth spots: A hemorrhage in the retina with a white center. Roth spots are often associated with bacterial endocarditis.

Russell sign: Callus on dorsum of the hand secondary to self-induced vomiting.

S_4 gallop: An S_4 gallop is a presystolic atrial sound that immediately precedes the first heart sound (S_1). This finding on auscultation of the heart can be indicative of myocardial disease.

Salicylism: Poisoning by salicylic acid or any of its compounds.

Salpingo-oophorectomy: Surgical removal of the ovaries and fallopian tubes.

Sarcoidosis: Sarcoidosis is a multisystem granulomatous disorder of unknown etiology characterized histologically by noncaseating epithelioid granulomas involving various organs or tissues, with symptoms dependent on the site and degree of involvement.

Scale: Flake of stratum corneum.

Scar: Fibrous tissue formed during healing of injury to skin.

Schizophrenia: A chronic disorder of thought and affect encompassing different constellations of symptoms (i.e., positive symptoms, negative symptoms, cognitive dysfunction), with the individual having a significant disturbance in interpersonal relationships and ability to function in society on a daily basis.

Scleritis: Inflammation of the white portion of the eyeball, which can be superficial (episcleritis) or involve deeper layers of the eye.

Scleroderma: Scleroderma is a diffuse connective tissue disease characterized by changes in the skin, blood vessels, skeletal muscles, and internal organs.

Sebaceous gland: Gland that secretes sebum.

Sebosuppressive: Decreasing amount of sebum produced by the sebaceous gland.

Sebum: Oil produced by the sebaceous gland.

Second-generation antipsychotic (atypical antipsychotic): An antipsychotic medication that has pharmacodynamic and clinical properties different than the first generation (typical or traditional) antipsychotics that act primarily by having high levels of binding to dopamine-2 (D_2) receptors. Although definitions of atypicality vary, all second-generation antipsychotics share the property of causing a much lower incidence of extrapyramidal side effects.

Secondary amenorrhea: Cessation of menses in a woman previously menstruating for 6 months or more.

Secondary brain injury: A complex sequence of pathophysiologic events precipitated by the initial or primary brain injury that disrupts the normal central nervous system balance between oxygen supply and demand resulting in a worsened patient outcome.

Secondary hypertension: Persistently elevated blood pressure that results from a known pathophysiologic etiology or drug-induced cause.

Secondary hypogonadism: Failure of hypothalamus or pituitary gland to produce adequate amount of luteinizing hormone-releasing hormone (LHRH) or luteinizing hormone (LH). Thus, testicular production of testosterone is reduced.

Secondary prophylaxis (or suppressive therapy): Refers to administration of systemic antifungal agents (generally prior to and throughout the period of granulocytopenia) to prevent relapse of a documented invasive fungal infection that was treated during a previous episode of granulocytopenia.

Secondary resistance: Develops on exposure to an antifungal agent and can be either reversible, because of transient adaptation, or acquired as a result of one or more genetic alterations.

Secondary-progressive multiple sclerosis: Often follows relapsing-remitting multiple sclerosis whereby attacks become continuously progressive over time. It is sometimes accompanied by acute relapses.

Seizure: Paroxysmal disorder of central nervous system, characterized by abnormal neuronal discharges with or without loss of consciousness. They vary in cause, presentation, consequences, duration, and management.

Selection bias: Systematic differences in characteristics between those selected for study and those who are not. See also *Information bias.*

Sepsis: The systemic inflammatory response syndrome (SIRS) secondary to infection. See also *Systemic inflammatory response syndrome.*

Septic shock: Sepsis with persistent hypotension despite fluid resuscitation, along with the presence of perfusion abnormalities. Patients who are on inotropic or vasopressor agents might not be hypotensive at the time perfusion abnormalities are measured.

Serotonin (5-hydroxytryptamine [5-HT]): An inhibitory neurotransmitter present in the raphe nucleus of the brainstem, platelets, carcinoid tumors, and other tissues. It is a vasoconstrictor and neurochemical involved in mood and sleep.

Serum urea nitrogen (SUN): See *Blood urea nitrogen.*

Severe sepsis: Sepsis associated with organ dysfunction, hypoperfusion, or hypotension. Hypoperfusion and perfusion abnormalities can include, but are not limited to, lactic acidosis, oliguria, or acute alteration in mental status.

Short stature: A broad term describing a condition commonly defined by a physical height that is more than two standard deviations below the population mean and lower than the third percentile for height in a specific age group.

Sickle cell disease: A group of inherited red blood cell (RBC) disorder in which sickle cell hemoglobin (HbS) is present. Hemolytic anemia and painful vasoocclusion are the main features.

Simple partial seizure: A seizure beginning in one hemisphere of the brain. It is manifested by alterations in motor functions, sensory or somatosensory symptoms without loss of consciousness. It can progress to a complex partial seizure or to a secondarily generalized seizure with loss of consciousness.

Single-nephron GFR (SNGFR): The rate of filtration through a single glomerulus of a nephron; often reported in nL/min.

Sinus ostia: The pathways that drain the sinuses.

Sinusitis: An inflammation and/or infection of the paranasal sinus mucosa.

Sjögren's syndrome: An inflammatory process affecting the mucous membranes. Can cause dry mouth with difficulty swallowing. Can occur secondary to autoimmune diseases such as rheumatoid arthritis or systemic lupus erythematosus.

Sleep latency: The amount of time it takes to fall asleep.

Sleep spindles: Brief burst of electrical activity seen on the EEG, 12 to 14 Hz.

Slipped capital femoral epiphysis (SCFE): Increased width of the femoral plate observed during GH treatment resulting in hip or knee pain.

Social anxiety disorder (SAD): A disorder characterized by clinically significant anxiety provoked by exposure to certain types of social or performance situations, often leading to avoidance behavior.

Social phobia: See *Social anxiety disorder.*

Somatic pain: Pain arising from skin, bone, joint, muscle, or connective tissue.

Specific measures: Instruments intended to provide greater detail concerning particular outcomes, in terms of functioning and well-being, uniquely associated with a condition and/or its treatment.

Specific phobia: A phobia characterized by clinically significant anxiety provoked by exposure to a specific feared object or situation, often leading to avoidance behavior.

Spermicide: A substance (nonoxynol-9 in the United States) placed in the vagina to inhibit the activity of sperm, thus reducing the risk of pregnancy; available as vaginal creams, films, foams, gels, suppositories, sponges, and tablets.

Spirochete: The class of microorganism that is the agent of syphilis (*Treponema pallidum*).

Standard gamble: An approach to health-state preference elicitation in which the respondent is offered a choice between two alternatives: choice A—living in health state *i* (a health state between full health and death) with certainty, or choice B—taking a gamble on a new treatment for which the outcome is uncertain.

Status epilepticus: Any recurrent or continuous seizure activity lasting longer than 30 minutes in which the patient does not regain baseline mental status. The two most common types are generalized convulsive status epilepticus and nonconvulsive status epilepticus.

Steatorrhea: Excessive fat in stool.

Stereotypy: Persistent repetition of senseless acts or words.

Stevens–Johnson syndrome: A serious dermatologic reaction characterized by blistering of the mucous membranes (mouth, eyes, vagina) with patchy rashes that can cover most of the body. Patients can also experience fever, headache, and cough.

Stress-related mucosal damage: Superficial gastritis-like lesions associated with critical illness in hospitalized patients.

Striae: Linear, atrophic, pink, purple, or white lesions of skin secondary to changes in connective tissue.

Stricture: An area of narrowing or constriction in the gastrointestinal tract because of buildup of fibrotic tissue; often a result of long-standing inflammation.

Stroke: A sudden onset, focal neurologic deficit, of presumed vascular origin, lasting longer than 24 hours.

Stroke volume: The volume of blood ejected from the heart during systole.

Stromal tissue of the prostate: This portion of the prostate is composed of smooth muscle tissue, which is embedded with α-adrenergic receptors. When stimulated, the muscle contracts around the urethra. This comprises approximately 75% of the total volume of the enlarged prostate gland in patients with benign prostatic hyperplasia.

Subarachnoid hemorrhage: Accumulation of blood in the space (subarachnoid space) surrounding the brain that usually contains the cerebrospinal fluid. It is usually caused by rupture of an intracranial aneurysm or trauma. It is a type of hemorrhagic stroke and can cause focal neurologic deficits.

Substance abuse: A maladaptive pattern of substance use indicated by repeated adverse consequences related to the repeated use of the substance. Examples include failure to fulfill important obligations at work, school, or home; repeated use in situations in which it is physically dangerous, such as driving under the influence; legal problems; and social or interpersonal problems such as arguments and fights.

Substance dependence: The continued use of the substance despite adverse substance-related problems. The criteria for substance dependence are the same for each of the drugs or drug classes, varying only to fit the unique pharmacologic properties of each drug.

Substantia nigra: Area of the brain (basal ganglia) where cells produce dopamine; characterized by neuromelanin deposits.

Subtle status epilepticus: For patients with prolonged refractory SE. The electrographic seizures persist; however, the motor manifestations of the seizures might not be apparent. In such cases the patient is considered in subtle SE.

Sudden death: Also known as sudden cardiac death; an unexpected death because of cardiac causes occurring in a short time period (generally within 1 hour of symptom onset) in a person with known or unknown cardiac disease in whom no previously diagnosed fatal condition is apparent. Most cases are related to cardiac arrhythmias, particularly ventricular fibrillation.

SUN (serum urea nitrogen): See *Blood urea nitrogen*.

Suppressive therapy: See *Secondary prophylaxis*.

Surge capacity: A term that refers to a healthcare system's ability to handle a large influx of patients in the event of an epidemic or disaster.

SV2A: A presynaptic vesicle protein found in the hippocampus as well as other areas of the brain believed to be important in the mechanism of action of levetiracetam.

Swan–Ganz catheter: A catheter (tube) inserted into the heart to measure pressure and cardiac output.

Symptomatic intracerebral hemorrhage: Collection of blood in the brain, usually after an ischemic stroke, that is associated with neurologic worsening.

Symptomatic: SE occurring during the time of an acute neurological injury. This etiology is associated with a poorer prognosis.

Syncope: Fainting.

Synechiae: A *creeping* angle closure that sometimes occurs in patients between attacks of closed-angle glaucoma.

Synergism: The combination of two drugs (such as antibiotics) that produces an effect greater than the sum of the two drugs if used alone.

Synesthesias: The overflow of one sensory modality to another. For example, colors are heard, sounds are seen.

Synovitis: Inflammation of the synovial lining of the joint.

Synovium: Synovial membrane, the inner of the two layers of the articular capsule of a synovial joint, composed of loose connective tissue and having a free smooth surface that lines the joint cavity. It secretes the synovial fluid.

Systemic inflammatory response syndrome (SIRS): Systemic inflammatory response to a variety of clinical insults, which can be of infectious or noninfectious etiology.

Systemic vascular resistance (SVR): The resistance to blood flow that is primarily determined by the vascular tone of the arteriolar blood vessels.

Systolic blood pressure: The arterial blood pressure that occurs during cardiac contraction.

Systolic heart failure: Systolic heart failure is a condition characterized by a decrease in myocardial contractility, which results in a reduction in the cardiac output and left ventricular ejection fraction.

Tachy-brady syndrome: Tachy-brady syndrome, also known as sick sinus syndrome, is a condition in which the sinoatrial node is unable to perform as the pacemaker of the heart.

Tangential speech: Speech pattern whereby the connections between expressed ideas are unrelated or have little relationship to each other.

Taper: To gradually decrease the dosage of a drug over a period of time.

Tardive: A modifier used to describe movement disorders secondary to chronic antipsychotic treatment (duration of treatment must be greater than 3 months). The disorder must persist for greater than 4 weeks and exhibit masking and unmasking characteristics. Tardive dyskinesia, tardive chorea, tardive dystonia, and tardive akathisia are examples of tardive movement disorders.

Tendonitis: Inflammation of tendons.

Tenesmus: A painful spasm of the urogenital diaphragm with an urgent desire to evacuate the bowel or bladder, involuntary straining, and the passage of little fecal matter or urine.

Teratogenicity: Ability of an agent to cause a defect or malformation in a fetus.

TEWL (transepidermal water loss): The rate of water loss by evaporation from the skin.

Thalassemia: Any of a group of inherited disorders of hemoglobin metabolism in which there is impaired synthesis of one or more of the polypeptide chains of globin.

Third-spacing: The shift of fluid and protein into the peritoneal cavity and bowel wall lumen that occurs as a result of peritonitis.

Thought blocking: Interruption of a train of thought whereby the person stops speaking suddenly and without warning, even in the middle of a sentence. Person may report that the thoughts were taken out of his or her head.

Thought broadcasting: Belief that one's thoughts are audible to others.

Thrombin: The enzyme formed from prothrombin that converts fibrinogen to fibrin. It is the principle driving force in the clotting cascade.

Thrombogenesis: The process of forming a blood clot.

Thrombolysis: The process of enzymatically dissolving or breaking apart a blood clot.

Thrombolytic: An enzyme that dissolves or breaks apart blood clots.

Thromboplastin: A substance that triggers the coagulation cascade. Tissue factor is a naturally occurring thromboplastin and used in the prothrombin time (PT) test.

Thrombopoiesis: The process of platelet production from immature cells.

Thrombosis: The process of forming a thrombus.

Thrombotic thrombocytopenic purpura: A life-threatening disease involving embolism and thrombosis of the small blood vessels in the brain and kidney.

Thrombus: An aggregation of fibrin and platelets within a blood vessel. A thrombus often causes vessel obstruction, inflammation, and injury.

Thrush: Fungal infection of the oral mucosa.

Thyroid-stimulating hormone (TSH): A polypeptide hormone secreted by the anterior pituitary gland that stimulates iodine uptake and thyroid hormone synthesis.

Thyrotropin-releasing hormone (TRH): A trophic hormone released by the hypothalamus that stimulates release of thyroid-stimulating hormone (TSH).

Time trade-off: An approach to health-state preference elicitation in which the respondent is asked to trade off years of life in less than full health for a shorter number of years in full health.

Tinea barbae: Fungal infection of the hair follicles of the beard or mustache.

Tinea capitis: Fungal infection of the scalp, hair follicles, or adjacent skin.

Tinea corporis: Fungal infection of the glabrous skin of the trunk and extremities.

Tinea cruris: Fungal infection of the proximal thighs and buttocks.

Tinea manuum: Fungal infection of the palmar surface of the hands.

Tinea pedis: Fungal infection of the feet.

Tinnitus: A noise in the ears, as ringing, buzzing, roaring, clicking, etc. Such sounds can at times be heard by those other than the patient.

Tocolytic: Agent that stops labor contractions.

Tolerance: (1) A state of adaptation in which exposure to a drug induces changes that result in a diminution of one or more of the drug's effects over time. (2) The ability of the immune system to accept a transplanted allograft as part of *self*.

Tonic-clonic seizures: Sharp tonic contraction of muscles followed by a period of rigidity and clonic movement.

Tophi: Urate deposits.

Toxic epidermal necrolysis: A syndrome similar to Stevens-Johnson syndrome characterized by blistering of skin and mucous membranes in response to administration of a drug. Large areas of skin may peel off.

Toxic megacolon: A segmental or total colonic distension of >6 cm with acute colitis and signs of systemic toxicity.

Toxic shock syndrome: Sudden onset of fever, muscle ache, vomiting and diarrhea, accompanied by a peeling rash and followed by low body temperature and shock; caused by staphylococcal endotoxin, especially from infection of the vagina associated with tampon use.

Toxoplasmosis: Clinical infection with *Toxoplasma gondii.*

Transmural: Across the wall of an organ or structure; in the case of Crohn's disease, inflammation can extend through all four layers of the intestinal wall.

Transurethral incision of the prostate: In this surgical procedure, the bladder neck opening is widened by making incisions at various locations around the bladder neck with a resectoscope, which is inserted into the penis. Excess prostate tissue is not removed.

Transurethral prostatectomy: In this surgical procedure, an enlarged prostate core is removed from the inside out. That is, a resectoscope is inserted into the penis. A cutting blade at the end shaves out excess prostate tissue.

Transverse lie: The fetus is perpendicular to the mother. Usually the shoulder is the presenting part. Fetuses in this position must be delivered by cesarean section.

Transverse myelitis: Inflammation of the full width of the spinal cord that disrupts communication to the muscles, resulting in pain, weakness, and muscle paralysis.

Traveler's diarrhea: Diarrhea caused by contaminated food or water and usually attributed to enterotoxigenic *Escherichia coli* (ETEC), *Shigella*, *Campylobacter*, *Salmonella* species, or viruses.

Troponin: A protein found predominately in cardiac, but not skeletal, muscle, which regulates calcium-mediated interaction of actin and myosin. Troponin I and T are released into the blood from the myocytes at the time of myocardial cell necrosis secondary to infarction. These biochemical markers become elevated and are used in the diagnosis of myocardial infarction. Troponin I and T are more sensitive and specific for infarction than creatinine kinase, which is found in both skeletal and myocardial cells. The exact value of troponin I or T, which is diagnostic of infarction, differs based on assay.

Trousseau's sign: A hand spasm produced by placing a blood pressure cuff over the forearm and inflating the pressure above the systolic pressure for 3 minutes.

Tubule: Section of the nephron that is responsible for secretion and reabsorption of water, electrolytes, and drugs.

Tumor: Elevated, solid lesion.

Tumor necrosis factor-α (TNF-α): A proinflammatory cytokine.

Type I reaction: An immediate, immunoglobulin E (IgE)-mediated allergic reaction.

Ulcer: Loss of epidermis and dermis caused by sloughing of necrotic tissue.

Ultradian sleep-wake rhythm: A cycle of sleep and wake that repeats in less than 24 hours. Babies have an ultradian sleep-wake rhythm with multiple sleep and wake periods in a 24-hour period.

Ultrafiltration: The process of removing water from the blood during dialysis.

Umbilication: Slight, navel-like depression, or dimpling, of the center of a rounded body.

Unilateral: On either the right or left side, not crossing the midline. When used for defining sensory or motor disturbances of migraine aura, it includes complete or partial hemi-distribution.

Upper respiratory tract infection: Otitis media, sinusitis, pharyngitis, laryngitis (croup), rhinitis, or epiglottitis.

Urea: A waste product found in the blood and caused by the normal breakdown of protein in the body.

Uremia: An array of symptoms associated with accumulation of metabolic by-products and endogenous toxins in the blood due to impaired kidney function. Symptoms include nausea, vomiting, loss of appetite, weakness, and mental confusion.

Urethritis: Inflammation of the urethra.

Urinalysis: The diagnostic analysis of urine and its components; can be microscopic or macroscopic in nature.

Urinary incontinence: Involuntary leakage of urine; can result from urethral underactivity (stress urinary incontinence), urethral overactivity (overflow incontinence), or mixed pathophysiologic mechanisms.

Urine: Fluid waste resulting from filtration of blood by the kidneys; transferred to the bladder by ureters and expelled from the body through the urethra by the act of voiding or urinating.

Urticaria: A dermatologic reaction noted by elevated, erythematous patches that are pruritic.

Vacuum erection device: Medical device used to manually induce an erection.

Vagal nerve stimulator (VNS): A medical device that is surgically implanted in patients with refractory epilepsy.

Validity: An estimation of the extent to which an instrument is measuring what it is purported to be measuring.

Valsalva maneuver: The Valsalva maneuver is the expiratory effort against a closed glottis, which increases thoracic cavity pressure, which impedes venous return to the heart. This maneuver results in blood pressure and heart rate changes and is used to diagnose treat various cardiac conditions.

Vasculitis: Inflammation of blood vessels.

Vasopressin: A posterior pituitary hormone that controls fluid balance by acting on the renal collecting ducts to prevent water loss.

Vector: Carrier (person, animal, or insect) of disease.

Vegetation: Bacterial growth on heart valves.

Ventricular remodeling: Alterations in myocardial cells and the extracellular matrix that result in changes in the size, shape, structure, and function of the heart. The remodeling process leads to reductions in myocardial systolic and/or diastolic function that, in turn, leads to further myocardial injury, perpetuating the remodeling process and the decline in ventricular dysfunction and progression of heart failure.

Vesicle: Clear blister (<0.5 cm in diameter) filled with fluid.

Visceral pain: Pain arising from internal organs such as the large intestine or pancreas.

Visual analog scale: A response scale that is a line with the end points well defined (e.g., 0 = worst imaginable health state, and 100 = best imaginable health state).

Volume of distribution: A proportionality constant that relates the amount of drug in the body to its serum concentration.

Vomiting: Contraction of the abdominal muscles, descent of the diaphragm, and opening of the gastric cardia resulting in expulsion of stomach contents from the mouth.

Vulgaris: Ordinary, common.

Wearing-off phenomena: Also known as end-of-dose wearing-off or motor fluctuations. The waning of the effects of a dose of levodopa prior to the scheduled time for the next dose, resulting in return of parkinsonian features, such as, tremor, slowness, and rigidity.

Withdrawal: The development of a substance-specific syndrome after cessation of or reduction in intake of a substance that was used regularly by the individual to induce a state of intoxication. Withdrawal causes significant distress to the individual and is associated with impairment in social, occupational, or other areas of functioning. Withdrawal is usually associated with substance dependence. Withdrawal generally is also associated with a craving to readminister the drug to relieve the symptoms.

Withdrawal bleeding: The predictable bleeding that results from cessation of a progestogen.

Withdrawal syndrome: The onset of a predictable constellation of signs and symptoms involving alerted activity of the central nervous system after the abrupt discontinuation of, or rapid decrease in, dosage of a drug.

Xerosis: Dry skin.

Xerostomia: Dry mouth caused by decreased salivary production.

Yeasts: Oval or spherically shaped unicellular forms that generally produce pasty or mucoid colonies on agar media, similar to those observed with bacterial cultures. Yeasts have rigid cell walls that reproduce by budding, a process in which daughter cells arise from pinching off a portion of the parent cell.

Zeitgeber: Environmental cue.

Zollinger–Ellison syndrome: Gastric acid hypersecretory disease caused by a gastrin-secreting tumor and leading to multiple, severe duodenal ulcers.

INDEX

Note: Page numbers followed by "f" refer to illustrations; page numbers followed by "t" refer to tables; page numbers preceded by "O" refer to online page numbers accessible via the Pharmacotherapy Online Learning Center at www.pharmacotherapyonline.com.

H

J

INDEX

W

X

Y

Z

Laboratory	Conventional Units	Conversion Factor	SI Units
Haptoglobin	60–270 mg/dL	0.01	0.6–2.7 g/L
HBeAg	Negative		
HbsAg	Negative		
HBV DNA	Negative		
Hematocrit			
Male	40.7–50.3%	0.01	0.407–0.503
Female	36.1–44.3%	0.01	0.361–0.443
Hemoglobin (blood)			
Male	13.8–17.2 g/dL	10	138–172 g/L
		Alternate SI: 0.62	8.56–10.67 mmol/L
Female	12.1–15.1 g/dL	10	121–151 g/L
		Alternate SI: 0.62	7.5–9.36 mmol/L
Hemoglobin A1c	4.0–6.0%	0.01	0.04–0.06
Heparin			
Via protamine titration method	0.2–0.4 mcg/mL		
Via anti-factor Xa assay	0.3–0.7 mcg/mL		
High-density lipoprotein (HDL) cholesterol	Greater than 35 mg/dL	0.0259	Greater than 0.91 mmol/L
Homocysteine	3.3–10.4 μmol/L		
Ibuprofen			
Therapeutic	10–50 mcg/mL	4.85	49–243 μmol/L
Toxic	100–700 mcg/mL or more	4.85	485–3395 μmol/L or more
Imipramine, therapeutic	100–300 ng/mL or mcg/L	3.57	357–1071 nmol/L
Immunoglobulin A (IgA)	85–385 mg/dL	0.01	0.85–3.85 g/L
Immunoglobulin G (IgG)	565–1765 mg/dL	0.01	5.65–17.65 g/L
Immunoglobulin M (IgM)	53–375 mg/dL	0.01	0.53–3.75 g/L
Insulin (fasting)	2–20 microunits/mL or milliunits/L	7.175	14.35–143.5 pmol/L
International normalized ratio (INR), therapeutic	2.0–3.0 (2.5–3.5 for some indications)		
Iron			
Male	45–160 mcg/dL	0.179	8.1–31.3 μmol/L
Female	30–160 mcg/dL	0.179	5.4–31.3 μmol/L
Iron binding capacity (total)	220–420 mcg/dL	0.179	39.4–75.2 μmol/L
Iron saturation	15–50%	0.01	0.15–0.50
Lactate (plasma)	0.7–2.1 mEq/L	1	0.7–2.1 mmol/L
	6.3–18.9 mg/dL	0.111	
Lactate dehydrogenase	100–250 IU/L	0.01667	1.67–4.17 μkat/L
Lead	Less than 25 mcg/dL	0.0483	Less than 1.21 μmol/L
Leukocyte count	3.8–9.8 × 10³/μL	10⁶	3.8–9.8 × 10⁹/L
Lidocaine, therapeutic	1.5–6.0 mcg/mL or mg/L	4.27	6.4–25.6 μmol/L
Lipase	Less than 100 IU/L	0.01667	1.7 μkat/L
Lithium, therapeutic	0.5–1.25 mEq/L	1	0.5–1.25 mmol/L
Low-density lipoprotein (LDL) cholesterol			
Desirable	Less than 130 mg/dL	0.0259	Less than 3.36 mmol/L
Borderline high risk	130–159 mg/dL	0.0259	3.36–4.11 mmol/L
High risk	Greater than or equal to 160 mg/dL	0.0259	Greater than or equal to 4.13 mmol/L
Luteinizing hormone (LH)			
Male	1–8 milliunits/mL	1	1–8 units/L
Female			
Follicular phase	1–12 milliunits/mL	1	1–12 units/L
Midcycle	16–104 milliunits/mL	1	16–104 units/L
Luteal phase	1–12 milliunits/mL	1	1–12 units/L
Postmenopausal	16–66 milliunits/mL	1	16–66 units/L
Lymphocyte count	1.2–3.3 × 10³/μL	10⁶	1.2–3.3 × 10⁹/L
Magnesium	1.3–2.2 mEq/L	0.5	0.65–1.10 mmol/L
	1.58–2.68 mg/dL	0.411	0.65–1.10 mmol/L
Mean corpuscular volume	80.0–97.6 μm³	1	80.0–97.6 fL
Mononuclear cell count	0.2–0.7 × 10³/μL	10⁶	0.2–0.7 × 10⁹/L
Nortriptyline, therapeutic	50–150 ng/mL or mcg/L	3.8	190–570 nmol/L
NT-ProBNP (see Pro-BNP)			
Osmolality (serum)	275–300 mOsm/kg	1	275–300 mmol/kg
Osmolality (urine)	250–900 mOsm/kg	1	250–900 mmol/kg
Parathyroid hormone (PTH), intact	10–60 pg/mL or ng/L	0.107	1.1–6.4 pmol/L
Parathyroid hormone (PTH), N-terminal	8–24 pg/mL or ng/L		
Parathyroid hormone (PTH), C-terminal	50–330 pg/mL or ng/L		
Phenobarbital, therapeutic	15–40 mcg/mL or mg/L	4.31	65–172 μmol/L
Phenytoin, therapeutic	10–20 mcg/mL or mg/L	3.96	40–79 μmol/L
Phosphate	2.5–4.5 mg/dL	0.323	0.81–1.45 mmol/L
Platelet count	140–440 × 10³/μL	10⁶	140–440 × 10⁹/L
Potassium (plasma)	3.3–4.9 mEq/L	1	3.3–4.9 mmol/L
Prealbumin (adult)	19.5–35.8 mg/dL	10	195–358 mg/dL
Primidone, therapeutic	5–12 mcg/mL or mg/L	4.58	23–55 μmol/L
ProBNP	Less than 125 pg/mL or ng/L	0.118	Less than 14.75 pmol/L
Procainamide, therapeutic	4–10 mcg/mL or mg/L	4.23	17–42 μmol/L
Progesterone			
Male	13–97 ng/dL	0.0318	0.4–3.1 nmol/L
Female			
Follicular phase	15–70 ng/dL		0.5–2.2 nmol/L
Luteal phase	200–2500 ng/dL		6.4–79.5 nmol/L
Prolactin	Less than 20 ng/mL	1	Less than 20 mcg/L
Prostate-specific antigen (PSA)	Less than 4 ng/mL	1	Less than 4 mcg/L
Protein, total	6.0–8.0 g/dL	10	60–80 g/L
Prothrombin time (PT)	10–12 seconds		
Quinidine, therapeutic	2–5 mcg/mL or mg/L	3.08	6.2–15.4 μmol/L
Radioactive iodine uptake (RAIU)	Less than 6% in 2 hours		
Red blood cell (RBC) count (blood)			
Male	4–6.2 × 10⁶/μL	10⁶	4–6.2 × 10¹²/L
Female	4–6.2 × 10⁶/μL	10⁶	4–6.2 × 10¹²/L
Pregnant			
Trimester 1	4–5 × 10⁶/μL	10⁶	4–5 × 10¹²/L
Trimester 2	3.2–4.5 × 10⁶/μL	10⁶	3.2–4.5 × 10¹²/L
Trimester 3	3–4.9 × 10⁶/μL	10⁶	3–4.9 × 10¹²/L
Post partum	3.2–5 × 10⁶/μL	10⁶	3.2–5 × 10⁶/L

(continued)